Stockley's Drug Interactions

A source book of interactions, their mechanisms, clinical importance and management

Eleventh edition

Edited by

Claire L Preston

BPharm, PGDipMedMan, MRPharmS

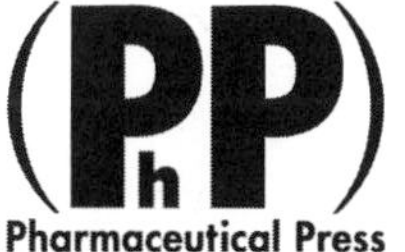

Published by Pharmaceutical Press
66–68 East Smithfield, London E1W 1AW, UK

First edition 1981
Second edition 1991
Third edition 1994
Fourth edition 1996
Fifth edition 1999
Sixth edition 2002
Seventh edition 2006
Eighth edition 2008
Ninth edition 2010
Tenth edition 2013
Eleventh edition 2016

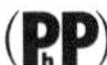 is a trade mark of Pharmaceutical Press

Pharmaceutical Press is the publishing division of the Royal Pharmaceutical Society

Typeset by Data Standards Ltd, Frome, Somerset
Printed in Italy by LEGO S.p.A

ISBN 978 0 85711 270 5

Disclaimer
Stockley's Drug Interactions (SDI) provides healthcare professionals with practical information on drug interactions and their management. SDI is published every three years and the Publisher works to ensure that the information is accurate and up-to-date as at the date of publication, but knowledge and best practice in this field change regularly. While considerable efforts have been made to check the material in this publication, neither the Publisher nor the authors accept any responsibility for errors or omissions. SDI is updated quarterly online at www.medicinescomplete.com

SDI is a reference text for drug interactions and it may not always include all information necessary for prescribing or dispensing. It is the responsibility of practitioners to interpret SDI in light of professional knowledge and relevant circumstances, and to supplement it as necessary with specialist publications and by reference to product literature, codes of conduct, and safety regulations.

To the fullest extent permitted by law the Publisher assumes no responsibility for any aspect of healthcare administered with the aid of this information or any other use of this information. The Publisher and authors do not exclude any liability for death or personal injury resulting from negligence, fraud, or any liability which cannot be excluded by applicable law.

A catalogue record for this book is available from the British Library

Contents

About the authors

Stockley's Drug Interactions is prepared within the Publications Division at the Royal Pharmaceutical Society under the editor, Claire L Preston. The editorial team of pharmacists draw on a wealth of experience in clinical and academic pharmacy to provide practising doctors, pharmacists, surgeons, nurses, and other healthcare professionals with unbiased, independent, and evaluated information on interactions with drugs and medicines in use around the world. The team uses extensive literature surveillance and modern information retrieval techniques to review the existing text and identify new areas of interest for inclusion.

Editor:

Claire L Preston, BPharm, PGDipMedMan, MRPharmS

Editorial Staff:

Lucía Camañas Sáez, MPharm, DipClinPharm, CertPsychTherap, MRPharmS
Elaina E Crehan, MChem
Samuel Driver, BSc
Chloë SAJ Hatwal, BSc, MRes
Claire Jones, BPharm, MRPharmS, DipPresSci
Stephanie L Jones, MPharm, MRPharmS
Bryony Jordan, BSc, DipPharmPrac
Sonia Z Khan, MPharm, PGCertPharmPrac
Rebecca E Luckhurst, BSc, MSc
John Martin, BPharm, PhD, MRPharmS
Christine Parry, BSc
Rebekah Raymond, BSc, DipPharmPrac, MRPharmS
Harpreet K Sandhu, MPharm, MRPharmS
Julia Sawyer, BPharm, DipPharmPrac
Sandra Sutton, BPharm, MSc Med, Cert ProjMngt
Julia A Webb, MPharm, PGCertPharmPrac, MRPharmS

Expert Contributors:

Karen Baxter, BSc, MSc, MRPharmS
C Rhoda Lee, BPharm, PhD, MRPharmS

Contact us

Email: phpeditorial@rpharms.com

Preface

In today's world of continually evolving drug data and unlimited access to information, healthcare professionals are now more in need of reliable, peer-reviewed, easy-to-access information on drug interactions than ever before. Pharmacists, doctors, nurses, and other healthcare professionals often cannot spare the time to search the rapidly expanding literature on drug interactions and to fully assess the evidence for themselves. They need a resource they can trust, and we believe that *Stockley's Drug Interactions* is the solution—the most authoritative and indispensable international resource available on drug interactions. It provides all busy healthcare professionals with the relevant information they need to help them treat and advise their patients, competently and confidently.

Based upon many thousands of published clinical papers and reports, *Stockley's Drug Interactions* provides a series of detailed, yet concise, monographs designed for quick and easy reference. A key strength of the publication is that we evaluate and include all of the published literature identified on any drug, regardless of the countries in which it is licensed. Furthermore, we review relevant information provided by regulatory bodies; in particular the MHRA in the UK, the European Medicines Agency, and the Food and Drug Administration in the US. This allows us to give our users the fullest possible view on interactions and ensures the international coverage of our publication.

Each monograph in *Stockley's Drug Interactions* contains the clinical evidence for the interaction under discussion, its probable mechanism, its clinical importance, and clear and practical guidance on the management of the interaction. There is also a brief summary of the interaction, which, when read together with the management advice for the interaction, provides the most relevant information to healthcare professionals who are under enormous time pressure. For those who wish to know the full picture, the clinical evidence and mechanism sections provide more detailed background on the interaction. Not only does *Stockley's Drug Interactions* include information on clinically relevant interactions, it also summarises the literature where clinically relevant interactions do not occur. The publication includes the interactions of herbal medicines for which clinical evidence is available.

Stockley's Drug Interactions is available in print, and also on MedicinesComplete (www.medicinescomplete.com) where it is updated quarterly. To meet the needs of healthcare professionals who need to make rapid, well-informed decisions about drug interactions in a clinical setting and those who prefer to use portable, hand-held devices to access drug information, we have developed the *Stockley's Interactions Checker.* Available via MedicinesComplete, the Checker is designed to be used in conjunction with *Stockley's Drug Interactions* and contains information derived from this full text publication. In essence it summarises drug-drug, drug-herb, and drug-food interactions in a few short lines to give quick guidance as to whether drugs can safely be taken together. Should they require more information, users can click through to the full details of the monograph in *Stockley's Drug Interactions*. Our sister publication, *Stockley's Herbal Medicines Interactions* (also available on MedicinesComplete) deals with the enormous numbers of theoretical and *in vitro* papers in this area, which do not fit with the clinically focussed philosophy of *Stockley's Drug Interactions*. For more details about our digital products please visit: www.pharmpress.com/stockleys.

Changes for the 11th edition of *Stockley's Drug Interactions*

Many of the existing interactions monographs have been reviewed, revalidated, and updated. Over 350 new monographs have been added, making a total of almost 4,500 monographs. Keeping the publication up to date is an on-going process, and the constantly expanding body of literature makes this a challenging task. We cite around 27,000 references, which we think is more than any other reference publication on drug interactions. Some notable changes for this edition include:

- A comprehensive update and restructure of the chapter on Antidiabetic drugs, in-line with published literature
- Addition of new advice regarding the concurrent use of aliskiren, ACE inhibitors, and angiotensin-II receptor antagonists
- An updated list of drugs that have a risk of prolonging the QT interval
- The addition of many new drugs, including apixaban, apremilast, dolutegravir, lomitapide, mirabegron, NS5A inhibitors (daclatasvir, ledipasvir, ombitasvir), NS5B inhibitors (dasabuvir, sofosbuvir), sodium-glucose co-transporter-2 inhibitors (canagliflozin, dapagliflozin, empagliflozin), and telavancin

Over the course of this edition, we have seen the handing over of the reins from one Editor to another. After more than 10 years as the Editor of *Stockley's Drug Interactions*, Karen Baxter has moved on to manage other publications within Pharmaceutical Press. The Editor would like to take this opportunity to thank Karen for all her years of hard work on *Stockley's Drug Interactions* and for developing this publication into the trusted resource that it continues to be today. We would also like to thank her for her continued invaluable advice and support.

The Editorial team have also had assistance from many other people in producing this publication, and the Editor gratefully acknowledges the assistance and guidance that they have provided. Alison Brayfield and the Martindale team continue to be a great source of advice and support, and in particular we derive much of our nomenclature from the Martindale databases. Thanks are also due to Jeremy Macdonald and his team, for their advice and support in the technical aspects of producing the *Stockley's Interactions Checker*, the integratable *Stockley's Interaction Alerts* product, and the MedicinesComplete platform, and to Heather Benson, for patiently handling the various aspects of producing our publications in print. We are also grateful for the support of our Managing Director, Alina Lourie.

Finally, thanks are due to those of you who take the time to provide us with feedback, either directly, or in the form of questions about the publication. We continue to value this input to evolve the publication and to ensure it meets the needs of its users. Anyone who wishes to contact the Stockley team can do so at the following address: phpeditorial@rpharms.com.

London, November 2015

Abbreviations

ACE—angiotensin-converting enzyme
ADP—adenosine diphosphate
AIDS—acquired immunodeficiency syndrome
ALT—alanine aminotransferase
am—ante meridiem (before noon)
aPTT—activated partial thromboplastin time
AST—aspartate aminotransferase
AUC—area under the time-concentration curve
AUC_{0-12}—area under the time-concentration curve measured over 0 to 12 hours
AV—atrioventricular
BCRP—breast cancer resistance protein (ABCG2)
BNF—British National Formulary
BP—blood pressure
BP—British Pharmacopoeia
BPC—British Pharmaceutical Codex
BPH—benign prostatic hyperplasia
bpm—beats per minute
BSEP—bile salt export pump
BUN—blood urea nitrogen
CAPD—continuous ambulatory peritoneal dialysis
CDC—Centers for Disease Control (USA)
CEPT—cholesteryl ester transfer protein
CHM—Commission on Human Medicines (UK)
CNS—central nervous system
COMT—catechol-*O*-methyl transferase
COPD—chronic obstructive pulmonary disease
COX—cyclo-oxygenase
CSF—cerebrospinal fluid
CSM—Committee on Safety of Medicines (UK) (now subsumed within the Commission on Human Medicines)
DNA—deoxyribonucleic acid
ECG—electrocardiogram
ECT—electroconvulsive therapy
ED_{50}—the dose at which 50% of subjects respond
EEG—electroencephalogram
e.g.—*exempli gratia* (for example)
EMEA—European Agency for the Evaluation of Medicinal Products
FDA—Food and Drug Administration (USA)
FEF_{25-75}—maximum expiratory flow over the middle 50% of the vital capacity
FEV_1—forced expiratory volume in one second
FSH—follicle stimulating hormone
FVC—forced vital capacity
g—gram(s)
GABA—gamma-aminobutyric acid
h—hour(s)
HAART—highly active antiretroviral therapy
HbA_{1c}—glycosylated (glycated) haemoglobin
HCV—hepatitis C virus
HIV—human immunodeficiency virus
HRT—hormone replacement therapy
ibid—*ibidem*, in the same place (journal or book)
i.e.—*id est* (that is)
INR—international normalised ratio
ITU—intensive therapy unit
IU—International Units
IUD—intra-uterine device
kg—kilogram(s)
L—litre(s)
LDL—low-density lipoprotein
LFT—liver function test
LH—luteinising hormone
LMWH—low-molecular-weight heparin
MAC—minimum alveolar concentration
MAO—monoamine oxidase
MAOI—monoamine oxidase inhibitor
MAO-A—monoamine oxidase, type A
MAO-B—monoamine oxidase, type B
MATE—multidrug and toxin extrusion proteins
MCA—Medicines Control Agency (UK) (now MHRA)
MHRA—Medicines and Healthcare products Regulatory Agency (UK)
MIC—minimum inhibitory concentration
MRP—multidrug-resistance proteins
mEq—milliequivalent(s)
mg—milligram(s)
mL—millilitre(s)
mmHg—millimetre(s) of mercury
mmol—millimole
mol—mole
MRSA—methicillin resistant *Staphylococcus aureus*
NICE—National Institute for Health and Clinical Excellence (UK) (formerly the National Institute for Clinical Excellence)
nM—nanomole
NNRTI—non-nucleoside reverse transcriptase inhibitor
NRTI—nucleoside reverse transcriptase inhibitor
NSAID—non-steroidal anti-inflammatory drug
NYHA—New York Heart Association
OATs—organic anion transporters
OATPs—organic anion-transporting polypeptides
OCTs—organic cation transporters
PABA—para-amino benzoic acid
PCP—pneumocystis pneumonia
pH—the negative logarithm of the hydrogen ion concentration
pm—*post meridiem* (after noon)
pO_2—plasma partial pressure (concentration) of oxygen
PPI—proton pump inhibitor
ppm—parts per million
PTT—partial thromboplastin time
RIMA—reversible inhibitor of monoamine oxidase type A
RNA—ribonucleic acid
sic—written exactly as it appears in the original
SNRI—serotonin and noradrenaline reuptake inhibitor
SSRI—selective serotonin reuptake inhibitor
SVT—supraventricular tachycardia
T3—Triiodothyronine
TPN—total parenteral nutrition
TSH—thyroid-stimulating hormone
UGT—uridine diphospho glucuronyltransferase
UK—United Kingdom
US and USA—United States of America
USP—United States Pharmacopeia

Before using the publication...

. . . you should read this short explanatory section so that you know how the drug interaction data have been set out here, and why - as well as the basic philosophy that has been followed in presenting it.

The monographs

This publication has almost 4200 monographs with a common format, which are subdivided into sections like these:
abstract or summary for quick reading.

- **Clinical evidence**, detailing one, two or more illustrative examples of the interaction, followed by most or all of other supportive clinical evidence currently available.
- **Mechanism**, in brief.
- **Importance and management**, a short discussion designed to aid rapid clinical decision making. For example:
  — Is the interaction established or not?
  — What is its incidence?
  — How important is it?
  — How can it be managed?
  And what, if any, are the non-interacting alternatives?
- **References**, a list of all of the relevant references. The length of the references list gives a very fair indication of the extent of the documentation. A long list indicates a well documented interaction, whereas a short list indicates poor documentation.

Some of the monographs have been compressed into fewer subsections instead of the more usual five, simply where information is limited or where there is little need to be more expansive.

The monographs do not carry the drug interaction Hazard/Severity ratings as used in the electronic Stockley Interactions Alerts, but what is written in each monograph should speak for itself.

Quality of information on interactions

The data on interactions are of widely varying quality and reliability. The best come from clinical studies carried out on large numbers of patients under scrupulously controlled conditions. The worst are anecdotal, uncontrolled, or based solely on *animal* studies. Sometimes they are no more than speculative and theoretical scaremongering guesswork, hallowed by repeated quotation until they become virtually set in stone.

The aim has been to filter out as much useless noise as possible, so wherever possible secondary references are avoided, and primary references which are available in good medical and scientific libraries are used instead - although sometimes unpublished, good quality, in-house reports on drug company files have been used where the drug company has kindly allowed access to the information. Product literature (the Summary of Product Characteristics in the UK and the Prescribing Information in the US) rather than the research reports that lie behind them are also cited because often they are the only source of published information about new drugs.

The quality of drug company literature is very variable. Some of it is excellent, helpful and very reliable, but regrettably a proportion contains a welter of speculative and self-protective statements, probably driven more by the company's medico-legal policy than anything else, and the nervousness of drug regulatory authorities. It is almost unbelievable (but true all the same) that drug companies that are scrupulous in the way they do their research come out with statements about possible interactions that are little more than guesswork.

When drawing your own conclusions

The human population is a total mixture, unlike selected batches of laboratory animals (same age, weight, sex, and strain etc.). For this reason human beings do not respond uniformly to one or more drugs. Our genetic make up, ethnic background, sex, renal and hepatic functions, diseases and nutritional states, ages and other factors (the route of administration, for example) all contribute towards the heterogeneity of our responses. This means that the outcome of giving one or more drugs to any individual for the first time is never totally predictable because it is a new and unique experiment . Even so, some idea of the probable outcome of using a drug or a pair of drugs can be based on what has been seen in other patients: the more extensive the data, the firmer the predictions.

The most difficult decisions concern isolated cases of interaction, many of which only achieved prominence because they were serious. Do you ignore them as idiosyncratic or do you, from that moment onwards, contraindicate the use of the two drugs totally?

There is no simple yes or no answer to these questions, but one simple rule-of-thumb is that isolated cases of interaction with old and very well-tried pairs of drugs are unlikely to be of general importance, whereas those with new drugs might be the tip of an emerging iceberg and should therefore initially be taken much more seriously until more is known. The delicate balance between these two has then to be set against the actual severity of the reaction reported and weighed up against how essential it is to use the drug combination in question.

When deciding the possible first-time use of any two drugs in any particular patient, you need to put what is currently known about these drugs against the particular profile of your patient. Read the monograph. Consider the facts and conclusions, and then set the whole against the backdrop of your patients unique condition (age, disease, general condition, and so forth) so that what you eventually decide to do is well thought out and soundly based. We do not usually have the luxury of knowing absolutely all the facts, so that an initial conservative approach is often the safest.

1

General considerations and an outline survey of some basic interaction mechanisms

Drug interactions overview

(a) What is a drug interaction?

An interaction is said to occur when the effects of one drug are changed by the presence of another drug, herbal medicine, food, drink or by some environmental chemical agent. Much more colourful and informal definitions by patients are that it is ". . . when medicines fight each other. . .", or ". . . when medicines fizz together in the stomach . . .", or ". . .what happens when one medicine falls out with another. . ."

The outcome can be harmful if the interaction causes an increase in the toxicity of the drug. For example, there is a considerable increase in risk of severe muscle damage if patients taking statins start taking azole antifungals (see 'Statins + Azoles', p.1322). Patients taking monoamine oxidase inhibitor antidepressants (MAOIs) may experience an acute and potentially life-threatening hypertensive crisis if they eat tyramine-rich foods such as cheese (see 'MAOIs or RIMAs + Food; Tyramine-containing', p.1389).

A reduction in efficacy due to an interaction can sometimes be just as harmful as an increase: patients taking warfarin who are given rifampicin (rifampin) need more warfarin to maintain adequate anticoagulation (see 'Coumarins + Antibacterials; Rifamycins', p.397), while patients taking tetracyclines or quinolones (see 'Tetracyclines + Food', p.360, and 'Quinolones + Dairy products', p.347, respectively) need to avoid antacids and milky foods (or separate their ingestion) because the effects of these antibacterials can be reduced or even abolished if admixture occurs in the gut.

These unwanted and unsought interactions are adverse and undesirable but there are other interactions that can be beneficial and valuable, such as the deliberate co-prescription of antihypertensive drugs and diuretics in order to achieve antihypertensive effects possibly not obtainable with either drug alone (see 'Antihypertensives + Other drugs that affect blood pressure', p.1054). The mechanisms of both types of interaction, whether adverse or beneficial, are often very similar, but the adverse interactions are the focus of this publication.

Definitions of a drug interaction are not rigidly adhered to in this publication because the subject inevitably overlaps into other areas of adverse reactions with drugs. So you will find in these pages some 'interactions' where one drug does not actually affect another at all, but the adverse outcome is the simple additive effects of two drugs with similar effects (for example the combined effects of two or more CNS depressants, or two drugs which affect the QT interval). Sometimes the term 'drug interaction' is used for the physico-chemical reactions that occur if drugs are mixed in intravenous fluids, causing precipitation or inactivation. The long-established and less ambiguous term is 'pharmaceutical incompatibilities'. Incompatibilities are not covered by this publication.

(b) What is the incidence of drug interactions?

The more drugs a patient takes the greater the likelihood that an adverse reaction will occur. One hospital study found that the rate was 7% in those taking 6 to 10 drugs but 40% in those taking 16 to 20 drugs, which represents a disproportionate increase.[1] A possible explanation is that the drugs were interacting.

Some of the early studies on the frequency of interactions uncritically compared the drugs that had been prescribed with lists of possible drug interactions, without appreciating that many interactions may be clinically trivial or simply theoretical. As a result, an unrealistically high incidence was suggested. Most of the later studies have avoided this error by looking at only potentially clinically important interactions, and incidences of up to 8.8% have been reported.[2-4] Even so, not all of these studies took into account the distinction that must be made between the incidence of potential interactions and the incidence of those where clinical problems actually arise. The simple fact is that some patients experience quite serious reactions while taking interacting drugs, while others appear not to be affected at all.

A screening of 2 422 patients over a total of 25 005 days revealed that 113 (4.7%) were taking combinations of drugs that could interact, but evidence of interactions was observed in only 7 patients, representing an incidence of 0.3%.[2] In another study of 44 hospital inpatients taking 10 to 17 drugs over a 5-day period, 77 potential drug interactions were identified, but only one probable and four possible adverse reactions (6.4%) were detected.[5] A further study, among patients taking antiepileptic drugs, found that 6% of the cases of toxicity were due to drug interactions.[6] These figures are low compared with those of a hospital survey that monitored 927 patients who had received 1004 potentially interacting drug combinations. Changes in drug dose were made in 44% of these cases.[7] A review of these and other studies found that the reported incidence rates ranged from 2.2 to 70.3%, and the percentage of patients actually experiencing problems was less than 11.1%. Another review of 639 elderly patients found a 37% incidence of interactions.[8] Yet another review of 236 geriatric patients found an 88% incidence of clinically significant interactions, and a 22% incidence of potentially serious and life-threatening interactions.[9] A 4.1% incidence of drug interactions on prescriptions presented to community pharmacists in the US was found in a further survey,[10] whereas the incidence was only 2.9% in another American study,[11] and just 1.9% in a Swedish study.[12] An Australian study found that about 10% of hospital admissions were drug-related, of which 4.4% were due to drug interactions.[13] A very high incidence (47 to 50%) of potential drug interactions was found in a study carried out in an Emergency Department in the US.[14] One French study found that 16% of the prescriptions for a group of patients taking antihypertensive drugs were contraindicated or unsuitable,[15] whereas another study in a group of geriatric patients found only a 1% incidence.[16] The incidence of problems would be expected to be higher in the elderly because ageing affects the functioning of the kidneys and liver.[17,18]

These discordant figures need to be put into the context of the under-reporting of adverse reactions of any kind by medical professionals, for reasons that may include pressure of work or the fear of litigation. Both doctors and patients may not recognise adverse reactions and interactions, and some patients simply stop taking their drugs without saying why. None of these studies give a clear answer to the question of how frequently drug interactions occur, but even if the incidence is as low as some of the studies suggest, it still represents a very considerable number of patients who appear to be at risk when one thinks of the large numbers of drugs prescribed and taken every day.

(c) How seriously should interactions be regarded and handled?

It would be very easy to conclude after browsing through this publication that it is extremely risky to treat patients with more than one drug at a time, but this would be an over-reaction. The figures quoted in the previous section illustrate that many drugs known to interact in some patients, simply fail to do so in others. This partially explains why some quite important drug interactions remained virtually unnoticed for many years, a good example of this being the increase in serum digoxin levels seen with quinidine (see 'Digoxin and related drugs + Quinidine', p.1108).

Examples of this kind suggest that patients apparently tolerate adverse interactions remarkably well, and that many experienced physicians accommodate the effects (such as rises or falls in serum drug levels) without consciously recognising that what they are seeing is the result of an interaction.

One of the reasons it is often difficult to detect an interaction is that, as already mentioned, patient variability is considerable. We now know many of the predisposing and protective factors that determine whether or not an interaction occurs but in practice it is still very difficult to predict what will happen when an individual patient is given two potentially interacting drugs.

Table 1.1 Some drug absorption interactions

Drug affected	*Interacting drugs*	*Effect of interaction*
Ciclosporin (Cyclosporine)	Orlistat, p.1237	Orlistat inhibits the absorption of dietary fats and therefore also lipophilic molecules such as ciclosporin
Digoxin	Metoclopramide, p.1102 Propantheline, p.1107	Reduced digoxin absorption Increased digoxin absorption (due to changes in gut motility)
Digoxin, p.1090 Levothyroxine, p.1524 Warfarin, p.414	Colestyramine	Reduced absorption due to binding/complexation with colestyramine
Ketoconazole	Antacids, p.235 H_2-receptor antagonists, p.237 Proton pump inhibitors, p.238	Reduced ketoconazole absorption due to reduced dissolution
Penicillamine	Antacids (containing Al^{3+} and/or Mg^{2+}), p.1578, iron compounds, p.1579, food, p.1579	Formation of less soluble penicillamine chelates resulting in reduced absorption of penicillamine
Methotrexate, p.693	Neomycin	Neomycin-induced malabsorption state
Quinolones	Antacids (containing Al^{3+} and/or Mg^{2+}), p.343, milk, p.347, Zn^{2+} (?), p.350, Fe^{2+}, p.350	Formation of poorly absorbed complexes
Tetracyclines	Antacids (containing Al^{3+}, Ca^{2+}, Mg^{2+}, and/or Bi^{2+}), p.359, milk, p.360, Zn^{2+}, Fe^{2+}, p.361	Formation of poorly soluble chelates resulting in reduced antibacterial absorption (see Fig. 1.1, p.3)

An easy solution to this practical problem is to choose a non-interacting alternative, but if none is available, it is frequently possible to give interacting drugs together, if appropriate precautions are taken. If the effects of the interaction are well-monitored they can often be allowed for, often simply by adjusting the doses of the interacting drugs. Many interactions are dose-related so that if the dose of the causative drug is reduced, the effects on the other drug will be reduced accordingly. Thus a non-prescription dose of cimetidine may not inhibit the metabolism of phenytoin, whereas a larger dose may clearly increase phenytoin levels (see 'Phenytoin + H_2-receptor antagonists', p.602).

The dose of the affected drug may also be critical. For example, isoniazid causes the levels of phenytoin to rise, particularly in those individuals who are slow acetylators of isoniazid, and levels may become toxic. If the serum phenytoin levels are monitored and its dose reduced appropriately, the concentrations can be kept within the therapeutic range (see 'Phenytoin + Antimycobacterials', p.593). Some interactions can be accommodated by using another member of the same group of drugs. For example, the serum levels of doxycycline can become subtherapeutic if phenytoin, barbiturates or carbamazepine are given, but other tetracyclines do not seem to be affected (see 'Tetracyclines + Antiepileptics; Enzyme-inducing', p.360). Erythromycin causes serum lovastatin levels to rise because it inhibits its metabolism, but does not affect pravastatin levels because these two statins are metabolised in different ways (see *Statins* under 'Lipid regulating drugs', p.1309). It is therefore clearly important not to uncritically extrapolate the interactions seen with one drug to all members of the same group.

It is interesting to note in this context that a study in two hospitals in Maryland, US, found that when interacting drugs were given with warfarin (but not theophylline) the length of hospital stay increased by a little over 3 days, with a rise in general costs because of the need to do more tests to get the balance right.[19] So it may be easier, quicker and cheaper to use a non-interacting alternative drug (always provided that its price is not markedly greater).

The variability in patient response has lead to some extreme responses among prescribers. Some clinicians have become over-anxious about interactions so that their patients are denied useful drugs that they might reasonably be given if appropriate precautions are taken. This attitude is exacerbated by some of the more alarmist lists and charts of interactions, which fail to make a distinction between interactions that are very well documented and well established, and those that have only been encountered in a single patient, and which in the final analysis are probably totally idiosyncratic. 'One swallow does not make a summer', nor does a serious reaction in a single patient mean that the drugs in question should never again be given to anyone else.

At the other extreme, there are some health professionals who, possibly because they have personally encountered few interactions, fail to consider drug interactions, so that some of their patients are potentially put at risk. An example of this is the fact that cisapride continued to be prescribed with known interacting drugs, even after the rare risk of fatal torsade de pointes arrhythmias, which can cause sudden death, was well established.[20] The responsible position lies between these two extremes, because a very substantial number of interacting drugs can be given together safely, if the appropriate precautions are taken. There are relatively few pairs of drugs that should always be avoided.

1. Smith JW, Seidl LG, Cluff LE. Studies on the epidemiology of adverse drug reactions. V. Clinical factors influencing susceptibility. *Ann Intern Med* (1969) 65, 629.
2. Puckett WH, Visconti JA. An epidemiological study of the clinical significance of drug-drug interaction in a private community hospital. *Am J Hosp Pharm* (1971) 28, 247.
3. Shinn AF, Shrewsbury RP, Anderson KW. Development of a computerized drug interaction database (Medicom) for use in a patient specific environment. *Drug Inf J* (1983) 17, 205.
4. Ishikura C, Ishizuka H. Evaluation of a computerized drug interaction checking system. *Int J Biomed Comput* (1983) 14, 311.
5. Schuster BG, Fleckenstein L, Wilson JP, Peck CC. Low incidence of adverse reactions due to drug-drug interaction in a potentially high risk population of medical inpatients. *Clin Res* (1982) 30, 258A.
6. Manon-Espaillat R, Burnstine TH, Remler B, Reed RC, Osorio I. Antiepileptic drug intoxication: factors and their significance. *Epilepsia* (1991) 32, 96–100.
7. Haumschild MJ, Ward ES, Bishop JM, Haumschild MS. Pharmacy-based computer system for monitoring and reporting drug interactions. *Am J Hosp Pharm* (1987) 44, 345.
8. Manchon ND, Bercoff E, Lamarchand P, Chassagne P, Senant J, Bourreille J. Fréquence et gravité des interaction médicamenteuses dans une population âgée: étude prospective concernant 639 malades. *Rev Med Interne* (1989) 10, 521–5.
9. Lipton HL, Bero LA, Bird JA, McPhee SJ. The impact of clinical pharmacists' consultations on physicians' geriatric drug prescribing. *Med Care* (1992) 30, 646–58.
10. Rupp MT, De Young M, Schondelmeyer SW. Prescribing problems and pharmacist interventions in community practice. *Med Care* (1992) 30, 926–40.
11. Rotman BL, Sullivan AN, McDonald T, DeSmedt P, Goodnature D, Higgins M, Suermond HJ, Young CY, Owens DK. A randomized evaluation of a computer-based physician's workstation; design considerations and baseline results. *Proc Annu Symp Comput Appl Med Care* (1995) 693–7.
12. Linnarsson R. Drug interactions in primary health care. A retrospective database study and its implications for the design of a computerized decision support system. *Scand J Prim Health Care* (1993) 11, 181–6.
13. Stanton LA, Peterson GM, Rumble RH, Cooper GM, Polack AE. Drug-related admissions to an Australian hospital. *J Clin Pharm Ther* (1994) 19, 341–7.
14. Goldberg RM, Mabee J, Chan L, Wong S. Drug-drug and drug-disease interactions in the ED; analysis of a high-risk population. *Am J Emerg Med* (1996) 14, 447–50.
15. Paille R, Pissochet P. L'ordonnance et les interactions medicamenteuses: etude prospective chez 896 patients traites pour hypertension arterielle en medicine generale. *Therapie* (1995) 50, 253–8.
16. Di Castri A, Jacquot JM, Hemmi P, Moati L, Rouy JM, Compan B, Nachar H, Bossy-Vassal A. Interactions medicamenteuses: etude de 409 ordannances etablies a l'issue d'une hospitalisation geriatrique. *Therapie* (1995) 50, 259–64.
17. Cadieux RJ. Drug interactions in the elderly. *Postgrad Med* (1989) 86, 179–86.
18. Tinawi M, Alguire P. The prevalence of drug interactions in hospitalized patients. *Clin Res* (1992) 40, 773A.
19. Jankel CA, McMillan JA, Martin BC. Effect of drug interactions on outcomes of patient receiving warfarin or theophylline. *Am J Hosp Pharm* (1994) 51, 661–6.
20. Smalley W, Shatin D, Wysowski DK, Gurwitz J, Andrade SE, Goodman M, Chan KA, Platt R, Schech SD, Ray WA. Contraindicated use of cisapride: impact of food and drug administration regulatory action. *JAMA* (2000) 284, 3036–9.

Mechanisms of drug interactions

Some drugs interact together in totally unique ways, but as the many examples in this publication amply illustrate, there are certain mechanisms of interaction that are encountered time and time again. Some of these common mechanisms are discussed here in greater detail than space will allow in the individual monographs, so that only the briefest reference need be made there.

Mechanisms that are unusual or peculiar to particular pairs of drugs are detailed within the monographs. Very many drugs that interact do so, not by a single mechanism, but often by two or more mechanisms acting in concert, although for clarity most of the mechanisms are dealt with here as though they occur in isolation. For convenience, the mechanisms of interactions can be subdivided into those that involve the pharmacokinetics of a drug, and those that are pharmacodynamic.

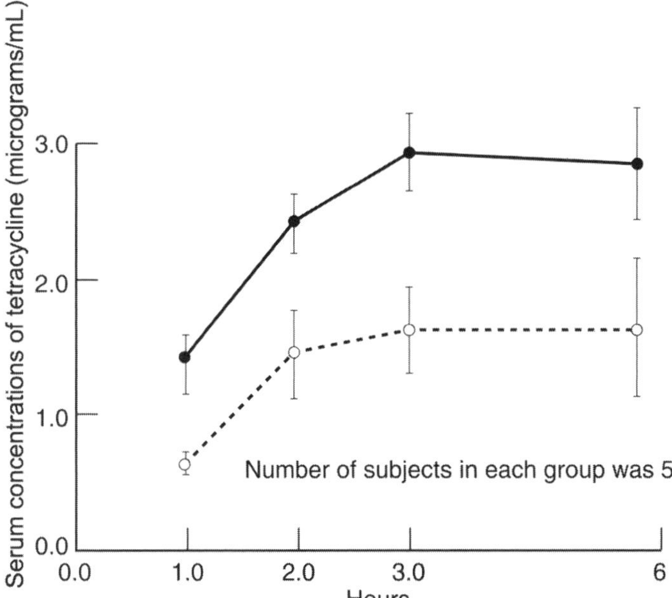

Fig. 1.1 A drug chelation interaction
Tetracycline forms a less-soluble chelate with iron if the two drugs are allowed to mix within the gut. This reduces the absorption and depresses the serum levels and the antibacterial effects (after Neuvonen PJ, *BMJ* (1970) 4, 532, with permission). The same interaction can occur with other ions such as Al^{3+}, Ca^{2+}, Mg^{2+}, Bi^{2+} and Zn^{2+}.

Pharmacokinetic interactions

Pharmacokinetic interactions are those that can affect the processes by which drugs are absorbed, distributed, metabolised and excreted (the so-called ADME interactions).

Drug absorption interactions

Most drugs are given orally for absorption through the mucous membranes of the gastrointestinal tract, and the majority of interactions that go on within the gut result in reduced rather than increased absorption. A clear distinction must be made between those that decrease the *rate* of absorption and those that alter the *total amount* absorbed. For drugs that are given long-term, in multiple doses (e.g. warfarin) the rate of absorption is usually unimportant, provided the total amount of drug absorbed is not markedly altered. On the other hand for drugs that are given as single doses, intended to be absorbed rapidly (e.g. analgesics such as paracetamol (acetaminophen)), where a rapidly achieved high concentration is needed, a reduction in the rate of absorption may result in failure to achieve an adequate effect. 'Table 1.1', p.2, lists some of the drug interactions that result from changes in absorption.

(a) Effects of changes in gastrointestinal pH

The passage of drugs through mucous membranes by simple passive diffusion depends upon the extent to which they exist in the non-ionised lipid-soluble form. Absorption is therefore governed by the pKa of the drug, its lipid-solubility, the pH of the contents of the gut and various other parameters relating to the pharmaceutical formulation of the drug. Thus the absorption of salicylic acid by the stomach is much greater at low pH than at high. On theoretical grounds it might be expected that alterations in gastric pH caused by drugs such as the H_2-receptor antagonists would have a marked effect on absorption, but in practice the outcome is often uncertain because a number of other mechanisms may also come into play, such as chelation, adsorption and changes in gut motility, which can considerably affect what actually happens. However, in some cases the effect can be significant. Rises in pH due to the proton pump inhibitors (see 'Azoles + Proton pump inhibitors', p.238), and the H_2-receptor antagonists (see 'Azoles + H_2-receptor antagonists', p.237), can markedly reduce the absorption of ketoconazole.

(b) Adsorption, chelation and other complexing mechanisms

Activated charcoal is intended to act as an adsorbing agent within the gut for the treatment of drug overdose or to remove other toxic materials, but inevitably it can affect the absorption of drugs given in therapeutic doses. Antacids can also adsorb a large number of drugs, but often other mechanisms of interaction are also involved. For example, the tetracycline antibacterials can chelate with a number of divalent and trivalent metallic ions, such as calcium, aluminium, bismuth and iron, to form complexes that are both poorly absorbed and have reduced antibacterial effects (see 'Figure 1.1', above). These metallic ions are found in dairy products and antacids. Separating the doses by 2 to 3 hours goes some way towards reducing the effects of this type of interaction. The marked reduction in the bioavailability of penicillamine caused by some antacids seems also to be due to chelation, although adsorption may have some part to play. Colestyramine, an anionic exchange resin intended to bind bile acids and cholesterol metabolites in the gut, binds to a considerable number of drugs (e.g. digoxin, warfarin, levothyroxine), thereby reducing their absorption. 'Table 1.1', p.2, lists some drugs that chelate, complex or adsorb other drugs.

(c) Changes in gastrointestinal motility

As most drugs are largely absorbed in the upper part of the small intestine, drugs that alter the rate at which the stomach empties can affect absorption. Propantheline, for example, delays gastric emptying and reduces paracetamol (acetaminophen) absorption, see 'Paracetamol (Acetaminophen) + Antimuscarinics', p.204, whereas metoclopramide, see 'Paracetamol (Acetaminophen) + Antiemetics', p.203, has the opposite effect. However, the total amount of drug absorbed remains unaltered. Drugs with antimuscarinic effects decrease the motility of the gut, thus the tricyclic antidepressants can increase the absorption of other drugs, probably because they increase the time available for dissolution and absorption but in the case of levodopa (see 'Levodopa + Tricyclic antidepressants', p.770), they may reduce the absorption, possibly because the exposure time to intestinal mucosal metabolism is increased. The same reduced levodopa absorption has also been seen with homatropine (see 'Levodopa + Antimuscarinics', p.762. These examples illustrate that what actually happens is sometimes very unpredictable because the final outcome may be the result of several different mechanisms.

(d) Induction or inhibition of drug transporter proteins

The oral bioavailability of some drugs is limited by the action of drug transporter proteins, which eject drugs that have diffused across the gut lining back into the gut. At present, the most well characterised drug transporter is P-glycoprotein (for more information, see under 'Drug transporter proteins', p.13). Digoxin is a substrate of P-glycoprotein, and drugs that induce this protein, such as rifampicin (rifampin), may reduce the bioavailability of digoxin, see 'Digoxin and related drugs + Rifampicin (Rifampin)', p.1109.

(e) Malabsorption caused by drugs

Neomycin causes a malabsorption syndrome, similar to that seen with non-tropical sprue. The effect is to impair the absorption of a number of drugs including digoxin and methotrexate (see under 'Digoxin + Aminoglycosides', p.1080, and 'Methotrexate + Antibacterials; Aminoglycosides, oral', p.693, respectively).

Drug distribution interactions

(a) Protein-binding interactions

After absorption, drugs are rapidly distributed around the body by the circulation. Some drugs are totally dissolved in the plasma water, but many others are transported with some proportion of their molecules in solution and the rest bound to plasma proteins, particularly the albumins. The extent of this binding varies enormously but some drugs are extremely highly bound. For example, dicoumarol has only four out of every 1000 molecules remaining unbound at serum concentrations of 0.5 mg%. Drugs can also become bound to albumin in the interstitial fluid, and some, such as digoxin, can bind to the heart muscle tissue.

The binding of drugs to the plasma proteins is reversible, an equilibrium being established between those molecules that are bound and those that are not. Only the unbound molecules remain free and pharmacologically active, while those that are bound form a circulating but pharmacologically inactive reservoir which, in the case of drugs with a low-extraction ratio, is temporarily protected from metabolism and excretion. As the free molecules become metabolised, some of the bound molecules become unbound and pass into solution to exert their normal pharmacological actions, before they, in their turn are metabolised and excreted.

Depending on the concentrations and their relative affinities for the binding sites, one drug may successfully compete with another and displace it from the sites it is already occupying. The displaced (and now active) drug molecules pass into the plasma water where their concentration rises. So for example, a drug that reduces the binding from 99% to 95% would increase the unbound concentration of free and active drug from 1% to 5% (a fivefold increase). This displacement is only likely to raise the number of free and active molecules significantly if the majority of the drug is within the plasma rather than the tissues, so that only drugs with a low apparent volume of distribution (V_d) will be affected. Examples include the sulfonylureas, such as tolbutamide (96% bound, V_d 10 litres), oral anticoagulants, such as warfarin (99% bound, V_d 9 litres), and phenytoin (90% bound, V_d 35 litres). However, another important factor is clearance. Clinically important protein-binding interactions are unlikely if only a small proportion of the drug is eliminated during a single-passage through the eliminating organ (low-extraction ratio drugs), as any increase in free fraction will be effectively cleared. Most drugs that are extensively bound to plasma proteins and subject to displacement reactions (e.g. warfarin, sulfonylureas, phenytoin, methotrexate, and valproate) have low-extraction ratios, and drug exposure is therefore independent of protein-binding.

An example of displacement of this kind happens when patients stabilised on warfarin are given cloral hydrate because its major metabolite, trichloroacetic acid, is a highly bound compound that successfully displaces warfarin. This effect is only very short-lived because the now free and active warfarin molecules become exposed to metabolism as the blood flows through the liver, and the amount of drug rapidly falls. This transient increase in free warfarin levels is unlikely to change the anticoagulant effect of warfarin because the clotting factor complexes that are produced when warfarin is taken have a very long half-life, and thus take a long time to reach a new steady state. Normally no change in the warfarin dose is needed (see 'Coumarins + Cloral hydrate and related drugs', p.418).

In vitro many commonly used drugs are capable of being displaced by others but in the body the effects seem almost always to be buffered so effectively that the outcome is not normally clinically important. It would therefore seem that the importance of this interaction mechanism has been grossly over-emphasised.[1-3] It is difficult to find an example of a clinically important interaction due to this mechanism alone. It has been suggested that this interaction mechanism is likely to be important only for drugs given intravenously that have a high-extraction ratio, a short pharmacokinetic-pharmacodynamic half-life and a narrow therapeutic index. Lidocaine has been given as an example of a drug fitting these criteria.[3] Some drug interactions that were originally assumed to be due to changes in protein binding have subsequently been shown to have other interaction mechanisms involved. For example, inhibition of metabolism has subsequently been shown to be important in the interactions between warfarin and phenylbutazone (see 'Coumarins and related drugs + NSAIDs; Phenylbutazone and related drugs', p.455), and tolbutamide and sulfonamides (see 'Sulfonylureas + Antibacterials; Sulfonamides and/or Trimethoprim', p.542).

However, knowledge of altered protein binding is important in therapeutic drug monitoring. Suppose for example a patient taking phenytoin was given a drug that displaced phenytoin from its binding sites. The amount of free phenytoin would rise but this would be quickly eliminated by metabolism and excretion thereby keeping the amount of free active phenytoin the same. However, the total amount of phenytoin would now be reduced. Therefore if phenytoin was monitored using an assay looking at total phenytoin levels it may appear that the phenytoin is subtherapeutic and that the dose may therefore need increasing. However, as the amount of free active phenytoin is unchanged this would not be necessary and may even be dangerous.

Basic drugs as well as acidic drugs can be highly protein bound, but clinically important displacement interactions do not seem to have been described. The reasons seem to be that the binding sites within the plasma are different from those occupied by acidic drugs (alpha-1-acid glycoprotein rather than albumin) and, in addition, basic drugs have a large V_d with only a small proportion of the total amount of drug being within the plasma.

(b) Induction or inhibition of drug transporter proteins

It is increasingly being recognised that distribution of drugs into the brain, and some other organs such as the testes, is limited by the action of drug transporter proteins such as P-glycoprotein. These proteins actively transport drugs out of cells when they have passively diffused in. Drugs that are inhibitors of these transporters could therefore increase the uptake of drug substrates into the brain, which could either increase adverse CNS effects, or be beneficial. For more information, see 'Drug transporter proteins', p.13.

1. MacKichan JJ. Protein binding drug displacement interactions. Fact or fiction? *Clin Pharmacokinet* (1989) 16, 65–73.
2. Sansom LN, Evans AM. What is the true clinical significance of plasma protein binding displacement interactions? *Drug Safety* (1995) 12, 227–33.
3. Benet LZ, Hoener B-A. Changes in plasma protein binding have little clinical relevance. *Clin Pharmacol Ther* (2002) 71, 115–121.

Drug metabolism interactions

Although a few drugs are cleared from the body simply by being excreted unchanged in the urine, most are chemically altered within the body to less lipid-soluble compounds, which are more easily excreted by the kidneys. If this were not so, many drugs would persist in the body and continue to exert their effects for a long time. This chemical change has been referred to as metabolism, biotransformation, biochemical degradation or sometimes detoxification. Some drug metabolism goes on in the serum, the kidneys, the skin, and the intestines, but the greatest proportion is carried out by enzymes that are found in the membranes of the endoplasmic reticulum of the liver cells. If liver is homogenised and then centrifuged, the reticulum breaks up into small sacs called microsomes which carry the enzymes, and it is for this reason that the metabolising enzymes of the liver are frequently referred to as liver microsomal enzymes.

Drugs are metabolised by two major types of reaction. The first, so-called phase I reactions (involving oxidation, reduction, or hydrolysis), result in metabolites that are more polar compounds (which are usually inactive), while phase II reactions involve coupling drugs and/or their phase I metabolites with some other substance (e.g. glucuronic acid, known as glucuronidation) to make polar metabolites, which are also usually inactive.

The majority of phase I oxidation reactions are carried out by the haem-containing enzyme cytochrome P450. Cytochrome P450 is not a single entity, but is a very large family of related isoenzymes. However, in practice, only a few specific subfamilies seem to be responsible for most (about 90%) of the metabolism of the commonly used drugs. The most important isoenzyme is CYP3A4, followed by CYP2D6 and CYP2C9, with CYP1A2, CYP2C8, and CYP2C19 also being important. Fewer drugs are known to be metabolised by CYP2B6 and CYP2E1. Other enzymes involved in phase I metabolism include monoamine oxidases and epoxide hydrolases.

Relatively less is known about the enzymes responsible for phase II conjugation reactions. Glucuronidation by UDP-glucuronyltransferases (UGTs), sulfation via sulfotransferases, methylation by methyltransferases, acetylation by N-acetyltransferases (NATs), and glutathione conjugation by glutathione S-transferases appear to be the main examples. UGTs are the subject of much study and are becoming increasingly important in explaining the mechanisms behind a number of drug interactions.

Although metabolism is very important for the body to remove drugs, it is increasingly recognised that drugs can be adsorbed, distributed, or eliminated by transporter proteins, the most well understood being P-glycoprotein (see *P-glycoprotein* under 'Drug transporter proteins', p.13 for further details).

It is also important to note that some drugs are given as inactive prodrugs, which are metabolised to the active drug, and some drugs have active metabolites that are more potent than the parent drug, and are considered principally responsible for the pharmacological effect.

(a) Changes in first-pass metabolism

1. Changes in rate of blood flow through the liver. After absorption in the intestine, the portal circulation takes drugs directly to the liver before they are distributed by the blood flow around the rest of the body. A number of highly lipid-soluble drugs undergo substantial biotransformation during this first-pass through the gut wall and liver and there is limited evidence that some drugs can have a marked effect on the extent of first pass metabolism by altering the rate of blood flow through the liver. However, there are few clinically relevant examples of this, and many can be explained by other mechanisms, usually altered hepatic metabolism (see *Inhibition or induction of first-pass metabolism*, below). One possible example is the increase in the rate of absorption of dofetilide with verapamil, which has resulted in an increased incidence of torsade de pointes (see 'Dofetilide + Verapamil', p.271). Another is the increase in bioavailability of high-extraction beta blockers with hydralazine, possibly caused by altered hepatic blood flow, or altered metabolism (see 'Beta blockers + Hydralazine', p.1014).

2. Inhibition or induction of first-pass metabolism. The gut wall and liver contain metabolising enzymes, principally cytochrome P450 isoenzymes. There is substantial evidence that some drugs can have a marked effect on the extent of first-pass metabolism of other drugs by inhibiting or inducing the cytochrome P450 isoenzymes in the gut wall and/or in the liver. A good example of this is the effect of grapefruit juice, which inhibits CYP3A4, mainly in the gut, and therefore reduces the first-pass metabolism of some oral calcium-channel blockers resulting in increased exposure, with the greatest effect being seen for those with the lowest bioavailability (see 'Calcium-channel blockers + Grapefruit juice', p.1037). Although altering the amount of drug absorbed, these interactions are usually considered drug metabolism interactions rather than drug absorption interactions (see 'Drug absorption interactions', p.3). The effect of grapefruit on the metabolism of other drugs is discussed further under 'Drug-food interactions', p.16.

Table 1.2 Classification of inhibitors, inducers and substrates of CYP1A2 using clinical pharmacokinetic data

Inhibitors[a] *Classification*		*Drug*	
Potent		≈Enoxacin 400 mg daily, p.1426 Fluvoxamine, p.1428	
Moderate		≈Ciprofloxacin, p.1426 ≈Combined hormonal contraceptives, p.1424 Enoxacin 100 or 200 mg daily, p.1426 Methoxsalen, oral, p.1426 ≈Mexiletine, p.1424 Pipemidic acid, p.1426 ≈Tiabendazole, p.1428	
Weak		Cimetidine, p.1423 Disulfiram, p.1424 Norfloxacin, p.1426 Pefloxacin, p.1426 Propafenone, p.1424 Verapamil, p.1429	
Unclassified[b] (inadequate data to attempt to classify)		Aciclovir, likely to be weak, p.1435 Diltiazem, likely to be weak, p.1439 Tacrine, likely to be weak, p.1436 Ticlopidine, likely to be weak, p.1441 Zileuton, likely to be weak to moderate, p.1463	
Inducers[a] *Classification*		*Drug*	
Potent			
Moderate		Phenytoin, p.1423	
Weak			
Unclassified[b] (inadequate data to attempt to classify)		Pentobarbital, likely to be weak, p.1437 Phenobarbital, likely to be weak, p.1437 Rifampicin (Rifampin), weak to moderate, p.1458 Ritonavir, likely to be weak to moderate, p.1446 Tobacco smoke, potentially moderate, p.1462	
Substrates[c,d] *Sensitive*	*Moderate*	*Minor*	*Unclassified*[e] *(inadequate data to attempt to classify)*
Alosetron, p.1488 Caffeine*, p.1428 Duloxetine, p.1478 Melatonin, p.1413 Tacrine, p.370 Tizanidine, p.1588	Clozapine, p.855 Olanzapine, p.869 Ropivacaine, p.119 Theophylline*, p.1459	Mexiletine, p.286	Amitriptyline, p.1515 Clomipramine, p.1515 Flecainide, p.277 Imipramine, p.1515 Rasagiline, potentially sensitive, p.773 Ropinirole, potentially sensitive, p.775 Zolmitriptan, p.650

* Considered the preferred *in vivo* substrates, see Bjornsson TD, Callaghan JT, Einolf HJ, *et al.* The conduct of *in vitro* and *in vivo* drug-drug interaction studies: a PhRMA perspective. *J Clin Pharmacol* (2003) 43, 443–69.
≈ There is some uncertainty about the classification because of deficiencies in available data.
a. Classified using caffeine
b. Data for caffeine unavailable, suggested classifications based on an extrapolation from data with other less sensitive CYP1A2 substrates
c. Classified using fluvoxamine
d. Note that for drugs where there are no specific studies of the metabolic pathways, CYP1A2 might not be the mechanism or might not be the sole mechanism, because fluvoxamine is also a potent inhibitor of CYP2C19 and a weak inhibitor of CYP2C9.
e. Data for fluvoxamine unavailable, suggested classifications based on an extrapolation from data with other less potent CYP1A2 inhibitors

(b) Enzyme induction

The phenomenon of enzyme induction is well demonstrated by the barbiturates which, when they were widely used as hypnotics, were found to be required in increasing doses as time went by to achieve the same hypnotic effect. The reason for this is that the barbiturates increase the synthesis of the microsomal enzymes responsible for their own metabolism (known as auto-induction), so that the extent of metabolism and excretion increases. This not only explains the need for an increased barbiturate dose, but also highlights the implications of enzyme induction if another drug that is metabolised by the same range of enzymes is also present: that is, its enzymatic metabolism will be similarly increased and larger doses will be needed to maintain the same therapeutic effect. Note that not all enzyme-inducing drugs also induce their own metabolism.

The metabolic pathway that is most commonly induced is phase I oxidation mediated by the cytochrome P450 isoenzymes. There are relatively few drugs that act as enzyme inducers, compared with the number of enzyme inhibitors, and many are not specific to a given isoenzyme. Rifampicin (rifampin) is the most studied enzyme inducer and induces most of the important drug metabolising cytochrome P450 isoenzymes to varying extents. However, it also induces other enzymatic processes, such as glucuronidation, and also various drug transporter proteins. The main drugs responsible for clinically relevant induction of CYP1A2 are listed in 'Table 1.2', above, CYP2B6 in 'Table 1.3', p.6, CYP2C8 in 'Table 1.4', p.6, CYP2C9 in 'Table 1.5', p.7, CYP2C19 in 'Table 1.6', p.8, CYP2D6 in 'Table 1.7', p.9, CYP2E1 in 'Table 1.8', p.10, and of CYP3A4 in 'Table 1.9', p.11.

The timing and extent of enzyme induction depends on the half-life of the inducing drug, its dose and the rate of turnover of the enzyme being induced. Therefore, broadly speaking, it can take days or even 2 to 3 weeks to develop fully, and might persist for a similar length of time when the enzyme inducer is stopped. This means that enzyme induction interactions can be delayed in onset and slow to resolve. Enzyme induction is a fairly common mechanism of interaction and can be caused by a number of substances, such as the chlorinated hydrocarbon insecticides (e.g. dicophane and lindane) and tobacco smoke.

If one drug reduces the effects of another by enzyme induction, it is often possible to accommodate the interaction simply by increasing the dose of the drug affected, but this requires good monitoring, and there can be hazards if the inducing drug is eventually stopped without remembering to reduce the

Table 1.3 Classification of inhibitors, inducers and substrates of CYP2B6 using clinical pharmacokinetic data

Inhibitors[a] *Classification*		*Drug*	
Potent			
Moderate			
Weak		Clopidogrel, p.1468 Ticlopidine, p.1468	
Unclassified[b] (inadequate data to attempt to classify)		Thiotepa, p.674	
Inducers[a] *Classification*		*Drug*	
Potent			
Moderate		Lopinavir boosted with ritonavir, p.1468 Rifampicin (Rifampin), p.1470 Ritonavir 600 mg daily, p.1468	
Weak			
Unclassified[b] (inadequate data to attempt to classify)			
Substrates[c] *Sensitive*	*Moderate*	*Minor*	*Unclassified*[d]
			Bupropion*, p.1468 Cyclophosphamide, p.670 Ifosfamide, p.670 Methadone, p.197 Tramadol, p.197

* Considered the preferred *in vivo* substrates, see Bjornsson TD, Callaghan JT, Einolf HJ, *et al.* The conduct of *in vitro* and *in vivo* drug-drug interaction studies: a PhRMA perspective. *J Clin Pharmacol* (2003) 43, 443–69.
a. Classified using bupropion
b. Data for bupropion unavailable, suggested classifications based on an extrapolation from data with other less sensitive CYP2B6 substrates
c. Note that for drugs where there are no specific studies of the metabolic pathways, CYP2B6 might not be the mechanism or might not be the sole mechanism.
d. The substrates cannot be classified due to the lack of a suitable inhibitor of CYP2B6.

Table 1.4 Classification of inhibitors, inducers and substrates of CYP2C8 using clinical pharmacokinetic data

Inhibitors[a] *Classification*		*Drug*	
Potent		Gemfibrozil*, p.528	
Moderate		Deferasirox, p.1573	
Weak		Trimethoprim, p.531	
Unclassified (inadequate data to attempt to classify)			
Inducers[a] *Classification*		*Drug*	
Potent			
Moderate		Rifampicin (Rifampin), p.550	
Weak			
Unclassified (inadequate data to attempt to classify)			
Substrates[b] *Sensitive*	*Moderate*	*Minor*	*Unclassified*
Repaglinide, p.528	Loperamide, p.1148 Pioglitazone, p.555 Rosiglitazone, p.555		Paclitaxel[c], p.718

* Gemfibrozil is also an inhibitor of some transport proteins including OATP, and therefore an interaction with gemfibrozil cannot be taken to mean that the drug is a substrate of CYP2C8 in the absence of specific data on its route of metabolism.
a. Classified using repaglinide
b. Classified using gemfibrozil
c. Paclitaxel is often listed as a CYP2C8 substrate based on *in vitro* data, but clinical data supporting this is lacking.

Table 1.5 Classification of inhibitors, inducers and substrates of CYP2C9 using clinical pharmacokinetic data

Inhibitors[a] *Classification*		*Drug*	
Potent			
Moderate		≈Amiodarone, p.381 ≈Benzbromarone, p.411 Fluconazole 200 mg and 400 mg daily, p.408 Miconazole, oral tablets, p.409 Sitaxentan, p.425 ≈Sulfinpyrazone, p.475	
Weak		Fluconazole 100 mg daily, p.408 Fluvastatin 80 mg daily, p.471 Fluvoxamine[b] 150 mg daily, p.551 Sulfinpyrazone, p.475 ≈Voriconazole[b], p.148 Zafirlukast, p.443	
Unclassified (inadequate data to attempt to classify)			
Inducers[a] *Classification*		*Drug*	
Potent			
Moderate		Rifampicin (Rifampin), p.397	
Weak		≈Aprepitant, p.542 Bosentan, p.425	
Unclassified (inadequate data to attempt to classify)			
Substrates[c,d] *Sensitive*	*Moderate*	*Minor*	*Unclassified*[e]
	Celecoxib, p.148 Glimepiride, p.543 *S*-warfarin*, p.408	Flurbiprofen, p.148 Fluvastatin, p.1322 Ibuprofen, p.148 Irbesartan, p.43 Losartan, p.43 Nateglinide, p.530 Phenytoin, p.595	Chlorpropamide, potentially minor, p.543 Diclofenac, potentially moderate, p.148 Glibenclamide (Glyburide), potentially minor, p.543 Gliclazide, potentially minor, p.543 Tolbutamide*, potentially minor, p.543

* Considered the preferred *in vivo* substrates, see Bjornsson TD, Callaghan JT, Einolf HJ, *et al.* The conduct of *in vitro* and *in vivo* drug-drug interaction studies: a PhRMA perspective. *J Clin Pharmacol* (2003) 43, 443–69.
≈ There is some uncertainty about the classification because of deficiencies in available data or because the effects are borderline.
a. Classified using warfarin, unless otherwise indicated
b. Classified using diclofenac or tolbutamide
c. Classified using fluconazole 200 mg or 400 mg daily, unless otherwise stated
d. Note that for drugs where there are no specific studies of the metabolic pathways, CYP2C9 might not be the mechanism or might not be the sole mechanism.
e. Data for fluconazole 200 mg or 400 mg daily unavailable, suggested classifications based on an extrapolation from data with other weaker CYP2C9 inhibitors.

dose again. That is, the increased drug dose might be an overdose when drug metabolism has returned to normal. It is also worth remembering that if a drug is *activated* by metabolism, enzyme induction might increase its effects.

(c) Enzyme inhibition

More common than enzyme induction is enzyme inhibition. This results in the reduced metabolism of an affected drug, so that it might begin to accumulate within the body, the effect usually being essentially the same as when the dose is increased. Unlike enzyme induction, which can take several days or even weeks to develop fully, enzyme inhibition can occur rapidly, often within 2 to 3 days, resulting in the rapid development of toxicity; however, the effects might not be maximal until the inhibiting drug reaches steady-state. The faster onset of enzyme inhibition is because this process often involves the drug binding with the enzyme, thereby preventing its function, whereas enzyme induction requires increased synthesis of the enzyme (a slower process). Some inhibitors have reversible effects (that is, their binding to the enzyme is reversible). Reversible inhibitors (such as the azoles) might compete with the substrate for the enzyme binding site, when they are known as competitive inhibitors, or bind to the enzyme without preventing the substrate also binding, when they are known as non-competitive inhibitors. Other inhibitors bind irreversibly to the enzyme (usually due to a reactive intermediate in their metabolism), requiring synthesis of new enzyme before activity is restored, a form of this is known as mechanism-based inhibition. Examples of mechanism-based inhibitors include the macrolides, clarithromycin and erythromycin.

The metabolic pathway that has been most studied and is most well understood is inhibition of phase I oxidation by cytochrome P450 isoenzymes. The ability of drugs to inhibit specific isoenzymes is principally determined in validated *in vitro* studies using relevant probe substrates. Subsequently, the clinical relevance of the inhibition is determined in a clinical pharmacokinetic study with a probe substrate of the isoenzyme in question. From a clinical perspective, inhibitors of cytochrome P450 isoenzymes can be classified according to the degree of inhibition they cause, as measured by the increase in exposure (AUC) or decrease in clearance of a known substrate. A universally accepted classification is still evolving, but definitions based on guidance for the pharmaceutical industry issued by the European Medicines Agency[1] and FDA,[2] and pharmacokinetic data, have been adopted in modified form in this publication. Using this classification, the main drugs responsible for clinically relevant inhibition of CYP1A2 are listed in 'Table 1.2', p.5, CYP2B6 in 'Table 1.3', p.6, CYP2C8 in 'Table 1.4', p.6, CYP2C9 in 'Table 1.5', above, CYP2C19 in 'Table 1.6', p.8, CYP2D6 in 'Table 1.7', p.9, CYP2E1 in 'Table 1.8', p.10, and of CYP3A4 in 'Table 1.9', p.11. Substrates of these isoenzymes are also included in these tables (and 'Table 1.10', p.12, for substrates of CYP3A4), with the drugs classified by how extensively they are metabolised by that isoenzyme. The clinical relevance of the increases in exposure of a substrate drug with a given inhibitor depends on the therapeutic range of the substrate. For a drug with a narrow therapeutic range and for which doses are individually adjusted and monitored (e.g. warfarin), even a small increase in exposure with a weak inhibitor could be clinically important. However, for a drug for which there is a very wide therapeutic range and for which there is no individualised dose (e.g. omeprazole), then even a marked rise with a potent inhibitor might not be clinically important. Furthermore, the sensitivity of a drug for the isoenzyme in question will also play a part. Bear in mind also that there are some

Table 1.6 Classification of inhibitors, inducers and substrates of CYP2C19 using clinical pharmacokinetic data

Inhibitors[a] *Classification*		*Drug*	*Effect on substrate*
Potent		Fluconazole 100 mg daily, p.238	6.3-fold increase in omeprazole exposure
		Fluvoxamine, p.1154	6-fold increase in omeprazole exposure
		Ticlopidine, p.1156	5- to 6-fold increase in omeprazole exposure
Moderate		Moclobemide, p.1406	2.1-fold increase in omeprazole exposure
		≈Omeprazole[b] 40 mg daily, p.834	54% decrease in diazepam clearance
		Voriconazole, p.238	4-fold increase in omeprazole exposure
Weak		Armodafinil, p.222	38% increase in omeprazole exposure
		Esomeprazole[b] 30 mg daily, p.834	81% increase in diazepam exposure
		Isoniazid[b], p.827	26% decrease in diazepam clearance
		Modafinil, p.222	Potency based on effect of armodafinil on omeprazole
		Omeprazole[b] 20 mg daily, p.834	27% decrease in diazepam clearance
Unclassified (inadequate data to attempt to classify)		Cimetidine, p.254	
Inducers[a] *Classification*		*Drug*	*Effect on substrate*
Potent			
Moderate		Rifampicin (Rifampin)[b], p.836	77% decrease in diazepam exposure
Weak		≈Artemisinin, p.1151	35% decrease in omeprazole exposure
Unclassified (inadequate data to attempt to classify)			
Substrates[c] *Sensitive*	*Moderate*	*Minor*	*Unclassified*
Omeprazole*, p.1154	Citalopram, p.1154	Cilostazol, p.784	≈Clopidogrel, p.788
	Diazepam, p.838	Phenytoin, p.605	
	Lansoprazole, p.1154	Proguanil, p.254	
	Moclobemide, p.1406		
	Rabeprazole, p.1154		

* Considered the preferred *in vivo* substrates, see Bjornsson TD, Callaghan JT, Einolf HJ, *et al.* The conduct of *in vitro* and *in vivo* drug-drug interaction studies: a PhRMA perspective. *J Clin Pharmacol* (2003) 43, 443–69.
≈ There is some uncertainty about the classification because of deficiencies in available data or because the effects are borderline.
a. Classifed using omeprazole unless otherwise indicated
b. Classified using diazepam
c. Note that for drugs where there are no specific studies of the metabolic pathways, CYP2C19 might not be the mechanism or might not be the sole mechanism.

drugs that are metabolised to form metabolites with greater activity. For these drugs, inhibition of metabolism might lead to reduced efficacy, for example, see 'Opioids; Codeine and related drugs + Quinidine', p.194.

An example of inhibition of phase I hydrolytic metabolism, is the inhibition of epoxide hydrolase by valpromide, which increases the levels of carbamazepine, see 'Carbamazepine and related drugs + Valproate', p.580. Phase II conjugative metabolism can also be inhibited. Examples are the inhibition of carbamazepine glucuronidation by sodium valproate, see 'Carbamazepine and related drugs + Valproate', p.580, and the inhibition of methyltransferase by aminosalicylates causing increased plasma concentrations of azathioprine, see 'Thiopurines + 5-Aminosalicylates', p.721.

Alteration of cytochrome P450 activity by therapeutic proteins. It has generally been perceived that therapeutic proteins such as interferons and monoclonal antibodies are unlikely to cause drug interactions via the cytochrome P450 isoenzyme system, principally because of their size and the fact they are not metabolised by this system. However, some unexplained interactions have been seen, for example interferons increase the exposure of theophylline, a drug extensively metabolised by CYP1A2, see 'Theophylline + Interferons', p.1447. The mechanism for these interactions is not fully understood, but might be due to changes in transcription factor activity for enzyme expression or changes in enzyme stability. This cannot be studied in the usual *in vitro* tests for cytochrome P450 isoenzyme inhibition or induction, and is an evolving area of research.[3,4]

(d) Genetic factors in drug metabolism

An increased understanding of genetics has shown that some of the cytochrome P450 isoenzymes are subject to genetic polymorphism, which simply means that at least 1% of the population have a variant gene for the isoenzyme that might result in important variability in drug metabolising capacity. The best known example is CYP2D6, for which a small proportion of the population have a variant with little or no activity (caused by the presence of two non-functional alleles in the CYP2D6 gene). Such individuals are described as poor metabolisers (or as possessing the poor metaboliser phenotype), and make up about 5 to 10% of Caucasians. Individuals with normal enzyme activity (resulting from the presence of two alleles with normal function in the gene) are described as extensive metabolisers. Such individuals make up the majority (70 to 80%) of Caucasians. In addition, for CYP2D6, it is now known that there are ultrarapid metabolisers who have more than one extra functional gene (3 to 5% of Caucasians) and also intermediate metabolisers who usually have one functional and one non-functional allele (10 to 17% of Caucasians). The metaboliser status (or phenotype) of any given individual is genetically determined and distribution varies greatly amongst ethnic groups, resulting in variable percentages within a given population. It is possible to find out the phenotype of an individual by looking at the way a single dose of a test or probe drug is metabolised (often dextromethorphan for CYP2D6). This varying ability to metabolise certain drugs might explain why some patients develop toxicity when given an interacting drug while others remain symptom free. CYP2C9 and CYP2C19 also show polymorphism, whereas CYP3A4 does not, although there is still some broad variation in the population without there being distinct groups. CYP2C19 polymorphism is discussed in more detail elsewhere (see under 'Gastrointestinal drugs', p.1135).

Such genetic variability means that when studying drug interactions mediated via CYP2D6, CYP2C19, and CYP2C9 it can be important to know which phenotype the subjects are, because for example, a CYP2D6 inhibitor would have little effect in those who are CYP2D6 poor metabolisers.[5] Looking at the differences in drug exposure between subjects with

Table 1.7 Classification of inhibitors, inducers and substrates of CYP2D6 using clinical pharmacokinetic data

Inhibitors[a] *Classification*		*Drug*	*Effect on substrate*
Potent		Bupropion, p.1504 Cinacalcet, p.1565 ≈Fluoxetine, p.1515 Paroxetine, p.1515 Quinidine, p.1513	5-fold increase in desipramine exposure 11.4-fold increase in dextromethorphan exposure up to 6.3-fold increase in desipramine exposure 5.2-fold increase in desipramine exposure 85% decrease in desipramine clearance
Moderate		Duloxetine, p.1514 Mirabegron, p.1512 ≈Propafenone, p.1019 Ritonavir high dose (500 mg twice daily), p.1509 Terbinafine, p.1517	2.9-fold increase in desipramine exposure 3.4-fold increase in desipramine exposure 51% decrease in metoprolol clearance 2.5-fold increase in desipramine exposure 4.9-fold increase in desipramine exposure
Weak		≈Amiodarone, p.1001 Celecoxib, p.1003 Cimetidine, p.1011 Citalopram, p.1515 Cobicistat, p.1506 Diphenhydramine, p.1009 ≈Escitalopram, p.1515 ≈Ritonavir low dose (100 mg daily), p.1509 Sertraline, p.1515	81% increase in metoprolol exposure 64% increase in metoprolol exposure 61% increase in metoprolol exposure 50% increase in desipramine exposure 65% increase in desipramine exposure 61% increase in metoprolol exposure 2-fold increase in desipramine exposure 26% increase in desipramine exposure 23% to 37% increase in desipramine exposure
Unclassified (inadequate data to attempt to classify)		Dextropropoxyphene (Propoxyphene), potentially moderate, p.1009 Moclobemide, p.1387 Quinine, p.1513 Ranolazine, potentially weak, p.1073 Venlafaxine, p.1482	
Inducers[a] *Classification*		*Drug*	*Effect on substrate*
Potent			
Moderate			
Weak		Carbamazepine, p.1505 Rifampicin (Rifampin), p.1021	31% increase in desipramine clearance 33% decrease in metoprolol exposure
Unclassified (inadequate data to attempt to classify)			
Substrates[c] *Sensitive*	*Moderate*	*Minor*	*Unclassified*
Atomoxetine, p.219 Desipramine*, p.1515 Dextromethorphan*, p.1565 Metoprolol, p.1022 Perphenazine, p.874	Nortriptyline, p.1513 Propranolol, p.1020 Tolterodine, p.1550	Carvedilol, p.1022 Darifenacin, p.1550 Duloxetine, p.1478 Flecainide, p.276 Galantamine, p.370 Imipramine, p.1513 Mexiletine, p.286 Pindolol, p.1022 Propafenone, p.292	Amitriptyline, p.1515 Clomipramine, p.1515 Clozapine, potentially minor, p.855 Codeine, p.194 Dihydrocodeine, p.194 Donepezil, p.370 Hydrocodone, p.194 Oxycodone, p.194 Risperidone, potentially moderate, p.887 Tamoxifen, p.712 Thioridazine, p.874 Trimipramine, p.1515 Venlafaxine, p.1482

* Considered the preferred *in vivo* substrates, see Bjornsson TD, Callaghan JT, Einolf HJ, *et al.* The conduct of *in vitro* and *in vivo* drug-drug interaction studies: a PhRMA perspective. *J Clin Pharmacol* (2003) 43, 443–69.
≈ There is some uncertainty about the classification because of deficiencies in available data or because the effects are borderline.
a. Classified using desipramine, dextromethorphan or metoprolol.
b. Note that some sources suggest that CYP2D6 is not inducible.
c. Note that for drugs where there are no specific studies of the metabolic pathways, CYP2D6 may not be the mechanism or may not be the sole mechanism.

different phenotypes of CYP2D6, CYP2C9, and CYP2C19 might be used as way of predicting what will happen with drugs that are inhibitors of these isoenzymes. For example, the difference in exposure of a particular drug between CYP2C19 extensive metabolisers and CYP2C19 poor metabolisers is likely to represent the greatest effect that could be expected for a potent inhibitor of CYP2C19 given with that drug. If this is unlikely to be clinically relevant, it might make interaction studies with strong inhibitors unnecessary.[3] At present, genotyping of cytochrome P450 isoenzymes is primarily a research tool and is not widely used clinically.

Similarly, acetylation by N-acetyltransferases (NATs) is also subject to genetic polymorphism. Individuals with the slow acetylator phenotype are slower to metabolise drugs (such as hydralazine, isoniazid, procainamide, and sulfasalazine) by this pathway, and these individuals generally experience greater toxicity from these drugs. Those individuals with the fast acetylator

Table 1.8 Classification of inhibitors, inducers and substrates of CYP2E1 using clinical pharmacokinetic data

Inhibitors[a] *Classification*		*Drug*	
Potent		Disulfiram, p.1559	
Moderate		Isoniazid, p.1559 see also inducers, below	
Weak			
Unclassified (inadequate data to attempt to classify)			
Inducers[a] *Classification*		*Drug*	
Potent			
Moderate			
Weak		Isoniazid, p.1559 see also inhibitors, above	
Unclassified (inadequate data to attempt to classify)		Alcohol, p.79	
Substrates *Sensitive*	*Moderate*	*Minor*	*Unclassified*
Chlorzoxazone*, p.1559			

* Considered the preferred *in vivo* substrates, see Bjornsson TD, Callaghan JT, Einolf HJ, *et al.* The conduct of *in vitro* and *in vivo* drug-drug interaction studies: a PhRMA perspective. *J Clin Pharmacol* (2003) 43, 443–69.
a. Classified using chlorzoxazone.

phenotype metabolise these drugs more quickly, and as a result might need higher doses. For an example of how acetylator status affects phenytoin exposure in patients given isoniazid, see 'Phenytoin + Antimycobacterials', p.593.

(e) Cytochrome P450 isoenzymes and predicting drug interactions

It is interesting to know which particular isoenzyme is responsible for the metabolism of drugs because by doing *in vitro* tests with human liver enzymes it is often possible to explain why and how some drugs interact. For example, midazolam is metabolised by CYP3A4, and rifampicin (rifampin) is a known, potent inducer of this isoenzyme, whereas ketoconazole inhibits its activity, so that it comes as no surprise that rifampicin reduces the exposure to midazolam and ketoconazole increases it.

What is very much more important than retrospectively finding out why two drugs interact, is the knowledge such *in vitro* tests can provide about forecasting which other drugs could also interact. This has the potential to reduce the numbers of expensive clinical studies in subjects and patients and avoids waiting until important drug interactions are observed in clinical use. A lot of effort is being put into this area of drug development.[1,2,6-11] If a drug does not inhibit a given isoenzyme in an established *in vitro* test, it can be concluded with certainty that it will not interact *via this mechanism* clinically. For example, if a drug does not inhibit CYP3A4 *in vitro* then it will not increase the exposure of drugs that are CYP3A4 substrates via this mechanism. However, at present, if a drug inhibits an isoenzyme *in vitro* at a clinically relevant concentration and in an established test, then it cannot be directly inferred that this will occur clinically because of unknown factors in absorption, distribution and metabolism of the drug, such as other routes of metabolism that might come into play. For this reason, if a drug is shown to be an inhibitor or inducer of a P450 isoenzyme *in vitro*, then a clinical pharmacokinetic study with a relevant probe substrate is currently necessary to determine the clinical relevance of the interaction.[1,2] Sometimes a 'cocktail' study is undertaken with a number of probe substrates given simultaneously as a single dose before and after the new drug has been taken for a relevant time period. However, it is worth bearing in mind that controlled clinical pharmacokinetic studies are not always considered ethical for some drugs, for example cytotoxic antineoplastics, and, in this situation, it might be necessary to advise precautions based on *in vitro* data, despite the limitations.

The tables of enzyme inducers, inhibitors and substrates (referred to above, under *Enzyme inhibition*) are lists of drugs that have been shown to be inhibitors, inducers, or substrates of the clinically important cytochrome P450 isoenzymes, in clinical studies. Each drug has a cross reference to a monograph describing a drug interaction thought to occur by that mechanism. If a new drug is shown to be an inducer, or an inhibitor, and/or a substrate of a given isoenzyme in clinical studies, these tables could be used to predict likely drug interactions. As stated above, if there is only *in vitro* data for the new drug, then some caution is needed in predicting interactions.

Sometimes, interactions occur that are the opposite from that predicted from *in vitro* data. For example, ritonavir is a well-known potent inhibitor of CYP3A4, and in clinical use increases the exposure to many drugs that are substrates of this isoenzyme. Methadone is a minor substrate of CYP3A4, and some *in vitro* data show that ritonavir (predictably) increased methadone concentrations. However, unexpectedly, in clinical use the HIV-protease inhibitors seem to *decrease* methadone concentrations, by an uncertain mechanism (see, 'Opioids; Methadone + HIV-protease inhibitors', p.182). Similarly, ritonavir *reduces* the exposure to ethinylestradiol and some progestogens in combined hormonal contraceptives (see, 'Combined hormonal contraceptives + HIV-protease inhibitors', p.1177).

Another factor complicating the understanding of metabolic drug interactions is the finding that there is a large overlap between the inhibitors, inducers and substrates of the drug transporter protein P-glycoprotein and those of CYP3A4. Therefore, both mechanisms might be involved in many of the drug interactions previously thought to be due to effects on CYP3A4. See *P-glycoprotein* under 'Drug transporter proteins', p.13 for further details.

1. EMA. Guidance on the investigation of drug interactions. Draft. 22 April 2010. Available at: http://www.ema.europa.eu/docs/en_GB/document_library/Scientific_guideline/2010/05/WC500090112.pdf (accessed 08/09/15).
2. US FDA. Guidance for industry. Drug interaction studies—study design, data analysis, implications for dosing, and labelling recommendations. Draft guidance, February 2012. Available at: http://www.fda.gov/downloads/Drugs/GuidanceComplianceRegulatoryInformation/Guidances/UCM292362.pdf (accessed 08/09/15).
3. Huang S-M, Strong JM, Zhang L, Reynolds KS, Nallani S, Temple R, Abraham S, Habet SA, Baweja RK, Burckart GJ, Chung S, Colangelo P, Frucht D, Green MD, Hepp P, Karnaukhova E, Ko HS, Lee JI, Marroum PJ, Norden JM, Qiu W, Rahman A, Sobel S, Stifano T, Thummel K, Wei XX, Yasuda S, Zheng JH, Zhao H, Lesko LJ. New era in drug interaction evaluation: US Food and Drug Administration update on CYP enzymes, transporters, and the guidance process. *J Clin Pharmacol* (2008) 48, 662–70.
4. Lee JI, Zhang L, Men AY, Kenna LA, Huang S-M. CYP-mediated therapeutic protein-drug interactions: clinical findings, proposed mechanisms and regulatory implications. *Clin Pharmacokinet* (2010) 49, 295–310.
5. Lee LS, Nafziger AN, Bertino JS. Evaluation of inhibitory drug interactions during drug development: genetic polymorphisms must be considered. *Clin Pharmacol Ther* (2005) 78, 1–6.
6. Bjornsson TD, Callaghan JT, Einolf HJ, Fischer V, Gan L, Grimm S, Kao J, King SP, Miwa G, Ni L, Kumar G, McLeod J, Obach RS, Roberts S, Roe A, Shah A, Snikeris F, Sullivan JT, Tweedie D, Vega JM, Walsh J, Wrighton SA. The conduct of in vitro and in vivo drug-drug interaction studies: a PhRMA perspective. *J Clin Pharmacol* (2003) 43, 443–69.
7. Bachmann KA, Ghosh R. The use of *in vitro* methods to predict *in vivo* pharmacokinetics and drug interactions. *Curr Drug Metab* (2001) 2, 299–314.
8. Venkatakrishnan K, von Moltke LL, Obach RS, Greenblatt DJ. Drug metabolism and drug interactions: application and clinical value of *in vitro* models. *Curr Drug Metab* (2003) 4, 423–59.
9. Brown HS, Galetin A, Hallifax D, Houston JB. Prediction of in vivo drug-drug interactions from in vitro data: factors affecting prototypic drug-drug interactions involving CYP2C9, CYP2D6 and CYP3A4. *Clin Pharmacokinet* (2006) 45, 1035–50.
10. Foti RS, Wahlstrom JL. Prediction of CYP-mediated drug interactions in vivo using in vitro data. *IDrugs* (2008) 11, 900–905.
11. Zhang L, Zhang Y, Zhao P, Huang S-M. Predicting drug–drug interactions: an FDA perspective. AAPS J. (2009) 11, 300–306.

Table 1.9 Classification of inhibitors and inducers of CYP3A4 using clinical pharmacokinetic data

Inhibitors[a] *Classification*	*Drug*	*Increase in oral midazolam exposure*
Potent*	Boceprevir, p.824	5.3-fold
	Clarithromycin, p.827	8-fold
	Cobicistat[c], p.820	9.8- to 19-fold
	HIV-protease inhibitors boosted with ritonavir[b,c], p.825	10- to 13-fold
	Itraconazole, p.814	6- to 10-fold
	Ketoconazole[c], p.825	11- to 17-fold
	Nelfinavir, p.1345	Potency based on simvastatin data
	Ritonavir 100 mg twice daily[c], p.825	≈26-fold
	Saquinavir, p.825	5.2-fold
	Telaprevir, p.824	9-fold
	Telithromycin, p.827	6.1-fold
	Voriconazole[c], p.817	10.3-fold
Moderate*	Aprepitant, p.813 see also inducers, below	2.3- to 3.3-fold
	Conivaptan, p.1592	3-fold
	Crizotinib, p.842	3.7-fold
	Diltiazem, p.818	≈4-fold
	Erythromycin, p.827	2- to 4.4-fold
	Fluconazole, p.814	3.5-fold
	Imatinib, p.1357	Potency based on simvastatin data
	Nefazodone, p.830	4.6-fold
	Posaconazole, p.816	4.5-fold
	Verapamil, p.818	≈3-fold
Weak*	Cimetidine, p.822	≈0 to 100%
	Fluvoxamine, p.838	39%
	Fosaprepitant, p.813	up to 80%
	Grapefruit juice, p.822	52 to 65%
	Lapatinib, p.842	45%
	Lomitapide, p.1318	Potency based on simvastatin data
	Pazopanib, p.842	30%
	Ranolazine, p.1355	Potency based on simvastatin data
	Roxithromycin, p.827	47%
Unclassified (inadequate data to attempt to classify)	Delavirdine, p.956	
	Indinavir, potentially moderate, p.181	
Inducers[a] *Classification*	*Drug*	*Decrease in oral midazolam exposure*
Potent*	Carbamazepine[d], p.819	≈94%[e]
	Fosphenytoin, p.833	Potency based on effect of phenytoin
	Phenytoin[d], p.833	≈94%[e]
	Rifampicin (Rifampin)[d], p.836	96%
Moderate*	Bosentan, p.1541	Potency based on sildenafil data
	Efavirenz, p.1352	Potency based on simvastatin data
	St John's wort (*Hypericum perforatum*), p.839	50%
Weak*	Aprepitant, p.813, effects appear transient see also inhibitors, above	22%
	Armodafinil, p.830	32%
	Modafinil, p.830	Potency based on effect of armodafinil
	Rufinamide, p.613	Potency based on triazolam data
Unclassified (inadequate data to properly classify)	Nevirapine, potentially moderate, p.953	
	Phenobarbital (and probably other barbiturates and primidone), potentially potent, p.1043	
	Rifabutin, potentially weak, p.195	
	Rifapentine[f], potentially potent, although generally considered moderate, p.836	

* Consider also 'Unclassified' drugs
≈ There is some uncertainty about the value, either because the inhibitor was not given for sufficient time to ensure a maximal effect, or because the study was not well-controlled.
a. Classified using midazolam, the preferred *in vivo* probe substrate.
Where midazolam data is lacking, other potential substrates have been used, but the magnitude of effect is not stated as it is not comparable to the effects on midazolam.
b. This general classification is based on data for lopinavir, saquinavir, and tipranavir but other HIV-protease inhibitors boosted with ritonavir would be expected to behave similarly.
c. These drugs increase oral midazolam exposure more than 10-fold. In some circumstances there is merit to considering them as very potent inhibitors.
d. These drugs decrease oral midazolam exposure by more than 90%. In some circumstances there is merit to considering them as very potent inducers.
e. Data for these drugs not analysed separately.
f. Data for rifapentine from controlled studies is limited and conflicting; data from experience suggests that its effects might be moderate rather than potent.

Drug excretion interactions

With the exception of the inhalational anaesthetics, most drugs are excreted either in the bile or in the urine. Blood entering the kidneys along the renal arteries is, first of all, delivered to the glomeruli of the tubules where molecules small enough to pass through the pores of the glomerular membrane (e.g. water, salts, some drugs) are filtered through into the lumen of the tubules. Larger molecules, such as plasma proteins, and blood cells are retained within the blood. The blood flow then passes to the remaining parts of the kidney tubules where active energy-using transport systems are able to remove drugs and their metabolites from the blood and secrete them into the tubular filtrate. The renal tubular cells additionally possess active and passive transport systems for the reabsorption of drugs. Interference by drugs

Table 1.10 Classification of CYP3A4 substrates using clinical pharmacokinetic data[a]

Sensitive[b]	*Moderate*[b]	*Minor*[b]	*Unclassified*[b]	*Substrates that are themselves inhibitors or inducers of CYPs*[c]
Alfentanil, p.181	Alprazolam, p.814	Almotriptan, p.643	Bromocriptine (potentially moderate), p.758	Amiodarone, p.264
Bosutinib, p.728	Atorvastatin, p.1322	Aripiprazole, p.808	Ciclosporin (potentially moderate to sensitive), p.1209	Amprenavir, p.941
Budesonide (oral), p.1247	Bosentan, p.1059	Buprenorphine, p.165	Cisapride (potentially moderate to sensitive), p.1140	Aprepitant, p.1138
Buspirone*, p.844	Budesonide (inhaled), p.1246	Donepezil, p.368	Cyclophosphamide (potentially minor), p.670	Atazanavir, p.941
Darifenacin, p.1548	Cabergoline, p.758	Erlotinib, p.728	Disopyramide, p.268	Carbamazepine, p.574
Dasatinib, p.728	≈Cilostazol, p.783	Fentanyl (intravenous)[e], p.181	Dutasteride (potentially minor), p.1536	Darunavir, p.941
Eletriptan, p.643	Crizotinib, p.728	Galantamine, p.368	Ergot derivatives (potentially sensitive), p.642	Diltiazem, p.1041
Eplerenone, p.1129	Dexamethasone, p.1246	Gefitinib, p.728	Irinotecan (potentially moderate), p.686	Fosaprepitant, p.1138
Felodipine[d], p.1033	Docetaxel, p.718	Haloperidol, p.859	Risperidone, p.883	Fosamprenavir, p.941
Fluticasone (intranasal), p.1252	Domperidone, p.1140	Imatinib, p.728	Temsirolimus (intravenous, potentially moderate), p.1307	Indinavir, p.941
Ivacaftor, p.1574	Eszopiclone, p.814	Lidocaine (oral), p.279	Toremifene, p.725	Itraconazole, p.330
Lercanidipine, p.1033	Fesoterodine, p.1548	Methadone, p.165	Vinblastine, p.744	Nelfinavir, p.941
Lomitapide, p.1318	Fluticasone (inhaled), p.1247	Reboxetine, p.1475	Vincristine, p.744	Rifabutin, p.939
Lovastatin, p.1322*	Lapatinib, p.728	Sibutramine, p.223		Ritonavir, p.941
Maraviroc, p.949	Loperamide, p.1148	Sunitinib, p.728		Saquinavir, p.941
Midazolam* (intravenous less sensitive than oral), p.814	Methylprednisolone, p.1246	Zolpidem, p.814		Tipranavir, p.934
Nisoldipine, p.1033	Nilotinib, p.728	Zopiclone, p.814		Voriconazole, p.954
Quetiapine, p.880	Oxybutynin, p.1548			Verapamil, p.1041
Salmeterol, p.1421	Pimozide, p.879			
Sildenafil, p.1543	Quinidine, p.294			
Simvastatin*, p.1322	Ranolazine, p.1073			
Sirolimus, p.1280	Solifenacin, p.1548			
Temsirolimus (oral), p.1307	Tacrolimus, p.1289			
Triazolam, p.814	Tadalafil, p.1540			
Vardenafil, p.1543	Tolterodine, p.1548			
	Trazodone, p.1499			

* Considered the preferred *in vivo* substrates, see Bjornsson TD, Callaghan JT, Einolf HJ, *et al.* The conduct of *in vitro* and *in vivo* drug-drug interaction studies: a PhRMA perspective. *J Clin Pharmacol* (2003) 43, 443–69.
≈ There is some uncertainty about the classification because of deficiencies in the available data.
a. Using potent or very potent inhibitors of CYP3A4 (see Table 1.9 for a list).
b. Note that there is a crossover between inhibition of CYP3A4 and the drug transporter protein P-glycoprotein, therefore, it is possible that for drugs where there are no specific studies of the metabolic pathways, CYP3A4 might not be the mechanism or might not be the sole mechanism.
c. Substrates of CYP3A4 that are themselves inhibitors or inducers of CYPs have been listed separately, because these drugs can alter their own metabolism, and the additional effect of adding another CYP3A4 inhibitor/inducer is not always straightforward.
d. Has been considered a preferred substrate for CYP3A4, but note that this drug has also been used to assess P-glycoprotein induction and inhibition.
e. Sensitivity of fentanyl given by other routes unclear.

with renal tubular fluid pH, with active transport systems and with blood flow to the kidney can alter the excretion of other drugs.

(a) Changes in urinary pH

As with drug absorption in the gut, passive reabsorption of drugs depends upon the extent to which the drug exists in the non-ionised lipid-soluble form, which in its turn depends on its pKa and the pH of the urine. Only the non-ionised form is lipid-soluble and able to diffuse back through the lipid membranes of the tubule cells. Therefore, at high pH values (alkaline), weakly acid drugs (pKa 3 to 7.5) largely exist as ionised lipid-insoluble molecules, which are unable to diffuse into the tubule cells and will therefore remain in the urine and be removed from the body. The converse will be true for weak bases with pKa values of 7.5 to 10.5. Therefore pH changes that increase the amount of drug in the ionised form (alkaline urine for acidic drugs, acid urine for basic drugs) will increase the loss of the drug, whereas

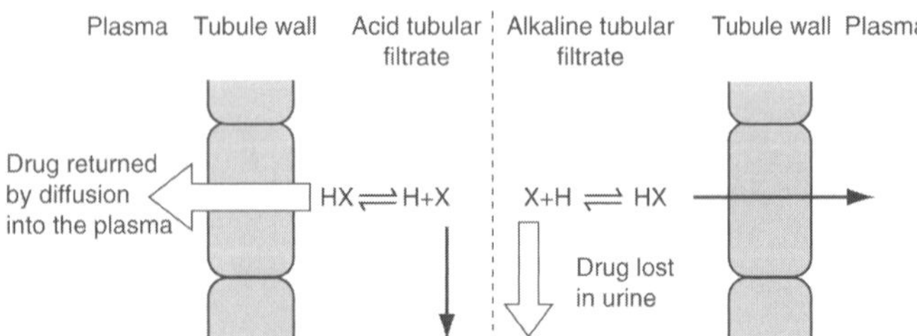

Fig. 1.2 An excretion interaction
If the tubular filtrate is acidified, most of the molecules of weakly acid drugs (HX) exist in an un-ionised lipid-soluble form and are able to return through the lipid membranes of the tubule cells by simple diffusion. Thus they are retained. In alkaline urine most of the drug molecules exist in an ionised non-lipid soluble form (X). In this form the molecules are unable to diffuse freely through these membranes and are therefore lost in the urine.

moving the pH in the opposite direction will increase their retention. 'Figure 1.2', above, illustrates the situation with a weakly acidic drug. The clinical significance of this interaction mechanism is small, because although a very large number of drugs are either weak acids or bases, almost all are largely metabolised by the liver to inactive compounds and few are excreted in the urine unchanged. In practice, therefore, only a handful of drugs seem to be affected by changes in urinary pH: possible exceptions include changes in the excretion of quinidine (see 'Quinidine + Antacids or Urinary alkalinisers', p.293) or analgesic-dose aspirin (see 'Aspirin or other Salicylates + Antacids', p.140) due to alterations in urinary pH caused by antacids, and the increase in the clearance of methotrexate (see 'Methotrexate + Urinary alkalinisers', p.704) with urinary alkalinisers. In cases of overdose, deliberate manipulation of urinary pH has been used to increase the removal of drugs such as methotrexate and salicylates.

(b) Changes in active renal tubular excretion

Drugs that use the same active transport systems in the renal tubules can compete with one another for excretion. For example, probenecid reduces the excretion of penicillin and other drugs. With the increasing understanding of drug transporter proteins in the kidneys, it is now known that probenecid inhibits the renal secretion of many other anionic drugs by organic anion transporters (OATs).[1] Probenecid possibly also inhibits some of the ATP-binding cassette (ABC) transporters in the kidneys. The ABC transporter, P-glycoprotein, is also present in the kidneys, and drugs that alter this might alter renal drug elimination. See, 'Drug transporter proteins', p.13, for further discussion. Some examples of drugs that possibly interact by alterations in renal transport are given in 'Table 1.11', p.13.

(c) Changes in renal blood flow

The flow of blood through the kidney is partially controlled by the production of renal vasodilatory prostaglandins. If the synthesis of these prostaglandins is inhibited the renal excretion of some drugs might be reduced. An interaction where this is the suggested mechanism is the rise in serum lithium seen with some NSAIDs, see 'Lithium + NSAIDs', p.1374.

Table 1.11 Examples of interactions probably due to changes in renal transport

Drug affected	*Interacting drug*	*Result of interaction*
Cephalosporins, p.311 Dapsone Methotrexate Penicillins Quinolones	Probenecid	Serum levels of drug affected raised; possibility of toxicity with some drugs
Methotrexate, p.700	Salicylates and some other NSAIDs	Methotrexate serum levels raised; serious methotrexate toxicity possible
Pramipexole	Cimetidine	Serum levels of drug affected raised

(d) Biliary excretion and the entero-hepatic shunt

1. Enterohepatic recirculation. A number of drugs are excreted in the bile, either unchanged or conjugated (e.g. as the glucuronide) to make them more water soluble. Some of the conjugates are metabolised to the parent compound by the gut flora and are then reabsorbed. This recycling process prolongs the stay of the drug within the body, but if the gut flora are diminished by the presence of an antibacterial, the drug is not recycled and is lost more quickly. This was thought to explain the rare failure of the hormonal contraceptives that can be brought about by the concurrent use of penicillins or tetracyclines, but see *Mechanism* in 'Combined hormonal contraceptives + Antibacterials', p.1162. In addition, colestyramine, which is known to bind with a number of other drugs, can affect the enterohepatic recirculation of the bound drug and therefore affect its overall exposure. This appears to be the case with mycophenolate, see 'Mycophenolate + Colestyramine', p.1274.

2. Drug transporter proteins. Increasing research shows that numerous drug transporter proteins (both from the ABC family and solute carrier superfamily (SLC), see 'Drug transporter proteins', p.13) are involved in the hepatic extraction and secretion of drugs into the bile.[2] The relevance of many of these to drug interactions is still unclear, but the bile salt export pump (ABCB11) is known to be inhibited by a variety of drugs including ciclosporin, glibenclamide, and bosentan. Inhibition of this pump might increase the risk of cholestasis, and these drugs should be avoided in patients taking bosentan (see 'Sulfonylureas + Bosentan', p.545, and 'Ciclosporin + Endothelin receptor antagonists', p.1227).

1. Lee W, Kim RB. Transporters and renal drug elimination. *Annu Rev Pharmacol Toxicol* (2004) 44, 137–66.
2. Faber KN, Müller M, Jansen PLM. Drug transport proteins in the liver. *Adv Drug Deliv Rev* (2003) 55, 107–24.

Drug transporter proteins

Drugs and endogenous substances are known to cross biological membranes, not just by passive diffusion, but by carrier-mediated processes: these carriers are often known as drug transporter proteins. Significant advances in the identification of various transporters have been made, although the contribution of many of these to drug interactions, in particular, is still unclear.[1,2] The most well-known is P-glycoprotein, which is a product of the MDR1 gene (ABCB1 gene) and a member of the ATP-binding cassette (ABC) family of efflux transporters.[1] Other transporters that are involved in some drug interactions are members of the solute carrier superfamily (SLC) of transporters. In a similar way to cytochrome P450, the individual members of the ABC and SLC subfamilies are numbered.

P-glycoprotein interactions

P-glycoprotein is an efflux pump found in the membranes of certain cells and is thought to fulfil a protective function, by actively pushing substances and drugs out of these cells. As a result, it can have an impact on the extent of drug absorption (in the intestine), distribution (to the brain, lymphocytes, testes, or placenta) and elimination (in the urine and bile). It is also expressed in some cancer cells, which is where it was first identified. Specifically, the P-glycoprotein in the cells lining the gut wall can eject some already absorbed drug molecules back into the lumen of the intestine, resulting in a reduction in the total amount of drug absorbed. The P-glycoprotein in the endothelial cells of the blood-brain barrier can eject certain drugs from the brain, thus limiting CNS distribution and reducing central effects. Similarly, distribution of drugs to lymphocytes and cancer cells can also be reduced by P-glycoprotein-mediated efflux. It is easy to see how this could be both beneficial in terms of reducing the adverse effects of some drugs, but also detrimental in terms of limiting distribution to the desired site of action. The latter is of particular importance for anticancer drugs and antiretrovirals reaching their site of action.

Drug interactions occur because some drugs can induce the expression of P-glycoprotein (that is, increase the amount of P-glycoprotein), or inhibit its activity. Such interactions are generally unintentional and these are the focus here; however, the effect can be exploited to achieve clinical goals (such as development of the P-glycoprotein inhibitor valspodar, with the aim of improving the penetration of cytotoxic drugs into cancer cells). So, for example, the induction of P-glycoprotein by rifampicin (rifampin) that occurs within the cells of the gut lining increases the ejection of digoxin into the lumen of the intestine. This results in a reduction in the plasma concentrations of digoxin (see 'Digoxin and related drugs + Rifampicin (Rifampin)', p.1109). In contrast, verapamil appears to inhibit the activity of P-glycoprotein, and is well known to increase digoxin concentrations (see 'Digoxin and related drugs + Calcium-channel blockers; Verapamil', p.1088). Ketoconazole also has P-glycoprotein inhibitory effects, and has been shown to increase the CSF concentrations of ritonavir, possibly by preventing the efflux of ritonavir from the CNS (see 'HIV-protease inhibitors + Azoles; Ketoconazole', p.923). Thus the induction or inhibition of P-glycoprotein can have an impact on the pharmacokinetics of some drugs, depending on, or influenced by, the site of the P-glycoprotein affected and the interplay with CYP3A4.

1. Interplay between P-glycoprotein and CYP3A4. It has been shown that the tissue distribution of CYP3A4 and P-glycoprotein is similar and that there is also considerable overlap between CYP3A4 and P-glycoprotein inhibitors, inducers, and substrates. There is evidence that the two systems operate in a coordinated way and, in the intestine particularly, P-glycoprotein might influence the extent of intestinal CYP3A4-mediated metabolism. It is suggested that P-glycoprotein-mediated efflux increases the intestinal residence time of a drug, increasing its exposure to CYP3A4 resulting in extensive intestinal metabolism and decreased bioavailability. If a drug inhibits both CYP3A4 and P-glycoprotein in the intestine, metabolism will be decreased and plasma concentrations will be increased. In contrast, an inducer of both systems in the intestine will result in greater metabolism and reduced plasma concentrations. The interplay in the liver is suggested to be the reverse of that in the intestine. There are also thought to be similarities in the mechanisms of induction of both CYP3A4 and P-glycoprotein and there is some evidence for the coordination of expression and induction via the pregnane X receptor, but this requires further study.

Additional confounding factors in determining the interplay between P-glycoprotein and CYP3A4 are numerous, but include simultaneous versus separate administration of drugs, single versus multiple doses of drugs, and differing effects on CYP3A4 and P-glycoprotein. As a result, the exact nature of the interplay between these two systems and its involvement in drug interactions is not yet clear and is the subject of much research. However, it does seem that the relative affinities of drugs for CYP3A4 or P-glycoprotein and the relative size of the individual effects of each system, ultimately dictates the resulting net effect of interactions involving dual CYP3A4 and P-glycoprotein substrates, inhibitors, and inducers.

This interplay seems likely to be involved in many of the drug interactions traditionally thought to be due to changes in CYP3A4 activity and might help to explain differences in the effects of drugs previously thought to affect CYP3A4 to similar extents. For example, see 'Sirolimus + Calcium-channel blockers', p.1282. 'Table 1.12', p.14, lists some examples of P-glycoprotein inhibitors, inducers, and substrates that have been associated with clinically important interactions and where there is reasonable evidence to relate this to the involvement of P-glycoprotein. This table can be compared with 'Table 1.9', p.11, which lists inhibitors and inducers of CYP3A4. However, note that drugs that are considered potent inhibitors of CYP3A4 might not necessarily be potent inhibitors of P-glycoprotein.

Digoxin and talinolol are examples of the few drugs that are substrates for P-glycoprotein but not CYP3A4, and they are therefore useful as probe drugs in studying interactions that occur specifically as a result of P-glycoprotein-mediated effects. Digoxin is generally considered the preferred *in vivo* substrate, although this has been debated.

2. Genetic polymorphism. It is widely recognised that P-glycoprotein is subject to genetic polymorphism (that is, variations in the expression of P-glycoprotein), but the influence of these variations on the functional capacity of P-glycoprotein and their clinical importance in relation to drug disposition is unclear.

Other drug transporter proteins

P-glycoprotein is not the only ABC transporter of relevance to drug interactions. Other examples include the bile salt export pump (BSEP or ABCB11), breast cancer resistance protein (BCRP or ABCG2), and multidrug-resistance proteins (MRP).

Table 1.12 Drugs affecting or transported by P-glycoprotein

Drug/Effect	*Comments*
Inducers	
Carbamazepine	Effect possibly clinically relevant, based on the effect on fexofenadine, p.630.
Rifampicin (Rifampin)	Effect clinically relevant, based on the effect on digoxin, p.1109.
St John's wort (*Hypericum perforatum*)	Effect clinically relevant, based on the effect on digoxin, p.1111.
Tipranavir	Effect possibly clinically relevant, based on the effect on loperamide, p.1148.
Inhibitors	
Amiodarone	Effect clinically relevant, based on the effect on digoxin, p.1080.
Azithromycin	Effect possibly clinically relevant, based on the effect on fexofenadine, p.635.
Ciclosporin	Effect likely to be clinically relevant, based on the effect on aliskiren, p.1051, but CYP3A4 effects cannot be excluded.
Clarithromycin	Effect clinically relevant, based on the effect on digoxin, p.1100.
Conivaptan	Effect clinically relevant, based on the effect on digoxin, p.1116.
Dronedarone	Effect clinically relevant, based on the effect on digoxin, p.272.
Erythromycin	Effect possibly clinically relevant, based on the effect on fexofenadine, p.635.
Lapatinib	Effect clinically relevant, based on the effect on digoxin, p.742.
Lopinavir boosted with ritonavir	Effect possibly clinically relevant, based on the effect on fexofenadine, p.634.
Itraconazole	Effect clinically relevant, based on the effect on digoxin, p.1083.
Ketoconazole	Effect likely to be clinically relevant, based on the effect on aliskiren, p.1051, but CYP3A4 effects cannot be excluded.
Quinidine	Effect clinically relevant, based on the effect on digoxin, p.1108.
Ranolazine	Effect clinically relevant, based on the effect on digoxin, p.1074.
Ritonavir	Effect clinically relevant at a ritonavir dose of 300 mg twice daily, based on the effect on digoxin, p.1098. Lower ritonavir doses might have less clinically relevant effects.
Saquinavir boosted with ritonavir	Effect clinically relevant, based on the effect on digoxin, p.1098.
Telaprevir	Effect clinically relevant, based on the effect on digoxin, p.1098.
Valspodar	Effect clinically relevant, based on the effect on digoxin, p.1115.
Verapamil	Effect clinically relevant, based on the effect on digoxin, p.1088.
Substrates	
Aliskiren	Likely substrate, based on the interaction with ciclosporin, p.1051, but other mechanisms cannot be excluded.
Colchicine	Likely substrate, based on the interaction with ciclosporin, p.1223, but other mechanisms cannot be excluded.

Continued

Table 1.12 Drugs affecting or transported by P-glycoprotein (continued)

Drug/Effect	*Comments*
Dabigatran	Likely substrate, based on the interaction with quinidine, p.493, but other mechanisms cannot be excluded.
Digoxin	Considered the preferred *in vivo* substrate for assessing the effects of other drugs on P-glycoprotein.
Edoxaban	Likely substrate, based on the interaction with quinidine, p.376, but other mechanisms cannot be excluded.
Everolimus	Likely substrate, based on the interaction with ciclosporin, p.1262, but other mechanisms cannot be excluded.
Fexofenadine	Considered a potential substrate for assessing the effects of other drugs on P-glycoprotein.
Loperamide	Likely substrate, based on the interaction with quinidine, p.1149, but other mechanisms cannot be excluded.
Paclitaxel	Likely substrate, based on the interaction with ciclosporin, p.714, but other mechanisms can not be excluded and clinical relevance unclear as data relate to the *oral* use of paclitaxel.
Sirolimus	Likely substrate, based on the interaction with ciclosporin, p.1282, but other mechanisms cannot be excluded.
Talinolol	Considered a potential substrate for assessing the effects of other drugs on P-glycoprotein.
Topotecan	Likely substrate, based on the interaction with ciclosporin, p.723, but other mechanisms can not be excluded and clinical relevance unclear as data relate to the *oral* use of topotecan.

The role of BSEP is less well defined than that of P-glycoprotein[1] and it has been suggested that inhibition of this pump might increase the risk of cholestasis, see *Drug transporter proteins* under 'Drug excretion interactions', p.11. BCRP is an efflux transporter that is found in the gastrointestinal tract, liver, and kidneys.[3] Inhibition of this transporter appears to increase the exposure to rosuvastatin, see 'Statins + Eltrombopag', p.1334. MRP2 (or ABCC2) is located in the membranes of cells in the liver, intestines, and the kidney. It is involved in the heptobiliary and renal elimination of many anionic substrates, including drugs.[4] It might be involved in increasing vincristine toxicity on concurrent use with piperacillin, see 'Vinca alkaloids; Vincristine + Piperacillin with Tazobactam', p.750.

Other transporters that are involved in some drug interactions are members of the solute carrier superfamily (SLC) of transporters,[1] and they are becoming increasingly important in explaining the mechanisms of a number of interactions previously not well understood. Examples include the organic anion transporters (OATs), organic anion-transporting polypeptides (OATPs), organic cation transporters (OCTs), and multidrug and toxin extrusion (MATE) proteins.

One example of a drug known to be an OAT inhibitor is probenecid, which affects OAT expression in the kidneys, and therefore affects the renal excretion of a number of drugs, see *Changes in active renal tubular excretion* under 'Drug excretion interactions', p.11. OATs are also expressed in a number of other sites, such as the intestine and in hepatocytes, and, in contrast to P-glycoprotein, are *influx* transporters, so, rather than ejecting drugs from cells, they facilitate drug uptake into cells. OATP1B1 (also known as SLCO1B1 or OATP2) appears to play a particularly important role in the transport of the statins, see 'Statins + Rifampicin (Rifampin)', p.1355. Inhibition of this transporter, by drugs such as ciclosporin, appears to lead to profound increases in the concentrations of some statins, see 'Statins + Ciclosporin', p.1327. The hepatic uptake of ambrisentan and bosentan by OATP1B3 appears to be inhibited by rifampicin, see 'Endothelin receptor antagonists + Rifampicin (Rifampin)', p.1060. MATE (or SLC47) proteins are involved in the renal and/or biliary excretion of drugs,[4] such as metformin (see 'Metformin + Pyrimethamine', p.534).

As with P-glycoprotein, some of these transporters are subject to genetic polymorphism[4] (that is, variations in their expression), but the clinical importance of this in relation to drug disposition is currently unclear.

1. Mizuno N, Niwa T, Yotsumoto Y, Sugiyama Y. Impact of drug transporter studies on drug discovery and development. *Pharmacol Rev* (2003) 55, 425–61.
2. Lin JH, Yamazaki M. Clinical relevance of P-glycoprotein in drug therapy. *Drug Metab Rev* (2003) 35, 417–54.

3. US FDA. Guidance for industry. Drug interaction studies—study design, data analysis, implications for dosing, and labelling recommendations. Draft guidance, February 2012. Available at: http://www.fda.gov/downloads/Drugs/GuidanceComplianceRegulatoryInformation/Guidances/UCM292362.pdf (accessed 08/09/15).
4. Hillgren KM, Keppler D, Zur AA, Giacomini KM, Stieger B, Cass CE, Zhang L; International Transporter Consortium. Emerging transporters of clinical importance: an update from the International Transporter Consortium. *Clin Pharmacol Ther* (2013) 94, 52–63.

Pharmacodynamic interactions

Pharmacodynamic interactions are those where the effects of one drug are changed by the presence of another drug at its site of action. Sometimes the drugs directly compete for particular receptors (e.g. $beta_2$ agonists, such as salbutamol, and beta blockers, such as propranolol) but often the reaction is more indirect and involves interference with physiological mechanisms. These interactions are much less easy to classify neatly than those of a pharmacokinetic type.

Additive or synergistic interactions

If two drugs that have the same pharmacological effect are given together the effects can be additive. For example, alcohol depresses the CNS and, if taken in moderate amounts with normal therapeutic doses of any of a large number of drugs (e.g. anxiolytics, hypnotics, etc.), can cause excessive drowsiness. Strictly speaking (as pointed out earlier) these are not interactions within the definition given in the section 'Drug interactions overview', p.1. Nevertheless, it is convenient to consider them within the broad context of the clinical outcome of giving two drugs together.

Additive effects can occur with both the main effects of the drugs as well as their adverse effects, thus an additive interaction can occur with antimuscarinic antiparkinson drugs (main effect) or butyrophenones (adverse effect) that can result in serious antimuscarinic toxicity (see 'Antipsychotics + Antimuscarinics', p.805).

Sometimes the additive effects are solely toxic (e.g. additive ototoxicity, nephrotoxicity, bone marrow depression, QT interval prolongation, serotonin syndrome). Examples of these reactions are listed in 'Table 1.13', above. It is common to use the terms 'additive', 'summation', 'synergy', or 'potentiation' to describe what happens if two or more drugs behave like this. These words have precise pharmacological definitions but they are often used rather loosely as synonyms because in practice it is often very difficult to know the extent of the increased activity, that is to say whether the effects are greater or smaller than the sum of the individual effects.

Table 1.13 Additive, synergistic or summation interactions

Drugs	*Result of interaction*
Antipsychotics + Antimuscarinics, p.805	Increased antimuscarinic effects; heat stroke in hot and humid conditions, paralytic ileus, toxic psychoses
Antihypertensives + Drugs that cause hypotension (e.g. Phenothiazines, p.1070, Sildenafil, p.1545)	Increased antihypertensive effects; orthostasis
Beta-agonist bronchodilators + Potassium-depleting drugs, p.1422	Hypokalaemia
CNS depressants + CNS depressants Alcohol + Antihistamines, p.54 Benzodiazepines + Anaesthetics, general, p.102 Opioids + Benzodiazepines, p.169	Impaired psychomotor skills, reduced alertness, drowsiness, stupor, respiratory depression, coma, death
Drugs that prolong the QT interval + Other drugs that prolong the QT interval Amiodarone + Disopyramide, p.263	Additive prolongation of QT interval, increased risk of torsade de pointes
Methotrexate + Co-trimoxazole, p.693	Bone marrow megaloblastosis due to folic acid antagonism
Nephrotoxic drugs + Nephrotoxic drugs (e.g. Aminoglycosides, p.305, Ciclosporin, p.1208, Cisplatin, p.668, Vancomycin, p.305)	Increased nephrotoxicity
Neuromuscular blockers + Drugs with neuromuscular blocking effects (e.g. Aminoglycosides, p.119)	Increased neuromuscular blockade; delayed recovery, prolonged apnoea
Potassium supplements + Potassium-sparing drugs (e.g. ACE inhibitors, p.41, Angiotensin II receptor antagonists, p.48, Potassium-sparing diuretics, p.1128)	Hyperkalaemia
Drugs that cause serotonin syndrome + Other drugs that cause serotonin syndrome MAOIs or RIMAs + Opioids; Pethidine (Meperidine), p.1399	Increased risk of serotonin syndrome; clonus, agitation, diaphoresis, tremor, and hyperreflexia

Table 1.14 Opposing or antagonistic interactions

Drug affected	*Interacting drugs*	*Results of interaction*
ACE inhibitors, p.38 or Loop diuretics, p.1120	NSAIDs	Antihypertensive effects opposed
Anticoagulants, p.484	Vitamin K	Anticoagulant effects opposed
Antidiabetics, p.507	Glucocorticoids	Blood glucose-lowering effects opposed
Antineoplastics, p.658	Megestrol	Antineoplastic effects possibly opposed
Levodopa, p.762	Antipsychotics (those with dopamine antagonist effects)	Antiparkinsonian effects opposed

Antagonistic or opposing interactions

In contrast to additive interactions, there are some pairs of drugs with activities that are opposed to one another. For example the coumarins can prolong the blood clotting time by competitively inhibiting the effects of dietary vitamin K. If the intake of vitamin K is increased, the effects of the coumarin are opposed and the prothrombin time can return to normal, thereby cancelling out the therapeutic benefits of anticoagulant treatment (see 'Coumarins and related drugs + Food; Vitamin K_1-rich', p.432). Other examples of this type of interaction are listed in 'Table 1.14', above.

Drug or neurotransmitter uptake interactions

A number of drugs with actions that occur at adrenergic neurones can be prevented from reaching those sites of action by the presence of other drugs. The tricyclic antidepressants prevent the re-uptake of noradrenaline (norepinephrine) into peripheral adrenergic neurones. Thus patients taking tricyclics and given parenteral noradrenaline have a markedly increased response (hypertension, tachycardia); see 'Tricyclic and related antidepressants + Inotropes and Vasopressors', p.1510. Similarly, the uptake of guanethidine (and related drugs guanoclor, betanidine, debrisoquine, etc.) is blocked by a number of antipsychotics including chlorpromazine, haloperidol, tiotixene (see 'Guanethidine + Antipsychotics', p.1061), a number of amfetamine-like drugs (see 'Guanethidine + Amfetamines and related drugs', p.1061), and the tricyclic antidepressants (see 'Guanethidine + Tricyclic and related antidepressants', p.1062), so that the antihypertensive effect is prevented. The antihypertensive effects of clonidine are also prevented by the tricyclic antidepressants, one possible reason being that the uptake of clonidine within the CNS is blocked (see 'Clonidine and related drugs + Tricyclic and related antidepressants', p.1057). Some of these interactions at adrenergic neurones are illustrated in 'Figure 1.3', p.16.

Drug-herb interactions

The market for herbal medicines and supplements in the Western world has markedly increased in recent years, and, not surprisingly, reports of interactions with 'conventional' drugs have arisen. The most well known and documented example is the interaction of St John's wort (*Hypericum perforatum*) with a variety of drugs, see below. There have also been isolated reports of other herb-drug interactions, attributable to various mechanisms, including additive pharmacological effects.

Based on these reports, there are a growing number of reviews of herbal medicine interactions, which seek to predict likely interactions based on the,

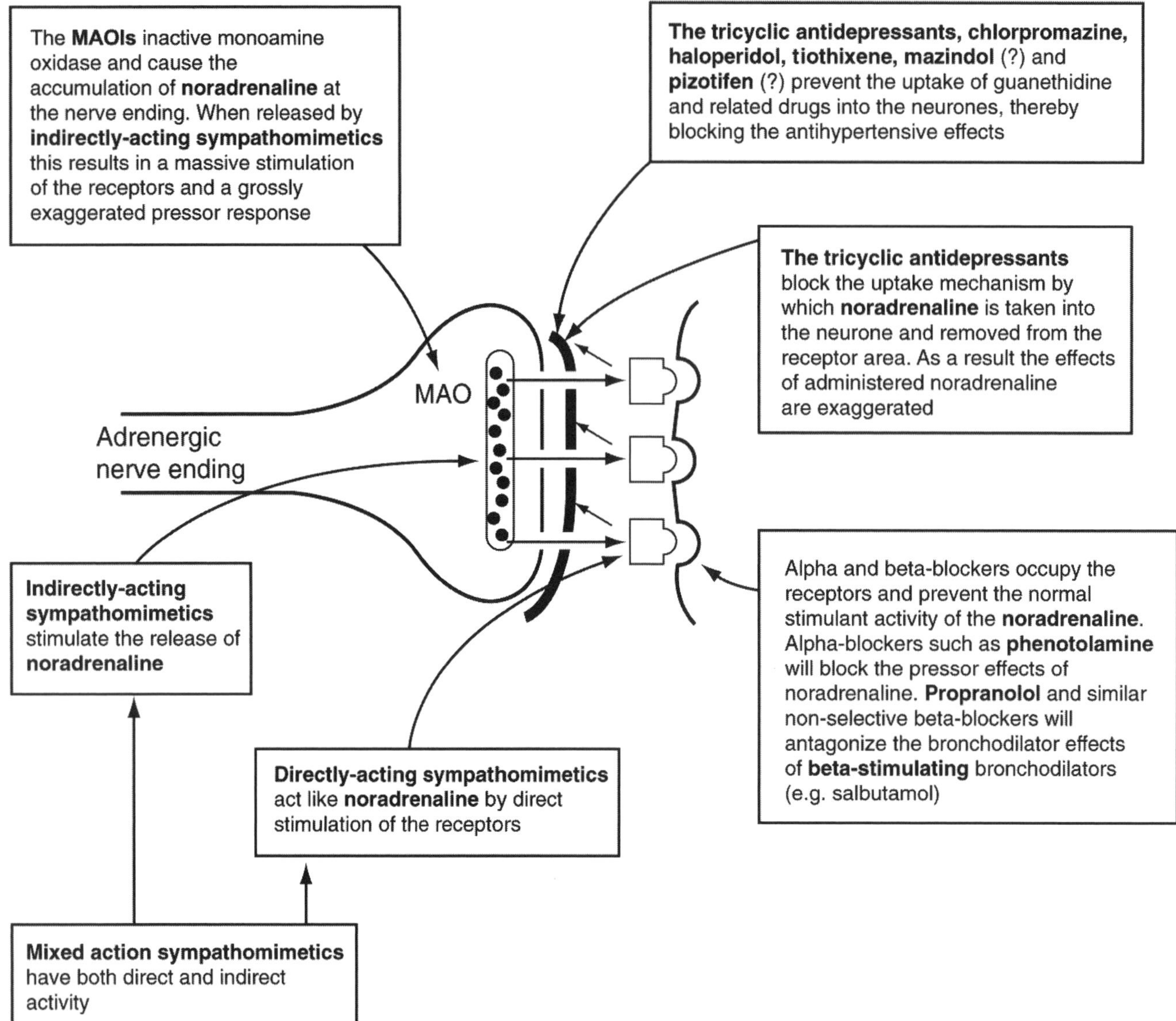

Fig. 1.3 Interactions at adrenergic neurones
A highly simplified composite diagram of an adrenergic neurone (molecules of noradrenaline (norepinephrine) indicated as (•) contained in a single vesicle at the nerve-ending) to illustrate in outline some of the different sites where drugs can interact. More details of these interactions are to be found in individual monographs.

often hypothesised, actions of various herbs. Many of these predictions seem tenuous at best.

Rather than add to the volume of predicted interactions, at present, *Stockley's Drug Interactions* includes only those interactions for which there are published reports. Our sister publication, *Stockley's Herbal Medicines Interactions*, attempts to deal with these interactions in much greater depth, assessing the theoretical as well as the clinical evidence for the interactions of herbal medicines, dietary supplements and nutraceuticals.

To aid collection of data in this area, health professionals should routinely ask patients about their use of herbal medicines and supplements, and report any unexpected responses to treatment.

An additional problem in interpreting these interactions, is that the interacting constituent of the herb is usually not known and is therefore not standardised for. It could vary widely between different products, and batches of the same product.

St John's wort (Hypericum perforatum)

An increasing number of reports have implicated St John's wort (*Hypericum perforatum*) in drug interactions. Evidence has shown that the herb can induce the cytochrome P450 isoenzyme CYP3A4, and can also induce P-glycoprotein (see *P-glycoprotein interactions*, under 'Drug transporter proteins', p.13). Hence St John's wort decreases the levels of ciclosporin (see 'Ciclosporin + St John's wort (*Hypericum perforatum*)', p.1242), and digoxin (see 'Digoxin + St John's wort (*Hypericum perforatum*)', p.1111). Other less certain evidence suggests that CYP2E1 and CYP1A2 may also be induced. St John's wort has serotonergic properties, and this has resulted in a pharmacodynamic interaction with the SSRIs (see 'SSRIs + St John's wort (*Hypericum perforatum*)', p.1496), namely the development of serotonin syndrome. St John's wort contains many possible constituents that could be responsible for its pharmacological effects. The major active constituents are currently considered to be hyperforin (a phloroglucinol) and hypericin (a naphthodianthrone). Hypericin is the only constituent that is standardised for, and then only in some St John's wort preparations.

1. Miller LG. Herbal medicinals. Selected clinical considerations focusing on known or potential drug-herb interactions. *Arch Intern Med* (1998) 158, 2200–11.
2. Fugh-Berman A. Herb-drug interactions. *Lancet* (2000) 355, 134–8. Correction. ibid. 1020.
3. Wang Z, Gorski JC, Hamman MA, Huang S-M, Lesko LJ, Hall SD. The effects of St John's wort (*Hypericum perforatum*) on human cytochrome P450 activity. *Clin Pharmacol Ther* (2001) 70, 317–26.
4. Williamson EM. Drug interactions between herbal and prescription medicines. *Drug Safety* (2003) 26, 1075–92.
5. Henderson L, Yue QY, Bergquist C, Gerden B, Arlett P. St John's wort (*Hypericum perforatum*): drug interactions and clinical outcomes. *Br J Clin Pharmacol* (2002) 54, 349–56.
6. Gurley BJ, Gardner SF, Hubbard MA, Williams DK, Gentry WB, Cui Y, Ang CYW. Cytochrome P450 phenotypic ratios for predicting herb-drug interactions in humans. *Clin Pharmacol Ther* (2002) 72, 276–87.
7. Dresser GK, Schwarz UI, Wilkinson GR, Kim RB. Coordinate induction of both cytochrome P4503A and MDR1 by St John's wort in healthy subjects. *Clin Pharmacol Ther* (2003) 73, 41–50.

Drug-food interactions

It is well established that food can cause clinically important changes in drug absorption through effects on gastrointestinal motility or by drug binding, see 'Drug absorption interactions', p.3. In addition, it is well known that tyramine (present in some foodstuffs) may reach toxic concentrations in patients taking MAOIs (see 'MAOIs or RIMAs + Food; Tyramine-containing', p.1389). With the growth in understanding of drug metabolism mechanisms, it has been increasingly recognised that some foods can alter drug metabolism. Currently, grapefruit juice causes the most clinically relevant of these interactions, see *Grapefruit juice*, below.

(a) Cruciferous vegetables and charcoal-broiled meats

Cruciferous vegetables, such as brussels sprouts, cabbage, and broccoli, contain substances that are inducers of the cytochrome P450 isoenzyme CYP1A2. Chemicals formed by 'burning' meats additionally have these properties. These foods do not appear to cause any clinically important drug interactions in their own right, but their consumption can add another variable to drug interaction studies, so complicating interpretation. In drug interaction studies where alteration of CYP1A2 is a predicted mechanism, it might be better for patients to avoid these foods during the study.

(b) Grapefruit juice

By chance, grapefruit juice was chosen to mask the taste of alcohol in a study of the effect of alcohol on felodipine, which led to the discovery that grapefruit juice itself moderately increased felodipine exposure, see 'Calcium-channel blockers + Grapefruit juice', p.1037. In general, grapefruit juice inhibits intestinal CYP3A4, and only slightly affects hepatic CYP3A4. This is demonstrated by the fact that intravenous preparations of drugs that are metabolised by CYP3A4 are not much affected, whereas oral preparations of the same drugs are. These interactions result in increased drug exposure.

Some drugs that are not metabolised by CYP3A4 have decreased exposure with grapefruit juice, such as fexofenadine (see 'Antihistamines + Grapefruit and other fruit juices', p.633. The probable reason for this is that grapefruit juice is an inhibitor of some drug transporters (see 'Drug transporter proteins', p.13), and possibly affects organic anion-transporting polypeptides (OATPs), although inhibition of P-glycoprotein has also been suggested.

The active constituent of grapefruit juice is uncertain. Grapefruit contains naringin, which degrades during processing to naringenin, a substance known to inhibit CYP3A4. Because of this, it has been assumed that whole grapefruit will not interact, but that processed grapefruit juice will. However, subsequently some reports have implicated the whole fruit. Other possible active constituents in the whole fruit include bergamottin and dihydroxybergamottin.

1. Ameer B, Wientraub RA. Drug interactions with grapefruit juice. *Clin Pharmacokinet* (1997) 33, 103–21.

Conclusions

It is now quite impossible to remember all the known clinically important interactions and how they occur, which is why this publication has been produced, but there are some broad general principles that need little memorising:

- Be on the alert with any drugs that have a narrow therapeutic window or where it is necessary to keep serum levels at or above a suitable level (e.g. certain anticoagulants, antidiabetic drugs, antiepileptics, antihypertensives, anti-infectives, antineoplastic cytotoxics, digitalis glycosides, immunosuppressants, etc.).
- Remember some of those drugs that are key enzyme inducers (e.g. phenytoin, barbiturates, rifampicin (rifampin), etc) or enzyme inhibitors (e.g. azole antifungals, HIV-protease inhibitors, erythromycin, SSRIs).
- Think about the basic pharmacology of the drugs under consideration so that obvious problems (additive CNS depression for example) are not overlooked, and try to think of what might happen if drugs that affect the same receptors are used together. Don't forget that many drugs affect more than one type of receptor.
- Keep in mind that the elderly are at risk because of reduced liver and renal function on which drug clearance depends.

2

ACE inhibitors and Angiotensin II receptor antagonists

ACE (angiotensin-converting enzyme) inhibitors prevent the production of angiotensin II from angiotensin I. The angiotensin II receptor antagonists are more selective, and target the angiotensin II type I (AT_1) receptor, which is responsible for the pressor actions of angiotensin II. 'Table 2.1', below, lists the ACE inhibitors and the angiotensin II receptor antagonists.

Angiotensin II is involved in the renin-angiotensin-aldosterone system, which regulates blood pressure, sodium and water homoeostasis by the kidneys, and cardiovascular function. Angiotensin II stimulates the synthesis and secretion of aldosterone and raises blood pressure via a direct vasoconstrictor effect.

ACE is identical to bradykinase, so ACE inhibitors might additionally reduce the degradation of bradykinin and affect enzymes involved in the production of prostaglandins.

Many of the interactions of the ACE inhibitors and angiotensin II receptor antagonists involve other drugs that affect blood pressure. Consequently, in most cases, the result is either an increase in the hypotensive effect (e.g. alcohol, see 'Alcohol + Antihypertensives', p.55) or a decrease in the hypotensive effect (e.g. indometacin, see 'ACE inhibitors + NSAIDs', p.38).

In addition, due to their effects on aldosterone, the ACE inhibitors and angiotensin II antagonists might increase plasma potassium levels and can therefore have additive hyperkalaemic effects with other drugs that cause elevated plasma potassium levels. Furthermore, drugs that affect renal function can potentiate the adverse effects of ACE inhibitors and angiotensin II antagonists on the kidneys.

Most ACE inhibitor and angiotensin II receptor antagonist interactions are pharmacodynamic, that is, interactions that result in an alteration in drug effects rather than drug disposition, so in most cases interactions of individual drugs will be applicable to the group. *In vitro* experiments suggest that the role of cytochrome P450 isoenzymes in the metabolism and interactions of the angiotensin II receptor antagonists (candesartan, eprosartan, irbesartan, losartan and valsartan) is small, although losartan, irbesartan, and to a minor extent, candesartan, are metabolised by CYP2C9. Only losartan and irbesartan were considered to have a theoretical potential for pharmacokinetic drug interactions involving CYP2C9,[1] see 'Angiotensin II receptor antagonists + Azoles', p.43. The ACE inhibitors do not appear to undergo interactions via cytochrome P450 isoenzymes.

1. Taavitsainen P, Kiukaanniemi K, Pelkonen O. In vitro inhibition screening of human hepatic P_{450} enzymes by five angiotensin-II receptor antagonists. *Eur J Clin Pharmacol* (2000) 56, 135–40.

Table 2.1 ACE inhibitors and Angiotensin II receptor antagonists

Group	*Drugs*
ACE inhibitors	Alacepril, Benazepril, Captopril, Cilazapril, Delapril, Enalapril, Fosinopril, Imidapril, Lisinopril, Moexipril, Perindopril, Quinapril, Ramipril, Spirapril, Temocapril, Trandolapril, Zofenopril
Angiotensin II receptor antagonists	Candesartan, Eprosartan, Irbesartan, Losartan, Olmesartan, Telmisartan, Valsartan

ACE inhibitors + Aliskiren

The concurrent use of ramipril and aliskiren does not result in a clinically relevant pharmacokinetic interaction, although additive blood pressure-lowering effects occur. The concurrent use of aliskiren and ACE inhibitors appears to increase the risk of hyperkalaemia.

Clinical evidence

In a study, 17 healthy subjects were given **ramipril** 2.5 mg daily, titrated to 10 mg daily by day 3, and aliskiren 300 mg daily, either alone or together for periods of 6 or 7 days. **Ramipril** increased the maximum concentration and AUC of aliskiren by 31% and 12%, respectively. Aliskiren increased the AUC of **ramipril** by 22%, but did not affect its plasma concentration. The AUC of the active metabolite of **ramipril**, ramiprilat, was unchanged, but its maximum plasma concentration decreased by 15%.[1] The concurrent use of **ramipril** with aliskiren results in additive blood pressure reduction.[2]

A subgroup analysis of patients taking aliskiren with an ACE inhibitor found an increase in the risk of hyperkalaemia and hypotension when compared with patients taking an ACE inhibitor alone.[3] In one study, where aliskiren was given with an ACE inhibitor to patients with diabetes, increases in serum potassium were more frequent (5.5%) compared with an incidence of about 2.5% with either drug alone.[4] In contrast, in a Canadian retrospective case-control study, aliskiren use was not associated with an increased risk of hospitalisation for hyperkalaemia, acute kidney injury, or stroke in patients aged 66 or older, who were also taking an ACE inhibitor or angiotensin II receptor antagonist.[5]

Mechanism

Both ACE inhibitors and the renin inhibitor aliskiren act on the renin-angiotensin-aldosterone system, and can increase the risk of hypotension and hyperkalaemia when given alone. This risk might be further increased when they are given together.

Importance and management

The evidence for a pharmacokinetic interaction between the ACE inhibitors and aliskiren is limited to one study with ramipril, but the pharmacokinetic changes seen are unlikely to be clinically relevant and, on this basis, dose adjustments would not be expected to be needed on concurrent use.[1] A pharmacokinetic interaction would not be expected between aliskiren and other ACE inhibitors, but this ideally needs confirmation. However, concurrent use of an ACE inhibitor with aliskiren might increase the risk of hypotension and hyperkalaemia. In September 2014, the European Medicines Agency issued guidance stating that the combination of an ACE inhibitor and aliskiren is not recommended in any patient, and is strictly contraindicated in patients with diabetic nephropathy or moderate to severe renal impairment (eGFR less than 60 mL/minute/1.73 m^2). In patients where it is considered absolutely necessary, an ACE inhibitor and aliskiren should only be given together under specialist supervision, with close monitoring of blood pressure, renal function, and electrolyte and fluid balance.[6]

1. Vaidyanathan S, Valencia J, Kemp C, Zhao C, Yeh C-M, Bizot M-N, Denouel J, Dieterich HA, Dole WP. Lack of pharmacokinetic interactions of aliskiren, a novel direct renin inhibitor for the treatment of hypertension, with the antihypertensives amlodipine, valsartan, hydrochlorothiazide (HCTZ) and ramipril in healthy volunteers. *Int J Clin Pract* (2006) 60, 1343–56.
2. O'Brien E, Barton J, Nussberger J, Mulcahy D, Jensen C, Dicker P, Stanton A. Aliskiren reduces blood pressure and suppresses plasma renin activity in combination with a thiazide diuretic, an angiotensin-converting enzyme inhibitor, or an angiotensin receptor blocker. *Hypertension* (2007) 49, 276–84.
3. Makani H, Bangalore S, Desouza KA, Shah A, Messerli FH. Efficacy and safety of dual blockade of the renin-angiotensin system: meta-analysis of randomised trials. *BMJ* (2013) 346, f360.
4. Uresin Y, Taylor AA, Kilo C, Tschöpe D, Santonastaso M, Ibram G, Fang H, Satlin A. Efficacy and safety of the direct renin inhibitor aliskiren and ramipril alone or in combination in patients with diabetes and hypertension. *J Renin Angiotensin Aldosterone Syst* (2007) 8, 190–8.
5. Gilbert CJ, Gomes T, Mamdani MM, Hellings C, Yao Z, Garg AX, Wald R, Harel Z, Juurlink DN. No increase in adverse events during aliskiren use among Ontario patients receiving angiotensin-converting enzyme inhibitors or angiotensin-receptor blockers. *Can J Cardiol* (2013) 29, 586–91.
6. European Medicines Agency. Restriction of combined use of medicines affecting the renin-angiotensin system (RAS), September 2014. Available at: http://www.ema.europa.eu/docs/en_GB/document_library/Referrals_document/Renin-angiotensin_system_(RAS)-acting_agents/European_Commission_final_decision/WC500175069.pdf (accessed 21/10/15).

ACE inhibitors + Allopurinol

A case of hypersensitivity has been attributed to the use of captopril with allopurinol. Anaphylaxis and myocardial infarction occurred when one man taking enalapril was given allopurinol. The concurrent use of ACE inhibitors and allopurinol might increase the risk of leucopenia and serious infection, especially in renal impairment.

Clinical evidence

No significant pharmacokinetic changes were seen in 12 healthy subjects given allopurinol and **captopril** alone and in combination.[1] A report describes fever, arthralgia and myalgia in a diabetic man with chronic renal failure who was also given **captopril** and allopurinol. He improved when the **captopril** was withdrawn.[2] A man taking **enalapril** had an acute anaphylactic reaction with severe coronary spasm, culminating in myocardial infarction, within 20 minutes of taking allopurinol 100 mg. He recovered and continued to take **enalapril** without allopurinol.[3]

The UK manufacturer of **captopril** also warns that neutropenia and agranulocytosis, resulting in serious infection, have occurred in patients taking **captopril** and other ACE inhibitors, and that the concurrent use of allopurinol might be a complicating factor, especially in those with renal impairment.[4]

Mechanism

Not understood. It is uncertain whether these are interactions because allopurinol alone can cause severe hypersensitivity reactions, particularly in the presence of renal impairment. Captopril can also induce a hypersensitivity reaction.

Importance and management

These interactions are not clearly established, and the reaction appears to be rare and unpredictable. All that can be constructively said is that patients taking both drugs should be very closely monitored for any signs of hypersensitivity (e.g. skin reactions) or a low white cell count (e.g. sore throat, fever), especially if they have renal impairment. The UK manufacturer of captopril recommends that differential white blood cell counts should be performed before adding allopurinol, then every 2 weeks during the first 3 months of treatment, and periodically thereafter.[4] Similar caution and advice is given by the UK manufacturers of several other ACE inhibitors.

For other possible interactions with ACE inhibitors that might result in an increased risk of leucopenia see also 'ACE inhibitors + Azathioprine', p.24 and 'ACE inhibitors + Procainamide', p.41.

1. Duchin KL, McKinstry DN, Cohen AI, Migdalof BH. Pharmacokinetics of captopril in healthy subjects and in patients with cardiovascular diseases. *Clin Pharmacokinet* (1988) 14, 241–59.
2. Samanta A, Burden AC. Fever, myalgia, and arthralgia in a patient on captopril and allopurinol. *Lancet* (1984) i, 679.
3. Ahmad S. Allopurinol and enalapril. Drug induced anaphylactic coronary spasm and acute myocardial infarction. *Chest* (1995) 108, 586.
4. Capoten (Captopril). E. R. Squibb & Sons Ltd. UK Summary of product characteristics, June 2010.

ACE inhibitors + Angiotensin II receptor antagonists

The concurrent use of ACE inhibitors and angiotensin II receptor antagonists increases the risk of hypotension, renal impairment, and hyperkalaemia. Telmisartan can increase the exposure to ramipril.

Clinical evidence

(a) Candesartan

In one randomised clinical study in patients with heart failure taking ACE inhibitors (74% taking **enalapril**, **lisinopril**, **captopril**, or **ramipril**), the addition of candesartan resulted in higher rates of withdrawals for renal impairment (increase in creatinine 7.8% versus 4.1% with placebo) and hyperkalaemia (3.4% versus 0.7% with placebo).[1]

Another study in patients with hypertension not controlled with **lisinopril** 20 mg daily found that either an increase in the **lisinopril** dose to 40 mg daily, or the addition of candesartan 16 mg daily for 2 weeks then 32 mg daily, controlled hypertension in 37% and 43% of patients, respectively. Eleven patients taking **lisinopril** and 9 patients taking **lisinopril** with candesartan developed hyperkalaemia resulting in discontinuation in 4 patients taking **lisinopril** with candesartan.[2]

(b) Irbesartan

A placebo-controlled study in 24 patients with diabetic nephropathy taking **enalapril** 40 mg daily found that the addition of irbesartan 300 mg daily had a greater effect on reduction of albuminuria and blood pressure than **enalapril** alone. Plasma potassium concentrations of greater than 5.2 mmol/L occurred in one patient taking **enalapril** alone and in one patient taking irbesartan with **enalapril**. Six patients taking both drugs experienced transient hypotension or tiredness.[3]

(c) Telmisartan

In the ONTARGET study, patients with vascular disease or high-risk diabetes without heart failure were given either **ramipril** 10 mg daily (8 576 patients), telmisartan 80 mg daily (8 542 patients), or both drugs (8 502 patients). The use of **ramipril** with telmisartan reduced the average systolic blood pressure by up to 5 mmHg, but did not have an additive effect on the renin-angiotensin system. The combination was associated with more adverse effects including hypotensive symptoms, syncope, renal impairment, and hyperkalaemia without an increase in benefit. Discontinuation of treatment because of hypotensive symptoms occurred in 406 patients taking both drugs, compared with 149 taking **ramipril** alone and 229 taking telmisartan alone. In patients at high vascular risk, the use of both drugs reduced proteinuria to a greater extent than **ramipril** alone, but overall worsened major renal outcomes.[4-6]

The US manufacturer of telmisartan notes that, in a study in healthy subjects given **ramipril** 10 mg and telmisartan 80 mg daily, the steady-state AUC and maximum plasma concentration of **ramipril** were increased 2.1- and 2.3-fold, respectively. The steady-state AUC and maximum concentration of ramiprilat were increased by 50% and 2.4-fold, respectively. The AUC and maximum plasma concentration of telmisartan were reduced by 16% and 31%, respectively. The effects of concurrent **ramipril** and telmisartan might be due to additive pharmacodynamic effects and because of increased **ramipril** concentrations in the presence of telmisartan.[7]

(d) Valsartan

In another double-blind study in patients with heart failure, the concurrent use of valsartan and **captopril** resulted in a higher incidence of adverse events leading to a dose reduction or a discontinuation of study treatment than either drug alone. Due to hypotension, treatment was discontinued in 90 patients (1.9%) taking both drugs, 70 patients (1.4%) taking valsartan, and 41 patients (0.8%) taking **captopril**. For renal causes, treatment was discontinued in 61 patients (1.3%) taking both drugs, 53 patients

(1.1%) taking valsartan and 40 patients (0.8%) taking **captopril**; and because of hyperkalaemia, treatment was discontinued in 12 patients (0.2%) taking both drugs, 7 patients (0.1%) taking valsartan and 4 patients (0.1%) taking **captopril**.[8]

(e) Unspecified angiotensin II receptor antagonists

A subgroup analysis of patients taking an ACE inhibitor and an angiotensin II receptor antagonist found an increase in the risk of hyperkalaemia and renal failure compared with an ACE inhibitor alone, and an increase in the risk of hypotension and of withdrawal due to adverse effects when compared with either an ACE inhibitor or an angiotensin II receptor antagonist alone.[9]

Mechanism

ACE inhibitors and angiotensin II receptor antagonists both act on the renin-angiotensin-aldosterone system, and can increase the risk of hypotension, renal impairment, and hyperkalaemia when given alone. These risks can be further increased when they are given together. The mechanism behind the pharmacokinetic interaction between ramipril and telmisartan is unknown.

Importance and management

The evidence for a pharmacokinetic interaction between the ACE inhibitors and angiotensin II receptor antagonists is limited to one study with telmisartan and ramipril, but the UK manufacturer[10] of telmisartan notes that the clinical relevance of this is not known, however both the UK and US manufacturers advise against concurrent use.[7,10] The concurrent use of an ACE inhibitor and angiotensin II receptor antagonist might increase the risk of hyperkalaemia, renal failure, and hypotension. Dose reduction or discontinuation of either or both drugs might be required, however in September 2014 the European Medicines Agency issued guidance stating that the combination of an ACE inhibitor and an angiotensin II receptor antagonist is not recommended in any patient, and it is strictly contraindicated in patients with diabetic nephropathy or moderate to severe renal impairment (eGFR less than 60 mL/minute/1.73 m^2). In patients where it is considered absolutely necessary, an ACE inhibitor and an angiotensin II receptor antagonist should only be given together under specialist supervision, with close monitoring of blood pressure, renal function, and electrolyte and fluid balance.[11]

1. McMurray JJV, Östergren J, Swedberg K, Granger CB, Held P, Michelson EL, Olofsson B, Yusuf S, Pfeffer MA; CHARM Investigators and Committees. Effects of candesartan in patients with chronic heart failure and reduced left-ventricular systolic function taking angiotensin-converting-enzyme inhibitors: the CHARM-Added trial. *Lancet* (2003) 362, 767–71.
2. Izzo JL, Weinberg MS, Hainer JW, Kerkering J, Tou CKP. Antihypertensive efficacy of candesartan-lisinopril in combination vs. up-titration of lisinopril: the AMAZE trials. *J Clin Hypertens (Greenwich)* (2004) 6, 485–93.
3. Jacobsen P, Andersen S, Rossing K, Jensen BR, Parving H-H. Dual blockade of the renin-angiotensin system versus maximal recommended dose of ACE inhibition in diabetic nephropathy. *Kidney Int* (2003) 63, 1874–80.
4. ONTARGET Investigators, Yusuf S, Teo KK, Pogue J, Dyal L, Copland I, Schumacher H, Dagenais G, Sleight P, Anderson C. Telmisartan, ramipril, or both in patients at high risk for vascular events. *N Engl J Med* (2008) 358, 1547–59.
5. Mann JFE, Schmieder RE, McQueen M, Dyal L, Schumacher H, Pogue J, Wang X, Maggioni A, Budaj A, Chaithiraphan S, Dickstein K, Keltai M, Metsärinne K, Oto A, Parkhomenko A, Piegas LS, Svendsen TL, Teo KK, Yusuf S; ONTARGET investigators. Renal outcomes with telmisartan, ramipril, or both, in people at high vascular risk (the ONTARGET study): a multicentre, randomised, double-blind, controlled trial. *Lancet* (2008) 372, 547–53.
6. Guthrie RM. Review of ONTARGET: treating patients at high risk for vascular events with telmisartan, ramipril, or both. *Postgrad Med* (2009) 121, 202–4.
7. Micardis (Telmisartan). Boehringer Ingelheim Pharmaceuticals Inc. US Prescribing information, October 2012.
8. Pfeffer MA, McMurray JJV, Velazquez EJ, Rouleau J-L, Køber L, Maggioni AP, Solomon SD, Swedberg K, Van de Werf F, White H, Leimberger JD, Henis M, Edwards S, Zelenkofske S, Sellers MA, Califf RM; Valsartan in Acute Myocardial Infarction Trial Investigators. Valsartan, captopril, or both in myocardial infarction complicated by heart failure, left ventricular dysfunction, or both. *N Engl J Med* (2003) 349, 1893–1906.
9. Makani H, Bangalore S, Desouza KA, Shah A, Messerli FH. Efficacy and safety of dual blockade of the renin-angiotensin system: meta-analysis of randomised trials. *BMJ* (2013) 346, f360.
10. Micardis 80 mg tablets (Telmisartan). Boehringer Ingelheim Ltd. UK Summary of product characteristics, September 2014.
11. European Medicines Agency. Restriction of combined use of medicines affecting the renin-angiotensin system (RAS), September 2014. Available at: http://www.ema.europa.eu/docs/en_GB/document_library/Referrals_document/Renin-angiotensin_system_(RAS)-acting_agents/European_Commission_final_decision/WC500175069.pdf (accessed 22/10/15).

ACE inhibitors + Antacids

Aluminium/magnesium hydroxide-containing antacids reduce the exposure to captopril by 40% and reduce the bioavailability of fosinopril by about one-third. The pharmacokinetics of the active metabolite of ramipril do not appear to be affected by an unnamed antacid.

Clinical evidence

In 10 healthy subjects an antacid containing **aluminium/magnesium hydroxide** and **magnesium carbonate** reduced the AUC of a single 50-mg dose of **captopril** by about 40%, when compared with the fasting state. However, this did not alter the extent of the reduction in blood pressure in response to **captopril**.[1]

Another study found that *Mylanta* [**aluminium/magnesium hydroxide** and simeticone[2]] reduced the bioavailability of **fosinopril** 20 mg by about one-third.[3]

It is briefly noted in a review that antacid use did not affect the pharmacokinetics of ramiprilat, the active metabolite of **ramipril**.[4]

Mechanism

The mechanism of this interaction is uncertain, but is unlikely to be due to elevated gastric pH as cimetidine did not have a similar effect.[3]

Importance and management

Evidence about interactions between ACE inhibitors and antacids is limited. Greater decreases in captopril bioavailability (see 'ACE inhibitors + Food', p.35) were found not to be clinically relevant, and therefore it is unlikely that the change seen with antacids will be clinically important. However, with fosinopril, the manufacturers[2,5] suggest separating administration of antacids by at least 2 hours.

The UK manufacturers of **moexipril**,[6] **quinapril**,[7] and **trandolapril**[8] also warn that antacids might reduce the bioavailability of ACE inhibitors, quite possibly based on the way that captopril and fosinopril interact, but there seems to be no evidence of a clinically significant interaction in practice.

1. Mäntylä R, Männistö PT, Vuorela A, Sundberg S, Ottoila P. Impairment of captopril bioavailability by concomitant food and antacid intake. *Int J Clin Pharmacol Ther Toxicol* (1984) 22, 626–9.
2. Monopril (Fosinopril sodium). Bristol-Myers Squibb Company. US Prescribing information, July 2008.
3. Moore L, Kramer A, Swites B, Kramer P, Tu J. Effect of cimetidine and antacid on the kinetics of the active diacid of fosinopril in healthy subjects. *J Clin Pharmacol* (1988) 28, 946.
4. Todd PA, Benfield P. Ramipril. A review of its pharmacological properties and therapeutic efficacy in cardiovascular disorders. *Drugs* (1990) 39, 110–35.
5. Staril (Fosinopril sodium). E. R. Squibb & Sons Ltd. UK Summary of product characteristics, January 2009.
6. Perdix (Moexipril hydrochloride). UCB Pharma Ltd. UK Summary of product characteristics, August 2010.
7. Accupro (Quinapril hydrochloride). Pfizer Ltd. UK Summary of product characteristics, June 2009.
8. Gopten (Trandolapril). Abbott Laboratories Ltd. UK Summary of product characteristics, July 2010.

ACE inhibitors + Antipsychotics

Marked postural hypotension occurred in a patient given chlorpromazine and captopril. The hypotensive adverse effects of antipsychotics such as the phenothiazines might be additive with the effects of ACE inhibitors.

Clinical evidence, mechanism, importance and management

A patient fainted and developed marked postural hypotension (standing blood pressure 66/48 mmHg) when given **captopril** 6.25 mg twice daily and **chlorpromazine** 200 mg three times daily. He had previously taken **chlorpromazine** with nadolol, prazosin and hydrochlorothiazide without any problems, although his blood pressure was poorly controlled by these drugs. As the patient's blood pressure was elevated when taking **chlorpromazine** or **captopril** alone, there appeared to be a synergistic hypotensive effect between the two drugs.[1]

The manufacturers of several ACE inhibitors warn that these drugs can enhance the hypotensive effects of certain antipsychotics, and that postural hypotension might occur. This has been seen with clozapine. see 'Clozapine + Antihypertensives', p.848. Some of these warnings are based, not unreasonably, on the adverse reactions seen with other ACE inhibitors,[2] but not necessarily on direct observations. If postural hypotension occurs advise patients to lie down and elevate their legs if they feel faint or dizzy, and, when recovered, to get up slowly. Dose adjustments might be necessary to accommodate this interaction.

1. White WB. Hypotension with postural syncope secondary to the combination of chlorpromazine and captopril. *Arch Intern Med* (1986) 146, 1833–4.
2. Knoll Ltd. Personal communication, 1993.

ACE inhibitors + Aprotinin

A retrospective study in patients undergoing cardiopulmonary bypass surgery found that pre-operative ACE inhibitor use with intra-operative aprotinin use increased the risk of renal failure.

Clinical evidence

The effects of pre-operative ACE inhibitor use and/or intra-operative use of aprotinin were studied in a retrospective analysis of risk factors for acute renal failure in 1 209 patients who underwent coronary artery bypass graft, valve, or combined procedures. Patients with pre-operative renal impairment were excluded from the study, and only those with a low baseline risk of renal complications and no immediately identifiable cause of acute renal failure were included. Multivariate analysis indicated that risk factors for acute renal failure in the study patients were increasing age, valve procedures, red blood cell and platelet transfusions, lowest haematocrit during cardiopulmonary bypass, and the combination of ACE inhibitor and aprotinin use. The use of either an ACE inhibitor alone or aprotinin alone was not a significant predictor of acute renal failure.[1]

Mechanism

Aprotinin is a proteolytic enzyme inhibitor that has many actions including antagonism of the kallikrein-kinin system, which in turn affects bradykinins and renin. It would therefore be expected to have complex interactions with the ACE inhibitors,[2] which also affect these proteins.

It has been suggested that ACE inhibitors promote vasodilation of the efferent arteriole of the glomerulus, which reduces glomerular perfusion pressure. This can be compensated by vasodilation of the afferent arteriole to preserve glomerular perfusion pressure. Aprotinin might counter this compensatory response by causing vasocon-

Table 2.2 Sub-group analyses of clinical studies assessing the interaction between aspirin and ACE inhibitors

Study and patients	*Aspirin dose*	*ACE inhibitor*	*Follow-up*	*Finding*	*Refs*
Evidence of an interaction					
SOLVD 6512 patients treated for heart failure or prevention of heart failure	Not reported	Enalapril	37 to 41 months	Combined treatment associated with reduced benefits compared with enalapril alone.	1
CONSENSUS II 6090 patients with acute MI	Not reported	Enalapril	6 months	Effect of enalapril less favourable in those taking aspirin at baseline.	2
GUSTO-I 31622 post-MI patients without heart failure	Not reported	Not reported	11 months (starting 30 days post MI)	Combined use associated with higher mortality than aspirin alone (mortality rates 3.3% vs 1.6%).	3
EPILOG 2619 patients undergoing coronary angioplasty	325 mg daily	Not reported	12 months	Combined use associated with higher mortality than aspirin alone (mortality rates 3.7% vs 1.2%).	3
AIRE 1986 patients after acute MI, with heart failure	Not reported	Ramipril 2.5 to 5 mg twice daily started 3 to 10 days after MI	15 months (average)	Trend towards greater benefit of ramipril in those not receiving aspirin.	4
No evidence of an interaction					
BIP Secondary prevention of MI in 1197 patients with coronary artery disease	250 mg daily	Captopril or enalapril	5 years (average)	Lower death rate in those on combined therapy than those on ACE inhibitor alone (19% vs 27%).	5
SAVE 2231 patients with left ventricular dysfunction after MI	Not reported	Captopril 75 to 150 mg daily	42 months (average)	Trend towards greater benefits of captopril when taken with aspirin.	6
HOPE Prevention of cardiovascular events in 9297 patients without left ventricular dysfunction or heart failure	Not reported	Ramipril 10 mg daily	About 4.5 years	Benefits of ramipril not affected by aspirin.	7
CATS Early treatment of acute MI in 298 patients	80 to 100 mg daily	Captopril	1 year	Benefits of captopril not affected by aspirin. Better prognosis in those on aspirin.	8
ISIS-4 Early treatment of acute MI in 58050 patients	Not reported	Captopril 100 mg daily	At 5 weeks and 1 year	Benefits of captopril not affected by aspirin.	9
Meta-analysis of AIRE, SAVE, SOLVD and TRACE 12763 patients with left ventricular dysfunction or heart failure with or without MI	Not reported	Captopril, enalapril, ramipril, trandolapril	35 months (average)	Benefits of ACE inhibitors observed even if aspirin given.	10
Meta-analysis of CCS-1, CONSENSUS II, GISSI-3, and ISIS-4 Early treatment of MI in 96712 patients	160 to 325 mg daily	Captopril, enalapril, lisinopril	30 days	ACE inhibitor reduced 30-day mortality from 15.1% to 13.8%. ACE inhibitor plus aspirin reduced 30-day mortality from 6.7% to 6.3%.	11
TRACE 1749 patients with left ventricular dysfunction after acute MI	Not reported	Trandolapril 1 to 4 mg daily	24 to 50 months	Trend towards greater benefit of trandolapril in those receiving aspirin (mortality of 45% with ACE inhibitor, and 34% with ACE inhibitor plus aspirin).	12
SMILE 1556 patients with acute MI	Not reported	Zofenopril 7.5 mg increasing to 30 mg twice daily for 6 weeks	At 6 weeks and 1 year	Benefits of zofenopril not significantly affected by aspirin.	13
Meta-analysis of AIRE, HOPE, SAVE, SOLVD, and TRACE 22060 patients with either; left ventricular dysfunction or heart failure without MI, coronary artery disease without left ventricular dysfunction, or acute MI	Not reported	Captopril, enalapril, ramipril, trandolapril	More than 3 years	Benefits of ACE inhibitors observed even if aspirin given.	14

1. Al-Khadra AS, Salem DN, Rand WM, Udelson JE, Smith JJ, Konstam MA. Antiplatelet agents and survival: a cohort analysis from the Studies of Left Ventricular Dysfunction (SOLVD) trial. *J Am Coll Cardiol* (1998) 31, 419-25.
2. Nguyen KN, Aursnes I, Kjekshus J. Interaction between enalapril and aspirin on mortality after acute myocardial infarction: subgroup analysis of the Cooperative New Scandanavian Enalapril Survival Study II (CONSENSUS II). *Am J Cardiol* (1997) 79, 115-19.

Continued

Table 2.2 Sub-group analyses of clinical studies assessing the interaction between aspirin and ACE inhibitors (continued)

3. Peterson JG, Topol EJ, Sapp SK, Young JB, Lincoff AM, Lauer MS. Evaluation of the effects of aspirin combined with angiotensin-converting enzyme inhibitors in patients with coronary artery disease. *Am J Med* (2000) 109, 371-7.
4. The Acute Infarction Ramipril Efficacy (AIRE) Study Investigators. Effect of ramipril on mortality and morbidity of survivors of acute myocardial infarction with clinical evidence of heart failure. *Lancet* (1993) 342, 821-8.
5. Leor J, Reicher-Reiss H, Goldbourt U, Boyko V, Gottlieb S, Battler A, Behar S. Aspirin and mortality in patients treated with angiotensin-converting enzyme inhibitors. A cohort study of 11,575 patients with coronary artery disease. *J Am Coll Cardiol* (1999) 33, 1920-5.
6. Pfeffer MA, Braunwald E, Moyé LA, Basta L, Brown EJ, Cuddy TE, Davis BR, Geltman EM, Goldman S, Flaker GC, Klein M, Lamas GA, Packer M, Rouleau J, Rouleau JL, Rutherford J, Wertheimer JH, Hawkins CM, on behalf of the SAVE Investigators. Effect of captopril on mortality and morbidity in patients with left ventricular dysfunction after myocardial infarction. Results of the survival and ventricular enlargement trial. *N Engl J Med* (1992) 327, 669-77.
7. The Heart Outcomes Prevention Evaluation Study Investigators. Effect of an angiotensin-converting-enzyme inhibitor, ramipril, on cardiovascular events in high-risk patients. *N Engl J Med* (2000) 342, 145-53.
8. Oosterga M, Anthonio RL, de Kam PJ, Kingma JH, Crijns HJ, van Gilst WH. Effects of aspirin on angiotensin-converting enzyme inhibition and left ventricular dilation one year after myocardial infarction. *Am J Cardiol* (1998) 81, 1178-81.
9. ISIS-4 (Fourth International Study of Infarct Survival) Collaborative Group. ISIS-4: a randomised factorial trial assessing early oral captopril, oral mononitrate, and intravenous magnesium sulphate in 58,050 patients with suspected acute myocardial infarction. *Lancet* (1995) 345; 669-85.
10. Flather MD, Yusuf S, Køber L, Pfeffer M, Hall A, Murray G, Trop-Pedersen C, Ball S, Pogue J, Moyé L, Braunwald E, for the ACE-inhibitor Myocardial Infarction Collaborative. Long-term ACE-inhibitor therapy in patients with heart failure or left-ventricular dysfunction: a systematic overview of data from individual patients. *Lancet* (2000) 335, 1575-81.
11. Latini R, Tognoni G, Maggioni AP, Baigent C, Braunwald E, Chen Z-M, Collins R, Flather M, Franzosi MG, Kjekshus J, Køber L, Liu L-S, Peto R, Pfeffer M, Pizzetti F, Santoro E, Sleight P, Swedberg K, Tavazzi L, Wang W, Yusuf S. Clinical effects of early angiotensin-converting enzyme inhibitor treatment for myocardial infarction are similar in the presence and absence of aspirin. *J Am Coll Cardiol* (2000) 35 1801-7.
12. Køber L, Torp-Pedersen C, Carlsen JE, Bagger H, Eliasen P, Lyngborg K, Videbæk J, Cole DS, Auclert L, Pauly NC, Aliot E, Persson S, Camm AJ, for the Trandolapril Cardiac Evaluation (TRACE) Study Group. A clinical trial of the angiotensin-converting-enzyme inhibitor trandolapril in patients with left ventricular dysfunction after myocardial infarction. *N Engl J Med* (1995) 333, 1670-6.
13. Ambrosioni E, Borghi C, Magnani B, for the Survival of Myocardial Infarction Long-Term Evaluation (SMILE) Study Investigators. The effect of the angiotensin-converting-enzyme inhibitor zofenopril on mortality and morbidity after anterior myocardial infarction. *N Engl J Med* (1995) 332, 80-5.
14. Teo KK, Yusuf S, Pfeffer M, Kober L, Hall A, Pogue J, Latini R, Collins R, for the ACE Inhibitors Collaborative Group. Effects of long-term treatment with angiotensin-converting-enzyme inhibitors in the presence or absence of aspirin: a systematic review. *Lancet* (2002) 360, 1037-43.

striction of the afferent arteriole, which reduces glomerular perfusion pressure and reduces renal excretory function. It was also suggested that this might not be generally clinically relevant, but in a situation such as cardiopulmonary bypass surgery, where there are altered haemodynamics, there is the theoretical possibility of affecting renal haemodynamics.[1]

Importance and management

Patients taking ACE inhibitors could potentially be at increased risk of renal failure following cardiac surgery if aprotinin is used intra-operatively. The authors suggest more study is needed, but do advise the avoidance of aprotinin in such patients. They suggest that consideration should be given to stopping the ACE inhibitor for 2 to 3 days before surgery.[1] For information about the peri-operative use of ACE inhibitors, consider also 'Anaesthetics, general + ACE inhibitors or Angiotensin II receptor antagonists', p.99.

1. Kincaid EH, Ashburn DA, Hoyle JR, Reichert MG, Hammon JW, Kon ND. Does the combination of aprotinin and angiotensin-converting enzyme inhibitor cause renal failure after cardiac surgery? *Ann Thorac Surg* (2005) 80, 1388–93.
2. Waxler B, Rabito SF. Aprotinin: a serine protease inhibitor with therapeutic actions: its interaction with ACE inhibitors. *Curr Pharm Des* (2003) 9, 777–87.

ACE inhibitors + Aspirin

The antihypertensive efficacy of captopril and enalapril can be reduced by high-dose aspirin in about 50% of patients. Low-dose aspirin (less than or equal to 100 mg daily) appears to have little effect. It is unclear whether aspirin attenuates the benefits of ACE inhibitors in heart failure. The likelihood of an interaction possibly depends on disease state and its severity.

Clinical evidence

A. Effects on blood pressure

(a) Captopril

In 8 patients with essential hypertension, aspirin 600 mg every 6 hours for 5 doses did not alter the blood pressure response to a single 25- to 100-mg dose of captopril. However, the prostaglandin response to captopril was blocked and the blood pressure response to captopril was blunted in 4 of the 8 patients.[1] In another study, in 15 patients with hypertension, aspirin 75 mg daily did not alter the antihypertensive effects of captopril 25 mg twice daily.[2]

(b) Enalapril

Two groups of 26 patients, one with mild to moderate hypertension taking enalapril 20 mg twice daily and the other with severe primary hypertension taking enalapril 20 mg twice daily (with nifedipine 30 mg and atenolol 50 mg daily), were given test doses of aspirin 100 mg and 300 mg daily for 5 days. The 100-mg dose of aspirin did not alter the efficacy of the antihypertensive drugs, but the 300-mg dose reduced the antihypertensive efficacy in about half the patients in both groups. In these patients, the antihypertensive effects were diminished by 63% in those with mild to moderate hypertension and by 91% in those with severe hypertension.[3] In contrast, another study in 7 patients with hypertension taking enalapril (mean daily dose 12.9 mg) found that aspirin 81 mg or 325 mg daily for 2 weeks did not affect blood pressure.[4] A further study in 18 patients also found that aspirin 100 mg daily for 2 weeks did not alter the antihypertensive effect of enalapril 20 or 40 mg daily.[5]

(c) Unspecified ACE inhibitors

In a randomised study, the use of low-dose aspirin 100 mg daily for 3 months did not alter blood pressure control in patients taking ACE inhibitors, when compared with placebo.[6] Similarly, in a re-analysis of data from the Hypertension Optimal Treatment (HOT) study, long-term low-dose aspirin 75 mg daily did not interfere with the blood pressure-lowering effects of the antihypertensive drugs studied, when compared with placebo. Of 18 790 treated hypertensive patients, 41% received an ACE inhibitor, usually in combination with felodipine.[7]

B. Effects in coronary artery disease and heart failure

Various pharmacological studies have looked at the *short-term* effects of the combination of ACE inhibitors and aspirin on haemodynamic parameters. In one study in 40 patients with decompensated heart failure, aspirin 300 mg given on the first day and 100 mg daily thereafter antagonised the short-term haemodynamic effects of **captopril** 50 mg given every 8 hours for 4 days. The **captopril**-induced increase in cardiac index and the reduction in peripheral vascular resistance and pulmonary wedge pressure were all abolished.[8] A placebo-controlled study in 9 patients with chronic heart failure found that aspirin 75 mg daily for 7 days inhibited both the arterial and venous dilator responses to a single 25-mg dose of **captopril**.[9] In another study, in 15 patients with chronic heart failure receiving treatment with ACE inhibitors (mainly **enalapril** 10 mg twice daily), aspirin in doses as low as 75 mg impaired vasodilatation induced by arachidonic acid.[10] In yet another study, aspirin 325 mg daily worsened pulmonary diffusion capacity and made the ventilatory response to exercise less effective in patients taking **enalapril** 10 mg twice daily, but did not exert this effect in the absence of ACE inhibitors.[11] However, results from studies are inconsistent. In a review,[12] five of 7 studies reported that aspirin did not alter the haemodynamic effects of ACE inhibitors whereas the remaining two did. In one of these studies showing an adverse interaction between aspirin and **enalapril**, **ticlopidine** did not interact with **enalapril**.[13]

A number of large clinical studies of ACE inhibitors, mostly post-myocardial infarction, have been re-examined to see if there was a difference in outcome between those receiving aspirin at baseline, and those not. The results are summarised in 'Table 2.2', p.21. However, in addition to the problems of retrospective analysis of non-randomised parameters, the studies vary in the initiation and duration of aspirin and ACE inhibitor treatment and the length of follow-up, the degree of heart failure or ischaemia, the prognosis of the patients, and the final end point (whether compared with placebo or with the benefits of aspirin or ACE inhibitors). The conclusions are therefore conflicting, and, although two meta-analyses of these studies found no interaction, an editorial[14] disputes the findings of one of these analyses.[15]

In addition to these sub-group analyses, there have been a number of retrospective cohort studies. The results are summarised in 'Table 2.3', p.23 and again the results are conflicting, in part this is due to the limitations of this type of study.[16]

C. Effects on renal function

Acute renal failure developed in a woman taking **captopril** when she started to take aspirin for arthritis. Renal function improved when both were stopped.[17] However, in a re-analysis of data from the Hypertension Optimal Treatment (HOT) study involving 18 790 treated hypertensive patients of whom 41% were treated with an ACE inhibitor, long-term low-dose aspirin 75 mg daily had no effect on changes in serum creatinine, estimated creatinine clearance or the number of patients developing renal impairment, when compared with placebo.[7] A study in 10 patients with chronic congestive heart failure, due to ischaemic heart disease, taking ACE inhibitors (**captopril**, **cilazapril**, **enalapril**, **ramipril**) and aspirin 75 to 125 mg daily found that when they were given a single 50-mg dose of diclofenac or placebo, after aspirin had been discontinued for at least one week, diclofenac caused a deterioration in renal function compared with placebo or aspirin. Compared with placebo, both aspirin and

Table 2.3 Retrospective cohort studies assessing the interaction between aspirin and ACE inhibitors

Trial and patients	*Aspirin dose*	*ACE inhibitor*	*Follow-up*	*Finding*	*Refs*
Evidence of increased risk with combination					
576 patients with heart failure requiring hospitalisation 179 taking ACE Inhibitors without, 199 taking ACE inhibitors with aspirin	Not reported	Not specified	30 days	Trend towards increased incidence of early readmissions with combined treatment compared with ACE inhibitors alone (16% vs 10%) and the increase was statistically significant (23%) in patients without coronary artery disease	1
344 patients with heart failure taking ACE inhibitors 235 taking ACE Inhibitors without, 109 taking ACE inhibitors with aspirin	Low dose aspirin (≤160 mg daily) in 45 and high dose aspirin (≥325 mg daily) 64	Not specified	Mean of 37.6 months	Compared with patients not taking aspirin, the use of high dose aspirin with an ACE inhibitor was associated with a small but statistically significant increase in the risk of death whereas low-dose aspirin was not	2
Evidence of improved outcome with combination					
430 patients with heart failure 134 taking ACE Inhibitors without, 138 taking ACE inhibitors with aspirin	Not reported	Not specified	0.1 to 59 months (median 28 months)	Long-term survival was not affected by combined treatment. However, in patients with coronary artery disease, trend towards improved mortality with combined treatment compared with ACE inhibitor alone (40% vs 56%)	3
14129 patients aged ≥65 years and post myocardial infarction; 2799 taking ACE Inhibitors without, 5380 taking ACE inhibitors with aspirin	Not reported	Not specified	1 year	No adverse interaction between ACE inhibitor and aspirin. Slightly lower mortality risk with combined therapy than with either ACE inhibitor or aspirin alone (not statistically significant)	4
Evidence for lack of additional effect of aspirin on ACE inhibitor activity					
7352 patients (mean age 75 years) discharged after first hospitalisation for heart failure Numbers taking ACE inhibitors with or without aspirin not specified	Mean dose 286 mg daily 77% patients prescribed 325 mg daily	Not specified	1 year	No dose-dependent interactions between ACE inhibitors and aspirin. Compared with non-users, ACE inhibitor treatment resulted in lower mortality and less hospital readmissions; aspirin alone did not affect mortality or rate of hospital readmission and did not attenuate the benefits of ACE inhibitors	5
12703 patients aged ≥65 years with heart failure treated with an ACE inhibitor and resident in nursing homes 10657 taking ACE Inhibitors without, 2046 taking ACE Inhibitors with aspirin	More than 90% taking at least 325 mg daily	Captopril 51%, Enalapril 33%, Lisinopril 9%, with the rest taking Benazepril, Fosinopril, Quinapril or Ramipril	1 year	Mortality rate, hospitalisation rate, or rate of decline in physical function, not decreased by use of aspirin. Findings not affected by presence of ischaemic heart disease or type or dose of ACE inhibitor	6
755 patients with stable left ventricular systolic dysfunction 287 taking aspirin and ACE Inhibitor at start of study	317 patients receiving aspirin (mean dose 183 mg daily; 74% of patients received ≤200 mg daily)	Not specified	1 and 2 years	No interaction between the use of aspirin and survival in patients taking ACE Inhibitors.	7
Hospitalised patients with heart failure 1442 taking ACE Inhibitors without, 1615 taking ACE Inhibitors with aspirin	Not reported	Not specified	60- to 90-days post discharge	When combined with either an ACE inhibitor or angiotensin II receptor antagonist, aspirin had no effect on intermediate-term post discharge outcomes for patients with ischaemic or non-ischaemic heart failure	8

1. Harjai KJ, Nunez E, Turgut T, Newman J. Effect of combined aspirin and angiotensin-converting enzyme inhibitor therapy versus angiotensin-converting enzyme inhibitor therapy alone on readmission rates in heart failure. *Am J Cardiol* (2001) 87, 483–7.
2. Guazzi M, Brambilla R, Rèina G, Tumminello G, Guazzi MD. Aspirin-angiotensin-converting enzyme inhibitor coadministration and mortality in patients with heart failure: a dose-related adverse effect of aspirin. *Arch Intern Med* (2003) 163, 1574–9.
3. Harjai KJ, Solis S, Prasad A, Loupe J. Use of aspirin in conjunction with angiotensin-converting enzyme inhibitors does not worsen long-term survival in heart failure. *Int J Cardiol* (2003) 88, 207–14.
4. Krumholz HM, Chen Y-T, Wang Y, Radford MJ. Aspirin and angiotensin-converting enzyme inhibitors among elderly survivors of hospitalization for an acute myocardial infarction. *Arch Intern Med* (2001) 161, 538–44.
5. McAlister FA, Ghali WA, Gong Y, Fang J, Armstrong PW, Tu JV. Aspirin use and outcomes in a community-based cohort of 7352 patients discharged after first hospitalization for heart failure. *Circulation* (2006) 113, 2572–8.
6. Lapane KL, Hume AL, Barbour MM, Lipsitz LA. Does aspirin attenuate the effect of angiotensin-converting enzyme inhibitors on health outcomes of very old patients with heart failure? *J Am Geriatr Soc* (2002) 50, 1198–204.
7. Aumégeat V, Lamblin N, de Groote P, Mc Fadden EP, Millaire A, Bauters C, Lablanche J-M. Aspirin does not adversely affect survival in patients with stable congestive heart failure treated with angiotensin-converting enzyme inhibitors. *Chest* (2003) 124, 1250–8.
8. Levy PD, Nandyal D, Welch RD, Sun JL, Pieper K, Ghali JK, Fonarrow GC, Gheorghiade M, O'Connor CM. Does aspirin use adversely influence intermediate-term postdischarge outcomes for hospitalized patients who are treated with angiotensin-converting enzyme inhibitors or angiotensin receptor blockers? Findings from Organized Program to Facilitate Life-Saving Treatment in Hospitalized Patients with Heart Failure (OPTIMIZE-HF). *Am Heart J* (2010) 159, 222–30.

diclofenac caused slight increases in serum creatinine. However, there was no overall change in renal function (determined by glomerular filtration rate, urine flow, osmolality clearance, and sodium and potassium excretion) between placebo and low-dose aspirin. Long-term, low-dose aspirin appeared not to worsen renal function in patients with heart failure taking ACE inhibitors.[18]

D. Pharmacokinetic studies

A single-dose study in 12 healthy subjects found that the pharmacokinetics of **benazepril** 20 mg and aspirin 325 mg were not affected by concurrent use.[19]

Mechanism

Some, but not all the evidence suggests that prostaglandins might be involved in the hypotensive action of ACE inhibitors, and that aspirin, by inhibiting prostaglandin synthesis, might partially antagonise the effect of ACE inhibitors on blood pressure. This effect appears to depend on the dose of aspirin and could also be dependent on sodium status and plasma renin, and therefore it does not occur in all patients.

The beneficial effects of ACE inhibitors in heart failure and ischaemic heart disease are thought to be due, in part, to the inhibition of the breakdown of kinins, which are important regulators of prostaglandin and nitric oxide synthesis. Such inhibition promotes vasodilatation and afterload reduction. Aspirin might block these beneficial effects by inhibiting cyclo-oxygenase and thus prostaglandin synthesis, causing vasoconstriction, decreased cardiac output and worsening heart failure.[12,16]

Importance and management

Low-dose aspirin (less than or equal to 100 mg daily) does not alter the **antihypertensive efficacy** of captopril and enalapril. No special precautions would therefore seem to be required with ACE inhibitors and these low doses of aspirin. A high dose of aspirin (2.4 g daily) has been reported to interact in 50% of patients in a single study. Aspirin 300 mg daily has been reported to interact in about 50% of patients in another study, whereas 325 mg daily did not interact in further study. Thus, at present, it appears that if an ACE inhibitor is used with aspirin in doses higher than 300 mg daily, blood pressure should be monitored more closely, and the ACE inhibitor dose raised if necessary. Intermittent use of aspirin should be considered as a possible cause of erratic control of blood pressure in patients taking ACE inhibitors.

Both ACE inhibitors and aspirin are often taken by patients with **coronary artery disease**, and ACE inhibitors are used in **chronic heart failure**, which is often associated with coronary heart disease. The information about a possible interaction between ACE inhibitors and aspirin in heart failure is conflicting. This could be due to much of the clinical data being obtained from retrospective non-randomised analyses.[16] It might also be a factor of different disease states. For example, an interaction may be less likely to be experienced in patients with heart failure of ischaemic aetiology than those with non-ischaemic causes, because of the added benefits of aspirin in ischaemic heart disease.[20] However, one study suggests that aspirin with an ACE inhibitor (or angiotensin receptor II antagonist) had no adverse effect on intermediate outcomes for patients with ischaemic *or* non-ischaemic heart failure.[21] The available data, and its implications, have been extensively reviewed and commented on.[12,14,16,20,22-29] Some commentators have advised that, if possible, aspirin should be avoided in patients requiring long-term treatment for heart failure, particularly if heart failure is severe.[14,24] Others suggest avoiding aspirin in heart failure unless there are clear indications, such as atherosclerosis.[12,16,25,26] The use of lower doses of aspirin (80 to 100 mg daily, rather than 325 mg daily or more) in those with heart failure taking ACE inhibitors has also been suggested.[20,22,25]

US guidelines from 2005 on chronic heart failure[30] state that, "Many physicians believe the data justify prescribing aspirin and ACE inhibitors together when there is an indication for use of aspirin", while recognising that not all physicians agree. The guidelines say that further study is needed. The 2005 update of the European Society of Cardiology (ESC) guidelines stated that there was little evidence to support using ACE inhibitors and aspirin together in heart failure. The guidelines said aspirin could be used as prophylaxis after myocardial infarction, but that it should be avoided in patients with recurrent hospitalisation for worsening heart failure.[31] However, the ESC guidelines published in 2008 do not comment on the use of ACE inhibitors and aspirin. They note that antiplatelet drugs are not as effective as warfarin in reducing the risk of thromboembolism in patients with atrial fibrillation and that there is no evidence that antiplatelet drugs reduce atherosclerotic risk in patients with heart failure.[32] NICE guidelines in the UK state that all patients with heart failure due to left ventricular systolic dysfunction should be considered for treatment with an ACE inhibitor, and that aspirin (75 to 150 mg daily) should be prescribed for patients with the combination of heart failure and atherosclerotic arterial disease (including coronary heart disease).[33] Data from ongoing randomised studies might provide further insight. Until these are available, low-dose aspirin and ACE inhibitors may continue to be used where there is a clear indication for both.

An increased risk of deterioration in **renal function** or **acute renal failure** appears to occur rarely with the combination of aspirin and ACE inhibitors. The routine monitoring of renal function, which is advised with ACE inhibitors, should be sufficient to detect any interaction.

1. Moore TJ, Crantz FR, Hollenberg NK, Koletsky RJ, Leboff MS, Swartz SL, Levine L, Podolsky S, Dluhy RG, Williams GH. Contribution of prostaglandins to the antihypertensive action of captopril in essential hypertension. *Hypertension* (1981) 3, 168–73.
2. Smith SR, Coffman TM, Svetkey LP. Effect of low-dose aspirin on thromboxane production and the antihypertensive effect of captopril. *J Am Soc Nephrol* (1993) 4, 1133–9.
3. Guazzi MD, Campodonico J, Celeste F, Guazzi M, Santambrogio G, Rossi M, Trabattoni D, Alimento M. Antihypertensive efficacy of angiotensin converting enzyme inhibition and aspirin counteraction. *Clin Pharmacol Ther* (1998) 63, 79–86.
4. Nawarskas JJ, Townsend RR, Cirigliano MD, Spinler SA. Effect of aspirin on blood pressure in hypertensive patients taking enalapril or losartan. *Am J Hypertens* (1999) 12, 784–9.
5. Polónia J, Boaventura I, Gama G, Camões I, Bernardo F, Andrade P, Nunes JP, Brandão F, Cerqueira-Gomes M. Influence of non-steroidal anti-inflammatory drugs on renal function and 24 h ambulatory blood pressure-reducing effects of enalapril and nifedipine gastrointestinal therapeutic system in hypertensive patients. *J Hypertens* (1995) 13, 925–31.
6. Avanzini F, Palumbo G, Alli C, Roncaglioni MC, Ronchi E, Cristofari M, Capra A, Rossi S, Nosotti L, Costantini C, Pietrofeso R. Collaborative Group of the Primary Prevention Project (PPP)–Hypertension study. Effects of low-dose aspirin on clinic and ambulatory blood pressure in treated hypertensive patients. *Am J Hypertens* (2000) 13, 611–16.
7. Zanchetti A, Hansson L, Leonetti G, Rahn K-H, Ruilope L, Warnold I, Wedel H. Low-dose aspirin does not interfere with the blood pressure-lowering effects of antihypertensive therapy. *J Hypertens* (2002) 20, 1015–22.
8. Viecili PR, Pamplona D, Park M, Silva SR, Ramires JAF, da Luz PL. Antagonism of the acute hemodynamic effects of captopril in decompensated congestive heart failure by aspirin administration. *Braz J Med Biol Res* (2003) 36, 771–80.
9. MacIntrye IM, Jhund PS, McMurray JJV. Aspirin inhibits the acute arterial and venous vasodilator response to captopril in patients with chronic heart failure. *Cardiovasc Drugs Ther* (2005) 19, 261–5.
10. Davie AP, Love MP, McMurray JJV. Even low-dose aspirin inhibits arachidonic acid-induced vasodilation in heart failure. *Clin Pharmacol Ther* (2000) 67, 530–7.
11. Guazzi M, Pontone G, Agostoni P. Aspirin worsens exercise performance and pulmonary gas exchange in patients with heart failure who are taking angiotensin-converting enzyme inhibitors. *Am Heart J* (1999) 138, 254–60.
12. Mahé I, Meune C, Diemer M, Caulin C, Bergmann J-F. Interaction between aspirin and ACE inhibitors in patients with heart failure. *Drug Safety* (2001) 24, 167–82.
13. Spaulding C, Charbonnier B, Cohen-Solal A, Juillière Y, Kromer EP, Benhamda K, Cador R, Weber S. Acute hemodynamic interaction of aspirin and ticlopidine with enalapril. Results of a double-blind, randomized comparative trial. *Circulation* (1998) 98, 757–65.
14. Hall D. The aspirin—angiotensin-converting enzyme inhibitor tradeoff: to halve and halve not. *J Am Coll Cardiol* (2000) 35, 1808–12.
15. Latini R, Tognoni G, Maggioni AP, Baigent C, Braunwald E, Chen Z-M, Collins R, Flather M, Franzosi MG, Kjekshus J, Køber L, Liu L-S, Peto R, Pfeffer M, Pizzetti F, Santoro E, Sleight P, Swedberg K, Tavazzi L, Wang W, Yusuf S, on behalf of the Angiotensin-converting Enzyme Inhibitor Myocardial Infarction Collaborative Group. Clinical effects of early angiotensin-converting enzyme inhibitor treatment for acute myocardial infarction are similar in the presence and absence of aspirin. Systematic overview of individual data from 96,712 randomized patients. *J Am Coll Cardiol* (2000) 35 1801–7.
16. Massie BM, Teerlink JR. Interaction between aspirin and angiotensin-converting enzyme inhibitors: real or imagined. *Am J Med* (2000) 109, 431–3.
17. Seelig CB, Maloley PA, Campbell JR. Nephrotoxicity associated with concomitant ACE inhibitor and NSAID therapy. *South Med J* (1990) 83, 1144–8.
18. Juhlin T, Björkman S, Gunnarsson B, Fyge Å, Roth B, Höglund P. Acute administration of diclofenac, but possibly not long term low dose aspirin, causes detrimental renal effects in heart failure patients treated with ACE-inhibitors. *Eur J Heart Fail* (2004) 6, 909–16.
19. Sioufi A, Pommier F, Gauducheau N, Godbillon J, Choi L, John V. The absence of a pharmacokinetic interaction between aspirin and the angiotensin-converting enzyme inhibitor benazepril in healthy volunteers. *Biopharm Drug Dispos* (1994) 15, 451–61.
20. Nawarskas JJ, Spinler SA. Update on the interaction between aspirin and angiotensin-converting enzyme inhibitors. *Pharmacotherapy* (2000) 20, 698–710.
21. Levy PD, Nandyal D, Welch RD, Sun JL, Pieper K, Ghali JK, Fonarrow GC, Gheorghiade M, O'Connor CM. Does aspirin use adversely influence intermediate-term postdischarge outcomes for hospitalized patients who are treated with angiotensin-converting enzyme inhibitors or angiotensin receptor blockers? Findings from Organized Program to Facilitate Life-Saving Treatment in Hospitalized Patients with Heart Failure (OPTIMIZE-HF). *Am Heart J* (2010) 159, 222–30.
22. Stys T, Lawson WE, Smaldone GC, Stys A. Does aspirin attenuate the beneficial effects of angiotensin-converting enzyme inhibition in heart failure? *Arch Intern Med* (2000) 160, 1409–13.
23. Barbash IM, Goldbourt U, Gottlieb S, Behar S, Leor J. Possible interaction between aspirin and ACE inhibitors: update on unresolved controversy. *Congest Heart Fail* (2000) 6, 313–18.
24. Cleland JGF, John J, Houghton T. Does aspirin attenuate the effect of angiotensin-converting enzyme inhibitors in hypertension or heart failure? *Curr Opin Nephrol Hypertens* (2001) 10, 625–31.
25. Peterson JG, Lauer MS. Using aspirin and ACE inhibitors in combination: why the hullabaloo? *Cleve Clin J Med* (2001) 68, 569–74.
26. Olson KL. Combined aspirin/ACE inhibitor treatment for CHF. *Ann Pharmacother* (2001) 35, 1653–8.
27. Park MH. Should aspirin be used with angiotensin-converting enzyme inhibitors in patients with chronic heart failure? *Congest Heart Fail* (2003) 9, 206–11.
28. Konstam MA. Aspirin and heart failure: square evidence meets a round patient. *Congest Heart Fail* (2003) 9, 203–5.
29. Brunner-La Rocca HP. Interaction of angiotensin-converting enzyme inhibition and aspirin in congestive heart failure: long controversy finally resolved? *Chest* (2003) 124, 1192–4.
30. Hunt SA, Abraham WT, Chin MH, Feldman AM, Francis GS, Ganiats TG, Jessup M, Konstam MA, Mancini DM, Michl K, Oates JA, Rahko PS, Silver MA, Stevenson LW, Yancy CW, Antman EM, Smith SC Jr, Adams CD, Anderson JL, Faxon DP, Fuster V, Halperin JL, Hiratzka LF, Hunt SA, Jacobs AK, Nishimura R, Ornato JP, Page RL, Riegel B; American College of Cardiology; American Heart Association Task Force on Practice Guidelines; American College of Chest Physicians; International Society for Heart and Lung Transplantation; Heart Rhythm Society. ACC/AHA 2005 Guideline Update for the Diagnosis and Management of Chronic Heart Failure in the Adult: a report of the American College of Cardiology/American Heart Association Task Force on Practice Guidelines (Writing Committee to Update the 2001 Guidelines for the Evaluation and Management of Heart Failure): developed in collaboration with the American College of Chest Physicians and the International Society for Heart and Lung Transplantation: endorsed by the Heart Rhythm Society. *Circulation* (2005) 112, e154–235. Available at: http://circ.ahajournals.org/content/112/12/e154.full.pdf (accessed 21/10/15).
31. Swedberg K, Cleland J, Dargie H, Drexler H, Follath F, Komajda M, Tavazzi L, Smiseth OA, Gavazzi A, Haverich A, Hoes A, Jaarsma T, Korewicki J, Lévy S, Linde C, Lopez-Sendon J-L, Nieminen MS, Piérard L, Remme WJ; The Task Force for the Diagnosis and Treatment of CHF of the European Society of Cardiology. Guidelines for the diagnosis and treatment of chronic heart failure: full text (update 2005): The Task Force for the Diagnosis and Treatment of Chronic Heart Failure of the European Society of Cardiology. *Eur Heart J* (2005) 26, 1115–40.
32. Dickstein K, Cohen-Solal A, Filippatos G, McMurray JJV, Ponikowski P, Poole-Wilson PA, Strömberg A, van Veldhuisen DJ, Atar D, Hoes AW, Keren A, Mebazaa A, Nieminen M, Priori SG, Swedberg K. ESC Guidelines for the diagnosis and treatment of acute and chronic heart failure 2008: The Task Force for the Diagnosis and Treatment of Acute and Chronic Heart Failure 2008 of the European Society of Cardiology. Developed in collaboration with the Heart Failure Association of the ESC (HFA) and endorsed by the European Society of Intensive Care Medicine (ESICM). *Eur Heart J* (2008) 29, 2388–442.
33. National Institute for Clinical Excellence. Chronic heart failure in adults: management (issued August 2010). Available at: http://www.nice.org.uk/guidance/cg108 (accessed 21/10/15).

ACE inhibitors + Azathioprine

Anaemia has developed patients given azathioprine with enalapril or captopril. Leucopenia occasionally occurs when captopril is given with azathioprine.

Clinical evidence

(a) Anaemia

Nine out of 11 kidney transplant patients taking ACE inhibitors (**enalapril** or **captopril**) had a fall in their haematocrit from 34% to 27%, and a fall in their haemoglobin from 11.6 g/dL to 9.5 g/dL when ciclosporin was replaced by azathioprine. Two patients were switched back to ciclosporin, and had a prompt rise in their haematocrit. Another 10 patients taking both drugs were also found to have developed a degree of anaemia when compared with 10 patients not taking an ACE inhibitor (haematocrit of 33% compared with 41%, and a haemoglobin of 11.5 g/dL compared with 13.9 g/dL).[1] A later study by the same group of workers (again in patients taking **enalapril** or **captopril**) confirmed these findings; however, no pharmacokinetic interaction was found between **enalapril** and azathioprine.[2]

In contrast, a more recent study suggests that renal failure and female sex, but neither azathioprine (compared with mycophenolate mofetil) nor ACE inhibitors, were identified as predisposing factors for chronic anaemia post-heart transplant.[3]

(b) Leucopenia

A patient whose white cell count fell sharply when taking both **captopril** 50 mg daily and azathioprine 150 mg daily, did not develop leucopenia when each drug was given separately.[4] Another patient who was given **captopril** (increased to 475 mg daily (sic) then reduced to 100 mg daily) immediately after discontinuing azathioprine, developed leucopenia. She was later successfully treated with **captopril** 4 to 6 mg daily (sic).[5] Other patients have similarly developed leucopenia when given both drugs:[6,7] in one case this did not recur when the patient was rechallenged with **captopril** alone (at a lower dose).[7]

Mechanism

The anaemia appears to be due to suppression of erythropoietin by the ACE inhibitors, and azathioprine might cause patients to be more susceptible to this effect.[2] The cause of the leucopenia is unknown. It could be due to the additive effects of both drugs.

Importance and management

Anaemia caused by captopril and enalapril has developed in kidney transplant patients and in dialysis patients (see 'ACE inhibitors + Epoetins', p.33). The evidence that this effect can be potentiated by azathioprine is limited, but it would be prudent to monitor well if these drugs are used together.

Evidence to suggest that the concurrent use of ACE inhibitors and azathioprine increases the risk of leucopenia is also limited. However, the UK manufacturer of captopril recommends that it should be used with extreme caution in patients receiving **immunosuppressants**, especially if there is renal impairment. They advise that in such patients differential white blood cell counts should be performed before starting captopril, then every 2 weeks in the first 3 months of treatment, and periodically thereafter.[8] The UK manufacturers of a number of other ACE inhibitors also state that the use of ACE inhibitors with **cytostatic** or **immunosuppressive drugs** might lead to an increased risk of leucopenia.

For other potential interactions with ACE inhibitors that might lead to an increased risk of leucopenia, see also 'ACE inhibitors + Allopurinol', p.19, and 'ACE inhibitors + Procainamide', p.41.

1. Gossmann J, Kachel H-G, Schoeppe W, Scheuermann E-H. Anemia in renal transplant recipients caused by concomitant therapy with azathioprine and angiotensin-converting enzyme inhibitors. *Transplantation* (1993) 56, 585–9.
2. Gossmann J, Thürmann P, Bachmann T, Weller S, Kachel H-G, Schoeppe W, Scheuermann E-H. Mechanism of angiotensin converting enzyme inhibitor-related anemia in renal transplant recipients. *Kidney Int* (1996) 50, 973–8.
3. Cursack GC, Crespo-Leiro MG, Paniagua-Martín MJ, Muñiz J, Naya C, Grille Z, Rodríguez JA, Marzoa R, Barge E, Rios R, Estévez F, Cuenca JJ, Juffé-Stein A, Castro-Beiras A. Anemia crónica en el trasplante cardiaco. Prevalencia, factores predisponentes y significado pronóstico. *Rev Esp Cardiol* (2007) 60, 1144–50.
4. Kirchertz EJ, Gröne HJ, Rieger J, Hölscher M, Scheler F. Successful low dose captopril rechallenge following drug-induced leucopenia. *Lancet* (1981) i, 1363.
5. Case DB, Whitman HH, Laragh JH, Spiera H. Successful low dose captopril rechallenge following drug-induced leucopenia. *Lancet* (1981) i, 1362–3.
6. Elijovisch F, Krakoff LR. Captopril associated granulocytopenia in hypertension after renal transplantation. *Lancet* (1980), i, 927–8.
7. Edwards CRW, Drury P, Penketh A, Damluji SA. Successful reintroduction of captopril following neutropenia. *Lancet* (1981) i, 723.
8. Capoten (Captopril). E. R. Squibb & Sons Ltd. UK Summary of product characteristics, June 2010.

ACE inhibitors + Beta blockers

The combination of an ACE inhibitor with a beta blocker is in established clinical use. Enhanced blood pressure-lowering effects occur, as would be expected. Although not all combinations have been studied, no clinically relevant pharmacokinetic interactions appear to occur between the ACE inhibitors and beta blockers.

Clinical evidence

(a) Atenolol

In a double-blind, crossover study in hypertensive subjects, the combination of atenolol 50 mg daily and **enalapril** 20 mg daily increased the hypotensive effect of either drug alone, but the effect was 30 to 50% less than additive.[1] In another double-blind, crossover study, the combination of atenolol 25 mg and **lisinopril** 5 mg produced a greater decrease in blood pressure than either drug alone.[2]

(b) Bisoprolol

In a single-dose, placebo-controlled, crossover study in 16 healthy men, bisoprolol 5 mg given with **imidapril** 10 mg did not affect the pharmacokinetics of its active metabolite imidaprilat to a clinically relevant extent, and the pharmacodynamic effects, including blood pressure and heart rate reductions, were mainly additive.[3]

(c) Propranolol

In 10 healthy subjects propranolol 80 mg three times daily did not affect the pharmacokinetics of a single 20-mg dose of **quinapril**.[4] In another study the pharmacokinetics of **ramipril** 5 mg daily were unaffected by propranolol 40 mg twice daily.[5] Similarly, the UK manufacturer of **fosinopril** reports that the bioavailability of fosinoprilat, its active metabolite, was not altered by propranolol.[6] Another study found no pharmacokinetic interaction between **cilazapril** 2.5 mg daily and propranolol 120 mg daily in healthy subjects, but the reductions in blood pressure were roughly doubled and long-lasting in 6 healthy subjects and in 13 patients with hypertension.[7,8] A later report by the same authors found similar results in 17 patients.[9]

Mechanism, importance and management

Both ACE inhibitors and beta blockers lower blood pressure by different mechanisms, and therefore the enhanced blood pressure-lowering effects of the combination would be expected. No pharmacokinetic interactions have been demonstrated. The combination of an ACE inhibitor and a beta blocker is clinically useful in a number of cardiovascular disorders.

1. Wing LMH, Chalmers JP, West MJ, Russell AE, Morris MJ, Cain MD, Bune AJC, Southgate DO. Enalapril and atenolol in essential hypertension: attenuation of hypotensive effects in combination. *Clin Exp Hypertens* (1988) 10, 119–33.
2. Wald DS, Law M, Mills S, Bestwick JP, Morris JK, Wald NJ. A 16-week, randomized, double-blind, placebo-controlled, crossover trial to quantify the combined effect of an angiotensin-converting enzyme inhibitor and a β-blocker on blood pressure reduction. *Clin Ther* (2008) 30, 2030–9.
3. Breithaupt-Grögler K, Ungethüm W, Meurer-Witt B, Belz GG. Pharmacokinetic and dynamic interactions of the angiotensin-converting enzyme inhibitor imidapril with hydrochlorothiazide, bisoprolol and nilvadipine. *Eur J Clin Pharmacol* (2001) 57, 275–84.
4. Horvath AM, Pilon D, Caillé G, Colburn WA, Ferry JJ, Frank GJ, Lacasse Y, Olson SC. Multiple-dose propranolol administration does not influence the single dose pharmacokinetics of quinapril and its active metabolite (quinaprilat). *Biopharm Drug Dispos* (1990) 11, 191–6.
5. van Griensven JMT, Seibert-Grafe M, Schoemaker HC, Frölich M, Cohen AF. The pharmacokinetic and pharmacodynamic interactions of ramipril with propranolol. *Eur J Clin Pharmacol* (1993) 45, 255–60.
6. Fosinopril sodium. Actavis UK Ltd. UK Summary of product characteristics, August 2009.
7. Belz GG, Essig J, Kleinbloesem CH, Hoogkamer JFW, Wiegand UW, Wellstein A. Interactions between cilazapril and propranolol in man; plasma drug concentrations, hormone and enzyme responses, haemodynamics, agonist dose-effect curves and baroreceptor reflex. *Br J Clin Pharmacol* (1988) 26, 547–56.
8. Belz GG, Essig J, Erb K, Breithaupt K, Hoogkamer JFW, Kneer J, Kleinbloesem CH. Pharmacokinetic and pharmacodynamic interactions between the ACE inhibitor cilazapril and β-adrenoceptor antagonist propranolol in healthy subjects and in hypertensive patients. *Br J Clin Pharmacol* (1989) 27, 317S–322S.
9. Erb KA, Essig J, Breithaupt K, Belz GG. Clinical pharmacodynamic studies with cilazapril and a combination of cilazapril and propranolol. *Drugs* (1991) 41 (Suppl 1) 11–17.

ACE inhibitors + Calcium-channel blockers

The combination of an ACE inhibitor and a dihydropyridine calcium-channel blocker is in established clinical use for hypertension, and, although only certain combinations have been studied, no clinically relevant pharmacokinetic interactions appear to occur between these groups of drugs.

Clinical evidence

(a) Amlodipine

A study in 12 healthy subjects indicated that there was no pharmacokinetic interaction between single doses of amlodipine 5 mg and **benazepril** 10 mg.[1]

(b) Felodipine

In healthy subjects, no pharmacokinetic interaction occurred between single doses of felodipine 10 mg and **ramipril** 5 mg. The blood pressure-lowering effect of the combination was greater, and **ramipril** attenuated the reflex tachycardia caused by felodipine.[2]

(c) Manidipine

In a single-dose crossover study in 18 healthy subjects, the concurrent use of manidipine 10 mg and **delapril** 30 mg did not affect the pharmacokinetics of either drug or their main metabolites to a clinically relevant extent.[3]

(d) Nicardipine

In a study in 12 patients with hypertension taking **enalapril** 20 mg daily, the addition of nicardipine 30 mg three times daily for 2 weeks did not alter the pharmacokinetics of **enalapril**.[4] The manufacturer of **spirapril** briefly noted in a review that the concurrent use of spirapril and nicardipine increased **spirapril** plasma levels by about 25% and increased the levels of its active metabolite, spiraprilat, by about 45%. The bioavailability of nicardipine was reduced by 30%. It was assumed that the interaction took place at the absorption site. However, the changes were not considered clinically relevant.[5]

(e) Nifedipine

No evidence of either a pharmacokinetic or adverse pharmacodynamic interaction was seen in 12 healthy subjects given single doses of slow-release nifedipine 20 mg and **lisinopril** 20 mg; the effects on blood pressure were additive.[6] Similarly, in healthy subjects, there was no pharmacokinetic interaction between single doses of slow-release nifedipine 20 mg and **benazepril** 10 mg; the effects on blood pressure were additive and the tachycardic effect of nifedipine was attenuated by benazepril.[7] The UK manufacturer of **fosinopril** notes that the bioavailability of fosinoprilat, the active metabolite of **fosinopril**, was not altered by nifedipine.[8] Similarly, the manufacturer of **moexipril** notes that in healthy subjects no clinically important pharmacokinetic interaction occurred between **moexipril** and nifedipine.[9]

(f) Nilvadipine

In a single-dose, placebo-controlled study in 16 healthy subjects, no pharmacokinetic interaction occurred between nilvadipine 8 mg and **imidapril** 10 mg, and the pharmacodynamic effects, including the reduction in blood pressure and the decrease in total peripheral resistance, were mostly additive.[10]

Mechanism

No pharmacokinetic interactions are expected. Enhanced blood pressure-lowering effects occur, as would be expected.

Importance and management

No clinically important pharmacokinetic interactions have been demonstrated. The combination of an ACE inhibitor and a dihydropyridine calcium-channel blocker is clinically useful in the treatment of hypertension. A number of products combining an ACE inhibitor with a calcium-channel blocker are available. It is generally advised that these combination products are only used in patients who have already been stabilised on the individual components in the same proportions.

1. Sun JX, Cipriano A, Chan K, John VA. Pharmacokinetic interaction study between benazepril and amlodipine in healthy subjects. *Eur J Clin Pharmacol* (1994) 47, 285–9.
2. Bainbridge AD, MacFadyen RJ, Lees KR, Reid JL. A study of the acute pharmacodynamic interaction of ramipril and felodipine in normotensive subjects. *Br J Clin Pharmacol* (1991) 31, 148–53.
3. Stockis A, Gengler C, Goethals F, Jeanbaptiste B, Lens S, Poli G, Acerbi D. Single oral dose pharmacokinetic interaction study of manidipine and delapril in healthy volunteers. *Arzneimittelforschung* (2003) 53, 627–34.
4. Donnelly R, Elliott HL, Reid JL. Nicardipine combined with enalapril in patients with essential hypertension. *Br J Clin Pharmacol* (1986) 22, 283S–287S.
5. Grass P, Gerbeau C, Kutz K. Spirapril: pharmacokinetic properties and drug interactions. *Blood Pressure* (1994) 3 (Suppl 2), 7–13.
6. Lees KR, Reid JL. Lisinopril and nifedipine: no acute interaction in normotensives. *Br J Clin Pharmacol* (1988) 25, 307–13.
7. Jakobsen J, Glaus L, Graf P, Degen P, Maurice NP, Bellet M, Ménard J. Unmasking of the hypotensive effect of nifedipine in normotensives by addition of the angiotensin converting enzyme inhibitor benazepril. *J Hypertens* (1992) 10, 1045–51.
8. Fosinopril sodium. Actavis UK Ltd. UK Summary of product characteristics, August 2009.
9. Perdix (Moexipril hydrochloride). UCB Pharma Ltd. UK Summary of product characteristics, August 2010.
10. Breithaupt-Grögler K, Ungethüm W, Meurer-Witt B, Belz GG. Pharmacokinetic and dynamic interactions of the angiotensin-converting enzyme inhibitor imidapril with hydrochlorothiazide, bisoprolol and nilvadipine. *Eur J Clin Pharmacol* (2001) 57, 275–84.

ACE inhibitors + Capsaicin

An isolated report describes a woman taking an ACE inhibitor who developed a cough each time she used a topical cream containing capsaicin.

Clinical evidence, mechanism, importance and management

A 53-year-old woman who had been taking an unnamed ACE inhibitor for several years, complained of cough each time she applied *Axsain*, a cream containing capsaicin 0.075%, to her lower extremities. Whether this reaction would have occurred without the ACE inhibitor was not determined,[1] but cough is a recognised adverse effect of ACE inhibitors and pre-treatment with an ACE inhibitor has been shown to enhance the cough caused by *inhaled* capsaicin.[1] Topical application of capsaicin can, rarely, result in coughing due to irritation of the mucous membranes of the respiratory tract.[2] This potential interaction is probably of little general clinical importance.

1. Hakas JF. Topical capsaicin induces cough in patient receiving ACE inhibitor. *Ann Allergy* (1990) 65, 322.
2. Axsain Cream (Capsaicin). Cephalon (UK) Ltd. UK Summary of product characteristics, March 2011.

ACE inhibitors + Cefradine

No clinically relevant pharmacokinetic interaction appears to occur between captopril and cefradine.

Clinical evidence, mechanism, importance and management

No clinically relevant pharmacokinetic interaction was noted in a single-dose study in 9 healthy subjects given **captopril** 25 mg and cefradine 500 mg.[1] **Captopril** and cefradine are both thought to be absorbed through common transport pathways, by intestinal peptide transporters, and as such it was considered that they might impair or delay the absorption of each other.[1] However, an *in vitro* study found that peptide transporters do not control intestinal absorption and renal reabsorption of ACE inhibitors and therefore other proteins or other mechanisms might be involved in the intestinal transport of ACE inhibitors.[2] No particular precautions seem necessary on concurrent use.

1. Foster DR, Yee S, Bleske BE, Carver PL, Shea MJ, Menon SS, Ramachandran C, Welage LS, Amidon GL. Lack of interaction between the peptidomimetic substrates captopril and cephradine. *J Clin Pharmacol* (2009) 49, 360–7.
2. Knütter I, Wollesky C, Kottra G, Hahn MG, Fischer W, Zebisch K, Neubert RHH, Daniel H, Brandsch M. Transport of angiotensin-converting enzyme inhibitors by H^+/peptide transporters revisited. *J Pharmacol Exp Ther* (2008) 327, 432–41.

ACE inhibitors + Clonidine

Potentiation of the antihypertensive effect of clonidine by ACE inhibitors can be clinically useful.[1] However, limited evidence suggests that the effects of captopril might be delayed when patients are switched from clonidine.[2] Note that sudden withdrawal of clonidine can cause rebound hypertension.

1. Catapres Tablets (Clonidine hydrochloride). Boehringer Ingelheim Ltd. UK Summary of product characteristics, July 2009.
2. Gröne H-J, Kirchertz EJ, Rieger J. Mögliche Komplikationen und Probleme der Captoprилtherapie bei Hypertonikern mit ausgeprägten Gefäßschäden. *Therapiewoche* (1981) 31, 5280–7.

ACE inhibitors + Colloids

Acute hypotension has been seen in a few patients taking enalapril when they were given a rapid infusion of albumin-containing stable plasma protein solution (SPPS). Another case occurred in an infant taking captopril when given albumin 4%. A few other cases have been described with gelatin-type colloids in patients taking ACE inhibitors (cilazapril, enalapril, lisinopril).

Clinical evidence

(a) Albumin

A woman taking **enalapril** 10 mg in the morning, underwent surgery for groin lymph node resection under spinal and general anaesthesia. When she was given a rapid infusion of 500 mL of the albumin solution, stable plasma protein solution (SPPS, *Commonwealth Serum Laboratories, Melbourne, Australia*), her pulse rose to 90 to 100 bpm, systolic blood pressure fell from 100 mmHg to 60 mmHg, and a red flush was noted on all exposed skin. The blood pressure was controlled at 90 to 95 mmHg with metaraminol 4.5 mg, given over 10 minutes. When the SPPS was finished, the blood pressure and pulse rate spontaneously restabilised.[1] SPPS is a 5% plasma protein solution prepared by the cold ethanol fractionation process and pasteurisation from human plasma (volunteer donors). It contains sodium octanoate as a stabiliser.[1] Two very similar cases have been recorded in patients taking **enalapril** when given SPPS.[2,3] The manufacturer of SPPS notes that **captopril** has also been involved in this hypotensive interaction.[4]

A 20-month-old infant taking **captopril** was haemodynamically stable for 35 minutes after induction of anaesthesia while awaiting a donor kidney, but then developed hypotension after a bolus dose of 20 mL of albumin 4% (*Albumex*) was given. This was reversed with a dopamine infusion.[5]

(b) Gelatin-based colloids

A report describes 3 cases of severe hypotension in patients taking ACE inhibitors (**lisinopril**, **enalapril**) while undergoing joint replacement surgery, and after they had been given a gelatin-based plasma expander (*Gelofusin*), which contains 4% succinylated gelatin in saline. The hypotension was resistant to ephedrine and methoxamine, and responded to adrenaline (epinephrine) or dobutamine, which was required for 24 hours and 3 days, respectively, in two cases. Anaphylactoid reactions were excluded as a cause of the hypotension.[6] In another similar case, a patient taking **cilazapril** developed hypotension refractory to sodium chloride 0.9% after induction of anaesthesia, and this worsened when a gelatin-type colloid (*Gelafundina*) was given.[7]

Mechanism

Not fully established, but it is believed that SPPS contains low levels of pre-kallikrein activator, which stimulates the production of bradykinin, which can cause vasodilatation and hypotension. Normally the bradykinin is destroyed by kininase II (ACE), but this is delayed by the ACE inhibitor so that the hypotensive effects are exaggerated and prolonged.[3,8] In the case with albumin 4%, a sample of the albumin used was analysed, and it was found to contain less prekallikrein activating factor than maximum permissible levels.[5] It was suggested that the infusion of gelatin-based colloids somehow resulted in raised plasma kinin levels associated with inhibition of ACE.[6]

Importance and management

The interaction between SPPS and captopril would appear to be established and of clinical importance, and would be expected to apply to all ACE inhibitors. The author of one report suggested that if rapid expansion of intravascular volume is needed in patients taking ACE inhibitors, an artificial colloid might be a safer choice than SPPS.[1] The manufacturer of SPPS also recommended using an alternative plasma volume expander, including other albumin solutions.[4] It should be noted that following these reports SPPS was withdrawn from the Australasian market.[9] However, note that a case has also occurred with albumin 4%, and cases have also been attributed to synthetic colloid solutions containing gelatin. It might be that this is an unpredictable effect of colloids in patients taking ACE inhibitors.

For discussion of the marked hypotension sometimes seen during the induction of anaesthesia in patients taking ACE inhibitors, see also 'Anaesthetics, general + ACE inhibitors or Angiotensin II receptor antagonists', p.99.

1. McKenzie AJ. Possible interaction between SPPS and enalapril. *Anaesth Intensive Care* (1990) 18, 124–6.
2. Young K. Enalapril and SPPS. *Anaesth Intensive Care* (1990) 18, 583.
3. Young K. Hypotension from the interaction of ACE inhibitors with stable plasma protein solution. *Anaesthesia* (1993) 48, 356.
4. Schiff P. SPPS, hypotension and ACE inhibitors. *Med J Aust* (1992) 156, 363.
5. Fong SY, Hansen TG. Perioperative hypotension following plasma volume expansion with albumin in an angiotensin-converting enzyme inhibited infant. *Br J Anaesth* (2000) 84, 537–8.
6. Powell CG, Unsworth DJ, McVey FK. Severe hypotension associated with angiotensin-converting enzyme inhibition in anaesthesia. *Anaesth Intensive Care* (1998) 26, 107–9.

7. Barber L, Barrio J, de Rojas MD, Ibañez F, Añó C, Alepuz R, Montero R. Hipotensión refractaria y sostenida durante une anestesia general asociada al tratamiento crónico con inhibidores de la enzima conversiva de la angiotensina. *Rev Esp Anestesiol Reanim* (2001) 48, 34–7.
8. Bönner G, Preis S, Schunk U, Toussaint C, Kaufmann W. Hemodynamic effects of bradykinin on systemic and pulmonary circulation in healthy and hypertensive humans. *J Cardiovasc Pharmacol* (1990) 15 (Suppl 6), S46–S56.
9. McKenzie AJ. ACE inhibitors, colloid infusions and anaesthesia. *Anaesth Intensive Care* (1998) 26, 330.

ACE inhibitors or Angiotensin II receptor antagonists + Co-trimoxazole or Trimethoprim

Studies suggest that concurrent use of an ACE inhibitor or an angiotensin II receptor antagonist with co-trimoxazole might increase the risk of hyperkalaemia and/or sudden death. Case reports describe hyperkalaemia, apparently caused by the use of co-trimoxazole and enalapril, benazepril, and quinapril, some in association with renal impairment.

Clinical evidence

A case-control study of patients aged 66 years or over and taking either an ACE inhibitor or an angiotensin II receptor antagonist found that of 4 148 admissions to hospital involving hyperkalaemia during the 14-year study period, 371 admissions occurred within 14 days of antibacterial exposure (co-trimoxazole (trimethoprim with sulfamethoxazole), amoxicillin, ciprofloxacin, norfloxacin, or nitrofurantoin). Using matched controls, and compared with **amoxicillin**, co-trimoxazole was found to be associated with a nearly 7-fold increase in risk of hyperkalaemia-associated hospitalisation. No such risk was found with the use of the other antibacterials.[1] In a similar study by the same authors, of 39 879 sudden deaths while taking either an ACE inhibitor or an angiotensin II receptor antagonist during the 18-year study period, 1 027 occurred within 7 days of antibacterial exposure (co-trimoxazole, amoxicillin, ciprofloxacin, norfloxacin, or nitrofurantoin). Using matched controls, and compared with **amoxicillin**, co-trimoxazole was found to be associated with a 1.4-fold increase in the risk of sudden death. The risk with **ciprofloxacin** was increased by 1.3-fold, but neither **norfloxacin** nor **nitrofurantoin** were associated with such a risk.[2] A retrospective analysis of medical records for patients who received co-trimoxazole during a 5-year period, found that of 6 162 patients, there were 91 cases of hyperkalaemia. Of the cases of hyperkalaemia, 45% were also taking an ACE inhibitor compared with 15% in the 6 071 patients who did not develop hyperkalaemia. There was no difference among those taking an angiotensin II receptor antagonist. Further, the use of an ACE inhibitor was independently associated with a 3.3-fold increased risk of hyperkalaemia, and use of high-dose co-trimoxazole (greater than 5 mg/kg daily) with an ACE inhibitor resulted in 9% of patients developing hyperkalaemia compared with about 2% with standard-dose co-trimoxazole (less than 5 mg/kg daily).[3]

Several case reports describe hyperkalaemia in patients taking co-trimoxazole and an ACE inhibitor. A 40-year-old woman with a lung transplant whose medication included **enalapril**, developed hyperkalaemia (serum potassium 6.8 mmol/L) when she was given high-dose co-trimoxazole 120 mg/kg daily for suspected pneumocystis pneumonia. The co-trimoxazole and **enalapril** were stopped and she was given sodium chloride 0.9%, mannitol, and furosemide. After 12 hours, her serum potassium had decreased to 4.6 mmol/L and she began to recover over a period of a week, but she then developed fatal septic shock with multi-organ failure.[4]

In two other cases, patients taking **quinapril** 20 mg daily,[5] and **benazepril** 10 mg daily,[6] were found to have hyperkalaemia (serum potassium of 7 to 7.4 mmol/L and 6.3 mmol/L) 20 days and 4 days, respectively, after starting to take co-trimoxazole. After stopping the co-trimoxazole and quinapril or benazepril the hyperkalaemia resolved within 36[5] and 48 hours[6] of treatment, respectively.

Mechanism

Hyperkalaemia has been reported in patients taking co-trimoxazole alone.[7] This is attributed to the trimethoprim component, which can have a potassium-sparing effect on the distal part of the kidney tubules. ACE inhibitors reduce aldosterone synthesis, which results in reduced renal loss of potassium. The interaction is probably due to the additive effects of these two mechanisms, compounded by impaired renal function.[4,5]

Importance and management

Evidence for an interaction between trimethoprim or co-trimoxazole and an ACE inhibitor or angiotensin II receptor antagonist is limited. However, the studies cited suggest that there might be an increased risk of hyperkalaemia and/or sudden death with the concurrent use of these drugs. Although, it is important to note that confounding factors and limitations of methodology within these studies might have influenced the results. Clinical examples of an interaction between trimethoprim or co-trimoxazole and an ACE inhibitor or angiotensin II receptor antagonist seem to be rare, but hyperkalaemia with trimethoprim, ACE inhibitors, or angiotensin II receptor antagonists alone, particularly in the presence of other factors, such as renal impairment, is well documented. Thus, taken together, the results of the studies and the few case reports, suggest that it would be prudent to monitor potassium concentrations on concurrent use. It has been suggested that trimethoprim and co-trimoxazole should probably be avoided where possible in elderly patients with, or without, chronic renal impairment taking ACE inhibitors or angiotensin II receptor antagonists,[1,2,5] and that patients with AIDS taking an ACE inhibitor for associated nephropathy should probably discontinue the ACE inhibitor during the use of high-dose co-trimoxazole.[5]

1. Antoniou T, Gomes T, Juurlink DN, Loutfy MR, Glazier RH, Mamdani MM. Trimethoprim-sulfamethoxazole-induced hyperkalemia in patients receiving inhibitors of the renin-angiotensin system: a population-based study. *Arch Intern Med* (2010) 170, 1045–9.
2. Fralick M, Macdonald EM, Gomes T, Antoniou T, Hollands S, Mamdani MM, Juurlink DN. Co-trimoxazole and sudden death in patients receiving inhibitors of renin-angiotensin system: population based study. *BMJ* (2014) 349, g6196.
3. Gentry CA, Nguyen AT. An evaluation of hyperkalemia and serum creatinine elevation associated with different dosage levels of outpatient trimethoprim-sulfamethoxazole with and without concomitant medications. *Ann Pharmacother* (2013) 47, 1618–26.
4. Bugge JF. Severe hyperkalaemia induced by trimethoprim in combination with an angiotensin-converting enzyme inhibitor in a patient with transplanted lungs. *J Intern Med* (1996) 240, 249–52.
5. Thomas RJ. Severe hyperkalemia with trimethoprim-quinapril. *Ann Pharmacother* (1996) 30, 413–14.
6. Marinella MA. Trimethoprim-sulfamethoxazole associated with hyperkalaemia. *West J Med* (1997) 167, 356–8.
7. Alappan R, Perazella MA, Buller GK. Hyperkalemia in hospitalized patients treated with trimethoprim-sulfamethoxazole. *Ann Intern Med* (1996) 124, 316–20.

ACE inhibitors + Dialysis or Transfusion membranes

An anaphylactoid reaction can occur in patients taking ACE inhibitors within a few minutes of starting haemodialysis using high-flux polyacrylonitrile membranes ('AN69') or modified ST-AN69 membranes. Anaphylactoid reactions have also been reported in patients taking ACE inhibitors undergoing low-density lipoprotein apheresis.

Hypotensive reactions associated with blood transfusions through leucoreduction filters have occurred in patients taking ACE inhibitors.

Clinical evidence, mechanism, importance and management

(a) Apheresis

1. Low-density lipoprotein (LDL) apheresis. Anaphylactoid reactions occurred in 2 patients taking **captopril** or **enalapril** during removal of low-density lipoproteins (LDL apheresis) with dextran sulfate adsorption.[1] Further reactions were reported in 6 patients taking either **captopril** or **enalapril** and undergoing dextran sulfate apheresis. When the interval between the last dose of the ACE inhibitor and the apheresis was prolonged to 12 to 30 hours no further adverse reactions occurred.[2] However, other workers found lengthening the interval to be ineffective in one patient.[3]

A report describes a patient who experienced an anaphylactoid reaction while taking **ramipril** (but not when taking losartan) and undergoing dextran sulfate LDL apheresis.[4] Another patient given **imidapril** had blurred vision and lacrimation with hypotension during dextran sulfate apheresis. When this patient was given losartan instead of **imidapril** during LDL apheresis, blood pressure reduction was mild and adverse effects were absent.[5]

The manufacturer of **enalapril** suggests temporarily withholding the ACE inhibitor before each apheresis,[6] whereas other manufacturers of ACE inhibitors recommend using a different class of antihypertensive drug[7,8] or changing the method of lipoprotein reduction.[7,9]

2. Therapeutic plasma exchange. In a review of 299 patients undergoing therapeutic plasma exchange, all 14 patients taking ACE inhibitors experienced hypotension and/or flushing. The ACE inhibitors taken were **enalapril** (8 patients), **captopril** (6 patients): 2 of the patients also received **lisinopril** or **benazepril**. In addition, 20 of 285 patients not taking ACE inhibitors experienced similar adverse effects. Therefore the patients taking ACE inhibitors accounted for 14 of 34 (41%) of patients experiencing these reactions. The 14 patients taking ACE inhibitors underwent 186 apheresis procedures. In 53 of these procedures an ACE inhibitor was given in the 24 hours before the procedure and hypotension and/or flushing occurred in 41 of the 53 procedures. Six of the 14 patients also underwent apheresis while not taking an ACE inhibitor. One patient experienced transient hypotension and no reactions occurred in the other 5 patients. The authors recommended that ACE inhibitors should be withheld for at least 24 hours before apheresis.[10]

(b) High-flux dialysis

In a retrospective study, 9 of 236 haemodialysis patients dialysed using high-flux polyacrylonitrile membranes ('AN69') were found to have had anaphylactoid reactions (severe hypotension, flushing, swelling of face and/or tongue, and dyspnoea) within 5 minutes of starting haemodialysis. Treatment with an ACE inhibitor had been recently started in all 9 patients (7 taking **enalapril**, the other 2 taking **captopril** or **lisinopril**). The anaphylactoid reactions resolved in all 6 patients who discontinued the ACE inhibitor. Two other patients were given a filter rinsing procedure (the 'Bioprime' rinse method) and a new dialysis membrane, and in the final patient, further anaphylactoid reactions were prevented by cellulose-triacetate haemofiltration while the ACE inhibitor was continued.[11] Similar reactions have been reported elsewhere and are thought to be bradykinin mediated.[12-14]

The CSM in the UK has advised that the combination of ACE inhibitors and such membranes should be avoided, either by substituting an alternative membrane or an alternative antihypertensive drug.[15] Modified AN69 membranes (surface-treated AN69 membranes; ST-AN69), which reduce the generation of bradykinin, have been developed and used in patients taking ACE inhibitors. However, there are reports of anaphylactoid reactions in 5 patients taking ACE inhibitors during haemodialysis with these modified membranes.[16,17]

(c) Transfusion reactions

A report describes 8 patients taking ACE inhibitors and given blood transfusions through bedside **leucoreduction filters**, who experienced severe hypotensive reactions. The reactions were attributed to bradykinin generation during blood filtration and prevention of bradykinin breakdown due to the ACE inhibitors. Six of the patients tolerated subsequent transfusions, but 3 patients had discontinued their medication the day before the planned transfusion and one received washed (plasma-depleted) components. One patient experienced a second reaction, but then received washed red cells and had no reaction.[18]

1. Olbricht CJ, Schaumann D, Fischer D. Anaphylactoid reactions, LDL apheresis with dextran sulphate, and ACE inhibitors. *Lancet* (1992) 340, 908–9.
2. Keller C, Grützmacher P, Bahr F, Schwarzbeck A, Kroon AA, Kiral A. LDL-apheresis with dextran sulphate and anaphylactoid reactions to ACE inhibitors. *Lancet* (1993) 341, 60–1.
3. Davidson DC, Peart I, Turner S, Sangster M. Prevention with icatibant of anaphylactoid reactions to ACE inhibitor during LDL apheresis. *Lancet* (1994) 343, 1575.
4. Elicio N, Bertolini S, Garbarini R, Nardiello G, Elicio A, Aimale V. LDL apheresis with dextran sulfate and angiotensin receptor antagonist (losartan). *Artif Organs* (1997) 21, 334–5.
5. Kojima S, Shida M, Takano H, Inami S, Yodogawa K, Yokoyama H, Kuramochi M. Effects of losartan on blood pressure and humoral factors in a patient who suffered from anaphylactoid reactions when treated with ACE inhibitors during LDL apheresis. *Hypertens Res* (2001) 24, 595–8.
6. Innovace (Enalapril maleate). Merck Sharp & Dohme Ltd. UK Summary of product characteristics, January 2011.
7. Capoten (Captopril). E. R. Squibb & Sons Ltd. UK Summary of product characteristics, June 2010.
8. Perdix (Moexipril hydrochloride). UCB Pharma Ltd. UK Summary of product characteristics, August 2010.
9. Accupro (Quinapril hydrochloride). Pfizer Ltd. UK Summary of product characteristics, June 2009.
10. Owen HG, Brecher ME. Atypical reactions associated with use of angiotensin-converting enzyme inhibitors and apheresis. *Transfusion* (1994) 34, 891–4.
11. Verresen L, Waer M, Vanrenterghem Y, Michielsen P. Angiotensin-converting-enzyme inhibitors and anaphylactoid reactions to high-flux membrane dialysis. *Lancet* (1990) 336, 1360–2.
12. Tielemans C, Madhoun P, Lenaers M, Schandene L, Goldman M, Vanherweghem JL. Anaphylactoid reactions during hemodialysis on AN69 membranes in patients receiving ACE inhibitors. *Kidney Int* (1990) 38, 982–4.
13. Tielemans C, Vanherweghem JL, Blumberg A, Cuvelier R, de Fremont JF, Dehout F, Dupont P, Richard C, Stolear JC, Wens R. ACE inhibitors and anaphylactoid reactions to high-flux membrane dialysis. *Lancet* (1991) 337, 370–1.
14. Kammerl MC, Schaefer RM, Schweda F, Schreiber M, Riegger GAJ, Krämer BK. Extracorporal therapy with AN69 membranes in combination with ACE inhibition causing severe anaphylactoid reactions: still a current problem? *Clin Nephrol* (2000) 53, 486–8.
15. Committee on Safety of Medicines. Anaphylactoid reactions to high-flux polyacrylonitrile membranes in combination with ACE inhibitors. *Current Problems* (1992) 33, 2.
16. Peces R. Anaphylactoid reaction induced by ACEI during haemodialysis with a surface-treated AN69 membrane. *Nephrol Dial Transplant* (2002) 17, 1859–60.
17. Roux VD, Plaisance M. Une série de réactions indésirables associées à l'utilisation concomitante d'une membrane AN69-ST et d'un IECA. Anaphylactoid reactions with the use of ST-AN69 dialysers in patients taking ACE inhibitors. *Nephrol Ther* (2008) 4, 335–8.
18. Quillen K. Hypotensive transfusion reactions in patients taking angiotensin-converting-enzyme inhibitors. *N Engl J Med* (2000) 343, 1422–3.

ACE inhibitors + Diuretics; Loop, Thiazide and related

The combination of captopril or another ACE inhibitor with a loop or thiazide diuretic is normally safe and effective, but first-dose hypotension (dizziness, lightheadedness, fainting) can occur, particularly if the dose of diuretic is high, and often in association with various predisposing conditions. Renal impairment, and even acute renal failure, have been reported. Diuretic-induced hypokalaemia can still occur if an ACE inhibitor is used with these potassium-depleting diuretics.

Clinical evidence

(a) First dose hypotensive reaction

The concurrent use of **captopril** or other ACE inhibitors and loop or thiazide diuretics is normally safe and effective, but some patients experience first-dose hypotension (i.e. dizziness, lightheadedness, fainting) after taking the first one or two doses of the ACE inhibitor. This appears to be associated with, and exaggerated by, certain conditions (such as heart failure, renovascular hypertension, haemodialysis, high levels of renin and angiotensin, low-sodium diet, dehydration, diarrhoea or vomiting) and/or hypovolaemia and sodium depletion caused by diuretics, particularly in high doses. A study describes one woman whose blood pressure of 290/150 mmHg did not respond to a 10-mg intravenous dose of **furosemide**. After 30 minutes she was given **captopril** 50 mg orally and within 45 minutes her blood pressure fell to 135/60 mmHg and she required an infusion of saline to maintain her blood pressure.[1] In another study, a man taking **captopril** developed severe postural hypotension shortly after **furosemide** was given.[2]

Starting with a low dose of the ACE inhibitor reduces the risk of first-dose hypotension. In a study in 8 patients with hypertension who had been taking a diuretic (mainly **furosemide** or **hydrochlorothiazide**) for at least 4 weeks, **captopril** was started in small, increasing doses, from 6.25 mg. Symptomatic postural hypotension was seen in 2 of the 8 patients, but it was only mild and transient.[3]

Hypotension is more common in patients with heart failure who are taking large doses of diuretics. In a study in 124 patients with severe heart failure, all taking **furosemide** (mean dose 170 mg daily; range 80 to 500 mg daily) and 90 patients also receiving the potassium-sparing diuretic spironolactone, the addition of **captopril** caused transient symptomatic hypotension in 44% of subjects. The **captopril** dose had to be reduced, and in 8 patients, it was later discontinued. In addition, 4 patients developed symptomatic hypotension after one to 2 months of concurrent use, and **captopril** was discontinued.[4]

There is some evidence that in patients with heart failure the incidence of marked orthostatic hypotension requiring treatment discontinuation in the first 36 hours was lower with **perindopril** 2 mg daily than **captopril** 6.25 mg three times daily (6 of 357 cases versus 16 of 368 cases, respectively).[5] However, the effect of other drugs, such as antihypertensives, vasodilators and diuretics, being taken by the patients was not assessed in this study.

(b) Hypokalaemia

In one study, the reduction in plasma potassium levels was greater with **hydrochlorothiazide** 25 mg daily than with **hydrochlorothiazide** given with **cilazapril** 2.5 mg daily, showing that cilazapril reduced the potassium-depleting effect of **hydrochlorothiazide**.[6] In a placebo-controlled study in hypertensive patients given **quinapril** 2.5 mg, 10 mg or 40 mg daily, **hydrochlorothiazide** 6.25 mg, 12.5 mg, or 25 mg daily, or one of nine possible combinations of **quinapril** and **hydrochlorothiazide** with these doses, minimal changes in serum potassium occurred with **quinapril** or placebo alone. The percentage of patients with decreases in serum potassium of 0.5 mmol or more increased with the dose of **hydrochlorothiazide** alone. The degree of attenuation of the hypokalaemic effect of **hydrochlorothiazide** was related to the dose of **quinapril**, with the 2.5-mg dose attenuating the hypokalaemic effect of **hydrochlorothiazide** 6.25 or 12.5 mg, but not that of **hydrochlorothiazide** 25 mg. At doses of **quinapril** 40 mg daily, dose-related decreases in serum potassium were not apparent.[7]

In one analysis, 7 of 21 patients taking potassium-depleting diuretics and given ACE inhibitors for heart failure developed hypokalaemia. This was corrected by potassium supplementation in 2 cases, an increase in the ACE inhibitor dose in 3 cases, and the use of a potassium-sparing diuretic in the remaining 2 cases.[8] In another report, a woman taking **furosemide** 80 to 120 mg daily remained hypokalaemic despite also taking **ramipril** 10 mg daily and spironolactone 50 to 200 mg daily.[9] However, note that the addition of spironolactone to ACE inhibitors and loop or thiazide diuretics has generally resulted in an increased incidence of hyperkalaemia. For further information on this effect, see 'ACE inhibitors + Diuretics; Potassium-sparing', p.29.

(c) Hyponatraemia

An isolated report describes a patient taking **enalapril** 20 mg daily and atenolol 100 mg daily who developed severe hyponatraemia 3 days after **bendroflumethiazide** 10 mg daily was started. However, on two other occasions she developed only mild hyponatraemia when given **bendroflumethiazide** alone.[10] An earlier study reported changes in sodium balance due to **captopril** in all 6 patients with renovascular hypertension and in 11 of 12 patients with essential hypertension: sodium loss occurred in 12 of the 18 patients.[1]

(d) Renal impairment

The risk of ACE inhibitor-induced renal impairment in patients with or without renovascular disease can be potentiated by diuretics.[11-14] In an analysis of 74 patients taking **captopril** or **lisinopril**, reversible acute renal failure was more common in those who were also taking a diuretic (**furosemide** and/or **hydrochlorothiazide**) than those who were not (11 of 33 patients compared with 1 of 41 patients).[13] Similarly, in a prescription-event monitoring study, **enalapril** was associated with raised creatinine or urea in 75 patients and it was thought to have contributed to the deterioration in renal function and subsequent deaths in 10 of these patients. However, 9 of these 10 were also receiving loop or thiazide diuretics, sometimes in high doses.[15] Retrospective analysis of a controlled study in patients with hypertensive nephrosclerosis identified 8 of 34 patients who developed reversible renal impairment when given **enalapril** and various other antihypertensives including a diuretic (**furosemide** or **hydrochlorothiazide**). In contrast, 23 patients given placebo and various other antihypertensives did not develop renal impairment. Subsequently, **enalapril** was tolerated by 7 of the 8 patients without deterioration in renal function and 6 of these patients later received diuretics.[16] One patient was subsequently given **enalapril** with a recurrence of renal impairment, but discontinuation of the diuretics (**furosemide**, **hydrochlorothiazide**, and triamterene) led to an improvement in renal function despite the continuation of **enalapril**.[17]

Renal impairment in patients taking ACE inhibitors and diuretics has also been described in patients with heart failure. A patient with congestive heart failure and pre-existing moderate renal impairment developed acute non-oliguric renal failure while taking **enalapril** 20 mg daily and **furosemide** 60 to 80 mg daily, which resolved when the sodium balance was restored.[18] In a study involving 90 patients with severe congestive heart failure who were receiving **furosemide** and spironolactone, a decline in renal function occurred in 18 patients during the first month after initiation of **captopril**: mean serum creatinine levels rose from 220 micromol/L to 300 micromol/L. All patients were receiving high daily doses of **furosemide** and all had renal impairment before receiving the first dose of **captopril**.[4]

Acute, fatal, renal failure developed in 2 patients with cardiac failure within 4 weeks of starting to take **enalapril** with **furosemide**, and in 2 similar patients renal impairment developed over a longer period.[19] Reversible renal failure developed in a patient with congestive heart failure when **captopril** and **metolazone** were given.[20]

(e) Pharmacokinetic and diuresis studies

1. Furosemide. A study in healthy subjects given single doses of **enalapril** and furosemide found no evidence of any pharmacokinetic interaction between these drugs.[21] Another study in hypertensive patients found that **captopril** did not affect the urinary excretion or the diuretic effects of furosemide.[22] However, a further study in healthy subjects found that, although **captopril** did not alter the urinary excretion of furosemide, it did reduce diuresis.[23] Yet another study in healthy subjects found that **captopril** reduced the urinary excretion of furosemide, halved the diuretic response during the first 20 minutes and decreased the natriuretic response to almost 30%, whereas **enalapril** and **ramipril** did not significantly alter the diuretic effects of furosemide.[24] In one single-dose study in healthy subjects, the concurrent use of **benazepril** and furosemide reduced the urinary excretion of furosemide by 10 to 20%: **benazepril** pharmacokinetics were unaffected.[25] In one study, **lisinopril** did not alter the plasma levels or urinary excretion of furosemide, nor did it alter urinary electrolyte excretion.[26] Similarly, furosemide did not affect the pharmacokinetics of **lisinopril** either in single-dose or multiple-dose regimens.[27]

2. Hydrochlorothiazide. In a single-dose, randomised, crossover study in 19 elderly patients, the pharmacokinetics of **enalapril** 10 mg were unaffected by hydrochlorothiazide 25 mg. However, there was a reduction in renal clearance and an increase in the AUC of its metabolite, enalaprilat, resulting in higher serum levels of the active drug. This acute interaction was not thought to be clinically significant for long-term use.[28]

No pharmacokinetic interaction occurred between **cilazapril** and hydrochlorothiazide in healthy subjects or patients with hypertension.[6] Similarly, no pharmacokinetic interaction occurred between **imidapril** and hydrochlorothiazide in healthy subjects[29] and neither **captopril** nor **ramipril** altered the diuresis induced by hydrochlorothiazide.[24] The manufacturer of **spirapril** briefly noted in a review that there was no clinically relevant pharmacokinetic interaction between spirapril and hydrochlorothiazide.[30] Furthermore no pharmacokinetic interaction was found when **spirapril** and hydrochlorothiazide were given together as a bi-layer tablet.[31] In a single-dose study in healthy subjects there was no clinically important pharmacokinetic interaction when **moexipril** was given with hydrochlorothiazide.[32]

Mechanism

The first dose hypotension interaction is not fully understood. One suggestion is that if considerable amounts of salt and water have already been lost as a result of using a diuretic, the resultant depletion in the fluid volume (hypovolaemia) transiently exaggerates the hypotensive effects of the ACE inhibitor.

The cases of hypokalaemia are simply a result of the potassium-depleting effects of the diuretics outweighing the potassium-conserving effects of the ACE inhibitor. The converse can also occur.

Thiazides can cause hyponatraemia, but the enhanced effect might have been due to an alteration in renal haemodynamics caused by the ACE inhibitor: sustained angiotensin-converting enzyme blockade can produce natriuresis.[1]

Marked decreases in blood pressure can affect renal function, and in addition, the renin-angiotensin system plays an important role in the maintenance of the glomerular filtration rate when renal artery pressure is diminished.[12] However, diuretic-induced sodium depletion might also be an important factor in the renal impairment that sometimes occurs with ACE inhibitors.

Importance and management

The interaction between ACE inhibitors and diuretics that results in **first-dose hypotension** is well established. The BNF in the UK notes that the risk is higher when the dose of diuretic is greater than furosemide 80 mg daily or equivalent,[33] and suggests that, in patients taking these doses of diuretics, ACE inhibitors should be initiated under close supervision, and consideration should be given to temporarily stopping the diuretic, or reducing its dose at least 24 hours before the ACE inhibitor is added. If this is not considered clinically appropriate, the response to the first dose of the ACE inhibitor should be monitored for at least 2 hours, or until blood pressure has stabilised. In all patients taking diuretics, an ACE inhibitor should be started at a very low dose, even in patients at low risk (e.g. those with uncomplicated essential hypertension taking low-dose thiazides). To be on the safe side, all patients should be given a simple warning about what can happen and what to do when they first start concurrent use. The immediate problem (dizziness, lightheadedness, faintness), if it occurs, can usually be solved by the patient lying down. Taking the first dose of the ACE inhibitor just before bedtime is also preferable. Any marked hypotension is normally transient, but if problems persist it might be necessary temporarily to reduce the diuretic dose. There is usually no need to avoid the combination just because an initially large hypotensive response has occurred. A number of products combining an ACE inhibitor with a thiazide diuretic are available for the treatment of hypertension. These products should be used only in those patients who have been stabilised on the individual components in the same proportions.

The use of ACE inhibitors in patients taking potassium-depleting diuretics does not always prevent **hypokalaemia** developing. Serum potassium should be monitored.

There is only one isolated report of **hyponatraemia**, but be aware that ACE inhibitors can affect the natriuresis caused by diuretics.

The cases of **renal impairment** cited emphasise the need to monitor renal function in patients taking ACE inhibitors and diuretics. If increases in blood urea and creatinine occur, a dose reduction and/or discontinuation of the diuretic and/or ACE inhibitor might be required. In a statement, the American Heart Association comments that acute renal failure complicating the use of an ACE inhibitor is almost always reversible, and repletion of extracellular fluid volume and discontinuation of the diuretic is the most effective approach. In addition, withdrawing the interacting drugs, supportive management of fluid and electrolytes, and temporary dialysis, where indicated, are the mainstays of treatment.[14] The concurrent use of ACE inhibitors, diuretics and NSAIDs might be particularly associated with an increased risk of renal failure, see 'ACE inhibitors + NSAIDs', p.38. The possibility of undiagnosed renal artery stenosis should also be considered.

None of the **pharmacokinetic** changes observed appear to be clinically significant.

1. Case DB, Atlas SA, Laragh JH, Sealey JE, Sullivan PA, McKinstry DN. Clinical experience with blockade of the renin-angiotensin-aldosterone system by an oral converting-enzyme inhibitor (SQ 14,225, captopril) in hypertensive patients. *Prog Cardiovasc Dis* (1978) 21, 195–206.
2. Ferguson RK, Vlasses PH, Koplin JR, Shirinian A, Burke JF, Alexander JC. Captopril in severe treatment-resistant hypertension. *Am Heart J* (1980) 99, 579–85.
3. Koffer H, Vlasses PH, Ferguson RK, Weis M, Adler AG. Captopril in diuretic-treated hypertensive patients. *JAMA* (1980) 244, 2532–5.
4. Dahlström U, Karlsson E. Captopril and spironolactone therapy for refractory congestive heart failure. *Am J Cardiol* (1993) 71, 29A–33A.
5. Haïat R, Piot O, Gallois H, Hanania G. Blood pressure response to the first 36 hours of heart failure therapy with perindopril versus captopril. French General Hospitals National College of Cardiologists. *J Cardiovasc Pharmacol* (1999) 33, 953–9.
6. Nilsen OG, Sellevold OFM, Romfo OS, Smedsrud A, Grynne B, Williams PEO, Kleinbloesem CH. Pharmacokinetics and effects on renal function following cilazapril and hydrochlorothiazide alone and in combination in healthy subjects and hypertensive patients. *Br J Clin Pharmacol* (1989) 27 (Suppl 2), 323S–328S.
7. Canter D, Frank GJ, Knapp LE, Phelps M, Quade M, Texter M, and the Quinapril Investigator Group. Quinapril and hydrochlorothiazide combination for control of hypertension: assessment by factorial design. *J Hum Hypertens* (1994) 8, 155–62.
8. D'Costa DF, Basu SK, Gunasekera NPR. ACE inhibitors and diuretics causing hypokalaemia. *Br J Clin Pract* (1990) 44, 26–7.
9. Jolobe OM. Severe hyperkalaemia induced by trimethoprim in combination with an angiotensin-converting enzyme inhibitor in a patient with transplanted lungs. *J Intern Med* (1997) 242, 88–9.
10. Collier JG, Webb DJ. Severe thiazide-induced hyponatraemia during treatment with enalapril. *Postgrad Med J* (1987) 63, 1105–6.
11. Watson ML, Bell GM, Muir AL, Buist TAS, Kellett RJ, Padfield PL. Captopril/diuretic combinations in severe renovascular disease: a cautionary note. *Lancet* (1983) ii, 404–5.
12. Hoefnagels WHL, Strijk SP, Thien T. Reversible renal failure following treatment with captopril and diuretics in patients with renovascular hypertension. *Neth J Med* (1984) 27, 269–74.
13. Mandal AK, Markert RJ, Saklayen MG, Mankus RA, Yokokawa K. Diuretics potentiate angiotensin converting enzyme inhibitor-induced acute renal failure. *Clin Nephrol* (1994) 42, 170–4.
14. Schoolwerth AC, Sica DA, Ballermann BJ, Wilcox CS. Renal considerations in angiotensin converting enzyme inhibitor therapy. A statement for healthcare professionals from the Council on the Kidney in Cardiovascular Disease and the Council for High Blood Pressure Research of the American Heart Association. *Circulation* (2001) 104, 1985–91.
15. Speirs CJ, Dollery CT, Inman WHW, Rawson NSB, Wilton LV. Postmarketing surveillance of enalapril. II: Investigation of the potential role of enalapril in deaths with renal failure. *BMJ* (1988) 297, 830–2.
16. Toto RD, Mitchell HC, Lee H-C, Milam C, Pettinger WA. Reversible renal insufficiency due to angiotensin converting enzyme inhibitors in hypertensive nephrosclerosis. *Ann Intern Med* (1991) 115, 513–19.
17. Lee H-C, Pettinger WA. Diuretics potentiate the angiotensin converting-enzyme inhibitor-associated acute renal dysfunction. *Clin Nephrol* (1992) 38, 236–7.
18. Funck-Brentano C, Chatellier G, Alexandre J-M. Reversible renal failure after combined treatment with enalapril and frusemide in a patient with congestive heart failure. *Br Heart J* (1986) 55, 596–8.
19. Stewart JT, Lovett D, Joy M. Reversible renal failure after combined treatment with enalapril and frusemide in a patient with congestive heart failure. *Br Heart J* (1986) 56, 489–90.
20. Hogg KJ, Hillis WS. Captopril/metolazone induced renal failure. *Lancet* (1986) 1, 501–2.
21. Van Hecken AM, Verbesselt R, Buntinx A, Cirillo VJ, De Schepper PJ. Absence of a pharmacokinetic interaction between enalapril and frusemide. *Br J Clin Pharmacol* (1987) 23, 84–7.
22. Fujimura A, Shimokawa Y, Ebihara A. Influence of captopril on urinary excretion of furosemide in hypertensive subjects. *J Clin Pharmacol* (1990) 30, 538–42.
23. Sommers De K, Meyer EC, Moncrieff J. Acute interaction of furosemide and captopril in healthy salt-replete man. *S Afr Tydskr Wet* (1991) 87, 375–7.
24. Toussaint C, Masselink A, Gentges A, Wambach G, Bönner G. Interference of different ACE-inhibitors with the diuretic action of furosemide and hydrochlorothiazide. *Klin Wochenschr* (1989) 67, 1138–46.
25. De Lepeleire I, Van Hecken A, Verbesselt R, Kaiser G, Barner A, Holmes I, De Schepper PJ. Interaction between furosemide and the converting enzyme inhibitor benazepril in healthy volunteers. *Eur J Clin Pharmacol* (1988) 34, 465–8.
26. Sudoh T, Fujimura A, Shiga T, Tateishi T, Sunaga K, Ohashi K, Ebihara A. Influence of lisinopril on urinary electrolytes excretion after furosemide in healthy subjects. *J Clin Pharmacol* (1993) 33, 640–3.
27. Beermann B. Pharmacokinetics of lisinopril. *Am J Med* (1988) 85 (Suppl 3B) 25–30.
28. Weisser K, Schloos J, Jakob S, Mühlberg W, Platt D, Mutschler E. The influence of hydrochlorothiazide on the pharmacokinetics of enalapril in elderly patients. *Eur J Clin Pharmacol* (1992) 43, 173–7.
29. Breithaupt-Grögler K, Ungethüm W, Meurer-Witt B, Belz GG. Pharmacokinetic and dynamic interactions of the angiotensin-converting enzyme inhibitor imidapril with hydrochlorothiazide, bisoprolol and nilvadipine. *Eur J Clin Pharmacol* (2001) 57, 275–84.
30. Grass P, Gerbeau C, Kutz K. Spirapril: pharmacokinetic properties and drug interactions. *Blood Pressure* (1994) 3 (Suppl 2), 7–13.
31. Schürer M, Erb K, Junge K, Schäfer HF, Schulz H-U, Amschler S, Krupp S, Hermann R. Drug interaction of spirapril hydrochloride monohydrate and hydrochlorothiazide. *Arzneimittelforschung* (2003) 53, 414–19.
32. Hutt V, Michaelis K, Verbesselt R, De Schepper PJ, Salomon P, Bonn R, Cawello W, Angehrn JC. Lack of a pharmacokinetic interaction between moexipril and hydrochlorothiazide. *Eur J Clin Pharmacol* (1996) 51, 339–44.
33. Joint Formulary Committee. *British National Formulary.* 70 ed. London: BMJ Group and Pharmaceutical Press; 2015. p.124.

ACE inhibitors + Diuretics; Potassium-sparing

The concurrent use of ACE inhibitors and potassium-sparing diuretics (e.g. amiloride), including the aldosterone antagonists (eplerenone, spironolactone) can result in clinically relevant or severe hyperkalaemia, particularly if other important risk factors are present.

Clinical evidence

It is generally accepted that the use of an ACE inhibitor and a potassium diuretic increases the risk of hyperkalaemia, and the effect can be quite marked. A 7-year, case-control study in elderly patients found that patients taking ACE inhibitors, and admitted to hospital with hyperkalaemia, were about 20 times more likely to have also been taking a potassium-sparing diuretic (adjusted odds ratio, 20.3) in the previous week, compared with control patients receiving ACE inhibitors who were not admitted for hyperkalaemia.[1] Reports involving the use of named potassium-sparing diuretics are described 'Table 2.4', p.30, and in the sections below.

(a) Amiloride

The serum potassium levels of 2 patients taking furosemide and unnamed potassium-sparing diuretics and potassium supplements rose by 18% and 24%, respectively, when they were given **captopril** 37.5 to 75 mg daily. The rises occurred within one or two days. No clinical signs or symptoms of hyperkalaemia were seen, but one of the patients had an increase in serum potassium levels to above the upper limits of normal.[2] In a study, there was no difference in serum potassium levels in 19 patients with normal renal function taking amiloride and furosemide and a similar group of 16 patients also taking **enalapril**.[3]

In a post-marketing survey, 2 patients who had **enalapril**-associated renal impairment and died were also receiving amiloride and furosemide; one was also taking potassium supplements.[4]

(b) Eplerenone

In the large Eplerenone Post-Acute Myocardial Infarction Heart Failure Efficacy and Survival Study (EPHESUS)[5] the rate of serious hyperkalaemia (defined as serum potassium 6 mmol/L or greater) was 5.5% in patients randomised to eplerenone 25 mg to 50 mg daily (mean 43 mg daily[6]) compared with 3.9% in those receiving placebo: this represented a 40% increase. More eplerenone recipients required hospitalisation for serious hyperkalaemia than placebo recipients (12 versus 3). The risk of serious hyperkalaemia was increased in those with a baseline creatinine clearance of less than

Table 2.4 Occurrence of hyperkalaemia with concurrent use of ACE inhibitors and Potassium-sparing diuretics

Study and patients	*ACE inhibitor*	*Diuretic*	*Hyperkalaemia*	*Other symptoms*	*Presence of other risk factors*	*Refs*
Unnamed potassium-sparing drugs						
Case review of serious hyperkalaemia in patients taking enalapril	Enalapril	One or more unnamed potassium-sparing drugs	47 serious cases of hyperkalaemia and in 25 also taking potassium-sparing drugs (and in 8 taking potassium supplements)		One or more factors present in all 47 cases: aged over 65 years (30 patients); renal impairment (17) and hyperkalaemia in association with acute renal impairment (23); baseline hyperkalaemia (4); diabetes (5); history of gout (3); steroid therapy (2)	1
Amiloride						
Retrospective review of 4 patients aged over 50 years taking ACE inhibitor	Enalapril	Amiloride (with *hydrochlorothiazide) added	Life-threatening hyperkalaemia (potassium 9.4-11 mmol/L) within 8-18 days	Severe cardiac arrhythmias and deterioration in renal function; 2 suffered fatal cardiac arrests	Diabetes; renal impairment; gouty arthritis and NSAID use	2
Retrospective review of 1 patient aged 55 years taking an ACE inhibitor	Captopril	Amiloride (with *hydrochlorothiazide) added	Life-threatening hyperkalaemia (potassium 6.8 mmol/L) within 8 days		Diabetes	2
Case report of 1 patient aged 65 years	Enalapril	Amiloride (with *furosemide)	Potassium 6.2 mmol/L	Cardiac arrest	Diabetes; renal impairment	3
Retrospective comparison of 35 patients with congestive heart failure	Enalapril (16 patients)	Amiloride (with *furosemide); also 19 patients taking amiloride/ furosemide without enalapril	No hyperkalaemia (potassium levels about 4 mmol/L)		Did not include patients with renal impairment or those taking other drugs likely to affect potassium levels	4
Eplerenone						
Double-blind, parallel group study in 153 patients with left ventricular atrophy; study period at least 3 months	Enalapril 40 mg alone or 10 mg with eplerenone	Eplerenone 200 mg daily	Serious hyperkalaemia (max. plasma potassium $\geq$6 mmol/L) in: 7 patients taking eplerenone (10.9%), 2 taking enalapril (2.8%) & 3 taking both (4.5%)		Some patients also given *hydrochlorothiazide at week 8, but effects on potassium not noted	5
Spironolactone						
Study in 44 patients with congestive heart failure, hospitalised with life-threatening hyperkalaemia	Benazepril, Captopril, Enalapril, Moexipril or Ramipril (39 patients); Angiotensin II receptor antagonists (6 patients)	Spironolactone mainly 25 – 200 mg daily (mean dose 88 mg daily)	Mean plasma potassium, 7.7 mmol/L	Symptoms on admission included vomiting (19), diarrhoea (8), bradyarrhythmia (14), muscle weakness and paralysis (27), severe dehydration (28). Haemodialysis was given to 37 patients; renal function did not recover in 6 and 2 died (of other causes)	Diabetes (35 patients); reduced renal function; elderly (mean age 76 years); spironolactone dose above 25 mg daily	6
Prospective 3-month study involving 112 patients with hyperkalaemia (including 40 drug-related cases) during hospitalisation	Unnamed	Spironolactone $\leq$25 mg (5 patients); 26-50 mg (1); >50 mg (4); 8 of these also taking an ACE inhibitor	Potassium levels at least 6 mmol/L	Increased creatinine in 67% of those with hyperkalaemia	Elderly (average age 73 years); renal impairment and diabetes in some patients	7
Retrospective study in 69 patients with chronic heart failure treated for 12 months	Enalapril 5 mg daily	Spironolactone 25 or 50 mg daily (with *furosemide)	Potassium levels >5.5 mmol/L at 12 months in 4 patients; 2 patients had hypokalaemia (potassium levels $\leq$3.5 mmol/L)		Spironolactone dose above 25 mg daily	8

* Consider also ACE inhibitors + Diuretics: Loop, Thiazide and related (p.28)

Continued

Table 2.4 Occurrence of hyperkalaemia with concurrent use of ACE inhibitors and Potassium-sparing diuretics (continued)

Study and patients	*ACE inhibitor*	*Diuretic*	*Hyperkalaemia*	*Other symptoms*	*Presence of other risk factors*	*Refs*
Post-marketing survey; 4 cases of hyperkalaemia	Enalapril 10 or 20 mg daily	Spironolactone 75 mg with *furosemide (1 patient) or 100 mg daily *bumetanide, *hydroflumethiazide or *furosemide & metolazone (3 patients)	Potassium levels, mean 6.6 mmol/L	Deterioration in renal function and death	Mean age, 71 years; pre-existing renal disease; spironolactone dose above 25 mg daily	9
Case report	Enalapril 5 mg daily	Spironolactone 100 mg daily (with *furosemide 120 mg daily)	Potassium level 7.3 mmol/L	Transient loss of consciousness, bradycardia, hypotension; widened QRS complexes; death from complete heart block	Age 85 years; spironolactone dose above 25 mg daily	10
Case report	Captopril 25 mg three times daily	Spironolactone 50 mg (with *hydroflumethiazide 50 mg) daily	Potassium level 8.5 mmol/L	Dizziness	Age 72 years; spironolactone dose above 25 mg daily	11
Case report	Lisinopril 10 mg daily	Spironolactone 25 mg daily (added to *furosemide 10 mg daily)	Potassium level 8.9 mmol/L	Decreased consciousness	Moderately impaired renal function; diabetes. Note: age 43 years and dose of spironolactone just 25 mg	12
Four case reports in hospitalised patients:			Potassium level:		Age 85 to 89 years; various degrees of renal impairment; spironolactone dose above 25 mg daily	13
i.	Captopril 25 mg three times daily	Spironolactone 100 mg daily (with *furosemide 40 mg on day 1)	6.9 mmol/L	Generalised weakness		
ii.	Lisinopril 10 mg daily	Spironolactone 50 mg daily	9.2 mmol/L	Major weakness; pulmonary oedema		
iii.	Lisinopril 20 mg daily	Spironolactone 100 mg daily (with *furosemide 40 mg daily)	6.9 mmol/L	Fall & hip fracture		
iv. initial admission	Lisinopril 20 mg daily	Spironolactone 100 mg daily	6.3 mmol/L	Weakness		
re-admission after 5 months	Lisinopril 20 mg daily	Spironolactone 100 mg daily (with *furosemide 40 mg daily)	9.6 mmol/L	Falls; pulmonary oedema		
2nd re-admission after further 3 months	Lisinopril 10 mg daily	Spironolactone 50 mg daily (with *furosemide 40 mg daily)	7.6 mmol/L	Weakness		
Open study in 124 patients with NYHA class III or IV heart failure, given captopril in addition to existing treatments	Captopril 18.75 to 150 mg per day, in three divided doses	Spironolactone (90 patients) 50 to 100 mg daily (mean dose 73 mg daily)	Overall, mean serum potassium increased from 4.1 mmol/L to 4.3 mmol/L; 6 patients taking spironolactone developed hyperkalaemia	Patients developing hyperkalaemia also had a deterioration in renal function	Mean age 68 years; spironolactone dose above 25 mg daily	14
Retrospective cohort study in 100 patients with class III or IV chronic heart failure treated with ACE inhibitor plus spironolactone (49 patients) or ACE inhibitor alone (51)	Captopril (mean 46 mg daily) or enalapril (mean 15 mg daily)	Spironolactone mean 37 mg daily (with *furosemide mean 69 or 62 mg daily)	ACE inhibitor + Spironolactone: 16 cases of hyperkalaemia (potassium $\geq$5.5 mmol/L); 7 cases of severe hyperkalaemia (potassium >6 mmol/L); ACE inhibitor alone: 1 case of hyperkalaemia.	Increases in creatinine following treatment	Diabetes; spironolactone dose above 25 mg daily	15

* Consider also ACE inhibitors + Diuretics: Loop, Thiazide and related (p.28)

1. Brown C, Rush J. Risk factors for the development of hyperkalemia in patients treated with enalapril for heart failure. *Clin Pharmacol Ther* (1989) 45, 167.
2. Chiu T-F, Bullard MJ, Chen J-C, Liaw S-J, Ng C-J. Rapid life-threatening hyperkalemia after addition of amiloride HCl/hydrochlorothiazide to angiotensin-converting enzyme inhibitor therapy. *Ann Emerg Med* (1997) 30, 612–15.

Continued

Table 2.4 Occurrence of hyperkalaemia with concurrent use of ACE inhibitors and Potassium-sparing diuretics (continued)

3. Johnston RT, de Bono DP, Nyman CR. Preventable sudden death in patients receiving angiotensin converting enzyme inhibitors and loop/potassium sparing diuretic combinations. *Int J Cardiol* (1992) 34, 213–15.
4. Radley AS, Fitzpatrick RW. An evaluation of the potential interaction between enalapril and amiloride. *J Clin Pharm Ther* (1987) 12, 319–23.
5. Pitt B, Reichek N, Willenbrock R, Zannad F, Phillips RA, Roniker B, Kleiman J, Krause S, Burns D, Williams GH. Effects of eplerenone, enalapril, and eplerenone/enalapril in patients with essential hypertension and left ventricular hypertrophy. The 4E–Left Ventricular Hypertrophy Study. *Circulation* (2003) 108, 1831–8.
6. Wrenger E, Müller R, Moesenthin M, Welte T, Frölich JC, Neumann KH. Interaction of spironolactone with ACE inhibitors or angiotensin receptor blockers: analysis of 44 cases. *BMJ* (2003) 327, 147–9.
7. Onno C, Rémignon H, Lagarce L, Bruhat C, Tourmen Y, Subra J-F, Lainé-Cessac P. Étude prospective observationnelle des hyperkaliémies médicamenteuses chez des adultes non dialysés hospitalisés. *Therapie* (2007) 62, 55–60.
8. Saito M, Takada M, Hirooka K, Isobe F, Yasumura Y. Serum concentration of potassium in chronic heart failure patients administered spironolactone plus furosemide and either enalapril maleate, losartan potassium or candesartan cilexetil. *J Clin Pharm Ther* (2005) 30, 603–10.
9. Speirs CJ, Dollery CT, Inman WHW, Rawson NSB, Wilton LV. Postmarketing surveillance of enalapril. II: Investigation of the potential role of enalapril in deaths with renal failure. *BMJ* (1988) 297, 830–2.
10. Lakhani M. Complete heart block induced by hyperkalaemia associated with treatment with a combination of captopril and spironolactone. *BMJ* (1986) 293, 271.
11. Lo TCN, Cryer RJ. Complete heart block induced by hyperkalaemia associated with treatment with a combination of captopril and spironolactone. *BMJ* (1986) 292, 1672.
12. Odawara M, Asano M, Yamashita K. Life-threatening hyperkalaemia caused by angiotensin-converting enzyme inhibitor and diuretics. *Diabet Med* (1997) 14, 169–70.
13. Vanpee D, Swine C. Elderly heart failure patients with drug-induced serious hyperkalemia. *Aging Clin Exp Res* (2000) 12, 315–19.
14. Dahlström U, Karlsson E. Captopril and spironolactone therapy for refractory congestive heart failure. *Am J Cardiol* (1993) 71, 29A–33A.
15. Cruz CS, Cruz ÁA, Marcílio de Souza CA. Hyperkalaemia in congestive heart failure patients using ACE inhibitors and spironolactone. *Nephrol Dial Transplant* (2003) 18, 1814–19.

50 mL/minute (10.1% in the eplerenone group and 5.9% in the placebo group). Eplerenone reduced the risk of serious hypokalaemia (defined as serum potassium 3.5 mmol/L or less) by 60% (8.4% versus 13.1%). About 86% of patients in this study were also receiving an ACE inhibitor or an angiotensin II receptor antagonist, and about 60% were receiving a (loop[6]) diuretic.[5] However, the US manufacturer states that the rate of maximum potassium levels greater than 5.5 mmol/L were similar in EPHESUS regardless of the use of ACE inhibitor or angiotensin II receptor antagonist.[6] Nevertheless, they mention another study in diabetics with microalbuminuria, where a higher dose of eplerenone 200 mg given with **enalapril** 10 mg increased the frequency of hyperkalaemia (defined as serum potassium greater than 5.5 mmol/L) from 17% with enalapril alone to 38% with the combination: this represented a 2.2-fold increase.[6]

(c) Spironolactone

Twenty-five of 262 patients taking ACE inhibitors and spironolactone, and admitted to hospital for medical emergencies, were found to have serious hyperkalaemia (defined as serum potassium levels greater than 6 mmol/L: 11 patients had levels of at least 8 mmol/L). These 25 patients were elderly (mean age 74 years) and being treated for hypertension, heart failure, diabetic nephropathy, proteinuria, or nephrotic syndrome; 22 had associated renal impairment and 12 had signs of volume depletion. Concurrent use of the ACE inhibitor and spironolactone had been started an average of 25 weeks before admission. The ACE inhibitors involved were **enalapril**, **captopril**, **lisinopril** or **perindopril,** and the average dose of spironolactone used was 57 mg daily; 10 patients were also receiving a loop or thiazide diuretic. Nineteen patients had ECG changes associated with hyperkalaemia; 2 of them died, another 2 required temporary pacing for third-degree heart block, and 2 others survived after sustained ventricular tachycardia and fibrillation. Of the 19 patients with ECG changes, 17 required at least one haemodialysis session and 12 were admitted to intensive care.[7] Other authors reported a higher 36% incidence of hyperkalaemia (serum potassium levels greater than 5 mmol/L) in 42 patients hospitalised for heart failure and prescribed spironolactone. It was suggested that this could be due to the excessively large doses of spironolactone prescribed,[8] although the specific doses were not mentioned. One of the factors that affects the incidence of hyperkalaemia appears to be the dose of spironolactone. In a preliminary investigation for the Randomised Aldactone Evaluation Study (RALES), 214 patients with congestive heart failure taking an ACE inhibitor and a loop diuretic, with or without digitalis, were randomised to receive placebo or various doses of spironolactone for 12 weeks. The incidence of hyperkalaemia (defined as serum potassium level of 5.5 mmol/L or greater) was 5% for the placebo group, whereas it was 5%, 13%, 20%, and 24% when spironolactone was given in single daily doses of 12.5 mg, 25 mg, 50 mg, or 75 mg, respectively.[9] The main RALES study involving 1 663 patients found a 30% reduction in the risk of mortality in patients with severe heart failure when they were given spironolactone in addition to treatment including an ACE inhibitor, a loop diuretic and in most cases digoxin. During the first year of follow-up, the median creatinine concentration in the spironolactone group increased by about 4 to 9 micromol/L and the median potassium level increased by 0.03 mmol/L, but there was a low incidence of serious hyperkalaemia (2% in the spironolactone group compared with 1% in the placebo group). However, the dose of spironolactone was fairly low (mean dose 26 mg daily; range 25 mg every other day to 50 mg daily depending on serum potassium levels and response). In addition, patients with a serum creatinine of more than 221 micromol/L or a serum potassium of more than 5 mmol/L were excluded.[10] In a Canadian population-based time-series analysis, the increase in use of spironolactone for heart failure in patients taking ACE inhibitors after publication of the RALES study was found be associated with 50 additional hospitalisations for hyperkalaemia for every 1 000 additional prescriptions for spironolactone, and there was a 6.7-fold increase in the number of patients dying from hyperkalaemia. The authors state that spironolactone-related hyperkalaemia is a much greater problem in every day practice than in the setting of a clinical study, and give a number of reasons for this, including less frequent monitoring of potassium levels, the presence of conditions predisposing to hyperkalaemia, failure to detect subsequent development of renal impairment, inappropriately high doses of spironolactone, increase in dietary potassium intake, and the use of spironolactone in heart failure with causes not included in the RALES study.[11] In another study, the use of spironolactone with ACE inhibitors in patients with class IV chronic heart failure was associated with a 14.6 odds ratio for developing hyperkalaemia when compared with ACE inhibitors alone. Predictors for hyperkalaemia included increases in creatinine following treatment, and diabetes.[12]

(d) Triamterene

A retrospective analysis found that **captopril**, given to 6 patients taking *Dyazide* (hydrochlorothiazide with triamterene), had not increased potassium levels.[13]

Mechanism

ACE inhibitors reduce the levels of aldosterone, which results in the retention of potassium. This would be expected to be additive with the potassium-retaining effects of amiloride and triamterene and aldosterone antagonists such as spironolactone and eplerenone, leading to hyperkalaemia, but usually only if other risk factors are present (see *Importance and management*, below).

Importance and management

Hyperkalaemia with ACE inhibitors and potassium-sparing diuretics, and particularly the aldosterone antagonist spironolactone, is well documented and well established. If it occurs it can be serious and potentially life threatening. Its incidence depends on the presence of other risk factors, and clinically important hyperkalaemia usually only appears to develop if one or more of these are also present, particularly renal impairment. Other risk factors for hyperkalaemia in patients with heart failure include:

- advanced age;[14]
- diabetes[15,16] (hyperkalaemia has been found to be relatively common in both non-insulin-dependent and insulin-dependent diabetics);[17]
- spironolactone in doses greater than 25 mg daily.

A retrospective study in hospitalised patients who developed hyperkalaemia found that risk factors associated with a rapid rate of increase in serum potassium levels in *decreasing order* of importance were:

- the use of potassium supplements,
- severe renal impairment,
- the use of ACE inhibitors or angiotensin II receptor antagonists,
- the use of potassium-sparing diuretics,
- diabetes mellitus.

Further, the presence of two or more of these risk factors was associated with an even faster development of hyperkalaemia. As the speed at which hyperkalaemia develops is also correlated with its severity, the authors recommend close monitoring in patients with two or more risk factors, and that a rapid increase in serum potassium (greater than 0.5 mmol/L per day) should prompt the identification and possible removal of any risk factors for hyperkalaemia.[18]

It is generally recommended that ACE inhibitors and potassium-sparing diuretics, such as **amiloride** and **triamterene**, should normally not be given concurrently. If, however, the use of both drugs is thought to be appropriate, the serum potassium levels should be closely monitored, particularly in those patients with additional risk factors, so that any problems can be quickly identified. Similar caution seems warranted on the concurrent use of **eplerenone** and an ACE inhibitor.

The combination of an ACE inhibitor and **spironolactone** can be beneficial in some types of heart failure, but close monitoring of serum potassium and renal function is needed, especially with any changes in treatment or the patient's clinical condition. The combination should be avoided in patients with renal impairment with a glomerular filtration rate of less than 30 mL/minute.[16] In addition, the dose of spironolactone should not exceed 25 mg daily.[16]

Note that the concurrent use of a potassium-depleting diuretic (a loop or thiazide diuretic) with the potassium-sparing diuretic may not necessarily prevent the development of hyperkalaemia (see also 'ACE inhibitors + Diuretics; Loop, Thiazide and related', p.28).

1. Juurlink DN, Mamdani M, Kopp A, Laupacis A, Redelmeier DA. Drug-drug interactions among elderly patients hospitalized for drug toxicity. *JAMA* (2003) 289, 1652–8.

2. Burnakis TG, Mioduch HJ. Combined therapy with captopril and potassium supplementation. A potential for hyperkalemia. *Arch Intern Med* (1984) 144, 2371–2.
3. Radley AS, Fitzpatrick RW. An evaluation of the potential interaction between enalapril and amiloride. *J Clin Pharm Ther* (1987) 12, 319–23.
4. Speirs CJ, Dollery CT, Inman WHW, Rawson NSB, Wilton LV. Postmarketing surveillance of enalapril. II: Investigation of the potential role of enalapril in deaths with renal failure. *BMJ* (1988) 297, 830–2.
5. Pitt B, Remme W, Zannad F, Neaton J, Martinez F, Roniker B, Bittman R, Hurley S, Kleiman J, Gatlin M; Eplerenone Post-Acute Myocardial Infarction Heart Failure Efficacy and Survival Study Investigators. Eplerenone, a selective aldosterone blocker, in patients with left ventricular dysfunction after myocardial infarction. *N Engl J Med* (2003) 348, 1309–21.
6. Inspra (Eplerenone). Pfizer Inc. US Prescribing information, April 2008.
7. Schepkens H, Vanholder R, Billiouw J-M, Lameire N. Life-threatening hyperkalemia during combined therapy with angiotensin-converting enzyme inhibitors and spironolactone: an analysis of 25 cases. *Am J Med* (2001) 110, 438–41.
8. Berry C, McMurray J. Life-threatening hyperkalemia during combined therapy with angiotensin-converting enzyme inhibitors and spironolactone. *Am J Med* (2001) 111, 587.
9. The RALES Investigators. Effectiveness of spironolactone added to an angiotensin-converting enzyme inhibitor and a loop diuretic for severe chronic congestive heart failure (The Randomized Aldactone Evaluation Study [RALES]). *Am J Cardiol* (1996) 78, 902–7.
10. Pitt B, Zannad F, Remme WJ, Cody R, Castaigne A, Perez A, Palensky J, Wittes J, for the Randomized Aldactone Evaluation Study Investigators. The effect of spironolactone on morbidity and mortality in patients with severe heart failure. *N Engl J Med* (1999) 341, 709–17.
11. Juurlink DN, Mamdani MM, Lee DS, Kopp A, Austin PC, Laupacis A, Redelmeier DA. Rates of hyperkalemia after publication of the Randomized Aldactone Evaluation Study. *N Engl J Med* (2004) 351, 543–51.
12. Cruz CS, Cruz ÁA, Marcílio de Souza CA. Hyperkalaemia in congestive heart failure patients using ACE inhibitors and spironolactone. *Nephrol Dial Transplant* (2003) 18, 1814–19.
13. Schuna AA, Schmidt GR, Pitterle ME. Serum potassium concentrations after initiation of captopril therapy. *Clin Pharm* (1986) 5, 920–3.
14. Vanpee D, Swine C. Elderly heart failure patients with drug-induced serious hyperkalemia. *Aging Clin Exp Res* (2000) 12, 315–19.
15. Wrenger E, Müller R, Moesenthin M, Welte T, Frölich JC, Neumann KH. Interaction of spironolactone with ACE inhibitors or angiotensin receptor blockers: analysis of 44 cases. *BMJ* (2003) 327, 147–9.
16. Palmer BF. Managing hyperkalemia caused by inhibitors of the renin-angiotensin-aldosterone system. *N Engl J Med* (2004) 351, 585–92.
17. Jarman PR, Keheley AM, Mather HM. Life-threatening hyperkalaemia caused by ACE inhibitor and diuretics. *Diabet Med* (1997) 14, 808.
18. Indermitte J, Burkolter S, Drewe J, Krähenbühl S, Hersberger KE. Risk factors associated with a high velocity of the development of hyperkalaemia in hospitalised patients. *Drug Safety* (2007) 30, 71–80.

ACE inhibitors + Epoetins

Epoetins can cause hypertension and therefore reduce the effects of antihypertensive drugs. It is not entirely clear whether ACE inhibitors affect the efficacy of epoetins or not, but any interaction could take many months to develop. An additive hyperkalaemic effect is theoretically possible on the concurrent use of ACE inhibitors and epoetins.

Clinical evidence

(a) Decreased epoetin effects

For a summary of the studies showing a decrease in the effects of epoetin in patients taking ACE inhibitors, see 'Table 2.5', p.34. In general, the studies show that increased epoetin doses are required in patients also taking an ACE inhibitor.

In a prospective study, 15 patients in whom ACE inhibitors (**enalapril**, **captopril**, or **perindopril**) were withdrawn and replaced with amlodipine, felodipine or doxazosin, had an increase in their mean haematocrit value and a decrease in their mean epoetin dose requirement.[1]

(b) No interaction

A prospective study carried out over a 6-month period in more than 10 000 patients found that ACE inhibitors did not interfere with the haemoglobin concentration, or epoetin dose, in haemodialysis patients. The findings did not exclude the possibility that individual patients might need more epoetin during the use of an ACE inhibitor or that haemoglobin concentrations might rise after withdrawal of the ACE inhibitor.[2] A short report of a study in 252 haemodialysis patients receiving epoetin found no reduction in the response to epoetin in 48 of the patients who were also taking ACE inhibitors.[3]

A number of other studies show a lack of effect with specific ACE inhibitors, as follows:

- No change in epoetin dose requirements or reduced haematocrit were seen with **captopril**,[4-6] **enalapril**,[4-6] or **lisinopril**.[6]
- No change in the response to epoetin was seen with **enalapril**,[7,8] **fosinopril**,[7] or **lisinopril**.[7]
- No effect on haematocrit was seen with **alacepril**, **benazepril**, **captopril**, **cilazapril**, **delapril**, **enalapril**, or **lisinopril**.[9]

(c) ACE inhibitors compared with Angiotensin II receptor antagonists

Two cross-sectional studies in over 1 000 haemodialysis patients found no difference between ACE inhibitor or angiotensin II receptor antagonist use and epoetin dose or resistance,[10] nor an association between their use and increased epoetin requirements.[11] However, a follow-up to a retrospective study found that in patients from countries where only 60 to 70% of patients had a haemoglobin concentration of greater than or equal to 11 g/dL, taking angiotensin II receptor antagonists reduced their response to epoetin (higher epoetin doses and lower haemoglobin response rates). This was not the case in countries where more than 70% of patients had similar haemoglobin concentrations, nor for ACE inhibitors in any patients.[12]

The findings of studies comparing the effects of specific ACE inhibitors and angiotensin II receptor antagonists on epoetin effects are summarised in 'Table 2.6', p.35.

Mechanism

It has been argued that ACE inhibitors might possibly reduce the efficacy of epoetin in haemodialysis patients for several reasons. A dose-dependent decrease in haematocrit is regularly observed when patients are given ACE inhibitors. In most patients this decrease is small and not clinically important. However, in conditions such as erythrocytosis associated with renovascular hypertension or renal transplantation, the haematocrit-lowering effects of these drugs could be notable.[13] Furthermore, ACE inhibitors can reduce the polycythaemia that occurs following renal transplantation, and ACE inhibitors reduce the plasma concentrations of endogenous erythropoietin.[4,14,15] Another suggestion is that ACE inhibitors might reduce testosterone concentrations in men receiving haemodialysis, but not in women, and this might be associated with resistance to epoetin.[16] As suppression of angiotensin II concentrations has been found in dialysis patients receiving epoetin, it has been suggested that the effect of ACE inhibitors on erythropoietin might be associated with a feedback loop between erythropoietin and the renin-angiotensin system.[17] Many other factors have also been proposed.[17,18]

Importance and management

Antihypertensive effects

A frequent adverse effect of epoetins is hypertension, possibly associated with the haemodynamic changes produced by the increase in haematocrit.[19] It is therefore important to control any existing hypertension before epoetin is started. Blood pressure should be routinely monitored before and during the use of epoetins, and if necessary antihypertensives should be started or increased if blood pressure rises occur.[20-22] This routine monitoring would seem sufficient to detect any interaction that affects the blood pressure-lowering effects of the ACE inhibitors. The dose of ACE inhibitor might need to be increased, but if blood pressure rises cannot be controlled, a transient interruption of the use of epoetin is recommended (the manufacturers contraindicate epoetin in uncontrolled hypertension).[20-22]

Epoetin efficacy

The overall picture of the effect of ACE inhibitors on epoetin efficacy is unclear, and it would seem that an interaction, if it happens, takes a long time to develop. The dose of both the ACE inhibitor and the epoetin might be important factors for the development of epoetin resistance, with the effect possibly being most apparent with high doses of ACE inhibitor, particularly if the patient is given low-dose epoetin. It has been suggested that any epoetin resistance due to high-dose ACE inhibitor should be counteracted by an increased dose of epoetin.[23]

Hyperkalaemia

Drugs that block angiotensin II reduce the concentration of aldosterone, which results in the retention of potassium. The manufacturers of epoetin alfa and beta state that increased potassium concentrations have been reported in a few patients with chronic renal failure receiving epoetin, although they note that it is not an established adverse effect of epoetin.[20,21] An additive hyperkalaemic effect is therefore theoretically possible in patients given epoetin and also taking ACE inhibitors. Serum electrolytes, including potassium, should be routinely monitored in patients on concurrent use. If potassium concentrations rise, consider withholding epoetin until the potassium concentration is corrected.[20,21]

1. Ertürk Ş, Nergizoğlu G, Ateş K, Duman N, Erbay B, Karatan O, Ertuğ AE. The impact of withdrawing ACE inhibitors on erythropoietin responsiveness and left ventricular hypertrophy in haemodialysis patients. *Nephrol Dial Transplant* (1999) 14, 1912–16.
2. Hörl WH, Jacobs C, Macdougall IC, Valderrábano F, Parrondo I, Thompson K, Carveth BG. European Best Practice Guidelines 14-16: inadequate response to epoetin. *Nephrol Dial Transplant* (2000) 15 (Suppl 4), 43–50.
3. Sánchez Tomero JA. ACE inhibitors do not decrease rHuEpo response in patients with end-stage renal failure. *Nephrol Dial Transplant* (1995) 10, 1476–7.
4. Conlon PJ, Albers F, Butterly D, Schwab SJ. ACE inhibitors do not affect erythropoietin efficacy in haemodialysis patients. *Nephrol Dial Transplant* (1994) 9, 1358.
5. Schwenk MH, Jumani AQ, Rosenberg CR, Kulogowski JE, Charytan C, Spinowitz BS. Potential angiotensin-converting enzyme inhibitor–epoetin alfa interaction in patients receiving chronic hemodialysis. *Pharmacotherapy* (1998) 18, 627–30.
6. Abu-Alfa AK, Cruz D, Perazella MA, Mahnensmith RL, Simon D, Bia MJ. ACE inhibitors do not induce recombinant human erythropoietin resistance in hemodialysis patients. *Am J Kidney Dis* (2000) 35, 1076–82.
7. Cruz DN, Perazella MA, Abu-Alfa AK, Mahnensmith RL. Angiotensin-converting enzyme inhibitor therapy in chronic hemodialysis patients: any evidence of erythropoietin resistance? *Am J Kidney Dis* (1996) 28, 535–40.
8. Charytan C, Goldfarb-Rumyantzev A, Wang YF, Schwenk MH, Spinowitz BS. Effect of angiotensin-converting enzyme inhibitors on response to erythropoietin therapy in chronic dialysis patients. *Am J Nephrol* (1998) 18, 498–503.
9. Hayashi K, Hasegawa K, Kobayashi S. Effects of angiotensin-converting enzyme inhibitors on the treatment of anemia with erythropoietin. *Kidney Int* (2001) 60, 1910–16.
10. Saudan P, Halabi G, Perneger T, Wasserfallen JB, Wauters J-P, Martin P-Y; Western Switzerland Dialysis Group. ACE inhibitors or angiotensin II receptor blockers in dialysed patients and erythropoietin resistance. *J Nephrol* (2006) 19, 91–6.
11. Yano S, Suzuki K, Iwamoto M, Urushidani Y, Yokogi H, Kusakari M, Aoki A, Sumi M, Kitamura K, Sanematsu H, Gohbara M, Imamura S, Sugimoto T. Association between erythropoietin requirements and antihypertensive agents. *Nephron Clin Pract* (2008) 109, c33–c39.
12. Jacobs C. Frei D, Perkins AC. Results of the European Survey on Anaemia Management 2003 (ESAM 2003): current status of anaemia management in dialysis patients, factors affecting epoetin dosage and changes in anaemia management over the last 5 years. *Nephrol Dial Transplant* (2005) 20 (Suppl 3), iii3–iii24.
13. Marathias KP, Agroyannis B, Mavromoustakos T, Matsoukas J, Vlahakos DV. Hematocrit-lowering effect following inactivation of renin-angiotensin system with angiotensin converting enzyme inhibitors and angiotensin receptor blockers. *Curr Top Med Chem* (2004) 4, 483–6.
14. Walter J. Does captopril decrease the effect of human recombinant erythropoietin in haemodialysis patients? *Nephrol Dial Transplant* (1993) 8, 1428.
15. Pratt MC, Lewis-Barned NJ, Walker RJ, Bailey RR, Shand BI, Livesey J. Effect of angiotensin converting enzyme inhibitors on erythropoietin concentrations in healthy volunteers. *Br J Clin Pharmacol* (1992) 34, 363–5.

Table 2.5 Studies into the effects of the concurrent use of ACE inhibitors or angiotensin II receptor antagonists and epoetins

Study type	*Study duration*	*ACE inhibitor(s)*	*Key findings*	*Refs*
Retrospective study of 43 haemodyalysis patients, 20 also taking an ACE inhibitor	About 10 months	Captopril (average dose 64.7 mg daily)	Similar epoetin doses resulted in lower haemoglobin concentrations and lower haematocrit with ACE inhibitor use.	1
Comparison of 108 haemodialysis patients, 49 also taking an ACE inhibitor	Single point of comparison	Benazapril, captopril, cilazapril, enalapril, imidapril, and temocapril (doses not stated)	Haematocrit the same between groups but weekly epoetin dose higher in those taking an ACE inhibitor (101.7 units/kg) than in those not taking an ACE inhibitor (79.2 units/kg).	2
Retrospective study of 40 dialysis patients given epoetin doses to achieve a target haematocrit of 30 to 35%, 20 also receiving an ACE inhibitor	18 months	Captopril (12.5 to 75 mg daily), enalapril (2.5 to 20 mg daily), fosinopril (10 to 20 mg daily)	Statistically significant difference in epoetin dose noted after 15 months; epoetin dose almost doubled in patients receiving an ACE inhibitor.	3
A prospective study of 60 haemodialyis patients, 20 taking an ACE inhibitor, 20 taking nifedipine and 20 patients without hypertension	12 months	Enalapril (5 to 20 mg daily)	To maintain the same haemoglobin concentration the weekly epoetin dose in those taking ACE inhibitors increased (from 84 units/kg to 138 units/kg) over the duration of the study, when compared with those taking nifedipine or without an antihypertensive. Epoetin dose returned to baseline 4 months after ACE inhibitor stopped.	4
Study of 49 haemodialysis patients, 22 also receiving an ACE inhibitor	Two points of comparison, 3 months apart	Captopril (12.5 to 37.5 mg daily), lisinopril (2.5 to 20 mg daily), perindopril 4 mg daily, ramipril 2.5 mg daily)	To achieve the same haematocrit, weekly epoetin doses were higher in the patients taking an ACE inhibitor (56 units/kg) compared with patients not taking an ACE inhibitor (36 units/kg).	5
Retrospective study of 47 haemodialysis patients, 23 also taking an ACE inhibitor	Single point of comparison after 3 months of ACE inhibitor use	Captopril (25 to 75 mg daily), enalapril (20 to 40 mg daily),	Patients defined as responders (median weekly epoetin dose 100 units/kg) or non-responders to epoetin (weekly epoetin dose exceeded 200 units/kg). Of the 22 non-responders, 17 were also taking an ACE inhibitor. Haematocrit was 23.6% in the non-reponders compared with 33.8% in the responders.	6
Study in 55 patients receiving CAPD, during the course of the study 7 patients were given epoetins alone, 11 patients were given an ACE inhibitor alone and 27 patients were given an epoetin and an ACE inhibitor	Up to 52 months	Captopril, enalapril and perindopril (doses not stated).	The dose of ACE inhibitor was correlated with the dose of epoetin, which might have been related either to epoetin affecting blood pressure or ACE inhibitors affecting epoetin efficacy.	7
Prospective study in 100 haemodialysis patients receiving epoetin, 48 also taking an ACE inhibitor or angiotensin II receptor antagonist	4 months	Captopril (25 to 75 mg daily), enalapril 2.5 to [20] mg daily), lisinopril 5 to 20 mg daily, losartan 50 mg daily, valsartan 160 mg daily.	The monthly increase in haematocrit over 4 months was less in patients given ACE inhibitors or angiotensin II receptor antagonists than in those given other antihypertensives, such as calcium-channel blockers or beta blockers.	8
Prospective study in 10 peritoneal dialysis patients receiving epoetin, 5 also taking an ACE inhibitor	One year	Captopril (25 to 75 mg daily), ramipril (2.5 to 5 mg daily)	Haemoglobin concentrations gradually decreased after the ACE inhibitor was started, and the difference was statistically significant from 6 months. Epoetin dose was statistically significantly higher in patients taking ACE inhibitors after 8 months.	9

1. Walter J. Does captopril decrease the effect of human recombinant erythropoietin in haemodialysis patients? *Nephrol Dial Transplant* (1993) 8, 1428.
2. Matsumura M, Nomura H, Koni I, Mabuchi H, for the Risks of Cardiac Disease in Dialysis Patients Study Group. Angiotensin-converting enzyme inhibitors are associated with the need for increased recombinant human erythropoietin maintenance doses in hemodialysis patients. *Nephron* (1997) 77, 164–8.
3. Heß E, Sperschneider H, Stein G. Do ACE inhibitors influence the dose of human recombinant erythropoietin in dialysis patients? *Nephrol Dial Transplant* (1996) 11, 749–51.
4. Albitar S, Genin R, Fen-Chong M, Serveaux M-O, Bourgeon B. High dose enalapril impairs the response to erythropoietin treatment in haemodialysis patients. *Nephrol Dial Transplant* (1998) 13, 1206–10.
5. Dhondt AW, Vanholder RC, Ringoir SMG. Angiotensin-converting enzyme inhibitors and higher erythropoietin requirement in chronic haemodialysis patients. *Nephrol Dial Transplant* (1995) 10, 2107–9.
6. Ertürk Ş, Ateş K, Duman N, Karatan O, Erbay B, Ertuğ E. Unresponsiveness to recombinant human erythropoietin in haemodialysis patients: possible implications of angiotensin-converting enzyme inhibitors. *Nephrol Dial Transplant* (1996) 11, 396–7.
7. Grzegorzewska AE, Leander M. Lymphocyte subsets counts in CAPD patients in relation to administration of recombinant human erythropoietin and angiotensin-converting enzyme inhibitors. *Perit Dial Int* (2002) 22, 635–8.
8. Qureshi IZ, Abid K, Ambreen F, Qureshi AL. Angiotensin converting enzyme inhibitors impair recombinant human erythropoietin induced erythropoiesis in patients with chronic renal failure. *Saudi Med J* (2007) 28, 193–6.
9. Navarro JF, Macía ML, Mora-Fernández C, Gallego E, Chahin J, Méndez ML, del Castillo N, Rivero A, García J. Effects of angiotensin-converting enzyme inhibitors on anemia and erythropoietin requirements in peritoneal dialysis patients. *Adv Perit Dial* (1997) 13, 257–59.

Table 2.6 Summary of studies assessing the comparative effects of ACE inhibitors and angiotensin II receptor antagonists on epoetin efficacy and dose

Study	ACE inhibitor and daily dose	Angiotensin II receptor antagonist and daily dose	Study duration	Effect of ACE inhibitor		Effect of angiotensin II receptor antagonist		Refs
				Epoetin dose	Haemoglobin or haematocrit levels	Epoetin dose	Haemoglobin or haematocrit levels	
Prospective, haemodialysis patients	Captopril 37.5 mg to 150 mg daily	Losartan 25 mg to 50 mg daily	6 months	Increased	Haematocrit: decreased from 27% to 24%	Not statistically significant	Not statistically significant	1
Prospective, 25 haemodialysis pts	Temocapril 2 mg	Losartan 25 mg to 50 mg		Increased from 76 units/kg per week to 121 units/kg per week	Decrease from 9.8 g/dL to 9 g/dL at 6 months	Not statistically significant	No change	2

1. Schiffl H, Lang SM. Angiotensin-converting enzyme inhibitors but not angiotensin II AT 1 receptor antagonists affect erythropoiesis in patients with anemia of end-stage renal disease. *Nephron* (1999) 81, 106–8.
2. Kato A, Takita T, Furuhashi M, Takahashi T, Maruyama Y, Hishida A. No effect of losartan on response to erythropoietin therapy in patients undergoing hemodialysis. *Nephron* (2000) 86, 538–9.

16. DeLong M, Logan JL, Yong K-C, Lien Y-HH. Renin-angiotensin blockade reduces serum free testosterone in middle-aged men on haemodialysis and correlates with erythropoietin resistance. *Nephrol Dial Transplant* (2005) 20, 585–90.
17. Gossmann J, Thürmann P, Bachmann T, Weller S, Kachel H-G, Schoeppe W, Scheuermann E-H. Mechanism of angiotensin converting enzyme inhibitor-related anemia in renal transplant recipients. *Kidney Int* (1996) 50, 973–8.
18. Macdougall IC. ACE inhibitors and erythropoietin responsiveness. *Am J Kidney Dis* (2001) 38, 649–51.
19. *Martindale. The Complete Drug Reference*, [online] London: Pharmaceutical Press. http://www.medicinescomplete.com/mc/martindale/current/ms-16635-r.htm (accessed 19/10/15).
20. NeoRecormon Solution for Injection in a Pre-filled Syringe (Epoetin beta). Roche Products Ltd. UK Summary of product characteristics, October 2011..
21. Eprex Pre-filled Syringe (Epoetin alfa). Janssen-Cilag Ltd. UK Summary of product characteristics, November 2012.
22. Epogen (Epoetin alfa). Amgen Inc. US Prescribing information, July 2012.
23. Macdougall IC. The role of ACE inhibitors and angiotensin II receptor blockers in the response to epoetin. *Nephrol Dial Transplant* (1999) 14, 1836–41.

ACE inhibitors + Food

Food has little or no effect on the extent of absorption of cilazapril, enalapril, fosinopril, lisinopril, quinapril, ramipril, spirapril, and trandolapril although the rate of absorption might be decreased. Food reduced the absorption of imidapril and moexipril, reduced the conversion of perindopril to perindoprilat, and might reduce the absorption of captopril.

Clinical evidence, mechanism, importance and management

(a) Captopril

Although food reduced the AUC of captopril 25 to 100 mg by up to 56%[1-4] this had no effect on the maximum decrease in blood pressure.[1,3,4] One study in 10 healthy subjects reported that food caused a one-hour delay in the maximum hypotensive effect of captopril.[1] Another study, in 10 hypertensive patients, found that the extent and duration of the antihypertensive efficacy of captopril 50 mg twice daily for one month was not affected by whether it was taken before or after food.[5] However, decreasing the dose of an ACE inhibitor might reduce the duration of the hypotensive effect and it has been suggested that these results should be confirmed with lower doses of captopril.[5]

(b) Moexipril

In one study, food reduced the AUC of the active metabolite of moexipril (moexiprilat) by 40 to 50%.[6] Food did not reduce moexipril-induced ACE-inhibition and therefore the reduced bioavailability was not expected to be clinically relevant.[7]

(c) Perindopril

Although food did not notably affect the pharmacokinetics of a single 4-mg dose of perindopril, the AUC of its active metabolite perindoprilat was reduced by 44%.[8] The blood pressure-lowering effects were not assessed, but it seems possible that they would not be affected (see *Captopril*, above). Nevertheless, the UK manufacturer recommends that perindopril should be taken in the morning before a meal.[9]

(d) Other ACE inhibitors

Single-dose studies have found that food has no statistically significant effect on the pharmacokinetics of **lisinopril**,[10] or **enalapril**, and its active metabolite, enalaprilat.[11] Similarly, food had minimal effects on the pharmacokinetics of **cilazapril** (AUC decreased by only 14%).[12] Food caused small increases in the time to reach maximum plasma levels of **quinapril** and its active metabolite. However, as the increase was less than 30 minutes this is not expected to alter the therapeutic effect.[13] Likewise, the manufacturers of **spirapril** briefly mention in a review that food delayed its absorption by one hour, but it did not affect the bioavailability of **spirapril** or spiraprilat, its active metabolite.[14] The US manufacturers of **fosinopril**,[15] **ramipril**,[16] and **trandolapril**[17] state that food might slow their absorption, but both the UK[18-20] and US[15-17] manufacturers state that the extent of absorption is unaffected.

The UK manufacturer of **imidapril** states that a fat-rich meal significantly reduces the absorption of **imidapril**, and recommends that the drug be taken at the same time each day, about 15 minutes before a meal.[21]

1. Mäntylä R, Männistö PT, Vuorela A, Sundberg S, Ottoila P. Impairment of captopril bioavailability by concomitant food and antacid intake. *Int J Clin Pharmacol Ther Toxicol* (1984) 22, 626–9.
2. Singhvi SM, McKinstry DN, Shaw JM, Willard DA, Migdalof BH. Effect of food on the bioavailability of captopril in healthy subjects. *J Clin Pharmacol* (1982) 22, 135–40.
3. Öhman KP, Kågedal B, Larsson R, Karlberg BE. Pharmacokinetics of captopril and its effects on blood pressure during acute and chronic administration and in relation to food intake. *J Cardiovasc Pharmacol* (1985) 7 (Suppl 1), S20–S24.
4. Müller H-M, Overlack A, Heck I, Kolloch R, Stumpe KO. The influence of food intake on pharmacodynamics and plasma concentration of captopril. *J Hypertens* (1985) 3 (Suppl 2), S135–S136.
5. Salvetti A, Pedrinelli R, Magagna A, Abdel-Haq B, Graziadei L, Taddei S, Stornello M. Influence of food on acute and chronic effects of captopril in essential hypertensive patients. *J Cardiovasc Pharmacol* (1985) 7 (Suppl 1), S25–S29.
6. Perdix (Moexipril). Schwarz Pharma. Product monograph, October 1995.
7. Stimpel M, Cawello W. Pharmacokinetics and ACE-inhibition of the new ACE-inhibitor moexipril: is coadministration with food of clinical relevance? *Hypertension* (1995) 25, 1384.
8. Lecocq B, Funck-Brentano C, Lecocq V, Ferry A, Gardin M-E, Devissaguet M, Jaillon P. Influence of food on the pharmacokinetics of perindopril and the time course of angiotensin-converting enzyme inhibition in serum. *Clin Pharmacol Ther* (1990) 47, 397–402.
9. Coversyl Arginine (Perindopril arginine). Servier Laboratories Ltd. UK Summary of product characteristics, December 2009.
10. Mojaverian P, Rocci ML, Vlasses PH, Hoholick C, Clementi RA, Ferguson RK. Effect of food on the bioavailability of lisinopril, a nonsulfhydryl angiotensin-converting enzyme inhibitor. *J Pharm Sci* (1986) 75, 395–7.
11. Swanson BN, Vlasses PH, Ferguson RK, Bergquist PA, Till AE, Irvin JD, Harris K. Influence of food on the bioavailability of enalapril. *J Pharm Sci* (1984) 73, 1655–7.
12. Massarella JW, DeFeo TM, Brown AN, Lin A, Wills RJ. The influence of food on the pharmacokinetics and ACE inhibition of cilazapril. *Br J Clin Pharmacol* (1989) 27, 205S–209S.
13. Ferry JJ, Horvath AM, Sedman AJ, Latts JR, Colburn WA. Influence of food on the pharmacokinetics of quinapril and its active diacid metabolite, CI-928. *J Clin Pharmacol* (1987) 27, 397–9.
14. Grass P, Gerbeau C, Kutz K. Spirapril: pharmacokinetic properties and drug interactions. *Blood Pressure* (1994) 3 (Suppl 2), 7–13.
15. Monopril (Fosinopril sodium). Bristol-Myers Squibb Company. US Prescribing information, July 2008.
16. Altace (Ramipril). King Pharmaceuticals, Inc. US Prescribing information, July 2008.
17. Mavik (Trandolapril). Abbott Laboratories. US Prescribing information, September 2011.
18. Fosinopril sodium. Actavis UK Ltd. UK Summary of product characteristics, August 2009.
19. Tritace (Ramipril). Sanofi-Aventis. UK Summary of product characteristics, November 2010.
20. Gopten (Trandolapril). Abbott Laboratories Ltd. UK Summary of product characteristics, July 2010.
21. Tanatril (Imidapril hydrochloride). Chiesi Ltd. UK Summary of product characteristics, May 2010.

ACE inhibitors + Garlic

In a single report, a patient taking lisinopril developed marked hypotension and became faint after taking garlic capsules.

Clinical evidence, mechanism, importance and management

A man whose blood pressure was 135/90 mmHg while taking **lisinopril** 15 mg daily began to take garlic 4 mg daily (*Boots odourless garlic oil capsules*). After 3 days he became faint on standing and was found to have a blood pressure of 90/60 mmHg. Stopping the garlic restored his blood pressure to 135/90 mmHg within a week. The garlic on its own did not lower his blood pressure. The reasons for this interaction are not known, although garlic has been reported to cause vasodilatation and reduce blood pressure.[1] This seems to be the first and only report of this reaction, so its general importance is small. There seems to be nothing documented about garlic and any of the other ACE inhibitors.

1. McCoubrie M. Doctors as patients: lisinopril and garlic. *Br J Gen Pract* (1996) 46, 107.

ACE inhibitors + Glucagon-like peptide-1 receptor agonists

Exenatide does not alter the pharmacokinetics or the efficacy of lisinopril. Liraglutide and dulaglutide do not appear to alter the pharmaco-

kinetics of lisinopril, and lixisenatide does not appear to alter the pharmacokinetics of ramipril.

Clinical evidence, mechanism, importance and management

(a) Dulaglutide

The UK and US manufacturers briefly report that, in a study, multiple doses of dulaglutide (dose not stated) had no effect on the pharmacokinetics of steady-state **lisinopril**, but, on days 3 and 24, the time to maximum concentration was delayed by 1 hour.[1,2] This delay in absorption would not be expected to be clinically relevant, and no lisinopril dose adjustment would seem necessary on concurrent use.

(b) Exenatide

In a randomised, crossover study in 19 hypertensive patients, exenatide 10 micrograms twice daily did not alter the steady-state AUC or maximum concentration of **lisinopril** 5 to 20 mg daily, but it did delay the time to maximum concentration by 2 hours. Exenatide did not alter the blood pressure-lowering effect of **lisinopril**.[3] The delay in absorption was not clinically relevant, and no lisinopril dose adjustment would seem necessary on concurrent use.

(c) Liraglutide

A preliminary report of a randomised, crossover study in 40 healthy subjects, states that steady-state liraglutide 1.8 mg daily decreases the AUC of a single 20-mg dose of **lisinopril**, given at the same time, by 15% and decreased the maximum concentration by 27%, with a delay in time to maximum concentration of 2 hours.[4] These pharmacokinetic changes are unlikely to be clinically relevant, and no adjustment of the lisinopril dose is expected to be needed in patients also given liraglutide.

(d) Lixisenatide

The UK manufacturer of lixisenatide briefly notes that, giving lixisenatide 20 micrograms and **ramipril** 5 mg for 6 days resulted in a 21% increase in the AUC of ramipril and a 63% decrease in its maximum concentration. The AUC and maximum concentration of ramiprilat, the active metabolite of ramipril, were unaffected. The time to maximum concentration of ramipril and ramiprilat were delayed by about 2.5 hours. No ramipril dose adjustment appears necessary on concurrent use.[5]

For the conflicting data on the possible increased risk of hypoglycaemia when some antidiabetics are used with ACE inhibitors, see 'Antidiabetics + ACE inhibitors', p.499.

1. Trulicity (Dulaglutide). Eli Lilly and Company Ltd. UK Summary of product characteristics, November 2014.
2. Trulicity (Dulaglutide). Eli Lilly and Company. US Prescribing information, March 2015.
3. Linnebjerg H, Kothare P, Park S, Mace K, Mitchell M. The effect of exenatide on lisinopril pharmacodynamics and pharmacokinetics in patients with hypertension. *Int J Clin Pharmacol Ther* (2009) 47, 651–8.
4. Malm-Erjefalt M, Ekblom M, Brondsted L, Vouis J, Lennernas H, Zdravkovic M. A randomized, double-blind, cross-over trial investigating the effect of liraglutide on the absorption pharmacokinetics of concomitantly administered oral drugs in healthy subjects. *Diabetes* (2008) 57 (Suppl 1), A130.
5. Lyxumia (Lixisenatide). Sanofi. UK Summary of product characteristics, October 2014.

ACE inhibitors + Gold

Peripheral vasodilatation has occurred in some patients given ACE inhibitors and gold. Isolated cases of loss of consciousness, cardiovascular collapse and cerebrovascular accident have been reported. In some patients the reaction occurred soon after the ACE inhibitor was started, while in others there appeared to be a lag time of several months or more.

Clinical evidence

A retrospective analysis of patients given gold compounds at one clinic from 1996 to 2000 identified 8 patients who had experienced a nitritoid reaction (adverse effects associated with the use of gold compounds, consisting of facial flushing, nausea, dizziness, and occasionally, hypotension, as a result of peripheral vasodilatation) of which one was considered serious. They had been given weekly doses of **sodium aurothiomalate** 25 to 50 mg for between 13 months and 13 years before the reaction occurred. However, in 2 of the patients who had been receiving gold for 2 years and 13 years, respectively, the nitritoid reaction occurred one to 4 weeks after starting the ACE inhibitor (**ramipril** in one patient; not specified in the other).[1]

A report describes 4 patients receiving long-term gold for rheumatoid arthritis who developed nitritoid reactions. These reactions occurred soon after starting an ACE inhibitor (**captopril**, **enalapril**, or **lisinopril**). All the patients had been given a monthly injection of **sodium aurothiomalate** 50 mg for at least 2 years and none had ever had such a reaction before. The reactions were controlled by changing treatment to **aurothioglucose**, discontinuing the ACE inhibitor, or reducing the dose of **sodium aurothiomalate** to 25 mg.[2]

Another report notes 2 further cases observed by one of the authors of the earlier report[2] and also describes a patient given a weekly and then monthly intramuscular injection of **sodium aurothiomalate** 50 mg for 4 months before she started taking **lisinopril** 20 mg daily. Seven months later she experienced paraesthesiae in her hands and tongue and palpitations a few minutes after the **sodium aurothiomalate** injection; mild paraesthesiae occurred again after her next injection. The following four injections were without any adverse effects, but then within 5 to 10 minutes of the next injection she became dizzy and flushed with nausea and vomiting and collapsed, requiring cardiopulmonary resuscitation. One day later she developed bloody diarrhoea and, the following day, a peeling erythematous rash, which gradually resolved over a few weeks: these were possible adverse effects of the gold. **Sodium aurothiomalate** was replaced with hydroxychloroquine and **lisinopril** was continued.[3]

Two patients who had been given **sodium aurothiomalate** 50 mg per month for over 20 years without adverse effects developed nitritoid reactions. One of the patients, who had been taking **ramipril** 10 mg daily for about 15 months, experienced nausea, angina, and hypotension 10 minutes after an injection of **sodium aurothiomalate**. Although it was concluded that the reaction was due to a vasovagal episode, secondary to the injection and possibly exaggerated by atenolol, on review of the case, it was considered that an interaction with **ramipril** was also a possibility. About 10 months after the second patient had started taking **perindopril** (2 mg daily gradually increased to 6 mg daily), he lost consciousness whilst driving his car 20 minutes after an injection of **sodium aurothiomalate**. On admission to hospital it was concluded that he had experienced a vasovagal attack secondary to ischaemic heart disease. A month later he developed chest pain 10 minutes after the gold injection and he remained conscious but was hypotensive with a heart rate of 40 bpm. Both patients had been receiving **sodium aurothiomalate** for many years, and the possibility of an interaction occurring several months after starting an ACE inhibitor was suggested.[4] A further report describes a patient who had taken **enalapril** for 3 years and **sodium aurothiomalate** for 6 years who experienced mild nitritoid symptoms following two successive injections of **sodium aurothiomalate** and then a cerebrovascular accident within several hours of her next injection.[5] Another patient who was given intramuscular **sodium aurothioglucose** started taking **perindopril** about 3 months later. After a further 4 months, she was inadvertently given **sodium aurothiomalate** 50 mg instead of **sodium aurothioglucose**. She became cyanotic immediately after the injection, with diaphoresis, absent peripheral pulses and unrecordable blood pressure. She also developed bronchospasm, abdominal pain and diarrhoea, and an ECG showed premature ventricular contractions. She recovered after treatment with intravenous fluids, corticosteroids and promethazine.[6]

Mechanism

Not understood. The nitritoid reaction is a recognised reaction that can occur in patients receiving gold compounds. Most reactions are associated with sodium aurothiomalate (incidence of about 5%), but they have also been reported with **auranofin** and **sodium aurothioglucose**.[5,7] It has been suggested that the difference in frequency with sodium aurothiomalate compared with other gold compounds could be related to differences in bioavailability, with the aqueous sodium aurothiomalate being rapidly absorbed, whereas the oil-based aurothioglucose or auranofin are absorbed more slowly.[1,5]

ACE inhibitors prevent bradykinin breakdown, so patients taking ACE inhibitors might have higher bradykinin levels.[1] It has been suggested that ACE inhibitors might 'unmask' a hypersensitivity reaction, possibly by potentiation of kinins, resulting in an exaggerated inflammatory response.[3] However, reactions involving bradykinin can be delayed for several months after starting an ACE inhibitor.[4] An *in vitro* study found that captopril binds strongly with gold, ejecting thiomalate into solution.[8]

Importance and management

Although the nitritoid reaction is an established adverse effect of gold compounds, patients also taking ACE inhibitors might be at an increased risk of this adverse reaction. A possible interaction should be borne in mind if a patient experiences these reactions and is also taking an ACE inhibitor. The manufacturer of sodium aurothiomalate advises caution in patients also taking ACE inhibitors because of an increased risk of severe anaphylactoid reaction.[9] The cases reported indicate that reactions can occur soon after starting an ACE inhibitor or there might be a lag time of several months or more. It has been recommended that patients taking ACE inhibitors who require gold compounds should, if possible, be given aurothioglucose. If this is not available, a 50% reduction in the sodium aurothiomalate dose is recommended, with the patient in the recumbent position, and under observation for 20 minutes following the next few injections.[1]

1. Arthur AB, Klinkhoff A, Teufel A. Nitritoid reactions: case reports, review, and recommendations for management. *J Rheumatol* (2001) 28, 2209–12.
2. Healey LA, Backes MB, Mason V. Nitritoid reactions and angiotensin-converting-enzyme inhibitors. *N Engl J Med* (1989) 321, 763.
3. Ching DWT, McClintock AD. Nitritoid reaction in a patient on ACE inhibitor and Myocrisin treatments. *Aust N Z J Med* (1997) 27, 343.
4. Nixon J, Pande I. Gold, nitritoid reactions and angiotensin-converting enzyme inhibitors. *Rheumatology (Oxford)* (2006) 45, 118–19.
5. Hill C, Pile K, Henderson D, Kirkham B. Neurological side effects in two patients receiving gold injections for rheumatoid arthritis. *Br J Rheumatol* (1995) 34, 989–90.
6. Karrer AA, El Ramahi KM, Al Jishi F. Intramuscular gold, angiotensin converting enzyme inhibitor and anaphylactic reactions. *J Rheumatol* (1996) 23, 200–1.
7. Ho M, Pullar T. Vasomotor reactions with gold. *Br J Rheumatol* (1997) 36, 154–6.
8. Isab AA. A reaction between captopril (a high blood pressure drug) and gold(I)-thiomalate. *J Inorg Biochem* (1987) 30, 69–75.
9. Myocrisin (Sodium aurothiomalate). Sanofi-Aventis. UK Summary of product characteristics, July 2010.

ACE inhibitors + H_2-receptor antagonists

In general, no clinically relevant interactions appear to occur between the H_2-receptor antagonists (including cimetidine) and the ACE inhibitors. However, cimetidine slightly reduces the bioavailability of temocapril.

Clinical evidence, mechanism, importance and management

In studies in healthy subjects, **cimetidine** did not appear to alter the pharmacokinetics or pharmacological effects of **captopril**[1] or **enalapril**;[2] or the pharmacokinetics of **fosinopril**[3] or **quinapril**.[4] The manufacturers of **cilazapril** state that no clinically significant interactions have occurred with H_2-receptor antagonists (not specifically named)[5] and the manufacturers of **benazepril**,[6] **moexipril**,[7] **ramipril**,[8] and **trandolapril**[9] state that no clinically relevant pharmacokinetic interaction occurred with **cimetidine**. The manufacturers of **spirapril** briefly note, in a review, that **cimetidine** did not alter the plasma concentrations of **spirapril** or its active metabolite spiraprilat.[10] None of these pairs of drugs appears to interact to a clinically relevant extent, and no particular precautions therefore appear to be necessary on their concurrent use.

Preliminary findings of a study in 18 healthy subjects suggest that **cimetidine** 400 mg twice daily has no effect on the metabolism of **temocapril** 20 mg daily, but the AUC was reduced by 26% on the fifth day of concurrent use.[11] The clinical relevance of this has not been established, but changes of this magnitude with other ACE inhibitors have often not been clinically relevant and therefore a clinically relevant interaction is not expected.

1. Richer C, Bah M, Cadilhac M, Thuillez C, Giudicelli JF. Cimetidine does not alter free unchanged captopril pharmacokinetics and biological effects in healthy volunteer. *J Pharmacol* (1986) 17, 338–42.
2. Ishizaki T, Baba T, Murabayashi S, Kubota K, Hara K, Kurimoto F. Effect of cimetidine on the pharmacokinetics and pharmacodynamics of enalapril in normal volunteers. *J Cardiovasc Pharmacol* (1988) 12, 512–9.
3. Moore L, Kramer A, Swites B, Kramer P, Tu J. Effect of cimetidine and antacid on the kinetics of the active diacid of fosinopril in healthy subjects. *J Clin Pharmacol* (1988) 28, 946.
4. Ferry JJ, Cetnarowski AB, Sedman AJ, Thomas RW, Horvath AM. Multiple-dose cimetidine administration does not influence the single-dose pharmacokinetics of quinapril and its active metabolite (CI-928). *J Clin Pharmacol* (1988) 28, 48–51.
5. Vascace (Cilazapril monohydrate). Roche Products Ltd. UK Summary of product characteristics, July 2010.
6. Lotensin (Benazepril hydrochloride). Novartis Pharmaceuticals Corporation. US Prescribing information, May 2011.
7. Perdix (Moexipril hydrochloride). UCB Pharma Ltd. UK Summary of product characteristics, August 2010.
8. Altace (Ramipril). King Pharmaceuticals, Inc. US Prescribing information, July 2008.
9. Mavik (Trandolapril). Abbott Laboratories. US Prescribing information, September 2011.
10. Grass P, Gerbeau C, Kutz K. Spirapril: pharmacokinetic properties and drug interactions. *Blood Pressure* (1994) 3 (Suppl 2), 7–13.
11. Trenk D, Schaefer A, Eberle E, Jähnchen E. Effect of cimetidine on the pharmacokinetics of the ACE-inhibitor temocapril. *Eur J Clin Pharmacol* (1996) 50, 556.

ACE inhibitors or Angiotensin II receptor antagonists + Heparins

Heparin might increase the risk of hyperkalaemia with ACE inhibitors or angiotensin II receptor antagonists.

Clinical evidence, mechanism, importance and management

An extensive review of the literature found that heparin (both **unfractionated** and **low-molecular-weight heparins**) and **heparinoids** inhibit the secretion of aldosterone, and this can cause hyperkalaemia.[1] The CSM in the UK suggests that plasma potassium levels should be measured in all patients with risk factors (including those taking potassium-sparing drugs) before starting heparin, and monitored regularly thereafter, particularly if heparin is to be continued for more than 7 days.[2] Note that ACE inhibitors and angiotensin II receptor antagonists are potassium sparing, via their effects on aldosterone. Some workers[1] have suggested that the monitoring interval should probably be no greater than 4 days in patients at a relatively high risk of hyperkalaemia. Other risk factors include renal impairment, diabetes mellitus, pre-existing acidosis or raised plasma potassium.[2]

If hyperkalaemia occurs, the offending drugs should be stopped (although this might not be practical in the case of heparin). When the hyperkalaemia has been corrected (by whatever medical intervention is deemed appropriate) the drugs can cautiously be reintroduced.

1. Oster JR, Singer I, Fishman LM. Heparin-induced aldosterone suppression and hyperkalemia. *Am J Med* (1995) 98, 575–86.
2. Committee on Safety of Medicines/Medicines Control Agency. Suppression of aldosterone secretion by heparin. *Current Problems* (1999) 25, 6.

ACE inhibitors + Insect allergen extracts

A few case reports describe severe anaphylactoid reactions in patients receiving ACE inhibitors during desensitisation with bee or wasp venom.

Clinical evidence

A report describes 2 cases of anaphylactoid reactions during **wasp venom immunotherapy** in patients taking **enalapril**. In one patient, generalised pruritus and severe hypotension occurred within a few minutes of the first venom injection. Desensitisation was achieved after the **enalapril** was stopped, and then the immunotherapy was maintained by discontinuing the **enalapril** 24 hours before the monthly venom injection. However, on one occasion, when the **enalapril** had not been stopped, the patient experienced a severe anaphylactoid reaction 30 minutes after the venom injection. In the other patient, an anaphylactoid reaction occurred after the second dose of venom. The ACE inhibitor was replaced with nifedipine so that venom immunotherapy could be continued. However, **enalapril** was reintroduced a few months later and subsequent venom administration induced an anaphylactoid reaction. **Enalapril** was stopped again so that desensitisation could be maintained.[1]

In another report, a 43-year-old man who had been taking ACE inhibitors for 2 years (**lisinopril** 40 mg daily for the previous 5 months) had a hypotensive reaction to an insect sting. After skin testing, he was given venom immunotherapy. About 4 months later, he had a severe anaphylactic reaction 5 minutes after being given a maintenance dose of **wasp venom** and **mixed vespid venom**. The ACE inhibitor was replaced with a calcium-channel blocker, and he subsequently tolerated full-strength venom immunotherapy injections.[2]

A retrospective review of patients evaluated for **Hymenoptera venom** allergy, at a single medical centre from 2000 to 2005, identified 79 patients undergoing venom immunotherapy. ACE inhibitors (**lisinopril**, **ramipril**, or **benazepril**) were taken by 17 patients (21%): 7 patients continued to take the ACE inhibitor when immunotherapy was started and 10 began to take an ACE inhibitor after starting immunotherapy. None of the patients taking ACE inhibitors had systemic reactions during venom immunotherapy (compared with 13 of 62 patients not taking an ACE inhibitor). However, the patients taking ACE inhibitors were older (mean age 56 years versus 36 years) and had received immunotherapy for longer (mean 72 months versus 30 months) than those who were not taking an ACE inhibitor. Twelve of the 17 patients (71%) taking an ACE inhibitor reported having field stings, but none of these patients had a systemic reaction. One patient did have a reaction to a field sting early in his venom immunotherapy treatment, before he started to take an ACE inhibitor, but he did not experience a reaction on rechallenge while taking an ACE inhibitor.[3]

Further, in a study in 962 patients with established bee or wasp venom allergy who had a systemic reaction after a field sting, the reaction was classed as a severe reaction (anaphylactic shock, loss of consciousness, or cardiopulmonary arrest) in 206 patients (21.4%). The frequency of severe reactions after a field sting was associated with higher serum tryptase levels. Other factors were wasp venom allergy, one or more previous field stings with less severe reaction, older age, male sex, and the use of an ACE inhibitor.[4]

Mechanism

ACE inhibitors alone can cause angioedema, possibly as a result of kinin potentiation.[5] They might therefore potentiate the hypotension associated with anaphylactic reactions by inhibiting the breakdown of bradykinin and decreasing concentrations of the vasoconstrictor angiotensin II.[6] It has also been suggested that similar reactions can occur after an insect sting.[6] This is supported by a case report that describes a woman who had generalised angioedema in response to bee stings on at least three occasions while taking captopril and then cilazapril, but experienced only localised swelling before and after treatment with an ACE inhibitor.[7]

Further, it has been suggested that patients allergic to hymenoptera venom who have anaphylactic reactions during hyposensitisation or after a field sting have lower renin, angiotensinogen, and angiotensin I and II levels than non-allergic controls or those who tolerate immunotherapy. In such patients, the renin-angiotensin system might be unable to provide sufficient angiotensin II to counter the symptoms of anaphylaxis.[8]

Importance and management

One retrospective review[3] suggested that ACE inhibitors do not increase the risk of anaphylaxis to venom immunotherapy; however, isolated reactions, especially following reintroduction of an ACE inhibitor in two cases mentioned above,[1] suggest that in some patients ACE inhibitors might increase the risk of anaphylaxis. On the basis of these few reports, it cannot be said with certainty that an interaction occurs, but it is possible that ACE inhibitors could exacerbate the response to both insect venoms and insect venom immunotherapy.

The use of ACE inhibitors in patients with **Hymenoptera venom** allergy (bee, wasp or stinging ant allergy) or patients undergoing venom immunotherapy requires caution because of the potential severity of the reaction. If an ACE inhibitor is considered necessary, appropriate measures should be put in place. These include minimising the risk of exposure to insect stings e.g. by physical protection, and ensuring the patient carries adrenaline (epinephrine) [such as an *EpiPen*] for emergency self-treatment.[6] The authors of one report suggest that as a preventative measure in patients with bee or wasp allergy, consideration should be given to replacing the ACE inhibitor with alternative medication.[4] It has been suggested that angiotensin II receptor antagonists might be associated with a lower anaphylactic risk than ACE inhibitors,[9] but there is insufficient evidence to make any recommendations about their use in patients with Hymenoptera venom allergy.[9,10]

Some authors[1,2,6] and manufacturers advise temporarily withholding the ACE inhibitor before each desensitisation (24 hours was sufficient in one case[1]), while others suggest temporary substitution of a different antihypertensive e.g. a calcium-channel blocker. ACE inhibitors with active metabolites with prolonged terminal half-lives (including **benazepril**, **quinapril**, and **ramipril**) might require discontinuation for longer periods.[6,11]

Note that some evidence suggests that anaphylactic shock in patients taking beta blockers might be resistant to treatment with adrenaline (epinephrine), see 'Beta blockers + Inotropes and Vasopressors', p.1014. Therefore beta blockers are probably not a suitable alternative.

1. Tunon-de-Lara JM, Villanueva P, Marcos M, Taytard A. ACE inhibitors and anaphylactoid reactions during venom immunotherapy. *Lancet* (1992) 340, 908.
2. Ober AI, MacLean JA, Hannaway PJ. Life-threatening anaphylaxis to venom immunotherapy in a patient taking an angiotensin-converting enzyme inhibitor. *J Allergy Clin Immunol* (2003) 112, 1008–9.
3. White KM, England RW. Safety of angiotensin-converting enzyme inhibitors while receiving venom immunotherapy. *Ann Allergy Asthma Immunol* (2008) 101, 426–30.
4. Rueff F, Przybilla B, Biló MB, Müller U, Scheipl F, Aberer W, Birnbaum J, Bodzenta-Lukaszyk A, Bonifazi F, Bucher C, Campi P, Darsow U, Egger C, Haeberli G, Hawranek T, Körner M, Kucharewicz I, Küchenhoff H, Lang R, Quercia O, Reider N, Severino M, Sticherling M, Sturm GJ, Wüthrich B. Predictors of severe systemic anaphylactic reactions in patients with Hymenoptera venom allergy: importance of baseline serum tryptase–a study of the European Academy of Allergology and Clinical Immunology Interest Group on Insect Venom Hypersensitivity. *J Allergy Clin Immunol* (2009) 124, 1047–54.
5. Pillans PI, Coulter DM, Black P. Angiooedema and urticaria with angiotensin converting enzyme inhibitors. *Eur J Clin Pharmacol* (1996) 51, 123–6.
6. Stumpf JL, Shehab N, Patel AC. Safety of angiotensin-converting enzyme inhibitors in patients with insect venom allergies. *Ann Pharmacother* (2006) 40, 699–703.
7. Black PN, Simpson IJ. Angio-oedema and ACE inhibitors. *Aust N Z J Med* (1995) 25, 746.

8. Hermann K, Ring J. The renin-angiotensin system in patients with repeated anaphylactic reactions during Hymenoptera venom hyposensitization and sting challenge. *Int Arch Allergy Immunol* (1997) 112, 251–6.
9. Rueff F, Biló MB, Müller U, Przybilla B. Reply. *J Allergy Clin Immunol* (2010) 125, 1171.
10. Caviglia AG, Passalacqua G, Senna G. Risk of severe anaphylaxis for patients with Hymenoptera venom allergy: are angiotensin-receptor blockers comparable to angiotensin-converting enzyme inhibitors? *J Allergy Clin Immunol* (2010) 125, 1171.
11. Melamed J. Response to life-threatening anaphylaxis to venom immunotherapy in a patient taking an angiotensin-converting enzyme inhibitor. *J Allergy Clin Immunol* (2004) 113, 1224.

ACE inhibitors + Interleukin-3

Marked hypotension occurred when three patients taking ACE inhibitors were given interleukin-3.

Clinical evidence, mechanism, importance and management

Twenty-six patients with ovarian or small-cell undifferentiated cancers were given chemotherapy followed by recombinant human interleukin-3. Three of the 26 were taking ACE inhibitors (not named) and all three developed marked hypotension (WHO toxicity grade 2 or 3) within one to 4 hours of the first interleukin-3 injection. Their blood pressures returned to normal while continuing the interleukin-3 when the ACE inhibitors were stopped. When the interleukin-3 was stopped, they once again needed the ACE inhibitors to control their blood pressure. None of the other 23 patients had hypotension, except one who did so during a period of neutropenic fever.[1] The authors of the report suggest (and present some supporting evidence) that the drugs act synergistically to generate large amounts of nitric oxide in the blood vessel walls. This relaxes the smooth muscle in the blood vessel walls causing vasodilatation and consequent hypotension.[1] Information seems to be limited to this single report, but it would be prudent to monitor blood pressure even more closely if patients taking ACE inhibitors are given interleukin-3.

1. Dercksen MW, Hoekman K, Visser JJ, ten Bokkel Huinink WW, Pinedo HM, Wagstaff J. Hypotension induced by interleukin-3 in patients on angiotensin-converting enzyme inhibitors. *Lancet* (1995) 345, 448.

ACE inhibitors + Iron compounds

Serious systemic reactions occurred when three patients taking enalapril were given infusions of ferric sodium gluconate; however, there was no increase in the incidence of such adverse reactions in patients taking ACE inhibitors in a very large clinical study. Oral ferrous sulfate might slightly decrease the absorption of captopril.

Clinical evidence

(a) Intravenous iron

A man with iron-deficiency anaemia taking furosemide and digoxin was given 125 mg of **ferric sodium gluconate** (*Ferlixit*[1]) intravenously in 100 mL of saline daily. Four days later, **enalapril** 5 mg daily was started. After the infusion of only a few drops of his next dose of **ferric sodium gluconate**, he developed diffuse erythema, abdominal cramps, hypotension, nausea and vomiting. He recovered after being given hydrocortisone 200 mg. Three days later, in the absence of **enalapril**, he restarted the iron infusions for a further 10 days without problems, and was later treated uneventfully with **enalapril**.[2] Two other patients taking **enalapril** reacted similarly when given intravenous infusions of **ferric sodium gluconate**. Neither was given any more intravenous iron and later had no problems while taking **enalapril** alone. During the same 13-month period in which these three cases occurred, 15 other patients, who were not taking ACE inhibitors, also received intravenous iron with no adverse reactions.[2]

An interim report of a randomised, crossover study involving 1 117 dialysis patients given placebo or a single 125-mg intravenous dose of **ferric sodium gluconate complex** (*Ferrlecit*) in sucrose, found no evidence of a greater incidence of immediate allergic reactions or other adverse reactions to iron in the 308 patients also taking ACE inhibitors.[3] The findings of the full study, which included 707 patients taking ACE inhibitors, were the same.[4] Similarly, longer-term follow-up of patients from this study who continued to receive intravenous **ferric sodium gluconate complex**, found that there was no difference in the incidence or severity of adverse events in 372 patients taking ACE inhibitors, when compared with 949 patients who were not taking ACE inhibitors.[5]

(b) Oral iron

A double-blind study in 7 healthy subjects, given a single 300-mg dose of **ferrous sulfate** or placebo with **captopril** 25 mg, found that the AUC of unconjugated plasma **captopril** (the active form) was reduced by 37% although the maximum plasma levels were not substantially changed. The AUC of total plasma **captopril** was increased by 43%, although this was not statistically significant. There were no notable differences in blood pressure between treatment and placebo groups.[6]

Mechanism

Uncertain. Intravenous iron can cause a variety of systemic reactions including fever, myalgia, arthralgia, hypotension, and nausea and vomiting, which are believed to be due to the release of various inflammatory mediators such as bradykinin, caused by iron-catalysed toxic free radicals. The authors of one report suggest that ACE inhibitors decrease the breakdown of kinins so that the toxic effects of the iron become exaggerated.[2]

The reduced levels of unconjugated captopril seen in the presence of oral iron are probably due to reduced absorption resulting from a chemical interaction between ferric ions and captopril in the gut producing a captopril disulfide dimer and ferrous iron.[6]

Importance and management

The interaction between the ACE inhibitors and intravenous iron is not firmly established because up to 25% of all patients given iron by this route develop a variety of systemic reactions, ranging from mild to serious anaphylactoid reactions. In addition, information from the large clinical study indicates that there is no increased risk of such a reaction to iron in patients taking ACE inhibitors. This suggests that no additional precautions are required if intravenous iron is given to patients taking an ACE inhibitor.

There is limited evidence that oral iron might reduce the absorption of captopril. The clinical relevance of this is unknown, but probably small as blood pressure appeared unaffected in the study. Information about the effect of oral iron on other ACE inhibitors is lacking.

1. Rolla G. Personal communication, 1994.
2. Rolla G, Bucca C, Brussino L. Systemic reactions to intravenous iron therapy in patients receiving angiotensin converting enzyme inhibitor. *J Allergy Clin Immunol* (1994) 93, 1074–5.
3. Warnock DG, Adkinson F, Coyne DW, Strobos J, Ferrlecit® Safety Study Group. ACE inhibitors and intravenous sodium ferric gluconate complex in sucrose (SFGC): lack of any significant interaction. *J Am Soc Nephrol* (2000) 11, 170A.
4. Michael B, Coyne DW, Fishbane S, Folkert V, Lynn R, Nissenson AR, Agarwal R, Eschbach JW, Fadem SZ, Trout JR, Strobos J, Warnock DG; Ferrlecit Publication Committee. Sodium ferric gluconate complex in hemodialysis patients: adverse reactions compared to placebo and iron dextran. *Kidney Int* (2002) 61, 1830–9.
5. Michael B, Coyne DW, Folkert VW, Dahl NV, Warnock DG; Ferrlecit Publication Committee. Sodium ferric gluconate complex in haemodialysis patients: a prospective evaluation of long-term safety. *Nephrol Dial Transplant* (2004) 19, 1576–80.
6. Schaefer JP, Tam Y, Hasinoff BB, Tawfik S, Peng Y, Reimche L, Campbell NRC. Ferrous sulphate interacts with captopril. *Br J Clin Pharmacol* (1998) 46, 377–81.

ACE inhibitors + Moracizine

Moracizine causes some slight alterations in the pharmacokinetics of captopril.

Clinical evidence, mechanism, importance and management

In a pharmacokinetic study, 19 healthy subjects were given moracizine 250 mg or **captopril** 50 mg, both every 8 hours, either alone or together, for 22 doses. When taken together the pharmacokinetics of the moracizine and total **captopril** remained unchanged, but the maximum blood levels of free **captopril** and its AUC decreased by 32% and 14%, respectively. The half-life of free **captopril** was reduced by 44%.[1] These slight changes are unlikely to be clinically relevant.

1. Pieniaszek HJ, Shum L, Widner P, Garner DM, Benedek IH. Pharmacokinetic interaction of moricizine and captopril in healthy volunteers. *J Clin Pharmacol* (1993) 33, 1005.

ACE inhibitors + NSAIDs

There is evidence that most NSAIDs can increase blood pressure in patients taking antihypertensives, including ACE inhibitors, although some studies have not found the increase to be clinically relevant. Some variation between drugs possibly occurs, with indometacin appearing to have the most substantial effect. The combination of an NSAID and an ACE inhibitor can increase the risk of renal impairment and hyperkalaemia.

Clinical evidence

A. Effects on blood pressure

Various large epidemiological studies and meta-analyses of clinical studies have been conducted to assess the effect of NSAIDs on blood pressure in patients taking antihypertensives, and the findings of these are summarised in 'Table 23.2', p.1031. In these studies, NSAIDs were not always associated with an increase in blood pressure, and the maximum increase was 6.2 mmHg. The effect has been shown for both coxibs and non-selective NSAIDs. In two meta-analyses,[1,2] the effects were evaluated by NSAID. The confidence intervals for all the NSAIDs overlapped, showing that there was no statistically significant difference between them, with the exception of the comparison between **indometacin** and **sulindac** in one analysis.[2] Nevertheless, an attempt was made at ranking the NSAIDs based on the means. In one analysis,[1] the effect was said to be greatest for **piroxicam**, **indometacin**, and **ibuprofen**, intermediate for **naproxen**, and least for **sulindac** and **flurbiprofen**. In the other meta-analysis,[2] the effect was said to be greatest for **indometacin** and **naproxen**, intermediate for **piroxicam**, and least for **ibuprofen** and **sulindac**. An attempt was also made to evaluate the effect by antihypertensive.[1] The mean effect was greatest for beta blockers, intermediate for vasodilators (this group included ACE inhibitors and calcium-channel blockers), and least for diuretics. However, the differences between the groups were not significant.

The findings of individual studies that have studied the effects of specific NSAIDs on ACE inhibitors are outlined in the subsections below.

(a) Celecoxib

In a double-blind study in hypertensive patients taking **lisinopril** 10 to 40 mg daily, celecoxib did not have a clinically or statistically significant effect on blood pressure. The 24-hour blood pressure increased by 2.6/1.5 mmHg in 91 patients taking celecoxib 200 mg twice daily for 4 weeks compared with 1/0.3 mmHg in 87 patients taking placebo.[3] In another large study in 810 elderly patients with osteoarthritis and controlled hypertension given either celecoxib 200 mg or rofecoxib 25 mg daily for 6 weeks, approximately 40% of the patients randomised to the celecoxib group were receiving ACE inhibitors. Systolic blood pressure increased by a clinically relevant amount (greater than 20 mmHg) in 11% of patients receiving celecoxib,[4] while in another study, only 4 of 87 (4.6%) of hypertensive patients taking ACE inhibitors had clinically relevant increases in blood pressure after taking celecoxib 200 mg twice - daily for 4 weeks.[5] A further study in 25 hypertensive patients with osteoarthritis taking **trandolapril** (with or without hydrochlorothiazide) found that the 24-hour blood pressure was not significantly increased by celecoxib 200 mg daily, but, at its peak activity, celecoxib increased blood pressure by about 5/4 mmHg.[6] In another randomised study, 16% of 138 patients given celecoxib 200 mg daily developed hypertension within 6 weeks (defined as a 24-hour systolic blood pressure greater than 135 mmHg). These patients had well-controlled hypertension at baseline; 83% were receiving an ACE inhibitor and 64% an additional antihypertensive.[7] The proportion of patients who developed hypertension was similar to that with naproxen (19%) and less than that with rofecoxib (30%).

(b) Ibuprofen

In 90 patients taking ACE inhibitors, giving ibuprofen for 4 weeks resulted in clinically relevant increases in blood pressure in 15 of the patients. For the group as a whole, diastolic blood pressure was increased by 3.5 mmHg.[5] In one single-dose study in 8 healthy subjects, ibuprofen 800 mg or indometacin 50 mg abolished the hypotensive effect of **captopril** 50 mg when they received a high sodium diet, but not when they received a low sodium diet.[8] A case report describes attenuation of the antihypertensive effects of **captopril** by ibuprofen in an elderly woman.[9] However, two studies in African women found that ibuprofen 800 mg three times daily for one month did not alter the antihypertensive effect of either **fosinopril** 10 to 40 mg daily or **lisinopril** 10 to 40 mg daily (given with hydrochlorothiazide 25 mg daily).[10,11] It was thought that the diuretic might have enhanced salt depletion and renin stimulation making the antihypertensive action of the combination less prostaglandin dependent.[10]

(c) Indometacin

1. Captopril. In a randomised, double-blind study, 105 patients with hypertension were given captopril 25 to 50 mg twice daily for 6 weeks, which reduced their blood pressure by a mean of 8.6/5.6 mmHg. Indometacin 75 mg daily was then added for one week, which caused a rise in blood pressure in the group as a whole of 4.6/2.7 mmHg (an attenuation of the effect of captopril of about 50%). Clear attenuation was seen in 67% of the patients, and occurred regardless of baseline blood pressure.[12] This same interaction has been described in numerous earlier studies, in both patients with hypertension and healthy subjects, given indometacin.[8,13-20] A man whose blood pressure was well controlled with captopril 75 mg daily had a rise in his blood pressure from 145/80 mmHg to 220/120 mmHg when he started using indometacin suppositories 200 mg daily.[21] In contrast, a randomised, placebo-controlled, crossover study in 11 patients found that indometacin 50 mg twice daily did not alter the antihypertensive efficacy of captopril 50 mg twice daily.[22]

2. Enalapril. In 9 patients with hypertension, indometacin 50 mg twice daily for one week reduced the antihypertensive effect of enalapril 20 to 40 mg daily by about 18 to 22%.[23] In another study in 18 patients, indometacin 25 mg three times daily attenuated the antihypertensive effect of enalapril 20 to 40 mg daily. The reduction in hypotensive effect was about 42% when assessed by 24-hour ambulatory blood pressure monitoring (9.4/4.1 mmHg increase in blood pressure with indometacin), and 12 to 23% when assessed by clinic blood pressure monitoring.[24] Similar results were found in other studies.[25-28] A further study in 10 normotensive subjects receiving a fixed sodium intake and enalapril 20 mg daily, with or without indometacin 50 mg twice daily for one week, found that indometacin reduced the natriuretic response to the ACE inhibitor.[29] A single case report describes a patient taking enalapril 10 mg daily whose hypertension was not controlled when indometacin 100 mg daily in divided doses was added.[30] However, other studies found that indometacin did not notably alter the blood pressure response to enalapril.[19,22,31]

3. Lisinopril. In a placebo-controlled, crossover study in 56 patients taking lisinopril 10 to 20 mg daily, indometacin 50 mg twice daily for 2 weeks produced mean blood pressure increases of 5.5/3.2 mmHg.[32] Similarly, results of an earlier study suggested that indometacin increased the blood pressure of 9 patients taking lisinopril.[26] In contrast in a placebo-controlled study in 16 patients, indometacin 50 mg twice daily for 4 weeks was found to have little effect on the antihypertensive efficacy of lisinopril 40 mg daily.[33]

4. Other ACE inhibitors. A placebo-controlled, randomised, crossover study in 16 hypertensive patients found that indometacin 50 mg twice daily reduced the blood pressure-lowering effects of **cilazapril** 2.5 mg daily. The reduction was greater when **cilazapril** was added to indometacin than when indometacin was added to **cilazapril** (approximately 60% versus 30% reduction in hypotensive effect measured 3 hours after the morning dose).[34] In 10 hypertensive patients the antihypertensive effects of **perindopril** 4 to 8 mg daily were also found to be reduced by about 30% by indometacin 50 mg twice daily.[35] A brief mention is made in a review that, in healthy subjects, the pharmacodynamics of **ramipril** were unaffected by indometacin (dose not stated) given for 3 days.[36] Indometacin 25 mg three times daily did not alter the hypotensive effects of **trandolapril** 2 mg daily in 17 hypertensive patients.[37]

(d) Naproxen

In a randomised study, 19% of 130 patients given naproxen 500 mg twice daily developed hypertension within 6 weeks (defined as a 24-hour systolic blood pressure greater than 135 mmHg). These patients had well-controlled hypertension at baseline; 83% were receiving an ACE inhibitor and 66% an additional antihypertensive.[7] The proportion of patients who developed hypertension was similar to that with celecoxib (16%) and less than that with rofecoxib (30%).

(e) Rofecoxib

The manufacturer of rofecoxib noted that in patients with mild-to-moderate hypertension, rofecoxib 25 mg daily, taken with **benazepril** 10 to 40 mg daily, for 4 weeks, was associated with a small attenuation of the antihypertensive effect (average increase in mean arterial pressure of 2.8 mmHg).[38] Similarly, a case report describes a patient taking **lisinopril** 10 mg daily whose blood pressure rose from 127/78 mmHg to 143/89 mmHg when he was given rofecoxib 25 mg daily. His blood pressure was controlled by increasing the dose of **lisinopril** to 20 mg daily.[39]

In another study, in 810 elderly patients with osteoarthritis and controlled hypertension given either celecoxib 200 mg or rofecoxib 25 mg daily for 6 weeks, approximately 29% of the patients randomised to the rofecoxib group were receiving ACE inhibitors. Systolic blood pressure increased by a clinically relevant amount (greater than 20 mmHg) in 17% of the patients receiving rofecoxib.[4] In another similar randomised study, 30% of 138 patients given rofecoxib 25 mg daily developed hypertension within 6 weeks (defined as a 24-hour systolic blood pressure greater than 135 mmHg). These patients had well-controlled hypertension at baseline; 84% were receiving an ACE inhibitor and 62% an additional antihypertensive.[7] The proportion of patients who developed hypertension was greater than with celecoxib (16%) or naproxen (19%).

(f) Sulindac

In one study, sulindac 200 mg twice daily given to patients taking **captopril** 100 to 200 mg twice daily caused only a small rise in blood pressure (from 132/92 mmHg to 137/95 mmHg).[15] Sulindac 150 mg twice daily did not attenuate the blood pressure response to **captopril** when it was substituted for ibuprofen in an elderly woman.[9] Similarly, sulindac 200 mg twice daily did not blunt the antihypertensive effect of **enalapril** in 9 patients with hypertension.[31] Two studies in black women also found that sulindac 200 mg twice daily for one month did not alter the antihypertensive effect of **fosinopril** 10 to 40 mg daily or **lisinopril** 10 to 40 mg daily (given with hydrochlorothiazide 25 mg daily).[10,11]

(g) Other NSAIDs

In 6 hypertensive patients taking **enalapril**, a single 8-mg dose of **lornoxicam** was found to have no effect on systolic blood pressure, but a small rise in diastolic pressure (from 88.2 mmHg to 93.3 mmHg) occurred after 2 hours.[25] In 29 patients with hypertension **oxaprozin** 1.2 g daily for 3 weeks did not affect the pharmacodynamics of **enalapril** 10 to 40 mg daily.[40]

Twenty-five hypertensive patients with osteoarthritis taking **trandolapril** 2 to 4 mg daily (with or without hydrochlorothiazide) had an increase in blood pressure of about 3/4 mmHg when they were given **diclofenac** 75 mg twice daily.[6] However, **diclofenac** 75 mg twice daily for one month did not alter the antihypertensive effect of **lisinopril** 10 to 40 mg daily (given with hydrochlorothiazide).[11]

A study found that only 5 of 91 (5.5%) hypertensive patients stable taking ACE inhibitors had clinically relevant increases in blood pressure when they were given **nabumetone** 1 g twice daily for 4 weeks.[5] A study in 17 black women found that **nabumetone** 1 g twice daily for one month did not alter the antihypertensive effect of **fosinopril** 10 to 40 mg daily (given with hydrochlorothiazide).[10]

B. Effects on renal function

A case report describes a patient with heart failure treated intermittently with **ibuprofen** and later with **naproxen** and **indometacin** for gout, who developed acute renal failure when also given **captopril**. Treatment with an NSAID alone was without adverse effects on renal function and treatment with **captopril** alone appeared to improve his renal function.[41] In a retrospective analysis, 3 of 162 patients who had been taking ACE inhibitors and NSAIDs developed reversible renal failure, compared with none of 166 patients taking ACE inhibitors alone and none of 2116 patients taking NSAIDs alone. One patient was taking **naproxen** or **salsalate** and had a progressive decline in renal function over 19 months after **captopril** was started. Another man taking unnamed NSAIDs developed reversible renal failure 4 days after starting to take **captopril**.[42] In another similar analysis, in patients aged over 75 years, 2 out of 12 patients given an ACE inhibitor and an NSAID developed acute renal failure (one died) and a further 4 patients had a deterioration in their renal function. All of these 6 patients were also taking diuretics (see 'ACE inhibitors + Diuretics; Loop, Thiazide and related', p.28), but of the 6 with unaffected renal function, only two were taking diuretics.[43] A randomised, crossover study in 17 black patients receiving **fosinopril** with hydrochlorothiazide and NSAIDs for a month, found that acute renal failure (a decrease in glomerular filtration rate of greater than or equal to 25%) occurred in 4 of the 17 patients when receiving **ibuprofen**, 1 of 17 when receiving **sulindac** and 0 of 17 when receiving **nabumetone**.[10]

In a multivariate analysis, the use of ACE inhibitors or angiotensin II receptor antagonists with NSAIDs or diuretics was associated with significant renal impairment when two or more drugs from these groups was taken.[44] In a nested case-control study using the UK General Practice Research Database, the relative risk of acute renal failure was 3.2 with NSAID use, 3.5 with ACE inhibitor use, and 10.6 with NSAIDs and a cardiovascular drug. The risk was not more than additive with NSAIDs and ACE inhibitors.[45] In a case-control study, recently starting an NSAID was associated with a 2.2-fold increased risk of hospitalisation for renal impairment in patients taking ACE inhibitors.[46] In 2002, 28 of 129 reports to the Australian Adverse Drug Reactions

Advisory Committee of acute renal failure were associated with the concurrent use of ACE inhibitors (or angiotensin II receptor antagonists), diuretics, and NSAIDs (including coxibs), and these cases had a fatality rate of 10%. In patients taking this triple combination, renal failure appeared to be precipitated by mild stress such as diarrhoea or dehydration. In other patients, the addition of a third drug (usually an NSAID) to a stable combination of the other two, resulted in acute renal failure.[47]

A placebo-controlled study in 10 patients with chronic congestive heart failure taking an ACE inhibitor (**captopril**, **cilazapril**, **enalapril**, **ramipril**), and aspirin 75 to 125 mg daily (for ischaemic heart disease) found that when they were given a single 50-mg dose of **diclofenac** after aspirin had been discontinued for at least one week, there was a deterioration in renal function compared with placebo or aspirin. Compared with placebo, both aspirin and **diclofenac** caused slight increases in serum creatinine.[48]

In contrast, a retrospective analysis found no evidence that the adverse effects of ACE inhibitors on renal function were greater in those taking NSAIDs.[49] A further study in 17 hypertensive patients with normal baseline renal function, found that **indometacin** 25 mg three times daily did not adversely affect renal function when it was given with **trandolapril** 2 mg daily for 3 weeks.[50]

C. Hyperkalaemia

Hyperkalaemia, resulting in marked bradycardia, was attributed to the use of **loxoprofen** in an elderly woman taking **imidapril**.[51] A 77-year-old woman with mild hypertension and normal renal function taking **enalapril** 2.5 mg daily arrested and died 5 days after starting to take **rofecoxib** for leg pain. Her potassium was found to be 8.8 mmol/L. Infection and dehydration could have contributed to the hyperkalaemia in this patient.[52]

D. Pharmacokinetic studies

The manufacturer of **spirapril** briefly noted in a review that there was no relevant pharmacokinetic interaction between spirapril and **diclofenac**.[53] In 29 patients with hypertension, **oxaprozin** 1.2 g daily for 3 weeks did not affect the pharmacokinetics of **enalapril** 10 to 40 mg daily.[40] A brief mention is made in a review that, in healthy subjects, the pharmacokinetics of **ramipril** were unaffected by **indometacin** [dose not stated] given for 3 days.[36]

Mechanism

Some, but not all the evidence suggests that prostaglandins might be involved in the hypotensive action of ACE inhibitors, and that NSAIDs, by inhibiting prostaglandin synthesis, might partially antagonise the effect of ACE inhibitors. Another suggestion is that NSAIDs promote sodium retention and so blunt the blood pressure lowering effects of several classes of antihypertensive drugs, including ACE inhibitors. This interaction might be dependent on sodium status and on plasma renin, and so drugs that affect sodium status e.g. diuretics can potentially influence the effect. Therefore, the interaction does not occur in all patients. It could also depend on the NSAID, with indometacin being frequently implicated, and sulindac less so, as well as on the dosing frequency.[6]

Both NSAIDs and ACE inhibitors alone can cause renal impairment. In patients whose kidneys are underperfused, they might cause further deterioration in renal function when used together.[54] Impaired renal function is a risk factor for hyperkalaemia with ACE inhibitors.

Importance and management

The interaction between indometacin and ACE inhibitors is well established, with several studies showing that indometacin can reduce the **blood pressure-lowering** effect of a number of ACE inhibitors. The interaction might not occur in all patients. If indometacin is required in a patient taking any ACE inhibitor, it would be prudent to monitor blood pressure. In a few small comparative studies, indometacin has been shown to have less effect on the calcium-channel blockers amlodipine, felodipine, and nifedipine, than on enalapril.[24,27,28] Therefore, a calcium-channel blocker may sometimes be an alternative to an ACE inhibitor in a patient requiring indometacin. Consider also, 'Calcium-channel blockers + Aspirin or NSAIDs', p.1030.

Limited information suggests that sulindac has little or no effect on ACE inhibitors, and might therefore be less likely to cause a problem, but further study is needed. The coxibs appear to have similar or greater effects on ACE inhibitors than conventional NSAIDs.

Although information about other NSAIDs is limited, the mechanism suggests that all of them are likely to interact similarly. Until more is known, it would seem prudent to increase blood pressure monitoring when any NSAID is added or discontinued in a patient taking any ACE inhibitor, and intermittent use of NSAIDs should be considered as a possible cause of erratic control of blood pressure. In addition, sodium status and therefore diuretic use might affect any interaction. However, some consider that the clinical importance of an interaction between NSAIDs and antihypertensives is less than has previously been suggested.[55] While their findings do not rule out a 2/1 mmHg increase in blood pressure with NSAIDs in treated hypertensives, they suggest that if patients in primary care have inadequate control of blood pressure, other reasons might be more likely than any effect of concurrent NSAIDs.[55] Further study is needed. For the effects of NSAIDs on other antihypertensive drug classes see 'Beta blockers + Aspirin or NSAIDs', p.1003, 'Calcium-channel blockers + Aspirin or NSAIDs', p.1030, and 'Thiazide diuretics + NSAIDs', p.1132.

There is an increased risk of **deterioration in renal function** or acute renal failure with the combination of NSAIDs and ACE inhibitors, especially if poor renal perfusion is present. Renal function should be monitored periodically in patients taking ACE inhibitors with NSAIDs, particularly in volume depleted patients. In a statement, the American Heart Association comments that acute renal failure complicating the use of an ACE inhibitor is almost always reversible and repletion of extracellular fluid volume and discontinuation of any diuretic is the best approach. In addition, withdrawal of interacting drugs, supportive management of fluid and electrolytes, and temporary dialysis, where indicated, are the mainstays of treatment.[56] The Australian Adverse Drug Reactions Advisory Committee consider that the triple combination of ACE inhibitors, diuretics and NSAIDs (including coxibs) should be avoided if possible, and that great care should be taken when giving ACE inhibitors and NSAIDs to patients with renal impairment.[47] Deterioration in renal function increases the risk of **hyperkalaemia**.

1. Johnson AG, Nguyen TV, Day RO. Do nonsteroidal anti-inflammatory drugs affect blood pressure? A meta-analysis. *Ann Intern Med* (1994) 121, 289–300.
2. Pope JE, Anderson JJ, Felson DT. A meta-analysis of the effects of nonsteroidal anti-inflammatory drugs on blood pressure. *Arch Intern Med* (1993) 153, 477–84.
3. White WB, Kent J, Taylor A, Verburg K, Lefkowith JB, Whelton A. Effects of celecoxib on ambulatory blood pressure in hypertensive patients on ACE inhibitors. *Hypertension* (2002) 39, 929–34.
4. Whelton A, Fort JG, Puma JA, Normandin D, Bello AE, Verburg KM, for the SUCCESS VI Study Group. Cyclooxygenase-2-specific inhibitors and cardiorenal function: a randomized, controlled trial of celecoxib and rofecoxib in older hypertensive osteoarthritis patients. *Am J Ther* (2001) 8, 85–95.
5. Palmer R, Weiss R, Zusman RM, Haig A, Flavin S, MacDonald B. Effects of nabumetone, celecoxib, and ibuprofen on blood pressure control in hypertensive patients on angiotensin converting enzyme inhibitors. *Am J Hypertens* (2003) 16, 135–9.
6. Izhar M, Alausa T, Folker A, Hung E, Bakris GL. Effects of COX inhibition on blood pressure and kidney function in ACE inhibitor-treated blacks and hispanics. *Hypertension* (2004) 43, 573–7.
7. Sowers JR, White WB, Pitt B, Whelton A, Simon LS, Winer N, Kivitz A, van Ingen H, Brabant T, Fort JG; Celecoxib Rofecoxib Efficacy and Safety in Comorbidities Evaluation Trial (CRESCENT) Investigators. *Arch Intern Med* (2005) 165, 161–8.
8. Goldstone R, Martin K, Zipser R, Horton R. Evidence for a dual action of converting enzyme inhibitor on blood pressure in normal man. *Prostaglandins* (1981) 22, 587–98.
9. Espino DV, Lancaster MC. Neutralization of the effects of captopril by the use of ibuprofen in an elderly woman. *J Am Board Fam Pract* (1992) 5, 319–21.
10. Thakur V, Cook ME, Wallin JD. Antihypertensive effect of the combination of fosinopril and HCTZ is resistant to interference by nonsteroidal antiinflammatory drugs. *Am J Hypertens* (1999) 12, 925–8.
11. Bhagat K. Effects of non-steroidal anti-inflammatory drugs on hypertension control using angiotensin converting enzyme inhibitors and thiazide diuretics. *East Afr Med J* (2001) 78, 507–9.
12. Conlin PR, Moore TJ, Swartz SL, Barr E, Gazdick L, Fletcher C, DeLucca P, Demopoulos L. Effect of indomethacin on blood pressure lowering by captopril and losartan in hypertensive patients. *Hypertension* (2000) 36, 461–5.
13. Moore TJ, Crantz FR, Hollenberg NK, Koletsky RJ, Leboff MS, Swartz SL, Levine L, Podolsky S, Dluhy RG, Williams GH. Contribution of prostaglandins to the antihypertensive action of captopril in essential hypertension. *Hypertension* (1981) 3, 168–73.
14. Swartz SL, Williams GH. Angiotensin-converting enzyme inhibition and prostaglandins. *Am J Cardiol* (1982) 49, 1405–9.
15. Salvetti A, Pedrinelli R, Magagna A, Ugenti P. Differential effects of selective and non-selective prostaglandin-synthesis inhibition on the pharmacological responses to captopril in patients with essential hypertension. *Clin Sci* (1982) 63, 261S–263S.
16. Silberbauer K, Stanek B, Templ H. Acute hypotensive effect of captopril in man modified by prostaglandin synthesis inhibition. *Br J Clin Pharmacol* (1982) 14, 87S–93S.
17. Witzgall H, Hirsch F, Scherer B, Weber PC. Acute haemodynamic and hormonal effects of captopril are diminished by indomethacin. *Clin Sci* (1982) 62, 611–15.
18. Ogihara T, Maruyama A, Hata T, Mikami H, Nakamaru M, Naka T, Ohde H, Kumahara Y. Hormonal responses to long-term converting enzyme inhibition in hypertensive patients. *Clin Pharmacol Ther* (1981) 30, 328–35.
19. Koopmans PP, Van Megen T, Thien T, Gribnau FWJ. The interaction between indomethacin and captopril or enalapril in healthy volunteers. *J Intern Med* (1989) 226, 139–42.
20. Fujita T, Yamashita N, Yamashita K. Effect of indomethacin on antihypertensive action of captopril in hypertensive patients. *Clin Exp Hypertens* (1981) 3, 939–52.
21. Robles Iniesta A, Navarro de León MC, Morales Serna JC. Bloqueo de la acción antihipertensiva del captoprilo por indometacina. *Med Clin (Barc)* (1991) 96, 438.
22. Gerber JG, Franca G, Byyny RL, LoVerde M, Nies AS. The hypotensive action of captopril and enalapril is not prostacyclin dependent. *Clin Pharmacol Ther* (1993) 54, 523–32.
23. Salvetti A, Abdel-Haq B, Magagna A, Pedrinelli R. Indomethacin reduces the antihypertensive action of enalapril. *Clin Exp Hypertens A* (1987) 9, 559–67.
24. Polónia J, Boaventura I, Gama G, Camões I, Bernardo F, Andrade P, Nunes JP, Brandão F, Cerqueira-Gomes M. Influence of non-steroidal anti-inflammatory drugs on renal function and 24 h ambulatory blood pressure-reducing effects of enalapril and nifedipine gastrointestinal therapeutic system in hypertensive patients. *J Hypertens* (1995) 13, 925–31.
25. Walden RJ, Owens CWI, Graham BR, Snape A, Nutt J, Prichard BNC. NSAIDs and the control of hypertension: a pilot study. *Br J Clin Pharmacol* (1992) 33, 241P.
26. Duffin D, Leahey W, Brennan G, Johnston GD. The effects of indomethacin on the antihypertensive responses to enalapril and lisinopril. *Br J Clin Pharmacol* (1992) 34, 456P.
27. Morgan T, Anderson A. Interaction of indomethacin with felodipine and enalapril. *J Hypertens* (1993) 11 (Suppl 5), S338–S339.
28. Morgan TO, Anderson A, Bertram D. Effect of indomethacin on blood pressure in elderly people with essential hypertension well controlled on amlodipine or enalapril. *Am J Hypertens* (2000), 13, 1161–7.
29. Fricker AF, Nussberger J, Meilenbrock S, Brunner HR, Burnier M. Effect of indomethacin on the renal response to angiotensin II receptor blockade in healthy subjects. *Kidney Int* (1998) 54, 2089–97.
30. Ahmad S. Indomethacin-enalapril interaction: an alert. *South Med J* (1991) 84, 411–2.
31. Oparil S, Horton R, Wilkins LH, Irvin J, Hammett DK. Antihypertensive effect of enalapril in essential hypertension: role of prostacyclin. *Am J Med Sci* (1987) 294, 395–402.
32. Fogari R, Zoppi A, Carretta R, Veglio F, Salvetti A: Italian Collaborative Study Group. Effect of indomethacin on the antihypertensive efficacy of valsartan and lisinopril: a multicentre study. *J Hypertens* (2002) 20: 1007–14.
33. Shaw W, Shapiro D, Antonello J, Cressman M, Vlasses P, Oparil S. Indomethacin does not blunt the antihypertensive effect of lisinopril. *Clin Pharmacol Ther* (1987) 41, 219.
34. Kirch W, Stroemer K, Hoogkamer JFW, Kleinbloesem CH. The influence of prostaglandin inhibition by indomethacin on blood pressure and renal function in hypertensive patients treated with cilazapril. *Br J Clin Pharmacol* (1989) 27, 297S–301S.
35. Abdel-Haq B, Magagna A, Favilla S, Salvetti A. Hemodynamic and humoral interactions between perindopril and indomethacin in essential hypertensive subjects. *J Cardiovasc Pharmacol* (1991) 18 (Suppl 7), S33–S36.
36. Todd PA, Benfield P. Ramipril: a review of its pharmacological properties and therapeutic efficacy in cardiovascular disorders. *Drugs* (1990) 39, 110–35.
37. Pritchard G, Lyons D, Webster J, Petrie JC, MacDonald TM. Indomethacin does not attenuate the hypotensive effect of trandolapril. *J Hum Hypertens* (1996) 10, 763–7.
38. Vioxx (Rofecoxib). Merck Sharp & Dohme Ltd. UK Summary of product characteristics, July 2004.
39. Brown CH. Effect of rofecoxib on the antihypertensive activity of lisinopril. *Ann Pharmacother* (2000) 34, 1486.
40. Noveck RJ, McMahon FG, Bocanegra T, Karem A, Sugimoto D, Smith M. Effects of oxaprozin on enalapril and enalaprilat pharmacokinetics, pharmacodynamics: blood pressure, heart rate, plasma renin activity, aldosterone and creatinine clearances, in hypertensive patients. *Clin Pharmacol Ther* (1997), 61, 208.
41. Hawkins MM, Seelig CB. A case of acute renal failure induced by the co-administration of NSAIDs and captopril. *N C Med J* (1990) 51, 291–2.
42. Seelig CB, Maloley PA, Campbell JR. Nephrotoxicity associated with concomitant ACE inhibitor and NSAID therapy. *South Med J* (1990) 83, 1144–8.

43. Adhiyaman V, Asghar M, Oke A, White AD, Shah IU. Nephrotoxicity in the elderly due to co-prescription of angiotensin converting enzyme inhibitors and nonsteroidal anti-inflammatory drugs. *J R Soc Med* (2001) 94, 512–14.
44. Loboz KK, Shenfield GM. Drug combinations and impaired renal function –the 'triple whammy'. *Br J Clin Pharmacol* (2005) 59, 239–43.
45. Huerta C, Castellsague J, Varas-Lorenzo C, García Rodríguez LA. Nonsteroidal anti-inflammatory drugs and risk of ARF in the general population. *Am J Kidney Dis* (2005) 45, 531–9.
46. Bouvy ML, Heerdink ER, Hoes AW, Leufkens HGM. Effects of NSAIDs on the incidence of hospitalisations for renal dysfunction in users of ACE inhibitors. *Drug Safety* (2003) 26, 983–9.
47. ADRAC. ACE inhibitor, diuretic and NSAID: a dangerous combination. *Aust Adverse Drug React Bull* (2003) 22, 14–15. Available at: http://www.tga.gov.au/hp/aadrb.htm (accessed 21/10/15).
48. Juhlin T, Björkman S, Gunnarsson B, Fyge Å, Roth B, Höglund P. Acute administration of diclofenac, but possibly not long term low dose aspirin, causes detrimental renal effects in heart failure patients treated with ACE-inhibitors. *Eur J Heart Fail* (2004) 6, 909–16.
49. Stürmer T, Erb A, Keller F, Günther K-P, Brenner H. Determinants of impaired renal function with use of nonsteroidal anti-inflammatory drugs: the importance of half-life and other medications. *Am J Med* (2001) 111, 521–7.
50. Pritchard G, Lyons D, Webster J, Petrie JC, MacDonald TM. Do trandolapril and indomethacin influence renal function and renal functional reserve in hypertensive patients? *Br J Clin Pharmacol* (1997) 44, 145–9.
51. Kurata C, Uehara A, Sugi T, Yamazaki K. Syncope caused by nonsteroidal anti-inflammatory drugs and angiotensin-converting enzyme inhibitors. *Jpn Circ J* (1999) 63, 1002–3.
52. Hay E, Derazon H, Bukish N, Katz L, Kruglyakov I, Armoni M. Fatal hyperkalaemia related to combined therapy with a COX-2 inhibitor, ACE inhibitor and potassium rich diet. *J Emerg Med* (2002) 22, 349–52.
53. Grass P, Gerbeau C, Kutz K. Spirapril: pharmacokinetic properties and drug interactions. *Blood Pressure* (1994) 3 (Suppl 2), 7–13.
54. Sturrock NDC, Struthers AD. Non-steroidal anti-inflammatory drugs and angiotensin converting enzyme inhibitors: a commonly prescribed combination with variable effects on renal function. *Br J Clin Pharmacol* (1993) 35, 343–8.
55. Sheridan R, Montgomery AA, Fahey T. NSAID use and BP in treated hypertensives: a retrospective controlled observational study. *J Hum Hypertens* (2005) 19, 445–50.
56. Schoolwerth AC, Sica DA, Ballermann BJ, Wilcox CS. Renal considerations in angiotensin converting enzyme inhibitor therapy. A statement for healthcare professionals from the Council on the Kidney in Cardiovascular Disease and the Council for High Blood Pressure Research of the American Heart Association. *Circulation* (2001) 104, 1985–91.

ACE inhibitors + Potassium compounds

ACE inhibitors maintain serum potassium levels. Hyperkalaemia is therefore possible if potassium supplements or potassium-containing salt substitutes are also given, particularly in those patients where other risk factors are present.

Clinical evidence

(a) Potassium levels increased by concurrent use

1. Potassium supplements. The serum potassium levels of a patient taking a potassium supplement rose by 66% when **captopril** was added, with signs of a deterioration in renal function. Four other patients taking potassium supplements and furosemide (2 also taking unnamed potassium-sparing diuretics) had rises in their potassium levels of only 8 to 24% when given **captopril**. The rises occurred within one or 2 days. No clinical signs or symptoms of hyperkalaemia were seen, but 3 of the 5 patients had rises to above the upper limits of normal.[1] A post-marketing survey identified 10 patients in whom **enalapril** appeared to have been associated with renal impairment and death. Eight of them were also taking potassium supplements and/or potassium-sparing diuretics, and hyperkalaemia appeared to have been the immediate cause of death in two of them.[2] In a review of 47 patients taking **enalapril** for heart failure who experienced serious hyperkalaemia, 8 had also received potassium supplements.[3]

In another survey of 53 patients taking ACE inhibitors who had hyperkalaemia in the absence of significant renal impairment, less than 5% were taking a potassium supplement, but 30% were using a potassium-containing salt substitute (see *Dietary potassium*, below).[4]

2. Dietary potassium. Two patients with renal impairment, one taking **lisinopril** and the other taking **enalapril**, developed marked hyperkalaemia shortly after starting to take '*Lo salt*' (a salt substitute containing 34.6 g potassium in every 100 g). One developed a life-threatening arrhythmia.[5] A similar report describes a man taking **captopril** who developed hyperkalaemia and collapsed 2 weeks after starting to use a salt substitute containing potassium.[6] In a further report, severe hyperkalaemia occurred in a patient receiving a very-low-calorie diet with a protein supplement who was taking **lisinopril** 10 mg daily. The protein supplement contained 48 mmol of potassium, and salad topped with lemon juice and potassium chloride salt added at least another 72 mmol of potassium daily.[7] In 53 patients taking ACE inhibitors, who had hyperkalaemia in the absence of significant renal impairment, 30% were using a salt substitute, and 72% were eating a moderate-to-high potassium diet, consisting of 2 or more servings of a potassium-rich food daily.[4] Hyperkalaemia and acute renal failure has also been reported in a diabetic patient taking **lisinopril** 20 mg twice daily following the use of a potassium-based water softener.[8]

(b) Potassium levels unaltered by concurrent use

A retrospective analysis of 14 patients without renal impairment taking potassium supplements and either furosemide or hydrochlorothiazide, found that the levels of serum potassium, during a 4-year period, had not notably increased after the addition of **captopril**.[9] Another study in 6 healthy subjects found that intravenous potassium chloride caused virtually the same rise in serum potassium levels in those given **enalapril** as in those given a placebo.[10]

Mechanism

The potassium-retaining effects of the ACE inhibitors (due to reduced aldosterone levels) are additive with an increased intake of potassium, particularly when there are other contributory factors such as poor renal function or diabetes.

Importance and management

The documentation of the interaction between ACE inhibitors and potassium compounds is well established. In practice, a clinically relevant rise in potassium levels usually occurs only if other factors are also present, the most important of which is impaired renal function. In general, because ACE inhibitors have potassium-sparing effects, potassium supplements should not routinely be given concurrently. If a supplement is needed, serum potassium should be closely monitored. This is especially important where other possible contributory risk factors are known to be present. A retrospective study in hospitalised patients who developed hyperkalaemia found that risk factors associated with a rapid rate of increase in serum potassium levels, in decreasing order of importance, were: the use of potassium supplements, severe renal impairment, the use of ACE inhibitors or angiotensin II receptor antagonists, the use of potassium-sparing diuretics, and diabetes mellitus. Further, the presence of two or more of these risk factors (e.g. the use of an ACE inhibitor and a potassium supplement) was associated with an even faster rate of development of hyperkalaemia. As the rate of development of hyperkalaemia is also correlated with its severity, the authors recommend close monitoring in patients with two or more risk factors, and that a rapid increase in serum potassium (greater than 0.5 mmol/L per day) should prompt the identification and possible removal of any risk factors for hyperkalaemia.[11]

Other sources of dietary potassium should also be borne in mind. Patients with heart disease and hypertension are often told to reduce their salt (sodium) intake. One way of doing this is to use potassium-containing salt substitutes. However, it appears that there is some risk associated with excess use of these substitutes, especially in patients taking ACE inhibitors.

1. Burnakis TG, Mioduch HJ. Combined therapy with captopril and potassium supplementation. A potential for hyperkalemia. *Arch Intern Med* (1984) 144, 2371–2.
2. Speirs CJ, Dollery CT, Inman WHW, Rawson NSB, Wilton LV. Postmarketing surveillance of enalapril. II: Investigation of the potential role of enalapril in deaths with renal failure. *BMJ* (1988) 297, 830–2.
3. Brown C, Rush J. Risk factors for the development of hyperkalemia in patients treated with enalapril for heart failure. *Clin Pharmacol Ther* (1989) 45, 167.
4. Good CB, McDermott L, McCloskey B. Diet and serum potassium in patients on ACE inhibitors. *JAMA* (1995) 274, 538.
5. Ray KK, Dorman S, Watson RDS. Severe hyperkalaemia due to the concomitant use of salt substitutes and ACE inhibitors in hypertension: a potentially life threatening interaction. *J Hum Hypertens* (1999) 13, 717–20.
6. Packer M, Lee WH. Provocation of hyper- and hypokalemic sudden death during treatment with and withdrawal of converting-enzyme inhibition in severe chronic congestive heart failure. *Am J Cardiol* (1986) 57, 347–8.
7. Stoltz ML, Andrews CE. Severe hyperkalemia during very-low-calorie diets and angiotensin converting enzyme use. *JAMA* (1990) 264, 2737–8.
8. Graves JW. Hyperkalemia due to a potassium-based water softener. *N Engl J Med* (1998) 339,1790–1.
9. Schuna AA, Schmidt GR, Pitterle ME. Serum potassium concentrations after initiation of captopril therapy. *Clin Pharm* (1986) 5, 920–3.
10. Scandling JD, Izzo JL, Pabico RC, McKenna BA, Radke KJ, Ornt DB. Potassium homeostasis during angiotensin-converting enzyme inhibition with enalapril. *J Clin Pharmacol* (1989) 29, 916–21.
11. Indermitte J, Burkolter S, Drewe J, Krähenbühl S, Hersberger KE. Risk factors associated with a high velocity of the development of hyperkalaemia in hospitalised patients. *Drug Safety* (2007) 30, 71–80.

ACE inhibitors + Probenecid

Probenecid decreases the renal clearance of captopril and enalapril.

Clinical evidence, mechanism, importance and management

In 4 healthy subjects, the steady-state levels of unchanged and total **captopril**, given by intravenous infusion, were slightly increased (by 14% and 36%, respectively) by the use of probenecid. Renal clearance of unchanged **captopril** decreased by 44%, but total clearance was reduced by only 19%.[1] These changes are unlikely to be clinically important.

In 12 healthy subjects, probenecid 1 g twice daily for 5 days increased the AUC of a single 20-mg oral dose of **enalapril** and its active metabolite, enalaprilat, by about 50%. The renal clearance of **enalapril** was decreased by 73%.[2] A moderate increase in the hypotensive effects of **enalapril** might be expected, but there do not appear to be any reports of adverse effects.

1. Singhvi SM, Duchin KL, Willard DA, McKinstry DN, Migdalof BH. Renal handling of captopril: effect of probenecid. *Clin Pharmacol Ther* (1982) 32, 182–9.
2. Noormohamed FH, McNabb WR, Lant AF. Pharmacokinetic and pharmacodynamic actions of enalapril in humans: effect of probenecid pretreatment. *J Pharmacol Exp Ther* (1990) 253, 362–8.

ACE inhibitors + Procainamide

The combination of captopril or other ACE inhibitors and procainamide possibly increases the risk of leucopenia. No pharmacokinetic interaction occurs between captopril and procainamide.

Clinical evidence, mechanism, importance and management

In 12 healthy subjects the concurrent use of **captopril** 50 mg twice daily and procainamide 250 mg every 3 hours did not affect the pharmacokinetics of either drug.[1] A study in 9 patients with heart failure, including 8 who were taking ACE inhibitors, found that there was no statistically significant difference in the pharmacokinetics of a single intravenous dose of procainamide 750 mg and its metabolite *N*-acetylprocainamide between these subjects and 7 matched control subjects without left ventricular dysfunction (one taking an ACE inhibitor). However, there was wider interpatient variation in pharmacokinetic parameters in the patients with heart failure.[2] The US manufacturer of one brand of **captopril** noted that in patients with heart failure who developed neutropenia, about 50% had a serum creatinine of about 140 micromol/L or greater, and more than 75% were also receiving procainamide.[3] Similarly, the

UK manufacturer of **captopril** notes that neutropenia or agranulocytosis and serious infection have occurred in patients taking **captopril**, and that the concurrent use of procainamide might be a complicating factor, especially if the ACE inhibitor is used at higher than the recommended dose. They state that the combination should be used with caution, especially in patients with renal impairment and note that differential white blood cell counts should be performed before concurrent use, then every 2 weeks in the first 3 months of treatment and periodically thereafter.[4]

Although evidence for other ACE inhibitors is generally lacking, many UK manufacturers suggest that the concurrent use of ACE inhibitors and procainamide might lead to an increased risk of leucopenia.

For reports of other possible interactions with ACE inhibitors that might result in an increased risk of leucopenia see also 'ACE inhibitors + Allopurinol', p.19 and 'ACE inhibitors + Azathioprine', p.24.

1. Levinson B, Sugerman AA, McKown J. Lack of kinetic interaction of captopril (CP) and procainamide (PA) in healthy subjects. *J Clin Pharmacol* (1985) 25, 460.
2. Tisdale JE, Rudis MI, Padhi ID, Borzak S, Svensson CK, Webb CR, Acciaioli J, Ware JA, Krepostman A, Zarowitz BJ. Disposition of procainamide in patients with chronic congestive heart failure receiving medical therapy. *J Clin Pharmacol* (1996) 36, 35–41.
3. Capoten (Captopril). Par Pharmaceutical, Inc. US Prescribing information, June 2003.
4. Capoten (Captopril). E. R. Squibb & Sons Ltd. UK Summary of product characteristics, June 2010.

ACE inhibitors + Rifampicin (Rifampin)

An isolated report describes a rise in blood pressure in one hypertensive patient, which was attributed to an interaction between enalapril and rifampicin. Rifampicin reduces the plasma levels of the active metabolites of imidapril and spirapril.

Clinical evidence

A man taking **enalapril** and a variety of other drugs (warfarin, acebutolol, bendroflumethiazide, dipyridamole, metoclopramide and *Gaviscon*) developed a fever. He was given streptomycin, oxytetracycline and rifampicin, because of a probable *Brucella abortus* infection, whereupon his blood pressure rose from 164/104 mmHg to 180/115 mmHg over the next 5 to 6 days. It was suspected that an interaction with the rifampicin was possibly responsible. Subsequent studies in the same patient found that rifampicin reduced the AUC_{0-7} of enalaprilat, the active metabolite of **enalapril**, by 31%, although the AUC of **enalapril** was unchanged.[1] There is also the hint of this interaction in another report, where **enalapril** did not control blood pressure in a patient taking rifampicin.[2]

The manufacturer of **imidapril** notes that rifampicin reduces the plasma levels of imidaprilat, the active metabolite of **imidapril**.[3]

The manufacturer of **spirapril** briefly noted in a review that the use of rifampicin with **spirapril** decreased the plasma levels of **spirapril** and its active metabolite, spiraprilat.[4]

Mechanism

The mechanism of this interaction is not clear, because rifampicin is an enzyme inducer, which might have been expected to cause the production of more, rather than less, of the active metabolites of these ACE inhibitors. However, the authors of one of the reports postulated that rifampicin might have increased the loss of enalaprilat in the urine,[1] and others suggested that rifampicin causes a non-specific stimulation of the elimination of spiraprilat.[4]

Importance and management

The general importance of these interactions between rifampicin and enalapril, imidapril and spirapril is uncertain. The isolated reports with enalapril suggest minor clinical relevance. The manufacturers of spirapril did not consider the pharmacokinetic changes to be clinically relevant.[4] However, the manufacturers of imidapril state that rifampicin might reduce the antihypertensive efficacy of imidapril,[3] but this awaits clinical assessment.

1. Kandiah D, Penny WJ, Fraser AG, Lewis MJ. A possible drug interaction between rifampicin and enalapril. *Eur J Clin Pharmacol* (1988) 35, 431–2.
2. Tada Y, Tsuda Y, Otsuka T, Nagasawa K, Kimura H, Kusaba T, Sakata T. Case report: nifedipine-rifampicin interaction attenuates the effect on blood pressure in a patient with essential hypertension. *Am J Med Sci* (1992) 303, 25–7.
3. Tanatril (Imidapril hydrochloride). Chiesi Ltd. UK Summary of product characteristics, May 2010.
4. Grass P, Gerbeau C, Kutz K. Spirapril: pharmacokinetic properties and drug interactions. *Blood Pressure* (1994) 3 (Suppl 2), 7–13.

ACE inhibitors + Sevelamer

Sevelamer did not alter the pharmacokinetics of enalapril in one study.

Clinical evidence, mechanism, importance and management

In 28 healthy subjects the concurrent use of a single 2.418-g dose of sevelamer hydrochloride (equivalent to 6 capsules) did not alter the AUC of a single 20-mg dose of **enalapril** or its active metabolite, enalaprilat.[1] Thus it appears that sevelamer does not bind to **enalapril** within the gut to reduce its absorption. Other ACE inhibitors would not be expected to interact with sevelamer, but this needs confirmation.

1. Burke SK, Amin NS, Incerti C, Plone MA, Lee JW. Sevelamer hydrochloride (Renagel®), a phosphate-binding polymer, does not alter the pharmacokinetics of two commonly used antihypertensives in healthy volunteers. *J Clin Pharmacol* (2001) 41, 199–205.

ACE inhibitors + Sibutramine

Sibutramine has only a minimal effect on the blood pressure control of patients taking ACE inhibitors.

Clinical evidence, mechanism, importance and management

In a randomised, double-blind study over 52 weeks, in 220 obese patients whose hypertension was well controlled with an ACE inhibitor (**benazepril**, **enalapril** or **lisinopril**) with or without a thiazide diuretic, two-thirds of the patients were also given sibutramine and one-third were given placebo. Sibutramine 20 mg daily caused small increases in mean blood pressure compared with placebo (133.1/85.5 mmHg compared with 130.4/82.8 mmHg, at 52 weeks, respectively), but overall, hypertension remained well controlled.[1] Another double-blind, placebo-controlled study in 86 obese patients taking ACE inhibitors and/or other antihypertensives, found that sibutramine 10 mg daily for 6 months reduced ventricular mass, but caused no alterations in blood pressure, although average heart rate increased from 78 bpm to 82 bpm.[2] No particular precautions therefore seem necessary if patients taking ACE inhibitors are given sibutramine.

1. McMahon FG, Weinstein SP, Rowe E, Ernst KR, Johnson F, Fujioka K, and the Sibutramine in Hypertensives Clinical Study Group. Sibutramine is safe and effective for weight loss in obese patients whose hypertension is well controlled with angiotensin-converting enzyme inhibitors. *J Hum Hypertens* (2002) 16, 5–11.
2. Faria AN, Ribeiro Filho FF, Lerário DDG, Kohlmann N, Ferreira SRG, Zanella MT. Effects of sibutramine on the treatment of obesity in patients with arterial hypertension. *Arq Bras Cardiol* (2002) 78, 176–80.

Angiotensin II receptor antagonists + Aliskiren

Irbesartan does not appear to alter the pharmacokinetics of aliskiren, and the concurrent use of valsartan with aliskiren does not appear to result in a clinically relevant pharmacokinetic interaction. However, the concurrent use of aliskiren and angiotensin II receptor antagonists might increase the risk of hyperkalaemia, and is likely to result in a greater reduction in blood pressure.

Clinical evidence

In a study, 11 patients with mild to moderate renal impairment and 17 healthy subjects were given aliskiren 300 mg daily for 7 days. **Irbesartan** 300 mg daily was then started, and both drugs were given for a further 7 days. The steady-state pharmacokinetics of aliskiren were not affected by the concurrent use of **irbesartan**.[1]

In a study in 23 patients with hypertension, the addition of aliskiren 75 or 150 mg daily to **irbesartan** 150 mg for 3 weeks resulted in lower night-time blood pressures, when compared with **irbesartan** alone, and there was a non-statistically significant reduction in daytime blood pressure with aliskiren 75 mg daily. There was a trend for both daytime and night-time blood pressures to increase rather than decrease when the dose of aliskiren was increased from 75 mg daily to 150 mg daily, but these changes were not statistically significant. The plasma concentrations of aliskiren were not affected by **irbesartan**.[2]

In another study, 18 healthy subjects were given **valsartan** 320 mg daily with aliskiren 300 mg daily for 4 days. When compared with the use of either drug alone, **valsartan** decreased the AUC and maximum plasma concentration of aliskiren by 26% and 28%, respectively, and aliskiren decreased the AUC and maximum plasma concentration of **valsartan** by 14% and 12%, respectively.[3] These pharmacokinetic changes were not considered to be clinically relevant.[3]

A subgroup analysis of patients taking aliskiren with an angiotensin II receptor antagonist found an increase in the risk of hyperkalaemia when compared with patients taking an angiotensin II receptor antagonist alone.[4] In contrast, in a Canadian retrospective case-control study, aliskiren use was not associated with an increased risk of hospitalisation for hyperkalaemia, acute kidney injury, or stroke in patients aged 66 or older, who were also taking an ACE inhibitor or angiotensin II receptor antagonist.[5]

Mechanism

Both angiotensin II receptor antagonists and the renin inhibitor aliskiren act on the renin-angiotensin-aldosterone system, and can increase the risk of hyperkalaemia when given alone. This risk can be further increased when they are given together.

Importance and management

The evidence for a pharmacokinetic interaction between the angiotensin II receptor antagonists and aliskiren is limited to the studies with irbesartan and valsartan. **Irbesartan** does not appear to alter the pharmacokinetics of aliskiren, and the concurrent use of aliskiren and **valsartan** does not appear to result in a clinically relevant pharmacokinetic interaction. However, as would be expected, concurrent use does appear to result in an increased blood pressure-lowering effect. Taking an angiotensin II receptor antagonist with aliskiren might also increase the risk of hyperkalaemia. Guidance from the European Medicines Agency issued in September 2014 states that the combination of an angiotensin II receptor antagonist and aliskiren is not recommended in any patient, and is strictly contraindicated in patients with diabetic nephropathy or moderate to severe renal impairment (eGFR less than 60 mL/minute/1.73 m^2). In patients where it is considered absolutely necessary, an angiotensin II receptor antagonist and aliskiren should only be given together under specialist supervision, with close monitoring of blood pressure, renal function, and electrolyte and fluid balance.[6]

1. Vaidyanathan S, Bigler H, Yeh CM, Bizot M-N, Dieterich HA, Howard D, Dole WP. Pharmacokinetics of the oral direct renin inhibitor aliskiren alone and in combination with irbesartan in renal impairment. *Clin Pharmacokinet* (2007) 46, 661–75.
2. O'Brien E, Barton J, Nussberger J, Mulcahy D, Jensen C, Dicker P, Stanton A. Aliskiren reduces blood pressure and suppresses plasma renin activity in combination with a thiazide diuretic, an angiotensin-converting enzyme inhibitor, or an angiotensin receptor blocker. *Hypertension* (2007) 49, 276–84.
3. Vaidyanathan S, Valencia J, Kemp C, Zhao C, Yeh C-M, Bizot M-N, Denouel J, Dieterich HA, Dole WP. Lack of pharmacokinetic interactions of aliskiren, a novel direct renin inhibitor for the treatment of hypertension, with the antihypertensives amlodipine, valsartan, hydrochlorothiazide (HCTZ) and ramipril in healthy volunteers. *Int J Clin Pract* (2006) 60, 1343–56.
4. Makani H, Bangalore S, Desouza KA, Shah A, Messerli FH. Efficacy and safety of dual blockade of the renin-angiotensin system: meta-analysis of randomised trials. *BMJ* (2013) 346, f360.
5. Gilbert CJ, Gomes T, Mamdani MM, Hellings C, Yao Z, Garg AX, Wald R, Harel Z, Juurlink DN. No increase in adverse events during aliskiren use among Ontario patients receiving angiotensin-converting enzyme inhibitors or angiotensin-receptor blockers. *Can J Cardiol* (2013) 29, 586–91.
6. European Medicines Agency. Restriction of combined use of medicines affecting the renin-angiotensin system (RAS), September 2014. Available at: http://www.ema.europa.eu/docs/en_GB/document_library/Referrals_document/Renin-angiotensin_system_(RAS)-acting_agents/European_Commission_final_decision/WC500175069.pdf (accessed 21/10/15).

Angiotensin II receptor antagonists + Antacids

Aluminium/magnesium hydroxide-containing antacids have a negligible effect on irbesartan and olmesartan exposure.

Clinical evidence, mechanism, importance and management

(a) Irbesartan

In a single-dose, crossover study in 18 healthy subjects, 10 mL of an antacid containing **aluminium/magnesium hydroxide** given with, or 2 hours before, a single 300-mg dose of irbesartan had little effect on irbesartan pharmacokinetics. The only difference was that the AUC of irbesartan was reduced by 10% when the antacid was given 2 hours before the irbesartan, when compared with irbesartan alone. However, this change is not considered to be clinically relevant.[1]

(b) Olmesartan

The steady-state AUC of olmesartan 20 mg daily was 12% lower when it was given 15 minutes after a daily dose of an **aluminium/magnesium hydroxide** antacid, when compared with olmesartan alone, but this was not considered to be clinically relevant.[2]

1. Marino MR, Vachharajani NN. Drug interactions with irbesartan. *Clin Pharmacokinet* (2001) 40, 605–14.
2. Laeis P, Püchler K, Kirch W. The pharmacokinetic and metabolic profile of olmesartan medoxomil limits the risk of clinically relevant drug interaction. *J Hypertens* (2001) 19 (Suppl 1), S21–S32.

Angiotensin II receptor antagonists + Aspirin or NSAIDs

Indometacin might attenuate the antihypertensive effect of losartan, valsartan, or other angiotensin II receptor antagonists. However, low-dose aspirin does not appear to alter the antihypertensive effect of losartan. No clinically relevant *pharmacokinetic* interactions occur between telmisartan and ibuprofen, or between valsartan and indometacin. The combination of an NSAID and angiotensin II receptor antagonist can increase the risk of renal impairment and hyperkalaemia.

Clinical evidence

In 2002, 28 of 129 reports to the Australian Adverse Drug Reactions Advisory Committee of acute renal failure were associated with the concurrent use of ACE inhibitors or angiotensin II receptor antagonists, diuretics, and NSAIDs (including coxibs), and these cases had a fatality rate of 10%. In patients taking this triple combination, renal failure appeared to be precipitated by mild stress such as diarrhoea or dehydration. In other patients, the addition of a third drug (usually an NSAID) to a stable combination of the other two, resulted in acute renal failure.[1] In a multivariate analysis, the use of an ACE inhibitor or angiotensin II receptor antagonist, and NSAIDs or diuretics was associated with significant renal impairment when two or more drugs from these groups was taken.[2]

Various large epidemiological studies and meta-analyses of clinical studies have been conducted to assess the effect of NSAIDs on blood pressure in patients taking antihypertensives, and the findings of these are summarised in 'Table 23.2', p.1031. In these studies, NSAIDs were not always associated with an increase in blood pressure, and the maximum increase was 6.2 mmHg.

Further data relating to specific pairs of drugs is given in the subsections below.

(a) Aspirin

A double-blind, placebo-controlled study in 10 patients with hypertension taking **losartan** (mean daily dose 47.5 mg) found that both aspirin 81 mg daily and aspirin 325 mg daily for 2 weeks did not affect blood pressure.[3]

(b) Ibuprofen

In a crossover study in 12 healthy subjects, **telmisartan** 120 mg daily had no effect on the pharmacokinetics of ibuprofen 400 mg three times daily for 7 days. Similarly, the pharmacokinetics of **telmisartan** were unaffected by the concurrent use of ibuprofen, when compared with previous studies of telmisartan alone.[4]

(c) Indometacin

1. Losartan. In a study in 111 patients with hypertension, losartan 50 mg daily for 6 weeks reduced their blood pressure by a mean of 7.9/5.3 mmHg. Indometacin 75 mg daily was then added for one week and this caused a rise in blood pressure in the group as a whole of 3.8/2.2 mmHg (reduction of about 45% in the effect of losartan). A rise in ambulatory diastolic blood pressure was seen in 69% of the patients taking losartan during indometacin use.[5] In contrast, a much smaller study in 10 patients with essential hypertension taking losartan found that indometacin 50 mg twice daily for one week caused sodium and fluid retention, but did not attenuate the antihypertensive effects of losartan.[6]

2. Valsartan. In a placebo-controlled, crossover study in 56 hypertensive patients whose blood pressure was adequately controlled by valsartan 80 to 160 mg daily, the addition of indometacin 50 mg twice daily for 2 weeks produced an increase in mean blood pressure of 2.1/1.9 mmHg.[7] A study in normotensive subjects given a fixed sodium intake and valsartan 80 mg daily, with or without indometacin 50 mg twice daily for one week, found that indometacin reduced the natriuretic response to angiotensin receptor blockade.[8]

In 12 healthy subjects, there was no statistically significant effect on the pharmacokinetics of single oral doses of valsartan 160 mg or indometacin 100 mg when the drugs were given together, although the pharmacokinetics of valsartan showed wide variations between subjects.[9]

Mechanism

Some evidence suggests that prostaglandins might be partially involved in the hypotensive action of angiotensin II receptor antagonists, and that NSAIDs, by inhibiting prostaglandin synthesis, might antagonise their effects. However, a non-specific mechanism such as sodium retention could also be involved, as indometacin has been shown to reduce the hypotensive effect of other classes of antihypertensive drugs.[7,8] Both NSAIDs and angiotensin II receptor antagonists alone can cause renal impairment: in patients whose kidneys are underperfused, they might cause further deterioration in renal function if they are used together. Renal impairment increases the risk of hyperkalaemia.

Importance and management

As with other antihypertensives, the **blood pressure-lowering effect** of angiotensin II receptor antagonists can be attenuated by NSAIDs such as indometacin. Patients taking losartan or valsartan or other angiotensin II receptor antagonists, who require indometacin and probably other NSAIDs, should be monitored for alterations in blood pressure control. Low-dose aspirin is unlikely to alter the blood pressure-lowering effect of angiotensin II receptor antagonists. Further, one study suggests that aspirin with an angiotensin receptor II antagonist (or an ACE inhibitor) had no adverse effect on intermediate outcomes for patients with ischaemic or non-ischaemic heart failure.[10] However, for a discussion of the controversy as to whether low-dose aspirin might attenuate the benefits of *ACE inhibitors* in patients with heart failure, see 'ACE inhibitors + Aspirin', p.22.

Poor renal perfusion can increase the risk of **renal failure** if angiotensin II receptor antagonists are given with NSAIDs and so regular hydration of the patient and monitoring of renal function is recommended.[11] The Australian Adverse Drug Reactions Advisory Committee consider that the triple combination of angiotensin II receptor antagonists or ACE inhibitors with diuretics and NSAIDs (including coxibs) should be avoided if possible.[1]

1. ADRAC. ACE inhibitor, diuretic and NSAID: a dangerous combination. *Aust Adverse Drug React Bull* (2003) 22, 14–15. Available at: http://www.tga.gov.au/hp/aadrb.htm (accessed 21/10/15).
2. Loboz KK, Shenfield GM. Drug combinations and impaired renal function –the 'triple whammy'. *Br J Clin Pharmacol* (2005) 59, 239–43.
3. Nawarskas JJ, Townsend RR, Cirigliano MD, Spinler SA. Effect of aspirin on blood pressure in hypertensive patients taking enalapril or losartan. *Am J Hypertens* (1999) 12, 784–9.
4. Stangier J, Su C-APF, Fraunhofer A, Tetzloff W. Pharmacokinetics of acetaminophen and ibuprofen when coadministered with telmisartan in healthy volunteers. *J Clin Pharmacol* (2000) 40, 1338–46.
5. Conlin PR, Moore TJ, Swartz SL, Barr E, Gazdick L, Fletcher C, DeLucca P, Demopoulos L. Effect of indomethacin on blood pressure lowering by captopril and losartan in hypertensive patients. *Hypertension* (2000) 36, 461–5.
6. Olsen ME, Thomsen T, Hassager C, Ibsen H, Dige-Petersen H. Hemodynamic and renal effects of indomethacin in losartan-treated hypertensive individuals. *Am J Hypertens* (1999) 12, 209–16.
7. Fogari R, Zoppi A, Carretta R, Veglio F, Salvetti A: Italian Collaborative Study Group. Effect of indomethacin on the antihypertensive efficacy of valsartan and lisinopril: a multicentre study. *J Hypertens* (2002) 20: 1007–14.
8. Fricker AF, Nussberger J, Meilenbrock S, Brunner HR, Burnier M. Effect of indomethacin on the renal response to angiotensin II receptor blockade in healthy subjects. *Kidney Int* (1998) 54, 2089–97.
9. Ciba. Data on file. Protocol 43.
10. Levy PD, Nandyal D, Welch RD, Sun JL, Pieper K, Ghali JK, Fonarrow GC, Gheorghiade M, O'Connor CM. Does aspirin use adversely influence intermediate-term postdischarge outcomes for hospitalized patients who are treated with angiotensin-converting enzyme inhibitors or angiotensin receptor blockers? Findings from Organized Program to Facilitate Life-Saving Treatment in Hospitalized Patients with Heart Failure (OPTIMIZE-HF). *Am Heart J* (2010) 159, 222–30.
11. Olmetec (Olmesartan medoxomil). Daiichi Sankyo UK Ltd. UK Summary of product characteristics, October 2009.

Angiotensin II receptor antagonists + Azoles

Fluconazole reduces the conversion of losartan to its active metabolite and decreases the metabolism of irbesartan but does not appear to affect the pharmacokinetics of eprosartan. Voriconazole might interact with these angiotensin II receptor antagonists in the same way as fluconazole.

Itraconazole does not have a clinically relevant effect on the pharmacokinetics or antihypertensive effects of losartan, and ketoconazole does not affect the pharmacokinetics of eprosartan or losartan.

Clinical evidence

(a) Fluconazole

1. Eprosartan. In a study, 16 healthy subjects were given eprosartan 300 mg twice-daily for 20 days, with fluconazole 200 mg daily on days 11 to 20. Fluconazole had no effect on the pharmacokinetics of eprosartan.[1]

2. Irbesartan. A study in 15 healthy subjects given irbesartan 150 mg daily for 20 days found that fluconazole 200 mg daily on days 11 to 20 increased the steady-state AUC and maximum levels by about 55% and 18%, respectively.[2]

3. Losartan. In a study, 16 healthy subjects were given losartan 100 mg daily (16 subjects) for 20 days, with fluconazole 200 mg daily on days 11 to 20. Fluconazole increased the AUC and maximum plasma levels of losartan by 69% and 31%, respectively, and reduced those of E-3174, the active metabolite of losartan, by 41% and 54%, respectively.[1] In a randomised, crossover study, 11 healthy subjects were given a single 50-mg dose of losartan after taking fluconazole (400 mg on day one and 200 mg daily on days 2 to 4). The AUC of losartan was increased by 27% while its maximum plasma level was reduced by 23%. The AUC and the maximum plasma levels of E-3174 were reduced by 47% and 77%, respectively. However, no clinically relevant changes in the hypotensive effect of losartan were noted.[3]

(b) Itraconazole

In 11 healthy subjects the pharmacokinetics and hypotensive effects of a single 50-mg dose of **losartan** and its active metabolite, E-3174, were not affected by itraconazole 200 mg daily for 4 days.[3]

(c) Ketoconazole

1. Eprosartan. In a study in 13 healthy subjects, ketoconazole 200 mg daily for 5 days was found to have no effect on the pharmacokinetics of eprosartan.[4]

2. Losartan. A placebo-controlled, crossover study in 11 healthy subjects given a single 30-mg intravenous dose of losartan, found that ketoconazole 400 mg daily for 4 days did not affect the conversion of losartan to its active metabolite, E-3174, or the plasma clearance of losartan.[5] The plasma clearance of a 20-mg intravenous dose of E-3174, the active metabolite of losartan, was also unaffected by pretreatment with ketoconazole.[5] Similarly, in a study in 14 healthy subjects, ketoconazole 200 mg daily for 5 days was found to have no effect on the pharmacokinetics of losartan and its active metabolite.[4]

Mechanism

It is thought that fluconazole inhibits the conversion of losartan to its active metabolite, mainly by inhibiting CYP2C9, although other isoenzymes might play a minor role. Similarly, irbesartan is primarily metabolised by CYP2C9 and is therefore also affected by fluconazole. Inhibition of CYP3A4 alone (caused by itraconazole and ketoconazole) does not appear to prevent the conversion of losartan to E-3174.

Importance and management

Evidence for an interaction between the azoles and the angiotensin II receptor antagonists appears to be limited to the studies cited, but what is known is in line with the expected pharmacokinetic interactions between these groups of drugs. **Ketoconazole** does not appear to affect the pharmacokinetics of either eprosartan or losartan, and therefore seems unlikely to affect the pharmacokinetics of other angiotensin II receptor antagonists. **Itraconazole** and **posaconazole** would be expected to behave in the same was as ketoconazole, and this suggestion is born out by the lack of effect of itraconazole on losartan pharmacokinetics.

In contrast, **fluconazole** does increase the exposure to losartan and irbesartan, but the study with losartan found that this did not result in changes in blood pressure. It therefore seems unlikely that a clinically relevant interaction will occur, although a note of caution might still be warranted as all the studies were in healthy subjects. Consider the possibility of an interaction if the blood pressure is undesirably lowered. Fluconazole does not appear to affect the pharmacokinetics of eprosartan. There appears to be no direct evidence regarding the use of **voriconazole** with the angiotensin II receptor antagonists, but it seems likely to behave in the same way as fluconazole.

1. Kazierad DJ, Martin DE, Blum RA, Tenero DM, Ilson B, Boike SC, Etheredge R, Jorkasky DK. Effect of fluconazole on the pharmacokinetics of eprosartan and losartan in healthy male volunteers. *Clin Pharmacol Ther* (1997) 62, 417–25.
2. Kovacs SJ, Wilton JH, Blum RA. Steady state pharmacokinetics of irbesartan alone and in combination with fluconazole. *Clin Pharmacol Ther* (1999) 65, 132.
3. Kaukonen K-M, Olkkola KT, Neuvonen PJ. Fluconazole but not itraconazole decreases the metabolism of losartan to E-3174. *Eur J Clin Pharmacol* (1998) 53, 445–9.
4. Blum RA, Kazierad DJ, Tenero DM. A review of eprosartan pharmacokinetic and pharmacodynamic drug interaction studies. *Pharmacotherapy* (1999) 19, 79S–85S.
5. McCrea JB, Lo MW, Furtek CI, Ritter MA, Carides A, Waldman SA, Bjornsson TD, Goldberg MR. Ketoconazole does not effect the systemic conversion of losartan to E-3174. *Clin Pharmacol Ther* (1996) 59, 169.

Angiotensin II receptor antagonists + Beta blockers

There appears to be no clinically relevant pharmacokinetic interaction between atenolol and either olmesartan or valsartan, and, as expected, concurrent use enhances blood pressure-lowering effects. The combination of angiotensin II receptor antagonists and beta blockers is in established clinical use.

Clinical evidence, mechanism, importance and management

A study in 18 healthy subjects given **olmesartan** 20 mg daily, **atenolol** 50 mg daily or both drugs together for 7 days found no clinically relevant pharmacokinetic interaction between **olmesartan** and **atenolol**.[1] In a single-dose, crossover study in 12 healthy subjects, the pharmacokinetics of **valsartan** 160 mg and **atenolol** 100 mg were not altered to a clinically relevant extent by concurrent use. The combination had some additive effects on resting blood pressure.[2]

Although pharmacokinetic information is apparently limited to these drug pairs, no clinically relevant adverse pharmacokinetic interaction would be expected between angiotensin II receptor antagonists and beta blockers, and the combination is clinically useful in a number of cardiovascular disorders.

1. Bolbrinker J, Huber M, Scholze J, Kreutz R. Pharmacokinetics and safety of olmesartan medoxomil in combination with either amlodipine or atenolol compared to respective monotherapies in healthy subjects. *Fundam Clin Pharmacol* (2009) 23, 767–74.
2. Czendlik CH, Sioufi A, Preiswerk G, Howald H. Pharmacokinetic and pharmacodynamic interaction of single doses of valsartan and atenolol. *Eur J Clin Pharmacol* (1997) 52, 451–9.

Angiotensin II receptor antagonists + Calcium-channel blockers

No clinically relevant pharmacokinetic interactions occur between nifedipine and candesartan or irbesartan, or between amlodipine and olmesartan, telmisartan or valsartan. Nisoldipine increases the exposure to telmisartan. Calcium-channel blockers have been given uneventfully with eprosartan, irbesartan, losartan, and telmisartan.

Clinical evidence, mechanism, importance and management

(a) Amlodipine

1. Losartan. A double-blind study in 198 patients with hypertension found that a fixed combination of amlodipine 5 mg with losartan 100 mg compared favourably in terms of blood pressure control and tolerability with either amlodipine 10 mg or losartan 100 mg given alone.[1]

2. Olmesartan. A study in 18 healthy subjects given olmesartan 20 mg daily, amlodipine 5 mg daily or both for 7 days found no clinically significant pharmacokinetic interaction between olmesartan and amlodipine.[2] Analysis of data from four phase I studies in healthy subjects and one phase III study in patients with hypertension found that the clearance of olmesartan and amlodipine were not affected to a clinically significant extent by concurrent use. The blood pressure lowering effect of both drugs in combination was greater than either drug alone, but slightly less than the sum of the effects of each drug.[3]

3. Telmisartan. In a study in 12 healthy subjects, telmisartan 120 mg daily had no clinically relevant effect on the pharmacokinetics of amlodipine 10 mg daily for 9 days, and there was no evidence of any notable effect of amlodipine on the pharmacokinetics of telmisartan. Although there were no serious adverse effects, mild to moderate adverse events (most commonly headache) occurred slightly more frequently with the combination, compared with amlodipine alone (19 events versus 12 events).[4] A placebo-controlled study in patients with moderate or severe hypertension found that combinations of telmisartan 40 to 80 mg with amlodipine 5 to 10 mg were effective at lowering blood pressure and the number of patients with adverse effects was comparable between combination and monotherapy groups.[5]

4. Valsartan. In 12 healthy subjects the pharmacokinetics of single oral doses of valsartan 160 mg and amlodipine 5 mg were not altered to a statistically significant extent by concurrent use, although the pharmacokinetics of valsartan showed wide variations between subjects.[6] A case report describes a 75-year-old woman who developed profound toxicity associated with the ingestion of a 'handful' of amlodipine 10 mg and valsartan 80 mg tablets. She had loss of vascular selectivity and prolonged hypotension associated with amlodipine that was refractory to conventional vasopressors. In addition, persistent loss of peripheral vasomotor tone attributed to valsartan probably increased the severity of the amlodipine toxicity.[7]

(b) Nifedipine

In 12 healthy subjects nifedipine 30 mg daily did not affect the pharmacokinetics of **candesartan** 16 mg daily to a clinically relevant extent.[8]

A randomised, crossover study in 11 healthy subjects given **irbesartan** 300 mg daily alone or with nifedipine 30 mg daily for 4 days, found that nifedipine did not alter the pharmacokinetics of **irbesartan**.[9] The UK manufacturer states that **irbesartan** has been safely given with antihypertensives, such as long-acting calcium-channel blockers.[10] Similarly the UK manufacturer of **eprosartan** notes that it has been safely given with calcium-channel blockers (such as sustained-release nifedipine).[11]

(c) Nisoldipine

In a study, 37 patients with hypertension were given **telmisartan** 40 mg daily, nisoldipine 10 mg daily or both drugs together for 3 weeks. The doses were then increased to **telmisartan** 80 mg daily, nisoldipine 20 mg daily, or a combination of **telmisartan** 80 mg daily and nisoldipine 10 mg daily for a further 3 weeks. The AUC of **telmisartan** 80 mg was increased by 132% when it was given with nisoldipine 10 mg and its clearance was lower, compared with telmisartan alone. There was a non-significant trend towards higher maximum plasma levels and AUC of nisoldipine when it was given with **telmisartan**. **Telmisartan** alone or with nisoldipine reduced blood pressure (reduction of 7 mmHg and 8.2 mmHg, respectively) whereas, in this study, nisoldipine alone had a smaller effect on blood pressure (reduction of 3.9 mmHg, which was not statistically significant). More study is required to confirm whether this pharmacokinetic interaction enhances antihypertensive efficacy with unchanged tolerability.[12]

1. Kohlmann O, Oigman W, Mion D, Rocha JC, Gomes MAM, Salgado N, Feitosa GS, Dallaverde E, Ribeiro AB. Estudo "LOTHAR": avaliação de eficácia e tolerabilidade da combinação fixa de anlodipino e losartana no tratamento da hipertensão arterial primária. The "LOTHAR" study: evaluation of efficacy and tolerability of the fixed combination of amlodipine and losartan in the treatment of essential hypertension. *Arq Bras Cardiol* (2006) 86, 39–51.
2. Bolbrinker J, Huber M, Scholze J, Kreutz R. Pharmacokinetics and safety of olmesartan medoxomil in combination with either amlodipine or atenolol compared to respective monotherapies in healthy subjects. *Fundam Clin Pharmacol* (2009) 23, 767–74.
3. Rohatagi S, Carrothers TJ, Kshirsagar S, Khariton T, Lee J, Salazar D. Evaluation of population pharmacokinetics and exposure-response relationship with coadministration of amlodipine besylate and olmesartan medoxomil. *J Clin Pharmacol* (2008) 48, 823–36.
4. Stangier J, Su C-APF. Pharmacokinetics of repeated oral doses of amlodipine and amlodipine plus telmisartan in healthy volunteers. *J Clin Pharmacol* (2000) 40, 1347–54.
5. Littlejohn TW, Majul CR, Olvera R, Seeber M, Kobe M, Guthrie R, Oigman W, on behalf of the study investigators. Telmisartan plus amlodipine in patients with moderate or severe hypertension: results from a subgroup analysis of a randomized, placebo-controlled, parallel-group, 4x 4 factorial study. *Postgrad Med* (2009) 121, 5–14.
6. Novartis Pharmaceuticals Ltd. Data on file. Protocol 37.
7. Smith SW, Ferguson KL, Hoffman RS, Nelson LS, Greller HA. Prolonged severe hypotension following combined amlodipine and valsartan ingestion. *Clin Toxicol* (2008) 46, 470–4.
8. Jonkman JHG, van Lier JJ, van Heiningen PNM, Lins R, Sennewald R, Högemann A. Pharmacokinetic drug interaction studies with candesartan cilexetil. *J Hum Hypertens* (1997) 11 (Suppl 2), S31–S35.
9. Marino MR, Hammett JL, Ferreira I, Ford NF, Uderman HD. Effect of nifedipine on the steady-state pharmacokinetics and pharmacodynamics of irbesartan in healthy subjects. *J Cardiovasc Pharmacol Ther* (1998) 3, 111–17.
10. Aprovel (Irbesartan). Sanofi Pharma Bristol-Myers Squibb SNC. UK Summary of product characteristics, June 2011.
11. Teveten (Eprosartan mesilate). Abbott Healthcare Products Ltd. UK Summary of product characteristics, September 2011.
12. Bajcetic M, Benndorf RA, Appel D, Schwedhelm E, Schulze F, Riekhof D, Maas R, Böger RH. Pharmacokinetics of oral doses of telmisartan and nisoldipine, given alone and in combination, in patients with essential hypertension. *J Clin Pharmacol* (2007) 47, 295–304.

Angiotensin II receptor antagonists + Dialysis or Transfusion membranes

An anaphylactoid reaction can possibly occur in patients taking losartan within a few minutes of starting haemodialysis using high-flux polyacrylonitrile membranes ('AN69') or modified ST-AN69 membranes. One study found no evidence of hypersensitivity reactions in patients taking either candesartan or valsartan and undergoing haemodialysis with AN69 membranes.

Clinical evidence, mechanism, importance and management

(a) Low-density lipoprotein (LDL) apheresis

A patient who experienced an anaphylactoid reaction while taking ramipril and undergoing dextran sulfate LDL apheresis took **losartan** 12.5 mg daily instead of ramipril without any reaction during the next four LDL apheresis procedures.[1] A patient taking imidapril had blurred vision and lacrimation with hypotension during dextran sulfate apheresis but when he was given **losartan** 50 mg daily instead of imidapril during LDL apheresis, blood pressure reduction was mild and he did not experience noticeable adverse effects. The blood pressure reduction was attributed to the effect of **losartan** on angiotensin receptors, but as bradykinin levels were increased (by the **losartan**) this could also have contributed.[2] The authors concluded that low-dose **losartan** appears to be safe in patients undergoing LDL apheresis with dextran sulfate,[1,2] despite an increase in bradykinin levels.[2]

(b) High-flux dialysis

A study in 11 patients with end-stage renal failure who had been receiving haemodialysis with AN69 membranes for at least 3 months found that the addition of either **valsartan** or **candesartan** did not result in any hypersensitivity reactions during 1 188 subsequent haemodialysis sessions.[3]

In a multicentre study, 324 of 406 haemodialysis patients who were given an initial dose of **losartan** 25 mg daily, increased after one week to 50 mg daily for 6 months, completed the study. Ninety-six patients were dialysed with AN69 membranes. Two of these patients had possible anaphylactoid reactions. One of them became hypotensive 13 minutes after the start of a haemodialysis session and developed malaise, nausea, vomiting, dysaesthesia and generalised heat sensation, severe enough to stop the dialysis session. The second patient had mild generalised heat sensation and dysaesthesia within one minute of the start of haemodialysis but did not require discontinuation of the dialysis. The symptoms did not occur on subsequent haemodialysis even though **losartan** was continued and an AN69 membrane was used. Neither patient developed signs of hypersensitivity such as oedema, bronchospasm, pruritus, or urticaria. Also, 9 of the patients who had an anaphylactoid reaction while taking ACE inhibitors during haemodialysis with AN69 membranes did not have anaphylactoid reactions when taking **losartan** and dialysed with these membranes.[4] Another patient taking **losartan** and undergoing haemodialysis developed breathlessness and became agitated with profuse sweating about one hour after the start of his first dialysis after changing from a *Haemophan* (COBE 400) membrane to an AN69 membrane in an attempt to improve the efficacy of dialysis.[5] However, it has been suggested that in this latter case, the adverse effects were not the result of an anaphylactoid reaction mediated by bradykinin.[6]

There are few reports of anaphylactoid-like reactions involving angiotensin II receptor antagonists and the use of AN69 membranes. The authors of one report found **losartan** to be a safe drug in haemodialysis patients and its use with AN69 was not associated with an increase in anaphylactoid reactions.[4] However, other authors advise caution.[5,6]

1. Elicio N, Bertolini S, Garbarini R, Nardiello G, Elicio A, Aimale V. LDL apheresis with dextran sulfate and angiotensin receptor antagonist (losartan). *Artif Organs* (1997) 21, 334–5.
2. Kojima S, Shida M, Takano H, Inami S, Yodogawa K, Yokoyama H, Kuramochi M. Effects of losartan on blood pressure and humoral factors in a patient who suffered from anaphylactoid reactions when treated with ACE inhibitors during LDL apheresis. *Hypertens Res* (2001) 24, 595–8.
3. Tepel M, van der Giet M, Zidek W. Efficacy and tolerability of angiotensin II type 1 receptor antagonists in dialysis patients using AN69 dialysis membranes. *Kidney Blood Press Res* (2001) 24, 71–4.
4. Saracho R, Martin-Malo A, Martinez I, Aljama P, Montenegro J. Evaluation of the losartan in hemodialysis (ELHE) study. *Kidney Int* (1998) 54 (Suppl 68) S-125–S-129.
5. John B, Anijeet HKI, Ahmad R. Anaphylactic reaction during haemodialysis on AN69 membrane in a patient receiving angiotensin II receptor antagonist. *Nephrol Dial Transplant* (2001) 16, 1955–6.
6. Krieter DH, Canaud B. Anaphylactic reaction during haemodialysis on AN69 membrane in a patient receiving angiotensin II receptor antagonist. *Nephrol Dial Transplant* (2002) 17, 943–4.

Angiotensin II receptor antagonists + Diuretics; Loop, Thiazide and related

Symptomatic hypotension can occur when an angiotensin II receptor antagonist is started in a patient taking high-dose diuretics. Potassium levels can be either increased, decreased or not affected by the concurrent use of an angiotensin II receptor antagonist and a loop or thiazide diuretic.

No clinically relevant pharmacokinetic interactions appear to occur between candesartan, eprosartan, irbesartan, losartan, olmesartan, telmisartan or valsartan and hydrochlorothiazide. Similarly, there is no clinically relevant pharmacokinetic interaction between valsartan and furosemide.

Clinical evidence

(a) Candesartan

In 18 healthy subjects, the concurrent use of hydrochlorothiazide 25 mg daily and candesartan 12 mg daily for 7 days increased the AUC and maximum serum levels of candesartan by 18% and 23%, respectively, and reduced the AUC of hydrochlorothiazide by 14%, but these changes were not considered to be clinically relevant.[1]

(b) Eprosartan

In 18 healthy subjects, eprosartan 800 mg decreased the AUC of hydrochlorothiazide 25 mg by about 20%, but this was not considered to be clinically relevant. In addition, hydrochlorothiazide had no effect on eprosartan pharmacokinetics.[2]

(c) Irbesartan

In a study, 12 patients with either hypertension or heart failure taking torasemide 10 mg daily for at least one week, were given irbesartan 150 mg daily. Irbesartan increased the AUC and half-life of torasemide by 13%, which was not considered to be clinically relevant.[3]

No clinically relevant pharmacokinetic interactions have been found between irbesartan and hydrochlorothiazide.[4]

(d) Losartan

In a study in 12 patients with mild or moderate hypertension given losartan 50 mg alone or with hydrochlorothiazide 12.5 mg daily for 7 days, the AUC of hydrochlorothiazide was decreased by 17% during concurrent use (not clinically relevant) while the pharmacokinetics of losartan were unchanged.[5]

In a study, in 12 patients with either hypertension or heart failure taking torasemide 10 mg (or for one patient 20 mg) daily for at least one week, the addition of losartan 50 mg on day one then 100 mg daily did not affect the pharmacokinetics of torasemide.[3]

(e) Olmesartan

No clinically relevant pharmacokinetic interactions have been found between olmesartan and hydrochlorothiazide.[6]

(f) Telmisartan

In a randomised, crossover study in 13 healthy subjects, telmisartan 160 mg daily was given with hydrochlorothiazide 25 mg daily for 7 days. There was no difference in AUC and maximum plasma concentrations of either drug, compared with when they were given alone.[7]

(g) Valsartan

In 12 healthy subjects, the relative bioavailability of furosemide 40 mg was reduced by about 26% when it was given with valsartan 160 mg. However, this pharmacokinetic interaction had no influence on the diuretic effect of furosemide. The simultaneous use of valsartan and furosemide did not modify the pharmacokinetics of valsartan.[8]

A single-dose study in 12 healthy subjects found that valsartan 160 mg reduced the AUC of hydrochlorothiazide 25 mg by 31%, but the mean amount of hydrochlorothiazide excreted in the urine does not appear to be notably changed. The pharmacokinetics of valsartan were not affected by hydrochlorothiazide.[9]

Mechanism, importance and management

No clinically relevant pharmacokinetic interaction appears to occur between angiotensin II receptor antagonists and loop or thiazide diuretics, although not all combinations have been studied. Probably of more clinical relevance than any pharmacokinetic effect is the potential for additive effects on blood pressure. Angiotensin II receptor antagonists and thiazide or related diuretics have useful additive effects in the control of hypertension and are generally well tolerated. For example, in one double-blind, placebo-controlled study in 604 patients with hypertension, losartan 50 mg given with hydrochlorothiazide 12.5 mg daily produced an additive reduction in trough sitting systolic and diastolic blood pressure, and the incidence of dizziness and headache was not notably different from placebo.[10] However, symptomatic hypotension, especially after the first dose, can occur when angiotensin II receptor antagonists are started in patients with heart failure or those with hypertension who also have sodium and/or volume depletion, such as those taking high-dose diuretics. It is recommended that any volume and/or sodium depletion should be corrected before the angiotensin II receptor antagonist is given. In some situations it might be appropriate to reduce the dose of the diuretic and/or use a lower starting dose of the angiotensin II receptor antagonist. A similar problem occurs with the ACE inhibitors, see 'ACE inhibitors + Diuretics; Loop, Thiazide and related', p.28. Further, angiotensin receptor II antagonists are potassium sparing, whereas loop and thiazide diuretics are potassium depleting. Giving an angiotensin receptor II antagonist with a diuretic could result in an increase, a decrease, or no change to the potassium levels, although logically adding an angiotensin II receptor antagonist to established treatment with a diuretic would seem more likely to raise potassium levels, and vice versa. Serum potassium should be routinely monitored when angiotensin II antagonists are used in patients with heart failure, renal impairment, or in the elderly.

1. Jonkman JHG, van Lier JJ, van Heiningen PNM, Lins R, Sennewald R, Högemann A. Pharmacokinetic drug interaction studies with candesartan cilexetil. *J Hum Hypertens* (1997) 11 (Suppl 2), S31–S35.
2. Blum RA, Kazierad DJ, Tenero DM. A review of eprosartan pharmacokinetic and pharmacodynamic drug interaction studies. *Pharmacotherapy* (1999) 19, 79S–85S.
3. Werner D, Werner U, Meybaum A, Schmidt B, Umbreen S, Grosch A, Lestin HG, Graf B, Zolk O, Fromm MF. Determinants of steady-state torasemide pharmacokinetics: impact of pharmacogenetic factors, gender and angiotensin II receptor blockers. *Clin Pharmacokinet* (2008) 47, 323–32.
4. Marino MR, Vachharajani NN. Drug interactions with irbesartan. *Clin Pharmacokinet* (2001) 40, 605–14.
5. McCrea JB, Lo M-W, Tomasko L, Lin CC, Hsieh JY-K, Capra NL, Goldberg MR. Absence of a pharmacokinetic interaction between losartan and hydrochlorothiazide. *J Clin Pharmacol* (1995) 35, 1200–6.
6. Kreutz R, Bolbrinker J, Huber M. Pharmacokinetics of olmesartan medoxomil plus hydrochlorothiazide combination in healthy subjects. *Clin Drug Invest* (2006) 26, 29–34.
7. Yong C-L, Dias VC, Stangier J. Multiple-dose pharmacokinetics of telmisartan and of hydrochlorothiazide following concurrent administration in healthy subjects. *J Clin Pharmacol* (2000) 40, 1323–30.
8. Bindschedler M, Degen P, Flesch G, de Gasparo M, Preiswerk G. Pharmacokinetic and pharmacodynamic interaction of single oral doses of valsartan and furosemide. *Eur J Clin Pharmacol* (1997) 52, 371–8.
9. Novartis Pharmaceuticals Ltd. Data on file. Protocol 07.
10. MacKay JH, Arcuri KE, Goldberg AI, Snapinn SM, Sweet CS. Losartan and low-dose hydrochlorothiazide in patients with essential hypertension. A double-blind, placebo-controlled trial of concomitant administration compared with individual components. *Arch Intern Med* (1996) 156, 278–85.

Angiotensin II receptor antagonists + Diuretics; Potassium-sparing

There is an increased risk of hyperkalaemia if angiotensin II receptor antagonists are given with potassium-sparing diuretics (such as amiloride and the aldosterone antagonists, eplerenone and spironolactone).

Clinical evidence

In a study in 13 hypertensive patients aged 61 to 83 years with mild chronic heart failure, the concurrent use of **valsartan** 80 mg daily and spironolactone 100 mg daily was considered to be effective and safe. However in one patient, the serum potassium level increased from 4.3 mmol/L to 5.8 mmol/L.[1]

An 84-year-old woman, taking several drugs including **losartan** 50 mg daily and **spironolactone** 25 mg daily, developed hyperkalaemia (potassium level 8.4 mmol/L), bradycardia, drowsiness and respiratory depression. She recovered after haemodialysis and ventilatory assistance.[2] There is also a report of life-threatening hyperkalaemia (9.4 mmol/L) in a patient with mild renal impairment given **candesartan** 8 mg daily and spironolactone 25 mg daily. Hyperkalaemia did not recur when she was given **candesartan** and a loop diuretic.[3]

Life-threatening hyperkalaemia occurred in 6 patients with congestive heart failure who were taking **spironolactone** and an angiotensin II receptor antagonist (**candesartan, losartan** or **telmisartan**).[4]

A study in patients with chronic heart failure taking **spironolactone** 25 or 50 mg daily, furosemide and either enalapril, **candesartan** 8 mg daily, or **losartan** 50 mg daily, for 12 months, found that hyperkalaemia occurred in about 9% of patients In patients given furosemide 40 mg and **spironolactone** 25 mg daily, *hypokalaemia* occurred in 14.3% and 6.5% of patients taking **losartan** or **candesartan**, respectively, but did not occur when patients were given **spironolactone** 50 mg daily.[5]

Mechanism

Angiotensin II receptor antagonists reduce the levels of aldosterone, which results in the retention of potassium. This would be expected to be additive with the potassium-retaining effects of amiloride, triamterene, spironolactone and eplerenone, leading to hyperkalaemia, but usually only if other risk factors are present.

Importance and management

The concurrent use of potassium-sparing diuretics (namely amiloride, triamterene and the aldosterone antagonists eplerenone and spironolactone) can increase serum potassium levels. Analysis of the patients in one of the studies cited, together with another 38 similar patients who had received ACE inhibitors,[4] identified certain conditions that could lead to the development of severe hyperkalaemia, which were:

- advanced age;
- dose of spironolactone greater than 25 mg;
- reduced renal function;
- type 2 diabetes.

Heart failure might also be contributory. Furthermore, a retrospective study in hospitalised patients who developed hyperkalaemia found that risk factors associated with a rapid rate of increase in serum potassium levels, in decreasing order of importance were:

- the use of potassium supplements;
- severe renal impairment;
- the use of ACE inhibitors or angiotensin II receptor antagonists;
- the use of potassium-sparing diuretics;
- diabetes mellitus.

The presence of two or more of these risk factors is associated with an even faster development of hyperkalaemia. As the rate at which hyperkalaemia develops is also correlated with its severity, the authors recommend close monitoring in patients with two or more risk factors, and that a rapid increase in serum potassium (greater than 0.5 mmol/L per day) should prompt the identification and possible removal of any risk factors for hyperkalaemia.[6]

Some consider that angiotensin II receptor antagonists and **amiloride** or **triamterene** should not normally be given concurrently. If, however, the use of both drugs is thought to be appropriate, the serum potassium levels should be closely monitored, particularly in those patients with additional risk factors, so that any problems can be quickly identified. Similar caution seems warranted on the concurrent use of **eplerenone** and an ACE inhibitor.

Aldosterone antagonists such as **spironolactone** can be useful in heart failure, but the concurrent use of an angiotensin II receptor antagonist requires increased monitoring of serum potassium. Note that the combination should be avoided in patients with a glomerular filtration rate of less than 30 mL/minute.[7] Hyperkalaemia associated with spironolactone is dose-related, but in the presence of an angiotensin II receptor antagonist, its occurrence might increase even if the dose of spironolactone is as low as 25 mg daily.[5] It has been recommended that the dose of spironolactone should not exceed 25 mg daily if an angiotensin II receptor antagonist is also given.[7]

1. Leone A, Bertanelli F, Mori L. Treatment of hypertension with valsartan combined with spironolactone. *Int Urol Nephrol* (2000) 32, 161–3.
2. Kauffmann R, Orozco R, Venegas JC. Hiperkalemia grave asociada a drogas que actúan sobre el sistema renina, angiotensina, aldosterona: un problema que requiere atención. Caso clínico. Severe hyperkalemia associated to the use of losartan and spironolactone. Case report. *Rev Med Chil* (2005) 133, 947–52.
3. Fujii H, Nakahama H, Yoshihara F, Nakamura S, Inenaga T, Kawano Y. Life-threatening hyperkalemia during a combined therapy with the angiotensin receptor blocker candesartan and spironolactone. *Kobe J Med Sci* (2005) 51, 1–6.
4. Wrenger E, Müller R, Moesenthin M, Welte T, Frölich JC, Neumann KH. Interaction of spironolactone with ACE inhibitors or angiotensin receptor blockers: analysis of 44 cases. *BMJ* (2003) 327, 147–9.
5. Saito M, Takada M, Hirooka K, Isobe F, Yasumura Y. Serum concentration of potassium in chronic heart failure patients administered spironolactone plus furosemide and either enalapril maleate, losartan potassium or candesartan cilexetil. *J Clin Pharm Ther* (2005) 30, 603–10.
6. Indermitte J, Burkolter S, Drewe J, Krähenbühl S, Hersberger KE. Risk factors associated with a high velocity of the development of hyperkalaemia in hospitalised patients. *Drug Safety* (2007) 30, 71–80.
7. Palmer BF. Managing hyperkalemia caused by inhibitors of the renin-angiotensin-aldosterone system. *N Engl J Med* (2004) 351, 585–92

Angiotensin II receptor antagonists + Epoetins

Epoetins can cause hypertension and therefore reduce the effects of antihypertensive drugs. It is not entirely clear whether angiotensin II receptor antagonists affect the efficacy of epoetins or not, but any interaction might take many months to develop. An additive hyperkalaemic effect is theoretically possible on the concurrent use of angiotensin II receptor antagonists and epoetins.

Clinical evidence

(a) Decreased epoetin effects

A crossover study in 33 proteinuric patients with preserved renal function treated for 6-week periods with placebo, **losartan** 100 mg daily, or **losartan** with hydrochlorothiazide 25 mg daily, found that the haemoglobin concentration was lowered by **losartan**, when given alone and with hydrochlorothiazide, but the erythropoietin concentration was decreased by **losartan** with hydrochlorothiazide only, but not by losartan alone.[1]

In a prospective study, hypertensive patients undergoing haemodialysis for more than 12 months and receiving epoetin were given either **losartan** 50 mg daily increased to 100 mg daily (20 patients) or amlodipine (20 patients) for 12 months. Twenty normotensive haemodialysis patients receiving epoetin were included as controls. It was found that the patients in the **losartan** group, but not those in the amlodipine or control groups, required higher doses of epoetin to maintain the same haemoglobin concentrations. This was apparent at 6 months, and at 12 months the epoetin dose had increased from the pre-study level of 90 units/kg per week to 129.5 units/kg per week.[2]

In one retrospective analysis of dialysis patients, 18 of 24 patients receiving **losartan** had decreases in haemoglobin concentrations, and 14 of these were using epoetin. A 3- to 4-fold increase in the epoetin dose was required in these patients to restore their haemoglobin concentration.[3] Consider also 'Table 2.5', p.34, for a study in which the effects of angiotensin II receptor antagonists and ACE inhibitors were considered collectively.

(b) No interaction

A prospective study in 15 haemodialysis patients found that **losartan** 50 to 100 mg daily for 3 months did not affect endogenous erythropoietin concentrations or affect the dose requirements of epoetin.[4] Another study in 14 haemodialysis patients found no difference in epoetin requirements between patients taking **losartan** 25 mg daily or placebo,[5] but the **losartan** was only given for 3 months.

(c) ACE inhibitors compared with Angiotensin II receptor antagonists

For a discussion of the studies comparing the effects of the angiotensin II receptor antagonists and ACE inhibitors on epoetin efficacy, see 'ACE inhibitors + Epoetins', p.33.

Mechanism

It has been argued that angiotensin II receptor antagonists might possibly reduce the efficacy of epoetin in haemodialysis patients for several reasons. A dose-dependent decrease in haematocrit is regularly observed when patients are given angiotensin II receptor antagonists. In most patients this decrease is small and not clinically important. However, in conditions such as erythrocytosis associated with renovascular hypertension or renal transplantation, the haematocrit-lowering effects of these drugs can be notable.[6] Another suggestion is that angiotensin II receptor antagonists might reduce testosterone concentrations in men receiving haemodialysis, but not in women, and this might be associated with resistance to epoetin.[7]

Importance and management

Antihypertensive effects

A frequent adverse effect of epoetins is an increase in blood pressure, possibly associated with the haemodynamic changes produced by the increase in haematocrit.[8] It is therefore important to control any existing hypertension before epoetin is started (the manufacturers contraindicate epoetin in uncontrolled hypertension). Blood pressure should be routinely monitored before and during the use of epoetins, and if necessary antihypertensives should be started or increased if the blood pressure rises.[9-11] This routine monitoring would seem sufficient to detect any interaction that affects the blood pressure-lowering effects of angiotensin II receptor antagonists. The dose of angiotensin II receptor antagonists might need to be increased, but if blood pressure rises cannot be controlled, a transient interruption of the use of epoetin is recommended.[9-11]

Reduced epoetin efficacy

There is limited evidence that angiotensin II receptor antagonists reduce epoetin efficacy, although one study suggests that epoetin resistance could develop in patients given high-dose losartan for 6 months or more.[2] It also is possible that the duration of the studies reporting no interaction was insufficient to detect an effect.

As the epoetin dose is governed by clinical response, no immediate intervention is generally necessary. More long-term study is needed. Compare also the effect of ACE inhibitors, see 'ACE inhibitors + Epoetins', p.33).

Hyperkalaemia

Drugs that block angiotensin II reduce the concentrations of aldosterone, which results in the retention of potassium. The manufacturers of epoetin alfa and beta comment that increased potassium concentrations have been reported in a few patients with chronic renal failure receiving epoetin, although they note that it is not an established adverse effect of epoetin.[9,10] An additive hyperkalaemic effect is therefore theoretically possible in patients given epoetin and also taking angiotensin II receptor antagonists. Serum electrolytes, including potassium, should be routinely monitored in patients using epoetin, and if potassium concentrations rise, consider withholding the epoetin until the potassium concentration is corrected.[9,10]

1. Erythropoietin is reduced by combination of diuretic therapy and RAAS blockade in proteinuric renal patients with preserved renal function. *Nephrol Dial Transplant* (2010) 25, 3256–60.
2. Odabas AR, Cetinkaya R, Selcuk Y, Keles S, Bilen H. The effect of high dose losartan on erythropoietin resistance in patients undergoing haemodialysis. *Panminerva Med* (2003) 45, 59–62.
3. Schwarzbeck A, Wittenmeier KW, Hällfritzsch U. Anaemia in dialysis patients as a side-effect of sartanes. *Lancet* (1998) 352, 286.
4. Lang SM, Schiffl H. Losartan and anaemia of end-stage renal disease. *Lancet* (1998) 352, 1708.
5. Chew CG, Weise MD, Disney APS. The effect of angiotensin II receptor antagonist on the exogenous erythropoietin requirement of haemodialysis patients. *Nephrol Dial Transplant* (1999) 14, 2047–9.
6. Marathias KP, Agroyannis B, Mavromoustakos T, Matsoukas J, Vlahakos DV. Hematocrit-lowering effect following inactivation of renin-angiotensin system with angiotensin converting enzyme inhibitors and angiotensin receptor blockers. *Curr Top Med Chem* (2004) 4, 483–6.
7. DeLong M, Logan JL, Yong K-C, Lien Y-HH. Renin-angiotensin blockade reduces serum free testosterone in middle-aged men on haemodialysis and correlates with erythropoietin resistance. *Nephrol Dial Transplant* (2005) 20, 585–90.
8. *Martindale. The Complete Drug Reference*, [online] London: Pharmaceutical Press. http://www.medicinescomplete.com/mc/martindale/current/ms-16635-r.htm (accessed 19/10/15).
9. NeoRecormon Solution for Injection in a Pre-filled Syringe (Epoetin beta). Roche Products Ltd. UK Summary of product characteristics, October 2011.
10. Eprex Pre-filled Syringe (Epoetin alfa). Janssen-Cilag Ltd. UK Summary of product characteristics, November 2012.
11. Epogen (Epoetin alfa). Amgen Inc. US Prescribing information, July 2012.

Angiotensin II receptor antagonists + Food

Food decreases eprosartan levels and slightly reduces the AUC of valsartan. Food has a negligible effect, or no effect, on the AUCs or bioavailability of candesartan, irbesartan, losartan, olmesartan, and telmisartan.

Clinical evidence, mechanism, importance and management

(a) Candesartan

A study in 18 healthy subjects found that a high-fat breakfast does not affect the bioavailability of a single 8-mg dose candesartan given 30 minutes later,[1] and therefore candesartan can be taken with or without food.

(b) Eprosartan

A study in 18 healthy subjects given a single oral dose of eprosartan found that a high-fat meal delays but does not affect the extent of eprosartan absorption. Eprosartan maximum plasma concentrations were decreased by about 25%.[2] The UK manufacturer recommends that eprosartan is given with food,[3] but the US manufacturer suggests that the change in bioavailability is not clinically relevant, and that eprosartan can be taken with or without food.[4]

(c) Irbesartan

In a study in 16 healthy men, a high-fat breakfast had no clinically relevant effects on the bioavailability of a single 300-mg dose of irbesartan,[5] and therefore irbesartan can be taken with or without food.

(d) Losartan

In a crossover study in healthy subjects, the AUC and maximum levels of a single 100-mg dose of losartan, given 30 minutes before a high-fat breakfast, was increased by 17% and 35%, respectively, when compared with the fasted state. Food caused a less than 10% decrease in AUC and maximum level of the losartan metabolite, E-3174.[6] These minor changes are unlikely to be clinically relevant, and the manufacturers state that losartan can be given with or without food.[7,8]

(e) Olmesartan

Food does not affect the bioavailability of olmesartan, and the manufacturers state that it can be given with or without food.[9,10]

(f) Telmisartan

Food reduces the AUC of telmisartan by about 6 to 20%, depending on dose, but this would not be expected to cause a reduction in therapeutic efficacy, and telmisartan can be taken with or without food.[11,12]

(g) Valsartan

Food decreased the AUC of valsartan by 40%, but the manufacturers state that it may be taken with or without food.[13,14]

1. Riddell JG. Bioavailability of candesartan is unaffected by food in healthy volunteers administered candesartan cilexetil. *J Hum Hypertens* (1997) 11 (Suppl 2) S29–S30.
2. Tenero D, Martin D, Ilson B, Jushchyshyn J, Boike S, Lundberg D, Zariffa N, Boyle D, Jorkasky D. Pharmacokinetics of intravenously and orally administered eprosartan in healthy males: absolute bioavailability and effect of food. *Biopharm Drug Dispos* (1998) 19, 351–6.
3. Teveten (Eprosartan mesilate). Abbott Healthcare Products Ltd. UK Summary of product characteristics, September 2011.
4. Teveten (Eprosartan mesylate). Abbott Laboratories. US Prescribing information, September 2012.
5. Vachharajani NN, Shyu WC, Mantha S, Park J-S, Greene DS, Barbhaiya RH. Lack of effect of food on the oral bioavailability of irbesartan in healthy male volunteers. *J Clin Pharmacol* (1998) 38, 433–6.
6. Marier J-F, Guilbaud R, Kambhampati SRP, Mathew P, Moberly J, Lee J, Salazar DE. The effect of AST-120 on the single-dose pharmacokinetics of losartan and losartan acid (E-3174) in healthy subjects. *J Clin Pharmacol* (2006) 46, 310–20.
7. Cozaar (Losartan potassium). Merck Sharp & Dohme Ltd. UK Summary of product characteristics, September 2011.
8. Cozaar (Losartan potassium). Merck & Co., Inc. US Prescribing information, July 2011.
9. Benicar (Olmesartan medoxomil). Daiichi Sankyo, Inc. US Prescribing information, June 2011.
10. Olmetec (Olmesartan medoxomil). Daiichi Sankyo UK Ltd. UK Summary of product characteristics, October 2009.
11. Micardis (Telmisartan). Boehringer Ingelheim Pharmaceuticals Inc. US Prescribing information, October 2012.
12. Micardis (Telmisartan). Boehringer Ingelheim Ltd. UK Summary of product characteristics, May 2011.
13. Diovan (Valsartan). Novartis. US Prescribing information, April 2011.
14. Diovan (Valsartan). Novartis Pharmaceuticals UK Ltd. UK Summary of product characteristics, March 2011.

Angiotensin II receptor antagonists + H_2-receptor antagonists

Cimetidine does not appear to have a clinically relevant effect on the pharmacokinetics of losartan or valsartan, and ranitidine does not appear to have a clinically relevant effect on the pharmacokinetics of eprosartan.

Clinical evidence, mechanism, importance and management

(a) Eprosartan

A single 400-mg dose of eprosartan was given to 17 healthy subjects, both alone and after **ranitidine** 150 mg twice daily for 3 days. The maximum plasma concentration and AUC of eprosartan were reduced by about 7% and 11%, respectively, but these changes were not statistically significant.[1]

(b) Losartan

In a randomised, crossover study in 8 healthy subjects, giving losartan 100 mg after **cimetidine** 400 mg four times daily for 6 days did not affect the pharmacokinetics and pharmacodynamics of losartan and its active metabolite, E-3174, to a clinically relevant extent, although there was a minor increase of 18% in the AUC of losartan.[2] No particular precautions are needed if these drugs are used concurrently.

(c) Valsartan

In a single-dose, crossover study, **cimetidine** 800 mg, given one hour before valsartan 160 mg, increased the initial rate of absorption of valsartan (attributed to a raised gastric pH) resulting in a roughly 50% increase in its maximum plasma concentration. However, the AUC was only slightly increased and there were large inter-subject variations in the pharmacokinetics of valsartan.[3] The changes in valsartan pharmacokinetics seen with **cimetidine** are unlikely to be clinically relevant.

1. Tenero DM, Martin DE, Ilson BE, Boyle DA, Boike SC, Carr AM, Lundberg DE, Jorkasky DK. Effect of ranitidine on the pharmacokinetics of orally administered eprosartan, an angiotensin II antagonist, in healthy male volunteers. *Ann Pharmacother* (1998) 32, 304–8.
2. Goldberg MR, Lo M-W, Bradstreet TE, Ritter MA, Höglund P. Effects of cimetidine on pharmacokinetics and pharmacodynamics of losartan, an AT_1-selective non-peptide angiotensin II receptor antagonist. *Eur J Clin Pharmacol* (1995) 49, 115–19.
3. Schmidt EK, Antonin K-H, Flesch G, Racine-Poon A. An interaction study with cimetidine and the new angiotensin II antagonist valsartan. *Eur J Clin Pharmacol* (1998) 53, 451–8.

Angiotensin II receptor antagonists + Mannitol

A report describes mannitol-induced acute renal failure in a patient with diabetes taking losartan.

Clinical evidence, mechanism, importance and management

A man with diabetic nephropathy taking **losartan** 25 mg twice daily for hypertension developed acute renal failure after being given a total of 420 g of intravenous mannitol over 4 days for haemorrhagic glaucoma. The patient recovered after the mannitol and **losartan** were discontinued, and after receiving haemodialysis.[1] It is not fully understood why this combination caused acute renal failure, but it might result in a marked decrease in glomerular filtration rate. The general relevance of this isolated case in unclear, but the authors of the report recommend caution on concurrent use.[1]

1. Matsumura M. Mannitol-induced toxicity in a diabetic patient receiving losartan. *Am J Med* (2001) 110, 331.

Angiotensin II receptor antagonists + Potassium compounds

Hyperkalaemia might develop if angiotensin II receptor antagonists are given with potassium supplements or potassium-containing salt substitutes, particularly in those patients where other risk factors are present.

Clinical evidence, mechanism, importance and management

Angiotensin II receptor antagonists are potassium-sparing, as a result of their effects on aldosterone, and their potential to cause clinically important hyperkalaemia is well established. The incidence of hyperkalaemia varies depending on the clinical indication and other disease conditions, being lowest in essential hypertension, and highest in heart failure, diabetes, and renal impairment. For example, the incidence of hyperkalaemia in clinical studies in patients with hypertension was 0.9% with **eprosartan**;[1,2] in those with heart failure the incidence was 6.3% with **candesartan**,[3] and in patients with type 2 diabetes with nephropathy, the incidence was 9.9% with **losartan**[4] and 18.6% with **irbesartan**.[5]

A retrospective study in hospitalised patients who developed hyperkalaemia found that risk factors associated with a rapid rate of increase in serum potassium levels, in decreasing order of importance, were: the use of potassium supplements, severe renal impairment, the use of ACE inhibitors or angiotensin II receptor antagonists, the use of potassium-sparing diuretics, and diabetes mellitus. Further, the presence of two or more of these risk factors was associated with an even faster rate of development of hyperkalaemia. As the rate of development of hyperkalaemia is also correlated with its severity, the authors recommend close monitoring in patients with two or more risk factors (which would include those taking potassium supplements with angiotensin II receptor antagonists), and that a rapid increase in serum potassium (greater than 0.5 mmol/L per day) should prompt the identification and possible removal of any risk factors for hyperkalaemia.[6]

Potassium supplements are generally unlikely to be needed in patients taking angiotensin II receptor antagonists, particularly if they have other risk factors for hyperkalaemia, and it might be prudent for such patients to be told to avoid using potassium-containing salt substitutes. If concurrent use is considered necessary, potassium levels should be closely monitored.

1. Teveten (Eprosartan mesilate). Abbott Healthcare Products Ltd. UK Summary of product characteristics, September 2011.
2. Teveten (Eprosartan mesylate). Abbott Laboratories. US Prescribing information, September 2012.
3. Atacand (Candesartan cilexetil). AstraZeneca. US Prescribing information, April 2011.
4. Cozaar (Losartan potassium). Merck Sharp & Dohme Ltd. UK Summary of product characteristics, September 2011.
5. Avapro (Irbesartan). Bristol-Myers Squibb Company. US Prescribing information, December 2011.
6. Indermitte J, Burkolter S, Drewe J, Krähenbühl S, Hersberger KE. Risk factors associated with a high velocity of the development of hyperkalaemia in hospitalised patients. *Drug Safety* (2007) 30, 71–80.

Angiotensin II receptor antagonists + Rifampicin (Rifampin)

Rifampicin slightly reduces the exposure to losartan and its active metabolite, E-3174. It seems possible that certain other angiotensin II receptor antagonists might be similarly affected.

Clinical evidence, mechanism, importance and management

Ten healthy subjects were given **losartan** 50 mg daily for a week and then, after a 6-day washout period, **losartan** 50 mg daily with rifampicin 300 mg twice daily for a week. It was found that rifampicin reduced the AUC of **losartan** by 36%, reduced its half-life from 2 hours to 0.9 hours, and increased its clearance by 60%. The AUC of the active metabolite, E3174, was reduced by 41% and its half-life was reduced from 5.1 hours to 2.5 hours. Diastolic blood pressure was reduced by **losartan** alone, but not by the combination.[1] The presumed reason for this interaction is that rifampicin (a recognised enzyme inducer) increases the metabolism of **losartan** to its active metabolite by CYP2C9.

The clinical importance of this interaction awaits assessment, but it seems possible that the antihypertensive effects of **losartan** could be reduced by rifampicin. If both drugs are used, be alert for the need to increase the **losartan** dose. There seems to be no information regarding other angiotensin II receptor antagonists, but note that **irbesartan**, and to a limited extent **candesartan**, are also metabolised by CYP2C9 (see under 'ACE inhibitors and Angiotensin II receptor antagonists', p.18) and so their exposure might also be reduced by rifampicin.

1. Williamson KM, Patterson JH, McQueen RH, Adams KF, Pieper JA. Effects of erythromycin or rifampin on losartan pharmacokinetics in healthy volunteers. *Clin Pharmacol Ther* (1998) 63, 316–23.

Angiotensin II receptor antagonists; Losartan + Amodiaquine

Amodiaquine inhibits the metabolism of losartan to its active metabolite, E-3174.

Clinical evidence, mechanism, importance and management

A study in 12 healthy subjects found that amodiaquine 600 mg, taken 2 to 3 hours before a single 25-mg dose of losartan, increased the metabolic ratio of losartan to its metabolite by 72% compared with baseline values for losartan. This was due to decreases in the metabolism of losartan to its active metabolite, E-3174, by amodiaquine and/or its metabolite, *N*-desethylamodiaquine, which inhibit CYP2C9.[1]

The clinical relevance of the findings of this study is unclear. The reduction in metabolism of losartan to its active metabolite might suggest that the therapeutic effects of losartan could be reduced. However, note that the effect of fluconazole (see 'Angiotensin II receptor antagonists + Azoles', p.43), which is a known potent inhibitor of CYP2C9, is probably not clinically relevant, which suggests the effect of amodiaquine is also unlikely to be clinically relevant.

1. Wennerholm A, Nordmark A, Pihlsgård M, Mahindi M, Bertilsson L, Gustafsson LL. Amodiaquine, its desethylated metabolite, or both, inhibit the metabolism of debrisoquine (CYP2D6) and losartan (CYP2C9) in vivo. *Eur J Clin Pharmacol* (2006) 62, 539–46.

Angiotensin II receptor antagonists; Losartan + AST-120

AST-120 has only a slight effect on the pharmacokinetics of losartan.

Clinical evidence, mechanism, importance and management

When a single 100-mg dose of losartan was given 30 minutes before a high-fat breakfast, with AST-120 3 g three times daily for 48 hours started 30 minutes after the breakfast, there was no statistically significant effect on the AUC of losartan, whereas there was a minor 12% decrease in the maximum losartan level. Similarly, various other schedules (losartan with breakfast, then AST-120 started 30 minutes later, or AST-120 started 30 minutes after breakfast, then losartan given 30 minutes after that), did not have a statistically significant effect on the AUC of losartan, when compared with losartan given 30 minutes before breakfast. However, there were slight increases in the AUC of losartan (of up to 37%) when these schedules were compared with losartan given in the fasting state, which was attributed to the effect of food.[1]

AST-120 is a predominantly carbon-based oral absorbent, and might therefore interfere with absorption of other drugs. Data from this pharmacokinetic study indicate that AST-120 has slight effects on the pharmacokinetics of losartan and so the authors suggest that giving AST-120 one hour after losartan might be preferred.[1] However, alterations in losartan exposure of this magnitude would not usually be expected to be clinically relevant.

1. Marier JF, Guilbaud R, Kambhampati SR, Mathew P, Moberly J, Lee J, Salazar DE. The effect of AST-120 on the single-dose pharmacokinetics of losartan and losartan acid (E-3174) in healthy subjects. *J Clin Pharmacol* (2006) 46, 310–20.

Angiotensin II receptor antagonists; Losartan + Erythromycin

The pharmacokinetics and blood pressure-lowering effect of losartan do not seem to be affected by erythromycin.

Clinical evidence, mechanism, importance and management

When 10 healthy subjects were given losartan 50 mg daily for a week and then, after a 6-day washout period, losartan 50 mg daily with erythromycin 500 mg four times daily for a week, it was found that erythromycin had no significant effect on the pharmacokinetics of losartan or its active metabolite, E-3174. In addition, erythromycin did not alter the blood pressure-lowering effect of losartan.[1] CYP3A4 inhibition alone does not appear to prevent the conversion of losartan to E-3174. There would therefore appear to be no reason to take any particular precautions if both drugs are used concurrently.

1. Williamson KM, Patterson JH, McQueen RH, Adams KF, Pieper JA. Effects of erythromycin or rifampin on losartan pharmacokinetics in healthy volunteers. *Clin Pharmacol Ther* (1998) 63, 316–23.

Angiotensin II receptor antagonists; Losartan + Fluorouracil

Fluorouracil inhibits the metabolism of losartan to its active metabolite, E-3174. The extent of inhibition appears to increase as the total cumulative dose of fluorouracil increases.

Clinical evidence, mechanism, importance and management

In a study, 17 patients with colorectal cancer, receiving fluorouracil 425 mg/m^2 and folinic acid as a one-hour infusion for at least 3 consecutive days for each cycle of treatment, were given a single 25-mg dose of losartan at least 2 days before the start of the first cycle of fluorouracil, and a further 25-mg dose on the last day of the cycle. Five of the patients were also given losartan 25 mg at the end of the third cycle. The ratio of losartan to its active metabolite, E-3174, increased from an average of 0.5 to 0.64 (28%) after the first cycle of fluorouracil, but there was large interpatient variation (ranging between a 71% decrease and a 223% increase) with increases in 10 patients and no change in one patient. The metabolic ratio increased after the third cycle of fluorouracil from 0.44 to 2.32 (a 5.3-fold increase) even though in 2 of the 5 patients the ratio had decreased after the first cycle of fluorouracil.

Fluorouracil appears to inhibit the metabolism of losartan to E-3174 by CYP2C9 and the inhibition becomes more pronounced as the cumulative dose of fluorouracil is increased.[1]

The clinical relevance of the findings of this study is unclear. The reduction in the metabolism of losartan to its active metabolite might suggest that the therapeutic effects of losartan could be reduced, but this remains to be established.

1. Gunes A, Coskun U, Boruban C, Gunel N, Babaoglu MO, Sencan O, Bozkurt A, Rane A, Hassan M, Zengil H, Yasar U. Inhibitory effect of 5-fluorouracil on cytochrome P450 2C9 activity in cancer patients. *Basic Clin Pharmacol Toxicol* (2006) 98, 197–200.

Angiotensin II receptor antagonists; Losartan + Grapefruit juice

Grapefruit juice has a negligible effect on the exposure to losartan and its active metabolite, E-3174.

Clinical evidence, mechanism, importance and management

In a study in 9 healthy subjects, grapefruit juice approximately doubled the time for a single 50-mg dose of losartan to be detected in the serum (from 40 minutes to 1.3 hours) and reduced the AUC of its active metabolite, E-3174, by 21%. Losartan is partly metabolised by CYP3A4 and transported by P-glycoprotein, both of which can be affected by grapefruit juice. This may explain the minor changes seen.[1] However, these pharmacokinetic changes are negligible and therefore this interaction is unlikely to be clinically relevant.

1. Zaidenstein R, Soback S, Gips M, Avni B, Dishi V, Weissgarten Y, Golik A, Scapa E. Effect of grapefruit juice on the pharmacokinetics of losartan and its active metabolite E3174 in healthy volunteers. *Ther Drug Monit* (2001) 23, 369–73.

Angiotensin II receptor antagonists; Losartan + Milk thistle

An extract of milk thistle containing silymarin appears to inhibit the metabolism of losartan to its active metabolite, E-3174.

Clinical evidence

In a study, 12 healthy subjects were given milk thistle capsules (standardised milk thistle extract, equivalent to **silymarin** 140 mg) or placebo three times daily for 15 days, with a single 50-mg dose of losartan on day 15. The AUC of losartan was increased about twofold in CYP2C9 extensive metabolisers (that is, those with normal levels of this isoenzyme) but not CYP2C9 poor metabolisers (that is, those lacking or deficient in CYP2C9). The AUC of the active metabolite of losartan, E-3174, was decreased by 17% and 13%, in the extensive metabolisers and the poor metabolisers, respectively.[1]

Mechanism

Silymarin appears to inhibit CYP2C9, the main isoenzyme involved in the metabolism of losartan. Losartan pharmacokinetics are affected in only the extensive metabolisers and not the poor metabolisers, as the poor metabolisers have minimal CYP2C9 activity.

Importance and management

Evidence for an interaction between milk thistle and losartan appears to be limited to this study, which did not assess the clinical relevance of the pharmacokinetic changes noted. However, a clinically relevant interaction seems unlikely, as changes of a similar magnitude (and greater, when considering the active metabolite) that occurred when fluconazole (a known CYP2C9 inhibitor) was given with losartan did not result in clinically relevant effects on blood pressure, see 'Angiotensin II receptor antagonists + Azoles', p.43.

1. Han Y, Guo D, Chen Y, Chen Y, Tan Z-R, Zhou H-H. Effect of silymarin on the pharmacokinetics of losartan and its active metabolite E-3174 in healthy Chinese volunteers. *Eur J Clin Pharmacol* (2009) 65, 585–91.

Angiotensin II receptor antagonists; Losartan + Phenobarbital

Phenobarbital has a negligible effect on the exposure to losartan and its active metabolite.

Clinical evidence, mechanism, importance and management

In a placebo-controlled study, 15 healthy subjects were given phenobarbital 100 mg daily for 16 days with a single 100-mg dose of losartan. Phenobarbital reduced the AUC of losartan and its active metabolite, E-3174, by about 20%, but this was not considered to be clinically important.[1]

1. Goldberg MR, Lo MW, Deutsch PJ, Wilson SE, McWilliams EJ, McCrea JB. Phenobarbital minimally alters plasma concentrations of losartan and its active metabolite E-3174. *Clin Pharmacol Ther* (1996) 59, 268–74.

Angiotensin II receptor antagonists; Losartan + Phenytoin

Phenytoin inhibits the metabolism of losartan to its active metabolite, E-3174.

Clinical evidence, mechanism, importance and management

In a crossover study in 16 healthy subjects, the concurrent use of phenytoin and losartan 50 mg daily for 10 days reduced the AUC of the active metabolite of losartan, E-3174, by 63%, but did not have a statistically significant effect on the AUC of losartan, and phenytoin did not alter the effect of losartan on blood pressure. The pharmacokinetics of phenytoin were not affected by losartan. In this study phenytoin was given at a dose of 4 mg/kg rounded to the nearest 100 mg, not to exceed 400 mg daily, and the dose was adjusted on the fourth day, if necessary, based on serum phenytoin levels. The effect of phenytoin appeared to be CYP2C9 genotype-specific, with increases in losartan AUC seen in the 14 subjects who were CYP2C9 extensive metabolisers (that is, those with normal levels of this isoenzyme) and decreases in the 2 subjects who were poor metabolisers (that is those lacking this isoenzyme).[1]

Both phenytoin and losartan are substrates for CYP2C9; however, it appears that phenytoin has an inhibitory effect on losartan metabolism. The conversion of losartan to E-3174 represents about 5 to 15% of the clearance of an oral losartan dose,[1] but E-3174 is much more pharmacologically active than losartan.

Although this study found that phenytoin did not affect blood pressure control in response to losartan, the moderate decrease in E-3174 exposure might be expected to have a clinically relevant effect in some patients. Therefore, until more is known, it might be prudent to suspect an interaction if blood pressure control is reduced in a patient taking losartan who is started on phenytoin.

1. Fischer TL, Pieper JA, Graff DW, Rodgers JE, Fischer JD, Parnell KJ, Goldstein JA, Greenwood R, Patterson JH. Evaluation of potential losartan-phenytoin drug interactions in healthy volunteers. *Clin Pharmacol Ther* (2002) 72, 238–46.

Angiotensin II receptor antagonists; Losartan + Tamoxifen

Tamoxifen might inhibit the metabolism of losartan to its active metabolite, E-3174.

Clinical evidence

In a study, 13 patients were given a single 25-mg dose of losartan 2 days before and 2 weeks after starting to take tamoxifen 20 mg daily. The metabolism of losartan was reduced in 10 patients (as assessed by an increase in the losartan to E-3174 metabolic ratio), but there was a wide inter-individual variation. The change in metabolic ratio in the 13 patients ranged from a decrease of 11% to an increase of 532%, with a median increase of 127%.[1]

Mechanism

Losartan is metabolised to its active metabolite, E-3174, by CYP2C9, and this study indicates that tamoxifen might inhibit this isoenzyme.

Importance and management

The clinical relevance of the findings of this study is unclear. The reduction in metabolism of losartan to its active metabolite might suggest that the therapeutic effects of losartan could be reduced. However, note that the effect of fluconazole (see 'Angiotensin II receptor antagonists + Azoles', p.43), which is a known potent inhibitor of CYP2C9, was probably not clinically relevant, which suggests the effect of tamoxifen is also unlikely to be clinically relevant.

1. Boruban MC, Yasar U, Babaoglu MO, Sencan O, Bozkurt A. Tamoxifen inhibits cytochrome P450 2C9 activity in breast cancer patients. *J Chemother* (2006) 18, 421–4.

Angiotensin II receptor antagonists; Telmisartan + Paracetamol (Acetaminophen)

No pharmacokinetic interaction occurs between telmisartan and paracetamol.

Clinical evidence, mechanism, importance and management

In a single-dose study in 12 healthy subjects telmisartan 120 mg had no effect on the pharmacokinetics of paracetamol 1 g. The pharmacokinetics of telmisartan were also unaffected by paracetamol, when compared with previous studies of telmisartan alone.[1]

1. Stangier J, Su C-APF, Fraunhofer A, Tetzloff W. Pharmacokinetics of acetaminophen and ibuprofen when coadministered with telmisartan in healthy volunteers. *J Clin Pharmacol* (2000) 40, 1338–46.

3

Alcohol

For social and historical reasons alcohol is usually bought from a store or in a bar or restaurant, rather than from a pharmacy, because it is considered to be a drink and not a drug. However, pharmacologically it is a drug that depresses the central nervous system. Objective tests show that as blood-alcohol levels rise, the ability to perform a number of skilled tasks gradually deteriorates as the brain becomes progressively disorganised. The myth that alcohol is a stimulant has arisen because at parties and social occasions it helps people to lose some of their inhibitions and it allows them to relax and unwind. Professor JH Gaddum put it amusingly and succinctly when, describing the early effects of moderate amounts of alcohol, he wrote that "logical thought is difficult but after dinner speeches easy." The expansiveness and loquaciousness that are socially acceptable can lead on, with increasing amounts of alcohol, to unrestrained behaviour in normally well-controlled individuals, through to drunkenness, unconsciousness, and finally death from respiratory failure. These effects are all a reflection of the progressive and deepening depression of the CNS.

'Table 3.1', p.52, gives an indication in very broad terms of the reactions of men and women to different amounts and concentrations of alcohol.

On the whole women have a higher proportion of fat in which alcohol is not very soluble, their body fluids represent a smaller proportion of their total body mass, and their first-pass metabolism of alcohol is less than men because they have less alcohol dehydrogenase in their stomach walls. Consequently if a man and woman of the same weight matched each other, drink for drink, the woman would finish up with a blood-alcohol level about 50% higher than the man. The values shown assume that the drinkers regularly drink, have had a meal and weigh between 9 and 11 stones (55 to 70 kg). Higher blood-alcohol levels would occur if alcohol was drunk on an empty stomach and lower values in much heavier individuals. The liver metabolises about one unit of alcohol per hour so the values will fall with time.

As alcohol impairs the skills needed to drive safely, almost all national and state authorities have imposed maximum legal blood alcohol limits. In a number of countries this has been set at 80 mg/100 mL (35 micrograms per 100 mL in the breath) but impairment is clearly detectable at lower concentrations, for which reason some countries have imposed much lower legal limits, even down to 0 mg/100 mL in some cases. Even within countries the legal limit can vary, depending on the type of vehicle being driven and the age of the driver.

Alcohol can interact with many drugs both by pharmacokinetic and/or pharmacodynamic mechanisms. The quantity and frequency of alcohol consumption can affect the bioavailability of alcohol and other drugs. Several hepatic enzymes are important in the metabolism of alcohol; primarily alcohol dehydrogenases convert alcohol into acetaldehyde, but other enzymes, in particular CYP2E1, are also involved, especially in moderate to heavy alcohol consumption. CYP3A4 and CYP1A2 might also have a role in the metabolism of alcohol.

Alcohol can induce CYP2E1 (and possibly other isoenzymes) after prolonged heavy intake, and this can result in an increased metabolic rate and lower blood levels of drugs metabolised by this isoenzyme. Conversely, short term binge drinking is likely to cause inhibition of this enzyme group by direct competition for binding sites and therefore decrease the metabolism of other drugs.

Probably the most common drug interaction of all occurs if alcohol is drunk by those taking other drugs that have CNS depressant activity, the result being even further CNS depression. Blood-alcohol levels well within the legal driving limit can, in the presence of other CNS depressants, be equivalent to blood-alcohol levels at or above the legal limit in terms of worsened driving and other skills. This can occur with some antihistamines, antidepressants, anxiolytics, hypnotics, opioids, and others. This section contains a number of monographs that describe the results of formal studies of alcohol combined with a number of recognised CNS depressants, but there are still many other drugs that await study of this kind, and which undoubtedly represent a real hazard.

A less common interaction that can occur between alcohol and some drugs, chemical agents, and fungi, is the flushing (*Antabuse*) reaction. This is exploited in the case of disulfiram (*Antabuse*) as a drink deterrent (see 'Alcohol + Disulfiram', p.67); however, it can occur unexpectedly with some other drugs, such as some antifungals and cephalosporins, chlorpropamide and metronidazole, and can be both unpleasant and possibly frightening, but it is not usually dangerous.

Table 3.1 Reactions to different concentrations of alcohol in the blood

Amounts of alcohol drunk ***Man 11 stones (70 kg)***	***Woman 9 stones (55 kg)***	***Blood-alcohol levels mg% (mg per 100 mL)***	***Reactions to different % of alcohol in the blood***
2 units	1 unit	25 to 30	Sense of well-being enhanced. Reaction times reduced
4 units	2 units	50 to 60	Mild loss of inhibition, judgement impaired, increased risk of accidents at home, at work and on the road; no overt signs of drunkenness
5 units	3 units	75 to 80	Physical co-ordination reduced, more marked loss of inhibition; noticeably under the influence; at the maximum legal limit for driving in some countries
7 units	4 units	100 or more	Clumsiness, loss of physical control, tendency to extreme responses; definite intoxication
10 units	6 units	150	Slurred speech, possible loss of memory the following day, probably drunk and disorderly
24 units	14 units	360	Dead drunk, sleepiness, possible loss of consciousness
33 units	20 units	500	Coma and possibly death

1 unit	= half a pint (300 mL medium strength beer)	= glass of wine (100 mL)	= single sherry or martini (50 mL)	= single spirit (25 mL)
	alcohol 3 to 4%	alcohol 11%	alcohol 17 to 20%	alcohol 37 to 40%

After Which? October 1984, page 447 and others.

Alcohol + Alpha blockers

The plasma levels of both indoramin and alcohol might be raised by concurrent use, and the combination has been reported to increase drowsiness. Prazosin appears to enhance the hypotensive effects of alcohol.

Clinical evidence

(a) Indoramin

When 10 healthy subjects were given a single 50-mg oral dose of indoramin together with alcohol 0.5 g/kg in 600 mL of alcohol-free lager, the AUC of indoramin was increased by 25% and its peak plasma levels were raised by 58%.[1,2] When the subjects were given a single 175-microgram/kg intravenous dose of indoramin together with the same oral dose of alcohol, a 26% rise in blood-alcohol levels occurred during the first 1.25 hours after dosing, but no change in indoramin pharmacokinetics were seen. The combination of alcohol and indoramin caused more sedation than either drug alone.[2]

(b) Prazosin

A study in 10 Japanese hypertensive patients found that alcohol 1 mL/kg decreased blood pressure for several hours. Treatment with prazosin 1 mg three times daily reduced blood pressure and enhanced alcohol-induced hypotension.[3]

Mechanism

Uncertain. Increased absorption of indoramin from the gut or reduced liver metabolism might be responsible for the raised indoramin serum levels. The increase in sedation would appear to be due to the additive sedative effects of the two drugs. The effects might be restricted to Oriental/Asian patients because the alcohol flush syndrome, caused by accumulation of vasodilative acetaldehyde due to a genetic alteration in aldehyde dehydrogenase, is rare in whites and blacks.[3]

Importance and management

Information is limited but the interaction between indoramin and alcohol appears to be established. The clinical importance of the raised levels of both drugs is uncertain. However as indoramin sometimes causes drowsiness when it is first given, there is the possibility that alertness will be reduced, which could increase the risks of driving or handling machinery. Patients should be warned. The clinical relevance of the drop in blood pressure with prazosin and alcohol is uncertain, as the dose of prazosin was relatively small and the dose of alcohol was relatively large; therefore these findings might not apply to more moderate drinking or higher doses of prazosin. Note that chronic moderate to heavy drinking can decrease the effects of antihypertensives, see 'Alcohol + Antihypertensives', p.55.

1. Abrams SML, Pierce DM, Franklin RA, Johnston A, Marrott PK, Cory EP, Turner P. Effect of ethanol on indoramin pharmacokinetics. *Br J Clin Pharmacol* (1984) 18, 294P–295P.
2. Abrams SML, Pierce DM, Johnston A, Hedges A, Franklin RA, Turner P. Pharmacokinetic interaction between indoramin and ethanol. *Hum Toxicol* (1989) 8, 237–41.
3. Kawano Y, Abe H, Kojima S, Takishita S, Omae T. Interaction of alcohol and an α_1-blocker on ambulatory blood pressure in patients with essential hypertension. *Am J Hypertens* (2000) 13, 307–12.

Alcohol + Amfetamines and related drugs

Dexamfetamine can reduce the deleterious effects of alcohol to some extent, but some impairment still occurs. Ecstasy can reduce subjective sedation associated with alcohol, without reversing the effects of alcohol on impulsivity or psychomotor skills. The combination of metamfetamine and alcohol produces an increase in perceived total intoxication, and might also increase cardiac adverse effects.

Alcohol can enhance the transient immune dysfunction associated with ecstasy. The concurrent use of alcohol and ecstasy results in very small changes in the pharmacokinetics of both drugs.

Clinical evidence

(a) Dexamfetamine

In 12 healthy subjects alcohol 0.85 g/kg (2 mL/kg of 100 proof vodka in orange juice) worsened the performance of a SEDI task (Simulator Evaluation of Drug Impairment).[1] This task is believed to parallel the skills needed to drive safely, and involves tests of attention, memory, recognition, decision making and reaction times. When the subjects were also given dexamfetamine 90 or 180 micrograms/kg, there was a dose-related improvement in the performance of the SEDI task, but the subjective assessment of intoxication was unchanged. Blood-alcohol levels reached a maximum of about 100 mg% at approximately one hour, and the bioavailability of alcohol was somewhat increased.[1]

Earlier reports using different testing methods found that in some tests dexamfetamine modified the effects of alcohol,[2,3] but the total picture was complex. Other reports found no antagonism.[4,5] Another study found that in stress situations, where relief of fatigue or boredom alone will not produce improved performance, dexamfetamine did not improve attentive motor performance impaired by alcohol.[6]

A 20-year-old-man had an acute myocardial infarction after drinking alcohol and taking a double dose of *Adderall XR* 30 mg (mixed salts of dexamfetamine and **amfetamine**). He had taken *Adderall XR* 15 mg alone before without any problems. Myocardial infarction can occur rarely with *Adderall XR* alone; however, in this case the high dose of the amphetamine and the concurrent use of alcohol were considered possible contributing factors.[7]

(b) Ecstasy (MDMA, Methylenedioxymethamfetamine)

1. Effect on behaviour or psychomotor skills. A study in 9 healthy subjects found that the combination of alcohol 0.8 g/kg and ecstasy 100 mg induced a longer lasting euphoria and sense of well-being than either ecstasy or alcohol alone. Ecstasy reversed the subjective feelings of sedation associated with alcohol, but did not reverse feelings of drunkenness, or the effects of alcohol on psychomotor performance.[8] Similarly, in a placebo-controlled, crossover study in 18 recreational users of ecstasy, alcohol-induced impairment in response inhibition tasks was not affected by single 75- or 100-mg doses of ecstasy. This indicated that the CNS-stimulating effects of ecstasy do not overcome alcohol-induced impairment of impulse-control or risk-taking behaviour.[9] In a placebo-controlled study, 18 healthy subjects were given a single 75- or 100-mg dose of ecstasy with sufficient alcohol to give a blood-alcohol level of 5 mg%. Alcohol alone impaired the performance of some psychomotor tests and driving performance. The addition of ecstasy improved the performance in some, but not all, of these tests. Subjects reported that the combined use of ecstasy and alcohol counteracted the feelings of sedation and lethargy caused by alcohol alone.[10] Another report also indicates that although ecstasy can reduce sedation in response to alcohol, it does not reduce the impairment of psychomotor skills caused by alcohol.[11] A further study found that the combination of ecstasy and alcohol reversed alcohol-induced sedation. Ecstasy alone increased psychomotor speed but did not affect psychomotor accuracy and alcohol alone impaired both. However, concurrent use improved psychomotor speed but impaired psychomotor accuracy,when compared with placebo.[12]

In a placebo-controlled study in 14 healthy subjects given a single 100-mg dose of ecstasy followed after 30 minutes by an infusion of alcohol 10%, given over 3 hours to maintain a blood-alcohol level of 60 mg%, concurrent use did not exacerbate the impairment of neuropsychological performance seen with either drug alone.[13]

2. Effect on immune system. A study in 6 healthy subjects found that a single dose of ecstasy produced a time-dependent immune dysfunction. Ecstasy impaired CD4 T-cell function, which is responsible for cellular immunity. Alcohol alone might produce a decrease in T-helper cells and in B lymphocytes, which are responsible for humoral immunity. Concurrent ecstasy and alcohol increased the suppressive effect of ecstasy on CD4 T-cells and increased natural killer cells.[14]

3. Pharmacokinetic studies. A study in 9 healthy subjects found that alcohol 0.8 g/kg increased the maximum plasma levels of a single 100-mg dose of ecstasy by 13%, with no change in its AUC. The AUC and maximum plasma levels of alcohol were reduced by 9% and 15%, respectively, after ecstasy use.[8] Another single-dose study in 18 recreational users of ecstasy found a similar decrease in mean blood-alcohol levels and a small increase in ecstasy levels when the two drugs were given together, but the results were not statistically significant.[9]

4. Other effects. A study in 14 healthy subjects found that a single 100-mg dose of ecstasy followed after 30 minutes by an infusion of alcohol 10%, given over 3 hours to maintain a blood-alcohol level of 60 mg%, did not affect cardiovascular function when compared with the effects of ecstasy alone. In addition alcohol attenuated the fluid retention associated with ecstasy and there was a trend for attenuation of ecstasy-induced temperature increase.[15]

(c) Metamfetamine

One study found that, while the combination of alcohol and metamfetamine diminished the subjective feelings of alcohol intoxication, there was actually an increase in feelings of total intoxication.[16] The combination of alcohol and metamfetamine might increase cardiac toxicity.[16]

Mechanism

Not understood. Although alcohol is a CNS depressant and the amfetamines are CNS stimulants, there is no simple antagonism between the two.[3]

Importance and management

Clear-cut conclusions regarding the potential interactions between alcohol and amfetamines cannot be drawn from the evidence presented in the reported studies. There is some evidence that the effects of alcohol are modified or reduced by amfetamines, but driving skills appear to remain impaired to some extent. The study using ecstasy suggests that this interaction could have implications for road safety, as subjects might consider they are driving better when actual performance is impaired by alcohol.[8] However, some studies used low amounts of alcohol and it has been suggested that the reported effects on neurophysiological functions might not reflect what happens with more commonly ingested amounts of alcohol.[17] The increase in perceived total intoxication noted in one report has been suggested as a possible reason for the popularity of the illicit use of the combination.[16]

Information about an increase in cardiac toxicity with the combination of an amfetamine and alcohol is limited, and no general conclusions can be drawn.

The effects of ecstasy and alcohol on immune function require more study; however, it has been suggested that the transient defect in immunological homoeostasis could have clinical consequences such as increased susceptibility to infectious diseases.[14]

1. Perez-Reyes M, White WR, McDonald SA, Hicks RE. Interaction between ethanol and dextroamphetamine: effects on psychomotor performance. *Alcohol Clin Exp Res* (1992) 16, 75–81.
2. Kaplan HL, Forney RB, Richards AB, Hughes FW. Dextro-amphetamine, alcohol, and dextro-amphetamine-alcohol combination and mental performance. In: Harger RN, ed. Alcohol and traffic safety. Bloomington, Indiana: Indiana Univ Press; 1966 p. 211–14.

3. Wilson L, Taylor JD, Nash CW, Cameron DF. The combined effects of ethanol and amphetamine sulfate on performance of human subjects. *Can Med Assoc J* (1966) 94, 478–84.
4. Hughes FW, Forney RB. Dextro-amphetamine, ethanol and dextro-amphetamine-ethanol combinations on performance of human subjects stressed with delayed auditory feedback (DAF). *Psychopharmacologia* (1964) 6, 234–8.
5. Newman HW, Newman EJ. Failure of dexedrine and caffeine as practical antagonists of the depressant effect of ethyl alcohol in man. *Q J Stud Alcohol* (1956) 17, 406–10.
6. Brown DJ, Hughes FW, Forney RB, Richards AB. Effect of d-amphetamine and alcohol on attentive motor performance in human subjects. In: Harger RN, ed. Alcohol and traffic safety. Bloomington, Indiana: Indiana Univ Press; 1966 p. 215–19.
7. Jiao X, Velez S, Ringstad J, Eyma V, Miller D, Bleiberg M. Myocardial infarction associated with Adderall XR and alcohol use in a young man. *J Am Board Fam Med* (2009) 22, 197–201.
8. Hernández-López C, Farré M, Roset PN, Menoyo E, Pizarro N, Ortuño J, Torrens M, Camí J, de la Torre R. 3,4-Methylenedioxymethamphetamine (Ecstasy) and alcohol interactions in humans: psychomotor performance, subjective effects, and pharmacokinetics. *J Pharmacol Exp Ther* (2002) 300, 236–44.
9. Ramaekers JG, Kuypers KPC. Acute effects of 3,4-methylenedioxymethamphetamine (MDMA) on behavioral measures of impulsivity: alone and in combination with alcohol. *Neuropsychopharmacology* (2006) 31, 1048–55.
10. Kuypers KPC, Samyn N, Ramaekers JG. MDMA and alcohol effects, combined and alone, on objective and subjective measures of actual driving performance and psychomotor function. *Psychopharmacology (Berl)* (2006) 187, 467–75.
11. Dumont GJH, Valkenberg MMGJ, Schoemaker R, Buitelaar JK, van Gerven JMA, Verkes RJ. Acute MDMA and ethanol interaction effects on psychomotor performance. *Br J Clin Pharmacol* (2007) 63, 503–8.
12. Dumont GJH, Schoemaker RC,Touw RC, Sweep FCGJ, Buitelaar JK, van Gerven JMA, Verkes RJ. Acute psychomotor effects of MDMA and ethanol (co-) administration over time in healthy volunteers. *J Psychopharmacol* (2010) 24, 155–64.
13. Dumont GJH, Wezenberg E, Valkenberg MMGJ, de Jong CAJ, Buitelaar JK, van Gerven JMA, Verkes RJ. Acute neuropsychological effects of MDMA and ethanol (co-) administration in healthy volunteers. *Psychopharmacology (Berl)* (2008) 197, 465–74.
14. Pacifici R, Zuccaro P, Hernández López C, Pichini S, Di Carlo S, Farré M, Roset PN, Ortuño J, Segura J, de la Torre R. Acute effects of 3,4-methylenedioxymethamphetamine alone and in combination with ethanol on the immune system in humans. *J Pharmacol Exp Ther* (2001) 296, 207–15.
15. Dumont GJH, Kramers C, Sweep FCGJ, Willemsen JJ, Touw DJ, Schoemaker RC, van Gerven JMA, Buitelaar JK, Verkes RJ. Ethanol co-administration moderates 3,4-methylenedioxymethamphetamine effects on human physiology. *J Psychopharmacol* (2010) 24, 165–74.
16. Mendelson J, Jones RT, Upton R, Jacob P. Methamphetamine and ethanol interactions in humans. *Clin Pharmacol Ther* (1995) 57, 559–68.
17. Cassel J-C, Hamida SB, Jones BC. Ethanol and MDMA: a comment on the paper by Dumont et al. *Psychopharmacology (Berl)* (2008) 200, 305–6.

Alcohol + Aminosalicylic acid

Alcohol can abolish the lipid-lowering effects of aminosalicylic acid.

Clinical evidence, mechanism, importance and management

The effectiveness of purified aminosalicylic acid recrystallised in vitamin C (PAS-C) and diet on the treatment of hyperlipidaemia types IIa and IIb was studied in a group of 63 subjects. It was noted that when 3 of the subjects drank unstated amounts of alcohol (beer or cocktails), the effects of the PAS-C on lowering serum cholesterol, triglyceride and LDL-cholesterol levels were completely abolished.[1] The reasons are not understood.

There seems to be no evidence that alcohol affects the treatment of tuberculosis with aminosalicylic acid.

1. Kuo PT, Fan WC, Kostis JB, Hayase K. Combined para-aminosalicylic acid and dietary therapy in long-term control of hypercholesterolemia and hypertriglyceridemia (types II_a and II_b hyperlipoproteinemia). *Circulation* (1976) 53, 338–41.

Alcohol + Amisulpride

No pharmacokinetic interaction appears to occur between amisulpride and alcohol. However, an isolated case report describes Pisa syndrome, which developed after an alcohol-dependent patient took amisulpride.

Clinical evidence, mechanism, importance and management

No clinically significant pharmacokinetic interactions were seen in 18 healthy subjects given single 50- and 200-mg doses of amisulpride with alcohol 0.8 g/kg, nor were the detrimental effects of alcohol on performance increased by amisulpride.[1]

An isolated case report describes a 57-year-old man with a history of alcohol dependence and liver cirrhosis who developed Pisa syndrome (a rare axial dystonia producing a postural disturbance) after taking amisulpride 200 mg daily for 10 days. Amisulpride was discontinued and symptoms resolved within 2 days. The authors suggested that alcohol dependence and liver cirrhosis might have contributed to the development of Pisa syndrome in this case via their effects on the dopamine system.[2]

The manufacturer states that the central effects of alcohol might be enhanced by amisulpride, and does not recommend the combination.[3]

1. Mattila MJ, Patat A, Seppälä T, Kalska H, Jalava M-L, Vanakoski J, Lavanant C. Single oral doses of amisulpride do not enhance the effects of alcohol on the performance and memory of healthy subjects. *Eur J Clin Pharmacol* (1996) 51, 161–6.
2. Kuo S-C, Yeh Y-W, Chen C-Y, Chen C-L. Low dose amisulpride induced Pisa syndrome in an alcohol-dependent patient with liver cirrhosis. *Prog Neuropsychopharmacol Biol Psychiatry* (2009) 33, 1080–1.
3. Solian Tablets (Amisulpride). Sanofi-Aventis. UK Summary of product characteristics, November 2011.

Alcohol + Antiepileptics

Moderate social drinking does not appear to cause a clinically relevant alteration in the serum levels of carbamazepine, ethosuximide, gabapentin, phenobarbital, phenytoin, sodium valproate or tiagabine. However, the adverse effects of both alcohol and some antiepileptics, such as enhanced sedation, could be additive.

Clinical evidence, mechanism, importance and management

A study in 29 non-drinking patients with epilepsy found that when they drank 1 to 3 glasses of an alcoholic beverage (1 to 3 units) over a 2-hour period, twice a week for 16 weeks, the serum levels of **carbamazepine**, **ethosuximide** and **phenytoin** were unchanged, when compared with a control group of 23 patients with epilepsy given drinks without alcohol. There was a marginal change in **phenobarbital** levels, and some increase in serum **valproate** levels. However, this effect is hard to interpret as **valproate** levels are known to fluctuate and are hard to reproduce. Other antiepileptics used were **clonazepam**, **primidone** and **sultiame**, but too few patients used these drugs to allow valid statistical analysis. Maximum blood-alcohol levels ranged from 5 to 33 mg%. More important than any changes that occurred in serum antiepileptic levels, was the finding that social drinking had no effect on the frequency of tonic-clonic convulsions, partial complex seizures, or on epileptic activity as measured by EEGs.[1]

In a study of patients with head injuries the clearance of unbound **valproate** was found to be increased (by up to 14%) in subjects who had measurable alcohol levels at the time of admission, when compared with those without detectable alcohol levels.[2] Another study in healthy subjects excluded any pharmacodynamic or pharmacokinetic interaction between **tiagabine** and alcohol. In this study, **tiagabine** 4 mg three times daily did not alter the effect of a single dose of alcohol, as assessed in a range of cognitive tests.[3] A study in 17 subjects who were considered to be heavy drinkers (average 34 drinks per week), found that **gabapentin** in doses of 1 g and 2 g did not affect the pharmacokinetics of alcohol, nor did it affect a number of subjective, physiological or performance measures, when compared with alcohol alone. However, the increase in heart rate seen with alcohol was increased to a statistically significant extent by gabapentin (exact figures not given).[4]

For the effect of chronic heavy drinking on the pharmacokinetics of carbamazepine or phenytoin, see 'Alcohol + Carbamazepine', p.64 and 'Alcohol + Phenytoin', p.81.

There are very few studies of alcohol use in patients with epilepsy, but there seem to be no reasons for these patients to avoid alcohol in moderate social amounts (1 or 2 drinks per occasion; no more than 3 to 6 drinks per week).[5] However, patients who drink moderate to heavy amounts of alcohol (3 to 4 drinks or more per occasion) should be warned that they are at increased risk of seizures, with the greatest risk occurring 7 to 48 hours after the last drink.[5] The British Epilepsy Association comments that drinking small or modest amounts of alcohol does not generally increase the risk of seizures, however some people (such as those with a history of alcohol abuse or those who have had alcohol-related seizures in the past) find that even a small amount of alcohol triggers their seizures.[6] Patients who drink heavily might also develop alcohol-withdrawal seizures, and binge drinking has been associated with seizures even in people who do not have epilepsy. The British Epilepsy Association also state that patients taking antiepileptics could be more sensitive to the effects of alcohol and alcohol can worsen the adverse effects of some antiepileptics.[6] A number of antiepileptics, such as **carbamazepine**, **clonazepam**, **phenobarbital** (see 'Alcohol + Barbiturates', p.59), **primidone**, and **topiramate**, have sedative effects, which could be additive with the CNS depressant effects of alcohol.

Individuals need to decide what level of alcohol intake is appropriate for them, and be aware that a change in medication, or an increase in the dose of their antiepileptic medication, could make them more susceptible to the effects of alcohol. Patients should also be made aware that drinking alcohol when taking antiepileptics might reduce their ability to perform certain skilled tasks, such as driving.

1. Höppener RJ, Kuyer A, van der Lugt PJM. Epilepsy and alcohol: the influence of social alcohol intake on seizures and treatment in epilepsy. *Epilepsia* (1983) 24, 459–71.
2. Anderson GD, Temkin NR, Awan AB, Winn HR. Effect of time, injury, age and ethanol on interpatient variability in valproic acid pharmacokinetics after traumatic brain injury. *Clin Pharmacokinet* (2007) 46, 307–318.
3. Kastberg H, Jansen JA, Cole G, Wesnes K. Tiagabine: absence of kinetic or dynamic interactions with ethanol. *Drug Metabol Drug Interact* (1998) 14, 259–73.
4. Bisaga A, Evans SM. The acute effects of gabapentin in combination with alcohol in heavy drinkers. *Drug Alcohol Depend* (2006) 83, 25–32.
5. Gordon E, Devinsky O. Alcohol and marijuana: effects on epilepsy and use by patients with epilepsy. *Epilepsia* (2001) 42, 1266–72.
6. British Epilepsy Association. Epilepsy and alcohol. Available at: https://www.epilepsy.org.uk/info/alcohol (accessed 21/10/15).

Alcohol + Antihistamines

Some antihistamines cause drowsiness, which can be increased by alcohol. The detrimental effects of alcohol on driving skills are considerably increased by the use of the more sedative antihistamines and appear to be minimally affected by the non-sedating antihistamines.

Clinical evidence

(a) Non-sedating antihistamines

Acrivastine 4 mg and 8 mg, given with and without alcohol, was found in a study to behave like terfenadine (which interacts minimally or not at all).[1] Other studies have shown that **desloratadine**,[2] **ebastine** 20 mg,[3] **fexofenadine** 120 to 240 mg,[4,5] **levocabastine** 2 nasal puffs of 0.5 mg/mL,[6] **loratadine** 10 to 20 mg[7,8] and **mizolastine** 10 mg[9] do not interact with alcohol. **Cetirizine** 10 mg did not appear to interact with alcohol in two studies[9,10] but some slight additive effects were detected in other studies.[8,11] Similarly, a single oral dose of **rupatadine** 10 mg did not interact with alcohol, but a 20-mg dose given with alcohol produced more cognitive and psychomotor impairment than alcohol alone.[11]

(b) Sedating antihistamines

The effects of alcohol (blood levels about 50 mg%) and antihistamines, alone or together, on the performance of tests designed to assess mental and motor performance were studied in 16 subjects. **Clemizole** 40 mg alone or **tripelennamine** 50 mg alone did not notably affect the performance under the stress of delayed auditory feedback, neither did they potentiate the effect of alcohol.[12] **Clemastine** in 3-mg doses had some additive detrimental effects with alcohol on co-ordination, whereas **clemastine** 1.5 mg and 1 mg did not.[13,14] A study in 5 subjects found that the detrimental effects of 100 mL of whisky on the performance of driving tests on a racing car simulator (blood-alcohol level estimated as less than 80 mg%) were not increased by **cyclizine** 50 mg.[15] However 3 of the subjects experienced drowsiness after **cyclizine**, and other studies have shown that **cyclizine** alone causes drowsiness in the majority of subjects.[16] Impairment of psychomotor performance was seen in healthy subjects given **chlorphenamine** 12 mg with alcohol 0.5 g/kg.[17] A further study similarly found impairment in driving skills when **chlorphenamine** was given with alcohol, see under *Significantly-sedating antihistamines*, below. In 13 healthy subjects alcohol 0.75 g/kg given with **dexchlorpheniramine** 4 mg/70 kg impaired the performance of a number of tests (standing steadiness, reaction time, manual dexterity, perception, etc.).[18] A study in 17 subjects found that **mebhydrolin** 0.71 mg/kg enhanced the alcohol-induced deficits in the performance of a number of tests of perceptual, cognitive and motor functions.[19] No interaction was detected in one study of the combined effects of **pheniramine aminosalicylate** 50 mg or **cyproheptadine hydrochloride** 4 mg and alcohol 0.95 mL/kg.[20] **Triprolidine** 10 mg alone can affect driving performance,[7] and marked deterioration in driving skills has been seen with 10 mL of *Actifed Syrup* (**triprolidine** with pseudoephedrine) alone and with a double whiskey.[21]

(c) Significantly-sedating antihistamines

Diphenhydramine in doses of 25 or 50 mg was shown to increase the detrimental effects of alcohol on the performance of choice reaction and co-ordination tests in subjects who had taken 0.5 g/kg of alcohol.[13] The interaction between **diphenhydramine** in doses of 50, 75 or 100 mg and alcohol 0.5 to 0.75 g/kg has been confirmed in other reports.[12,22-25] **Emedastine**, in oral doses of 2 or 4 mg twice daily, was found to be sedating and impair driving ability in 19 healthy subjects. The addition of alcohol increased this impairment.[26] A marked interaction can also occur with **hydroxyzine**[5,11] or **promethazine**.[27] A very marked deterioration in driving skills was clearly demonstrated in a test of car drivers given 20 mL of *Beechams Night Nurse* (**promethazine** with dextromethorphan), 10 mL of *Benylin* (**diphenhydramine** with dextromethorphan), or 30 mL of *Lemsip Night time flu medicine* (**chlorphenamine** with dextromethorphan). Very poor scores were seen when they were also given a double Scotch whisky about 1.5 hours later.[21]

Mechanism

When an interaction occurs it appears to be due to the combined or additive central nervous depressant effects of both the alcohol and the antihistamine. The highly-sedating antihistamines are highly lipophilic and readily cross the blood-brain barrier; consequently they have considerable sedative effects that can persist into the next day. The sedating antihistamines do not cross the blood-brain barrier so readily, and are therefore less sedating. Most of the non-sedating antihistamines, such as fexofenadine, do not appear to cross the blood-brain barrier,[5] and would therefore not be expected to cause much, if any, sedation. The authors of one study found that the sedating effects of cetirizine and emedastine were more marked in women than in men, and they noted that they had also previously seen this with acrivastine, clemastine and mizolastine.[26] The reason for this is not established although it has been suggested that a smaller volume of distribution in women might result in higher plasma antihistamine levels.

Importance and management

An adverse interaction between alcohol and the **highly-sedating antihistamines** (see 'Table 15.1', p.628, for a list) is well established and clinically important. Marked drowsiness can occur with these antihistamines taken alone, which makes driving or handling other potentially dangerous machinery much more hazardous. This can be further worsened by alcohol. Patients should be warned. Remember that some of these antihistamines are present in non-prescription products licensed as antiemetics and sedatives, and as components of cough, cold, and influenza remedies (e.g. some preparations of *Benylin*, *Lemsip*, and *Night Nurse*). Emedastine can also cause marked sedation when used orally, but it is usually given as eye drops, and its use by this route would not be expected to result in a clinically relevant interaction with alcohol.

The situation with some of the **sedating antihistamines** (see 'Table 15.1', p.628, for a list) is less clear cut, and tests with some of them did not detect an interaction with normal doses and moderate amounts of alcohol; however, it has been clearly seen with *Actifed Syrup* (containing triprolidine). It would therefore be prudent to issue some cautionary warning, particularly if the patient is likely to drive.

The **non-sedating antihistamines** (see 'Table 15.1', p.628, for a list) seem to cause little or no drowsiness in most patients and the risks if taken alone or with alcohol appear to be minimal or absent. However, the incidence of sedation varies with the non-sedating antihistamine (e.g. sedation appears to be lower with fexofenadine and loratadine than with acrivastine or cetirizine)[28] and with the individual (e.g. women might be more affected than men).[26] Therefore, patients should be advised to be alert to the possibility of drowsiness if they have not taken the drug before. Any drowsiness would be apparent after the first few doses.

The possible interactions of alcohol with other antihistamines not cited here do not seem to have been formally studied, but increased drowsiness and increased driving risks would be expected with any that cause some sedation. Patients should be warned about drinking alcohol when taking sedative antihistamines. The risks with antihistamines given as eye drops or nasal spray (e.g. **azelastine**, **epinastine**) are probably minimal, but this needs confirmation.

1. Cohen AF, Hamilton MJ, Peck AW. The effects of acrivastine (BW825C), diphenhydramine and terfenadine in combination with alcohol on human CNS performance. *Eur J Clin Pharmacol* (1987) 32, 279–88.
2. Scharf M, Berkowitz. Effects of desloratadine and alcohol coadministration on psychomotor performance. *Curr Med Res Opin* (2007) 23, 313–21.
3. Mattila MJ, Kuitunen T, Plétan Y. Lack of pharmacodynamic and pharmacokinetic interactions of the antihistamine ebastine with ethanol in healthy subjects. *Eur J Clin Pharmacol* (1992) 43, 179–84.
4. Vermeeren A, O'Hanlon JF. Fexofenadine's effects, alone and with alcohol, on actual driving and psychomotor performance. *J Allergy Clin Immunol* (1998) 101, 306–11.
5. Ridout F, Shamsi Z, Meadows R, Johnson S, Hindmarch I. A single-center, randomized, double-blind, placebo-controlled, crossover investigation of the effects of fexofenadine hydrochloride 180 mg alone and with alcohol, with hydroxyzine hydrochloride 50 mg as a positive internal control, on aspects of cognitive and psychomotor function related to driving a car. *Clin Ther* (2003) 25, 1518–38.
6. Nicholls A, Janssens M, James R. The effects of levocabastine and ethanol on psychomotor performance in healthy volunteers. *Allergy* (1993) 48 (Suppl 16), 34.
7. O'Hanlon JF. Antihistamines and driving performance: The Netherlands. *J Respir Dis* (1988) (Suppl), S12–S17.
8. Ramaekers JG, Uiterwijk MMC, O'Hanlon JF. Effects of loratadine and cetirizine on actual driving and psychometric test performance, and EEG during driving. *Eur J Clin Pharmacol* (1992) 42, 363–9.
9. Patat A, Stubbs D, Dunmore C, Ulliac N, Sexton B, Zieleniuk I, Irving A, Jones W. Lack of interaction between two antihistamines, mizolastine and cetirizine, and ethanol in psychomotor and driving performance in healthy subjects. *Eur J Clin Pharmacol* (1995) 48, 143–50.
10. Doms M, Vanhulle G, Baelde Y, Coulie P, Dupont P, Rihoux J-P. Lack of potentiation by cetirizine of alcohol-induced psychomotor disturbances. *Eur J Clin Pharmacol* (1988) 34, 619–23.
11. Barbanoj MJ, García-Gea C, Antonijoan R, Izquierdo I, Donado E, Pérez I, Solans A, Jané F. Evaluation of the cognitive, psychomotor and pharmacokinetic profiles of rupatadine, hydroxyzine and cetirizine, in combination with alcohol, in healthy volunteers. *Hum Psychopharmacol* (2006) 21, 13–26.
12. Hughes FW, Forney RB. Comparative effect of three antihistaminics and ethanol on mental and motor performance. *Clin Pharmacol Ther* (1964) 5, 414–21.
13. Linnoila M. Effects of antihistamines, chlormezanone and alcohol on psychomotor skills related to driving. *Eur J Clin Pharmacol* (1973) 5, 247–54.
14. Franks HM, Hensley VR, Hensley WJ, Starmer GA, Teo RKC. The interaction between ethanol and antihistamines. 2. Clemastine. *Med J Aust* (1979) 1, 185–6.
15. Hughes DTD, Cramer F, Knight GJ. Use of a racing car simulator for medical research. The effects of marzine and alcohol on driving performance. *Med Sci Law* (1967) 7, 200–4.
16. Brand JJ, Colquhoun WP, Gould AH, Perry WLM. (–)-Hyoscine and cyclizine as motion sickness remedies. *Br J Pharmacol Chemother* (1967) 30, 463–9.
17. Hindmarch I, Bhatti JZ. Psychomotor effects of astemizole and chlorpheniramine, alone and in combination with alcohol. *Int Clin Psychopharmacol* (1987) 2, 117–19.
18. Franks HM, Hensley VR, Hensley WJ, Starmer GA, Teo RKC. The interaction between ethanol and antihistamines. 1: Dexchlorpheniramine. *Med J Aust* (1978) 1, 449–52.
19. Franks HM, Lawrie M, Schabinsky VV, Starmer GA, Teo RKC. Interaction between ethanol and antihistamines. 3. mebhydrolin. *Med J Aust* (1981) 2, 477–9.
20. Landauer AA, Milner G. Antihistamines, alone and together with alcohol, in relation to driving safety. *J Forensic Med* (1971) 18, 127–39.
21. Carter N. Cold cures drug alert. *Auto Express* (1992) November Issue 218, 15–16.
22. Moser L, Hüther KJ, Koch-Weser J, Lundt PV. Effects of terfenadine and diphenhydramine alone or in combination with diazepam or alcohol on psychomotor performance and subjective feelings. *Eur J Clin Pharmacol* (1978) 14, 417–23.
23. Baugh R, Calvert RT. The effect of diphenhydramine alone and in combination with ethanol on histamine skin response and mental performance. *Eur J Clin Pharmacol* (1977) 12, 201–4.
24. Burns M, Moskowitz H. Effects of diphenhydramine and alcohol on skills performance. *Eur J Clin Pharmacol* (1980) 17, 259–66.
25. Burns M. Alcohol and antihistamine in combination: effects on performance. *Alcohol Clin Exp Res* (1989) 13, 341.
26. Vermeeren A, Ramaekers JG, O'Hanlon JF. Effects of emedastine and cetirizine, alone and with alcohol, on actual driving of males and females. *J Psychopharmacol* (2002) 16, 57–64.
27. Hedges A, Hills M, Maclay WP, Newman-Taylor AJ, Turner P. Some central and peripheral effects of meclastine, a new antihistaminic drug, in man. *J Clin Pharmacol* (1971) 11, 112–19.
28. Mann RD, Pearce GL, Dunn N, Shakir S. Sedation with "non-sedating" antihistamines: four prescription-event monitoring studies in general practice. *BMJ* (2000) 320, 1184–6.

Alcohol + Antihypertensives

Chronic moderate to heavy drinking raises blood pressure and reduces, to some extent, the effectiveness of antihypertensive drugs. A few patients experience postural hypotension, dizziness and fainting shortly after having drunk alcohol. Alpha blockers might enhance the hypotensive effect of alcohol in subjects susceptible to the alcohol flush syndrome.

Clinical evidence, mechanism, importance and management

(a) Hypertensive reaction

A study in 40 men with essential hypertension (taking **beta blockers**, **captopril**, **diuretics**, **methyldopa**, **prazosin** or **verapamil**) who were moderate to heavy drinkers, found that when they reduced their drinking over a 6-week period from an average of 450 mL of alcohol weekly (about 6 drinks daily) to 64 mL of alcohol weekly, their average blood pressure fell by 5/3 mmHg.[1] The reasons for this effect are uncertain.

The Atherosclerosis Risk in Communities (ARIC) study involving 8 334 subjects who were free from hypertension at baseline and were assessed after 6 years, found that higher levels of consumption of alcoholic beverages (210 g or more of alcohol per week; approximately 3 drinks or more per day) were associated with a higher risk of hypertension. Low to moderate consumption of alcohol (up to 3 drinks daily) was associated with an increase in blood pressure in black, but not in white men.[2] A study in Japanese men found that the effect of alcohol intake on the risk of developing hypertension was dose-dependent, starting at low-to-moderate levels of alcohol (less than 23 g daily).[3]

These findings are consistent with those of other studies in hypertensive[4] and normotensive[5] subjects. It seems likely that this effect will occur with any antihypertensive. Patients with hypertension who are moderate to heavy drinkers should be encouraged to reduce their intake of alcohol. It might then become possible to reduce the dose of the antihypertensive. It should be noted that epidemiological studies show that regular light to moderate alcohol consumption is associated with a *lower* risk of cardiovascular disease.[6]

(b) Hypotensive reaction

A few patients taking some antihypertensives feel dizzy or begin to 'black out' or faint if they stand up quickly or after exercise. This orthostatic and exertional hypotension might be exaggerated in some patients shortly after drinking alcohol, possibly because it can lower the cardiac output (noted in patients with various types of heart disease[7,8]). Patients should be warned. For other reports of postural hypotension with alcohol, see 'Alcohol + Alpha blockers', p.53, and 'Alcohol + Calcium-channel blockers', p.63.

(c) CNS and other effects

For mention of the possibility of increased sedation with alcohol and clonidine or indoramin, see 'Clonidine and related drugs + CNS depressants', p.1056, and 'Alcohol + Alpha blockers', p.53.

For the possible CNS effects of beta blockers and alcohol, see 'Alcohol + Beta blockers', p.61.

For mention of the disulfiram-like reaction when tolazoline is given with alcohol, see 'Alcohol + Tolazoline', p.86.

1. Puddey IB, Beilin LJ, Vandongen R. Regular alcohol use raises blood pressure in treated hypertensive subjects. A randomised controlled trial. *Lancet* (1987) i, 647–51.
2. Fuchs FD, Chambless LE, Whelton PK, Nieto FJ, Heiss G. Alcohol consumption and the incidence of hypertension. The Atherosclerosis Risk in Communities Study. *Hypertension* (2001) 37, 1242–50.
3. Nakanishi N, Yoshida H, Nakamura K, Suzuki K, Tatara K. Alcohol consumption and risk for hypertension in middle-aged Japanese men. *J Hypertens* (2001) 19, 851–5.
4. Potter JF, Beevers DG. Pressor effect of alcohol in hypertension. *Lancet* (1984) i, 119–22.
5. Puddey IB, Beilin LJ, Vandongen R, Rouse IL, Rogers P. Evidence for a direct effect of alcohol on blood pressure in normotensive men — a randomized controlled trial. *Hypertension* (1985) 7, 707–13.
6. Sesso HD. Alcohol and cardiovascular health: recent findings. *Am J Cardiovasc Drugs* (2001) 1, 167–72.
7. Gould L, Zahir M, DeMartino A, Gomprecht RF. Cardiac effects of a cocktail. *JAMA* (1971) 218, 1799–1802.
8. Conway N. Haemodynamic effects of ethyl alcohol in patients with coronary heart disease. *Br Heart J* (1968) 30, 638–44.

Alcohol + Antimuscarinics

Propantheline does not appear to affect blood-alcohol levels, whereas atropine might cause a negligible reduction in blood-alcohol levels. Marked impairment of attention can occur if alcohol is taken in the presence of atropine or glycopyrronium (glycopyrrolate). No adverse interaction usually appears to occur with hyoscine (scopolamine) and alcohol, although hyoscine hydrobromide presents more of a theoretical risk than hyoscine butylbromide.

Clinical evidence, mechanism, importance and management

(a) Atropine

In a study in 3 subjects, a single 3-mg oral dose of atropine, given 2 hours before alcohol reduced the AUC of alcohol by 20%.[1] Another study in healthy subjects found that oral atropine 500 micrograms given with alcohol 0.5 g/kg either did not affect or improved reaction times and co-ordination; however, there was a marked impairment of attention, which was large enough to make driving more hazardous.[2] Patients should be warned.

(b) Glycopyrronium

A study in healthy subjects found that glycopyrronium 1 mg given with alcohol 0.5 g/kg either did not affect or improved reaction times and co-ordination; however, there was a marked impairment of attention, which was large enough to make driving more hazardous.[2] Patients should be warned.

(c) Hyoscine (Scopolamine)

A double-blind, crossover study in 12 healthy subjects found that a transdermal hyoscine preparation (*Scopoderm-TTS*) did not alter the effects of alcohol on the performance of several psychometric tests (Critical Flicker Fusion Frequency, Choice Reaction Tasks), nor was the clearance of alcohol or hyoscine changed. Blood-alcohol levels of up to 80 mg%, and 130 mg%, were studied.[3] In a study investigating the metabolism of alcohol, 10 patients were given hyoscine butylbromide 20 mg with oral alcohol 0.225 g/kg. Peak serum alcohol levels were not notably altered, but were delayed from about 23 minutes to 50 minutes by the hyoscine, when compared with alcohol alone. Gastric emptying time was also increased, from about 44 minutes to 71 minutes.[4] Although the evidence would seem to suggest that a clinically significant pharmacokinetic interaction is unlikely, the manufacturer of *Scopoderm-TTS* suggests caution in patients taking drugs that act on the CNS, and advises that patients should not drink alcohol.[5] This is presumably because drowsiness and other CNS adverse effects have occasionally been reported with transdermal hyoscine.[5,6] The manufacturers of travel tablets and injections containing hyoscine hydrobromide recommend avoiding alcohol.[7,8] However, unlike hyoscine and hyoscine hydrobromide, the quaternary derivatives, such as hyoscine butylbromide or hyoscine methobromide, do not readily pass the blood-brain barrier,[9] and would therefore be expected to be less likely to cause additive adverse effects with alcohol.

(d) Propantheline

In a study in 3 subjects oral propantheline (15 mg four times daily or 30 mg three times daily for 5 days, with 30 mg or 60 mg two hours before alcohol) did not affect blood-alcohol levels.[1]

1. Gibbons DO, Lant AF. Effects of intravenous and oral propantheline and metoclopramide on ethanol absorption. *Clin Pharmacol Ther* (1975) 17, 578–84.
2. Linnoila M. Drug effects on psychomotor skills related to driving: interaction of atropine, glycopyrrhonium and alcohol. *Eur J Clin Pharmacol* (1973) 6, 107–12.
3. Gleiter CH, Antonin K-H, Schoenleber W, Bieck PR. Interaction of alcohol and transdermally administered scopolamine. *J Clin Pharmacol* (1988) 28, 1123–7.
4. Oneta CM, Simanowski UA, Martinez M, Allali-Hassani A, Parés X, Homann N, Conradt C, Waldherr R, Fiehn W, Coutelle C, Seitz HK. First pass metabolism of ethanol is strikingly influenced by the speed of gastric emptying. *Gut* (1998) 43, 612–19.
5. Scopoderm TTS (Hyoscine). Novartis Consumer Health. UK Summary of product characteristics, December 2008.
6. Transderm Scop (Scopolamine). Novartis Consumer Health Inc. US Prescribing information, March 2006.
7. Joy-rides Tablets (Hyoscine hydrobromide). GlaxoSmithKline Consumer Healthcare. UK Summary of product characteristics, September 2008.
8. Hyoscine Injection (Hyoscine hydrobromide). UCB Pharma Ltd. UK Summary of product characteristics, April 2009.
9. *Martindale. The Complete Drug Reference*, [online] London: Pharmaceutical Press. http://www.medicinescomplete.com/mc/martindale/current/ms-11415-z.htm (accessed 19/10/15).

Alcohol + Antimycobacterials

The hepatotoxicity of some antimycobacterials might be increased by high alcohol consumption. Alcohol could increase the risk of epileptic episodes in patients taking cycloserine. A psychotoxic reaction in a patient taking ethionamide was attributed to concurrent heavy alcohol consumption. Isoniazid slightly increases the hazards of driving after drinking alcohol. Isoniazid-induced hepatitis might also be increased by alcohol, and the effects of isoniazid are possibly reduced in some heavy drinkers. Acute alcohol intake does not appear to affect the pharmacokinetics of a single-dose of isoniazid.

Clinical evidence, mechanism, importance and management

(a) Combined antitubercular regimens

Hepatotoxicity can occur with several antimycobacterial drugs including **ethionamide**, **isoniazid**, **pyrazinamide** and **rifampicin** and high alcohol consumption/chronic alcoholism has been reported to increase the risk.[1,2] However, one study in patients with active tuberculosis taking **rifampicin** and **pyrazinamide** found that of the 14 patients who developed hepatotoxicity, only 5 of these reported alcohol use (not quantified), and alcohol was not found to be associated with an increased risk of hepatotoxicity.[3] Similarly, another study found that alcohol consumption was not a risk factor for antimycobacterial-induced hepatotoxicity.[4]

(b) Cycloserine

A study in 45 healthy subjects given cycloserine 500 mg, 1000 mg or placebo, 4 hours before alcohol 0.8 g/kg, found that cycloserine did not affect breath- or blood-alcohol levels. Sedative effects occurred with cycloserine and alcohol alone: these effects were not additive. Both cycloserine and alcohol impaired memory and impaired verbal fluency: these effects were additive.[5] A brief report describes an enhancement of the effects of alcohol in 2 patients taking cycloserine.[6] The clinical relevance of these findings is unclear. However, the UK manufacturer of cycloserine states that it is 'incompatible' with alcohol because of an increased risk of epileptic episodes, and contraindicates its use in alcohol abuse.[7]

(c) Ethionamide

A psychotoxic reaction seen in a patient taking ethionamide was attributed to the concurrent heavy consumption of alcohol.[8] It is unclear whether this represents a clinically meaningful interaction but it appears to be the only case on record. However, because of this reaction, the UK manufacturer advises that patients should avoid drinking excessive amounts of alcohol while taking ethionamide.[9]

(d) Isoniazid

The effects of isoniazid 750 mg with alcohol 0.5 g/kg were examined in 100 subjects given various psychomotor tests, and in a further 50 drivers using a driving simulator. No major interaction was seen in the psychomotor tests, but the number of drivers who drove off the road on the simulator was increased.[10,11] There would therefore appear to be some extra risks for patients taking isoniazid who drink and drive, but the effect does not appear to be large. Patients should nevertheless be warned.

The incidence of severe progressive liver damage due to isoniazid is said to be higher in those who drink alcohol regularly,[1,12,13] and the clinical effects of isoniazid are also said to be reduced by heavy drinking in some patients.[12] The manufacturer advises care if giving isoniazid to patients with chronic alcoholism.[14]

Acute alcohol intake in 16 healthy subjects did not have any effect on the pharmacokinetics of a single 200-mg dose of isoniazid.[15] Alcohol is metabolised to acetaldehyde in the liver and isoniazid has been found to interact with acetaldehyde *in vitro*. The clinical importance of this is unknown, but if this binding occurs *in vivo*, it could lead to decreased bioavailability of isoniazid and possibly the acetaldehyde-modified drug formed could mediate some adverse effects.[16]

1. Wada M. The adverse reactions of anti-tuberculosis drugs and its management. *Nippon Rinsho* (1998) 56, 3091–5.
2. Fernández-Villar A, Sopeña B, Fernández-Villar J, Vázquez-Gallardo R, Ulloa F, Leiro V, Mosteiro M, Piñeiro L. The influence of risk factors on the severity of anti-tuberculosis drug-induced hepatotoxicity. *Int J Tuberc Lung Dis* (2004) 8, 1499–1505.
3. Lee AM, Mennone JZ, Jones RC, Paul WS. Risk factors for hepatotoxicity associated with rifampin and pyrazinamide for the treatment of latent tuberculosis infection: experience from three public health tuberculosis clinics. *Int J Tuberc Lung Dis* (2002) 6, 995–1000.
4. Døssing M, Wilcke JTR, Askgaard DS, Nybo B. Liver injury during antituberculosis treatment: an 11-year study. *Tubercle Lung Dis* (1996) 77, 335–40.
5. Trevisan L, Petrakis IL, Pittman B, Gueorguieva R, D'Souza DC, Perry E, Limoncelli D, Krystal JH. Absence of significant interactive effects of high-dose d-cycloserine and ethanol in healthy human subjects: preliminary insights into ethanol actions at the glycine$_B$ site of NMDA glutamate receptors. *Alcohol Clin Exp Res* (2008) 32, 36–42.

6. Glaß F, Mallach HJ, Simsch A. Beobachtungen und Untersuchungen über die gemeinsame Wirkung von Alkohol und D-Cycloserin. *Arzneimittelforschung* (1965) 15, 684–8.
7. Cycloserine. King Pharmaceuticals Ltd. UK Summary of product characteristics, March 2007.
8. Lansdown FS, Beran M, Litwak T. Psychotoxic reaction during ethionamide therapy. *Am Rev Respir Dis* (1967) 95, 1053–5.
9. Trecator (Ethionamide). Wyeth Pharmaceuticals Inc. US Prescribing information, November 2007.
10. Linnoila M, Mattila MJ. Effects of isoniazid on psychomotor skills related to driving. *J Clin Pharmacol* (1973) 13, 343–50.
11. Linnoila M, Mattila MJ. Interaction of alcohol and drugs on psychomotor skills as demonstrated by a driving simulator. *Br J Pharmacol* (1973) 47, 671P–672P.
12. Anon. Interactions of drugs with alcohol. *Med Lett Drugs Ther* (1981) 23, 33–4.
13. Kopanoff DE, Snider DE, Caras GJ. Isoniazid-related hepatitis. *Am Rev Respir Dis* (1978) 117, 991–1001.
14. Isoniazid Tablets. UCB Pharma Ltd. UK Summary of product characteristics, July 2009.
15. Dattani RG, Harry F, Hutchings AD, Routledge PA. The effects of acute ethanol intake on isoniazid pharmacokinetics. *Eur J Clin Pharmacol* (2004) 60, 679–82.
16. Nuñez-Vergara LJ, Yudelevich J, Squella JA, Speisky H. Drug-acetaldehyde interactions during ethanol metabolism *in vitro*. *Alcohol Alcohol* (1991) 26, 139–46.

Alcohol + Antipsychotics

The detrimental effects of alcohol on the skills related to driving are exacerbated by chlorpromazine, and, to a lesser extent, by flupentixol, sulpiride and thioridazine. Small or single-dose studies with haloperidol or tiapride suggest that any interaction would seem to be mild; nevertheless, all antipsychotic drugs that cause drowsiness have the potential to enhance the effects of alcohol. There is also some evidence to suggest that drinking can precipitate the emergence of extrapyramidal adverse effects in patients taking antipsychotics.

Clinical evidence

(a) Effect on driving and other skills

Twenty-one subjects had a marked deterioration in the performance of a number of skills related to driving when they were given **chlorpromazine** 200 mg daily and alcohol (blood-alcohol levels 42 mg%). Many complained of feeling sleepy, lethargic, dull, groggy, and poorly coordinated; and most considered themselves more unsafe to drive than with alcohol alone.[1] A later study confirmed these findings with **chlorpromazine** 1 mg/kg and blood-alcohol levels of 80 mg%.[2] Increased sedation was clearly seen in another study with alcohol and **chlorpromazine**,[3] and their concurrent use clearly impairs the psychomotor skills related to driving.[4]

Single 500-microgram doses of **haloperidol** or **flupentixol** strongly impaired attention, but did not notably interact with alcohol in one study.[5] However, a double-blind study in subjects given **flupentixol** 500 micrograms three times a day for 2 weeks found that, when they were also given alcohol 0.5 g/kg, their performance of a number of tests (choice reaction, coordination, attention) was impaired to such an extent that driving or handling other potentially dangerous machinery could be hazardous.[6]

Sulpiride 50 mg three times daily for 2 weeks caused a mild decrease in psychomotor skills with alcohol in healthy subjects, but not as much as that seen with **chlorpromazine** and alcohol.[4,7] **Thioridazine** 25 mg caused some additive effects with alcohol, with a moderately deleterious effect on attention.[5] Another study found that **thioridazine** and alcohol affected skills related to driving, but not as much as the effects seen with **chlorpromazine**.[2] A further study found no difference between the effects of **thioridazine** and a placebo with alcohol.[4,8]

A study in 9 alcoholics given **tiapride** 400 to 600 mg daily found that wakefulness was not impaired when alcohol 0.5 g/kg was also given, and in fact appeared to be improved, but the effect on driving skills was not studied.[9]

(b) Precipitation of extrapyramidal adverse effects

A report describes 7 patients who developed acute extrapyramidal adverse effects (akathisia, dystonia) while taking **trifluoperazine**, **fluphenazine**, **perphenazine**, or **chlorpromazine** and drinking alcohol.[10] The author stated that these were examples of numerous such alcohol-induced toxicity reactions observed by him over an 18-year period involving phenothiazines and butyrophenones. Elsewhere he describes the emergence of drug-induced parkinsonism in a woman taking **perphenazine** and amitriptyline when she began to drink alcohol.[11] Eighteen cases of **haloperidol**-induced extrapyramidal reactions among young drug abusers, in most instances associated with the ingestion of alcohol, have also been described.[12] Similarly, a study involving 41 patients with schizophrenia found that those with a substance use disorder (alcohol or cannabis with or without cocaine) displayed more extrapyramidal symptoms compared with non-abusing patients.[13]

(c) Toxicity

A study involving 332 fatal poisonings in Finland found that alcohol was present in 65% of cases involving **promazine**, and when alcohol was present, relatively small overdoses of **promazine** could result in fatal poisoning.[14] It appears that **promazine** and possibly **levomepromazine** might be more toxic when given with alcohol.[15]

(d) Pharmacokinetic studies

A study in 12 patients taking **chlorpromazine** 600 mg to 1.2 g daily long-term, found that **chlorpromazine** had no apparent effect on alcohol metabolism. However, about half of the patients had a decrease (of up to 33%) in the urinary excretion of **chlorpromazine** and its metabolites during the 24-hour period following the consumption of 50 to 75 mL of alcohol.[16]

A study in 7 patients with schizophrenia found that when they were given 40 g of alcohol to drink at about the same time as their regular injection of **fluphenazine decanoate** (25 to 125 mg every 2 weeks), their serum **fluphenazine** levels were reduced by 30% at 2 hours and by 16% at 12 hours.[17]

Mechanism

Uncertain. Additive CNS depressant effects are one explanation of this interaction. One suggestion to account for the emergence of the drug adverse effects is that alcohol lowers the threshold of resistance to the neurotoxicity of these drugs. Also alcohol might impair the activity of tyrosine hydroxylase so that the dopamine/acetylcholine balance within the corpus striatum is upset.[11] In addition, chlorpromazine has been found to inhibit alcohol dehydrogenase, which could facilitate the formation of biogenic amines that have been implicated in extrapyramidal adverse effects.[18]

Pharmacokinetic interactions between acute and chronic alcohol ingestion, and single or multiple doses of antipsychotic drug are complex; acute alcohol intake can decrease metabolic clearance, whereas chronic intake can increase clearance.[19] Alcohol might also affect the peripheral circulation and membrane permeability, which might affect absorption from an injection site.[17]

Importance and management

Evidence for an interaction between alcohol and antipsychotics appears to mostly relate to the use of chlorpromazine; however, what is known is in line with what would be anticipated if alcohol is given with antipsychotics with a sedative potential. Warn patients that if they drink alcohol while taking chlorpromazine, and to a lesser extent flupenthixol, sulpiride or thioridazine (probably other related drugs as well), they might become drowsy, and should not drive or handle other potentially dangerous machinery. Some risk is possible with any antipsychotic that causes drowsiness, including those used as antiemetics, such as **prochlorperazine**.

The authors of the reports describing the emergence of serious adverse effects to antipsychotics in those who drink alcohol consider that patients should routinely be advised to abstain from alcohol during antipsychotic treatment.

It has been suggested that a less dangerous alternative to promazine, and possibly levomepromazine, should be chosen when indications of alcohol abuse or suicide risk are present.[15]

The clinical importance of the pharmacokinetic studies is uncertain, but the changes observed were generally small and seem unlikely to be clinically relevant.

1. Zirkle GA, King PD, McAtee OB. Van Dyke R. Effects of chlorpromazine and alcohol on coordination and judgement. *JAMA* (1959) 171, 1496–9.
2. Milner G, Landauer AA. Alcohol, thioridazine and chlorpromazine effects on skills related to driving behaviour. *Br J Psychiatry* (1971) 118, 351–2.
3. Sutherland VC, Burbridge TN, Adams JE, Simon A. Cerebral metabolism in problem drinkers under the influence of alcohol and chlorpromazine hydrochloride. *J Appl Physiol* (1960) 15, 189–96.
4. Seppälä T, Saario I, Mattila MJ. Two weeks' treatment with chlorpromazine, thioridazine, sulpiride, or bromazepam: actions and interactions with alcohol on psychomotor skills related to driving. *Mod Probl Pharmacopsychiatry* (1976) 11, 85–90.
5. Linnoila M. Effects of diazepam, chlordiazepoxide, thioridazine, haloperidole, flupenthixole and alcohol on psychomotor skills related to driving. *Ann Med Exp Biol Fenn* (1973) 51, 125–32.
6. Linnoila M, Saario I, Olkoniemi J, Liljequist R, Himberg JJ, Mäki M. Effect of two weeks' treatment with chlordiazepoxide or flupenthixole, alone or in combination with alcohol, on psychomotor skills related to driving. *Arzneimittelforschung* (1975) 25, 1088–92.
7. Seppälä T. Effect of chlorpromazine or sulpiride and alcohol on psychomotor skills related to driving. *Arch Int Pharmacodyn Ther* (1976) 223, 311–23.
8. Saario I. Psychomotor skills during subacute treatment with thioridazine and bromazepam, and their combined effects with alcohol. *Ann Clin Res* (1976) 8, 117–23.
9. Vandel B, Bonin B, Vandel S, Blum D, Rey E, Volmat R. Étude de l'interaction entre le tiapride et l'alcool chez l'homme. *Sem Hop Paris* (1984) 60, 175–7.
10. Lutz EG. Neuroleptic-induced akathisia and dystonia triggered by alcohol. *JAMA* (1976) 236, 2422–3.
11. Lutz EG. Neuroleptic-induced parkinsonism facilitated by alcohol. *J Med Soc New Jers* (1978) 75, 473–4.
12. Kenyon-David D. Haloperidol intoxication. *N Z Med J* (1981) 93, 165.
13. Potvin S, Pampoulova T, Mancini-Marië A, Lipp O, Bouchard R-H, Stip E. Increased extrapyramidal symptoms in patients with schizophrenia and a comorbid substance use disorder. *J Neurol Neurosurg Psychiatry* (2006) 77, 796–8.
14. Koski A, Vuori E, Ojanperä I. Relation of postmortem blood alcohol and drug concentrations in fatal poisonings involving amitriptyline, propoxyphene and promazine. *Hum Exp Toxicol* (2005) 24, 389–96.
15. Koski A, Ojanperä I, Vuori E. Interaction of alcohol and drugs in fatal poisonings. *Hum Exp Toxicol* (2003) 22, 281–7.
16. Forrest F-M, Forrest I-S, Finkle B-S. Alcohol-chlorpromazine interaction in psychiatric patients. *Agressologie* (1972) 13, 67–74.
17. Soni SD, Bamrah JS, Krska J. Effects of alcohol on serum fluphenazine levels in stable chronic schizophrenics. *Hum Psychopharmacol* (1991) 6, 301–6.
18. Messiha FS. Cerebral and peripheral neurotoxicity of chlorpromazine and ethanol interaction: implications for alcohol and aldehyde dehydrogenase. *Neurotoxicology* (1991) 12, 559–70.
19. Tanaka E. Toxicological interactions involving psychiatric drugs and alcohol: an update. *J Clin Pharm Ther* (2003) 28, 81–95.

Alcohol + Antiretrovirals

Heavy alcohol intake might affect the virological response to HAART. Theoretically, alcohol consumption can induce liver enzymes, which interfere with the metabolism of some antivirals such as the HIV-protease inhibitors. Alcohol reduces the metabolism of abacavir.

Clinical evidence, mechanism, importance and management

(a) Alcohol and HAART regimens

A study of 94 HIV-positive patients receiving HAART, which included 2 **nucleoside analogues** with either **indinavir**, **ritonavir**, **saquinavir**, **nelfinavir**, or **saquinavir boosted with ritonavir**, found that the amount of alcohol consumed did not affect the antiviral response. However, the proportion of complete responders was slightly lower (57%) in heavy drinkers (more than 60 g of alcohol per day) compared with 68% in both non-drinkers and moderate drinkers (less than 60 g of alcohol per day), although this was not a statistically significant finding. There was also a high prevalence of infection with hepatitis C virus, and liver decompensation occurred in 2 patients (both heavy drinkers).[1]

Alcohol might affect thymus-induced immune repletion in HIV-positive patients and it has been reported that heavy alcohol users taking antiretrovirals are twice as likely not to achieve a positive virological response, compared with those who do not drink alcohol.[2]

It has been suggested that alcohol consumption might induce CYP3A4, resulting in concern that HAART might not be as effective in some individuals who consume alcohol.[3] CYP3A4 is involved in the metabolism of the HIV-protease inhibitors **amprenavir**, **fosamprenavir**, **indinavir**, **lopinavir**, **nelfinavir**, **ritonavir**, and **saquinavir** and the NNRTIs **delavirdine**, **efavirenz**, and **nevirapine**, and therefore CYP3A4 induction might result in enhanced drug metabolism and reduced therapeutic concentrations.[4] Avoidance of alcohol has been suggested for HIV-positive patients receiving HIV-protease inhibitors,[3,4] but at present there does not seem to be any clinical data to support this. Furthermore, one study of HIV-positive patients found that 18% of drinkers occasionally stopped taking their antiretrovirals while drinking because of beliefs about the possible toxicity of the combination. The authors suggested that although patients should be advised to avoid excessive drinking, they should also be advised to continue taking their antiretrovirals even when drinking alcohol.[5] Note that some preparations of **ritonavir** contain alcohol, see 'Alcohol + Disulfiram', p.67.

(b) Effect of alcohol on abacavir

A study in 24 HIV-positive patients found that alcohol 0.7 g/kg increased the AUC of a single 600-mg dose of abacavir by 41%. The half-life of abacavir was increased by 26%, from 1.42 hours to 1.79 hours. The pharmacokinetics of alcohol were not affected by abacavir.[6] Alcohol might inhibit the formation of abacavir carboxylate resulting in a trend towards increased abacavir glucuronide formation and reduced abacavir metabolism. The increase in exposure to abacavir was not considered to be clinically relevant, as it is within concentrations seen in other studies using higher doses, which demonstrated no additional safety concerns at doses of up to three times the recommended daily dose of abacavir.[6] No special precautions therefore appear to be necessary.

1. Fabris P, Tositti G, Manfrin V, Giordani MT, Vaglia A, Cattelan AM, Carlotto A. Does alcohol intake affect highly active antiretroviral therapy (HAART) response in HIV-positive patients? *J Acquir Immune Defic Syndr* (2000) 25, 92–3.
2. Miguez MJ, Burbano X, Morales G, Shor-Posner G. Alcohol use and HIV infection in the HAART era. *Am Clin Lab* (2001) 20, 20–3.
3. Flexner CW, Cargill VA, Sinclair J, Kresina TF, Cheever L. Alcohol use can result in enhanced drug metabolism in HIV pharmacotherapy. *AIDS Patient Care STDS* (2001) 15, 57–8.
4. Kresina TF, Flexner CW, Sinclair J, Correia MA, Stapleton JT, Adeniyi-Jones S, Cargill V, Cheever LW. Alcohol use and HIV pharmacotherapy. *AIDS Res Hum Retroviruses* (2002) 18, 757–70.
5. Kalichman SC, Amaral CM, White D, Swetsze C, Pope H, Kalicjman MO, Cherry C, Eaton L. Prevalence and clinical implications of interactive toxicity beliefs regarding mixing alcohol and antiretroviral therapies among people living with HIV/AIDS. *AIDS Patient Care STDS* (2009) 23, 449–54.
6. McDowell JA, Chittick GE, Stevens CP, Edwards KD, Stein DS. Pharmacokinetic interaction of abacavir (1592U89) and ethanol in human immunodeficiency virus-infected adults. *Antimicrob Agents Chemother* (2000) 44, 1686–90.

Alcohol + Apomorphine

Apomorphine can increase the effects of alcohol and the hypotensive adverse effects of apomorphine might be increased by alcohol.

Clinical evidence, mechanism, importance and management

In a study, 12 healthy subjects were given alcohol-containing drinks to give a blood-alcohol level of about 100 mg%, followed by a single 5-mg dose of apomorphine. Subjective and objective measures of drunkenness were increased by apomorphine, but the peak blood-alcohol levels were not altered.[1]

The manufacturer of a preparation of apomorphine used for erectile dysfunction stated that interaction studies in subjects given apomorphine found that alcohol increased the incidence and extent of hypotension (one of the adverse effects of apomorphine). They also pointed out that alcohol can diminish sexual performance.[2] The US manufacturer of a preparation of apomorphine for the treatment of parkinsonism advises the avoidance of alcohol.[3] It might be prudent to warn patients they might feel dizzy if they drink alcohol when receiving apomorphine, and advise them to sit or lay down until the effects pass.

1. Alkana RL, Parker ES, Malcolm RD, Cohen HB, Birch H, Noble EP. Interaction of apomorphine and amantadine with ethanol in men. *Alcohol Clin Exp Res* (1982) 6, 403–11.
2. Uprima (Apomorphine hydrochloride). Abbott Laboratories Ltd. UK Summary of product characteristics, September 2004.
3. Apokyn (Apomorphine hydrochloride). Tercica Inc. US Prescribing information, February 2012.

Alcohol + Aspirin or other Salicylates

A small increase in the gastrointestinal blood loss caused by aspirin occurs if individuals also drink alcohol, but any increased damage to the lining of the stomach is small and appears usually to be of minimal importance in most healthy individuals. The risks might be greater in heavy drinkers. Some limited information suggests that aspirin can raise or lower blood-alcohol levels, and alcohol might cause some small changes in salicylate levels.

Clinical evidence

(a) Gastrointestinal effects

In 13 healthy men, the mean daily blood loss from the gut was 0.4 mL while they were taking no medication, 3.2 mL while they were taking 2.1 g of soluble unbuffered aspirin (*Disprin*) and 5.3 mL while they were taking aspirin with 180 mL of Australian whisky (alcohol 31.8%). In this study, alcohol alone did not cause gastrointestinal bleeding.[1] Similar results were reported in another study in healthy subjects.[2]

An epidemiological study of patients admitted to hospital with gastrointestinal haemorrhage found a statistical association between bleeding and the ingestion of aspirin alone, and the combination with alcohol produced a synergistic effect.[3] A large case-controlled study found similar results: the overall relative risk of bleeding with regular use of aspirin, at doses greater than 325 mg, was 7 among drinkers and 5.1 among people who never drank alcohol. For those who drank less than 1 to 20 drinks a week there was no evidence of a trend of increasing or decreasing relative risk as levels of alcohol consumption increased, but among those who consumed 21 or more drinks a week there was a large association with upper gastrointestinal bleeding (crude estimated risk 27). For regular aspirin use at doses of 325 mg or less, the overall relative risk among all current drinkers and among people who never drank alcohol was 2.8 and 2.2, respectively.[4] Another case-control study suggested that the odds ratio for gastrointestinal complications in those regularly consuming more than 5 drinks during a drinking session was increased from 2.8 to 8.1 when aspirin was also taken. This was also increased when compared with the use of aspirin alone (odds ratio 3).[5]

Endoscopic examination revealed that aspirin and alcohol have additive damaging effects on the gastric mucosa (not on the duodenum), but the extent is small.[6] A further case-control study found that large amounts of red wine (roughly over 500 mL of wine daily) increased the risk of upper gastrointestinal bleeding associated with low-dose aspirin; however, small amounts of red wine (roughly less than 200 mL of wine daily) reduced this risk.[7] Another study, using gastric mucosal potential difference as a measure of mucosal damage, found that aspirin with alcohol caused additive damage to the mucosa.[8] In a review of the evidence, it was considered that while more study was needed, data available are highly suggestive that the gastrointestinal toxicity of alcohol and aspirin are combined in individuals who are heavy daily drinkers and heavy aspirin users.[9]

No increased gastrointestinal bleeding occurred in 22 healthy subjects given three double gins or whiskies (equivalent to 142 mL of alcohol 40%) and 728 mg of buffered sodium acetylsalicylate (*Alka-Seltzer*).[10]

(b) Effect on blood-alcohol levels

In a study, 28 healthy subjects were given a midday meal (two sandwiches and a cup of tea or coffee), followed 90 minutes later by 600 mg of aspirin or a placebo, and then 30 minutes later by two standard drinks (35.5 mL of vodka 37.5% (21.6 g of alcohol) with 60 mL of orange juice), which were drunk within a 15-minute period. The blood-alcohol levels of the men were raised by 31% after one hour (from about 24 mg% to 32 mg%) and by 18% (from about 21 mg% to 25 mg%) after 2 hours. The blood-alcohol levels of the women were raised by 32% (from about 37 mg% to 49 mg%) after one hour and by 21% (from about 38 mg% to 46 mg%) after 2 hours.[11]

Five healthy subjects were given a standard breakfast with and without aspirin 1 g followed one hour later by alcohol 0.3 g/kg. Aspirin increased the peak blood-alcohol levels by 39% and increased the AUC of alcohol by 26%.[12] However, in what was essentially a repeat of this study, in 12 healthy subjects, aspirin did not appear to affect blood-alcohol levels.[5] A crossover study in 10 healthy male subjects found that after taking aspirin 75 mg daily for one week, their mean blood alcohol AUC following a 0.3 g/kg-dose was not notably altered. However, individual *maximum* blood levels varied; one subject showed a rise, two were unchanged, and five were lowered: overall the reduction was 23%.[13]

(c) Effect on salicylate levels

One study in 12 healthy subjects found that alcohol reduced peak aspirin levels by 25%.[5] In a study in 5 healthy subjects the AUC and maximum levels of a single 500-mg dose of aspirin were found to be increased by a modest 11% by 50 mL of 40% alcohol, but decreased by 13% and 17%, respectively, when taken with 200 mL of beer.[14]

Mechanism

Aspirin and alcohol can damage the mucosal lining of the stomach, one measure of the injury being a fall in the gastric potential difference. Once the protective mucosal barrier is breached, desquamation of the cells occurs and damage to the capillaries follows. Aspirin causes a marked prolongation in bleeding times, and this can be increased by alcohol.[15] The total picture is complex.

The increased blood-alcohol levels in the presence of food and aspirin might occur because the aspirin reduces the enzymic oxidation of the alcohol by alcohol dehydrogenase in the gastric mucosa, so that more remains available for absorption.[12] Any decreases with low-dose aspirin may possibly be due to delayed gastric emptying.[13]

It is possible that several mechanisms are involved in the alteration of aspirin bioavailability by alcohol, including increased dissolution and altered gastric emptying.[14]

Importance and management

The combined effect of aspirin and alcohol on the stomach wall is established. Aspirin 3 g daily for a period of 3 to 5 days induces an average blood loss of about 5 mL or so. Some increased loss undoubtedly occurs with alcohol, but it seems to be quite small and unlikely to be of much importance in most healthy individuals using moderate salicylate doses and drinking moderate amounts of alcohol. In one study it was found that alcohol was a mild damaging agent or a mild potentiating agent for other drugs that damaged the gastrointestinal mucosa.[6] However, it should be remembered that chronic and/or gross overuse of salicylates and alcohol can result in gastric ulceration. People who consume at least 3 or more alcoholic drinks daily and who regularly take more than 325 mg of aspirin have been shown to have a high risk of bleeding.[16] The FDA in the US has ruled that non-prescription pain relievers and fever reducers, containing aspirin or salicylates, must carry a warning label advising people who consume moderate amounts of alcohol to consult their doctor before using these drugs, and that stomach bleeding might occur with these drugs.[17] However, the Australian Medicines Evaluation Committee has decided against such action as, for most people with mild to moderate alcohol intake, there is little risk especially if the aspirin is taken only as needed.[16]

Information about the increase in blood-alcohol levels caused by aspirin after food is very limited and contradictory, and of uncertain practical importance. However, no practically relevant interaction has been seen with other drugs, such as the H_2-receptor antagonists, which have been extensively studied, and which appear to interact by the same mechanism (see 'Alcohol + H_2-receptor antagonists', p.71). The pattern for these drugs is that the increases in blood-alcohol levels are appreciable with small amounts of alcohol, but usually they become proportionately too small to matter with larger amounts of alcohol (i.e. those that give blood and breath levels at or around the legal driving limit in the UK).

The change in salicylate levels with alcohol is almost certainly too small to be of clinical relevance.

1. Goulston K, Cooke AR. Alcohol, aspirin, and gastrointestinal bleeding. *BMJ* (1968) 4, 664–5.
2. DeSchepper PJ, Tjandramaga TB, De Roo M, Verhaest L, Daurio C, Steelman SL, Tempero KF. Gastrointestinal blood loss after diflunisal and after aspirin: effect of ethanol. *Clin Pharmacol Ther* (1978) 23, 669–76.
3. Needham CD, Kyle J, Jones PF, Johnston SJ, Kerridge DF. Aspirin and alcohol in gastrointestinal haemorrhage. *Gut* (1971) 12, 819–21.
4. Kaufman DW, Kelly JP, Wiholm B-E, Laszlo A, Sheehan JE, Koff RS, Shapiro S. The risk of acute major upper gastrointestinal bleeding among users of aspirin and ibuprofen at various levels of alcohol consumption. *Am J Gastroenterol* (1999) 94, 3189–96.
5. Melander O, Lidén A, Melander A. Pharmacokinetic interactions of alcohol and acetylsalicylic acid. *Eur J Clin Pharmacol* (1995) 48, 151–3.
6. Lanza FL, Royer GL, Nelson RS, Rack MF, Seckman CC. Ethanol, aspirin, ibuprofen, and the gastroduodenal mucosa: an endoscopic assessment. *Am J Gastroenterol* (1985) 80, 767–9.
7. Lanas A, Serrano P, Bajador E, Fuentes J, Guardia J, Sainz R. Effect of red wine and low dose aspirin on the risk or upper gastrointestinal bleeding. A case-control study. *Gastroenterology* (2000) 118 (Suppl. 2) A251.
8. Murray HS, Strottman MP, Cooke AR. Effect of several drugs on gastric potential difference in man. *BMJ* (1974) 1, 19–21.
9. Pfau PR, Lichtenstein GR. NSAIDs and alcohol: never the twain shall mix? *Am J Gastroenterol* (1999) 94, 3098–3101.
10. Bouchier IAD, Williams HS. Determination of faecal blood-loss after combined alcohol and sodium acetylsalicylate intake. *Lancet* (1969) i, 178–80.
11. Sharma SC, Feeley J. The influence of aspirin and paracetamol on blood concentrations of alcohol in young adults. *Br J Clin Pharmacol* (1996) 41, 467P.
12. Roine R, Gentry T, Hernández-Munõz R, Baraona E, Lieber CS. Aspirin increases blood alcohol concentrations in humans after ingestion of ethanol. *JAMA* (1990) 264, 2406–8.
13. Kechagias S, Jönsson K-Å, Norlander B, Carlsson B, Jones AW. Low-dose aspirin decreases blood alcohol concentrations by delaying gastric emptying. *Eur J Clin Pharmacol* (1997) 53, 241–6.
14. Odou P, Barthélémy C, Robert H. Influence of seven beverages on salicylate disposition in humans. *J Clin Pharm Ther* (2001) 26, 187–93.
15. Rosove MH, Harwig SSL. Confirmation that ethanol potentiates aspirin-induced prolongation of the bleeding time. *Thromb Res* (1983) 31, 525–7.
16. Newgreen DB. Should consumers be warned about aspirin, alcohol and gastric bleeding? *Aust Prescriber* (2005) 28, 18–19.
17. Food and Drug Administration. Questions and answers on final rule for labeling changes to over-the-counter pain relievers. Available at: http://www.fda.gov/Drugs/NewsEvents/ucm144068.htm (accessed 22/10/15).

Alcohol + Barbiturates

Alcohol and the barbiturates are CNS depressants, which together can have additive and possibly even synergistic effects on the CNS. Alcohol might continue to interact the next day if the barbiturate has hangover effects.

Clinical evidence

A study in healthy subjects of the effects of a single 0.5-g/kg dose of alcohol, taken in the morning after a dose of **amobarbital** 100 mg every night for 2 weeks, found that the performance of co-ordination skills was much more impaired than with either drug alone.[1] This increased CNS depression due to the combined use of alcohol and barbiturates has been described in other clinical studies with **phenobarbital**.[2,3] However, a study in healthy subjects found that although **phenobarbital** 45 mg daily for one week and alcohol (35 to 45 mg%) affected some perceptual-motor tests when given separately, these effects were not always found when they were given together.[4] Nevertheless, high doses of **phenobarbital** can affect driving skills[5] and increased CNS depression has featured very many times in coroners' reports of fatal accidents and suicides involving barbiturates and alcohol.[6] A study of the fatalities due to this interaction indicated that with some barbiturates the CNS depressant effects are more than additive.[7] There is also some evidence that blood-alcohol levels can be reduced in the presence of a barbiturate.[8,9]

For the interaction between thiopental and alcohol, see 'Anaesthetics, general + Alcohol', p.99.

Mechanism

Both alcohol and the barbiturates are CNS depressants, and simple additive CNS depression provides part of the explanation. Acute alcohol ingestion might inhibit the liver enzymes concerned with the metabolism of barbiturates, such as phenobarbital and **pentobarbital**, but chronic exposure to alcohol increases hepatic microsomal enzyme activity and might reduce sedation from barbiturates in patients without liver impairment.[10,11] Similarly, chronic exposure to a barbiturate, such as phenobarbital, can increase alcohol metabolism due to enzyme induction and consequently reduce blood-alcohol levels.[7]

Importance and management

Few formal studies in normal clinical situations have been made of the interactions between alcohol and the barbiturates, and most of these studies are old and involved barbiturates used as hypnotics. However, the effects (particularly those that result in fatalities) are very well established, serious, and of clinical importance. The most obvious hazards are increased drowsiness, lack of alertness, and impaired co-ordination, which make the handling of potentially dangerous machinery (e.g. car driving), and even the performance of everyday tasks (e.g. walking downstairs) more difficult and dangerous. Only amobarbital and phenobarbital appear to have been specifically studied, but this interaction would be expected with all of the barbiturates. Some barbiturate hangover effects might be present the next morning and could therefore continue to interact with alcohol. Patients should be warned.

For comments on the use of alcohol in epileptic patients taking drugs including phenobarbital, see 'Alcohol + Antiepileptics', p.54.

1. Saario I, Linnoila M. Effect of subacute treatment with hypnotics, alone or in combination with alcohol, on psychomotor skills relating to driving. *Acta Pharmacol Toxicol (Copenh)* (1976) 38, 382–92.
2. Kielholz P, Goldberg L, Obersteg JI, Pöldinger W, Ramseyer A, Schmid P. Fahrversuche zur Frage der Beeinträchtigung der Verkehrstüchtigkeit durch Alkohol, Tranquilizer und Hypnotika. *Dtsch Med Wochenschr* (1969) 94, 301–6.
3. Morselli PL, Veneroni E, Zaccala M, Bizzi A. Further observations on the interaction between ethanol and psychotropic drugs. *Arzneimittelforschung* (1971) 21, 20–3.
4. Michiels W, Fryc O, Meyer JJ. Effet du tétrabamate, du phénobarbital et d'une faible quantité d'alcool sur quelques aspects perceptivo-moteurs en relation avec la conduite automobile. *Schweiz Med Wochenschr* (1978) 108, 640–6.
5. Cary PL, Johnson CA, Foltz RL, Pape BE. Driving under the influence of phenobarbital. *J Forensic Sci* (1983) 28, 502–4.
6. Gupta RC, Kofoed J. Toxicological statistics for barbiturates, other sedatives, and tranquillizers in Ontario: a 10-year survey. *Can Med Assoc J* (1966) 94, 863–5.
7. Stead AH, Moffat AC. Quantification of the interaction between barbiturates and alcohol and interpretation of fatal blood concentrations. *Hum Toxicol* (1983) 2, 5–14.
8. Mould GP, Curry SH, Binns TB. Interaction of glutethimide and phenobarbitone with ethanol in man. *J Pharm Pharmacol* (1972) 24, 894–9.
9. Mezey E, Robles EA. Effects of phenobarbital administration on rates of ethanol clearance and on ethanol-oxidizing enzymes in man. *Gastroenterology* (1974) 66, 248–53.
10. Rubin E, Gang H, Misra PS, Lieber CS. Inhibition of drug metabolism by acute ethanol intoxication. A hepatic microsomal mechanism. *Am J Med* (1970) 49, 801–6.
11. Weller RA, Preskorn SH. Psychotropic drugs and alcohol: pharmacokinetic and pharmacodynamic interactions. *Psychosomatics* (1984) 25, 301–3, 305–6, 309.

Alcohol + Benzodiazepines and related drugs

Benzodiazepines and related anxiolytics and hypnotics increase the CNS depressant effects of alcohol to some extent. Some benzodiazepines used at night for sedation are still present in appreciable amounts the next day and therefore could continue to interact. Alcohol might also increase the plasma levels of brotizolam, clobazam, diazepam, and possibly triazolam, whereas alprazolam might increase blood-alcohol levels. Alcohol has been reported to increase aggression or amnesia and/or reduce the anxiolytic effects of some benzodiazepines.

Clinical evidence

(a) Additive CNS depressant effects

It is very difficult to assess and compare the results of the many studies of this interaction because of differences between the tests, their duration, the doses of the benzodiazepines and alcohol used, whether the drugs were given chronically or acutely, and a number of other variables. However, the overall picture seems to be that benzodiazepines and related drugs including **diazepam**,[1-12] **alprazolam**,[13-15] **bromazepam**,[16] **brotizolam**,[17] **chlordiazepoxide**,[12,18-22] **clobazam**,[23] **dipotassium clorazepate**,[24] **flunitrazepam**,[25,26] **flurazepam**,[27-31] **loprazolam**,[28,32] **lorazepam**,[10,33-36] **lormetazepam**,[37] **medazepam**,[38] **midazolam**,[39] **nitrazepam**,[3,40,41] **oxazepam**,[6] **temazepam**,[41-43] **triazolam**,[29,42,44-46] and **zopiclone**[46] enhance the effects of alcohol i.e. cause increased drowsiness, impaired performance and driving skills.

Patients taking benzodiazepines including **lorazepam**[34] or **triazolam**[44] could be unaware of the extent of the impairment that occurs. Furthermore, changes in CNS functioning might occur in heavy social drinkers; a placebo-controlled study in 20-year-olds suggested that **lorazepam** 2 mg had more impairment on delayed auditory verbal memory performance in those who were heavy social drinkers (more than 20 drinks; 200 g of alcohol per week) than light social drinkers (20 g or less of alcohol per week).[47]

One study found the combination of an intermediate or long-acting benzodiazepines with alcohol resulted in a greater risk of an unsafe driving action (OR 1.38 and 1.18, respectively) than the combination of a short-acting benzodiazepine and alcohol, which carried a similar risk to alcohol alone.[48] Some of the benzodiazepines and related drugs that are used primarily to aid sleep, such as **flunitrazepam**,[25,26] **flurazepam**,[27,28,30,31,49] **nitrazepam**,[3,40] and **temazepam**,[49,50] when taken the night before alcohol or in the evening with alcohol, can still interact with alcohol the next morning. However, **midazolam**,[39] **loprazolam**,[28] **lormetazepam**,[37] **triazolam**,[31,46] **zolpidem**,[51] and **zopiclone**[25,30,46] have been reported not to do so. The sedative effects of **midazolam** alone, and **midazolam** with fentanyl have been shown to have dissipated within 4 hours, and to not be affected by alcohol after this time.[52,53] However, some patients metabolise **midazolam** more slowly and so an interaction could still be possible,[54] especially in older patients or those taking additional drugs.[55]

Some contrasting effects have also been reported. One study suggested that alcohol might mitigate the effects of **loprazolam** on psychological performance.[32] Similarly, some antagonism has been reported between **chlordiazepoxide** and alcohol, but this is unlikely to be of practical importance.[18,19] The development of tolerance between benzodiazepines and alcohol with chronic use has also been suggested.[56,57]

(b) Increased aggression, anxiety, or amnesia

The anxiolytic effects of **lorazepam**[35] and possibly **chlordiazepoxide**[20] might be opposed by alcohol. **Alprazolam** and alcohol together might increase behavioural aggression.[58] Similarly, **flunitrazepam** abuse can cause violent behaviour, impulsive decision-making and anterograde amnesia: a report looking at violent crimes committed by abusers of **flunitrazepam** found that alcohol was almost always also present.[59] Alcoholic drinks also enhance the effects of **flunitrazepam** when it is used as a 'date rape' drug.[60]

(c) Pharmacokinetic effects

Several studies have reported that alcohol increases the plasma levels of **diazepam**[13,61] and that alcohol accelerates the absorption of **diazepam**,[5] but others have suggested that alcohol has no significant effect on **diazepam** pharmacokinetics.[9,11,62] Plasma levels of **brotizolam**[17] and **clobazam**[23] might be increased by alcohol. One study reported that the plasma levels of **triazolam** were increased by alcohol,[44] but other studies have found only a minimal pharmacokinetic interaction.[45,46] Another pharmacokinetic study suggested that there was no interaction between alcohol and **flunitrazepam**.[26] Alcohol appears to have minimal effects on the pharmacokinetics of **alprazolam**,[13] and **zopiclone**.[46,63]

The pharmacokinetics of alcohol do not appear to be affected to a clinically relevant extent by **diazepam**,[11] **flunitrazepam**,[26] **zolpidem**,[51] or **zopiclone**,[46] but **alprazolam**[13] might increase blood-alcohol levels.

Mechanism

The CNS depressant actions of the benzodiazepines and alcohol are mainly additive and it appears that different aspects of CNS processing could be involved.[41,64]

A pharmacokinetic interaction can sometimes occur, but the mechanisms seem to be quite complex. Acute alcohol intake increases the absorption and raises the serum levels of some benzodiazepines.[23,61] It has been suggested that clearance of benzodiazepines via phase I metabolism, by *N*-demethylation and/or hydroxylation, tends to be more affected by alcohol intake than that of drugs such as lorazepam, oxazepam or lormetazepam that only undergo phase II conjugation. In addition, phase I metabolism is inhibited or decreases with increasing age and liver disease.[65] However, phase I metabolism is *increased* by chronic administration of substances that induce the cytochrome P450 isoenzyme system, such as alcohol.[65]

Importance and management

Extensively studied, well established and clinically important interactions. The overall picture is that the benzodiazepines and related drugs worsen the detrimental effects of alcohol.[66] Up to a 20 to 30% increase in the impairment of psychomotor function has been suggested.[44] The deterioration in skills will depend on the particular drug in question, its dose and the amounts of alcohol taken. With modest amounts of alcohol the effects can be quite small in most patients (although a few might be more markedly affected[11]), but anyone taking any of these drugs should be warned that their usual response to alcohol might be greater than expected, and their ability to drive a car, or carry out any other tasks requiring alertness, might be impaired. They can be quite unaware of the deterioration or that the effects might still be present the following day. Benzodiazepines and alcohol are frequently found in the blood of car drivers involved in traffic accidents, which suggests that the risks are real.[57,66-69] Furthermore, alcohol has contributed to fatal poisonings and other deaths involving benzodiazepines, particularly diazepam[70-73] and temazepam.[74] Alcohol might contribute to drug-related accidents and deaths due to a disregard for safety;[69,75] and there is also an association between alcohol and benzodiazepines and violence-related accidents.[69]

1. Morselli PL, Veneroni E, Zaccala M, Bizzi A. Further observations on the interaction between ethanol and psychotropic drugs. *Arzneimittelforschung* (1971) 21, 20–3.
2. Linnoila M, Häkkinen S. Effects of diazepam and codeine, alone and in combination with alcohol, on simulated driving. *Clin Pharmacol Ther* (1974) 15, 368–73.
3. Linnoila M. Drug interaction on psychomotor skills related to driving: hypnotics and alcohol. *Ann Med Exp Biol Fenn* (1973) 51, 118–24.
4. Missen AW, Cleary W, Eng L, McMillan S. Diazepam, alcohol and drivers. *N Z Med J* (1978) 87, 275–7.
5. Laisi U, Linnoila M, Seppälä T, Himberg J-J, Mattila MJ. Pharmacokinetic and pharmacodynamic interactions of diazepam with different alcoholic beverages. *Eur J Clin Pharmacol* (1979) 16, 263–70.
6. Molander L, Duvhök C. Acute effects of oxazepam, diazepam and methylperone, alone and in combination with alcohol on sedation, coordination and mood. *Acta Pharmacol Toxicol (Copenh)* (1976) 38, 145–60.
7. Curry SH, Smith CM. Diazepam-ethanol interaction in humans: addition or potentiation? *Commun Psychopharmacol* (1979) 3, 101–13.
8. Smiley A, Moskowitz H. Effects of long-term administration of buspirone and diazepam on driver steering control. *Am J Med* (1986) 80 (Suppl 3B), 22–9.
9. Erwin CW, Linnoila M, Hartwell J, Erwin A, Guthrie S. Effects of buspirone and diazepam, alone and in combination with alcohol, on skilled performance and evoked potentials. *J Clin Psychopharmacol* (1986) 6, 199–209.
10. Aranko K, Seppälä T, Pellinen J, Mattila MJ. Interaction of diazepam or lorazepam with alcohol. Psychomotor effects and bioassayed serum levels after single and repeated doses. *Eur J Clin Pharmacol* (1985) 28, 559–65.
11. van Steveninck AL, Gieschke R, Schoemaker HC, Pieters MSM, Kroon JM, Breimer DD, Cohen AF. Pharmacodynamic interactions of diazepam and intravenous alcohol at pseudo steady state. *Psychopharmacology (Berl)* (1993) 110, 471–8.
12. Hughes FW, Forney RB, Richards AB. Comparative effect in human subjects of chlordiazepoxide, diazepam, and placebo on mental and physical performance. *Clin Pharmacol Ther* (1965) 6, 139–45.
13. Linnoila M, Stapleton JM, Lister R, Moss H, Lane E, Granger A, Eckardt MJ. Effects of single doses of alprazolam and diazepam, alone and in combination with ethanol, on psychomotor and cognitive performance and on autonomic nervous system reactivity in healthy volunteers. *Eur J Clin Pharmacol* (1990) 39, 21–8.
14. Rush CR, Griffiths RR. Acute participant-rated and behavioral effects of alprazolam and buspirone, alone and in combination with ethanol, in normal volunteers. *Exp Clin Psychopharmacol* (1997) 5, 28–38.
15. Bond AJ, Silveira JC, Lader MH. The effects of alprazolam alone and combined with alcohol on central integrative activity. *Eur J Clin Pharmacol* (1992) 42, 495–8.
16. Seppälä T, Saario I, Mattila MJ. Two weeks' treatment with chlorpromazine, thioridazine, sulpiride, or bromazepam: actions and interactions with alcohol on psychomotor skills relating to driving. *Mod Probl Pharmacopsychiatry* (1976) 11, 85–90.
17. Scavone JM, Greenblatt DJ, Harmatz JS, Shader RI. Kinetic and dynamic interaction of brotizolam and ethanol. *Br J Clin Pharmacol* (1986) 21, 197–204.
18. Dundee JW, Isaac M. Interaction of alcohol with sedatives and tranquillisers (a study of blood levels at loss of consciousness following rapid infusion). *Med Sci Law* (1970) 10, 220–4.
19. Linnoila M. Effects of diazepam, chlordiazepoxide, thioridazine, haloperidole, flupenthixole and alcohol on psychomotor skills related to driving. *Ann Med Exp Biol Fenn* (1973) 51, 125–32.
20. Linnoila M, Saario I, Olkoniemi J, Liljequist R, Himberg JJ, Mäki M. Effect of two weeks' treatment with chlordiazepoxide or flupenthixole, alone or in combination with alcohol, on psychomotor skills related to driving. *Arzneimittelforschung* (1975) 25, 1088–92.
21. Hoffer A. Lack of potentiation by chlordiazepoxide (Librium) of depression or excitation due to alcohol. *Can Med Assoc J* (1962) 87, 920–1.
22. Kielholz P, Goldberg L, Obersteg JI, Pöldinger W, Ramseyer A, Schmid P. Fahrversuche zur Frage der Beeinträchtigung der Verkehrstüchtigkeit durch Alkohol, Tranquilizer und Hypnotika. *Dtsch Med Wochenschr* (1969) 94, 301–6.
23. Taeuber K, Badian M, Brettel HF, Royen T, Rupp K, Sittig W, Uihlein M. Kinetic and dynamic interaction of clobazam and alcohol. *Br J Clin Pharmacol* (1979) 7, 91S-97S.
24. Staak M, Raff G, Nusser W. Pharmacopsychological investigations concerning the combined effects of dipotassium clorazepate and ethanol. *Int J Clin Pharmacol Biopharm* (1979) 17, 205–12.
25. Seppälä T, Nuotto E, Dreyfus JF. Drug–alcohol interactions on psychomotor skills: zopiclone and flunitrazepam. *Pharmacology* (1983) 27 (Suppl 2), 127–35.
26. Linnoila M, Erwin CW, Brendle A, Logue P. Effects of alcohol and flunitrazepam on mood and performance in healthy young men. *J Clin Pharmacol* (1981) 21, 430–5.
27. Saario I, Linnoila M. Effect of subacute treatment with hypnotics, alone or in combination with alcohol, on psychomotor skills related to driving. *Acta Pharmacol Toxicol (Copenh)* (1976) 38, 382–92.
28. Hindmarch I, Gudgeon AC. Loprazolam (HR158) and flurazepam with ethanol compared on tests of psychomotor ability. *Eur J Clin Pharmacol* (1982) 23, 509–12.
29. Hill SY, Goodwin DW, Reichman JB, Mendelson WB, Hopper S. A comparison of two benzodiazepine hypnotics administered with alcohol. *J Clin Psychiatry* (1982) 43, 408–10.
30. Mamelak M, Buck L, Csima A, Price V, Smiley A. Effects of flurazepam and zopiclone on the performance of chronic insomniac patients: a study of ethanol-drug interaction. *Sleep* (1987) 10 (Suppl 1), 79–87.
31. Mendelson WB, Goodwin DW, Hill SY, Reichman JD. The morning after: residual EEG effects of triazolam and flurazepam, alone and in combination with alcohol. *Curr Ther Res Clin Exp* (1976) 19, 155–63.
32. McManus IC, Ankier SI, Norfolk J, Phillips M, Priest RG. Effects on psychological performance of the benzodiazepine, loprazolam, alone and with alcohol. *Br J Clin Pharmacol* (1983) 16, 291–300.
33. Allen D, Baylav A, Lader M. A comparative study of the interaction of alcohol with alpidem, lorazepam and placebo in normal subjects. *Int Clin Psychopharmacol* (1988) 3, 327–41.
34. Seppälä T, Aranko K, Mattila MJ, Shrotriya RC. Effects of alcohol on buspirone and lorazepam actions. *Clin Pharmacol Ther* (1982) 32, 201–7.
35. Lister RG, File SE. Performance impairment and increased anxiety resulting from the combination of alcohol and lorazepam. *J Clin Psychopharmacol* (1983) 3, 66–71.
36. Soo-Ampon S, Wonqwitdecha N, Plasen S, Hindmarch I, Boyle J. Effects of word frequency on recall memory following lorazepam, alcohol, and lorazepam alcohol interaction in healthy volunteers. *Psychopharmacology (Berl)* (2004) 176, 420–5.
37. Willumeit H-P, Ott H, Neubert W, Hemmerling K-G, Schratzer M, Fichte K. Alcohol interaction of lormetazepam, mepindolol sulphate and diazepam measured by performance on the driving simulator. *Pharmacopsychiatry* (1984) 17, 36–43.
38. Landauer AA, Pocock DA, Prott FW. The effect of medazepam and alcohol on cognitive and motor skills used in car driving. *Psychopharmacologia* (1974) 37, 159–68.
39. Hindmarch I, Subhan Z. The effects of midazolam in conjunction with alcohol on sleep, psychomotor performance and car driving ability. *Int J Clin Pharmacol Res* (1983) 3, 323–9.
40. Saario I, Linnoila M, Mäki M. Interaction of drugs with alcohol on human psychomotor skills related to driving: effect of sleep deprivation or two weeks' treatment with hypnotics. *J Clin Pharmacol* (1975) 15, 52–9.
41. Taberner PV, Roberts CJC, Shrosbree E, Pycock CJ, English L. An investigation into the interaction between ethanol at low doses and the benzodiazepines nitrazepam and temazepam on psychomotor performance in normal subjects. *Psychopharmacology (Berl)* (1983) 81, 321–26.
42. Simpson CA, Rush CR. Acute performance-impairing and subject-rated effects of triazolam and temazepam, alone and in combination with ethanol, in humans. *J Psychopharmacol* (2002) 16, 23–34.
43. Lehmann W, Liljenberg B. Effect of temazepam and temazepam-ethanol on sleep. *Eur J Clin Pharmacol* (1981) 20, 201–5.
44. Dorian P, Sellers EM, Kaplan HL, Hamilton C, Greenblatt DJ, Abernethy D. Triazolam and ethanol interaction: kinetic and dynamic consequences. *Clin Pharmacol Ther* (1985) 37, 558–62.
45. Ochs HR, Greenblatt DJ, Arendt RM, Hübbel W, Shader RI. Pharmacokinetic noninteraction of triazolam and ethanol. *J Clin Psychopharmacol* (1984) 4,106–7.
46. Kuitunen T, Mattila MJ, Seppala T. Actions and interactions of hypnotics on human performance: single doses of zopiclone, triazolam and alcohol. *Int Clin Psychopharmacol* (1990) 5 (Suppl 2), 115–30.
47. Nichols JM, Martin F. The effect of lorazepam on long-term verbal recall in heavy and light social drinkers. *Alcohol* (1997) 14, 455–61.
48. Maxwell HG, Dubois S, Weaver B, Bédard M. The additive effects of alcohol and benzodiazepines on driving. *Can J Public Health* (2010) 101, 353–7.
49. Betts TA, Birtle J. Effect of two hypnotic drugs on actual driving performance next morning. *BMJ* (1982) 285, 852.
50. Hindmarch I. The effects of repeated doses of temazepam taken in conjunction with alcohol on aspects of psychomotor performance the morning following night time medication. *Arzneimittelforschung* (1978) 28, 2357–60.
51. Wilkinson CJ. The acute effects of zolpidem, administered alone and with alcohol, on cognitive and psychomotor function. *J Clin Psychiatry* (1995) 56, 309–18.
52. Lichtor JL, Zacny J, Korttila K, Apfelbaum JL, Lane BS, Rupani G, Thisted RA, Dohrn C. Alcohol after midazolam sedation: does it really matter? *Anesth Analg* (1991) 72, 661–6.
53. Lichtor JL, Zacny J, Apfelbaum JL, Lane BS, Rupani G, Thisted RA, Dohrn C, Korttila K. Alcohol after sedation with i.v. midazolam–fentanyl: effects on psychomotor functioning. *Br J Anaesth* (1991) 67, 579–84.
54. Dundee JW. Safety of alcohol after midazolam. *Anesth Analg* (1991) 73, 829.
55. Lichtor JL, Zacny J, Korttila K, Apfelbaum JL. Safety of alcohol after midazolam. Response. *Anesth Analg* (1991) 73, 829.
56. Palva ES, Linnoila M, Saario I, Mattila MJ. Acute and subacute effects of diazepam on psychomotor skills: interaction with alcohol. *Acta Pharmacol Toxicol (Copenh)* (1979) 45, 257–64.
57. Chan AWK. Effects of combined alcohol and benzodiazepine: a review. *Drug Alcohol Depend* (1984) 13, 315–41.
58. Bond AJ, Silveira JC. Behavioural aggression following the combination of alprazolam and alcohol. *J Psychopharmacol* (1990) 4, 315.
59. Dåderman AM, Fredriksson B, Kristiansson M, Nilsson L-H, Lidberg L. Violent behavior, impulsive decision-making, and anterograde amnesia while intoxicated with flunitrazepam and alcohol or other drugs: a case study in forensic psychiatric patients. *J Am Acad Psychiatry Law* (2002) 30, 238–51.
60. Schwartz RH, Milteer R, LeBeau MA. Drug-facilitated sexual assault ('date rape'). *South Med J* (2000) 93, 558–61.
61. MacLeod SM, Giles HG, Patzalek G, Thiessen JJ, Sellers EM. Diazepam actions and plasma concentrations following ethanol ingestion. *Eur J Clin Pharmacol* (1977) 11, 345–9.
62. Divoll M, Greenblatt DJ. Alcohol does not enhance diazepam absorption. *Pharmacology* (1981) 22, 263–8.
63. Larivière L, Caillé G, Elie R. The effects of low and moderate doses of alcohol on the pharmacokinetic parameters of zopiclone. *Biopharm Drug Dispos* (1986) 7, 207–10.

64. Martin FH, Siddle DA. The interactive effects of alcohol and temazepam on P300 and reaction time. *Brain Cogn* (2003) 53, 58–65.
65. Tanaka E, Misawa S. Pharmacokinetic interactions between acute alcohol ingestion and single doses of benzodiazepines, and tricyclic and tetracyclic antidepressants–an update. *J Clin Pharm Ther* (1998) 23, 331–6.
66. Schuster R, Bodem M. Evaluation of ethanol-benzodiazepine-interactions using blood sampling protocol data. *Blutalkohol* (1997) 34, 54–65.
67. Staub C, Lacalle H, Fryc O. Présence de psychotropes dans le sang de conducteurs responsables d'accidents de la route ayant consommé en même temps de l'alcool. *Soz Praventivmed* (1994) 39, 143–9.
68. Longo MC, Hunter CE, Lokan RJ, White JM, White MA. The prevalence of alcohol, cannabinoids, benzodiazepines and stimulants amongst injured drivers and their role in driver culpability. Part II: The relationship between drug prevalence and drug concentration, and driver culpability. *Accid Anal Prev* (2000) 32, 623–32.
69. Kurzthaler I, Wambacher M, Golser K, Sperner G, Sperner-Unterweger B, Haidekker A, Pavlic M, Kemmler G, Fleischhacker WW. Alcohol and/or benzodiazepine use: different accidents – different impacts? *Hum Psychopharmacol* (2005) 20, 583–9.
70. Serfaty M, Masterton G. Fatal poisonings attributed to benzodiazepines in Britain during the 1980s. *Br J Psychiatry* (1993) 163, 386–93.
71. Kovac C. Airline passenger dies after being sedated by doctor. *BMJ* (1999) 318, 12.
72. Macdonald HA. Airline passenger dies after being sedated. Death may have been due to positional asphyxia. *BMJ* (1999) 318, 1491.
73. Samer Abdalla M. Airline passenger dies after being sedated. …or to potentiating effects on diazepam. *BMJ* (1999) 318, 1491.
74. Koski A, Ojanperä I, Vuori E. Alcohol and benzodiazepines in fatal poisonings. *Alcohol Clin Exp Res* (2002) 26, 956–9.
75. Gable RS. Acute toxic effects of club drugs. *J Psychoactive Drugs* (2004) 36, 303–13.

Alcohol + Beta blockers

The haemodynamic and pharmacokinetic effects of atenolol and metoprolol in healthy subjects do not appear to be changed by alcohol. There is some evidence that alcohol modestly reduces the haemodynamic effects of propranolol, and some of the effects of sotalol might also be changed by alcohol. Some evidence suggests that the effects of alcohol and atenolol with chlortalidone, or propranolol, are additive on the performance of some psychomotor tests.

Clinical evidence

(a) Atenolol

In 12 healthy subjects the performance of a number of psychomotor tests was found to be impaired by alcohol 0.6 g/kg and by one tablet of *Tenoretic* (atenolol 100 mg with chlortalidone 25 mg). When alcohol and *Tenoretic* were taken together there was some evidence of additive effects but the practical importance of this is not clear.[1] In 8 healthy subjects the pharmacokinetics of single 100-mg doses of atenolol or **metoprolol** were unaffected 6 hours after they had drunk the equivalent of 200 mL of absolute alcohol. No clinically significant changes in blood pressure or pulse rate were seen.[2] A similar study in 23 healthy subjects found that atenolol 100 mg did not affect the pharmacokinetics of alcohol 1 g/kg. However, alcohol increased the reduction in heart rate and blood pressure in response to atenolol (from 60 bpm to 56 bpm and from 124/82 mmHg to about 109/76 mmHg at 2 and 3 hours after ingestion).[3]

(b) Propranolol

In 12 healthy subjects propranolol 40 mg every 6 hours had no effect on the impairment of performance of a number of psychomotor tests caused by 50 mL/70 kg of alcohol, except that propranolol antagonised the effect of alcohol in one test (pursuit meter).[4] However, in another study, propranolol enhanced the effects of alcohol on some tests (inebriation and divided attention).[5] A study in 6 healthy subjects found that alcohol (sufficient to maintain blood-alcohol levels of 80 mg%) raised the mean AUC of a single 80-mg oral dose of propranolol by about 17% in 5 subjects and decreased it by 37% in the other subject, but this was considered unlikely to be clinically important. No changes in heart rate or blood pressure were seen.[6] In contrast, a double-blind study in 14 healthy subjects found that alcohol (equivalent to 32 to 72 mL of absolute alcohol) increased the clearance of a single 80-mg dose of propranolol and diminished its ability to lower blood pressure. Propranolol was not able to abolish the alcohol-induced rise in heart rate.[7] Similarly, another study found that alcohol decreased the rate of absorption and increased the rate of elimination of propranolol, but the clinical significance of this small alteration was not assessed.[8] Other studies have found that propranolol enhances the decrease in blood pressure seen with alcohol,[9,10] but attenuates[9] or does not alter[10] its effects on heart rate. Furthermore, in this study alcohol increased peak propranolol levels 2- to 3.5-fold.[10]

(c) Sotalol

A study in 6 healthy subjects found that although the blood-pressure lowering effects of sotalol 160 mg were increased by alcohol, sotalol did not cancel out the alcohol-induced rise in heart rate.[7]

Mechanism

Both the beta blockers and alcohol can affect blood pressure, and it appears that these effects can be additive.

Importance and management

Evidence for an interaction between alcohol and the beta blockers appears to be limited to just a few of the beta blockers. In general, alcohol appears to enhance the response to the blood-pressure lowering effects of the beta blockers, an effect that is in common with most antihypertensive drugs, see 'Alcohol + Antihypertensives', p.55. Some, but not all studies suggest that alcohol might enhance any effect of the beta blockers on the skills related to driving, but evidence is limited and of unclear general relevance.

1. Gerrard L, Wheeldon NM, McDevitt DG. Psychomotor effects of combined atenolol/chlorthalidone administration: interaction with alcohol. *Br J Clin Pharmacol* (1994) 37, 517P–518P.
2. Kirch W, Spahn H, Hutt HJ, Ohnhaus EE, Mutschler E. Interaction between alcohol and metoprolol or atenolol in social drinking. *Drugs* (1983) 25 (Suppl 2), 152.
3. Kupari M, Heikkilä J, Tolppanen E-M,. Nieminen MS, Ylikahri R. Acute effects of alcohol, beta blockade, and their combination on left ventricular function and hemodynamics in normal man. *Eur Heart J* (1983) 4, 463–71.
4. Lindenschmidt R, Brown D, Cerimele B, Walle T, Forney RB. Combined effects of propranolol and ethanol on human psychomotor performance. *Toxicol Appl Pharmacol* (1983) 67, 117–21.
5. Alkana RL, Parker ES, Cohen HB, Birch H, Noble EP. Reversal of ethanol intoxication in humans: an assessment of the efficacy of propranolol. *Psychopharmacology (Berl)* (1976) 51, 29–37.
6. Dorian P, Sellers EM, Carruthers G, Hamilton C, Fan T. Propranolol-ethanol pharmacokinetic interaction. *Clin Pharmacol Ther* (1982) 31, 219.
7. Sotaniemi EA, Anttila M, Rautio A, Stengård J, Saukko P, Järvensivu P. Propranolol and sotalol metabolism after a drinking party. *Clin Pharmacol Ther* (1981) 29, 705–10.
8. Grabowski BS, Cady WJ, Young WW, Emery JF. Effects of acute alcohol administration on propranolol absorption. *Int J Clin Pharmacol Ther Toxicol* (1980) 18, 317–19.
9. Kawano Y, Abe H, Kojima S, Takishita S, Omae T. Effects of propranolol on cardiovascular and neurohumoral actions of alcohol in hypertensive patients. *Blood Pressure* (1999) 8, 37–42.
10. Chakrabarti A, Garg SK, Sharma PL. A preliminary study on the interaction between ethanol and propranolol in normal human subjects. *Indian J Physiol Pharmacol* (1992) 36, 209–212.

Alcohol + Bicalutamide, Flutamide, or Nilutamide

Alcohol intolerance has been reported in patients taking nilutamide, but not in those taking bicalutamide or flutamide.

Clinical evidence, mechanism, importance and management

Several studies have described alcohol intolerance (facial flushes, malaise, hypotension) in patients taking nilutamide.[1-4] The incidence has been reported to be between 3 and 19%.[1,3,5] It is recommended that patients who experience this reaction should avoid drinking alcohol.[5]

Flutamide and bicalutamide have not been reported to produce these effects when patients drink alcohol,[3] and so in some cases they might be considered as an alternative option to nilutamide.

1. Boccardo F, Decensi AU, Guarneri D, Martorana G, Fioretto L, Mini E, Macaluso MP, Giuliani L, Santi L, Periti P; the Italian Prostatic Cancer Project. Anandron (RU 23908) in metastatic prostate cancer: preliminary results of a multicentric Italian study. *Cancer Detect Prev* (1991), 15, 501–3.
2. Decensi AU, Boccardo F, Guarneri D, Positano N, Paoletti MC, Costantini M, Martorana G, Giuliani L; for the Italian Prostatic Cancer Project. Monotherapy with nilutamide, a pure nonsteroidal antiandrogen, in untreated patients with metastatic carcinoma of the prostate. *J Urol (Baltimore)* (1991) 146, 377–81.
3. McLeod DG. Tolerability of nonsteroidal antiandrogens in the treatment of advanced prostate cancer. *Oncologist* (1997) 2, 18–27.
4. Du Plessis DJ. Castration plus nilutamide vs castration plus placebo in advanced prostate cancer. *Urology* (1991) 37 (2 Suppl), 20–24.
5. Nilandron (Nilutamide). Sanofi-Aventis US LLC. US Prescribing information, June 2006.

Alcohol + Bromocriptine

Some very limited evidence suggests that the adverse effects of bromocriptine might be increased by alcohol.

Clinical evidence, mechanism, importance and management

Intolerance to alcohol, which improved on continued treatment, has been briefly mentioned in a report about patients taking bromocriptine for acromegaly.[1] In another report, 2 patients with high prolactin levels were said to have developed bromocriptine adverse effects, even at low bromocriptine doses, while continuing to drink. When they abstained from alcohol, the frequency and the severity of the adverse effects was reduced, even with higher doses of bromocriptine.[2] This, it is suggested, could be due to some alcohol-induced increase in the sensitivity of dopamine receptors.[2] There would seem to be little reason, on the basis of this extremely sparse evidence, to advise all patients taking bromocriptine not to drink alcohol, but if adverse effects develop, it would be reasonable to advise them to try avoiding alcohol.

1. Wass JAH, Thorner MO, Morris DV, Rees LH, Mason AS, Jones AE, Besser GM. Long-term treatment of acromegaly with bromocriptine. *BMJ* (1977) 1, 875–8.
2. Ayres J, Maisey MN. Alcohol increases bromocriptine's side effects. *N Engl J Med* (1980) 302, 806.

Alcohol + Bupropion

The concurrent use of bupropion and alcohol does not appear to affect the pharmacokinetics of either drug; however, adverse CNS effects might occur on concurrent use.

Clinical evidence, mechanism, importance and management

Single-dose studies in healthy subjects found that the pharmacokinetics of bupropion 100 mg were not affected by the concurrent use of alcohol, and bupropion did not affect blood-alcohol levels.[1,2] However, rare cases of adverse neuropsychiatric events and reduced alcohol tolerance have been reported in patients who drink alcohol while taking bupropion.[3,4] Because of this, the manufacturers recommend that the consumption of alcohol should be minimised or avoided.[3,4] Moreover, because abrupt withdrawal from alcohol is a risk factor for seizures, and there is a small dose-related risk of seizures with bupropion, the manufacturers contraindicate the use of bupropion in patients undergoing abrupt withdrawal from alcohol, and advise caution with its use in alcohol abuse.[3,4]

1. Posner J, Bye A, Jeal S, Peck AW, Whiteman P. Alcohol and bupropion pharmacokinetics in healthy male volunteers. *Eur J Clin Pharmacol* (1984) 26, 627–30.
2. Hamilton MJ, Bush MS, Peck AW. The effect of bupropion, a new antidepressant drug, and alcohol and their interaction in man. *Eur J Clin Pharmacol* (1984) 27, 75–80.
3. Zyban (Bupropion hydrochloride). GlaxoSmithKline UK. UK Summary of product characteristics, November 2013.
4. Zyban (Bupropion hydrochloride). GlaxoSmithKline. US Prescribing information, March 2014.

Alcohol + Buspirone

The use of buspirone with alcohol can cause drowsiness and weakness.

Clinical evidence, mechanism, importance and management

A study in 12 healthy subjects found that, in contrast to lorazepam, buspirone 10 or 20 mg did not appear to interact with alcohol (i.e. worsen the performance of certain psychomotor tests), but it did make the subjects feel drowsy and weak.[1,2] Similarly, another study in 13 healthy subjects found that giving buspirone (15 and 30 mg/70 kg) with alcohol caused sedation, but very little impairment of performance. In this study, the sedative effects were broadly similar to those seen with alprazolam and alcohol, but alprazolam and alcohol clearly impaired performance.[3] Similar findings were reported in another earlier comparison with diazepam.[4] A further study reported that single 5- to 15-mg doses of buspirone had a minimal effect on performance in both light and moderate female social drinkers.[5]

The UK manufacturer notes that there is no information on higher therapeutic doses of buspirone given with alcohol, and they suggest that it would be prudent to avoid alcohol while taking buspirone.[6] They also state that patients should be warned of the potential hazards of driving or handling other potentially dangerous machinery until they are certain that buspirone does not adversely affect them.[6] The evidence would appear to support this suggestion.

1. Mattila MJ, Aranko K, Seppala T. Acute effects of buspirone and alcohol on psychomotor skills. *J Clin Psychiatry* (1982) 43, 56–60.
2. Seppälä T, Aranko K, Mattila MJ, Shrotriya RC. Effects of alcohol on buspirone and lorazepam actions. *Clin Pharmacol Ther* (1982) 32, 201–7.
3. Rush CR, Griffiths RR. Acute participant-rated and behavioral effects of alprazolam and buspirone, alone and in combination with ethanol, in normal volunteers. *Exp Clin Psychopharmacol* (1997) 5, 28–38.
4. Erwin CW, Linnoila M, Hartwell J, Erwin A, Guthrie S. Effects of buspirone and diazepam, alone and in combination with alcohol, on skilled performance and evoked potentials. *J Clin Psychopharmacol* (1986) 6, 199–209.
5. Evans SM, Levin FR. The effects of alprazolam and buspirone in light and moderate female social drinkers. *Behav Pharmacol* (2002) 13, 427–39.
6. Buspirone hydrochloride. Actavis UK Ltd. UK Summary of product characteristics, January 2009.

Alcohol + Butyraldoxime

A disulfiram-like reaction can occur in those exposed to butyraldoxime if they drink alcohol.

Clinical evidence, mechanism, importance and management

Workers in a printing company complained of flushing of the face, neck and upper trunk, shortness of breath, tachycardia and drowsiness very shortly after drinking alcohol (about 45 mL of whiskey), and were found to have increased levels of acetaldehyde in their blood. The reason appeared to be that the printing ink they were using contained butyraldoxime, an antioxidant which, like disulfiram (see 'Alcohol + Disulfiram', p.67) can inhibit the metabolism of alcohol causing acetaldehyde to accumulate.[1] It is possible that it is a metabolite of butyraldoxime that causes this effect, rather than butyraldoxime itself.[2] This reaction would seem to be more unpleasant and socially disagreeable than serious. No treatment normally seems necessary.

1. Lewis W, Schwartz L. An occupational agent (N-butyraldoxime) causing reaction to alcohol. *Med Ann Dist Columbia* (1956) 25, 485–90.
2. DeMaster EG, Redfern B, Shirota FN, Crankshaw DL, Nagasawa HT. Metabolic activation of *n*-butyraldoxime by rat liver microsomal cytochrome P450. A requirement for the inhibition of aldehyde dehydrogenase. *Biochem Pharmacol* (1993) 46, 117–23.

Alcohol + Caffeine

Objective tests show that caffeine might counteract some of the effects of alcohol. However, it does not completely sober up those who have drunk too much, and could even make them more accident-prone.

Clinical evidence

(a) Effect on skills related to driving

A study in a large number of healthy subjects given a cup of **coffee** containing caffeine 300 mg/70 kg, either alone or immediately after drinking alcohol 0.75 g/kg, found that caffeine did not antagonise the deleterious effect of alcohol on the performance of psychomotor skill tests. Only reaction times were reversed.[1] Two other studies also found that caffeine did not antagonise the effects of alcohol in a variety of tests.[2,3] In one study in 26 healthy male subjects, drinking an energy drink (*Red Bull*) containing caffeine 1.14 mg/kg reduced the perception of headache, weakness, dry mouth ,and motor co-ordination, but it did not counteract most of the objectively measured effects of alcohol (0.6 g/kg or 1 g/kg) in tests of motor co-ordination and reaction time.[4]

A further study in 8 subjects found that, contrary to expectations, caffeine increased the frequency of errors in the performance of a serial reaction time task,[5] although a later study did not find this effect.[6] Caffeine has also been reported to *increase* the detrimental effects of alcohol.[7] In contrast, other studies (usually using caffeine in capsule form) have found that some of the performance-impairing effects of alcohol, such as increased reaction time,[8-10] increased errors with four choice reaction time,[11] impaired performance of divided attention tasks,[6] sedation,[12] and slowing of psychomotor speed,[11] can be antagonised if caffeine is given with alcohol. However, caffeine does not appear to affect most subjective effects e.g. feelings of drunkenness.[8,12,13]

One study found that giving alcohol with caffeine typically altered the effects of caffeine alone rather than altering the effects of alcohol alone. For example the addition of alcohol reduced the jitteriness and alertness produced by caffeine, and although caffeine modestly antagonised alcohol impairment of driving, there was still a 9% increase in brake-response time, when compared with placebo.[13]

(b) Pharmacokinetic effects

In a placebo-controlled, crossover study in 8 healthy subjects, the AUC of a 400-mg dose of caffeine (given as a capsule) was 30% greater when it was taken with alcohol 0.8 g/kg than when taken alone. Blood-alcohol levels were not affected by caffeine use.[8] Similarly, other studies reported that alcohol increases serum-caffeine levels[2] and that blood-alcohol levels[1,2,9] and breath-alcohol levels[4] were not modified by caffeine. However, one study in 8 healthy subjects reported that caffeine 3.3 mg/kg reduced blood-alcohol levels, measured 30 minutes after a single 0.7-g/kg dose of ethanol, from 38 mg% to 26 mg%.[10]

Mechanism

Not fully understood. Caffeine is a CNS stimulant, which seems to oppose some of the CNS depressant effects of alcohol. It appears that only those objective tests able to detect an enhancement due to a CNS stimulant show the clearest antagonistic effects.[8]

Alcohol appears to modestly inhibit the hepatic metabolism of caffeine.[2]

Importance and management

It is not known why some studies report that caffeine antagonises some of the detrimental effects of alcohol and others report no interaction. However, the type of psychomotor tests, the amount of alcohol and caffeine consumed, and the timing and administration of the caffeine might affect the results.

Caffeine does appear to improve some of the detrimental effects of alcohol in some psychomotor tests, which is probably why there is a long-standing and time-hallowed belief in the value of strong black coffee to sober up those who have drunk too much. However, it seems that it is not effective in all aspects of alcohol impairment, particularly subjective effects. In addition, caffeine does not reduce blood-alcohol levels. **Coffee** and other sources of caffeine such as caffeine-containing energy drinks do not make it safe to drive or handle dangerous machinery, and could even make drivers more accident-prone.

1. Franks HM, Hagedorn H, Hensley VR, Hensley WJ, Starmer GA. The effect of caffeine on human performance, alone and in combination with alcohol. *Psychopharmacologia* (1975) 45, 177–81.
2. Nuotto E, Mattila MJ, Seppälä T, Konno K. Coffee and caffeine and alcohol effects on psychomotor function. *Clin Pharmacol Ther* (1982) 31, 68–76.
3. Newman HW, Newman EJ. Failure of dexedrine and caffeine as practical antagonists of the depressant effect of ethyl alcohol in man. *Q J Stud Alcohol* (1956) 17, 406–10.
4. Ferreira SE, de Mello MT, Pompéia S, de Souza-Formigoni MLO. Effects of energy drink ingestion on alcohol intoxication. *Alcohol Clin Exp Res* (2006) 30, 598–605.
5. Lee DJ, Lowe G. Interaction of alcohol and caffeine in a perceptual-motor task. *IRCS Med Sci* (1980) 8, 420.
6. Marczinski CA, Fillmore MT. Clubgoers and their trendy cocktails: implications of mixing caffeine into alcohol on information processing and subjective reports of intoxication. *Exp Clin Psychopharmacol* (2006) 14, 450–8.
7. Oborne DJ, Rogers Y. Interactions of alcohol and caffeine on human reaction time. *Aviat Space Environ Med* (1983) 54, 528–34.
8. Azcona O, Barbanoj MJ, Torrent J, Jané F. Evaluation of the central effects of alcohol and caffeine interaction. *Br J Clin Pharmacol* (1995) 40, 393–400.
9. Marczinski CA, Fillmore MT. Dissociative antagonistic effects of caffeine on alcohol-induced impairment of behavioral control. *Exp Clin Psychopharmacol* (2003) 11, 228–36.
10. Hasenfratz M, Bunge A, Dal Prá G, Bättig K. Antagonistic effects of caffeine and alcohol on mental performance parameters. *Pharmacol Biochem Behav* (1993) 46, 463–5.
11. Mackay M, Tiplady B, Scholey AB. Interactions between alcohol and caffeine in relation to psychomotor speed and accuracy. *Hum Psychopharmacol* (2002) 17, 151–6.
12. Drake CL, Roehrs T, Turner L, Scofield HM, Roth T. Caffeine reversal of ethanol effects on the multiple sleep latency test, memory, and psychomotor performance. *Neuropsychopharmacology* (2003) 28, 371–8.
13. Liguori A, Robinson JH. Caffeine antagonism of alcohol-induced driving impairment. *Drug Alcohol Depend* (2001) 63, 123–9.

Alcohol + Calcium carbimide

Alcohol causes a disulfiram-like reaction in patients taking calcium carbimide. Calcium carbimide has been used as an alcohol deterrent.

Clinical evidence, mechanism, importance and management

Calcium carbimide interacts with alcohol in a similar way to disulfiram and by a similar mechanism[1] (see 'Alcohol + Disulfiram', p.67). Like disulfiram it is used to deter alcoholics from continuing to drink.[1,2] Both of these drugs bind to aldehyde dehydrogenase, but calcium carbimide is said to have fewer adverse effects because it does not bind to dopamine beta hydroxylase.[2] However, marked cardiovascular effects and fatalities have occurred in those who drank alcohol while taking calcium carbimide.[3-6]

1. Peachey JE, Brien JF, Roach CA, Loomis CW. A comparative review of the pharmacological and toxicological properties of disulfiram and calcium carbimide. *J Clin Psychopharmacol* (1981) 1, 21–6.
2. Monteiro MG. Pharmacological treatment of alcoholism. *Aust N Z J Med* (1992) 22, 220–3.

3. Kupari M, Hillbom M, Lindros K, Nieminen M. Possible cardiovascular hazards of the alcohol-calcium carbimide interaction. *J Toxicol Clin Toxicol* (1982) 19, 79–86.
4. Brien JF, Peachey JE, Loomis CW. Calcium carbimide–ethanol interaction. *Clin Pharmacol Ther* (1980) 27, 426–33.
5. Kojima T, Nagasawa N, Yashiki M, Iwasaki Y, Kubo H, Kimura N. A fatal case of drinking and cyanimide intake. *Jpn J Leg Med* (1997) 51, 111–15.
6. González Fernández C, González Castro A, López Sánchez M, Rodriguez Borregán JC. Intento autolítico por abuso de carbimida y alcohol con resultado fatal. *Med Clin (Barc)* (2009) 132, 683–4.

Alcohol + Calcium-channel blockers

Blood-alcohol levels can be raised and might remain elevated for a much longer period of time in patients taking verapamil. Alcohol might also increase the exposure to felodipine and nifedipine, but amlodipine appears not to interact with alcohol. Alcohol might increase the rate of release of diltiazem from a prolonged-release formulation. An increased incidence of postural hypotension has been reported in patients who took felodipine with alcohol.

Clinical evidence

(a) Amlodipine

A study in 30 healthy subjects found that single and multiple doses of amlodipine 10 mg for 15 days (with or without lisinopril and simvastatin) had no effect on the pharmacokinetics of alcohol 0.8 g/kg, and subjective psychological performance was unaffected. Alcohol did not alter the pharmacokinetics of amlodipine.[1]

(b) Felodipine

A study in 8 healthy subjects given enough alcohol to maintain their blood levels at 80 to 120 mg% found that the exposure to a single 10-mg dose of felodipine was increased (AUC increased by 77%) and its maximum blood levels were also increased (by 98%). Diuresis was approximately doubled and heart rates were increased.[2]

In a study, 8 non-smoking, healthy subjects were given a single 10-mg dose of an extended-release preparation of felodipine, with 250 mL of red wine, on an empty stomach and 4 hours before a meal. Red wine reduced felodipine levels for the first 4 hours of the study, when compared with 250 mL of water, but felodipine levels rose rapidly 5 hours after dosing, resulting in a peak level that was higher with red wine than with water.[3]

Another study suggested that alcohol increased the haemodynamic effects of felodipine (lower total peripheral resistance, lower blood pressure, higher heart rate) and increased the rate of adverse effects (e.g. postural lightheadedness).[4] However, the alcohol was given in grapefruit juice, which is known to increase felodipine levels; indeed, felodipine levels were reported as being higher than expected in this study, so it is possible these effects were, at least in part, due to an interaction with grapefruit juice (see 'Calcium-channel blockers + Grapefruit juice', p.1037).

(c) Isradipine

In a placebo-controlled study, 9 healthy subjects were given isradipine 5 or 10 mg followed by alcohol 0.5 or 1 g/kg. The performance impairment in response to alcohol was not affected by isradipine. However, increases in heart rate, and decreases in blood pressure appeared to be enhanced when both drugs were taken together. Furthermore, isradipine 10 mg caused a small decrease in breath-alcohol levels.[5]

(d) Nifedipine

Alcohol (75 mL of 94% alcohol with 75 mL of orange juice) given to 10 healthy subjects increased the AUC of a single 20-mg dose of nifedipine by 54%, but no statistically significant changes in heart rate or blood pressure were seen.[6] Another study, involving 226 patients taking sustained-release nifedipine, found that reported alcohol use was associated with a lower nifedipine clearance (8.6 mL/minute per kg compared with 10.8 mL/minute per kg for alcohol use and no alcohol, respectively).[7] In another study no evidence was found that nifedipine 10 or 20 mg antagonised the effects of alcohol.[8]

(e) Nimodipine

In a randomised study in 6 healthy subjects, a single 30- or 60-mg dose of nimodipine had no effect on the subjective or psychomotor response to a single oral 0.7-g/kg dose of alcohol, and there were no clinically significant changes in blood pressure or heart rate. Nimodipine 60 mg reduced the peak breath-alcohol level by 20 mg%, but this was considered slight.[9]

(f) Verapamil

In one study, 10 healthy subjects were given verapamil 80 mg three times daily for 6 days with alcohol 0.8 g/kg on day 6. Peak blood-alcohol levels were found to be raised by almost 17% (from about 106 mg% to 124 mg%) and the AUC_{0-12} was raised by almost 30%. The time that blood-alcohol levels exceeded 100 mg% was prolonged from 0.2 hours to 1.3 hours and the subjects said they felt more intoxicated.[10] Another study found that verapamil 80 or 160 mg did not antagonise the intoxicating effects of alcohol.[8] A further randomised study in 6 healthy subjects found that a single 80-mg dose of verapamil had no effect on the subjective or psychomotor response to a single oral 0.7-g/kg dose of alcohol, and no clinically significant changes were noted in blood pressure or heart rate. The pharmacokinetics of alcohol were not affected by verapamil.[9]

Mechanism

Not understood. It seems possible that verapamil inhibits the metabolism of alcohol by the liver, thereby reducing its loss from the body. Alcohol also appears to inhibit the metabolism of nifedipine, and to increase the bioavailability of felodipine. Red wine might have caused "dose dumping" of felodipine from the extended-release preparation, which altered its pharmacokinetic profile, but the reason why the felodipine levels remained low until after a meal is unclear.[3] An *in vitro* study suggested that alcohol inhibited the oxidative metabolism of nifedipine by the cytochrome P450 subfamily CYP3A.[11]

Importance and management

Information regarding an interaction between alcohol and calcium-channel blockers seems to be limited to these reports. Information regarding **verapamil** is conflicting, with one study finding no pharmacokinetic interaction and another finding an almost 17% increase in blood-alcohol levels. This increase could be enough to raise legal blood levels to illegal levels if driving. Moreover the intoxicant effects of alcohol persisted for a much longer period of time (five times longer) in this study. Therefore, despite the conflicting findings, it would be prudent to bear the possibility of an interaction in mind. The decreases in breath-alcohol levels with **felodipine** and **nimodipine** were small, and unlikely to be of clinical significance because performance indicators were not altered. However, the bioavailability of felodipine and **nifedipine** appear to be increased by alcohol. The manufacturers of some calcium-channel blockers warn that inter-individual variations in the response to these drugs can occur and the ability of some patients to drive or operate machinery might be impaired, particularly at the start of treatment and in conjunction with alcohol.[12,13] Patients should therefore be advised about these effects. The manufacturers of a prolonged-release **diltiazem** preparation (*Adizem*) similarly warn that alcohol might increase the rate of diltiazem release, and therefore suggest that alcohol should not be taken at the same time as this preparation.[14]

Note that long-term moderate to heavy drinking can impair the efficacy of antihypertensives, see 'Alcohol + Antihypertensives', p.55.

1. Vincent J, Colangelo P, Baris B, Willavize S. Single and multiple doses of amlodipine do not alter the pharmacokinetics of alcohol in man. *Therapie* (1995) (Suppl) 50, 509.
2. Pentikainen PJ, Virolainen T, Tenhunen R, Aberg J. Acute alcohol intake increases the bioavailability of felodipine. *Clin Pharmacol Ther* (1994) 55, 148.
3. Bailey DG, Dresser GK, Bend JR. Bergamottin, lime juice, and red wine as inhibitors of cytochrome P450 3A4 activity: Comparison with grapefruit juice. *Clin Pharmacol Ther* (2003) 73, 529–37.
4. Bailey DG, Spence JD, Edgar B, Bayliff CD, Arnold JMO. Ethanol enhances the hemodynamic effects of felodipine. *Clin Invest Med* (1989) 12, 357–62.
5. Rush CR, Pazzaglia PJ. Pretreatment with isradipine, a calcium-channel blocker, does not attenuate the acute behavioral effects of ethanol in humans. *Alcohol Clin Exp Res* (1998) 22, 539–47.
6. Qureshi S, Laganière S, Caillé G, Gossard D, Lacasse Y, McGilveray I. Effect of an acute dose of alcohol on the pharmacokinetics of oral nifedipine in humans. *Pharm Res* (1992) 9, 683–6.
7. Krecic-Shepard ME, Park K, Barnas C, Slimko J, Kerwin DR, Schwartz JB. Race and sex influence clearance of nifedipine: results of a population study. *Clin Pharmacol Ther* (2000) 68, 130–42.
8. Perez-Reyes M, White WR, Hicks RE. Interaction between ethanol and calcium channel blockers in humans. *Alcohol Clin Exp Res* (1992) 16, 769–75.
9. Zacny JP, Yajnik S. Effects of calcium channel inhibitors on ethanol effects and pharmacokinetics in healthy volunteers. *Alcohol* (1993) 10, 505–9.
10. Bauer LA, Schumock G, Horn J, Opheim K. Verapamil inhibits ethanol elimination and prolongs the perception of intoxication. *Clin Pharmacol Ther* (1992) 52, 6–10.
11. Patki KC, Greenblatt DJ, von Moltke LL. Ethanol inhibits in-vitro metabolism of nifedipine, triazolam and testosterone in human liver microsomes. *J Pharm Pharmacol* (2004) 56, 963–6.
12. Adalat Retard (Nifedipine). Bayer plc. UK Summary of product characteristics, April 2012.
13. Univer (Verapamil hydrochloride). Cephalon (UK) Ltd. UK Summary of product characteristics, March 2012.
14. Adizem-XL Capsules (Diltiazem hydrochloride). Napp Pharmaceuticals Ltd. UK Summary of product characteristics, November 2011.

Alcohol + Cannabis

The detrimental effects of drinking alcohol and smoking cannabis might be additive on some aspects of driving performance. However, there is some evidence that regular cannabis use *per se* does not potentiate the effects of alcohol. Smoking cannabis can alter the bioavailability of alcohol.

Clinical evidence and mechanism

(a) CNS effects

Simultaneous use of alcohol and oral Δ^9-tetrahydrocannabinol (THC, the major active ingredient of cannabis) reduced the performance of psychomotor tests, suggesting that those who use both drugs together should expect the deleterious effects to be additive.[1] Additive effects were found in other studies,[2,3] but in one,[3] additive effects occurred mainly in the first 40 minutes, but in later test periods (at 100 and 160 minutes) the depressant effects of oral Δ^9-tetrahydrocannabinol were not as marked as expected and for some tests, including standing steadiness, the effect of Δ^9-tetrahydrocannabinol alone was greater than that when it was given with alcohol, suggesting an antagonistic effect.[3]

In a placebo-controlled study, subjects smoked cannabis containing 100 or 200 micrograms/kg of Δ^9-tetrahydrocannabinol and drank alcohol (to achieve an initial blood level of 70 mg%, with further drinks taken to maintain levels at 40 mg%) 30 minutes before driving. They found that cannabis, even in low to moderate doses, negatively affected driving performance in real traffic situations. Further, the effect of combining moderate doses of both alcohol and cannabis resulted in dramatic performance impairment as great as that observed with blood-alcohol levels of 140 mg% alone.[4,5] Similar results (including a suggestion of a synergistic impairment of performance[6]) have been found in a number of other studies,[6-9] including different doses of cannabis and regular cannabis users.[7]

A study in 22 healthy subjects, who occasionally used cannabis cigarettes and drank moderate amounts of alcohol, found that the number of euphoric events in response to a cannabis cigarette was greater after alcohol ingestion, and the duration of euphoric events was longer. The speed of onset of the effects of cannabis was also faster when it was smoked after the ingestion of alcohol.[10]

One study in 14 regular cannabis users (long-term daily use) and 14 infrequent cannabis users found that regular use reduced the disruptive effects of alcohol on some psychomotor skills relevant to driving, whereas infrequent use did not have this effect. In this study, neither group had smoked any cannabis in the 12 hours before the alcohol test.[11] Another study found that moderate doses of alcohol and cannabis, consumed either alone or in combination, did not produce significant behavioural or subjective impairment the following day.[12]

A study in 12 healthy subjects who regularly used both cannabis and alcohol found that alcohol 0.5 g/kg increased break latency without affecting body sway, whereas cannabis given as a cigarette containing tetrahydrocannabinol 3.33%, increased body sway but did not affect brake latency. There were no notable additive effects on brake latency, body sway, or mood when the two drugs were used together.[13] A population-based study of 2 777 drivers involved in fatal road crashes, who drank alcohol and/or used cannabis, found that although both cannabis and alcohol increased the risk of being responsible for a fatal crash, no statistically significant interaction was observed between the two drugs.[14]

(b) Pharmacokinetic studies

Fifteen healthy subjects given alcohol 0.7 g/kg developed peak plasma alcohol levels of about 78 mg% at 50 minutes, but if they smoked a cannabis cigarette 30 minutes after the drink, their peak plasma alcohol levels were only 55 mg% and they occurred 55 minutes later. In addition, their subjective experience of the drugs decreased when they were used together.[15] However, another study found that smoking cannabis 10 minutes before alcohol consumption did not affect blood-alcohol levels.[12] A further study found smoking cannabis following alcohol consumption did not affect alcohol levels.[8] Other studies have found that blood-alcohol levels were not affected by Δ^9-tetrahydrocannabinol given orally one hour before alcohol.[1-3] A study in 22 healthy subjects, who occasionally used cannabis cigarettes and drank moderate amounts of alcohol, found that plasma Δ^9-tetrahydrocannabinol levels were higher when alcohol was consumed before smoking a cannabis cigarette.[10]

Importance and management

Several studies have found that cannabis and alcohol produce additive detrimental effects on driving performance, but other studies have not found any potentiation. This is probably due to the variety of simulated driving tests used and possibly the time lag between the administration of alcohol and cannabis; behavioural impairment after cannabis has been reported to peak within 30 minutes of smoking.[12] Nevertheless, both drugs have been shown to affect some aspects of driving performance and increase the risk of fatal car accidents. Of concern, one study found that drivers are willing to drive despite being aware of the effects of alcohol and/or cannabis and the only consideration that affected their risk taking was the urgency of the drive.[9] Concurrent use of cannabis and alcohol before driving should be avoided.

1. Bird KD, Boleyn T, Chesher GB, Jackson DM, Starmer GA, Teo RKC. Intercannabinoid and cannabinoid-ethanol interactions and their effects on human performance. *Psychopharmacology (Berl)* (1980) 71, 181–8.
2. Belgrave BE, Bird KD, Chesher GB, Jackson DM, Lubbe KE, Starmer GA, Teo RKC. The effect of (−) trans-Δ^9-tetrahydrocannabinol, alone and in combination with ethanol, on human performance. *Psychopharmacology (Berl)* (1979) 62, 53–60.
3. Chesher GB, Franks HM, Jackson DM, Starmer GA, Teo RKC. Ethanol and Δ^9-tetrahydrocannabinol interactive effects on human perceptual, cognitive and motor functions. II. *Med J Aust* (1977) 1, 478–81.
4. National Highway Traffic Safety Administration. Marijuana and alcohol combined severely impede driving performance. *Ann Emerg Med* (2000) 35, 398–9.
5. Jolly BT. Commentary: drugged driving—different spin on an old problem. *Ann Emerg Med* (2000) 35, 399–400.
6. Perez-Reyes M, Hicks RE, Burnberry J, Jeffcoat AR, Cook CE. Interaction between marihuana and ethanol: effects on psychomotor performance. *Alcohol Clin Exp Res* (1988) 12, 268–76.
7. Marks DF, MacAvoy MG. Divided attention performance in cannabis users and non-users following alcohol and cannabis separately and in combination. *Psychopharmacology (Berl)* (1989) 99, 397–401.
8. Hansteen RW, Miller RD, Lonero L, Reid LD, Jones B. Effects of cannabis and alcohol on automobile driving and psychomotor tracking. *Ann N Y Acad Sci* (1976) 282, 240–56.
9. Ronen A, Chassidim HS, Gershon P, Parmet Y, Rabinovich A, Bar-Hamburger R, Cassuto Y, Shinar D. The effect of alcohol, THC and their combination on perceived effects, willingness to drive and performance of driving and non-driving tasks. *Accid Anal Prev* (2010) 42, 1855–65.
10. Lukas SE, Orozco S. Ethanol increases plasma Δ^9-tetrahydrocannabinol (THC) levels and subjective effects after marihuana smoking in human volunteers. *Drug Alcohol Depend* (2001) 64, 143–9.
11. Wright KA, Terry P. Modulation of the effects of alcohol on driving-related psychomotor skills by chronic exposure to cannabis. *Psychopharmacology (Berl)* (2002) 160, 213–19.
12. Chait LD, Perry JL. Acute and residual effects of alcohol and marijuana, alone and in combination, on mood and performance. *Psychopharmacology (Berl)* (1994) 115, 340–9.
13. Liguori A, Gatto CP, Jarrett DB. Separate and combined effects of marijuana and alcohol on mood, equilibrium and simulated driving. *Psychopharmacology (Berl)* (2002) 163, 399–405.
14. Laumon B, Gadeqbeku B, Martin J-L, Biecheler M-B; the SAM Group. Cannabis intoxication and fatal road crashes in France: population based case-control study. *BMJ* (2005) 331, 1371–6. Correction. ibid. (2006) 332, 1298.
15. Lukas SE, Benedikt R, Mendelson JH, Kouri E, Sholar M, Amass L. Marihuana attenuates the rise in plasma ethanol levels in human subjects. *Neuropsychopharmacology* (1992) 7, 77–81.

Alcohol + Carbamazepine

Moderate social drinking does not affect the serum levels of carbamazepine. Heavy drinking might increase the metabolism of carbamazepine, and this could be further increased in alcoholics who abstain from drinking alcohol.

Clinical evidence, mechanism, importance and management

(a) Heavy drinking and alcohol withdrawal

A study in 7 alcoholics who consumed a mean dose of 750 mL of spirits (240 g of alcohol) daily found that the early (0 to 4 hours) bioavailability of a single 400-mg dose of carbamazepine was not affected by 9 days of controlled alcohol withdrawal. However, over the 4- to 12-hour period, carbamazepine levels were higher, and those of its epoxy metabolite lower, in alcoholics following alcohol exposure, when compared with abstinence. This effect was thought to be due to the acute inhibition of carbamazepine metabolism by alcohol and/or accelerated carbamazepine metabolism in the abstinence phase. The absorption rate of carbamazepine in alcoholics appeared to be slower, when compared with 8 healthy subjects, probably due to alcoholism-induced chronic gastrointestinal changes; however, this did not affect the maximum serum levels of alcohol. However, adverse effects occurred in all of the healthy subjects but in none of the alcoholics, possibly indicating that long-term alcohol exposure might make the patient less sensitive to acute carbamazepine exposure.[1]

The long-term use of alcohol can induce hepatic enzymes possibly resulting in increased metabolism and reduced plasma levels of carbamazepine. The risk of seizures might also increase on tapering or stopping alcohol because of an increase in metabolism and elimination caused by the relative lack of a competing substrate.[2]

(b) Moderate social drinking

Alcohol 25 g did not affect the bioavailability of carbamazepine in 8 healthy subjects.[1] A study in non-drinking patients with epilepsy (21 in the experimental alcohol group, 18 in the control group) found that the serum levels of carbamazepine were unchanged by moderate drinking (1 to 3 glasses of an alcoholic beverage, containing 9.85 g of alcohol, twice weekly), and there was no influence on tonic-clonic convulsions or partial complex seizures.[3]

For comment on moderate social drinking in patients with epilepsy and also the possible increased sedative effect of carbamazepine with alcohol, see 'Alcohol + Antiepileptics', p.54.

1. Sternebring B, Lidén A, Andersson K, Melander A. Carbamazepine kinetics and adverse effects during and after ethanol exposure in alcoholics and in healthy volunteers. *Eur J Clin Pharmacol* (1992) 43, 393–7.
2. Gordon E, Devinsky O. Alcohol and marijuana: effects on epilepsy and use by patients with epilepsy. *Epilepsia* (2001) 42, 1266–72.
3. Höppener RJ, Kuyer A, van der Lugt PJM. Epilepsy and alcohol: the influence of social alcohol intake on seizures and treatment in epilepsy. *Epilepsia* (1983) 24, 459–71.

Alcohol + Carmofur

A disulfiram-like reaction occurred in a patient taking carmofur when he was given a coeliac plexus blockade with alcohol.

Clinical evidence, mechanism, importance and management

A man with pancreatic carcinoma taking carmofur 500 mg daily for 25 days experienced a disulfiram-like reaction (facial flushing, diaphoresis, hypotension with blood pressure of 60/30 mmHg, and tachycardia of 128 bpm) within 30 minutes of being given a coeliac plexus alcohol blockade for pain relief. Blood-acetaldehyde levels were found to have risen sharply, supporting the belief that the underlying mechanism is similar to the disulfiram-alcohol interaction (see 'Alcohol + Disulfiram', p.67, for further explanation). It is suggested that alcohol blockade should be avoided for 7 days after treatment with carmofur.[1]

1. Noda J, Umeda S, Mori K, Fukunaga T, Mizoi Y. Disulfiram-like reaction associated with carmofur after celiac plexus alcohol block. *Anesthesiology* (1987) 67, 809–10.

Alcohol + Cephalosporins

Disulfiram-like reactions can occur in those who take cefamandole, cefmenoxime, cefoperazone, cefotetan, latamoxef (moxalactam) and possibly cefonicid, and drink alcohol. This is not a general reaction of the cephalosporins, but is confined to those with particular chemical structures.

Clinical evidence

A young man with cystic fibrosis was given **latamoxef** 2 g intravenously every 8 hours for pneumonia. After 3 days of treatment he drank, as was his custom, a can of beer with lunch. He rapidly became flushed with a florid macular eruption over his face and chest. This faded over the next 30 minutes but he complained of severe nausea and headache. Similarly, a patient taking **latamoxef** became flushed, diaphoretic and nauseated after drinking a cocktail of vodka and tomato juice.[1] This reaction has also been described in two subjects who drank alcohol while receiving **latamoxef**,[2] two of 10 subjects given **latamoxef** and alcohol,[3] and a patient taking **latamoxef** given theophylline elixir containing alcohol 20%.[4] It has also been seen in a patient taking **latamoxef** following the injection of alcohol into the para-aortic space for coeliac plexus block.[5] The symptoms experienced by these patients have included flushing of the face, arms and neck, shortness of breath, headache, tachycardia, dizziness, hypertension, hypotension, and nausea and vomiting.

Similar reactions have been described in patients or subjects receiving **cefamandole**,[6,7] **cefoperazone**,[8-15] **cefmenoxime**,[16] **cefonicid**[17] and **cefotetan**,[18] after drinking wine, beer, other alcoholic drinks, or after the ingestion of an 8.5% alcoholic elixir.[16]

This disulfiram-like reaction is not a general reaction of all the cephalosporins. One study found no interaction in those taking **cefpirome** and alcohol,[19] and in another, **ceftizoxime** was reported not to interact with alcohol.[20] No interaction was seen with **cefonicid** and alcohol in one placebo-controlled study;[21] however, a case report describes a disulfiram-like reaction in one patient taking alcohol with **cefonicid**.[17]

Mechanism

These reactions appear to have the same pharmacological basis as the reaction in those who drink alcohol while taking disulfiram (see 'Alcohol + Disulfiram', p.67). Three of these cephalosporins (latamoxef, cefamandole and cefoperazone) can raise blood acetaldehyde levels in *rats* when alcohol is given, but to a lesser extent than disulfiram.[2,11,22] It appears that any reaction normally only occurs with cephalosporins that possess a methyltetrazolethiol group in the 3-position on the cephalosporin molecule,[11,23] but the reaction has also been seen with cefonicid, which possesses a sulfanylmethyltetrazolethiol group instead.[17] Some amine-containing cephalosporins (**cefalexin**, **cefadroxil** and **cefradine**) have also been reported to interact with acetaldehyde *in vitro*, but the clinical relevance of this is unknown.[24]

Importance and management

The interactions between alcohol and a number of the cephalosporins are established but unpredictable, and of varying incidence. In studies, two out of 10 subjects taking latamoxef and alcohol reacted,[3] five out of 8 taking cefotetan reacted,[18] and 8 out of 9 taking cefoperazone reacted.[14,15] The reaction appears normally to be more embarrassing or unpleasant and frightening than serious, with the symptoms subsiding spontaneously after a few hours. There is evidence that the severity varies; in one study cefoperazone was said to be worse than latamoxef, which in turn was said to be worse than **cefmetazole**.[25] Treatment is not usually needed but there are two reports[4,6] of elderly patients who needed treatment for hypotension, which was life-threatening in one case;[4] plasma expanders and dopamine have been used as treatment.[4,6]

Because the reaction is unpredictable, warn all patients taking these potentially interacting cephalosporins (cefamandole, cefmenoxime, cefmetazole, cefonicid, cefoperazone, cefotetan, latamoxef) that it can occur during and up to 3 days after the course of treatment is over. Advise them to avoid alcohol. Those with renal or hepatic impairment in whom the drug clearance is prolonged should avoid alcohol for a week. It should not be forgotten that some foods and pharmaceuticals contain substantial amounts of alcohol, and a reaction with some topically applied alcohol-containing products cannot be excluded (see 'Alcohol + Disulfiram', p.67).

A number of other cephalosporins are possible candidates for this reaction because they possess the methyltetrazolethiol group in the 3-position. These include, **ceforanide**, **cefotiam**, and **cefpiramide**,[11,25] but there do not appear to be any reports of an interaction between alcohol and these drugs.

1. Neu HC, Prince AS. Interaction between moxalactam and alcohol. *Lancet* (1980), i, 1422.
2. Buening MK, Wold JS, Israel KS, Kammer RB. Disulfiram-like reaction to β-lactams. *JAMA* (1981) 245, 2027–8.
3. Elenbaas RM, Ryan JL, Robinson WA, Singsank MJ, Harvey MJ, Klaasen CD. On the disulfiram-like activity of moxalactam. *Clin Pharmacol Ther* (1982) 32, 347–55.
4. Brown KR, Guglielmo BJ, Pons VG, Jacobs RA. Theophylline elixir, moxalactam, and a disulfiram-like reaction. *Ann Intern Med* (1982) 97, 621–2.
5. Umeda S, Arai T. Disulfiram-like reaction to moxalactam after celiac plexus alcohol block. *Anesth Analg* (1985) 64, 377.
6. Portier H, Chalopin JM, Freysz M, Tanter Y. Interaction between cephalosporins and alcohol. *Lancet* (1980), ii, 263.
7. Drummer S, Hauser WE, Remington JS. Antabuse-like effect of β-lactam antibiotics. *N Engl J Med* (1980) 303, 1417–18.
8. Foster TS, Raehl CL, Wilson HD. Disulfiram-like reaction associated with parenteral cephalosporin. *Am J Hosp Pharm* (1980) 37, 858–9.
9. Allaz A-F, Dayer P, Fabre J, Rudhardt M, Balant L. Pharmacocinétique d'une nouvelle céphalosporine, la céfopérazone. *Schweiz Med Wochenschr* (1979), 109, 1999–2005.
10. Kemmerich B, Lode H. Cefoperazone – another cephalosporin associated with a disulfiram type alcohol incompatibility. *Infection* (1981) 9, 110.
11. Uri JV, Parks DB. Disulfiram-like reaction to certain cephalosporins. *Ther Drug Monit* (1983) 5, 219–24.
12. Bailey RR, Peddie B, Blake E, Bishop V, Reddy J. Cefoperazone in the treatment of severe or complicated infections. *Drugs* (1981) 22 (Suppl 1), 76–86.
13. Ellis-Pegler RB, Lang SDR. Cefoperazone in Klebsiella meningitis: A case report. *Drugs* (1981) 22 (Suppl 1), 69–71.
14. Reeves DS, Davies AJ. Antabuse effect with cephalosporins. *Lancet* (1980) ii, 540.
15. McMahon FG. Disulfiram-like reaction to a cephalosporin. *JAMA* (1980), 243, 2397.
16. Kannangara DW, Gallagher K, Lefrock JL. Disulfiram-like reactions with newer cephalosporins: cefmenoxime. *Am J Med Sci* (1984) 287, 45–7.
17. Marcon G, Spolaor A, Scevola M, Zolli M, Carlassara GB. Effetto disulfiram-simile da cefonicid: prima segnalazione. *Recenti Prog Med* (1990) 81, 47–8.
18. Kline SS, Mauro VF, Forney RB, Freimer EH, Somani P. Cefotetan-induced disulfiram-type reactions and hypoprothrombinemia. *Antimicrob Agents Chemother* (1987) 31, 1328–31.
19. Lassman HB, Hubbard JW, Chen B-L, Puri SK. Lack of interaction between cefpirome and alcohol. *J Antimicrob Chemother* (1992) 29 (Suppl A), 47–50.
20. McMahon FG, Noveck RJ. Lack of disulfiram-like reactions with ceftizoxime. *J Antimicrob Chemother* (1982) 10 (Suppl C), 129–33.
21. McMahon FG, Ryan JR, Jain AK, LaCorte W, Ginzler F. Absence of disulfiram-type reactions to single and multiple doses of cefonicid: a placebo-controlled study. *J Antimicrob Chemother* (1987) 20, 913–8.
22. Yanagihara M, Okada K, Nozaki M, Tsurumi K, Fujimura H. Cephem antibiotics and alcohol metabolism. Disulfiram-like reaction resulting from intravenous administration of cephem antibiotics. *Folia Pharmacol Japon* (1982) 79, 551–60.
23. Norrby SR. Adverse reactions and interactions with newer cephalosporin and cephamycin antibiotics. *Med Toxicol* (1986) 1, 32–46.
24. Nuñez-Vergara LJ, Yudelevich J, Squella JA, Speisky H. Drug-acetaldehyde interactions during ethanol metabolism *in vitro*. *Alcohol Alcohol* (1991) 26, 139–46.
25. Nakamura K, Nakagawa A, Tanaka M, Masuda H, Hayashi Y, Saionji K. Effects of cephem antibiotics on ethanol metabolism. *Folia Pharmacol Japon* (1984) 83, 183–91.

Alcohol + Ciprofloxacin

Ciprofloxacin does not notably affect the pharmacokinetics of alcohol or its effects on psychomotor performance. There is an isolated report of a cutaneous reaction to ciprofloxacin, which might have been precipitated by alcohol consumption.

Clinical evidence, mechanism, importance and management

In a study in 12 healthy subjects, ciprofloxacin 500 mg twice daily for 3 days had no statistically significant effect on the pharmacokinetics of a single 30-g oral dose of alcohol (75 mL of vodka), and the performance of a number of psychomotor tests was unaffected.[1] A study in 8 healthy male subjects found that ciprofloxacin 750 mg twice daily for 7 days decreased the elimination rate of alcohol 0.63 g/kg by about 10% and increased its AUC by 11%, which would not be expected to be clinically significant. It was suggested that ciprofloxacin reduced the number of aerobic bacteria in the gut, which reduced alcohol dehydrogenase activity and therefore reduced ethanol metabolism.[2]

There is an isolated report of red blotches developing on the face and body of a tetraplegic patient taking ciprofloxacin 250 mg twice daily, which developed within 10 minutes of drinking 2 cans of beer containing alcohol 4.7%. He did not feel unwell or drowsy, and the blotches faded over a period of 30 minutes. Previous courses of ciprofloxacin had not produced any adverse effects and the same brand of alcohol caused no problems in the absence of ciprofloxacin.[3] The general clinical importance of this report is unknown, but it seems likely to be small.

1. Kamali F. No influence of ciprofloxacin on ethanol disposition: a pharmacokinetic-pharmacodynamic interaction study. *Eur J Clin Pharmacol* (1994) 47, 71–4.
2. Tillonen J, Homann N, Rautio M, Jousimies-Somer H, Salaspuro M. Ciprofloxacin decreases the rate of ethanol elimination in humans. *Gut* (1999) 44, 347–52.
3. Vaidyanathan S, Singh G, Sett P, Watt JWH, Soni BM, Oo T. Cutaneous adverse reaction to ciprofloxacin precipitated by ingestion of alcohol in a tetraplegic patient. *Spinal Cord* (1999) 37, 663–4. Correction. ibid. 807.

Alcohol + Clomethiazole

Clomethiazole has been successfully used to treat alcohol withdrawal, but the long-term use of alcohol with clomethiazole can cause serious CNS depression. This is potentially fatal, even with short-term use in alcoholics with cirrhosis. The bioavailability of clomethiazole might be increased by alcohol.

Clinical evidence, mechanism, importance and management

(a) Enhanced adverse effects and bioavailability

The following is taken from an editorial in the British Medical Journal, which was entitled 'Chlormethiazole and alcohol: a lethal cocktail'.[1]

Clomethiazole is commonly used to treat withdrawal from alcohol because of its hypnotic, anxiolytic and anticonvulsant effects. It is very effective if a rapidly reducing dosage regimen is followed over six days, but if it is used long-term and drinking continues it carries several serious risks.

Alcoholics readily transfer dependency to clomethiazole and may visit several practitioners and hospitals to get their supplies. Tolerance develops so that very large amounts may need to be taken (up to 25 g daily). Often alcohol abuse continues and the combination of large amounts of alcohol and clomethiazole can result in coma and even fatal respiratory depression, due mainly to simple additive CNS depression.[1]

Other factors contributing to the increase in CNS depression seen include increases in the bioavailability of clomethiazole, probably caused by alcohol impairing first pass metabolism,[2] and, in the case of those with alcoholic cirrhosis, the systemic bioavailability of clomethiazole can be increased tenfold because of venous shunting.[3] A randomised study in 8 healthy subjects found that alcohol 0.8 g/kg increased the AUC of a single 192-mg dose of clomethiazole by 82%.[2] However, one study in 6 healthy subjects reported that intravenous alcohol 0.8 mL/kg given acutely had no effect on the disposition or elimination of clomethiazole. It was proposed that alcohol given orally might affect the absorption or rate of uptake of clomethiazole.[4]

Clomethiazole should not be given long-term for alcohol withdrawal states[1] or to those who continue to drink alcohol.[5] Use for more than 9 days is not recommended.[5,6] It has been said that if prescribers choose to manage detoxification at home, it should be done under very close supervision, issuing prescriptions for only one day's supply to ensure daily contact and to minimise the risk of abuse. Further, if the patient shows evidence of tolerance or clomethiazole dependency or of continuing to drink alcohol, the only safe policy is rapid admission for inpatient care.[1] The manufacturer warns that alcohol given with clomethiazole particularly in alcoholics with cirrhosis can lead to fatal respiratory depression, even with short-term use.[5]

(b) Effects on driving and related skills

There do not appear to be any studies on the combined effects of clomethiazole and alcohol on driving and related skills, but concurrent use would be expected to increase the risks. One report describes a man who had a blood-alcohol level of 23 mg% who was driving dangerously and caused a traffic accident. The clinical signs of impairment were far greater than expected and further analysis of the blood sample identified a high level of clomethiazole (5 mg/L). In 13 other impaired driving cases where clomethiazole was detected in blood samples, the concentrations ranged from 0.3 to

3.3 mg/L.[7] The manufacturer warns that clomethiazole can potentiate or be potentiated by CNS depressant drugs, including alcohol.[5]

1. McInnes GT. Chlormethiazole and alcohol: a lethal cocktail. *BMJ* (1987) 294, 592.
2. Neuvonen PJ, Pentikäinen PJ, Jostell KG, Syvälahti E. Effect of ethanol on the pharmacokinetics of chlormethiazole in humans. *Int J Clin Pharmacol Ther Toxicol* (1981) 19, 552–60.
3. Pentikäinen PJ, Neuvonen PJ, Tarpila S, Syvälahti E. Effect of cirrhosis of the liver on the pharmacokinetics of chlormethiazole. *BMJ* (1978) 2, 861–3.
4. Bury RW, Desmond PV, Mashford ML, Westwood B, Shaw G, Breen KJ. The effect of ethanol administration on the disposition and elimination of chlormethiazole. *Eur J Clin Pharmacol* (1983) 24, 383–5.
5. Heminevrin Capsules (Clomethiazole). AstraZeneca UK Ltd. UK Summary of product characteristics, August 2009.
6. Morgan MY. The management of alcohol withdrawal using chlormethiazole. *Alcohol Alcohol* (1995) 30, 771–4.
7. Jones, AW. Driving under the influence of chlormethiazole. *Forensic Sci Int* (2005) 153, 213–17.

Alcohol + Cloral hydrate

Both alcohol and cloral hydrate are CNS depressants, and their effects could be additive, or possibly even synergistic. Some patients might experience a disulfiram-like flushing reaction if they drink alcohol after taking cloral hydrate for several days.

Clinical evidence

Studies in 5 healthy subjects given cloral hydrate 15 mg/kg and alcohol 0.5 g/kg found that both drugs given alone impaired their ability to carry out complex motor tasks. When taken together, the effects were additive, and possibly even more than additive. After taking cloral hydrate for 7 days, one of the subjects experienced a disulfiram-like reaction (bright red-purple flushing of the face, tachycardia, hypotension, anxiety and persistent headache) after drinking alcohol.[1,2]

The disulfiram-like reaction has been described in other reports.[3] Note that the earliest report was published in 1872 and described two patients taking cloral hydrate who experienced this reaction after drinking half a bottle of beer.[2]

Mechanism

Alcohol, cloral and trichloroethanol (to which cloral hydrate is metabolised) are all CNS depressants. During concurrent use, the metabolic pathways used for their elimination are mutually inhibited: blood-alcohol levels rise because the trichloroethanol competitively depresses the oxidation of alcohol to acetaldehyde, while trichloroethanol levels also rise because its production from cloral hydrate is increased and its further conversion and clearance as the glucuronide is inhibited. As a result the rises in the blood levels of alcohol and trichloroethanol are exaggerated, and their effects are accordingly greater.[1,2,4,5] In one subject, blood levels of acetaldehyde during the use of cloral hydrate with alcohol were only 50% of those after alcohol alone, so that the flushing reaction, despite its resemblance to the disulfiram reaction, might have a partially different basis.[2]

Importance and management

The interaction between alcohol and cloral hydrate is a well-documented and established interaction, which has been comprehensively reviewed.[1,2] Only a few references are given here. Patients given cloral hydrate should be warned about the extensive CNS depression that can occur if they drink alcohol, and of the disulfiram-like reaction that can occur if they drink after taking cloral hydrate for a period of time. Its incidence is uncertain. The legendary Mickey Finn, which is concocted of cloral hydrate and alcohol, is reputed to be so potent that deep sleep can be induced in an unsuspecting victim within minutes of ingestion, but the evidence seems to be largely anecdotal. Very large doses of both drugs would be likely to cause serious and potentially life-threatening CNS depression.

It seems likely that **cloral betaine, triclofos** and other compounds closely related to cloral hydrate will interact with alcohol in a similar manner, but this requires confirmation.

1. Sellers EM, Lang M, Koch-Weser J, LeBlanc E, Kalant H. Interaction of chloral hydrate and ethanol in man. I. Metabolism. *Clin Pharmacol Ther* (1972) 13, 37–49.
2. Sellers EM, Carr G, Bernstein JG, Sellers S, Koch-Weser J. Interaction of chloral hydrate and ethanol in man. II. Hemodynamics and performance. *Clin Pharmacol Ther* (1972) 13, 50–8.
3. Bardodĕj Z. Intolerance alkoholu po chloralhydrátu. *Cesk Farm* (1965) 14, 478–81.
4. Wong LK, Biemann K. A study of drug interaction by gas chromatography–mass spectrometry—synergism of chloral hydrate and ethanol. *Biochem Pharmacol* (1978) 27, 1019–22.
5. Weller RA, Preskorn SH. Psychotropic drugs and alcohol: pharmacokinetic and pharmacodynamic interactions. *Psychosomatics* (1984) 25, 301–3, 305–6, 309.

Alcohol + Cocaine

Alcohol increases the plasma levels of cocaine and its active metabolite cocaethylene. Subjective effects such as euphoria are enhanced and some of the CNS depressant effects of alcohol, such as sedation, are attenuated by cocaine. The combination is potentially more toxic, with increased cardiovascular effects.

Clinical evidence

A study in 8 cocaine users found that intranasal cocaine 100 mg and alcohol 0.8 g/kg produced a greater euphoria and feeling of well-being than cocaine alone, and reduced alcohol sedation without altering the feeling of drunkenness. Compared with placebo, the peak heart-rate was increased by 17 bpm, 23 bpm, and 41 bpm, with alcohol, cocaine, or the combination, respectively. In addition, the combination resulted in higher plasma levels of cocaine and the appearance of cocaethylene, an active and potentially toxic metabolite produced by the interaction of the two drugs.[1] Other similar studies have reported comparable findings.[2,3] A further study found that intranasal cocaine 96 mg/70 kg improved behavioural performance, measured by the digit symbol substitution test (DSST), whereas alcohol 1 g/kg decreased DSST performance. The combination of alcohol 1 g/kg with intranasal cocaine 48 or 96 mg/70 kg reduced the DSST below that found with cocaine alone. The combination also additively increased heart rate and diastolic blood pressure. Blood-alcohol levels were not notably affected by the concurrent use of intranasal cocaine.[4] A study in 6 male subjects found that alcohol 0.85 g/kg, taken 30 minutes after snorting cocaine, did not alter the effect of cocaine on heart rate, did not alter cocaine levels or blood-alcohol levels, and did not affect subjective ratings of drunkenness.[5]

In contrast, a study in 11 healthy male subjects found that when alcohol 0.85 g/kg was given 15 minutes before snorting cocaine (either 1.25 mg/kg or 1.9 mg/kg), the bioavailability of cocaine was increased, and there were increases in heart rate, cardiac output, and blood pressure.[6]

Mechanism

In the presence of alcohol, cocaine is metabolised in the liver to cocaethylene, which appears to have the same stimulant effects as cocaine, but a longer half-life (2 hours compared with about 38 minutes for cocaine). *Animal* studies suggest that this metabolite is more toxic than cocaine.[7] In addition, chronic alcohol exposure might facilitate the metabolism of cocaine, promoting the formation of intermediate metabolites that can cause liver damage, potentiating the hepatotoxic properties of alcohol.[8] It has been suggested that the ingestion of alcohol before snorting cocaine results in greater absorption of cocaine through the nasal vasculature due to increased dilatation by alcohol.[5]

Importance and management

It has been suggested that the enhanced psychological effects associated with alcohol and cocaine could lead to the use of larger amounts of the combination with an increased risk for toxic effects,[2] such as cardiotoxicity.[1] It has been reported that users of alcohol and cocaine who also have coronary artery disease have 21.5 times the risk for sudden death than users of cocaine alone.[7] The longer half-life of the metabolite cocaethylene explains why many people who experience cocaine-related heart attacks and strokes do so when the cocaine levels in their blood are low, as cocaethylene can remain active in the body for 7 hours after cocaine has disappeared.[7] Patients with coronary artery disease or alcoholics appear to be particularly vulnerable to the combined toxic effects of alcohol and cocaine.

1. Farré M, de la Torre R, González ML, Terán MT, Roset PN, Menoyo E, Camí J. Cocaine and alcohol interactions in humans: neuroendocrine effects and cocaethylene metabolism. *J Pharmacol Exp Ther* (1997) 283, 164–76.
2. McCance-Katz EF, Kosten TR, Jatlow P. Concurrent use of cocaine and alcohol is more potent and potentially more toxic than use of either alone–a multiple-dose study. *Biol Psychiatry* (1998) 44, 250–9.
3. Farré M, de la Torre R, Llorente M, Lamas X, Ugena B, Segura J, Camí J. Alcohol and cocaine interactions in humans. *J Pharmacol Exp Ther* (1993) 266, 1364–73.
4. Higgins ST, Rush CR, Bickel WK, Hughes JR, Lynn M, Capeless MA. Acute behavioral and cardiac effects of cocaine and alcohol combinations in humans. *Psychopharmacology (Berl)* (1993) 111, 285–94.
5. Perez-Reyes M. The order of drug administration: its effects on the interaction between cocaine and ethanol. *Life Sci* (1994) 55, 541–50.
6. Perez-Reyes M, Jeffcoat AR. Ethanol/cocaine interaction: cocaine and cocaethylene plasma concentrations and their relationship to subjective and cardiovascular effects. *Life Sci* (1992) 51, 553–63.
7. Randall T. Cocaine, alcohol mix in body to form even longer lasting, more lethal drug. *JAMA* (1992) 267, 1043–4.
8. Hoyumpa AM. Alcohol interactions with benzodiazepines and cocaine. *Adv Alcohol Subst Abuse* (1984) 3, 21–34.

Alcohol + Codergocrine mesilate (Ergoloid mesylates)

Codergocrine mesilate causes a very small reduction in blood-alcohol levels.

Clinical evidence, mechanism, importance and management

Thirteen subjects were given 0.5 g/kg of alcohol 25% in orange juice after breakfast, before and after taking 4.5 mg of codergocrine mesilate (ergoloid mesylates, *Hydergine*) every 8 hours for nine doses. The codergocrine caused a very small reduction in blood-alcohol levels (maximum serum levels reduced from 59 mg% to 55.7 mg%), and its clearance was reduced by 11%.[1] The reason is not understood. This interaction is almost certainly not of clinical importance.

1. Savage IT, James IM. The effect of Hydergine on ethanol pharmacokinetics in man. *J Pharm Pharmacol* (1993) 45 (Suppl 2), 1119.

Alcohol + Co-trimoxazole

A disulfiram-like reaction has been reported when two patients taking co-trimoxazole drank beer.

Clinical evidence, mechanism, importance and management

A 31-year-old man who had been taking prophylactic double-strength co-trimoxazole twice daily for 3 days experienced flushing, palpitations, dyspnoea, headache and nausea 10 to 20 minutes after drinking about 780 mL of beer. Symptoms resolved gradually over 2 to 3 hours, but occurred again the next day when he drank about 170 mL of beer. A similar experience occurred in another man taking double-strength co-trimoxazole after drinking one litre of beer. However, on the previous day, he drank 4 to 5 beers (approximately 1.4 L) without a problem, even though he had taken co-trimoxazole.[1] The clinical relevance of these case reports is unknown as there do not appear to be any other reports of this interaction. Further, note that some formulations of co-trimoxazole contain ethanol.

1. Heelon MW, White M. Disulfiram-cotrimoxazole reaction. *Pharmacotherapy* (1998) 18, 869–70.

Alcohol + Cyproterone

Excessive alcohol consumption might reduce the antiandrogenic effect of cyproterone in the treatment of hypersexuality, but the relevance of this effect in prostate cancer is not known; there seems to be no evidence that normal social amounts of alcohol interact.

Clinical evidence, mechanism, importance and management

The UK manufacturer of cyproterone (*Androcur*) states that alcohol appears to reduce its effects, and so it is of no value in chronic alcoholics.[1] This appears to be based solely on a simple and unelaborated statement in an abstract of studies[2] in 84 men whose hyper- or abnormal sexuality was treated with cyproterone acetate, which stated that "antiandrogens do not inhibit male sexual behaviour during alcohol excess."

The suggested reasons for this reaction are unknown, but it might be due to several factors. These include enzyme induction by alcohol, which could possibly increase the metabolism and clearance of cyproterone; increased sexual drive caused by alcohol, which might oppose the effects of cyproterone; and reduced compliance by alcoholic patients, who forget to take their tablets while drinking to excess.[3]

It seems therefore that cyproterone might not be effective in alcoholic patients, but there is nothing to suggest that the effects of cyproterone are opposed by normal moderate social amounts of alcohol. The relevance of this in prostate cancer is not known; nevertheless, it has been suggested that the use of alcohol during treatment with cyproterone is not advisable.[4] In the absence of further information it would seem prudent to limit alcohol intake in patients taking cyproterone.

1. Androcur (Cyproterone acetate). Schering Health Care Ltd. UK Summary of product characteristics, January 2011.
2. Laschet U, Laschet L. Three years clinical results with cyproterone-acetate in the inhibiting regulation of male sexuality. *Acta Endocrinol (Copenh)* (1969) 138 (Suppl), 103.
3. Schering Health Care Limited. Personal communication, January 1997.
4. Androcur (Cyproterone acetate). Bayer Inc. Canadian Product Monograph, February 2011.

Alcohol + Dimethylformamide

A disulfiram-like reaction can occur in workers exposed to dimethylformamide vapour if they drink alcohol. Alcohol might enhance the toxic effects of dimethylformamide on liver function.

Clinical evidence

A 3-year study in a chemical plant where dimethylformamide was used found that about 20% (19 out of 102 men) exposed to dimethylformamide vapour experienced flushing of the face, and often of the neck, arms, hands, and chest, after drinking alcohol. Sometimes dizziness, nausea, and tightness of the chest also occurred. A single glass of beer was enough to induce a flush lasting 2 hours. The majority of the men experienced the reaction within 24 hours of exposure to dimethylformamide, but it could occur even after 4 days.[1] Three further cases of this interaction are described in other reports.[2,3]

Another study, in 126 factory workers exposed to dimethylformamide and 54 workers who had no contact with dimethylformamide, indicated that dimethylformamide adversely affected liver function, and that concurrent alcohol had a synergistic effect (both drugs are hepatotoxic), although individual differences in tolerance to the interaction were observed. Flush symptoms after alcohol consumption were reported by 86 out of 126 (approximately 70%) of workers exposed to dimethylformamide, compared with 2 out of 54 (4%) of controls.[4]

Mechanism

Subjects exposed to dimethylformamide vapour develop substantial amounts of dimethylformamide and its metabolite (*N*-methylformamide) in their blood and urine.[1] This latter compound in particular has been shown in *rats* given alcohol to raise their blood acetaldehyde levels by a factor of five, so it would seem probable that the *N*-methylformamide is similarly responsible for this disulfiram-like reaction in man.[5] For more details of this mechanism, see under 'Alcohol + Disulfiram', below.

Importance and management

The interaction between alcohol and dimethylformamide is established, with the incidence reported to be between about 20% and 70%.[1] Those who come into contact with dimethylformamide, even in very low concentrations, should be warned of this possible interaction with alcohol. It would appear to be more unpleasant than serious in most instances, and normally requires no treatment; however the hepatotoxic effects are clearly more of a concern.

1. Lyle WH, Spence TWM, McKinneley WM, Duckers K. Dimethylformamide and alcohol intolerance. *Br J Ind Med* (1979) 36, 63–6.
2. Chivers CP. Disulfiram effect from inhalation of dimethylformamide. *Lancet* (1978) i, 331.
3. Reinl W, Urban HJ. Erkrankungen durch dimethylformamid. *Int Arch Gewerbepathol Gewerbehyg* (1965) 21, 333–46.
4. Wrbitzky R. Liver function in workers exposed to *N,N*-dimethylformamide during the production of synthetic textiles. *Int Arch Occup Environ Health* (1999) 72, 19–25.
5. Hanasono GK, Fuller RW, Broddle WD, Gibson WR. Studies on the effects of *N,N'*-dimethylformamide on ethanol disposition and monoamine oxidase activity in rats. *Toxicol Appl Pharmacol* (1977) 39, 461–72.

Alcohol + Dimethyl sulfoxide (DMSO)

Dimethyl sulfoxide appears to increase the psychomotor impairment that occurs in response to alcohol.

Clinical evidence, mechanism, importance and management

A case report describes a man who had applied 'relatively large' amounts of dimethyl sulfoxide to his hands in the course of his work, for 2 days before, and while drinking 6 or 7 bottles of beer over 6 hours. Seven hours after he had drunk the last bottle of beer he was noted to be driving erratically, and a positive alcohol breath test was recorded (details not given). The amount of alcohol ingested and the timescale was not expected to result in a positive breath test, and an interaction with DMSO was suspected.[1] Anecdotal reports imply that this is not the only case of increased psychomotor impairment that has been attributed to this interaction.[1,2]

A study in 30 healthy subjects found that the absorption of oral alcohol 0.75 g/kg was not affected by DMSO applied topically, either one hour before or with the alcohol. However, even though DMSO appeared to increase the clearance of alcohol, the subjects developed twice the psychomotor impairment, when compared with alcohol alone.[2]

Although the effect of DMSO on blood-alcohol levels is unclear (the study only measured clearance, which was increased, and the case only reported breath-alcohol levels, which were increased), it seems that the concurrent use of both drugs increases psychomotor impairment. Those applying DMSO should be reminded that gloves should be worn and those being treated with DMSO should be warned of the potential consequences of consuming alcohol.

1. Doig PA, Dimethyl sulfoxide and alcohol – a potentially dangerous combination. *Can Vet J* (1999) 40, 755–6.
2. Mallach HJ. Interaction of DMSO and alcohol. *Ann N Y Acad Sci* (1967) 141, 457–62.

Alcohol + Disopyramide

In healthy subjects, the renal clearance of disopyramide might be very slightly increased by alcohol-induced diuresis.

Clinical evidence, mechanism, importance and management

A crossover study in 6 healthy subjects found that the half-life and total body clearance of disopyramide were not affected by alcohol, but the amount of the metabolite mono-*N*-dealkylated disopyramide excreted in the urine was reduced. Alcohol increased diuresis in 5 of the 6 subjects, and the renal clearance of disopyramide was increased by 19% in these subjects.[1] The overall clinical effect of these changes is likely to be minimal.

1. Olsen H, Bredesen JE, Lunde PKM. Effect of ethanol intake on disopyramide elimination by healthy volunteers. *Eur J Clin Pharmacol* (1983) 25, 103–5.

Alcohol + Disulfiram

Drinking alcohol while taking disulfiram will result in flushing and fullness of the face and neck, tachycardia, breathlessness, giddiness, hypotension, and nausea and vomiting. This is called the disulfiram reaction. It is used to deter alcoholic patients from drinking. A mild flushing reaction of the skin can occur in particularly sensitive individuals if alcohol is applied to the skin or if alcohol vapour is inhaled.

Clinical evidence

(a) Alcoholic drinks

One of the earliest descriptions of a disulfiram-like interaction with alcohol was made in 1937 by Dr EE Williams[1] who noted it amongst workers in the rubber industry who were handling **tetramethylthiuram disulphide**:

"Even beer will cause a flushing of the face and hands, with rapid pulse, and some of the men describe palpitations and a terrible fullness of the face, eyes and head. After a glass of beer the blood pressure falls about 10 points, the pulse is slightly accelerated and the skin becomes flushed in the face and wrists. In 15 minutes the blood pressure falls another 10 points, the heart is more rapid, and the patient complains of fullness in the head."

The later observation of the same reaction with the ethyl congener of **tetramethylthiuram disulphide**, disulfiram, led to its introduction as an alcoholic drink deterrent.[2] Patients experience throbbing in the head and neck, giddiness, sweating, nausea, vomiting, thirst, chest pain, difficulty in breathing, and headache. The severity of the reaction can depend upon the amount of alcohol consumed, but some individuals are extremely sensitive. Respiratory depression, cardiovascular collapse, cardiac arrhythmias, unconsciousness, and convulsions can occur. There have been fatalities.[3,4]

An unusually severe reaction has been described in a number of case reports. A 27-year-old man developed hypotension (blood pressure 63/15 mmHg), tachycardia of

140 bpm, and ST depression after drinking a can of beer 2 weeks after starting to take disulfiram; he needed noradrenaline (norepinephrine) to maintain an adequate blood pressure.[5] In a second case, a 53-year-old man who had taken disulfiram (initially 250 mg for one week, then 500 mg daily) developed severe hypotension (blood pressure 35/20 mmHg) and had an ischaemic stroke after drinking approximately 300 mL of wine 2 to 3 hours after taking disulfiram 500 mg on day 9.[6] A third report describes a case of acute myocardial infarction in a 22-year-old patient with chronic alcoholism who developed severe chest pain and hypotension (blood pressure 80/50 mmHg) 2 hours after taking disulfiram 500 mg with a large amount of alcohol (amount not specified).[7]

Another unusual and isolated report describes painful, intermittent and transient myoclonic jerking of the arms and legs as the predominant manifestation of the disulfiram reaction in one patient.[8] A further unusual case has been reported in which a woman with a history of bipolar disorder and alcoholism, who was taking disulfiram, was admitted to hospital with a 3- to 4-day history of changes in her mental state, including difficulties with orientation, concentration and visual hallucinations. The confusional state was attributed to alcohol consumption while taking disulfiram, and the probability of this was supported by an earlier similar, though shorter, episode experienced by the patient.[9] Some alcoholics find that disulfiram potentiates the euphoric effects of low doses of alcohol, which alone would be relatively ineffective.[10]

(b) Products containing alcohol

A mild disulfiram reaction is said to occur in some patients who apply alcohol to the skin, but it is probably largely due to inhalation of the vapour.[11] It has been reported after using **after-shave lotion** (50% alcohol),[11] **tar gel** (33% alcohol)[12] and a **beer-containing shampoo** (3% alcohol).[13] A **contact lens wetting solution** (containing **polyvinyl alcohol**) used to irrigate the eye has also been implicated in a reaction,[14,15] although the probability of an interaction with this secondary alcohol has been disputed.[16] It has also been described in a patient who inhaled vapour from paint in a poorly ventilated area and from the inhalation of '**mineral spirits**'.[17] A 36-year-old man with no known cardiac disorders, taking disulfiram 500 mg daily, had a myocardial infarction, which was attributed to **fermented vinegar** in a salad dressing and the use of an **after-shave lotion**.[18]

Furthermore, an unusual case describes a woman taking disulfiram who reported vaginal stinging and soreness during sexual intercourse, and similar discomfort to her husband's penis, which seemed to be related to the disulfiram dose and how intoxicated her husband was.[19]

The UK manufacturer of the oral solution of **ritonavir** (*Norvir*) states that as it contains alcohol 43% v/v (which they say is about equivalent to 27 mL of wine per dose) the preparation should not be taken with disulfiram or other drugs such as **metronidazole** because a disulfiram-like reaction is possible.[20] The oral concentrate of sertraline (*Zoloft oral concentrate*) is contraindicated with disulfiram due to the alcohol content (12%).[21]

Mechanism

Partially understood. Alcohol is normally rapidly metabolised within the liver, firstly by alcohol dehydrogenase to acetaldehyde, then by acetaldehyde dehydrogenase, and then by a series of biochemical steps to water and carbon dioxide. Disulfiram inhibits the enzyme acetaldehyde dehydrogenase so that the acetaldehyde accumulates.[3] The authors of the report of a case of myocardial infarction suggest that an increased acetaldehyde level in the blood may have caused cause coronary vasospasm and myocardial infarction.[18]

Although the symptoms of the disulfiram-alcohol reaction are due partly to the high levels of acetaldehyde, not all of the symptoms can be reproduced by injecting acetaldehyde, so that some other biochemical mechanism(s) must also be involved. The conversion of dopamine to noradrenaline is also inhibited and the depletion of noradrenaline in the heart and blood vessels allows acetaldehyde to act directly on these tissues to cause flushing, tachycardia and hypotension.[22] Prostaglandin release might also be involved.[23] It has been suggested that the mild skin flush that can occur if alcohol is applied to the skin is not a true disulfiram reaction.[24]

However, some individuals appear to be more sensitive than others, which might be partially due to liver function and variations in the metabolism of disulfiram to its active metabolite by cytochrome P450 isoenzymes.[25,26] Genetic variation in the alcohol metabolising enzymes alcohol and acetaldehyde dehydrogenase have been shown to influence the breakdown of alcohol and formation of acetaldehyde and influence drinking behaviour and the risk of developing alcoholism in certain populations.[27,28] This might partly explain differences in response to disulfiram.

Importance and management

The interaction between alcohol and disulfiram is an extremely well-documented and important interaction, which is exploited therapeutically to deter alcoholics from drinking alcohol. Initial treatment should be closely supervised because an extremely intense and potentially serious reaction occurs in a few individuals, even with quite small doses of alcohol. Apart from the usual warnings about drinking alcohol, patients should also be warned about unwitting contact with alcohol in some pharmaceutical preparations.[29] The risk of a reaction is real. It has been seen following a single-dose of an alcohol-containing **cough mixture**,[30] whereas the ingestion of small amounts of **communion wine** and the absorption of alcohol from a **bronchial nebuliser spray** or **ear drops** did not result in any reaction in 3 individuals.[31] The severity of the reaction is reported to be proportional to the dose of both disulfiram and alcohol.[32] Patients should also be warned about the exposure to alcohol from some foods, cosmetics, solvents etc. The manufacturers advise that certain foods (sauces and vinegars), liquid medicines, remedies (cough mixtures, tonics, back rubs), and toiletries (aftershave, perfumes and aerosol sprays) might contain sufficient alcohol to elicit a reaction.[22,32] Caution should also be exercised with low-alcohol and "non-alcohol" or "alcohol-free" beers and wines, which could provoke a reaction when consumed in sufficient quantities.[22] Disulfiram is eliminated slowly from the body and therefore drinking alcohol might produce unpleasant symptoms up to 14 days after taking the last dose of disulfiram.[32]

Treatment

The disulfiram reaction can be treated, if necessary, with ascorbic acid. A dose of 1 g given orally is reported to be effective in mild cases (heart rate less than 100 bpm and general condition good). It works within 30 to 45 minutes. Moderately severe cases (heart rate 100 to 150 bpm, blood pressure 150/100 mmHg) can be treated with 1 g of intravenous ascorbic acid and this is effective within 2 to 5 minutes. Critically ill patients could need other standard supportive emergency measures.[33]

1. Williams EE. Effects of alcohol on workers with carbon disulfide. *JAMA* (1937) 109, 1472.
2. Hald J, Jacobsen E, Larsen V. The sensitizing effects of tetraethylthiuramdisulphide (Antabuse) to ethylalcohol. *Acta Pharmacol* (1948) 4, 285–96.
3. Kwentus J, Major LF. Disulfiram in the treatment of alcoholism: a review. *J Stud Alcohol* (1979) 40, 428–46.
4. Stransky G, Lambing MK, Simmons GT, Robinson A. Methemolglobinemia in a fatal case of disufiram-ethanol reaction. *J Anal Toxicol* (1997) 21, 178–9.
5. Milne HJ, Parke TRJ. Hypotension and ST depression as a result of disulfiram ethanol reaction. *Eur J Emerg Med* (2007) 14, 228–9.
6. Prancheva MG, Krasteva SA, Tufkova SG, Karaivanova TP, Nizamova VV, Iliev YT. Severe hypotension and ischemic stroke after disulfiram-ethanol reaction. *Folia Med (Plovdiv)* (2010) 52, 70–73.
7. Tayyareci Y, Acarel E. Acute myocardial infarction associated with disulfiram-alcohol interaction in a young man with normal coronary arteries. *Turk Kardiyol Dern Ars* (2009) 37, 48–50.
8. Syed J, Moarefi G. An unusual presentation of a disulfiram-alcohol reaction. *Del Med J* (1995) 67, 183.
9. Park CW, Riggio S. Disulfiram-ethanol induced delirium. *Ann Pharmacother* (2001) 35, 32–5.
10. Brown ZW, Amit Z, Smith BR, Sutherland EA, Selvaggi N. Alcohol-induced euphoria enhanced by disulfiram and calcium carbimide. *Alcohol Clin Exp Res* (1983) 7, 276–8.
11. Mercurio F. Antabuse®-alcohol reaction following the use of after-shave lotion. *JAMA* (1952) 149, 82.
12. Ellis CN, Mitchell AJ, Beardsley GR. Tar gel interaction with disulfiram. *Arch Dermatol* (1979) 115, 1367–8.
13. Stoll D, King LE. Disulfiram-alcohol skin reaction to beer-containing shampoo. *JAMA* (1980) 244, 2045.
14. Newsom SR, Harper BS. Disulfiram-alcohol reaction caused by contact lens wetting solution. *Contact Intraocul Lens Med J* (1980) 6, 407–8.
15. Newsom SR. Letter to the editor. *Contact Intraocul Lens Med J* (1981) 7, 172.
16. Refojo MF. Letter to Editor. *Contact Intraocul Lens Med J* (1981) 7, 172.
17. Scott GE, Little FW. Disulfiram reaction to organic solvents other than ethanol. *N Engl J Med* (1985) 312, 790.
18. Altun G, Altun A, Erdogan O. Acute myocardial infarction due to disulfiram (Antabus) – alcohol interaction. *Cardiovasc Drugs Ther* (2006) 20, 391–2.
19. Chick JD. Disulfiram reaction during sexual intercourse. *Br J Psychiatry* (1988) 152, 438.
20. Norvir Oral Solution (Ritonavir). AbbVie Ltd. UK Summary of product characteristics, September 2012.
21. Zoloft (Sertraline hydrochloride). Pfizer Inc. US Prescribing information, August 2014.
22. Antabuse (Disulfiram). Actavis UK Ltd. UK Summary of product characteristics, December 2011.
23. Truitt EB, Gaynor CR, Mehl DL. Aspirin attenuation of alcohol-induced flushing and intoxication in oriental and occidental subjects. *Alcohol Alcohol* (1987) 22 (Suppl 1), 595–9.
24. Haddock NF, Wilkin JK. Cutaneous reactions to lower aliphatic alcohols before and during disulfiram therapy. *Arch Dermatol* (1982) 118, 157–9.
25. Poikolainen K. The disulfiram-ethanol reaction (DER) experience. *Addiction* (2004) 99, 26.
26. Beyeler C, Fisch H-U, Preisig R. The disulfiram-alcohol reaction: factors determining and potential tests predicting severity. *Alcohol Clin Exp Res* (1985) 9, 118–24.
27. Scott DM, Taylor RE. Health-related effects of genetic variations of alcohol-metabolizing enzymes in African Americans. *Alcohol Res Health* (2007) 30, 18–21.
28. Thomasson HR, Edenberg HJ, Crabb DW, Mai X-L, Jerome RE, Li T-K, Wang S-P, Lin Y-T, Lu R-B, Yin S-J. Alcohol and aldehyde dehydrogenase genotypes and alcoholism in Chinese men. *Am J Hum Genet* (1991) 48, 677–81.
29. Parker WA. Alcohol-containing pharmaceuticals. *Am J Drug Alcohol Abuse* (1982–3) 9, 195–209.
30. Koff RS, Papadimas I, Honig EG. Alcohol in cough medicines: hazard to disulfiram user. *JAMA* (1971) 215, 1988–9.
31. Rothstein E. Use of disulfiram (Antabuse) in alcoholism. *N Engl J Med* (1970) 283, 936.
32. Antabuse (Disulfiram). Odyssey Pharmaceuticals, Inc. US Prescribing information, December 2003.
33. McNichol RW, Sowell JM, Logsdon SA, Delgado MH, McNichol J. Disulfiram: a guide to clinical use in alcoholism treatment. *Am Fam Physician* (1991) 44, 481–4.

Alcohol + Edible fungi

A disulfiram-like reaction can occur if alcohol is taken after eating the smooth ink(y) cap fungus (*Coprinus atramentarius*) or certain other edible fungi.

Clinical evidence

A man who drank 3 pints of beer 2 hours after eating a meal of freshly picked and fried **ink(y) caps** (***Coprinus atramentarius***) developed facial flushing and a blotchy red rash over the upper half of his body. His face and hands swelled, and he became breathless, sweated profusely, and vomited during the 3 hours when the reaction was most severe. On admission to hospital he was tachycardic and 12 hours later he was in atrial fibrillation, which lasted for 60 hours. The man's wife, who ate the same meal but without an alcoholic drink, did not show the reaction.[1]

This reaction has been described on many occasions in medical and pharmacological reports[2-7] and in books devoted to descriptions of edible and poisonous fungi. Only a few are listed here. Mild hypotension and "alarming orthostatic features" are said to be common symptoms[8] but the arrhythmia seen in the case cited above[1] appears to be rare. Recovery is usually spontaneous and uncomplicated.

A similar reaction has been described after eating ***Boletus luridus***,[6,9] ***Lepiota aspera***,[10] and other fungi including ***Coprinus micaceus***, ***Clitocybe claviceps*** and certain **morels**.[9,11] An African relative of ***Coprinus atramentarius***, ***Coprinus africanus***, which also causes this reaction, is called the **Ajeimutin** fungus by the Nigerian Yoruba people. The literal translation of this name is the 'eat-without-drinking-alcohol' mushroom.[12]

Mechanism

An early and attractive idea was that the reaction with *Coprinus atramentarius* (ink caps; also known as tippler's bane) was due to the presence of disulfiram (one group of workers actually claimed to have isolated it from the fungus[13]), but this was not confirmed by later work,[14,15] and it now appears that the active ingredient is coprine (*N*-5-(1-hydroxycyclopropyl)-glutamine).[16,17] This is metabolised in the body to 1-aminocyclopropanol, which appears, like disulfiram, to inhibit aldehyde dehydrogenase (see 'Alcohol + Disulfiram', p.67). The active ingredients in the other fungi are unknown.

Importance and management

The interaction between alcohol and these fungi is established and well-documented. It is said to occur up to 24 hours after eating the fungus. The intensity depends upon the quantity of fungus and alcohol consumed, and the time interval between them.[1,4,18] Despite the widespread consumption of edible fungi and alcohol, reports of this reaction in the medical literature are few and far between, suggesting that even though it can be very unpleasant and frightening, the outcome is usually uncomplicated. Treatment appears normally not to be necessary.

The related fungus ***Coprinus comatus*** (the **'shaggy ink cap'** or **'Lawyers wig'**) is said not to interact with alcohol,[8,19] nor is there anything to suggest that it ever occurs with the **common field mushroom** (***Agaricus campestris***) or the cultivated variety (***Agaricus bisporis***).[19]

1. Caley MJ, Clarke RA. Cardiac arrhythmia after mushroom ingestion. *BMJ* (1977) 2, 1633.
2. Reynolds WA, Lowe FH. Mushrooms and a toxic reaction to alcohol: report of four cases. *N Engl J Med* (1965) 272, 630–1.
3. Wildervanck LS. Alcohol en de kale inktzwam. *Ned Tijdschr Geneeskd* (1978) 122, 913–14.
4. Buck RW. Mushroom toxins—a brief review of the literature. *N Engl J Med* (1961) 265, 681–6.
5. Marty H. Von Pilzen und Schnäpsen. *Schweiz Med Wochenschr* (1998) 128, 598.
6. Flammer R. Brechdurchfälle als Leitsymptom – Pilze und Alkohol. Emesis and diarrhea – mushrooms and alcohol. *Schweiz Rundsch Med Prax* (1985) 74, 992–6.
7. Oteo Revuelta JA, Grandival García R, Olarte Arce A. Reaccíon disulfiram-like por ingesta de hongos [Disulfiram-like reaction caused by mushroom ingestion]. *Rev Clin Esp* (1989) 184, 394–5.
8. Broadhurst-Zingrich L. Ink caps and alcohol. *BMJ* (1978) 1, 511.
9. Budmiger H, Kocher F. Hexenröhrling (Boletus luridus) mit Alkohol: ein kasuistischer beitrag. *Schweiz Med Wochenschr* (1982) 112, 1179–81.
10. Haberl B, Pfab R, Berndt S, Greifenhagen C, Zilker T. Case series: alcohol intolerance with coprine-like syndrome after consumption of the mushroom *Lepiota aspera* (Pers.:Fr.) Quél., 1886 (Freckled Dapperling). *Clin Toxicol* (2011) 49, 113–14.
11. Cochran KW, Cochran MW. *Clitocybe clavipes:* antabuse-like reaction to alcohol. *Mycologia* (1978) 70, 1124–6.
12. Oso BA. Mushrooms and the Yoruba people of Nigeria. *Mycologia* (1975) 67, 311–19.
13. Simandl J, Franc J. Isolace tetraethylthiuramdisulfidu z hníku inko ustového (*Coprinus atramentarius*). *Chem Listy* (1956) 50, 1862–3.
14. Vanhaelen M, Vanhaelen-Fastré R, Hoyois J, Mardens Y. Reinvestigation of disulfiram-like biological activity of *Coprinus atramentarius* (Bull. *ex* Fr.) Fr. extracts. *J Pharm Sci* (1976) 65, 1774–6.
15. Wier JK, Tyler VE. An investigation of *Coprinus atramentarius* for the presence of disulfiram. *J Am Pharm Assoc* (1960) 49, 426–9.
16. Hatfield GM, Schaumberg JP. Isolation and structural studies of coprine, the disulfiram-like constituent of *Coprinus atramentarius*. *Lloydia* (1975) 38, 489–96.
17. Lindberg P, Bergman R, Wickberg B. Isolation and structure of coprine, the *in vivo* aldehyde dehydrogenase inhibitor in *Coprinus atramentarius*; syntheses of coprine and related cyclopropanone derivatives. *J Chem Soc* (1977) (6) 684–91.
18. Fujiyama Y, Naitoh M, Nakamura M, Minezaki K, Shigeta Y, Okubo M. [Mushroom poisoning whose symptoms were relevant to the amount of alcohol taken]. *Nippon Naika Gakkai Zasshi* (2002) 91, 2189–91.
19. Radford AP. Ink caps and mushrooms. *BMJ* (1978) 1, 112.

Alcohol + Erythromycin

Alcohol can cause a small reduction in the absorption of erythromycin ethylsuccinate. Some evidence suggests that intravenous erythromycin can raise blood-alcohol levels.

Clinical evidence, mechanism, importance and management

(a) Effects on alcohol

A study in 10 healthy subjects found that erythromycin base 500 mg three times daily did not alter the pharmacokinetics of oral alcohol 0.8 g/kg, and the subjects' perception of intoxication was unaltered.[1] In contrast, another study in 8 healthy subjects, primarily investigating the effects of intravenous erythromycin lactobionate 3 mg/kg on gastric emptying, found that when they were given a liquid meal of orange juice, alcohol 0.5 g/kg and lactulose 10 g immediately after a solid meal, the mean peak blood-alcohol levels were raised by about 40% and the AUC over the first hour was increased by 33%. After that the curve was virtually the same as that seen with a saline placebo. The authors suggest that the increased blood-alcohol levels are a result of erythromycin causing more rapid gastric emptying, so that the alcohol is exposed to metabolism by the gastric mucosa for a shorter time.[2]

What this means in terms of an increase in the effects of alcohol (e.g. on driving) is not known.

(b) Effects on erythromycin

When a single 500-mg dose of erythromycin ethylsuccinate was taken by 9 healthy subjects with two 150-mL alcoholic drinks (one immediately and the other 2.5 hours later) the AUC of erythromycin was decreased by about 27% and erythromycin absorption was delayed. One subject had a 185% *increase* in absorption. The alcoholic drink was pisco sour, which contains lemon juice, sugar and pisco (a brandy-like liqueur). Blood-alcohol levels achieved were about 50 mg%.[3]

The reason for the reduced absorption of erythromycin is not understood but it is suggested that the slight delay occurs because alcohol delays gastric emptying, resulting in erythromycin reaching its absorption site in the duodenum a little later.[3] The extent to which this reduction in absorption might alter the antibacterial effects of erythromycin is uncertain, but it seems likely to be small.

1. Min DI, Noormohamed SE, Flanigan MJ. Effect of erythromycin on ethanol's pharmacokinetics and perception of intoxication. *Pharmacotherapy* (1995) 15, 164–9.
2. Edelbroek MAL, Horowitz M, Wishart JM, Akkermans LMA. Effects of erythromycin on gastric emptying, alcohol absorption and small intestinal transit in normal subjects. *J Nucl Med* (1993) 34, 582–8.
3. Morasso MI, Chávez J, Gai MN, Arancibia A. Influence of alcohol consumption on erythromycin ethylsuccinate kinetics. *Int J Clin Pharmacol Ther Toxicol* (1990) 28, 426–9.

Alcohol + Fluvastatin

Alcohol does not affect the pharmacokinetics of fluvastatin to a clinically relevant extent.

Clinical evidence, mechanism, importance and management

Ten healthy subjects took a single 40-mg dose of fluvastatin and 70 g of alcohol diluted in lemonade. This acute ingestion of alcohol had no effect on the peak serum levels of fluvastatin or its AUC, but the half-life was reduced by almost one-third.[1] In a second related study, 20 patients with hypercholesterolaemia were given 40 mg of fluvastatin and 20 g of alcohol daily for 6 weeks. The AUC of fluvastatin was slightly increased and the half-life was increased by almost one-third, but the lipid profile with fluvastatin and alcohol was little different from fluvastatin alone.[1,2] The conclusion was reached that although long-term moderate drinking has some small effect on the pharmacokinetics of fluvastatin, its safety and efficacy are unaltered.[1] There would seem to be no reason for patients taking fluvastatin to avoid alcohol.

1. Smit JWA, Wijnne HJA, Schobben F, Sitsen A, de Bruin TWA, Erkelens DW. Effects of alcohol consumption on pharmacokinetics, efficacy, and safety of fluvastatin. *Am J Cardiol* (1995) 76, 89A–96A.
2. Smit JW, Wijnne HJ, Schobben F, Sitsen A, De Bruin TW, Erkelens DW. Effects of alcohol and fluvastatin on lipid metabolism and hepatic function. *Ann Intern Med* (1995) 122, 678–80.

Alcohol + Food

Food and milk decrease the absorption of alcohol and meals increase the metabolism of alcohol. The concentration and carbonation of alcoholic drinks can alter the rate of absorption of alcohol. Foods rich in serotonin (e.g. bananas) taken with alcohol might produce adverse effects such as diarrhoea and headache. Previous alcohol consumption and the glycaemic load of a meal appear to interact to influence both mood and memory.

Clinical evidence, mechanism, importance and management

(a) Alcohol absorption and metabolism

In one study 10 subjects were given 25 mL of alcohol (equivalent to a double whisky) after drinking about 850 mL of water or **milk** during the previous 90 minutes. Blood-alcohol levels at 90 minutes were reduced by about 40%, and at 120 minutes by about 25% by the presence of the **milk**. The intoxicant effects of the alcohol were also clearly reduced.[1]

In a randomised, crossover study, 24 healthy subjects were given alcohol 0.3 g/kg either one hour before or after an evening meal. It was found that the maximum alcohol levels were increased by 87% from 21.3 mg% to 39.9 mg%, and the AUC was increased by 63% when alcohol was given in the fasting rather than the fed state. However there was large inter and intra-individual variability in alcohol bioavailability.[2] Other studies have shown similar effects,[3-5] and have found that this is not limited to specific components of food,[4,5] as well as demonstrating that food reduces the feeling of intoxication and reduces the time required to eliminate alcohol from the body.[3] After food, the rate of gastric emptying is slower, and hepatic blood flow and the activities of alcohol-metabolising enzymes are increased, which allows greater first-pass metabolism of alcohol. Thus, the effects of alcohol are greatest when taken on an empty stomach.

A study in 21 healthy subjects found that 20 of the 21 subjects absorbed vodka diluted with a still water mixer (alcohol 18.75%) more rapidly than neat (undiluted) vodka (alcohol 37.5%). Dilution of vodka with carbonated rather than still water increased the alcohol absorption rate in 14 subjects, while 7 subjects showed no change or a decreased rate of absorption. Overall the mean absorption of the dilute vodka was greater with a carbonated mixer than with a still mixer.[6]

In a randomised, crossover study, 30 healthy subjects consumed an average of 1.06 g/kg of alcohol (wine, beer or vodka) over a 2-hour test period. On a second test day they were given either 250-mL of *Outox* (containing fructose 50 g as a soft drink) or a placebo 15 minutes after completing the same alcohol intake. *Outox* did not increase alcohol elimination. However, following *Outox* consumption, there was a statistically significant reduction in blood- and breath-alcohol concentrations of 10.3% and 14.3%, respectively, due to slower gastric absorption rather than increased elimination.[7]

(b) Dietary serotonin

Serotonin (5-hydroxytryptamine, 5-HT) is excreted in the urine as 5-hydroxyindole-3-acetic acid (5-HIAA) and 5-hydroxytryptophol (5-HTOL). The ratio of 5-HTOL to 5-HIAA is normally very low (less than 0.01). A study in 10 healthy subjects found that, 4 hours after the ingestion of alcohol 0.5 g/kg, the ratio was increased by about 70-fold. When the same amount of alcohol was given with 3 bananas, a food rich in serotonin, the ratio was increased about 100-fold at 4 hours and was still raised at

24 hours. Within 4 hours, 7 of the 10 subjects experienced adverse effects including diarrhoea, headache and fatigue. The symptoms were attributed to high levels of 5-HTOL, which is usually a minor metabolite of serotonin. Other foods rich in serotonin such as pineapple, kiwi fruit or walnuts might produce similar effects if taken with even moderate amounts of alcohol.[8]

(c) Glycaemic load

Breakfasts that release glucose at different speeds were found to interact with alcohol drunk the previous evening to influence cognition and mood. When less than 4.5 g of alcohol had been drunk, a breakfast high in rapidly available glucose was associated with better memory later in the morning. In contrast, when more than 4.5 g of alcohol had been drunk, a breakfast high in slowly available glucose resulted in better memory. After a high glycaemic-load lunch, the rapidly available glucose breakfast resulted in a more confused feeling than the slowly available glucose breakfast or fasting, in those who had drunk more than 4.5 g of alcohol the previous evening.[9]

1. Miller DS, Stirling JL, Yudkin J. Effect of ingestion of milk on concentrations of blood alcohol. *Nature* (1966) 212, 1051.
2. Fraser AG, Rosalki SB, Gamble GD, Pounder RE. Inter-individual and intra-individual variability of ethanol concentration-time profiles: comparison of ethanol ingestion before or after an evening meal. *Br J Clin Pharmacol* (1995) 40, 387–92.
3. Jones AW, Jönsson KÅ. Food-induced lowering of blood-ethanol profiles and increased rate of elimination immediately after a meal. *J Forensic Sci* (1994) 39, 1084–93.
4. Jones AW, Jönsson KÅ, Kechagias S. Effect of high-fat, high-protein, and high-carbohydrate meals on the pharmacokinetics of a small dose of ethanol. *Br J Clin Pharmacol* (1997) 44, 521–6.
5. Ramchandani VA, Kwo PY, Li T-K. Effect of food and food composition on alcohol elimination rates in healthy men and women. *J Clin Pharmacol* (2001) 41, 1345–50.
6. Roberts C, Robinson SP. Alcohol concentration and carbonation of drinks: The effect on blood alcohol levels. *J Forensic Leg Med* (2007) 14, 398–405.
7. Pavlic M, Libiseller K, Grubweiser P, Ulmer H, Sauper T, Rabl W. Another 'soberade' on the market: does Outox keep its promise? *Wien Klin Wochenschr* (2007) 119, 104–11.
8. Helander A, Some M. Dietary serotonin and alcohol combined may provoke adverse physiological symptoms due to 5-hydroxytryptophol. *Life Sci* (2000) 67, 799–806.
9. Benton D, Nabb S. Breakfasts that release glucose at different speeds interact with previous alcohol intake to influence cognition and mood before and after lunch. *Behav Neurosci* (2004) 118, 936–43.

Alcohol + Furazolidone

A disulfiram-like reaction might occur in patients taking furazolidone if they drink alcohol.

Clinical evidence

A patient taking furazolidone 200 mg four times daily complained of facial flushing, lachrymation, conjunctivitis, weakness, and light-headedness within 10 minutes of drinking beer. These effects occurred on several occasions and lasted 30 to 45 minutes.[1] A man prescribed furazolidone 100 mg four times daily and who had taken only three doses, developed intense facial flushing, wheezing and dyspnoea (lasting one hour), within one hour of drinking about 60 mL of brandy. The same thing happened again the next day after drinking a *Martini* cocktail. No treatment was given.[2] A report originating from the manufacturers of furazolidone stated that by 1976, 43 cases of a disulfiram-like reaction had been reported, of which 14 were produced experimentally using above-normal doses of furazolidone.[3] A later study in 1986 described 9 out of 47 patients (19%) who complained of a disulfiram-like reaction after drinking alcohol while taking furazolidone 100 mg four times daily for 5 days.[4]

Mechanism

Uncertain. It seems possible that furazolidone acts like disulfiram by inhibiting the activity of acetaldehyde dehydrogenase, see *Mechanism*, under 'Alcohol + Disulfiram', p.67.

Importance and management

The interaction between furazolidone and alcohol is established and clinically important, but of uncertain incidence. One report suggests that about 1 in 5 patients might be affected.[4] Reactions of this kind appear to be more unpleasant and possibly frightening than serious, and normally need no treatment; however, patients should be warned about what might happen if they drink alcohol.

1. Calesnick B. Antihypertensive action of the antimicrobial agent furazolidone. *Am J Med Sci* (1958) 236, 736–46.
2. Kolodny AL. Side-effects produced by alcohol in a patient receiving furazolidone. *Md State Med J* (1962) 11, 248.
3. Chamberlain RE. (Eaton Laboratories, Norwich Pharmacal Co.) Chemotherapeutic properties of prominent nitrofurans. *J Antimicrob Chemother* (1976) 2, 325–36.
4. DuPont HL, Ericsson CD, Reves RR, Galindo E. Antimicrobial therapy for travelers' diarrhea. *Rev Infect Dis* (1986) 8, (Suppl 2), S217–S222.

Alcohol + Ginseng

***Panax ginseng* (Asian ginseng) increases the clearance of alcohol and lowers blood-alcohol levels.**

Clinical evidence

Fourteen healthy subjects, each acting as their own control, were given alcohol (72 g/65 kg as a 25% solution) with and without a *Panax ginseng* (Asian ginseng) extract (3 g/65 kg) mixed in with it. They drank the alcohol or the alcohol/ginseng mixture over a 45-minute period in 7 portions, the first four at 5-minute intervals and the next three at 10-minute intervals. Measurements taken 40 minutes later found that the presence of the ginseng lowered blood-alcohol levels by an average of about 39%. The alcohol levels of 10 subjects were lowered by 32 to 51% by the ginseng, 3 showed reductions of 14 to 18%, and one showed no changes at all.[1]

Mechanism

The reasons for this interaction are uncertain, but it is suggested that *Panax ginseng* possibly increases the activity of the enzymes (alcohol and aldehyde dehydrogenase)[2] that are concerned with the metabolism of alcohol, thereby increasing the clearance of alcohol.

Importance and management

Evidence for an interaction between alcohol and ginseng appears to be limited to the report cited, involving *Panax ginseng* (Asian ginseng), which found a reduction in blood-alcohol levels. What this reduction means in practical terms is not clear but the authors of the report suggest the possibility of using ginseng to treat alcoholic patients and those with acute alcohol intoxication;[1] however, this needs confirmation in further clinical studies. The available data suggests that the concurrent use of alcohol and *Panax ginseng* is unlikely to be detrimental.

1. Lee FC, Ko JH, Park KJ, Lee JS. Effect of *Panax ginseng* on blood alcohol clearance in man. *Clin Exp Pharmacol Physiol* (1987) 14, 543–6.
2. Choi CW, Lee SI, Huh K. Effect of ginseng on the hepatic alcohol metabolizing enzyme system activity in chronic alcohol-treated mice. *Korean J Pharmacol* (1984) 20, 13–21.

Alcohol + Glyceryl trinitrate (Nitroglycerin)

Patients who take glyceryl trinitrate while drinking alcohol might feel faint and dizzy.

Clinical evidence, mechanism, importance and management

The results of studies[1,2] on the combined haemodynamic effects of alcohol and glyceryl trinitrate give support to earlier claims that their concurrent use increases the risk of exaggerated hypotension and fainting.[3,4] Their vasodilatory effects would appear to be additive.[5] The greatest effect was seen when glyceryl trinitrate was taken one hour or more after starting to drink alcohol.[1] It is suggested that this increased susceptibility to postural hypotension should not be allowed to stop patients from using glyceryl trinitrate if they have been drinking alcohol, but they should be warned about the possible effects and told what to do if they feel faint and dizzy (i.e. sit or lie down).[1]

1. Kupari M, Heikkilä J, Ylikahri R. Does alcohol intensify the hemodynamic effects of nitroglycerin? *Clin Cardiol* (1984) 7, 382–6.
2. Abrams J, Schroeder K, Raizada V, Gibbs D. Potentially adverse effects of sublingual nitroglycerin during consumption of alcohol. *J Am Coll Cardiol* (1990) 15, 226A.
3. Shafer N. Hypotension due to nitroglycerin combined with alcohol. *N Engl J Med* (1965) 273, 1169.
4. Opie. LH. Drugs and the heart. II. Nitrates. *Lancet* (1980) i, 750–3.
5. Allison RD, Kraner JC, Roth GM. Effects of alcohol and nitroglycerin on vascular responses in man. *Angiology* (1971) 22, 211–22.

Alcohol + Griseofulvin

An isolated case report describes a severe disulfiram-like reaction when a man taking griseofulvin drank a can of beer. Other isolated reports describe flushing and tachycardia, or increased alcohol effects, when patients taking griseofulvin consumed alcohol.

Clinical evidence

A man took griseofulvin 500 mg daily for about 2 weeks without problems. Subsequently he drank a can of beer, took his usual dose of griseofulvin about one hour later, and within 30 to 60 minutes developed a severe disulfiram-like reaction (flushing, severe nausea, vomiting, diarrhoea, hypotension, and paraesthesias of all extremities). He was successfully treated with intravenous sodium chloride 0.9%, potassium, dopamine, and intramuscular promethazine.[1] Another isolated case of flushing and tachycardia has been attributed to the concurrent use of alcohol and griseofulvin; rechallenge produced the same effects.[2]

It has been suggested that griseofulvin can increase the effects of alcohol, but the descriptions of this response are very brief. One report describes a man who had a decreased tolerance to alcohol and emotional instability manifested by crying and nervousness, which was said to be so severe that the drug was stopped.[3] Another report states that this effect has been noted in a very small number of patients, but gives no further information.[4]

Mechanism

Not understood. The reaction described above might possibly have the same pharmacological basis as the interaction between disulfiram and alcohol, see 'Alcohol + Disulfiram', p.67.

Importance and management

The documentation regarding an interaction between alcohol and griseofulvin is extremely sparse, which would seem to suggest that adverse interactions are uncommon; however, the disulfiram-like reaction described in one patient was unusually severe. Concurrent use need not be avoided but it might be prudent to warn patients about the possible effects (e.g. flushing and tachycardia).

1. Fett DL, Vukov LF. An unusual case of severe griseofulvin-alcohol interaction. *Ann Emerg Med* (1994) 24, 95–7.
2. Robinson MM. Griseofulvin therapy of superficial mycoses. *Antibiot Annu* (1959–60) 7, 680–6.
3. Drowns BV, Fuhrman DL, Dennie CC. Use, abuse and limitations of griseofulvin. *Mo Med* (1960) 57, 1473–6.
4. Simon HJ, Randz LA. Untoward reactions to antimicrobial agents. *Annu Rev Med* (1961) 12, 111–34.

Alcohol + H_2-receptor antagonists

Although some studies have found that blood-alcohol levels can be raised to some extent and possibly remain elevated for longer than usual in those taking an H_2-receptor antagonist, others report that no clinically relevant interaction occurs. Drinking could worsen the gastrointestinal disease for which these H_2-receptor antagonists are being given. Hypoglycaemia associated with alcohol might be enhanced by H_2-receptor antagonists.

Clinical evidence

(a) Cimetidine

A double-blind study in 6 healthy subjects found that cimetidine 300 mg four times daily for 7 days, increased the peak plasma levels of alcohol 0.8 g/kg by about 12% (from 146 mg% to 163 mg%) and increased its AUC by about 7%. The subjects assessed themselves as being more intoxicated while taking cimetidine and alcohol than with alcohol alone.[1] An essentially similar study[2,3] found that blood-alcohol levels were raised by 17% (from 73 mg% to 86 mg%) by cimetidine, and another study found that cimetidine almost doubled peak blood-alcohol levels.[4] A study in 6 healthy subjects also found that cimetidine 400 mg twice daily for one week approximately doubled the AUC of a single 0.15-g/kg oral dose of alcohol and raised peak alcohol levels by about 33%. No changes were seen when the alcohol was given intravenously.[5] A further study in healthy subjects given cimetidine for only 2 days found that peak plasma alcohol levels were raised by 17%, and the time that blood levels remained above the 80 mg% mark (the legal driving limit in some countries) was prolonged by about one-third.[6]

A study in 6 subjects given 0.75 g/kg of alcohol found that a single 800-mg dose of cimetidine, raised blood-alcohol levels at 45 minutes by 32% (from about 76 mg% to 100 mg%), and the AUC at 120 minutes was increased by 25%. Each of the subjects said they felt more inebriated after taking cimetidine.[7]

In subjects with substantial first-pass metabolism of alcohol, cimetidine increased the blood levels of repeated small drinks of alcohol to a greater degree than that which occurred after an equivalent single dose. The levels reached were associated with psychomotor impairment.[8]

In contrast, another study found that a combination of chlorphenamine (which blocks H_1-receptors) and cimetidine reduced the rate of absorption and peak blood-alcohol levels, and suppressed alcohol-induced flushing.[9]

A study in 10 healthy subjects given alcohol 0.5 g/kg before and after cimetidine 400 mg twice daily for 7 days, found that hypoglycaemia following alcohol ingestion was enhanced.[10]

In contrast to these findings a number of studies, using a variety of doses of cimetidine, and a variety of types of alcohol, have found that no interaction occurs.[11-21]

(b) Famotidine

Two studies that found an interaction between other H_2-receptor antagonists and alcohol found that famotidine had no notable effect on blood-alcohol levels.[4,7] Similarly a number of other studies, using a variety of doses of famotidine, and a variety of types of alcohol, have found no interaction occurs.[14-16,18,19,21] However, a study in 10 healthy subjects given alcohol 0.5 g/kg before and after famotidine 40 mg once daily for 7 days, found that marked hypoglycaemia occurred following alcohol ingestion.[10]

(c) Nizatidine

A study in subjects given 0.75 g/kg of alcohol found that a single 300-mg dose of nizatidine raised blood-alcohol levels at 45 minutes by 20% (from about 76 mg% to 90 mg%), and increased the AUC of alcohol at 120 minutes by 20%.[7]

Another report briefly mentions that nizatidine has similar effects on alcohol absorption to cimetidine,[22] whereas two other studies found no interaction between nizatidine and alcohol.[21,23]

(d) Ranitidine

A placebo-controlled study in 8 healthy subjects found that ranitidine 300 mg daily for 7 days did not affect the peak plasma levels of alcohol 0.8 g/kg.[2,3] However, another study found that ranitidine 150 mg twice daily for 8 days increased the peak levels of a 0.3 g/kg oral dose of alcohol by 34%.[4] A further study in healthy subjects given ranitidine for only 2 days found that peak plasma alcohol levels were raised by 28%, and the time that blood levels remained above the 80 mg% mark (the legal driving limit in some countries) was prolonged by about one-third.[6]

A study in subjects given 0.75 g/kg of alcohol found that a single 300-mg dose of ranitidine raised blood-alcohol levels at 45 minutes by 6% (from about 75 mg% to 81 mg%), and the AUC at 120 minutes was increased by 10%.[7]

Ranitidine 150 mg twice daily for 7 days considerably increased blood-alcohol levels and the high levels persisted for longer in social drinkers (with substantial first-pass metabolism) receiving 4 drinks of 0.15 g/kg of alcohol at 45-minute intervals.[24] Another report briefly mentions that ranitidine has similar effects on alcohol absorption to cimetidine.[22]

A study in 10 healthy subjects given alcohol 0.5 g/kg before and after ranitidine 150 mg twice daily for 7 days, found that hypoglycaemia following alcohol ingestion was enhanced.[10]

In contrast to these findings a number of studies, using a variety of doses of ranitidine, and a variety of types of alcohol, have found that no interaction occurs.[12,14,16-21,25-27]

Mechanism

It would appear that the interacting H_2-receptor antagonists inhibit the activity of alcohol dehydrogenase (ADH) in the gastric mucosa so that more alcohol passes unmetabolised into the circulation, thereby raising the levels.[28-32] Most of the studies assessing the interaction of H_2-receptor antagonists with larger quantities of alcohol have not found an interaction. The decrease in first pass metabolism with increasing amounts of alcohol could explain this, as it implies that an interaction with H_2-receptor antagonists would be more likely with smaller quantities of alcohol.[8,33] Other factors that affect the first pass metabolism of alcohol, such as fasting, chronic alcoholism and female gender could also affect the outcome. The increase in blood-alcohol levels with cimetidine or ranitidine and a small amount of alcohol might also be explained by the effect of H_2-receptor antagonists or alcohol on gastric emptying times.[27,33] In one study the decrease in first-pass metabolism correlated with a ranitidine-induced increase in the rate of gastric emptying and an increase in blood-alcohol levels.[34] However, with small quantities of alcohol the magnitude of the effect on peak levels might be too small to increase effects on psychomotor performance,[33,35] although two studies suggested that an effect could occur.[8]

The hypoglycaemic effect is not considered to be due to effects on alcohol absorption but might be an effect of H_2-receptor antagonists on glucose metabolism.[10]

Importance and management

The contrasting and apparently contradictory results cited here clearly show that an interaction between alcohol and H_2-receptor antagonists is by no means established. Extensive reviews of the data concluded that the interaction is not, in general, clinically relevant.[32,33,36-38] Under conditions mimicking social drinking there is some evidence that H_2-receptor antagonists might[10,24] or might not[20] increase blood-alcohol levels to those associated with impairment of psychomotor skills. However, as yet, there are insufficient grounds to justify any general warning regarding alcohol and H_2-receptor antagonists. However, note that many of the conditions for which H_2-receptor antagonists are used could be made worse by alcohol, so restriction of alcohol intake might be prudent. Other factors that can affect this interaction are discussed under *Mechanism*, above.

1. Feely J, Wood AJJ. Effects of cimetidine on the elimination and actions of alcohol. *JAMA* (1982) 247, 2819–21.
2. Seitz HK, Bösche J, Czygan P, Veith S, Simon B, Kommerell B. Increased blood ethanol levels following cimetidine but not ranitidine. *Lancet* (1983) i, 760.
3. Seitz HK, Veith S, Czygan P, Bösche J, Simon B, Gugler R, Kommerell B. *In vivo* interactions between H_2-receptor antagonists and ethanol metabolism in man and in rats. *Hepatology* (1984) 4, 1231–4.
4. DiPadova C, Roine R, Frezza M, Gentry T, Baraona E, Lieber CS. Effects of ranitidine on blood alcohol levels after ethanol ingestion: comparison with other H_2-receptor antagonists. *JAMA* (1992) 267, 83–6.
5. Caballeria J, Baraona E, Rodamilans M, Lieber CS. Effects of cimetidine on gastric alcohol dehydrogenase activity and blood ethanol levels. *Gastroenterology* (1989) 96, 388–92.
6. Webster LK, Jones DB, Smallwood RA. Influence of cimetidine and ranitidine on ethanol pharmacokinetics. *Aust N Z J Med* (1985) 15, 359–60.
7. Guram M, Howden CW, Holt S. Further evidence for an interaction between alcohol and certain H_2-receptor antagonists. *Alcohol Clin Exp Res* (1991) 15, 1084–5.
8. Gupta AM, Baraona E, Lieber CS. Significant increase of blood alcohol by cimetidine after repetitive drinking of small alcohol doses. *Alcohol Clin Exp Res* (1995) 19, 1083–7.
9. Tan OT, Stafford TJ, Sarkany I, Gaylarde PM, Tilsey C, Payne JP. Suppression of alcohol-induced flushing by a combination of H_1 and H_2 histamine antagonists. *Br J Dermatol* (1982) 107, 647–52.
10. Czyżyk A, Lao B, Szutowski M, Szczepanik Z, Muszyński J. Enhancement of alcohol-induced hypoglycaemia by H_2-receptor antagonists. *Arzneimittelforschung* (1997) 47, 746–9.
11. Smith Kline and French. Personal communication, February 1989.
12. Dobrilla G, de Pretis G, Piazzi L, Chilovi F, Comberlato M, Valentini M, Pastorino A, Vallaperta P. Is ethanol metabolism affected by oral administration of cimetidine and ranitidine at therapeutic doses? *Hepatogastroenterology* (1984) 31, 35–7.
13. Johnson KI, Fenzl E, Hein B. Einfluß von Cimetidin auf den Abbau und die Wirkung des Alkohols. *Arzneimittelforschung* (1984) 34, 734–6.
14. Tanaka E, Nakamura K. Effects of H_2-receptor antagonists on ethanol metabolism in Japanese volunteers. *Br J Clin Pharmacol* (1988) 26, 96–9.
15. Holtmann G, Singer MV. Histamine H_2 receptor antagonists and blood alcohol levels. *Dig Dis Sci* (1988) 33, 767–8.
16. Fraser AG, Prewett EJ, Hudson M, Sawyerr AM, Rosalki SB, Pounder RE. The effect of ranitidine, cimetidine or famotidine on low-dose post-prandial alcohol absorption. *Aliment Pharmacol Ther* (1991) 5, 263–72.
17. Jönsson K-Å, Jones AW, Boström H, Andersson T. Lack of effect of omeprazole, cimetidine, and ranitidine on the pharmacokinetics of ethanol in fasting male volunteers. *Eur J Clin Pharmacol* (1992) 42, 209–12.
18. Fraser AG, Hudson M, Sawyerr AM, Smith M, Rosalki SB, Pounder RE. Ranitidine, cimetidine, famotidine have no effect on post-prandial absorption of ethanol 0.8 g/kg taken after an evening meal. *Aliment Pharmacol Ther* (1992) 6, 693–700.
19. Kendall MJ, Spannuth F, Walt RP, Gibson GJ, Hale KA, Braithwaite R, Langman MJS. Lack of effect of H2-receptor antagonists on the pharmacokinetics of alcohol consumed after food at lunchtime. *Br J Clin Pharmacol* (1994) 37, 371–4.
20. Brown ASJM, James OFW. Omeprazole, ranitidine and cimetidine have no effect on peak blood ethanol concentrations, first pass metabolism or area under the time–ethanol curve under 'real-life' drinking conditions. *Aliment Pharmacol Ther* (1998) 12, 141–5.
21. Raufman J-P, Notar-Francesco V, Raffaniello RD, Straus EW. Histamine-2 receptor antagonists do not alter serum ethanol levels in fed, non-alcoholic men. *Ann Intern Med* (1993) 118, 488–94.
22. Palmer RH. Cimetidine and alcohol absorption. *Gastroenterology* (1989) 97, 1066–8.
23. Hindmarch I, Gilburt S. The lack of CNS effects of nizatidine, with and without alcohol, on psychomotor ability and cognitive function. *Hum Psychopharmacol* (1990) 5, 25–32.
24. Arora S, Baraona E, Lieber CS. Alcohol levels are increased in social drinkers receiving ranitidine. *Am J Gastroenterol* (2000) 95, 208–13.
25. Fraser AG, Prewett EJ, Hudson M, Sawyerr AM, Rosalki SB, Pounder RE. Ranitidine has no effect on post-prandial absorption of alcohol (0.6 g/kg) after an evening meal. *Eur J Gastroenterol Hepatol* (1992) 4, 43–7.
26. Pipkin GA, Mills JG, Wood JR. Does ranitidine affect blood alcohol concentrations? *Pharmacotherapy* (1994) 14, 273–81.

27. Bye A, Lacey LF, Gupta S, Powell JR. Effect of ranitidine hydrochloride (150 mg twice daily) on the pharmacokinetics of increasing doses of ethanol (0.15, 0.3, 0.6 g kg^{-1}). *Br J Clin Pharmacol* (1996) 41, 129–33.
28. Caballería J. Interactions between alcohol and gastric metabolizing enzymes: practical implications. *Clin Ther* (1991) 13, 511–20.
29. Fiatarone JR, Bennett MK, Kelly P, James OFW. Ranitidine but not gastritis or female sex reduces the first pass metabolism of ethanol. *Gut* (1991) 32, A594.
30. Caballería J, Baraona E, Deulofeu R, Hernández-Muñoz R, Rodés J, Lieber CS. Effects of H_2-receptor antagonists on gastric alcohol dehydrogenase activity. *Dig Dis Sci* (1991) 36, 1673–9.
31. Brown ASJM, Fiaterone JR, Day CP, Bennett MK, Kelly PJ, James OFW. Ranitidine increases the bioavailability of postprandial ethanol by the reduction of first pass metabolism. *Gut* (1995) 37, 413–17.
32. Gugler R. H_2-antagonists and alcohol: Do they interact? *Drug Safety* (1994) 10, 271–80.
33. Fraser AG. Is there an interaction between H_2-antagonists and alcohol? *Drug Metabol Drug Interact* (1998) 14, 123–145.
34. Amir I, Anwar N, Baraona E, Lieber CS. Ranitidine increases the bioavailability of imbibed alcohol by accelerating gastric emptying. *Life Sci* (1996) 58, 511–18.
35. Baraona E, Gentry RT, Lieber CS. Bioavailability of alcohol: role of gastric metabolism and its interaction with other drugs. *Dig Dis* (1994) 12, 351–57.
36. Levitt MD. Review article: lack of clinical significance of the interaction between H_2-receptor antagonists and ethanol. *Aliment Pharmacol Ther* (1993) 7, 131–8.
37. Monroe ML, Doering PL. Effect of common over-the-counter medications on blood alcohol levels. *Ann Pharmacother* (2001) 35, 918–24.
38. Weinberg DS, Burnham D, Berlin JA. Effect of histamine-2 receptor antagonists on blood alcohol levels: a meta-analysis. *J Gen Intern Med* (1998) 13, 594–9.

Alcohol + Hormonal contraceptives or HRT

Alcohol does not affect the pharmacokinetics of ethinylestradiol. Estradiol does not affect blood-alcohol levels, but alcohol clearance might be reduced in women taking combined hormonal contraceptives. The acute ingestion of alcohol increases the levels of circulating estradiol in women using oral HRT; a smaller increase is seen with transdermal HRT. In addition, alcohol intake appears to increase the risk of breast cancer in women receiving HRT.

Clinical evidence

(a) Effect of oestrogens on alcohol

A controlled study in 54 women found that those taking an oral combined hormonal contraceptive (30, 35, or 50 micrograms of oestrogen) unexpectedly tolerated the effects of alcohol better than those not taking oral contraceptives (as measured by a reaction-time test and a bead-threading test), but their blood-alcohol levels and its rate of alcohol clearance were unchanged.[1] Similarly, a study in 12 healthy postmenopausal women found that HRT (**estradiol** 1 mg daily and **medroxyprogesterone acetate** 10 mg daily for 10 out of each 25 days) did not affect blood-alcohol levels.[2] A study of 214 postmenopausal women suggested that small amounts of alcohol might enhance visuospatial processes (improved cognitive function measured by block design performance). HRT also appeared to be linked with better visuospatial performance, but only when the task was difficult. There was a trend (not statistically significant) towards improved performance with alcohol consumption (up to approximately half a standard drink per day) and oestrogen replacement therapy.[3]

(b) Effect of alcohol on oestrogens

Alcohol ingestion did not have a statistically significant effect on **ethinylestradiol** pharmacokinetics in 9 healthy women taking an oral combined hormonal contraceptive (ethinylestradiol 30 micrograms with gestodene 75 micrograms). In this study, alcohol was given as a single 0.4-g/kg dose (equivalent to 2 to 3 standard drinks) on day 14 then 0.4 g/kg twice daily for 7 days. In contrast, 12 healthy postmenopausal women receiving HRT (**estradiol** 1 mg daily and **medroxyprogesterone acetate** 10 mg daily for 10 out of each 25 days) were given an alcoholic drink (0.7 g/kg, a dose shown to achieve mean peak serum-alcohol levels of about 97 mg% after about one hour) during the oestrogen-only phase of the HRT cycle. It was found that their peak **estradiol** levels rose threefold and were above the baseline for 5 hours. No clinically significant increases in the levels of circulating estrone (an oestrogen secreted by the ovaries) were seen.[2] A similar, smaller 20% increase in peak **estradiol** levels was seen in another study when women using **transdermal estradiol** were given alcohol.[4]

(c) Risk of breast cancer

Both alcohol and HRT are linked with a small increase in breast cancer risk, and it has therefore been suggested that the combination of HRT and alcohol could have additive risks.[5] A prospective study of 51 847 postmenopausal women confirmed an association with alcohol intake and breast cancer risk (for oestrogen receptor-positive (ER+) tumours, but not oestrogen receptor-negative (ER−) tumours). Furthermore, among women who consumed alcohol, postmenopausal hormone use was associated with an increased risk for the development of ER+ tumours. For women with the highest alcohol intake (10 g (approximately one drink) or more daily) the relative risk of developing oestrogen receptor-positive/progesterone receptor-positive (ER+PR+) breast cancer was 1.2 and 1.8 for non-users and users of HRT, respectively, compared with non-drinkers who had never used postmenopausal hormones; the relative risk of developing ER+PR− tumours was even greater, being approximately 2.5 and 3.5, respectively.[6] Another study also reported a similar increased risk of developing ER+PR+ tumours with alcohol and oestrogen replacement therapy, but only a slight risk for ER+PR− tumours; the risk for ER−PR− breast cancer was, however, greatest.[7] The Women's Health Study found that an alcohol intake of greater than 10 g of alcohol per day and postmenopausal hormone use was associated with a relative risk of developing breast cancer of 1.84, compared with those who did not consume alcohol or take postmenopausal hormones.[8]

In contrast to these findings of an enhanced risk of breast cancer, the European Prospective Investigation into Cancer and Nutrition (EPIC) using data from 274 688 women found no evidence of a synergistically enhanced risk of breast cancer associated with alcohol intake and concurrent HRT. Further, no difference in the risk of breast cancer was found between users and non-users of HRT who drink alcohol, although this study did not include information on ER status.[9]

Mechanism

The reasons for the changes in estradiol levels with alcohol use are not understood. Alcohol can increase *endogenous* estradiol levels in postmenopausal women, although the findings are variable. Another possible explanation is altered clearance of estradiol in women who drink alcohol.[10] The effects on ethinylestradiol are in contrast. This might be because the ethinyl group in ethinylestradiol confers protection from the effects of alcohol.[11]

Importance and management

The evidence for an interaction between alcohol and oestrogens is variable. The authors of one study, which found that alcohol was better tolerated in those taking oral combined hormonal contraceptives state that they do not recommend women taking these contraceptives should attempt to drink more alcohol than usual, because even if alcohol is tolerated better, blood-alcohol levels are not reduced.[1] However, two other studies suggest that peak blood-alcohol levels might be reduced in those taking oral contraceptives, but alcohol clearance is also reduced and so alcohol could be present for longer in women who are taking oral contraceptives.[12,13]

Regular consumption of alcohol as low as 1 to 2 drinks per day might contribute to a modest increased risk of some types of breast cancer,[10] and it has been suggested that women taking HRT should limit their alcohol intake;[5] about one drink or less per day has been proposed.[10] More study is needed to confirm the amount and frequency of alcohol consumption associated with an increased risk of breast cancer and any additional deleterious effect of alcohol in women who use HRT.

1. Hobbes J, Boutagy J, Shenfield GM. Interactions between ethanol and oral contraceptive steroids. *Clin Pharmacol Ther* (1985) 38, 371–80.
2. Ginsburg ES, Mello NK, Mendelson JH, Barbieri RL, Teoh SK, Rothman M, Gao X, Sholar JW. Effects of alcohol ingestion on estrogens in postmenopausal women. *JAMA* (1996) 276, 1747–51.
3. Tivis LJ, Green MD, Nixon SJ, Tivis RD. Alcohol, estrogen replacement therapy, and visuospatial processes in postmenopausal women. *Alcohol Clin Exp Res* (2003) 27, 1055–63.
4. Ginsburg ES, Walsh BW, Gao X, Gleason RE, Feltmate C, Barbieri RL. The effect of acute ethanol ingestion on estrogen levels in postmenopausal women using transdermal estradiol. *J Soc Gynecol Investig* (1995) 2, 26–9.
5. Gorins A. Responsabilité croisée des estrogènes et de l'alcool dans le cancer du sein. *Presse Med* (2000) 29, 670–2.
6. Suzuki R, Ye W, Rylander-Rudqvist T, Saji S, Colditz GA, Wolk A. Alcohol and postmenopausal breast cancer risk defined by estrogen and progesterone receptor status: a prospective cohort study. *J Natl Cancer Inst* (2005) 97, 1601–8.
7. Gapstur SM, Potter JD, Drinkard C, Folsom AR. Synergistic effect between alcohol and estrogen replacement therapy on risk of breast cancer differs by estrogen/progesterone receptor status in the Iowa Women's Health Study. *Cancer Epidemiol Biomarkers Prev* (1995) 4, 313–18.
8. Zhang SM, Lee I-M, Manson JE, Cook NR, Willett WC, Buring JE. Alcohol consumption and breast cancer risk in the Women's Health Study. *Am J Epidemiol* (2007) 165, 667–76.
9. Tjønneland A, Christensen J, Olsen A, Stripp C, Thomsen BL, Overvad K, Peeters PHM, van Gils CH, Bueno-de-Mesquita HB, Ocké MC, Thiebaut A, Fournier A, Clavel-Chapelon F, Berrino F, Palli D, Tumino R, Panico S, Vineis P, Agudo A, Ardanaz E, Martinez-Garcia C, Amiano P, Navarro C, Quirós JR, Key TJ, Reeves G, Khaw K-T, Bingham S, Trichopoulou A, Trichopoulos D, Naska A, Nagel G, Chang-Claude J, Boeing H, Lahmann PH, Manjer J, Wirfält E, Hallmans G, Johansson I, Lund E, Skeie G, Hjartåker A, Ferrari P, Slimani N, Kaaks R, Riboli E. Alcohol intake and breast cancer risk: the European prospective investigation into cancer and nutrition (EPIC). *Cancer Causes Control* (2007) 18, 361–73.
10. Singletary KW, Gapstur SM. Alcohol and breast cancer. Review of epidemiologic and experimental evidence and potential mechanisms. *JAMA* (2001) 286, 2143–51.
11. Sarkola T, Ahola L, von der Pahlen B, Eriksson CJP. Lack of effect of alcohol on ethinylestradiol in premenopausal women. *Contraception* (2001) 63, 19–23.
12. Jones MK, Jones BM. Ethanol metabolism in women taking oral contraceptives. *Alcohol Clin Exp Res* (1984) 8, 24–8.
13. Zeiner AR, Kegg PS. Menstrual cycle and oral contraceptive effects on alcohol pharmacokinetics in caucasian females. *Curr Alcohol* (1981) 8, 47–56.

Alcohol + Inotropes and Vasopressors

Alcohol does not affect the cardiovascular response to isoprenaline. Alcohol increases the plasma levels of noradrenaline, but reduces its effects on diastolic blood pressure. Similarly alcohol reduces the increase in blood pressure in response to methoxamine.

Clinical evidence, mechanism, importance and management

(a) Isoprenaline (Isoproterenol)

A study in 21 healthy subjects found that a 1-mL/kg oral dose of 20% alcohol did not alter the effects of isoprenaline, given in doses of up to 1.78 micrograms, on blood pressure and heart rate.[1]

(b) Methoxamine

In a placebo-controlled study, 8 subjects were given 1 mL/kg of 20% alcohol, followed after 90 to 150 minutes by an infusion of methoxamine 200, 400, 800, 1600, and 2000 micrograms per minute, each for one minute. The increase in blood pressure was reduced after a cumulative 5 mg dose of methoxamine (from about 33/31 mmHg to 19/11 mmHg), but heart rate was not notably affected.[2] This study suggests that patients who have drunk alcohol might require higher doses of methoxamine.

(c) Noradrenaline (Norepinephrine)

In a placebo-controlled study, 8 subjects were given 1 mL/kg of 20% alcohol, followed after 45 minutes by an infusion of noradrenaline 24, 48 and 90 nanograms/kg per minute, each for 20 minutes. There was an increase in plasma noradrenaline levels after the ingestion of alcohol at the lower two doses of noradrenaline. Systolic blood pressure was not notably affected, but there was an approximately twofold decrease in diastolic blood pressure at each dosing level. Heart rate was not affected.[2] This study suggests that patients who have drunk alcohol might require higher doses of noradrenaline; however, as noradrenaline is titrated to effect, this interaction seems unlikely to be clinically relevant.

1. Eisenhofer G, Lambie DG, Johnson RH. No effect of ethanol ingestion on β-adrenoceptor-mediated circulatory responses to isoprenaline in man. *Br J Clin Pharmacol* (1985) 20, 684–7.
2. Eisenhofer G, Lambie DG, Johnson RH. Effects of ethanol ingestion on α-adrenoceptor-mediated circulatory responses in man. *Br J Clin Pharmacol* (1984) 18, 581–6.

Alcohol + Interferons

Studies have found a reduced response to interferon in patients who drink alcohol. Those who drink the most seem to exhibit the lowest response to interferon.

Clinical evidence, mechanism, importance and management

In a study involving 245 patients, alcohol intake and its effect on treatment were retrospectively evaluated, between 1 and 3 years after diagnosis of hepatitis C virus-related chronic liver disease. Less than 50% of the patients who drank alcohol stopped after being diagnosed with liver disease, despite being advised to abstain from alcohol. Alcohol intake affected both fibrosis (especially in women) and the response to interferon. Seventeen out of 65 patients (26.1%) who were given **interferon alfa** had a sustained response. However, the number of responders decreased as alcohol intake increased; there were more drinkers (63.1%) than abstainers (10.7%) among the 73.8% of patients who did not respond.[1] A study in non-drinkers, light drinkers (less than 70 g of alcohol per day) and heavy drinkers (more than 70 g of alcohol per day), with hepatitis C, assessed the response to **interferon** (**alfa** and **beta**). It was found that drinking reduced the response to interferon; with 47%, 57%, and 100% of subjects not responding in the non-drinking group, moderate drinking group, and heavy drinking group, respectively.[2] Other studies have found similar results,[3,4] with one study finding that heavy drinkers, who abstained from drinking for at least 6 months before receiving interferon, had similar outcomes to infrequent drinkers.[3]

One manufacturer notes that hepatotoxicity has been reported with **interferon beta-1a**. They state the potential additive toxicity with hepatotoxic drugs such as alcohol has not been determined, and further state that caution is warranted.[5]

There appears to be insufficient information to suggest that patients receiving interferons should avoid alcohol completely; however, alcohol intake, particularly heavy drinking, might increase the risk of hepatotoxicity and reduce the response to treatment with interferon.

1. Loguercio C, Di Pierro M, Di Marino MP, Federico A, Disalvo D, Crafa E, Tuccillo C, Baldi F, del Vecchio Blanco C. Drinking habits of subjects with hepatitis C virus-related chronic liver disease: prevalence and effect on clinical, virological and pathological aspects. *Alcohol Alcohol* (2000) 35, 296–301.
2. Okazaki T, Yoshihara H, Suzuki K, Yamada Y, Tsujimura T, Kawano K, Yamada Y, Abe H. Efficacy of interferon therapy in patients with chronic hepatitis C. Comparison between non-drinkers and drinkers. *Scand J Gastroenterol* (1994) 29, 1039–43.
3. Ohnishi K, Matsuo S, Matsutani K, Itahashi M, Kakihara K, Suzuki K, Ito S, Fujiwara K. Interferon therapy for chronic hepatitis C in habitual drinkers: comparison with chronic hepatitis C in infrequent drinkers. *Am J Gastroenterol* (1996) 91, 1374–9.
4. Mochida S, Ohnishi K, Matsuo S, Kakihara K, Fujiwara K. Effect of alcohol intake on the efficacy of interferon therapy in patients with chronic hepatitis C as evaluated by multivariate logistic regression analysis. *Alcohol Clin Exp Res* (1996) 20 (Suppl), 371A–377A.
5. Avonex (Interferon beta-1a). Biogen Idec Ltd. UK Summary of product characteristics, May 2014.

Alcohol + Ivermectin

Alcohol might increase the bioavailability of ivermectin.

Clinical evidence, mechanism, importance and management

Anecdotal reports from Nigeria suggest that ivermectin is more potent when taken with palm wine, a local alcoholic drink, and a few cases of ataxia and postural hypotension occurring with ivermectin were considered to be due to an interaction with alcohol.[1] Ivermectin formulated as an alcoholic solution has been found to have about twice the systemic availability of tablets and capsules.[2] In one study, 20 healthy subjects were given ivermectin 150 micrograms/kg with either 750 mL of beer (alcohol 4.5%) or 750 mL of water. Beer increased the plasma levels of ivermectin at 1 to 4 hours by about 51 to 66% when compared with water. No adverse effects were reported in either group.[1] The evidence suggests that concurrent use could be of benefit, if adverse effects such as postural hypotension are not troublesome; this type of adverse effect might be more of a problem in those with pre-existing heart disease.

1. Shu EN, Onwujekwe EO, Okonkwo PO. Do alcoholic beverages enhance availability of ivermectin? *Eur J Clin Pharmacol* (2000) 56, 437–8.
2. Edwards G, Dingsdale A, Helsby N, Orme MLE, Breckenridge AM. The relative systemic bioavailability of ivermectin after administration as capsule, tablet, and oral solution. *Eur J Clin Pharmacol* (1988) 35, 681–4.

Alcohol + Kava

There is some evidence that kava might worsen the CNS depressant effects of alcohol. The concurrent use of alcohol has been suggested as a possible contributing factor in some cases of kava hepatotoxicity.

Clinical evidence, mechanism, importance and management

Forty healthy subjects underwent a number of cognitive and visuomotor tests after taking alcohol alone, kava alone, or both together. The subjects took 0.75 g/kg of alcohol (enough to give blood-alcohol levels above 50 mg%) and the kava dose was 1 g/kg. The kava drink was made by mixing middle grade Fijian kava (Kava-Kava; the pepper plant *Piper methysticum*) with water and straining it to produce about 350 mL of kava liquid. It was found that kava alone had no effect on the tests, but when the kava was given with alcohol it potentiated both the perceived and measured impairment that occurred with alcohol alone.[1] However, another study found that a kava extract (WS 1490) did not enhance the negative effects of alcohol on performance tests.[2]

No very strong conclusions can be drawn from the results of these studies, but it is possible that driving and handling other machinery could be more hazardous if kava and alcohol are taken together. However, note that the use of kava is restricted in the UK because of reports of idiosyncratic hepatotoxicity.[3] It has been suggested that hepatotoxicity occurring in subjects taking alcohol with kava might involve the contribution of reactive metabolites generated by CYP2E1 during chronic alcohol intake or by hepatic enzyme induction during acute alcohol ingestion leading to increased exposure to kavalactones, the active ingredients of kava;[4] however further evidence is needed to support this suggestion.

1. Foo H, Lemon J. Acute effects of kava, alone or in combination with alcohol, on subjective measures of impairment and intoxication and on cognitive performance. *Drug Alcohol Rev* (1997) 16, 147–55.
2. Herberg K-W. Zum Einfluß von Kava-Spezialextrakt WS 1490 in Kombination mit Ethylalkohol auf sicherheitsrelevante Leistungsparameter. The influence of kava-special extract WS 1490 on safety-relevant performance alone and in combination with ethyl alcohol. *Blutalkohol* (1993) 30, 96–105.
3. Committee on Safety of Medicines/Medicines and Healthcare Regulatory Authority. Kava-kava and hepatotoxicity. *Current Problems* (2003) 29, 8.
4. Li XZ, Ramzan I. Role of ethanol in kava hepatotoxicity. *Phytother Res* (2010) 24, 475–80.

Alcohol + Ketoconazole

A few cases of disulfiram-like reactions have been reported in patients who drank alcohol while taking ketoconazole.

Clinical evidence, mechanism, importance and management

One patient (an alcoholic), out of a group of 12 patients with Candida infections taking ketoconazole 200 mg daily, experienced a disulfiram-like reaction (nausea, vomiting, facial flushing) after drinking alcohol.[1] No further details are given, and the report does not state whether any of the other subjects drank alcohol. A woman taking ketoconazole 200 mg daily developed a disulfiram-like reaction when she drank alcohol.[2] Another report describes a transient 'sunburn-like' rash or flush on the face, upper chest and back of a patient taking ketoconazole 200 mg daily when she drank modest quantities of wine or beer.[3]

The reasons for the reactions are not known but it seems possible that ketoconazole might act like disulfiram and inhibit the activity of acetaldehyde dehydrogenase (see *Mechanism*, under 'Alcohol + Disulfiram', p.67). The incidence of this reaction appears to be very low (these appear to be the only reports) and the manufacturers note that symptoms resolve within a few hours.[4] Nevertheless, to avoid these effects, the manufacturer advises avoidance of alcohol while taking ketoconazole.[5] However, note that reactions of this kind are usually more unpleasant than serious and normally require no treatment.

1. Fazio RA, Wickremesinghe PC, Arsura EL. Ketoconazole treatment of *Candida esophagitis*—a prospective study of 12 cases. *Am J Gastroenterol* (1983) 78, 261–4.
2. Meyboom RHB, Pater BW. Overgevoeligheid voor alcoholische dranken tijdens behandeling met ketoconazol. *Ned Tijdschr Geneeskd* (1989) 133, 1463–4.
3. Magnasco AJ, Magnasco LD. Interaction of ketoconazole and ethanol. *Clin Pharm* (1986) 5, 522–3.
4. Nizoral Tablets (Ketoconazole). Janssen-Cilag Ltd. UK Summary of product characteristics, June 2010.
5. Nizoral Tablets (Ketoconazole). Janssen-Cilag Ltd. UK Patient information leaflet, June 2010.

Alcohol + Leflunomide or Teriflunomide

The concurrent use of alcohol with leflunomide might increase the risk of hepatotoxicity, although limited alcohol consumption appears to have little effect on liver enzyme values in patients. Teriflunomide might have a similar effect.

Clinical evidence, mechanism, importance and management

The UK manufacturer of leflunomide states that because of the potential for additive hepatotoxic effects, it is recommended that alcohol should be avoided by patients taking leflunomide.[1] However, one study suggested that self-reported alcohol consumption had no influence on ALT concentrations in rheumatoid arthritis patients taking leflunomide,[2] and the British Society for Rheumatology guidelines recommend that patients taking leflunomide should be asked to limit alcohol intake to 4 to 8 units a week.[3] The UK manufacturer of teriflunomide (the active metabolite of leflunomide) recommends that it should be used with caution in patients who consume substantial quantities of alcohol [not defined].[4]

1. Arava (Leflunomide). Sanofi. UK Summary of product characteristics, September 2014.
2. Rajakulendran S, Gadsby K, Deighton C. Rheumatoid arthritis, alcohol, leflunomide and methotrexate. Can changes to the BSR guidelines for leflunomide and methotrexate on alcohol consumption be justified? *Musculoskeletal Care* (2008) 6, 233–45.
3. Chakravarty K, McDonald H, Pullar T, Taggart A, Chalmers R, Oliver S, Mooney J, Somerville M, Bosworth A, Kennedy T, on behalf of the British Society for Rheumatology, British Health Professionals in Rheumatology Standards, Guidelines and Audit Working Group in consultation with the British Association of Dermatologists. BSR/BHPR guideline for disease-modifying anti-rheumatic drug (DMARD) therapy in consultation with the British Association of Dermatologists. *Rheumatology (Oxford)* (2008) 47, 924–5. Available at: http://rheumatology.oxfordjournals.org/cgi/data/kel216a/DC1/1 (accessed 21/10/15).
4. Aubagio (Teriflunomide). Genzyme Therapeutics. UK Summary of product characteristics, September 2014.

Alcohol + Levamisole

The Brazilian manufacturer of levamisole notes that a disulfiram-like reaction has been reported when levamisole was given with alcohol.[1] Reactions of this kind are usually more unpleasant than serious; and symptoms often resolve within a few hours. It would seem prudent to warn patients of the possibility.

1. Ascaridil (Cloridrato de levamisole). Janssen-Cilag (Brazil). Brazilian Prescribing information, March 2008.

Alcohol + Levosimendan

Levosimendan does not appear to interact with alcohol.

Clinical evidence, mechanism, importance and management

A double-blind, randomised, crossover study in 12 healthy subjects given oral alcohol 0.8 g/kg with intravenous levosimendan 1 mg found no clinically relevant pharmacokinetic or pharmacodynamic interactions.[1] There therefore seems no reason to avoid the use of levosimendan in patients who have recently consumed alcohol.

1. Antila S, Järvinen A, Akkila J, Honkanen T, Karlsson M, Lehtonen L. Studies on psychomotoric effects and pharmacokinetic interactions of the new calcium sensitizing drug levosimendan and ethanol. *Arzneimittelforschung* (1997) 47, 816–20.

Alcohol + Lithium

The concurrent use of alcohol and lithium does not notably affect the levels of either drug, but some limited evidence suggests that the combination might impair psychomotor skills.

Clinical evidence, mechanism, importance and management

In 9 out of 10 healthy subjects alcohol 0.5 g/kg raised the serum levels of a single 600-mg dose of lithium carbonate by 16%. Four subjects had at least a 25% increase in lithium levels. However these rises were not considered to be clinically important.[1] Two studies suggest that lithium does not affect blood-alcohol levels.[2,3]

In a study, 20 healthy subjects were given lithium carbonate (to achieve lithium serum levels of 0.75 mmol/L) and alcohol 0.5 g/kg, and undertook various psychomotor tests to assess any impairment of skills related to driving. Lithium carbonate alone prolonged reaction times and increased the inaccuracy of responses, whereas alcohol alone increased the number of mistakes in tests of co-ordination and attention; both drugs together were therefore considered to present extra risks than either drug alone.[2] In a placebo-controlled study, 35 alcoholic patients were given about 1.25 g/kg of alcohol after taking lithium for 14 days (mean serum lithium level of 0.89 mmol/L). Patients considered themselves to be less intoxicated when taking lithium with alcohol (compared with placebo) and there was an improvement in performance in 3 of the 6 cognitive tests used, but not in the tests of skills related to driving.[3]

Information is limited but patients should be warned about the possible increased risk of driving or other potentially hazardous activities when taking lithium and drinking alcohol.

1. Anton RF, Paladino JA, Morton A, Thomas RW. Effect of acute alcohol consumption on lithium kinetics. *Clin Pharmacol Ther* (1985) 38, 52–5.
2. Linnoila M, Saario I, Maki M. Effect of treatment with diazepam or lithium and alcohol on psychomotor skills related to driving. *Eur J Clin Pharmacol* (1974) 7, 337–42.
3. Judd LL, Huey LY. Lithium antagonizes ethanol intoxication in alcoholics. *Am J Psychiatry* (1984) 141, 1517–21.

Alcohol + *Liv 52*

***Liv 52*, an Ayurvedic herbal remedy, appears to reduce hangover symptoms after drinking, reducing blood-alcohol and acetaldehyde levels at 12 hours. However *Liv 52* also raises the blood-alcohol levels of moderate drinkers for the first few hours after drinking.**

Clinical evidence

Nine healthy subjects who normally drank socially (alcohol 40 to 100 g weekly) took *Liv 52* two hours before drinking alcohol (four 60 mL doses of Indian whisky, equivalent to 90 g of alcohol). After taking 6 tablets of *Liv 52* their one-hour blood-alcohol levels were increased by 15% (from 75 mg% to 86.2 mg%), and after taking 3 tablets of *Liv 52* daily for 2 weeks, their one-hour blood-alcohol levels were raised by 27% (from 75 mg% to 95.3 mg%).[1] Acetaldehyde levels in the blood and urine were lowered at 12 hours, and hangover symptoms seemed to be reduced.[1] In a similar study, the blood-alcohol levels of 9 moderate drinkers were raised over the first 2 hours by about 28 to 44% after taking three tablets of *Liv 52* twice daily for 2 weeks, and by 17 to 19% over the following 2 hours.[2] In 8 occasional drinkers, the increase in blood-alcohol levels was very small.[2]

Mechanism

Not understood. The *Liv 52* preparation in this study was said to contain the active principles from *Capparis spinosa*, *Cichorium intybus*, *Solanum nigrum*, *Cassia occidentalis*, *Terminalia arjuna*, *Achillea millefolium*, *Tamarix gallica* and *Phyllanthus amarus*.[1] These appear to increase the absorption of alcohol, or reduce its metabolism by the liver, thereby raising blood-alcohol levels. It is suggested that the reduced hangover effects might occur because *Liv 52* prevents the binding of acetaldehyde to cell proteins allowing a more rapid elimination.[1]

Importance and management

Direct pharmacokinetic evidence seems to be limited to the two studies cited, but *Liv 52* appears to reduce the hangover effects after drinking; however, it can also increase the blood-alcohol levels of moderate drinkers for the first few hours after drinking. Increases of up to 30% might be enough to raise blood-alcohol levels from legal to illegal, when driving. Moderate drinkers should be warned. Occasional drinkers appear to develop higher blood-alcohol levels than moderate drinkers but *Liv 52* does not seem to increase them to a clinically relevant extent.

1. Chauhan BL, Kulkarni RD. Alcohol hangover and Liv.52. *Eur J Clin Pharmacol* (1991) 40, 187–8.
2. Chauhan BL, Kulkarni RD. Effect of Liv.52, a herbal preparation, on absorption and metabolism of ethanol in humans. *Eur J Clin Pharmacol* (1991) 40, 189–91.

Alcohol + MAOIs or RIMAs

The hypotensive adverse effects of the MAOIs could be exaggerated in a few patients by alcohol, and they might experience dizziness and faintness after drinking relatively modest amounts of alcohol. Moclobemide does not appear to have a clinically relevant effect on the psychomotor effects of alcohol.

Clinical evidence, mechanism, importance and management

(a) MAOIs

In one report, a patient taking an MAOI describes drinking gin and orange and then becoming unsteady when standing up, and hitting her head on a wall.[1] Some degree of hypotension can occur in patients taking MAOIs and this could be exaggerated by the vasodilation and reduced cardiac output caused by alcohol. Patients taking MAOIs should therefore be warned of the possibility of orthostatic hypotension and fainting if they drink alcohol. They should be advised not to stand up too quickly, and to remain sitting or lying if they feel faint or begin to 'black out'.

For a discussion of the interaction of MAOIs with tyramine present in some alcoholic drinks, see 'MAOIs or RIMAs + Food; Tyramine-containing', p.1389.

(b) Moclobemide

The possibility that alcohol-induced deterioration in psychomotor skills (i.e. those associated with safe driving) might be increased by the RIMAs has been studied. In three controlled studies in healthy subjects, moclobemide, given as single doses of either 100 mg or 300 mg, or as 200 mg three times daily for 5 days, with alcohol, appeared to have only a minor and clinically unimportant effect on the adverse effects of alcohol.[2,3]

For a discussion of the interaction of RIMAs with tyramine present in some alcoholic drinks, see 'MAOIs or RIMAs + Food; Tyramine-containing', p.1389.

1. Anon. MAOIs — a patient's tale. *Pulse* (1981) December 5th, 69.
2. Berlin I, Cournot A, Zimmer R, Pedarriosse A-M, Manfredi R, Molinier P, Puech AJ. Evaluation and comparison of the interaction between alcohol and moclobemide or clomipramine in healthy subjects. *Psychopharmacology (Berl)* (1990) 100, 40–5.
3. Tiller JWG. Antidepressants, alcohol and psychomotor performance. *Acta Psychiatr Scand* (1990) (Suppl 360), 13–17.

Alcohol + Mefloquine

Mefloquine does not normally appear to interact with alcohol, although excessive alcohol intake might contribute to the hepatic adverse effects of mefloquine. An isolated report describes two incidents of severe psychosis and depression when a man taking mefloquine drank large quantities of alcohol.

Clinical evidence, mechanism, importance and management

Mefloquine 250 mg or placebo was given to two groups of 20 healthy subjects on three occasions, each time the day before they drank enough alcohol to achieve blood levels of about 35 mg%. Mefloquine did not affect blood-alcohol levels, nor did it increase the effects of alcohol on two real-highway driving tests, or on psychomotor tests done in the laboratory. In fact, the mefloquine group actually drove better than the placebo group.[1]

A 40-year-old man with no previous psychiatric history, taking mefloquine 250 mg weekly for malaria prophylaxis, had no problems with the first 2 doses. However, on two separate occasions when taking the third and fourth doses he also drank about half a litre of whisky, whereupon he developed severe paranoid delusions, hallucinations and became suicidal. When he stopped drinking he had no further problems while taking subsequent doses of mefloquine. He was used to drinking large amounts of alcohol and had experienced no problems while previously taking proguanil and chloroquine.[2]

The broad picture is that mefloquine appears not to worsen the psychomotor effects of moderate amounts of alcohol. Just why an unusual toxic reaction developed in one individual is not known, although mefloquine alone can increase the risk of psychiatric events.[3,4] It has been suggested that many of the adverse effects of mefloquine are associated with liver damage, and concurrent insults to the liver, such as from alcohol and dehydration, might be related to the development of severe or prolonged adverse reactions to mefloquine. In a review of 516 published case reports of mefloquine adverse effects, 11 cited alcohol as a possible contributing factor.[4] One group of authors suggested that travellers taking mefloquine should avoid alcohol, particularly within 24 hours of their weekly mefloquine dose.[4] However, the manufacturer has not issued such a warning.[5]

1. Vuurman EFPM, Muntjewerff ND, Uiterwijk MMC, van Veggel LMA, Crevoisier C, Haglund L, Kinzig M, O'Hanlon JF. Effects of mefloquine alone and with alcohol on psychomotor and driving performance. *Eur J Clin Pharmacol* (1996) 50, 475–82.
2. Wittes RC, Saginur R. Adverse reaction to mefloquine associated with ethanol ingestion. *Can Med Assoc J* (1995) 152, 515–17.
3. van Riemsdijk MM, Sturkenboom MCJM, Pepplinkhuizen L, Stricker BHC. Mefloquine increases the risk of serious psychiatric events during travel abroad: a nationwide case-control study in the Netherlands. *J Clin Psychiatry* (2005) 66, 199–204.
4. Croft AM, Herxheimer A. Hypothesis: Adverse effects of the antimalaria drug, mefloquine: due to primary liver damage with secondary thyroid involvement? *BMC Public Health* (2002) 2:6.
5. Lariam (Mefloquine hydrochloride). Roche Products Ltd. UK Summary of product characteristics, November 2011.

Alcohol + Meprobamate

The intoxicant effects of alcohol can be considerably increased by the presence of meprobamate.

Clinical evidence

A study in 22 subjects, given meprobamate 400 mg four times daily for one week, found that with blood-alcohol levels of 50 mg% the performance of a number of coordination and judgement tests was much more impaired than with either drug alone.[1] Four of the subjects were quite obviously drunk while taking both meprobamate and alcohol, and showed marked incoordination and social disinhibition. Two could not walk without assistance. The authors stated this effect was much greater than anything seen with alcohol alone. Other studies confirm this interaction, although the effects appeared to be less pronounced.[2-6]

Mechanism

Both meprobamate and alcohol are CNS depressants, which appear to have additive effects. There is also some evidence that alcohol might inhibit or increase meprobamate metabolism, depending on whether it is taken acutely or chronically, but the contribution of this to the enhanced CNS depression is uncertain.[7,8] Meprobamate does not appear to increase blood-alcohol levels.[5]

Importance and management

The interaction between meprobamate and alcohol is well-documented and potentially serious. Normal daily doses of meprobamate in association with relatively moderate blood-alcohol levels, well within the UK legal limit for driving, can result in obviously hazardous intoxication. Patients should be warned; the patient information leaflet for meprobamate states that the concurrent use of alcohol should be avoided.[9]

1. Zirkle GA, McAtee OB, King PD, Van Dyke R. Meprobamate and small amounts of alcohol: effects on human ability, coordination, and judgement. *JAMA* (1960) 173, 1823–5.
2. Reisby N, Theilgaard A. The interaction of alcohol and meprobamate in man. *Acta Psychiatr Scand* (1969) 208 (Suppl), 5–204.
3. Forney RB, Hughes FW. Meprobamate, ethanol or meprobamate-ethanol combinations on performance of human subjects under delayed audiofeedback (DAF). *J Psychol* (1964) 57, 431–6.
4. Ashford JR, Cobby JM. Drug interactions. The effects of alcohol and meprobamate applied singly and jointly in human subjects. III. The concentrations of alcohol and meprobamate in the blood and their effects on performance; application of mathematical models. *J Stud Alcohol* (1975) (Suppl 7), 140–61.
5. Cobby JM, Ashford JR. Drug interactions. The effects of alcohol and meprobamate applied singly and jointly in human subjects. IV. The concentrations of alcohol and meprobamate in the blood. *J Stud Alcohol* (1975) (Suppl 7), 162–76.
6. Ashford JR, Carpenter JA. Drug interactions. The effect of alcohol and meprobamate applied singly and jointly in human subjects. V. Summary and conclusions. *J Stud Alcohol* (1975) (Suppl 7), 177–87.
7. Misra PS, Lefèvre A, Ishii H, Rubin E, Lieber CS. Increase of ethanol, meprobamate and pentobarbital metabolism after chronic ethanol administration in man and in rats. *Am J Med* (1971) 51, 346–51.
8. Rubin E, Gang H, Misra PS, Lieber CS. Inhibition of drug metabolism by acute ethanol intoxication: a hepatic microsomal mechanism. *Am J Med* (1970) 49, 801–6.
9. Meprobamate. Genus Pharmaceuticals. UK Patient information leaflet, July 2009.

Alcohol + Methotrexate

Some inconclusive evidence suggests that the consumption of alcohol might increase the risk of methotrexate-induced hepatic cirrhosis and fibrosis.

Clinical evidence, mechanism, importance and management

It has been claimed that alcohol can increase the hepatotoxic effects of methotrexate,[1] and two reports of patients treated for psoriasis support this suggestion. In one report, 3 out of 5 patients with methotrexate-induced cirrhosis were reported to have drunk alcohol concurrently (2 patients greater than 85 g of alcohol per week, one patient 25 to 85 g of alcohol per week):[2] in the other report, the subject was known to drink excessively.[3] The evidence is by no means conclusive and no direct causal relationship has been established. However, one manufacturer of methotrexate advises the avoidance of drugs, including alcohol, which have hepatotoxic potential,[4] and another contraindicates the use of methotrexate in patients with alcoholism or alcoholic liver disease.[5]

1. Almeyda J, Barnardo D, Baker H. Drug reactions XV. Methotrexate, psoriasis and the liver. *Br J Dermatol* (1971) 85, 302–5.
2. Tobias H, Auerbach R. Hepatotoxicity of long-term methotrexate therapy for psoriasis. *Arch Intern Med* (1973) 132, 391–400.
3. Pai SH, Werthamer S, Zak FG. Severe liver damage caused by treatment of psoriasis with methotrexate. *N Y State J Med* (1973) 73, 2585–7.
4. Methotrexate Tablets. Hospira UK Ltd. UK Summary of product characteristics, January 2008.
5. Rheumatrex (Methotrexate sodium). Stada Pharmaceuticals Inc. US Prescribing information, July 2009.

Alcohol + Methylphenidate

Alcohol can increase methylphenidate levels and exacerbate some of its CNS effects.

Clinical evidence, mechanism, importance and management

In 17 subjects who had taken methylphenidate orally or intranasally with alcohol on at least 10 separate occasions, the primary reason for concurrent use was given as an alteration in psychotropic effects with increased euphoria and energy and a diminished sense of drunkenness. In addition, a minority of subjects also reported occasionally experiencing unpleasant adverse effects such as increased nausea (3 subjects), insomnia (2), and jaw clenching (1).[1] In a study in 20 subjects, alcohol 0.6 g/kg was given either 30 minutes before or 30 minutes after a single 0.3-mg/kg dose of methylphenidate. Alcohol increased the AUC and maximum serum levels of methylphenidate, regardless of the timing of administration, by about 25% and 40%, respectively.[2]

In a similar study in 9 healthy subjects, alcohol 0.8 g/kg, given either 30 minutes before or 30 minutes after a single 20-mg dose of methylphenidate, did not affect the pharmacokinetics of methylphenidate. However, plasma levels of the inactive metabolite ritalinic acid were reduced, whereas levels of ethylphenidate, a minor active metabolite were increased.[3] Methylphenidate has a short half-life mainly due to conversion to the inactive metabolite ritalinic acid, but the concurrent use of alcohol and methylphenidate has been reported to result in production of a minor metabolite, ethylphenidate, which has CNS activity.[4,5] However, a further study found that the ethylphenidate formed is predominantly of the inactive enantiomer, so is unlikely to contribute to the additive CNS effects of alcohol and methylphenidate.[2]

The UK manufacturer of methylphenidate advises that alcohol might exacerbate the CNS effects of methylphenidate and therefore recommends that alcohol should be avoided during treatment.[6] In addition, methylphenidate should be given cautiously to patients with a history of drug dependence or alcoholism because of its potential for abuse.[1,6,7]

1. Barrett SP, Pihl RO. Oral methylphenidate-alcohol co-abuse. *J Clin Psychopharmacol* (2002) 22, 633–4.
2. Patrick KS, Straughn AB, Minhinnett RR, Yeatts SD, Herrin AE, DeVane CL, Malcolm R, Janis GC, Markowitz JS. Influence of ethanol and gender on methylphenidate pharmacokinetics and pharmacodynamics. *Clin Pharmacol Ther* (2007) 81, 346–53.
3. Koehm M, Kauert GF, Toennes SW. Influence of ethanol on the pharmacokinetics of methylphenidate's metabolites ritalinic acid and ethylphenidate. *Arzneimittelforschung* (2010) 60, 238–44.
4. Markowitz JS, DeVane CL, Boulton DW, Nahas Z, Risch SC, Diamond F, Patrick KS. Ethylphenidate formation in human subjects after the administration of a single dose of methylphenidate and ethanol. *Drug Metab Dispos* (2000) 28, 620–4.
5. Markowitz JS, Logan BK, Diamond F, Patrick KS. Detection of the novel metabolite ethylphenidate after methylphenidate overdose with alcohol coingestion. *J Clin Psychopharmacol* (1999) 19, 362–6.
6. Ritalin (Methylphenidate hydrochloride). Novartis Pharmaceuticals UK Ltd. UK Summary of product characteristics, May 2011.
7. Ritalin (Methylphenidate hydrochloride). Novartis. US Prescribing information, December 2010.

Alcohol + Metoclopramide

Some evidence suggests that metoclopramide can increase the rate of alcohol absorption, raise maximum blood-alcohol levels, and possibly increase alcohol-related sedation.

Clinical evidence, mechanism, importance and management

A study in 5 healthy subjects found that 20 mg of intravenous metoclopramide increased the rate of alcohol absorption, and raised peak blood-alcohol levels, from 55 mg% to 86 mg%.[1] Increases in blood-alcohol levels were also seen in 2 healthy subjects[1] and in a small study[2] in which metoclopramide was given orally.[1] Another study in 7 healthy subjects found that 10 mg of intravenous metoclopramide accelerated the rate of absorption of alcohol 70 mg/kg given orally, and increased its peak levels, but not to a statistically significant extent. Blood-alcohol levels remained below 12 mg%. More importantly the sedative effects of the alcohol were increased.[3] The reasons for this effect are not fully understood, but it appears to be related to an increase in gastric emptying. These studies were done to find out more about intestinal absorption mechanisms rather than to identify daily practicalities of concurrent use, so the importance of their findings is uncertain. However, it seems possible that the effects of alcohol will be increased by metoclopramide. Note that metoclopramide alone can sometimes cause drowsiness, and if affected, patients should not drive or operate machinery.

1. Gibbons DO, Lant AF. Effects of intravenous and oral propantheline and metoclopramide on ethanol absorption. *Clin Pharmacol Ther* (1975) 17, 578–84.
2. Oneta CM, Simanowski UA, Martinez M, Allali-Hassani A, Parés X, Homann N, Conradt C, Waldherr R, Fiehn W, Coutelle C, Seitz HK. First pass metabolism of ethanol Is strikingly influenced by the speed of gastric emptying. *Gut* (1998) 43, 612–19.
3. Bateman DN, Kahn C, Mashiter K, Davies DS. Pharmacokinetic and concentration-effect studies with intravenous metoclopramide. *Br J Clin Pharmacol* (1978) 6, 401–7.

Alcohol + Metronidazole and related drugs

A number of patients taking oral metronidazole have developed a disulfiram-like reaction after drinking alcohol. There is one report of its

occurrence when metronidazole was applied as a vaginal insert, and another when metronidazole was given intravenously. Some clinical studies have not confirmed the interaction, and its existence is disputed in some reports. The interaction has been seen in one case with ornidazole, and is alleged to occur with all other 5-nitroimidazoles (e.g. tinidazole).

Clinical evidence

(a) Metronidazole

A man who had been in a drunken stupor for 3 days was given two metronidazole tablets (a total of 500 mg) one hour apart by his wife in the belief that they might sober him up. Twenty minutes after the first tablet he was awake and complaining that he had been given disulfiram (which he had taken some months before). Immediately after the second tablet, he took another drink and developed a classic disulfiram-like reaction with flushing of the face and neck, nausea and epigastric discomfort.[1] Other individual cases have been reported,[2] including a reaction with a metronidazole vaginal insert.[3]

In a test of the value of metronidazole 250 mg twice daily as a possible drink-deterrent, all 10 alcoholic patients studied experienced some disulfiram-like reactions of varying intensity (facial flushing, headaches, sensation of heat, fall in blood pressure, vomiting) when given alcohol.[4] In another study in 60 alcoholic patients, given metronidazole 250 to 750 mg daily, most developed mild to moderate disulfiram-like reactions during an alcohol tolerance test.[5] A lower incidence of this reaction, between 2 and 24%, has also been reported.[6-8]

Pharmaceutical preparations containing alcohol have also been implicated. A 2-year-old child became flushed and dyspnoeic when metronidazole was given with both *Stopayne* syrup (an analgesic/sedative combination) and a phenobarbital syrup, both of which contained alcohol.[9] Another reaction has been seen in a patient receiving intravenous metronidazole and a co-trimoxazole preparation containing alcohol 10%.[10] A further patient who had just finished a 7-day course of metronidazole developed severe, prolonged nausea and vomiting postpartum: she had received a single 800-mg dose of prophylactic clindamycin intravenously before the birth and it was thought that the benzyl alcohol present in the clindamycin preparation could have caused the reaction. However, other factors such as intrathecal anaesthesia could have also contributed to the adverse effects.[11] For mention of other products containing alcohol, which have the potential to interact, see 'Alcohol + Disulfiram', p.67.

An interaction has also been reported in association with metabolic acidosis in an intoxicated man 4 hours after he was given intravenous metronidazole as prophylaxis following injury.[12] A fatality occurred in a frail 31-year old woman, which was attributed to cardiac arrhythmias caused by acetaldehyde toxicity resulting from the interaction between alcohol and metronidazole, linked to autonomic distress caused by a physical assault.[13] Alcohol is also said to taste unpleasant[1,4] or to be less pleasurable[8] while taking metronidazole. Some drug abusers apparently exploit the reaction for 'kicks'.[14]

Not all studies have found an interaction. A study in 207 patients with inflammatory bowel disease, assessed using a phone survey, the presence of adverse reactions to alcohol in patients taking chronic metronidazole and/or mercaptopurine or neither drug; all of the patients consumed less than 4 alcoholic beverages per day. There was a trend towards more adverse effects in both the metronidazole and mercaptopurine study groups, but no statistically significant interaction between alcohol and metronidazole was found.[15] There are other reports, including two well-controlled studies, showing that metronidazole has no disulfiram-like effects.[16-18]

(b) Ornidazole

An isolated case report describes a disulfiram-like reaction in a 48-year-old man with a history of chronic alcohol abuse taking ornidazole 500 mg and ofloxacin 200 mg, both twice daily, for diarrhoea and vomiting. He drank alcohol about 2 hours after taking the antibacterials and, about 45 minutes later, developed severe restlessness, palpitations, facial flushing and sweating. The patient was given oxygen and intravenous fluids as well as diazepam for anxiety. Symptoms improved within 2 hours and the patient was discharged after 3 days.[19]

Mechanism

Not understood. In the disulfiram reaction, the accumulation of acetaldehyde appears to be responsible for most of the symptoms, see *Mechanism*, under 'Alcohol + Disulfiram', p.67. Some workers have reported an increase in acetaldehyde levels due to the interaction between metronidazole and alcohol,[13] but others have reported no effect[18] or a reduction in plasma acetaldehyde levels.[20] Furthermore, some studies with metronidazole indicate a lack of a disulfiram-like reaction,[16,17] and it has been suggested that if such a reaction does occur it might be by a mechanism other than the inhibition of hepatic acetaldehyde dehydrogenase.[18] It appears that metronidazole, like disulfiram, can inhibit other enzymes related to alcohol metabolism including xanthine oxidase and alcohol dehydrogenase.[21,22] Inhibition of xanthine oxidase might cause noradrenaline excess, and inhibition of alcohol dehydrogenase can lead to activation of microsomal enzyme oxidative pathways that generate ketones and lactate, which could produce acidosis.[12]

Importance and management

The interaction between alcohol and metronidazole is reasonably well studied, but it remains a controversial issue. The incidence is variously reported as between 0 and 100%, with more recent reports disputing its existence.[18,20] Nevertheless because of the uncertainty, all patients given metronidazole should be warned about what might happen if they drink alcohol. The manufacturers recommend avoiding alcohol when metronidazole is taken, and for at least 48 hours after it has been stopped (UK) or 24 hours after it has been stopped (US).[23,24] In the US, for the capsules, and extended-release preparation, 72 hours is recommended.[25,26] However, the authors of one report suggest a cautious trial of alcohol in patients that are starting and will be taking metronidazole on a long-term basis.[15]

The reaction, when it occurs, normally seems to be more unpleasant and possibly frightening than serious, and usually requires no treatment, although one report describes a serious reaction when intravenous metronidazole was given to an intoxicated man,[12] and one possible fatality has been reported.[13] The risk of a reaction with metronidazole used intravaginally seems to be small because the absorption is low (about 20% compared with about 100% orally), but evidently it can happen, even if only rarely.[3] Patients should be warned.

It has been alleged that the disulfiram-like reaction with alcohol occurs with all of the related 5-nitroimidazoles,[27,28] One report describes this interaction with ornidazole, but there do not appear to be any published reports of it occurring with **nimorazole**, **secnidazole** or **tinidazole**. The manufacturer of **tinidazole** notes that, as with related compounds, there is a possibility of a disulfiram-like reaction with alcoholic beverages, and recommends that alcohol should be avoided until 72 hours after discontinuing tinidazole.[29] Until more is known it would seem prudent to consider the possibility of an effect with all 5-nitroimidazoles.

1. Taylor JAT. Metronidazole—a new agent for combined somatic and psychic therapy for alcoholism: a case study and preliminary report. *Bull Los Angel Neuro Soc* (1964) 29, 158–62.
2. Alexander I. 'Alcohol—Antabuse' syndrome in patients receiving metronidazole during gynaecological treatment. *Br J Clin Pract* (1985) 39, 292–3.
3. Plosker GL. Possible interaction between ethanol and vaginally administered metronidazole. *Clin Pharm* (1987) 6, 189 and 192–3.
4. Ban TA, Lehmann HE, Roy P. Rapport préliminaire sur l'effect thérapeutique du Flagyl dans l'alcoolisme. *Union Med Can* (1966) 95, 147–9.
5. Sansoy OM. Evaluation of metronidazole in the treatment of alcoholism. A comprehensive three-year study comprising 60 cases. *Rocky Mtn Med J* (1970) 67, 43–7.
6. de Mattos H. Relações entre o alcoolismo e aparelho digestivo. Experiência com metronidazol. *Hospital (Rio J)* (1968) 74, 1669–76.
7. Channabasavanna SM, Kaliaperumal VG, Mathew G, Itty A. Metronidazole in the treatment of alcoholism: a controlled trial. *Indian J Psychiatry* (1979) 21, 90–3.
8. Penick SB, Carrier RN, Sheldon JB. Metronidazole in the treatment of alcoholism. *Am J Psychiatry* (1969) 125, 1063–6.
9. Tunguy-Desmarais GP. Interaction between alcohol and metronidazole. *S Afr Med J* (1983) 63, 836.
10. Edwards DL, Fink PC, Van Dyke PO. Disulfiram-like reaction associated with intravenous trimethoprim–sulfamethoxazole and metronidazole. *Clin Pharm* (1986) 5, 999–1000.
11. Krulewitch CJ. An unexpected adverse drug effect. *J Midwifery Womens Health* (2003) 48, 67–8.
12. Harries DP, Teale KFH, Sunderland G. Metronidazole and alcohol: potential problems. *Scott Med J* (1990) 35, 179–180.
13. Cina SJ, Russell RA, Conradi SE. Sudden death due to metronidazole/ethanol interaction. *Am J Forensic Med Pathol* (1996) 17, 343–6.
14. Giannini AJ, DeFrance DT. Metronidazole and alcohol—potential for combinative abuse. *J Toxicol Clin Toxicol* (1983) 20, 509–15.
15. Ginzburg L, Present DH. Alcohol is well tolerated in IBD patients taking either metronidazole or 6-mercaptopurine. *Am J Gastroenterol* (2003) 98 (Suppl), S241.
16. Goodwin DW. Metronidazole in the treatment of alcoholism: a negative report. *Am J Psychiatry* (1967) 123, 1276–8.
17. Gelder MG, Edwards G. Metronidazole in the treatment of alcohol addiction: a controlled trial. *Br J Psychiatry* (1968) 114, 473–5.
18. Visapää J-P, Tillonen JS, Kaihovaara PS, Salaspuro MP. Lack of disulfiram-like reaction with metronidazole and ethanol. *Ann Pharmacother* (2002) 36, 971–4.
19. Sharma V, Sharma A, Kumar V, Aggarwal S. Disulfiram-like reaction with ornidazole. *J Postgrad Med* (2009) 55, 292–3.
20. Williams CS, Woodcock KR. Do ethanol and metronidazole interact to produce a disulfiram-like reaction? *Ann Pharmacother* (2000) 34, 255–7.
21. Fried R, Fried LW. The effect of Flagyl on xanthine oxidase and alcohol dehydrogenase. *Biochem Pharmacol* (1966) 15, 1890–4.
22. Gupta NK, Woodley CL, Fried R. Effect of metronidazole on liver alcohol dehydrogenase. *Biochem Pharmacol* (1970) 19, 2805–8.
23. Flagyl Tablets (Metronidazole). Zentiva. UK Summary of product characteristics, May 2011.
24. Flagyl (Metronidazole). Pfizer Inc. US Prescribing information, April 2010.
25. Flagyl 375 (Metronidazole). Pfizer Inc. US Prescribing information, April 2010.
26. Flagyl ER (Metronidazole). Pfizer Inc. US Prescribing information, September 2010.
27. Ralph ED. Nitroimidazoles. In: Koren G, Prober CG, Gold R, eds. Antimicrobial therapy in infants and children. New York: Marcel Dekker; 1988 p. 729–45.
28. Andersson KE. Pharmacokinetics of nitroimidazoles. Spectrum of adverse reactions. *Scand J Infect Dis* (1981) 26 (Suppl), 60–7.
29. Fasigyn (Tinidazole). Pfizer Ltd. UK Summary of product characteristics, December 2008.

Alcohol + Mirtazapine

The sedative effects of mirtazapine might be increased by alcohol.

Clinical evidence, mechanism, importance and management

In 6 healthy subjects alcohol (equivalent to 60 g) had a minimal effect on the plasma levels of mirtazapine 15 mg.[1] Furthermore, mirtazapine does not affect the absorption of alcohol.[2] However the sedation and CNS impairment seen with mirtazapine is additive with that produced by alcohol, and the manufacturers therefore recommend avoiding concurrent use.[1,3]

1. Remeron (Mirtazapine). Merck Sharp & Dohme Corp. US Prescribing information, January 2014.
2. Sitsen JMA, Zivkov M. Mirtazapine: clinical profile. *CNS Drugs* (1995) 4 (Suppl 1), 39–48.
3. Zispin SolTab (Mirtazapine). Merck Sharp & Dohme Ltd. UK Summary of product characteristics, February 2015.

Alcohol + Muscle relaxants

The concurrent use of small or moderate amounts of alcohol with muscle relaxants can increase drowsiness and reduce alertness. Three reported

cases of modest overdose with methocarbamol and alcohol resulted in death due to CNS depression.

Clinical evidence, mechanism, importance and management

(a) Baclofen

The manufacturer of baclofen warns that it might enhance the sedative effect of alcohol.[1] However, tolerance to the sedative effect of baclofen has been reported in alcohol-addicted patients after a period of abstinence, as well as after a relapse.[2]

(b) Dantrolene

The manufacturer of dantrolene advises caution if it is given with alcohol[3] and the patient information leaflet suggests that alcohol should be avoided because it might increase dizziness or drowsiness.[4]

(c) Methocarbamol

Fatal cerebral anoxia produced by CNS respiratory depression occurred in a 31-year-old man after he took significant amounts of methocarbamol and alcohol. Two other lethal overdoses have been reported with these two drugs. In all three cases the methocarbamol doses exceeded the recommended daily doses, but were estimated to be less than the reported maximum tolerated single dose of 12 g. Acute alcohol intoxication in conjunction with methocarbamol usage can lead to CNS depression, which might be sufficient to cause death.[5] The manufacturers of methocarbamol warn that it might potentiate the effects of alcohol.[6,7]

(d) Other muscle relaxants

For enhanced CNS effects with alcohol with other muscle relaxants, see 'Alcohol + Benzodiazepines and related drugs', p.59, 'Alcohol + Meprobamate', p.75, and 'Tizanidine + Miscellaneous', p.1589.

1. Lioresal Tablets (Baclofen). Novartis Pharmaceuticals UK Ltd. UK Summary of product characteristics, February 2013.
2. Addolorato G, Leggio L, Abenavoli L, Caputo F, Gasbarrini G. Tolerance to baclofen's sedative effect in alcohol-addicted patients: no dissipation after a period of abstinence. *Psychopharmacology (Berl)* (2005) 178, 351–2.
3. Dantrium Capsules (Dantrolene sodium). SpePharm UK Ltd. UK Summary of product characteristics, January 2012.
4. Dantrium Capsules (Dantrolene sodium). SpePharm UK Ltd. UK Patient information leaflet, December 2009.
5. Ferslew KE, Hagardorn AN, McCormick WF. A fatal interaction of methocarbamol and ethanol in an accidental poisoning. *J Forensic Sci* (1990) 35, 477–82.
6. Robaxin-750 (Methocarbamol). Almirall Ltd. UK Summary of product characteristics, March 2010.
7. Methocarbamol Tablets USP. Watson Laboratories Inc. US Prescribing information, March 2008.

Alcohol + Nefazodone

In one study nefazodone 400 mg was found not to increase the sedative-hypnotic effects of alcohol.[1]

1. Frewer LJ, Lader M. The effects of nefazodone, imipramine and placebo, alone and combined with alcohol, in normal subjects. *Int Clin Psychopharmacol* (1993) 8, 13–20.

Alcohol + Niclosamide

Alcohol might increase the adverse effects of niclosamide.

Clinical evidence, mechanism, importance and management

The manufacturer of niclosamide advises avoiding alcohol while taking niclosamide. The reasoning behind this is that, while niclosamide is virtually insoluble in water, it is slightly soluble in alcohol. Therefore taking niclosamide with alcohol might increase its absorption by the gut, resulting in an increase in its adverse effects. There are no formal reports of this interaction in practice but the manufacturer states that they have some anecdotal information that is consistent with this suggestion.[1]

1. Bayer. Personal communication, July 1992.

Alcohol + Nicotine

Nicotine (as a patch) might enhance the effect of alcohol on heart rate and reduce the time to peak alcohol levels. The concurrent use of alcohol and a nicotine nasal spray does not affect the pharmacokinetics of either drug.

Clinical evidence, mechanism, importance and management

A placebo-controlled study in 12 otherwise healthy tobacco smokers found that alcohol-induced increases in heart rate were enhanced by pretreatment with a 21-mg nicotine transdermal patch. The time to peak alcohol levels with a 0.4 g/kg dose of alcohol was faster with nicotine pretreatment (43 minutes) compared with 52 minutes in the absence of nicotine; however, this effect was not seen with a 0.7 g/kg dose of alcohol.[1] Another study in 12 otherwise healthy tobacco smokers found that although alcohol 0.4 or 0.8 g/kg (equivalent to approximately 2 or 4 drinks, respectively) influenced selected subjective responses and heart rate, pretreatment with alcohol did not affect the subjects responses to low-dose nicotine 3 to 20 micrograms/kg given as a nasal spray (20 microgram/kg dose is equivalent to about one-half of a cigarette). The concurrent use of nicotine and alcohol did not influence the blood levels of either drug.[2]

1. Kouri EM, McCarthy EM, Faust AH, Lukas SE. Pretreatment with transdermal nicotine enhances some of ethanol's acute effects in men. *Drug Alcohol Depend* (2004) 75, 55–65.
2. Perkins KA, Fonte C, Blakesley-Ball R, Stolinski A, Wilson AS. The influence of alcohol pre-treatment on the discriminative stimulus, subjective, and relative reinforcing effects of nicotine. *Behav Pharmacol* (2005) 16, 521–9.

Alcohol + Nicotinic acid (Niacin)

An isolated report describes delirium and metabolic acidosis when a patient taking nicotinic acid for hypercholesterolaemia drank about one litre of wine. The manufacturers state that the concurrent use of nicotinic acid and alcohol might result in an increase in adverse effects such as flushing and pruritus, and possibly liver toxicity.

Clinical evidence, mechanism, importance and management

An isolated report describes delirium and metabolic acidosis after a patient taking nicotinic acid 3 g daily for hypercholesterolaemia drank about one litre of wine. Delirium had occurred on a previous similar occasion after he drank a large quantity of beer while taking nicotinic acid. It is suggested that the nicotinic acid might have caused liver impairment, which was exacerbated by the large amount of alcohol. The patient did have some elevations in liver enzymes.[1] Acidosis has been associated with alcohol intoxication[2] (although the frequency of this association has been disputed[3]) and there has been a report of lactic acidosis associated with the use of high-dose (3 g daily) nicotinic acid,[4] and therefore a combined effect would seem possible. However, no general conclusions can be drawn from this single case.

Hepatic toxicity can occur with nicotinic acid and the manufacturers advise caution in patients who consume substantial quantities of alcohol. They also suggest avoiding alcohol around the time that nicotinic acid is taken, as the adverse effects of flushing and pruritus might be increased by concurrent use.[5,6]

1. Schwab RA, Bachhuber BH. Delirium and lactic acidosis caused by ethanol and niacin coingestion. *Am J Emerg Med* (1991) 9, 363–5.
2. Zehtabchi S, Sinert R, Baron BJ, Paladino L, Yadav K. Does ethanol explain the acidosis commonly seen in ethanol-intoxicated patients? *Clin Toxicol* (2005) 43, 161–6.
3. Ginsburg BY, Porter R, Nelson LS. Is acidosis commonly seen in patients with elevated ethanol levels? *Clin Toxicol* (2006) 44, 193.
4. Earthman TP, Odom L, Mullins CA. Lactic acidosis associated with high-dose niacin therapy. *South Med J* (1991) 84, 496–7.
5. Niaspan (Nicotinic acid). Abbott Laboratories Ltd. UK Summary of product characteristics, December 2010.
6. Niaspan (Niacin). Abbott Laboratories. US Prescribing information, April 2015.

Alcohol + Nitrofurantoin

There appears to be no good clinical evidence for an alleged interaction between alcohol and nitrofurantoin.

Clinical evidence, mechanism, importance and management

Despite claims in some books and reviews, an extensive literature search was unable to find any experimental or clinical evidence for an alleged disulfiram-like reaction between alcohol and nitrofurantoin.[1] A study in healthy subjects did not demonstrate any such interaction[2] and a survey of the reports in the manufacturer's database have also been unable to find good evidence for alcohol intolerance.[3] It is concluded that this 'interaction' is erroneous.[1]

1. Rowles B, Worthen DB. Clinical drug information: a case of misinformation. *N Engl J Med* (1982) 306, 113–4.
2. Miura K, Reckendorf HK. The nitrofurans. *Prog Med Chem* (1967) 5, 320–81.
3. D'Arcy PF. Nitrofurantoin. *Drug Intell Clin Pharm* (1985) 19, 540–7.

Alcohol + Nitrous oxide

In a double-blind study in 11 healthy subjects there were several instances when alcohol 0.25 to 0.5 g/kg (equivalent to 1 to 3 drinks) enhanced the effects of nitrous oxide 30% in oxygen, inhaled for 35 minutes. Some effects seen on concurrent use were not seen with either drug alone; these included subjective effects and delayed free recall.[1] For mention of the effect of alcohol following anaesthesia, see 'Anaesthetics, general + Alcohol', p.99.

1. Zacny JP, Camarillo VM, Sadeghi P, Black M. Effects of ethanol and nitrous oxide, alone and in combination, on mood, psychomotor performance and pain reports in healthy volunteers. *Drug Alcohol Depend* (1998) 52, 115–23.

Alcohol + NSAIDs

Alcohol might increase the risk of gastrointestinal haemorrhage associated with NSAIDs. The skills related to driving are impaired by indometacin and phenylbutazone and this is made worse if patients drink alcohol while taking phenylbutazone, but this does not appear to occur with indometacin. A few isolated reports attribute acute renal

failure following the use of NSAIDs and acute excessive alcohol consumption.

Clinical evidence, mechanism, importance and management

(a) Gastrointestinal complications

In healthy subjects the concurrent use of alcohol with **ibuprofen** 2.4 g over 24 hours increased the damaging effect of **ibuprofen** on the stomach wall, although this did not reach statistical significance.[1] A case-control study, involving 1 224 patients admitted to hospital with upper gastrointestinal bleeding and 2 945 controls, found that alcohol consumption was associated with a threefold increase in the incidence of acute upper gastrointestinal haemorrhage from light drinking (less than one alcoholic drink per week) to heavy drinking (21 alcoholic drinks or more per week). There was some evidence to suggest that the risk of upper gastrointestinal bleeding was increased by the concurrent use of **ibuprofen.**[2] Another case-control study suggested that the odds ratio for gastrointestinal complications in those regularly consuming more than 5 drinks during a drinking session was increased from 2.8 to 6 when an NSAID was also taken. This was also increased when compared with the use of an NSAID alone (odds ratio 3.8).[3] A third case-control study found that the use of prescription NSAIDs or non-prescription **naproxen** or **ibuprofen** in those with a history of alcohol abuse produced a risk ratio of adverse gastrointestinal effects that was greater than the expected additive risk. Both NSAID use and excessive alcohol consumption carry the risk of gastrointestinal adverse effects. This information suggests that NSAIDs should be used with caution in heavy drinkers.[4] The FDA in the US has ruled that non-prescription pain relievers and fever reducers containing **ibuprofen**, **ketoprofen**, or **naproxen** must carry a warning label advising people who consume moderate amounts of alcohol to consult their doctor before using these drugs, and that stomach bleeding can occur with these drugs.[5]

(b) Psychomotor skills and alcohol levels

A study in a large number of healthy subjects found that the performance of various psychomotor skills related to driving (choice reaction, coordination, divided attention tests) were impaired by single doses of **indometacin** 50 mg or **phenylbutazone** 200 mg. Alcohol 0.5 g/kg made things worse in those taking **phenylbutazone**, but the performance of those taking **indometacin** was improved to some extent.[6] The reasons are not understood. The study found that the subjects were subjectively unaware of the adverse effects of **phenylbutazone**. Information is very limited, and the general relevance of the findings is unclear.

In two studies, **ibuprofen** 800 mg had no statistically significant effect on blood-alcohol levels of healthy subjects.[7,8] The pharmacokinetics of alcohol 1 g/kg and the results of performance tests were found to be similar in subjects given **dipyrone** 1 g or a placebo.[9]

(c) Renal complications

A healthy young woman with no history of renal disease developed acute renal failure after taking **ibuprofen** 400 mg the evening before, 400 mg the following morning, and then 375 mL of **rum** later in the day, followed by two further 400-mg tablets of **ibuprofen.**[10] Another similar case was reported in a 22-year-old woman who had taken **ibuprofen** 1.2 g the morning after binge drinking.[11] Both recovered.[10,11] A further case describes renal impairment in a young woman, which was associated with the use of **ketoprofen** 600 mg and binge drinking.[12] It is suggested that volume depletion caused by the alcohol (and compounded by vomiting) predisposed these patients to NSAID-induced renal toxicity.[11,12] The general importance of these isolated cases remains to be determined.

1. Lanza FL, Royer GL, Nelson RS, Rack MF, Seckman CC. Ethanol, aspirin, ibuprofen, and the gastroduodenal mucosa: an endoscopic assessment. *Am J Gastroenterol* (1985) 80, 767–9.
2. Kaufman DW, Kelly JP, Wiholm B-E, Laszlo A, Sheehan JE, Koff RS, Shapiro S. The risk of acute major upper gastrointestinal bleeding among users of aspirin and ibuprofen at various levels of alcohol consumption. *Am J Gastroenterol* (1999) 94, 3189–96.
3. Henry D, Dobson A, Turner C. Variability in the risk of major gastrointestinal complications from nonaspirin nonsteroidal anti-inflammatory drugs. *Gastroenterology* (1993) 105, 1078–88.
4. Neutel CI, Appel WC. The effect of alcohol abuse on the risk of NSAID-related gastrointestinal events. *Ann Epidemiol* (2000) 10, 246–50.
5. Food and Drug Administration. Questions and answers on final rule for labeling changes to over-the-counter pain relievers. Available at: http://www.fda.gov/Drugs/NewsEvents/ucm144068.htm (accessed 21/10/15).
6. Linnoila M, Seppälä T, Mattila MJ. Acute effect of antipyretic analgesics, alone or in combination with alcohol, on human psychomotor skills related to driving. *Br J Clin Pharmacol* (1974) 1, 477–84.
7. Barron SE, Perry JR, Ferslew KE. The effect of ibuprofen on ethanol concentration and elimination rate. *J Forensic Sci* (1992) 37, 432–5.
8. Melander O, Lidén A, Melander A. Pharmacokinetic interactions of alcohol and acetylsalicylic acid. *Eur J Clin Pharmacol* (1995) 48, 151–3.
9. Badian LM, Rosenkrantz B. Quoted as personal communication by Levy M, Zylber-Katz E, Rosenkranz B. Clinical pharmacokinetics of dipyrone and its metabolites. *Clin Pharmacokinet* (1995) 28, 216–34.
10. Elsasser GN, Lopez L, Evans E, Barone EJ. Reversible acute renal failure associated with ibuprofen ingestion and binge drinking. *J Fam Pract* (1988) 27, 221–2.
11. Johnson GR, Wen S-F. Syndrome of flank pain and acute renal failure after binge drinking and nonsteroidal anti-inflammatory drug ingestion. *J Am Soc Nephrol* (1995) 5, 1647–52.
12. Galzin M, Brunet P, Burtey S, Dussol B, Berland Y. Nécrose tubulaire après prise d'anti-inflammatoire non stéroïdien et intoxication éthylique aiguë. *Nephrologie* (1997) 18, 113–15.

Alcohol + Olanzapine

Postural hypotension and possibly drowsiness might be increased when olanzapine is given with alcohol.

Clinical evidence, mechanism, importance and management

The manufacturers state that patients taking olanzapine have shown an increased heart rate and accentuated postural hypotension when given a single-dose of alcohol.[1,2] In a study, 9 of 11 subjects experienced orthostatic hypotension when they drank alcohol one hour after taking olanzapine 10 mg, but no pharmacokinetic interaction was seen.[3] In practical terms this means that patients should be warned of the risk of faintness and dizziness if they stand up quickly, and advised to sit or lie down if this occurs. The manufacturers of olanzapine state that drowsiness is a common adverse effect of olanzapine, and they advise caution in patients taking other products that can cause CNS depression, including alcohol.[2,4] The US manufacturer advises that patients should avoid alcohol while taking olanzapine.[2]

1. Zyprexa (Olanzapine). Eli Lilly. Clinical and Laboratory Experience: A Comprehensive Monograph, August 1996.
2. Zyprexa (Olanzapine). Eli Lilly and Company. US Prescribing information, June 2011.
3. Callaghan JT, Bergstrom RF, Ptak LR, Beasley CM. Olanzapine. Pharmacokinetic and pharmacodynamic profile. *Clin Pharmacokinet* (1999) 37, 177–93.
4. Zyprexa Tablets (Olanzapine). Eli Lilly and Company Ltd. UK Summary of product characteristics, November 2011.

Alcohol + Ondansetron

Ondansetron does not appear to affect the pharmacokinetics of alcohol, but it might increase subjective measures of alcohol intoxication.

Clinical evidence, mechanism, importance and management

In a placebo-controlled study, 12 healthy subjects were given ondansetron 8 mg with an oral dose of alcohol (0.65 and 0.75 [g/kg] for women and men, respectively). It was found that ondansetron did not alter the pharmacokinetics of alcohol or increase the objective measures of sedation that occurred in response to alcohol. However, *subjective* measures of impairment and intoxication caused by alcohol were increased by ondansetron.

It therefore seems unlikely that a particularly detrimental effect occurs if patients receiving ondansetron drink alcohol, but they could feel more intoxicated.[1]

1. Swift RM, Davidson D, Whelihan W, Kuznetsov O. Ondansetron alters human alcohol intoxication. *Biol Psychiatry* (1996) 40, 514–21.

Alcohol + Opioids

In general the opioid analgesics can enhance the CNS depressant effects of alcohol, which has resulted in fatalities in some cases: this appears to be a particular problem with dextropropoxyphene. This could be related to that fact that the bioavailability of dextropropoxyphene is increased by alcohol. Alcohol has been associated with rapid release of hydromorphone and morphine from extended-release preparations, which could result in potentially fatal doses. The acute use of alcohol and methadone appears to result in lower blood-alcohol levels.

Clinical evidence

(a) Buprenorphine

A study in 12 patients taking buprenorphine found that alcohol 14.7 g/70 kg produced a lower blood-alcohol level, when compared with a group of patients not taking buprenorphine (56 mg% compared with 40 mg%), but this was not statistically significant.[1] See also, *Methadone*, below.

(b) Codeine

Double-blind studies in a large number of professional army drivers found that 50 mg of codeine and alcohol 0.5 g/kg, both alone and together, impaired their ability to drive safely on a static driving simulator. The number of collisions, neglected instructions and the times they drove off the road were increased.[2,3] Alcohol does not appear to affect the pharmacokinetics of codeine.[4] See also, *Controlled-release opioids*, below.

(c) Dextropropoxyphene

In a study in 8 healthy subjects, alcohol alone (blood levels of 50 mg%) impaired the performance of various psychomotor tests (motor co-ordination, mental performance and stability of stance) more than dextropropoxyphene 65 mg alone. When given together there was some evidence that the effects were greater than with either drug alone, but in some instances the impairment was no greater than with alcohol alone. The effect of alcohol clearly predominated.[5] In contrast, other studies have found that dextropropoxyphene does not enhance the psychomotor impairment seen with alcohol,[6,7] but the bioavailability of the dextropropoxyphene has been reported to be raised by 25 to 31% by alcohol.[7,8] A retrospective study involving 332 fatal poisonings in Finland found that alcohol was present in 73% of cases involving dextropropoxyphene and, when alcohol was present, relatively small overdoses of dextropropoxyphene could result in fatal poisoning.[9] Further reports describe alcohol reducing the lethal dose of dextropropoxyphene.[10-12]

(d) Hydromorphone

A young man died from the combined cardiovascular and respiratory depressant effects of hydromorphone and alcohol.[13] He fell asleep, the serious nature of which was not recognised by those around him. Post-mortem analysis revealed alcohol and hydromorphone concentrations of 90 mg% and 100 nanograms/mL, respectively, neither of which is particularly excessive. A study in 9 healthy subjects found that pre-treatment with hydromorphone 1 or 2 mg did not notably affect the subject-rated effects of alcohol 0.5 or 1 g/kg. However, hydromorphone enhanced the sedative scores of alcohol on the adjective rating scale.[14] See also, *Controlled-release opioids*, below.

(e) Methadone

A study in 21 opioid-dependent subjects who had been taking methadone or **buprenorphine** for 3 months, and 21 matched non-drug-using controls, found that although alcohol (target blood-alcohol level around 50 mg%) resulted in decreased driving performance, there appeared to be no difference in simulated driving tests in the opioid-treated patients, when compared with controls. It was suggested that restrictions on opioids and driving are not necessary in stabilised patients receiving maintenance **buprenorphine** or methadone treatment, but little is known about the effects in the initial treatment period. This study also found that blood-alcohol levels were lower in the opioid-treated patients, when compared with the controls, despite both groups receiving the same amount of alcohol.[15] A study in 14 patients taking methadone also found that alcohol 14.7 g/70 kg produced a lower blood-alcohol level, when compared with a group of patients not taking methadone (56 mg% compared with 40 mg%).[1]

However, clinical anecdotal reports have indicated that taking methadone with alcohol produces an additive and/or synergistic response,[16] which can result in serious respiratory depression and hypotension.[17]

(f) Controlled-release opioids

Pharmacokinetic data in healthy subjects have shown that consuming alcohol with a particular 24-hour extended-release formulation of **hydromorphone** *(Palladone XL Capsules; Purdue Pharma, USA)* could lead to rapid release (dose dumping) and absorption of a potentially fatal dose of hydromorphone.[18,19] Although no reports of serious problems had been received, the FDA in the US asked for the product to be withdrawn from the market.[20] Health Canada warned that this interaction might occur with other slow-release opioid analgesics.[21] However, the Canadian distributor of hydromorphone has commented that the controlled-release technology employed in *Palladone XL* is not the same as that of many other controlled-release opioid formulations. Dose-dumping with alcohol is said not to occur with:

- **morphine** sustained-release tablets: *MS Contin*,[22,23] *MST Continus* suspension and tablets, *MXL* capsules,[23] *KADIAN* capsules,[24]
- **codeine** controlled-release tablets: *Codeine Contin*,[22,23]
- **dihydrocodeine** controlled-release tablets: *DHC Continus* tablets,[23]
- **hydromorphone** controlled-release capsules: *Hydromorph Contin*,[22] *Palladone SR*,[23]
- **oxycodone** controlled-release tablets: *OxyContin*,[22,23]
- **tramadol** once daily and twice daily formulations*Dromadol SR, Zamadol SR*, [23]

In contrast, in laboratory studies, an extended-release capsule preparation of **morphine** (*Avinza; King Pharmaceuticals, USA*) was found to release morphine earlier than expected when exposed to alcohol, and this effect increased dramatically with increasing alcohol concentration.[25,26] The product literature for *Avinza* now carries a warning to avoid alcohol, including medications containing alcohol, while taking this preparation.[26]

Mechanism

Both opioids and alcohol are CNS depressants, which together might result in enhanced suppression of the medullary respiratory control centre.[10-12] The acute use of alcohol appears to increase methadone effects due to inhibition of hepatic microsomal enzymes, but chronic alcoholism reduces the AUC and half-life of methadone because cytochrome P450 isoenzymes are induced.[16]

Importance and management

The reports describing increased sedation and even fatalities in those consuming alcohol while taking dextropropoxyphene emphasise the importance of warning patients about the potentially hazardous consequences of drinking while taking potent CNS depressants like the opioids. This seems to be a particular risk with dextropropoxyphene overdose, and it has been suggested that a less dangerous alternative could be chosen when indications of alcohol abuse or suicide risk are present.[27] There is less information about therapeutic doses of dextropropoxyphene with moderate social drinking. In general it is suggested that alcohol intake should be avoided where possible, or limited in those taking opioids, but some manufacturers actually contraindicate alcohol. The objective evidence is that the interaction with moderate doses of alcohol and opioids is quite small (with the exception of the dose dumping effect). It would seem prudent to warn patients that opioids can cause drowsiness and this may be exaggerated to some extent by alcohol. They should be warned that driving or handling potentially hazardous machinery can be more risky, but total abstinence from alcohol does not seem to be necessary. Smaller doses, such as those available without a prescription, would be expected to have a smaller effect, but this does not appear to have been studied.

1. Clark NC, Dietze P, Lenné MG, Redman JR. Effect of opioid substitution therapy on alcohol metabolism. *J Subst Abuse Treat* (2006) 30, 191–6.
2. Linnoila M, Häkkinen S. Effects of diazepam and codeine, alone and in combination with alcohol, on simulated driving. *Clin Pharmacol Ther* (1974) 15, 368–73.
3. Linnoila M, Mattila MJ. Interaction of alcohol and drugs on psychomotor skills as demonstrated by a driving simulator. *Br J Pharmacol* (1973) 47, 671P–672P.
4. Bodd E, Beylich KM, Christophersen AS, Mørland J. Oral administration of codeine in the presence of ethanol: a pharmacokinetic study in man. *Pharmacol Toxicol* (1987) 61, 297–300.
5. Kiplinger GF, Sokol G, Rodda BE. Effects of combined alcohol and propoxyphene on human performance. *Arch Int Pharmacodyn Ther* (1974) 212, 175–80.
6. Edwards C, Gard PR, Handley SL, Hunter M, Whittington RM. Distalgesic and ethanol-impaired function. *Lancet* (1982) ii, 384.
7. Girre C, Hirschhorn M, Bertaux L, Palombo S, Dellatolas F, Ngo R, Moreno M, Fournier PE. Enhancement of propoxyphene bioavailability by ethanol: relation to psychomotor and cognitive function in healthy volunteers. *Eur J Clin Pharmacol* (1991) 41, 147–52.
8. Sellers EM, Hamilton CA, Kaplan HL, Degani NC, Foltz RL. Pharmacokinetic interaction of propoxyphene with ethanol. *Br J Clin Pharmacol* (1985) 19, 398–401.
9. Koski A, Vuori E, Ojanperä I. Relation of postmortem blood alcohol and drug concentrations in fatal poisonings involving amitriptyline, propoxyphene and promazine. *Hum Exp Toxicol* (2005) 24, 389–96.
10. Carson DJL, Carson ED. Fatal dextropropoxyphene poisoning in Northern Ireland: review of 30 cases. *Lancet* (1977) i, 894–7.
11. Whittington RM, Barclay AD. The epidemiology of dextropropoxyphene (Distalgesic) overdose fatalities in Birmingham and the West Midlands. *J Clin Hosp Pharm* (1981) 6, 251–7.
12. Williamson RV, Galloway JH, Yeo WW, Forrest ARW. Relationship between blood dextropropoxyphene and ethanol levels in fatal co-proxamol overdosage. *Br J Clin Pharmacol* (2000) 50, 388–9.
13. Levine B, Saady J, Fierro M, Valentour J. A hydromorphone and ethanol fatality. *J Forensic Sci* (1984) 29, 655–9.
14. Rush CR. Pretreatment with hydromorphone, a μ-opioid agonist, does not alter the acute behavioral and physiological effects of ethanol in humans. *Alcohol Clin Exp Res* (2001) 25, 9–17.
15. Lenné MG, Dietze P, Rumbold GR, Redman JR, Triggs TJ. The effects of the opioid pharmacotherapies methadone, LAAM and buprenorphine, alone and in combination with alcohol, on simulated driving. *Drug Alcohol Depend* (2003) 72, 271–8.
16. Schlatter J, Madras JL, Saulnier JL, Poujade F. Interactions médicamenteuses avec la méthadone. *Presse Med* (1999) 28, 1381–4.
17. Methadone Hydrochloride Oral Solution. Rosemont Pharmaceuticals Ltd. UK Summary of product characteristics, September 2014.
18. Palladone (Hydromorphone hydrochloride). Purdue Pharma L.P. US Prescribing information, November 2004.
19. Murray S, Wooltorton E. Alcohol-associated rapid release of a long-acting opioid. *CMAJ* (2005) 173, 756.
20. FDA News. FDA asks Purdue Pharma to withdraw Palladone for safety reasons (issued 13th July 2005). Available at: http://www.fda.gov/NewsEvents/Newsroom/PressAnnouncements/2005/ucm108460.htm (accessed 20/10/15).
21. Health Canada. Potentially fatal interaction between slow-release opioid painkillers and alcohol (issued 3rd August 2005). Available at: http://www.healthycanadians.gc.ca/recall-alert-rappel-avis/hc-sc/2005/13702a-eng.php (accessed 20/10/15).
22. Darke AC. Controlled-release opioids and alcohol. *CMAJ* (2006) 174, 352.
23. Walden M, Nicholls FA, Smith KJ, Tucker GT. The effect of ethanol on the release of opioids from oral prolonged-release preparations. *Drug Dev Ind Pharm* (2007) 33, 1101–11.
24. Johnson F, Wagner G, Sun S, Stauffer J. Effect of concomitant ingestion of alcohol on the in vivo pharmacokinetics of KADIAN (morphine sulfate extended-release) capsules. *J Pain* (2008) 9, 330–6.
25. FDA Patient Safety News. Potentially hazardous interaction between Avinza and alcohol (issued March 2006). Available at: http://www.fda.gov/downloads/Safety/FDAPatientSafetyNews/UCM417829.pdf (accessed 20/10/15).
26. Avinza (Morphine sulfate extended-release capsules). King Pharmaceuticals, Inc. US Prescribing information, April 2014.
27. Koski A, Ojanperä I, Vuori E. Interaction of alcohol and drugs in fatal poisonings. *Hum Exp Toxicol* (2003) 22, 281–7.

Alcohol + Orlistat

A study in healthy subjects found that orlistat 120 mg three times daily for 6 days had no effect on the pharmacokinetics of alcohol. Alcohol at plasma levels of less than 80 mg% did not affect the activity of orlistat as measured by inhibition of dietary fat absorption.[1] There is nothing to suggest that alcohol should be avoided while taking orlistat.

1. Melia AT, Zhi J, Zelasko R, Hartmann D, Güzelhan C, Guerciolini R, Odink J. The interaction of the lipase inhibitor orlistat with ethanol in healthy volunteers. *Eur J Clin Pharmacol* (1998) 54, 773–7.

Alcohol + Paracetamol (Acetaminophen)

Many case reports describe severe liver damage, sometimes fatal, in some alcoholics and persistent heavy drinkers who take only moderate doses of paracetamol. However, other controlled studies have found no association between alcohol intake and paracetamol-induced hepatotoxicity. There is controversy about the use of paracetamol in alcoholics. Some consider standard therapeutic doses can be used, whereas others recommend the dose of paracetamol should be reduced, or paracetamol avoided. Occasional and light to moderate drinkers do not seem to be at any extra risk.

Clinical evidence

(a) Increased hepatotoxicity

Three chronic alcoholic patients developed severe liver damage after taking paracetamol. They had AST levels of about 7 000 to 10 000 units. Two of them had taken 10 g of paracetamol over 24 or 48 hours before admission, and the third patient had taken about 50 g of paracetamol over 72 hours. One of them developed hepatic encephalopathy and died, and subsequent post-mortem revealed typical paracetamol toxicity. Two of them also developed renal failure.[1] A case of severe liver impairment has also been reported in a moderate social drinker who regularly drank 3 glasses of wine with dinner, but had stopped drinking alcohol while taking paracetamol for a viral infection.[2]

There are numerous other case reports of liver toxicity in alcoholics or chronic heavy alcohol users attributed to the concurrent use of alcohol and paracetamol. In the reports cited here, which include a total of about 30 patients, about one-third had been taking daily paracetamol doses of up to 4 g daily, and one-third had taken doses within the range of 4 to 8 g daily.[3-19] Fasting possibly makes things worse.[20] A later survey reviewed a total of 94 cases from the literature, and described a further 67 patients who were regular users of alcohol, 64% of whom were alcoholics, who developed liver toxicity after taking paracetamol. In 60% of cases the paracetamol dose did not exceed

6 g daily and in 40% of cases the dose did not exceed 4 g daily. More than 90% of the patients developed AST levels ranging from 3 000 to 48 000 units.[21]

(b) No effect on hepatotoxicity

In a retrospective review of 553 cases of paracetamol-induced severe hepatotoxicity treated at a liver failure unit over a 7-year period, there was no association between the level of alcohol consumption and the severity of the hepatotoxicity (mean INR and serum creatinine levels in the first 7 days after overdose). Alcohol consumption was categorised into 4 groups ranging from non-drinkers to heavy drinkers (greater than 60 g of alcohol daily in men and 40 g daily in women).[22]

In a randomised, placebo-controlled study, there was no difference in measures of hepatotoxicity (mean AST levels, mean INR) between 102 alcoholic patients who took paracetamol 1 g four times daily for 2 days, and 99 alcoholic patients who were given placebo. In this study, patients had entered an alcohol detoxification centre, and were given paracetamol immediately after stopping alcohol use[23] (the assumed time of greatest susceptibility, see *Mechanism*, below). A systematic review by the same research group concluded that the use of therapeutic doses of paracetamol in alcoholic patients is not associated with hepatic injury.[24]

(c) Effect on alcohol levels

Paracetamol 1 g was found to have no effect on the single-dose pharmacokinetics of alcohol in 12 healthy subjects.[25] Another study found that blood-alcohol levels were raised by 1 g of paracetamol but this was not statistically significant.[26]

Mechanism

Uncertain. The interaction between paracetamol and alcohol is complex, because acute and chronic alcohol consumption can have opposite effects.[27,28] Paracetamol is usually predominantly metabolised by the liver to non-toxic sulfate and glucuronide conjugates. Persistent heavy drinking appears to stimulate a normally minor biochemical pathway involving CYP2E1, and possibly the CYP3A subfamily, which allows the production of unusually large amounts of highly hepatotoxic metabolites via oxidation.[20,28,29] Unless sufficient glutathione is present to detoxify these metabolites (alcoholics often have an inadequate intake of protein), they become covalently bound to liver macromolecules and damage results. Fasting might also make things worse by reducing the availability of glucose, and thus shifting paracetamol metabolism from glucuronidation towards microsomal oxidation.[20] However, most studies have been unable to demonstrate an increase in hepatotoxic metabolites in alcoholics.[27,30] In fact alcoholics might be most susceptible to toxicity during alcohol withdrawal because, while drinking, alcohol potentially competes with paracetamol for metabolism, and might even inhibit paracetamol metabolism. Acute ingestion of alcohol by non-alcoholics could possibly protect them against damage because the damaging biochemical pathway is inhibited rather than stimulated. The relative timing of alcohol and paracetamol intake is therefore critical;[27] for example, a study in 10 healthy subjects found that ingestion of 500 mg of paracetamol 8 hours after an intravenous infusion of alcohol (roughly equivalent to a bottle of wine) resulted in an increased production of the toxic metabolite of paracetamol, *N*-acetyl-*p*-benzoquinoneimine (NABQI), when compared with dextrose 5%.[31]

Importance and management

The incidence of unexpected paracetamol toxicity in chronic alcoholics is uncertain, but possibly fairly small, bearing in mind the very widespread use of paracetamol and alcohol. Note that most of the evidence for an interaction comes from anecdotal case reports and case series, albeit in large numbers. However, the damage, when it occurs, can be serious and therefore some have advised that alcoholics and those who persistently drink heavily should avoid paracetamol or limit their intake considerably.[21] The normal daily recommended 'safe' maximum of 4 g is said to be too high in some alcoholics.[21] Because of this, the FDA in the US have required that all paracetamol-containing non-prescription products bear the warning that those consuming 3 or more alcoholic drinks every day should ask their doctor whether they should take paracetamol.[32] However, others consider that the evidence does not prove that there is an increase in paracetamol hepatotoxicity in alcoholics,[24,27] and is insufficient to support any change in paracetamol use or dose in alcoholics.[24,33] They note that the alternatives, aspirin and NSAIDs, are associated with a greater risk of gastrointestinal adverse effects in alcoholics,[24] see 'Alcohol + Aspirin or other Salicylates', p.58, and 'Alcohol + NSAIDs', p.77'. The risk for non-alcoholics, moderate drinkers and those who very occasionally drink a lot appears to be low, although some chronic moderate social drinkers might be at risk, especially if alcohol intake is abruptly stopped.[34]

Note that chronic alcohol intake increases the risk of hepatotoxicity after paracetamol *overdose*.

1. McClain CJ, Kromhout JP, Peterson FJ, Holtzman JL. Potentiation of acetaminophen hepatotoxicity by alcohol. *JAMA* (1980) 244, 251–3.
2. Slattery JT, Nelson SD, Thummel KE. The complex interaction between ethanol and acetaminophen. *Clin Pharmacol Ther* (1996) 60, 241–6.
3. Emby DJ, Fraser BN. Hepatotoxicity of paracetamol enhanced by ingestion of alcohol. *S Afr Med J* (1977) 51, 208–9.
4. Goldfinger R, Ahmed KS, Pitchumoni CS, Weseley SA. Concomitant alcohol and drug abuse enhancing acetaminophen toxicity. *Am J Gastroenterol* (1978) 70, 385–8.
5. Barker JD, de Carle DJ, Anuras S. Chronic excessive acetaminophen use and liver damage. *Ann Intern Med* (1977) 87, 299–301.
6. O'Dell JR, Zetterman RK, Burnett DA. Centrilobular hepatic fibrosis following acetaminophen-induced hepatic necrosis in an alcoholic. *JAMA* (1986) 255, 2636–7.
7. McJunkin B, Barwick KW, Little WC, Winfield JB. Fatal massive hepatic necrosis following acetaminophen overdosage. *JAMA* (1976) 236, 1874–5.
8. LaBrecque DR, Mitros FA. Increased hepatotoxicity of acetaminophen in the alcoholic. *Gastroenterology* (1980) 78, 1310.
9. Johnson MW, Friedman PA, Mitch WE. Alcoholism, nonprescription drugs and hepatotoxicity. The risk from unknown acetaminophen ingestion. *Am J Gastroenterol* (1981) 76, 530–3.
10. Licht H, Seeff LB, Zimmerman HJ. Apparent potentiation of acetaminophen hepatotoxicity by alcohol. *Ann Intern Med* (1980) 92, 511.
11. Black M, Cornell JF, Rabin L, Shachter N. Late presentation of acetaminophen hepatotoxicity. *Dig Dis Sci* (1982) 27, 370–4.
12. Fleckenstein JL. *Nyquil* and acute hepatic necrosis. *N Engl J Med* (1985) 313, 48.
13. Gerber MA, Kaufmann H, Klion F, Alpert LI. Acetaminophen associated hepatic injury: report of two cases showing unusual portal tract reactions. *Hum Pathol* (1980) 11, 37–42.
14. Leist MH, Gluskin LE, Payne JA. Enhanced toxicity of acetaminophen in alcoholics: report of three cases. *J Clin Gastroenterol* (1985) 7, 55–9.
15. Himmelstein DU, Woolhandler SJ, Adler RD. Elevated SGOT/SGPT ratio in alcoholic patients with acetaminophen hepatotoxicity. *Am J Gastroenterol* (1984) 79, 718–20.
16. Levinson M. Ulcer, back pain and jaundice in an alcoholic. *Hosp Pract* (1983) 18, 48N, 48S.
17. Seeff LB, Cuccherini BA, Zimmerman HJ, Adler E, Benjamin SB. Acetaminophen hepatotoxicity in alcoholics. A therapeutic misadventure. *Ann Intern Med* (1986) 104, 399–404.
18. Florén C-H, Thesleff P, Nilsson Å. Severe liver damage caused by therapeutic doses of acetaminophen. *Acta Med Scand* (1987) 222, 285–8.
19. Edwards R, Oliphant J. Paracetamol toxicity in chronic alcohol abusers – a plea for greater consumer awareness. *N Z Med J* (1992) 105, 174–5.
20. Whitcomb DC, Block GD. Association of acetaminophen hepatotoxicity with fasting and ethanol use. *JAMA* (1994) 272, 1845–50.
21. Zimmerman HJ, Maddrey WC. Acetaminophen (paracetamol) hepatotoxicity with regular intake of alcohol: analysis of instances of therapeutic misadventure. *Hepatology* (1995) 22, 767–73.
22. Makin A, Williams R. Paracetamol hepatotoxicity and alcohol consumption in deliberate and accidental overdose. *Q J Med* (2000) 93, 341–9.
23. Kuffner EK, Dart RC, Bogdan GM, Hill RE, Casper E, Darton L. Effect of maximal daily doses of acetaminophen on the liver of alcoholic patients: a randomized, double-blind, placebo-controlled trial. *Arch Intern Med* (2001) 161, 2247–52.
24. Dart RC, Kuffner EK, Rumack BH. Treatment of pain or fever with paracetamol (acetaminophen) in the alcoholic patient: a systematic review. *Am J Ther* (2000) 7, 123–4.
25. Melander O, Lidén A, Melander A. Pharmacokinetic interactions of alcohol and acetylsalicylic acid. *Eur J Clin Pharmacol* (1995) 48, 151–3.
26. Sharma SC, Feely J. The influence of aspirin and paracetamol on blood concentrations of alcohol in young adults. *Br J Clin Pharmacol* (1996) 41, 467P.
27. Prescott LF. Paracetamol, alcohol and the liver. *Br J Clin Pharmacol* (2000) 49, 291–301.
28. Tanaka E, Yamazaki K, Misawa S. Update: the clinical importance of acetaminophen hepatotoxicity in non-alcoholic and alcoholic subjects. *J Clin Pharm Ther* (2000) 25, 325–32.
29. Buckley NA, Srinivasan J. Should a lower treatment line be used when treating paracetamol poisoning in patients with chronic alcoholism? A case for. *Drug Safety* (2002) 25, 619–24.
30. Dargan PI, Jones AL. Should a lower treatment line be used when treating paracetamol poisoning in patients with chronic alcoholism? A case against. *Drug Safety* (2002) 25, 625–32.
31. Thummel KE, Slattery JT, Ro H, Chien JY, Nelson SD, Lown KE, Watkins PB. Ethanol and production of the hepatotoxic metabolite of acetaminophen in healthy adults. *Clin Pharmacol Ther* (2000) 67, 591–9.
32. Food and Drug Administration. Acetaminophen information (in Acetaminophen final rule). Available at: http://www.fda.gov/Drugs/DrugSafety/InformationbyDrugClass/ucm165107.htm (accessed 22/10/15).
33. Rumack BH. Acetaminophen hepatotoxicity: the first 35 years. *J Toxicol Clin Toxicol* (2002) 40, 3–20.
34. Draganov P, Durrence H, Cox C, Reuben A. Alcohol-acetaminophen syndrome. Even moderate social drinkers are at risk. *Postgrad Med* (2000) 107, 189–95.

Alcohol + Paraldehyde

Both alcohol and paraldehyde have CNS depressant effects, which can be additive. The use of paraldehyde in the treatment of acute alcohol intoxication has caused fatalities.

Clinical evidence, mechanism, importance and management

A report describes 9 patients who died suddenly and unexpectedly after treatment for acute alcohol intoxication with 30 to 90 mL of paraldehyde (the authors quote a normal dose range of 8 to 30 mL; fatal dose 120 mL or more, usually preceded by coma). None of the patients had hepatic impairment, although one did have some fatty changes.[1] Both drugs are CNS depressants and might therefore be expected to have additive effects at any dose, although an *animal* study suggested that the effect might be less than additive,[2] and cross-tolerance could occur as paraldehyde is pharmacologically similar to alcohol.[3] Nevertheless, it would seem prudent to avoid giving paraldehyde to intoxicated patients wherever possible.

1. Kaye S, Haag HB. Study of death due to combined action of alcohol and paraldehyde in man. *Toxicol Appl Pharmacol* (1964) 6, 316–20.
2. Gessner PK, Shakarjian MP. Interactions of paraldehyde with ethanol and chloral hydrate. *J Pharmacol Exp Ther* (1985) 235, 32–6.
3. Weller RA, Preskorn SH. Psychotropic drugs and alcohol: pharmacokinetic and pharmacodynamic interactions. *Psychosomatics* (1984) 25, 301–9.

Alcohol + Penicillins

No clinically relevant pharmacokinetic interaction appears to occur between alcohol and phenoxymethylpenicillin or amoxicillin.

Clinical evidence, mechanism, importance and management

A long-standing and very common belief among members of the general public (presumably derived from advice given by doctors and pharmacists) is that alcohol should be strictly avoided while taking any antibacterial. It has been claimed that alcohol increases the degradation of penicillin in the gut and reduces the amount available for absorption.[1] However, one study showed that the pharmacokinetics of **phenoxymethylpenicillin (penicillin V)** were unaffected by alcoholic drinks,[2] and another study found that alcohol delayed the absorption of **amoxicillin** but did not affect the total amount absorbed.[3] An *in vitro* study did report that acetaldehyde, at concentrations occurring *in vivo* during alcohol metabolism, reacted with amine containing penicillins (**amoxicillin**, **ampicillin**, and **ciclacillin**), which theoretically could lead to decreased drug bioavailability and possibly adverse effects.[4] However, there seems to be no clinical evidence to support claims of an adverse interaction.

1. Kitto W. Antibiotics and ingestion of alcohol. *JAMA* (1965) 193, 411.
2. Lindberg RLP, Huupponen RK, Viljanen S and Pihlajamäki KK. Ethanol and the absorption of oral penicillin in man. *Int J Clin Pharmacol Ther Toxicol* (1987) 25, 536–8.

3. Morasso MI, Hip A, Márquez M, González C, Arancibia A. Amoxicillin kinetics and ethanol ingestion. *Int J Clin Pharmacol Ther Toxicol* (1988) 26, 428–31.
4. Nuñez-Vergara LJ, Yudelevich J, Squella JA, Speisky H. Drug-acetaldehyde interactions during ethanol metabolism *in vitro*. *Alcohol Alcohol* (1991) 26, 139–46.

Alcohol + Phenytoin

Acute alcohol intake and moderate social drinking appear to have little or no effect on serum phenytoin levels. However, chronic heavy drinking reduces serum phenytoin levels so that above-average doses of phenytoin might be needed to maintain adequate levels.

Clinical evidence

(a) Acute alcohol ingestion

The metabolism of a single dose of phenytoin was not affected in one study in healthy subjects by the acute ingestion of alcohol.[1]

(b) Heavy drinking

In a group of 15 drinkers (consuming a minimum of 200 g of ethanol daily for at least 3 months) phenytoin levels measured 24 hours after the last dose of phenytoin were approximately half of those in 76 non-drinkers. The phenytoin half-life was reduced by 30%.[2] Another study confirmed that alcoholics without liver disease have lower than expected plasma levels of phenytoin while drinking.[3] Two reports describe a chronic alcoholic who was resistant to large doses of phenytoin;[4] and seizures, which developed in a man when an increase in his alcohol consumption appeared to cause a reduction in his serum phenytoin levels.[5]

(c) Moderate social drinking

A study in non-drinking patients with epilepsy (17 in the experimental group, 14 in the control group) found that the serum levels of phenytoin were unchanged by moderate drinking, and there was no influence on tonic-clonic convulsions or partial complex seizures. The experimental group drank 1 to 3 glasses of an alcoholic beverage (equivalent to a glass of beer containing 9.85 g of ethanol) over a 2-hour period, twice a week, for 16 weeks, and their maximum blood-alcohol levels ranged from 5 to 33 mg%.[6]

Mechanism

Supported by *animal* data,[7] the evidence suggests that repeated exposure to large amounts of alcohol induces liver microsomal enzymes so that the rate of metabolism and clearance of phenytoin is increased. Conversely, acute alcohol intake might decrease the hepatic metabolism of phenytoin.[8]

Importance and management

The interaction between alcohol and phenytoin appears to be established and clinically important, although the documentation is limited. Heavy drinkers might need above-average doses of phenytoin to maintain adequate serum levels. However, be aware that patients with liver impairment usually need lower doses of phenytoin, so the picture might be more complicated. Note that, the manufacturers of phenytoin suggest that acute alcohol intake can increase phenytoin levels,[9,10] but a single-dose study[1] found that no interaction occurs. Moderate drinking appears to be without notable problems in those taking phenytoin.[6] Consider also 'Alcohol + Antiepileptics', p.54.

1. Schmidt D. Effect of ethanol intake on phenytoin metabolism in volunteers. *Experientia* (1975) 31, 1313–14.
2. Kater RMH, Roggin G, Tobon F, Zieve P, Iber FL. Increased rate of clearance of drugs from the circulation of alcoholics. *Am J Med Sci* (1969) 258, 35–9.
3. Sandor P, Sellers EM, Dumbrell M, Khouw V. Effect of short- and long-term alcohol use on phenytoin kinetics in chronic alcoholics. *Clin Pharmacol Ther* (1981) 30, 390–7.
4. Birkett DJ, Graham GG, Chinwah PM, Wade DN, Hickie JB. Multiple drug interactions with phenytoin. *Med J Aust* (1977) 2, 467–8.
5. Bellibas SE, Tuglular I. A case of phenytoin-alcohol interaction. *Therapie* (1995) 50, 487–8.
6. Höppener RJ, Kuyer A, van der Lugt PJM. Epilepsy and alcohol: the influence of social alcohol intake on seizures and treatment in epilepsy. *Epilepsia* (1983) 24, 459–71.
7. Rubin E, Lieber CS. Hepatic microsomal enzymes in man and rat: induction and inhibition by ethanol. *Science* (1968) 162, 690–1.
8. Tanaka E. Toxicological interactions involving psychiatric drugs and alcohol: an update. *J Clin Pharm Ther* (2003) 28, 81–95.
9. Epanutin Capsules (Phenytoin sodium). Pfizer Ltd. UK Summary of product characteristics, February 2012.
10. Dilantin Kapseals (Phenytoin sodium). Pfizer Inc. US Prescribing information, April 2009.

Alcohol + Phosphodiesterase type-5 inhibitors

Sildenafil, tadalafil, and vardenafil do not usually alter the effects of alcohol on blood pressure, although postural hypotension has been seen in some subjects given tadalafil and alcohol, and headache and flushing has been reported in one patient taking sildenafil and alcohol. Avanafil appears to enhance the hypotensive effects of alcohol. Alcohol does not affect the pharmacokinetics of tadalafil or vardenafil.

Clinical evidence, mechanism, importance and management

(a) Avanafil

The UK manufacturer briefly reports that, in a crossover study in healthy subjects the mean maximum decrease in diastolic blood pressure was considerably greater (figures not stated) following administration of avanafil 200 mg and alcohol (dose not stated), compared with either avanafil alone (3.2 mmHg) or alcohol alone (5 mmHg).[1] Similarly, the US manufacturer briefly notes an additional decrease in supine blood pressure of 3.5/4.5 mmHg and an increase in heart rate (9.3 beats/minute) following administration of a single 200-mg dose of avanafil and 0.5 g/kg of alcohol, compared with alcohol alone; however, avanafil did not alter the plasma concentration of alcohol.[2] Both manufacturers state that as the vasodilatory effects of alcohol and avanafil can be additive, the risk of symptoms such as hypotension, dizziness, or syncope is increased if used together.[1,2] The UK manufacturer recommends that patients should be advised about these symptoms, and what to do should they occur, .[1] while the US manufacturer indicates that the likelihood for postural hypotension increases after consumption of more than 3 units of alcohol.[2] Note that aside from any interaction, alcoholic drink can worsen erection difficulties.

(b) Sildenafil

The UK and US manufacturers briefly report that sildenafil 50 mg did not potentiate the hypotensive effect of 0.5 g/kg[3] of alcohol (mean maximum blood-alcohol concentration of 80 mg/dL or 0.08%) in healthy subjects.[3,4] A study in 8 healthy subjects also found that sildenafil 100 mg did not affect the haemodynamic effects of red wine (such as heart rate, mean arterial pressure).[5] However, a case report describes potentiation of the adverse effects of sildenafil when alcohol was consumed within one hour of taking the drug: a 36-year-old patient with hypertension taking amlodipine was given sildenafil 25 mg, which he took 3 times a week without any adverse effects. However, after having 2 drinks of whiskey (55.2 g of alcohol) he experienced severe headache and flushing about 15 minutes after taking sildenafil. The next day he took sildenafil 25 mg without any alcohol and no symptoms developed, but one week later, a challenge dose of sildenafil was given after a single 30-mL drink of whiskey and similar symptoms of severe headache and flushing occurred.[6] Note that aside from any interaction, alcoholic drink can worsen erection difficulties.

(c) Tadalafil

A study in 48 healthy subjects given a single 20-mg dose of tadalafil followed by alcohol 0.6 mg/kg found that standing and supine blood pressure, and heart rate were not notably altered, when compared with placebo and alcohol.[7] Similar or the same work is quoted by the UK and US manufacturers. In addition the UK manufacturer notes that some subjects given both alcohol and tadalafil experienced dizziness and postural hypotension, and the effects of alcohol on cognitive function were unchanged by tadalafil 10 mg.[8] The plasma concentrations of tadalafil 10 or 20 mg and alcohol were also unaffected by concurrent use.[8,9] However, the US manufacturer states that because both alcohol and tadalafil can cause peripheral vasodilation, additive blood pressure-lowering effects (which could result in postural hypotension, increased heart rate, dizziness and headache) are possible, especially with substantial amounts of alcohol (5 units or more).[9] Note that aside from any interaction, alcoholic drink can worsen erection difficulties.

(d) Vardenafil

A placebo-controlled study in 12 healthy subjects found that when alcohol 0.5 g/kg was given with vardenafil 20 mg the pharmacokinetics of both drugs were not altered, and there were no clinically relevant changes in systolic or diastolic blood pressure. Both alcohol and vardenafil alone increased heart rate, and the use of both drugs further increased heart rate, but this was only statistically significant when compared with vardenafil alone.[10] Note that aside from any interaction, alcoholic drink can worsen erection difficulties.

1. Spedra (Avanafil). A. Menarini Farmaceutica Internazionale SRL. UK Summary of product characteristics, January 2015.
2. Stendra (Avanafil). Vivus, Inc. US Prescribing information, January 2015.
3. Viagra (Sildenafil citrate). Pfizer Inc. US Prescribing information, March 2015.
4. Viagra (Sildenafil citrate). Pfizer Ltd. UK Summary of product characteristics, June 2015.
5. Leslie SJ, Atkins G, Oliver JJ, Webb DJ. No adverse hemodynamic interaction between sildenafil and red wine. *Clin Pharmacol Ther* (2004) 76, 365–70.
6. Bhalla A. Is sildenafil safe with alcohol? *J Assoc Physicians India* (2003) 51, 1125–6.
7. Mitchell M, Sanderson B, Payne C, Bedding A. Pharmacodynamic interaction between alcohol and tadalafil in healthy volunteers. *Int J Impot Res* (2002) 14, S64.
8. Cialis (Tadalafil). Eli Lilly and Company Ltd. UK Summary of product characteristics, March 2013.
9. Cialis (Tadalafil). Eli Lilly and Company. US Prescribing information, April 2014.
10. Wensing G, Bauer R, Unger S, Rohde G, Heinig R. Simultaneous administration of vardenafil and alcohol does not result in a pharmacodynamic or pharmacokinetic interaction in healthy male subjects. *Int J Clin Pharmacol Ther* (2006) 44, 216–24.

Alcohol + Procainamide

Alcohol might slightly increase the clearance of procainamide.

Clinical evidence, mechanism, importance and management

In a study in 11 healthy subjects, alcohol 0.73 g/kg followed by alcohol 0.11 g/kg every hour, increased the clearance and decreased the elimination half-life of a single 10-mg/kg oral dose of procainamide by 34% and 25%, respectively. This was due to increased acetylation of procainamide to its active metabolite *N*-acetylprocainamide.[1] The clinical relevance of these slight changes is probably small.

1. Olsen H, Mørland J. Ethanol-induced increase in procainamide acetylation in man. *Br J Clin Pharmacol* (1982) 13, 203–8.

Alcohol + Procarbazine

A flushing reaction has been seen when patients taking procarbazine drank alcohol.

Clinical evidence

One report describes 5 patients taking procarbazine whose faces became very red and hot for a short time after drinking wine.[1] Another report states that flushing occurred in 3 patients taking procarbazine after they drank beer.[2] In a third study, 2 out of 40 patients taking procarbazine complained of facial flushing after taking a small alcoholic drink, and one patient thought that the effects of alcohol were markedly increased.[3] Yet another study describes a 'flush syndrome' in 3 out of 50 patients who drank alcohol while taking procarbazine.[4]

Mechanism

Unknown. Animal studies[5] suggest that procarbazine might inhibit acetaldehyde dehydrogenase in the liver causing a disulfiram-like reaction (see 'Alcohol + Disulfiram', p.67).

Importance and management

The interaction between alcohol and procarbazine is established but of uncertain incidence. It seems to be more embarrassing and possibly frightening, than serious, and if it occurs it is unlikely to require treatment; however, patients should be warned. The manufacturer of procarbazine states that alcohol should not be used concurrently.[6] Note that some alcoholic beverages contain significant amounts of tyramine (see 'Table 32.2', p.1390), so there is a slight possibility that the tyramine reaction might occur if a patient taking procarbazine consumes significant quantities of these beverages, as procarbazine is a weak inhibitor of MAO, see 'Procarbazine + Sympathomimetics', p.709.

1. Mathé G, Berumen L, Schweisguth O, Brule G, Schneider M, Cattan A, Amiel JL, Schwarzenberg L. Methyl-hydrazine in the treatment of Hodgkin's disease and various forms of haematosarcoma and leukaemia. *Lancet* (1963) ii, 1077–80.
2. Dawson WB. Ibenzmethyzin in the management of late Hodgkin's disease. In Jelliffe AM, Marks J, eds. 'Natulan, Ibenzmethyzin'. Report of the proceedings of a symposium, Downing College, Cambridge, June 1965. Bristol: John Wright; 1965 p. 31–4.
3. Todd IDH. Natulan in management of late Hodgkin's disease, other lymphoreticular neoplasms, and malignant melanoma. *BMJ* (1965) 1, 628–31.
4. Brulé G, Schlumberger JR, Griscelli C. *N*-isopropyl-α-(2-methylhydrazino)-*p*-toluamide, hydrochloride (NSC-77213) in treatment of solid tumors. *Cancer Chemother Rep* (1965) 44, 31–8.
5. Vasiliou V, Malamas M, Marselos M. The mechanism of alcohol intolerance produced by various therapeutic agents. *Acta Pharmacol Toxicol (Copenh)* (1986) 58, 305–10.
6. Matulane (Procarbazine hydrochloride). Sigma-tau Pharmaceuticals Inc. US Prescribing information, March 2008.

Alcohol + Proton pump inhibitors

Lansoprazole, omeprazole and pantoprazole do not affect blood-alcohol levels: other proton pump inhibitors therefore seem unlikely to interact with alcohol.

Clinical evidence

(a) Lansoprazole

A study in 30 healthy subjects given 0.6 g/kg of alcohol before and after taking lansoprazole 30 mg daily for 3 days found that the pharmacokinetics of alcohol were not affected, and blood-alcohol levels were not raised, by lansoprazole.[1]

(b) Omeprazole

A number of studies have shown that omeprazole does not affect blood-alcohol levels.[2-6]

(c) Pantoprazole

In a placebo-controlled study 16 healthy subjects were given pantoprazole 40 mg daily for 7 days, with alcohol 0.5 g/kg in 200 mL of orange juice 2 hours after a standard breakfast on day 7. The maximum blood levels and the AUC of alcohol were not notably affected by pantoprazole.[7]

Mechanism

The proton pump inhibitors do not affect alcohol dehydrogenase activity[3,8] and would not be expected to alter the first-pass metabolism of alcohol.

Importance and management

The proton pump inhibitors do not appear to affect blood-alcohol levels, and no particular precautions are necessary on their concurrent use. However, note that some of the conditions for which these drugs are used can be made worse by alcohol, so restricting alcohol intake might be prudent.

1. Girre C, Coutelle C, David P, Fleury B, Thomas G, Palmobo S, Dally S, Couzigou P. Lack of effect of lansoprazole on the pharmacokinetics of ethanol in male volunteers. *Gastroenterology* (1994) 106, A504.
2. Guram M, Howden CW, Holt S. Further evidence for an interaction between alcohol and certain H_2-receptor antagonists. *Alcohol Clin Exp Res* (1991) 15, 1084–5.
3. Roine R, Hernández-Muñoz R, Baraona E, Greenstein R, Lieber CS. Effect of omeprazole on gastric first-pass metabolism of ethanol. *Dig Dis Sci* (1992) 37, 891–6.
4. Jönsson K-Å, Jones AW, Boström H, Andersson T. Lack of effect of omeprazole, cimetidine, and ranitidine on the pharmacokinetics of ethanol in fasting male volunteers. *Eur J Clin Pharmacol* (1992) 42, 209–212.
5. Minocha A, Rahal PS, Brier ME, Levinson SS. Omeprazole therapy does not affect pharmacokinetics of orally administered ethanol in healthy male subjects. *J Clin Gastroenterol* (1995) 21, 107–9.
6. Brown ASM, James OFW. Omeprazole, ranitidine, and cimetidine have no effect on peak blood ethanol concentrations, first pass metabolism or area under the time-ethanol curve under 'real-life' drinking conditions. *Aliment Pharmacol Ther* (1998) 12, 141–5.
7. Heinze H, Fischer R, Pfützer R, Teyssen S, Singer MV. Lack of interaction between pantoprazole and ethanol: a randomised, double-blind, placebo-controlled study in healthy volunteers. *Clin Drug Invest* (2001) 21, 345–51.
8. Battiston L, Tulissi P, Moretti M, Pozzato G. Lansoprazole and ethanol metabolism: comparison with omeprazole and cimetidine. *Pharmacol Toxicol* (1997) 81, 247–52.

Alcohol + Quetiapine

Postural hypotension and possibly drowsiness might be increased when quetiapine is given with alcohol. Quetiapine does not appear to affect the pharmacokinetics of alcohol.

Clinical evidence, mechanism, importance and management

A randomised, crossover study in 8 men with psychotic disorders found that quetiapine 250 mg three times daily did not affect the mean breath-alcohol concentration after they took 0.8 g/kg of alcohol in orange juice. Some statistically significant changes in the performance of psychomotor tests were seen, but these were considered to have little clinical relevance.[1] However, the US manufacturers of quetiapine state that, in clinical studies, the motor and cognitive effects of alcohol were potentiated by quetiapine.[2] They therefore advise avoiding alcohol, whereas the UK manufacturer[3] advises caution with the concurrent use of alcohol. Note that drowsiness is the most common adverse effect of quetiapine, occurring in over 10% of patients (over 30% in some studies).[2,3] Quetiapine might occasionally induce postural hypotension,[2,3] which could be exacerbated by alcohol. In practical terms this means that patients should be warned of the risk of faintness and dizziness if they stand up quickly, and advised to sit or lie down if this occurs.

1. Zeneca Pharma. Personal communication, October 1997.
2. Seroquel (Quetiapine fumarate). AstraZeneca. US Prescribing information, December 2011.
3. Seroquel (Quetiapine fumarate). AstraZeneca UK Ltd. UK Summary of product characteristics, April 2012.

Alcohol + Reboxetine

A study in 10 healthy subjects found that reboxetine does not affect cognitive or psychomotor function, and there is no interaction with alcohol.[1]

1. Kerr JS, Powell J, Hindmarch I. The effects of reboxetine and amitriptyline, with and without alcohol on cognitive function and psychomotor performance. *Br J Clin Pharmacol* (1996) 42, 239–41.

Alcohol + Retinoids

The consumption of alcohol can increase the serum levels of etretinate in patients taking acitretin. Alcohol did not affect the pharmacokinetics of isotretinoin in one study; however, a single case report describes a marked reduction in the effects of isotretinoin following the acute intake of alcohol.

Clinical evidence, mechanism, importance and management

(a) Acitretin

A study, in 10 patients with psoriasis taking acitretin, found that the concurrent use of alcohol seemed to be associated with an increase in the formation of etretinate, a metabolite that has a much longer half-life than acitretin.[1] A later study by some of the same authors, in 86 patients taking acitretin, similarly found that alcohol increases the levels of etretinate and the magnitude of the increase appeared to be related to the amount of alcohol that they drank.[2] The implications of these studies are not known, but it is suggested that it might have some bearing on the length of the period after acitretin therapy during which women are advised not to conceive.[1,2]

(b) Isotretinoin

A study, in 11 patients with severe acne or rosacea taking isotretinoin 30 to 50 mg daily for 3 months, found that the concurrent use of alcohol did not influence the metabolism and pharmacokinetics of isotretinoin and its main metabolites. Alcohol intake was described as considerable in 7 of the patients (150 to 250 g per week in 4 subjects and 300 to 1400 g per week in 3 subjects).[3]

A case report describes a former alcoholic, who no longer drank alcohol, and who was treated for acne conglobata, with some success, with isotretinoin 60 mg daily for 3 months. When for 2 weeks he briefly started to drink alcohol again as part of his job (he was a sherry taster) his skin lesions reappeared and the isotretinoin adverse effects (mucocutaneous dryness) vanished. When he stopped drinking alcohol his skin lesions became controlled again and the drug adverse effects re-emerged. The following year, while taking another course of isotretinoin, the same thing happened when he started and stopped drinking alcohol. The reasons are not known, but one suggestion is that the alcohol briefly induced the liver microsomal enzymes responsible for the metabolism of isotretinoin, thereby reducing both its therapeutic and adverse effects.[4] The general relevance of this apparent interaction is not known.

1. Larsen FG, Jakobsen P, Knudsen J, Weismann K, Kragballe K, Nielsen-Kudsk F. Conversion of acitretin to etretinate in psoriatic patients is influenced by ethanol. *J Invest Dermatol* (1993) 100, 623–7.

2. Grønhøj Larsen F, Steinkjer B, Jakobsen P, Hjorter A, Brockhoff PB, Nielsen-Kudsk F. Acitretin is converted to etretinate only during concomitant alcohol intake. *Br J Dermatol* (2000) 1164–9.
3. Grønhøj Larsen F, Jakobsen P, Grønhøj Larsen C, Heidenheim M, Held E, Nielsen-Kudsk F. The metabolism and pharmacokinetics of isotretinoin in patients with acne and rosacea are not influenced by ethanol. *Br J Dermatol* (2009) 161, 664–70.
4. Soria C, Allegue F, Galiana J, Ledo A. Decreased isotretinoin efficacy during acute alcohol intake. *Dermatologica* (1991) 182, 203.

Alcohol + Salbutamol (Albuterol)

A patient with high blood-alcohol levels developed lactic acidosis after being exposed to smoke from a fire and receiving salbutamol.

Clinical evidence, mechanism, importance and management

An isolated report describes a 49-year-old male alcoholic who developed severe lactic acidosis after he was exposed to smoke from a fire and given salbutamol for bronchospasm. The correction of lactic acidosis following salbutamol withdrawal and a transitory increase in lactate after salbutamol re-introduction suggested hypersensitivity to salbutamol. However, the patient also had a very high plasma-alcohol level (240 mg%), and the metabolism of alcohol was thought to have competed with the conversion of lactate to pyruvate, resulting in reduced lactate clearance, and thereby potentiating the acidosis caused by the salbutamol.[1] The general relevance of this report is unclear as beta agonist-induced exacerbation of lactic acidosis has been reported in asthmatics, both adults and children. The authors of the report suggest close monitoring of lactate levels in alcoholic patients receiving beta agonists.[1]

1. Taboulet P, Clemessy J-L, Fréminet A, Baud FJ. A case of life-threatening lactic acidosis after smoke inhalation – interference between ß-adrenergic agents and ethanol? *Intensive Care Med* (1995) 21, 1039–42.

Alcohol + Sibutramine

Sibutramine does not appear to notably alter the psychomotor response to alcohol.

Clinical evidence, mechanism, importance and management

In a randomised study, 20 healthy subjects were given sibutramine 20 mg, with 0.5 g/kg of alcohol diluted in ginger beer or placebo. Sibutramine did not potentiate the cognitive or psychomotor effects of alcohol, and in one test sibutramine slightly reduced the impairment caused by alcohol.[1] However, before the withdrawal of the drug from the UK market, the manufacturer noted that the consumption of alcohol is generally not compatible with the dietary modifications that are recommended in those given sibutramine.[2]

1. Wesnes KA, Garratt C, Wickens M, Gudgeon A, Oliver S. Effects of sibutramine alone and with alcohol on cognitive function in healthy volunteers. *Br J Clin Pharmacol* (2000) 49, 110–17.
2. Reductil (Sibutramine hydrochloride monohydrate). Abbott Laboratories Ltd. UK Summary of product characteristics, December 2009.

Alcohol + SNRIs

No important psychomotor interaction normally appears to occur between desvenlafaxine, duloxetine or venlafaxine and alcohol. Duloxetine and milnacipran might be associated with liver injury.

Clinical evidence and mechanism

(a) Desvenlafaxine

The US manufacturer of desvenlafaxine briefly notes that in a study, the impairment of mental and motor skills induced by alcohol was not increased by desvenlafaxine.[1]

(b) Duloxetine

In a single-dose study in healthy subjects, duloxetine 60 mg, and alcohol given in a dose sufficient to produce blood-alcohol concentrations of about 100 mg%, did not worsen the psychomotor impairment observed with alcohol alone.[2]

(c) Levomilnacipran

The US manufacturer of levomilnacipran briefly notes that in an *in vitro* study, the extended release properties of levomilnacipran capsules were affected by alcohol.[3]

(d) Venlafaxine

In a study in 15 healthy subjects, venlafaxine 50 mg every 8 hours was found to have some effect on psychomotor tests (digit symbol substitution, divided attention reaction times, profile of mood scales), but these changes were small and not considered to be clinically important. No pharmacodynamic or pharmacokinetic interactions occurred when alcohol 0.5 g/kg was also given.[4]

Importance and management

Although evidence is limited, the studies reported above suggest that no pharmacodynamic interactions occur between most SNRIs and alcohol, although some small effects were seen with venlafaxine. However, most manufacturers of SNRIs advise that concurrent use with alcohol should be avoided.[1,5,6] This is presumably because both drugs act on the CNS and also because of the increased risk of alcohol abuse in depressed patients. Pharmacokinetic data is lacking, but based on *in vitro* data, alcohol might accelerate the release of levomilnacipran from its formulation, hence the US manufacturer recommends that it should not be taken with alcohol.[3]

The US manufacturers of duloxetine and **milnacipran** warn that concurrent use with alcohol might aggravate pre-existing liver disease, hence these should not be given to patients with substantial alcohol use or evidence of chronic liver disease.[7,8]

1. Pristiq (Desvenlafaxine succinate). Wyeth Pharmaceuticals Inc. US Prescribing information, July 2014.
2. Skinner MH, Weerakkody G. Duloxetine does not exacerbate the effects of alcohol on psychometric tests. *Clin Pharmacol Ther* (2002) 71, 53.
3. Fetzima (Levomilnacipran hydrochloride). Forest Pharmaceuticals Inc. US Prescribing information, July 2014.
4. Troy SM, Turner MB, Unruh M, Parker VD, Chiang ST. Pharmacokinetic and pharmacodynamic evaluation of the potential drug interaction between venlafaxine and ethanol. *J Clin Pharmacol* (1997) 37, 1073–81.
5. Efexor XL (Venlafaxine hydrochloride). Pfizer Ltd. UK Summary of product characteristics, December 2013.
6. Effexor XR (Venlafaxine hydrochloride). Wyeth Pharmaceuticals Inc. US Prescribing information, March 2014.
7. Cymbalta (Duloxetine hydrochloride). Eli Lilly and Company. US Prescribing information, July 2014.
8. Savella (Milnacipran hydrochloride). Forest Pharmaceuticals Inc. US Prescribing information, November 2013.

Alcohol + Sodium cromoglicate (Cromolyn sodium)

No adverse interaction occurs between sodium cromoglicate and alcohol.

Clinical evidence, mechanism, importance and management

A double-blind, crossover study in 17 healthy subjects found that the inhalation of 40 mg of sodium cromoglicate had little or no effect on the performance of a number of tests on human perceptual, cognitive, and motor skills, whether taken alone or with alcohol 0.75 g/kg. Nor did it affect blood-alcohol levels.[1] This is in line with the common experience of patients, and no special precautions seem to be necessary if patients taking sodium cromoglicate want to drink alcohol.

1. Crawford WA, Franks HM, Hensley VR, Hensley WJ, Starmer GA, Teo RKC. The effect of disodium cromoglycate on human performance, alone and in combination with ethanol. *Med J Aust* (1976) 1, 997–9.

Alcohol + Sodium oxybate

The concurrent use of sodium oxybate and alcohol appears to increase respiratory depression, lead to an increase in adverse effects, and is expected to increase sedation.

Clinical evidence, mechanism, importance and management

In a randomised, placebo-controlled study, 16 healthy subjects were given alcohol 0.3 g/kg with sodium oxybate 50 mg/kg. The study found that concurrent use did not have a statistically significant effect on the pharmacokinetics of both drugs and sodium oxybate did not alter the effects of alcohol on blood pressure and heart rate, although there were two episodes of postural hypotension (systolic blood pressure 71 to 73 mmHg). Vomiting occurred more frequently compared with alcohol or gamma-hydroxybutyric acid alone, and oxygen saturations were decreased by just over 2% by the combination (modest effect), which was greater than the effect of alcohol alone, suggesting that the combination increases respiratory depression.[1]

Sodium oxybate is the sodium salt of gamma hydroxybutyrate (GHB) a CNS depressant substance with well known abuse potential. When used clinically it is predicted to have additive effects with alcohol and other CNS depressants and the manufacturers specifically state that it should not be used with these drugs.[2,3] Patients should be warned not to drink alcohol while taking sodium oxybate.[2,3] In light of the findings the manufacturers recommendations appear cautious, but prudent.

1. Thai D, Dyer JE, Benowitz NL, Haller CA. Gamma-hydroxybutyrate and ethanol effects and interactions in humans. *J Clin Psychopharmacol* (2006) 26, 524–9.
2. Xyrem (Sodium oxybate). UCB Pharma Ltd. UK Summary of product characteristics, April 2011.
3. Xyrem (Sodium oxybate). Jazz Pharmaceuticals, Inc. US Prescribing information, November 2005.

Alcohol + SSRIs

There is no pharmacokinetic interaction between fluoxetine and alcohol, but a modest increase in sedation might occur if alcohol is given with fluvoxamine or paroxetine. No change in psychomotor performance appears to occur with sertraline and alcohol. Alcohol does not appear to affect the pharmacokinetics of vilazodone. No pharmacodynamic interaction is expected to occur between escitalopram or citalopram and alcohol.

Clinical evidence and mechanism

(a) Citalopram

The manufacturers of citalopram state that no pharmacodynamic[1,2] or pharmacokinetic[1] interactions have been noted when citalopram was given with alcohol.

(b) Escitalopram

The manufacturers of escitalopram state that no pharmacokinetic or pharmacodynamic interactions are expected between alcohol and escitalopram.[3]

(c) Fluoxetine

In a study in healthy subjects the concurrent use of fluoxetine 30 to 60 mg and alcohol (about 120 mL of whiskey) did not affect the pharmacokinetics of either drug, and fluoxetine did not alter the effect of alcohol on psychomotor activity (stability of stance, motor performance, manual co-ordination).[4] Similarly, in 12 healthy subjects, blood-alcohol concentrations of 80 mg% impaired the performance of a number of psychomotor tests but the addition of fluoxetine 40 mg daily, taken for 6 days before the alcohol, had little further effect.[5] Another study also found no change in the performance of a number of psychophysiological tests when fluoxetine was given with alcohol.[6] No problems were found in a study of 20 alcohol-dependent patients taking fluoxetine 60 mg daily when they drank alcohol, or in approximately 31 patients taking fluoxetine 20 mg daily who drank unspecified small quantities of alcohol.[7]

(d) Fluvoxamine

One study found that fluvoxamine 150 mg daily with alcohol impaired alertness and attention more than alcohol alone.[8] However, another study in subjects given 40 g of alcohol (blood-alcohol concentrations up to 70 mg%) found no evidence to suggest that the addition of fluvoxamine 50 mg twice daily worsened the performance of the psychomotor tests, and it even appeared to reverse some of the effects. The pharmacokinetics of alcohol were hardly affected by fluvoxamine, but the steady-state maximum plasma concentrations of fluvoxamine were increased by 20%, although the AUC of fluvoxamine was unchanged. It was suggested that alcohol might have promoted the dissolution of fluvoxamine and increased the absorption rate without affecting bioavailability.[9] Another study also found that fluvoxamine did not appear to enhance the detrimental effects of alcohol on the performance of psychomotor tests.[10]

(e) Paroxetine

Studies have found that paroxetine alone caused little impairment of a series of psychomotor tests related to car driving, and with alcohol the effects were unchanged, except for a decrease in attentiveness and an increase in reaction time.[11,12] Another study suggested that the alcohol-induced sedation was antagonised by paroxetine.[13]

(f) Sertraline

Sertraline (in doses of up to 200 mg for 9 days) was found not to impair cognitive or psychomotor performance, and it also appeared not to increase the effects of alcohol.[14]

(g) Vilazodone

The US manufacturer of vilazodone briefly notes that there is no change in the pharmacokinetics of vilazodone on concurrent use with alcohol.[15]

Importance and management

The results of the few studies reported above suggest that no pharmacokinetic or pharmacodynamic interactions occur between most SSRIs and alcohol, although some small effects were seen with fluvoxamine and possibly paroxetine. However, most manufacturers of SSRIs suggest that concurrent use with alcohol is not advisable. This is presumably because both drugs act on the CNS and also because of the risk of alcohol abuse in depressed patients.[16]

1. Cipramil Tablets (Citalopram hydrobromide). Lundbeck Ltd. UK Summary of product characteristics, July 2015.
2. Celexa (Citalopram hydrobromide). Forest Pharmaceuticals, Inc. US Prescribing information, July 2014.
3. Cipralex Tablets (Escitalopram oxalate). Lundbeck Ltd. UK Summary of product characteristics, September 2013.
4. Lemberger L, Rowe H, Bergstrom RF, Farid KZ, Enas GG. Effect of fluoxetine on psychomotor performance, physiologic response, and kinetics of ethanol. *Clin Pharmacol Ther* (1985) 37, 658–64.
5. Allen D, Lader M, Curran HV. A comparative study of the interactions of alcohol with amitriptyline, fluoxetine and placebo in normal subjects. *Prog Neuropsychopharmacol Biol Psychiatry* (1988) 12, 63–80.
6. Schaffler K. Study on performance and alcohol interaction with the antidepressant fluoxetine. *Int Clin Psychopharmacol* (1989) 4 (Suppl 1), 15–20.
7. Florkowski A, Gruszczyński W. Alcohol problems and treating patients with fluoxetine. *Pol J Pharmacol* (1995) 47, 547.
8. Duphar Laboratories. Data on file. Study of the effects of the antidepressant fluvoxamine on driving skills and its interaction with alcohol. 1981.
9. van Harten J, Stevens LA, Raghoebar M, Holland RL, Wesnes K, Cournot A. Fluvoxamine does not interact with alcohol or potentiate alcohol-related impairment of cognitive function. *Clin Pharmacol Ther* (1992) 52, 427–35.
10. Linnoila M, Stapleton JM, George DT, Lane E, Eckardt MJ. Effects of fluvoxamine, alone and in combination with ethanol, on psychomotor and cognitive performance and on autonomic nervous system reactivity in healthy volunteers. *J Clin Psychopharmacol* (1993) 13, 175–80.
11. Cooper SM, Jackson D, Loudon JM, McClelland GR, Raptopoulos P. The psychomotor effects of paroxetine alone and in combination with haloperidol, amylobarbitone, oxazepam, or alcohol. *Acta Psychiatr Scand* (1989) 80 (Suppl 350), 53–55.
12. Hindmarch I, Harrison C. The effects of paroxetine and other antidepressants in combination with alcohol on psychomotor activity related to car driving. *Acta Psychiatr Scand* (1989) 80 (Suppl 350), 45.
13. Kerr JS, Fairweather DB, Mahendran R, Hindmarch I. The effects of paroxetine, alone and in combination with alcohol on psychomotor performance and cognitive function in the elderly. *Int Clin Psychopharmacol* (1992) 7, 101–8.
14. Warrington SJ. Clinical implications of the pharmacology of sertraline. *Int Clin Psychopharmacol* (1991) 6 (Suppl 2), 11–21.
15. Viibryd (Vilazodone hydrochloride). Forest Pharmaceuticals Inc. US Prescribing information, March 2015.
16. Eli Lilly and Company Ltd. Personal communication, October 2006.

Alcohol + Sulfiram

Disulfiram-like reactions have been seen in at least three patients who drank alcohol after using a topical solution of sulfiram.

Clinical evidence

A man who used undiluted *Tetmosol* (a solution of sulfiram) for 3 days on the skin all over his body developed a disulfiram-like reaction (flushing, sweating, skin swelling, severe tachycardia and nausea) on the third day, after drinking 3 double whiskies. The same thing happened on two subsequent evenings again after he drank 3 double whiskies.[1] Similar reactions have been described in 2 other patients who drank alcohol while using *Tetmosol* or *Ascabiol* (also containing sulfiram).[2,3]

Mechanism

Sulfiram (tetraethylthiuram *monosulphide*) is closely related to disulfiram (tetraethylthiuram *disulphide*) and can apparently undergo photochemical conversion to disulfiram when exposed to light. The longer it is stored, the higher the concentration.[4,5] The reaction with alcohol appears therefore to be largely due to the presence of disulfiram,[6] see 'Alcohol + Disulfiram', p.67.

Importance and management

An established interaction. It has been suggested that alcohol should be avoided before, and for at least 48 hours after the application of sulfiram, but this might not always be necessary. The author of a letter,[7] commenting on one of the cases cited,[1] wrote that he had never encountered this reaction when using a diluted solution of *Tetmosol* on patients at the Dreadnought Seamen's Hospital in London who he described as "not necessarily abstemious". This would suggest that the reaction is normally uncommon and unlikely to occur if the solution is correctly diluted (usually with 2 to 3 parts of water), thereby reducing the amount absorbed through the skin. However, one unusually sensitive patient is said to have had a reaction (flushing, sweating, tachycardia) after using diluted *Tetmosol*, but without drinking alcohol. It was suggested that she reacted to the alcohol base of the formulation passing through her skin.[8]

1. Gold S. A skinful of alcohol. *Lancet* (1966) ii, 1417.
2. Dantas W. Monosulfiram como causa de síndrome do acetaldeído. *Arq Cat Med* (1980) 9, 29–30.
3. Blanc D, Deprez Ph. Unusual adverse reaction to an acaricide. *Lancet* (1990) 335, 1291–2.
4. Lipsky JJ, Mays DC, Naylor S. Monosulfiram, disulfiram, and light. *Lancet* (1994) 343, 304.
5. Mays DC, Nelson AN, Benson LM, Johnson KL, Naylor S, Lipsky JJ. Photolysis of monosulfiram: a mechanism for its disulfiram-like reaction. *Clin Pharmacol Ther* (1994) 55, 191.
6. Lipsky JJ, Nelson AN, Dockter EC. Inhibition of aldehyde dehydrogenase by sulfiram. *Clin Pharmacol Ther* (1992) 51, 184.
7. Erskine D. A skinful of alcohol. *Lancet* (1967) i, 54.
8. Burgess I. Adverse reactions to monosulfiram. *Lancet* (1990) 336, 873.

Alcohol + Tacrolimus or Pimecrolimus

Alcohol can cause facial flushing or erythema in patients using tacrolimus ointment; this reaction appears to be fairly common. Alcohol intolerance has been reported rarely with pimecrolimus cream.

Clinical evidence

Six patients reported facial flushing with small quantities of beer or wine during facial treatment with tacrolimus ointment. Re-exposure to tacrolimus 0.1% ointment, applied to the face twice daily for 4 days, followed by 100 mL of white wine on the fifth day, resulted in a facial flush reaction in all the patients, which occurred within 5 to 15 minutes of alcohol ingestion. The intensity of the erythema varied among the patients and was not confined to the treated areas, but started to fade after 30 minutes; a slight headache occurred in one patient. Forearm skin was also exposed to a patch containing 70 mg of tacrolimus 0.1% ointment, but these sites remained unchanged following alcohol exposure. After a tacrolimus washout period of at least 4 weeks, controlled exposure to alcohol in 2 patients was uneventful.[1] Another report describes one patient using tacrolimus ointment for mild eyelid eczema who experienced erythema, limited to the area the tacrolimus ointment was applied, after drinking wine. Two other patients experienced an erythematous rash after drinking alcohol when using topical tacrolimus; areas affected included the elbows, ears, eyes and face. The response to alcohol disappeared within 2 weeks of discontinuing tacrolimus ointment.[2]

Three patients experienced application site erythema following the consumption of alcohol after using topical tacrolimus or pimecrolimus for the treatment of facial dermatoses. Two of the patients then participated in a double-blind, controlled evaluation of the reaction. Both patients consumed alcohol (240 mL of red or white wine) without experiencing flushing, but following tacrolimus or pimecrolimus application, they experienced moderate or severe facial flushing (limited to the area of application) 5 to 10 minutes after alcohol consumption. The intensity of the erythema was sharply reduced after taking aspirin 325 mg twice daily for 3 days before alcohol consumption, but cetirizine 10 mg daily with cimetidine 400 mg twice daily for 3 days appeared to have little effect.[3]

In a study in 25 patients with chronic-stable localised vitiligo (13 given pimecrolimus and 12 given tacrolimus, both locally), 2 patients using pimecrolimus and 5 patients using tacrolimus developed erythematous flushing of the face after they consumed small quantities of alcohol (amounts not stated).[4]

There are other reports of this interaction between tacrolimus and alcohol,[3,5-9] including 3 cases in children aged 6 months to 3.5 years who were given oral medicines containing alcohol while using tacrolimus ointment.[9] The reaction is usually confined to the face[5,9] and the intensity might be related to the amount of alcohol ingested.[5] In an open study of 316 patients, alcohol intolerance (facial flushing) was observed in 19% of the patients using tacrolimus 0.1% ointment[7] and in a controlled study, 6.9% of patients experienced the reaction with tacrolimus 0.1% ointment, and 3.4% of patients experienced the reaction with tacrolimus 0.03% ointment.[6] A number of case reports have described a similar reaction in patients using pimecrolimus. One report describes a 54-year-old woman who had been using topical pimecrolimus for 2 weeks when she experienced episodes of intense facial flushing after drinking alcohol.[10] A 34-year-old patient with seborrhoeic dermatitis using pimecrolimus 1% cream reported flushing in the areas to which he had applied the cream, 10 minutes after drinking beer. The reaction did not occur with alcohol after pimecrolimus was discontinued. Two similar cases have been reported.[11]

Mechanism

The mechanism of this interaction is not understood. It has been proposed that tacrolimus might act on the same biochemical pathway as alcohol, potentiating a capsaicin-mediated release of neuropeptides, which increase vasodilatory effects. Alternatively, cutaneous aldehyde dehydrogenase inhibition in areas where tacrolimus has been applied might increase cutaneous aldehyde levels that, through prostaglandins as mediators, could lead to vasodilation following alcohol consumption.[1,5]

Importance and management

The interaction between topical tacrolimus and alcohol is established and appears to occur in about 6 to 7% of patients using tacrolimus 0.1% ointment. Patients should be warned of the possibility of a flushing reaction with alcohol and that consumption of alcohol should perhaps be avoided if this occurs. It has been suggested that aspirin might reduce the symptoms of this reaction,[3] but this needs further study. Alcohol intolerance with pimecrolimus has been reported,[3,12] but appears to be rare.[13]

1. Milingou M, Antille C, Sorg O, Saurat J-H, Lübbe J. Alcohol intolerance and facial flushing in patients treated with topical tacrolimus. *Arch Dermatol* (2004) 140, 1542–4.
2. Knight AK, Boxer M, Chandler MJ. Alcohol-induced rash caused by topical tacrolimus. *Ann Allergy Asthma Immunol* (2005) 95, 291–2.
3. Ehst BD, Warshaw EM. Alcohol-induced application site erythema after topical immunomodulator use and its inhibition by aspirin. *Arch Dermatol* (2004) 140, 1014–15.
4. Stinco G, Piccirillo F, Sallustio M, Patrone P. Facial flush reaction after alcohol ingestion during topical pimecrolimus and tacrolimus treatment. *Dermatology* (2009) 218, 71–2.
5. Morales-Molina JA, Mateu-de Antonio J, Grau S, Ferrández O. Alcohol ingestion and topical tacrolimus: a disulfiram-like interaction? *Ann Pharmacother* (2005) 39, 772–3.
6. Soter NA, Fleischer AB, Webster GF Monroe E, Lawrence I; the Tacrolimus Ointment Study Group. Tacrolimus ointment for the treatment of atopic dermatitis in adult patients: part II, safety. *J Am Acad Dermatol* (2001) 44 (Suppl 1), S39–S46.
7. Reitamo S, Wollenberg A, Schöpf E, Perrot JL, Marks R, Ruzicka T, Christophers E, Kapp A, Lahfa M, Rubins A, Jablonska S, Rustin M.; the European Tacrolimus Ointment Study Group. Safety and efficacy of 1 year of tacrolimus ointment monotherapy in adults with atopic dermatitis. *Arch Dermatol* (2000) 136, 999–1006.
8. Lübbe J, Milingou M. Tacrolimus ointment, alcohol, and facial flushing. *N Engl J Med* (2004) 351, 2740.
9. Calza A-M, Lübbe J. Tacrolimus ointment-associated alcohol intolerance in infants receiving ethanol-containing medication. *Br J Dermatol* (2005) 152, 569.
10. de la Torre C. Alcohol intolerance with facial flushing due to topical pimecrolimus treatment. *Actas Dermosifiliogr* (2008) 99, 419–27.
11. Ogunleye T, James WD. Ethanol-induced flushing with topical pimecrolimus use. *Dermatitis* (2008) 19, E1–E2.
12. Elidel (Pimecrolimus). Novartis Pharmaceuticals Corp. US Prescribing information, August 2010.
13. Elidel (Pimecrolimus). Meda Pharmaceuticals. UK Summary of product characteristics, January 2012.

Alcohol + Tetracyclic antidepressants

Mianserin and maprotiline can cause drowsiness, which is worsened by alcohol. Giving alcohol with these antidepressants impairs the performance of psychomotor tests.

Clinical evidence

(a) Maprotiline

A double-blind, crossover study in 12 healthy subjects found that a single 75-mg oral dose of maprotiline subjectively caused drowsiness, which was increased by 1 g/kg of alcohol. The performance of a number of psychomotor tests was also worsened after the addition of alcohol.[1] However, in a later study, the same group found that maprotiline 50 mg twice daily for 15 days did not increase the detrimental effects of alcohol.[2] A case report attributes two epileptic seizures in a 21-year-old woman taking maprotiline 125 mg daily to an increase in her alcohol intake during the preceding week (3 to 4 beers or 3 to 4 glasses of champagne each night). She was also taking alprazolam 500 micrograms four times daily.[3]

(b) Mianserin

A double-blind, crossover study in 13 healthy subjects given 10 to 30 mg of mianserin twice daily for 8 days, with and without alcohol 1 g/kg, found that their performance in a number of psychomotor tests (choice reaction, coordination, critical flicker frequency) were impaired both by mianserin alone and by the concurrent use of alcohol. The subjects were aware of feeling drowsy, muzzy, and less able to carry out the tests.[4] These results confirm the findings of other studies.[5,6]

Mechanism

The CNS depressant effects of mianserin, and possibly maprotiline, appear to be additive with those of alcohol. In the case report it was suggested that the seizures occurred due to high levels of maprotiline caused by the alcohol intake.[3]

Importance and management

Drowsiness is a frequently reported adverse effect of mianserin, particularly during the first few days of treatment. Patients should be warned that driving or handling dangerous machinery will be made more hazardous if they drink alcohol. It would also be prudent to warn patients taking maprotiline of the possible increased risk if they drink.[2] The general relevance of the case of seizures with maprotiline and alcohol is unclear.

1. Strömberg C, Seppälä T, Mattila MJ. Acute effects of maprotiline, doxepin and zimeldine with alcohol in healthy volunteers. *Arch Int Pharmacodyn Ther* (1988) 291, 217–228.
2. Strömberg C, Suokas A, Seppälä T. Interaction of alcohol with maprotiline or nomifensine: echocardiographic and psychometric effects. *Eur J Clin Pharmacol* (1988) 35, 593–99.
3. Strawn SK, Pederson CA, Evans DL. Alcohol precipitation of maprotiline-associated seizures. *South Med J* (1988) 81, 1205–6.
4. Seppälä T, Strömberg C, Bergman I. Effects of zimeldine, mianserin and amitriptyline on psychomotor skills and their interaction with ethanol: a placebo controlled cross-over study. *Eur J Clin Pharmacol* (1984) 27, 181–9.
5. Seppälä T. Psychomotor skills during acute and two-week treatment with mianserin (Org GB 94) and amitriptyline, and their combined effects with alcohol. *Ann Clin Res* (1977) 9, 66–72.
6. Strömberg C, Mattila MJ. Acute comparison of clovoxamine and mianserin, alone and in combination with ethanol, on human psychomotor performance. *Pharmacol Toxicol* (1987) 60, 374–9.

Alcohol + Tetracyclines

Doxycycline serum levels might fall below minimum therapeutic levels in alcoholic patients, but tetracycline is not affected. There is nothing to suggest that moderate amounts of alcohol have a clinically relevant effect on the serum levels of any tetracycline in non-alcoholic subjects.

Clinical evidence

(a) Alcoholic patients

A study into the effects of alcohol on **doxycycline** and **tetracycline** pharmacokinetics found that the half-life of **doxycycline** was 10.5 hours in 6 alcoholics (with normal liver function) compared with 14.7 hours in 6 healthy subjects. The serum **doxycycline** levels of 3 of the alcoholic patients fell below the generally accepted minimum inhibitory concentration at 24 hours. The half-life of **tetracycline** was the same in both groups. All of the subjects were given **doxycycline** 100 mg daily after a 200-mg loading dose, and **tetracycline** 500 mg twice daily after an initial 750-mg loading dose.[1]

(b) Non-alcoholic patients

Single 500-mg doses of **tetracycline** were given to 9 healthy subjects with water or alcohol 2.7 g/kg. The alcohol caused a 33% rise in the maximum serum levels of **tetracycline**, from 9.3 micrograms/mL to 12.4 micrograms/mL, and a 50% rise in the AUC of **tetracycline**.[2] The clinical relevance of this rise is unknown.

Another study in healthy subjects found that cheap red wine, but not whisky (both 1 g/kg) delayed the absorption of **doxycycline**, probably because of the presence of acetic acid, which slows gastric emptying. However, the total absorption was not affected. The authors concluded that acute intake of alcoholic beverages has no clinically relevant effects on the pharmacokinetics of **doxycycline**.[3]

Mechanism

Heavy drinkers can metabolise some drugs much more quickly than non-drinkers due to the enzyme-inducing effects of alcohol.[4] The interaction with doxycycline would seem to be due to this effect, possibly allied with some reduction in absorption from the gut.

Importance and management

Information is limited, but the interaction between doxycycline and alcohol appears to be established and of clinical significance in alcoholics but not in non-alcoholic individuals. One possible solution to the problem of enzyme induction is to give alcoholic subjects double the dose of doxycycline,[5] or in some cases tetracycline might be a suitable non-interacting alternative. There is nothing to suggest that moderate or even occasional heavy drinking has a clinically relevant effect on any of the tetracyclines in non-alcoholic subjects.

1. Neuvonen PJ, Penttilä O, Roos M, Tirkkonen J. Effect of long-term alcohol consumption on the half-life of tetracycline and doxycycline in man. *Int J Clin Pharmacol Biopharm* (1976) 14, 303–7.
2. Seitz C, Garcia P, Arancibia A. Influence of ethanol ingestion on tetracycline kinetics. *Int J Clin Pharmacol Ther* (1995) 33, 462–4.
3. Mattila MJ, Laisi U, Linnoila M, Salonen R. Effect of alcoholic beverages on the pharmacokinetics of doxycycline in man. *Acta Pharmacol Toxicol (Copenh)* (1982) 50, 370–3.
4. Misra PS, Lefèvre A, Ishii H, Rubin E, Lieber CS. Increase of ethanol, meprobamate and pentobarbital metabolism after chronic ethanol administration in man and in rats. *Am J Med* (1971) 51, 346–51.
5. Neuvonen PJ, Penttilä O, Lehtovaara R and Aho K. Effect of antiepileptic drugs on the elimination of various tetracycline derivatives. *Eur J Clin Pharmacol* (1975) 9, 147–54.

Alcohol + Thiopurines

Alcohol has been well tolerated in patients taking mercaptopurine. A single case report describes liver toxicity in a patient taking azathioprine, which was attributed to the concurrent use of alcohol.

Clinical evidence, mechanism, importance and management

A study in 207 patients with inflammatory bowel disease assessed (using a phone survey) the presence of adverse reactions to alcohol in patients taking **mercapto-**

purine and/or metronidazole long-term, or neither drug. All of the patients consumed less than 4 alcoholic beverages per day. The proportion of patients experiencing any clinically significant adverse effects was: metronidazole group 16.3%, **mercaptopurine** group 14.5%, control group (not taking either drug) 8.97%. Although there was a trend towards more adverse effects in the drug study groups, this was not statistically significant. The authors suggest a cautious trial of alcohol is advisable in patients that are starting and will be taking either of the medications on a long-term basis.[1]

A case report describes a man taking **azathioprine** for Crohn's disease, who developed peliosis hepatis (liver toxicity) several months after three episodes of excessive alcohol consumption. The patient's liver function returned to normal after stopping **azathioprine**. **Azathioprine** alone is rarely associated with peliosis hepatis, which has been suggested to occur as a result of glutathione depletion. The authors considered that the excessive alcohol intake in this patient led to glutathione depletion, which increased **azathioprine** toxicity, resulting in the liver damage seen.[2] This appears to be an isolated case, but it reinforces the need for cautious alcohol use in patients taking thiopurines.

1. Ginzburg L, Present DH. Alcohol is well tolerated in IBD patients taking either metronidazole or 6-mercaptopurine. *Am J Gastroenterol* (2003) 98 (Suppl), S241.
2. Elsing C, Placke J, Herrmann T. Alcohol binging causes peliosis hepatis during azathioprine therapy in Crohn's disease. *World J Gastroenterol* (2007) 13, 4646–8.

Alcohol + Tianeptine

In one study alcohol reduced the absorption of tianeptine and lowered its plasma levels.

Clinical evidence, mechanism, importance and management

In 12 healthy subjects the absorption and peak plasma levels of a single 12.5-mg dose of tianeptine were reduced by about 30% by alcohol. The subjects were given vodka diluted in orange juice to give blood-alcohol levels of 64 to 77 mg%. The plasma levels of the major metabolite of tianeptine were unchanged.[1] No behavioural studies were done so that the clinical significance of these studies is uncertain; however, the changes reported were small and seem unlikely to be clinically relevant.

1. Salvadori C, Ward C, Defrance R, Hopkins R. The pharmacokinetics of the antidepressant tianeptine and its main metabolite in healthy humans — influence of alcohol co-administration. *Fundam Clin Pharmacol* (1990) 4, 115–25.

Alcohol + Tolazoline

A disulfiram-like reaction might occur in patients taking tolazoline if they drink alcohol.

Clinical evidence, mechanism, importance and management

Seven healthy subjects were given tolazoline 25 mg daily for 4 days. Within 15 to 90 minutes of drinking 90 mL of port wine (alcohol 18.2%), 2 hours after the last dose of tolazoline, 6 experienced tingling over the head, and 4 developed warmth and fullness of the head.[1] The reasons are not understood, but this reaction is not unlike a mild disulfiram reaction, and might have a similar mechanism (see *Mechanism*, under 'Alcohol + Disulfiram', p.67). Patients given tolazoline should be warned about this reaction if they drink alcohol, and advised to limit their consumption. Reactions of this kind with drugs other than disulfiram are usually more unpleasant or frightening than serious, and treatment is rarely needed. In infants given tolazoline, it would seem sensible to avoid preparations containing alcohol, where possible.

1. Boyd EM. A search for drugs with disulfiram-like activity. *Q J Stud Alcohol* (1960) 21, 23–5.

Alcohol + Trazodone

Trazodone impairs performance in some psychomotor tests. Performance can be further impaired if alcohol is also given.

Clinical evidence, mechanism, importance and management

A study in 6 healthy subjects comparing the effects of single-doses of amitriptyline 50 mg and trazodone 100 mg found that both drugs impaired the performance of a number of psychomotor tests, causing drowsiness and reducing 'clearheadedness' to approximately the same extent. Only manual dexterity was further impaired when the subjects taking trazodone were given sufficient alcohol to give blood-alcohol levels of about 40 mg%.[1]

Another study similarly found that the impairment of psychomotor performance by trazodone was increased by alcohol.[2] This appears to be due to simple additive depression of the CNS. This is an established interaction, and of practical importance. Patients should be warned that their ability to drive, handle dangerous machinery or to do other tasks needing complex psychomotor skills might be impaired by trazodone, and further worsened by alcohol.

1. Warrington SJ, Ankier SI, Turner P. Evaluation of possible interactions between ethanol and trazodone or amitriptyline. *Neuropsychobiology* (1986) 15 (Suppl 1), 31–7.
2. Tiller JWG. Antidepressants, alcohol and psychomotor performance. *Acta Psychiatr Scand* (1990) (Suppl 360), 13–17.

Alcohol + Trichloroethylene

A flushing skin reaction similar to a mild disulfiram reaction can occur in those who drink alcohol following exposure to trichloroethylene. Alcohol might also increase the risk of liver toxicity due to trichloroethylene exposure.

Clinical evidence

An engineer from a factory where trichloroethylene was being used as a degreasing agent, developed facial flushing, a sensation of increased pressure in the head, lachrymation, tachypnoea and blurred vision within 12 minutes of drinking 85 mL of bourbon whiskey. The reaction did not develop when he was no longer exposed to trichloroethylene. Other workers in the same plant reported the same experience.[1] Vivid red blotches, in a symmetrical pattern on the face, neck, shoulders and back, were seen in other workers when they drank about 2 pints of beer[2] after having been exposed for a few hours each day for 3 weeks to increasing concentrations of trichloroethylene vapour (up to 200 ppm). Note that this was twice the maximum permissible level for trichloroethylene in air at that time.[3] This reaction has been described as the "degreasers' flush".[2] A later study involving 188 workers occupationally exposed to trichloroethylene found a statistically significant synergistic toxic interaction between trichloroethylene and alcohol. There were 30 cases (15.9%) of degreasers' flush and 10 cases (5.3%) of clinical liver impairment.[4]

There is also some evidence that short-term exposure to the combination might possibly reduce mental capacity, although in this study the concentration of trichloroethylene was quite high (200 ppm).[5]

Another study investigated the metabolism of trichloroethylene in 5 healthy subjects who inhaled trichloroethylene 50 ppm for 6 hours per day for 5 days and then again 2 weeks later in the presence of alcohol. Inhalation of trichloroethylene with blood-alcohol levels of 60 mg% resulted in increased blood and expired air concentrations of trichloroethylene 2 to 3 times greater than without alcohol.[6] A simulation study suggested that drinking moderate amounts of alcohol (0.23 to 0.92 g/kg) before the start of work or at lunchtime, but not at the end of work, could cause pronounced increases in blood-trichloroethylene levels and decreases in the urinary excretion rates of trichloroethylene metabolites. However, when alcohol was consumed the previous evening there was a negligible effect on the metabolism of trichloroethylene (exposure below 100 ppm).[7]

Mechanism

Uncertain. One suggested mechanism is a disulfiram-like inhibition of acetaldehyde metabolism by trichloroethylene (see *Mechanism*, under 'Alcohol + Disulfiram', p.67). Another suggested mechanism is inhibition of trichloroethylene metabolism in the presence of alcohol, resulting in increased plasma levels and possibly an accumulation of trichloroethylene in the CNS.[6]

Importance and management

The flushing reaction that occurs when those exposed to trichloroethylene drink alcohol is an established interaction that has been reported to occur in about 16% of workers who are exposed. It would seem to be more unpleasant and socially disagreeable than serious, and normally requires no treatment. However, the hepatotoxicity of trichloroethylene and other organic solvents might be increased by alcohol; increased body fat has been reported to increase the risk of solvent toxicity and heavy alcohol consumption might further increase the risk of liver toxicity.[8]

1. Pardys S, Brotman M. Trichloroethylene and alcohol: a straight flush. *JAMA* (1974) 229, 521–2.
2. Stewart RD, Hake CL, Peterson JE. "Degreasers' Flush": dermal response to trichloroethylene and ethanol. *Arch Environ Health* (1974) 29, 1–5.
3. Smith GF. Trichloroethylene: a review. *Br J Ind Med* (1966) 23, 249–62.
4. Barret L, Faure J, Guilland B, Chomat D, Didier B, Debru JL. Trichloroethylene occupational exposure: elements for better prevention. *Int Arch Occup Environ Health* (1984) 53, 283–9.
5. Windemuller FJB, Ettema JH. Effects of combined exposure to trichloroethylene and alcohol on mental capacity. *Int Arch Occup Environ Health* (1978) 41, 77–85.
6. Müller G, Spassowski M, Henschler D. Metabolism of trichloroethylene in man. III. Interaction of trichloroethylene and ethanol. *Arch Toxicol* (1975) 33, 173–89.
7. Sato A, Endoh K, Kaneko T, Johanson G. Effects of consumption of ethanol on the biological monitoring of exposure to organic solvent vapours: a simulation study with trichloroethylene. *Br J Ind Med* (1991) 48, 548–56.
8. Brautbar N, Williams J. Industrial solvents and liver toxicity: risk assessment, risk factors and mechanisms. *Int J Hyg Environ Health* (2002) 205, 479–91.

Alcohol + Tricyclic antidepressants

Amitriptyline, and to a lesser extent, doxepin and imipramine impair psychomotor skills, particularly during the first few days of treatment. This impairment can be increased by alcohol. Amoxapine, clomipramine, desipramine, and nortriptyline appear to interact with alcohol only minimally. The toxicity of some tricyclics might be increased by alcohol.

Clinical evidence

(a) Amitriptyline

A single-dose, crossover study in 5 healthy subjects found that the plasma levels of amitriptyline 25 mg over an 8-hour period were increased by alcohol (blood-alcohol level maintained at approximately 80 mg%). Compared with amitriptyline alone, the AUC_{0-8} increased by a mean of 44% following alcohol consumption, and was associated with decreased standing steadiness, recent memory and alertness.[1] Amitriptyline 800 micrograms/kg impaired the performance of three motor skills tests related to driving in 21 healthy subjects. When alcohol, to produce blood levels of about 80 mg%, was also given the performance was even further impaired.[2] Similar results have been clearly demonstrated in considerable numbers of subjects using a variety of psychomotor skill tests,[1-6] the interaction being most marked during the first few days of treatment, but tending to wane as treatment continues.[5] Unexplained blackouts lasting a few hours have been described in 3 women who had been taking amitriptyline or imipramine for a month after they drank only modest amounts of alcohol.[7]

A study involving 332 fatal poisonings in Finland found that alcohol was present in 67% of cases involving amitriptyline, and when alcohol was present, relatively small overdoses of amitriptyline could result in fatal poisoning.[8] It appears that amitriptyline might be more toxic when given with alcohol, and it has been suggested that a less dangerous alternative could be chosen when indications of alcohol abuse or suicide risk are present.[9]

(b) Amoxapine

The interaction between amoxapine and alcohol affecting psychomotor skills is said to be slight,[10] but two patients experienced reversible extrapyramidal symptoms (parkinsonism, akathisia) while taking amoxapine, which was apparently caused by drinking alcohol.[11]

(c) Clomipramine

Studies in subjects with blood-alcohol levels of 40 to 60 mg% found that clomipramine had only slight or no effect on various choice reaction, coordination, memory and learning tests.[4,12,13] A case describes a fatal poisoning in a chronic alcoholic patient taking clomipramine for depression. The ultimate toxic effect was thought to be due to alcohol-induced decreased biotransformation of clomipramine, as post-mortem examination revealed toxic liver damage, and low levels of the metabolite were found in blood and hair samples.[14]

(d) Desipramine

Plasma desipramine levels were transiently, but not significantly increased after healthy subjects drank alcohol, and breath-alcohol concentrations were not affected by desipramine. Further, skilled performance tests in subjects given desipramine 100 mg indicated that no notable interaction occurred with alcohol.[15]

(e) Doxepin

A placebo-controlled, crossover study in 20 healthy subjects given various combinations of alcohol and doxepin found that with blood-alcohol levels of 40 to 50 mg% their choice reaction test times were prolonged and the number of mistakes increased. Coordination was obviously impaired after 7 days of treatment with doxepin, but not after 14 days.[4] In an earlier study doxepin appeared to cancel out the deleterious effects of alcohol on the performance of a simulated driving test.[16] It appears that doxepin might be more toxic when given with alcohol, and it has been suggested that a less dangerous alternative could be chosen when indications of alcohol abuse or suicide risk are present.[9]

(f) Imipramine

Imipramine 150 mg daily has been reported to enhance some of the hypno-sedative effects of alcohol,[17] and unexplained blackouts lasting a few hours have been described in 3 women who had been taking amitriptyline or imipramine for only a month after they drank only modest amounts of alcohol.[7]

(g) Nortriptyline

Studies in subjects with blood-alcohol levels of 40 to 60 mg% found that nortriptyline had only slight or no effects on various choice reaction, coordination, memory and learning tests,[4,12,18] although the acute use of alcohol with nortriptyline impaired learning in one study.[12]

Mechanism

Part of the explanation for the increased CNS depression is that both alcohol and some of the tricyclics, particularly amitriptyline, cause drowsiness and other CNS depressant effects, which can be additive with the effects of alcohol.[6] The sedative effects have been reported to be greatest with amitriptyline, then doxepin and imipramine, followed by nortriptyline, and least with amoxapine, clomipramine, desipramine, and **protriptyline**.[19-22] In addition acute alcohol intake causes increases (of 100 to 200%) in the plasma levels of amitriptyline, probably by inhibiting its first-pass metabolism.[1,23] Alcohol-induced liver damage could also result in impaired amitriptyline metabolism.[21]

Importance and management

Increased CNS depression resulting from the interaction between amitriptyline and alcohol is well documented and clinically important. The interaction between alcohol and doxepin or imipramine is less well documented and the information is conflicting. Amoxapine, clomipramine, desipramine, and nortriptyline appear to interact only minimally with alcohol. Direct information about other tricyclics seems to be lacking, but there appear to be no particular reasons for avoiding concurrent use, although tricyclics with greater sedative effects, such as **trimipramine**, seem more likely to interact. During the first 1 to 2 weeks of treatment many tricyclics (without alcohol) can temporarily impair the skills related to driving.[10] Therefore it would seem prudent to warn any patient given a tricyclic that driving or handling dangerous machinery might be made more hazardous if they drink alcohol, particularly during the first few days of treatment, but the effects of the interaction diminish during continued use. Most manufacturers of tricyclic antidepressants warn that the effects of alcohol may be enhanced by tricyclics and several suggest avoiding the concurrent use of alcohol.

1. Dorian P, Sellers EM, Reed KL, Warsh JJ, Hamilton C, Kaplan HL, Fan T. Amitriptyline and ethanol: pharmacokinetic and pharmacodynamic interaction. *Eur J Clin Pharmacol* (1983) 25, 325–31.
2. Landauer AA, Milner G, Patman J. Alcohol and amitriptyline effects on skills related to driving behavior. *Science* (1969) 163, 1467–8.
3. Seppälä T. Psychomotor skills during acute and two-week treatment with mianserin (ORG GB 94) and amitriptyline, and their combined effects with alcohol. *Ann Clin Res* (1977) 9, 66–72.
4. Seppälä T, Linnoila M, Elonen E, Mattila MJ, Mäki M. Effect of tricyclic antidepressants and alcohol on psychomotor skills related to driving. *Clin Pharmacol Ther* (1975) 17, 515–22.
5. Seppälä T, Strömberg C, Bergman I. Effects of zimeldine, mianserin and amitriptyline on psychomotor skills and their interaction with ethanol: a placebo controlled cross-over study. *Eur J Clin Pharmacol* (1984) 27, 181–9.
6. Scott DB, Fagan D, Tiplady B. Effects of amitriptyline and zimelidine in combination with alcohol. *Psychopharmacology (Berl)* (1982) 76, 209–11.
7. Hudson CJ. Tricyclic antidepressants and alcoholic blackouts. *J Nerv Ment Dis* (1981) 169, 381–2.
8. Koski A, Vuori E, Ojanperä I. Relation of postmortem blood alcohol and drug concentrations in fatal poisonings involving amitriptyline, propoxyphene and promazine. *Hum Exp Toxicol* (2005) 24, 389–96.
9. Koski A, Ojanperä I, Vuori E. Interaction of alcohol and drugs in fatal poisonings. *Hum Exp Toxicol* (2003) 22, 281–7.
10. Wilson WH, Petrie WM, Ban TA, Barry DE. The effects of amoxapine and ethanol on psychomotor skills related to driving: a placebo and standard controlled study. *Prog Neuropsychopharmacol* (1981) 5, 263–70.
11. Shen WW. Alcohol, amoxapine, and akathisia. *Biol Psychiatry* (1984) 19, 929–30.
12. Liljequist R, Linnoila M, Mattila M. Effect of two weeks' treatment with chlorimipramine and nortriptyline, alone or in combination with alcohol, on learning and memory. *Psychopharmacologia* (1974) 39, 181–6.
13. Berlin I, Cournot A, Zimmer R, Pedarriosse A-M, Manfredi R, Molinier P, Puech AJ. Evaluation and comparison of the interaction between alcohol and moclobemide or clomipramine in healthy subjects. *Psychopharmacology (Berl)* (1990) 100, 40–5.
14. Kłys M, Ścisłowski M, Rojek S, Kołodziej J. A fatal clomipramine intoxication case of a chronic alcoholic patient: application of postmortem hair analysis method of clomipramine and ethyl glucuronide using LC/APCI/MS. *Leg Med* (2005) 7, 319–25.
15. Linnoila M, Johnson J, Dubyoski K, Buchsbaum MS, Schneinin M, Kilts C. Effects of antidepressants on skilled performance. *Br J Clin Pharmacol* (1984) 18, 109S–120S.
16. Milner G, Landauer AA. The effects of doxepin, alone and together with alcohol, in relation to driving safety. *Med J Aust* (1973) 1, 837–41.
17. Frewer LJ, Lader M. The effects of nefazodone, imipramine and placebo, alone and combined with alcohol, in normal subjects. *Int Clin Psychopharmacol* (1993) 8, 13–20.
18. Hughes FW, Forney RB. Delayed audiofeedback (DAF) for induction of anxiety: effect of nortriptyline, ethanol, or nortriptyline-ethanol combinations on performance with DAF. *JAMA* (1963) 185, 556–8.
19. Marco LA, Randels RM. Drug interactions in alcoholic patients. *Hillside J Clin Psychiatry* (1981) 3, 27–44.
20. Linnoila M, Seppala T. Antidepressants and driving. *Accid Anal Prev* (1985) 17, 297–301.
21. Weathermon R, Crabb DW. Alcohol and medication interactions. *Alcohol Res Health* (1999) 23, 40–54.
22. Weller RA, Preskorn SH. Psychotropic drugs and alcohol: pharmacokinetic and pharmacodynamic interactions. *Psychosomatics* (1984) 25, 301–3, 305–6, 309.
23. Fraser AG. Pharmacokinetic interactions between alcohol and other drugs. *Clin Pharmacokinet* (1997) 33, 79–90.

Alcohol + Trinitrotoluene

Men exposed to trinitrotoluene (TNT) in a munitions factory were found to have a greater risk of TNT-induced liver damage if they had a long history of heavy alcohol drinking than if they were non-drinkers.[1]

1. Li J, Jiang Q-G, Zhong W-D. Persistent ethanol drinking increases liver injury induced by trinitrotoluene exposure: an in-plant case-control study. *Hum Exp Toxicol* (1991) 10, 405–9.

Alcohol + Triptans

Alcohol does not appear to alter the pharmacokinetics of almotriptan, frovatriptan, naratriptan or sumatriptan.

Clinical evidence, mechanism, importance and management

In a study in 16 healthy subjects, the rate and extent of exposure to a single 12.5-mg dose of **almotriptan** was not altered when it was given 30 minutes after alcohol (dose targeted to achieve plasma levels of 0.8 g/kg).[1]

In a retrospective analysis of data from 178 healthy subjects involved in phase I studies, alcohol consumption did not affect the pharmacokinetics of **frovatriptan**.[2]

In a study in 16 healthy subjects, the pharmacokinetics of a single 5-mg dose of **naratriptan** were not altered when it was given 30 minutes after alcohol (amount not specified).[3]

A single 0.8-g/kg dose of alcohol was given to 16 healthy subjects, followed 30 minutes later by 200 mg of **sumatriptan**. No statistically significant changes were seen in the pharmacokinetics of **sumatriptan**.[4]

There is nothing to suggest that alcohol needs to be avoided in patients taking **almotriptan**, **frovatriptan**, **naratriptan** or **sumatriptan**.

1. Cabarrocas X, Salva M, Pavesi M, Costa J. Ethanol does not significantly affect the bioavailability of almotriptan: an open randomized, crossover, single-dose, phase I clinical trial in healthy volunteers. *Int J Clin Pharmacol Ther* (2006) 44, 443–8.
2. Buchan P, Wade A, Ward C, Oliver SD, Stewart AJ, Freestone S. Frovatriptan: a review of drug-drug interactions. *Headache* (2002) 42 (Suppl 2), S63–S73.
3. GlaxoSmithKline. Data on file. A study to investigate whether alcohol has an effect on the safety, tolerability, pharmacokinetics or pharmacodynamics of GR85548 (Study C93-087). 1994. Available at: http://www.gsk-clinicalstudyregister.com/ (accessed 21/10/15).
4. Kempsford RD, Lacey LF, Thomas M, Fowler PA. The effect of alcohol on the pharmacokinetic profile of oral sumatriptan. *Fundam Clin Pharmacol* (1991) 5, 470.

Alcohol + Vitamin A (Retinol)

Heavy consumption of alcohol might increase betacarotene levels and affect vitamin A metabolism; there have been reports of possible increased toxicity.

Clinical evidence, mechanism, importance and management

A study involving 30 abstinent male alcoholics found that 5 of 15 given high-dose vitamin A (10 000 units daily by mouth) for 4 months developed liver abnormalities during treatment, compared with 1 of 15 patients given placebo. Two of the 6 patients admitted intermittent alcohol consumption. Five of these patients continued with vitamin A and in 4 of these patients the abnormal liver function tests resolved.[1]

The interaction between alcohol and vitamin A is complex. They have overlapping metabolic pathways; a similar 2-step process is involved in the metabolism of both alcohol and vitamin A, with alcohol dehydrogenases and acetaldehyde dehydrogenases being implicated in the conversion of vitamin A to retinoic acid.[2,3] Alcohol appears to act as a competitive inhibitor of vitamin A oxidation.[2,4] In addition, chronic alcohol intake can induce cytochrome P450 isoenzymes that appear to increase the breakdown of vitamin A (retinol and retinoic acid) into more polar metabolites in the liver, which can cause hepatocyte death. Chronic alcohol consumption might therefore enhance the intrinsic hepatotoxicity of high-dose vitamin A. Alcohol has also been shown to alter retinoid homoeostasis by increasing vitamin A mobilisation from the liver to extrahepatic tissues, which could result in depletion of hepatic stores of vitamin A.[2,3]

It appears that consumption of substantial amounts of alcohol is associated with vitamin A deficiency partially due to poor nutrition and also the direct effects of alcohol on the metabolism of vitamin A. Vitamin A supplementation might therefore be indicated in heavy drinkers, but is complicated by the hepatotoxicity associated with large amounts of vitamin A, which might be potentiated by alcohol.[3] It would therefore seem reasonable to try to control alcohol consumption when vitamin A supplementation is required. Patients who consume alcohol, particularly heavy drinkers or alcoholics, should be questioned about their use of vitamin supplements as some non-prescription vitamin A and D supplements contain substantial amounts of vitamin A.

1. Worner TM, Gordon GG, Leo MA, Lieber CS. Vitamin A treatment of sexual dysfunction in male alcoholics. *Am J Clin Nutr* (1988) 48, 1431–5.
2. Wang X-D. Alcohol, vitamin A, and cancer. *Alcohol* (2005) 35, 251–8.
3. Leo MA, Lieber CS. Alcohol, vitamin A, and ß-carotene: adverse interactions, including hepatotoxicity and carcinogenicity. *Am J Clin Nutr* (1999) 69, 1071–85.
4. Crabb DW, Pinairs J, Hasanadka R, Fang M, Leo MA, Lieber CS, Tsukamoto H, Motomura K, Miyahara T, Ohata M, Bosron W, Sanghani S, Kedishvili N, Shiraishi H, Yokoyama H, Miyagi M, Ishii H, Bergheim I, Menzl I, Parlesak A, Bode C. Alcohol and retinoids. *Alcohol Clin Exp Res* (2001) 25 (5 Suppl ISBRA), 207S–217S.

Alcohol + Xylene

Some individuals exposed to xylene vapour, who subsequently drink alcohol, might experience dizziness and nausea. A flushing skin reaction has also been seen.

Clinical evidence, mechanism, importance and management

Studies in subjects exposed to *m*-xylene vapour at concentrations of approximately 145 or 280 ppm for 4 hours who were then given 0.4 or 0.8 g/kg of alcohol found that about 10 to 20% experienced dizziness and nausea.[1,2] One subject exposed to 300 ppm of *m*-xylene vapour developed a conspicuous dermal flush on his face, neck, chest and back. He also developed some erythema with alcohol alone.[3] A study using a population-based pharmacokinetic and pharmacodynamic model predicted that the probability of experiencing CNS effects following exposure to xylene at the current UK occupational exposure standard (100 ppm time-weighted average over 8 hours) increased markedly with alcohol dose; the effects were non-linear.[4]

The reasons for these reactions are not fully understood, but it is possible that xylene plasma levels are increased because alcohol impairs its metabolic clearance by CYP2E1.[4] After alcohol intake, blood-xylene levels have been reported to rise by about 50 to 100%;[2] acetaldehyde levels might also be transiently increased.[2]

Alcoholic beverages are quite often consumed during lunchtime or after work, and as the excretion of xylene is delayed by its high solubility and storage in lipid-rich tissues, the simultaneous presence of xylene and alcohol in the body is probably not uncommon and could result in enhancement of the toxicity of xylene.[5]

1. Savolainen K, Riihimäki V, Vaheri E, Linnoila M. Effects of xylene and alcohol on vestibular and visual functions in man. *Scand J Work Environ Health* (1980) 6, 94–103.
2. Riihimäki V, Savolainen K, Pfäffli P, Pekari K, Sippel HW, Laine A. Metabolic interaction between m-xylene and ethanol. *Arch Toxicol* (1982) 49, 253–63.
3. Riihimäki V, Laine A, Savolainen K, Sippel H. Acute solvent-ethanol interactions with special reference to xylene. *Scand J Work Environ Health* (1982) 8, 77–9.
4. MacDonald AJ, Rostami-Hodjegan A, Tucker GT, Linkens DA. Analysis of solvent central nervous system toxicity and ethanol interactions using a human population physiologically based kinetic and dynamic model. *Regul Toxicol Pharmacol* (2002) 35, 165–76.
5. Lieber CS. Microsomal ethanol-oxidizing system. *Enzyme* (1987) 37, 45–56.

4

Alpha blockers

The term alpha blockers covers a range of drugs, but for the purposes of this section it is primarily used to describe the selective alpha blockers that are mainly used for managing hypertension and benign prostatic hyperplasia. Other drugs that have alpha-blocking actions are covered elsewhere in this publication. The selective and non-selective alpha blockers are categorised and listed in 'Table 4.1', below.

The principal interactions of the alpha blockers are those relating to enhanced hypotensive effects. Early after the introduction of the selective alpha blockers it was discovered that, in some individuals, they can cause a rapid reduction in blood pressure on starting treatment (also called the 'first-dose effect' or 'first-dose hypotension'). The risk of this might be higher in patients already taking other antihypertensive drugs. A similar hypotensive effect can occur when the dose of the alpha blocker is increased, or if treatment is interrupted for a few days and then re-introduced.

The first-dose effect has been minimised by starting with a very low dose of the alpha blocker, and then escalating the dose slowly over a couple of weeks. Some manufacturers recommend giving the first dose on retiring to bed, or if not, avoiding tasks that are potentially hazardous if syncope occurs (such as driving) for the first 12 hours. If symptoms such as dizziness, fatigue, or sweating develop, patients should be warned to lie down, and to remain lying flat until they abate completely.

It is unclear whether there are any real differences between the alpha blockers in their propensity to cause this first-dose effect. However, tamsulosin is reported to have some selectivity for the alpha receptor 1A subtype, which are found mostly in the prostate and so have less effect on blood pressure: an initial titration of the dose is therefore not considered to be necessary. Nevertheless, it would be prudent to exercise caution with all the drugs in this class.

Other alpha blockers are also used to increase urinary flow-rate and improve obstructive symptoms in benign prostatic hyperplasia. In this setting, their effects on blood pressure are more of an adverse effect, and their additive hypotensive effect with other antihypertensives might not be beneficial.

Some alpha blockers (e.g. alfuzosin, doxazosin, silodosin, tamsulosin) are in part metabolised by the cytochrome P450 isoenzyme system, particularly by CYP3A4, and therefore potent CYP3A4 inhibitors might increase their exposure, see 'Alpha blockers + Ketoconazole and other CYP3A4 inhibitors', p.93. Some alpha blockers form conjugates and the potential for interactions with drugs that inhibit glucuronidation has been noted for silodosin, see 'Alpha blockers + Miscellaneous', p.94.

Drowsiness or increased somnolence has been reported as an adverse effect of many alpha blockers. However, with the exception of indoramin (see 'Alcohol + Alpha blockers', p.53), there appear to be no reports of alpha blocker interactions associated with additive CNS depressant effects. This is probably because sedation occurs more frequently with indoramin than with other alpha blockers and is one of its commonest adverse effects.

Table 4.1 Alpha blockers

Drug	*Principal indications*
Selective $alpha_1$ blockers (Alpha blockers)	
Alfuzosin	BPH
Bunazosin	Hypertension
Doxazosin	BPH; Hypertension
Indoramin	BPH; Hypertension; Migraine
Prazosin	BPH; Heart failure; Hypertension; Raynaud's syndrome
Silodosin	BPH
Tamsulosin	BPH
Terazosin	BPH; Hypertension
Other drugs with alpha-blocking actions	
Moxisylyte	Peripheral vascular disease; Erectile dysfunction
Phenoxybenzamine	Hypertensive episodes in phaeochromocytoma
Tolazoline	Peripheral vascular disease; Pulmonary hypertension
Phentolamine	Erectile dysfunction; Hypertensive episodes in phaeochromocytoma
Urapidil	Hypertension

Alpha blockers + ACE inhibitors or Angiotensin II receptor antagonists

The first-dose effect seen with alpha blockers (particularly alfuzosin, prazosin, and terazosin) is likely to be potentiated by ACE inhibitors and probably angiotensin II receptor antagonists. There is no pharmacokinetic interaction between doxazosin and enalapril, and the hypotensive effects appear to be additive. In one small study tamsulosin did not have any clinically relevant effects on blood pressure that was already well controlled by enalapril.

Clinical evidence

(a) Bunazosin

A patient taking **enalapril** developed severe first-dose hypotension after being given bunazosin, resulting in this interaction being further studied in 6 healthy subjects. When **enalapril** 10 mg or bunazosin 2 mg was given, the mean blood pressure over 6 hours was reduced by 9.5/6.7 mmHg. When bunazosin was given one hour after **enalapril** the blood pressure fell by 27/28 mmHg. Blood pressure still fell (by 19/22 mmHg) even when the dose of **enalapril** was reduced to 2.5 mg.[1]

(b) Doxazosin

In a study in 12 healthy normotensive subjects given either **enalapril** 10 mg daily or doxazosin 1 mg daily, the pharmacokinetics of both drugs were not affected during steady-state administration of the second drug. The antihypertensive effects of the drugs in normotensive subjects were additive.[2] For comment that doxazosin appeared to have less effect on blood pressure in patients with BPH receiving ACE inhibitors than in those taking beta blockers or diuretics, see 'Alpha blockers + Beta blockers', below.

(c) Tamsulosin

In a placebo-controlled study in 6 hypertensive men with blood pressure well controlled by **enalapril**, the addition of tamsulosin 400 micrograms daily for 7 days, then 800 micrograms daily for a further 7 days, had no clinically relevant effects on blood pressure (assessed after 6 and 14 days of tamsulosin). In addition, no first-dose hypotensive effect was seen on the day tamsulosin was started, or on the day the tamsulosin dose was increased.[3]

(d) Terazosin

Retrospective analysis of a large multinational study in patients with BPH given terazosin 5 or 10 mg daily found that terazosin only affected the blood pressure of patients taking ACE inhibitors (**enalapril**, **lisinopril**, or **perindopril**) if the blood pressure was uncontrolled. No change in blood pressure was seen in those with normal blood pressure (i.e. those without hypertension and those with hypertension controlled by ACE inhibitors). The most common adverse effect in the 10-week terazosin phase was dizziness, and the incidence of this appeared to be lower in those taking antihypertensives (13 to 16%) than in those not taking antihypertensives (21 to 25%).[4] Similarly, another, subsequent retrospective analysis found that terazosin did not affect the blood pressure of hypertensive men whose blood pressure was controlled with an ACE inhibitor.[5] However, the UK manufacturer of terazosin notes that the incidence of dizziness in patients taking terazosin was higher when they were also receiving an ACE inhibitor.[6]

Mechanism

The first-dose effect of alpha blockers (see 'Alpha blockers', p.89) might be potentiated by ACE inhibitors. Tamsulosin possibly has less effect on blood pressure since it has some selectivity for alpha receptors in the prostate.

Importance and management

Direct information about the interaction between alpha blockers and ACE inhibitors is limited, but what is known is in line with the way alpha blockers interact with other antihypertensive drugs. Acute hypotension (dizziness, fainting) sometimes occurs unpredictably with the first dose of some alpha blockers, particularly, alfuzosin, prazosin, and terazosin; but there is insufficient evidence to suggest that the alpha blockers differ in their propensity to cause this effect. Note that the acute hypotensive reaction appears to be short-lived.

When starting an alpha blocker it is often recommended that those already taking an antihypertensive should have their dose reduced to a maintenance level, while initiating the alpha blocker at a low dose, with the first dose taken just before going to bed. Patients should also be warned about the possibility of postural hypotension and how to manage it (i.e. lay down, raise the legs, and, when recovered, get up slowly). Similarly, when adding an antihypertensive to an alpha blocker, it might be prudent to decrease the dose of the alpha blocker and re-titrate as necessary.

There is limited evidence that tamsulosin and possibly terazosin might not cause an additional hypotensive effect when given in the longer term in patients with BPH who have hypertension already well controlled with ACE inhibitors. Nevertheless, caution should be exercised in this situation, and a dose reduction of the ACE inhibitor might be required.

Angiotensin II receptor antagonists would be expected to interact in the same way as ACE inhibitors. Some manufacturers of angiotensin II receptor antagonists state that enhanced hypotensive effects can occur with other antihypertensive drugs, but alpha blockers do not appear to be specifically mentioned.

1. Baba T, Tomiyama T, Takebe K. Enhancement by an ACE inhibitor of first-dose hypotension caused by an alpha$_1$-blocker. *N Engl J Med* (1990) 322, 1237.
2. Bainbridge AD, Meredith PA, Elliott HL. A clinical pharmacological assessment of doxazosin and enalapril in combination. *Br J Clin Pharmacol* (1993) 36, 599–602.
3. Lowe FC. Coadministration of tamsulosin and three antihypertensive agents in patients with benign prostatic hyperplasia: pharmacodynamic effect. *Clin Ther* (1997) 19, 730–42.
4. Kirby RS. Terazosin in benign prostatic hyperplasia: effects on blood pressure in normotensive and hypertensive men. *Br J Urol* (1998) 82, 373–9.
5. Lowe F, Olson PJ, Padley RJ. Effects of terazosin therapy on blood pressure in men with benign prostatic hyperplasia concurrently treated with other antihypertensive medications. *Urology* (1999) 54, 81–5.
6. Hytrin (Terazosin monohydrochloride dihydrate). Amdipharm Mercury Company Ltd. UK Summary of product characteristics, June 2009.

Alpha blockers + Aspirin or NSAIDs

Indometacin reduces the blood pressure lowering effects of prazosin in some individuals. However, indometacin does not appear to interact adversely with other alpha blockers.

Clinical evidence

(a) Doxazosin

The UK manufacturer of doxazosin states that it has been given without any evidence of adverse interaction to patients taking NSAIDs.[1]

(b) Prazosin

A study in 9 healthy subjects found that **indometacin** 50 mg twice daily for 3 days had no statistically significant effect on the hypotensive effect of a single 5-mg dose of prazosin. However, in 4 subjects it was noted that the maximum fall in the mean standing blood pressure due to prazosin was 20 mmHg less when they were taking **indometacin**. Three of these 4 felt faint when given prazosin alone, but not while they were also taking **indometacin**.[2] The manufacturer states that prazosin has, in clinical experience, been given with **indometacin** (and also **aspirin** and **phenylbutazone**) without any adverse interaction.[3]

(c) Terazosin

The UK manufacturer of terazosin states that no adverse interactions have been reported between terazosin and analgesics/anti-inflammatories.[4]

Mechanism

Not established. It seems probable that indometacin inhibits the production of hypotensive prostaglandins by the kidney, resulting in an increase in blood pressure in some cases and reducing the hypotensive effect of prazosin.

Importance and management

Information about the interactions between alpha blockers and NSAIDs or aspirin appears to be limited, but the general picture suggests that no interaction of clinical importance occurs. A possible exception is the use of indometacin with prazosin, which is consistent with the way indometacin reduces the effects of many other different antihypertensives (e.g. see 'ACE inhibitors + NSAIDs', p.38, and 'Beta blockers + Aspirin or NSAIDs', p.1003). This interaction apparently does not affect every patient. If indometacin is added to established treatment with prazosin, be alert for a reduced antihypertensive response. It is not known exactly what happens in patients taking both drugs long-term, but note that with other interactions between antihypertensives and NSAIDs the effects seem to be modest.

1. Cardura XL (Doxazosin mesilate). Pfizer Ltd. UK Summary of product characteristics, August 2012.
2. Rubin P, Jackson G, Blaschke T. Studies on the clinical pharmacology of prazosin. II: The influence of indomethacin and of propranolol on the action and disposition of prazosin. *Br J Clin Pharmacol* (1980) 10, 33–9.
3. Hypovase (Prazosin hydrochloride). Pfizer Ltd. UK Summary of product characteristics, June 2009.
4. Hytrin (Terazosin monohydrochloride dihydrate). Amdipharm Mercury Company Ltd. UK Summary of product characteristics, June 2009.

Alpha blockers + Beta blockers

The risk of first-dose hypotension with prazosin is higher if the patient is already taking a beta blocker. This is also likely to be true of other alpha blockers, particularly alfuzosin and terazosin. Alpha blockers and beta blockers can be given together for additional lowering of blood pressure in patients with hypertension, and studies with patients taking beta blockers suggest that silodosin or tamsulosin can be used concurrently without adverse effects on blood pressure.

Clinical evidence

(a) Alfuzosin

In a single-dose study in 8 healthy subjects no pharmacokinetic interaction occurred when alfuzosin 2.5 mg was given with **atenolol** 100 mg.[1] However, the manufacturer reports that, in a similar study, **atenolol** increased the maximum plasma concentration and AUC of alfuzosin by 28% and 21%, respectively, and alfuzosin increased atenolol concentrations by 26% and 14%, respectively. There were also significant reductions in mean blood pressure and heart rate,[2] but these were not quantified.

(b) Doxazosin

A study involving 2 363 patients, with hypertension controlled with a single antihypertensive drug, investigated the effects of adding doxazosin for BPH. The dose of doxazosin was increased gradually to 4 mg daily and then the patients were monitored for 14 weeks. The addition of doxazosin was found to be well tolerated, and adverse effects mainly occurred early after the onset of treatment or in patients with lower systolic and diastolic blood pressure. However, the antihypertensive effect was more marked in patients taking beta blockers or diuretics than in patients taking ACE inhibitors or calcium-channel blockers.[3] The UK and US manufacturers of doxazosin state that no adverse drug interaction has been observed between doxazosin and beta blockers,[4,5] although they do note that the most common adverse reactions associated with doxazosin are of a postural hypotension type.[4]

(c) Prazosin

A marked hypotensive reaction (dizziness, pallor, sweating) occurred in 3 out of 6 hypertensive patients taking **alprenolol** 400 mg twice daily when they were given the first 500-microgram dose of prazosin. In all 6 patients the reduction in blood pressure was greater after the first prazosin dose than after 2 weeks of treatment with prazosin 500 micrograms three times daily with no beta blocker (mean reduction 22/11 mmHg compared with 4/4 mmHg). A further 3 patients already taking prazosin 500 micrograms three times daily had no unusual decrease in blood pressure when they were given a 200-mg dose of **alprenolol**.[6] The severity and the duration of the first-dose effect of prazosin were also found to be increased in healthy subjects given a single dose of **propranolol**.[7]

Two studies have shown that the pharmacokinetics of prazosin are not affected by either **alprenolol**[6] or **propranolol**.[8]

(d) Silodosin

In a crossover study, 24 healthy subjects were given either a single 8-mg dose of silodosin, or placebo, with a single 50-mg dose of metoprolol. There was no clinically relevant effect on orthostatic blood pressure or heart rate on concurrent use.[9]

(e) Tamsulosin

In a placebo-controlled study in 8 men with hypertension well controlled by **atenolol**, the addition of tamsulosin 400 micrograms daily for 7 days, then 800 micrograms daily for a further 7 days, had no clinically relevant effect on blood pressure (assessed after 6 and 14 days of tamsulosin). No hypotension was seen with the first dose of tamsulosin or when the dose of tamsulosin was increased.[10]

(f) Terazosin

Retrospective analysis of a large multinational study, in patients with BPH given terazosin 5 or 10 mg daily, found that terazosin only affected the blood pressure of patients taking beta blockers (**atenolol**, **labetalol**, **metoprolol**, **sotalol**, and **timolol**) if the blood pressure was uncontrolled. No change in blood pressure was seen in those with normal blood pressure (i.e. those without hypertension and those with hypertension controlled by beta blockers). The most common adverse effect in the 10-week terazosin phase was dizziness, and the incidence of this appeared to be lower in those taking antihypertensives (13 to 16%) than in those not taking antihypertensives (21 to 25%).[11] Another retrospective analysis similarly found a statistically significant decrease in both systolic and diastolic blood pressure when patients with hypertension controlled by a beta blocker were given terazosin for BPH.[12]

Mechanism

The normal cardiovascular response (a compensatory increase in cardiac output and heart rate) that should follow the first-dose hypotensive reaction to alpha blockers is apparently compromised by the presence of a beta blocker. The problem is usually only short lasting because some physiological compensation occurs within hours or days, and this allows the blood pressure to be lowered without falling precipitously. Tamsulosin possibly has less effect on blood pressure because it has some selectivity for alpha receptors in the prostate.

Importance and management

The interaction between the alpha blockers and the beta blockers is established. Some patients experience acute postural hypotension, tachycardia, and palpitations when they begin to take prazosin or other alpha blockers. A few patients even collapse in a sudden faint within 30 to 90 minutes, and this can be exacerbated if they are already taking a beta blocker. The evidence seems to suggest that this is greater with alfuzosin and terazosin, but it is unclear whether there are any real differences between the alpha blockers in their propensity to cause these effects.

In general, when starting an alpha blocker it is recommended that those already taking a beta blocker should have their dose of the beta blocker reduced to a maintenance dose and begin with a low dose of the alpha blocker, with the first dose taken just before going to bed. They should also be warned about the possibility of postural hypotension and how to manage it (i.e. lay down, raise the legs, and, when recovered, get up slowly). Similarly, when adding a beta blocker to an alpha blocker, it might be prudent to decrease the dose of the alpha blocker and re-titrate as necessary. There is limited evidence that tamsulosin and possibly terazosin might not cause an additional hypotensive effect when taken long term by patients with BPH who have hypertension already well controlled with beta blockers. Nevertheless, caution should be exercised in this situation, and a dose reduction of the beta blocker might still be required.

1. Bianchetti G, Padovani P, Coupez JM, Guinebault P, Hermanns P, Coupez-Lopinot R, Guillet P, Thénot JP, Morselli PL. Pharmacokinetic interactions between hydrochlorothiazide, atenolol, and alfuzosin: a new antihypertensive drug. *Acta Pharmacol Toxicol (Copenh)* (1986) 59 (Suppl 5), 197.
2. Uroxatral (Alfuzosin hydrochloride extended-release tablets). Sanofi-Aventis US LLC. US Prescribing information, October 2011.
3. Martell N, Luque M, on behalf of the HT-BPH Group. Doxazosin added to single-drug therapy in hypertensive patients with benign prostatic hypertrophy. *J Clin Hypertens* (2001) 3, 218–23.
4. Cardura XL (Doxazosin mesilate). Pfizer Ltd. UK Summary of product characteristics, August 2012.
5. Cardura (Doxazosin mesylate). Pfizer Inc. US Prescribing information, November 2013.
6. Seideman P, Grahnén A, Haglund K, Lindström B, von Bahr C. Prazosin first dose phenomenon during combined treatment with a β-adrenoceptor in hypertensive patients. *Br J Clin Pharmacol* (1982) 13, 865–70.
7. Elliott HL, McLean K, Sumner DJ, Meredith PA, Reid JL. Immediate cardiovascular reponses to oral prazosin—effects of concurrent β-blockers. *Clin Pharmacol Ther* (1981) 29, 303–9.
8. Rubin P, Jackson G, Blaschke T. Studies on the clinical pharmacology of prazosin. II: The influence of indomethacin and of propranolol on the action and the disposition of prazosin. *Br J Clin Pharmacol* (1980) 10, 33–9.
9. Vargas R, Olsen S, Thomas H, Dahl NV. Pharmacodynamic interaction of the unique alpha-1A-adrenoceptor antagonist silodosin and the antihypertensive agent metoprolol. *Clin Pharmacol Ther* (2010) 87, S14.
10. Lowe FC. Coadministration of tamsulosin and three antihypertensive agents in patients with benign prostatic hyperplasia: pharmacodynamic effect. *Clin Ther* (1997) 19, 730–42.
11. Kirby RS. Terazosin in benign prostatic hyperplasia: effects on blood pressure in normotensive and hypertensive men. *Br J Urol* (1998) 82, 373–9.
12. Lowe F, Olson PJ, Padley RJ. Effects of terazosin therapy on blood pressure in men with benign prostatic hyperplasia concurrently treated with other antihypertensive medications. *Urology* (1999) 54, 81–5.

Alpha blockers + Calcium-channel blockers

Alpha blockers and calcium-channel blockers can be given together for additional blood pressure lowering in patients with hypertension. Blood pressure might decrease sharply when calcium-channel blockers are first given to patients already taking alpha blockers (particularly prazosin and terazosin), and *vice versa*. In a small study, tamsulosin did not have any clinically relevant effects on blood pressure well controlled by nifedipine. Verapamil might increase the exposure to prazosin and terazosin, and might also increase the adverse effects related to tamsulosin. The concurrent use of diltiazem and alfuzosin can increase the concentrations of both drugs.

Clinical evidence

(a) Alfuzosin

The US manufacturer of alfuzosin notes that when **diltiazem** 240 mg daily was given with alfuzosin 2.5 mg three times daily, the maximum serum concentrations and AUC of alfuzosin were increased by 50% and 30%, respectively, and the maximum serum concentrations and AUC of **diltiazem** were increased by 40%. However, no changes in blood pressure were seen.[1]

(b) Doxazosin

In a study, 6 normotensive subjects were given **nifedipine** 20 mg twice daily for 20 days with doxazosin 2 mg daily for the last 10 days. Although there was a tendency for first-dose hypotension, no serious adverse events or postural symptoms were seen. The same results were noted in 6 other normotensive subjects given the drugs in the opposite order, and no pharmacokinetic interactions were found.[2]

In a study in healthy subjects given doxazosin 2 mg daily, alone or with extended-release **nifedipine** 20 mg twice daily, the AUC and maximum plasma concentration of nifedipine were increased by 13% and 23%, respectively; and the AUC and maximum plasma concentration of doxazosin were decreased by 17% and 14%, respectively. As would be expected, blood pressures were lower when both drugs were given.[3]

For comment that doxazosin appeared to have less effect on blood pressure in patients with BPH receiving calcium-channel blockers than in those taking beta blockers or diuretics, see 'Alpha blockers + Beta blockers', p.90.

(c) Prazosin

1. Nifedipine. In a placebo-controlled, crossover study, 12 subjects with hypertension were given nifedipine 20 mg and prazosin 2 mg, separated by one hour. The combination of the two drugs reduced blood pressure more than either drug alone, although the effects of prazosin were delayed when it was given after nifedipine.[4] Another study similarly found that prazosin, given 2 hours before nifedipine, caused an enhanced hypotensive effect.[5]

Two patients with severe hypertension given prazosin 4 or 5 mg experienced a sharp decrease in blood pressure shortly after being given nifedipine *sublingually*. One of them complained of dizziness and had a reduction in standing blood pressure from 232/124 mmHg to 88/48 mmHg about 20 minutes after taking nifedipine 10 mg. However, in a further 8 patients with hypertension taking prazosin, the reduction in blood pressure 20 minutes after the addition of *sublingual* nifedipine was smaller (mean reduction of 25/12 mmHg when lying and 24/17 mmHg when standing).[6] It is not clear what contribution prazosin had to the effect seen with *sublingual* nifedipine, because the experiment was not repeated using a prazosin placebo, but blood pressure in these patients had earlier remained unchanged one hour after taking prazosin alone. It should also be noted that *sublingual* nifedipine alone can cause a dangerous drop in blood pressure.

2. Verapamil. A study in 8 normotensive subjects given a single 1-mg dose of prazosin found that the peak serum prazosin concentrations were increased by 85% (from 5.2 nanograms/mL to 9.6 nanograms/mL) and the prazosin AUC was increased by 62% when it was given with a single 160-mg dose of verapamil. The standing blood pressure 4 hours after dosing was unchanged after verapamil alone, but fell from 114/82 mmHg to 99/73 mmHg with prazosin alone, and was further reduced to 89/68 mmHg when both drugs were given together.[7] A similar pharmacokinetic interaction was noted in another study in hypertensive patients.[8] In this study, the first 1-mg dose of prazosin alone caused a 23 mmHg fall in standing systolic blood pressure, and half of the patients (3 of 6) experienced symptomatic postural hypotension. A similar reduction in blood pressure occurred when the first 1-mg dose of prazosin was given to 6 patients who had been taking verapamil for 5 days: 2 patients experienced symptomatic postural hypotension.[8]

(d) Tamsulosin

1. Nifedipine. In a placebo-controlled study in 8 men with hypertension well controlled by nifedipine, the addition of tamsulosin 400 micrograms daily for 7 days, then 800 micrograms daily for a further 7 days, had no clinically relevant effect on blood pressure (assessed after 6 and 14 days of tamsulosin). In addition, no first-dose hypotension was seen on the first day of tamsulosin, or when the tamsulosin dose was increased.[9]

2. Verapamil. A study into the safety of tamsulosin, with particular regard to the use of other medications, found that the concurrent use of verapamil increased the risk of adverse events related to tamsulosin 3-fold. The use of other calcium-channel blockers (not specified) did not appear to increase adverse effects, although there was a trend towards an increase.[10]

(e) Terazosin

1. Dihydropyridine calcium-channel blockers. Retrospective analysis of a large multinational study, in patients with BPH given terazosin 5 or 10 mg daily, found that terazosin only affected the blood pressure of patients taking calcium-channel blockers (**amlodipine**, **felodipine**, **flunarizine**, **isradipine**, and **nifedipine**) if the blood pressure was uncontrolled. No change in blood pressure was seen in those with normal blood pressure (i.e. those without hypertension and those with hypertension controlled by calcium-channel blockers). The most common adverse effect in the 10-week terazosin phase was dizziness, and the incidence of this appeared to be lower in those taking antihypertensives (13 to 16%) than in those not taking antihypertensives (21 to 25%).[11] Similarly, another subsequent retrospective analysis found that terazosin did not affect the blood pressure of hypertensive men whose blood pressure was controlled with a calcium-channel blocker.[12]

2. Verapamil. When verapamil 120 mg twice daily was given to 12 patients with hypertension taking terazosin 5 mg daily, the maximum plasma concentrations and the AUC of terazosin were increased by about 25%. In contrast, in another 12 patients taking verapamil 120 mg twice daily, the addition of terazosin (1 mg increased to 5 mg daily) did not affect verapamil pharmacokinetics.[13] Both groups of patients had a statistically significant reduction in standing blood pressure when they first started taking both drugs. Symptomatic orthostatic hypotension (which lessened within about 3 weeks) occurred in 4 patients when verapamil was first added to terazosin, and in 2 patients when terazosin was first added to verapamil.[13]

Mechanism

Not fully understood. It would seem that the vasodilatory effects of the alpha blockers and the calcium-channel blockers can be additive or synergistic, particularly after the first dose.[2,5,14] Tamsulosin possibly has less effect on blood pressure because it has some selectivity for alpha receptors in the prostate. It has been suggested that the interaction between tamsulosin and verapamil occurs because verapamil has alpha antagonist effects,[10] but as tamsulosin is, in part, metabolised by CYP3A4,[15] which verapamil moderately inhibits, there might be a pharmacokinetic component to the interaction.

The reduction in blood pressure seen with prazosin or terazosin and verapamil might, in part, result from a pharmacokinetic interaction, involving reduced hepatic metabolism, although the exact mechanism is not certain.[7,13,14] The pharmacokinetic interaction between alfuzosin and diltiazem appears to occur because diltiazem is a moderate inhibitor of CYP3A4, which is the principal enzyme involved in the hepatic metabolism of alfuzosin.[1]

Importance and management

The interaction between calcium-channel blockers and alpha blockers would appear to be established and of clinical importance, although the documentation is limited. Marked additive hypotensive effects can occur when concurrent use is first started, and the effects might be increased if a pharmacokinetic interaction also occurs (for example with alfuzosin and diltiazem, and prazosin or terazosin with verapamil). When starting an alpha blocker it is recommended that patients already taking a calcium-channel blocker should have their dose of calcium-channel blocker reduced and begin with a low-dose of alpha blocker, with the first dose taken just before going to bed. Caution should also be taken when calcium-channel blockers are added to established treatment with an alpha blocker. Patients should be warned about the possibilities of exaggerated hypotension, and told what to do if they feel faint and dizzy (i.e. lay down, raise the legs, and, when recovered, get up slowly). There is limited evidence that tamsulosin and possibly terazosin might not cause an additional hypotensive effect when taken longer term in patients with BPH who have hypertension already well controlled with calcium-channel blockers. Nevertheless, caution should be exercised in this situation, and a dose reduction of the calcium-channel blocker might be required. It seems likely that any pharmacokinetic interaction will be accounted for by this dose titration. However, in some situations the pharmacokinetic interactions of tamsulosin with moderate CYP3A4 inhibitors such as diltiazem and verapamil might be of more clinical relevance. For further information, see 'Alpha blockers + Ketoconazole and other CYP3A4 inhibitors', p.93.

1. Uroxatral (Alfuzosin hydrochloride extended-release tablets). Sanofi-Aventis US LLC. US Prescribing information, October 2011.
2. Donnelly R, Elliott HL, Meredith PA, Howie CA, Reid JL. The pharmacodynamics and pharmacokinetics of the combination of nifedipine and doxazosin. *Eur J Clin Pharmacol* (1993) 44, 279–82.
3. Adalat CC (Nifedipine). Bayer HealthCare. US Prescribing information, April 2011.
4. Kiss I, Farsang C. Nifedipine-prazosin interaction in patients with essential hypertension. *Cardiovasc Drugs Ther* (1989) 3, 413–15.
5. Sluiter HE, Huysmans FTM, Thien TA, Koene RAP. The influence of alpha$_1$-adrenergic blockade on the acute antihypertensive effect of nifedipine. *Eur J Clin Pharmacol* (1985) 29, 263–7.
6. Jee LD, Opie LH. Acute hypotensive response to nifedipine added to prazosin in treatment of hypertension. *BMJ* (1983) 287, 1514.
7. Pasanisi F, Elliott HL, Meredith PA, McSharry DR, Reid JL. Combined alpha adrenoceptor antagonism and calcium channel blockade in normal subjects. *Clin Pharmacol Ther* (1984) 36, 716–23.
8. Elliott HL, Meredith PA, Campbell L, Reid JL. The combination of prazosin and verapamil in the treatment of essential hypertension. *Clin Pharmacol Ther* (1988) 43, 554–60.
9. Starkey LP, Yasukawa K, Trenga C, Miyazawa Y, Ito Y. Study of possible pharmacodynamic interaction between tamsulosin and nifedipine in subjects with essential hypertension. *J Clin Pharmacol* (1994) 34, 1019.
10. Michel MC, Bressel H-U, Goepel M, Rübben H. A 6-month large-scale study into the safety of tamsulosin. *Br J Clin Pharmacol* (2001) 51, 609–14.
11. Kirby RS. Terazosin in benign prostatic hyperplasia: effects on blood pressure in normotensive and hypertensive men. *Br J Urol* (1998) 82, 373–9.
12. Lowe F, Olson PJ, Padley RJ. Effects of terazosin therapy on blood pressure in men with benign prostatic hyperplasia concurrently treated with other antihypertensive medications. *Urology* (1999) 54, 81–5.
13. Lenz ML, Pool JL, Laddu AR, Varghese A, Johnston W, Taylor AA. Combined terazosin and verapamil therapy in essential hypertension. Hemodynamic and pharmacokinetic interactions. *Am J Hypertens* (1995) 8, 133–45.
14. Meredith PA, Elliott HL. An additive or synergistic drug interaction: application of concentration-effect modeling. *Clin Pharmacol Ther* (1992) 51, 708–14.
15. Flomax (Tamsulosin hydrochloride). Astellas Pharma Inc. US Prescribing information, May 2012.

Alpha blockers + Cimetidine

No clinically important interaction occurs between cimetidine and either alfuzosin or doxazosin in healthy subjects. Tamsulosin does not appear to have a clinically significant interaction with cimetidine.

Clinical evidence

(a) Alfuzosin

In 10 healthy subjects cimetidine 1 g daily in divided doses for 20 days was found to have minimal effects on the pharmacokinetics of a single 5-mg dose of alfuzosin. The maximum serum concentrations and AUC of alfuzosin were increased by up to 24% (not statistically significant) and the half-life was shortened by 14%. Cimetidine did not appear to increase the incidence of postural hypotension seen with alfuzosin.[1]

(b) Doxazosin

The UK and US manufacturers of doxazosin note that, in a placebo-controlled study in healthy subjects, cimetidine 400 mg twice daily increased the AUC of a single 1-mg dose of doxazosin given on day 4 by 10%.[2,3]

(c) Tamsulosin

A study in 10 healthy subjects found that giving cimetidine 400 mg four times daily with a single 400-microgram dose of tamsulosin resulted in a 44% increase in the AUC of tamsulosin and a 26% reduction in tamsulosin clearance. Adverse events were not increased by concurrent use.[4]

Mechanism

Cimetidine is a non-specific inhibitor of cytochrome P450. It is therefore possible that the negligible increase in alfuzosin exposure occurs due to inhibition of its metabolism by this enzyme system. Doxazosin and tamsulosin are also metabolised by cytochrome P450 isoenzymes and their exposure is therefore also increased by cimetidine. Other **H_2-receptor antagonists** do not inhibit cytochrome P450 isoenzymes to a clinically relevant extent and therefore would not be expected to affect the pharmacokinetics of these alpha blockers.

Importance and management

Although the studies with alfuzosin, doxazosin, and tamsulosin suggest that cimetidine might interact, the increases in the exposure to these alpha blockers were negligible to slight and not thought to be clinically relevant. There would seem to be no reason for avoiding concurrent use. Nevertheless, some have very cautiously suggested that as the bioavailability of alfuzosin is generally increased in elderly patients, even a small increase in exposure might be clinically relevant.[1]

The UK manufacturer of tamsulosin considers that no dose adjustment is necessary in the presence of cimetidine;[5] however, the US manufacturer advises caution, particularly with tamsulosin doses greater than 400 micrograms.[6] In practice this probably means being aware that an increase in the adverse effects of tamsulosin (e.g. dizziness, headache, postural hypotension) might occur as a result of this interaction.

Other H_2-receptor antagonists would not be expected to interact (see *Mechanism*, above).

For mention of an interaction between tolazoline and cimetidine or ranitidine, see 'Tolazoline + H_2-receptor antagonists', p.1076.

1. Desager JP, Harvengt C, Bianchetti G, Rosenzweig P. The effect of cimetidine on the pharmacokinetics of single oral doses of alfuzosin. *Int J Clin Pharmacol Ther Toxicol* (1993) 31, 568–71.
2. Cardura XL (Doxazosin mesylate). Pfizer Inc. US Prescribing information, July 2011.
3. Cardura XL (Doxazosin mesilate). Pfizer Ltd. UK Summary of product characteristics, August 2012.
4. Miyazawa Y, Forrest A, Schentag JJ, Kamimura H, Swarz H, Ito Y. Effect of concomitant administration of cimetidine hydrochloride on the pharmacokinetic and safety profile of tamsulosin hydrochloride 0.4 mg in healthy subjects. *Curr Ther Res* (2002) 63, 15–26.
5. Flomaxtra XL (Tamsulosin hydrochloride). Astellas Pharma Ltd. UK Summary of product characteristics, May 2013.
6. Flomax (Tamsulosin hydrochloride). Astellas Pharma Inc. US Prescribing information, May 2012.

Alpha blockers + Ketoconazole and other CYP3A4 inhibitors

Ketoconazole, a potent CYP3A4 inhibitor, moderately increases the exposure to alfuzosin, silodosin, and tamsulosin: other potent CYP3A4 inhibitors would be expected to interact similarly. *In vitro* studies suggest that the metabolism of doxazosin might also be inhibited by potent CYP3A4 inhibitors.

Clinical evidence, mechanism, importance and management

(a) Alfuzosin

The UK and US manufacturers of an extended-release preparation of alfuzosin briefly mention a study in which ketoconazole 400 mg daily for 8 days increased the AUC and maximum concentration of a 10-mg dose of alfuzosin 3-fold and 2.3-fold, respectively. Similarly, a lower dose of ketoconazole of 200 mg daily increased the AUC of alfuzosin 2.5-fold.[1,2] The US manufacturer[1] therefore contraindicates the concurrent use of potent CYP3A4 inhibitors. For a list of potent CYP3A4 inhibitors, see 'Table 1.9', p.11. Based on the information available, this contraindication with alfuzosin seems somewhat cautious; however, note that the US manufacturers of the HIV-protease inhibitors generally contraindicate their concurrent use with alfuzosin because the increased alfuzosin concentrations could result in hypotension.

If any potent CYP3A4 inhibitor is given with alfuzosin, it would seem prudent to use the minimum dose of the alpha blocker and titrate the dose as necessary, monitoring for adverse effects, particularly hypotension, when the dose is increased. Be aware that the risks are likely to be greater in patients also taking other antihypertensives.

(b) Doxazosin

Doxazosin is extensively metabolised in the liver, and *in vitro* studies suggest that CYP3A4 is the primary isoenzyme involved, although CYP2D6 and CYP2C19 also contribute to its metabolism.[3] The US manufacturer[3] advises caution when a potent CYP3A4 inhibitor is given with doxazosin. For a list of potent CYP3A4 inhibitors, see 'Table 1.9', p.11. The clinical relevance of these predictions is unclear, but until more is known some caution seems prudent. If concurrent use is undertaken, be aware that the adverse effects of doxazosin (such as dizziness, headache, postural hypotension) might be increased.

(c) Silodosin

The US manufacturer of silodosin reports that in a study, ketoconazole 400 mg daily for 4 days increased the maximum plasma concentration and AUC of a single 8-mg dose of silodosin 3.8-fold and 3.2-fold, respectively. In another study, a lower dose of ketoconazole of 200 mg daily for 4 days caused a similar increase in the AUC of a single 4-mg dose of silodosin (2.9-fold). Other potent inhibitors of CYP3A4 (see 'Table 1.9', p.11, for a list) are expected to interact similarly, and the manufacturer contraindicates concurrent use.[4] The manufacturer also states that the concurrent use of silodosin with moderate CYP3A4 inhibitors (see 'Table 1.9', p.11, for a list) has not been evaluated. However, as they might increase silodosin exposure, the manufacturer advises caution and monitoring for adverse effects (e.g. dizziness, diarrhoea, orthostatic hypotension) on concurrent use.[4]

(d) Tamsulosin

In a pharmacokinetic study in 24 healthy subjects, ketoconazole 400 mg daily for 5 days increased the AUC of a single 400-microgram dose of tamsulosin (taken on day 4) 2.8-fold. However, this increase in exposure did not alter systolic or diastolic blood pressure during orthostatic stress testing. All of the subjects in this study had normal CYP2D6 isoenzyme activity (extensive metabolisers).[5]

The moderate increase in tamsulosin exposure with ketoconazole did not result in any clinically relevant adverse effects in this study. However, the authors considered the increase was equivalent to doubling the tamsulosin dose,[5] an increase that would be expected to be clinically important in some patients. Note that as 400 micrograms is the smallest dose form available, it is not easy to reduce the dose of tamsulosin if adverse effects did occur. In addition, although there are no data, the tamsulosin exposure in CYP2D6 poor metabolisers (those lacking or deficient in this isoenzyme) given ketoconazole would be expected to be greater than that seen in this study. For this reason, the UK manufacturer states that tamsulosin should not be given with potent CYP3A4 inhibitors, such as ketoconazole, in patients who are CYP2D6 poor metabolisers. In other patients, they advise caution.[6] Because CYP2D6 metaboliser status is generally unknown, the US manufacturer states that tamsulosin 400 micrograms daily should not be given with potent CYP3A4 inhibitors. The manufacturers also suggest that tamsulosin should be used with caution with moderate inhibitors of CYP3A4,[6,7] particularly at doses higher than 400 micrograms daily.[7] If concurrent use is undertaken, be aware that the adverse effects of tamsulosin (e.g. dizziness, headache, postural hypotension) might be increased. For a list of moderate and potent CYP3A4 inhibitors, see 'Table 1.9', p.11.

1. Uroxatral (Alfuzosin hydrochloride extended-release tablets). Sanofi-Aventis US LLC. US Prescribing information, October 2011.
2. Xatral XL (Alfuzosin hydrochloride). Sanofi. UK Summary of product characteristics, August 2013.
3. Cardura XL (Doxazosin mesylate). Pfizer Inc. US Prescribing information, July 2011.
4. Rapaflo (Silodosin). Watson Pharma, Inc. US Prescribing information, January 2013.
5. Troost J, Tatami S, Tsuda Y, Mattheus M, Mehlburger L, Wein M, Michel MC. Effects of strong CYP2D6 and 3A4 inhibitors, paroxetine and ketoconazole, on the pharmacokinetics and cardiovascular safety of tamsulosin. *Br J Clin Pharmacol* (2011) 72, 247–56.
6. Flomaxtra XL (Tamsulosin hydrochloride). Astellas Ltd. UK Summary of product characteristics, May 2013.
7. Flomax (Tamsulosin hydrochloride). Astellas Pharma Inc. US Prescribing information, May 2012.

Alpha blockers + Dapoxetine

The concurrent use of tamsulosin and dapoxetine does not appear to affect the pharmacokinetics of either drug. The manufacturers predict that the concurrent use of dapoxetine and an alpha blocker might have additive effects on blood pressure.

Clinical evidence

In a crossover study, 54 patients taking **tamsulosin** in doses of at least 400 micrograms daily for BPH were also given either dapoxetine 30 or 60 mg, or placebo, daily for 7 days. The pharmacokinetics of **tamsulosin** and dapoxetine were similar to those previously reported and were not affected by concurrent use. The orthostatic effects of **tamsulosin** were not affected by dapoxetine.[1]

Mechanism

Dapoxetine and tamsulosin are both extensively metabolised, mainly by CYP2D6 and CYP3A4, but it appears that the potential competition for metabolism does not result in a pharmacokinetic interaction.

Importance and management

The study suggests that an interaction between tamsulosin and dapoxetine that results in clinically relevant hypotension is unlikely. However, the Swedish manufacturer of dapoxetine notes that dapoxetine alone can cause syncope and orthostatic hypotension, and therefore recommends caution when it is given with drugs that can cause vasodilation, such as the alpha blockers, because of a possibility of an increase in these adverse effects.[2] Although tamsulosin is less associated with orthostatic hypotension than many other alpha blockers, until more is known this might be prudent.

1. Modi NB, Kell S, Aquilina J, Rivas D. Effect of dapoxetine on the pharmacokinetics and hemodynamic effects of tamsulosin in men on a stable dose of tamsulosin. *J Clin Pharmacol* (2008) 48, 1438–50.
2. Priligy (Dapoxetine hydrochloride). Janssen–Cilag AB. Swedish Summary of product characteristics, February 2010.

Alpha blockers + Diuretics

As would be expected, the use of an alpha blocker with a diuretic might result in an additive hypotensive effect, but aside from first-dose hypotension, this usually seems to be a beneficial interaction in patients with hypertension. The effects in patients with congestive heart failure might be more severe.

Clinical evidence

(a) Alfuzosin

In a single-dose study in 8 healthy subjects no pharmacokinetic interaction occurred when alfuzosin 5 mg was given with **hydrochlorothiazide** 25 mg.[1]

(b) Doxazosin

A study, involving 2 363 patients with hypertension controlled with a single antihypertensive drug, investigated the effects of adding doxazosin for BPH. The dose of doxazosin was increased gradually to 4 mg daily and then the patients were monitored for a further 14 weeks of treatment. The addition of doxazosin was found to be well tolerated, and adverse effects mainly occurred early after the onset of treatment, or in patients with lower systolic and diastolic blood pressure. However, the antihypertensive effect was more marked in patients taking diuretics or beta blockers than in patients taking ACE inhibitors or calcium-channel blockers.[2] The UK and US manufacturers of doxazosin notes that no adverse drug interaction has been seen between doxazosin and **thiazides** or **furosemide**.[3] However, they state that doxazosin doses of greater then 4 mg daily increase the likelihood of adverse effects such as postural hypotension and syncope.[4]

(c) Tamsulosin

The US manufacturer of tamsulosin[5] notes that when 10 healthy subjects taking tamsulosin 800 micrograms daily were given a single 20-mg intravenous dose of **furosemide** the AUC of tamsulosin was reduced by about 12%.

(d) Terazosin

A study in 296 patients with hypertension found that terazosin 5 mg daily lowered the supine and standing blood pressure by 4.8/8.1 mmHg and 2.6/6.1 mmHg, respectively, when compared with placebo. When **methyclothiazide** 5 mg daily was also given, the blood pressure was reduced by 20.6/14.4 mmHg and 23.3/14.6 mmHg, respectively, when compared with placebo. A similar reduction in blood pressure (17.3/12.4 mmHg and 16/11.2 mmHg, respectively) occurred when the dose of **methyclothiazide** was halved. The concurrent use of both drugs, starting with terazosin and then adding a thiazide diuretic, was considered to be effective and well tolerated.[6]

Retrospective analysis of a large multinational study, in patients with BPH given terazosin 5 or 10 mg daily, found that terazosin only affected the blood pressure of patients taking diuretics (**amiloride**, **bendroflumethiazide**, **chlortalidone**, **hydrochlorothiazide**, and **spironolactone**) if the blood pressure was uncontrolled. No change in blood pressure was seen in those with normal blood pressure (i.e. those without hypertension and those with hypertension controlled by diuretics). The most common adverse effect in the 10-week terazosin phase was dizziness, and the incidence of this appeared to be lower in those taking antihypertensives (13 to 16%) than in those not taking antihypertensives (21 to 25%).[7] However, in clinical studies in patients with hypertension, a higher proportion of patients experienced dizziness when they took terazosin with a diuretic, than when they took a placebo with a diuretic (20% versus 13%).[8]

Mechanism, importance and management

The acute first-dose hypotension that can occur with alpha blockers can be exacerbated by beta blockers (see 'Alpha blockers + Beta blockers', p.90) and calcium-channel blockers (see 'Alpha blockers + Calcium-channel blockers', p.91), but there seems to be no direct evidence that diuretics normally do the same. However, the UK manufacturer of **prazosin** suggests that it is particularly important that patients with congestive heart failure who have undergone vigorous diuretic treatment should be started on the lowest dose of prazosin (500 micrograms two to four times daily), with the initial dose given at bedtime. The reason is that left ventricular filling pressure might decrease in these patients with a resultant fall in cardiac output and systemic blood pressure.[9] There seems to be no reason for avoiding concurrent use if these precautions are taken. The only other direct evidence of a possible interaction is with **terazosin**, and the UK manufacturer of terazosin states that when it is added to a diuretic, dose reduction and re-titration might be necessary.[10] The pharmacokinetic interaction between **tamsulosin** and furosemide would not be expected to be clinically relevant, and both the UK and US manufacturers of tamsulosin specifically note that as concentrations remained within the normal range, no change in dose is necessary.[5,11]

No specific guidance is given on the concurrent use of diuretics with the other alpha blockers, but as most manufacturers note that postural hypotension is a possibility, it would be prudent to warn patients about the possibilities of exaggerated hypotension, and tell them what to do if they feel faint and dizzy (i.e. lay down, raise the legs, and, when recovered, get up slowly).

1. Bianchetti G, Padovani P, Coupez JM, Guinebault P, Hermanns P, Coupez-Lopinot R, Guillet P, Thénot JP, Morselli PL. Pharmacokinetic interactions between hydrochlorothiazide, atenolol, and alfuzosin: a new antihypertensive drug. *Acta Pharmacol Toxicol (Copenh)* (1986) 59 (Suppl 5), 197.
2. Martell N, Luque M, on behalf of the HT-BPH Group. Doxazosin added to single-drug therapy in hypertensive patients with benign prostatic hypertrophy. *J Clin Hypertens* (2001) 3, 218–23.
3. Cardura XL (Doxazosin mesilate). Pfizer Ltd. UK Summary of product characteristics, August 2012.
4. Cardura XL (Doxazosin mesylate). Pfizer Inc. US Prescribing information, July 2011.
5. Flomax (Tamsulosin hydrochloride). Astellas Pharma Inc. US Prescribing information, May 2012.
6. Black HR, Chrysant SG, Curry CL, Frishman WH, Grimm RH, Lasseter KC, Okun R, Pool JL, Raizada V, Vlachakis ND, Wombolt DG, Hosmane BS, Jackson LA, Juan D, Laddu AR. Antihypertensive and metabolic effects of concomitant administration of terazosin and methyclothiazide for the treatment of essential hypertension. *J Clin Pharmacol* (1992) 32, 351–9.
7. Kirby RS. Terazosin in benign prostatic hyperplasia: effects on blood pressure in normotensive and hypertensive men. *Br J Urol* (1998) 82, 373–9.
8. Rudd P. Cumulative experience with terazosin administered in combination with diuretics. *Am J Med* (1986) 80 (Suppl 5B), 49–54.
9. Hypovase (Prazosin hydrochloride). Pfizer Ltd. UK Summary of product characteristics, June 2009.
10. Hytrin (Terazosin monohydrochloride dihydrate). Amdipharm Mercury Company Ltd. UK Summary of product characteristics, June 2009.
11. Flomaxtra XL (Tamsulosin hydrochloride). Astellas Pharma Ltd. UK Summary of product characteristics, May 2013.

Alpha blockers + Dutasteride or Finasteride

No clinically important interaction has been found to occur between finasteride and doxazosin. In one study terazosin did not interact with finasteride, but in another there was a suggestion of modestly increased finasteride concentrations. No clinically relevant interaction appears to occur between dutasteride and tamsulosin or terazosin.

Clinical evidence, mechanism, importance and management

(a) Dutasteride

A study in 24 subjects given dutasteride 500 micrograms daily for 14 days found that when they were also given **tamsulosin** 400 micrograms daily or **terazosin** (titrated to 10 mg daily) for 14 days, the pharmacokinetics of the alpha blockers remained unchanged.[1] Although the concurrent use of **tamsulosin** and dutasteride is beneficial and generally well tolerated, it might modestly increase adverse effects (24% for concurrent use compared with 18% for dutasteride and 16% for **tamsulosin**).[2] A further sub-analysis of 325 Asian patients,[3,4] and 2 925 European patients (983 taking both drugs),[5] found a similar modest increase in adverse effects on concurrent use.

(b) Finasteride

In a parallel study, 48 healthy subjects were divided into three groups. One group took **terazosin** 10 mg daily for 18 days, another took finasteride 5 mg daily for 18 days, and the third group took both drugs. The pharmacokinetics and pharmacodynamics of both drugs remained unchanged, and the serum concentrations of testosterone and dihydrotestosterone were also unaltered by concurrent use.[6] However, another study, comparing groups of healthy subjects taking finasteride and **doxazosin** or **terazosin**, found that after 10 days of concurrent use, the maximum finasteride concentration and AUC were increased by 16% and 31%, respectively, in the presence of **terazosin**, whereas the exposure to both finasteride and **doxazosin** was not significantly affected by concurrent use. The clinical significance of the possible modest increased finasteride exposure with **terazosin** is not clear,[7] but is likely to be small.

1. GlaxoSmithKline. Personal Communication, August 2003.
2. Roehrborn CG, Siami P, Barkin J, Damião R, Major-Walker K, Morrill B, Montorsi F; the CombAT Study Group. The effect of dutasteride, tamsulosin and combination therapy on lower urinary tract symptoms in men with benign prostatic hyperplasia and prostatic enlargement:2-year results from the CombAT study. *J Urol (Baltimore)* (2008) 179, 616–21.
3. Chung B-H, Roehrborn CG, Siami P, Major-Walker K, Morrill BB, Wilson TH, Montorsi F; the CombAT Study Group. Efficacy and safety of dutasteride, tamsulosin and their combination in a subpopulation of the CombAT study: 2-year results in Asian men with moderate to severe BPH. *Prostate Cancer Prostatic Dis* (2009) 12, 152–9.
4. Chung BH, Lee SH, Roehrborn CG, Siami PF, Major-Walker K, Wilson TH, Montorsi F, CombAT Study Group. Comparison of the response to treatment between Asian and Caucasian men with benign prostatic hyperplasia: long-term results from the combination of dutasteride and tamsulosin study. *Int J Urol* (2012), 19, 1031–35.
5. Haillot O, Fraga A, Maciukiewicz P, Pushkar D, Tammela T, Höfner K, Chantada V, Gagnier P, Morrill B. The effects of combination therapy with dutasteride plus tamsulosin on clinical outcomes in men with symptomatic BPH: 4-year *post hoc* analysis of European men in the CombAT study. *Prostate Cancer Prostatic Dis* (2011) 14, 302–306.
6. Samara E, Hosmane B, Locke C, Eason C, Cavanaugh J, Granneman GR. Assessment of the pharmacokinetic-pharmacodynamic interaction between terazosin and finasteride. *J Clin Pharmacol* (1996) 36, 1169–78.
7. Vashi V, Chung M, Hilbert J, Lawrence V, Phillips K. Pharmacokinetic interaction between finasteride and terazosin, but not finasteride and doxazosin. *J Clin Pharmacol* (1998) 38, 1072–6.

Alpha blockers + Food

Food does not appear to have a clinically relevant effect on the pharmacokinetics of alfuzosin, doxazosin, or terazosin; however, food might affect the absorption from some extended-release preparations of these alpha blockers. The bioavailability of silodosin and tamsulosin is reduced by food.

Clinical evidence, mechanism, importance and management

(a) Alfuzosin

The manufacturers of alfuzosin state that its pharmacokinetics are not affected by food,[1] but the extent of absorption of the extended-release preparation is 50% lower under fasting conditions.[2] Therefore extended-release preparations should be taken immediately after a meal.[2,3]

(b) Doxazosin

In a crossover study in 12 hypertensive subjects, the maximum plasma concentration and AUC of doxazosin were not notably affected by food. However, when compared with the fasting state, food increased the maximum concentration and AUC of extended-release doxazosin (*Cardura XL*) by 32% and 18%, respectively.[4] The US manufacturer states that, in order to provide the most consistent exposure, *Cardura XL* should be given with breakfast,[4] whereas the UK manufacturers of *Cardura XL* (modified release) and *Colixil XL* (prolonged release) state that they can be taken with or without food.[5,6]

(c) Silodosin

The US manufacturer of silodosin states that in three studies, the effect of moderate fat, moderate calorie meals on silodosin pharmacokinetics was variable, with its maximum plasma concentration and AUC decreased by about 18 to 43% and 4 to 49%, respectively. They recommend that silodosin is taken with food.[7]

(d) Tamsulosin

The US manufacturer of tamsulosin states that under fasted conditions, there is a 30% increase in its bioavailability and a 40 to 70% increase in its maximum concentration, when compared with fed conditions.[8] However, some manufacturers recommend that, for uniformity of absorption, tamsulosin should be taken after the same meal each day.[8,9] With other formulations (e.g. the prolonged-release tablet, *Flomaxtra XL*) the rate and extent of absorption of tamsulosin is not affected by food and the UK manufacturer of this product states that it can be taken with or without food.[10]

(e) Terazosin

The UK manufacturer of terazosin states that food has little or no effect on its bioavailability.[11]

1. Xatral (Alfuzosin hydrochloride). Sanofi. UK Summary of product characteristics, September 2013.
2. Uroxatral (Alfuzosin hydrochloride extended-release tablets). Sanofi-Aventis US LLC. US Prescribing information, October 2011.
3. Xatral XL (Alfuzosin hydrochloride). Sanofi. UK Summary of product characteristics, August 2013.
4. Cardura XL (Doxazosin mesylate). Pfizer Inc. US Prescribing information, July 2011.
5. Cardura XL (Doxazosin mesilate). Pfizer Ltd. UK Summary of product characteristics, August 2012.
6. Colixil XL (Doxazosin mesilate prolonged-release tablets). Sandoz Ltd. UK Summary of product characteristics, October 2012.
7. Rapaflo (Silodosin). Watson Pharma, Inc. US Prescribing information, January 2013.
8. Flomax (Tamsulosin hydrochloride). Astellas Pharma Inc. US Prescribing information, May 2012.
9. Stronazon MR (Tamsulosin hydrochloride modified-release capsules). Actavis UK Ltd. UK Summary of product characteristics, January 2013.
10. Flomaxtra XL (Tamsulosin hydrochloride). Astellas Pharma Ltd. UK Summary of product characteristics, May 2013.
11. Hytrin (Terazosin monohydrochloride dihydrate). Amdipharm Mercury Company Ltd. UK Summary of product characteristics, June 2009.

Alpha blockers + Miscellaneous

Fluconazole, probenecid, and valproate are predicted to increase silodosin exposure. A large number of drugs are not expected to interact with alpha blockers, and the data for this are summarised here.

Clinical evidence, mechanism, importance and management

The US manufacturer of **silodosin** predicts that giving silodosin with inhibitors of the enzyme UGT2B7 (they name **fluconazole**, **probenecid**, and **valproate**) might in-

Table 4.2 Drugs that are not expected to interact with alpha blockers as listed by the manufacturers

	Doxazosin[1,2]	*Prazosin*[3]	*Tamsulosin*[4,5,6]	*Terazosin*[7]
Amitriptyline			No expected interaction (*in vitro* study)	
Analgesics	No expected interaction with codeine or paracetamol (acetaminophen)	No expected interaction with dextropropoxyphene (propoxyphene) or phenylbutazone		No expected interaction
Antacids	No expected interaction			
Antiarrhythmics		No expected interaction with procainamide or quinidine		No expected interaction
Antibacterials	No expected interaction with amoxicillin, co-trimoxazole, or erythromycin			No expected interaction
Antidiabetic drugs	No expected interaction with oral hypoglycaemic drugs	No expected interaction with chlorpropamide, insulin, tolazamide, or tolbutamide	No expected interaction with glibenclamide (glyburide) (*in vitro* study)	No expected interaction
Antigout drugs	No expected interaction with uricosuric drugs	No expected interaction with allopurinol, colchicine, or probenecid		No expected interaction
Anxiolytics and Hypnotics	No expected interaction with diazepam	No expected interaction with chlordiazepoxide or diazepam	No expected interaction with diazepam (*in vitro* study)	No expected interaction
Chlorphenamine	No expected interaction			
Cold and flu remedies	No expected interaction			
Corticosteroids	No expected interaction			
Phenobarbital		No expected interaction		
Phenytoin	No expected interaction (*in vitro* study)			
Salbutamol (Albuterol)			No expected interaction (*in vitro* study)	
Simvastatin			No expected interaction (*in vitro* study)	

1. Cardura (Doxazosin mesylate). Pfizer Inc. US Prescribing information, July 2009.
2. Cardura (Doxazosin mesilate). Pfizer Ltd. UK Summary of product characteristics, June 2012.
3. Hypovase (Prazosin hydrochloride). Pfizer Ltd. UK Summary of product characteristics, June 2009.
4. Stronazon MR Capsules (Tamsulosin hydrochloride). Actavis UK Ltd. UK Summary of product characteristics, January 2013.
5. Flomaxtra XL (Tamsulosin hydrochloride). Astellas Pharma Ltd. UK Summary of product characteristics, May 2013.
6. Flomax (Tamsulosin hydrochloride). Astellas Pharma Inc. US Prescribing information, May 2012.
7. Hytrin Tablets 1 mg (Terazosin monohydrochloride dihydrate). Amdipharm Mercury Company Ltd. UK Summary of product characteristics, June 2009.

crease the exposure to silodosin. These drugs might inhibit the formation of the main metabolite of silodosin which is a glucuronide conjugate, formed by direct conjugation by UGT2B7.[1] However, there appears to be no clinical evidence to support this prediction, and its clinical relevance is therefore unknown. Until more is known it would be prudent to be alert for **silodosin** adverse effects (e.g. dizziness, diarrhoea, orthostatic hypotension) on the concurrent use of these drugs.

The manufacturers of several alpha blockers also provide lists of drugs that are *not* expected to interact. These are shown in 'Table 4.2', above. In some cases these predictions are based on *in vitro* studies or from observation of clinical use. Although this type of data can provide a guide, remember that it gives only the broadest indication of whether or not a drug interacts.

1. Rapaflo (Silodosin). Watson Pharma, Inc. US Prescribing information, January 2013.

Alpha blockers + Nitrates

There might be an enhanced hypotensive effect if alpha blockers are given with nitrates.

Clinical evidence, mechanism, importance and management

The UK manufacturer of **alfuzosin** states that it might interact with nitrates.[1] Although this interaction is not specifically mentioned for other alpha blockers, most manufacturers warn of enhanced hypotensive effects with other drugs that can lower blood pressure. Consider also 'Antihypertensives + Other drugs that affect blood pressure', p.1054.

The UK manufacturer of **prazosin** states that when prazosin is initially given to patients with congestive heart failure who have undergone vigorous diuretic or other vasodilator treatment, the resultant decrease in left ventricular filling pressure might be associated with a clinically relevant decrease in cardiac output and systemic blood pressure. Observance of the recommended starting dose of **prazosin** followed by gradual dose increase is particularly important in such patients.[2]

1. Xatral XL (Alfuzosin hydrochloride). Sanofi. UK Summary of product characteristics, August 2013.
2. Hypovase (Prazosin hydrochloride). Pfizer Ltd. UK Summary of product characteristics, June 2009.

Alpha blockers; Bunazosin + Rifampicin (Rifampin)

Rifampicin reduces bunazosin serum concentrations, which reduces both the adverse and beneficial effects of bunazosin.

Clinical evidence, mechanism, importance and management

In 15 healthy subjects, rifampicin 600 mg daily for 7 days reduced the maximum serum concentrations of bunazosin 6 mg daily by 82% (from 11.6 nanograms/mL to 2.1 nanograms/mL). The AUC of bunazosin was reduced more than 7-fold. The duration of the blood pressure lowering effect of bunazosin was shortened, the heart rate increase was less pronounced, and some adverse effects of bunazosin (fatigue, headache) disappeared.[1,2] The probable reason is that rifampicin (a known enzyme inducer) increases the metabolism of bunazosin so that its concentrations are reduced, and its effects therefore diminished.

The evidence for an interaction between bunazosin and rifampicin seems to be limited to this study, but anticipate the need to increase the bunazosin dose if rifampicin is added. Information about other alpha blockers does not seem to be available.

1. Al-Hamdan Y, Otto U, Kirch W. Interaction of rifampicin with bunazosin, an alpha$_1$-adrenoceptor antagonist. *J Clin Pharmacol* (1993) 33, 998.
2. Nokhodian A, Halabi A, Ebert U, Al-Hamdan Y, Kirch W. Interaction of rifampicin with bunazosin, an α_1-adrenoceptor antagonist, in healthy volunteers. *Drug Invest* (1993) 6, 362–4.

Alpha blockers; Indoramin + MAOIs

It has been predicted that the concurrent use of indoramin and MAOIs might lead to hypertension.

Clinical evidence, mechanism, importance and management

The concurrent use of MAOIs is contraindicated by the UK manufacturers of indoramin.[1,2] This contraindication was included in the datasheet at the time indoramin was first licensed, and was based on a theoretical suggestion that the effects of noradrenaline (norepinephrine) might be potentiated by indoramin,[3] leading to vasoconstriction, and resulting in a possible increase in blood pressure. However, the pharmacology of these drugs suggests just the opposite; namely that hypotension is the more likely outcome. In addition, the hypertensive effects of noradrenaline (norepinephrine) can be treated with a non-selective alpha blocker such as phentolamine, and the MAOIs are not contraindicated with any of the other alpha blockers. A clinically relevant interaction resulting in hypertension therefore seems unlikely.

1. Doralese Tiltab (Indoramin hydrochloride).Chemidex Pharma Ltd. UK Summary of product characteristics, January 2011.
2. Baratol (Indoramin hydrochloride). Amdipharm. UK Summary of product characteristics, August 2009.
3. GlaxoSmithKline. Personal communication, August 2003.

Alpha blockers; Tamsulosin + Paroxetine and other CYP2D6 inhibitors

Paroxetine, a potent CYP2D6 inhibitor, slightly increases tamsulosin exposure. Other potent inhibitors of CYP2D6 are expected to interact similarly.

Clinical evidence

In a pharmacokinetic study in healthy subjects, paroxetine (10 mg daily for 3 days then 20 mg once daily for 9 days) increased the AUC of tamsulosin by 65% when a single 400 microgram dose of tamsulosin was taken on day 11. All subjects in this study were CYP2D6 extensive metabolisers (that is, they had normal activity of this isoenzyme). This slight increase in tamsulosin exposure did not alter systolic or diastolic blood pressure during orthostatic stress testing.[1]

Mechanism

Tamsulosin is partially metabolised by CYP2D6, of which paroxetine is a potent inhibitor. Concurrent use therefore leads to an increase in tamsulosin exposure.

Importance and management

The slight increase in tamsulosin exposure in the presence of paroxetine is unlikely to be clinically important. However, the US manufacturer[2] suggests that tamsulosin should be used with caution with moderate and potent CYP2D6 inhibitors (see 'Table 1.7', p.9, for a list), particularly at doses higher than 400 micrograms daily. A greater increase in exposure would be expected if CYP3A4 inhibitors were also given, see 'Alpha blockers + Ketoconazole and other CYP3A4 inhibitors', p.93.

1. Troost J, Tatami S, Tsuda Y, Mattheus M, Mehlburger L, Wein M, Michel MC. Effects of strong CYP2D6 and 3A4 inhibitors, paroxetine and ketoconazole, on the pharmacokinetics and cardiovascular safety of tamsulosin. *Br J Clin Pharmacol* (2011) 72, 247–56.
2. Flomax (Tamsulosin hydrochloride). Astellas Pharma Inc. US Prescribing information, May 2012.

5

Anaesthetics and Neuromuscular blockers

Many patients undergoing anaesthesia may be taking long-term medication, which may affect their haemodynamic status during anaesthesia. This section is limited to drug interactions and therefore does not cover the many precautions relating to patients taking long-term medication and undergoing anaesthesia.

(a) General anaesthetics

In general anaesthesia a balanced approach is often used to meet the main goals of the anaesthetic procedure. These goals are unconsciousness/amnesia, analgesia, muscle relaxation, and maintenance of homoeostasis. Therefore general anaesthesia often involves the use of several drugs, including benzodiazepines, opioids, and anticholinesterases, as well as general anaesthetics (sometimes more than one) and neuromuscular blockers. The use of several different types of drugs in anaesthesia means that there is considerable potential for drug interactions to occur in the peri-operative period, but this section concentrates on the effects of drugs on general anaesthetics and neuromuscular blockers. The interactions of other drugs used peri-operatively, such as the anticholinesterases, benzodiazepines and opioids are mainly covered under 'Anticholinesterases', p.365, 'Antipsychotics, Anxiolytics, and Hypnotics', p.803, and 'Analgesics and NSAIDs', p.138.

There may be difficulty in establishing which of the drugs being used in a complex regimen are involved in a suspected interaction. It should also be borne in mind that disease processes and the procedure for which anaesthesia is used may also be factors to be taken into account when evaluating a possible interaction.

Some established interactions are advantageous and are employed clinically. For example, the hypnotic and anaesthetic effects of propofol and midazolam (see "'Anaesthetics, general + Anaesthetics, general', p.99).

The general anaesthetics mentioned in this section are listed in 'Table 5.1', p.98. Barbiturates used as anaesthetics (e.g. thiopental) are largely covered here, whereas barbiturates used predominantly for their antiepileptic or sedative properties (e.g. phenobarbital or secobarbital) are dealt with in the appropriate sections.

Many anaesthetics have been associated with arrhythmias, due to their sensitising effects on the myocardium. A suggested listing of inhalational anaesthetics in order of decreasing sensitising effect on the myocardium is as follows: cyclopropane, halothane, enflurane/methoxyflurane, desflurane/isoflurane/sevoflurane.

(b) Local anaesthetics

The interactions discussed in this section mainly involve the interaction of drugs with local anaesthetics used for epidural or spinal anaesthesia. The interactions of lidocaine used as an antiarrhythmic is dealt with in 'Antiarrhythmics', p.260. The local anaesthetics mentioned in this section are listed in 'Table 5.1', p.98.

(c) Neuromuscular blockers

The competitive (non-depolarising) neuromuscular blockers and depolarising neuromuscular blockers mentioned in this section are listed in 'Table 5.2', p.98. The modes of action of the two types of neuromuscular blocker are discussed in the monograph 'Neuromuscular blockers + Neuromuscular blockers', p.132. It should be noted that mivacurium (a competitive blocker) and suxamethonium (a depolarising blocker) are hydrolysed by cholinesterase, so share some interactions in common that are not relevant to other competitive neuromuscular blockers.

Table 5.1 Anaesthetics

General anaesthetics			
Halogenated inhalational anaesthetics	**Miscellaneous inhalational anaesthetics**	**Barbiturate parenteral anaesthetics**	**Miscellaneous parenteral anaesthetics**
Chloroform Desflurane Enflurane Halothane Isoflurane Methoxyflurane Sevoflurane Trichloroethylene	Anaesthetic ether Cyclopropane Nitrous oxide Xenon	Methohexital Thiamylal Thiopental	Etomidate Ketamine Propofol
Local anaesthetics			
Amide-type	**Ester-type (ester of benzoic acid)**	**Ester-type (ester of para-aminobenzoic acid)**	
Articaine Bupivacaine Etidocaine Levobupivacaine Lidocaine Mepivacaine Prilocaine Ropivacaine	Cocaine	Chloroprocaine Procaine Propoxycaine Tetracaine	

Table 5.2 Neuromuscular blockers

Competitive (Non-depolarising) blockers - Aminosteroid type	*Competitive (Non-depolarising) blockers - Benzylisoquinolinium type*	*Depolarising blockers*
Pancuronium Pipecuronium Rapacuronium Rocuronium Vecuronium	Alcuronium Atracurium Cisatracurium Doxacurium Gallamine Metocurine Mivacurium Tubocurarine (d-Tubocurarine)	Suxamethonium (Succinylcholine)

Anaesthetics, general + ACE inhibitors or Angiotensin II receptor antagonists

The concurrent use of general anaesthetics and antihypertensives generally need not be avoided but it should be recognised that the normal homoeostatic responses of the cardiovascular system will be impaired. For example, marked hypotension has been seen in patients taking ACE inhibitors or angiotensin-II receptor antagonists during anaesthetic induction.

Clinical evidence, mechanism, importance and management

(a) ACE inhibitors

Marked hypotension (systolic BP 75 mmHg), which did not respond to surgical stimulation, occurred in a 42-year-old man taking **enalapril** when he was anaesthetised with **propofol**. He responded slowly to the infusion of one litre of Hartmann's solution.[1] Severe and unexpected hypotension has been seen during anaesthetic induction in patients taking **captopril**.[2] In a randomised clinical study, the incidence of hypotension during anaesthetic induction was higher in patients who had taken **captopril** or **enalapril** on the day of surgery than in those who had stopped these drugs 12 or 24 hours before surgery.[3] In 18 patients induction of anaesthesia for coronary artery bypass surgery resulted in a significant reduction in blood pressure and heart rate, irrespective of whether or not they were taking ACE inhibitors. The patients taking ACE inhibitors showed a marked decrease in cardiac index but no changes in systemic vascular resistance compared with the patients not taking ACE inhibitors.[4] In another study in patients undergoing coronary artery bypass surgery, short-lasting hypotensive episodes (less than 60 seconds) occurred in 9 of 16 patients receiving **captopril**, **enalapril**, **perindopril** or **lisinopril**, compared with 2 of 16 patients who were not taking ACE inhibitors. The patients experiencing hypotension required additional intravenous fluids and vasoconstrictors to maintain haemodynamic stability.[5] Similar findings are reported in another study, which included patients taking **captopril**, **enalapril**, **ramipril**, or **lisinopril**.[6] Another experimental study found that a single dose of **captopril** at induction of anaesthesia caused a small reduction in cerebral blood flow, when compared with control patients or patients given metoprolol.[7]

Particular care would seem to be needed with patients taking ACE inhibitors, but there is insufficient evidence to generally recommend discontinuing ACE inhibitors before surgery. Whether ACE inhibitors are discontinued or continued, haemodynamic instability may occur after induction of anaesthesia.[8]

One recommendation is that intravenous fluids should be given to all patients taking ACE inhibitors who are anaesthetised.[1] If hypotension occurs, blood pressure can be restored in most patients by giving sympathomimetics such as phenylephrine.[8] However, sympathomimetics may not be fully effective in treating hypotension due to ACE inhibitors and anaesthesia because ACE inhibitor administration may result in a decrease in the adrenergic vasoconstrictive response.[5,9] Terlipressin (a vasopressin analogue that has some effects as a vasopressin agonist) is reported to be an effective treatment for refractory hypotension during anaesthesia in patients taking ACE inhibitors.[8,10,11] One study found that severe hypotension during anaesthetic induction in patients chronically taking ACE inhibitors could be controlled with an intravenous injection of angiotensin II (*Hypertensine*).[12]

(b) Angiotensin II receptor antagonists

A study in 12 hypertensive patients taking angiotensin II receptor antagonists found that hypotension occurred in all patients after induction of anaesthesia. This was more frequent than that found in matched groups of hypertensive patients receiving either beta blockers and/or calcium-channel blockers (27 out of 45) or ACE inhibitors (18 of 27). The magnitude of hypotension was also significantly greater in those treated with angiotensin II receptor antagonists and it was less responsive to ephedrine and phenylephrine.[10] Terlipressin has been found to be effective in patients with refractory hypotension taking angiotensin II receptor antagonists.[10,11]

1. Littler C, McConachie I, Healy TEJ. Interaction between enalapril and propofol. *Anaesth Intensive Care* (1989) 17, 514–15.
2. McConachie I, Healy TEJ. ACE inhibitors and anaesthesia. *Postgrad Med J* (1989) 65, 273–4.
3. Coriat P, Richer C, Douraki T, Gomez C, Hendricks K, Giudicelli J-F, Viars P. Influence of chronic angiotensin-converting enzyme inhibition on anesthetic induction. *Anesthesiology* (1994) 81, 299–307.
4. Ryckwaert F, Colson P. Hemodynamic effects of anesthesia in patients with ischemic heart failure chronically treated with angiotensin-converting enzyme inhibitors. *Anesth Analg* (1997) 84, 945–9.
5. Licker M, Schweizer A, Höhn L, Farinelli C, Morel DR. Cardiovascular responses to anesthetic induction in patients chronically treated with angiotensin-converting enzyme inhibitors. *Can J Anaesth* (2000) 47, 433–40.
6. Colson P, Saussine M, Séguin JR, Cuchet D, Chaptal P-A, Roquefeuil B. Hemodynamic effects of anesthesia in patients chronically treated with angiotensin-converting enzyme inhibitors. *Anesth Analg* (1992) 74, 805–8.
7. Jensen K, Bunemann L, Riisager S, Thomsen LJ. Cerebral blood flow during anaesthesia: influence of pretreatment with metoprolol or captopril. *Br J Anaesth* (1989) 62, 321–3.
8. Colson P, Ryckwaert F, Coriat P. Renin angiotensin system antagonists and anesthesia. *Anesth Analg* (1999) 89, 1143–55.
9. Licker M, Neidhart P, Lustenberger S, Valloton MB, Kalonji T, Fathi M, Morel DR. Long-term angiotensin-converting enzyme inhibitor treatment attenuates adrenergic responsiveness without altering hemodynamic control in patients undergoing cardiac surgery. *Anesthesiology* (1996) 84, 789–800.
10. Brabant SM, Bertrand M, Eyraud D, Darmon P-L, Coriat P. The hemodynamic effects of anesthetic induction in vascular surgical patients chronically treated with angiotensin II receptor antagonists. *Anesth Analg* (1999) 88, 1388–92.
11. Eyraud D, Brabant S, Nathalie D, Fléron M-H, Gilles G, Bertrand M, Coriat P. Treatment of intraoperative refractory hypotension with terlipressin in patients chronically treated with an antagonist of the renin-angiotensin system. *Anesth Analg* (1999) 88, 980–4.
12. Eyraud D, Mouren S, Teugels K, Bertrand M, Coriat P. Treating anesthesia-induced hypotension by angiotensin II in patients chronically treated with angiotensin-converting enzyme inhibitors. *Anesth Analg* (1998) 86, 259–63.

Anaesthetics, general + Alcohol

Those who regularly drink alcohol may need more thiopental or propofol than those who do not. In theory, alcohol may increase the risk of renal damage with sevoflurane. It is also probably unwise to drink for several hours following anaesthesia because of the combined central nervous depressant effects.

Clinical evidence, mechanism, importance and management

A study in 532 healthy patients, aged from 20 to over 80 years, found that those who normally drank alcohol (more than 40 g weekly, roughly 400 mL of wine) needed more **thiopental** to achieve anaesthesia than non-drinkers. After adjusting for differences in age and weight distribution, men and women who were heavy drinkers (more than 40 g alcohol daily) needed 33% and 44% more **thiopental**, respectively, for induction than non-drinkers.[1] Chronic alcohol intake is known to increase barbiturate metabolism by cytochrome P450 enzymes,[2] see 'Alcohol + Barbiturates', p.59.

Another study found that 26 chronic alcoholics (drinkers of about 40 g of alcohol daily, with no evidence of liver impairment) needed about one-third more **propofol** to induce anaesthesia than another 20 patients who only drank socially. However, there was great interindividual variation in the amount of **propofol** needed in the alcoholic group.[3]

When 12 healthy subjects were given 0.7 g/kg of alcohol 4 hours after receiving 5 mg/kg of **thiopental** 2.5%, body sway and lightheadedness were accentuated.[4] This suggests that an interaction may occur if an ambulatory patient drinks alcohol within 4 hours of receiving an induction dose of **thiopental**. Patients should be cautioned not to drink alcohol following anaesthesia and surgery.

The manufacturer of **sevoflurane** notes that its metabolism may be increased by known inducers of the cytochrome P450 isoenzyme CYP2E1 including alcohol.[5,6] This may increase the risk of renal damage because of an increase in plasma fluoride; however, no cases appear to have been reported.

1. Dundee JW, Milligan KR. Induction dose of thiopentone: the effect of alcohol intake. *Br J Clin Pharmacol* (1989) 27, 693P–694P.
2. Weathermon R, Crabb DW. Alcohol and medication interactions. *Alcohol Res Health* (1999) 23, 40–54.
3. Fassoulaki A, Farinotti R, Servin F, Desmonts JM. Chronic alcoholism increases the induction dose of propofol in humans. *Anesth Analg* (1993) 77, 553–6.
4. Lichtor JL, Zacny JP, Coalson DW, Flemming DC, Uitvlugt A, Apfelbaum JL, Lane BS, Thisted RA. The interaction between alcohol and the residual effects of thiopental anesthesia. *Anesthesiology* (1993) 79, 28–35.
5. Sevoflurane. Abbott Laboratories Ltd. UK Summary of product characteristics, June 2007.
6. Ultane (Sevoflurane). Abbott Laboratories. US Prescribing information, September 2006.

Anaesthetics, general + Alpha blockers

The UK manufacturers of alfuzosin note that the use of general anaesthetics in patients taking alfuzosin could cause profound hypotension, and they recommend that alfuzosin should be withdrawn 24 hours before surgery.[1]

1. Xatral (Alfuzosin hydrochloride). Sanofi. UK Summary of product characteristics, September 2013.

Anaesthetics, general + Anaesthetics, general

In general, the effects of the combined use of general anaesthetics are at least additive. See 'Table 5.3', p.100, for specific comments about pairs of anaesthetics.

Anaesthetics, general + Anaesthetics, local

An isolated report describes convulsions associated with the use of propofol with topical cocaine Arrhythmias have been reported in patients given propofol and topical cocaine. Cocaine abuse may increase the risk of cardiovascular complications during inhalational anaesthesia. Abstinence from cocaine or the avoidance of anaesthetics with sympathomimetic properties has been suggested.

The dosage of propofol may need to be reduced after the use of bupivacaine, ropivacaine, or lidocaine (e.g. during regional anaesthetic techniques). Similarly, epidural lidocaine reduces sevoflurane requirements, and is likely to have the same effect on other inhalational anaesthetics.

Clinical evidence, mechanism, importance and management

Note that drugs such as adrenaline (epinephrine), which are used with local anaesthetics, may interact with inhalational anaesthetics such as halothane to increase the risk of arrhythmias, see 'Anaesthetics, general + Inotropes and Vasopressors', p.106.

(a) Bupivacaine

In a placebo-controlled study of patients undergoing minor gynaecological surgery, giving intramuscular bupivacaine 0.5% 30 minutes before induction of anaesthesia

Table 5.3 Effects of the concurrent use of anaesthetics

Anaesthetic	*Effect*	*Refs*
Ketamine		
Barbiturate anaesthetics	Effects of ketamine prolonged. Recovery may be delayed.	1,2
Nitrous oxide		
Inhalational anaesthetics	Nitrous oxide usually reduces the MAC of inhalational anaesthetics in a simple additive manner; an inspired concentration of 60 to 70% nitrous oxide is commonly used with volatile anaesthetics.	3
Barbiturate anaesthetics	Reduces the required dose of intravenous barbiturate anaesthetics.	4
Propofol	Concurrent use produces a deeper sedation than that produced by propofol alone. Reduced propofol dose may be required.	5,6
Sevoflurane	Reduces the required dose of sevoflurane.	7
Propofol		
Inhalational anaesthetics	Generally expected to increase the effects of propofol. Reduced propofol dose may be required.	5
Halothane	Serum propofol concentrations raised by about 20% during the maintenance of general anaesthesia. Propofol effects expected to be increased.	5,8
Isoflurane	Serum propofol concentrations raised by about 20% during the maintenance of general anaesthesia. Propofol effects expected to be increased.	5,8
Intravenous anaesthetics	Generally expected to increase the effects of propofol. Reduced propofol dose may be required.	5
Etomidate	Synergistic effect: patients given induction doses of either etomidate or propofol alone required about a 15% higher dose than those given half etomidate and half propofol in sequence.	9
Sevoflurane		
Intravenous anaesthetics	Lower concentrations may be required following the use of an intravenous anaesthetic.	10
Propofol	In a study in surgical patients concurrent use was found to be additive (loss of consciousness and movement to skin incision assessed). Lower sevoflurane concentrations may be required following the use of propofol. Concurrent use in ECT results in a longer recovery time, probably due to deeper anaesthesia, but results in smaller increases in heart rate and blood pressure than with sevoflurane alone and a shorter seizure duration than with propofol alone. (Note that the UK manufacturers of propofol do not recommend its use in ECT.)	10-13

1. Ketalar (Ketamine hydrochloride). Pfizer Ltd. UK Summary of product characteristics, May 2009.
2. Ketalar (Ketamine hydrochloride). JHP Pharmaceuticals, LLC. US Prescribing information, December 2007.
3. Dale O. Drug interactions in anaesthesia: focus on desflurane and sevoflurane. *Baillieres Clin Anaesthesiol* (1995) 9, 105–17.
4. Aitkenhead AR, ed. Textbook of anaesthesia. 4th ed. Edinburgh: Churchill Livingstone; 2001 p. 172–4.
5. Diprivan (Propofol). AstraZeneca. US Prescribing information, August 2005.
6. Kakinohana M, Miyata Y, Tomiyama H, Sugahara K. Nitrous oxide can enhance the hypnotic effect, but not the suppression of spinal motor neuron excitability by propofol in humans. *J Anesth* (2006) 20, 173–8.
7. Ultane (Sevoflurane). Abbott Laboratories. US Prescribing information, July 2009.
8. Grundmann U, Ziehmer M, Kreienmeyer J, Larsen R, Altmayer P. Propofol and volatile anaesthetics. *Br J Anaesth* (1994) 72 (Suppl 1), 88.
9. Drummond GB, Cairns DT. Do propofol and etomidate interact kinetically during induction of anaesthesia? *Br J Anaesth* (1994) 73, 272P.
10. Sevoflurane. Abbott Laboratories Ltd. UK Summary of product characteristics, June 2007.
11. Wajima Z, Shiga T, Yoshikawa T, Ogura A. Inoue T, Ogawa R. Propofol alone, sevoflurane alone, and combined propofol-sevoflurane anaesthesia in electroconvulsive therapy. *Anaesth Intensive Care* (2003) 31, 396–400.
12. Diprivan (Propofol). AstraZeneca UK Ltd. UK Summary of product characteristics, July 2009.
13. Harris RS, Lazar O, Johansen JW, Sebel PS. Interaction of propofol and sevoflurane on loss of consciousness and movement to skin incision during general anesthesia. *Anesthesiology* (2006) 104, 1170–5.

significantly enhanced the hypnotic effect of intravenous **propofol** in a dose-dependent manner. Only the lowest dose of bupivacaine tested (250 micrograms/kg) lacked a significant effect on the hypnotic dose of **propofol**. The highest dose of bupivacaine (1 mg/kg) reduced the hypnotic requirements for **propofol** by about 40%. The dose of **propofol** should therefore be modified after the intramuscular use of bupivacaine.[1] The UK manufacturer of **propofol** also notes that required doses may be lower when general anaesthesia is used in association with regional anaesthetic techniques.[2]

(b) Cocaine

A patient with no history of epilepsy, undergoing septorhinoplasty for cosmetic reasons, was premedicated with papaveretum and hyoscine, and intubated after **propofol** and suxamethonium (succinylcholine) were given. Anaesthesia was maintained with **nitrous oxide**/oxygen and **isoflurane** 2%. During anaesthesia a paste containing cocaine 10% was applied to the nasal mucosa. During recovery the patient experienced a dystonic reaction, which developed into a generalised convulsion. The authors of the report suggest that a possible interaction between the **propofol** and cocaine might have been responsible, although they also suggest that the convulsions may have been an adverse effect of the propofol.[3]

In one study, **thiopental** with either 5 mL of lidocaine 4% or 3 mL of cocaine 5%, was found to be an effective anaesthetic when performing a laryngoscopy and biopsy. However, the procedure for applying cocaine topically in these circumstances prolongs the procedure and hence increases **thiopental** requirements. Also serious cardiac arrhythmias (bigeminal rhythms and ectopic ventricular contractions) occurred in 7 of 20 patients given cocaine (which resolved, either without treatment or with intravenous propranolol). Arrhythmias did not occur in those given lidocaine.[4] In another study, **thiopental** and suxamethonium were used to induce anaesthesia in 45 patients and anaesthesia was maintained with **nitrous oxide**/oxygen and **halothane**. When a stable level of anaesthesia had been obtained, topical cocaine 20, 35, or 50 mg in 2 mL of water was sprayed into both nostrils to shrink the nasal mucosa before nasal surgery. Two patients who received cocaine 35 mg developed atrial and ventricular extrasystoles. Two other cases of AV nodal rhythm and two cases of bradycardia, which responded to atropine, were also observed.[5] However, in another study in 20 patients, topical application of cocaine (1 mL of 25% paste or 4 mL of 4% solution) with or without adrenaline (epinephrine) 0.1%, after induction of anaesthesia with **thiopental**, did not cause any cardiac toxicity.[6]

Reviews of the anaesthetic implications of illicit drug use have stated that anaesthetists should be aware of the medical complications of cocaine abuse, such as myocardial ischaemia, hypertension and tachycardia due to sympathetic nervous system stimulation.[7,8] It was suggested that the concurrent use of cocaine and inhalational anaesthetics, such as **halothane**, that are known to significantly sensitise the myocardium to circulating catecholamines, should be avoided, and that other halogenated anaesthetics should be used with caution.[7,8] Theoretically, **isoflurane** would be a better choice of inhalational anaesthetic since it has less cardiovascular effects.[7] **Ketamine** should also be avoided because of its sympathomimetic effects. **Nitrous oxide**, **thiopental** and fentanyl were considered to be useful for general anaesthesia in patients who regularly abuse cocaine.[7,8] Although it has been suggested that anaesthesia is safe for patients with chronic cocaine abuse after abstinence for 24 hours, the occurrence of ventricular fibrillation in one such patient during anaesthesia with **thiopental** and **isoflurane**, led the authors of the case report to conclude that there should be a cocaine-free interval of at least one week before elective surgical procedures. They also suggest that if an emergency operation is required during acute cocaine intoxication, all sympathomimetic anaesthetic drugs should be avoided.[9]

(c) Lidocaine

A double-blind, randomised study of 17 patients requiring ventilatory support demonstrated that hourly laryngotracheal instillation of 5 mL of 1% lidocaine significantly reduced the dose of **propofol** required to maintain adequate sedation (overall reduction of 50%) when compared with pre-study values.[10]

In a placebo-controlled study of patients undergoing minor gynaecological surgery, giving intramuscular lidocaine 4% 10 minutes before induction of anaesthesia significantly enhanced the hypnotic effect of intravenous **propofol** in a dose-dependent manner. Only the lowest dose of lidocaine tested (500 micrograms/kg) lacked a significant effect on the hypnotic dose of **propofol**. The highest dose of lidocaine (3 mg/kg) reduced the hypnotic requirements for **propofol** by about 34%. The dose of **propofol** should therefore be modified after the intramuscular use of lidocaine or bupivacaine.[1] The UK manufacturer of **propofol** also notes that required doses may be lower when general anaesthesia is used in association with regional anaesthetic techniques.[2]

An *in vitro* study using liver microsomes found that **propofol** inhibited the metabolism of lidocaine by cytochrome P450 isoenzymes.[11] However, a further study by the same authors in 31 patients undergoing anaesthesia with either **propofol** or **sevoflurane**, and receiving epidural lidocaine, found that, compared with **sevoflurane** (which does not inhibit lidocaine metabolism), **propofol** did not affect the metabolism of epidural lidocaine. The lack of interaction in the latter study could be due to the lower doses of **propofol** involved and because other isoenzymes or extrahepatic metabolism of lidocaine might possibly be involved.[12] A study in patients undergoing surgery found that a single 2-mg/kg dose of **propofol** did not affect serum lidocaine levels in subjects who smoked and consumed alcohol chronically. Enzyme inhibition by **propofol** may be countered by enzyme induction associated with cigarette smoking and alcohol, but it is probable in this study, that the single dose of **propofol** was insufficient to produce enzyme inhibition.[13]

A randomised, double-blind, placebo-controlled study involving 44 patients found that lidocaine epidural anaesthesia (15 mL of 2% plain lidocaine) reduced the MAC of **sevoflurane** required for general anaesthesia by approximately 50% (from 1.18 to 0.52%). This implies that a lower dose of **inhalational anaesthetic** provides adequate anaesthesia during combined epidural-general anaesthesia than for general anaesthesia alone.[14]

(d) Ropivacaine

In an *in vitro* study using liver microsomes, **propofol** inhibited the cytochrome P450 isoenzyme CYP3A4-mediated metabolism of ropivacaine.[15]

1. Ben-Shlomo I, Tverskoy M, Fleyshman G, Cherniavsky G. Hypnotic effect of i.v. propofol is enhanced by i.m. administration of either lignocaine or bupivacaine. *Br J Anaesth* (1997) 78, 375–7.
2. Diprivan (Propofol). AstraZeneca UK Ltd. UK Summary of product characteristics, July 2009.
3. Hendley BJ. Convulsions after cocaine and propofol. *Anaesthesia* (1990) 45, 788–9.
4. Orr D, Jones I. Anaesthesia for laryngoscopy: a comparison of the cardiovascular effects of cocaine and lignocaine. *Anaesthesia* (1968) 23, 194–202.
5. Anderton JM, Nassar WY. Topical cocaine and general anaesthesia: an investigation of the efficacy and side effects of cocaine on the nasal mucosae. *Anaesthesia* (1975) 30, 809–17.
6. Lips FJ, O'Reilly J, Close D, Beaumont GD, Clapham M. The effects of formulation and addition of adrenaline to cocaine for haemostasis in intranasal surgery. *Anaesth Intensive Care* (1987) 15, 141–6.
7. Voigt L. Anesthetic management of the cocaine abuse patient. *J Am Assoc Nurse Anesth* (1995) 63, 438–43.
8. Culver JL, Walker JR. Anesthetic implications of illicit drug use. *J Perianesth Nurs* (1999) 14, 82–90.
9. Vagts DA, Boklage C, Galli C. Intraoperatives Kammerflimmern bei einer Patientin mit chronischem Kokainmissbrauch – Eine Kasuistik. Intraoperative ventricular fibrillation in a patient with chronic cocaine abuse – a case report. *Anaesthesiol Reanim* (2004) 29, 19–24.
10. Mallick A, Smith SN, Bodenham AR. Local anaesthesia to the airway reduces sedation requirements in patients undergoing artificial ventilation. *Br J Anaesth* (1996) 77, 731–4.
11. Inomata S, Nagashima A, Osaka Y, Kazama T, Tanaka E, Sato S, Toyooka H. Propofol inhibits lidocaine metabolism in human and rat liver microsomes. *J Anesth* (2003) 17, 246–50.
12. Nakayama S, Miyabe M, Kakiuchi Y, Inomata S, Osaka Y, Fukuda T, Kohda Y, Toyooka H. Propofol does not inhibit lidocaine metabolism during epidural anesthesia. *Anesth Analg* (2004) 99, 1131–5.
13. Elmas T, Mavioglu O, Oztekin S, Elar Z, Guven H. The effect of propofol (anesthetic and inhibitor of CYP3A4) on serum lidocaine concentrations in smokers and chronic alcohol consumers. *Int J Clin Pharmacol Ther* (2003) 41, 182–4.
14. Hodgson PS, Liu SS, Gras TW. Does epidural anesthesia have general anesthetic effects? *Anesthesiology* (1999) 91, 1687–92.
15. Osaka Y, Inomata S, Tanaka E, Nakamura T, Honda K, Miyabe M, Toyooka H, Tanaka M. Effect of propofol on ropivacaine metabolism in human liver microsomes. *J Anesth* (2006) 20; 60–3.

Anaesthetics, general + Anthracyclines

Pretreatment with anthracyclines may result in prolongation of the QT interval during isoflurane anaesthesia.

Clinical evidence, mechanism, importance and management

A study in women with breast cancer found that the QTc interval was prolonged (to more than 440 milliseconds) during anaesthesia with **isoflurane** (end-tidal concentration 0.5 vol%) in more than half of the 20 patients who had received chemotherapy, compared with only 1 of 20 patients who had not previously received chemotherapy. However, QTc intervals of 600 milliseconds and above, which may be associated with serious arrhythmias, were not observed. The chemotherapy, which was given about 1 month before surgery, consisted of fluorouracil and cyclophosphamide and either **doxorubicin** or **epirubicin**. Anthracyclines (such as **doxorubicin** and **epirubicin**) and **isoflurane** can prolong the QT interval. The patients had also received midazolam, which is reported to reduce QTc prolongation induced by other anaesthetics. It was noted that the use of higher **isoflurane** concentrations in patients given anthracyclines could result in greater QTc interval prolongation.[1] Several drugs used in anaesthesia may affect the QT interval. For example **thiopental** and **sufentanil** are also reported to prolong the QT interval, while **propofol** and **halothane** are said to shorten it.[1] This should be borne in mind if patients treated with anthracyclines or other drugs that prolong the QT interval undergo anaesthesia.

1. Owczuk R, Wujtewicz MA, Sawicka W, Wujtewicz M, Swierblewski M. Is prolongation of the QTc interval during isoflurane anaesthesia more prominent in women pretreated with anthracyclines for breast cancer? *Br J Anaesth* (2004) 92, 658–61.

Anaesthetics, general + Anticholinesterases

Inhalation anaesthetics may impair the efficacy of anticholinesterases in reversing neuromuscular blockade, although propofol does not affect the reversal of rocuronium block by neostigmine. Physostigmine pre-treatment increased propofol requirements by 20% in one study.

Clinical evidence, mechanism, importance and management

(a) Neostigmine

Inhalational anaesthetics can impair neostigmine reversal of neuromuscular blockade. In one study, neostigmine took longer to reverse pancuronium blockade after anaesthesia with **enflurane**, when compared with fentanyl or **halothane**.[1] Another study found that the reversal of vecuronium block with neostigmine 40 micrograms/kg was more dependent on the concentration of **sevoflurane** than the degree of block present. At the lowest concentration of **sevoflurane** (0.2 MAC), adequate reversal was obtained in all patients within 15 minutes, but with increasing concentrations (up to 1.2 MAC) satisfactory restoration of neuromuscular function was not achieved within 15 minutes, probably because of a greater contribution of **sevoflurane** to the degree of block.[2] In another randomised study, 120 patients were given **sevoflurane**, **isoflurane** (adjusted to 1.5 MAC), or intravenous **propofol** 6 to 12 mg/kg per hour for maintenance of anaesthesia. Neuromuscular block was induced with rocuronium and monitored using train-of-four stimulation (TOF) of the ulnar nerve. Neostigmine was given when the first response in TOF had recovered to 20 to 25%. At this point **isoflurane** or **sevoflurane** was stopped, or the **propofol** dose reduced, in half of the patients in each of the three groups. The times to recovery of the TOF ratio to 0.8 were 12 minutes and 6.8 minutes in the **sevoflurane** continued and stopped groups, respectively, 9 minutes and 5.5 minutes in the **isoflurane** continued and stopped groups, respectively, and 5.2 minutes and 4.7 minutes in the **propofol** continued and reduced groups, respectively. Only 9/20 and 15/20 patients in the **sevoflurane** and **isoflurane** continued groups, respectively, achieved a TOF ratio of 0.8 within 15 minutes. This showed that the reversal of rocuronium block by neostigmine is slowed by **sevoflurane** and to a lesser extent by **isoflurane**, but not significantly affected by **propofol**.[3] The manufacturers of neostigmine injection[4] and tablets[5] state that neostigmine should not be given during **cyclopropane** or **halothane** anaesthesia, but may be given after the withdrawal of these anaesthetics.

Note that inhalation anaesthetics potentiate neuromuscular blockers, see 'Anaesthetics, general + Neuromuscular blockers', p.108.

(b) Physostigmine

A study of 40 patients found that physostigmine pre-treatment (2 mg intravenously 5 minutes before induction of anaesthesia) increased **propofol** requirements by 20%.[6]

1. Delisle S, Bevan DR. Impaired neostigmine antagonism of pancuronium during enflurane anaesthesia in man. *Br J Anaesth* (1982) 54, 441–5.
2. Morita T, Kurosaki D, Tsukagoshi H, Shimada H, Sato H, Goto F. Factors affecting neostigmine reversal of vecuronium block during sevoflurane anaesthesia. *Anaesthesia* (1997) 52, 538–43.
3. Reid JE, Breslin DS, Mirakhur RK, Hayes AH. Neostigmine antagonism of rocuronium block during anesthesia with sevoflurane, isoflurane or propofol. *Can J Anaesth* (2001) 48, 351–5.
4. Neostigmine methylsulphate injection. Hameln Pharmaceuticals Ltd. UK Summary of product characteristics, September 2007.
5. Neostigmine bromide tablets. Cambridge Laboratories. UK Summary of product characteristics, January 2001.
6. Fassoulaki A, Sarantopoulos C, Derveniotis C. Physostigmine increases the dose of propofol required to induce anaesthesia. *Can J Anaesth* (1997) 44, 1148–51.

Anaesthetics, general + Antiemetics

Metoclopramide pre-treatment reduces the dosage requirements of propofol and thiopental. Droperidol, but not ondansetron, reduces the dose requirements of thiopental.

Clinical evidence

(a) Metoclopramide or Droperidol

A randomised, placebo-controlled study of 60 surgical patients, half of whom were given metoclopramide 150 micrograms/kg 5 minutes before induction, found that the induction dose of **propofol** was reduced by 24% in the group given metoclopramide.[1] Similar results were seen in another study of 21 patients, in which metoclopramide 10 or 15 mg reduced the dose requirements of **propofol** by about 25% and 41%, respectively.[2] In a randomised, placebo-controlled study in 96 female patients, both metoclopramide and droperidol reduced the amount of **thiopental** needed to induce anaesthesia by about 45%.[3]

(b) Ondansetron

In a randomised, placebo-controlled study of 168 female patients ondansetron 100 or 200 micrograms/kg given intravenously 5 minutes before **thiopental** induction did not influence the hypnotic requirements of **thiopental**.[4]

Mechanism

The exact mechanism by which metoclopramide reduces propofol or thiopental dose requirements is unclear, but it appears to involve the blockade of dopamine (D_2) receptors. Droperidol probably interacts with thiopental by a similar mechanism.

Importance and management

Although the evidence is limited these interactions between metoclopramide and thiopental or propofol, and between droperidol and thiopental would appear to be established. Droperidol has not been studied with propofol, but, on the basis of other interactions it would be expected to behave like metoclopramide. When patients are pretreated with either metoclopramide or droperidol, be alert for the need to use less propofol and thiopental to induce anaesthesia. If the mechanism is correct, it seems likely that other dopamine antagonists used as antiemetics, such as **haloperidol**, will interact similarly, although this does not appear to have been studied. Ondansetron appears not to interact.

1. Page VJ, Chhipa JH. Metoclopramide reduces the induction dose of propofol. *Acta Anaesthesiol Scand* (1997) 41, 256–9.
2. Santiveri X, Castillo J, Buil JA, Escolano F, Castaño J. Efectos de la metoclopramida sobre las dosis hipnóticas de propofol. *Rev Esp Anestesiol Reanim* (1996) 43, 297–8.
3. Mehta D, Bradley EL, Kissin I. Metoclopramide decreases thiopental hypnotic requirements. *Anesth Analg* (1993) 77, 784–7.
4. Kostopanagiotou G, Pouriezis T, Theodoraki K, Kottis G, Andreadou I, Smyrniotis V, Papadimitriou L. Influence of ondansetron on thiopental hypnotic requirements. *J Clin Pharmacol* (1998) 38, 825–9.

Anaesthetics, general + Antipsychotics

An isolated report describes a grand mal seizure in a man taking chlorpromazine and flupentixol when he was anaesthetised with enflurane. Another report describes delayed recovery from anaesthesia in a patient taking clozapine, but the use of alprazolam may have been a contributory factor. The sedative properties of antipsychotics may be enhanced by thiopental. Lower etomidate doses are recommended in patients taking antipsychotics.

Clinical evidence, mechanism, importance and management

An isolated report[1] describes an unexpected grand mal seizure in a schizophrenic patient without a history of epilepsy when he was given **enflurane** anaesthesia. He was taking **chlorpromazine** 50 mg three times daily (irregularly) and **flupentixol** 40 mg intramuscularly every 2 weeks. The suggested reason is that the **enflurane** had a synergistic effect with the two antipsychotics, all of which are known to lower the seizure threshold. The general importance of this interaction is not known. Another isolated report[2] describes delayed recovery in a patient taking **clozapine** after short duration (1 hour) anaesthesia induced by **thiopental**, sufentanil and atracurium and maintained with **desflurane** and nitrous oxide/oxygen. However, the patient was also taking alprazolam which may also have contributed to the delayed recovery, see 'Anaesthetics, general + Benzodiazepines', below.

The manufacturer of thiopental notes that, as would be expected, the sedative properties of antipsychotics may be potentiated by **thiopental**.[3] The manufacturer of **etomidate** recommends that the dose of **etomidate** should be reduced in patients taking antipsychotics.[4] **Droperidol** and other drugs with dopamine antagonist properties, such as many of the antipsychotics, may reduce the dose requirements of **thiopental**, see 'Anaesthetics, general + Antiemetics', p.101.

In general, drugs with sedative properties, including many antipsychotics, have the potential to enhance the sedative effects of general anaesthetics, which may result in delayed recovery. However, there appear to be no reports of a problem in practice, and so it would seem reasonable to conclude that, in most patients, any effect is modest.

1. Vohra SB. Convulsions after enflurane in a schizophrenic patient receiving neuroleptics. *Can J Anaesth* (1994) 41, 420–2.
2. Geeraerts T, Moghrabi Z, Benhamou D. Delayed recovery after short-duration, general anesthesia in a patient chronically treated with clozapine. *Anesth Analg* (2006) 103, 1618.
3. Thiopental Injection. Link Pharmaceuticals Ltd. UK Summary of product characteristics, January 2003.
4. Hypnomidate (Etomidate). Janssen-Cilag Ltd. UK Summary of product characteristics, March 2009.

Anaesthetics, general + Aspirin

The anaesthetic dosage of thiopental is reduced by pretreatment with aspirin.

Clinical evidence

In a study in patients undergoing surgery, intravenous lysine aspirin increased mean free **thiopental** levels in the plasma by 39%, and 3 of 7 patients fell asleep again during recovery from **thiopental** anaesthesia.[1] Another study[2] in patients about to undergo surgery found that pretreatment with aspirin 1 g (given as intravenous lysine aspirin) one minute before induction reduced the dosage of **thiopental** by 34%, from 5.3 to 3.5 mg/kg.

Mechanism

Not understood. It has been suggested that aspirin increases the amount of free (and active) thiopental in the plasma since it competes for the binding sites on the plasma albumins.[1,2]

Importance and management

Information is limited but what is known shows that the effects of thiopental are increased by aspirin. Be alert for the need to reduce the dosage. However, note also that regular aspirin use may increase the risk of bleeding during surgery, and it is often recommended that aspirin should not be taken in the week before surgery.[3]

1. Hu OY-P, Chu KM, Liu HS, Chiao SF, Ho W, Ho ST. Reinduction of the hypnotic effects of thiopental with NSAIDs by decreasing thiopental plasma protein binding in humans. *Acta Anaesthesiol Scand* (1993) 37, 258–61.
2. Dundee JW, Halliday NJ, McMurray TJ. Aspirin and probenecid pretreatment influences the potency of thiopentone and the onset of action of midazolam. *Eur J Anaesthesiol* (1986) 3, 247–51.
3. Anon. Drugs in the peri-operative period: 4 – Cardiovascular drugs. *Drug Ther Bull* (1999) 37, 89–92.

Anaesthetics, general + Baclofen

A patient taking baclofen had severe seizures during induction of anaesthesia with propofol.

Clinical evidence, mechanism, importance and management

A 48-year-old man with a cyst in his spinal cord taking baclofen for flexor spasms underwent surgery for the relief of obstructive hydrocephalus. His last dose of baclofen was 6 hours before induction of anaesthesia with pethidine (meperidine) 40 mg followed by **propofol**. After he had received about 60 mg of **propofol** he developed severe myoclonic seizures, which lasted about 3 minutes. The patient was given additional **propofol** 40 mg because he appeared to be awakening, and severe generalised seizures lasting 2 minutes occurred. He was then given vecuronium, and anaesthesia was maintained with isoflurane and nitrous oxide/oxygen without further problem.[1]

Seizures have been reported in patients with and without epilepsy receiving **propofol**. They mainly occur at induction or emergence or are delayed after anaesthesia, suggesting changes in cerebral levels of **propofol** may be causal.[2] Baclofen can cause acute desensitisation of $GABA_B$ receptors producing persistent epileptiform discharges.[1] It was suggested that in this patient the seizures were mediated by both baclofen and **propofol**.[1] Opioid analgesics may induce seizures and opisthotonos has been reported in patients given opioids and **propofol** (see 'Anaesthetics, general + Opioids', p.109). However, generalised seizures attributed to pethidine are probably due to a metabolite. The time course therefore makes pethidine an unlikely cause of the seizure in this patient.[1]

1. Manikandan S, Sinha PK, Neema PK, Rathod RC. Severe seizures during propofol induction in a patient with syringomyelia receiving baclofen. *Anesth Analg* (2005) 100, 1468–9.
2. Walder B, Tramèr MR, Seeck M. Seizure-like phenomena and propofol. A systematic review. *Neurology* (2002) 58, 1327–32.

Anaesthetics, general + Benzodiazepines

Midazolam markedly potentiates the anaesthetic action of halothane. Similarly, the effects of propofol or thiopental are greater than would be expected by simple addition when midazolam is given concurrently, although the extent varies between the end-points measured (analgesic, motor, hypnotic). Quazepam reduces induction time for propofol anaesthesia and premedication with diazepam reduces the dose of ketamine required.

Clinical evidence

(a) Halothane

In a study in 50 women undergoing surgery, **midazolam** markedly potentiated the anaesthetic action of halothane: a mean **midazolam** dose of 278 micrograms/kg reduced the halothane MAC by about 51%.[1]

(b) Ketamine

A study in patients undergoing major abdominal surgery found that in 10 patients premedicated with rectal **diazepam** one hour before induction, the haemodynamic effects of ketamine (increases in heart rate and blood pressure) were significantly reduced, when compared with 31 controls. Also, a lower rate of ketamine infusion was required during the initial 30 minutes of anaesthesia, the half-life of ketamine was significantly increased, and the plasma levels of the hydroxylated metabolites of ketamine were reduced. These findings suggest that both pharmacodynamic and pharmacokinetic interactions exist between **diazepam** and ketamine. In the same study, 3 patients were given 20 mg of intravenous **clorazepate** about one hour before induction of anaesthesia, but this did not affect either the dose of ketamine required or its pharmacokinetics.[2]

(c) Propofol

Two studies found that if propofol and **midazolam** were given together, the hypnotic and anaesthetic effects were greater than would be expected by the simple additive effects of both drugs.[3,4] In one of these studies, the ED_{50} (the dose required for 50% of the patients to respond) for hypnosis was 44% less than that expected with the individual drugs and the addition of **midazolam** 130 micrograms/kg caused a 52% reduction in the ED_{50} of propofol required for anaesthesia.[3] A pharmacokinetic study found a very modest 20% increase in the levels of free **midazolam** in the plasma when it was given with propofol, but this was considered too small to explain the considerable synergism.[5] In a further placebo-controlled study in 24 patients, premedication with intravenous **midazolam**, 50 micrograms/kg given 20 minutes before induction of anaesthesia, reduced the propofol dose requirements for multiple anaesthetic end-points, including hypnotic, motor, EEG and analgesia. However, the potentiating effect and the mechanism of the interaction appeared to vary with the anaesthetic end-point and the dose of propofol. Notably, the interaction was most marked for analgesia.[6] Another placebo-controlled study in 60 children aged 1 to 3 years found that oral **midazolam** 500 micrograms/kg approximately 30 minutes before the induction of anaesthesia delayed early recovery from anaesthesia, which was induced with propofol and maintained with **sevoflurane** and **nitrous oxide/oxygen**. However, the time to hospital discharge was not prolonged.[7]

A further placebo-controlled study in 24 patients found that propofol decreased the clearance of **midazolam** by 37% and increased its elimination half-life by 61%.[8]

A study in 33 patients found that **quazepam** 15 or 30 mg given the night before induction of anaesthesia with propofol and fentanyl reduced the induction time when compared with a third group of patients not given a hypnotic. **Quazepam** did not affect blood pressure or heart rate, but the 30 mg dose of **quazepam** did increase anterograde amnesia.[9]

(d) Thiopental

Thiopental has been shown to act synergistically with **midazolam** at induction of anaesthesia in two studies.[10,11] In one of these studies, **midazolam** reduced the dose of thiopental required to produce anaesthesia by 50%.[11] In a further placebo-controlled study in 23 patients, premedication with intravenous **midazolam** 50 micrograms/kg, given 20 minutes before the induction of anaesthesia, reduced the thiopental dose requirements for multiple anaesthetic end-points, including hypnotic, motor, EEG and analgesia. Potentiation was greatest for the motor end-point (about 40%) and smallest for analgesia (18%).[12]

Mechanism

Propofol, barbiturates and halothane appear to interact with benzodiazepines through their effects on the GABA receptor.

Diazepam appears to undergo similar oxidative processes as ketamine and therefore competitively inhibits ketamine metabolism.[2] Clorazepate is only slowly decarboxylated and is therefore not affected.[2]

An *in vitro* study suggests that propofol may reduce the clearance of midazolam by inhibition of the cytochrome P450 isoenzyme CYP3A4.[8]

Importance and management

The interactions between propofol or thiopental and midazolam are well established. This synergy has been utilised for the induction of anaesthesia.[13] Midazolam also reduces the dose requirements of halothane. Other benzodiazepines may also potentiate the effects of general anaesthetics. In general this may reduce the dose of anaesthetic required and/or slow recovery from the anaesthetic. In many cases this interaction is exploited clinically.

1. Inagaki Y, Sumikawa K, Yoshiya I. Anesthetic interaction between midazolam and halothane in humans. *Anesth Analg* (1993) 76, 613–17.
2. Idvall J, Aronsen KF, Stenberg P, Paalzow L. Pharmacodynamic and pharmacokinetic interactions between ketamine and diazepam. *Eur J Clin Pharmacol* (1983) 24, 337–43.
3. Short TG, Chui PT. Propofol and midazolam act synergistically in combination. *Br J Anaesth* (1991) 67, 539–45.
4. McClune S, McKay AC, Wright PMC, Patterson CC, Clarke RSJ. Synergistic interactions between midazolam and propofol. *Br J Anaesth* (1992) 69, 240–5.
5. Teh J, Short TG, Wong J, Tan P. Pharmacokinetic interactions between midazolam and propofol: an infusion study. *Br J Anaesth* (1994) 72, 62–5.
6. Wilder-Smith OHG, Ravussin PA, Decosterd LA, Despland PA, Bissonnette B. Midazolam premedication reduces propofol dose requirements for multiple anesthetic endpoints. *Can J Anesth* (2001) 48, 439–45.
7. Viitanen H, Annila P, Viitanen M, Yli-Hankala A. Midazolam premedication delays recovery from propofol-induced sevoflurane anesthesia in children 1-3 yr. *Can J Anesth* (1999) 46, 766–71.
8. Hamaoka N, Oda Y, Hase I, Mizutani K, Nakamoto T, Ishizaki T, Asada A. Propofol decreases the clearance of midazolam by inhibiting CYP3A4: in vivo and in vitro study. *Clin Pharmacol Ther* (1999) 66, 110–17.
9. Imamachi N, Saito Y, Sakura S, Doi K, Nomura T. Effects of quazepam given the night before surgery on amnesia and induction and recovery characteristics of propofol anesthesia. Annual Meeting of the American Society of Anesthesiologists, Orlando USA, 2002. Abstract A-444.
10. Tverskoy M, Fleyshman G, Bradley EL, Kissin I. Midazolam–thiopental anesthetic interaction in patients. *Anesth Analg* (1988) 67, 342–5.
11. Short TG, Galletly DC, Plummer JL. Hypnotic and anaesthetic action of thiopentone and midazolam alone and in combination. *Br J Anaesth* (1991) 66, 13–19.
12. Wilder-Smith OHG, Ravussin PA, Decosterd LA, Despland PA, Bissonnette B. Midazolam premedication and thiopental induction of anaesthesia: interactions at multiple end-points. *Br J Anaesth* (1999) 83, 590–5.
13. Orser BA, Miller DR. Propofol-benzodiazepine interactions: insights from a "bench to bedside" approach. *Can J Anesth* (2001) 48, 431–4.

Anaesthetics, general + Beta-agonist bronchodilators

Arrhythmias developed in two patients anaesthetised with halothane when terbutaline was given.

Clinical evidence, mechanism, importance and management

Two patients developed ventricular arrhythmias while anaesthetised with **halothane** and nitrous oxide/oxygen when given **terbutaline** 250 to 350 micrograms subcutaneously for wheezing. Both developed unifocal premature ventricular contractions followed by bigeminy, which responded to lidocaine.[1] **Halothane** was replaced by **enflurane** in one case, which allowed the surgery to be completed without further incident.[1]

Halothane is known to cause arrhythmias and it has been suggested that it may increase susceptibility to the adverse cardiac effects of beta-agonist bronchodilators,[2] which can cause arrhythmias. A number of inhalational anaesthetics have been associated with arrhythmias. For a list, in order of arrhythmogenic potential, see 'Anaesthetics and Neuromuscular blockers', p.97. This interaction is therefore, in theory, possible with any of these anaesthetics and a beta$_2$-agonist bronchodilator, although the case above appears to be the only one reported.

1. Thiagarajah S, Grynsztejn M, Lear E, Azar I. Ventricular arrhythmias after terbutaline administration to patients anesthetized with halothane. *Anesth Analg* (1986) 65, 417–8.
2. Combivent UDVs (Ipratropium bromide monohydrate/Salbutamol sulfate). Boehringer Ingelheim Ltd. UK Summary of product characteristics, February 2009.

Anaesthetics, general + Beta blockers

Anaesthesia in the presence of beta blockers normally appears to be safer than withdrawal of the beta blocker before anaesthesia, provided certain inhalational anaesthetics are avoided (methoxyflurane, cyclopropane, trichloroethylene) and atropine is used to prevent bradycardia. Bradycardia and marked hypotension occurred in a man using timolol eye drops when he was anaesthetised.

Acute peri-operative administration of beta blockers may reduce the dose of anaesthetic required for induction and may result in deeper anaesthesia.

Clinical evidence and mechanism

A. Cardiac depressant effects

It used to be thought that beta blockers should be withdrawn from patients before surgery because of the risk that their cardiac depressant effects would be additive with those of inhalational anaesthetics, resulting in a reduction in cardiac output and blood pressure, but it seems that any effect depends on the anaesthetic used.[1] It has been suggested that the ranking order of compatibility (from the least to the most compatible with beta blockers) is as follows: **methoxyflurane, cyclopropane, trichloroethylene, enflurane, halothane, isoflurane.**[1] This review pre-dated the advent of newer anaesthetics, such as sevoflurane.

(a) Cyclopropane, Methoxyflurane, and Trichloroethylene

A risk of cardiac depression certainly seems to exist with cyclopropane because its depressant effects on the heart are normally counteracted by the release of catecholamines, which would be blocked by the presence of a beta blocker. There is also some evidence (clinical and/or *animal*) that unacceptable cardiac depression may occur with methoxyflurane and trichloroethylene when a beta blocker is present. This has been the subject of two reviews.[2,3] For these three inhalational anaesthetics it has been stated that an absolute indication for their use should exist before giving them in combination with a beta blocker.[1]

(b) Enflurane, Halothane, and Isoflurane

Although a marked reduction in cardiac performance has been described in a study in *dogs* given **propranolol** and enflurane (discussed in two reviews[2,3]) these drugs have been widely used without apparent difficulties.[1] Normally beta blockers and halothane or isoflurane appear to be safe.

(c) Methohexital and Propofol

A study on the effects of adding a beta blocker to anaesthesia was undertaken in 80 patients who were given oxycodone and atropine as pre-medication and then anaesthetised with either methohexital or propofol, either alone or with **esmolol**. The QTc intervals were recorded before any drugs were given and after the administration of propofol or methohexital alone or with esmolol. The addition of **esmolol** to either methohexital or propofol significantly shortened the QTc interval. The heart rate tended to decrease in the propofol plus **esmolol** group. Blood pressure decreased significantly in all four groups but diastolic pressure was significantly lower in the propofol plus **esmolol** group, when compared with the other groups. It was concluded that haemodynamic responses were controlled with methohexital plus **esmolol** or propofol alone, but that propofol plus **esmolol** tended to cause haemodynamic depression.[4]

(d) Unnamed general anaesthetic

A 75-year-old man being treated with **timolol** eye drops for glaucoma developed bradycardia and severe hypotension when anaesthetised and responded poorly to intravenous atropine, dextrose-saline infusion and elevation of his feet.[5] It would seem that there was sufficient systemic absorption of the **timolol** for its effects to be additive with the anaesthetic and cause marked cardiodepression.

B. Reduction of anaesthetic requirements

(a) Atenolol

Intra-operative intravenous atenolol given in 5 mg stepwise doses (median dose 20 mg; range 10 to 80 mg) was found to reduce the **isoflurane** requirement by about 40% without affecting the bispectral index (a predictor of the depth of anaesthesia). Patients also received on average 21% less fentanyl compared with control patients who were not given atenolol.[6]

(b) Esmolol

Several studies have found that the use of esmolol reduces the required dose of **isoflurane** or **propofol**, or results in a deeper anaesthesia (as measured by BIS), but only in the presence of an opioid.[7-11] As there appears to be no pharmacokinetic interaction between esmolol and **propofol**[7,9] it has been suggested that esmolol could be interacting with the opioid.[7,11]

However, in one study 60 patients were given one of three treatments before induction of anaesthesia with **propofol**: esmolol 1 mg/kg followed by an infusion of 250 micrograms/kg per minute; midazolam; or placebo (sodium chloride 0.9%). No opioids were given. Esmolol and midazolam reduced the required induction doses of **propofol** by 25% and 45%, respectively. Esmolol reduced the mean heart rate by 7.6 bpm in the pre-induction period, when compared with placebo, and the only adverse effect noted was a transient episode of bradycardia (44 bpm) in one patient receiving esmolol.

Esmolol reduces cardiac output by reduction of heart rate and stroke volume and this possibly reduces the required induction dose of **propofol** by changing its distribution.[12]

Another study found that a single 80-mg dose of esmolol after induction of anaesthesia with **propofol** and either fentanyl or placebo did not affect the depth of anaesthesia (measured by bispectral index; a predictor of the depth of anaesthesia) in either group of patients, even though cardiovascular effects were seen (reduction in systolic arterial pressure and heart rate).[13]

Importance and management

The consensus of opinion is that beta blockers should not be withdrawn before anaesthesia and surgery[14,15] because of the advantages of maintaining beta-blockade, and because the risks accompanying withdrawal are considerable. But, if inhalational anaesthetics are used, it is important to select the safest anaesthetics (isoflurane, halothane), and avoid those that appear to be most risky (methoxyflurane, cyclopropane, trichloroethylene: most of which are no longer regularly used), as well as ensuring that the patient is protected against bradycardia by atropine. The manufacturers of celiprolol, labetalol, nadolol and sotalol recommend avoiding anaesthetics such as ether, cyclopropane and trichloroethylene,[16-19] as they cause myocardial depression,[16] and note that labetalol may increase the hypotensive effects of halothane.[16]

Although most manufacturers do not contraindicate the continuation of beta blockers during anaesthesia, many do recommend a specific withdrawal period if a clinical decision is made to discontinue beta blockade:

- **Acebutolol,**[20] **atenolol,**[21] **labetalol,**[16] **nebivolol,**[22] **propranolol,**[23] and **timolol**[24] should be discontinued for at least 24 hours before the procedure.
- The dose of **metoprolol**[25,26] should be gradual reduced and stopped at least 24 to 48 hours before anaesthesia.
- The dose of **bisoprolol,**[27] **celiprolol**[19] and **oxprenolol**[28] should be gradually reduced and stopped at least 48 hours before anaesthesia.
- One manufacturer of **sotalol**[17] advises that it may be stopped 4 days before surgery.
- **Nadolol**[18] and **pindolol**[29] should be gradually withdrawn several days before surgery.

The manufacturers of nadolol state that in no circumstances should beta blockers be discontinued before surgery in patients with phaeochromocytoma or thyrotoxicosis.[18]

The authors of the report[5] concerning topically applied beta blockers suggest that if such patients are to be anaesthetised, low concentrations of timolol should be used (possibly withhold the drops pre-operatively), and that "induction agents should be used judiciously and beta-blocking antagonists kept readily available." It is easy to overlook the fact that systemic absorption from eye drops can be high enough to cause adverse interactions.

There appear to be considerable benefits to be gained from the continued use of beta blockers during anaesthesia. Their sudden withdrawal from patients treated for angina or hypertension can result in the development of acute and life-threatening cardiovascular complications whether the patient is undergoing surgery or not. In the peri-operative period patients benefit from beta blockade because it can minimise the effects of sympathetic overactivity of the cardiovascular system during anaesthesia and surgery (for example during endotracheal intubation, laryngoscopy, bronchoscopy and various surgical manoeuvres), which can cause cardiac arrhythmias and hypertension.

Although several studies suggest that beta blockers, such as atenolol and esmolol, given before induction reduce the anaesthetic dose requirement and may potentiate hypnosis there are concerns that reducing the dose of anaesthetic may increase the risk of intra-operative awareness, and it has been suggested that the use of BIS to predict the depth of anaesthesia in the presence of beta blockers may not be valid.[30] There is a possibility that acute as well as chronic administration of beta blockers may prevent peri-operative cardiac complications,[13,15] but more study is needed on this.[15,30]

1. Lowenstein E. Beta-adrenergic blockers. In: Smith NT, Miller RD, Corbascio AN, eds. Drug Interactions in Anesthesia. Philadelphia: Lea and Febiger; 1981 p. 83–101.
2. Foëx P, Cutfield GR, Francis CM. Interactions of cardiovascular drugs with inhalational anaesthetics. *Anasth Intensivmed* (1982) 150, 109–28.
3. Foëx P, Francis CM, Cutfield GR. The interactions between β-blockers and anaesthetics. Experimental observations. *Acta Anaesthesiol Scand* (1982) (Suppl 76), 38–46.
4. Korpinen R, Klemola U-M, Simola M, Toivonen H. The electrocardiographic and hemodynamic effect of methohexital and propofol with and without esmolol. *Acta Anaesthesiol Scand* (2006) 50, 188–192.
5. Mostafa SM, Taylor M. Ocular timolol and induction agents during anaesthesia. *BMJ* (1985) 290, 1788.
6. Zaugg M, Tagliente T, Silverstein JH, Lucchinetti E. Atenolol may not modify anesthetic depth indicators in elderly patients – a second look at the data. *Can J Anaesth* (2003) 50, 638–42.
7. Johansen JW, Flaishon R. Sebel PS. Esmolol reduces anesthetic requirement for skin incision during propofol/nitrous oxide/morphine anesthesia. *Anesthesiology* (1997) 86, 364–71.
8. Johansen JW, Schneider G, Windsor AM, Sebel PS. Esmolol potentiates reduction of minimum alveolar isoflurane concentration by alfentanil. *Anesth Analg* (1998) 87, 671–6.
9. Johansen JW. Esmolol promotes electroencephalographic burst suppression during propofol/alfentanil anesthesia. *Anesth Analg* (2001) 93, 1526–31.
10. Menigaux C, Guignard B, Adam F, Sessler DI, Joly V, Chauvin M. Esmolol prevents movement and attenuates the BIS response to orotracheal intubation. *Br J Anaesth* (2002) 89, 857–62.
11. Orme R, Leslie K, Umranikar A, Ugoni A. Esmolol and anesthetic requirement for loss of responsiveness during propofol anesthesia. *Anesth Analg* (2002) 93, 112–16.
12. Wilson ES, McKinlay S, Crawford JM, Robb HM. The influence of esmolol on the dose of propofol required for induction of anaesthesia. *Anaesthesia* (2004) 59, 122–6.
13. Berkenstadt H, Loebstein R, Faibishenko I, Halkin H, Keidan I, Perel A. Effect of a single dose of esmolol on the bispectral index scale (BIS) during propofol/fentanyl anaesthesia. *Br J Anaesth* (2002) 89, 509–11.
14. Anon. Drugs in the peri-operative period: 4 – Cardiovascular drugs. *Drug Ther Bull* (1999) 37, 89–92.
15. Howell SJ, Sear JW, Foex P. Peri-operative β-blockade: a useful treatment that should be greeted with cautious enthusiasm. *Br J Anaesth* (2001) 86, 161–4.
16. Trandate (Labetalol). UCB Pharma Ltd. UK Summary of product characteristics, June 2005.
17. Beta-Cardone (Sotalol). UCB Pharma Ltd. UK Summary of product characteristics, June 2005.
18. Corgard (Nadolol). Sanofi-Aventis. UK Summary of product characteristics, October 2006.
19. Celectol (Celiprolol hydrochloride). Winthrop Pharmaceuticals UK Ltd. UK Summary of product characteristics, March 2009.
20. Sectral Tablets (Acebutolol hydrochloride). Sanofi-Aventis. UK Summary of product characteristics, February 2007.
21. Tenormin (Atenolol). AstraZeneca UK Ltd. UK Summary of product characteristics, December 2007.
22. Nebilet (Nebivolol). A. Merarini Pharma UK SRL. UK Summary of product characteristics, August 2007.
23. Inderal LA (Propranolol). AstraZeneca UK Ltd. UK Summary of product characteristics, June 2007.
24. Betim (Timolol). Valeant Pharmaceuticals Ltd. UK Summary of product characteristics, July 2006.
25. Lopresor SR (Metoprolol tartrate). Novartis Pharmaceuticals UK Ltd. UK Summary of product characteristics, July 2008.
26. Betaloc SA (Metoprolol). AstraZeneca UK Ltd. UK Summary of product characteristics, March 2007.
27. Cardicor (Bisoprolol hemifumarate). Merck Serono. UK Summary of product characteristics, February 2010.
28. Trasicor (Oxprenolol hydrochloride). Amdipharm. UK Summary of product characteristics, September 2005.
29. Visken Tablets (Pindolol). Amdipharm. UK Summary of product characteristics, January 2005.
30. Yang H, Fayad A. Are β-blockers anesthetics?/Les β-bloquants sont-ils des anesthésiques? *Can J Anaesth* (2003) 50, 627–30.

Anaesthetics, general + Calcium-channel blockers

Impaired myocardial conduction has been seen in two patients taking diltiazem after they were anaesthetised with enflurane, and prolonged anaesthesia has been seen when patients taking verapamil were anaesthetised with etomidate, but it has been suggested that chronic administration of oral calcium-channel blockers up to the day of surgery is usually beneficial. Intravenous dihydropyridines have been used to control peri-operative hypertension, but the use of intravenous verapamil is not recommended in patients anaesthetised with either halothane or enflurane.

Clinical evidence, mechanism, importance and management

(a) Dihydropyridines

Enhanced hypotension was seen in a study in which patients were given intravenous **nimodipine** during general anaesthesia involving **halothane** or **isoflurane**.[1]

The presence of low concentrations of **isoflurane** (0.6%) or **sevoflurane** (0.9%) are reported not to have a marked effect on the pharmacological action of **nicardipine**.[2] In one study intravenous **nicardipine** 17 micrograms/kg was given to 30 neurosurgical patients anaesthetised with either **enflurane**, **isoflurane** or **sevoflurane**. Peak reductions in blood pressure occurred 3 minutes after **nicardipine** was given, and were greatest in the group receiving **sevoflurane**. However, with **isoflurane** peak reductions in blood pressure persisted for longer (30 minutes), as did increases in heart rate, even though the clearance of **nicardipine** was most rapid in patients given **isoflurane**.[3]

Some caution is clearly appropriate, especially with intravenous calcium-channel blockers given during surgery, but general experience suggests that long-term treatment with *oral* dihydropyridine calcium-channel blockers need not be avoided in most patients undergoing anaesthesia, and may be continued until the day of surgery. Further, *intravenous* dihydropyridines have been reported to be safe and effective for the control of peri-operative hypertension.[4]

(b) Diltiazem or Verapamil

The author of a review about calcium-channel blockers and anaesthetics concludes that their concurrent use in patients with reasonable ventricular function is normally beneficial, except where there are other complicating factors. Thus he warns about possible decreases in ventricular function in patients undergoing open chest surgery given *intravenous* verapamil or diltiazem.[5] A report describes a patient taking diltiazem and atenolol who had impaired AV and sinus node function before anaesthesia, which worsened following the use of **enflurane**.[6] Another patient taking diltiazem (and atenolol) had to be paced due to bradycardia of 35 bpm at induction, but despite this he developed severe sinus bradycardia, which progressed to asystole when **enflurane** was given.[6] The authors of this latter report suggest that **enflurane** and diltiazem can have additive depressant effects on myocardial conduction. The presence of low concentrations of **isoflurane** (0.6%) or **sevoflurane** (0.9%) are reported not to have a marked effect on the pharmacological action of diltiazem.[2] Two cases of prolonged anaesthesia and Cheyne-Stokes respiration have been reported in patients who were undergoing cardioversion. Both received verapamil and were induced with **etomidate**.[7] The UK manufacturer of verapamil states that the doses of verapamil and inhalational anaesthetics should be titrated carefully to avoid any adverse cardiac effects (such as bradycardia and hypotension).[8]

The authors of a review concluded that *intravenous* verapamil or diltiazem are not recommended in patients anaesthetised with either **halothane** or **enflurane**, especially if the patients have cardiac failure or conduction disturbances.[9]

1. Müller H, Kafurke H, Marck P, Zierski J, Hempelmann G. Interactions between nimodipine and general anaesthesia – clinical investigations in 124 patients during neurosurgical operations. *Acta Neurochir (Wien)* (1988) 45 (Suppl), 29–35.
2. Fukusaki M, Tomiyasu S, Tsujita T, Ogata K, Goto Y. Interaction of cardiovascular effect of calcium channel blocking drugs and those of inhalation anesthetics in humans. *Masui* (1993) 42, 848–55.

3. Nishiyama T, Matsukawa T, Hanaoka K, Conway CM. Interactions between nicardipine and enflurane, isoflurane, and sevoflurane. *Can J Anaesth* (1997) 44, 1071–6.
4. Tobias JD. Nicardipine: applications in anesthesia practice. *J Clin Anesth* (1995) 7, 525–33.
5. Merin RG. Calcium channel blocking drugs and anesthetics: is the drug interaction beneficial or detrimental? *Anesthesiology* (1987) 66, 111–13.
6. Hantler CB, Wilton N, Learned DM, Hill AEG, Knight PR. Impaired myocardial conduction in patients receiving diltiazem therapy during enflurane anesthesia. *Anesthesiology* (1987) 67, 94–6.
7. Moore CA, Hamilton SF, Underhill AL, Fagraeus L. Potentiation of etomidate anesthesia by verapamil: a report of two cases. *Hosp Pharm* (1989) 24, 24–5.
8. Univer (Verapamil hydrochloride). Cephalon (UK) Ltd. UK Summary of product characteristics, March 2012.
9. Durand P-G, Lehot J-J, Foëx P. Calcium-channel blockers and anaesthesia. *Can J Anaesth* (1991) 38, 75–89.

Anaesthetics, general + Clonidine

Clonidine significantly attenuates the responses to hypercapnia in patients anaesthetised with propofol, but not with isoflurane. Clonidine reduces the dose of thiamylal required for induction of anaesthesia.

Clinical evidence, mechanism, importance and management

Note that additive hypotensive effects are theoretically possible in patients taking clonidine who are given general anaesthetics.

(a) Propofol or Isoflurane

In a study, 60 patients were premedicated with famotidine or famotidine with clonidine 5 micrograms/kg, and anaesthesia was induced with propofol and vecuronium, and maintained with either isoflurane or propofol. The cardiovascular responses (mean arterial pressure, heart rate and cardiac index) to hypercapnia were significantly attenuated in the patients given clonidine and propofol, when compared with those given propofol without clonidine or isoflurane with or without clonidine.[1]

(b) Thiamylal

In a double-blind study 60 children were given either oral clonidine 2 micrograms/kg, 4 micrograms/kg or placebo, 105 minutes before induction of anaesthesia with thiamylal 1% at a rate of 1 mg/kg every 15 seconds until completion of induction (assessed by loss of eyelash reflex). The thiamylal dose required for induction was 5.4 mg/kg, 4.5 mg/kg, and 3.4 mg/kg in the placebo, clonidine 2 micrograms/kg and clonidine 4 micrograms/kg groups respectively, indicating a dose-dependent clonidine reduction in thiamylal requirements. Systolic blood pressure decreased by 6.8%, 5.6%, and 6.6% and heart rate increased by 5.7%, 4.8%, and 4.1% with placebo, clonidine 2 micrograms/kg and 4 micrograms/kg, respectively. The authors note that smaller doses of thiamylal may be needed if given as a bolus dose rather than by incremental administration.[2] In an earlier report, there was a greater decrease in blood pressure in children given a bolus dose of thiamylal 5 mg/kg with clonidine 4 micrograms/kg than those given thiamylal with diazepam.[3]

1. Uchida M, Iida H, Osawaa Y, Tanahashi S, Kumazawa M, Sumi K, Dohi S. Clonidine attenuates the hemodynamic responses to hypercapnia during propofol anesthesia. *Can J Anesth* (2004) 51, 188–9.
2. Nishina K, Mikawa K, Maekawa N, Takao Y, Obara H. Clonidine decreases the dose of thiamylal required to induce anesthesia in children. *Anesth Analg* (1994) 79, 766–8.
3. Mikawa K, Maekawa N, Nishina K, Takao Y, Yaku H, Obara H. Efficacy of oral clonidine premedication in children. *Anesthesiology* (1993) 79, 926–31.

Anaesthetics, general + Dexmedetomidine

Dexmedetomidine may reduce the dose requirements of thiopental, isoflurane, propofol and probably other anaesthetics. In an *animal* study, the analgesic effects of nitrous oxide were increased by dexmedetomidine.

Clinical evidence, mechanism, importance and management

Dexmedetomidine reduced the **thiopental** dose requirement for EEG burst suppression by 30% in 7 patients, when compared with 7 control patients given placebo. In this study, dexmedetomidine was given for 35 minutes before anaesthesia and during anaesthesia at a dose of 100 nanograms/kg per minute for the first 10 minutes, 30 nanograms/kg per minute for the following 15 minutes, and 6 nanograms/kg per minute thereafter. There was no pharmacodynamic synergism, and pharmacokinetic analysis showed that dexmedetomidine significantly reduced the **thiopental** distribution, probably due to reduced cardiac output and decreased regional blood flow.[1]

A placebo-controlled study in women undergoing abdominal hysterectomy found that a dexmedetomidine infusion started 15 minutes before induction of anaesthesia caused a dose-dependent reduction in the **isoflurane** MAC (by 35% and 47%, with dexmedetomidine plasma levels maintained at 0.37 nanograms/mL and 0.69 nanograms/mL, respectively).[2] In another study, in 9 healthy subjects, dexmedetomidine reduced the ED_{50} dose requirement of **isoflurane** for anaesthesia (motor response). Dexmedetomidine plasma levels of 0.35 nanograms/mL and 0.75 nanograms/mL reduced the requirements for **isoflurane** by about 30% and 50%, respectively. Subjects who had received dexmedetomidine took longer to wake up.[3]

In a study, 9 healthy subjects were given stepwise increases in **propofol** concentrations (1 to 13.8 micrograms/mL) 45 minutes after the start of either dexmedetomidine or placebo infusions.[4] Dexmedetomidine did not significantly affect the pharmacokinetics of **propofol**; however, the concurrent use of dexmedetomidine reduced the **propofol** concentration required for sedation by 65 to 80% and reduced the **propofol** concentration required for suppression of motor responses by 40%. It was suggested that the **propofol** dose for sedation and induction may have to be reduced in the presence of dexmedetomidine.[4] Another study in 40 patients given a mean dose of intravenous dexmedetomidine of 63 nanograms/kg found that concurrent use reduced the concentration and dose of **propofol** required to produce loss of consciousness.[5]

An *animal* study found that the analgesic effects of **nitrous oxide** were enhanced by dexmedetomidine.[6]

Dexmedetomidine has sedative, analgesic and anxiolytic effects[7] and therefore, like other sedatives, may reduce the dose requirements of anaesthetics. However, it may also affect the distribution of **thiopental** and possibly other **intravenous anaesthetics**.

1. Bührer M, Mappes A, Lauber R, Stanski DR, Maitre PO. Dexmedetomidine decreases thiopental dose requirement and alters distribution pharmacokinetics. *Anesthesiology* (1994) 80, 1216–27.
2. Aantaa R, Jaakola M-L, Kallio A, Kanto J. Reduction of the minimum alveolar concentration of isoflurane by dexmedetomidine. *Anesthesiology* (1997) 86, 1055–60.
3. Khan ZP, Munday IT, Jones RM, Thornton C, Mant TG, Amin D. Effects of dexmedetomidine on isoflurane requirements in healthy volunteers. 1: Pharmacodynamic and pharmacokinetic interactions. *Br J Anaesth* (1999) 83, 372–80.
4. Dutta S, Karol MD, Cohen T, Jones RM, Mant T. Effect of dexmedetomidine on propofol requirements in healthy subjects. *J Pharm Sci* (2001) 90, 172–81.
5. Peden CJ, Cloote AH, Stratford N, Prys-Roberts C. The effect of intravenous dexmedetomidine premedication on the dose requirement of propofol to induce loss of consciousness in patients receiving alfentanil. *Anaesthesia* (2001) 56, 408–13.
6. Dawson C, Ma D, Chow A, Maze M. Dexmedetomidine enhances analgesic action of nitrous oxide: mechanisms of action. *Anesthesiology* (2004) 100, 894–904.
7. Bhana N, Goa KL, McClellan KJ. Dexmedetomidine. *Drugs* (2000) 59, 263–8.

Anaesthetics, general + Enzyme inducers

A child developed phenytoin toxicity following halothane anaesthesia, a near fatal hepatic reaction occurred in a woman given rifampicin (rifampin) after halothane anaesthesia, and hepatitis occurred in a patient taking phenobarbital who was given halothane anaesthesia.

Clinical evidence

A 10-year-old girl receiving long-term treatment with phenytoin 300 mg daily was found to have **phenytoin** plasma levels of 25 micrograms/mL before surgery. Three days after anaesthesia with **halothane** her plasma **phenytoin** levels had risen to 41 micrograms/mL and she had marked signs of **phenytoin** toxicity.[1]

A woman taking promethazine and **phenobarbital** 60 mg three times daily died from **halothane**-associated hepatitis within 6 days of being given **halothane** for the first time.[2]

A nearly fatal, shock-producing hepatic reaction occurred in a woman 4 days after she was given **halothane** anaesthesia immediately followed by a course of **rifampicin** 600 mg daily and isoniazid 300 mg daily.[3]

Mechanism

It seems possible that the general adverse hepatotoxic effects of halothane can slow the normal rate of phenytoin metabolism. One suggested explanation for the increased adverse effects on the liver is that, just as in *animals*, pre-treatment with phenobarbital and phenytoin increases the rate of drug metabolism and therefore increases the levels of the hepatotoxic metabolites of halothane and other halogenated hydrocarbons.[4,5] As well as increased metabolism, the halothane-rifampicin interaction might also involve additive hepatotoxicity.

Importance and management

No firm conclusions can be drawn from these isolated cases, but they serve to emphasise the potential hepatotoxicity when halogenated anaesthetics are given to patients taking these drugs. It has been suggested that enzyme induction could present a risk factor for serious toxicity with halogenated anaesthetics,[6] and this could reasonably be expected to include the use of drugs such as phenobarbital and phenytoin. Consider also 'Anaesthetics, general + Isoniazid', p.106, and 'Anaesthetics, general; Methoxyflurane + Miscellaneous', p.114.

1. Karlin JM, Kutt H. Acute diphenylhydantoin intoxication following halothane anesthesia. *J Pediatr* (1970) 76, 941–4.
2. Patial RK, Sarin R, Patial SB. Halothane associated hepatitis and phenobarbitone. *J Assoc Physicians India* (1989) 37, 480.
3. Most JA, Markle GB. A nearly fatal hepatotoxic reaction to rifampin after halothane anesthesia. *Am J Surg* (1974) 127, 593–5.
4. Garner RC, McLean AEM. Increased susceptibility to carbon tetrachloride poisoning in the rat after pretreatment with oral phenobarbitone. *Biochem Pharmacol* (1969) 18, 645–50.
5. Jenner MA, Plummer JL, Cousins MJ. Influence of isoniazid, phenobarbital, phenytoin, pregnenolone 16-α carbonitrile, and β-naphthoflavone on halothane metabolism and hepatotoxicity. *Drug Metab Dispos* (1990) 18, 819–22.
6. *Martindale. The Complete Drug Reference*, [online] London: Pharmaceutical Press. http://www.medicinescomplete.com/mc/martindale/current/3101-x.htm (accessed 19/10/15).

Anaesthetics, general + Herbal medicines

There are two isolated reports, of profound hypotension during anaesthesia, and of prolonged anaesthesia, following the long-term use of St John's wort. A report describes increased bleeding, which was tentatively attributed to the concurrent use of sevoflurane and aloe vera. The

American Society of Anesthesiologists recommends that all herbal medicines should be stopped two weeks before elective surgery.

Clinical evidence and mechanism

(a) Aloe vera

A case report describes a 35-year-old woman undergoing surgery for a haemangioma of the left thigh, who had twice the expected intra-operative blood loss. The patient had been taking 4 tablets of aloe vera for 2 weeks before surgery, and so the blood loss was attributed to an interaction between the herbal medicine and **sevoflurane**, which was used to maintain anaesthesia.[1] **Sevoflurane** can inhibit platelet aggregation by inhibiting thromboxane A_2, and aloe vera affects prostaglandin synthesis, which may also impair platelet aggregation. However, it should be noted that the patient's aPTT and INR were not assessed pre-operatively and the authors do state that the vascularity and size of the haemangioma were the most important factors in the blood loss,[1] so an interaction is by no means proven.

(b) Kava

There is one case report of kava potentiating the effect of benzodiazepines (see 'Benzodiazepines + Kava', p.827), and it has been suggested that it could potentiate other CNS depressants including **barbiturates**[2,3] (e.g. **thiopental**), and may prolong or potentiate the effects of anaesthetics.[4-6] Kava may act via GABA receptors, and kavalactones (one group of active constituents) also have skeletal muscle relaxant and local anaesthetic properties.[2,3] Toxic doses can produce muscle weakness and paralysis.[2,3]

(c) St John's wort (Hypericum perforatum)

It has been suggested that St John's wort may prolong anaesthesia.[4-7] The prediction appears to have been based on the possibility that St John's wort acts as an MAOI,[5,7,8] (although this has been disputed[9]) and the limited evidence that MAOIs may cause hepatic enzyme inhibition and potentiate the effects of barbiturates (see 'MAOIs + Barbiturates', p.1385). However, there is now increasing evidence that St John's wort induces hepatic enzymes, and might therefore increase the metabolism of barbiturates (see 'Antiepileptics + St John's wort (*Hypericum perforatum*)', p.566). This suggests that it could in fact increase requirements for **thiopental** anaesthesia. However, prolonged anaesthesia has been reported in a 21-year-old woman who had been taking St John's wort 1 g three times daily for 3 months before general anaesthetics were given for the surgical removal of an abscess. Anaesthesia was induced by intravenous **fentanyl citrate** 1 microgram/kg and **propofol** 3 mg/kg, and maintained throughout the procedure by **sevoflurane** and **nitrous oxide** using a face mask.[10]

The possible MAOI activity of St John's wort has led to the recommendation that the same considerations apply as for other MAOIs and general anaesthetics,[7,8] see 'Anaesthetics, general + MAOIs and related drugs', p.107.

Another case report describes a healthy 23-year-old woman who had been taking St John's wort on a daily basis for 6 months, who developed severe hypotension (BP 60/20 mmHg) during general anaesthesia, which responded poorly to ephedrine and phenylephrine (BP increased to 70/40 mmHg). It was suggested that the St John's wort might have caused adrenergic desensitisation with decreased responsiveness to the vasopressors.[11]

Importance and management

Not established. The evidence presented suggests that some caution may be warranted in patients using kava, or St John's wort if they are given general anaesthetics. The situation with aloe vera is less clear. Many other herbs have the potential to cause problems in the care of patients undergoing surgery (other than via drug interactions with anaesthetics) and these have been reviewed.[5-7] Because of the limited information, the American Society of Anesthesiologists have recommended discontinuation of all herbal medicines 2 weeks before an elective anaesthetic[4,6] and if there is any doubt about the safety of a product, this may be a prudent precaution.[5]

1. Lee A, Chui PT, Aun CST, Gin T, Lau ASC. Possible interaction between sevoflurane and aloe vera. *Ann Pharmacother* (2004) 38, 1651–4.
2. Anon. Piper methysticum (kava kava). *Altern Med Rev* (1998) 3, 458–60.
3. Pepping J. Kava: *Piper methysticum*. *Am J Health-Syst Pharm* (1999) 56, 957–8 and 960.
4. Larkin, M. Surgery patients at risk for herb–anaesthesia interactions. *Lancet* (1999) 354, 1362.
5. Cheng B, Hung CT, Chiu W. Herbal medicine and anaesthesia. *Hong Kong Med J* (2002) 8, 123–30.
6. Leak JA. Perioperative considerations in the management of the patient taking herbal medicines. *Curr Opin Anaesthesiol* (2000) 13, 321–5.
7. Lyons TR. Herbal medicines and possible anesthesia interactions. *AANA J* (2002) 70, 47–51.
8. Klepser TB, Klepser ME. Unsafe and potentially safe herbal therapies. *Am J Health-Syst Pharm* (1999) 56, 125–38.
9. Miller LG. Herbal medicinals. Selected clinical considerations focusing on known or potential drug-herb interactions. *Arch Intern Med* (1998) 158, 2200–11.
10. Crowe S, McKeating K. Delayed emergence and St. John's wort [case reports]. *Anesthesiology* (2002) 96, 1025–7.
11. Irefin S, Sprung J. A possible cause of cardiovascular collapse during anesthesia: long-term use of St John's wort. *J Clin Anesth* (2000) 12, 498–9.

Anaesthetics, general + Inotropes and Vasopressors

Patients anaesthetised with inhalational anaesthetics (particularly cyclopropane and halothane, and to a lesser extent desflurane, enflurane, isoflurane, methoxyflurane, and sevoflurane) can develop cardiac arrhythmias if they are given adrenaline (epinephrine) or noradrenaline (norepinephrine), unless the dosages are very low. Children appear to be less susceptible to this interaction. The addition of adrenaline to intrathecal tetracaine enhances the sedative effects of propofol.

Clinical evidence, mechanism, importance and management

As early as 1895, it was noted that an adrenal extract could cause ventricular fibrillation in a *dog* anaesthetised with **chloroform**,[1] and it is now very well recognised that similar cardiac arrhythmias can be caused by **adrenaline (epinephrine)** and **noradrenaline (norepinephrine)** in humans anaesthetised with **inhalational anaesthetics**. The mechanism appears to be a sensitisation of the myocardium to β-adrenergic stimulation, caused by the **inhalational anaesthetic**. The likelihood of arrhythmias is increased by hypoxia and marked hypercapnia. It has been reported that the highest incidence of complications has been in patients anaesthetised with **cyclopropane**, but that the incidence is also high with **trichloroethylene** and **halothane**.[2] A suggested listing of inhalational anaesthetics in order of decreasing sensitising effect on the myocardium is as follows:[3] **cyclopropane**, **halothane**, **enflurane/methoxyflurane**, **isoflurane**. **Sevoflurane**[4] and **desflurane**[5] appear to behave like **isoflurane**. Similarly, others consider that if **adrenaline** is used for haemostasis during surgery, **isoflurane** or **sevoflurane** carry less risk of cardiac arrhythmias than **halothane**.[6]

It has been recommended that if **adrenaline** is used to reduce surgical bleeding in patients anaesthetised with **halothane/nitrous oxide/oxygen**, the dosage of **adrenaline** should not exceed 10 mL of 1:100 000 in any given 10 minute period, or 30 mL per hour (i.e. about a 100 microgram bolus or 1.5 micrograms/kg per 10 minutes for a 70 kg person), and adequate alveolar ventilation must be assured.[7] This dosage guide should also be safe for use with other inhalational anaesthetics since **halothane** is more arrhythmogenic than the others,[3] with the exception of **cyclopropane**, which is no longer widely used. However, some have suggested that the concurrent use of **halothane** and **adrenaline** may have been a contributing factor in 3 deaths in patients undergoing tooth implant surgery.[8] Solutions containing **lidocaine** 0.5% with **adrenaline** 1:200 000 also appear to be safe because lidocaine may help to control the potential dysrhythmic effects. For example, a study in 19 adult patients anaesthetised with **halothane** found that the dose of **adrenaline** needed to cause three premature ventricular contractions in half the group was 2.11 micrograms/kg when it was given in sodium chloride 0.9% but 3.69 micrograms/kg when it was given in **lidocaine** 0.5%. Note that both these values were less than that in 16 patients anaesthetised with **isoflurane** (6.72 micrograms/kg), demonstrating that **isoflurane** was still safer.[9] It should be borne in mind that the arrhythmogenic effects of **adrenaline** are increased if sympathetic activity is increased, and in hyperthyroidism and hypercapnia.[3]

Children appear to be much less susceptible to these effects than adults. A retrospective study of 28 children found no evidence of arrhythmia during **halothane** anaesthesia, with **adrenaline** doses of up to 8.8 micrograms/kg, and a subsequent study in 83 children (aged 3 months to 17 years) found that 10 micrograms/kg doses of **adrenaline** were safe.[10]

A study in 20 patients undergoing spinal anaesthesia with tetracaine found that **propofol** sedation (as measured by bispectral index monitoring (BIS)) was enhanced when **adrenaline** was added to the intrathecal tetracaine.[11] A study in *sheep* found that **adrenaline**, **noradrenaline** and **dopamine** decreased **propofol** concentrations during a continuous propofol infusion, with the result that **propofol** anaesthesia was reversed. This was thought to be due to increased first pass clearance of **propofol** secondary to increased cardiac output. It was concluded that this could be of clinical importance if **propofol** is used in hyperdynamic circulatory conditions induced by catecholamine infusions or disease states such as sepsis.[12]

1. Oliver G, Schäfer EA. The physiological effects of extracts of the suprarenal capsules. J Physiol (1895) 18, 230–76.
2. Gibb D. Drug interactions in anaesthesia. *Clin Anaesthesiol* (1984) 2, 485–512.
3. Wong KC. Sympathomimetic drugs. In: Smith NT, Miller RD, Corbascio AN, eds. Drug Interactions in Anesthesia. Philadelphia: Lea and Febiger; 1981 p. 55–82.
4. Navarro R, Weiskopf RB, Moore MA, Lockhart S, Eger EI, Koblin D, Lu G, Wilson C. Humans anesthetized with sevoflurane or isoflurane have similar arrhythmic response to epinephrine. *Anesthesiology* (1994) 80, 545–9.
5. Moore MA, Weiskopf RB, Eger EI, Wilson C, Lu G. Arrhythmogenic doses of epinephrine are similar during desflurane or isoflurane anesthesia in humans. *Anesthesiology* (1993) 79, 943–7.
6. Ransom ES, Mueller RA. Safety considerations in the use of drug combinations during general anaesthesia. *Drug Safety* (1997) 16, 88–103.
7. Katz RL, Matteo RS, Papper EM. The injection of epinephrine during general anesthesia with halogenated hydrocarbons and cyclopropane in man. 2. Halothane. *Anesthesiology* (1962) 23, 597–600.
8. Buzik SC. Fatal interaction? Halothane, epinephrine and tooth implant surgery. *Can Pharm J* (1990) 123, 68–9 and 81.
9. Johnston RR, Eger EI, Wilson C. A comparative interaction of epinephrine with enflurane, isoflurane, and halothane in man. *Anesth Analg* (1976) 55, 709–12.
10. Karl HW, Swedlow DB, Lee KW, Downes JJ. Epinephrine–halothane interactions in children. *Anesthesiology* (1983) 58, 142–5.
11. Yotsui T, Kitamura A, Ogawa R. Addition of epinephrine to intrathecal tetracaine augments depression of the bispectral index during intraoperative propofol sedation. *J Anesth* (2004) 18, 147–50.
12. Myburgh JA, Upton RN, Grant C, Martinez A. Epinephrine, norepinephrine and dopamine infusions decrease propofol concentrations during continuous propofol infusion in an ovine model. *Intensive Care Med* (2001) 27, 276–82.

Anaesthetics, general + Isoniazid

Isoniazid may increase the metabolism of enflurane, isoflurane or sevoflurane and thereby increase plasma-fluoride concentrations.

Clinical evidence, mechanism, importance and management

A 46-year-old woman underwent anaesthesia for renal transplantation 6 days after starting to take isoniazid 300 mg daily. Anaesthesia was induced with intravenous thiopental and maintained for 4 hours with 60% nitrous oxide, fentanyl and **isoflurane**. Serum fluoride ions increased, from 4.3 micromol preoperatively, to approximately 30 micromol between 2 and 8 hours after starting **isoflurane**. However, no impairment of renal function occurred. A second patient who was given 5 times the first patient's exposure to **isoflurane** and who had received isoniazid for 13 years had no increase in serum fluoride concentrations over preoperative values, but did show an increase in tri*fluoro*acetic acid levels.[1]

When **enflurane** was given to 20 patients who had been taking isoniazid 300 mg daily for between one week and one year, 9 had an increase in peak fluoride ion levels. These 9 patients had a fourfold higher fluoride level than both 36 control subjects not taking isoniazid and 11 other subjects taking isoniazid only. By 48 hours after anaesthesia, there was no difference in fluoride levels. Despite the increase in fluoride levels, there was no change in renal function.[2]

Isoniazid may increase the metabolism of **enflurane**, **isoflurane** or **sevoflurane**[3,4] in some patients (probably related to isoniazid acetylator phenotype[2]) and so increase the release of fluoride ions that may cause nephrotoxicity. However, there do not appear to be any reports of this resulting in a significant clinical effect on renal function.

1. Gauntlett IS, Koblin DD, Fahey MR, Konopka K, Gruenke LD, Waskell L, Eger EI. Metabolism of isoflurane in patients receiving isoniazid. *Anesth Analg* (1989) 69, 245–9.
2. Mazze RI, Woodruff RE, Heerdt ME. Isoniazid-induced enflurane defluorination in humans. *Anesthesiology* (1982) 57, 5–8.
3. Sevoflurane. Abbott Laboratories Ltd. UK Summary of product characteristics, June 2007.
4. Ultane (Sevoflurane). Abbott Laboratories. US Prescribing information, September 2006.

Anaesthetics, general + Levothyroxine

Two patients taking levothyroxine developed marked hypertension and tachycardia when they were given ketamine.

Clinical evidence, mechanism, importance and management

Two patients taking levothyroxine developed severe hypertension (240/140 mmHg and 210/130 mmHg, respectively) and tachycardia (190 bpm and 150 bpm) when they were given **ketamine**. Both were effectively treated with 1 mg of intravenous propranolol.[1] It was not clear whether this was an interaction or simply a particularly exaggerated response to **ketamine**, but care is clearly needed if **ketamine** is given to patients receiving thyroid replacement therapy.

1. Kaplan JA, Cooperman LH. Alarming reactions to ketamine in patients taking thyroid medication — treatment with propranolol. *Anesthesiology* (1971) 35, 229–30.

Anaesthetics, general + MAOIs and related drugs

Individual cases of both hypo- and hypertension have been seen and MAOIs can interact dangerously with other drugs sometimes used during surgery (particularly pethidine (meperidine) and ephedrine).

Clinical evidence

The absence of problems during emergency general anaesthesia in 2 patients taking MAOIs prompted further study in 6 others receiving long-term treatment with unnamed MAOIs. All 6 were premedicated with 10 to 15 mg of diazepam 2 hours before surgery, induced with **thiopental**, given suxamethonium (succinylcholine) before intubation, and maintained with **nitrous oxide/oxygen** with either **halothane** or **isoflurane**. Pancuronium was used for muscle relaxation, and morphine was given postoperatively. One patient experienced hypotension that responded to repeated 100-microgram intravenous doses of phenylephrine without hypertensive reactions. No other untoward events occurred either during or after the anaesthesia.[1]

A retrospective review of 32 patients taking **isocarboxazid** 10 mg daily who underwent elective surgery (involving **thiopental** or **ketamine** for induction of anaesthesia and maintenance with an inhalation anaesthetic with or without a muscle relaxant or analgesic) found that 5 patients experienced intra-operative hypotension, another patient developed hypertension, and bradycardia occurred in 4 patients. No postoperative complications were attributed to the interaction between the MAOI and the drugs given peri-operatively.[2]

Unexplained hypertension has been described in a patient taking **tranylcypromine** when **etomidate** and atracurium were given.[3] Severe and prolonged cardiovascular collapse occurred in one patient in whom long-term **tranylcypromine** 10 mg four times daily was discontinued 20 days before surgery. During surgery **etomidate** and suxamethonium were given for induction, and **isoflurane** and **nitrous oxide/oxygen** for maintenance, as well as epidural anaesthesia with bupivacaine, but without an opioid.[4]

Further reports describe a lack of adverse reactions in:

- 27 patients taking MAOIs (**tranylcypromine, phenelzine, isocarboxazid, pargyline**) when they were anaesthetised,[5]
- 2 patients taking **phenelzine** and anaesthetised with **propofol**,[6,7]
- 3 patients taking **tranylcypromine** or **phenelzine** and anaesthetised with **propofol** (and alfentanil),[8,9]
- one patient taking **tranylcypromine** when **ketamine** was given,[10]
- one patient taking **phenelzine** when anaesthetised with **sevoflurane**, then **isoflurane**, and an infusion of remifentanil.[11]

Further case reports describe the uneventful use of selective MAOIs in patients undergoing general anaesthesia: one patient taking **selegiline** was uneventfully anaesthetised with fentanyl, **isoflurane** and midazolam,[12] and **moclobemide** was stopped on the morning of surgery in a patient who was anaesthetised with **propofol** and later **isoflurane** in **nitrous oxide** and oxygen. Atracurium, morphine and droperidol were also used.[13]

Mechanism, importance and management

There seems to be little documentary evidence that the withdrawal of MAOIs before giving an anaesthetic is normally necessary. Scrutiny of reports[14] alleging an adverse reaction usually shows that what happened could be attributed to an interaction between the MAOI and other drugs used during the surgery (e.g. either 'inotropes and vasopressors', p.1392, 'pethidine (meperidine)', p.1399, or 'fentanyl', p.1397) rather than with the anaesthetics.

The authors of two of the reports cited here offer the opinion that 'general and regional anaesthesia may be provided safely without discontinuation of MAOI therapy, provided proper monitoring, adequate preparation, and prompt treatment of anticipated reactions are utilised'.[1,5] This implies that the possible interactions between the MAOI and other drugs are fully recognised, but be alert for the rare unpredictable response. The conclusion of another report was that patients on low-dose MAOIs could be safely anaesthetised.[2]

1. El-Ganzouri A, Ivankovich AD, Braverman B, Land PC. Should MAOI be discontinued preoperatively? *Anesthesiology* (1983) 59, A384.
2. Ebrahim ZY, O'Hara J, Borden L, Tetzlaff J. Monoamine oxidase inhibitors and elective surgery. *Cleve Clin J Med* (1993) 60, 129–30.
3. Sides CA. Hypertension during anaesthesia with monoamine oxidase inhibitors. *Anaesthesia* (1987) 42, 633–5.
4. Sprung J, Distel D, Grass J, Bloomfield EL, Lavery IC. Cardiovascular collapse during anesthesia in a patient with preoperatively discontinued chronic MAO inhibitor therapy. *J Clin Anesth* (1996) 8, 662–5.
5. El-Ganzouri AR, Ivankovich AD, Braverman B, McCarthy R. Monoamine oxidase inhibitors: should they be discontinued preoperatively? *Anesth Analg* (1985) 64, 592–6.
6. Hodgson CA. Propofol and mono-amine oxidase inhibitors. *Anaesthesia* (1992) 47, 356.
7. Fischer SP, Mantin R, Brock-Utne JG. Ketorolac and propofol anesthesia in a patient taking chronic monoamine oxidase inhibitors. *J Clin Anesth* (1996) 8, 245–7.
8. Powell H. Use of alfentanil in a patient receiving monoamine oxidase inhibitor therapy. *Br J Anaesth* (1990) 64, 528–9.
9. Beresford BJ, Glick D, Dinwiddie SH. Combination propofol-alfentanil anesthesia for electroconvulsive therapy in patients receiving monoamine oxidase inhibitors. *J ECT* (2004) 20, 120–2.
10. Doyle DJ. Ketamine induction and monoamine oxidase inhibitors. *J Clin Anesth* (1990) 2, 324–5.
11. Ure DS, Gillies MA, James KS. Safe use of remifentanil in a patient treated with the monoamine oxidase inhibitor phenelzine. *Br J Anaesth* (2000) 84, 414–16.
12. Noorily SH, Hantler CB, Sako EY. Monoamine oxidase inhibitors and cardiac anesthesia revisited. *South Med J* (1997) 90, 836–8.
13. McFarlane HJ. Anaesthesia and the new generation monoamine oxidase inhibitors. *Anaesthesia* (1994) 49, 597–9.
14. Stack CG, Rogers P, Linter SPK. Monoamine oxidase inhibitors and anaesthesia: a review. *Br J Anaesth* (1988) 60, 222–7.

Anaesthetics, general + Melatonin

Melatonin slightly reduces the dose of propofol needed for the induction of anaesthesia.

Clinical evidence

A study in 45 adult patients found that the induction dose of intravenous **propofol**, as measured by bispectral index and loss of eyelash reflex, was 15% lower in patients who had received a single 3- or 5-mg oral dose of melatonin 100 minutes preoperatively, compared with patients who had received placebo. The time to recover from the anaesthetic was not affected by premedication with melatonin. **Propofol** was given in an incremental dose fashion in this study so that any difference could be assessed, but is usually given as a bolus dose.[1]

Mechanism

Melatonin appears to have anxiolytic and sedative effects, which might reduce the required induction dose of propofol.

Importance and management

This study was conducted to assess the clinical value of using melatonin premedication, which is not an established use. The reduction in required dose of propofol was small, and on the basis of these data, it is unlikely that any untoward effects would be seen in the situation where a patient who had recently taken a melatonin supplement was anaesthetised with propofol.

1. Turkistani A, Abdullah KM, Al-Shaer AA, Mazen KF, Alkatheri K. Melatonin premedication and the induction dose of propofol. *Eur J Anaesthesiol* (2007) 24, 399–402.

Anaesthetics, general + Methylphenidate

A single report described difficulty in sedating a child taking methylphenidate, and a possible delayed interaction between ketamine and methylphenidate, which resulted in nausea, vomiting and dehydration. The use of methylphenidate after ketamine anaesthesia increased the incidence of vomiting, excessive talking, and limb movements in one study. Methylphenidate should probably be withheld before anaesthesia

with inhalational anaesthetics, because of the potential risk of hypertension and/or arrhythmias.

Clinical evidence, mechanism, importance and management

A 6-year-old boy weighing 22 kg, who was taking methylphenidate 5 mg twice daily for attention deficit disorder, was found to be difficult to sedate for an echocardiogram. Sedation was attempted with oral cloral hydrate 75 mg/kg without success. One week later he received midazolam 20 mg orally, but was only mildly sedated 20 minutes later and would not lie still. Despite an additional oral dose of midazolam 10 mg mixed with oral **ketamine** 60 mg the child was still alert and uncooperative 20 minutes later. He was finally given intravenous glycopyrronium (glycopyrrolate) 100 micrograms followed by intravenous midazolam 5 mg given over 5 minutes and was successfully sedated. He recovered from sedation uneventfully, but developed nausea, vomiting and lethargy after discharge from hospital, which responded to rehydration treatment.[1] In a double-blind study, methylphenidate was given as a single 20-mg intravenous dose to try to speed recovery at the end of **ketamine** anaesthesia for short urological procedures. However, methylphenidate did not improve recovery, and increased the incidence of vomiting, excessive talking, and limb movements.[2]

In the first case, the stimulant effect of methylphenidate was thought to have antagonised the sedative effect of the midazolam and **ketamine**. It has been suggested that methylphenidate may also have delayed the absorption of the oral drugs, and inhibited liver microsomal enzymes delaying the elimination of both **ketamine** and midazolam. These effects may have resulted in hazardous plasma concentrations;[1] however, the study did not find evidence of these effects.

These appear to be the only reports, so any effect is not established. Be aware that methylphenidate may possibly antagonise the effect of sedative drugs, and may also be associated with an increased incidence of vomiting. Note that methylphenidate is an indirectly-acting sympathomimetic, and as such might be expected to increase the risk of hypertension and arrhythmias if used with **inhalational anaesthetics** (consider 'Anaesthetics, general + Inotropes and Vasopressors', p.106). Because of this, the manufacturer of one brand of methylphenidate recommends that, if surgery with halogenated anaesthetics is planned, methylphenidate treatment should not be given on the day of surgery.[3] Taken together, these reports suggest this advice may be a prudent precaution for any form of sedation and/or general anaesthesia.

1. Ririe DG, Ririe KL, Sethna NF, Fox L. Unexpected interaction of methylphenidate (Ritalin®) with anaesthetic agents. *Paediatr Anaesth* (1997) 7, 69–72.
2. Attalah MM, Saied MMA, Yahya R, Ibrahiem EI. Ketamine anesthesia for short transurethral urologic procedures. *Middle East J Anesthesiol* (1993) 12, 123–33.
3. Concerta XL (Methylphenidate hydrochloride). Janssen-Cilag Ltd. UK Summary of product characteristics, November 2009.

Anaesthetics, general + Neuromuscular blockers

Many inhalational anaesthetics increase the effects of the neuromuscular blockers, and in some cases this allows for a dosage reduction of the neuromuscular blocker. Nitrous oxide appears not to interact significantly and halothane seems less likely to interact. Propofol and xenon are reported not to interact with mivacurium or rocuronium. Bradycardia has been reported with combinations of anaesthetics (propofol, etomidate or thiopental) and neuromuscular blockers (atracurium, suxamethonium or vecuronium), particularly in the presence of an opioid.

Clinical evidence, mechanism, importance and management

The effects of neuromuscular blockers are increased by inhalational anaesthetics, the greater the dosage of the anaesthetic the greater the increase in blockade. In broad terms **desflurane**, **ether**, **enflurane**, **isoflurane**, **methoxyflurane** and **sevoflurane** have a greater effect than **halothane**, which is more potent than **cyclopropane**, whereas **nitrous oxide** appears not to interact significantly with competitive blockers.[1-7]

The mechanism is not fully understood but seems to be multifactorial. It has been suggested that the anaesthetic may:

- have an effect via the CNS (including depression of spinal motor neurones);
- have an effect on the neuromuscular junction (including a decrease in the release of acetylcholine and in the sensitivity of the motor end-plate to acetylcholine);
- affect the muscle tissue itself.[6,8]

The duration of exposure to the anaesthetic and the duration of effect of the various neuromuscular blockers also appear to affect the degree of potentiation that occurs.[8,9]

Reports pertaining to interactions between specific neuromuscular blockers and anaesthetics are discussed in the subsections below.

(a) Atracurium

In a study in which the muscle relaxant was given about 5 minutes after the start of inhalational anaesthesia, **enflurane** prolonged the action of atracurium. It was suggested that more prolonged exposure to the anaesthetic, allowing equilibration of the anaesthetic to the tissues, might result in more significant potentiation of the neuromuscular blockers.[9] Similarly, in another study, **ketamine** prolonged the duration of neuromuscular blockade induced by atracurium.[10] In contrast, **halothane** did not significantly prolong the clinical duration of atracurium.[9]

The dosage of atracurium can be reduced by 25 to 30% if, instead of balanced anaesthesia (with **thiopental**, fentanyl and **nitrous oxide**/oxygen),[11] **enflurane** is used, and by up to 50% if **isoflurane** or **desflurane** are used.[4,12,13] Another study recommended reduced doses of neuromuscular blockers such as atracurium and **tubocurarine** in children undergoing anaesthesia with **enflurane** or **isoflurane**.[14]

Bradycardia and asystole have been reported in a patient given **propofol**, fentanyl and atracurium.[15]

(b) Cisatracurium

A myasthenic patient developed marked potentiation of neuromuscular block following the combination of **sevoflurane** and a small dose of cisatracurium 25 micrograms/kg.[16]

(c) Mivacurium

It has been suggested that higher plasma levels of mivacurium, especially of the potent *trans-trans* isomer, occur in the presence of **isoflurane**, and these could contribute to the enhanced neuromuscular blockade observed in patients given this combination. Lower infusion rates of mivacurium were required in those given **isoflurane** rather than **propofol** (which does not appear to interact).[17]

Xenon is reported not to affect the onset time, duration and recovery from mivacurium.[18]

(d) Pancuronium

In a study in which the muscle relaxant was given about 5 minutes after the start of inhalational anaesthesia, **enflurane** prolonged the action of pancuronium. It was suggested that more prolonged exposure to the anaesthetic, allowing equilibration of the anaesthetic to the tissues, might result in more significant potentiation of the neuromuscular blocker.[9] In this study, **halothane** did not significantly prolong the clinical duration of pancuronium;[9] however, in an early study, **halothane** was found to *shorten* the recovery from pancuronium.[19,20]

(e) Pipecuronium

In a study in which the muscle relaxant was given about 5 minutes after the start of inhalational anaesthesia, **enflurane** prolonged the action of pipecuronium. It was suggested that more prolonged exposure to the anaesthetic, allowing equilibration of the anaesthetic to the tissues, might result in more significant potentiation of the neuromuscular blockers.[9] In this study, **halothane** did not significantly prolong the clinical duration of pipecuronium.[9]

(f) Rapacuronium

One study demonstrated considerable prolongation of neuromuscular blockade with rapacuronium in the presence of **sevoflurane**; the recovery times were approximately doubled compared with those given in the published literature using **thiopental**/opioid-**nitrous oxide** anaesthesia. This led to the study being prematurely terminated as spontaneous recovery of neuromuscular function was required after short surgical procedures.[21]

(g) Rocuronium

The rate of infusion of rocuronium (0.39 mg/kg per hour) was significantly less in 10 patients anaesthetised with **isoflurane** and **nitrous oxide** when compared with the rate (0.61 to 0.67 mg/kg per hour) in 50 other patients anaesthetised with **etomidate**, fentanyl, midazolam, **propofol**, or **thiopental** and **nitrous oxide**.[22]

In one study when the volatile anaesthetics were given about 10 minutes before the neuromuscular blocker, **sevoflurane** was reported to increase and prolong the blockade of rocuronium more than **isoflurane** or **propofol**.[23] However, another study found that after a 40-minute equilibration period of the inhalation anaesthetic (steady-state conditions), there was no significant difference between **desflurane**, **isoflurane** and **sevoflurane** in relation to potency, infusion requirements or recovery characteristics of rocuronium; the potency of rocuronium was increased by 25 to 40% under inhalational anaesthesia, when compared with **propofol**.[24]

It is reported that the neuromuscular blocking effects of rocuronium are not prolonged by **xenon**.[25]

In *animals*, **ketamine** and **thiopental** potentiated the neuromuscular blocking effects of rocuronium, whereas **propofol** had no effect.[26]

(h) Suxamethonium (Succinylcholine)

Although it is generally assumed that **nitrous oxide** does not affect the potency of neuromuscular blockers, one study found that **nitrous oxide** did increase suxamethonium neuromuscular blockade.[27]

In children receiving suxamethonium, those anaesthetised with **halothane** had much higher levels of serum myoglobin than those undergoing intravenous induction with **thiopental** followed by **halothane**. This suggests that prior use of **halothane** may have potentiated suxamethonium-induced muscle damage.[28]

In one study, **ketamine** did not influence suxamethonium-induced neuromuscular blockade.[29] However, the UK manufacturers of suxamethonium still warn of a possible interaction because they say that **ketamine** may reduce normal plasma cholinesterase activity.[30]

Serious sinus bradycardia (heart rates of 30 to 40 bpm) developed rapidly in two young women when they were anaesthetised with a slow intravenous injection of **propofol** 2.5 mg/kg, followed by suxamethonium 1.5 mg/kg. This was controlled with 600 micrograms of intravenous atropine. Four other patients premedicated with 600 micrograms of intramuscular atropine given 45 minutes before induction of anaesthesia did not develop bradycardia.[31] It would appear that **propofol** lacks central vagolytic activity and can exaggerate the muscarinic effects of suxamethonium.[31] Another report describes a woman who became asystolic when given an anaesthetic induction sequence of fentanyl, **propofol** and suxamethonium.[32] The authors of this report suggest that atropine or glycopyrronium (glycopyrrolate) pretreatment should attenuate or prevent such reactions.[32] Bradycardia and asystole has also been seen following the sequential use of **propofol** and fentanyl in 2 patients.[33,34] All of these three drugs (fentanyl, **propofol**, suxamethonium) alone have been associated with bradycardia and their effects can apparently be additive.

(i) Vecuronium

In a study in which the muscle relaxant was given about 5 minutes after the start of inhalational anaesthesia, **enflurane** did not significantly affect vecuronium. It was suggested that the duration of effect of the vecuronium may have been too short for interaction with a volatile anaesthetic that had not had time to equilibrate with the tissues.[9] In this study, **halothane** did not significantly prolong the clinical duration of vecuronium.[9] One study in children found that the potentiation of vecuronium was greater with **isoflurane** than with **enflurane**, and **halothane** had a lesser effect.[35] In another study, **enflurane** and **isoflurane** reduced the vecuronium infusion rate requirements by as much as 70%, when compared with fentanyl anaesthesia.[36] Another study found that although **halothane** and **isoflurane** could both increase the neuromuscular potency of vecuronium, only **isoflurane** prolonged the recovery from neuromuscular blockade.[37]

The duration of exposure to **sevoflurane** also influences the dose-response of vecuronium, but it has been suggested that **sevoflurane**-induced potentiation of neuromuscular blockers might be more rapid than with other inhalational anaesthetics.[8]

Xenon is reported to have less effect on recovery from vecuronium-induced neuromuscular block than **sevoflurane**.[38]

The original formulation of **propofol** in *Cremophor* was found to increase the blockade due to vecuronium,[39] but the more recent formulation in soybean oil and egg phosphatide has been found in an extensive study not to interact with vecuronium.[40]

Bradycardia occurring during anaesthetic induction with vecuronium and **etomidate**, or to a lesser extent **thiopental**, has also been reported, particularly in patients also receiving fentanyl.[41] Consider also 'Neuromuscular blockers + Opioids', p.133.

1. Schuh FT. Differential increase in potency of neuromuscular blocking agents by enflurane and halothane. *Int J Clin Pharmacol Ther Toxicol* (1983) 21, 383–6.
2. Fogdall RP, Miller RD. Neuromuscular effects of enflurane, alone and combined with *d*-tubocurarine, pancuronium, and succinylcholine, in man. *Anesthesiology* (1975) 42, 173–8.
3. Miller RD, Way WL, Dolan WM, Stevens WC, Eger EI. Comparative neuromuscular effects of pancuronium, gallamine, and succinylcholine during Forane and halothane anesthesia in man. *Anesthesiology* (1971) 35, 509–14.
4. Lee C, Kwan WF, Chen B, Tsai SK, Gyermek L, Cheng M, Cantley E. Desflurane (I-653) potentiates atracurium in humans. *Anesthesiology* (1990) 73, A875.
5. Izawa H, Takeda J, Fukushima K. The interaction between sevoflurane and vecuronium and its reversibility by neostigmine in man. *Anesthesiology* (1992) 77, A960.
6. Østergaard D, Engbaek J, Viby-Mogensen J. Adverse reactions and interactions of the neuromuscular blocking drugs. *Med Toxicol Adverse Drug Exp* (1989) 4, 351–68.
7. Vanlinthout LEH, Booij LHDJ, van Egmond J, Robertson EN. Effect of isoflurane and sevoflurane on the magnitude and time course of neuromuscular block produced by vecuronium, pancuronium and atracurium. *Br J Anaesth* (1996) 76, 389–95.
8. Suzuki T, Iwasaki K, Fukano N, Hariya S, Saeki S, Ogawa S. Duration of exposure to sevoflurane affects dose–response relationship of vecuronium. *Br J Anaesth* (2000) 85, 732–4.
9. Swen J, Rashkovsky OM, Ket JM, Koot HWJ, Hermans J, Agoston S. Interaction between nondepolarizing neuromuscular blocking agents and inhalational anesthetics. *Anesth Analg* (1989) 69, 752–5.
10. Toft P, Helbo-Hansen S. Interaction of ketamine with atracurium. *Br J Anaesth* (1989) 62, 319–20.
11. Ramsey FM, White PA, Stullken EH, Allen LL, Roy RC. Enflurane potentiation of neuromuscular blockade by atracurium. *Anesthesiology* (1982) 57, A255.
12. Sokoll MD, Gergis SD, Mehta M, Ali NM, Lineberry C. Safety and efficacy of atracurium (BW33A) in surgical patients receiving balanced or isoflurane anesthesia. *Anesthesiology* (1983) 58, 450–5.
13. Smiley RM, Ornstein E, Mathews D, Matteo RS. A comparison of the effects of desflurane and isoflurane on the action of atracurium in man. *Anesthesiology* (1990) 73, A882.
14. Lynas AGA, Fitzpatrick KTJ, Black GW, Mirakhur RK, Clarke RSJ. Influence of volatile anaesthetics on the potency of tubocurarine and atracurium. *Br J Clin Pharmacol* (1988) 26, 617P–618P.
15. Ricós P, Trillo L, Crespo MT, Guilera N, Puig MM. Bradicardia y asistolia asociadas a la administración simultánea de propofol y fentanilo en la inducción anestésica. *Rev Esp Anestesiol Reanim* (1994) 41, 194–5.
16. Baraka AS, Taha SK, Kawkabani NI. Neuromuscular interaction of sevoflurane - cisatracurium in a myasthenic patient. *Can J Anesth* (2000) 47, 562–5.
17. Ledowski T, Wulf H, Ahrens K, Weindlmayr-Goettel M, Kress H-G, Geldner G, Scholz J. Neuromuscular block and relative concentrations of mivacurium isomers under isoflurane versus propofol anaesthesia. *Eur J Anaesthesiol* (2003) 20, 821–5.
18. Kunitz O, Baumert H-J, Hecker K, Coburn M, Beeker T, Zühlsdorff A, Fassl J, Rossaint R. Xenon does not modify mivacurium induced neuromuscular block. *Can J Anesth* (2005) 52, 940–3.
19. Barth L. Paradoxical interaction between halothane and pancuronium. *Anaesthesia* (1973) 28, 514–20.
20. Feldman SA, Andrew D. Paradoxical interaction between halothane and pancuronium. *Anaesthesia* (1974) 29, 100–2.
21. Cara DM, Armory P, Mahajan RP. Prolonged duration of neuromuscular block with rapacuronium in the presence of sevoflurane. *Anesth Analg* (2000) 91, 1392–3.
22. Olkkola KT, Tammisto T. Quantitation of the interaction of rocuronium bromide with etomidate, fentanyl, midazolam, propofol, thiopentone, and isoflurane using closed-loop feedback control of infusion of rocuronium. *Eur J Anaesthesiol* (1994) 11 (Suppl 9), 99–100.
23. Lowry DW, Mirakhur RK, McCarthy GJ, Carroll MT, McCourt KC. Neuromuscular effects of rocuronium during sevoflurane, isoflurane, and intravenous anesthesia. *Anesth Analg* (1998) 87, 936–40.
24. Bock M, Klippel K, Nitsche B, Bach A, Martin E, Motsch J. Rocuronium potency and recovery characteristics during steady-state desflurane, sevoflurane, isoflurane or propofol anaesthesia. *Br J Anaesth* (2000) 84, 43–7.
25. Kunitz O, Baumert J-H, Hecker K, Beeker T, Coburn M, Zühlsdorff A, Rossaint R. Xenon does not prolong neuromuscular block of rocuronium. *Anesth Analg* (2004) 99, 1398–1401.
26. Muir AW, Anderson KA, Pow E. Interaction between rocuronium bromide and some drugs used during anaesthesia. *Eur J Anaesthesiol* (1994) 11 (Suppl 9), 93–8.
27. Szalados JE, Donati F, Bevan DR. Nitrous oxide potentiates succinylcholine neuromuscular blockade in humans. *Anesth Analg* (1991) 72, 18–21.
28. Laurence AS, Henderson P. Serum myoglobin after suxamethonium administration to children: effect of pretreatment before i.v. and inhalation induction. *Br J Anaesth* (1986) 58, 126P.
29. Helbo-Hansen HS, Toft P, Kirkegaard Neilsen H. Ketamine does not affect suxamethonium-induced neuromuscular blockade in man. *Eur J Anaesthesiol* (1989) 6, 419–23.
30. Anectine (Suxamethonium). GlaxoSmithKline UK. UK Summary of product characteristics, September 2008.
31. Baraka A. Severe bradycardia following propofol-suxamethonium sequence. *Br J Anaesth* (1988) 61, 482–3.
32. Egan TD, Brock-Utne JG. Asystole after anesthesia induction with a fentanyl, propofol, and succinylcholine sequence. *Anesth Analg* (1991) 73, 818–20.
33. Guise PA. Asystole following propofol and fentanyl in an anxious patient. *Anaesth Intensive Care* (1991) 19, 116–18.
34. Dorrington KL. Asystole with convulsion following a subanaesthetic dose of propofol plus fentanyl. *Anaesthesia* (1989) 44, 658–9.
35. Lynas AGA, Fitzpatrick KTJ, Black GW, Mirakhur RK. Influence of volatile anaesthetics on the potency of vecuronium in children. *Br J Anaesth* (1988) 61, 506P.
36. Cannon JE, Fahey MR, Castagnoli KP, Furuta T, Canfell PC, Sharma M, Miller RD. Continuous infusion of vecuronium: the effect of anesthetic agents. *Anesthesiology* (1987) 67, 503–6.
37. Pittet J-F, Melis A, Rouge J-C, Morel DR, Gemperle G, Tassonyi E. Effect of volatile anesthetics on vecuronium-induced neuromuscular blockade in children. *Anesth Analg* (1990) 70, 248–52.
38. Nakata Y, Goto T, Morita S. Vecuronium-induced neuromuscular block during xenon or sevoflurane anaesthesia in humans. *Br J Anaesth* (1998) 80, 238–40.
39. Robertson EN, Fragen RJ, Booij LHDJ, van Egmond J, Crul JF. Some effects of diisopropyl phenol (ICI 35 868) on the pharmacodynamics of atracurium and vecuronium in anaesthetized man. *Br J Anaesth* (1983) 55, 723–7.
40. McCarthy GJ, Mirakhur RK, Pandit SK. Lack of interaction between propofol and vecuronium. *Anesth Analg* (1992) 75, 536–8.
41. Inoue K, El-Banayosy A, Stolarski L, Reichelt W. Vecuronium induced bradycardia following induction of anaesthesia with etomidate or thiopentone, with or without fentanyl. *Br J Anaesth* (1988) 60, 10–17.

Anaesthetics, general + Opioids

The effects of inhalational anaesthetics may be enhanced by opioid analgesics, and the dose requirements of desflurane, etomidate, propofol and thiopental may be lower after opioid use. The respiratory depressant effects of ketamine and morphine may be additive. Opisthotonos or grand mal seizures have rarely been associated with the use of propofol with alfentanil and/or fentanyl.

Clinical evidence, mechanism, importance and management

(a) Inhalational anaesthetics

Opioid analgesics have been reported to reduce the MAC values of inhalational anaesthetics. For example, **fentanyl** has been shown to lower the MAC value of **desflurane**, probably in a dose-dependent manner, and this has been the subject of a review.[1] The manufacturer notes that lower doses of **desflurane** are required in patients receiving opioids.[2] **Remifentanil** at a target-controlled plasma level of 1 nanogram/mL was found to decrease the MAC of **sevoflurane** with **nitrous oxide** by 60%, and **remifentanil** 3 nanograms/mL produced a further 30% decrease in the MAC of **sevoflurane**.[3] Another study found that **remifentanil** dose-dependently decreased the level of **sevoflurane** required to maintain anaesthesia.[4] However, 100 microgram/kg doses of **morphine** given during anaesthesia did not alter the awakening concentration of **sevoflurane**.[5]

(b) Intravenous anaesthetics

1. Etomidate. The manufacturer of etomidate recommends that the dose of etomidate should be reduced in patients who have already received opioids.[6]

2. Ketamine. A study in 11 healthy subjects found that the combination of ketamine and **morphine** almost abolished windup-like pain (progressive increase in pain intensity on repeated stimulation) in a skin burn injury. This effect was not found with either drug alone. Further, although ketamine alone reduced the area of secondary hyperalgesia of the local burn and increased the pain threshold, the combination did not appear to enhance this effect. The reduction of wind-up pain may be due to ketamine-induced prevention of acute tolerance to **morphine**.[7] Ketamine is a respiratory depressant like **morphine**, but less potent. Nevertheless its effects can be additive with morphine.[8]

Another study in healthy subjects using various experimental pain models found that ketamine *antagonised* the respiratory depressant effect of **remifentanil**. **Remifentanil** alone produced analgesic effects with all pain tests, but ketamine only enhanced the effect of **remifentanil** on intramuscular electrical stimulation. Acute **remifentanil**-induced hyperalgesia and tolerance were detected only by the pressure pain test and were not suppressed by ketamine. The combined effects of **remifentanil** and ketamine probably depend on the type of pain.[9]

The manufacturer notes that a prolonged recovery time may occur if opioids are used with ketamine.[10]

3. Propofol. A 71-year-old man undergoing a minor orthopaedic operation was given a 500-microgram intravenous injection of **alfentanil** followed by a slow injection of propofol 2.5 mg/kg. Approximately 15 seconds after the propofol, the patient developed strong bilateral fits and grimaces, which lasted for 10 seconds. Anaesthesia was maintained with nitrous oxide/oxygen and halothane and there were no other intra- or postoperative complications. The patient had no history of convulsions.[11] There is a further report of opisthotonos during recovery from anaesthesia with **alfentanil**, propofol and nitrous oxide.[12] Propofol has been associated with opisthotonos (a spasm where the head and heels bend backwards and the body arches forwards) in two patients given **fentanyl** with or without **alfentanil**,[13] and seizures have been reported in patients with and without epilepsy receiving propofol. They mainly occur during induction and emergence or are delayed after anaesthesia, suggesting that they may be caused by changes in cerebral levels of propofol,[14] and post-anaesthetic opisthotonos may be due to a propofol-induced tolerance to inhibitory transmitters (glycine and GABA).[12] Any association with the opioid remains unknown, although it has been suggested that opioids may aggravate propofol-induced opisthotonos by antagonising the actions of glycine.[12]

Alfentanil has been found to reduce the amount of propofol needed for loss of eyelash reflex and loss of consciousness, as well as enhancing the reduction in blood pressure produced by propofol.[15] Propofol inhibits both **alfentanil** and **sufentanil** metabolism causing an increase in plasma concentrations of these opioids, while **alfentanil** also increases propofol concentrations (which has been the subject of a review[16] and also described in more recent reports[17-20]). Pretreatment with **fentanyl** may also decrease the propofol requirements for induction of anaesthesia,[16] and increase blood concentrations of propofol.[21] However, another study was unable to confirm that **fentanyl** had an effect on blood propofol concentrations.[22]

A study in 2 groups of 20 patients undergoing similar types of surgery with similar propofol consumption, the duration of clinical anaesthesia with **remifentanil** and propofol was longer than with **fentanyl** and propofol.[23] **Remifentanil** has been reported to reduce the dose of propofol needed for anaesthesia and also to reduce the recovery time.[24,25] Further, propofol and **remifentanil** caused dose-dependent respiratory-depression, which, during combined use, was synergistic.[26] One study using EEG-controlled dosing of propofol and **remifentanil** for anaesthesia found their pharmacodynamic effects were no more than additive.[27] Although **remifentanil** alone appears to be ineffective at countering the response to stimuli, a study in healthy subjects has found that **remifentanil** can significantly reduce the levels of propofol required to remove a response to shouting, shaking or laryngoscopy (synergistic effect), but the effects on EEG measures were additive.[28] In another study in healthy subjects given **remifentanil** and propofol, the synergy that occurred for both analgesic and hypnotic endpoints was found to be greatest at lower levels of the drugs, which for each drug alone would not be producing maximal effects.[29] Another study found changes in BIS (bispectral index) that suggested that **remifentanil** may have some hypnotic properties or that it can potentiate the hypnotic effect of propofol.[30] It has been suggested that the increased hypnotic effects may be due to a dose-dependent decrease in cardiac output by **remifentanil**, resulting in an increase in arterial and brain propofol with increased anaesthetic effect.[31] One pharmacokinetic study found that the levels of **remifentanil** may be increased during concurrent propofol infusion,[32] while another study found that concurrent propofol reduced volume of distribution and distribution clearance of **remifentanil** by 41%. It was concluded that although propofol affects **remifentanil** bolus dose pharmacokinetics, maintenance infusion rates and recovery times would not be significantly affected.[33]

The manufacturer notes that the required induction dose of propofol may be reduced in patients who have received opioids, and that these drugs may increase the anaesthetic and sedative effects of propofol, and also cause greater reductions in blood pressure and cardiac output. They also state that propofol requirements for maintenance of anaesthesia may be reduced in the presence of opioids.[34]

Two reviews have discussed the use of opioids and propofol in anaesthesia, their pharmacokinetic and pharmacodynamic interactions, and administration and monitoring techniques.[35,36]

4. Thiopental. Opioid analgesics would be expected to potentiate the respiratory depressant effects of barbiturate anaesthetics. A study has found that the dose of thiopental required to induce anaesthesia was reduced by pretreatment with **fentanyl**.[37] The manufacturer recommends reduced doses of thiopental in patients premedicated with opioids.[38]

1. Dale O. Drug interactions in anaesthesia: focus on desflurane and sevoflurane. *Baillieres Clin Anaesthesiol* (1995) 9, 105–17.
2. Suprane (Desflurane). Baxter Healthcare Corporation. US Prescribing information, November 2005.
3. Albertin A, Casati A, Bergonzi P, Fano G, Torri G. Effects of two target-controlled concentrations (1 and 3 ng/ml) of remifentanil on MAC_{BAR} of sevoflurane. *Anesthesiology* (2004) 100, 255–9.
4. Coltura MJ-J, Van Belle K, Van Hemelrijck JH. Influence of remifentanil (Ultiva, Glaxo Wellcome) and nitrous oxide on sevoflurane (Sevorane, Abbott) requirement during surgery. 2001 Annual Meeting of the American Society of Anesthesiologists, New Orleans USA, 2002. Abstract A-462.
5. Katoh T, Suguro Y, Kimura T, Ikeda K. Morphine does not affect the awakening concentration of sevoflurane. *Can J Anaesth* (1993) 40, 825–8.
6. Hypnomidate (Etomidate). Janssen-Cilag Ltd. UK Summary of product characteristics, March 2009.
7. Schulte H, Sollevi A, Segerdahl M. The synergistic effect of combined treatment with systemic ketamine and morphine on experimentally induced windup-like pain in humans. *Anesth Analg* (2004) 98, 1574–80.
8. Bourke DL, Malit LA, Smith TC. Respiratory interactions of ketamine and morphine. *Anesthesiology* (1987) 66, 153–6.
9. Luginbühl M, Gerber A, Schnider TW, Petersen-Felix S, Arendt-Nielsen L, Curatolo M. Modulation of remifentanil-induced analgesia, hyperalgesia, and tolerance by small-dose ketamine in humans. *Anesth Analg* (2003) 96, 726–32.
10. Ketalar (Ketamine hydrochloride). Pfizer Ltd. UK Summary of product characteristics, January 2006.
11. Wittenstein U, Lyle DJR. Fits after alfentanil and propofol. *Anaesthesia* (1989) 44, 532–3.
12. Ries CR, Scoates PJ, Puil E. Opisthotonos following propofol: a nonepileptic perspective and treatment strategy. *Can J Anaesth* (1994) 41, 414–19.
13. Laycock GJA. Opisthotonos and propofol: a possible association. *Anaesthesia* (1988) 43, 257.
14. Walder B, Tramèr MR, Seeck M. Seizure-like phenomena and propofol. A systematic review. *Neurology* (2002) 58, 1327–32.
15. Vuyk J, Griever GER, Engbers FHM, Burm AGL, Bovill JG, Vletter AA. The interaction between propofol and alfentanil during induction of anesthesia. *Anesthesiology* (1994) 81, A400.
16. Vuyk J. Pharmacokinetic and pharmacodynamic interactions between opioids and propofol. *J Clin Anesth* (1997) 9, 23S–26S.
17. Ihmsen H, Albrecht S, Fechner J, Hering W, Schuttler J. The elimination of alfentanil is decreased by propofol. 2000 Annual Meeting of the American Society of Anesthesiologists, San Francisco USA, 2002. Abstract 531.
18. Mertens MJ, Vuyk J, Olofsen E, Bovill JG, Burm AGL. Propofol alters the pharmacokinetics of alfentanil in healthy male volunteers. *Anesthesiology* (2001) 94, 949–57.
19. Mertens MJ, Olofsen E, Burm AGL, Bovill JG, Vuyk J. Mixed-effects modeling of the influence of alfentanil on propofol pharmacokinetics. *Anesthesiology* (2004) 100, 795–805.
20. Schwilden H, Fechner J, Albrecht S, Hering W, Ihmsen H, Schüttler J. Testing and modelling the interaction of alfentanil and propofol on the EEG. *Eur J Anaesthesiol* (2003) 20, 363–72.
21. Cockshott ID, Briggs LP, Douglas EJ, White M. Pharmacokinetics of propofol in female patients. Studies using single bolus injections. *Br J Anaesth* (1987) 59, 1103–10.
22. Dixon J, Roberts FL, Tackley RM, Lewis GTR, Connell H, Prys-Roberts C. *Br J Anaesth* (1990) 64, 142–7.
23. Ferreira TA, Rama-Maceiras P, Molins N, Rey-Rilo T. Potenciación de una dosis única de rocuronio por fentanilo o remifentanilo en pacientes anestesiados con propofol. Evaluación por acelerometría. *Rev Esp Anestesiol Reanim* (2004) 51; 190–4.
24. O'Hare R, Reid J, Breslin D, Hayes A, Mirakhur RK. Propofol–remifentanil interaction: influence on recovery. *Br J Anaesth* (1999) 83, 180P.
25. Drover DR, Litalien C, Wellis V, Shafer SL, Hammer GB. Determination of the pharmacodynamic interaction of propofol and remifentanil during esophagogastroduodenoscopy in children. *Anesthesiology* (2004) 100, 1382–6.
26. Nieuwenhuijs, DJF, Olofsen E, Romberg RR, Sarton E, Ward D, Engbers F, Vuyk J, Mooren R, Teppema LJ, Dahan A. Response surface modeling of remifentanil-propofol interaction on cardiorespiratory control and bispectral index. *Anesthesiology* (2003) 98, 312–22.
27. Fechner J, Hering W, Ihmsen H, Palmaers T, Schüttler J, Albrecht S. Modelling the pharmacodynamic interaction between remifentanil and propofol by EEG-controlled dosing. *Eur J Anaesthesiol* (2003) 20, 373–9.
28. Bouillon TW, Bruhn J, Radulescu L, Andresen C, Shafer TJ, Cohane C, Shafer SL. Pharmacodynamic interaction between propofol and remifentanil regarding hypnosis, tolerance of laryngoscopy, bispectral index and electroencephalographic approximate entropy. *Anesthesiology* (2004) 100, 1353–72.
29. Kern SE, Xie G, White JL, Egan TD. Opioid-hypnotic synergy. *Anesthesiology* (2004) 100, 1373–81.
30. Koitabashi T, Johansen JW, Sebel PS. Remifentanil dose/electroencephalogram bispectral response during combined propofol/regional anesthesia. *Anesth Analg* (2002) 94, 1530–3.
31. Ludbrook GL, Upton RN. Pharmacokinetic drug interaction between propofol and remifentanil? *Anesth Analg* (2003) 97, 924–5.
32. Crankshaw DP, Chan C, Leslie K, Bjorksten AR. Remifentanil concentration during target-controlled infusion of propofol. *Anaesth Intensive Care* (2002) 30, 578–83.
33. Bouillon T, Bruhn J, Radu-Radulescu L, Bertaccini E, Park S, Shafer S. Non-steady state analysis of the pharmacokinetic interaction between propofol and remifentanil. *Anesthesiology* (2002) 97, 1350–62.
34. Diprivan (Propofol). AstraZeneca. US Prescribing information, August 2005.
35. Lichtenbelt B-J, Mertens M, Vuyk J. Strategies to optimise propofol-opioid anaesthesia. *Clin Pharmacokinet* (2004) 43, 577–93.
36. Vuyk J. Clinical interpretation of pharmacokinetic and pharmacodynamic propofol-opioid interactions. *Acta Anaesthesiol Belg* (2001) 52, 445–51.
37. Wang LP, Hermann C, Westrin P. Thiopentone requirements in adults after varying pre-induction doses of fentanyl. *Anaesthesia* (1996) 51, 831–5.
38. Thiopental Injection. Link Pharmaceuticals Ltd. UK Summary of product characteristics, January 2003.

Anaesthetics, general + Parecoxib

Limited evidence suggests parecoxib does not affect the pharmacokinetics or clinical effects of propofol. Parecoxib does not appear to interact with nitrous oxide and isoflurane.

Clinical evidence, mechanism, importance and management

A randomised, placebo-controlled, crossover study in 12 healthy subjects found that pretreatment with 40 mg of intravenous parecoxib, given one hour before a 2 mg/kg intravenous bolus of **propofol**, did not significantly affect the pharmacokinetics of **propofol**. Moreover, parecoxib did not alter the clinical effects of **propofol** (e.g. the time to loss of consciousness or the speed of awakening).[1] These limited data suggest that no special precautions should be required during concurrent use.

The UK manufacturer of parecoxib says that no formal interaction studies have been done with inhalational anaesthetics, but in surgical studies, where parecoxib was given preoperatively, there was no evidence of pharmacodynamic interactions in patients who had been given **nitrous oxide** and **isoflurane**.[2]

1. Ibrahim A, Park S, Feldman J, Karim A, Kharasch ED. Effects of parecoxib, a parenteral COX-2-specific inhibitor, on the pharmacokinetics and pharmacodynamics of propofol. *Anesthesiology* (2002) 96, 88–95.
2. Dynastat (Parecoxib sodium). Pfizer Ltd. UK Summary of product characteristics, June 2013.

Anaesthetics, general + Phenylephrine, topical

Phenylephrine eye drops given to patients undergoing general anaesthesia caused marked cyanosis and bradycardia in a baby, and hypertension in a woman.

Clinical evidence, mechanism, importance and management

A 3-week-old baby anaesthetised with **halothane** and **nitrous oxide/oxygen** became cyanosed shortly after 2 drops of phenylephrine 10% solution were put into one eye. The heart rate decreased from 160 to 60 bpm, ST-segment and T-wave changes were seen, and blood pressure measurements were unobtainable. The baby recovered uneventfully when anaesthesia was stopped and oxygen given. It was suggested that the phenylephrine caused severe peripheral vasoconstriction, cardiac failure and reflex bradycardia.[1] A 54-year-old woman anaesthetised with **isoflurane** developed hypertension (a rise from 125/70 to 200/90 mmHg) shortly after having two drops of phenylephrine 10% solution put into one eye. The hypertension responded to nasal glyceryl trinitrate (nitroglycerin) and increasing concentrations of isoflurane.[1] The authors of this report consider that general anaesthesia may have contributed to the systemic absorption of the phenylephrine. They suggest that phenylephrine should be given 30 to 60 minutes before anaesthesia, and not during anaesthesia; however, if it is necessary to give phenylephrine, use the lowest concentration (2.5%). They also point out that the following are effective mydriatics: single drop combinations of cyclopentolate 0.5% and phenylephrine 2.5%, or tropicamide 0.5% and phenylephrine 2.5%.

Phenylephrine is a sympathomimetic, and as such may carry some risk of potentiating arrhythmias if it is used with inhalational anaesthetics such as halothane – see 'Anaesthetics, general + Inotropes and Vasopressors', p.106. However, it is considered that it is much less likely than adrenaline (epinephrine) to have this effect, since it has primarily alpha-agonist activity.[2]

1. Van der Spek AFL, Hantler CB. Phenylephrine eyedrops and anesthesia. *Anesthesiology* (1986) 64, 812–14.
2. Wong KC. Sympathomimetic drugs. In: Smith NT, Miller RD, Corbascio AN, eds. Drug Interactions in Anesthesia. Philadelphia: Lea and Febiger; 1981 p. 55–82.

Anaesthetics, general + Probenecid

The anaesthetic dosage of thiopental is reduced, and its effects prolonged by pretreatment with probenecid.

Clinical evidence

A study[1] in patients about to undergo surgery found that probenecid 1 g given one hour before anaesthesia reduced the thiopental dosage by 23%, from 5.3 to 4.1 mg/kg.

A further double-blind study[2] in 86 women found that probenecid given 3 hours before surgery prolonged the duration of anaesthesia with thiopental:

- In patients premedicated with atropine 7.5 micrograms/kg, pethidine (meperidine) 1 mg/kg, and 500 mg of probenecid, the duration of anaesthesia with thiopental 7 mg/kg was prolonged by 65%,
- In patients premedicated with atropine 7.5 micrograms/kg, pethidine 1 mg/kg, and *1 g of probenecid*, the duration of anaesthesia with thiopental 7 mg/kg was prolonged by 46%,
- In patients premedicated with atropine 7.5 micrograms/kg (*no pethidine*) and 500 mg of probenecid, the duration of anaesthesia with thiopental 7 mg/kg was prolonged by 26%,
- In patients premedicated with atropine 7.5 micrograms/kg (*no pethidine*) and 500 mg of probenecid, and *no surgical stimulus* the duration of anaesthesia with *thiopental 4 mg/kg* was prolonged by 109%.

Mechanism

Not understood. It has been suggested that probenecid increases the amount of free (and active) thiopental in the plasma since it competes for the binding sites on the plasma albumins.[1]

Importance and management

Information is limited but what is known shows that the effects of thiopental are increased by probenecid. As the change in propofol requirements is modest, and because the dose would be expected to be titrated to effect, this interaction seems likely to be of minimal clinical relevance.

1. Dundee JW, Halliday NJ, McMurray TJ. Aspirin and probenecid pretreatment influences the potency of thiopentone and the onset of action of midazolam. *Eur J Anaesthesiol* (1986) 3, 247–51.
2. Kaukinen S, Eerola M, Ylitalo P. Prolongation of thiopentone anaesthesia by probenecid. *Br J Anaesth* (1980) 52, 603–7.

Anaesthetics, general + Sparteine sulfate

Patients given thiamylal sodium had a marked increase in cardiac arrhythmias when they were given intravenous sparteine sulfate, but those given thiopental or etomidate did not.

Clinical evidence, mechanism, importance and management

A group of 109 women undergoing dilatation and curettage were premedicated with atropine and fentanyl, and given either **thiamylal sodium** 2% (5 mg/kg), **etomidate** 0.2% (0.3 mg/kg) or **thiopental** 2.5% (4 mg/kg) to induce anaesthesia, which was maintained with **nitrous oxide/oxygen**. During the surgical procedure they were given a slow intravenous injection of sparteine sulfate 100 mg. Fourteen out of 45 patients given **thiamylal sodium** developed cardiac arrhythmias; 10 had bigeminy and 4 had frequent ventricular premature contractions. Only two patients given **etomidate** or **thiopental** developed any cardiac arrhythmias. It is not understood why sparteine should interact with **thiamylal sodium** in this way. Although the arrhythmias were effectively treated with lidocaine, the authors of this report suggest that the concurrent use of sparteine and **thiamylal sodium** should be avoided.[1]

1. Cheng C-R, Chen S-Y, Wu K-H, Wei T-T. Thiamylal sodium with sparteine sulfate inducing dysrhythmia in anesthetized patients. *Ma Zui Xue Za Zhi* (1989) 27, 297–8.

Anaesthetics, general + SSRIs

One patient had a seizure when she was given methohexital while taking paroxetine. Spontaneous movements have been seen in two patients taking fluoxetine when they were anaesthetised with propofol.

Clinical evidence, mechanism, importance and management

(a) Methohexital

A generalised tonic-clonic seizure occurred in a 42-year-old woman immediately after she was anaesthetised with 120 mg of intravenous methohexital for the last in a series of six electroconvulsive therapies. She had been receiving **paroxetine** 40 mg daily throughout the series.[1] The authors suggest that paroxetine should be given with caution to patients receiving ECT or methohexital anaesthesia.[1] Note that this appears to be an isolated report.

(b) Propofol

Two women in their mid-twenties, who had been taking **fluoxetine** 20 mg daily for 4 to 6 months, had pronounced involuntary upper limb movements lasting 20 to 30 seconds immediately after anaesthetic induction with 180 mg of propofol (2 to 2.5 mg/kg). The movements ceased spontaneously and the rest of the anaesthesia and surgery were uneventful. Neither had any history of epilepsy or movement disorders. It is not clear whether this was an interaction between propofol and **fluoxetine** or just a rare (but previously reported) reaction to propofol.[2]

1. Folkerts H. Spontaneous seizure after concurrent use of methohexital anesthesia for electroconvulsive therapy and paroxetine: a case report. *J Nerv Ment Dis* (1995) 183, 115–16.
2. Armstrong TSH, Martin PD. Propofol, fluoxetine and spontaneous movement. *Anaesthesia* (1997) 52, 809–10.

Anaesthetics, general + Sulfonamides

The anaesthetic effects of thiopental are increased, but shortened, by sulfafurazole. Phenobarbital appears not to affect the pharmacokinetics of sulfafurazole or sulfisomidine.

Clinical evidence

A study in 48 patients found that intravenous **sulfafurazole** 40 mg/kg reduced the required anaesthetic dosage of **thiopental** by 36%, but the duration of action was shortened.[1] This interaction has also been observed in *animal* experiments.[2] A study in children found that **phenobarbital** did not affect the pharmacokinetics of **sulfafurazole** or **sulfisomidine**.[3]

Mechanism

It has been suggested that sulfafurazole successfully competes with thiopental for plasma protein binding sites,[4] the result being that more free and active barbiturate molecules remain in circulation to exert their anaesthetic effects and therefore smaller doses are required.

Importance and management

The evidence for an interaction between sulfafurazole and thiopental is limited, but it appears to be strong. Less thiopental than usual may be required to achieve adequate anaesthesia, but since the awakening time is shortened repeated doses may be needed.

Phenobarbital does not appear to affect the pharmacokinetics of the sulfonamides.

1. Csögör SI, Kerek SF. Enhancement of thiopentone anaesthesia by sulphafurazole. *Br J Anaesth* (1970) 42, 988–90.
2. Csögör SI, Pálffy B, Feszt G, Papp J. Influence du sulfathiazol sur l'effet narcotique du thiopental et de l'hexobarbital. *Rev Roum Physiol* (1971) 8, 81–5.
3. Krauer B. Vergleichende Untersuchung der Eliminationskinetik zweier Sulfonamide bei Kindern mit und ohne Phenobarbitalmedikation. *Schweiz Med Wochenschr* (1971) 101, 668–71.
4. Csögör SI, Papp J. Competition between sulphonamides and thiopental for the binding sites of plasma proteins. *Arzneimittelforschung* (1970) 20, 1925–7.

Anaesthetics, general + Theophylline

Cardiac arrhythmias can develop during the concurrent use of halothane and aminophylline. One report attributes seizures to an interaction between ketamine and aminophylline. Theophylline would be expected to interact similarly.

Clinical evidence, mechanism, importance and management

(a) Development of arrhythmias

A number of reports describe arrhythmias apparently due to an interaction between **halothane** and theophylline or aminophylline. One describes intraoperative arrhythmias in three out of 45 adult asthmatics who had received preoperative theophylline or aminophylline followed by **halothane** anaesthesia.[1] Nine other patients developed heart rates exceeding 140 bpm when given aminophylline and **halothane**, whereas tachycardia did not occur in 22 other patients given only **halothane**.[1] There are other reports of individual adult and child patients who developed ventricular tachycardias attributed to this interaction.[2-5] One child had a cardiac arrest.[5] The same interaction has been reported in *animals*.[6,7] One suggested reason for the interaction with **halothane** is that theophylline causes the release of endogenous catecholamines (adrenaline (epinephrine), noradrenaline (norepinephrine)), which are known to sensitise the myocardium, see 'Anaesthetics, general + Inotropes and Vasopressors', p.106. For a report describing supraventricular tachycardia, in a patient taking aminophylline who was anaesthetised with thiopental and fentanyl and then given pancuronium, see 'Neuromuscular blockers + Theophylline', p.135.

The authors of one of the reports advise avoiding concurrent use, and suggest waiting approximately 13 hours after the last dose of aminophylline before using **halothane**[2] but another[8] says that: "my own experience with the liberal use of these drugs has convinced me of the efficacy and wide margin of safety associated with their use in combination." For a list of inhalational anaesthetics, in order of arrhythmogenic potential, see 'Anaesthetics and Neuromuscular blockers', p.97.

(b) Development of seizures

Over a period of 9 years, tachycardia and extensor-type seizures were observed in 4 patients taking theophylline or aminophylline, who were initially anaesthetised with **ketamine**, and then given **halothane** or **enflurane**.[9] Based on a subsequent study in *mice*, the authors attributed the seizures to an interaction between **ketamine** and theophylline or aminophylline, and they suggest that the combination should perhaps be avoided in some, or antiepileptic premedication be given to patients at risk. However, these cases come from one isolated report. Note that, in *mice*, **ketamine** had no effect on aminophylline-induced seizures.[10]

1. Barton MD. Anesthetic problems with aspirin-intolerant patients. *Anesth Analg* (1975) 54, 376–80.
2. Roizen MF, Stevens WC. Multiform ventricular tachycardia due to the interaction of aminophylline and halothane. *Anesth Analg* (1978) 57, 738–41.
3. Naito Y, Arai T, Miyake C. Severe arrhythmias due to the combined use of halothane and aminophylline in an asthmatic patient. *Jpn J Anesthesiol* (1986) 35, 1126–9.
4. Bedger RC, Chang J-L, Larson CE, Bleyaert AL. Increased myocardial irritability with halothane and aminophylline. *Anesth Prog* (1980) 27, 34–6.
5. Richards W, Thompson J, Lewis G, Levy DS, Church JA. Cardiac arrest associated with halothane anesthesia in a patient receiving theophylline. *Ann Allergy* (1988) 61, 83–4
6. Takaori M, Loehning RW. Ventricular arrhythmias induced by aminophylline during halothane anaesthesia in dogs. *Can Anaesth Soc J* (1967) 14, 79–86.

7. Stirt JA, Berger JM, Roe SD, Ricker SM, Sullivan SF. Halothane-induced cardiac arrhythmias following administration of aminophylline in experimental animals. *Anesth Analg* (1981) 60, 517–20.
8. Zimmerman BL. Arrhythmogenicity of theophylline and halothane used in combination. *Anesth Analg* (1979) 58, 259–60.
9. Hirshman CA, Krieger W, Littlejohn G, Lee R, Julien R. Ketamine-aminophylline-induced decrease in seizure threshold. *Anesthesiology* (1982) 56, 464–7.
10. Czuczwar SJ, Janusz W, Wamil A, Kleinrok Z. Inhibition of aminophylline-induced convulsions in mice by antiepileptic drugs and other agents. *Eur J Pharmacol* (1987) 144, 309–15.

Anaesthetics, general + Tizanidine

Premedication with oral tizanidine appears to reduce the MAC of sevoflurane.

Clinical evidence, mechanism, importance and management

In a study, 52 patients were given either oral tizanidine 4 mg or placebo 70 minutes before induction of anaesthesia with **sevoflurane** 5%. The MAC of **sevoflurane** was 2.2% and 1.8% in the control and tizanidine-treated groups, respectively. The sedation score in the tizanidine group was higher than in the placebo group, and the time to loss of consciousness in the tizanidine and control groups was about 60 seconds and 74 seconds, respectively. Tizanidine therefore exerted a hypnotic effect and reduced the MAC of **sevoflurane** by 18%. No tizanidine-related adverse effects, such as hypotension, were reported.[1] The general relevance is not yet established, but the changes seen were minimal and therefore would not be expected to clinically significant.

1. Wajima Z, Yoshikawa T, Ogura A, Imanaga K, Shiga T, Inoue T, Ogawa R. Oral tizanidine, an α_2-adrenoceptor agonist, reduces the minimum alveolar concentration of sevoflurane in human adults. *Anesth Analg* (2002) 95, 393–6.

Anaesthetics, general + Topiramate

Topiramate and may reduce the anaesthetic properties of amobarbital. One study suggests that topiramate may attenuate the effects of ketamine, whereas another did not find an interaction.

Clinical evidence, mechanism, importance and management

(a) Amobarbital

In a retrospective study, it was found that 11 of 56 epileptic patients who had undergone the intracarotid amobarbital procedure (IAP) recovered very rapidly from the anaesthetic (within 60 seconds) or had anaesthetic failure. Seven of the 11 were taking topiramate and one had recently discontinued topiramate at the time of the procedure. The other 3 patients had been taking **zonisamide** (2), or furosemide (1). A further 2 patients taking topiramate or hydrochlorothiazide had a rapid recovery (within 90 seconds).

It was suggested that the anaesthetic effect of amobarbital may be affected by the carbonic anhydrase-inhibiting activity of these drugs. No anaesthetic failures were reported in patients taking combinations of antiepileptics such as carbamazepine, phenytoin and valproate but without drugs with carbonic anhydrase-inhibiting effects.[1] The mechanism is not understood but may be due to interference with the activity of amobarbital on $GABA_A$ receptors by effects on electrochemical gradients across cell membranes or via metabolic acidosis.

The authors recommend that topiramate, **zonisamide** or other carbonic anhydrase inhibitors should be discontinued at least 8 weeks before the IAP.[1] Similar findings are reported in a review of 40 other patients.[2]

(b) Ketamine

A study in 36 healthy subjects found that a single 50-mg dose of topiramate slightly decreased the effect of sub-anaesthetic doses of ketamine (slow intravenous injection of 120 micrograms/kg followed by 500 micrograms/kg over one hour) on a cognitive performance test (anti-saccade test). Pharmacokinetic analysis also found that ketamine levels were increased by about 25% in the subjects given topiramate.[3] A follow-up, placebo-controlled study by the same authors in 36 healthy subjects found that pretreatment with a single 50-mg dose of topiramate did not significantly affect the reaction time to ketamine (same dose as the previous study).[4] The general significance of these results in patients taking topiramate and undergoing sedation or anaesthesia with ketamine is unclear. Further study is needed.

1. Bookheimer S, Schrader LM, Rausch R, Sankar R, Engel J. Reduced anesthetization during intracarotid amobarbital (Wada) test in patients taking carbonic anhydrase-inhibiting medications. *Epilepsia* (2005) 46, 236–43.
2. Ringman JM, Grant AC. Carbonic anhydrase inhibitors and amobarbital resistance. *Epilepsia* (2005) 46, 1333.
3. Gavaudan G, Micallef-Roll J, Hasbroucq T, Masson G, Lançon, Blin O. Does topiramate blunt N-methyl-D-aspartate receptor antagonists effects in healthy humans? *Eur Arch Psychiatry Clin Neurosci* (2003) 253 (Suppl 1) I/16.
4. Micallef J, Gavaudan G, Burle B, Blin O, Hasbroucq T. A study of a topiramate pre-treatment on the effects induced by a subanaesthetic dose of ketamine on human reaction time. *Neurosci Lett* (2004) 369, 99–103.

Anaesthetics, general + Trichloroethane

Two patients had evidence of chronic cardiac toxicity after repeated exposure to trichloroethane There was circumstantial evidence in both cases of a deterioration in cardiac function following halothane anaesthesia.

Clinical evidence, mechanism, importance and management

Two patients, who had been repeatedly exposed to trichloroethane; one during solvent abuse including *Tipp-Ex* typewriter correcting fluid thinner and the other due to industrial exposure including *Genklene* for degreasing steel, showed evidence of chronic cardiac toxicity. In both cases there was circumstantial evidence of cardiac deterioration after routine anaesthesia with **halothane**. Some **solvents** have a close chemical similarity to **inhalational anaesthetic** drugs, particularly the halogenated hydrocarbons, and these related compounds might have a toxic interaction.[1]

1. McLeod AA, Marjot R, Monaghan MJ, Hugh-Jones P, Jackson G. Chronic cardiac toxicity after inhalation of 1,1,1-trichloroethane. *BMJ* (1987) 294, 727–9.

Anaesthetics, general and/or Neuromuscular blockers + Tricyclic and related antidepressants

Tricyclic antidepressants may increase the risk of arrhythmias and hypotension during anaesthesia. Tachyarrhythmias have been seen in patients taking imipramine who were given halothane and pancuronium. Some very limited evidence suggests that amitriptyline may increase the likelihood of enflurane-induced seizure activity. A man taking maprotiline and lithium developed a tonic-clonic seizure when given propofol. Tricyclics may cause an increase in the duration of barbiturate anaesthesia.

Clinical evidence, mechanism, importance and management

(a) Development of arrhythmias

Two patients who were taking **nortriptyline** (one also taking fluphenazine) developed prolonged cardiac arrhythmias during general anaesthesia with **halothane**.[1] Two further patients taking **imipramine** developed marked tachyarrhythmias when anaesthetised with **halothane** and given **pancuronium**.[2] This adverse interaction was subsequently clearly demonstrated in *dogs*.[2] The authors concluded on the basis of their studies that:

- **pancuronium** should be given with caution to patients taking any **tricyclic antidepressant** if **halothane** is used;
- **gallamine** probably should be avoided but **tubocurarine** may be an acceptable alternative to **pancuronium**;
- **pancuronium** is probably safe in the presence of a tricyclic if **enflurane** is used.

However, this last conclusion does not agree with that reached by the authors of another report[3], who found that the combination of **pancuronium** and **enflurane** increased the risk of seizures.

One manufacturer[4] has recommended stopping tricyclics several days before elective surgery where possible. However, the BNF advises that tricyclic antidepressants need not be stopped, but there may be an increased risk of arrhythmias and hypotension (and dangerous interactions with vasopressor drugs, see 'Tricyclic and related antidepressants + Inotropes and Vasopressors', p.1510). Therefore, the anaesthetist should be informed if they are not stopped.[5]

(b) Development of seizures

1. Enflurane + Tricyclics. Two patients taking **amitriptyline** developed clonic movements of the leg, arm and hand during surgery while anaesthetised with enflurane and **nitrous oxide**. The movements stopped when the enflurane was replaced by **halothane**.[3] A possible reason is that **amitriptyline** can lower the threshold at which enflurane-induced seizure activity occurs. It is suggested that it may be advisable to avoid enflurane in patients needing tricyclic antidepressants, particularly in those who have a history of seizures, or when hyperventilation or high concentrations of enflurane are likely to be used.[3]

2. Propofol + Maprotiline. A man with a bipolar disorder taking maprotiline 200 mg four times daily and lithium carbonate 300 mg daily, underwent anaesthesia during which he received fentanyl, **tubocurarine** and propofol 200 mg. Shortly after the injection of the propofol the patient complained of a burning sensation in his face. He then became rigid, his back and neck extended and his eyes turned upwards. After 15 seconds, rhythmic twitching developed in his eyes, arms and hands. This apparent seizure lasted for about one minute until suxamethonium (succinylcholine) was given. The patient regained consciousness after several minutes and the surgery was cancelled.[6] It is not known whether the reaction was due to an interaction between propofol and the antidepressants, or due to just one of the drugs, because both propofol[7,8] and maprotiline[9] have been associated with seizures. However, the authors of this report suggest that it would now be prudent to avoid using propofol in patients taking drugs that significantly lower the convulsive threshold, and this would be expected to include tricyclic antidepressants. More study of this possible interaction is needed.

(c) Increased duration of anaesthesia

A study in *dogs* found that **imipramine** caused about a 50% increase in the duration of **thiopental**-induced sleep.[10] In an early review of electroconvulsive therapy and anaesthesia, it was noted that tricyclics interact with **barbiturates** resulting in an increased sleep time and duration of anaesthesia, and therefore it was suggested that lower doses of barbiturate anaesthetics such as **thiopental** should be given to patients taking tricyclics.[11] However, in a later review, it was noted that no complications have been attributed to the use of ECT (which has often been undertaken using **methohexital** or possibly **propofol**) in patients taking tricyclic antidepressants.[12] Apart from the study in *animals,*[10] there seems little published information to suggest that tricyclics interact significantly with barbiturate anaesthetics, but even if there is an interaction, as the dose of barbiturate should be carefully adjusted according to the patient's response any interaction will probably be accounted for by standard anaesthetic procedures. Consider also 'Tricyclic and related antidepressants + Barbiturates or Phenytoin', p.1503.

1. Plowman PE, Thomas WJW. Tricyclic antidepressants and cardiac dysrhythmias during dental anaesthesia. *Anaesthesia* (1974) 29, 576–8.
2. Edwards RP, Miller RD, Roizen MF, Ham J, Way WL, Lake CR, Roderick L. Cardiac responses to imipramine and pancuronium during anesthesia with halothane or enflurane. *Anesthesiology* (1979) 50, 421–5.
3. Sprague DH, Wolf S. Enflurane seizures in patients taking amitriptyline. *Anesth Analg* (1982) 61, 67–8.
4. Amitriptyline Oral Solution. Rosemont Pharmaceuticals Ltd. UK Summary of product characteristics, March 2008.
5. Joint Formulary Committee. *British National Formulary.* 70 ed. London: BMJ Group and Pharmaceutical Press; 2015. p. 1094.
6. Orser B, Oxorn D. Propofol, seizure and antidepressants. *Can J Anaesth* (1994) 41, 262.
7. Bevan JC. Propofol-related convulsions. *Can J Anaesth* (1993) 40, 805–9.
8. Committee on Safety of Medicines. Propofol – convulsions, anaphylaxis and delayed recovery from anaesthesia. *Current Problems* (1989) 26.
9. Jabbari B, Bryan GE, Marsh EE, Gunderson CH. Incidence of seizures with tricyclic and tetracyclic antidepressants. *Arch Neurol* (1985) 42, 480–1.
10. Dobkin AB. Potentiation of thiopental anesthesia by derivatives and analogues of phenothiazine. *Anesthesiology* (1960) 21, 292–6.
11. Gaines GY, Rees DI. Electroconvulsive therapy and anesthetic considerations. *Anesth Analg* (1986) 65, 1345–56.
12. Wagner KJ, Möllenberg O, Rentrop M, Werner C, Kochs EF. Guide to anaesthetic selection for electroconvulsive therapy. *CNS Drugs* (2005) 19, 745–58.

Anaesthetics, general; Esketamine + Clarithromycin

Clarithromycin moderately increases the exposure to oral esketamine.

Clinical evidence

In a crossover study in 10 healthy subjects, clarithromycin 500 mg twice daily for 4 days increased the AUC of ketamine 2.6-fold and increased its maximum plasma concentration 3.6-fold, when a single oral 200-microgram/kg dose of esketamine (the *S*-isomer of ketamine) was given one hour after the morning dose of clarithromycin on day 4. There was a reduction in the formation of the metabolite, norketamine. Self-rated esketamine-induced drowsiness and impaired performance were increased by clarithromycin, but not its analgesic effects.[1]

Mechanism

As clarithromycin is a potent CYP3A4 inhibitor, and this isoenzyme is involved in the metabolism of esketamine, it was assumed that this was why clarithromycin increased the exposure to esketamine.[1] However, in a more recent study by this same research group, another potent CYP3A4 inhibitor, itraconazole, had no effect on esketamine exposure (see 'Anaesthetics, general; Esketamine + Itraconazole', below), raising doubts as to the proposed mechanism here. Further study of the mechanism is needed.

Importance and management

The pharmacokinetic interaction of clarithromycin with oral esketamine would appear to be established, and some caution might be appropriate on concurrent use. Consider decreasing the oral esketamine dose as necessary. Until more is known about the mechanism, it is not possible to assess whether this interaction is also likely with intravenous esketamine or **ketamine**. Be aware of the possibility.

1. Hagelberg NM, Peltoniemi MA, Saari TI, Kurkinen KJ, Laine K, Neuvonen PJ, Olkkola KT. Clarithromycin, a potent inhibitor of CYP3A, greatly increases exposure to oral S-ketamine. *Eur J Pain* (2010) 14, 625–9.

Anaesthetics, general; Esketamine + Grapefruit juice

Grapefruit juice moderately increases the exposure to oral esketamine.

Clinical evidence

In a crossover study in 12 healthy subjects, grapefruit juice 200 mL three times daily for 5 days and 150 mL given at the same time as a single 200-microgram/kg oral dose of esketamine on day 5, increased the AUC of esketamine 3-fold. There was a reduction in the formation of the metabolite, norketamine. However, self-rated esketamine-induced relaxation was decreased, and performance was increased, by grapefruit juice.[1]

Mechanism

Grapefruit juice inhibits intestinal CYP3A4, which is involved in the metabolism of esketamine, and therefore probably impairs the oral absorption of esketamine by this route. Although the exact role of CYP3A4 in the metabolism of esketamine is not clear, as other known potent CYP3A4 inhibitors have been shown to have conflicting effects in studies by the same group of researchers (see 'Anaesthetics, general; Esketamine + Clarithromycin', above and 'Anaesthetics, general; Esketamine + Itraconazole', below).

Importance and management

The pharmacokinetic interaction between grapefruit juice and oral esketamine would appear to be established, and it might be prudent to avoid grapefruit juice with oral esketamine. If the proposed mechanism is correct, this interaction would not be expected to be relevant with intravenous esketamine or **ketamine**.

1. Peltoniemi MA, Saari TI, Hagelberg NM, Laine K, Neuvonen PJ, Olkkola KT. S-ketamine concentrations are greatly increased by grapefruit juice. *Eur J Clin Pharmacol* (2012) 68, 979–86.

Anaesthetics, general; Esketamine + Itraconazole

Itraconazole has no effect on oral esketamine exposure.

Clinical evidence

In a crossover study in 11 healthy subjects, itraconazole 200 mg once daily for 6 days did not alter the AUC or half-life of a single oral 200-microgram/kg dose of esketamine. However, there was a small reduction in the formation of the metabolite, norketamine. Also, self-reported esketamine-induced drowsiness and impaired performance were increased to a minor extent by itraconazole, but not its analgesic effects.[1]

Mechanism

Itraconazole is a potent inhibitor of CYP3A4, which is involved in the metabolism of esketamine. Based on the interaction of esketamine with clarithromycin, which is also a potent CYP3A4 inhibitor (see 'Anaesthetics, general; Esketamine + Clarithromycin', p.113), itraconazole was expected to increase esketamine exposure. The mechanism for the differing effects of itraconazole and clarithromycin on esketamine exposure is not understood and requires further investigation.

Importance and management

The pharmacokinetic data here unexpectedly show no effect on oral esketamine by itraconazole, suggesting that no clinically relevant pharmacokinetic interaction occurs. No interaction would therefore be expected with other routes of esketamine administration. A pharmacokinetic interaction with **ketamine** (the racemic drug) cannot be ruled out because this might be metabolised differently.[2]

1. Peltoniemi MA, Saari TI, Hagelberg NM, Reponen P, Turpeinen M, Laine K Neuvonen PJ, Olkkola KT. Exposure to oral S-ketamine is unaffected by itraconazole but greatly increased by ticlopidine. *Clin Pharmacol Ther* (2011) 90, 296–302.
2. Portmann S, Kwan HY, Theurillat R, Schmitz A, Mevissen M, Thormann W. Enantioselective capillary electrophoresis for identification and characterization of human cytochrome P450 enzymes which metabolize ketamine and norketamine in vitro. *J Chromatogr A* (2010) 1217, 7942–8.

Anaesthetics, general; Esketamine + Rifampicin (Rifampin)

Rifampicin negligibly reduces the exposure to intravenous esketamine.

Clinical evidence

In a crossover study in 20 healthy subjects, rifampicin 600 mg once daily for 6 days decreased the AUC of a 2-hour infusion of esketamine 20 or 40 mg/70 kg hourly, by 10%. The AUC of the norketamine metabolite was moderately reduced by 50%. In a modelling study, these pharmacokinetic changes had little effect on the analgesic efficacy of esketamine.[1]

Mechanism

The data suggest that rifampicin minimally induces the metabolism of esketamine and has a greater inductive effect on the norketamine metabolite (possibly by CYP2B6 or CYP3A4). This was unexpected.[1]

Importance and management

Evidence for a pharmacokinetic interaction between esketamine and rifampicin is limited to this one study, which showed that rifampicin has some effect on intravenous esketamine metabolism, although the clinical relevance of this is likely to be minimal. A pharmacokinetic interaction with **ketamine** (the racemic drug) cannot be ruled out because this might be metabolised differently.[2]

1. Noppers I, Olofsen E, Niesters M, Aarts L, Mooren R, Dahan A, Kharasch E, Sarton E. Effect of rifampicin on S-ketamine and S-norketamine plasma concentrations in healthy volunteers after intravenous S-ketamine administration. *Anesthesiology* (2011) 114, 1435–45.
2. Portmann S, Kwan HY, Theurillat R, Schmitz A, Mevissen M, Thormann W. Enantioselective capillary electrophoresis for identification and characterization of human cytochrome P450 enzymes which metabolize ketamine and norketamine in vitro. *J Chromatogr A* (2010) 1217, 7942–8.

Anaesthetics, general; Esketamine + Ticlopidine

Ticlopidine moderately increases the exposure to oral esketamine.

Clinical evidence

In a crossover study in 11 healthy subjects, ticlopidine 250 mg twice daily for 6 days increased the AUC of a single oral 200-microgram/kg dose of esketamine 2.4-fold. There was a reduction in the formation of the metabolite, norketamine. Self-reported esketamine-induced drowsiness and impaired performance were increased by ticlopidine, but not its analgesic effects.[1]

Mechanism

Ticlopidine is known to inhibit CYP2B6 and probably inhibits the metabolism of esketamine via hepatic CYP2B6, resulting in increased exposure.[1] Further study is needed.

Importance and management

The pharmacokinetic interaction between ticlopidine with oral esketamine would appear to be established, and a modest increase in oral esketamine exposure should be expected on concurrent use, with a possible increase in sedative effects. Given the suggested mechanism, it is likely that this interaction will apply to all routes of esketamine administration. It would be prudent to consider reducing the dose of esketamine in patients taking ticlopidine, or to monitor the outcome of concurrent use carefully. It is anticipated that the interaction will also apply to **ketamine** (which is the racemic mixture), but the magnitude requires confirmation as *R*-ketamine might be metabolised differently.[2]

1. Peltoniemi MA, Saari TI, Hagelberg NM, Reponen P, Turpeinen M, Laine K, Neuvonen PJ, Olkkola KT. Exposure to oral S-ketamine is unaffected by itraconazole but greatly increased by ticlopidine. *Clin Pharmacol Ther* (2011) 90, 296–302.
2. Portmann S, Kwan HY, Theurillat R, Schmitz A, Mevissen M, Thormann W. Enantioselective capillary electrophoresis for identification and characterization of human cytochrome P450 enzymes which metabolize ketamine and norketamine in vitro. *J Chromatogr A* (2010) 1217, 7942–8.

Anaesthetics, general; Methoxyflurane + Miscellaneous

The nephrotoxic effects of methoxyflurane appear to be increased by the use of tetracyclines, and possibly some aminoglycoside antibacterials and barbiturates.

Clinical evidence, mechanism, importance and management

Methoxyflurane has been withdrawn in many countries because it is nephrotoxic. This damage can be exacerbated by the concurrent use of other nephrotoxic drugs or possibly by the chronic use of hepatic enzyme-inducing drugs. Five out of 7 patients anaesthetised with methoxyflurane who had been given **tetracycline** before or after surgery had rises in blood urea nitrogen, and three died. Post-mortem examination found pathological changes (oxalosis) in the kidneys.[1] Another study identified renal tubular necrosis associated with calcium oxalate crystals in 6 patients who had been anaesthetised with methoxyflurane and given **tetracycline** (4 patients) and **penicillin** with **streptomycin** (2 patients).[2] Other reports support the finding of increased nephrotoxicity with **tetracycline** and methoxyflurane.[3-5] Another study suggested that **penicillin, streptomycin** and **chloramphenicol** appear not to increase the renal toxicity of methoxyflurane,[1] but **gentamicin** and **kanamycin** possibly do so.[6] There is also some evidence that **barbiturates** can exacerbate the renal toxicity because they enhance the metabolism of the methoxyflurane and increase the production of nephrotoxic metabolites.[7,8]

The risk of nephrotoxicity with methoxyflurane would therefore appear to be increased by some of these drugs and the concurrent use of **tetracycline** or **nephrotoxic antibiotics** should be avoided. Similarly, methoxyflurane should only be used with great caution, if at all, following the chronic use of hepatic enzyme-inducing drugs.

1. Kuzucu EY. Methoxyflurane, tetracycline, and renal failure. *JAMA* (1970) 211, 1162–4.
2. Dryden GE. Incidence of tubular degeneration with microlithiasis following methoxyflurane compared with other anesthetic agents. *Anesth Analg* (1974) 53, 383–5.
3. Albers DD, Leverett CL, Sandin JH. Renal failure following prostatovesiculectomy related to methoxyflurane anesthesia and tetracycline—complicated by Candida infection. *J Urol (Baltimore)* (1971) 106, 348–50.
4. Proctor EA, Barton FL. Polyuric acute renal failure after methoxyflurane and tetracycline. *BMJ* (1971) 4, 661–2.
5. Stoelting RK, Gibbs PS. Effect of tetracycline therapy on renal function after methoxyflurane anesthesia. *Anesth Analg* (1973) 52, 431–5.
6. Cousins MJ, Mazze RI. Tetracycline, methoxyflurane anaesthesia, and renal dysfunction. *Lancet* (1972) i, 751–2.
7. Churchill D, Yacoub JM, Siu KP, Symes A, Gault MH. Toxic nephropathy after low-dose methoxyflurane anesthesia: drug interaction with secobarbital? *Can Med Assoc J* (1976) 114, 326–33.
8. Cousins MJ, Mazze RI. Methoxyflurane nephrotoxicity: a study of dose response in man. *JAMA* (1973) 225, 1611–16.

Anaesthetics, local + Acetazolamide

In a study in 6 healthy subjects, the mean procaine half-life was increased by 66% (from 1.46 to 2.43 minutes) 2 hours after they were given acetazolamide 250 mg orally. This appears to be because the hydrolysis of the procaine is inhibited by the acetazolamide.[1] As the evidence for this interaction is limited to one report, its general significance is unclear.

1. Calvo R, Carlos R, Erill S. Effects of disease and acetazolamide on procaine hydrolysis by red blood cell enzymes. *Clin Pharmacol Ther* (1980) 27, 179–83.

Anaesthetics, local + Alcohol and/or Antirheumatics

Limited evidence suggests that the failure rate of spinal anaesthesia with bupivacaine may be markedly increased in patients who are receiving antirheumatic drugs and/or who drink alcohol.

Clinical evidence, mechanism, importance and management

The observation that regional anaesthetic failures seemed to be particularly high among patients undergoing orthopaedic surgery who were suffering from rheumatic joint diseases, prompted further study of a possible interaction. It was found that the failure rate of low-dose spinal anaesthesia with **bupivacaine** 0.5% (average volume of 2 mL) increased from 5% in the control group (no alcohol or long-term treatment) to 32% to 42% in those who had been taking antirheumatic drugs (**indometacin** or unspecified) for at least 6 months or who drank at least 80 g of ethanol daily, or both. The percentage of those patients who had a reduced response (i.e. an extended latency period and/or a reduced duration of action) also increased from 3% up to 39 to 42%.[1] The reasons are not understood. This appears to be the only report of such an effect.

1. Sprotte G, Weis KH. Drug interaction with local anaesthetics. *Br J Anaesth* (1982) 54, 242P–243P.

Anaesthetics, local + Anaesthetics, local

Mixtures of local anaesthetics are sometimes used to exploit the most useful characteristics of each drug. This normally seems to be safe although it is sometimes claimed that it increases the risk of toxicity. There is a case report of a man who developed toxicity when bupivacaine and mepivacaine were mixed together. Spinal bupivacaine followed by epidural ropivacaine may also interact to produce profound motor blockade. However, the effectiveness of bupivacaine in epidural anaesthesia may be reduced if it is preceded by chloroprocaine.

Clinical evidence and mechanism

(a) Evidence of no interaction

A study designed to assess the possibility of adverse interactions retrospectively studied the records of 10 538 patients over the period 1952 to 1970 who had been given **tetracaine** combined with **chloroprocaine, lidocaine, mepivacaine, prilocaine** or **propoxycaine** for caudal, epidural, or peripheral nerve block. The incidence of systemic toxic reactions was found to be no greater than when used singly and the conclusion was reached that combined use was advantageous and safe.[1] An *animal* study using combinations of **bupivacaine, lidocaine** and **chloroprocaine** also found no evidence that the toxicity was greater than if the anaesthetics were used singly.[2]

A study investigating the use of **chloroprocaine** 3%, **bupivacaine** 0.5% or a mixture of **chloroprocaine** 1.5% with **bupivacaine** 0.375% in obstetric epidural anaesthesia found that the time to onset of analgesia, the time to maximum analgesia, and the effectiveness of analgesia were similar irrespective of the treatment regimen. **Bupivacaine** 0.5% alone had a longer duration of action than **chloroprocaine** or the mixture of anaesthetics.[3] Another study found that **lidocaine** did not affect the pharmacokinetics of **bupivacaine.**[4]

(b) Evidence of reduced analgesia

A study designed to examine the clinical impression that **bupivacaine** given epidurally did not relieve labour pain effectively if preceded by **chloroprocaine** confirmed that this was so. Using an initial 10-mL dose of **chloroprocaine** 2% followed by an 8-mL dose of **bupivacaine** 0.5%, given when pain recurred, the pain relief was less and the block took longer to occur, had a shorter duration of action and had to be augmented more frequently than if only **bupivacaine** was used.[5] This interaction could not be corrected by adjusting the pH of the local anaesthetics.[6]

(c) Evidence of enhanced effect/toxic interaction

An isolated case report describes a patient given **bupivacaine** 0.75% and **mepivacaine** 2% who demonstrated lethargy, dysarthria and mild muscle tremor. The authors of the report suggested that this correlated with a marked increase in the percentage of unbound (active) **mepivacaine**, which was attributed to its displacement from protein binding sites by **bupivacaine.**[7] **Bupivacaine** has also been shown *in vitro* to displace **lidocaine** from α_1-acid glycoprotein.[8] Two cases of prolonged, profound motor blockade, have occurred in patients receiving patient-controlled epidural analgesia with **ropivacaine** 0.1% following spinal **bupivacaine** for caesarean section. Including these 2 patients, a total of 11 out of 23 patients given regional anaesthesia with **bupivacaine** had clinical evidence of motor weakness 8 hours after subsequently starting **ropivacaine.**[9]

Importance and management

Well studied interactions. The overall picture is that combined use does not normally result in increased toxicity, although there may be some exceptions. For example, until more is known, caution should be exercised when giving epidural ropivacaine postoperatively to patients who have had bupivacaine spinal anaesthesia, as unexpected motor block may occur.[9] Reduced effectiveness might be seen if bupivacaine is preceded by chloroprocaine.

1. Moore DC, Bridenbaugh LD, Bridenbaugh PO, Thompson GE, Tucker GT. Does compounding of local anesthetic agents increase their toxicity in humans? *Anesth Analg* (1972) 51, 579–85.
2. de Jong RH, Bonin JD. Mixtures of local anesthetics are no more toxic than the parent drugs. *Anesthesiology* (1981) 54, 177–81.
3. Cohen SE, Thurlow A. Comparison of a chloroprocaine–bupivacaine mixture with chloroprocaine and bupivacaine used individually for obstetric epidural analgesia. *Anesthesiology* (1979) 51, 288–92.
4. Freysz M, Beal JL, D'Athis P, Mounie J, Wilkening M, Escousse A. Pharmacokinetics of bupivacaine after axillary brachial plexus block. *Int J Clin Pharmacol Ther Toxicol* (1987) 25, 392–5.
5. Hodgkinson R, Husain FJ, Bluhm C. Reduced effectiveness of bupivacaine 0.5% to relieve labor pain after prior injection of chloroprocaine 2%. *Anesthesiology* (1982) 57, A201.
6. Chen B-J, Kwan W-F. pH is not a determinant of 2-chloroprocaine-bupivacaine interaction: a clinical study. *Reg Anesth* (1990) 15 (Suppl 1), 25.
7. Hartrick CT, Raj PP, Dirkes WE, Denson DD. Compounding of bupivacaine and mepivacaine for regional anesthesia. A safe practice? *Reg Anesth* (1984) 9, 94–7.
8. Goolkasian DL, Slaughter RL, Edwards DJ, Lalka D. Displacement of lidocaine from serum α_1-acid glycoprotein binding sites by basic drugs. *Eur J Clin Pharmacol* (1983) 25, 413–17.
9. Buggy DJ, Allsager CM, Coley S. Profound motor blockade with epidural ropivacaine following spinal bupivacaine. *Anaesthesia* (1999) 54, 895–8.

Anaesthetics, local + Antihypertensives

Severe hypotension and bradycardia have been seen in patients taking captopril or verapamil when they were given epidural anaesthesia with bupivacaine. Verapamil does not appear to interact with epidural lidocaine. Acute hypotension occurred in a man taking prazosin when he was given epidural anaesthesia with bupivacaine.

Clinical evidence

(a) ACE inhibitors

An 86-year-old man who had been receiving **captopril** 25 mg twice daily and bendroflumethiazide 25 mg daily [sic] for hypertension, underwent a transurethral resection of his prostate under spinal anaesthesia using 3 to 3.5 mL of heavy **bupivacaine** 0.5%. At the end of surgery, he was returned to the supine position and he suddenly developed severe sinus bradycardia (35 bpm), his arterial blood pressure fell to 65/35 mmHg and he became unrousable. Treatment with head-down tilt, oxygen and atropine 1.2 mg produced rapid improvement in cardiovascular and cerebral function. A further hypotensive episode (without bradycardia) occurred approximately one hour later, which responded rapidly to methoxamine 4 mg.[1]

(b) Alpha blockers

A man taking **prazosin** 5 mg three times daily for hypertension developed marked hypotension (BP 60/40 mmHg) within 3 to 5 minutes of receiving **bupivacaine** 100 mg through an L3–4 lumbar epidural catheter.[2] He was unresponsive to intravenous phenylephrine (five 100-microgram boluses) but his blood pressure rose within 3 to 5 minutes of starting a 0.05-micrograms/kg per minute infusion of adrenaline (epinephrine).

(c) Beta blockers

See 'Anaesthetics, local + Beta blockers', below, for reports of cardiotoxicity in patients given beta blockers with local anaesthetics.

(d) Calcium-channel blockers

Four patients taking long-term **verapamil** developed severe hypotension (systolic pressure as low as 60 mmHg) and bradycardia (48 bpm) 30 to 60 minutes after an epidural block with **bupivacaine** 0.5% and adrenaline (epinephrine). This was totally resistant to atropine and ephedrine, and responded only to calcium gluconate or calcium chloride. No such interaction was seen in a similar group of patients when epidural **lidocaine** was used.[3]

(e) Clonidine

See 'Anaesthetics, local + Clonidine', p.116.

Mechanism

Spinal anaesthesia can produce bradycardia and a fall in cardiac output resulting in arterial hypotension, which may be magnified by the action of the antihypertensive drug, and by hypovolaemia. Other factors probably contributed to the development of this interaction in these particular patients.

Importance and management

Direct information seems to be limited to the reports cited. Their general relevance is uncertain, but they serve to emphasise the importance of recognising that all antihypertensive drugs interfere in some way with the normal homoeostatic mechanisms that control blood pressure, so that the normal physiological response to hypotension during epidural anaesthesia may be impaired. Intravenous calcium effectively controls the hypotension and bradycardia produced by verapamil toxicity by reversing its calcium-channel blocking effects.[3,4]

Accidental intravenous administration of local anaesthetics during spinal anaesthesia may cause cardiovascular collapse and, on theoretical grounds, the serious cardiac depressant effects could be enhanced in patients taking antihypertensives, and it has been suggested that this may be a particular risk in elderly patients with impaired cardiovascular function.[5] Particular care would seem to be important with any patient given epidural anaesthesia while taking antihypertensives.

1. Williams NE. Profound bradycardia and hypotension following spinal anaesthesia in a patient receiving an ACE inhibitor: an important 'drug' interaction? *Eur J Anaesthesiol* (1999) 16, 796–8.
2. Lydiatt CA, Fee MP, Hill GE. Severe hypotension during epidural anesthesia in a prazosin-treated patient. *Anesth Analg* (1993) 76, 1152–3.
3. Collier C. Verapamil and epidural bupivacaine. *Anaesth Intensive Care* (1984) 13, 101–8.
4. Coaldrake LA. Verapamil overdose. *Anaesth Intensive Care* (1984) 12, 174–5.
5. Howie MB, Mortimer W, Candler EM, McSweeney TD, Frolicher DA. Does nifedipine enhance the cardiovascular depressive effects of bupivacaine? *Reg Anesth* (1989) 14, 19–25.

Anaesthetics, local + Benzodiazepines

Diazepam may increase the maximum plasma concentrations of bupivacaine, but the rate of bupivacaine elimination may also be increased. Midazolam has been reported to cause a modest decrease in lidocaine, but not mepivacaine, levels. Spinal anaesthesia with bupivacaine, lidocaine, or tetracaine may increase the sedative effects of midazolam. A case of possible lidocaine toxicity has been described when a woman taking sertraline was given flurazepam and then intraoperative lidocaine.

Clinical evidence

(a) Diazepam

Twenty-one children aged 2 to 10 years were given a single 1-mL/kg caudal injection of a mixture of **lidocaine** 0.5% and **bupivacaine** 0.125% for regional anaesthesia. Pretreatment with diazepam 10 mg rectally half-an-hour before the surgery had no significant effect on the plasma levels of **lidocaine**, but the AUC and maximum plasma **bupivacaine** levels were increased by 70 to 75%.[1] In another study in adult patients giving intravenous diazepam slightly, but not significantly, increased the mean maximum plasma levels of subsequent epidural **bupivacaine** or **etidocaine**. However, the elimination half-lives of both anaesthetics were significantly decreased, by about a half.[2]

(b) Flurazepam

A single report describes possible **lidocaine** toxicity following tumescent liposuction in a patient given perioperative sedation with flurazepam 30 mg orally. Ten hours after the completion of the procedure, in which a total of 58 mg/kg of lidocaine was used, the patient developed nausea and vomiting, an unsteady gait, mild confusion, and speech impairment. Her lidocaine level was 6.3 mg/L (levels greater than 6 mg/L were considered to be associated with an increased risk of toxicity). The patient was also taking sertraline.[3]

(c) Midazolam

In a study, 20 children aged 2 to 7 years were given a caudal block with 1 mL/kg of a solution containing **lidocaine** 0.5% and **bupivacaine** 0.125%, with midazolam 400 micrograms/kg given rectally half-an-hour before surgery. Midazolam caused a slight but non-significant reduction in the AUC and plasma levels of **bupivacaine**, whereas the AUC of **lidocaine** was reduced by 24%,[4] which would not be expected to be clinically significant. In another study, midazolam 400 micrograms/kg given rectally as a premedication was found to have no significant effect on plasma **mepivacaine** levels.[5] In a further study in which patients were given intravenous midazolam following an intramuscular injection of either **bupivacaine**, **lidocaine** or sodium chloride 0.9%, it was found that both anaesthetics enhanced the effect of midazolam. This effect was dose-dependent and it was concluded that the use of **lidocaine** or **bupivacaine** for regional blocks or local infiltration could alter the effect of midazolam from sedative to hypnotic.[6]

Twenty patients undergoing surgery were given repeated 1-mg intravenous doses of midazolam as induction anaesthesia every 30 seconds until they failed to respond to three repeated commands to squeeze the anaesthetist's hand. This was considered as the induction end-point 'titrated' dose. It was found that the 10 patients who had previously been given spinal anaesthesia with **tetracaine** 12 mg needed only half the dose of midazolam (7.6 mg) than the 10 other patients who had not received **tetracaine** (14.7 mg). The reasons are not known.[7]

Mechanism

The reasons for the pharmacokinetic interaction between diazepam and bupivacaine are not understood. The authors of the case report[3] describing lidocaine toxicity with flurazepam suggested that the flurazepam and sertraline inhibited lidocaine metabolism by the cytochrome P450 isoenzyme CYP3A4. However, note that flurazepam and sertraline are not usually considered to have inhibitory effects on this isoenzyme.

Both benzodiazepines and local anaesthetics are CNS depressants and therefore their concurrent use may result in additive CNS depression.

Importance and management

The clinical importance of these interactions is uncertain, but be aware that increased bupivacaine plasma levels have been seen with diazepam. One Canadian manufacturer of bupivacaine[8] suggests that reduced doses should be given if bupivacaine is given with sedatives. Note that, as with the use of any two CNS depressant drugs, consideration should be given to the potential for increased sedation.

1. Giaufre E, Bruguerolle B, Morisson-Lacombe G, Rousset-Rouviere B. The influence of diazepam on the plasma concentrations of bupivacaine and lignocaine after caudal injection of a mixture of the local anaesthetics in children. *Br J Clin Pharmacol* (1988) 26, 116–18.
2. Giasi RM, D'Agostino E, Covino BG. Interaction of diazepam and epidurally administered local anesthetic agents. *Reg Anesth* (1980) 5, 8–11.
3. Klein JA, Kassarjdian N. Lidocaine toxicity with tumescent liposuction: a case report of probable drug interactions. *Dermatol Surg* (1997) 23, 1169–74.
4. Giaufre E, Bruguerolle B, Morrison-Lacombe G, Rousset-Rouviere B. The influence of midazolam on the plasma concentrations of bupivacaine and lidocaine after caudal injection of a mixture of the local anesthetics in children. *Acta Anaesthesiol Scand* (1990) 34, 44–6.
5. Giaufre E, Bruguerolle B, Morisson-Lacombe G, Rousset-Rouviere B. Influence of midazolam on the plasma concentrations of mepivacaine after lumbar epidural injection in children. *Eur J Clin Pharmacol* (1990) 38, 91–2.
6. Ben-Shlomo I, Tverskoy M, Fleyshman G, Melnick V, Katz Y. Intramuscular administration of lidocaine or bupivacaine alters the effect of midazolam from sedation to hypnosis in a dose-dependent manner. *J Basic Clin Physiol Pharmacol* (2003) 14, 257–63.
7. Ben-David B, Vaida S, Gaitini L. The influence of high spinal anesthesia on sensitivity to midazolam sedation. *Anesth Analg* (1995) 81, 525–8.
8. Marcaine 0.5% with Epinephrine 1:200,000 Injection (Bupivacaine hydrochloride and Epinephrine bitartrate). Cooke-Waite. Canadian Prescribing information, March 2007.

Anaesthetics, local + Beta blockers

Propranolol reduces the clearance of bupivacaine and so theoretically the toxicity of bupivacaine may be increased. There has been a single

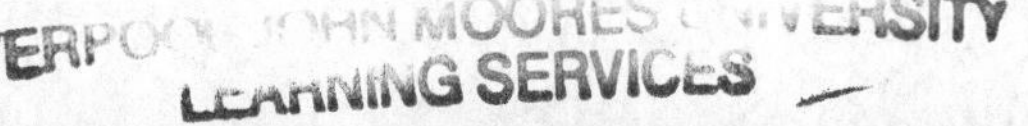

report of enhanced bupivacaine cardiotoxicity in a patient also receiving metoprolol and digoxin. The coronary vasoconstriction caused by cocaine is increased by propranolol. Nadolol appears to increase the duration of anaesthesia seen with lidocaine combined with adrenaline but not with lidocaine alone. Transient hypertension has been reported in a patient taking propranolol and given mepivacaine with corbadrine.

Clinical evidence, mechanism, importance and management

(a) Bupivacaine

1. Metoprolol. A case report describes enhanced bupivacaine cardiotoxicity in a patient taking enalapril 5 mg daily, metoprolol 25 mg twice daily and **digoxin** 250 micrograms four times daily (serum digoxin level 1.1 nanograms/mL). Cardiac arrest occurred 15 minutes after the injection of bupivacaine 0.5% with adrenaline (epinephrine) for intercostal nerve block (total bupivacaine dose 100 mg). The cardiodepressant effects of metoprolol, **digoxin** and bupivacaine were thought to have combined to produce toxicity at a dose of bupivacaine not usually considered toxic. The authors suggest that patients taking **digoxin** with a beta blocker and/or calcium-channel blocker should be considered at higher risk for bupivacaine cardiotoxicity.[1] See also 'Anaesthetics, local + Antihypertensives', p.115, for further discussion of the use of local anaesthetics in patients receiving antihypertensives.

2. Propranolol. In a study in 6 healthy subjects, the clearance of bupivacaine was modestly reduced by about 35% when they were given bupivacaine 30 to 50 mg intravenously over 10 to 15 minutes after taking propranolol 40 mg every 6 hours for one day. It was suggested that propranolol inhibited the activity of the liver microsomal enzymes by changing hepatic blood flow, thereby reducing the metabolism of the bupivacaine. Changes in blood flow to the liver are unlikely to affect bupivacaine metabolism substantially because it is relatively poorly extracted from the blood. The clinical importance of this interaction is uncertain, but it is suggested that an increase in local anaesthetic toxicity might occur and caution should be exercised if multiple doses of bupivacaine are given.[2] See also 'Anaesthetics, local + Antihypertensives', p.115, for further discussion of the use of local anaesthetics in patients receiving antihypertensives.

(b) Cocaine

A study in 30 patients being evaluated for chest pain found that 2 mg/kg of an intranasal solution of cocaine 10% reduced coronary sinus flow by about 14% and coronary artery diameter by 6 to 9%. The coronary vascular resistance increased by 22%. The addition of **propranolol** 400 micrograms/minute by intracoronary infusion (to a total of 2 mg) reduced coronary sinus flow by a further 15% and increased the coronary vascular resistance by 17%. These effects were thought to occur because cocaine stimulates the alpha receptors of the coronary blood vessels causing vasoconstriction. When the beta receptors are blocked by **propranolol**, the resultant unopposed alpha-adrenergic stimulation may lead to enhanced coronary vasoconstriction (see also 'Beta blockers + Inotropes and Vasopressors', p.1014). The clinical importance of these findings is uncertain but the authors of the report suggest that beta blockers should be avoided in patients with myocardial ischaemia or infarction associated with the use of cocaine.[3]

(c) Local anaesthetics with vasoconstrictors

In a randomised, placebo-controlled, crossover study in 10 healthy subjects, the upper lateral incisor teeth were anaesthetised using **lidocaine** with or without **adrenaline** (epinephrine). The mean duration of anaesthesia using 1 mL of lidocaine 2% containing 1:100 000 adrenaline was increased by 58% (17 minutes) for pulpal anaesthesia and 19% (16.5 minutes) for soft-tissue anaesthesia in subjects pretreated with **nadolol** 80 mg orally. Pretreatment with the beta blocker did not affect the duration of anaesthesia when lidocaine without adrenaline was used.[4] It seems likely that the combined effects of **adrenaline** (epinephrine) and **nadolol** caused increased local vasoconstriction, which resulted in the lidocaine persisting for longer. Therefore when a small amount of local anaesthetic with adrenaline is injected for dental procedures an increased duration of analgesia may result. Also note that a case report describes a transient hypertensive reaction in a patient taking **propranolol** when injections of **mepivacaine** 2% with **corbadrine** 1:20 000 were given for dental anaesthesia.[5] Larger doses of adrenaline have resulted in serious hypertension and bradycardia because of the interaction between non-selective beta blockers and adrenaline (see 'Beta blockers + Inotropes and Vasopressors', p.1014). It has been suggested that, for dental procedures, the minimum amount of local anaesthetic containing the lowest concentration of adrenaline should be used. Alternatively, if excessive bleeding is unlikely, a local anaesthetic without adrenaline is preferred.[4]

Propranolol and some other beta blockers are known to reduce the metabolism of intravenous and possibly oral lidocaine, see 'Lidocaine + Beta blockers', p.280. Note that this interaction is not expected to be important when lidocaine is given as a throat spray.[6]

1. Roitman K, Sprung J, Wallace M, Matjasko J. Enhancement of bupivacaine cardiotoxicity with cardiac glycosides and β-adrenergic blockers: a case report. *Anesth Analg* (1993) 76, 658–61.
2. Bowdle TA, Freund PR, Slattery JT. Propranolol reduces bupivacaine clearance. *Anesthesiology* (1987) 66, 36–8.
3. Lange RA, Cigarroa RG, Flores ED, McBride W, Kim AS, Wells PJ, Bedotto JB, Danziger RS, Hillis LD. Potentiation of cocaine-induced coronary vasoconstriction by beta-adrenergic blockade. *Ann Intern Med* (1990) 112, 897–903.
4. Zhang C, Banting DW, Gelb AW, Hamilton JT. Effect of β-adrenoreceptor blockade with nadolol on the duration of local anesthesia. *J Am Dent Assoc* (1999) 130, 1773–80.
5. Mito RS, Yagiela JA. Hypertensive response to levonordefrin in a patient receiving propranolol: report of a case. *J Am Dent Assoc* (1988) 116, 55–7.
6. Xylocaine Spray (Lidocaine). AstraZeneca UK Ltd. UK Summary of product characteristics, April 2012.

Anaesthetics, local + Clonidine

Studies suggest that the plasma levels of lidocaine (after epidural use) may be reduced in patients given clonidine. The addition of clonidine to bupivacaine spinal block shortens the onset time and increases the duration of sensory and motor block.

Clinical evidence

A study in 35 children undergoing ureteroneocystostomy found that the addition of clonidine 1 microgram/kg increased the duration of caudal block with **bupivacaine** 0.125% (with adrenaline (epinephrine) 1:400 000) and reduced the postoperative morphine requirements.[1] In a study in patients undergoing transurethral resection of prostate or bladder tumours patients were given spinal anaesthesia with hyperbaric **bupivacaine** 12 mg (**bupivacaine** 0.75% and glucose 82.5 mg) alone or with clonidine 30 micrograms. Onset time of motor block was shorter in the patients given **bupivacaine** with clonidine, when compared with those given **bupivacaine** alone (time to reach Bromage 3 motor block 11.7 minutes and 20.7 minutes, respectively). The duration of the sensory and motor block was longer in those given clonidine. No differences in the heart rate or mean arterial pressures were found between the groups.[2]

Another study, in children, found that oral premedication with clonidine 4 micrograms/kg reduced the plasma levels of epidural **lidocaine** by 25 to 50%.[3] Similar findings are reported in another study in which clonidine was given with epidural **lidocaine**.[4]

Mechanism

Not fully understood. An *in vitro* study using liver microsomes found that clonidine, at clinical levels, is unlikely to affect the metabolism of lidocaine.[5] However, the haemodynamic effects of clonidine may lead to decreased hepatic blood flow and reduced metabolism.[5]

Importance and management

Evidence of an interaction between bupivacaine and clonidine appears to be limited to two studies, which suggest that clonidine may increase the response to bupivacaine without causing adverse cardiac effects. This interaction may be beneficial.

Evidence for an interaction between lidocaine and clonidine is also limited, but what is known suggests that clonidine may reduce the levels of lidocaine appearing in the plasma, following epidural administration. This interaction may also be beneficial.

Note that clonidine used as an antihypertensive could, theoretically, cause severe hypotension if given with local anaesthetics. See also 'Anaesthetics, local + Antihypertensives', p.115.

1. Tripi PA, Palmer JS, Thomas S, Elder JS. Clonidine increases duration of bupivacaine caudal analgesia for ureteroneocystostomy: a double-blind prospective trial. *J Urol (Baltimore)* (2005) 174, 1081–3.
2. Kanazi GE, Aouad MT, Jabbour-Khoury SI, Al Jazzar MD, Alameddine MM, Al-Yaman R, Bulbul M, Baraka AS. Effect of low dose dexmedetomidine or clonidine on the characteristics of bupivacaine spinal block. *Acta Anaesthesiol Scand* (2006) 50, 222–7.
3. Inomata S, Tanaka E, Miyabe M, Kakiuchi Y, Nagashima A, Yamasaki Y, Nakayama S, Baba Y, Toyooka H, Okuyama K, Kohda Y. Plasma lidocaine concentrations during continuous thoracic epidural anesthesia after clonidine premedication in children. *Anesth Analg* (2001) 93, 1147–51.
4. Mazoit JX, Benhamou D, Veillette Y, Samii K. Clonidine and or adrenaline decrease lignocaine plasma peak concentration after epidural injection. *Br J Clin Pharmacol* (1996) 42, 242–5.
5. Inomata S, Nagashima A, Osaka Y, Tanaka E, Toyooka H. Effects of clonidine on lidocaine metabolism in human or rat liver microsomes. *J Anesth* (2003) 17, 281–3.

Anaesthetics, local + CYP3A4 inhibitors

Itraconazole may reduce the clearance of bupivacaine. Itraconazole, ketoconazole or clarithromycin may slightly decrease ropivacaine clearance.

Clinical evidence, mechanism, importance and management

(a) Bupivacaine

In a placebo-controlled, crossover study in 7 healthy subjects pretreatment with **itraconazole** 200 mg daily for 4 days reduced the clearance of bupivacaine (300 micrograms/kg given intravenously over 60 minutes) by 20 to 25%.[1] It seems unlikely that a decrease of this magnitude in the clearance of bupivacaine will be clinically relevant.

(b) Ropivacaine

In a study in 8 healthy subjects, pretreatment with **itraconazole** 200 mg daily or **clarithromycin** 250 mg twice daily for 4 days did not significantly affect the pharmacokinetics of intravenous ropivacaine 600 microgram/kg. However, there was considerable interindividual variation in the findings. A small but statistically insignificant 20% increase in the AUC of ropivacaine occurred, and the peak plasma concentrations of the metabolite 2′,6′-pipecoloxylidide were decreased by **clarithromycin** and **itraconazole**, by 44% and 74%, respectively. Both **itraconazole** and **clarithromycin** inhibit the formation of this metabolite by the cytochrome P450 isoenzyme CYP3A4.[2] Similar results were found with **ketoconazole** and ropivacaine.[3] Potent inhibitors of CYP3A4 appear to cause only a minor decrease in clearance of ropivacaine, which is unlikely to be of clinical relevance.[3] For a report of erythromycin, an inhibitor of CYP3A4, enhancing the effect of fluvoxamine, an inhibitor of

CYP1A2, on the clearance of ropivacaine, see 'Anaesthetics, local; Ropivacaine + Fluvoxamine', p.119.

1. Palkama VJ, Neuvonen PJ, Olkkola KT. Effect of itraconazole on the pharmacokinetics of bupivacaine enantiomers in healthy volunteers. *Br J Anaesth* (1999) 83, 659–61.
2. Jokinen MK, Ahonen J, Neuvonen PJ, Olkkola KT. Effect of clarithromycin and itraconazole on the pharmacokinetics of ropivacaine. *Pharmacol Toxicol* (2001) 88, 187–91.
3. Arlander E, Ekström G, Alm C, Carrillo JA, Bielenstein M, Böttiger Y, Bertilsson L, Gustafsson LL. Metabolism of ropivacaine in humans is mediated by CYP1A2 and to a minor extent by CYP3A4: An interaction study with fluvoxamine and ketoconazole as in vivo inhibitors. *Clin Pharmacol Ther* (1998) 64, 484–91.

Anaesthetics, local + H_2-receptor antagonists

Some studies suggest that both cimetidine and ranitidine can modestly raise the plasma levels of bupivacaine, whereas other evidence suggests that no significant interaction occurs. Some studies found that cimetidine does not affect lidocaine when used as an anaesthetic, whereas others found that cimetidine increased plasma lidocaine levels. Ranitidine and probably famotidine do not appear to significantly affect the pharmacokinetics of lidocaine.

Clinical evidence

(a) Bupivacaine

1. Cimetidine. In a study in 16 women undergoing caesarean section, pretreatment with cimetidine 300 mg intramuscularly 1 to 4 hours before epidural anaesthesia with bupivacaine 0.5% had no effect on the pharmacokinetics of bupivacaine in either the women or the neonates, when compared with 20 control women, although the maternal unbound bupivacaine plasma levels rose by 22%.[1] These findings were confirmed in two similar studies in which women receiving bupivacaine were pretreated with cimetidine before caesarean section,[2,3] and a further study in 7 healthy subjects (6 women and one man) given two oral doses of cimetidine 400 mg before intramuscular bupivacaine.[4] However, in a further study in 4 healthy male subjects, the AUC of bupivacaine was increased by 40% (when compared to placebo) by cimetidine. In this study cimetidine 400 mg was given at 10 pm and 8 am the following day, with a 50-mg infusion of bupivacaine given at 11 am.[5]

2. Ranitidine. In a study in 10 subjects given extradural anaesthesia for caesarean section, pretreatment with oral ranitidine 150 mg 1.5 to 2 hours before bupivacaine increased the maximum plasma levels of bupivacaine by about 36%, when compared with 10 patients given no pretreatment.[3] A further study in 9 patients also found that pretreatment with ranitidine 150 mg increased plasma bupivacaine levels.[6] Another study found that two oral doses of ranitidine 150 mg caused a 25% increase in the mean AUC of bupivacaine, but this was not statistically significant.[5] No increased bupivacaine toxicity was described in any of these reports. However, two other studies in 36 and 28 women undergoing caesarean section found no measurable effect on the bupivacaine disposition when ranitidine 150 mg was given the night before and on the morning of anaesthesia,[2] or when ranitidine 50 mg was given intramuscularly 2 hours before anaesthesia, respectively.[7]

(b) Lidocaine

1. Cimetidine. In 5 women given epidural anaesthesia for caesarean section, the pharmacokinetics of 400 mg of lidocaine 2% (with adrenaline (epinephrine) 1:200 000) were unchanged by a single 400-mg oral dose of cimetidine given about 2 hours preoperatively.[8] Another very similar study in 9 women found no statistically significant rises in whole blood lidocaine levels (although they tended to be higher), in the presence of cimetidine 300 mg, given intramuscularly, at least one hour preoperatively.[9] However, in patients pretreated with cimetidine (200 mg orally on the night before surgery and 400 mg one hour before induction) peak plasma levels of epidural lidocaine 2% (with adrenaline 1:200 000) were 3.2 micrograms/mL. Lidocaine levels in patients who did not receive pretreatment with H_2-receptor antagonists were 2.3 micrograms/mL.[10]

2. Famotidine. In patients pretreated with famotidine (20 mg orally on the night before surgery plus 20 mg intramuscularly one hour before induction), peak plasma levels of epidural lidocaine 2% (with adrenaline 1:200 000) were 2.4 micrograms/mL. Lidocaine levels in patients who did not receive pretreatment with H_2-receptor antagonists were 2.3 micrograms/mL.[10] In another study, the effects of famotidine on lidocaine were found to be less than those of cimetidine, but greater than in patients not given an H_2-receptor antagonist.[11]

3. Ranitidine. In 7 women given epidural anaesthesia for caesarean section the pharmacokinetics of 400 mg of lidocaine 2%, (with adrenaline (epinephrine) 1:200 000) were unchanged after a single 150-mg oral dose of ranitidine given about 2 hours preoperatively.[8] A similar study in 8 women also found no statistically significant rises in whole blood lidocaine levels in the presence of ranitidine 150 mg given orally at least 2 hours preoperatively.[9]

Mechanism

Not understood. It has been suggested that cimetidine reduces the hepatic metabolism of bupivacaine and lidocaine. Protein binding displacement has also been suggested.

Importance and management

A confusing situation. No clinically important interaction has been established, but be alert for any evidence of increased bupivacaine toxicity resulting from raised total plasma levels and rises in unbound bupivacaine levels during the concurrent use of cimetidine. Ranitidine may modestly increase the levels of bupivacaine but this does not appear to be clinically significant.

Cimetidine (but not ranitidine) has been shown to raise plasma lidocaine levels when lidocaine is used as an antiarrhythmic (see 'Lidocaine + H_2-receptor antagonists', p.281), but some of the studies cited above found cimetidine did not affect lidocaine levels when lidocaine is used as a local anaesthetic. However, in the studies comparing the effects of cimetidine and famotidine, cimetidine was found to increase lidocaine levels and it was suggested that famotidine may be preferable to cimetidine as pretreatment before epidural lidocaine.[10,11]

1. Kuhnert BR, Zuspan KJ, Kuhnert PM, Syracuse CD, Brashear WT, Brown DE. Lack of influence of cimetidine on bupivacaine levels during parturition. *Anesth Analg* (1987) 66, 986–90.
2. O'Sullivan GM, Smith M, Morgan B, Brighouse D, Reynolds F. H_2 antagonists and bupivacaine clearance. *Anaesthesia* (1988) 43, 93–5.
3. Flynn RJ, Moore J, Collier PS, McClean E. Does pretreatment with cimetidine and ranitidine affect the disposition of bupivacaine? *Br J Anaesth* (1989) 62, 87–91.
4. Pihlajamäki KK, Lindberg RLP, Jantunen ME. Lack of effect of cimetidine on the pharmacokinetics of bupivacaine in healthy subjects. *Br J Clin Pharmacol* (1988) 26, 403–6.
5. Noble DW, Smith KJ, Dundas CR. Effects of H-2 antagonists on the elimination of bupivacaine. *Br J Anaesth* (1987) 59, 735–7.
6. Wilson CM, Moore J, Ghaly RG, McClean E, Dundee JW. Plasma bupivacaine concentrations associated with extradural anaesthesia for caesarean section: influence of pretreatment with ranitidine. *Br J Anaesth* (1986) 58, 1330P–1331P.
7. Brashear WT, Zuspan KJ, Lazebnik N, Kuhnert BR, Mann LI. Effect of ranitidine on bupivacaine disposition. *Anesth Analg* (1991) 72, 369–76.
8. Flynn RJ, Moore J, Collier PS, Howard PJ. Single dose oral H_2-antagonists do not affect plasma lidocaine levels in the parturient. *Acta Anaesthesiol Scand* (1989) 33, 593–6.
9. Dailey PA, Hughes SC, Rosen MA, Healey K, Cheek DBC, Shnider SM. Effect of cimetidine and ranitidine on lidocaine concentrations during epidural anesthesia for cesarean section. *Anesthesiology* (1988) 69, 1013–17.
10. Kishikawa K, Namiki A, Miyashita K, Saitoh K. Effects of famotidine and cimetidine on plasma levels of epidurally administered lignocaine. *Anaesthesia* (1990) 45, 719–21.
11. Sabatakaki A, Daifotis Z, Karayannacos P, Danou K, Kaniaris P. La famotidine ne modifie pas les taux plasmatiques de la lidocaïne pour rachianesthésie. Étude comparative de la famotidine et de la cimétidine. *Cah Anesthesiol* (1992) 40, 317–20.

Anaesthetics, local + Rifampicin (Rifampin)

Rifampicin increases the metabolism of ropivacaine.

Clinical evidence, mechanism, importance and management

A study in 10 healthy non-smokers and 8 otherwise healthy smokers given ropivacaine 600 micrograms/kg by intravenous infusion over 30 minutes found that pretreatment with rifampicin 600 mg daily for 5 days increased the clearance of the metabolite 3-hydroxyropivacaine and decreased the urinary excretion of 2′,6′-pipecoloxylidide by 93% and 46%, respectively, decreased the AUC by 52% and 38%, respectively, and decreased the half-life of ropivacaine in both non-smokers and smokers.[1] Ropivacaine undergoes oxidative hepatic metabolism mainly by the cytochrome P450 isoenzymes CYP1A2 and CYP3A4. The elimination of ropivacaine may be considerably accelerated by rifampicin, which is a potent cytochrome P450 enzyme inducer. However, in clinical use the local anaesthetic is given near the nerves to be desensitised and induction of these isoenzymes is not likely to affect the local anaesthetic before it enters the systemic blood circulation.[1] This interaction is therefore of little clinical relevance.

Rifampicin may also increase the metabolism of lidocaine to a minor extent, see 'Lidocaine + Rifampicin (Rifampin)', p.284.

1. Jokinen MJ, Olkkola KT, Ahonen J, Neuvonen PJ. Effect of rifampin and tobacco smoking on the pharmacokinetics of ropivacaine. *Clin Pharmacol Ther* (2001) 70, 344–50.

Anaesthetics, local + Tobacco

Smoking appears to have only a minor effect on ropivacaine pharmacokinetics. Tobacco smoking may enhance cocaine-associated myocardial ischaemia.

Clinical evidence, mechanism, importance and management

(a) Cocaine

In a study in 42 smokers (36 with proven coronary artery disease), the mean product of the heart rate and systolic arterial pressure increased by 11% after intranasal cocaine 2 mg/kg, by 12% after one cigarette and by 45% after both cocaine use and one cigarette. Compared with baseline measurements, the diameters of non-diseased coronary arterial segments decreased on average by 7% after cocaine use, 7% after smoking and 6% after cocaine and smoking. However, the diameters of diseased segments decreased by 9%, 5% and 19%, respectively.[1] Cigarette smoking increases myocardial oxygen demand and induces coronary-artery vasoconstriction through an alpha-adrenergic mechanism similar to cocaine and therefore tobacco smoking may enhance cocaine-associated myocardial ischaemia.[1,2]

(b) Ropivacaine

A study in 10 healthy non-smokers and 8 otherwise healthy smokers given ropivacaine 600 micrograms/kg by intravenous infusion over 30 minutes found that smoking increased the urinary excretion of the metabolite 3-hydroxyropivacaine and decreased the urinary excretion of the metabolite 2′,6′-pipecoloxylidide by 62%, but did not significantly affect the ropivacaine AUC.[3]

Ropivacaine undergoes oxidative hepatic metabolism mainly by the cytochrome P450 isoenzymes CYP1A2 and CYP3A4. Cigarette smoking is known to induce CYP1A2 and may therefore increase the metabolism of ropivacaine. However, in clinical use the local anaesthetic is given near the nerves to be desensitised and induction of isoenzymes is not likely to affect the local anaesthetic before it enters the systemic blood circulation.[3] This interaction is therefore of little clinical relevance.

Note that smoking may reduce the bioavailability of *oral* lidocaine, see 'Lidocaine + Tobacco', p.284.

1. Moliterno DJ, Willard JE, Lange RA, Negus BH, Boehrer JD, Glamann DB, Landau C, Rossen JD, Winniford MD, Hillis LD. Coronary-artery vasoconstriction induced by cocaine, cigarette smoking, or both. *N Engl J Med* (1994) 330, 454–9.
2. Hollander JE. The management of cocaine-associated myocardial ischemia. *N Engl J Med* (1995) 333, 1267–72.
3. Jokinen MJ, Olkkola KT, Ahonen J, Neuvonen PJ. Effect of rifampin and tobacco smoking on the pharmacokinetics of ropivacaine. *Clin Pharmacol Ther* (2001) 70, 344–50.

Anaesthetics, local; Bupivacaine + Antipsychotics

Exaggerated hypotension occurred in a patient taking risperidone when she was given spinal anaesthesia with bupivacaine.

Clinical evidence, mechanism, importance and management

A patient with bipolar disorder, taking lithium 600 mg twice daily and **risperidone** 2 mg at bedtime, was given spinal anaesthesia with hyperbaric bupivacaine 0.75% (12 mg), fentanyl 10 micrograms and morphine 200 micrograms for an elective caesarean section. Within a few minutes, her blood pressure decreased from 120/50 mmHg to 70/30 mmHg, for which she was given ephedrine 50 mg and Ringer's lactate solution. Her heart rate increased from about 80 bpm to 130 bpm, with little improvement in the hypotension until phenylephrine 600 micrograms was given, after which her vital signs gradually improved over 10 minutes. A previous caesarean section in the same patient, while taking lithium but not **risperidone** and using the same epidural anaesthesia, had been accompanied by hypotension to about 80/50 mmHg which had rapidly normalised with ephedrine 20 mg and phenylephrine 40 micrograms.

Hypotension is a common adverse effect of bupivacaine and lithium may cause hypotension in toxicity. However, the patient's lithium level was subtherapeutic on the morning of the caesarean section. **Risperidone** is an antagonist of alpha-adrenergic receptors, which the authors believe contributed to the difficulty in treating the peri-operative hypotension seen in the case report above. Further, it was suggested that the tachycardia without improvement in the hypotension after ephedrine was given may have been due to the beta-adrenergic effects of ephedrine combined with the alpha-adrenergic antagonism of risperidone.[1]

The general importance of this isolated case is unclear; however, it serves as a reminder that the adverse hypotensive effects that are common to many antipsychotics, could be additive with the hypotensive effects of bupivacaine.

1. Williams JH, Hepner DL. Risperidone and exaggerated hypotension during a spinal anesthetic. *Anesth Analg* (2004) 98, 240–1.

Anaesthetics, local; Bupivacaine + Dexmedetomidine

The addition of dexmedetomidine to bupivacaine spinal block shortens the onset time and increases the duration of sensory and motor block.

Clinical evidence, mechanism, importance and management

In a study in patients undergoing transurethral resection of prostate or bladder tumours patients were given spinal anaesthesia with hyperbaric bupivacaine 12 mg (bupivacaine 0.75% and glucose 82.5 mg) alone or with dexmedetomidine 3 micrograms. Onset time of motor block was shorter in the patients given bupivacaine with dexmedetomidine, when compared with those given bupivacaine alone (time to reach Bromage 3 motor block, 13.2 minutes and 20.7 minutes, respectively). The duration of the sensory and motor block was significantly longer in those given the combination. No differences in the heart rate or mean arterial pressures were found between the groups.[1]

Evidence appears to be limited to this study, but it demonstrates that concurrent use may be beneficial.

1. Kanazi GE, Aouad MT, Jabbour-Khoury SI, Al Jazzar MD, Alameddine MM, Al-Yaman R, Bulbul M, Baraka AS. Effect of low dose dexmedetomidine or clonidine on the characteristics of bupivacaine spinal block. *Acta Anaesthesiol Scand* (2006) 50, 222–7.

Anaesthetics, local; Cocaine + Adrenaline (Epinephrine)

Arrhythmias occurred in three patients given a concentrated nasal paste containing cocaine and adrenaline (epinephrine).

Clinical evidence, mechanism, importance and management

Two children and one adult patient undergoing general anaesthesia[1] developed arrhythmias shortly after nasal application of a paste containing cocaine 25% and adrenaline (epinephrine) 0.18%. All 3 patients received doses of cocaine that exceeded the usual maximum total dose (1.5 mg/kg) recommended for nasal application in healthy adults.[2]

Cocaine has sympathomimetic actions (tachycardia, peripheral vasoconstriction, and hypertension). Combined use with sympathomimetics such as adrenaline increases these effects, and the risk of life-threatening arrhythmias. This risk may be further increased if halothane anaesthesia is used (two of the above patients received halothane[1]). See also 'Anaesthetics, general + Anaesthetics, local', p.99, and 'Anaesthetics, general + Inotropes and Vasopressors', p.106.

The use of adrenaline with topical cocaine is controversial. Some consider that the addition of adrenaline is of doubtful value and that the combination should not be used, especially in the form of a concentrated paste.[1] However, others consider the combination to be safe and useful.[3] Note also that the use of local anaesthetics containing adrenaline should be avoided in patients who abuse cocaine, unless it is certain that they have not used cocaine for at least 24 hours.[4]

1. Nicholson KEA, Rogers JEG. Cocaine and adrenaline paste: a fatal combination? *BMJ* (1995) 311, 250–1.
2. *Martindale. The Complete Drug Reference*, [online] London: Pharmaceutical Press. https://www.medicinescomplete.com/mc/martindale/current/ms-7619-y.htm (accessed 19/10/15).
3. De R, Uppal HS, Shehab ZP, Hilger AW, Wilson PS, Courteney-Harris R. Current practices of cocaine administration by UK otorhinolaryngologists. *J Laryngol Otol* (2003) 117, 109–12.
4. Goulet J-P, Pérusse R, Turcotte J-Y. Contraindications to vasoconstrictors in dentistry: part III. *Oral Surg Oral Med Oral Pathol* (1992) 74, 692–7.

Anaesthetics, local; Cocaine + Disulfiram

Disulfiram increases plasma levels of inhaled and intravenous cocaine. Disulfiram increases the cardiovascular effects associated with inhaled, but not intravenous cocaine, whereas it does not significantly affect the behavioural responses to inhaled cocaine but decreases the behavioural responses to intravenous cocaine.

Clinical evidence

A preliminary study in 6 subjects taking cocaine by inhalation found that disulfiram 250 mg daily significantly increased plasma levels of cocaine 1 mg/kg by threefold and increased the plasma levels of cocaine 2 mg/kg by greater than fourfold, respectively. Concurrent treatment also increased the heart rate and blood pressure but did not affect 'high' and 'nervous' ratings.[1]

In a further study by the same authors, 7 subjects from the initial study were given disulfiram 250 mg, disulfiram 500 mg or placebo daily for 5 days. Intranasal cocaine 1 or 2 mg/kg or placebo was started after the third disulfiram dose. Following treatment with disulfiram 250 or 500 mg, the AUC of cocaine was increased three- to sixfold and plasma cocaine levels were increased two- to threefold. Increases in heart rate with disulfiram alone just reached significance, but disulfiram treatment significantly increased the heart rate responses to inhaled cocaine. Disulfiram alone had no significant effect on blood pressure. However, systolic and diastolic blood pressure increased after disulfiram 500 mg daily with cocaine 2 mg/kg, and tended to increase after the disulfiram 250 mg dose. Disulfiram had no significant effects on the behavioural responses to cocaine.[2]

In a further study, cocaine-dependent subjects were given disulfiram 62.5 mg, disulfiram 250 mg or placebo daily for 6 days, with intravenous cocaine 250 micrograms/kg (9 subjects), 500 micrograms/kg (3 subjects) or placebo, taken 2 hours after the disulfiram dose, on days 4 to 6. Disulfiram 62.5 mg and 250 mg increased the AUC of cocaine 250 micrograms/kg by 67 to 84%. Larger increases were seen with the cocaine 500 microgram/kg dose, although these did not reach statistical significance. The clearance of cocaine was also reduced. Disulfiram did not affect the cardiovascular responses to either dose of intravenous cocaine. The behavioural responses to cocaine 250 micrograms/kg ('highs', 'rush') were significantly decreased by disulfiram; similar effects were seen with the larger dose but this did not reach statistical significance due to the small sample size.[3]

The studies above differed in the routes of administration of cocaine (intranasal versus intravenous) and the latter study noted that the dose of intravenous cocaine used produced lower overall levels of cocaine than the intranasal dose studied.[3]

Of interest, a report of a cost-effectiveness study looking at the benefits of using disulfiram to treat cocaine use in methadone-maintained opioid addicts, found that disulfiram use was associated with a reduction in the amount of cocaine used.[4]

Mechanism

Disulfiram has been reported to inhibit carboxylesterases and plasma cholinesterase, which are enzymes involved in the metabolism of cocaine.[3]

Importance and management

It would appear that disulfiram may significantly increase the plasma levels and reduce the clearance of both intranasal and intravenous cocaine. There is conflicting data as to whether this enhances the cardiovascular and behavioural effects of cocaine use. Overall, it would be prudent to exercise caution when giving disulfiram to patients using cocaine as the increase in cocaine levels may result in cocaine toxicity.

1. McCance-Katz EF, Kosten TR, Jatlow P. Chronic disulfiram treatment effects on intranasal cocaine administration: initial results. *Biol Psychiatry* (1998) 43, 540–3.
2. McCance-Katz EF, Kosten TR, Jatlow P. Disulfiram effects on acute cocaine administration. *Drug Alcohol Depend* (1998) 52, 27–39.
3. Baker JR, Jatlow P, McCance-Katz EF. Disulfiram effects on responses to intravenous cocaine administration. *Drug Alcohol Depend* (2007) 87, 202–9.
4. Jofre-Bonet M, Sindelar JL, Petrakis IL, Nich C, Frankforter T, Rounsaville BJ, Carroll KM. Cost effectiveness of disulfiram: treating cocaine use in methadone-maintained patients. *J Subst Abuse Treat* (2004) 26, 225–232.

Anaesthetics, local; Cocaine + Progesterone

There is some evidence to suggest that progesterone may attenuate some of the cardiovascular and subjective effects of smoked or intravenous cocaine, but not the effects of intranasal cocaine.

Clinical evidence, mechanism, importance and management

A preliminary, placebo-controlled study in 5 female cocaine-dependent subjects found that a single 200-mg dose of progesterone, given during days 3 to 9 of the menstrual cycle, attenuated the subjective effects of smoked cocaine.[1] In a further placebo-controlled study by the same authors, 6 male and 4 female cocaine-dependent subjects were given two doses of progesterone 200 mg at 10 pm the day before, and at 8 am on the morning of, intravenous cocaine administration. The initial dose of cocaine 300 micrograms/kg was given 2 hours after the second progesterone dose. Subjects then started a self-administration period in which 5 optional doses of cocaine were available in a 2.5-hour period. Progesterone attenuated cocaine-induced increases in diastolic blood pressure but did not affect systolic blood pressure or heart rate increases. Progesterone also attenuated subjective ratings of 'high' and 'feel the effect of the last dose' in response to cocaine, but did not affect self-administration behaviour.[2]

In a pilot study, male methadone-stabilised cocaine users were given either placebo (15 subjects) or progesterone (dose gradually increased from 100 mg to 300 mg twice daily over 4 weeks; 30 subjects) for 10 weeks. Cocaine positive urine tests showed a slight decrease in cocaine use in the progesterone group and a slight increase in use in the placebo group. However, at weeks 9 and 10, the placebo group showed a significantly lower use of cocaine (as measured by the cocaine positive urine test), when compared with the group given progesterone, suggesting a lack of efficacy of progesterone as a treatment for cocaine dependence in male users.[3]

These findings are probably more relevant to the potential use of progesterone in cocaine dependence, but they do demonstrate that the concurrent use of progesterone in patients taking cocaine is unlikely to result in an adverse outcome.

1. Sofuoglu M, Babb D, Hatsukami DK. Effects of progesterone treatment on smoked cocaine response in women. *Pharmacol Biochem Behav* (2002) 72, 431–5.
2. Sofuoglu M, Mitchell E, Kosten TR. Effects of progesterone treatment on cocaine responses in male and female cocaine users. *Pharmacol Biochem Behav* (2004) 78, 699–705.
3. Sofuoglu M, Poling J, Gonzalez G, Gonsai K, Oliveto A, Kosten TR. Progesterone effects on cocaine use in male cocaine users maintained on methadone: a randomized, double-blind, pilot study. *Exp Clin Psychopharmacol* (2007) 15, 453–60.

Anaesthetics, local; Lidocaine + Ondansetron

Ondansetron may reduce the efficacy of the sensory block induced by lidocaine.

Clinical evidence, mechanism, importance and management

In a placebo-controlled study oral ondansetron 4 mg was given to patients the evening before surgery, followed by intravenous ondansetron 4 mg given over 15 minutes before subarachnoid anaesthesia with lidocaine 5% in dextrose 8%. Ondansetron significantly reduced the sensory block measured at 30 minutes. Motor block was unaffected. In this study 54 patients were enrolled, but not all patients were assessed for both motor and sensory block.[1]

Evidence appears to be limited to this one study, but, until more is known, it may be prudent to monitor closely for a reduction in the efficacy of the sensory block with lidocaine if ondansetron is also given.

1. Fassoulaki A, Melemeni A, Zotou M, Sarantopoulos C. Systemic ondansetron antagonizes the sensory block produced by intrathecal lidocaine. *Anesth Analg* (2005) 100, 1817–21.

Anaesthetics, local; Ropivacaine + Fluvoxamine

Fluvoxamine inhibits the clearance of ropivacaine.

Clinical evidence, mechanism, importance and management

In a randomised, crossover study in 12 healthy subjects fluvoxamine decreased the mean total plasma clearance of ropivacaine by 68%, and almost doubled the half-life of ropivacaine. Fluvoxamine was given at a dose of 25 mg twice daily for 2 days, and a single 40-mg intravenous dose of ropivacaine was given over 20 minutes one hour after the morning dose of fluvoxamine on the second day.[1]

Fluvoxamine is a potent inhibitor of the cytochrome P450 isoenzyme CYP1A2 and so reduces the metabolism of ropivacaine to its major metabolite 3-hydroxyropivacaine. In one study in healthy subjects the combination of fluvoxamine with **erythromycin**, an inhibitor of CYP3A4, which on its own has little effect on the pharmacokinetics of ropivacaine, was found to decrease the clearance of ropivacaine more than fluvoxamine alone.[2]

The UK manufacturer recommends that the prolonged use of ropivacaine should be avoided in patients given potent CYP1A2 inhibitors, such as fluvoxamine.[3] Be aware that CYP3A4 inhibitors, such as erythromycin, in combination with CYP1A2 inhibitors may further reduce ropivacaine clearance.[2]

1. Arlander E, Ekström G, Alm C, Carrillo JA, Bielenstein M, Böttiger Y, Bertilsson L, Gustafsson LL. Metabolism of ropivacaine in humans is mediated by CYP1A2 and to a minor extent by CYP3A4: An interaction study with fluvoxamine and ketoconazole as in vivo inhibitors. *Clin Pharmacol Ther* (1998) 64, 484–91.
2. Jokinen MJ, Ahonen J, Neuvonen PJ, Olkkola KT. The effect of erythromycin, fluvoxamine, and their combination on the pharmacokinetics of ropivacaine. *Anesth Analg* (2000) 91, 1207–12.
3. Naropin (Ropivacaine hydrochloride monohydrate). AstraZeneca UK Ltd. UK Summary of product characteristics, August 2008.

Anaesthetics, local; Ropivacaine + Quinolones

Ciprofloxacin may decrease the clearance of ropivacaine. It is also likely that enoxacin will inhibit the metabolism of ropivacaine.

Clinical evidence, mechanism, importance and management

A study in 9 healthy subjects found that **ciprofloxacin** 500 mg twice daily decreased the mean clearance of a single 600-microgram/kg intravenous dose of ropivacaine by 31%, but there was considerable inter-individual variation in the effects of **ciprofloxacin**. The reduction in clearance probably occurs because **ciprofloxacin** inhibits the cytochrome P450 isoenzyme CYP1A2, which metabolises ropivacaine to its major metabolite 3-hydroxyropivacaine. For some patients concurrent use may cause toxicity.[1] Bear the potential for an interaction in mind if ropivacaine is given to a patient taking **ciprofloxacin**.

On the basis of data with fluvoxamine (see 'Anaesthetics, local; Ropivacaine + Fluvoxamine', above) the UK manufacturer of ropivacaine has recommended that the prolonged use of ropivacaine should be avoided in patients taking potent CYP1A2 inhibitors such as **enoxacin**.[2]

1. Jokinen MJ, Olkkola KT, Ahonen J, Neuvonen PJ. Effect of ciprofloxacin on the pharmacokinetics of ropivacaine. *Eur J Clin Pharmacol* (2003) 58, 653–7.
2. Naropin (Ropivacaine hydrochloride monohydrate). AstraZeneca UK Ltd. UK Summary of product characteristics, August 2008.

Neuromuscular blockers + Aminoglycosides

The aminoglycoside antibacterials possess neuromuscular blocking activity. Appropriate measures should be taken to accommodate the increased neuromuscular blockade and the prolonged and potentially fatal respiratory depression that can occur if these antibacterials are used with conventional neuromuscular blocking drugs.

Clinical evidence

Two examples from many:

A 38-year-old patient anaesthetised with cyclopropane experienced severe respiratory depression after being given intraperitoneal **neomycin** 500 mg. She had also received **suxamethonium** (**succinylcholine**) and **tubocurarine**. This antibacterial-induced neuromuscular blockade was resistant to treatment with edrophonium.[1]

A 71-year-old woman received a standard bowel preparation consisting of oral erythromycin and **neomycin** (a total of 3 g). Surgery was postponed for one day and she received a second similar bowel preparation pre-operatively. Anaesthesia was induced with sufentanil and etomidate and maintained with isoflurane and sufentanil. **Rocuronium** (total dose of 60 mg over 2 hours) was used to facilitate tracheal intubation and maintain muscle relaxation. Despite clinical appearance of a reversal of the neuromuscular blockade by neostigmine 3.5 mg and glycopyrronium (glycopyrrolate) 400 micrograms, the patient complained of dyspnoea and required reintubation twice. The effects of additional doses of neostigmine were inconsistent and the use edrophonium 50 mg or calcium chloride 500 mg intravenously did not result in an improvement.[2]

Many other reports confirm that some degree of respiratory depression or paralysis can occur if aminoglycosides are given to anaesthetised patients. When a conventional neuromuscular blocker is also used, the blockade is deepened and recovery prolonged. If the antibacterial is given towards the end of surgery the result can be that a patient who is recovering normally from neuromuscular blockade suddenly develops serious apnoea, which can lead to prolonged and in some cases fatal respiratory depression.

A review of the literature[3] lists more than 100 cases over the period 1956 to 1970 involving:

- **tubocurarine** with **neomycin** or **streptomycin,**
- **gallamine** with **neomycin**, **kanamycin** or **streptomycin**,
- **suxamethonium** with **neomycin**, **kanamycin** or **streptomycin**.

The routes of antibacterial administration were oral, intraperitoneal, oesophageal, intraluminal, retroperitoneal, intramuscular, intrapleural, cystic, beneath skin flaps, extradural and intravenous.

Later reports involve:

- **pancuronium**; with **amikacin**,[4] **gentamicin**,[5] **neomycin**,[6] or **streptomycin**,[7,8]
- **pipecuronium** with **netilmicin**,[9]
- **suxamethonium** with **dibekacin**,[10]
- **tubocurarine**; with **amikacin**,[11] **dibekacin**,[10,12] **framycetin** (eye irrigation),[13] **ribostamycin**,[10,12] or **tobramycin**,[14]
- **vecuronium**; with **amikacin/polymyxin**,[15] **gentamicin**,[16-18] **gentamicin/clindamycin**,[19] **neomycin/clindamycin**,[20] or **tobramycin**.[17,21]

Aminoglycosides and neuromuscular blockers that have been reported not to interact are:

- **alcuronium** with **tobramycin**,[22]
- **atracurium** with **gentamicin** or **tobramycin**,[17]
- **suxamethonium** with **tobramycin** or **ribostamycin**.[10]

Mechanism

The aminoglycosides appear to reduce or prevent the release of acetylcholine at neuromuscular junctions (related to an impairment of calcium influx) and they may also lower the sensitivity of the post-synaptic membrane, thereby reducing transmission. These effects would be additive with those of conventional neuromuscular blockers, which act at the post-synaptic membrane.

Importance and management

Extremely well documented, very long established, clinically important and potentially serious interactions. Ten out of the 111 cases in one review[3] were fatal, related directly or indirectly to aminoglycoside-induced respiratory depression. Concurrent use need not be avoided, but be alert for increased and prolonged neuromuscular blockade with every aminoglycoside and neuromuscular blocker, although the potencies of the aminoglycosides differ to some extent. In *animal* studies, at concentrations representing the maximum therapeutic levels, the neuromuscular blocking potency of various aminoglycosides was rated (from highest to lowest): neomycin, streptomycin, gentamicin, kanamycin.[23] The postoperative recovery period should also be closely monitored because of the risk of recurarisation if the aminoglycoside is given during surgery. High-risk patients appear to be those with renal disease and hypocalcaemia, who may have elevated serum antibacterial levels, and those with pre-existing muscular weakness. Treatment of the increased blockade with anticholinesterases and calcium has met with variable success because the response seems to be inconsistent.

1. LaPorte J, Mignault G, L'Allier R, Perron P. Un cas d'apnée à la néomycine. *Union Med Can* (1959) 88, 149–52.
2. Hasfurther DL, Bailey PL. Failure of neuromuscular blockade reversal after rocuronium in a patient who received oral neomycin. *Can J Anaesth* (1996) 43, 617–20.
3. Pittinger CB, Eryasa Y, Adamson R. Antibiotic-induced paralysis. *Anesth Analg* (1970) 49, 487–501.
4. Monsegur JC, Vidal MM, Beltrán J, Felipe MAN. Parálisis neuromuscular prolongada tras administración simultánea de amikacina y pancuronio. *Rev Esp Anestesiol Reanim* (1984) 31, 30–3.
5. Regan AG, Perumbetti PPV. Pancuronium and gentamicin interaction in patients with renal failure. *Anesth Analg* (1980) 59, 393.
6. Giala M, Sareyiannis C, Cortsaris N, Paradelis A, Lappas DG. Possible interaction of pancuronium and tubocurarine with oral neomycin. *Anaesthesia* (1982) 37, 776.
7. Giala MM, Paradelis AG. Two cases of prolonged respiratory depression due to interaction of pancuronium with colistin and streptomycin. *J Antimicrob Chemother* (1979) 5, 234–5.
8. Torresi S, Pasotti EM. Su un caso di curarizzazione prolungata da interazione tra pancuronio e streptomicina. *Minerva Anestesiol* (1984) 50, 143–5.
9. Stanley JC, Mirakhur RK, Clarke RSJ. Study of pipecuronium-antibiotic interaction. *Anesthesiology* (1990) 73, A898.
10. Arai T, Hashimoto Y, Shima T, Matsukawa S, Iwatsuki K. Neuromuscular blocking properties of tobramycin, dibekacin and ribostamycin in man. *Jpn J Antibiot* (1977) 30, 281–4.
11. Singh YN, Marshall IG, Harvey AL. Some effects of the aminoglycoside antibiotic amikacin on neuromuscular and autonomic transmission. *Br J Anaesth* (1978) 50, 109–17.
12. Hashimoto Y, Shima T, Matsukawa S, Iwatsuki K. Neuromuscular blocking properties of some antibiotics in man. *Tohoku J Exp Med* (1975) 117, 339–400.
13. Clark R. Prolonged curarization due to intraocular soframycin. *Anaesth Intensive Care* (1975) 3, 79–80.
14. Waterman PM, Smith RB. Tobramycin-curare interaction. *Anesth Analg* (1977) 56, 587–8.
15. Kronenfeld MA, Thomas SJ, Turndorf H. Recurrence of neuromuscular blockade after reversal of vecuronium in a patient receiving polymyxin/amikacin sternal irrigation. *Anesthesiology* (1986) 65, 93–4.
16. Harwood TN, Moorthy SS. Prolonged vecuronium-induced neuromuscular blockade in children. *Anesth Analg* (1989) 68, 534–6.
17. Dupuis JY, Martin R, Tétrault J-P. Atracurium and vecuronium interaction with gentamicin and tobramycin. *Can J Anaesth* (1989) 36, 407–11.
18. Dotan ZA, Hana R, Simon D, Geva D, Pfeffermann RA, Ezri T. The effect of vecuronium is enhanced by a large rather than a modest dose of gentamicin as compared with no preoperative gentamicin. *Anesth Analg* (2003) 96, 750–4.
19. Jedeikin R, Dolgunski E, Kaplan R, Hoffman S. Prolongation of neuromuscular blocking effect of vecuronium by antibiotics. *Anaesthesia* (1987) 42, 858–60.
20. Gilbert TB, Jacobs SC, Quaddoura AA. Deafness and prolonged neuromuscular blockade following single-dose peritoneal neomycin irrigation. *Can J Anaesth* (1998) 45, 568–70.
21. Vanacker BF, Van de Walle J. The neuromuscular blocking action of vecuronium in normal patients and in patients with no renal function and interaction vecuronium-tobramycin in renal transplant patients. *Acta Anaesthesiol Belg* (1986) 37, 95–9.
22. Boliston TA, Ashman R. Tobramycin and neuromuscular blockade. *Anaesthesia* (1978) 33, 552.
23. Caputy AJ, Kim YI, Sanders DB. The neuromuscular blocking effects of therapeutic concentrations of various antibiotics on normal rat skeletal muscle: a quantitative comparison. *J Pharmacol Exp Ther* (1981) 217, 369–78.

Neuromuscular blockers + Anaesthetics, local

The neuromuscular blockade due to suxamethonium (succinylcholine) can be increased and prolonged by procaine. Increased toxicity occurred when mivacurium and prilocaine were given together for regional anaesthesia. Local anaesthetics have some neuromuscular blocking activity and may theoretically also enhance the block produced by competitive neuromuscular blockers.

Clinical evidence

A study found that **procaine** prolonged the apnoea following the use of **suxamethonium** 700 micrograms/kg. A dose-relationship was established. The duration of apnoea was approximately doubled by 2.2 mg/kg of procaine intravenously, and tripled by 11.2 mg/kg, although the effects of procaine at higher doses were more marked.[1]

In a study in 10 healthy subjects, prolonged muscle weakness and symptoms of local anaesthetic toxicity were experienced after deflation of the tourniquet when 40 mL of **prilocaine** 0.5% and **mivacurium** 600 micrograms were used together for intravenous regional anaesthesia of the forearm. Giving **prilocaine** or **mivacurium** alone did not produce these effects. The slow recovery suggested that **mivacurium** was not broken down in the ischaemic limb,[2] but inhibition of plasma cholinesterase by **prilocaine** would not fully explain the prolonged weakness once the cuff was deflated.[3]

Mechanism

Uncertain. Some local anaesthetics (ester-type[4]) such as procaine appear to inhibit plasma cholinesterase,[5] which might prolong the activity of suxamethonium. There may additionally be competition between suxamethonium and procaine for hydrolysis by plasma cholinesterase, which metabolises them both.[1,6] These effects are particularly important in patients with abnormal plasma cholinesterase.[7] This may also partially explain the interaction with mivacurium.

All local anaesthetics have some neuromuscular blocking activity and may enhance the block produced by competitive neuromuscular blockers if given in sufficient doses.[7,8]

Importance and management

Information is limited but the interaction between suxamethonium and procaine appears to be established and of clinical importance. Be alert for signs of increased blockade and/or recurarisation with apnoea during the recovery period from suxamethonium, although note that in the study cited, procaine was given intravenously, and local administration would be expected to produce less dramatic effects.

In general, local anaesthetics (e.g. **lidocaine**, procaine) have some neuromuscular blocking activity and may also enhance the block produced by competitive neuromuscular blockers if given in sufficient doses. However, again, there seems to be an absence of reports of this, probably because the amount of local anaesthetic absorbed into the circulation following a local block is usually modest.[8]

Some local anaesthetics (e.g. lidocaine) are also used as antiarrhythmics. For the use of lidocaine and other antiarrhythmics with neuromuscular blockers, see 'Neuromuscular blockers + Antiarrhythmics', below.

1. Usubiaga JE, Wikinski JA, Morales RL, Usubiaga LEJ. Interaction of intravenously administered procaine, lidocaine and succinylcholine in anesthetized subjects. *Anesth Analg* (1967) 46, 39–45.
2. Torrance JM, Lewer BMF, Galletly DC. Low-dose mivacurium supplementation of prilocaine i.v. regional anaesthesia. *Br J Anaesth* (1997) 78, 222–3.
3. Torrance JM, Lewer BMF, Galletly DC. Interactions between mivacurium and prilocaine. *Br J Anaesth* (1997) 79, 262.
4. *Martindale. The Complete Drug Reference*, [online] London: Pharmaceutical Press. https://www.medicinescomplete.com/mc/martindale/current/7600-a6-a.htm (accessed 19/10/15).
5. Reina RA, Cannavà N. Interazione di alcuni anestetici locali con la succinilcolina. *Acta Anaesthesiol Ital* (1972) 23, 1–10
6. Kambam JR, Naukam RJ, Sastry BVR. The effect of procainamide on plasma cholinesterase activity. *Can J Anaesth* (1987) 34, 579–81.
7. Østergaard D, Engbaek J, Viby-Mogensen J. Adverse reactions and interactions of the neuromuscular blocking drugs. *Med Toxicol Adverse Drug Exp* (1989) 4, 351–68.
8. Feldman S, Karalliedde L. Drug interactions with neuromuscular blockers. *Drug Safety* (1996) 15, 261–73.

Neuromuscular blockers + Antiarrhythmics

The neuromuscular blockade due to suxamethonium (succinylcholine) can be increased and prolonged by lidocaine and possibly procainamide. These drugs have some neuromuscular blocking activity and may theoretically also enhance the block produced by competitive neuromuscular blockers.

Clinical evidence

A patient anaesthetised with fluroxene and nitrous oxide demonstrated 100% blockade with **suxamethonium (succinylcholine)** and **tubocurarine**. About 50 minutes later, when twitch height had fully returned and tidal volume was 400 mL, she was given **lidocaine** 50 mg intravenously for premature ventricular contractions. She immediately stopped breathing and the twitch disappeared. About 45 minutes later the tidal volume was 450 mL. Later it was found that the patient had a dibucaine number (a measure of cholinesterase activity) of 23%.[1]

A study has confirmed that **lidocaine** prolongs the apnoea following the use of **suxamethonium** 700 micrograms/kg. A dose-relationship was established, with the duration of apnoea approximately doubled by intravenous lidocaine 5 mg/kg, and tripled by lidocaine 16.6 mg/kg.[2]

Procainamide has been reported to increase the effects of **suxamethonium** in *animals*,[3] increase muscle weakness in a myasthenic patient,[4] and reduce plasma cholinesterase activity in *in vitro* plasma samples from healthy subjects.[5]

Mechanism

Uncertain. Therapeutic procainamide plasma concentrations of 5 to 10 micrograms/mL have been found to inhibit cholinesterase activity by 19 to 32%. Procainamide also has acetylcholine receptor channel blocking activity.[6]

Importance and management

Information is limited but the interaction between suxamethonium (succinylcholine) and lidocaine appears to be established and of clinical importance. Be alert for signs of increased blockade and/or recurarisation with apnoea during the recovery period from suxamethonium in patients given intravenous lidocaine.

Despite the potential for an interaction between suxamethonium and procainamide, no marked interaction has yet been reported. Nevertheless be aware that some increase in the neuromuscular blocking effects is possible.

Lidocaine and procainamide both have some neuromuscular blocking activity and may also enhance the block produced by competitive neuromuscular blockers. However, again, there seems to be an absence of reports of this effect in practice.

1. Miller RD. Neuromuscular blocking agents. In: Smith NT, Miller RD, Corbascio AN, eds. Drug Interactions in Anesthesia. Philadelphia: Lea and Febiger; 1981 p. 249–69.
2. Usubiaga JE, Wikinski JA, Morales RL, Usubiaga LEJ. Interaction of intravenously administered procaine, lidocaine and succinylcholine in anesthetized subjects. *Anesth Analg* (1967) 46, 39–45.
3. Cuthbert MF. The effect of quinidine and procainamide on the neuromuscular blocking action of suxamethonium. *Br J Anaesth* (1966) 38, 775–9.
4. Drachman DA, Skom JH. Procainamide—a hazard in myasthenia gravis. *Arch Neurol* (1965) 13, 316–20.
5. Kambam JR, Naukam RJ, Sastry BVR. The effect of procainamide on plasma cholinesterase activity. *Can J Anaesth* (1987) 34, 579–81.
6. Feldman S, Karalliedde L. Drug interactions with neuromuscular blockers. *Drug Safety* (1996) 15, 261–73.

Neuromuscular blockers + Anticholinesterases

Anticholinesterases oppose the actions of competitive neuromuscular blockers (e.g. tubocurarine) and can therefore be used as an antidote to restore muscular activity following their use. Conversely, anticholinesterases increase and prolong the actions of the depolarising neuromuscular blockers (e.g. suxamethonium (succinylcholine)). Anticholinesterases used to treat Alzheimer's disease may also interact with neuromuscular blockers.

Clinical evidence, mechanism, importance and management

There are two main types of neuromuscular blockers: competitive (non-depolarising) and depolarising (i.e. suxamethonium (succinylcholine)), see 'Table 5.2', p.98.

(a) Competitive (non-depolarising) neuromuscular blockers

Competitive (non-depolarising) neuromuscular blockers (e.g. **tubocurarine**) compete with acetylcholine for receptors on the motor endplate. Anticholinesterases (e.g. **ambenonium**, **edrophonium**, **neostigmine**, **physostigmine**, **pyridostigmine**, etc.) can be used as an antidote to this kind of neuromuscular blockade, because they inhibit the enzymes that destroy acetylcholine so that the concentration of acetylcholine at the neuromuscular junction builds up. In this way the competition between the molecules of the blocker and the acetylcholine for occupancy of the receptors swings in favour of the acetylcholine so that transmission is restored. These drugs are used routinely following surgery to reactivate paralysed muscles. However, note that the **aminoglycosides** can act as neuromuscular blockers (see 'Neuromuscular blockers + Aminoglycosides', p.119) and therefore the use of an aminoglycoside may unintentionally antagonise the effects of the anticholinesterases.

Some inhalational anaesthetics can impair the effect of anticholinesterases on neuromuscular blockers (see 'Anaesthetics, general + Anticholinesterases', p.101).

(b) Suxamethonium (Succinylcholine)

The depolarising neuromuscular blockers (such as suxamethonium) act like acetylcholine to depolarise the motor endplate, but unlike acetylcholine, they are not immediately removed by cholinesterase. The anticholinesterase drugs increase the concentration of acetylcholine at the neuromuscular junction, which enhances and prolongs this type of blockade, and therefore anticholinesterases cannot be used as an antidote for this kind of blocker. Care should be taken if an anticholinesterase has been given to antagonise a competitive neuromuscular block before the use of suxamethonium, as the duration of the suxamethonium block may be prolonged.[1]

(c) Tacrine and other centrally-acting anticholinesterases

1. Competitive (non-depolarising) neuromuscular blockers. Tacrine, like other anticholinesterases, has been used *intravenously* in anaesthetic practice to reverse the effects of competitive (non-depolarising) blockers such as **tubocurarine**.[2] However, tacrine is now more commonly used *orally* for its central effects in the treatment of Alzheimer's disease. Therefore be alert for a reduction in the effects of any competitive neuromuscular blocker in patients taking tacrine. Other centrally acting anticholinesterases (including **galantamine**, **rivastigmine** and possibly **donepezil**) would be expected to behave like tacrine.

The clinical relevance of this warning is supported by a case report, which describes prolonged **suxamethonium**-induced relaxation in a 75-year-old man who had been taking **donepezil** for 14 months. In this patient the effect of **atracurium** was found to be inadequate even at higher than usual doses, based on the patient's weight.[3]

2. Suxamethonium (Succinylcholine). Tacrine, like other anticholinesterases, has been used *intravenously* in anaesthetic practice to prolong the effects of depolarising blockers such as suxamethonium.[2,4-7] For example, one study found that only one-third of the normal dosage of suxamethonium was needed in the presence of 15 mg of intravenous tacrine.[8] However, tacrine is now more commonly used *orally* for its central effects in the treatment of Alzheimer's disease. Therefore be alert for an increase in the effects of suxamethonium in patients taking tacrine. Other centrally acting anticholinesterases (including **galantamine**, **rivastigmine** and possibly **donepezil**) would be expected to behave like tacrine.

There is a report of such an interaction in a 72-year-old woman taking **donepezil** who had prolonged paralysis after induction of anaesthesia with propofol and suxamethonium. It is possible that levels of **donepezil** in this patient were high due to the concurrent use of fluoxetine (see 'Anticholinesterases; Centrally acting + SSRIs', p.370), and this may have contributed to the prolonged action of suxamethonium.[9] Another report describes an 85-year-old woman taking **donepezil**, who developed prolonged neuromuscular blockade after she was given neostigmine to reverse the effects of pancuronium (she had also received suxamethonium). This patient probably had atypical pseudocholinesterase activity, and the authors suggest the interaction may not be clinically relevant in patients with normal enzyme activity.[10]

(d) Organophosphorus compounds

Organophosphorus compounds are potent anticholinesterases, see 'Neuromuscular blockers + Organophosphorus compounds', p.133.

1. Fleming NW, Macres S, Antognini JF, Vengco J. Neuromuscular blocking action of suxamethonium after antagonism of vecuronium by edrophonium, pyridostigmine or neostigmine. *Br J Anaesth* (1996) 77, 492–5.
2. Hunter AR. Tetrahydroaminacrine in anaesthesia. *Br J Anaesth* (1965) 37, 505–13.
3. Sánchez Morillo J, Demartini Ferrari A, Roca de Togores López A. Interacción entre donepezilo y bloqueantes musculares en la enfermedad de Alzheimer. *Rev Esp Anestesiol Reanim* (2003) 50, 97–100.
4. Oberoi GS, Yaubihi N. The use of tacrine (THA) and succinylcholine compared with alcuronium during laparoscopy. *P N G Med J* (1990) 33, 25–8.
5. Davies-Lepie SR. Tacrine may prolong the effect of succinylcholine. *Anesthesiology* (1994) 81, 524.
6. Norman J, Morgan M. The effect of tacrine on the neuromuscular block produced by suxamethonium in man. *Br J Anaesth* (1975) 47, 1027.
7. Lindsay PA, Lumley J. Suxamethonium apnoea masked by tetrahydroaminacrine. *Anaesthesia* (1978) 33, 620–2.
8. El-Kammah BM, El-Gafi SH, El-Sherbiny AM, Kader MMA. Biochemical and clinical study for the role of tacrine as succinylcholine extender. *J Egypt Med Assoc* (1975) 58, 559–67.
9. Crowe S, Collins L. Suxamethonium and donepezil: a cause of prolonged paralysis. *Anesthesiology* (2003) 98, 574–5.
10. Sprung J, Castellani WJ, Srinivasan V, Udayashankar S. The effects of donepezil and neostigmine in a patient with unusual pseudocholinesterase activity. *Anesth Analg* (1998) 87, 1203–5.

Neuromuscular blockers + Antineoplastics

The effects of suxamethonium (succinylcholine) can be increased and prolonged in patients receiving cyclophosphamide because their plasma cholinesterase levels are depressed. Respiratory insufficiency and prolonged apnoea have been reported. Irinotecan may prolong the neuromuscular blocking effects of suxamethonium and antagonise that of non-depolarising drugs. *Animal* data suggests that thiotepa may also enhance the effects of suxamethonium. An isolated report describes a marked increase in the neuromuscular blocking effects of pancuronium in a myasthenic patient who was given thiotepa, but normally it appears not to interact with competitive neuromuscular blockers.

Clinical evidence

(a) Cyclophosphamide

Respiratory insufficiency and prolonged apnoea occurred in a patient taking cyclophosphamide on two occasions, both during anaesthesia during which **suxamethonium (succinylcholine)** and **tubocurarine** were given. Plasma cholinesterase levels were found to be low. Anaesthesia without the **suxamethonium** was uneventful. Seven out of 8 patients subsequently examined also showed depressed plasma cholinesterase levels while taking cyclophosphamide.[1]

Respiratory depression and low plasma cholinesterase levels have been described in other reports in patients taking cyclophosphamide.[2-5] Similarly, in the discussion of an *in vitro* study, the authors report preliminary results from a study in patients, showing a 35 to 70% reduction in cholinesterase activity, which lasted for several days after cyclophosphamide use.[2] See also *Mechanism*, below.

(b) Irinotecan

The manufacturer of irinotecan warns that it could possibly prolong the neuromuscular blocking effects of suxamethonium (succinylcholine) and antagonise the neuromuscular blockade of competitive (non-depolarising) drugs.[6] This is based on the fact that irinotecan has anticholinesterase activity.[6,7] See 'Neuromuscular blockers + Anticholinesterases', above, for an explanation of this mechanism.

(c) Thiotepa

A myasthenic patient developed very prolonged respiratory depression very shortly after being given thiotepa intraperitoneally, following the use of **pancuronium**.[8] Thiotepa has also been shown to increase the duration of **suxamethonium (succinylcholine)** neuromuscular blockade in *dogs*.[9] However, an *in vitro* study showed that thiotepa was a poor inhibitor of plasma cholinesterase.[2] See also *Mechanism*, below.

Mechanism

Cyclophosphamide inhibits the activity of plasma cholinesterase,[4] and as a result the metabolism of the suxamethonium is reduced and its actions are enhanced and prolonged. Other alkylating agents are also reported to reduce plasma cholinesterase activity.[10] An *in vitro* study found that human motor endplate or red blood cell acetylcholinesterase was inhibited by alkylating antineoplastics, with chlormethine exerting the greatest effect, followed by dacarbazine, nimustine, cyclophosphamide and ifosfamide. Chlormethine and cyclophosphamide inhibited plasma pseudocholinesterase most strongly, followed by thiotepa, nimustine, dacarbazine, ifosfamide, and carmustine.[10]

Importance and management

The interaction between suxamethonium (succinylcholine) and cyclophosphamide is well documented and established. It is of clinical importance, but whether all patients are affected to the same extent is uncertain. The depression of the plasma cholinesterase levels may last several days, possibly weeks, so that ideally plasma cholinesterase levels should be checked before using suxamethonium. In patients taking cyclophosphamide, suxamethonium should certainly be used with caution, and the dosage should be reduced.[2] Some have suggested that concurrent use should be avoided.[1] Irinotecan may possibly enhance the effects of suxamethonium and antagonise the effects of non-depolarising drugs. *Animal* data suggest thiotepa may enhance the effects of suxamethonium, while *in vitro* data and a case report in a patient with myasthenia,[11] suggest some other antineoplastics may also have an effect. The general silence in the literature would seem to indicate that no special precautions are generally necessary. However, patients with malignant tumours often have a reduced plasma cholinesterase activity, so care is warranted in these patients.[12]

1. Walker IR, Zapf PW, Mackay IR. Cyclophosphamide, cholinesterase and anaesthesia. *Aust N Z J Med* (1972) 3, 247–51.
2. Zsigmond EK, Robins G. The effect of a series of anti-cancer drugs on plasma cholinesterase activity. *Can Anaesth Soc J* (1972) 19, 75–82.
3. Mone JG, Mathie WE. Qualitative and quantitative defects of pseudocholinesterase activity. *Anaesthesia* (1967) 22, 55–68.
4. Wolff H. Die Hemmung der Serumcholinesterase durch Cyclophosphamid (Endoxan®). *Klin Wochenschr* (1965) 43, 819–21.
5. Koseoglu V, Chiang J, Chan KW. Acquired pseudocholinesterase deficiency after high-dose cyclophosphamide. *Bone Marrow Transplant* (1999) 24, 1367–8.
6. Campto (Irinotecan hydrochloride trihydrate). Pfizer Ltd. UK Summary of product characteristics, May 2009.
7. Hyatt JL, Tsurkan L, Morton CL, Yoon KJP, Harel M, Brumshtein B, Silman I, Sussman JL, Wadkins RM, Potter PM. Inhibition of acetylcholinesterase by the anticancer prodrug CPT-11. *Chem Biol Interact* (2005) 157–8, 247–52.
8. Bennett EJ, Schmidt GB, Patel KP, Grundy EM. Muscle relaxants, myasthenia, and mustards? *Anesthesiology* (1977) 46, 220–1
9. Cremonesi E, Rodrigues I de J. Interação de agentes curarizantes com antineoplásico. *Rev Bras Anestesiol* (1982) 32, 313–15.
10. Fujii M, Ohnoshi T, Namba T, Kimura I. Inhibitory effect of antineoplastic agents on human cholinesterases. *Gan To Kagaku Ryoho* (1982) 9, 831–5.
11. Ng CVT. Myasthenia gravis and a rare complication of chemotherapy. *Med J Aust* (2005) 182, 120.
12. Viby Mogensen J. Cholinesterase and succinylcholine. *Dan Med Bull* (1983) 30, 129–50.

Neuromuscular blockers + Antipsychotics

An isolated report describes prolonged apnoea in a patient given promazine while recovering from neuromuscular blockade with suxamethonium (succinylcholine). The use of intravenous chlorpromazine before suxamethonium was found not to affect the activity of suxamethonium. Recovery from the neuromuscular blocking effects of suxamethonium is prolonged by fentanyl with droperidol.

Clinical evidence

(a) Chlorpromazine

In a study in 50 patients undergoing elective ophthalmic surgery, intravenous chlorpromazine 100 micrograms/kg given 3 minutes before **suxamethonium (succinylcholine)** 500 micrograms/kg did not significantly affect time to maximum neuromuscular block or reappearance and complete recovery of the twitch response, when compared with patients who had not been given chlorpromazine.[1]

(b) Fentanyl with Droperidol

The observation that patients who had received *Innovar* (fentanyl with droperidol) before anaesthesia appeared to have prolonged **suxamethonium (succinylcholine)** effects, seen as apnoea, prompted further study of this possible interaction.[2] An average delay in recovery from neuromuscular blockade of 36% to 80% was seen in two studies.[2,3] Another study[4] showed that the droperidol component of *Innovar* was probably responsible for this interaction.

(c) Promazine

A woman recovering from surgery during which she had received **suxamethonium (succinylcholine)**, was given promazine 25 mg intravenously for sedation. Within 3 minutes she had become cyanotic and apnoeic, and required assisted respiration for 4 hours.[5]

Mechanism

Not understood. It has been suggested that promazine[5] and droperidol[4] depress plasma cholinesterase levels, which would reduce the metabolism of the suxamethonium and thereby prolong recovery. It has also been suggested that droperidol might act as a membrane stabiliser at neuromuscular junctions.[4]

Importance and management

Some caution would seem appropriate if promazine is given to any patient who has been given suxamethonium (succinylcholine). The use of intravenous chlorpromazine just before suxamethonium appears not to affect suxamethonium activity. There seems to be no information about other phenothiazines and other neuromuscular blockers.

Delayed recovery should be anticipated in patients given suxamethonium if droperidol is used. This is an established interaction.

1. McLoughlin CC, Mirakhur RK, MCCarthy GJ. Neuromuscular effects of succinylcholine following different pretreatments. *J Clin Anesth* (1993) 5, 50–3.
2. Wehner RJ. A case study: the prolongation of Anectine® effect by Innovar®. *J Am Assoc Nurse Anesth* (1979) 47, 576–9.
3. Moore GB, Ciresi S, Kallar S. The effect of Innovar® versus droperidol or fentanyl on the duration of action of succinylcholine. *J Am Assoc Nurse Anesth* (1986) 54, 130–6.
4. Lewis RA. A consideration of prolonged succinylcholine paralysis with Innovar®: is the cause droperidol or fentanyl? *J Am Assoc Nurse Anesth* (1982) 50, 55–9.
5. Regan AG, Aldrete JA. Prolonged apnea after administration of promazine hydrochloride following succinylcholine infusion. *Anesth Analg* (1967) 46, 315–18.

Neuromuscular blockers + Aprotinin

Apnoea developed in a number of patients after they were given aprotinin while recovering from neuromuscular blockade with suxamethonium (succinylcholine), either alone or with tubocurarine.

Clinical evidence

Three patients undergoing surgery who had received **suxamethonium (succinylcholine)**, either alone or with **tubocurarine**, were given aprotinin intravenously in doses of 2500 to 12 000 KIU (kallikrein inactivator units) at the end of, or shortly after, the operation when spontaneous breathing had resumed. In each case respiration rapidly became inadequate and apnoea lasting periods of 7, 30 and 90 minutes occurred.[1] Seven other cases have been reported elsewhere.[2]

Mechanism

Not fully understood. Aprotinin is only a very weak inhibitor of serum cholinesterase (100 000 KIU caused a maximal 16% inhibition)[3] and on its own would have little effect on the metabolism of suxamethonium. However, it might tip the balance in those whose cholinesterase was already very depressed.

Importance and management

The incidence of this interaction is uncertain but probably low. Only a few cases have been reported. It seems probable that it only affects those whose plasma cholinesterase levels are already very low for other reasons. No difficulties should arise in those whose plasma cholinesterase levels are normal.

1. Chasapakis G, Dimas C. Possible interaction between muscle relaxants and the kallikrein-trypsin inactivator "Trasylol". *Br J Anaesth* (1966) 38, 838–9.
2. Marcello B, Porati U. Trasylol e blocco neuromuscolare. *Minerva Anestesiol* (1967) 33, 814–15.
3. Doenicke A, Gesing H, Krumey I, Schmidinger St. Influence of aprotinin (Trasylol) on the action of suxamethonium. *Br J Anaesth* (1970) 42, 948–60.

Neuromuscular blockers + Benzodiazepines

A few studies report that diazepam and other benzodiazepines increase the effects of neuromuscular blockers, but many others have not found an interaction. If an interaction does occur, the response is likely to be little different from the individual variations in response of patients to neuromuscular blockers.

Clinical evidence

(a) Increased blockade

A comparative study of 10 patients given **gallamine** and 4 others given **gallamine** with intravenous **diazepam** 150 to 200 micrograms/kg found that **diazepam** prolonged the duration of activity of **gallamine** by a factor of three, and doubled the depression of the twitch response.[1] Persistent muscle weakness and respiratory depression was seen in two other patients given **tubocurarine** after premedication with **diazepam**.[2] A small reduction (approximately 10%) in neuromuscular blocker requirement has been described when **diazepam** was given with **tubocurarine**[3] or **suxamethonium (succinylcholine)**, but see also (b) below.[4] In a study in 10 patients, giving **diazepam** 200 micrograms/kg 3 minutes before **vecuronium** 100 micrograms/kg during anaesthetic induction shortened the time to onset of **vecuronium** and prolonged its duration of action, when compared with the activity of **vecuronium** in a similar group of patients not given **diazepam**.[5]

Another study found that recovery to 25% and 75% of the twitch height after **vecuronium** was prolonged by about 25% by 15 mg of intravenous **midazolam**, when compared with control patients.[6] The same study found that **midazolam** prolonged the recovery from the effects of **atracurium** by about 20%. However, the increased recovery time due to **midazolam** was not statistically significant when compared with control patients, but was significantly longer when compared with patients receiving 20 mg of intravenous **diazepam**.[6] See also (b) below.

(b) Reduced blockade or no interaction

The duration of paralysis due to **suxamethonium** was reduced in one study by 20% when **diazepam** (150 micrograms/kg) was also given, and the recovery time was shortened.[1] **Diazepam** also slightly reduced the time to 25% and 75% recovery of twitch height in patients given **vecuronium** by about 15% (not statistically significant).[6] In *animals*, **diazepam** increased the mean dose of **rocuronium** required by 13%, but this was not statistically significant.[7]

In other studies **diazepam** was found to have no significant effect on the neuromuscular blockade due to **alcuronium**,[8] **atracurium**,[6] **gallamine**,[9] **pancuronium**,[8,10] **suxamethonium**[8,11] or **tubocurarine**.[8,9,11,12] **Lorazepam** and **lormetazepam** have been reported to have little or no effects on **atracurium** or **vecuronium**,[6] and **midazolam** has been reported to have no effect on **suxamethonium**, **pancuronium**,[13] **rocuronium**[14] or **vecuronium**.[15,16]

Mechanism

Not understood. One suggestion is that where some alteration in response is seen it may be a reflection of a central depressant action rather than a direct effect on the myoneural junction.[9] Another study suggests that a direct action on the muscle may be responsible.[17]

Importance and management

What is known shows that the benzodiazepines may sometimes unpredictably alter the depth and prolong the recovery period from neuromuscular blockade, but the extent may not be very great and may possibly be little different from the individual variations in the response of patients to neuromuscular blockers.

Given that benzodiazepines are commonly given as premedication it seems likely that any significant interaction would have come to light by now.

1. Feldman SA, Crawley BE. Interaction of diazepam with the muscle-relaxant drugs. *BMJ* (1970) 2, 336–8.
2. Feldman SA, Crawley BE. Diazepam and muscle relaxants. *BMJ* (1970) 1, 691.
3. Stovner J, Endresen R. Intravenous anaesthesia with diazepam. *Acta Anaesthesiol Scand* (1966) 24 (Suppl), 223–7.
4. Jörgensen H. Premedicinering med diazepam, Valium®. Jämförelse med placebo i en dubbel-blind-undersökning. *Nord Med* (1964) 72, 1395–9.
5. Yuan H-B, Yang M-W, Chan K-H, Lee T-Y. The interaction of diazepam with vecuronium: a clinical study. *Zhonghua Yi Xue Za Zhi (Taipei)* (1994) 54, 259–64.
6. Driessen JJ, Crul JF, Vree TB, van Egmond J, Booij LHDJ. Benzodiazepines and neuromuscular blocking drugs in patients. *Acta Anaesthesiol Scand* (1986) 30, 642–6.
7. Muir AW, Anderson KA, Pow E. Interaction between rocuronium bromide and some drugs used during anaesthesia. *Eur J Anaesthesiol* (1994) 11 (Suppl 9), 93–8.
8. Bradshaw EG, Maddison S. Effect of diazepam at the neuromuscular junction. A clinical study. *Br J Anaesth* (1979) 51, 955–60.
9. Dretchen K, Ghoneim MM, Long JP. The interaction of diazepam with myoneural blocking agents. *Anesthesiology* (1971) 34, 463–8.
10. Asbury AJ, Henderson PD, Brown BH, Turner DJ, Linkens DA. Effect of diazepam on pancuronium-induced neuromuscular blockade maintained by a feedback system. *Br J Anaesth* (1981) 53, 859–63.
11. Stovner J, Endresen R. Diazepam in intravenous anaesthesia. *Lancet* (1965) ii, 1298–9.
12. Hunter AR. Diazepam (Valium) as a muscle relaxant during general anaesthesia: a pilot study. *Br J Anaesth* (1967) 39, 633–7.
13. Tassonyi E. Effects of midazolam (Ro 21-3981) on neuromuscular block. *Pharmatherapeutica* (1984) 3, 678–81.
14. Olkkola KT, Tammisto T. Quantitation of the interaction of rocuronium bromide with etomidate, fentanyl, midazolam, propofol, thiopentone, and isoflurane using closed-loop feedback control of infusion of rocuronium. *Eur J Anaesthesiol* (1994) 11 (Suppl 9), 99–100.
15. Husby P, Vamnes JS, Rodt SÅ, Rørvik K, Koller M-E, Gramstad L. Midazolam does not potentiate the effect of vecuronium in patients. *Acta Anaesthesiol Scand* (1989) 33, 280–2.
16. Okuda T, Sakaguchi M, Tsuchiya N, Wakita K, Tanaka K, Suekane K. Interaction of midazolam and vecuronium in anesthetized patients. *Masui* (1993) 42, 1153–6.
17. Ludin HP, Dubach K. Action of diazepam on muscular contraction in man. *Z Neurol* (1971) 199, 30–8.

Neuromuscular blockers + Beta-agonist bronchodilators

Bambuterol can prolong the recovery time from neuromuscular blockade with suxamethonium (succinylcholine) or mivacurium. A case report describes modestly enhanced neuromuscular blockade when pancuronium or vecuronium were given after intravenous salbutamol.

Clinical evidence

(a) Bambuterol

A double-blind study in 25 patients found that the recovery time from neuromuscular blockade with **suxamethonium (succinylcholine)** was prolonged by about 30% in those who had been given 10 mg of bambuterol 10 to 16 hours before surgery, and by about 50% in those who had been given 20 mg of bambuterol.[1]

This confirms two previous studies,[2,3] one of which found that 30 mg of bambuterol given about 10 hours before surgery approximately doubled the duration of **suxamethonium** blockade.[2] Furthermore, in 7 patients who had abnormal plasma cholinesterase levels, 20 mg of bambuterol taken 2 hours before surgery prolonged **suxamethonium** blockade two- to threefold, and in 4 patients a phase II block occurred.[4]

Similar results have been found in a study involving 27 patients given **mivacurium**. A marked decrease in plasma cholinesterase activity, leading to reduced clearance and prolonged elimination half-life of **mivacurium,** occurred when oral bambuterol 20 mg was given 2 hours before induction of anaesthesia. The duration of action of **mivacurium** was prolonged three- to fourfold, when compared with placebo.[5]

(b) Salbutamol

A case report describes a 28-year-old man undergoing elective surgery who was given three intravenous doses of salbutamol 125 micrograms over 3.5 hours for the treatment and prophylaxis of bronchospasm. Muscle relaxation was maintained with **pancuronium** and then **vecuronium**. The neuromuscular blockade (measured by the force of contraction of the adductor pollicis in response to ulnar nerve stimulation) increased after the salbutamol injection, from 45% to 66% during **pancuronium** blockade and from 66% to 86% following **vecuronium**. In addition, recovery of neuromuscular function with neostigmine appeared to be slower than expected.[6]

Mechanism

Bambuterol is an inactive prodrug, which is slowly converted enzymatically in the body to its active form, terbutaline. The carbamate groups that are split off can selectively inhibit the plasma cholinesterase that is necessary for the metabolism of suxamethonium and mivacurium. As a result, the metabolism of these neuromuscular blockers is reduced and their effects are thereby prolonged. The effect appears to be related to the dose of the bambuterol and the time lag after administration; maximal depression of plasma cholinesterase activity appears to occur about 2 to 6 hours following oral administration, but is still markedly depressed after 10 hours.[2]

The effect of intravenous salbutamol was probably a direct effect at the neuromuscular junction.[6]

Importance and management

The interaction with bambuterol is an established interaction. It may be more important where other factors reduce plasma cholinesterase activity or affect the extent of blockade in other ways (e.g. subjects with abnormal plasma cholinesterase levels). This interaction only applies to beta agonists that are metabolised to carbamic acid (bambuterol appears to be the only one available).

The interaction between intravenous salbutamol and pancuronium or vecuronium appears to be limited to the one report cited, and is probably of only minor clinical importance.

1. Staun P, Lennmarken C, Eriksson LI, Wirén J-E. The influence of 10 mg and 20 mg of bambuterol on the duration of succinylcholine-induced neuromuscular blockade. *Acta Anaesthesiol Scand* (1990) 34, 498–500.
2. Fisher DM, Caldwell JE, Sharma M, Wirén J-E. The influence of bambuterol (carbamylated terbutaline) on the duration of action of succinylcholine-induced paralysis in humans. *Anesthesiology* (1988) 69, 757–9.
3. Bang U, Viby-Mogensen J, Wirén JE, Skovgaard LT. The effect of bambuterol (carbamylated terbutaline) on plasma cholinesterase activity and suxamethonium-induced neuromuscular blockade in genotypically normal patients. *Acta Anaesthesiol Scand* (1990) 34, 596–9.
4. Bang U, Viby-Mogensen J, Wirén JE. The effect of bambuterol on plasma cholinesterase activity and suxamethonium-induced neuromuscular blockade in subjects heterozygous for abnormal plasma cholinesterase. *Acta Anaesthesiol Scand* (1990) 34, 600–4.
5. Østergaard D, Rasmussen SN, Viby-Mogensen J, Pedersen NA, Boysen R. The influence of drug-induced low plasma cholinesterase activity on the pharmacokinetics and pharmacodynamics of mivacurium. *Anesthesiology* (2000) 92, 1581–7.
6. Salib Y, Donati F. Potentiation of pancuronium and vecuronium neuromuscular blockade by intravenous salbutamol. *Can J Anaesth* (1993) 40, 50–3.

Neuromuscular blockers + Beta blockers

Increases or decreases (often only modest) in the extent of neuromuscular blockade have been seen in patients taking beta blockers. The bradycardia and hypotension sometimes caused by anaesthetics and beta blockers is not counteracted by atracurium.

Clinical evidence

(a) Alcuronium

Bradycardia and hypotension were seen in a patient given alcuronium while using **timolol** eye drops for glaucoma.[1]

(b) Atracurium

Eight out of 42 patients taking unnamed beta blockers given atracurium developed bradycardia (less than 50 bpm) and hypotension (systolic pressure less than 80 mmHg). Most of them had been premedicated with diazepam, induced with methohexital, and maintained with droperidol, fentanyl and nitrous oxide/oxygen. A further 24 developed bradycardia, associated with hypotension on 9 occasions. All responded promptly to 300 to 600 micrograms of intravenous atropine.[2]

A patient using **timolol** 0.5% eye drops for glaucoma developed bradycardia and hypotension when atracurium was given.[3] Bradycardia and hypotension have also been seen in a patient, who was given atracurium while taking **atenolol** for hypertension.[1]

(c) Rocuronium

A study of 16 patients who had been taking various beta blockers (**propranolol** 5, **atenolol** 5, **metoprolol** 2, **bisoprolol** 2, **oxprenolol** 1, **celiprolol** 1) for longer than one month found no difference in the onset and duration of action of rocuronium, when compared with a control group not taking beta blockers.[4]

(d) Suxamethonium (Succinylcholine)

In a study in 8 patients, the effects of suxamethonium were slightly, but not significantly, reduced by a 1-mg/15 kg intravenous dose of **propranolol**, given 15 minutes pre-operatively.

In 8 patients, intravenous **esmolol** 300 to 500 micrograms/kg per minute reduced the increase in heart rate during intubation, and slightly but significantly prolonged the recovery from blockade with suxamethonium by approximately 3 minutes, when compared with 8 patients given placebo.[5] In another study, intra-operative **esmolol** did not affect the onset and recovery time from suxamethonium blockade in patients with normal plasma cholinesterase (pseudocholinesterase) activity.[6]

(e) Tubocurarine

In a study in 8 patients, **propranolol**, given intravenously 20 to 40 minutes after the onset of action of tubocurarine, shortened the recovery from tubocurarine.[7] Another study described a shortened recovery period from tubocurarine due to **oxprenolol** or **propranolol**, but **pindolol** only slightly affected recovery in a few subjects.[8] Two patients with thyrotoxicosis showed prolonged neuromuscular blockade with tubocurarine after they had taken **propranolol** 120 mg daily for 14 days before surgery.[9]

(f) Vecuronium

For reports of bradycardia associated with vecuronium and opioids in patients also receiving beta blockers, see 'Neuromuscular blockers + Opioids', p.133.

Mechanism

The changes in the degree of blockade are not understood but the interaction appears to occur at the neuromuscular junction. It has been seen in *animal* studies.[10,11] The bradycardia and hypotension were probably due to the combined depressant effects on the heart of the anaesthetics and the beta blocker not being offset by atracurium, which has little or no effect on the vagus nerve at doses within the recommended range. Note that neuromuscular blockers with vagolytic activity can cause tachycardia and hypotension.

Importance and management

Information is fairly sparse, but these interactions appear normally to be of relatively minor importance. Be aware that changes in neuromuscular blockade (increases or decreases) can occur if beta blockers are used, but they seem to be unpredictable, and then often only modest in extent. The possible combined cardiac depressant effects of beta blockade and anaesthesia are well known (see 'Anaesthetics, general + Beta blockers', p.103). These effects may not be prevented when a neuromuscular blocker is used that has little or no effect on the vagus (such as atracurium or vecuronium).

1. Yate B, Mostafa SM. Drug interaction? *Anaesthesia* (1984) 39, 728–9.
2. Rowlands DE. Drug interaction? *Anaesthesia* (1984) 39, 1252.
3. Glynne GL. Drug interaction? *Anaesthesia* (1984) 39, 293.
4. Loan PB, Connolly FM, Mirakhur RK, Kumar N, Farling P. Neuromuscular effects of rocuronium in patients receiving beta-adrenoreceptor blocking, calcium entry blocking and anticonvulsant drugs. *Br J Anaesth* (1997) 78, 90–1.
5. Murthy VS, Patel KD, Elangovan RG, Hwang T-F, Solochek SM, Steck JD, Laddu AR. Cardiovascular and neuromuscular effects of esmolol during induction of anesthesia. *J Clin Pharmacol* (1986) 26, 351–7.
6. McCammon RL, Hilgenberg JC, Sandage BW, Stoelting RK. The effect of esmolol on the onset and duration of succinylcholine-induced neuromuscular blockade. *Anesthesiology* (1985) 63, A317.
7. Varma YS, Sharma PL, Singh HW. Effect of propranolol hydrochloride on the neuromuscular blocking action of d-tubocurarine and succinylcholine in man. *Indian J Med Res* (1972) 60, 266–72.
8. Varma YS, Sharma PL, Singh HW. Comparative effect of propranolol, oxprenolol and pindolol on neuromuscular blocking action of d-tubocurarine in man. *Indian J Med Res* (1973) 61, 1382–6.
9. Rozen MS, Whan FM. Prolonged curarization associated with propranolol. *Med J Aust* (1972) 1, 467–8.
10. Usubiaga JE. Neuromuscular effects of beta-adrenergic blockers and their interaction with skeletal muscle relaxants. *Anesthesiology* (1968) 29, 484–92.
11. Harrah MD, Way WL, Katzung BG. The interaction of d-tubocurarine with antiarrhythmic drugs. *Anesthesiology* (1970) 33, 406–10.

Neuromuscular blockers + Calcium-channel blockers

Limited evidence indicates that intra-operative intravenous diltiazem, nicardipine, nifedipine and verapamil can decrease the requirements for vecuronium and other competitive neuromuscular blockers. Intravenous nimodipine did not alter vecuronium effects in one study.

An isolated case report describes potentiation of tubocurarine and pancuronium by oral verapamil. However, long-term oral nifedipine did not alter vecuronium or atracurium effects, and long-term therapy with various calcium-channel blockers did not interact with rocuronium. Calcium-channel blockers do not increase the plasma potassium rise due to suxamethonium (succinylcholine).

Clinical evidence

(a) Intravenous calcium-channel blockers

A study in 24 surgical patients[1] anaesthetised with nitrous oxide and isoflurane found that **diltiazem** 5 or 10 microgram/kg per minute decreased the **vecuronium** requirements by up to 50%. Another study in 24 surgical patients found that **diltiazem** (5 mg bolus followed by a 4-microgram/kg per minute infusion) decreased **vecuronium** requirements by 45%, when compared with a control group (no **diltiazem**), or those receiving **diltiazem** at half the infusion dose.[2] Reductions in the requirements for **vecuronium** were also noted in other surgical patients receiving intravenous **diltiazem** or **nicardipine**.[3] A study in patients given **vecuronium** 100 micrograms/kg for tracheal intubation found that **nicardipine** 10 micrograms/kg shortened the onset of blockade, making it the same as in other patients given **vecuronium** 150 micrograms/kg alone. Recovery times were unaffected by the **nicardipine**.[4] Yet another study showed that **nicardipine** reduced the requirements for **vecuronium** in a dose-dependent manner: nicardipine 1, 2 and 3 micrograms/kg per minute reduced the vecuronium dose requirement to 79%, 60% and 53% of the control, respectively.[5] A study in 44 patients anaesthetised with isoflurane in nitrous oxide/oxygen found that 1 mg of intravenous **nifedipine** prolonged the neuromuscular blockade due to **atracurium** from 29 minutes to 40 minutes, and increased the neuromuscular blockade of **atracurium** or **vecuronium** from 75% to 90%.[6] In contrast, a study in 20 patients found that an intravenous infusion of **nimodipine** had no significant effect on the time course of action of **vecuronium**.[7]

A 66-year-old woman with renal impairment, receiving 5 mg of intravenous **verapamil** three times daily for supraventricular tachycardia, underwent abdominal surgery during which she was initially anaesthetised with thiopental and then maintained on nitrous oxide/oxygen with fentanyl. **Vecuronium** was used as the muscle relaxant. The effects of the **vecuronium** were increased and prolonged, and at the end of surgery reversal of the blockade using neostigmine was difficult and extended.[8] Intravenous **verapamil** alone has caused respiratory failure in a patient with poor neuromuscular transmission (Duchenne's dystrophy).[9] Note that *in vitro* and *animal* studies have confirmed that the neuromuscular blocking effects of **tubocurarine, pancuronium, vecuronium, atracurium** and **suxamethonium (succinylcholine)** are increased by **diltiazem, verapamil** and **nifedipine**.[9-11]

(b) Oral calcium-channel blockers

A report describes increased neuromuscular blockade in a patient taking long-term **verapamil** 40 mg three times daily who was given **pancuronium** 2 mg and **tubocurarine** 5 mg. The neuromuscular blockade was difficult to reverse with neostigmine, but responded well to edrophonium.[12] However, the authors of this report say that many patients taking long-term **verapamil** do not show a clinically significant increase in sensitivity to muscle relaxants.[12] This case also contrasts with another study in which 30 predominantly elderly patients taking long-term **nifedipine** (mean daily dose 33 mg) showed no changes in the time to onset of maximum block nor the duration of clinical relaxation in response to **atracurium** or **vecuronium**, when compared with 30 control patients not taking nifedipine.[13] Similarly, a study in 17 patients taking calcium-channel blockers (**nifedipine** 12, **diltiazem** 2, **nicardipine** 2, **amlodipine** 1) found no changes in the neuromuscular blocking effects of **rocuronium**.[14]

A comparative study in 21 patients taking calcium-channel blockers long term (**diltiazem, nifedipine, verapamil**) and 15 other patients not taking calcium-channel blockers found that, although **suxamethonium (succinylcholine)** caused a modest average peak rise of 0.5 mmol/L in plasma potassium levels, there were no differences between the two groups.[15]

Mechanism

Not fully understood. One suggested explanation is that nerve impulses arriving at nerve endings release calcium ions, which in turn causes the release of acetylcholine. Calcium-channel blockers can reduce the concentration of calcium ions within the nerve so that less acetylcholine is released. This would be additive with the effects of a neuromuscular blocker.[11,12]

Importance and management

Direct information so far seems to be limited. Increased neuromuscular blockade seems possible in any patient given an intravenous calcium-channel blocker (except possibly nimodipine) during surgery, but it seems likely that any effect will be managed by routine dose titration of the neuromuscular blocker and standard pre- and post-operative monitoring. From the limited evidence available it appears that increased blockade is not likely in patients taking long-term oral calcium-channel blockers, although one case has been reported with verapamil.

It would also seem that patients taking chronic calcium-channel blocker treatment are at no greater risk of hyperkalaemia with suxamethonium than other patients.

1. Sumikawa K, Kawabata K, Aono Y, Kamibayashi T, Yoshiya I. Reduction in vecuronium infusion dose requirements by diltiazem in humans. *Anesthesiology* (1992) 77, A939.
2. Takasaki Y, Naruoka Y, Shimizu C, Ochi G, Nagaro T, Arai T. Diltiazem potentiates the neuromuscular blockade by vecuronium in humans. *Jpn J Anesthesiol* (1995) 44, 503–7.
3. Takiguchi M, Takaya T. Potentiation of neuromuscular blockade by calcium channel blockers. *Tokai J Exp Clin Med* (1994) 19, 131–7.
4. Yamada T, Takino Y. Can nicardipine potentiate vecuronium induced neuromuscular blockade? *Jpn J Anesthesiol* (1992) 41, 746–50.
5. Kawabata K, Sumikawa K, Kamibayashi T, Kita T, Takada K, Mashimo T, Yoshiya I. Decrease in vecuronium infusion dose requirements by nicardipine in humans. *Anesth Analg* (1994) 79, 1159–64.
6. Jelen-Esselborn S, Blobner M. Wirkungsverstärkung von nichtdepolarisierenden Muskelrelaxanzien durch Nifedipin i.v. in Inhalationsanaesthesie. *Anaesthesist* (1990) 39, 173–8.
7. Aysel İ, HepağuŞlar H, Balcioğlu T, Uyar M. The effects of nimodipine on vecuronium-induced neuromuscular blockade. *Eur J Anaesthesiol* (2000) 17, 383–9.
8. van Poorten JF, Dhasmana KM, Kuypers RSM, Erdmann W. Verapamil and reversal of vecuronium neuromuscular blockade. *Anesth Analg* (1984) 63, 155–7.
9. Durant NN, Nguyen N, Katz RL. Potentiation of neuromuscular blockade by verapamil. *Anesthesiology* (1984) 60, 298–303.
10. Bikhazi GB, Leung I, Foldes FF. Interaction of neuromuscular blocking agents with calcium channel blockers. *Anesthesiology* (1982) 57, A268.
11. Wali FA. Interactions of nifedipine and diltiazem with muscle relaxants and reversal of neuromuscular blockade with edrophonium and neostigmine. *J Pharmacol* (1986) 17, 244–53.
12. Jones RM, Cashman JN, Casson WR, Broadbent MP. Verapamil potentiation of neuromuscular blockade: failure of reversal with neostigmine but prompt reversal with edrophonium. *Anesth Analg* (1985) 64, 1021–5.
13. Bell PF, Mirakhur RK, Elliott P. Onset and duration of clinical relaxation of atracurium and vecuronium in patients on chronic nifedipine therapy. *Eur J Anaesthesiol* (1989) 6, 343–6.
14. Loan PB, Connolly FM, Mirakhur RK, Kumar N, Farling P. Neuromuscular effects of rocuronium in patients receiving beta-adrenoreceptor blocking, calcium entry blocking and anticonvulsant drugs. *Br J Anaesth* (1997) 78, 90–1.
15. Rooke GA, Freund PR, Tomlin J. Calcium channel blockers do not enhance increases in plasma potassium after succinylcholine in humans. *J Clin Anesth* (1994) 6, 114–18.

Neuromuscular blockers + Carbamazepine

The effects of many competitive neuromuscular blockers are reduced and shortened if carbamazepine is given for longer than one week, but they may be increased if carbamazepine is given acutely (e.g. during surgery). Carbamazepine does not appear not to interact with mivacurium.

Clinical evidence

(a) Carbamazepine given long-term

1. Atracurium or Cisatracurium. One study found that the recovery time from intravenous atracurium 500 micrograms/kg was shorter in 14 patients taking long-term carbamazepine (5.93 minutes) than in 21 non-epileptic patients (8.02 minutes). This was assessed using the recovery index (time between 25% and 75% recovery of baseline electromyogram values).[1] However, carbamazepine has also been reported to have no effect on atracurium.[2,3]

A study found that the recovery time from intravenous cisatracurium was shorter in patients taking carbamazepine or phenytoin than in patients not receiving carbamazepine or phenytoin; the recovery index (times between 25% and 75% recovery) was 16.2 minutes and 21.2 minutes, respectively. Clearance of cisatracurium was increased by about 25% in patients taking carbamazepine or phenytoin, and the steady-state plasma level of cisatracurium required to maintain 95% block was increased by 20%, indicating increased resistance to the action of cisatracurium.[4]

2. Doxacurium. In a study, 9 patients taking carbamazepine for at least one week and undergoing surgery were given doxacurium. These patients took 66 minutes to reach

50% recovery compared with 161 minutes in a control group not taking carbamazepine.[5] Similar findings were obtained in another study.[6]

3. Mivacurium. In contrast to other neuromuscular blockers, the long-term (greater than 4 weeks) use of carbamazepine does not appear to affect mivacurium-induced neuromuscular blockade.[7] Similarly, a study in 32 patients who had been taking carbamazepine alone or with phenytoin or **valproic acid** for greater than 2 weeks found no resistance to mivacurium,[8] although an earlier preliminary study by the same research group found a trend towards a shorter recovery from mivacurium in 13 patients taking unspecified antiepileptics (not statistically significant).[9]

4. Pancuronium. In 18 patients undergoing craniotomy for tumours, seizure foci or cerebrovascular surgery, the recovery from neuromuscular blockade with pancuronium was on average 65% shorter in those patients taking carbamazepine.[10]

5. Pipecuronium. The effects of pipecuronium are reduced by carbamazepine.[11,12] In one study it was found that the *onset* time for pipecuronium blockade was lengthened (although this was not statistically significant) in patients with therapeutic plasma concentrations of carbamazepine, but not in those with subtherapeutic levels. However, a shorter duration of action was seen regardless of antiepileptic levels.[12]

6. Rapacuronium. A reduced duration of action has been reported with rapacuronium in a patient taking carbamazepine.[13]

7. Rocuronium. Several reports and studies have found that rocuronium has a shorter duration of action following long-term carbamazepine use,[14-17] although preliminary investigations found no effect.[18,19]

8. Suxamethonium (Succinylcholine). Eight patients who had been taking phenytoin and/or carbamazepine for at least one month took longer to recover from suxamethonium blockade, than 9 control patients; the time for return to baseline twitch height was 14.3 minutes and 10 minutes, respectively.[20]

9. Vecuronium. Several studies have found that carbamazepine shortens the recovery time from vecuronium blockade in adults[2] and in children.[21]

(b) Carbamazepine given short-term

An *in vitro* study found that the acute neuromuscular effects of **carbamazepine** reduced the concentrations required for 50% paralysis with both a depolarising neuromuscular blocker (**suxamethonium (succinylcholine)**) and a competitive neuromuscular blocker (**atracurium**) by about 30%.[22]

Mechanism

Not fully understood, but it appears to be multifactorial. The acute use of carbamazepine may result in neuromuscular block and potentiation of the action of competitive (non-depolarising) blockers.[22]

The long-term use of carbamazepine may produce subclinical neuromuscular blockade thought to be due to modest blockade of acetylcholine effects and a decrease in acetylcholine release; this antagonism may induce changes at the neuromuscular junction including an increased number of acetylcholine receptors on the muscle membrane (up-regulation), with decreased sensitivity.[20,21] Other suggestions to account for the reduced response with the long-term use of carbamazepine include induction of liver enzyme activity (carbamazepine is a potent inducer of cytochrome P450 isoenzymes), which would increase the metabolism and clearance of the neuromuscular blocker; and changes in plasma protein binding.[20,21] It has been shown that carbamazepine doubles the clearance of vecuronium.[21,23]

Importance and management

Established and clinically important interactions. Anticipate the need to use a larger dose of the neuromuscular blocker in patients who have taken carbamazepine for more than one week, and expect an accelerated recovery. The neuromuscular blockers appear to interact to differing extents, with mivacurium apparently unaffected.

Although evidence is limited, if carbamazepine is given acutely, it may be prudent to anticipate the need to use a smaller neuromuscular blocker dosage, or prepare for a longer recovery time.

1. Tempelhoff R, Modica PA, Jellish WS, Spitznagel EL. Resistance to atracurium-induced neuromuscular blockade in patients with intractable seizure disorders treated with anticonvulsants. *Anesth Analg* (1990) 71, 665–9.
2. Ebrahim Z, Bulkley R, Roth S. Carbamazepine therapy and neuromuscular blockade with atracurium and vecuronium. *Anesth Analg* (1988) 67, S55.
3. Spacek A, Neiger FX, Spiss CK, Kress HG. Atracurium-induced neuromuscular block is not affected by chronic anticonvulsant therapy with carbamazepine. *Acta Anaesthesiol Scand* (1997) 41, 1308–11.
4. Richard A, Girard F, Girard DC, Boudreault D, Chouinard P, Moumdjian R, Bouthilier A, Ruel M, Couture J, Varin F. Cisatracurium-induced neuromuscular blockade is affected by chronic phenytoin or carbamazepine treatment in neurosurgical patients. *Anesth Analg* (2005) 100, 538–44.
5. Ornstein E, Matteo RS, Weinstein JA, Halevy JD, Young WL, Abou-Donia MM. Accelerated recovery from doxacurium-induced neuromuscular blockade in patients receiving chronic anticonvulsant therapy. *J Clin Anesth* (1991) 3, 108–11.
6. Desai P, Hewitt PB, Jones RM. Influence of anticonvulsant therapy on doxacurium and pancuronium-induced paralysis. *Anesthesiology* (1989) 71, A784.
7. Spacek A, Neiger FX, Spiss CK, Kress HG. Chronic carbamazepine therapy does not influence mivacurium-induced neuromuscular block. *Br J Anaesth* (1996) 77, 500–2.
8. Jellish WS, Thalji Z, Brundidge PK, Tempelhoff R. Recovery from mivacurium-induced neuromuscular blockade is not affected by anticonvulsant therapy. *J Neurosurg Anesthesiol* (1996) 8, 4–8.
9. Thalji Z, Jellish WS, Murdoch J, Tempelhoff R. The effect of chronic anticonvulsant therapy on recovery from mivacurium induced paralysis. *Anesthesiology* (1993) 79 (Suppl 3A), A965.
10. Roth S, Ebrahim ZY. Resistance to pancuronium in patients receiving carbamazepine. *Anesthesiology* (1987) 66, 691–3.
11. Jellish WS, Modica PA, Tempelhoff R. Accelerated recovery from pipecuronium in patients treated with chronic anticonvulsant therapy. *J Clin Anesth* (1993) 5, 105–8.
12. Hans P, Ledoux D, Bonhomme V, Brichant JF. Effect of plasma anticonvulsant level on pipecuronium-induced neuromuscular blockade: preliminary results. *J Neurosurg Anesthesiol* (1995) 7, 254–8.
13. Tobias JD, Johnson JO. Rapacuronium administration to patients receiving phenytoin or carbamazepine. *J Neurosurg Anesthesiol* (2001) 13, 240–2.
14. Baraka A, Idriss N. Resistance to rocuronium in an epileptic patient on long-term carbamazepine therapy. *Middle East J Anesthesiol* (1996) 13, 561–4.
15. Loan PB, Connolly FM, Mirakhur RK, Kumar N, Farling P. Neuromuscular effects of rocuronium in patients receiving beta-adrenoreceptor blocking, calcium entry blocking and anticonvulsant drugs. *Br J Anaesth* (1997) 78, 90–1.
16. Spacek A, Neiger FX, Krenn CG, Hoerauf K, Kress HG. Rocuronium-induced neuromuscular block is affected by chronic carbamazepine therapy. *Anesthesiology* (1999) 90, 109–12.
17. Soriano SG, Kaus SJ, Sullivan LJ, Martyn JAJ. Onset and duration of action of rocuronium in children receiving chronic anticonvulsant therapy. *Paediatr Anaesth* (2000) 10, 133–6.
18. Spacek A, Neiger FX, Katz RL, Watkins WD, Spiss CK. Chronic carbamazepine therapy does not affect neuromuscular blockade by rocuronium. *Anesth Analg* (1995) 80 (Suppl 2), S463.
19. Spacek A, Neiger FX, Krenn C-G, Spiss CK, Kress HG. Does chronic carbamazepine therapy influence neuromuscular blockade by rocuronium? *Anesthesiology* (1997) 87, A833.
20. Melton AT, Antognini JF, Gronert GA. Prolonged duration of succinylcholine in patients receiving anticonvulsants: evidence for mild up-regulation of acetylcholine receptors? *Can J Anaesth* (1993) 40, 939–42.
21. Soriano SG, Sullivan LJ, Venkatakrishnan K, Greenblatt DJ, Martyn JAJ. Pharmacokinetics and pharmacodynamics of vecuronium in children receiving phenytoin or carbamazepine for chronic anticonvulsant therapy. *Br J Anaesth* (2001) 86, 223–9.
22. Nguyen A, Ramzan I. Acute in vitro neuromuscular effects of carbamazepine and carbamazepine-10,11-epoxide. *Anesth Analg* (1997) 84, 886–90.
23. Alloul K, Whalley DG, Shutway F, Ebrahim Z, Varin F. Pharmacokinetic origin of carbamazepine-induced resistance to vecuronium neuromuscular blockade in anesthetized patients. *Anesthesiology* (1996) 84, 330–9.

Neuromuscular blockers + Chloroquine and related drugs

A report describes respiratory insufficiency during the recovery period following surgery, which was attributed to the use of chloroquine diorotate. Hydroxychloroquine would be expected to interact similarly. An isolated report describes recurarisation and dyspnoea in a patient given intravenous quinine after recovering from neuromuscular blockade with suxamethonium (succinylcholine) and pancuronium.

Clinical evidence, mechanism, importance and management

(a) Chloroquine

Studies were carried out on the possible neuromuscular blocking actions of chloroquine diorotate in *animals,* because it was noticed that when it was used in the peritoneal cavity to prevent adhesions following abdominal surgery in man, it caused respiratory insufficiency during the recovery period. These studies found that it had a non-depolarising blocking action at the neuromuscular junction, which was opposed by neostigmine.[1] It would seem therefore that during the recovery period the effects of the chloroquine can be additive with the residual effects of the conventional neuromuscular blocker used during the surgery.

Although this appears to be the only report of this interaction, it is consistent with the way chloroquine can unmask or aggravate myasthenia gravis, or oppose the effects of drugs used in its treatment. Be alert for this reaction if chloroquine is used. Note that **hydroxychloroquine** would be expected to interact similarly.

(b) Quinine

A 47-year-old man with acute pancreatitis, taking quinine 600 mg three times daily, was given penicillin and gentamicin intravenously before undergoing surgery, during which **pancuronium** and **suxamethonium (succinylcholine)** were used uneventfully. After surgery the neuromuscular blockade was reversed with neostigmine and atropine, and the patient awoke and was breathing well. A 6-hour intravenous infusion of quinine 500 mg was started 90 minutes postoperatively. Within 10 minutes (after receiving about 15 mg of quinine) he became dyspnoeic, his breathing became totally ineffective and he needed re-intubation. Muscle flaccidity persisted for 3 hours.[2] The reason for this reaction is not fully understood. A possible explanation is that it may have been the additive neuromuscular blocking effects of the gentamicin (well recognised as having neuromuscular blocking activity; see 'Neuromuscular blockers + Aminoglycosides', p.119) and the quinine (an optical isomer of quinidine; see 'Neuromuscular blockers + Quinidine', p.135) and the residual effects of the **pancuronium** and **suxamethonium**.

There seem to be no other reports of problems in patients receiving neuromuscular blockers with quinine, but this isolated case serves to emphasise the importance of being alert for any signs of recurarisation in patients given drugs possessing some neuromuscular blocking activity, particularly during the postoperative recovery period.

1. Jui-Yen T. Clinical and experimental studies on mechanism of neuromuscular blockade by chloroquine diorotate. *Jpn J Anesthesiol* (1971) 20, 491–503.
2. Sher MH, Mathews PA. Recurarization with quinine administration after reversal from anaesthesia. *Anaesth Intensive Care* (1983) 11, 241–3.

Neuromuscular blockers + Corticosteroids

Long-term use of prednisolone delays the onset and shortens the duration of action of rocuronium, and shortens the duration of action of atracurium. Two reports describe antagonism of the neuromuscular blocking effects of pancuronium by high-dose prednisone, or prednisolone, and hydrocortisone. A third report in a patient with adrenocortical insufficiency describes reversal of the pancuronium block by hydrocortisone. Some evidence suggests the dose of vecuronium might need to be increased in those receiving intramuscular betamethasone. However,

prolonged use of high-dose corticosteroids with neuromuscular blockers can increase the risk of myopathy, resulting in prolonged paralysis following the discontinuation of the neuromuscular blocker.

Clinical evidence

(a) Neuromuscular blocking effects

In a study in 40 patients with inflammatory bowel disease, the onset of action of **rocuronium** was delayed (from 187 to 253 seconds) and its duration of action shorter (25.7 compared with 34.7 minutes) in 20 patients taking **prednisolone** than in 20 patients not receiving any corticosteroid.[1] A shorter duration of action, but not a delayed onset, was reported for **atracurium** in an almost identical study by the same research group.[2] A man undergoing surgery who was taking oral **prednisone** 250 mg daily, had good muscular relaxation in response to intravenous **pancuronium** 8 mg (100 micrograms/kg) early in the operation, but one hour later he began to show signs of inadequate relaxation, and continued to do so for the next 75 minutes despite being given four additional 2-mg doses of **pancuronium**.[3] Another patient taking large doses of **hydrocortisone**, **prednisolone**, and aminophylline proved to be resistant to the effects of **pancuronium**.[4] A man who had undergone a hypophysectomy and was taking **cortisone** developed profound paralysis when given **pancuronium**, which was rapidly reversed with 100 mg of **hydrocortisone sodium succinate**.[5]

Inadequate neuromuscular blockade with **vecuronium** (presenting as unexpected movements) occurred in 2 patients during neurosurgery. They had both been given a preoperative course of **betamethasone** 4 mg four times daily to reduce raised intracranial pressure.[6] This prompted a retrospective search of the records of 50 other patients, which revealed that those given intramuscular **betamethasone** preoperatively had needed almost double the dose of **vecuronium** (134 micrograms/kg per hour compared with 76 micrograms/kg per hour).[6]

These reports contrast with another, in which 25 patients who had no adrenocortical dysfunction or histories of corticosteroid use were given **pancuronium**, **metocurine**, **tubocurarine**, or **vecuronium**. Neuromuscular blockade was not altered when a single intravenous dose of **dexamethasone** 400 micrograms/kg or **hydrocortisone** 10 mg/kg was given.[7]

(b) Increased risk of myopathy

A report describes 3 patients in status asthmaticus who developed acute reversible myopathy after treatment with high-dose intravenous **methylprednisolone** 320 to 750 mg daily and steroidal neuromuscular blockers (**vecuronium** or **pancuronium**), used concurrently for at least 8 days.[8] A review of the literature from 1977 to 1995 found over 75 cases of prolonged weakness associated with combined use of neuromuscular blockers and **corticosteroids**.[9] This condition has been referred to as 'blocking agent–corticosteroid myopathy' (BACM). Before 1994, virtually all cases involved either **pancuronium** or **vecuronium**, leading some authors to suggest that **atracurium** might be safer as it does not have the steroidal structure of these neuromuscular blockers.[8] However, there have since been reports of prolonged paralysis associated with extended treatment with high-dose **corticosteroids** and **atracurium**[10,11] or **cisatracurium**.[12]

Mechanism

Not understood. For the partial reversal of neuromuscular blockade, one suggestion, based on *animal* studies, is that adrenocortical insufficiency causes a defect in neuromuscular transmission, which is reversed by the corticosteroids.[5] Another suggestion is that the effects seen are connected in some way with the steroid nucleus of the pancuronium and vecuronium, and are mediated presynaptically.[6,13]

The increased myopathy might be due to an additive effect, as both neuromuscular blockers and corticosteroids can cause myopathy. Results of an *in vitro* study suggested that the combination of vecuronium and methylprednisolone might augment pharmacologic denervation, which might lead to myopathy and contribute to the prolonged weakness observed in some critically ill patients.[14]

Importance and management

The evidence for antagonism of neuromuscular-blocking effects seems to be limited to the studies and reports cited. The effects seen in the studies with atracurium and rocuronium were minor, and probably of little clinical relevance. However, the few cases and retrospective review suggest that greater effects have occurred with pancuronium and vecuronium. Bear in mind the possibility of an interaction if competitive neuromuscular blockers are used in patients who have been treated with corticosteroids, being alert for the need to increase the dosage of the neuromuscular blocker. Note that *animal* studies suggest that atracurium might also possibly be affected by betamethasone to the same extent as vecuronium.[13] However, also be aware that prolonged use of competitive neuromuscular blockers with corticosteroids, particularly in patients in intensive care, can result in a marked prolongation of muscle weakness (several months of rehabilitation have been needed in some cases[8]). The complex state of the critically ill patient means that the effects of neuromuscular blockers can be unpredictable.

1. Soltész S, Mencke T, Stunz M, Diefenbach C, Ziegeler S, Molter GP. Attenuation of a rocuronium-induced neuromuscular block in patients receiving prednisolone. *Acta Anaesthesiol Scand* (2009) 53, 443–8.
2. Soltész S, Mencke T, Mey C, Röhrig S, Diefenbach C, Molter GP. Influence of a continuous prednisolone medication on the time course of neuromuscular block of atracurium in patients with chronic inflammatory bowel disease. *Br J Anaesth* (2008) 100, 798–802.
3. Laflin MJ. Interaction of pancuronium and corticosteroids. *Anesthesiology* (1977) 47, 471–2.
4. Azar I, Kumar D, Betcher AM. Resistance to pancuronium in an asthmatic patient treated with aminophylline and steroids. *Can Anaesth Soc J* (1982) 29, 280–2.
5. Meyers EF. Partial recovery from pancuronium neuromuscular blockade following hydrocortisone administration. *Anesthesiology* (1977) 46, 148–50.
6. Parr SM, Galletly DC, Robinson BJ. Betamethasone-induced resistance to vecuronium: a potential problem in neurosurgery? *Anaesth Intensive Care* (1991) 19, 103–5.
7. Schwartz AE, Matteo RS, Ornstein E, Silverberg PA. Acute steroid therapy does not alter nondepolarizing muscle relaxant effects in humans. *Anesthesiology* (1986) 65, 326–7.
8. Griffin D, Fairman N, Coursin D, Rawsthorne L, Grossman JE. Acute myopathy during treatment of status asthmaticus with corticosteroids and steroidal muscle relaxants. *Chest* (1992) 102, 510–14.
9. Fischer JR, Baer RK. Acute myopathy associated with combined use of corticosteroids and neuromuscular blocking agents. *Ann Pharmacother* (1996) 30, 1437–45.
10. Branney SW, Haenel JB, Moore FA, Tarbox BB, Schreiber RH, Moore EE. Prolonged paralysis with atracurium infusion: a case report. *Crit Care Med* (1994) 22, 1699–1701.
11. Meyer KC, Prielipp RC, Grossman JE, Coursin DB. Prolonged weakness after infusion of atracurium in two intensive care unit patients. *Anesth Analg* (1994) 78, 772–4.
12. Fodale V, Praticò C, Girlanda P, Baradello A, Lucanto T, Rodolico C, Nicolosi C, Rovere V, Santamaria LB, Dattola R. Acute motor axonal polyneuropathy after a cisatracurium infusion and concomitant corticosteroid therapy. *Br J Anaesth* (2004) 92, 289–93.
13. Robinson BJ, Lee E, Rees D, Purdie GL, Galletly DC. Betamethasone-induced resistance to neuromuscular blockade: a comparison of atracurium and vecuronium in vitro. *Anesth Analg* (1992) 74, 762–5.
14. Kindler CH, Verotta D, Gray AT, Gropper MA, Yost CS. Additive inhibition of nicotinic acetylcholine receptors by corticosteroids and the neuromuscular blocking drug vecuronium. *Anesthesiology* (2000) 92, 821–32.

Neuromuscular blockers + Dantrolene

In one patient dantrolene increased the effects of vecuronium, whereas two other patients were unaffected.

Clinical evidence, mechanism, importance and management

A 60-year-old woman, given a total of 350 mg of dantrolene orally during the 28 hours before surgery to prevent malignant hyperthermia, developed increased neuromuscular blockade and a slow recovery rate when **vecuronium** was subsequently given.[1] This report contrasts with another describing two patients taking long-term dantrolene 20 to 50 mg daily who had no changes in **vecuronium**-induced neuromuscular blockade during or after surgery.[2] Dantrolene is a muscle relaxant that acts directly on the muscle by lowering intracellular calcium concentrations in skeletal muscle; it reduces the release of calcium from the sarcoplasmic reticulum. It may also possibly inhibit calcium-dependent presynaptic neurotransmitter release.[3]

Evidence of an interaction appears to be limited to this one case but, given the potential mechanism, it may be prudent to be alert for any increased effects if dantrolene is given with vecuronium, and possibly other neuromuscular blockers. These case reports indicate that the effects could be dose-related, and so patients receiving higher doses of dantrolene may be at greater risk, although more study is needed to confirm this.

1. Driessen JJ, Wuis EW, Gielen MJM. Prolonged vecuronium neuromuscular blockade in a patient receiving orally administered dantrolene. *Anesthesiology* (1985) 62, 523–4.
2. Nakayama M, Iwasaki H, Fujita S, Narimatsu E, Namiki A. Neuromuscular effects of vecuronium in patients receiving long-term administration of dantrolene. *Jpn J Anesthesiol* (1993) 42, 1508–10.
3. Dantrium Capsules (Dantrolene sodium). SpePharm UK Ltd. UK Summary of product characteristics, January 2012.

Neuromuscular blockers + Dexmedetomidine

Dexmedetomidine caused a minor increase in plasma rocuronium levels in one study.

Clinical evidence, mechanism, importance and management

A study in 10 healthy subjects under general anaesthesia with alfentanil, propofol and nitrous oxide/oxygen, found that an intravenous infusion of dexmedetomidine (950 to 990 nanograms/kg) increased plasma **rocuronium** levels by 7.6%, which was not clinically significant, and decreased the twitch tension from 51% to 44% after 45 minutes. Dexmedetomidine also decreased finger blood flow and increased systemic blood pressure. It was suggested these pharmacokinetic changes occurred due to peripheral vasoconstriction,[1] and therefore seem possible with other neuromuscular blockers. However, the effects are unlikely to be of clinical significance.

1. Talke PO, Caldwell JE, Richardson CA, Kirkegaard-Nielsen H, Stafford M. The effects of dexmedetomidine on neuromuscular blockade in human volunteers. *Anesth Analg* (1999) 88, 633–9.

Neuromuscular blockers + Disopyramide

An isolated case report suggests that disopyramide may oppose the effects of neostigmine used to reverse neuromuscular blockade with vecuronium.

Clinical evidence, mechanism, importance and management

A case report[1] suggests that the normal antagonism of **vecuronium** neuromuscular blockade by neostigmine may be opposed by therapeutic serum levels of disopyramide (5 micrograms/mL). Disopyramide has also been shown to decrease neostigmine-induced antagonism of the neuromuscular blockade of **tubocurarine** on the *rat* phrenic nerve-diaphragm preparation.[2] The general clinical importance of these observations is not known.

1. Baurain M, Barvais L, d'Hollander A, Hennart D. Impairment of the antagonism of vecuronium-induced paralysis and intra-operative disopyramide administration. *Anaesthesia* (1989) 44, 34–6.
2. Healy TEJ, O'Shea M, Massey J. Disopyramide and neuromuscular transmission. *Br J Anaesth* (1981) 53, 495–8.

Neuromuscular blockers + Diuretics

The effects of some neuromuscular blockers (e.g. pancuronium, tubocurarine) have been both increased and decreased by furosemide.

Clinical evidence

(a) Increased neuromuscular blockade

Three patients receiving kidney transplants[1] developed increased neuromuscular blockade with **tubocurarine** (seen as a pronounced decrease in twitch tension) when given furosemide 40 or 80 mg and mannitol 12.5 g intravenously. One of them had the same reaction when later given only 40 mg of furosemide but no mannitol. The residual blockade was easily antagonised with pyridostigmine 14 mg or neostigmine 3 mg with atropine 1.2 mg.

(b) Decreased neuromuscular blockade

Ten neurosurgical patients given furosemide 1 mg/kg 10 minutes before induction of anaesthesia, took 14.7 minutes to recover from 95 to 50% blockade with **pancuronium** (as measured by a twitch response) compared with 21.8 minutes in 10 similar patients who had not received furosemide.[2]

Mechanism

Uncertain. *Animal* studies indicate that what happens probably depends on the dosage of furosemide: 0.1 to 10 micrograms/kg increased the blocking effects of tubocurarine and **suxamethonium** (succinylcholine) whereas 1 to 4 mg/kg opposed the blockade.[3] One suggestion is that low doses of furosemide may inhibit protein kinase causing a reduction in neuromuscular transmission, whereas higher doses cause inhibition of phosphodiesterase resulting in increased cyclic AMP activity and causing antagonism of neuromuscular blockade. It has also been suggested that large doses of loop diuretics may affect the renal excretion of neuromuscular blockers that are cleared by this route, resulting in more rapid recovery from the blockade.[3]

Importance and management

The documentation is very limited. Be aware of changes in the response to any neuromuscular blocker if furosemide is used, although it seems likely that any effect will be detected as part of routine monitoring. Note that the manufacturers of *Moduretic* (amiloride/**hydrochlorothiazide**) suggest that these diuretics may interact similarly, and enhance the effects of the non-depolarising (competitive) neuromuscular blockers.[4] This prediction appears to be based on some old experimental data using thiazides in *animals*.

1. Miller RD, Sohn YJ, Matteo RS. Enhancement of *d*-tubocurarine neuromuscular blockade by diuretics in man. *Anesthesiology* (1976) 45, 442–5.
2. Azar I, Cottrell J, Gupta B, Turndorf H. Furosemide facilitates recovery of evoked twitch response after pancuronium. *Anesth Analg* (1980) 59, 55–7.
3. Scappaticci KA, Ham JA, Sohn YJ, Miller RD, Dretchen KL. Effects of furosemide on the neuromuscular junction. *Anesthesiology* (1982) 57, 381–8.
4. Moduretic (Amiloride/Hydrochlorothiazide). Bristol-Myers Squibb Pharmaceuticals Ltd. UK Summary of product characteristics, September 2006.

Neuromuscular blockers + Ecothiopate iodide

The neuromuscular blocking effects of suxamethonium (succinylcholine) are markedly increased and prolonged in patients receiving ecothiopate iodide.

Clinical evidence

In 1965 a study showed that ecothiopate iodide eye drops could markedly lower pseudocholinesterase levels.[1] It was noted that "within a few days of commencing therapy, levels are reached at which protracted apnoea could occur, should these patients require general anaesthesia in which muscle relaxation is obtained with **succinylcholine**". Cases of apnoea due to this interaction were reported the following year,[2,3] and other cases have been subsequently reported.[4,5] In one case, a woman given **suxamethonium (succinylcholine)** 200 mg had apnoea for 5.5 hours.[2] Other studies have confirmed that ecothiopate given orally[6] or as eye drops[7] markedly reduced the levels of plasma cholinesterase, and can prolong recovery after **suxamethonium**.[6]

One report describes the successful and uneventful use of **atracurium** in a patient receiving ecothiopate.[5]

Mechanism

Suxamethonium is metabolised in the body by plasma cholinesterase. Ecothiopate iodide depresses the levels of this enzyme so that the metabolism of the suxamethonium is reduced and its effects are thereby enhanced and prolonged.[3,6] One study in 71 patients found that two drops of ecothiopate iodide 0.06% three times a week in each eye caused a twofold reduction in plasma cholinesterase (pseudocholinesterase) activity in about one-third of the patients, and a fourfold reduction in 1 in 7 patients.[8] It has been reported that, on discontinuing ecothiopate, it takes between several weeks and 2 months for enzyme activity to return to normal.[7]

Importance and management

An established, adequately documented and clinically important interaction. The dosage of suxamethonium should be reduced appropriately because of the reduced plasma cholinesterase levels caused by ecothiopate. The study cited above[8] suggests that prolonged apnoea is likely in about 1 in 7 patients. One report describes the successful use of approximately one-fifth of the normal dosage of suxamethonium in a patient receiving ecothiopate 0.125% iodide solution, one drop twice a day in both eyes, and with a plasma cholinesterase activity 62% below normal. Recovery from the neuromuscular blockade was rapid and uneventful.[9] **Mivacurium** is also metabolised by plasma cholinesterase, and would be expected to interact with ecothiopate in the same way as suxamethonium.[10]

1. McGavi DDM. Depressed levels of serum-pseudocholinesterase with ecothiophate-iodide eyedrops. *Lancet* (1965) ii, 272–3.
2. Gesztes T. Prolonged apnoea after suxamethonium injection associated with eye drops containing an anticholinesterase agent. *Br J Anaesth* (1966) 38, 408–409.
3. Pantuck EJ. Ecothiopate iodide eye drops and prolonged response to suxamethonium. *Br J Anaesth* (1966) 38, 406–407.
4. Mone JG, Mathie WE. Qualitative and quantitative defects of pseudocholinesterase activity. *Anaesthesia* (1967) 22, 55–68.
5. Messer GJ, Stoudemire A, Knos G, Johnson GC. Electroconvulsive therapy and the chronic use of pseudocholinesterase-inhibitor (echothiophate iodide) eye drops for glaucoma. A case report. *Gen Hosp Psychiatry* (1992) 14, 56–60.
6. Cavallaro RJ, Krumperman LW, Kugler F. Effect of echothiophate therapy on the metabolism of succinylcholine in man. *Anesth Analg* (1968) 47, 570–4.
7. de Roetth A, Dettbarn W-D, Rosenberg P, Wilensky JG, Wong A. Effect of phospholine iodide on blood cholinesterase levels of normal and glaucoma subjects. *Am J Ophthalmol* (1965) 59, 586–92.
8. Eilderton TE, Farmati O, Zsigmond EK. Reduction in plasma cholinesterase levels after prolonged administration of echothiophate iodide eyedrops. *Can Anaesth Soc J* (1968) 15, 291–6.
9. Donati F, Bevan DR. Controlled succinylcholine infusion in a patient receiving echothiophate eye drops. *Can Anaesth Soc J* (1981) 28, 488–90.
10. Feldman S, Karalliedde L. Drug interactions with neuromuscular blockers. *Drug Safety* (1996) 15, 261–73.

Neuromuscular blockers + Ephedrine

Ephedrine may reduce the onset time of rocuronium and suxamethonium (succinylcholine), Some, but not all studies suggest ephedrine has a similar effect on cisatracurium and vecuronium, but possibly not on atracurium.

Clinical evidence

(a) Atracurium

A study in 40 patients found that premedication with ephedrine 10 mg did not significantly alter the onset time of atracurium.[1]

(b) Cisatracurium

In a study in 30 patients, ephedrine 70 micrograms/kg or sodium chloride 0.9%, was given 5 seconds before the patients were anaesthetised with sufentanil and propofol, and followed by cisatracurium 150 micrograms/kg after loss of consciousness. The onset time of cisatracurium was found to be shorter after ephedrine was given with cisatracurium, than when sodium chloride 0.9% was given with cisatracurium (167 seconds compared with 235 seconds, respectively). Neuromuscular block at intubation was also greater in the patients given ephedrine, and the frequency of excellent intubating conditions was higher after ephedrine (87%) than after sodium chloride 0.9% (40%). No significant differences in haemodynamic parameters were noted between the two groups, although a trend towards a slightly higher heart rate and blood pressure was seen in the ephedrine group.[2] In contrast, another study in 60 patients found that the addition of ephedrine 0.5 mg/mL or 1 mg/mL to anaesthesia with remifentanil, propofol and cisatracurium 150 micrograms/kg had no significant effects on the onset time of cisatracurium.[3] Slight increases in the heart rate, blood pressure and overall mean arterial pressure were seen; however, no adverse cardiac events occurred.[3]

(c) Rocuronium

The effects of pretreatment with ephedrine 75, 100, or 150 micrograms/kg or sodium chloride 0.9% on intubation conditions and haemodynamics were studied in 100 patients given propofol and rocuronium 600 micrograms/kg. A significant increase in heart rate and mean arterial pressure occurred in patients pretreated with ephedrine 75 or 150 micrograms/kg. However, the overall hypotensive effect of the anaesthesia was not completely abolished. Intubation conditions were also significantly better in those pretreated with ephedrine 75 or 100 micrograms/kg but less so in the group who received ephedrine 150 micrograms/kg.[4] Similarly, ephedrine pretreatment was found to improve intubating conditions in another study in patients given propofol and rocuronium. A significant increase in the mean arterial pressure and heart rate was seen in those patients given both ephedrine and propofol in this study although no clinically significant adverse cardiac events, such as arrhythmias, occurred in this group.[5] A study in 60 patients found that ephedrine 70 micrograms/kg given with thiopental anaesthesia reduced the onset time of rocuronium 600 micrograms/kg, with no adverse cardiac effects,[6] and another study, in 40 patients, found that premedication with ephedrine 10 mg reduced the onset time of rocuronium by roughly 30%.[1]

One study in 60 patients found that the onset of rocuronium was 22% shorter after ephedrine 500 micrograms/kg was given (but 26% longer after esmolol, which decreases cardiac output).[7]

(d) Suxamethonium (Succinylcholine)

A study in patients given either ephedrine 70 micrograms/kg or sodium chloride 0.9% three minutes before the induction of anaesthesia with propofol and remifentanil, found that the onset time of suxamethonium was shorter in the ephedrine group than the sodium chloride group (26 seconds compared with 43 seconds, respectively). The heart rate and mean arterial pressure were increased in the ephedrine group at one minute; however, there were no other significant differences at all other measurement times and no adverse cardiac effects were reported.[8]

(e) Vecuronium

In a study, 119 patients were pretreated with ephedrine 30, 70 or 110 micrograms/kg or sodium chloride 0.9%, anaesthetised with fentanyl and propofol and tracheal intubation was performed 2 minutes after vecuronium 100 micrograms/kg was given. The onset time of vecuronium was shorter, intubating conditions were improved and neuromuscular blockade was greater in the patients who received ephedrine but the higher dose was associated with adverse haemodynamic effects (tachycardia and an increase in the mean arterial pressure of more than 30%). No arrhythmias occurred in the ephedrine-treated patients. It was suggested that ephedrine 70 micrograms/kg was a suitable dose to improve tracheal intubation conditions at 2 minutes after vecuronium, by increasing cardiac output but without adverse haemodynamic effects.[9] In contrast, in another study in 53 patients maintained under anaesthesia with propofol, the onset time of neuromuscular block with vecuronium 100 micrograms/kg was not affected by pretreatment with ephedrine 210 micrograms/kg when compared with sodium chloride, despite an increase in systolic blood pressure and the cardiac index (around 17%). However, the authors suggest that because vecuronium was given 10 minutes after the start of the propofol infusion this may have affected the result,[10] whereas ephedrine was given immediately before or just after propofol induction in the studies that found a beneficial effect on the onset of neuromuscular block.[2,4,5,9]

Mechanism

The onset time of neuromuscular blockers is partly dependent on circulatory factors such as muscle blood flow and cardiac output. Ephedrine is thought to decrease the onset times of neuromuscular blockers by increasing cardiac output and improving circulation time of the neuromuscular blocker to the muscle.[9,11] However, other studies that found a reduced onset time of neuromuscular blockade with ephedrine found no difference in haemodynamic parameters.[2,6] It has also been suggested that neuromuscular blockers with a fast onset of action are more likely to be affected by changes in cardiac output and blood flow than those with an intermediate onset of action such as atracurium.[11]

Importance and management

Some studies[1,2,7,9] suggest that small doses of ephedrine reduce the onset time of some neuromuscular blockers and improve intubating conditions. However, other studies[1,3,10] found that ephedrine did not significantly decrease the onset time of neuromuscular blockers. Its use may also be associated with increases in blood pressure and heart rate[3-5,10] and may lead to adverse haemodynamic affects, such as tachycardia, particularly at higher doses.[9] It should be noted that, in the studies above, no patients developed significant arrhythmias, although in most cases patients with pre-existing cardiac disease were excluded. These haemodynamic changes may be of more clinical significance in at-risk patients such as those with ischaemic heart disease.

1. Santiveri X, Mansilla R, Pardina B, Navarro J, Álvarez JC, Castillo J. La efedrina acorta el inicio de acción del rocuronio pero no del atracurio. *Rev Esp Anestesiol Reanim* (2003) 50, 176–81.
2. Albert F, Hans P, Bitar Y, Brichant JF, Dewandre PY, Lamy M. Effects of ephedrine on the onset time of neuromuscular block and intubating conditions after cisatracurium: preliminary results. *Acta Anaesthesiol Belg* (2000) 51, 167–71.
3. Moro ET, Nakamura G, de Martino RS, Nakamoto ML, Rodrigues GR, Ganem EM, Módolo NSP. Efeito do propofol associado à efedrina no tempo de latência do cisatracúrio. *Rev Assoc Med Bras* (2007) 53, 272–5.
4. Gopalakrishna MD, Krishna HM, Shenoy UK. The effect of ephedrine on intubating conditions and haemodynamics during rapid tracheal intubation using propofol and rocuronium. *Br J Anaesth* (2007) 99, 191–4.
5. Leykin Y, Pellis T, Lucca M, Gullo A. Effects of ephedrine on intubating conditions following priming with rocuronium. *Acta Anaesthesiol Scand* (2005) 49, 792–7.
6. Muñoz HR, González AG, Dagnino JA, González JA, Pérez AE. The effect of ephedrine on the onset time of rocuronium. *Anesth Analg* (1997) 85, 437–40.
7. Szmuk P, Ezri T, Chelly JE, Katz J. The onset time of rocuronium is slowed by esmolol and accelerated by ephedrine. *Anesth Analg* (2000) 90, 1217–19.
8. Ganidagli S, Cengiz M, Baysal Z. Effect of ephedrine on the onset time of succinylcholine. *Acta Anaesthesiol Scand* (2004) 48, 1306–9.
9. Kim KS, Cheong MA, Jeon JW, Lee JH, Shim JC. The dose effect of ephedrine on the onset time of vecuronium. *Anesth Analg* (2003) 96, 1042–6.
10. Komatsu R, Nagata O, Ozaki M, Sessler DI. Ephedrine fails to accelerate the onset of neuromuscular block by vecuronium. *Anesth Analg* (2003) 97, 480–3.
11. Simhi E, Brandom W. Cardiac output and onset time of different muscle relaxants. *Anesth Analg* (1998) 86, 1145.

Neuromuscular blockers + H_2-receptor antagonists

Isolated reports suggest that the effects of suxamethonium (succinylcholine) and vecuronium are prolonged by cimetidine. *Animal* studies suggest that the effects of tubocurarine and pancuronium may also be increased by cimetidine. Other reports suggest that no interaction generally occurs between neuromuscular blockers and other H_2-receptor antagonists, but not all combinations have been studied.

Clinical evidence

(a) Cimetidine

A study in 10 patients given cimetidine 300 mg orally at bedtime and another 300 mg 2 hours before anaesthesia, found that while the onset of action of **suxamethonium (succinylcholine)** 1.5 mg/kg intravenously was unchanged, when compared with 10 control patients, the time to recover 50% of the twitch height was prolonged 2- to 2.5-fold (from 8.6 to 20.3 minutes). One patient took 57 minutes to recover. His plasma cholinesterase levels were found to be normal.[1] It was later reported that some patients were also taking metoclopramide, which is known to interact in this way.[2] See also 'Neuromuscular blockers + Metoclopramide', p.131.

A study in 10 patients given 400 mg of cimetidine orally at bedtime and again 90 minutes before anaesthesia found no evidence of an effect on the neuromuscular blockade caused by **suxamethonium**, nor on its duration or recovery period, when compared with 10 control patients.[3] Another controlled study in patients given cimetidine 300 mg the night before and 1 to 2 hours before surgery, found no evidence that the duration of action of **suxamethonium** or the activity of plasma cholinesterase were altered.[2] Other studies similarly suggest that cimetidine does not alter the neuromuscular blocking effects of **suxamethonium**.[4,5]

Another study[6] in 16 patients found that cimetidine 400 mg significantly prolonged the recovery (T1–25 period) from **vecuronium**, but few patients had any response to cimetidine 200 mg. This slight prolongation of action of **vecuronium** due to cimetidine 400 mg was confirmed in another placebo-controlled study (mean time to return of T1 was 30 versus 22.5 minutes).[7] A study using a *rat* phrenic nerve hemi-diaphragm preparation found that, at clinically relevant concentrations, cimetidine produces neuromuscular paralysis and may potentiate the response to **vecuronium.**[8] A similar study using a *rat* phrenic nerve diaphragm preparation found that cimetidine increased the neuromuscular blocking effects of **tubocurarine** and **pancuronium**, but there seem to be no reports confirming this in man.[9]

Cimetidine appears not to alter the effects of **atracurium** or **rocuronium**.[10]

(b) Other H_2-receptor antagonists

A study in 8 patients found that the response to vecuronium was generally unchanged by **ranitidine** 100 mg, although some patients did show a slight prolongation in recovery.[6] A study using a *rat* phrenic nerve hemi-diaphragm preparation found that, at clinically relevant concentrations, **ranitidine** produced neuromuscular paralysis and may potentiate the response to **vecuronium**, but low concentrations of **ranitidine** may antagonise the effects of **vecuronium.**[8] Another controlled study in patients given **ranitidine** 150 mg the night before and 1 to 2 hours before surgery, found no evidence that the duration of action of **suxamethonium (succinylcholine)** or the activity of plasma cholinesterase were altered.[2] Other studies suggest that **ranitidine** and **famotidine** do not alter the neuromuscular blocking effects of suxamethonium.[4,5]

Ranitidine does not appear to alter the effects of **atracurium**[10] or **vecuronium.**[7] Another study found that premedication with **ranitidine** did not affect **vecuronium** blockade in postpartum patients, but that the neuromuscular blockade was prolonged in these patients, when compared with non-pregnant controls.[11] A study using a *rat* phrenic nerve hemi-diaphragm preparation found that **famotidine** lacked significant neuromuscular effects and did not alter the response to **vecuronium.**[8]

Mechanism

Not understood. Studies with human plasma failed to find any evidence that cimetidine in therapeutic concentrations inhibits the metabolism of suxamethonium.[2,12] However, metoclopramide may do and therefore is possibly the drug responsible for any interaction seen. *In vitro* studies with very high cimetidine concentrations found inhibition of plasma cholinesterase (pseudocholinesterase) activity.[13] The interaction between cimetidine and vecuronium is not understood, but it has been suggested that cimetidine may reduce the hepatic metabolism of vecuronium.[7]

Importance and management

Information seems to be limited to the reports cited. The most likely explanation for the discord between the results from studies with suxamethonium (succinylcholine) is that in the one study reporting increased suxamethonium effects[1] some of the patients were also given metoclopramide, which can inhibit plasma cholinesterase and prolong the effects of suxamethonium[2,5] (see also 'Neuromuscular blockers + Metoclopramide', p.131). In four other studies, cimetidine and other H_2-receptor antagonists did not alter suxamethonium effects. Therefore, it seems unlikely that an interaction exists. There is some evidence that cimetidine may slightly prolong the effects of vecuronium, but ranitidine appears not to interact. Atracurium and rocuronium appear not to be affected. Overall these possible interactions seem to be of little clinical significance.

1. Kambam JR, Dymond R, Krestow M. Effect of cimetidine on duration of action of succinylcholine. *Anesth Analg* (1987) 66, 191–2.
2. Woodworth GE, Sears DH, Grove TM, Ruff RH, Kosek PS, Katz RL. The effect of cimetidine and ranitidine on the duration of action of succinylcholine. *Anesth Analg* (1989) 68, 295–7.
3. Stirt JA, Sperry RJ, DiFazio CA. Cimetidine and succinylcholine: potential interaction and effect on neuromuscular blockade in man. *Anesthesiology* (1988) 69, 607–8.
4. Bogod DG, Oh TE. The effect of H_2 antagonists on duration of action of suxamethonium in the parturient. *Anaesthesia* (1989) 44, 591–3.
5. Turner DR, Kao YJ, Bivona C. Neuromuscular block by suxamethonium following treatment with histamine type 2 antagonists or metoclopramide. *Br J Anaesth* (1989) 63, 348–50.
6. Tryba M, Wruck G. Interaktionen von H_2-Antagonisten und nichtdepolarisierenden Muskelrelaxantien. *Anaesthesist* (1989) 38, 251–4.
7. McCarthy G, Mirakhur RK, Elliott P, Wright J. Effect of H_2-receptor antagonist pretreatment on vecuronium- and atracurium-induced neuromuscular block. *Br J Anaesth* (1991) 66, 713–15.
8. Mishra Y, Torda T, Ramzan I, Graham G. In-vitro interaction between H_2 antagonists and vecuronium. *J Pharm Pharmacol* (1994) 46, 205–8.
9. Galatulas I, Bossa R, Benvenuti C. Cimetidine increases the neuromuscular blocking activity of aminoglycoside antibiotics: antagonism by calcium. *Chem Indices Mec Proc Symp* (1981) 321–5.
10. Latorre F, de Almeida MCS, Stanek A, Weiler N, Kleemann PP. Beeinflussung der Pharmakodynamik von Rocuronium durch Cimetidin. *Anaesthesist* (1996) 45, 900–2.
11. Hawkins JL, Adenwala J, Camp C, Joyce TH. The effect of H_2-receptor antagonist premedication on the duration of vecuronium-induced neuromuscular blockade in postpartum patients. *Anesthesiology* (1989) 71, 175–7.
12. Cook DR, Stiller RL, Chakravorti S, Mannenhira T. Cimetidine does not inhibit plasma cholinesterase activity. *Anesth Analg* (1988) 67, 375–6.
13. Hansen WE, Bertl S. The inhibition of acetylcholinesterase and pseudocholinesterase by cimetidine. *Arzneimittelforschung* (1983) 33, 161–3.

Neuromuscular blockers + Immunosuppressants

There is limited evidence to suggest that the neuromuscular blocking effects of atracurium, pancuronium and vecuronium may be increased in some patients taking ciclosporin. There is also some evidence of reduced neuromuscular blockade with azathioprine and antilymphocyte immunoglobulins, but other evidence suggests that there is no clinically relevant interaction with azathioprine.

Clinical evidence

(a) Azathioprine or Antilymphocyte immunoglobulins

A retrospective study found that patients taking azathioprine or antilymphocyte immunoglobulins following organ transplantation needed an increased dosage of unspecified **muscle relaxants** to achieve satisfactory muscle relaxation.[1] A control group of 74 patients not receiving immunosuppression needed 0 to 10 mg of a **competitive (non-depolarising) muscle relaxant**; 13 patients taking azathioprine needed 12.5 to 25 mg; 11 patients receiving antilymphocyte immunoglobulins (antilymphocyte globulin) needed 10 to 20 mg and two patients taking azathioprine and guanethidine needed 55 and 90 mg.[1] However, a controlled study of 28 patients undergoing renal transplantation, who were receiving **atracurium**, **pancuronium** or **vecuronium** at a constant infusion rate, found that an injection of azathioprine 3 mg/kg given over 3 minutes caused a rapid, but only small and transient decrease of neuromuscular blockade. Ten minutes after the end of the azathioprine injection, a residual interaction was only detectable in those patients who had been given **pancuronium**.[2]

(b) Ciclosporin

A retrospective study found that 4 of 36 patients receiving **atracurium** and 4 of 29 patients receiving **vecuronium** experienced prolonged neuromuscular blockade after anaesthesia for renal transplantation. Respiratory failure occurred more often in patients who were given intravenous ciclosporin during surgery.[3] Extended recovery times after **atracurium** and **vecuronium** are described in another report in renal transplant patients who had been taking oral ciclosporin.[4] Similarly, a prolonged duration of action of **vecuronium** was noted in 7 renal transplant recipients, when compared with patients with normal renal function, and ciclosporin was considered to be a factor in this.[5] Two case reports describe prolonged neuromuscular blockade, which was attributed to intravenous ciclosporin. In the first report,[6] a woman with a 2-year renal transplant underwent surgery during which **pancuronium** 5.5 mg was used as the neuromuscular blocker. She was also given intravenous ciclosporin before and after surgery. The surgery lasted for 4 hours and no additional doses of **pancuronium** were given. Residual paralysis was inadequately reversed with neostigmine and atropine, and so edrophonium was given before extubation. However, she had to be re-intubated 20 minutes later because of increased respiratory distress. In the second report,[7] a 15-year-old girl receiving intravenous ciclosporin with serum levels of 138 micrograms/L was anaesthetised using fentanyl, thiopental and **vecuronium** 100 micrograms/kg. Anaesthesia was maintained with nitrous oxide, oxygen and isoflurane. Attempts were later made to reverse the blockade with edrophonium, atropine and neostigmine but full neuromuscular function was not restored until 3 hours and 20 minutes after the **vecuronium** was given. Another report describes a prolongation of the effects of **vecuronium** in a renal-transplant recipient taking oral ciclosporin, azathioprine, and prednisolone.[8]

Mechanism

The reasons for the reduction in neuromuscular blockade with azathioprine and antilymphocyte immunoglobulins are not understood. It has been suggested that azathioprine may inhibit phosphodiesterase at the motor nerve terminal resulting in increased release of acetylcholine.[9]

The ciclosporin interaction may be partly due to the vehicle used in intravenous preparations. One idea is that *Cremophor*, a surfactant which has been used as a solvent for ciclosporin, may increase the effective concentration of pancuronium at the neuromuscular junction.[6] In *animal* studies both compounds have been observed to increase vecuronium blockade,[10] and *Cremophor* has also been seen to decrease the onset time of pancuronium blockade in patients given *Cremophor*-containing anaesthetics.[11] However, this is not the entire answer because the interaction has also been seen with oral ciclosporin, which does not contain *Cremophor*.[8]

Importance and management

Direct information seems to be limited to the reports cited, and the interactions are not established. Although retrospective data suggest that azathioprine and antilymphocyte immunoglobulins can cause a reduction in the effects of neuromuscular blockers, and in some cases the dosage may need to be increased two- to fourfold,[1] the only prospective study found that the interaction with azathioprine was not clinically significant.[2] The general importance of the ciclosporin interaction is also uncertain, but be aware that the effects of atracurium, pancuronium or vecuronium may be increased in any patient receiving ciclosporin. Not all patients appear to develop this interaction.[3] Any effects seem likely to be managed by routine dose titration of the neuromuscular blocker and standard post-operative monitoring.

1. Vetten KB. Immunosuppressive therapy and anaesthesia. *S Afr Med J* (1973) 47, 767–70.
2. Gramstad L. Atracurium, vecuronium and pancuronium in end-stage renal failure. Dose-response properties and interactions with azathioprine. *Br J Anaesth* (1987) 59, 995–1003.
3. Sidi A, Kaplan RF, Davis RF. Prolonged neuromuscular blockade and ventilatory failure after renal transplantation and cyclosporine. *Can J Anaesth* (1990) 37, 543–8.
4. Lepage JY, Malinowsky JM, de Dieuleveult C, Cozian A, Pinaud M, Souron R. Interaction cyclosporine atracurium et vecuronium. *Ann Fr Anesth Reanim* (1989) 8 (Suppl), R135.
5. Takita K, Goda Y, Kawahigashi H, Okuyama A, Kubota M, Kemmotsu O. Pharmacodynamics of vecuronium in the kidney transplant recipient and the patient with normal renal function. *Jpn J Anesthesiol* (1993) 42, 190–4.
6. Crosby E, Robblee JA. Cyclosporine-pancuronium interaction in a patient with a renal allograft. *Can J Anaesth* (1988) 35, 300–2.
7. Wood GG. Cyclosporine-vecuronium interaction. *Can J Anaesth* (1989) 36, 358.
8. Ganjoo P, Tewari P. Oral cyclosporine-vecuronium interaction. *Can J Anaesth* (1994) 41, 1017.
9. Viby-Mogensen J. Interaction of other drugs with muscle relaxants. *Semin Anesth* (1985) 4, 52–64.
10. Gramstad L, Gjerløw JA, Hysing ES, Rugstad HE. Interaction of cyclosporin and its solvent, cremophor, with atracurium and vecuronium: studies in the cat. *Br J Anaesth* (1986) 58, 1149–55.
11. Gramstad L, Lilleaasen P, Minsaas B. Onset time for alcuronium and pancuronium after cremophor-containing anaesthetics. *Acta Anaesthesiol Scand* (1981) 25, 484–6.

Neuromuscular blockers + Lithium

The concurrent use of neuromuscular blockers and lithium is normally safe and uneventful, but four patients taking lithium experienced prolonged blockade and respiratory difficulties after receiving standard doses of pancuronium and/or suxamethonium (succinylcholine).

Clinical evidence

A manic depressive woman taking lithium carbonate, with a lithium level of 1.2 mmol/L, underwent surgery and was given thiopental, **suxamethonium (succinylcholine)** 310 mg over a period of 2 hours, and **pancuronium** 500 micrograms. Prolonged neuromuscular blockade with apnoea occurred.[1]

Three other patients taking lithium experienced enhanced neuromuscular blockade when given **pancuronium**,[2] or **pancuronium** with **suxamethonium**.[3,4] The authors of one of these reports[4] also suggest that they have seen several other cases where of the neuromuscular blockade produced by **suxamethonium** was potentiated in patients taking lithium carbonate, but give no further details. In contrast, a retrospective analysis of data from 17 patients taking lithium carbonate who received **suxamethonium** during a total of 78 ECT treatments, did not reveal any instances of unusually prolonged recovery.[5] Interactions between lithium and pancuronium[1] or suxamethonium[6,7] have been demonstrated in *dogs*, and an interaction between lithium and **tubocurarine** has been demonstrated in *cats*,[8] but no clear interaction has been demonstrated with any other neuromuscular blocker.[7,9] A case of lithium toxicity has been described in a woman taking lithium who was given **suxamethonium**, but it is doubtful if it arose because of an interaction.[10]

Mechanism

Uncertain. One suggestion is that, when an interaction occurs, it may be due to changes in the electrolyte balance caused by the lithium, which results in changes in the release of acetylcholine at the neuromuscular junction.[8,11]

Importance and management

Information is limited. There are only four definite reports of this interaction in man, and good evidence that no adverse interaction normally occurs. The concurrent use of lithium and neuromuscular blockers need not be avoided, and, on the rare occurrence an interaction occurs, it seems likely that it will be managed by routine intra-operative and post-operative monitoring.

1. Hill GE, Wong KC, Hodges MR. Potentiation of succinylcholine neuromuscular blockade by lithium carbonate. *Anesthesiology* (1976) 44, 439–42.
2. Borden H, Clarke MT, Katz H. The use of pancuronium bromide in patients receiving lithium carbonate. *Can Anaesth Soc J* (1974) 21, 79–82.
3. Rabolini V, Gatti G. Potenziamento del blocco neuro-muscolare di tipo depolarizzante da sali di litio (relazione su un caso). *Anest Rianim* (1988) 29, 157–9.
4. Rosner TM, Rosenberg M. Anesthetic problems in patients taking lithium. *J Oral Surg* (1981) 39, 282–5.
5. Martin BA, Kramer PM. Clinical significance of the interaction between lithium and a neuromuscular blocker. *Am J Psychiatry* (1982) 139, 1326–8.
6. Reimherr FW, Hodges MR, Hill GE, Wong KC. Prolongation of muscle relaxant effects by lithium carbonate. *Am J Psychiatry* (1977) 134, 205–6.
7. Hill GE, Wong KC, Hodges MR. Lithium carbonate and neuromuscular blocking agents. *Anesthesiology* (1977) 46, 122–6.
8. Basuray BN, Harris CA. Potentiation of d-tubocurarine (d-Tc) neuromuscular blockade in cats by lithium chloride. *Eur J Pharmacol* (1977) 45, 79–82.
9. Waud BE, Farrell L, Waud DR. Lithium and neuromuscular transmission. *Anesth Analg* (1982) 61, 399–402.
10. Jephcott G, Kerry RJ. Lithium: an anaesthetic risk. *Br J Anaesth* (1974) 46, 389–90.
11. Dehpour AR, Samadian T, Roushanzamir F. Interaction of aminoglycoside antibiotics and lithium at the neuromuscular junctions. *Drugs Exp Clin Res* (1992) 18, 383–7.

Neuromuscular blockers + Magnesium compounds

The effects of cisatracurium, mivacurium, pancuronium, rocuronium, tubocurarine, vecuronium, and probably other competitive neuromuscular blockers can be increased and prolonged by magnesium sulfate given parenterally. There is some evidence that magnesium might interact similarly with suxamethonium (succinylcholine), but also evidence from well-controlled studies to suggest that it does not.

Clinical evidence

(a) Competitive (non-depolarising) neuromuscular blockers

1. Cisatracurium. A study in 20 patients undergoing elective cardiac surgery found that magnesium sulfate, 70 mg/kg given before induction of anaesthesia, followed by 30 mg/kg per hour, prolonged the neuromuscular blockade of cisatracurium by just over 30 minutes.[1] A patient given cisatracurium 14 mg during induction of anaesthesia was then given intravenous magnesium sulfate 2 g over 5 minutes for atrial fibrillation, which had developed about 15 minutes after the end of surgery. Within a few minutes of receiving magnesium, recurarisation occurred (despite the patient having been given 2 doses of neostigmine and glycopyrronium (glycopyrrolate) postoperatively), and the patient required re-intubation and artificial ventilation for about 20 minutes.[2]

2. Mivacurium. The infusion rate of mivacurium required to obtain relaxation in women undergoing a caesarean section was about 3-fold lower in 12 women who had received magnesium sulfate for pre-eclampsia than in 12 women who had not.[3] In another study in 10 hypertensive patients undergoing caesarean section and given magnesium sulfate 30 or 60 mg/kg at induction, the action of mivacurium was prolonged when compared with normotensive controls or hypertensive controls not given magnesium.[4]

3. Pancuronium. In two patients who underwent cardiac surgery, neuromuscular blockade with either pancuronium, or pancuronium and **rocuronium** was prolonged by more than 10 hours. This was attributed to the effects of high doses of neuromuscular blockers being potentiated by magnesium sulfate 2.5 g. Moderate renal impairment might also have been a factor.[5]

4. Rapacuronium. Prolonged neuromuscular blockade with rapacuronium has been reported in a patient undergoing emergency caesarean section who received magnesium sulfate and clindamycin,[6] although the clindamycin was thought to be mainly responsible (see also 'Neuromuscular blockers + Miscellaneous anti-infectives', p.131).

5. Rocuronium. A 4-fold increase in the duration of neuromuscular blockade of rocuronium 0.9 mg/kg was reported in a pregnant woman given magnesium sulfate.[7] A further randomised, placebo-controlled study confirmed that pretreatment with magnesium sulfate 60 mg/kg increased the duration of neuromuscular blockade produced by rocuronium (time to initial recovery increased from about 25 minutes to 42 minutes), but the onset time was not affected.[8] In another controlled study in children with cerebral palsy undergoing orthopaedic surgery, intravenous magnesium sulfate reduced the required dose of rocuronium by 31%, from 0.42 to 0.29 mg/kg.[9] For a case of very prolonged neuromuscular blockade when rocuronium and pancuronium were used in a patient also given intravenous magnesium sulfate, see under *Pancuronium*, above.

6. Tubocurarine. Prolonged neuromuscular blockade has been described in three women with pre-eclampsia who were given magnesium sulfate and either tubocurarine alone or with suxamethonium (succinylcholine).[10,11] Increased blockade by magnesium has been demonstrated with tubocurarine in *animals*.[10,12]

7. Vecuronium. A pregnant 40-year-old with severe pre-eclampsia and receiving magnesium sulfate by infusion, underwent emergency caesarean section during which she was initially anaesthetised with thiopental, maintained with nitrous oxide/oxygen and enflurane, and given firstly suxamethonium (succinylcholine) and later vecuronium as muscle relaxants. At the end of surgery she rapidly recovered from the anaesthesia but the neuromuscular blockade was very prolonged (an 8-fold increase in duration).[13] In a series of randomised studies involving 125 patients, pretreatment with intravenous magnesium sulfate 40 mg/kg reduced the dose requirement of vecuronium by 25%, approximately halved the time to the onset of action, and prolonged the duration of action from about 25 minutes to 43 minutes.[14] Another study found that pretreatment with magnesium sulfate 40 mg/kg decreased the onset and prolonged the recovery time from vecuronium blockade, but a lower dose of magnesium sulfate of 20 mg/kg had no effect.[15] Evidence of enhanced vecuronium neuromuscular blockade by magnesium sulfate is described in one other study,[16] and case report.[17] A further study in 20 patients found that recurarisation (sufficient to compromise respiration) occurred when magnesium sulfate 60 mg/kg was given in the postoperative period, shortly after recovery from neuromuscular blockade with vecuronium.[18] In a randomised study, neostigmine-induced recovery from vecuronium blockade was attenuated by about 30% in patients pretreated with magnesium sulfate. The authors demonstrated this was due to slower spontaneous recovery and not decreased response to neostigmine.[19]

(b) Suxamethonium (Succinylcholine)

An early study in 59 women undergoing caesarean section found that those given magnesium sulfate for eclampsia and pre-eclampsia needed less suxamethonium than control patients (4.73 compared with 7.39 mg/kg per hour).[20] Prolonged neuromuscular blockade has been described in three women with pre-eclampsia who were given magnesium sulfate and either tubocurarine alone or with suxamethonium.[10,11] A 71-year-old woman given magnesium sulfate and lidocaine for ventricular tachycardia underwent emergency cardioversion and had a delayed onset and prolonged neuromuscular blockade when she was given suxamethonium.[21] Increased blockade by magnesium has been seen with suxamethonium in *animals*.[10,12]

However, a randomised study involving 20 patients found that pretreatment with a single 60-mg/kg bolus dose of magnesium sulfate did not significantly affect the onset of neuromuscular blockade, or prolong the blockade produced by suxamethonium.[22] Similar results were found in a non-randomised study[16] and in a double-blind, randomised study.[23] In randomised studies, the use of magnesium sulfate has also been reported to reduce suxamethonium-associated fasciculations[23] and reduce the increase in serum potassium concentrations produced by suxamethonium.[22]

Mechanism

Magnesium sulfate has direct neuromuscular blocking activity by inhibiting the normal release of acetylcholine from nerve endings, reducing the sensitivity of the postsynaptic membrane and depressing the excitability of the muscle membranes. These effects are seen when serum magnesium concentrations rise above the normal range (hypermagnesaemia) and are possibly simply additive (or perhaps more than additive) with the effects of competitive neuromuscular blockers.

Importance and management

The interaction between competitive (non-depolarising) neuromuscular blockers and parenteral magnesium is established. Magnesium may decrease the time to onset of neuromuscular blockade, prolong the duration of action, and reduce the dose requirement of competitive neuromuscular blockers. Be alert for an increase in the effects of any competitive neuromuscular blocker if intravenous magnesium sulfate has been used, and anticipate the need to reduce the dose. Some have suggested that the decreased time to onset with vecuronium may be of use clinically to improve the intubating conditions for rapid sequence induction if suxamethonium is not suitable.[14] Intravenous calcium gluconate was used to assist recovery in one case of prolonged blockade.[10] Also be aware that recurarisation can occur when intravenous magnesium compounds are used in the postoperative period.[2,18] The authors of one report suggest that magnesium sulfate should be avoided for at least 30 minutes after reversal of residual neuromuscular blockade, to minimise the risk of recurarisation.[2] Hypermagnesaemia can occur in patients receiving magnesium in antacids, enemas, or parenteral nutrition, especially if there is impaired renal function, but an interaction with neuromuscular blockers would not normally be expected, as oral magnesium compounds generally result in lower systemic concentrations than intravenous magnesium due to poor absorption.[24]

The interaction between magnesium and suxamethonium is not established. Although some *animal* and clinical evidence suggests potentiation of suxamethonium can occur, well-controlled studies have not confirmed this. Therefore some authors consider that magnesium sulfate does not have a clinically relevant effect on the response to suxamethonium.[16,25]

1. Pinard AM, Donati F, Martineau R, Denault AY, Taillefer J, Carrier M. Magnesium potentiates neuromuscular blockade with cisatracurium during cardiac surgery. *Can J Anesth* (2003) 50, 172–8.
2. Fawcett WJ, Stone JP. Recurarization in the recovery room following the use of magnesium sulphate. *Br J Anaesth* (2003) 91, 435–8.
3. Ahn EK, Bai SJ, Cho BJ, Shin Y-S. The infusion rate of mivacurium and its spontaneous neuromuscular recovery in magnesium-treated parturients. *Anesth Analg* (1998) 86, 523–6.
4. Hodgson RE, Rout CC, Rocke D, Louw NJ. Mivacurium for caesarean section in hypertensive parturients receiving magnesium sulphate therapy. *Int J Obstet Anesth* (1998) 7, 12–17.
5. Olivieri L, Plourde G. Prolonged (more than ten hours) neuromuscular blockade after cardiac surgery: report of two cases. *Can J Anesth* (2005) 52, 88–93.
6. Sloan PA, Rasul M. Prolongation of rapacuronium neuromuscular blockade by clindamycin and magnesium. *Anesth Analg* (2002) 94, 123–4.
7. Gaiser RR, Seem EH. Use of rocuronium in a pregnant patient with an open eye injury, receiving magnesium medication, for preterm labour. *Br J Anaesth* (1996) 77, 669–71.
8. Kussman B, Shorten G, Uppington J, Comunale ME. Administration of magnesium sulphate before rocuronium: effects on speed of onset and duration of neuromuscular block. *Br J Anaesth* (1997) 79, 122–4.
9. Na HS, Lee JH, Hwang JY, Ryu JH, Han SH, Jeon YT, Do SH. Effects of magnesium sulphate on intraoperative neuromuscular blocking agent requirements and postoperative analgesia in children with cerebral palsy. *Br J Anaesth* (2010) 104, 344–50.
10. Ghoneim MM, Long JP. The interaction between magnesium and other neuromuscular blocking agents. *Anesthesiology* (1970) 32, 23–7.
11. de Silva AJC. Magnesium intoxication: an uncommon cause of prolonged curarization. *Br J Anaesth* (1973) 45, 1228–9.
12. Giesecke AH, Morris RE, Dalton MD, Stephen CR. Of magnesium, muscle relaxants, toxemic parturients, and cats. *Anesth Analg* (1968) 47, 689–95.
13. Sinatra RS, Philip BK, Naulty JS, Ostheimer GW. Prolonged neuromuscular blockade with vecuronium in a patient treated with magnesium sulfate. *Anesth Analg* (1985) 64, 1220–2.
14. Fuchs-Buder T, Wilder-Smith OHG, Borgeat A, Tassonyi E. Interaction of magnesium sulphate with vecuronium-induced neuromuscular block. *Br J Anaesth* (1995) 74, 405–9.
15. Okuda T, Umeda T, Takemura M, Shiokawa Y, Koga Y. Pretreatment with magnesium sulphate enhances vecuronium-induced neuromuscular block. *Jpn J Anesthesiol* (1998) 47, 704–8.
16. Baraka A, Yazigi A. Neuromuscular interaction of magnesium with succinylcholine-vecuronium sequence in the eclamptic parturient. *Anesthesiology* (1987) 67, 806–8.
17. Hino H, Kaneko I, Miyazawa A, Aoki T, Ishizuka B, Kosugi K, Amemiya A. Prolonged neuromuscular blockade with vecuronium in patient with triple pregnancy treated with magnesium sulfate. *Jpn J Anesthesiol* (1997) 46, 266–70.
18. Fuchs-Buder T, Tassonyi E. Magnesium sulphate enhances residual neuromuscular block induced by vecuronium. *Br J Anaesth* (1996) 76, 565–6.
19. Fuchs-Buder T, Ziegenfuß T, Lysakowski K, Tassonyi E. Antagonism of vecuronium-induced neuromuscular block in patients pretreated with magnesium sulphate: dose-effect relationship of neostigmine. *Br J Anaesth* (1999) 82, 61–5.
20. Morris R, Giesecke AH. Potentiation of muscle relaxants by magnesium sulfate therapy in toxemia of pregnancy. *South Med J* (1968) 61, 25–8.
21. Ip-Yam C, Allsop E. Abnormal response to suxamethonium in a patient receiving magnesium therapy. *Anaesthesia* (1994) 49, 355–6.
22. James MFM, Cork RC, Dennett JE. Succinylcholine pretreatment with magnesium sulfate. *Anesth Analg* (1986) 65, 373–6.
23. Stacey MRW, Barclay K, Asai T, Vaughan RS. Effects of magnesium sulphate on suxamethonium-induced complications during rapid-sequence induction of anaesthesia. *Anaesthesia* (1995) 50, 933–6.
24. Cammu G. Interactions of neuromuscular blocking drugs. *Acta Anaesthesiol Belg* (2001) 52, 357–63.
25. Guay J, Grenier Y, Varin F. Clinical pharmacokinetics of neuromuscular relaxants in pregnancy. *Clin Pharmacokinet* (1998) 34, 483–96.

Neuromuscular blockers + MAOIs

The effects of suxamethonium (succinylcholine) were enhanced in three patients taking phenelzine.

Clinical evidence, mechanism, importance and management

Two patients, one taking **phenelzine** and the other who had ceased to do so 6 days previously, developed apnoea following ECT during which **suxamethonium (succinylcholine)** was used. Both responded to injections of nikethamide and positive pressure ventilation with oxygen.[1] A later study observed the same response in another patient taking **phenelzine**.[2] This would appear to be explained by the finding that **phenelzine** caused a reduction in the levels of plasma cholinesterase (pseudocholinesterase) in 4 out of 10 patients studied. Since the metabolism of **suxamethonium** depends on this enzyme, reduced levels of the enzyme would result in a reduced rate of **suxamethonium** metabolism and in a prolongation of its effects. None of 12 other patients taking **tranylcypromine, isocarboxazid** or **mebanazine** had reduced plasma cholinesterase levels.[2]

It would clearly be prudent to be on the alert for this interaction in patients taking **phenelzine. Phenelzine** may be anticipated to react similarly with **mivacurium** as it is also metabolised by plasma cholinesterase.[3]

1. Bleaden FA, Czekanska G. New drugs for depression. *BMJ* (1960) 1, 200.
2. Bodley PO, Halwax K, Potts L. Low serum pseudocholinesterase levels complicating treatment with phenelzine. *BMJ* (1969) 3, 510–12.
3. Feldman S, Karalliedde L. Drug interactions with neuromuscular blockers. *Drug Safety* (1996) 15, 261–73.

Neuromuscular blockers + Metoclopramide

The neuromuscular blocking effects of suxamethonium (succinylcholine) and mivacurium can be increased and prolonged in patients taking metoclopramide.

Clinical evidence

Metoclopramide 10 mg given intravenously 1 to 2 hours before induction of anaesthesia prolonged the time to 25% recovery after **suxamethonium (succinylcholine)** by 1.83 minutes (23%) in 19 patients, when compared with 21 control patients.[1,2] A larger 20-mg dose of metoclopramide prolonged the time to recovery by 56% in a further 10 patients.[1] In another study by the same research group, the recovery from neuromuscular blockade (time from 95% to 25% suppression of the activity of the adductor pollicis muscle) due to **suxamethonium** was prolonged by 67% in 11 patients who were given metoclopramide 10 mg intravenously during surgery, one - minute before the **suxamethonium.**[3]

A randomised, placebo-controlled study in 30 patients found that intravenous metoclopramide 150 micrograms/kg given about 10 minutes before anaesthetic induction with **mivacurium** 150 micrograms/kg prolonged the duration of action of **mivacurium** by about 30%.[4] Another report found that infusion rates of **mivacurium** were reduced by up to about 80% in patients given metoclopramide 10 or 20 mg intravenously, 5 minutes before induction, and metoclopramide delayed complete recovery from neuromuscular block after **mivacurium** by 36% (10 mg dose) and 50% (20 mg dose).[5] Metoclopramide 20 mg delayed the recovery from **mivacurium** block by 78% in another study.[6]

Mechanism

It has been suggested that metoclopramide may reduce the activity of plasma cholinesterase, which is responsible for the metabolism of suxamethonium and mivacurium. One *in vitro* study found that a metoclopramide level of 800 nanograms/mL inhibited plasma cholinesterase activity by 50%. However, a 10-mg dose of metoclopramide in adult patients weighing 50 to 70 kg produces peak plasma levels five times less than this (140 nanograms/mL).[7] Further, in an *in vivo* study, metoclopramide had only minimal inhibitory effects on plasma cholinesterase, and there was no difference in plasma cholinesterase levels in patients who had received metoclopramide and those who had not.[4]

Importance and management

The interaction between metoclopramide and suxamethonium is an established but not extensively documented interaction of only moderate or minor clinical importance. However, some enhancement of blockade can occur. The authors of the suxamethonium reports also point out that plasma cholinesterase activity is reduced in pregnancy and so suxamethonium sensitivity is more likely in obstetric patients.

The interaction between metoclopramide and mivacurium has only more recently been demonstrated. Metoclopramide appears to allow a reduction in the infusion rate of mivacurium and it causes a significant delay in recovery from neuromuscular block. Care is recommended during combined use.[5]

Ester-type local anaesthetics also depend on plasma cholinesterase activity for metabolism[1,7] and their effects would therefore be expected to be additive with the effects of metoclopramide, see 'Neuromuscular blockers + Anaesthetics, local', p.120.

1. Kao YJ, Tellez J, Turner DR. Dose-dependent effect of metoclopramide on cholinesterases and suxamethonium metabolism. *Br J Anaesth* (1990) 65, 220–4.
2. Turner DR, Kao YJ, Bivona C. Neuromuscular block by suxamethonium following treatment with histamine type 2 antagonists or metoclopramide. *Br J Anaesth* (1989) 63, 348–50.
3. Kao YJ, Turner DR. Prolongation of succinylcholine block by metoclopramide. *Anesthesiology* (1989) 70, 905–8.
4. Skinner HJ, Girling KJ, Whitehurst A, Nathanson MH. Influence of metoclopramide on plasma cholinesterase and duration of action of mivacurium. *Br J Anaesth* (1999) 82, 542–5.
5. El Ayass N, Hendrickx P. Decreased mivacurium infusion rate and delayed neuromuscular recovery after metoclopramide: a randomized double blind placebo-controlled study. *Eur J Anaesthesiol* (2005) 22, 197–201.
6. Motamed C, Kirov K, Combes X, Dhonneur G, Duvaldestin P. Effect of metoclopramide on mivacurium-induced neuromuscular block. *Acta Anaesthesiol Scand* (2002) 46, 214–16.
7. Kambam JR, Parris WCV, Franks JJ, Sastry BVR, Naukam R, Smith BE. The inhibitory effect of metoclopramide on plasma cholinesterase activity. *Can J Anaesth* (1988) 35, 476–8.

Neuromuscular blockers + Miscellaneous anti-infectives

Colistin, colistimethate sodium, polymyxin B, clindamycin, lincomycin, some penicillins (apalcillin, azlocillin, mezlocillin, piperacillin) and vancomycin possess some neuromuscular blocking activity. Increased and prolonged neuromuscular blockade is possible if these antibacterials are used with neuromuscular blocking drugs. In theory amphotericin B might also interact. No clinically significant interaction has been seen with cefoxitin, cefuroxime, or metronidazole.

Clinical evidence

(a) Amphotericin B

Amphotericin B can induce hypokalaemia resulting in muscle weakness,[1] which might be expected to enhance the effects of neuromuscular blockers, but there appear to be no reports in the literature confirming that a clinically significant interaction actually occurs.

(b) Cephalosporins

In a controlled study, intravenous **cefuroxime**, given shortly before **pipecuronium**[2] or **rocuronium**[3] did not alter the neuromuscular-blocking effects of these drugs. Similarly, intravenous **cefoxitin** given before, during and after surgery was not associated with a clinically important prolongation of **vecuronium** blockade.[4]

(c) Clindamycin and Lincomycin

Enhanced blockade has been seen in patients given **pancuronium** and lincomycin, which was reversed by neostigmine.[5] Respiratory paralysis was seen 10 minutes after lincomycin 600 mg was given intramuscularly to a man recovering from neuromuscular blockade with **tubocurarine**[6] and this interaction was confirmed in another report.[7] Other case reports[8-10] and clinical studies[11] describe minor to marked increases in neuromuscular blockade in patients receiving **pancuronium**,[9] **pipecuronium**,[11] **rapacuronium**[10] or **suxamethonium (succinylcholine)**[8] when they were given clindamycin. One patient developed very prolonged blockade after being unintentionally given clindamycin 2.4 g instead of 600 mg shortly after recovery from **suxamethonium** and **tubocurarine**.[12] Prolongation of the neuromuscular blocking effects of **vecuronium** has also been reported in a patient who received both clindamycin and gentamicin.[13]

(d) Metronidazole

An increase in the neuromuscular blocking effects of **vecuronium** with metronidazole has been reported in *cats*;[14] however, a later study in patients found no evidence of an interaction,[15] and another study with **rocuronium** also found no evidence of an interaction with metronidazole.[3] Similarly, no interaction was seen with **rocuronium** and metronidazole/cefuroxime,[3] and another study found no significant interaction between **pipecuronium** and metronidazole.[2]

(e) Penicillins

A study in patients found that the neuromuscular blocking effects of **vecuronium** were prolonged by a number of penicillins: **apalcillin** 26%, **azlocillin** 55%, **mezlocillin** 38%, and **piperacillin** 46%.[16] Reinstitution of neuromuscular blockade and respiratory failure occurred in a postoperative patient given **piperacillin** 3 g by intravenous infusion following the reversal of **vecuronium** blockade.[17] However, a randomised, study in 30 patients found that **piperacillin** or cefoxitin, given by intravenous infusion, pre- and intraoperatively, were not associated with clinically important prolongation of the neuromuscular block induced by **vecuronium**. Of 27 patients who could be evaluated, 22 showed a modest overall decrease in recovery time and 2 patients given **piperacillin** exhibited a slight prolongation in recovery time, but these patients all responded readily to neostigmine or other anticholinesterases and subsequent recurarisation did not occur.[4]

(f) Polymyxins

A literature review of interactions between antibacterials and neuromuscular blockers identified 17 cases over the period 1956 to 1970 in which **colistin (polymyxin E)** or **colistimethate sodium**, with or without conventional neuromuscular blockers, were responsible for the development of increased blockade and respiratory muscle paralysis. Some of the patients had renal disease.[18] A later report describes prolonged respiratory depression in a patient receiving **pancuronium** and **colistin**. Calcium gluconate was found to reverse the blockade.[19] A placebo-controlled study found that one million units of **colistin** considerably prolonged the recovery time from **pipecuronium** blockade.[11] Six cases of enhanced neuromuscular blockade involving **polymyxin B** have also been reported.[18] An increase in the blockade due to **pancuronium** by **polymyxin B** and bacitracin wound irrigation is described in another report; pyridostigmine, neostigmine and edrophonium were ineffective antagonists of this block and only partial improvement occurred after calcium chloride was given.[20] Prolonged and fatal apnoea occurred in another patient given **suxamethonium** when his peritoneal cavity was instilled with a solution containing 100 mg of **polymyxin B** and 100 000 units of bacitracin.[21]

(g) Vancomycin

A man recovering from neuromuscular blockade with **suxamethonium** (with some evidence of residual Phase II block) developed almost total muscle paralysis and apnoea when given an intravenous infusion of vancomycin. He recovered spontaneously when the vancomycin was stopped, but it took several hours.[22] The neuromuscular blockade due to **vecuronium** was increased in a patient who was given an infusion of vancomycin (1 g in 250 mL of sodium chloride 0.9% over 35 minutes).[23] Transient apnoea and apparent cardiac arrest have also been described in a patient following a 1-g intravenous injection of vancomycin given over 2 minutes.[24] However, in both of these cases[23,24] the vancomycin was given more rapidly than the current recommendations. It is now known that rapid infusion of vancomycin can provoke histamine release, which can result in apnoea, hypotension, anaphylaxis and muscular spasm, effects similar to those seen in these two patients.

Mechanism

Not fully understood but several sites of action at the neuromuscular junction (pre and/or post, effects on ion-channels or receptors) have been suggested.

The neuromuscular blocking properties of the polymyxins (polymyxin B, colistin, colistimethate sodium) involve a number of mechanisms, which may explain the difficulty in reversing the blockade.[25]

Importance and management

The interactions involving polymyxin B, colistin, colistimethate sodium, lincomycin, and clindamycin are established and clinically important. The incidence is uncertain. Concurrent use need not be avoided, but be alert for increased and prolonged neuromuscular blockade. The recovery period should be well monitored because of the risk of recurarisation. There seem to be no reports of an interaction with amphotericin B, but it may be prudent to be aware of a potential for interaction during the recovery period.

No interaction would be expected with cefuroxime, cefoxitin, or metronidazole, but some caution would seem appropriate with azlocillin, mezlocillin and piperacillin.

The situation with vancomycin is less clear. The evidence does suggest a link between vancomycin and increased neuromuscular blockade following the use of suxamethonium, and possibly vecuronium. However, vancomycin is given routinely as antibacterial prophylaxis before surgical procedures. The sparsity of reports therefore suggests that, in practice, vancomycin rarely causes a clinically significant interaction with neuromuscular blockers.

Consider also 'Neuromuscular blockers + Aminoglycosides', p.119.

1. Drutz DJ, Fan JH, Tai TY, Cheng JT, Hsieh WC. Hypokalemic rhabdomyolysis and myoglobinuria following amphotericin B therapy. *JAMA* (1970) 211, 824–6.
2. Stanley JC, Mirakhur RK, Clarke RSJ. Study of pipecuronium-antibiotic interaction. *Anesthesiology* (1990) 73, A898.
3. Cooper R, Maddineni VR, Mirakhur RK. Clinical study of interaction between rocuronium and some commonly used antimicrobial agents. *Eur J Anaesthesiol* (1993) 10, 331–5.
4. Condon RE, Munshi CA, Arfman RC. Interaction of vecuronium with piperacillin or cefoxitin evaluated in a prospective, randomized, double-blind clinical trial. *Am Surg* (1995) 61, 403–6.
5. Booij LHDJ, Miller RD, Crul JF. Neostigmine and 4-aminopyridine antagonism of lincomycin-pancuronium neuromuscular blockade in man. *Anesth Analg* (1978) 57, 316–21.
6. Samuelson RJ, Giesecke AH, Kallus FT, Stanley VF. Lincomycin-curare interaction. *Anesth Analg* (1975) 54, 103–5.
7. Hashimoto Y, Iwatsuki N, Shima T, Iwatsuki K. Neuromuscular blocking properties of lincomycin and Kanendomycin® in man. *Jpn J Anesthesiol* (1971) 20, 407–11.
8. Avery D, Finn R. Succinylcholine-prolonged apnea associated with clindamycin and abnormal liver function tests. *Dis Nerv Syst* (1977) 38, 473–5.
9. Fogdall RP, Miller RD. Prolongation of a pancuronium-induced neuromuscular blockade by clindamycin. *Anesthesiology* (1974) 41, 407–8.
10. Sloan PA, Rasul M. Prolongation of rapacuronium neuromuscular blockade by clindamycin and magnesium. *Anesth Analg* (2002) 94, 123–4.
11. de Gouw NE, Crul JF, Vandermeersch E, Mulier JP, van Egmond J, Van Aken H. Interaction of antibiotics on pipecuronium-induced neuromuscular blockade. *J Clin Anesth* (1993) 5, 212–15.
12. Al Ahdal O, Bevan DR. Clindamycin-induced neuromuscular blockade. *Can J Anaesth* (1995) 42, 614–7.
13. Jedeikin R, Dolgunski E, Kaplan R, Hoffman S. Prolongation of neuromuscular blocking effect of vecuronium by antibiotics. *Anaesthesia* (1987) 42, 858–60.
14. McIndewar IC, Marshall RJ. Interactions between the neuromuscular blocking drug ORG NC 45 and some anaesthetic, analgesic and antimicrobial agents. *Br J Anaesth* (1981) 53, 785–92.
15. d'Hollander A, Agoston S, Capouet V, Barvais L, Bomblet JP, Esselen M. Failure of metronidazole to alter a vecuronium neuromuscular blockade in humans. *Anesthesiology* (1985) 63, 99–102.
16. Tryba M. Wirkungsverstärkung nicht-depolarisierender Muskelrelaxantien durch Acylaminopenicilline. Untersuchungen am Beispiel von Vecuronium. *Anaesthesist* (1985) 34, 651–55.
17. Mackie K, Pavlin EG. Recurrent paralysis following piperacillin administration. *Anesthesiology* (1990) 72, 561–3.
18. Pittinger CB, Eryasa Y, Adamson R. Antibiotic-induced paralysis. *Anesth Analg* (1970) 49, 487–501.
19. Giala MM, Paradelis AG. Two cases of prolonged respiratory depression due to interaction of pancuronium with colistin and streptomycin. *J Antimicrob Chemother* (1979) 5, 234–5.
20. Fogdall RP, Miller RD. Prolongation of a pancuronium-induced neuromuscular blockade by polymyxin B. *Anesthesiology* (1974) 40, 84–7.
21. Small GA. Respiratory paralysis after a large dose of intraperitoneal polymyxin B and bacitracin. *Anesth Analg* (1964) 43, 137–9.
22. Albrecht RF, Lanier WL. Potentiation of succinylcholine-induced phase II block by vancomycin. *Anesth Analg* (1993) 77, 1300–1302.
23. Huang KC, Heise A, Shrader AK, Tsueda K. Vancomycin enhances the neuromuscular blockade of vecuronium. *Anesth Analg* (1990) 71, 194–6.
24. Glicklich D, Figura I. Vancomycin and cardiac arrest. *Ann Intern Med* (1984) 101, 880–1.
25. Østergaard D, Engbaek J, Viby-Mogensen J. Adverse reactions and interactions of the neuromuscular blocking drugs. *Med Toxicol Adverse Drug Exp* (1989) 4, 351–68.

Neuromuscular blockers + Neuromuscular blockers

Combinations of competitive neuromuscular blockers may have additive or synergistic effects. However, the sequence of administration may also affect the interaction. The previous use of a small dose of a competitive neuromuscular blocker (e.g. vecuronium) generally reduces the effects of suxamethonium (succinylcholine), but if suxamethonium is given during recovery from a competitive neuromuscular blocker, antagonism, enhancement or a combination of the two may occur. The effects of a competitive blocker may be increased if it is given after suxamethonium.

Clinical evidence, mechanism, importance and management

Neuromuscular blockers are of two types: competitive (non-depolarising) and depolarising. The competitive or non-depolarising blockers (**atracurium** and others listed in 'Table 5.2', p.98) compete with acetylcholine for the receptors on the endplate of the neuromuscular junction. Thus the receptors fail to be stimulated and muscular paralysis results. **Suxamethonium (succinylcholine)**, a depolarising neuromuscular blocker, also occupies the receptors on the endplate but it acts like acetylcholine to cause depolarisation. However, unlike acetylcholine, it is not immediately removed by cholinesterase so that the depolarisation persists and the muscle remains paralysed.

(a) Combinations of competitive (non-depolarising) neuromuscular blockers

Combinations of competitive (non-depolarising) neuromuscular blockers may have additive or synergistic effects. Structural differences between the interacting neuromuscular blockers may have an effect; it has been suggested that structurally similar neuromuscular blockers tend to produce an additive response, whereas structurally different blockers may be synergistic.[1,2] For a list of competitive neuromuscular blockers by structural type, see 'Table 5.2', p.98.

Additive effects have been found with the following structurally similar combinations:

- **atracurium** and **cisatracurium**[3] or **mivacurium**,[4]
- **pancuronium** and **vecuronium**,[5]
- **pipecuronium** and **vecuronium**,[6]
- **tubocurarine** and **metocurine**.[1]

Synergism has been reported with the following structurally similar combinations:

- **cisatracurium** and **mivacurium**,[3]
- **tubocurarine** and **atracurium**.[7]

Potentiation of neuromuscular blockade or synergy has been reported with the following structurally different combinations:

- **atracurium** and **vecuronium**,[8]
- **cisatracurium** and **rocuronium**,[3,9,10] or **vecuronium**,[3]
- **metocurine** and **pancuronium**,[1]
- **mivacurium** and **pancuronium**[2,11] or **rocuronium**,[12]
- **tubocurarine** and **pancuronium**[1] or **vecuronium**.[7]

In addition to affecting response, the initial blocker may modify the duration of action of the supplemental blocker.[13,14] The blocking action of **pancuronium** was shortened when it was given during **vecuronium**-induced partial neuromuscular blockade.[14] Conversely, the duration of action of **mivacurium**[2,15] or **vecuronium**[14] was lengthened when they were given after **pancuronium**-induced neuromuscular block. Therefore, care should be taken if a small dose of a short-acting blocker is given near the end of an operation in which a longer-acting blocker has already been given.

(b) Competitive neuromuscular blocker given first

The combination of a competitive neuromuscular blocker and **suxamethonium (succinylcholine)** has an intrinsic antagonistic effect. This interaction has been used clinically to reduce muscle fasciculations caused by **suxamethonium**. A small dose of competitive neuromuscular blocker given shortly before **suxamethonium** generally reduces its effects and duration of action.[16] **Suxamethonium** would be expected to antagonise competitive neuromuscular blockers due to their opposite mechanisms of action (**suxamethonium** exerts a receptor agonist-type activity whereas competitive blockers exhibit receptor antagonism). However, **suxamethonium** may also reverse a competitive block by enhancing the effect of acetylcholine postsynaptically.[17,18]

The neuromuscular blockade will also be affected by the competitive neuromuscular blocker used and whether or not an anticholinesterase has been given.[19,20] See also, 'Neuromuscular blockers + Anticholinesterases', p.121.

1. Atracurium. If suxamethonium is given during the recovery from a paralysing dose of atracurium, the resultant neuromuscular block is influenced by the depth of residual block and the dose of suxamethonium used.[19,20] In a study in 38 patients recovering from atracurium 400 micrograms/kg, lower intravenous doses of suxamethonium 0.25 to 1 mg/kg mainly antagonised the partial block, whereas higher doses (1.5 to 3 mg/kg) usually enhanced the blockade.[19] However, the degree of recovery from the underlying block also influences the effects of suxamethonium: early on when the residual block is still considerable, suxamethonium may appear to have no effect or produce a partial antagonism of the block, but later, a biphasic response may be seen (antagonism of the competitive block initially before superimposing a depolarising block); a combination of antagonism and enhancement may also occur in different muscle groups.[20]

2. Pancuronium. Following pancuronium pretreatment, the duration of suxamethonium blockade appears to be prolonged,[16] and this is probably due to the inhibition of cholinesterase by pancuronium.[21]

(c) Suxamethonium (Succinylcholine) given first

In general, when a competitive blocker is given following suxamethonium, the onset time may be reduced and the potency or duration of the block may be increased, although not always significantly. In a study in 350 patients, the previous use of suxamethonium 1 mg/kg significantly accelerated the onset of neuromuscular blockade with **atracurium**, **pancuronium**, **pipecuronium** and **vecuronium**, when these were given after full recovery from the suxamethonium block. However, the duration of blockade was only significantly prolonged with **vecuronium**.[22]

It has been suggested that suxamethonium may have a presynaptic action resulting in reduced acetylcholine output.[17] Although not always clinically significant, be aware that a reduction in the dose of competitive blocker may be necessary following the use of a depolarising neuromuscular blocker.

1. Atracurium. A study showed that the effect of the previous use of suxamethonium on atracurium neuromuscular block appears to depend on the level of recovery from suxamethonium. As with previous studies, the onset of atracurium blockade was shortened when given after full recovery from the suxamethonium. However, this effect was less apparent when the atracurium was given before full suxamethonium recovery.[23]

2. Cisatracurium. Pretreatment with suxamethonium reduced the time to onset of cisatracurium block, but did not potentiate it or prolong recovery.[24]

3. Pancuronium or Vecuronium. One study found potentiation of vecuronium when it was given up to 30 minutes after full recovery from a single 1-mg/kg intravenous dose of suxamethonium.[25] Another study found that the effects of vecuronium or pancuronium were potentiated for at least 2 hours after full recovery from an intubating dose of suxamethonium.[26]

4. Rocuronium. Pretreatment with suxamethonium decreased the onset time and increased the duration of action or rocuronium.[27]

1. Lebowitz PW, Ramsey FM, Savarese JJ, Ali HH. Potentiation of neuromuscular blockade in man produced by combinations of pancuronium and metocurine or pancuronium and *d*-tubocurarine. *Anesth Analg* (1980) 59, 604–9.
2. Kim KS, Shim JC, Kim DW. Interactions between mivacurium and pancuronium. *Br J Anaesth* (1997) 79, 19–23.
3. Kim KS, Chun YS, Chon SU, Suh JK. Neuromuscular interaction between cisatracurium and mivacurium, atracurium, vecuronium or rocuronium administered in combination. *Anaesthesia* (1998) 53, 872–8.
4. Naguib M, Abdulatif M, Al-Ghamdi A, Selim M, Seraj M, El-Sanbary M, Magboul MA. Interactions between mivacurium and atracurium. *Br J Anaesth* (1994) 73, 484–9.
5. Ferres CJ, Mirakhur RK, Pandit SK, Clarke RSJ, Gibson FM. Dose-response studies with pancuronium, vecuronium and their combination. *Br J Clin Pharmacol* (1984) 18, 947–50.
6. Smith I, White PF. Pipecuronium-induced prolongation of vecuronium neuromuscular block. *Br J Anaesth* (1993) 70, 446–8.
7. Middleton CM, Pollard BJ, Healy TEJ, Kay B. Use of atracurium or vecuronium to prolong the action of tubocurarine. *Br J Anaesth* (1989) 62, 659–63.
8. Steinberg D. Revisión de la interacción entre vecuronio y atracurio por la adaptación de un método alterno. *Rev Esp Anestesiol Reanim* (2004) 51, 583–88.
9. Naguib M, Samarkandi AH, Ammar A, Elfaqih SR, Al-Zahrani S, Turkistani A. Comparative clinical pharmacology of rocuronium, cisatracurium, and their combination. *Anesthesiology* (1998) 89, 1116–24.
10. Breslin DS, Jiao K, Habib AS, Schultz J, Gan TJ. Pharmacodynamic interactions between cisatracurium and rocuronium. *Anesth Analg* (2004) 98, 107–10.
11. Motamed C, Menad R, Farinotti R, Kirov K, Combes X, Bouleau D, Feiss P, Duvaldestin P. Potentiation of mivacurium blockade by low dose of pancuronium. A pharmacokinetic study. *Anesthesiology* (2003) 98, 1057–62.
12. Naguib M. Neuromuscular effects of rocuronium bromide and mivacurium chloride administered alone and in combination. *Anesthesiology* (1994) 81, 388–95.
13. Okamoto T, Nakai T, Aoki T, Satoh T. Interaction between vecuronium and pancuronium. *Jpn J Anesthesiol* (1993) 42, 534–9.
14. Rashkovsky OM, Agoston S, Ket JM. Interaction between pancuronium bromide and vecuronium bromide. *Br J Anaesth* (1985) 57, 1063–6.
15. Erkola O, Rautoma P, Meretoja OA. Mivacurium when preceded by pancuronium becomes a long-acting muscle relaxant. *Anesthesiology* (1996) 84, 562–5.
16. Ferguson A, Bevan DR. Mixed neuromuscular block. The effect of precurarization. *Anaesthesia* (1981) 36, 661–6.
17. Feldman S, Fauvel N. Potentiation and antagonism of vecuronium by decamethonium. *Anesth Analg* (1993) 76, 631–4.
18. Braga MFM, Rowan EG, Harvey AL, Bowman WC. Interactions between suxamethonium and non-depolarizing neuromuscular blocking drugs. *Br J Anaesth* (1994) 72, 198–204.
19. Scott RPF, Norman J. Effect of suxamethonium given during recovery from atracurium. *Br J Anaesth* (1988) 61, 292–6.
20. Black AMS. Effect of suxamethonium given during recovery from atracurium. *Br J Anaesth* (1989) 62, 348–9.
21. Stovner J, Oftedal N, Holmboe J. The inhibition of cholinesterases by pancuronium. *Br J Anaesth* (1975) 47, 949–54.
22. Swen J, Koot HWJ, Bencini A, Ket JM, Hermans J, Agoston S. The interaction between suxamethonium and the succeeding non-depolarizing neuromuscular blocking agent. *Eur J Anaesthesiol* (1990) 7, 203–9.
23. Roed J, Larsen PB, Olsen JS, Engbæk J. The effect of succinylcholine on atracurium-induced neuromuscular block. *Acta Anaesthesiol Scand* (1997) 41, 1331–4.
24. Pavlin EG, Forrest AP, Howard M, Quessy S, McClung C. Prior administration of succinylcholine does not affect the duration of Nimbex (51W89) neuromuscular blockade. *Anesth Analg* (1995) 80, S374.
25. d'Hollander AA, Agoston S, De Ville A, Cuvelier F. Clinical and pharmacological actions of a bolus injection of suxamethonium: two phenomena of distinct duration. *Br J Anaesth* (1983) 55, 131–4.
26. Ono K, Manabe N, Ohta Y, Morita K, Kosaka F. Influence of suxamethonium on the action of subsequently administered vecuronium or pancuronium. *Br J Anaesth* (1989) 62, 324–6.
27. Robertson EN, Driessen JJ, Booij LHDJ. Suxamethonium administration prolongs the duration of action of subsequent rocuronium. *Eur J Anaesthesiol* (2004) 21, 734–7.

Neuromuscular blockers + Ondansetron

Ondansetron does not affect atracurium-induced neuromuscular blockade.

Clinical evidence, mechanism, importance and management

A double-blind, placebo-controlled study in 30 patients undergoing elective surgery found that intravenous ondansetron 8 or 16 mg given over 5 minutes had no effect on subsequent neuromuscular blockade with **atracurium**.[1] No special precautions would therefore seem necessary. The authors suggest that no interaction is likely with other non-depolarising neuromuscular blockers, but this needs confirmation.

1. Lien CA, Gadalla F, Kudlak TT, Embree PB, Sharp GJ, Savarese JJ. The effect of ondansetron on atracurium-induced neuromuscular blockade. *J Clin Anesth* (1993) 5, 399–403.

Neuromuscular blockers + Opioids

A woman experienced hypertension and tachycardia when she was given pancuronium after induction of anaesthesia with morphine and nitrous oxide/oxygen. Bradycardia has been reported when vecuronium was given with alfentanil, fentanyl, or sufentanil, sometimes in patients taking beta blockers and/or calcium-channel blockers.

Clinical evidence, mechanism, importance and management

(a) Pancuronium

A woman about to receive a coronary by-pass graft was premedicated with **morphine** 10 mg and hyoscine 400 micrograms, intramuscularly, one hour before the induction of anaesthesia. **Morphine** 1 mg/kg was then slowly infused while the patient was ventilated with 50% nitrous oxide/oxygen. With the onset of neuromuscular relaxation with pancuronium 150 micrograms/kg, her blood pressure rose sharply from 120/60 mmHg to 200/110 mmHg and her pulse rate increased from 54 bpm to 96 bpm, persisting for several minutes but restabilising when halothane 1% was added.[1] The suggested reason for this reaction is that pancuronium can antagonise the vagal tone (heart slowing) induced by the **morphine**, thus allowing the blood pressure and heart rate to rise. The authors of the report point out the undesirability of this in those with coronary heart disease.

(b) Vecuronium

Two patients, one aged 72 years and the other aged 84 years, undergoing elective carotid endarterectomy developed extreme bradycardia following induction with **alfentanil** and vecuronium; both were premedicated with **morphine**. The first was taking **propranolol** 20 mg every 8 hours and, as the drugs were injected, his heart rate fell from 50 bpm to 35 bpm and his blood pressure fell from 160/70 mmHg to 75/35 mmHg. He responded to atropine, ephedrine and phenylephrine. The other patient was taking nifedipine and quinidine. His heart rate fell from 89 bpm to 43 bpm, and his blood pressure dropped from 210/80 mmHg to 120/45 mmHg. Both heart rate and blood pressures recovered following skin incision.[2]

Bradycardia in the presence of vecuronium has been seen during anaesthetic induction with other drugs including **fentanyl**,[3,4] and **sufentanil** (in 3 patients taking beta blockers with or without diltiazem).[5] The lack of vagolytic effects associated with vecuronium may mean that opioid-induced bradycardia is unopposed.[4,5] The beta blockers and diltiazem may also have played a part in the bradycardia seen in some of these patients[5] (see also 'Neuromuscular blockers + Beta blockers', p.123, and 'Neuromuscular blockers + Calcium-channel blockers', p.124). Be alert for this effect if vecuronium is given with any of these drugs. Atropine 500 micrograms given intravenously at the time of induction may prevent the bradycardia.[4]

For reports of bradycardia occurring with atracurium or suxamethonium used with propofol and fentanyl, see 'Anaesthetics, general + Neuromuscular blockers', p.108.

1. Grossman E, Jacobi AM. Hemodynamic interaction between pancuronium and morphine. *Anesthesiology* (1974) 40, 299–301.
2. Lema G, Sacco C, Urzúa J. Bradycardia following induction with alfentanil and vecuronium. *J Cardiothorac Vasc Anesth* (1992) 6, 774–5.
3. Mirakhur RK, Ferres CJ, Clarke RSJ, Bali IM, Dundee JW. Clinical evaluation of Org NC 45. *Br J Anaesth* (1983) 55, 119–24.
4. Inoue K, El-Banayosy A, Stolarski L, Reichelt W. Vecuronium induced bradycardia following induction of anaesthesia with etomidate or thiopentone, with or without fentanyl. *Br J Anaesth* (1988) 60, 10–17.
5. Starr NJ, Sethna DH, Estafanous FG. Bradycardia and asystole following the rapid administration of sufentanil with vecuronium. *Anesthesiology* (1986) 64, 521–3.

Neuromuscular blockers + Organophosphorus compounds

Exposure to organophosphorus insecticides such as malathion and dimpylate (diazinon) can markedly prolong the neuromuscular blocking effects of suxamethonium (succinylcholine).

Clinical evidence

A man admitted to hospital for an appendectomy became apnoeic during the early part of the operation when given **suxamethonium** (**succinylcholine**) 100 mg to facilitate tracheal intubation. He remained apnoeic throughout the 40 minutes of surgery. Restoration of neuromuscular activity occurred about 180 minutes after he had received the **suxamethonium**. Later studies showed that he had an extremely low plasma cholinesterase activity (3 to 10%), even though he had a normal phenotype for this enzyme. It subsequently turned out that he had been working with **malathion** for 11 weeks without any protection.[1]

Another report describes a man whose recovery from neuromuscular blockade with **suxamethonium** was very prolonged. He had attempted suicide approximately 2 weeks earlier with **dimpylate** (**diazinon**), a household insecticide. His pseudocholinesterase was found to be 2.5 units/L (normal values 7 to 19 units/L) and his dibucaine number (a measurement of cholinesterase activity) was too low to be measured.[2]

Other cases of prolonged **suxamethonium**-induced paralysis associated with organophosphate poisoning have been reported.[3-7] These cases have involved accidental ingestion of **chlorpyrifos**[3] or **dichlorvos**[7] in children, and one case resulted from subclinical exposure to **chlorpyrifos** and **propetamphos** following the treatment of carpets for pests.[4] Also, prolonged **suxamethonium**-induced paralysis has occurred following suicide attempts in adults with **chlorpyrifos**[6] or *Diazinon* [**dimpylate**].[5] In one report a patient was given ECT 2 weeks after attempted suicide with **chlorpyrifos** and, despite low plasma cholinesterase levels, paralysis with **suxamethonium** was carried out successfully using one-fifth of the normal dose.[6]

Mechanism

Malathion, dimpylate, and other organophosphorus insecticides inhibit the activity of plasma cholinesterase, thereby reducing the metabolism of the suxamethonium and prolonging its effects.

Importance and management

An established and well understood interaction. The organophosphorus pesticides are potent anticholinesterases used in agriculture and horticulture to control insects on crops, and in veterinary practice to control various ectoparasites. They are applied as sprays and dips. Anyone who is exposed to these toxic pesticides may therefore show changes in their responses to neuromuscular blockers. Widely used organophosphorus pesticides are said to include **azamethiphos, bromophos, chlorpyrifos, clofenvinfos, coumafos, cythioate, dichlorvos, dimethoate, dimpylate, dioxation, ethion, famphur, fenitrothion, fenthion, heptenophos, iodofenphos, malathion, naled, parathion, phosmet, phoxim, pirimiphos-methyl, propetamphos, pyraclofos, temefos.**[8] A number of the **nerve gases** (such as **sarin, soman, tabun** and **VX**) are also potent anticholinesterases.

1. Guillermo FP, Pretel CMM, Royo FT, Macias MJP, Ossorio RA, Gomez JAA, Vidal CJ. Prolonged suxamethonium-induced neuromuscular blockade associated with organophosphate poisoning. *Br J Anaesth* (1988) 61, 233–6.
2. Ware MR, Frost ML, Berger JJ, Stewart RB, DeVane CL. Electroconvulsive therapy complicated by insecticide ingestion. *J Clin Psychopharmacol* (1990) 10, 72–3.
3. Selden BS, Curry SC. Prolonged succinylcholine-induced paralysis in organophosphate insecticide poisoning. *Ann Emerg Med* (1987) 16, 215–17.
4. Weeks DB, Ford D. Prolonged suxamethonium-induced neuromuscular block associated with organophosphate poisoning. *Br J Anaesth* (1989) 62, 237.
5. Jaksa RJ, Palahniuk RJ. Attempted organophosphate suicide: a unique cause of prolonged paralysis during electroconvulsive therapy. *Anesth Analg* (1995) 80, 832–3.
6. Dillard M, Webb J. Administration of succinylcholine for electroconvulsive therapy after organophosphate poisoning: a case study. *AANA J* (1999) 67, 513–17.
7. Sener EB, Ustun E, Kocamanoglu S, Tur A. Prolonged apnea following succinylcholine administration in undiagnosed acute organophosphate poisoning. *Acta Anaesthesiol Scand* (2002) 46, 1046–8.
8. *Martindale. The Complete Drug Reference*, [online] London: Pharmaceutical Press. https://www.medicinescomplete.com/mc/martindale/current/3560-a4-b.htm (accessed 19/10/15).

Neuromuscular blockers + Phenytoin

The effects of many competitive neuromuscular blockers are reduced and shortened if phenytoin is given for longer than one week, but they appear to be increased if phenytoin is given acutely (e.g. during surgery). Phenytoin appears not to interact with mivacurium.

Clinical evidence

(a) Phenytoin given long-term

1. Atracurium. A reduced recovery time from atracurium-induced neuromuscular blockade was found in one study in patients taking long-term antiepileptics including phenytoin.[1] In contrast, other studies suggest that atracurium is normally minimally affected by phenytoin.[2-4]

2. Cisatracurium. A study found that the recovery time from intravenous cisatracurium was shorter in patients taking carbamazepine or phenytoin than in patients not receiving carbamazepine or phenytoin; the recovery index (times between 25% and 75% recovery) was 16.2 minutes and 21.2 minutes, respectively. Clearance of cisatracurium was increased by about 25% in patients taking carbamazepine or phenytoin. Furthermore, the steady-state plasma level of cisatracurium required to maintain 95% block was increased by 20%, indicating increased resistance to the action of cisatracurium.[5]

3. Mivacurium. A study in 32 patients who had been taking carbamazepine alone or with phenytoin or valproic acid for greater than 2 weeks found no resistance to mivacurium,[6] although an earlier preliminary study by the same research group found a trend towards a shorter recovery from mivacurium in 13 patients taking unspecified antiepileptics (not statistically significant).[7]

4. Pancuronium. In the preliminary report of a study, the reduction in the time to recover from 25 to 75% of the response to ulnar nerve stimulation, in patients who had received phenytoin for longer than one week was 40% for pancuronium.[4] In another study about 80% more pancuronium was needed in 9 patients taking long-term phenytoin (58 micrograms/kg per hour) than in 18 others not receiving phenytoin (32 micrograms/kg per hour).[8] Resistance to pancuronium and a shortening of the recovery period due to long-term phenytoin[9,10] or unspecified antiepileptics[11] has also been described in other reports.

5. Pipecuronium. Some reports suggest that the recovery period from pipecuronium is reduced by phenytoin.[12,13] In one study it was found that the *onset* time for pipecuronium blockade was lengthened (although this was not statistically significant) for patients with therapeutic plasma concentrations of phenytoin or carbamazepine, but not in those with subtherapeutic levels. However, a shorter duration of action occurred regardless of the level of the antiepileptic drug.[13]

6. Suxamethonium (Succinylcholine). Eight patients who had been taking phenytoin and/or carbamazepine for at least one month took longer to recover from suxamethonium blockade, compared with 9 control patients; the time for return to baseline twitch height was 14.3 minutes and 10 minutes, respectively.[14]

7. Miscellaneous neuromuscular blockers. In the preliminary report of a study, the reduction in the time to recover from 25 to 75% of the response to ulnar nerve stimulation, in patients who had received phenytoin for longer than one week was 58% for **metocurine**. Some reduction in response was seen with **tubocurarine** but this was not statistically significant.[4] The **metocurine** results are published in full elsewhere.[15] The recovery period from **doxacurium,**[9,16] **rapacuronium** (case report),[17] **rocuronium**[18,19] and **vecuronium**[2,20-23] is also reduced by phenytoin.

(b) Phenytoin given short-term

A retrospective review of 8 patients taking long-term phenytoin (greater than 2 weeks) and 3 others given phenytoin within 8 hours of surgery found that the average doses of **vecuronium** used from induction to extubation were 155 micrograms/kg per hour (long-term use) and 61.5 micrograms/kg per hour (acute use).[24] Others have reported similar results.[21] Short-term phenytoin use may have been a contributing factor in the prolonged clearance of **vecuronium** in another patient.[25,26] Another study found that the sensitivity of patients to **vecuronium** was increased by phenytoin given intravenously during surgery,[27] and this has also been seen in *animal* studies using **tubocurarine** and phenytoin.[28] Similarly, a study of 20 patients undergoing craniotomy found that phenytoin (10 mg/kg over about 30 minutes) given during the operation augmented the neuromuscular block produced by **rocuronium.**[29]

Mechanism

Not fully understood, but it appears to be multifactorial. The acute use of phenytoin may result in neuromuscular block and potentiation of the action of competitive (non-depolarising) blockers.

The long-term use of phenytoin may produce subclinical neuromuscular blockade thought to be due to modest blockade of acetylcholine effects and a decrease in acetylcholine release; this antagonism may induce changes at the neuromuscular junction including increased number of acetylcholine receptors on the muscle membrane (up-regulation), with decreased sensitivity.[14,20,30] Other suggestions to account for the reduced response with chronic antiepileptics include: induction of liver enzyme activity (phenytoin is a potent inducer of cytochrome P450 isoenzymes), which would increase the metabolism and clearance of the neuromuscular blocker; and changes in plasma protein binding.[14,20,30] It has been shown that phenytoin possibly increases the plasma clearance of pancuronium[10] and rocuronium.[18]

Importance and management

Established and clinically important interactions. Anticipate the need to use more (possibly up to twice as much) doxacurium, metocurine, pancuronium, pipecuronium, rocuronium and vecuronium in patients who have taken phenytoin for more than a week,[21] and expect an accelerated recovery. The effects on tubocurarine and atracurium appear only to be small or moderate, whereas mivacurium appears not to interact.

In patients are given phenytoin acutely, anticipate the need to use a smaller neuromuscular blocker dosage, or prepare for a longer recovery time.

1. Tempelhoff R, Modica PA, Jellish WS, Spitznagel EL. Resistance to atracurium-induced neuromuscular blockade in patients with intractable seizure disorders treated with anticonvulsants. *Anesth Analg* (1990) 71, 665–9.
2. Ornstein E, Matteo RS, Schwartz AE, Silverberg PA, Young WL, Diaz J. The effect of phenytoin on the magnitude and duration of neuromuscular block following atracurium or vecuronium. *Anesthesiology* (1987) 67, 191–6.
3. deBros F, Okutani R, Lai A, Lawrence KW, Basta S. Phenytoin does not interfere with atracurium pharmacokinetics and pharmacodynamics. *Anesthesiology* (1987) 67, A607.
4. Ornstein E, Matteo RS, Silverberg PA, Schwartz AE, Young WL, Diaz J. Chronic phenytoin therapy and nondepolarizing muscular blockade. *Anesthesiology* (1985) 63, A331.
5. Richard A, Girard F, Girard DC, Boudreault D, Chouinard P, Moumdjian R, Bouthilier A, Ruel M, Couture J, Varin F. Cisatracurium-induced neuromuscular blockade is affected by chronic phenytoin or carbamazepine treatment in neurosurgical patients. *Anesth Analg* (2005) 100, 538–44.
6. Jellish WS, Thalji Z, Brundidge PK, Tempelhoff R. Recovery from mivacurium-induced neuromuscular blockade is not affected by anticonvulsant therapy. *J Neurosurg Anesthesiol* (1996) 8, 4–8.
7. Thalji Z, Jellish WS, Murdoch J, Tempelhoff R. The effect of chronic anticonvulsant therapy on recovery from mivacurium induced paralysis. *Anesthesiology* (1993) 79 (Suppl 3A), A965.
8. Chen J, Kim YD, Dubois M, Kammerer W, Macnamara TE. The increased requirement of pancuronium in neurosurgical patients receiving Dilantin chronically. *Anesthesiology* (1983) 59, A288.
9. Desai P, Hewitt PB, Jones RM. Influence of anticonvulsant therapy on doxacurium and pancuronium-induced paralysis. *Anesthesiology* (1989) 71, A784.
10. Liberman BA, Norman P, Hardy BG. Pancuronium-phenytoin interaction: a case of decreased duration of neuromuscular blockade. *Int J Clin Pharmacol Ther Toxicol* (1988) 26, 371–4.
11. Messick JM, Maass L, Faust RJ, Cucchiara RF. Duration of pancuronium neuromuscular blockade in patients taking anticonvulsant medication. *Anesth Analg* (1982) 61, 203–4.
12. Jellish WS, Modica PA, Tempelhoff R. Accelerated recovery from pipecuronium in patients treated with chronic anticonvulsant therapy. *J Clin Anesth* (1993) 5, 105–8.
13. Hans P, Ledoux D, Bonhomme V, Brichant JF. Effect of plasma anticonvulsant level on pipecuronium-induced neuromuscular blockade: preliminary results. *J Neurosurg Anesthesiol* (1995) 7, 254–8.
14. Melton AT, Antognini JF, Gronert GA. Prolonged duration of succinylcholine in patients receiving anticonvulsants: evidence for mild up-regulation of acetylcholine receptors? *Can J Anaesth* (1993) 40, 939–42.
15. Ornstein E, Matteo RS, Young WL, Diaz J. Resistance to metocurine-induced neuromuscular blockade in patients receiving phenytoin. *Anesthesiology* (1985) 63, 294–8.
16. Ornstein E, Matteo RS, Weinstein JA, Halevy JD, Young WL, Abou-Donia MM. Accelerated recovery from doxacurium-induced neuromuscular blockade in patients receiving chronic anticonvulsant therapy. *J Clin Anesth* (1991) 3, 108–11.
17. Tobias JD, Johnson JO. Rapacuronium administration to patients receiving phenytoin or carbamazepine. *J Neurosurg Anesthesiol* (2001) 13, 240–2.
18. Szenohradszky J, Caldwell JE, Sharma ML, Gruenke LD, Miller RD. Interaction of rocuronium (ORG 9426) and phenytoin in a patient undergoing cadaver renal transplantation: a possible pharmacokinetic mechanism? *Anesthesiology* (1994) 80, 1167–70.
19. Hernández-Palazón J, Tortosa JA, Martínez-Lage JF, Pérez-Ayala M. Rocuronium-induced neuromuscular blockade is affected by chronic phenytoin therapy. *J Neurosurg Anesthesiol* (2001) 13, 79–82.
20. Soriano SG, Sullivan LJ, Venkatakrishnan K, Greenblatt DJ, Martyn JAJ. Pharmacokinetics and pharmacodynamics of vecuronium in children receiving phenytoin or carbamazepine for chronic anticonvulsant therapy. *Br J Anaesth* (2001) 86, 223–9.
21. Platt PR, Thackray NM. Phenytoin-induced resistance to vecuronium. *Anaesth Intensive Care* (1993) 21, 185–91.
22. Caldwell JE, McCarthy GJ, Wright PMC, Szenohradszky J, Sharma ML, Gruenke LD, Miller RD. Influence of chronic phenytoin administration on the pharmacokinetics and pharmacodynamics of vecuronium. *Br J Anaesth* (1999) 83, 183P–184P.
23. Wright PMC, McCarthy G, Szenohradszky J, Sharma ML, Caldwell JE. Influence of chronic phenytoin administration on the pharmacokinetics and pharmacodynamics of vecuronium. *Anesthesiology* (2004) 100, 626–33.
24. Baumgardner JE, Bagshaw R. Acute versus chronic phenytoin therapy and neuromuscular blockade. *Anaesthesia* (1990) 45, 493–4.
25. Kainuma M, Miyake T, Kanno T. Extremely prolonged vecuronium clearance in a brain death case. *Anesthesiology* (2001) 95, 1023–4.

26. Gronert GA. Vecuronium sensitivity in part due to acute use of phenytoin. *Anesthesiology* (2002) 97, 1035.
27. Gray HSJ, Slater RM, Pollard BJ. The effect of acutely administered phenytoin on vecuronium-induced neuromuscular blockade. *Anaesthesia* (1989) 44, 379–81.
28. Gandhi IC, Jindal MN, Patel VK. Mechanism of neuromuscular blockade with some antiepileptic drugs. *Arzneimittelforschung* (1976) 26, 258–61.
29. Spacek A, Nickl S, Neiger FX, Nigrovic V, Ullrich O-W, Weindlmayr-Goettel M, Schwall B, Taeger K, Kress HG. Augmentation of the rocuronium-induced neuromuscular block by the acutely administered phenytoin. *Anesthesiology* (1999) 90, 1551–5.
30. Kim CS, Arnold FJ, Itani MS, Martyn JAJ. Decreased sensitivity to metocurine during long-term phenytoin therapy may be attributable to protein binding and acetylcholine receptor changes. *Anesthesiology* (1992) 77, 500–6.

Neuromuscular blockers + Quinidine

The effects of both depolarising neuromuscular blockers (e.g. suxamethonium (succinylcholine)) and competitive neuromuscular blockers (e.g. tubocurarine) can be increased by quinidine. Recurarisation and apnoea have been seen in patients when quinidine was given during the recovery period from neuromuscular blockade.

Clinical evidence

A patient given **metocurine** during surgery regained her motor functions and was able to talk coherently during the recovery period. However, within 15 minutes of being given quinidine sulfate 200 mg by injection she developed muscular weakness and respiratory depression. She needed intubation and assisted respiration for a period of two and a half hours. Edrophonium and neostigmine were used to aid recovery.[1]

This interaction has also been described in case reports involving **tubocurarine**[2] and **suxamethonium (succinylcholine)**,[3,4] and has been confirmed in *animal* studies.[5-7]

Mechanism

Not fully understood, but it has been shown that quinidine can inhibit the enzyme (choline acetyltransferase), which is concerned with the synthesis of acetylcholine at nerve endings.[8] Neuromuscular transmission would be expected to be reduced if the synthesis of acetylcholine is reduced. Quinidine also inhibits the activity of plasma cholinesterase, which is concerned with the metabolism of suxamethonium.[4]

Importance and management

The interaction between quinidine and neuromuscular blockers is an established interaction of clinical importance, but the documentation is limited. The incidence is uncertain, but it was seen in one report cited to a greater or lesser extent in 5 of the 6 patients studied.[3] It has only been reported clinically with metocurine, tubocurarine and suxamethonium, but it occurs in *animals* with **gallamine**, and it seems possible that it could occur clinically with any depolarising or non-depolarising neuromuscular blocker. Be alert for increased neuromuscular blocking effects, particularly after surgery.

1. Schmidt JL, Vick NA, Sadove MS. The effect of quinidine on the action of muscle relaxants. *JAMA* (1963) 183, 669–71.
2. Way WL, Katzung BG, Larson CP. Recurarization with quinidine. *JAMA* (1967) 200, 163–4.
3. Grogono AW. Anaesthesia for atrial defibrillation: effect of quinidine on muscular relaxation. *Lancet* (1963) ii, 1039–40.
4. Kambam JR, Franks JJ, Naukam R, Sastry BVR. Effect of quinidine on plasma cholinesterase activity and succinylcholine neuromuscular blockade. *Anesthesiology* (1987) 67, 858–60.
5. Miller RD, Way WL, Katzung BG. The neuromuscular effects of quinidine. *Proc Soc Exp Biol Med* (1968) 129, 215–18.
6. Miller RD, Way WL, Katzung BG. The potentiation of neuromuscular blocking agents by quinidine. *Anesthesiology* (1967) 28, 1036–41.
7. Cuthbert MF. The effect of quinidine and procainamide on the neuromuscular blocking action of suxamethonium. *Br J Anaesth* (1966) 38, 775–9.
8. Kambam JR, Day P, Jansen VE, Sastry BVR. Quinidine inhibits choline acetyltransferase activity. *Anesthesiology* (1989) 71, A819.

Neuromuscular blockers + Testosterone

An isolated report describes marked resistance to the effects of suxamethonium (succinylcholine) and vecuronium, apparently due to the long-term use of testosterone. Another case reports resistance to vecuronium in a patient with elevated plasma testosterone levels.

Clinical evidence, mechanism, importance and management

A transsexual who had been receiving testosterone enantate 200 mg intramuscularly twice monthly for 10 years was resistant to intravenous **suxamethonium (succinylcholine)** 100 mg and needed intravenous **vecuronium** 100 micrograms/kg for effective tracheal intubation before surgery. During the surgery it was found necessary to use a total of 22 mg of **vecuronium** over a 50-minute period to achieve acceptable relaxation of the abdominal muscles for a hysterectomy and salpingo-oophorectomy to be carried out.[1] Considerably higher than usual doses of **vecuronium** were required in a patient with testicular feminisation and elevated plasma testosterone levels.[2]

The reasons are not understood. However, it has been suggested that the close structural similarity between testosterone and **vecuronium**, with respect to their common steroidal core, might mean that they share similar metabolic pathways (see also 'Neuromuscular blockers + Corticosteroids', p.125). Chronic elevation of circulating testosterone may up-regulate the hepatic metabolism of steroidal molecules in general, and so enhance the hepatic elimination of **vecuronium.**[2]

1. Reddy P, Guzman A, Robalino J, Shevde K. Resistance to muscle relaxants in a patient receiving prolonged testosterone therapy. *Anesthesiology* (1989) 70, 871–3.
2. Lee HT, Appel MI. Increased tolerance to vecuronium in a patient with testicular feminization. *J Clin Anesth* (1998) 10, 156–9.

Neuromuscular blockers + Theophylline

Supraventricular tachycardia occurred in a patient taking aminophylline when pancuronium was given. Isolated cases suggest that the effects of pancuronium, but not vecuronium, can be opposed by aminophylline. Theophylline would be expected to interact similarly.

Clinical evidence, mechanism, importance and management

A report describes supraventricular tachycardia in a patient taking aminophylline who was anaesthetised with thiopental and fentanyl, and then given **pancuronium**. Three minutes later his heart rate rose to 180 bpm and an ECG revealed supraventricular tachycardia.[1] The authors of this report attributed this reaction to an interaction between the **pancuronium** and the aminophylline, because previous surgery with these drugs in the absence of aminophylline had been without incident.[1] Marked resistance to the effects of **pancuronium** (but not **vecuronium**) was seen in one patient receiving an aminophylline infusion.[2] Two other patients are reported to have shown a similar resistance to **pancuronium** but they had also been given hydrocortisone, which could have had a similar effect[3,4] (see also 'Neuromuscular blockers + Corticosteroids', p.125). These appear to be the only clinical reports of such an interaction and their general relevance is unclear. Note that, any interaction would also be expected to apply to theophylline, although this needs confirmation.

1. Belani KG, Anderson WW, Buckley JJ. Adverse drug interaction involving pancuronium and aminophylline. *Anesth Analg* (1982) 61, 473–4.
2. Daller JA, Erstad B, Rosado L, Otto C, Putnam CW. Aminophylline antagonizes the neuromuscular blockade of pancuronium but not vecuronium. *Crit Care Med* (1991) 19, 983–5.
3. Doll DC, Rosenberg H. Antagonism of neuromuscular blockage by theophylline. *Anesth Analg* (1979) 58, 139–40.
4. Azar I, Kumar D, Betcher AM. Resistance to pancuronium in an asthmatic patient treated with aminophylline and steroids. *Can Anaesth Soc J* (1982) 29, 280–2.

Neuromuscular blockers + Tobacco

There is some evidence that smokers may need more vecuronium and possibly more rocuronium, but less atracurium to achieve the same effects as non-smokers. However, results are variable and another study found that rocuronium appeared to be unaffected by smoking. Passive-smoking children appear to require less rocuronium than those not exposed to environmental tobacco smoke.

Clinical evidence, mechanism, importance and management

Variable results have been reported on the effect of smoking on neuromuscular blockers. The amount of **atracurium** required was about 25% lower in smokers, when compared with non-smokers.[1] However, in another study, smokers required more **vecuronium** than non-smokers (96.8 micrograms/kg per hour compared with 72.11 micrograms/kg per hour, respectively; a 34% increase).[2] Similarly another study in patients undergoing minor surgery found that the 20 smokers required about 20% more **rocuronium** than the 20 non-smokers.[3] However, this study has been criticised for having too few patients, which meant that it was unable to properly detect a statistically significant difference between the smokers and non-smokers.[4] In yet another study, the onset and recovery times from the neuromuscular blocking effects of **rocuronium** 600 micrograms/kg were reported to be not significantly affected by smoking more than 10 cigarettes daily.[5] In another study in children aged 4 to 10 years, those with a history of passive smoking required less **rocuronium** during similar anaesthesia than those without a familial smoking history.[6]

Tobacco smoke contains many different compounds and has enzyme-inducing properties, which may affect the dose requirements of neuromuscular blockers. In addition, the time interval in refraining from smoking will affect plasma **nicotine** concentrations; small doses of nicotine may stimulate the neuromuscular junction, but larger doses may block transmission.[2]

Although an interaction is established it seems unlikely to be generally important, as the dose of neuromuscular blocker is individualised and titrated to effect.

1. Kroeker KA, Beattie WS, Yang H. Neuromuscular blockade in the setting of chronic nicotine exposure. *Anesthesiology* (1994) 81, A1120.
2. Teiriä H, Rautoma P, Yli-Hankala A. Effect of smoking on dose requirements for vecuronium. *Br J Anaesth* (1996) 76, 154–5.
3. Rautoma P, Svartling N. Smoking increases the requirement for rocuronium. *Can J Anaesth* (1998) 45, 651–4.
4. Pühringer FK, Benzer A, Keller P, Luger TJ. Does smoking really increase the requirements for rocuronium? *Can J Anaesth* (1999) 46, 513.
5. Latorre F, de Almeida MCS, Stanek A, Kleemann PP. Die Wechselwirkung von Rocuronium und Rauchen. Der Einfluß des Rauchens auf die neuromuskuläre Übertragung nach Rocuronium. *Anaesthesist* (1997) 46, 493–5.
6. Reisli R, Apilliogullari S, Reisli I, Tuncer S, Erol A, Okesli S. The effect of environmental tobacco smoke on the dose requirements of rocuronium in children. *Pediatr Anesth* (2004) 14, 247–50.

Neuromuscular blockers + Trimetaphan

Trimetaphan can increase the effects of suxamethonium (succinylcholine), which may result in prolonged apnoea. This may possibly occur with other neuromuscular blocking drugs, such as alcuronium.

Clinical evidence

A man undergoing neurosurgery was given **tubocurarine** and **suxamethonium (succinylcholine)**. Neuromuscular blockade was prolonged postoperatively, lasting about 2.5 hours, and this was attributed to the concurrent use of trimetaphan 4.5 g, given over a 90-minute period. Later, when he underwent further surgery using essentially the same anaesthetic techniques and drugs, but with a very much smaller dose of trimetaphan (35 mg over a 10-minute period), the recovery was normal.[1]

Nine out of 10 patients receiving ECT and given **suxamethonium** had an almost 90% prolongation in apnoea (from 142 seconds to 265 seconds) when trimetaphan 10 to 20 mg was used instead of 1.2 mg of atropine.[2] Prolonged apnoea has been seen in another patient given **suxamethonium** and trimetaphan.[3] On the basis of an *in vitro* study it was calculated that a typical dose of trimetaphan would double the duration of paralysis due to **suxamethonium**.[4] Prolonged neuromuscular blockade was also seen in a man given **alcuronium** and trimetaphan.[5]

Mechanism

Not fully understood. Trimetaphan can inhibit plasma cholinesterase to some extent,[2,5] which would reduce the metabolism of suxamethonium and thereby prolong its activity. Studies in *rats*[6,7] and case reports[8] also indicate that trimetaphan has direct neuromuscular blocking activity. Its effects are at least additive with the neuromuscular blocking effects of the **aminoglycosides**.[7]

Importance and management

Information is limited but the interaction appears to be established. If trimetaphan and suxamethonium (succinylcholine) are used concurrently, be alert for enhanced and prolonged neuromuscular blockade. This has also been seen with alcuronium, and trimetaphan may interact with other competitive neuromuscular blockers.[5] Respiratory arrest has been seen when large doses of trimetaphan were given in the absence of a neuromuscular blocker, so that caution is certainly needed.[8] *Animal* studies suggested that the blockade might not be reversed by neostigmine or calcium chloride,[7] but neostigmine and calcium gluconate were successfully used to reverse the effects of alcuronium and trimetaphan in one case.[5]

1. Wilson SL, Miller RN, Wright C, Hasse D. Prolonged neuromuscular blockade associated with trimethaphan: a case report. *Anesth Analg* (1976) 55, 353–6.
2. Tewfik GI. Trimetaphan. Its effect on the pseudo-cholinesterase level of man. *Anaesthesia* (1957) 12, 326–9.
3. Poulton TJ, James FM, Lockridge O. Prolonged apnea following trimethaphan and succinylcholine. *Anesthesiology* (1979) 50, 54–6.
4. Sklar GS, Lanks KW. Effects of trimethaphan and sodium nitroprusside on hydrolysis of succinylcholine *in vitro*. *Anesthesiology* (1977) 47, 31–3.
5. Nakamura K, Koide M, Imanaga T, Ogasawara H, Takahashi M, Yoshikawa M. Prolonged neuromuscular blockade following trimetaphan infusion. *Anaesthesia* (1980) 35, 1202–7.
6. Pearcy WC, Wittenstein ES. The interactions of trimetaphan (Arfonad), suxamethonium and cholinesterase inhibitor in the rat. *Br J Anaesth* (1960) 32, 156–9.
7. Paradelis AG, Crassaris LG, Karachalios DN, Triantaphyllidis CJ. Aminoglycoside antibiotics: interaction with trimethaphan at the neuromuscular junctions. *Drugs Exp Clin Res* (1987) 13, 233–6.
8. Dale RC, Schroeder ET. Respiratory paralysis during treatment of hypertension with trimethaphan camsylate. *Arch Intern Med* (1976) 136, 816–18.

Neuromuscular blockers + Ulinastatin

Ulinastatin delays the onset and hastens the recovery from vecuronium neuromuscular block.

Clinical evidence, mechanism, importance and management

A randomised, placebo-controlled study in 60 patients found that a 5000 unit/kg intravenous bolus dose of ulinastatin given before induction of anaesthesia, and again 2 minutes before intravenous **vecuronium** 100 micrograms/kg, delayed the onset of neuromuscular blockade, when compared with placebo (250 seconds compared with 214 seconds). The recovery from neuromuscular block (measured as return of post-tetanic count) was significantly shorter after ulinastatin than placebo (11 minutes compared with 17.7 minutes). The effects of ulinastatin were thought to be due to an increase in the release of acetylcholine at the neuromuscular junction and enhanced **vecuronium** elimination due to increases in liver blood flow and urine volume.[1]

If the mechanism of interaction is correct, it seems possible that other neuromuscular blockers could interact similarly. However, the clinical relevance of this interaction seems likely to be small, as any effect is likely to be detected by routine monitoring.

1. Saitoh Y, Fujii Y, Oshima T. The ulinastatin-induced effect on neuromuscular block caused by vecuronium. *Anesth Analg* (1999) 89, 1565–9.

Neuromuscular blockers; Atracurium + Danazol or Tamoxifen

Two isolated case reports describe prolonged atracurium effects, which were attributed to the use of tamoxifen or danazol.

Clinical evidence, mechanism, importance and management

A case report describes a 67-year-old mastectomy patient taking methyldopa, hydrochlorothiazide, triamterene and long-term tamoxifen 10 mg twice daily who developed prolonged neuromuscular blockade after a single 500-microgram/kg dose of atracurium, which the authors suggest might be due to an interaction between atracurium and tamoxifen.[1] There is an earlier report[2] of prolonged atracurium blockade where the patient was taking danazol, another antioestrogenic drug. These interactions are probably not of general importance.

1. Naguib M, Gyasi HK. Antiestrogenic drugs and atracurium – a possible interaction? *Can Anaesth Soc J* (1986) 33, 682–3.
2. Bizzarri-Schmid MD, Desai SP. Prolonged neuromuscular blockade with atracurium. *Can Anaesth Soc J* (1986) 33, 209–12.

Neuromuscular blockers; Botulinum toxin + Miscellaneous

Theoretically, the neuromuscular blocking effects of botulinum toxin can be increased by other drugs with neuromuscular blocking effects, such as the aminoglycosides and muscle relaxants, but no such interactions appear to have been reported.

Clinical evidence, mechanism, importance and management

A case report describes a 5-month-old baby boy who was admitted to hospital because of lethargy, poor feeding, constipation and muscle weakness (later identified as being due to a *Clostridium botulinum* infection). One hour after starting intravenous treatment with ampicillin and **gentamicin** 7.5 mg/kg daily (in divided doses every 8 hours) for presumed sepsis, he stopped breathing and died. The reason appeared to be the additive neuromuscular blocking effects of the systemic botulinum toxin produced by the *Clostridium botulinum* infection and the **gentamicin**.[1] *Animal* studies confirm that **gentamicin** and **tobramycin** potentiate the neuromuscular blocking effects of systemic botulinum toxin (used to mimic botulism),[1] and there is every reason to believe that any of the other drugs known to cause neuromuscular blockade (such as the **aminoglycosides** and conventional **neuromuscular blockers**) will behave similarly. However, note that clinically, botulinum A toxin is injected for its local effect in specific muscles, and is not used systemically; and so the situation is not analogous to that described in the case of the child with systemic botulism. Nevertheless, several manufacturers prudently advise caution if drugs that affect neuromuscular transmission are given concurrently.[2-4] **Aminoglycosides**, **anticholinesterases**, lincosamides (such as **clindamycin** and **lincomycin**), **magnesium sulphate**, polymixins (such as **colistin** and **polymixin B**), **quinidine**, **spectinomycin**, and **neuromuscular blockers** are specifically named.[2-4]

1. Santos JI, Swensen P, Glasgow LA. Potentiation of *Clostridium botulinum* toxin by aminoglycoside antibiotics: clinical and laboratory observations. *Pediatrics* (1981) 68, 50–4.
2. Botox (Botulinum A toxin). Allergan Ltd. UK Summary of product characteristics, September 2011.
3. NeuroBloc (Botulinum B toxin). Eisai Ltd. UK Summary of product characteristics, November 2010.
4. Myobloc (Botulinum B toxin). Solstice Neurosciences Inc. US Prescribing information, May 2010.

Neuromuscular blockers; Suxamethonium (Succinylcholine) + Dexpanthenol

An isolated report describes an increase in the neuromuscular blocking effects of suxamethonium, which was attributed to the concurrent use of dexpanthenol, but a further study using pantothenic acid (the main metabolite of dexpanthenol) failed to confirm this interaction.

Clinical evidence, mechanism, importance and management

A study in 6 patients under general anaesthesia found that their response to suxamethonium was unaffected by the infusion of 500 mg of **pantothenic acid**.[1] This study was conducted in response to an earlier case report, which reported respiratory depression requiring re-intubation following the use of intramuscular dexpanthenol (which is converted to pantothenic acid in the body) shortly after stopping a suxamethonium infusion.[1]

Apart from the single unconfirmed report there seems to be little other reason for avoiding concurrent use or for taking particular precautions. However, the US manufacturer of dexpanthenol recommends that it should not be given within one hour of suxamethonium.[2]

1. Smith RM, Gottshall SC, Young JA. Succinylcholine-pantothenyl alcohol: a reappraisal. *Anesth Analg* (1969) 48, 205–208.
2. Dexpanthenol Injection. American Regent, Inc. US Prescribing information, January 2003.

Neuromuscular blockers; Vecuronium + Clonidine

There is limited evidence to suggest that clonidine modestly increases the duration of action of vecuronium.

Clinical evidence, mechanism, importance and management

In a study in 16 surgical patients, 8 patients took oral clonidine 4 micrograms/kg to 5.5 micrograms/kg 90 minutes before their operation. Anaesthesia was induced by thiamylal, and maintained with nitrous oxide/oxygen and isoflurane supplemented by fentanyl. Clonidine increased the duration of neuromuscular blockade following the use of vecuronium by 26%, when compared with the patients not taking clonidine.[1]

The reasons for this modest increase in neuromuscular blockade are not understood. The clinical importance of this interaction would appear to be small.

1. Nakahara T, Akazawa T, Kinoshita Y, Nozaki J. The effect of clonidine on the duration of vecuronium-induced neuromuscular blockade in humans. *Jpn J Anesthesiol* (1995) 44, 1458–63.

Neuromuscular blockers; Vecuronium + Lansoprazole

There is some evidence to suggest that lansoprazole increases the duration of action of vecuronium.

Clinical evidence, mechanism, importance and management

In a study of 50 adult surgical patients, half of whom received lansoprazole 30 mg the night before their operation, it was found that there was no difference between the time to onset of neuromuscular blockade by vecuronium in the two groups, but lansoprazole increased the duration of neuromuscular blockade by about 34%.[1] This interaction needs confirmation and the clinical relevance requires assessment, although given patients would be routinely monitored it seems likely to be small.

1. Ahmed SM, Panja C, Khan RM, Bano S. Lansoprazole potentiates vecuronium paralysis. *J Indian Med Assoc* (1997) 95, 422–3.

6

Analgesics and NSAIDs

The drugs dealt with in this section include aspirin and other salicylates, NSAIDs, opioid analgesics, and the miscellaneous analgesics, such as nefopam and paracetamol. 'Table 6.1', p.139 contains a listing, with a further classification of the NSAIDs.

Interactions

(a) Aspirin and NSAIDs

Aspirin and the NSAIDs generally undergo few clinically significant pharmacokinetic interactions. The majority are highly protein bound, and have the potential to interact with other drugs via this mechanism. However, with a few exceptions, most of these interactions are not clinically important (see 'Protein-binding interactions', p.3).

Of the newer NSAIDs, celecoxib is metabolised by the cytochrome P450 isoenzyme CYP2C9, and inhibits CYP2D6. Rofecoxib, now withdrawn, inhibits CYP1A2, see 'Tizanidine + CYP1A2 inhibitors', p.1588. Nevertheless, most of the important interactions with NSAIDs and aspirin are pharmacodynamic. Aspirin and all non-selective NSAIDs inhibit platelet aggregation, and so can increase the risk of bleeding and interact with other drugs that have this effect. NSAIDs that are highly selective for cyclo-oxygenase-2 (COX-2) do not inhibit platelet aggregation.

Aspirin and all NSAIDs (including COX-2 selective NSAIDs) affect the synthesis of renal prostaglandins, and so can cause salt and water retention. This can increase blood pressure and affect antihypertensive therapy.

Aspirin and non-selective NSAIDs inhibit the mechanisms that protect the gastrointestinal mucosa and so cause gastrointestinal toxicity. COX-2 selective NSAIDs (coxibs) are less likely to have this effect, but they can still cause gastrointestinal toxicity.

(b) Opioids

Morphine is metabolised by glucuronidation by UDP-glucuronosyltransferases, mainly to one active and one inactive metabolite. The glucuronidation of morphine can be induced or inhibited by various drugs. Morphine is not notably affected by cytochrome P450 isoenzymes. The semi-synthetic morphine analogues, hydromorphone and oxymorphone, are metabolised similarly. Buprenorphine is metabolised by CYP3A4, and tramadol is metabolised by CYP3A4 and CYP2D6, although the importance of CYP3A4 in tramadol metabolism is unclear. Pethidine (meperidine) is metabolised by several cytochrome P450 isoenzymes. If the metabolism of pethidine is increased it can lead to increased production of the potentially neurotoxic metabolite, norpethidine, and increased CNS adverse effects.

1. Codeine and related drugs. Codeine, dihydrocodeine, and hydrocodone are thought to be prodrugs, and require metabolic activation, possibly by CYP2D6 or glucuronosyltransferases. Inhibitors of these enzymes might therefore reduce their efficacy. Oxycodone is also metabolised by CYP2D6 and CYP3A4. See 'Opioids; Codeine and related drugs + Quinidine', p.194 for further discussion and for the effect of metaboliser status.

2. Fentanyl and related drugs. Alfentanil is extensively metabolised by CYP3A4, and has been used as a probe drug for assessing CYP3A4 activity. Fentanyl and sufentanil are also metabolised by CYP3A4, but because they are high hepatic-extraction drugs (see 'Changes in first-pass metabolism', p.4) they are less affected by inhibitors or inducers of CYP3A4, although in some instances this might still lead to clinically important effects.

3. Methadone. The metabolism of methadone is unclear. Historically several cytochrome P450 isoenzymes were implicated, including CYP3A4, CYP2B6, and CYP2D6, with CYP2C8, CYP2C9, and CYP2C19 also possibly being involved. However, the role of CYP3A4 has become less certain (see 'Opioids; Methadone + HIV-protease inhibitors', p.182 for an unexpected effect of ritonavir), and that of CYP2B6 is emerging (see 'Opioids + Ticlopidine', p.197).

(c) Paracetamol

Paracetamol is not absorbed from the stomach, and the rate of absorption is well correlated with the gastric emptying rate. Paracetamol has therefore been used as a marker drug in studies of gastric emptying. Paracetamol is primarily metabolised by the liver to a variety of metabolites, principally the glucuronide and sulfate conjugates. Hepatotoxicity of paracetamol is thought to be due to a minor metabolite, *N*-acetyl-p-benzoquinone imine (NAPQI), which is inactivated with glutathione and excreted as mercapturate and cysteine conjugates. When the liver stores of glutathione are depleted, and the rate of production of NAPQI exceeds the rate of production of glutathione, excess NAPQI attaches to liver proteins and causes liver damage. CYP2E1 may be involved in the formation of this hepatotoxic metabolite.

1. Brouwers JRBJ, de Smet PAGM. Pharmacokinetic-pharmacodynamic drug interactions with nonsteroidal anti-inflammatory drugs. *Clin Pharmacokinet* (1994) 27, 462–5.
2. Rumack BH. Acetaminophen hepatotoxicity: the first 35 years. *J Toxicol Clin Toxicol* (2002) 40, 3–20.
3. Armstrong AC, Cozza KL. Pharmacokinetic drug interactions of morphine, codeine, and their derivatives: theory and clinical reality, Part I. *Psychosomatics* (2003) 44, 167–71.
4. Armstrong AC, Cozza KL. Pharmacokinetic drug interactions of morphine, codeine, and their derivatives: theory and clinical reality, Part II. *Psychosomatics* (2003) 44, 515–20.
5. Shiran MR, Lennard MS, Iqbal MZ, Lagundoye O, Seivewright N, Tucker GT, Rostami-Hodjegan A. Contribution of the activities of CYP3A, CYP2D6, CYP1A2 and other potential covariates to the disposition of methadone in patients undergoing methadone maintenance treatment. *Br J Clin Pharmacol* (2009) 67, 29–37.
6. Kharasch ED, Stubbert K. Role of cytochrome P4502B6 in methadone metabolism and clearance. *J Clin Pharmacol* (2013) 53, 305–13.

Table 6.1 Analgesics and NSAIDs

Group	*Drugs*
Aspirin and oral salicylates	Aloxiprin, Aspirin, Benorilate, Choline salicylate, Diflunisal, Ethenzamide, Lysine aspirin, Magnesium salicylate, Salsalate, Sodium salicylate
NSAIDs	
Fenamates	Floctafenine, Flufenamic acid, Meclofenamic acid, Mefenamic acid, Tolfenamic acid
Indole- and indene-acetic acids	Acemetacin, Etodolac, Indometacin, Sulindac
Oxicams	Lornoxicam, Meloxicam, Piroxicam, Tenoxicam
Phenylacetic acid derivatives	Aceclofenac, Alclofenac, Diclofenac
Propionic acid derivatives	Dexibuprofen, Dexketoprofen, Fenbufen, Fenoprofen, Flurbiprofen, Ibuprofen, Ketoprofen, Naproxen, Oxaprozin, Tiaprofenic acid
Pyrazolone derivatives	Azapropazone, Feprazone, Kebuzone, Metamizole sodium (Dipyrone), Oxyphenbutazone, Phenylbutazone
Selective inhibitors of cyclo-oxygenase-2 (Coxibs)	Celecoxib, Etoricoxib, Lumiracoxib, Meloxicam (see under *Oxicams*), Parecoxib, Rofecoxib, Valdecoxib
Other	Benzydamine hydrochloride, Felbinac, Ketorolac, Nabumetone, Nimesulide, Phenazone (Antipyrine), Tolmetin
Opioid and related analgesics	
Anaesthetic adjuncts	Alfentanil, Fentanyl, Remifentanil, Sufentanil
Mild to moderate pain	Codeine, Dextropropoxyphene (Propoxyphene), Dihydrocodeine
Moderate to severe pain:	
Partial agonists and agonists/antagonists	Buprenorphine (also used for opioid dependence), Butorphanol, Meptazinol, Nalbuphine, Pentazocine
Pure agonists	Dextromoramide, Diamorphine (Heroin), Dipipanone, Hydrocodone, Hydromorphone, Methadone (also used for opioid dependence), Morphine, Oxycodone, Oxymorphone, Papaveretum, Pethidine (Meperidine), Tapentadol, Tramadol
Miscellaneous	Nefopam, Paracetamol (Acetaminophen)

Aspirin or other Salicylates + Antacids

The serum salicylate levels of patients taking large, anti-inflammatory doses of aspirin or other salicylates can be reduced to subtherapeutic levels by some antacids. The maximum plasma levels of single doses of aspirin may be increased by giving an antacid, although the extent of absorption is unaltered.

Clinical evidence

A study in 10 healthy subjects found that the mean maximum plasma level of a single 650-mg dose of aspirin was about 70% higher when it was given 10 minutes after an antacid (**aluminium/magnesium hydroxide**), when compared with aspirin alone. However, there was no change in the time to reach the peak level or the AUC. There were also no significant changes in the pharmacokinetics of the metabolites, salicylic acid and salicyluric acid.[1]

A child with rheumatic fever taking aspirin 600 mg five times daily had a serum salicylate level of between 82 and 118 mg/L while taking 30 mL of *Maalox* (**aluminium/magnesium hydroxide** suspension). When the *Maalox* was withdrawn, the urinary pH fell from a range of 7 to 8 down to a range of 5 to 6.4, whereupon the serum salicylate level rose three- to fourfold to about 380 mg/L, which required a dose reduction.[2] An associated study in 13 healthy subjects taking aspirin 4 g daily for a week found that **sodium bicarbonate** 4 g daily reduced serum salicylate levels by 44%, from 270 mg/L to 150 mg/L. This reflected a rise in the urinary pH from a range of 5.6 to 6.1 up to around 6.2 to 6.9.[2,3]

Similar changes have been reported in other studies with:

- aspirin or **choline salicylate** and **aluminium/magnesium hydroxide**;
- aspirin and **magnesium trisilicate/aluminium hydroxide**;
- aspirin or **sodium salicylate** and **sodium bicarbonate**.[4-8]

There is some evidence to suggest that this effect does not occur at low serum salicylate levels,[5,6] or if the pH of the urine is unchanged by the antacid.[6]

Mechanism

Aspirin and other salicylates are acidic compounds that are excreted by the kidney tubules and are ionised in solution. In alkaline solution, much of the drug exists in the ionised form, which is not readily reabsorbed, and therefore is lost in the urine. If the urine is made more acidic (e.g. with ammonium chloride), much more of the drug exists in the un-ionised form, which is readily reabsorbed, so that less is lost in the urine and the drug is retained in the body.[7,8]

In vitro data show that magnesium oxide and aluminium hydroxide strongly adsorb aspirin and sodium salicylate.[9] However, in three of the studies above aluminium hydroxide-containing antacids had no effect on the extent of absorption of salicylate,[1,4,6] although the rate of absorption may be increased as a result of an increase in the solubility of salicylate in a less acidic gastric environment.[1]

Importance and management

A well established and clinically important interaction for those receiving long-term treatment with large doses of salicylates, because the serum salicylate level may become subtherapeutic. This interaction can occur with both 'systemic' antacids (e.g. sodium bicarbonate) as well as some 'non-systemic' antacids (e.g. aluminium/magnesium hydroxide), but only appears to occur if there is an increase in the urinary pH. Care should be taken to monitor serum salicylate levels if any antacid is started or stopped in patients where the control of salicylate levels is critical.

No important adverse interaction would be expected in those taking occasional doses of aspirin for analgesia. Some aspirin formulations actually include antacids as buffering agents to increase absorption rates and raise peak serum levels,[10] which gives more rapid analgesia, and/or in an attempt to decrease gastric irritation. Note that antacids may also increase the rate of absorption of aspirin given as enteric-coated tablets.[11]

1. Itthipanichpong C, Sirivongs P, Wittayalertpunya S, Chaiyos N. The effect of antacid on aspirin pharmacokinetics in healthy Thai volunteers. *Drug Metabol Drug Interact* (1992) 10, 213–28.
2. Levy G. Interaction of salicylates with antacids. In: Blondheim SH, Alkan WJ, Brunner D, eds. Frontiers of Internal Medicine. 12th Int Congr Intern Med, Tel Aviv, 1974. Basel: Karger; 1975 p. 404–8.
3. Levy G, Leonards JR. Urine pH and salicylate therapy. *JAMA* (1971) 217, 81.
4. Levy G, Lampman T, Kamath BL, Garrettson LK. Decreased serum salicylate concentration in children with rheumatic fever treated with antacid. *N Engl J Med* (1975) 293, 323–5.
5. Hansten PD, Hayton WL. Effect of antacid and ascorbic acid on serum salicylate concentration. *J Clin Pharmacol* (1980) 20, 326–31.
6. Shastri RA. Effect of antacids on salicylate kinetics. *Int J Clin Pharmacol Ther Toxicol* (1985) 23, 480–4.
7. Macpherson CR, Milne MD, Evans BM. The excretion of salicylate. *Br J Pharmacol* (1955) 10, 484–9.
8. Hoffman WS, Nobe C. The influence of urinary pH on the renal excretion of salicyl derivatives during aspirin therapy. *J Lab Clin Med* (1950) 35, 237–48.
9. Naggar VF, Khalil SA, Daabis NA. The in-vitro adsorption of some antirheumatics on antacids. *Pharmazie* (1976) 31, 461–5.
10. Nayak RK, Smyth RD, Polk A, Herczeg T, Carter V, Visalli AJ, Reavey-Cantwell NH. Effect of antacids on aspirin dissolution and bioavailability. *J Pharmacokinet Biopharm* (1977) 5, 597–613.
11. Feldman S, Carlstedt BC. Effect of antacid on absorption of enteric-coated aspirin. *JAMA* (1974) 227, 660–1.

Aspirin + Bile-acid binding resins

Colestyramine and colestipol do not appear to have any clinically important effects on the absorption of aspirin.

Clinical evidence, mechanism, importance and management

(a) Colestipol

In 12 healthy subjects the extent of absorption of a single 650-mg dose of aspirin was unaffected by colestipol 10 g. However, the rate of aspirin absorption was increased by colestipol: at 60 minutes after the dose the plasma level was increased by about 40%.[1] No particular precautions seem to be necessary during concurrent use.

(b) Colestyramine

A study in 3 healthy subjects and 3 patients, and a later study in 7 healthy subjects, found that colestyramine 4 g delayed the absorption of a single 500-mg dose of aspirin (time to peak levels extended from 30 to 60 minutes) but the total amount absorbed was only reduced by 5 to 6%. Some of the subjects had slightly higher serum aspirin levels while taking colestyramine.[2] Similar results were reported in another study (a 31% lower plasma aspirin level at 60 minutes, but no difference in total absorption).[1] There would seem to be little reason for avoiding concurrent use unless rapid analgesia is needed.

1. Hunninghake DB, Pollack E. Effect of bile acid sequestering agents on the absorption of aspirin, tolbutamide, and warfarin. *Fedn Proc* (1977) 35, 996.
2. Hahn K-J, Eiden W, Schettle M, Hahn M, Walter E, Weber E. Effect of cholestyramine on the gastrointestinal absorption of phenprocoumon and acetylosalicylic acid in man. *Eur J Clin Pharmacol* (1972) 4, 142–5.

Aspirin or other Salicylates + Carbonic anhydrase inhibitors

A severe and even life-threatening toxic reaction can occur in patients taking high-dose salicylates if they are given carbonic anhydrase inhibitors, such as acetazolamide or diclofenamide.

Clinical evidence

An 8-year-old boy with chronic juvenile arthritis, taking prednisolone, indometacin and **aloxiprin**, was admitted to hospital with drowsiness, vomiting and hyperventilation (diagnosed as metabolic acidosis) within a month of the **aloxiprin** dose being increased from 3 to 3.6 g daily and starting to take **diclofenamide** 25 mg three times daily for glaucoma.[1]

Other cases of toxicity (metabolic acidosis) have included a 22-year-old woman taking **salsalate** with **acetazolamide** 250 mg four times daily,[1] and two elderly women taking large doses of aspirin with **acetazolamide** or **diclofenamide**.[2] A 50-year-old woman taking **acetazolamide** for glaucoma was admitted to hospital with confusion and cerebellar ataxia, associated with hyperchloraemic acidosis, 14 days after starting to take aspirin for acute pericarditis.[3] A man taking **diclofenamide** developed salicylate poisoning within 10 days of starting to take aspirin 3.9 g daily.[4] Coma developed in an 85-year-old woman taking aspirin 3.9 g daily when her dosage of **acetazolamide** was increased from 500 mg to 1 g daily,[5,6] and toxicity was seen in a very elderly man given both drugs: levels of unbound **acetazolamide** were found to be unusually high.[6] An elderly man became confused, lethargic, incontinent and anorexic while taking **acetazolamide** and **salsalate**. He needed intravenous hydration.[7]

Mechanism

Not fully established. One idea is that these carbonic anhydrase inhibitors (acetazolamide, diclofenamide) affect the plasma pH, so that more of the salicylate exists in the un-ionised (lipid-soluble) form, which can enter the CNS and other tissues more easily, leading to salicylate toxicity.[2] However, carbonic anhydrase inhibitors also make the urine more alkaline, which increases the loss of salicylate[8] (see also 'Aspirin or other Salicylates + Antacids', p.140). *Animal* studies confirm that carbonic anhydrase inhibitors increase the lethal toxicity of aspirin.[4] An alternative suggestion is that because salicylate inhibits the plasma protein binding of acetazolamide and its excretion by the kidney, acetazolamide toxicity, which mimics salicylate toxicity, may occur.[6]

Importance and management

Although there are few clinical reports on record, the interaction between carbonic anhydrase inhibitors and salicylates is established, well confirmed by *animal* studies, and potentially serious. One study recommended that carbonic anhydrase inhibitors should probably be avoided in those receiving high-dose salicylate treatment.[6] If they are used, the patient should be well monitored for any evidence of toxicity (confusion, lethargy, hyperventilation, tinnitus) because the interaction may develop slowly and insidiously.[2] In this context NSAIDs may be a safer alternative. Naproxen proved to be a satisfactory substitute in one case.[1] The authors of one study suggest that **methazolamide** may possibly be a safer alternative to acetazolamide because it is minimally bound to plasma proteins. They also suggest paracetamol (acetaminophen) as an alternative to salicylate in patients taking acetazolamide.[6] The reports cited here concern carbonic anhydrase inhibitors given orally, not as eye drops. It is not known whether the latter interact similarly, but there appear to be no reports.

1. Cowan RA, Hartnell GG, Lowdell CP, McLean Baird I, Leak AM. Metabolic acidosis induced by carbonic anhydrase inhibitors and salicylates in patients with normal renal function. *BMJ* (1984) 289, 347–8.
2. Anderson CJ, Kaufman PL, Sturm RJ. Toxicity of combined therapy with carbonic anhydrase inhibitors and aspirin. *Am J Ophthalmol* (1978) 86, 516–19.
3. Hazouard E, Grimbert M, Jonville-Berra A-P, De Toffol M-C, Legras A. Salicylisme et glaucome: augmentation réciproque de la toxicité de l'acétazolamide et de l'acide acétyl salicylique. *J Fr Ophtalmol* (1999) 22, 73–5.
4. Hurwitz GA, Wingfield W, Cowart TD, Jollow DJ. Toxic interaction between salicylates and a carbonic anhydrase inhibitor: the role of cerebral edema. *Vet Hum Toxicol* (1980) 22 (Suppl), 42–4.
5. Chapron DJ, Brandt JL, Sweeny KR, Olesen-Zammett L. Interaction between acetazolamide and aspirin — a possible unrecognized cause of drug-induced coma. *J Am Geriatr Soc* (1984) 32, S18.
6. Sweeney KR, Chapron DJ, Brandt JL, Gomolin IH, Feig PU, Kramer PA. Toxic interaction between acetazolamide and salicylate: case reports and a pharmacokinetic explanation. *Clin Pharmacol Ther* (1986) 40, 518–24.
7. Rousseau P, Fuentevilla-Clifton A. Acetazolamide and salicylate interaction in the elderly: a case report. *J Am Geriatr Soc* (1993) 41, 868–9.
8. Macpherson CR, Milne MD, Evans BM. The excretion of salicylate. *Br J Pharmacol* (1955) 10, 484–9.

Aspirin or other Salicylates + Corticosteroids or Corticotropin

Serum salicylate levels are reduced by the corticosteroids. This appears to be of most consequence if the corticosteroid is withdrawn. Concurrent use increases the risk of gastrointestinal bleeding and ulceration.

Clinical evidence

A 5-year-old boy taking long-term **prednisone** in doses of at least 20 mg daily, was given **choline salicylate** 3.6 g daily, and the **prednisone** was gradually tapered off to 3 mg daily over a 3-month period. Severe salicylate toxicity developed, and in a retrospective investigation of the cause, using frozen serum samples drawn for other purposes, it was found that the serum salicylate levels had risen from less than 100 mg/L up to 880 mg/L during the withdrawal of the **prednisone**.[1] Later studies in 3 other patients taking **choline salicylate** or aspirin and either **prednisone** or another unnamed corticosteroid, found about a threefold rise in salicylate levels during corticosteroid withdrawal.[1] **Hydrocortisone** was also found to increase the clearance of **sodium salicylate** in 4 other patients.[1] A serum salicylate rise has been described in a patient taking **aloxiprin** when **prednisolone** was withdrawn.[2] Other studies in both adults and children show that **prednisone**, **methylprednisolone**, **betamethasone** and **corticotropin** reduce serum salicylate levels.[3-5] Two studies also found that intra-articular **dexamethasone**, **methylprednisolone**, and **triamcinolone** transiently reduced serum salicylate levels in patients given enteric-coated aspirin.[6,7] However one study in patients found that **prednisone** 12 to 60 mg daily had no effect on the clearance of single doses of **sodium salicylate**.[8]

Mechanism

Uncertain. One idea is that the presence of the corticosteroid increases the glomerular filtration rate, which increases salicylate clearance. When the corticosteroid is withdrawn, the clearance returns to normal and the salicylate accumulates. Another suggestion is that the corticosteroids increase the metabolism of the salicylate.[3]

Importance and management

Well established interactions. Patients should be monitored to ensure that salicylate levels remain adequate when corticosteroids are added[4] and do not become excessive if they are withdrawn. It should also be remembered that concurrent use may increase the incidence of gastrointestinal bleeding and ulceration. See also 'Corticosteroids + NSAIDs', p.1256.

1. Klinenberg JR, Miller F. Effect of corticosteroids on blood salicylate concentration. *JAMA* (1965) 194, 601–4.
2. Muirden KD, Barraclough DRE. Drug interactions in the management of rheumatoid arthritis. *Aust N Z J Med* (1976) 6 (Suppl 1), 14–17.
3. Graham GG, Champion GD, Day RO, Paull PD. Patterns of plasma concentrations and urinary excretion of salicylate in rheumatoid arthritis. *Clin Pharmacol Ther* (1977) 22, 410–20.
4. Bardare M, Cislaghi GU, Mandelli M, Sereni F. Value of monitoring plasma salicylate levels in treating juvenile rheumatoid arthritis. *Arch Dis Child* (1978) 53, 381–5.
5. Koren G, Roifman C, Gelfand E, Lavi S, Suria D, Stein L. Corticosteroids-salicylate interaction in a case of juvenile rheumatoid arthritis. *Ther Drug Monit* (1987) 9, 177–9.
6. Edelman J, Potter JM, Hackett LP. The effect of intra-articular steroids on plasma salicylate concentrations. *Br J Clin Pharmacol* (1986) 21, 301–7.
7. Baer PA, Shore A, Ikeman RL. Transient fall in serum salicylate levels following intraarticular injection of steroid in patients with rheumatoid arthritis. *Arthritis Rheum* (1987) 30, 345–7.
8. Day RO, Harris G, Brown M, Graham GG, Champion GD. Interaction of salicylate and corticosteroids in man. *Br J Clin Pharmacol* (1988) 26, 334–7.

Aspirin + Dapsone

Dapsone does not significantly affect the pharmacokinetics of aspirin.

Clinical evidence, mechanism, importance and management

A comparison of the pharmacokinetics of aspirin in 8 healthy subjects and 8 patients with uncomplicated lepromatous leprosy found that the pharmacokinetics of a single 600-mg dose of aspirin was not affected by either leprosy, or by treatment with dapsone 100 mg daily for 8 days.[1] No aspirin dose adjustments would seem likely to be needed on concurrent use.

1. Garg SK, Kumar B, Shukla VK, Bakaya V, Lal R, Kaur S. Pharmacokinetics of aspirin and chloramphenicol in normal and leprotic patients before and after dapsone therapy. *Int J Clin Pharmacol Ther Toxicol* (1988) 26, 204–5.

Aspirin + Food

Food delays the absorption of aspirin.

Clinical evidence, mechanism, importance and management

A study in 25 subjects given aspirin 650 mg in five different preparations found that food roughly halved their serum salicylate levels (measured 10 and 20 minutes later), compared with those seen when the same dose of aspirin was given while fasting.[1] Similar results were found in subjects given calcium aspirin 1.5 g.[2] In another study in 8 healthy subjects who were given effervescent aspirin 900 mg, serum salicylate levels at 15 minutes were roughly halved by food, but were more or less unchanged at one hour.[3]

A further study in 16 healthy subjects found that the extent of absorption of a single 900-mg dose of soluble aspirin was not significantly affected by a high-fat meal. The rate of absorption was reduced by food and the maximum plasma level was reduced by 18%, which was not considered to be clinically significant. Furthermore, there was no statistically significant change in the time to maximum plasma levels (20 minutes fasted; 30 minutes fed).[4]

A possible reason for the reduced rate of absorption is that food delays gastric emptying. Thus, if rapid analgesia is needed, aspirin should be taken without food, but if aspirin is needed long-term, giving it with food is thought to help to protect the gastric mucosa.

1. Wood JH. Effect of food on aspirin absorption. *Lancet* (1967) ii, 212.
2. Spiers ASD, Malone HF. Effect of food on aspirin absorption. *Lancet* (1967) i, 440.
3. Volans GN. Effects of food and exercise on the absorption of effervescent aspirin. *Br J Clin Pharmacol* (1974) 1, 137–41.
4. Stillings M, Havlik I, Chetty M, Clinton C, Schall R, Moodley I, Muir N, Little S. Comparison of the pharmacokinetic profiles of soluble aspirin and solid paracetamol tablets in fed and fasted volunteers. *Curr Med Res Opin* (2000) 16, 115–24.

Aspirin + Griseofulvin

An isolated report describes a marked fall in the serum salicylate levels of a child given aspirin and griseofulvin.

Clinical evidence, mechanism, importance and management

An 8-year-old boy with rheumatic fever taking aspirin 110 mg/kg daily and furosemide, digoxin, captopril, potassium, aluminium/magnesium hydroxide and iron, had a very marked fall in his serum salicylate levels (from a range of 18.3 to 30.6 mg/dL to less than 0.2 mg/dL) within 2 days of starting griseofulvin 10 mg/kg daily. Two days after the griseofulvin was stopped, the salicylate levels were back to their former levels. The reasons for this effect are not known, but it was suggested that the salicylate absorption was impaired in some way.[1] This appears to be the first and only report of this interaction so that its general importance is uncertain.

1. Phillips KR, Wideman SD, Cochran EB, Becker JA. Griseofulvin significantly decreases serum salicylate concentrations. *Pediatr Infect Dis J* (1993) 12, 350–2.

Aspirin + Kaolin-pectin

Kaolin-pectin causes a small reduction in the absorption of aspirin.

Clinical evidence, mechanism, importance and management

In 10 healthy subjects the absorption of aspirin 975 mg was reduced by 5 to 10% by 30 or 60 mL of kaolin-pectin.[1] A likely explanation is that the aspirin becomes adsorbed by the kaolin so that the amount available for absorption through the gut wall is reduced. However, this small reduction in absorption is unlikely to be of clinical importance.

1. Juhl RP. Comparison of kaolin-pectin and activated charcoal for inhibition of aspirin absorption. *Am J Hosp Pharm* (1979) 36, 1097–8.

Aspirin + Laxatives

Sodium sulfate and castor oil used as laxatives can cause a modest reduction in aspirin absorption.

Clinical evidence, mechanism, importance and management

In an experimental study of the possible effects of laxatives on drug absorption, healthy subjects were given 10 to 20 g of oral **sodium sulfate** and 20 g of **castor oil** (doses sufficient to provoke diarrhoea). Absorption, measured by the amount of drug excreted in the urine, was decreased at 4 hours. The reduction was 21% for **castor oil** and aspirin, and 27% for **sodium sulfate** and aspirin. However, serum levels of aspirin were relatively unchanged. The overall picture was that while these laxatives can alter the pattern of absorption, they do not seriously impair the total amount of drug absorbed.[1]

1. Mattila MJ, Takki S, Jussila J. Effect of sodium sulphate and castor oil on drug absorption from the human intestine. *Ann Clin Res* (1974) 6, 19–24.

Aspirin + Levamisole

The salicylate levels of a patient taking aspirin rose when levamisole was given, but this effect was not confirmed in a subsequent controlled study.

Clinical evidence, mechanism, importance and management

A preliminary report of a patient who had an increase in salicylate levels (magnitude not stated) when levamisole was given with aspirin 5.4 g daily[1] prompted a study in 9 healthy subjects of this possible interaction. Sustained-release aspirin 3.9 g daily in two divided doses was given over a period of 3 weeks, with levamisole 50 mg three times daily for a week, each subject acting as his own control. No significant changes in plasma salicylate levels were found.[2] The reasons for the increase in salicylate levels in the case report are unclear. No interaction would generally be expected.

1. Laidlaw D'A. Rheumatoid arthritis improved by treatment with levamisole and L-histidine. *Med J Aust* (1976) 2, 382–5.
2. Rumble RH, Brooks PM, Roberts MS. Interaction between levamisole and aspirin in man. *Br J Clin Pharmacol* (1979) 7, 631–3.

Aspirin + Pentazocine

A man regularly taking large doses of aspirin developed renal papillary necrosis when he was given pentazocine.

Clinical evidence, mechanism, importance and management

An isolated report describes a man, regularly taking aspirin 1.8 to 2.4 g daily, who developed renal papillary necrosis within 6 months of also starting to take pentazocine 800 to 850 mg daily. He developed abdominal pain, nausea and vomiting, and passed tissue via his urethra. Before starting the pentazocine and after it was stopped, no necrosis was apparent. The postulated reason for this reaction is that a pentazocine-induced reduction in blood flow through the kidney potentiated the adverse effects of chronic aspirin use.[1] The general importance of this isolated case is uncertain and no general recommendations can be made.

1. Muhalwas KK, Shah GM, Winer RL. Renal papillary necrosis caused by long-term ingestion of pentazocine and aspirin. *JAMA* (1981) 246, 867–8.

Aspirin + Phenylbutazone

Phenylbutazone reduces the uricosuric effects of high-dose aspirin. Concurrent use is likely to be associated with an increased risk of gastrointestinal damage.

Clinical evidence

The observation that several patients given aspirin and phenylbutazone developed elevated serum urate levels, prompted a study in 4 patients without gout. The study found that aspirin 2 g daily had little effect on the excretion of uric acid in the urine, but marked uricosuria occurred with aspirin 5 g daily. When phenylbutazone 200, 400 and then 600 mg daily (over 3 days) was also given the uricosuria was abolished. Serum uric acid levels rose from an average of about 40 mg/L to 60 mg/L. The interaction was confirmed in a patient with tophaceous gout. The retention of uric acid also occurs if the phenylbutazone is given first.[1]

Mechanism

Not understood. Phenylbutazone is structurally related to sulfinpyrazone, which interacts similarly, see 'Uricosuric drugs + Aspirin or other Salicylates', p.1590.

Importance and management

An established but sparsely documented interaction. The potential problems arising from this interaction should be recognised in any patient given aspirin and phenylbutazone. The concurrent use of aspirin and NSAIDs increases the risk of gastrointestinal damage and is not recommended. Although there does not appear to be any specific evidence for phenylbutazone, it would be expected to interact in the same way as other NSAIDs, see 'NSAIDs + Aspirin', p.145.

1. Oyer JH, Wagner SL, Schmid FR. Suppression of salicylate-induced uricosuria by phenylbutazone. *Am J Med Sci* (1966) 225, 39–45.

Nefopam + Miscellaneous

The concurrent use of nefopam and an MAOI might result in a potentially fatal hypertensive crisis. Nefopam can cause seizures and antimuscarinic adverse effects, which might be additive with other drugs that have these effects, such as the tricyclics. The intensity and incidence of adverse effects (such as sedation) are somewhat increased when nefopam is given with codeine, pentazocine or dextropropoxyphene (propoxyphene), and the CNS depressant effect of dihydrocodeine might have contributed to a fatal overdose with nefopam.

Clinical evidence, mechanism, importance and management

(a) Antidepressants

The UK manufacturer advises caution if nefopam is given with a **tricyclic**[1] presumably as nefopam alone can cause convulsions and the tricyclics can also lower the convulsive threshold. In addition, the antimuscarinic adverse effects of nefopam could be additive with those of the tricyclics and other drugs with antimuscarinic effects[1] (see 'Antimuscarinics + Antimuscarinics', p.754). For example, the CSM in the UK has a number of reports of urinary retention caused by nefopam,[2] which would be expected to be worsened by the concurrent use of other drugs with antimuscarinic activity, such as the tricyclics.

Nefopam appears to have sympathomimetic activity, and therefore the manufacturers state that caution should be used when prescribing other drugs with sympathomimetic effects.[1]

The concurrent use of nefopam with an MAOI might be expected to result in hypertensive crisis (see 'MAOIs or RIMAs + Nasal decongestants and related drugs', p.1396), and the UK manufacturer[1] contraindicates the use of nefopam with an **MAOI**.

(b) Other drugs

The incidence of sedation with nefopam has been reported as 20 to 30% which, depending on the circumstances, could increase the risk of sedation if it is given with other **sedative drugs**.[3] A report describes a fatal overdose with nefopam, which was complicated by the CNS depressant effect of **dihydrocodeine**.[4]

In a study in patients undergoing orthopaedic surgery, intravenous nefopam had a **morphine**-sparing effect (up to 35% dose reduction).[5] However, a further study found that the effects were less than additive.[6] A study in 72 surgical patients found that the use of nefopam with **ketoprofen** had a synergistic analgesic effect.[7]

A study was conducted in 45 healthy subjects divided into nine groups of five, each given oral nefopam 60 mg three times daily for 3 days with **aspirin** 650 mg, **codeine** 60 mg, **diazepam** 5 mg, **dextropropoxyphene (propoxyphene)** 65 mg, **hydroxyzine** 50 mg, **indometacin** 25 mg, **pentazocine** 50 mg, **phenobarbital** 60 mg, or placebo (all three times daily). The only changes were a possible additive increase in the intensity and incidence of adverse effects with nefopam and **codeine**, **pentazocine** or **dextropropoxyphene**. There was no evidence that the bioavailability of nefopam was changed by the other drugs.[8]

1. Acupan (Nefopam hydrochloride). Meda Pharmaceuticals. UK Summary of product characteristics, February 2010.
2. Committee on Safety of Medicines (CSM). Nefopam hydrochloride (Acupan). Current Problems No 24, January 1989.
3. Heel RC, Brogden RN, Pakes GE, Speight TM, Avery GS. Nefopam: a review of its pharmacological properties and therapeutic efficacy. *Drugs* (1980) 19, 249–67.
4. Urwin SC, Smith HS. Fatal nefopam overdose. *Br J Anaesth* (1999) 83, 501–2.
5. Du Manoir B, Aubrun F, Langlois M, Le Guern ME, Alquier C, Chauvin M, Fletcher D. Randomized prospective study of the analgesic effect of nefopam after orthopaedic surgery. *Br J Anaesth* (2003) 91, 836–41.
6. Beloeil H, Delage N, Nègre I, Mazoit J-X, Benhamou D. The median effective dose of nefopam and morphine administered intravenously for postoperative pain after minor surgery: a prospective randomized double-blinded isobolographic study of their analgesic action. *Anesth Analg* (2004) 98, 395–400.
7. Delage N, Maaliki H, Beloeil H, Benhamou D, Mazoit J-X. Median effective dose (ED_{50}) of nefopam and ketoprofen in postoperative patients: a study of interaction using sequential analysis and isobolographic analysis. *Anesthesiology* (2005) 102, 1211–16.
8. Lasseter KC, Cohen A, Back EL. Nefopam HCl interaction study with eight other drugs. *J Int Med Res* (1976) 4, 195–201.

NSAIDs + Allopurinol

Allopurinol does not affect indometacin clearance or phenylbutazone levels.

Clinical evidence, mechanism, importance and management

In a study in 8 patients, allopurinol 300 mg each morning was given with **indometacin** 50 mg every 8 hours for 5 days. The allopurinol had no significant effect on the AUC of **indometacin** and the amounts of **indometacin** excreted in the urine were not significantly altered.[1]

Allopurinol 100 mg three times daily for a month had no effect on the elimination of **phenylbutazone** 200 mg daily in 6 healthy subjects, and no effect on the steady-state plasma levels of **phenylbutazone** 200 or 300 mg daily in 3 patients.[2] In another study in 8 patients with acute gouty arthritis it was found that allopurinol 100 mg every 8 hours produced a small but clinically unimportant effect on the half-life of **phenylbutazone** 6 mg/kg.[3]

There seems to be no pharmacokinetic reason for avoiding the concurrent use of these NSAIDs and allopurinol.

1. Pullar T, Myall O, Haigh JRM, Lowe JR, Dixon JS, Bird HA. The effect of allopurinol on the steady-state pharmacokinetics of indomethacin. *Br J Clin Pharmacol* (1988) 25, 755–7.
2. Rawlins MD, Smith SE. Influence of allopurinol on drug metabolism in man. *Br J Pharmacol* (1973) 48, 693–8.
3. Horwitz D, Thorgeirsson SS, Mitchell JR. The influence of allopurinol and size of dose on the metabolism of phenylbutazone in patients with gout. *Eur J Clin Pharmacol* (1977) 12, 133–6.

NSAIDs + Amoxicillin

A study in healthy subjects found that diclofenac increased the clearance of amoxicillin. An isolated report describes acute interstitial nephritis with nephrotic syndrome associated with the use of naproxen and amoxicillin.

Clinical evidence, mechanism, importance and management

(a) Diclofenac

In a study in 20 healthy subjects, diclofenac 100 mg caused a slight reduction in the AUC and a slight increase in the mean renal clearance of a single 2-g dose of amoxicillin.[1] It should be noted that there was considerable individual variation and overlapping between the two groups, and the clinical significance of this finding is unclear.

(b) Naproxen

A man without any previous renal problems developed acute interstitial nephritis with nephrotic syndrome after taking naproxen for 4 days (total 4 g) and amoxicillin for 10 days (total 24 g). He appeared to recover when the drugs were stopped, but 3 months later he developed renal failure and needed haemodialysis.[2] Acute interstitial nephritis is not only a rare syndrome (reported to be only 55 cases in the world literature in 1988)[2] but this is the first case involving both of these drugs. No special precautions would normally seem to be necessary.

1. de Cássia Bergamaschi C, Motta RHL, Franco GCN, Cogo K, Montan MF, Ambrosano GMB, Rosalen PL, de Sá Del Fiol F, Groppo FC. Effect of sodium diclofenac on the bioavailability of amoxicillin. *Int J Antimicrob Agents* (2006) 27, 417–22.
2. Nortier J, Depierreux M, Bourgeois V, Dupont P. Acute interstitial nephritis with nephrotic syndrome after intake of naproxen and amoxycillin. *Nephrol Dial Transplant* (1990) 5, 1055.

NSAIDs + Anabolic steroids

Serum oxyphenbutazone levels are raised by methandienone (methandrostenolone). Phenylbutazone appears to be unaffected.

Clinical evidence

The serum levels of **oxyphenbutazone** 300 to 400 mg daily for 2 to 5 weeks were raised by 43% (range 5 to 100%) in 6 subjects given **methandienone** (**methandrostenolone**).[1] Two other studies confirm this interaction with **oxyphenbutazone**.[2,3] One of them found no interaction with **phenylbutazone**.[2]

Mechanism

Uncertain. One idea is that the anabolic steroids alter the distribution of oxyphenbutazone between the tissues and plasma so that more remains in circulation. There may also possibly be some changes in metabolism.

Importance and management

The interaction is established but its importance is uncertain. There seem to be no reports of toxicity arising from concurrent use but the possibility should be borne in mind.

1. Weiner M, Siddiqui AA, Shahani RT, Dayton PG. Effect of steroids on disposition of oxyphenbutazone in man. *Proc Soc Exp Biol Med* (1967) 124, 1170–3.
2. Hvidberg E, Dayton PG, Read JM, Wilson CH. Studies of the interaction of phenylbutazone, oxyphenbutazone and methandrostenolone in man. *Proc Soc Exp Biol Med* (1968) 129, 438–43.
3. Weiner M, Siddiqui AA, Bostanci N, Dayton PG. Drug interactions.The effect of combined administration on the half-life of coumarin and pyrazolone drugs in man. *Fedn Proc* (1965) 24, 153.

NSAIDs; Azapropazone + Antacids or Laxatives

A study in 15 patients taking azapropazone 300 mg three times daily found that antacids (dihydroxyaluminium sodium carbonate, aluminium magnesium silicate), bisacodyl or anthraquinone laxatives only caused a minor (5 to 7%) reduction in azapropazone plasma levels.[1] No special precautions would seem to be needed if any of these drugs are given together with azapropazone.

1. Faust-Tinnefeldt G, Geissler HE, Mutschler E. Azapropazon-Plasmaspiegel unter Begleitmedikation mit einem Antacidum oder Laxans. *Arzneimittelforschung* (1977) 27, 2411–14.

NSAIDs; Coxibs + Antacids

Aluminium/magnesium-containing antacids had no clinically significant effect on the bioavailability of celecoxib,[1,2] or lumiracoxib.[3] Aluminium/magnesium hydroxides or calcium carbonate had no clinically significant effect on the pharmacokinetics of etoricoxib.[4]

Antacids do not appear to affect meloxicam pharmacokinetics, see 'NSAIDs; Oxicam derivatives + Antacids', p.145.

1. Celebrex (Celecoxib). Pfizer Ltd. UK Summary of product characteristics, January 2013.
2. Celebrex (Celecoxib). Pfizer Inc. US Prescribing information, June 2009.
3. Scott G, Vinluan Reynolds C, Milosavljev S, Langholff W, Shenouda M, Rordorf C. Lack of effect of omeprazole or of an aluminium hydroxide/magnesium hydroxide antacid on the pharmacokinetics of lumiracoxib. *Clin Pharmacokinet* (2004) 43, 341–8.
4. Schwartz JI, Agrawal NGB, Kher UA, DeSmet M, Cavanaugh PF, Guillaume M, Ebel DL, Merschman SA, Wagner JA. Lack of effect of antacids on single-dose pharmacokinetics of etoricoxib. *J Clin Pharmacol* (2007) 47, 1342–6.

NSAIDs; Diclofenac + Antacids

The absorption of diclofenac is not affected by aluminium hydroxide and/or magnesium hydroxide.

Clinical evidence, mechanism, importance and management

In a study in 7 healthy subjects, about 10 mL of a 5.8% suspension of **aluminium hydroxide** had no effect on the bioavailability of a single 50-mg dose of diclofenac.[1] In another study, in 6 healthy, fasted subjects, 10 mL of **magnesium hydroxide** suspension (850 mg) was found to have no significant effect on the rate or extent of absorption of a single 50-mg dose of diclofenac.[2] However, there was a tendency to an increased rate of absorption. *Aluco Gel* (**aluminium/magnesium hydroxide**) had no effect on the extent of absorption of enteric-coated diclofenac, but it may have reduced the rate of absorption.[3] No particular precautions would seem to be needed if these antacids are given with diclofenac.

1. Schumacher A, Faust-Tinnefeldt G, Geissler HE, Gilfrich HJ, Mutschler E. Untersuchungen potentieller Interaktionen von Diclofenac-Natrium (Voltaren) mit einem Antazidum und mit Digitoxin. *Therapiewoche* (1983) 33, 2619–25.
2. Neuvonen PJ. The effect of magnesium hydroxide on the oral absorption of ibuprofen, ketoprofen and diclofenac. *Br J Clin Pharmacol* (1991) 31, 263–6.
3. Sioufi A, Stierlin H, Schweizer A, Botta L, Degen PH, Theobald W, Brechbühler S. Recent findings concerning clinically relevant pharmacokinetics of diclofenac sodium. In: Voltarol — New Findings, ed Kass E. Proc Int Symp Voltarol, Paris June 22nd, 1981. 15th Int Congress of Rheumatology. p 19–30.

NSAIDs; Diflunisal + Antacids

Antacids containing aluminium with or without magnesium can reduce the absorption of diflunisal by up to 40%, but no important interaction occurs if food is taken at the same time. Magnesium hydroxide can increase the rate of diflunisal absorption.

Clinical evidence

A study in 4 healthy, fasted subjects found that when a single 500-mg oral dose of diflunisal was given 2 hours before, together with, and 2 hours after three 15-mL doses of *Aludrox* (**aluminium hydroxide**), the diflunisal AUC was reduced by about 40%.[1] Another study found that the AUC of a single 500-mg dose of diflunisal was reduced by 13% when it was given with a single 30-mL dose of *Maalox* (**aluminium/magnesium hydroxide**), by 21% when it was given 1 hour after the antacid, and by 32% when the antacid was given four times daily.[2] However, in another study, **aluminium/magnesium hydroxide** had no effect on the AUC diflunisal when the diflunisal was given 30 minutes after food.[3] This study also found that the AUC of diflunisal was reduced by 26% by 15 mL of **aluminium hydroxide** gel in fasted subjects, but was not affected in fed subjects.[3] **Magnesium hydroxide** suspension markedly increased the rate of diflunisal absorption in fasted subjects. The plasma diflunisal level was increased by 130% at 30 minutes, and by 64% at one hour but the AUC was only increased by a modest 10%.[3]

Mechanism

It is unclear how aluminium antacids reduce the absorption of diflunisal, but adsorption or the formation of insoluble salts has been suggested. Food appears to diminish the effect of antacids on diflunisal absorption.[3] By raising the pH, magnesium hydroxide may promote the dissolution of diflunisal, so increasing its absorption.[3]

Importance and management

Aluminium-containing antacids appear to reduce the absorption of diflunisal in the fasted state, but not if the diflunisal is taken with food. NSAIDs should be taken with or after food to minimise gastrointestinal adverse effects, and so it would appear that this interaction has little clinical relevance.

Magnesium hydroxide increases the absorption of diflunisal in the fasted state, which may improve the onset of analgesia. However, note that magnesium hydroxide increased the endoscopically-detected gastric toxicity of ibuprofen in one study, see 'NSAIDs; Ibuprofen and related drugs + Antacids', p.144.

1. Verbeeck R, Tjandramaga TB, Mullie A, Verbesselt R, De Schepper PJ. Effect of aluminium hydroxide on diflunisal absorption. *Br J Clin Pharmacol* (1979) 7, 519–22.
2. Holmes GI, Irvin JD, Schrogie JJ, Davies RO, Breault GO, Rogers JL, Huber PB, Zinny MA. Effects of Maalox on the bioavailability of diflunisal. *Clin Pharmacol Ther* (1979) 25, 229.
3. Tobert JA, DeSchepper P, Tjandramaga TB, Mullie A, Buntinx AP, Meisinger MAP, Huber PB, Hall TLP, Yeh KC. Effect of antacids on the bioavailability of diflunisal in the fasting and postprandial states. *Clin Pharmacol Ther* (1981) 30, 385–9.

NSAIDs; Fenamates + Antacids

Magnesium hydroxide increases the rate of absorption of mefenamic acid and tolfenamic acid in fasted subjects. The rate of tolfenamic acid absorption is reduced by aluminium hydroxide alone or combined with

magnesium hydroxide/magnesium carbonate, but is not affected by sodium bicarbonate.

Clinical evidence

Studies in 6 healthy, fasted subjects given a single dose of **mefenamic acid** 500 mg or **tolfenamic acid** 400 mg found that **magnesium hydroxide** increased the rate of the absorption of both drugs (the **mefenamic acid** AUC after 1 hour was increased threefold and the **tolfenamic acid** AUC was increased sevenfold) but the total bioavailability was only slightly increased. In contrast, **aluminium hydroxide**, alone and in combination with **magnesium hydroxide/magnesium carbonate** (*Medisan Forte*), markedly *reduced* the rate of absorption of **tolfenamic acid**, but similarly, the total amount absorbed was not markedly changed. In this study **sodium bicarbonate** 1 g did not significantly alter the absorption of **tolfenamic acid**.[1]

Mechanism

Uncertain. It is suggested that magnesium hydroxide increases the solubility of acidic drugs such as the fenamates, possibly by forming a soluble salt and therefore enhancing their dissolution. In contrast, aluminium antacids may form insoluble salts of the drug. Note that food may reduce these effects, see 'NSAIDs; Diflunisal + Antacids', p.143.

Importance and management

Information is limited but it would appear that if rapid analgesia is needed with either mefenamic acid or tolfenamic acid, magnesium hydroxide can be given concurrently but aluminium hydroxide should be avoided. However, note that this applies to the fasted state, whereas NSAIDs are usually taken with or after food. Also note that magnesium hydroxide increased the endoscopically-detected gastric toxicity of ibuprofen in one study, see 'NSAIDs; Ibuprofen and related drugs + Antacids', below. Sodium bicarbonate does not interact.

1. Neuvonen PJ, Kivistö KT. Effect of magnesium hydroxide on the absorption of tolfenamic and mefenamic acids. *Eur J Clin Pharmacol* (1988) 35, 495–501.

NSAIDs; Ibuprofen and related drugs + Antacids

Magnesium hydroxide increased the initial absorption of ibuprofen and flurbiprofen, but had no effect on ketoprofen absorption. Unexpectedly, a pharmacodynamic study found increased gastric erosions when ibuprofen was formulated with magnesium hydroxide.

The absorption of dexketoprofen, fenoprofen, flurbiprofen and ibuprofen were not significantly affected by aluminium/magnesium hydroxide. Aluminium phosphate had no effect on ketoprofen absorption. Aluminium hydroxide caused a small reduction in ketoprofen absorption but had no effect on the bioavailability of tiaprofenic acid.

The rate of naproxen absorption is increased by sodium bicarbonate and aluminium/magnesium hydroxide, but decreased by aluminium hydroxide and magnesium oxide.

Simeticone did not affect ketoprofen bioavailability.

Clinical evidence

(a) Dexketoprofen

In 24 healthy subjects an **aluminium/magnesium hydroxide** antacid (*Maalox*) had no effect on the rate or extent of absorption of a single 25-mg dose of dexketoprofen, although the maximum level was slightly (13%) lower.[1]

(b) Fenoprofen

In a study in 6 subjects plasma levels of a single 600-mg dose of fenoprofen were not affected by a single 30-mL dose of *Maalox* (**aluminium/magnesium hydroxide**).[2]

(c) Flurbiprofen

In a group of young and old fasting healthy subjects, *Maalox* (**aluminium/magnesium hydroxide**) 30 mL, taken 30 minutes before a single 100-mg dose of flurbiprofen, was found to affect neither the rate nor extent of flurbiprofen absorption. Similarly, *Maalox* had no effect on steady-state pharmacokinetics of flurbiprofen when both drugs were given 90 minutes before food.[3] Another study, in fasted subjects, found that **magnesium hydroxide** increased the AUC_{0-2} of flurbiprofen by 61%, but the AUC_{0-8} was not changed, which indicated an increased rate of flurbiprofen absorption.[4]

(d) Ibuprofen

In 8 healthy, fasted subjects an antacid containing **aluminium/magnesium hydroxide**, given before, with, and after a single 400-mg dose of ibuprofen, did not alter the pharmacokinetics of ibuprofen.[5] In another study, the absorption of ibuprofen formulated with **aluminium** was delayed and reduced, when compared to that of ibuprofen without **aluminium**.[6]

A study in 6 healthy fasted subjects found that **magnesium hydroxide** 850 mg increased the AUC_{0-1} and the peak levels of a single 400-mg dose of ibuprofen by 65% and 31%, respectively. The time to the peak was shortened by about 30 minutes but the total bioavailability was unchanged.[7] In a pharmacodynamic study in healthy subjects, a 400-mg ibuprofen tablet buffered with 200 mg of **magnesium hydroxide**, given at a dose of two tablets three times daily for 5 days resulted in about a threefold increase in number of endoscopically-detected gastric erosions, when compared with the same dose of conventional ibuprofen tablets.[8]

A **sodium/potassium salt** (kanwa), often taken as an antacid in some West African countries, appeared to reduce the absorption of ibuprofen. The bioavailability of ibuprofen 400 mg given to 6 healthy subjects with a millet meal containing the salt extract (pH of 8.9) was reduced by about 80%, when compared with either the millet meal alone (pH 5.3) or following overnight fasting.[9]

(e) Ketoprofen

Five healthy, fasted subjects had a 22% reduction in the absorption of a 50-mg dose of ketoprofen (as measured by the amount excreted in the urine) when they were given a 1-g dose of **aluminium hydroxide**.[10] In 10 patients, **aluminium phosphate** 11 g (as a single then a daily dose) had no effect on the pharmacokinetics of ketoprofen 100 mg.[11]

A study in 12 healthy, fasted subjects showed that [activated] dimeticone (**simeticone**) did not significantly affect the bioavailability of a single 100-mg dose of ketoprofen.[12]

In one study, 10 mL of **magnesium hydroxide** suspension (equivalent to 850 mg) was found to have no significant effect on the rate or extent of absorption of ketoprofen 50 mg in fasted subjects, although the rate of ketoprofen absorption was already noted to be fast.[7]

(f) Naproxen

In a study in 14 healthy, fasted subjects, **sodium bicarbonate** 700 mg or 1.4 g increased the rate of absorption of a single 300-mg dose of naproxen, whereas **magnesium oxide** or **aluminium hydroxide** 700 mg reduced the rate of absorption. **Magnesium carbonate** had little effect.[13] On the other hand when 15 or 60 mL of **aluminium/magnesium hydroxide** (*Maalox*) was given, the rate and extent of absorption of naproxen were slightly increased.[13]

(g) Tiaprofenic acid

In a study in 7 healthy subjects, **aluminium hydroxide** did not affect the pharmacokinetics of **tiaprofenic acid**.[14]

Mechanism

Magnesium hydroxide appears to improve the rate of absorption of some acidic NSAIDs (which become more soluble as the pH rises) such as ibuprofen and flurbiprofen. An *in vitro* study found that magnesium hydroxide increased ibuprofen solubility, and increased the dissolution rate of 3 ibuprofen tablet formulations, with the greatest increase occurring with the slowest dissolving product.[15] Why this increased the gastric toxicity of ibuprofen in the one pharmacodynamic study is unclear.[8] Sodium bicarbonate appears to have a similar effect on rate of absorption. An *in vitro* study found that an insoluble ibuprofen salt was formed in the presence of aluminium ions[15] and this may explain why the rate/extent of absorption of some NSAIDs is reduced.

Importance and management

It would appear that the initial absorption of both ibuprofen and flurbiprofen is increased by magnesium hydroxide, but not if aluminium hydroxide is present as well. Thus if rapid analgesia is needed, consider using an antacid containing magnesium hydroxide but without aluminium hydroxide. However, the unexpected finding that magnesium hydroxide increased the endoscopically-detected gastric toxicity of ibuprofen[8] suggests that caution may be warranted, particularly on long-term use. Further study is needed.

The rate of naproxen absorption appears to be increased by sodium bicarbonate and decreased by aluminium hydroxide. However, note that these effects were seen in the fasted state, and may not apply when the NSAID is taken with or after food (as is recommended), as is the case with diflunisal (see 'NSAIDs; Diflunisal + Antacids', p.143).

No particular precautions would seem to be needed if simeticone, aluminium phosphate or magnesium hydroxide are given with ketoprofen, and it seems doubtful if the effects of ketoprofen will be reduced to any great extent by aluminium hydroxide.

1. McEwen J, De Luca M, Casini A, Gich I, Barbanoj MJ, Tost D, Artigas R, Mauleón D. The effect of food and an antacid on the bioavailability of dexketoprofen trometamol. *J Clin Pharmacol* (1998) 38 (Suppl), 41S–45S.
2. Chernish SM, Rubin A, Rodda BE, Ridolfo AS, Gruber CM. The physiological disposition of fenoprofen in man. IV. The effects of position of subject, food ingestion and antacid ingestion on the plasma levels of orally administered fenoprofen. *J Med* (1972) 3, 249–57.
3. Caillé G, du Souich P, Vézina M, Pollock SR, Stalker DJ. Pharmacokinetic interaction between flurbiprofen and antacids in healthy volunteers. *Biopharm Drug Dispos* (1989) 10, 607–15.
4. Rao TRK, Ravisekhar K, Shobha JC, Sekhar EC, Naidu MUR, Krishna DR. Influence of magnesium hydroxide on the oral absorption of flurbiprofen. *Drug Invest* (1992) 4, 473–6.
5. Gontarz N, Small RE, Comstock TJ, Stalker DJ, Johnson SM, Willis HE. Effect of antacid suspension on the pharmacokinetics of ibuprofen. *Clin Pharm* (1987) 6, 413–16.
6. Laska EM, Sunshine A, Marrero I, Olson N, Siegel C, McCormick N. The correlation between blood levels of ibuprofen and clinical analgesic response. *Clin Pharmacol Ther* (1986) 40, 1–7.
7. Neuvonen PJ. The effect of magnesium hydroxide on the oral absorption of ibuprofen, ketoprofen and diclofenac. *Br J Clin Pharmacol* (1991) 31, 263–6.
8. Mäenpää J, Tarpila A, Jouhikainen T, Ikävalko H, Löyttyniemi E, Perttunen K, Neuvonen PJ, Tarpila S. Magnesium hydroxide in ibuprofen tablet reduces the gastric mucosal tolerability of ibuprofen. *J Clin Gastroenterol* (2004) 38, 41–5.
9. Yakasai IA. Effect of sodium/potassium salt (potash) on the bioavailability of ibuprofen in healthy human volunteers. *Eur J Drug Metab Pharmacokinet* (2003) 28, 93–9.
10. Ismail FA, Khalafallah N, Khalil SA. Adsorption of ketoprofen and bumadizone calcium on aluminium-containing antacids and its effect on ketoprofen bioavailability in man. *Int J Pharmaceutics* (1987) 34, 189–96.
11. Brazier JL, Tamisier JN, Ambert D, Bannier A. Bioavailability of ketoprofen in man with and without concomitant administration of aluminium phosphate. *Eur J Clin Pharmacol* (1981) 19, 305–7.

12. Presle N, Lapicque F, Gillet P, Herrmann M-A, Bannwarth B, Netter P. Effect of dimethicone (polysilane gel) on the stereoselective pharmacokinetics of ketoprofen. *Eur J Clin Pharmacol* (1998) 54, 351–4.
13. Segre EJ, Sevelius H, Varady J. Effects of antacids on naproxen absorption. *N Engl J Med* (1974) 291, 582–3.
14. Mareček N, Lücker PW, Penth B, Altmayer P, Wetzelsberger K. Zur Pharmakokinetik von Tiaprofensäure und zur Frage der Interaktion mit ASS und Aluminiumhydroxid. *Arzneimittelforschung* (1981) 31, 116–20.
15. Parojčić J, Corrigan OI. Rationale for ibuprofen co-administration with antacids: potential interaction mechanisms affecting drug absorption. *Eur J Pharm Biopharm* (2008) 69, 640–7.

NSAIDs; Indometacin or Sulindac + Antacids

A variety of different antacids have been found to slightly alter the absorption of indometacin. Aluminium/magnesium hydroxide does not affect sulindac absorption.

Clinical evidence

In 12 healthy, fasted subjects the AUC of a single 50-mg dose of indometacin was reduced by 35% when formulated with 80% *Mergel* and by 18% when taken with 90% *Mergel*. *Mergel* contains **aluminium/magnesium hydroxide** and **magnesium carbonate**.[1]

In another single-dose study, in 6 healthy, fasted subjects, **aluminium hydroxide** suspension 700 mg reduced the rate of indometacin absorption, and reduced the peak indometacin plasma levels. Conversely, **sodium bicarbonate** 1.4 g appeared to increase the rate of absorption, but this did not reach significance because of wide inter-individual variation.[2] In a further study 30 mL of **aluminium/magnesium hydroxide** caused only slight changes in the absorption of a 50-mg dose of indometacin in fasted subjects.[3]

The manufacturer of sulindac notes that an antacid (**aluminium/magnesium hydroxide** suspension) had no effect on the extent of the absorption of sulindac.[4]

Mechanism

Not known. Aluminium compounds might form insoluble salts with indometacin.[2] Food might reduce this effect, see 'NSAIDs; Diflunisal + Antacids', p.143.

Importance and management

Adequately but not extensively documented interactions. Some reduction in indometacin levels is possible with some aluminium-containing antacids, but given the magnitude of this effect this interaction is unlikely to be clinically relevant. Sulindac absorption is not affected.

1. Galeazzi RL. The effect of an antacid on the bioavailability of indomethacin. *Eur J Clin Pharmacol* (1977) 12, 65–8.
2. Garnham JC, Kaspi T, Kaye CM and Oh VMS. The different effects of sodium bicarbonate and aluminium hydroxide on the absorption of indomethacin in man. *Postgrad Med J* (1977) 53, 126–9.
3. Emori HW, Paulus H, Bluestone R, Champion GD, Pearson C. Indomethacin serum concentrations in man. Effects of dosage, food and antacid. *Ann Rheum Dis* (1976) 35, 333–8.
4. Clinoril (Sulindac). Merck & Co., Inc. US Prescribing information, August 2009.

NSAIDs; Miscellaneous + Antacids

The rate and extent of absorption of ketorolac, dipyrone and tolmetin were not significantly affected by aluminium/magnesium hydroxide. Nabumetone absorption was not affected by aluminium hydroxide, and an unspecified antacid did not affect etodolac absorption.

Clinical evidence

(a) Dipyrone (Metamizole sodium)

The concurrent use of 20 mL of *Maaloxan* (**aluminium/magnesium hydroxide** gel) was reported to have had no effect on the pharmacokinetics of the metabolites of dipyrone.[1]

(b) Etodolac

A study in 18 healthy, fasted subjects found that when they were given a single 400-mg dose of etodolac with 30 mL of an unnamed antacid both the rate and the extent of etodolac absorption were unchanged.[2]

(c) Ketorolac

In 12 healthy, fasted subjects the AUC of oral ketorolac 10 mg was found to be reduced by 11% (not statistically significant) when it was taken with an unstated amount of **aluminium/magnesium hydroxide** suspension (*Maalox*). The rate of absorption was not affected.[3]

(d) Nabumetone

In 15 healthy, fasted subjects, the absorption of a single 1-g dose of nabumetone (as assessed by AUC and maximum plasma level) was not significantly altered by 160 mL of **aluminium hydroxide** suspension (*Aludrox*).[4]

(e) Tolmetin

A pharmacokinetic study in 24 healthy, fasted subjects found that **aluminium/magnesium hydroxide** suspension (*Maalox*), given as a single 20-mL dose four times daily for 3 days, had no significant effect on the absorption of a single 400-mg dose of **tolmetin**.[5]

Mechanism

None.

Importance and management

Although information is limited, no particular precautions would seem to be needed if aluminium or aluminium/magnesium antacids are given with any of these antacids. Note that antacids have been frequently given with NSAIDs to reduce their gastric irritant effects.

1. Levy M, Zylber-Katz E, Rosenkranz B. Clinical pharmacokinetics of dipyrone and its metabolites. *Clin Pharmacokinet* (1995) 28, 216–34.
2. Troy S, Sanda M, Dressler D, Chiang S, Latts J. The effect of food and antacid on etodolac bioavailability. *Clin Pharmacol Ther* (1990) 47, 192.
3. Mroszczak EJ, Jung D, Yee J, Bynum L, Sevelius H, Massey I. Ketorolac tromethamine pharmacokinetics and metabolism after intravenous, intramuscular, and oral administration in humans and animals. *Pharmacotherapy* (1990) 10 (Suppl 6), 33S–39S.
4. von Schrader HW, Buscher G, Dierdorf D, Mügge H, Wolf D. Nabumetone — a novel anti-inflammatory drug: the influence of food, milk, antacids, and analgesics on bioavailability of single oral doses. *Int J Clin Pharmacol Ther Toxicol* (1983) 21, 311–21.
5. Ayres JW, Weidler DJ, MacKichan J, Sakmar E, Hallmark MR, Lemanowicz EF, Wagner JG. Pharmacokinetics of tolmetin with and without concomitant administration of antacid in man. *Eur J Clin Pharmacol* (1977) 12, 421–8.

NSAIDs; Oxicam derivatives + Antacids

The pharmacokinetics of lornoxicam, meloxicam, piroxicam and tenoxicam are not affected by aluminium/magnesium hydroxide antacids. Lornoxicam pharmacokinetics were also not altered by tripotassium dicitratobismuthate or aluminium hydroxide with calcium carbonate.

Clinical evidence, mechanism, importance and management

(a) Lornoxicam

In a study in 18 healthy, fasted subjects, either 10 mL of *Maalox* (**aluminium/magnesium hydroxide**) or 10 g of *Solugastril* (**aluminium hydroxide** with **calcium carbonate**) had no effect on the pharmacokinetics of a 4-mg lornoxicam film-coated tablet.[1] A later study similarly found no changes in the absorption or pharmacokinetics of a lornoxicam film-coated tablet given with **tripotassium dicitratobismuthate** 120 mg twice daily.[2] There would seem to be no reason for avoiding concurrent use.

(b) Meloxicam

In a randomised, crossover study 9 healthy, fasted subjects were given meloxicam 30 mg alone or with *Maalox* suspension (**aluminium/magnesium hydroxide** 900/600 mg) four times daily for 4 days. *Maalox* had no significant effect on the pharmacokinetics of meloxicam.[3] Therefore no adjustments of the dose of meloxicam are needed if given with this type of antacid.

(c) Piroxicam

A multiple-dose study in 20 healthy subjects found that *Mylanta* (**aluminium/magnesium hydroxide**) and *Amphojel* (**aluminium hydroxide**) did not significantly affect the bioavailability of piroxicam 20 mg daily taken after food.[4] Concurrent use need not be avoided.

(d) Tenoxicam

The bioavailability of tenoxicam 20 mg was found to be unaffected in 12 healthy subjects by **aluminium hydroxide** (*Amphojel*) or **aluminium/magnesium hydroxide** (*Mylanta*) whether taken before, with, or after the tenoxicam, and in the fasted state or with food.[5] No special precautions seem necessary.

1. Dittrich P, Radhofer-Welte S, Magometschnigg D, Kukovetz WR, Mayerhofer S, Ferber HP. The effect of concomitantly administered antacids on the bioavailability of lornoxicam, a novel highly potent NSAID. *Drugs Exp Clin Res* (1990) 16, 57–62.
2. Ravic M, Johnston A, Turner P, Foley K, Rosenow D. Does bismuth chelate influence lornoxicam absorption? *Hum Exp Toxicol* (1992) 11, 59–60.
3. Busch U, Heinzel G, Narjes H, Nehmiz G. Interaction of meloxicam with cimetidine, Maalox or aspirin. *J Clin Pharmacol* (1996) 36, 79–84.
4. Hobbs DC, Twomey TM. Piroxicam pharmacokinetics in man: aspirin and antacid interaction studies. *J Clin Pharmacol* (1979) 19, 270–81.
5. Day RO, Lam S, Paull P, Wade D. Effect of food and various antacids on the absorption of tenoxicam. *Br J Clin Pharmacol* (1987) 24, 323–8.

NSAIDs + Aspirin

There is some evidence that non-selective NSAIDs such as ibuprofen antagonise the antiplatelet effects of low-dose aspirin, but that COX-2-selective NSAIDs (coxibs) do not. Some, but not other, epidemiological studies have shown that non-selective NSAIDs reduce the cardioprotective effects of low-dose aspirin. Furthermore, some NSAIDs (particularly coxibs) are associated with increased thrombotic risk and possibly increased risk of death if used in patients with a history of myocardial infarction. The combined use of NSAIDs and low-dose aspirin increases the risk of gastrointestinal bleeds. This seems to apply equally to coxibs.

The combined use of analgesic-dose aspirin and NSAIDs increases the risk of gastrointestinal damage. There are numerous early pharmacoki-

Table 6.2 Summary of studies on the effect of NSAIDs on the cardioprotective effect of antiplatelet-dose aspirin

Study type	*Criteria*	*Outcome*	*Drugs (Number of patients)*	*Comments*	*Refs*
Studies showing a decrease in the cardioprotection of aspirin with NSAIDs					
Retrospective cohort	Discharge after CVD	Mortality	Aspirin alone (6285) Aspirin with Ibuprofen (187) Aspirin with Diclofenac (206) Aspirin with other NSAID (429)	Increased all-cause mortality and cardiovascular mortality in those taking aspirin with ibuprofen compared with the other groups.	1
Subgroup analysis of an RCT	Male physicians randomised to aspirin 325 mg on alternate days or placebo	First MI	Aspirin alone (5273) Aspirin with intermittent NSAID (5147) Aspirin with regular NSAID (598)	Use of NSAIDs for 60 days or more per year was associated with an increased risk of MI in those taking aspirin.	2
Case-control		First non-fatal MI	Aspirin alone (694) Aspirin with NSAIDs (170) NSAIDs alone (128)	Both aspirin alone, and NSAIDs alone were associated with a reduced risk of MI, but combined use was not.	3
Studies showing no effect of NSAIDs on the cardioprotection of aspirin					
Retrospective cohort	Discharge after MI	Death in first year	Aspirin alone (36211) NSAID alone (736) Aspirin with NSAID (2096) Neither (9541)	Risk of death reduced to a similar extent by aspirin, NSAIDs, and the combination.	4
Retrospective cohort	Discharge after MI and on aspirin	Death in first year	Aspirin alone (66739) Aspirin with Ibuprofen (844) Aspirin with other NSAID (2733)	Risk of death comparable between the 3 groups.	5
Retrospective cohort	General Practice Research Database	Acute MI or death from coronary heart disease	NSAID alone (417) NSAID with Aspirin (163) Aspirin alone (1119) Non-NSAID users (1878)	Incidence of acute MI unaffected by NSAID alone. NSAID with aspirin similar to aspirin alone.	6
Studies showing an increase in the cardioprotection of aspirin with NSAIDs					
Retrospective cohort	Two consecutive prescriptions for aspirin or ibuprofen	Biochemical evidence of MI	Aspirin alone (10239) Aspirin with Ibuprofen (3859)	The aspirin alone group experienced 0.0044 MIs per patient month, compared with 0.0026 in the aspirin with ibuprofen group.	7

1. MacDonald TM, Wei L. Effect of ibuprofen on cardioprotective effect of aspirin. *Lancet* (2003) 361, 573-4.
2. Kurth T, Glynn RJ, Walker AM, Chan KA, Buring JE, Hennekens CH, Gaziano JM. Inhibition of clinical benefits of aspirin on first myocardial infarction by nonsteroidal antiinflammatory drugs. *Circulation* (2003) 108, 1191-5.
3. Kimmel SE, Berlin JA, Reilly M, Jaskowiak J, Kishel L, Chittams J, Strom BL. The effects of nonselective non-aspirin non-steroidal anti-inflammatory medications on the risk of nonfatal myocardial infarction and their interaction with aspirin. *J Am Coll Cardiol* (2004) 43, 985-90.
4. Ko D, Wang Y, Berger AK, Radford MJ, Krumholz HM. Nonsteroidal antiinflammatory drugs after acute myocardial infarction. *Am Heart J* (2002) 143, 475-81.
5. Curtis JP, Wang Y, Portnay EL, Masoudi FA, Havranek EP, Krumholz HM. Aspirin, ibuprofen, and mortality after myocardial infarction: retrospective cohort study. *BMJ* (2003) 327, 1322-3.
6. García Rodríguez LA, Varas-Lorenzo C, Maguire A, González-Pérez A. Nonsteroidal antiinflammatory drugs and the risk of myocardial infarction in the general population. *Circulation* (2004) 109, 3000-6.
7. Patel TN,Goldberg KC. Use of aspirin and ibuprofen compared with aspirin alone and the risk of myocardial infarction. *Arch Intern Med* (2004) 164, 852-6.

netic studies of aspirin and NSAIDs, many of which found that aspirin reduced the levels of NSAIDs.

Clinical evidence

A. Cardioprotective effects

A number of pharmacodynamic studies have investigated whether or not NSAIDs affect the antiplatelet effects of low-dose aspirin. **Celecoxib** 200 mg twice daily,[1-3] **diclofenac** 75 mg twice daily,[4] **etoricoxib** 120 mg daily,[5] **lumiracoxib** 400 mg daily,[6] **meloxicam** 15 mg daily,[7] **parecoxib** 40 mg twice daily,[8] **rofecoxib** 25 mg daily,[4] and **sulindac** 200 mg twice daily[3] have all been shown not to alter the antiplatelet effects of aspirin in doses of 75 to 325 mg daily. **Naproxen**,[3,9] **indometacin**,[3] and **tiaprofenic acid**[3] may antagonise the antiplatelet effects of aspirin. The effects of **ibuprofen** are less clear, and may be related to the order of drug administration.[4]

As a consequence of the evidence from a number of pharmacodynamic studies, various cohort/case-control studies or sub-group analyses have been conducted to see if **ibuprofen** and/or other NSAIDs reduce the cardioprotective effect of low-dose aspirin in patients, see 'Table 6.2', above. Because these studies are neither prospective nor randomised, their findings are only suggestive, nevertheless they provide some useful insight. In addition to these studies, there are a number of controlled studies that specifically investigated the effects of using aspirin and ibuprofen.

Ibuprofen

A placebo-controlled, randomised study in patients taking aspirin 100 mg daily long-term for its cardioprotective effects found that ibuprofen 600 mg three times daily for 7 days reduced the antiplatelet effects of aspirin.[2] Further, another placebo-controlled study in healthy subjects found that ibuprofen 400 mg every 12 hours for 3 doses antagonised the antiplatelet effects of a 300-mg dose of soluble aspirin.[3] In a prospective, randomised study, 47 healthy subjects were given aspirin 81 mg daily for 8 days, and then either ibuprofen 400 mg or placebo three times daily (1, 7 and 13 hours after the aspirin dose) for 10 days. No clinically meaningful loss of the cardioprotective effects of low-dose aspirin (as measured by thromboxane B_2 inhibition) occurred with this ibuprofen regimen. However, the authors noted that the continued use of ibuprofen for longer than 10 days might possibly have resulted in a clinically relevant interaction.[10]

B. Gastrointestinal effects

(a) Low-dose aspirin

Low-dose aspirin alone (300 mg or less daily) was associated with an increased risk of hospitalisation for bleeding peptic ulcer in a case-control study. The odds ratios were 2.3 for aspirin 75 mg daily, 3.2 for aspirin 150 mg daily, and 3.9 for aspirin 300 mg daily. Use of NSAIDs combined with low-dose aspirin was associated with a greater risk of bleeding (odds ratio 7.7) than use of either NSAIDs alone (5.4) or low-dose aspirin alone (3.3).[11] Similar findings were reported in a cohort study (rate ratio for gastrointestinal bleed for low-dose aspirin 2.6, and for combined use with NSAIDs 5.6).[12]

A case-control study found that coxib use alone was associated with a lower risk of upper gastrointestinal bleeding than that found with non-selective NSAIDs. However, when coxibs were given with low-dose aspirin, the gastrointestinal advantage tended to disappear.[13] Patients taking low-dose aspirin (325 mg or less daily) with **celecoxib** had a higher frequency of gastrointestinal complications than those taking **celecoxib** alone. Moreover, there was no difference in the frequency of gastrointestinal complications between those taking low-dose aspirin with **celecoxib** and those taking low-dose aspirin with **ibuprofen** or **diclofenac**. This was despite **celecoxib** alone being associated with a lower frequency of gastrointestinal adverse effects than **ibuprofen** or **diclofenac** alone.[14] Similar results were found with **rofecoxib** 25 mg daily, which increased the incidence of ulcers in patients taking enteric-coated aspirin 81 mg daily.[15]

(b) Analgesic-dose aspirin

In a case-control study of data from 1993 to 1998 in the UK General Practice Research Database the risk of upper gastrointestinal bleeding or perforation was increased by slightly more than an additive effect in patients taking both aspirin and NSAIDs (8.2-fold), when compared with aspirin alone (2.4-fold), or NSAIDs alone (3.6-fold). The specific NSAIDs were not mentioned.[16] Another study provided similar findings,[17] as have studies specifically looking at low-dose aspirin (325 mg or less daily), see above. Analysis of Yellow Card reports to the CSM in the UK of gastrointestinal perforation/obstruction, ulceration or bleeding with **diclofenac**, **naproxen**, and **ibuprofen** revealed that 28% of the patients were receiving concurrent aspirin (dose not stated).[18]

The one pharmacodynamic study (see below), that also measured gastrointestinal blood loss, found increased bleeding when anti-inflammatory doses of aspirin were given with **sodium meclofenamate**.[6]

A case report described acute ulcerative colitis in a woman taking **rofecoxib** 25 mg daily who also took aspirin.[19]

C. Pharmacokinetic and Pharmacodynamic studies

Early studies evaluating non-aspirin NSAIDs in rheumatoid arthritis commonly permitted the concurrent use of aspirin, which was then in wide use for this condition. The unexpected finding that **indometacin** was no more effective than placebo in patients taking aspirin in one study led to a number of pharmacokinetic studies with this combination (see *Indometacin*, below), and subsequently other NSAID/aspirin combinations. These studies generally have little clinical relevance to current clinical practice where anti-inflammatory doses of aspirin should not be used in combination with NSAIDs because of the increased risk of gastrointestinal bleeding (see above) and lack of proven additional benefit. However, the pharmacokinetic studies are briefly summarised below.

(a) Diclofenac

Aspirin 900 mg reduced the AUC of diclofenac 50 mg by about one-third in a single-dose study.[20] In a clinical study, there was no significant difference in efficacy between diclofenac 50 mg three times daily alone or with aspirin 900 mg three times daily.[21]

(b) Fenamates

A study in 20 healthy subjects given aspirin 600 mg and **sodium meclofenamate** 100 mg both three times daily for 14 days found no significant reductions in plasma salicylate levels, but plasma **meclofenamate** levels were reduced to some extent. However, gastrointestinal blood loss was approximately doubled compared with either drug alone.[22]

(c) Ibuprofen and related drugs

Aspirin 1.3 to 3.6 g daily more than halved the serum levels of ibuprofen 800 mg to 2.4 g daily,[23,24] without affecting salicylate levels.[24] There was little additional clinical benefit from the combination.[24] Similarly, aspirin reduced the AUC of **flurbiprofen** by about two-thirds,[25] but without any clear changes in clinical effectiveness.[26] The pharmacokinetics of the aspirin were unchanged by **flurbiprofen**.[25] Aspirin 3.9 g daily also virtually halved the AUC of **fenoprofen** 2.4 g daily,[27] and reduced the AUC of **ketoprofen** 200 mg daily[28] by about one-third. The AUC of **naproxen** was only minimally reduced (by 10 to 15%).[29,30] **Choline magnesium trisalicylate** increased the clearance of **naproxen** by 56% and decreased its serum levels by 26% in one study.[31]

(d) Indometacin

The overall picture with aspirin and indometacin is confusing and contradictory. One early study found that indometacin had no additional benefit in patients already taking aspirin.[32] Consequently, a number of studies were conducted to see if there was a drug interaction. Some studies reported that aspirin reduced serum indometacin levels[27,33-35] or its efficacy,[36] or that the combination was no more effective than either drug alone.[37] Others report that no change in indometacin levels occurred.[38-40] Further studies using buffered aspirin claimed that it increased the rate of absorption of indometacin and was associated with an increase in adverse effects (tiredness, lack of coordination).[41,42] One study found that indometacin 50 mg given as suppositories at night was found to have a significant additive effect when given with slow-release aspirin 2 or 4.5 g daily, estimated by articular index and subjective ratings of pain and morning stiffness. However, the dose of aspirin (most often the 4.5 g dose) had to be reduced in 7 of the 24 treatment periods due to adverse effects.[43]

(e) Oxicams

Aspirin 3 g daily increased the maximum plasma levels of **meloxicam** 30 mg daily by 25% and its AUC by 10%.[44] Plasma levels of **piroxicam** 40 mg then 20 mg daily were not significantly affected by aspirin 3.9 g daily, and salicylate levels were unaffected by **piroxicam**.[45] Aspirin 2.6 to 3.9 g daily more than halved the serum levels of **tenoxicam** 20 mg daily.[46]

(f) Miscellaneous NSAIDs

Aspirin 600 mg four times daily caused a 15% reduction in the plasma levels of **diflunisal** 250 mg twice daily for 3 days.[47] Single-dose studies have shown that the absorption of **nabumetone** 1 g is not significantly altered by aspirin 1.5 g.[48] The plasma levels of **tolmetin** 1.2 g daily were slightly reduced by aspirin 3.9 g daily.[49]

Mechanism

Aspirin irreversibly blocks the production of thromboxane A2 by binding to cyclo-oxygenase (COX-1) in platelets, and so inhibits platelet aggregation. The beneficial cardiovascular effects are attributed to this effect. Other NSAIDs that are COX-1 inhibitors also have this effect, but it is more short-lived since they bind reversibly. These NSAIDs can therefore competitively inhibit the binding of aspirin to platelets (a fact that was shown *in vitro* as early as the 1980s[50]). When these NSAIDs are present in sufficient quantities when a daily low-dose of aspirin is given, they therefore reduce its antiplatelet effect. *In vitro* study confirms that COX-2 selective NSAIDs have less effect.[51]

The damaging effects of aspirin and NSAIDs on the gut appear to be additive. This occurs even at the low doses of aspirin used for antiplatelet effects (doses as low as 75 mg daily).[11] The mechanisms behind the pharmacokinetic changes have not been resolved. Changes in the rates of absorption and renal clearance and competition for plasma protein binding have been proposed.

Importance and management

A. Cardioprotective effects

The evidence currently available on the antagonism of the antiplatelet effects of aspirin by ibuprofen is conflicting. However, the FDA in the US warn that ibuprofen may interfere with the antiplatelet effects of low-dose aspirin and reduce its cardioprotective benefits. Until definitive clinical information is available, they recommend that patients taking immediate-release, low-dose aspirin (81 mg daily) should take the aspirin 30 minutes before or 8 hours after taking ibuprofen to prevent any possible interaction. The recommendation applies to patients taking ibuprofen chronically but does not apply to those taking enteric-coated aspirin formulations.[52] Others have concluded that ibuprofen is more likely to interact with aspirin than not, and that the interaction is more likely to occur in those who take ibuprofen long-term and more importantly in those at high cardiovascular risk.[53] It has also been suggested that non-selective NSAIDs should be avoided in patients taking low-dose aspirin, or that it may be advisable to replace aspirin with an alternative antiplatelet drug.[54] A coxib has been suggested as an alternative to non-selective NSAIDs in patients taking low-dose aspirin for cardioprotection who require long-term NSAIDs for inflammatory conditions,[55] but the subsequent findings of an increased risk of serious cardiovascular effects with the coxibs (as a class[56]) probably precludes this. In 2006 the CHM in the UK advised that there may be a small increased risk of thrombotic events with the non-selective NSAIDs, particularly when used at high doses and for long-term treatment.[57] In addition, the European Society of Cardiology guidelines recommend that patients resistant to antiplatelet treatment should not be given either coxibs or non-selective NSAIDs with either aspirin or clopidogrel.[58]

Further, a retrospective analysis of 58 432 patients discharged from hospital after a first myocardial infarction found that the subsequent use of coxibs in all doses and non-selective NSAIDs in high doses resulted in increased mortality.[59] On the basis of this and other studies, the European Society of Cardiology guidelines recommend that coxibs and NSAIDs should not be used in the post myocardial infarction period.[58] Some have concluded that when patients taking low-dose aspirin for cardioprotection require long-term NSAIDs for inflammatory conditions, the use of diclofenac would seem preferable to ibuprofen.[55] However, a review by the European Medicines Agency identified a small increased risk of arterial thrombotic events with diclofenac, compared with other NSAIDs. In some cases this has resulted in heart attack or stroke, particularly if diclofenac is used at a high-dose or for long-term treatment. They state that the risk is similar to that for coxibs, and therefore contraindicate the use of diclofenac in patients with ischaemic heart disease, peripheral arterial disease, cerebrovascular disease, or congestive heart failure.[60]

For further information on the concurrent use of NSAIDs with other antiplatelet drugs, such as clopidogrel, see 'Clopidogrel and related drugs + NSAIDs', p.788.

B. Gastrointestinal effects

The additive risk of gastrointestinal damage from combining aspirin and NSAIDs is established. Because of this, and because of the lack of clear benefit from the combination, the use of anti-inflammatory/analgesic doses of aspirin with NSAIDs should be avoided. With antiplatelet-dose aspirin, from a gastrointestinal perspective, the lowest dose of aspirin should be used (75 mg).[11] However, when combined with low-dose aspirin, the available evidence indicates that there is no gastrointestinal benefit to be obtained from using a coxib instead of diclofenac or ibuprofen.[14] Note that the CSM in the UK advised that the combination of a non-aspirin NSAID and low-dose aspirin should be used only if absolutely necessary.[18,61] They stated that patients taking long-term aspirin should be reminded to avoid NSAIDs, including those bought without prescription.[61] If concurrent use is necessary, where appropriate, the use of a proton pump inhibitor may be considered for prophylaxis of NSAID-induced gastro-intestinal damage. Note also that the European Society of Cardiology advises against the use of anti-inflammatory drugs post-myocardial infarction (see A above).

1. Wilner KD, Rushing M, Walden C, Adler R, Eskra J, Noveck R, Vargas R. Celecoxib does not affect the antiplatelet activity of aspirin in healthy volunteers. *J Clin Pharmacol* (2002) 42, 1027–30.
2. Renda G, Tacconelli S, Capone ML, Sacchetta D, Santarelli F, Sciulli MG, Zimarino M, Grana M, D'Amelio E, Zurro M, Price TS, Patrono C, De Caterina R, Patrignani P. Celecoxib, ibuprofen, and the antiplatelet effect of aspirin in patients with osteoarthritis and ischemic heart disease. *Clin Pharmacol Ther* (2006) 80, 264–74.
3. Gladding PA, Webster MWI, Farrell HB, Zeng ISL, Park R, Ruijne N. The antiplatelet effect of six non-steroidal anti-inflammatory drugs and their pharmacodynamic interaction with aspirin in healthy volunteers. *Am J Cardiol* (2008) 101, 1060–3.
4. Catella-Lawson F, Reilly MP, Kapoor SC, Cucchiara AJ, De Marco S, Tournier B, Vyas SN, FitzGerald GA. Cyclooxygenase inhibitors and the antiplatelet effects of aspirin. *N Engl J Med* (2001) 345, 1809–17.
5. Arcoxia (Etoricoxib). Merck Sharp & Dohme Ltd. UK Summary of product characteristics, May 2012.
6. Jermany J, Branson J, Schmouder R, Guillaume M, Rordorf C. Lumiracoxib does not affect the ex vivo antiplatelet aggregation activity of low-dose aspirin in healthy subjects. *J Clin Pharmacol* (2005) 45, 1172–8.
7. Van Ryn J, Kink-Eiband M, Kuritsch I, Feifel U, Hanft G, Wallenstein G, Trummlitz G, Pairet M. Meloxicam does not affect the antiplatelet effect of aspirin in healthy male and female volunteers. *J Clin Pharmacol* (2004) 44, 777–84.
8. Noveck RJ, Kuss ME, Qian J, North J, Hubbard RC. Parecoxib sodium, injectable COX-2 specific inhibitor, does not affect aspirin-mediated platelet function. *Reg Anesth Pain Med* (2001) 26 (Suppl), 19.
9. Capone ML, Sciulli MG, Tacconelli S, Grana M, Ricciotti E, Renda G, Di Gregorio P, Merciaro G, Patrignani P. Pharmacodynamic interaction of naproxen with low-dose aspirin in healthy subjects. *J Am Coll Cardiol* (2005) 45, 1295–1301.

10. Cryer B, Berlin RG, Cooper SA, Hsu C, Wason S. Double-blind, randomized, parallel, placebo-controlled study of ibuprofen effects on thromboxane B_2 concentrations in aspirin-treated healthy adult volunteers. *Clin Ther* (2005) 27, 185–91.
11. Weil J, Colin-Jones D, Langman M, Lawson D, Logan R, Murphy M, Rawlins M, Vessey M, Wainwright P. Prophylactic aspirin and risk of peptic ulcer bleeding. *BMJ* (1995) 310, 827–30.
12. Sorensen HT, Mellemkjaer L, Blot WJ, Nielsen GL, Steffensen FH, McLaughlin JK, Olsen JH. Risk of upper gastrointestinal bleeding associated with use of low-dose aspirin. *Am J Gastroenterol* (2000) 95, 2218–24.
13. Lanas A, García-Rodríguez LA, Arroyo MT, Gomollón F, Feu F, González-Pérez A, Zapata E, Bástida G, Rodrigo L, Santolaria S, Güell M, de Argila CM, Quintero E, Borda F, Piqué JM, on behalf of the Investigators of the Asociación Española de Gastroenterología (AEG). Risk of upper gastrointestinal ulcer bleeding associated with selective cyclo-oxygenase-2 inhibitors, traditional non-aspirin non-steroidal anti-inflammatory drugs, aspirin and combinations. *Gut* (2006) 55, 1731–8.
14. Silverstein FE, Faich G, Goldstein JL, Simon LS, Pincus T, Whelton A, Makuch R, Eisen G, Agrawal NM, Stenson WF, Burr AM, Zhao WW, Kent JD, Lefkowith JB, Verburg KM, Geis GS. Gastrointestinal toxicity with celecoxib vs nonsteroidal anti-inflammatory drugs for osteoarthritis and rheumatoid arthritis: the CLASS study: a randomized controlled trial. *JAMA* (2000) 284, 1247–55.
15. Laine L, Maller ES, Yu C, Quan H, Simon T. Ulcer formation with low-dose enteric-coated aspirin and the effect of COX-2 selective inhibition: a double-blind trial. *Gastroenterology* (2004) 127, 395–402.
16. García Rodríguez LA, Hernández-Díaz S. The risk of upper gastrointestinal complications associated with nonsteroidal anti-inflammatory drugs, glucocorticoids, acetaminophen, and combinations of these agents. *Arthritis Res* (2001) 3, 98–101.
17. Mellemkjaer L, Blot WJ, Sørensen HT, Thomassen L, McLaughlin JK, Nielsen GL, Olsen JH. Upper gastrointestinal bleeding among users of NSAIDs: a population-based cohort study in Denmark. *Br J Clin Pharmacol* (2002) 53, 173–81.
18. Committee on Safety of Medicines/Medicines Control Agency. Non-steroidal anti-inflammatory drugs (NSAIDs) and gastrointestinal safety. *Current Problems* (2002) 28, 5.
19. Charachon A, Petit T, Lamarque D, Soulé J-C. Colite aiguë hémorragique chez une malade traitée par rofécoxib associé à une auto-médication par aspirine. *Gastroenterol Clin Biol* (2003) 27, 511–13.
20. Willis JV, Kendall MJ, Jack DB. A study of the effect of aspirin on the pharmacokinetics of oral and intravenous diclofenac sodium. *Eur J Clin Pharmacol* (1980) 18, 415–18.
21. Bird HA, Hill J, Leatham P, Wright V. A study to determine the clinical relevance of the pharmacokinetic interaction between aspirin and diclofenac. *Agents Actions* (1986) 18, 447–9.
22. Baragar FD, Smith TC. Drug interaction studies with sodium meclofenamate (Meclomen®). *Curr Ther Res* (1978) 23 (April Suppl), S51–S59.
23. Albert KS, Gernaat CM. Pharmacokinetics of ibuprofen. *Am J Med* (1984) 77(1A), 40–6.
24. Grennan DM, Ferry DG, Ashworth ME, Kenny RE, Mackinnon M. The aspirin-ibuprofen interaction in rheumatoid arthritis. *Br J Clin Pharmacol* (1979) 8, 497–503.
25. Kaiser DG, Brooks CD, Lomen PL. Pharmacokinetics of flurbiprofen. *Am J Med* (1986) 80 (Suppl 3A), 10–15.
26. Brooks PM, Khong TK. Flurbiprofen-aspirin interaction: a double-blind crossover study. *Curr Med Res Opin* (1977) 5, 53–7.
27. Rubin A, Rodda BE, Warrick P, Gruber CM, Ridolfo AS. Interactions of aspirin with nonsteroidal antiinflammatory drugs in man. *Arthritis Rheum* (1973) 16, 635–45.
28. Williams RL, Upton RA, Buskin JN, Jones RM. Ketoprofen-aspirin interactions. *Clin Pharmacol Ther* (1981) 30, 226–31.
29. Segre EJ, Chaplin M, Forchielli E, Runkel R, Sevelius H. Naproxen-aspirin interactions in man. *Clin Pharmacol Ther* (1974) 15, 374–9.
30. Segre E, Sevelius H, Chaplin M, Forchielli E, Runkel R, Rooks W. Interaction of naproxen and aspirin in the rat and in man. *Scand J Rheumatol* (1973) (Suppl 2), 37–42.
31. Furst DE, Sarkissian E, Blocka K, Cassell S, Dromgoole S, Harris ER, Hirschberg JM, Josephson N, Paulus HE. Serum concentrations of salicylate and naproxen during concurrent therapy in patients with rheumatoid arthritis. *Arthritis Rheum* (1987) 30, 1157–61.
32. The Cooperating Clinics Committee of the American Rheumatism Association. A three-month trial of indomethacin in rheumatoid arthritis, with special reference to analysis and inference. *Clin Pharmacol Ther* (1967) 8, 11–37.
33. Kaldestad E, Hansen T, Brath HK. Interaction of indomethacin and acetylsalicylic acid as shown by the serum concentrations of indomethacin and salicylate. *Eur J Clin Pharmacol* (1975) 9, 199–207.
34. Jeremy R, Towson J. Interaction between aspirin and indomethacin in the treatment of rheumatoid arthritis. *Med J Aust* (1970) 3, 127–9.
35. Kwan KC, Breault GO, Davis RL, Lei BW, Czerwinski AW, Besselaar GH, Duggan DE. Effects of concomitant aspirin administration on the pharmacokinetics of indomethacin in man. *J Pharmacokinet Biopharm* (1978) 6, 451–76.
36. Pawlotsky Y, Chales G, Grosbois B, Miane B, Bourel M. Comparative interaction of aspirin with indomethacin and sulindac in chronic rheumatic diseases. *Eur J Rheumatol Inflamm* (1978) 1, 18–20.
37. Brooks PM, Walker JJ, Bell MA, Buchanan WW, Rhymer AR. Indomethacin—aspirin interaction: a clinical appraisal. *BMJ* (1975) 3, 69–71.
38. Champion D, Mongan E, Paulus H, Sarkissian E, Okun R, Pearson C. Effect of concurrent aspirin (ASA) administration on serum concentrations of indomethacin (I). *Arthritis Rheum* (1971) 14, 375.
39. Lindquist B, Jensen KM, Johansson H, Hansen T. Effect of concurrent administration of aspirin and indomethacin on serum concentrations. *Clin Pharmacol Ther* (1974) 15, 247–52.
40. Barraclough DRE, Muirden KD, Laby B. Salicylate therapy and drug interaction in rheumatoid arthritis. *Aust N Z J Med* (1975) 5, 518–23.
41. Turner P,Garnham JC. Indomethacin-aspirin interaction. *BMJ* (1975) 2, 368.
42. Garnham JC, Raymond K, Shotton E, Turner P. The effect of buffered aspirin on plasma indomethacin. *Eur J Clin Pharmacol* (1975) 8, 107–13.
43. Alván G, Ekstrand R. Clinical effects of indomethacin and additive clinical effect of indomethacin during salicylate maintenance therapy. *Scand J Rheumatol* (1981) Suppl 39, 29–32.
44. Busch U, Heinzel G, Narjes H, Nehmiz G. Interaction of meloxicam with cimetidine, Maalox or aspirin. *J Clin Pharmacol* (1996) 36, 79–84.
45. Hobbs DC, Twomey TM. Piroxicam pharmacokinetics in man: aspirin and antacid interaction studies. *J Clin Pharmacol* (1979) 19, 270–81.
46. Day RO, Paull PD, Lam S, Swanson BR, Williams KM, Wade DN. The effect of concurrent aspirin upon plasma concentrations of tenoxicam. *Br J Clin Pharmacol* (1988) 26, 455–62.
47. Schulz P, Perrier CV, Ferber-Perret F, VandenHeuvel WJA, Steelman SL. Diflunisal, a new-acting analgesic and prostaglandin inhibitor: effect of concomitant acetylsalicylic acid therapy on ototoxicity and on disposition of both drugs. *J Int Med Res* (1979) 7, 61–8.
48. von Schrader HW, Buscher G, Dierdorf D, Mügge H, Wolf D. Nabumetone — a novel anti-inflammatory drug: the influence of food, milk, antacids, and analgesics on bioavailability of single oral doses. *Int J Clin Pharmacol Ther Toxicol* (1983) 21, 311–21.
49. Cressman WA, Wortham GF, Plostnieks J. Absorption and excretion of tolmetin in man. *Clin Pharmacol Ther* (1976) 19, 224–33.
50. Parks WM, Hoak JC, Czervionke RL. Comparative effect of ibuprofen on endothelial and platelet prostaglandin synthesis. *J Pharmacol Exp Ther* (1981) 219, 415–19.
51. Ouellet M, Riendeau D, Percival MD. A high level of cyclooxygenase-2 inhibitor selectivity is associated with a reduced interference of platelet cyclooxygenase-1 inactivation by aspirin. *Proc Natl Acad Sci U S A* (2001) 98, 14583–8.
52. Ellison J, Dager W. Recent FDA warning of the concomitant use of aspirin and ibuprofen and the effects on platelet aggregation. *Prev Cardiol* (2007), 10, 61–3.
53. MacDonald M, Wei L. Is there an interaction between the cardiovascular protective effects of low-dose aspirin and ibuprofen? *Basic Clin Pharmacol Toxicol* (2006) 98, 275–80.
54. Flipo R-M. Les AINS sont-ils susceptibles de compromettre l'efficacité cardiopréventive de l'aspirine? *Presse Med* (2006) 35, (Suppl 1) 53–60.
55. FitzGerald GA. Parsing an enigma: the pharmacodynamics of aspirin resistance. *Lancet* (2003) 361, 542–4.
56. FitzGerald GA. Coxibs and cardiovascular disease. *N Engl J Med* (2004) 351, 1709–11.
57. Commission on Human Medicines. NSAIDs letter to healthcare professionals: Safety of selective and non-selective NSAIDs. October 2006. Available at: http://webarchive.nationalarchives.gov.uk/20141205150130/http://www.mhra.gov.uk/home/groups/pl-p/documents/websiteresources/con2025036.pdf (accessed 22/10/15).
58. Bassand J-P, Hamm CW, Ardissino D, Boersma E, Budaj A, Fernández-Avilés F, Fox KAA, Hasdai D, Ohman EM, Wallentin L, Wijns W: The Task Force for the Diagnosis and Treatment of Non-ST-Segment Elevation Acute Coronary Syndromes of the European Society of Cardiology. Guidelines for the diagnosis and treatment of non-ST-segment elevation acute coronary syndromes. *Eur Heart J* (2007) 28, 1598–1660.
59. Gislason GH, Jacobsen S, Rasmussen JN, Rasmussen S, Buch P, Friberg J, Schramm TK, Abildstrom SZ, Køber L, Madsen M, Torp-Pedersen C. Risk of death or reinfarction associated with the use of selective cyclooxygenase-2 inhibitors and nonselective nonsteroidal antiinflammatory drugs after acute myocardial infarction. *Circulation* (2006) 113, 2906–13.
60. European Medicines Agency. PRAC recommends the same cardiovascular precautions for diclofenac as for selective COX-2 inhibitors. June 2013. Available at: http://www.ema.europa.eu/docs/en_GB/document_library/Press_release/2013/06/WC500144451.pdf (accessed 10/07/13).
61. Committee on Safety of Medicines/Medicines and Healthcare products Regulatory Agency. Reminder: Gastrointestinal toxicity of NSAIDs. *Current Problems* (2003) 29, 8–9.

NSAIDs + Azoles

Fluconazole markedly raises celecoxib levels, whereas ketoconazole has no effect on celecoxib levels. Fluconazole and ketoconazole moderately increase the levels of valdecoxib (the main metabolite of parecoxib). Ketoconazole moderately raises etoricoxib plasma levels. Fluconazole has no clinically relevant effect on lumiracoxib pharmacokinetics. Voriconazole markedly raises diclofenac and ibuprofen levels and fluconazole raises flurbiprofen and ibuprofen levels.

Clinical evidence

(a) Coxibs

1. Celecoxib. The manufacturer notes that **fluconazole** 200 mg daily increased the AUC of a single 200-mg dose of celecoxib by 130% and increased the maximum level by 60%. Conversely, **ketoconazole** had no effect on the pharmacokinetics of celecoxib.[1]

2. Etoricoxib. A single 60-mg dose of etoricoxib was given to healthy subjects on day 7 of an 11-day course of **ketoconazole** 400 mg daily. The AUC of etoricoxib was increased by 43% and its maximum plasma level was increased by 29%.[2]

3. Lumiracoxib. A placebo-controlled, crossover study in 13 healthy subjects[3] found that **fluconazole** 400 mg on day 1 and 200 mg on days 2 to 4 had no clinically relevant effect on the pharmacokinetics of a single 400-mg dose of lumiracoxib given on day[4].

4. Parecoxib. The manufacturer of parecoxib reports a study in which **fluconazole** increased the plasma levels of valdecoxib (the main metabolite of parecoxib) by 19% and raised its AUC by 62%.[4] **Ketoconazole** had a similar, but more moderate effect on the levels of valdecoxib (maximum plasma levels increased by 24%, AUC increased by 38%).[4]

(b) Diclofenac

In a randomised, crossover study, 10 healthy subjects were given either diclofenac 50 mg alone or one hour after the last dose of **voriconazole** (400 mg twice daily on the first day, 200 mg twice daily on the second day). The AUC of diclofenac was increased by 78% in the presence of **voriconazole**, its peak plasma level was approximately doubled and its renal clearance was decreased by 47%.[5]

(c) Ibuprofen and related drugs

1. Flurbiprofen. In a study, 14 healthy subjects were given a single 100-mg dose of flurbiprofen either alone or 30 minutes after two doses of **fluconazole** 200 mg. **Fluconazole** increased the peak plasma level and AUC of flurbiprofen by 23% and 81%, respectively, reduced its clearance by about 45% and prolonged its half-life from 3.3 hours to 5.3 hours. The AUC of the metabolite 4-hydroxyflurbiprofen was significantly reduced.[6]

2. Ibuprofen. In a study, 12 healthy subjects were given ibuprofen 400 mg, alone or one hour after the last dose of **voriconazole** (400 mg twice daily on the first day, 200 mg twice daily on the second day) or **fluconazole** (400 mg on the first day and 200 mg on the second day). **Voriconazole** increased the peak plasma level of S-ibuprofen by 22%, doubled its AUC, and increased its elimination half-life by 43%. **Fluconazole** increased the peak plasma level and AUC of S-ibuprofen by 16% and 83%, respectively, and increased its elimination half-life by 34%. **Voriconazole** and **fluconazole** had only weak effects on the pharmacokinetics of R-ibuprofen.[7]

Mechanism

Fluconazole is an inhibitor of the cytochrome P450 isoenzyme CYP2C9 and ketoconazole inhibits CYP3A4. Celecoxib is extensively metabolised by CYP2C9, and therefore shows marked rises in plasma levels when given with fluconazole but not ketoconazole. Etoricoxib is partially metabolised by CYP3A4, and therefore shows moderate rises in plasma levels with ketoconazole. Valdecoxib is metabolised by both CYP2C9 and CYP3A4, and therefore it is modestly affected by both fluconazole and ketoconazole. Parecoxib is a valdecoxib prodrug, and interacts similarly. From the study with lumiracoxib it appears that its pharmacokinetics are unlikely to be affected by inhibitors of CYP2C9, because, even though lumiracoxib is largely metabolised by CYP2C9, other pathways are also important (e.g. glucuronidation).[3] Voriconazole probably increased the levels of diclofenac by inhibiting its metabolism by CYP2C9 and possibly by CYP3A4,[5] and the metabolism of flurbiprofen and the *S*-enantiomer of ibuprofen by CYP2C9 is inhibited by fluconazole and voriconazole.[6,7]

Importance and management

The pharmacokinetic interactions between the coxibs and azoles are established, although their effect in clinical practice has not been assessed. The marked rise in celecoxib levels with fluconazole could be important, and the UK manufacturer recommends that the dose of celecoxib should be halved in patients receiving fluconazole,[1] whereas the US manufacturer suggests starting with the lowest recommended dose.[8] The rise in valdecoxib levels with fluconazole is less marked; nevertheless, the manufacturer recommends that for parecoxib the dose should be reduced (but they do not suggest by how much).[4] No dose adjustments are thought to be necessary if etoricoxib or parecoxib are given with ketoconazole, and if lumiracoxib is given with fluconazole.

The clinical importance of the interaction between voriconazole and diclofenac is not known, but lower doses of diclofenac may be adequate for patients also taking voriconazole.[5] Similarly, lower doses of ibuprofen,[7] or possibly flurbiprofen, may be adequate if they are given with either fluconazole or voriconazole, especially if the initial NSAID dose is high.[7]

1. Celebrex (Celecoxib). Pfizer Ltd. UK Summary of product characteristics, January 2013.
2. Agrawal NGB, Matthews CZ, Mazenko RS, Woolf EJ, Porras AG, Chen X, Miller JL, Michiels N, Wehling M, Schultz A, Gottlieb AB, Kraft WK, Greenberg HE, Waldman SA, Curtis SP, Gottesdiener KM. The effects of modifying in vivo cytochrome P450 3A (CYP3A) activity on etoricoxib pharmacokinetics and of etoricoxib administration on CYP3A activity. *J Clin Pharmacol* (2004) 44, 1125–31.
3. Scott G, Yih L, Yeh C-M, Milosavljev S, Laurent A, Rordorf C. Lumiracoxib: pharmacokinetic and pharmacodynamic profile when coadministered with fluconazole in healthy subjects. *J Clin Pharmacol* (2004) 44, 193–9.
4. Dynastat (Parecoxib sodium). Pfizer Ltd. UK Summary of product characteristics, June 2013.
5. Hynninen V-V, Olkkola KT, Leino K, Lundgren S, Neuvonen PJ, Rane A, Valtonen M, Laine K. Effect of voriconazole on the pharmacokinetics of diclofenac. *Fundam Clin Pharmacol* (2007) 21, 651–6.
6. Greenblatt DJ, von Moltke LL, Perloff ES, Luo Y, Harmatz JS, Zinny MA. Interaction of flurbiprofen with cranberry juice, grape juice, tea, and fluconazole: in vitro and clinical studies. *Clin Pharmacol Ther* (2006) 79, 125–33.
7. Hynninen V-V, Olkkola KT, Leino K, Lundgren S, Neuvonen PJ, Rane A, Valtonen M, Vyyryläinen H, Laine K. Effects of the antifungals voriconazole and fluconazole on the pharmacokinetics of S-(+)- and R-(−)-ibuprofen. *Antimicrob Agents Chemother* (2006) 50, 1967–72.
8. Celebrex (Celecoxib). Pfizer Inc. US Prescribing information, June 2009.

NSAIDs + Bile-acid binding resins

The simultaneous use of colestyramine markedly reduced the absorption of diclofenac and sulindac, modestly reduced the absorption of ibuprofen, but only delayed and did not reduce the extent of naproxen absorption. Giving colestyramine three or more hours after oral sulindac, piroxicam, or tenoxicam still markedly reduced their plasma levels. Markedly reduced NSAID levels have also been found when colestyramine is given after intravenous meloxicam or tenoxicam.

The simultaneous use of colestipol modestly reduced the oral absorption of diclofenac, but had no effect on ibuprofen absorption.

Clinical evidence

(a) Diclofenac

A single-dose, crossover study in 6 healthy, fasting subjects found that the simultaneous use of **colestyramine** 8 g markedly reduced the AUC of a single 100-mg oral dose of enteric-coated diclofenac by 62% and reduced its maximum plasma levels by 75%. **Colestipol** 10 g reduced the AUC of diclofenac by 33% and reduced its maximum plasma levels by 58%.[1]

(b) Ibuprofen

A single-dose, crossover study in 6 healthy fasting subjects found that the simultaneous use of **colestyramine** 8 g modestly reduced the AUC of a single 400-mg oral dose of ibuprofen by 26% and reduced its maximum plasma levels by 34%. The rate of absorption was also reduced. Conversely, **colestipol** 10 g had no significant effect on the pharmacokinetics of ibuprofen.[2]

(c) Meloxicam

A study in 12 healthy subjects found that **colestyramine** 4 g taken 2 hours before a 30-mg *intravenous* dose of meloxicam increased its clearance by 49% and reduced its mean residence time in the body by 39%.[3]

(d) Naproxen

In a study in 8 healthy fasting subjects the absorption of a single 250-mg dose of naproxen was delayed but not reduced by the simultaneous use of **colestyramine** 4 g in 100 mL of orange juice. The amount of naproxen absorbed after 2 hours was reduced from 96% to 51%, but was complete after 5 hours.[4]

(e) Piroxicam or Tenoxicam

A study in 8 healthy subjects found that **colestyramine** increased the clearance of a single 20-mg oral dose of piroxicam and a single 20-mg *intravenous* dose of tenoxicam by 52% and 105%, respectively, and reduced their half-lives by 40% and 52%, respectively. In this study, **colestyramine** 4 g three times daily was started 2 hours before the intravenous tenoxicam and 3.5 hours after the oral piroxicam.[5] In another multiple-dose study **colestyramine**, given 4 hours after oral piroxicam or oral tenoxicam, gave similar results,[6] as did a study starting **colestyramine** 24 hours after the last dose of a 14-day course of **piroxicam** 20 mg daily [which has a long half-life].[7] The elimination half-life of both analgesics was roughly doubled by **colestyramine** 24 g daily.[6]

(f) Sulindac

In 6 healthy subjects **colestyramine** 4 g twice daily with meals was found to reduce the AUC of a single 400-mg dose of sulindac (given simultaneously) by 78%, and reduced the AUC of the sulfide metabolite of sulindac by 84%. Even when sulindac was given 3 hours before **colestyramine**, the AUCs of the sulindac and its sulphide metabolite were reduced by 44% and 55%, respectively.[8]

Mechanism

The studies of simultaneous oral use suggest that the anion-exchange resin colestyramine, and to a lesser extent colestipol, bind anionic NSAIDs (e.g. diclofenac) in the gut, so reducing their absorption. The studies that found reduced plasma levels when colestyramine was given after intravenous oxicams or separated by at least 3 hours from some oral NSAIDs, suggest that colestyramine can reduce the enterohepatic recirculation of these drugs.

Importance and management

Established interactions. Colestyramine markedly reduces the initial absorption of some NSAIDs (seen with diclofenac), and if these NSAIDs also undergo enterohepatic recirculation, their clearance will also be increased (seen with meloxicam, piroxicam, sulindac, and tenoxicam). This latter interaction cannot be avoided by separating the doses, and it may be best not to use colestyramine with these NSAIDs. Colestyramine can be used to speed the removal of piroxicam and tenoxicam following overdosage.[4] Diclofenac has been formulated with colestyramine in an attempt to reduce gastric mucosal damage by reducing direct mucosal contact: 140 mg of diclofenac-colestyramine is considered equivalent to 70 mg of diclofenac.[9]

Any interaction between colestyramine and naproxen or ibuprofen is probably not clinically important, although colestyramine delayed the absorption of both drugs, which may be relevant if they are being taken for the management of acute pain. Information on many other NSAIDs appears to be lacking. *Animal* studies suggest that **mefenamic acid**, **flufenamic acid** and **phenylbutazone** will also be affected by colestyramine.[10,11] Note that it is usually recommended that other drugs are given 1 hour before or 4 to 6 hours after colestyramine.

The reduction in diclofenac absorption with colestipol may be clinically relevant; if the combination is required, monitor well. Note that it is usually recommended that other drugs are given 1 hour before or 4 hours after colestipol.

1. Al-Balla SR, El-Sayed YM, Al-Meshal MA, Gouda MW. The effects of cholestyramine and colestipol on the absorption of diclofenac in man. *Int J Clin Pharmacol Ther* (1994) 32, 441–5.
2. Al-Meshal MA, El-Sayed YM, Al-Balla SR, Gouda MW. The effect of colestipol and cholestyramine on ibuprofen bioavailability in man. *Biopharm Drug Dispos* (1994) 15, 463–71.
3. Busch U, Heinzel G, Narjes H. The effect of cholestyramine on the pharmacokinetics of meloxicam, a new non-steroidal anti-inflammatory drug (NSAID), in man. *Eur J Clin Pharmacol* (1995) 48, 269–72.
4. Calvo MV, Dominguez-Gil A. Interaction of naproxen with cholestyramine. *Biopharm Drug Dispos* (1984) 5, 33–42.
5. Guentert TW, Defoin R, Mosberg H. The influence of cholestyramine on the elimination of tenoxicam and piroxicam. *Eur J Clin Pharmacol* (1988) 34, 283–9.
6. Benveniste C, Striberni R, Dayer P. Indirect assessment of the enterohepatic recirculation of piroxicam and tenoxicam. *Eur J Clin Pharmacol* (1990) 38, 547–9.
7. Ferry DG, Gazeley LR, Busby WJ, Beasley DMG, Edwards IR, Campbell AJ, Enhanced elimination of piroxicam by administration of activated charcoal or cholestyramine. *Eur J Clin Pharmacol* (1990) 39, 599–601.
8. Malloy MJ, Ravis WR, Pennell AT, Hagan DR, Betagari S, Doshi DH. Influence of cholestyramine resin administration on single dose sulindac pharmacokinetics. *Int J Clin Pharmacol Ther* (1994) 32, 286–9.
9. Suárez-Otero R, Robles-San Román M, Jaimes-Hernández J, Oropeza-de la Madrid E, Medina-Peñaloza RM, Rosas-Ramos R, Castañeda-Hernández G. Efficacy and safety of diclofenac-cholestyramine and celecoxib in osteoarthritis. *Proc West Pharmacol Soc* (2002) 45, 26–8.
10. Rosenberg HA, Bates TR. Inhibitory effect of cholestyramine on the absorption of flufenamic and mefenamic acids in rats. *Proc Soc Exp Biol Med* (1974) 145, 93–8.
11. Gallo D G, Bailey K R, Sheffner A L. The interaction between cholestyramine and drugs. *Proc Soc Exp Biol Med* (1965) 120, 60–5.

NSAIDs or Aspirin + Caffeine

Caffeine modestly increases the bioavailability, rate of absorption and plasma levels of aspirin. Adding caffeine to diclofenac may improve its efficacy in the treatment of migraine.

Clinical evidence, mechanism, importance and management

In a study in healthy subjects, caffeine citrate 120 mg given with a single 650-mg dose of aspirin increased the AUC of aspirin 36%, increased its maximum plasma levels by 15%, and increased its rate of absorption by 30%.[1] This confirms the results of previous studies.[2,3] These studies suggest that caffeine may modestly potentiate the efficacy of aspirin by a pharmacokinetic mechanism. However, a meta-analysis of randomised, controlled studies concluded that there was no therapeutic advantage to adding caffeine to analgesic doses of aspirin in patients experiencing postoperative pain.[4]

In a placebo-controlled study in patients with migraine, there was a non-significant trend towards improved analgesic effect in patients receiving **diclofenac** softgel capsules 100 mg and caffeine 100 mg, when compared with diclofenac alone, although the sample size was too small to provide meaningful results.[5]

1. Thithapandha A. Effect of caffeine on the bioavailability and pharmacokinetics of aspirin. *J Med Assoc Thai* (1989) 72, 562–6.
2. Yoovathaworn KC, Sriwatanakul K, Thithapandha A. Influence of caffeine on aspirin pharmacokinetics. *Eur J Drug Metab Pharmacokinet* (1986) 11, 71–6.
3. Dahanukar SA, Pohujani S, Sheth UK. Bioavailability of aspirin and interacting influence of caffeine. *Indian J Med Res* (1978) 68, 844–8.
4. Zhang WY, Po ALW. Do codeine and caffeine enhance the analgesic effect of aspirin?–A systematic overview. *J Clin Pharm Ther* (1997) 22, 79–97.

5. Peroutka SJ, Lyon JA, Swarbrick J, Lipton RB, Kolodner K, Goldstein J. Efficacy of diclofenac sodium softgel 100 mg with or without caffeine 100 mg in migraine without aura: a randomized, double-blind, crossover study. *Headache* (2004) 44, 136–41.

NSAIDs + Febuxostat

Febuxostat does not affect the pharmacokinetics of indometacin and naproxen. Naproxen, but not indometacin, increases the plasma levels of febuxostat.

Clinical evidence, mechanism, importance and management

A crossover study in 26 healthy subjects found that the concurrent use of febuxostat 80 mg daily and **indometacin** 50 mg twice daily did not affect the pharmacokinetics of either drug.[1] In a further study, 25 healthy subjects were given febuxostat 80 mg daily, **naproxen** 500 mg twice daily, or both drugs together. **Naproxen** increased the peak plasma level and AUC of febuxostat by about 28% and 40%, respectively, but this was not expected to be clinically significant. Febuxostat did not affect the pharmacokinetics of **naproxen** (24 subjects evaluated). It was concluded that febuxostat may be given with either **indometacin** or **naproxen** without dose adjustments.[1]

1. Khosravan R, Wu J-T, Joseph-Ridge N, Vernillet L. Pharmacokinetic interactions of concomitant administration of febuxostat and NSAIDs. *J Clin Pharmacol* (2006) 46, 855–66.

NSAIDs + Food

In general, food has no clinically significant effect on the absorption of the NSAIDs; however, the delay in absorption that occurs may be important if NSAIDs are given in acute pain management.

Clinical evidence

(a) Celecoxib

A study in 50 children found that high-fat food, increased the maximum plasma concentration of a single 250-mg/m^2 dose of celecoxib by 82% and increased its AUC by 60%. When steady-state levels were achieved with celecoxib 250 mg/m^2 twice daily, food increased its maximum plasma concentration by 99% and increased its AUC by 75%.[1] The manufacturers of celecoxib note that a high-fat meal delayed celecoxib absorption by about one to 2 hours[2,3] and the total absorption was increased by 10% to 20%.[3]

(b) Dexketoprofen

The absorption of a single 25-mg dose of dexketoprofen was delayed by food (maximum level reduced by 45% and time to maximum level delayed by about 1 hour), but the AUC was not affected.[4]

(c) Diclofenac

In a study, 13 healthy subjects were given a single 105-mg dose of diclofenac potassium suspension (*Flogan*) while fasting and after food. The pharmacokinetics of diclofenac were not changed to a clinically relevant extent by food, except that absorption was delayed (time to maximum level increased by about 30 minutes).[5] Similar findings (an increase in time to maximum level of 1.5 to 3 hours) were reported for single doses of enteric-coated diclofenac tablets.[6] However, there was no difference in the steady-state levels of diclofenac 50 mg twice daily when given before or after food.[6]

(d) Etodolac

When 18 healthy subjects were given etodolac 400 mg after a high-fat meal, peak serum levels were roughly halved, and delayed, from 1.4 hours to 3.8 hours, but the total amount absorbed was not markedly changed, when compared to the fasting state.[7]

(e) Etoricoxib

A high-fat meal reduced the maximum level of a 120-mg dose of etoricoxib by 36% and delayed it by 2 hours, without affecting the extent of absorption.[8]

(f) Flurbiprofen

Food slightly increased the maximum plasma level and AUC of sustained-release flurbiprofen (*Froben SR*) by 15% and 25%, respectively, but delayed the time to achieve the maximum level by about 5 hours.[9]

(g) Ibuprofen

Food had no effect on the pharmacokinetics of the *S*- and *R*-enantiomers of ibuprofen in one study.[10] However, in another study, food delayed the absorption of both enantiomers of ibuprofen, and slightly increased the ratio of the *S*- to *R*-enantiomer.[11] A study considering the effect of food on ibuprofen pharmacokinetics found that the maximum level of a single 400-mg dose of a standard release ibuprofen tablet and two readily soluble preparations (ibuprofen lysinate and ibuprofen extrudate), was consistently lower and appeared later when the dose was given after a standardised breakfast; the extent of ibuprofen absorption was also reduced by food for all three formulations.[12] However, in a further study, food increased the maximum plasma level of sustained-release ibuprofen (*Brufen Retard*) by 42% without affecting the time to achieve the maximum level or the bioavailability.[9]

(h) Indometacin

Studies in patients and healthy subjects, given single or multiple oral doses of indometacin have found that food delays and reduces peak serum indometacin levels, but the fluctuations in levels are somewhat reduced.[13]

(i) Ketoprofen

Food significantly decreased the rate and extent of absorption of ketoprofen in both single and multiple dose studies in healthy subjects. The AUC was decreased by about 40% and the time to maximum levels decreased by about 5 hours.[14] A further study found that the rate of absorption and the peak plasma levels of ketoprofen were reduced by food, although the AUC was unaltered.[15] In another study, the absorption of ketoprofen (200 mg daily, as a gastric-juice resistant, sustained-release formulation, given 4 hours before the first meal of the day) was about 15 to 24% greater when 16 healthy subjects were given a low-calorie/low-fat diet rather than a high-calorie/high-fat diet.[16] In a further study in 4 healthy subjects, which measured the urinary excretion of ketoprofen after a single 50-mg dose given with water, whole skimmed milk, or a traditional Egyptian breakfast, it was concluded that the rate and extent of absorption of ketoprofen had been reduced by the presence of food, and the extent of absorption was also reduced by milk.[17]

(j) Meloxicam

In one study, the rate (time to peak serum levels) and extent of absorption (AUC) of meloxicam 30 mg was not altered by food intake.[18]

(k) Nabumetone

The absorption of a single 1-g dose of nabumetone was increased by food and milk, as shown by an increase of about 50% in the maximum levels and a 40% increase in the AUC_{0-24}. However, the AUC_{0-72} was not significantly increased.[19]

(l) Naproxen

Food did not have any clinically relevant effect on the pharmacokinetics of sustained-release naproxen in two studies.[20,21] Taking a single 550-mg dose of naproxen sodium with a meal had no effect on its analgesic efficacy in postoperative pain, when compared with the fasted state.[22] However, the rate of absorption of a single 550-mg dose of *S*-naproxen betainate sodium salt monohydrate was found to be reduced by a high-fat meal, when compared with the fasting state.[23]

(m) Piroxicam

Food caused some delay in the time to reach maximum levels of piroxicam in a single-dose study, but had no effect on total absorption.[24] In another study, the steady-state plasma levels of piroxicam 20 mg daily were unaffected by food.[25]

(n) Tenoxicam

In a study in 12 healthy subjects, the bioavailability of tenoxicam 20 mg was unaffected by food, although the time taken to reach peak serum levels was delayed by about 4 hours.[26]

Mechanism

Food delays gastric emptying, therefore frequently affects the rate, but not the extent, of absorption of the NSAIDs.

Importance and management

Food reduces the rate of absorption but has little or no effect on the extent of absorption of most of the NSAIDs studied. The effect of food was seen to vary with different formulations of NSAIDs; however, these changes in absorption will have little clinical relevance when these drugs are being used regularly to treat chronic pain and inflammation. If these drugs are being used for the treatment of acute pain, giving them on an empty stomach would be preferable in terms of onset of effect, and is suggested by the manufacturers of dexketoprofen[27] and etoricoxib.[8] However, it is usually recommended that NSAIDs are given with or after food in an attempt to minimise their gastrointestinal adverse effects.

Although food delayed the absorption of celecoxib, the UK manufacturer says that it can be taken with or without food.[2] However, high-fat food may increase the total absorption of celecoxib and the US manufacturer suggests that higher doses (400 mg twice daily) should be given with food to improve absorption.[3]

1. Stempak D, Gammon J, Halton J, Champagne M, Koren G, Baruchel S. Modulation of celecoxib pharmacokinetics by food in pediatric patients. *Clin Pharmacol Ther* (2005) 77, 226–8.
2. Celebrex (Celecoxib). Pfizer Ltd. UK Summary of product characteristics, January 2013.
3. Celebrex (Celecoxib). Pfizer Inc. US Prescribing information, June 2009.
4. McEwen J, De Luca M, Casini A, Gich I, Barbanoj MJ, Tost D, Artigas R, Mauleón D. The effect of food and an antacid on the bioavailability of dexketoprofen trometamol. *J Clin Pharmacol* (1998) 38 (Suppl), 41S–45S.
5. Poli A, Moreno RA, Ribiero W, Dias HB, Moreno H, Muscara MN, De Nucci G. Influence of gastric acid secretion blockade and food intake on the bioavailability of a potassium diclofenac suspension in healthy male volunteers. *Int J Clin Pharmacol Ther* (1996) 34, 76–9.
6. Sioufi A, Stierlin H, Schweizer A, Botta L, Degen PH, Theobald W, Brechbühler S. Recent findings concerning clinically relevant pharmacokinetics of diclofenac sodium. In: Voltarol — New Findings, ed Kass E. Proc Int Symp Voltarol, Paris June 22nd, 1981. 15th Int Congress of Rheumatology. p 19–30.
7. Troy S, Sanda M, Dressler D, Chiang S, Latts J. The effect of food and antacid on etodolac bioavailability. *Clin Pharmacol Ther* (1990) 47, 192.
8. Arcoxia (Etoricoxib). Merck Sharp & Dohme Ltd. UK Summary of product characteristics, May 2012.
9. Pargal A, Kelkar MG, Nayak PJ. The effect of food on the bioavailability of ibuprofen and flurbiprofen from sustained release formulation. *Biopharm Drug Dispos* (1996) 17, 511–19.
10. Levine MA, Walker SE, Paton TW. The effect of food or sucralfate on the bioavailability of S(+) and R(-) enantiomers of ibuprofen. *J Clin Pharmacol* (1992) 32, 1110–14.
11. Siemon D, de Vries JX, Stötzer F, Walter-Sack I, Dietl R. Fasting and postprandial disposition of R(-)- and S(+)-ibuprofen following oral administration of racemic drug in healthy individuals. *Eur J Med Res* (1997) 2, 215–19.
12. Klueglich M, Ring A, Scheuerer S, Trommeshauser D, Schuijt C, Liepold B, Berndl G. Ibuprofen extrudate, a novel, rapidly dissolving ibuprofen formulation: relative bioavailability compared to ibupro-

fen lysinate and regular ibuprofen, and food effect on all formulations. *J Clin Pharmacol* (2005) 45, 1055–61.
13. Emori HW, Paulus H, Bluestone R, Champion GD, Pearson C. Indomethacin serum concentrations in man. Effects of dosage, food, and antacid. *Ann Rheum Dis* (1976) 35, 333–8.
14. Caillé G, du Souich P, Besner JG, Gervais P, Vèzina M. Effects of food and sucralfate on the pharmacokinetics of naproxen and ketoprofen in humans. *Am J Med* (1989) 86 (Suppl 6A) 38–44. Correction. ibid. (1990) 89, 838.
15. Bannwarth B, Lapicque F, Netter P, Monot C, Tamisier JN, Thomas P, Royer RJ. The effect of food on the systemic availability of ketoprofen. *Eur J Clin Pharmacol* (1988) 33, 643–5.
16. Le Liboux A, Teule M, Frydman A, Oosterhuis B, Jonkman JHG. Effect of diet on the single- and multiple-dose pharmacokinetics of sustained-release ketoprofen. *Eur J Clin Pharmacol* (1994) 47, 361–6.
17. Eshra AG, Etman MA, Naggar VF. Effect of milk and food on the bioavailability of ketoprofen in man. *Int J Pharmaceutics* (1988) 44, 9–14.
18. Busch U, Heinzel G, Narjes H. Effect of food on pharmacokinetics of meloxicam, a new non steroidal anti-inflammatory drug (NSAID). *Agents Actions* (1991) 32, 52–3.
19. von Schrader HW, Buscher G, Dierdorf D, Mügge H, Wolf D. Nabumetone — a novel anti-inflammatory drug: the influence of food, milk, antacids, and analgesics on bioavailability of single oral doses. *Int J Clin Pharmacol Ther Toxicol* (1983) 21, 311–21.
20. Mroszczak E, Yee JP, Bynum L. Absorption of naproxen controlled-release tablets in fasting and postprandial volunteers. *J Clin Pharmacol* (1988) 28, 1128–31.
21. Palazzini E, Cristofori M, Babbini M. Bioavailability of a new controlled-release oral naproxen formulation given with and without food. *Int J Clin Pharmacol Res* (1992) 12, 179–84.
22. Forbes JA, Sandberg RÅ, Bood-Björklund L. The effect of food on bromfenac, naproxen sodium, and acetaminophen in postoperative pain after orthopedic surgery. *Pharmacotherapy* (1998) 18, 492–503.
23. Marzo A, Dal Bo L, Wool C, Cerutti R. Bioavailability, food effect and tolerability of S-naproxen betainate sodium salt monohydrate in steady state. *Arzneimittelforschung* (1998) 48, 935–40.
24. Ishizaki T, Nomura T, Abe T. Pharmacokinetics of piroxicam, a new nonsteroidal anti-inflammatory agent, under fasting and postprandial states in man. *J Pharmacokinet Biopharm* (1979) 7, 369–81.
25. Tilstone WJ, Lawson DH, Omara F, Cunningham F. The steady-state pharmacokinetics of piroxicam: effect of food and iron. *Eur J Rheumatol Inflamm* (1981) 4, 309–13.
26. Day RO, Lam S, Paull P, Wade D. Effect of food and various antacids on the absorption of tenoxicam. *Br J Clin Pharmacol* (1987) 24, 323–8.
27. Keral (Dexketoprofen trometamol). A.Menarini Pharma U.K. S.R.L. UK Summary of product characteristics, March 2007.

NSAIDs + Ginkgo (*Ginkgo biloba*)

An isolated case describes fatal intracerebral bleeding in a patient taking ginkgo with ibuprofen, and another case describes prolonged bleeding and subdural haematomas in another patient taking ginkgo and rofecoxib. Studies with diclofenac and flurbiprofen showed that ginkgo had no effect on the pharmacokinetics of these drugs.

Clinical evidence

A case of fatal intracerebral bleeding has been reported in a 71-year-old patient taking a ginkgo supplement (*Gingium*) 4 weeks after he started to take **ibuprofen** 600 mg daily.[1] A 69-year-old man taking a ginkgo supplement and **rofecoxib** had a subdural haematoma after a head injury, then recurrent small spontaneous haematomas. He was subsequently found to have a prolonged bleeding time, which returned to normal one week after stopping the ginkgo supplement and **rofecoxib**, and remained normal after restarting low-dose **rofecoxib**.[2]

A placebo-controlled study in 11 healthy subjects who were given ginkgo leaf (*Ginkgold*) 120 mg twice daily for three doses, followed by a single 100-mg dose of **flurbiprofen**, found that the pharmacokinetics of flurbiprofen were unchanged.[3]

A study in 12 healthy subjects who were given **diclofenac** 50 mg twice daily for 14 days, with ginkgo extract (*Ginkgold*) 120 mg twice daily on days 8 to 15, found no alteration in the AUC or oral clearance of diclofenac.[4]

Mechanism

The reason for the bleeding is not known, but ginkgo extract contains ginkgolide B, a potent inhibitor of platelet-activating factor *in vitro*, which is needed for arachidonate-independent platelet aggregation. However, in one controlled study in healthy subjects, taking a ginkgo preparation alone for two weeks had no effect on platelet function.[5] Nevertheless, there are case reports of ginkgo supplements, on their own, being associated with prolonged bleeding times,[6,7] left and bilateral subdural haematomas,[6,8] a right parietal haematoma,[9] post-laparoscopic cholecystectomy bleeding,[10] and subarachnoid haemorrhage.[7] Ibuprofen is an inhibitor of platelet aggregation, but selective inhibitors of COX-2 such as rofecoxib have no effect on platelets and would not be expected to potentiate any bleeding effect of ginkgo.

The pharmacokinetic studies involving diclofenac and flurbiprofen were designed to identify whether ginkgo exerted an inhibitory effect on the cytochrome P450 isoenzyme CYP2C9, which is involved in the metabolism of these NSAIDs.

Importance and management

The evidence from these reports is too slim to forbid patients to take NSAIDs and ginkgo concurrently, but some do recommend caution.[11] Medical professionals should be aware of the possibility of increased bleeding tendency with ginkgo, and report any suspected cases.[9] Consider also 'Antiplatelet drugs + Ginkgo (*Ginkgo biloba*)', p.779.

1. Meisel C, Johne A, Roots I. Fatal intracerebral mass bleeding associated with *Ginkgo biloba* and ibuprofen. *Atherosclerosis* (2003) 167, 367.
2. Hoffman T. Ginko, Vioxx and excessive bleeding – possible drug-herb interactions: case report. *Hawaii Med J* (2001) 60, 290.
3. Greenblatt DJ, von Moltke LL, Luo Y, Perloff ES, Horan KA, Bruce A, Reynolds RC, Harmatz JS, Avula B, Khan IA, Goldman P. Ginkgo biloba does not alter clearance of flurbiprofen, a cytochrome P450-2C9 substrate. *J Clin Pharmacol* (2006) 46, 214–21.
4. Mohutsky MA, Anderson GD, Miller JW, Elmer GW. *Ginkgo biloba:* evaluation of CYP2C9 drug interactions in vitro and in vivo. *Am J Ther* (2006) 13, 24–31.
5. Beckert BW, Concannon MJ, Henry SL, Smith DS, Puckett CL. The effect of herbal medicines on platelet function: an in vivo experiment and review of the literature. *Plast Reconstr Surg* (2007) 120, 2044–50.
6. Rowin J, Lewis SL. Spontaneous bilateral subdural hematomas associated with chronic *Ginkgo biloba* ingestion. *Neurology* (1996) 46, 1775–6.
7. Vale S. Subarachnoid haemorrhage associated with *Ginkgo biloba*. *Lancet* (1998) 352, 36.
8. Gilbert GJ. *Ginkgo biloba*. *Neurology* (1997) 48, 1137.
9. Benjamin J, Muir T, Briggs K, Pentland B. A case of cerebral haemorrhage – can *Ginkgo biloba* be implicated? *Postgrad Med J* (2001) 77, 112–13.
10. Fessenden JM, Wittenborn W, Clarke L. Gingko biloba: a case report of herbal medicine and bleeding postoperatively from a laparoscopic cholecystectomy. *Am Surg* (2001) 67, 33–5.
11. Griffiths J, Jordan S, Pilon S. Natural health products and adverse reactions. *Can Adverse React News* (2004) 14, 2–3.

NSAIDs or Aspirin + Gold

Gold appears to increase the risk of aspirin-induced liver damage. The use of gold with fenoprofen seems to be safer with regard to liver toxicity. An isolated report suggested that naproxen may have contributed to gold-induced pneumonitis.

Clinical evidence, mechanism, importance and management

A study in patients with rheumatoid arthritis given aspirin 3.9 g or **fenoprofen** 2.4 g daily suggested that gold induction therapy (**sodium aurothiomalate**, by intramuscular injection, to a total dose of 985 mg over 6 months) increased aspirin-induced hepatotoxicity. Levels of AST, lactate dehydrogenase, and alkaline phosphatase were higher in those taking aspirin than in those taking **fenoprofen**. These indicators of liver impairment suggest that **fenoprofen** is safer than aspirin in this context. The concurrent use of gold and NSAIDs was more effective than the NSAIDs alone.[1]

A patient with rheumatoid arthritis taking gold (**sodium aurothiomalate**) developed pneumonitis soon after **naproxen** 500 mg twice daily was added. An *in vitro* study suggested the pneumonitis was due to hypersensitivity to gold. However, the patient's condition continued to deteriorate despite stopping the gold, then showed marked improvement when the **naproxen** was also stopped. The authors suggest that the **naproxen** may have altered the patient's immune system in some way to make them more sensitive to the gold.[2] This appears to be the only report of such an effect, and it is therefore unlikely to be of general relevance.

1. Davis JD, Turner RA, Collins RL, Ruchte IR, Kaufmann JS. Fenoprofen, aspirin, and gold induction in rheumatoid arthritis. *Clin Pharmacol Ther* (1977) 21, 52–61.
2. McFadden RG, Fraher LJ, Thompson JM. Gold-naproxen pneumonitis: a toxic drug interaction? *Chest* (1989) 96, 216–18.

NSAIDs or Aspirin + H_2-receptor antagonists

The H_2-receptor antagonists have no effect or cause only modest and normally clinically unimportant changes in the serum levels of aspirin and NSAIDs. More importantly H_2-receptor antagonists may protect the gastric mucosa from the irritant effects of the NSAIDs.

Clinical evidence

(a) Aspirin

Cimetidine 300 mg, given one hour before a single 1.2-g dose of aspirin caused only a modest increase in the serum salicylate levels of 3 out of 6 healthy subjects.[1] When 13 patients with rheumatoid arthritis taking enteric-coated aspirin were given **cimetidine** 300 mg four times daily for 7 days the total amount of aspirin absorbed was unaltered, but aspirin levels were slightly raised, from 161 micrograms/mL to 180 micrograms/mL.[2] The pharmacokinetics of a single 1-g dose of aspirin were largely unchanged in 6 healthy subjects given **ranitidine** 150 mg twice daily for a week.[3] However, a study in 10 healthy subjects found that the antiplatelet effects of aspirin were reduced when it was given with **ranitidine**. This was unexpected as **ranitidine** alone may cause a modest decrease in platelet aggregation so it would be expected to enhance the marked antiplatelet effects of aspirin. The reduced effect was attributed to reduced blood levels of salicylate possibly due to changes in the absorption conditions of aspirin in the presence of **ranitidine**.[4] **Famotidine** has been found to cause some small changes in the pharmacokinetics of aspirin, but this is of doubtful clinical importance.[5]

(b) Azapropazone

A randomised, pharmacokinetic study in 12 healthy subjects found that **cimetidine** 300 mg every 6 hours for 6 days increased the AUC of a single 600-mg dose of azapropazone by 25%. The AUC of **cimetidine** was altered by less than 20%. No significant changes in laboratory values (blood counts, enzyme levels) were seen, and adverse effects were minor (headaches in 3 subjects).[6]

(c) Diclofenac

In 14 healthy subjects, **famotidine** 40 mg raised the peak plasma levels of enteric-coated diclofenac 100 mg from 5.84 mg/L to 7.04 mg/L. Peak plasma diclofenac levels also occurred more rapidly (2 hours versus 2.75 hours). The extent of diclofenac absorption was unchanged.[7] Diclofenac did not affect the pharmacokinetics of **ranitidine** nor its ability to suppress gastric pH.[8] Another study also found that the pharmacokinetics of diclofenac were unaffected by **ranitidine**.[9]

(d) Dipyrone (Metamizole)

In a study in 12 patients with confirmed duodenal ulcer, but no gastrointestinal bleeding, **cimetidine** 200 mg was given three times daily with another 400 mg at night for 20 days. A single 1.5-g or 750-mg dose of dipyrone was given on days 8 and 13. In the presence of **cimetidine**, the AUC of the active metabolite of dipyrone, 4-methyl-amino-antipyrine (4-MAA), was increased by 74%, with dipyrone doses of 1.5 g, but the renal clearance of 4-MAA remained unchanged.[10]

(e) Flurbiprofen

In 30 patients with rheumatoid arthritis, **cimetidine** 300 mg three times daily for 2 weeks increased the maximum serum level of flurbiprofen 150 to 300 mg daily, but **ranitidine** 150 mg twice daily had no effect. The efficacy of the flurbiprofen (assessed by Ritchie score, 50 foot walking time, grip strength) was not altered.[11] Another study in healthy subjects found that **cimetidine** 300 mg four times daily slightly increased the serum levels of a single 200-mg dose of flurbiprofen, and raised the flurbiprofen AUC by 13%.[12] No statistically significant interaction occurred with **ranitidine** 150 mg twice daily.[12] Although the activity of flurbiprofen is thought to be related to the *S*-enantiomer, neither **cimetidine** nor **ranitidine** were shown to interact preferentially with one enantiomer over the other.[13]

(f) Ibuprofen

Cimetidine 400 mg three times daily raised the peak serum levels and AUC of a 600-mg dose of ibuprofen by 14% and 6%, respectively. No changes were seen with **ranitidine** 300 mg daily.[14] Another study found that the AUC of *R*-ibuprofen and *S*-ibuprofen increased by 37% and 19%, respectively, but these changes were not statistically significant.[15] However, five other studies with ibuprofen found no interaction with **cimetidine** or **ranitidine**,[16-20] or **nizatidine**.[17] However, analysis of the results of one study showed that peak serum ibuprofen levels in black American subjects were 54% higher and occurred sooner, whereas in white American subjects they were 27% lower and delayed.[18,21]

(g) Indometacin

Cimetidine 1.2 g daily for 2 weeks was given to 10 patients with rheumatoid arthritis taking steady-state indometacin 100 to 200 mg daily. The plasma indometacin levels fell by 18%, but there was no significant change in the clinical effectiveness of the anti-inflammatory treatment (as measured by articular index, pain, grip strength and erythrocyte sedimentation rate).[22] Another study found no changes in the pharmacokinetics of indometacin in healthy subjects given **ranitidine**.[23] In a single-dose study in healthy subjects, indometacin did not markedly affect the bioavailability of either **cimetidine** or **ranitidine**.[24]

(h) Ketoprofen

In a study in 12 healthy subjects, **cimetidine** 600 mg twice daily did not affect the pharmacokinetics of enteric-coated ketoprofen 100 mg twice daily.[25]

(i) Lornoxicam

In 12 healthy subjects, **cimetidine** 400 mg twice daily increased the maximum serum levels and AUC of lornoxicam 8 mg twice daily by 28% and 9%, respectively. **Ranitidine** 150 mg twice daily had no significant effect on lornoxicam pharmacokinetics in these same subjects, except that one subject had a very marked increase in serum lornoxicam levels while taking both drugs. He dropped out of the study after 6 days because of severe gastric irritation. It is not clear what part, if any, the **ranitidine** had to play in this effect.[26]

(j) Meloxicam

In a randomised, crossover study, a group of 9 healthy subjects was given meloxicam 30 mg either alone, or with **cimetidine** 200 mg four times daily for 5 days. **Cimetidine** had no significant effect on the pharmacokinetics of the meloxicam.[27]

(k) Naproxen

One study found no adverse interaction between naproxen and **cimetidine** and no alteration in the beneficial effects of **cimetidine** on gastric acid secretion,[28] but another study found that cimetidine caused a moderate 39 to 60% decrease in the half-life of naproxen,[29,30] and a 20% reduction in the AUC of naproxen.[30] In one of these studies the half-life of naproxen was reduced by about 40% by **ranitidine** and by 50% by **famotidine**.[30] A further study found that **nizatidine** does not affect the pharmacokinetics of naproxen.[31]

(l) Oxaprozin

In a study in 12 healthy subjects, peak plasma levels, time to peak level and elimination half-lives of a single 1.2-g dose of oxaprozin were not significantly affected by either **cimetidine** 300 mg four times daily or **ranitidine** 150 mg twice daily. Oxaprozin clearance was reduced by 20% by both **cimetidine** and **ranitidine**.[32]

(m) Piroxicam

In 10 healthy subjects, **cimetidine** 300 mg four times daily for 7 days slightly increased the half-life and the AUC of a single 20-mg dose of piroxicam, by 8% and 16%, respectively.[33] Another study found that **cimetidine** caused a 15% rise in the AUC of piroxicam.[34] In 12 healthy subjects the half-life and AUC of a single-dose of piroxicam were increased by 41% and 31%, respectively, by **cimetidine** 200 mg three times daily, and the plasma levels were raised accordingly.[35] For example, at 4 hours they were raised by almost 25%.[35] **Ranitidine** was not found to affect the pharmacokinetics of piroxicam.[36] No clinically significant changes occurred in the steady-state serum levels of piroxicam in a further study when either **cimetidine** or **nizatidine** were given.[37]

(n) Tenoxicam

The pharmacokinetics of a single 20-mg oral dose of tenoxicam was unaltered in 6 healthy subjects after they took **cimetidine** 200 mg three times daily and 400 mg at night for 7 days.[38]

Mechanism

Uncertain. Azapropazone, 4-MAA (the active metabolite of dipyrone), lornoxicam, and piroxicam serum levels are possibly increased because their metabolism via the cytochrome P450 system is reduced by cimetidine.[6,10,26,35] There may also be some effects on renal excretion.[6]

Importance and management

Most of the interactions between the NSAIDs and cimetidine, famotidine, nizatidine or ranitidine appear to be of no particular clinical importance. The general relevance of the isolated case of increased lornoxicam levels and severe gastric irritation with ranitidine is uncertain, but probably small. The H_2-receptor antagonists as a group may protect the gastric mucosa from the irritant effects of the NSAIDs and concurrent use may therefore be generally advantageous.

1. Khoury W, Geraci K, Askari A, Johnson M. The effect of cimetidine on aspirin absorption. *Gastroenterology* (1979) 76, 1169.
2. Willoughby JS, Paton TW, Walker SE, Little AH. The effect of cimetidine on enteric-coated ASA disposition. *Clin Pharmacol Ther* (1983) 33, 268.
3. Corrocher R, Bambara LM, Caramaschi P, Testi R, Girelli M, Pellegatti M, Lomeo A. Effect of ranitidine on the absorption of aspirin. *Digestion* (1987) 37, 178–83.
4. Lev EI, Ramabadran RS, Guthikonda S, Patel R, Kleiman A, Granada JF, DeLao T, Kleiman NS. Effect of ranitidine on the antiplatelet effects of aspirin in healthy human subjects. *Am J Cardiol* (2007), 99, 124–8.
5. Domecq C, Fuentes A, Hurtado C, Arancibia A. Effect of famotidine on the bioavailability of acetylsalicylic acid. *Med Sci Res* (1993) 21, 219–20.
6. Maggon KK, Lam GM. Azapropazone: 20 years of clinical use. Rainsford KD, ed. Kluwer Academic Pub; 1989 p. 136–45.
7. Suryakumar J, Chakrapani T, Krishna DR. Famotidine affects the pharmacokinetics of diclofenac sodium. *Drug Invest* (1992) 4, 66–8.
8. Blum RA, Alioth C, Chan KKH, Furst DE, Ziehmer BA, Schentag JJ. Diclofenac does not affect the pharmacodynamics of ranitidine. *Clin Pharmacol Ther* (1992) 51, 192.
9. Dammann HG, Simon-Schultz J, Steinhoff I, Damaschke A, Schmoldt A, Sallowsky E. Differential effects of misoprostol and ranitidine on the pharmacokinetics of diclofenac and gastrointestinal symptoms. *Br J Clin Pharmacol* (1993) 36, 345–9.
10. Bacracheva N, Tyutyulkova N, Drenska A, Gorantcheva J, Schinzel S, Scholl T, Stoinov A, Tchakarski I, Tentcheva J, Vlahov V. Effect of cimetidine on the pharmacokinetics of the metabolites of metamizol. *Int J Clin Pharmacol Ther* (1997) 35, 275–81.
11. Kreeft JH, Bellamy N, Freeman D. Do H_2-antagonists alter the kinetics and effects of chronically-administered flurbiprofen in rheumatoid arthritis? *Clin Invest Med* (1987) 10 (4 Suppl B), B58.
12. Sullivan KM, Small RE, Rock WL, Cox SR, Willis HE. Effects of cimetidine or ranitidine on the pharmacokinetics of flurbiprofen. *Clin Pharm* (1986) 5, 586–9.
13. Small RE, Cox SR, Adams WJ. Influence of H_2 receptor antagonists on the disposition of flurbiprofen enantiomers. *J Clin Pharmacol* (1990) 30, 660–4.
14. Ochs HR, Greenblatt DJ, Matlis R, Weinbrenner J. Interaction of ibuprofen with the H-2 receptor antagonists ranitidine and cimetidine. *Clin Pharmacol Ther* (1985) 38, 648–51.
15. Li G, Treiber G, Klotz U. The ibuprofen-cimetidine interaction. Stereochemical considerations. *Drug Invest* (1989) 1, 11–17.
16. Conrad KA, Mayersohn M, Bliss M. Cimetidine does not alter ibuprofen kinetics after a single dose. *Br J Clin Pharmacol* (1984) 18, 624–6.
17. Forsyth DR, Jayasinghe KSA, Roberts CJC. Do nizatidine and cimetidine interact with ibuprofen? *Eur J Clin Pharmacol* (1988) 35, 85–8.
18. Stephenson DW, Small RE, Wood JH, Willis HE, Johnson SM, Karnes HT, Rajasekharaiah K. Effect of ranitidine and cimetidine on ibuprofen pharmacokinetics. *Clin Pharm* (1988) 7, 317–21.
19. Evans AM, Nation RL, Sansom LN. Lack of effect of cimetidine on the pharmacokinetics of R(-)- and S (+)-ibuprofen. *Br J Clin Pharmacol* (1989) 28, 143–9.
20. Small RE, Wilmot-Pater MG, McGee BA, Willis HE. Effects of misoprostol or ranitidine on ibuprofen pharmacokinetics. *Clin Pharm* (1991) 10, 870–2.
21. Small RE, Wood JH. Influence of racial differences on effects of ranitidine and cimetidine on ibuprofen pharmacokinetics. *Clin Pharm* (1989) 8, 471–2.
22. Howes CA, Pullar T, Sourindhrin I, Mistra PC, Capel H, Lawson DH, Tilstone WJ. Reduced steady-state plasma concentrations of chlorpromazine and indomethacin in patients receiving cimetidine. *Eur J Clin Pharmacol* (1983) 24, 99–102.
23. Kendall MJ, Gibson R, Walt RP. Co-administration of misoprostol or ranitidine with indomethacin: effects on pharmacokinetics, abdominal symptoms and bowel habit. *Aliment Pharmacol Ther* (1992) 6, 437–46.
24. Delhotal-Landes B, Flouvat B, Liote F, Abel L, Meyer P, Vinceneux P, Carbon C. Pharmacokinetic interactions between NSAIDs (indomethacin or sulindac) and H_2-receptor antagonists (cimetidine or ranitidine) in human volunteers. *Clin Pharmacol Ther* (1988) 44, 442–52.
25. Verbeeck RK, Corman CL, Wallace SM, Herman RJ, Ross SG, Le Morvan P. Single and multiple dose pharmacokinetics of enteric coated ketoprofen: effect of cimetidine. *Eur J Clin Pharmacol* (1988) 35, 521–7.
26. Ravic M, Salas-Herrera I, Johnston A, Turner P, Foley K, Rosenow DE. A pharmacokinetic interaction between cimetidine or ranitidine and lornoxicam. *Postgrad Med J* (1993) 69, 865–66.
27. Busch U, Heinzel G, Narjes H, Nehmiz G. Interaction of meloxicam with cimetidine, Maalox or aspirin. *J Clin Pharmacol* (1996) 36, 79–84.
28. Holford NHG, Altman D, Riegelman S, Buskin JN, Upton RA. Pharmacokinetic and pharmacodynamic study of cimetidine administered with naproxen. *Clin Pharmacol Ther* (1981) 29, 251–2.
29. Vree TB, van den Biggelaar-Martea M, Verwey-van Wissen CPWGM, Vree ML, Guelen PJM. The pharmacokinetics of naproxen, its metabolite *O*-desmethylnaproxen, and their acyl glucuronides in humans. Effect of cimetidine. *Br J Clin Pharmacol* (1993) 35, 467–72.
30. Vree TB, van den Biggelaar-Martea M, Verwey-van Wissen CPWGM, Vree ML, Guelen PJM. The effects of cimetidine, ranitidine and famotidine on the single-dose pharmacokinetics of naproxen and its metabolites in humans. *Int J Clin Pharmacol Ther Toxicol* (1993) 31, 597–601.
31. Satterwhite JH, Bowsher RR, Callaghan JT, Cerimele BJ, Levine LR. Nizatidine: lack of drug interaction with naproxen. *Clin Res* (1992) 40, 706A.
32. Scavone JM, Greenblatt DJ, Matlis R, Harmatz JS. Interaction of oxaprozin with acetaminophen, cimetidine, and ranitidine. *Eur J Clin Pharmacol* (1986) 31, 371–4.
33. Mailhot C, Dahl SL, Ward JR. The effect of cimetidine on serum concentrations of piroxicam. *Pharmacotherapy* (1986) 6, 112–17.
34. Freeman DJ, Danter WR, Carruthers SG. Pharmacokinetic interaction between cimetidine and piroxicam in normal subjects. *Clin Invest Med* (1988) 11, C19.
35. Said SA, Foda AM. Influence of cimetidine on the pharmacokinetics of piroxicam in rat and man. *Arzneimittelforschung* (1989) 39, 790–2.
36. Dixon JS, Lacey LF, Pickup ME, Langley SJ, Page MC. A lack of pharmacokinetic interaction between ranitidine and piroxicam. *Eur J Clin Pharmacol* (1990) 39, 583–6.
37. Milligan PA, McGill PE, Howden CW, Kelman AW, Whiting B. The consequences of H_2 receptor antagonist-piroxicam coadministration in patients with joint disorders. *Eur J Clin Pharmacol* (1993) 45, 507–12.
38. Day RO, Geisslinger G, Paull P, Williams KM. Neither cimetidine nor probenecid affect the pharmacokinetics of tenoxicam in normal volunteers. *Br J Clin Pharmacol* (1994) 37, 79–81.

NSAIDs or Aspirin + Hormonal contraceptives or HRT

Oral hormonal contraceptives increase diflunisal clearance in women, but only to the level normally seen in men. One study found modestly reduced levels of ibuprofen with oral hormonal contraceptives, but

another study did not. Oral hormonal contraceptives reduce the levels of aspirin, decrease the clearance of phenazone (antipyrine), but do not appear to affect the pharmacokinetics of phenylbutazone. Conjugated oestrogens have no clinically relevant effects on the pharmacokinetics of oxaprozin or phenazone (antipyrine).

Clinical evidence, mechanism, importance and management

(a) Aspirin

The AUCs of single 300- and 600-mg doses of aspirin were lower in 10 women after they started to take an oral combined hormonal contraceptive (**ethinylestradiol/norethisterone** 30 micrograms/1 mg). After the contraceptive had been discontinued, the pharmacokinetics of aspirin returned to baseline values.[1]

(b) Coxibs

For a report of pulmonary embolism in a patient taking valdecoxib with an oral combined hormonal contraceptive, and for the effects of coxibs on contraceptive metabolism, see 'Combined hormonal contraceptives + Coxibs', p.1172.

(c) Diflunisal

The clearance of a single 250-mg dose of diflunisal was 53% higher in 6 women taking oral hormonal contraceptives than in 6 control women, but was similar to the clearance in 6 men.[2] This difference is unlikely to be of clinical importance.

(d) Ibuprofen

In one study, the pharmacokinetics of *R*-ibuprofen did not differ between women taking oral combined hormonal contraceptives and two control groups (one women and one men).[3] However, in another study, the median AUC_{0-12} of *S*-ibuprofen lysinate was 29% lower in users of oral contraceptives, and pain-intensity was higher (although this was possibly due to reduced pain tolerance).[4]

(e) Oxaprozin

There was no difference in the pharmacokinetics of a single 1.2-g dose of oxaprozin in 11 women taking **conjugated oestrogens** (*Premarin*) and in 11 women not taking oestrogens, except that the time to peak concentration was shorter (4 hours versus 8.9 hours).[5] This difference is unlikely to be of clinical importance.

(f) Phenazone (Antipyrine)

In a study, 12 healthy women taking an oral hormonal contraceptives were given a single 1-g intravenous dose of phenazone. When compared with 26 similar women not taking oral hormonal contraceptives, the clearance of phenazone was found to be 28% lower and its half-life was 3.4 hours greater, suggesting that oral hormonal contraceptives have modest effects on hepatic enzymes.[6] In another study in healthy women, the use of **conjugated oestrogens** for at least 3 months did not affect the clearance of single 1- to 1.2-g intravenous doses of phenazone.[7]

(g) Phenylbutazone

The pharmacokinetics of a single 400-mg dose of phenylbutazone did not change in 10 women after they started to take an oral combined hormonal contraceptive containing **ethinylestradiol/norethisterone** 30 micrograms/1 mg.[1]

1. Gupta KC, Joshi JV, Hazari K, Pohujani SM, Satoskar RS. Effect of low estrogen combination oral contraceptive on metabolism of aspirin and phenylbutazone. *Int J Clin Pharmacol Ther Toxicol* (1982) 20, 511–13.
2. Macdonald JI, Herman RJ, Verbeeck RK. Sex-difference and the effects of smoking and oral contraceptive steroids on the kinetics of diflunisal. *Eur J Clin Pharmacol* (1990) 38, 175–9.
3. Knights KM, McLean CF, Tonkin AL, Miners JO. Lack of effect of gender and oral contraceptive steroids on the pharmacokinetics of (R)-ibuprofen in humans. *Br J Clin Pharmacol* (1995) 40, 153–6.
4. Warnecke J, Pentz R, Siegers C-P. Effects of smoking and contraceptives on the pharmacokinetics and pharmacodynamics of S(+)-ibuprofen lysinate in humans. *Naunyn Schmiedebergs Arch Pharmacol* (1996) 354 (Suppl 1), R33.
5. Scavone JM, Ochs HR, Greenblatt DJ, Matlis R. Pharmacokinetics of oxaprozin in women receiving conjugated estrogen. *Eur J Clin Pharmacol* (1988) 35, 105–8.
6. Scavone JM, Greenblatt DJ, Abernethy DR, Luna BG, Harmatz JS, Shader RI. Influence of oral contraceptive use and cigarette smoking, alone and together, on antipyrine pharmacokinetics. *J Clin Pharmacol* (1997) 37, 437–41.
7. Scavone JM, Greenblatt DJ, Blyden GT. Antipyrine pharmacokinetics in women receiving conjugated estrogens. *J Clin Pharmacol* (1988) 28, 463–6.

NSAIDs or Salicylates + Mazindol

Mazindol does not appear to interact adversely with indometacin or salicylates.

Clinical evidence, mechanism, importance and management

In an 8-week, placebo-controlled study, mazindol was given to 26 patients with obesity and arthritis, 15 of whom were taking salicylates, 11 were taking **indometacin** and one was taking dextropropoxyphene (propoxyphene) with paracetamol (acetaminophen). Additional analgesic and anti-inflammatory drugs used were ibuprofen (4 patients), phenylbutazone (1), dextropropoxyphene (7) and paracetamol (3). No symptoms attributable to salicylism or **indometacin** toxicity (gastric intolerance, headache) were observed.[1]

1. Thorpe PC, Isaac PF, Rodgers J. A controlled trial of mazindol (Sanjorex, Teronac) in the management of obese rheumatic patients. *Curr Ther Res* (1975) 17, 149–55.

NSAIDs or Aspirin + Metoclopramide

Metoclopramide increases the rate of absorption of aspirin and tolfenamic acid. Conversely, metoclopramide reduces the bioavailability of ketoprofen.

Clinical evidence

(a) Aspirin

In one study, intramuscular metoclopramide given before oral effervescent aspirin increased the rate of aspirin absorption during a migraine attack to that seen when aspirin was given alone to subjects who were headache free.[1] Similarly, in another study, intramuscular or oral metoclopramide 10 mg increased the rate of absorption of aspirin in patients with migraine.[2] However, in healthy subjects metoclopramide did not alter the pharmacokinetics of aspirin.[3] In addition, in one clinical study there was no difference in analgesic efficacy between aspirin with metoclopramide (*Migravess*) and aspirin alone (*Alka-Seltzer*) for migraine attacks.[4]

(b) Ketoprofen

In a single-dose study in 4 healthy subjects, metoclopramide 10 mg reduced the AUC of a 50-mg capsule of ketoprofen by 28%. The maximum plasma levels of ketoprofen were almost halved and the time to reach this maximum was prolonged by 30%.[5]

(c) Tolfenamic acid

Rectal metoclopramide 20 mg, given to 8 healthy subjects 30 minutes before oral tolfenamic acid 300 mg, caused a threefold increase in the serum tolfenamic acid levels at 45 minutes. However, there was no change in the maximum level or the AUC.[6] In another study, rectal metoclopramide similarly enhanced the rate of oral absorption of tolfenamic acid when it was given during a migraine attack.[7]

Mechanism

Metoclopramide speeds up gastric emptying. The relatively poorly soluble ketoprofen spends less time in the stomach where it dissolves, and as a result less is available for absorption in the small intestine. Conversely, the absorption rate of tolfenamic acid is increased, without a change in the extent of absorption.

Importance and management

The clinical importance of the reduction in ketoprofen levels is unknown, but the authors of the study recommend that ketoprofen (and possibly other NSAIDs that are poorly soluble) should be taken 1 to 2 hours before metoclopramide. Conversely, for aspirin, tolfenamic acid, and other NSAIDs, metoclopramide can be used to increase the rate of absorption, and therefore possibly speed up the onset of analgesic effect in conditions such as migraine.

1. Volans GN. The effect of metoclopramide on the absorption of effervescent aspirin in migraine. *Br J Clin Pharmacol* (1975) 2, 57–63.
2. Ross-Lee LM, Eadie MJ, Heazlewood V, Bochner F, Tyrer JH. Aspirin pharmacokinetics in migraine: the effect of metoclopramide. *Eur J Clin Pharmacol* (1983) 24, 777–85.
3. Manniche PM, Dinneen LC, Langemark M. The pharmacokinetics of the individual constituents of an aspirin-metoclopramide combination ('Migravess'). *Curr Med Res Opin* (1984) 9, 153–6.
4. Tfelt-Hansen P, Olesen J. Effervescent metoclopramide and aspirin (Migravess) versus effervescent aspirin or placebo for migraine attacks: a double-blind study. *Cephalalgia* (1984) 4, 107–11.
5. Etman MA, Ismail FA, Nada AH. Effect of metoclopramide on ketoprofen pharmacokinetics in man. *Int J Pharmaceutics* (1992) 88, 433–5.
6. Tokola RA, Anttila V-J, Neuvonen PJ. The effect of metoclopramide on the absorption of tolfenamic acid. *Int J Clin Pharmacol Ther Toxicol* (1982) 20, 465–8.
7. Tokola RA, Neuvonen PJ. Effects of migraine attack and metoclopramide on the absorption of tolfenamic acid. *Br J Clin Pharmacol* (1984) 17, 67–75.

NSAIDs + NSAIDs

The concurrent use of two or more NSAIDs increases the risk of gastrointestinal damage. Diflunisal raises serum indometacin levels about twofold but does not affect naproxen levels. The concurrent use of indometacin and flurbiprofen does not appear to affect the pharmacokinetics of either drug. Floctafenine does not alter diclofenac levels. Indometacin caused renal impairment in a patient recovering from phenylbutazone-induced acute renal failure.

Clinical evidence

(a) Gastrointestinal effects

The risk of serious upper gastrointestinal bleeding was increased by the use of more than one NSAID in a meta-analysis of data from three case-controlled studies (odds ratio 4.9 with one NSAID and 10.7 with two NSAIDs).[1] Another study provided similar findings: the odds ratio was 7.1 with one NSAID and 12.3 with two or more NSAIDs.[2] Similar findings have been reported with aspirin and NSAIDs, see 'NSAIDs + Aspirin', p.145. Analysis of yellow card reports to the CSM in the UK, of gastrointestinal perforation, obstruction, ulceration or bleeding with **diclofenac**, **naproxen**, and **ibuprofen**, revealed that 6% of the patients were receiving another non-aspirin NSAID.[3]

One pharmacodynamic study in healthy subjects found that gastric instillation of a solution of **diflunisal** before an **indometacin** solution prevented the fall in transmucosal potential difference seen with **indometacin** alone. This was interpreted as evidence that **diflunisal** protects the human gastric mucosa against the damaging effects of **indometacin**.[4] However, the relevance of this test to the adverse effects of NSAIDs used clinically is unknown. Note that fatal gastrointestinal haemorrhage has been reported in a patient taking **diflunisal** and **indometacin**.[5]

(b) Pharmacokinetic studies

No clinically significant changes in the pharmacokinetics of either **indometacin** 75 mg daily or **flurbiprofen** 150 mg daily occurred when both drugs were given together.[6]

Diflunisal 250 mg twice daily had no effect on plasma levels or urinary excretion of **naproxen** 250 mg twice daily.[7]

A study in 16 healthy subjects found that **diflunisal** 500 mg twice daily raised the steady-state plasma levels and the AUC of **indometacin** 50 mg twice daily about twofold. Combined use was associated with more gastrointestinal and CNS adverse effects, but there was no clear effect on blood loss in the faeces.[8] Another study produced similar findings.[9]

No change in free **diclofenac** levels was seen when 6 healthy subjects were given **floctafenine** 400 mg with **diclofenac** 75 mg daily for a week.[10]

(c) Renal effects

An isolated report describes deterioration in renal function in a patient during recovery from **phenylbutazone**-induced renal failure when **indometacin** 25 mg three times a day was given. The **indometacin** was discontinued with improvement of renal function.[11]

Mechanism

The damaging effects of the NSAIDs on the gut appear to be additive. Diflunisal may inhibit the glucuronidation of indometacin, or could compete for renal clearance with unmetabolised indometacin.[9] All NSAIDs have the propensity to cause renal impairment.

Importance and management

The gastrointestinal toxicity of the NSAIDs is well documented, and it appears that combined use increases this risk. The CSM in the UK have suggested that the concurrent use of more than one NSAID should be avoided.[3,12] The marked rise in the plasma levels of indometacin with diflunisal gives an additional reason why this combination in particular should not be used. Some NSAIDs cause more gastrointestinal toxicity than others; a suggested broad 'rank order' of seven NSAIDs is as follows: highest risk (azapropazone); intermediate risk (diclofenac, indometacin, ketoprofen and naproxen, with piroxicam more risky); lowest risk (ibuprofen),[12] which has been borne out in another analysis.[3] The ranking was based on epidemiological studies and the yellow card database. **Ketorolac** may also be particularly associated with gastrointestinal bleeding, and concurrent use with other NSAIDs has been identified as a risk factor,[13] therefore the manufacturer of ketorolac specifically contraindicates its use with other NSAIDs.[14]

1. Lewis SC, Langman MJS, Laporte J-R, Matthews JNS, Rawlins MD, Wiholm B-E. Dose-response relationships between individual nonaspirin nonsteroidal anti-inflammatory drugs (NANSAIDs) and serious upper gastrointestinal bleeding: a meta-analysis based on individual patient data. *Br J Clin Pharmacol* (2002) 54, 320–6.
2. Anon. Do not combine several NSAIDs. *Prescrire Int* (2003) 12, 20.
3. Committee on Safety of Medicines/Medicines Control Agency. Non-steroidal anti-inflammatory drugs (NSAIDs) and gastrointestinal safety. *Current Problems* (2002) 28, 5.
4. Cohen MM. Diflunisal protects human gastric mucosa against damage by indomethacin. *Dig Dis Sci* (1983) 28, 1070–77.
5. Edwards IR. Medicines Adverse Reactions Committee: eighteenth annual report, 1983. *N Z Med J* (1984) 97, 729–32.
6. Rudge SR, Lloyd-Jones JK, Hind ID. Interaction between flurbiprofen and indomethacin in rheumatoid arthritis. *Br J Clin Pharmacol* (1982) 13, 448–51.
7. Dresse A, Gerard MA, Quinaux N, Fischer P, Gerardy J. Effect of diflunisal on human plasma levels and on the urinary excretion of naproxen. *Arch Int Pharmacodyn Ther* (1978) 236, 276–84.
8. Van Hecken A, Verbesselt R, Tjandra-Maga TB, De Schepper PJ. Pharmacokinetic interaction between indomethacin and diflunisal. *Eur J Clin Pharmacol* (1989) 36, 507–12.
9. Eriksson L-O, Wåhlin-Boll E, Liedholm H, Seideman P, Melander A. Influence of chronic diflunisal treatment on the plasma levels, metabolism and excretion of indomethacin. *Eur J Clin Pharmacol* (1989) 37, 7–15.
10. Sioufi A, Stierlin H, Schweizer A, Botta L, Degen PH, Theobald W, Brechbühler S. Recent findings concerning clinically relevant pharmacokinetics of diclofenac sodium. In: Voltarol — New Findings, ed Kass E. Proc Int Symp Voltarol, Paris June 22nd, 1981. 15th Int Congress of Rheumatology. p 19–30.
11. Kimberly R, Brandstetter RD. Exacerbation of phenylbutazone-related renal failure by indomethacin. *Arch Intern Med* (1978) 138, 1711–12.
12. Committee on the Safety of Medicines/Medicines Control Agency. Relative safety of oral non-aspirin NSAIDs. *Current Problems* (1994) 20, 9–11.
13. Committee on Safety of Medicines/Medicines Control Agency. Ketorolac: new restrictions on dose and duration of treatment. *Current Problems* (1993) 19, 5–6.
14. Toradol (Ketorolac trometamol). Roche Products Ltd. UK Summary of product characteristics, July 2009.

NSAIDs or Aspirin + Paracetamol (Acetaminophen)

Paracetamol levels are increased by diflunisal. Aspirin, diclofenac, nabumetone and sulindac pharmacokinetics do not appear to be affected by paracetamol. There is no pharmacokinetic interaction between ibuprofen and paracetamol. Propacetamol, and possibly paracetamol, increase the antiplatelet effects of diclofenac, although the evidence is limited and the clinical relevance of this is uncertain.

One epidemiological study found that paracetamol alone, and particularly when combined with NSAIDs, was associated with an increased risk of gastrointestinal bleeding, but other studies have not found such an effect. Case reports describe renal toxicity in patients taking ibuprofen or flurbiprofen in which paracetamol use was a theoretical contributing factor.

Clinical evidence, mechanism, importance and management

(a) Antiplatelet effects

In healthy subjects giving single doses of intravenous **propacetamol** 30 mg/kg and **diclofenac** 1.1 mg/kg augmented the platelet inhibitory effect of **diclofenac** by about one-third at 90 minutes post dose. At 5 minutes, the platelet inhibitory effect of both **diclofenac** alone and the combination was 100%, and by 22 to 24 hours, neither **diclofenac** alone nor the combination had any platelet inhibitory effect.[1] In a previous study, the authors had found that **propacetamol** (which is hydrolysed to paracetamol) also inhibited platelet function, and they suggested that the effects of **diclofenac** and **propacetamol** were additive.[1] The clinical relevance of these findings is unclear, but the authors say it should be considered when assessing the risk of surgical bleeding.[1] Further study is needed.

An *in vitro* study suggested that high doses of paracetamol, and a combination of paracetamol and **diclofenac**, may cause platelet inhibition and may increase the risk of bleeding, particularly post-surgery.[2]

In 18 healthy subjects, intravenous **parecoxib** 40 mg given with intravenous paracetamol 1 g, was found not to alter platelet function when compared with paracetamol alone.[3]

(b) Gastrointestinal damage

In a case-control study of the UK General Practice Research Database from 1993 to 1998 the risk of upper gastrointestinal bleeding or perforation was slightly increased in those taking both aspirin and paracetamol (relative risk 3.3), when compared with aspirin alone (2.4), or paracetamol alone (2.4). Moreover, the risk was markedly increased in those taking NSAIDs and paracetamol (16.6), when compared with NSAIDs alone (3.6). The paracetamol doses used were at least 2 g daily. Paracetamol in doses of less than 2 g daily was not associated with an increased risk. Other drug doses and specific NSAIDs were not mentioned.[4] However, other epidemiological studies have not found any increased risk of upper gastrointestinal bleeding with paracetamol at any dose.[5] Paracetamol is usually considered not to increase the risk of upper gastrointestinal adverse effects, and the results of this case-control study are probably insufficient to change prescribing practice. Further studies are needed, controlled for the dose of the NSAID and indication for treatment.

(c) Pharmacokinetic studies

1. Aspirin. In a study in 6 healthy subjects, two doses of dextropropoxyphene with paracetamol 65 mg/650 mg, given one hour before and 3 hours after a single 1.2-g dose of soluble aspirin did not affect the plasma salicylate levels. A reduction in plasma salicylate levels was seen in one subject after a single 1.2-g dose of enteric-coated aspirin was taken with dextropropoxyphene and paracetamol, although the authors suggested that this was related to erratic absorption rather than a pharmacokinetic interaction.[6]

2. Diclofenac. In 6 healthy subjects, diclofenac 25 mg given with paracetamol 500 mg, both three times daily for 14 days, had no effect on the pharmacokinetics of diclofenac.[7]

3. Diflunisal. In a study in healthy subjects, diflunisal significantly raised serum paracetamol levels by 50% but the total bioavailability was unchanged; diflunisal levels were not affected.[8,9] This interaction has not been shown to be clinically important. Nevertheless, the manufacturer of diflunisal recommended that the combination should be used with caution, because of the association of high levels of paracetamol with hepatotoxicity.[9]

4. Ibuprofen. In a crossover study in 20 healthy subjects, ibuprofen 400 mg given with paracetamol 650 mg, both every 6 hours for 2 days, had no effect on the pharmacokinetics of either drug.[10]

5. Nabumetone. In a single-dose study, the absorption of nabumetone 1 g was not significantly altered by paracetamol 1.5 g.[11]

(d) Renal effects

Two children (aged 12 and 14 years) developed acute flank pain and reversible renal impairment during the short-term use of **flurbiprofen** or **ibuprofen**. They had also taken paracetamol.[12] Similarly, a 14-month-old infant with febrile status epilepticus was given an alternating regimen of paracetamol and **ibuprofen**, and subsequently developed acute renal failure.[13] NSAIDs can cause renal toxicity, whereas paracetamol is less likely to cause renal toxicity, except perhaps in overdose.[14] The authors of the first case report proposed that tubular toxicity of NSAIDs and paracetamol are theoretically synergistic.[12] This is because NSAIDs inhibit the production of glutathione (needed to prevent the accumulation of toxic metabolites of paracetamol) and renal ischaemia (possibly induced by NSAIDs, or by dehydration) might lead to the accumulation of paracetamol in the renal medulla.[12]

A review concluded that the available evidence does not support an increased risk of renal toxicity with the use of combination products of aspirin and paracetamol when compared with either drug alone.[15] Paracetamol is often combined with NSAIDs in the management of chronic pain. In addition, paracetamol and **ibuprofen** are often used concurrently (as alternating doses) in the management of fever, particularly in children. This latter practice has become controversial. Opponents cite the lack of efficacy data to support combined use (rather than appropriate doses of individual drugs), and the theoretical increased risk of overdose and renal toxicity.[16,17] Others consider that, in the absence of true safety issues, professional judgement should be used for recommending combined use.[18] Further study is clearly needed.

1. Munsterhjelm E, Niemi TT, Syrjälä MT, Ylikorkala O, Rosenberg PH. Propacetamol augments inhibition of platelet function by diclofenac in volunteers. *Br J Anaesth* (2003) 91, 357–62.
2. Munsterhjelm E, Niemi TT, Ylikorkala O, Silvanto M, Rosenberg PH. Characterization of inhibition of platelet function by paracetamol and its interaction with diclofenac *in vitro*. *Acta Anaesthesiol Scand* (2005) 49, 840–6.
3. Munsterhjelm E, Niemi TT, Ylikorkala O, Neuvonen PJ, Rosenberg PH. Influence on platelet aggregation of i.v. parecoxib and acetaminophen in healthy volunteers. *Br J Anaesth* (2006) 97, 226–31.
4. García Rodríguez LA, Hernández-Díaz S. The risk of upper gastrointestinal complications associated with nonsteroidal anti-inflammatory drugs, glucocorticoids, acetaminophen, and combinations of these agents. *Arthritis Res* (2001) 3, 98–101.
5. Lewis SC, Langman MJS, Laporte J-R, Matthews JNS, Rawlins MD, Wiholm B-E. Dose-response relationships between individual nonaspirin nonsteroidal anti-inflammatory drugs (NANSAIDs) and serious upper gastrointestinal bleeding: a meta-analysis based on individual patient data. *Br J Clin Pharmacol* (2002) 54, 320–6.
6. Hemming JD, Bird HA, Pickup ME, Saunders A, Lowe JR, Dixon JS. Bioavailability of aspirin in the presence of dextropropoxyphene/paracetamol combination. *Pharmatherapeutica* (1981) 2, 543–6.
7. Sioufi A, Stierlin H, Schweizer A, Botta L, Degen PH, Theobald W, Brechbühler S. Recent findings concerning clinically relevant pharmacokinetics of diclofenac sodium. In: Voltarol — New Findings, ed Kass E. Proc Int Symp Voltarol, Paris June 22nd, 1981. 15th Int Congress of Rheumatology. p 19–30.
8. Merck Sharp & Dohme Ltd. Personal communication, 1988.
9. Dolobid (Diflunisal). Merck Sharp & Dohme Ltd. UK Summary of product characteristics, March 2000.
10. Wright CE, Antal EJ, Gillespie WR, Albert KS. Ibuprofen and acetaminophen kinetics when taken concurrently. *Clin Pharmacol Ther* (1983) 34, 707–10.
11. von Schrader HW, Buscher G, Dierdorf D, Mügge H, Wolf D. Nabumetone — a novel anti-inflammatory drug: the influence of food, milk, antacids, and analgesics on bioavailability of single oral doses. *Int J Clin Pharmacol Ther Toxicol* (1983) 21, 311–21.
12. McIntire SC, Rubenstein RC, Gartner JC, Gilboa N, Ellis D. Acute flank pain and reversible renal dysfunction associated with nonsteroidal anti-inflammatory drug use. *Pediatrics* (1993) 92, 459–60.
13. Del Vecchio MT, Sundel ER. Alternating antipyretics: is this an alternative? *Pediatrics* (2001) 108, 1236–7.
14. Whelton A. Renal effects of over-the-counter analgesics. *J Clin Pharmacol* (1995) 35, 454–63.
15. Bach PH, Berndt WO, Delzell E, Dubach U, Finn WF, Fox JM, Hess R, Michielsen P, Sandler DP, Trump B, Williams G. A safety assessment of fixed dose combinations of acetaminophen and acetylsalicylic acid, coformulated with caffeine. *Ren Fail* (1998) 20, 749–62.
16. Carson SM. Alternating acetaminophen and ibuprofen in the febrile child: examination of the evidence regarding efficacy and safety. *Pediatr Nurs* (2003) 29, 379–82.
17. Anon. No evidence for practice of alternating doses of paracetamol and ibuprofen in children with fever. *Pharm J* (2004) 272, 4.
18. Conroy S, Tomlin S, Soor S. Unsubstantiated alarmist declarations need to be examined. *Pharm J* (2004) 272, 152.

NSAIDs + Pentoxifylline

A review of bleeding events associated with the use of postoperative ketorolac revealed that a small number of patients were also taking pentoxifylline.[1] The UK manufacturer therefore, rather cautiously, contraindicates concurrent use,[2] whereas the US manufacturer[3] made no mention of this tentative interaction. The manufacturer of dexketoprofen similarly predicts that the concurrent use of pentoxifylline increases the risk of bleeding.[4] There seems to be no evidence regarding this interaction with other NSAIDs, but as non-selective NSAIDs have antiplatelet effects and pentoxifylline can cause bleeding events, it would be prudent to be alert for this possible interaction with any of the non-selective NSAIDs.

1. Syntex Pharmaceuticals Limited. Personal communication, January 1995.
2. Toradol (Ketorolac trometamol). Roche Products Ltd. UK Summary of product characteristics, July 2009.
3. Toradol (Ketorolac tromethamine). Roche Pharmaceuticals. US Prescribing information, September 2002.
4. Keral (Dexketoprofen trometamol). A.Menarini Pharma U.K. S.R.L. UK Summary of product characteristics, March 2007.

NSAIDs + Pesticides

Chronic exposure to lindane and other chlorinated pesticides can slightly increase the rate of metabolism of phenazone (antipyrine) and phenylbutazone.

Clinical evidence, mechanism, importance and management

(a) Phenazone (Antipyrine)

A study in 26 men occupationally exposed to a mixture of insecticides, predominantly **DDT [clofenotane]**, **chlordane** and **lindane**, found that the half-life of phenazone 10 or 15 mg/kg was reduced from 13.1 hours, in a group of 33 unexposed subjects, to 7.7 hours in the exposed group.[1] The significance of this is unclear as changes in working practices have reduced occupational exposure to such chemicals.

(b) Phenylbutazone

The plasma half-life of phenylbutazone in a group of men who regularly used **chlorinated insecticide** sprays (mainly **lindane**) as part of their work, was found to be 20% shorter (51 hours) than in a control group (64 hours), due, it is believed, to the enzyme-inducing effects of the pesticides.[2] This modest increase in rate of metabolism is of doubtful direct clinical importance, but it illustrates the changed metabolism that can occur in those exposed to environmental chemical agents.

1. Kolmodin B, Azarnoff DL, Sjöqvist F. Effect of environmental factors on drug metabolism: decreased plasma half-life of antipyrine in workers exposed to chlorinated hydrocarbon insecticides. *Clin Pharmacol Ther* (1969) 10, 638–42.
2. Kolmodin-Hedman B. Decreased plasma half-life of phenylbutazone in workers exposed to chlorinated pesticides. *Eur J Clin Pharmacol* (1973) 5, 195–8.

NSAIDs + Phenobarbital

Phenobarbital modestly decreases the AUC of fenoprofen and increases the clearance of phenylbutazone.

Clinical evidence, mechanism, importance and management

In 6 healthy subjects pretreatment with phenobarbital 15 or 60 mg every 6 hours for 10 days reduced the AUC of a single 200-mg dose of **fenoprofen** by 23% and 37%, respectively.[1]

In 5 healthy subjects the half-life of a single 6-mg/kg dose of **phenylbutazone** was reduced by 38% after pretreatment with phenobarbital 2 to 3 mg/kg daily for 3 weeks.[2] Other studies confirm that phenobarbital increases the clearance of **phenylbutazone**.[3,4]

The probable reason for the increased clearance or decreased exposure to these NSAIDs is that phenobarbital increases their metabolism by the liver. **Phenazone** is metabolised by mixed function oxidase enzymes in the liver, for which reason it is extensively used as a model drug for studying whether other drugs induce or inhibit liver enzymes. In one study phenobarbital caused about a 40% reduction in the half-life of **phenazone** thereby demonstrating that liver enzymes were being stimulated to metabolise **phenazone** more rapidly.[5]

The clinical importance of these interactions is uncertain, but given the magnitude of the effects it seems likely to be small. Nevertheless if the effects of these NSAIDs are reduced if phenobarbital is added it would seem prudent to consider an interaction as a possible cause.

1. Helleberg L, Rubin A, Wolen RL, Rodda BE, Ridolfo AS, Gruber CM. A pharmacokinetic interaction in man between phenobarbitone and fenoprofen, a new anti-inflammatory agent. *Br J Clin Pharmacol* (1974) 1, 371–4.
2. Anderson KE, Peterson CM, Alvares AP, Kappas A. Oxidative drug metabolism and inducibility by phenobarbital in sickle cell anemia. *Clin Pharmacol Ther* (1977) 22, 580–7.
3. Levi AJ, Sherlock S, Walker D. Phenylbutazone and isoniazid metabolism in patients with liver disease in relation to previous drug therapy. *Lancet* (1968) i, 1275–9.
4. Whittaker JA, Price Evans DA. Genetic control of phenylbutazone metabolism in man. *BMJ* (1970) 4, 323–8.
5. Vesell ES, Page JG. Genetic control of the phenobarbital-induced shortening of plasma antipyrine half-lives in man. *J Clin Invest* (1969) 48, 2202–9.

NSAIDs + Probenecid

Probenecid reduces the clearance of diflunisal, indometacin (toxicity seen), ketoprofen, ketorolac, naproxen, meclofenamate, tenoxicam and tiaprofenic acid and raises their levels. The uricosuric effects of probenecid are not affected by indometacin but may be slightly reduced by sulindac.

Clinical evidence

(a) Diflunisal

In 8 healthy subjects probenecid 500 mg twice daily increased the steady-state plasma levels of diflunisal 250 mg twice daily by 65%, and reduced the clearances of its glucuronide metabolites.[1]

(b) Indometacin

A study in 28 patients with osteoarthritis, taking indometacin 50 to 150 mg daily orally or rectally, found that probenecid 500 mg to 1 g daily roughly doubled indometacin plasma levels and this paralleled increased effectiveness (relief of morning stiffness, joint tenderness and raised grip strength indices). However, 4 patients developed indometacin toxicity.[2]

Other studies have also found that probenecid causes a marked rise in plasma indometacin levels.[3-5] Clear signs of indometacin toxicity (nausea, headache, tinnitus, confusion and a rise in blood urea) occurred when a woman with stable mild renal impairment was given probenecid.[6] The uricosuric effects of probenecid were not altered.[3]

(c) Ketoprofen

In 6 healthy subjects probenecid 500 mg every 6 hours reduced the clearance of ketoprofen 50 mg every 6 hours by 67%.[7]

(d) Ketorolac

In a study in 8 subjects, probenecid 500 mg four times daily for 4 days increased the total AUC of a single 10-mg dose of ketorolac by more than threefold, increased its half-life from 6.6 hours to 15.1 hours, raised its maximum plasma levels by 24% and reduced its clearance by 67%.[8]

(e) Meclofenamate

Single-dose studies in 6 healthy subjects on the pharmacokinetics of sodium meclofenamate 100 mg found that pretreatment with probenecid (dosage unstated) increased its AUC and reduced its apparent plasma clearance by 60%, primarily due to a decrease in non-renal clearance.[9]

(f) Naproxen

In 12 healthy subjects, probenecid 500 mg twice daily increased the plasma levels of naproxen 250 mg twice daily by 50%.[10]

(g) Sulindac

The manufacturer of sulindac notes that probenecid increased plasma levels of sulindac and its sulfone metabolite, but had little effect on the active sulfide metabolite. Sulindac produced a modest reduction in the uricosuric action of probenecid,[11] which is said not to be clinically significant in most circumstances.[11]

(h) Tenoxicam

Probenecid 1 g twice daily for 4 days increased the maximum serum levels of a single 20-mg oral dose of tenoxicam by 25%. None of the other pharmacokinetic parameters was significantly altered.[12]

(i) Tiaprofenic acid

Probenecid appeared to reduce the urinary excretion of tiaprofenic acid in one healthy subject. The maximum urinary excretion rate was reduced by 66% and delayed by 2 hours.[13]

Mechanism

Probenecid is a known substrate for renal glucuronidation, and possibly competitively inhibits the renal glucuronidation of these NSAIDs.[14]

Importance and management

The interaction between indometacin and probenecid is established and adequately documented. Concurrent use should be well monitored because, while clinical improvement can undoubtedly occur, some patients may develop indometacin toxicity (headache, dizziness, light-headedness, nausea, etc.). This is particularly likely in those with some renal impairment. Reduce the indometacin dose as necessary. Information about other NSAIDs is not as well documented, but these interactions also appear to be established. The clinical importance of most of them is uncertain, but probably small. Reports of adverse effects seem to be lacking, but it would still be prudent to be alert for any evidence of increased adverse effects. Reduce the NSAID dose if necessary. The exception is ketorolac, which its manufacturer[15] contraindicates with probenecid.

1. Macdonald JI, Wallace SM, Herman RJ, Verbeeck RK. Effect of probenecid on the formation and elimination kinetics of the sulphate and glucuronide conjugates of diflunisal. *Eur J Clin Pharmacol* (1995) 47, 519–23.
2. Brooks PM, Bell MA, Sturrock RD, Famaey JP, Dick WC. The clinical significance of indomethacin-probenecid interaction. *Br J Clin Pharmacol* (1974) 1, 287–90.
3. Skeith MD, Simkin PA, Healey LA. The renal excretion of indomethacin and its inhibition by probenecid. *Clin Pharmacol Ther* (1968) 9, 89–93.
4. Emori W, Paulus HE, Bluestone R, Pearson CM. The pharmacokinetics of indomethacin in serum. *Clin Pharmacol Ther* (1973) 14, 134.
5. Baber N, Halliday L, Littler T, Orme ML'E, Sibeon R. Clinical studies of the interaction between indomethacin and probenecid. *Br J Clin Pharmacol* (1978) 5, 364P.
6. Sinclair H, Gibson T. Interaction between probenecid and indomethacin. *Br J Rheumatol* (1986) 25, 316–17.
7. Upton RA, Williams RL, Buskin JN, Jones RM. Effects of probenecid on ketoprofen kinetics. *Clin Pharmacol Ther* (1982) 31, 705–12.
8. Mroszczak EJ, Combs DL, Goldblum R, Yee J, McHugh D, Tsina I, Fratis T. The effect of probenecid on ketorolac pharmacokinetics after oral dosing of ketorolac tromethamine. *Clin Pharmacol Ther* (1992) 51, 154.
9. Waller ES. The effect of probenecid on the disposition of meclofenamate sodium. *Drug Intell Clin Pharm* (1983) 17, 453–4.
10. Runkel R, Mroszczak E, Chaplin M, Sevelius H, Segre E. Naproxen-probenecid interaction. *Clin Pharmacol Ther* (1978) 24, 706–13.
11. Clinoril (Sulindac). Merck & Co., Inc. US Prescribing information, August 2009.
12. Day RO, Geisslinger G, Paull P, Williams KM. Neither cimetidine nor probenecid affect the pharmacokinetics of tenoxicam in normal volunteers. *Br J Clin Pharmacol* (1994) 37, 79–81.
13. Jamali F, Russell AS, Lehmann C, Berry BW. Pharmacokinetics of tiaprofenic acid in healthy and arthritic subjects. *J Pharm Sci* (1985) 74, 953–6.
14. Vree TB, van den Biggelaar-Martea M, Verwey-van Wissen CPWGM, van Ewijk-Beneken Kolmer EWJ. Probenecid inhibits the glucuronidation of indomethacin and *O*-desmethylindomethacin in humans: a pilot experiment. *Pharm World Sci* (1994) 16, 22–6.
15. Toradol (Ketorolac trometamol). Roche Products Ltd. UK Summary of product characteristics, July 2009.

NSAIDs or Aspirin + Prostaglandins

Misoprostol increases the incidence of abdominal pain and diarrhoea when used with diclofenac or indometacin. Isolated cases of neurological adverse effects have been seen when naproxen or phenylbutazone were given with misoprostol. However, no important pharmacokinetic interactions seem to occur between misoprostol and aspirin, diclofenac, ibuprofen or indometacin. NSAIDs are reported not to affect the abortive effects of intravaginal misoprostol.

Clinical evidence, mechanism, importance and management

A. Oral misoprostol

(a) Gastrointestinal adverse effects

A higher incidence of abdominal pain, diarrhoea, nausea and dyspepsia occurred when **diclofenac** was given with misoprostol.[1,2] Concurrent use of **indometacin** and misoprostol also resulted in an increase in the frequency and severity of abdominal symptoms, frequency of bowel movements, and a decrease in faecal consistency.[3] The most frequent adverse effect of misoprostol alone is diarrhoea, and this may limit the dose tolerated. When using misoprostol with NSAIDs, warn patients about the possibility of increased stomach pain and diarrhoea. However, note that preparations containing **diclofenac** or **naproxen** with misoprostol are available.

(b) Neurological adverse effects

A man with rheumatoid arthritis taking long-term **naproxen** developed ataxic symptoms a few hours after starting to take misoprostol. He said he felt drunk, staggering about and vomiting. He rapidly improved when he stopped the misoprostol but the adverse symptoms recurred on two further occasions when he restarted misoprostol.[4]

Adverse effects developed in 3 patients taking **phenylbutazone** 200 to 400 mg daily when they took misoprostol 400 to 800 micrograms daily.[5] One had headaches, dizziness and ambulatory instability that disappeared and then reappeared when the misoprostol was stopped and then restarted. No problems occurred when the **phenylbutazone** was replaced by **etodolac** 400 mg daily. The other 2 patients developed symptoms including headache, dizziness, hot flushes and transient diplopia.[5,6] No problems developed when one of them was given **naproxen** and misoprostol.[6] The reasons for this reaction are not understood but theoretically it could be due to a potentiation of the adverse effects of **phenylbutazone**. The general relevance of these few reports is unclear, but bear them in mind should unexpected neurological effects occur.

(c) Other studies

No clinically important pharmacokinetic interactions have been found to occur between **aspirin** 975 mg and misoprostol 200 micrograms,[7] or between **ibuprofen** and misoprostol.[8] One study found that misoprostol 800 micrograms daily decreased the AUC of a single 100-mg dose of **diclofenac** by a modest 20%.[2] However, other studies have found that misoprostol had no effect on steady-state **diclofenac** pharmacokinetics.[9] One study found that misoprostol 200 micrograms raised the steady-state levels of **indometacin** 50 mg three times daily by about 30%,[10] whereas another found that misoprostol 400 micrograms twice daily reduced the AUC of **indometacin** 50 mg twice daily by 13% after one dose and reduced the maximum steady-state plasma concentration by 24%.[3] These modest changes in **diclofenac** and **indometacin** levels are not expected to be clinically important.

Women undergoing second trimester medical terminations of pregnancy were given oral mifepristone 600 mg on day one, then 36 to 48 hours later, intravaginal misoprostol 800 micrograms. Starting 3 hours later, misoprostol 400 micrograms was given orally every 3 hours until expulsion, up to a maximum of nine oral doses of misoprostol. The women were randomised to receive a single dose of either paracetamol 1 g with dihydrocodeine 20 mg (n=38) or **diclofenac** 100 mg (n=36), given at the time of the intravaginal dose of misoprostol. The use of **diclofenac** did not increase either the time required for termination, or the amount of misoprostol needed.[11]

B. Vaginal prostaglandins

NSAIDs and aspirin are frequently avoided before the use of **prostaglandins** for induction of uterine contractions, because of the theoretical concern that they may inhibit efficacy.[12] For example, the UK manufacturer of **dinoprostone** says that NSAIDs including aspirin should be stopped before giving intravaginal **dinoprostone** for induction of labour.[13] However, a study involving 416 women given intravaginal **misoprostol** to induce early abortion found that the concurrent use of oral NSAIDs did not interfere with the efficacy of misoprostol,[12] and the US manufacturer of **dinoprostone** does not list NSAIDs or aspirin as possible interacting drugs.[14]

1. Gagnier P. Review of the safety of diclofenac/misoprostol. *Drugs* (1993) 45 (Suppl 1), 31–5.
2. Dammann HG, Simon-Schultz J, Steinhoff I, Damaschke A, Schmoldt A, Sallowsky E. Differential effects of misoprostol and ranitidine on the pharmacokinetics of diclofenac and gastrointestinal symptoms. *Br J Clin Pharmacol* (1993) 36, 345–9.
3. Kendall MJ, Gibson R, Walt RP. Co-administration of misoprostol or ranitidine with indomethacin: effects on pharmacokinetics, abdominal symptoms and bowel habit. *Aliment Pharmacol Ther* (1992) 6, 437–46.
4. Huq M. Neurological adverse effects of naproxen and misoprostol combination. *Br J Gen Pract* (1990) 40, 432.
5. Jacquemier JM, Lassoued S, Laroche M, Mazières B. Neurosensory adverse effects after phenylbutazone and misoprostol combined treatment. *Lancet* (1989) 2, 1283.
6. Chassagne Ph, Humez C, Gourmelen O, Moore N, Le Loet X, Deshayes P. Neurosensory adverse effects after combined phenylbutazone and misoprostol. *Br J Rheumatol* (1991) 30, 392.
7. Karim A, Rozek LF, Leese PT. Absorption of misoprostol (Cytotec), an antiulcer prostaglandin, or aspirin is not affected when given concomitantly to healthy human subjects. *Gastroenterology* (1987) 92, 1742.
8. Small RE, Wilmot-Pater MG, McGee BA, Willis HE. Effects of misoprostol or ranitidine on ibuprofen pharmacokinetics. *Clin Pharm* (1991) 10, 870–2.
9. Karim A. Pharmacokinetics of diclofenac and misoprostol when administered alone or as a combination product. *Drugs* (1993) 45 (Suppl 1), 7–14.
10. Rainsford KD, James C, Hunt RH, Stetsko PI, Rischke JA, Karim A, Nicholson PA, Smith M, Hantsbarger G. Effects of misoprostol on the pharmacokinetics of indomethacin in human volunteers. *Clin Pharmacol Ther* (1992) 51, 415–21.
11. Fiala C, Swahn ML, Stephansson O, Gemzell-Danielsson K. The effect of non-steroidal anti-inflammatory drugs on medical abortion with mifepristone and misoprostol at 13-22 weeks gestation. *Hum Reprod* (2005) 20, 3072–7.
12. Creinin MD, Shulman T. Effect of nonsteroidal anti-inflammatory drugs on the action of misoprostol in a regimen for early abortion. *Contraception* (1997) 56, 165–8.
13. Propess (Dinoprostone). Ferring Pharmaceuticals Ltd. UK Summary of product characteristics, February 2007.
14. Prostin E2 (Dinoprostone). Pfizer Inc. US Prescribing information, April 2006.

NSAIDs or Aspirin + Proton pump inhibitors

The antiplatelet activity and the pharmacokinetics of aspirin do not appear to be affected by omeprazole. There was no clinically relevant pharmacokinetic interaction between omeprazole and diclofenac, enteric-coated ketoprofen, naproxen, or piroxicam; or between pantoprazole

and diclofenac or naproxen; or between esomeprazole and naproxen or rofecoxib.

Clinical evidence

(a) Aspirin

In a preliminary study in 11 healthy subjects, **omeprazole** 20 mg daily for 2 days reduced the serum levels of the salicylic acid metabolite of aspirin at 30 and 90 minutes after a single 650-mg dose of aspirin by 40% and 52%, respectively.[1] However, another study in 14 healthy subjects given **omeprazole** 20 mg daily for 4 days, with a final dose one hour before a single 125-mg dose of aspirin, found that **omeprazole** did not significantly affect the plasma levels of either aspirin or salicylic acid. **Omeprazole** also did not affect the antiplatelet effects of aspirin.[2] Similarly, **omeprazole** had no effect on the bioavailability of aspirin (uncoated or enteric-coated tablets) in another study, although it increased the rate of absorption of aspirin from enteric-coated tablets.[3]

(b) Diclofenac

In a study in 13 healthy subjects, a single 105-mg dose of diclofenac potassium suspension (*Flogan*) was given during fasting and after gastric acid secretion blockade with **omeprazole**. The pharmacokinetics of the diclofenac were not changed to a clinically relevant extent by **omeprazole**.[4] Similarly, in 14 healthy subjects, the concurrent use of **omeprazole** 20 mg daily and diclofenac 50 mg twice daily for one week had no effect on the pharmacokinetics of either drug.[5]

In another study in 24 healthy subjects, the concurrent use of a single 40-mg oral dose of **pantoprazole** and diclofenac 100 mg (as enteric-coated *Voltarol*) did not affect the pharmacokinetics of either drug.[6]

(c) Ketoprofen

One study found that there were no significant changes in the pharmacokinetics of enteric-coated ketoprofen, given with or without **omeprazole**, although a trend towards higher plasma concentrations with omeprazole was noted, indicating the possibility of increased drug release in the stomach in the presence of an elevated pH.[7]

(d) Naproxen

Naproxen 250 mg twice daily, given to healthy subjects with **omeprazole** 20 mg daily,[5] **pantoprazole** 40 mg daily,[8] or **esomeprazole** 40 mg daily[9] for one week, had no effect on the pharmacokinetics of either naproxen or the proton pump inhibitor.

(e) Phenazone (Antipyrine)

In one study, the pharmacokinetics of **pantoprazole** 40 mg orally daily for 8 days was not altered to a clinically relevant extent by a single 5-mg/kg oral dose of phenazone given on day 8. **Pantoprazole** did not affect the pharmacokinetics of phenazone.[10]

(f) Piroxicam

In a study in 24 healthy subjects, the concurrent use of **omeprazole** 20 mg daily and piroxicam 10 mg daily for one week had no effect on the pharmacokinetics of either drug.[5]

(g) Rofecoxib

In a study in 30 healthy subjects, the concurrent use of **esomeprazole** 40 mg daily and rofecoxib 12.5 mg daily for one week had no effect on the pharmacokinetics of either drug, apart from a slight increase in the maximum level and AUC of rofecoxib, which was not thought to be clinically relevant.[9]

Mechanism

Data from *animal* studies suggest that the absorption and thus the effects of aspirin and NSAIDs can be reduced by omeprazole and H_2-receptor antagonists by a pH dependent mechanism.[11,12] However, note that clinical studies have not found H_2-receptor antagonists to have any important effect on the pharmacokinetics of aspirin or NSAIDs, see 'NSAIDs or Aspirin + H_2-receptor antagonists', p.151. It has been suggested that reducing gastric acidity with omeprazole results in the earlier disruption of enteric-coated tablets, and an increased absorption rate.[3]

Importance and management

The interaction between aspirin and omeprazole is not established. The balance of evidence suggests that omeprazole is unlikely to have an important effect on the pharmacokinetics and efficacy of aspirin. However, it would be of benefit to confirm this in further studies.[2,13]

No clinically significant pharmacokinetic interactions have been identified between any of the other NSAIDs and the proton pump inhibitors cited here, and no special precautions are needed during concurrent use. However, for mention that valdecoxib raises the plasma levels of omeprazole see 'NSAIDs; Parecoxib + Miscellaneous', p.161.

Note that omeprazole and other proton pump inhibitors are widely used in the management of the gastrointestinal complications of aspirin and NSAIDs.

1. Anand BS, Sanduja SK, Lichtenberger LM. Effect of omeprazole on the bioavailability of aspirin: a randomized controlled study on healthy volunteers. *Gastroenterology* (1999) 116: A371.
2. Iñarrea P, Esteva F, Cornudella R, Lanas A. Omeprazole does not interfere with the antiplatelet effect of low-dose aspirin in man. *Scand J Gastroenterol* (2000) 35, 242–6.
3. Nefesoglu FZ, Ayanoglu-Dülger G, Ulusoy NB, Imeryüz N. Interaction of omeprazole with enteric-coated salicylate tablets. *Int J Clin Pharmacol Ther* (1998) 36, 549–53.
4. Poli A, Moreno RA, Ribeiro W, Dias HB, Moreno H, Muscara MN, De Nucci G. Influence of gastric acid secretion blockade and food intake on the bioavailability of a potassium diclofenac suspension in healthy male volunteers. *Int J Clin Pharmacol Ther* (1996) 34, 76–9.
5. Andersson T, Bredberg E, Lagerström P-O, Naesdal J, Wilson I. Lack of drug-drug interaction between three different non-steroidal anti-inflammatory drugs and omeprazole. *Eur J Clin Pharmacol* (1998) 54, 399–404.
6. Bliesath H, Huber R, Steinijans VW, Koch HJ, Wurst W, Mascher H. Lack of pharmacokinetic interaction between pantoprazole and diclofenac. *Int J Clin Pharmacol Ther* (1996) 34, 152–6.
7. Qureshi SA, Caillé G, Lacasse Y, McGilveray IJ. Pharmacokinetics of two enteric-coated ketoprofen products in humans with or without coadministration of omeprazole and comparison with dissolution findings. *Pharm Res* (1994) 11, 1669–72.
8. Schulz H-U, Hartmann M, Krupp S, Schuerer M, Huber R, Luehmann R, Bethke T, Wurst W. Pantoprazole lacks interaction with the NSAID naproxen. *Gastroenterology* (2000) 118 (Suppl 2), A1304.
9. Hassan-Alin M, Naesdal J, Nilsson-Pieschl C, Långström G, Andersson T. Lack of pharmacokinetic interaction between esomeprazole and the nonsteroidal anti-inflammatory drugs naproxen and rofecoxib in healthy subjects. *Clin Drug Invest* (2005) 25, 731–40.
10. De Mey C, Meineke I, Steinijans VW, Huber R, Hartmann M, Bliesath H, Wurst W. Pantoprazole lacks interaction with antipyrine in man, either by inhibition or induction. *Int J Clin Pharmacol Ther* (1994) 32, 98–106.
11. Lichtenberger LM, Ulloa C, Romero JJ, Vanous AL, Illich PA, Dial EJ. Nonsteroidal anti-inflammatory drug and phospholipid prodrugs: combination therapy with antisecretory agents in rats. *Gastroenterology* (1996) 111, 990–5.
12. Giraud M-N, Sanduja SK, Felder TB, Illich PA, Dial EJ, Lichtenberger LM. Effect of omeprazole on the bioavailability of unmodified and phospholipid-complexed aspirin in rats. *Aliment Pharmacol Ther* (1997) 11, 899–906.
13. Fernández-Fernández FJ. Might proton pump inhibitors prevent the antiplatelet effects of low- or very low-dose aspirin? *Arch Intern Med* (2002) 162, 2248.

NSAIDs + Rifampicin (Rifampin)

The plasma levels of celecoxib, diclofenac, and etoricoxib are reduced by rifampicin, but piroxicam does not appear to be affected. Dipyrone increased the maximum level of rifampicin in one study.

Clinical evidence

(a) Celecoxib

In 12 healthy subjects pretreatment with rifampicin 600 mg daily for 5 days reduced the AUC of a single 200-mg dose of celecoxib by 64% and increased its clearance by 185%.[1] A preliminary report of another study found broadly similar results.[2]

(b) Diclofenac

A study in 6 healthy subjects found that, after taking rifampicin 450 mg daily for 6 days, the maximum serum level of diclofenac, measured 8 hours after a single 100-mg dose of an enteric-coated tablet, was reduced by 43% and the AUC was reduced by 67%.[3]

(c) Dipyrone (Metamizole sodium)

A study in untreated patients with leprosy found that the pharmacokinetics of a single 600-mg dose of rifampicin were not markedly changed by 1 g of dipyrone, but peak serum rifampicin levels occurred sooner (at 3 instead of 4 hours) and were about 50% higher.[4]

(d) Etoricoxib

Rifampicin 600 mg daily for 12 days reduced the AUC of a single 60-mg dose of etoricoxib given on day 8 by 65%. The maximum plasma concentration of etoricoxib was reduced by 40%.[5]

(e) Phenazone (Antipyrine)

Rifampicin 600 mg daily for 13 days reduced the plasma concentrations of a single 1.2-g oral dose of phenazone. The mean AUC of phenazone was reduced by 59% and had not returned to the pre-rifampicin level 13 days after the final rifampicin dose.[6]

(f) Piroxicam

A study in 6 healthy subjects given a single 40-mg dose of piroxicam before and after a 7-day course of rifampicin 600 mg daily found that rifampicin did not significantly alter the pharmacokinetics of piroxicam.[7]

Mechanism

Rifampicin is a potent inducer of hepatic enzymes, and it is likely that it increased the metabolism of the affected NSAIDs.

Importance and management

Although information is limited, these pharmacokinetic interactions appear to be established. Their clinical relevance remains to be determined, but it seems likely that the efficacy of these NSAIDs will be reduced by rifampicin. Combined use should be well monitored, and the NSAID dosage increased if necessary, or an alternative analgesic considered. The clinical relevance of the increase in rifampicin maximum levels with metamizole is uncertain, but as it was only this pharmacokinetic parameter that was altered, it seems likely to be small.

1. Jayasagar G, Krishna Kumar M, Chandrasekhar K, Madhusudan RY. Influence of rifampicin pretreatment on the pharmacokinetics of celecoxib in healthy male volunteers. *Drug Metabol Drug Interact* (2003) 19, 287–95.
2. Porras AG, Gertz B, Buschmeier A, Constanzer M, Gumbs C, Gottesdiener K, Waldman S, Gelmann A, Greenberg H, Schwartz J. The effects of metabolic induction by rifampin (Rf) on the elimination of celecoxib (CXB) and the effect of CXB on CYP2D6 metabolism. *Clin Pharmacol Ther* (2001) 69, P58.
3. Kumar JS, Mamidi NVSR, Chakrapani T, Krishna DR. Rifampicin pretreatment reduces bioavailability of diclofenac sodium. *Indian J Pharmacol* (1995) 27, 183–5.
4. Krishna DR, Appa Rao AVN, Ramanakar TV, Reddy KSC, Prabhakar MC. Pharmacokinetics of rifampin in the presence of dipyrone in leprosy patients. *Drug Dev Ind Pharm* (1984) 10, 101–110.
5. Agrawal NGB, Matthews CZ, Mazenko RS, Woolf EJ, Porras AG, Chen X, Miller JL, Michiels N, Wehling M, Schultz A, Gottlieb AB, Kraft WK, Greenberg HE, Waldman SA, Curtis SP, Gottesdiener KM. The effects of modifying in vivo cytochrome P450 3A (CYP3A) activity on etoricoxib pharmacokinetics and of etoricoxib administration on CYP3A activity. *J Clin Pharmacol* (2004) 44, 1125–31.

6. Bennett PN, John VA, Whitmarsh VB. Effect of rifampicin on metoprolol and antipyrine kinetics. *Br J Clin Pharmacol* (1982) 13, 387–91.
7. Patel RB, Shah GF, Jain SM. The effect of rifampicin on piroxicam kinetics. *Indian J Physiol Pharmacol* (1988) 32, 226–228.

NSAIDs + SSRIs

SSRIs might increase the risk of gastrointestinal bleeding, especially upper gastrointestinal bleeding, and the risk appears to be further increased by the concurrent use of NSAIDs.

Clinical evidence

A large number of studies have found that SSRIs alone increase the risk of gastro-intestinal bleeding, mainly from the upper gastrointestinal tract. One review of 15 epidemiological studies found that the relative risk of upper gastrointestinal bleeding with SSRIs compared with non-use, ranged from 1.2 to 3.6, which was statistically significant in 11 of the studies. The pooled estimate of the 14 studies that provided an odds ratio compared with non-users was 1.7, but note that there was a lack of consistency between the studies.[1] A meta-analysis[2] of 4 observational studies including 153 000 patients, calculated an odds ratio of 2.36 for SSRI-associated upper gastrointestinal bleeding with number needed to harm per year of 411. Another review concludes that overall the risk is small, but it is important because of the potential clinical consequences of gastrointestinal bleeding.[3] A retrospective cohort study in elderly patients taking antidepressants with greater inhibition of serotonin reuptake, found that after controlling for age, the risk of upper gastrointestinal bleeding increased by 10.7% and the risk was greatest in octogenarians.[4]

A number of studies also show that the risk of gastrointestinal bleeding with SSRIs is further increased by the concurrent use of NSAIDs. The meta-analysis[2] of 4 observational studies including 153 000 patients, found that the odds ratio for upper gastrointestinal bleeding increased to 6.33 for concurrent SSRI and NSAID use, with a number needed to harm per year of 106. A review of 11 epidemiological studies into the potential interaction between SSRIs and NSAIDs, found that six of these showed an effect that was greater than the sum of the SSRIs or NSAIDs alone. The relative risk of combined use ranged from 4.2 to 15.6, compared with 1.3 to 3.6 for SSRIs alone and 2.8 to 4.5 for NSAIDs alone.[1]

One of the studies that showed no effect, reported that both SSRIs and NSAIDs were associated with a 2-fold increase in risk of gastrointestinal bleeding, but that the risk of bleeding was not substantially increased when both drugs were taken together (odds ratio for NSAIDs was 2.19, SSRIs was 2.63 and combined use was 2.93).[5] A further study found that the incidence of upper gastrointestinal bleeding in patients taking an SSRI and an NSAID was similar to that in those taking NSAIDs alone (odds ratio for NSAIDs was 7.82 and combined use was 8.32), with the SSRI alone having little risk.[6] Some other workers have also disagreed with the suggestion of increased risk with combined use, and found no evidence to suggest that SSRIs are more likely to cause gastrointestinal bleeding than other drugs.[7]

Mechanism

Serotonin is not synthesised by platelets but is taken up into platelets from the bloodstream. Serotonin released from platelets has an important role in regulating the haemostatic response to injury as it potentiates platelet aggregation. At therapeutic doses, SSRIs can block this reuptake of serotonin by platelets leading to serotonin depletion, impairment of haemostatic function and an increased risk of bleeding.[4,8-10]

Importance and management

Serotonin released by platelets plays an important role in haemostasis and there appears to be an association between the use of antidepressant drugs that interfere with serotonin reuptake and the occurrence of bleeding, including gastrointestinal bleeding. In addition, the concurrent use of an NSAID can potentiate the risk of bleeding. Therefore, in general, caution is recommended in patients taking SSRIs with NSAIDs or other drugs that affect coagulation or platelet function, such as aspirin (see 'Antiplatelet drugs + SSRIs or SNRIs', p.780). Alternatives such as paracetamol (acetaminophen) or less gastrotoxic NSAIDs, such as ibuprofen, should be considered, but if the combination of an SSRI and NSAID cannot be avoided, prescribing of gastroprotective drugs, such as proton pump inhibitors, H_2-receptor antagonists, or prostaglandin analogues, should be considered, especially in elderly patients, who seem to be at greater risk of SSRI-associated bleeding, or those with a history of gastrointestinal bleeding. Patients, particularly those taking multiple drugs that can cause bleeding, should be advised to seek informed medical opinion before using non-prescription drugs, such as ibuprofen, on a regular basis.

1. de Abajo FJ. Effects of selective serotonin reuptake inhibitors on platelet function: mechanisms, clinical outcomes and implications for use in elderly patients. *Drugs Aging* (2011) 28, 345–67.
2. Meta-analysis: gastrointestinal bleeding due to interaction between selective serotonin uptake inhibitors and non-steroidal anti-inflammatory drugs. *Aliment Pharmacol Ther* (2008) 27, 31–40.
3. Andrade C, Sandarsh S, Chethan KB, Nagesh KS. Serotonin reuptake inhibitor antidepressants and abnormal bleeding: a review for clinicians and a reconsideration of mechanisms. *J Clin Psychiatry* (2010) 71, 1565–75.
4. Van Walraven C, Mamdani MM, Wells PS, Williams JI. Inhibition of serotonin reuptake by antidepressants and upper gastrointestinal bleeding in elderly patients: retrospective cohort study. *BMJ* (2001) 323, 655–8.
5. Tata LJ, Fortun PJ, Hubbard RB, Smeeth L, Hawkey CJ, Smith CJ, Whitaker HJ, Farrington CP, Card TR, West J. Does concurrent prescription of selective serotonin reuptake inhibitors and non-steroidal anti-inflammatory drugs substantially increase the risk of upper gastrointestinal bleeding? *Aliment Pharmacol Ther* (2005) 22, 175–81.
6. Vidal X, Ibáñez L, Vendrell L, Conforti A, Laporte J-R, Spanish-Italian Collaborative Group for the Epidemiology of Gastrointestinal Bleeding. Risk of upper gastrointestinal bleeding and the degree of serotonin reuptake inhibition by antidepressants: a case-control study. *Drug Safety* (2008) 31, 159–68.
7. Dunn NR, Pearce GL, Shakir SAW. Association between SSRIs and upper gastrointestinal bleeding. SSRIs are no more likely than other drugs to cause such bleeding. *BMJ* (2000) 320, 1405.
8. De Abajo FJ, Rodríguez LAG, Montero D. Association between selective serotonin reuptake inhibitors and upper gastrointestinal bleeding population based case-control study. *BMJ* (1999) 319, 1106–9.
9. Serebruany VL. Selective serotonin reuptake inhibitors and increased bleeding risk: are we missing something? *Am J Med* (2006) 119, 113–6.
10. Dalton SO, Sørensen HT, Johansen C. SSRIs and upper gastrointestinal bleeding. What is known and how should it influence prescribing? *CNS Drugs* (2006) 20, 143–51.

NSAIDs or Aspirin + Sucralfate

Sucralfate appears not to have a clinically important effect on the pharmacokinetics of aspirin, choline-magnesium trisalicylate, diclofenac, ibuprofen, indometacin, ketoprofen, naproxen or piroxicam.

Clinical evidence, mechanism, importance and management

Sucralfate 2 g was given to 18 healthy subjects 30 minutes before single-doses of **ketoprofen** 50 mg, **indometacin** 50 mg, or **naproxen** 500 mg. Some statistically significant changes were seen (modestly reduced maximum plasma levels of **ketoprofen**, **indometacin**, and **naproxen**, reduced the rate of absorption of **naproxen** and **indometacin**, and increased the time to achieve maximum plasma levels with **indometacin**) but no alterations in bioavailability occurred.[1] A delay, but no reduction in the total absorption of **naproxen** is described in two studies.[2,3] Sucralfate 1 g four times daily for 2 days was found not to decrease the rate of absorption of a single 400-mg dose of **ibuprofen**[4] or of a single 650-mg dose of **aspirin**.[5] Sucralfate 5 g in divided doses did not significantly alter the absorption of a single 600-mg dose of **ibuprofen**.[6] Similarly, another study also found that sucralfate had no important effect on the pharmacokinetics of **ibuprofen** enantiomers.[7] In one study, sucralfate 2 g was found not to affect significantly the pharmacokinetics of either **piroxicam** 20 mg or **diclofenac** 50 mg.[8] In another study, sucralfate 2 g twice daily modestly reduced the AUC_{0-8} and maximum serum levels of a single 105-mg dose of **diclofenac potassium** by 20% and 38%, respectively.[9] Sucralfate 1 g every 6 hours was found not to affect the pharmacokinetics of **choline-magnesium trisalicylate** 1.5 g every 12 hours.[10]

Single-dose studies do not necessarily reliably predict what will happen when patients take drugs regularly, but most of the evidence available suggests that the effects of sucralfate are modest at most, and it is therefore unlikely to have an adverse effect on treatment with these NSAIDs.

1. Caillé G, Du Souich P, Gervais P, Besner J-G. Single dose pharmacokinetics of ketoprofen, indomethacin, and naproxen taken alone or with sucralfate. *Biopharm Drug Dispos* (1987) 8, 173–83.
2. Caille G, du Souich P, Gervais P, Besner JG, Vezina M. Effects of concurrent sucralfate administration on pharmacokinetics of naproxen. *Am J Med* (1987) 83 (Suppl 3B), 67–73.
3. Lafontaine D, Mailhot C, Vermeulen M, Bissonnette B, Lambert C. Influence of chewable sucralfate or a standard meal on the bioavailability of naproxen. *Clin Pharm* (1990) 9, 773–7.
4. Anaya AL, Mayersohn M, Conrad KA, Dimmitt DC. The influence of sucralfate on ibuprofen absorption in healthy adult males. *Biopharm Drug Dispos* (1986) 7, 443–51.
5. Lau A, Chang C-W, Schlesinger PK. Evaluation of a potential drug interaction between sucralfate and aspirin. *Clin Pharmacol Ther* (1986) 39, 151–5.
6. Pugh MC, Small RE, Garnett WR, Townsend RJ, Willis HE. Effect of sucralfate on ibuprofen absorption in normal volunteers. *Clin Pharm* (1984) 3, 630–3.
7. Levine MAH, Walker SE, Paton TW. The effect of food or sucralfate on the bioavailability of S(+) and R(-) enantiomers of ibuprofen. *J Clin Pharmacol* (1992) 32, 1110–14.
8. Ungethüm W. Study on the interaction between sucralfate and diclofenac/piroxicam in healthy volunteers. *Arzneimittelforschung* (1991) 41, 797–800.
9. Pedrazzoli J, Pierossi M de A, Muscará MN, Dias HB, da Silva CMF, Mendes FD, de Nucci G. Short-term sucralfate administration alters potassium diclofenac absorption in healthy male volunteers. *Br J Clin Pharmacol* (1997) 43, 104–8.
10. Schneider DK, Gannon RH, Sweeney KR, DeFusco PA. Influence of sucralfate on trilisate bioavailability. *J Clin Pharmacol* (1991) 31, 377–9.

NSAIDs or Aspirin + *Tamarindus indica*

***Tamarindus indica* (tamarind) fruit extract markedly increases the absorption and plasma levels of aspirin and ibuprofen.**

Clinical evidence, mechanism, importance and management

(a) Aspirin

A study in 6 healthy subjects found that the bioavailability of a single 600-mg dose of aspirin was increased when it was taken with a millet meal containing *Tamarindus indica* (tamarind) fruit extract, compared with the millet meal alone or following overnight fasting. The aspirin AUC rose sixfold, the maximum plasma levels rose almost threefold (from about 10 micrograms/mL with the meal or fasting to about 29 micrograms/mL with the *Tamarindus indica* extract) and the half-life increased moderately (from about 1.04 to 1.5 hours).[1] The reasons are not known, nor has the clinical importance of these large increases been evaluated, but this interaction should be borne in mind if high (analgesic or anti-inflammatory) doses of aspirin are taken with this fruit extract. There would seem to be the possible risk of aspirin toxicity.

(b) Ibuprofen

A study in 6 healthy subjects found that the bioavailability of a single 400-mg dose of ibuprofen was increased when it was taken with a millet meal containing *Tamarindus indica* (tamarind) fruit extract compared with the millet meal alone, or following overnight fasting. The ibuprofen AUC rose approximately twofold and the maximum plasma levels rose from about 38 micrograms/mL to 45 micrograms/mL. There was also an increase in the plasma levels of the metabolites of ibuprofen. Ingestion of the meal containing *Tamarindus indica* was thought to favour the absorption of ibuprofen. This might result in an increased risk of toxicity.[2]

1. Mustapha A, Yakasai IA, Aguye IA. Effect of *Tamarindus indica* L. on the bioavailability of aspirin in healthy human volunteers. *Eur J Drug Metab Pharmacokinet* (1996) 21, 223–6.
2. Garba M, Yakasai IA, Bakare MT, Munir HY. Effect of *Tamarindus indica* L. on the bioavailability of ibuprofen in healthy human volunteers. *Eur J Drug Metab Pharmacokinet* (2003) 28, 179–84.

NSAIDs + Tobacco

The clearance of diflunisal, phenazone (antipyrine) and phenylbutazone is greater in smokers than in non-smokers.

Clinical evidence, mechanism, importance and management

(a) Diflunisal

The clearance of a single 250-mg dose of diflunisal was 35% higher in 6 women who smoked 10 to 20 cigarettes a day than in 6 non-smoking women.[1] This change does not appear to be large enough to be of clinical importance.

(b) Phenazone (Antipyrine)

When a single 1-g dose of phenazone was given intravenously, its clearance was increased by 63% and its half-life reduced from 13.2 hours to 8 hours in 10 healthy women who smoked cigarettes, when compared with a control group of 26 non-smoking women.[2] Similar results were reported in another study.[3] This is likely to be as a result of cigarette smoking causing induction of CYP1A2, the enzyme involved in the metabolism of phenazone.[2]

This suggests that smokers may need larger doses of phenazone to achieve the same effects as non-smokers.

(c) Phenylbutazone

The half-life of a single 6-mg/kg dose of phenylbutazone was 37 hours in a group of smokers (10 or more cigarettes daily for 2 years) compared with 64 hours in a group of non-smokers. The metabolic clearance was roughly doubled.[4] The conclusion to be drawn is that those who smoke may possibly need larger or more frequent doses of phenylbutazone to achieve the same therapeutic response, but this needs confirmation.

1. Macdonald JI, Herman RJ, Verbeeck RK. Sex-difference and the effects of smoking and oral contraceptive steroids on the kinetics of diflunisal. *Eur J Clin Pharmacol* (1990) 38, 175–9.
2. Scavone JM, Greenblatt DJ, Abernethy DR, Luna BG, Harmatz JS, Shader RI Influence of oral contraceptive use and cigarette smoking, alone and together, on antipyrine pharmacokinetics. *J Clin Pharmacol* (1997) 37, 437–41.
3. Scavone JM, Greenblatt DJ, LeDuc BW, Blyden GT, Luna BG, Harmatz JS. Differential effect of cigarette smoking on antipyrine oxidation versus acetaminophen conjugation. *Pharmacology* (1990) 40, 77–84.
4. Garg SK, Kiran TNR. Effect of smoking on phenylbutazone disposition. *Int J Clin Pharmacol Ther Toxicol* (1982) 20, 289–90.

NSAIDs + Tricyclic antidepressants

An isolated report describes desipramine toxicity when ibuprofen was also given. The tricyclic antidepressants can delay the absorption of phenylbutazone and oxyphenbutazone from the gut.

Clinical evidence, mechanism, importance and management

(a) Ibuprofen

A 15-year-old patient with attention deficit disorder and depression treated with **desipramine**, which because of compliance problems was taken as a single 300-mg dose at bedtime, had **desipramine** levels of 164 nanograms/mL. The dose was increased to 375 mg at bedtime because of missed doses once or twice a week. He developed chest wall pain one week later, but an ECG at this time was normal. He was given ibuprofen 600 mg three times daily for the chest pain, but one week later developed blurred vision, clouding of consciousness and a grand mal seizure. He had a second seizure and ventricular tachycardia and was unresponsive until treated with physostigmine. Tricyclic toxicity was confirmed by a desipramine level of 657 nanograms/mL. This toxic level could have been due to the increase in **desipramine** dose, but as the ECG was normal one week after the increase and the fact that toxicity did not occur until 2 weeks after the dose increase and one week after starting ibuprofen, it was suggested that the toxicity might be due to inhibition of **desipramine** metabolism by ibuprofen.[1] This case is isolated and unconfirmed, and as such, no general recommendations can be made as a result of it.

(b) Oxyphenbutazone and Phenylbutazone

The absorption of a single 400-mg dose of phenylbutazone in 4 depressed women was considerably delayed (time to maximum level, 4 to 10 hours compared with 2 hours), but the total amount absorbed (measured by the urinary excretion of oxyphenbutazone) remained unchanged when they were pretreated with **desipramine** 75 mg daily for 7 days.[2] In another 5 depressed women the half-life of oxyphenbutazone was found to be unaltered by 75 mg of **desipramine** or **nortriptyline** daily.[3] *Animal* studies have confirmed that the absorption of phenylbutazone and oxyphenbutazone are delayed by the tricyclic antidepressants, probably because their antimuscarinic effects reduce gut motility,[4,5] but there seems to be no direct clinical evidence that the antirheumatic effects of either drug are reduced by this interaction. No particular precautions appear to be needed.

1. Gillette DW. Desipramine and ibuprofen. *J Am Acad Child Adolesc Psychiatry* (1998) 37, 1129.
2. Consolo S, Morselli PL, Zaccala M, Garattini S. Delayed absorption of phenylbutazone caused by desmethylimipramine in humans. *Eur J Pharmacol* (1970) 10, 239–42.
3. Hammer W, Mårtens S, Sjöqvist F. A comparative study of the metabolism of desmethylimipramine, nortriptyline, and oxyphenylbutazone in man. *Clin Pharmacol Ther* (1969) 10, 44–9.
4. Consolo S. An interaction between desipramine and phenylbutazone. *J Pharm Pharmacol* (1968) 20, 574–5.
5. Consolo S, Garattini S. Effect of desipramine on intestinal absorption of phenylbutazone and other drugs. *Eur J Pharmacol* (1969) 6, 322–6.

NSAIDs; Acemetacin + Miscellaneous

Acemetacin is a glycolic acid ester of indometacin, and its major metabolite is indometacin. Therefore acemetacin would be expected to interact in a similar way to indometacin.

NSAIDs; Azapropazone + Chloroquine

The plasma levels of azapropazone are not significantly altered by chloroquine.

Clinical evidence, mechanism, importance and management

A study in 12 subjects given azapropazone 300 mg three times daily found that the plasma levels of azapropazone, measured at 4 hours, were not affected by chloroquine 250 mg daily for 7 days.[1] No azapropazone dose adjustment would seem to be needed if these drugs are given together.

1. Faust-Tinnefeldt G, Geissler HE. Azapropazon und rheumatologische Basistherapie mit Chloroquin unter dem Aspekt der Arzneimittelinteraktion. *Arzneimittelforschung* (1977) 27, 2170–4.

NSAIDs; Celecoxib + Selenium

Selenium enriched baker's yeast does not appear to affect the pharmacokinetics of celecoxib.

Clinical evidence, mechanism, importance and management

In a study in 73 healthy subjects, celecoxib 400 mg was given daily for 2 weeks, then selenium enriched baker's yeast (*Saccharomyces cerevisiae*) 200 micrograms daily or matched placebo were added for 30 days. Following blood chemistry analysis (urea and electrolytes, full blood count etc), there were no clinically significant changes from baseline, nor were there any changes in celecoxib steady-state plasma levels.[1]

1. Frank DH, Roe DJ, Chow H-HS, Guillen JM, Choquette K, Gracie D, Francis J, Fish A, Alberts DS. Effects of a high-selenium yeast supplement on celecoxib plasma levels: a randomized phase II trial. *Cancer Epidemiol Biomarkers Prev* (2004) 13, 299–303.

NSAIDs; Diclofenac + Fluvastatin

Fluvastatin slightly increases the exposure to diclofenac.

Clinical evidence

A study in 14 healthy subjects given fluvastatin 40 mg daily for 8 days and a single 25-mg dose of **diclofenac** found that fluvastatin increased the peak plasma level and AUC of diclofenac by 60% and 25%, respectively, although there was considerable inter-individual variation in these results. The clearance of **diclofenac** was decreased by about 15%.[1] In a crossover study, 12 healthy subjects were given single doses of diclofenac 50 mg and fluvastatin 40 mg, alone and together. The AUC and maximum plasma concentration of both drugs were unaffected by concurrent use.[2]

Mechanism

Diclofenac is extensively metabolised by CYP2C9. Fluvastatin is a weak inhibitor of CYP2C9, and therefore may be expected to inhibit the metabolism of diclofenac by this route.

Importance and management

The available evidence for an interaction between diclofenac and fluvastatin is somewhat conflicting, with a single dose study finding no pharmacokinetic interaction and a multiple dose study finding that fluvastatin slightly increased the exposure to diclofenac. However, as this increase would not be expected to be clinically relevant, no dose adjustments would appear necessary when diclofenac and fluvastatin are taken together.

1. Transon C, Leemann T, Vogt N, Dayer P. In vivo inhibition profile of cytochrome P450TB (CYP2C9) by (±)-fluvastatin. *Clin Pharmacol Ther* (1995) 58, 412–17.
2. Andersson TB, Bredberg E, Ericsson H, Sjöberg H. An evaluation of the in vitro metabolism data for predicting the clearance and drug-drug interaction potential of CYP2C9 substrates. *Drug Metab Dispos* (2004) 32, 715–21.

NSAIDs; Diclofenac topical + Miscellaneous

Topical diclofenac intended for use on the skin is very unlikely to interact adversely with any of the drugs known to interact with diclofenac given orally.

Clinical evidence, mechanism, importance and management

The manufacturer of *Pennsaid* (a topical solution containing diclofenac 16 mg/mL in dimethyl sulfoxide) says that when the maximum dosage of 1 mL is used on the skin, the maximum plasma levels of diclofenac achieved are less than 10 nanograms/mL.[1] This is 50 times lower than the maximum plasma levels achieved with oral diclofenac 25 mg. Despite these very low concentrations, the manufacturer lists all the interactions that have been observed after systemic administration of diclofenac sodium (including **aspirin, digoxin, lithium, oral hypoglycaemic agents, diuretics, NSAIDs** including other **diclofenac** preparations, **methotrexate, ciclosporin, quinolones** and **antihypertensives**).[1] They note that the risk of these interactions in association with topical use is not known, but is probably low.[1] None of the drugs listed have yet been reported to interact with topical diclofenac.

The manufacturers of other topical preparations (*Solaraze* 3% w/w gel and *Voltarol* 1% w/w gel patch) state that interactions are not anticipated due to the low level of systemic absorption,[2,3] although one manufacturer still warns not to give, by either the topical or systemic route, any other medicinal product containing diclofenac or other NSAIDs.[3]

1. Pennsaid (Diclofenac sodium). Dimethaid International. UK Summary of product characteristics, February 2004.
2. Solaraze 3% Gel (Diclofenac sodium). Almirall Ltd. UK Summary of product characteristics, February 2009.
3. Voltarol Gel Patch (Diclofenac epolamine). Novartis Consumer Health. UK Summary of product characteristics, November 2005.

NSAIDs; Etoricoxib + Miscellaneous

The manufacturer of etoricoxib recommends care when using etoricoxib with drugs that are metabolised by human sulfotransferases (they name oral salbutamol and minoxidil). This is because etoricoxib is an inhibitor of human sulfotransferase activity, and may increase the levels of these drugs. The increase in ethinylestradiol levels with etoricoxib is thought to occur as a result of this mechanism,[1] see 'Combined hormonal contraceptives + Coxibs', p.1172.

1. Arcoxia (Etoricoxib). Merck Sharp & Dohme Ltd. UK Summary of product characteristics, May 2012.

NSAIDs; Flurbiprofen + Cranberry juice

Limited evidence suggests that cranberry juice does not appear to affect the pharmacokinetics of flurbiprofen.

Clinical evidence

In a study in 14 healthy subjects, 230 mL of cranberry juice taken the night before, and 30 minutes before a single 100-mg dose of flurbiprofen, had no significant effect on the pharmacokinetics of flurbiprofen. Fluconazole, used as a positive control, increased the flurbiprofen AUC by about 80%.[1] In this study, the cranberry juice used was *Ocean Spray* cranberry juice cocktail from concentrate containing 27% cranberry juice.

Mechanism

Flurbiprofen is metabolised by the cytochrome P450 isoenzyme CYP2C9, and the clinical study appears to suggest that cranberry has no clinically relevant effect on this particular isoenzyme, despite the fact that it had some weak inhibitory effects *in vitro*.[1]

Importance and management

Evidence is limited, but what is known suggests that no pharmacokinetic interaction occurs between flurbiprofen and cranberry juice. Therefore no dose adjustment appears to be necessary if patients taking flurbiprofen wish to drink cranberry juice.

1. Greenblatt DJ, von Moltke LL, Perloff ES, Luo Y, Harmatz JS, Zinny MA. Interaction of flurbiprofen with cranberry juice, grape juice, tea, and fluconazole: in vitro and clinical studies. *Clin Pharmacol Ther* (2006) 79, 125–33.

NSAIDs; Ibuprofen + Moclobemide

Moclobemide did not alter the pharmacokinetics of ibuprofen, or ibuprofen-induced faecal blood loss in one study. Ibuprofen does not affect the pharmacokinetics of moclobemide.

Clinical evidence, mechanism, importance and management

A study in 24 healthy subjects found that moclobemide 150 mg three times daily for 7 days had no effect on the steady-state pharmacokinetics of ibuprofen 600 mg three times daily, and the amount of ibuprofen-induced faecal blood loss was unaffected.[1] Ibuprofen did not affect the pharmacokinetics of moclobemide. No special precautions appear to be required during concurrent use.

1. Güntert TW, Schmitt M, Dingemanse J, Jonkman JHG. Influence of moclobemide on ibuprofen-induced faecal blood loss. *Psychopharmacology (Berl)* (1992) 106, S40–S42.

NSAIDs; Ibuprofen + Nitric oxide

The manufacturer of ibuprofen injection, which is used to treat patent ductus arteriosus in preterm newborn infants, warns that its use with nitric oxide, which is used to treat hypoxic respiratory failure in neonates, may in theory increase the risk of bleeding as both drugs inhibit platelet function.[1] The clinical significance of this proposed interaction is unclear, but it may be prudent to be alert for any evidence of bruising or bleeding if both drugs are given.

1. Pedea Injection (Ibuprofen). Orphan Europe (UK) Ltd. UK Summary of product characteristics, July 2004.

NSAIDs; Ibuprofen + St John's wort (*Hypericum perforatum*)

St John's wort does not affect the pharmacokinetics of ibuprofen.

Clinical evidence

Eight healthy male subjects were given an oral dose of ibuprofen 400 mg before, and at the end of, a 21 day course of St John's wort 300 mg three times daily. The pharmacokinetics of ibuprofen were unaffected by St John's wort. The St John's wort extract was standardised to contain hypericin (probably 0.3%) and a minimum of 4% hyperforin.[1]

Mechanism

As ibuprofen is a substrate for the cytochrome P450 isoenzymes CYP2C9 and CYP2C8, the authors of the study suggest that the lack of interaction is evidence that St John's wort has no significant effects on these isoenzymes.[1]

Importance and management

St John's wort does not appear to interact with ibuprofen and therefore no special precautions seem necessary on concurrent use.

1. Bell EC, Ravis WR, Lloyd KB, Stokes TJ. Effects of St. John's wort supplementation on ibuprofen pharmacokinetics. *Ann Pharmacother* (2007) 41, 229–34.

NSAIDs; Indometacin + Cocaine

An isolated report describes marked oedema, anuria and haematemesis in a premature child attributed to an interaction between cocaine and indometacin, which were taken by the mother before the birth.

Clinical evidence, mechanism, importance and management

A woman who was a cocaine user and who was in premature labour was unsuccessfully treated with terbutaline and magnesium sulfate. Indometacin proved to be more effective, but after being given 400 mg over 2 days she gave birth to a boy estimated at 34 to 35 weeks. Before birth the child was noted to be anuric and at birth showed marked oedema, and later haematemesis.

It was suggested that the anuria and oedema were due to renal vascular constriction of the foetus caused by the cocaine combined with an adverse effect of indometacin on ADH-mediated water reabsorption. Both drugs can cause gastrointestinal bleeding, which would account for the haematemesis. The authors of this report point out that one of the adverse effects of cocaine is premature labour, and that the likelihood is high that indometacin may be used to control it. They advise screening likely addicts in premature labour for evidence of cocaine usage before indometacin is given.[1]

1. Carlan SJ, Stromquist C, Angel JL, Harris M, O'Brien WF. Cocaine and indomethacin: fetal anuria, neonatal edema and gastrointestinal bleeding. *Obstet Gynecol* (1991) 78, 501–3.

NSAIDs; Indometacin + Vaccines

Some very limited evidence suggests that the response to immunisation with live vaccines may be more severe than usual in the presence of indometacin.

Clinical evidence, mechanism, importance and management

A man with ankylosing spondylitis taking indometacin 25 mg three times daily had a strong primary-type reaction 12 days after **smallpox vaccination**. He experienced 3 days of severe malaise, headache and nausea, as well as enlarged lymph nodes. The scab that formed was unusually large (3 cm in diameter) but he suffered no long term ill-effects.[1] The suggestion was that indometacin alters the response of the body to viral infections, whether originating from vaccines or not.[1] This suggestion is supported by the case of a child taking indometacin who developed haemorrhagic chickenpox during a ward outbreak of the disease.[2] However, these appear to be isolated and relatively old reports, and are therefore probably of little general importance. Note that NSAIDs such as indometacin may mask some of the signs and symptoms of infection.

1. Maddocks AC. Indomethacin and vaccination. *Lancet* (1973) ii, 210–11.
2. Rodriguez RS, Barbabosa E. Hemorrhagic chickenpox after indomethacin. *N Engl J Med* (1971) 285, 690.

NSAIDs; Ketorolac + Vancomycin

An isolated report describes temporary acute renal failure and gastrointestinal bleeding following the use of ketorolac and vancomycin.

Clinical evidence, mechanism, importance and management

A previously healthy middle-aged man developed acute renal failure and subsequent gastrointestinal bleeding following uncomplicated surgery and treatment with ketorolac trometamol and vancomycin. The reason for the temporary renal failure is not known, but the authors of the report suggest that ketorolac inhibited the normal production of the vasodilatory renal prostaglandins so that renal blood flow was reduced. This would seem to have been additive with the nephrotoxic effects of vancomycin. Note that a vancomycin level taken on postoperative day 3 was found to be above the normal therapeutic range (although the timing of the sample was not stated).[1] Ketorolac alone can cause dose-related and transient renal impairment. The gastrointestinal bleeding appeared to be due to the direct irritant effects of the ketorolac, possibly made worse by the previous use of piroxicam[1] (see also 'NSAIDs + NSAIDs', p.153). The general importance of this interaction is uncertain. As renal function should be routinely monitored in patients given vancomycin no additional precautions seem necessary, but if renal impairment develops in a patient taking both drugs, consider an interaction as a possible cause.

1. Murray RP, Watson RC. Acute renal failure and gastrointestinal bleed associated with postoperative Toradol and vancomycin. *Orthopedics* (1993) 16, 1361–3.

NSAIDs; Naproxen + Diphenhydramine

No significant pharmacokinetic interaction appears to occur between diphenhydramine and naproxen.

Clinical evidence, mechanism, importance and management

In a study in 27 healthy subjects, diphenhydramine hydrochloride 50 mg had no clinically significant effect on the pharmacokinetics of a single 220-mg dose of naproxen sodium. The pharmacokinetics of diphenhydramine were similarly unaffected by naproxen.[1] No dose adjustment of either drug appears to be necessary on concurrent use.

1. Toothaker RD, Barker SH, Gillen MV, Helsinger SA, Kindberg CG, Hunt TL, Powell JH. Absence of pharmacokinetic interaction between orally co-administered naproxen sodium and diphenhydramine hydrochloride. *Biopharm Drug Dispos* (2000) 21, 229–33.

NSAIDs; Naproxen + Sulglicotide

Sulglicotide does not affect the absorption of naproxen.

Clinical evidence, mechanism, importance and management

In a study in 12 healthy subjects, sulglicotide 200 mg had no significant effects on the pharmacokinetics of a single 500-mg dose of naproxen.[1] Sulglicotide may therefore be used to protect the gastric mucosa from possible injury by naproxen without altering its absorption.

1. Berté F, Feletti F, De Bernardi di Valserra M, Nazzari M, Cenedese A, Cornelli U. Lack of influence of sulglycotide on naproxen bioavailability in healthy volunteers. *Int J Clin Pharmacol Ther Toxicol* (1988) 26, 125–8.

NSAIDs; Naproxen + Zileuton

No clinically significant pharmacokinetic or pharmacodynamic interaction appears to occur between naproxen and zileuton.

Clinical evidence, mechanism, importance and management

In a randomised, placebo-controlled study, 24 healthy subjects were given zileuton 800 mg every 12 hours with naproxen 500 mg every 12 hours for 6 days. No clinically significant change was found in the pharmacokinetics of either drug. Naproxen did not affect the inhibitory effect of zileuton on leukotriene B_4 levels and similarly zileuton did not affect the inhibitory effect of naproxen on thromboxane B_2. The inhibition of the 5-lipoxygenase pathway by zileuton did not appear to worsen the gastrointestinal effects associated with naproxen. No special precautions would seem necessary if both drugs are given.[1]

1. Awni WM, Braeckman RA, Cavanaugh JH, Locke CS, Linnen PJ, Granneman GR, Dube LM. The pharmacokinetic and pharmacodynamic interactions between the 5-lipoxygenase inhibitor zileuton and the cyclo-oxygenase inhibitor naproxen in human volunteers. *Clin Pharmacokinet* (1995) 29 (Suppl 2) 112–24.

NSAIDs; Parecoxib + Miscellaneous

As parecoxib is rapidly metabolised to valdecoxib, the interactions are usually considered to be due to the effects of valdecoxib. The manufacturer of parecoxib cautions the concurrent use of carbamazepine, dexamethasone, phenytoin and rifampicin (rifampin). Valdecoxib increases the levels of dextromethorphan and omeprazole. Because of these interactions, caution is advised with drugs that are metabolised by the same isoenzymes.

Clinical evidence, mechanism, importance and management

Parecoxib is a parenteral drug that is rapidly metabolised in the liver to the active COX-2 inhibitor valdecoxib. Valdecoxib is predominantly metabolised by the cytochrome P450 isoenzymes CYP3A4 and CYP2C9. The interactions therefore are usually considered to be due to the effects of valdecoxib.

(a) CYP2C19 substrates

The manufacturers say that the AUC of **omeprazole** 40 mg was increased by 46% by valdecoxib 40 mg twice daily for a week. This indicates that valdecoxib is an inhibitor of CYP2C19, and although the manufacturers consider it to be a weak inhibitor,[1] they advise caution if valdecoxib is given with other drugs that are known to be metabolised by CYP2C19. They name **diazepam**, **imipramine** and **phenytoin**.[2] The implication is that the serum levels of these drugs and their effects may possibly be increased by the use of parecoxib.

(b) CYP2D6 substrates

The manufacturers say that valdecoxib 40 mg twice daily for a week caused a threefold increase in the serum levels of **dextromethorphan**. This indicates that valdecoxib is an inhibitor of CYP2D6, and therefore the manufacturers[1] suggest that caution should be observed with drugs that have a narrow therapeutic margin and are known to be predominantly metabolised by CYP2D6. They list **flecainide**, **metoprolol** and **propafenone**.[2] The implication is that the serum levels of these drugs and their effects may possibly be increased by the use of parecoxib; however, a study with metoprolol and valdecoxib did not find any clinically relevant interaction, see 'Beta blockers + Aspirin or NSAIDs', p.1003.

(c) Enzyme inducers

The manufacturer of parecoxib[2] warns that, although they have not been studied, enzyme inducers (they name **carbamazepine**, **dexamethasone**, **phenytoin** and **rifampicin (rifampin)**) may increase the metabolism of valdecoxib. It may therefore be prudent to monitor the outcome of concurrent use for valdecoxib efficacy. However, note that dexamethasone does not usually appear to interact to a clinically relevant extent by this mechanism.

1. Pharmacia Ltd. Personal communication, May 2002.
2. Dynastat (Parecoxib sodium). Pfizer Ltd. UK Summary of product characteristics, June 2013.

NSAIDs; Phenylbutazone + Methylphenidate

Methylphenidate significantly increased the serum levels of phenylbutazone 200 to 400 mg daily in 5 out of 6 patients, due, it is suggested, to inhibition of liver metabolising enzymes.[1] The clinical importance of effect this is uncertain, especially as the report does not indicate the magnitude of the interaction.

1. Dayton PG, Perel JM, Israili ZH, Faraj BA, Rodewig K, Black N, Goldberg LI. Studies with methylphenidate: drug interactions and metabolism. In: Sellers EM ed. Clinical Pharmacology of Psychoactive Drugs. Ontario: Addiction Research Foundation, 1973. p183–202.

NSAIDs; Sulindac + Dimethyl sulfoxide (DMSO)

Isolated case reports describe serious peripheral neuropathy, which occurred when DMSO was applied to the skin of two patients taking sulindac.

Clinical evidence, mechanism, importance and management

A man with a long history of degenerative arthritis took sulindac 400 mg daily uneventfully for 6 months until, without his doctor's knowledge, he began regularly to apply a topical preparation containing DMSO 90% to his upper and lower extremities. Soon afterwards he began to experience pain, weakness in all his extremities, and difficulty in standing or walking. He was found to have both segmental demyelination and axonal neuropathy. He made a partial recovery but was unable to walk without an artificial aid.[1]

A second case describes a 68-year-old man with a history of mild osteoarthritis of the knees who was taking sulindac 150 mg twice daily. He later started to apply aqueous solutions of DMSO to his lower extremities, whilst continuing to take sulindac. Within 3 months he reported difficulty in climbing stairs, and myalgia of the thighs and legs. Over the next 5 months he experienced a progressive loss of gait, wasting of thigh and leg muscles, and more intense myalgia, cramps and fasciculations. Nerve conduction studies revealed damage to the nerves. During the year after discontinuing the DMSO, and supplementing his diet with vitamins B_6 and B_{12}, the patient had an improvement in the myalgia and physical disabilities, and a return to normal muscle strength. He continued to take the sulindac at a dose of 200 mg twice daily.[2]

The reason for this reaction is not known, but studies in *rats* have shown that DMSO can inhibit a reductase enzyme by which sulindac is metabolised,[3] and it may be that the high concentrations of unmetabolised sulindac increased the neurotoxic activity of the DMSO. Although there are only these two cases on record, its seriousness suggests that patients should not use sulindac and DMSO-containing preparations concurrently.

1. Reinstein L, Mahon R, Russo GL. Peripheral neuropathy after concomitant dimethyl sulfoxide use and sulindac therapy. *Arch Phys Med Rehabil* (1982) 63, 581–4.
2. Swanson BN, Ferguson RK, Raskin NH, Wolf BA. Peripheral neuropathy after concomitant administration of dimethyl sulfoxide and sulindac. *Arthritis Rheum* (1983) 26, 791–3.
3. Swanson BN, Mojaverian P, Boppana VK, Dudash M. Dimethylsulfoxide (DMSO) interaction with sulindac (SO). *Pharmacologist* (1981) 23, 196.

Opioids + Amfetamines and related drugs

Dexamfetamine and methylphenidate increase the analgesic effects of morphine and other opioids but reduce their sedative and respiratory depressant effects.

Clinical evidence, mechanism, importance and management

In a single-dose controlled study in 450 patients receiving postoperative analgesia[1] intramuscular **dexamfetamine** increased the analgesic effect of intramuscular **morphine** and appeared to reduce its sedative effect.[1] In another controlled study in 7 healthy subjects, intravenous **dexamfetamine** reduced the respiratory depressant effects of intravenous morphine to some extent.[2] **Methylphenidate** 15 mg daily similarly increased the analgesic effects of various opioids (**morphine**, **hydromorphone**, **levorphanol**, **oxycodone**) and reduced the sedative effects in 28 patients with chronic pain due to advanced cancer when compared with placebo.[3] Similarly, the US manufacturers of several amfetamines advise that amfetamines potentiate the analgesic effects of **pethidine (meperidine)**.[4,5] Therefore, the analgesic dose of an opioid might be lower than expected in patients taking amfetamines. The manufacturers also note that, in cases of **dextropropoxyphene (propoxyphene)** *overdose*, amfetamine CNS stimulation is potentiated and fatal convulsions can occur.[4,5]

For mention of a study where use of stimulants including cocaine and amfetamines with **methadone** was associated with a longer QT interval, see 'Opioids + Cocaine', p.174.

Note that both the amfetamines and some opioids (see 'Table 35.3', p.1472) have serotonergic effects, and concurrent use might lead to the serotonin syndrome. Serotonin syndrome is a rare adverse effect, but because of its severity, some caution is warranted if both drugs are given. For more information on serotonin syndrome and its management, see 'Drugs that cause serotonin syndrome + Other drugs that cause serotonin syndrome', p.1471.

1. Forrest WH, Brown BW, Brown CR, Defalque R, Gold M, Gordon HE, James KE, Katz J, Mahler DL, Schroff P, Teutsch G. Dextroamphetamine with morphine for the treatment of postoperative pain. *N Engl J Med* (1977) 296, 712–15.
2. Bourke DL, Allen PD, Rosenberg M, Mendes RW, Karabelas AN. Dextroamphetamine with morphine: respiratory effects. *J Clin Pharmacol* (1983) 23, 65–70.
3. Bruera E, Chadwick S, Brenneis C, Hanson J, MacDonald RN. Methylphenidate associated with narcotics for the treatment of cancer pain. *Cancer Treat Rep* (1987) 71, 67–70.
4. Adderall XR (Mixed salts of amphetamine and dextroamphetamine). Shire US Inc. US Prescribing information, April 2015.
5. Dexedrine (Dextroamphetamine sulfate). Amedra Pharmaceuticals, LLC. US Prescribing information, October 2013.

Opioids + Anaesthetics, local

Chloroprocaine might reduce the efficacy of epidural morphine and fentanyl analgesia. Fentanyl and sufentanil might enhance the local anaesthetic effect of bupivacaine, but do not appear to affect respiratory depression. Similarly, extradural lidocaine does not appear to increase respiratory depression with extradural morphine. However, one case of respiratory depression has been reported with submucosal lidocaine and alphaprodine.

Clinical evidence, mechanism, importance and management

(a) Bupivacaine

A study in 50 elderly patients undergoing spinal anaesthesia, found that those given bupivacaine 7.5 mg and **sufentanil** 5 micrograms had a reduced incidence of hypotension requiring treatment with ephedrine, when compared with the patients who received bupivacaine 15 mg alone. None of the patients developed respiratory depression.[1] A study involving 40 elderly patients undergoing spinal anaesthesia found that bupivacaine 9 mg, with **fentanyl** 20 micrograms reduced the incidence of hypotension, when compared with bupivacaine 11 mg alone. Respiratory rates were not depressed in either group. The rate of failed spinal block and discomfort was similar in both groups. The addition of fentanyl allowed a reduction in the minimum dose of bupivacaine required to produce an adequate block, and consequently the incidence of hypotension was reduced.[2]

(b) Chloroprocaine

1. Fentanyl. A controlled study in women undergoing caesarean section found that following spinal anaesthesia with chloroprocaine, the duration and effectiveness of postoperative analgesia with fentanyl was less than after spinal anaesthesia with lidocaine (mean duration 20 minutes vs 149 minutes).[3] In another study using low-doses of chloroprocaine and lidocaine to test the epidural catheter tip location prior to spinal analgesia with bupivacaine, fentanyl and epinephrine, the duration of analgesia was shorter in those women who received chloroprocaine than in those who received lidocaine (91 minutes vs 164 minutes).[4] In contrast, the addition of fentanyl to epidural chloroprocaine (used in this study as analgesia), resulted in a 40% lower minimum local analgesic concentration (the median effective concentration) of chloroprocaine when compared with chloroprocaine alone.[5] The mechanism behind these findings is unclear, with two studies suggesting antagonism,[3,4] and one suggesting synergy.[5] An *in-vitro* study suggests that epidural fentanyl is antagonised by chloroprocaine by acting at opioid receptors.[6] Further study is required.

2. Morphine. A controlled study in women undergoing caesarean section found that following spinal anaesthesia with bupivacaine and fentanyl, the effectiveness and duration of postoperative analgesia from epidural morphine, was no different after administration of chloroprocaine 15 minutes previously, than after placebo.[7] Other studies in women undergoing caesarean section, using varying spinal anaesthesia regimens, have found both similar and conflicting results. In one study there was no difference in the duration of epidural morphine analgesia when chloroprocaine or lidocaine were used as spinal anaesthesia,[8] but in another study the morphine requirements were much higher in women who had received chloroprocaine for spinal anaesthesia than in those who had received lidocaine.[9] In a study using low-doses of chloroprocaine and lidocaine to test the epidural catheter tip location prior to spinal anaesthesia with bupivacaine, the duration of epidural morphine analgesia was shorter in those women who received chloroprocaine than in those who received lidocaine (16 hours vs 24 hours).[10] The authors of one of the studies suggest that chloroprocaine should be avoided if epidural morphine is used.[10] However, it is important to note that any differences in morphine-induced analgesia seen, could be related to the spinal anaesthesia chosen, or the shorter duration of effect of chloroprocaine, rather than an antagonism of the effect of morphine by chloroprocaine.[7] The results of another study suggest that the timing of administration may also be important; in women undergoing post-partum obstetric surgery the administration of chloroprocaine 30 minutes after epidural morphine resulted in a longer duration of analgesia than when the choroprocaine was administered before the morphine, and was comparable to that seen when lidocaine was given before morphine.[11]

(c) Lidocaine

In a study in 24 patients, giving extradural lidocaine with extradural **morphine** did not increase the risk of respiratory depression associated with morphine.[12] However, respiratory depression occurred in a 3-year-old boy given lidocaine with adrenaline (epinephrine) about 5 minutes after a submucosal injection of the narcotic **alphaprodine**. Naloxone reversed the respiratory depression.[13]

For further information on the interaction of opioids with *intravenous* lidocaine used to treat arrhythmias, see 'Lidocaine + Opioids', p.283.

1. Olofsson C, Nygårds E-B, Bjersten A-B, Hessling A. Low-dose bupivacaine with sufentanil prevents hypotension after spinal anesthesia for hip repair in elderly patients. *Acta Anaesthesiol Scand* (2004) 48, 1240–4.
2. Martyr JW, Stannard KJD, Gillespie G. Spinal-induced hypotension in elderly patients with hip fracture. A comparison of glucose-free bupivacaine with glucose-free bupivacaine and fentanyl. *Anaesth Intensive Care* (2005) 33, 64–8.
3. Camann WR, Hartigan PM, Gilbertson LI, Johnson MD, Datta S. Chloroprocaine antagonism of epidural opioid analgesia: a receptor-specific phenomenon? *Anesthesiology* (1990) 73, 860–3.
4. Grice SC, Eisenach JC, Dewan DM. Labor analgesia with epidural bupivacaine plus fentanyl: enhancement with epinephrine and inhibition with 2-chloroprocaine. *Anesthesiology* (1990) 72, 623–8.
5. Polley LS, Columb MO, Lyons G, Nair SA. The effect of epidural fentanyl on the minimum local analgesic concentration of epidural chloroprocaine in labor. *Anesth Analg* (1996) 83, 987–90.
6. Coda B, Bausch S, Haas M, Chavkin C. The hypothesis that antagonism of fentanyl analgesia by 2-chloroprocaine is mediated by direct action on opioid receptors. *Reg Anesth* (1997) 22, 43–52.
7. Hess PE, Snowman CE, Hahn CJ, Kunze LJ, Ingold VJ, Pratt SD. Chloroprocaine may not affect epidural morphine for postcesarean delivery analgesia. *J Clin Anesth* (2006) 18, 29–33.
8. Phan CQ, Azar I, Osborn IP, Salter OR, Lear E. The quality of epidural morphine analgesia following epidural anesthesia with lidocaine or chloroprocaine for cesarean delivery. *Anesth Analg* (1988) 67, S172.
9. Karambelkar DJ, Ramanathan S. 2-Chloroprocaine antagonism of epidural morphine analgesia. *Acta Anaesthesiol Scand* (1997) 41, 774–8.
10. Eisenach JC, Schlairet TJ, Dobson CE, Hood DH. Effect of prior anesthetic solution on epidural morphine analgesia. *Anesth Analg* (1991) 73, 119–23.
11. Toledo P, McCarthy RJ, Ebarvia MJ, Huser CJ, Wong CA. The interaction between epidural 2-chloroprocaine and morphine: a randomized controlled trial of the effect of drug administration timing on the efficacy of morphine analgesia. *Anesth Analg* (2009) 109, 168–73.
12. Saito Y, Sakura S, Kaneko M, Kosaka Y. Interaction of extradural morphine and lignocaine on ventilatory response. *Br J Anaesth* (1995) 75, 394–8.
13. Moore PA. Local anesthesia and narcotic drug interaction in pediatric dentistry. *Anesth Prog* (1988) 35, 17.

Opioids + Antiemetics; Droperidol

The use of droperidol with opioids can improve postsurgical analgesia, but an increase in sedation appears to occur. A case of early respiratory depression (not reversed by naloxone) was seen when droperidol was used before epidural hydromorphone.

Clinical evidence

(a) Fentanyl

Epidural droperidol given with epidural fentanyl improved postsurgical analgesia following anorectal surgery and there was less nausea compared with fentanyl alone.[1]

(b) Hydromorphone

Early respiratory depression has been reported when droperidol was given 10 minutes before epidural hydromorphone 1.25 mg; the patient became apnoeic 15 minutes after the epidural was given. Naloxone did not reverse the respiratory depression, but spontaneous ventilation resumed within 3 minutes of a 1-mg intravenous dose of physostigmine.[2]

(c) Morphine

In a double-blind study in 179 patients following abdominal hysterectomy, droperidol 50 micrograms given with morphine 1 mg on demand via patient-controlled analgesia (PCA) provided a morphine-sparing effect and reduced the frequency of postoperative nausea and vomiting, when compared with morphine PCA alone.[3] However, in a study of 107 patients undergoing caesarean section, intravenous droperidol 2.5 mg given just after delivery reduced the incidence and severity of epidural morphine-induced pruritus, but the incidence of nausea and vomiting was not affected. Furthermore, somnolence was greater in the droperidol-treated patients (17% versus 2% in the control group) but it was never incapacitating.[4] Similar sedative effects were seen with spinal morphine and intravenous droperidol in another study.[5]

Mechanism

Droperidol can enhance adverse effects such as sedation, and in some cases respiratory depression, possibly through opioid and other receptor sites in the CNS.[1] In one case, the respiratory depression was not reversed by naloxone, suggesting that droperidol was at least partially if not completely responsible.[2] Opioids can also cause hypotension and the risk of this could be increased by droperidol.[6]

Importance and management

The opioid-sparing effect of droperidol is a useful interaction, but the increased sedation and possible respiratory depression and hypotension should be borne in mind. Note that the use of droperidol has been restricted in some countries because of its potential to cause QT prolongation, and this risk also be additive with that of high-dose **methadone**, see also 'Drugs that prolong the QT interval + Other drugs that prolong the QT interval', p.272.

1. Kotake Y, Matsumoto M, Ai K, Morisaki H, Takeda J. Additional droperidol, not butorphanol, augments epidural fentanyl analgesia following anorectal surgery. *J Clin Anesth* (2000) 12, 9–13.
2. Cohen SE, Rothblatt AJ, Albright GA. Early respiratory depression with epidural narcotic and intravenous droperidol. *Anesthesiology* (1983) 59, 559–60.
3. Lo Y, Chia Y-Y, Liu K, Ko N-H. Morphine sparing with droperidol in patient-controlled analgesia. *J Clin Anesth* (2005) 17, 271–5.
4. Horta ML, Horta BL. Inhibition of epidural morphine-induced pruritus by intravenous droperidol. *Reg Anesth* (1993) 18, 118–20.
5. Horta ML, Morejon LCL, da Cruz AW, dos Santos GR, Welling LC, Terhorst L, Costa RC, Alam RUZ. Study of the prophylactic effect of droperidol, alizapride, propofol and promethazine on spinal morphine-induced pruritus. *Br J Anaesth* (2006) 96, 796–800.
6. DepoDur (Morphine). SkyePharma Inc, US Prescribing information, February 2007.

Opioids + Antiemetics; Metoclopramide

Metoclopramide increases the rate of absorption of oral morphine and increases its rate of onset and sedative effects. Intravenous metoclopramide appears to increase the incidence of sedation with intravenous tramadol. Opioids might antagonise the effects of metoclopramide on gastric emptying. Metoclopramide does not appear to affect the pharmacokinetics of butorphanol or tapentadol.

Clinical evidence

(a) Butorphanol

In a study in 24 healthy women, the pharmacokinetics of a single 1-mg intranasal dose of butorphanol were unaffected by a single 10-mg oral dose of metoclopramide. The pharmacokinetics of metoclopramide were also not affected, except for a delay in the time to reach maximum plasma concentrations (increased from one hour to 2 hours), which was probably due to reduction of gastrointestinal motility by butorphanol.[1] Metoclopramide reduced the nausea associated with butorphanol, probably by antagonism of central and peripheral dopamine receptors.[2]

(b) Morphine

A single 10-mg dose of oral metoclopramide, given to 10 patients before surgery, greatly increased the extent and speed of sedation due to a 20-mg oral dose of modified-release morphine (*MST Continus Tablets*) in the first 1.5 hours after the dose. The time to maximum plasma concentrations of morphine was almost halved, but maximum plasma morphine concentrations and the total absorption remained unaltered.[2] A study involving 40 patients found that intravenous metoclopramide 10 mg antagonised the reduction in gastric emptying caused by premedication with intramuscular morphine 10 mg, given 20 minutes earlier. However, intramuscular metoclopramide given at the same time as the morphine had no effect on the reduced gastric emptying.[3]

(c) Tapentadol

The UK and US manufacturers briefly note, that in an interaction study metoclopramide had no effect on the pharmacokinetics of tapentadol.[4,5]

(d) Tramadol

In a small controlled study in patients receiving patient-controlled analgesia, the addition of metoclopramide to tramadol reduced the incidence of nausea and vomiting, but increased the incidence of sedation (7 out of 20 patients compared with 1 out of 20 for tramadol alone).[6]

Mechanism

Metoclopramide increases the rate of gastric emptying so that the rate of morphine absorption from the small intestine is increased. An alternative mechanism is that both drugs act additively on opiate receptors to increase sedation.[2] The increased sedation seen with the combination of tramadol and metoclopramide could be due to additive effects, as metoclopramide alone can cause sedation.

Importance and management

The effect of metoclopramide on oral morphine absorption is an established interaction that can be usefully exploited in anaesthetic practice, but the increased sedation can also present a problem if the morphine is being given long-term.

Morphine appears to antagonise the effects of metoclopramide on gastric emptying. As a reduction in gastric motility occurs with all opioids they would all be expected to interact with metoclopramide and other motility stimulants, such as **domperidone**. However, these drugs are commonly used together and the clinical importance of such effects is not clear.

Metoclopramide appears not to affect the pharmacokinetics of butorphanol or tapentadol. When used in intravenous patient-controlled analgesia, metoclopramide appears to increase the incidence of sedation with tramadol. It might therefore be prudent to bear this in mind if this combination is used in this way.

Note that some sedating antihistamines, such as **cyclizine**, are also used as antiemetics, and additive sedation is likely to occur on concurrent use.

Consider also 'Opioids + Antiemetics; Ondansetron', below.

1. Vachharajani NN, Shyu WC, Barbhaiya RH. Pharmacokinetic interaction between butorphanol nasal spray and oral metoclopramide in healthy women. *J Clin Pharmacol* (1997) 37, 979–85.
2. Manara AR, Shelly MP, Quinn K, Park GR. The effect of metoclopramide on the absorption of oral controlled release morphine. *Br J Clin Pharmacol* (1988) 25, 518–21.
3. McNeill MJ, Ho ET, Kenny GNC. Effect of i.v. metoclopramide on gastric emptying after opioid premedication. *Br J Anaesth* (1990) 64, 450–2.
4. Palexia (Tapentadol hydrochloride). Grünenthal Ltd. UK Summary of product characteristics, July 2014.
5. Nucynta (Tapentadol). PriCara. US Prescribing information, July 2013.
6. Pang WW, Wu HS, Lin CH, Chang DP, Huang MH. Metoclopramide decreases emesis but increases sedation in tramadol patient-controlled analgesia. *Can J Anaesth* (2002) 49, 1029–33.

Opioids + Antiemetics; Ondansetron

Ondansetron reduced the analgesic efficacy of tramadol in four controlled clinical studies, at least doubling the tramadol dose required in one of these studies. In contrast, in a larger controlled study, ondansetron had no effect on the required dose of tramadol. Ondansetron does not alter the pharmacokinetics of tramadol.

In studies in healthy subjects, ondansetron had no effect on the analgesic effects of morphine and alfentanil, and had no effect on the pharmacokinetics of morphine.

Clinical evidence

(a) Alfentanil

In a study in healthy subjects, single 8- or 16-mg doses of intravenous ondansetron were found to have no effect on the sedation or ventilatory depression due to alfentanil (a continuous infusion of 0.25 to 0.75 micrograms/kg following a 5-micrograms/kg bolus dose) and had no effect on the rate of recovery.[1] Similarly, in another study, intravenous ondansetron 8 mg did not oppose the analgesic effect of intramuscular alfentanil 30 micrograms/kg on experimentally-induced pain stimuli.[2]

(b) Morphine

A double-blind, placebo-controlled study in 12 healthy subjects found that a single 16-mg intravenous dose of ondansetron given 30 minutes after a single 10-mg intravenous dose of morphine did not alter the pharmacokinetics of morphine or its metabolites, morphine-3-glucuronide and morphine-6-glucuronide. The analgesic effect of morphine (as measured by a contact thermode system) was also unaffected by ondansetron.[3]

(c) Tramadol

In a randomised study, 20 patients who were given a single 4-mg dose of ondansetron, one minute before induction of anaesthesia, required 26 to 35% more intravenous tramadol by patient controlled analgesia (PCA) from one to 4 hours postoperatively than 20 patients who received placebo.[4] Similarly, in another randomised study, a 1-mg/hour ondansetron infusion increased the dose of postoperative intravenous tramadol given using a PCA pump by 2- to 3-fold in 30 patients, when compared with 29 patients who received placebo. Moreover, in this study, the group receiving ondansetron actually experienced more vomiting, probably because they used more tramadol, which caused an emetic effect not well controlled by the ondansetron.[5] Two other randomised placebo-controlled studies reported similar findings.[6,7] In contrast, in a larger placebo-controlled randomised study in 179 patients, there was no difference in the analgesic efficacy of tramadol (assessed by amount administered via patient-controlled analgesia) between 60 patients receiving intravenous ondansetron, 59 receiving metoclopramide, and 60 receiving placebo. In addition, postoperative nausea and vomiting was lower in patients receiving ondansetron than those receiving placebo, and was similar to that in patients receiving metoclopramide.[8]

The US manufacturer of ondansetron briefly notes that there is no pharmacokinetic interaction between ondansetron and tramadol.[9]

Mechanism

On theoretical grounds ondansetron (a 5-HT_3-receptor antagonist) might be expected to decrease the effects of drugs that reduce pain transmission, because serotonin (5-HT) is thought to affect pain responses via presynaptic 5-HT_3 receptors in the spinal dorsal horn. This has been demonstrated for tramadol, which is not a pure opioid and also acts by enhancing the effects of serotonin and noradrenaline (norepinephrine). However, ondansetron had no effect on alfentanil or morphine analgesia in healthy subjects.

Importance and management

The pharmacodynamic interaction between ondansetron and tramadol is not established. Of five controlled studies, four demonstrated an interaction whereas the fifth larger study did not. Bear in mind the possibility that ondansetron might increase the dose requirement of tramadol, resulting in reduced pain control.

Ondansetron appears to have no effect on alfentanil or morphine analgesia.

1. Dershwitz M, Di Biase PM, Rosow CE, Wilson RS, Sanderson PE, Joslyn AF. Ondansetron does not affect alfentanil-induced ventilatory depression or sedation. *Anesthesiology* (1992) 77, 447–52.
2. Petersen-Felix S, Arendt-Nielsen L, Bak P, Bjerring P, Breivik H, Svensson P, Zbinden AM. Ondansetron does not inhibit the analgesic effect of alfentanil. *Br J Anaesth* (1994) 73, 326–30.
3. Crews KR, Murthy BP, Hussey EK, Passannante AN, Palmer JL, Maixner W, Brouwer KLR. Lack of effect of ondansetron on the pharmacokinetics and analgesic effects of morphine and metabolites after single-dose morphine administration in healthy volunteers. *Br J Clin Pharmacol* (2001) 51, 309–16.
4. De Witte JL, Schoenmaekers B, Sessler DI, Deloof T. The analgesic efficacy of tramadol is impaired by concurrent administration of ondansetron. *Anesth Analg* (2001) 92, 1319–21.
5. Arcioni R, della Rocca M, Romanò S, Romano R, Pietropaoli P, Gasparetto A. Ondansetron inhibits the analgesic effects of tramadol: a possible 5-HT_3 spinal receptor involvement in acute pain in humans. *Anesth Analg* (2002) 94, 1553–7.
6. Vale C, Oliveira F, Assunção J, Fontes-Ribeiro C, Pereira F. Co-administration of ondansetron decreases the analgesic efficacy of tramadol in humans. *Pharmacology* (2011) 88, 182–7.
7. Cubukçu Z, Ozbek H, Güneş Y, Gündüz M, Ozcengiz D, Işik G. Effect of ondansetron in lower extremity bone surgery on morphine and tramadol consumption using patient controlled analgesia [In Turkish]. *Agri* (2007) 19, 36–41.
8. Rauers NI, Stüber F, Lee EH, Musshoff F, Fimmers R, Barann M, Stamer UM. Antagonistic effects of ondansetron and tramadol? A randomized placebo and active drug controlled study. *J Pain* (2010) 11, 1274–81.
9. Zofran (Ondansetron hydrochloride). GlaxoSmithKline. US Prescribing information, September 2011.

Opioids + Antiepileptics; Carbamazepine

Patients taking carbamazepine alone or in combination with phenytoin appear to need more fentanyl than those not taking these antiepileptics. Carbamazepine appears to increase the production of a more potent metabolite of codeine, normorphine. Carbamazepine reduces tramadol concentrations, appears to reduce oxycodone concentrations, and is predicted to reduce the concentrations and efficacy of buprenorphine.

Clinical evidence

(a) Buprenorphine

Although interaction studies have not been performed, buprenorphine is partially metabolised by CYP3A4 and therefore drugs that induce this isoenzyme such as carbamazepine are expected to induce the metabolism and increase the clearance of buprenorphine.[1,2]

(b) Codeine

An experimental study in 7 patients with epilepsy, to find out if carbamazepine induces the enzymes concerned with the metabolism of codeine, found that carbamazepine increased *N*-demethylation (to norcodeine and normorphine) 2- to 3-fold, but did not affect *O*-demethylation (to morphine). The patients were given a single 25-mg dose of codeine before, and 3 weeks after, starting to take carbamazepine 400 to 600 mg daily.[3]

(c) Dextropropoxyphene (Propoxyphene)

Dextropropoxyphene increases carbamazepine concentrations and has caused carbamazepine toxicity, see 'Carbamazepine and related drugs + Dextropropoxyphene (Propoxyphene)', p.570.

(d) Fentanyl

Forty-one patients, undergoing craniotomy for seizure focus excision and receiving long-term treatment with antiepileptics in various combinations, needed 65% to 2.9-fold more maintenance fentanyl during anaesthesia than a control group of 20 patients who were not taking antiepileptics, although the required loading dose did not differ.[4] The fentanyl maintenance requirements were:

- 2.6 micrograms/kg per hour in the control group;
- 4.3 micrograms/kg per hour in 16 patients taking carbamazepine alone;
- 5.4 micrograms/kg per hour in 12 patients taking carbamazepine and either **phenytoin** or **valproate**;
- 7.6 micrograms/kg per hour in 13 patients taking carbamazepine, **valproate** and either **phenytoin** or **primidone**.

(e) Methadone

Methadone concentrations can be reduced by carbamazepine, See 'Opioids; Methadone + Antiepileptics; Enzyme-inducing', p.165.

(f) Oxycodone

In a regression analysis of oxycodone concentrations in cancer patients, use of carbamazepine in 3 patients and **phenobarbital** in one patient was associated with 84% lower oxycodone concentrations than in patients not taking these drugs.[5]

(g) Tramadol

An unpublished study by the US manufacturers found that the maximum plasma concentration and the elimination half-life of a single 50-mg dose of tramadol were reduced by 50% by **carbamazepine** 400 mg twice daily for 9 days.[6]

Mechanism

Carbamazepine is a known enzyme-inducer, particularly of CYP3A4. It is likely that carbamazepine increases the metabolism of codeine, fentanyl, and tramadol, and it is predicted to increase metabolism of buprenorphine. For codeine, this results in increased concentrations of an active metabolite, whereas for fentanyl and tramadol this might reduce analgesic efficacy. For fentanyl, changes in the state of opiate receptors induced by long-term antiepileptic exposure might also be involved.[4]

Importance and management

The clinical relevance of the increased metabolism of **codeine** to normorphine, an active metabolite, is unknown. The authors suggest that patients taking both codeine and carbamazepine might experience a stronger analgesic effect.[3] However, this needs further study. There would seem to be no reason for avoiding concurrent use.

Conversely, carbamazepine might reduce the efficacy of **buprenorphine**[1,2,7] and, the US manufacturers advise that if concurrent use is necessary patients should be closely monitored and dose adjustments should be considered.[2] Similarly, an increase in **fentanyl** requirements would be anticipated in any patient receiving long-term treatment with carbamazepine, and probably also barbiturates, such as **primidone**, and **phenytoin** (and probably **fosphenytoin**, which is a prodrug of phenytoin).

Carbamazepine also increases **tramadol** metabolism, and the UK and US manufacturers state that the analgesic effectiveness of tramadol[8,9] and its duration of action would be expected to be reduced.[6,9] The US manufacturer recommends avoidance of concurrent use because of the increased metabolism and also the seizure risk associated with tramadol,[8] although not all patients will be taking carbamazepine for its antiepileptic effects. The UK manufacturer states that patients with a history of epilepsy or those susceptible to seizures should only be given tramadol if there are compelling reasons.[9] Monitor carefully if tramadol and carbamazepine are required.

Carbamazepine appears to reduce **oxycodone** concentrations, which might reduce oxycodone efficacy. Bear this possibility in mind.

1. Temgesic Sublingual Tablets (Buprenorphine hydrochloride). RB Pharmaceuticals Ltd. UK Summary of product characteristics, September 2010.
2. Suboxone (Buprenorphine with naloxone). Reckitt Benckiser Pharmaceuticals Inc. US Prescribing information, August 2012.
3. Yue Q-Y, Tomson T, Säwe J. Carbamazepine and cigarette smoking induce differentially the metabolism of codeine in man. *Pharmacogenetics* (1994) 4, 193–8.
4. Tempelhoff R, Modica PA, Spitznagel EL. Anticonvulsant therapy increases fentanyl requirements during anaesthesia for craniotomy. *Can J Anaesth* (1990) 37, 327–32.
5. Andreassen TN, Klepstad P, Davies A, Bjordal K, Lundström S, Kaasa S, Dale O. Influences on the pharmacokinetics of oxycodone: a multicentre cross-sectional study in 439 adult cancer patients. *Eur J Clin Pharmacol* (2011) 67, 493–506.
6. GD Searle. Personal Communication, November 1994.
7. Subutex (Buprenorphine hydrochloride). RB Pharmaceuticals Ltd. UK Summary of product characteristics, September 2014.
8. Ultram ER (Tramadol hydrochloride). PriCara. US Prescribing information, June 2009.
9. Zydol SR Tabs (Tramadol hydrochloride). Grünenthal Ltd. UK Summary of product characteristics, January 2011.

Opioids + Antiepileptics; Phenytoin

A pharmacokinetic study confirms that phenytoin increases the production of the toxic metabolite of pethidine (meperidine) and toxicity has occurred following their concurrent use. Phenytoin is predicted to increase the metabolism of buprenorphine. Fosphenytoin would be expected to interact similarly to phenytoin.

Clinical evidence

(a) Buprenorphine

Although interaction studies have not been performed, buprenorphine is partially metabolised by CYP3A4 and therefore drugs that induce this isoenzyme, such as phenytoin, are expected to induce the metabolism and increase the clearance of buprenorphine.[1,2]

(b) Dextropropoxyphene (Propoxyphene)

For mention of a case report of phenytoin toxicity in a patient given dextropropoxyphene, see 'Phenytoin + Dextropropoxyphene (Propoxyphene)', p.600.

(c) Fentanyl

For mention that fentanyl requirements during anaesthesia were higher in patients taking carbamazepine with other antiepileptics including phenytoin, see 'Opioids + Antiepileptics; Carbamazepine', above.

(d) Methadone

Methadone concentrations can be reduced by phenytoin. See 'Opioids; Methadone + Antiepileptics; Enzyme-inducing', p.165.

(e) Pethidine (Meperidine)

A small study in 4 healthy subjects found that phenytoin 300 mg daily for 9 days decreased the elimination half-life of pethidine (100 mg orally and 50 mg intravenously) from 6.4 hours to 4.3 hours, and the systemic clearance increased by 27%. Phenytoin increased production of the metabolite norpethidine (AUC increased by 25 to 53%).[3] There is an isolated case of a 61-year-old man with cancer and chronic renal failure who was taking pethidine 5 to 10 g weekly and phenytoin, and who developed repeated seizures and myoclonus when he increased his pethidine dose. The problem resolved when both drugs were stopped.[4]

Mechanism

Phenytoin is a known enzyme inducer, including of CYP3A4 by which a number of opioids are at least partially metabolised. For pethidine, induction of its metabolism increases production of the active metabolite norpethidine;[5] however, accumulation of this metabolite is believed to be responsible for pethidine neurotoxicity (such as, seizures,[5] myoclonus, tremors).

Importance and management

The UK and US manufacturers of **buprenorphine** state that inducers of CYP3A4, such as phenytoin, might reduce the efficacy of buprenorphine and therefore concurrent therapy should be well monitored:[2,6] if necessary, dose adjustments should be considered.[6] The same advice should therefore probably apply to **fosphenytoin**, which is a prodrug of phenytoin.

Limited evidence suggests that phenytoin induces the metabolism of **pethidine** and could therefore decrease its analgesic efficacy. Bear the possibility of this in mind if phenytoin or **fosphenytoin** are given with pethidine. The general relevance of the case report of toxicity in a patient with renal failure taking phenytoin and large doses of pethidine is uncertain.

1. Temgesic Sublingual Tablets (Buprenorphine hydrochloride). RB Pharmaceuticals Ltd. UK Summary of product characteristics, September 2010.
2. Suboxone (Buprenorphine with naloxone). Reckitt Benckiser Pharmaceuticals Inc. US Prescribing information, August 2012.
3. Pond SM, Kretschzmar KM. Effect of phenytoin on meperidine clearance and normeperidine formation. *Clin Pharmacol Ther* (1981) 30, 680–6.
4. Hochman MS. Meperidine-associated myoclonus and seizures in long-term hemodialysis patients. *Ann Neurol* (1983) 14, 593.
5. Demerol (Meperidine hydrochloride). Sanofi-Aventis US LLC. US Prescribing information, July 2014.
6. Subutex (Buprenorphine hydrochloride). RB Pharmaceuticals Ltd. UK Summary of product characteristics, September 2014.

Opioids; Methadone + Antiepileptics; Enzyme-inducing

Methadone concentrations can be reduced by carbamazepine, phenobarbital, or phenytoin, and withdrawal symptoms have occurred. Eslicarbazepine, fosphenytoin, primidone, and oxcarbazepine are expected to interact similarly. A single report suggests that valproate does not appear to interact with methadone. The CNS depressant effects of barbiturates are predicted to be additive with those of methadone.

Clinical evidence

A study in 37 patients taking methadone maintenance found that the 10 patients taking enzyme-inducing drugs (**carbamazepine**, **phenobarbital**, or **phenytoin**) had low methadone minimum concentrations of less than 100 nanograms/mL. One patient taking **carbamazepine** complained of daily withdrawal symptoms and had signs of opioid withdrawal.[1]

Methadone withdrawal symptoms have been seen in other patients taking **carbamazepine**,[2] **phenobarbital**,[3] and **phenytoin**.[1,2,4-6] In one of these reports, methadone withdrawal symptoms developed in 5 patients within 3 to 4 days of starting to take **phenytoin** 300 to 500 mg daily. Methadone plasma concentrations were reduced by about 60%. The withdrawal symptoms disappeared within 2 to 3 days of stopping **phenytoin** and the methadone plasma concentrations returned to their former values.[6] In another of these reports, 2 patients who had methadone withdrawal symptoms while taking phenytoin 300 to 400 mg daily, and one of them later when taking carbamazepine 600 mg daily, became free from withdrawal symptoms when they were given **valproate** instead. It was also found possible to virtually halve their daily methadone dose.[2] A further patient experienced methadone-induced respiratory depression after stopping **carbamazepine**.[7]

Mechanism

Not fully established, but carbamazepine, phenobarbital, and phenytoin are recognised inducers of CYP3A4, by which methadone is, in part, metabolised. Therefore concurrent use increases methadone metabolism and results in reduced plasma concentrations. In one study it was found that phenytoin increased the urinary excretion of the main metabolite of methadone.[6]

Importance and management

Information is limited but the interaction between methadone and the enzyme-inducing antiepileptics carbamazepine, phenobarbital, and phenytoin appears to be established and of clinical importance. Anticipate the need to increase the methadone dose in patients taking these antiepileptics. It might be necessary to give the methadone twice daily to prevent withdrawal symptoms appearing towards the end of the day. It seems probable that **primidone** and **fosphenytoin** will interact similarly because they are metabolised to phenobarbital and phenytoin, respectively. **Eslicarbazepine** and **oxcarbazepine**, both inducers of CYP3A4, would also be expected to increase the metabolism of methadone, and similar precautions would seem prudent. A single report indicates that **valproate** appears not to interact in the same way.

Note that barbiturates such as phenobarbital are CNS depressants and therefore might have additive CNS depressant effects with methadone, so come caution might be appropriate on concurrent use.

1. Bell J, Seres V, Bowron P, Lewis J, Batey R. The use of serum methadone levels in patients receiving methadone maintenance. *Clin Pharmacol Ther* (1988) 43, 623–9.
2. Saxon AJ, Whittaker S, Hawker CS. Valproic acid, unlike other anticonvulsants, has no effect on methadone metabolism: two cases. *J Clin Psychiatry* (1989) 50, 228–9.
3. Liu S-J, Wang RIH. Case report of barbiturate-induced enhancement of methadone metabolism and withdrawal syndrome. *Am J Psychiatry* (1984) 141, 1287–8.
4. Finelli PF. Phenytoin and methadone tolerance. *N Engl J Med* (1976) 294, 227.
5. Knoll B, Haefeli WE, Ladewig D, Stohler R. Early recurrence of withdrawal symptoms under phenytoin and chronic alcohol use. *Pharmacopsychiatry* (1997) 30, 72–3.
6. Tong TG, Pond SM, Kreek MJ, Jaffery NF, Benowitz NL. Phenytoin-induced methadone withdrawal. *Ann Intern Med* (1981) 94, 349–51.
7. Benítez-Rosario MA, Salinas Martín A, Gómez-Ontañón E, Feria M. Methadone-induced respiratory depression after discontinuing carbamazepine administration. *J Pain Symptom Manage* (2006) 32, 99–100.

Opioids + Antihistamines

Increased respiratory depression has been seen when hydroxyzine was given with pethidine and when fentanyl was given with chlorphenamine.

Clinical evidence, mechanism, importance and management

Increased respiratory depression has been seen with **hydroxyzine** and **pethidine (meperidine)** in one study in healthy subjects,[1] but not in two others.[2,3] A woman receiving epidural **fentanyl** with bupivacaine following a caesarean section developed somnolence and severe respiratory depression (4 breaths/minute) 35 minutes after receiving intramuscular **chlorphenamine** 10 mg for opioid-induced pruritus.[4]

All sedating antihistamines (see "Opioids + Phenothiazines', p.193.

1. Reier CE, Johnstone RE. Respiratory depression: narcotic versus narcotic-tranquilizer combinations. *Anesth Analg* (1970) 49, 119–124.
2. Zsigmond EK, Flynn K, Shively JG. Effect of hydroxyzine and meperidine on arterial blood gases in healthy human volunteers. *J Clin Pharmacol* (1989) 29, 85–90.
3. Zsigmond EK, Flynn K, Shively JG. Effect of hydroxyzine and meperidine on arterial blood gases in patients with chronic obstructive pulmonary disease. *Int J Clin Pharmacol Ther Toxicol* (1993) 31, 124–9.
4. Anwari JS, Iqbal S. Antihistamines and potentiation of opioid induced sedation and respiratory depression. *Anaesthesia* (2003) 58, 494–5.

Opioids + Azoles

Ketoconazole slightly increases sublingual buprenorphine exposure, but does not appear to affect the pharmacokinetics of transdermal buprenorphine. Itraconazole caused a negligible increase in morphine exposure, without altering its sedative effects. Itraconazole appears not to alter tramadol exposure.

Clinical evidence

(a) Buprenorphine

The UK manufacturers of sublingual buprenorphine briefly state that, in a study, **ketoconazole** increased the AUC of buprenorphine by about 50% and increased its maximum concentration by about 70%. The concentration of the metabolite, norbuprenorphine, was also affected but to a lesser extent.[1] In contrast, in a placebo-controlled study in 20 healthy subjects, there was no change in the AUC or maximum concentrations of buprenorphine when oral **ketoconazole** 200 mg twice daily for 7 days was taken while a buprenorphine transdermal patch was in use (one 10 micrograms/hour patch for 7 days).[2]

(b) Fentanyl and related drugs

The azoles can increase and prolong the effects of alfentanil and possibly fentanyl, see 'Opioids; Fentanyl and related drugs + Azoles', p.166.

(c) Methadone

The azoles can increase the exposure to methadone, resulting in serious toxicity in some cases, see 'Opioids; Methadone + Azoles', p.167.

(d) Morphine

In a placebo-controlled, crossover study in 12 healthy subjects given a single 300-microgram/kg oral dose of morphine, pretreatment with **itraconazole** 200 mg daily for 4 days increased the $AUC_{0\text{-}48}$ of morphine by 22% and increased its maximum plasma concentration by 28%. **Itraconazole** did not affect the pharmacokinetics of the metabolites morphine-3-glucuronide or morphine-6-glucuronide, nor did it affect the pharmacodynamic effects of morphine as assessed using visual analogue scales, the digit symbol substitution test and the critical flicker fusion test.[3]

(e) Oxycodone

The azoles can increase the exposure to oxycodone and alter the exposure to its metabolites, see 'Opioids; Oxycodone + Azoles', p.167.

(f) Tramadol

In a crossover study, 12 healthy subjects were given ticlopidine 250 mg twice daily for 5 days with a single 50-mg dose of tramadol on day 4, with or without **itraconazole**

200 mg daily. Itraconazole had no effect on the AUC and maximum plasma concentration of tramadol when compared with ticlopidine and tramadol alone.[4] For details of the effect of ticlopidine on tramadol exposure, see 'Opioids + Ticlopidine', p.197.

Mechanism

Buprenorphine is partially metabolised by CYP3A4,[5] an isoenzyme inhibited by ketoconazole and other azoles. Concurrent use therefore decreases buprenorphine metabolism and increases its exposure. The apparent lack of interaction when buprenorphine is given transdermally is possibly because this route avoids intestinal CYP3A4.[2]

The authors of the study assessing the effect of itraconazole on morphine, suggest that the increase in morphine concentrations seen is a result of inhibition of intestinal P-glycoprotein by itraconazole. They also comment that the lack of effect on the pharmacodynamics of morphine might mean that itraconazole did not inhibit P-glycoprotein at the blood-brain barrier, although this lack of effect might be related to limitations in the tests used.[3]

Importance and management

Evidence for an interaction between the azoles and **buprenorphine** is limited, but is consistent with the known metabolism of both these drugs. Ketoconazole appears to slightly increase sublingual buprenorphine exposure. Although the clinical relevance of this interaction has not been assessed, monitor patients given ketoconazole with sublingual buprenorphine closely for an increase in buprenorphine adverse effects (such as drowsiness, nausea, and vomiting), and consider a dose reduction if necessary; one manufacturer recommends that the dose of sublingual buprenorphine for treating opioid addiction should be halved when starting treatment with ketoconazole.[1] Itraconazole and voriconazole are also potent inhibitors of CYP3A4, and would be expected to interact similarly; posaconazole is a moderate CYP3A4 inhibitor and would be expected to interact to a lesser extent. In contrast, ketoconazole did not interact to a clinically relevant extent with transdermal buprenorphine,[6] therefore no precaution appears to be necessary in patients using transdermal buprenorphine with these azoles. If the proposed mechanism is correct (bypassing gastrointestinal CYP3A4), then intravenous buprenorphine should also be little affected on concurrent use with the azoles.

The small change in **morphine** concentrations seen with concurrent use of itraconazole suggests that this interaction is unlikely to be clinically important.

The US manufacturers of **tramadol** suggest that CYP3A4 inhibitors, such as ketoconazole, might increase the risk of tramadol adverse effects, such as seizures and serotonin syndrome by inhibiting its metabolism[7]. However, the evidence with itraconazole suggests that potent inhibitors of CYP3A4 (see 'Table 1.9', p.11 for a list) will not alter tramadol exposure. No special precautions would seem necessary on concurrent use.

1. Subutex (Buprenorphine hydrochloride). RB Pharmaceuticals Ltd. UK Summary of product characteristics, September 2014.
2. Kapil RP, Cipriano A, Michels GH, Perrino P, O'Keefe SA, Shet MS, Colucci SV, Noveck RJ, Harris SC. Effect of ketoconazole on the pharmacokinetic profile of buprenorphine following administration of a once-weekly buprenorphine transdermal system. *Clin Drug Investig* (2012) 32, 583–92.
3. Heiskanen T, Backman JT, Neuvonen M, Kontinen VK, Neuvonen PJ, Kalso E. Itraconazole, a potent inhibitor of P-glycoprotein, moderately increases plasma concentrations of oral morphine. *Acta Anaesthesiol Scand* (2008) 52, 1319–26.
4. Hagelberg NM, Saarikoski T, Saari TI, Neuvonen M, Neuvonen PJ, Turpeinen M, Scheinin M, Laine K, Olkkola KT. Ticlopidine inhibits the O-demethylation and renal clearance of tramadol, increasing the exposure to it, but itraconazole has no marked effect on the tramadol-ticlopidine interaction. *Eur J Clin Pharmacol* (2013) 69, 867–75.
5. Iribarne C, Picart D, Dréano Y, Bail J-P, Berthou F. Involvement of cytochrome P450 3A4 in N-dealkylation of buprenorphine in human liver microsomes. *Life Sci* (1997) 60, 1953–64.
6. BuTrans (Buprenorphine transdermal patch). Napp Pharmaceuticals Ltd. UK Summary of product characteristics, November 2008.
7. Ultram ER (Tramadol hydrochloride). PriCara. US Prescribing information, June 2009.

Opioids; Fentanyl and related drugs + Azoles

Ketoconazole and voriconazole moderately to markedly increase intravenous alfentanil exposure, whereas fluconazole slightly to moderately increases intravenous alfentanil exposure. Fluconazole negligibly increased and voriconazole slightly increased intravenous fentanyl exposure, whereas single-dose itraconazole had no effect. A fatality, possibly due to an interaction between fluconazole and transdermal fentanyl, has been reported, as has a case of opioid toxicity when itraconazole was used with transdermal fentanyl.

Clinical evidence

(a) Alfentanil

1. Fluconazole. A crossover study in 9 healthy subjects given intravenous alfentanil 20 micrograms/kg after receiving fluconazole 400 mg, orally or by infusion, found that fluconazole moderately reduced alfentanil clearance by about 60%. Both the alfentanil-induced ventilatory depression and its subjective effects were increased.[1] In another study in healthy subjects (assessing the suitability of alfentanil for use as a CYP3A4 probe substrate), single oral doses of **fluconazole** of 100 mg, 200 mg, and 400 mg were given 3 hours before intravenous or oral alfentanil. The AUC of intravenous alfentanil 15 micrograms/kg was increased by 20% and 60%, and 2.2-fold by increasing doses of fluconazole, respectively. The AUC of oral alfentanil 40 micrograms/kg was increased to a greater extent by 80% and 2.9-fold and 4.9-fold, respectively.[2]

2. Ketoconazole. In a crossover study in healthy subjects, ketoconazole 400 mg daily for 3 to 4 days increased the AUC of a single intravenous dose of alfentanil 4.8- to 5-fold, and increased the AUC of a single oral dose of alfentanil 9.2- to 12-fold.[3]

3. Voriconazole. A crossover study in 12 healthy subjects found that oral voriconazole (400 mg twice daily on the first day and 200 mg twice daily on the second day) caused about a 5-fold increase in the mean AUC of intravenous alfentanil 20 micrograms/kg, given one hour after the last dose of the antifungal. The mean plasma clearance of alfentanil was decreased by 85% and its elimination half-life was prolonged from 1.5 hours to 6.6 hours. Visual adverse effects, nausea, and vomiting occurred in 6, 5, and 4 subjects, respectively.[4]

(b) Fentanyl

Fluconazole. In a study in 12 healthy subjects, oral fluconazole (400 mg on day one followed by 200 mg on day 2) reduced the clearance of a single 3-micrograms/kg dose of intravenous fentanyl by 16% and reduced the AUC of norfentanyl by 56%.[5]

A patient receiving transdermal fentanyl 150 micrograms/hour for at least 3 weeks started taking oral fluconazole 50 mg daily but died 3 days later. Post-mortem analysis found a toxic concentration of fentanyl in the patient's blood and a high concentration of fluconazole, which the authors of this report attribute to an interaction between the fluconazole and fentanyl.[6]

Itraconazole. In a crossover study in 10 healthy subjects the pharmacokinetics and pharmacodynamics of a single 3-micrograms/kg intravenous dose of fentanyl were not altered by itraconazole 200 mg daily for 4 days.[7]

However, a case report describes a man with cancer and severe oropharyngeal candidiasis receiving transdermal fentanyl 50 micrograms/hour who developed signs of opioid toxicity (agitated delirium, bilateral myoclonus of muscles in the hand) the day after starting oral itraconazole 200 mg twice daily.[8]

Voriconazole. A study in 12 healthy subjects reported that oral voriconazole (400 mg twice daily on day one followed by 200 mg twice daily on day 2) reduced the clearance of a single intravenous dose of fentanyl 5 micrograms/kg by 23% and increased the AUC of fentanyl by 39% and decreased that of its metabolite, norfentanyl, by 56%.

Mechanism

The azoles, to varying degrees, inhibit CYP3A4 (see 'Table 1.9', p.11), which is involved in the metabolism of alfentanil and fentanyl. Fentanyl has a high hepatic extraction and so is more affected by changes in hepatic blood flow (see 'Changes in first-pass metabolism', p.4), than changes in the isoenzymes responsible for its metabolism, and it is therefore less affected by CYP3A4 inhibitors than alfentanil. **Sufentanil** is metabolised similarly to fentanyl, and so would be expected to interact in more or less the same way. Alfentanil is affected to a greater extent when given by the oral route (not used therapeutically) than by the intravenous route because the intravenous route bypasses intestinal CYP3A4.

Importance and management

The pharmacokinetic interaction between **alfentanil** and the azoles is established, and is likely to be clinically important, particularly for those that are potent inhibitors of CYP3A4 (itraconazole, ketoconazole, and voriconazole). It is considered unlikely that a small, single dose of alfentanil will need adjustment.[4] However, multiple doses or continuous infusions of alfentanil should be given with care to patients taking these azoles, as the clearance of alfentanil might be markedly reduced and its effects increased; consider using a lower alfentanil dose.[4] Be alert for evidence of prolonged alfentanil effects, particularly respiratory depression, even after a single dose. Although the interaction is not as great with fluconazole, a moderate CYP3A4 inhibitor at higher doses, some caution would also seem appropriate on concurrent use. **Posaconazole**, another moderate CYP3A4 inhibitor would be expected to interact similarly.

Itraconazole had no effect on the pharmacokinetics of intravenous **fentanyl** in one single-dose study, and 2 days of fluconazole and voriconazole had only a negligible to slight effect on intravenous fentanyl exposure, respectively. Nevertheless, there are a couple of case reports of possible interactions of fluconazole and itraconazole with transdermal fentanyl, which introduce a note of caution. It might therefore seem prudent to use similar precautions to those advised for alfentanil if intravenous fentanyl is given with any of the azoles, particularly in multiple doses. Several manufacturers of transdermal fentanyl do not recommend concurrent use with potent CYP3A4 inhibitors (itraconazole, ketoconazole, and voriconazole) unless the patient is closely monitored, and some extend this to moderate CYP3A4 inhibitors, which would include fluconazole and **posaconazole**. Caution should similarly be used if azoles are given concurrently with fentanyl by other routes, such as the oral transmucosal route, and a fentanyl dose adjustment should be considered. Close monitoring is recommended.

1. Palkama VJ, Isohanni MH, Neuvonen PJ, Olkkola KT. The effect of intravenous and oral fluconazole on the pharmacokinetics and pharmacodynamics of intravenous alfentanil. *Anesth Analg* (1998) 87, 190–4.
2. Kharasch ED, Walker A, Hoffer C, Sheffels P. Sensitivity of intravenous and oral alfentanil and pupillary miosis as minimally invasive and noninvasive probes for hepatic and first-pass CYP3A activity. *J Clin Pharmacol* (2005) 45, 1187–97.
3. Kharasch ED, Vangveravong S, Buck N, London A, Kim T, Blood J, Mach RH. Concurrent assessment of hepatic and intestinal cytochrome P450 3A activities using deuterated alfentanil. *Clin Pharmacol Ther* (2011) 89, 562–70.
4. Saari TI, Laine K, Leino K, Valtonen M, Neuvonen PJ, Olkkola KT. Voriconazole, but not terbinafine, markedly reduces alfentanil clearance and prolongs its half-life. *Clin Pharmacol Ther* (2006) 80, 502–8.
5. Saari TI, Laine K, Neuvonen M, Neuvonen PJ, Olkkola KT. Effect of voriconazole and fluconazole on the pharmacokinetics of intravenous fentanyl. *Eur J Clin Pharmacol* (2008) 64, 25–30.
6. Hallberg P, Martén L, Wadelius M. Possible fluconazole-fentanyl interaction — a case report. *Eur J Clin Pharmacol* (2006) 62, 491–2.
7. Palkama VJ, Neuvonen PJ, Olkkola KT. The CYP3A4 inhibitor itraconazole has no effect on the pharmacokinetics of i.v. fentanyl. *Br J Anaesth* (1998) 81, 598–600.

8. Mercadante S, Villari P, Ferrera P. Itraconazole–fentanyl interaction in a cancer patient. *J Pain Symptom Manage* (2002) 24, 284–6.

Opioids; Methadone + Azoles

Methadone exposure was slightly increased by fluconazole and slightly to moderately increased by voriconazole. Cases of torsade de pointes have been reported with concurrent use of high-dose methadone and itraconazole or voriconazole, and a case of respiratory depression occurred with methadone and fluconazole.

Clinical evidence

(a) Fluconazole

A randomised, placebo-controlled study in 25 patients taking maintenance methadone 20 to 90 mg daily found that fluconazole 200 mg daily for 2 weeks increased the steady-state serum methadone concentration and slightly increased the AUC by about 30%, but no signs of methadone overdose were seen and no changes in the methadone dose were needed.[1]

However, a case report describes a man with advanced cancer who had been taking methadone 65 to 75 mg daily for 10 days, who rapidly developed respiratory depression of 4 breaths per minute and became unresponsive 4 days after starting fluconazole 100 mg daily, initially orally, then intravenously. Within a few minutes of receiving naloxone he regained consciousness and his respiratory rate increased.[2]

(b) Itraconazole

A case report describes a 44-year-old woman receiving high-dose maintenance methadone 120 mg daily, who presented to hospital with chest discomfort and an episode of syncope after taking two 200-mg doses of itraconazole. ECG monitoring showed a prolonged QTc interval of 520 milliseconds, leading to torsade de pointes which resolved spontaneously. After admission for cardiac monitoring, the ECG returned to normal once the methadone was stopped and buprenorphine given. Follow up after 3 months showed no further cardiac symptoms or ECG changes.[3]

(c) Voriconazole

In a study in 16 patients taking maintenance methadone 30 to 100 mg daily, voriconazole 400 mg twice daily for one day then 200 mg twice daily for 4 days slightly increased the steady-state AUC of *R*-methadone (active) by 47% and moderately increased the AUC of *S*-methadone (no opioid activity) 2-fold compared with baseline values. Seven additional patients randomised to receive placebo had no change in their methadone pharmacokinetics. Methadone appeared to have no effect on voriconazole pharmacokinetics, when compared with a reference study in healthy subjects. There were no important signs or symptoms of opioid withdrawal or overdose. A total of 10 patients had QT prolongation during the study, but the incidence did not appear to be higher in patients given voriconazole than in those given placebo, although the numbers were small for this comparison.[4]

Torsade de pointes has been reported in two patients receiving methadone maintenance therapy and voriconazole.[5,6] In both cases the patients were HIV-positive, cocaine abusers, and were receiving voriconazole 200 mg daily with high-dose methadone 125 mg daily. The QTc interval exceeded 600 milliseconds and required insertion of an implantable cardioverter-defibrillator. Note that these cases are complicated by numerous factors which could also explain the effects seen.

A case of ventricular bigeminy has been reported in a 26-year-old woman 4 days after she started taking methadone 30 mg daily, voriconazole (900 mg and then 300 mg twice daily), and esomeprazole 20 mg daily. Plasma concentrations of voriconazole and methadone were 3- to 4-fold higher than the upper limit of the respective therapeutic ranges, but decreased after esomeprazole was stopped. The methadone dose was reduced to 20 mg and voriconazole was withheld for two doses; cardiac arrhythmias also ceased. No further episodes of bigeminy occurred in the following 9 months. The authors suggested that this was due to an interaction between voriconazole and esomeprazole that further enhanced the interaction between voriconazole and methadone,[7] see 'Azoles + Proton pump inhibitors', p.238, for further details.

Mechanism

The metabolism of methadone is, in part, mediated by CYP3A4, and therefore methadone clearance can be decreased by drugs that inhibit CYP3A4, such as the azoles. Methadone alone has been associated with QT prolongation, particularly at doses higher than 100 mg daily. Therefore, it is possible that the azoles that are potent inhibitors of CYP3A4 might increase the risk of QT prolongation by increasing methadone exposure.

Importance and management

Several studies have documented an interaction between methadone and a number of the azoles, However, the pharmacokinetic interaction between methadone and **fluconazole** results in only a slight increase in methadone exposure and therefore seems unlikely to be clinically important. Nevertheless, the serious case report of respiratory depression with fluconazole and methadone introduces a note of caution. **Voriconazole** also slightly increases the exposure to *R*-methadone without appearing to increase opioid toxicity; however, it did double the exposure to *S*-methadone, and there is some evidence that *S*- methadone might cause greater QT-prolongation than *R*-methadone.[8] The cases of torsade de pointes with voriconazole and high-dose methadone suggest that caution should also be used if both drugs are given, and that a reduction in the methadone dose might be required. A similar case occurred with high-dose methadone and **itraconazole**, and the same precautions would seem prudent. **Ketoconazole** would be expected to interact similarly.

The UK manufacturer recommends ECG monitoring in those given methadone (particularly with methadone doses greater than 100 mg) with drugs that inhibit CYP3A4. They also recommend that patients requiring methadone in doses greater than 100 mg should have ECG monitoring before, and 7 days after, dose titration, irrespective of other drugs they are taking.[9] For more information on QT-interval prolongation, see 'Drugs that prolong the QT interval + Other drugs that prolong the QT interval', p.272.

1. Cobb MN, Desai J, Brown LS, Zannikos PN, Rainey PM. The effect of fluconazole on the clinical pharmacokinetics of methadone. *Clin Pharmacol Ther* (1998) 63, 655–62.
2. Tarumi Y, Pereira J, Watanabe S. Methadone and fluconazole: respiratory depression by drug interaction. *J Pain Symptom Manage* (2002) 23, 148–53.
3. NoorZurani MH, Vicknasingam B, Narayanan S. Itraconazole-induced torsade de pointes in a patient receiving methadone substitution therapy. *Drug Alcohol Rev* (2009) 28, 688–90.
4. Liu P, Foster G, Labadie R, Somoza E, Sharma A. Pharmacokinetic interaction between voriconazole and methadone at steady state in patients on methadone therapy. *Antimicrob Agents Chemother* (2007) 51, 110–18.
5. Reinhold JA, Sanoski CA, Russo AM, Cooper JM, Spinler SA. Torsades de pointes associated with methadone and voriconazole. *BMJ Case Rep* (2009) Epub.
6. Prosser JM, Mills A, Rhim ES, Perrone J. Torsade de pointes caused by polypharmacy and substance abuse in a patient with human immunodeficiency virus. *Int J Emerg Med* (2008) 1, 217–20.
7. Scholler J, Nivoix Y, Herbrecht R, Kemmel V, Levêque D. Ventricular bigeminy associated with voriconazole, methadone and esomeprazole. *Int J Clin Pharmacol* (2011) 33, 905–8.
8. Ansermot N, Albayrak O, Schläpfer J, Crettol S, Croquette-Krokar M, Bourquin M, Déglon JJ, Faouzi M, Scherbaum N, Eap CB. Substitution of (R,S)-methadone by (R)-methadone: Impact on QTc interval. *Arch Intern Med* (2010) 170, 529–36.
9. Methadone Hydrochloride Oral Solution. Rosemont Pharmaceuticals Ltd. UK Summary of product characteristics, September 2014.

Opioids; Oxycodone + Azoles

Voriconazole moderately increases oxycodone exposure, itraconazole and ketoconazole slightly to moderately increase oxycodone exposure, and miconazole slightly increases oxycodone exposure. The effect of itraconazole was greater on oral oxycodone than intravenous oxycodone. Fluconazole might increase oxycodone exposure.

Clinical evidence

(a) Fluconazole

In a regression analysis of oxycodone concentrations in cancer patients, use of CYP3A4 inhibitors in 23 patients (which included fluconazole in 15 patients, verapamil in 3, clarithromycin in 2, and **itraconazole**, nelfinavir, and diltiazem in 1 each) was associated with higher oxycodone concentrations compared with patients not taking these drugs (approximately 60% higher).[1]

(b) Itraconazole

In a placebo-controlled, crossover study, 12 healthy subjects were given a single 0.1-mg/kg intravenous dose of oxycodone or a single 10-mg oral dose on day 4 of a 5-day course of itraconazole 200 mg daily. Itraconazole increased the AUC of intravenous oxycodone by 50% and increased that of oral oxycodone 2.4-fold. The maximum plasma concentration of the metabolite, noroxycodone, was decreased by 64% and 71%, respectively, after intravenous and oral administration, and the AUC was decreased by 54% and 49%, respectively. Itraconazole had no effect on oxycodone analgesia in heat or cold pain tests.[2] Two other placebo-controlled, crossover studies by the same authors, also in healthy subjects given the same intravenous[3] and oral[4] doses of oxycodone on day 4 of a 5-day course of paroxetine with itraconazole 200 mg daily, found that the AUC of oxycodone was increased 2-fold and 2.9-fold after intravenous and oral oxycodone, respectively. The AUC of noroxycodone was not affected after oral or intravenous oxycodone administration, but its maximum plasma concentrations were decreased by 63% and 46%, respectively. The pharmacokinetics of oxymorphone were unaffected when oxycodone was given by either route. No effect on oxycodone analgesia was seen, as assessed using the cold pressor test.[3,4] The effect of the combination of paroxetine and itraconazole was greater than paroxetine alone (see 'SSRIs + Opioids', p.1492).

(c) Ketoconazole

In a placebo-controlled, crossover study, 10 healthy subjects were given a single 0.2-mg/kg oral dose of oxycodone 2 hours after a single 400-mg dose of ketoconazole. Ketoconazole increased the AUC_∞ of oxycodone by 80% and increased the AUC_∞ of the metabolite, oxymorphone, 3.5-fold. Ketoconazole also decreased the $AUC_{0\text{-}1.5}$ of the metabolite, noroxycodone, by 78%, but the AUC_∞ was unaffected. When ketoconazole was given with a single 100-mg oral dose of quinidine, the AUC_∞ of oxycodone was increased 3.2-fold and the AUC_∞ of the metabolite, oxymorphone, was not affected. However, the AUC_∞ of the metabolite, noroxycodone, was increased 3-fold.[5] In a further study by the same authors, using the same doses of oxycodone and ketoconazole, all pharmacodynamic assessments (e.g. pain tolerance as assessed using the cold pressor test) were enhanced by ketoconazole use, except for pupil size, and concurrent use with quinidine was no different to ketoconazole use alone. The use of ketoconazole was associated with a greater risk of adverse effects than placebo or oxycodone, and this seemed to be especially evident in ultrarapid CYP2D6 metabolisers (that is, those with higher than usual isoenzyme activity).[6] In another study, 12 healthy subjects who were all CYP2D6 extensive metabolisers (that is, they had normal isoenzyme activity), were given ketoconazole 200 mg daily for 3 doses followed by a single 0.2-mg/kg oral dose of oxycodone. Ketoconazole increased the AUC of oxycodone 2.4-fold, decreased the maximum plasma concentration of noroxycodone by 45%, but had no effect on the maximum plasma concentration of oxymorphone. Ketoconazole was also associated with an increased effect on oxycodone-induced miosis and analgesia (as assessed using the cold pressor test), and also adverse effects.[7]

(d) Miconazole

In a crossover study, 12 healthy subjects were given miconazole oral gel 85 mg three times daily for 4 days (held in the mouth for one minute and then swallowed), with a single 10-mg oral dose of oxycodone on day 4. The maximum plasma concentration and AUC of oxycodone were increased by 31% and 63%, respectively. The maximum plasma concentration and AUC of the metabolite, noroxycodone, were decreased by 20% and increased by 30%, respectively. However, the maximum plasma concentration and AUC of the metabolite, oxymorphone, were both decreased, by 66% and 83%, respectively. No differences in the effects of oxycodone were seen.[8]

(e) Voriconazole

In a crossover study in 12 healthy subjects given voriconazole for 4 days (as 400 mg on day one, 400 mg and 200 mg on day 2, and 200 mg twice daily on days 3 and 4), the AUC of a single 10-mg oral dose of oxycodone given on day 3 was increased 3.6-fold and its maximum plasma concentration was increased by 70%. The maximum plasma concentration and AUC of the metabolite, noroxycodone, were decreased by 87% and 67%, respectively. The maximum plasma concentration and AUC of the metabolite, oxymorphone, were increased 2-and 7-fold. The analgesic effects of oxycodone were unaffected.[9]

A case report of a 41-year-old man with Burkitt's lymphoma and a retrospective case series of 8 other patients, describe enhanced analgesic effects and adverse effects mostly developing within one to 4 days of the concurrent use of voriconazole and oxycodone. In one case, an oxycodone dose reduction was required as a result of vomiting and sweating, and in another, analgesia was inadequate after voriconazole was discontinued.[10]

Mechanism

Oxycodone is principally metabolised to noroxycodone by CYP3A4, and to a lesser extent, to oxymorphone by CYP2D6. The azoles are all known to inhibit CYP3A4 (to varying extents) and therefore reduce noroxycodone concentrations. CYP2D6 is subject to genetic polymorphism (that is, the activity of this isoenzyme varies between individuals), meaning that the effects of azoles are possibly of greater importance in individuals who are CYP2D6 poor metabolisers (that is patients with little or no activity of this isoenzyme) than in extensive metabolisers (that is, those with normal isoenzyme activity). Note too, that the concurrent use of a CYP2D6 inhibitor such as paroxetine or quinidine, effectively renders an individual a poor metaboliser and the importance of CYP3A4 for metabolism appears to be increased, meaning that the effect of both CYP2D6 and CYP3A4 inhibition seems to be greater than CYP2D6 inhibition alone.

The authors of the miconazole study conclude from the metabolite profile that miconazole produced its effect principally by inhibiting CYP2D6, and to a lesser extent CYP3A4, although note that this appears to be the first evidence of miconazole as a CYP2D6 inhibitor.[8]

Importance and management

A pharmacokinetic interaction between the azoles and oxycodone is established, but its general clinical importance is still uncertain. Note that the effect is possibly greater in CYP2D6 poor metabolisers than extensive metabolisers, but metaboliser status is rarely known in clinical practice. Both itraconazole and miconazole appear to have no effect on oxycodone analgesia, but, in contrast, ketoconazole and voriconazole appear to enhance the analgesic effect of oxycodone and to increase oxycodone adverse effects (such as drowsiness, nausea). The concurrent use of azoles and oxycodone need not be avoided, and no oxycodone dose adjustment would generally seem necessary, but be alert for increased adverse effects.

1. Andreassen TN, Klepstad P, Davies A, Bjordal K, Lundström S, Kaasa S, Dale O. Influences on the pharmacokinetics of oxycodone: a multicentre cross-sectional study in 439 adult cancer patients. *Eur J Clin Pharmacol* (2011) 67, 493–506.
2. Saari TI, Grönlund J, Hagelbergb NM, Neuvonen M, Laine K, Neuvonen PJ, Olkkola KT. Effects of itraconazole on the pharmacokinetics and pharmacodynamics of intravenously and orally administered oxycodone. *Eur J Clin Pharmacol* (2010) 66, 387–97.
3. Grönlund J, Saari TI, Hagelberg NM, Neuvonen PJ, Laine K, Olkkola KT. Effect of inhibition of cytochrome P450 enzymes 2D6 and 3A4 on the pharmacokinetics of intravenous oxycodone: a randomized, three-phase, crossover, placebo-controlled study. *Clin Drug Investig* (2011) 31, 143–53.
4. Grönlund J, Saari TI, Hagelberg NM, Neuvonen PJ, Olkkola KT, Laine K. Exposure to oral oxycodone is increased by concomitant inhibition of CYP2D6 and 3A4 pathways, but not by inhibition of CYP2D6 alone. *Br J Clin Pharmacol* (2010) 70, 78–87.
5. Samer CF, Daali Y, Wagner M, Hopfgartner G, Eap CB, Rebsamen MC, Rossier MF, Hochstrasser D, Dayer P, Desmeules JA. The effects of CYP2D6 and CYP3A activities on the pharmacokinetics of immediate release oxycodone. *Br J Pharmacol* (2010) 160, 907–18.
6. Samer CF, Daali Y, Wagner M, Hopfgartner G, Eap CB, Rebsamen MC, Rossier MF, Hochstrasser D, Dayer P, Desmeules JA. Genetic polymorphisms and drug interactions modulating CYP2D6 and CYP3A activities have a major effect on oxycodone analgesic efficacy and safety. *Br J Pharmacol* (2010) 160, 919–30.
7. Kummer O, Hammann F, Moser C, Schaller O, Drewe J, Krähenbühl S. Effect of the inhibition of CYP3A4 or CYP2D6 on the pharmacokinetics and pharmacodynamics of oxycodone. *Eur J Clin Pharmacol* (2011) 67, 63–71.
8. Grönlund J, Saari TI, Hagelberg N, Neuvonen PJ, Olkkola KT, Laine K. Miconazole oral gel increases exposure to oral oxycodone by inhibition of CYP2D6 and CYP3A4. *Antimicrob Agents Chemother* (2011) 55, 1063–7.
9. Hagelberg NM, Nieminen TH, Saari TI, Neuvonen M, Neuvonen PJ, Laine K, Olkkola KT. Voriconazole drastically increases exposure to oral oxycodone. *Eur J Clin Pharmacol* (2009) 65, 263–71.
10. Watanabe M, Homma M, Momo K, Okoshi Y, Wada T, Hara A, Chiba S, Kohda Y. Effects of voriconazole co-administration on oxycodone-induced adverse events: a case in the retrospective survey. *Eur J Clin Pharmacol* (2011) 67, 859–61.

Opioids + Baclofen

The analgesic effects of fentanyl and morphine, but probably not pentazocine, might be increased by baclofen. Increased sedation can occur and the risk of respiratory depression might increase if opioids are given with baclofen.

Clinical evidence, mechanism, importance and management

A study in three groups of 10 patients found that pretreatment with baclofen 600 micrograms/kg, either in four intramuscular doses for 5 days, or intravenously in 100 mL of glucose 5%, 45 minutes before surgery, prolonged the duration of **fentanyl** analgesia from 18 minutes to 30 minutes. Baclofen also reduced the amount of **fentanyl** needed by 30 to 40%.[1]

In a placebo-controlled study in 69 patients undergoing surgery for the removal of third molar teeth, oral baclofen (5 mg three times daily for 3 days and then a 10-mg dose, 6 hours before surgery and again immediately before surgery) enhanced the postoperative analgesic effect of intravenous **morphine** 6 mg. However, analgesia due to intravenous **pentazocine** 30 mg was not enhanced.[2]

These limited reports suggest that baclofen might potentiate the effects of **fentanyl** and **morphine**. The reasons for this effect are not understood, but it could be connected in some way with the action of baclofen on GABA receptors, as the spinal cord circuits that are important in opioid analgesia contain GABAergic receptors.[1,2] It appears that baclofen enhances the analgesic effect of **fentanyl** and **morphine**, which are pure opioid agonists that act primarily through μ-opioid receptors, whereas it does not affect pentazocine, a predominantly <kappa>-opioid analgesic.[2]

The UK manufacturer of baclofen warns that increased sedation could occur if baclofen is taken with synthetic opioids and that the risk of respiratory depression is also increased. Careful monitoring of respiratory and cardiovascular functions is essential.[3]

1. Panerai AE, Massei R, De Silva E, Sacerdote P, Monza G, Mantegazza P. Baclofen prolongs the analgesic effect of fentanyl in man. *Br J Anaesth* (1985) 57, 954–5.
2. Gordon NC, Gear RW, Heller PH, Paul S, Miaskowski C, Levine JD. Enhancement of morphine analgesia by the $GABA_B$ agonist baclofen. *Neuroscience* (1995) 69, 345–9.
3. Lioresal Tablets (Baclofen). Novartis Pharmaceuticals UK Ltd. UK Summary of product characteristics, February 2013.

Opioids + Barbiturates

A case of increased sedation with severe CNS toxicity has been reported with concurrent use of pethidine (meperidine) and phenobarbital. The analgesic effects of pethidine can be reduced by barbiturates. Secobarbital increases the respiratory depressant effects of morphine. Other barbiturates would also be expected to increase the CNS depressant effects of opioids. Phenobarbital is predicted to induce the metabolism of buprenorphine and tapentadol.

Clinical evidence

(a) Codeine

A study in pain-free patients found that codeine 60 mg increased the hypnotic actions of **secobarbital** 100 mg resulting in synergism in the sedative effects.[1]

(b) Dextropropoxyphene (Propoxyphene)

For mention that dextropropoxyphene increased **phenobarbital** concentrations, see 'Phenobarbital + Dextropropoxyphene (Propoxyphene)', p.590.

(c) Fentanyl

For mention that fentanyl requirements during anaesthesia were higher in patients taking carbamazepine with other antiepileptics including **primidone**, see 'Opioids + Antiepileptics; Carbamazepine', p.164.

(d) Methadone

Methadone concentrations can be reduced by **phenobarbital**, see 'Opioids; Methadone + Antiepileptics; Enzyme-inducing', p.165.

(e) Morphine

In a study in 30 healthy subjects, both intravenous **secobarbital** and intravenous morphine depressed respiration when given alone, and a much greater and more prolonged respiratory depression occurred when they were given together.[2]

(f) Pethidine (Meperidine)

1. Increased pethidine toxicity. A woman whose pain had been satisfactorily controlled with pethidine without particular CNS depression, had prolonged sedation with severe CNS toxicity when she was given pethidine after taking **phenobarbital** 30 mg four times daily for 2 weeks.[3]

2. Pethidine effects reduced. Studies in women undergoing dilatation and curettage found that **thiopental** and **pentobarbital** increased their sensitivity to pain, and opposed the analgesic effects of pethidine.[4] This confirmed the findings of previous studies.[5] A large reduction in the analgesic effect of pethidine has been seen for up to 5 hours after high doses (6 to 10 mg/kg) of **thiopental**.[4] This reduction in efficacy also occurred with **phenobarbital**.[4]

Mechanism

Studies suggest that phenobarbital induces the liver enzymes concerned with the metabolism (*N*-demethylation) of pethidine (meperidine) so that the production of its more toxic metabolite (norpethidine) is increased. The toxicity seen appears to be the combined effects of this compound and the directly sedative effects of the barbiturate.[3,6] Phenobarbital is also likely to induce the metabolism of other opioids that are metabolised by the cytochrome P450 isoenzyme system (see Opioids in the 'Introduction', p.138). Both barbiturates and opioids have CNS depressant effects, and these are likely to be additive.

Importance and management

Although phenobarbital has been seen to alter the metabolism of **pethidine** (meperidine) there is only one report of toxicity. The general clinical importance of this interaction is therefore uncertain. It has also been suggested that if pethidine is continued but phenobarbital is suddenly withdrawn, the toxic concentrations of norpethidine might lead to convulsions in the absence of an antiepileptic.[3] Note that the metabolite, norpethidine, is a less effective analgesic than pethidine and its increased production may increase the risk of CNS toxicity. Concurrent use should therefore be undertaken with care.

Both the barbiturates and the opioids have CNS depressant effects, which would be expected to be additive. The manufacturers of several opiates specifically mention that barbiturates can potentiate the adverse effects of opioids, such as sedation and respiratory depression. Care is therefore warranted on concurrent use. Be aware that, because of their enzyme-inducing effects, the barbiturates might reduce the analgesic effects of the opioids, but the clinical relevance of this is unclear. Any effect is probably of most relevance in patients that have been titrated to stable doses of opioids. A reduction in efficacy with the concurrent use of barbiturates, such as phenobarbital has been predicted by the manufacturers of **buprenorphine**[7,8] and of **tapentadol**.[9] For these drugs, monitor their effect on concurrent use with barbiturates, and consider adjusting the dose.

1. Bellville JW, Forrest WH, Shroff P, Brown BW. The hypnotic effects of codeine and secobarbital and their interaction in man. *Clin Pharmacol Ther* (1971) 12, 607–12.
2. Zsigmond EK, Flynn K. Effect of secobarbital and morphine on arterial blood gases in healthy human volunteers. *J Clin Pharmacol* (1993) 33, 453–7.
3. Stambaugh JE, Wainer IW, Hemphill DM, Schwartz I. A potentially toxic drug interaction between pethidine (meperidine) and phenobarbitone. *Lancet* (1977) i, 398–9.
4. Dundee JW. Alterations in response to somatic pain associated with anaesthesia. II. The effect of thiopentone and pentobarbitone. *Br J Anaesth* (1960) 32, 407–14.
5. Clutton-Brock J. Some pain threshold studies with particular reference to thiopentone. *Anaesthesia* (1960) 15, 71–2.
6. Stambaugh JE, Wainer IW, Schwartz I. The effect of phenobarbital on the metabolism of meperidine in normal volunteers. *J Clin Pharmacol* (1978) 18, 482–90.
7. Suboxone (Buprenorphine with naloxone). Reckitt Benckiser Pharmaceuticals Inc. US Prescribing information, August 2014.
8. Subutex (Buprenorphine hydrochloride). RB Pharmaceuticals Ltd. UK Summary of product characteristics, September 2014.
9. Palexia (Tapentadol hydrochloride). Grünenthal Ltd. UK Summary of product characteristics, July 2014.

Opioids + Benzodiazepines

The concurrent use of opioids and benzodiazepines generally results in enhanced sedation and respiratory depression; however, in one case benzodiazepines have antagonised the respiratory depressant effects of opioids. An additive effect on pain control has been seen, but, conversely, diazepam has been shown to antagonise the analgesic effect of morphine. Opioids delay the oral absorption of diazepam. Dextropropoxyphene appears to slightly reduce alprazolam clearance, but not to alter diazepam or lorazepam pharmacokinetics. Oxymorphone does not alter midazolam pharmacokinetics.

Clinical evidence

A. Analgesia

(a) Fentanyl and related drugs

For the effect of midazolam on the analgesic effect of fentanyl and related drugs, see 'Opioids; Fentanyl and related drugs + Benzodiazepines', p.170.

(b) Morphine

In one study, low-dose **midazolam** (given to achieve a concentration of 50 nanograms/mL) reduced the dose of morphine required for postoperative analgesia in the first 12 hours.[1] However, in another study postoperative pain scores were higher in patients premedicated with oral **diazepam** 10 mg than with placebo, although morphine consumption did not differ.[2] Similarly, in another study, the benzodiazepine antagonist flumazenil enhanced morphine analgesia in patients who had been premedicated with **diazepam**.[3]

B. CNS depression

(a) Overdose

Sudden deaths in patients who abuse opioids are frequently associated with ingestion of other CNS depressants, particularly benzodiazepines. The pharmacodynamic interaction of additive CNS depression resulting in coma and respiratory depression is clearly a factor in these cases. However, various authors have suggested that a pharmacokinetic interaction might have contributed in cases occurring with **buprenorphine**,[4-6] **oxycodone**,[7] and **tramadol**[4] based on the fact that these opioids and some benzodiazepines are substrates for the cytochrome P450 isoenzyme system and might therefore inhibit each other's metabolism. Note that this is not an established mechanism for pharmacokinetic drug interactions, and substrates of a given isoenzyme do not cause clinically relevant interactions via that isoenzyme unless they are also an inhibitor of the isoenzyme. *In vitro* studies with buprenorphine show it is unlikely to be a clinically relevant CYP3A4 inhibitor,[5,6] and there are no known interactions of buprenorphine via this mechanism.

(b) Respiratory depression

1. Diamorphine. A 14-year-old boy with staphylococcal pneumonia secondary to influenza developed adult respiratory distress syndrome. It was decided to suppress his voluntary breathing with opioids and use assisted ventilation and he was therefore given **phenoperidine** and **diazepam** for 11 days, and later diamorphine with **lorazepam**. Despite receiving diamorphine 19.2 mg in 24 hours his respiratory drive was not suppressed. On day 17, despite serum morphine and **lorazepam** concentrations of 320 micrograms/mL and 5.3 micrograms/mL, respectively, he remained conscious and his pupils were not constricted.[8] Later *animal* studies suggested that **lorazepam** opposed the respiratory depressant effects of **morphine**.[8]

2. Fentanyl and related drugs. For the respiratory depressant effect of concurrent benzodiazepines and fentanyl, see 'Opioids; Fentanyl and related drugs + Benzodiazepines', p.170.

3. Pethidine (meperidine). Intravenous **diazepam** 150 micrograms/kg did not alter the respiratory depressant effect of intravenous pethidine 1.5 mg/kg in a study in healthy subjects[9] or in patients with chronic obstructive pulmonary disease.[10]

(c) Sedation

1. Buprenorphine. Single oral doses of **diazepam** 10 or 20 mg given to 8 patients taking buprenorphine increased subjective effects, such as sedation and strength of drug effects, and also caused a deterioration in performance measures, such as cancellation time, compared with placebo.[11] A further study by the same authors found similar effects when subjects stabilised taking buprenorphine were given a single 40-mg dose of oral diazepam.[12]

2. Fentanyl and related drugs. For mention that concurrent use of midazolam and alfentanil increased sedation, see 'Opioids; Fentanyl and related drugs + Benzodiazepines', p.170.

3. Methadone. For the increased sedation seen with diazepam and methadone, see 'Opioids; Methadone + Benzodiazepines', p.171.

4. Morphine. The sedative effects of **midazolam** and morphine were additive in a study in patients given these drugs intravenously before surgery.[13]

5. Pethidine (meperidine). A prospective study in 80 patients undergoing elective endoscopy found that deep sedation occurred frequently (68% of patients) with pethidine and **midazolam** used with the intent of moderate sedation.[14]

C. Pharmacokinetics

(a) Dextropropoxyphene (propoxyphene)

A study in healthy subjects found that dextropropoxyphene 65 mg every 6 hours prolonged the **alprazolam** half-life from 11.6 hours to 18.3 hours, and decreased its clearance by 38% (from 1.3 to 0.8 mL/minute per kg). The pharmacokinetics of single doses of **diazepam** and **lorazepam** were not affected by dextropropoxyphene.[15]

(b) Fentanyl and related drugs

For mention that fentanyl slightly reduced midazolam clearance, see 'Opioids; Fentanyl and related drugs + Benzodiazepines', p.170.

(c) Methadone

For mention of the lack of a pharmacokinetic interaction between methadone and diazepam, see 'Opioids; Methadone + Benzodiazepines', p.171.

(d) Morphine

In a study in 12 female patients, intramuscular morphine 10 mg delayed the absorption of oral **diazepam** 10 mg, taken 60 minutes after the opioid. Diazepam concentrations were found to be lower and maximum concentrations were not reached in the 90-minute study period, when compared with the maximum concentration at 60 minutes in the control group.[16]

(e) Oxymorphone

In a controlled study in healthy subjects, neither high-dose extended-release oxymorphone 60 mg twice daily plus naltrexone nor low-dose extended-release oxymorphone 10 to 20 mg daily had any effect on the pharmacokinetics of oral **midazolam**.[17]

(f) Pethidine (meperidine)

In a study in 10 female patients, intramuscular pethidine 100 mg delayed the absorption of oral **diazepam** 10 mg, taken 60 minutes after the opioid. Diazepam concentrations were found to be lower and maximum concentrations were not reached in the 90-minute study period, when compared with the maximum concentration at 60 minutes in the control group.[16]

Mechanism

A. Analgesia

Benzodiazepines are generally not thought to possess analgesic properties independent of their CNS depressant effect, but this indirect effect would be expected to be additive with that of opioids. Nevertheless, data from the two diazepam studies suggests that benzodiazepines can actually antagonise the analgesic effect of opioids via their effect on supraspinal GABA receptors.[3]

B. CNS Depression

Both opioids and benzodiazepines cause CNS and respiratory depression, which would be expected to be additive or synergistic on concurrent use. The reason for the lack of additive respiratory depressant effect, or possible antagonism of respiratory depressant effect in the case report and a few of the studies cited is uncertain. In the case of overdose with oxycodone and clonazepam, it was suggested that the two drugs might have inhibited each other's metabolism.[7] However, neither oxycodone nor clonazepam are known to be inhibitors of drug metabolism, so this explanation seems unlikely. It was also considered that the woman might have had impaired liver function, which would have reduced the clearance of both drugs.[7]

C. Pharmacokinetics

Opioid analgesics delay gastric emptying thereby reducing the rate of absorption of oral diazepam. It would seem that dextropropoxyphene inhibits the hydroxylation of alprazolam by the liver, thereby reducing its clearance from the body, but has little or no effect on the *N*-demethylation or glucuronidation of diazepam or lorazepam, respectively.

Importance and management

A. Analgesia

The sedative and CNS depressant effect of benzodiazepines might be expected to diminish the perception of pain and therefore be additive with analgesics. However, from the studies with diazepam, it seems possible that benzodiazepines might have some antagonistic effect against the analgesic action of opioids. The authors suggest that short-acting benzodiazepines might be preferred for use premedication than long-acting agents, such as **diazepam**, so that any effect will have diminished by the time that postoperative analgesia is needed.[3] Benzodiazepines and opioids are commonly used in surgical anaesthesia, and short-acting oral forms of benzodiazepines are usual in current premedication regimens. The relevance of the findings for use of benzodiazepines with opioids in patients with chronic pain is unknown.

B. CNS Depression

Both opioids and benzodiazepines can cause sedation and respiratory depression, and the effects are likely to be additive on combined use. However, there are a few studies and reports where an additive respiratory depressant effect was not seen. Despite these few reports, it would be prudent to assume that the respiratory depressant effects of benzodiazepines and opioids are likely to be additive, and to take any necessary precautions relevant to the clinical setting of concurrent use. Similarly, as shown in the few studies cited, the sedative effect of opioids and benzodiazepines are likely to be greater on concurrent use. The effect can be beneficial and intentional in the setting of induced sedation for medical procedures or anaesthetic protocols. However, in other clinical settings the likely increased sedation is an adverse effect. The degree of impairment will depend on the individual patient, the doses used, and the particular drugs. Warn all patients of the potential adverse effects on driving and other skilled tasks.

Note that co-abuse of both opioids and benzodiazepines is common and sudden deaths in patients who abuse opioids are frequently associated with ingestion of benzodiazepines. Severe CNS depression is a feature of these cases.

C. Pharmacokinetics

The maximal effect of oral **diazepam** might be expected to be delayed in patients receiving opioids, but the clinical relevance of this is uncertain. Other oral benzodiazepines might be similarly affected. The slight reduction in **alprazolam** clearance by dextropropxyphene is of uncertain clinical importance, but the inference to be drawn is that the CNS depressant effects of alprazolam will be increased, over and above the simple additive CNS depressant effects likely when other benzodiazepines and dextropropoxyphene are taken together. More study is needed, but in the meantime it would be prudent to monitor for an increase in adverse effects on concurrent use.

Oxymorphone does not alter the pharmacokinetics of **midazolam**, so no extra precautions would be required on concurrent use other than those relating to additive CNS depression. Midazolam is a sensitive probe substrate for CYP3A4, and these data therefore shown that oxymorphone is not an inhibitor or inducer of CYP3A4.

1. Gilliland HE, Prasad BK, Mirakhur RK, Fee JPH. An investigation of the potential morphine sparing effect of midazolam. *Anaesthesia* (1996) 51, 808–11.
2. Caumo W, Hidalgo MPL, Schmidt AP, Iwamoto CW, Adamatti LC, Bergmann J, Ferreira MBC. Effect of pre-operative anxiolysis on postoperative pain response in patients undergoing total abdominal hysterectomy. *Anaesthesia* (2002) 57, 740–6.
3. Gear RW, Miaskowski C, Heller PH, Paul SM, Gordon NC, Levine JD. Benzodiazepine mediated antagonism of opioid analgesia. *Pain* (1997) 71, 25–9.
4. Clarot F, Goullé JP, Vaz E, Proust B. Fatal overdoses of tramadol: is benzodiazepine a risk factor of lethality? *Forensic Sci Int* (2003) 134, 57–61.
5. Ibrahim RB, Wilson JG, Thorsby ME, Edwards DJ. Effect of buprenorphine on CYP3A activity in rat and human liver microsomes. *Life Sci* (2000) 66, 1293–8.
6. Kilicarslan T, Sellers EM. Lack of interaction of buprenorphine with flunitrazepam metabolism. *Am J Psychiatry* (2000) 157, 1164–6.
7. Burrows DL, Hagardorn AN, Harlan GC, Wallen EDB, Ferslew KE. A fatal drug interaction between oxycodone and clonazepam. *J Forensic Sci* (2003) 48, 683–6.
8. McDonald CF, Thomson SA, Scott NC, Scott W, Grant IWB, Crompton GK. Benzodiazepine-opiate antagonism — a problem in intensive-care therapy. *Intensive Care Med* (1986) 12, 39–42.
9. Zsigmond EK, Flynn K, Martinez OA. Diazepam and meperidine on arterial blood gases in healthy volunteers. *J Clin Pharmacol* (1974) 14, 377–81.
10. Zsigmond EK, Shively JG, Flynn K. Diazepam and meperidine on arterial blood gases in patients with chronic obstructive pulmonary disease. *J Clin Pharmacol* (1975) 15, 464–69.
11. Lintzeris N, Mitchell TB, Bond A, Nestor L, Strang J. Interactions on mixing diazepam with methadone or buprenorphine in maintenance patients. *J Clin Psychopharmacol* (2006) 26, 274–83.
12. Lintzeris N, Mitchell TB, Bond AJ, Nestor L, Strang J. Pharmacodynamics of diazepam co-administered with methadone or buprenorphine under high dose conditions in opioid dependent patients. *Drug Alcohol Depend* (2007) 91, 187–94.
13. Tverskoy M, Fleyshman G, Ezry J, Bradley EL, Kissin I. Midazolam-morphine sedative interaction in patients. *Anesth Analg* (1989) 68, 282–5.
14. Patel S, Vargo JJ, Khandwala F, Lopez R, Trolli P, Dumot JA, Conwell DL, Zuccaro G. Deep sedation occurs frequently during elective endoscopy with meperidine and midazolam. *Am J Gastroenterol* (2005) 100, 2689–95.
15. Abernethy DR, Greenblatt DJ, Morse DS, Shader RI. Interaction of propoxyphene with diazepam, alprazolam and lorazepam. *Br J Clin Pharmacol* (1985) 19, 51–7.
16. Gamble JAS, Gaston JH, Nair SG, Dundee JW. Some pharmacological factors influencing the absorption of diazepam following oral administration. *Br J Anaesth* (1976) 48, 1181–5.
17. Adams M, Pieniaszek HJ, Gammaitoni AR, Ahdieh H. Oxymorphone extended release does not affect CYP2C9 or CYP3A4 metabolic pathways. *J Clin Pharmacol* (2005) 45, 337–45.

Opioids; Fentanyl and related drugs + Benzodiazepines

In general the concurrent use of benzodiazepines with alfentanil or fentanyl in anaesthesia is synergistic but might also result in additive adverse effects, such as respiratory depression and/or hypotension. Single-dose intravenous fentanyl slightly increased single-dose intravenous midazolam exposure. Retrospective evidence suggests that midazolam can increase the dose requirement of sufentanil, but midazolam did not alter the analgesic efficacy of fentanyl in healthy subjects.

Clinical evidence

(a) Anaesthetic induction

Giving **midazolam** with **alfentanil** or **fentanyl** for the induction of anaesthesia reduces the dose required of both the benzodiazepine and the opioid, when compared with either drug alone.[1-3] The interaction is synergistic.[2]

(b) Analgesic effects

An analysis of 43 patients who were mechanically ventilated following major trauma, and who were given infusions of **sufentanil** alone or **sufentanil** with **midazolam**, found that midazolam appeared to reduce the analgesic efficacy of sufentanil. The rate of sufentanil infusion in the group given both drugs (21 patients) was increased by more than 50%, when compared with the group given sufentanil alone (22 patients). It was found possible to reduce the sufentanil infusion in 8 of the patients given sufentanil alone, whereas this was possible in only one patient given both drugs.[4]

Conversely, in a study in healthy subjects, intravenous **midazolam** 500 micrograms to 2 mg per 70 kg did not affect the analgesia produced by intravenous **fentanyl** 100 micrograms per 70 kg in a cold pressor test.[5]

(c) Hypotension and respiratory depression

1. Neonates. Hypotension occurred in 6 neonates with respiratory distress who were given **midazolam** (a bolus of 200 micrograms/kg and/or an infusion of 60 micrograms/kg per hour) for sedation during the first 12 to 36 hours of life. Five of them were also given **fentanyl** either as an infusion (1 to 2 micrograms/kg per hour) or a bolus (1.5 to 2.5 micrograms/kg), or both. Blood pressures decreased from an average of 55/40 mmHg to 36/24 mmHg in 5 of the neonates, and from 42/28 mmHg to less than 20 mmHg in the other neonate.[6] Another report describes respiratory arrest in a child of 14 months who was given both drugs.[7]

2. Adults. In a study in 12 healthy subjects, **midazolam** 50 micrograms/kg alone caused no episodes of apnoea or hypoxaemia, whereas **fentanyl** 2 micrograms/kg alone caused hypoxaemia in 6 subjects but no apnoea. When both drugs were given together 6 subjects had apnoea and 11 subjects had hypoxaemia.[8] Similarly, in a study in 12 healthy subjects, **fentanyl** with **diazepam** caused more respiratory depression than either drug alone.[9] Hypotension has also been seen in adults given fentanyl with **midazolam**[10] or **diazepam**.[11]

Acute hypotension occurred in a man receiving clonidine, captopril, and furosemide who

was premedicated with intramuscular **midazolam** 5 mg and anaesthetised with **sufentanil** 150 micrograms.[12] This is consistent with another report of sudden hypotension during anaesthetic induction in 4 patients given high-dose **sufentanil** who had been given **lorazepam** before induction.[13]

(d) Pharmacokinetics

In a single-dose, placebo-controlled study in 30 patients undergoing orthopaedic surgery, intravenous **fentanyl** 200 micrograms given one minute before intravenous **midazolam** 200 micrograms/kg decreased the systemic clearance of midazolam by 30% and increased midazolam exposure by 54%. The elimination half-life of midazolam was prolonged by about 50%.[14]

(e) Sedation

A study in patients undergoing an abdominal hysterectomy under **alfentanil** and **midazolam** anaesthesia found that although the pharmacokinetics of midazolam were unchanged, postoperative sedation was more pronounced, when compared with a group of patients that did not receive alfentanil.[15]

Mechanism

Uncertain. The concurrent use of two or more CNS depressants can produce additive respiratory depressant and sedative effects. Why midazolam appeared to increase the analgesic dose requirement for sufentanil is unknown. An *in-vitro* study found that high concentrations of fentanyl slightly inhibited the metabolism of midazolam by CYP3A4,[16] but fentanyl is not usually considered to be a CYP3A4 inhibitor.

Importance and management

A pharmacodynamic interaction between alfentanil, fentanyl, or sufentanil and the benzodiazepines would appear to be established. Not all pairs appear to have been studied, but they would all be expected to interact similarly, to a greater or lesser extent. Increased sedative and respiratory depressant effects are to be expected on concurrent use, and hypotension might also occur. Increased sedation can be beneficial and intentional in the setting of induced sedation for medical procedures or anaesthetic protocols. However, in other clinical settings it is an adverse effect. It would therefore seem prudent to be alert for CNS depression and hypotension in all patients given alfentanil, fentanyl, or sufentanil and a benzodiazepine, and to take any necessary precautions relevant to the clinical setting of concurrent use.. The US manufacturer of a transdermal fentanyl product indicated for chronic pain suggests that if benzodiazepines are also given the dose of one or both drugs should be reduced.[17]

The sedative and CNS depressant effect of benzodiazepines might be expected to diminish the perception of pain and therefore be additive with analgesics. The reduced analgesic efficacy of sufentanil in patients given both midazolam and sufentanil in the intensive care setting is therefore unexpected, and its clinical relevance unclear. See also 'Opioids + Benzodiazepines', p.169 for the possible antagonism of morphine analgesia with diazepam.

1. Ben-Shlomo I, Abd-El-Khalim H, Ezry J, Zohar S, Tverskoy M. Midazolam acts synergistically with fentanyl for induction of anaesthesia. *Br J Anaesth* (1990) 64, 45–7.
2. Vinik HR, Bradley EL, Kissin I. Midazolam–alfentanil synergism for anesthetic induction in patients. *Anesth Analg* (1989) 69, 213–17.
3. Kissin I, Vinik HR, Castillo R, Bradley EL. Alfentanil potentiates midazolam-induced unconsciousness in subanalgesic doses. *Anesth Analg* (1990) 71, 65–9.
4. Luger TJ, Hill HF, Schlager A. Can midazolam diminish sufentanil analgesia in patients with major trauma? A retrospective study with 43 patients. *Drug Metabol Drug Interact* (1992) 10, 177–84.
5. Zacny JP, Coalson DW, Klafta JM, Klock PA, Alessi R, Rupani G, Young CJ, Patil PG, Apfelbaum JL. Midazolam does not influence intravenous fentanyl-induced analgesia in healthy volunteers. *Pharmacol Biochem Behav* (1996) 55, 275–80.
6. Burtin P, Daoud P, Jacqz-Aigrain E, Mussat P, Moriette G. Hypotension with midazolam and fentanyl in the newborn. *Lancet* (1991) 337, 1545–6.
7. Yaster M, Nichols DG, Deshpande JK, Wetzel RC. Midazolam-fentanyl intravenous sedation in children: case report of respiratory arrest. *Pediatrics* (1990) 86, 463–7.
8. Bailey PL, Moll JWB, Pace NL, East KA, Stanley TH. Respiratory effects of midazolam and fentanyl: potent interaction producing hypoxemia and apnea. *Anesthesiology* (1988) 69, 3A, A813.
9. Bailey PL, Andriano KP, Pace NL, Westenskow DR, Stanley TH. Small doses of fentanyl potentiate and prolong diazepam induced respiratory depression. *Anesth Analg* (1984) 63, 183.
10. Heikkilä J, Jalonen J, Arola M, Kanto J, Laaksonen V. Midazolam as adjunct to high-dose fentanyl anaesthesia for coronary artery bypass grafting operation. *Acta Anaesthesiol Scand* (1984) 28, 683–9.
11. Tomicheck RC, Rosow CE, Philbin DM, Moss J, Teplick RS, Schneider RC. Diazepam-fentanyl interaction — hemodynamic and hormonal effects in coronary artery surgery. *Anesth Analg* (1983) 62, 881–4.
12. West JM, Estrada S, Heerdt M. Sudden hypotension associated with midazolam and sufentanil. *Anesth Analg* (1987) 66, 693–4.
13. Spiess BD, Sathoff RH, El-Ganzouri ARS, Ivankovich AD. High-dose sufentanil: four cases of sudden hypotension on induction. *Anesth Analg* (1986) 65, 703–5.
14. Hase I, Oda Y, Tanaka K, Mizutani K, Nakamoto T, Asada A. I.v. fentanyl decreases the clearance of midazolam. *Br J Anaesth* (1997) 79, 740 –3.
15. Persson MP, Nilsson A, Hartvig P. Relation of sedation and amnesia to plasma concentrations of midazolam in surgical patients. *Clin Pharmacol Ther* (1988) 43, 324–31.
16. Oda Y, Mizutani K, Hase I, Nakamoto T, Hamaoka N, Asada A. Fentanyl inhibits metabolism of midazolam: competitive inhibition of CYP3A4 *in vitro*. *Br J Anaesth* (1999) 82, 900–3.
17. Duragesic (Fentanyl transdermal system). Janssen Pharmaceuticals, Inc. US Prescribing information, July 2012.

Opioids; Methadone + Benzodiazepines

Patients taking methadone who are given diazepam might experience increased drowsiness and possibly enhanced opioid effects. Temazepam could have contributed to the sudden death of a patient taking methadone. Diazepam appears not to alter methadone pharmacokinetics.

Clinical evidence

(a) CNS effects

1. Diazepam. In a study in 5 patients taking maintenance methadone, the opioid effects of methadone (subjective effects and pupil constriction) appeared to be enhanced by acute administration of diazepam and this was statistically significant with high-dose methadone (150% of the maintenance dose) and diazepam 40 mg.[1] Similarly, a further study in 8 patients taking methadone found that single oral doses of diazepam 10 or 20 mg, which are within the usual therapeutic range, increased the subjective effects such as sedation, strength of drug effects and euphoria, and also caused a significant deterioration in performance measures such as reaction time, when compared with placebo.[2] A study in 4 patients stabilised on methadone found that diazepam 40 mg increased the intensity of subjective effects, such as sedation, and decreased psychological performance, such as reaction times and digit symbol substitution test (DSST), generally independent of the methadone dose administered. However, high-dose methadone was associated with a reduction in oxygen saturation levels.[3] A study in patients taking methadone noted that diazepam abuse was prevalent, and that many patients reported that diazepam boosted the effects of methadone.[4]

In contrast, in a study in four addicts taking methadone for at least 6 months and given diazepam 300 micrograms/kg for 9 days, the opioid effects of methadone appeared to be unchanged, although all addicts were sedated while taking diazepam.[5]

2. Temazepam. A 39-year-old man taking methadone 60 mg daily and temazepam 20 mg twice daily was found dead. Blood concentrations of methadone and temazepam were not particularly high, and revealed that amitriptyline had also been taken.[6] The cause of death was therefore considered to be accidental owing to methadone toxicity enhanced by the additive CNS depressant effects of both temazepam and amitriptyline.

(b) Pharmacokinetics

The pharmacokinetics of methadone were not apparently changed by **diazepam** in 4 patients taking maintenance methadone.[5] Similarly, analysis of blood samples from another study[1] confirmed that there is no pharmacokinetic interaction between methadone and **diazepam**.[7]

Mechanism

A pharmacodynamic interaction of additive or synergistic CNS and respiratory depression would be expected on concurrent use of methadone and benzodiazepines.

There is no known mechanism whereby benzodiazepines might be expected to alter methadone pharmacokinetics. Competition of substrates for CYP3A4 metabolism has been suggested, but this is not a clinically relevant mechanism of pharmacokinetic interactions.

Importance and management

The concurrent use of methadone with diazepam and other benzodiazepines need not be avoided, but patients given both drugs are likely to experience increased drowsiness and reduced psychomotor performance, and should be warned against driving or operating machinery under these circumstances. The possibility of opioid enhancement should also be borne in mind. Bear in mind that the concurrent use of benzodiazepines appears to be a risk factor in sudden death in patients taking methadone.

1. Preston KL, Griffiths RR, Stitzer ML, Bigelow GE, Liebson IA. Diazepam and methadone interactions in methadone maintenance. *Clin Pharmacol Ther* (1984) 36, 534–41.
2. Lintzeris N, Mitchell TB, Bond A, Nestor L, Strang J. Interactions on mixing diazepam with methadone or buprenorphine in maintenance patients. *J Clin Psychopharmacol* (2006) 26, 274–83.
3. Lintzeris N, Mitchell TB, Bond AJ, Nestor L, Strang J. Pharmacodynamics of diazepam co-administered with methadone or buprenorphine under high dose conditions in opioid dependent patients. *Drug Alcohol Depend* (2007) 91, 187–94.
4. Stitzer ML, Griffiths RR, McLellan AT, Grabowski J, Hawthorne JW. Diazepam use among methadone maintenance patients: patterns and dosages. *Drug Alcohol Depend* (1981) 8, 189–9.
5. Pond SM, Tong TG, Benowitz NL, Jacob P, Rigod J. Lack of effect of diazepam on methadone metabolism in methadone-maintained addicts. *Clin Pharmacol Ther* (1982) 31, 139–43.
6. Fahey T, Law F, Cottee H, Astley P. Sudden death in an adult taking methadone: lessons for general practice. *Br J Gen Pract* (2003) 53, 471–2.
7. Preston KL, Griffiths RR, Cone EJ, Darwin WD, Gorodetzky CW. Diazepam and methadone blood levels following concurrent administration of diazepam and methadone. *Drug Alcohol Depend* (1986) 18, 195–202.

Opioids + Calcium-channel blockers

Diltiazem slightly increased alfentanil exposure and prolonged its effects in one study, but had no effect on requirements for parenteral fentanyl in another study. A case of exacerbated delirium, after the addition of diltiazem to intravenous fentanyl, has been described. Neither diltiazem nor verapamil altered morphine analgesia or its subjective, psychomotor or physiological effects. The effect of nifedipine and nimodipine on the analgesic effects of morphine is conflicting, with enhanced effects, no effect, and possible reduced effects reported. Neither nifedipine nor nimodipine altered morphine concentrations. Bradycardia and hypotension are predicted to be enhanced in patients given remifentanil with calcium-channel blockers.

Clinical evidence

(a) Dihydropyridines

1. Morphine. Calcium-channel blockers have been investigated for their ability to enhance opioid analgesia. In some studies, an enhanced effect has been seen. For example, in a controlled study in 26 patients undergoing surgery, two doses of slow-release **nifedipine** 20 mg given on the day preceding surgery and a further dose given 60 to 90 minutes before surgery increased the analgesic effect of the first postoperative dose of morphine.[1] Similarly, in 30 patients with cancer taking oral morphine, addition of **nimodipine** allowed the morphine dose to be reduced when compared with placebo.[2]

In contrast, in other studies, calcium-channel blockers have had no effect on morphine analgesia, or possibly even led to increased morphine requirements. For example, in a study in 9 healthy subjects, **nimodipine** 60 mg taken 120 minutes before intravenous morphine had no effect on morphine analgesia in the cold-pressor test when compared with placebo.[3] Similarly, in a controlled study in patients undergoing surgery, neither oral **nifedipine** 60 mg nor **nimodipine** 30 micrograms/kg over 20 hours reduced postoperative morphine requirements, and morphine consumption in the **nifedipine** group was actually higher.[4] Furthermore, in a placebo-controlled study in 40 patients undergoing knee arthroplasty, 20 patients given oral **nimodipine** 90 mg one hour before surgery followed by 30 mg every 6 hours for 48 hours postoperatively had increased intravenous morphine consumption via patient-controlled analgesia (PCA). No difference in pain scores was reported between the groups.[5] In two of these studies, pharmacokinetics were assessed and neither **nifedipine**[1] nor **nimodipine**[2] altered morphine concentrations. In the study in healthy subjects, **nimodipine** did not alter the subjective, psychomotor or physiological (e.g. heart rate, blood pressure) effects of morphine.[3]

(b) Diltiazem

1. Alfentanil. In a study, 15 patients were anaesthetised with midazolam, isoflurane, propofol, and alfentanil (induced with 50 micrograms/kg, then maintained with 1 microgram/kg per minute). The AUC and half-life of alfentanil were increased by 24% and 50%, respectively, by diltiazem 60 mg, given orally 2 hours before induction and then as an infusion for 23 hours starting at induction. Tracheal extubation was performed on average 2.5 hours later in the patients receiving diltiazem than in a placebo group.[6]

2. Fentanyl. In a study in 30 patients who had undergone lower abdominal gynaecological surgery, a continuous infusion of diltiazem 1 microgram/kg per minute for 24 hours after surgery, did not alter the consumption of fentanyl by patient-controlled analgesia (PCA), when compared with placebo.[7]

A case report describes an exacerbation of delirium in an 85-year-old patient receiving intravenous fentanyl 25 micrograms/hour, 3 days after diltiazem (dose unknown) was added for treatment of supraventricular tachycardia. Within hours of fentanyl being stopped the patient became more alert and 2 days later was discharged alert and lucid. The authors attributed the exacerbation of delirium to fentanyl toxicity as a result of an interaction with diltiazem, but also noted the potential contribution of other factors such as infection.[8]

3. Morphine. In a study in 9 healthy subjects, diltiazem 30 mg taken 120 minutes before intravenous morphine had no effect on morphine analgesia in the cold-pressor test, neither did it alter the subjective, psychomotor, or physiological effects (such as heart rate, blood pressure) of morphine when compared with placebo.[3]

(c) Verapamil

1. Morphine. In a study in 9 healthy subjects, verapamil 80 mg taken 120 minutes before intravenous morphine had no effect on morphine analgesia in the cold-pressor test, neither did it alter the subjective, psychomotor, or physiological effects (such as heart rate, blood pressure) of morphine when compared with placebo.8

Mechanism

Diltiazem is a moderate inhibitor of CYP3A4, which is responsible for the metabolism of alfentanil and fentanyl, and so concurrent use can increase the concentrations of these opioids. Note that fentanyl has a high hepatic extraction and so is more affected by changes in hepatic blood flow than effects on the isoenzymes responsible for its metabolism (see 'Changes in first-pass metabolism', p.4); it is therefore less affected by CYP3A inhibitors than alfentanil. **Sufentanil** is similarly metabolised like fentanyl and so might be expected to interact in the same way.

Verapamil is also a moderate inhibitor of CYP3A4 and so might be expected to affect these opioids in the same way as diltiazem, although this needs confirmation.

Pre-clinical evidence suggests that calcium ions are involved in the signalling of pain in the nervous system, and suggests that calcium channel blockers might enhance opioid analgesia. However, the clinical evidence is conflicting and the reason for this is not known.

Importance and management

Although information about an interaction between diltiazem or verapamil and these opioids is limited, an interaction between **alfentanil** and diltiazem would appear to be established. Caution is required on their concurrent use as there could be an increased risk of prolonged or delayed respiratory depression. Monitor closely and adjust the alfentanil dose accordingly. It would seem prudent to be alert for similar effects with verapamil (see *Mechanism*, above).

Information for an interaction between **fentanyl** and diltiazem is limited, but the study suggests that in general any effect on the pharmacokinetics of fentanyl given parenterally is not clinically relevant. The case report is of unknown general relevance as other factors might have had a part to play, but perhaps introduces a note of caution. The use of fentanyl by other routes, such as the transdermal patch or oral transmucosal preparation, does not appear to have been studied. It is possible that the buccal route might be affected to a greater extent by diltiazem if appreciable fentanyl is swallowed as this does not bypass CYP3A4, but this is theoretical and requires study. Note that some manufacturers of oral transmucosal or transdermal fentanyl preparations recommend close monitoring for respiratory depression with concurrent use of CYP3A4 inhibitors and name diltiazem and/or verapamil.[9-13] Parenterally administered **sufentanil** is anticipated to interact similarly to fentanyl (see *Mechanism*, above), suggesting a clinically relevant interaction is unlikely.

The effect of calcium-channel blockers on the analgesic efficacy of morphine is unclear, and the available information conflicting. No general recommendations can be made. Neither nifedipine nor nimodipine altered morphine concentrations.

The UK manufacturer of **remifentanil** states that cardiovascular effects (bradycardia and hypotension) might be greater in patients also taking calcium-channel blockers.[14]

1. Carta F, Bianchi M, Argenton S, Cervi D, Marolla G, Tamburini M, Breda M, Fantoni A, Panerai AE. Effect of nifedipine on morphine-induced analgesia. *Anesth Analg* (1990) 70, 493–8.
2. Santillán R, Hurlé MA, Armijo JA, de los Mozos R, Flórez J. Nimodipine-enhanced opiate analgesia in cancer patients requiring morphine dose escalation: a double-blind, placebo-controlled study. *Pain* (1998) 76, 17–26.
3. Hasegawa AE, Zacny JP. The influence of three L-type calcium channel blockers on morphine effects in healthy volunteers. *Anesth Analg* (1997) 85, 633–8.
4. Zarauza R, Sáez-Fernández AN, Iribarren MJ, Carrascosa F, Adame M, Fidalgo I, Monedero P. A comparative study with oral nifedipine, intravenous nimodipine, and magnesium sulfate in postoperative analgesia. *Anesth Analg* (2000) 91, 938–43.
5. Casey G, Nortcliffe S-A, Sharpe P, Buggy DJ. Perioperative nimodipine and postoperative analgesia. *Anesth Analg* (2006) 102, 504–8.
6. Ahonen J, Olkkola KT, Salmenperä M, Hynynen M, Neuvonen PJ. Effect of diltiazem on midazolam and alfentanil disposition in patients undergoing coronary artery bypass grafting. *Anesthesiology* (1996) 85, 1246–52.
7. Nitahara K, Matsunaga M, Katori K, Yotsui H, Higuchi H, Higa K. Effect of continuous low-dose intravenous diltiazem on epidural fentanyl analgesia after lower abdominal surgery. *Br J Anaesth* (2003) 90, 507–9.
8. Levin TT, Bakr MH, Nikolova T. Case report: delirium due to a diltiazem-fentanyl CYP3A4 drug interaction. *Gen Hosp Psychiatry* (2010) 32, e9–e10.
9. Actiq (Fentanyl citrate lozenge). Teva Pharmaceuticals Ltd. UK Summary of product characteristics, June 2015.
10. Actiq (Fentanyl citrate lozenge). Cephalon, Inc. US Prescribing information, December 2011.
11. Effentora (Fentanyl citrate buccal tablet). Teva Pharmaceuticals Ltd. UK Summary of product characteristics, February 2015.
12. Fentora (Fentanyl citrate buccal tablet). Cephalon, Inc. US Prescribing information, December 2011.
13. Durogesic DTrans (Fentanyl transdermal patch). Janssen-Cilag Ltd. UK Summary of product characteristics, July 2015.
14. Ultiva (Remifentanil hydrochloride). GlaxoSmithKline UK. UK Summary of product characteristics, December 2010.

Opioids + Cannabis and cannabinoids

Vaporised cannabis reduced pain in patients with chronic pain taking morphine or oxycodone in one study, but had no effect on the pharmacokinetics of these opioids. Low doses of cannabis also enhanced the effect of morphine in three patients. Dronabinol with and without cannabidiol appears to reduce pain in patients taking opioids. Additive sedation and CNS depression can occur with concurrent use of cannabis or cannabinoids, such as dronabinol and nabilone, with opioids.

Clinical evidence

(a) Cannabis

1. Methadone. Cannabis use in methadone-maintained patients did not appear to affect treatment progress, although some psychological difficulties were slightly more prevalent.[1] However, others have suggested that heavy cannabis use is associated with a poorer progress when methadone is given in the treatment of opioid addiction.[2] In a retrospective regression analysis, cannabis use appeared to be associated with lower minimum methadone concentrations.[3]

2. Morphine or Oxycodone. In a study, 21 patients with chronic pain taking stable doses of sustained-release morphine (10 patients) or oxycodone (11 patients) twice daily, were given inhaled vaporised cannabis (900 mg) once on day one, three times daily on days 2 to 4, and once on day 5. There were no differences in the AUCs for morphine or oxycodone after cannabis use, and overall pain scores were decreased by an average of 27%. Note that the reduction in pain scores for those taking oxycodone was not statistically significant. All patients in this study had previous experience of smoking cannabis.[4] Similarly, a report of 3 patients with chronic pain (due to multiple sclerosis, HIV-related peripheral neuropathy, and lumbar spinal damage) found that small doses of smoked cannabis potentiated the analgesic effects of morphine. The patients were able to decrease the dose of opioid by 60 to 100%.[5]

(b) Dronabinol

In a controlled study in 63 patients with neuropathic pain, 40 were taking an opioid analgesic (**codeine**, **dihydrocodeine**, **dextropropoxyphene**, **methadone**, **morphine**, **oxycodone**, **pethidine**, or **tramadol**). The mean pain score was 22% lower than at baseline when *Sativex* (dronabinol and **cannabidiol**) was added, compared with 8% in the placebo group. Objective measures of psychomotor performance were no different between the groups.[6] In an open study in patients with chronic non-cancer pain taking stable doses of opioids (**hydrocodone**, **hydromorphone**, **methadone**, **morphine**, or **oxycodone**), after the addition of dronabinol (starting at 5 mg twice daily and titrated according to response, up to 20 mg three times daily), there was a decrease in average pain scores from baseline (from an average of about 7 at baseline to about 5.25 at week 4).[7]

(c) Nabilone

The UK and US manufacturers of nabilone briefly note that additive CNS depression was shown with single doses of nabilone 2 mg and **codeine** 65 mg in healthy subjects.[8,9]

Mechanism

Studies in *animals* have shown that dronabinol (Δ^9-tetrahydrocannabinol), the major psychoactive constituent of cannabis, enhances the analgesic potency of opioids such as morphine, codeine, hydromorphone, methadone, oxymorphone, and pethidine (meperidine).[10-12] It has been suggested that low doses of dronabinol given with low doses of morphine might increase opioid potency without increasing adverse effects.[13] However, additive CNS depression has been shown with concurrent use of cannabis or cannabinoids and opioids.

Importance and management

From the limited available clinical evidence, it is unclear whether **cannabis** has additive effects with opioids for pain relief, but the **cannabinoids** dronabinol and cannabidiol might improve pain relief. Similarly, it is uncertain what effect cannabis has on methadone use for opioid addiction. However, combined use of cannabis or cannabinoids and opioids is likely to have additive sedative effects, and some consider that patients requiring both medicinal cannabis and opioids should not operate a motor vehicle.[14] Similarly, the manufacturers of various **cannabinoids** for buccal or oral use advise that additive sedation and CNS depression can occur on the concurrent use of these cannabinoids and opioids.[8,9] The US manufacturer of oral **nabilone** also notes reports of cross-tolerance and mutual potentiation with cannabinoids and opioids.[8]

1. Epstein DH, Preston KL. Does cannabis use predict poor outcome for heroin-dependent patients on maintenance treatment? Past findings and more evidence against. *Addiction* (2003) 98, 269–79. Erratum. ibid., 538.
2. Nixon LN. Cannabis use and treatment outcome in methadone maintenance. *Addiction* (2003) 98, 1321–2.
3. Hallinan R, Crettol S, Agho K, Attia J, Besson J, Croquette-Krokar M, Hämmig R, Déglon JJ, Byrne A, Ray J, Somogyi AA, Eap CB. Cannabis and benzodiazepines as determinants of methadone trough plasma concentration variability in maintenance treatment: a transnational study. *Eur J Clin Pharmacol* (2009) 65, 1113–20.
4. Abrams DI, Couey P, Shade SB, Kelly ME, Benowitz NL. Cannabinoid-opioid interaction in chronic pain. *Clin Pharmacol Ther* (2011) 90, 844–51.
5. Lynch ME, Clark AJ. Cannabis reduces opioid dose in the treatment of chronic non-cancer pain. *J Pain Symptom Manage* (2003) 25, 496–8.
6. Nurmikko TJ, Serpell MG, Hoggart B, Toomey PJ, Morlion BJ, Haines D. Sativex successfully treats neuropathic pain characterised by allodynia: a randomised, double-blind, placebo-controlled clinical trial. *Pain* (2007) 133, 210–20.
7. Narang S, Gibson D, Wasan AD, Ross EL, Michna E, Nedeljkovic SS, Jamison RN. Efficacy of dronabinol as an adjuvant treatment for chronic pain patients on opioid therapy. *J Pain* (2008) 9, 254–64.
8. Cesamet (Nabilone). Meda Pharmaceuticals Inc. US Prescribing information, April 2011.
9. Nabilone capsules. Meda Pharmaceuticals. UK Summary of product characteristics, June 2009.
10. Smith FL, Cichewicz D, Martin ZL, Welch SP. The enhancement of morphine antinociception in mice by Δ^9-tetrahydrocannabinol. *Pharmacol Biochem Behav* (1998) 60, 559–66.
11. Cichewicz DL, Martin ZL, Smith FL, Welch SP. Enhancement of μ opioid antinociception by oral Δ^9-tetrahydrocannabinol: dose-response analysis and receptor identification. *J Pharmacol Exp Ther* (1999) 289, 859–67.
12. Cichewicz DL, McCarthy EA. Antinociceptive synergy between Δ^9-tetrahydrocannabinol and opioids after oral administration. *J Pharmacol Exp Ther* (2003) 304, 1010–15.
13. Cichewicz DL. Synergistic interactions between cannabinoid and opioid analgesics. *Life Sci* (2004) 74, 1317–24.
14. Reisfield GM. Medical cannabis and chronic opioid therapy. *J Pain Palliat Care Pharmacother* (2010) 24, 356–61.

Opioids + Carisoprodol

Carisoprodol might enhance the CNS depressant effects of the opioids.

Clinical evidence

(a) Dextropropoxyphene (propoxyphene)

In a retrospective review of deaths recorded in Jefferson County over a 12-year period, carisoprodol was present in the blood of 24 cases, but was never the sole drug detected; dextropropoxyphene was also present in 8 of the 24 cases. Respiratory depression was a major cause of death, and as carisoprodol causes respiratory depression, it was considered to be probably responsible, in part, for these deaths.[1]

(b) Oxycodone

In a single-dose controlled study in 15 healthy subjects, giving carisoprodol 350 mg and oxycodone 10 mg one hour apart resulted in greater subjective and psychomotor effects in some tests than when each drug was administered alone. For example when taken together patients experienced a higher incidence of difficulty concentrating, light-headedness, and itchy skin. A dose of carisoprodol 700 mg was initially used in some subjects, but was withdrawn because of excessive sedation.[2]

A 49-year-old woman who had been taking oxycodone (*OxyContin*) 40 mg twice daily for more than one year was given carisoprodol 350 mg (one tablet) four times daily to treat muscle spasm and uncontrolled pain. After taking this regimen for one week without relief, she increased the dose of carisoprodol to 8 to 10 tablets daily, which is more than twice the recommended dose. She was found unconscious, was responsive only to painful stimuli, and her respiration was also depressed. She rapidly returned to full alertness when she was given naloxone 2 mg intravenously, although she had not taken any extra oxycodone tablets. The adverse effects were thought to be due to additive CNS depressant effects of both oxycodone and carisoprodol.[3]

Mechanism

Carisoprodol has sedative properties, which are additive with those of opioids.

Importance and management

Evidence for an interaction between carisoprodol and the opioids is limited, however because of the risk of additive CNS depression, concurrent use should be undertaken with caution. Patients should be warned against driving or operating machinery. Note that the manufacturer of carisoprodol recommends a maximum duration of use of carisoprodol of two to three weeks.[4]

1. Davis GG, Alexander CB. A review of carisoprodol deaths in Jefferson County, Alabama. *South Med J* (1998) 91, 726–30.
2. Zacny JP, Paice JA, Coalson DW. Subjective and psychomotor effects of carisoprodol in combination with oxycodone in healthy volunteers. *Drug Alcohol Depend* (2012) 120, 229–32.
3. Reeves RR, Mack JE. Possible dangerous interaction of OxyContin and carisoprodol. *Am Fam Physician* (2003) 67, 941–2.
4. Soma (Carisoprodol). Meda Pharmaceuticals Inc. US Prescribing information, January 2013.

Opioids + Chlorobutanol

Chlorobutanol, used as a preservative in some intravenous formulations of methadone, might have contributed to the QT prolongation seen with methadone in one study. Somnolence in a patient given high-dose intravenous morphine was attributed to the associated high intake of chlorobutanol preservative in the morphine injection.

Clinical evidence, mechanism, importance and management

(a) Methadone

A study in 47 patients receiving intravenous methadone for cancer pain found an approximately linear relationship between the log-dose of methadone and QTc measurements. In addition, methadone and chlorobutanol (a preservative in the methadone preparation) were both found to block cardiac potassium ion channels *in vitro*, and chlorobutanol potentiated this effect with methadone.[1] High doses of methadone alone have been reported to cause torsade de pointes, but this study suggests that chlorobutanol used as a preservative in some methadone injections might contribute to the QT prolongation.[1]

(b) Morphine

A report describes a 19-year-old woman who required increasing doses of intravenous morphine to control pain, reaching a peak of 275 mg/hour, which was maintained for 4 days. After palliative radiotherapy the rate was reduced to 100 to 150 mg/hour, but only partial pain relief was achieved; however the patient was somnolent, which was attributed to the chlorobutanol preservative content of the morphine injection (1 mg of chlorobutanol for every 3 mg of morphine). At doses of morphine 275 mg/hour, chlorobutanol intake was 90 mg/hour, which is in excess of the dose that has been used to aid sleep (150 mg); chlorobutanol accumulation might also have occurred as it has a long half-life.[2] This appears to be an isolated report, the general importance of which is unknown.

1. Kornick CA, Kilborn MJ, Santiago-Palma J, Schulman G, Thaler HT, Keefe DL, Katchman AN, Pezzullo JC, Ebert SN, Woosley RL, Payne R, Manfredi PL. QTc interval prolongation associated with intravenous methadone. *Pain* (2003) 105, 499–506.
2. DeChristoforo R, Corden BJ, Hood JC, Narang PK, Magrath IT. High-dose morphine infusion complicated by chlorobutanol-induced somnolence. *Ann Intern Med* (1983) 98, 335–6.

Opioids + Cobicistat

Cobicistat slightly increases buprenorphine and norbuprenorphine exposure, but does not affect methadone exposure. Naloxone exposure is slightly decreased by cobicistat. The pharmacokinetics of cobicistat are not affected by buprenorphine, naloxone, or methadone.

Clinical evidence

(a) Buprenorphine

In a study, 17 HIV-negative subjects, stable taking buprenorphine 16 to 24 mg daily with naloxone 4 to 6 mg daily, were given cobicistat 150 mg once daily (as a pharmacokinetic enhancer with elvitegravir 150 mg once daily) for 10 days. The AUC and maximum concentration of buprenorphine were increased by 35% and 11%, respectively, and the AUC and maximum concentration of norbuprenorphine were increased by 42% and 24%, respectively. No clinical consequences of these increased exposures were observed. The AUC and maximum concentration of naloxone were decreased by 21% and 34%, respectively. The pharmacokinetics of cobicistat were no different to historical controls.[1]

(b) Methadone

In a study in 11 HIV-negative subjects stable taking methadone 80 to 120 mg once daily, and given cobicistat 150 mg once daily (as a pharmacokinetic enhancer with elvitegravir 150 mg once daily) for 10 days, the AUC and maximum concentration of *R*- and *S*-methadone were unaltered, and the pharmacokinetics of cobicistat were no different to historical controls.[2]

Mechanism

Buprenorphine is a substrate of CYP3A4, which is inhibited by cobicistat, and hence concurrent use results in its increased exposure. Methadone is partially metabolised by CYP3A4, with involvement of a number of other cytochrome P450 isoenzymes, most of which do not appear to be affected by cobicistat, and hence overall there is no effect on methadone exposure. The reasons for the increase in norbuprenorphine exposure and decrease in naloxone exposure are not known.

Importance and management

A pharmacokinetic interaction between buprenorphine and cobicistat is established, but the increase in buprenorphine exposure was only slight and is therefore unlikely to be of clinical importance. No dose adjustments would seem necessary on concurrent use. No pharmacokinetic interaction occurs between cobicistat and methadone and no dose adjustments are necessary on their concurrent use.

1. Bruce RD, Winkle P, Custudio JM, Wei LX, Rhee MS, Kearney BP, Ramanathan S, Friedland GH. The pharmacokinetic and pharmacodynamic interactions between buprenorphine/naloxone and elvitegravir/cobicistat in subjects receiving chronic buprenorphine/naloxone treatment. *J Acquir Immune Defic Syndr* (2013) 63, 480–4.
2. Bruce RD, Winkle P, Custudio JM, Wei X, Rhee MS, Kearney BP, Ramanathan S, Friedland GH. Investigation of the interactions between methadone and elvitegravir-cobicistat in subjects receiving chronic methadone maintenance. *Antimicrob Agents Chemother* (2013) 57, 6154–7.

Opioids + Cocaine

A case of cocaine-related torsade de pointes occurred in a patient taking methadone. Some analyses have found that cocaine is associated with longer QTc intervals in methadone maintenance patients. Ventricular arrhythmias and increased cardiovascular effects have been reported when patients taking methadone were given cocaine. Cocaine appears to have negligible effects on methadone pharmacokinetics and appears to slightly reduce buprenorphine exposure. The cardiovascular effects of single-dose cocaine with maintenance buprenorphine or single-dose morphine appear to be similar to those seen with cocaine alone.

Clinical evidence

(a) Buprenorphine

In a study in opioid dependent patients, there was no difference in the cardiovascular or respiratory effect of a single intravenous dose of cocaine when given alone or with sublingual buprenorphine 4 or 8 mg daily for 21 days.[1]

In a retrospective analysis in patients on maintenance buprenorphine with naloxone, the AUC of buprenorphine was 34% lower in regular cocaine users than in patients who used cocaine intermittently or not at all.[2]

(b) Methadone

1. Cardiovascular effects. In a study, 155 methadone maintenance patients underwent ECG monitoring for QT prolongation. Use of cocaine or **amfetamines** (41 patients), was associated with longer QTc intervals, as was higher methadone dose.[3] In another similar study, recent cocaine use showed a statistically significant correlation with QTc prolongation in patients on methadone maintenance treatment.[4] However, in a third study in such patients, the presence of cocaine metabolites in urine was not associated with an increase in QTc interval.[5]

A 46-year-old woman, who had been taking methadone 80 mg daily for over one year, started abusing cocaine by inhalation and injection and subsequently developed frequent self-limiting episodes of syncope. These syncopal events consistently occurred within an hour of cocaine use. She was admitted to hospital after collapsing and becoming comatose, and was found to have torsade de pointes. She developed irreversible anoxic brain injury secondary to cardiac arrest. Although methadone can cause QT prolongation, her serum methadone concentration was well within the therapeutic range and it was felt that several factors might have contributed to the arrhythmias including cocaine abuse.[6] Another patient taking methadone was withdrawn from a study due to the occurrence of premature ventricular contractions for several minutes after a single 32-mg/70 kg intravenous dose of cocaine.[7] Furthermore, increased cardiovascular effects (e.g. increased diastolic pressure and heart rate) have been reported when cocaine is given to patients taking methadone.[7]

2. Pharmacokinetics. In a retrospective analysis in patients on maintenance methadone, the minimum methadone concentration was 21% lower in 16 regular cocaine users than in 23 patients who used cocaine intermittently or not at all. In addition, the AUC of methadone was 16% lower, a difference which was not statistically significant.[8] However, in a non-comparative study in patients taking methadone maintenance who chronically abused cocaine, methadone serum concentrations were found to be inadequate (less than 100 nanograms/mL), 24 hours after a single 100-mg dose in 48 of 67 patients tested.[9] However, since this study did not have a control group of methadone maintenance patients not using cocaine, the finding is difficult to interpret.

(c) Morphine

A study in 9 healthy subjects found that although the combination of single intravenous doses of morphine and cocaine produced clinically relevant cardiovascular and subjective effects, for the most part, the cardiovascular effects were similar to those produced by cocaine alone. Neither cocaine nor morphine altered the plasma concentrations of the other drug.[10] However, note that single-dose studies do not rule out interactions at steady-state if the mechanism is altered metabolism.

Mechanism

Both cocaine and methadone are considered to have effects on the QTc interval and both are potassium-channel blockers. The authors of one study suggested that the combination of these two drugs creates a potentially dangerous risk of torsade de pointes.[11] There is no known mechanism for a pharmacokinetic interaction between cocaine and methadone or buprenorphine.

Importance and management

Methadone (in doses greater than 100 mg) is associated with some risk of prolonging the QT interval and causing torsade de pointes, and concurrent use of cocaine might independently add to the risk. A pharmacokinetic interaction between cocaine and methadone is not established. The apparent differences in methadone pharmacokinetics in cocaine users in the one comparative study[9] are very small and not likely to be clinically important.

A single intravenous dose of cocaine had no adverse physiological interaction with **buprenorphine**. The clinical relevance of the apparent slight reduction in buprenorphine exposure with cocaine use is of uncertain clinical relevance and requires confirmation in a controlled study.

There does not appear to be any interaction between single doses of **morphine** and cocaine, but how this relates to longer term use is uncertain.

1. Teoh SK, Mendelson JH, Mello NK, Kuehnle J, Sintavanarong P, Rhoades EM. Acute interactions of buprenorphine with intravenous cocaine and morphine: an investigational new drug phase I safety evaluation. *J Clin Psychopharmacol* (1993) 13, 87–99.
2. McCance-Katz EF, Rainey PM, Moody DE. Effect of cocaine use on buprenorphine pharmacokinetics in humans. *Am J Addict* (2010) 19, 38–46.
3. Mayet S, Gossop M, Lintzeris N, Markides V, Strang J. Methadone maintenance, QTc and torsade de pointes: who needs an electrocardiogram and what is the prevalence of QTc prolongation? *Drug Alcohol Rev* (2011) 30, 388–96.
4. Fareed A, Vayalapalli S, Byrd-Sellers J, Casarella J, Drexler K, Amar R, Smith-Cox J, Lutchman TS. Onsite QTc interval screening for patients in methadone maintenance treatment. *J Addict Dis* (2010) 29, 15–22.
5. Roy AK, McCarthy C, Kiernan G, McGorrian C, Keenan E, Mahon NG, Sweeney B. Increased incidence of QT interval prolongation in a population receiving lower doses of methadone maintenance therapy. *Addiction* (2012) 107, 1132–9.
6. Krantz MJ, Rowan SB, Mehler PS. Cocaine-related torsade de pointes in a methadone maintenance patient. *J Addict Dis* (2005) 24, 53–60.
7. Foltin RW, Christiansen I, Levin FR, Fischman MW. Effects of single and multiple intravenous cocaine injections in humans maintained on methadone. *J Pharmacol Exp Ther* (1995) 275, 38–47.
8. McCance-Katz EF, Jatlow P, Rainey PM. Effect of cocaine use on methadone pharmacokinetics in humans. *Am J Addict* (2010) 19, 47–52.
9. Tennant F, Shannon J. Cocaine abuse in methadone maintenance patients is associated with low serum methadone concentrations. *J Addict Dis* (1995)14, 67–74.
10. Foltin RW, Fischman MW. The cardiovascular and subjective effects of intravenous cocaine and morphine combinations in humans. *J Pharmacol Exp Ther* (1992) 261, 623–32.
11. Krantz MJ, Baker WA, Schmittner J. Cocaine and methadone: parallel effects on the QTc interval. *Am J Cardiol* (2006) 98, 1121.

Opioids + Dextromethorphan

Dextromethorphan does not appear to alter the pharmacokinetics of morphine. Dextromethorphan might be a useful adjunct to opioid analgesia, postoperatively.

Clinical evidence, mechanism, importance and management

(a) Pharmacodynamic effects

Evidence for the use of dextromethorphan as an adjunct to opioids to reduce pain and opioid requirements is both extensive and conflicting, and detailed discussion is outside the scope of this monograph. However, a recent systematic review of 28 controlled studies found that there was a tendency for patients to report less pain than with placebo, and require less opioid analgesia postoperatively, but the consistency of these effects was varied, and the clinical importance was questionable. In addition there was a suggestion that the route of administration of the dextromethorphan might influence its effects.[1] The role of dextromethorphan as an opioid adjunct remains to be established.

(b) Pharmacokinetic effects

In a study in patients undergoing spinal surgery, the plasma concentrations of **morphine** and its glucuronide metabolites, were no different in the group receiving dextromethorphan before and after surgery (30 patients), than in another group of 30 patients receiving placebo before and after surgery.[2] This study suggests that dextromethorphan does not alter the pharmacokinetics of **morphine**.

For a report of dextromethorphan-induced delirium attributed to an interaction with methadone, see 'Dextromethorphan + Methadone', p.1566.

1. Duedahl TH, Rømsing J, Møiniche S, Dahl JB. A qualitative systematic review of peri-operative dextromethorphan in post-operative pain. *Acta Anaesthesiol Scand* (2006) 50, 1–13.
2. Suski M, Bujak-Gizycka B, Madej J, Kacka K, Dobrogowski J, Woron J, Olszanecki R, Korbut R. Co-administration of dextromethorphan and morphine: reduction of post-operative pain and lack of influence on morphine metabolism. *Basic Clin Pharmacol Toxicol* (2010) 107, 680–4.

Opioids + Food

Food can delay the absorption of dextropropoxyphene (propoxyphene), but the total amount absorbed might be slightly increased. Food slightly increases the morphine exposure of from an oral solution, but delays the absorption of some controlled-release preparations of morphine without appreciably affecting morphine exposure. Food can negligibly to slightly increase the AUC of immediate-release hydromorphone and oxycodone solution, but sustained-release preparations of hydromorphone, oxycodone, and tramadol do not appear to be affected by food. Tapentadol exposure is not affected by food.

Clinical evidence, mechanism, importance and management

(a) Dextropropoxyphene (Propoxyphene)

A study in healthy subjects given a single 130-mg dose of dextropropoxyphene (as capsules) found that while fasting, the maximum plasma concentrations of dextropropoxyphene were reached after about 2 hours. High-fat and high-carbohydrate meals delayed the time to maximum plasma concentration by about one hour, and high protein meals delayed the time to maximum plasma concentration by about 2 hours. Both the protein and carbohydrate meals caused a 25 to 30% increase in the total amount of dextropropoxyphene absorbed.[1] The delay in absorption probably occurs because food delays gastric emptying. Avoid food if rapid analgesic effects are needed.

(b) Hydromorphone

A crossover study in 24 healthy subjects found that food reduced the maximum plasma concentration of a single 8-mg dose of immediate-release hydromorphone and increased its AUC by 30%. However, these changes were not considered to be of clinical importance.[2]

A study in 24 healthy subjects found that food had no effect on the AUC of an extended-release once-daily hydromorphone capsule.[3] Similarly, two other studies in healthy subjects found that food had no effect on the AUC of hydromorphone from a 24-hour controlled-release preparation that utilised an *OROS* osmotic pump delivery system (*Exalgo* or *Jurnista*).[4,5]

(c) Morphine

Twelve patients with chronic pain were given oral morphine hydrochloride 50 mg in 200 mL of water either while fasting or after a high-fat breakfast (fried eggs and bacon, toast with butter, and milk). The maximum blood morphine concentration and the time to achieve this was not altered by the presence of the food, but the AUC was increased by 34% and blood morphine concentrations were maintained at higher levels over the period from 4 to 10 hours after the morphine had been given.[6] The reasons for this effect are not understood. However, this slight increase in morphine exposure is unlikely to be clinically relevant.

Some differences in pharmacokinetic parameters have also been reported between the fed and fasted states for controlled-release formulations of morphine, but these are not necessarily translated into measurable differences in the pharmacodynamic effects of pain relief and adverse effects.[7] The effects also appear to vary by preparation. Studies have found that, compared with the fasting state, food:

- slightly increases the AUC and maximum plasma concentration and delays the time to maximum concentration of morphine from *MST Continus*;[8]
- slightly increases the AUC and delays the time to maximum concentration with little effect on the maximum concentration of morphine from *Oramorph SR*;[8]
- has no effect on the extent (AUC), but reduces the rate (reduced maximum concentration and delayed time to maximum concentration) of morphine absorption from *Kapanol*,[9,10] and *Embeda*;[11]
- reduces the rate (maximum concentration and time to maximum concentration) and negligibly reduces the extent (AUC) of morphine absorption from *MXL* capsules;[10]
- does not affect the rate (maximum concentration) or extent (AUC) of morphine absorption from *MS Contin* (Purdue Frederick Company, USA).[12]

Most of these studies used single doses in healthy subjects and food was given in the form of a high-fat breakfast and, although it appears that there might be some delay in the absorption of some sustained-release preparations of morphine with food, the overall effect is unlikely to be clinically important.

Studies in *animals* suggest that ingestion of **sucrose** for a short duration might activate the endogenous opioid system and might modify morphine withdrawal.[13,14] Sucrose ingestion has also been shown to alleviate pain and distress in infants and adults.[13]

(d) Oxycodone

In a study in 22 healthy subjects given oxycodone as an immediate-release solution, the AUC was increased by 20% and the maximum plasma concentration was decreased by 18%, when compared with the fasted state.[15] A study in healthy subjects using a preparation containing oxycodone 5 mg and ibuprofen 400 mg found no change in the rate of absorption of oxycodone between the fasted state and after a high-fat breakfast, and only a 20% increase in the AUC in the fed state.[16] Yet another study using an immediate-release tablet reported a similar negligible 21% increase in oxycodone AUC.[17] However, there was no effect of food on the AUC of oxycodone given as a controlled-release tablet.[15] None of these changes are clinically important.

(e) Tapentadol

The UK and US manufacturers state that the AUC and maximum plasma concentration of tapentadol were increased by 25% and 16% respectively, after a high-fat, high-calorie breakfast. These changes were not considered to be clinically relevant and tapentadol may be given without regard to food.[18,19]

(f) Tramadol

In an open, crossover study in 24 healthy subjects, a formulation of tramadol sustained-release capsules were found to be bioequivalent with and without concurrent food intake (a high-fat breakfast).[20]

1. Musa MN, Lyons LL. Effect of food and liquid on the pharmacokinetics of propoxyphene. *Curr Ther Res* (1976) 19, 669–74.
2. Durnin C, Hind ID, Channon E, Yates DB, Cross M. Effect of food on the pharmacokinetics of oral immediate-release hydromorphone (Dilaudid® IR). *Proc West Pharmacol Soc* (2001) 44, 75–6.
3. Vashi V, Harris S, El-Tahtawy A, Wu D, Cipriano A. Clinical pharmacology and pharmacokinetics of once-daily hydromorphone hydrochloride extended-release capsules. *J Clin Pharmacol* (2005) 45, 547–54.
4. Sathyan G, Xu E, Thipphawong J, Gupta SK. Pharmacokinetic profile of a 24-hour controlled-release OROS® formulation of hydromorphone in the presence and absence of food. *BMC Clin Pharmacol* (2007) 7, 2.
5. Moore KT, St-Fleur D, Marricco NC, Ariyawansa J, Pagé V, Natarajan J, Morelli G, Richarz U. A randomized study of the effects of food on the pharmacokinetics of once-daily extended-release hydromorphone in healthy volunteers. *J Clin Pharmacol* (2011) 51, 1571–9.
6. Gourlay GK, Plummer JL, Cherry DA, Foate JA, Cousins MJ. Influence of a high-fat meal on the absorption of morphine from oral solutions. *Clin Pharmacol Ther* (1989) 46, 463–8.
7. Gourlay GK. Sustained relief of chronic pain. Pharmacokinetics of sustained release morphine. *Clin Pharmacokinet* (1998) 35, 173–90.
8. Drake J, Kirkpatrick CT, Aliyar CA, Crawford FE, Gibson P, Horth CE. Effect of food on the comparative pharmacokinetics of modified-release morphine tablet formulations: Oramorph SR and MST Continus. *Br J Clin Pharmacol* (1996) 41, 417–20.
9. Kaiko RF. The effect of food intake on the pharmacokinetics of sustained-release morphine sulfate capsules. *Clin Ther* (1997) 19, 296–303.
10. Broomhead A, West R, Eglinton L, Jones M, Bubner R, Sienko D, Knox K. Comparative single-dose pharmacokinetics of sustained-release and modified-release morphine sulfate capsules under fed and fasting conditions. *Clin Drug Invest* (1997) 13, 162–70.
11. Johnson F, Ciric S, Boudriau S, Swearingen D, Stauffer J. Food effects on the pharmacokinetics of morphine sulfate and naltrexone hydrochloride extended release capsules. *Adv Therapy* (2010) 27, 846–58.
12. Kaiko RF, Lazarus H, Cronin C, Grandy R, Thomas G, Goldenheim P. Controlled-release morphine bioavailability (MS Contin® tablets) in the presence and absence of food. *Hosp J* (1990) 6, 17–30.
13. Bhattacharjee M, Mathur R. Antinociceptive effect of sucrose ingestion in the human. *Indian J Physiol Pharmacol* (2005) 49, 383–94.
14. Jain R, Mukherjee K, Singh R. Influence of sweet tasting solutions on opioid withdrawal. *Brain Res Bull* (2004) 64, 319–22.
15. Benziger DP, Kaiko RF, Miotto JB, Fitzmartin RD, Reder RF, Chasin M. Differential effects of food on the bioavailability of controlled-release oxycodone tablets and immediate-release oxycodone solution. *J Pharm Sci* (1996) 85, 407–10.
16. Kapil R, Nolting A, Roy P, Fiske W, Benedek I, Abramowitz W. Pharmacokinetic properties of combination oxycodone plus racemic ibuprofen: two randomized, open-label, crossover studies in healthy adult volunteers. *Clin Ther* (2004) 26, 2015–25.
17. Bass A, Stark JG, Pixton GC, Sommerville KW, Zamora CA, Leibowitz M, Rolleri R. Dose proportionality and the effects of food on bioavailability of an immediate-release oxycodone hydrochloride tablet designed to discourage tampering and its relative bioavailability compared with a marketed oxycodone tablet under fed conditions: a single-dose, randomized, open-label, 5-way crossover study in healthy volunteers. *Clin Ther* (2012) 34, 1601–12.
18. Palexia (Tapentadol hydrochloride). Grünenthal Ltd. UK Summary of product characteristics, July 2014.
19. Nucynta (Tapentadol). PriCara. US Prescribing information, July 2013.
20. Raber M, Schulz H-U, Schürer M, Bias-Imhoff U, Momberger H. Pharmacokinetic properties of tramadol sustained release capsules. 2nd communication: investigation of relative bioavailability and food interaction. *Arzneimittelforschung* (1999) 49, 588–93.

Opioids + Gabapentin and Pregabalin

Morphine slightly increases gabapentin exposure, whereas hydrocodone had a negligible effect. Gabapentin had no effect on morphine exposure and slightly decreased hydrocodone exposure. However, gabapentin enhanced the analgesic effects of morphine. The impairment of cognitive and gross motor function caused by oxycodone appears to be additive with pregabalin, but there was no pharmacokinetic interaction.

Clinical evidence

(a) Gabapentin

1. Hydrocodone. In a study mentioned by the US manufacturer,[1] low-dose gabapentin 500 mg decreased the AUC of hydrocodone by 22%, whereas a very low dose of gabapentin of 125 mg had little effect (4% decrease). The hydrocodone increased the AUC of gabapentin by 14%. It is unclear if this study was single-dose, and the effects of higher therapeutic doses of gabapentin were not assessed.

2. Morphine. A single-dose, placebo-controlled study in 12 healthy subjects given controlled-release morphine 60 mg found that gabapentin 600 mg, given after an interval of 2 hours, had no effect on the pharmacokinetics of morphine, morphine-3- and morphine-6-glucuronides. In the presence of morphine the gabapentin AUC increased by 44% and its oral clearance and apparent renal clearance decreased by 23% and 16%, respectively. The analgesic effect of morphine and gabapentin was evaluated by changes in the area under the curve of pain tolerance. Gabapentin with placebo had no appreciable analgesic effect, but an increase in the pain threshold and pain tolerance was found when gabapentin was given with morphine, when compared with placebo. The adverse effect profiles were similar for both the gabapentin with morphine and the morphine with placebo groups.[2]

(b) Pregabalin

The UK and US manufacturers of pregabalin briefly note that there was no clinically relevant pharmacokinetic interaction between pregabalin and **oxycodone**, and that there was no clinically important effect on respiration. However, pregabalin appeared to cause an additive impairment in cognitive and gross motor function when given with **oxycodone**.[3,4]

Mechanism

Uncertain. The absorption of gabapentin might be increased by reduced intestinal motility caused by morphine. The increased morphine analgesia was thought to be due to a pharmacodynamic effect, as morphine pharmacokinetics were not changed.[2]

Importance and management

The negligible to slight pharmacokinetic interaction seen between hydrocodone and gabapentin is unlikely to be clinically relevant. Similarly, the slight increase in gabapentin exposure seen in the study with morphine is unlikely to require a gabapentin dose adjustment or to be clinically relevant. However, note that the UK and US manufacturers of gabapentin warn that patients should be carefully observed for signs of CNS depression such as somnolence, and the dose of gabapentin or **morphine** should be reduced appropriately.[1,5] Similarly be aware that concurrent use of pregabalin and **oxycodone** and other opioids might result in increased CNS depression. Reviews of clinical studies have reported that gabapentin[6-8] and pregabalin[9] used in conjunction with opioids probably have an analgesic and opioid-sparing effect in acute postoperative pain management[6,7,9] and neuropathic pain.[8]

1. Neurotonin (Gabapentin). Pfizer, Inc. US Prescribing information, July 2012.
2. Eckhardt K, Ammon S, Hofmann U, Riebe A, Gugeler N, Mikus G. Gabapentin enhances the analgesic effect of morphine in healthy volunteers. *Anesth Analg* (2000) 91, 185–91.
3. Lyrica (Pregabalin). Pfizer Ltd. UK Summary of product characteristics, April 2013.
4. Lyrica (Pregabalin). Pfizer, Inc. US Prescribing information, June 2012.

5. Neurontin (Gabapentin). Pfizer Ltd. UK Summary of product characteristics, April 2012.
6. Ho K-Y, Gan TJ, Habib AS. Gabapentin and postoperative pain–a systematic review of randomised controlled trials. *Pain* (2006) 126, 91–101.
7. Turan A, White PF, Karamanlioğlu B, Memis D, Taşdoğan M, Pamukçu Z, Yavuz E. Gabapentin: an alternative to the cyclooxygenase-2 inhibitors for perioperative pain management. *Anesth Analg* (2006) 102, 175–81.
8. Vadalouca A, Siafaka I, Argyra E, Vrachnou E, Moka E. Therapeutic management of chronic neuropathic pain: an examination of pharmacologic treatment. *Ann N Y Acad Sci* (2006) 1088, 164–86.
9. Zhang J, Ho KY, Wang Y. Efficacy of pregabalin in acute postoperative pain: a meta-analysis. *Br J Anaesth* (2011) 106, 454–62.

Opioids + Grapefruit juice

Grapefruit juice slightly increases the exposure to oral oxycodone and negligibly increases oral methadone exposure. Oral alfentanil exposure is slightly to moderately increased by grapefruit juice, but grapefruit juice does not affect intravenous alfentanil exposure or transmucosal fentanyl exposure.

Clinical evidence

(a) Alfentanil

A study in 10 healthy subjects found that grapefruit juice given at bedtime and then in the morning had no effect on the pharmacokinetics of a single *intravenous* dose of alfentanil given one hour after the grapefruit juice was taken in the morning.[1] However, using the same study design, the clearance of *oral* alfentanil was reduced by about 40%, and its maximum plasma concentration and AUC were increased by about 40% and 60%, respectively.[1] In another similar study by the same research group, the AUC of *intravenous* alfentanil was unaffected by grapefruit juice, whereas that of *oral* alfentanil was increased by 70% to 2-fold.[2]

(b) Fentanyl

In a study in 12 healthy subjects, grapefruit juice given at bedtime and then in the morning had no effect on the AUC of a single oral transmucosal fentanyl lozenge given one hour after the grapefruit juice in the morning, despite about 75% of the dose being swallowed and absorbed enterally.[3]

(c) Methadone

A study in 8 patients taking methadone found that 200 mL of grapefruit juice given 30 minutes before, and also with, their daily dose of methadone for 5 days was associated with a 17% increase in methadone AUC.[4] A further study in healthy subjects found that grapefruit juice caused a 19% increase in methadone AUC following oral methadone, but had no effect on intravenous methadone AUC.[5]

(d) Oxycodone

In a randomised, crossover study, 12 healthy subjects (10 of whom were CYP2D6 extensive metabolisers, that is they had normal isoenzyme activity), were given 200 mL of grapefruit juice three times daily for 5 days with a single 10-mg oral dose of oxycodone on day 4. Grapefruit juice increased the AUC of oxycodone by 67% and increased its maximum plasma concentration by 48%. The maximum plasma concentration of the metabolite noroxycodone was decreased by 24%, but its AUC was unchanged. Both the AUC and maximum concentration of the metabolite oxymorphone were increased, by 47% and 22%, respectively. No difference in analgesic effect was seen, but there was an increase in self-reported performance impairment with grapefruit juice.[6]

Mechanism

Grapefruit juice is a weak inhibitor of CYP3A4, of which alfentanil is a sensitive substrate. Oral alfentanil is affected to a greater extent than intravenous alfentanil because of inhibition of intestinal CYP3A by grapefruit juice.[1] Fentanyl would not be expected to be affected to the same extent because it is a high hepatic extraction drug. Oxycodone is principally metabolised to noroxycodone by CYP3A4, and to a lesser extent, to oxymorphone by CYP2D6. As grapefruit juice inhibits CYP3A4 it would be expected to reduce oxycodone metabolism.

Importance and management

Grapefruit juice has no effect on intravenous **alfentanil** exposure, therefore no precautions are necessary. The exposure to oral alfentanil was slightly to moderately increased; however, since alfentanil is not used orally in clinical practice, this information is of academic interest only. The studies using oral administration were conducted to assess the suitability of alfentanil for use as a probe substrate for CYP3A4 in pharmacokinetic studies.

Grapefruit juice had no effect on **fentanyl** exposure from a lozenge. However, the UK and US manufacturers of fentanyl products for oral mucosal administration suggest that grapefruit juice might increase fentanyl concentrations and therefore either advise caution or avoiding concurrent use.[7-10] This seems overly cautious. Note that intravenous and transdermal fentanyl are unlikely to be affected since they bypass intestinal CYP3A4.

The negligible increase in **methadone** exposure is not clinically relevant. On the basis of this evidence dose adjustments of methadone seem unlikely to be necessary in the presence of grapefruit juice.

On the basis of the slight increase in **oxycodone** exposure, it would not seem necessary to adjust the oxycodone dose in patients who drink grapefruit juice, but be alert for the possibility of increased effects and if these become troublesome, consider advising the avoidance of grapefruit juice.

1. Kharasch ED, Walker A, Hoffer C, Sheffels P. Intravenous and oral alfentanil as in vivo probes for hepatic and first-pass cytochrome P450 3A activity: noninvasive assessment by use of papillary miosis. *Clin Pharmacol Ther* (2004) 76, 452–66..
2. Kharasch ED, Vangveravong S, Buck N, London A, Kim T, Blood J, Mach RH. Concurrent assessment of hepatic and intestinal cytochrome P450 3A activities using deuterated alfentanil. *Clin Pharmacol Ther* (2011) 89, 562–70.
3. Kharasch ED, Whittington D, Hoffer C. Influence of hepatic and intestinal cytochrome P4503A activity on the acute disposition and effects of oral transmucosal fentanyl citrate. *Anesthesiology* (2004) 101, 729–37.
4. Benmebarek M, Devaud C, Gex-Fabry M, Powell Golay K, Brogli C, Baumann P, Gravier B, Eap CB. Effects of grapefruit juice on the pharmacokinetics of the enantiomers of methadone. *Clin Pharmacol Ther* (2004) 76, 55–63.
5. Kharasch ED, Hoffer C, Whittington D, Sheffels P. Role of hepatic and intestinal cytochrome P450 3A and 2B6 in the metabolism, disposition, and miotic effects of methadone. *Clin Pharmacol Ther* (2004) 76, 250–69.
6. Nieminen TH, Hagelberg NM, Saari TI, Neuvonen M, Neuvonen PJ, Laine K, Olkkola KT. Grapefruit juice enhances the exposure to oral oxycodone. *Basic Clin Pharmacol Toxicol* (2010) 107, 782–8.
7. Actiq (Fentanyl citrate lozenge). Teva Pharmaceuticals Ltd. UK Summary of product characteristics, June 2015.
8. Actiq (Fentanyl citrate lozenge). Cephalon, Inc. US Prescribing information, December 2011.
9. Effentora (Fentanyl citrate buccal tablet). Teva Pharmaceuticals Ltd. UK Summary of product characteristics, February 2015.
10. Fentora (Fentanyl citrate buccal tablet). Cephalon, Inc. US Prescribing information, December 2011.

Opioids + H_2-receptor antagonists

No pharmacokinetic interaction appears to occur between cimetidine and butorphanol (intranasal), hydromorphone, morphine, pethidine (meperidine) or tramadol; between famotidine and hydromorphone; or between ranitidine and hydromorphone, morphine or pethidine (meperidine). However, reports describe adverse reactions in patients taking cimetidine with methadone, morphine, mixed opium alkaloids, or pethidine, and in patients taking ranitidine with morphine.

Clinical evidence

(a) Butorphanol

In a study in 16 healthy subjects given intranasal butorphanol 1 mg every 6 hours and oral **cimetidine** 300 mg every 6 hours alone and then concurrently for 4 days, there was no change in the pharmacokinetics of butorphanol. The only change in the pharmacokinetics of cimetidine was a small increase in the elimination half-life of **cimetidine**, but note that there was no increase in cimetidine AUC.[1]

(b) Hydromorphone

When it was available, one US manufacturer of hydromorphone stated that the concurrent use of H_2-receptor antagonists (**cimetidine, famotidine, ranitidine**) had no significant effect on hydromorphone steady-state pharmacokinetics.[2]

(c) Fentanyl and related drugs

For the interactions of alfentanil and fentanyl with H_2-receptor antagonists, see 'Opioids; Fentanyl and related drugs + H_2-receptor antagonists', p.177.

(d) Methadone

An *in vitro* study briefly mentions an elderly patient receiving methadone 25 mg daily who developed apnoea 2 days after starting **cimetidine** 1.2 g daily.[3] Another elderly patient taking oral methadone 5 mg every 8 hours and subcutaneous **morphine** 8 mg every 3 hours also developed apnoea (respiratory rate of 2 breaths per minute) after receiving intravenous **cimetidine** 300 mg every 6 hours for 6 days. This was controlled with naloxone. It is unclear why the patient developed adverse effects on this occasion as no adverse effects occurred on the previous use of these drugs.[4]

(e) Morphine

1. Cimetidine. In a placebo-controlled study in 118 patients undergoing major abdominal surgery and given analgesia with morphine, preoperative or postoperative intravenous cimetidine 4 mg/kg did not affect postoperative pain intensity, sedation score, cumulative morphine consumption, or the incidence of adverse effects.[5] In a study in 7 healthy subjects, cimetidine 300 mg four times daily for 4 days had no effect on the pharmacokinetics of a single 10-mg dose of intravenous morphine. The extent and duration of the morphine-induced pupillary miosis were also unchanged.[6] In other healthy subjects, cimetidine 600 mg, given one hour before a 10-mg dose of intramuscular morphine prolonged the respiratory depression due to morphine, but the extent was small and not considered to be clinically relevant.[7]

In contrast, an acutely ill patient with grand mal epilepsy, gastrointestinal bleeding and an intertrochanteric fracture, who was undergoing haemodialysis three times a week, was taking cimetidine 300 mg three times daily. After being given the sixth dose of intramuscular morphine (15 mg every 4 hours) he became apnoeic (three breaths per minute), which was managed with naloxone. He remained confused and agitated for the next 80 hours with muscular twitching and further periods of apnoea controlled with naloxone. He had received nine 10-mg intramuscular doses of morphine on a previous occasion in the absence of cimetidine without problems. About a month later he experienced the same adverse reactions when given opium alkaloids while still taking cimetidine (see below).[8] Apnoea has also been reported in a patient receiving morphine, methadone and cimetidine, see under *Methadone*, above.

2. Ranitidine. A study in 8 healthy subjects taking ranitidine 150 mg twice daily for 7 doses followed by a single 10-mg dose of oral morphine mixture suggested that ranitidine might slightly increase the bioavailability of morphine, although the increase was not statistically significant.[9] A man with terminal cancer receiving intravenous ranitidine 150 mg every 8 hours became confused, disorientated, and agitated when given ranitidine after an intravenous infusion of morphine 50 mg daily was started. When the ranitidine was stopped his mental state improved, but it worsened when he was given ranitidine again 8 hours and 16 hours later. He again improved when the ranitidine was stopped.[10] In another case, severe symptoms of morphine overdose requiring prolonged naltrexone infusion occurred in an elderly man with metastatic lung cancer when he was hospitalised for daily dose titration of oral morphine and also given amitriptyline and ranitidine. The authors attributed the effect, in part, to an interaction with amitriptyline and, secondarily, with ranitidine.[11] Similarly, another report describes hallucinations in a patient receiving ranitidine and sustained-release morphine followed by rectal **methadone**, but the author discounted the possibility of an interaction.[12]

(f) Opium alkaloids, mixed

A patient taking **cimetidine** 150 mg twice daily developed apnoea, confusion, and muscle twitching after receiving 7 doses of intramuscular *Pantopon* (hydrochlorides of mixed opium alkaloids) postoperatively. He required 4 doses of naloxone over the next 24 hours.[8]

(g) Pethidine (Meperidine)

In a study in 8 healthy subjects, **cimetidine** 600 mg twice daily for one week reduced the total body clearance of a single 70-mg intravenous dose of pethidine by 22%.[13] In a similar study by the same research group, **ranitidine** 150 mg twice daily had no effect on pethidine pharmacokinetics.[14] In a review of 6 cases of pethidine-induced delirium, concurrent cimetidine was considered to be a risk factor.[15]

(h) Tramadol

In an unpublished study in healthy subjects on file with the manufacturers, **cimetidine** increased the AUC of tramadol by 15 to 27% and decreased the total body clearance by 14 to 22%.[16]

Mechanism

Cimetidine inhibits the activity of liver enzymes concerned with the *N*-demethylation of methadone[3] and the oxidation of pethidine (meperidine),[13,14] reducing their metabolism, so they could accumulate in the body, thereby exaggerating their respiratory depressant effects. However, cimetidine is a weak inhibitor at best, so any effects are likely to be minimal. A reduction in liver function might possibly have contributed towards, or even been largely responsible for the cases with methadone, because both patients were elderly. In addition to an interaction via CYP3A4 inhibition, the manufacturers of methadone also suggest that H_2-receptor antagonists, such as cimetidine, can reduce the protein binding of methadone resulting in increased opiate action,[17,18] but altered protein binding does not usually result in clinically important drug interactions, see 'Protein binding interactions', p.3.

The isolated case reports of possible interactions between morphine and H_2-receptor antagonists remain unexplained,[8,10] but both patients were seriously ill. *In vitro* studies have reported that the conjugation of morphine does not appear to be affected by cimetidine or ranitidine.[19]

Importance and management

The evidence generally suggests that **morphine** does not interact with cimetidine: those cases describing an interaction involved seriously ill patients. Concurrent use normally causes only a slight, and normally unimportant, prolongation of the respiratory depression due to morphine, but it might possibly have some importance in patients with pre-existing respiratory disorders. Several manufacturers note that cimetidine may inhibit the metabolism of morphine, although they do not give any specific advice regarding the management of this interaction. Some US manufacturers warn that, because of the isolated report (see under *Morphine*, above), patients should be monitored for increased respiratory and CNS depression.[20-22] However, it should be noted that this patient was undergoing haemodialysis, and probably does not reflect the effects of this interaction in the general population. In contrast, one of the UK manufacturers gives no mention of a possible interaction with cimetidine.[23]

In-vitro evidence suggests that ranitidine is unlikely to interact with morphine,[8] although the one pharmacokinetic study was inconclusive as to whether ranitidine might increase morphine concentrations.[9] Again, the case reports are probably not of general relevance given the widespread use of both of these drugs.

Information about the interaction between **pethidine (meperidine)** and cimetidine is limited. A minor pharmacokinetic interaction appears to occur, but is probably unlikely to be clinically relevant. Nevertheless, some manufacturers advise caution on concurrent use because of the pharmacokinetic interaction.[24] Ranitidine has been shown not to affect the pharmacokinetics of pethidine.

It also seems doubtful whether the theoretical pharmacokinetic interaction between **methadone** and cimetidine is of general importance, when the two reports cited here are viewed against the background of the widespread use of both drugs over many years and the lack of other published adverse reports.

The UK manufacturer of **oxycodone** suggests that cimetidine might inhibit its metabolism.[25] However, cimetidine is only a weak inhibitor of CYP3A4 and CYP2D6, by which oxycodone is partially metabolised, therefore any effects would be expected to be minimal.

No clinically relevant pharmacokinetic interaction appears to occur between intranasal **butorphanol** and oral cimetidine, or between **hydromorphone** and the H_2-receptor antagonists. Similarly, the minor changes in **tramadol** pharmacokinetics caused by cimetidine are unlikely to be of clinical relevance.

1. Shyu WC, Barbhaiya RH. Lack of pharmacokinetic interaction between butorphanol nasal spray and cimetidine. *Br J Clin Pharmacol* (1996) 42, 513–17.
2. Palladone (Hydromorphone hydrochloride). Purdue Pharma L.P. US Prescribing information, November 2004.
3. Dawson GW, Vestal RE. Cimetidine inhibits the *in vitro* N-demethylation of methadone. *Res Commun Chem Pathol Pharmacol* (1984) 46, 301–4.
4. Sorkin EM, Ogawa GS. Cimetidine potentiation of narcotic action. *Drug Intell Clin Pharm* (1983) 17, 60–1.
5. Chia Y-Y, Chiang H-L, Liu K, Ko N-H. Randomized, double-blind study comparing postoperative effects of treatment timing with histamine H_2-receptor antagonist cimetidine. *Acta Anaesthesiol Scand* (2005) 49, 865–9.
6. Mojaverian P, Fedder IL, Vlasses PH, Rotmensch HH, Rocci ML, Swanson BN, Ferguson RK. Cimetidine does not alter morphine disposition in man. *Br J Clin Pharmacol* (1982) 14, 809–13.
7. Lam AM, Clement JL. Effect of cimetidine premedication on morphine-induced ventilatory depression. *Can Anaesth Soc J* (1984) 31, 36–43.
8. Fine A, Churchill DN. Potentially lethal interaction of cimetidine and morphine. *Can Med Assoc J* (1981) 124, 1434–6.
9. Aasmundstad TA, Størset P. Influence of ranitidine on the morphine-3-glucuronide to morphine-6-glucuronide ratio after oral administration of morphine in humans. *Hum Exp Toxicol* (1998) 17, 347–52.
10. Martinez-Abad M, Delgado Gomis F, Ferrer JM, Morales-Olivas FJ. Ranitidine-induced confusion with concomitant morphine. *Drug Intell Clin Pharm* (1988) 22, 914–15.
11. Upadhyay S, Jain R, Chauhan H, Gupta D, Mishra S, Bhatnagar S. Oral morphine overdose in a cancer patient antagonized by prolonged naloxone infusion. *Am J Hosp Palliat Care* (2008) 25, 401–5.
12. Jellema JG. Hallucination during sustained-release morphine and methadone administration. *Lancet* (1987) ii, 392.
13. Guay DRP, Meatherall RC, Chalmers JL, Grahame GR. Cimetidine alters pethidine disposition in man. *Br J Clin Pharmacol* (1984) 18, 907–14.
14. Guay DRP, Meatherall RC, Chalmers JL, Grahame GR, Hudson RJ. Ranitidine does not alter pethidine disposition in man. *Br J Clin Pharmacol* (1985) 20, 55–9.
15. Eisendrath SJ, Goldman B, Douglas J, Dimatteo L, Van Dyke C. Meperidine-induced delirium. *Am J Psychiatry* (1987) 144, 1062–5.
16. Raffa RB, Nayak RK, Liao S, Minn FL. The mechanism(s) of action and pharmacokinetics of tramadol hydrochloride. *Rev Contemp Pharmacother* (1995) 6, 485–97.
17. Methadose (Methadone hydrochloride). Rosemont Pharmaceuticals Ltd. UK Summary of product characteristics, April 2012.
18. Methadone Solution for Injection (Methadone hydrochloride). Martindale Pharmaceuticals Ltd. UK Summary of product characteristics, December 2010.
19. Knodell RG, Holtzman JL, Crankshaw DL, Steele NM, Stanley LN. Drug metabolism by rat and human hepatic microsomes in response to interaction with H_2-receptor antagonists. *Gastroenterology* (1982) 82, 84–8.
20. Avinza (Morphine sulfate extended-release capsules). King Pharmaceuticals, Inc. US Prescribing information, April 2014.
21. MS Contin (Morphine sulfate). Purdue Pharma L.P. US Prescribing information, June 2014.
22. Kadian (morphine sulfate). Actavis Pharma Inc. US Prescribing information, August 2014.
23. Zomorph (Morphine sulphate). Archimedes Pharma UK Ltd. UK Summary of product characteristics, October 2011.
24. Demerol (Meperidine hydrochloride). Sanofi-Aventis US LLC. US Prescribing information, July 2014.
25. OxyContin (Oxycodone hydrochloride). Napp Pharmaceuticals Ltd. UK Summary of product characteristics, May 2011.

Opioids; Fentanyl and related drugs + H_2-receptor antagonists

Cimetidine, but not ranitidine, increases the plasma concentrations of alfentanil. Some preliminary observations suggest that the effects of fentanyl might be increased by cimetidine.

Clinical evidence, mechanism, importance and management

(a) Alfentanil

In a pharmacokinetic study in 19 intensive care patients, intravenous **cimetidine** 1.2 g daily for 2 days was given with a single 125-microgram/kg intravenous dose of alfentanil. When compared with either an aluminium/magnesium hydroxide antacid or intravenous **ranitidine** 300 mg daily, **cimetidine** increased the alfentanil half-life by 75% and 61%, respectively, and reduced the clearance by 64% and 54%, respectively. The alfentanil plasma concentrations were notably increased by the **cimetidine**, probably because **cimetidine** inhibits the metabolism of the alfentanil.[1] Whether the effects of alfentanil are increased to a clinically important extent awaits assessment. However, be alert for increased alfentanil effects because pharmacokinetic changes of this size are known to be clinically important in some patients (see 'Opioids; Fentanyl and related drugs + Macrolides', p.187, and 'Opioids; Fentanyl and related drugs + Azoles', p.166). The UK manufacturer of alfentanil warns that alfentanil is metabolised mainly by CYP3A4, and therefore inhibitors of this isoenzyme, including **cimetidine**, could increase the risk of prolonged or delayed respiratory depression. The concurrent use of such drugs requires special patient care and observation; it may be necessary to lower the dose of alfentanil.[2] **Ranitidine** does not appear to interact.[1]

(b) Fentanyl

The terminal half-life of fentanyl 100 micrograms/kg was reported to be more than doubled, from 155 minutes to 340 minutes, by pretreatment with **cimetidine** (10 mg/kg the night before and 5 mg/kg 90 minutes before the fentanyl dose). This increase in half-life probably occurs because **cimetidine** inhibits the metabolism of fentanyl by the liver, thereby delaying its clearance from the body.[3] The clinical importance of this interaction has not been assessed, but if both drugs are used concurrently, be alert for increased and prolonged fentanyl effects.

1. Kienlen J, Levron J-C, Aubas S, Roustan J-P, du Cailar J. Pharmacokinetics of alfentanil in patients treated with either cimetidine or ranitidine. *Drug Invest* (1993) 6, 257–62.
2. Rapifen Solution for Injection or Infusion (Alfentanil hydrochloride). Janssen-Cilag Ltd. UK Summary of product characteristics, April 2013.
3. Maurer PM, Barkowski RR. Drug interactions of clinical significance with opioid analgesics. *Drug Safety* (1993) 8, 30–48.

Opioids + Haloperidol

A patient taking long-term haloperidol and morphine experienced extrapyramidal symptoms when naloxone was given. Haloperidol decreased

the dose requirements of sufentanil for sedation in one study. The use of haloperidol and methadone might increase the risk of torsade de pointes.

Clinical evidence, mechanism, importance and management

(a) Morphine

An 18-year-old woman with nasopharyngeal carcinoma who had been receiving long-term haloperidol and morphine developed profound extrapyramidal adverse effects during an attempt to reverse an intrathecal morphine overdose with naloxone. It was suggested that the long-term use of morphine might suppress haloperidol-induced extrapyramidal symptoms through its antimuscarinic and dopaminergic effects. Abrupt opioid withdrawal could be potentially hazardous in patients who are also taking haloperidol.[1]

See also 'Opioids; Morphine + Miscellaneous', p.201, for limited evidence that haloperidol may increase the risk of myoclonus with morphine.

(b) Methadone

Note that both methadone and haloperidol are associated with an increased risk of QT prolongation when used alone, an effect which might be additive if used together, and increase the risk of torsade de pointes. See 'Drugs that prolong the QT interval + Other drugs that prolong the QT interval', p.272 for further information on the concurrent use of two or more drugs that prolong the QT interval.

(c) Sufentanil

A study involving 30 patients in an intensive care unit investigated the effects of adding haloperidol 3 mg/hour to a sufentanil infusion. The study found that haloperidol decreased the dose requirements of sufentanil when compared with sufentanil infusion alone. No differences in adverse effects were reported between the two groups.[2]

1. Guo S-L, Lin C-J, Huang H-H, Chen L-K, Sun W-Z. Reversal of morphine with naloxone precipitates haloperidol-induced extrapyramidal side effects. *J Pain Symptom Manage* (2006) 31, 391–2.
2. Tukenmez B, Memis D, Pamukcu Z. The addition of haloperidol, propofol, or midazolam to sufentanil for intravenous sedation in the intensive care unit using bispectral index. *J Opioid Manag* (2008) 4, 34–40.

Opioids + HCV-protease inhibitors

Telaprevir and boceprevir negligibly to slightly reduce the exposure to methadone, and do not appear to notably affect the pharmacokinetics of buprenorphine or naloxone. Simeprevir and paritaprevir appear not to affect the pharmacokinetics of methadone. Paritaprevir might slightly increase exposure to buprenorphine, but appears to have no effect on the pharmacokinetics of naloxone. Simeprevir is predicted to interact similarly. Telaprevir is predicted to increase the effects of fentanyl and alfentanil. The pharmacokinetics of boceprevir and paritaprevir boosted with ritonavir (in a fixed-dose combination) do not appear to be altered by methadone or buprenorphine with naloxone. Similarly, the pharmacokinetics of telaprevir do not appear to be altered by methadone to a clinically relevant extent.

Clinical evidence

(a) Buprenorphine

1. Boceprevir. The UK and US manufacturers briefly report that, in a study in subjects taking buprenorphine 8 to 24 mg daily with naloxone 2 to 6 mg daily, and given boceprevir 800 mg three times daily for 6 days, the plasma concentrations of both buprenorphine and naloxone were very slightly increased.[1,2] The US manufacturer also reports that the maximum concentration of boceprevir was decreased by 18%, but there was no effect on the AUC or minimum concentration.[1]

2. Paritaprevir. The UK and US manufacturers briefly report that, in a study in 10 subjects taking buprenorphine 4 to 24 mg daily and naloxone 1 to 6 mg daily, and given paritaprevir 150 mg daily (in a fixed-dose combination with ombitasvir and ritonavir, and given with dasabuvir), the dose-normalised AUC and maximum concentration of buprenorphine were increased around 2-fold and 2.2-fold, respectively. The dose-normalised AUC and maximum concentration of norbuprenorphine (the active metabolite of buprenorphine) were increased by 84% and 2-fold, respectively.[3,4] The pharmacokinetics of naloxone were unaffected,[3,4] and neither were the pharmacokinetics of paritaprevir according to a cross-study comparison.[3] Furthermore, the UK manufacturer also reports that similar changes were seen when the combination was given without dasabuvir.[3]

3. Telaprevir. In a study in 13 subjects stable on buprenorphine with naloxone, telaprevir 750 mg three times daily for 7 days decreased the maximum plasma concentration of buprenorphine by 20%, but had no effect on the AUC or minimum plasma concentration. The pharmacokinetics of its metabolite, norbuprenorphine, and of naloxone were not affected. Three subjects had mild withdrawal symptoms, one of whom had their buprenorphine dose adjusted, but this subject's pharmacokinetic data were not included in the results. No subject had moderate or severe signs or symptoms of opioid withdrawal.[5]

(b) Methadone

1. Boceprevir. The UK and US manufacturers briefly report that, in a study in subjects taking methadone 20 to 150 mg daily and given boceprevir 800 mg three times daily for 6 days, the AUC of *R*-methadone was decreased by 15%, but the maximum and minimum concentrations were unaffected. The minimum concentration and AUC of *S*-methadone were decreased by 26% and 22%, respectively, but the maximum concentration was unaffected.[1,2] The US manufacturer also reports that the maximum concentration and AUC of boceprevir were decreased by 38% and 20%, respectively, but the minimum concentration was not affected.[1]

2. Paritaprevir. The UK manufacturer briefly reports that, in a study in subjects taking methadone 20 to 120 mg daily and given paritaprevir 150 mg daily (in a fixed-dose combination with ombitasvir and ritonavir, and given with and without dasabuvir), the dose-normalised pharmacokinetics of *R*- and *S*-methadone were unaltered, as were those of paritaprevir according to a cross-study comparison.[3]

3. Simeprevir. The UK and US manufacturers briefly report that, in a study in 16 subjects stable on methadone maintenance therapy (30 to 150 mg daily) and given simeprevir 150 mg daily for 7 days, the pharmacokinetics of *R*-methadone were unaffected.[6,7]

4. Telaprevir. In a study, 15 subjects stable taking methadone 40 to 120 mg daily were given telaprevir 750 mg every 8 hours for 7 days. Telaprevir reduced the AUC and minimum plasma concentration of *R*-methadone by 29% and 31%, respectively, and also reduced the AUC and minimum plasma concentration of *S*-methadone by 36% and 40%, respectively. Although the free fraction of *R*-methadone was increased by 26%, the unbound fraction of *R*-methadone was not altered by telaprevir. The pharmacokinetics of telaprevir did not differ, when compared with historical controls. Fewer subjects had signs of opioid withdrawal on concurrent use, when compared with methadone alone.[8]

Mechanism

Boceprevir, simeprevir, and telaprevir are (to varying extents) inhibitors of CYP3A4, by which methadone is partially metabolised, and so would be expected to lead to an *increase* in methadone exposure. However, the opposite effect was seen with boceprevir and telaprevir, and the authors of one study suggested that this was due to displacement of bound methadone from plasma proteins by telaprevir.[8] Further study is required. The increase in buprenorphine exposure seen with paritaprevir boosted with ritonavir (in a fixed-dose combination) might be due to the CYP3A4-inhibitory effects of the ritonavir, used as a pharmacokinetic enhancer, as paritaprevir itself does not appear to affect this isoenzyme. However, the role of glucuronosyltransferase, UGT1A1, cannot be ruled out as paritaprevir inhibits this enzyme, which has some involvement in the metabolism of buprenorphine. Note that other components of the combination (ombitasvir and dasabuvir) might also have similar effects and their involvement also cannot be ruled out.

Importance and management

A pharmacokinetic interaction between boceprevir and telaprevir, and **methadone** would appear to be established, but is unlikely to be clinically important. The reduction in methadone exposure was slight at worst, and fewer cases of opioid withdrawal were reported on concurrent use with telaprevir. No initial methadone dose adjustment is considered likely to be needed in patients also taking telaprevir. However, the UK and US manufacturers suggest that some patients might need their methadone dose adjusting during maintenance therapy, and so they recommend monitoring concurrent use.[9,10] The UK and US manufacturers of boceprevir advise that no methadone dose adjustment is necessary, but some patients might require additional titration of their methadone dose when boceprevir is started or stopped, to maintain clinical benefit.[1,2]

Simeprevir and paritaprevir boosted with ritonavir (in a fixed-dose combination with ombitasvir, with and without dasabuvir) had no effect on methadone pharmacokinetics and so no dose adjustments are necessary.

Note that boceprevir and telaprevir have been reported to cause some prolongation of the QT interval and as high-dose methadone can also prolong the QT interval, some caution on concurrent use would seem prudent (see 'Drugs that prolong the QT interval + Other drugs that prolong the QT interval', p.272). No clinically relevant effect on boceprevir pharmacokinetics was seen and so no boceprevir dose adjustment would seem necessary on concurrent use with methadone.

No clinically relevant pharmacokinetic interaction occurs between boceprevir, paritaprevir boosted with ritonavir (in a fixed-dose combination with ombitasvir, with and without dasabuvir) or telaprevir and **buprenorphine** or **naloxone**, and so no dose adjustments are needed on concurrent use. However, the UK manufacturer of boceprevir, and the US manufacturer of paritaprevir boosted with ritonavir (in a fixed-dose combination with ombitasvir, and given with dasabuvir), advise that because of the increase in buprenorphine exposure patients should be monitored for signs of opiate toxicity,[2] or sedation and cognitive effects.[4] The UK and US manufacturers of simeprevir predict that this will also be the case if it is used concurrently with buprenorphine and naloxone, and similarly advise that no dose adjustment is necessary.[6,7] The pharmacokinetics of boceprevir and paritaprevir were not altered to a clinically relevant extent by buprenorphine and so no dose adjustments would seem necessary on concurrent use.

As **alfentanil** and to a lesser extent, **fentanyl**, are metabolised by CYP3A4, the UK and US manufacturers of telaprevir advise that careful monitoring of therapeutic and adverse effects (such as respiratory depression) is necessary on their concurrent use.[9,10] This includes oral, buccal, and nasal use,[9] as well as extended-release transdermal or transmucosal use.[9,10] The UK manufacturer warns that this might be especially important on starting alfentanil or fentanyl, and a dosage adjustment might be necessary. The greatest effect is expected with oral, nasal, and buccal/sublingual use.[9]

1. Victrelis (Boceprevir). Merck & Co., Inc. US Prescribing information, July 2014.
2. Victrelis (Boceprevir). Merck Sharp & Dohme Ltd. UK Summary of product characteristics, August 2014.
3. Viekirax (Ombitasvir, paritaprevir, ritonavir). AbbVie Ltd. UK Summary of product characteristics, January 2015.

4. Viekira Pak (Ombitasvir, paritaprevir, ritonavir co-packaged with dasabuvir sodium monohydrate). AbbVie Inc. US Prescribing information, December 2014.
5. Luo X, Trevejo J, van Heeswijk RPG, Smith F, Garg V. Effect of telaprevir on the pharmacokinetics of buprenorphine in volunteers on stable buprenorphine/naloxone maintenance therapy. *Antimicrob Agents Chemother* (2012) 56, 3641–7.
6. Olysio (Simeprevir sodium). Janssen-Cilag Ltd. UK Summary of product characteristics, May 2014.
7. Olysio (Simeprevir sodium). Janssen Products, LP. US Prescribing information, November 2014.
8. van Heeswijk R, Verboven P, Vandevoorde A, Vinck P, Snoeys J, Boogaerts G, De Paepe E, Van Solingen-Ristea R, Witek J, Garg V. Pharmacokinetic interaction between telaprevir and methadone. *Antimicrob Agents Chemother* (2013) 57, 2304–9.
9. Incivo (Telaprevir). Janssen-Cilag Ltd. UK Summary of product characteristics, July 2014.
10. Incivek (Telaprevir). Vertex Pharmaceuticals Inc. US Prescribing information, October 2013.

Opioids + Herbal medicines; Miscellaneous

Some herbal teas contain opioids and could theoretically cause additive CNS depression if taken with other opioids.

Clinical evidence, mechanism, importance and management

Some herbal preparations contain opioids; the **morphine** content of two herbal teas containing *Papaveris fructus* was found to be 10.4 micrograms/mL and 31.5 micrograms/mL, respectively. Furthermore, **morphine** was detected in the urine of 5 healthy subjects one hour after drinking 2 cups of either of the herbal teas, and was maximal at 4 to 6 hours: positive urine samples were detected up to 6 to 9 hours after drinking the teas.[1] Therefore, in theory at least, it might be expected that additive CNS depressant effects will occur if such teas are taken with other opioid preparations.

1. Van Thuyne W, Van Eenoo P, Delbeke FT. Urinary concentrations of morphine after the administration of herbal teas containing *Papaveris fructus* in relation to doping analysis. *J Chromatogr B Analyt Technol Biomed Life Sci* (2003) 785, 245–51.

Opioids + HIV-integrase inhibitors

No pharmacokinetic interaction occurs between buprenorphine and raltegravir, and buprenorphine does not affect the pharmacokinetics of elvitegravir. No pharmacokinetic interaction occurs between methadone and dolutegravir, elvitegravir, or raltegravir.

Clinical evidence, mechanism, importance and management

(a) Buprenorphine

1. Elvitegravir. In a study in 17 HIV-negative subjects stable taking buprenorphine 16 to 24 mg daily with naloxone 4 to 6 mg daily, and given elvitegravir boosted with cobicistat 150/150 mg daily for 10 days, the pharmacokinetics of elvitegravir were no different to historical controls.[1] No elvitegravir dose adjustment is necessary on concurrent use.

2. Raltegravir. In a study in 12 HIV-negative subjects stable taking buprenorphine 16 to 32 mg daily with naloxone 4 to 8 mg daily, and given raltegravir 400 mg twice daily, the AUC and maximum concentration of buprenorphine and naloxone were unaltered, and the pharmacokinetics of raltegravir were no different to historical controls.[2] No dose adjustments are necessary on concurrent use.

(b) Methadone

1. Dolutegravir. In a study in 11 subjects stable taking methadone 16 to 150 mg daily, and given dolutegravir 50 mg twice daily, the AUC and maximum concentration of *R*- and *S*-methadone were unaltered, and the pharmacokinetics of dolutegravir were no different to historical controls.[3] No dose adjustments are necessary on concurrent use.

2. Elvitegravir. In a study in 11 subjects stable taking methadone 80 to 120 mg daily, and given elvitegravir boosted with cobicistat 150/150 mg daily for 10 days, the AUC and maximum concentration of *R*- and *S*-methadone were unaltered, and the pharmacokinetics of elvitegravir were no different to historical controls.[4] No dose adjustments are necessary on concurrent use.

3. Raltegravir. A crossover study in 9 patients maintained on methadone for at least 4 weeks, found that raltegravir 400 mg twice daily for 10 days did not alter the pharmacokinetics of methadone. The pharmacokinetics of raltegravir were also found to be no different to historical controls.[5] No dose adjustments are therefore necessary on the concurrent use of these drugs.

1. Bruce RD, Winkle P, Custudio JM, Wei LX, Rhee MS, Kearney BP, Ramanathan S, Friedland GH. The pharmacokinetic and pharmacodynamic interactions between buprenorphine/naloxone and elvitegravir/cobicistat in subjects receiving chronic buprenorphine/naloxone treatment. *J Acquir Immune Defic Syndr* (2013) 63, 480–4.
2. Bruce RD, Moody DE, Chodkowski D, Andrews L, Fang WB, Morrison J, Parsons TL, Friedland GH. Pharmacokinetic interactions between buprenorphine/naloxone and raltegravir in subjects receiving chronic buprenorphine/naloxone treatment. *Am J Drug Alcohol Abuse* (2013) 39, 80–5.
3. Song I, Mark S, Chen S, Savina P, Wajima T, Peppercorn A, Bala U, Geoffroy P, Piscitelli S. Dolutegravir does not affect methadone pharmacokinetics in opioid-dependent, HIV-seronegative subjects. *Drug Alcohol Depend* (2013) 133, 781–4.
4. Bruce RD, Winkle P, Custudio JM, Wei X, Rhee MS, Kearney BP, Ramanathan S, Friedland GH. Investigation of the interactions between methadone and elvitegravir-cobicistat in subjects receiving chronic methadone maintenance. *Antimicrob Agents Chemother* (2013) 57, 6154–7.
5. Anderson MS, Mabalot Luk JA, Hanley WD, Jin B, Riesenberg RA, Wenning LA, Chodakewitz JA, Wagner JA, Iwamoto M. Effect of raltegravir on the pharmacokinetics of methadone. *J Clin Pharmacol* (2010) 50, 1461–6.

Opioids + HIV-protease inhibitors

Ritonavir and lopinavir boosted with ritonavir moderately increase the exposure to oxycodone. Ritonavir moderately decreases pethidine (meperidine) exposure and slightly increases that of its active metabolite, norpethidine. Ritonavir might increase the metabolism of morphine, and decrease the metabolism of codeine, dihydrocodeine, dextropropoxyphene (propoxyphene), and tramadol.

Clinical evidence

(a) Buprenorphine

For the interactions of the HIV-protease inhibitors with buprenorphine, see 'Opioids; Buprenorphine + HIV-protease inhibitors', p.180.

(b) Fentanyl and related drugs

For the interactions of the HIV-protease inhibitors with alfentanil or fentanyl, see 'Opioids; Fentanyl and related drugs + HIV-protease inhibitors', p.181.

(c) Methadone

For the interactions of the HIV-protease inhibitors with methadone, see 'Opioids; Methadone + HIV-protease inhibitors', p.182.

(d) Oxycodone

In a crossover study, 12 healthy subjects were given either **ritonavir** 300 mg alone, **lopinavir** boosted with ritonavir 400/100 mg, or placebo twice daily for 4 days, with oxycodone 10 mg as a single-dose on day 3. Ritonavir alone increased the AUC and maximum plasma concentration of oxycodone 3-fold and by 70%, respectively. Lopinavir with ritonavir increased the AUC and maximum plasma concentration of oxycodone 2.6-fold and by 40%, respectively. The AUC of the oxycodone metabolites, noroxycodone and noroxymorphone, were reduced by 51% and 81%, respectively, by ritonavir alone, and by 56% and 76%, respectively, by lopinavir with ritonavir. The AUC of the oxymorphone metabolite was increased 2.7-fold by lopinavir with ritonavir but was unaffected by ritonavir alone. Self-reported drug effects (such as alert or drowsy, good or poor performance) were also increased during concurrent use.[1]

(e) Pethidine (Meperidine)

A study in 8 healthy subjects given a single 50-mg oral dose of pethidine before and after **ritonavir** 500 mg twice daily for 10 days found that the AUC was decreased by 62% and the AUC of its metabolite, norpethidine, was increased by 47%.[2]

Mechanism

Ritonavir is a potent inhibitor of CYP3A4 and a weak to moderate inhibitor of CYP2D6 (depending on the dose used). It can also induce glucuronidation, and other cytochrome P450 isoenzymes, such as CYP1A2 and CYP2B6.

Lopinavir is also an inhibitor of CYP3A4 and when given with ritonavir in a boosted-regimen, potently inhibits CYP3A4. **Oxycodone** is principally metabolised by CYP3A4 to noroxycodone, but CYP2D6 is also involved, to produce oxymorphone (which has some analgesic activity). Both metabolites are further metabolised to noroxymorphone by CYP3A4 and/or CYP2D6. The concurrent use of oxycodone and ritonavir or lopinavir boosted ritonavir increases the exposure to oxycodone and reduces that of its noroxycodone metabolite.

Pethidine is metabolised by several cytochrome P450 isoenzymes. The reduction in exposure seen with ritonavir possibly suggests induction of its metabolism, but if this is correct, the route by which this occurs is not known. Further study is needed.

Importance and management

Evidence for interactions between the HIV-protease inhibitors and opioids (other than buprenorphine, fentanyl and related drugs, and methadone, which are discussed elsewhere), is limited to the studies with **oxycodone** and **pethidine** (**meperidine**). A pharmacokinetic interaction between ritonavir, or lopinavir boosted with ritonavir, and **oxycodone** is established, and the moderate increases in oxycodone exposure seen are likely to be clinically relevant. It would therefore be prudent to monitor for increased oxycodone effects and consider an oxycodone dose reduction if these drugs are used together. Other HIV-protease inhibitors boosted with ritonavir would be expected to interact similarly. The interaction between ritonavir and **pethidine** appears to be established, and in particular the slight increase in exposure to the active metabolite, norpethidine, which can cause CNS effects such as seizures, might be clinically important. Some UK and US manufacturers contraindicate or advise against the concurrent use of **pethidine** with ritonavir because of the risk of norpethidine toxicity.[3-5] The long-term use of pethidine with other HIV-protease inhibitors that are boosted with low-dose ritonavir is also not recommended.

Codeine and **dihydrocodeine** are metabolised by CYP2D6 (and codeine also undergoes some glucuronidation[6]), but the consequences of inhibition of CYP2D6 are most pronounced for **codeine**. CYP2D6 inhibition by higher doses of ritonavir might lead to decreased concentrations of the morphine metabolite of codeine and therefore, perhaps contrary to expectation, a reduced effect. The concentrations of **dihydrocodeine** are also increased by CYP2D6 inhibition, and might be increased by higher doses of ritonavir, but note that the increases seen with the potent CYP2D6 inhibitor, quinidine, did not appear to be clinically important. The effects of CYP2D6 inhibition on codeine and dihydrocodeine are discussed in greater detail in 'Opioids; Codeine and related drugs + Quinidine', p.194.

Similarly, because **tramadol** is metabolised by both CYP3A4 and CYP2D6, its concentrations would be expected to be increased by ritonavir, and dose reductions might be necessary. But note the clinical importance of CYP2D6 inhibition on tramadol effects is not clear (see 'Opioids + Quinidine', p.194), and the potent CYP3A4 inhibitor, itraconazole, had no effect on tramadol pharmacokinetics (see 'Opioids + Azoles', p.165). Nevertheless, until more is known it would seem prudent to monitor for tramadol adverse effects, such as sedation.

As *low-dose* ritonavir (i.e. the dose used as a pharmacokinetic booster with other HIV-protease inhibitors) has a less potent effect on CYP2D6, dose reductions of opioids metabolised by CYP2D6 would not generally be expected to be necessary if this dose of ritonavir is given concurrently.

Dextropropoxyphene (**propoxyphene**) is metabolised by CYP3A4, and the UK manufacturer of ritonavir contraindicates concurrent use as increased dextropropoxyphene concentrations seem likely to occur, which would increase the risk of serious respiratory depression or other serious adverse events.[4] However, the US manufacturer only suggests that a dose decrease of dextropropoxyphene might be needed.[3] If both drugs are given it would seem prudent to monitor for adverse effects, such as sedation, and decrease the dextropropoxyphene dose accordingly.

Morphine undergoes glucuronidation, and the morphine metabolite [morphine-6 glucuronide] is believed to contribute to the analgesic effects of morphine. However, the outcome of taking ritonavir with **morphine** is less clear, but it is expected that its concentrations will be decreased.[4] It would seem prudent to monitor concurrent use closely to ensure morphine is effective in patients taking ritonavir. More study is needed.

1. Nieminen TH, Hagelberg NM, Saari TI, Neuvonen M, Neuvonen PJ, Laine K, Olkkola KT. Oxycodone concentrations are greatly increased by the concomitant use of ritonavir or lopinavir/ritonavir. *Eur J Clin Pharmacol* (2010) 66, 977–85.
2. Piscitelli SC, Kress DR, Bertz RJ, Pau A, Davey R. The effect of ritonavir on the pharmacokinetics of meperidine and normeperidine. *Pharmacotherapy* (2000) 20, 549–53.
3. Norvir Capsules (Ritonavir). AbbVie Inc. US Prescribing information, November 2013.
4. Norvir Tablets (Ritonavir). AbbVie Ltd. UK Summary of product characteristics, December 2013.
5. Demerol (Meperidine hydrochloride). Sanofi-Aventis US LLC. US Prescribing information, July 2014.
6. Lötsch J, Skarke C, Tegeder I, Geisslinger G. Drug interactions with patient-controlled analgesia. *Clin Pharmacokinet* (2002) 41, 31–57.

Opioids; Buprenorphine + HIV-protease inhibitors

Ritonavir (low-dose) and atazanavir (boosted and unboosted) slightly increase the exposure to buprenorphine, and slightly and moderately increase the concentration of its active metabolite, respectively. Darunavir, fosamprenavir, lopinavir, and tipranavir (all boosted with ritonavir) and nelfinavir do not affect buprenorphine exposure, but concentrations of the active metabolite might be affected.

Clinical evidence

(a) Pharmacokinetic interactions

1. Atazanavir. In a study showing increased exposure to buprenorphine and norbuprenorphine by atazanavir alone, and when boosted with ritonavir, (see 'Table 6.3', p.181 for the effects on buprenorphine), buprenorphine had no effects on the pharmacokinetics of atazanavir or ritonavir, when compared with healthy non-opioid-dependent controls.[1] In a prospective study of 181 HIV-positive, opioid-dependent patients, there were no differences in the mean buprenorphine dose between those taking atazanavir (38 patients, 27 with ritonavir) and those taking other antiretrovirals (drugs not stated).[2] Atazanavir plasma concentrations were found to be lower after sublingual buprenorphine (16 mg) was added, in one patient taking a regimen containing atazanavir boosted with ritonavir 300/100 mg daily.[3]

One report describes 3 HIV-positive patients who experienced increased buprenorphine adverse effects (e.g. daytime sleepiness, dizziness, and reduced mental function) within about 2 days of starting to take atazanavir boosted with ritonavir. When the dose of buprenorphine was reduced there was a reduction in sedative symptoms, although in one case this led to an increase in opioid cravings.[4]

2. Darunavir. In 2 studies, darunavir boosted with ritonavir had no effect on the pharmacokinetics of buprenorphine (see 'Table 6.3', p.181).[5,6] There was a small increase in the AUC of the active metabolite, norbuprenorphine, in one of these studies, but opioid withdrawal and toxicity were reported as being mild, at worst, during the study and no dose adjustment of buprenorphine with naloxone was needed.[5] In both studies the pharmacokinetics of darunavir were no different than when compared with historical data,[5] or in a control group taking darunavir boosted with ritonavir alone.[6] The pharmacokinetics of ritonavir were not affected when compared with historical data, and the pharmacokinetics of naloxone were also unaffected.[5]

3. Fosamprenavir. In a study showing no effect of fosamprenavir boosted with ritonavir on the pharmacokinetics of buprenorphine or the active metabolite, norbuprenorphine (see 'Table 6.3', p.181), the pharmacokinetics of fosamprenavir were no different than in a control group taking fosamprenavir boosted with ritonavir alone.[6]

4. Lopinavir. In 2 studies, lopinavir boosted with ritonavir had no effect on the pharmacokinetics of buprenorphine, but caused a small decrease in the maximum plasma concentration of the active metabolite, norbuprenorphine (see 'Table 6.3', p.181).[7,8] However, no signs of opioid withdrawal were seen.[7] The AUC of lopinavir was 18% higher in the buprenorphine with naloxone group than in a control group of 15 patients taking lopinavir boosted with ritonavir alone in one of the studies,[7] but did not differ from historical controls in the other study.[8] See also, *QT interval prolongation*, below.

5. Nelfinavir. In a study nelfinavir had no effect on the pharmacokinetics of buprenorphine, the maximum plasma concentration of the active metabolite, norbuprenorphine, was decreased (see 'Table 6.3', p.181), but no signs of opioid withdrawal were seen. The maximum plasma concentration of nelfinavir was 40% lower in the buprenorphine with naloxone group than in a control group of 16 patients taking nelfinavir alone.[7] See also, *QT interval prolongation*, below.

6. Ritonavir. In a study with low-dose ritonavir there was a small increase in the AUCs of buprenorphine and its active metabolite, norbuprenorphine (see 'Table 6.3', p.181), but no increase in adverse effects or opioid withdrawal was seen. The pharmacokinetics of ritonavir were no different in the buprenorphine with naloxone group than in a control group of 15 patients taking ritonavir alone.[7] See also, *QT interval prolongation*, below.

7. Tipranavir. In a study, tipranavir boosted with ritonavir had no effect on the pharmacokinetics of buprenorphine, but caused a decrease in the AUC of the active metabolite, norbuprenorphine (see 'Table 6.3', p.181). Tipranavir also decreased the AUC and maximum plasma concentration of naloxone by 43% and 36%, respectively. The maximum plasma concentration of tipranavir was 25% lower than in 161 historical controls, but the minimum plasma concentration was relatively unchanged. No subjects developed any signs of opioid withdrawal or toxicity, and no buprenorphine dose adjustments were necessary.[9] The US manufacturer states that the concurrent use of buprenorphine has resulted in 40% lower minimum concentrations of tipranavir than historical controls.[10]

(b) QT-interval prolongation

In a study in opioid-dependent patients taking sublingual buprenorphine and naloxone, patients were given an antiretroviral (**nelfinavir**, **lopinavir** boosted with ritonavir, **ritonavir**, delavirdine, or efavirenz) for 5 to 15 days to investigate the effect of these drugs on the QT interval. Buprenorphine with naloxone alone did not notably alter the QT interval, but when an antiretroviral was also given there was a statistically significant, but probably not clinically relevant, increase in the QT interval. Of the HIV-protease inhibitors, **ritonavir** 100 mg twice daily (a low dose, used as a pharmacokinetic enhancer) resulted in the greatest increase in QTc interval.[11]

Mechanism

Buprenorphine is metabolised by CYP3A4 and also undergoes glucuronidation. Ritonavir is a well-known potent inhibitor of CYP3A4, and other HIV-protease inhibitors also inhibit this isoenzyme. Ritonavir also induces glucuronidation. Inhibition of CYP3A4 by the HIV-protease inhibitors would therefore be expected to lead to increased buprenorphine concentrations, and this has been seen with atazanavir boosted with ritonavir and ritonavir alone, but not with darunavir, fosamprenavir, lopinavir, and tipranavir (all boosted with ritonavir) or nelfinavir.

The increased concentrations of the glucuronide metabolite, buprenorphine-3-glucuronide, seen with darunavir, fosamprenavir, and tipranavir, have been suggested to be due to induction of glucuronidation by the HIV- protease inhibitor,[6,12] but this requires confirmation. Note also, that ritonavir did not affect the concentrations of this metabolite.

The exact mechanism for the unexpected increase in the concentrations of the active metabolite, norbuprenorphine, reported with atazanavir and ritonavir is unclear, although the authors of one study suggest that atazanavir alone or with ritonavir might increase the gastrointestinal bioavailability of swallowed buprenorphine, thereby leading to an apparent increase in metabolite concentrations.[1]

Importance and management

A pharmacokinetic interaction between the HIV-protease inhibitors boosted with ritonavir and buprenorphine is established but its clinical relevance is less clear. One UK manufacturer of buprenorphine[13] suggests that the buprenorphine dose should be halved in patients taking CYP3A4 inhibitors, such as the HIV-protease inhibitors (see 'Table 1.9', p.11), when it is used for opioid dependence. Evidence of increased exposure to the active metabolite, norbuprenorphine, with atazanavir and darunavir would appear to support this, although note that no dose adjustment was reported to be necessary in the darunavir study. Another study[7] suggests that this interaction might not be of clinical importance in opioid-tolerant patients given low-dose ritonavir alone with buprenorphine. Furthermore, the studies with lopinavir, nelfinavir, and tipranavir, showed reduced concentrations of the active metabolite which could possibly result in reduced effects, although this was not reported in any of the studies and no buprenorphine dose adjustments were required. Evidence with fosamprenavir is limited, but what is known suggests that an effect on buprenorphine pharmacokinetics would not be expected.

If buprenorphine is given with any HIV-protease inhibitor it would seem prudent to monitor the outcome of concurrent use and adjust the dose of buprenorphine accordingly.

1. McCance-Katz EF, Moody DE, Morse GD, Ma Q, DiFrancesco R, Friedland G, Pade P, Rainey PM. Interaction between buprenorphine and atazanavir or atazanavir/ritonavir. *Drug Alcohol Depend* (2007) 91, 269–78.
2. Vergara-Rodriguez P, Tozzi MJ, Botsko M, Nandi V, Altice F, Egan JE, O'Connor PG, Sullivan LE, Fiellin DA. Hepatic safety and lack of antiretroviral interactions with buprenorphine/naloxone in HIV-infected opioid-dependent patients. *J Acquir Immune Defic Syndr* (2011) 56 (Suppl 1), S62–7.
3. DiFrancesco R, Fischl MA, Donnelly J, Zingman BS, McCance-Katz EF, Moody DE, Reichman RC, Gripshover B, Morse GD. Buprenorphine assay and plasma concentration monitoring in HIV-infected substance users. *J Pharm Biomed Anal* (2007) 44, 188–95.
4. Bruce RD, Altice FL. Three case reports of a clinical pharmacokinetic interaction with buprenorphine and atazanavir plus ritonavir. *AIDS* (2006) 20, 783–4.
5. Sekar V, Tomaka F, Lefebvre E, De Pauw M, Vangeneugden T, van den Brink W, Hoetelmans R. Pharmacokinetic interactions between darunavir/ritonavir and opioid maintenance therapy using methadone or buprenorphine/naloxone. *J Clin Pharmacol* (2011) 51, 271–8.
6. Gruber VA, Rainey PM, Moody DE, Morse GD, Ma Q, Prathikanti S, Pade PA, Avanzo AA, McCance-Katz EF. Interactions between buprenorphine and the protease inhibitors darunavir-ritonavir and fosamprenavir-ritonavir. *Clin Infect Dis* (2012) 54, 414–23.

Table 6.3 Summary of the effect of the HIV-protease inhibitors on the pharmacokinetics of oral buprenorphine

HIV-protease inhibitor	*Dose*	*Study subjects*	*Effect on buprenorphine AUC (unless stated otherwise)*	*Effect on buprenorphine maximum concentration (unless stated otherwise)*	*Refs*
Atazanavir	400mg daily for 5 days	10 opioid-dependent patients stable on buprenorphine with naloxone	93% increase Norbuprenorphine: 76% increase	64% increase Norbuprenorphine: 36% increase	1
Atazanavir boosted with ritonavir	300/100mg daily for 5 days	10 opioid-dependent patients stable on buprenorphine with naloxone	67% increase Norbuprenorphine: 2-fold increase	37% increase Norbuprenorphine: 61% increase	1
Darunavir boosted with ritonavir	600/100mg twice daily for 8 days	17 HIV-negative patients stable on buprenorphine with naloxone	No effect Norbuprenorphine: 46% increase	No effect Norbuprenorphine: 36% increase, and 71% increase in minimum concentration	2
	800/100mg daily for 15 days	11 opioid-dependent patients stable on buprenorphine with naloxone	No effect Norbuprenorphine: no effect Buprenorphine-3-glucuronide: 69% increase	No effect Norbuprenorphine: no effect	3
Fosamprenavir boosted with ritonavir	1400/200mg daily for 15 days	10 opioid-dependent patients stable on buprenorphine with naloxone	No effect Norbuprenorphine: no effect Buprenorphine-3-glucuronide: 63% increase	No effect Norbuprenorphine: no effect	3
Lopinavir boosted with ritonavir	400/100mg twice daily for 7 days	10 opioid-dependent patients stable on buprenorphine with naloxone	No effect	No effect Norbuprenorphine: 31% decrease Buprenorphine-3-glucuronide: 2-fold increase	4
	800/200mg daily for 10 days	12 opioid-dependent patients stable on buprenorphine with naloxone	No effect	No effect Norbuprenorphine: 41% decrease	5
Nelfinavir	1.25g twice daily for 5 days	10 opioid-dependent patients stable on buprenorphine with naloxone		Norbuprenorphine: 40% decrease	4
Ritonavir	100mg twice daily for 7 days	10 opioid-dependent patients stable on buprenorphine with naloxone	57% increase Norbuprenorphine: 33% Buprenorphine-3-glucuronide: no effect		4
Tipranavir boosted with ritonavir	500/200mg twice daily for 7 days	10 opioid-dependent patients stable on buprenorphine with naloxone	No effect Norbuprenorphine: 79% decrease	No effect Norbuprenorphine: 80% decrease	6
	500/200mg twice daily for at least 7 days	10 opioid-dependent patients stable on buprenorphine with naloxone	Buprenorphine-3-glucuronide: 88% increase		7

1. McCance-Katz EF, Moody DE, Morse GD, Ma Q, DiFrancesco R, Friedland G, Pade P, Rainey PM. Interaction between buprenorphine and atazanavir or atazanavir/ritonavir. *Drug Alcohol Depend* (2007) 91, 269–78.
2. Sekar V, Tomaka F, Lefebvre E, De Pauw M, Vangeneugden T, van den Brink W, Hoetelmans R. Pharmacokinetic interactions between darunavir/ritonavir and opioid maintenance therapy using methadone or buprenorphine/naloxone. *J Clin Pharmacol* (2011) 51, 271–8.
3. Gruber VA, Rainey PM, Moody DE, Morse GD, Ma Q, Prathikanti S, Pade PA, Avanzo AA, McCance-Katz EF. Interactions between buprenorphine and the protease inhibitors darunavir-ritonavir and fosamprenavir-ritonavir. *Clin Infect Dis* (2012) 54, 414–23.
4. McCance-Katz EF, Moody DE, Smith PF, Morse GD, Friedland G, Pade P, Baker J, Alvanzo A, Jatlow P, Rainey PM. Interactions between buprenorphine and antiretrovirals. II. The protease inhibitors nelfinavir, lopinavir/ritonavir, and ritonavir. *Clin Infect Dis* (2006) 43 (Suppl 4), S235–46.
5. Bruce RD, Altice FL, Moody DE, Morse GD, Andrews L, Lin S-N, Fang WB, Ma Q, Friedland GH. Pharmacokinetic interactions between buprenorphine/naloxone and once-daily lopinavir/ritonavir. *J Acquir Immune Defic Syndr* (2010) 54, 511–4.
6. Bruce RD, Altice FL, Moody DE, Lin S-N, Fang WB, Sabo JP, Wruck JM, Piliero PJ, Conner C, Andrews L, Friedland GH. Pharmacokinetic interactions between buprenorphine/naloxone and tipranavir/ritonavir in HIV-negative subjects chronically receiving buprenorphine/naloxone. *Drug Alcohol Depend* (2009) 105, 234–9.
7. Bruce RD, Moody DE, Fang WB, Chodkowski D, Andrews L, Friedland GH. Tipranavir/ritonavir induction of buprenorphine glucuronide metabolism in HIV-negative subjects chronically receiving buprenorphine/naloxone. *Am J Drug Alcohol Abuse* (2011) 37, 224–8.

7. McCance-Katz EF, Moody DE, Smith PF, Morse GD, Friedland G, Pade P, Baker J, Alvanzo A, Jatlow P, Rainey PM. Interactions between buprenorphine and antiretrovirals. II. The protease inhibitors nelfinavir, lopinavir/ritonavir, and ritonavir. *Clin Infect Dis* (2006) 43 (Suppl 4), S235–46.
8. Bruce RD, Altice FL, Moody DE, Morse GD, Andrews L, Lin S-N, Fang WB, Ma Q, Friedland GH. Pharmacokinetic interactions between buprenorphine/naloxone and once-daily lopinavir/ritonavir. *J Acquir Immune Defic Syndr* (2010) 54, 511–4.
9. Bruce RD, Altice FL, Moody DE, Lin S-N, Fang WB, Sabo JP, Wruck JM, Piliero PJ, Conner C, Andrews L, Friedland GH. Pharmacokinetic interactions between buprenorphine/naloxone and tipranavir/ritonavir in HIV-negative subjects chronically receiving buprenorphine/naloxone. *Drug Alcohol Depend* (2009) 105, 234–9.
10. Aptivus (Tipranavir). Boehringer Ingelheim Pharmaceuticals, Inc. US Prescribing information, April 2012.
11. Baker JR, Best AM, Pade PA, McCance-Katz EF. Effect of buprenorphine and antiretroviral agents on the QT interval in opioid-dependent patients. *Ann Pharmacother* (2006) 40, 392–6.
12. Bruce RD, Moody DE, Fang WB, Chodkowski D, Andrews L, Friedland GH. Tipranavir/ritonavir induction of buprenorphine glucuronide metabolism in HIV-negative subjects chronically receiving buprenorphine/naloxone. *Am J Drug Alcohol Abuse* (2011) 37, 224–8.
13. Subutex (Buprenorphine hydrochloride). RB Pharmaceuticals Ltd. UK Summary of product characteristics, September 2014.

Opioids; Fentanyl and related drugs + HIV-protease inhibitors

Ritonavir very markedly and moderately decreases the clearance of oral and intravenous alfentanil, respectively, and moderately decreases that of intravenous fentanyl. Indinavir alone moderately decreases the clearance of oral and intravenous alfentanil, but when boosted with ritonavir its effects are very marked. Similarly, nelfinavir moderately reduces

alfentanil clearance. Other HIV-protease inhibitors would be expected to have a similar effect.

Clinical evidence

(a) Alfentanil

1. Indinavir. A crossover study in 12 healthy subjects found that steady-state indinavir boosted with ritonavir 800/100 mg twice daily reduced the clearance of both intravenous and oral alfentanil by 92% and 97%, respectively. Acute administration (3 days) of indinavir boosted with ritonavir had a similar effect on the clearance of oral alfentanil. The oral bioavailability of alfentanil was increased from 34% to 81%, and alfentanil-induced miosis was increased and prolonged.[1] Another crossover study in 12 healthy subjects found that indinavir 800 mg three times daily for 21 days reduced the clearance of intravenous and oral alfentanil by 50% and 70%, respectively. The oral bioavailability of alfentanil was increased from 51% to 78%, and overall these changes led to increased and prolonged miosis.[2]

2. Nelfinavir. A crossover study in 12 healthy subjects found that nelfinavir 1.25 g twice daily reduced the clearance of intravenous and oral alfentanil by 50% and 76% respectively. The oral bioavailability of alfentanil was increased from 41% to 71% and maximum miosis increased.[3]

3. Ritonavir. A crossover study in 11 healthy subjects found that steady-state ritonavir reduced the clearance of both intravenous and oral alfentanil by 73% and 90%, respectively. The oral bioavailability of alfentanil was increased from 37% to 95% by ritonavir and alfentanil-induced miosis was also increased.[4] The same or a similar study has been reported elsewhere.[5]

(b) Fentanyl

In a crossover study in healthy subjects, **ritonavir** 200 mg increased to 300 mg three times daily for a total of 7 doses increased the AUC of a single 5-mg/kg intravenous dose of fentanyl by 83%, decreased its clearance by 67%, and increased its elimination half-life 2-fold.[6]

Mechanism

Both fentanyl and alfentanil are metabolised by CYP3A4. Fentanyl has a high hepatic extraction and so is more affected by changes in hepatic blood flow (see 'Changes in first-pass metabolism', p.4), than changes in the isoenzymes responsible for its metabolism, and it is therefore less affected by CYP3A4 inhibitors than alfentanil. Ritonavir, indinavir, and other HIV-protease inhibitors are CYP3A4 inhibitors and they therefore reduce the metabolism of these opioids, which results in reduced clearance and increased effects. Note that, alfentanil is affected to a greater extent when given by the oral route (not used therapeutically) than by the intravenous route because the intravenous route bypasses intestinal CYP3A4.

Importance and management

The evidence for an interaction between alfentanil or fentanyl and the HIV-protease inhibitors is relatively limited, but an interaction is established. The reduction in intravenous alfentanil clearance is clinically important, particularly with indinavir boosted with ritonavir which very markedly decreased its clearance, and the effects of alfentanil were demonstrably increased. If alfentanil is given with indinavir, nelfinavir, or ritonavir it would be prudent to consider reducing the dose of alfentanil and monitoring closely for increased and prolonged sedation. Similarly, caution is required in patients taking ritonavir who are given fentanyl by any route (oral, parenteral, or transdermal) and similar precautions are advisable.

Evidence about other HIV-protease inhibitors is lacking, but as they are all known to inhibit CYP3A4 and are generally given with ritonavir as a pharmacokinetic enhancer, it would seem prudent to apply the same precautions recommended above.

1. Kharasch ED, Hoffer C, Whittington D, Walker A, Bedynek PS. Methadone pharmacokinetics are independent of cytochrome P4503A (CYP3A) activity and gastrointestinal drug transport: insights from methadone interactions with ritonavir/indinavir. *Anesthesiology* (2009) 110, 660–72.
2. Kharasch ED, Bedynek PS, Hoffer C, Walker A, Whittington D. Lack of indinavir effects on methadone disposition despite inhibition of hepatic and intestinal cytochrome P4503A (CYP3A). *Anesthesiology* (2012) 116, 432–47.
3. Kharasch ED, Walker A, Whittington D, Hoffer C, Bedynek PS. Methadone metabolism and clearance are induced by nelfinavir despite inhibition of cytochrome P4503A (CYP3A) activity. *Drug Alcohol Depend* (2009) 101, 158–68.
4. Kharasch ED, Bedynek PS, Walker A, Whittington D, Hoffer C. Mechanism of ritonavir changes in methadone pharmacokinetics and pharmacodynamics: II. Ritonavir effects on CYP3A and P-glycoprotein activities. *Clin Pharmacol Ther* (2008) 84, 506–12.
5. Kharasch ED, Hoffer C. Assessment of ritonavir effects on hepatic and first-pass CYP3A activity and methadone disposition using noninvasive pupillometry. *Clin Pharmacol Ther* (2004) 75, P96.
6. Olkkola KT, Palkama VJ, Neuvonen PJ. Ritonavir's role in reducing fentanyl clearance and prolonging its half-life. *Anesthesiology* (1999) 91, 681–5.

Opioids; Methadone + HIV-protease inhibitors

Methadone exposure can be reduced by amprenavir, nelfinavir, and high-dose ritonavir; as well as darunavir, lopinavir, saquinavir, and tipranavir boosted with ritonavir. Fosamprenavir and indinavir (both boosted with ritonavir), and possibly unboosted atazanavir or saquinavir, do not appear to have clinically important effects on methadone pharmacokinetics. Amprenavir and lopinavir concentrations might be reduced by methadone. Cases of QT prolongation and torsade de pointes have been reported in patients taking HIV-protease inhibitors and methadone.

Clinical evidence

(a) Amprenavir

In a study in 5 patients, methadone concentrations were reduced by 35% (range 28 to 87%) within 17 days of starting to take amprenavir 1.2 g twice daily and abacavir 600 mg twice daily. Two patients reported nausea before their daily methadone dose, which can be a sign of opioid withdrawal.[1] Note that abacavir might reduce methadone concentrations, and could therefore have contributed to this effect, see 'Opioids + NRTIs', p.190. In a study showing a slight decrease in methadone exposure with amprenavir (see 'Table 6.4', p.183), symptoms of opioid withdrawal were not detected. In this study, a 30% lower amprenavir AUC was seen in opioid-dependent patients taking amprenavir and methadone, than in non-matched historical controls.[2]

(b) Atazanavir

In a study showing no effect of atazanavir on methadone pharmacokinetics (see 'Table 6.4', p.183), symptoms of opiate withdrawal or excess were not detected.[3] Similarly, in a study in HIV-positive drug users, in the group taking atazanavir, the mean methadone requirement remained the same.[4]

Two studies in HIV-positive patients taking atazanavir boosted with ritonavir 300/100 mg daily found that the plasma concentrations of atazanavir were lower in patients taking methadone than in those not taking methadone. In one study the *maximum* plasma concentration was 46% lower,[5] and in another the *minimum* plasma concentration was 56% lower.[6]

A case of torsade de pointes has been reported in a patient taking methadone and atazanavir boosted with ritonavir 300/100 mg daily (although the patient admitted poor compliance). The HIV-protease inhibitors were withdrawn and the QT interval prolongation was reversed over the next 48 hours.[7] Ventricular tachycardia with QT interval prolongation has been described in 2 patients receiving atazanavir boosted with ritonavir 300/100 mg daily and methadone. In both cases the QT interval prolongation reduced after atazanavir was stopped, and in one of the patients, increased again on rechallenge with atazanavir.[8]

(c) Darunavir

In the study into the effects of darunavir boosted with ritonavir on methadone pharmacokinetics (see 'Table 6.4', p.183), four subjects had mild symptoms of methadone withdrawal, but the methadone dose did not need to be adjusted. The pharmacokinetics of darunavir and ritonavir were not affected by methadone, when compared with historical data.[9]

(d) Fosamprenavir

In the study into the effects of fosamprenavir boosted with ritonavir on methadone pharmacokinetics (see 'Table 6.4', p.183), the small changes in the pharmacokinetics of both the *R*- and *S*-enantiomers of methadone did not result in any serious adverse effects or any notable changes in cognitive performance. None of the patients experienced opioid withdrawal and no methadone dose adjustments were required. The concentrations of amprenavir, derived from fosamprenavir, were unaffected, when compared with historical control data.[10]

(e) Indinavir

A randomised, crossover study in 12 patients taking methadone and indinavir 800 mg every 8 hours for 8 days, found a small decrease in indinavir maximum concentrations and a small increase in minimum concentrations, when compared with historical controls.[11]

Two reports describe patients whose methadone concentrations appeared to be unaltered while taking indinavir, but who later had reduced concentrations when taking nelfinavir, or saquinavir with ritonavir (see *Nelfinavir*, and *Saquinavir*, below).[12,13] These would seem to confirm that indinavir does not have a clinically relevant effect on methadone concentrations. Another case report describes a patient who presented with symptoms which included chills, sweating, yawning, runny nose, back pain, diarrhoea, mydriasis, vomiting, restlessness, anxiety and hypertension within 4 days of his antiretroviral medication being changed to indinavir with stavudine, ritonavir and nevirapine, despite taking his usual dose of methadone. His methadone concentration was found to be low and a dose increase was required.[14] For other pharmacokinetic studies, see 'Table 6.4', p.183.

(f) Lopinavir

In the study finding reduced exposure to methadone with lopinavir boosted with ritonavir (see 'Table 6.4', p.183), 4 of the 15 patients had clinically important increases in opioid-withdrawal scores, and were found to have sub-therapeutic minimum methadone concentrations.[15] However, in another study finding reduced methadone exposure, none of the patients experienced methadone withdrawal during the study or the 6 weeks of follow-up.[16] In a study that did not measure methadone concentrations, none of the 18 patients experienced methadone withdrawal during the 28 days after starting lopinavir boosted with ritonavir.[17] In a further study, in HIV-positive drug users, in the group taking lopinavir the mean methadone requirement remained the same.[4]

In one study methadone appeared to have no effect on the pharmacokinetics of lopinavir or ritonavir (given together),[18] but in another, lopinavir minimum plasma concentrations were 75% lower in patients taking methadone than in those not taking methadone.[6] A case of prolonged QT interval associated with torsade de pointes has been reported in an HIV-positive patient taking long-term methadone when lopinavir boosted with ritonavir was stopped.[19]

Table 6.4 Summary of the effect of the HIV-protease inhibitors on the pharmacokinetics of oral methadone

HIV-protease inhibitor	*Dose*	*Study subjects*	*Effect on methadone AUC*	*Effect on methadone maximum concentration (unless stated otherwise)*	*Refs*
Amprenavir	1.2 g twice daily for 10 days	16 opioid-dependent, HIV-negative subjects	*R*-methadone: 13% decrease *S*-methadone: 40% decrease	*R*-methadone: 25% decrease *S*-methadone: 48% decrease	1
Atazanavir	400 mg daily for 14 days	16 opiate-dependent, HIV-negative subjects	Not statistically significant	Not statistically significant	2
Darunavir boosted with ritonavir	600/100 mg twice daily for 8 days	16 HIV-negative subjects stabilised on methadone	*R*-methadone: 16% decrease *S*-methadone: 36% decrease	*R*-methadone: 24% decrease *S*-methadone: 44% decrease	3
Fosamprenavir boosted with ritonavir	700/100 mg twice daily for 14 days	19 opioid dependent, HIV-negative subjects	*R*-methadone: 18% decrease *S*-methadone: 43% decrease	*R*-methadone: 21% decrease *S*-methadone: 43% decrease	4
Indinavir	800 mg 8-hourly for 8 days	12 subjects stabilised on methadone	Not statistically significant	Not reported	5
	Not stated	6 HIV-positive subjects taking methadone	Not reported	No change in minimum plasma concentration	6
	800 mg three times daily for 14 days	12 healthy subjects	Not statistically significant	Not statistically significant	7
Indinavir boosted with ritonavir	800/100 mg twice daily for 14 days	12 healthy subjects	Not statistically significant	Not statistically significant	8
Lopinavir boosted with ritonavir	400/100 mg twice daily for 10 days	At least 12 healthy subjects	53% decrease	Not reported	9
	400/100 mg twice daily for 7 days	15 HIV negative subjects maintained on methadone	26% decrease	28% decrease	10
	Not stated	8 HIV-positive subjects taking methadone	36% decrease	44% decrease	11
Nelfinavir	1.25 g twice daily for 8 days	13 HIV-negative subjects taking methadone	*R*-methadone: 43% decrease *S*-methadone: 51% decrease	*R*-methadone: 43% decrease *S*-methadone: 50% decrease	12
	1.25 g twice daily for 5 days	17 opioid-dependent, HIV-negative subjects	38% decrease	43% decrease	13
	Not stated	2 HIV-positive subjects taking methadone	Not reported	50 to 60% decrease in minimum plasma concentration	6
	1.25 g twice daily for 14 days	6 subjects stabilised on methadone	56% decrease	55% decrease	14
	1.25 g twice daily for at least 2 weeks	12 healthy, HIV-negative subjects	*R*-methadone: 40% decrease *S*-methadone: 50% decrease	*R*-methadone: 15% decrease *S*-methadone: 27% decrease	15
	1.25 g twice daily for 4 weeks	7 HIV-positive subjects stabilised on methadone	Not reported	37% decrease in minimum plasma concentration	16
Ritonavir	Not stated	One HIV-positive patient taking methadone	Not reported	56% decrease in minimum plasma concentration	6
	200 mg three times daily on day one, then 300 mg twice daily for 6 days, then 400 mg twice daily for 2 weeks	12 healthy subjects, given single doses of intravenous and oral methadone	For short-term use and steady state: *R*-methadone: 32% and 49% decrease, respectively *S*-methadone: 43% and 50% decrease, respectively	*R*-methadone: 25% and 33% decrease *S*-methadone: 38% and 43% decrease	17
	Dose not stated, for 14 days	11 healthy subjects, given single oral methadone dose on day 11	36% decrease	38% decrease	18
	100 mg twice daily for 7 days	15 HIV negative subjects maintained on methadone	Not statistically significant	Not statistically significant	10
Saquinavir	Not stated	One HIV-positive subject taking methadone	Not reported	No change in minimum plasma concentration	6
Saquinavir boosted with ritonavir	1600/100 mg daily for 14 days	12 HIV-negative subjects taking methadone	Not statistically significant for both *R*- and *S*-methadone	Not statistically significant for both *R*- and *S*-methadone	19
	1000/100 mg twice daily for 14 days	12 HIV-negative subjects stabilised on methadone	*R*-methadone: 19% decrease *S*-methadone: 21% decrease	*R*-methadone: 20% decrease *S*-methadone: 20% decrease	20

Continued

Table 6.4 Summary of the effect of the HIV-protease inhibitors on the pharmacokinetics of oral methadone (continued)

HIV-protease inhibitor	*Dose*	*Study subjects*	*Effect on methadone AUC*	*Effect on methadone maximum concentration (unless stated otherwise)*	*Refs*
Saquinavir and ritonavir	400 mg twice daily with ritonavir 400 mg twice daily, for 15 days	12 HIV-positive subjects stabilised on methadone	*R*-methadone: 32% (20% corrected for protein binding) decrease *S*-methadone: 40% (25% corrected for protein binding) decrease	Not reported	21

1. Hendrix CW, Wakeford J, Wire MB, Lou Y, Bigelow GE, Martinez E, Christopher J, Fuchs EJ, Snidow JW. Pharmacokinetics and pharmacodynamics of methadone enantiomers after coadministration with amprenavir in opioid-dependent subjects. *Pharmacotherapy* (2004) 24, 1110–21.
2. Friedland G, Andrews L, Schreibman T, Agarwala S, Daley L, Child M, Shi J, Wang Y, O'Mara E. Lack of an effect of atazanavir on steady-state pharmacokinetics of methadone in patients chronically treated for opiate addiction. *AIDS* (2005) 19, 1635–41.
3. Sekar V, Tomaka F, Lefebvre E, De Pauw M, Vangeneugden T, van den Brink W, Hoetelmans R. Pharmacokinetic interactions between darunavir/ritonavir and opioid maintenance therapy using methadone or buprenorphine/naloxone. *J Clin Pharmacol* (2011) 51, 271–8 .
4. Cao Y-J, Smith PF, Wire MB, Lou Y, Lancaster CT, Causon RC, Bigelow GE, Martinez E, Fuchs EJ, Radebaugh C, McCabe S, Hendrix CW. Pharmacokinetics and pharmacodynamics of methadone enantiomers after coadministration with fosamprenavir-ritonavir in opioid-dependent subjects. *Pharmacotherapy* (2008) 28, 863–74.
5. Cantilena L, McCrea J, Blazes D, Winchell G, Carides A, Royce C, Deutsch P. Lack of a pharmacokinetic interaction between indinavir and methadone. *Clin Pharmacol Ther* (1999) 65, 135.
6. Beauverie P, Taburet A-M, Dessalles M-C, Furlan V, Touzeau D. Therapeutic drug monitoring of methadone in HIV-infected patients receiving protease inhibitors. *AIDS* (1998) 12, 2510–11.
7. Kharasch ED, Bedynek PS, Hoffer C, Walker A, Whittington D. Lack of indinavir effects on methadone disposition despite inhibition of hepatic and intestinal cytochrome P4503A (CYP3A). *Anesthesiology* (2012) 116, 432–47.
8. Kharasch ED, Hoffer C, Whittington D, Walker A, Bedynek PS. Methadone pharmacokinetics are independent of cytochrome P4503A (CYP3A) activity and gastrointestinal drug transport: insights from methadone interactions with ritonavir/indinavir. *Anesthesiology* (2009) 110, 660–72.
9. Bertz R, Hsu A, Lam W, Williams L, Renz C, Karol M, Dutta S, Carr R, Zhang Y, Wang Q, Schweitzer S, Foit C, Andre A, Bernstein B, Granneman GR, Sun E. Pharmacokinetic interactions between lopinavir/ritonavir (ABT-378r) and other non-HIV drugs [abstract P291]. *AIDS* (2000) 14 (Suppl 4), S100.
10. McCance-Katz EF, Rainey PM, Friedland G, Jatlow P. The protease inhibitor lopinavir-ritonavir may produce opiate withdrawal in methadone-maintained patients. *Clin Infect Dis* (2003) 37, 476–82.
11. Clarke S, Mulcahy F, Bergin C, Reynolds H, Boyle N, Barry M, Back DJ. Absence of opioid withdrawal symptoms in patients receiving methadone and the protease inhibitor lopinavir-ritonavir. *Clin Infect Dis* (2002) 34, 1143–5.
12. Hsyu P-H, Lillibridge J, Daniels E, Kerr BM. Pharmacokinetic interaction of nelfinavir and methadone in intravenous drug users. *Biopharm Drug Dispos* (2006) 27, 61–8.
13. McCance-Katz EF, Rainey PM, Smith P, Morse G, Friedland G, Gourevitch M, Jatlow P. Drug interactions between opioids and antiretroviral medications: interaction between methadone, LAAM, and nelfinavir. *Am J Addict* (2004) 13, 163–80.
14. Clarke S, Mulcahy F, Bergin C, Tjia J, Brown R, Barry M, Back DJ. The pharmacokinetic interaction between methadone and nelfinavir [abstract P276]. *AIDS* (2000) 14 (Suppl 4), S95.
15. Kharasch ED, Walker A, Whittington D, Hoffer C, Bedynek PS. Methadone metabolism and clearance are induced by nelfinavir despite inhibition of cytochrome P4503A (CYP3A) activity. *Drug Alcohol Depend* (2009) 101, 158–68.
16. Marco A, Deig E, Cadafalch J, Fuster M, Valls I Pedrol E. Interacciones clínicas y farmacocinéticas entre methadone y nelfinavir (studio Nemesia). *Med Clin (Barc)* (2006) 127, 47–9.
17. Kharasch ED, Bedynek PS, Park S, Whittington D, Walker A, Hoffer C. Mechanism of ritonavir changes in methadone pharmacokinetics and pharmacodynamics: I. Evidence against CYP3A mediation of methadone clearance. *Clin Pharmacol Ther* (2008) 84, 497–505.
18. Hsu A, Granneman GR, Carothers L, Dennis S, Chiu Y-L, Valdes J, Sun E. Ritonavir does not increase methadone exposure in healthy volunteers. 5th Conference on Retroviruses and Opportunistic Infection, Chicago, Feb 1–5, 1998, abstract 342.
19. Shelton MJ, Cloen D, DiFrancesco R, Berenson CS, Esch A, de Caprariis PJ, Palic B, Schur JL, Buggé CJL, Ljungqvist A, Espinosa O, Hewitt RG. The effects of once-daily saquinavir/minidose ritonavir on the pharmacokinetics of methadone. *J Clin Pharmacol* (2004) 44, 293–304.
20. Jamois C, Smith P, Morrison R, Riek M, Patel A, Schmitt C, Morcos PN, Zhang X. Effect of saquinavir/ritonavir (1000/100 mg bid) on the pharmacokinetics of methadone in opiate-dependent HIV-negative patients on stable methadone maintenance therapy. *Addict Biol* (2009) 14, 321–7.
21. Gerber JG, Rosenkranz S, Segal Y, Aberg J, D'Amico R, Mildvan D, Gulick R, Hughes V, Flexner C, Aweeka F, Hsu A, Gal J. Effect of ritonavir/saquinavir on stereoselective pharmacokinetics of methadone: Results of AIDS Clinical Trials Group (ACTG) 401. *J Acquir Immune Defic Syndr* (2001) 27, 153–60.

(g) Nelfinavir

In a study finding reduced methadone exposure with nelfinavir (see 'Table 6.4', p.183), none of the subjects developed opioid withdrawal symptoms or required methadone dose alterations. The methadone concentrations increased during the 14-day period after nelfinavir was stopped, but to a slightly lower level than before nelfinavir was added. Nelfinavir pharmacokinetics were not affected by methadone, when compared with historical data.[20] In a study looking at the concentrations of nelfinavir and its active metabolite M8, methadone had no effect on the AUC of nelfinavir, but the AUC_{0-12} of M8 was reduced by 48%.[21]

An HIV-positive man who had been taking methadone 100 mg daily for several years with indinavir 800 mg and zalcitabine 750 micrograms three times daily, developed opioid withdrawal symptoms within 6 weeks of starting to take stavudine and nelfinavir 750 mg three times daily. His methadone dose was increased to 285 mg daily before therapeutic serum concentrations were achieved. When his antiretroviral treatment was withdrawn, his methadone dose was successfully reduced to 125 mg daily.[13] Similarly, in a study finding reduced methadone exposure, within 5 to 7 days of starting nelfinavir-based therapy, symptoms of methadone withdrawal were seen in 4 of 6 patients and a mean increase in the methadone dose of 15% was required.[22]

A retrospective study of HIV-positive patients taking methadone reported that 5 out of 30 patients (17%) required methadone dose adjustments (mean 26 mg). The use of nelfinavir with methadone was effective and well tolerated.[23] A further study by the same authors reported that the mean methadone dose was increased by 10.6 mg with concurrent nelfinavir, when compared with methadone doses before nelfinavir was started.[24] A patient receiving methadone experienced torsade de pointes after starting to take nelfinavir.[25]

(h) Ritonavir

A patient receiving methadone experienced an opioid withdrawal syndrome when ritonavir was added to an antiretroviral regimen which included lamivudine and zidovudine.[26] A similar case is described in a patient, 4 days after the antiretroviral regimen was changed to ritonavir with indinavir, stavudine and nevirapine. A methadone dose increase was required.[14]

In a study, methadone apparently increased ritonavir exposure by 60%, when given alone, but had no effect on ritonavir pharmacokinetics when it was given with lopinavir.[18] Similarly, the pharmacokinetics of ritonavir 100 mg daily (given with atazanavir 300 mg daily) were no different between patients given methadone and matched controls in one study,[5] nor when given with saquinavir (1 g twice daily) and compared with historical controls.[27]

In healthy subjects, the miosis caused by oral and intravenous methadone was increased by the acute use of ritonavir for 3 days but returned to below baseline after longer-term use for 14 days. It appeared that acute ritonavir inhibited, but chronic ritonavir caused a small increase in methadone elimination.[28] A case of torsade de pointes has been reported in a patient taking methadone, atazanavir and ritonavir, see *Atazanavir*, above. For other pharmacokinetic studies, see 'Table 6.4', p.183.

(i) Saquinavir

In contrast to a study that found that methadone serum concentrations were not affected by saquinavir (see 'Table 6.4', p.183), an HIV-positive patient taking indinavir, lamivudine, and zidovudine, stabilised on methadone 90 mg daily, developed withdrawal symptoms and was hospitalised within a week of switching to saquinavir 400 mg with ritonavir 400 mg, and stavudine 40 mg twice daily. The patient was eventually re-stabilised on methadone 130 mg daily.[12] In the studies showing small or no reductions in exposure to *R*- and *S*-methadone (see 'Table 6.4', p.183), none of the subjects experienced methadone withdrawal,[27,29,30] or required a change in their methadone dose.[29]

In one study, the pharmacokinetics of saquinavir boosted with ritonavir 1000/100 mg were unchanged by methadone, when compared with historical controls.[27]

(j) Tipranavir

The manufacturers of tipranavir briefly note that in a study, the AUC and maximum plasma concentration of a single 5-mg dose of methadone were reduced by about 50% by tipranavir boosted with ritonavir 500/200 mg twice daily for 16 doses.[31,32]

Mechanism

Not known. The findings are the opposite of those originally predicted based on *in vitro* data showing *inhibition* of methadone metabolism (principally mediated by the subfamily CYP3A).[33] A 40 to 50% increase in the renal clearance of methadone has been reported with ritonavir, but this does not appear to be mediated by CYP3A as this occurred despite more than 70% inhibition of CYP3A by ritonavir.[34] It is possible that the HIV-protease inhibitors induce the activity of other isoenzymes or act by other mechanisms (e.g. glucuronosyltransferases). The reduction in methadone concentrations has not always correlated with clinical effects, and it has been suggested that this might be because the pharmacokinetics of the enantiomers (one of which is inactive) are affected differently, and/or altered protein binding occurs.[10,21,34]

Importance and management

Information is limited but the interactions of methadone with **amprenavir**, **nelfinavir**, **ritonavir**; and **darunavir**, **lopinavir**, **saquinavir**, and **tipranavir** (all boosted with ritonavir) would appear to be established. However, the picture seems to be that not all patients experience withdrawal symptoms if given these drugs. Therefore, in methadone-maintained patients, care should be taken if any of these HIV-protease inhibitors is started or stopped. It has been suggested that patients taking methadone who are given an HIV-protease inhibitor should be screened for opioid withdrawal beginning on the fourth day of the new medication. If symptoms develop, the methadone dose should be increased by 10 mg every 2 to 3 days until symptoms abate.[35] However, others have suggested dose increments should be made at one-week intervals to avoid overdose, as methadone has a long half-life (reported to range from 13 to 47 hours).[25] If the HIV-protease inhibitor is stopped the methadone dose should be gradually reduced to pretreatment amounts over the course of one to 2 weeks.[35]

The concentrations of methadone are minimally affected by **fosamprenavir** boosted with ritonavir and no withdrawal signs were reported in one study. However, despite noting that the interaction does not appear to be clinically relevant, the manufacturers still advise monitoring patients given both drugs for signs of opioid withdrawal, as a precaution.[36,37]

Amprenavir plasma concentrations might be reduced by methadone. The US manufacturer noted that amprenavir could be less effective if taken concurrently with methadone and suggested that alternative antiretroviral therapy should be considered.[38] In contrast, amprenavir concentrations from fosamprenavir boosted with ritonavir were not affected by the concurrent use of methadone.[10]

Indinavir appears not to interact with methadone, and very limited evidence suggests that **atazanavir** and **saquinavir** alone do not interact either.

The HIV-protease inhibitors appear to have contributed to the cases of QT prolongation and torsade de pointes reported above, and a retrospective study in HIV-positive patients reported that nelfinavir and methadone were independently associated with an increased risk of QTc prolongation.[39] Patients taking methadone in doses greater than 100 mg and with additional risk factors for QT prolongation (including taking other drugs that can prolong the QT interval) should be carefully monitored due to the risk of torsade de pointes, see 'Drugs that prolong the QT interval + Other drugs that prolong the QT interval', p.272.

1. Bart P-A, Rizzardi PG, Gallant S, Golay KP, Baumann P, Pantaleo G, Eap CB. Methadone blood concentrations are decreased by the administration of abacavir plus amprenavir. *Ther Drug Monit* (2001) 23, 553–5.
2. Hendrix CW, Wakeford J, Wire MB, Lou Y, Bigelow GE, Martinez E, Christopher J, Fuchs EJ, Snidow JW. Pharmacokinetics and pharmacodynamics of methadone enantiomers after coadministration with amprenavir in opioid-dependent subjects. *Pharmacotherapy* (2004) 24, 1110–21.
3. Friedland G, Andrews L, Schreibman T, Agarwala S, Daley L, Child M, Shi J, Wang Y, O'Mara E. Lack of an effect of atazanavir on steady-state pharmacokinetics of methadone in patients chronically treated for opiate addiction. *AIDS* (2005) 19, 1635–41.
4. Tossonian HK, Raffa JD, Grebely J, Trotter B, Viljoen M, Mead A, Khara M, McLean M, Duncan F, Fraser C, DeVlaming S, Conway B. Methadone dosing strategies in HIV-infected injection drug users enrolled in a directly observed therapy program. *J Acquir Immune Defic Syndr* (2007) 45, 324–7.
5. Haberl A, Moesch M, Nisius G, Stephan C, Bickel M, Khaykin P, Kurowski M, Brodt R, von Hentig N. Atazanavir plasma concentrations are impaired in HIV-1-infected adults simultaneously taking a methadone oral solution in a once-daily observed therapy setting. *Eur J Clin Pharmacol* (2010) 66, 375–81
6. Higgins N, Zingman BS, Slish J, Reichman RC, Fischl MA, Gripshover B, Tooley K, Boston N, Forrest A, Brazeau D, Catanzaro LM, DiFrancesco R, Lliguicota F, Ma Q, Morse GD. Factors associated with altered pharmacokinetics in substance users and non-substance users receiving lopinavir and atazanavir. *Am J Addict* (2007) 16, 488–94.
7. Falconer M, Molloy D, Ingerhaug J, Barry M. Methadone induced torsade de pointes in a patient receiving antiretroviral therapy. *Ir Med J* (2007) 100, 631–2.
8. Gallagher DP, Kieran J, Sheehan G, Lambert J, Mahon N, Mallon PWG. Ritonavir-boosted atazanavir, methadone, and ventricular tachycardia: 2 case reports. *Clin Infect Dis* (2008) 47, e36–e38.
9. Sekar V, Tomaka F, Lefebvre E, De Pauw M, Vangeneugden T, van den Brink W, Hoetelmans R. Pharmacokinetic interactions between darunavir/ritonavir and opioid maintenance therapy using methadone or buprenorphine/naloxone. *J Clin Pharmacol* (2011) 51, 271–8.
10. Cao Y-J, Smith PF, Wire MB, Lou Y, Lancaster CT, Causon RC, Bigelow GE, Martinez E, Fuchs EJ, Radebaugh C, McCabe S, Hendrix CW. Pharmacokinetics and pharmacodynamics of methadone enantiomers after coadministration with fosamprenavir-ritonavir in opioid-dependent subjects. *Pharmacotherapy* (2008) 28, 863–74.
11. Cantilena L, McCrea J, Blazes D, Winchell G, Carides A, Royce C, Deutsch P. Lack of a pharmacokinetic interaction between indinavir and methadone. *Clin Pharmacol Ther* (1999) 65, 135.
12. Geletko SM, Erickson AD. Decreased methadone effect after ritonavir initiation. *Pharmacotherapy* (2000) 20, 93–4.
13. McCance-Katz EF, Farber S, Selwyn PA, O'Connor A. Decrease in methodone levels with nelfinavir mesylate. *Am J Psychiatry* (2000) 157, 481.
14. de la Cruz Pellín M, Esteban J, Gimeno C, Mora E. Interaction between methadone and antiretrovirals (stavudine, indinavir, ritonavir, nevirapine). *Med Clin (Barc)* (2003) 121, 439.
15. McCance-Katz EF, Rainey PM, Friedland G, Jatlow P. The protease inhibitor lopinavir-ritonavir may produce opiate withdrawal in methadone-maintained patients. *Clin Infect Dis* (2003) 37, 476–82.
16. Clarke S, Mulcahy F, Bergin C, Reynolds H, Boyle N, Barry M, Back DJ. Absence of opioid withdrawal symptoms in patients receiving methadone and the protease inhibitor lopinavir-ritonavir. *Clin Infect Dis* (2002) 34, 1143–5.
17. Stevens RC, Rapaport S, Maroldo-Connelly L, Patterson JB, Bertz R. Lack of methadone dose alterations or withdrawal symptoms during therapy with lopinavir/ritonavir. *J Acquir Immune Defic Syndr* (2003) 33, 650–1.
18. Smith P, McCance-Katz E, Sarlo J, Di Francesco R, Morse GD. Methadone increases ritonavir (RTV) exposure when administered alone but not lopinavir/RTV combination. *Intersci Conf Antimicrob Agents Chemother* (2003) 43, 339.
19. Lüthi B, Huttner A, Speck RF, Mueller NJ. Methadone-induced torsade de pointes after stopping lopinavir-ritonavir. *Eur J Clin Microbiol Infect Dis* (2007) 26, 367–9.
20. Hsyu P-H, Lillibridge J, Daniels E, Kerr BM. Pharmacokinetic interaction of nelfinavir and methadone in intravenous drug users. *Biopharm Drug Dispos* (2006) 27, 61–8.
21. McCance-Katz EF, Rainey PM, Smith P, Morse G, Friedland G, Gourevitch M, Jatlow P. Drug interactions between opioids and antiretroviral medications: interaction between methadone, LAAM, and nelfinavir. *Am J Addict* (2004) 13, 163 –80.
22. Clarke S, Mulcahy F, Bergin C, Tjia J, Brown R, Barry M, Back DJ. The pharmacokinetic interaction between methadone and nelfinavir [abstract P276]. *AIDS* (2000) 14 (Suppl 4), S95.
23. Brown LS, Chu M, Aug C, Dabo S. The use of nelfinavir and two nucleosides concomitantly with methadone is effective and well-tolerated in HepC co-infected patients. *Intersci Conf Antimicrob Agents Chemother* (2001) 41, 311.
24. Brown LS, Kritz S, Chu M, Madray C. Safety, efficacy, and tolerability of nelfinavir-containing antiretroviral therapy for patients coinfected with HIV and hepatitis C undergoing methadone maintenance. *J Subst Abuse Treat* (2006) 30, 331–5.
25. Anon. Torsades de pointes with methadone. *Prescrire Int* (2005) 14, 61–2.
26. Jiménez-Lerma JM, Iraurgi I. Probable síndrome de abstinencia a opiáceos tras la administración de ritonavir en un paciente en tratamiento con metadona. *Rev Clin Esp* (1999) 199, 188–9.
27. Jamois C, Smith P, Morrison R, Riek M, Patel A, Schmitt C, Morcos PN, Zhang X. Effect of saquinavir/ritonavir (1000/100 mg bid) on the pharmacokinetics of methadone in opiate-dependent HIV-negative patients on stable methadone maintenance therapy. *Addict Biol* (2009) 14, 321–7.
28. Kharasch ED, Hoffer C. Assessment of ritonavir effects on hepatic and first-pass CYP3A activity and methadone disposition using noninvasive pupillometry. *Clin Pharmacol Ther* (2004) 75, P96.
29. Gerber JG, Rosenkranz S, Segal Y, Aberg J, D'Amico R, Mildvan D, Gulick R, Hughes V, Flexner C, Aweeka F, Hsu A, Gal J. Effect of ritonavir/saquinavir on stereoselective pharmacokinetics of methadone: Results of AIDS Clinical Trials Group (ACTG) 401. *J Acquir Immune Defic Syndr* (2001) 27, 153–60.
30. Shelton MJ, Cloen D, DiFrancesco R, Berenson CS, Esch A, de Caprariis PJ, Palic B, Schur JL, Buggé CJL, Ljungqvist A, Espinosa O, Hewitt RG. The effects of once-daily saquinavir/minidose ritonavir on the pharmacokinetics of methadone. *J Clin Pharmacol* (2004) 44, 293–304.
31. Aptivus Soft Capsules (Tipranavir). Boehringer Ingelheim Ltd. UK Summary of product characteristics, December 2013.
32. Aptivus (Tipranavir). Boehringer Ingelheim Pharmaceuticals, Inc. US Prescribing information, April 2012.
33. Iribarne C, Berthou F, Carlhant D, Dreano Y, Picart D, Lohezic F, Riche C. Inhibition of methadone and buprenorphine *N*-dealkylations by three HIV-1 protease inhibitors. *Drug Metab Dispos* (1998) 26, 257–60.
34. Kharasch ED, Bedynek PS, Park S, Whittington D, Walker A, Hoffer C. Mechanism of ritonavir changes in methadone pharmacokinetics and pharmacodynamics: I. Evidence against CYP3A mediation of methadone clearance. *Clin Pharmacol Ther* (2008) 84, 497–505.
35. Bruce RD, Altice FL, Gourevitch MN, Friedland GH. Pharmacokinetic drug interactions between opioid agonist therapy and antiretroviral medications: implications and management for clinical practice. *J Acquir Immune Defic Syndr* (2006) 41, 563–72.
36. Telzir (Fosamprenavir calcium). ViiV Healthcare UK Ltd. UK Summary of product characteristics, October 2013.
37. Lexiva (Fosamprenavir calcium). ViiV Healthcare. US Prescribing information, April 2013.
38. Agenerase (Amprenavir). GlaxoSmithKline. US Prescribing information, May 2005.
39. Chinello P, Lisena FP, Angeletti C, Boumis E, Papetti F, Petrosillo N. Role of antiretroviral treatment in prolonging QTc interval in HIV-positive patients. *J Infect* (2007) 54, 597–602.

Opioids + Hormonal contraceptives

The clearance of morphine is roughly doubled by oral combined hormonal contraceptives. Oral combined hormonal contraceptives do not appear to alter the pharmacokinetics of pethidine (meperidine). Gestodene is predicted to increase the exposure to buprenorphine.

Clinical evidence, mechanism, importance and management

(a) Buprenorphine

An *in vitro* study reported that **gestodene** inhibited the metabolism of buprenorphine to norbuprenorphine by CYP3A4 by about 60 to 70%.[1] Based on data from a study with the CYP3A4 inhibitor ketoconazole, where the AUC of buprenorphine was increased by about 50% (see 'Opioids + Azoles', p.165), the UK manufacturer predicts that other CYP3A4 inhibitors might also increase the exposure to buprenorphine, and they specifically name **gestodene**. They advise that a buprenorphine dose reduction should be considered when initiating treatment.[2] Halving the starting dose of buprenorphine has been suggested for patients taking CYP3A4 inhibitors and receiving buprenorphine as a substitute for opioid dependence.[2] However, the same manufacturer suggests that, as the magnitude of an inhibitory effect is unknown, such drug combinations should be avoided when buprenorphine is used parenterally or sublingually as a strong analgesic.[3,4] Also note that there appear to be no clinical cases or studies reporting interactions where **gestodene** is acting as a clinically relevant CYP3A4 inhibitor or has specifically affected the metabolism of buprenorphine or other opioids, so the appropriateness of any dose adjustment remains to be established.

(b) Morphine

The clearance of intravenous morphine 1 mg and oral morphine 10 mg was increased by 75% and 120%, respectively, in 6 young women taking an oral combined hormonal contraceptive.[5] It was suggested that the oestrogen component of the contraceptive increases the activity of the liver enzyme (glucuronyltransferase) concerned with the metabolism of morphine, which results in an increased clearance. This implies that the dose of morphine would need to be increased to achieve the same degree of analgesia. Whether this is required in practice needs confirmation; however as the dose of morphine is usually titrated to effect, the clinical relevance of any effect seems likely to be small.

(c) Pethidine (Meperidine)

One early study suggested that 4 of 5 women taking an oral combined hormonal contraceptive (**mestranol** with **noretynodrel** or **norethisterone**) excreted more unchanged pethidine in the urine than a control group of 4 women not taking contraceptives, who were found to excrete more of the demethylated metabolite.[6] However a later, well-controlled, comparative study in 24 healthy subjects (8 women taking **ethinylestradiol** 50 micrograms with **norgestrel** 500 micrograms, and 8 women and 8 men not taking contraceptives) found no differences between the plasma concentrations or excretion patterns of pethidine between the three groups.[7] No special precautions therefore appear to be needed if pethidine is given to women taking combined hormonal contraceptives.

1. Iribarne C, Picart D, Dréano Y, Bail J-P, Berthou F. Involvement of cytochrome P450 3A4 in N-dealkylation of buprenorphine in human liver microsomes. *Life Sci* (1997) 60, 1953–64.
2. Subutex (Buprenorphine hydrochloride). RB Pharmaceuticals Ltd. UK Summary of product characteristics, September 2014.
3. Temgesic Injection (Buprenorphine hydrochloride). RB Pharmaceuticals Ltd. UK Summary of product characteristics, September 2010.
4. Temgesic Sublingual Tablets (Buprenorphine hydrochloride). RB Pharmaceuticals Ltd. UK Summary of product characteristics, September 2010.
5. Watson KJR, Ghabrial H, Mashford ML, Harman PJ, Breen KJ, Desmond PV. The oral contraceptive pill increases morphine clearance but does not increase hepatic blood flow. *Gastroenterology* (1986) 90, 1779.
6. Crawford JS, Rudofsky S. Some alterations in the pattern of drug metabolism associated with pregnancy, oral contraceptives, and the newly-born. *Br J Anaesth* (1966) 38, 446–54.
7. Stambaugh JE, Wainer IW. Drug interactions I: meperidine and combination oral contraceptives. *J Clin Pharmacol* (1975) 15, 46–51.

Opioids + Interferons

Peginterferon alfa-2a and alfa-2b do not affect the pharmacokinetics of methadone, but an isolated report describes a patient who relapsed to heroin use following treatment with peginterferon. Methadone maintenance does not appear to affect the pharmacokinetics of peginterferon alfa-2a. Neither methadone nor buprenorphine maintenance appear to alter the virological response to interferons used to treat hepatitis C.

Clinical evidence and mechanism

A study involving 22 patients with chronic hepatitis C who had been receiving **methadone** maintenance for at least 3 months found that subcutaneous **peginterferon alfa-2a** 180 micrograms once weekly for 4 weeks increased the methadone AUC by 10 to 15%. The pharmacokinetics of **peginterferon alfa-2a** did not appear to be altered by **methadone** when compared with values from other patients.[1] Similarly, a study involving 20 patients with chronic hepatitis C and taking **methadone** for at least 3 months reported an increase in the AUC and maximum concentration of methadone of about 15% when **peginterferon alfa-2b** 1.5 micrograms/kg per week for 4 weeks was also given.[2] Another study in 9 patients with hepatitis C and HIV infections taking **methadone** 40 to 200 mg daily for at least 8 weeks, found that two doses of **peginterferon alfa-2b** 1.5 micrograms/kg, given one week apart, had no effect on the pharmacokinetics of methadone. Similarly, no evidence of opiate toxicity or withdrawal occurred during concurrent use. Subjects were not taking HIV medication known to interact with methadone (such as ritonavir).[3] However, a case report describes a patient who stopped taking **methadone** and then relapsed to heroin use approximately 5 months after completing treatment for chronic hepatitis C with peginterferon 180 micrograms per week and ribavirin.[4]

Note that a number of clinical studies suggest that the use of opioids (**buprenorphine**[5,6] and **methadone**[5-12]) has no effect on the outcome of treatment with interferon or peginterferon in patients with chronic hepatitis C, although one study suggests that opioids might facilitate the outbreak of infections through immunomodulating effects on the immune response against a virus.[7]

Importance and management

Interferon does not affect the pharmacokinetics of methadone to a clinically relevant extent. Despite the minor changes reported, the UK manufacturers of peginterferon alfa-2a and alfa-2b advise monitoring for methadone toxicity,[13] such as increased sedation and respiratory depression with concurrent use.[14] Note that patients taking methadone might experience increased cravings while receiving antiviral therapy as the adverse effects of interferons can mimic opioid withdrawal symptoms, and cravings can be secondary to mood changes caused by antiviral therapy, or be related to the use of needles used to deliver interferon.[4] It might therefore, be necessary to increase the dose of methadone during interferon treatment.[4,5] Note also, that as alfa interferons are associated with a risk of psychiatric disturbance and suicide, the US manufacturer of interferon alfa-2b advises that opioids should be used with caution.[15]

There appears to be no specific pharmacokinetic data relating to the use of other interferons with methadone or other opioids. It has been suggested that interferons might theoretically reduce the activity of hepatic cytochrome P450 and hence increase the exposure to drugs metabolised by this route. However, clinical evidence of such an effect is lacking, and so the general relevance of this potential interaction is unknown. Further study is needed.

1. Sulkowski M, Wright T, Rossi S, Arora S, Lamb M, Wang K, Gries J-M, Yalamanchili S. Peginterferon alfa-2a does not alter the pharmacokinetics of methadone in patients with chronic hepatitis C undergoing methadone maintenance therapy. *Clin Pharmacol Ther* (2005) 77, 214–24.
2. Gupta SK, Sellers E, Somoza E, Angles L, Kolz K, Cutler DL. The effect of multiple doses of peginterferon alfa-2b on the steady-state pharmacokinetics of methadone in patients with chronic hepatitis C undergoing methadone maintenance therapy. *J Clin Pharmacol* (2007) 47, 604–12. Correction. ibid., (2007) 47, 1061.
3. Berk SI, Litwin AH, Arnsten JH, Du E, Soloway I, Gourevitch MN. Effects of pegylated interferon alfa-2b on the pharmacokinetic and pharmacodynamic properties of methadone: a prospective, nonrandomized, crossover study in patients coinfected with hepatitis C and HIV receiving methadone maintenance treatment. *Clin Ther* (2007) 29, 131–8.
4. Matthews AM, Fireman M, Zucker B, Sobel M, Hauser P. Relapse to opioid use after treatment of chronic hepatitis C with pegylated interferon and ribavirin. *Am J Psychiatry* (2006) 163, 1342–7.
5. Verrando R, Robaeys G, Mathei C, Buntinx F. Methadone and buprenorphine maintenance therapies for patients with hepatitis C virus infected after intravenous drug use. *Acta Gastroenterol Belg* (2005) 68, 81–5.
6. Belfiori B, Ciliegi P, Chiodera A, Bacosi D, Tosti A, Baldelli F, Francisci D. Peginterferon plus ribavarin for chronic hepatitis C in opiate addicts on methadone/buprenorphine maintenance therapy. *Dig Liver Dis* (2009) 41, 303–7.
7. Sergio N, Salvatore T, Gaetano B, Davide P, Claudio I, Massimo L, Barbara M, Giuseppe A, Stefano C, Danila C, Aikaterini T, Luca I, Daniela C, Luciano C. Immune response in addicts with chronic hepatitis C treated with interferon and ribavirin. *J Gastroenterol Hepatol* (2007) 22, 74–9.
8. Mauss S, Berger F, Goelz J, Jacob B, Schmutz G. A prospective controlled study of interferon-based therapy of chronic hepatitis C in patients on methadone maintenance. *Hepatology* (2004) 40, 120–4.
9. Van Thiel DH, Anantharaju A, Creech S. Response to treatment of hepatitis C in individuals with a recent history of intravenous drugs abuse. *Am J Gastroenterol* (2003) 98, 2281–8.
10. Neukam K, Mira JA, Gilabert I, Claro E, Vázquez MJ, Cifuentes C, García-Rey S, Merchante N, Almeida C, Macías J, Pineda JA. Efficacy of chronic hepatitis C therapy with pegylated interferon and ribavirin in patients on methadone maintenance treatment. *Eur J Clin Microbiol Infect Dis* (2012) 31, 1225–32.
11. Litwin AH, Harris KA, Nahvi S, Zamor PJ, Soloway IJ, Tenore PL, Kaswan D, Gourevitch MN, Arnsten JH. Successful treatment of chroni hepatitis C with pegylated interferon in combination with ribavirin in a methadone maintenance treatment program. *J Subst Abuse Treat* (2009) 37, 32–40.
12. Bonkovsky HL, Tice AD, Yapp RG, Bodenheimer HC, Monto A, Rossi SJ, Sulkowski MS. Efficacy and safety of peginterferon alfa-2a/ribavirin in methadone maintenance patients: randomized comparison of direct observed therapy and self-administration. *Am J Gastroenterol* (2008) 103, 2757–65.
13. Pegasys (Peginterferon alfa-2a). Roche Products Ltd. UK Summary of product characteristics, October 2013.
14. ViraferonPeg (Peginterferon alfa-2b). Merck Sharp and Dohme Ltd. UK Summary of product characteristics, May 2013.
15. Intron A (Interferon alfa-2b). Merck and Co. Inc. US Prescribing information, November 2013.

Opioids + Levothyroxine

Two case reports describe increased morphine and oxycodone requirements after levothyroxine dose increases.

Clinical evidence, mechanism, importance and management

A report describes 2 patients with chronic pain and hypothyroidism, who experienced increased pain and an increased requirement for pain control, following an increase in their levothyroxine doses. In one case, the patient was taking controlled-release **oxycodone** 20 mg three times daily, with 15 mg four times daily as needed. She reported exacerbations of pain necessitating increased use of oxycodone, and had pain scores about double those measured previously, 2 months after her levothyroxine dose was increased from 225 micrograms daily to 300 micrograms daily. The other patient was taking controlled-release **morphine** 50 mg three to four times daily with **oxycodone**/acetaminophen 10/325 mg three times daily as needed. Similarly, she reported exacerbation of her pain requiring increased use of analgesia after her levothyroxine dose was increased by 100 to 122 micrograms daily.[1] Note that both patients had complex medical histories and numerous concurrent medicines, but the only changes noted were in levothyroxine dose (and hence thyroid status).

It is not clear whether the effects seen here represent a drug-drug interaction, or are in fact the result of a drug-disease interaction, that is, whether changes in thyroid status alter opioid pharmacokinetics or pain nociception. Further study is needed.

1. Matoushek TA, Kearney TC, Lindsay TJ, Herndon CM. Loss of antinociceptive effectiveness of morphine and oxycodone following titration of levothyroxine: case reports and a brief review of published literature. *J Opioid Manag* (2012) 8, 193–8.

Opioids + Macrolides

Clarithromycin and telithromycin decrease the metabolism of oxycodone, and erythromycin might interact similarly. Macrolides that inhibit CYP3A4 are predicted to increase buprenorphine bioavailability. It has been suggested that the metabolism of methadone could be decreased by some macrolides, but there do not appear to be any clinical reports confirming this. QT-interval prolongation has been reported in a patient taking methadone with azithromycin.

Clinical evidence, mechanism, importance and management

(a) Buprenorphine

Although no data from clinical studies are available, the UK and US manufacturers of buprenorphine predict that inhibitors of CYP3A4, such as the macrolides, could increase buprenorphine concentrations. One manufacturer recommends close monitoring and possibly a dose reduction,[1] while another specifically suggests using half the dose of buprenorphine if CYP3A4 inhibitors are given.[2] This would be expected to include **erythromycin**, **clarithromycin**, and **telithromycin**.

(b) Fentanyl and related drugs

For the interactions of the macrolides with alfentanil, fentanyl, or sufentanil, see 'Opioids; Fentanyl and related drugs + Macrolides', p.187.

(c) Methadone

Methadone is metabolised, at least in part, by CYP3A4, and one UK manufacturer warns that its clearance might be decreased if it is given with drugs that inhibit CYP3A4 activity, such as some macrolides.[3] Note that decreased methadone metabolism has been seen with some of the azoles (see 'Opioids + Azoles', p.165), which are well-known CYP3A4 inhibitors. Until more is known, it might be prudent to monitor concurrent use for increased and prolonged sedation if **erythromycin**, **clarithromycin**, or **telithromycin** is given with methadone, and adjust the dose of methadone accordingly.

A case report describes QT prolongation in a 47-year-old man taking methadone 30 mg three times daily, 3 days after **azithromycin** was started. The patient had no risk factors for QT prolongation and opiate overdose was ruled out. The authors of the report suggested that because of the timing of the QT prolongation in relation to the azithromycin, the case might have been a result of the additive effects of methadone and azithromycin on the QT interval.[4] Note that **azithromycin** does not inhibit CYP3A4, although no methadone concentrations were measured in the report. Methadone in doses greater than 100 mg has some risk of prolonging the QT interval. Patients taking more than methadone 100 mg and with additional risk factors for QT prolongation (including taking other drugs that can prolong the QT interval, such as some macrolides) should be carefully monitored due to the risk of torsade de pointes, see 'Drugs that prolong the QT interval + Other drugs that prolong the QT interval', p.272.

(d) Oxycodone

In a randomised, crossover study, 11 healthy subjects were given **telithromycin** 800 mg daily or placebo for 4 days, with a single 10-mg dose of oxycodone on day 3. **Telithromycin** increased the AUC of oxycodone by almost 80% and decreased its oral clearance by 43%. In addition, **telithromycin** decreased subject-rated measures of performance, increased subject-rated measures of drug effect, and decreased pupil size.[5] In another randomised, crossover study, 20 healthy subjects (10 young and 10 elderly) were given **clarithromycin** 500 mg twice daily or placebo for 5 days with a single 10-mg oral dose of oxycodone on day 4. The AUC of oxycodone was increased 2-fold and 2.3-fold in young and elderly subjects, respectively. The pharmacological response to oxycodone (e.g. pupil size, performance in psychometric tests) was not altered in any of the subjects.[6] Oxycodone is principally metabolised by CYP3A4, of which **clarithromycin** and **telithromycin** are known inhibitors. Concurrent use therefore decreases oxycodone metabolism, leading to increased exposure and increased effects. The authors of the **telithromycin** study suggest that repeated use of oxycodone in patients taking **telithromycin** might lead to greater effects, and suggest that a dose decrease of 25 to 50% could be necessary, with further titration according to response. The authors of the study with **clarithromycin** suggest that oxycodone dose reductions might be necessary in the most sensitive patients if oxycodone is given with **clarithromycin**. Both pieces of advice would seem prudent. Information about other macrolides is lacking, but **erythromycin** is also known to inhibit CYP3A4 and might therefore be expected to interact similarly. Until more is known, similar precautions to those suggested for **telithromycin** and **clarithromycin** would seem prudent.

(e) Tramadol

Some UK and US manufacturers of tramadol predict that inhibitors of CYP3A4 such as erythromycin might inhibit the metabolism of tramadol and that of its active metabolite.[7-9] Further, some suggest that this might increase the risk of tramadol adverse effects such as seizures and serotonin syndrome.[7,8] There is an isolated case of visual-auditory hallucinations that occurred two days after starting tramadol and **clarithromycin** that was attributed to a drug interaction.[10] However, there appears to be no other evidence of any interactions of tramadol with erythromycin or other macrolides that are inhibitors of CYP3A4. As such, a clinically relevant pharmacokinetic interaction would not be expected.

1. Buprenorphine Hydrochloride Injection. American Regent Inc. US Prescribing information, December 2009.
2. Subutex (Buprenorphine hydrochloride). RB Pharmaceuticals Ltd. UK Summary of product characteristics, September 2014.
3. Synastone (Methadone hydrochloride). Auden McKenzie (Pharma Division) Ltd. UK Summary of product characteristics, June 2015.
4. Winton JC, Twilla JD. Sudden cardiac arrest in a patient on chronic methadone after the addition of azithromycin. *Am J Med Sci* (2013) 345, 160–2.
5. Grönlund J, Saari T, Hagelberg N, Martikainen IK, Neuvonen PJ, Olkkola KT, Laine K. Effect of telithromycin on the pharmacokinetics and pharmacodynamics of oral oxycodone. *J Clin Pharmacol* (2010) 50, 101–108.
6. Liukas A, Hagelberg NM, Kuusniemi K, Neuvonen PJ, Olkkola KT. Inhibition of cytochrome P450 3A by clarithromycin uniformly affects the pharmacokinetics and pharmacodynamics of oxycodone in young and elderly volunteers. *J Clin Psychopharmacol* (2011) 31, 302–8.
7. Rybix ODT (Tramadol hydrochloride). Shionogi Inc. US Prescribing information, August 2011
8. Ultram ER (Tramadol hydrochloride). PriCara. US Prescribing information, June 2009.
9. Zydol (Tramadol hydrochloride). Grünenthal Ltd. UK Summary of product characteristics, August 2013.
10. Kovács G, Péter L. Komplex hallucináció (vizuális-auditív) tramadol és clarithromycin együttadása során. *Neuropsychopharmacol Hung* (2010) 12, 309–12.

Opioids; Fentanyl and related drugs + Macrolides

Some patients might experience prolonged and increased alfentanil effects if they are given erythromycin. Two cases of serious respiratory depression have been described in patients receiving transdermal fentanyl, after clarithromycin was added. Erythromycin appears not to interact with sufentanil.

Clinical evidence

(a) Clarithromycin

A case report describes an 81-year-old man with advanced COPD, stabilised on transdermal fentanyl 200 micrograms/hour for chronic pain, who developed serious respiratory depression (hypoventilation, respiratory rate of 2 breaths per minute, and unresponsive to verbal or tactile stimuli) within 36 hours of starting clarithromycin 500 mg twice daily for *H. pylori* eradication. He recovered consciousness after he was given naloxone and his respiratory rate increased. The fentanyl patch was discontinued and opioid withdrawal symptoms were managed with morphine. The following day he was alert, conversive, and had a normal respiratory rate and oxygen saturation. The clarithromycin was stopped and the fentanyl restarted at 50% of his dose at admission, without increased pain or opioid toxicity.[1] Similarly, another case report describes respiratory arrest in a 72-year-old woman, 2 days after clarithromycin 500 mg twice daily was added to existing medication which included transdermal fentanyl 87 micrograms/hour. She was treated with naloxone and the fentanyl was stopped until the course of clarithromycin had been completed. The fentanyl was then restarted without event.[2]

(b) Erythromycin

Erythromycin 500 mg twice daily for 7 days increased the half-life of **alfentanil** in 6 subjects by 55% (from 84 minutes to 131 minutes) and decreased its clearance by 26%. There was notable variability between the subjects, with considerable changes in both half-life and clearance in the two most sensitive subjects after only one day of erythromycin, which were maintained over the 7-day study period. The other 4 subjects showed more modest changes.[3] A 32-year-old man undergoing an exploratory laparotomy was given erythromycin 1 g and neomycin 1 g, both three times daily, on the day before surgery. During the induction and maintenance of anaesthesia he received a total of 20.9 mg of **alfentanil**. One hour after recovery he was found to be unrousable, with a respiratory rate of only 5 breaths per minute. He was successfully treated with naloxone.[4] Another patient given **alfentanil** and erythromycin is said to have developed respiratory arrest during recovery.[5]

In 6 healthy subjects erythromycin 500 mg twice daily for 7 days did not affect the pharmacokinetics of intravenous **sufentanil** 3 micrograms/kg in the 9 hours following administration.[6] Two of the subjects were the same as those who had an interaction with alfentanil and erythromycin, as cited above.

Mechanism

Erythromycin and clarithromycin inhibit CYP3A4 in the liver, which is involved in the metabolism of alfentanil, fentanyl, and sufentanil. Alfentanil is a low-extraction drug cleared mainly by hepatic metabolism,[7] whereas fentanyl and sufentanil are high-extraction drugs (see 'Changes in first-pass metabolism', p.4), and so are more affected by changes in hepatic blood flow than effects on the isoenzymes responsible for their metabolism; they are therefore less affected by CYP3A inhibitors than alfentanil. Alterations in intestinal or hepatic CYP3A activity also appear to have little influence on oral transmucosal fentanyl absorption and onset of effect; however, a large proportion (approximately 75%) is swallowed and its systemic clearance can be decreased by CYP3A inhibitors.[8,9]

Importance and management

The interaction of **alfentanil** with erythromycin appears to be established and clinically important. Clarithromycin and telithromycin are also CYP3A4 inhibitors (and are more potent than erythromycin), and so would be expected to interact similarly or possibly have a greater effect. Alfentanil should be given in reduced amounts or avoided in those who are taking, or who have recently taken any of these drugs.[3] Be alert for evidence of prolonged alfentanil effects and respiratory depression. Note that the interaction appears not to affect all patients given erythromycin. Alternatively, **sufentanil** in doses of 3 micrograms/kg or less might be used with erythromycin, but much larger doses of sufentanil should be given with caution.[6] It would seem prudent to apply similar advice to the concurrent use of sufentanil with clarithromycin and telithromycin. Based on the interaction with alfentanil and sufentanil, intravenous **fentanyl** can probably be used safely with erythromycin, but until more is known, it might be prudent to apply some caution to the use of oral transmucosal fentanyl, which could be swallowed in sufficient quantities to provoke an interaction. Fentanyl by any route of administration should probably be used with caution with clarithromycin and telithromycin. Therefore, if fentanyl is given with clarithromycin or telithromycin, and if erythromycin is given with oral transmucosal fentanyl, monitor for increased and prolonged effects, particularly sedation, and adjust the fentanyl dose accordingly.

1. Horton R, Barber C. Opioid-induced respiratory depression resulting from transdermal fentanyl-clarithromycin drug interaction in a patient with advanced COPD. *J Pain Symptom Manage* (2009) 37, e2–e5.
2. Cronnolly B, Pegrum H. Fentanyl-clarithromycin interaction. *BMJ Case Rep* (2012) Epub.
3. Bartkowski RR, Goldberg ME, Larijani GE, Boerner T. Inhibition of alfentanil metabolism by erythromycin. *Clin Pharmacol Ther* (1989) 46, 99–102.
4. Bartkowski RR, McDonnell TE. Prolonged alfentanil effect following erythromycin administration. *Anesthesiology* (1990) 73, 566–8.
5. Yate PM, Thomas D, Short SM, Sebel PS, Morton J. Comparison of infusions of alfentanil or pethidine for sedation of ventilated patients on the ITU. *Br J Anaesth* (1986) 58, 1091–9.
6. Bartkowski RR, Goldberg ME, Huffnagle S, Epstein RH. Sufentanil disposition. Is it affected by erythromycin administration? *Anesthesiology* (1993) 78, 260–5.
7. Kharasch ED, Walker A, Hoffer C, Sheffels P. Intravenous and oral alfentanil as in vivo probes for hepatic and first-pass cytochrome P450 3A activity: non-invasive assessment by use of pupillary miosis. *Clin Pharmacol Ther* (2004) 76, 452–66.
8. Kharasch ED, Whittington D, Hoffer C. Influence of hepatic and intestinal cytochrome P4503A activity on the acute disposition and effects of oral transmucosal fentanyl citrate. *Anesthesiology* (2004) 101, 729–37.
9. Actiq (Fentanyl citrate lozenge). Teva Pharmaceuticals Ltd. UK Summary of product characteristics, June 2015.

Opioids + Magnesium compounds

Magnesium compounds can potentiate opioid analgesia, although some studies have failed to find an effect. Magnesium sulfate may also reduce opioid requirements during anaesthesia. Magnesium can delay the onset of spinal anaesthesia in patients given fentanyl with bupivacaine.

Clinical evidence, mechanism, importance and management

Three meta-analyses of randomised studies involving the perioperative use of intravenous magnesium, generally conclude that such use reduces postoperative opioid consumption,[1-3] but its effect on pain scores is not conclusive; with 2 reviews finding minimal effects on pain scores,[2,3] and one finding a reduction.[1] One review additionally concluded that the reduction in opioid consumption does not necessarily result in reduced opioid adverse effects.[2] Several clinical studies not included in these analyses have also found that magnesium enhances the analgesic effect of opioids, including intrathecal magnesium with intrathecal **fentanyl**,[4] and intravenous magnesium with intravenous **fentanyl**.[5] Magnesium sulfate infusion has also been reported to decrease **sufentanil** requirements for sedation.[6] In contrast, other studies have reported no beneficial effect with peri- or postoperative use of magnesium on postoperative **morphine** or **pethidine (meperidine)** requirements.[7,8]

Respiratory depression occurred in a patient with congenital myopathy following intramuscular administration of morphine for pain relief during labour and the subsequent administration of magnesium for hypertension and proteinuria. This was possibly due to an interaction between the magnesium and morphine; however, other factors could also have contributed.[9]

In general, no additional serious adverse effects were reported in these studies, although one study found that the perioperative use of intravenous magnesium sulfate appeared to increase intraoperative blood loss at caesarean delivery. However, as magnesium is a tocolytic and can cause uterine atony, an increase in bleeding would be expected.[7]

Intrathecal magnesium sulfate prolonged the period of spinal anaesthesia induced by bupivacaine and **fentanyl** without additional adverse effects, but the onset of anaesthesia was also notably delayed.[10]

Divalent cations appear to be involved in the pain pathway and magnesium sulfate can potentiate the opioid analgesic effect,[6] possibly by antagonism of *N*-methyl-D-aspartate receptor ion channels.[6,11] It has been suggested that as magnesium ions do not easily cross the blood brain barrier, the intrathecal use of magnesium could modulate pain relief via central effects, whereas the intravenous route mainly affects peripheral mechanisms.[12] If anything, these interactions appear to be generally beneficial, and no particular precautions seem necessary.

1. De Oliveira GS, Castro-Alves LJ, Khan JH, McCarthy RJ. Perioperative systemic magnesium to minimize postoperative pain: a meta-analysis of randomized controlled trials. *Anesthesiology* (2013) 119, 178–90.
2. Murphy JD, Paskaradevan J, Eisler LL, Ouanes JPP, Tomas VA, Freck EZ, Wu CL. Analgesic efficacy of continuous intravenous magnesium infusion as an adjuvant to morphine for postoperative analgesia: a systematic review and meta-analysis. *Middle East J Anesthesiol* (2013) 22, 11–20.
3. Albrecht E, Kirkham KR, Liu SS, Brull R. Peri-operative intravenous administration of magnesium sulphate and postoperative pain: a meta-analysis. *Anaesthesia* (2013) 68, 79–90. PMID:
4. Buvanendran A, McCarthy RJ, Kroin JS, Leong W, Perry P, Tuman KJ. Intrathecal magnesium prolongs fentanyl analgesia: a prospective, randomized, controlled trial. *Anesth Analg* (2002) 95, 661–6.
5. Gupta K, Vohra V, Sood J. The role of magnesium as an adjuvant during general anaesthesia. *Anaesthesia* (2006) 61, 1058–63.
6. Memiş D, Turan A, Karamanlioğlu B, Oğuzhan N, Pamukçu Z. Comparison of sufentanil with sufentanil plus magnesium sulphate for sedation in the intensive care unit using bispectral index. *Crit Care* (2003) 7, R123–R128.
7. Paech MJ, Magann EF, Doherty DA, Verity LJ, Newnham JP. Does magnesium sulfate reduce the short- and long-term requirements for pain relief after caesarean delivery? A double-blind placebo-controlled trial. *Am J Obstet Gynecol* (2006) 194, 1596–1603.
8. Machowska B, Duda K. [Does intravenous administration of magnesium affect postoperative analgesia?]. *Folia Med Cracov* (2001) 42, 255–62.
9. Robins K, Lyons G. Opioid-related narcosis in a woman with myopathy receiving magnesium. *Int J Obstet Anesth* (2007) 16, 367–9.
10. Özalevli M, Cetin TO, Unlugenc H, Guler T, Isik G. The effect of adding intrathecal magnesium sulphate to bupivacaine-fentanyl spinal anaesthesia. *Acta Anaesthesiol Scand* (2005) 49, 1514–19.
11. Ünlügenç H, Gündüz M, Özalevli M, Akman H. A comparative study on the analgesic effect of tramadol, tramadol plus magnesium, and tramadol plus ketamine for postoperative pain management after major abdominal surgery. *Acta Anaesthesiol Scand* (2002) 46, 1025–30.
12. Steinlechner B, Dworschak M, Birkenberg B, Grubhofer G, Weigl M, Schiferer A, Lang T, Rajek A. Magnesium moderately decreases remifentanil dosage required for pain management after cardiac surgery. *Br J Anaesth* (2006) 96, 444–9.

Opioids; Alfentanil + NNRTIs; Efavirenz

Efavirenz slightly decreases the exposure to intravenous alfentanil and moderately reduces the exposure to oral alfentanil.

Clinical evidence, mechanism, importance and management

In a crossover study, 12 healthy subjects were given a single 43-micrograms/kg oral dose of alfentanil, and a single 15-micrograms/kg intravenous dose of alfentanil, on day 15 and 16 respectively, of a course of efavirenz 600 mg daily. The AUC of oral alfentanil was reduced by 78%, and the AUC of intravenous alfentanil was reduced by 46%. The clearance was increased 5-fold and 2-fold for oral and intravenous administration, respectively.[1] Efavirenz is a known inducer of CYP3A4 in the liver, which is involved in the metabolism of alfentanil; concurrent use therefore leads to an increase in the clearance of alfentanil. These results are from a larger study designed to investigate the effects of efavirenz on methadone pharmacokinetics, with the effect of efavirenz on hepatic and intestinal CYP3A4 being studied using alfentanil as a probe substrate, but they also provide good evidence that alfentanil is likely to be less effective in patients taking efavirenz. A larger dose of alfentanil will almost certainly be needed. Note that the greater effect on exposure to oral alfentanil is of little clinical relevance as it is not given by this route in practice.

1. Kharasch ED, Whittington D, Ensign D, Hoffer C, Bedynek PS, Campbell S, Stubbert K, Crafford A, London A, Kim T. Mechanism of efavirenz influence on methadone pharmacokinetics and pharmacodynamics. *Clin Pharmacol Ther* (2012) 91, 673–84.

Opioids; Buprenorphine + NNRTIs

Delavirdine moderately increases, and efavirenz moderately decreases, buprenorphine exposure. Nevirapine might also decrease buprenorphine exposure. Preliminary evidence suggests that buprenorphine is unlikely to affect the pharmacokinetics of delavirdine, efavirenz, or nevirapine.

Delavirdine given with buprenorphine and naloxone appears to slightly prolong the QT interval.

Clinical evidence

(a) Pharmacokinetic interactions

A study in 20 opioid-dependent subjects taking **buprenorphine** with naloxone found that **efavirenz** 600 mg daily for 15 days decreased the AUC of buprenorphine and its metabolite, norbuprenorphine, by 51% and 71%, respectively. **Delavirdine** 600 mg twice daily for 7 days caused a 4.2-fold increase in the AUC of buprenorphine, but the AUC of norbuprenorphine was decreased by 61%.[1] In this study the pharmacokinetics of **delavirdine** were not different to matched controls, nor were the pharmacokinetics of **efavirenz** when compared with historical controls.[1] In another study by the same authors, in 7 opioid-dependent patients maintained on **buprenorphine** with naloxone, the addition of **nevirapine** 200 mg daily for 15 days resulted in minor reductions in the AUC of buprenorphine and its three main metabolites, but none of these was statistically significant. No clinical consequences of reduced buprenorphine exposure were observed. In addition, the pharmacokinetics of **nevirapine** were no different to historical controls.[2]

(b) QT interval prolongation

A study in 50 opioid-dependent patients given sublingual buprenorphine with naloxone alone for at least 2 weeks and then also given an antiretroviral (**delavirdine**, **efavirenz**, nelfinavir, lopinavir boosted with ritonavir, or ritonavir alone) for 5 to 15 days, investigated the effect of these drugs on the QT interval. Buprenorphine with naloxone alone did not notably affect the QT interval; however, when antiretrovirals were given there was a statistically significant, but probably not clinically relevant, increase in the QT interval. Overall, the greatest increase in the QTc interval was seen in patients taking **delavirdine** 600 mg twice daily.[3]

Mechanism

Buprenorphine is a substrate for CYP3A4. **Efavirenz** is an inducer of CYP3A4 and therefore increases metabolism via this route resulting in a decrease in the exposure to buprenorphine. **Nevirapine** is also an inducer of CYP3A4 and so would be expected to decrease buprenorphine exposure. In contrast, **delavirdine** is an inhibitor of CYP3A4 and so reduces the metabolism of buprenorphine to norbuprenorphine by this route, resulting in an increase in its exposure.

Importance and management

Evidence for an interaction between buprenorphine and the NNRTIs is limited. In the study with **efavirenz**, buprenorphine exposure was moderately decreased, but no opioid withdrawal symptoms, cognitive effects, or adverse effects were reported, even though such a decrease might have been expected to be clinically relevant. However, only patients without HIV infection were included in the study and it has been suggested that any interaction might be of more clinical relevance in HIV-positive patients.[4] Therefore, until more is known it would seem prudent to monitor the outcome of the concurrent use of efavirenz and buprenorphine, adjusting the buprenorphine dose if necessary.

The changes in buprenorphine pharmacokinetics in the study with **nevirapine** were not statistically significant. Although this might have been due to the small sample size used, the changes were not of a magnitude to have been clinically relevant, and so an interaction seems unlikely. Nevertheless, as in the study with efavirenz, the subjects were not HIV-positive, and so it is not possible to exclude the possibility of a greater effect in clinical practice.

Delavirdine, a CYP3A4 inhibitor, appears to moderately increase buprenorphine exposure and therefore it would seem prudent to monitor for increased buprenorphine adverse effects (such as drowsiness and respiratory depression). For details on the manufacturers' warnings and dose recommendations for buprenorphine with CYP3A4 inhibitors, see 'Opioids + Azoles', p.165.

The increase in the QT interval reported with the concurrent use of buprenorphine and delavirdine or efavirenz is not considered to be clinically important.[3]

1. McCance-Katz EF, Moody DE, Morse GD, Friedland G, Pade P, Baker J, Alvanzo A, Smith P, Ogundele A, Jatlow P, Rainey PM. Interactions between buprenorphine and antiretrovirals. I: The nonnucleoside reverse-transcriptase inhibitors efavirenz and delavirdine. *Clin Infect Dis* (2006) 43 (Suppl 4), S224–S234.
2. McCance-Katz EF, Moody DE, Morse GD, Ma Q, Rainey PM. Lack of clinically significant interactions between nevirapine and buprenorphine. *Am J Addict* (2010) 19, 30–7.
3. Baker JR, Best AM, Pade PA, McCance-Katz EF. Effect of buprenorphine and antiretroviral agents on the QT interval in opioid-dependent patients. *Ann Pharmacother* (2006) 40, 392–6.
4. Bruce RD, McCance-Katz E, Kharasch ED, Moody DE, Morse GD. Pharmacokinetic interactions between buprenorphine and antiretroviral medications. *Clin Infect Dis* (2006) 43 (Suppl 4), S216–S223.

Opioids; Methadone + NNRTIs

Methadone exposure can be moderately reduced by efavirenz or nevirapine, and opioid withdrawal symptoms requiring, sometimes large, dose increases have been seen. Rilpivirine negligibly reduces methadone exposure, whereas etravirine and delavirdine negligibly increase methadone exposure.

Clinical evidence

(a) Delavirdine

The pharmacokinetics of delavirdine 600 mg twice daily did not differ between 16 subjects taking methadone and 15 healthy control subjects.[1] In another study methadone did not affect delavirdine pharmacokinetics. However, delavirdine decreased methadone clearance and increased its AUC by 19%.[2]

(b) Efavirenz

A retrospective case series of 6 patients stabilised on methadone and started on efavirenz, found that methadone doses needed to be increased from a mean of 120 mg daily to a mean of 224 mg daily (range 29% to 6-fold) in order to alleviate the withdrawal symptoms experienced. Plasma methadone concentrations, as well as symptoms, were used to guide dose increases.[3] Other individual case reports describe similar effects. An HIV-positive woman who had been taking methadone for over one year began to complain of discomfort within 4 weeks of having nelfinavir replaced by efavirenz 600 mg daily, and by 8 weeks typical methadone withdrawal symptoms were occurring late in the afternoon. It was found that the concentrations of *R*-methadone (the active enantiomer) had decreased from 168 nanograms/mL to 90 nanograms/mL, and those of *S*-methadone had decreased from 100 nanograms/mL to 28 nanograms/mL. The methadone dose had to be increased from 100 mg to 180 mg daily before the symptoms disappeared.[4] Another report describes a man taking methadone, who, stopped taking efavirenz 600 mg daily because of the occurrence of withdrawal symptoms, despite having had his methadone dose increased.[5] A further report describes a man who required a 2.3-fold increase in his methadone dose over 4 weeks after starting efavirenz, and mentions two other patients who complained of opioid withdrawal shortly after starting efavirenz. They also required methadone dose increases.[6]

In a crossover study, 12 healthy subjects were given a single 11-mg oral dose, and a single 6-mg intravenous dose, of methadone on day 17 of a course of efavirenz 600 mg daily. The AUCs of *R*-methadone and *S*-methadone were reduced by 46% and 60%, respectively, after intravenous administration, and by 55% and 69%, respectively, after oral administration.[7] In another study, 11 patients taking methadone 35 to 100 mg daily were given efavirenz 600 mg daily for 2 to 3 weeks with two nucleoside analogues. The methadone AUC was reduced by 57% and the maximum plasma concentration by 48%. Nine of the patients developed methadone withdrawal symptoms and needed a mean dose increase of 22% (15 to 30 mg).[8] Similar results have been seen in other studies: 20%,[9] 87%,[10] and 61%[11] of patients required mean methadone dose increases of 52%,[9] 8% to 200%,[10] and a median increase of 7.5 mg daily.[11]

(c) Etravirine

In a study, 16 subjects taking methadone for at least 14 days were also given etravirine 100 mg twice daily for 14 days. The AUC of active *R*-methadone was increased (by about 6% by day 14) and that of *S*-methadone was reduced (by about 11%) by etravirine. Similarly, methadone had no apparent effect on the pharmacokinetics of etravirine when compared with historical controls. No relevant signs or symptoms of opioid withdrawal were reported.[12]

(d) Nevirapine

A retrospective review revealed 7 cases of patients taking methadone who developed withdrawal symptoms after starting regimens including nevirapine. The symptoms developed within 4 to 8 days, and methadone dose increases of 21 to 186% were required. Despite this, 3 patients did not respond. They elected to discontinue nevirapine, and in 2 patients somnolence developed within 2 weeks, so the methadone dose was reduced. Methadone plasma concentrations were available in 2 patients, and these suggested that nevirapine decreased methadone concentrations by about 90%.[13] Similarly, a retrospective case series of 3 patients stabilised on methadone and started on nevirapine found that methadone doses needed to be increased from a mean of 150 mg daily to a mean of 338 mg daily (range 30% to 4-fold) in order to alleviate the withdrawal symptoms experienced. Plasma methadone concentrations were used to guide dose increases, as well as symptoms.[3] Other studies have similarly reported the need for methadone dose increases with nevirapine in some patients: 30% of patients in one study,[14] and 86%[11] and 80%[15] in others. Where stated, increases of a median of 20 mg daily,[11] and 33% and 100%[15] were necessary. Three other similar cases have been reported.[5,16,17]

In a pharmacokinetic study, 8 patients taking methadone 30 to 120 mg daily had methadone plasma concentrations measured before and 14 days after starting an antiretroviral regimen including nevirapine 200 mg daily. The AUC of methadone decreased by 52%, and its maximum plasma concentration decreased by 36%. Six patients complained of symptoms of methadone withdrawal, and required a mean increase in their methadone dose of 16%.[18] Similarly, in 20 HIV-positive subjects stabilised on once-daily doses of racemic methadone or *R*-methadone, the addition of nevirapine decreased the mean dose-adjusted AUC of methadone by 41%. This decrease resulted in symptoms of opioid withdrawal in 14 patients, which required additional doses of methadone.[19] Another pharmacokinetic study in 10 patients stabilised on methadone for at least 15 days found that nevirapine 200 mg daily reduced the AUC and maximum concentration of methadone by about 63% and 55%, respectively, but when the dose of nevirapine was increased to 400 mg daily there was no additional decrease in these pharmacokinetic parameters.[20]

(e) Rilpivirine

In a study in 12 HIV-negative patients taking methadone 60 to 100 mg daily, rilpivirine 25 mg daily for 11 days reduced the AUC of both enantiomers of methadone by 16%, and their maximum plasma concentrations by about 13%. Methadone had no apparent effect on the pharmacokinetics of rilpivirine, when compared with historical control data.[21]

Mechanism

Efavirenz and nevirapine induce the metabolism of methadone (possibly by CYP3A4 although data for efavirenz show that induction of CYP2B6 is the likely mechanism[7]), which results in reduced plasma concentrations and effects. In contrast, delavirdine is an *inhibitor* of various cytochrome P450 isoenzymes, and might therefore be expected to inhibit the metabolism of methadone, although the effects appear small.

Importance and management

The interaction between methadone and **efavirenz** or **nevirapine** is established and of clinical importance. Some authors have found that the dose increase required is much less than that predicted based on the reduction in methadone concentrations,[8,18] whereas others have questioned this.[6,22] It seems important not to confuse the adverse effects of the NNRTIs with opioid withdrawal symptoms.[3,8] It has been suggested that patients taking methadone who are given these drugs should be screened for opioid withdrawal beginning on the fourth day of the new medication. If symptoms develop, the methadone dose should be increased by 10 mg every 2 to 3 days until symptoms abate.[23] However, others have suggested dose increments should be made at one-week intervals to avoid overdose, as methadone has a long half-life (reported to range 13 to 47 hours).[24] Note that some patients might require an increase in methadone dose frequency to twice daily.[3,15] Measuring methadone maximum and minimum concentrations might be of more value in guiding an appropriate methadone dose than just titration based on symptoms.[3] If efavirenz or nevirapine is stopped, the methadone dose should be gradually reduced to the pretreatment dose over the course of one to 2 weeks.[23]

The decrease in methadone exposure seen with **rilpivirine** was negligible and would not be expected to clinically relevant. No initial methadone dose adjustment is necessary on concurrent use; however, the UK and US manufacturers advise monitoring as it is possible that some patients taking rilpivirine might need an increase in their maintenance dose of methadone.[25,26] No methadone dose adjustments are usually needed on the concurrent use of **etravirine**. However, despite this, the US manufacturer advises that patients are still monitored for signs of opioid withdrawal as the maintenance dose of methadone might need to be altered in some patients.[27]

The US manufacturer of **delavirdine**[28] suggests that the methadone dose might need to be reduced if delavirdine is started; however, the effects in the study reported are negligible, and would not be expected to be of any clinical relevance.

1. Booker B, Smith P, Forrest A, DiFrancesco R, Morse G, Cottone P, Murphy M, McCance-Katz E. Lack of effect of methadone on the pharmacokinetics of delavirdine & N-delavirdine. *Intersci Conf Antimicrob Agents Chemother* (2001) 41, 14.
2. McCance-Katz EF, Rainey PM, Smith P, Morse GD, Friedland G, Boyarsky B, Gourevitch M, Jatlow P. Drug interactions between opioids and antiretroviral medications: interaction between methadone, LAAM, and delavirdine. *Am J Addict* (2006) 15, 23–34.
3. Pelet A, Favrat B, Cavassini M, Eap CB, Besson J, Monnat M. Usefulness of methadone plasma concentration measurement in patients receiving nevirapine or efavirenz. *Am J Drug Alcohol Abuse* (2011) 37, 264–8.
4. Marzolini C, Troillet N, Telenti A, Baumann P, Decosterd LA, Eap CB. Efavirenz decreases methadone blood concentrations. *AIDS* (2000) 14, 1291–2.
5. Pinzani V, Faucherre V, Peyriere H, Blayac J-P. Methadone withdrawal symptoms with nevirapine and efavirenz. *Ann Pharmacother* (2000) 34, 405–7.
6. Boffito M, Rossati A, Reynolds HE, Hoggard PG, Back DJ, di Perri G. Undefined duration of opiate withdrawal induced by efavirenz in drug users with HIV infection and undergoing chronic methadone treatment. *AIDS Res Hum Retroviruses* (2002) 18, 341–2.
7. Kharasch ED, Whittington D, Ensign D, Hoffer C, Bedynek PS, Campbell S, Stubbert K, Crafford A, London A, Kim T. Mechanism of efavirenz influence on methadone pharmacokinetics and pharmacodynamics. *Clin Pharmacol Ther* (2012) 91, 673–84.
8. Clarke SM, Mulcahy FM, Tjia J, Reynolds HE, Gibbons SE, Barry MG, Back DJ. The pharmacokinetics of methadone in HIV-positive patients receiving the non-nucleoside reverse transcriptase inhibitor efavirenz. *Br J Clin Pharmacol* (2001) 51, 213–17.
9. McCance-Katz EF, Gourevitch MN, Arnsten J, Sarlo J, Rainey P, Jatlow P. Modified directly observed therapy (MDOT) for injection drug users with HIV disease. *Am J Addict* (2002) 11, 271–8.
10. Tashima K, Bose T, Gormley J, Sousa H, Flanigan TP. The potential impact of efavirenz on methadone maintenance. Poster presented at 9th European Conference on Clinical Microbiology and Infectious Diseases, Berlin, March 23rd 1999 (Poster PO552).
11. Tossonian HK, Raffa JD, Grebely J, Trotter B, Viljoen M, Mead A, Khara M, McLean M, Duncan F, Fraser C, DeVlaming S, Conway B. Methadone dosing strategies in HIV-infected injection drug users enrolled in a directly observed therapy program. *J Acquir Immune Defic Syndr* (2007) 45, 324–7.
12. Schöller-Gyüre M, van den Brink W, Kakuda TN, Woodfall B, De Smedt G, Vanaken H, Stevens T, Peeters M, Vandermeulen K, Hoetelmans RMW. Pharmacokinetic and pharmacodynamic study of concomitant administration of methadone and TMC125 in HIV-negative volunteers. *J Clin Pharmacol* (2008) 48, 322–9.
13. Altice FL, Friedland GH, Cooney EL. Nevirapine induced opiate withdrawal among injection drug users with HIV infection receiving methadone. *AIDS* (1999) 13, 957–62.
14. Staszewski S, Haberl A, Gute P, Nisius G, Miller V, Carlebach A. Nevirapine/didanosine/lamivudine once daily in HIV-1-infected intravenous drug users. *Antivir Ther* (1998) 3 (Suppl 4), 55–6.
15. Otero M-J, Fuertes A, Sánchez R, Luna G. Nevirapine-induced withdrawal symptoms in HIV patients on methadone maintenance programme: an alert. *AIDS* (1999) 13, 1004–5.
16. Heelon MW, Meade LB. Methadone withdrawal when starting an antiretroviral regimen including nevirapine. *Pharmacotherapy* (1999) 19, 471–2.
17. de la Cruz Pellin M, Esteban J, Gimeno C, Mora E. Interacción entre metadona y antirretrovirales (estavudina, indinavir, ritonavir, nevirapina). *Med Clin (Barc)* (2003) 121, 439.
18. Clarke SM, Mulcahy FM, Tjia J, Reynolds HE, Gibbons SE, Barry MG, Back DJ. Pharmacokinetic interactions of nevirapine and methadone and guidelines for use of nevirapine to treat injection drug users. *Clin Infect Dis* (2001) 33, 1595–7.
19. Stocker H, Kruse G, Kreckel P, Herzmann C, Arastéh K, Claus J, Jessen H, Cordes C, Hintsche B, Schlote F, Schneider L, Kurowski M. Nevirapine significantly reduces the levels of racemic methadone and (*R*)-methadone in human immunodeficiency virus-infected patients. *Antimicrob Agents Chemother* (2004) 48, 4148–53.
20. Arroyo E, Valenzuela B, Portilla J, Climent-Grana E, Pérez-Ruixo JJ, Merino E. Pharmacokinetics of methadone in human-immunodeficiency-virus-infected patients receiving nevirapine once daily. *Eur J Clin Pharmacol* (2007) 63, 669–75.
21. Crauwels HM, Rolf PG, van Heeswijk RP, Vandevoorde A, Buelens A, Stevens M, Hoetelmans RMW. The effect of rilpivirine on the pharmacokinetics of methadone in HIV-negative volunteers. *J Clin Pharmacol* (2013) 54, 133–40
22. Calvo R, Lukas JC, Rodriguez M, Carlos MA, Suarez E. Pharmacokinetics of methadone in HIV-positive patients receiving the non-nucleoside reverse transcriptase efavirenz. *Br J Clin Pharmacol* (2002) 53, 212–14.
23. Bruce RD, Altice FL, Gourevitch MN, Friedland GH. Pharmacokinetic drug interactions between opioid agonist therapy and antiretroviral medications: implications and management for clinical practice. *J Acquir Immune Defic Syndr* (2006) 41, 563–72.
24. Anon. Torsades de pointes with methadone. *Prescrire Int* (2005) 14, 61–2.
25. Edurant (Rilpivirine hydrochloride). Janssen-Cilag Ltd. UK Summary of product characteristics, December 2013.
26. Edurant (Rilpivirine hydrochloride). Tibotec Pharmaceuticals. US Prescribing information, June 2013.
27. Intelence (Etravirine). Tibotec, Inc. US Prescribing information, February 2013.
28. Rescriptor (Delavirdine mesylate). ViiV Healthcare. US Prescribing information, August 2012.

Opioids + NRTIs

Case reports describe patients who needed methadone dose increases after starting zidovudine or abacavir. Didanosine, stavudine, tenofovir, and a single dose of zidovudine with lamivudine do not appear to affect methadone pharmacokinetics.

Methadone can increase zidovudine concentrations, and reduce the concentrations of abacavir and stavudine, and didanosine from the tablet formulation, but not the enteric-coated capsule preparation.

The concurrent use of didanosine, lamivudine, or tenofovir and buprenorphine does not appear to affect the pharmacokinetics of any of these drugs. The pharmacokinetics of zidovudine are not affected by buprenorphine.

Clinical evidence

(a) Buprenorphine

1. Didanosine. In a study in 10 opioid-dependent patients taking buprenorphine with naloxone sublingually, didanosine 400 mg daily for 5 days (enteric-coated formulation) had no clinically relevant effect on the pharmacokinetics of buprenorphine or its metabolites, and none of the patients showed signs of opiate withdrawal. There was also no difference in the pharmacokinetics of didanosine when compared with matched controls.[1]

2. Lamivudine. In a study in 7 opioid-dependent patients taking buprenorphine with naloxone sublingually, lamivudine 300 mg daily for 5 days had no effect on the pharmacokinetics of buprenorphine and none of the patients showed any signs of opiate withdrawal. There was no difference in the pharmacokinetics of lamivudine when compared with historical controls.[1]

3. Tenofovir. In a study in 10 opioid-dependent patients taking buprenorphine with naloxone sublingually, tenofovir disoproxil fumarate 300 mg daily for 5 days had no effect on the pharmacokinetics of buprenorphine or its metabolites. There was no difference in the pharmacokinetics of tenofovir when compared with matched controls.[1]

4. Zidovudine. In one study, there was no difference in the pharmacokinetics of oral zidovudine between patients receiving buprenorphine and control subjects.[2]

(b) Methadone

1. Abacavir. Eleven patients given methadone with abacavir had a 23% increase in the rate of methadone clearance but no change in its half-life or renal clearance. In addition, there was a delay, and a 34% decrease, in the maximum concentration of abacavir, but no change in its clearance or half-life.[3] Of 3 patients taking methadone who started taking abacavir, lamivudine, and zidovudine, 2 patients required methadone dose increases (of 31% and 46%). Abacavir was thought to be responsible for this effect.[4] A patient taking methadone experienced torsade de pointes when abacavir, lamivudine, and zidovudine were also taken.[5]

See also 'Opioids; Methadone + HIV-protease inhibitors', p.182, for a report of a decrease in methadone concentrations in patients taking abacavir with amprenavir.

2. Didanosine. A study in 17 subjects taking methadone found that the AUC and maximum concentrations of didanosine tablets were 57% and 66% lower, respectively, when compared with 10 control subjects. Methadone minimum concentrations did not differ from historical controls, suggesting that didanosine had no effect on methadone pharmacokinetics.[6] A later study found that there was no reduction in the AUC of didanosine given as enteric-coated capsules when methadone was also given.[7]

3. Stavudine. A study in 17 subjects taking methadone found that the AUC and maximum concentration of stavudine were 23% and 44% lower, respectively, when compared with 10 control subjects. Methadone minimum concentrations did not differ from historical controls suggesting that stavudine had no effect on methadone pharmacokinetics.[6]

4. Tenofovir. In a study in 13 healthy subjects receiving methadone, tenofovir 300 mg daily for 2 weeks did not alter the pharmacokinetics of methadone, and no symptoms of opioid toxicity or opioid withdrawal were detected.[8]

5. Zidovudine. A patient with AIDS needed an increase in his **levomethadone** (*R*-methadone) dose from 40 to 60 mg daily, within one month of starting to take zidovudine 1 g daily.[9] In contrast, a study found no evidence of any change in the pharmacokinetics of methadone in HIV-positive patients taking methadone 14 days after they started to take zidovudine 200 mg every 4 hours. No methadone withdrawal symptoms occurred.[10] Another study in 16 patients taking methadone found that a single-dose of a fixed combination of zidovudine 300 mg with lamivudine 150 mg had no effect on the pharmacokinetics of methadone, and there was no evidence of withdrawal or toxicity.[11]

The effect of methadone on the pharmacokinetics of zidovudine has also been studied. In one study, the AUC of zidovudine was increased by 43% by methadone, and in 4 of 9 patients it was doubled.[10] Another study, in 8 HIV-positive patients starting methadone, found a 29% increase in the AUC of zidovudine given orally and a 41% increase in the AUC of zidovudine given intravenously. Three of the 8 patients stopped zidovudine because of adverse effects or haematological toxicity.[12] Decreased zidovudine clearance in patients taking methadone is described in another report.[13]

Mechanism

Uncertain. It appears that methadone reduces the exposure to didanosine, and to a lesser extent, stavudine, possibly because it delays gastric emptying. Thus, the enteric-coated didanosine preparation appears not to be affected.[6,7] Conversely, methadone apparently reduces the glucuronidation of zidovudine by the liver, resulting in an increase in its exposure.[14] Methadone might also reduce the renal clearance of zidovudine.[12]

Importance and management

Methadone

Evidence for an interaction between methadone and NRTIs is limited or lacking. However, the increase in **zidovudine** concentrations with methadone is established. The clinical relevance of this increase is uncertain, but be alert for any increase in zidovudine adverse effects. The balance of evidence for an effect of zidovudine on methadone, suggests that zidovudine is unlikely to reduce methadone concentrations. The one case reported remains unexplained, although note that some of the adverse effects of zidovudine could be mistaken for opioid withdrawal effects.

The reduction in **didanosine** concentrations with methadone might be clinically relevant, and the authors suggest increasing the dose of the tablet formulation. It would also be prudent to monitor virological response. Note that the enteric-coated didanosine preparation is not affected and it might therefore be worth considering using this preparation instead. Limited evidence suggests that didanosine does not affect methadone concentrations and so no methadone dose adjustment would seem to be necessary on concurrent use. Further study is required to confirm this.

The reduction in **stavudine** concentrations with methadone is probably not clinically relevant, but further data are required. As with didanosine, limited evidence suggests that stavudine also does not affect methadone concentrations, and no methadone dose adjustment would appear to be necessary on concurrent use.

The change in **abacavir** maximum concentration with methadone was small, and given that the exposure was not affected, this change would not be expected to be clinically relevant.[15] The reports suggest that it would be prudent to monitor for signs of opioid withdrawal and adjust the methadone dose if needed, when abacavir is also given.

Tenofovir does not appear to affect methadone concentrations.

Buprenorphine

Didanosine (enteric coated formulation), **lamivudine**, and **tenofovir** do not affect buprenorphine pharmacokinetics, and the pharmacokinetics of these NRTIs seem to be unaffected by buprenorphine. Buprenorphine does not alter the pharmacokinetics of **zidovudine**. No dose adjustments would seem necessary on concurrent use of any of these NRTIs with buprenorphine.

1. Baker J, Rainey PM, Moody DE, Morse GD, Ma Q, McCance-Katz EF. Interactions between buprenorphine and antiretrovirals: nucleos(t)ide reverse transcriptase inhibitors (NRTI) didanosine, lamivudine and tenofovir. *Am J Addict* (2010) 19, 17–29.
2. McCance-Katz EF, Rainey PM, Friedland G, Kosten TR, Jatlow P. Effect of opioid dependence pharmacotherapies on zidovudine disposition. *Am J Addict* (2001) 10, 296–307.
3. Sellers E, Lam R, McDowell J, Corrigan B, Hedayetullah N, Somer G, Kirby L, Kersey K, Yuen G. The pharmacokinetics of abacavir and methadone following coadministration: CNAA1012. *Intersci Conf Antimicrob Agents Chemother* (1999) 39, 663.
4. Pardo López MA, Cuadrado Pastor JM, Pérez Hervás MP, Fernández Villalba E. Síndrome de abstinencia a opiáceos tras la administración de zidovudina + lamivudina + abacavir en pacientes infectados por el virus de la inmunodeficiencia humana en tratamiento con metadona. *Rev Clin Esp* (2003) 203, 407–8.
5. Anon. Torsades de pointes with methadone. *Prescrire Int* (2005) 14, 61–2.
6. Rainey PM, Friedland G, McCance-Katz EF, Andrews L, Mitchell SM, Charles C, Jatlow P. Interaction of methadone with didanosine and stavudine. *J Acquir Immune Defic Syndr* (2000) 24, 241–8.
7. Friedland G, Rainey P, Jatlow P, Andrews L, Damle B, McCance-Katz E. Pharmacokinetics of didanosine from encapsulated enteric coated bead formulation vs chewable tablet formulation in patients on chronic methadone therapy. XIV International AIDS Conference, Barcelona, 2002. Abstract TuPeB4548.
8. Smith PF, Kearney BP, Liaw S, Cloen D, Bullock JM, Haas CE, Yale K, Booker BM, Berenson CS, Coakley DF, Flaherty JF. Effect of tenofovir disoproxil fumarate on the pharmacokinetics and pharmacodynamics of total, R-, and S-methadone. *Pharmacotherapy* (2004) 24, 970–77.
9. Brockmeyer NH, Mertins L, Goos M. Pharmacokinetic interaction of antimicrobial agents with levomethadon in drug-addicted AIDS patients. *Klin Wochenschr* (1991) 69, 16–18.
10. Schwartz EL, Brechbühl A-B, Kahl P, Miller MA, Selwyn PA, Friedland GH. Pharmacokinetic interactions of zidovudine and methadone in intravenous drug-using patients with HIV infection. *J Acquir Immune Defic Syndr* (1992) 5, 619–26.
11. Rainey PM, Friedland GH, Snidow JW, McCance-Katz EF, Mitchell SM, Andrews L, Lane B, Jatlow P. The pharmacokinetics of methadone following co-administration with a lamivudine/zidovudine combination tablet in opiate-dependent subjects. *Am J Addict* (2002) 11, 66–74.
12. McCance-Katz EF, Rainey PM, Jatlow P, Friedland G. Methadone effects on zidovudine disposition (AIDS clinical trials group 262). *J Acquir Immune Defic Syndr Hum Retrovirol* (1998) 18, 435–43.
13. Burger DM, Meenhorst PL, ten Napel CHH, Mulder JW, Neef C, Koks CHW, Bult A, Beijnen JH. Pharmacokinetic variability of zidovudine in HIV-infected individuals: subgroup analysis and drug interactions. *AIDS* (1994) 8, 1683–9.
14. Cretton-Scott E, de Sousa G, Nicolas F, Rahmani R, Sommadossi J-P. Methadone and its metabolite N-demethyl methadone, inhibit AZT glucuronidation in vitro. *Clin Pharmacol Ther* (1996) 59, 168.
15. Ziagen (Abacavir sulfate). ViiV Healthcare UK Ltd. UK Summary of product characteristics, August 2013.

Opioids + NS5A inhibitors

No interaction occurs between daclatasvir and buprenorphine with naloxone or methadone. Buprenorphine with naloxone and methadone do not appear to alter the pharmacokinetics of ombitasvir. Ombitasvir might increase exposure to buprenorphine, but appears to have no effect on the pharmacokinetics of methadone. Ledipasvir does not appear to

affect the pharmacokinetics of methadone, and methadone is not expected to affect the exposure to ledipasvir.

Clinical evidence, mechanism, importance and management

(a) Buprenorphine

1. Daclatasvir. The preliminary report of a study in 11 opioid dependent subjects taking buprenorphine 8 to 24 mg daily with naloxone 2 to 6 mg daily, notes that daclatasvir 60 mg daily had no effect on the pharmacokinetics of buprenorphine or naloxone.[1] The UK manufacturer also notes that the pharmacokinetics of daclatasvir were no different to historical controls.[2] No dose adjustments are therefore necessary on concurrent use.

2. Ombitasvir. The UK and US manufacturers briefly report that, in a study in 10 subjects taking buprenorphine 4 to 24 mg daily with naloxone 1 to 6 mg daily, and given ombitasvir 25 mg daily (in a fixed-dose combination with paritaprevir and ritonavir, and given with and without dasabuvir), the dose-normalised AUC and maximum concentration of buprenorphine were increased 2-fold and 2.2-fold, respectively. The dose-normalised AUC and maximum concentration of norbuprenorphine were increased by 84% and 2-fold, respectively.[3,4] The pharmacokinetics of naloxone were unaffected,[3,4] as were the pharmacokinetics of ombitasvir.[4] The mechanism behind the increase in buprenorphine exposure is unclear, but could be a result of inhibition of the glucuronosyltransferase, UGT1A1, which is involved in the metabolism of buprenorphine, by ombitasvir. Other components of the combination could also be involved. No dose adjustments on concurrent use are recommended by the UK manufacturer,[4] but the US manufacturer advises that patients should be closely monitored for sedation and cognitive effects.[3]

(b) Methadone

1. Daclatasvir. The preliminary report of a study in 14 opioid dependent subjects taking methadone 40 to 120 mg daily, notes that daclatasvir 60 mg daily had no effect on the pharmacokinetics of *R*-methadone.[1] The UK manufacturer also notes that the pharmacokinetics of daclatasvir were no different to historical controls.[2] No dose adjustments are therefore necessary on concurrent use.

2. Ledipasvir. The UK manufacturer of ledipasvir (in a fixed-dose combination with sofosbuvir) predicts that ledipasvir exposure will be unaffected by methadone.[5] The US manufacturer states that no change was seen in the pharmacokinetics of methadone when given with ledipasvir.[6] No dose adjustments are necessary on concurrent use.

3. Ombitasvir. The UK manufacturer briefly reports that, in a study in subjects taking methadone 20 to 120 mg daily, and given ombitasvir 25 mg daily (in a fixed-dose combination with paritaprevir and ritonavir, and given with and without dasabuvir), the pharmacokinetics of ombitasvir and *R*- and *S*-methadone were not affected.[4] No dose adjustments are necessary on concurrent use.

1. Garimella T, Wang R, Luo WL, Wastall P, Kandoussi H, Demicco M, Bruce D, Hwang C, Bertz R, Bifano M. Evaluation of drug-drug interaction between daclatasvir and methadone or buprenorphine/naloxone. *J Int AIDS Soc* (2014) 17 (Suppl 3), 19628. Abstract P096.
2. Daklinza (Daclatasvir dihydrochloride). Bristol-Myers Squibb Pharmaceutical Ltd. UK Summary of product characteristics, September 2014.
3. Viekira Pak (Ombitasvir, paritaprevir, ritonavir co-packaged with dasabuvir sodium monohydrate). AbbVie Inc. US Prescribing information, December 2014.
4. Viekirax (Ombitasvir, paritaprevir, ritonavir). AbbVie Ltd. UK Summary of product characteristics, January 2015.
5. Harvoni (Ledipasvir, sofosbuvir). Gilead Sciences Ltd. UK Summary of product characteristics, November 2014.
6. Harvoni (Ledipasvir, sofosbuvir). Gilead Sciences, Inc. US Prescribing information, March 2015.

Opioids + NS5B inhibitors

Dasabuvir might slightly increase the exposure to buprenorphine, but appears to have no effect on the pharmacokinetics of naloxone or methadone. The pharmacokinetics of dasabuvir do not appear to be affected by buprenorphine with naloxone or methadone. No interaction appears to occur between sofosbuvir and methadone.

Clinical evidence, mechanism, importance and management

(a) Buprenorphine

The UK and US manufacturers of **dasabuvir** briefly reports that, in a study in 10 subjects taking buprenorphine 4 to 24 mg daily with naloxone 1 to 6 mg daily, and given dasabuvir 250 or 400 mg twice daily (with a fixed-dose combination of ombitasvir and paritaprevir boosted with ritonavir), the dose-normalised AUC and maximum concentration of buprenorphine were increased 2- and 2.2-fold, respectively. The dose-normalised AUC and maximum concentration of norbuprenorphine were increased by 84% and 2-fold, respectively.[1,2] The pharmacokinetics of naloxone were unaffected, as were the pharmacokinetics of dasabuvir.[1,2] The mechanism behind the increase in buprenorphine exposure is unclear, but could be a result of inhibition of the glucuronosyltransferase, UGT1A1, which is involved in the metabolism of buprenorphine, by dasabuvir. Other components of the combination could also be involved. No dose adjustments on concurrent use are recommended by the UK manufacturer,[1] but the US manufacturer advises that patients should be closely monitored for sedation and cognitive effects.[2]

(b) Methadone

1. Dasabuvir. The UK manufacturer briefly reports that, in a study in subjects taking methadone 20 to 120 mg daily, and given dasabuvir 250 or 400 mg twice daily (with a fixed-dose combination of paritaprevir boosted with ritonavir, and ombitasvir), the pharmacokinetics of dasabuvir and *R*- and *S*-methadone were not affected.[1] No dose adjustments are necessary on concurrent use.

2. Sofosbuvir. The preliminary report of a study in 14 subjects taking methadone 30 to 105 mg daily, and given sofosbuvir 400 mg once daily, notes that the pharmacokinetics of *R*- and *S*-methadone were unaffected, and those of sofosbuvir and its major inactive metabolite, were no different to historical controls.[3] No dose adjustments are therefore necessary on concurrent use.

1. Exviera (Dasabuvir sodium monohydrate). AbbVie Ltd. UK Summary of product characteristics, January 2015.
2. Viekira Pak (Ombitasvir, paritaprevir, ritonavir co-packaged with dasabuvir sodium monohydrate). AbbVie Inc. US Prescribing information, December 2014.
3. Denning JM, Cornpropst M, Clemons D, Fang L, Sale M, Berrey MM, Symonds WT. Lack of effect of the nucleotide analog polymerase inhibitor PSI-7977 on methadone pharmacokinetics and pharmacodynamics. *Hepatology* (2011) 54 (Suppl S1), 544A. Abstract 372.

Opioids + NSAIDs

In general, the concurrent use of NSAIDs and opioids is beneficial (improved pain relief, decreased adverse effects, reduced opioid requirements), and clinically relevant pharmacokinetic interactions are lacking. However, there is some conflicting evidence as to whether respiratory depression is increased or decreased in those given diclofenac and morphine. A single case report describes notable respiratory depression in a man given buprenorphine when ketorolac was added. An isolated report describes grand mal seizures in a patient given diclofenac and pentazocine.

Clinical evidence, mechanism, importance and management

NSAIDs are often given with opioids because they usually reduce the opioid requirements and some of the opioid-induced adverse effects.[1] A recent systematic review of 60 clinical studies found that NSAIDs reduced morphine consumption from patient-controlled analgesia, by a mean of 10.2 mg when compared with placebo. This was better than with paracetamol, and comparable to the coxibs. The effect on morphine-related adverse effects was largely inconclusive.[2]

Enhanced pain relief has been reported with various combinations including **dextromethorphan** with **ketorolac**[3] or **tenoxicam**,[4] **fentanyl** with **flurbiprofen**,[5] **oxycodone** with **ibuprofen**,[6] and **tramadol** with **ketorolac**[7] without increased adverse effects. Consider also 'Opioids + NSAIDs; Coxibs', p.192.

However, cases of respiratory depression have been reported, see *Morphine* below, and myoclonus has been reported with high doses of morphine given with NSAIDs, see 'Opioids; Morphine + Miscellaneous', p.201.

(a) Buprenorphine

A man underwent thoracotomy for carcinoma of the middle third of his oesophagus. One hour after transfer to the recovery ward he complained of severe pain at the operative site and was given epidural buprenorphine 150 micrograms (3 micrograms/kg), and 2 hours later intramuscular **ketorolac** 30 mg because of continued pain. During the next hour he became more drowsy, stopped obeying commands and his respiratory rate dropped to 6 breaths per minute. He recovered after 6 hours of mechanical ventilation. The authors of this report suggest that it might be necessary to use less buprenorphine in the presence of ketorolac to avoid the development of these respiratory depressant effects.[8] This appears to be the only report of this possible interaction, and, as with other opioids, NSAIDs such as **etodolac** have been used with buprenorphine to reduce the postoperative pain score without increasing adverse effects.[9]

(b) Codeine

A study in 12 healthy subjects found that a single 50-mg dose of **diclofenac** did not have a clinically important effect on the pharmacokinetics of a single 100-mg dose of codeine phosphate when compared with placebo. There was no effect on the metabolic clearance of morphine, and only a negligible (about 5 to 10%) increase in the concentrations of glucuronide metabolites. In addition, **diclofenac** did not alter the analgesic effects of codeine as assessed in a cold pressor test (a test in which opioids, but not NSAIDs, are effective).[10] These findings in healthy subjects suggest that no special precautions are required during the concurrent use of **diclofenac** and codeine.

Single oral-dose studies in 24 healthy subjects found that the bioavailability of both codeine phosphate 25 mg and **ibuprofen** 200 mg were unaffected by concurrent use.[11] A systematic review of 4 clinical studies (involving 443 subjects) to assess the analgesic efficacy of single oral dose ibuprofen with codeine found that 64% of subjects taking ibuprofen 400 mg with codeine 25.6 to 60 mg achieved at least 50% maximum pain relief compared with 18% of subjects taking placebo. However in other studies using different doses, the effect of the combination was barely better than ibuprofen alone, but did appear to be better than codeine alone.[12]

(c) Dextropropoxyphene (Propoxyphene)

In healthy subjects the concurrent use of dextropropoxyphene 260 mg daily and **sodium meclofenamate** 400 mg daily for one week was found to have no effect on the plasma concentrations of either drug.[13]

The UK manufacturer of **sulindac** notes that dextropropoxyphene had no effect on the plasma concentrations of sulindac or its sulfide metabolite.[14]

(d) Methadone

In a study in 16 patients with cancer-related pain, intramuscular **diclofenac** 75 mg twice daily given for 5 days with oral methadone solution every 8 hours had no effect on the AUC or the maximum plasma concentration of methadone.[15] Therefore, no methadone dose adjustments appear to be necessary during concurrent use.

(e) Morphine

In a study in 11 healthy subjects, an infusion of **ketoprofen** 1.5 mg/kg with morphine 100 micrograms/kg reduced the respiratory depression associated with morphine alone. There was no change in the plasma concentration of morphine.[16] Another study in 6 patients found that intramuscular **diclofenac** 75 mg twice daily for 5 days did not affect the half-life and AUC of oral morphine solution.[17] Other studies have reported superior pain relief with morphine and NSAIDs, including **lornoxicam**,[3] **ketoprofen**,[18] and **ketorolac**,[19] with fewer adverse effects. Consider also 'Opioids + NSAIDs; Coxibs', below.

However, in contrast to these reports, a study in 7 patients on the first post-operative day after spinal surgery found that, although rectal **diclofenac** 100 mg reduced patient-controlled morphine consumption by 20%, respiratory rates were considerably lower after the **diclofenac**, and minimal at about 200 minutes. Concentrations of an active metabolite, morphine-6-glucuronide did not appreciably decrease until 420 minutes post-dose.[20]

NSAIDs are frequently used with opioids because of their lack of respiratory depression and opioid-sparing effects. However, this study demonstrates that there might be a risk of respiratory depression and other adverse effects due to persistently high concentrations of morphine-6-glucuronide for a number of hours after receiving an NSAID. During this time period, patients should be more closely monitored.[20]

For mention of an increased incidence of myoclonus when high-dose morphine was given with NSAIDs, see 'Opioids; Morphine + Miscellaneous', p.201.

(f) Oxycodone

A study involving 23 healthy subjects found that the single-dose pharmacokinetics of **ibuprofen** 400 mg and oxycodone 5 mg were similar when given alone or in combination.[21] A systematic review of 3 clinical studies, involving 1 202 subjects, to assess the analgesic efficacy of a single oral dose of ibuprofen plus oxycodone, found that the combination of ibuprofen 400 mg with oxycodone 5 mg provided equivalent analgesia at 6 hours to ibuprofen alone, but greater than oxycodone alone. Fewer patients required rescue analgesia when taking the combination than when talking either drug alone, but there was no difference in the adverse effect profile between the combination and either drug alone.[22]

(g) Pentazocine

A man with Buerger's disease had a grand mal seizure while watching television 2 hours after being given a single 50-mg suppository of **diclofenac**. He was also taking pentazocine 50 mg three times daily. He might have had a previous seizure some months before after taking a single 100-mg slow-release **diclofenac** tablet.[10] The reasons for this reaction are not known, but on rare occasions **diclofenac** alone has been associated with seizures (incidence said to be 1 in 100 000) and seizures have also been seen with pentazocine alone. It is not clear what part the disease itself, or watching television, had in the development of this adverse reaction.[23] Therefore no interaction between **diclofenac** and pentazocine is established, but be aware of this case if concurrent use is being considered, particularly in patients who are known to be seizure-prone.

(h) Tapentadol

A crossover study in 34 healthy subjects found that **naproxen** 500 mg twice daily for 4 doses, increased the AUC of a single 80-mg dose of tapentadol given after the third naproxen dose, by 17%, but there was no effect on the maximum plasma concentration.[24] The change in bioavailability seen was just outside the limits set for equivalence and was not felt to be clinically important. No tapentadol dose adjustment would seem necessary on its concurrent use with naproxen.

1. Kehlet H. Postoperative opioid sparing to hasten recovery: what are the issues? *Anesthesiology* (2005) 102, 1083–5.
2. McCaid C, Maund E, Rice S, Wright K, Jenkins B, Woolacott N. Paracetamol and selective and non-selective anti-inflammatory drugs (NSAIDs) for the reduction of morphine-related side effects after major surgery: a systematic review. *Health Technol Assess* (2010) 14, 1–153. Available at: http://www.journalslibrary.nihr.ac.uk/__data/assets/pdf_file/0014/65300/FullReport-hta14170.pdf (accessed 19/08/15).
3. Lu C-H, Liu J-Y, Lee M-S, Borel CO, Yeh C-C, Wong C-S, Wu C-T. Preoperative cotreatment with dextromethorphan and ketorolac provides an enhancement of pain relief after laparoscopic-assisted vaginal hysterectomy. *Clin J Pain* (2006) 22, 799–804.
4. Yeh C-C, Wu C-T, Lee M-S, Yu J-C, Yang C-P, Lu C-H, Wong C-S. Analgesic effects of preincisional administration of dextromethorphan and tenoxicam following laparoscopic cholecystectomy. *Acta Anaesthesiol Scand* (2004) 48, 1049–53.
5. Liu ZF, Chai XQ, Chen KZ. Flurbiprofen axetil enhances analgesic effect of fentanyl associated with increase in β-endorphin levels. *J Anesth* (2011) 25, 679–84.
6. Oldfield V, Perry CM. Oxycodone/ibuprofen combination tablet: a review of its use in the management of acute pain. *Drugs* (2005) 65, 2337–54.
7. Lepri A, Sia S, Catinelli S, Casali R, Novelli G. Patient-controlled analgesia with tramadol *versus* tramadol plus ketorolac. *Minerva Anestesiol* (2006) 72, 59–67.
8. Jain PN, Shah SC. Respiratory depression following combination of epidural buprenorphine and intramuscular ketorolac. *Anaesthesia* (1993) 48, 898–9.
9. Koizuka S, Saito S, Obata H, Sasaki M, Nishikawa K, Takahashi K, Saito Y, Goto F. Oral etodolac, a COX-2 inhibitor, reduces postoperative pain immediately after fast-track cardiac surgery. *J Anesth* (2004) 18, 9–13.
10. Ammon S, Marx C, Behrens C, Hofmann U, Mürdter T, Griese E-U, Mikus G. Diclofenac does not interact with codeine metabolism in vivo: a study in healthy volunteers. *BMC Clin Pharmacol* (2002) 2, 2.
11. Laneury JP, Duchene P, Hirt P, Delarue A, Gleizes S, Houin G, Molinier P. Comparative bioavailability study of codeine and ibuprofen after administration of the two products alone or in association to 24 healthy volunteers. Eur J Drug Metab Pharmacokinet. (1998) 23, 185–9.
12. Derry S, Karlin SM, Moore RA. Single dose oral ibuprofen plus codeine for acute postoperative pain in adults. Available in The Cochrane Database of Systematic Reviews; Issue 3. Chichester: John Wiley; 2013. Available at: http://onlinelibrary.wiley.com/doi/10.1002/14651858.CD010107.pub2/pdf (accessed 03/03/14).
13. Baragar FD, Smith TC. Drug interaction studies with sodium meclofenamate (Meclomen®). *Curr Ther Res* (1978) 23 (April Suppl), S51–S59.
14. Clinoril (Sulindac). Merck Sharp & Dohme Ltd. UK Summary of product characteristics, February 2008.
15. Bianchi M, Clavenna A, Groff L, Zecca E, Ripamonti C. Diclofenac dose not modify methadone bioavailability in cancer patients. *J Pain Symptom Manage* (1999) 17, 227–9.
16. Moren J, Francois T, Blanloeil Y, Pinaud M. The effects of a nonsteroidal antiinflammatory drug (ketoprofen) on morphine respiratory depression: a double-blind, randomized study in volunteers. *Anesth Analg* (1997) 85, 400–5.
17. De Conno F, Ripamonti C, Bianchi M, Ventafridda V, Panerai AE. Diclofenac does not modify morphine bioavailability in cancer patients. *Pain* (1992) 48, 401–2.
18. Karaman S, Gunusen I, Uyar M, Firat V. The effect of pre-operative lornoxicam and ketoprofen application on the morphine consumption of post-operative patient-controlled analgesia. *J Int Med Res* (2006) 34, 168–75.
19. Safdar B, Degutis LC, Landry K, Vedere SR, Moscovitz HC, D'Onofrio G. Intravenous morphine plus ketorolac is superior to either drug alone for treatment of acute renal colic. *Ann Emerg Med* (2006) 48, 173–81.
20. Tighe KE, Webb AM, Hobbs GJ. Persistently high plasma morphine-6-glucuronide levels despite decreased hourly patient-controlled analgesia morphine use after single-dose diclofenac: potential for opioid-related toxicity. *Anesth Analg* (1999) 88, 1137–42.
21. Kapil R, Nolting A, Roy P, Fiske W, Benedek I, Abramowitz W. Pharmacokinetic properties of combination oxycodone plus racemic ibuprofen: two randomized, open-label, crossover studies in healthy adult volunteers. *Clin Ther* (2004) 26, 2015–25.
22. Derry S, Derry CJ, Moore RA. Single dose oral ibuprofen plus oxycodone for acute postoperative pain in adults. Available in The Cochrane Database of Systematic Reviews; Issue 6. Chichester: John Wiley; 2013. Available at: http://onlinelibrary.wiley.com/doi/10.1002/14651858.CD010289.pub2/pdf (accessed 19/08/15).
23. Heim M, Nadvorna H, Azaria M. Grand mal seizures following treatment with diclofenac and pentazocine. *S Afr Med J* (1990) 78, 700–1.
24. Smit JW, Oh C, Rengelshausen J, Terlinden R, Ravenstijn PGM, Wang SS, Upmalis D, Mangold B. Effects of acetaminophen, naproxen and acetylsalicylic acid on tapentadol pharmacokinetics: results of two randomized, open-label, crossover, drug-drug interaction studies. *Pharmacotherapy* (2010) 25–34.

Opioids + NSAIDs; Coxibs

Parecoxib has no effect on the pharmacokinetics of alfentanil or fentanyl, and celecoxib does not appear to affect the pharmacokinetics of tramadol. Coxibs can reduce the perioperative opioid requirement, but adverse effects are not necessarily reduced.

Clinical evidence, mechanism, importance and management

(a) Pharmacokinetic studies

In a crossover study in 12 healthy subjects, intravenous **parecoxib** 40 mg, given one hour before and 12 hours after an infusion of **alfentanil** 15 micrograms/kg or **fentanyl** 5 micrograms/kg, had no effect on the pharmacokinetics of these opioids.[1] Pupil diameter versus time curves were not affected by **parecoxib**. This interaction was investigated because both valdecoxib (the main metabolite of **parecoxib**) and **alfentanil** are substrates of CYP3A4. However, there is no clinical evidence that two drugs that are solely substrates of the same isoenzyme will cause a relevant interaction by competing for metabolism by that isoenzyme.

Analysis of data from a study in patients receiving stable doses of **celecoxib** or rofecoxib, found that the clearance of **tramadol** (given with paracetamol) did not differ between the coxibs.[2] **Tramadol** is metabolised by CYP2D6 (of which **celecoxib** is a weak inhibitor) and CYP3A4, but these results suggest that no pharmacokinetic interaction occurs between tramadol and celecoxib.

(b) Pharmacodynamic studies

Many studies have reported reduced opioid requirements and reduced opioid-related adverse effects when coxibs are given perioperatively or postoperatively with various opioids. Examples include the coxibs, **celecoxib**,[3] and **parecoxib**,[4] and the opioids, **hydrocodone**[3] and **morphine**.[5] Other studies exist but are not cited here. A recent systematic review of 60 clinical studies found that coxibs reduced morphine consumption from patient-controlled analgesia, by a mean of 10.9 mg when compared with placebo. This was better than with paracetamol, and comparable to the NSAIDs (consider also 'Opioids + NSAIDs', p.191). The effect on morphine-related adverse effects was largely inconclusive.[6] The timing of the administration of the coxib appears to affect opioid-induced analgesia and post-infusion increases in sensitivity to pain. One study in healthy subjects found that pretreatment with **parecoxib** increased the analgesic effects of a **remifentanil** infusion and notably diminished the increased sensitivity to pain after remifentanil was withdrawn. Giving parecoxib at the start of the remifentanil infusion did not alter its analgesic effects.[7]

In a double-blind, placebo-controlled study in 72 patients undergoing laparoscopic cholecystectomy, oral **etoricoxib** 120 mg given 1.5 hours before surgery reduced the need for postoperative patient controlled analgesia (PCA) with **fentanyl**, but opioid-related adverse effects were not reduced.[8]

1. Ibrahim AE, Feldman J, Karim A, Kharasch ED. Simultaneous assessment of drug interactions with low- and high-extraction opioids. Application to parecoxib effects on the pharmacokinetics and pharmacodynamics of fentanyl and alfentanil. *Anesthesiology* (2003) 98, 853–61.
2. Punwani NG. Tramadol pharmacokinetics and its possible interactions with cyclooxygenase 2-selective nonsteroidal anti-inflammatory drugs. *Clin Pharmacol Ther* (2004) 75, 363–5.
3. Ekman EF, Wahba M, Ancona F. Analgesic efficacy of perioperative celecoxib in ambulatory arthroscopic knee surgery: a double-blind, placebo-controlled study. *Arthroscopy* (2006) 22, 635–42.
4. Nussmeier NA, Whelton AA, Brown MT, Joshi GP, Langford RM, Singla NK, Boye ME, Verburg KM. Safety and efficacy of the cyclooxygenase-2 inhibitors parecoxib and valdecoxib after noncardiac surgery. *Anesthesiology* (2006) 104, 518–26.
5. Riest G, Peters.J, Weiss M, Pospiech J, Hoffmann O, Neuhauser M, Beiderlinden M, Eikermann M. Does perioperative administration of rofecoxib improve analgesia after spine, breast and orthopaedic surgery? *Eur J Anaesthesiol* (2006) 23, 219-26.
6. McCaid C, Maund E, Rice S, Wright K, Jenkins B, Woolacott N. Paracetamol and selective and non-selective anti-inflammatory drugs (NSAUIDs) for the reduction of morphine-related side effects after major surgery: a systematic review. *Health Technol Assess* (2010) 14, 1–153. Available at: http://www.journalslibrary.nihr.ac.uk/__data/assets/pdf_file/0014/65300/FullReport-hta14170.pdf (accessed 19/08/15).
7. Tröster A, Sittl R, Singler B, Schmelz M, Schüttler J, Koppert W. Modulation of remifentanil-induced analgesia and postinfusion hyperalgesia by parecoxib in humans. *Anesthesiology* (2006) 105, 1016–23.
8. Puura A, Puolakka P, Rorarius M, Salmelin R, Lindgren L. Etoricoxib pre-medication for post-operative pain after laparoscopic cholecystectomy. *Acta Anaesthesiol Scand* (2006) 50, 688–93.

Opioids + Opioids

The concurrent use of two opioid agonists may have enhanced effects, although acute opioid tolerance may also occur. Opioids with mixed agonist/antagonist properties (e.g. buprenorphine, butorphanol, nalbuphine, pentazocine) might precipitate opioid withdrawal symptoms in patients taking pure opioid agonists (e.g. fentanyl, methadone, morphine). Methadone might reduce the efficacy of codeine.

Clinical evidence, mechanism, importance and management

(a) Pharmacodynamic effects

Many of the opioids used clinically act primarily at μ-opioid receptors including **codeine**, **diamorphine**, **fentanyl**, **methadone**, and **morphine** (see 'Table 6.1', p.139, for a classification), but they often have pharmacological differences, and patients tolerant to one opioid can frequently be switched to another opioid (opioid rotation) at doses lower than predicted by relative potencies.[1] Studies in *animals* have found synergistic or additive effects between μ-opioids.[1] The majority of studies in patients have reported enhanced analgesic effects with opioid combinations,[2,3] although combined opioids are not always beneficial;[4] in some cases adverse effects were increased and acute opioid tolerance has also occurred.[3] For example, a study in 69 patients who had undergone abdominal surgery and were receiving **morphine** found that the addition of a **tramadol** infusion was associated with improved patient-controlled analgesia (PCA) and smaller **morphine** requirements with no increase in adverse effects.[2] However, another study found that the effects of this combination were less than additive.[5] Furthermore, the incidence of dry mouth was greater and it was concluded that the use of two μ-opioid agonists in combination might only increase the number of adverse effects.[5] A case report describes catatonia in a patient given intravenous **tramadol** and single 25-mg dose of **pethidine** (**meperidine**) injection was given.[6] Other studies have found that transdermal **fentanyl** reduced **morphine** requirements after hysterectomy[7,8] without affecting sedation scores.[7] However, the combination of **fentanyl** and **morphine** resulted in more pronounced respiratory depression than morphine alone.[7,8] In contrast, in a study of 49 patients undergoing major abdominal surgery, relatively large doses of intraoperative **remifentanil** (mean remifentanil infusion rate 300 nanograms/kg per minute) were reported to almost double **morphine** requirements in the first 24 hours postoperatively. The results suggested that **remifentanil** caused the development of acute opioid tolerance and excessive sensitivity to pain.[9] This result was not replicated in a study in 45 cardiac surgery patients given the same high intraoperative **remifentanil** doses followed by **oxycodone** postoperatively. There was no difference in oxycodone consumption or pain scores between the remifentanil group and the placebo group.[10] The reason for the differences in effect seen in these 2 studies[9,10] is unclear. So, although some opioid combinations are useful, clinical studies are needed to ascertain the benefits and safety of specific combinations.[4]

Opioids with mixed agonist/antagonist properties (e.g. **buprenorphine**, **butorphanol**, **nalbuphine**, **pentazocine**) might precipitate opioid withdrawal symptoms in patients taking pure opioid agonists such as **fentanyl**, **methadone**, and **morphine** (see 'Table 6.1', p.139, for a classification). An example of this occurred in a 60-year-old woman who was taking slow-release **morphine** 90 mg twice daily for cancer pain and was additionally given **nalbuphine** 30 mg intravenously in an ambulance following a fractured femur. She became agitated and experienced involuntary movements, tachycardia, hypertension, and sweating (typical of opioid withdrawal). Her management was further complicated by resistance to intravenous **morphine**, necessitating a femoral nerve block. The agitation, which lasted for about 4 hours after she was given the **nalbuphine**, was controlled with lorazepam.[11]

Note that some opioids (see 'Table 35.3', p.1472) have serotonergic effects, and concurrent use might lead to the serotonin syndrome. Serotonin syndrome is a rare adverse effect, but because of its severity, some caution is warranted if both drugs are given. For more information on serotonin syndrome and its management, see 'Drugs that cause serotonin syndrome + Other drugs that cause serotonin syndrome', p.1471.

(b) Pharmacokinetic effects

In a study, patients maintained on either **methadone** or **buprenorphine**, and who were extensive CYP2D6 metabolisers (that is, they had normal activity of CYP2D6), were given a single 60-mg dose of **codeine**. The plasma concentrations of codeine and its metabolite norcodeine were almost 2-fold and 6-fold higher, respectively, in the methadone group when compared with those taking buprenorphine. The plasma concentrations of the glucuronide metabolite of codeine, codeine-6-glucuronide was 44% lower, and the plasma concentrations of the glucuronide metabolites of morphine, morphine-3-glucuronide (inactive) and morphine-6-glucuronide (active), were 60% and 70% lower, respectively, in the methadone group when compared with those taking buprenorphine. The authors concluded that this was a result of methadone inhibiting the CYP2D6 conversion of codeine to morphine, and inhibiting the glucuronidation (via UGT2B4 and UGT2B7) of codeine to codeine-6-glucuronide, and of morphine to its glucuronide metabolites. The conversion of codeine to norcodeine via CYP3A4 was not affected. Furthermore, they suggested that this might result in reduced efficacy of codeine as an analgesic in patients taking methadone.[12] Bear the possibility of an interaction in mind in the case of reduced codeine efficacy on concurrent use with methadone. For a discussion of the potential analgesic effects of CYP2D6 inhibition, see 'Opioids; Codeine and related drugs + Quinidine', p.194.

1. Bolan EA, Tallarida RJ, Pasternak GW. Synergy between μ opioid ligands: evidence for functional interactions among μ opioid receptor subtypes. *J Pharmacol Exp Ther* (2002) 303, 557–62.
2. Webb AR, Leong S, Myles PS, Burn SJ. The addition of a tramadol infusion to morphine patient-controlled analgesia after abdominal surgery: a double-blinded, placebo-controlled randomized trial. *Anesth Analg* (2002) 95, 1713–18.
3. Lötsch J, Skarke C, Tegeder I, Geisslinger G. Drug interactions with patient-controlled analgesia. *Clin Pharmacokinet* (2002) 41, 31–57.
4. Davis MP, LeGrand SB, Lagman R. Look before leaping: combined opioids may not be the rave. *Support Care Cancer* (2005) 13, 769–74.
5. Marcou TA, Marque S, Mazoit J-X, Benhamou D. The median effective dose of tramadol and morphine for postoperative patients: a study of interactions. *Anesth Analg* (2005) 100, 469–74.
6. Huang SS, Jou SH, Chiu NY. Catatonia associated with coadministration of tramadol and meperidine. *J Formos Med Assoc* (2007) 106, 323–6.
7. Broome IJ, Wright BM, Bower S, Reilly CS. Postoperative analgesia with transdermal fentanyl following lower abdominal surgery. *Anaesthesia* (1995) 50, 300–3.
8. Sandler AN, Baxter AD, Katz J, Samson B, Friedlander M, Norman P, Koren G, Roger S, Hull K, Klein J. A double-blind, placebo-controlled trial of transdermal fentanyl after abdominal hysterectomy. Analgesic, respiratory, and pharmacokinetic effects. *Anesthesiology* (1994), 81, 1169–80.
9. Guignard B, Bossard AE, Coste C, Sessler DI, Lebrault C, Alfonsi P, Fletcher D, Chauvin M. Acute opioid tolerance: intraoperative remifentanil increases postoperative pain and morphine requirement. *Anesthesiology* (2000) 93, 409–17.
10. Lahtinen P, Kokki H, Hynynen M. Remifentanil infusion does not induce opioid tolerance after cardiac surgery. *J Cardiothorac Vasc Anesth* (2008) 22, 225–9.
11. Smith J, Guly H. Nalbuphine and slow release morphine. *BMJ* (2004) 328, 1426.
12. Gelston EA, Coller JK, Lopatko OV, James HM, Schmidt H, White JM, Somogyi AA. Methadone inhibits CYP2D6 and UGT2B7/2B4 *in vivo*: a study using codeine in methadone- and buprenorphine-maintained subjects. *Br J Clin Pharmacol* (2012) 73, 786–94.

Opioids + Phenothiazines

Levomepromazine does not appear to inhibit the conversion of codeine to morphine, except in homozygous extensive metabolisers of CYP2D6. Chlorpromazine has been reported to increase the analgesic effect of pethidine (meperidine), but increased respiratory depression, sedation, CNS toxicity, and hypotension can also occur. Other phenothiazines such as levomepromazine, promethazine, prochlorperazine, propiomazine, and thioridazine might also interact with pethidine to cause some of these effects. Additive CNS depressant effects would be expected when opioids are given with phenothiazines.

Clinical evidence

(a) Codeine

In a randomised study, 22 patients hospitalised for acute back pain who were extensive CYP2D6 metabolisers (that is, they had normal isoenzyme activity), were given either codeine with paracetamol (60 mg and 1 g, respectively) four times daily, alone or with levomepromazine for 24 hours. There was no difference in the O-demethylation of codeine to morphine between the 2 groups, but there was a difference when analysed by CYP2D6 genotype: those who were *homozygous* extensive metabolisers had lower O-demethylation ratios when taking codeine with levomepromazine than when taking codeine alone, but there was no difference between the groups in those who were *heterozygous* extensive metabolisers.[1]

(b) Pethidine (Meperidine)

>In a single-dose study in healthy subjects, **chlorpromazine** had no effect on the pharmacokinetics of pethidine. However, the excretion of the metabolites of pethidine was increased, and symptoms of light-headedness, dry mouth, and lethargy were considerably increased: 4 subjects experienced such marked debilitation that they required assistance to continue the study. Systolic and diastolic blood pressures were also reduced.[2]

Chlorpromazine 25 mg/70 kg given alone had no consistent effect on respiratory function in 6 healthy subjects but the respiratory depression produced by pethidine 100 mg/70 kg was exacerbated when the two drugs were given together. One subject had marked respiratory depression, beginning about 30 minutes after both drugs were given, and lasting 2 hours.[3]

The respiratory depressant effects of pethidine can be increased by **promethazine** with pentobarbital,[4] **propiomazine**,[5,6] and **levomepromazine**[7], but the effects of **prochlorperazine**[8] with pethidine on respiration were not statistically significant.

A 12-year-old patient taking long-term **thioridazine** 50 mg twice daily and given premedication with pethidine, diphenhydramine and glycopyrrolate, was very lethargic after surgery and stopped breathing. He responded to naloxone.[9] Promethazine may also decrease the dose requirements of pethidine during surgery, see under *Other opioids*, below.

(c) Other opioids

There have been conflicting data as to whether or not phenothiazines potentiate narcotic analgesia,[10] and it has been suggested that some patients treated with an opioid and a phenothiazine are merely too sedated to report pain.[11] However, some studies have found that **promethazine** reduces opioid requirements. The maintenance doses of a variety of opioid analgesics (**morphine**, **pethidine** (**meperidine**), **oxymorphone**, **hydromorphone**, **fentanyl**, **pentazocine**) required during surgical anaesthesia were reduced by 28 to 46% when 132 patients were premedicated with intramuscular **promethazine** 50 mg/70 kg, when compared with control patients. Similarly, on-demand **pentazocine** requirements post-caesarean section were reduced by 32% in women given **promethazine** as soon as the cord was clamped.[12] In a randomised, placebo-controlled study in 90 patients undergoing abdominal hysterectomy, the preoperative use of intravenous **promethazine** 100 micrograms/kg (given over 30 minutes, starting 30 minutes before induction), reduced the 24-hour postoperative **morphine** consumption by about 30%, when compared with placebo or postoperative **promethazine** use. Postoperative nausea and vomiting were reduced by both pre- and postoperative **promethazine**, when compared with placebo.[13]

Mechanism

The O-demethylation of codeine to morphine is mediated by CYP2D6 and is inhibited by levomepromazine, although only in homozygous extensive metabolisers (see

'Genetic factors in drug metabolism', p.8 for further details).[1] There is evidence that chlorpromazine can increase the activity of liver microsomal enzymes so that the metabolism of pethidine (meperidine) to norpethidine and norpethidinic acid are increased. These metabolites probably account for the lethargy and hypotension seen in one study.[2] The effects of the phenothiazines on pethidine-induced respiratory depression may be related. Both the opioids and the phenothiazines are CNS depressants, and their effects can be additive.

Importance and management

Evidence for a pharmacokinetic interaction between opioids and phenothiazines is limited. For codeine, one study suggests that the CYP2D6 conversion of codeine to morphine is inhibited by levomepromazine, but only in individuals who are homozygous extensive metabolisers. The authors suggest that in such patients, the amount of morphine produced might be insufficient to produce analgesic efficacy.[1] However, the application of this finding to clinical practice is limited, as determining the metaboliser status of an individual is a research tool rather than a clinical one. Further study is needed.

Evidence for a pharmacodynamic interaction is more extensive, and phenothiazines might enhance the hypotensive, sedative, and respiratory depressant effects of opioids. Patients should be monitored carefully on concurrent use, and opioid dose reductions made if necessary. However note that one UK manufacturer of **methadone** suggests that the concurrent use of other CNS depressants is not advised.[14] Although lower analgesic doses of pethidine (meperidine) have been used with chlorpromazine,[15] a marked increase in respiratory depression can occur in some susceptible individuals[3] and the authors of one study[2] suggested that the risks of giving pethidine with chlorpromazine outweighed the advantages. Information about other adverse interactions between pethidine and the phenothiazines seems to be very limited: the interaction with thioridazine seems to be the only one reported. Increased analgesia might occur but it might be accompanied by increased respiratory depression, which is undesirable in patients with existing respiratory insufficiency. The US manufacturer advises that concurrent use of pethidine with phenothiazines might also result in severe hypotension, profound sedation, or coma if usual doses of pethidine are used. They suggest that the dose of pethidine should be proportionally reduced (usually by 25 to 50%) when it is given with phenothiazines.[16]

For mention of myoclonus associated with high doses of morphine and chlorpromazine, see 'Opioids; Morphine + Miscellaneous', p.201.

1. Vevelstad M, Petterson S, Tallaksen C, Brørs O. O-demethylation of codeine to morphine inhibited by low-dose levomepromazine. *Eur J Clin Pharmacol* (2009) 65, 795–801.
2. Stambaugh JE, Wainer IW. Drug interaction: meperidine and chlorpromazine, a toxic combination. *J Clin Pharmacol* (1981) 21, 140–6.
3. Lambertsen CJ, Wendel H, Longenhagen JB. The separate and combined respiratory effects of chlorpromazine and meperidine in normal men controlled at 46 mmHg alveolar pCO_2. *J Pharmacol Exp Ther* (1961) 131, 381–93.
4. Pierce JA, Garofalvo ML. Preoperative medication and its effect on blood gases. *JAMA* (1965) 194, 487–90.
5. Hoffman JC, Smith TC. The respiratory effects of meperidine and propiomazine in man. *Anesthesiology* (1970) 32, 325–31.
6. Reier CE, Johnstone RE. Respiratory depression: narcotic versus narcotic-tranquilizer combinations. *Anesth Analg* (1970) 49, 119–124.
7. Zsigmond EK, Flynn K. The effect of methotrimeprazine on arterial blood gases in human volunteers. *J Clin Pharmacol* (1988) 28, 1033–7.
8. Steen SN, Yates M. The effects of benzquinamide and prochlorperazine, separately and combined, on the human respiratory center. *Anesthesiology* (1972) 36, 519–20.
9. Grothe DR, Ereshefsky L, Jann MW, Fidone GS. Clinical implications of the neuroleptic-opioid interaction. *Drug Intell Clin Pharm* (1986) 20, 75–7.
10. Warfield CA. Phenothiazines and analgesic potentiation. Reply. *Hosp Pract* (1984) 19, 24.
11. Creek K. Phenothiazines and analgesic potentiation. *Hosp Pract* (1984) 19, 22, 24.
12. Keèri-Szàntò M. The mode of action of promethazine in potentiating narcotic drugs. *Br J Anaesth* (1974) 46, 918–24.
13. Chia YY, Lo Y, Liu K, Tan PH, Chung NC, Ko NH. The effect of promethazine on postoperative pain: a comparison of preoperative, postoperative, and placebo administration in patients following total abdominal hysterectomy. *Acta Anaesthesiol Scand* (2004) 48, 625–30.
14. Synastone (Methadone hydrochloride). Auden McKenzie (Pharma Division) Ltd. UK Summary of product characteristics, June 2015.
15. Sadove MS, Levin MJ, Rose RF, Schwartz L, Witt FW. Chlorpromazine and narcotics in the management of pain of malignant lesions. *JAMA* (1954) 155, 626–8.
16. Demerol (Meperidine hydrochloride). Sanofi-Aventis US LLC. US Prescribing information, July 2014.

Opioids + Quinidine

Quinidine appears to increase the oral absorption and effects of fentanyl, methadone, and morphine, but does not alter the opioid-induced miosis when these opioids are given intravenously. Care should be taken if high-dose methadone is used with quinidine as cardiac conduction might possibly be affected. Quinidine might slightly increase the exposure to tramadol.

Clinical evidence

(a) Codeine and related drugs

For the interactions of quinidine with codeine, dihydrocodeine, hydrocodone and oxycodone, see 'Opioids; Codeine and related drugs + Quinidine', p.194.

(b) Fentanyl

In a study in healthy subjects, quinidine sulfate 600 mg given one hour before an intravenous infusion of fentanyl 2.5 micrograms/kg did not alter fentanyl-induced miosis. However, the same dose of quinidine given before oral fentanyl 2.5 micrograms/kg (with ondansetron as an antiemetic) increased fentanyl-induced miosis. This increase was considered proportionate to the increase in the AUC of fentanyl (2.6-fold). There was no change in the elimination half-life of fentanyl.[1]

(c) Methadone

In a study in healthy subjects, quinidine sulfate 600 mg, given one hour before intravenous methadone hydrochloride 10 mg, did not alter methadone-induced miosis. However, the same dose of quinidine given before oral methadone hydrochloride 10 mg (with ondansetron as an antiemetic) increased the peak methadone-induced miosis by 34%. The plasma concentrations of oral methadone in the absorption phase were increased, but the maximum plasma concentration or AUC of methadone were not affected.[2]

(d) Morphine

In a study in healthy subjects, quinidine sulfate 600 mg, given one hour before intravenous morphine sulfate 150 micrograms/kg, did not alter morphine-induced miosis. However, the same dose of quinidine given before oral morphine sulfate 30 mg (with ondansetron as an antiemetic) increased morphine-induced miosis by 56%. This increase was considered proportionate to the increase in morphine AUC (60%) and maximum concentration (88%). There was no change in the elimination half-life of morphine.[3] Similarly, in another study in healthy subjects, quinidine 800 mg given one hour before intravenous morphine 7.5 mg did not alter the respiratory depressant or miotic effects of morphine, and there was no change in plasma morphine or morphine glucuronide concentrations.[4]

(e) Tramadol

A placebo-controlled study in 12 healthy subjects found that quinidine 50 mg had virtually no effect on the analgesic effect of tramadol 100 mg but it inhibited the effect of tramadol on pupil size.[5] The US manufacturer reports that, in a single-dose study, quinidine 200 mg taken 2 hours before extended-release tramadol 100 mg increased the exposure to tramadol by 50 to 60%, and decreased the exposure to its active *O*-desmethyl metabolite (M1) by a similar amount.[6]

Mechanism

Quinidine increased the effects of orally administered fentanyl, methadone, and morphine, but had a lack of effect when these opioids were given intravenously, indicating that quinidine has an effect other than on the hepatic metabolism of these opioids. Fentanyl, methadone, and morphine are P-glycoprotein substrates *in vitro*,[1-3] and quinidine is a known inhibitor of P-glycoprotein. This might explain the increase in fentanyl, methadone, and morphine concentrations seen, as a result of increased intestinal absorption.[1-3] The lack of effect on miosis after intravenous administration suggests that quinidine does not alter the brain distribution of these opioids, or that other factors are also important in determining the access of these opioids to the brain. Further study is needed.

Tramadol is partially metabolised to the active metabolite, *O*-desmethyltramadol, by CYP2D6, which is inhibited by quinidine. However, this appears to have little effect on the analgesic efficacy of tramadol.[5]

Importance and management

The clinical importance of the increase in absorption of oral **fentanyl**, **morphine**, and **methadone** caused by quinidine is unknown. However, note that both high doses of methadone and quinidine can affect the QT interval, see 'Drugs that prolong the QT interval + Other drugs that prolong the QT interval', p.272 for further discussion. The clinical importance of a possible interaction with oral transmucosal fentanyl citrate (of which a considerable proportion is swallowed) remains to be determined, but be aware that its effects could be increased.

The general importance of the interaction between quinidine and **tramadol** is unclear, although it would be prudent to bear in mind the possibility of an interaction should a patient taking both drugs develop an increase in tramadol adverse effects (such as sedation).

1. Kharasch ED, Hoffer C, Altuntas TG, Whittington D. Quinidine as a probe for the role of P-glycoprotein in the intestinal absorption and clinical effects of fentanyl. *J Clin Pharmacol* (2004) 44, 224–33.
2. Kharasch ED, Hoffer C, Whittington D. The effect of quinidine, used as a probe for the involvement of P-glycoprotein, on the intestinal absorption and pharmacodynamics of methadone. *Br J Clin Pharmacol* (2004) 57, 600–10.
3. Kharasch ED, Hoffer C, Whittington D, Sheffels. Role of P-glycoprotein in the intestinal absorption and clinical effects of morphine. *Clin Pharmacol Ther* (2003) 74, 543–54.
4. Skarke C, Jarrar M, Erb K, Schmidt H, Geisslinger G, Lötsch J. Respiratory and miotic effects of morphine in healthy volunteers when P-glycoprotein is blocked by quinidine. *Clin Pharmacol Ther* (2003) 74, 303–11.
5. Collart L, Luthy C, Dayer P. Multimodal analgesic effect of tramadol. *Clin Pharmacol Ther* (1993) 53, 223.
6. Ultram ER (Tramadol hydrochloride). PriCara. US Prescribing information, June 2009.

Opioids; Codeine and related drugs + Quinidine

The analgesic effects of codeine, and probably also hydrocodone, appear to be reduced or abolished by quinidine. Other potent inhibitors of CYP2D6 would be expected to interact similarly. Quinidine alters the pharmacokinetics of dihydrocodeine and oxycodone, but this does not appear to alter their analgesic effects.

Clinical evidence

(a) Codeine

Codeine 100 mg was given to 16 healthy CYP2D6 extensive metabolisers (that is, those with normal isoenzyme activity) with and without a single 200-mg dose of quinidine. Quinidine reduced the morphine maximum concentrations by about 80% (from 18 nanomol/L to less than 4 nanomol/L). Codeine given alone increased the pain threshold (pin-prick pain test using an argon laser) but no notable analgesic effects were detectable when quinidine was also present.[1] Another study found that the respiratory depressant, psychomotor and miotic effects of codeine in healthy CYP2D6 extensive metabolisers who were given quinidine, were virtually the same as codeine alone in healthy CYP2D6 poor metabolisers (that is, those lacking or deficient in CYP2D6).[2] These studies confirm the preliminary findings of an earlier study in healthy subjects using codeine 100 mg and quinidine 50 mg, which found that quinidine reduced the maximum morphine plasma concentrations by more than 90% (by 92% in 7 extensive metabolisers, and by 97% in one poor metaboliser) and similarly abolished its analgesic effects.[3]

(b) Dihydrocodeine

A study in which four healthy CYP2D6 extensive metabolisers (that is, those with normal isoenzyme activity) were given dihydrocodeine 40 or 60 mg found that, when they were pretreated with quinidine 200 mg, almost none of the morphinoid metabolites of dihydrocodeine normally present in the serum could be detected.[4] The same authors found essentially similar results in a later study in ten healthy CYP2D6 extensive metabolisers given dihydrocodeine 60 mg and quinidine 50 mg.[5] However, a single-dose study involving 10 healthy subjects who were CYP2D6 extensive metabolisers investigated the effect of quinidine on the visceral and somatic analgesic effects of dihydrocodeine and its metabolite, dihydromorphine. It was found that although quinidine reduced dihydromorphine plasma concentrations (by inhibiting CYP2D6 and thereby reducing the metabolism of dihydrocodeine to dihydromorphine), this did not result in diminished pain tolerance thresholds. This suggested that the metabolism of dihydrocodeine to dihydromorphine might not be clinically important for analgesia.[6]

(c) Hydrocodone

In a comparative study in healthy subjects, 5 extensive metabolisers and 6 poor metabolisers of CYP2D6 (that is, those with normal isoenzyme activity, or those lacking or deficient in this isoenzyme, respectively) were given hydrocodone, and another four CYP2D6 extensive metabolisers were given hydrocodone after pretreatment with quinidine. The metabolism of the hydrocodone to its active metabolite, hydromorphone, was found to be high in the extensive metabolisers who described the opioid effects as good, but low in the poor metabolisers and the extensive metabolisers pretreated with quinidine who described the opioid effects as poor.[7]

(d) Oxycodone

Quinidine 200 mg, given 3 hours before and quinidine 100 mg given 6 hours after a single 20-mg dose of oxycodone almost completely inhibited the formation of the metabolite, oxymorphone, in 10 healthy CYP2D6 extensive metabolisers (that is, those with normal isoenzyme activity). Despite this, the psychomotor and subjective effects of oxycodone were not altered (note that analgesia was not assessed). The AUC of the metabolite noroxycodone was increased about 85%, and the oxycodone AUC was increased by 13%.[8] In a placebo-controlled, crossover study, 10 healthy subjects were given a single 0.2-mg/kg oral dose of oxycodone 2 hours after a single 100-mg dose of quinidine. Quinidine increased the AUC_∞ of oxycodone by 40% and the AUC_∞ of the metabolite noroxycodone by 70%. Quinidine also decreased the AUC_{0-3} of the metabolite oxymorphone by 40%. The increase in noroxycodone exposure was most pronounced in the ultrarapid CYP2D6 metabolisers (that is, those with higher than usual isoenzyme activity) and least pronounced in the poor metabolisers (that is, those lacking or deficient in this isoenzyme). When quinidine was given with a single 400-mg oral dose of ketoconazole, the AUC_∞ of oxycodone was increased 3.1-fold and the AUC_∞ of the metabolite oxymorphone was not affected. However, the AUC_{0-3} of the metabolite noroxycodone was decreased by 60%.[9] In a further study in healthy subjects by the same authors, using the same doses of oxycodone and quinidine, in some tests of analgesic effect oxycodone was no different to placebo after the addition of quinidine, but quinidine did enhance the effect on the cold pressor test and pupil size. The effect of quinidine and ketoconazole was greater than quinidine alone.[10] Similar results were found in the preliminary report of another study in healthy subjects.[11]

Mechanism

The evidence available shows that the conversion of codeine, dihydrocodeine, and hydrocodone to their metabolites, morphine, morphinoid metabolites, and hydromorphone, respectively, depends upon the activity of CYP2D6, which is potently inhibited by quinidine. If these metabolites are responsible for the analgesic effects, efficacy of these opioids might be reduced or abolished by quinidine. This interaction is only likely to occur in extensive metabolisers (that is, those with normal isoenzyme activity), and not in poor metabolisers, who have minimal CYP2D6 activity, and who therefore might only derive minimal benefit from analgesics such as codeine in any case. However, one study in healthy subjects has suggested that the analgesic effect of dihydrocodeine does not necessarily depend on its systemic metabolism to dihydromorphine.[6] Similarly, although quinidine also blocks the conversion of oxycodone to oxymorphone, it appears that this is not important for the pharmacodynamic effects of this drug. Moreover, there is some evidence that codeine analgesia is not due to the minor metabolite morphine, but to codeine-6-glucuronide, which is formed by glucuronidation.[12]

Importance and management

The pharmacokinetic interaction between **codeine** and quinidine is well established, and appears to result in reduced analgesic effects in healthy subjects, suggesting it is likely to be clinically important. This suggests that codeine will be virtually ineffective as an analgesic in CYP2D6 extensive metabolisers (the majority of patients) taking quinidine. No interaction would be expected in poor metabolisers (about 7% of Caucasians), but, if the metabolism of codeine by CYP2D6 is essential for efficacy, codeine is probably unlikely to be effective in these patients in any case. Monitor for reduced analgesic efficacy if codeine is given to a patient taking quinidine, and consider using an alternative analgesic. Whether the antitussive effects of codeine are similarly affected is not established, but it seems likely. Note that this interaction has been used clinically in an attempt to treat codeine dependence, but this was not successful.[13] Other potent inhibitors of CYP2D6 (for a list see 'Table 1.7', p.9) would be expected to interact similarly to quinidine.

The interaction of **hydrocodone** is less well established, but the evidence suggests that its analgesic effect might similarly be reduced or lost if quinidine is given. Further study is needed.

The available evidence suggests that, although there is a pharmacokinetic interaction, the analgesic effect of **dihydrocodeine** or **oxycodone** does not seem to be affected by quinidine. This suggests that a clinically relevant interaction might not occur, but this needs confirmation.

1. Sindrup SH, Arendt-Nielsen L, Brøsen K, Bjerring P, Angelo HR, Eriksen B, Gram LF. The effect of quinidine on the analgesic effect of codeine. *Eur J Clin Pharmacol* (1992) 42, 587–92.
2. Caraco Y, Sheller J, Wood AJ. Pharmacogenetic determination of the effects of codeine and prediction of drug interactions. *J Pharmacol Exp Ther* (1996) 278, 1165–74.
3. Desmeules J, Dayer P, Gascon M-P, Magistris M. Impact of genetic and environmental factors on codeine analgesia. *Clin Pharmacol Ther* (1989) 45, 122.
4. Hufschmid E, Theurillat R, Martin U, Thormann W. Exploration of the metabolism of dihydrocodeine via determination of its metabolites in human urine using micellar electrokinetic capillary chromatography. *J Chromatogr B Biomed Appl* (1995) 668, 159–70.
5. Hufschmid E, Theurillat R, Wilder-Smith CH, Thormann W. Characterization of the genetic polymorphism of dihydrocodeine O-demethylation in man via analysis of urinary dihydrocodeine and dihydromorphine by micellar electrokinetic capillary chromatography. *J Chromatogr B Biomed Appl* (1996) 678, 43–51.
6. Wilder-Smith CH, Hufschmid E, Thormann W. The visceral and somatic antinociceptive effects of dihydrocodeine and its metabolite, dihydromorphine. A cross-over study with extensive and quinidine-induced poor metabolizers. *Br J Clin Pharmacol* (1998) 45, 575–81.
7. Otton SV, Schadel M, Cheung SW, Kaplan, Busto UE, Sellers EM. CYP2D6 phenotype determines the metabolic conversion of hydrocodone to hydromorphone. *Clin Pharmacol Ther* (1993) 54, 463–72.
8. Heiskanen T, Olkkola KT, Kalso E. Effects of blocking CYP2D6 on the pharmacokinetics and pharmacodynamics of oxycodone. *Clin Pharmacol Ther* (1998) 64, 603–11.
9. Samer CF, Daali Y, Wagner M, Hopfgartner G, Eap CB, Rebsamen MC, Rossier MF, Hochstrasser D, Dayer P, Desmeules JA. The effects of CYP2D6 and CYP3A activities on the pharmacokinetics of immediate release oxycodone. *Br J Pharmacol* (2010) 160, 907–18.
10. Samer CF, Daali Y, Wagner M, Hopfgartner G, Eap CB, Rebsamen MC, Rossier MF, Hochstrasser D, Dayer P, Desmeules JA. Genetic polymorphisms and drug interactions modulating CYP2D6 and CYP3A activities have a major effect on oxycodone analgesic efficacy and safety. *Br J Pharmacol* (2010) 160, 919–30.
11. Colucci R, Kaiko R, Grandy R. Effects of quinidine on the pharmacokinetics and pharmacodynamics of oxycodone. *Clin Pharmacol Ther* (1998) 63, 141.
12. Vree TB, van Dongen RT, Koopman-Kimenai PM. Codeine analgesia is due to codeine-6-glucuronide, not morphine. *Int J Clin Pract* (2000) 54, 395–8.
13. Fernandes LC, Kilicarslan T, Kaplan HL, Tyndale RF, Sellers EM, Romach MK. Treatment of codeine dependence with inhibitors of cytochrome P450 2D6. *J Clin Psychopharmacol* (2002) 22, 326–9.

Opioids + Rifamycins

Rifampicin increases the metabolism of buprenorphine, codeine, morphine, and intravenous and oral oxycodone and tramadol. Rifampicin is predicted to induce the metabolism of tapentadol. Rifabutin increases the metabolism of buprenorphine, but to a lesser extent than rifampicin; rifapentine would also be expected to increase the metabolism of buprenorphine.

Clinical evidence, mechanism, importance and management

(a) Buprenorphine

In a controlled study in 12 opioid-dependent subjects taking buprenorphine with naloxone, **rifampicin** 600 mg daily for 15 days decreased the AUC and maximum concentration of buprenorphine by 70% and 38%, respectively. Opiate withdrawal was experienced by 50% of the subjects. Similarly, in another group of 9 opioid-dependent subjects taking buprenorphine with naloxone, **rifabutin** 300 mg daily for 15 days decreased the AUC and maximum concentration of buprenorphine by 35% and 21%, respectively, but no subjects experienced opiate withdrawal.[1]

Buprenorphine is metabolised by CYP3A4 to norbuprenorphine, which is induced by both rifampicin and rifabutin, although rifampicin is a more potent inducer and therefore has greater effects. The moderate reduction in buprenorphine exposure seen with rifampicin was clinically important, and buprenorphine dose increases might therefore be required on concurrent use, to avoid withdrawal symptoms. The slight reduction in buprenorphine exposure with rifabutin did not result in clinically important effects, and no buprenorphine dose adjustment would appear necessary. Rifabutin might be a suitable alternative to rifampicin, where appropriate. **Rifapentine**, which is generally considered to be a moderate inducer of CYP3A4, would also be expected to reduce buprenorphine exposure and some caution on concurrent use might be warranted.

(b) Codeine

A study in 15 healthy subjects found that after taking **rifampicin** 600 mg daily for 3 weeks, the metabolism of a single 120-mg oral dose of codeine phosphate was increased. The AUC of codeine was decreased by about 80% and both the *N*-demethylation and glucuronidation metabolic pathways were induced. Of the 15 subjects, 9 were CYP2D6 extensive metabolisers (that is, those with normal activity of this isoenzyme) and 6 were CYP2D6 poor metabolisers (those with little or no CYP2D6 activity). The *O*-demethylation of codeine to its main active metabolite, morphine is mediated by CYP2D6, and so was induced only in the extensive metabolisers. In these subjects there was a 56% reduction in the AUC of morphine, and a 2.7-fold increase in the AUC of normorphine (another active metabolite). Note that morphine and its metabolites were not detected in poor metabolisers, either before or after **rifampicin** was given, because they have little or no CYP2D6 activity. **Rifampicin** reduced the respiratory and psychomotor effects of codeine in extensive metabolisers, but not in poor metabolisers. In contrast, rifampicin decreased the pupillary effect of codeine in poor metabolisers, but it was not altered in extensive metabolisers, possibly due to the increase in the AUC of normorphine.[2] The question of whether, and to what extent, the analgesic effects of the codeine were reduced by this interaction was not addressed by this study. However, some reduction in the effects of codeine might be expected. Therefore, if these drugs are given concurrently, be alert for the need to increase the codeine dose, or use an alternative analgesic.

(c) Fentanyl and related drugs

For the interactions of alfentanil and fentanyl with rifampicin, see 'Opioids; Fentanyl and related drugs + Rifampicin (Rifampin)', p.196.

(d) Methadone

For the interactions of methadone with rifabutin and rifampicin, see 'Opioids; Methadone + Rifamycins', p.197.

(e) Morphine

In a crossover study in 10 healthy subjects **rifampicin** 600 mg daily for 13 days increased the clearance of a single 10-mg dose of morphine by 49%, and its analgesic effects (using a modified cold pressor test) were abolished.[3] A case report describes very low serum morphine concentrations in a 51-year-old man taking **rifampicin** 600 mg daily, 7 days after sustained-release morphine 75 mg three times daily was started. The concentration was about 78% less than would have been expected, given the dose the patient was taking.[4] The mechanism of this interaction is uncertain as morphine is principally metabolised by glucuronidation, and the findings of the study could not be attributed to induction of glucuronosyltransferases by rifampicin.[3] However, the role of P-glycoprotein (which can be induced by rifampicin and could therefore reduce the absorption of morphine) could not be excluded by either groups of authors.[3,4] Further study is needed, but whatever the mechanism of this interaction, it would be prudent to be alert for the need to use an increased dose of morphine in patients taking rifampicin.

(f) Oxycodone

A 60-year-old man who was taking **rifampicin** as well as oxycodone had three consecutive negative urine oxycodone screens in a 2-month period, which would normally suggest that he was not taking the oxycodone. However, oxycodone metabolites were found in his urine confirming compliance with his medication. An interaction between rifampicin and oxycodone was suspected and his oxycodone dose was increased to optimise his pain control.[5] A pharmacokinetic study in 12 healthy subjects (11 of whom were CYP2D6 extensive metabolisers, that is they had normal activity of this isoenzyme) also showed a similar effect. Pretreatment with **rifampicin** 600 mg daily for 6 days reduced the AUC of oxycodone by 53% and 86% after administration of a single 0.1-mg/kg intravenous dose and a single 15-mg oral dose of oxycodone, respectively. The AUC of the oxycodone metabolite, oxymorphone, was reduced by 95% and 92%, after intravenous and oral administration, respectively, and the maximum plasma concentration of the metabolite, noroxycodone, was increased 2.5- and 1.8-fold, respectively. **Rifampicin** also reduced the analgesic effect of oxycodone after oral but not intravenous administration, as assessed using the cold pressor test.[6]

Oxycodone is principally metabolised to noroxycodone by CYP3A4 and, to a lesser extent, to oxymorphone by CYP2D6. As **rifampicin** is a known non-specific enzyme inducer, it would be expected to increase oxycodone metabolism and possibly reduce its analgesic efficacy (when given orally), particularly by CYP3A4. Be aware that the dose of oxycodone might need adjusting in patients taking rifampicin.

(g) Tapentadol

The UK manufacturer of tapentadol states that caution is necessary if a potent enzyme inducer, such as **rifampicin**, is started or stopped in a patient taking tapentadol, as this might lead to decreased efficacy or an increased risk of adverse effects.[7] The mechanism of this proposed interaction is unclear as tapentadol is principally metabolised by a number of glucuronosyltransferases and rifampicin is not known to be an inducer of these particular isoforms. Further study is required. Until more is known, be aware that the dose of tapentadol might need to be adjusted in patients taking rifampicin.

(h) Tramadol

In a crossover study in 11 healthy subjects, pretreatment with **rifampicin** 600 mg daily for 5 days, decreased the AUC of tramadol by 42% and 59%, after a 50-mg intravenous dose and a 100-mg oral dose, respectively. The AUC of its main active metabolite, M1, was also reduced by 58% and 54%, respectively. The pharmacodynamic effects of tramadol (as assessed using visual analogue scales for drowsiness, cold pain threshold and pain intensity) were not affected.[8]

Tramadol is metabolised by CYP3A4 and CYP2D6, both of which can be induced by rifampicin. Concurrent use of rifampicin would therefore be expected to reduce tramadol exposure. The importance of CYP3A4 in tramadol metabolism is unclear, as the potent CYP3A4 *inhibitor*, itraconazole, had no effect on its pharmacokinetics (see 'Opioids + Azoles', p.165). It is possible that the effect seen here is largely due to induction of CYP2D6, although further study is required. The size of the reduction in exposure is only slight and no effect was seen on the effects of tramadol, suggesting that no clinically important reduction in tramadol effects would be expected on concurrent use, and no dose increase would seem necessary. Nevertheless, it might be prudent to bear the possibility of an interaction in mind should a patient taking both drugs experience a reduction in pain control.

1. McCance-Katz EF, Moody DE, Prathikanti S, Friedland G, Rainey PM. Rifampin, but not rifabutin, may produce opiate withdrawal in buprenorphine-maintained patients. *Drug Alcohol Depend* (2011) 118, 326–34.
2. Caraco Y, Sheller J, Wood AJJ. Pharmacogenetic determinants of codeine induction by rifampin: the impact on codeine's respiratory, psychomotor and miotic effects. *J Pharmacol Exp Ther* (1997) 281, 330–6.
3. Fromm MF, Eckhardt K, Li S, Schänzle G, Hofmann U, Mikus G, Eichelbaum M. Loss of analgesic effect of morphine due to coadministration of rifampin. *Pain* (1997) 72, 261–7.
4. Fudin J, Fontanelle DV, Payne A. Rifampin reduces oral morphine absorption: a case of transdermal buprenorphine selection based on morphine pharmacokinetics. *J Pain Palliat Care Pharmacother* (2012) 26, 362–7.
5. Lee HK, Lewis LD, Tsongalis GJ, McMullin M, Schur BC, Wong SH, Yeo K-TJ. Negative urine opioid screening caused by rifampin-mediated induction of oxycodone hepatic metabolism. *Clin Chim Acta* (2006) 367, 196–200.
6. Nieminen TH, Hagelberg NM, Saari TI, Pertovaara A, Neuvonen M, Laine K, Neuvonen PJ, Olkkola KT. Rifampin greatly reduces the plasma concentrations of intravenous and oral oxycodone. *Anesthesiology* (2009) 110, 1371–8.
7. Palexia (Tapentadol hydrochloride). Grünenthal Ltd. UK Summary of product characteristics, July 2014.
8. Saarikoski T, Daari TI, Hagelberg NM, Neuvonen M, Neuvonen PJ, Scheinin M, Olkkola KT, Laine K. Rifampicin markedly decreases exposure to oral and intravenous tramadol. *Eur J Clin Pharmacol* (2013) 69, 1293–301.

Opioids; Fentanyl and related drugs + Rifampicin (Rifampin)

The serum concentrations and effects of transdermal fentanyl were decreased in two patients when they took rifampicin. Studies in healthy subjects have found that the bioavailability of oral transmucosal fentanyl is reduced by rifampicin. The exposure to intravenous alfentanil is moderately decreased by rifampicin, but the exposure to oral alfentanil is very markedly decreased.

Clinical evidence, mechanism, importance and management

(a) Alfentanil

A crossover study in 9 healthy subjects found that when they were given intravenous alfentanil 20 micrograms/kg after taking rifampicin 600 mg orally for 5 days, alfentanil clearance was increased 2.8-fold.[1] In another study by the same research group in 6 healthy subjects, rifampicin 600 mg daily for 5 to 6 days decreased the AUC of intravenous alfentanil 1 mg by about 65%, and decreased the AUC of oral alfentanil 4 mg by about 95%.[2] Rifampicin is a known potent inducer of CYP3A4, which is involved in the metabolism of alfentanil; concurrent use therefore leads to an increase in alfentanil clearance. These studies were primarily designed to investigate the role of CYP3A4 in the metabolism of alfentanil, but also provide good evidence that alfentanil is likely to be less effective in patients taking rifampicin. A larger dose of alfentanil will almost certainly be needed, although note that the much greater effect on oral alfentanil is not of clinical relevance as it is not given by this route in practice. A further study using lower doses of rifampicin (up to 75 mg daily for 5 days) also confirms this.[3]

(b) Fentanyl

In a study in 12 healthy subjects, the maximum plasma concentrations and maximum miosis after oral transmucosal fentanyl 10 micrograms/kg were minimally affected by oral rifampicin 600 mg daily for 5 days, but the AUC of fentanyl was decreased by 63%; the AUC of its metabolite, norfentanyl, was increased by 73%, and the AUC_{0-10} of miosis was decreased by 54%.[4]

A patient with lung metastases was given transdermal fentanyl (1.67 mg patch every 3 days). Serum fentanyl concentrations measured after 48 and 72 hours of treatment were 0.9 nanograms/mL and 0.77 nanograms/mL, respectively (within the reported minimum effective therapeutic range of 0.2 to 1.2 nanograms/mL). On day 5, due to insufficient pain control, the fentanyl patch was increased to 2.5 mg every 3 days. However, on day 7, oral rifampicin 300 mg daily, isoniazid and ethambutol were started for pulmonary tuberculosis. The following day severe pain developed and the fentanyl serum concentrations at 48 and 72 hours were 0.53 nanograms/mL and 0.21 nanograms/mL, respectively, despite the large increase in the fentanyl dose. Even after the dose was increased again up to 7.5 mg every 3 days, the patient still complained of moderate pain and the fentanyl serum concentration 72 hours after treatment was only 0.69 nanograms/mL, less than the concentration achieved with the 1.67 mg dose in the absence of rifampicin.[5]

A patient with colon cancer taking rifampicin 450 mg daily, isoniazid 300 mg daily and ethambutol 750 mg daily was started on a transdermal fentanyl patch at a dose of 600 micrograms daily. However, this did not control his pain and neither did titration of the fentanyl dose up to 2.5 mg daily. The patient was changed to an equivalent dose of morphine, which provided effective pain relief.[6]

Fentanyl is metabolised by CYP3A4 and rifampicin, a potent inducer of CYP3A4, appears to reduce its serum concentrations and analgesic effects. Thus an increase in fentanyl dose is likely to be needed in patients using fentanyl patches and taking rifampicin. The situation with other routes of fentanyl administration is less clear, but until more is known it would be prudent to be alert for a reduction in the effects of fentanyl given by any route in patients also taking rifampicin.

1. Kharasch ED, Russell M, Mautz D, Thummel KE, Kunze KL, Bowdle TA, Cox K. The role of cytochrome P450 3A4 in alfentanil clearance: implications for interindividual variability in disposition and perioperative drug interactions. *Anesthesiology* (1997) 87, 36–50.
2. Kharasch ED, Vangveravong S, Buck N, London A, Kim T, Blood J, Mach RH. Concurrent assessment of hepatic and intestinal cytochrome P450 3A activities using deuterated alfentanil. *Clin Pharmacol Ther* (2011) 89, 562–70.

3. Kharasch ED, Francis A, London A, Frey K, Kim T, Blood J. Sensitivity of intravenous and oral alfentanil and pupillary miosis as minimal and noninvasive probes for hepatic and first-pass CYP3A induction. *Clin Pharmacol Ther* (2011) 90, 100–8.
4. Kharasch ED, Whittington D, Hoffer C. Influence of hepatic and intestinal cytochrome P4503A activity on the acute disposition and effects of oral transmucosal fentanyl citrate. *Anesthesiology* (2004) 101, 729–37.
5. Takane H, Nosaka A, Wakushima H, Hosokawa K, Ieiri I. Rifampin reduces the analgesic effect of transdermal fentanyl. *Ann Pharmacother* (2005) 39, 2139–40.
6. Morii H, Chiba M, Konishi H, Endo Y, Yamaji A. Failure of pain control using transdermal fentanyl during rifampicin treatment. *J Pain Symptom Manage* (2007) 33, 5–6.

Opioids; Methadone + Rifamycins

Rifampicin (rifampin) appears to cause large reductions in the plasma concentrations of methadone. Rifabutin might interact similarly, but any effect is much smaller than that of rifampicin.

Clinical evidence

(a) Rifabutin

A study in 24 HIV-positive patients taking methadone found that rifabutin 300 mg daily for 13 days had only minimal effects on the pharmacokinetics of methadone, and although 75% of the patients reported at least one mild symptom of methadone withdrawal it was not enough for any of them to withdraw from the study. Only 3 of them asked for and received an increase in their methadone dose. The authors offered the opinion that over-reporting of withdrawal symptoms was likely to be due to the warnings that the patients had received.[1]

(b) Rifampicin (Rifampin)

The observation that former diamorphine addicts taking methadone complained of withdrawal symptoms when given rifampicin, prompted a study[2] in 30 patients taking methadone. Withdrawal symptoms developed in 21 of the 30 patients within one to 33 days of starting rifampicin 600 to 900 mg daily and isoniazid. In 6 of the 7 patients most severely affected, the symptoms developed within one week, and their plasma methadone concentrations were reduced by 33 to 68%. Of 56 other patients taking methadone with other antitubercular drugs (which included isoniazid but not rifampicin), none developed withdrawal symptoms.[2-4] Other cases of this interaction have been reported.[5-9] Some patients needed 2- to 3-fold increases in their methadone dose while taking rifampicin in order to control the withdrawal symptoms.[6,7,9]

Mechanism

Rifampicin is an enzyme inducer, which increases the activity of the intestinal and liver cytochrome P450 isoenzymes concerned with the metabolism of methadone, resulting in a large decrease in its concentrations.[10] In 4 patients in the study cited, the urinary excretion of the major metabolite of methadone increased 2.5-fold.[2] Rifabutin is a less potent enzyme-inducer than rifampicin and therefore the effects are not as great.

Importance and management

The interaction between methadone and rifampicin is established, adequately documented, and of clinical importance. The incidence is high: two-thirds (21) of the opioid-dependent patients in one study[2] developed this interaction, 14 of whom were able to continue treatment. Withdrawal symptoms can develop within 24 hours. The analgesic effects of methadone would also be expected to be reduced. Concurrent use need not be avoided, but the effects should be monitored and appropriate methadone dose increases (as much as 2- to 3-fold) made where necessary.

Rifabutin appears to interact to a lesser extent than rifampicin, so that fewer, if any, patients are likely to need a methadone dose increase. Rifabutin might therefore be considered as an alternative to rifampicin, where appropriate.

1. Brown LS, Sawyer RC, Li R, Cobb MN, Colborn DC, Narang PK. Lack of a pharmacologic interaction between rifabutin and methadone in HIV-infected former injecting drug users. *Drug Alcohol Depend* (1996) 43, 71–7.
2. Kreek MJ, Garfield JW, Gutjahr CL, Giusti LM. Rifampin-induced methadone withdrawal. *N Engl J Med* (1976) 294, 1104–6.
3. Garfield JW, Kreek MJ, Giusti L. Rifampin-methadone relationship. 1. The clinical effects of rifampin-methadone interaction. *Am Rev Respir Dis* (1975) 111, 926.
4. Kreek MJ, Garfield JW, Gutjahr CL, Bowen D, Field F, Rothschild M. Rifampin-methadone relationship. 2. Rifampin effects on plasma concentration, metabolism, and excretion of methadone. *Am Rev Respir Dis* (1975) 111, 926–7.
5. Bending MR, Skacel PO. Rifampicin and methadone withdrawal. *Lancet* (1977) i, 1211.
6. Van Leeuwen DJ. Rifampicine leidt tot onthoudingsverschijnselen bij methadongebruikers. *Ned Tijdschr Geneeskd* (1986) 130, 548–50.
7. Brockmeyer NH, Mertins L, Goos M. Pharmacokinetic interaction of antimicrobial agents with levo-methadon in drug-addicted AIDS patients. *Klin Wochenschr* (1991) 69, 16–18.
8. Holmes VF. Rifampin-induced methadone withdrawal in AIDS. *J Clin Psychopharmacol* (1990) 10, 443–4.
9. Raistrick D, Hay A, Wolff K. Methadone maintenance and tuberculosis treatment. *BMJ* (1996) 313, 925–6.
10. Kharasch ED, Hoffer C, Whittington D, Sheffels P. Role of hepatic and intestinal cytochrome P450 3A and 2B6 in the metabolism, disposition, and miotic effects of methadone. *Clin Pharmacol Ther* (2004) 76, 250–69.

Opioids + St John's wort (*Hypericum perforatum*)

St John's wort moderately reduced the exposure to oxycodone, and appears to reduce the plasma concentrations of methadone. St John's wort is predicted to induce the metabolism of tapentadol, and concurrent use might increase the risk of serotonin syndrome.

Clinical evidence

(a) Methadone

In a study in 4 patients taking methadone, St John's wort (*Jarsin*) 900 mg daily for 14 to 47 days decreased methadone plasma concentration-to-dose ratios (indicating decreased methadone concentrations) by 19 to 60%. Two patients reported symptoms that suggested a withdrawal syndrome.[1]

(b) Oxycodone

In a crossover study in 12 healthy subjects, St John's wort (*Jarsin* containing hyperforin 2 to 6%) 300 mg three times daily was given for 15 days, with a single 15-mg oral dose of oxycodone on day 14. The AUC and maximum plasma concentration of oxycodone were reduced by 50% and 29%, respectively, and the AUC and maximum plasma concentration of the oxycodone metabolite, noroxycodone, were increased by 13% and 50%, respectively. The AUC of another metabolite, oxymorphone, was reduced by 52%, but its maximum plasma concentration was not notably affected. St John's wort reduced the self-reported analgesic effect of oxycodone (using visual analogue scales), but had no effect on cold pain intensity and threshold, as assessed using the cold pressor test. All but two of the subjects were extensive CYP2D6 metabolisers (that is, they had normal CYP2D6 activity).[2]

(c) Tapentadol

The US manufacturer of tapentadol warns of an increased risk of serotonin syndrome when it is given with other serotonergic drugs,[3] which would include St John's wort.

Mechanism

St John's wort is a known inducer of CYP3A4, and so can affect the plasma concentrations of drugs metabolised by this isoenzyme, such as methadone.[1] Oxycodone is metabolised to noroxycodone by CYP3A4, and to oxymorphone by CYP2D6. St John's wort therefore increases the metabolism of oxycodone to noroxycodone, increasing its exposure.

Importance and management

St John's wort appears to reduce the plasma concentrations of methadone causing withdrawal symptoms in some patients. Therefore concurrent use should be avoided. It might be prudent to follow the same advice for other opioids[4] that are mainly metabolised by CYP3A4, such as **buprenorphine**, **fentanyl**, or **alfentanil**. Exposure to oxycodone is moderately reduced by St John's wort, but its analgesic effects do not appear to be notably altered. Concurrent use need not be avoided, but consider this interaction in the case of any unexpected reduction in analgesic effect, and adjust the oxycodone dose accordingly.

The UK manufacturer of **tapentadol** states that caution is necessary if a potent enzyme inducer (they name St John's wort) is started or stopped in a patient taking tapentadol, as this might lead to decreased efficacy or an increased risk of adverse effects.[5] However, the mechanism by which this might occur is unclear, as tapentadol is principally metabolised by a number of glucuronidases which is not the known mechanism by which St John's wort usually interacts (see *Mechanism* above). *In vitro* and *animal* studies suggest that some constituents of St. John's wort can alter the activity of glucuronidases, but the *in vivo* consequences of this effect are unknown,[6] and so the clinical importance of this prediction is unclear. Until more is known, be aware that the dose of tapentadol might need to be adjusted on concurrent use. Serotonin syndrome is a rare adverse effect, but because of its severity, some caution would be warranted if both **tapentadol** and St John's wort are given concurrently. Concurrent use of other opioids might also increase the risk of serotonin syndrome. For a list of serotonergic drugs, see 'Table 35.3', p.1472, and for more information on serotonin syndrome and its management, see 'Drugs that cause serotonin syndrome + Other drugs that cause serotonin syndrome', p.1471.

1. Eic-Höchli D, Oppliger R, Powell Golay K, Baumann P, Eap CB. Methadone maintenance treatment and St John's wort. *Pharmacopsychiatry* (2003) 36, 35–7.
2. Nieminen TH, Hagelberg NM, Saari TI, Neuvonen M, Laine K, Neuvonen PJ, Olkkola KT. St John's wort greatly reduces the concentrations of oral oxycodone. *Eur J Pain* (2010) 14, 854–9.
3. Nucynta (Tapentadol). Janssen Pharmaceuticals, Inc. US Prescribing information, July 2013.
4. Kumar NB, Allen K, Bel H. Perioperative herbal supplement use in cancer patients: potential implications and recommendations for presurgical screening. *Cancer Control* (2005) 12, 149–57.
5. Palexia (Tapentadol hydrochloride). Grünenthal Ltd. UK Summary of product characteristics, July 2014.
6. Mohamed M-EF, Frye RF. Effects of herbal supplements on drug glucuronidation. Review of clinical, animal, and *in vitro* studies. *Planta Med* (2011) 77, 311–21.

Opioids + Ticlopidine

Ticlopidine moderately increases the exposure to tramadol and slightly increases that of methadone.

Clinical evidence

(a) Methadone

In a crossover study in 12 healthy subjects, ticlopidine 250 mg twice daily was given for 9 days with a single 8-mg oral dose and a single 4-mg intravenous dose of methadone on day 4. The AUC of *S*-methadone was increased by 62% and 57%, after oral and intravenous administration, respectively.[1]

(b) Tramadol

In a crossover study in 12 healthy subjects, ticlopidine 250 mg twice daily was given for 5 days with a single 50-mg dose of tramadol on day 4. The AUC of tramadol was increased 2-fold and the maximum plasma concentration was increased 1.4-fold. The maximum plasma concentration of the active metabolite, O-desmethyltramadol (M1), was reduced by 40% but the AUC was unaffected. The analgesic effect of tramadol was not affected, as assessed by the cold pressor test.[2]

Mechanism

Ticlopidine is an inhibitor of CYP2B6, which is said to be involved in the metabolism of tramadol[2] and methadone.[1] Concurrent use therefore results in increased exposure.

Importance and management

A pharmacokinetic interaction between ticlopidine and tramadol and methadone is established, but the general clinical importance of this is unclear. It does not seem that the analgesic effects of **tramadol** are altered, but given the moderate increase in tramadol exposure, it would seem prudent to bear the possibility of an interaction in mind should a patient taking both drugs develop an increase in tramadol adverse effects (such as sedation or seizures). The effect on **methadone** exposure is smaller, and the resultant slight increase is unlikely to be clinically important in most patients. Nevertheless it would seem prudent to bear the possibility of an interaction in mind (especially in those patients taking high doses of methadone), should a patient taking both drugs develop an increase in methadone adverse effects (such as sedation and respiratory depression).

1. Kharasch ED, Stubbert K. Role of cytochrome P4502B6 in methadone metabolism and clearance. *J Clin Pharmacol* (2013) 53, 305–13.
2. Hagelberg NM, Saarikoski T, Saari TI, Neuvonen M, Neuvonen PJ, Turpeinen M, Scheinin M, Laine K, Olkkola KT. Ticlopidine inhibits the O-demethylation and renal clearance of tramadol, increasing the exposure to it, but itraconazole has no marked effect on the tramadol-ticlopidine interaction. *Eur J Clin Pharmacol* (2013) 69, 867–75.

Opioids + Tobacco

Smokers appear to require more opioid analgesics for postoperative pain control than non-smokers; this has been seen with both fentanyl and morphine patient-controlled analgesia. Atmospheric pollution and smoking has a similar effect on pentazocine. Codeine metabolism was not affected to a clinically relevant extent by smoking in one study. A case of methadone toxicity was attributed to reduced smoking.

Clinical evidence

A retrospective study of coronary artery bypass graft (CABG) patients found that 20 smokers required more postoperative opioid analgesics than 69 non-smokers. The opioid analgesics included **dextropropoxyphene (propoxyphene)**, **fentanyl**, **hydrocodone**, **oxycodone**, **morphine**, **nalbuphine**, and **pethidine (meperidine)**, but the most commonly used opioid was **fentanyl** (used in approximately two-thirds of the patients) given by patient-controlled analgesia (PCA). Smokers deprived of nicotine as a result of being hospitalised for CABG had an increase in opioid requirements (converted to morphine equivalents), during the first 48 hours after surgery, ranging from 29 to 33% (when normalised for body-weight or body mass index).[1] Similarly, another retrospective study in 171 women found that the average postoperative narcotic use over 12 hours (expressed as equivalent doses of morphine) was 10.9 mg for patients who had never smoked, 13 mg for former smokers, and 13.1 mg for current smokers.[2]

(a) Codeine

The metabolism of a single 25-mg dose of codeine did not differ between 9 heavy smokers (greater than 20 cigarettes daily) and 9 non-smoking control subjects, except that smokers had a slightly higher rate of codeine glucuronidation.[3] This is unlikely to be clinically important. Another study found no clinically important differences in the systemic availability of single 60-mg oral or intramuscular doses of codeine between 10 smokers and 12 non-smokers. There was no significant difference in the plasma half-life of codeine or in the conversion of codeine to morphine; however, there was a slightly higher plasma clearance of codeine in smokers than in non-smokers.[4] No differences in the efficacy of codeine are expected between smokers and non-smokers.

(b) Dextropropoxyphene (Propoxyphene)

A study in 835 patients who were given dextropropoxyphene for mild or moderate pain or headache found that its efficacy as an analgesic was decreased by smoking. The drug was rated as ineffective in about 10% of 335 non-smokers, 15% of 347 patients who smoked up to 20 cigarettes daily, and 20% of 153 patients who smoked more than 20 cigarettes daily.[5]

(c) Methadone

A patient who had been taking a stable dose of methadone 10 mg twice daily for 4 months for back pain was admitted with decreased respiratory rate and altered mental status. Methadone was temporarily stopped and his symptoms improved, and the symptoms were attributed to methadone toxicity. Over the past month he had reduced his cigarette smoking from one pack to half-a-pack daily, and it was suggested that this had reduced methadone metabolism.[6]

(d) Morphine

A study in 7 women during the acute post-caesarean recovery period found that intravenous morphine use over 24 hours (as patient-controlled analgesia; PCA) was greater in smokers compared with non-smokers: weight-adjusted morphine use was 1.8 mg/kg compared with 0.64 mg/kg, respectively). It was suggested that a history of nicotine use and/or short-term nicotine abstinence could modulate morphine use and analgesia during postoperative recovery.[7] Similarly, another retrospective study found increased morphine PCA requirements in smokers compared with non-smokers.[8]

(e) Pentazocine

A study in which pentazocine was used to supplement nitrous oxide relaxant anaesthesia found that patients who came from an urban environment needed about 50% more pentazocine than those who lived in the country (3.6 micrograms/kg per minute compared with 2.4 micrograms/kg per minute). Roughly the same difference was seen between those who smoked and those who did not (3.8 micrograms/kg per minute compared with 2.5 micrograms/kg per minute).[9] In another study it was found that pentazocine metabolism was 40% higher in smokers than in non-smokers.[10]

Mechanism

It is thought that tobacco smoke contains compounds that increase the activity of the liver enzymes concerned with the metabolism of dextropropoxyphene, methadone, pentazocine, and many other opioids, which increases their metabolism, decreases their concentrations, and diminishes their effectiveness as analgesics.[2,5,6] A patient taking regular opioids who stopped smoking might therefore have increased opiate effects.[6] Nicotine might also decrease pain perception (note that nicotine has been tried for use in post-operative pain relief[11]); therefore, stopping smoking before surgery might increase pain perception because of the lack of nicotine. In addition, because former smokers have also been found to have increased opioid requirements, it has been suggested that nicotine addiction and opioid requirements might be genetically linked.[2]

Importance and management

The interaction between tobacco smoking and opioids appears to be established. Prescribers should be aware that smokers might require a greater amount of opioids postoperatively than non-smokers, although as pain control is tailored to requirement, this is unlikely to be clinically important. However, as the case with methadone illustrates, adverse effects might possibly develop if smoking is decreased, and this should be borne in mind if patients taking opioids decide to give up smoking.

Codeine metabolism does not appear to be affected to a clinically relevant extent by smoking, but this lack of pharmacokinetic interaction does not rule out an interaction if the mechanism is pharmacodynamic.

1. Creekmore FM, Lugo RA, Weiland KJ. Postoperative opiate analgesia requirements of smokers and nonsmokers. *Ann Pharmacother* (2004) 38, 949–53.
2. Woodside JR. Female smokers have increased postoperative narcotic requirements. *J Addict Dis* (2000) 19, 1–10.
3. Yue Q-Y, Tomson T, Säwe J. Carbamazepine and cigarette smoking induce differentially the metabolism of codeine in man. *Pharmacogenetics* (1994) 4, 193–8.
4. Hull JH, Findlay JWA, Rogers JF, Welch RM, Butz RF, Bustrack JA. An evaluation of the effects of smoking on codeine pharmacokinetics and bioavailability in normal human volunteers. *Drug Intell Clin Pharm* (1982) 16, 849–54.
5. Boston Collaborative Drug Surveillance Program. Decreased clinical efficacy of propoxyphene in cigarette smokers. *Clin Pharmacol Ther* (1973) 14, 259–63.
6. Wahawisan J, Kolluru S, Nguyen T, Molina C, Speake J. Methadone toxicity due to smoking cessation—a case report on the drug-drug interaction involving cytochrome P450 isoenzyme 1A2. *Ann Pharmacother* (2011) 45, e34.
7. Marco AP, Greenwald MK, Higgins MS. A preliminary study of 24-hour post-cesarean patient controlled analgesia: postoperative pain reports and morphine requests/utilization are greater in abstaining smokers than non-smokers. *Med Sci Monit* (2005) 11, CR255–CR261.
8. Glasson JC, Sawyer WT, Lindley CM, Ginsberg B. Patient-specific factors affecting patient-controlled analgesia dosing. *J Pain Palliat Care Pharmacother* (2002) 16, 5–21.
9. Keeri-Szanto M, Pomeroy JR. Atmospheric pollution and pentazocine metabolism. *Lancet* (1971) i, 947–9.
10. Vaughan DP, Beckett AH, Robbie DS. The influence of smoking on the intersubject variation in pentazocine elimination. *Br J Clin Pharmacol* (1976) 3, 279–83.
11. Jankowski CJ, Weingarten TN, Martin DP, Whalen FX, Gebhart JB, Liedl LM, Danielson DR, Nadeau AM, Schroeder DR, Warner DO, Sprung J. Randomised trial of intranasal nicotine and postoperative pain, nausea and vomiting in non-smoking women. *Eur J Anaesthesiol* (2011) 28, 585–91.

Opioids + Tricyclic and related antidepressants

In general, the concurrent use of most opioids and tricyclics is uneventful, although lethargy, sedation, and respiratory depression have been reported. The concurrent use of tramadol with tricyclic antidepressants might increase the possible risk of seizures and serotonin syndrome. Concurrent use of tapentadol with tricyclics might also increase the risk of serotonin syndrome. Dextropropoxyphene might cause small increases in the serum concentrations of amitriptyline, nortriptyline, and possibly doxepin, and methadone might modestly increase desipramine concentrations. The exposure and degree of analgesia of oral morphine are increased by clomipramine, desipramine, and possibly amitriptyline.

Clinical evidence

(a) Buprenorphine

A study in 12 healthy subjects found that both sublingual buprenorphine 400 micrograms and oral **amitriptyline** 50 mg impaired the performance of a number of psychomotor tests (digit symbol substitution, flicker fusion, Maddox wing, hand-to-eye co-ordination, reactive skills), and the subjects felt drowsy, feeble, mentally slow, and muzzy. When **amitriptyline** 30 mg, increased to 75 mg daily, was given for 4 days before a single dose of buprenorphine, the psychomotor effects were not increased, but the respiratory depressant effects of buprenorphine were enhanced.[1]

(b) Dextropropoxyphene (Propoxyphene)

An elderly man taking **doxepin** 150 mg daily developed lethargy and daytime sedation when he started to take dextropropoxyphene 65 mg every 6 hours. His plasma **doxepin** concentrations increased almost 2.5-fold (from 20 to 48.5 nanograms/mL) and desmethyldoxepin concentrations were similarly increased (from 8.8 to 20.7 nanograms/mL).[2]

The **amitriptyline** concentration to dose ratio in 12 patients given **amitriptyline** and dextropropoxyphene was increased by about 20% (suggesting increased amitriptyline concentrations), when compared with other patients taking **amitriptyline** alone. Similarly, the plasma concentration of the **amitriptyline** metabolite, nortriptyline, was increased by about 30% in 14 patients given dextropropoxyphene;[3] and in another study, **nortriptyline** plasma concentrations were increased by 16% by dextropropoxyphene.[3]

Fifteen patients with rheumatoid arthritis given a single 25-mg dose of **amitriptyline** and dextropropoxyphene (up to 65 mg three times daily) experienced some drowsiness and mental slowness. They complained of being clumsier and had more pain, but these effects were said to be mild.[4]

(c) Methadone

The mean serum concentrations of **desipramine** 2.5 mg/kg daily were approximately doubled in 5 men who took methadone 500 micrograms/kg daily for 2 weeks. Previous observations in patients given both drugs had shown that **desipramine** concentrations were higher than expected and adverse effects developed at relatively low doses.[5] Further evidence of an increase in plasma **desipramine** concentrations due to methadone is described in another study.[6]

(d) Morphine

In a study in 24 patients with cancer-related pain, **clomipramine** or **amitriptyline**, in doses of 20 or 50 mg daily, increased the AUC of oral morphine by 28 to 111%. The half-life of morphine was also prolonged.[7] A previous study[8] found that **desipramine**, but not **amitriptyline**, increased and prolonged morphine analgesia, and a later study by the same group confirmed this potentially beneficial effect of **desipramine**.[9] A case of severe symptoms of morphine overdose requiring prolonged naltrexone infusion occurred in an elderly man with metastatic lung cancer hospitalised for daily dose titration of oral morphine, when his dose of **amitriptyline** was increased from 25 to 50 mg daily. The authors attributed the effect, in part, to an interaction with amitriptyline and, secondarily, with ranitidine.[10] See also, 'Opioids; Morphine + Miscellaneous', p.201, for limited evidence that amitriptyline and **doxepin** might increase the risk of myoclonus with morphine.

(e) Oxycodone

In a study in 9 healthy subjects, pretreatment with **amitriptyline** 10 mg increased to 50 mg daily for 4 days caused no major changes in the psychomotor effects of a single 280-microgram/kg oral dose of oxycodone.[11] Respiratory effects were not assessed.

(f) Pentazocine

Both pentazocine and **amitriptyline** given alone caused 11 healthy subjects to feel drowsy, muzzy, and clumsy, and reduced the performance of a number of psychomotor tests. However, when the same subjects were given intramuscular pentazocine 30 mg after taking **amitriptyline** 50 mg daily for one week, the combination of drugs appeared not to impair driving or occupational skills more than either drug given alone.[12] Respiratory depression was increased more by concurrent use than by either drug alone. **Amitriptyline** decreased pentazocine plasma concentrations by about 20% at 1.5 hours and 3.5 hours post-dose.[12]

(g) Tapentadol

The US manufacturer of tapentadol warns of an increased risk of serotonin syndrome when tapentadol is given with a tricyclic antidepressant.[13]

(h) Tramadol

The CSM in the UK has publicised 27 reports of convulsions and one of worsening epilepsy with tramadol, a reporting rate of 1 in 7000 patients. Some of the patients were given doses well in excess of those recommended, and 8 patients were also taking tricyclic antidepressants, which are known to lower the convulsive threshold.[14] Similarly, the FDA in the US has received 124 reports of seizures associated with tramadol, 28 of which included the concurrent use of tricyclic antidepressants,[15] and the Australian Adverse Drug Reaction Advisory Committee (ADRAC) has received 26 cases of convulsions associated with tramadol, some of which included the concurrent use of tricyclic antidepressants.[16] ADRAC have also received reports of serotonin syndrome, which were associated with the use of tramadol and tricyclic antidepressants.[16] Furthermore, two case reports suggest that tramadol might have contributed to the development of serotonin syndrome: one report was of a patient abusing tramadol, moclobemide, and **clomipramine**,[17] and the other was of a 79-year-old patient taking morphine *(MST)*, co-proxamol (dextropropoxyphene with paracetamol (acetaminophen)) and **amitriptyline**, after she started to take tramadol.[18,19] In both of these cases the patient died. For another case of serotonin syndrome in a patient taking doxepin and tramadol with milnacipran and fluoxetine, see 'SNRIs + SSRIs', p.1478.

Mechanism

The CNS depressant effects of the opioids and the tricyclic antidepressants are expected to be additive. The reasons for the increased morphine exposure and analgesic effects that occur with some tricyclics are not understood. However, it has been suggested that the increased analgesia might be due not only to the increased exposure to morphine, but possibly also to some alteration in the way the morphine affects its receptors. Dextropropoxyphene probably inhibits the metabolism of some tricyclic antidepressants[3] by inhibiting CYP2D6, and as a result the serum concentrations of the tricyclic antidepressants increase. It is suggested that methadone may possibly inhibit the hydroxylation of desipramine, thereby increasing its concentrations.[6] Note that, on the basis of *in-vitro* study, the US manufacturers of tramadol include amitriptyline as an inhibitor of CYP2D6 that might increase tramadol concentrations. However, amitriptyline is not considered an inhibitor of CYP2D6 in clinical use.

Importance and management

The majority of the evidence, and general clinical experience, suggests that in most cases, the use of opioids with tricyclic antidepressants is uneventful. Furthermore, limited evidence suggests that concurrent use may be beneficial in pain management. However, the CNS depressant effects of both these classes of drugs should be considered when prescribing the combination, especially as there is some evidence to suggest that the respiratory depressant effects are increased: this may be clinically important in patients with a restricted respiratory capacity.[12]

Certain opioids appear to have a greater propensity to interact. Both **tramadol** and the tricyclics can lower the seizure threshold and cause serotonin syndrome when used alone. Concurrent use can result in additive effects, and therefore particular caution is warranted with this combination, especially in patients with epilepsy or those already taking other drugs that affect serotonin. Be aware that **dextropropoxyphene** and **methadone** might increase tricyclic concentrations: however, the general clinical relevance of these interactions is uncertain but be alert for any evidence of increased CNS depression and increased tricyclic antidepressant adverse effects (such as dry mouth, constipation, and urinary retention). In this context it is worth noting that one study reported that the incidence of hip fractures in the elderly was found to be increased by a factor of 1.6 in those taking dextropropoxyphene, and further increased to 2.6 when antidepressants, benzodiazepines or antipsychotics were added.[20] Serotonin syndrome is a rare adverse effect, but because of its severity, some caution would be warranted if both **tapentadol** and a tricyclic antidepressant are given concurrently. Concurrent use of other opioids might also increase the risk of serotonin syndrome. For more information on serotonin syndrome and its management, see 'Drugs that cause serotonin syndrome + Other drugs that cause serotonin syndrome', p.1471.

1. Saarialho-Kere U, Mattila MJ, Paloheimo M, Seppälä T. Psychomotor, respiratory and neuroendocrinological effects of buprenorphine and amitriptyline in healthy volunteers. *Eur J Clin Pharmacol* (1987) 33, 139–46.
2. Abernethy DR, Greenblatt DJ, Steel K. Propoxyphene inhibition of doxepin and antipyrine metabolism. *Clin Pharmacol Ther* (1982) 31, 199.
3. Jerling M, Bertilsson L, Sjöqvist F. The use of therapeutic drug monitoring data to document kinetic drug interactions: an example with amitriptyline and nortriptyline. *Ther Drug Monit* (1994) 16, 1–12.
4. Saarialho-Kere U, Julkunen H, Mattila MJ, Seppälä T. Psychomotor performance of patients with rheumatoid arthritis: cross-over comparison of dextropropoxyphene, dextropropoxyphene plus amitriptyline, indomethacin and placebo. *Pharmacol Toxicol* (1988) 63, 286–92.
5. Maany I, Dhopesh V, Arndt IO, Burke W, Woody G, O'Brien CP. Increase in desipramine serum levels associated with methadone treatment. *Am J Psychiatry* (1989) 146, 1611–13.
6. Kosten TR, Gawin FH, Morgan C, Nelson JC, Jatlow P. Desipramine and its 2-hydroxy metabolite in patients taking or not taking methadone. *Am J Psychiatry* (1990) 147, 1379–80.
7. Ventafridda V, Ripamonti C, De Conno F, Bianchi M, Pazzuconi F, Panerai AE. Antidepressants increase bioavailability of morphine in cancer patients. *Lancet* (1987) i, 1204.
8. Levine JD, Gordon NC, Smith R, McBryde R. Desipramine enhances opiate postoperative analgesia. *Pain* (1986) 27, 45–9.
9. Gordon NC, Heller PH, Gear RW, Levine JD. Temporal factors in the enhancement of morphine analgesia by desipramine. *Pain* (1993) 53, 273–6.
10. Upadhyay S, Jain R, Chauhan H, Gupta D, Mishra S, Bhatnagar S. Oral morphine overdose in a cancer patient antagonized by prolonged naloxone infusion. *Am J Hosp Palliat Care* (2008) 25, 401–5.
11. Pöyhiä R, Kalso E, Seppälä T. Pharmacodynamic interactions of oxycodone and amitriptyline in healthy volunteers. *Curr Ther Res* (1992) 51, 739–49.
12. Saarialho-Kere U, Mattila MJ, Seppälä T. Parenteral pentazocine: effects on psychomotor skills and respiration, and interactions with amitriptyline. *Eur J Clin Pharmacol* (1988) 35, 483–9.
13. Nucynta (Tapentadol). Janssen Pharmaceuticals, Inc. US Prescribing information, July 2013.
14. Committee on Safety of Medicines/Medicines Control Agency. In focus—tramadol. *Current Problems* (1996) 22, 11.
15. Kahn LH, Alderfer RJ, Graham DJ. Seizures reported with tramadol. *JAMA* (1997) 278, 1661.
16. Adverse Drug Reactions Advisory Committee (ADRAC). Tramadol – four years' experience. *Aust Adverse Drug React Bull* (2003) 22, 2.
17. Hernandez AF, Montero MN, Pla A, Villanueva E. Fatal moclobemide overdose or death caused by serotonin syndrome? *J Forensic Sci* (1995) 40, 128–30.
18. Kitson R, Carr B. Tramadol and severe serotonin syndrome. *Anaesthesia* (2005) 60, 934–5.
19. Gillman K. A response to 'Tramadol and severe serotonin syndrome'. *Anaesthesia* (2006) 61, 76. Author reply. Ibid., 76–77.
20. Shorr RI, Griffin MR, Daugherty JR, Ray WA. Opioid analgesics and the risk of hip fracture in the elderly: codeine and propoxyphene. *J Gerontol* (1992) 47, M111–M115.

Opioids + Urinary acidifiers or alkalinisers

Urinary methadone clearance is increased if the urine is made acidic (e.g. by giving ammonium chloride) and reduced if it is made alkaline (e.g. by giving sodium bicarbonate). The urinary clearance of dextropropoxyphene (propoxyphene) and pethidine (meperidine) might also be increased by acidification of the urine.

Clinical evidence

(a) Dextropropoxyphene (Propoxyphene)

A study in 6 healthy subjects found that the cumulative 72-hour urinary excretion of unchanged dextropropoxyphene was increased 6-fold by acidification of the urine with oral **ammonium chloride** and reduced by 95% by alkalinisation with **sodium bicarbonate**; the half-life of dextropropoxyphene was also shortened by ammonium chloride. The excretion of the active metabolite, norpropoxyphene, was much less dependent on urinary pH. However, the cumulative excretion of dextropropoxyphene and norpropoxyphene, even into acidic urine, accounted for less than 25% of the dose during 72 hours.[1]

(b) Methadone

A study in patients taking methadone found that the urinary clearance in those with a urinary pH of less than 6 was greater than those with a higher urinary pH.[2] When the urinary pH of one subject was lowered from 6.2 to 5.5, the loss of unchanged methadone in the urine was nearly doubled.[3] A pharmacokinetic study in 5 healthy subjects given a 10-mg intramuscular dose of methadone found that the plasma half-life was 19.5 hours when the urine was made acidic (pH 5.2) with **ammonium chloride**, compared with 42.1 hours when the urine was made alkaline (pH 7.8) with **sodium bicarbonate**. The clearance of methadone decreased from 134 mL/minute to 91.9 mL/minute when the urine was changed from acidic to alkaline.[4]

(c) Pethidine (Meperidine)

A study in 6 healthy subjects given intravenous pethidine 21.75 mg found that the 48-hour urinary recovery of pethidine and norpethidine was increased by urinary acidification with **ammonium chloride**, when compared with no urinary pH control. Recovery of pethidine increased from about 7% to 20%, and recovery of norpethidine increased from about 12% to 24%. Urinary alkalinisation reduced the urinary recovery of pethidine and norpethidine to less than 1% and 7%, respectively. These pronounced effects had inconsequential effects on the blood concentration/time profiles.[5] A study in 10 healthy Chinese subjects given intravenous pethidine 150 micrograms/kg found large variations in the 48-hour urinary recovery of pethidine and norpethidine depending on urinary pH; mean urinary recovery values under acidic conditions were 24% and 33%, respectively, and under alkaline conditions were 0.4% and 4%, respectively. The bioavailability was slightly lower under acidic urinary conditions due to the greater renal clearance of the drug.[6]

Mechanism

Methadone is eliminated from the body both by liver metabolism and excretion of unchanged methadone in the urine. Above pH 6 the urinary excretion is less important, but with urinary pH below 6 the half-life becomes dependent on both excretion (30%) and metabolism (70%).[3,4,7] Methadone is a weak base (pKa 8.4) so that in acidic urine little of the drug is in the non-ionised form and little is reabsorbed by simple passive diffusion. On the other hand, in alkaline solution most of the drug is in the non-ionised form, which is readily reabsorbed by the kidney tubules, and little is lost in the urine.

Acidification of the urine might also increase the renal clearance of unchanged pethidine (meperidine) and norpethidine, probably also due to reduced reabsorption in the renal tubule.[6] Dextropropoxyphene (propoxyphene) appears to be similarly affected, although this appears to be a minor route for dextropropoxyphene elimination.

Importance and management

The effect of urinary pH on the clearance of methadone is an established interaction, but, given the lack of reports in the published literature over the past 30 or so years, it would seem that it is not of clinical importance. Theoretically, urinary alkalinisers, such as sodium bicarbonate and **acetazolamide**, might increase the effect of methadone. However, note that sodium bicarbonate might be employed in the management of rhabdomyolysis occurring after methadone toxicity.

Similarly, the urinary clearance of dextropropoxyphene (propoxyphene) and pethidine (norpethidine) appear to be increased to some extent by acidification of the urine, although their bioavailabilities do not appear to be notably affected. As with methadone above, the lack of recent published literature describing this, suggests this is not a clinically important effect.

1. Kärkkäinen S, Neuvonen PJ. Effect of oral charcoal and urine pH on dextropropoxyphene pharmacokinetics. *Int J Clin Pharmacol Ther Toxicol* (1985) 23, 219–25.
2. Bellward GD, Warren PM, Howald W, Axelson JE, Abbott FS. Methadone maintenance: effect of urinary pH on renal clearance in chronic high and low doses. *Clin Pharmacol Ther* (1977) 22, 92–9.
3. Inturrisi CE, Verebely K. Disposition of methadone in man after a single oral dose. *Clin Pharmacol Ther* (1972) 13, 923–30.
4. Nilsson M-I, Widerlöv E, Meresaar U, Änggård E. Effect of urinary pH on the disposition of methadone in man. *Eur J Clin Pharmacol* (1982) 22, 337–42.
5. Verbeeck RK, Branch RA, Wilkinson GR. Meperidine disposition in man: influence of urinary pH and route of administration. *Clin Pharmacol Ther* (1981) 30, 619–28.
6. Chan K, Tse J, Jennings F, Orme ML'E. Influence of urinary pH on pethidine kinetics in healthy volunteer subjects. 2. A study of ten Chinese subjects. *Methods Find Exp Clin Pharmacol* (1987) 9, 49–54.
7. Baselt RC, Casarett LJ. Urinary excretion of methadone in man. *Clin Pharmacol Ther* (1972) 13, 64–70.

Opioids; Alfentanil + Reserpine

An isolated report describes ventricular arrhythmias when a patient taking reserpine was given alfentanil during anaesthesia.

Clinical evidence, mechanism, importance and management

A hypertensive woman taking reserpine 250 micrograms daily was given intravenous alfentanil 800 micrograms over 5 minutes, before anaesthesia with thiopental and suxamethonium (succinylcholine). During surgery she was given nine 100-microgram doses of alfentanil and 70% nitrous oxide/oxygen. Bradycardia developed and frequent unifocal premature ventricular contractions occurred throughout the surgery, but they disappeared 3 to 4 hours afterwards. The arrhythmia was attributed to an interaction between reserpine and alfentanil, but just why this should occur is not understood.[1] This is an isolated report and its general relevance is unclear.

1. Jahr JS, Weber S. Ventricular dysrhythmias following an alfentanil anesthetic in a patient on reserpine for hypertension. *Acta Anaesthesiol Scand* (1991) 35, 788–9.

Opioids; Alfentanil + Statins

Atorvastatin does not appear to alter the pharmacokinetics of alfentanil.

Clinical evidence, mechanism, importance and management

In a study, 7 matched pairs of patients undergoing elective surgery were given alfentanil 80 micrograms/kg per hour as a bolus dose followed by an intravenous infusion of 0.67 micrograms/kg per minute for 90 minutes. Half of the patients had been receiving **atorvastatin** for at least 4 months. There were no differences in the pharmacokinetics of alfentanil between the groups.[1] No alfentanil dose adjustments would appear to be necessary on concurrent use with atorvastatin.

Alfentanil is metabolised by CYP3A4, and as none of the statins are known to be clinically important CYP3A4 inhibitors or inducers, no pharmacokinetic interaction would be expected if any of these drugs are given with alfentanil.

1. McDonnell CG, Malkan D, Van Pelt FD, Shorten GD. Elimination of alfentanil delivered by infusion is not altered by the chronic administration of atorvastatin. *Eur J Anaesthesiol* (2003) 20, 662–7.

Opioids; Alfentanil + Terbinafine

No pharmacokinetic interaction occurs between terbinafine and alfentanil.

Clinical evidence, mechanism, importance and management

In a crossover study in 12 healthy subjects, terbinafine 250 mg daily for 3 days had no effect on the pharmacokinetics of intravenous alfentanil 20 micrograms/kg, given one hour after the last dose of the antifungal.[1] Therefore, no alfentanil dose adjustment is necessary on concurrent use.

1. Saari TI, Laine K, Leino K, Valtonen M, Neuvonen PJ, Olkkola KT. Voriconazole, but not terbinafine, markedly reduces alfentanil clearance and prolongs its half-life. *Clin Pharmacol Ther* (2006) 80, 502–8.

Opioids; Codeine + Kaolin

The bioavailability of codeine might be reduced by kaolin.

Clinical evidence, mechanism, importance and management

An isolated report describes patients suffering from chronic diarrhoea, who were stabilised taking codeine phosphate, but who experienced a relapse when the codeine was added to *Kaolin Mixture*. An *in vitro* study suggested the bioavailability of codeine might be reduced by adsorption onto kaolin.[1] The general importance of this finding is unknown but bear this report in mind should a patient taking a kaolin-containing product report a reduced effect from codeine.

1. Yu SKS, Oppenheim RC, Stewart NF. Codeine phosphate adsorbed by kaolin. *Aust J Pharm* (1976) 57, 468.

Opioids; Codeine + Somatostatin analogues

Lanreotide and octreotide appear to partially inhibit the metabolism of codeine, which theoretically could reduce its analgesic effects.

Clinical evidence, mechanism, importance and management

A study in 6 patients with gastrointestinal carcinoid tumours found that **lanreotide** or **octreotide** 750 micrograms subcutaneously three times daily for 3 days decreased the partial metabolic clearance of codeine by *N*-demethylation (by the cytochrome P450 subfamily CYP3A) by an average of 44%, and the *O*-demethylation (by CYP2D6) by 35%. However, the partial clearance by 6-glucuronidation and the total systemic clearance of codeine were not consistently changed. All patients were extensive CYP2D6 metabolisers (that is, they had normal CYP2D6 activity). The authors suggested that the effects of the somatostatins were mediated by a suppression of growth hormone secretion as alterations in growth hormone secretion have been shown to alter the hepatic cytochrome P450 enzyme system in *animals* and humans. Further, they suggest that the reduction in *O*-demethylation could reduce concentrations of morphine, which is an active metabolite of codeine, and result in a reduction in the analgesic effect of the drug.[1] The clinical relevance of this does not appear to have been studied, and further study into the proposed mechanism is required.

1. Rasmussen E, Eriksson B, Öberg K, Bondesson U, Rane A. Selective effects of somatostatin analogs on human drug-metabolizing enzymes. *Clin Pharmacol Ther* (1998) 64, 150–9.

Opioids; Dextropropoxyphene (Propoxyphene) + Orphenadrine

An alleged adverse interaction between dextropropoxyphene and orphenadrine, which is said to cause mental confusion, anxiety, and tremors, seems to be very rare, if indeed it ever occurs.

Clinical evidence, mechanism, importance and management

The manufacturers of orphenadrine used to state in their package insert that mental confusion, anxiety, and tremors have been reported in patients receiving both orphenadrine and dextropropoxyphene. The manufacturers of dextropropoxyphene issued a similar warning. However, in correspondence with both manufacturers the basis of these statements was identified as 6 anecdotal reports from clinicians to one manufacturer and 7 to the other (some could represent the same cases). Of the 7 cases to one manufacturer, 4 occurred where patients had received twice the recommended dose of orphenadrine. In every case the adverse reactions seen were similar to those reported with either drug alone.[1] A brief study in 5 patients given both drugs to investigate this alleged interaction did not identify an adverse interaction.[2] One case has been reported separately.[3]

The documentation is therefore sparse, and no case of an interaction has been firmly established. At the time, the investigators calculated that the two drugs were probably being used together on 300 000 prescriptions a year, and that these few cases would be less than significant.[1] There therefore seems little reason for avoiding concurrent use.

1. Pearson RE, Salter FJ. Drug interaction? — Orphenadrine with propoxyphene. *N Engl J Med* (1970) 282, 1215.
2. Puckett WH, Visconti JA. Orphenadrine and propoxyphene (cont.). *N Engl J Med* (1970) 283, 544.
3. Renforth W. Orphenadrine and propoxyphene. *N Engl J Med* (1970) 283, 998.

Opioids; Methadone + Aromatase inhibitors; Letrozole

Letrozole appears to negligibly increase methadone exposure.

Clinical evidence, mechanism, importance and management

In a study, 15 postmenopausal women were given a single 2-mg intravenous dose of methadone before and after **letrozole** 2.5 mg daily for 7 days. The clearance of methadone was decreased by 22%, and the AUC was increased by 23%. However, there was wide interindividual variability in the AUC, with increases up to 3-fold also seen.[1] The alterations in methadone pharmacokinetics seen here are negligible and are unlikely to be clinically important. No methadone dose adjustment would be expected to be necessary on concurrent use.

1. Lu WJ, Thong N, Flockhart DA. Reduced methadone clearance during aromatase inhibition. *J Clin Psychopharmacol* (2012) 32, 511–7.

Opioids; Methadone + Disulfiram

No adverse interaction was seen when patients taking methadone were given disulfiram.

Clinical evidence, mechanism, importance and management

Seven opioid addicts, without chronic alcoholism or liver disease, and who were receiving methadone maintenance treatment (45 to 65 mg daily) had an increase in the urinary excretion of the major pyrrolidine metabolite of methadone (an indicator of increased *N*-demethylation) when given disulfiram 500 mg daily for 7 days. However, there was no effect on the degree of opioid intoxication, nor were opioid withdrawal symptoms experienced.[1] No special precautions would therefore seem to be necessary if both drugs are given.

1. Tong TG, Benowitz NL, Kreek MJ. Methadone-disulfiram interaction during methadone maintenance. *J Clin Pharmacol* (1980) 20, 506–13.

Opioids; Methadone + Fusidic acid

Fusidic acid might affect the clearance of levomethadone (*R*-methadone), and a case of opioid withdrawal has been reported following the concurrent use of these drugs. However, another study found no evidence of an interaction.

Clinical evidence, mechanism, importance and management

A patient with AIDS needed an increase in his levomethadone (*R*-methadone) dose from 60 to 80 mg daily within 6 months of starting to take fusidic acid 1.5 g daily.[1] The patient had evidence of liver enzyme induction (using antipyrine as a marker), from which it was concluded that fusidic acid had increased the metabolism and loss of methadone from the body.[1] A subsequent study in 10 patients taking levomethadone confirmed that fusidic acid 500 mg daily for 28 days increased antipyrine clearance and some patients developed clinical signs of under dosing. In contrast, fusidic acid 500 mg daily for 14 days had no effect in another 10 patients taking levomethadone.[2]

Information appears to be limited to these reports. Bear them in mind in the event of any unexpected reduction in efficacy of levomethadone (and probably methadone) in a patient taking long-term fusidic acid.

1. Brockmeyer NH, Mertins L, Goos M. Pharmacokinetic interaction of antimicrobial agents with levomethadon in drug-addicted AIDS patients. *Klin Wochenschr* (1991) 69, 16–18.
2. Reimann G, Barthel B, Rockstroh JK, Spatz D, Brockmeyer NH. Effect of fusidic acid on the hepatic cytochrome P450 enzyme system. *Int J Clin Pharmacol* (1999) 37, 562–6.

Opioids; Methadone + Lofexidine

The concurrent use of methadone and low-dose lofexidine can cause clinically important hypotension and additional CNS depression.

Clinical evidence, mechanism, importance and management

A small study in 14 subjects taking stable doses of methadone 80 mg daily for 3 weeks, found that the addition of lofexidine 400 micrograms daily had clinically important effects on blood pressure and cognitive function. Systolic and diastolic blood pressures were reduced by an average of 27 mmHg and 15 mmHg, respectively. Two female subjects became drowsy, with low blood pressure readings of 88/55 mmHg and 80/48 mmHg, respectively, which required discontinuation of lofexidine. Cognitive tests such as simple reaction times, memory tests, and mathematical processing were also affected, although only the effect on mathematical processing reached statistical significance for overall dose effect. Two patients also developed asymptomatic, transient QTc prolongation after a single dose of lofexidine, which resolved when lofexidine was stopped.[1] Further study of the concurrent use of lofexidine and methadone in the management of opioid withdrawal is needed. Patients given both drugs should be closely monitored for adverse effects, in particular reductions in blood pressure and cognitive changes.

Note that cases of QT prolongation have been reported with lofexidine, and this is predicted to be additive with other drugs that might cause QT prolongation, such as methadone. See 'Drugs that prolong the QT interval + Other drugs that prolong the QT interval', p.272, for more information on the use of two or more drugs that prolong the QT interval.

1. Schroeder JR, Schmittner J, Bleiberg J, Epstein DH, Krantz MJ, Preston KL. Hemodynamic and cognitive effects of lofexidine and methadone coadministration: a pilot study. *Pharmacotherapy* (2007) 27, 1111–19.

Opioids; Methadone + Olanzapine

Olanzapine does not appear to alter the pharmacokinetics of methadone.

Clinical evidence, mechanism, importance and management

A study in 15 patients taking methadone maintenance for cocaine abuse, found that the addition of olanzapine 5 to 10 mg daily did not appear to alter the methadone concentration-to-dose ratio.[1] This study suggests that olanzapine does not alter the pharmacokinetics of methadone and that no dose adjustment would appear necessary on concurrent use.

1. Baño MD, Micó JA, Agujetas M, López ML, Guillén JL. Olanzapine efficacy in the treatment of cocaine abuse in methadone maintenance patients. Interaction with plasma levels. *Actas Esp Psiquiatr* (2001) 29, 215–20.

Opioids; Methadone + Quetiapine

In one study, quetiapine caused small increases in the concentrations of methadone.

Clinical evidence, mechanism, importance and management

In a study, 14 patients taking methadone maintenance for at least one month were given an average dose of quetiapine of 138 mg daily for an average of 30 days. The addition of quetiapine increased the mean *R*-methadone plasma concentration to dose ratio by 21%, although there was considerable interpatient variability (range 23% decrease to 85% increase). No notable effects on the *S*-methadone enantiomer were seen, and there were no reports of methadone overdose or toxicity in any of the patients. Some minor differences in the metabolism of *R*-methadone were seen when patients were assessed for difference in the expression of CYP2D6 and P-glycoprotein, but these were not statistically significant. However, because some changes were seen, the authors suggest that one or both of these mechanisms might be responsible for the interaction.[1]

Evidence appears to be limited to this study, in which only small, clinically unimportant increases in methadone concentrations were seen. However, as the dose of quetiapine was relatively low, and the patient numbers were small, further study is needed to establish these findings.

1. Uehlinger C, Crettol S, Chassot P, Brocard M, Koeb L, Brawand-Amey M, Eap CB. Increased (*R*)-methadone plasma concentrations by quetiapine in cytochrome P450s and *ABCB1* genotyped patients. *J Clin Psychopharmacol* (2007) 27, 273–8.

Opioids; Morphine + Miscellaneous

Limited evidence suggests that some antidepressants, antipsychotics, NSAIDs, and thiethylperazine might increase the myoclonus caused by high doses of morphine.

Clinical evidence, mechanism, importance and management

In 19 patients with malignant disease taking high doses of morphine (daily doses of 500 mg or more orally or 250 mg or more parenterally), an analysis was made of the relationship between myoclonus and the use of supplemental drugs. In the 12 patients with myoclonus, 8 patients were taking antidepressants (**amitriptyline**, **doxepin**) or antipsychotics (**chlorpromazine**, **haloperidol**), compared with none of 6 patients without myoclonus. In addition, there was a higher use of NSAIDs (**indometacin**, **naproxen**, **piroxicam**, **aspirin**) and an antiemetic (**thiethylperazine**).[1] The reasons are not understood, and the findings of this paper have been questioned.[2]

1. Potter JM, Reid DB, Shaw RJ, Hackett P, Hickman PE. Myoclonus associated with treatment with high doses of morphine: the role of supplemental drugs. *BMJ* (1989) 299, 150–3.
2. Quinn N. Myoclonus associated with high doses of morphine. *BMJ* (1989) 299, 683–4.

Opioids; Pethidine (Meperidine) + Aciclovir

An isolated report describes pethidine toxicity associated with the use of high-dose aciclovir.

Clinical evidence, mechanism, importance and management

A man with Hodgkin's disease was given high-dose intravenous aciclovir for localised herpes zoster, with intramuscular pethidine, oral methadone, and levodopa with carbidopa. On the second day he experienced nausea, vomiting, and confusion, and later dysarthria, lethargy, and ataxia. Despite vigorous treatment he later died. It was concluded that some of the adverse effects were due to pethidine toxicity arising from norpethidine accumulation, associated with renal impairment caused by the aciclovir.[1] The US manufacturer of pethidine states that plasma concentrations of pethidine, and its metabolite norpethidine, might be increased by aciclovir, thus caution should be used if both drugs are given;[2] however, evidence for such an effect is sparse and the general relevance of any interaction remains to be established.

1. Johnson R, Douglas J, Corey L, Krasney H. Adverse effects with acyclovir and meperidine. *Ann Intern Med* (1985) 103, 962–3.
2. Demerol (Meperidine hydrochloride). Sanofi-Aventis US LLC. US Prescribing information, July 2014.

Opioids; Tapentadol + Aspirin

Aspirin does not appear to affect the pharmacokinetics of tapentadol.

Clinical evidence, mechanism, importance and management

A crossover study in 36 healthy subjects found that aspirin 325 mg daily for two doses had no effect on the pharmacokinetics of a single 80-mg dose of tapentadol.[1] No tapentadol dose adjustment would appear to be necessary on concurrent use.

1. Smit JW, Oh C, Rengelshausen J, Terlinden R, Ravenstijn PGM, Wang SS, Upmalis D, Mangold B. Effects of acetaminophen, naproxen and acetylsalicylic acid on tapentadol pharmacokinetics: results of two randomized, open-label, crossover, drug-drug interaction studies. *Pharmacotherapy* (2010) 30, 25–34.

Opioids; Tapentadol + Miscellaneous

Omeprazole does not affect the pharmacokinetics of tapentadol. Probenecid increases tapentadol exposure but does not affect its maximum plasma concentration.

Clinical evidence, mechanism, importance and management

(a) Omeprazole

The UK and US manufacturers briefly note that omeprazole does not affect the pharmacokinetics of tapentadol.[1,2] No tapentadol dose adjustments are therefore necessary on concurrent use.

(b) Probenecid

The UK and US manufacturers briefly note that, in a study probenecid 500 mg twice daily for 2 days increased the AUC of tapentadol by 57% but there was no effect on its maximum plasma concentration. The manufacturers did not consider the increase in AUC to be clinically important[1,2] and no tapentadol dose adjustment is therefore necessary on concurrent use.

1. Palexia (Tapentadol hydrochloride). Grünenthal Ltd. UK Summary of product characteristics, July 2014.
2. Nucynta (Tapentadol). Janssen Pharmaceuticals, Inc. US Prescribing information, July 2013.

Opioids; Tramadol + Mirtazapine

Concurrent use of tramadol and mirtazapine might lead to seizures and possibly serotonin syndrome, and has been found to be associated with an increased risk of restless leg syndrome.

Clinical evidence, mechanism, importance and management

Seizures and serotonin syndrome have been reported in a woman who took mirtazapine with tramadol, but this might have been due to over-use of the tramadol rather than an interaction.[1] Similarly, a man taking tramadol and mirtazapine (with alprazolam, amisulpride, and paracetamol (acetaminophen)) experienced fluctuating confusion and cognitive impairment during a period of 2 years, which only improved after tramadol was discontinued.[2] However, the patient had slightly higher than normal tramadol serum concentrations, and confessed to regularly taking high doses of tramadol which he had not reported previously, so this case might also not be related to a possible interaction with mirtazapine. Lethargy, confusion, hypotension, bronchospasm, and hypoxia has also been seen following the use of tramadol and mirtazapine, which resolved within hours of both drugs being stopped.[3] A retrospective analysis of 14 patients who developed restless leg syndrome while taking mirtazapine, found that the concurrent use of tramadol greatly increased the risk of developing the condition (odds ratio 8.61).[4]

Mirtazapine and tramadol can lower the seizure threshold, and the use of mirtazapine with other drugs that alter serotonin transmission, which includes tramadol, can lead to serotonin syndrome (and might contribute to restless leg syndrome[4]). Particular caution is warranted with this combination, especially in patients with epilepsy or those already taking other drugs that affect serotonin.

1. Freeman WD, Chabolla DR. 36-Year-old woman with loss of consciousness, fever, and tachycardia. *Mayo Clin Proc* (2005) 80, 667–70.
2. Künig G, Dätwyler S, Eschen A, Schreiter Gasser U. Unrecognised long-lasting tramadol-induced delirium in two elderly patients. A case report. *Pharmacopsychiatry* (2006) 39, 194–9.
3. Gnanadesigan N, Espinoza RT, Smith R, Israel M, Reuben DB. Interaction of serotonergic antidepressants and opioid analgesics: is serotonin syndrome going undetected? *J Am Med Dir Assoc* (2005) 6, 265–9.
4. Kim SW, Shin IS, Kim JM, Park KH, Youn T, Yoon JS. Factors potentiating the risk of mirtazapine-associated restless legs syndrome. *Hum Psychopharmacol* (2008) 23, 615–20.

Opioids; Tramadol + Pseudoephedrine

An isolated report describes ischaemic colitis when a patient taking tramadol took a decongestant containing pseudoephedrine.

Clinical evidence, mechanism, importance and management

Acute, self-limiting ischaemic colitis occurred in a 46-year-old patient taking regular tramadol, celecoxib, and diazepam for back pain, who had self-medicated with an oral decongestant containing pseudoephedrine. He had taken the maximum recommended dose of pseudoephedrine (240 mg daily) for 7 days. A similar, but milder abdominal discomfort had occurred 3 months earlier when he had used the same medication for one week. The colitis was thought to be due to pseudoephedrine, but the concurrent use of tramadol might possibly have contributed by increasing adrenergic vasoconstriction.[1] Note also that post-marketing reports of colitis or aggravated colitis have been made for celecoxib alone,[2] although the relevance of this to this case is unknown. The general importance of this isolated case is unclear.

1. Traino AA, Buckley NA, Bassett ML. Probable ischemic colitis caused by pseudoephedrine with tramadol as a possible contributing factor. *Ann Pharmacother* (2004) 38, 2068–70.
2. Celebrex (Celecoxib). Pfizer Ltd. UK Summary of product characteristics, January 2013.

Paracetamol (Acetaminophen) + Amantadine

Amantadine had no clinically significant effect on the pharmacokinetics of a single dose of paracetamol in one study.

Clinical evidence, mechanism, importance and management

In a study, a single 650-mg dose of paracetamol was given to 5 healthy subjects after amantadine 200 mg daily for 42 days, and also after a single dose of amantadine. Although the apparent volume of distribution of paracetamol was very slightly larger following the long-term use of amantadine, no other pharmacokinetic parameters were altered. Therefore, from this limited information, it appears that no change in the dose of paracetamol is necessary if these two drugs are given together.[1] Consider also 'Paracetamol (Acetaminophen) + Antimuscarinics', p.204.

1. Aoki FY, Sitar DS. Effects of chronic amantadine hydrochloride ingestion on its and acetaminophen pharmacokinetics in young adults. *J Clin Pharmacol* (1992) 32, 24–7.

Paracetamol (Acetaminophen) + Antidiabetics

The rate and extent of paracetamol (acetaminophen) absorption is decreased by exenatide, even when the paracetamol is given up to 4 hours after the exenatide. Liraglutide, lixisenatide, and pramlintide also slow gastric emptying, but to a lesser extent than exenatide, and do not affect the extent of absorption. Steady-state dulaglutide does not appear to alter the pharmacokinetics of paracetamol.

Clinical evidence

(a) Dulaglutide

The UK manufacturer briefly reports that, in a study, the first 1 and 3 mg doses of dulaglutide decreased the maximum concentration of paracetamol by 36% and 50%, respectively, and increased the time to maximum concentration. However, dulaglutide up to 3 mg at steady state had no effect on the pharmacokinetics of paracetamol.[1]

(b) Exenatide

In a randomised, crossover study, 39 healthy subjects were given a single 10-microgram dose of subcutaneous exenatide before breakfast, and one hour before a single 1-g oral dose of paracetamol. The maximum plasma concentration of paracetamol was decreased by 56% and the time to maximum concentration increased from 0.6 hours to 4.2 hours. The overall extent of absorption was decreased (a 23% decrease in the AUC of paracetamol). This effect was seen when paracetamol was given at the same time as exenatide, and also 2 and 4 hours after exenatide, although the extent of the interaction was smaller. It was not seen when paracetamol was given one hour *before* exenatide.[2] In two other studies in patients with type 2 diabetes, the mean plasma concentration of paracetamol was decreased by 58%[3] and about 60% when given with exenatide.[4]

(c) Liraglutide

In a randomised, crossover study in 18 patients with type 2 diabetes, subcutaneous liraglutide 1.8 mg daily in the evening did not alter the overall exposure (AUC) of a single 1-g oral dose of paracetamol given 8 hours later. The maximum concentration of paracetamol was decreased by 31% and the median time to maximum concentration increased by 15 minutes.[5] A similar study found that subcutaneous liraglutide 1.2 mg and 1.8 mg (given once daily in the evening) decreased the AUC of a single 1.5-mg dose of paracetamol (given with a standardised breakfast) by 43% and 30%, respectively, and the maximum plasma concentration by 31% and 23%, respectively. However, only liraglutide 1.2 mg decreased the overall exposure to paracetamol (by 17%). Liraglutide 0.6 mg did not alter exposure to paracetamol or delay gastric emptying.[6] In another study, liraglutide 1.8 mg (given once daily in the evening) decreased the AUC and maximum plasma concentration of a single 1-g dose of paracetamol (given about one hour before breakfast) by around 30% and 20%, respectively.[7]

(d) Lixisenatide

The UK manufacturer of lixisenatide briefly reports that, in a study, the AUC of a single 1-g oral dose of paracetamol was unaltered by lixisenatide 10 micrograms, when it was given before or after the lixisenatide. When the paracetamol was given 1 or 4 hours after the lixisenatide, its maximum concentration was decreased by 29% and 31%, respectively, and the time to maximum concentration was delayed by 2 hours and 1.75 hours, respectively. There was no effect on maximum concentration or time to maximum concentration when the paracetamol was administered 1 hour *before* the lixisenatide.[8]

(e) Pramlintide

In a randomised, crossover study in 24 patients with type 2 diabetes, a single 120-microgram dose of subcutaneous pramlintide, given immediately before breakfast, increased the time to maximum plasma concentration of a single 1-g oral dose of paracetamol by 48 to 72 minutes, and decreased the maximum concentration by 14 to 29%, without altering the overall extent of absorption (AUC), when compared with placebo. This effect was seen when paracetamol was given at the same time as pramlintide, and for up to 2 hours after pramlintide. It was not seen when paracetamol was given one to 2 hours before pramlintide.[9] In a similar study in 9 adolescents with type 1 diabetes, subcutaneous pramlintide 15 micrograms or 30 micrograms was given immediately before a standardised breakfast and a single 1-g oral dose of paracetamol. The time to maximum plasma concentration of paracetamol was delayed by 2 and 3 hours, respectively, but the overall exposure (AUC) to paracetamol was not affected, compared with placebo.[10]

Mechanism

Paracetamol (acetaminophen) can be used as a marker of gastric emptying and hence can be used to assess the potential effects of drugs on the absorption of other drugs. These studies therefore show that exenatide considerably slows gastric emptying, and has the potential to delay, and/or decrease the extent of the absorption of other drugs. Liraglutide, lixisenatide, and pramlintide delayed gastric emptying to a lesser degree than exenatide, and did not decrease the extent of absorption.

Importance and management

Studies using paracetamol (acetaminophen) as a marker of gastric emptying, show that exenatide, liraglutide, lixisenatide, and pramlintide all delay gastric emptying, albeit to varying degrees, but that dulaglutide at steady state does not appear to have an effect. Exenatide has the greatest effect, and also decreased the extent of paracetamol absorption. Exenatide, liraglutide, lixisenatide, and pramlintide therefore have the potential to delay the absorption of other oral drugs, and exenatide might additionally decrease the extent of absorption. They could also, theoretically, oppose the effects of **metoclopramide**, which increases gastric emptying. However, the actual clinical relevance of any such effects has not been assessed. Nevertheless, the manufacturers of exenatide[11,12] and lixisenatide[8] recommend caution in patients receiving oral drugs that require rapid gastrointestinal absorption, but do not give any specific examples. Despite the lack of effect of steady-state dulaglutide on paracetamol pharmacokinetics, the UK manufacturer gives the same warning,[1] whereas the US manufacturer advises caution with all oral drugs,[13] which seems unnecessarily cautious. Where a rapid effect of an oral drug is required, for example, an analgesic for acute pain or fever, it might be prudent to give the drug at least one hour before the antidiabetic. Concurrent use of drugs with a narrow therapeutic window should also be used with caution, and these are recommended to be given in a standardised manner [to avoid fluctuations].[8,12] The US manufacturer of dulaglutide advises that the concentrations of drugs with a narrow therapeutic window should be adequately monitored if given concurrently.[13]

Further, the manufacturers also suggest that exenatide and lixisenatide should be used with caution in patients receiving oral drugs that are dependent on threshold concentrations for efficacy. They give **antibacterials** as an example (but no drugs are specifically named), and recommend that they should be taken at least one hour before exenatide,[11,12] or 1 hour before, or 4 hours, after lixisenatide.[8] Whether this is clinically necessary remains to be shown. The US manufacturer of exenatide additionally mentions oral contraceptives as an example,[11] but see 'Combined hormonal contraceptives + Glucagon-like peptide-1 receptor agonists', p.1174 for a discussion of the clinical relevance of this effect in this case.

For drugs that are formulated as gastric-resistant formulations, or that are sensitive to degradation by gastric acid, it is recommended that they are taken one hour before, or at least 4 hours after, exenatide[12] or lixisenatide.[8]

The UK manufacturer of liraglutide states that the small delay of gastric emptying with liraglutide might influence absorption of oral medicinal products given concurrently. Note that they also state that severe diarrhoea has been reported in a few patients given liraglutide, and that diarrhoea might affect the absorption of oral medicinal products given concurrently.[14] The UK manufacturer of dulaglutide also advises that concurrent use might increase the release of other drugs from some prolonged release formulations as a result of increased gastric residence time, and might slightly increase drug exposure.[1]

For pramlintide, the US manufacturer notes that if a rapid onset of action is required (for example when giving an oral **analgesic**), the drug should be given at least one hour before or 2 hours after pramlintide.[15] Furthermore, because of the delay in gastric emptying, the manufacturer recommends that pramlintide should not be used in patients taking other drugs that alter gastrointestinal motility. They specifically name **antimuscarinics**, such as **atropine**,[15] which also delay gastric emptying. Pramlintide is also not recommended in patients taking agents that slow the intestinal absorption of nutrients and they specifically mention **alpha-glucosidase inhibitors**.[15]

For **albiglutide**, the US manufacturer warns that it might slow gastric emptying and hence decrease drug absorption, and advises caution on concurrent administration with all oral drugs,[16] which seems overly cautious.

1. Trulicity (Dulaglutide). Eli Lilly and Company Ltd. UK Summary of product characteristics, November 2014.
2. Blase E, Taylor K, Gao H, Wintle M, Fineman M. Pharmacokinetics of an oral drug (acetaminophen) administered at various times in relation to subcutaneous injection of exenatide (exendin-4) in healthy subjects. *J Clin Pharmacol* (2005) 45, 570–7.
3. Cervera A, Wajcberg E, Sriwijitkamol A, Fernandez M, Zuo P, Triplitt C, Musi N, DeFronzo RA, Cersosimo E. Mechanism of action of exenatide to reduce postprandial hyperglycemia in type 2 diabetes. *Am J Physiol Endocrinol Metab* (2008) 294, E846–52.
4. Kolterman OG, Buse JB, Fineman MS, Gaines E, Heintz S, Bicsak TA, Taylor K, Kim D, Aisporna M, Wang Y, Baron AD. Synthetic Exendin-4 (exenatide) significantly reduces postprandial and fasting plasma glucose in subjects with type 2 diabetes. *J Clin Endocrinol Metab* (2003) 88, 3082–9.
5. Kapitza C, Zdravkovic M, Hindsberger C, Flint A. The effect of the once-daily human glucagon-like peptide 1 analog liraglutide on the pharmacokinetics of acetaminophen. *Adv Therapy* (2011) 28, 650–60.
6. Flint A, Kapitza C, Hinsberger C, Zdravkovic M. The once-daily human glucagon-like peptide-1 (GLP-1) analogue liraglutide improves postprandial glucose levels in type 2 diabetes patients. *Adv Therapy* (2011) 28, 213–26.
7. Horowitz M, Flint A, Jones KL, Hindsberger C, Rasmussen MF, Kapitza C, Doran S, Jax T, Zdravkovic M, Chapman IM. Effect of the once-daily human GLP-1 analogue liraglutide on appetite, energy intake, energy expenditure and gastric emptying in type 2 diabetes. *Diabetes Res Clin Pract* (2012) 97, 258–66.
8. Lyxumia (Lixisenatide). Sanofi. UK Summary of product characteristics, October 2014.
9. Kellmeyer TA, Kesty NC, Wang Y, Frias JP, Fineman MS. Pharmacokinetics of an oral drug (acetaminophen) administered at various times relative to subcutaneous injection of pramlintide in subjects with type 2 diabetes. *J Clin Pharmacol* (2007) 47, 798–805.
10. Chase HP, Lutz K, Pencek R, Zhang B, Porter L. Pramlintide lowered glucose excursions and was well-tolerated in adolescents with type 1 diabetes: results from a randomized, single-blind, placebo-controlled, crossover study. *J Pediatr* (2009) 155, 369–73.
11. Byetta (Exenatide). AstraZeneca Pharmaceuticals LP. US Prescribing information, February 2015
12. Byetta (Exenatide). AstraZeneca UK Ltd. UK Summary of product characteristics, January 2015.
13. Trulicity (Dulaglutide). Eli Lilly and Company. US Prescribing information, March 2015.
14. Victoza (Liraglutide). Novo Nordisk Ltd. UK Summary of product characteristics, March 2015.
15. Symlin (Pramlintide acetate). AstraZeneca Pharmaceuticals LP. US Prescribing information, February 2015.
16. Tanzeum (Albiglutide). GlaxoSmithKline LLC. US Prescribing information, May 2015.

Paracetamol (Acetaminophen) + Antiemetics

Metoclopramide increases the rate of paracetamol absorption. Similarly, domperidone might increase the rate of absorption of paracetamol.

Clinical evidence

In a study in 5 healthy subjects (slow absorbers of paracetamol), intravenous metoclopramide 10 mg increased the maximum plasma levels of a single 1.5-g dose of paracetamol by 64% and increased its rate of absorption (maximum levels reached in 48 minutes instead of 120 minutes), but the total amount absorbed remained virtually unaltered.[1] Oral metoclopramide also increases the rate of paracetamol absorption.[2].

In a study, 10 critically ill patients intolerant to enteral feeding (because of reduced gastric emptying) were given a single 975-mg dose of liquid paracetamol before and after 4 doses of intravenous metoclopramide 10 mg every 6 hours. Metoclopramide increased the maximum plasma level and AUC_{0-60} of paracetamol by 46% and 115%, respectively, indicating an increase in the rate of gastric emptying. However, after 3 hours there was a 38% increase in the AUC of paracetamol, which was not statistically significant, suggesting minimal effects on overall paracetamol absorption.[3] The pharmacokinetics of paracetamol in the presence of metoclopramide in this study were similar to those found in 10 patients who were absorbing enteral feed and were not given a prokinetic,[4] suggesting that the use of metoclopramide in patients with reduced gastric emptying restores paracetamol absorption to that seen in patients with normal gastric emptying.

Mechanism

Paracetamol absorption is closely related to gastric emptying. Increasing the rate of gastric emptying with a prokinetic, such as metoclopramide, therefore increases the rate of paracetamol absorption.

Importance and management

Evidence for an interaction between paracetamol and metoclopramide appears to be limited to these studies, all of which were in patients with a reduced rate of gastric emptying. The findings illustrate that the use of metoclopramide in those with reduced gastric emptying restores the rate of paracetamol absorption to that seen in patients with normal rates of gastric emptying, without having a notable effect on the overall amount of paracetamol absorbed. This interaction is exploited in *Paramax* (a proprietary oral preparation containing both paracetamol and metoclopramide) to increase the effectiveness and onset of analgesia for the treatment of migraine. This is obviously an advantageous interaction in this situation. As **domperidone** increases gastric emptying in the same way as metoclopramide, it seems likely that it also have a similar effect on paracetamol absorption.

For the effect of other antiemetics, consider also 'Paracetamol (Acetaminophen) + 5-HT_3-receptor antagonists', p.208.

1. Nimmo J, Heading RC, Tothill P, Prescott LF. Pharmacological modification of gastric emptying: effects of propantheline and metoclopramide on paracetamol absorption. *BMJ* (1973) 1, 587–9.
2. Crome P, Kimber GR, Wainscott G, Widdop B. The effect of the simultaneous administration of oral metoclopramide on the absorption of paracetamol in healthy volunteers. *Br J Clin Pharmacol* (1981) 11, 430P–431P.
3. MacLaren R, Kiser TH, Fish DN, Wischmeyer PE. Erythromycin vs metoclopramide for facilitating gastric emptying and tolerance to intragastric nutrition in critically ill patients. *J Parenter Enteral Nutr* (2008) 32, 412–19.
4. Landzinski J, Kiser TH, Fish DN, Wischmeyer PE, MacLaren R. Gastric motility function in critically ill patients tolerant *vs* intolerant to gastric nutrition. *J Parenter Enteral Nutr* (2008) 32, 45–50.

Paracetamol (Acetaminophen) + Antiepileptics; Enzyme-inducing

The metabolism of paracetamol is increased in patients taking enzyme-inducing antiepileptics (carbamazepine, phenytoin, phenobarbital, primidone). Isolated reports describe unexpected hepatotoxicity in patients taking phenobarbital, phenytoin, or carbamazepine after taking paracetamol. Paracetamol does not appear to affect the levels of phenytoin or carbamazepine.

Clinical evidence

The AUC of oral paracetamol 1 g was found to be 40% lower (and when given intravenously, 31% lower) in 6 patients with epilepsy than in 6 healthy subjects. Five of the patients were taking at least two antiepileptics (combinations of **carbamazepine**, **phenobarbital**, **primidone**, and **phenytoin**), and one was taking **phenytoin** alone.[1] Similar findings (a 38% decrease in AUC) were reported in another study in 13 patients taking enzyme-inducing antiepileptics and 2 patients taking rifampicin (rifampin). In these patients, the amount of glucuronide, but not sulfate, metabolites of paracetamol were higher than the controls, but the amount of the potentially hepatotoxic metabolite (assessed by mercapturic acid and cysteine conjugates) was not raised.[2] Similar changes in the metabolites of paracetamol were reported in Chinese patients taking **phenytoin** alone. However, in those taking **carbamazepine** alone there was no change in the metabolites of paracetamol, when compared with control subjects.[3] Other studies have also reported a greater rate of paracetamol glucuronidation and unchanged paracetamol sulfation in patients taking **phenytoin** alone[4] and patients taking **phenytoin** and/or **carbamazepine**.[5] The latter study found an increase in the clearance of the glutathione-derived conjugates (mercapturic and cysteine conjugates), which might indicate an increased risk of paracetamol hepatotoxicity.[5]

A woman with epilepsy taking **phenobarbital** 100 mg daily developed hepatitis after taking paracetamol 1 g daily for 3 months for headaches. Within 2 weeks of stopping paracetamol her serum transaminase levels had fallen to within the reference range, which implied drug-induced liver damage.[6] Another patient taking **phenobarbital** developed liver and kidney toxicity after taking 9 g of paracetamol over 48 hours.[7] Similarly, **phenobarbital** also appeared to have increased the toxic effects of paracetamol in an adolescent who took an overdose of both drugs, which resulted in fatal hepatic encephalopathy.[8]

Other case reports describe unexpected paracetamol hepatotoxicity in three patients taking **phenytoin**,[9-11] four patients taking **carbamazepine**,[12-15] and a patient taking **phenytoin** and **primidone**.[16] Another analysis of patients with paracetamol-induced fulminant hepatic failure suggested that mortality was higher in the group of patients receiving enzyme-inducing antiepileptics (including **phenytoin**, **phenobarbital**, **carbamazepine**, **primidone** and valproate alone or in combination).[17]

In a study in 10 patients with epilepsy, paracetamol 1.5 g daily, taken for 3 days, had no statistically significant effect on the serum levels of **phenytoin** and **carbamazepine**.[18]

Mechanism

The increased paracetamol clearance seen with carbamazepine, phenobarbital, primidone, and phenytoin is due to the well-recognised enzyme-inducing effects of these antiepileptics, which increase paracetamol metabolism (glucuronidation and oxidation) and clearance. It has been suggested that this could result in an increase in the production of the hepatotoxic oxidative metabolite of paracetamol, *N*-acetyl-*p*-benzoquinone imine. If this toxic metabolite then exceeds the normal glutathione binding capacity, liver damage could occur (see *Paracetamol* under 'Analgesics and NSAIDs', p.138). The production of the toxic metabolite *in vitro* in *animals* and in humans seems to depend on several isoenzymes, but the available evidence indicates that CYP2E1 is the primary isoenzyme involved in humans.[19] Therefore, because these enzyme-inducing antiepileptics do not induce this isoenzyme, some consider that the few possible cases described merely represent idiosyncratic effects.[19] However, others have suggested that, when several drugs, including phenobarbital or phenytoin are taken, inhibition of glucuronyltransferases by one of these drugs can lead to decreased glucuronidation, increased systemic exposure, and paracetamol toxicity.[20]

Importance and management

Information on the interaction between paracetamol and enzyme-inducing antiepileptics is limited and their clinical importance is not established. Paracetamol is possibly a less effective analgesic in patients taking enzyme-inducing antiepileptics (carbamazepine, phenobarbital, primidone, and phenytoin) as plasma paracetamol levels seem likely to be reduced. However, levels of the potentially hepatotoxic metabolites might be increased. Some believe that the evidence indicates that the risk of liver damage after paracetamol overdose is increased, and they suggest that patients taking enzyme-inducing antiepileptics should be treated with antidotes at lower plasma levels of paracetamol.[9,11,12,16] In addition, some suggest that therapeutic doses of paracetamol should be used with caution in patients receiving enzyme-inducing antiepileptics.[10,11,17] Conversely, others consider that therapeutic doses of paracetamol are not associated with an increased risk of toxicity when used with enzyme-inducers. Moreover, phenytoin, by increasing glucuronidation, might actually have some hepato-protective effects.[19,21] The differences stem from different understandings of which mechanism and isoenzyme(s) are important in the production of the hepatotoxic metabolite of paracetamol[10,19] (see *Mechanism*, above).

Note that, there appears to be no evidence regarding an interaction between paracetamol and **fosphenytoin**, but as fosphenytoin is a prodrug of phenytoin, it would be expected to interact in much the same way.

1. Perucca E, Richens A. Paracetamol disposition in normal subjects and in patients treated with antiepileptic drugs. *Br J Clin Pharmacol* (1979) 7, 201–6.
2. Prescott LF, Critchley JAJH, Balali-Mood M, Pentland B. Effects of microsomal enzyme induction on paracetamol metabolism in man. *Br J Clin Pharmacol* (1981) 12, 149–53.
3. Tomlinson B, Young RP, Ng MCY, Anderson PJ, Kay R, Critchley JAJH. Selective liver enzyme induction by carbamazepine and phenytoin in Chinese epileptics. *Eur J Clin Pharmacol* (1996) 50, 411–15.
4. Bock KW, Wiltfang J, Blume R, Ullrich D, Bircher J. Paracetamol as a test drug to determine glucuronide formation in man. Effects of inducers and of smoking. *Eur J Clin Pharmacol* (1987) 31, 677–83.
5. Miners JO, Attwood J, Birkett DJ. Determinants of acetaminophen metabolism: effect of inducers and inhibitors of drug metabolism on acetaminophen's metabolic pathways. *Clin Pharmacol Ther* (1984) 35, 480–6.
6. Pirotte JH. Apparent potentiation by phenobarbital of hepatotoxicity from small doses of acetaminophen. *Ann Intern Med* (1984) 101, 403.
7. Marsepoil T, Mahassani B, Roudiak N, Sebbah JL, Caillard G. Potentialisation de la toxicité hépatique et rénale du paracétamol par le phénobarbital. *JEUR* (1989) 2, 118–20.
8. Wilson JT, Kasantikul V, Harbison R, Martin D. Death in an adolescent following an overdose of acetaminophen and phenobarbital. *Am J Dis Child* (1978) 132, 466–73.
9. McClements BM, Hyland M, Callender ME, Blair TL. Management of paracetamol poisoning complicated by enzyme induction due to alcohol or drugs. *Lancet* (1990) 335, 1526.
10. Brackett CC, Bloch JD. Phenytoin as a possible cause of acetaminophen hepatotoxicity: case report and review of the literature. *Pharmacotherapy* (2000) 20, 229–33.
11. Suchin SM, Wolf DC, Lee Y, Ramaswamy G, Sheiner PA, Facciuto M, Marvin MR, Kim-Schluger L, Lebovics E. Potentiation of acetaminophen hepatotoxicity by phenytoin, leading to liver transplantation. *Dig Dis Sci* (2005) 50, 1836–8.
12. Smith JAE, Hine ID, Beck P, Routledge PA. Paracetamol toxicity: is enzyme-induction important? *Hum Toxicol* (1986) 5, 383–5.
13. Young CR, Mazure CM. Fulminant hepatic failure from acetaminophen in an anorexic patient treated with carbamazepine. *J Clin Psychiatry* (1998) 59, 622.
14. Parikh S, Dillon LC, Scharf SL. Hepatotoxicity possibly due to paracetamol with carbamazepine. Intern Med J. (2004) 34, 441–2.
15. Jickling G, Heino A, Ahmed SN. Acetaminophen toxicity with concomitant use of carbamazepine. *Epileptic Disord* (2009) 11, 329–32.
16. Minton NA, Henry JA, Frankel RJ. Fatal paracetamol poisoning in an epileptic. *Hum Toxicol* (1988) 7, 33–4.
17. Bray GP, Harrison PM, O'Grady JG, Tredger JM, Williams R. Long-term anticonvulsant therapy worsens outcome in paracetamol-induced fulminant hepatic failure. *Hum Exp Toxicol* (1992) 11, 265–70.
18. Neuvonen PJ, Lehtovaara R, Bardy A, Elomaa E. Antipyretic analgesics in patients on antiepileptic drug therapy. *Eur J Clin Pharmacol* (1979) 15, 263–8.
19. Rumack BH. Acetaminophen hepatotoxicity: the first 35 years. *J Toxicol Clin Toxicol* (2002) 40, 3–20.
20. Kostrubsky SE, Sinclair JF, Strom SC, Wood S, Urda E, Stolz DB, Wen YH, Kulkarni S, Mutlib A. Phenobarbital and phenytoin increased acetaminophen hepatotoxicity due to inhibition of UDP-glucuronosyltransferases in cultured human hepatocytes. *Toxicol Sci* (2005) 87, 146–55.
21. Cook MD, Williams SR, Clark RF. Phenytoin-potentiated hepatotoxicity following acetaminophen overdose? A closer look. *Dig Dis Sci* (2007) 52, 208–9.

Paracetamol (Acetaminophen) + Antimuscarinics

Propantheline reduces the rate, but not the extent, of paracetamol absorption. Other antimuscarinic drugs would be expected to interact similarly. However, one study found that diphenhydramine did not appear to affect the absorption of paracetamol, although one report suggests that an effect might occur in overdose.

Clinical evidence

(a) Diphenhydramine

One study in 10 healthy subjects reported that diphenhydramine 250 mg, taken with paracetamol 5 g (simulated paracetamol overdose), had little effect on the absorption of paracetamol.[1] However, a case has been described where the diphenhydramine component of a paracetamol product (*Tylenol PM*) taken in overdose (paracetamol 7.5 g and diphenhydramine 375 mg) delayed the absorption of paracetamol, so that the peak serum-paracetamol level did not occur until 8 hours after ingestion (usual maximum is 2 hours).[2]

(b) Propantheline

In a study in 6 convalescent patients, propantheline 30 mg, given intravenously, delayed the peak serum levels of paracetamol 1.5 g from about one hour to 3 hours. The peak levels of paracetamol were lowered by about one-third, but the total amount absorbed was unchanged.[3]

Mechanism

Paracetamol absorption is delayed by propantheline and probably diphenhydramine because both drugs have antimuscarinic effects, which slow the rate at which the stomach empties, so that the rate of absorption of paracetamol in the gut is reduced.

Importance and management

Evidence for an interaction between paracetamol and antimuscarinic drugs appears to be limited to these reports with propantheline and diphenhydramine, but the findings of the study with propantheline and the case with diphenhydramine are in line with what would theoretically be expected to happen. All antimuscarinic drugs would be expected to interact similarly (see 'Table 18.2', p.754, for a list of drugs with known antimuscarinic effects); however, one study with amantadine found no clinically relevant effect (see 'Paracetamol (Acetaminophen) + Amantadine', p.202). Therefore the precise outcome of concurrent use is not clear.

The practical consequence of any delay to paracetamol absorption seems likely to be a delay and possibly a reduction in rapid pain relief with single doses of paracetamol but this needs clinical confirmation. If paracetamol is being taken in repeated doses over extended periods this seems unlikely to be an important interaction because the total amount absorbed is unchanged. However, one situation where the effect might be of importance is in assessing paracetamol overdose: when assessing treatment options it is worth noting that maximum plasma levels might be delayed.

1. Halcomb SE, Sivilotti ML, Goklaney A, Mullins ME. Pharmacokinetic effects of diphenhydramine or oxycodone in simulated acetaminophen overdose. *Acad Emerg Med* (2005) 12, 169–72.
2. Tsang WO, Nadroo AM. An unusual case of acetaminophen overdose. *Pediatr Emerg Care* (1999) 15, 344–6.
3. Nimmo J, Heading RC, Tothill P, Prescott LF. Pharmacological modification of gastric emptying: effects of propantheline and metoclopramide on paracetamol absorption. *BMJ* (1973) 1, 587–9.

Paracetamol (Acetaminophen) + Caffeine

Caffeine appears to increase the rate of absorption of paracetamol, and has been reported to increase the bioavailability of paracetamol, although one study found a decrease and another found no change in paracetamol bioavailability.

Clinical evidence, mechanism, importance and management

In a study in 10 healthy subjects, caffeine citrate 120 mg increased the AUC of a single 500-mg dose of paracetamol by 29%, increased its maximum plasma levels by 15% and decreased its total body clearance by 32%. The decrease in time to maximum level and increase in absorption rate were not statistically significant.[1] A randomised, crossover study in 24 healthy subjects compared the effects of a single 1-g dose of paracetamol alone and with caffeine 130 mg. The overall bioavailability was the same with or without caffeine, but paracetamol had a faster rate of absorption in the presence of caffeine, shown by an increase in the AUC of paracetamol over the first 20 minutes.[2] There was also an increase in analgesic effects (using a pain model) throughout the observation period from about one to 3.5 hours.[2] In another study, although caffeine increased the rate of absorption of paracetamol, it had no effect on the extent of absorption.[3] However, a further study states that caffeine *decreased* both the plasma levels and AUC of paracetamol, and increased paracetamol elimination in healthy men.[4]

Caffeine is commonly included in paracetamol preparations as an analgesic adjuvant, although its potential benefits and the exact mechanism for its action are still unclear. However, note that if paracetamol formulated with caffeine is given there is the potential for additive caffeine adverse effects (such as headache, jitteriness, restlessness, and insomnia) with dietary caffeine. Caffeine intake should be reduced if this occurs.

1. Iqbal N, Ahmad B, Janbaz KH, Gilani A-UH, Niazi SK. The effect of caffeine on the pharmacokinetics of acetaminophen in man. *Biopharm Drug Dispos* (1995) 16, 481–7.
2. Renner B, Clarke G, Grattan T, Beisel A, Mueller C, Werner U, Kobal G, Brune K. Caffeine accelerates absorption and enhances the analgesic effect of acetaminophen. *J Clin Pharmacol* (2007) 47, 715–26.
3. Tukker JJ, Sitsen JMA, Gusdorf CF. Bioavailability of paracetamol after oral administration to healthy volunteers. Influence of caffeine on rate and extent of absorption. *Pharm Weekbl (Sci)* (1986) 8, 239–43.
4. Raińska-Giezek T. Influence of caffeine on toxicity and pharmacokinetics of paracetamol [Article in Polish]. *Ann Acad Med Stetin* (1995) 41, 69–85.

Paracetamol (Acetaminophen) + Chloroquine

Chloroquine very slightly increases the exposure to paracetamol, and chloroquine very slightly increases the exposure to paracetamol.

Clinical evidence, mechanism, importance and management

In a single-dose study, intravenous chloroquine increased the peak plasma levels and AUC of paracetamol by 47% and 22%, respectively.[1] Another single-dose study in 8 healthy subjects found that paracetamol 500 mg increased the maximum plasma level and AUC of chloroquine 600 mg by 17% and 24%, respectively.[2] These changes were thought unlikely to be clinically significant.[1] A further study, in 5 healthy subjects, found that the pharmacokinetics of a single 300-mg dose of chloroquine were not affected by a single 1-g dose of paracetamol.[3] This evidence suggests that no dose adjustments would be expected to be necessary when paracetamol is given with chloroquine.

1. Adjepon-Yamoah KK, Woolhouse NM, Prescott LF. The effect of chloroquine on paracetamol disposition and kinetics. *Br J Clin Pharmacol* (1986) 21, 322–4.
2. Raina RK, Bano G, Amla V, Kapoor V, Gupta KL. The effect of aspirin, paracetamol and analgin on pharmacokinetics of chloroquine. *Indian J Physiol Pharmacol* (1993) 37, 229–31.
3. Essien EE, Ette EI, Brown-Awala EA. Evaluation of the effect of co-administered paracetamol on the gastro-intestinal absorption and disposition of chloroquine. *J Pharm Biomed Anal* (1988) 6, 521–6.

Paracetamol (Acetaminophen) + Ciprofloxacin

Paracetamol does not appear to have a clinically relevant effect on the pharmacokinetics of ciprofloxacin. Ciprofloxacin might delay the onset of action of paracetamol, but does not affect its overall exposure.

Clinical evidence

In a randomised study, 10 healthy subjects were given a single 500-mg dose of oral ciprofloxacin alone or as a combination preparation also containing 500-mg of paracetamol. In the presence of paracetamol, the AUC and maximum plasma level of ciprofloxacin were 16% and 4% greater, respectively; however, this was not statistically significant. However, the authors note that there was a statistically significant increase in plasma ciprofloxacin levels at several (but not all) time points between 30 minutes and 4 hours after dosing,[1] but these changes appear slight, and would not be expected to be clinically relevant.

A single-dose study in 10 healthy subjects who were given a 1-g dose of oral paracetamol alone, or taken at the same time as ciprofloxacin 500 mg, found that ciprofloxacin decreased the maximum salivary level of paracetamol by 30%, and increased the time to maximum level by about 40 minutes; however, the extent of absorption was unchanged.[2]

Mechanism

Unknown. It has been suggested that ciprofloxacin could have formed an insoluble complex with paracetamol, reducing its absorption from the intestine.[2]

Importance and management

The evidence regarding an interaction between paracetamol and ciprofloxacin is limited. In the first study it was suggested that the doses of paracetamol and ciprofloxacin should be separated, but the pharmacokinetic data suggests that any effect is very slight and unlikely to be of clinical relevance: therefore separating the doses seems overly cautious. The other study, which was by the same authors, found a slight delay in the maximum salivary levels of paracetamol and it is unclear whether this would be clinically relevant, particularly if regular doses of paracetamol were given. These findings do not appear to provide sufficient evidence to suggest that particular precautions are necessary if ciprofloxacin is given with paracetamol.

1. Issa MM, Nejem RM, El-Abadla NS, El-Naby MK, Roshdy AA, Kheiralla ZA. Effects of paracetamol on the pharmacokinetics of ciprofloxacin in plasma using a microbiological assay. *Clin Drug Investig* (2007) 27, 463–7.
2. Issa MM, Nejem RM, El-Abadla NS. Oral ciprofloxacin affects the pharmacokinetics of paracetamol in saliva. *Clin Drug Investig* (2006) 26, 223–6.

Paracetamol (Acetaminophen) + Colestyramine

The absorption of paracetamol might be reduced if colestyramine is given simultaneously, but the reduction in absorption is small if colestyramine is given one hour after paracetamol.

Clinical evidence

In a study in 4 healthy subjects the absorption of a 2-g dose of paracetamol was reduced by 60% (range 30 to 98%) at 2 hours by the simultaneous use of colestyramine 12 g, but the results were not statistically significant. When colestyramine was given one hour after paracetamol, the absorption was reduced by only 16%.[1]

Mechanism

Colestyramine is an ion-exchange resin, intended to bind with bile acids in the gut, but it can also bind with drugs, leading to a reduction in their absorption. This appears to occur with paracetamol, thereby reducing its absorption. Separating the doses minimises mixing in the gut and reduces the effect.

Importance and management

Information regarding an interaction between paracetamol and colestyramine is limited, and although the findings in the study were not statistically significant this might have been due to the very small numbers of patients. The available information suggests that colestyramine should not be given within one hour of paracetamol if maximal analgesia is to be achieved. It is usually recommended that other drugs are given one hour before or 4 to 6 hours after colestyramine.

1. Dordoni B, Willson RA, Thompson RPH, Williams R. Reduction of absorption of paracetamol by activated charcoal and cholestyramine: a possible therapeutic measure. *BMJ* (1973) 3, 86–7.

Paracetamol (Acetaminophen) + Disulfiram

Disulfiram had no notable effect on the metabolism of paracetamol in one study, but decreased the production of the glutathione (hepatotoxic) metabolites of paracetamol in another.

Clinical evidence, mechanism, importance and management

In a study in 5 healthy subjects without liver disease and 5 others with alcoholic liver cirrhosis, disulfiram 200 mg daily for 5 days reduced the clearance of a single 500-mg intravenous dose of paracetamol by about 10%, but did not alter the fractional clearance of paracetamol to its glucuronide, sulfate and glutathione metabolites.[1] In contrast, another study found that the pretreatment of healthy subjects with a single 500-mg dose of disulfiram 10 hours before a single 500-mg oral dose of paracetamol reduced the recovery of glutathione metabolites (a measure of the production of the hepatotoxic metabolite, see *Paracetamol*, under 'Analgesics and NSAIDs', p.138) by 69%.[2]

Disulfiram is an inhibitor of CYP2E1, which is involved in the metabolism of paracetamol. Previously, the authors of the first study[1] had shown that in *rats*, high doses of disulfiram protected against the hepatotoxicity of paracetamol. Therefore, it was suggested that disulfiram might be useful in reducing the risks of paracetamol overdose. However, the authors of the first study concluded that disulfiram, at doses used clinically, is unlikely to have any beneficial (or adverse) effect on paracetamol metabolism.[1] In contrast, the authors of the second study consider that disulfiram might be useful in reducing the formation of the hepatotoxic metabolite of paracetamol in some situations.[2] Further study is needed to establish this.

1. Poulson HE, Ranek L, Jørgensen L. The influence of disulfiram on acetaminophen metabolism in man. *Xenobiotica* (1991) 21, 243–9.
2. Manyike PT, Kharasch ED, Kalhorn TF, Slattery JT. Contribution of CYP2E1 and CYP3A to acetaminophen reactive metabolite formation. *Clin Pharmacol Ther* (2000) 67, 275–82.

Paracetamol (Acetaminophen) + Erythromycin

Erythromycin increases the rate of gastric emptying and might increase paracetamol absorption.

Clinical evidence

In a study in 10 healthy subjects, intravenous erythromycin 0.75 to 3 mg/kg accelerated gastric emptying in a dose-dependent manner and increased the absorption of a 1.5-g dose of paracetamol (given with an enteral feed).[1] In clinical studies in patients, the rate of paracetamol absorption has been used as a way of measuring the improvement in gastric emptying in response to a prokinetic, such as erythromycin. In one study, 10 critically ill patients intolerant to enteral feeding (because of reduced gastric emptying) were given a single 975-mg dose of liquid paracetamol before and after a total of 4 doses of intravenous erythromycin 250 mg every 6 hours. Erythromycin increased the maximum plasma level and AUC_{0-60} of paracetamol by 86% and more than 3.5-fold, respectively,[2] indicating an increase in the rate of gastric emptying. However, after 3 hours the AUC of paracetamol, was only increased by 73%, suggesting only moderate effects on overall paracetamol absorption. The pharmacokinetics of paracetamol in the presence of erythromycin in this study were similar to those found in 10 patients who were absorbing enteral feed and were not given a prokinetic,[3] suggesting that the use of metoclopramide in patients with reduced gastric emptying restores paracetamol to that seen in patients with normal gastric emptying.

A study in 7 healthy subjects found that a single 250-mg dose of intravenous erythromycin promoted gastric emptying of solids during acute pain, but had no statistically significant effect on the pharmacokinetics of paracetamol 1 g in 150 mL of water.[4] Another study found that intravenous erythromycin 200 mg, given to promote gastrointestinal motility, did not alter the pharmacokinetics of a 1.3-g oral dose of extended-release paracetamol.[5] A further study in 7 healthy subjects reported that the pharmacokinetics of a single 1-g oral dose of paracetamol were not affected by pretreatment with oral erythromycin 250 mg four times daily for 7 days.[6]

Mechanism

Paracetamol absorption is closely related to gastric emptying. Increasing the rate of gastric emptying with a prokinetic, such as erythromycin, therefore increases the rate of paracetamol absorption.

Importance and management

An interaction between erythromycin and paracetamol is relatively well documented, with the majority of studies in healthy subjects suggesting that erythromycin is unlikely to have a clinically relevant effect on overall paracetamol absorption in healthy subjects. However, in those with reduced gastric motility, erythromycin appears to restore paracetamol absorption to a similar extent to that seen in patients with normal gastric motility, and so any interaction is likely to be beneficial in this patient group. Note that erythromycin has been used in clinical practice to increase gastric emptying and enteral nutrition absorption in those with reduced gastric motility.

1. Boivin MA, Carey MC, Levy H. Erythromycin accelerates gastric emptying in a dose-response manner in healthy subjects. *Pharmacotherapy* (2003) 23, 5–8.
2. MacLaren R, Kiser TH, Fish DN, Wischmeyer PE. Erythromycin vs metoclopramide for facilitating gastric emptying and tolerance to intragastric nutrition in critically ill patients. *J Parenter Enteral Nutr* (2008) 32, 412–19.
3. Landzinski J, Kiser TH, Fish DN, Wischmeyer PE, MacLaren R. Gastric motility function in critically ill patients tolerant *vs* intolerant to gastric nutrition. *J Parenter Enteral Nutr* (2008) 32, 45–50.
4. Bouvet L, Duflo F, Bleyzac N, Mion F, Boselli E, Allaouchiche B, Chassard D. Erythromycin promotes gastric emptying during acute pain in volunteers. *Anesth Analg* (2006) 102, 1803–8.
5. Amato CS, Wang RY, Wright RO, Linakis JG. Evaluation of promotility agents to limit the gut bioavailability of extended-release acetaminophen. *J Toxicol Clin Toxicol* (2004) 42, 73–7.
6. Ridtitid W, Wongnawa M, Mahathanatrakul W, Rukthai D, Sunbhanich M. Effect of erythromycin administration alone or coadministration with cimetidine on the pharmacokinetics of paracetamol in healthy volunteers. *Asia Pac J Pharmacol* (1998) 13, 19–23.

Paracetamol (Acetaminophen) + Food

Food slows the rate of absorption of paracetamol, but the overall bioavailability is not usually affected. However, in some individuals food might delay and reduce peak paracetamol-plasma levels, and a high-fat meal might slightly reduce the extent of paracetamol absorption. Certain foods, such as cabbage and brussels sprouts, might also affect the metabolism of paracetamol.

Clinical evidence

(a) Absorption of paracetamol

Several studies have demonstrated that food slows the rate of absorption of paracetamol, but the overall bioavailability is not affected[1-5] and some studies have also reported that food has no effect on the analgesic efficacy of paracetamol[6] or its onset of action.[7] Carbohydrate,[2] fat,[2] **guar gum** and **pectin**,[5] protein,[1] and particularly **fibre**,[2,4] can delay the absorption of paracetamol. Furthermore, the rate and extent of absorption, and the peak plasma levels of a single dose of paracetamol have been found to be impaired in vegetarians compared with non-vegetarians.[8] A high-fat diet has also been reported to slightly reduce the extent of absorption.[2]

Although the overall bioavailability of paracetamol is not usually affected by food, there might be a delay in reaching therapeutic plasma levels, particularly following a single dose of paracetamol. A reduction in the maximum plasma level of paracetamol has been reported when it is given after food, when compared with the fasted state:[3,9] in one study, in some individuals, the maximum plasma level of paracetamol did not reach the level reported to be required for effective analgesia.[9] The dosage form will also affect the absorption: many of the studies have used conventional paracetamol tablets, but some formulations (for example paracetamol with sodium bicarbonate)[3,7] are more rapidly absorbed and, although food might reduce the rate of absorption,[3,4] one study found that there was no difference in the onset of analgesia between the fed and fasted states.[7] Another study found that diet composition did not affect the systemic availability of paracetamol in a liquid dosage form, whereas absorption of the tablet was delayed by a **fibre**-enriched diet.[4]

(b) Metabolism of paracetamol

In a crossover study in 10 healthy subjects, a 10-day balanced diet including cabbage 100 g and brussels sprouts 150 g at lunch and dinner was found to stimulate the metabolism of paracetamol. Compared with a control diet (which included instead, lettuce, cucumber, green beans and peas), cabbage and brussels sprouts induced a 16% decrease in the mean AUC of paracetamol, a 17% increase in the mean metabolic clearance rate, and an 8% increase in the mean 24-hour urinary recovery of the glucuronide metabolite.[10] Consumption of watercress caused a decrease in the levels of plasma and urinary oxidative metabolites of paracetamol, but the urinary excretion of paracetamol, or its glucuronide and sulfate were not notably altered.[11] However, charcoal-broiled beef (which accelerates the oxidative metabolism of some drugs) did not affect paracetamol metabolism.[12]

(c) Toxicity of paracetamol

A prospective study found that, of 49 patients with paracetamol hepatotoxicity, all had taken more than the recommended limit of 4 g of paracetamol daily. Paracetamol hepatotoxicity after a dose of 4 to 10 g daily was associated with fasting, and less commonly with alcohol use, and it was suggested that paracetamol hepatotoxicity after an overdose appears to be enhanced by fasting in addition to alcohol ingestion.[13] The metabolism of a lower 2-g dose of paracetamol was not, however, affected by food restriction in obese patients.[14]

Mechanism

The absorption of paracetamol is affected by the rate of gastric emptying and most foods delay this. Cabbage and brussels sprouts are thought to enhance the glucuronidation of paracetamol. Fasting might possibly contribute to paracetamol toxicity by shunting paracetamol detoxification from the conjugative to the potentially toxic oxidative pathways.[14]

Importance and management

The effect of food on paracetamol absorption appears to have been well studied, but the clinical importance of these findings is uncertain. It appears that rapid pain relief with single doses of paracetamol tablets could possibly be delayed and reduced by food in some individuals, but liquid or rapidly absorbed preparations are less likely to be affected. If paracetamol is taken in repeated doses, the interaction with food is unlikely to be clinically important as the total amount absorbed is usually unchanged. It seems unlikely that specific foods, such as watercress and charcoal-broiled beef, would have a significant clinical effect, except perhaps cabbage and brussels sprouts if eaten to excess.

Consider also, the food preservative sodium nitrate, see 'Paracetamol (Acetaminophen) + Sodium nitrate', p.210.

1. Robertson DRC, Higginson I, Macklin BS, Renwick AG, Waller DG, George CF. The influence of protein containing meals on the pharmacokinetics of levodopa in healthy volunteers. *Br J Clin Pharmacol* (1991) 31, 413–17.
2. Wessels JC, Koeleman HA, Boneschans B, Steyn HS. The influence of different types of breakfast on the absorption of paracetamol among members of an ethnic group. *Int J Clin Pharmacol Ther Toxicol* (1992) 30, 208–13.
3. Rostami-Hodjegan A, Shiran MR, Ayesh R, Grattan TJ, Burnett I, Darby-Dowman A, Tucker GT. A new rapidly absorbed paracetamol tablet containing sodium bicarbonate. I. A four-way crossover study to compare the concentration-time profile of paracetamol from the new paracetamol/sodium bicarbonate tablet and a conventional paracetamol tablet in fed and fasted volunteers. *Drug Dev Ind Pharm* (2002) 28, 523–31.
4. Walter-Sack IE, de Vries JX, Nickel B, Stenzhorn G, Weber E. The influence of different formula diets and different pharmaceutical formulations on the systemic availability of paracetamol, gallbladder size, and plasma glucose. *Int J Clin Pharmacol Ther Toxicol* (1989) 27, 544–50.
5. Holt S, Heading RC, Carter DC, Prescott LF, Tothill P. Effect of gel fibre on gastric emptying and absorption of glucose and paracetamol. *Lancet* (1979) 1, 636–9.
6. Forbes JA, Sandberg RA, Bood-Bjorklund L. The effect of food on bromfenac, naproxen sodium, and acetaminophen in postoperative pain after orthopedic surgery. *Pharmacotherapy* (1998) 18, 492–503.
7. Burnett I, Schachtel B, Sanner K, Bey M, Grattan T, Littlejohn S. Onset of analgesia of a paracetamol tablet containing sodium bicarbonate: a double-blind, placebo-controlled study in adult patients with acute sore throat. *Clin Ther* (2006) 28, 1273–8.
8. Prescott LF, Yoovathaworn K, Makarananda K, Saivises R, Sriwatanakul K. Impaired absorption of paracetamol in vegetarians. *Br J Clin Pharmacol* (1993) 36, 237–40.
9. Stillings M, Havlik I, Chetty M, Clinton C, Schall R, Moodley I, Muir N, Little S. Comparison of the pharmacokinetic profiles of soluble aspirin and solid paracetamol tablets in fed and fasted volunteers. *Curr Med Res Opin* (2000) 16, 115–24.
10. Pantuck EJ, Pantuck CB, Anderson KE, Wattenberg LW, Conney AH, Kappas A. Effect of brussels sprouts and cabbage on drug conjugation. *Clin Pharmacol Ther* (1984) 35, 161–9.
11. Chen L, Mohr SN, Yang CS. Decrease of plasma and urinary oxidative metabolites of acetaminophen after consumption of watercress by human volunteers. *Clin Pharmacol Ther* (1996) 60, 651–60.

12. Anderson KE, Schneider J, Pantuck EJ, Pantuck CB, Mudge GH, Welch RM, Conney AH, Kappas A. Acetaminophen metabolism in subjects fed charcoal-broiled beef. *Clin Pharmacol Ther* (1983) 34, 369–74.
13. Whitcomb DC, Block GD. Association of acetaminophen hepatotoxicity with fasting and ethanol use. *JAMA* (1994) 272, 1845–50.
14. Schenker S, Speeg KV, Perez A, Finch J. The effects of food restriction in man on hepatic metabolism of acetaminophen. *Clin Nutr* (2001) 20, 145–50.

Paracetamol (Acetaminophen) + Garlic

A study in healthy subjects found that garlic did not have a clinically relevant effect on the pharmacokinetics of single-dose paracetamol.

Clinical evidence

A study in 16 healthy subjects found that the use of an aged garlic extract (approximately equivalent to 6 to 7 cloves of garlic daily) for 3 months had little effect on the metabolism of a single 1-g oral dose of paracetamol.[1]

Mechanism

The study found that there was a very slight increase in glucuronidation of a therapeutic dose of paracetamol after the long-term use of garlic, and some evidence that sulfate conjugation was enhanced, but there did not appear to be any effect on the oxidative metabolism of paracetamol.

Importance and management

The evidence regarding an interaction between paracetamol and garlic is limited, but what is known suggests that no clinically significant interaction would be expected if paracetamol is taken with garlic. *Animal* data suggest that it is possible that some garlic constituents, or substances derived from them, might protect against the hepatotoxicity from higher than therapeutic doses of paracetamol,[2] but this requires further study.

1. Gwilt PR, Lear CL, Tempero MA, Birt DD, Grandjean AC, Ruddon RW, Nagel DL. The effect of garlic extract on human metabolism of acetaminophen. *Cancer Epidemiol Biomarkers Prev* (1994) 3, 155–60.
2. Lin MC, Wang E-J, Patten C, Lee M-J, Xiao F, Reuhl KR, Yang CS. Protective effect of diallyl sulfone against acetaminophen-induced hepatotoxicity in mice. *J Biochem Toxicol* (1996) 11, 11–20.

Paracetamol (Acetaminophen) + H_2-receptor antagonists

Cimetidine, nizatidine, and ranitidine do not appear to alter the pharmacokinetics of paracetamol to a clinically relevant extent.

Clinical evidence

(a) Cimetidine

In a study in 4 healthy subjects, cimetidine (given as a single 200-mg dose or as 1 g daily in divided doses for 7 days) had no statistically significant effect on the pharmacokinetics of a single 750-mg dose of paracetamol.[1] Similarly, in another study in 10 healthy subjects, a single 800-mg dose of cimetidine given one hour before paracetamol 1 g had no effect on the half-life or plasma clearance of paracetamol, and no effect on the urinary excretion of its principal metabolites (glucuronide, sulfate, mercapturate).[2] Furthermore, a study in 10 patients found that the pharmacokinetics of a single 1-g dose of paracetamol were not altered by cimetidine 400 mg twice daily given for 2 months. The only difference in urinary metabolites was a modest 37% decrease in paracetamol mercapturate (indicating a reduction in the hepatotoxic metabolite).[2] Other studies have found that cimetidine does not alter the clearance[3-5] or metabolic pathways of paracetamol.[3,5]

In contrast, one study reported that cimetidine 300 mg every 6 hours decreased the fractional clearance of the oxidised metabolites (mercapturate and cysteine conjugates) of paracetamol in healthy subjects.[6] Another study found that a single 400-mg dose of cimetidine given one hour before paracetamol 1 g in fasting subjects delayed the absorption of paracetamol (for instance, there was a 37% reduction in peak salivary level and a 63% increase in time to peak level). This effect was not seen when the two drugs were given simultaneously.[7]

(b) Nizatidine

In a study in 5 healthy subjects, nizatidine 300 mg taken with paracetamol 1 g modestly increased the AUC of paracetamol in the first 3 hours by 25%. Over this time period, there was also a 4% reduction in the formation of paracetamol glucuronide, and this reached statistical significance at 30 minutes and 45 minutes. Nizatidine 150 mg had a similar, but smaller, effect.[8]

(c) Ranitidine

In a study in 8 healthy subjects, ranitidine 300 mg twice daily for 4 days had no effect on the clearance and half-life of single 1-g intravenous and oral doses of paracetamol, given one hour after the dose of ranitidine. In addition, there was no difference in the urinary excretion of the paracetamol metabolites.[9,10] Another study reported similar findings when ranitidine 300 mg was given one hour before paracetamol 1 g. However, when the two drugs were given simultaneously, the AUC_{0-3} of paracetamol was increased by 63%, and the AUC_{0-3} of paracetamol glucuronide was decreased by 35%, but there was no change in paracetamol sulfate levels.[11]

An isolated case describes a man who noted his urine was dark 3 weeks after starting to take ranitidine 150 mg twice daily and paracetamol 1.3 to 2 g daily. He was found to have raised liver enzyme levels (alkaline phosphatase 708 units/L; AST 196 mIU/mL), which returned to normal on discontinuing ranitidine.[12]

Mechanism

Cimetidine appears to inhibit the oxidative metabolism of paracetamol by cytochrome P450 isoenzymes, resulting in a reduction in the hepatotoxic metabolite, see *Paracetamol*, under 'Analgesics and NSAIDs', p.138. It was suggested that cimetidine delayed paracetamol absorption by reducing gastric emptying.[7] Nizatidine might cause a minor inhibition of glucuronyltransferases.[8] Ranitidine might also inhibit paracetamol glucuronyltransferases when given simultaneously, but this was not seen when the drugs were given one hour apart.

Importance and management

Any changes in the pharmacokinetics of paracetamol with these H_2-receptor antagonists do not appear to be clinically relevant. Thus, no particular precautions seem to be necessary when paracetamol is given with cimetidine, nizatidine or ranitidine. The effect of cimetidine on the oxidative metabolism of paracetamol has been investigated as a means of reducing paracetamol hepatotoxicity. However, it appears that cimetidine is not effective for this purpose.[13]

1. Chen MM, Lee CS. Cimetidine-acetaminophen interaction in humans. *J Clin Pharmacol* (1985) 25, 227–9.
2. Vendemiale G, Altomare E, Trizio T, Leandro G, Manghisi OG, Albano O. Effect of acute and chronic cimetidine administration on acetaminophen metabolism in humans. *Am J Gastroenterol* (1987) 82, 1031–4.
3. Slattery JT, McRorie TI, Reynolds R, Kalhorn TF, Kharasch ED, Eddy AC. Lack of effect of cimetidine on acetaminophen disposition in humans. *Clin Pharmacol Ther* (1989) 46, 591–7.
4. Abernethy DR, Greenblatt DJ, Divoll M, Ameer B, Shader RI. Differential effect of cimetidine on drug oxidation (antipyrine and diazepam) *vs* conjugation (acetaminophen and lorazepam): prevention of acetaminophen toxicity by cimetidine. *J Pharmacol Exp Ther* (1983) 224, 508–13.
5. Miners JO, Attwood J, Birkett DJ. Determinants of acetaminophen metabolism: effect of inducers and inhibitors of drug metabolism on acetaminophen's metabolic pathways. *Clin Pharmacol Ther* (1984) 35, 480–6.
6. Mitchell MC, Schenker S, Speeg KV. Selective inhibition of acetaminophen oxidation and toxicity by cimetidine and other histamine H_2-receptor antagonists in vivo and in vitro in rat and in man. *J Clin Invest* (1984) 73, 383–91.
7. Garba M, Odunola MT, Ahmed BH. Effect of study protocol on the interactions between cimetidine and paracetamol in man. *Eur J Drug Metab Pharmacokinet* (1999) 24, 159–62.
8. Itoh H, Nagano T, Takeyama M. Effect of nizatidine on paracetamol and its metabolites in human plasma. *J Pharm Pharmacol* (2002) 54, 869–73.
9. Thomas M, Michael MF, Andrew P, Scully N. A study to investigate the effects of ranitidine on the metabolic disposition of paracetamol in man. *Br J Clin Pharmacol* (1988) 25, 671P.
10. Jack D, Thomas M, Skidmore IF. Ranitidine and paracetamol metabolism. *Lancet* (1985) ii, 1067.
11. Itoh H, Nagano T, Hayashi T, Takeyama M. Ranitidine increases bioavailability of acetaminophen by inhibiting the first-pass glucuronidation in man. *Pharm Pharmacol Commun* (2000) 6, 495–500.
12. Bredfeldt JE, von Huene C. Ranitidine, acetaminophen, and hepatotoxicity. *Ann Intern Med* (1984) 101, 719.
13. Kaufenberg AJ, Shepherd MF. Role of cimetidine in the treatment of acetaminophen poisoning. *Am J Health-Syst Pharm* (1998) 55, 1516–19.

Paracetamol (Acetaminophen) + Hibiscus (*Hibiscus sabdariffa*)

Hibiscus extract does not appear to affect the pharmacokinetics of single-dose paracetamol to a clinically relevant extent.

Clinical evidence, mechanism, importance and management

A study in 6 healthy subjects found that Zobo drink (*Hibiscus sabdariffa* water extract) given 78 minutes before a single 1-g dose of paracetamol did not affect the absorption or AUC of paracetamol, but the total body clearance increased by 12%.[1] This is not expected to be clinically relevant.

1. Kolawole JA, Maduenyi A. Effect of Zobo drink (Hibiscus sabdariffa water extract) on the pharmacokinetics of acetaminophen in human volunteers. *Eur J Drug Metab Pharmacokinet* (2004) 29, 25–9.

Paracetamol (Acetaminophen) + Hormonal contraceptives or HRT

Paracetamol clearance is increased in women taking oral hormonal contraceptives. Paracetamol very slightly increases the exposure to ethinylestradiol. HRT containing conjugated oestrogens does not appear to affect the pharmacokinetics of paracetamol.

Clinical evidence

(a) Contraceptives

In a study in 7 healthy women taking oral combined hormonal contraceptives (containing **ethinylestradiol**), the plasma clearance of a single 1.5-g dose of paracetamol was 64% higher and its elimination half-life was 30% lower, when compared with 7 healthy women not taking these contraceptives. The fractional clearance by glucuronidation and of the cysteine conjugate was increased, but that of sulfation and the mercapturic acid conjugate were unchanged.[1] Similarly, other studies have found higher paracetamol clearances of 30 to 49%, and corresponding lower paracetamol half-lives, in women taking oral hormonal contraceptives, when compared with control subjects.[2-4]

In a study in 6 healthy women, a single 1-g oral dose of paracetamol increased the AUC of **ethinylestradiol** (from an oral combined hormonal contraceptive) by 22%, and decreased the AUC of its metabolite, ethinylestradiol sulfate, by 41%. The plasma levels of **levonorgestrel** were not affected.[5]

(b) HRT

One study found that the pharmacokinetics of a single 650-mg intravenous dose of paracetamol did not differ between women who had taken **conjugated oestrogens** for at least 3 months and control subjects.[6]

Mechanism

The evidence suggests that oral hormonal contraceptives increase the metabolism (both oxidation and glucuronidation) of paracetamol by the liver.[3] The increased absorption of ethinylestradiol probably occurs because paracetamol reduces its metabolism by the gut wall.[5] It has been suggested that the differences between the effects of oral hormonal contraceptives and conjugated oestrogens on paracetamol might be attributable to the influence of progestogens on glucuronide and sulfate conjugation.[6] This needs confirmation.

Importance and management

The very slight to slight effect of the oral hormonal contraceptives on the pharmacokinetics of paracetamol appears to be established, but its clinical importance has not been directly studied. Based on the pharmacokinetic changes reported any effect seems likely to be of minimal clinical relevance. The clinical importance of the modest increase in ethinylestradiol absorption is also uncertain, but it is likely to be minor. HRT does not appear to interact with paracetamol.

1. Mitchell MC, Hanew T, Meredith CG, Schenker S. Effects of oral contraceptive steroids on acetaminophen metabolism and elimination. *Clin Pharmacol Ther* (1983) 34, 48–53.
2. Abernethy DR, Divoll M, Ochs HR, Ameer B, Greenblatt DJ. Increased metabolic clearance of acetaminophen with oral contraceptive use. *Obstet Gynecol* (1982) 60, 338–41.
3. Miners JO, Attwood J, Birkett DJ. Influence of sex and oral contraceptive steroids on paracetamol metabolism. *Br J Clin Pharmacol* (1983) 16, 503–9.
4. Mucklow JC, Fraser HS, Bulpitt CJ, Kahn C, Mould G, Dollery CT. Environmental factors affecting paracetamol metabolism in London factory and office workers. *Br J Clin Pharmacol* (1980) 10, 67–74.
5. Rogers SM, Back DJ, Stevenson PJ, Grimmer SFM, Orme ML'E. Paracetamol interaction with oral contraceptive steroids: increased plasma concentration of ethinyloestradiol. *Br J Clin Pharmacol* (1987) 23, 721–5.
6. Scavone JM, Greenblatt DJ, Blyden GT, Luna BG, Harmatz JS. Acetaminophen pharmacokinetics in women receiving conjugated estrogen. *Eur J Clin Pharmacol* (1990) 38, 97–8.

Paracetamol (Acetaminophen) + 5-HT$_3$-receptor antagonists

Tropisetron and granisetron blocked the analgesic effects of paracetamol in one study in healthy subjects, whereas, in another study in patients, ondansetron did not reduce the analgesic or opioid-sparing effects of paracetamol.

Clinical evidence, mechanism, importance and management

(a) Granisetron and Tropisetron

A placebo-controlled, crossover study in 26 healthy subjects found that both intravenous granisetron 3 mg and tropisetron 5 mg blocked the analgesic effect of a single 1-g oral dose of paracetamol given 90 minutes later. The pharmacokinetics of paracetamol were unaffected by the two drugs. This interaction was thought to involve the serotonergic system,[1] see *Mechanism*, under 'Opioids + Antiemetics; Ondansetron', p.163, for further explanation of this effect. Until more is known, it would be prudent to consider the possibility of an interaction should a patient fail to respond to paracetamol. If an interaction is suspected, consider giving alternative analgesics.

(b) Ondansetron

A randomised, placebo-controlled study in 120 patients undergoing laparoscopic hysterectomy, given oxycodone patient-controlled analgesia, evaluated the effect of a single 4-mg dose of [intravenous] ondansetron, given at the end of surgery, on the analgesic and opioid-sparing effect of intravenous paracetamol 1 g (given before, and at 6-, 12- and 18-hours after the induction of anaesthesia). When 40 patients receiving paracetamol and ondansetron were compared with 80 control patients, the addition of ondansetron to paracetamol had no effect on the time to first oxycodone dose or on the total dose of oxycodone required, suggesting that the analgesic and opioid-sparing effects of paracetamol were unchanged by ondansetron. The authors of this study suggest that the difference in outcomes between this study and the study with granisetron and tropisetron, which found a reduction in the effects of paracetamol, might be due to several factors, including the use of a comparatively lower dose of the 5-HT$_3$-receptor antagonist, possible changes in the organisation of the serotonergic system due to tissue injury from the surgery, or that oxycodone blocked the effect of ondansetron on paracetamol.[2]

1. Pickering G, Loriot M-A, Libert F, Eschalier A, Beaune P, Dubray C. Analgesic effect of acetaminophen in humans: first evidence of a central serotonergic mechanism. *Clin Pharmacol Ther* (2006) 79, 371–8.
2. Jokela R, Ahonen J, Seitsonen E, Marjakangas P, Korttila K. The influence of ondansetron on the analgesic effect of acetaminophen after laparoscopic hysterectomy. *Clin Pharmacol Ther* (2010) 87, 672–78.

Paracetamol (Acetaminophen) + Isoniazid

A number of reports suggest that the toxicity of paracetamol might be increased by isoniazid so that normal analgesic doses (4 g daily) might not be safe in some individuals. Pharmacokinetic studies suggest that isoniazid usually inhibits the metabolism of paracetamol, but that metabolism to toxic metabolites might be induced shortly after stopping isoniazid, or late in the isoniazid dose-interval in fast acetylators of isoniazid.

Clinical evidence

A 21-year-old woman who had been taking isoniazid 300 mg for 6 months developed marked evidence of liver damage (prolonged prothrombin time, elevated ammonia, transaminases, hyperbilirubinaemia) within about 6 hours of taking 3.25 g of paracetamol for abdominal cramping.[1]

A young woman taking isoniazid who had taken up to 11.5 g of paracetamol in a suicide attempt, developed life-threatening hepatic and renal toxicity despite the fact that her serum paracetamol levels were only 15 micromol/L 13 hours after ingestion (toxicity normally associated with levels above 26 micromol/L).[2]

Three other similar cases have been reported in patients taking isoniazid, rifampicin (rifampin) and pyrazinamide who had taken only 2 to 6 g of paracetamol daily.[3] Three other possible cases of this toxic interaction have also been described.[4]

However, in a pharmacokinetic study in 10 healthy subjects (including both slow and fast acetylators of isoniazid), isoniazid 300 mg daily for 7 days decreased the total clearance of a single 500-mg dose of paracetamol by 15%. Moreover, the clearance of paracetamol to oxidative metabolites was decreased.[5] Similarly, in a further study, in 10 healthy slow acetylators of isoniazid, the formation of paracetamol thioether metabolites and oxidative metabolites was reduced by 63% and 49%, respectively, by isoniazid 300 mg daily. However, one day after stopping isoniazid, the formation of thioether metabolites was *increased* by 56%, and this returned to pretreatment values 3 days after the discontinuation of isoniazid.[6] In yet another study in 10 healthy subjects taking isoniazid as prophylaxis, the formation clearance of paracetamol to *N*-acetyl-*p*-benzoquinone imine (NAPQI) was inhibited by 56% when paracetamol was given simultaneously with the daily dose of isoniazid, but when paracetamol was taken 12 hours after isoniazid, there was no difference in NAPQI formation clearance, compared with the control phase (one to 2 weeks after isoniazid had been discontinued). However, when the results were analysed by isoniazid acetylator status, it appeared that the NAPQI formation clearance was *increased* in fast acetylators taking paracetamol 12 hours after the dose of isoniazid.[7]

Mechanism

Not established. A possible reason for the altered paracetamol metabolism is that isoniazid induces CYP2E1 by stabilisation.[8] This means that while isoniazid is present, the metabolism of substrates such as paracetamol is inhibited. However, when isoniazid levels drop sufficiently (as could be the case late in the dosing interval in fast acetylators), metabolism might be induced resulting in a greater proportion of paracetamol being converted into toxic metabolites than would normally occur.[7]

Importance and management

Information is limited, but it would now seem prudent to consider warning patients taking isoniazid to limit their use of paracetamol because it seems that some individuals risk possible paracetamol-induced liver toxicity, even with normal recommended doses of paracetamol. Pharmacokinetic studies suggest that it is possible that the risk is greatest shortly after stopping isoniazid. The risk might also be higher if paracetamol is taken late in the isoniazid dosing interval, particularly in fast acetylators of isoniazid. More study is needed to clarify the situation.

1. Crippin JS. Acetaminophen hepatotoxicity: potentiation by isoniazid. *Am J Gastroenterol* (1993) 88, 590–2.
2. Murphy R, Swartz R, Watkins P B. Severe acetaminophen toxicity in a patient receiving isoniazid. *Ann Intern Med* (1990) 113, 799–800.
3. Nolan CM, Sandblom RE, Thummel KE, Slattery JT, Nelson SD. Hepatotoxicity associated with acetaminophen usage in patients receiving multiple drug therapy for tuberculosis. *Chest* (1994) 105, 408–11.
4. Moulding TS, Redeker AG, Kanel GC. Acetaminophen, isoniazid, and hepatic toxicity. *Ann Intern Med* (1991) 114, 431.
5. Epstein MM, Nelson SD, Slattery JT, Kalhorn TF, Wall RA, Wright JM. Inhibition of the metabolism of paracetamol by isoniazid. *Br J Clin Pharmacol* (1991) 31, 139–42.
6. Zand R, Nelson SD, Slattery JT, Thummel KE, Kalhorn TF, Adams SP, Wright JM. Inhibition and induction of cytochrome P4502E1-catalyzed oxidation by isoniazid in humans. *Clin Pharmacol Ther* (1993) 54, 142–9.
7. Chien JY, Peter RM, Nolan CM, Wartell C, Slattery JT, Nelson SD, Carithers RL, Thummel KE. Influence of polymorphic *N*-acetyltransferase phenotype on the inhibition and induction of acetaminophen bioactivation with long-term isoniazid. *Clin Pharmacol Ther* (1997) 61, 24–34.
8. Chien JY, Thummel KE, Slattery JT. Pharmacokinetic consequences of induction of CYP2E1 by ligand stabilization. *Drug Metab Dispos* (1997) 25, 1165–75.

Paracetamol (Acetaminophen) + Kakkonto

Kakkonto extract does not appear to affect the pharmacokinetics of a single dose of paracetamol

Clinical evidence, mechanism, importance and management

A study in 6 healthy subjects found that 5 g of Kakkonto extract (a Chinese herbal medicine containing extracts of *Puerariae*, *Ephedrae*, *Zingiberis*, *Cinnamomi*, *Glycyrrhizae*, *Paeoniae* and *Zizphi* spp.) had no effects on the pharmacokinetics of a single 12-mg/kg dose of paracetamol. A further study (by the same authors) in 19 healthy subjects found that 1.25 g of Kakkonto had no effect on the pharmacokinetics of paracetamol 150 mg (from a preparation also containing salicylamide, caffeine and promethazine methylene disalicylate). Because in *animal* studies high doses of Kakkonto for 7 days were found to increase the serum levels of paracetamol, the authors concluded that further investigations were required to assess the safety and efficacy of concurrent use.[1]

1. Qi J, Toyoshima A, Honda Y, Mineshita S. Pharmacokinetic study on acetaminophen: interaction with a Chinese medicine. *J Med Dent Sci* (1997) 44, 31–5.

Paracetamol (Acetaminophen) + Lamotrigine

Paracetamol very slightly reduces the exposure to lamotrigine.

Clinical evidence, mechanism, importance and management

A study in 8 healthy subjects found that paracetamol 2.7 g daily very slightly reduced the AUC of a 300-mg dose of lamotrigine by 20% and reduced its half-life by 15%.[1] It is unlikely that this reduction in lamotrigine exposure is of clinical importance.

1. Depot M, Powell JR, Messenheimer JA, Cloutier G, Dalton MJ. Kinetic effects of multiple oral doses of acetaminophen on a single oral dose of lamotrigine. *Clin Pharmacol Ther* (1990) 48, 346–55.

Paracetamol (Acetaminophen) + Opioids

Diamorphine, morphine, oxycodone, pentazocine and pethidine (meperidine) delay gastric emptying so that the rate of absorption of oral paracetamol is reduced. No pharmacokinetic interaction occurs between codeine and paracetamol, but the combination may not always result in increased analgesia. Paracetamol does not appear to alter the pharmacokinetics of tapentadol.

Clinical evidence

(a) Codeine

A study in 6 healthy subjects found that paracetamol 1 g every 8 hours for 7 doses had no effect on the pharmacokinetics of a single 30-mg oral dose of codeine, or its metabolites.[1] Similarly in other studies, codeine had no effect on the pharmacokinetics of paracetamol.[2,3] Paracetamol and codeine are often given together because the combination is more effective than either drug given alone. However, note that not all studies have found this. For example, in one clinical study of surgical removal of impacted third molar teeth, there was no difference in analgesic efficacy between patients given paracetamol alone (800 mg given 3, 6, and 9 hours after surgery, then 400 mg four times daily for 2 days) and those given the same dose of paracetamol with the addition of codeine phosphate 30 mg. Moreover, patients given codeine experienced more adverse effects (nausea, dizziness, drowsiness).[4]

(b) Diamorphine, Pethidine (Meperidine) and Pentazocine

A study in 8 healthy subjects reported that the absorption of a single 20-mg/kg oral dose of paracetamol solution given 30 minutes after an intramuscular injection of either pethidine 150 mg or diamorphine 10 mg was markedly delayed and reduced. Peak plasma paracetamol levels were reduced by 31% and 74%, respectively, and delayed from 22 minutes to 114 minutes and 142 minutes, respectively.[5] This interaction was also observed, by the same study group, in women in labour who had been given paracetamol tablets after receiving pethidine, diamorphine or pentazocine.[6]

(c) Fentanyl

An *in vitro* study found that paracetamol inhibited the oxidation of fentanyl to norfentanyl, but the concentrations of paracetamol used were greater than those found therapeutically. A potential interaction was thought possible because fentanyl is metabolised by CYP3A4 and paracetamol is also partially metabolised by the CYP3A family.[7]

(d) Morphine

A study in healthy subjects, who remained in the supine position, investigated the effect of morphine syrup (4 doses of 10 mg given every 4 hours) on the absorption of paracetamol. The time to the maximum plasma paracetamol level, for conventional tablets, was increased from 51 minutes to 160 minutes by morphine, whereas the time to the maximum plasma paracetamol level for dispersible tablets was only increased from 14 minutes to 15 minutes.[8]

(e) Oxycodone

A crossover study in 10 healthy subjects investigated the effect of oxycodone 500 micrograms/kg on the absorption kinetics of a simulated paracetamol overdose (5 g). The maximum serum paracetamol level was reduced by 40%, the time to maximum level was increased by 68%, and the AUC_{0-8} was 27% lower, when compared with paracetamol alone.[9]

(f) Tapentadol

A crossover study in 20 healthy subjects found that paracetamol 1 g every 6 hours for 7 doses had no effect on the pharmacokinetics of a single 80 mg-dose of tapentadol, given after the fifth dose of paracetamol.[10]

Mechanism, importance and management

The underlying mechanism of these interactions is that the opioid analgesics delay gastric emptying so that the rate of absorption of paracetamol is reduced, but the total amount absorbed is not affected. These were largely investigational studies in healthy subjects, where paracetamol was used as a measure of gastric emptying, and any clinical relevance has not been determined. Reducing the rate of paracetamol absorption would be expected to reduce the onset of analgesic effect, but this is probably not relevant in patients who are receiving regular doses of paracetamol. However, if speed of onset of action is important, one study[8] suggested that the use of dispersible paracetamol might help to reduce the delay in reaching therapeutic plasma levels.

In paracetamol overdose, it has been suggested that when an opioid is present there may be a potential role for the use of activated charcoal beyond one-hour post-ingestion, because of the delay in the absorption of paracetamol.[9] When assessing treatment options it is also worth noting that maximum plasma levels may be delayed.

1. Somogyi A, Bochner F, Chen ZR. Lack of effect of paracetamol on the pharmacokinetics and metabolism of codeine in man. *Eur J Clin Pharmacol* (1991) 41, 379–82.
2. Bajorek P, Widdop B, Volans G. Lack of inhibition of paracetamol absorption by codeine. *Br J Clin Pharmacol* (1978) 5, 346–8.
3. Sonne J, Poulsen HE, Loft S, Døssing M, Vollmer-Larsen A, Simonsen K, Thyssen H, Lundstrøm K. Therapeutic doses of codeine have no effect on acetaminophen clearance or metabolism. *Eur J Clin Pharmacol* (1988) 35, 109–11.
4. Skjelbred P, Løkken P. Codeine added to paracetamol induced adverse effects but did not increase analgesia. *Br J Clin Pharmacol* (1982) 14, 539–43.
5. Nimmo WS, Heading RC, Wilson J, Tothill P, Prescott LF. Inhibition of gastric emptying and drug absorption by narcotic analgesics. *Br J Clin Pharmacol* (1975) 2, 509–13.
6. Nimmo WS, Wilson J, Prescott LF. Narcotic analgesics and delayed gastric emptying during labour. *Lancet* (1975) i, 890–3.
7. Feierman DE. The effect of paracetamol (acetaminophen) on fentanyl metabolism *in vitro*. *Acta Anaesthesiol Scand* (2000) 44, 560–3.
8. Kennedy JM, Tyers NM, Davey AK. The influence of morphine on the absorption of paracetamol from various formulations in subjects in the supine position, as assessed by TDx measurement of salivary paracetamol concentrations. *J Pharm Pharmacol* (2003) 55, 1345–50.
9. Halcomb SE, Sivilotti ML, Goklaney A, Mullins ME. Pharmacokinetic effects of diphenhydramine or oxycodone in simulated acetaminophen overdose. *Acad Emerg Med* (2005) 12, 169–72.
10. Smit JW, Oh C, Rengelshausen J, Terlinden R, Ravenstijn PGM, Wang SS, Upmalis D, Mangold B. Effects of acetaminophen, naproxen and acetylsalicylic acid on tapentadol pharmacokinetics: results of two randomized, open-label, crossover, drug-drug interaction studies. *Pharmacotherapy* (2010) 30, 25–34.

Paracetamol (Acetaminophen) + Probenecid

Probenecid reduces the clearance of paracetamol.

Clinical evidence, mechanism, importance and management

A single-dose study in 10 healthy subjects found that the clearance of paracetamol 1.5 g was almost halved (from 6.23 mL/minute per kg to 3.42 mL/minute per kg) when it was taken one hour after a 1-g dose of probenecid. The amount of unchanged paracetamol in the urine stayed the same, but the amount of the glucuronide metabolite fell sharply.[1] Another study in 11 subjects also found that probenecid 500 mg every 6 hours almost halved the clearance of a 650-mg intravenous dose of paracetamol (from 329 mL/minute to 178 mL/minute). The urinary excretion of the glucuronide metabolite was decreased by 68% and the excretion of the sulfate metabolite was increased by 49%.[2]

These studies suggest that probenecid inhibits paracetamol glucuronidation, possibly by inhibiting glucuronyltransferases. The clinical relevance of this interaction is uncertain but there seem to be no reports of an adverse reaction.

1. Kamali F. The effect of probenecid on paracetamol metabolism and pharmacokinetics. *Eur J Clin Pharmacol* (1993) 45, 551–3.
2. Abernethy DR, Greenblatt DJ, Ameer B, Shader RI. Probenecid impairment of acetaminophen and lorazepam clearance: direct inhibition of ether glucuronide formation. *J Pharmacol Exp Ther* (1985) 234, 345–9.

Paracetamol (Acetaminophen) + Propranolol

Propranolol causes a negligible decrease in the clearance of paracetamol.

Clinical evidence, mechanism, importance and management

In a study in 10 healthy subjects, propranolol 80 mg twice daily for 4 days increased the half-life of a single 1.5-g dose of paracetamol by 25% and lowered its clearance by 14%. The partial clearance of paracetamol to its cysteine and mercapturate derivatives was decreased by 16% and 32%, respectively, and the clearance to the glucuronide conjugate was decreased by 27%, but the sulfate metabolite was not significantly affected.[1] Similarly, an earlier study found that propranolol 40 mg four times daily for one week increased the maximum plasma level of a single 1.5-g dose of paracetamol and reduced the time to peak plasma level. However, the increased rate of absorption of paracetamol was not thought to be clinically important.[2] In contrast, a study in 6 subjects found that a relatively small dose of propranolol (80 mg daily for 6 days) did not affect the pharmacokinetics of paracetamol.[3] Another study found that long-term propranolol use in patients with chronic liver disease did not influence the clearance of total or unconjugated paracetamol.[4] The pharmacokinetic changes described here appear to be negligible, and are therefore unlikely to be clinically relevant.

1. Baraka OZ, Truman CA, Ford JM, Roberts CJC. The effect of propranolol on paracetamol metabolism in man. *Br J Clin Pharmacol* (1990) 29, 261–4.
2. Clark RA, Holdsworth CD, Rees MR, Howlett PJ. The effect on paracetamol absorption of stimulation and blockade of β-adrenoceptors. *Br J Clin Pharmacol* (1980) 10, 555–9.
3. Sanchez-Martinez V, Tucker GT, Jackson PR, Lennard MS, Bax NDS, Woods HF. Lack of effect of propranolol on the kinetics of paracetamol in man. *Br J Clin Pharmacol* (1985) 20, 548P.
4. Hayes PC, Bouchier IAD. Effect of acute and chronic propranolol administration on antipyrine and paracetamol clearance in patients with chronic liver disease. *Am J Gastroenterol* (1989) 84, 723–6.

Paracetamol (Acetaminophen) + Proton pump inhibitors

Lansoprazole increased the rate, but not the extent, of absorption of a paracetamol solution in one study. Omeprazole does not appear to have

any effect on the metabolism of paracetamol or phenacetin (which is metabolised to paracetamol) .

Clinical evidence

(a) Lansoprazole

In a study in 6 healthy subjects, lansoprazole 30 mg daily for 3 days increased the peak level of paracetamol (given as a single 1-g dose in solution) by 43%, and decreased the time to peak paracetamol levels by half (from about 35 minutes to 17.5 minutes). However, lansoprazole had no effect on the AUC and elimination half-life of paracetamol.[1]

(b) Omeprazole

In a study in 10 healthy subjects, omeprazole 20 mg daily for 8 days had no effect on the pharmacokinetics of **phenacetin**, or paracetamol derived from **phenacetin**, except that the peak plasma level of **phenacetin** was higher. There was no change in the metabolism (oxidative and conjugative) of **phenacetin** or derived paracetamol.[2] In another study in 10 subjects, omeprazole 40 mg daily for 7 days had no effect on the formation of the thioether metabolites of paracetamol.[3]

Mechanism

Lansoprazole might increase the absorption of paracetamol by indirectly increasing the rate of gastric emptying.[1] Phenacetin is metabolised to paracetamol by CYP1A2, and it has been suggested that omeprazole can induce CYP1A2, and possibly increase the formation of the hepatotoxic metabolites of paracetamol. However, the findings of the study suggest that omeprazole has no important effect on CYP1A2, or on phenacetin or paracetamol metabolism.

Importance and management

The findings from these studies suggest that neither lansoprazole nor omeprazole cause any clinically important changes in the pharmacokinetics of paracetamol. No paracetamol dose adjustment appears to be needed on the concurrent use of either omeprazole or lansoprazole. Other proton pump inhibitors would also not be expected to interact, but this needs confirmation. Similarly, omeprazole has no clinically relevant effect on the pharmacokinetics of phenacetin.

1. Sanaka M, Kuyama Y, Mineshita S, Qi J, Hanada Y, Enatsu I, Tanaka H, Makino H, Yamanaka M. Pharmacokinetic interaction between acetaminophen and lansoprazole. *J Clin Gastroenterol* (1999) 29, 56–8.
2. Xiaodong S, Gatti G, Bartoli A, Cipolla G, Crema F, Perucca E. Omeprazole does not enhance the metabolism of phenacetin, a marker of CYP1A2 activity, in healthy volunteers. *Ther Drug Monit* (1994) 16, 248–50.
3. Sarich T, Kalhorn T, Magee S, Al-Sayegh F, Adams S, Slattery J, Goldstein J, Nelson S, Wright J. The effect of omeprazole pretreatment on acetaminophen metabolism in rapid and slow metabolizers of S-mephenytoin. *Clin Pharmacol Ther* (1997) 62, 21–8.

Paracetamol (Acetaminophen) + Rifampicin (Rifampin)

Rifampicin increases the metabolism of paracetamol. An isolated report describes liver failure, which might have been due to an interaction between paracetamol and rifampicin.

Clinical evidence, mechanism, importance and management

In a study in 10 patients taking rifampicin 600 mg daily, the metabolite to paracetamol ratio for glucuronides was twice as high as that of 14 healthy control subjects. In contrast, the ratio for sulfates did not differ between the two groups.[1] In a crossover study in healthy subjects, rifampicin 600 mg daily for one week, given before paracetamol 500 mg, had no effect on the formation of *N*-acetyl-*p*-benzoquinone imine (NAPQI) or the recovery of thiol metabolites formed by conjugation of NAPQI with glutathione.[2]

The clinical importance of these studies awaits further clarification, but they suggest that rifampicin might reduce the efficacy of paracetamol. They also suggest that rifampicin induces the glucuronidation of paracetamol, but that it does not increase the formation of the hepatotoxic metabolites of paracetamol. However, a 32-year-old woman, who had taken paracetamol 2 to 4 g daily for several weeks, and who had not responded to doxycycline or clarithromycin for suspected cat scratch fever, became confused and agitated 2 days after starting to take rifampicin 600 mg twice daily. Her INR increased from 1.1 to 5.2 and her liver enzymes became raised. Rifampicin and paracetamol were stopped, she was treated with vitamin K and acetylcysteine, and her liver function returned to normal. Paracetamol hepatotoxicity, in doses not normally associated with such effects, occurred only after the addition of rifampicin. It was suggested that rifampicin, which alone can cause hepatitis, had in this case induced the metabolism of paracetamol to its hepatotoxic metabolites.[3] The general relevance of this isolated case is unknown.

1. Bock KW, Wiltfang J, Blume R, Ullrich D, Bircher J. Paracetamol as a test drug to determine glucuronide formation in man. Effects of inducers and of smoking. *Eur J Clin Pharmacol* (1987) 31, 677–83.
2. Manyike PT, Kharasch ED, Kalhorn TF, Slattery JT. Contribution of CYP2E1 and CYP3A to acetaminophen reactive metabolite formation. *Clin Pharmacol Ther* (2000) 67, 275–82.
3. Stephenson I, Qualie M, Wiselka MJ. Hepatic failure and encephalopathy attributed to an interaction between acetaminophen and rifampicin. *Am J Gastroenterol* (2001) 96, 1310–1.

Paracetamol (Acetaminophen) + Sodium nitrate

An isolated report describes severe methaemoglobinaemia in a patient who had taken paracetamol after a meal consisting of 'yuke' (raw beef preserved with sodium nitrate). Both paracetamol and sodium nitrate may cause methaemoglobinaemia, so an interaction resulting in additive effects might possibly have occurred, but a genetic cause was also considered to be a possibility.[1] This is an isolated report and its general relevance is therefore unknown.

1. Kobayashi T, Kawabata M, Tanaka S, Maehara M, Mishima A, Murase T. Methemoglobinemia induced by combined use of sodium nitrate and acetoaminophen. *Intern Med* (2000) 39, 860.

Paracetamol (Acetaminophen) + Sucralfate

Sucralfate does not affect the absorption of paracetamol.

Clinical evidence mechanism, importance and management

In a placebo-controlled study in 6 healthy subjects, the bioavailability of paracetamol 1 g (using salivary paracetamol levels over 4 hours as a measure of paracetamol absorption) was found to be unchanged by sucralfate 1 g.[1] This suggests that paracetamol absorption is unlikely to be affected by sucralfate. No particular precautions appear to be necessary if both drugs are given.

1. Kamali F, Fry JR, Smart HL, Bell GD. A double-blind placebo-controlled study to examine effects of sucralfate on paracetamol absorption. *Br J Clin Pharmacol* (1985) 19, 113–14.

Paracetamol (Acetaminophen) + Sulfinpyrazone

Sulfinpyrazone increases the clearance of paracetamol.

Clinical evidence, mechanism, importance and management

In a study in 12 healthy subjects, sulfinpyrazone 200 mg every 6 hours for one week increased the clearance of a single 1-g dose of paracetamol by 23%. There was a 26% increase in the metabolic clearance of the glucuronide conjugate of paracetamol, and a 43% increase in the glutathione-derived conjugates (indicating an increased production of the hepatotoxic metabolite), but no change in sulfation.[1] It has therefore been suggested that, in patients taking sulfinpyrazone, the risk of liver damage might be increased after paracetamol overdose and perhaps during prolonged consumption,[1] but there seem to be no reports of an adverse effect. The clinical importance of these findings awaits further study.

1. Miners JO, Attwood J, Birkett DJ. Determinants of acetaminophen metabolism: effect of inducers and inhibitors of drug metabolism on acetaminophen's metabolic pathways. *Clin Pharmacol Ther* (1984) 35, 480–6.

Paracetamol (Acetaminophen) + Tobacco

Heavy, but not moderate, tobacco smoking might increase the metabolism of paracetamol. The clearance of phenacetin (which is metabolised to paracetamol) also appears to be increased in smokers. There is some evidence that smokers are at risk of a poorer outcome after paracetamol overdose.

Clinical evidence, mechanism, importance and management

A study in 6 otherwise healthy smokers (more than 15 cigarettes per day) and 6 healthy non-smokers found no difference in the clearance of a single 1-g dose of paracetamol or its metabolites between the two groups.[1] Similarly, another study found no difference in the pharmacokinetics of a single 650-mg intravenous dose of paracetamol between 14 otherwise healthy smokers (range 8 to 35 cigarettes per day) and 15 non-smokers.[2] In contrast, in another study, the glucuronide metabolite to paracetamol ratio was 83% higher in 9 heavy smokers (about 40 cigarettes daily), suggesting increased paracetamol metabolism, than in 14 healthy non-smokers. However, it was not higher in moderate smokers (about 10 cigarettes daily).[3] A retrospective study of patients treated for paracetamol poisoning found that there was a much higher proportion of smokers than in the general population (70% versus 31%). Moreover, smoking was independently associated with an increased risk of hepatic encephalopathy (odds ratio 2.68) and death (odds ratio 3.64) following paracetamol overdose.[4]

A study in 36 healthy Chinese subjects given a single 900-mg dose of **phenacetin** (which is metabolised to paracetamol) found that subjects who smoked cigarettes (7 to 40 daily; mean 20 daily) had a 2.5-fold higher phenacetin apparent oral clearance, when compared with non-smokers. Paracetamol plasma levels were also lower in the smokers.[5]

Cigarette smoke appears to induce the metabolism of **phenacetin** by CYP1A2, and also appears to increase the metabolism of paracetamol, either by stimulating a minor pathway involving CYP1A2 oxidation or by stimulating the conversion of phenacetin to compounds other than paracetamol.[5]

An interaction between paracetamol and tobacco smoking is not established, but the above studies suggest that heavy smoking might increase the metabolism of paracetamol. The retrospective study also suggests that smoking is associated with a poorer outcome after paracetamol overdose. Further study is needed to establish the general relevance of these findings.

1. Miners JO, Attwood J, Birkett DJ. Determinants of acetaminophen metabolism: effect of inducers and inhibitors of drug metabolism on acetaminophen's metabolic pathways. *Clin Pharmacol Ther* (1984) 35, 480–6.
2. Scavone JM, Greenblatt DJ, LeDuc BW, Blyden GT, Luna BG, Harmatz JS. Differential effect of cigarette smoking on antipyrine oxidation versus acetaminophen conjugation. *Pharmacology* (1990) 40, 77–84.
3. Bock KW, Wiltfang J, Blume R, Ullrich D, Bircher J. Paracetamol as a test drug to determine glucuronide formation in man. Effects of inducers and of smoking. *Eur J Clin Pharmacol* (1987) 31, 677–83.
4. Schmidt LE, Dalhoff K. The impact of current tobacco use on the outcome of paracetamol poisoning. *Aliment Pharmacol Ther* (2003) 18, 979–85.
5. Dong SX , Ping ZZ, Xiao WZ, Shu CC, Bartoli A, Gatti G, D'Urso S, Perucca E. Effect of active and passive cigarette smoking on CYP1A2-mediated phenacetin disposition in Chinese subjects. *Ther Drug Monit* (1998) 20, 371–5.

Paracetamol (Acetaminophen) + Valproate

Valproate does not appear to affect the pharmacokinetics of paracetamol.

Clinical evidence, mechanism, importance and management

In a study in 3 patients with epilepsy, stable taking carbamazepine and phenytoin, steady-state valproate had no effect on the pharmacokinetics of a single 10-mg/kg dose of paracetamol.[1] As a large proportion of valproate metabolism occurs by glucuronide conjugation, this study was designed to determine whether valproate would affect the disposition of other drugs that are dependent on this mechanism. However, from this study, valproate does not appear to affect the metabolism of paracetamol, and so no particular precautions seem necessary on concurrent use.

1. Kapetanović IM, Kupferberg HJ, Theodore W, Porter RJ. Lack of effect of valproate on paracetamol (acetaminophen) disposition in epileptic patients. *Br J Clin Pharmacol* (1981) 11, 391–3.

Ziconotide + Miscellaneous

The use of ziconotide with intrathecal morphine increases the risk of neuropsychiatric adverse effects. Additive CNS depression could occur if ziconotide is given with other CNS depressants: ziconotide appears to increase the risk of somnolence in patients also taking baclofen, clonidine, propofol or bupivacaine. ACE inhibitors and HIV-protease inhibitors do not appear to affect ziconotide exposure.

Clinical evidence, mechanism, importance and management

(a) Opioids

Intrathecal ziconotide appears to increase the incidence of neuropsychiatric adverse effects (confusion, paranoia, hallucinations, abnormal gait) as well as vomiting, anorexia and peripheral oedema in patients receiving *intrathecal* **morphine**.[1] Intrathecal **morphine** given to patients established on ziconotide might be better tolerated, although pruritus has been reported.[1] If an opioid and ziconotide are needed, patients should be closely monitored for adverse effects. If adverse effects occur, consideration should be given to discontinuing one or both drugs, or decreasing their doses. The US manufacturer advises against the use of *intrathecal* opioids with ziconotide as this has not been fully studied in placebo-controlled clinical studies.[2]

The UK manufacturer notes that there is no data on the concurrent use of partial opioid agonists such as **buprenorphine** with ziconotide.[1]

(b) CNS depressants

The use of ziconotide with other CNS depressant drugs could increase the risk of CNS adverse effects, including confusion and dizziness.[2] Note that respiratory depression does not appear to occur with ziconotide.[1,2] Ziconotide might cause loss of consciousness or stupor, and the manufacturers recommend that, should this occur, the concurrent use of other CNS depressants should be reviewed and ziconotide discontinued until the patient regains full consciousness.[1,2] The US manufacturer notes that patients also taking antiepileptics, sedatives or diuretics are at higher risk of this loss of consciousness occurring.[2] Note that increased somnolence has been seen in patients given ziconotide with systemic **baclofen**, **clonidine**, **propofol** or **bupivacaine**.[1] See also *Opioids*, above.

(c) Miscellaneous

The manufacturers of ziconotide note that, based on limited data, ACE inhibitors (**benazepril**, **lisinopril** and **moexipril** specifically named) and HIV-protease inhibitors (**ritonavir**, **saquinavir** and **indinavir** specifically named) are not expected to affect the plasma exposure to ziconotide.[1]

Note that ziconotide is given intrathecally, and is therefore contraindicated with intrathecal **chemotherapy**. The UK manufacturers also note that only a small number of patients have received systemic chemotherapy and intrathecal ziconotide, and therefore caution is advised on concurrent use.[1]

1. Prialt (Ziconotide acetate). Eisai Ltd. UK Summary of product characteristics, July 2011.
2. Prialt (Ziconotide). Elan Pharmaceuticals Inc. US Prescribing information, May 2010.

7

Anorectics and Stimulants

This section covers the drugs used in the management of obesity (such as orlistat, rimonabant and sibutramine) as well as the older drugs, such as the amfetamines, which are now no longer widely indicated for this condition and are now more generally considered as drugs of abuse. However, it should not be forgotten that the amfetamines (largely dexamfetamine and more recently, lisdexamfetamine) still have a limited therapeutic role in the management of narcolepsy and refractory attention deficit hyperactivity disorder (ADHD).

Ecstasy (MDMA, methylenedioxymethamfetamine), a drug of abuse that is structurally related to amfetamine, is also included in this section. The amfetamines are sympathomimetics, a diverse group, which have a number of interactions. The mechanism of action and classification of sympathomimetics is discussed in 'Cardiovascular drugs, miscellaneous', p.1049.

Other stimulant drugs discussed in this section include atomoxetine, methylphenidate, and its d-isomer, dexmethylphenidate (also sympathomimetics), and armodafinil and modafinil. These drugs have a role in ADHD or narcolepsy.

Amfetamines and related drugs + Antiretrovirals

A man taking ritonavir suffered a fatal serotonergic reaction after taking ecstasy (MDMA, methylenedioxymethamfetamine). A similar fatal reaction has occurred with metamfetamine and ritonavir. An isolated case of haemolytic anaemia has been reported in a patient taking indinavir and ecstasy. The effectiveness of antiretroviral therapy (particularly NNRTIs) has been found to be reduced in users of metamfetamine.

Clinical evidence

(a) Ecstasy (MDMA, Methylenedioxymethamfetamine)

An HIV-positive man taking lamivudine and zidovudine was also given **ritonavir** 600 mg twice daily. About 2 weeks later he went to a club and took ecstasy, in a dose estimated to be about 180 mg. He soon became unwell, and when seen by a nurse in the club, was hypertonic, tachypnoeic (45 breaths per minute), tachycardic (more than 140 bpm), cyanosed and diaphoretic. He had a tonic-clonic seizure, his pulse rose to 200 bpm, he then vomited, had a cardiorespiratory arrest and died. A post-mortem showed blood-alcohol concentrations of 24 mg% and an ecstasy concentration of 4.56 micrograms/mL, which was almost 10 times greater than might have been expected from the dose he had taken. The authors say that death was consistent with a severe serotonergic reaction.[1] Another report verifies that high ecstasy concentrations (4.05 micrograms/mL) may result in these life-threatening symptoms.[2]

In another case, a patient with AIDS, taking **ritonavir** and **saquinavir**, experienced agitation that lasted for over a day, following a small dose of ecstasy. He then experienced a nearly fatal reaction to a small dose of **sodium oxybate** (**GHB, gamma-hydroxybutyrate, γ-hydroxybutyrate**), becoming unresponsive within 20 minutes of ingestion of the drug and exhibiting a brief episode of repetitive clonic contractions.[3]

Another case describes an HIV-positive man, well established on HAART (zidovudine, lamivudine and **indinavir**), who experienced transient haemolytic anaemia thought to be a toxic reaction to taking three ecstasy tablets, the effects of which may have been potentiated by the indinavir.[4]

(b) Metamfetamine

A 49-year-old HIV-positive man taking HIV-protease inhibitors was found dead after injecting himself twice with metamfetamine as well as sniffing **amyl nitrate**. He had been taking an antiretroviral regimen of **ritonavir** 400 mg twice daily, **saquinavir** 400 mg twice daily and stavudine 40 mg twice daily for 4 months and it was considered that the HIV-protease inhibitors may have interacted with the recreational drugs. Toxicology analyses detected blood metamfetamine concentrations of 500 nanograms/mL, which were considered to be in the fatal range, especially when used with other drugs (unnamed). Cannabinoids and traces of diazepam and nordiazepam were also found in this patient.[5]

An analysis of 133 patients who were receiving HAART, found that HAART effectively lowered viral loads in *former* metamfetamine users, but not in *active* metamfetamine users.[6] Further, a retrospective case analysis of 300 patients assessed the association of metamfetamine use with resistance to HIV-protease inhibitors, NRTIs and NNRTIs. A significant association was established between frequent metamfetamine use (defined as use on a weekly or more intensive basis) and resistance to NNRTIs; no association was noted between any frequency of metamfetamine use and resistance to either HIV-protease inhibitors or NRTIs.[7]

Mechanism

Ritonavir inhibits the cytochrome P450 isoenzyme CYP2D6, which is responsible for the demethylenation of ecstasy, so concurrent use leads to a sharp rise in ecstasy plasma concentrations. Metamfetamine is also metabolised by CYP2D6 and its concentrations would therefore similarly be raised by ritonavir. Poor liver function (due to alcoholism) may have been a contributory factor in one patient,[1] and further inhibition of cytochrome P450 by nitric oxide (the metabolite of amyl nitrate) may have contributed to another case.[5] An additional factor is that ecstasy may show non-linear pharmacokinetics.[8]

It was suggested that the increase in virus load in metamfetamine users receiving HAART might be due to poor adherence or altered metabolism of the antiretroviral medications.[6] Studies have found that chronic metamfetamine use leads to dopamine transport reduction and this is associated with motor and cognitive impairment, although some alterations may be reversed by protracted metamfetamine abstinence.[9,10] Further, HIV infection is reported to be associated with changes in brain metabolites and therefore there may be additive neurotoxicity due to amfetamine use and HIV infection.[11] It has further been suggested that metamfetamine induces increases in extracellular dopamine, which in turn might activate HIV replication.[11] In addition, metamfetamine use can undermine the general health of the user.[12]

Importance and management

Although there are few reported cases of interactions between amfetamines or related drugs and HIV-protease inhibitors, what happens is consistent with the known toxic effects and pharmacology of the drugs concerned.

It has been suggested that patients who are prescribed any HIV-protease inhibitor should be made aware of the potential risks of using any form of recreational drugs metabolised by CYP2D6,[5] but note that ritonavir and tipranavir appear to be the only HIV-protease inhibitors that inhibit CYP2D6 to a clinically relevant extent. In particular, some authors recommend that patients taking ritonavir should avoid using ecstasy and other amfetamines, particularly metamfetamine.[13] Open discussions of illicit drug use would enable carers to warn patients that the use of these drugs may be even more dangerous while taking HIV-protease inhibitors. Appropriate precautions, apart from avoidance, include a reduction of the usual dose of ecstasy to about 25%, taking breaks from dancing, checking that a medical team are on site, maintaining adequate hydration by avoiding alcohol, and replenishing fluids regularly.[13]

1. Henry JA, Hill IR. Fatal interaction between ritonavir and MDMA. *Lancet* (1998) 352, 1751–2.
2. Roberts L, Wright H. Survival following intentional massive overdose of 'Ecstasy'. *J Accid Emerg Med* (1993) 11, 53–4.
3. Harrington RD, Woodward JA, Hooton TM, Horn JR. Life-threatening interactions between HIV-1 protease inhibitors and the illicit drugs MDMA and γ-hydroxybutyrate. *Arch Intern Med* (1999) 159, 2221–4.
4. Goorney BP, Scholes P. Transient haemolytic anaemia due to ecstasy in a patient on HAART. *Int J STD AIDS* (2002) 13, 651.
5. Hales G, Roth N, Smith D. Possible fatal interaction between protease inhibitors and methamphetamine. *Antivir Ther* (2000) 5, 19.
6. Ellis RJ, Childers ME, Cherner M, Lazzaretto D, Letendre S, Grant I, and the HIV Neurobehavioral Research Center Group. Increased human immunodeficiency virus loads in active methamphetamine users are explained by reduced effectiveness of antiretroviral therapy. *J Infect Dis* (2003) 188, 1820–6.
7. Colfax GN, Vittinghoff E, Grant R, Lum P, Spotts G, Hecht FM. Frequent methamphetamine use is associated with primary non-nucleoside reverse transcriptase inhibitor resistance. *AIDS* (2007) 21, 239–41.
8. de la Torre R, Ortuño J, Mas M, Farré M, Segura J. Fatal MDMA intoxication. *Lancet* (1999) 353, 593.
9. Volkow ND, Chang L, Wang G-J, Fowler JS, Leonido-Yee M, Franceschi D, Sedler MJ, Gatley SJ, Hitzemann R, Ding Y-S, Logan J, Wong C, Miller EN. Association of dopamine transporter reduction with psychomotor impairment in methamphetamine abusers. *Am J Psychiatry* (2001) 158, 377–82.
10. Volkow ND, Chang L, Wang G-J, Fowler JS, Franceschi D, Sedler M, Gatley SJ, Miller E, Hitzemann R, Ding Y-S, Logan J. Loss of dopamine transporters in methamphetamine abusers recovers with protracted abstinence. *J Neurosci* (2001) 21, 9414–18.
11. Chang L, Ernst T, Speck O, Grob CS. Additive effects of HIV and chronic methamphetamine use on brain metabolite abnormalities. *Am J Psychiatry* (2005) 162, 361–9.
12. Huff B. Methamphetamine and HIV. *BETA* (2006) 18, 42–7.
13. Antoniou T, Tseng AL. Interactions between recreational drugs and antiretroviral agents. *Ann Pharmacother* (2002) 36, 1598–1613.

Amfetamines + Caffeine

A man who took a mixture of amfetamines and caffeine intranasally had an ischaemic stroke, and a girl receiving dexamfetamine experienced acute onset myoclonus after taking a caffeine-containing preparation.

Clinical evidence, mechanism, importance and management

A 37-year-old man experienced an ischaemic stroke after the nasal use of amfetamines and caffeine. Three hours after he took the mixture, his blood pressure was 230/130 mmHg and pulse rate 120 bpm, but there was no neurological deficit. However, 6 hours later he had developed motor aphasia, right hemiplegia and right facial nerve palsy, and his blood pressure was 200/100 mmHg. It was thought that the nasal use of a mixture of amfetamines and caffeine caused the stroke, probably through the rapid rise in blood pressure combined with cerebral vasoconstriction.[1]

A 16-year-old girl with attention deficit hyperactivity disorder (ADHD) well controlled with **dexamfetamine** 10 mg daily, experienced a severe headache and then, on the following day, palpitations and acute onset myoclonus, which ceased spontaneously within 4 to 5 hours. The patient then revealed that she had taken *Excedrin* (paracetamol (acetaminophen), aspirin and caffeine) for headaches, both the day before and on the day of the abnormal movements; the last dose had been taken about 30 minutes before the jerking movements began. The combination of the CNS stimulant effects of caffeine and **dexamfetamine** were thought to have caused the CNS toxicity.[2]

These appear to be the only documented cases of an interaction and so their general relevance is unclear. However, given the severity of the outcome, it may be prudent to consider potential caffeine intake in anyone receiving amfetamines.

1. Lambrecht GLY, Malbrain MLNG, Chew SL, Baeck E, Verbraeken H. Intranasal caffeine and amphetamine causing stroke. *Acta Neurol Belg* (1993) 93, 146–9.
2. Jafri SH, Cook JW, Reed RR, Beebe DK. Acute onset of bilateral myoclonus in a 16-year-old female. *J Miss State Med Assoc* (2004) 45, 169–72.

Amfetamines + Calcium-channel blockers

Diltiazem attenuated the increase in blood pressure caused by dexamfetamine, and isradipine had similar effects with metamfetamine. The subjective changes or changes in reaction time associated with dexamfetamine were not affected by diltiazem. However, isradipine, both alone and with metamfetamine, tended to modestly decrease cognitive performance and in some circumstances may reduce some of the subjective effects of metamfetamine.

Clinical evidence, mechanism, importance and management

In a placebo-controlled study in 10 healthy subjects, pretreatment with a single 60-mg oral dose of **diltiazem** significantly attenuated the increase in diastolic blood pressure caused by a single 20-mg oral dose of **dexamfetamine**. The increase in systolic blood pressure was also attenuated, but the effect of **diltiazem** wore off over the 4-hour study period. The subjective changes or changes in reaction time associated with **dexamfetamine** were not affected by **diltiazem**.[1] A placebo-controlled study in 19 **metamfetamine**-dependent subjects found that pretreatment with **isradipine** reduced intravenous metamfetamine-associated increases in all measures of blood pressure except pulse pressure, but tended to enhance the effect of metamfetamine on heart rate.[2] Furthermore, another study found that **isradipine** tended to modestly decrease cognitive performance both with and without **metamfetamine**.[3] A further crossover study in 18 **metamfetamine**-dependent subjects found that in those subjects who had initially received **metamfetamine** after placebo, subsequently giving **isradipine** before **metamfetamine** reduced some of the positive subjective and reinforcing effects of **metamfetamine.**[4]

The clinical relevance of these effects is unclear; the interaction between **dexamfetamine** and **diltiazem** may be beneficial, but the effects of **isradipine** on **metamfetamine** may be detrimental in some subjects. More study is needed. Note that the amfetamines are predicted to attenuate the blood pressure-lowering effects of the antihypertensives, see 'Amfetamines + Miscellaneous', p.215.

1. Fabian JE, Silverstone PH. Diltiazem, a calcium antagonist, partly attenuates the effects of dextroamphetamine in healthy volunteers. *Int Clin Psychopharmacol* (1997) 12, 113–20.
2. Johnson BA, Wells LT, Roache JD, Wallace C, Ait-Daoud N, Wang Y. Isradipine decreases the hemodynamic response of cocaine and methamphetamine: results from two human laboratory studies. *Am J Hypertens* (2005) 18, 813–22.
3. Johnson BA, Roache JD, Ait-Daoud N, Wallace C, Wells LT, Wang Y. Effects of isradipine on methamphetamine-induced changes in attentional and perceptual-motor skills of cognition. *Psychopharmacology (Berl)* (2005) 178, 296–302.
4. Johnson BA, Roache JD, Ait-Daoud N, Wallace C, Wells L, Dawes M, Wang Y. Effects of isradipine, a dihydropyridine-class calcium-channel antagonist, on d-methamphetamine's subjective and reinforcing effects. *Int J Neuropsychopharmacol* (2005) 8, 203–13.

Amfetamines + Cannabis

Cannabis opposes the stimulant effects of ecstasy, but long-term users of both drugs may potentially experience cumulative CNS impairment and additive immunomodulation. The effects of ecstasy and Δ^9-tetrahydrocannabinol on heart rate may be additive and Δ^9-tetrahydrocannabinol may prolong the hyperthermic effects of ecstasy. A report describes severe arterial ischaemia in a patient who regularly abused amfetamines and cannabis. The concurrent use of amfetamines and synthetic cannabinoids may lead to adverse cardiac effects.

Clinical evidence

In a study, 16 healthy subjects who were regular users of ecstasy (MDMA, methylenedioxymethamfetamine) were given a single 100-mg oral dose of **ecstasy** or placebo and inhaled Δ^9-tetrahydrocannabinol (THC, the major active ingredient of cannabis) 4 mg to ensure tolerability. Subsequent doses of Δ^9-tetrahydrocannabinol 6 mg were given by inhalation 90 and 120 minutes after **ecstasy** 100 mg. Heart rate was increased by both substances (ecstasy 20.4 bpm; Δ^9-tetrahydrocannabinol 14.2 bpm), and this effect appeared to be roughly additive on concurrent use (29.9 bpm). **Ecstasy**-induced temperature increases (about 0.3 C over time) were not prevented by Δ^9-tetrahydrocannabinol but it delayed the onset and prolonged the duration of temperature elevation.[1]

In a study in 23 cannabis users, 37 cannabis and **ecstasy** users and a control group of 34 subjects who used neither drug, there was enhanced immunomodulation in those who used both **ecstasy** and cannabis, similar to that induced in stress conditions or mediated by other drugs of abuse. Cannabis alone produced less immunomodulation. A higher rate of mild infections was found in regular users of **ecstasy** and cannabis compared with occasional users, those who used cannabis only, and those who did not use either drug.[2]

A study in 18 cannabis users, 11 cannabis and **ecstasy** users, and 31 subjects who had used neither drug, found that users of cannabis and users of cannabis with **ecstasy** performed similarly in most CNS tests. However, these subjects performed less well than non-drug users on tests of memory, learning, word fluency, speed of processing and manual dexterity. Furthermore, the deficits were more closely related to cannabis usage than **ecstasy** usage.[3] Similar results were reported in another study.[4] A further self-rated study found that moderate cannabis use might help to improve or mask **ecstasy**-induced aggression and somatic symptoms (e.g. headache, chronic tiredness). However, heavy cannabis and **ecstasy** use appeared to be associated with problems such as paranoia or cognitive disorders, which might emerge after a period of abstinence from both drugs.[5] Another study found that self-reported psychological problems in **ecstasy** users were predominantly attributable to concurrent cannabis use. Abstinence from cannabis was found to be a predictor for remission of psychological problems in **ecstasy** users.[6]

A 22-year-old woman who smoked cigarettes and had regularly abused amfetamine derivatives such as **metamfetamine** and **ecstasy** together with cannabis, experienced severe arterial ischaemia leading to claudication and ulceration of the feet.[7]

Mechanism

Both cannabis and ecstasy may cause additive CNS impairment. Enhanced immunomodulation due to regular use of both ecstasy and cannabis may result in poorer general health and increased susceptibility to infection.[2] The additive effects of ecstasy appear to be due the effects of ecstasy on catecholamines and the direct cannabinoid (CB_1) agonism in cardiac tissue.[1]

In the case report describing ischaemia it was suggested that the amfetamine derivatives might have induced vasculitis of the arteries with cannabis possibly adding to the effect on the microcirculation.[7]

Importance and management

The majority of recreational ecstasy users (up to 98%[8]) also take cannabis and this combined drug usage appears to reflect the opposing effects of the two drugs: ecstasy is a powerful stimulant whereas cannabis is a relaxant. Therefore cannabis may modulate the acute reactions to ecstasy.[8] Ecstasy is hyperthermic and although cannabis is reported to be hypothermic,[8] one study suggests Δ^9-tetrahydrocannabinol may prolong the duration of ecstasy-associated temperature increases.[1] Ecstasy increases oxidative stress whereas cannabinoids are antioxidant, but one report suggests enhanced immunomodulation on concurrent use.[2] The chronic effects of each drug may be functionally damaging, so that using both drugs may be associated with a variety of psychological problems.[8,9] Furthermore, regular cannabis use seems to be necessary for the development and maintenance of symptoms of mental illness in ecstasy users.[6,9]

Note that synthetic cannabinoids are available as licenced medicinal products. The manufacturers of two such products, nabilone and dronabinol (synthetic Δ^9-tetrahydrocannabinol), suggest that the concurrent use of amfetamines may lead to additive hypertension, tachycardia, and possible cardiotoxicity.[10,11] The clinical relevance of these predictions does not appear to have been studied, and therefore, until more is known, it would be prudent to monitor the cardiac effects of concurrent use, particularly in those with pre-existing cardiovascular disease.

1. Dumont GJ, Kramers C, Sweep FC, Touw DJ, van Hasselt JG, de Kam M, van Gerven JM, Buitelaar JK, Verkes RJ. Cannabis coadministration potentiates the effects of "ecstasy" on heart rate and temperature in humans. *Clin Pharmacol Ther* (2009) 86, 160–6.
2. Pacifici R, Zuccaro P, Farré M, Poudevida S, Abanades S, Pichini S, Langohr K, Segura J, de la Torre R. Combined immunomodulating properties of 3,4-methylenedioxymethamphetamine (MDMA) and cannabis in humans. *Addiction* (2007) 102, 931–6.
3. Croft RJ, Mackay AJ, Mills ATD, Gruzelier JGH. The relative contributions of ecstasy and cannabis to cognitive impairment. *Psychopharmacology (Berl)* (2001) 153, 373–9.
4. Fisk JE, Montgomery C, Wareing M, Murphy PN. The effects of concurrent cannabis use among ecstasy users: neuroprotective or neurotoxic? *Hum Psychopharmacol* (2006) 21, 355–66.
5. Milani RM, Parrott AC, Schifano F, Turner JJD. Pattern of cannabis use in ecstasy polydrug users: moderate cannabis use may compensate for self-rated aggression and somatic symptoms. *Hum Psychopharmacol* (2005) 20, 249–61.
6. Daumann J, Hensen G, Thimm B, Rezk M, Till B, Gouzoulis-Mayfrank E. Self-reported psychopathological symptoms in recreational ecstasy (MDMA) users are mainly associated with regular cannabis use: further evidence from a combined cross-sectional/longitudinal investigation. *Psychopharmacology (Berl)* (2004) 173, 398–404.
7. Leithäuser B, Langheinrich AC, Rau WS, Tillmanns H, Matthias FR. A 22-year-old woman with lower limb arteriopathy. Buerger's disease, or methamphetamine- or cannabis-induced arteritis? *Heart Vessels* (2005) 20, 39–43.
8. Parrott AC, Milani RM, Gouzoulis-Mayfrank E, Daumann J. Cannabis and ecstasy/MDMA (3,4-methylenedioxymethamphetamine): an analysis of their neuropsychobiological interactions in recreational users. *J Neural Transm* (2007) 114, 959–68.
9. Sala M, Braida D. Endocannabinoids and 3,4-methylenedioxymethamphetamine (MDMA) interaction. *Pharmacol Biochem Behav* (2005) 81, 407–16.
10. Cesamet (Nabilone). Meda Pharmaceuticals Inc. US Prescribing information, April 2011.
11. Marinol (Dronabinol). AbbVie Inc. US Prescribing information, February 2013.

Amfetamines + Cocaine

An ischaemic stroke occurred in a patient who was abusing amfetamine and cocaine. Convulsions and cardiovascular adverse effects occurred in an infant exposed to an amfetamine and cocaine.

Clinical evidence, mechanism, importance and management

A 16-year-old boy developed unsteadiness and double vision 5 minutes after intranasal inhalation of a small amount of **amfetamine** 'cut' with cocaine. Cranial magnetic resonance imaging (MRI) revealed a mesencephalic lesion that was seen to have decreased 12 days later, and he became symptom-free after 3 weeks. The ischaemic lesion was thought to be due to vasospasm caused by synergistic stimulation of the sympathetic nervous system: **amfetamine** causes the release of adrenaline (epinephrine) and noradrenaline (norepinephrine), while cocaine prevents their reuptake.[1]

An 11-month-old infant experienced apparent generalised convulsions and cardiovascular adverse effects after accidental ingestion of **ecstasy** (MDMA, methylenedioxymethamfetamine) and chronic exposure to cocaine. It was suggested that, as both drugs are neurotoxic and have similar mechanisms of action, the combination could increase the risk of serious medical consequences.[2]

An *in vitro* study showed that cocaine (an inhibitor of the cytochrome P450 isoenzyme CYP2D6) inhibited the metabolism (demethylenation) of **ecstasy** by CYP2D6. Therefore, theoretically, the use of cocaine would be expected to increase plasma and CNS **ecstasy** levels[3] but it is not known if this is clinically significant.

Evidence is currently limited, but it would appear that the concurrent use of amfetamines and cocaine may have adverse CNS consequences.

1. Strupp M, Hamann GF, Brandt T. Combined amphetamine and cocaine abuse caused mesencephalic ischemia in a 16-year-old boy – due to vasospasm? *Eur Neurol* (2000) 43, 181–2.
2. Garcia-Algar O, López N, Bonet M, Pellegrini M, Marchei E, Pichini S. 3,4-Methylenedioxymethamphetamine (MDMA) intoxication in an infant chronically exposed to cocaine. *Ther Drug Monit* (2005) 27, 409–11.
3. Ramamoorthy Y, Yu A, Suh N, Haining RL, Tyndale RF, Sellers EM. Reduced (±)-3,4-methylenedioxymethamphetamine ("Ecstasy") metabolism with cytochrome P450 2D6 inhibitors and pharmacogenetic variants *in vitro*. *Biochem Pharmacol* (2002) 63, 2111–19.

Amfetamines and related drugs + Lithium

The stimulant and/or cardiovascular effects of the amfetamines have been shown to be opposed by lithium in some, but not all studies.

Clinical evidence

Two depressed patients stopped abusing **metamfetamine** and cannabis, or **phenmetrazine** and 'other diet pills' because, while taking lithium carbonate, they were unable to get 'high'. Another patient complained that she felt no effects from amfetamines taken for weight reduction, including no decrease in appetite, until lithium carbonate was withdrawn.[1] A controlled study in 9 depressed patients confirmed that lithium carbonate taken for 10 days attenuated the subjective stimulant effects of **dexamfe-**

tamine or **levamfetamine**.[2] Another study found similar results with **dexamfetamine** in patients with schizophrenia.[3] However, in a further study, the stimulant effects of **amfetamine** were attenuated in only 4 of 8 subjects given lithium. However, lithium attenuated the increase in systolic blood pressure caused by amfetamine (from an average increase of 31/15 mmHg down to 20/9 mmHg).[4]

In contrast, in a placebo-controlled study in healthy subjects, lithium 1.2 g daily for 7 days did not alter the subjective or cardiovascular effects of a single 20-mg dose of **dexamfetamine**.[5] In another controlled study, in 9 subjects, the only significant effect of pretreatment with lithium 900 mg for 14 days was to attenuate the feeling of happiness induced by **dexamfetamine**.[6]

Mechanism

The reasons for these reactions, when they occur, are not known. One study found that pretreatment of healthy subjects with lithium for 14 days attenuated dexamfetamine-induced decreases in brain activation when performing cognitive tasks.[7] In addition, it has been suggested that amfetamines and lithium have mutually opposing pharmacological actions on dopamine and noradrenaline (norepinephrine) release and uptake at adrenergic neurones.[1,7]

Importance and management

Information regarding an interaction between the amfetamines and related stimulants and lithium is contradictory, and therefore an interaction is not fully established. Nevertheless, it may be prudent to be alert for evidence of reduced amfetamine effects in the presence of lithium.

Note that both the amfetamines and lithium have serotonergic effects, and concurrent use might lead to the serotonin syndrome. Serotonin syndrome is a rare adverse effect, but because of its severity, some caution is warranted if both drugs are given. For more information on serotonin syndrome and its management, see 'Drugs that cause serotonin syndrome + Other drugs that cause serotonin syndrome', p.1471.

1. Flemenbaum A. Does lithium block the effects of amphetamine? A report of three cases. *Am J Psychiatry* (1974) 131, 820–1.
2. van Kammen DP, Murphy DL. Attenuation of the euphoriant and activating effects of *d*- and *l*-amphetamine by lithium carbonate treatment. *Psychopharmacologia* (1975) 44, 215–24.
3. van Kammen DP, Docherty JP, Marder SR, Rosenblatt JE, Bunney WE. Lithium attenuates the activation-euphoria but not the psychosis induced by *d*-amphetamine in schizophrenia. *Psychopharmacology (Berl)* (1985) 87, 111–15.
4. Angrist B, Gershon S. Variable attenuation of amphetamine effects by lithium. *Am J Psychiatry* (1979) 136, 806–10.
5. Silverstone PH, Pukhovsky A, Rotzinger S. Lithium does not attenuate the effects of D-amphetamine in healthy volunteers. *Psychiatry Res* (1998) 9, 219–26.
6. Willson MC, Bell EC, Dave S, Asghar SJ, McGrath BM, Silverstone PH. Valproate attenuates dextroamphetamine-induced subjective changes more than lithium. *Eur Neuropsychopharmacol* (2005) 15, 633–9.
7. Bell EC, Willson MC, Wilman AH, Dave S, Asghar SJ, Silverstone PH. Lithium and valproate attenuate dextroamphetamine-induced changes in brain activation. *Hum Psychopharmacol* (2005) 20, 87–96.

Amfetamines + Miscellaneous

Amfetamines may counter the sedative effects of antihistamines and antagonise the hypotensive effects of antihypertensives. One manufacturer suggests that propranolol may antagonise the effects of dexamfetamine. Delavirdine and disulfiram are predicted to inhibit the metabolism of amphetamines, and drugs that increase gastrointestinal acidity are predicted to decrease the absorption of amfetamines. Dexamfetamine may reduce and delay the absorption of hyoscine.

Clinical evidence, mechanism, importance and management

(a) Antihistamines

The US manufacturers of **lisdexamfetamine**, **dexamfetamine**, and **amfetamine** with **dexamfetamine** note that the amfetamines may oppose the sedative effects of the antihistamines.[1-3]

(b) Antihypertensives

The US manufacturers of several amfetamines give general warnings that amfetamines may antagonise the hypotensive effects of antihypertensives.[1-4] However, there is some evidence that drugs such as **diltiazem** may attenuate the increase in blood pressure seen with the amfetamines, see 'Amfetamines + Calcium-channel blockers', p.213. Therefore the effect on blood pressure would appear to be a balance of the effects of both drugs, the outcome of which is not certain, but it would seem prudent to consider the contribution of the amfetamine if a patient taking an amfetamine and an antihypertensive has inadequate blood pressure control.

The US manufacturers of several amfetamines also give general warnings that the effects of adrenergic blockers (presumably adrenergic neurone blockers) are inhibited by amfetamines,[1-3] and this effect has been seen with **guanethidine**, see 'Guanethidine + Amfetamines and related drugs', p.1061.

The UK manufacturer of **dexamfetamine** also warns that the concurrent use of beta blockers may result in severe hypertension and in addition states that adrenoceptor blocking drugs such as **propranolol** may antagonise the effects of **dexamfetamine** (a sympathomimetic).[5] This is similar to the effects seen with vasopressor sympathomimetics, see 'Beta blockers + Inotropes and Vasopressors', p.1014. It would therefore seem prudent to monitor blood pressure if amfetamines are given to patients taking beta blockers, and consider the contribution of the amfetamine if a patient taking an amfetamine and an antihypertensive has inadequate blood pressure control.

(c) Delavirdine

The NNRTI, delavirdine, is an inhibitor of CYP3A and other isoenzymes including CYP2D6. The US manufacturer of delavirdine suggests that the amfetamines are metabolised by these isoenzymes and therefore suggests caution if delavirdine is used with amfetamines because the amfetamine levels may be increased.[6]

(d) Disulfiram

Studies in *animals* have indicated that disulfiram may inhibit the metabolism of amfetamines.[7] The UK manufacturer of **dexamfetamine** says that disulfiram may inhibit the metabolism and excretion of **dexamfetamine**. In addition, they contraindicate the use of **dexamfetamine** in patients with a history of alcohol abuse.[5]

(e) Drugs that affect gastric acidity

The manufacturers note that drugs or substances that increase gastrointestinal acidity (they name **glutamic acid hydrochloride**, **ascorbic acid**, **fruit juices**) could lower the absorption of amfetamines and might therefore lower their blood levels and efficacy.[1,2,5]

(f) Hyoscine

In a single-dose study, 12 healthy subjects were given oral dexamfetamine 10 mg with oral hyoscine 800 micrograms. The maximum plasma level of hyoscine was reported to be similar, irrespective of dexamfetamine use, whereas the time taken to achieve peak hyoscine levels was prolonged in the presence of dexamfetamine. In addition, the bioavailability of hyoscine was reported to be reduced in the presence of dexamfetamine.[8]

1. Dexedrine (Dextroamphetamine sulfate). Amedra Pharmaceuticals, LLC. US Prescribing information, October 2013.
2. Adderall XR (Mixed salts of amphetamine and dextroamphetamine). Shire US Inc. US Prescribing information, April 2015.
3. Vyvanse (Lisdexamfetamine dimesylate). Shire US Inc. US Prescribing information, January 2012.
4. Didrex (Benzphetamine hydrochloride). Pfizer, Inc. US Prescribing information, August 2010.
5. Dexamfetamine sulphate tablets. Auden McKenzie (Pharma Division) Ltd. UK Summary of product characteristics, March 2010.
6. Rescriptor (Delavirdine mesylate). ViiV Healthcare. US Prescribing information, August 2012.
7. Antabuse (Disulfiram). Actavis UK Ltd. UK Summary of product characteristics, December 2011.
8. Boyd JL, Du B, Vaksman Z, Locke JP, Putcha L. Relative bioavailability of scopolamine dosage forms and interaction with dextroamphetamine. *J Gravit Physiol* (2007) 14, P-107–P-108.

Amfetamines + Ondansetron

Ondansetron appears to attenuate the effects of amfetamine and dexamfetamine on subjective feelings such as light-headedness, but not the effects of amfetamine on psychomotor tests. One study found that ondansetron did not affect most physiological responses to dexamfetamine, but might attenuate blood pressure increases, although another study found ondansetron had no effect on amfetamine-induced increases in blood pressure. Ondansetron appears not to decrease any of the measures of metamfetamine dependence.

Clinical evidence, mechanism, importance and management

In a placebo-controlled study, when 9 healthy subjects were given **amfetamine** 15 mg, they reported an increase in subjective feelings such as light-headedness or 'high' and a decrease in hunger. The use of **amfetamine** also caused an increase in systolic blood pressure and a decrease in the mean time to complete psychomotor tests. When ondansetron 4 mg was given every 12 hours for 3 doses, with the last dose 30 minutes before the amfetamine, the effects of **amfetamine** on hunger and subjective state were diminished, but its effects on blood pressure and psychomotor performance tests were not altered.[1] These findings have also been published elsewhere.[2]

In another placebo-controlled study, in 10 healthy subjects, pretreatment with ondansetron 150, 50 or 15 micrograms/kg reduced the increases in prolactin associated with intravenous **dexamfetamine** 500 micrograms/kg, but did not affect other neuroendocrine responses (increased plasma levels of cortisol and growth hormone) or most physiological responses (elevated pulse and temperature). However, the lower doses of ondansetron attenuated amfetamine-induced increases in diastolic blood pressure. Mild/moderate euphoria/activation induced by **dexamfetamine** was only minimally affected by pretreatment with ondansetron, but ondansetron did attenuate the responses in subjects with robust euphoria/activation.[3]

A placebo-controlled study in 150 **metamfetamine**-dependent subjects given ondansetron 0.25, 1, or 4 mg twice daily for 8 weeks found that ondansetron did not decrease any of the measures of **metamfetamine** use, withdrawal, craving or severity of dependence.[4]

It is suggested that ondansetron may attenuate some catecholamine-mediated effects of **amfetamine**, but a pharmacokinetic interaction has not yet been excluded.[1,2] However, analysis of the plasma levels in 4 subjects found that ondansetron did not significantly alter mean **dexamfetamine** levels, or the time taken to reach peak dexamfetamine levels.[3]

These studies were mainly designed to establish whether or not ondansetron altered the responses to amfetamines. They suggest that no clinically relevant adverse interaction occurs, but more study is needed to establish the absence of a pharmacokinetic interaction.

1. Silverstone PH, Oldman D, Johnson B, Cowen PJ. Ondansetron, a 5-HT_3 receptor antagonist, partially attenuates the effects of amphetamine: a pilot study in healthy volunteers. *Int Clin Psychopharmacol* (1992) 7, 37–43.
2. Silverstone PH, Johnson B, Cowen PJ. Does ondansetron attenuate amphetamine-induced behaviour in human volunteers? *Psychopharmacology (Berl)* (1992) 107, 140–1.
3. Grady TA, Broocks A, Canter SK, Pigott TA, Dubbert B, Hill JL, Murphy DL. Biological and behavioral responses to d-amphetamine, alone and in combination with the serotonin$_3$ receptor antagonist ondansetron, in healthy volunteers. *Psychiatry Res* (1996) 64, 1–10.

4. Johnson BA, Ait-Daoud N, Elkashef AM, Smith EV, Kahn R, Vocci F, Li S-H, Bloch DA; Methamphetamine Study Group. A preliminary randomized, double-blind, placebo-controlled study of the safety and efficacy of ondansetron in the treatment of methamphetamine dependence. *Int J Neuropsychopharmacol* (2008) 11, 1–14.

Amfetamines and related drugs + Phenothiazines

The appetite suppressant and other effects of amfetamines, chlorphentermine and phenmetrazine are opposed by chlorpromazine. It seems possible that other phenothiazines will interact similarly. Dexamfetamine can oppose the antipsychotic effects of chlorpromazine, and in one case dexamfetamine exacerbated a perphenazine-related withdrawal dyskinesia.

Clinical evidence

In a placebo-controlled study, 10 obese patients with schizophrenia who were taking drugs including **chlorpromazine, thioridazine**, imipramine and chlordiazepoxide did not respond to treatment with **dexamfetamine** for obesity. The expected sleep disturbance in response to **dexamfetamine** was also not seen.[1] In a double-blind, placebo-controlled study in 76 patients, **chlorpromazine** was found to diminish the weight-reducing effect of **phenmetrazine**,[2] and, in another study, 30 obese patients taking **chlorpromazine** did not experience the expected weight loss when they were given **phenmetrazine** or **chlorphentermine**.[3] Similarly, antagonism of the effects of amfetamines by **chlorpromazine** has been described in other reports,[4,5] and this interaction has been deliberately exploited, with success, in the treatment of 22 children poisoned with various amfetamines or related compounds (**amfetamine, dexamfetamine, metamfetamine, phenmetrazine**).[4]

The amfetamines may also affect the efficacy of the phenothiazines. One study in 462 patients taking **chlorpromazine** 200 to 600 mg daily found that the addition of **dexamfetamine** 10 to 60 mg daily had a detrimental effect on the control of their schizophrenic symptoms.[6]

A 9-year-old boy taking **perphenazine, dexamfetamine**, fluoxetine and diphenhydramine had all drugs, with the exception of **dexamfetamine**, discontinued. Two - days after the **perphenazine** was stopped the patient began to have repeated tongue protrusions, which progressed to abnormal involuntary movements involving his upper and lower extremities. It was suspected that **dexamfetamine** was aggravating the movement disorder and so it was tapered over 2 days and stopped, resulting in an immediate and dramatic improvement.[7]

Mechanism

Not fully understood. It is known that chlorpromazine can inhibit adrenergic and dopaminergic activity, which could explain some part of the antagonism of the amfetamines, the euphoriant effects of which are said to be mediated by central dopamine receptors.

The severe extrapyramidal movement disorder described in the case report might have occurred due to the patient developing dopamine supersensitivity as a result of long-term antipsychotic therapy. On antipsychotic withdrawal, an increased number of postsynaptic dopamine receptors were available to the dopamine agonist effects of continued amfetamine treatment, resulting in the extrapyramidal movement disorder, which did not subside until the dopamine agonist was withdrawn.[7]

Importance and management

Established interactions. These reports suggest that it is not beneficial to attempt to treat patients taking chlorpromazine with amfetamines, such as dexamfetamine, or other central stimulants such as phenmetrazine. Although in one study, thioridazine also appeared to interact it is not clear whether this interaction takes place with antipsychotics other than chlorpromazine. However, it seems possible that this interaction may occur with all phenothiazines, especially if the suggested mechanism is correct. Note that central stimulants are no longer recommended for the treatment of obesity.

The case of dyskinesia suggests that central stimulants may exacerbate symptoms caused by antipsychotic withdrawal. See also 'Methylphenidate + Risperidone', p.221.

1. Modell W, Hussar AE. Failure of dextroamphetamine sulfate to influence eating and sleeping patterns in obese schizophrenic patients: clinical and pharmacological significance. *JAMA* (1965) 193, 275–8.
2. Reid AA. Pharmacological antagonism between chlorpromazine and phenmetrazine in mental hospital patients. *Med J Aust* (1964) 10, 187–8.
3. Sletten IW, Ognjanov V, Menendez S, Sundland D, El-Toumi A. Weight reduction with chlorphentermine and phenmetrazine in obese psychiatric patients during chlorpromazine therapy. *Curr Ther Res* (1967) 9, 570–5.
4. Espelin DE, Done AK. Amphetamine poisoning: effectiveness of chlorpromazine. *N Engl J Med* (1968) 278, 1361–65.
5. Jönsson L-E. Pharmacological blockade of amphetamine effects in amphetamine dependent subjects. *Eur J Clin Pharmacol* (1972) 4, 206–11.
6. Casey JF, Hollister LE, Klett CJ, Lasky JJ, Caffey EM. Combined drug therapy of chronic schizophrenics. Controlled evaluation of placebo, dextro-amphetamine, imipramine, isocarboxazid and trifluoperazine added to maintenance doses of chlorpromazine. *Am J Psychiatry* (1961) 117, 997–1003.
7. Connor DF, Benjamin S, Ozbayrak KR. Case study: neuroleptic withdrawal dyskinesia exacerbated by ongoing stimulant treatment. *J Am Acad Child Adolesc Psychiatry* (1995) 34, 1490–4.

Amfetamines + Pimozide

Two studies suggest that pimozide attenuates the stimulant effects of amfetamine or dexamfetamine, but in two other studies with dexamfetamine the effects were inconsistent.

Clinical evidence, mechanism, importance and management

Pimozide, a dopamine antagonist, given in single oral doses of 5, 10 or 20 mg, or repeated doses of 5 mg daily, reduced the euphoriant effects of large (200 mg) intravenous doses of **amfetamine** in subjects with a history of **amfetamine** abuse. The blood pressure response to **amfetamine** was also reduced.[1] Similarly, a placebo-controlled study in 8 healthy subjects found that pimozide 2 mg attenuated the stimulant action of **dexamfetamine** 10 mg, but had no effect on **dexamfetamine**-induced anorexia.[2]

In contrast, in a placebo-controlled study, 10 healthy subjects were given **dexamfetamine** 10 or 20 mg two hours after pimozide 1 or 2 mg. Pimozide was found to be inconsistent in antagonising the subjective responses to **dexamfetamine.**[3] In a further study by the same authors, pimozide 8 mg did not consistently antagonise the effects of **dexamfetamine**, although pimozide 8 mg alone did produce effects opposite to those of **dexamfetamine.**[4]

The results are inconsistent, and therefore more study would be beneficial to establish an interaction, and its clinical relevance.

1. Jönsson L-E. Pharmacological blockade of amphetamine effects in amphetamine dependent subjects. *Eur J Clin Pharmacol* (1972) 4, 206–11.
2. Silverstone T, Fincham J, Wells B, Kyriakides M. The effect of the dopamine receptor blocking drug pimozide on the stimulant and anorectic actions of dextroamphetamine in man. *Neuropharmacology* (1980) 19, 1235–7.
3. Brauer LH, de Wit H. Subjective responses to d-amphetamine alone and after pimozide pre-treatment in normal, healthy volunteers. *Biol Psychiatry* (1996) 39, 26–32.
4. Brauer LH, De Wit H. High dose pimozide does not block amphetamine-induced euphoria in normal volunteers. *Pharmacol Biochem Behav* (1997) 56, 265–72.

Amfetamines and related drugs + SSRIs

The psychological effects of ecstasy (MDMA, methylenedioxymethamfetamine) and its effects on heart rate may be reduced if citalopram, fluoxetine or paroxetine have previously been given. Other SSRIs are expected to interact similarly. There may be an increased risk of serotonergic effects and neurotoxic reactions if amfetamines or related drugs are given with SSRIs. Fluoxetine and paroxetine may decrease the metabolism of amfetamines and ecstasy: amfetamine toxicity and phentermine toxicity have been reported.

Clinical evidence

(a) Dexamfetamine

A patient who developed serotonin syndrome while taking venlafaxine with dexamfetamine (see 'SNRIs; Venlafaxine + Amfetamines', p.1480) had a second episode when **citalopram** was taken with dexamfetamine.[1]

(b) Ecstasy (MDMA, Methylenedioxymethamfetamine)

1. Citalopram. A placebo-controlled psychometric study in 16 healthy subjects found that oral ecstasy 1.5 mg/kg produced an emotional state with heightened mood, increased self-confidence and extroversion, moderate derealisation and an intensification of sensory perception. Most of these effects were found to be markedly reduced by pretreatment with intravenous citalopram 40 mg, although their duration was prolonged by up to 2 hours.[2]

When a man taking citalopram 60 mg daily also took unknown amounts of ecstasy he became aggressive, agitated, severely grandiose, restless and performed compulsive movements in a peculiar and joyless dance-like manner. He lacked normal movement control and said he could see little bugs. He was treated with haloperidol and chlordiazepoxide, and improved within 2 days of replacing the citalopram with promazine.[3]

A case report describes a patient taking citalopram 20 mg daily who did not experience any effects from ecstasy after starting the SSRI.[4]

2. Fluoxetine. A study in 8 ecstasy users found that fluoxetine 20 mg daily for at least 5 days attenuated most of the positive subjective effects associated with ecstasy (e.g. arousal, elation, positive mood, vigour etc.). In addition, heart rate but not blood pressure increases were reduced.[5] However, an account of 4 ecstasy users who had taken fluoxetine 20 mg before taking ecstasy 100 to 250 mg, reported that they still experienced the subjective effects of euphoria, but one commented that the overall acute experience was "slightly calmer". Some of the adverse effects such as jaw clenching and insomnia were also attenuated and recovery was more rapid.[6]

3. Paroxetine. A study found that pretreatment with oral paroxetine 20 mg daily for 3 days decreased both the physiological and subjective effects of a single 100-mg oral dose of ecstasy.[7]

In a placebo-controlled, randomised study, 7 healthy subjects were given ecstasy 100 mg on the last day of taking paroxetine 20 mg daily for 3 days. Paroxetine raised the maximum serum levels and AUC of ecstasy by 17% and 27%, respectively.[8] Another study also found that pretreatment with paroxetine resulted in similar increases in the maximum plasma levels and AUC of ecstasy (16% and 22%, respectively), and reductions in those of the metabolite, 3-methoxy-4-hydroxy-methamfetamine (49% and 38%, respectively).[7]

A case report describes a patient taking paroxetine 20 mg daily who did not experience any effects from ecstasy after starting the SSRI.[4]

(c) Unnamed amfetamines

A man who had taken a small, unspecified, but previously tolerated dose of amfetamines developed signs of amfetamine overdose (restlessness, agitation, hyperventilation, etc.) while taking **fluoxetine** 60 mg daily. Another man taking **fluoxetine** 20 mg daily developed symptoms of schizophrenia after taking two unspecified doses of amfetamines.[9]

(d) Phentermine

A 22-year-old woman who had successfully and uneventfully taken **fluoxetine** 20 mg daily for 3 months, stopped the **fluoxetine** and then 8 days later took a single 30-mg tablet of phentermine. Within a few hours she experienced racing thoughts, stomach cramps, palpitations (pulse 84 bpm), tremors, dry eyes and diffuse hyperreflexia. The problems had all resolved the following day after she took lorazepam 1.5 mg. The authors of this report suggested that the residual inhibitory effects of the **fluoxetine** on liver cytochrome P450 enzymes led to decreased phentermine metabolism, resulting in increased phentermine levels and sympathetic hyperstimulation. It is known that **fluoxetine** and its active metabolite have a long half-life and can persist for weeks. The authors also alternatively wondered whether some of the symptoms might have fitted those of serotonin syndrome.[10]

Mechanism

Complex. It has been suggested that the psychological and neurotoxic effects of ecstasy may be caused by serotonin release in the brain.[6,11] This could potentially be blocked by serotonin reuptake inhibitors (such as citalopram) resulting in reduced ecstasy effects. However, ecstasy is also thought to inhibit serotonin reuptake,[11] so its use with the SSRIs could increase serotonergic effects, which could result in neurotoxicity.[12] Other amfetamines also affect catecholamines such as dopamine, noradrenaline (norepinephrine) and serotonin in the brain, so they have the potential to interact with SSRIs, although they differ in their affinity for these neurotransmitters (for example metamfetamine primarily affects dopamine).[13]

In addition, some SSRIs (to varying degrees) inhibit the cytochrome P450 isoenzyme CYP2D6, by which amfetamine, metamfetamine and ecstasy are metabolised, so concurrent use (as demonstrated in *animal* studies with fluoxetine and ecstasy[14]) could result in increased levels of the amfetamine.

Importance and management

The available evidence suggests that patients already taking citalopram, fluoxetine or paroxetine may not be able to get as 'high' on usual doses of ecstasy, and some adverse effects of ecstasy may also be reduced. If the proposed mechanism of interaction is correct, the same is also likely to be true with any SSRI. Also be aware of possible pharmacokinetic interactions with some SSRIs that are CYP2D6 inhibitors (e.g. paroxetine, see 'Table 35.2', p.1465), which may increase the levels of ecstasy, or possibly other amfetamines, many of which appear to be metabolised by CYP2D6. Marked decreases in the effects of these drugs could lead users to take higher doses, which might produce potentially life-threatening toxic effects, especially if plasma levels are raised as a result of a pharmacokinetic interaction. This interaction has been investigated for its potential to aid amfetamine abstinence,[15,16] but the results have not been promising, and the incidence of adverse effects may be increased.

Some case reports suggest that there may be a risk of increased serotonergic activity if SSRIs are given with amfetamines, and concurrent use might lead to the serotonin syndrome. Serotonin syndrome is a rare adverse effect, but because of its severity, some caution is warranted if both drugs are given. For more information on serotonin syndrome and its management, see 'Drugs that cause serotonin syndrome + Other drugs that cause serotonin syndrome', p.1471. The other neurotoxic reactions cited seem to be isolated cases but they illustrate some of the risks attached to using anorectic, stimulant or 'recreational' drugs by patients already taking other medications, particularly antidepressant and psychotropic drugs that affect the same receptors in the CNS. Furthermore, as with the other interactions discussed here, toxic reactions may be more likely if the plasma levels of the amfetamine are increased by the SSRI.

1. Prior FH, Isbister GK, Dawson AH, Whyte IM. Serotonin toxicity with therapeutic doses of dexamphetamine and venlafaxine. *Med J Aust* (2002) 176, 240–1.
2. Liechti ME, Baumann C, Gamma A, Vollenweider FX. Acute psychological effects of 3,4-methylenedioxymethamphetamine (MDMA, "Ecstasy") are attenuated by the serotonin uptake inhibitor citalopram. *Neuropsychopharmacology* (2000) 22, 513–21.
3. Lauerma H, Wuorela M, Halme M. Interaction of serotonin reuptake inhibitor and 3,4-methylenedioxymethamphetamine? *Biol Psychiatry* (1998) 43, 929.
4. Stein DJ, Rink J. Effects of "ecstasy" blocked by serotonin reuptake inhibitors. *J Clin Psychiatry* (1999) 60, 485.
5. Tancer M, Johanson C-E. The effects of fluoxetine on the subjective and physiological effects of 3,4-methylenedioxymethamphetamine (MDMA) in humans. *Psychopharmacology (Berl)* (2007) 189, 565–73.
6. McCann UD, Ricaurte GA. Reinforcing subjective effects of (±) 3,4-methylenedioxymethamphetamine ("Ecstasy") may be separable from its neurotoxic actions: clinical evidence. *J Clin Psychopharmacol* (1993) 13, 214–17.
7. Farré M, Abanades S, Roset PN, Peiró AM, Torrens M, O'Mathúna B, Segura M, de la Torre R. Pharmacological interaction between 3,4-methylenedioxymethamphetamine (ecstasy) and paroxetine: pharmacological effects and pharmacokinetics. *J Pharmacol Exp Ther* (2007) 323, 954–62.
8. Segura M, Farré M, Pichini S, Peiró AM, Roset PN, Ramírez A, Ortuño J, Pacifici R, Zuccaro P, Segura J, de la Torre R. Contribution of cytochrome P450 2D6 to 3,4-methylenedioxymethamphetamine disposition in humans: use of paroxetine as a metabolic inhibitor probe. *Clin Pharmacokinet* (2005) 44, 649–60.
9. Barrett J, Meehan O, Fahy T. SSRI and sympathomimetic interaction. *Br J Psychiatry* (1996) 168, 253.
10. Bostwick JM, Brown TM. A toxic reaction from combining fluoxetine and phentermine. *J Clin Psychopharmacol* (1996) 16, 189–90.
11. Lyles J, Cadet JL. Methylenedioxymethamphetamine (MDMA, Ecstasy) neurotoxicity: cellular and molecular mechanisms. *Brain Res Brain Res Rev* (2003) 42, 155–68.
12. Oesterheld JR, Armstrong SC, Cozza KL. Ecstasy: pharmacodynamic and pharmacokinetic interactions. *Psychosomatics* (2004) 45, 84–7.
13. Clemens KJ, McGregor IS, Hunt GE, Cornish JL. MDMA, methamphetamine and their combination: possible lessons for party drug users from recent preclinical research. *Drug Alcohol Rev* (2007) 26, 9–15.
14. Upreti VV, Eddington ND. Fluoxetine pretreatment effects pharmacokinetics of 3,4-methylenedioxymethamphetamine (MDMA, *ECSTASY*) in rat. *J Pharm Sci* (2008) 97, 1593–1605.
15. Shoptaw S, Huber A, Peck J, Yang X, Liu J, Dang J, Roll J, Shapiro B, Rotheram-Fuller E, Ling W. Randomized, placebo-controlled trial of sertraline and contingency management for the treatment of methamphetamine dependence. *Drug Alcohol Depend* (2006) 85, 12–18.
16. Piasecki MP, Steinagel GM, Thienhaus OJ, Kohlenberg BS. An exploratory study: the use of paroxetine for methamphetamine craving. *J Psychoactive Drugs* (2002) 34, 301–4.

Amfetamines + Topiramate

A case report describes lack of euphoric effects in a subject who took ecstasy during treatment with topiramate. Topiramate does not affect the haemodynamic response to metamfetamine, although some aspects of metamfetamine-induced positive cognitive performance and subjective mood may be increased.

Clinical evidence, mechanism, importance and management

A 28-year-old man who had regularly used **ecstasy** (MDMA; methylenedioxymethamfetamine) 2 to 4 times weekly was given topiramate for about 3 months, starting with a dose of 50 mg daily, titrated to 200 mg daily during the second week of treatment. He took **ecstasy** once while also taking topiramate and reported that, in contrast to previous use without topiramate, there was no feeling of euphoria when **ecstasy** was taken during treatment with topiramate.[1]

A study in 10 metamfetamine-dependent subjects, given intravenous **metamfetamine** 15 or 30 mg, found that topiramate 100 or 200 mg appeared to accentuate some aspects of **metamfetamine**-induced positive subjective mood, although topiramate alone showed a non-significant trend towards mild reductions in positive mood and reinforcement.[2] A placebo-controlled study in the same subjects found that intravenous **metamfetamine** 15 or 30 mg was associated with increased psychomotor performance and attention. Pretreatment with topiramate 100 or 200 mg orally in two divided doses tended to enhance **metamfetamine**-induced increases in attention and concentration, but decreased perceptual motor function.[3] A further study in the same subjects found that **metamfetamine**-associated increases in haemodynamic response (blood pressure, heart rate) were not significantly affected by pretreatment with topiramate. However, there was a non-significant trend for topiramate to increase plasma **metamfetamine** levels, possibly due to alkalinisation of the urine by topiramate.[4]

These studies were primarily designed to assess the potential use of topiramate in amfetamine abuse. However, they indicate that a clinically significant pharmacokinetic interaction seems unlikely, and that concurrent use does not appear to be associated with any clinically significant adverse effects.

1. Akhondzadeh S, Hampa AD. Topiramate prevents ecstasy consumption: a case report. *Fundam Clin Pharmacol* (2005) 19, 601–2.
2. Johnson BA, Roache JD, Ait-Daoud N, Wells LT, Wallace CL, Dawes MA, Liu L, Wang X-Q. Effects of acute topiramate dosing on methamphetamine-induced subjective mood. *Int J Neuropsychopharmacol* (2007) 10, 85–98.
3. Johnson BA, Roache JD, Ait-Daoud N, Wells LT, Wallace CL, Dawes MA, Liu L, Wang X-Q. Effects of topiramate on methamphetamine-induced changes in attentional and perceptual-motor skills of cognition in recently abstinent methamphetamine-dependent individuals. *Prog Neuropsychopharmacol Biol Psychiatry* (2007) 31, 123–30.
4. Johnson BA, Wells LT, Roache JD, Wallace CL, Ait-Daoud N, Dawes MA, Liu L, Wang X-Q, Javors MA. Kinetic and cardiovascular effects of acute topiramate dosing among non-treatment-seeking, methamphetamine-dependent individuals. *Prog Neuropsychopharmacol Biol Psychiatry* (2007) 31, 455–61.

Amfetamines + Urinary acidifiers or alkalinisers

The urinary excretion of amfetamines is increased by urinary acidifiers (ammonium chloride) and reduced by urinary alkalinisers (acetazolamide, sodium bicarbonate).

Clinical evidence

A study in 6 healthy subjects given **dexamfetamine** 10 to 15 mg found that when the urine was made alkaline (pH of about 8) by giving **sodium bicarbonate**, only 3% of the original dose of amfetamine was excreted over a 16-hour period, compared with 55% when the urine was made acidic (pH of about 5) by taking **ammonium chloride**.[1] Similar results have been reported elsewhere for **amfetamine**, **dexamfetamine** and **metamfetamine**.[2-5] A further study found that the effects of **amfetamine** were increased and prolonged in subjects with alkaline urine,[6] and psychoses resulting from **amfetamine** retention in patients with alkaline urine have been described.[7]

Mechanism

Amfetamines are bases, which are excreted by the kidneys. If the urine is alkaline most of the drug exists in the un-ionised form, which is readily reabsorbed by the kidney tubules, so that little is lost. In acid urine, little of the drug is in the un-ionised form so that little can be reabsorbed and much of it is lost. For more detail on this mechanism, see *Changes in urinary pH*, under 'Drug excretion interactions', p.11.

Importance and management

The interaction between the amfetamines and urinary acidifiers or alkalinisers is well established and well understood but reports of problems in practice seem rare. Nevertheless, there is still the possibility that therapeutic doses of amfetamines may be excreted too rapidly if urinary acidifying drugs are given. This interaction has been exploited to increase the clearance of amfetamines in cases of overdose, but although amfetamine excretion is increased, acidification of the urine is believed to increase the risk of acute renal failure if myoglobinuria is present.[8-10] Only amfetamine, dexamfetamine and metamfetamine appear to have been studied, but similar effects are expected with all amfetamines, and the interaction is predicted by the manufacturers of **benzfetamine**[11] and **lisdexamfetamine**.[10]

Care is needed to ensure that amfetamine toxicity does not develop if the urine is made alkaline with sodium bicarbonate or another urinary alkaliniser such as **acetazolamide**, or **sodium phosphate**.[9,10,12] Note that sodium bicarbonate may also increase the absorption of amfetamines, by decreasing gastrointestinal acidity, and one manufacturer says that gastrointestinal alkalinising agents such as **antacids** should be avoided with amfetamines.[12]

1. Beckett AH, Rowland M, Turner P. Influence of urinary pH on excretion of amphetamine. *Lancet* (1965) i, 303.
2. Rowland M, Beckett AH. The amphetamines: clinical and pharmacokinetic implications of recent studies of an assay procedure and urinary excretion in man. *Arzneimittelforschung* (1966) 16, 1369–73.
3. Beckett AH, Salmon JA, Mitchard M. The relation between blood levels and urinary excretion of amphetamine under controlled acidic and under fluctuating urinary pH values using [^{14}C]amphetamine. *J Pharm Pharmacol* (1969) 21, 251–8.
4. Davis JM, Kopin IJ, Lemberger L, Axelrod J. Effects of urinary pH on amphetamine metabolism. *Ann N Y Acad Sci* (1971) 179, 493–501.
5. Wan SH, Matin SB, Azarnoff DL. Kinetics, salivary excretion of amphetamine isomers, and effect of urinary pH. *Clin Pharmacol Ther* (1978) 23, 585–90.
6. Smart JV, Turner P. Influence of urinary pH on the degree and duration of action of amphetamine on the critical flicker fusion frequency in man. *Br J Pharmacol* (1966) 26, 468–72.
7. Änggård E, Jönsson L-E, Hogmark A-L, Gunne L-M. Amphetamine metabolism in amphetamine psychosis. *Clin Pharmacol Ther* (1973) 14, 870–80.
8. Desoxyn (Methamphetamine hydrochloride). Lundbeck Inc. US Prescribing information, May 2009.
9. Dexedrine (Dextroamphetamine sulfate). Amedra Pharmaceuticals, LLC. US Prescribing information, October 2013.
10. Vyvanse (Lisdexamfetamine dimesylate). Shire US Inc. US Prescribing information, January 2012.
11. Didrex (Benzphetamine hydrochloride). Pfizer, Inc. US Prescribing information, August 2010.
12. Adderall XR (Mixed salts of amphetamine and dextroamphetamine). Shire US Inc. US Prescribing information, April 2015.

Amfetamines; Dexamfetamine + Risperidone

Blepharospasm occurred in a child during treatment with dexamfetamine and risperidone.

Clinical evidence, mechanism, importance and management

A 9-year-old girl with attention deficit hyperactivity disorder (ADHD), who also had anxiety and aggressive symptoms, was taking sertraline 25 mg daily (reduced from 50 mg daily because of an increase in angry outbursts) and risperidone 250 micrograms in the morning and 500 micrograms at bedtime, which mildly reduced aggression. When she was also given extended-release dexamfetamine 5 mg daily her aggression was further decreased. The dose of dexamfetamine was therefore increased to 10 mg daily, and 4 days later the dose of risperidone was increased to 500 micrograms twice daily. One week later she developed bilateral blepharospasm, which completely resolved when the doses of both dexamfetamine and risperidone were reduced to the starting doses. The dose of dexamfetamine was then gradually increased to 15 mg daily without the occurrence of dystonic symptoms.[1]

This appears to be the only case of a possible interaction between risperidone and dexamfetamine. Risperidone alone commonly causes dystonias, which may present as blepharospasm. As the risperidone was not given alone at the higher dose it is not possible to say whether what occurred was as a result of an interaction, or simply an adverse effect of the risperidone. Furthermore, the patient had stopped methylphenidate shortly before the dose increase of risperidone and this has been associated with the onset of dystonias, see 'Methylphenidate + Risperidone', p.221. Therefore an interaction is not established and no general recommendations can be made on the basis of this case.

1. Levine JB, Deneys ML, Benjamin S. Dystonia with combined antipsychotic and stimulant treatment. *J Am Acad Child Adolesc Psychiatry* (2007) 46, 665–6.

Amfetamines; Dexamfetamine + Valproate

Valproate appears to attenuate the effects of dexamfetamine on mood changes, some cognitive tasks, and blood pressure.

Clinical evidence, mechanism, importance and management

In a placebo-controlled study, 12 healthy subjects were given sodium valproate 500 mg daily for 3 days, then 1 g daily for 11 days, followed by a single 25-mg dose of **dexamfetamine**. Pretreatment with valproate was found to significantly attenuate the effects of **dexamfetamine** on mood (happiness, energy, alertness) and attenuated the increases in diastolic blood pressure associated with **dexamfetamine**.[1] The reasons for these reactions are not known. One study found that pretreating 12 healthy subjects with sodium valproate for 14 days (500 mg daily for 3 days, then 1 g daily for 11 days) attenuated **dexamfetamine**-induced regional decreases in brain activation when the subjects performed cognitive tasks.[2]

It has been suggested that amfetamines and valproate have mutually opposing pharmacological actions on dopamine and noradrenaline (norepinephrine) release and uptake at adrenergic neurones,[2] possibly partially due to opposing effects on the phosphoinositol second messenger system.[1,2]

The clinical significance of these changes is unclear, but the effects on blood pressure are, if anything, likely to be beneficial. It is unclear whether other amfetamines are affected similarly.

1. Willson MC, Bell EC, Dave S, Asghar SJ, McGrath BM, Silverstone PH. Valproate attenuates dextroamphetamine-induced subjective changes more than lithium. *Eur Neuropsychopharmacol* (2005) 15, 633–9.
2. Bell EC, Willson MC, Wilman AH, Dave S, Asghar SJ, Silverstone PH. Lithium and valproate attenuate dextroamphetamine-induced changes in brain activation. *Hum Psychopharmacol* (2005) 20, 87–96.

Amfetamines; Levamfetamine + Phenylpropanolamine

The effects of levamfetamine were attenuated in a hyperactive child by a nasal decongestant containing chlorphenamine and phenylpropanolamine.

Clinical evidence, mechanism, importance and management

The use of **levamfetamine succinate** 42 mg daily in was found to be ineffective a 12-year-old hyperactive boy on two occasions when he took *Contac* cold capsules and *Allerest* tablets for colds. Both of these proprietary nasal decongestants contain **phenylpropanolamine** and **chlorphenamine**.[1] The reason for this interaction is not understood and there is too little information to make any statement about its general importance.

1. Huestis RD, Arnold LE. Possible antagonism of amphetamine by decongestant-antihistamine compounds. *J Pediatr* (1974) 85, 579–80.

Amfetamines; Lisdexamfetamine + Food

The bioavailability of lisdexamfetamine is not affected by food.

Clinical evidence, mechanism, importance and management

In a crossover study, 18 healthy subjects were given a single 70-mg dose of lisdexamfetamine (a pro-drug of dexamfetamine) as a capsule formulation under fasting conditions or after a high-fat meal; or as a solution of the capsule contents under fasting conditions. All subjects were fasted for at least 4 hours after drug administration, and then given standard meals. The lisdexamfetamine AUC was similar when it was taken under fasting or fed conditions. Absorption of lisdexamfetamine and dexamfetamine was delayed and peak levels of lisdexamfetamine were decreased when it was taken with food, but food appears not to have a significant effect on either lisdexamfetamine or dexamfetamine bioavailability,[1] and the US manufacturers of lisdexamfetamine state that it may be taken with or without food.[2]

1. Krishnan S, Zhang Y. Relative bioavailability of lisdexamfetamine 70-mg capsules in fasted and fed healthy adult volunteers and in solution: a single-dose, crossover pharmacokinetic study. *J Clin Pharmacol* (2008) 48, 293–302.
2. Vyvanse (Lisdexamfetamine dimesylate). Shire US Inc. US Prescribing information, January 2012.

Atomoxetine + Amfetamines

The use of atomoxetine in patients taking amfetamines may lead to adverse effects, such as psychosis and movement disorders. In addition, a study in healthy subjects found that atomoxetine may attenuate some of the physiological and subjective effects of dexamfetamine.

Clinical evidence

A 77 kg, 9-year-old boy with attention deficit hyperactivity disorder (ADHD) who had been taking clonidine 300 micrograms twice daily and **amfetamine** with **dexamfetamine** (*Adderall XR*) 60 mg daily for several years, developed psychosis, abnormal involuntary movements, and insomnia when atomoxetine 25 mg daily was added to his treatment.[1]

In a study, atomoxetine 40 mg daily or placebo was given to 10 healthy subjects for 4 days, with a single 20-mg/70 kg dose of **dexamfetamine** on day 4. **Dexamfetamine**-induced increases in blood pressure, plasma cortisol levels, and the self-ratings of 'stimulated', 'high' and 'good drug effects' were all reduced by atomoxetine.[2]

Mechanism

The authors of the case report[1] suggested that the addition of atomoxetine to moderately high, stable doses of dexamfetamine and the alpha$_2$-adrenergic agonist clonidine triggered the adverse symptoms via additive effects on noradrenaline (norepinephrine) and possibly dopamine. The study in healthy subjects suggested that atomoxetine attenuates some of dexamfetamine's physiological and subjective effects via its effects as a noradrenaline transport inhibitor.[2,3]

Importance and management

Evidence for an interaction between atomoxetine and the amfetamines appears to be limited. As the study found an attenuation of some of the effects of dexamfetamine, further study is suggested to assess atomoxetine for the treatment of stimulant addiction.[2,3] However, the manufacturer recommends caution when atomoxetine is given with other drugs that affect noradrenaline (norepinephrine), because of the potential for additive or synergistic pharmacological effects.[4] If atomoxetine is given with an amfetamine, be aware that adverse CNS effects may develop, and consider reducing the doses or stopping one of the drugs should this occur.

1. Bond GR, Garro AC, Gilbert DL. Dyskinesias associated with atomoxetine in combination with other psychoactive drugs. *Clin Toxicol* (2007) 45, 182–5.
2. Sofuoglu M, Poling J, Hill K, Kosten T. Atomoxetine attenuates dextroamphetamine effects in humans. *Am J Drug Alcohol Abuse* (2009) 35, 412–16.
3. Sofuoglu M, Sewell RA. Norepinephrine and stimulant addiction. *Addict Biol* (2009) 14, 119–29.
4. Strattera (Atomoxetine hydrochloride). Eli Lilly and Company Ltd. UK Summary of product characteristics, October 2012.

Atomoxetine + CYP2D6 inhibitors

Paroxetine (a CYP2D6 inhibitor) markedly increases atomoxetine exposure in extensive metabolisers of CYP2D6. Fluoxetine and other CYP2D6 inhibitors are expected to interact similarly and one small study with fluoxetine supports this suggestion.

Clinical evidence

(a) Fluoxetine

Following a small-scale study in which atomoxetine was given with fluoxetine without any adverse effects, 127 children with attention deficit hyperactivity disorder (ADHD) were randomised to receive fluoxetine 20 mg daily and 46 to receive placebo. After 3 weeks atomoxetine (starting at 0.5 mg/kg daily, increasing over 5 weeks to a maximum of 1.8 mg/kg daily) was also given to both groups. The fluoxetine group had 3.3-fold higher maximum concentration of atomoxetine than the placebo group. However, despite a trend towards a greater incidence of decreased appetite with the combination (20% versus 6.8%), there was no significant difference in adverse events between the two groups.[1]

(b) Paroxetine

In one study, 22 healthy subjects who were extensive metabolisers of CYP2D6 (that is, those with normal CYP2D6 activity) were given paroxetine 20 mg daily for 17 days, with atomoxetine 20 mg twice daily on the last 5 days. Paroxetine increased the AUC of atomoxetine 6.5-fold, increased its maximum plasma concentration 3.5-fold, and increased its elimination half-life 2.5-fold, when compared with atomoxetine alone. No changes in paroxetine pharmacokinetics were seen.[2] The pharmacokinetics of atomoxetine with paroxetine in these subjects was similar to that previously seen with atomoxetine alone in poor metaboliser subjects (that is, those lacking or with low activity of this isoenzyme).[2,3]

A case report describes a 38-year-old man, with attention deficit hyperactivity disorder (ADHD), in whom this interaction was exploited for clinical benefit: the addition of paroxetine to atomoxetine 30 mg three times daily increased the maximum concentration of atomoxetine up to 3-fold, with a corresponding improvement in his clinical condition.[4]

Mechanism

Atomoxetine is extensively metabolised by CYP2D6,[5] an isoenzyme that shows polymorphism, with up to 10% of the population lacking an active form (poor metabolisers). Paroxetine inhibits CYP2D6, and thereby increases atomoxetine concentrations in those with an extensive metaboliser phenotype. It would not be expected to have any effect in poor metabolisers because of the absence of functional isoenzyme. Fluoxetine can also inhibit CYP2D6 and therefore interacts similarly.

Importance and management

An established pharmacokinetic interaction. Paroxetine effectively changes patients from extensive metabolisers into poor metabolisers, markedly increasing atomoxetine exposure. Although the clinical relevance of this effect has not been directly assessed, the manufacturer notes that in clinical studies some adverse effects of atomoxetine were up to twice as frequent in poor metabolisers.[3] Both manufacturers suggest that, in patients already taking CYP2D6 inhibitors, dose adjustment and slower titration of atomoxetine might be necessary,[3,6] with the dose increased only if symptoms fail to improve and if the initial dose is well tolerated.[3] This seems a sensible precaution. Note that in the fluoxetine study, which found that the concurrent use of atomoxetine was generally well tolerated, dose increases were made on a weekly basis, from 0.5 mg/kg to 0.8 mg/kg and then 1.2 mg/kg daily at the start of the third week.[1] The US manufacturer suggests a starting dose of atomoxetine 0.5 mg/kg daily (40 mg per day in those over 70 kg) and only increasing the dose to 1.2 mg/kg daily (or 80 mg per day) if symptoms do not improve after 4 weeks and the initial dose is well tolerated.[3] The UK manufacturers say that the initial dose should be maintained for a minimum of 7 days before increasing it, if necessary.[6]

It would also seem prudent to be alert to the possibility of an increase in adverse effects if CYP2D6 inhibitors are given to patients taking atomoxetine, and the manufacturers specifically name fluoxetine, paroxetine, **quinidine**,[3,6] and **terbinafine**.[6] If one of these drugs is given they suggest that the clinical response and tolerability should be re-evaluated and a dose adjustment may be necessary.[6] For a list of CYP2D6 inhibitors, see 'Table 1.7', p.9.

Extra caution would seem prudent with paroxetine or fluoxetine in those with epilepsy, as both atomoxetine and the SSRIs can lower the seizure threshold, and this risk appears to be increased by higher atomoxetine concentrations.[3] The UK manufacturer[6] notes that patients might also be more at risk of QT interval prolongation when atomoxetine is given with CYP2D6 inhibitors; however, the US manufacturer[3] gives no such warning. See 'Drugs that prolong the QT interval + Other drugs that prolong the QT interval', p.272, for further information on the concurrent use of two or more drugs that prolong the QT interval.

1. Kratochvil CJ, Newcorn JH, Arnold LE, Duesenberg D, Emslie GJ, Quintana H, Sarkis EH, Wagner KD, Gao H, Michelson D, Biederman J. Atomoxetine alone or combined with fluoxetine for treating ADHD with comorbid depressive or anxiety symptoms. *J Am Acad Child Adolesc Psychiatry* (2005) 44, 915–24.
2. Belle DJ, Ernest CS, Sauer J-M, Smith BP, Thomasson HR, Witcher JW. Effect of potent CYP2D6 inhibition by paroxetine on atomoxetine pharmacokinetics. *J Clin Pharmacol* (2002) 42, 1219–27.
3. Strattera (Atomoxetine hydrochloride). Eli Lilly and Company. US Prescribing information, August 2012.
4. Paulzen M, Clement H-W, Gründer G. Enhancement of atomoxetine serum levels by co-administration of paroxetine. *Int J Neuropsychopharmacol* (2008) 11, 289–91.
5. Sauer J-M, Ponsler GD, Mattiuz EL, Long AJ, Witcher JW, Thomasson HR, Desante KA. Disposition and metabolic fate of atomoxetine hydrochloride: the role of CYP2D6 in human disposition and metabolism. *Drug Metab Dispos* (2003) 31, 98–107.
6. Strattera (Atomoxetine hydrochloride). Eli Lilly and Company Ltd. UK Summary of product characteristics, October 2012.

Atomoxetine + Miscellaneous

The manufacturer of atomoxetine contraindicates the concurrent use of MAOIs. Atomoxetine is predicted to have additive effects with pressor drugs and other sympathomimetics and in one study has been seen to potentiate the increase in heart rate and blood pressure caused by intravenous salbutamol. However, no increase in cardiovascular effects was seen when atomoxetine was given with methylphenidate. Atomoxetine is also said to have the potential for an interaction with drugs that lower the seizure threshold.

Atomoxetine does not alter desipramine or midazolam pharmacokinetics and would therefore not be expected to affect other substrates of CYP2D6 or CYP3A4. Antacids, omeprazole and food do not alter atomoxetine bioavailability.

Clinical evidence, mechanism, importance and management

(a) Antacids or Omeprazole

In a study in 20 subjects, the use of **aluminium/magnesium hydroxide** (*Maalox*) or omeprazole did not affect the bioavailability of atomoxetine 40 mg.[1] No special precautions appear to be necessary on concurrent use.

(b) CYP2D6 substrates

In a study[2] in 21 subjects who were extensive metabolisers of CYP2D6 (that is, those with normal activity of this isoenzyme), atomoxetine 40 or 60 mg twice daily for 13 days had no effect on the pharmacokinetics of a single 50-mg dose of **desipramine** given on day 4.

Desipramine is extensively metabolised by CYP2D6, and can be used as a probe drug for the assessment of the effect of drugs on this isoenzyme (see 'Genetic factors in drug metabolism', p.8). It was therefore concluded that atomoxetine, even at the maximum recommended dose, does not cause clinically relevant inhibition of CYP2D6 *in vivo*, and so will not affect the pharmacokinetics of other CYP2D6 substrates.[2]

(c) CYP3A4 substrates

Atomoxetine 60 mg twice daily for 12 days was given to 6 subjects who were poor metabolisers of CYP2D6 (that is, those with low activity or totally lacking activity of this isoenzyme), with a single 5-mg oral dose of **midazolam** on days 6 and 12. Atomoxetine increased the maximum concentration and AUC of **midazolam** by about 16%, which was not statistically or clinically significant.[2]

Midazolam is extensively metabolised by CYP3A4, and can be used as a probe drug for assessment of the effect of drugs on this isoenzyme. Poor metabolisers of CYP2D6 were chosen for this study, because they have much higher concentrations of atomoxetine than extensive metabolisers of CYP2D6. It was concluded that atomoxetine, even at the maximum recommended dose, does not cause clinically relevant inhibition of CYP3A4 *in vivo*, and so will not affect the pharmacokinetics of other CYP3A4 substrates.[2]

(d) Drugs that lower the seizure threshold

Seizures are a potential risk with atomoxetine and caution is advised if drugs that lower the seizure threshold (such as **antidepressants**, **antipsychotics**, **chloroquine**, **mefloquine**, **bupropion**, or **tramadol**) are given concurrently.[3] Note that both atomoxetine and a number of these drugs are also associated with an increased risk of QT interval prolongation, see 'Drugs that prolong the QT interval + Other drugs that prolong the QT interval', p.272, for further information on the concurrent use of two or more drugs that prolong the QT interval.

(e) Food

In a study in 25 healthy subjects given atomoxetine under fasting or fed conditions, it was found that food decreased the maximum plasma concentration of atomoxetine by 37% and delayed the time to maximum concentrations by 3 hours, but did not affect its overall bioavailability.[1]

(f) MAOIs

The manufacturers contraindicate the use of atomoxetine with an MAOI, or within 2 weeks of stopping an MAOI,[3,4] because other drugs that affect brain monoamine levels have caused serious reactions (including symptoms of serotonin syndrome or symptoms similar to neuroleptic malignant syndrome) when taken with an MAOI.[4]

(g) Methylphenidate

In a placebo-controlled, crossover study, 12 healthy subjects were given atomoxetine 60 mg twice daily or methylphenidate 60 mg daily for 5 days, with the other drug added for the final 2 days. No additional changes in blood pressure or heart rate were seen when the drugs were given together, and concurrent use did not increase the frequency of adverse effects.[5]

(h) Pressor drugs

Atomoxetine is a sympathomimetic that acts as a noradrenaline reuptake inhibitor. As such, it causes a modest increase in pulse and/or blood pressure in many patients.[3,4] The manufacturer recommends caution if atomoxetine is given concurrently with pressor drugs (e.g. **dopamine, dobutamine**)[4] because of the possible additive effects on blood pressure.[3,4]

(i) Salbutamol (Albuterol)

The manufacturer notes that atomoxetine 60 mg twice daily for 5 days potentiated the increase in heart rate and blood pressure caused by an infusion of salbutamol 600 micrograms, given over 2 hours.[4] Because of this, they recommend caution when atomoxetine is used in patients receiving intravenous or oral salbutamol or other **beta$_2$ agonists**[3,4] (for a list, see 'Table 34.1', p.1419). The UK manufacturer also extends this precaution to high-dose nebulised salbutamol.[3] However, the effects on heart rate and blood pressure were not seen in another study when 21 healthy Asian subjects, who were extensive CYP2D6 metabolisers (that is, those with normal isoenzyme activity), were given salbutamol 200 to 800 micrograms daily with atomoxetine 80 mg daily, for 5 days.[4]

(j) Miscellaneous

The UK manufacturer recommends caution when atomoxetine is given concurrently with other drugs that affect noradrenaline (norepinephrine), because of the potential for additive or synergistic pharmacological effects. They name antidepressants such as **imipramine**, **mirtazapine** and venlafaxine, and the decongestants **pseudoephedrine** or **phenylephrine**.[3] This would seem a sensible precaution, particularly as neurological complications have been reported in one patient given atomoxetine and venlafaxine, see 'SNRIs; Venlafaxine + Atomoxetine', p.1480 and a child given atomoxetine and dexamfetamine, see 'Atomoxetine + Amfetamines', p.218.

1. DeSante KA, Long AJ, Smith BP, Thomasson HR, Sauer JM, Agbo F, Abeyratne A, Riggio AL, Sheets BA, Witcher JW. Atomoxetine absolute bioavailability and effects of food, Maalox or omeprazole on atomoxetine bioavailability. *AAPS PharmSci* (2001) 3 (S1).
2. Sauer J-M, Long AJ, Ring B, Gillespie JS, Sanburn NP, DeSante KA, Petullo D, VandenBranden MR, Jensen CB, Wrighton SA, Smith BP, Read HA, Witcher JW. Atomoxetine hydrochloride: clinical drug-drug interaction prediction and outcome. *J Pharmacol Exp Ther* (2004) 308, 410–18.
3. Strattera (Atomoxetine hydrochloride). Eli Lilly and Company Ltd. UK Summary of product characteristics, October 2012.
4. Strattera (Atomoxetine hydrochloride). Eli Lilly and Company. US Prescribing information, August 2012.
5. Kelly RP, Yeo KP, Teng C-H, Smith BP, Lowe S, Soon D, Read HA, Wise SD. Hemodynamic effects of acute administration of atomoxetine and methylphenidate. *J Clin Pharmacol* (2005) 45, 851–55.

Dexfenfluramine or Fenfluramine + Anorectics

Fenfluramine and dexfenfluramine have generally been withdrawn worldwide because of the occurrence of serious and sometimes fatal valvular heart disease and pulmonary hypertension, which occurred when they were taken alone and when taken with phentermine. Some herbal preparations may, however, still contain fenfluramine and related drugs. There is an isolated case of cardiomyopathy attributed to the use of fenfluramine and mazindol.

Clinical evidence, mechanism, importance and management

Fenfluramine and dexfenfluramine have generally been withdrawn worldwide because of the occurrence of serious and sometimes fatal valvular heart disease (aortic, mitral, tricuspid or mixed valve disease). Pulmonary hypertension has also sometimes been seen. These serious adverse effects occurred when these drugs were taken alone, and when taken with **phentermine** as *Fen-phen* and *Dexfen-phen*, but not with phentermine alone.[1-6]

Before the withdrawal of the drug from the market, the manufacturer of fenfluramine recommended that concurrent use with other centrally-acting anorectics should be avoided.[7]

Case reports suggest that severe cardiac adverse effects may occur when fenfluramine is given with other drugs. In one report, a patient developed cardiomyopathy, which was attributed to the use of fenfluramine with **mazindol**.[8] For a report of bradycardia and hypotension in a patient taking fenfluramine, **phentermine** and fluoxetine, see 'Amfetamines and related drugs + SSRIs', p.216.

Note that some unlicensed traditional Chinese medicines have been found to contain **nitrosofenfluramine** (known to be toxic to the liver) and fenfluramine. Reports suggest that other products for weight loss may also contain undeclared fenfluramine and **nitrosofenfluramine**.[9]

1. Committee on Safety of Medicines/Medicines Control Agency. Fenfluramine and dexfenfluramine withdrawn. *Current Problems* (1997) 23, 13.
2. Food and Drugs Administration. FDA announces withdrawal fenfluramine and dexfenfluramine (Fen-Phen). September 15th, 1997.
3. Connolly HM, Crary JL, McGoon MD, Hensrud DD, Edwards BS, Edwards WD, Schaff HV. Valvular heart disease associated with fenfluramine-phentermine. *N Engl J Med* (1997) 337, 581–8.
4. Mark EJ, Patalas ED, Chang HT, Evans RJ, Kessler SC. Fatal pulmonary hypertension associated with short-term use of fenfluramine and phentermine. *N Engl J Med* (1997) 337, 602–6.
5. Graham DJ, Green L. Further cases of valvular heart disease associated with fenfluramine-phentermine. *N Engl J Med* (1997) 337, 635.
6. Fleming RM, Boyd LB. The longitudinal effects of fenfluramine-phentermine use. *Angiology* (2007) 58, 353–9.
7. Ponderax Pacaps (Fenfluramine). Servier Laboratories Limited. ABPI Compendium of Datasheets and Summaries of Product Characteristics 1997–8, 1307.
8. Gillis D, Wengrower D, Witztum E, Leitersdorf E. Fenfluramine and mazindol: acute reversible cardiomyopathy associated with their use. *Int J Psychiatry Med* (1985) 15, 197–200.
9. MHRA. Letter from R Woodfield, Group Manager Herbal Policy, to Herbal Interest Groups: Shubao Slimming Capsules containing fenfluramine and nitrosofenfluramine, 28 April 2004. Available at: http://webarchive.nationalarchives.gov.uk/20141205150130/http://www.mhra.gov.uk/home/groups/es-herbal/documents/websiteresources/con009291.pdf (accessed 21/10/15).

Methylphenidate + Carbamazepine

Carbamazepine may reduce methylphenidate levels.

Clinical evidence, mechanism, importance and management

A 7-year-old boy with attention deficit disorder taking carbamazepine 1 g daily for grand mal epilepsy was referred because of unmanageable behaviour. He did not respond to methylphenidate in doses of up to 30 mg every 4 hours, and his blood levels of both methylphenidate and its metabolites were undetectable. The authors of the report attributed this to an interaction with the carbamazepine.[1] Similarly, symptoms of attention deficit hyperactivity disorder (ADHD) worsened in a 13-year-old girl taking methylphenidate after she also took carbamazepine. Methylphenidate serum levels decreased markedly and the dose of methylphenidate had to be increased from 20 mg three times daily to 60 mg three times daily to regain a benefit similar to that achieved before the addition of carbamazepine.[2] However, another report describes 4 out of 7 children taking methylphenidate and carbamazepine in whom the combination was successful. Blood levels of methylphenidate were apparently not measured.[3]

Despite the scarcity of the information, and the cases of apparently successful use, it would seem wise to consider carbamazepine as a possible cause if patients do not respond adequately to methylphenidate. If this occurs, consider increasing the methylphenidate dose. However, note that methylphenidate may lower the seizure threshold and should be used with caution in patients with epilepsy. If seizure frequency increases or new onset seizures occur, methylphenidate should be discontinued.[4]

1. Behar D, Schaller J, Spreat S. Extreme reduction of methylphenidate levels by carbamazepine. *J Am Acad Child Adolesc Psychiatry* (1998) 37, 1128–9.
2. Schaller JL, Behar D. Carbamazepine and methylphenidate in ADHD. *J Am Acad Child Adolesc Psychiatry* (1999) 38, 112–13.
3. Gross-Tsur V. Carbamazepine and methylphenidate. *J Am Acad Child Adolesc Psychiatry* (1999) 38, 637.
4. Ritalin (Methylphenidate hydrochloride). Novartis Pharmaceuticals UK Ltd. UK Summary of product characteristics, May 2011.

Methylphenidate + Clonidine

Much publicised fears about the serious consequences of using methylphenidate with clonidine appear to be unfounded. There is some evidence to suggest that concurrent use can be both safe and effective.

Clinical evidence, mechanism, importance and management

There have been fears about serious adverse events when methylphenidate is taken with clonidine,[1] due to reports of three deaths in children taking both drugs. One child died from ventricular fibrillation due to cardiac abnormalities, one from cardiac arrest attributed to an overdose of fluoxetine, and the third death was unexplained. Studies of these cases and one further case did not establish any link between the use of methylphenidate with clonidine and these deaths; the final broad conclusion being that the event was largely a media-inspired scare story built on inconclusive evidence.[2,3] However, there are theoretical reasons to be concerned about giving clonidine with methylphenidate (which have opposing adrenergic effects), because missed doses, extra doses, or mistimed doses can lead to significant hypertension and/or tachycardia or hypotension and/or bradycardia.[2] These adverse responses have been reported in children given clonidine alone and in combination with methylphenidate.[4,5] Furthermore, one study suggested a potential pharmacokinetic interaction, with methylphenidate lowering clonidine plasma levels.[6] Nevertheless, over the 2 years following the initial adverse reports, there did not appear to be any more data to support an increase in deaths associated with concurrent use and the use of methylphenidate with clonidine appeared to be beneficial.[7] A small-scale pilot study in 24 patients suggested that concurrent use is both safe and effective for the treatment of attention deficit hyperactivity disorder (ADHD).[8] Similarly, a study in children with both ADHD and Tourette's syndrome found that clonidine used with methylphenidate was more effective than either drug alone, and only one child had evidence of adverse cardiac effects.[9] Furthermore, the manufacturers of one formulation of methylphenidate[1] said that, as of 2002, they were not aware of any reports describing adverse events when *Concerta XL* (methylphenidate) was used with clonidine.

1. Janssen-Cilag. Personal communication, April 2002.
2. Popper CW. Combining methylphenidate and clonidine: pharmacologic questions and news reports about sudden death. *J Child Adolesc Psychopharmacol* (1995) 5, 157–66.
3. Fenichel RR. Combining methylphenidate and clonidine: the role of post-marketing surveillance. *J Child Adolesc Psychopharmacol* (1995) 5, 155–6.
4. Swanson JM, Flockhart D, Udrea D, Cantwell D, Connor D, Williams L. Clonidine in the treatment of ADHD: questions about safety and efficacy. *J Child Adolesc Psychopharmacol* (1995) 5, 301–4.
5. Cantwell DP, Swanson J, Connor DF. Case study: adverse response to clonidine. *J Am Acad Child Adolesc Psychiatry* (1997) 36, 539–44.
6. Hunt RD, Cohen DJ, Anderson G, Clark L. Possible change in noradrenergic receptor sensitivity following methylphenidate treatment: growth hormone and MHPG response to clonidine challenge in children with attention deficit disorder and hyperactivity. *Life Sci* (1984) 35, 885–97.
7. Wilens TE, Spencer TJ. Combining methylphenidate and clonidine: a clinically sound medication option. *J Am Acad Child Adolesc Psychiatry* (1999) 38, 614–16.
8. Connor DF, Barkley RA, Davis HT. A pilot study of methylphenidate, clonidine, or the combination in ADHD comorbid with aggressive oppositional defiant or conduct disorder. *Clin Pediatr (Phila)* (2000) 39, 15–25.
9. Tourette's Syndrome Study Group. Treatment of ADHD in children with tics: a randomized controlled trial. *Neurology* (2002) 58, 527–36.

Methylphenidate + Cocaine

Methylphenidate does not appear to alter the pharmacokinetics or physiological effects of cocaine to a clinically significant extent.

Clinical evidence, mechanism, importance and management

A placebo-controlled study in 7 otherwise healthy cocaine-dependent subjects found that methylphenidate 60 or 90 mg was well tolerated, did not significantly affect the pharmacokinetics of intravenous cocaine 20 or 40 mg, and did not have a clinically significant effect on the physiological effects of cocaine. However, some of the positive subjective effects of cocaine (desire for cocaine and good drug effects) were decreased. The results suggested that although both drugs can cause cardiovascular and CNS stimulation, in the doses studied, methylphenidate could be given to active cocaine users without any serious adverse reaction.[1]

1. Winhusen T, Somoza E, Singal BM, Harrer J, Apparaju S, Mezinskis J, Desai P, Elkashef A, Chiang CN, Horn P. Methylphenidate and cocaine: a placebo-controlled drug interaction study. *Pharmacol Biochem Behav* (2006) 85, 29–38.

Methylphenidate + Disulfiram

A psychotic episode occurred when a patient taking disulfiram was also given methylphenidate.

Clinical evidence

A 33-year-old man who was taking disulfiram 400 mg daily, without any noticeable adverse effects, experienced a psychotic-like episode after receiving a single 36-mg dose of modified-release methylphenidate. He discontinued the methylphenidate, but continued to take the disulfiram, and when assessed 2 months later there was no clinical evidence of psychosis, anxiety or depression. After a further 3 months, the disulfiram was discontinued and he took methylphenidate without any adverse effect or recurrence of the psychotic experience.[1]

Mechanism

It was suggested that an interaction might have occurred as disulfiram blocks dopamine-beta-hydroxylase. Low levels of this enzyme have been associated with psychotic symptoms.

Importance and management

Evidence of an interaction appears to be limited to this case report. As the effects of disulfiram persist for up to 2 weeks this interaction may occur even after the disulfiram is stopped. It has been suggested that there should be a significant washout period before starting methylphenidate; alternatively, it may be preferable to choose a non-dopaminergic drug for the treatment of attention deficit hyperactivity disorder (ADHD) if disulfiram is being taken.[1] Note that caution is advised when using methylphenidate in emotionally unstable patients, such as those with a history of alcoholism, because of the potential for abuse or misuse.[2-4]

1. Caci H, Baylé F. A case of disulfiram-methylphenidate interaction: implications for treatment. *Am J Psychiatry* (2007) 164, 1759.
2. Concerta XL (Methylphenidate hydrochloride). Janssen-Cilag Ltd. UK Summary of product characteristics, November 2009.
3. Ritalin (Methylphenidate hydrochloride). Novartis Pharmaceuticals UK Ltd. UK Summary of product characteristics, May 2011.
4. Concerta (Methylphenidate hydrochloride). McNeil Pediatrics. US Prescribing information, November 2009.

Methylphenidate + Risperidone

The use of methylphenidate with risperidone may possibly increase the risk of dyskinesias. Furthermore, there may be an increased risk of adverse effects if methylphenidate is started following risperidone withdrawal or if methylphenidate is withdrawn after concurrent use.

Clinical evidence

Although clinical studies have suggested that the use of risperidone with a psychostimulant (including methylphenidate) is safe, effective, and does not increase the incidence of adverse effects,[1] a limited case series suggested that children taking a psychostimulant and an atypical antipsychotic had a higher propensity for movement abnormalities.[2] A number of case reports support this suggestion. For example, a case of extrapyramidal symptoms occurred in a child taking methylphenidate, risperidone, sertraline and tropisetron. He recovered when given benzatropine.[3]

A number of reports describe adverse effects when risperidone has been replaced by methylphenidate. For example, a 7-year-old boy experienced acute dyskinesia, overactivity, distress, headache, fatigue and vomiting within 8 hours of starting to take modified-release methylphenidate 36 mg in place of risperidone 1.5 mg daily, which was stopped abruptly 12 hours earlier. Similar but less severe symptoms were seen 5 months later when modified-release methylphenidate 18 mg daily was started 6 days after the end of a course of risperidone, which had been reduced over 4 weeks.[4] Another case report describes three children who developed severe behavioural adverse reactions when switching from risperidone to methylphenidate. In one of these cases, a 5-year-old boy who had been taking risperidone 1 mg daily for 8 months became agitated, irritable, vigilant and violent when risperidone was abruptly withdrawn and methylphenidate 15 mg daily started 2 days later. The methylphenidate was discontinued and the severe behavioural reactions disappeared. After a 6-week drug-free period, methylphenidate was restarted at the same dose, with beneficial effects on attention and hyperactivity. A similar reaction occurred in a 6-year-old girl when risperidone 1 mg daily was discontinued abruptly and methylphenidate 15 mg daily was started. Another report describes a 15-year-old girl who was given risperidone 1 mg daily to alleviate the symptoms of attention deficit hyperactivity disorder (ADHD). When risperidone was stopped for one week withdrawal symptoms were not seen, but irritability and agitation were reported when methylphenidate 18 mg daily was started.[5]

Other reports describe adverse effects when methylphenidate is stopped in patients taking risperidone. One report describes a 9-year-old boy taking methylphenidate 15 mg and risperidone 1.5 mg, both three times daily, who developed acute dystonia when the methylphenidate was withdrawn. He recovered when given benzatropine.[6] A similar report describes an 11-year-old girl taking methylphenidate 30 mg daily and risperidone 1.75 mg daily, which was increased to 2 mg daily when she became increasingly aggressive. After 4 days of persistent aggressive behaviour, it was decided to reduce the dose of methylphenidate, but instead it was abruptly stopped and within a day the patient had developed generalised dystonia, with torsion movements of trunk and axial muscles, and torticollis. She recovered when given intramuscular diphenhydramine.[7]

Mechanism

Antipsychotics and psychostimulants have conflicting mechanisms of action in the CNS; risperidone is a combined serotonin and dopamine antagonist whereas methylphenidate is a dopamine agonist.[1,2] It has been suggested that adverse effects develop because stopping risperidone removes the dopaminergic blockade, which results in supersensitive dopamine receptors. Over-stimulation then occurs when methylphenidate is started.[4]

The dystonia that occurred when methylphenidate was abruptly withdrawn may be due to decreased dopamine transmission.[7]

Importance and management

Information regarding an interaction between risperidone and methylphenidate seems limited to case reports. However, the available data suggest that the combination of risperidone and methylphenidate carries the risk of drug-induced dyskinesias and particular care should be taken if one of the drugs is discontinued. Slow antipsychotic withdrawal, followed by a drug-free interval has been suggested when switching from risperidone to methylphenidate.[4,5] Methylphenidate should then be initiated at a low dose and withdrawn immediately if a dyskinesia appears.[4]

1. Aman MG, Binder C, Turgay A. Risperidone effects in the presence/absence of psychostimulant medicine in children with ADHD, other disruptive behavior disorders, and subaverage IQ. *J Child Adolesc Psychopharmacol* (2004) 14, 243–54.
2. Sharp B, Perdue C. Abnormal motor movements associated with combining psychostimulants and atypical antipsychotics in children. *CNS Spectr* (2007) 12, 659–62.
3. Teoh L, Allen H, Kowalenko N. Drug-induced extrapyramidal reactions. *J Paediatr Child Health* (2002) 38, 95–7.
4. Hollis CP, Thompson A. Acute dyskinesia on starting methylphenidate after risperidone withdrawal. *Pediatr Neurol* (2007) 37, 287–8.
5. Sabuncuoglu O. Risperidone-to-methylphenidate switch reaction in children: three cases. *J Psychopharmacol* (2007) 21, 216–19.
6. Benjamin E, Salek S. Stimulant-atypical antipsychotic interaction and acute dystonia. *J Am Acad Child Adolesc Psychiatry* (2005) 44, 510–12. Erratum. ibid., 960.
7. Levine JB, Deneys ML, Benjamin S. Dystonia with combined antipsychotic and stimulant treatment. *J Am Acad Child Adolesc Psychiatry* (2007) 46, 665–6.

Methylphenidate + St John's wort (*Hypericum perforatum*)

St John's wort may decrease the efficacy of methylphenidate in the treatment of attention deficit hyperactivity disorder.

Clinical evidence, mechanism, importance and management

A 22-year-old man who had been successfully treated with methylphenidate 20 mg daily for attention deficit hyperactivity disorder (ADHD) for 6 months started to take St John's wort 600 mg daily. Over the next 4 months the efficacy of methylphenidate decreased, but 3 weeks after St John's wort was stopped, methylphenidate became more effective. No adverse effects were seen during the concurrent use of the herbal medicine and the drug.[1]

This is an isolated case report and therefore no general recommendations can be made. However, if the efficacy of methylphenidate becomes reduced, it may be worth questioning the patient about St John's wort use, and giving consideration to stopping the herb.

1. Niederhofer H. St John's wort may diminish methylphenidate's efficacy in treating patients suffering from attention deficit hyperactivity disorder. *Med Hypotheses* (2007) 68, 1189.

Modafinil + Cocaine

Modafinil does not appear to alter the haemodynamic effects of cocaine, but it may blunt cocaine-induced euphoria and increase some cocaine-related minor adverse effects. Armodafinil would be expected to interact in a similar way to modafinil.

Clinical evidence, mechanism, importance and management

In a placebo-controlled study in 7 subjects, pretreatment with modafinil 200 or 400 mg daily for 4 days did not affect the increase in blood pressure, pulse, temperature, or changes in ECG, produced by a single 30-mg intravenous dose of cocaine. However, subjective cocaine-induced euphoria was blunted.[1] A similar lack of any significant haemodynamic interaction was found in 12 cocaine-dependent subjects who were given modafinil 400 or 800 mg daily and infusions of 20 or 40 mg of cocaine.[2] No serious adverse events were reported in a study of cocaine abstinence in 30 cocaine-dependent patients given modafinil 200 to 400 mg daily for 8 weeks, when compared with 32 patients given placebo. However, modafinil increased the incidence of minor adverse events including nausea, dizziness, anxiety and tachycardia, which required a dose reduction from 400 mg to 300 or 200 mg daily in 6 patients.[3]

In a placebo-controlled study in 12 cocaine-dependent subjects, modafinil 400 or 800 mg daily for 7 days reduced the peak plasma levels of intravenous cocaine 40 mg, given over one minute. The $AUC_{0\text{-}3}$ of cocaine was reduced by about 20% by modafinil, but there were no statistically significant changes in the total AUC, clearance, or elimination half-life of cocaine.[4] **Armodafinil**, the *R*-isomer of modafinil, would be expected to interact in a similar way and it would seem prudent to follow the same precautions given for modafinil.

Note that the manufacturer of modafinil[5] advises caution and the manufacturer of armodafinil[6] advises close monitoring (e.g. of drug-seeking behaviour) if modafinil is given to patients with history of drug or illicit substance abuse.

1. Dackis CA, Lynch KG, Yu E, Samaha FF, Kampman KM, Cornish JW, Rowan A, Poole S, White L, O'Brien CP. Modafinil and cocaine: a double-blind, placebo-controlled drug interaction study. *Drug Alcohol Depend* (2003) 70, 29–37.
2. Malcolm R, Swayngim K, Donovan JL, DeVane CL, Elkashef A, Chiang N, Khan R, Mojsiak J, Myrick DL, Hedden S, Cochran K, Woolson RF. Modafinil and cocaine interactions. *Am J Drug Alcohol Abuse* (2006) 32, 577–87.
3. Dackis CA, Kampman KM, Lynch KG, Pettinati HM, O'Brien CP. A double-blind, placebo-controlled trial of modafinil for cocaine dependence. *Neuropsychopharmacology* (2005) 30, 205–11.
4. Donovan JL, DeVane CL, Malcolm RJ, Mojsiak J, Chiang CN, Elkashef A, Taylor RM. Modafinil influences the pharmacokinetics of intravenous cocaine in healthy cocaine-dependent volunteers. *Clin Pharmacokinet* (2005) 44, 753–65.
5. Provigil (Modafinil). Cephalon (UK) Ltd. UK Summary of product characteristics, August 2013.
6. Nuvigil (Armodafinil). Cephalon, Inc. US Prescribing information, June 2013.

Modafinil + Dexamfetamine

No pharmacokinetic interaction appears to occur between modafinil (and therefore armodafinil, the *R*-isomer of modafinil) and dexamfetamine.

Clinical evidence, mechanism, importance and management

In a steady-state study, 23 healthy subjects were given modafinil 200 mg daily for 7 days, then 400 mg daily for 3 weeks. During the last week, 10 of the subjects were also given dexamfetamine 20 mg daily, 7 hours after their modafinil dose. Dexamfetamine caused no significant change in the pharmacokinetics of modafinil and concurrent use was well tolerated. In addition, the pharmacokinetics of dexamfetamine did not appear to be affected by modafinil, when compared with values reported in the literature.[1] Similar results were found in a single-dose study.[2] No dose adjustments therefore appear to be necessary on concurrent use.

There appears to be no specific data regarding an interaction between **armodafinil**, the *R*-isomer of modafinil, and dexamfetamine, but it would be expected to behave in the same way as modafinil.

1. Hellriegel ET, Arora S, Nelson M, Robertson P. Steady-state pharmacokinetics and tolerability of modafinil administered alone or in combination with dextroamphetamine in healthy volunteers. *J Clin Pharmacol* (2002) 42, 448–58.
2. Wong YN, Wang L, Hartman L, Simcoe D, Chen Y, Laughton W, Eldon R, Markland C, Grebow P. Comparison of the single-dose pharmacokinetics and tolerability of modafinil and dextroamphetamine administered alone or in combination in healthy male volunteers. *J Clin Pharmacol* (1998) 38, 971–8.

Modafinil + Methylphenidate

No pharmacokinetic interaction appears to occur between modafinil (and therefore armodafinil, the *R*-isomer of modafinil) and methylphenidate.

Clinical evidence, mechanism, importance and management

In a single-dose study in healthy subjects, modafinil 200 mg and methylphenidate 40 mg were given together without any clinically relevant changes in the pharmacokinetics of either drug.[1] In a steady-state study, 30 healthy subjects were given modafinil 200 mg daily for 7 days, then 400 mg daily for 3 weeks. During the last week, 16 of the subjects were also given methylphenidate 20 mg daily, taken 8 hours after their modafinil dose. Methylphenidate caused no significant change in the pharmacokinetics of modafinil. In addition, the pharmacokinetics of methylphenidate did not appear to be affected by modafinil, when compared with values reported in the literature.[2] No dose adjustments would therefore appear to be necessary on concurrent use. There appears to be no specific data regarding an interaction between **armodafinil**, the *R*-isomer of modafinil, and methylphenidate, but it would be expected to behave in the same way as modafinil.

1. Wong YN, King SP, Laughton WB, McCormick GC, Grebow PE. Single-dose pharmacokinetics of modafinil and methylphenidate given alone or in combination in healthy male volunteers. *J Clin Pharmacol* (1998) 38, 276–82.
2. Hellriegel ET, Arora S, Nelson M, Robertson P. Steady-state pharmacokinetics and tolerability of modafinil given alone or in combination with methylphenidate in healthy volunteers. *J Clin Pharmacol* (2001) 41, 895–904.

Modafinil + Miscellaneous

The manufacturers of modafinil advise caution if CYP3A4 inducers, particularly phenytoin, are given with modafinil. Caution is also advised with CYP3A4 inhibitors (e.g. ketoconazole). There is speculation, based on *in vitro* studies, about some possible interactions with other drugs, such as CYP2C19 substrates (e.g. omeprazole). Modafinil is a weak inducer of CYP3A4 and therefore may be expected to interact with substrates of this isoenzyme (e.g. the calcium-channel blockers). Armodafinil, the *R*-isomer of modafinil, would be expected to interact in a similar way to modafinil.

Clinical evidence, mechanism, importance and management

(a) CYP2C19 substrates

In a study in 24 healthy subjects, the AUC and peak plasma concentration of a single 40-mg dose of **omeprazole** were increased by about 38% when it was given 2 hours after a single 400-mg dose of armodafinil, the *R*-isomer of modafinil. The AUC and peak plasma concentration of 5′-hydroxyomeprazole, the main metabolite of **omeprazole**, were decreased by 8% and 25%, respectively. **Omeprazole** clearance was decreased by about 37%. Armodafinil is an inhibitor of CYP2C19, by which omeprazole is metabolised. Concurrent use therefore leads to increases in **omeprazole** concentrations.[1]

The manufacturers of modafinil[2,3] and armodafinil[4] note that the concentrations of other drugs that are CYP2C19 substrates (they name drugs including **omeprazole, phenytoin** and **propranolol**) may be increased by modafinil and armodafinil and they state that dose reductions of these drugs may be required. Until more is known, it may be prudent to be alert for an increase in the adverse effects of **phenytoin** (e.g. blurred vision, nystagmus, ataxia or drowsiness). However, note that CYP2C19 is only of minor relevance in the metabolism of **propranolol**, and **omeprazole** has a very wide therapeutic margin, so a clinically relevant interaction with these drugs seems unlikely. See also *Phenytoin*, below.

(b) CYP3A4 inducers and inhibitors

Modafinil and armodafinil are CYP3A4 substrates, and the manufacturers therefore reasonably suggest that their metabolism will be increased by known CYP3A4 inducers such as **carbamazepine**,[2-4] **phenobarbital**,[2-4] [and therefore probably **primidone**] and **rifampicin (rifampin)**.[3,4] See also *Phenytoin*, below.

Similarly, inhibitors of CYP3A4 (**itraconazole**, **ketoconazole**,[2-4] and **erythromycin**[4] are specifically named) are predicted to increase armodafinil and modafinil concentrations.[3,4] However, clinically relevant interactions with either CYP3A4 inducers or inhibitors seem unlikely because CYP3A4 is not the only cytochrome P450 isoenzyme that is involved in the metabolism of modafinil and armodafinil. Nevertheless, until this is established it may be prudent to monitor for modafinil or armodafinil efficacy with any CYP3A4 inducer, and modafinil or armodafinil adverse effects (e.g. headache, insomnia, confusion) with any CYP3A4 inhibitors.

(c) CYP3A4 substrates

Modafinil and armodafinil are inducers of CYP3A4 (see 'Benzodiazepines + Modafinil', p.830). The manufacturers therefore predict that it may reduce the concentrations of drugs that are CYP3A4 substrates,[2-4] particularly those that undergo significant presystemic metabolism.[2] The UK manufacturer of modafinil[2] specifically names drugs including **buspirone**, the **HIV-protease inhibitors**, and most of the **calcium-channel blockers** and **statins**. However, note that only some statins, namely atorvastatin, lovastatin and simvastatin, are CYP3A4 substrates, and although the **HIV-protease inhibitors** are *substrates* of CYP3A4, many are potent *inhibitors* of this isoenzyme, and therefore, if anything, an interaction affecting modafinil concentrations (see under *CYP3A4 inducers and inhibitors*, above) seems more likely.

For a list of substrates of CYP3A4, see 'Table 1.10', p.12.

(d) Food

The manufacturer of armodafinil states that the peak concentrations of armodafinil are attained after about 2 hours when it is taken in the fasting state, but are delayed by 2 to 4 hours and increased when it is given with food.[4] However, as food has only minimal effects on the overall bioavailability of armodafinil, a clinically important interaction is unlikely.

(e) Phenytoin

In vitro evidence indicates that modafinil may possibly inhibit the metabolism of phenytoin by CYP2C9 and CYP2C19; therefore there is some reason for monitoring concurrent use for evidence of increased phenytoin effects and toxicity.[2,3] Nevertheless, modafinil did not have any clinically relevant inhibitory effect on CYP2C9 using warfarin as a substrate (see 'Coumarins + Modafinil', p.446).

Note that phenytoin is also an inducer of CYP3A4, and so may be expected to reduce modafinil concentrations, see under *CYP3A4 inducers and inhibitors*, above.

It may be prudent to expect **fosphenytoin**, a prodrug of phenytoin, to interact in the same way as phenytoin, and armodafinil to interact with phenytoin and **fosphenytoin** in the same way as modafinil.

1. Darwish M, Kirby M, Robertson P, Hellriegel ET. Interaction profile of armodafinil with medications metabolized by cytochrome P450 enzymes 1A2, 3A4 and 2C19 in healthy subjects. *Clin Pharmacokinet* (2008) 47, 61–74.
2. Provigil (Modafinil). Cephalon (UK) Ltd. UK Summary of product characteristics, August 2013.
3. Provigil (Modafinil). Cephalon, Inc. US Prescribing information, October 2010.
4. Nuvigil (Armodafinil). Cephalon, Inc. US Prescribing information, June 2013.

Orlistat + Anorectics

Orlistat does not appear to affect the bioavailability or adverse effects of phentermine or the metabolites or adverse effects of sibutramine.

Clinical evidence, mechanism, importance and management

In two pharmacokinetic studies, healthy subjects were given phentermine 37.5 mg daily for 7 days or sibutramine 10 mg daily for 7 days with orlistat 120 mg three times daily for 6 or 7 days. Orlistat did not affect the bioavailability of phentermine or the active metabolites of sibutramine, and concurrent use did not appear to increase the incidence of adverse effects, or cause significant changes in vital signs (e.g. heart rate, blood pressure).[1] No particular precautions therefore appear to be necessary if either of these drugs is given with orlistat.

1. Zhi J, Moore R, Kanitra L, Mulligan TE. Pharmacokinetic evaluation of the possible interaction between selected concomitant medications and orlistat at steady state in healthy subjects. *J Clin Pharmacol* (2002) 42, 1011–19.

Orlistat + Sucrose polyesters

A single case report suggests that the concurrent use of orlistat and sucrose polyesters (*Olestra* – used in some foods as a fat substitute) can result in additive gastrointestinal adverse effects (soft, fatty/oily stools, increased flatus and abdominal pain). In the case in question, symptoms resolved when the patient stopped eating *Olestra*-containing food while continuing to take orlistat.[1]

1. Heck AM, Calis KA, McDuffie JR, Carobene SE, Yanovski JA. Additive gastrointestinal effects with concomitant use of olestra and orlistat. *Ann Pharmacother* (2002) 36, 1003–5.

Phenmetrazine + Barbiturates

The CNS adverse effects and the weight reducing effects of phenmetrazine are reduced by amobarbital. Psychotic episodes occurred in two patients taking barbiturates and phenmetrazine.

Clinical evidence, mechanism, importance and management

A comparative study in 50 overweight adults, of the effects of phenmetrazine 25 mg three times daily with or without **amobarbital** 30 mg three times daily, found that although the adverse CNS effects, particularly insomnia, headache and nervousness, were decreased by the presence of the barbiturate, the weight reducing effects were also decreased (by 65%).[1]

A case report describes two cases of psychoses induced by the long-term use of barbiturates in combination with phenmetrazine, which resolved when the barbiturates or phenmetrazine were withdrawn.[2]

1. Hadler AJ. Phenmetrazine vs. phenmetrazine with amobarbital for weight reduction: a double-blind study. *Curr Ther Res* (1969) 11, 750–4.
2. Vina<r-CZ/V>ová E, Vina<r-CZ/V> O. Psychotické epizody, vyvolané kombinací barbiturát<u-ANG-STROM> s fenmetrazinem. *Cesk Psychiatr* (1971) 67, 284–91.

Rimonabant + Miscellaneous

Ketoconazole, a potent CYP3A4 inhibitor, doubles the AUC of rimonabant; other potent CYP3A4 inhibitors are expected to interact similarly, whereas potent CYP3A4 inducers are expected to lower rimonabant levels. Rimonabant may slightly increase ciclosporin exposure but does not appear to affect the levels of oral contraceptives, digoxin, midazolam, tacrolimus or warfarin. Alcohol, lorazepam, and orlistat do not appear to alter rimonabant levels.

Clinical evidence, mechanism, importance and management

(a) Ciclosporin and Tacrolimus

In a study in stable kidney transplant patients taking either ciclosporin (10 patients) or tacrolimus (8 patients), the use of rimonabant 20 mg daily for 2 months increased the AUC of ciclosporin by about 20%, but had no significant effect on tacrolimus pharmacokinetics. The effect on ciclosporin pharmacokinetics was probably of marginal clinical relevance as trough levels were not affected to a statistically significant extent, although they were increased by 36%. However, possibly because the small study size may have masked an effect on ciclosporin trough levels, it was suggested that ciclosporin levels should be more closely monitored if rimonabant is also given.[1]

(b) CYP3A4 inducers and inhibitors

Rimonabant is partly metabolised by the cytochrome P450 isoenzyme CYP3A4. **Ketoconazole**, a potent CYP3A4 inhibitor, doubles the AUC of rimonabant. The manufacturer therefore predicted that other potent CYP3A4 inhibitors (they named **clarithromycin**, **itraconazole**, **nefazodone**, **ritonavir**, and **telithromycin**) will also raise rimonabant levels, and they therefore advised caution on their concurrent use.[2] It would seem prudent to be alert for rimonabant adverse effects (e.g. nausea, dizziness or insomnia). The manufacturer similarly suggested that potent CYP3A4 inducers (such as **carbamazepine**, **phenobarbital** (and therefore probably **primidone**, which is metabolised to phenobarbital), **phenytoin** (and therefore probably **fosphenytoin**, a prodrug of phenytoin), **rifampicin** (**rifampin**) and **St John's wort**) may lower rimonabant plasma levels.[2] If concurrent use is necessary, monitor to ensure that rimonabant remains effective. See 'Table 1.9', p.11, for a list of clinically relevant CYP3A4 inducers and inhibitors.

(c) Miscellaneous

In clinical studies, **digoxin**, **midazolam**, and **warfarin** were given with rimonabant to assess the effect of rimonabant on P-glycoprotein, CYP3A4 and CYP2C9, respectively. As rimonabant did not interact with these drugs, the manufacturer stated that this confirms *in vitro* evidence that rimonabant has no effect on these isoenzymes or drug transporter, and would not be expected to interact with other substrates of P-glycoprotein, CYP3A4 or CYP2C9. The manufacturer also noted that rimonabant had no effect on the pharmacokinetics of an oral hormonal contraceptive containing **ethinylestradiol** and **levonorgestrel**, and that **alcohol**, **lorazepam**, and **orlistat** did not affect the plasma levels of rimonabant.[2]

1. Amundsen R, Asberg A, Robertsen I, Vethe NT, Bergan S, Hartmann A, Midtvedt K. Rimonabant affects cyclosporine a, but not tacrolimus pharmacokinetics in renal transplant recipients. *Transplantation* (2009) 87, 1221–4.
2. Acomplia (Rimonabant). Sanofi-Aventis. UK Summary of product characteristics, October 2007.

Sibutramine + Azoles

Ketoconazole, a potent CYP3A4 inhibitor, modestly increases the steady-state levels of sibutramine and its active metabolites. Other azoles that potently inhibit CYP3A4 are expected to interact similarly.

Clinical evidence, mechanism, importance and management

In a study, 12 obese patients were given sibutramine 20 mg daily for 14 days, with **ketoconazole** 200 mg twice daily for the last 7 days. **Ketoconazole** caused moderate increases in the serum levels of sibutramine and its two metabolites (AUC and maximum serum level increases of 58% and 36%, respectively, for metabolite M_1, and 20% and 19%, respectively, for metabolite M_2). Small increases in heart rates were seen (2.5 bpm at 4 hours and 1.4 bpm at 8 hours), while ECG parameters were unchanged.[1] **Ketoconazole** probably raised sibutramine levels by inhibiting the cytochrome P450 isoenzyme CYP3A4, by which sibutramine is metabolised. Sibutramine alone can cause an increase in heart rate, and a rate increase of 10 bpm is an indication to withdraw the drug. Therefore, the manufacturer in the UK[2] suggested that caution should be exercised when sibutramine is used with **ketoconazole**. They also suggested that, due to its ability to inhibit CYP3A4, **itraconazole** should also be used with caution. Note that, of the azoles, **posaconazole** and **voriconazole** are also potent CYP3A4 inhibitors and any caution applied to **ketoconazole** or **itraconazole** as a result of CYP3A4 inhibition is probably also appropriate with these drugs.

A clinically relevant interaction between sibutramine and any of these azoles seems unlikely; however, until more is known it may be prudent to be alert for an increase in sibutramine adverse effects (e.g. dry mouth, headache, insomnia, and constipation) and adjust treatment accordingly.

1. Hinson JL, Leone MB, Kisiki MJ, Moult JT, Trammel JT, Faulkner RD. Steady-state interaction study of sibutramine (Meridia) and ketoconazole in uncomplicated obese subjects. *Pharm Res* (1996) 13 (9 Suppl), S116.
2. Reductil (Sibutramine hydrochloride monohydrate). Abbott Laboratories Ltd. UK Summary of product characteristics, December 2009.

Sibutramine + Food

Food may delay the time to peak plasma levels of sibutramine and its metabolites. The bioavailability of sibutramine and possibly its M_1 metabolite may be increased by food.

Clinical evidence, mechanism, importance and management

A study in 6 healthy subjects found that, compared with the fasted state, a high-fat meal increased the AUC and maximum plasma level of sibutramine 15 mg by about fivefold and threefold, respectively, and delayed its peak plasma level by 2 to 4 hours. The AUC and maximum plasma level of the M_1 metabolite was increased twofold, but the M_2 metabolite was not affected.[1] In contrast, another study found that giving a single 20-mg dose of sibutramine with a standard breakfast modestly reduced the peak levels of the active metabolites M_1 and M_2 by 27% and 32%, respectively, and delayed their peak levels by about 3 hours. However, the AUCs of M_1 and M_2 were not significantly altered.[2] Despite the large increases in sibutramine levels the manufacturers have stated that it may be given with or without food.[2,3] This is presumably because sibutramine is rapidly metabolised to its active metabolites, which are only modestly affected by food.

1. Abolfathi Z, Couture J, Vallée F, LeBel M, Tanguay M, Masson É. A pilot study to evaluate the pharmacokinetics of sibutramine in healthy subjects under fasting and fed conditions. *J Pharm Pharm Sci* (2004) 7, 345–9.
2. Meridia (Sibutramine hydrochloride monohydrate). Abbott Laboratories. US Prescribing information, January 2010.
3. Reductil (Sibutramine hydrochloride monohydrate). Abbott Laboratories Ltd. UK Summary of product characteristics, December 2009.

Sibutramine + Macrolides

The UK manufacturer of sibutramine suggested that clarithromycin, erythromycin and troleandomycin may interact with sibutramine. However, a study suggests that erythromycin does not affect the pharmacokinetics of sibutramine.

Clinical evidence, mechanism, importance and management

Twelve obese patients were given sibutramine 20 mg daily for 14 days, with **erythromycin** 500 mg three times daily for the last 7 days. It was found that, apart from some slight and unimportant changes in the pharmacokinetics of the metabolites of sibutramine (probably caused by some inhibition of the cytochrome P450 isoenzyme CYP3A4), the pharmacokinetics of sibutramine were not significantly altered by **erythromycin**. No blood pressure changes were seen and only very small and clinically irrelevant increases in the QTc interval and heart rate occurred.[1] The extent of any interaction appears to be too small to matter,[1] and there would seem to be no reason for avoiding the concurrent use of these two drugs. Nevertheless, the UK manufacturer suggested that caution should be exercised if both drugs are given, probably because sibutramine is principally metabolised by CYP3A4.[2] They also extrapolated their caution to other macrolides that inhibit CYP3A4, and named **clarithromycin** and **troleandomycin**.

1. Hinson JL, Leone MB, Leese PT, Moult JT, Carter FJ, Faulkner RD. Steady-state interaction study of sibutramine (Meridia) and erythromycin in uncomplicated obese subjects. *Pharm Res* (1996) 13 (9 Suppl), S116.
2. Reductil (Sibutramine hydrochloride monohydrate). Abbott Laboratories Ltd. UK Summary of product characteristics, December 2009.

Sibutramine + Miscellaneous

The manufacturers of sibutramine have contraindicated its use with MAOIs and centrally-acting appetite suppressants; the UK manufacturers also contraindicated antipsychotics. The manufacturers also suggest that sibutramine should not be given with serotonergic drugs or given with caution to patients taking nasal decongestants. The plasma levels of sibutramine are moderately increased by olanzapine and omeprazole, and are predicted to be increased by grapefruit juice. Conversely, sibutramine levels are predicted to be reduced by CYP3A4 inducers (e.g. rifampicin). Cimetidine has no clinically relevant effect on the pharmacokinetics of sibutramine and sibutramine does not affect inhibition of ovulation in response to an oral hormonal contraceptive. No clinically relevant pharmacokinetic interaction has been seen between sibutramine and simvastatin.

Clinical evidence, mechanism, importance and management

(a) Centrally-acting appetite suppressants and Nasal Decongestants

The manufacturers have stated that the concurrent use of sibutramine and other centrally-acting appetite suppressants is contraindicated.[1,2] This may be expected to include drugs such as **diethylpropion, phentermine** and the **amfetamines**. Note that both sibutramine and the **amfetamines** have serotonergic effects, and concurrent use might lead to the serotonin syndrome (see under *Serotonergic drugs*, below). No work appears to have been done to see what happens if sibutramine is given with sympathomimetics, including certain **decongestants, cough, cold** and **allergy medications**, but the manufacturers advise caution because of the risk of raised blood pressure or heart rate. The manufacturers in the UK and US both list **ephedrine** and **pseudoephedrine**,[1,2] while in the UK **xylometazoline** is also specifically named.[2] It would therefore also seem prudent to apply this caution to the related drug, **oxymetazoline**.

(b) Cimetidine

In a study, 12 healthy subjects were given cimetidine 400 mg twice daily was given with sibutramine 15 mg daily. Cimetidine raised the maximum serum levels and AUCs of the combined sibutramine metabolites by 3.4% and 7.3%, respectively.[1] These changes are too small to be of clinical significance.

(c) CYP3A4 inducers

The UK manufacturer stated that **carbamazepine, dexamethasone, phenobarbital** [and therefore probably **primidone**, which is metabolised to phenobarbital], **phenytoin** [and therefore probably **fosphenytoin**, a prodrug of phenytoin] and **rifampicin (rifampin)** are all inducers of CYP3A4, an isoenzyme involved in the metabolism of sibutramine.[2] These drugs might therefore increase the metabolism of sibutramine resulting in a fall in its serum levels. However, this has not been studied experimentally and, at the present time, the existence, the extent and the possible clinical relevance of any such interaction is unknown. Furthermore, clinically relevant interactions occurring as a result of **dexamethasone** inducing CYP3A4 appear rare.

(d) Grapefruit juice

Grapefruit juice is predicted to interact with sibutramine by inhibiting its metabolism by the cytochrome P450 isoenzyme CYP3A4.[3] It has been suggested that, as the manufacturer of sibutramine advises caution if CYP3A4 inhibitors such as ketoconazole are given, it might also be appropriate to suggest avoidance of grapefruit juice, especially as patients might consider the 'grapefruit diet' as an adjunct to weight reduction.[3] However, only modest increases in sibutramine levels were seen with the potent CYP3A4 inhibitor, ketoconazole, see 'Sibutramine + Azoles', p.223, and therefore a clinically relevant interaction with grapefruit juice would not generally be anticipated.

(e) MAOIs

There are no reports of adverse reactions between sibutramine and the MAOIs. However, sibutramine inhibits serotonin reuptake, and because the serious serotonin syndrome can occur when MAOIs and SSRIs are used together, the manufacturers have contraindicated the concurrent use of sibutramine and MAOIs. They state that 14 days should elapse between stopping either drug and starting the other.[1,2] The US manufacturer includes **selegiline** in this warning.[1] For more information on serotonin syndrome and its management, see 'Drugs that cause serotonin syndrome + Other drugs that cause serotonin syndrome', p.1471.

(f) Olanzapine

In a study in healthy subjects, olanzapine moderately increased the AUC and maximum plasma levels of sibutramine by 63% and 47%, respectively, whereas sibutramine had no significant effect on olanzapine pharmacokinetics.[1] However, the UK manufacturer of sibutramine contraindicated its use both with and for 2 weeks after the use of antipsychotics.[2]

(g) Omeprazole

In a study in 26 healthy subjects, omeprazole 20 mg daily for 7 days increased the maximum plasma level and AUC of sibutramine by 57% and 67%, respectively, and increased the levels of the active M_1 metabolite of sibutramine by 30% and 40%, respectively. The pharmacokinetics of the M_2 metabolite of sibutramine were not significantly affected. Sibutramine had no significant effect on omeprazole pharmacokinetics.[1] These changes are modest, and no dose adjustment would be expected to be necessary on concurrent use.

(h) Oral hormonal contraceptives

A crossover study in 12 subjects found that sibutramine 15 mg daily, given for 8 weeks, had no clinically significant effect on the inhibition of ovulation caused by an oral hormonal contraceptive, and it was concluded that there is no need to use alternative contraceptive methods while taking sibutramine.[1]

(i) Serotonergic drugs

Because sibutramine inhibits serotonin uptake, and because the serious serotonin syndrome has been seen when serotonergic drugs were taken with SSRIs, the manufacturers have stated that sibutramine should not be taken with any serotonergic drugs.[1,2] They name **dextromethorphan, dihydroergotamine, fentanyl, pentazocine, pethidine (meperidine)**, SSRIs, **sumatriptan**, and **tryptophan**. Possible cases have been reported for sibutramine and the SSRIs, see 'SSRIs + Sibutramine', p.1495. The US manufacturer also includes **lithium** in their list.[1] Note that this list is not exhaustive (see *MAOIs*, above) and a case of serotonin syndrome has been seen when **venlafaxine** was given with sibutramine, see 'SNRIs; Venlafaxine + Sibutramine', p.1483. The extent of the risk with these serotonergic drugs is not known, but because of the potential severity of the reaction this warning would seem to be a prudent precaution. For more information about serotonin syndrome and its management, see 'Drugs that cause serotonin syndrome + Other drugs that cause serotonin syndrome', p.1471.

(j) Simvastatin

In a study in 27 healthy subjects, giving simvastatin 20 mg daily in the evening and sibutramine 15 mg daily in the morning for 7 days resulted in a slight decrease in the maximum plasma levels and AUC of sibutramine of 14% and 21%, respectively. The plasma levels of the active M_1 and M_2 metabolites of sibutramine combined were not significantly affected, although the plasma levels of the M_1 metabolite were slightly reduced. Sibutramine decreased the maximum levels and AUC of simvastatin by 25% and 15%, respectively, but the AUC of the active metabolite of simvastatin, simvastatin acid, was increased by 7%.[1] These changes are not expected to be clinically significant.

1. Meridia (Sibutramine hydrochloride monohydrate). Abbott Laboratories. US Prescribing information, January 2010.
2. Reductil (Sibutramine hydrochloride monohydrate). Abbott Laboratories Ltd. UK Summary of product characteristics, December 2009.
3. Bailey DG, Dresser GK. Interactions between grapefruit juice and cardiovascular drugs. *Am J Cardiovasc Drugs* (2004) 4, 281–97.

8

Anthelmintics, Antifungals and Antiprotozoals

'Table 8.1', p.226, lists the drugs covered in this section by therapeutic group and drug class. If the anti-infective is the drug causing the interaction, the interaction is generally dealt with under the affected drug. Also note that drugs such as the 5-nitroimidazoles (e.g. metronidazole), which have actions against more than one type of organism (e.g. bacteria and protozoa), are covered under Antibacterials.

(a) Amphotericin B

Intravenous amphotericin B causes important pharmacodynamic interactions via additive nephrotoxicity and myelotoxicity, and might increase the cardiotoxicity of other drugs because of amphotericin-induced hypokalaemia. No important pharmacokinetic interactions are known. Lipid formulations of amphotericin B are less nephrotoxic than non-lipid formulations, and would therefore be expected to interact less frequently. Orally administered amphotericin B is not absorbed systemically, and no interactions are established.

(b) Azoles

The most important interactions affecting and caused by the azoles are those resulting from inhibition and induction of cytochrome P450 isoenzymes.

- **Fluconazole** is principally (80%) excreted unchanged in the urine, so is less affected by enzyme inducers and inhibitors than some other azoles. Fluconazole is a potent inhibitor of CYP2C19, a dose-dependent weak to moderate inhibitor of CYP2C9, and it moderately inhibits CYP3A4. Interactions are less likely with single doses used for genital candidiasis than with longer term use.
- **Itraconazole** is extensively metabolised by CYP3A4, and its metabolism might become saturated with multiple dosing. Itraconazole and its major metabolite, hydroxy-itraconazole, are potent inhibitors of CYP3A4. Itraconazole is also known to inhibit P-glycoprotein, as demonstrated by its effects on digoxin (see 'Digoxin + Azoles; Itraconazole or Ketoconazole', p.1083).
- **Ketoconazole** is extensively metabolised, particularly by CYP3A4. It is also a potent inhibitor of CYP3A4. Ketoconazole is also known to inhibit P-glycoprotein (see 'Digoxin + Azoles; Itraconazole or Ketoconazole', p.1083).
- **Miconazole** is a moderate inhibitor of CYP2C9. Because this azole is generally used topically as pessaries, cream, or an oral gel, it is less likely to cause interactions, although it should be noted that at maximum doses of the oral gel, a sufficient quantity might be absorbed to cause systemic effects, see 'Coumarins and related drugs + Azoles; Miconazole', p.409.
- **Posaconazole** is metabolised via UDP-glucuronidation, and might also be a substrate for P-glycoprotein. Posaconazole is a moderate inhibitor of CYP3A4.
- **Voriconazole** is metabolised by a number of pathways including CYP3A4. Voriconazole is an inhibitor of CYP2C9 (weak to moderate), CYP2C19 (moderate), and CYP3A4 (potent).

A number of other azoles are only used topically in the form of creams or intravaginal preparations, and have not been associated with drug interactions, presumably since their systemic absorption is so low, see 'Azoles; Topical + Miscellaneous', p.242.

Fluconazole, ketoconazole, and voriconazole have been associated with prolongation of the QT interval, although generally not to a clinically relevant extent. However, they might also raise the plasma concentration of other drugs that prolong the QT interval, and these combinations are often contraindicated, see 'Antihistamines + Azoles', p.630.

1. Venkatakrishnan K, von Moltke LL, Greenblatt DJ. Effects of the antifungal agents on oxidative drug metabolism: clinical relevance. *Clin Pharmacokinet* (2000) 38, 111–80.

Table 8.1 Anthelmintics, antifungals and antimalarials and other antiprotozoals

Group	*Drugs*
Anthelmintics	
Benzimidazole derivatives	Albendazole, Flubendazole, Mebendazole, Tiabendazole (Thiabendazole)
Organophosphorous compounds	Metrifonate (Metriphonate)
Other	Diethylcarbamazine, Ivermectin, Levamisole, Niclosamide, Oxamniquine, Piperazine, Praziquantel, Pyrantel
Antifungals	
Allylamines	Naftifine, Terbinafine
Azoles:	
Imidazoles	Bifonazole,* Butoconazole,* Chlormidazole,* Clotrimazole,* Econazole,* Fenticonazole,* Isoconazole,* Ketoconazole, Miconazole, Oxiconazole,* Sertaconazole,* Sulconazole,* Tioconazole*
Triazoles	Fluconazole, Itraconazole, Posaconazole, Terconazole,* Voriconazole
Echinocandins	Anidulafungin, Caspofungin, Micafungin
Polyene antibacterials	Amphotericin B, Natamycin,* Nystatin*
Other	Amorolfine,* Butenafine,* Ciclopirox,* Flucytosine, Griseofulvin, Tolnaftate*
Antimalarials	
4-aminoquinolines	Amodiaquine, Chloroquine, Hydroxychloroquine
8-aminoquinolines	Primaquine
4-methanolquinolines	Mefloquine, Quinine
Artemisinin derivatives	Artemether, Artemotil, Artesunate, Artemether with Lumefantrine
Other	Atovaquone, Doxycycline,† Halofantrine, Lumefantrine, Proguanil, Pyrimethamine with Sulfadoxine, Tetracycline†
Antiprotozoals	
Antimony compounds	Sodium stibogluconate
Arsenicals	Melarsoprol
5-nitroimidazoles†	Metronidazole, Ornidazole, Tinidazole
Nitrofuran	Furazolidone, Nifurtimox
Other	Atovaquone, Diiodohydroxyquinoline, Diloxanide furoate, Eflornithine, Mepacrine, Nitazoxanide, Pentamidine, Pyrimethamine with Sulfadiazine, Suramin

* Mainly used by topical application
† Covered under Antibacterials

Albendazole or Mebendazole + Antiepileptics; Enzyme-inducing

Carbamazepine, phenytoin, and phenobarbital lower the plasma concentrations of albendazole and mebendazole.

Clinical evidence

(a) Albendazole

In one study, 32 patients with intraparenchymatous neurocysticercosis were given albendazole 7.5 mg/kg every 12 hours for 8 days. Some of these patients were also taking antiepileptics: either **phenytoin** 200 to 300 mg daily (9 patients), **carbamazepine** 600 to 1200 mg daily (9 patients), or **phenobarbital** 100 to 300 mg daily (5 patients) all for at least 3 months. A control group (9 patients) did not receive any antiepileptics. The AUCs for (+)-albendazole sulfoxide were 49%, 66%, and 61% lower than the control group for the **carbamazepine**, **phenytoin**, and **phenobarbital** groups, respectively. The maximum plasma concentrations of (+)-albendazole sulfoxide were 50 to 63% lower and the half-lives about 3 to 4 hours shorter. The AUCs, maximum plasma concentrations and half-life of (−)-albendazole sulfoxide (present in much lower amounts than the (+)-isomer) were similarly reduced by the antiepileptics.[1]

(b) Mebendazole

A retrospective analysis found that patients with echinococcosis taking mebendazole and **phenytoin** or **carbamazepine** tended to have lower plasma mebendazole concentrations than patients not taking these antiepileptics.[2] However, the plasma concentration of mebendazole was only measured once in each patient and the sample size was too small to provide meaningful results. Some patients had a clinically important rise in mebendazole concentration when they were switched from **phenytoin** or **carbamazepine** to valproic acid,[2] although this increase would be expected when the enzyme-inducing drug is stopped.

Mechanism

Carbamazepine, phenytoin, and phenobarbital appear to induce the oxidative metabolism of albendazole by CYP3A to roughly the same extent, resulting in reduced concentrations of albendazole sulfoxide, the active metabolite of albendazole. Mebendazole is similarly affected.

Importance and management

The pharmacokinetic interactions between albendazole or mebendazole and the enzyme-inducing antiepileptics are established, and are likely to be clinically important when these anthelmintics are used to treat systemic worm infections. It might be necessary to increase the albendazole or mebendazole dose in patients also taking phenytoin (and therefore probably **fosphenytoin**), carbamazepine, or phenobarbital (and therefore **primidone**). Monitor the outcome of concurrent use.

These interactions are of no importance when albendazole or mebendazole are used for intestinal worm infections (where they have a local effect on the worms in the gut).

1. Lanchote VL, Garcia FS, Dreossi SAC, Takayanagui OM. Pharmacokinetic interaction between albendazole sulfoxide enantiomers and antiepileptic drugs in patients with neurocysticercosis. *Ther Drug Monit* (2002) 24, 338–45.
2. Luder PJ, Siffert B, Witassek F, Meister F, Bircher J. Treatment of hydatid disease with high oral doses of mebendazole. Long-term follow-up of plasma mebendazole levels and drug interactions. *Eur J Clin Pharmacol* (1986) 31, 443–8.

Albendazole with Ivermectin + Azithromycin

The combination of albendazole and ivermectin with azithromycin results in moderate changes in the pharmacokinetics of all three drugs.

Clinical evidence, mechanism, importance and management

In a three-way crossover study, 18 healthy subjects were given single doses of either azithromycin 500 mg alone, ivermectin 200 micrograms/kg (to the nearest 3 mg) with albendazole 400 mg, or all three drugs together. The combination of all three drugs increased the AUC and maximum concentration of azithromycin by 13% and 20%, respectively, and increased the AUC and maximum concentration of ivermectin by 31% and 27%, respectively. In addition, the AUC and maximum concentration of albendazole sulfoxide (active metabolite of albendazole) were reduced by 16% and 14%, respectively. No serious adverse effects were reported.[1] These changes are unlikely to be of clinical importance, although the authors note that large inter-individual variability was seen in the pharmacokinetics of these drugs, suggesting that some patients might experience greater effects. However, a pharmacokinetic model analysis of the data from this study suggests that the maximum ivermectin concentration that might be seen when it is given with azithromycin is lower than that previously shown to be safe.[2] Nonetheless, further clinical study is needed to establish the safety and efficacy of concurrent use.

Note that a study has found no pharmacokinetic interaction between albendazole and ivermectin, see 'Albendazole + Ivermectin', p.228.

1. Amsden GW, Gregory TB, Michalak CA, Glue P, Knirsch CA. Pharmacokinetics of azithromycin and the combination of ivermectin and albendazole when administered alone and concurrently in healthy volunteers. *Am J Trop Med Hyg* (2007) 76, 1153–7.
2. El-Tahtawy A, Glue P, Andrews EN, Mardekian J, Amsden GW, Knirsch CA. The effect of azithromycin on ivermectin pharmacokinetics – a population pharmacokinetic model analysis. *PLoS Negl Trop Dis* (2008) 2, e236.

Albendazole or Mebendazole + Cimetidine

Cimetidine raises the serum concentration of mebendazole, and prolongs the half-life of albendazole sulfoxide, the active metabolite of albendazole.

Clinical evidence

(a) Albendazole

In a study, 6 healthy subjects were given cimetidine 10 mg/kg twice daily for 48 hours before, and 36 hours after, [a single] 20-mg/kg dose of albendazole. Cimetidine inhibited the metabolism of the active sulfoxide metabolite of albendazole, as indicated by an increase in its elimination half-life from 7.4 hours to 19 hours. Cimetidine decreased the inter-individual variability in the maximum plasma concentration of albendazole sulfoxide by about 50%, although this was not statistically significant. In addition, the inter-individual variability in the AUC of albendazole sulfoxide was also decreased without being altered to a statistically significant extent.[1] A similar study by the same authors[2] also found that cimetidine reduced the increase in the albendazole sulfoxide concentration produced by grapefruit juice (see 'Albendazole + Grapefruit juice', p.228). Another study in patients with cystic echinococcosis given albendazole 20 mg/kg daily, for three 4-week courses separated by intervals of 10 days, found that concentrations of albendazole sulfoxide were higher in bile and hydatid cyst fluid in 7 patients who were also given cimetidine 10 mg/kg daily. The therapeutic benefit of concurrent use was reported to be greater than that of albendazole alone.[3]

(b) Mebendazole

A study in 8 patients (5 with peptic ulcers and 3 with hydatid cysts) taking mebendazole 1.5 g three times daily found that cimetidine 400 mg three times daily for 30 days increased the maximum plasma mebendazole concentration by 48%. The previously unresponsive hepatic hydatid cysts resolved totally.[4] However, a previous study had found smaller increases in the serum mebendazole concentration with cimetidine 1 g daily in divided doses, which were considered too small to be clinically useful.[5]

Mechanism

It is suggested that the interaction is caused by the enzyme inhibitory actions of cimetidine, which result in a reduction in the metabolism of albendazole (to its active metabolite albendazole sulfoxide)[1] and mebendazole.[4] However, as cimetidine might also inhibit the metabolism of albendazole sulfoxide to its inactive sulfone metabolite, any reduction in the concentration of albendazole sulfoxide are compensated for by its prolonged elimination half-life.[1] Cimetidine might also reduce albendazole absorption and minimise inter-patient variability by reducing gastric acidity,[1,2] but the reduction in absorption appears to be outweighed by the enzyme-inhibitory effects.

Importance and management

The pharmacokinetic interactions between cimetidine and albendazole or mebendazole appear to be established, but their clinical relevance is uncertain. Increased efficacy has been shown in some studies for systemic worm infections. There would seem to be no reason for avoiding concurrent use, but increased monitoring for efficacy and toxicity might be prudent.

1. Schipper HG, Koopmans RP, Nagy J, Butter JJ, Kager PA, Van Boxtel CJ. Effect of dose increase or cimetidine co-administration on albendazole bioavailability. *Am J Trop Med Hyg* (2000) 63, 270–3.
2. Nagy J, Schipper HG, Koopmans RP, Butter JJ, Van Boxtel CJ, Kager PA. Effect of grapefruit juice or cimetidine coadministration on albendazole bioavailability. *Am J Trop Med Hyg* (2002) 260–3.
3. Wen H, Zhang HW, Muhmut M, Zou PF, New RRC, Craig PS. Initial observation on albendazole in combination with cimetidine for the treatment of human cystic echinococcosis. *Ann Trop Med Parasitol* (1994) 88, 49–52.
4. Bekhti A, Pirotte J. Cimetidine increases serum mebendazole concentrations. Implications for treatment of hepatic hydatid cysts. *Br J Clin Pharmacol* (1987) 24, 390–2.
5. Luder PJ, Siffert B, Witassek F, Meister F, Bircher J. Treatment of hydatid disease with high oral doses of mebendazole. Long-term follow-up of plasma mebendazole levels and drug interactions. *Eur J Clin Pharmacol* (1986) 31, 443–8.

Albendazole + Dexamethasone

Dexamethasone can increase the plasma concentration of the active metabolite of albendazole, albendazole sulfoxide.

Clinical evidence

In one study albendazole 15 mg/kg daily in three divided doses was given to 8 patients with neurocysticercosis. The plasma concentration of the active metabolite of albendazole (albendazole sulfoxide) was found to be increased by about 50% by the use of dexamethasone 8 mg every 8 hours.[1] Another study did not detect a statistically significant increase in the maximum plasma concentration of albendazole sulfoxide when dexamethasone was given, but its AUC was increased twofold, and there was a decrease in its clearance.[2]

Mechanism

Uncertain. It has been suggested that dexamethasone is an inducer of CYP3A4, which is involved in the metabolism of albendazole. Concurrent use might therefore be expected to increase the concentration of the active metabolite, albendazole sulfoxide, but direct evidence to support this proposed mechanism appears to be lacking.

Dexamethasone appears not to alter the rate of formation of albendazole sulfoxide, but decreases its elimination.[2]

Importance and management

Information regarding an interaction between albendazole and the corticosteroids seems to be limited to this study with dexamethasone, but the interaction would appear to be established and potentially clinically important. The evidence suggests that albendazole can be given with dexamethasone without compromising treatment.[3]

1. Jung H, Hurtado M, Tulio Medina M, Sanchez M, Sotelo J. Dexamethasone increases plasma levels of albendazole. *J Neurol* (1990) 237, 279–80.
2. Takayanagui OM, Lanchote VL, Marques MPC, Bonato PS. Therapy for neurocysticercosis: pharmacokinetic interaction of albendazole sulfoxide with dexamethasone. *Ther Drug Monit* (1997) 19, 51–5.
3. Sotelo J, Jung H. Pharmacokinetic optimisation of the treatment of neurocysticercosis. *Clin Pharmacokinet* (1998) 34, 503–15.

Albendazole + Diethylcarbamazine

There appears to be no pharmacokinetic interaction between albendazole and diethylcarbamazine.

Clinical evidence, mechanism, importance and management

The pharmacokinetics of single doses of diethylcarbamazine 6 mg/kg and albendazole 400 mg were no different when groups of 14 amicrofilaraemic subjects given either drug alone were compared with another group of 14 subjects given both drugs.[1] This study suggests that there is no pharmacokinetic interaction between albendazole and diethylcarbamazine, and the lack of adverse events[1] suggests that concurrent use is safe.

1. Shenoy RK, Suma TK, John A, Arun SR, Kumaraswami V, Fleckenstein LL, Na-Bangchang K. The pharmacokinetics, safety and tolerability of the co-administration of diethylcarbamazine and albendazole. *Ann Trop Med Parasitol* (2002) 96, 603–14.

Albendazole + Food

Giving albendazole with a fatty meal markedly increases the plasma concentration of its active metabolite, albendazole sulfoxide.

Clinical evidence, mechanism, importance and management

A study in Sudanese men found that giving a single 400-mg dose of albendazole with a meal resulted in a 7.9-fold higher plasma concentration of the active metabolite, albendazole sulfoxide, than when albendazole was given in the fasted state.[1] Similarly, a further study in healthy subjects found that when albendazole 10 mg/kg was given with a fatty meal, rather than with water, the maximum plasma concentration of albendazole sulfoxide was increased more than 6-fold and the half-life decreased from 8.8 hours to 8.2 hours.[2] A study in 16 healthy subjects given a single 800-mg dose of albendazole after a fatty meal found that the maximum concentration and AUC of albendazole sulfoxide were increased sevenfold and eightfold, respectively, when compared with the fasted state.[3] Similarly, in two further studies in patients with echinococcosis or onchocerciasis, a fatty breakfast resulted in about a 4-fold increase in the plasma concentration of albendazole sulfoxide when compared with the fasting state.[4,5] Administration of a soybean emulsion of albendazole, rather than a tablet formulation, resulted in about a 60% increase in the maximum plasma concentration and AUC of albendazole sulfoxide.[6]

Albendazole absorption is poor and if it is being used for systemic infections, it is advisable to take it with a meal. For the treatment of intestinal parasites, giving albendazole on an empty stomach would enhance its local effect.[4]

1. Homeida M, Leahy W, Copeland S, Ali MMM, Harron DWG. Pharmacokinetic interaction between praziquantel and albendazole in Sudanese men. *Ann Trop Med Parasitol* (1994) 88, 551–9.
2. Nagy J, Schipper HG, Koopmans RP, Butter JJ, Van Boxtel CJ, Kager PA. Effect of grapefruit juice or cimetidine coadministration on albendazole bioavailability. *Am J Trop Med Hyg* (2002) 66, 260–3.
3. Mares SS, Jung CH, López AT, González-Esquivel DF. Influence of a Mexican diet on the bioavailability of albendazole. *Basic Clin Pharmacol Toxicol* (2005) 97, 122–4.
4. Lange H, Eggers R, Bircher J. Increased systemic availability of albendazole when taken with a fatty meal. *Eur J Clin Pharmacol* (1988) 34, 315–7.
5. Awadzi K, Hero M, Opoku NO, Büttner DW, Coventry PA, Prime MA, Orme MLE, Edwards G. The chemotherapy of onchocerciasis XVII. A clinical evaluation of albendazole in patients with onchocerciasis; effects of food and pretreatment with ivermectin on drug response and pharmacokinetics. *Trop Med Parasitol* (1994) 45, 203–8.
6. Mingjie W, Shuhua X, Junjie C, Bin L, Cheng F, Weixia S, Hotez P. Albendazole–soybean oil emulsion for the treatment of human cystic echinococcosis: evaluation of bioavailability and bioequivalence. *Acta Trop* (2002) 83, 177–81.

Albendazole + Grapefruit juice

Grapefruit juice increases the plasma concentration of albendazole sulfoxide, the active metabolite of albendazole.

Clinical evidence

In a study in 6 healthy subjects, 250 mL of double-strength grapefruit juice increased the peak plasma concentration of albendazole sulfoxide 3.2-fold and shortened its half-life by 46%. When cimetidine 10 mg/kg was also given, the effect of the grapefruit juice was diminished: the peak plasma concentration of albendazole sulfoxide was almost 50% lower than when albendazole was given with grapefruit juice alone. However, the peak plasma concentration of albendazole sulfoxide was still 2.7-fold greater in the presence of cimetidine and grapefruit juice than that achieved when albendazole was given with water.[1]

Mechanism

It has been suggested that grapefruit juice inhibits the metabolism of albendazole in the intestinal mucosa by CYP3A4, raising the plasma concentration of albendazole. The addition of cimetidine might decrease this effect as cimetidine inhibits the metabolism of albendazole to its active metabolite, and the changes in gastric pH caused by cimetidine might also reduce albendazole absorption (see 'Albendazole or Mebendazole + Cimetidine', p.227).[1]

Importance and management

Evidence for an interaction between albendazole and grapefruit juice appears to be limited to this study, and the clinical outcome of the change in albendazole sulfoxide concentration with grapefruit juice is uncertain. For systemic infections, increased absorption might be beneficial (although adverse effects could be increased), but the decrease in half-life might be detrimental. Further study is required to establish the clinical importance of this interaction.

1. Nagy J, Schipper HG, Koopmans RP, Butter JJ, Van Boxtel CJ, Kager PA. Effect of grapefruit juice or cimetidine coadministration on albendazole bioavailability. *Am J Trop Med Hyg* (2002) 66, 260–3.

Albendazole + Ivermectin

No pharmacokinetic interaction occurs between albendazole and ivermectin.

Clinical evidence, mechanism, importance and management

In a placebo-controlled study, 42 patients with onchocerciasis were given single doses of either ivermectin 200 micrograms/kg, albendazole 400 mg, or both drugs together. The pharmacokinetics of both drugs were not changed by concurrent use, and although the combination seemed to offer no advantage over ivermectin alone for the treatment on onchocerciasis, the combination appeared safe.[1] Another earlier study by the same research group found no change in the pharmacokinetics of albendazole sulfoxide given 5 to 7 days after ivermectin.[2] Similarly, no additive benefit was seen and the combination was well tolerated. No dose adjustments would be required during the concurrent use of albendazole and ivermectin.[1]

1. Awadzi K, Edwards G, Duke BOL, Opoku NO, Attah SK, Addy ET, Ardrey AE, Quarty BT. The co-administration of ivermectin and albendazole— safety, pharmacokinetics and efficacy against *Onchocerca volvulus*. *Ann Trop Med Parasitol* (2003) 97, 165–78.
2. Awadzi K, Hero M, Opoku NO, Büttner DW, Coventry PA, Prime MA, Orme ML'E, Edwards G. The chemotherapy of onchocerciasis XVII. A clinical evaluation of albendazole in patients with onchocerciasis; effects of food and pretreatment with ivermectin on drug response and pharmacokinetics. *Trop Med Parasitol* (1994) 45, 203–8.

Albendazole + Levamisole

In one study, levamisole moderately lowered the exposure to albendazole sulfoxide, the active metabolite of albendazole, when compared with historical data, and albendazole slightly decreased the exposure to levamisole.

Clinical evidence, mechanism, importance and management

A study in 28 healthy subjects given levamisole 2.5 mg/kg, alone or with albendazole 400 mg, found that albendazole produced a 34% reduction in the AUC of levamisole but no other pharmacokinetic parameters were affected. However, the AUC of the active sulfoxide metabolite of albendazole was 75% lower in the presence of levamisole, when compared with historical values in subjects who had received albendazole alone.[1] An associated study in 44 patients found that levamisole, with or without albendazole, was not effective against *Onchocerca volvulus* infections. A similar number of adverse effects were seen in both groups.[1] The clinical relevance of these findings is unclear, but they suggest that caution is needed if a patient is given albendazole and levamisole for systemic worm infections as there might be a risk of treatment failure.

1. Awadzi K, Edwards G, Opoku NO, Ardrey AE, Favager S, Addy ET, Attah SK, Yamuah LK, Quartey BT. The safety, tolerability and pharmacokinetics of levamisole alone, levamisole plus ivermectin, and levamisole plus albendazole, and their efficacy against *Onchocerca volvulus*. *Ann Trop Med Parasitol* (2004) 98, 595–614.

Albendazole + Praziquantel

Albendazole does not alter the bioavailability of praziquantel. Praziquantel increases the bioavailability of the active metabolite of albendazole, albendazole sulfoxide, in fasted subjects, but has a much smaller effect when albendazole is given with food.

Clinical evidence, mechanism, importance and management

In a study, Sudanese men were given a single 400-mg dose of albendazole with praziquantel 40 mg/kg while fasting. The pharmacokinetics of praziquantel were not affected by albendazole, whereas the AUC of albendazole sulfoxide, the active metabolite of albendazole, was increased 4.5-fold by praziquantel. However, this difference was much less notable (only a 1.5-fold increase) when the drugs were given with food.[1] The reasons for these changes and their practical consequences are not known, but the increase in the plasma concentration of albendazole sulfoxide did not cause any adverse effects.[1]

In a randomised study, 23 healthy subjects were given albendazole 400 mg and ivermectin 200 micrograms/kg, with or without praziquantel 40 mg/kg. The addition of praziquantel increased the AUC and maximum plasma concentration of albendazole sulfoxide by 31% and 8%, respectively, although there was wide inter-individual variability in these results. No serious adverse effects were reported.[2]

In another randomised study, 21 children treated for giardiasis were given a single 400-mg dose of albendazole, either alone or with a single 20-mg/kg dose of praziquantel. It was found that the maximum plasma concentration of albendazole was increased by 80% (not statistically significant) when it was given with praziquantel and 200 mL of milk, one hour after breakfast. There were wide inter-individual variations in the plasma concentration and AUC of albendazole sulfoxide, but these were similar whether albendazole was given alone or with praziquantel.[3]

If both drugs are given with food (see 'Albendazole + Food', p.228, and 'Praziquantel + Food', p.253), any interaction is modest. On the basis of these studies, there do not seem to be any reasons why the concurrent use of albendazole and praziquantel should be avoided.

1. Homeida M, Leahy W, Copeland S, Ali MMM, Harron DWG. Pharmacokinetic interaction between praziquantel and albendazole in Sudanese men. *Ann Trop Med Parasitol* (1994) 88, 551–9.
2. Na-Bangchang K, Kietinun S, Pawa KK, Hanpitakpong W, Na-Bangchang C, Lazdins J. Assessments of pharmacokinetic drug interactions and tolerability of albendazole, praziquantel and ivermectin combinations. *Trans R Soc Trop Med Hyg* (2006) 100, 335–45.
3. Pengsaa K, Na-Bangchang K, Limkittikul K, Kabkaew K, Lapphra K, Sirivichayakul C, Wisetsing P, Pojjaroen-Anant C, Chanthavanich P, Subchareon A. Pharmacokinetic investigation of albendazole and praziquantel in Thai children infected with *Giardia intestinalis*. *Ann Trop Med Parasitol* (2004) 98, 349–57.

Albendazole or Mebendazole + Ritonavir

Ritonavir reduces the exposure to albendazole, its active metabolite, albendazole sulfoxide, and mebendazole.

Clinical evidence

A study in 16 healthy subjects given single oral doses of albendazole 400 mg (8 subjects) or mebendazole 1 g (8 subjects) found that short-term use of ritonavir (200 mg twice daily for 2 doses) did not alter the pharmacokinetics of albendazole, its active sulfoxide metabolite, or mebendazole. However, long-term ritonavir use (200 mg twice daily for 8 days) reduced the AUC and maximum concentrations of mebendazole by about 60%. The AUCs of albendazole and albendazole sulfoxide were both reduced by about 75% and their maximum concentrations were reduced by 60% and 40%, respectively.[1]

Mechanism

Uncertain. Both albendazole and mebendazole undergo extensive first pass metabolism. Ritonavir is a known enzyme inducer, and the authors suggest that this might have played a part in the reduced concentrations seen.

Importance and management

Evidence for an interaction between ritonavir and albendazole or mebendazole is limited to this one study, but ritonavir is an established enzyme inducer. The reductions in the albendazole and mebendazole concentrations seen are likely to be clinically important when used to treat systemic worm infections. It might be necessary to increase the albendazole or mebendazole dose when treating systemic worm infections in patients taking ritonavir. Monitor the outcome of concurrent use.

The interaction is of no importance when these anthelmintics are used for intestinal worm infections (where they have a local effect on the worms in the gut).

1. Corti N, Heck A, Rentsch K, Zingg W, Jetter A, Stieger B, Pauli-Magnus C. Effect of ritonavir on the pharmacokinetics of the benzimidazoles albendazole and mebendazole: an interaction study in healthy volunteers. *Eur J Clin Pharmacol* (2009) 65, 999–1006.

Amodiaquine + Artesunate

The concurrent use of amodiaquine and artesunate does not affect the pharmacokinetics of either drug, but the concentrations of their active metabolites, desethylamodiaquine and dihydroartemisinin, are reduced.

Clinical evidence, mechanism, importance and management

In a crossover study, 12 healthy subjects were given single oral doses of artesunate 4 mg/kg and amodiaquine 10 mg/kg alone and in combination. The pharmacokinetics of artesunate were unaffected by amodiaquine, but the AUC and maximum plasma concentration of its active metabolite, dihydroartemisinin, were reduced by about one-third and one-half, respectively. The half-life of dihydroartemisinin was increased by 50%. Likewise, the pharmacokinetics of amodiaquine were unaffected by artesunate, but the AUC and time to maximum concentration of its active metabolite, desethylamodiaquine, were reduced by about 33% and 40%, respectively. When amodiaquine was given with artesunate, there was also a trend towards lower desethylamodiaquine concentrations at day 7, although this was not statistically significant. Clinically important adverse effects (raised AST, neutropenia, or hypersensitivity) were reported in about 25% of subjects, but ECG changes were not seen.[1] The clinical importance of these findings is unclear, as this was a single-dose study in healthy subjects. However, the authors suggest that the reduced desethylamodiaquine concentrations at day 7 might result in reduced efficacy, although they note that extensive clinical study data show that the concurrent use of artesunate and amodiaquine is more effective than amodiaquine alone.[1] Indeed, this combination is recommended by the WHO for the treatment of uncomplicated falciparum malaria.[2]

1. Orrell C, Little F, Smith P, Folb P, Taylor W, Olliaro P, Barnes KI. Pharmacokinetics and tolerability of artesunate and amodiaquine alone and in combination in healthy volunteers. *Eur J Clin Pharmacol* (2008) 64, 683–90.
2. World Health Organization. Guidelines for the treatment of malaria - 3rd edition. Available at: https://extranet.who.int/iris/restricted/bitstream/10665/162441/1/9789241549127_eng.pdf (accessed 21/10/15)

Amodiaquine + Chlorphenamine

Chlorphenamine might improve the efficacy of amodiaquine.

Clinical evidence, mechanism, importance and management

In a randomised study, 103 children with acute uncomplicated falciparum malaria were given amodiaquine 10 mg/kg daily for 3 days, either alone or with chlorphenamine (6 mg or 8 mg loading dose followed by 4 mg or 6 mg every 8 hours if under 5-years-old or over 5-years-old, respectively) for 7 days. The combination showed improved cure rates compared with amodiaquine alone, but no pharmacokinetic data for either drug were reported. Drowsiness was only reported in 3 of the patients, all of whom were taking the combination.[1] A smaller study in 5 children treated unsuccessfully for acute uncomplicated falciparum malaria with amodiaquine, also found that the addition of chlorphenamine (same doses as above), improved the antimalarial efficacy and cure rate of amodiaquine. Drowsiness after the first dose of the combination was the only reported common adverse effect, occurring in all children. Similarly, no pharmacokinetic data were reported.[2]

The use of chlorphenamine with amodiaquine might improve the efficacy of amodiaquine; however, the mechanism of this is not understood, particularly as no pharmacokinetic data were collected in either study. It is therefore unclear whether this combination might increase the risk of amodiaquine adverse effects. It would seem prudent that if amodiaquine and chlorphenamine are used concurrently, patients should be advised about the potential risk of drowsiness.

1. Falade CO, Micahel SO, Oduola AMJ. Enhanced efficacy of amodiaquine and chlorpheniramine combination over amodiaquine alone in the treatment of acute uncomplicated *Plasmodium falciparum* malaria in children. *Med Princ Pract* (2008) 17, 197–201.
2. Sowunmi A, Gbotosho GP, Happi CT, Adedeji AA, Bolaji OM, Fehintola FA, Oduola AMJ. Enhancement of the antimalarial efficacy of amodiaquine by chlorpheniramine in vivo. *Mem Inst Oswaldo Cruz* (2007) 102, 417–19.

Amodiaquine or Artesunate + Efavirenz

Some very limited evidence suggests that efavirenz might increase the exposure to amodiaquine. The concurrent use of amodiaquine, artesunate, and efavirenz might cause liver toxicity.

Clinical evidence

Two healthy subjects were given amodiaquine and artesunate (doses not stated) for 3 days and then for another 3 days during a course of efavirenz (dose not stated). Efavirenz increased the AUC of amodiaquine in the two subjects by 114% and 302% and decreased the AUC of desethylamodiaquine (the active metabolite of amodiaquine) by 24% and 9%. The AUC of efavirenz was raised, when compared with historical data, in one subject. ALT and AST were normal throughout the study period, but 5 to 6 weeks after the study was completed both subjects had sizeable increases in these enzymes but were asymptomatic. ALT and AST slowly returned to normal over the course of the following 3 to 5 months.[1]

Mechanism

Uncertain. Amodiaquine is metabolised to its active metabolite, desethylamodiaquine, by CYP2C8. An *in vitro* study showed that efavirenz inhibits CYP2C8 at therapeutic concentrations,[2] which could lead to the increase in plasma concentration of amodiaquine and the decrease in plasma concentration of desethylamodiaquine seen.

Importance and management

Evidence of an interaction between amodiaquine and efavirenz is limited, and the clinical importance of the findings is unclear. The short-term use of amodiaquine, artesunate, or efavirenz is not generally associated with hepatotoxicity. However, the prolonged use of amodiaquine has been associated with hepatitis and so it is possible that the hepatotoxicity seen in this study[1] was due to the increased exposure to amodiaquine. The authors suggest that patients requiring amodiaquine or artesunate while taking efavirenz should be monitored for liver toxicity, and this would seem a sensible precaution, as would monitoring for other signs of amodiaquine toxicity (such as agranulocytosis).

1. German P, Greenhouse B, Coates C, Dorsey G, Rosenthal PJ, Charlebois E, Lindegardh N, Havlir D, Aweeka FT. Hepatotoxicity due to a drug interaction between amodiaquine plus artesunate and efavirenz. *Clin Infect Dis* (2007) 44, 889–91.
2. Parikh S, Ouedraogo J-B, Goldstein JA, Rosenthal PJ, Kroetz DL. Amodiaquine metabolism is impaired by common polymorphisms in CYP2C8: implications for malaria treatment in Africa. *Clin Pharmacol Ther* (2007) 82, 197–203.

Amodiaquine with Artesunate + Food

A high-fat meal appears to increase exposure to amodiaquine and its active metabolite, desethylamodiaquine, and delay the time to maximum concentration. In contrast, maximum concentrations of artesunate and its active metabolite, dihydroartemisinin, appear to be reduced by a high-fat meal.

Clinical evidence, mechanism, importance and management

In a crossover study in 22 healthy subjects, a single oral dose of amodiaquine 540 mg and artesunate 200 mg (given as a combination preparation) was given after an overnight fast and 30 minutes after a high-fat breakfast. After the high-fat breakfast, the AUC and maximum plasma concentration of amodiaquine were increased by about 60% and 20%, compared with the fasted state. Slightly smaller increases in these parameters were seen for desethylamodiaquine, the active metabolite of amodiaquine. In the fed state, the time to maximum concentration was also increased, from 0.75 hours to 1 hour for amodiaquine and from 1.67 hours to 4 hours for desethylamodiaquine. For artesunate, the maximum concentration was reduced by two-thirds, but the AUC and time to maximum concentration were unaffected by food. A smaller effect was seen for the active metabolite of artesunate, dihydroartemisinin, with the maximum concentration reduced by one-half in the fed state. The AUC was similarly unaffected, but the time to maximum concentration was increased about 2-fold in the fed state. No adverse events were reported which required treatment to be stopped and no clinically important changes in ECG measurements were noted.[1]

This is an isolated study and as such, the general clinical importance of these changes is not known. The authors suggest that the slight delay in the time to reach maximum concentrations of amodiaquine and desethylamodiaquine is unlikely to be clinically important because the role of amodiaquine is to provide longer-term killing of parasites after artesunate has exerted its effect. They also comment that the possibility of reduced efficacy of artesunate cannot be ruled out, and it is unknown whether this reduction in efficacy can be compensated for by the increased exposure to amodiaquine and its metabolite.[1] Further study is required, but until more is know it would seem prudent to avoid giving amodiaquine with artesunate after a high-fat meal.

1. Fitoussi S, Thang C, Lesauvage E, Barré J, Charron B, Filali-Ansary A, Lameyre V. Bioavailability of a co-formulated combination of amodiaquine and artesunate under fed and fasted conditions. Arzneimittelforschung. (2009) 59, 370–6.

Amphotericin B + Azoles

The effects of amphotericin B and the azoles would be expected to be antagonistic, and there is some clinical evidence that supports this suggestion. An isolated study found that amphotericin B reduced the serum concentration of itraconazole, and the combination might increase the incidence of hepatotoxicity.

Clinical evidence

There are numerous *in vitro* and *animal* studies of the potential interaction of azoles with amphotericin B, which show conflicting results from antagonism to additive or synergistic effects, some of which have been the subject of a review.[1] Many of the studies into the use of azoles with amphotericin B investigate potential therapeutic uses and are therefore outside the scope of this monograph; however, there are some clinical reports of reduced efficacy and adverse effects, and these are discussed below.

In one study, 4 out of 6 patients did not respond to amphotericin B while also taking **ketoconazole**, whereas treatment with amphotericin B was successful in 6 others, 5 of whom had stopped taking prophylactic **miconazole** or **ketoconazole**. The authors suggested that the numbers are too small to draw any definite conclusions, but antagonism is certainly a possibility.[2] Similarly, the antifungal effects of **miconazole** and amphotericin B were found to be antagonistic in one small study.[3] In contrast, two randomised studies, in patients with candidaemia or HIV-positive subjects with cryptococcal meningitis, found that the use of amphotericin B with **fluconazole** might be slightly more effective than the use of **fluconazole** or amphotericin B alone.[4,5]

A comparative study found that patients given **itraconazole** and amphotericin B had **itraconazole** serum concentrations of less than 1 microgram/mL, whereas those given **itraconazole** alone had **itraconazole** serum concentrations of 3.75 micrograms/mL, which suggests that amphotericin B might reduce **itraconazole** serum concentrations.[6]

A retrospective study of **itraconazole** use found that 11 of 12 leukaemic patients given amphotericin B and **itraconazole** had raised liver enzymes. These abnormalities resolved in 7 patients when the amphotericin B was discontinued. **Itraconazole** alone, given to another 8 patients, did not cause liver enzyme abnormalities even though it was used in high doses.[7]

Mechanism

Uncertain. In theory, the combination of an antifungal that binds to ergosterol in fungal cell membranes (amphotericin B) with one that inhibits the synthesis of ergosterol (azoles) would be expected to exert antagonistic effects.[1,8,9] *In vitro* studies with *Candida albicans* found that azole exposure might allow the generation of cells that are unaffected by subsequent exposure to amphotericin B. The degree of resistance appears to depend on the concentration and the azole involved, with itraconazole causing more resistance than fluconazole.[10] Resistance of *Candida* species to amphotericin B appears to depend on the duration of pre-exposure to fluconazole and is also greater when amphotericin B is subsequently used with fluconazole rather than alone.[9,11] Resistance might also depend on the organism involved and its sensitivity to azoles.[12,13]

Importance and management

Despite extensive *in vitro* and *animal* data, it is not entirely clear whether or not azoles inhibit the efficacy of amphotericin B.[8,14,15] The emergence of resistant strains of fungi, and the fact that antifungal therapy for invasive fungal infections remains suboptimal, has meant that combinations of antifungals have continued to be tried. Critically ill patients are often given empirical treatment with amphotericin B, with a subsequent change to fluconazole if the organism is sensitive. The Infectious Disease Society of America advises that a combination of amphotericin B and fluconazole might be an option in selected patients.[16] However, the concurrent use of azoles and amphotericin B should not be considered as routine practice, and until more is known, it may be better to limit concurrent use to specific cases. The outcome of concurrent use should be well monitored for both a reduced antifungal response and an increase in adverse effects. There are a number of reviews that have usefully discussed the topic of antifungal combinations.[17-19]

The evidence for a pharmacokinetic interaction between amphotericin B and the azoles is poor and appears to be limited to the single study with itraconazole reported above. Similarly evidence for an adverse hepatic interaction is sparse. Amphotericin B has only rarely been associated with adverse effects on the liver, although increases in liver enzymes can occur in patients given itraconazole. Given these findings, it might be prudent to closely monitor the outcome of concurrent use of amphotericin B and itraconazole for both a reduced antifungal response to itraconazole as well as an increase in adverse effects, such as a worsening of liver function tests.[7] Further study is needed to substantiate these results.

1. Sugar AM. Use of amphotericin B with azole antifungal drugs: what are we doing? *Antimicrob Agents Chemother* (1995) 39, 1907–12.
2. Meunier-Carpentier F, Cruciani M, Klastersky J. Oral prophylaxis with miconazole or ketoconazole of invasive fungal disease in neutropenic cancer patients. *Eur J Cancer Clin Oncol* (1983) 19, 43–8.
3. Schacter LP, Owellen RJ, Rathbun HK, Buchanan B. Antagonism between miconazole and amphotericin B. *Lancet* (1976) ii, 318.
4. Rex JH, Pappas PG, Karchmer AW, Sobel J, Edwards JE, Hadley S, Brass C, Vazquez JA, Chapman SW, Horowitz HW, Zervos M, McKinsey D, Lee J, Babinchak T, Bradsher RW, Cleary JD, Cohen DM, Danziger L, Goldman M, Goodman J, Hilton E, Hyslop NE, Kett DH, Lutz J, Rubin RH, Scheld WM, Schuster M, Simmons B, Stein DK, Washburn RG, Mautner L, Chu TC, Panzer H, Rosenstein RB, Booth J; National Institute of Allergy and Infectious Diseases Mycoses Study Group. A randomized and blinded multicenter trial of high-dose fluconazole plus placebo versus fluconazole plus amphotericin B as therapy for candidemia and its consequences in nonneutropenic subjects. Clin Infect Dis. (2003) 36, 1221–8.
5. Brouwer AE, Rajanuwong A, Chierakul W, Griffen GE, Larsen RA, White NJ, Harrison TS. Combination antifungal therapies for HIV-associated cryptococcal meningitis: a randomised trial. *Lancet* (2004) 363, 1764–7.
6. Pennick GJ, McGough DA, Barchiesi F, Rinaldi MG. Concomitant therapy with amphotericin B and itraconazole: Does this combination affect the serum concentration of itraconazole? *Intersci Conf Antimicrob Agents Chemother* (1994) 34, 39.
7. Persat F, Schwartzbrod PE, Troncy J, Timour Q, Maul A, Piens MA, Picot S. Abnormalities in liver enzymes during simultaneous therapy with itraconazole and amphotericin B in leukaemic patients. *J Antimicrob Chemother* (2000) 45, 928–30.
8. Pahls S, Schaffner A. *Aspergillus fumigatus* pneumonia in neutropenic patients receiving fluconazole for infection due to *Candida* species: is amphotericin B combined with fluconazole the appropriate answer? *Clin Infect Dis* (1994) 18, 484–5.
9. Ernst EJ, Klepser ME, Pfaller MA. In vitro interaction of fluconazole and amphotericin B administered sequentially against *Candida albicans*: effect of concentration and exposure time. *Diagn Microbiol Infect Dis* (1998) 32, 205–10.
10. Vazquez JA, Arganoza MT, Vaishampayan JK, Akins RA. In vitro interaction between amphotericin B and azoles in Candida albicans. *Antimicrob Agents Chemother* (1996) 40, 2511–16.
11. Louie A, Kaw P, Banerjee P, Liu W, Chen G, Miller MH. Impact of order of initiation of fluconazole and amphotericin B in sequential or combination therapy on killing of Candida albicans in vitro and in rabbit model of endocarditis and pyelonephritis. *Antimicrob Agents Chemother* (2001) 45, 485–510.
12. Louie A, Banerjee P, Drusano GL, Shayegani M, Miller MH. Interaction between fluconazole and amphotericin B in mice with systemic infection due to fluconazole-susceptible or –resistant strains of Candida albicans. *Antimicrob Agents Chemother* (1999) 43, 2841–7.
13. LeMonte AM, Washum KE, Smedema ML, Schnizlein-Bick C, Kohler SM, Wheat LJ. Amphotericin B combined with itraconazole or fluconazole for treatment of histoplasmosis. *J Infect Dis* (2000) 182, 545–50.
14. Meis JF, Donnelly JP, Hoogkamp-Korstanje JA, De Pauw BE. Reply. *Clin Infect Dis* (1994) 18, 485–6.
15. Scheven M, Scheven M-L. Interaction between azoles and amphotericin B in the treatment of candidiasis. *Clin Infect Dis* (1995) 20, 1079.
16. Pappas PG, Rex JH, Sobel JD, Filler SG, Dismukes WE, Walsh TJ, Edwards JE. Infectious Disease Society of America: Guidelines for treatment of candidiasis. *Clin Infect Dis* (2004) 38,161–89.
17. Baddley JW, Pappas PG. Antifungal combination therapy: clinical potential. *Drugs* (2005) 65, 1461–80.
18. Sobel JD. Combination therapy for invasive mycoses: evaluation of past clinical trial designs. *Clin Infect Dis* (2004) 39 (Suppl 4), S224–S227.
19. Patterson TF. Advances and challenges in management of invasive mycoses. *Lancet* (2005) 366, 1013–25.

Amphotericin B + Drugs that lower potassium concentrations

The concurrent use of amphotericin B with drugs that can lower plasma-potassium concentrations (such as loop diuretics, thiazide diuretics, and corticosteroids) can lead to hypokalaemia.

Clinical evidence

(a) Corticosteroids

Four patients given amphotericin B and **hydrocortisone** 25 to 40 mg daily developed cardiac enlargement and congestive heart failure secondary to hypokalaemia. In these cases the plasma-potassium concentration decreased from about 5 mmol/L pre-treatment to between 2.3 and 3 mmol/L during amphotericin B therapy. The cardiac size decreased and the heart failure disappeared within 2 weeks of stopping **hydrocortisone**. The amphotericin B was continued successfully with the addition of potassium supplements in some cases.[1] A retrospective study reported an incidence of hypokalaemia of about 18% in patients prescribed amphotericin B and **hydrocortisone**.[2]

(b) Potassium-depleting diuretics

Amphotericin B and **loop diuretics**, or **thiazides and related diuretics**, can lower plasma-potassium concentrations, and their concurrent use might increase the risk of hypokalaemia. One retrospective study reports an incidence of hypokalaemia of about 36% in patients prescribed both amphotericin B and **furosemide**.[2] Conversely, potassium-sparing diuretics, such as **amiloride**, might reduce the incidence of hypokalaemia with amphotericin B.[3]

Mechanism

Amphotericin B causes potassium to be lost in the urine: the incidence of hypokalaemia with amphotericin B alone has been reported to be as high as 75 to 90%.[3] Potassium-depleting diuretics (such as the loop diuretics or thiazides and related diuretics) and corticosteroids can also increase potassium excretion. Corticosteroids can cause salt and water to be retained, and occasional instances of hypernatraemia with amphotericin B have also been seen. Together, these mechanisms could account for the hypokalaemic cardiomegaly and the circulatory overload that was seen.

Importance and management

Information about an interaction between amphotericin B and corticosteroids or diuretics is limited, but the interaction would seem to be established. The UK manufacturer of a non-lipid formulation of amphotericin B advises that corticosteroids should not be used concurrently unless they are necessary to control drug reactions.[4] However, in clinical practice, it is sometimes deemed necessary to use amphotericin B with either corticosteroids or diuretics, or all three together. In this situation, close monitoring of the patient's fluid balance, electrolytes (especially potassium, which should be closely monitored in patients receiving amphotericin B in any case), and renal and cardiovascular parameters is required. The elderly would seem to be particularly at risk of this interaction. One small study found that giving spironolactone 100 mg twice daily with amphotericin B reduced the need for potassium supplementation, and did not result in clinically important adverse effects.[5] Note that hypokalaemia increases the risk of adverse interactions with digitalis glycosides (see 'Digoxin and related drugs + Drugs that lower potassium concentrations', p.1095), and drugs that prolong the QT interval (see 'Drugs that prolong the QT interval + Drugs that lower potassium concentrations', p.272).

1. Chung D-K, Koenig MG. Reversible cardiac enlargement during treatment with amphotericin B and hydrocortisone. Report of three cases. *Am Rev Respir Dis* (1971) 103, 831–41.
2. Depont F, Vargas F, Dutronc H, Giauque E, Ragnaud J-M, Galpérine T, Abouelfath A, Valentino R, Dupon M, Hérbert G, Moore N. Drug-drug interactions with systemic antifungals in clinical practice. *Pharmacoepidemiol Drug Safety* (2007) 16, 1227–33.
3. Wazny LD, Brophy DF. Amiloride for the prevention of amphotericin B–induced hypokalemia and hypomagnesemia. *Ann Pharmacother* (2000) 34, 94–7.
4. Fungizone Intravenous (Amphotericin B). E. R. Squibb & Sons Ltd. UK Summary of product characteristics, February 2010.
5. Ural AU. Comment: spironolactone prevents amphotericin B-induced hypokalaemia in neutropenic patients. *Ann Pharmacother* (2000) 34, 1488.

Amphotericin B + Pentamidine

Acute renal failure and electrolyte disturbances might develop in patients taking amphotericin B if they are also given pentamidine.

Clinical evidence, mechanism, importance and management

A retrospective study between 1985 and 1988 identified 101 patients with AIDS who had been given amphotericin B for various systemic mycoses. The patients were given amphotericin B 600 micrograms/kg to 800 micrograms/kg daily for 7 to 10 days, then a dose three times each week for about 9 weeks. Nine patients were concurrently treated for pneumocystis pneumonia, and of these, the 4 who had been given pentamidine parenterally developed acute and rapid reversible renal impairment. In all 4 cases, renal function returned to normal when the drugs were withdrawn. No renal impairment was seen in two other patients given pentamidine by inhalation or three other patients given intravenous co-trimoxazole and the renal impairment in the first patients was therefore attributed to the additive nephrotoxicity of intravenous pentamidine with amphotericin.[1]

Both amphotericin B and intravenous pentamidine are known to be nephrotoxic. Reversible renal adverse effects might occur in up to 20% of patients given intravenous pentamidine alone and, rarely, renal impairment might also occur in patients given inhaled pentamidine.[2] However, it seems likely that no toxicity occurred in the patients mentioned above when the pentamidine was given by inhalation because the serum concentrations achieved were low.

Close monitoring of renal function should be routine when either drug is used (daily monitoring is recommended in the case of parenteral pentamidine[2]), and it is essential that this recommendation is adhered to if both drugs are given. It might be prudent to use liposomal amphotericin B rather than a non-lipid formulation of amphotericin B to reduce the risk of renal impairment. Anticipate the likelihood of renal impairment and consider the need to withdraw the drugs.

Note also that both drugs can cause significant electrolyte disturbances, such as hypomagnesaemia[2,3], and serum electrolytes should also be closely monitored during concurrent use.

1. Antoniskis D, Larsen RA. Acute, rapidly progressive renal failure with simultaneous use of amphotericin B and pentamidine. *Antimicrob Agents Chemother* (1990) 34, 470–2.
2. Pentacarinat (Pentamidine isetionate). Sanofi. UK Summary of product characteristics, March 2012.
3. Atsmon J, Dolev E. Drug-induced hypomagnesaemia: scope and management. *Drug Safety* (2005), 28, 763–88.

Amphotericin B; Oral + Miscellaneous

The UK manufacturer of amphotericin B for oral use[1] noted that its absorption from the gastrointestinal tract is negligible, and that no interactions have been noted with amphotericin B lozenges or other oral formulations. For a theoretical interaction with sucralfate, see 'Amphotericin B; Oral + Sucralfate', below.

1. Fungilin Lozenge, Oral Suspension, Oral Tablets (Amphotericin B). E. R. Squibb & Sons Ltd. UK Summary of product characteristics, May 2006.

Amphotericin B; Oral + Sucralfate

An *in vitro* study with amphotericin B found that it became irreversibly bound to sucralfate at the pH values found in the gut.

Clinical evidence, mechanism, importance and management

To simulate what might happen in the gut, amphotericin B 25 mg/L was mixed with sucralfate 500 mg in 40 mL of water at pH 3.5 and allowed to stand for 90 minutes at 25°C. Analysis of the solution found that the amphotericin B concentration fell rapidly and progressively over 90 minutes to about 20%. When the pH of the mixture was then raised to about 6.5 to 7 for 90 minutes, there was no change in the concentration of amphotericin B, suggesting that the interaction was irreversible.[1] The reason for this change is not known, but the suggestion is that sucralfate forms insoluble chelates with amphotericin B.[1]

It is not known how important this interaction is likely to be in practice, but the efficacy of amphotericin B for intestinal candidiasis or gut decontamination could be decreased. Separating the doses might not be effective in some postoperative patients because their gastric function may not return to normal for up to 5 days, and some sucralfate might still be present when the next dose is given.[1] No further clinical studies appear to have been conducted to establish this hypothesis. If both sucralfate and oral amphotericin B are required, it would seem prudent to monitor concurrent use carefully, being alert for any evidence of a reduction in efficacy.

1. Feron B, Adair CG, Gorman SP, McClurg B. Interaction of sucralfate with antibiotics used for selective decontamination of the gastrointestinal tract. *Am J Hosp Pharm* (1993) 50, 2550–3.

Artemether with Lumefantrine + CYP3A4 inhibitors

Ketoconazole slightly to moderately increases the AUCs of artemether and lumefantrine, and lopinavir boosted with ritonavir moderately increases the AUC of lumefantrine.

Clinical evidence

(a) Ketoconazole

In a study, 16 healthy subjects were given a single dose of artemether with lumefantrine 80/480 mg with a high-fat breakfast, followed by ketoconazole 400 mg on day one and then 200 mg daily for 4 days. Ketoconazole increased the AUC of artemether 2.4-fold, its active metabolite, dihydroartemisinin, 1.7-fold, and lumefantrine 1.7-fold.[1] The maximum concentrations of the drugs were also increased to a similar extent. The half-life of lumefantrine was unchanged by ketoconazole, but those of artemether and dihydroartemisinin were slightly increased.

(b) Lopinavir boosted with ritonavir

In a study in 10 healthy HIV-*negative* subjects, artemether with lumefantrine 80/480 mg twice daily for 3 days was given before and during a 26-day course of lopinavir boosted with ritonavir 400/100 mg twice daily.[2] Lopinavir boosted with ritonavir decreased the AUCs of dihydroartemisinin and artemether by 45% and about 35%, respectively. The decrease in artemether exposure was not statistically significant. The AUC of lumefantrine was increased 2.3-fold, but its half-life was not altered by lopinavir boosted with ritonavir. No changes in the pharmacokinetics of lopinavir or ritonavir were seen.

Mechanism

Ketoconazole and ritonavir are both inhibitors of intestinal and hepatic CYP3A4. The lack of effect on the half-life of lumefantrine suggests that its exposure might have been increased as a result of increased absorption due to inhibition of intestinal CYP3A4 by ketoconazole and ritonavir. The exposure to artemether might have been increased by inhibition of intestinal and/or hepatic CYP3A4. The decrease in artemether exposure seen in one study (all be it not statistically significant) may have been a result of autoinduction.

Importance and management

Although a pharmacokinetic interaction with ketoconazole and lopinavir boosted with ritonavir appears to be established, the clinical relevance of a 2-fold increase in artemether and lumefantrine exposure appears to be minimal and the effect is considerably smaller than that seen when artemether with lumefantrine is given with food, as is recommended (see 'Artemether with Lumefantrine + Food', p.232). In addition, one study reported no changes in ECG parameters or increases in adverse effects, and the pharmacokinetic changes seen are within the expected intersubject variability for these drugs.[1] The UK manufacturer[3] therefore advises that no dose adjustment is necessary when artemether with lumefantrine is given with ketoconazole or other potent inhibitors of CYP3A4 (which would include ritonavir, given at a dose used to boost other HIV-protease inhibitors).

1. Lefèvre G, Carpenter P, Souppart C, Schmidli H, McClean M, Stypinski D. Pharmacokinetics and electrocardiographic pharmacodynamics or artemether-lumefantrine (Riamet®) with concomitant administration of ketoconazole in healthy subjects. *Br J Clin Pharmacol* (2002) 54, 485–92.
2. German P, Parikh S, Lawrence J, Dorsey G, Rosenthal PJ, Havlir D, Charlebois E, Hanpithakpong W, Lindegardh N, Aweeka FT. Lopinavir/ritonavir affects pharmacokinetic exposure of artemether/lumefantrine in HIV-uninfected healthy volunteers. *J Acquir Immune Defic Syndr* (2009) 51, 424–9.
3. Riamet (Artemether with Lumefantrine). Novartis Pharmaceuticals UK Ltd. UK Summary of product characteristics, October 2011.

Artemether with Lumefantrine + Food

High-fat food and soya milk markedly increase the bioavailability of lumefantrine, and high-fat food moderately increases the bioavailability of artemether.

Clinical evidence

In a study in healthy Chinese subjects, a single dose of artemether with lumefantrine 80/480 mg was taken after a high-fat meal and in the fasted state. The relative bioavailabilities of artemether and its active metabolite, dihydroartemisinin, were increased more than 2-fold, and the bioavailability of lumefantrine was increased 16-fold by the meal.[1] Based on these data, the UK manufacturer notes that if 100% absorption is assumed for lumefantrine taken with a high-fat meal, then absorption in the fasted state is less than 10% of the dose.[2] In a clinical study in patients with malaria, intake of a light meal within one hour of lumefantrine increased the bioavailability by 48% and intake of a normal meal increased absorption 2-fold, when compared with liquids alone. After 24 to 48 hours, most patients were eating normally.[3]

A study in 11 healthy subjects to investigate the amount of fat required to maximise lumefantrine bioavailability found that giving increasing quantities of **soya milk** (up to 500 mL) significantly increased the AUC of lumefantrine more than 5-fold. The optimum quantity of fat to obtain 90% bioavailability of lumefantrine was 1.2 g (equivalent to 36 mL of **soya milk**).[4]

Mechanism

Not studied.

Importance and management

The effect of food on artemether is moderate, whereas the effect of food on the bioavailability of lumefantrine is marked. The associated increase in the plasma concentration of lumefantrine is clinically important because lumefantrine is critical in eliminating residual parasites remaining after artemether has been cleared from the body and thus in preventing recrudescence (reappearance of the disease after a period of inactivity). Therefore artemether with lumefantrine should be taken with food. However, patients with acute uncomplicated malaria are unlikely to tolerate food, and the UK manufacturer notes that patients should be encouraged to take artemether with lumefantrine with food as soon as this can be tolerated. Patients who remain averse to food during treatment should be closely monitored as they might be at greater risk of recrudescence.[2] One study[4] suggests that soya milk might be an option to improve lumefantrine bioavailability in those patients unable to tolerate a full meal.

1. Bindschedler M, Degen P, Lu ZL, Jiao XQ, Liu GY, Fan F. Comparative bioavailability of benflumetol after administration of single oral doses of co-artemether under fed and fasted conditions to healthy subjects. Cited in Lefèvre G, Thomsen MS. Clinical Pharmacokinetics of artemether and lumefantrine (Riamet®). *Clin Drug Invest* (1999) 18, 467–80.
2. Riamet (Artemether with Lumefantrine). Novartis Pharmaceuticals UK Ltd. UK Summary of product characteristics, October 2011.
3. Ezzet F, van Vugt M, Nosten F, Looareesuwan S, White NJ. Pharmacokinetics and pharmacodynamics of lumefantrine (Benflumetol) in acute falciparum malaria. *Antimicrob Agents Chemother* (2000) 44, 697–704.
4. Ashley EA, Stepniewska K, Lindegårdh N, Annerberg A, Kham A, Brockman A, Singhasivanon P, White NJ, Nosten F. How much fat is necessary to optimize lumefantrine oral bioavailability? *Trop Med Int Health* (2007) 12, 195–200.

Artemether + Grapefruit juice

Grapefruit juice increases the exposure to artemether.

Clinical evidence

In a crossover study, 6 healthy subjects were given a single 100-mg dose of artemether with water, after breakfast, then after a 7-day washout period the study was repeated, replacing water with 350 mL of double-strength grapefruit juice. Grapefruit juice increased the AUC of artemether almost 2-fold, and increased its maximum plasma concentration more than 2-fold. The pharmacokinetics of the active metabolite of artemether, dihydroartemisinin, were unaffected. No ECG changes were reported on concurrent use.[1] In a further multiple-dose study, artemether 100 mg was taken with water or 350 mL of double-strength grapefruit juice, daily for 5 days. The AUC of artemether given alone was lower on day 5 than on day 1 due to auto-induction of its metabolism. When grapefruit juice was also given, the AUC and maximum plasma concentration of artemether were increased 2-fold on both day one and day 5, with the day 5 AUC remaining lower than the day 1 AUC.[2]

Mechanism

These studies suggest that grapefruit juice might increase the plasma concentration of artemether by inhibiting intestinal CYP3A4, which is involved in the metabolism of artemether. As the effect was the same on day 1 and day 5 it appears that artemether auto-induction does not affect this process.

Importance and management

An interaction between artemether and grapefruit juice is established, but its clinical relevance does not appear to have been studied. However, based on the evidence for ketoconazole, a potent inhibitor of CYP3A4 (see 'Artemether with Lumefantrine + CYP3A4 inhibitors', p.231), it seems unlikely to result in adverse effects or ECG changes, and the UK manufacturer advises that no dose adjustments are needed when artemether with lumefantrine is given with potent CYP3A4 inhibitors.[3] The authors of the two studies[1,2] suggest that the use of grapefruit juice might improve the clinical efficacy of artemether in malaria, and might theoretically reduce recrudescence (the reappearance of a disease after a period of inactivity); however, note that artemether is used in combination with lumefantrine for this very reason.

1. van Agtmael MA, Gupta V, van der Wosten TH, Rutten JP, van Boxtel CJ. Grapefruit juice increases the bioavailability of artemether. *Eur J Clin Pharmacol* (1999) 55, 405–10.
2. van Agtmael MA, Gupta V, van der Graaf CAA, van Boxtel CJ. The effect of grapefruit juice on the time-dependent decline of artemether plasma levels in healthy subjects. *Clin Pharmacol Ther* (1999) 66, 408–14.
3. Riamet (Artemether with Lumefantrine). Novartis Pharmaceuticals UK Ltd. UK Summary of product characteristics, October 2011.

Atovaquone + Antiemetics

Preliminary evidence suggests that metoclopramide decreases the plasma concentration of atovaquone.

Clinical evidence, mechanism, importance and management

An analysis of 191 patients with AIDS, given atovaquone as part of efficacy studies, found that when normalised for plasma albumin, body-weight, and the absence of other drugs, the expected steady-state plasma concentration of atovaquone was 14.8 micrograms/mL. Steady-state plasma concentrations of atovaquone achieved in the presence of other drugs were examined in an attempt to identify possible interactions. **Metoclopramide** was associated with a decrease in the atovaquone concentration of 7.2 micrograms/mL. Antiemetics other than metoclopramide (individual drugs not named) were not associated with any change in the steady-state plasma concentration of atovaquone.[1,2]

This kind of analysis provides only the very broadest indication that a sizeable interaction might occur between atovaquone and **metoclopramide**, and there appear to be no further published studies to confirm this report of an interaction. However, it does highlight the need to be vigilant if **metoclopramide** is used concurrently, and the UK manufacturer of atovaquone suspension recommends caution on the concurrent use of **metoclopramide** until the interaction has been further studied.[2] The US manufacturer of atovaquone suspension does not mention **metoclopramide**.[3] If an antiemetic is required in patients taking atovaquone with proguanil, the US manufacturer suggests that **metoclopramide** should be given only if other antiemetics are unavailable,[4] whereas the UK manufacturer does not recommend concurrent use.[5]

1. Sadler BM, Blum MR. Relationship between steady-state plasma concentrations of atovaquone (C_{ss}) and the use of various concomitant medications in AIDS patients with *Pneumocystis carinii* pneumonia. *Int Conf AIDS* (1993): 9, 504.
2. Wellvone Oral Suspension (Atovaquone). GlaxoSmithKline UK. UK Summary of product characteristics, April 2010.
3. Mepron Suspension (Atovaquone). GlaxoSmithKline. US Prescribing information, May 2008.
4. Malarone (Atovaquone with Proguanil hydrochloride). GlaxoSmithKline. US Prescribing information, September 2009.
5. Malarone Tablets (Atovaquone with Proguanil hydrochloride). GlaxoSmithKline UK. UK Summary of product characteristics, August 2012.

Atovaquone with Proguanil + Artesunate

Artesunate did not affect the pharmacokinetics of atovaquone with proguanil in a single-dose study. In one small study, concurrent use did not cause cardiotoxicity.

Clinical evidence, mechanism, importance and management

In a pharmacokinetic study, a single dose of atovaquone with proguanil 1 g/400 mg was given to 12 healthy subjects with and without artesunate 250 mg. No change was noted in the pharmacokinetics of either atovaquone or proguanil and no unexpected adverse events were seen.[1] Although artesunate does not therefore appear to alter the pharmacokinetics of atovaquone with proguanil, this needs confirmation in a multiple-dose study.

A study in 42 patients, to investigate whether the addition of artesunate to atovaquone with proguanil increased the risk of cardiotoxicity, found that the QT_c interval was no different in those receiving all three drugs, when compared with those receiving atovaquone with proguanil alone.[2]

1. van Vugt M, Edstein MD, Proux S, Lay K, Ooh M, Looareesuwan S, White NJ, Nosten F. Absence of an interaction between artesunate and atovaquone – proguanil. *Eur J Clin Pharmacol* (1999) 55, 469–74.
2. Gupta RK, van Vugt M, Paiphun L, Slight T, Looareesuwan S, White NJ, Nosten F. Short Report: No evidence of cardiotoxicity of atovaquone-proguanil alone or in combination with artesunate. *Am J Trop Med Hyg* (2005) 73, 267–8.

Atovaquone + Co-trimoxazole

In one small study co-trimoxazole did not alter the plasma concentration of atovaquone, but atovaquone caused a minor decrease in the plasma concentration of co-trimoxazole.

Clinical evidence, mechanism, importance and management

As part of a larger study, 6 HIV-positive subjects received atovaquone 500 mg once daily, co-trimoxazole 960 mg (trimethoprim with sulfamethoxazole 160/800 mg) twice daily, or both co-trimoxazole and atovaquone, with food. There was no change in the steady-state plasma concentration of atovaquone but there was a minor 16% decrease in the steady-state plasma concentration of trimethoprim and a minor 10% decrease in the plasma concentration of sulfamethoxazole when both drugs were given together.[1]

This study shows there is no clinically important pharmacokinetic interaction between atovaquone and co-trimoxazole. No dose adjustments of either drug would be required on concurrent use.

1. Falloon J, Sargent S, Piscitelli SC, Bechtel C, LaFon SW, Sadler B, Walker RE, Kovacs JA, Polis MA, Davey RT, Lan HC, Masur H. Atovaquone suspension in HIV-infected volunteers: pharmacokinetics, pharmacodynamics, and TMP-SMX interaction study. *Pharmacotherapy* (1999) 19, 1050–6.

Atovaquone with Proguanil + Efavirenz

Atovaquone exposure appears to be moderately reduced by efavirenz. The effect of efavirenz on proguanil exposure is uncertain, with different types of studies finding different effects.

Clinical evidence

In a study in 20 HIV-positive patients taking efavirenz and given a single dose of atovaquone with proguanil, the AUC of atovaquone was 75% lower than in 18 healthy subjects given atovaquone with proguanil alone. The AUC of proguanil was also lower (by 43%) in the patients.[1] In contrast, in a crossover study in 15 healthy subjects given single 300-mg doses of proguanil, either alone or on day 9 of an 11-day course of efavirenz 400 mg daily, the maximum plasma concentration and AUC of proguanil were increased by 47% and 2-fold, respectively. The plasma concentration and AUC of the active metabolite of proguanil, cycloguanil, were decreased.[2]

Mechanism

Uncertain. Atovaquone is predominantly excreted as unchanged drug in the faeces and so the interaction is not due to induction of cytochrome P450 isoenzymes by efavirenz.

Proguanil is metabolised by CYP2C19 to its active metabolite, cycloguanil. *In vitro* studies suggest that efavirenz could be an inhibitor of CYP2C19,[3] which would explain the increased proguanil exposure seen in the crossover study. However, the *in vitro* effect of efavirenz on other isoenzymes is opposite to that seen clinically.[3] If this were the case with CYP2C19, efavirenz might induce this isoenzyme, which would explain the findings of the other study.

Importance and management

Evidence for an interaction between **proguanil** and efavirenz is limited, and the findings of the study that compared HIV-positive subjects with healthy subjects contrasted with those of the crossover study in healthy subjects. If efavirenz does reduce the exposure to the active metabolite of proguanil, cycloguanil, which is responsible for the antimalarial activity of proguanil, then the clinical efficacy of proguanil might be expected to be reduced. However, two studies suggest that proguanil efficacy is independent of cycloguanil exposure (see 'Proguanil + Fluvoxamine', p.254). This suggests that any interaction with efavirenz resulting in reduced cycloguanil exposure would be unlikely to be clinically relevant. In contrast, the patient study implied that increased cycloguanil exposure might be a possibility in patients taking efavirenz. As a result, further study is needed to establish the exact nature of the interaction. Until more is known, some caution might be appropriate if efavirenz is given with proguanil.

The situation with **atovaquone** is less clear, but the moderately reduced exposure seen in the crossover study would seem to suggest that the efficacy of atovaquone could be reduced if it is given with efavirenz. It would therefore seem prudent to avoid concurrent use.

1. van Luin M, Van der Ende ME, Richter C, Visser M, Faraj D, Van der Ven A, Gelinck L, Kroon F, Wit FW, Van Schaik RH, Kuks PF, Burger DM. Lower atovaquone/proguanil concentrations in patients taking efavirenz, lopinavir/ritonavir or atazanavir/ritonavir. *AIDS* (2010) 24, 1223–6.
2. Soyinka JO, Onyeji CO. Alteration of pharmacokinetics of proguanil in healthy volunteers following concurrent administration of efavirenz. *Eur J Pharm Sci* (2010) 39, 213–18.
3. Sustiva Film-coated Tablets (Efavirenz). Bristol Myers Squibb Pharmaceutical Ltd. UK Summary of product characteristics, March 2014.

Atovaquone + Food

Fatty foods moderately increase the exposure to atovaquone given as tablets or suspension.

Clinical evidence

(a) Suspension

A pharmacokinetic study in 12 HIV-positive subjects, designed to determine the dose of atovaquone suspension that would achieve a specific steady-state plasma concentration, found that high-fat food increased the bioavailability of atovaquone by 40%, when compared with the fasted state.[1] In another similar study, giving atovaquone suspension with food (23 g of fat) increased the average steady-state concentration by 30 to 70% with different dose regimens (using 500 mg to 1.5 g of atovaquone).[2]

In a single-dose study in healthy subjects, a high-fat breakfast (21 g of fat) increased the AUC of atovaquone suspension 2.4-fold, and an enteral nutritional supplement (*Sustacal Plus*, containing 28 g of fat) increased the AUC 2.7-fold, when compared with the fasted state.[3]

(b) Tablets

In a crossover study in 18 healthy subjects a single 500-mg dose of atovaquone given after a high-fat standard breakfast (23 g of fat) increased the AUC 3.3-fold, when compared with the fasted state.[4] In a further study of similar design, 2 slices of toast alone had no effect on the AUC of atovaquone, 2 slices of toast with 23 g of butter increased the AUC 3-fold, and 2 slices of toast with 56 g of butter increased the AUC 3.9-fold.[4]

Mechanism

Atovaquone is a highly lipophilic compound which shows considerable inter-individual variability in absorption. Dietary fat increases the rate and extent of atovaquone absorption from both the suspension and the tablets, probably by increasing its solubility in the gut. The suspension has about a 2-fold higher oral bioavailability than the tablets when given with food or when fasting.

Importance and management

The interaction between atovaquone and food is established and of clinical importance. Atovaquone suspension used for the treatment or prevention of pneumocystis pneumonia must be taken with food, as this is likely to increase the likelihood of successful treatment and survival.[5,6] Alternatively, an enteral nutritional supplement with a high-fat content appears to be suitable.[3] In the US, the manufacturer states that, for patients with pneumocystis pneumonia who have difficulty taking atovaquone suspension with food, parenteral treatment (with other drugs) should be considered.[6]

Similarly, atovaquone with proguanil tablets used for the treatment or prophylaxis of malaria should be taken with a milky drink or with food to maximise absorption.[7,8] Be aware that if patients are unable to tolerate food, the systemic exposure to atovaquone will be reduced.[7] In this situation, monitoring of parasitaemia to ensure efficacy would seem advisable.

1. Dixon R, Pozniak AL, Watt HM, Rolan P, Posner J. Single-dose and steady-state pharmacokinetics of a novel microfluidized suspension of atovaquone in human immunodeficiency virus-seropositive patients. *Antimicrob Agents Chemother* (1996) 40, 556–60.
2. Falloon J, Sargent S, Piscitelli SC, Bechtel C, LaFon SW, Sadler B, Walker RE, Kovacs JA, Polis MA, Davey RT, Lan HC, Masur H. Atovaquone suspension in HIV-infected volunteers: pharmacokinetics, pharmacodynamics, and TMP-SMX interaction study. *Pharmacotherapy* (1999) 19, 1050–6.
3. Freeman CD, Klutman NE, Lamp KC, Dall LH, Strayer AH. Relative bioavailability of atovaquone suspension when administered with an enteral nutrition supplement. *Ann Pharmacother* (1998) 32, 1004–7.
4. Rolan PE, Mercer AJ, Weatherley BC, Holdich T, Meire H, Peck RW, Ridout G, Posner J. Examination of some factors responsible for a food-induced increase in absorption of atovaquone. *Br J Clin Pharmacol* (1994) 37, 13–20.
5. Wellvone Oral Suspension (Atovaquone). GlaxoSmithKline UK. UK Summary of product characteristics, April 2010.
6. Mepron Suspension (Atovaquone). GlaxoSmithKline. US Prescribing information, May 2008.
7. Malarone Tablets (Atovaquone with Proguanil hydrochloride). GlaxoSmithKline UK. UK Summary of product characteristics, August 2012.
8. Malarone (Atovaquone with Proguanil hydrochloride). GlaxoSmithKline. US Prescribing information, September 2009.

Atovaquone + Macrolides

Azithromycin and erythromycin do not appear to interact with atovaquone.

Clinical evidence, mechanism, importance and management

(a) Azithromycin

In a small study, 8 HIV-positive children were given azithromycin suspension 5 mg/kg daily, either alone or with atovaquone suspension 30 mg/kg daily, for pneumocystis pneumonia. The maximum serum concentration and AUC_{0-24} of azithromycin were reduced by about 30% by atovaquone. However, due to the large inter-subject variability in azithromycin pharmacokinetics, there were insufficient patients for this reduction to be statistically significant.[1]

A study in 58 patients compared the efficacy of atovaquone 750 mg twice daily and azithromycin (500 mg on day one followed by 250 mg daily) with the standard treatment of clindamycin and quinine in patients with non-life threatening babesiosis (a tick-borne, malaria-like illness). The two combinations were of similar efficacy, and the frequency of adverse effects in the 40 patients taking azithromycin with atovaquone was considerably less than that in the 18 patients taking quinine and clindamycin (15% compared with 72%). However, no pharmacokinetic data were recorded.[2] There are also reports of the successful treatment of babesiosis with azithromycin and atovaquone in a further 2 patients.[3,4] Another efficacy study in HIV-positive children found that the combination of azithromycin with atovaquone was as effective as co-trimoxazole for the prophylaxis of bacterial infections, and that the adverse effect profiles were similar. However, the patients taking co-trimoxazole were known to have taken it without problem previously and this may explain differences between this study and an earlier one which reported a higher rate of adverse effects with co-trimoxazole than with atovaquone alone.[5]

Information on a possible pharmacokinetic interaction between atovaquone and azithromycin appears to be limited to one report.[1] However, the clinical studies[2-5] appear to indicate that the efficacy of neither drug is affected when used in combination. Therefore, no particular precautions appear to be necessary if both drugs are given.

(b) Erythromycin

A preliminary analysis of 191 patients with AIDS given atovaquone as part of efficacy studies, found that erythromycin was not associated with any change in the steady-state plasma concentration of atovaquone. Erythromycin was represented by fewer than 5 subjects.[6] However, note that this kind of analysis provides only the very broadest indication that interactions might or might not occur.

1. Ngo LY, Yogev R, Dankner WM, Hughes WT, Burchett S, Xu J, Sadler B, Unadkat JD for the ACTG 254 Team. Pharmacokinetics of azithromycin administered alone and with atovaquone in human immunodeficiency virus-infected children. *Antimicrob Agents Chemother* (1999) 43, 1516–19.
2. Krause PJ, Lepore T, Sikand VK, Gadbaw J, Burke G, Telford SR, Brassard P, Pearl D, Azlanzadeh J, Christianson D, McGrath D, Spielman A. Atovaquone and azithromycin for the treatment of babesiosis. *N Engl J Med* (2000) 343, 1454–8.
3. Raju M, Salazar JC, Leopold H, Krause PJ. Atovaquone and azithromycin treatment for babesiosis in an infant. *Pediatr Infect Dis J* (2007) 26, 181–3.
4. Bonoan JT, Johnson DH, Cunha BA. Life-threatening babesiosis in an asplenic patient treated with exchange transfusion, azithromycin and atovaquone. *Heart Lung* (1998) 27, 424–8.
5. Hughes WT, Dankner WM, Yogev R, Huang S, Paul ME, Flores MA, Kline MW, Wei L-J, for the Pediatric AIDS Clinical Trials Group (PACTG) 254 Team. Comparison of atovaquone and azithromycin with trimethoprim-sulfamethoxazole for the prevention of serious bacterial infections in children with HIV infection. *Clin Infect Dis* (2005) 40, 136–45.
6. Sadler BM, Blum MR. Relationship between steady-state plasma concentrations of atovaquone (C_{ss}) and the use of various concomitant medications in AIDS patients with *Pneumocystis carinii* pneumonia. *Int Conf AIDS* (1993): 9, 504.

Atovaquone + Miscellaneous

Preliminary evidence suggests that a number of drugs given in clinical studies do not interact with atovaquone.

Clinical evidence, mechanism, importance and management

An analysis of 191 patients with AIDS, given atovaquone as part of efficacy studies, found that when normalised for plasma albumin, body-weight, and the absence of other drugs, the expected steady-state plasma concentration of atovaquone was 14.8 micrograms/mL. The steady-state plasma concentrations of atovaquone achieved in the presence of other drugs were examined in an attempt to identify possible interactions. **Fluconazole** and **prednisone** were associated with increases of 2.5 micrograms/mL and 2.3 micrograms/mL, respectively, whereas **paracetamol (acetaminophen)**, **aciclovir**, **opioids**, **antidiarrhoeals**, **cephalosporins**, **benzodiazepines**, and **laxatives** were associated with decreases of 3.4 micrograms/mL or less. **Clofazimine**, **antacids**, **clotrimazole**, **NSAIDs**, **ketoconazole**, **hydroxyzine**, **megestrol**, **antiemetics** (other than metoclopramide, see 'Atovaquone + Antiemetics', p.232), **other systemic steroids**, and **H_2-receptor antagonists** were not associated with any change in the steady-state plasma concentration of atovaquone. **Clofazimine** was represented by fewer than 5 subjects.[1]

The kind of analysis described above[1] provides only the very broadest indication that interactions might or might not occur between atovaquone and these drugs; however, it would appear that no dose adjustments are necessary when these drugs are used with atovaquone. Clinical studies or case reports appear to confirm this for **ceftriaxone**,[2] **fluconazole**,[3] and **prednisone**.[4] The use of atovaquone with these drugs was not reported to cause adverse effects. The concurrent use of **fluconazole** with atovaquone for the treatment of visceral leishmaniasis (kala-azar) was more effective than atovaquone alone, but was not substantially more effective than fluconazole alone.[3]

1. Sadler BM, Blum MR. Relationship between steady-state plasma concentrations of atovaquone (C_{ss}) and the use of various concomitant medications in AIDS patients with *Pneumocystis carinii* pneumonia. *Int Conf AIDS* (1993): 9, 504.
2. Harvey WT, Martz D. Motor neurone disease recovery associated with IV ceftriaxone and anti-Babesia therapy. *Acta Neurol Scand* (2007) 115, 129–31.
3. Sundar S, Kumar P, Makharia M, Goyal A, Rogers M, Gibbs D, Murray H. Atovaquone alone or with fluconazole as oral therapy for Indian kala-azar. *Clin Infect Dis* (1998) 27, 215–16.
4. Pearson PA, Piracha AR, Sen HA, Jaffe GJ. Atovaquone for the treatment of toxoplasma retinochoroiditis in immunocompetent patients. *Ophthalmology* (1999) 106, 148–53.

Atovaquone + Proguanil

No pharmacokinetic interaction appears to occur between atovaquone and proguanil, although one study reported modest decreases in the exposure to cycloguanil, the active metabolite of proguanil, in some subjects.

Clinical evidence, mechanism, importance and management

Atovaquone did not affect the pharmacokinetics of proguanil in a comparative study of 4 patients taking proguanil 200 mg twice daily for 3 days and 12 patients taking proguanil 200 mg twice daily with atovaquone 500 mg twice daily for 3 days.[1] Similarly, no interaction was seen in 18 healthy subjects given proguanil 400 mg daily with atovaquone 1 g daily for 3 days.[2]

In contrast, in a longer study, 13 healthy subjects were given a single 250/100-mg dose of atovaquone with proguanil, then, after an interval of one week, they were given daily doses for 13 days. There was no change in the AUC of atovaquone from single dose to steady state, indicating that accumulation did not occur. However in 9 subjects who had normal CYP2C19 activity, the AUC of proguanil was increased at steady state and the AUC of the active metabolite, cycloguanil, was decreased: both changes were small. It was suggested that atovaquone might inhibit the production of cycloguanil by CYP3A4. However, as this study had no arm looking at each drug alone, it is impossible to determine whether these changes in pharmacokinetics were due to an interaction or not.[3]

A pharmacokinetic interaction is not established. However, any interaction is of little clinical relevance because the efficacy of the combination product for malaria prophylaxis is established (up to 12 weeks).[4]

1. Edstein MD, Looareesuwan S, Viravan C, Kyle DE. Pharmacokinetics of proguanil in malaria patients treated with proguanil plus atovaquone. *Southeast Asian J Trop Med Public Health* (1996) 27, 216–20.
2. Gillotin C, Mamet JP, Veronese L. Lack of pharmacokinetic interaction between atovaquone and proguanil. *Eur J Clin Pharmacol* (1999) 55, 311–15.
3. Thapar MM, Ashton M, Lindegardh N, Bergqvist Y, Nivelius S, Johansson I, Bjorkman A. Time-dependent pharmacokinetics and drug metabolism of atovaquone plus proguanil (Malarone) when taken as chemoprophylaxis. *Eur J Clin Pharmacol* (2002) 58, 19–27.
4. Srivastava IK, Vaidya AB. A mechanism for the synergistic antimalarial action of atovaquone and proguanil. *Antimicrob Agents Chemother* (1999) 43, 1334–9.

Atovaquone + Rifamycins

Rifampicin reduces the plasma concentration of atovaquone, and atovaquone raises the plasma concentration of rifampicin. Rifabutin interacts similarly, although to a lesser extent.

Clinical evidence

(a) Rifabutin

In a study in 24 healthy subjects, atovaquone 750 mg twice daily was given with rifabutin 300 mg daily for 14 days. There was a slight 34% decrease in the AUC of atovaquone and a small 19% decrease in the plasma concentration of rifabutin.[1]

(b) Rifampicin (Rifampin)

A steady-state study in 13 HIV-positive subjects found that the use of atovaquone 750 mg twice daily with rifampicin 600 mg daily for 14 days resulted in a more than 50% reduction in the AUC and plasma concentration of atovaquone, but a more than 30% rise in the AUC and plasma concentration of rifampicin.[2,3]

Mechanism

Uncertain. Atovaquone is predominantly excreted (greater than 90%) as unchanged drug in the faeces,[3,4] and would not therefore be expected to be affected by cytochrome P450 enzyme induction.

Importance and management

Although information is limited, the pharmacokinetic interactions between atovaquone and rifampicin or rifabutin appear to be established. It seems highly likely that the efficacy of atovaquone will be reduced in the presence of rifampicin, and concurrent use should therefore be avoided. The effect of rifabutin is smaller than that of rifampicin, and the authors of the above report suggest that no atovaquone dose adjustment is needed.[1] The UK and US manufacturers of atovaquone still consider that concurrent rifabutin use could result in subtherapeutic plasma concentrations of atovaquone in some patients,[3,4] and the UK manufacturer also advises against the concurrent use of this combination.[4]

1. Gillotin C, Grandpierre I, Sadler BM. Pharmacokinetic interaction between atovaquone (ATVQ) suspension and rifabutin (RFB). *Clin Pharmacol Ther* (1998) 63, 229.
2. Sadler BM, Caldwell P, Scott JD, Rogers M, Blum MR. Drug interaction between rifampin and atovaquone (Mepron®) in HIV+ asymptomatic volunteers. *Intersci Conf Antimicrob Agents Chemother* (1995) 35, 7.
3. Mepron Suspension (Atovaquone). GlaxoSmithKline. US Prescribing information, May 2008.
4. Wellvone Oral Suspension (Atovaquone). GlaxoSmithKline UK. UK Summary of product characteristics, April 2010.

Atovaquone + Tetracyclines

Tetracycline reduces the plasma concentration of atovaquone. Tetracycline and doxycycline might increase the antimalarial efficacy of atovaquone.

Clinical evidence, mechanism, importance and management

A study looking at the population pharmacokinetics of atovaquone in 24 Thai patients found that neither the oral clearance nor the volume of distribution of atovaquone were affected by the concurrent use of **tetracycline**.[1] This sort of data gives only the broadest indication of whether or not an interaction occurs, and the US manufacturer of atovaquone with proguanil[2] notes that **tetracycline** might reduce the plasma concentration of atovaquone by about 40%. The UK and US manufacturers therefore suggest that parasitaemia should be closely monitored in patients taking atovaquone with proguanil with **tetracycline**.[2,3] In the UK, the manufacturer of atovaquone suspension also states that **tetracycline** should be given with caution until the interaction has been further studied,[4] whereas the US manufacturer of atovaquone suspension does not mention **tetracycline**.[5]

In contrast, in a clinical study to assess the efficacy of atovaquone alone or in combination with other antimalarials, the addition of **tetracycline** or **doxycycline** to atovaquone achieved cure rates of greater than 90%, compared with a cure rate of about two-thirds for atovaquone alone. However, these cure rates were still less than those achieved with atovaquone and proguanil. No pharmacokinetic data were collected.[6]

There appears to be no information about the effect of **doxycycline** on the absorption of atovaquone. Information about other tetracyclines is also lacking.

1. Hussein Z, Eaves J, Hutchinson DB, Canfield CJ. Population pharmacokinetics of atovaquone in patients with acute malaria caused by *Plasmodium falciparum*. *Clin Pharmacol Ther* (1997) 61, 518–30.
2. Malarone (Atovaquone with Proguanil hydrochloride). GlaxoSmithKline. US Prescribing information, September 2009.
3. Malarone Tablets (Atovaquone with Proguanil hydrochloride). GlaxoSmithKline UK. UK Summary of product characteristics, August 2012.
4. Wellvone Oral Suspension (Atovaquone). GlaxoSmithKline UK. UK Summary of product characteristics, April 2010.
5. Mepron Suspension (Atovaquone). GlaxoSmithKline. US Prescribing information, May 2008.
6. Looareesuwan S, Viravan C, Webster HK, Kyle DE, Hutchinson DB, Canfield CJ. Clinical studies of atovaquone, alone or in combination with other antimalarial drugs, for treatment of acute uncomplicated malaria in Thailand. *Am J Trop Med Hyg* (1996) 54, 62–6.

Azoles + Antacids

The gastrointestinal absorption of itraconazole capsules and ketoconazole are moderately to markedly reduced by some antacids. Itraconazole solution, fluconazole, and posaconazole absorption appears not to be affected by antacids. Similarly, voriconazole is not expected to be affected by antacids.

Clinical evidence

(a) Fluconazole

In 14 healthy subjects, 20 mL of an **aluminium/magnesium hydroxide** suspension did not affect the absorption of a single 100-mg dose of fluconazole.[1]

(b) Itraconazole

In a randomised study, 12 healthy subjects were given 30 mL of an **aluminium/ magnesium hydroxide** suspension four times daily for 2 days before taking a single 200-mg dose of itraconazole capsules. The antacid reduced the maximum plasma concentration and AUC of itraconazole by 70% and 66%, respectively, and delayed absorption (time to maximum plasma concentration increased from 3 hours to 5.1 hours).[2] In contrast, a study in 204 liver transplant patients[3] comparing the antifungal efficacy of itraconazole oral solution with fluconazole reported that itraconazole minimum plasma concentrations were not affected in 16 patients also taking antacids, proton pump inhibitors (see ‘Azoles + Proton pump inhibitors’, p.238), or H_2-receptor antagonists (see ‘Azoles + H_2-receptor antagonists’, p.237).

For mention of a study in which some patients needed an increase in their itraconazole dose when they took ranitidine and an unnamed antacid, see ‘Azoles + H_2-receptor antagonists’, p.237.

(c) Ketoconazole

A haemodialysis patient did not respond to treatment with ketoconazole 200 mg daily while taking **cimetidine**, **sodium bicarbonate** 2 g daily, and **aluminium [hydr]oxide** 2.5 g daily. Only when the ketoconazole dose was increased to 200 mg four times daily did the plasma concentration rise. A later study in 3 healthy subjects found that when ketoconazole 200 mg was taken 2 hours after cimetidine 400 mg, its absorption was considerably reduced (AUC reduced by about 60%). When this was repeated with the addition of **sodium bicarbonate** 500 mg, the absorption of ketoconazole was reduced by about 95%. In contrast, when this was again repeated, but with the ketoconazole in an acidic solution, the absorption was increased by about 50%.[4]

A study in 4 patients found that the concurrent use of **aluminium/magnesium hydroxide** 30 mL reduced the absorption of ketoconazole, but this was not statistically significant.[5] An anecdotal report suggested that giving ketoconazole 2 hours before a stomatitis cocktail containing **aluminium/magnesium hydroxide** seemed to prevent the cocktail reducing ketoconazole effectiveness.[6]

(d) Posaconazole

A study in 12 healthy subjects found that **aluminium/magnesium hydroxide** 20 mL did not affect the bioavailability of a single 200-mg dose of posaconazole to a clinically relevant extent, when taken with food or when fasting.[7]

Mechanism

Ketoconazole is a poorly soluble base which must be converted by the acid in the stomach into the soluble hydrochloride salt before it can be absorbed. Drugs that reduce gastric acidity, such as antacids, H_2-receptor antagonists (see ‘Azoles + H_2-receptor antagonists’, p.237), and proton pump inhibitors (see ‘Azoles + Proton pump inhibitors’, p.238), raise the pH in the stomach so that the dissolution of the ketoconazole and its absorption are reduced. The absorption of itraconazole, and possibly posaconazole, is also affected by changes in gastric pH. Fluconazole absorption is minimally affected by changes in gastric acidity.

Importance and management

The interaction between antacids and **ketoconazole** is clinically important, but not extensively documented. Advise patients to take antacids not less than 2 to 3 hours before or after ketoconazole so that absorption can take place with minimal changes in the pH of the gastric contents. Monitor response to confirm that ketoconazole is effective.

The absorption of **itraconazole** from *capsules* appears to be reduced by antacids, and it would therefore be prudent to separate administration. The UK manufacturer of itraconazole capsules recommends taking antacids at least 2 hours after itraconazole.[8] In the US, the recommendation is to take antacids at least one hour before or 2 hours after itraconazole capsules.[9] Although the UK and US manufacturers of itraconazole *solution*[10,11] do not give any specific advice regarding concurrent use of antacids, the solution is already in a soluble form and is therefore unlikely to be affected.[12]

Antacids do not appear to affect the bioavailability of **posaconazole** or **fluconazole** to a clinically relevant extent. However, the UK manufacturer of posaconazole still considers that its absorption might be affected by drugs that affect gastric acidity, including antacids.[13] Note, they recommend avoiding concurrent administration with other acid reducing drugs,[14] such as H_2-receptor antagonists (see ‘Azoles + H_2-receptor antagonists’, p.237) and proton pump inhibitors (see ‘Azoles + Proton pump inhibitors’, p.238).

1. Thorpe JE, Baker N, Bromet-Petit M. Effect of oral antacid administration on the pharmacokinetics of oral fluconazole. *Antimicrob Agents Chemother* (1990) 34, 2032–3.
2. Lohitnavy M, Lohitnavy O, Thangkaettiyanon O, Srichai W. Reduced oral itraconazole bioavailability by antacid suspension. *J Clin Pharm Ther* (2005) 30, 201–6.
3. Winston DJ, Busuttil RW. Randomized controlled trial of oral itraconazole solution versus intravenous/ oral fluconazole for prevention of fungal infections in liver transplant recipients. *Transplantation* (2002) 74, 688–95.
4. Van der Meer JWM, Keuning JJ, Scheijgrond HW, Heykants J, Van Cutsem J, Brugmans J. The influence of gastric acidity on the bio-availability of ketoconazole. *J Antimicrob Chemother* (1980) 6, 552–4.
5. Brass C, Galgiani JN, Blaschke TF, Defelice R, O'Reilly RA, Stevens DA. Disposition of ketoconazole, an oral antifungal, in humans. *Antimicrob Agents Chemother* (1982) 21, 151–8.
6. Franklin MG. Nizoral and stomatitis cocktails may not mix. *Oncol Nurs Forum* (1991) 18, 1417.
7. Courtney R, Radwanski E, Lim J, Laughlin M. Pharmacokinetics of posaconazole coadministered with antacid in fasting or nonfasting healthy men. *Antimicrob Agents Chemother* (2004) 48, 804–8.
8. Sporanox Capsules (Itraconazole). Janssen-Cilag Ltd. UK Summary of product characteristics, October 2011.
9. Sporanox Capsules (Itraconazole). Ortho-McNeill-Janssen Pharmaceuticals, Inc. US Prescribing information, June 2011.
10. Sporanox Oral Solution (Itraconazole). Centocor Ortho Biotech. US Prescribing information, November 2011.
11. Sporanox Oral Solution (Itraconazole). Janssen-Cilag Ltd. UK Summary of product characteristics, July 2011.
12. Janssen-Cilag. Personal communication, March 2008.
13. Schering-Plough Ltd. Personal communication, March 2008.
14. Noxafil (Posaconazole). Merck Sharp & Dohme Ltd. UK Summary of product characteristics, September 2014.

Azoles + Carbonated beverages

Some carbonated beverages can temporarily lower the gastric pH of patients with achlorhydria or hypochlorhydria due to disease or acid-suppressing drugs. This improves the bioavailability of itraconazole, ketoconazole, and posaconazole.

Clinical evidence

(a) Itraconazole

A study in 8 healthy subjects given itraconazole 100 mg with either 325 mL of water or *Coca-Cola* (pH 2.5) found that the maximum plasma concentration of itraconazole was more than doubled by *Coca-Cola* and the AUC of itraconazole was increased by 80%, although two of the subjects did not show this effect.[1] Another study in 30 healthy subjects compared the bioavailability of itraconazole alone or after ranitidine, both with and without a cola drink. Ranitidine reduced the absorption of itraconazole but this effect was countered by the cola drink.[2] A study in 18 fasted patients with AIDS, who absorbed itraconazole poorly, found that the absorption was restored to that of fasted healthy subjects when itraconazole was given with a cola drink.[3]

(b) Ketoconazole

In a study in 9 healthy subjects, a single 200-mg dose of ketoconazole was given after pre-treatment with omeprazole 60 mg the night before (to simulate achlorhydria), with 240 mL of water or with 240 mL of *Coca-Cola Classic*. Pretreatment with omeprazole reduced the absorption of ketoconazole by 83%, whereas when the cola drink was also given, the absorption of ketoconazole was only reduced by 35%. However, in 2 subjects the cola drink had only minor effects on ketoconazole absorption.[4]

(c) Posaconazole

A crossover study in healthy subjects compared the bioavailability of a single 400-mg dose of posaconazole oral suspension either alone while fasting or after esomeprazole pretreatment, both with and without a carbonated beverage (ginger ale). The maximum plasma concentration and AUC of posaconazole were increased by 92% and 70% respectively, when given with about 355 mL of ginger ale. Esomeprazole reduced the absorption of posaconazole, but the ginger ale partially reversed this effect.[5]

Mechanism

Itraconazole and ketoconazole are poorly soluble bases, which must be transformed by the acid in the stomach into a soluble hydrochloride salt. Therefore any drug or condition that reduces gastric acidity (i.e. increases the pH) can reduce the dissolution and absorption of these antifungals. Acidic drinks, which lower the pH, can increase their absorption. Posaconazole might be similarly affected.

Importance and management

The interactions of itraconazole and ketoconazole with carbonated beverages that lower the gastric pH are established. The interaction can be exploited to improve the absorption of these antifungals in patients with achlorhydria or hypochlorhydria and those taking gastric acid suppressants, such as H_2-receptor antagonists (see ‘Azoles + H_2-receptor antagonists’, p.237) and proton pump inhibitors (see ‘Azoles + Proton pump inhibitors', p.238). This is recommended by some manufacturers of ketoconazole[6] and itraconazole.[7,8] *Coca-Cola Classic, Pepsi,* and *Canada Dry Ginger Ale* can be used because they can achieve stomach pH values of less than 3, but none of the other beverages examined in one study produced such a low pH. The authors suggest that these would be less effective, although they were not actually studied. They included *Diet Coca-Cola, Diet Pepsi, Diet 7-Up, Diet Canada Dry Ginger Ale, Diet Canada Dry Orange Juice, 7-Up,* and *Canada Dry Orange Juice*.[4] The acidic drug **glutamic acid** does not appear to increase the absorption of itraconazole in fasted or fed subjects, or increase the absorption of ketoconazole in subjects pre-treated with cimetidine. See 'Azoles + Food', below, and 'Azoles + H_2-receptor antagonists', p.237, respectively.

The absorption of posaconazole appears to be increased by ginger ale, but the effect is probably not sufficient to fully reverse the effects of proton pump inhibitors (see 'Azoles + Proton pump inhibitors', p.238) or H_2-receptor antagonists (see 'Azoles + H_2-receptor antagonists', p.237).

For a brief mention of the use of carbonated drinks to increase itraconazole levels and thereby increase ciclosporin levels, see 'Ciclosporin + Azoles; Itraconazole', p.1215.

1. Jaruratanasirikul S, Kleepkaew A. Influence of an acidic beverage (Coca-Cola) on absorption of itraconazole. *Eur J Clin Pharmacol* (1997) 52, 235–7.
2. Lange D, Pavao JH, Wu J, Klausner M. Effect of cola beverage on the bioavailability of itraconazole in the presence of H_2 blockers. *J Clin Pharmacol* (1997) 37, 535–40.
3. Hardin J, Lange D, Heykants J, Ding C, Van de Velde V, Slusser C, Klausner M. The effect of co-administration of a cola beverage on the bioavailability of itraconazole in AIDS patients. *Intersci Conf Antimicrob Agents Chemother* (1995) 35, 6.
4. Chin TWF, Loeb M, Fong IW. Effects of an acidic beverage (Coca-Cola) on absorption of ketoconazole. *Antimicrob Agents Chemother* (1995) 39, 1671–5.
5. Krishna G, Moton A, Ma L, Medlock MM, McLeod J. Pharmacokinetics and absorption of posaconazole oral suspension under various gastric conditions in healthy volunteers. *Antimicrob Agents Chemother* (2009) 53, 958–66.
6. Nizoral Tablets (Ketoconazole). Janssen-Cilag Ltd. UK Summary of product characteristics, June 2010.
7. Sporanox Capsules (Itraconazole). Janssen-Cilag Ltd. UK Summary of product characteristics, October 2011.
8. Sporanox Capsules (Itraconazole). Ortho-McNeill-Janssen Pharmaceuticals, Inc. US Prescribing information, June 2011.

Azoles + Food

Some foods increase the absorption of itraconazole from capsules or tablets; however, food decreases the absorption of itraconazole from solution. Food or nutritional supplements increase the absorption of posaconazole from suspension. Studies with ketoconazole have shown little effect of food on absorption, although one found a decrease. The bioavailability of voriconazole is reduced by food. Food does not appear to affect the bioavailability of fluconazole.

Clinical evidence

(a) Fluconazole

A study in 12 healthy subjects found that food had no clinically relevant effect on the pharmacokinetics of a single 100-mg dose of fluconazole in capsule form.[1]

(b) Itraconazole

A study in 24 patients with superficial dermatophyte, *Candida albicans*, and pityriasis versicolor infections, given itraconazole 50 or 100 mg daily, found that taking the drug with or after breakfast resulted in higher plasma concentrations and gave much better treatment results than taking the drug before breakfast.[2] A later study found that the relative bioavailability of itraconazole (given as a capsule) was 54% on an empty stomach, 86% after a light meal, and 100% after a full meal.[1] Similar results were found in other studies using itraconazole.[3,4] Another study investigated the absorption of itraconazole in 144 healthy subjects given itraconazole 100 mg (as tablets or capsules) either in the fasting state, or immediately after a bread- or rice-based meal. This study found that while a bread-based meal more than doubled the bioavailability of itraconazole, when compared with the fasting state, in contrast a rice-based meal reduced the bioavailability of itraconazole by 43 to 80%.[5]

Studies with itraconazole oral solution give different results. A study in 30 healthy males given itraconazole 200 mg daily (as an oral solution), either on an empty stomach or with a standard breakfast, found that the bioavailability was 29% higher when itraconazole was taken in the fasting state.[6] A similar increase in bioavailability in the fasting state was seen in another study using itraconazole 100 mg daily (as an oral solution).[7]

A study comparing itraconazole capsules with solution found that the bioavailability of the capsules given in the fed state (immediately after a standard breakfast) was comparable to that of the solution given in the fasting state (102% versus 100%).[8]

(c) Ketoconazole

A study in 10 healthy subjects found that the AUC and maximum serum concentrations of a single 200-mg dose of ketoconazole (as tablets) were reduced by about 40% when given after a standard meal.[9]

In contrast, one study found that high-carbohydrate and high-fat diets tend to reduce the rate, but not the overall amount, of ketoconazole absorbed from tablets.[10] Further, a study in 8 healthy subjects found that the absorption of single 200- or 800-mg doses of ketoconazole was not altered when they were taken after a standard breakfast, although the time taken to reach the maximum plasma concentration was delayed. The absorption of single 400- or 600-mg doses of ketoconazole were increased by up to 50% with food, but this was not statistically significant.[11]

(d) Posaconazole

In a crossover study, a single 400-mg dose of posaconazole (as oral suspension) was given 5 minutes before, halfway through, or 20 minutes after a high-fat meal (containing 50 g of fat). The maximum plasma concentrations of posaconazole were increased 96%, 3.4-fold, and 3.3-fold, respectively, when compared with the fasting state, and the AUC was increased 1.1-, 3.8-, and 3.8-fold, respectively.[12] In a further study in 20 healthy subjects, a single 200-mg dose of posaconazole (as oral suspension) was given with either a high-fat meal, a non-fat breakfast, or after a 10-hour fast. The AUC of posaconazole was increased fourfold by the high-fat meal and 2.7-fold by the non-fat breakfast, when compared with the fasting state.[13] Two crossover studies in 49 healthy subjects found that the maximum plasma concentration and AUC of a single 400-mg dose of posaconazole (as oral suspension) were increased 3.4- to 3.5-fold and 2.6- to 2.9-fold, respectively, by 240 mL of a nutritional supplement (*Boost Plus*), when compared with the fasting state.[14,15] In another study, posaconazole 400 mg twice daily (as oral suspension) was given with an unstated amount of a **nutritional supplement** (*Boost*) for 7 days. The maximum plasma concentration and AUC of posaconazole were increased by 66% and 65%, respectively, when compared with the fasting state. A much greater effect was seen when posaconazole was given in doses of 200 mg four times daily for 7 days with the same nutritional supplement. The maximum plasma concentration and AUC increased by 40% and 60%, respectively. Increases of a similar magnitude were also seen when posaconazole 200 mg four times daily was given in the fasting state.[12]

(e) Voriconazole

In a study, 12 healthy subjects were given voriconazole capsules 200 mg twice daily either with food or in the fasting state (2 hours before or after food). Food delayed the oral absorption of voriconazole by about one hour and reduced the AUC by 22%.[16]

Mechanism

Not understood, but several factors might be important. It is possible that the enhanced absorption seen with itraconazole capsules and posaconazole suspension in the presence of food is related to gastric pH, as both drugs are poorly soluble and require acidic conditions for absorption, although posaconazole possibly less so (see 'Azoles + Antacids', p.235, and 'Azoles + Carbonated beverages', p.235, for further discussion of pH effects). The fat content of food might also play a role, with higher fat meals possibly resulting in increased absorption as a result of delayed gastric emptying and/or increased bile production. A further suggestion for the effect of food on posaconazole in particular, is that because posaconazole is lipophilic, the fat content of food improves its solubility rather than delaying gastric emptying. This is based on a study where metoclopramide and loperamide did not affect the absorption of posaconazole.[12]

Importance and management

Itraconazole absorption from the capsule formulation is best when it is taken with or after food and patients should be advised of this. However, as one study[5] found a reduction in the bioavailability of itraconazole (as capsules or tablets) with a rice-based meal, further study is needed to clarify if other foods might have the opposite effect to that expected. It would be prudent to be aware that the choice of food taken with itraconazole might not always have a positive effect on its absorption, and bear this in mind in case of an unexpected response to treatment. The absorption of itraconazole from the acidic liquid formulation appears to be better when it is taken at least one hour before food, and this is recommended by the UK manufacturer.[17]

The absorption of **posaconazole** from the oral suspension is improved by food, and the UK manufacturer recommends that posaconazole should be taken with food (or with a nutritional supplement for those who cannot tolerate food).[18]

A confusing and conflicting picture is presented by the studies with **ketoconazole**; two showing no change in absorption with food, and one showing a decrease. However, the UK manufacturer of ketoconazole states that the absorption of ketoconazole is maximal when it is taken during a meal, as it depends on stomach acidity, and it should therefore always be taken with meals.[19]

The UK and US manufacturers of **voriconazole** tablets and the US manufacturer of voriconazole suspension recommend that it should be taken at least one hour before, or one hour after, a meal.[20,21] The UK manufacturer of voriconazole suspension suggests that it should be taken at least one hour before, or *2* hours after, a meal.[20]

There appears to be no clinically relevant interaction between food and **fluconazole**.

1. Zimmermann T, Yeates RA, Laufen H, Pfaff G, Wildfeuer A. Influence of concomitant food intake on the oral absorption of two triazole antifungal agents, itraconazole and fluconazole. *Eur J Clin Pharmacol* (1994) 46, 147–150.
2. Wishart JM. The influence of food on the pharmacokinetics of itraconazole in patients with superficial fungal infection. *J Am Acad Dermatol* (1987) 17, 220–3.
3. Carver P, Welage L, Kauffman C. The effect of food and gastric pH on the oral bioavailability of itraconazole in HIV+ patients. *Intersci Conf Antimicrob Agents Chemother* (1996) 36, 6.
4. Barone JA, Koh JG, Bierman RH, Colaizzi JL, Swanson KA, Gaffar MC, Moskovitz BL, Mechlinski W, Van De Velde V. Food interaction and steady-state pharmacokinetics of itraconazole capsules in healthy male volunteers. *Antimicrob Agents Chemother* (1993) 37, 778–84.
5. Yun H-Y, Baek MS, Park IS, Choi BK, Kwon K-I. Comparative analysis of the effects of rice and bread meals on bioavailability of itraconazole using NONMEM in healthy volunteers. *Eur J Clin Pharmacol* (2006) 62, 1033–9.
6. Barone JA, Moskovitz BL, Guarnieri J, Hassell AE, Colaizzi JL, Bierman RH, Jessen L. Food interaction and steady-state pharmacokinetics of itraconazole oral solution in healthy volunteers. *Pharmacotherapy* (1998) 18, 295–301.
7. Van de Velde VJS, Van Peer AP, Heykants JJP, Woestenborghs RJH, Van Rooy P, De Beule KL, Cauwenbergh GFMJ. Effect of food on the pharmacokinetics of a new hydroxypropyl-β-cyclodextrin formulation of itraconazole. *Pharmacotherapy* (1996) 16, 424–8.
8. Van Peer A, Woestenborghs R, Heykants J, Gasparini R, Gauwenbergh G. The effects of food and dose on the oral systemic availability of itraconazole in healthy subjects. *Eur J Clin Pharmacol* (1989) 36, 423–6.
9. Männistö PT, Mäntylä R, Nykänen S, Lamminsivu U, Ottoila P. Impairing effect of food on ketoconazole absorption. *Antimicrob Agents Chemother* (1982) 21, 730–33.

10. Lelawongs P, Barone JA, Colaizzi JL, Hsuan ATM, Mechlinski W, Legendre R, Guarnieri J. Effect of food and gastric acidity on absorption of orally administered ketoconazole. *Clin Pharm* (1988) 7, 228–35.
11. Daneshmend TK, Warnock DW, Ene MD, Johnson EM, Potten MR, Richardson MD, Williamson PJ. Influence of food on the pharmacokinetics of ketoconazole. *Antimicrob Agents Chemother* (1984) 25, 1–3.
12. Krishna G, Moton A, Ma L, Medlock MM, McLeod J. Pharmacokinetics and absorption of posaconazole oral suspension under various gastric conditions in healthy volunteers. *Antimicrob Agents Chemother* (2009) 53, 958–66.
13. Courtney R, Wexler D, Radwanski E, Lim J, Laughlin M. Effect of food on the relative bioavailability of two oral formulations of posaconazole in healthy adults. *Br J Clin Pharmacol* (2004) 57, 218–22.
14. Sansone-Parsons A, Krishna G, Calzetta A, Wexler D, Kantesaria B, Rosenberg MA, Saltzmann MA. Effect of a nutritional supplement on posaconazole pharmacokinetics following oral administration to healthy volunteers. *Antimicrob Agents Chemother* (2006) 50, 1881–3.
15. Krishna G, Ma L, Vickery D, Yu X, Wu I, Power E, Beresford E, Komjathy S. Effect of varying amounts of a liquid nutritional supplement on the pharmacokinetics of posaconazole in healthy volunteers. *Antimicrob Agents Chemother* (2009) 53, 4749–52.
16. Purkins L, Wood N, Kleinermans D, Greenhalgh K, Nichols D. Effect of food on the pharmacokinetics of multiple-dose oral voriconazole. *Br J Clin Pharmacol* (2003) 56 (Suppl 1) 17–23.
17. Sporanox Oral Solution (Itraconazole). Janssen-Cilag Ltd. UK Summary of product characteristics, July 2011.
18. Noxafil (Posaconazole). Merck Sharp & Dohme Ltd. UK Summary of product characteristics, September 2014.
19. Nizoral Tablets (Ketoconazole). Janssen-Cilag Ltd. UK Summary of product characteristics, June 2010.
20. VFEND (Voriconazole). Pfizer Ltd. UK Summary of product characteristics, October 2014.
21. VFEND (Voriconazole). Pfizer Inc. US Prescribing information, February 2014.

Azoles + H_2-receptor antagonists

H_2-receptor antagonists markedly reduce ketoconazole exposure, and slightly reduce that of itraconazole and posaconazole; whereas the absorption of fluconazole and voriconazole is not affected to a clinically relevant extent. Not all H_2-receptor antagonists have been studied, but all are expected to affect azole exposure in the same way.

Ketoconazole might increase the plasma concentration of ranitidine.

Clinical evidence

(a) Fluconazole

In a study in 6 healthy subjects, the AUC_{0-48} of fluconazole 100 mg was reduced by 13% by a single 400-mg dose of **cimetidine**.[1] Two other studies found that **cimetidine**[2] and **famotidine**[3] did not affect fluconazole absorption.

(b) Itraconazole

In one study, 12 healthy subjects were given **cimetidine** 400 mg twice daily or **ranitidine** 150 mg twice daily for 3 days before and after a single 200-mg dose of itraconazole. There was a negligible reduction in the AUC and maximum plasma concentration of itraconazole and there was large inter-individual variability. The largest changes were 20% reductions in the AUC and maximum plasma concentration with **ranitidine**.[4] A study in 204 liver transplant patients,[5] comparing the antifungal efficacy of itraconazole with fluconazole, reported that the minimum plasma concentrations of itraconazole were not affected in the 16 patients also taking H_2-receptor antagonists, proton pump inhibitors (see 'Azoles + Proton pump inhibitors', p.238), or antacids (see 'Azoles + Antacids', p.235).

In contrast, another study in 30 healthy subjects found that **ranitidine** 150 mg twice daily for 3 days reduced the AUC of a single 200-mg dose of itraconazole by 44%, and reduced its maximum plasma concentration by 52%.[6] A study of the bioavailability of itraconazole, in 12 lung transplant patients also given **ranitidine** 150 mg twice daily and an antacid four times daily, found that the plasma concentration of itraconazole was highly variable. Half of the patients required the dose of itraconazole to be increased from 200 to 400 mg daily to achieve a satisfactory plasma concentration.[7]

In 12 healthy subjects, the plasma concentration of a single 200-mg dose of itraconazole was reduced by about 50% when they were given two doses of **famotidine** 40 mg, one dose the night before and the second dose taken one hour before itraconazole.[3] In a further study **famotidine** 20 mg twice daily was given with itraconazole 200 mg daily for 10 days to 16 patients undergoing chemotherapy for haematological malignancies. The minimum plasma concentration of itraconazole was reduced by about 39%, and 8 patients did not achieve the concentrations considered necessary to protect neutropenic patients from fungal infections.[8]

In another study in 20 HIV-positive patients, **glutamic acid** 1360 mg, given to acidify the stomach, either with or without food, did not enhance itraconazole absorption.[9]

A study in 8 healthy subjects found that **itraconazole** 200 mg twice daily for 3 days increased the AUC of intravenous **cimetidine** (loading dose 0.2 mg/kg followed by an infusion of 36 mg/hour for 4 hours) by 25%.[10]

(c) Ketoconazole

A case report describes a haemodialysis patient who did not respond to treatment with ketoconazole 200 mg daily while taking **cimetidine**, sodium bicarbonate 2 g daily, and aluminium oxide 2.5 g daily. Only when the ketoconazole dose was increased to 200 mg four times daily did her plasma concentration of ketoconazole rise. A later study in 3 healthy subjects found that when ketoconazole 200 mg was taken 2 hours after **cimetidine** 400 mg, the absorption was considerably reduced (AUC reduced by about 60%). When these two drugs were given with the addition of sodium bicarbonate 500 mg, the absorption of ketoconazole was reduced by about 95%. In contrast, when cimetidine was given with ketoconazole in an acidic solution, the absorption of ketoconazole was increased by about 50%.[11]

The AUC of a single 200-mg oral dose of ketoconazole was reduced by 91% in 12 fasting subjects who were given **cimetidine** 300 mg two hours before ketoconazole and then sodium bicarbonate 2 g one hour before ketoconazole. This effect was only slightly reversed by the use of **glutamic acid**.[12] Another study[2] in 24 healthy subjects found that intravenous **cimetidine**, titrated to give a gastric pH of 6 or more, reduced the absorption of ketoconazole by 95%. Similarly, a study[13] in 6 healthy subjects found that **ranitidine** 150 mg given 2 hours before ketoconazole 400 mg reduced its AUC by about 95%.

A study in 12 healthy subjects found that pretreatment with **ketoconazole** 200 mg daily for 5 days affected the pharmacokinetics of a single 150-mg dose of **ranitidine**, taken 30 minutes before ketoconazole on day 5. Ketoconazole pretreatment increased the AUC, maximum plasma concentration, and half-life of ranitidine by 74%, 78%, and 56%, respectively. The effects of ranitidine on ketoconazole were not reported in this study.[14]

(d) Posaconazole

A placebo-controlled study in 12 healthy subjects found that **cimetidine** 400 mg every 12 hours, given with posaconazole 200 mg once daily for 10 days, reduced the AUC and maximum plasma concentration of posaconazole by about 40%.[15] A population pharmacokinetic model, using therapeutic drug monitoring data from 16 allogeneic stem cell transplant patients receiving prophylactic posaconazole, found that **ranitidine** did not alter the pharmacokinetics of posaconazole.[16]

(e) Voriconazole

A study in 12 healthy subjects found that **cimetidine** 400 mg twice daily given with voriconazole 200 mg twice daily increased the maximum plasma concentration and AUC of voriconazole by about 20%, but this is not considered sufficient to warrant a dose adjustment.[17] **Ranitidine** 150 mg twice daily had no effect on the AUC and maximum plasma concentration of voriconazole.[17]

Mechanism

Ketoconazole is a poorly soluble base, which must be converted by the acid in the stomach into the soluble hydrochloride salt. Drugs that reduce gastric acidity, such as H_2-receptor antagonists, proton pump inhibitors (see 'Azoles + Proton pump inhibitors', p.238), or antacids (see 'Azoles + Antacids', p.235), raise the pH in the stomach so that the dissolution of the ketoconazole and its absorption are reduced. Conversely, anything that increases the gastric acidity increases the dissolution and the absorption (see 'Azoles + Carbonated beverages', p.235). The absorption of itraconazole capsules, and possibly posaconazole, is similarly affected by changes in gastric pH. The absorption of fluconazole and voriconazole[18] are not affected by reductions in gastric acidity.

The slight increase in the plasma concentration of cimetidine in the presence of itraconazole might be due to inhibition of P-glycoprotein mediated renal tubular secretion of cimetidine,[10] and the increase in the bioavailability of ranitidine is thought to be due to inhibition of intestinal P-glycoprotein by ketoconazole.[14]

Importance and management

The interactions of the H_2-receptor antagonists with **ketoconazole** are clinically important but not extensively documented. The situation with **itraconazole** is not entirely clear, but some reduction in its exposure apparently occurs which might be of clinical significance. It would therefore be prudent to confirm that both itraconazole and ketoconazole remain effective in the presence of H_2-receptor antagonists. It has been suggested[6] that the reduction in bioavailability due to H_2-receptor antagonists can be minimised by giving itraconazole and ketoconazole with an acidic drink, such as cola (see 'Azoles + Carbonated beverages', p.235), and this is recommended by some manufacturers.[19-21] Although there appear to be no specific studies with itraconazole oral solution, the concurrent use of drugs that affect gastric acidity, such as H_2-receptor antagonists, would not be expected to have a similar effect. Studies with omeprazole (see 'Azoles + Proton pump inhibitors', p.238) have found no important reductions in the absorption of itraconazole oral solution. The UK manufacturer of itraconazole oral solution[22] does not give any specific advice on concurrent use of these drugs; however, the US manufacturer advises caution with concurrent use, although they expect the effect to be considerably less than that seen with itraconazole capsules.[23]

The bioavailability of **posaconazole** also appears to be reduced by cimetidine. There appear to be no data on the effects of other H_2-receptor antagonists such as ranitidine, famotidine, or nizatidine. If this reduction in absorption is due to the reduction in gastric acid, then it could be minimised by taking posaconazole with a carbonated beverage, such as a cola drink, as for ketoconazole and itraconazole. However, the UK manufacturer currently recommends that the use of posaconazole with cimetidine, or other H_2-receptor antagonists (as there are no data), should be avoided if possible.[24] Further study is needed.

Fluconazole only interacts to a small, and clinically irrelevant, extent with H_2-receptor antagonists and is therefore a possible alternative to ketoconazole and itraconazole. Similarly, **voriconazole** is not affected by drugs that increase gastric pH such as the H_2-receptor antagonists,[18] and no dose adjustments are necessary with concurrent use.[25]

The clinical significance of the increases in **ranitidine** bioavailability produced by ketoconazole in one isolated study[14] is unclear; however, as ranitidine has a wide therapeutic margin, dose-related toxicity arising from this interaction seems unlikely.

1. Lazar JD, Wilner KD. Drug interactions with fluconazole. *Rev Infect Dis* (1990) 12 (Suppl 3), S327–S333.
2. Blum RA, D'Andrea DT, Florentino BM, Wilton JH, Hilligoss DM, Gardner MJ, Henry EB, Goldstein H, Schentag JJ. Increased gastric pH and the bioavailability of fluconazole and ketoconazole. *Ann Intern Med* (1991) 114, 755–7.
3. Lim SG, Sawyerr AM, Hudson M, Sercombe J, Pounder RE. Short report: The absorption of fluconazole and itraconazole under conditions of low intragastric acidity. *Aliment Pharmacol Ther* (1993) 7, 317–21.
4. Stein AG, Daneshmend TK, Warnock DW, Bhaskar N, Burke J, Hawkey CJ. The effects of H_2-receptor antagonists on the pharmacokinetics of itraconazole, a new oral antifungal. *Br J Clin Pharmacol* (1989) 27, 105P–106P.
5. Winston DJ, Busuttil RW. Randomized controlled trial of oral itraconazole solution versus intravenous/oral fluconazole for prevention of fungal infections in liver transplant recipients. *Transplantation* (2002) 74, 688–95.

6. Lange D, Pavao JH, Wu J, Klausner M. Effect of a cola beverage on the bioavailability of itraconazole in the presence of H_2 blockers. *J Clin Pharmacol* (1997) 37, 535–40.
7. Patterson TF, Peters J, Levine SM, Anzueto A, Bryan CL, Sako EY, LaWayne Miller O, Calhoon JH, Rinaldi MG. Systemic availability of itraconazole in lung transplantation. *Antimicrob Agents Chemother* (1996) 40, 2217–20.
8. Kanda Y, Kami M, Matsuyama T, Mitani K, Chiba S, Yazaki Y, Hirai H. Plasma concentration of itraconazole in patients receiving chemotherapy for hematological malignancies: the effect of famotidine on the absorption of itraconazole. *Hematol Oncol* (1998) 16, 33–7.
9. Carver P, Welage L, Kauffman C. The effect of food and gastric pH on the oral bioavailability of itraconazole in HIV+ patients. *Intersci Conf Antimicrob Agents Chemother* (1996) 36, 6.
10. Karyekar CS, Eddington ND, Briglia A, Gubbins PO, Dowling TC. Renal interaction between itraconazole and cimetidine. *J Clin Pharmacol* (2004) 44, 919–27.
11. Van der Meer JWM, Keuning JJ, Scheijgrond HW, Heykants J, Van Cutsem J, Brugmans J. The influence of gastric acidity on the bio-availability of ketoconazole. *J Antimicrob Chemother* (1980) 6, 552–4.
12. Lelawongs P, Barone JA, Colaizzi JL, Hsuan ATM, Mechlinski W, Legendre R, Guarnieri J. Effect of food and gastric acidity on absorption of orally administered ketoconazole. *Clin Pharm* (1988) 7, 228–35.
13. Piscitelli SC, Goss TF, Wilton JH, D'Andrea DT, Goldstein H, Schentag JJ. Effects of ranitidine and sucralfate on ketoconazole bioavailability. *Antimicrob Agents Chemother* (1991) 35, 1765–71.
14. Machavaram KK, Gundu J, Yamsani MR. Effect of ketoconazole and rifampicin on the pharmacokinetics of ranitidine in healthy human volunteers: a possible role of P-glycoprotein. *Drug Metabol Drug Interact* (2006) 22, 47–65.
15. Courtney R, Wexler D, Statkevich P, Lim J, Batra V, Laughlin M. Effect of cimetidine on the pharmacokinetics of posaconazole in healthy volunteers. *Intersci Conf Antimicrob Agents Chemother* (2002) 42, 29.
16. Kohl V, Müller C, Cornely OA, Abduljalil K, Fuhr U, Vehreschild JJ, Schield C, Hallek M, Rüping MJGT. Factors influencing pharmacokinetics of prophylactic posaconazole in patients undergoing allogenic stem cell transplantation. *Antimicrob Agents Chemother* (2010) 54, 207–12.
17. Purkins L, Wood N, Kleinermans D, Nichols D. Histamine H_2-receptor antagonists have no clinically significant effect on the steady-state pharmacokinetics of voriconazole. *Br J Clin Pharmacol* (2003) 56, 51–5.
18. VFEND (Voriconazole). Pfizer Inc. US Prescribing information, February 2014.
19. Nizoral Tablets (Ketoconazole). Janssen-Cilag Ltd. UK Summary of product characteristics, June 2010.
20. Sporanox Capsules (Itraconazole). Janssen-Cilag Ltd. UK Summary of product characteristics, October 2011.
21. Sporanox Capsules (Itraconazole). Ortho-McNeill-Janssen Pharmaceuticals, Inc. US Prescribing information, June 2011.
22. Sporanox Oral Solution (Itraconazole). Janssen-Cilag Ltd. UK Summary of product characteristics, July 2011.
23. Sporanox Oral Solution (Itraconazole). Centocor Ortho Biotech. US Prescribing information, November 2011.
24. Noxafil (Posaconazole). Merck Sharp & Dohme Ltd. UK Summary of product characteristics, September 2014.
25. VFEND (Voriconazole). Pfizer Ltd. UK Summary of product characteristics, October 2014.

Azoles + Proton pump inhibitors

The bioavailability of ketoconazole, itraconazole capsules (but not oral solution), and posaconazole is reduced by omeprazole. Other proton pump inhibitors are expected to behave similarly with these azoles and a limited number of studies support this suggestion. The bioavailability of fluconazole does not appear to be affected by the proton pump inhibitors. Voriconazole exposure might be increased by omeprazole.

The exposure to esomeprazole and omeprazole is increased or likely to be increased by most azoles, although the extent of the interaction varies. Pantoprazole clearance might be lowered by fluconazole and voriconazole. Rabeprazole pharmacokinetics are not affected by ketoconazole.

Clinical evidence

(a) Esomeprazole

In a crossover study in healthy subjects, esomeprazole 40 mg daily for 3 days reduced the maximum plasma concentration and AUC of a single 400-mg dose of **posaconazole** given on day 3 by 46% and 32%, respectively. The half-life of **posaconazole** was unaffected.[1] Based on data for omeprazole, and the known acid-lowering effect of esomeprazole,[2] the manufacturers predict that esomeprazole might also reduce the absorption of **itraconazole**[2] and **ketoconazole**,[2,3] which depend on a low pH for optimal dissolution and absorption.

The UK and US manufacturers briefly note that exposure to esomeprazole might be more than doubled by **voriconazole**.[2,3]

(b) Omeprazole

1. Fluconazole. A study in 12 healthy subjects found that omeprazole 20 mg daily for 7 days did not affect the pharmacokinetics of a single 100-mg dose of fluconazole, given after a standard breakfast.[4] In another study in 18 healthy subjects, fluconazole 100 mg daily for 5 days increased the maximum plasma concentration and AUC of a single 20-mg dose of omeprazole 2.4-fold and 6.3-fold, respectively.[5]

2. Itraconazole. In a study, 11 healthy subjects were given omeprazole 40 mg daily for 14 days, with a single 200-mg dose of itraconazole [capsule] given after a standard breakfast on day 14. The AUC and maximum plasma concentration of itraconazole were both reduced by about 65% by omeprazole.[6] In contrast, another study in 15 healthy subjects found that omeprazole 40 mg daily did not affect the pharmacokinetics of single 400-mg doses of itraconazole or its metabolite, hydroxy-itraconazole, but in this study itraconazole was given as an oral solution, and there was a large interpatient variation in mean plasma concentrations.[7] Another study similarly reported that omeprazole had little effect on the pharmacokinetics of itraconazole oral solution.[8] A study in 204 liver transplant patients,[9] comparing the antifungal efficacy of itraconazole solution with fluconazole, reported that the minimum plasma concentration of itraconazole was not affected in 16 patients also taking proton pump inhibitors, H_2-receptor antagonists (see 'Azoles + H_2-receptor antagonists', p.237), or antacids (see 'Azoles + Antacids', p.235).

3. Ketoconazole. A three-way crossover study in 9 healthy fasting subjects found that omeprazole 60 mg reduced the AUC of ketoconazole 200 mg by about 80%.[10] Another study was undertaken in 10 healthy subjects to find the extent to which CYP3A4 is involved in the metabolism (sulfoxidation) of omeprazole. This revealed that ketoconazole 100 to 200 mg, a known inhibitor of CYP3A4, reduced the formation of omeprazole sulfone in both subjects with normal CYP2C19 activity and those deficient or totally lacking CYP2C19 (poor metabolisers). However, the plasma concentration of omeprazole was doubled in the poor metabolisers.[11]

4. Posaconazole. Esomeprazole reduces the plasma concentration and AUC of posaconazole (see under *Esomeprazole*, above). The UK manufacturer of posaconazole therefore considers that other proton pump inhibitors, such as omeprazole, might interact similarly.[12] This has been described in a 58-year-old man who had been taking posaconazole (dose unknown) for about 21 days, and whose minimum plasma concentration of posaconazole was approximately halved 3 days after omeprazole 40 mg daily was started. Omeprazole was discontinued and the plasma concentration of posaconazole returned to baseline over the course of the following 3 weeks.[13]

5. Voriconazole. A study in 18 healthy subjects found that omeprazole 40 mg daily for 7 days increased the maximum plasma concentration and AUC of voriconazole by 15% and 41%, respectively. Food was prohibited within one hour before, and after, each dose.[14] In another study, voriconazole 200 mg twice daily increased the maximum plasma concentration and AUC of omeprazole 40 mg once daily by about 2-fold and 4-fold, respectively.[15] In a therapeutic drug monitoring study in 52 patients, 7 of 16 (44%) patients with a minimum plasma concentration of voriconazole of greater than 5.5 mg/L were also taking omeprazole, and of these, 3 developed serious neurological adverse effects. These effects resolved completely in all 3 patients, 3 to 5 days after voriconazole was discontinued. No neurological adverse effects were seen in the patients with a plasma concentration of less than or equal to 5.5 mg/L (36 patients); 6 of these (17%) were also taking omeprazole.[16]

An isolated case report suggests that the use of omeprazole with voriconazole might have contributed to the 'unmasking' of an inherited long QT syndrome in a young female patient. In this case, the patient developed torsade de pointes and cardiac arrest (successfully resuscitated). However, voriconazole had been stopped 12 hours previously and this particular patient had many other contributing risk factors for the development of torsade de pointes, such as hypomagnesaemia and the use of other drugs that have been reported to increase the QT interval.[17]

(c) Pantoprazole

In a population pharmacokinetic analysis of intravenous pantoprazole in paediatric patients, the clearance of pantoprazole was reduced by 66% in 4 patients taking CYP2C19 inhibitors (including **fluconazole** and **voriconazole**).[18]

(d) Rabeprazole

In a randomised, placebo-controlled study, 18 healthy subjects were given **ketoconazole** 400 mg before, and after, taking rabeprazole 20 mg daily for 7 days.[19] Rabeprazole decreased the **ketoconazole** AUC and maximum plasma concentration by about 30%.[20] There was no evidence that **ketoconazole** affected rabeprazole metabolism.[19]

Mechanism

Ketoconazole and itraconazole are poorly soluble bases, which must be converted by the acid in the stomach into the soluble hydrochloride salt. Drugs that reduce gastric acidity, such as proton pump inhibitors, H_2-receptor antagonists (see 'Azoles + H_2-receptor antagonists', p.237), or antacids (see 'Azoles + Antacids', p.235), therefore reduce the dissolution and absorption of drugs such as itraconazole (in capsule form), ketoconazole, and posaconazole. Conversely, anything that increases the gastric acidity increases their dissolution and absorption.[10] For discussion of this effect see 'Azoles + Carbonated beverages', p.235.

In contrast, voriconazole absorption is not affected by changes in gastric pH. The increase in its plasma concentration seen with omeprazole might instead be via inhibition of CYP2C19, as the plasma concentration of voriconazole in poor metabolisers of CYP2C19 (a situation akin to the intake of an enzyme inhibitor) are about threefold higher than those in extensive metabolisers.[21]

Fluconazole and voriconazole almost certainly cause a rise in the plasma concentration of omeprazole and esomeprazole by inhibiting their metabolism by CYP2C19 and CYP3A4. Pantoprazole might be similarly affected. Ketoconazole inhibits CYP3A4 and not CYP2C19 and therefore causes a less marked rise in the plasma concentration of omeprazole, although in subjects deficient in CYP2C19, where the metabolism of omeprazole is more dependent on CYP3A4, ketoconazole has greater effects. Itraconazole would be expected to interact similarly to ketoconazole.

Importance and management

Fluconazole

Fluconazole pharmacokinetics are not affected by **omeprazole**, and are unlikely to be affected by other proton pump inhibitors. However, fluconazole markedly increases omeprazole exposure. The clinical relevance of these changes is uncertain, but not likely to be important for single-dose fluconazole regimens. More study is needed to establish whether it is advisable to reduce the omeprazole dose in those given both drugs longer-term. Note that these increases in omeprazole exposure are of a similar magnitude to those seen with voriconazole, and the UK manufacturer of omeprazole recommends dose adjustments in patients with hepatic impairment or on long-term use.[22]

The importance of the effect of fluconazole on **pantoprazole** clearance is unclear as the population pharmacokinetic analysis was in a very small number of patients, making it difficult to assess the validity of the finding. More study is needed.

Itraconazole

The interaction between itraconazole *capsules* and **omeprazole** appears to be established, but it appears that this can be minimised by using an oral itraconazole solution. As with ketoconazole, giving itraconazole capsules with an acidic drink such as cola (see 'Azoles + Carbonated beverages', p.235), would minimise the interaction, and this is recommended by the UK manufacturer of itraconazole capsules.[23] These might also be sensible strategies for the use of other proton pump inhibitors; however, one UK manufacturer of **lansoprazole** suggests that concurrent use should be avoided.[24] Any patient taking itraconazole should be monitored for antifungal efficacy if a proton pump inhibitor is also given.

The UK manufacturer of itraconazole *oral solution*[25] does not give any specific advice on concurrent use of drugs that reduce gastric acidity, such as the proton pump inhibitors. However the US manufacturers advise caution, although they expect the effect to be considerably less than that seen with itraconazole capsules.[26]

The effect of itraconazole on omeprazole is unknown, but it might be expected to increase the plasma concentration of omeprazole similarly to ketoconazole: any effect seems unlikely to be clinically important in the majority of patients.

Ketoconazole

The interaction between ketoconazole and **omeprazole** appears to be established and of clinical importance. Direct evidence seems to be limited to this study, but other drugs that raise the gastric pH have a similar effect (see 'Azoles + Antacids', p.235, or 'Azoles + H_2-receptor antagonists', p.237). Such a large reduction in the absorption of ketoconazole would be expected to result in the failure of treatment. Separating the doses of the two drugs is unlikely to be the answer because the effect of omeprazole is so prolonged. An alternative would simply be to monitor for any inadequate response to ketoconazole if omeprazole or **esomeprazole** is also given and to increase the dose if necessary. Giving ketoconazole with an acidic drink[10] such as cola (see 'Azoles + Carbonated beverages', p.235), appears to minimise the interaction, and is recommended by the UK manufacturer.[27] However, bear in mind that ketoconazole can also double the plasma concentration of omeprazole, although the clinical relevance of this is likely to be small for the majority of patients.

The interaction between ketoconazole and **rabeprazole** is also established, but the reduction in ketoconazole bioavailability is only small (30%) and it might be possible to accommodate any interaction by increasing the antifungal dose. There seem to be no reports about ketoconazole and other proton pump inhibitors but they are expected to interact similarly. It would therefore be prudent to monitor for a reduced effect if other proton pump inhibitors are used with ketoconazole. However, note that one manufacturer of **lansoprazole** suggests that concurrent use should be avoided.[24]

Posaconazole

Posaconazole exposure is reduced by esomeprazole (and therefore possibly by omeprazole). The UK manufacturer of posaconazole therefore recommends that concurrent use of proton pump inhibitors be avoided if possible.[12]

Voriconazole

The small increase in the bioavailability of voriconazole seen with **omeprazole** is not expected to be of general clinical importance, and no adjustment to the dose of voriconazole is required[15,28] on a pharmacokinetic basis. However, the report of serious neurological adverse effects in patients with very high minimum plasma concentrations of voriconazole, whilst taking omeprazole, warrants some consideration and should be borne in mind if such events occur in patients given both drugs. The clinical importance of the marked rise in the plasma concentration of omeprazole caused by voriconazole is not established, but the UK and US manufacturers of voriconazole recommend that the omeprazole dose be halved in patients taking omeprazole 40 mg or more.[15,28] The UK manufacturer of omeprazole does not recommend routine omeprazole dose adjustments with the concurrent use of voriconazole, but suggests that consideration is given to reducing the dose in patients with hepatic impairment or if long-term treatment is required.[22]

The increase in the **esomeprazole** exposure seen with voriconazole does not routinely require a dose adjustment of esomeprazole. However, patients taking esomeprazole in doses of more than 240 mg daily (e.g. for Zollinger-Ellison syndrome) might require a dose adjustment.[3]

The importance of the effect of voriconazole on **pantoprazole** clearance is unclear as the population pharmacokinetic analysis was in a very small number of patients, making it difficult to assess the validity of the finding. More study is needed.

1. Krishna G, Moton A, Ma L, Medlock MM, McLeod J. Pharmacokinetics and absorption of posaconazole oral suspension under various gastric conditions in healthy volunteers. *Antimicrob Agents Chemother* (2009) 53, 958–66.
2. Nexium Tablets (Esomeprazole magnesium trihydrate). AstraZeneca UK Ltd. UK Summary of product characteristics, August 2013.
3. Nexium (Esomeprazole magnesium). AstraZeneca Pharmaceuticals LP. US Prescribing information, November 2012.
4. Zimmermann T, Yeates RA, Riedel K-D, Lach P, Laufen H. The influence of gastric pH on the pharmacokinetics of fluconazole: the effect of omeprazole. *Int J Clin Pharmacol Ther* (1994) 32, 491–6.
5. Kang BC, Yang CQ, Cho HK, Suh OK, Shin WG. Influence of fluconazole on the pharmacokinetics of omeprazole in healthy volunteers. *Biopharm Drug Dispos* (2002) 23, 77–81.
6. Jaruratanasirikul S, Sriwiriyajan S. Effect of omeprazole on the pharmacokinetics of itraconazole. *Eur J Clin Pharmacol* (1998) 54, 159–61.
7. Johnson MD, Hamilton CD, Drew RH, Sanders LL, Pennick GJ, Perfect JR. A randomized comparative study to determine the effect of omeprazole on the peak serum concentration of itraconazole oral solution. *J Antimicrob Chemother* (2003) 51, 453–7.
8. Levron JC, Chwetzoff E, Le Moing JP, Lappereau-Gallot A, Chrétien P. Lack of interaction of antacid drug omeprazole on the bioavailability of itraconazole oral solution. *Blood* (1998) 92 (Suppl 1, part 2), 54b.
9. Winston DJ, Busuttil RW. Randomized controlled trial of oral itraconazole solution versus intravenous/oral fluconazole for prevention of fungal infections in liver transplant recipients. *Transplantation* (2002) 74, 688–95.
10. Chin TWF, Loeb M, Fong IW. Effects of an acidic beverage (Coca-Cola) on absorption of ketoconazole. *Antimicrob Agents Chemother* (1995) 39, 1671–5.
11. Böttiger Y, Tybring G, Götharson E, Bertilsson L. Inhibition of the sulfoxidation of omeprazole by ketoconazole in poor and extensive metabolizers of S-mephenytoin. *Clin Pharmacol Ther* (1997) 62, 384–91.
12. Noxafil (Posaconazole). Merck Sharp & Dohme Ltd. UK Summary of product characteristics, September 2014.
13. Alffenaar J-W, van Assen S, van der Werf TS, Kosterink JGW, Uges DRA. Omeprazole significantly reduces posaconazole serum trough level. *Clin Infect Dis* (2009) 15, 839.
14. Wood N, Tan K, Purkins L, Layton G, Hamlin J, Kleinermans D, Nichols D. Effect of omeprazole on the steady-state pharmacokinetics of voriconazole. *Br J Clin Pharmacol* (2003) 56, 56–61.
15. VFEND (Voriconazole). Pfizer Inc. US Prescribing information, February 2014.
16. Pascual A, Calandra T, Bolay S, Buclin T, Bille J, Marchetti O. Voriconazole therapeutic drug monitoring in patients with invasive mycoses improves efficacy and safety outcomes. *Clin Infect Dis* (2008) 15, 201–11.
17. Eiden C, Peyrière H, Tichit R, Cociglio M, Amedro P, Blayac J-P, Margueritte G, Hillaire-Buys D. Inherited long QT syndrome revealed by antifungals drug-drug interaction. *J Clin Pharm Ther* (2007) 31, 321–4.
18. Pettersen G, Mouksassi M-S, Théorêt Y, Labbé L, Faure C, Nguyen B, Litalien C. Population pharmacokinetics of intravenous pantoprazole in paediatric intensive care patients. *Br J Clin Pharmacol* (2009) 67, 216–27.
19. Humphries TJ, Nardi RV, Spera AC, Lazar JD, Laurent AL, Spanyers SA. Coadministration of rabeprazole sodium (E3810) and ketoconazole results in a predictable interaction with ketoconazole. *Gastroenterology* (1996) 110 (Suppl), A138.
20. Personal communication. Eisai Corporation of North America, October 1996.
21. Scholz I, Oberwittler H, Riedel K-D, Burhenne J, Weiss J, Haefeli WE, Mikus G. Pharmacokinetics, metabolism and bioavailability of the triazole antifungal agent voriconazole in relation to CYP2C19 genotype. *Br J Clin Pharmacol* (2009) 68, 906–15.
22. Losec Capsules (Omeprazole). AstraZeneca UK Ltd. UK Summary of product characteristics, May 2013.
23. Sporanox Capsules (Itraconazole). Janssen-Cilag Ltd. UK Summary of product characteristics, October 2011.
24. Lansoprazole Gastro-resistant Capsules. Zentiva. UK Summary of product characteristics, April 2015.
25. Sporanox Oral Solution (Itraconazole). Janssen-Cilag Ltd. UK Summary of product characteristics, July 2011.
26. Sporanox Oral Solution (Itraconazole). Centocor Ortho Biotech. US Prescribing information, November 2011.
27. Nizoral Tablets (Ketoconazole). Janssen-Cilag Ltd. UK Summary of product characteristics, June 2010.
28. VFEND (Voriconazole). Pfizer Ltd. UK Summary of product characteristics, October 2014.

Azoles + Rifabutin

Rifabutin moderately to markedly reduces the plasma concentration of itraconazole (and therefore possibly also ketoconazole), posaconazole, and voriconazole. Rifabutin does not affect the metabolism of fluconazole.

The plasma concentration of rifabutin is increased by fluconazole, posaconazole, voriconazole, possibly itraconazole (and therefore possibly also ketoconazole).

Clinical evidence

(a) Fluconazole

Twelve HIV-positive patients were given zidovudine 500 mg daily from day 1 to 44, fluconazole 200 mg daily from days 3 to 30, and rifabutin 300 mg daily from days 17 to 44. Rifabutin did not affect the pharmacokinetics of fluconazole,[1] but fluconazole increased the AUC of rifabutin by 82%, and increased the AUC of the rifabutin metabolite, LM565, by 216%.[1] In another study in 10 HIV-positive patients, fluconazole 200 mg daily increased the AUC of rifabutin 300 mg daily by 76% and increased its maximum plasma concentration by 91%. When the patients were also given clarithromycin 500 mg daily, the AUC of rifabutin was further increased, to 152%.[2] There is some evidence that fluconazole increases the prophylactic efficacy of rifabutin against *Mycobacterium avium* complex disease, although there was also an increase in the incidence of leucopenia.[3] Uveitis developed in 6 HIV-positive patients taking rifabutin 450 to 600 mg daily and fluconazole, 5 of whom were also taking clarithromyci,[4] which is also known to increase rifabutin exposure, see 'Macrolides + Rifamycins', p.332. Uveitis has been attributed to the concurrent use of rifabutin and fluconazole in other reports.[5,6]

Rifabutin does not appear to affect the metabolism of fluconazole.[7,8]

(b) Itraconazole

In a three-period study, 6 HIV-positive patients were given itraconazole 200 mg daily for 14 days, rifabutin 300 mg daily for 10 days, and then both drugs for 14 days. It was found that the rifabutin reduced the maximum plasma concentration of itraconazole by 71% and reduced its AUC by 74%.[9]

A 49-year-old HIV-positive man taking rifabutin 300 mg daily was also given itraconazole 600 mg daily. Because of low plasma concentrations after 3 weeks, the itraconazole dose was increased to 900 mg daily. One week later the patient developed anterior uveitis. It was found that the minimum plasma concentration of itraconazole was normal but the minimum plasma concentration of rifabutin was 153 nanograms/mL (expected to be less than 50 nanograms/mL after 24 hours). Rifabutin was stopped and the uveitis was treated. Symptoms resolved after 5 days.[10]

(c) Posaconazole

In a study in healthy subjects the concurrent use of posaconazole 200 mg daily and rifabutin 300 mg daily for 10 days increased the AUC of rifabutin by 72% and decreased the AUC of posaconazole by 51%, when compared with either drug alone.[11] Another study in 24 healthy subjects given posaconazole 200 mg daily for 10 days alone, or starting on day 8 of a 17-day course of rifabutin 300 mg daily, found that rifabutin reduced the maximum plasma concentration and AUC of posaconazole by 43% and 49%, respectively. Posaconazole increased the AUC and maximum plasma concentration of rifabutin by 72% and 31%, respectively. Adverse effects (headache, back pain, leucopenia, eye abnormalities) were more common with the concurrent use of posaconazole and rifabutin, leading to 4 subjects given both drugs being withdrawn from the study.[12]

(d) Voriconazole

The UK and US manufacturers describe a study in which rifabutin 300 mg daily decreased the AUC and maximum plasma concentration of voriconazole 200 mg twice daily by 79% and 67%, respectively.[13,14] Increasing the dose of voriconazole to 350 mg twice daily in the presence of rifabutin gave an AUC of 68% and maximum plasma concentration, which were more or less the same as that achieved with voriconazole 200 mg twice daily alone.[13] A case report describes a 30-year old woman receiving concurrent voriconazole and rifabutin therapy for multiple infections, who required an increase in voriconazole dose from 300 mg twice daily to 300 mg three times daily to achieve an adequate minimum plasma concentration of voriconazole. Subsequently her clinical condition improved dramatically. The authors also comment, that voriconazole may have affected the plasma concentration of rifabutin, as a lower dose was required to achieve target concentrations (150 mg daily rather than 300 mg daily).[15] At a dose of 400 mg twice daily, voriconazole increased the maximum plasma concentration and AUC of rifabutin 300 mg twice daily by about 3-fold and 4-fold, respectively.[13,14]

Mechanism

Rifabutin increases the metabolism of itraconazole and voriconazole, probably, at least in part, by inducing their metabolism by CYP3A4. Ketoconazole would be expected to be similarly affected. Rifabutin is also an inducer of P-glycoprotein and so would be expected to reduce the plasma concentration of posaconazole, which is a substrate for P-glycoprotein.[16] Fluconazole is largely excreted unchanged in the urine and so it is not affected by rifabutin.

The azoles apparently increase the plasma concentration of rifabutin by inhibiting its metabolism, probably by CYP3A4. Increased exposure to rifabutin can cause uveitis. An increase in the plasma concentration of rifabutin can cause uveitis.

Importance and management

The interaction between rifabutin and **fluconazole** is established, the general picture being that concurrent use can be advantageous. However, because of the increased risk of uveitis, the CSM in the UK stated that full consideration should be given to reducing the dose of rifabutin to 300 mg daily. The rifabutin should be stopped if uveitis develops and the patient referred to an ophthalmologist.[17] A later review suggests this 300 mg dose is associated with a reduced risk of uveitis and maintains efficacy.[18] The combination should be well monitored. Note that the effects of clarithromycin (see 'Macrolides + Rifamycins', p.332), are additive with those of fluconazole.

Information on the interaction between **itraconazole** and rifabutin is very limited, but if both drugs are given, monitor for reduced antifungal activity, raising the itraconazole dose as necessary, and be alert for an increase in the plasma concentration of rifabutin and toxicity (in particular uveitis). Note that the UK and US manufacturers do not recommend concurrent use.[19,20]

The UK manufacturer of **ketoconazole** does not recommend concurrent use with enzyme inducers, such as rifabutin.[21] However, if concurrent use is necessary, it would seem prudent to follow the same precautions suggested for itraconazole.

Similarly, the manufacturer of **posaconazole**, suggests that concurrent use should be avoided unless the benefit to the patient outweighs the risk.[16] If both drugs are used, monitor the efficacy of posaconazole and the toxicity of rifabutin, particularly full blood counts and uveitis.

The US manufacturer of **voriconazole** contraindicates its use with rifabutin.[14] However, the UK manufacturer permits concurrent use if the benefits outweigh the risks.[13] If used with rifabutin, the oral dose of voriconazole should be increased from 200 mg twice daily to 350 mg twice daily (and from 100 to 200 mg twice daily in patients under 40 kg). The intravenous dose should also be increased from 4 to 5 mg/kg twice daily. Importantly, the UK manufacturer advises careful monitoring for rifabutin adverse effects (e.g. check full blood counts, monitor for uveitis).[13]

1. Trapnell CB, Narang PK, Li R, Lavelle JP. Increased plasma rifabutin levels with concomitant fluconazole therapy in HIV-infected patients. *Ann Intern Med* (1996) 124, 573–6.
2. Jordan MK, Polis MA, Kelly G, Narang PK, Masur H, Piscitelli SC. Effects of fluconazole and clarithromycin on rifabutin and 25-*O*-desacetylrifabutin pharmacokinetics. *Antimicrob Agents Chemother* (2000) 44, 2170–2.
3. Narang PK, Trapnell CB, Schoenfelder JR, Lavelle JP, Bianchine JR. Fluconazole and enhanced effect of rifabutin prophylaxis. *N Engl J Med* (1994) 330, 1316–17.
4. Becker K, Schimkat M, Jablonowski H, Häussinger D. Anterior uveitis associated with rifabutin medication in AIDS patients. *Infection* (1996) 24, 34–6.
5. Fuller JD, Stanfield LED, Craven DE. Rifabutin prophylaxis and uveitis. *N Engl J Med* (1994) 330, 1315–16.
6. Kelleher P, Helbert M, Sweeney J, Anderson J, Parkin J, Pinching A. Uveitis associated with rifabutin and macrolide therapy for *Mycobacterium avium intracellulare* infections in AIDS patients. *Genitourin Med* (1996) 72, 419–21.
7. Mycobutin (Rifabutin). Pfizer Inc. US Prescribing information, October 2007.
8. Mycobutin (Rifabutin). Pfizer Ltd. UK Summary of product characteristics, December 2013.
9. Smith JA, Hardin TC, Patterson TF, Rinaldi MG, Graybill JR. Rifabutin (RIF) decreases itraconazole (ITRA) plasma levels in patients with HIV-infection. Am Soc Microbiol 2nd Nat Conf. Human retroviruses and related infections. Washington DC, Jan 29 – Feb 2 1995, 77.
10. Lefort A, Launay O, Carbon C. Uveitis associated with rifabutin prophylaxis and itraconazole therapy. *Ann Intern Med* (1996) 125, 939–40.
11. Courtney RD, Statkevich P, Laughlin M, Radwanski E, Lim J, Clement RP, Batra VK. Potential for a drug interaction between posaconazole and rifabutin. *Intersci Conf Antimicrob Agents Chemother* (2001) 41, 4–5.
12. Krishna G, Parsons A, Kantesaria B, Mant T. Evaluation of the pharmacokinetics of posaconazole and rifabutin following co-administration to healthy men. *Curr Med Res Opin* (2007) 23, 545–52.
13. VFEND (Voriconazole). Pfizer Ltd. UK Summary of product characteristics, October 2014.
14. VFEND (Voriconazole). Pfizer Inc. US Prescribing information, February 2014.
15. Schwiesow JN, Iseman MD, Peloquin CA. Concomitant use of voriconazole and rifabutin in a patient with multiple infections. *Pharmacotherapy* (2008) 28, 1076–80.
16. Noxafil (Posaconazole). Merck Sharp & Dohme Ltd. UK Summary of product characteristics, September 2014.
17. Committee on Safety of Medicines/Medicines Control Agency. Stop Press: Rifabutin (Mycobutin) — uveitis. *Current Problems* (1994) 20, 4.
18. Committee on the Safety of Medicines/Medicines Control Agency. Revised indications and drug interactions of rifabutin. *Current Problems* (1997) 23, 14.
19. Sporanox Capsules (Itraconazole). Janssen-Cilag Ltd. UK Summary of product characteristics, October 2011.
20. Sporanox Capsules (Itraconazole). Ortho-McNeill-Janssen Pharmaceuticals, Inc. US Prescribing information, June 2011.
21. Nizoral Tablets (Ketoconazole). Janssen-Cilag Ltd. UK Summary of product characteristics, June 2010.

Azoles + Rifampicin (Rifampin)

Rifampicin causes a negligible decrease in fluconazole exposure; however, cases of reduced fluconazole efficacy have been reported and larger effects have been seen with intravenous fluconazole. Rifampicin markedly or very markedly reduces the exposure to itraconazole, ketoconazole, and voriconazole, and had similar effects on posaconazole in one case.

Fluconazole does not appear to affect rifampicin pharmacokinetics, but the plasma concentration of rifampicin is reduced by ketoconazole.

Clinical evidence

(a) Fluconazole

1. Effects on fluconazole. In a study in healthy subjects rifampicin 600 mg daily for 19 days reduced the AUC of a single 200-mg dose of oral fluconazole by 23% and decreased its half-life by 19%.[1] Similarly, a study in patients with AIDS, taking fluconazole 400 mg daily for cryptococcal meningitis, found that the AUC and maximum plasma concentration of fluconazole were 22% and 17% lower, respectively, in 12 patients also taking rifampicin 600 mg daily, when compared with 12 similar patients not given rifampicin. There were no important changes in clinical outcome, although the subsequent use of a lower prophylactic dose of fluconazole 200 mg with rifampicin was found to result in plasma concentrations of fluconazole below the MIC of the infecting organism.[2] Another 3 patients with AIDS, taking fluconazole 400 mg daily for cryptococcal meningitis, relapsed when rifampicin was added.[3] Another report briefly states that one of 5 patients taking fluconazole needed an increased dose, or a replacement antifungal, when given rifampicin,[4] and a small study found that the AUC of *intravenous* fluconazole was 52% lower in 2 patients taking rifampicin, when compared with 3 patients not taking rifampicin.[5]

2. Effects on rifampicin (rifampin). A study in 11 patients with AIDS and cryptococcal meningitis found that fluconazole 200 mg twice daily for 14 days had no effect on the pharmacokinetics of rifampicin 300 mg daily.[6] Five patients with AIDS and tuberculosis, taking rifampicin and fluconazole, had normal plasma concentrations of rifampicin, when compared with 14 similar patients taking rifampicin alone, but in both groups the plasma concentrations of rifampicin were only about 28% of those predicted.[7]

3. Hypercalcaemia. An isolated report describes severe hypercalcaemia, which was attributed to the use of rifampicin and fluconazole, in a patient with tuberculosis and pneumocystosis.[8] The clinical relevance of this case is uncertain.

(b) Itraconazole

A patient receiving antitubercular treatment including rifampicin 600 mg and isoniazid 300 mg daily was also given itraconazole 200 mg daily. After 2 weeks of treatment the plasma concentration of itraconazole was very low (0.011 mg/L). Even when the itraconazole dose was doubled the plasma concentration only reached a maximum of 0.056 mg/L. When the antitubercular drugs were stopped the plasma concentration of itraconazole increased to 3.23 mg/L with a 300 mg daily dose, and 2.35 to 2.6 mg/L with a 200 mg daily dose.[9]

A later study in 8 other patients confirmed that the plasma concentration of itraconazole was reduced by rifampicin but the clinical outcome depended on the mycosis being treated. Four out of 5 patients responded to treatment for a *Cryptococcus neoformans* infection, despite undetectable itraconazole concentrations, apparently because of synergy between the two drugs (demonstrated *in vitro*). In contrast, 2 patients with coccidioidomycosis did not respond, and 2 others with cryptococcosis suffered a relapse or persistence of seborrhoeic dermatitis (possibly due to *M. furfur*), while taking both drugs.[10] A further study in 6 healthy subjects found that the AUC of a single 100-mg dose of itraconazole was reduced by 80% by rifampicin 600 mg daily for 3 days.[11] Large reductions in the plasma concentrations of itraconazole (undetectable in some instances) have been seen in other healthy subjects and patients with AIDS when they were given rifampicin.[12-14]

A retrospective review of the medical records of 2 patients given itraconazole and rifampicin indicated that itraconazole was not effective until rifampicin was stopped. This conclusion was based on the finding of continued weight loss while taking the combination and a clear weight gain after rifampicin was stopped.[15]

(c) Ketoconazole

1. Effects on ketoconazole. A study[16] in 6 healthy subjects found that rifampicin 600 mg daily reduced the AUC of ketoconazole 200 mg by 80%. Similarly, in another patient, the plasma concentration of ketoconazole 200 mg daily was roughly halved by rifampicin 600 mg. After 5 months of concurrent use with rifampicin and isoniazid 300 mg daily, there was a 9-fold decrease in the maximum plasma concentration, and the AUC was reduced by nearly 90%.[17]

A study in a 3-year-old child who had responded poorly to treatment, found that the maximum plasma concentration and AUC of ketoconazole were both reduced by about 65% to 80% by rifampicin and/or isoniazid. The interaction also occurred when the doses were separated by 12 hours. When all three drugs were given together the plasma concentration of ketoconazole was undetectable.[18] Other reports also confirm these findings.[19-23]

2. Effects on rifampicin (rifampin). A study in 6 healthy subjects found that the addition of ketoconazole 200 mg twice daily for one day, then 200 mg daily for 2 days to rifampicin 600 mg daily had little effect on the maximum plasma concentration and AUC of rifampicin.[16] In contrast, the plasma concentration of rifampicin in a child were roughly halved by ketoconazole, but when the rifampicin was given 12 hours after the ketoconazole, the plasma concentration of rifampicin was unaffected.[18] Other studies also show a reduction in the plasma concentration of rifampicin caused by ketoconazole,[21-23] one confirming that separation of the drugs by 12 hours minimised the interaction.[21]

(d) Posaconazole

A case report describes a 20-year-old man receiving vancomycin, ciprofloxacin, linezolid, and posaconazole 200 mg four times daily for multiple infections, including liver abscesses with MRSA and pulmonary fungal infections. Rifampicin (dose unstated) was started and, because of a suspected interaction, the plasma concentration of posaconazole was monitored. Posaconazole concentrations were 0.66 micrograms/mL 8 days after starting posaconazole, but had reduced by 80% (0.13 micrograms/mL) 21 days after rifampicin was started, and were still reduced (although they had risen to 0.28 micrograms/mL) after 33 days of concurrent use.[24]

(e) Voriconazole

A study investigating the steady-state pharmacokinetics of voriconazole reported a case where rifampicin was inadvertently started in a patient taking voriconazole 200 mg twice daily. The maximum plasma concentration of voriconazole was reduced from 3.92 micrograms/L to 0.038 micrograms/L and the AUC of voriconazole was reduced by 99%, after voriconazole was given with rifampicin (dose not stated) for 30 days.[25] The US manufacturer[26] notes that rifampicin 600 mg once daily decreased the maximum plasma concentration and AUC of voriconazole 200 mg twice daily for 7 days by about 95%. Even doubling the dose of voriconazole to 400 mg twice daily did not give adequate exposure.[26]

Mechanism

Rifampicin is an inducer of many cytochrome P450 isoenzymes, including CYP3A4, and therefore increases the metabolism of the azoles by these hepatic isoenzymes. However, as fluconazole (unlike ketoconazole, itraconazole, and voriconazole) is mainly excreted unchanged in the urine, changes to its metabolism would not be expected to have as marked an effect as on these other azoles. Furthermore, posaconazole is a substrate for P-glycoprotein and UDP-glucuronyltransferases. Rifampicin is an inducer of both this transporter system and glucuronidation, and therefore concurrent use reduces the plasma concentration of posaconazole.

The absorption of antitubercular drugs might be reduced in patients with AIDS and an increase in the plasma concentration of rifampicin could be due to increased absorption in the presence of fluconazole.[7] In contrast, it is suggested that ketoconazole impairs the absorption of rifampicin from the gut.

Importance and management

The interaction between rifampicin and **fluconazole** appears to be established and of clinical importance. Although rifampicin has only a negligible effect on the exposure to fluconazole, the cases of relapse cited above,[3] and the need for an increased dose,[4] indicate that this interaction can be clinically important. Monitor concurrent use and increase the fluconazole dose if necessary. One study suggests that, for serious infections, a 30% increase in the fluconazole dose may be considered if rifampicin is also given. This might be especially important during prophylaxis of cryptococcal meningitis with lower doses of fluconazole, such as 200 mg daily.[2]

The interaction between **itraconazole** and rifampicin is established and clinically important. The effect on the exposure to itraconazole can be very marked indeed, but the clinical importance of this interaction can apparently depend on the mycosis being treated. Therefore if the decision is taken to use both drugs, monitor the outcome closely and be alert for the need to increase the itraconazole dose. However, note that the UK and US manufacturers do not recommend the concurrent use of itraconazole and rifampicin, due to the magnitude of the effect on itraconazole.[27,28]

The interaction between **ketoconazole** and rifampicin appears to be established and of clinical importance. The effects on rifampicin can apparently be avoided by giving the ketoconazole at a different time (12 hours apart seems to be effective) but this does not solve the problem of the effects on ketoconazole: because of this the UK manufacturer suggests that concurrent use is not recommended.[29]

Evidence for an interaction between **posaconazole** and rifampicin appears to be limited to one case report, but what is known supports the prediction of reduced posaconazole exposure on concurrent use. The manufacturer of posaconazole suggests that the combination should be avoided unless the benefit to the patient outweighs the risk.[30]

The exposure to **voriconazole** is very markedly reduced by rifampicin and concurrent use is contraindicated.[26,31]

1. Apseloff G, Hilligoss M, Gardner MJ, Henry EB, Inskeep PB, Gerber N, Lazar JD. Induction of fluconazole metabolism by rifampin: *in vivo* study in humans. *J Clin Pharmacol* (1991) 31, 358–61.
2. Panomvana Na Ayudhya D, Thanompuangseree N, Tansuphaswadikul S. Effect of rifampicin on the pharmacokinetics of fluconazole in patients with AIDS. *Clin Pharmacokinet* (2004) 43, 725–32.
3. Coker RJ, Tomlinson DR, Parkin J, Harris JRW, Pinching AJ. Interaction between fluconazole and rifampicin. *BMJ* (1990) 301, 818.
4. Tett S, Carey D, Lee H-S. Drug interactions with fluconazole. *Med J Aust* (1992) 156, 365.
5. Nicolau DP, Crowe HM, Nightingale CH, Quintiliani R. Rifampin-fluconazole interaction in critically ill patients. *Ann Pharmacother* (1995) 29, 994–6.
6. Jaruratanasirikul S, Kleepaew A. Lack of effect of fluconazole on the pharmacokinetics of rifampicin in AIDS patients. *J Antimicrob Chemother* (1996) 38, 877–80.
7. Peloquin CA, Nitta AT, Burman WJ, Brudney KF, Miranda-Massari JR, McGuinness ME, Berning SE, Gerena GT. Low antituberculosis drug concentrations in patients with AIDS. *Ann Pharmacother* (1996) 30, 919–25.
8. Bani-Sadr F, Hoff J, Chiffoleau A, Allavena C, Raffi F. Hypercalcémie sévère chez une patiente traitée par fluconazole et rifampicine. *Presse Med* (1998) 27, 860.
9. Blomley M, Teare EL, de Belder A, Thway Y, Weston M. Itraconazole and anti-tuberculosis drugs. *Lancet* (1990) ii, 1255.
10. Tucker RM, Denning DW, Hanson LH, Rinaldi MG, Graybill JR, Sharkey PK, Pappagianis D, Stevens DA. Interaction of azoles with rifampin, phenytoin and carbamazepine: *in vitro* and clinical observations. *Clin Infect Dis* (1992) 14, 165–74.
11. Heykants J, Michiels M, Meuldermans W, Monbaliu J, Lavrijsen K, Van Peer A, Levron JC, Woestenborghs R, Cauwenbergh G. The pharmacokinetics of itraconazole in animals and man: an overview. In: Fromtling RA, ed. Recent Trends in the Discovery, Development and Evaluation of Antifungal Agents. SA: JR Prous Science Publishers, 1987 p 223–49.
12. Jaruratanasirikul S, Sriwiriyajan S. Effect of rifampicin on the pharmacokinetics of itraconazole in normal volunteers and AIDS patients. *Eur J Clin Pharmacol* (1998) 54, 155–8.
13. Drayton J, Dickinson G, Rinaldi MG. Coadministration of rifampin and itraconazole leads to undetectable levels of serum itraconazole. *Clin Infect Dis* (1994) 18, 266.
14. Hecht FM, Wheat J, Korzun AH, Hafner R, Skahan KJ, Larsen R, Limjoco MT, Simpson M, Schneider D, Keefer MC, Clark R, Lai KK, Jacobsen JM, Squires K, Bartlett JA, Powderly W. Itraconazole maintenance treatment for histoplasmosis in AIDS: a prospective, multicenter trial. *J Acquir Immune Defic Syndr Hum Retrovirol* (1997) 16, 100–107.
15. Todd JR, Arigala MR, Penn RL, King JW. Case report: possible clinically significant interaction of itraconazole plus rifampin. *AIDS Patient Care STDS* (2001) 15, 505–10.
16. Doble N, Shaw R, Rowland-Hill C, Lush M, Warnock DW, Keal EE. Pharmacokinetic study of the interaction between rifampicin and ketoconazole. *J Antimicrob Chemother* (1988) 21, 633–5.
17. Brass C, Galgiani JN, Blaschke TF, Defelice R, O'Reilly RA, Stevens DA. Disposition of ketoconazole, an oral antifungal, in humans. *Antimicrob Agents Chemother* (1982) 21, 151–8.
18. Engelhard D, Stutman HR,Marks MI. Interaction of ketoconazole with rifampin and isoniazid. *N Engl J Med* (1984) 311, 1681–3.
19. Drouhet E, Dupont B. Laboratory and clinical assessment of ketoconazole in deep-seated mycoses. *Am J Med* (1983) 74, 30–47.
20. Meunier F. Serum fungistatic and fungicidal activity in volunteers receiving antifungal agents. *Eur J Clin Microbiol* (1986) 5, 103–9.
21. Doble N, Hykin P, Shaw R, Keal EE. Pulmonary mycobacterium tuberculosis in acquired immune deficiency syndrome. *BMJ* (1985) 291, 849–50.
22. Abadie-Kemmerly S, Pankey GA, Dalvisio JR. Failure of ketoconazole treatment of *Blastomyces dermatidis* due to interaction of isoniazid and rifampin. *Ann Intern Med* (1988) 109, 844–5.
23. Pilheu JA, Galati MR, Yunis AS, De Salvo MC, Negroni R, Garcia Fernandez JC, Mingolla L, Rubio MC, Masana M, Acevedo C. Interaccion farmacocinetica entre ketoconazol, isoniacida y rifampicina. *Medicina (B Aires)* (1989) 49, 43–7.
24. Hohmann C, Kang EM, Jancel T. Rifampin and posaconazole coadministration leads to decreased serum posaconazole concentrations. *Clin Infect Dis* (2010) 50, 939–40.
25. Geist MJP, Egerer G, Burhenne J, Riedel K-D, Mikus G. Induction of voriconazole metabolism by rifampin in a patient with acute myeloid leukemia: importance of interdisciplinary communication to prevent treatment errors with complex medications. *Antimicrob Agents Chemother* (2007) 51, 3455–6.
26. VFEND (Voriconazole). Pfizer Inc. US Prescribing information, February 2014.
27. Janssen-Cilag Ltd. UK Summary of product characteristics, October 2011.
28. Sporanox Capsules (Itraconazole). Ortho-McNeill-Janssen Pharmaceuticals, Inc. US Prescribing information, June 2011.
29. Nizoral Tablets (Ketoconazole). Janssen-Cilag Ltd. UK Summary of product characteristics, June 2010.
30. Noxafil (Posaconazole). Merck Sharp & Dohme Ltd. UK Summary of product characteristics, September 2014.
31. VFEND (Voriconazole). Pfizer Ltd. UK Summary of product characteristics, October 2014.

Azoles + Sucralfate

The gastrointestinal absorption of ketoconazole is reduced by sucralfate, whereas the absorption of fluconazole does not appear to be affected.

Clinical evidence

(a) Fluconazole

Sucralfate 2 g was found to have no effect on the pharmacokinetics of a single 200-mg dose of fluconazole in 10 healthy subjects, confirming the results of an *in vitro* study.[1]

(b) Ketoconazole

A study[2] in 6 fasting healthy subjects found that sucralfate 1 g, given 2 hours before ketoconazole 400 mg, reduced the AUC of ketoconazole by about 20%. Another study in fasting healthy subjects found that sucralfate 1 g given with glutamic acid hydrochloride reduced the AUC and maximum plasma concentration of a single 100-mg dose of ketoconazole by about 25%, but no appreciable changes were seen when the ketoconazole was given 2 hours after sucralfate.[3]

Mechanism

There is *in vitro* evidence to suggest that an electrostatic interaction occurs between ketoconazole and sucralfate to form an ion pair that cannot pass through the gut wall.[4]

Importance and management

The interaction between sucralfate and ketoconazole is slight and therefore probably of limited clinical importance. Any interaction can be minimised by taking sucralfate not less than 2 to 3 hours before, or after, ketoconazole. No adjustments would be expected to be necessary if fluconazole is given with sucralfate.

1. Carver PL, Hoeschele JD, Partipilo L, Kauffman CA, Mercer BT, Pecoraro VL. Fluconazole: a model compound for in vitro and in vivo interactions with sucralfate. *Pharmacotherapy* (1994) 14, 347.
2. Piscitelli SC, Goss TF, Wilton JH, D'Andrea DT, Goldstein H, Schentag JJ. Effects of ranitidine and sucralfate on ketoconazole bioavailability. *Antimicrob Agents Chemother* (1991) 35, 1765–71.
3. Carver PL, Berardi RR, Knapp MJ, Rider JM, Kauffman CA, Bradley SF, Atassi M. In vivo interaction of ketoconazole and sucralfate in healthy volunteers. *Antimicrob Agents Chemother* (1994) 38, 326–9.
4. Hoeschele JD, Roy AK, Pecoraro VL, Carver PL. In vitro analysis of the interaction between sucralfate and ketoconazole. *Antimicrob Agents Chemother* (1994) 38, 319–25.

Azoles; Fluconazole + Hydrochlorothiazide

Hydrochlorothiazide slightly increases the exposure to fluconazole.

Clinical evidence, mechanism, importance and management

The UK and US manufacturers note that, in 13 healthy subjects, hydrochlorothiazide 50 mg daily increased the AUC and plasma concentration of fluconazole 100 mg daily for 10 days by about 40%.[1,2] They attribute these changes to a reduction in the renal clearance of fluconazole.[2] However they state that it is unlikely that a change in the fluconazole dose will be needed in patients taking diuretics, but that the interaction should be borne in mind.[1] Any interaction is almost certainly of no relevance in a patient taking a single dose of fluconazole (e.g. for genital candidiasis).

1. Diflucan (Fluconazole). Pfizer Ltd. UK Summary of product characteristics, June 2009.
2. Diflucan (Fluconazole). Pfizer Inc. US Prescribing information, June 2011.

Azoles; Itraconazole + Ciprofloxacin

In a study, the exposure to itraconazole was increased by ciprofloxacin. The pharmacokinetics of ciprofloxacin were unaffected by itraconazole.

Clinical evidence, mechanism, importance and management

In a pharmacokinetic study, 10 healthy subjects were given ciprofloxacin 500 mg twice daily for 7 days, alone, itraconazole 200 mg twice daily for 7 days, alone, and then both drugs together for 7 days. The AUC and maximum plasma concentration of itraconazole were increased 53% and 82% by ciprofloxacin. The pharmacokinetics of ciprofloxacin were not affected by itraconazole. The authors concluded that these increases were due to inhibition of the CYP3A4-mediated metabolism of itraconazole by ciprofloxacin.[1] However, note that ciprofloxacin is not known to be an inhibitor of CYP3A4, and so the reason for the altered itraconazole pharmacokinetics is not known. Note also, that the general clinical relevance of this study is likely to be small, given the widespread and long-standing use of both of these drugs.

1. Sriwiriyajan S, Samaeng M, Ridtitid W, Mahatthanatrakul W, Wongnawa M. Pharmacokinetic interactions between ciprofloxacin and itraconazole in healthy male volunteers. *Biopharm Drug Dispos* (2011) 32, 168–74.

Azoles; Itraconazole + Grapefruit and other fruit juices

Grapefruit juice impaired the absorption of itraconazole capsules in one study, but not in another. Grapefruit juice had no effect on the absorption of itraconazole oral solution. Orange juice impaired the absorption of itraconazole capsules in one study, but appeared to have no effect on itraconazole exposure when itraconazole was given as an oral solution.

Clinical evidence

(a) Capsules

In one study, 11 healthy subjects were given a single 200-mg dose of itraconazole (*Sporanox capsules, Janssen*) immediately after a standard breakfast. Either 240 mL of double-strength grapefruit juice or water were given with, and 2 hours after, the dose of itraconazole. Grapefruit juice unexpectedly decreased the AUC of itraconazole by 43% (range 81% reduction to 105% increase), with a similar decrease in the AUC of its active metabolite,hydroxy-itraconazole.[1] However, another similar study found that grapefruit juice had no effect on the pharmacokinetics of itraconazole capsules (*Itrizole, Janssen*). The only apparent differences in the studies were that the study where no interaction was detected used a lower dose of itraconazole (100 mg versus 200 mg) and a larger volume of less concentrated grapefruit juice (350 mL of single-strength grapefruit juice).[2] The latter study[2] also used **orange juice**, which was found to reduce the AUC of itraconazole by an average of 41%.

(b) Oral solution

In a study in 20 healthy subjects grapefruit juice caused a 17% increase in the AUC of itraconazole. In this study, regular strength grapefruit juice 240 mL was given alone three times daily for 2 days, then together with itraconazole oral solution 200 mg on the morning of the third day in the fasted state, and then again 2 hours later.[3] When itraconazole oral solution was mixed with **orange juice** to improve tolerability and treatment adherence, the plasma concentration of itraconazole did not differ from that achieved when it was given with water.[4]

Mechanism

Grapefruit juice is an inhibitor of intestinal CYP3A4, the major isoenzyme involved in itraconazole metabolism. It was therefore predicted that it would enhance itraconazole exposure, a prediction confirmed with itraconazole oral solution. However, studies with itraconazole capsules have found both a decrease and no change in the exposure to itraconazole. The mechanism is not known, but one plausible suggestion is that grapefruit juice might impair the absorption of itraconazole capsules by lowering the duodenal pH.[1]

Importance and management

Evidence for an interaction between itraconazole and grapefruit juice is limited and somewhat conflicting. The 40% reduction in the exposure to itraconazole from itraconazole *capsules* seen with grapefruit juice would be expected to be clinically relevant in some situations, but it was seen in only one of two single-dose studies. Similarly, the reduction in exposure with orange juice might be clinically relevant. However, at present, there is insufficient evidence to recommend avoiding concurrent use. Until more is known, in the event of an unexpected reduction in itraconazole efficacy or reduced itraconazole exposure, consider grapefruit juice or orange juice intake as a possible factor.

Itraconazole *oral solution*, which is better absorbed than the capsules, does not appear to be affected by grapefruit juice or orange juice.

1. Penzak SR, Gubbins PO, Gurley BJ, Wang P-L, Saccente M. Grapefruit juice decreases the systemic availability of itraconazole capsules in healthy volunteers. *Ther Drug Monit* (1999) 21, 304–309.
2. Kawakami M, Suzuki K, Ishizuka T, Hidaka T, Matsuki Y, Nakumara H. Effect of grapefruit juice on pharmacokinetics of itraconazole in healthy subjects. *Int J Clin Pharmacol Ther* (1998) 36, 306–308.
3. Gubbins PO, McConnell SA, Gurley BJ, Fincher TK, Franks AM, Williams DK, Penzak SR, Saccente M. Influence of grapefruit juice on the systemic availability of itraconazole oral solution in healthy adult volunteers. *Pharmacotherapy* (2004) 24, 460–7.
4. Adachi Y, Sumikuma T, Kagami R, Nishio A, Akasaka K, Tsunemine H, Kodaka T, Hiramatsu Y, Tada H. Improvement of patient adherence by mixing oral itraconazole solution with a beverage (orange juice). *Rinsho Ketsueki* (2010) 51, 315–19.

Azoles; Itraconazole + Valproate

An isolated case report describes very low itraconazole concentrations in a patient also taking valproate.

Clinical evidence, mechanism, importance and management

A case report describes a 55-year-old man with neuroparacoccidioidomycosis (NPCM) with an associated abdominal ulcerated granulomatous lesion, who started taking itraconazole 400 mg daily, while taking sodium valproate (400 mg in the morning and 200 mg in the evening) to avoid seizures. One month after starting itraconazole his clinical response was minimal, and his itraconazole concentrations were undetectable. The sodium valproate was switched to clonazepam 1 mg daily and itraconazole was continued at the same dose. Fifteen days later his itraconazole concentrations were 4.6 micrograms/mL and his dose was lowered to 300 mg daily. During the first 2 months after this dose alteration, the abdominal ulceration healed and other symptoms began to resolve. After 5 months his itraconazole concentration was 9.76 micrograms/mL and the dose was further reduced to 200 mg daily. The itraconazole was continued for a further year at this dose and the patient continued to make substantial improvements.[1]

This appears to be an isolated report, and the mechanism by which valproate might reduce itraconazole concentrations is unclear. The general relevance of this case is therefore unclear.

1. Villa LA, Tobón A, Restrepo A, Calle D, Rosero DS, Gómez BL, Restrepo A. Central nervous system paracoccidioidomycosis. Report of a case successfully treated with itraconazol (sic). *Rev Inst Med Trop Sao Paulo* (2000) 42, 231–4.

Azoles; Topical + Miscellaneous

Butoconazole, clotrimazole, econazole, and fenticonazole are absorbed very poorly from the vagina so that the risk of an interaction with other drugs given systemically is small. Similarly, econazole, oxiconazole, and sertaconazole are minimally absorbed through the skin, and would not be expected to cause drug interactions, although isolated cases have been reported.

Clinical evidence, mechanism, importance and management

(a) Intravaginal application

The US manufacturer notes that 1.3 to 2.2% of the dose of intravaginal **butoconazole** cream 2% was absorbed in a study in three women.[1]

Early studies with intravaginal **clotrimazole** revealed that only a small fraction (3 to 10% of the dose) was absorbed systemically, and that this was rapidly metabolised.[2]

A study in 14 women (5 of them healthy, 4 with relapsing vulvovaginal candidiasis, and 5 with cervical carcinoma) found that the systemic absorption of **fenticonazole** nitrate from a single 1-g pessary was very small indeed. The amount absorbed, based on the amount recovered from the urine and faeces over 5 days, ranged from 0.58 to 1.81% of the original dose.[3] **Econazole** is also poorly absorbed when given intravaginally.[4]

The risk of a clinically relevant interaction with other drugs that might be present in the body would therefore seem to be very small with these antifungals used vaginally. However, isolated cases of raised INRs in women taking oral anticoagulants while using intravaginal miconazole have occurred, see 'Coumarins and related drugs + Azoles; Miconazole', p.409.

(b) Topical application

Systemic **econazole** is known to inhibit cytochrome P450 isoenzymes but, because of the very low systemic availability after topical application, the UK manufacturer notes that clinically relevant interactions are rare.[5] However, for a case report of a raised INR in a man taking warfarin while using econazole cream, see 'Coumarins + Azoles; Bifonazole or Econazole', p.407.

The US manufacturer of **oxiconazole** notes that systemic absorption is low, and in healthy subjects less than 0.3% of the applied dose was recovered in the urine after topical application of the cream.[6]

The plasma concentration of **sertaconazole** was below the limit of detection (2.5 nanograms/mL) when 5 patients with interdigital tinea pedis applied sertaconazole cream 2% every 2 hours for a total of 13 doses.[7]

Based on this information the risk of a clinically relevant drug interaction with systemically administered drugs and these topical azoles would seem to be very small. However, for a case report of raised INR in a man taking warfarin while using miconazole cream for a groin infection, see 'Coumarins and related drugs + Azoles; Miconazole', p.409.

1. Gynazole-1 (Butoconazole nitrate). Ther-Rx Corp. US Prescribing information, December 2009.
2. Ritter W. Pharmacokinetic fundamentals of vaginal treatment with clotrimazole. *Am J Obstet Gynecol* (1985) 152, 945–7.
3. Novelli A, Periti E, Massi GB, Mazzei T, Periti P. Systemic absorption of 3H-fenticonazole after vaginal administration of 1 gram in patients. *J Chemother* (1991) 3, 23–7.
4. Gyno-Pevaryl Vaginal Pessaries (Econazole nitrate). Janssen-Cilag Ltd. UK Summary of product characteristics, March 2011.
5. Pevaryl Topical Cream (Econazole nitrate). Janssen-Cilag Ltd. UK Summary of product characteristics, February 2011.
6. Oxistat (Oxiconazole nitrate). PharmaDerm. US Prescribing information, August 2009.
7. Ertaczo (Sertaconazole nitrate). OrthoNeutrogena. US Prescribing information, November 2005.

Azoles; Voriconazole + St John's wort (*Hypericum perforatum*)

St John's wort, taken for two weeks, more than halved the AUC of a single dose of voriconazole.

Clinical evidence, mechanism, importance and management

In a study in 17 healthy subjects, a single 400-mg dose of oral voriconazole was given alone and on the first and last day of a 15-day course of St John's wort (*Jarsin, Lichtwer Pharma*), given at a dose of 300 mg three times daily. One day of St John's wort had no effect on the $AUC_{0-\infty}$ of voriconazole, but increased its maximum plasma concentration and AUC_{0-10} by 22%. However, when voriconazole was given on day 15, the AUC of voriconazole was decreased by 59% and there was a 2.4-fold increase in oral clearance.[1]

These results suggest that the short-term effect of St John's wort is to enhance the absorption of voriconazole, whereas the longer-term effect is to induce absorption-limiting transport proteins and intestinal metabolism by cytochrome P450 isoenzymes.[1]

The increase in voriconazole absorption with a single dose of St John's wort is small and therefore not clinically relevant. However, the reduction in the plasma concentration and AUC of voriconazole after 15 days of St John's wort could reduce clinical efficacy. For this reason, the UK and US manufacturers contraindicate the concurrent use of St John's wort and voriconazole.[2,3] Patients already taking voriconazole should therefore be advised not to start St John's wort. Patients requiring voriconazole should be asked about current or recent use of St John's wort, as this might indicate the need to use an increased voriconazole dose, at least initially, while the metabolic effects of the herb decline.

1. Rengelshausen J, Banfield M, Riedel KD, Burhenne J, Mikus G, et al. Opposite effects of short-term and long-term St John's wort on voriconazole pharmacokinetics. *Clin Pharmacol Ther* (2005) 78, 25–33.
2. VFEND (Voriconazole). Pfizer Ltd. UK Summary of product characteristics, October 2014.
3. VFEND (Voriconazole). Pfizer Inc. US Prescribing information, February 2014.

Chloroquine and related drugs + Antacids or Kaolin

The absorption of chloroquine is reduced by magnesium trisilicate and kaolin. Calcium carbonate and gerdiga might have a similar effect.

Hydroxychloroquine absorption is predicted to be similarly reduced.

Clinical evidence

Six healthy subjects were given chloroquine phosphate 1 g (equivalent to 620 mg of chloroquine base) with either **magnesium trisilicate** 1 g or **kaolin** 1 g after an overnight fast. **Magnesium trisilicate** reduced the AUC of chloroquine by about 18% and **kaolin** reduced it by about 29%.[1]

Related *in vitro* studies by the same authors using segments of *rat* intestine found that the absorption of chloroquine was decreased as follows: **magnesium trisilicate** 31%, **kaolin** 47%, **calcium carbonate** 52%, and **gerdiga** 36%. **Gerdiga** is a clay containing hydrated silicates with sodium and potassium carbonates and bicarbonates. It is used as an antacid and is similar to attapulgite.[2]

Mechanism

These antacid and antidiarrhoeal compounds adsorb chloroquine thereby reducing the amount available for absorption by the gut. Dissolution of chloroquine from tablets might also be delayed by adsorbent antacids, such as **aluminium hydroxide, magnesium oxide**, or magnesium trisilicate.[3]

Importance and management

The modest pharmacokinetic interactions between chloroquine and magnesium trisilicate or kaolin are established, but their clinical importance does not seem to have been assessed. One way to minimise any interaction is to separate the doses of the antimalarials and magnesium trisilicate or kaolin as much as possible (at least 2 to 3 hours has been effective with similar adsorption interactions) to reduce admixture in the gut. Note that one UK manufacturer of chloroquine[4] suggests that the concurrent use of antacids should be separated by at least 4 hours. There do not appear to be any clinical studies to see if other antacids behave similarly, but it might be prudent to separate the administration of any type of antacid.

The manufacturer of **hydroxychloroquine**[5] predicts that, as with chloroquine, antacids might decrease hydroxychloroquine absorption, and they recommend separating administration by 4 hours.

1. McElnay JC, Mukhtar HA, D'Arcy PF, Temple DJ, Collier PS. The effect of magnesium trisilicate and kaolin on the *in vivo* absorption of chloroquine. *J Trop Med Hyg* (1982) 85, 159–63.
2. McElnay JC, Mukhtar HA, D'Arcy PF, Temple DJ. *In vitro* experiments on chloroquine and pyrimethamine absorption in the presence of antacid constituents or kaolin. *J Trop Med Hyg* (1982) 85, 153–8.
3. Iwuagwu MA, Aloko KS. Adsorption of paracetamol and chloroquine phosphate by some antacids. *J Pharm Pharmacol* (1992) 44, 655–8.
4. Avloclor (Chloroquine phosphate). AstraZeneca UK Ltd. UK Summary of product characteristics, July 2010.
5. Plaquenil (Hydroxychloroquine sulfate). Sanofi-Aventis. UK Summary of product characteristics, July 2010.

Chloroquine + Antihistamines

Chlorphenamine appears to increase the levels and therapeutic efficacy of chloroquine. Intramuscular promethazine appears to increase the levels of intramuscular chloroquine and its metabolites, although no increase was seen when both drugs were given orally.

Clinical evidence and mechanism

(a) Chlorphenamine

A study in 8 children given chloroquine 25 mg/kg over 3 days found that the addition of chlorphenamine (8 mg as a loading dose then 4 mg three times daily for 7 days) markedly increased the AUC and peak concentration of chloroquine, when compared with 9 children given chloroquine alone. A shorter parasite clearance rate (reduced from 3.5 days to 2 days) and higher cure rate (increased from 67% to 88%) were reported with the combination.[1]

A study in 10 healthy subjects given chloroquine 10 mg/kg on days 1 and 2 and 5 mg/kg on day 3, alone or with chlorphenamine (8 mg as a single dose followed by 4 mg every 8 hours for 7 days), found that the combination of chloroquine with chlorphenamine increased the peak level of chloroquine in erythrocytes by about 25% and doubled the erythrocyte AUC and half-life, when compared with chloroquine alone. Increased erythrocyte bioavailability is thought to reduce resistance to chloroquine. However, the clinical efficacy of this increase was not studied.[2]

A study in 41 children found that the adverse cardiac effects (QT prolongation, PR interval prolongation) of chloroquine with chlorphenamine were similar to that of chloroquine alone and these effects were less severe and occurred in fewer children when compared with halofantrine alone.[3]

(b) Promethazine

A study in 20 healthy subjects found that *intramuscular* promethazine hydrochloride 25 mg increased the AUC of *intramuscular* chloroquine phosphate 200 mg and its metabolites by 85%. This may be due to promethazine enhancing the absorption of chloroquine from the injection site or displacing it and its metabolites from binding sites in the blood. The initial rate of excretion of chloroquine and the total drug excreted within 3 hours was unaffected by promethazine.[4] The increased bioavailability of chloroquine may improve its therapeutic effects but could also increase toxicity. A study in 10 healthy subjects given *oral* chloroquine 10 mg/kg on days 1 and 2, and 5 mg/kg on day 3, alone or with *oral* promethazine (25 mg followed by 12.5 mg every 8 hours for 5 days), found that promethazine had no effect on the plasma or erythrocyte bioavailability of chloroquine.[2]

See also 'Metronidazole + Chloroquine', p.334, for details of an isolated case of acute dystonia in a patient given chloroquine, promethazine and metronidazole.

Importance and management

Evidence is limited and many of the available studies were primarily designed to assess efficacy. Nevertheless, it would appear that the concurrent use of chloroquine and chlorphenamine, or possibly *intramuscular* promethazine, might result in a marked increase in chloroquine levels. This appears to improve the efficacy of chloroquine in malaria treatment without increasing serious adverse effects, particularly cardiac toxicity.

1. Okonkwo CA, Coker HAB, Agomo PU, Ogunbanwo JA, Mafe AG, Agomo CO, Afolabi BM. Effect of chlorpheniramine on the pharmacokinetics and response to chloroquine of Nigerian children with falciparum malaria. *Trans R Soc Trop Med Hyg* (1999) 93, 306–11.
2. Gbotosho GO, Happi CT, Sijuade A, Ogundahunsi OAT, Sowunmi A, Oduola AMJ. Comparative study of interactions between chloroquine and chlorpheniramine or promethazine in healthy volunteers: a potential combination-therapy phenomenon for resuscitating chloroquine for malaria treatment in Africa. *Ann Trop Med Parasitol* (2008) 102, 3–9.
3. Sowunmi A, Fehintola FA, Ogundahunsi OAT, Ofi AB, Happi TC, Oduola AMJ. Comparative cardiac effects of halofantrine and chloroquine plus chlorpheniramine in children with acute uncomplicated falciparum malaria. *Trans R Soc Trop Med Hyg* (1999) 93, 78–83.
4. Ehiemua AO, Komolafe OO, Oyedeji GA, Olamijulo SK. Effect of promethazine on the metabolism of chloroquine. *Eur J Drug Metab Pharmacokinet* (1988) 13, 15–17.

Chloroquine + Colestyramine

Colestyramine can slightly reduce the absorption of chloroquine.

Clinical evidence, mechanism, importance and management

In a study in 5 children aged 6 years to 13 years, colestyramine 4 g reduced the absorption of chloroquine 10 mg/kg by about 30%. Considerable inter-individual differences were seen.[1] This reduced absorption is consistent with the way colestyramine interacts with other drugs by binding to them in the gut. The clinical importance of this isolated report is uncertain but separating the doses is effective in minimising the interaction of colestyramine with other drugs, and this would seem to be a prudent precaution with chloroquine. It is generally advised that other drugs are given one hour before or 4 to 6 hours after colestyramine.

1. Gendrel D, Verdier F, Richard-Lenoble D, Nardou M. Interaction entre cholestyramine et chloroquine. *Arch Fr Pediatr* (1990) 47, 387–8.

Chloroquine and related drugs + H_2-receptor antagonists

Cimetidine reduces the metabolism and clearance of chloroquine. Hydroxychloroquine is predicted to interact with cimetidine in the same way as chloroquine. Ranitidine does not appear to interact with chloroquine.

Clinical evidence, mechanism, importance and management

Cimetidine 400 mg daily for 4 days approximately halved the clearance of a single 600-mg dose of chloroquine base in 10 healthy subjects. The elimination half-life was also prolonged from 3.11 to 4.62 days.[1] It was suggested that these effects occurred because **cimetidine** inhibits the metabolism of chloroquine by the liver. A similar study by the same authors found that **ranitidine** does not interact with chloroquine.[2] On the basis of the data for chloroquine and cimetidine, the manufacturer of **hydroxychloroquine** states that, even though specific reports have not appeared, **cimetidine** might inhibit **hydroxychloroquine** metabolism.[3]

The clinical importance of this interaction is uncertain, but it would seem prudent to be alert for any signs of chloroquine or hydroxychloroquine toxicity during the concurrent use of cimetidine. Ranitidine would appear to be a non-interacting alternative to cimetidine.

1. Ette EI, Brown-Awala EA, Essien EE. Chloroquine elimination in humans: effect of low-dose cimetidine. *J Clin Pharmacol* (1987) 27, 813–16.
2. Ette EI, Brown-Awala EA, Essien EE. Effect of ranitidine on chloroquine disposition. *Drug Intell Clin Pharm* (1987) 21, 732–4.
3. Plaquenil (Hydroxychloroquine sulfate). Sanofi-Aventis. UK Summary of product characteristics, July 2010.

Chloroquine + Imipramine

No pharmacokinetic interaction was seen in 6 healthy subjects given single doses of chloroquine 300 mg and imipramine 50 mg.[1]

1. Onyeji CO, Toriola TA, Ogunbona FA. Lack of pharmacokinetic interaction between chloroquine and imipramine. *Ther Drug Monit* (1993) 15, 43–6.

Chloroquine + Methylthioninium chloride (Methylene blue)

Methylthioninium chloride possibly reduces the exposure to chloroquine.

Clinical evidence, mechanism, importance and management

In a study in 12 healthy subjects given oral methylthioninium chloride (methylene blue) 130 mg twice daily for 3 days with a 3-day course of chloroquine, the AUC of chloroquine was about 20% lower than in a control group of 12 healthy subjects receiving chloroquine with placebo. This difference was not statistically significant and renal clearance was unaffected. This very slight difference would not be expected to be clinically relevant.[1]

1. Rengelshausen J, Burhenne J, Fröhlich M, Tayrouz Y, Kumar Singh S, Riedel K-D, Müller O, Hoppe-Tichy T, Haefeli WE, Mikus G, Walter-Sack I. Pharmacokinetic interaction of chloroquine and methylene blue combination against malaria. *Eur J Clin Pharmacol* (2004) 60, 709–15.

Chloroquine and related drugs + Rifampicin (Rifampin)

A single case report suggests that rifampicin might increase the metabolism of hydroxychloroquine. Data in *mice* suggest that chloroquine might interact similarly.

Clinical evidence, mechanism, importance and management

A woman with discoid lupus, controlled by hydroxychloroquine 200 mg daily, was given rifampicin, isoniazid, and pyrazinamide for tuberculosis. Within one to 2 weeks the discoid lupus flared-up but it rapidly responded when the hydroxychloroquine dose was doubled. The reason for this reaction is not established but the authors of the report suggest that rifampicin (a recognised enzyme inducer) increased the metabolism and clearance of hydroxychloroquine so that it was no longer effective.[1] It also seems possible that P-glycoprotein might have a part to play. It is already known that discoid lupus flare-ups can occur within 2 weeks of stopping hydroxychloroquine,[2] which supports the suggested mechanisms. Neither isoniazid nor pyrazinamide is likely to have been responsible for the relapse.

This seems to be the first and only report of this interaction, but these results are consistent with the way rifampicin interacts with many other drugs. If rifampicin is given with hydroxychloroquine, the outcome should be well monitored. Be alert for the need to increase the hydroxychloroquine dose. Data from *mice* suggest that chloroquine might interact similarly,[3] and therefore similar precautions would seem prudent.

1. Harvey CJ, Bateman NT, Lloyd ME, Hughes GRV. Influence of rifampicin on hydroxychloroquine. *Clin Exp Rheumatol* (1995) 13, 536.
2. The Canadian Hydroxychloroquine Study Group. A randomized study of the effect of withdrawing hydroxychloroquine sulfate in systemic lupus erythematosus. *N Engl J Med* (1991) 324, 150–4.
3. Hou LJ, Raju SS, Abdulah MS, Nor NM, Ravichandran M. Rifampicin antagonizes the effect of chloroquine on chloroquine-resistant Plasmodium berghei in mice. *Jpn J Infect Dis* (2004), 198–202.

Diethylcarbamazine + Urinary acidifiers or alkalinisers

Urinary alkalinisers can reduce the loss of diethylcarbamazine in the urine, whereas urinary acidifiers can increase the loss of diethylcarbamazine in the urine.

Clinical evidence

Two studies, one in healthy subjects[1] and the other in patients with onchocerciasis,[2] found that making the urine alkaline with **sodium bicarbonate** increased the retention of diethylcarbamazine. The urinary excretion of a 50-mg dose of diethylcarbamazine was about 62% and its elimination half-life 4 hours when the urine was made acidic (pH less than 5.5) by giving **ammonium chloride**, compared with about 5% and 9.6 hours, respectively, when the urine was made alkaline (pH more than 7.5) using **sodium bicarbonate**.[1]

Mechanism

In alkaline urine most of the diethylcarbamazine is non-ionised and is therefore easily reabsorbed in the kidney by simple diffusion through the lipid membrane. The opposite effect occurs with acidic urine.

Importance and management

The clinical importance of any unsought for changes in the urinary pH brought about by the use of other drugs during diethylcarbamazine treatment has not been assessed, but be aware that its pharmacokinetics, and possibly the severity of its adverse effects, can be changed. One study[2] concluded that, in practice, there would seem to be no advantage in making the urine alkaline in order to be able to use smaller doses of diethylcarbamazine. This was because the severity of adverse reactions (the Mazzotti reaction) was not reduced and the microfilarial counts, one month after completion of treatment, were of a similar order to those in subjects in whom urinary pH was not manipulated.

1. Edwards G, Breckenridge AM, Adjepon-Yamoah KK, Orme M L'E, Ward SA. The effect of variations in urinary pH on the pharmacokinetics of diethylcarbamazine. *Br J Clin Pharmacol* (1981) 12, 807–12.
2. Awadzi K, Adjepon-Yamoah KK, Edwards G, Orme M L'E, Breckenridge AM, Gilles HM. The effect of moderate urine alkalinisation on low dose diethylcarbamazine therapy in patients with onchocerciasis. *Br J Clin Pharmacol* (1986) 21, 669–76.

Echinocandins + Amphotericin B

Amphotericin B does not appear to alter the pharmacokinetics of anidulafungin, caspofungin, or micafungin. The pharmacokinetics of amphotericin B are not altered by caspofungin, but exposure to amphotericin B might be increased by micafungin.

Clinical evidence, mechanism, importance and management

(a) Anidulafungin

The US manufacturer of anidulafungin briefly notes that population pharmacokinetic analysis showed no difference in its pharmacokinetics in 27 patients who were also given liposomal amphotericin B, when compared with data from patients receiving anidulafungin alone.[1] This suggests that no dose adjustment of anidulafungin is required if it is given with amphotericin B.[1,2]

(b) Caspofungin

The UK and US manufacturers of caspofungin briefly note that there were no pharmacokinetic interactions between caspofungin and amphotericin B in clinical studies in healthy subjects.[3,4] Therefore no dose adjustments are likely to be needed on concurrent use.

(c) Micafungin

The UK and US manufacturers of micafungin briefly note that, in drug interaction studies in healthy subjects, no change in the pharmacokinetics of micafungin occurred with the concurrent use of amphotericin B.[5,6] Therefore no micafungin dose adjustments are likely to be needed with concurrent use. However, the UK manufacturer notes that giving micafungin with a non-lipid formulation of amphotericin B was associated with a 30% increase in amphotericin B exposure. Concurrent use is advised only if the benefits clearly outweigh the risks and with close monitoring of patients for signs of amphotericin B adverse effects.[6]

1. Eraxis (Anidulafungin). Pfizer Injectables. US Prescribing information, November 2013.
2. Ecalta (Anidulafungin). Pfizer Ltd. UK Summary of product characteristics, August 2014.
3. Cancidas (Caspofungin acetate). Merck Sharp & Dohme Ltd. UK Summary of product characteristics, June 2014.
4. Cancidas (Caspofungin acetate). Merck & Co., Inc. US Prescribing information, August 2013.
5. Mycamine (Micafungin sodium). Astellas Pharma US, Inc. US Prescribing information, June 2013.
6. Mycamine (Micafungin sodium). Astellas Pharma Ltd. UK Summary of product characteristics, December 2013.

Echinocandins + Azoles

No pharmacokinetic interaction appears to occur between anidulafungin and voriconazole, between caspofungin and itraconazole, or between micafungin and fluconazole or voriconazole. Micafungin causes a negligible increase the exposure to itraconazole.

Clinical evidence, mechanism, importance and management

(a) Anidulafungin

In a crossover study in 17 healthy subjects the steady-state maximum plasma concentration and AUC of both anidulafungin and **voriconazole** were not altered by concurrent use, when compared with either drug given with placebo. Intravenous anidulafungin was given at a dose of 200 mg on the first day, then 100 mg daily for 3 days. **Voriconazole** was given orally, at a dose of 400 mg every 12 hours on the first day, then 200 mg every 12 hours for 3 days.[1] No dose adjustment of either drug appears to be necessary when they are used concurrently.

(b) Caspofungin

Caspofungin 70 mg on day 1 and 50 mg for the next 13 days did not alter the pharmacokinetics of **itraconazole** 200 mg daily.[2] The pharmacokinetics of caspofungin were also unaltered. No dose adjustment of either drug appears to be necessary when they are used concurrently.

(c) Micafungin

A study in 35 healthy subjects found no evidence of a clinically relevant pharmacokinetic interaction when intravenous micafungin 150 mg was given daily for 14 days with oral **voriconazole** 400 mg twice daily on day 11 and then 200 mg twice daily on days 12 to 14.[3]

A study in 62 patients undergoing a bone marrow or stem cell transplant found that the pharmacokinetics of both **fluconazole** 400 mg daily and micafungin 12.5 mg to 200 mg daily for 7 days were unaffected by concurrent use. No increase in adverse effects was seen, when compared with the use of fluconazole alone. An unpublished study in 30 healthy subjects also found similar results.[4]

The manufacturers briefly note that in studies in healthy subjects, **fluconazole**, **itraconazole**, and **voriconazole** did not alter the pharmacokinetics of micafungin. Micafungin increased the AUC and maximum concentration of **itraconazole** by 22% and 11%, respectively. Although this small change is unlikely to be of clinical importance, the manufacturers of micafungin recommend that patients taking both drugs should be monitored for itraconazole toxicity and the dose of **itraconazole** reduced as necessary.[5,6] No dose adjustments appear to be necessary with the concurrent use of **fluconazole** or **voriconazole** and micafungin.

1. Dowell JA, Schranz J, Baruch A, Foster G. Safety and pharmacokinetics of coadministered voriconazole and anidulafungin. *J Clin Pharmacol* (2005) 45, 1373–82.
2. Stone JA, McCrea JB, Wickersham PJ, Holland SD, Deutsch PJ, Bi S, Cicero T, Greenberg H, Waldman SA. A phase I study of caspofungin evaluating the potential for drug interactions with itraconazole, the effect of gender and the use of a loading dose regimen. *Intersci Conf Antimicrob Agents Chemother* (2000) 40, 26.
3. Keirns J, Sawamoto T, Holum M, Buell D, Wisemandle W, Alak A. Steady-state pharmacokinetics of micafungin and voriconazole after separate and concomitant dosing in healthy adults. *Antimicrob Agents Chemother* (2007) 51, 787–90.
4. Hiemenz J, Cagnoni P, Simpson D, Devine S, Chao N, Keirns J, Lau W, Facklam D, Buell D. Pharmacokinetic and maximum tolerated dose study of micafungin in combination with fluconazole versus fluconazole alone for prophylaxis of fungal infections in adult patients undergoing a bone marrow or peripheral stem cell transplant. *Antimicrob Agents Chemother* (2005) 49, 1331–6.
5. Mycamine (Micafungin sodium). Astellas Pharma US, Inc. US Prescribing information, June 2013.
6. Mycamine (Micafungin sodium). Astellas Pharma Ltd. UK Summary of product characteristics, December 2013.

Echinocandins + Rifampicin (Rifampin) and other enzyme inducers

Rifampicin reduces the minimum plasma concentration of caspofungin. One case of caspofungin treatment failure has been reported in a patient taking rifampicin. The manufacturers suggest that enzyme inducers (such as carbamazepine) might interact similarly.

Rifampicin does not appear to alter anidulafungin clearance or affect the pharmacokinetics of micafungin.

Clinical evidence

(a) Anidulafungin

A population pharmacokinetic analysis of anidulafungin in patients with serious fungal infections found that the clearance of anidulafungin did not differ between 27 patients also taking rifampicin and 77 patients taking no known interacting drugs.[1]

(b) Caspofungin

A parallel-group study in healthy subjects looked at the effects of rifampicin on the pharmacokinetics of caspofungin. In the first group, rifampicin 600 mg daily was given with intravenous caspofungin 50 mg daily, started on the same day. It was found that the minimum plasma concentration and AUC of caspofungin were increased by 170% and 61%, respectively, on day one. However, after 2 weeks the AUC had returned to normal, and, when compared with subjects not taking rifampicin, there was a trend towards lower minimum plasma concentrations of caspofungin. In the second group of healthy subjects in this study, rifampicin 600 mg daily was given for 14 days alone and then for a further 14 days combined with caspofungin. No increase in the caspofungin AUC was seen on day one of concurrent use. On both day one and day 14, the minimum plasma concentration of caspofungin was reduced by about 30%, without any change in the AUC, similar to the findings on day 14 in the first group. In this second group, caspofungin did not alter the pharmacokinetics of rifampicin.[2]

A case report describes a neutropenic patient with fungaemia who did not respond to intravenous caspofungin (70 mg on the first day then 50 mg daily) while taking rifampicin 600 mg daily. Although this patient was given a standard dose of caspofungin, the authors note she weighed just 47 kg and did not show even an initial response. Susceptibility testing found that the isolate was not resistant to caspofungin. The patient was subsequently successfully treated with amphotericin B. The authors suggest that caspofungin doses of more than 70 mg daily would have been required for efficacy in their patient.[3]

(c) Micafungin

The UK and US manufacturers of micafungin state that, in drug interaction studies in healthy subjects, rifampicin did not affect the pharmacokinetics of micafungin.[4,5]

Mechanism

Caspofungin is a poor substrate for cytochrome P450 and is not a substrate for P-glycoprotein,[6] therefore these mechanisms are not thought to be involved in the interaction with rifampicin. It is possible that the modest effect of rifampicin on caspofungin is due to induction of tissue uptake transport proteins at steady-state.[2]

Importance and management

Evidence for an interaction between rifampicin and caspofungin appears limited. The UK manufacturer of caspofungin recommends that consideration should be given to increasing the dose from 50 to 70 mg daily in patients taking rifampicin,[6] whereas the US manufacturer specifically states that the higher dose should be used.[7] A 70-mg dose has been generally well tolerated in clinical studies.[2] However, bear in mind the case report of possible caspofungin failure, even at this dose. The manufacturers also state that a population pharmacokinetic analysis suggested that the concurrent use of other metabolic inducers (**carbamazepine**, **dexamethasone**, **efavirenz**, **nevirapine**, or **phenytoin**) might result in clinically meaningful reductions in the AUC of caspofungin.[6,7] They suggest giving consideration to increasing the dose of caspofungin from 50 to 70 mg daily if it is used with these enzyme inducers. However, further study is needed to verify these predictions as the mechanism for any interaction has not been established.

No dose adjustments for anidulafungin or micafungin appear to be necessary with the concurrent use of rifampicin.

1. Dowell J, Knebel W, Ludden T, Stogniew M, Krause D, Henkel T. Population pharmacokinetic analysis of anidulafungin, an echinocandin antifungal. *J Clin Pharmacol* (2004) 44, 590–8.
2. Stone JA, Migoya EM, Hickey L, Winchell GA, Deutsch PJ, Ghosh K, Freeman A, Bi S, Desai R, Dilzer SC, Lasseter KC, Kraft WK, Greenberg H, Waldman SA. Potential for interactions between caspofungin and nelfinavir or rifampin. *Antimicrob Agents Chemother* (2004) 48, 4306–14.
3. Belmares J, Colaizzi L, Parada JP, Johnson S. Caspofungin treatment failure in a patient with invasive candidiasis and concomitant rifampicin treatment. *Int J Antimicrob Agents* (2005) 26, 264–5.
4. Mycamine (Micafungin sodium). Astellas Pharma Ltd. UK Summary of product characteristics, December 2013.
5. Mycamine (Micafungin sodium). Astellas Pharma US, Inc. US Prescribing information, June 2013.
6. Cancidas (Caspofungin acetate). Merck Sharp & Dohme Ltd. UK Summary of product characteristics, June 2014.
7. Cancidas (Caspofungin acetate). Merck & Co., Inc. US Prescribing information, August 2013.

Echinocandins; Caspofungin + Nelfinavir

Nelfinavir has a negligible effect on caspofungin exposure.

Clinical evidence, mechanism, importance and management

In a parallel-group study, healthy subjects were given nelfinavir 1.25 g every 12 hours and intravenous caspofungin 50 mg daily, started on the same day. The AUC and minimum plasma concentration of caspofungin were 16% and 58% higher, respectively, on the first day, when compared with subjects receiving caspofungin alone. However, after 2 weeks of concurrent use, the AUC and minimum plasma concentration of caspofungin were similar in both groups of patients.[1] The authors note that their previous population pharmacokinetic analysis had shown that nelfinavir might decrease the AUC and minimum plasma concentration of caspofungin, which in the light of the controlled study, they consider to be a spurious finding.

It appears that nelfinavir does not have a clinically relevant effect on the pharmacokinetics of caspofungin, when both drugs are given in multiple doses, and therefore no dose adjustment of caspofungin is required on concurrent use.

1. Stone JA, Migoya EM, Hickey L, Winchell GA, Deutsch PJ, Ghosh K, Freeman A, Bi S, Desai R, Dilzer SC, Lasseter KC, Kraft WK, Greenberg H, Waldman SA. Potential for interactions between caspofungin and nelfinavir or rifampin. *Antimicrob Agents Chemother* (2004) 48, 4306–14.

Echinocandins; Micafungin + Miscellaneous

Micafungin might increase the exposure to nifedipine and sirolimus. Micafungin has no effect on the pharmacokinetics of prednisolone.

Nifedipine, prednisolone, ritonavir, and sirolimus do not affect the pharmacokinetics of micafungin.

Clinical evidence, mechanism, importance and management

(a) Nifedipine

The UK and US manufacturers briefly note that micafungin (at steady-state) increased the AUC and maximum concentration of nifedipine by 18% and 42%, respectively, when compared with nifedipine alone. Nifedipine did not affect the pharmacokinetics of micafungin in healthy subjects.[1,2]

The increase in the AUC and plasma concentration of nifedipine is minor and would not be expected to be clinically important in most patients. Nevertheless, the manufacturers advise increased monitoring for adverse effects and toxicity,[1,2] and, as the occasional patient might be affected, it would seem prudent to check that blood pressure is not excessively reduced when micafungin is started.

(b) Prednisolone

Prednisolone did not affect the pharmacokinetics of micafungin in clinical studies in healthy subjects. Similarly, both single and multiple doses of micafungin had no effect on the pharmacokinetics of prednisolone.[1,2]

(c) Ritonavir

Ritonavir did not affect the pharmacokinetics of micafungin in a clinical studies in healthy subjects.[1,2]

(d) Sirolimus

The UK and US manufacturers briefly reports that micafungin (at steady-state) increased the AUC of sirolimus by 21%; however, its maximum concentration was not affected. Sirolimus did not affect the pharmacokinetics of micafungin in healthy subjects.[1,2]

An increase in the AUC of sirolimus would not generally be expected to be clinically relevant. Nevertheless, the manufacturers of micafungin[1,2] advise increased monitoring for sirolimus adverse effects and toxicity on concurrent use. As a greater effect in patients cannot be excluded, consider monitoring the plasma concentration of sirolimus when micafungin is started.

1. Mycamine (Micafungin sodium). Astellas Pharma US, Inc. US Prescribing information, June 2013.
2. Mycamine (Micafungin sodium). Astellas Pharma Ltd. UK Summary of product characteristics, December 2013.

Flucytosine + Amphotericin B

For some fungal infections the combination of flucytosine with amphotericin B can be more effective than flucytosine alone, but amphotericin B increases the toxicity of flucytosine. An isolated report describes a case of cardiomyopathy with concomitant use.

Clinical evidence, mechanism, importance and management

The combined use of flucytosine and amphotericin B is more effective than the use of flucytosine alone in the treatment of cryptococcal meningitis, as demonstrated in an early study.[1] However, amphotericin B can cause deterioration in renal function, which reduces flucytosine elimination, and might increase the plasma concentration of flucytosine. In addition, amphotericin B might increase the cellular uptake of flucytosine.[2] Whatever the exact mechanism, concurrent use increases flucytosine bone marrow toxicity. A study of 194 patients randomised to either a 4-week or a 6-week course of low-dose amphotericin B (initially 0.3 mg/kg daily) and a maximal dose of flucytosine (150 mg/kg daily, adjusted for renal function) found that severe adverse effects were common. These included azotaemia (51 patients), blood dyscrasias (52 patients), and hepatitis (13 patients).[3] An isolated report describes a case of cardiomyopathy in a 55-year-old woman taking flucytosine and amphotericin B for recurrent cryptococcal laryngitis. Amphotericin B had been started 4 days before hospital admission, and flucytosine 2 days before. Six months after stopping both drugs the cardiomyopathy had resolved. The patient had no predisposing risk factors for cardiomyopathy, but the authors note that she did have impaired renal function, which might have increased the plasma concentration of flucytosine and contributed to the toxicity.[4] However, they also note that both drugs alone can cause cardiotoxicity and therefore an interaction is not established.

The concurrent use of flucytosine and amphotericin B is the recommended treatment for some systemic fungal infections.[5] Nevertheless, the plasma concentration of flucytosine and renal function should be very closely monitored when these drugs are used together. It may also be prudent to be alert for signs of cardiac toxicity.

1. Bennett JE, Dismukes WE, Duma RJ, Medoff G, Sande MA, Gallis H, Leonard J, Fields BT, Bradshaw M, Haywood H, McGee ZA, Cate TR, Cobbs CG, Warner JF, Alling DW. A comparison of amphotericin B alone and combined with flucytosine in the treatment of cryptoccal meningitis. *N Engl J Med* (1979) 301, 126–31.
2. Fungizone Intravenous (Amphotericin B). E. R. Squibb & Sons Ltd. UK Summary of product characteristics, February 2010.
3. Stamm AM, Diasio RB, Dismukes WE, Shadomy S, Cloud GA, Bowles CA, Karam GH, Espinel-Ingroff A and members of the National Institute of Allergy and Infectious Diseases Mycoses Study group. Toxicity of amphotericin B plus flucytosine in 194 patients with cryptococcal meningitis. *Am J Med* (1987) 83, 236–42.
4. Johnson RE, Campbell-Bright S, Raasch RH, Rodgers JE. Reversible cardiomyopathy following treatment with amphotericin B and flucytosine. *Int J Antimicrob Agents* (2008) 31, 582–4.
5. Pappas PG, Rex JH, Sobel JD, Filler SG, Dismukes WE, Walsh TJ, Edwards JE. IDSA Guidelines for treatment of candidiasis. *Clin Infect Dis* (2004) 38, 161–89.

Flucytosine + Antacids

Aluminium/magnesium hydroxide delays the absorption of flucytosine from the gut, but the total amount absorbed remains unaffected.[1] No additional precautions therefore appear to be needed if this antacid is given with oral flucytosine.

1. Cutler RE, Blair AD, Kelly MR. Flucytosine kinetics in subjects with normal and impaired renal function. *Clin Pharmacol Ther* (1978) 24, 333–42.

Flucytosine + Cytarabine

Some very limited evidence suggests that cytarabine might oppose the antifungal effects, or reduce the plasma concentration, of flucytosine. Theoretically, their bone marrow suppressant effects might be additive.

Clinical evidence, mechanism, importance and management

A man with Hodgkin's disease, given flucytosine 100 mg/kg daily for cryptococcal meningitis, had reduced plasma and CSF concentrations of flucytosine (from a range of 30 mg/L to 40 mg/L down to undetectable amounts) when he was given intravenous cytarabine. When cytarabine was replaced by procarbazine, the flucytosine concentrations returned to their former values. *In vitro* tests found that cytarabine 1 mg/L completely abolished the activity of up to 50 mg/L of flucytosine against the patient's strain of *Cryptococcus*, whereas procarbazine did not.[1] In another study in a patient with acute myeloid leukaemia, the pre-dose flucytosine concentration fell from 65 mg/L to 42 mg/L and the post-dose flucytosine concentration fell from 80 mg/L to 53 mg/L when cytarabine and daunorubicin were given. However, these concentrations were still within the therapeutic range and the decreases were attributed to an improvement in renal function rather than antagonism between flucytosine and cytarabine.[2]

In an *in vitro* study, the antifungal effects of flucytosine against 14 out of 16 wild isolates of *Cryptococcus* were not changed in the presence of cytarabine. In the remaining two isolates, an increase in effect was seen in one and a decrease was seen in the other.[2]

The evidence for any interaction between flucytosine and cytarabine is therefore very limited and its general clinical importance remains uncertain. The manufacturer of flucytosine advises that strict monitoring of the plasma concentration of flucytosine is required if both drugs are given,[3] whereas, despite the very limited evidence, the manufacturer of cytarabine recommends avoiding concurrent use.[4] It would seem prudent to closely monitor the efficacy and clinical response to flucytosine if both drugs are needed.

Of equal concern is the fact that both drugs are bone marrow suppressants, and this effect might be additive; however, it should be standard practice to closely monitor full blood counts if either of these drugs is given, and therefore additional monitoring seems unnecessary.

1. Holt RJ. Clinical problems with 5-fluorocytosine. *Mykosen* (1978) 21, 363–9.
2. Wingfield HJ. Absence of fungistatic antagonism between flucytosine and cytarabine *in vitro* and *in vivo*. *J Antimicrob Chemother* (1987) 20, 523–7.
3. Ancotil Solution for Infusion (Flucytosine). Meda Pharmaceuticals. UK Summary of product characteristics, December 2010.
4. Cytarabine. Pharmacia Ltd. UK Summary of product characteristics, January 2010.

Furazolidone + Miscellaneous

The concurrent use of furazolidone with amfetamines, nasal decongestants, or with tyramine-rich foods and drinks might be expected to result in a potentially serious rise in blood pressure. However, direct evidence of adverse reactions of this kind does not seem to have been reported.

The pressor effects of noradrenaline (norepinephrine) are unchanged by furazolidone.

Clinical evidence

A study in 4 hypertensive patients found that after 6 days of treatment with furazolidone 400 mg daily, the pressor responses to **tyramine** or **dexamfetamine** had increased two- to threefold, and after 13 days had increased about tenfold. These responses to furazolidone were about the same as those found in 2 other patients taking the MAOI pargyline.[1] The MAO-inhibitory activity of furazolidone was confirmed by measurements taken on jejunal mucosal samples.[2]

The pressor effects of **noradrenaline (norepinephrine)** were unchanged by furazolidone.[1]

Mechanism

The MAO-inhibitory activity of furazolidone is not immediate and might in fact be due to a metabolite of furazolidone.[3] It develops gradually so that, after 5 to 10 days of use, amfetamines and tyramine (indirectly-acting sympathomimetics) will interact with furazolidone in the same way as they do with other non-selective MAOIs.[2,4] More details of the mechanisms of this interaction are to be found elsewhere, see 'MAOIs or RIMAs + Food; Tyramine-containing', p.1389, and 'MAOIs or RIMAs + Nasal decongestants and related drugs', p.1396.

Importance and management

The MAO-inhibitory activity of furazolidone after 5 to 10 days of use is established, but reports of hypertensive crises either with sympathomimetics or tyramine-containing foods or drinks appear to be lacking. This might, in part, be a reflection of the fact that furazolidone can be given for just 2 to 5 days. However, a few UK manufacturers of pseudoephedrine-containing cold and influenza preparations contraindicate their use with furazolidone and other MAOIs.[5,6] It would seem prudent to warn patients given furazolidone not to take any of the drugs, foods, or drinks that are prohibited with non-selective MAOIs (see 'MAOIs', p.1382, and '"MAOIs or RIMAs + Inotropes and Vasopressors', p.1392), that are directly-acting sympathomimetics, such as noradrenaline (norepinephrine).

1. Pettinger WA, Oates JA. Supersensitivity to tyramine during monoamine oxidase inhibition in man. Mechanism at the level of the adrenergic neurone. *Clin Pharmacol Ther* (1968) 9, 341–4.
2. Pettinger WA, Soyangco FG, Oates JA. Inhibition of monoamine oxidase in man by furazolidone. *Clin Pharmacol Ther* (1968) 9, 442–7.
3. Stern IJ, Hollifield RD, Wilk S, Buzard JA. The anti-monoamine oxidase effects of furazolidone. *J Pharmacol Exp Ther* (1967) 156, 492–9.
4. Pettinger WA, Soyangco FG, Oates JA. Monoamine-oxidase inhibition by furazolidone in man. *Clin Res* (1966) 14, 258.
5. Meltus Decongestant (Pseudoephedrine hydrochloride) SSL International plc. UK Summary of product characteristics, January 2004.
6. Benadryl Plus Capsules (Pseudoephedrine hydrochloride and acrivastine). McNeil Products Ltd. UK Summary of product characteristics, October 2010.

Furazolidone + Proton pump inhibitors

Omeprazole reduces the maximum serum concentration of furazolidone. Other proton pump inhibitors could interact similarly.

Clinical evidence, mechanism, importance and management

A study in 18 healthy subjects found that **omeprazole** 20 mg twice daily for 5 days reduced the maximum serum concentration of a single 200-mg dose of furazolidone by about 30%. **Omeprazole** might alter the bioavailability of furazolidone by reducing its dissolution or increasing its degradation before it reaches the intestine and/or inducing its first-pass metabolism.[1] The clinical relevance of this small change is uncertain, as there are a large number of clinical studies describing the successful combination of furazolidone with **omeprazole** in regimens to eradicate *H. pylori*. However, there is some evidence that success rates are unacceptable if low-dose furazolidone (100 mg twice daily) rather than standard dose (200 mg twice daily) is used.[2] It is possible that a pharmacokinetic interaction could play a part in this finding. It might be prudent to be alert for a decrease in the effects of low doses of furazolidone if it is given with **omeprazole** outside of an established regimen. Other proton pump inhibitors do not appear to have been studied, but if the proposed mechanism is correct, it seems likely that they would interact similarly.

1. Calafatti SA, Ortiz RAM, Deguer M, Martinez M, Pedrazzoli J. Effect of acid secretion blockade by omeprazole on the relative bioavailability of orally administered furazolidone in healthy volunteers. *Br J Clin Pharmacol* (2001) 52, 205–9.
2. Fakheri H, Merat S, Hosseini C, Malekzadeh R. Low-dose furazolidone in triple and quadruple regimens for Helicobacter pylori eradication. *Aliment Pharmacol Ther* (2004) 19, 89–93.

Griseofulvin + Food

The rate, and probably the extent, of griseofulvin absorption is increased if it is taken with a high-fat meal.

Clinical evidence, mechanism, importance and management

A study in 5 healthy subjects found that the absorption of micronised griseofulvin 125 mg (*Fulcin*) was enhanced if it was given with a fatty meal rather than in the fasting state, as assessed by a 37% increase in griseofulvin urinary excretion.[1] Other studies similarly found that the absorption of griseofulvin at 4 hours and 8 hours was approximately doubled when it was taken with a high-fat meal.[2,3] A further study in 12 healthy subjects found that the higher the fat content of the meal, the higher the bioavailability of griseofulvin (70% increase in bioavailability with a low-fat meal and 120% increase with a high-fat meal, when compared with fasting state absorption).[4] However, another study found that although food increased the rate of absorption of micronised and PEG-ultramicronised griseofulvin, the extent of absorption was not changed.[5] Another report suggests that giving griseofulvin with food tends to reduce the differences in the bioavailability of griseofulvin from micronised and ultramicronised tablets.[6] Enhanced absorption was also found with a formulation of griseofulvin in a corn oil emulsion, when compared with tablets or an aqueous suspension.[7] The effect of a high-fat meal was found to be more pronounced for immediate-release griseofulvin tablets (*Fulvin*) than for a fast-disintegrating lyophilised dry emulsion tablet (prepared for the study).[8]

The interaction between griseofulvin and food is established and of clinical importance. The UK manufacturers advise that griseofulvin should be given after meals, otherwise absorption is likely to be inadequate.[9]

1. Khalafalla N, Elgholmy ZA, Khalil SA. Influence of a high fat diet on GI absorption of griseofulvin tablets in man. *Pharmazie* (1981) 36, 692–3.
2. Crounse RG. Human pharmacology of griseofulvin: the effect of fat intake on gastrointestinal absorption. *J Invest Dermatol* (1961) 37, 529–33.
3. Crounse RG. Effective use of griseofulvin. *Arch Dermatol* (1963) 87, 176–8.
4. Ogunbona FA, Smith IF, Olawoye OS. Fat contents of meals and bioavailability of griseofulvin in man. *J Pharm Pharmacol* (1985) 37, 283–4.
5. Aoyagi N, Ogata H, Kaniwa N, Ejima A. Effect of food on the bioavailability of griseofulvin from microsize and PEG ultramicrosize (GRIS-PEG) plain tablets. *J Pharmacobiodyn* (1982) 4, 120–4.
6. Bijanzadeh M, Mahmoudian M, Salehian P, Khazainia T, Eshghi L, Khosravy A. The bioavailability of griseofulvin from microsized and ultramicrosized tablets in nonfasting volunteers. *Indian J Physiol Pharmacol* (1990) 34, 157–61.
7. Bates TR, Sequeria JA. Bioavailability of micronized griseofulvin from corn oil-in-water emulsion, aqueous suspension, and commercial tablet dosage forms in humans. *J Pharm Sci* (1975) 64, 793–7.
8. Ahmed IS, Aboul-Einien MH, Mohamed OH, Farid SF. Relative bioavailability of griseofulvin lyophilized dry emulsion tablet vs. immediate release tablet: a single-dose, randomized, open-label, six-period, crossover study in healthy adult volunteers in the fasted and fed states. *Eur J Pharm Sci* (2008) 35, 219–25.
9. Fulsovin (Griseofulvin). Kappin Ltd. UK Summary of product characteristics, March 2010.

Griseofulvin + Liraglutide

Liraglutide had no effect on the pharmacokinetics of a single dose of griseofulvin.

Clinical evidence, mechanism, importance and management

A preliminary report of a randomised, crossover study in 27 healthy subjects, states that steady-state liraglutide 1.8 mg daily, increased the maximum concentration of a single 500-mg dose of griseofulvin given at the same time, by 37% without any change in median time to maximum concentration or in its overall exposure (AUC).[1] Therefore, no adjustment of the griseofulvin dose is likely to be needed in patients also given liraglutide.

1. Malm-Erjefalt M, Ekblom M, Brondsted L, Vouis J, Lennernas H, Zdravkovic M. A randomized, double-blind, cross-over trial investigating the effect of liraglutide on the absorption pharmacokinetics of concomitantly administered oral drugs in healthy subjects. *Diabetes* (2008) 57 (Suppl 1), A130.

Griseofulvin + Phenobarbital

The antifungal effects of griseofulvin can be reduced, or even abolished, by phenobarbital.

Clinical evidence

Two epileptic children taking phenobarbital 40 mg daily did not respond to long-term treatment for tinea capitis with griseofulvin 125 mg three times daily until the barbiturate was withdrawn.[1] Five other patients similarly did not respond to griseofulvin while taking phenobarbital (3 of the patients were also taking phenytoin).[2-4]

Two studies, with a total of 14 healthy subjects, found that phenobarbital 30 mg three times daily reduced the blood concentration of oral griseofulvin by roughly 33%,[5] and the absorption of griseofulvin was reduced from about 58% without phenobarbital to 41% in the presence of phenobarbital.[6]

Mechanism

Not fully understood. Initially it was thought that phenobarbital increased the metabolism and clearance of griseofulvin,[7] but it has also been suggested that phenobarbital reduces the absorption of griseofulvin from the gut.[6] It has variously been suggested that this is due to an increase in peristalsis reducing the opportunity for absorption,[6] the formation of a complex (which makes an already poorly soluble drug even less soluble and therefore less readily absorbed),[8] and a reduction in the amount of intestinal bile salts leading to reduced griseofulvin solubility.[9]

Importance and management

The interaction between griseofulvin and phenobarbital is established and of clinical importance, although the evidence seems to be limited to the reports cited. If phenobarbital must be given, it has been suggested that the griseofulvin should be given three times daily, in divided doses, to allow it a better chance of being absorbed;[6] however, griseofulvin was given in divided doses in one of the reports describing an interaction.[1] The effect of increasing the dose of griseofulvin appears not to have been studied. An alternative, where possible, is to use a non-interacting antiepileptic, such as valproate. This proved to be successful in one of the cases cited.[1]

1. Beurey J, Weber M, Vignaud J-M. Traitement des teignes microsporiques. Interférence métabolique entre phénobarbital et griséofulvine. *Ann Dermatol Venereol* (1982) 109, 567–70.
2. Lorenc E. A new factor in griseofulvin treatment failures. *Mo Med* (1967) 64, 32–3.
3. Stepanova ZV, Sheklakova AA. Liuminal kak prichina neudachi griseoful'vinoterapii bol'nogo mikrosporiei. *Vestn Dermatol Venerol* (1975) 12, 63–5.
4. Hay RJ, Clayton YM, Moore MK, Midgely G. An evaluation of itraconazole in the management of onychomycosis. *Br J Dermatol* (1988) 119, 359–66.
5. Busfield D, Child KJ, Atkinson RM, Tomich EG. An effect of phenobarbitone on blood-levels of griseofulvin in man. *Lancet* (1963) ii, 1042–3.
6. Riegelman S, Rowland M, Epstein WL. Griseofulvin-phenobarbital interaction in man. *JAMA* (1970) 213, 426–31.
7. Busfield D, Child KJ, Tomich EG. An effect of phenobarbitone on griseofulvin metabolism in the rat. *Br J Pharmacol* (1964) 22, 137–42.
8. Abougela IKA, Bigford DJ, McCorquodale I, Grant DJW. Complex formation and other physico-chemical interactions between griseofulvin and phenobarbitone. *J Pharm Pharmacol* (1976) 28, 44P.
9. Jamali F, Axelson JE. Griseofulvin–phenobarbital interaction: a formulation-dependent phenomenon. *J Pharm Sci* (1978) 67, 466–70.

Hydroxyquinoline (Oxyquinoline) + Zinc oxide

The presence of zinc oxide inhibits the therapeutic effects of hydroxyquinoline in ointments.

Clinical evidence

The observation that a patient had an allergic reaction to hydroxyquinoline in ointments with a paraffin base, but not a zinc oxide base, prompted further study of a possible incompatibility. The subsequent study in 13 patients confirmed that zinc oxide reduces the eczematogenic (allergic) properties of the hydroxyquinoline. However, it also inhibits the antibacterial and antimycotic effects of hydroxyquinoline, and appears to stimulate the growth of *Candida albicans*.[1]

Mechanism

It seems almost certain that the zinc ions and hydroxyquinoline form chelates, which have little, or no, antibacterial properties.[1,2]

Importance and management

The documentation is limited, but the interaction between hydroxyquinolone and zinc oxide appears to be established. There is no benefit in using zinc oxide to reduce the allergic properties of hydroxyquinoline if, at the same time, the therapeutic effects disappear.

1. Fischer T. On 8-hydroxyquinoline-zinc oxide incompatibility. *Dermatologica* (1974) 149, 129–35.
2. Albert A, Rubbo SD, Goldacre RJ, Balfour BG. The influence of chemical constitution on antibacterial activity. Part III: A study of 8-hydroxyquinoline (oxine) and related compounds. *Br J Exp Pathol* (1947) 28, 69–87.

Ivermectin + Food

The bioavailability of ivermectin is markedly increased by food.

Clinical evidence, mechanism, importance and management

In a study, 11 subjects were given ivermectin 30 mg after overnight fasting three times a week for one week and then a single 30-mg dose of ivermectin 20 minutes after a **high-fat breakfast**. Food increased the AUC and maximum plasma concentration of ivermectin about 2.6-fold and 3-fold, respectively.[1] The US manufacturers recommend that ivermectin is taken with water on an empty stomach.[2]

1. Guzzo CA, Furtek CI, Porras AG, Chen C, Tipping R, Clineschmidt CM, Sciberras DG, Hsieh JY-K, Lasseter KC,. Safety, tolerability, and pharmacokinetics of escalating high doses of ivermectin in healthy adult subjects. *J Clin Pharmacol* (2002) 42, 1122–33.
2. Stromectol (Ivermectin). Merck & Co., Inc. US Prescribing information, May 2010.

Ivermectin + Levamisole

Levamisole appears to increase the exposure to ivermectin. Ivermectin does not alter the pharmacokinetics of levamisole.

Clinical evidence, mechanism, importance and management

A study in 28 healthy subjects given levamisole 2.5 mg/kg, alone or with ivermectin 200 micrograms/kg, found that ivermectin had no effect on the AUC or maximum plasma concentration of levamisole. However, the AUC of ivermectin was twofold higher in patients given levamisole, when compared with historical values in subjects who had received ivermectin alone.[1] An associated study in 44 patients with *Onchocerca volvulus* infections found that levamisole given with ivermectin was neither macrofilaricidal, nor more effective against microfilariae and adult worms, than ivermectin alone. In addition, patients taking both drugs had a higher incidence of pruritus, arthralgia, and fever than those taking ivermectin alone.[1] Concurrent use need not be avoided, but it would seem prudent to be alert for an increase in adverse effects (such as orthostatic hypotension, dizziness, or pruritus) if both drugs are thought to be necessary.

1. Awadzi K, Edwards G, Opoku NO, Ardrey AE, Favager S, Addy ET, Attah SK, Yamuah LK, Quartey BT. The safety, tolerability and pharmacokinetics of levamisole alone, levamisole plus ivermectin, and levamisole plus albendazole, and their efficacy against *Onchocerca volvulus*. *Ann Trop Med Parasitol* (2004) 98, 595–614.

Ivermectin + Orange juice

Orange juice slightly reduces the bioavailability of ivermectin.

Clinical evidence, mechanism, importance and management

A study in 16 healthy subjects found that the AUC and maximum plasma concentration of a single 150-micrograms/kg dose of ivermectin were reduced by 36% and 39%, respectively, when ivermectin was given with orange juice (750 mL over 4 hours) rather than with water. The mechanism for the reduced bioavailability is not known but it does not seem related to P-glycoprotein activity.[1] The clinical relevance of these changes is uncertain, although with an AUC decrease of this size, a reduction in the efficacy of ivermectin given for systemic infections might be a possibility. Further study is needed to establish the clinical relevance of this interaction.

1. Vanapalli SR, Chen Y, Ellingrod VL, Kitzman D, Lee Y, Hohl RJ, Fleckenstein L. Orange juice decreases the oral bioavailability of ivermectin in healthy volunteers. *Clin Pharmacol Ther* (2003) 73, P94.

Ivermectin + Praziquantel

No pharmacokinetic interaction appears to occur between praziquantel and ivermectin.

Clinical evidence, mechanism, importance and management

In a pharmacokinetic study, 23 healthy subjects were given a single dose of praziquantel 40 mg/kg either alone, or with single doses of a combination of albendazole 400 mg and ivermectin 200 micrograms/kg. The pharmacokinetics of ivermectin and praziquantel were not affected by concurrent use. No serious adverse effects were reported.[1] Modest effects were seen on the pharmacokinetics of albendazole, see 'Albendazole + Praziquantel', p.228.

From this study it would appear that the concurrent use of ivermectin and praziquantel has no clinically significant effects on the pharmacokinetics of either drug. No additional precautions appear to be necessary if both drugs are given concurrently.

1. Na-Bangchang K, Kietinun S, Pawa KK, Hanpitakpong W, Na-Bangchang C, Lazdins J. Assessments of pharmacokinetic drug interactions and tolerability of albendazole, praziquantel and ivermectin combinations. *Trans R Soc Trop Med Hyg* (2006) 100, 335–45.

Lumefantrine + CYP2D6 substrates

***In vitro* data indicate that lumefantrine inhibits CYP2D6 and might therefore increase the exposure to drugs such as some tricyclics, metoprolol, and flecainide.**

Clinical evidence, mechanism, importance and management

The manufacturer of artemether with lumefantrine[1] states that *in vitro* data indicate that lumefantrine significantly inhibits CYP2D6. As a consequence, they contraindicate the use of artemether with lumefantrine in patients taking any drug that is metabolised by CYP2D6, and they give **flecainide**, **metoprolol**, **imipramine**, **amitriptyline**, and **clomipramine** as examples (for a list of CYP2D6 substrates, see 'Table 1.7', p.9). These contraindications seem unnecessarily restrictive, especially as none of the drugs they give as examples are contraindicated with other established inhibitors of CYP2D6. Until more is known, it would be prudent to closely monitor the effects of any CYP2D6 substrate in patients for whom artemether with lumefantrine is considered the antimalarial drug of choice.

1. Riamet (Artemether with Lumefantrine). Novartis Pharmaceuticals UK Ltd. UK Summary of product characteristics, October 2011.

Mefloquine + Ampicillin

Ampicillin increases the plasma concentrations of mefloquine and reduces its half-life.

Clinical evidence, mechanism, importance and management

In a study, 8 healthy subjects were given ampicillin 250 mg four times daily for 5 days with a single 750-mg dose of mefloquine on day 2. The maximum plasma concentration and 5-day AUC of mefloquine were increased by 34% and 49%, respectively, although the $AUC_{0-\infty}$ was not increased. Ampicillin reduced the half-life of mefloquine from 17.7 days to 15.3 days. No increase in adverse events was seen. These pharmacokinetic effects might be due to an increase in mefloquine bioavailability, possibly due to a reduction in its enterohepatic recycling.[1] The clinical relevance of these changes is uncertain, but the authors consider that the changes in elimination are unlikely to be clinically important because they occur after the resolution of malaria.[1]

1. Karbwang J, Na Bangchang K, Back DJ, Bunnag D. Effect of ampicillin on mefloquine pharmacokinetics in Thai males. *Eur J Clin Pharmacol* (1991) 40, 631–3.

Mefloquine + Artemisinin derivatives

Artemether pretreatment might slightly reduce the exposure to mefloquine. If mefloquine is given shortly after artesunate, its plasma concentration is lowered, whereas giving mefloquine two days after starting artesunate appears to slightly increase the exposure to mefloquine. The plasma concentration of lumefantrine is slightly reduced by mefloquine pretreatment, but the plasma concentrations of artemether and mefloquine are not affected. There is no pharmacokinetic interaction between artemisinin and mefloquine.

Clinical evidence, mechanism, importance and management

(a) Artemether

In a study, 15 patients with acute uncomplicated falciparum malaria were given a single 750-mg dose of mefloquine 24 hours after a single 300-mg dose of artemether. The AUC of mefloquine was 27% lower, when compared with 7 patients given a single 750-mg dose of mefloquine alone. However, the addition of artemether improved the rate of parasite clearance, and cure rates were similar between the groups.[1] Another study in 8 healthy subjects found the pharmacokinetics of single doses of artemether 300 mg and mefloquine 750 mg were not affected by concurrent use. No serious adverse effects were reported.[2]

(b) Artemether with Lumefantrine

In a study, 42 healthy subjects were given 6 doses of artemether with lumefantrine 80/480 mg over 60 hours, starting 12 hours after a short course of mefloquine (3 doses totalling 1 g given over 12 hours). The pharmacokinetics of mefloquine and artemether were unaffected by sequential use, but the maximum plasma concentration and AUC of lumefantrine were reduced by 29% and 41%, respectively. However, given that the plasma concentration of lumefantrine is usually highly variable, these changes were not thought to be large enough to affect the efficacy of treatment.[3]

In another study, similar sequential use of these drugs did not affect the QT interval, and drug concentrations were also considered adequate for treatment.[4] The authors considered that adverse effects on the QT interval are unlikely to occur if artemether with lumefantrine is given after mefloquine prophylaxis or treatment.

These data indicate that sequential use of mefloquine then artemether with lumefantrine is unlikely to require any special precautions. The manufacturer of artemether with lumefantrine notes that prolongation of the QT interval was seen in about 5% of patients in clinical studies, although they state that this could be disease related. They recommend, due to the limited data on safety and efficacy, that artemether with lumefantrine should not be given concurrently with any other antimalarial unless there is no other treatment option.[5]

(c) Artemisinin

A study in patients with falciparum malaria found no pharmacokinetic interaction between artemisinin and mefloquine. In this study, patients were given mefloquine 750 mg alone, or artemisinin 500 mg daily for 3 days, with a single 750-mg dose of mefloquine either on day 1 or day 4. There was no difference in overall efficacy between treatments, although those given artemisinin with mefloquine on the first day of treatment had the fastest parasite clearance rates.[6]

(d) Artesunate

A study in 20 patients with acute uncomplicated falciparum malaria given mefloquine (750 mg followed by 500 mg after 6 hours), found that the plasma concentration of mefloquine was reduced by 27% and its clearance rate was increased 2.6-fold when the doses of mefloquine were given 6 hours and 12 hours after artesunate 200 mg. However, the patients who received the combination had shorter fever-clearance and parasite-clearance times than those given mefloquine alone, although the cure rate was lower for concurrent use (66%) than for mefloquine alone (75%). To prevent the pharmacokinetic interaction resulting in a reduction in mefloquine efficacy, the authors of this study recommended that mefloquine should be given when artesunate and its metabolites have cleared the circulation (the authors suggest possibly 24 hours after a dose).[7] This suggestion is supported by a study looking at the efficacy of mefloquine with artesunate, which found that the AUC of mefloquine was about 30% higher in 22 children given mefloquine on day 2 of artesunate treatment, when compared with 24 children given mefloquine on day 0 (before artesunate was started). Both groups were given mefloquine without food.[8]

In a further study, 179 patients with falciparum malaria were given a single 4-mg/kg dose of artesunate with a single 15-mg/kg dose of mefloquine taken either with, 8 hours after, or 24 hours after the artesunate dose. The study found that the pharmacokinetics of mefloquine and artesunate were not affected by the timing of the doses.[9] Another pharmacokinetic study in 25 healthy subjects also found no evidence of an interaction when a single 250-mg dose of mefloquine was given at the same time as artesunate 200 mg daily for 3 days.[10]

The concurrent use of artesunate and mefloquine is one of the recommended treatment options in the WHO guidelines for the treatment of uncomplicated falciparum malaria, and for uncomplicated vivax malaria in selected areas.[11]

(e) Other artemisinin derivatives

In a single-dose crossover study, 10 healthy subjects were given either mefloquine 750 mg, dihydroartemisinin 300 mg (exact derivative not specified), or both drugs together. The pharmacokinetics of the drugs were unchanged on concurrent use, except for the rate of mefloquine absorption, which was increased. Also the activity of these drugs against *Plasmodium falciparum* was synergistic, rather than additive.[12] A study in 12 patients with acute uncomplicated falciparum malaria, given either two doses of dihydroartemisinin (exact derivative not specified) 300 mg 24 hours apart, with a single 750-mg dose of mefloquine either 6 hours after the first dose of dihydroartemisinin or with the last dose of dihydroartemisinin, found no evidence of a pharmacokinetic interaction.[13]

1. Na-Bangchang K, Karbwang J, Molunto P, Banmairuroi V, Thanavibul A. Pharmacokinetics of mefloquine, when given alone and in combination with artemether, in patients with uncomplicated falciparum malaria. *Fundam Clin Pharmacol* (1995) 9, 576–82.
2. Na-Bangchang K, Karbwang J, Ubalee R, Thanavibul A, Saenglertsilapachai S. Absence of significant pharmacokinetic and pharmacodynamic interactions between artemether and quinoline antimalarials. *Eur J Drug Metab Pharmacokinet* (2000) 25 171–8.
3. Lefèvre G, Bindschedler M, Ezzet F, Schaeffer N, Meyer I, Thomsen MS. Pharmacokinetic interaction trial between co-artemether and mefloquine. *Eur J Pharm Sci* (2000) 10, 141–51.
4. Bindschedler M, Lefèvre G, Ezzet F, Schaeffer N, Meyer I, Thomsen MS. Cardiac effects of co-artemether (artemether/lumefantrine) and mefloquine given alone or in combination to healthy volunteers. *Eur J Clin Pharmacol* (2000) 56, 375–81.
5. Riamet (Artemether with Lumefantrine). Novartis Pharmaceuticals UK Ltd. UK Summary of product characteristics, October 2011.
6. Svensson USH, Alin MH, Karlsson MO, Bergqvist Y, Ashton M. Population pharmacokinetic and pharmacodynamic modelling of artemisinin and mefloquine enantiomers in patients with falciparum malaria. *Eur J Clin Pharmacol* (2002) 58, 339–51.
7. Karbwang J, Na Bangchang K, Thanavibul A, Back DJ, Bunnag D, Harinasuta T. Pharmacokinetics of mefloquine alone or in combination with artesunate. *Bull WHO* (1994) 72, 83–7.
8. Price R, Simpson JA, Teja-Isavatharm P, Than MM, Luxemburger C, Heppner DG, Chongsuphajaisiddhi T, Nosten F, White NJ. Pharmacokinetics of mefloquine combined with artesunate in children with acute falciparum malaria. *Antimicrob Agents Chemother* (1999) 43, 341–6.
9. Hung le Q, De Vries PJ, Binh TQ, Giao PT, Nam NV, Holman R, Kager PA. Artesunate with mefloquine at various intervals for non-severe *Plasmodium falciparum* malaria. *Am J Trop Med Hyg* (2004) 71, 160–6.
10. Davis TME, England M, Dunlop A-M, Page-Sharp M, Cambon N, Keller TG, Heidecker JL, Ilett K. Assessment of the effect of mefloquine on artesunate pharmacokinetics in healthy male volunteers. *Antimicrob Agents Chemother* (2007) 51, 1099–1101.
11. World Health Organization. Guidelines for the treatment of malaria - 3rd edition. Available at: Guidelines for the treatment of malaria https://extranet.who.int/iris/restricted/bitstream/10665/162441/1/9789241549127_eng.pdf (accessed 28/10/15).
12. Na-Bangchang K, Tippawangkosol P, Thanavibul A, Ubalee R, Karbwang J. Pharmacokinetic and pharmacodynamic interactions of mefloquine and dihydroartemisinin. *Int J Clin Pharmacol Res* (1999) 19, 9–17.
13. Thuy le TD, Hung le N, Hung NC, Na-Bangchang K. Pharmacokinetics of mefloquine with dihydroartemisinin as 2-day regimens in patients with uncomplicated falciparum malaria. *Southeast Asian J Trop Med Public Health* (2007) 38, 205–12.

Mefloquine + Azoles

Ketoconazole increases the exposure to mefloquine.

Clinical evidence, mechanism, importance and management

In a study in healthy subjects given a single 500-mg dose of mefloquine on day 5 of a 10-day course of **ketoconazole** 400 mg daily, the AUC, maximum plasma concentration, and half-life of mefloquine were increased by 79%, 64%, and 34%, respectively, when compared with mefloquine alone. A 28% decrease in the AUC of the carboxylic metabolite of mefloquine was also seen. No significant adverse effects were reported.[1] It is probable that **ketoconazole** inhibits the metabolism of mefloquine by CYP3A4. Although the clinical relevance of this increase in mefloquine exposure is not known, it seems possible that it could increase the risk of adverse effects in some patients. In particular, the UK manufacturer of mefloquine warns of the risk of QT prolongation if **ketoconazole** is given with mefloquine, or within 15 weeks of the last dose of mefloquine.[2] Until more is known, it might be prudent to undertake concurrent use cautiously.

Note that many azoles have inhibitory effects on CYP3A4, see under *Azoles* in 'Anthelmintics, Antifungals, and Antiprotozoals', p.225, for further details. If the suggested mechanism is correct, these azoles might interact similarly, although there are no clinical reports of an interaction.

1. Ridtitid W, Wongnawa M, Mahatthanatrakul W, Raungsri N, Sunbhanich M. Ketoconazole increases plasma concentrations of antimalarial mefloquine in healthy human volunteers. *J Clin Pharm Ther* (2005) 30, 285–90.
2. Lariam (Mefloquine hydrochloride). Roche Products Ltd. UK Summary of product characteristics, November 2011.

Mefloquine + Cimetidine

The plasma concentration of mefloquine can be modestly increased, and/or its elimination modestly reduced, by cimetidine.

Clinical evidence, mechanism, importance and management

A single 500-mg dose of mefloquine was given to 10 healthy subjects before, and after, they took cimetidine 400 mg twice daily for 28 days. Cimetidine had no effect on the AUC or plasma concentration of mefloquine, but the mefloquine half-life increased by 50% (from 9.6 days to 14.4 days) and the oral clearance decreased by almost 40%.[1] In another study mefloquine was given to 6 healthy subjects and 6 patients with peptic ulcers before, and after, cimetidine 400 mg twice daily for 3 days. In contrast to the first study, cimetidine increased the maximum plasma concentration of mefloquine by about 42% and 20%, and increased the AUC by about 37% and 32%, in the healthy subjects and patients, respectively. The elimination half-life was increased, but this was not statistically significant.[2]

The findings of the first study suggest that cimetidine (a recognised enzyme inhibitor) reduces the metabolism of the mefloquine by the liver,[1] whereas the second study suggests that cimetidine may increase the rate of mefloquine absorption without notably inhibiting its elimination.[2]

These two studies produced different findings and an interaction is therefore not established. However, the changes seen in both studies were modest and unlikely to be clinically relevant in most patients taking lower doses of mefloquine for malaria prophylaxis. With higher doses of mefloquine used to treat malaria, prescribers should be alert for any evidence of increased mefloquine adverse effects (e.g. dizziness, nausea, vomiting, or abdominal pain) and psychiatric or neurological reactions during concurrent use. Note that the CSM in the UK state that any patient given mefloquine [for malaria prophylaxis] should be informed about its neurological adverse effects and advised, if these occur, to seek medical advice about the use of alternative antimalarials before the next dose is due.[3]

1. Sunbhanichi M, Ridtitid W, Wongnawa M, Akesiripong S, Chamnongchob P. Effect of cimetidine on an oral single-dose mefloquine pharmacokinetics in humans. *Asia Pac J Pharmacol* (1997) 12, 51–5.
2. Kolawole JA, Mustapha A, Abudu-Aguye I, Ochekpe N. Mefloquine pharmacokinetics in healthy subjects and in peptic ulcer patients after cimetidine administration. *Eur J Drug Metab Pharmacokinet* (2000) 25, 165–70.
3. Committee on Safety of Medicines/Medicines Control Agency. Mefloquine (Lariam) and neuropsychiatric reactions. *Current Problems* (1996) 22, 6.

Mefloquine + Metoclopramide

Metoclopramide increases the rate of absorption and maximum plasma concentration of a single-dose of mefloquine.

Clinical evidence, mechanism, importance and management

When 7 healthy subjects took a 10-mg dose of metoclopramide 15 minutes before a single 750-mg dose of mefloquine, the absorption half-life of the mefloquine was reduced from 3.2 hours to 2.4 hours and the maximum blood concentration was raised by 31%. In addition, the rate of absorption was increased, but the total amount absorbed was unchanged. A possible reason for these changes is that metoclopramide increases gastric emptying causing mefloquine to reach the small intestine more quickly, which would increase the rate of absorption. Despite these changes, the toxicity of mefloquine (e.g. dizziness, nausea, vomiting, and abdominal pain) was noted to be reduced.[1] The increase in the mefloquine maximum concentration is small, and probably not clinically relevant, especially with prophylactic mefloquine doses.

1. Na Bangchang K, Karbwang J, Bunnag D, Harinasuta T, Back DJ. The effect of metoclopramide on mefloquine pharmacokinetics. *Br J Clin Pharmacol* (1991) 32, 640–1.

Mefloquine + Miscellaneous

An isolated report describes cardiopulmonary arrest in a patient taking mefloquine with propranolol. Some warn that the concurrent use of mefloquine with drugs that prolong the QT interval might have additive effects on cardiac function.

Clinical evidence, mechanism, importance and management

The WHO,[1] and the UK[2] and US[3] manufacturers of mefloquine warn that its use with **antiarrhythmics** (such as **amiodarone** and **quinidine**), **antihistamines**, **beta blockers**, **calcium-channel blockers**, **digoxin**, **phenothiazines**, and **tricyclic antidepressants** might increase the risk of arrhythmias. The UK and US manufacturers also point out that the interactions are theoretical, and that clinically relevant QTc prolongation has not been found with mefloquine alone.[2,3] No formal studies on the possible adverse effects of combining any of the above drugs with mefloquine seem to have been carried out. One 1990 review[4] briefly mentions a single case of cardiopulmonary arrest when a patient taking **propranolol** was given a single dose of mefloquine. It has been suggested that the concurrent use of beta blockers and mefloquine might also lead to bradycardia, which is an uncommon adverse effect of mefloquine,[2,3] and a known effect of the beta blockers. However, there do not appear to be any reports of an adverse interaction in the literature. It remains to be confirmed whether the effects of mefloquine and these other drugs on cardiac function are normally additive, and whether the outcome is clinically important, although a case has been reported of the successful use of digoxin and sotalol in the treatment of mefloquine-induced atrial flutter with AV 1:1 conduction.[5] Until more is known it would seem prudent to follow the cautionary advice issued by the WHO and the manufacturers of mefloquine.

Drugs that can prolong the QT interval are listed in 'Table 9.2', p.273. Note that some quinolones can prolong the QT interval, and might also increase the risk of convulsions if given with mefloquine, see 'Mefloquine + Quinolones', p.251.

For mention that halofantrine should not be used with, or after, mefloquine because of a clinically relevant lengthening of the QT interval (which may be due to a pharmacokinetic interaction), see 'Halofantrine + Miscellaneous', p.1604. For mention of adverse cardiac effects when mefloquine is given with chloroquine, quinine, or quinidine, see 'Mefloquine + Quinine and related drugs', below.

1. WHO. Guidelines for the treatment of malaria-3rd edition. Available at: https://extranet.who.int/iris/restricted/bitstream/10665/162441/1/9789241549127_eng.pdf (accessed 21/10/15).
2. Lariam (Mefloquine hydrochloride). Roche Products Ltd. UK Summary of product characteristics, May 2014.
3. Mefloquine hydrochloride. Teva Pharmaceuticals USA. US Prescribing information, June 2013.
4. Anon. Mefloquine for malaria. *Med Lett Drugs Ther* (1990) 31, 13–14.
5. Fonteyne W, Bauwens A, Jordaens L. Atrial flutter with 1:1 conduction after administration of the antimalarial drug mefloquine. *Clin Cardiol* (1996) 19, 967–8.

Mefloquine + Primaquine

Although one study suggests that primaquine can increase both the maximum plasma concentration and adverse effects of mefloquine, other studies have generally found no important interaction.

Clinical evidence

A preliminary report of a randomised, crossover study in 14 healthy subjects given mefloquine 1 g, found that the addition of primaquine 15 mg or 30 mg increased the maximum plasma concentration of mefloquine by 48% and 29%, respectively. Those taking the larger dose of primaquine had a transient increase in its maximum plasma concentration, and the conversion to its inactive carboxyl metabolite was also increased. Clinically important CNS symptoms were also experienced by those taking the larger dose of primaquine.[1]

However, these results contrast with another single-dose study in 8 healthy subjects, who were given mefloquine 750 mg with primaquine 45 mg. No increased adverse effects attributable to concurrent use were seen, and mefloquine pharmacokinetics (including the maximum plasma concentration) were not altered by primaquine.[2] Similarly, in a study in patients with malaria, there was no change in mefloquine pharmacokinetics when it was given with primaquine.[3] In another group in this study, the only difference in mefloquine pharmacokinetics was an 11% shorter terminal elimination half-life in those taking primaquine with mefloquine and pyrimethamine with sulfadoxine, when compared with those taking mefloquine and pyrimethamine with sulfadoxine.[3] Similarly, in another study in children given mefloquine and pyrimethamine with sulfadoxine, the addition of primaquine had no effect on the pharmacokinetics of mefloquine, and there were no serious adverse effects.[4]

In a further study, the pharmacokinetics of a single 45-mg dose of primaquine were not altered by a single 10-mg/kg oral dose of mefloquine in healthy subjects.[5]

Mechanism

In vitro studies suggest that primaquine is a potent inhibitor of mefloquine metabolism.[6]

Importance and management

The bulk of the evidence suggests there is no important alteration in the pharmacokinetics or effect of mefloquine when it is given with primaquine. To prevent relapse after treatment of vivax malaria, the UK and US manufacturers of mefloquine advise that primaquine is used to eradicate hepatic parasites.[7,8]

1. Macleod CM, Trenholme GM, Nora MV, Bartley EA, Frischer H. Interaction of primaquine with mefloquine in healthy males. *Intersci Conf Antimicrob Agents Chemother* (1990) 30, 213.
2. Karbwang J, Na Bangchang K, Thanavibul A, Back DJ, Bunnag D. Pharmacokinetics of mefloquine in the presence of primaquine. *Eur J Clin Pharmacol* (1992) 42, 559–60.
3. Karbwang J, Back DJ, Bunnag D, Breckenridge AM. Pharmacokinetics of mefloquine in combination with sulfadoxine-pyrimethamine and primaquine in male Thai patients with falciparum malaria. *Bull WHO* (1990) 68, 633–8.
4. Singhasivanon V, Chongsuphajaisiddhi T, Sabchareon A, Attanath P, Webster HK, Edstein MD, Lika ID. Pharmacokinetic study of mefloquine in Thai children aged 5–12 years suffering from uncomplicated falciparum malaria treated with MSP or MSP plus primaquine. *Eur J Drug Metab Pharmacokinet* (1994) 19, 27–32.
5. Edwards G, McGrath CS, Ward SA, Supanaranond W, Pukrittayakamee S, Davis TM, White NJ. Interactions among primaquine, malaria infection and other antimalarials in Thai subjects. *Br J Clin Pharmacol* (1993) 35, 193–8.
6. Na Bangchang K, Karbwang J, Back DJ. Mefloquine metabolism by human liver microsomes. Effect of other antimalarial drugs. *Biochem Pharmacol* (1992) 43, 1957–61.
7. Lariam (Mefloquine hydrochloride). Roche Products Ltd. UK Summary of product characteristics, November 2011.
8. Mefloquine hydrochloride. West-Ward Pharmaceuticals. US Prescribing information, March 2010.

Mefloquine + Pyrimethamine with Sulfadoxine

Pyrimethamine with sulfadoxine does not appear to increase the exposure to mefloquine.

Clinical evidence, mechanism, importance and management

In healthy subjects, a comparison of the pharmacokinetic parameters of a single 750-mg dose of mefloquine, given alone or in combination with pyrimethamine with sulfadoxine, found that the only difference was a 33% increase in mean residence time and a 27% increase in the half-life of mefloquine.[1] However, in a further study in patients with malaria, there was no difference in any pharmacokinetic parameter of mefloquine 750 mg between 15 patients taking mefloquine alone and 16 patients taking mefloquine and pyrimethamine with sulfadoxine.[2] In both of these studies there was considerable inter-individual variability in the pharmacokinetics of mefloquine.[1,2] In another study in healthy subjects, the AUC of mefloquine was increased by 13% (not statistically significant) when mefloquine was given as a combination tablet (containing mefloquine, sulfadoxine, and pyrimethamine), when compared with mefloquine given alone.[3]

These studies suggest that any effect of pyrimethamine with sulfadoxine on mefloquine pharmacokinetics is small and unlikely to be clinically relevant, especially in view of the inter-individual variability in mefloquine pharmacokinetics.

1. Karbwang J, Bunnag D, Breckenridge AM, Back DJ. The pharmacokinetics of mefloquine when given alone or in combination with sulphadoxine and pyrimethamine in Thai male and female subjects. *Eur J Clin Pharmacol* (1987) 32, 173–7.
2. Karbwang J, Back DJ, Bunnag D, Breckenridge AM. Pharmacokinetics of mefloquine in combination with sulfadoxine-pyrimethamine and primaquine in male Thai patients with falciparum malaria. *Bull WHO* (1990) 68, 633–8.
3. Schwartz DE, Weidekamm E, Ranalder UB, Dubach UC, Forgo I, Weber B. Absence of pharmacokinetic interaction between Fansidar and mefloquine. *Trans R Soc Trop Med Hyg* (1986) 80, 1001–2.

Mefloquine + Quinine and related drugs

The plasma concentration of mefloquine might be increased by quinine. In theory, there is an increased risk of convulsions if mefloquine is given with quinine, quinidine, or chloroquine.

Clinical evidence, mechanism, importance and management

Mefloquine 750 mg was given to 7 healthy subjects either alone, or followed 24 hours later by quinine 600 mg. Concurrent use did not affect the pharmacokinetics of either drug, but the number of adverse effects and the period of QT interval prolongation was greater with the combination, although no symptomatic cardiotoxicity was seen.[1] Another study in 13 patients with uncomplicated falciparum malaria, given quinine dihydrochloride 10 mg/kg as a one-hour infusion and simultaneous oral mefloquine 15 mg/kg, found no evidence of a pharmacokinetic interaction, but postural hypotension was common. The QTc interval was prolonged by 12%, although no clinically important cardiovascular interaction was reported.[2] The absence of pharmacokinetic changes in these studies is contrary to earlier *in vitro* data and unpublished clinical observations,[3] which suggest that quinine might inhibit the metabolism of mefloquine, thereby raising its plasma concentration.

The UK and US manufacturers of mefloquine warn that concurrent use with quinine or related compounds (e.g. **quinidine**, **chloroquine**) could increase the risk of ECG abnormalities and convulsions.[4,5] The UK and US manufacturers suggest that, in patients initially given intravenous quinine for at least 2 to 3 days, the use of mefloquine should be delayed until at least 12 hours after the last dose of quinine to minimise interactions leading to adverse events.[4,5] However, there seem to be no documented adverse reports of this interaction leading to convulsions.

1. Na-Bangchang K, Tan-Ariya P, Thanavibul A, Reingchainam S, Shrestha SB, Karbwang J. Pharmacokinetic and pharmacodynamic interactions of mefloquine and quinine. *Int J Clin Pharmacol Res* (1999) 19, 73–82.
2. Supanaranond W, Suputtamongkol Y, Davis TME, Pukrittayakamee S, Teja-Isavadharm P, Webster HK, White NJ. Lack of a significant adverse cardiovascular effect of combined quinine and mefloquine therapy for uncomplicated malaria. *Trans R Soc Trop Med Hyg* (1997) 91, 694–6.
3. Na Bangchang K, Karbwang J, Back DJ. Mefloquine metabolism by human liver microsomes. Effect of other antimalarial drugs. *Biochem Pharmacol* (1992) 43, 1957–61.
4. Lariam (Mefloquine hydrochloride). Roche Products Ltd. UK Summary of product characteristics, November 2011.
5. Mefloquine hydrochloride. West-Ward Pharmaceuticals. US Prescribing information, March 2010.

Mefloquine + Quinolones

Three non-epileptic patients had convulsions when they were given mefloquine and a quinolone. Some quinolones, such as moxifloxacin, prolong the QT interval and concurrent use with mefloquine might theoretically result in additive effects.

Clinical evidence, mechanism, importance and management

A large scale survey in India of the adverse effects of mefloquine identified 3 cases of convulsions out of a total of 150 patients also taking **ciprofloxacin**, **ofloxacin**, or **sparfloxacin**. All 3 patients were not epileptic and had no family history of epilepsy. All were being treated for fever which was due to *P. vivax* in one case, *P. falciparum* in the second, and was not established in the third. None of the patients had severe or complicated malaria, which suggests that the convulsions were not solely a result of the disease state. **Ofloxacin** was given 2 days before mefloquine, and the other two quinolones were given together with mefloquine.[1] The reason for the seizures is not known, but seizures are among the recognised adverse effects of both mefloquine and these quinolones. These adverse, apparently additive, effects are rare but prescribers should be aware of the potential increased risk of convulsions when prescribing these drugs together.

Some quinolones (such as moxifloxacin) can cause clinically relevant prolongation of the QT interval, see 'Drugs that prolong the QT interval + Other drugs that prolong the QT interval', p.272. Although mefloquine alone has not been shown to cause a clinically relevant lengthening of the QT interval, caution is recommended when it is used concurrently with certain drugs that can prolong the QT interval, see 'Mefloquine + Miscellaneous', p.250. It would therefore be prudent to extend this caution to these quinolones.

1. Mangalvedhekar SS, Gogtay NJ, Wagh VR, Waran MS, Mane D, Kshirsagar NA. Convulsions in non-epileptics due to mefloquine-fluoroquinolone co-administration. *Natl Med J India* (2000) 13, 47.

Mefloquine + Rifampicin (Rifampin)

Rifampicin moderately reduces the exposure to mefloquine.

Clinical evidence, mechanism, importance and management

In a crossover study, 7 healthy subjects were given rifampicin 600 mg daily for 7 days with a single 500-mg dose of mefloquine on day 7. The maximum plasma concentration of mefloquine was decreased by 19% and its AUC was decreased by 68%. Rifampicin, a potent enzyme-inducer, was thought to have lowered the plasma concentration of mefloquine by inducing CYP3A4 in the liver and gut wall, thereby increasing mefloquine metabolism. The clinical relevance of this reduction in mefloquine exposure is uncertain, but the magnitude of the effect suggests that it is likely to be of note. The authors suggest that simultaneous use of rifampicin and mefloquine should be avoided to prevent treatment failure and the risk of *Plasmodium falciparum* resistance to mefloquine.[1] Until more is known, this would seem a sensible precaution.

1. Ridtitid W, Wongnawa M, Mahatthanatrakul W, Chaipol P, Sunbhanich M. Effect of rifampicin on plasma concentrations of mefloquine in healthy volunteers. *J Pharm Pharmacol* (2000) 52, 1265–9.

Mefloquine + Tetracycline

Mefloquine exposure is slightly increased by tetracycline.

Clinical evidence, mechanism, importance and management

In a study in 20 healthy Thai men, the maximum concentration of a single 750-mg dose of mefloquine was increased by 38% (from 1.16 mg/mL to 1.6 mg/mL) by tetracycline 250 mg four times daily for one week. The AUC was increased by 30% and the half-life reduced from 19.3 days to 14.4 days without any evidence of an increase in adverse effects. It is suggested that mefloquine pharmacokinetics are altered because its enterohepatic recycling is reduced by competition with tetracycline for biliary excretion.[1] The authors of the report concluded that concurrent use of mefloquine and tetracycline might be valuable for treating multi-drug resistant falciparum malaria because higher mefloquine concentrations are associated with a more effective response. However, more study is needed to confirm these findings. There seems to be no reason for avoiding concurrent use.

1. Karbwang J, Na Bangchang K, Back DJ, Bunnag D, Rooney W. Effect of tetracycline on mefloquine pharmacokinetics in Thai males. *Eur J Clin Pharmacol* (1992) 43, 567–9.

Metrifonate + Antacids or H_2-receptor antagonists

The pharmacokinetics of metrifonate do not appear to affected by an antacid containing aluminium/magnesium hydroxide, or by pretreatment with cimetidine or ranitidine.

Clinical evidence, mechanism, importance and management

(a) Antacids

A single-dose study in healthy subjects found that the AUC and maximum plasma concentration of metrifonate and its pharmacologically active metabolite were not altered by the concurrent use of an **aluminium/magnesium hydroxide**-containing antacid.[1] Therefore no special precautions seem necessary on their concurrent use.

(b) H_2-receptor antagonists

In a study in healthy subjects the AUC and maximum plasma concentration of metrifonate and its pharmacologically active metabolite were not altered by pretreatment with either **cimetidine** or **ranitidine**.[1] Based on these results it seems unlikely that other H_2-receptor antagonists will interact with metrifonate.

1. Heinig R, Boettcher M, Herman-Gnjidic Z, Pierce CH. Effects of magnesium/aluminium hydroxide-containing antacid, cimetidine or ranitidine on the pharmacokinetics of metrifonate and its metabolite DDVP. *Clin Drug Invest* (1999) 17, 67–77.

Nitazoxanide + Food

Food can almost double the exposure to nitazoxanide, depending on the formulation given.

Clinical evidence, mechanism, importance and management

In a randomised study in healthy subjects, giving increasing single oral doses of nitazoxanide tablets with a standardised breakfast, resulted in a mean increase in the AUC of the active metabolite tizoxanide, and of its glucuronide, of 82% and 93%, respectively, when compared with the fasted state.[1] The US manufacturer also briefly notes that when given as the oral suspension, the AUC of tizoxanide, and that of its glucuronide, were increased by 45 to 50%.[2] This increased bioavailability is considered to be clinically beneficial, and the manufacturers recommend that nitazoxanide be administered with food.[2]

1. Stockis A, Allemon AM, De Bruyn S, Gengler C. Nitazoxanide pharmacokinetics and tolerability in man using single ascending oral doses. *Int J Clin Pharmacol Ther* (2002) 40, 213–20.
2. Alinia (Nitazoxanide). Romark Laboratories, LC. US Prescribing information, October 2007.

Piperazine + Chlorpromazine

An isolated case of convulsions in a child was attributed to the use of piperazine followed by chlorpromazine.

Clinical evidence, mechanism, importance and management

A child given piperazine for pin worms developed convulsions when chlorpromazine was given several days later.[1] In a subsequent *animal* study using piperazine and chlorpromazine 4.5 mg/kg or 10 mg/kg, many of the *animals* died from respiratory arrest after severe clonic convulsions.[1] However, a later *animal* study did not confirm these findings[2] and it is unclear whether or not the adverse reaction in the child was due to an interaction. Given that both piperazine and chlorpromazine can cause convulsions, there is probably enough evidence to warrant caution if they are used concurrently.

1. Boulos BM, Davis LE. Hazard of simultaneous administration of phenothiazine and piperazine. *N Engl J Med* (1969) 280, 1245–6.
2. Armbrecht BH. Reaction between piperazine and chlorpromazine. *N Engl J Med* (1970) 282, 1490–1.

Praziquantel + Antiepileptics; Enzyme-inducing

Phenytoin, phenobarbital, and carbamazepine markedly reduce the exposure to praziquantel. Fosphenytoin would be expected to interact similarly.

Clinical evidence

(a) Carbamazepine, Phenobarbital, or Phenytoin

In a comparative study, patients taking long-term phenytoin or carbamazepine (10 in each group) and 10 healthy subjects not taking either antiepileptic were given a single 25-mg/kg oral dose of praziquantel. The AUC of praziquantel was about 74% and 90% lower, and its maximum plasma concentration 76% and 92% lower, in the phenytoin- and carbamazepine-treated patients, respectively, when compared with the healthy subjects.[1] Another study also reported low plasma concentrations of praziquantel (maximum concentrations of 42 nanograms/mL to 540 nanograms/mL with undetectable minimum concentrations) in patients given praziquantel 15 mg/kg three times daily for 15 days and also taking phenytoin (4 patients) or phenobarbital (8 patients). However, in this study praziquantel was still found to be very effective for neurocysticercosis, with all patients showing a marked improvement.[2]

(b) Phenytoin/Phenobarbital and Cimetidine

A patient with neurocysticercosis taking phenytoin and phenobarbital for a seizure disorder had no response to praziquantel (four courses in doses of up to 50 mg/kg daily). Praziquantel 50 mg/kg daily and dexamethasone 12 mg daily were started and, after one week, cimetidine 400 mg four times daily was added. The plasma concentration of praziquantel more than doubled with the addition of cimetidine (maximum plasma concentration increased from 350 nanograms/mL to 826 nanograms/mL); the AUC rose about 4-fold and became similar to that found in control subjects taking praziquantel alone. The patient showed marginal improvement and continued to slowly improve over the following 4 months.[3]

Mechanism

Not established. Praziquantel appears to be metabolised by CYP1A2, CYP2C19, and CYP3A4.[4] These antiepileptics have cytochrome P450 enzyme-inducing effects and might therefore increase the metabolism of praziquantel, resulting in a decrease in its exposure. However, the fact that praziquantel was still effective in one study suggests that praziquantel metabolites might be active.[2]

Importance and management

Direct information on an interaction between praziquantel and carbamazepine, phenobarbital, or phenytoin appears to be limited to the reports cited, but the pharmacokinetic interaction appears to be established. However, the clinical relevance of the interaction is uncertain. When treating systemic worm infections such as neurocysticercosis some authors advise increasing the praziquantel dose from 25 mg/kg to 50 mg/kg if potent enzyme inducers such as carbamazepine or phenytoin are being used, in order to reduce the risk of treatment failure.[1] A 45 mg/kg daily dose was effective in one study in 11 patients taking antiepileptics, despite a low plasma concentration of praziquantel,[2] but a 50 mg/kg daily dose was not effective in another case.[3] The recommended dose of praziquantel for the treatment of neurocysticercosis is 50 mg/kg daily in 3 divided doses.[5] Adding cimetidine might reduce the effect of enzyme-inducing antiepileptics. However, the authors of the case above[3] were not sure whether the improvement they saw was in fact due to the cimetidine or simply part of the natural history of the disease. It is clear that cimetidine alone can increase the plasma concentration of praziquantel (see 'Praziquantel + Cimetidine', below). Note that **fosphenytoin**, a prodrug of phenytoin, and **primidone**, which is metabolised to phenobarbital, would be expected to interact similarly, and similar precautions should be considered.

Note that the interaction with enzyme-inducing antiepileptics is of no importance when praziquantel is used for intestinal worm infections (where its action is a local effect on the worms in the gut).

1. Bittencourt PRM, Gracia CM, Martins R, Fernandes AG, Diekmann HW, Jung W. Phenytoin and carbamazepine decrease oral bioavailability of praziquantel. *Neurology* (1992) 42, 492–6.
2. Na-Bangchang K, Vanijanonta S, Karbwang J. Plasma concentrations of praziquantel during the therapy of neurocysticerosis with praziquantel, in the presence of antiepileptics and dexamethasone. *Southeast Asian J Trop Med Public Health* (1995) 26, 120–3.
3. Dachman WD, Adubofour KO, Bikin DS, Johnson CH, Mullin PD, Winograd M. Cimetidine-induced rise in praziquantel levels in a patient with neurocysticercosis being treated with anticonvulsants. *J Infect Dis* (1994) 169, 689–91.
4. Li X-Q, Björkman A, Andersson TB, Gustafsson LL, Masimirembwa CM. Identification of human cytochrome P_{450}s that metabolise anti-parasitic drugs and predictions of in vivo hepatic clearance from in vitro data. *Eur J Clin Pharmacol* (2003) 59, 429–42.
5. *Martindale. The Complete Drug Reference*, [online] London: Pharmaceutical Press. https://www.medicinescomplete.com/mc/martindale/current/13161-h.htm (accessed 19/10/15).

Praziquantel + Azoles

Ketoconazole increases the plasma concentration of praziquantel. Other azoles are predicted to interact similarly.

Clinical evidence

In a randomised, crossover study, 10 healthy subjects were given a single dose of praziquantel 20 mg/kg alone or after pretreatment with **ketoconazole** 400 mg daily for 5 days. **Ketoconazole** increased the AUC and maximum plasma concentration of praziquantel by 93% and 102%, respectively. The total clearance was decreased by 58% but the half-life was only slightly prolonged. No adverse effects were reported with praziquantel alone; however, mild headache and gastrointestinal adverse effects (including nausea and vomiting) were reported when patients were pretreated with **ketoconazole**.[1]

Mechanism

Praziquantel is metabolised by CYP3A4, which is potently inhibited by ketoconazole. Concurrent use therefore decreases praziquantel metabolism, resulting in an increase in plasma concentration. All azoles inhibit this isoenzyme (although the extent varies, see under *Azoles* in 'Anthelmintics, Antifungals, and Antiprotozoals', p.225), and would therefore be expected to interact.

Importance and management

Information on an interaction between the azoles and praziquantel is limited, but the findings of the one available study are in line with the known metabolism of praziquantel and the inhibitory effects of ketoconazole on CYP3A4. All azoles inhibit this isoenzyme and would therefore be expected to interact similarly, albeit to varying degrees (see *Mechanism* above). Although there is no direct information, it is possible that concurrent use might lead to an improved clinical outcome as has been reported for cimetidine, which also raises the plasma concentration of praziquantel (see 'Praziquantel + Cimetidine', below). However, the study with ketoconazole found that concurrent use increased adverse effects, and so it would seem prudent to monitor for praziquantel adverse effects if an azole is also given.

1. Pharmacokinetic interaction between ketoconazole and praziquantel in healthy volunteers. *J Clin Pharm Ther* (2007) 32, 585–93.

Praziquantel + Chloroquine

Chloroquine reduces the bioavailability of praziquantel.

Clinical evidence

A single 40-mg/kg oral dose of praziquantel was given to 8 healthy subjects, alone and 2 hours after chloroquine 600 mg. Chloroquine reduced the AUC and maximum plasma concentration of praziquantel by 65% and 59%, respectively. There were large individual variations in plasma concentrations, and one subject was not affected.[1]

Mechanism

Not understood.

Importance and management

Evidence for an interaction between praziquantel and chloroquine is limited to this one small study and the clinical importance is uncertain. The result of this interaction could be that some patients will not achieve a high enough plasma concentration of praziquantel to treat systemic worm infections, such as schistosomiasis. In the study, after taking chloroquine, the plasma concentration of praziquantel in 50% of subjects did not reach the threshold of 0.3 micrograms/mL for about 6 hours (which is required to effectively kill schistosomes), compared with only 25% during the control period. The authors conclude that an increased dose of praziquantel should be considered if chloroquine is given (they do not suggest how much), particularly in anyone who does not respond to initial treatment with praziquantel.[1] Further study of this interaction is needed to establish its clinical relevance.

Note that this interaction is of no importance when praziquantel is used for intestinal worm infections (where its action is a local effect on the worms in the gut).

1. Masimirembwa CM, Naik YS, Hasler JA. The effect of chloroquine on the pharmacokinetics and metabolism of praziquantel in rats and in humans. *Biopharm Drug Dispos* (1994) 15, 33–43.

Praziquantel + Cimetidine

Cimetidine can moderately increase the exposure to praziquantel.

Clinical evidence

In a randomised, crossover study, 8 healthy subjects were given three 25-mg/kg oral doses of praziquantel at 2-hourly intervals with cimetidine 400 mg given one hour before each dose of praziquantel. Cimetidine roughly doubled the AUC and plasma concentration of praziquantel.[1,2] A further study in patients with neurocysticercosis found that this short regimen of praziquantel with cimetidine (which increased the plasma concentration of praziquantel about 3-fold), had similar efficacy to the traditional regimen of 50 mg/kg daily in divided doses for 15 days.[3] Of the 6 patients receiving praziquantel with cimetidine, the clinical cure rate was 83%, compared with only 50% in 6 patients receiving praziquantel alone.[3]

Mechanism

Uncertain. An *in vitro* study has shown praziquantel to be a substrate for several cytochrome P450 isoenzymes including CYP1A2, CYP2C19, and CYP3A4.[4] Although cimetidine is an inhibitor of various cytochrome P450 isoenzymes, its effects are generally weak, and so this seems unlikely to explain the marked increase in exposure to praziquantel.

Importance and management

Direct information appears to be limited to the reports cited, but the interaction appears to be established. It is clear that cimetidine can markedly increase the exposure to praziquantel, and the authors state that concurrent use can reduce treatment for neurocysticercosis from 2 weeks to one day.[1,3] One case report suggests that the concurrent use of cimetidine contributed to the resolution of refractory neurocysticercosis in a patient treated with high-dose praziquantel 100 mg/kg daily, although no pharmacokinetic data for praziquantel were reported.[5]

Cimetidine has been used to try to reverse the effects of enzyme-inducing antiepileptics (see 'Praziquantel + Antiepileptics; Enzyme-inducing', p.251) and corticosteroids (see 'Praziquantel + Dexamethasone', below), which reduce the plasma concentration of praziquantel.

1. Jung H, Medina R, Castro N, Corona T, Sotelo J. Pharmacokinetic study of praziquantel administered alone and in combination with cimetidine in a single-day therapeutic regimen. *Antimicrob Agents Chemother* (1997) 41, 1256–9.
2. Castro N, González-Esquivel D, Medina R, Sotelo J, Jung H. The influence of cimetidine on plasma levels of praziquantel after a single day therapeutic regimen. *Proc West Pharmacol Soc* (1997) 40, 33–4.
3. Castro N, González-Esquivel DF, López M, Jung H. Análisis comparativo de la influencia de los alimentos y la cimetidina en los niveles plasmáticos de prazicuantel. *Rev Invest Clin* (2003) 55, 655–61.
4. Li X-Q, Björkman A, Andersson TB, Gustafsson LL, Masimirembwa CM. Identification of human cytochrome P_{450}s that metabolise anti-parasitic drugs and predictions of in vivo hepatic clearance from in vitro data. *Eur J Clin Pharmacol* (2003) 59, 429–42.
5. Yee T, Barakos JA, Knight RT. High-dose praziquantel with cimetidine for refractory neurocysticercosis: a case report with clinical and MRI follow-up. *West J Med* (1999), 170, 112–15.

Praziquantel + Dexamethasone

The continuous use of dexamethasone can halve the plasma concentration of praziquantel.

Clinical evidence

Eight patients with parenchymal brain cysticercosis taking praziquantel 50 mg/kg daily (in three divided doses every 8 hours) had a 50% reduction in the steady-state plasma concentration of praziquantel (from 3.13 micrograms/mL to 1.55 micrograms/mL) when given dexamethasone 8 mg every 8 hours.[1] Another patient with recurrent neurocysticercosis, who did not respond to praziquantel 50 mg/kg daily, was successfully treated with high-dose praziquantel 100 mg/kg daily, dexamethasone 12 mg daily, and cimetidine 800 mg daily. As dexamethasone was thought to reduce the plasma concentration of praziquantel, cimetidine was added to try to reverse this effect[2] as it has been reported to increase the bioavailability of praziquantel (see 'Praziquantel + Cimetidine', above). However, some patients have responded well to praziquantel, despite low plasma concentrations.[3]

Mechanism

Uncertain. Praziquantel is partly metabolised by CYP3A4 and it has been suggested that dexamethasone is an inducer of this isoenzyme. Dexamethasone might therefore reduce the plasma concentration of praziquantel by this route, although the size of the effect seen might raise questions about this.

Importance and management

Information about an interaction between praziquantel and the corticosteroids seems to be limited, but the pharmacokinetic interaction appears to be established. However, the extent to which it affects the clinical outcome of treatment for systemic worm infections, such as cysticercosis, is unknown as the optimum praziquantel concentration required is still uncertain and it is also possible that the metabolites of praziquantel might be active.[3] The authors of one report suggest that dexamethasone should not be given continuously with praziquantel but only used transiently to resolve inflammatory reactions to praziquantel treatment.[1] Alternatively, limited information suggests that the addition of cimetidine might allow dexamethasone to be used.[2]

The interaction with dexamethasone is of no importance when praziquantel is used for intestinal worm infections (where its action is a local effect on the worms in the gut).

1. Vazquez ML, Jung H, Sotelo J. Plasma levels of praziquantel decrease when dexamethasone is given simultaneously. *Neurology* (1987) 37, 1561–2.
2. Yee T, Barakos JA, Knight RT. High-dose praziquantel with cimetidine for refractory neurocysticercosis: a case report with clinical and MRI follow-up. *West J Med* (1999) 170, 112–15.
3. Na-Bangchang K, Vanijanonta S, Karbwang J. Plasma concentrations of praziquantel during the therapy of neurocysticerosis with praziquantel, in the presence of antiepileptics and dexamethasone. *Southeast Asian J Trop Med Public Health* (1995) 26, 120–3.

Praziquantel + Food

Food increases the bioavailability of praziquantel.

Clinical evidence, mechanism, importance and management

In a crossover study, the maximum plasma concentration and AUC of a single 1.8-g dose of praziquantel were increased 3.4-fold and 2.8-fold when it was given immediately after a high-fat meal, and 6.2-fold and 3.7-fold after a high-carbohydrate meal, respectively, when compared with the fasted state.[1] In another study in healthy Sudanese men, when praziquantel was given with food, the AUC was 2.6-fold higher than when it was given in the fasted state.[2]

A further study in patients with neurocysticercosis found that taking praziquantel 25 mg/kg every 2 hours for 3 doses with a high-carbohydrate diet increased the plasma concentration of praziquantel and provided an adequate clinical alternative to the traditional regimen of 50 mg/kg daily in divided doses for 15 days.[3] In 6 patients who took praziquantel with food, the clinical cure rate was 83%, compared with only 50% in 6 patients who took praziquantel while fasting.[3]

On the basis of the above studies, if praziquantel is used for systemic worm infections, administration with food is advisable.

1. Castro N, Medina R, Sotelo J, Jung H. Bioavailability of praziquantel increases with concomitant administration of food. *Antimicrob Agents Chemother* (2000) 44, 2903–4.
2. Homeida M, Leahy W, Copeland S, Ali MM, Harron DWG. Pharmacokinetic interaction between praziquantel and albendazole in Sudanese men. *Ann Trop Med Parasitol* (1994) 88, 551–9.
3. Castro N, González-Esquivel DF, López M, Jung H. Análisis comparativo de la influencia de los alimentos y la cimetidina en los niveles plasmáticos de prazicuantel. *Rev Invest Clin* (2003) 55, 655–61.

Praziquantel + Grapefruit juice

Grapefruit juice increases the exposure to praziquantel.

Clinical evidence, mechanism, importance and management

In a randomised, crossover study in 18 healthy subjects a single 1.8-g dose of praziquantel was given with 250 mL of grapefruit juice or water. Grapefruit juice increased the maximum plasma concentration and AUC of praziquantel by about 63% and 90%, respectively, when compared with water.[1] The authors suggest that grapefruit juice probably increases the absorption of praziquantel. The clinical effect of this interaction has not been assessed: it might lead to improved efficacy, but it might also lead to an increase in praziquantel adverse effects (e.g. headache, diarrhoea, dizziness, or drowsiness). Until more is known it might be prudent to be alert for an increase in praziquantel adverse effects in patients who drink grapefruit juice. When compared with other studies, the authors note that the effect of grapefruit juice is comparable to that of cimetidine (see 'Praziquantel + Cimetidine', p.252), but less than that of food (see 'Praziquantel + Food', above).

1. Castro N, Jung H, Medina R, González-Esquivel D, Lopez M, Sotelo J. Interaction between grapefruit juice and praziquantel in humans. *Antimicrob Agents Chemother* (2002) 46, 1614–16.

Praziquantel + Rifampicin (Rifampin)

Rifampicin reduces the plasma concentration of praziquantel.

Clinical evidence, mechanism, importance and management

A study in 10 subjects found that pretreatment with rifampicin 600 mg daily for 5 days reduced the maximum plasma concentration of a single 40-mg/kg dose of praziquantel, with 7 of the subjects having undetectable praziquantel concentrations (less than 12.5 nanograms/mL). In the other 3 subjects, there was an 85% reduction in the AUC of praziquantel. The same 10 subjects were then given three doses of praziquantel 25 mg/kg at intervals of 8 hours, alone and after pretreatment with rifampicin, as before. In this multiple-dose study, 5 of the 10 subjects had undetectable plasma concentrations of praziquantel and the remainder had an 80% reduction in the AUC of praziquantel.[1]

Praziquantel is metabolised by various cytochrome P450 isoenzymes. Rifampicin is a non-specific enzyme inducer which appears to induce the metabolism of praziquantel. Although the clinical relevance of the findings were not been assessed, the authors concluded that the plasma concentration of praziquantel after rifampicin pretreatment was less than that considered necessary for anthelmintic activity. They therefore recommend that the combination should be avoided,[1] a stance which is also taken by one of the manufacturers of praziquantel.[2]

1. Ridtitid W, Wongnawa M, Mahatthanatrakul W, Punyo J, Sunbhanich M. Rifampin markedly decreases plasma concentrations of praziquantel in healthy volunteers. *Clin Pharmacol Ther* (2002) 72, 505–13.
2. Biltricide (Praziquantel). Bayer Inc. Canadian Prescribing information, November 2007.

Primaquine + Artemether

No pharmacokinetic interaction appears to occur between primaquine and artemether.

Clinical evidence, mechanism, importance and management

A crossover study in 8 healthy subjects found that the pharmacokinetics of single oral doses of artemether 300 mg (a derivative of artemisinin) and primaquine 45 mg were not affected by concurrent use. No adverse effects were seen.[1] The WHO recommends the addition of primaquine to artemisinin-based combination therapy for the treatment of uncomplicated falciparum and uncomplicated vivax malaria.[2]

1. Na-Bangchang K, Karbwang J, Ubalee R, Thanavibul A, Saenglertsilapachai S. Absence of significant pharmacokinetic and pharmacodynamic interactions between artemether and quinoline antimalarials. *Eur J Drug Metab Pharmacokinet* (2000) 25 171–8.
2. World Health Organization. Guidelines for the treatment of malaria - 3rd edition. Available at: https://extranet.who.int/iris/restricted/bitstream/10665/162441/1/9789241549127_eng.pdf (accessed 21/101/15).

Primaquine + Food

Food causes a negligible increase in the bioavailability of primaquine.

Clinical evidence, mechanism, importance and management

A crossover study in 20 healthy subjects found that giving a single 30-mg dose of primaquine with food (two bread rolls and 30 g of butter) increased the AUC and maximum plasma concentration of primaquine by 14% and 26%, respectively, when compared with administration in the fasting state. These small increases are unlikely to increase the risk of adverse effects.[1] Primaquine should usually be taken with a meal to minimise gastrointestinal adverse effects, such as abdominal cramps, and it appears that this is unlikely to have a clinically relevant effect on bioavailability.

1. Cuong BT, Binh VQ, Dai B, Duy DN, Lovell CM, Rieckmann KH, Edstein MD. Does gender, food or grapefruit juice alter the pharmacokinetics of primaquine. *Br J Clin Pharmacol* (2006) 61, 682–9.

Primaquine + Grapefruit juice

Grapefruit juice might very slightly increase the exposure to primaquine. The effect might be greater in some individuals.

Clinical evidence, mechanism, importance and management

A crossover study in 20 healthy subjects found that 300 mL of grapefruit juice (concentrated grapefruit juice diluted to 50%) increased the mean AUC and maximum plasma concentration of primaquine by 19% and 23%, respectively. These changes are very slight; however, the authors note that although there was no interaction in some individuals, in others there was up to a twofold increase in primaquine bioavailability.[1]

Evidence is limited to this study and the general importance of this interaction is unclear. The authors of the study suggest that due to a lack of further information, particularly on the effects of more concentrated juice and the unpredictability of this interaction, it might be prudent to avoid drinking grapefruit juice while taking primaquine.[1] This would appear to be sensible advice until further evidence is available.

1. Cuong BT, Binh VQ, Dai B, Duy DN, Lovell CM, Rieckmann KH, Edstein MD. Does gender, food or grapefruit juice alter the pharmacokinetics of primaquine. *Br J Clin Pharmacol* (2006) 61, 682–9.

Primaquine + Mepacrine (Quinacrine)

Theoretically, mepacrine might be expected to elevate the plasma concentration of primaquine, but there do not seem to be any reports confirming or disproving this.

Clinical evidence, mechanism, importance and management

Patients given pamaquine (a formerly used antimalarial that was a predecessor of primaquine, and almost identical in structure) had grossly elevated plasma concentrations of pamaquine when they were also given mepacrine.[1,2] The reason for this interaction is unknown. On theoretical grounds primaquine might be expected to interact with mepacrine similarly, but there seem to be no reports confirming that a clinically important interaction actually takes place. However, the US manufacturer contraindicates the concurrent use of primaquine with mepacrine and also the use of primaquine in patients who have recently taken mepacrine.[3]

1. Zubrod CG, Kennedy TJ, Shannon JA. Studies on the chemotherapy of the human malarias. VIII. The physiological disposition of pamaquine. *J Clin Invest* (1948) 27 (Suppl), 114–120.
2. Earle DP, Bigelow FS, Zubrod CG, Kane CA. Studies on the chemotherapy of the human malarias. IX. Effect of pamaquine on the blood cells of man. *J Clin Invest* (1948) 27, (Suppl), 121–9.
3. Primaquine phosphate. Sanofi-Aventis. US Prescribing information, November 2010.

Primaquine + Quinine

Quinine does not appear to affect the pharmacokinetics of primaquine.

Clinical evidence, mechanism, importance and management

In a study in 7 subjects, quinine 10 mg/kg three times daily had no effect on the pharmacokinetics of a single 45-mg dose of primaquine, except for a 50% increase in the AUC of the carboxyprimaquine metabolite. The combination was effective for the treatment of malaria with no complications and no adverse effects reported.[1]

Usually, primaquine and quinine are unlikely to be taken together because quinine is used for the treatment of falciparum malaria and primaquine is used to eliminate the liver stages of vivax and ovale malarias. However, quinine may be used if the infective species is unknown, or if the infection is mixed, and then subsequent use of primaquine might be required. The limited data from the above study suggest that no special precautions would be required in this situation.

1. Edwards G, McGrath CS, Ward SA, Supanaranond W, Pukrittayakamee S, Davis TM, White NJ. Interactions among primaquine, malaria infection and other antimalarials in Thai subjects. *Br J Clin Pharmacol* (1993) 35, 193–8.

Proguanil + Antacids

The exposure to proguanil is moderately reduced by magnesium trisilicate. Other antacids such as aluminium hydroxide might interact similarly.

Clinical evidence

Magnesium trisilicate reduced the AUC of a single 200-mg dose of proguanil by about 65% in 8 healthy subjects, as assessed by the salivary concentration of proguanil.[1]

Mechanism

In vitro tests show that magnesium trisilicate adsorbs proguanil. Two other antacids, **aluminium hydroxide** and light **magnesium carbonate**, also adsorb proguanil, but to a lesser extent.[1] Therefore, antacids might reduce the amount of proguanil available for absorption by the gut.

Importance and management

Evidence for an interaction between proguanil and antacids is limited to this one small study. However, based on the known interactive potential of antacids, the interaction between proguanil and magnesium trisilicate appears to be established, but its clinical importance does not seem to have been assessed. Given the extent of the reduction in exposure, the antimalarial effects of proguanil might be expected to be reduced. One way to minimise the interaction is to separate the dose of proguanil and magnesium trisilicate as much as possible (2 to 3 hours has been shown to be sufficient with other drugs that interact with antacids in this way) to reduce admixture in the gut. There do not appear to be any clinical studies to see if other antacids behave similarly, but *in vitro* studies suggest aluminium hydroxide and magnesium carbonate might also interact with proguanil. Therefore similar precautions for these antacids might be prudent.

1. Onyeji CO, Babalola CP. The effect of magnesium trisilicate on proguanil absorption. *Int J Pharmaceutics* (1993) 100, 249–52.

Proguanil + Chloroquine

When given as antimalarial prophylaxis, chloroquine appears to increase the incidence of mouth ulcers in those taking proguanil by 50%.

Clinical evidence, mechanism, importance and management

Following the observation that mouth ulcers appeared to be common in those taking prophylactic antimalarials, an extensive study was undertaken in 628 servicemen in Belize. Of those taking proguanil 200 mg daily, 24% developed mouth ulcers, and in those also taking chloroquine base 150 to 300 mg weekly, 37% developed mouth ulcers. The incidence of diarrhoea was also increased from 63% among those who did not develop ulcers to 83% in those who did develop ulcers (any treatment). The reasons are not understood. The authors of the study suggested that these two drugs should not be given together unnecessarily for prophylaxis against falciparum malaria.[1] However, note that there appears to be no other published reports of an increased incidence of mouth ulcers with concurrent use, and the use of chloroquine with proguanil has been an established prophylactic regimen for many years and is still commonly recommended in regions where there is some resistance to chloroquine.

1. Drysdale SF, Phillips-Howard PA, Behrens RH. Proguanil, chloroquine, and mouth ulcers. *Lancet* (1990) 1, 164.

Proguanil + Drugs that affect gastric pH

There is some evidence that omeprazole and cimetidine can reduce the production of cycloguanil, the active metabolite of proguanil.

Clinical evidence

(a) Cimetidine

In one study, 4 patients with peptic ulcer disease and 6 healthy subjects were given a single 200-mg dose of proguanil on the last day of a 3-day course of cimetidine 400 mg twice daily. In both groups the half-life and AUC of proguanil were notably increased, but only the healthy subjects had an increase in the maximum plasma concentration (of 89%). In both groups these pharmacokinetic changes resulted in a decrease in the maximum plasma concentration of cycloguanil, the active metabolite of proguanil.[1] This decrease in cycloguanil exposure supported the findings of an earlier study, which had found a 30% decrease in the urinary recovery of cycloguanil when proguanil and cimetidine were given together.[2]

(b) Omeprazole

A steady-state study in 12 healthy subjects taking proguanil 200 mg daily found that omeprazole 20 mg daily roughly halved the AUC of cycloguanil, the active metabolite of proguanil.[3] However, an earlier study found that omeprazole 20 mg had no effect on the urinary recovery of cycloguanil (or proguanil) from a single 200-mg dose of proguanil.[2]

Mechanism

Cimetidine and omeprazole both increase the gastric pH which might lead to an increase in the absorption of proguanil. Cimetidine[1,2] and omeprazole[3] are also thought to inhibit the metabolism of proguanil due to their inhibitory effects on CYP2C19.

Importance and management

Evidence for an interaction between proguanil and cimetidine or omeprazole is limited, but roughly consistent with the known pharmacokinetic effects of these drugs. The differences between the healthy subjects and patients with peptic ulcer disease seen in one study might have been caused by the disease itself altering the effects of the cimetidine in some way.[1] Patients with peptic ulcer disease are also likely to have an increased gastric pH which will lead to altered proguanil absorption. The clinical relevance of all these findings is still unclear, although the implication is that a decrease in the plasma concentration of cycloguanil might lead to inadequate malaria prophylaxis. However, a subsequent clinical study reported that subjects who were lacking or had low CYP2C19 activity (and who therefore had relatively low plasma concentrations of cycloguanil) did not have an increased risk of failure of proguanil prophylaxis.[4] Similarly, treatment of malaria with proguanil was as effective in 62 patients who were deficient or lacking CYP2C19 as in 33 patients with normal CYP2C19 activity, independent of the plasma concentration of cycloguanil .[5] This suggests that any interaction with omeprazole or cimetidine by this mechanism would be unlikely to be clinically relevant, and therefore dose adjustments would not be expected to be necessary in patients given proguanil with cimetidine or omeprazole.

1. Kolawole JA, Mustapha A, Abdul-Aguye I, Ochekpe N, Taylor RB. Effects of cimetidine on the pharmacokinetics of proguanil in healthy subjects and in peptic ulcer patients. *J Pharm Biomed Anal* (1999) 20, 737–43.
2. Somogyi AA, Reinhard HA, Bochner F. Effects of omeprazole and cimetidine on the urinary metabolic ratio of proguanil in healthy volunteers. *Eur J Clin Pharmacol* (1996) 50, 417–19.
3. Funck-Bretano C, Becquemont L, Lenevu A, Roux A, Jaillon P, Beaune P. Inhibition by omeprazole of proguanil metabolism: mechanism of the interaction *in vitro* and prediction of *in vivo* results from the *in vitro* experiments. *J Pharmacol Exp Ther* (1997) 280, 730–8.
4. Mberu EK, Wansor T, Sato H, Nishikawa Y, Watkins WM. Japanese poor metabolizers of proguanil do not have an increased risk of malaria chemoprophylaxis breakthrough. Trans R Soc Trop Med Hyg. (1995) 89;658–9.
5. Kaneko A, Bergqvist Y, Takechi M, Kalkoa M, Kaneko O, Kobayakawa T, Ishizaki T, Bjorkman A. Intrinsic efficacy of proguanil against falciparum and vivax malaria independent of the metabolite cycloguanil. *J Infect Dis* (1999) 179; 974–9.

Proguanil + Fluvoxamine

The conversion of proguanil to its active metabolite, cycloguanil, is markedly inhibited by fluvoxamine in patients who have normal CYP2C19 activity.

Clinical evidence

Twelve healthy subjects, 6 of whom had normal CYP2C19 activity and 6 of whom were lacking or deficient in CYP2C19, were given proguanil 200 mg daily for 8 days, followed by fluvoxamine 100 mg for 8 days with a single 200-mg dose of proguanil on day 6. In the subjects with normal CYP2C19 activity it was found that fluvoxamine reduced the total clearance of proguanil by about 40%. The partial clearance of proguanil via its two metabolites was also reduced, by 85% for cycloguanil and by 89% for 4-chlorophenylbiguanide. The concentrations of these two metabolites in the plasma were hardly detectable while fluvoxamine was being taken. No pharmacokinetic interaction occurred in any of the subjects lacking or deficient in CYP2C19.[1]

Mechanism

Proguanil, which is thought to be a prodrug, is metabolised to its active metabolite, cycloguanil, by CYP2C19. This isoenzyme is inhibited by fluvoxamine and this prevents proguanil from being activated.[2]

Importance and management

Information about an interaction between fluvoxamine and proguanil appears to be limited to the studies cited, the purpose of which was to confirm that fluvoxamine is an inhibitor of CYP2C19. However, they also demonstrate that proguanil, which is a prodrug, will not be effectively converted into its active form in patients who have normal CYP2C19 activity (extensive metabolisers) if fluvoxamine is also being taken, making them effectively poor metabolisers (i.e. like those subjects lacking or deficient in CYP2C19). There do not appear to be any reports of treatment failures due to this interaction but if the activity of proguanil is virtually abolished by fluvoxamine, as the authors suggest,[2] then proguanil would also be expected to be ineffective in the proportion of the population that are poor metabolisers. However, a subsequent clinical study reported that subjects who were poor metabolisers of proguanil did not have an increased risk of failure of proguanil prophylaxis.[3] Similarly, treatment of malaria with proguanil was as effective in 62 patients who were CYP2C19 poor metabolisers as in 33 patients who were extensive metabolisers, independent of the plasma concentration of cycloguanil.[4] This suggests that any interaction with fluvoxamine might not be clinically relevant.

1. Jeppesen U, Rasmussen BB, Brøsen K. Fluvoxamine inhibits the CYP2C19-catalyzed bioactivation of chloroguanide. *Clin Pharmacol Ther* (1997) 62, 279–86.
2. Rasmussen BB, Nielsen TL, Brøsen K. Fluvoxamine inhibits the CYP2C19-catalysed metabolism of proguanil in vitro. *Eur J Clin Pharmacol* (1998) 54, 735–40.
3. Mberu EK, Wansor T, Sato H, Nishikawa Y, Watkins WM. Japanese poor metabolizers of proguanil do not have an increased risk of malaria chemoprophylaxis breakthrough. *Trans R Soc Trop Med Hyg* (1995) 89, 658–9.
4. Kaneko A, Bergqvist Y, Takechi M, Kalkoa M, Kaneko O, Kobayakawa T, Ishizaki T, Bjorkman A. Intrinsic efficacy of proguanil against falciparum and vivax malaria independent of the metabolite cycloguanil. *J Infect Dis* (1999) 179, 974–9.

Pyrantel + Piperazine

Piperazine is expected to oppose the anthelmintic actions of pyrantel.

Clinical evidence, mechanism, importance and management

Pyrantel acts as an anthelmintic because it depolarises the neuromuscular junctions of some intestinal nematodes causing the worms to contract. This paralyses the worms so that they are dislodged by peristalsis and expelled in the faeces. Piperazine also paralyses nematodes but it does so by causing hyperpolarisation of the neuromuscular junctions. These two pharmacological actions oppose one another, as was shown in two *in vitro* pharmacological studies. Strips of whole *Ascaris lumbricoides* (roundworm) contracted when exposed to pyrantel, but did not do so when also exposed to piperazine.[1] Parallel electrophysiological studies using *Ascaris* cells confirmed that the depolarisation due to pyrantel was opposed by piperazine.[1]

In practical terms this means that piperazine does not enhance the anthelmintic effect of pyrantel on *Ascaris* as might be expected, but opposes it. For this reason it is recommended that concurrent use should be avoided, but direct clinical evidence confirming that concurrent use is ineffective seems to be lacking.

It seems reasonable to extrapolate the results of these studies on *Ascaris lumbricoides* to the other gastrointestinal parasites for which pyrantel is used, i.e. *Enterobius vermicularis* (threadworm or pinworm), *Ancylostoma duodenale*, *Necator americanus* (hookworm), and *Trichostrongylus* spp. However, this does not appear to have been studied.

1. Aubry ML, Cowell P, Davey MJ, Shevde S. Aspects of the pharmacology of a new anthelmintic: pyrantel. *Br J Pharmacol* (1970) 38, 332–44.

Pyrimethamine + Antacids or Kaolin

***In vitro* data suggest that the absorption of pyrimethamine might be reduced by antacids or kaolin.**

Clinical evidence, mechanism, importance and management

In vitro studies using segments of *rat* intestine found that the absorption of pyrimethamine was decreased by the following antacids: **calcium carbonate** (32%), **gerdiga** (38%), and **magnesium trisilicate** (38%). **Gerdiga** is a clay containing hydrated silicates with sodium and potassium carbonates and bicarbonates and is similar to **attapulgite**. The study also found that **kaolin** decreased the absorption of pyrimethamine by 50%.[1]

A later *in vivo* study by the same authors, but only looking at effects on chloroquine (see 'Chloroquine and related drugs + Antacids or Kaolin', p.243), suggested that pyrimethamine might be similarly adsorbed by the antacids mentioned above and by kaolin. The authors suggest that administration should be separated by at least 4 hours to avoid reduced bioavailability.[2] However, there is no specific clinical information about an adverse interaction between pyrimethamine and antacids or kaolin, and although the UK manufacturer briefly notes the *in vitro* data, they do not suggest any precautions with concurrent use.[3]

1. McElnay JC, Mukhtar HA, D'Arcy PF, Temple DJ. *In vitro* experiments on chloroquine and pyrimethamine absorption in the presence of antacid constituents or kaolin. *J Trop Med Hyg* (1982) 85, 153–8.
2. McElnay JC, Mukhtar HA, D'Arcy PF, Temple DJ, Collier PS. The effect of magnesium trisilicate and kaolin on the *in vivo* absorption of chloroquine. *J Trop Med Hyg* (1982) 85, 159–63.
3. Daraprim (Pyrimethamine). GlaxoSmithKline UK. UK Summary of product characteristics, December 2005.

Pyrimethamine ± Sulfadoxine + Artemisinin derivatives

Artemether increases the plasma concentration of pyrimethamine. Artesunate does not appear to affect the pharmacokinetics of pyrimethamine or sulfadoxine.

Clinical evidence, mechanism, importance and management

(a) Artemether

In a crossover study, 8 healthy subjects were given a single dose of either artemether 300 mg, pyrimethamine 100 mg, or both drugs together. Although there were large inter-individual variations in the pharmacokinetics of pyrimethamine, its mean maximum plasma concentration was increased by 44%. As there was no corresponding increase in adverse effects the authors suggest that the interaction might be of benefit.[1] More study is warranted to confirm this result.

(b) Artesunate

A study in 16 healthy subjects found that artesunate (200 mg on day one then 100 mg daily for 4 days) had no effect on the pharmacokinetics of pyrimethamine with sulfadoxine 75 mg/1500 mg taken on day one. However, the pharmacokinetics of artesunate were not investigated in this study.[2] No particular dose adjustments of pyrimethamine with sulfadoxine appear to be required if artesunate is also given. Note that artesunate and pyrimethamine with sulfadoxine is one of the artemisinin-based combinations recommended by the WHO for the treatment of malaria.[3]

1. Tan-ariya P, Na-Bangchang K, Ubalee R, Thanavibul A, Thipawangkosol P, Karbwang J. Pharmacokinetic interaction or artemether and pyrimethamine in healthy male Thais. *Southeast Asian J Trop Med Public Health* (1998) 29, 18–23.
2. Minzi OMS, Gupta A, Haule AF, Kagashe GAB, Massele AY, Gustafsson LL. Lack of impact of artesunate on the disposition pharmacokinetics of sulfadoxine/pyrimethamine when the two drugs are concomitantly administered. *Eur J Clin Pharmacol* (2007) 63, 457–62.
3. World Health Organization. Guidelines for the treatment of malaria - 3rd edition. Available at: https://extranet.who.int/iris/restricted/handle/10665/162441 (accessed 21/10/15)

Pyrimethamine + Co-trimoxazole or Sulfonamides

Serious pancytopenia and megaloblastic anaemia have occasionally occurred in patients given pyrimethamine with co-trimoxazole or other sulfonamides.

Clinical evidence

A woman taking pyrimethamine 50 mg weekly as malaria prophylaxis, developed petechial haemorrhages and widespread bruising within 10 days of starting to take co-trimoxazole (trimethoprim 320 mg with sulfamethoxazole 800 mg) daily for a urinary-tract infection. She was found to have gross megaloblastic changes and pancytopenia in addition to being obviously pale and ill. After withdrawal of the two drugs she responded rapidly to hydroxocobalamin and folic acid. She was subsequently given chloroquine for malaria prophylaxis.[1]

Similar cases have been described in other patients taking pyrimethamine with co-trimoxazole,[2-4] **sulfafurazole (sulfisoxazole)**,[5] or other sulfonamides.[6]

Mechanism

Uncertain, but a reasonable surmise can be made. Pyrimethamine and **trimethoprim** are both **folate antagonists** and both selectively inhibit the actions of the enzyme dihydrofolate reductase, which leads to the eventual synthesis of the nucleic acids needed for the production of new cells. This might result in folate deficiency and the development of megaloblastic anaemia. The sulfonamides inhibit another part of the same synthetic chain. The adverse reactions seen would seem to reflect a gross reduction of the normal folate metabolism caused by the combined actions of both drugs. Megaloblastic anaemia and pancytopenia are among the adverse effects of both pyrimethamine and, more rarely, co-trimoxazole.

Importance and management

Information seems to be limited to the reports cited with a notable lack of recent information, but the interaction appears to be established although its incidence is unknown. Pyrimethamine is usually given with a sulfonamide for toxoplasmosis (**sulfadiazine**) and malaria (**sulfadoxine**). Caution should be used in prescribing these combinations, especially in the presence of other drugs, such as folate antagonists (see 'Pyrimethamine ± Sulfonamides + Miscellaneous', p.256), or disease states that can predispose to folate deficiency. Note that the US manufacturer of sulfadoxine with pyrimethamine (*Fansidar*) recommended that the concurrent use of folate antagonists, such as other sulfonamides, trimethoprim, co-trimoxazole, and some antiepileptics, should be avoided.[7] When high-dose pyrimethamine is used for the treatment of toxoplasmosis, the UK and US manufacturers recommend that all patients should receive a folate supplement, preferably calcium folinate, to reduce the risk of bone marrow depression.[8,9]

1. Fleming AF, Warrell DA, Dickmeiss H. Co-trimoxazole and the blood. *Lancet* (1974) ii, 284–5.
2. Ansdell VE, Wright SG, Hutchinson DBA. Megaloblastic anaemia associated with combined pyrimethamine and co-trimoxazole administration. *Lancet* (1976) ii, 1257.
3. Malfatti S, Piccini A. Anemia megaloblastica pancitopenica in corso di trattamento con pirimetamina, trimethoprim e sulfametossazolo. *Haematologica* (1976) 61, 349–57.
4. Borgstein A, Tozer RA. Infectious mononucleosis and megaloblastic anaemia associated with Daraprim and Bactrim. *Cent Afr J Med* (1974) 20, 185.
5. Waxman S, Herbert V. Mechanism of pyrimethamine-induced megaloblastosis in human bone marrow. *N Engl J Med* (1969) 280, 1316–19.
6. Weißbach G. Auswirkungen kombinierter Behandlung der kindlichen Toxoplasmose mit Pyrimethamin (Daraprim) und Sulfonamiden auf Blut und Knochenmark. *Z Arztl Fortbild (Berl)* (1965) 59, 10–22.
7. Fansidar (Sulfadoxine with Pyrimethamine). Roche Pharmaceuticals. US Prescribing information, August 2004.
8. Daraprim (Pyrimethamine). GlaxoSmithKline UK. UK Summary of product characteristics, December 2005.
9. Daraprim (Pyrimethamine). Amedra Pharmaceuticals. US Prescribing information, November 2010.

Pyrimethamine ± Sulfonamides + Miscellaneous

Serious pancytopenia and megaloblastic anaemia might occur in patients given pyrimethamine (with or without a sulfonamide) and other drugs that inhibit folate metabolism or cause bone marrow suppression.

Clinical evidence, mechanism, importance and management

(a) Drugs that affect folate metabolism

Pyrimethamine is known to inhibit folate metabolism, which is associated with a risk of adverse effects (in particular anaemias and pancytopenia). Pyrimethamine is usually given with a sulfonamide for toxoplasmosis (**sulfadiazine**) and malaria (**sulfadoxine**), which is known to further increase the risk of additive haematological toxicity. When **sulfadoxine** with pyrimethamine (*Fansidar*) was more widely available for the treatment of malaria, the US manufacturer recommended that the concurrent use of folate antagonists (they named other sulfonamides, **trimethoprim**, and some **antiepileptics**) should be avoided.[1] This seems a prudent precaution as adverse haematological effects have been seen with the use of pyrimethamine and sulfonamides (see 'Pyrimethamine + Co-trimoxazole or Sulfonamides', p.255) and folate deficiency is a known adverse effect of a number of antiepileptics (see 'Antiepileptics + Folinates', p.564). Other drugs known to be folate antagonists include **proguanil**, **methotrexate**, and **pemetrexed**, but note that methotrexate and pemetrexed are often given with folate supplements to limit their toxicity.

If the concurrent use of pyrimethamine and a drug that inhibits folate metabolism cannot be avoided, it would seem prudent to consider the use of a folate supplement, preferably folinic acid. This is recommended for all patients with toxoplasmosis taking high-dose pyrimethamine, to reduce the risk of bone marrow suppression.[2,3]

(b) Drugs that cause bone marrow suppression

The UK manufacturer of pyrimethamine briefly notes that cases of fatal bone marrow aplasia have been reported with the concurrent use of **daunorubicin**, **cytarabine**, and pyrimethamine in patients with acute myeloid leukaemia. They also warn of the additive risk if pyrimethamine is given with agents associated with myelosuppression.[2]

1. Fansidar (Sulfadoxine with Pyrimethamine). Roche Pharmaceuticals. US Prescribing information, August 2004.
2. Daraprim (Pyrimethamine). GlaxoSmithKline UK. UK Summary of product characteristics, December 2005.
3. Daraprim (Pyrimethamine). Amedra Pharmaceuticals. US Prescribing information, November 2010.

Pyrimethamine ± Sulfadoxine + Zidovudine

Pyrimethamine does not appear to alter zidovudine pharmacokinetics, and zidovudine does not appear to alter the prophylactic efficacy of pyrimethamine with sulfadoxine for toxoplasmosis. However, the combination of pyrimethamine and zidovudine might increase the risk of myelosuppression.

Clinical evidence, mechanism, importance and management

The addition of pyrimethamine (200 mg loading dose then 50 mg daily) and folinic acid 10 mg daily to zidovudine had no effect on zidovudine pharmacokinetics, based on data from 10 HIV-positive patients for whom zidovudine pharmacokinetics were available before, and after, starting pyrimethamine. Of 26 patients receiving the combination, 5 developed leucopenia and one discontinued treatment because of anaemia.[1]

A study in patients with AIDS found that zidovudine 250 mg four times daily did not adversely affect prophylaxis of toxoplasma encephalitis using pyrimethamine with sulfadoxine (*Fansidar*), one tablet twice weekly for up to 8 months.[2] *In vitro* and *animal* data have shown that the combination of zidovudine and pyrimethamine caused synergistic decreases in lymphocyte and neutrophil numbers.[3]

The UK and US manufacturers of pyrimethamine note that the concurrent use of zidovudine might increase the risk of bone marrow depression.[4,5] They state that if signs of folate deficiency develop, then pyrimethamine should be discontinued and folinic acid given. Note that the prophylactic use of a folate supplement, preferably folinic acid, is recommended for all patients with toxoplasmosis taking high-dose pyrimethamine, to reduce the risk of bone marrow suppression.[4,5]

1. Jacobson JM, Davidian M, Rainey PM, Hafner R, Raasch RH, Luft BJ. Pyrimethamine pharmacokinetics in human immunodeficiency virus-positive patients seropositive for *Toxoplasma gondii*. *Antimicrob Agents Chemother* (1996) 40, 1360–5.
2. Eljaschewitsch J, Schürmann D, Pohle HD, Ruf B. Zidovudine does not antagonize Fansidar in preventing toxoplasma encephalitis in HIV infected patients. 7th International Conference on AIDS; Science Challenging AIDS, Florence, Italy, 1991. Abstract W.B.2334.
3. Freund YR, Dabbs J, Creek MR, Phillips SJ, Tyson CA, MacGregor JT. Synergistic bone marrow toxicity of pyrimethamine and zidovudine in murine *in vivo* and *in vitro* models: mechanism of toxicity. *Toxicol Appl Pharmacol* (2002) 181, 16–26.
4. Daraprim (Pyrimethamine). GlaxoSmithKline UK. UK Summary of product characteristics, December 2005.
5. Daraprim (Pyrimethamine). Amedra Pharmaceuticals. US Prescribing information, November 2010.

Quinine + Artemisinin derivatives

No pharmacokinetic interaction appears to occur between quinine and artemether with lumefantrine or artemether alone. Quinine-induced QTc prolongation might be enhanced by artemether.

Clinical evidence

(a) Artemether

A crossover study in 8 healthy subjects found that the pharmacokinetics of single oral doses of artemether 300 mg and quinine 600 mg were not affected by concurrent use. No serious adverse effects were reported and no notable changes in ECG measurements were seen.[1]

(b) Artemether with Lumefantrine

In a placebo-controlled study in healthy subjects, 6 doses of artemether with lumefantrine 80 mg/480 mg were given to 14 subjects over a period of 60 hours, followed 2 hours after the last dose by intravenous quinine 10 mg/kg (to a maximum of 600 mg) over 2 hours. Two other groups, each with 14 subjects, received quinine or artemether with lumefantrine and placebo. The pharmacokinetics of lumefantrine and quinine were unaffected by concurrent use but the AUC and plasma concentration of artemether and its active metabolite, dihydroartemisinin, appeared to be lower when artemether with lumefantrine was given with quinine. However, the plasma concentration of artemether before quinine use in this group was also lower, and this reduction in plasma concentration in the presence of quinine was not considered clinically relevant. The transient prolongation of the QTc interval noted with quinine (average and maximum increases of 3 milliseconds and 6 milliseconds, respectively) was slightly greater when quinine was given after artemether with lumefantrine (average and maximum increases 7 milliseconds and 15 milliseconds, respectively).[2]

Mechanism

Both quinine and artemether are known to prolong the QT interval. Concurrent use might therefore result in additive effects.

Importance and management

In general, it is advised that the concurrent use of two or more drugs that prolong the QT interval should be avoided (see also 'Drugs that prolong the QT interval + Other drugs that prolong the QT interval', p.272). However, the authors of this study considered that the modest increased risk of QTc prolongation was outweighed by the potential benefit of the combined treatment in complicated or multidrug-resistant falciparum malaria.[2] The UK manufacturer of artemether with lumefantrine recommends close cardiac monitoring if it is given after quinine.[3]

1. Na-Bangchang K, Karbwang J, Ubalee R, Thanavibul A, Saenglertsilapachai S. Absence of significant pharmacokinetic and pharmacodynamic interactions between artemether and quinoline antimalarials. *Eur J Drug Metab Pharmacokinet* (2000) 25 171–8.
2. Lefèvre G, Carpenter P, Souppart C, Schmidli H, Martin JM, Lane A, Ward C, Amakye D. Interaction trial between artemether-lumefantrine (Riamet®) and quinine in healthy subjects. *J Clin Pharmacol* (2002) 42, 1147–58.
3. Riamet (Artemether with Lumefantrine). Novartis Pharmaceuticals UK Ltd. UK Summary of product characteristics, October 2011.

Quinine + Colestyramine

A single-dose study suggests that colestyramine might not alter the pharmacokinetics of quinine.

Clinical evidence, mechanism, importance and management

In a study in 8 healthy subjects, colestyramine 8 g did not alter the pharmacokinetics of quinine 600 mg. The authors warn that this lack of interaction might have been because only single doses were used, and suggest that continuing to separate the administration of the two drugs until a lack of interaction is demonstrated in a multiple dose study.[1] It is usually recommended that other drugs are taken one hour before, or 4 to 6 hours after, colestyramine.

1. Ridtitid W, Wongnawa M, Kleekaew A, Mahatthanatrakul W, Sunbhanich M. Cholestyramine does not significantly decrease the bioavailability of quinine in healthy volunteers. *Asia Pac J Pharmacol* (1998) 13, 123–7.

Quinine + Fluvoxamine

Fluvoxamine has no effect on the pharmacokinetics of quinine.

Clinical evidence, mechanism, importance and management

In a study in healthy subjects, fluvoxamine 25 mg was given both 12 hours and one hour before a single 500-mg dose of quinine hydrochloride, followed by a further 4 doses of fluvoxamine, given every 12 hours.[1] Fluvoxamine had no effect on the apparent oral clearance of quinine and caused a minor 6% increase in the AUC of 3-hydroxyquinine, with no effect on the AUC of various other metabolites.[1,2]

Fluvoxamine is a known inhibitor of CYP1A2 and to some extent CYP2C19, and it appears that this has little effect on the pharmacokinetics of quinine. No quinine dose adjustments are necessary with concurrent use of fluvoxamine.

1. Mirghani RA, Helllgren U, Westerberg PA, Ericsson O, Bertilsson L, Gustafsson LL. The roles of cytochrome P450 3A4 and 1A2 in the 3-hydroxylation of quinine in vivo. *Clin Pharmacol Ther* (1999) 66, 454–60.
2. Mirghani RA, Hellgren U, Bertilsson L, Gustafsson LL, Ericsson Ö. Metabolism and elimination of quinine in healthy volunteers. *Eur J Clin Pharmacol* (2003) 59, 423–7.

Quinine + Food

A study in 7 healthy subjects found that neither a low- nor a high-salt diet affected the pharmacokinetics of a single 600-mg dose of quinine sulfate.[1]

1. Newton P, Simpson A, Wanwimolruk S, Maliakal P, Villegas L, Kuypers D, White NJ. Oral quinine pharmacokinetics and dietary salt intake. *Eur J Clin Pharmacol* (2001) 57, 111–13.

Quinine + Grapefruit juice

Grapefruit juice had no effect on the pharmacokinetics of quinine in healthy subjects. An isolated case of torsade de pointes has been reported following the excessive intake of grapefruit juice and quinine-containing tonic water in a patient with a history of long QT syndrome.

Clinical evidence, mechanism, importance and management

In a study in 10 healthy subjects, 200 mL of full-strength grapefruit juice, half-strength grapefruit juice, or orange juice was given twice daily for 11 doses, with a single 600-mg dose of quinine sulfate given on day 6, with the last dose of fruit juice. There were no differences in the pharmacokinetics of quinine between the three groups although the maximum plasma concentration of the 3-hydroxymetabolite of quinine was reduced (by 19%) with full-strength grapefruit juice, when compared with orange juice or half-strength grapefruit juice.[1]

An isolated report describes a diabetic patient with a history of long QT syndrome who was found to have torsade de pointes after admission to hospital with polydipsia. It was discovered that, because of the polydipsia, she had been drinking excessive quantities of grapefruit juice and quinine-containing tonic water. Two days after discontinuing these drinks the torsade de pointes resolved.[2]

Grapefruit juice is a known inhibitor of intestinal CYP3A4 and it appears that this has little effect on the pharmacokinetics of quinine in healthy subjects. It would seem that, in general, patients taking quinine can safely drink grapefruit juice.[1] Although, the case report introduces an element of caution, it should be noted that its clinical relevance is unclear because the patient did not take quinine without grapefruit juice and so the arrhythmia might have been caused by the use of quinine in a patient with long QT syndrome, rather than an interaction.

1. Ho PC, Chalcroft SC, Coville PF, Wanwimolruk S. Grapefruit juice has no effect on quinine pharmacokinetics. *Eur J Clin Pharmacol* (1999) 55, 393–8.
2. Hermans K, Stockman D, Van den Branden F. Grapefruit and tonic: A deadly combination in a patient with the long QT syndrome. *Am J Med* (2003) 114, 511–12.

Quinine + H_2-receptor antagonists

The clearance of quinine is reduced by cimetidine, but not ranitidine.

Clinical evidence, mechanism, importance and management

In a crossover study in 6 healthy subjects, pretreatment with **cimetidine** 200 mg three times daily and 400 mg at night for one week reduced the oral clearance of a single 600-mg dose of quinine sulfate by 27%, increased its half-life from 7.6 hours to 11.3 hours, and increased its AUC by 42%. The maximum plasma concentration of quinine was unchanged. No interaction was seen when **cimetidine** was replaced by **ranitidine** 150 mg twice daily.[1] The probable reason for this effect is that **cimetidine** (a recognised non-specific enzyme inhibitor) reduces the hepatic metabolism of quinine by CYP3A4, which is responsible for the metabolism of quinine to its major metabolite, 3-hydroxyquinine. **Ranitidine** does not inhibit hepatic enzymes and therefore does not interact. It therefore seems likely that other H_2-receptor antagonists (that also lack enzyme-inhibitory effects) will not interact, although this needs confirmation.

The clinical importance of the slight interaction between cimetidine and quinine is uncertain, but be alert for any evidence of quinine adverse effects if cimetidine is also given. Ranitidine might be a suitable alternative.

1. Wanwimolruk S, Sunbhanich M, Pongmarutai M and Patamasucon P. Effects of cimetidine and ranitidine on the pharmacokinetics of quinine. *Br J Clin Pharmacol* (1986) 22, 346–50.

Quinine + HIV-protease inhibitors

Ritonavir moderately increases the exposure to quinine, whereas quinine has only very slight effects on ritonavir pharmacokinetics. Lopinavir boosted with ritonavir moderately reduces the exposure to quinine.

Clinical evidence

(a) Lopinavir

In a pharmacokinetic study, 12 healthy subjects were given a single 648-mg dose of quinine sulfate, before and after 22 doses of lopinavir boosted with ritonavir 400/100 mg twice daily for a total of 27 doses. Lopinavir boosted with ritonavir reduced the AUC of quinine by 50% and reduced its maximum plasma concentration by 48%. Similarly, the AUC and maximum plasma concentration of the active metabolite of quinine, 3-hydroxyquinine, were both reduced by 69%.[1]

(b) Ritonavir

In a pharmacokinetic study, 10 healthy subjects were given ritonavir 200 mg twice daily for 9 days, with a single 600-mg dose of quinine sulfate on day 8. Ritonavir increased the AUC and maximum plasma concentration of quinine 4.4-fold and 3.8-fold, respectively. Quinine modestly affected the pharmacokinetics of ritonavir, increasing its AUC and maximum plasma concentration by 21% and 15%, respectively.[2]

Mechanism

Ritonavir is a known, potent inhibitor of CYP3A4 by which quinine is metabolised. Concurrent use therefore decreases quinine metabolism, resulting in the increases in exposure seen. However, when lopinavir is also present, and ritonavir is given at a lower dose, quinine exposure is reduced. This might be because other mechanisms, such as glucuronidation, become more relevant and outweigh CYP3A4 inhibition.

The very slight effects of quinine on ritonavir metabolism were thought to be mostly due to an effect on its metabolism by CYP2D6,[2] although this remains to be determined as ritonavir is not known to be affected by recognised inhibitors of CYP2D6 to a clinically relevant extent (see 'SSRIs + HIV-protease inhibitors', p.1487).

Importance and management

Information regarding an interaction between ritonavir and quinine appears to be limited to two single-dose studies, one involving ritonavir alone and one involving lopinavir boosted with ritonavir. The findings with ritonavir alone are consistent with the way ritonavir is known to interact with other substrates of CYP3A4. The clinical importance of this interaction was not evaluated in the study; however, the exposure to quinine was moderately increased and this might lead to an increase in adverse effects. This is of particular importance because high-dose quinine can affect the QT interval, see 'Drugs that prolong the QT interval + Other drugs that prolong the QT interval', p.272. It might therefore be prudent to avoid concurrent use, although the risks will be lower with smaller doses of quinine, such as those used for leg cramps. If concurrent use is essential, patients should be monitored closely, being alert for an increase in quinine adverse effects (e.g. tinnitus, headache, vomiting, vertigo, or cardiac disorders). Reduce the dose of quinine as necessary.

The findings with lopinavir boosted with ritonavir are in contrast, and suggest that a reduction in the effects of quinine might occur. In this situation it would seem prudent to closely monitor quinine efficacy, adjusting treatment as necessary if quinine appears ineffective.

There appears to be no evidence regarding other HIV-protease inhibitors. Until more is known it would seem prudent to avoid the concurrent use of any HIV-protease inhibitor and quinine. If this is not possible, monitor the outcome of concurrent use carefully, for both a potential decrease in quinine efficacy and a potential increase in quinine toxicity.

1. Nyunt MM, Lu Y, Yu Q, El-Gasim M, Parsons TL, Petty BG, Hendrix CW. Effects of ritonavir-boosted lopinavir on the pharmacokinetics of quinine. *Clin Pharmacol Ther* (2012) 91, 889–95.
2. Soyinka JO, Onyeji CO, Omoruyi SI, Owalabi AR, Sarma PV, Cook JM. Pharmacokinetics interactions between ritonavir and quinine in healthy volunteers following concurrent administration. *Br J Clin Pharmacol* (2010) 69, 262–70.

Quinine + Isoniazid

In one small study, isoniazid did not affect the pharmacokinetics of quinine.

Clinical evidence, mechanism, importance and management

A study in 9 healthy subjects found that the pharmacokinetics of a single 600-mg dose of quinine sulfate were not affected by pretreatment with isoniazid 300 mg daily for one week, with the exception of the half-life, which was increased (from 11.1 hours to 14.2 hours).[1] No additional precautions would seem necessary if quinine is given with isoniazid; however, bear in mind that isoniazid is usually used in combination with rifampicin, which might reduce the efficacy of quinine (see 'Quinine + Rifampicin (Rifampin)', p.258).

1. Wanwimolruk S, Kang W, Coville PF, Viriyayudhakorn S, Thitiarchakul S. Marked enhancement by rifampicin and lack of effect of isoniazid on the elimination of quinine in man. *Br J Clin Pharmacol* (1995) 40, 87–91.

Quinine + Ketoconazole

Ketoconazole slightly decreases the clearance of quinine.

Clinical evidence, mechanism, importance and management

In a crossover study in healthy subjects, ketoconazole 100 mg twice daily was given for 3 days with a single 500-mg dose of quinine hydrochloride one hour after the second dose of ketoconazole. Ketoconazole decreased the apparent oral clearance of quinine by 31% and decreased the AUC of its major metabolite, 3-hydroxyquinine, by 30%,[1] with increases in the AUCs of various other metabolites.[2]

Ketoconazole inhibits CYP3A4, which is responsible for the metabolism of quinine to 3-hydroxyquinine. CYP3A5 might possibly also play some part.[3] This pharmacokinetic interaction would appear to be established, but of unknown clinical relevance. The slight decrease in exposure to 3-hydroxyquinine seen is probably unlikely to be of much importance.

1. Mirghani RA, Helllgren U, Westerberg PA, Ericsson O, Bertilsson L, Gustafsson LL. The roles of cytochrome P450 3A4 and 1A2 in the 3-hydroxylation of quinine in vivo. *Clin Pharmacol Ther* (1999) 66, 454–60.
2. Mirghani RA, Hellgren U, Bertilsson L, Gustafsson LL, Ericsson Ö. Metabolism and elimination of quinine in healthy volunteers. *Eur J Clin Pharmacol* (2003) 59, 423–7.
3. Allqvist A, Miura J, Bertilsson L, Mirghani RA. Inhibition of CYP3A4 and CYP3A5 catalyzed metabolism of alprazolam and quinine by ketoconazole as racemate and four different enantiomers. *Eur J Clin Pharmacol* (2007) 63, 173–9.

Quinine + Miscellaneous

Urinary alkalinisers can reduce the urinary excretion of quinine in man, and antacids can reduce the absorption of quinine in *animals*.

Clinical evidence, mechanism, importance and management

(a) Antacids

Aluminium/magnesium hydroxide gel reduces the absorption of quinine from the gut of *rats* and reduces the blood concentration of quinine by 50 to 70%.[1] This appears to occur because **aluminium hydroxide** slows gastric emptying and **magnesium hydroxide** forms an insoluble precipitate with quinine, both of which reduce quinine absorption. However, there seem to be no clinical reports of a reduction in the therapeutic effectiveness of quinine due to the concurrent use of antacids.

(b) Urinary alkalinisers

The excretion of unchanged quinine is virtually halved (from 17.4% to 8.9%) if the urine is alkalinised. This is because, in alkaline urine, more of the quinine exists in the non-ionised (lipid soluble) form, which is more easily reabsorbed by the kidney tubules.[2] However, there seem to be no reports of adverse effects arising from changes in excretion due to this interaction and no special precautions seem to be necessary.

1. Hurwitz A. The effects of antacids on gastrointestinal drug absorption. II. Effect of sulfadiazine and quinine. *J Pharmacol Exp Ther* (1971) 179, 485–9.
2. Haag HB, Larson PS, Schwartz JJ. The effect of urinary pH on the elimination of quinine in man. *J Pharmacol Exp Ther* (1943) 79, 136–9.

Quinine + Nevirapine

The exposure to quinine is decreased, and the plasma concentration of 3-hydroxyquinine, the major metabolite of quinine, is increased, by nevirapine.

Clinical evidence, mechanism, importance and management

A crossover study in 14 healthy subjects given a single 600-mg oral dose of quinine sulfate, found that pretreatment with nevirapine 200 mg twice daily for 8 days reduced the AUC, maximum plasma concentration, and half-life of quinine by 33%, 36%, and 25% respectively. The oral clearance of quinine was increased by 50%. In addition, the AUC and maximum plasma concentration of 3-hydroxyquinine, the major metabolite of quinine, were increased by 25% and 31%, respectively.[1]

Nevirapine induces CYP3A4, which is responsible for the formation of 3-hydroxyquinine from quinine. The clinical importance of the changes in quinine pharmacokinetics seen is unclear, but the reduced exposure to quinine and the increased plasma concentration of 3-hydroxyquine suggest that reduced efficacy and possibly increased toxicity (the metabolite is reported to be more toxic than quinine[1]) could result. Monitor for an increase in quinine adverse effects (such as tinnitus, headache, vomiting, vertigo, or cardiac disorders) and quinine efficacy, increasing the dose of quinine, if appropriate.

1. Soyinka JO, Onyeji CO, Omoruyi SI, Owolabi AR, Sarma PV, Cook JM. Effects of concurrent administration of nevirapine on the disposition of quinine in healthy volunteers. *J Pharm Pharmacol* (2009) 61, 439–43.

Quinine + Rifampicin (Rifampin)

Rifampicin induces the metabolism of quinine.

Clinical evidence

A study in 9 healthy subjects found that the clearance of a single 600-mg dose of quinine sulfate was increased more than 6-fold by pretreatment with rifampicin 600 mg daily for 2 weeks. The elimination half-life of quinine was decreased from about 11 hours to 5.5 hours.[1] In another study in patients with uncomplicated falciparum malaria, quinine sulfate 10 mg/kg three times daily was given either alone (30 patients) or with rifampicin 15 mg/kg daily (29 patients) for 7 days. Maximum plasma concentrations of quinine during monotherapy were attained within 2 days of treatment and remained within the therapeutic range for the 7-day treatment period. Plasma concentrations of the main metabolite of quinine, 3-hydroxyquinine, followed a similar pattern. In patients taking quinine with rifampicin, quinine was more extensively metabolised and, after the second day of treatment, the plasma concentration of quinine was sharply reduced to below therapeutic concentrations. Although patients who received rifampicin with quinine had shorter parasite clearance times than those who received quinine alone (suggesting rifampicin might enhance the antimalarial activity of quinine), recrudescence rates (the reappearance of the disease after a period of inactivity) were 5 times higher suggesting increased resistance to quinine treatment.[2]

A report describes a patient with myotonia, controlled with quinine, whose symptoms worsened within 3 weeks of starting to take rifampicin for the treatment of tuberculosis. The maximum plasma concentration of quinine was found to be low, but rose again when the rifampicin was stopped. Control of the myotonia was regained 6 weeks later.[3]

Mechanism

Acute malaria reduces the metabolic clearance of quinine (mainly by a reduction in hepatic CYP3A4 activity) and recovery from malaria is associated with a sharp decline in the plasma concentration of quinine. Rifampicin induces the cytochrome P450 isoenzymes and this probably antagonised their inhibition by acute malaria, resulting in increased quinine metabolism.

Importance and management

Although there is limited evidence, an interaction between rifampicin and quinine would appear to be of clinical importance. The authors of one of the studies[2] suggest that rifampicin should not be given with quinine for the treatment of malaria. Increased quinine doses should be considered if the concurrent use of rifampicin is considered essential.

1. Wanwimolruk S, Kang W, Coville PF, Viriyayudhakorn S, Thitiarchakul S. Marked enhancement by rifampicin and lack of effect of isoniazid on the elimination of quinine in man. *Br J Clin Pharmacol* (1995) 40, 87–91.
2. Pukrittayakamee S, Prakongpan S, Wanwimolruk S, Clemens R, Looareesuwan S, White NJ. Adverse effect of rifampin on quinine efficacy in uncomplicated falciparum malaria. *Antimicrob Agents Chemother* (2003) 47, 1509–13.
3. Osborn JE, Pettit MJ, Graham P. Interaction between rifampicin and quinine: case report. *Pharm J* (1989) 243, 704.

Quinine + Tetracyclines

Doxycycline does not appear to alter the pharmacokinetics of quinine. Tetracycline increases the plasma concentration of quinine.

Clinical evidence, mechanism, importance and management

(a) Doxycycline

In a study in 13 patients with acute falciparum malaria, giving intravenous doxycycline with intravenous quinine did not affect the pharmacokinetics of quinine, when compared with 13 patients taking quinine alone.[1] In contrast, *in vitro*, doxycycline appears to be a potent inhibitor of quinine metabolism.[2] However, given the evidence from the study, no special precautions would seem to be necessary on concurrent use and the combination is one of the second line treatments recommended in the WHO guidelines for the treatment of uncomplicated falciparum malaria.[3]

(b) Tetracycline

A study in patients with acute falciparum malaria given quinine sulfate 600 mg every 8 hours, found that the plasma concentration of quinine was about doubled by the concurrent use of tetracycline 250 mg every 6 hours, when compared with quinine alone. The plasma concentration of quinine was above the MIC for malaria when tetracycline was also given but not with quinine alone. Two of 8 patients treated with quinine alone had malaria recrudescence (the reappearance of the disease after a period of inactivity) compared with none of 8 patients receiving the combination.[4] *In vitro*, tetracycline is also a potent inhibitor of quinine metabolism.[2] The authors considered that this pharmacokinetic interaction might be part of the explanation why the combination of quinine and tetracycline has been found to be more effective than quinine alone.[4] Quinine with tetracycline is one of the second line combinations recommended by the WHO for the treatment of uncomplicated falciparum malaria.[3]

1. Couet W, Laroche R, Floch JJ, Istin B, Fourtillan JB, Sauniere JF. Pharmacokinetics of quinine and doxycycline in patients with acute falciparum malaria: a study in Africa. *Ther Drug Monit* (1991) 13, 496–501.
2. Zhao X-J, Ishizaki T. A further interaction study of quinine with clinically important drugs by human liver microsomes: determinations of inhibition constant (K_i) and type of inhibition. *Eur J Drug Metab Pharmacokinet* (1999) 24, 272–8.
3. World Health Organization. Guidelines for the treatment of malaria -3rd edition. Available at: https://extranet.who.int/iris/restricted/bitstream/10665/162441/1/9789241549127_eng.pdf (accessed 21/10/15).
4. Karbwang J, Molunto P, Bunnag D, Harinasuta T. Plasma quinine levels in patients with falciparum malaria given alone or in combination with tetracycline with or without primaquine. *Southeast Asian J Trop Med Public Health* (1991) 22, 72–6.

Quinine + Tobacco

Quinine pharmacokinetics and efficacy were unchanged by smoking in one study. In contrast, in another study, otherwise healthy smokers

appeared to clear quinine from the body much more quickly than non-smokers.

Clinical evidence

A comparative study found that in 10 smokers (averaging 17 cigarettes daily) the AUC of a single 600-mg dose of quinine sulfate was 44% lower, the clearance was 77% higher, and the half-life was shorter (7.5 hours and 12 hours, respectively), when compared with 10 non-smokers.[1] In contrast, in a study in patients with uncomplicated falciparum malaria taking quinine sulfate 10 mg/kg three times daily for 7 days, there was no notable difference in fever clearance time, parasite clearance time, and cure rate between 10 regular smokers and 12 non-smokers. In addition pharmacokinetic parameters did not differ between the smokers and non-smokers.[2]

Mechanism

Tobacco smoke contains polycyclic aromatic compounds, and other substances, which are potent inducers of the liver enzymes that metabolise quinine. It is not yet clear which cytochrome P450 isoenzymes are affected. Smoking induces the CYP1A subfamily, but the formation of the major metabolite of quinine, 3-hydroxyquinine, is catalysed by the CYP3A subfamily which suggests that other metabolic pathways of quinine are affected by smoking.[3]

Importance and management

Information about an interaction between tobacco smoking and quinine seems to be limited but the pharmacokinetic interaction would appear to be established in healthy subjects. However, the clinical study in patients with falciparum malaria suggests that any pharmacokinetic differences are more limited (probably due to the additional effect the disease has on quinine metabolism) and that smoking status does not appear to affect the clinical outcome of quinine treatment for malaria. The systemic clearance of quinine in acute falciparum malaria might be reduced by up to two-thirds, when compared with healthy subjects, as malaria reduces hepatic microsomal enzyme activity. The authors state that this reduction in the clearance of quinine outweighs the possible effects of smoking-induced clearance.[2]

1. Wanwimolruk S, Wong SM, Coville PF, Viriyayudhakorn S, Thitiarchakul S. Cigarette smoking enhances the elimination of quinine. *Br J Clin Pharmacol* (1993) 36, 610–14.
2. Pukrittayakamee S, Pitisuttithum P, Zhang H, Jantra A, Wanwimolruk S, White NJ. Effects of cigarette smoking on quinine pharmacokinetics in malaria. *Eur J Clin Pharmacol* (2002) 58, 315–19.
3. Wanwimolruk S, Wong S-M, Zhang H, Coville PF, Walker RJ. Metabolism of quinine in man: identification of a major metabolite, and effects of smoking and rifampicin pretreatment. *J Pharm Pharmacol* (1995) 47, 957–63.

Sodium stibogluconate + Amphotericin B

The use of amphotericin B shortly after sodium stibogluconate increases the risk of fatal cardiac disorders.

Clinical evidence, mechanism, importance and management

A study in patients with ECG changes following the use of sodium stibogluconate 20 mg/kg (to a maximum of 800 mg) for leishmaniasis was stopped early when, 3 of 7 patients recruited to group A (who had been given amphotericin B shortly after sodium stibogluconate) developed cardiac disorders (resulting in two deaths and one cardiac arrest), whilst those in group B (who received amphotericin 10 days after sodium stibogluconate, when any ECG changes had stabilised) did not develop cardiac disorders.[1] Subsequently, all of the remaining 18 patients in the study were given amphotericin B 10 days after sodium stibogluconate, without cardiac disorders.[1]

A series of three case studies also describes the development of arrhythmia and sudden cardiac death in paediatric patients with visceral leishmaniasis given amphotericin up to 15 days after sodium stibogluconate.[2]

The authors of the case series suggested that sodium stibogluconate might increase myocardial sensitivity to the effects of amphotericin B and recommend a 14-day rest period between treatments, which should be extended if ECG changes persist.[2] The same advice is given by the UK manufacturer of sodium stibogluconate, who also state that electrolyte imbalances should be corrected before amphotericin B is started.[3]

1. Thakur CP. Sodium antimony gluconate, amphotericin and myocardial damage. *Lancet* (1998) 351, 1928–9.
2. Maheshwari A, Seth A, Kaur A, Aneja S, Rath B Basu S, Patel R, Dutta AK. Cumulative cardiac toxicity of sodium stibogluconate and amphotericin B in treatment of Kala-azar. *Pediatr Infect Dis J* (2011) 30, 180–1.
3. Pentostam (Sodium stibogluconate). GlaxoSmithKline UK. UK Summary of product information, June 2012.

Terbinafine + Fluconazole

A single dose of fluconazole slightly increased terbinafine exposure in one study.

Clinical evidence, mechanism, importance and management

The US manufacturer of terbinafine briefly notes that, in a single-dose study, fluconazole 100 mg slightly increased the AUC of terbinafine by 69%. They consider that inhibition of both CYP2C9 and CYP3A4 is the reason for this effect.[1] However, note that single-dose simultaneous administration does not guarantee maximal inhibition of these isoenzymes, and a study using multiple dose fluconazole would be more conclusive.

The magnitude of the change in terbinafine exposure seen is unlikely to be clinically important, suggesting that single doses of fluconazole can be used with terbinafine without any particular precautions. For multiple doses and higher doses of fluconazole, some caution might be warranted because it is not possible to rule out a larger increase in exposure. The UK and US manufacturers of terbinafine state that caution is warranted on the concurrent use of other drugs that inhibit both CYP2C9 and CYP3A4, and they name **ketoconazole** and **amiodarone** as examples.[1,2] However, note that ketoconazole is not known to be an inhibitor of CYP2C9.

1. Lamisil Tablets (Terbinafine hydrochloride). Novartis. US Prescribing information, April 2012.
2. Lamisil Tablets (Terbinafine hydrochloride). Novartis Pharmaceuticals UK, Ltd. UK Summary of product characteristics, March 2012.

Terbinafine + H_2-receptor antagonists

Cimetidine slightly increases the exposure to terbinafine. Limited evidence suggests that ranitidine does not interact with terbinafine.

Clinical evidence, mechanism, importance and management

In a study in 12 healthy subjects **cimetidine** 400 mg twice daily for 5 days increased the AUC of a single 250-mg dose of terbinafine by 34% and reduced its clearance by 30%.[1] The likely reason is that **cimetidine** (a known non-specific enzyme inhibitor) reduces the metabolism of terbinafine by the liver. However, it seems that this slight increase in the exposure to terbinafine is of little or no clinical relevance. This is supported by a large scale post-marketing survey of patients taking terbinafine that found no interactions were reported in patients also taking **cimetidine** or **ranitidine** (number unknown).[2] The UK manufacturer of terbinafine recommends that the dose of terbinafine might need adjusting (presumably reduced) if drugs that inhibit cytochrome P450 are given,[3] but the evidence available suggests that this will not be necessary with cimetidine. Evidence regarding an interaction with other H_2-receptor antagonists is lacking, but there seems to be no reason to suspect that they will interact.

1. Jensen JC. Pharmacokinetics of Lamisil® in humans. *J Dermatol Treat* (1990) 1 (Suppl 2), 15–18.
2. Hall M, Monka C, Krupp P, O'Sullivan D. Safety of oral terbinafine. Results of a postmarketing surveillance study in 25 884 patients. *Arch Dermatol* (1997) 133, 1213–19.
3. Lamisil Tablets (Terbinafine hydrochloride). Novartis Pharmaceuticals UK Ltd. UK Summary of product characteristics, March 2012.

Terbinafine + Miscellaneous

Terbinafine might raise the plasma concentration of drugs that are substrates of CYP2D6, such as a number of beta blockers and some antiarrhythmics.

Clinical evidence, mechanism, importance and management

In vitro studies, and studies in healthy subjects using **dextromethorphan** as a probe substrate, suggest that terbinafine is a clinically relevant inhibitor of CYP2D6. It might therefore be expected to increase the plasma concentrations of other drugs that are substrates of this isoenzyme. The UK and US manufacturers[1,2] specifically mention this applies to certain members (none stated) of the following drug classes: tricyclic antidepressants, SSRIs, **beta blockers**, **antiarrhythmics** (including class Ia, Ib, and Ic), and **MAO-B inhibitors**.

Of these predictions, the tricyclic, desipramine, has been seen to interact markedly (see 'Tricyclic antidepressants + Terbinafine', p.1517) and the SSRI, paroxetine, has been seen to interact moderately (see 'SSRIs + Terbinafine', p.1496). For examples of **beta blockers** that are substrates of CYP2D6 and would be expected to interact, see 'Table 22.1', p.999.

The **antiarrhythmics** that are known to be clinically relevant CYP2D6 substrates and which would be expected to interact are **flecainide**, **mexiletine**, and **propafenone**.

There appear to be no reported interactions between **selegiline** or **rasagiline** and CYP2D6 inhibitors, so the clinical relevance of this prediction is unclear.

Until more is known it would seem wise to be aware of the possibility of an increase in adverse effects if any of these drugs is given with terbinafine and consider a dose reduction, if necessary. See 'Table 1.7', p.9, for a list of drugs that are known to be clinically relevant substrates of CYP2D6.

1. Lamisil Tablets (Terbinafine hydrochloride). Novartis Pharmaceuticals UK Ltd. UK Summary of product characteristics, March 2012.
2. Lamisil Tablets (Terbinafine hydrochloride). Novartis. US Prescribing information, April 2012.

Terbinafine + Rifampicin (Rifampin)

The exposure to terbinafine is reduced by rifampicin.

Clinical evidence, mechanism, importance and management

A study in 12 healthy subjects found that rifampicin 600 mg daily for 6 days halved the AUC of terbinafine and roughly doubled its clearance.[1] Rifampicin is a known enzyme inducer, which increases the metabolism of many drugs. Be alert, therefore, for the need to increase the dose of terbinafine if rifampicin is given.

1. Jensen JC. Pharmacokinetics of Lamisil® in humans. *J Dermatol Treat* (1990) 1 (Suppl 2), 15–18.

9

Antiarrhythmics

This section is mainly concerned with the class I antiarrhythmics, which also possess some local anaesthetic properties, and with class III antiarrhythmics. Antiarrhythmics that fall into other classes are dealt with elsewhere, see 'Beta blockers', p.999, 'Digitalis glycosides', p.1077, and 'Calcium-channel blockers', p.1029. Some antiarrhythmics that do not fit into the Vaughan Williams classification (see 'Table 9.1', below) are also included here, for example adenosine. This section is generally concerned with those drugs that affect the activity of antiarrhythmic drugs. Where the antiarrhythmic is the affecting drug, the interaction is dealt with elsewhere.

(a) Predicting interactions between two antiarrhythmics

It is difficult to know exactly what is likely to happen if two antiarrhythmics are used together. The hope is always that a combination will work better than just one drug, and many studies have confirmed that hope, but sometimes the combinations are unsafe. Predicting unsafe combinations is difficult, but there are some very broad general rules that can be applied if the general pharmacology of the drugs is understood.

If drugs with similar effects are used together, whether they act on the myocardium itself or on the conducting tissues, the total effect is likely to be increased (additive). The classification of the antiarrhythmics in 'Table 9.1', below, helps to predict what is likely to happen, but remember that the classification is not rigid, and therefore drugs in one class can share some characteristics with others. The following sections deal with some examples.

1. Combinations of antiarrhythmics from the same class. The drugs in class Ia can prolong the QT interval; combining drugs from this class would be expected to have an increased effect on the QT interval. This prolongation carries the risk of causing torsade de pointes (see 'Drugs that prolong the QT interval + Other drugs that prolong the QT interval', p.272). It would also be expected that the negative inotropic effects of quinidine would be additive with procainamide or any of the other drugs within class Ia. Therefore, for safety, it is sometimes considered best to avoid drugs that fall into the same class or only to use them together with caution.

2. Combinations of antiarrhythmics from different classes. Class III antiarrhythmics such as amiodarone can also prolong the QT interval; they would therefore be expected to interact with drugs in other classes that have the same effect, namely class Ia drugs (see 'Drugs that prolong the QT interval + Other drugs that prolong the QT interval', p.272). Verapamil (a class IV antiarrhythmic) has negative inotropic effects; it can therefore interact with other drugs having similar effects, such as sotalol (a class III antiarrhythmic). For safety, always consider the whole drug profile and take care with any two drugs, from any class, that share a common pharmacological action.

(b) Propafenone metabolism

The metabolism of propafenone is complex. Propafenone is principally metabolised by CYP2D6, with CYP3A4 and CYP1A2 also involved. Therefore inhibitors of CYP2D6 will have the greatest effect on propafenone metabolism, with the magnitude of their effect related to their inhibitory potency on this isoenzyme. Inhibitors of CYP3A4 and CYP1A2 will also decrease propafenone metabolism, but as this isoenzyme plays a smaller role in propafenone metabolism, even potent inhibitors of these isoenzymes might have only small effects on propafenone concentrations. The picture becomes more complex because CYP2D6 shows genetic polymorphism, with up to 10% of the Caucasian population deficient in this isoenzyme (described as poor metabolisers). In patients that are poor metabolisers the other pathways of propafenone metabolism become more important, and interactions with inhibitors or inducers of CYP3A4 and CYP1A2 become more likely to be clinically relevant. In clinical practice it is unlikely that the metaboliser status of the patient will be known, and therefore all patients will need to be monitored to detect these potential effects.

Table 9.1 Antiarrhythmics (modified Vaughan Williams classification)
Class I: Membrane stabilising drugs (a) Ajmaline, Cibenzoline,* Disopyramide, Hydroquinidine, Procainamide, Quinidine (b) Aprindine, Lidocaine, Mexiletine, Tocainide (c) Flecainide, Propafenone Class I, but not easily fitting the above subgroups – Moracizine
Class II: Beta blocker activity Atenolol, Bretylium,† Propranolol
Class III: Inhibitors of depolarisation Amiodarone, Azimilide, Bretylium,† Cibenzoline,* Dofetilide, Dronedarone, Ibutilide, Sotalol
Class IV: Calcium-channel blocker activity Cibenzoline,* Diltiazem, Verapamil
Drugs not fitting into this classification Adenosine

* Cibenzoline has class Ia, and also some class III and IV activity
† Bretylium has class II and III activity

Adenosine + Dipyridamole

Dipyridamole reduces the bolus dose of adenosine necessary to convert supraventricular tachycardia to sinus rhythm. Profound bradycardia occurred in one patient taking dipyridamole when an adenosine infusion was given for myocardial stress testing.

Clinical evidence

(a) Adenosine bolus for supraventricular tachycardia

Adenosine by rapid intravenous bolus (10 to 200 micrograms/kg in stepwise doses) was found to restore sinus rhythm in 10 of 14 episodes of tachycardia in 7 patients with supraventricular tachycardia (SVT). The mean dose required was 8.8 mg, compared with only 1 mg in 2 patients also taking oral dipyridamole.[1] Another study in 6 patients found that dipyridamole (560 microgram/kg intravenous bolus, followed by a continuous infusion of 5 micrograms/kg per minute) reduced the minimum effective bolus dose of intravenous adenosine required to stop the SVT from 68 micrograms/kg to 17 micrograms/kg in 5 patients. In the other patient, dipyridamole alone stopped the SVT.[2]

Other studies in healthy subjects have clearly shown that dipyridamole reduces the dose of adenosine required to produce an equivalent cardiovascular effect fourfold[3] or even six- to sixteenfold.[4] A brief report describes a woman with paroxysmal SVT who lost ventricular activity for 18 seconds when given adenosine 6 mg intravenously. She was also taking dipyridamole (dose unstated), which was considered to have contributed to the loss of ventricular function.[5] Another report describes 3 of 4 patients who had heart block of 3-, 9- and 21-second duration, respectively, when given adenosine 3 to 6 mg by central venous bolus. The patient with the most profound heart block was also receiving dipyridamole, which was thought to have contributed to the reaction.[6]

(b) Adenosine infusion for myocardial stress testing

A 79-year-old woman taking a combination of low-dose aspirin and extended-release dipyridamole *(Aggrenox)* became bradycardic (36 bpm), dizzy and almost fainted 2 minutes after the start of an adenosine infusion for radionuclide myocardial imaging. Adenosine was stopped, and she recovered within 2 minutes. The last dose of *Aggrenox* had been taken 12 hours previously.[7] However, note that bradycardia is a known adverse effect of adenosine,[8,9] and so the contribution of dipyridamole to the bradycardia in this patient is unclear.

Mechanism

Not fully understood. Part of the explanation is that dipyridamole increases the plasma levels of endogenous adenosine by inhibiting its uptake into cells.[2,4,10]

Importance and management

The interaction between adenosine and dipyridamole is established. Patients will need much less adenosine to treat arrhythmias while taking dipyridamole. It has been suggested that the initial dose of adenosine should be reduced twofold[5] or fourfold.[2] The UK manufacturers of adenosine suggest avoiding dipyridamole in patients being treated for supraventricular tachycardia,[8] and contraindicate the use of dipyridamole with adenosine for myocardial perfusion imaging.[9] In both cases if adenosine must be used, they state that the dipyridamole should be stopped 24 hours before use of adenosine, or the adenosine dose be greatly reduced.[8,9] This could be insufficient for extended-release dipyridamole preparations: the authors of one report recommend stopping dipyridamole several days before testing with adenosine.[7] Xanthines, such as intravenous aminophylline, have been used to terminate persistent adverse effects resulting from the use of adenosine infusions, see 'Adenosine + Xanthines', below.

1. Watt AH, Bernard MS, Webster J, Passani SL, Stephens MR, Routledge PA. Intravenous adenosine in the treatment of supraventricular tachycardia: a dose-ranging study and interaction with dipyridamole. *Br J Clin Pharmacol* (1986) 21, 227–30.
2. Lerman BB, Wesley RC, Belardinelli L. Electrophysiologic effects of dipyridamole on atrioventricular nodal conduction and supraventricular tachycardia. Role of endogenous adenosine. *Circulation* (1989) 80, 1536–43.
3. Biaggioni I, Onrot J, Hollister AS, Robertson D. Cardiovascular effects of adenosine infusion in man and their modulation by dipyridamole. *Life Sci* (1986) 39, 2229–36.
4. Conradson T-BG, Dixon CMS, Clarke B, Barnes PJ. Cardiovascular effects of infused adenosine in man: potentiation by dipyridamole. *Acta Physiol Scand* (1987) 129, 387–91.
5. Mader TJ. Adenosine: adverse interactions. *Ann Emerg Med* (1992) 21, 453.
6. McCollam PL, Uber WE, Van Bakel AB. Adenosine-related ventricular asystole. *Ann Intern Med* (1993) 118, 315–16.
7. Littmann L, Anderson JD, Monroe MH. Adenosine and Aggrenox: a hazardous combination. *Ann Intern Med* (2002) 137, W1.
8. Adenocor (Adenosine). Sanofi-Aventis. UK Summary of product characteristics, December 2011.
9. Adenoscan (Adenosine). Sanofi-Aventis. UK Summary of product characteristics, July 2011.
10. German DC, Kredich NM, Bjornsson TD. Oral dipyridamole increases plasma adenosine levels in human beings. *Clin Pharmacol Ther* (1989) 45, 80–4.

Adenosine + Nicotine

Nicotine appears to enhance the effects of adenosine.

Clinical evidence, mechanism, importance and management

In a study in 10 healthy subjects, **nicotine chewing gum** 2 mg (approximately equal to one cigarette) increased the circulatory effects of a 70 micrograms/kg per minute infusion of adenosine. The 5.5 bpm increase in heart rate due to nicotine was further increased to 14.9 bpm by adenosine, and the 7 mmHg diastolic blood pressure rise due to nicotine was reduced to 1.1 mmHg by adenosine.[1] In another study, in 7 healthy subjects, **nicotine chewing gum** 2 mg increased chest pain and the duration of AV block when it was given with intravenous bolus doses of adenosine.[2] What this means in practical terms is uncertain, but be aware that the effects of adenosine might be modified to some extent by nicotine-containing products (such as **tobacco smoking** and **nicotine gum**).

1. Smits P, Eijsbouts A, Thien T. Nicotine enhances the circulatory effects of adenosine in human beings. *Clin Pharmacol Ther* (1989) 46, 272–8.
2. Sylvén C, Beerman B, Kaijser L, Jonzon B. Nicotine enhances angina pectoris-like chest pain and atrioventricular blockade provoked by intravenous bolus of adenosine in healthy volunteers. *J Cardiovasc Pharmacol* (1990) 16, 962–5.

Adenosine + Xanthines

Caffeine and theophylline can inhibit the effects of adenosine infusions used in conjunction with radionuclide myocardial imaging. Aminophylline has been used to terminate persistent adverse effects of adenosine infusions, but adenosine might still be effective for terminating supraventricular tachycardia in patients taking xanthines.

Clinical evidence

(a) Adenosine bolus for supraventricular tachycardia

It is usually considered that an adenosine bolus for the termination of paroxysmal supraventricular tachycardia will be ineffective in patients taking xanthines. However, one case describes a man taking **theophylline** (serum level 8 nanograms/mL) in whom adenosine 9 mg terminated supraventricular tachycardia. Two previous adenosine doses, one of 3 mg and one of 6 mg had not been effective.[1] Another report found that high adenosine doses, of 400 to 800 micrograms/kg (usual dose 50 to 200 micrograms/kg), were required to revert supraventricular tachycardia in a preterm infant given **theophylline.**[2]

(b) Adenosine infusion

Experimental studies in healthy subjects, on the way xanthine drugs possibly interact with adenosine, have found that **caffeine** and **theophylline** reduced the increased heart rate and the changes in blood pressure caused by infusions of adenosine,[3-6] as well as attenuating adenosine-induced vasodilatation.[7,8] **Theophylline** also attenuated adenosine-induced respiratory effects and chest pain.[5,6] Similarly, an adenosine infusion antagonised the haemodynamic effects of a single dose of **theophylline** in healthy subjects, but did not reduce the metabolic effects (reductions in plasma potassium and magnesium concentrations).[5]

Mechanism

Caffeine and theophylline have an antagonistic effect on adenosine receptors.[9] They appear to have opposite effects on the circulatory system: caffeine and theophylline cause vasoconstriction whereas adenosine infusions generally cause vasodilatation.[3]

Importance and management

Adenosine bolus injections for the termination of paroxysmal supraventricular tachycardia might still be effective in patients receiving xanthines. The usual dose schedule should be followed. However, note that adenosine has induced bronchospasm. The US manufacturers[10,11] state that adenosine preparations, whether used for supraventricular tachycardia or myocardial imaging, should be avoided in patients with bronchoconstriction or bronchospasm (e.g. asthma), and used cautiously in those with obstructive pulmonary disease not associated with bronchospasm (e.g. emphysema, bronchitis). The UK manufacturers contraindicate the use of adenosine in chronic obstructive lung disease with evidence of bronchospasm and warn that adenosine may aggravate or precipitate bronchospasm.[12,13] Whether an adenosine bolus can stop theophylline-induced supraventricular tachycardia does not appear to have been studied.

The manufacturers of adenosine also state that theophylline, aminophylline and other xanthines should be avoided for 24 hours before administration of adenosine, and that xanthine-containing drinks (tea, coffee, chocolate, cola drinks etc.) should be avoided for at least 12 hours before administration.[12,13] In a recent study in 70 patients, measurable caffeine serum levels were found in 74% of patients after 12 hours of self-reported abstention from caffeine-containing products. Patients with caffeine serum levels of at least 2.9 mg/L had considerably fewer stress symptoms (chest tightness, chest pain, headache, dyspnoea, nausea, dizziness) than those with lower serum levels. The authors suggest that a 12-hour abstention from caffeine-containing products might be insufficient, and could result in false-negative results.[14] A study in 30 patients also found that caffeine serum levels were detectable in 43% of patients after 12 hours of self-reported abstention from caffeine-containing products. The same study also found that 200-mg of caffeine given 60 minutes before adenosine-stress testing, reduced the effect of adenosine compared with baseline, but that this could be overcome by increasing the dose of adenosine (from 140 micrograms/kg per minute to 210 micrograms/kg per minute).[15] Xanthines, such as intravenous aminophylline, have been used to terminate persistent adverse effects of adenosine infusion given for supraventricular tachycardia or myocardial imaging.[12,13]

1. Giagounidis AAN, Schäfer S, Klein RM, Aul C, Strauer BE. Adenosine is worth trying in patients with paroxysmal supraventricular tachycardia on chronic theophylline medication. *Eur J Med Res* (1998) 3, 380–2.
2. Berul CI. Higher adenosine dosage required for supraventricular tachycardia in infants treated with theophylline. *Clin Pediatr (Phila)* (1993) 32, 167–8.
3. Smits P, Schouten J, Thien T. Cardiovascular effects of two xanthines and the relation to adenosine antagonism. *Clin Pharmacol Ther* (1989) 45, 593–9.

4. Smits P, Boekema P, De Abreu R, Thien T, van 't Laar A. Evidence for an antagonism between caffeine and adenosine in the human cardiovascular system. *J Cardiovasc Pharmacol* (1987) 10, 136–43.
5. Minton NA, Henry JA. Pharmacodynamic interactions between infused adenosine and oral theophylline. *Hum Exp Toxicol* (1991) 10, 411–18.
6. Maxwell DL, Fuller RW, Conradson T-B, Dixon CMS, Aber V, Hughes JMB, Barnes PJ. Contrasting effects of two xanthines, theophylline and enprofylline, on the cardio-respiratory stimulation of infused adenosine in man. *Acta Physiol Scand* (1987) 131, 459–65.
7. Taddei S, Pedrinelli R, Salvetti A. Theophylline is an antagonist of adenosine in human forearm arterioles. *Am J Hypertens* (1991) 4, 256–9.
8. Smits P, Lenders JWM, Thien T. Caffeine and theophylline attenuate adenosine-induced vasodilation in humans. *Clin Pharmacol Ther* (1990) 48, 410–18.
9. Fredholm BB. On the mechanism of action of theophylline and caffeine. *Acta Med Scand* (1985) 217, 149–53.
10. Adenocard (Adenosine). Astellas Pharma Inc. US Prescribing information, May 2009.
11. Adenoscan (Adenosine). Astellas Pharma Inc. US Prescribing information, February 2011.
12. Adenocor (Adenosine). Sanofi-Aventis. UK Summary of product characteristics, December 2011.
13. Adenoscan (Adenosine). Sanofi-Aventis. UK Summary of product characteristics, July 2011.
14. Majd-Ardekani J, Clowes P, Menash-Bonsu V, Nunan TO. Time for abstention from caffeine before an adenosine myocardial perfusion scan. *Nucl Med Commun* (2000) 21, 361–4.
15. Reyes E, Loong CY, Harbinson M, Donovan J, Anagnostopoulos C, Underwood SR. High-dose adenosine overcomes the attenuation of myocardial perfusion reserve caused by caffeine. *J Am Coll Cardiol* (2008) 52, 2008–16.

Ajmaline + Miscellaneous

An isolated report describes cardiac failure in a patient given ajmaline with lidocaine. Quinidine causes a very considerable increase in ajmaline levels, whereas phenobarbital appears to cause an increase in ajmaline clearance.

Clinical evidence, mechanism, importance and management

(a) Lidocaine

A woman had a marked aggravation of her existing cardiac failure when she was given ajmaline orally and lidocaine intravenously for repeated ventricular tachycardias.[1] The general relevance of this isolated case is uncertain.

(b) Phenobarbital

The clearance of intravenous ajmaline was almost twice as high in 3 patients also taking phenobarbital when compared with 5 patients who were not taking phenobarbital. Therefore the clinical effects of ajmaline would be expected to be diminished in those taking phenobarbital.[2] The clinical relevance of this interaction does not appear to have been established. Nevertheless, it would seem prudent to monitor concurrent use to ensure ajmaline remains effective.

(c) Quinidine

A single-dose study[3] in 4 healthy subjects found that the concurrent use of quinidine 200 mg with ajmaline 50 mg increased the AUC of ajmaline 10- to 30-fold and increased its maximum plasma concentration from 18 nanograms/mL to 141 nanograms/mL. Another single-dose study in 5 healthy subjects found that the metabolism of ajmaline was inhibited by quinidine, possibly because the quinidine becomes competitively bound to the enzymes that metabolise ajmaline.[4] This marked rise in ajmaline levels is likely to increase its adverse effects, and concurrent use should probably be avoided.

1. Bleifeld W. Side effects of antiarrhythmics. *Naunyn Schmiedebergs Arch Pharmacol* (1971) 269, 282–97.
2. Köppel C, Wagemann A, Martens F. Pharmacokinetics and antiarrhythmic efficacy of intravenous ajmaline in ventricular arrhythmia of acute onset. *Eur J Drug Metab Pharmacokinet* (1989) 14, 161–7.
3. Hori R, Okumura K, Inui K-I, Yasuhara M, Yamada K, Sakurai T, Kawai C. Quinidine-induced rise in ajmaline plasma concentration. *J Pharm Pharmacol* (1984) 36, 202–4.
4. Köppel C, Tenczer J, Arndt I. Metabolic disposition of ajmaline. *Eur J Drug Metab Pharmacokinet* (1989) 14, 309–16.

Amiodarone + Anaesthesia

There is some evidence that the presence of amiodarone possibly increases the risk of complications (atropine-resistant bradycardia, hypotension, decreased cardiac output) during general anaesthesia. All of these cases were with fentanyl-based anaesthesia, but other studies have shown no problems with fentanyl-based anaesthesia.

Clinical evidence

(a) Evidence for complications

Several case reports[1-4] and two studies[5,6] suggest that severe intra-operative complications (atropine-resistant bradycardia, myocardial depression, hypotension) may occur in patients receiving amiodarone. One of the studies, a comparative retrospective review of patients (16 receiving amiodarone 300 to 800 mg daily and 30 controls) having operations under anaesthesia (mainly open-heart surgery), found that the incidence of slow nodal rhythm, complete heart block or pacemaker dependency rose from 17% in controls to 66% in amiodarone-treated patients. Intra-aortic balloon pump augmentation (reflecting poor cardiac output) was 50% in the amiodarone group compared with 7% in the control group, and a state of low systemic vascular resistance with normal to high cardiac output occurred in 13% of the amiodarone-treated patients, but not in the control patients. Overall there were 3 fatalities; all of these patients had received amiodarone and had been on cardiopulmonary bypass during surgery. **Fentanyl** was used for all of the patients, often combined with diazepam, and sometimes also **isoflurane**, **enflurane** or **halothane**.[5]

Another study of 37 patients receiving amiodarone (mean dose about 250 mg daily) found no problems in 8 patients undergoing non-cardiac surgery. Of the 29 patients undergoing cardiac surgery, 52% had postoperative arrhythmias and 24% required a pacemaker, which was not considered exceptional for the type of surgery. However, one patient having coronary artery bypass surgery had fatal vasoplegia (a hypotensive syndrome), which was considered to be amiodarone-related. This occurred shortly after he was taken off cardiopulmonary bypass. Anaesthesia in all patients was **fentanyl**-based.[6] It was suggested in one case report that serious hypotension in 2 patients taking amiodarone undergoing surgery may have been further compounded by the presence of an **ACE inhibitor**.[3] For interactions between ACE inhibitors and anaesthetics see 'Anaesthetics, general + ACE inhibitors or Angiotensin II receptor antagonists', p.99.

(b) Evidence for no complications

The preliminary report of a study in 21 patients taking amiodarone (mean dose 538 mg daily) and undergoing defibrillator implantation suggested that haemodynamic changes during surgery were not significantly different from those in matched controls not taking amiodarone.[7] Similarly, another study found no difference in haemodynamic status or pacemaker dependency between patients taking short-term amiodarone 600 mg daily for one week then 400 mg daily for 2 weeks before surgery and a control group not taking amiodarone, during valve replacement surgery with **thiopental-fentanyl** anaesthesia.[8] In a double-blind study, there was no significant difference in haemodynamic instability during **fentanyl-isoflurane** anaesthesia between patients randomised to receive short-term amiodarone (3.4 g over 5 days or 2.2 g over 24 hours) or placebo before cardiac surgery. In this study, haemodynamic instability was assessed by fluid balance, use of dopamine or other vasopressors, and use of a phosphodiesterase inhibitor or intra-aortic balloon pump.[9]

A case report describes the successful use of epidural anaesthesia with **fentanyl** then **chloroprocaine** during labour and caesarean section in a woman who had been taking amiodarone long-term. The only haemodynamic change of possible note was that the patient had a drop in systemic vascular resistance from high to almost normal levels shortly after receiving **fentanyl** during the first stage of labour, and again when **fentanyl** was given for postoperative pain relief.[10] Another case report describes the successful use of epidural anaesthesia using incremental doses of lidocaine 2% with adrenaline and **fentanyl** 100 micrograms for caesarean section in a woman receiving high-dose amiodarone (1600 mg daily) for fetal supraventricular tachycardia.[11]

Mechanism

In vitro and *in vivo* studies in *animals* suggest that amiodarone has additive cardio-depressant and vasodilator effects with volatile anaesthetics such as halothane, enflurane and isoflurane.[2,12] The manufacturer notes that fentanyl is a substrate for the cytochrome P450 isoenzyme CYP3A4, and that amiodarone might inhibit CYP3A4, thereby increasing the toxicity of fentanyl.[13]

Importance and management

The assessment of this interaction is complicated by the problem of conducting studies in anaesthesia, most being retrospective and using matched controls. The only randomised study used short-term amiodarone to assess its safety in the prevention of post-operative atrial fibrillation, and its findings may not be relevant to patients taking long-term amiodarone.[9] It appears that potentially severe complications may occur in some patients taking amiodarone who undergo general anaesthesia, including bradycardia unresponsive to atropine, hypotension, conduction disturbances, and decreased cardiac output. It has been suggested that anaesthetists should take particular care in patients taking amiodarone who undergo surgery on cardiopulmonary bypass.[14] Amiodarone persists in the body for many weeks, which usually means it cannot be withdrawn before surgery, especially if there are risks in delaying surgery,[6] or the amiodarone is being used for serious arrhythmias.[14] A possible pharmacokinetic interaction exists between fentanyl and amiodarone, which could contribute to the interactions seen, and further study is needed on this.

1. Gallagher JD, Lieberman RW, Meranze J, Spielman SR, Ellison N. Amiodarone-induced complications during coronary artery surgery. *Anesthesiology* (1981) 55, 186–8.
2. MacKinnon G, Landymore R, Marble A. Should oral amiodarone be used for sustained ventricular tachycardia in patients requiring open-heart surgery? *Can J Surg* (1983) 26, 355–7.
3. Mackay JH, Walker IA, Bethune DW. Amiodarone and anaesthesia: concurrent therapy with ACE inhibitors—an additional cause for concern? *Can J Anaesth* (1991) 38, 687.
4. Navalgund AA, Alifimoff JK, Jakymec AJ, Bleyaert AL. Amiodarone-induced sinus arrest successfully treated with ephedrine and isoproterenol. *Anesth Analg* (1986) 65, 414–16.
5. Liberman BA, Teasdale SJ. Anaesthesia and amiodarone. *Can Anaesth Soc J* (1985) 32, 629–38.
6. Van Dyck M, Baele P, Rennotte MT, Matta A, Dion R, Kestens-Servaye Y. Should amiodarone be discontinued before cardiac surgery? *Acta Anaesthesiol Belg* (1988) 39, 3–10.
7. Elliott PL, Schauble JF, Rogers MC, Reid PR. Risk of decompensation during anesthesia in presence of amiodarone. *Circulation* (1983) 68 (Suppl 3), 280.
8. Chassard D, George M, Guiraud M, Lehot JJ, Bastien O, Hercule C, Villard J, Estanove S. Relationship between preoperative amiodarone treatment and complications observed during anaesthesia for valvular cardiac surgery. *Can J Anaesth* (1990) 37, 251–4.
9. White CM, Dunn A, Tsikouris J, Waberski W, Felton K, Freeman-Bosco L, Giri S, Kluger J. An assessment of the safety of short-term amiodarone therapy in cardiac surgical patients with fentanyl-isoflurane anesthesia. *Anesth Analg* (1999) 89, 585–9.
10. Koblin DD, Romanoff ME, Martin DE, Hensley FA, Larach DR, Stauffer RA, Luck JC. Anesthetic management of the parturient receiving amiodarone. *Anesthesiology* (1987) 66, 551–3.
11. Fulgencio JP, Hamza J. Anaesthesia for caesarean section in a patient receiving high dose amiodarone for fetal supraventricular tachycardia. *Anaesthesia* (1994) 49, 406–8.
12. Rooney RT, Marijic J, Stommel KA, Bosnjak ZJ, Aggarwai A, Kampine JP, Stowe DF. Additive cardiac depression by volatile anesthetics in isolated hearts after chronic amiodarone treatment. *Anesth Analg* (1995) 80, 917–24.
13. Cordarone X (Amiodarone hydrochloride). Zentiva. UK Summary of product characteristics, April 2014.
14. Teasdale S, Downar E. Amiodarone and anaesthesia. *Can J Anaesth* (1990) 37, 151–5.

Amiodarone + Calcium-channel blockers

Increased cardiac depressant effects would be expected if amiodarone is used with diltiazem or verapamil. One case of sinus arrest and serious hypotension occurred in a woman taking diltiazem when she was given amiodarone.

Clinical evidence, mechanism, importance and management

A woman with compensated congestive heart failure, paroxysmal atrial fibrillation and ventricular arrhythmias was taking furosemide and **diltiazem** 90 mg every 6 hours. Four days after amiodarone 600 mg every 12 hours was added, she developed sinus arrest and a life-threatening low cardiac output state (systolic blood pressure 80 mmHg) with oliguria. **Diltiazem** and amiodarone were stopped and she was treated with pressor drugs and ventricular pacing. She had previously had no problems when taking **diltiazem** or **verapamil** alone, and later she took amiodarone 400 mg daily alone without incident. This reaction is thought to be caused by the additive effects of both drugs on myocardial contractility, and on sinus and atrioventricular nodal function.[1] Before this isolated case report was published, another author predicted this interaction with **diltiazem** or **verapamil** on theoretical grounds, and warned of the risks if dysfunction of the sinus node (bradycardia or sick sinus syndrome) is suspected, or if partial AV block exists.[2] The manufacturers state that amiodarone is not recommended,[3] or should be used with caution,[4] with certain calcium-channel blockers (**diltiazem**, **verapamil**) because potentiation of negative chronotropic properties and conduction-slowing effects may occur. Note that **diltiazem** has been used for rate control in patients developing postoperative atrial fibrillation despite the use of prophylactic amiodarone.[5] There do not appear to be any reports of adverse effects attributed to the use of amiodarone with the dihydropyridine class of calcium-channel blockers (e.g. **nifedipine**), which typically have little or no negative inotropic activity at usual doses.

1. Lee TH, Friedman PL, Goldman L, Stone PH, Antman EM. Sinus arrest and hypotension with combined amiodarone-diltiazem therapy. *Am Heart J* (1985) 109, 163–4.
2. Marcus FI. Drug interactions with amiodarone. *Am Heart J* (1983) 106, 924–30.
3. Cordarone X (Amiodarone hydrochloride). Zentiva. UK Summary of product characteristics, April 2014.
4. Cordarone (Amiodarone hydrochloride). Wyeth Pharmaceuticals Inc. US Prescribing information, December 2014.
5. Kim MH, Rachwal W, McHale C, Bruckman D, Decena BF, Russman P, Morady F, Eagle KA. Effect of amiodarone ± diltiazem ± beta blocker on frequency of atrial fibrillation, length of hospitalization, and hospital costs after coronary artery bypass grafting. *Am J Cardiol* (2002) 89, 1126–28.

Amiodarone + Chloroquine

In theory the concurrent use of chloroquine and amiodarone may increase the risk of torsade de pointes, but there appears to be no published cases of an interaction.

Clinical evidence, mechanism, importance and management

Some UK manufacturers of amiodarone and chloroquine contraindicate the concurrent use of these drugs because of the risk of torsade de pointes,[1,2] whereas another warns of an increased risk of arrhythmias.[3] Chloroquine may cause arrhythmias and ECG changes when used alone, particularly in high doses[2,3] and for prolonged periods (e.g. for rheumatoid arthritis);[2] however, chloroquine is not generally considered a high risk for causing cardiovascular toxicity, especially when given at the correct dose and administered appropriately.[4] There appears to be only one isolated report of QT prolongation in a patient taking chloroquine, but this was secondary to long term use (17 years) for systemic lupus erythematosus,[5] and no published cases of an interaction with amiodarone. Furthermore, the US manufacturers of amiodarone and chloroquine do not include any warnings about QT prolongation on concurrent use.[6,7] An interaction is therefore not established.

1. Cordarone X (Amiodarone hydrochloride). Zentiva. UK Summary of product characteristics, April 2014.
2. Avloclor (Chloroquine phosphate). AstraZeneca UK Ltd. UK Summary of product characteristics, July 2010.
3. Nivaquine Syrup (Chloroquine sulphate). Sanofi-Aventis. UK Summary of product characteristics, September 2008.
4. White NJ. Cardiotoxicity of antimalarial drugs. *Lancet Infect Dis* (2007) 7, 549–58.
5. Stas P, Faes D, Noyens P. Conduction disorder and QT prolongation secondary to long-term treatment with chloroquine. Int J Cardiol. (2008) 127, e80–e82.
6. Cordarone (Amiodarone hydrochloride). Wyeth Pharmaceuticals Inc. US Prescribing information, December 2014.
7. Aralen (Chloroquine phosphate). Sanofi-Aventis U.S LLC. US Prescribing information, September 2008.

Amiodarone + Cimetidine

Cimetidine possibly causes a modest rise in the serum levels of amiodarone in some patients.

Clinical evidence, mechanism, importance and management

The preliminary report of one study in 12 patients noted that the mean serum levels of amiodarone 200 mg twice daily rose by an average of 38%, from 1.4 micrograms/mL to 1.93 micrograms/mL, when cimetidine 1.2 g daily was given for a week. The desethylamiodarone levels rose by 54%. However, these increases were not statistically significant (possibly due to the small sample size), and only 8 of the 12 patients had any rise.[1]

It is possible that cimetidine (a non-specific enzyme inhibitor) may reduce the metabolism of amiodarone leading to the increased levels seen.

Information seems to be limited to this study but this interaction may be clinically important in some patients. Monitor the effects when cimetidine is started, being alert for amiodarone adverse effects (e.g. bradycardia, taste disturbances, tremor, nausea). Remember that amiodarone has a very long half-life of 25 to 100 days, so that the results of the one-week study cited here may possibly not adequately reflect the magnitude of this interaction. There does not appear to have been anything further published on this.

1. Hogan C, Landau S, Tepper D, Somberg J. Cimetidine-amiodarone interaction. *J Clin Pharmacol* (1988) 28, 909.

Amiodarone + Colestyramine

Colestyramine appears to reduce the serum levels of amiodarone.

Clinical evidence

In a study in 11 patients, 4 doses of colestyramine 4 g were given at one-hour intervals starting 1.5 hours after a single 400-mg dose of amiodarone. The serum amiodarone levels measured 7.5 hours later were reduced by about 50%.[1] In a further study, the amiodarone half-life was shorter in 3 patients given colestyramine 4 g daily after discontinuing long-term amiodarone (23.5, 29 and 32 days, respectively) compared with the half-life in 8 patients discontinuing amiodarone and not given colestyramine (35 to 58 days).[1]

Mechanism

This interaction probably occurs because colestyramine binds with amiodarone in the gut, thereby reducing its absorption. It may also affect the enterohepatic recirculation of amiodarone.[1] This is consistent with the way colestyramine interacts with other drugs.

Importance and management

Information is very limited but a reduced response to amiodarone may be expected. Separating the dosages to avoid admixture in the gut would reduce or prevent any effects on absorption from the gut, but not the effects due to reduced enterohepatic recirculation. Monitor concurrent use closely for amiodarone efficacy and consider an alternative to colestyramine, or raise the amiodarone dosage if necessary.

1. Nitsch J, Luderitz B. Beschleunigte elimination von Amiodaron durch Colestyramin. *Dtsch Med Wochenschr* (1986) 111, 1241–44.

Amiodarone + Co-trimoxazole

Some predict that co-trimoxazole (trimethoprim with sulfamethoxazole) increases the risk of QT prolongation and ventricular arrhythmias with amiodarone, but clinical evidence for this is sparse.

Clinical evidence, mechanism, importance and management

The UK manufacturer of amiodarone contraindicates the concurrent use of co-trimoxazole (trimethoprim with sulfamethoxazole), as they state that it prolongs the QT interval and increases the risk of torsade de pointes.[1] However, one UK manufacturer of co-trimoxazole similarly states that concurrent use increases the risk of ventricular arrhythmias, but does not specifically contraindicate concurrent use.[2] Co-trimoxazole is not generally associated with causing significant QT interval prolongation and torsade de pointes, and only three isolated cases appear to have been reported for co-trimoxazole alone,[3-5] of these, one was in a 90-year-old woman,[3] and another was in a patient genetically predisposed to QT prolongation.[4] Furthermore, the US manufacturer[6] of amiodarone and one other UK manufacturer[7] of co-trimoxazole make no mention of any possible interaction. An interaction is therefore not established.

1. Cordarone X (Amiodarone hydrochloride). Zentiva. UK Summary of product characteristics, April 2014.
2. Co-trimoxazole Tablets. Actavis UK Ltd. UK Summary of product characteristics, October 2009.
3. Lopez JA, Harold JG, Rosenthal MC, Oseran DS, Schapira JN, Peter T. QT prolongation and torsades de pointes after administration of trimethoprim-sulfamethoxazole. *Am J Cardiol* (1987) 59, 376–7.
4. Sesti F, Abbott GW, Wei J, Murray KT, Saksena S, Schwartz PJ, Priori SG, Roden DM, George AL, Goldstein SAN. A common polymorphism associated with antibiotic-induced cardiac arrhythmia. *Proc Natl Acad Sci U S A* (2000) 97, 10613–18.
5. Owens RC. Risk assessment for antimicrobial agent-induced QTc interval prolongation and torsades de pointes. *Pharmacotherapy* (2001) 21, 301–19.
6. Cordarone (Amiodarone hydrochloride). Wyeth Pharmaceuticals Inc. US Prescribing information, December 2014.
7. Septrin Tablets (Trimethoprim with Sulfamethoxazole). GlaxoSmithKline UK. UK Summary of product characteristics, July 2009.

Amiodarone + Disopyramide

The risk of QT interval prolongation and torsade de pointes is increased if amiodarone is given with disopyramide.

Clinical evidence

A brief report describes 2 patients who developed torsade de pointes when they were given amiodarone with disopyramide. Their QT intervals became markedly prolonged to somewhere between 500 and 600 milliseconds.[1] In another study, 2 patients who had been taking disopyramide 300 mg daily for a number of months developed prolonged QT intervals, increasing from 450 milliseconds to 640 milliseconds and from 390 milliseconds to 680 milliseconds respectively, and developed torsade de pointes 2 days and 5 days respectively, after starting amiodarone 800 mg daily.[2] However, one early report also described the successful and apparently safe use of amiodarone 100 to 600 mg daily with disopyramide 300 to 500 mg daily,[3] although the results of long-term follow-up were not reported in all cases.

Mechanism

Amiodarone is a class III antiarrhythmic and can prolong the QT interval. Disopyramide is a class Ia antiarrhythmic and also prolongs the QT interval. Their additive effects can result in the development of torsade de pointes.

Importance and management

An established and potentially serious interaction. In general, class Ia antiarrhythmics such as disopyramide (see 'Table 9.2', p.273) should be avoided or used with great caution with amiodarone because of their additive effects in delaying conduction. The manufacturers of amiodarone contraindicate[4] or urge caution[5] if it is used with class Ia antiarrhythmics. If amiodarone is started in a patient taking disopyramide, they suggest the dose of disopyramide should be reduced by 30 to 50% several days after the addition of amiodarone, and that the continued need for disopyramide should be monitored, and withdrawal attempted. If disopyramide is given to a patient already taking amiodarone, the initial dose of disopyramide should be about half of the usual recommended dose.[5]

See also 'Drugs that prolong the QT interval + Other drugs that prolong the QT interval', p.272, and for the interactions of other class Ia antiarrhythmics with amiodarone see 'Procainamide + Amiodarone', p.287, and 'Quinidine + Amiodarone', p.292.

1. Tartini R, Kappenberger L, Steinbrunn W. Gefährliche Interaktionen zwischen Amiodaron und Antiarrhythmika der Klass I. *Schweiz Med Wochenschr* (1982) 112, 1585–87.
2. Keren A, Tzivoni D, Gavish D, Levi J, Gottlieb S, Benhorin J, Stern S. Etiology, warning signs and therapy of torsade de pointes. A study of 10 patients. *Circulation* (1981) 64, 1167–74.
3. James MA, Papouchado M, Vann Jonec J. Combined therapy with disopyramide and amiodarone: a report of 11 cases. *Int J Cardiol* (1986) 13, 248–52.
4. Cordarone X (Amiodarone hydrochloride). Zentiva. UK Summary of product characteristics, April 2014.
5. Cordarone (Amiodarone hydrochloride). Wyeth Pharmaceuticals Inc. US Prescribing information, December 2014.

Amiodarone + Grapefruit juice

Grapefruit juice inhibited the metabolism of oral amiodarone, and *decreased* its effects on the PR and QTc interval.

Clinical evidence

A single 17-mg/kg oral dose of amiodarone was given to 11 healthy subjects on two occasions, once with water and once with grapefruit juice (300 mL taken three times on the same day). Grapefruit juice completely inhibited the metabolism of amiodarone to its major metabolite *N*-desethylamiodarone and increased the amiodarone AUC by 50% and increased its peak serum level by 84%. The effect of amiodarone on the PR and QTc intervals was *decreased*.[1]

Mechanism

It is likely that grapefruit juice inhibits the cytochrome P450 isoenzyme CYP3A4 in the intestinal mucosa, thus inhibiting the formation of *N*-desethylamiodarone from oral, but probably not intravenous, amiodarone.

Importance and management

The interaction between amiodarone and grapefruit juice appears to be established, but its clinical consequences remain to be determined. *N*-desethylamiodarone is known to be active, so this could possibly result in decreased activity. In addition, high amiodarone concentrations may increase toxicity. Conversely, a reduction in QT prolongation is potentially beneficial.[1] However, further study is needed to establish any beneficial effect. The US manufacturer recommends that grapefruit juice should not be taken during treatment with oral amiodarone.[2]

1. Libersa CC, Brique SA, Motte KB, Caron JF, Guédon-Moreau LM, Humbert L, Vincent A, Devos P, Lhermitte MA. Dramatic inhibition of amiodarone metabolism induced by grapefruit juice. *Br J Clin Pharmacol* (2000) 49, 373–8.
2. Cordarone (Amiodarone hydrochloride). Wyeth Pharmaceuticals Inc. US Prescribing information, December 2014.

Amiodarone + Haloperidol

A retrospective study describes QT prolongation on the concurrent use of amiodarone and haloperidol.

Clinical evidence, mechanism, importance and management

A retrospective analysis identified 49 patients who were given amiodarone (mean daily dose 771 mg) with haloperidol (mean daily dose 11 mg) and a total of 381 instances of concurrent use (classified as haloperidol administration by any route within 24 hours of amiodarone administration by any route). Most patients were already taking amiodarone when haloperidol (intravenous haloperidol in 96% of patients) was given, with a mean increase in the QTc interval of 9.8 milliseconds. No ventricular arrhythmias were reported.[1] Both drugs are known to prolong the QT interval, and concurrent use is contraindicated by the UK manufacturers of amiodarone and haloperidol.[2,3] In contrast, the US manufacturer of amiodarone does not contraindicate the use of haloperidol, but advises that the concurrent use of amiodarone and any QT-prolonging drugs should only be undertaken after careful risk assessment.[4] For a further discussion of the risks of QT prolongation and the concurrent use or two or more QT-prolonging drugs, see 'Drugs that prolong the QT interval + Other drugs that prolong the QT interval', p.272.

1. Bush SE, Hatton RC, Winterstein AG, Thomson MR, Woo GW. Effects of concomitant amiodarone and haloperidol on Q-Tc interval prolongation. *Am J Health-Syst Pharm* (2008) 65, 2232–6.
2. Cordarone X (Amiodarone hydrochloride). Zentiva. UK Summary of product characteristics, April 2014.
3. Haldol Tablets (Haloperidol). Janssen-Cilag Ltd. UK Summary of product characteristics, October 2009.
4. Cordarone (Amiodarone hydrochloride). Wyeth Pharmaceuticals Inc. US Prescribing information, December 2014.

Amiodarone + HIV-protease inhibitors

A case report describes increased amiodarone concentrations in a patient given indinavir. Other HIV-protease inhibitors are predicted to interact similarly.

Clinical evidence

A patient taking amiodarone 200 mg daily was also given zidovudine, lamivudine, and **indinavir** for 4 weeks, as post HIV-exposure prophylaxis after a needlestick injury. Amiodarone serum concentrations increased, from 0.9 mg/L before antiretroviral prophylaxis, to 1.3 mg/L during prophylaxis, and gradually decreased to 0.8 mg/L during the 77 days after stopping prophylaxis. Although the reference range for amiodarone concentrations is not established, these concentrations were not outside those usually considered to achieve good antiarrhythmic control.[1]

Mechanism

HIV-protease inhibitors such as indinavir are inhibitors of cytochrome P450 enzymes and pharmacokinetic interactions are therefore possible. It was considered that the increase in serum amiodarone in this case was due to decreased metabolism of amiodarone, although no decrease in the serum concentrations of desethylamiodarone were observed.[1]

Importance and management

Although in the case cited the interaction was not clinically relevant, the authors considered that it could be important in patients with higher initial amiodarone concentrations. They recommend monitoring amiodarone if indinavir is also given.[1] In general the UK manufacturers of HIV-protease inhibitors suggest that they may increase amiodarone concentrations, and contraindicate concurrent use. The exception is **atazanavir boosted with ritonavir**,[2] where caution and increased monitoring, including taking amiodarone concentrations, where possible, is recommended. Similarly the US manufacturers of the HIV-protease inhibitors generally contraindicate concurrent use. The exceptions are **amprenavir**,[3] **atazanavir**,[4] **darunavir boosted with ritonavir**,[5] **fosamprenavir**[6] and **lopinavir boosted with ritonavir**,[7] where the manufacturers recommend increased monitoring, including taking amiodarone concentrations, where possible. Amiodarone adverse effects include bradycardia, taste disturbances, tremor and nausea.

1. Lohman JJHM, Reichert LJM, Degen LPM. Antiretroviral therapy increases serum concentrations of amiodarone. *Ann Pharmacother* (1999) 33, 645–6.
2. Reyataz (Atazanavir sulfate). Bristol-Myers Squibb Pharmaceuticals Ltd. UK Summary of product characteristics, August 2012.
3. Agenerase (Amprenavir). GlaxoSmithKline. US Prescribing information, May 2005.
4. Reyataz (Atazanavir sulfate). Bristol-Myers Squibb. US Prescribing information, March 2012.
5. Prezista (Darunavir ethanolate). Janssen Pharmaceuticals, Inc. US Prescribing information, May 2012.
6. Lexiva (Fosamprenavir calcium). ViiV Healthcare. US Prescribing information, April 2013.
7. Kaletra (Lopinavir with Ritonavir). Abbott Laboratories. US Prescribing information, April 2012.

Amiodarone + Lithium

Hypothyroidism developed very rapidly in two patients taking amiodarone when lithium was added.

Clinical evidence, mechanism, importance and management

A patient who had taken amiodarone 400 mg daily for more than a year developed acute manic depression. He was given lithium 600 mg daily (salt unknown), but within 2 weeks he developed clinical signs of hypothyroidism, which were confirmed by clinical tests. He made a complete recovery within 3 weeks of stopping amiodarone while continuing lithium.[1] Similarly, another patient rapidly developed hypothyroidism, when taking amiodarone with lithium (dose and salt unknown). It resolved when the amiodarone was stopped.[1] Both lithium and amiodarone on their own can cause hypothyroidism (amiodarone can also cause hyperthyroidism). In these two cases the effects appear to have been additive, and very rapid.

These two cases appear to be the first and only reports of this interaction. Its general importance is therefore still uncertain. Note that lithium has been tried for the treatment of amiodarone-induced hyperthyroidism,[2,3] and monitoring of thyroid status is recommended before, and regularly throughout, amiodarone treatment.[4,5] It would therefore seem prudent to be extra vigilant for any signs of hypothyroidism (lethargy, weakness, depression, weight gain, hoarseness) in any patient given both drugs.

Lithium therapy has rarely been associated with cardiac QT prolongation, and consequently the UK manufacturer of amiodarone contraindicates combined use.[4] However, note that QT-prolongation associated with lithium is usually as a result of lithium toxicity. See also 'Drugs that prolong the QT interval + Other drugs that prolong the QT interval', p.272.

1. Ahmad S. Sudden hypothyroidism and amiodarone-lithium combination: an interaction. *Cardiovasc Drugs Ther* (1995) 9, 827–8.
2. Dickstein G, Shechner C, Adawi F, Kaplan J, Baron E, Ish-Shalom S. Lithium treatment in amiodarone-induced thyrotoxicosis. *Am J Med* (1997) 102, 454–8.
3. Boeving A, Cubas ER, Santos CM, de Carvalho GA, Graf H. O uso de carbonato de litio no tratamento da tireotoxicose induzida por amiodarona. *Arq Bras Endocrinol Metabol* (2005) 49, 991–5.
4. Cordarone X (Amiodarone hydrochloride). Zentiva. UK Summary of product characteristics, April 2014.
5. Cordarone (Amiodarone hydrochloride). Wyeth Pharmaceuticals Inc. US Prescribing information, December 2014.

Amiodarone + Macrolides

Torsade de pointes occurred in a man taking amiodarone when he was also given intravenous erythromycin. QT prolongation occurred in another patient when azithromycin was added to long-term amiodarone.

Clinical evidence

A 76-year-old man taking amiodarone 200 mg daily had a prolonged QT interval and a syncopal episode with torsade de pointes 24 hours after starting a course of intravenous **erythromycin lactobionate** (1 g every 6 hours). This occurred on rechallenge.[1] Marked QT prolongation and increased QT dispersion occurred when **azithromycin** was given to a patient taking amiodarone long-term, and resolved when the **azithromycin** was stopped.[2]

Mechanism

Amiodarone alone can prolong the QT interval and increase the risk of torsade de pointes. Of the macrolides, *intravenous* erythromycin is known to prolong the QT interval, and there is some evidence that clarithromycin might prolong the QT interval.[3] Azithromycin and telithromycin are also associated with an increased risk of QT interval prolongation. Amiodarone and these macrolides may therefore have additive effects on the QT interval.

Importance and management

In general the concurrent use of two or more drugs that prolong the QT interval should be avoided, because this increases the risk of torsade de pointes arrhythmias (see also 'Drugs that prolong the QT interval + Other drugs that prolong the QT interval', p.272). For this reason, the UK manufacturer of amiodarone contraindicates the concurrent use of *intravenous* erythromycin.[4] The authors of the above report suggest that the combination of azithromycin and amiodarone should be used with caution,[2] and this should probably also apply to **clarithromycin** and **telithromycin** until more is known. The US manufacturer recommends that a careful risk assessment should be undertaken if amiodarone is to be given with a macrolide.[5]

1. Nattel S, Ranger S, Talajic M, Lemery R, Roy D. Erythromycin-induced long QT syndrome: concordance with quinidine and underlying cellular electrophysiologic mechanism. *Am J Med* (1990) 89, 235–8.
2. Samarendra P, Kumari S, Evans SJ, Sacchi TJ, Navarro V. QT prolongation associated with azithromycin/amiodarone combination. *Pacing Clin Electrophysiol* (2001) 24, 1572–4.
3. Lee KL, Man-Hong J, Tang SC, Tai Y-T. QT-prolongation and torsades de pointes associated with clarithromycin. *Am J Med* (1998) 104, 395–6.
4. Cordarone X (Amiodarone hydrochloride). Zentiva. UK Summary of product characteristics, April 2014.
5. Cordarone (Amiodarone hydrochloride). Wyeth Pharmaceuticals Inc. US Prescribing information, December 2014.

Amiodarone + Metronidazole

An isolated report describes QT interval prolongation and torsade de pointes in a patient given metronidazole and amiodarone.

Clinical evidence, mechanism, importance and management

An elderly patient taking metronidazole 500 mg three times daily for antibacterial-associated colitis and amiodarone (as an initial bolus of 450 mg followed by 900 mg daily) for paroxysmal atrial fibrillation developed marked QTc interval prolongation and torsade de pointes. Metronidazole and amiodarone were withdrawn and defibrillation was required to restore sinus rhythm. The QTc interval gradually decreased to normal over 6 days.[1]

It was suggested that metronidazole may have inhibited the metabolism of amiodarone by the cytochrome P450 isoenzyme CYP3A4 resulting in higher levels which are associated with QT interval prolongation and torsade de pointes.[1] However, some pharmacokinetic studies have found that metronidazole is not an inhibitor of CYP3A4/5 and suggest that increases in plasma levels of CYP3A4 substrates in the presence of metronidazole are not the result of CYP3A4 inhibition.[2] Furthermore, amiodarone was not given alone, so it is unclear if the effects seen were as a result of an interaction, of simply an adverse effect of the amiodarone. No general conclusions can be drawn from this isolated case.

1. Kounas SP, Letsas K, Sideris A, Efraimidis M, Kardaras F. QT interval prolongation and torsades de pointes due to a coadministration of metronidazole and amiodarone. *Pacing Clin Electrophysiol* (2005) 28, 472–3.
2. Roedler R, Neuhauser MM, Penzak SR. Does metronidazole interact with CYP3A substrates by inhibiting their metabolism through this metabolic pathway? Or should other mechanisms be considered? *Ann Pharmacother* (2007) 41, 653–8.

Amiodarone + Orlistat

Orlistat modestly reduces the absorption of amiodarone.

Clinical evidence, mechanism, importance and management

A randomised, placebo-controlled study in 16 healthy subjects found that orlistat 120 mg three times daily reduced the AUC and peak serum level of a single 1.2-g dose of amiodarone by 23% and 27%, respectively. Levels of its active metabolite, desethylamiodarone, were similarly reduced. The half-life and time to maximum serum level were not significantly altered. It was suggested that orlistat, which inhibits dietary fat absorption, may also reduce the absorption of amiodarone, which is a lipophilic drug.[1]

Although this modest reduction in amiodarone levels is unlikely to be clinically relevant, the manufacturer of orlistat recommends clinical and ECG monitoring during concurrent use.[2]

1. Zhi J, Moore R, Kanitra L, Mulligan TE. Effects of orlistat, a lipase inhibitor, on the pharmacokinetics of three highly lipophilic drugs (amiodarone, fluoxetine, and simvastatin) in healthy volunteers. *J Clin Pharmacol* (2003) 43, 428–35.
2. Xenical (Orlistat). Roche Products Ltd. UK Summary of product characteristics, April 2014.

Amiodarone + Oxygen

High-dose oxygen may increase the risks of amiodarone-induced post-operative adult respiratory distress syndrome.

Clinical evidence, mechanism, importance and management

A retrospective review of 20 patients who underwent cardiac surgery found that pulmonary complications were more common in those receiving amiodarone (73% versus 25%). Moreover, the incidence of pulmonary complications in patients taking amiodarone was higher in those exposed to 100% oxygen (6 of 7) than those not exposed to this concentration of oxygen (2 of 4).[1]

Four other patients taking amiodarone (without preoperative amiodarone pulmonary toxicity), developed postoperative toxicity, and 2 patients died. The common intraoperative factor in the 4 patients was exposure to high inspired oxygen concentrations.[2] A further two reports describe 3 patients taking amiodarone who developed acute onset unilateral adult respiratory distress syndrome after receiving 100% oxygen ventilation of one lung during surgery.[3,4]

Life-threatening pulmonary complications occurred in 4 patients with diagnosed amiodarone pulmonary toxicity who subsequently underwent cardiothoracic surgery: 2 patients died. These 4 patients were compared with 13 other patients taking amiodarone (only one of whom had preoperative amiodarone pulmonary toxicity) who were undergoing similar surgery and who did not develop pulmonary complications. The comparison indicated that *preoperative* amiodarone pulmonary toxicity appears to be a risk factor in the development of pulmonary complications, but other additional factors could include pump-oxygenator time and oxygen toxicity.[5]

The UK manufacturer of amiodarone suggests caution in patients receiving high-dose oxygen,[6] and the US manufacturer recommends that the determinants of oxygen delivery to the tissues should be closely monitored.[7] Others have suggested that the concentration of oxygen should be maintained at the lowest possible level consistent with adequate oxygenation.[1,3,4]

1. Duke PK, Ramsay MAE, Herndon JC, Swygert TH, Cook AO. Acute oxygen induced amiodarone pulmonary toxicity after general anaesthesia. *Anesthesiology* (1991) 75, A228.
2. Kay GN, Epstein AE, Kirklin JK, Diethelm AG, Graybar G, Plumb VJ. Fatal postoperative amiodarone pulmonary toxicity. *Am J Cardiol* (1988) 62, 490–2.
3. Herndon JC, Cook AO, Ramsay AE, Swygert TH, Capehart J. Postoperative unilateral pulmonary edema: possible amiodarone pulmonary toxicity. *Anesthesiology* (1992) 76, 308–12.
4. Saussine M, Colson P, Alauzen M, Mary H. Postoperative acute respiratory distress syndrome. A complication of amiodarone associated with 100 percent oxygen ventilation. *Chest* (1992) 102, 980–1.
5. Nalos PC, Kass RM, Gang ES, Fishbein MC, Mandel WJ, Peter T. Life-threatening postoperative pulmonary complications in patients with previous amiodarone pulmonary toxicity undergoing cardiothoracic operations. *J Thorac Cardiovasc Surg* (1987) 93, 904–12.
6. Cordarone X (Amiodarone hydrochloride). Zentiva. UK Summary of product characteristics, April 2014.
7. Cordarone (Amiodarone hydrochloride). Wyeth Pharmaceuticals Inc. US Prescribing information, December 2014.

Amiodarone + Quinolones

Torsade de pointes has been reported in two patients taking amiodarone and levofloxacin, and in one patient given amiodarone, sotalol and ciprofloxacin. Post-marketing surveillance identified two similar cases with amiodarone and sparfloxacin. An increased risk of this arrhythmia would also be expected if amiodarone is used with gatifloxacin or moxifloxacin.

Clinical evidence

(a) Ciprofloxacin

A case report describes a 70-year old woman with new onset atrial fibrillation who received intravenous amiodarone (450 mg loading dose then 650 mg every 24 hours) and digoxin for about 48 hours until conversion to sinus rhythm, at which point she was given sotalol 40 mg twice daily. The day after the sotalol was started, she also received intravenous ciprofloxacin 400 mg twice daily for cholecystitis, and within 12 hours developed torsade de pointes requiring defibrillation. Before starting the ciprofloxacin, her QTc was 380 milliseconds and after resuscitation it was prolonged at 620 milliseconds. Within 3 days of stopping the sotalol and ciprofloxacin her QT interval had fallen to 420 milliseconds.[1] The authors attributed this case to ciprofloxacin (for which QT prolongation is rare); however, both amiodarone alone and sotalol alone are well known causes of QT prolongation, and therefore either or both cannot be excluded as causes (see also 'Beta blockers + Amiodarone', p.1001). In addition, this patient had a low potassium level of 3 mmol/L, which is also a risk factor for QT prolongation.

(b) Levofloxacin

Torsade de pointes occurred in a patient taking levofloxacin and amiodarone.[2] The same authors subsequently encountered a second case of this reaction.[3]

(c) Sparfloxacin

During post-marketing surveillance of sparfloxacin in France over a period of 8 months (about 750 000 patients) serious adverse cardiovascular effects were reported in 7 patients. All 7 patients had underlying risk factors including 3 patients who were also receiving amiodarone. Of these, 2 patients had documented QT prolongation and ventricular tachycardia.[4]

(d) Unspecified quinolones

The Adverse Events Reporting System database of the FDA in the US was reviewed for cases of torsade de pointes associated with quinolones up until May 2001. In total, 37 cases of torsade de pointes were identified, and 19 occurred in patients also taking other drugs known to prolong the QT interval. Of the 19 cases, 4 cases were noted in patients taking amiodarone and a quinolone (unspecified, but **ciprofloxacin, gatifloxacin, levofloxacin, moxifloxacin,** and **ofloxacin** were assessed).[5] These 4 cases possibly include the two with **levofloxacin** mentioned above.

Mechanism

Amiodarone can prolong the QT interval and increase the risk of torsade de pointes. Of the quinolones used clinically, gatifloxacin, moxifloxacin, and sparfloxacin are known to prolong the QT interval (see 'Table 9.2', p.273). There is also evidence that levofloxacin may prolong the QT interval.[3,5] The effect of amiodarone and the quinolones may be additive.

Importance and management

In general the concurrent use of two or more drugs that prolong the QT interval should be avoided, because this increases the risk of torsade de pointes arrhythmias (see also 'Drugs that prolong the QT interval + Other drugs that prolong the QT interval', p.272). The quinolones that prolong the QT interval (gatifloxacin, moxifloxacin, sparfloxacin) should probably be avoided in patients taking amiodarone: moxifloxacin is specifically contraindicated.[6] Ciprofloxacin appears to have less effect on the QT interval.[5] Nevertheless, in the UK the manufacturer of amiodarone suggests that the concurrent use of any quinolone should be avoided.[6]

1. Keivanidou A, Arnaoutoglou C, Krommydas A, Papanikolaou G, Tsiptses K, Chrisopoulos C, Kirpizidis C. Ciprofloxacin induced acquired long QT syndrome in a patient under class III antiarrhythmic therapy. *Cardiol J* (2009) 16, 172–4.
2. Iannini PB, Kramer H, Circiumaru I, Byazrova E, Doddamani S. QTc prolongation associated with levofloxacin. *Intersci Conf Antimicrob Agents Chemother* (2000) 40, 477.
3. Iannini P. Quinolone-induced QT interval prolongation: a not-so-unexpected class effect. *J Antimicrob Chemother* (2001) 47, 893–4.
4. Jaillon P, Morganroth J, Brumpt I, Talbot G, and the Sparfloxacin Safety Group. Overview of electrocardiographic and cardiovascular safety data for sparfloxacin. *J Antimicrob Chemother* (1996) 37 (Suppl A), 161–7.
5. Frothingham R. Rates of torsades de pointes associated with ciprofloxacin, ofloxacin, levofloxacin, gatifloxacin, and moxifloxacin. *Pharmacotherapy* (2001) 21, 1468–72.
6. Cordarone X (Amiodarone hydrochloride). Zentiva. UK Summary of product characteristics, April 2014.

Amiodarone + Rifampicin (Rifampin)

A case report suggests that rifampicin may decrease the serum levels of amiodarone and its metabolite *N*-desethylamiodarone.

Clinical evidence, mechanism, importance and management

A woman with congenital heart disease, and atrial and ventricular arrhythmias managed by an implanted cardioverter defibrillator, epicardial pacing and amiodarone 400 mg daily, experienced deterioration in the control of her condition. She developed palpitations and experienced a shock from the defibrillator. Her amiodarone serum levels were 40% lower than 2 months previously, and her *N*-desethylamiodarone levels were undetectable. It was noted that 5 weeks earlier rifampicin 600 mg daily had been started to treat an infection of the pacing system. The amiodarone dose was doubled, but the palpitations continued. Amiodarone and *N*-desethylamiodarone levels increased after rifampicin was discontinued.[1] Rifampicin is a potent enzyme inducer and it may have increased the metabolism and clearance of amiodarone. Evidence appears to be limited to this case, but it is in line with the way both drugs are known to interact with other substances. An interaction would therefore seem to be established. It would be prudent to monitor concurrent use for amiodarone efficacy, taking amiodarone and metabolite levels, where possible.

1. Zarembski DG, Fischer SA, Santucci PA, Porter MT, Costanzo MR, Trohman RG. Impact of rifampin on serum amiodarone concentrations in a patient with congenital heart disease. *Pharmacotherapy* (1999) 19, 249–51.

Amiodarone + Sertraline

In an isolated report, a slight to moderate rise in plasma amiodarone levels was attributed to the concurrent use of sertraline.

Clinical evidence, mechanism, importance and management

A depressed patient taking amiodarone 200 mg twice daily had his treatment with carbamazepine 200 mg twice daily and sertraline 100 mg daily stopped, just before ECT treatment. After 4 days it was noted that his plasma amiodarone levels had fallen by nearly 20%. The authors of the report drew the conclusion that while taking all three drugs, the amiodarone levels had become slightly raised due to the enzyme inhibitory effects of the sertraline, despite the potential enzyme-inducing activity of the carbamazepine.[1] The patient had no changes in his cardiac status while amiodarone levels were reduced. Furthermore, a change of 20% would usually be considered to be within the normal fluctuation of drug levels. Therefore an interaction, particularly a clinically relevant interaction, seems unlikely.

1. DeVane CL, Gill HS, Markowitz JS, Carson WH. Awareness of potential drug interactions may aid avoidance. *Ther Drug Monit* (1997) 19, 366–7.

Amiodarone + Tolvaptan

Tolvaptan does not appear to affect the pharmacokinetics of amiodarone.

Clinical evidence, mechanism, importance and management

In a study in 17 patients with stable arrhythmias taking amiodarone 200 mg daily, single 30- or 90-mg doses of tolvaptan had no effect on the AUC or maximum plasma concentrations of amiodarone or its metabolite, desethylamiodarone. The pharmacokinetics of tolvaptan did not appear to differ, when compared with historical control data. No clinically relevant ECG changes were reported on concurrent use.[1]

Therefore, no amiodarone dose adjustment would be expected to be needed on the concurrent use of tolvaptan.

1. Shoaf SE, Elizari MV, Wang Z, Sekar K, Grinfeld LR, Barbagelata NA, Lerman J, Bramer SL, Trongé J, Orlandi C. Tolvaptan administration does not affect steady state amiodarone concentrations in patients with cardiac arrhythmias. *J Cardiovasc Pharmacol Ther* (2005) 10, 165–71.

Amiodarone + Trazodone

Two reports describe the development of torsade de pointes in patients taking trazodone and amiodarone; in one case trazodone was added to amiodarone, and in the other case amiodarone was added to trazodone.

Clinical evidence, mechanism, importance and management

A 74-year-old woman with a pacemaker, taking nifedipine, furosemide, aspirin and amiodarone 200 mg daily, began to have dizzy spells but no loss of consciousness soon after starting trazodone (initially 50 mg and eventually 150 mg daily by the end of 2 weeks). Both the amiodarone and trazodone were stopped when she was hospitalised. She had a prolonged QTc interval and recurrent episodes of torsade de pointes, which were controlled by increasing the ventricular pacing rate. The QTc interval shortened and she was later discharged taking amiodarone without the trazodone, with an ECG similar to that seen 4 months before hospitalisation.[1] In a review of torsade de pointes in patients taking amiodarone long-term, one elderly female patient who had taken trazodone 50 mg daily for 2 years developed torsade de pointes 2 months after amiodarone 200 mg daily was added. The authors noted that hypokalaemia in this patient might have contributed to the arrhythmia.[2]

Note that QT prolongation has been associated with trazodone, and this could be additive with other drugs that might cause QT prolongation, such as amiodarone. See 'Drugs that prolong the QT interval + Other drugs that prolong the QT interval', p.272, for more information on the use of two or more drugs that prolong the QT interval.

1. Mazur A, Strasberg B, Kusniec J, Sclarovsky S. QT prolongation and polymorphous ventricular tachycardia associated with trasodone-amiodarone combination. *Int J Cardiol* (1995) 52, 27–9.
2. Antonelli D, Atar S, Freedberg NA, Rosenfeld T. Torsade de pointes in patients on chronic amiodarone treatment: contributing factors and drug interactions. *Isr Med Assoc J* (2005) 7,163–5.

Aprindine + Amiodarone

Serum aprindine levels can be increased by amiodarone.

Clinical evidence, mechanism, importance and management

The serum aprindine levels of 2 patients rose, accompanied by signs of toxicity (e.g. nausea, ataxia), when they were also given amiodarone. One of them, taking aprindine 100 mg daily, had a progressive rise in trough serum levels from 2.3 mg/L to 3.5 mg/L over a 5-week period, when given 1.2 g and later 600 mg of amiodarone daily. Even when the aprindine dose was reduced, serum levels remained higher than before amiodarone was started.[1] The authors say that those taking both drugs generally need less aprindine than those taking aprindine alone. This interaction has been briefly reported elsewhere.[2]

The reason for the rise in aprindine levels is not understood. Nevertheless it would seem prudent to monitor the effects of concurrent use and reduce the dose of aprindine as necessary.

1. Southworth W, Friday KJ, Ruffy R. Possible amiodarone-aprindine interaction. *Am Heart J* (1982) 104, 323.
2. Zhang Z, Wang G, Wang H, Zhang J. Effect of amiodarone on the plasma concentration of aprindine [Abstract 115: 197745u in Chemical Abstracts (1991) 115, 22]. *Zhongguo Yao Xue Za Zhi* (1991) 26, 156–9.

Azimilide + Miscellaneous

Ketoconazole (a CYP3A4 inhibitor) did not alter the pharmacokinetics of azimilide to a clinically relevant extent, and azimilide did not affect the pharmacokinetics of omeprazole (a CYP2C19 substrate) to a clinically relevant extent. Interactions with other CYP3A4 inhibitors and CYP2C19 substrates are therefore considered unlikely.

A case report describes QT prolongation in a patient given azimilide and ciprofloxacin. Azimilide does not appear to interact to a clinically relevant extent with digoxin or food, and its antiarrhythmic effects are unaffected by isoprenaline (isoproterenol).

Clinical evidence, mechanism, importance and management

(a) Ciprofloxacin

A patient with a history of myocardial infarction and with an implanted cardioverter-defibrillator (ICD) who was taking several drugs including azimilide 125 mg daily, was admitted to hospital because of worsening heart failure. On day 6 he developed a urinary-tract infection and was given ciprofloxacin 250 mg twice daily, but after 2 doses he developed QTc interval prolongation (increase from 470 milliseconds on admission to 754 milliseconds) and multiple episodes of torsade de pointes followed by ICD shocks. Azimilide and ciprofloxacin were withdrawn and he was given metoprolol but he also required ICD reprogramming. It was suggested that this occurred as a result of the additive effects of both drugs on the QT interval.[1]

(b) Digoxin

A study in 18 healthy subjects found that the concurrent use of azimilide and digoxin had only minor effects on the pharmacokinetics of both drugs (azimilide renal clearance increased by 36%, digoxin maximum serum level and AUC increased by 21% and 10%, respectively). In this study, azimilide 175 mg was given orally daily for 4 days then 100 mg on day 5 and digoxin was given as a loading dose of 750 micrograms on day one then as 250 micrograms daily for 4 days. Azimilide alone increased the QTc: this effect was decreased by 2 to 4% by digoxin. These effects are unlikely to be clinically relevant.[2]

(c) Food

A study in 30 healthy subjects given azimilide in the fasted state or after a high-fat meal found that the high-fat meal decreased the maximum serum levels of azimilide by 19%, but the extent of absorption was the same. Azimilide may be given without regard to meal times.[3]

(d) Isoprenaline (Isoproterenol)

In a placebo-controlled study, patients with cardiovascular disorders were given an infusion of isoprenaline, titrated from 0.5 micrograms/minute up to a maximum of 4 micrograms/minute until the heart rate reached 125% of baseline (up to a maximum 120 bpm). This dose of isoprenaline was then given again, but with an infusion of azimilide, as a loading dose of 4.5 mg/kg over 15 minutes followed by a continuous infusion of 0.625 mg/kg per hour. It was found that azimilide maintained its class III antiarrhythmic effect in the presence of isoprenaline, and at increased heart rate.[4]

(e) Ketoconazole

In a randomised, placebo-controlled study, 21 healthy subjects were given ketoconazole 200 mg daily with a single 125-mg dose of azimilide on day 8. Ketoconazole affected the AUC, maximum blood levels, half-life and clearance of azimilide by less than 20%. Azimilide is partly metabolised by the cytochrome P450 isoenzyme CYP3A4, which is inhibited by ketoconazole. The minor changes in azimilide pharmacokinetics with ketoconazole are not considered to be clinically important, and clinically significant pharmacokinetic interactions with other CYP3A4 inhibitors are not expected.[5]

(f) Omeprazole

In a randomised, placebo-controlled study, 40 healthy subjects (extensive metabolisers of the cytochrome P450 isoenzyme CYP2C19, that is, those that have normal levels of this isoenzyme) were given azimilide 125 mg every 12 hours for 3 days, then daily for 5 days. Azimilide reduced the AUC of a single 20-mg dose of omeprazole given on day 8 by 12%, which is not clinically relevant. There was no change in the metabolite-to-parent AUC suggesting that azimilide had no effect on the metabolism of omeprazole by CYP2C19.[6]

The authors note that *in vitro* studies suggested that of the cytochrome P450 isoenzymes, azimilide had the lowest inhibitory concentration against CYP2C19. On this basis they suggest that azimilide is also unlikely to interact with drugs metabolised by CYP1A2, CYP2C9, CYP2D6 and CYP3A4.[6]

1. Kaźmierczak J, Peregud-Pogorzelska M, Rzeuski R. QT interval prolongation and torsades de pointes due to a coadministration of ciprofloxacin and azimilide in a patient with implantable cardioverter–defibrillator. *Pacing Clin Electrophysiol* (2007) 30, 1043–6.
2. Toothaker RD, Corey AE, Valentine SN, Agnew JR, Parekh N, Moehrke W, Thompson GA, Powell JH. Influence of coadministration on the pharmacokinetics of azimilide dihydrochloride and digoxin. *J Clin Pharmacol* (2005) 45, 773–80.
3. Corey AE, Agnew JR, Valentine SN, Nesbitt JD, Wagner DL, Powell JH, Thompson GA. Comparative oral bioavailability of azimilide dihydrochloride in the fed and fasted states. *Br J Clin Pharmacol* (2000) 49, 279–82.
4. Dorian P, Dunnmon P, Elstun L, Newman D. The effect of isoproterenol on the class III effect of azimilide in humans. *J Cardiovasc Pharmacol Ther* (2002) 7, 211–17.
5. El Mouelhi M, Worley DJ, Kuzmak B, Destefano AJ, Thompson GA. Influence of ketoconazole on azimilide pharmacokinetics in healthy subjects. *Br J Clin Pharmacol* (2004) 58, 641–7.
6. El Mouelhi M, Worley DJ, Kuzmak B, Destefano AJ, Thompson GA. Influence of azimilide on CYP2C19-mediated metabolism. *J Clin Pharmacol* (2004) 44, 373–8.

Cibenzoline (Cifenline) + H_2-receptor antagonists

Cimetidine increases the plasma levels of cibenzoline. Ranitidine does not interact with cibenzoline.

Clinical evidence, mechanism, importance and management

In a study in 12 healthy subjects, **cimetidine** 1.2 g daily raised the maximum plasma levels of a single 160-mg dose of cibenzoline by 27%, increased its AUC by 44%, and prolonged its half-life by 30%. **Ranitidine** 300 mg daily had no effect.[1] The probable reason for the rise in cibenzoline levels is that **cimetidine**, an enzyme inhibitor, reduces the metabolism of the cibenzoline by the liver, whereas **ranitidine**, which is not an enzyme inhibitor, does not affect cibenzoline metabolism. The clinical importance of this interaction is not known but be alert for increased cibenzoline adverse effects.

1. Massarella JW, Defeo TM, Liguori J, Passe S, Aogaichi K. The effects of cimetidine and ranitidine on the pharmacokinetics of cifenline. *Br J Clin Pharmacol* (1991) 31, 481–3.

Disopyramide + Antacids

There is some inconclusive evidence that aluminium phosphate may possibly cause a small reduction in the absorption of disopyramide.

Clinical evidence, mechanism, importance and management

In a study in 10 patients, a single 11-g dose of an **aluminium phosphate** antacid had no statistically significant effect on the pharmacokinetics of a single 200-mg oral dose of disopyramide. However the antacid appeared to reduce the absorption of disopyramide to some extent in individual subjects.[1] The clinical importance of this interaction is uncertain, but probably small.

1. Albin H, Vincon G, Bertolaso D, Dangoumau J. Influence du phosphate d'aluminium sur la biodisponibilité de la procaïnamide et du disopyramide. *Therapie* (1981) 36, 541–6.

Disopyramide + Azoles

Ketoconazole increased the levels of disopyramide *in vitro*. Other azole antifungals would be expected to interact similarly.

Clinical evidence, mechanism, importance and management

An *in vitro* study[1] found that **ketoconazole** inhibits the metabolism of disopyramide, although there do not appear to be any case reports or clinical studies of an interaction. Disopyramide is metabolised by the cytochrome P450 isoenzyme CYP3A4, of which ketoconazole is an inhibitor. Therefore concurrent use would be expected to increase disopyramide levels and adverse effects. The UK manufacturer of **ketoconazole** contraindicates the concurrent use of disopyramide, as this increase in disopyramide levels may increase the risk of developing QT prolongation and torsade de pointes.[2] As **itraconazole** is also a potent inhibitor of CYP3A4, the UK manufacturer[3] contraindicates its concurrent use in patients taking disopyramide for non-life threatening indications, whereas the US manufacturer advises caution during concurrent use.[4] Other azole antifungals inhibit CYP3A4 to varying degrees (see *Azoles*, under 'Anthelmintics, Antifungals, and Antiprotozoals', p.225) and therefore they would also be expected to interact with disopyramide. If the concurrent use of disopyramide and an azole is necessary, it would seem prudent to monitor the patient for an increase in disopyramide adverse effects (such as dry mouth, blurred vision, urinary retention and nausea).

1. Zhang L, Fitzloff JF, Engel LC, Cook CS. Species difference in stereoselective involvement of CYP3A in the mono-*N*-dealkylation of disopyramide. *Xenobiotica* (2001) 31, 73–83.
2. Nizoral Tablets (Ketoconazole). Janssen-Cilag Ltd. UK Summary of product characteristics, June 2010.
3. Sporanox Capsules (Itraconazole). Janssen-Cilag Ltd. UK Summary of product characteristics, October 2011.
4. Sporanox Capsules (Itraconazole). Ortho-McNeill-Janssen Pharmaceuticals, Inc. US Prescribing information, June 2011.

Disopyramide + Beta blockers

Severe bradycardia has been described after the use of disopyramide with beta blockers including practolol, pindolol, and metoprolol; in some cases this was fatal. Atenolol modestly decreased disopyramide clearance in one study. Oral propranolol and disopyramide have been given

together without any increase in negative inotropic effects or pharmacokinetic changes in healthy subjects.

A patient given disopyramide and intravenous sotalol developed asystole. For more information on the effects of giving sotalol with disopyramide, see 'Drugs that prolong the QT interval + Other drugs that prolong the QT interval', p.272.

Clinical evidence

Two patients with supraventricular tachycardia (180 bpm) were given, firstly intravenous **practolol** (20 mg and 10 mg, respectively) and shortly afterwards with disopyramide (150 mg and 80 mg, respectively). The first patient rapidly developed sinus bradycardia of 25 bpm, lost consciousness and became profoundly hypotensive. He did not respond to 600 micrograms of atropine, but later his heart rate increased to 60 bpm while a temporary pacemaker was being inserted.[1] He was successfully treated with disopyramide 150 mg alone for a later episode of tachycardia. The second patient also developed severe bradycardia and asystole, despite the use of atropine. He was resuscitated with adrenaline (epinephrine) but later died.[1]

Severe bradycardia has been reported in another patient, also given intravenous **practolol** and then disopyramide.[2] Another patient developed severe bradycardia and died when given **pindolol** 5 mg and disopyramide 250 mg (both orally) for supraventricular tachycardia.[3] Another patient taking oral disopyramide 250 mg twice daily developed asystole when given a total of 60 mg of intravenous **sotalol**.[4]

A patient with hypertrophic obstructive cardiomyopathy and paroxysmal atrial fibrillation taking disopyramide 450 mg daily developed hypotension, bradycardia and cardiac conduction disturbances 5 days after starting **metoprolol** 50 mg daily.[5]

Atenolol 100 mg daily has been shown to increase the steady-state disopyramide levels from 3.46 micrograms/mL to 4.25 micrograms/mL and reduce the clearance of disopyramide by 16% in healthy subjects and patients with ischaemic heart disease.[6] None of the subjects developed any adverse reactions or symptoms of heart failure, apart from one of the subjects who had transient first degree heart block.[6]

In contrast, studies in healthy subjects have found that the negative inotropic effects were no greater when oral **propranolol** and disopyramide were used concurrently,[7] nor were the pharmacokinetics of either drug affected.[8]

Mechanism

Not understood. Both disopyramide and the beta blockers can depress the contractility and conductivity of the heart muscle.

Importance and management

An interaction between disopyramide and beta blockers is established. It seems to occur rarely, but is potentially very serious; fatalities have been reported. The US manufacturers of disopyramide suggest that the combination of disopyramide and beta blockers should generally be avoided, except in the case of life-threatening arrhythmias unresponsive to a single drug.[9]

Note that the concurrent use of sotalol presents a greater risk than that of other beta blockers, as it may prolong the QT interval. See also 'Drugs that prolong the QT interval + Other drugs that prolong the QT interval', p.272.

1. Cumming AD, Robertson C. Interaction between disopyramide and practolol. *BMJ* (1979) 2, 1264.
2. Gelipter D, Hazell M. Interaction between disopyramide and practolol. *BMJ* (1980) 1, 52.
3. Pedersen C, Josephsen P, Lindvig K. Interaktion mellem disopyramid og pindolol efter oral indgift. *Ugeskr Laeger* (1983) 145, 3266.
4. Bystedt T, Vitols S. Sotalol-disopyramid ledde till asystoli. *Lakartidningen* (1994) 91, 2241.
5. Pernat A, Pohar B, Horvat M. Heart conduction disturbances and cardiovascular collapse after disopyramide and low-dose metoprolol in a patient with hypertrophic obstructive cardiomyopathy. *J Electrocardiol* (1997) 30, 341–4.
6. Bonde J, Bødtker S, Angelo HR, Svendsen TL, Kampmann JP. Atenolol inhibits the elimination of disopyramide. *Eur J Clin Pharmacol* (1986) 28, 41–3.
7. Cathcart-Rake WF, Coker JE, Atkins FL, Huffman DH, Hassanein KM, Shen DD, Azarnoff DL. The effect of concurrent oral administration of propranolol and disopyramide on cardiac function in healthy men. *Circulation* (1980) 61, 938–45.
8. Karim A, Nissen C, Azarnoff DL. Clinical pharmacokinetics of disopyramide. *J Pharmacokinet Biopharm* (1982) 10, 465–94.
9. Norpace (Disopyramide). Pfizer Inc. US Prescribing information, September 2006.

Disopyramide + HIV-protease inhibitors

Disopyramide concentrations may be increased by ritonavir. Other HIV-protease inhibitors may interact similarly.

Clinical evidence, mechanism, importance and management

Direct, published evidence (from case reports or clinical studies) of an interaction between disopyramide and the HIV-protease inhibitors appears to be lacking; however, a review of HIV-protease inhibitor interactions reports that **ritonavir** may increase the plasma concentrations of disopyramide more than threefold.[1] Furthermore, the manufacturer of ritonavir states that cardiac adverse effects have been reported on the concurrent use of disopyramide.[2]

Disopyramide is partially metabolised by the cytochrome P450 isoenzyme CYP3A4, of which **ritonavir** is a potent inhibitor, and therefore concurrent use would be expected to result in raised disopyramide concentrations, which may increase the risk of arrhythmias and other adverse effects, Note that the HIV-protease inhibitors as a group are inhibitors of CYP3A4, to varying degrees, and may be expected to interact similarly.

An interaction between the HIV-protease inhibitors and disopyramide is therefore considered to be established, despite the general lack of direct data. The manufacturer of disopyramide states that concurrent use is not recommended, because the outcome of concurrent use is not known.[3] They also state that as the HIV-protease inhibitors (they name **ritonavir**, **indinavir** and **saquinavir**) are substrates of CYP3A4, they may compete with disopyramide for metabolism by CYP3A4, possibly resulting in increased serum concentrations of these drugs.[3] However, note that drug interactions by this mechanism do not generally result in a clinically relevant interaction. Other known inhibitors of CYP3A4, such as some macrolides (see 'Disopyramide + Macrolides', below) have been reported to increase disopyramide concentrations and this has resulted in serious adverse effects. It would therefore seem prudent to monitor any patient taking both disopyramide and a HIV-protease inhibitor for an increase in disopyramide adverse effects (such as dry mouth, blurred vision, urinary retention and nausea).

1. Burger DM, Hoetelmans RMW, Koopmans PP, Meenhorst PL, Mulder JW, Hekster YA, Beijnen JH. Clinically relevant drug interactions with antiretroviral agents. *Antivir Ther* (1997) 2, 149–165.
2. Norvir Soft Capsules (Ritonavir). Abbott Laboratories Ltd. UK Summary of product characteristics, October 2010.
3. Rythmodan Capsules (Disopyramide). Sanofi. UK Summary of product characteristics, August 2013.

Disopyramide + H_2-receptor antagonists

Cimetidine may slightly increase the serum levels of oral disopyramide, but does not affect the pharmacokinetics of intravenous disopyramide. Ranitidine appears not to interact with disopyramide.

Clinical evidence, mechanism, importance and management

In a study in 7 healthy subjects, oral **cimetidine** 400 mg twice daily for 14 days did not alter the pharmacokinetics of a single 150-mg intravenous dose of disopyramide.[1] Another study, in 6 healthy subjects, found that a single 400-mg dose of **cimetidine** increased the AUC of a single 300-mg oral dose of disopyramide by 9% and increased the maximum serum levels by 19%, but did not significantly affect the metabolism of disopyramide. **Ranitidine** 150 mg was found not to interact significantly.[2]

The reasons for the slight increase in disopyramide levels are not known, but the authors of the report suggest that **cimetidine** may have increased disopyramide absorption.[2] **Cimetidine** is only a weak inhibitor of disopyramide metabolism *in vitro*.[3] The changes described are unlikely to be clinically important, but this should probably be confirmed in a more clinically realistic situation, using multiple oral doses of both drugs.

1. Bonde J, Pedersen LE, Nygaard E, Ramsing T, Angelo HR, Kampmann JP. Stereoselective pharmacokinetics of disopyramide and interaction with cimetidine. *Br J Clin Pharmacol* (1991) 31, 708–10.
2. Jou M-J, Huang S-C, Kiang F-M, Lai M-Y, Chao P-DL. Comparison of the effects of cimetidine and ranitidine on the pharmacokinetics of disopyramide in man. *J Pharm Pharmacol* (1997) 49, 1072–5.
3. Echuzen H, Kawasaki H, Chiba K, Tani M. Ishizaki T. A potent inhibitory effect of erythromycin and other macrolide antibiotics on the mono-N-dealkylation metabolism of disopyramide with human liver microsomes. *J Pharmacol Exp Ther* (1993) 264, 1425–31.

Disopyramide + Macrolides

Erythromycin appears to increase disopyramide concentrations; concurrent use has led to QT prolongation, cardiac arrhythmias, and heart block. The concurrent use of clarithromycin and disopyramide has led to torsade de pointes, ventricular fibrillation, and severe hypoglycaemia, and the concurrent use of azithromycin and disopyramide has led to ventricular fibrillation.

Clinical evidence

(a) Azithromycin

A patient taking disopyramide 150 mg three times daily developed ventricular tachycardia requiring cardioversion 11 days after starting azithromycin 250 mg daily.[1] Her disopyramide concentration was found to have increased from 2.6 micrograms/mL to 11.1 micrograms/mL.

(b) Clarithromycin

A 74-year-old woman who had been taking disopyramide 200 mg twice daily for 7 years collapsed with ventricular fibrillation 6 days after starting to take omeprazole 40 mg, metronidazole 800 mg and clarithromycin 500 mg daily. After successful resuscitation, her QTc interval, which had never previously been above 440 milliseconds, was found to have increased to 625 milliseconds. Her disopyramide plasma concentration was also increased (4.6 micrograms/mL) and the half-life was markedly prolonged (40 hours). The QTc interval normalised as her plasma disopyramide concentrations decreased.[2] A 76-year old woman taking disopyramide developed torsade de pointes when given clarithromycin 200 mg twice daily. Hypokalaemia (potassium 2.8 mmol/L) probably contributed to this case.[3]

An episode of torsade de pointes occurred in another elderly woman taking disopyramide 5 days after starting clarithromycin 250 mg twice daily.[4]

A haemodialysis patient, receiving disopyramide 50 mg daily because of paroxysmal atrial fibrillation, was hospitalised with hypoglycaemic coma after also taking clarithromycin 600 mg daily. Serum disopyramide concentrations increased from 1.5 to 8 micrograms/mL during treatment with clarithromycin. QT and QTc intervals were prolonged, but torsade de pointes did not occur.[5] Hypoglycaemic coma has also been reported in another patient taking disopyramide with clarithromycin.[6]

(c) Erythromycin

A woman with ventricular ectopy taking disopyramide (300 mg alternating with 150 mg every 6 hours) developed new arrhythmias (ventricular asystoles and later torsade de pointes) within 36 hours of starting erythromycin lactobionate 1 g intravenously every 6 hours, and cefamandole. Her QTc interval had increased from 390 to 600 milliseconds and her serum disopyramide concentration was found to be 16 micromol/L. The problem resolved when the disopyramide was stopped and bretylium given, but returned again when disopyramide was restarted. It resolved again when the erythromycin was stopped.[7] Another patient with ventricular tachycardia, well controlled over 5 years with disopyramide 200 mg four times daily, developed polymorphic ventricular tachycardia within a few days of starting erythromycin 500 mg four times daily. His QTc interval had increased from 430 milliseconds to 630 milliseconds and serum disopyramide concentrations were found to be increased at 30 micromol/L. The problem resolved when both drugs were withdrawn and antiarrhythmics given.[7]

Mechanism

Not fully established. An *in vitro* study using human liver microsomes indicated that erythromycin inhibits the metabolism (mono-*N*-dealkylation) of disopyramide which, *in vivo*, would be expected to reduce its loss from the body and increase its serum levels.[8] Clarithromycin probably does the same. The increased disopyramide serum concentrations can result in adverse effects such as QT prolongation and torsade de pointes, and might result in enhanced insulin secretion and hypoglycaemia.[5,6] Azithromycin, intravenous erythromycin,[9] and clarithromycin[10] alone have been associated with prolongation of the QT interval and torsade de pointes. Therefore, disopyramide and macrolides might have additive effects on the QT interval in addition to the pharmacokinetic interaction.

Importance and management

An established interaction, although it is probably rare. Even so the effects of concurrent use should be well monitored if azithromycin, clarithromycin, or erythromycin is added to disopyramide, being alert for the development of increased plasma disopyramide concentrations and prolongation of the QT interval. The manufacturer of disopyramide[11] recommends avoiding the combination of disopyramide and macrolides that inhibit CYP3A4, and this would certainly be prudent in situations where close monitoring is not possible. Although direct clinical information is lacking, *in vitro* studies with human liver microsomes[8] indicate that **josamycin** is likely to interact similarly, and **telithromycin** might also be expected to interact in the same way. See also 'Drugs that prolong the QT interval + Other drugs that prolong the QT interval', p.272.

1. Granowitz EV, Tabor KJ, Kirchhoffer JB. Potentially fatal interaction between azithromycin and disopyramide. *Pacing Clin Electrophysiol* (2000) 23, 1433–5.
2. Paar D, Terjung B, Sauerbruch T. Life-threatening interaction between clarithromycin and disopyramide. *Lancet* (1997) 349, 326–7.
3. Hayashi Y, Ikeda U, Hashimoto T, Watanabe T, Mitsuhashi T, Shimada K. Torsade de pointes ventricular tachycardia induced by clarithromycin and disopyramide in the presence of hypokalaemia. *Pacing Clin Electrophysiol* (1999) 22, 672–4.
4. Choudhury L, Grais IM, Passman RS. Torsade de pointes due to drug interaction between disopyramide and clarithromycin. *Heart Dis* (1999) 1, 206–7.
5. Iida H, Morita T, Suzuki E, Iwasawa K, Toyo-oka T, Nakajima T. Hypoglycemia induced by interaction between clarithromycin and disopyramide. *Jpn Heart J* (1999) 40, 91–6.
6. Morlet-Barla N, Narbonne H, Vialettes B. Hypoglycémie grave et récidivante secondaire á l'interaction disopyramide-clarithromicine. *Presse Med* (2000) 29, 1351.
7. Ragosta M, Weihl AC, Rosenfeld LE. Potentially fatal interaction between erythromycin and disopyramide. *Am J Med* (1989) 86, 465–6.
8. Echizen H, Kawasaki H, Chiba K, Tani M. Ishizaki T. A potent inhibitory effect of erythromycin and other macrolide antibiotics on the mono-N-dealkylation metabolism of disopyramide with human liver microsomes. *J Pharmacol Exp Ther* (1993) 264, 1425–31.
9. Gitler B, Berger LS, Buffa SD. Torsades de pointes induced by erythromycin. *Chest* (1994) 105, 368–72.
10. Lee KL, Jim M-H, Tang SC, Tai Y-T. QT-prolongation and torsades de pointes associated with clarithromycin. *Am J Med* (1998) 104, 395–6.
11. Rythmodan Capsules (Disopyramide). Sanofi. UK Summary of product characteristics, August 2013.

Disopyramide + Phenobarbital

Serum disopyramide levels are reduced by phenobarbital.

Clinical evidence

In a study in 16 healthy subjects, phenobarbital 100 mg daily for 21 days reduced the half-life and AUC of a single 200-mg dose of disopyramide by about 35%. The apparent metabolic clearance more than doubled, and the fraction recovered in the urine as metabolite increased. There were no significant differences seen between subjects who smoked and non-smoking subjects.[1]

Mechanism

It seems probable that phenobarbital (a known enzyme inducer) increases the metabolism of disopyramide by the liver, and thereby increases its loss from the body.

Importance and management

This interaction between phenobarbital and disopyramide appears to be established, but its clinical importance is uncertain. The extent to which it would reduce the control of arrhythmias by disopyramide is unknown, but monitor the effects and, where possible, the serum levels of disopyramide if phenobarbital is added or withdrawn. The manufacturer of disopyramide[2] recommends avoiding using it in combination with inducers of the cytochrome P450 subfamily CYP3A, such as phenobarbital. Other **barbiturates** would be expected to interact similarly.

1. Kapil RP, Axelson JE, Mansfield IL, Edwards DJ, McErlane B, Mason MA, Lalka D, Kerr CR. Disopyramide pharmacokinetics and metabolism: effect of inducers. *Br J Clin Pharmacol* (1987) 24, 781–91.
2. Rythmodan Capsules (Disopyramide). Sanofi. UK Summary of product characteristics, August 2013.

Disopyramide + Phenytoin

Serum disopyramide levels are reduced by phenytoin and may fall below therapeutic levels.

Clinical evidence

Eight patients with ventricular tachycardia taking disopyramide 600 mg to 2 g daily had a 54% fall in their serum disopyramide levels (from a mean of 3.99 micrograms/mL to 1.82 micrograms/mL) when they were also given phenytoin 200 to 600 mg daily for a week. Two of the patients who responded to disopyramide and underwent Holter monitoring had a 53- and 2000-fold increase in ventricular premature beat frequency as a result of this interaction.[1]

In other reports, 3 patients who had low levels of disopyramide and high levels of its metabolite were noted to be taking phenytoin,[2] and one patient taking phenytoin required an unusually high dose of disopyramide.[3] A marked fall in serum disopyramide levels (75% in one case) was seen in 2 patients who took phenytoin 300 to 400 mg daily for up to 2 weeks.[4] Pharmacokinetic studies[3,5] in a total of 12 healthy subjects confirm this interaction. In addition, one healthy patient with epilepsy, taking phenytoin, had a disopyramide AUC and elimination half-life that were 50% lower than those in control subjects.[5]

Mechanism

Phenytoin, which is a known enzyme-inducer, increases the metabolism of the disopyramide by the liver. Although the major metabolite (*N*-dealkyldisopyramide) also possesses antiarrhythmic activity, the net effect is a reduction in arrhythmic control.[1]

Importance and management

The interaction between disopyramide and phenytoin is established and of clinical importance. Some loss of arrhythmic control can occur during concurrent use. Disopyramide adverse effects (e.g. dry mouth, blurred vision, urinary retention and nausea), because of the potential for high metabolite levels, and the antiarrhythmic response should be well monitored. An increase in the dose of disopyramide may be necessary. The interaction appears to resolve fully within 2 weeks of withdrawing the phenytoin. Note that the manufacturer of disopyramide[6] recommends avoiding using it in combination with inducers of the cytochrome P450 subfamily CYP3A, such as phenytoin.

1. Matos JA, Fisher JD, Kim SG. Disopyramide-phenytoin interaction. *Clin Res* (1981) 29, 655A.
2. Aitio M-L, Vuorenmaa T. Enhanced metabolism and diminished efficacy of disopyramide by enzyme induction? *Br J Clin Pharmacol* (1980) 9, 149–152.
3. Nightingale J, Nappi JM. Effect of phenytoin on serum disopyramide concentrations. *Clin Pharm* (1987) 6, 46–50.
4. Kessler JM, Keys PW, Stafford RW. Disopyramide and phenytoin interaction. *Clin Pharm* (1982) 1, 263–4.
5. Aitio M-L, Mansury L, Tala E, Haataja M, Aitio A. The effect of enzyme induction on the metabolism of disopyramide in man. *Br J Clin Pharmacol* (1981) 11, 279–85.
6. Rythmodan Capsules (Disopyramide). Sanofi. UK Summary of product characteristics, August 2013.

Disopyramide + Quinidine

Disopyramide serum levels may be slightly raised by quinidine. Both drugs prolong the QT interval, and this effect may be additive on combined use.

Clinical evidence, mechanism, importance and management

In a study in 16 healthy subjects, quinidine 200 mg four times daily increased the peak serum levels of a single 150-mg dose of disopyramide by 20% from 2.68 micrograms/mL to 3.23 micrograms/mL. The effect was smaller (14%) when disopyramide 150 mg four times daily was given. Serum quinidine levels were decreased by 26%. However, there was no change in the half-life of either drug. Both quinidine and disopyramide caused a slight lengthening of the QTc interval, and when quinidine was added to disopyramide additional lengthening of the QT interval occurred. The frequency of adverse effects such as dry mouth, blurred vision, urinary retention and nausea were also somewhat increased.[1]

The mechanism of the effect on serum levels is not understood. If both drugs are given, the antimuscarinic adverse effects of disopyramide may be increased; consider decreasing the disopyramide dose if these are troublesome. Disopyramide and quinidine are both class Ia antiarrhythmics that prolong the QT interval, and, in general, such combinations should be avoided (see also 'Drugs that prolong the QT interval + Other drugs that prolong the QT interval', p.272).

1. Baker BJ, Gammill J, Massengill J, Schubert E, Karin A, Doherty JE. Concurrent use of quinidine and disopyramide: evaluation of serum concentrations and electrocardiographic effects. *Am Heart J* (1983) 105, 12–15.

Disopyramide + Rifampicin (Rifampin)

The plasma levels of disopyramide can be reduced by rifampicin.

Clinical evidence

In a study in 11 patients with tuberculosis, rifampicin for 14 days approximately halved the plasma levels of a single 200- or 300-mg dose of disopyramide.[1] The disopyramide AUC was reduced by about two-thirds and the half-life was reduced from 5.9 to 3.25 hours. A woman who had been taking rifampicin for 2 weeks started taking disopyramide 100 mg every 8 hours but only achieved a subtherapeutic level of 0.9 micromol/L. The dose of disopyramide was increased to 300 mg every 8 hours, and the rifampicin was discontinued. Three days after discontinuing rifampicin the disopyramide level was 3.6 micromol/L and after 5 days it was 8.1 micromol/L. The patient was eventually stabilised taking disopyramide 250 mg every 8 hours.[2]

Mechanism

The most probable explanation is that rifampicin (a well-known enzyme inducer) increases the metabolism of the disopyramide by the liver so that it is cleared from the body much more quickly.

Importance and management

Information seems to be limited to these studies, but they indicate that the dosage of disopyramide will need to be increased in most patients taking rifampicin. Note that the manufacturer of disopyramide[3] recommends avoiding using it in combination with inducers of the cytochrome P450 subfamily CYP3A, such as rifampicin.

1. Aitio M-L, Mansury L, Tala E, Haataja M, Aitio A. The effect of enzyme induction on the metabolism of disopyramide in man. *Br J Clin Pharmacol* (1981) 11, 279–85.
2. Staum JM. Enzyme induction: rifampin-disopyramide interaction. *DICP Ann Pharmacother* (1990) 24, 701–3.
3. Rythmodan Capsules (Disopyramide). Sanofi. UK Summary of product characteristics, August 2013.

Disopyramide + Verapamil

Profound hypotension and collapse has occurred in a small number of patients taking verapamil who were also given disopyramide.

Clinical evidence, mechanism, importance and management

A group of clinicians who had used single 400-mg oral doses of disopyramide successfully and with few adverse effects for reverting acute supraventricular arrhythmias, reported 5 cases of profound hypotension and collapse. Three of the patients developed severe epigastric pain. All 5 had previous myocardial disease and/or were taking myocardial depressants, either beta blockers or verapamil in small quantities [not specified].[1]

On the basis of this report, reports of studies in *animals*,[2] and from the known risks associated with the concurrent use of beta blockers (see 'Disopyramide + Beta blockers', p.267), the UK manufacturer warns about combining disopyramide and other drugs [such as verapamil] that may have additive negative inotropic effects.[3] However, they do point out that in some specific circumstances combinations of antiarrhythmic drugs may be beneficial; they specifically name verapamil for the control of atrial fibrillation).[3] However, the US manufacturer advises that until more data is available, disopyramide should not be given within 48 hours before or 24 hours after verapamil.[4]

1. Manolas EG, Hunt D, Dowling JT, Luxton M, Vohra J. Collapse after oral administration of disopyramide. *Med J Aust* (1979) 1, 20.
2. Lee JT, Davy J-M, Kates RE. Evaluation of combined administration of verapamil and disopyramide in dogs. *J Cardiovasc Pharmacol* (1985) 7, 501–7.
3. Rythmodan Capsules (Disopyramide). Sanofi. UK Summary of product characteristics, August 2013.
4. Norpace (Disopyramide). Pfizer Inc. US Prescribing information, September 2006.

Dofetilide + Antacids

Antacids (aluminium/magnesium hydroxide) appear not to interact with dofetilide.

Clinical evidence, mechanism, importance and management

A study in 12 healthy subjects found that pretreatment with **aluminium/magnesium hydroxide** (*Maalox*) 30 mL, given 10 hours, 2 hours and 0.5 hours before dofetilide, did not affect the pharmacokinetics of a single 500-microgram dose of dofetilide, or the dofetilide-induced change in QTc interval.[1] No special precautions appear to be necessary.

1. Vincent J, Gardner MJ, Baris B, Willavize SA. Concurrent administration of omeprazole and antacid does not alter the pharmacokinetics and pharmacodynamic of dofetilide in healthy subjects. *Clin Pharmacol Ther* (1996) 59, 182.

Dofetilide + Diuretics

Hydrochlorothiazide and hydrochlorothiazide/triamterene modestly increase dofetilide plasma exposure. Concurrent use increased the QT interval prolongation seen with dofetilide alone.

Clinical evidence

The manufacturer notes that the concurrent use of dofetilide 500 micrograms twice daily with **hydrochlorothiazide** 50 mg daily for 7 days increased the dofetilide AUC by 14% and increased the QTc interval by 48 milliseconds.[1] Similar results were seen with the same dose of dofetilide given with **hydrochlorothiazide/triamterene** 50/100 mg daily (18% increase in AUC, and 38 millisecond increase in QTc).[1]

Mechanism

Triamterene might be expected to increase dofetilide plasma levels by competing for its renal tubular secretion (see 'Dofetilide + Miscellaneous', p.271), but the effect of its combination with hydrochlorothiazide was no greater than with hydrochlorothiazide alone. Why hydrochlorothiazide should increase dofetilide levels is unclear. An increase in dofetilide levels would be expected to increase the QT interval, but the increase seen here was much greater than expected by the change in plasma levels. The manufacturer suggests that a reduction in serum potassium could have contributed to the extent of QT prolongation.[1] This makes sense for hydrochlorothiazide (a potassium-depleting diuretic), but the combination with triamterene (a potassium-sparing diuretic) might therefore have been expected to have less effect on the QT interval.

Importance and management

On the basis of the above findings, the manufacturer contraindicates the use of dofetilide with hydrochlorothiazide alone or in combination with triamterene.[2] Given the increase in QT interval, a risk factor for torsade de pointes, this appears a prudent precaution. Further study is needed. Any diuretic that depletes serum potassium (such as the **loop diuretics**) might be expected to increase the risk of QT prolongation and torsade de pointes with dofetilide, and serum potassium should be monitored.[2]

1. Pfizer Global Pharmaceuticals. Personal Communication, June 2004.
2. Tikosyn (Dofetilide). Pfizer Labs. US Prescribing information, November 2006.

Dofetilide + H_2-receptor antagonists

Cimetidine markedly increases plasma dofetilide levels, and increases dofetilide-induced QT prolongation and the risk of torsade de pointes. Dofetilide appears not to interact with ranitidine.

Clinical evidence

A placebo-controlled study in 24 healthy subjects found that **cimetidine** 400 mg twice daily given with dofetilide 500 micrograms twice daily for 7 days decreased the renal clearance of dofetilide by 44%, increased its AUC by 58%, and increased its peak blood levels by 50%, without significantly altering the QTc interval.[1] In a further study it was found that **cimetidine** 100 mg twice daily or 400 mg twice daily for 4 days reduced the renal clearance of a single 500-microgram dose of dofetilide by 13% and 33%, respectively. In addition, the respective **cimetidine** doses increased the QTc interval by 22% and 33%. Conversely, **ranitidine** 150 mg twice daily did not significantly affect the pharmacokinetics or pharmacodynamics of dofetilide.[2]

Mechanism

At least 50% of a dofetilide dose is eliminated unchanged in the urine by an active renal tubular secretion mechanism.[3,4] Drugs that inhibit this mechanism, such as cimetidine, increase dofetilide plasma levels.[2,3] There is a linear relationship between plasma dofetilide concentrations and prolongation of the QT interval, which increases the risk of torsade de pointes.[3]

Importance and management

An established interaction. Because of the likely increased risk of torsade de pointes, the manufacturer contraindicates the use of cimetidine in patients taking dofetilide. This would seem to be a prudent precaution. This applies equally to cimetidine at non-prescription doses, and patients taking dofetilide should be warned to avoid this. No special precautions appear to be necessary with ranitidine.

1. Vincent J, Gardner MJ, Apseloff G, Baris B, Willavize S, Friedman HL. Cimetidine inhibits renal elimination of dofetilide without altering QTc activity on multiple dosing in healthy subjects. *Clin Pharmacol Ther* (1998) 63, 210.
2. Abel S, Nichols DJ, Brearly CJ, Eve MD. Effect of cimetidine and ranitidine on pharmacokinetics and pharmacodynamics of a single dose of dofetilide. *Br J Clin Pharmacol* (2000) 49, 64–71.
3. Tikosyn (Dofetilide). Pfizer Labs. US Prescribing information, November 2006.
4. Rasmussen HS, Allen MJ, Blackburn KJ, Butrous GS, Dalrymple HW. Dofetilide, a novel class III antiarrhythmic agent. *J Cardiovasc Pharmacol* (1992) 20 (Suppl 2), S96–S105.

Dofetilide + Ketoconazole

Ketoconazole markedly increases the plasma levels of dofetilide. This is likely to be associated with an increased risk of dofetilide-induced QT prolongation and torsade de pointes.

Clinical evidence

The manufacturer of dofetilide notes that ketoconazole 400 mg daily, given with dofetilide 500 micrograms twice daily for 7 days, increased the dofetilide peak levels by 53% in men and 97% in women, and increased the AUC by 41% in men and 69% in women.[1] Ketoconazole decreased the renal clearance of dofetilide by 31% and the non-renal clearance by 40%, resulting in a reduction in total clearance of 35%.[2]

Mechanism

Ketoconazole may inhibit the active renal tubular secretion mechanism by which dofetilide is eliminated, so reducing its loss from the body.[1,2] Ketoconazole also inhibits the metabolism of dofetilide[2] by the cytochrome P450 isoenzyme CYP3A4. Both of these mechanisms contribute to the increase in dofetilide plasma levels. There is a linear relationship between plasma dofetilide concentrations and prolongation of the QT interval, which increases the risk of torsade de pointes.[1]

Importance and management

An established interaction. Because of the likely increased risk of torsade de pointes, the manufacturer contraindicates the use of ketoconazole in patients taking dofetilide. This would seem to be a prudent precaution.

1. Tikosyn (Dofetilide). Pfizer Labs. US Prescribing information, November 2006.
2. Tikosyn (Dofetilide). Pfizer US Pharmaceuticals. Product monograph, March 2002.

Dofetilide + Miscellaneous

The manufacturer of dofetilide cautions about the use of various drugs that may have the potential to increase dofetilide plasma concentrations, so increasing the risk of QT prolongation and arrhythmias. Use with other drugs that prolong the QT interval should be avoided.

Clinical evidence, mechanism, importance and management

(a) Drugs that affect renal secretion

At least 50% of a dofetilide dose is eliminated unchanged in the urine by an active renal tubular secretion mechanism.[1,2] Some drugs that inhibit this mechanism have been shown to increase dofetilide plasma concentrations (e.g. see 'Dofetilide + H_2-receptor antagonists', p.270). The manufacturer contraindicates their concurrent use since there is a linear relationship between plasma dofetilide concentrations and prolongation of the QT interval, which is a risk factor for torsade de pointes.[1] The manufacturer also contraindicates the use of other drugs that may inhibit the renal mechanism by which dofetilide is eliminated, such as **prochlorperazine** and **megestrol**,[1] although these have not been directly studied. Furthermore, the manufacturer suggests[1] that there is a potential for dofetilide plasma concentrations to be increased by other drugs undergoing active renal secretion (e.g. **amiloride**, **metformin** and **triamterene**), but this needs confirmation in direct studies (see also 'Dofetilide + Diuretics', p.270). Until then, these drugs should be used cautiously with dofetilide.

(b) Inhibitors of hepatic metabolism

Dofetilide is partially metabolised by the liver, primarily by the cytochrome P450 isoenzyme CYP3A4.[3] The manufacturer suggests[1] that there is a potential for dofetilide plasma concentrations to be increased by inhibitors of CYP3A4, and this has been shown for ketoconazole (see 'Dofetilide + Ketoconazole', p.270). They recommend caution with other CYP3A4 inhibitors and specifically name **macrolides**, **azoles**, **HIV-protease inhibitors**, **amiodarone**, **diltiazem**, **grapefruit juice**, and **nefazodone**. They also name **SSRIs**, **cannabinoids**, **norfloxacin**, **quinine** and **zafirlukast**, but with the exception of the SSRI **fluvoxamine** (and possibly **fluoxetine**), these drugs do not usually appear to cause clinically relevant interactions by this mechanism.

(c) Other drugs that prolong the QT interval

Dofetilide is a class III antiarrhythmic that prolongs the QT interval and can cause torsade de pointes arrhythmia. In general, use of two or more drugs that prolong the QT interval should be avoided. See also 'Drugs that prolong the QT interval + Other drugs that prolong the QT interval', p.272.

(d) Other drugs

Studies in healthy subjects have shown that **amlodipine**, **glibenclamide**, and **HRT** (**conjugated oestrogens** plus **medroxyprogesterone**) do not affect the pharmacokinetics of dofetilide.[1] The pharmacokinetics of **propranolol** 40 mg twice daily and **oral contraceptives** are not affected by dofetilide.[1]

1. Tikosyn (Dofetilide). Pfizer Inc. US prescribing information, November 2006.
2. Rasmussen HS, Allen MJ, Blackburn KJ, Butrous GS, Dalrymple HW. Dofetilide, a novel class III antiarrhythmic agent. *J Cardiovasc Pharmacol* (1992) 20 (Suppl 2), S96–S105.
3. Walker DK, Alabaster CT, Congrave GS, Hargreaves MB, Hyland R, Jones BC, Reed LJ, Smith DA. Significance of metabolism in the disposition and action of the antidysrhythmic drug, dofetilide. *In vitro* studies and correlation with *in vivo* data. *Drug Metab Dispos* (1996) 24, 447–55.

Dofetilide + Omeprazole

Omeprazole appears not to interact with dofetilide.

Clinical evidence, mechanism, importance and management

A study in 12 healthy subjects found that pretreatment with omeprazole 40 mg (10 or 2 hours before dofetilide) did not affect the pharmacokinetics of a single 500-microgram dose of dofetilide or the dofetilide-induced change in QTc interval.[1] No special precautions appear to be necessary.

1. Vincent J, Gardner MJ, Baris B, Willavize SA. Concurrent administration of omeprazole and antacid does not alter the pharmacokinetics and pharmacodynamic of dofetilide in healthy subjects. *Clin Pharmacol Ther* (1996) 59, 182.

Dofetilide + Phenytoin

The concurrent use of dofetilide and phenytoin does not affect the pharmacokinetics of either drug.

Clinical evidence, mechanism, importance and management

In a placebo-controlled study, 24 healthy subjects were given phenytoin, to achieve steady-state plasma levels of 8 to 20 micrograms/mL, and then dofetilide 500 micrograms twice daily. No changes in phenytoin pharmacokinetics or cardiac effects were seen.[1] Another study by the same researchers in 24 subjects given dofetilide 500 micrograms every 12 hours found that phenytoin 300 mg daily did not have a clinically important effect on either the pharmacokinetics of dofetilide or on its cardiovascular pharmacodynamics (QTc, PR, QRS, RR intervals).[2] These findings confirm those of an *in vitro* study[3] showing that dofetilide did not inhibit the cytochrome P450 isoenzyme CYP2C9, thus suggesting that dofetilide is unlikely to affect the metabolism of phenytoin. No additional precautions therefore seem necessary on concurrent use.

1. Vincent J, Gardner M, Scavone J, Ashton H, Willavize S, Friedman HL. The effect of dofetilide on the steady-state PK and cardiac effects of phenytoin in healthy subjects. *Clin Pharmacol Ther* (1997) 61, 233.
2. Gardner MJ, Ashton HM, Willavize SA, Friedman HL, Vincent J. The effects of phenytoin on the steady-state PK and PD of dofetilide in healthy subjects. *Clin Pharmacol Ther* (1997) 61, 205.
3. Walker DK, Alabaster CT, Congrave GS, Hargreaves MB, Hyland R, Jones BC, Reed LJ, Smith DA. Significance of metabolism in the disposition and action of the antidysrhythmic drug, dofetilide. *In vitro* studies and correlation with *in vivo* data. *Drug Metab Dispos* (1996) 24, 447–55.

Dofetilide + Theophylline

The concurrent use of theophylline and dofetilide does not appear to affect the pharmacokinetics of either drug.

Clinical evidence, mechanism, importance and management

Studies in healthy subjects found that the concurrent use of theophylline 450 mg every 12 hours and dofetilide 500 micrograms every 12 hours did not alter the steady-state pharmacokinetics of either drug.[1,2] In addition, the increase in the QTc interval was no greater with the combination than with dofetilide alone.[1] No additional precautions appear to be necessary if both drugs are given. Aminophylline does not appear to have been studied, but it would be expected to behave in much the same way as theophylline.

1. Gardner MJ, Ashton HM, Willavize SA, Vincent J. The effects of concomitant dofetilide therapy on the pharmacokinetics and pharmacodynamics of theophylline. *Clin Pharmacol Ther* (1996) 59, 181.
2. Gardner MJ, Ashton HM, Willavize SA, Vincent J. The effects of orally administered theophylline on the pharmacokinetics and pharmacodynamics of dofetilide. *Clin Pharmacol Ther* (1996) 59, 182.

Dofetilide + Trimethoprim

Trimethoprim markedly increases the plasma levels of dofetilide. This is likely to be associated with an increased risk of dofetilide-induced QT prolongation and torsade de pointes.

Clinical evidence, mechanism, importance and management

The manufacturer of dofetilide notes that trimethoprim 160 mg (in combination with sulfamethoxazole 800 mg) twice daily given with dofetilide 500 micrograms twice daily for 4 days increased the peak levels of dofetilide by 93% and increased its AUC by 103%.[1] Trimethoprim inhibits the active renal tubular secretion mechanism by which dofetilide is eliminated, so reducing its loss from the body. There is a linear relationship between plasma dofetilide concentrations and prolongation of the QT interval, which increases the risk of torsade de pointes.[1] For this reason, the manufacturer contraindicates the use of trimethoprim in patients taking dofetilide. This would seem to be a prudent precaution.

1. Tikosyn (Dofetilide). Pfizer Labs. US Prescribing information, November 2006.

Dofetilide + Verapamil

Verapamil transiently increases dofetilide plasma levels and QTc prolongation, and has been associated with an increased risk of torsade de pointes.

Clinical evidence

A study in 12 healthy subjects found that verapamil 80 mg three times daily given with dofetilide 500 micrograms twice daily for 3 days caused a 42% increase in the peak plasma levels of dofetilide (from 2.4 nanograms/mL to 3.43 nanograms/mL). There was a 26% increase in the AUC_{0-4}, which was associated with a transient simultaneous increase in the QTc interval of 20 milliseconds for dofetilide alone and 26 milliseconds for the combination. However, the AUC_{0-8} was not significantly different.[1] The manufacturer notes that an analysis of clinical study data for dofetilide revealed a higher occurrence of torsade de pointes when verapamil was used with dofetilide.[2]

Mechanism

Verapamil is postulated to interact with dofetilide by increasing its rate of absorption by increasing hepatic blood flow.[1] There is a linear relationship between plasma dofetilide concentrations and prolongation of the QT interval, which is a risk factor for torsade de pointes.[2]

Importance and management

The use of verapamil with dofetilide appears to be associated with a transient increase in dofetilide plasma concentrations, and an increased risk of torsade de pointes. For this reason, the combination is contraindicated.

1. Johnson BF, Cheng SL, Venitz J. Transient kinetic and dynamic interactions between verapamil and dofetilide, a class III antiarrhythmic. *J Clin Pharmacol* (2001) 41, 1248–56.
2. Tikosyn (Dofetilide). Pfizer Labs. US Prescribing information, November 2006.

Dronedarone + Miscellaneous

CYP3A4 inhibitors (such as ketoconazole) appear to increase dronedarone exposure, whereas inducers of CYP3A4 (such as rifampicin (rifampin)) appear to decrease dronedarone exposure. Dronedarone increases the exposure to nisoldipine and nifedipine, and other calcium-channel blockers are predicted to be similarly affected. Dronedarone increases the exposure to digoxin, and other P-glycoprotein substrates are predicted to be similarly affected. Dronedarone is also predicted to increase the exposure to CYP2D6 substrates. Additive bradycardia and cardiac depression can occur with the concurrent use of dronedarone and digoxin, diltiazem, or verapamil. Pantoprazole and losartan do not appear to affect the pharmacokinetics of dronedarone, and dronedarone does not appear to affect the pharmacokinetics of hormonal contraceptives, theophylline, or losartan.

Clinical evidence, mechanism, importance and management

(a) Calcium-channel blockers

1. Dihydropyridines. Many dihydropyridine calcium-channel blockers are substrates for CYP3A4, of which dronedarone is an inhibitor, and it would therefore be expected to increase their exposure: dronedarone 400 mg twice daily increased the exposure of **nisoldipine** (by 50%[1]), and **nifedipine** exposure has also been increased (no figure stated).[2] **Nifedipine** 20 mg twice daily has also been seen to cause a negligible increase in dronedarone exposure (of about 20%),[1] which would not be expected to be clinically relevant. In clinical studies, 13% of patients received dronedarone and calcium-channel blockers, with no increase in hypotension, bradycardia, or heart failure.[1]

No dose adjustment of these calcium-channel blockers is therefore expected to be necessary on concurrent use with dronedarone.

2. Diltiazem and verapamil. Dronedarone is primarily metabolised by CYP3A4, and its exposure was increased by 70% by **diltiazem** 240 mg twice daily, and by 40% by **verapamil** 240 mg daily, both of which inhibit CYP3A4.[1] Dronedarone is also a CYP3A4 inhibitor, and when given at a dose of 400 mg twice daily, it increased the exposure to **verapamil** by about 40%.[1,2] Note that additive bradycardia and cardiac depression could also occur with the concurrent use of dronedarone and calcium-channel blockers that affect heart rate, such as **verapamil** or **diltiazem**. However, in clinical studies, 13% of patients received dronedarone and calcium-channel blockers, with no increase in hypotension, bradycardia, or heart failure.[1] Nevertheless, the UK and US manufacturers of dronedarone advise that calcium-channel blockers with cardiac depressant effects should be started at a low dose in patients taking dronedarone, and the dose should only be increased after an ECG has been checked.[1,2] If dronedarone is started in a patient already taking a calcium-channel blocker, the UK manufacturer advises that a baseline ECG should be carried out and the dose of the calcium-channel blocker should be adjusted if needed.[1]

(b) CYP2D6 substrates

Dronedarone is an inhibitor of CYP2D6 and as such might increase the exposure to drugs metabolised by this route. This has been seen with metoprolol, although the effect was only weak to moderate; see 'Beta blockers + Dronedarone', p.1009 for details.

(c) CYP3A4 inducers

Dronedarone is primarily metabolised by CYP3A4, and **rifampicin** (**rifampin**) 600 mg daily has been reported to decrease dronedarone exposure by 80%. The UK and US manufacturers of dronedarone therefore advise that the concurrent use of **rifampicin** and other inducers of CYP3A4 should be avoided.[1,2] For a list of CYP3A4 inducers, see 'Table 1.9', p.11.

(d) CYP3A4 inhibitors

1. Grapefruit juice. Grapefruit juice (repeated 300-mL quantities) increased the AUC and maximum plasma concentration of dronedarone 3-fold and 2.5-fold, respectively,[1] and the UK and US manufacturers state that it should be avoided in patients taking dronedarone.[1,2]

2. Moderate inhibitors. The AUC and maximum plasma concentration of dronedarone were increased 3.8-fold and about 3-fold, respectively, by **erythromycin** 500 mg three times daily for 10 days.[1,2] Other moderate CYP3A4 inhibitors are predicted to interact similarly,[1] see 'Table 1.9', p.11 for a list, but note that diltiazem and verapamil, which are moderate CYP3A4 inhibitors, only had slight effects on the pharmacokinetics of dronedarone (see *Calcium-channel blockers*, above) . Note also that the concurrent use of erythromycin with dronedarone is contraindicated because of the risk of torsade de pointes.[1,2]

3. Potent inhibitors. The AUC and maximum plasma concentration of dronedarone were increased 17-fold and 9-fold, respectively, by repeated doses of **ketoconazole** 200 mg daily.[1] Dronedarone is primarily metabolised by CYP3A4, of which ketoconazole is a potent inhibitor, and concurrent use leads to very marked increases in dronedarone exposure. The UK and US manufacturers of dronedarone therefore contraindicate its use with potent CYP3A4 inhibitors (see 'Table 1.9', p.11 for a list of known, clinically relevant CYP3A4 inhibitors).[1,2] In addition to the drugs listed in this table, they name posaconazole and nefazodone as potent inhibitors, however note that these drugs are generally considered moderate CYP3A4 inhibitors and so would be expected to behave more like diltiazem and verapamil (see *Calcium-channel blockers*, above).

(e) Digoxin and other P-glycoprotein substrates

The UK and US manufacturers of dronedarone state that the exposure to digoxin was increased 2.5-fold by dronedarone 400 mg twice daily.[1,2] Digoxin is a substrate of the drug transporter protein P-glycoprotein, which is inhibited by dronedarone. Furthermore, as both drugs can cause bradycardia, additive bradycardia and AV block might possibly occur. Because of this, the manufacturers advise that the need for digoxin should be reviewed:[2] if both drugs are considered necessary, they advise that the digoxin dose should be halved and its plasma concentration monitored closely. The patient should also be monitored for any signs of digoxin adverse effects (e.g. bradycardia).[1,2]

Digoxin can be used as a probe drug to assess the effects of other drugs on P-glycoprotein, and therefore the US manufacturer predicts that dronedarone might increase the concentrations of other P-glycoprotein substrates, see 'Table 1.12', p.14 for a list. For details of the interaction between dronedarone and the P-glycoprotein substrate **dabigatran**, see 'Thrombin inhibitors; Dabigatran + P-glycoprotein inhibitors', p.493.

(f) Hormonal contraceptives

The UK and US manufacturers of dronedarone state that, in healthy subjects, the concentrations of **ethinylestradiol** 30 micrograms and **levonorgestrel** 150 micrograms (given once daily as an oral combined hormonal contraceptive) were not affected by the concurrent use of dronedarone 800 mg twice daily.[1,2]

(g) Other drugs

The UK and US manufacturers of dronedarone state that **pantoprazole** 40 mg daily had no effect on the pharmacokinetics of dronedarone. Dronedarone 400 g twice daily had no effect on the steady-state exposure to **theophylline**.[1,2] No interaction has been reported between **losartan** and dronedarone, and on this basis, the UK manufacturer advises that an interaction with other **angiotensin II receptor antagonists** would not be expected.[1]

1. Multaq (Dronedarone hydrochloride). Sanofi. UK Summary of product characteristics, November 2013.
2. Multaq (Dronedarone). Sanofi-Aventis U.S. LLC. US Prescribing information, March 2014.

Drugs that prolong the QT interval + Drugs that lower potassium concentrations

The combined use of drugs that can cause hypokalaemia (e.g. amphotericin B, beta-agonist bronchodilators, corticosteroids, thiazide and loop diuretics, stimulant laxatives, and theophylline) and drugs that prolong the QT interval (e.g. class Ia and class III antiarrhythmics; see 'Table 9.2', p.273) should be well monitored because hypokalaemia increases the risk of torsade de pointes. There appear to be only a few reports of this interaction, for example, see 'Beta blockers + Potassium-depleting drugs', p.1019. Note that stimulant laxatives only tend to cause hypokalaemia in cases of misuse or overuse.

Drugs that prolong the QT interval + Other drugs that prolong the QT interval

The concurrent use of more than one drug that prolongs the QT interval increases the risk of torsade de pointes, which might lead to life-threatening ventricular arrhythmias. The risk varies with different combinations of drugs that prolong the QT interval, and with the presence of other risk factors for this effect.

Clinical evidence, mechanism, importance and management

If the QT interval on the ECG becomes excessively prolonged, ventricular arrhythmias can develop, in particular a type of polymorphic tachycardia known as torsade de pointes. On the ECG this arrhythmia can appear as an intermittent series of rapid spikes during which the heart fails to pump effectively, the blood pressure falls and the patient will feel dizzy and might lose consciousness. Usually the condition is self-limiting but it might progress and degenerate into ventricular fibrillation, which can cause sudden death.

There are a number of reasons why QT interval prolongation can occur. These include:

- increasing age
- female sex
- congenital long QT syndrome
- cardiac disease
- thyroid disease
- some metabolic disturbances (hypocalcaemia, hypokalaemia, hypomagnesaemia)

Another important cause is the use of various QT-prolonging drugs including some antiarrhythmics, antipsychotics, antihistamines, antimalarials and others.[1,2] These

Table 9.2 Drugs causing QT prolongation and torsade de pointes

High risk	*Some risk*	*Risk not categorised*
Antiarrhythmics, class Ia (ajmaline, cibenzoline, disopyramide, hydroquinidine, procainamide, quinidine)	Amisulpride	Amifampridine (no data but because of the arrhythmogenic potential of amifampridine other drugs that prolong the QT interval are contraindicated)
Antiarrhythmics, class III (amiodarone, azimilide, cibenzoline, dofetilide,† dronedarone, ibutilide,† sotalol†)	Bedaquiline (QTcF interval prolonged by 15.7 to 23.7 milliseconds)	Androgen antagonists (abiraterone, bicalutamide, enzalutamide, flutamide, nilutamide - lack of direct evidence but note, low testosterone concentrations are associated with an increase in the QT interval)
Arsenic trioxide (40% of patients had a QTc interval greater than 500 milliseconds)	Bosutinib (QTcF interval greater than 500 milliseconds reported in some patients, with greater than 60-millisecond increase in 0.9% of patients)	Asenapine (QTc interval increased by 2 to 5 milliseconds with 5 to 20 mg daily; nevertheless some advise caution or avoiding other QT prolonging drugs)
Artemisinin derivatives (artemisinin, artemether/ lumefantrine, artenimol - 5% of patients had an asymptomatic prolongation of QTc intervals by greater than 30 milliseconds, with an actual QTc of greater than 450 milliseconds in males and greater than 470 milliseconds in females)	Chlorpromazine	Atomoxetine (No significant change in QTc interval from baseline in a study; however because of post-marketing reports of QT interval prolongation, some advise caution with other QT prolonging drugs)
Halofantrine†	Citalopram (dose-dependent increase in QTcF interval of 7.5 to 18.5 milliseconds).	Azithromycin (because of post-marketing reports of QT interval prolongation, some advise caution with other QT prolonging drugs)
Haloperidol (risk increased in high doses and with intravenous use)	Crizotinib (QTcF interval greater than 500 milliseconds reported in some patients, with greater than 60-millisecond increase in 5% of patients)	Boceprevir (no effect seen in studies; nevertheless UK manufacturer advises caution with other drugs that prolong the QT interval)
Ketanserin (30% of patients had an increase of greater than 30 milliseconds in a clinical trial)	Dasatinib (increase in QTcF interval of 7 to 13.4 milliseconds)	Clarithromycin (increase in QTc interval of less than 5 milliseconds but because of rare case reports of torsade de pointes some advise caution with other QT prolonging drugs)
Mesoridazine†	Delamanid (QTcF interval increased by 7.6 to 12.1 milliseconds, with greater than 60-millisecond increase in 3% of patients)	Clozapine (because of post-marketing reports of QT interval prolongation, some advise caution with other drugs that prolong the QT interval)
Pimozide†	Dolasetron* (increase in QTcF interval of 14.1 milliseconds, larger increases have been seen in overdose; not all studies have found an increase)	Erythromycin (greater risk with intravenous use)
Sertindole†	Droperidol†	Gonadorelin analogues (buserelin, goserelin, histrelin, leuprorelin, triptorelin - lack of direct evidence but note, low testosterone concentrations are associated with an increase in the QT interval)
Thioridazine†	Eribulin (QTcF interval prolonged by 11.4 milliseconds on day 8 of use)	Gonadorelin antagonists (degarelix - lack of direct evidence but note, low testosterone concentrations are associated with an increase in the QT interval)
Vandetanib (QTcF prolonged by 35 milliseconds, with greater than 60 millisecond increase in QTcF interval in 36% of patients)	Escitalopram (QTcF interval prolonged by 10.7 milliseconds with 30 mg daily)	Lapatinib (small, dose-dependent prolongation of the QTc interval; magnitude not stated)
	Gatifloxacin (increase in QTc interval less than 10 milliseconds)	Lithium (can increase the QT interval particularly if concentrations increased therefore some advise caution with other QT prolonging drugs)
	Iloperidone (12 mg twice daily increased QTc interval by 9 milliseconds; greater increases if metabolism inhibited)	Lofexidine (because of post-marketing reports of QT interval prolongation, some advise caution with other QT prolonging drugs)
	Hydroxyzine	Olanzapine (studies suggest no effect but UK manufacturer advises caution on the basis that other antipsychotics have QT prolonging effects)
	Levomepromazine	Pentamidine (intravenous)
	Methadone (in doses greater than 100 mg)	Quetiapine (the available data neither proves nor disproves an effect, therefore some advise caution with other QT prolonging drugs)
	Moxifloxacin (increase in QTc interval less than 10 milliseconds)	Rilpivirine (dose-related QT-prolongation occurs, which is considered unlikely to be clinically relevant at the recommended dose; however, because of the limited information manufacturers advise caution)
	Nilotinib (QTc interval prolonged by 5 to 15 milliseconds)	
	Ondansetron* (dose-related prolongation of QTcF interval of up to 20 milliseconds)	
	Paliperidone (dose-dependent prolongation of 6.8 to 12.3 milliseconds)	
	Pasireotide (QTcF interval prolongation that equates to a 17.5 millisecond increase over placebo)	
	Pazopanib (QT interval of greater than 500 milliseconds in some patients)	

†indicates drug suspended/restricted in some countries because of this effect

* All 5-HT$_3$-receptor antagonists have been associated with QT-interval prolongation, but the evidence is variable; see 5-HT$_3$-receptor antagonists + Drugs that prolong the QT interval, p.1146.

This list is not exhaustive

Continued

Table 9.2 Drugs causing QT prolongation and torsade de pointes (continued)

High risk	*Some risk*	*Risk not categorised*
	Quinine (greater risk with higher doses and intravenous use)	Risperidone (lack of direct evidence but note, paliperidone is a metabolite of risperidone and so some advise caution with other QT prolonging drugs)
	Ranolazine (dose-related QTc interval prolonged by up to 15 milliseconds, or more if metabolism inhibited)	Sodium stibogluconate (dose-related QT interval prolongation occurs; magnitude not stated, therefore some advise caution with other QT prolonging drugs)
	Romidepsin (QTc interval prolongation of 14.4 milliseconds in lymphoma patients)	Solifenacin (QTcF interval prolonged by 2 milliseconds with a 10 mg dose; however, because of post-marketing reports of QT interval prolongation, some advise caution with other QT prolonging drugs)
	Saquinavir boosted with ritonavir (QTcS interval increased by 18.9 milliseconds with 1 g/100 mg twice daily)	Spiramycin
	Sildenafil (QT interval prolonged by 6 milliseconds with 50 mg dose; not all studies have found an increase)	Sulpiride (because of a few reports of QT interval prolongation, some do not recommend the use of other QT prolonging drugs)
	Sorafenib (QTcF interval prolonged by 9 milliseconds)	Tacrolimus (because of a few reports of QT interval prolongation, some advise caution with other QT prolonging drugs)
	Sparfloxacin (QTcF interval prolonged by 10 milliseconds in clinical studies)	Telavancin (increase in QTc of less than 5 miliseconds, but some advise caution with other QT prolonging drugs)
	Sultopride†	Telithromycin (minimal effects seen in some studies, but others suggest an effect similar to clarithromycin in small proportion of patients)
	Sunitinib (QTcF interval prolonged by 9.6 milliseconds)	Tizanidine (small *in vivo* studies suggest no increase in QT or QTc intervals; however, chronic toxicity studies in *dogs* have resulted in QT prolongation and therefore some advise caution with other QT prolonging drugs)
	Telaprevir (QT interval prolonged by 8 milliseconds)	Trazodone (because of post-marketing reports of QT interval prolongation, some advise caution with other QT prolonging drugs)
	Tolterodine (QTcF interval prolonged by up to 11.8 milliseconds)	Vinflunine (because of a few reports of QT interval prolongation, some do not recommend the use of other QT prolonging drugs)
	Toremifene (Dose-related effect; QT interval prolonged by 21 to 26 milliseconds with 80 mg dose)	Zotepine (dose-related QT prolongation said to occur, magnitude not stated)
	Tricyclics (prolongation of QTc interval greater than 10 milliseconds, most notable risk occurs with clomipramine, risk with other tricyclics largely seems to be in overdose)	Zuclopentixol (appears to cause QT prolongation in overdose; because of the known effects of other antipsychotics, some advise caution with other QT prolonging drugs)
	Vardenafil (QTcF interval prolonged by 8 milliseconds with 10 mg dose)	
	Ziprasidone (QTc interval prolonged by about 10 milliseconds with 160 mg dose)	

† Indicates drug suspended/restricted in some countries because of this effect

* All $5\text{-}HT_3$-receptor antagonists have been associated with QT-interval prolongation, but the evidence is variable; see $5\text{-}HT_3$-receptor antagonists + Drugs that prolong the QT interval, p.1146.

This list is not exhaustive

drugs all appear to cause this effect by blocking the rapid component of the delayed rectifier (repolarisation) potassium channel.

At what degree of prolongation of corrected QT (QTc) interval torsade de pointes is likely to develop is uncertain. However, a QTc interval exceeding 500 milliseconds is generally considered of particular concern, but this is not an exact figure. In addition, there is uncertainty about what constitutes an important change in QTc interval from baseline, although, in general, increases of 30 to 60 milliseconds should raise concern, and increases of over 60 milliseconds raise clear concerns about the potential for arrhythmias. Because of these uncertainties, historically, many drug manufacturers and regulatory agencies contraindicated the concurrent use of drugs known to prolong the QT interval, and a 'blanket' warning was often issued because the QT prolonging effects of the drugs are expected to be additive. However, regulatory guidance developed in 2005,[3,4] provides recommendations for the assessment of risk of a non-antiarrhythmic drug, and in particular outlines the criteria for studying these effects, in what is called a 'Thorough QT/QTc study' which is considered the definitive study design. One of the key criteria of such studies is that it should include use of a positive control, i.e. a drug known to cause an increase in QTc interval of about 5 milliseconds [moxifloxacin is often used for this purpose]. Further, the guidance states that drugs causing an increase in mean QT/QTc interval of around 5 milliseconds or less do not appear to cause torsade de pointes. Data on drugs causing mean increases of around 5 milliseconds and less than 20 milliseconds are inconclusive, and some drugs causing this have been associated with proarrhythmic risk. Drugs with an increase of more than 20 milliseconds have a substantially increased likelihood of being proarrhythmic.[3,4] The extent of the drug-induced prolongation usually depends on the dose of the drug and the particular drugs in question.

'Table 9.2', p.273 is a list of drugs that are known to prolong the QT interval and cause torsade de pointes. Note that this list is not exhaustive of all the drugs that have ever been reported to be associated with QT interval prolongation and torsade de pointes. For some of the drugs listed, QT prolongation is a fairly frequent effect when the drug is used alone, and it is well accepted that use of these drugs requires careful monitoring (e.g. a number of the antiarrhythmics). For other drugs, QT prolongation is rare, but because of the relatively benign indications for these drugs, the risk-benefit ratio is considered poor, and use of these drugs has been severely restricted or discontinued (e.g. astemizole, terfenadine, cisapride). For others there is less clear evidence of the risk of QT prolongation (e.g. clarithromycin, chlorpromazine). Drugs that have only been associated with isolated cases of torsade de pointes, and drugs that are commonly considered to cause QT prolongation, but for which there does not appear to be any published evidence to support this effect (e.g. **chloroquine**), are not usually included in this table. Specific reports of additive QT-prolonging effects with or without torsade de pointes are covered in individual monographs.

Drugs that do not themselves prolong the QT interval, but potentiate the effect of drugs that do (e.g. by pharmacokinetic mechanisms, lowering serum potassium, or by causing bradycardia) are not included in 'Table 9.2', p.273. The interactions of these drugs (e.g. azole antifungals with cisapride, astemizole, or terfenadine, and potassium-depleting diuretics with sotalol) are dealt with in individual monographs. However, note that some drugs, for example the macrolide antibacterials, might cause QT prolongation by dual mechanisms: they appear to have both the intrinsic ability to prolong the QT interval, and they might inhibit the metabolism of drugs that prolong the QT interval.[5]

General references discussing the problems of QT-prolongation are given below.[6-15]

The consensus of opinion is that the concurrent use of drugs that have a high risk of prolonging the QTc interval should be avoided because of the risk of additive effects, leading to the possible development of serious and potentially life-threatening torsade de pointes. However, under certain circumstances (e.g. in the treatment of life-threatening arrhythmias) concurrent use might be unavoidable. In this situation close ECG monitoring, and a careful consideration of other risk factors present is essential. With drugs that have some risk of prolonging the QTc interval, some caution is appropriate, particularly in patients with other risk factors for QTc prolongation.

1. Zeltzer D, Justo D, Halkin A, Prokhorov V, Heller K, Viskin S. Torsade de pointes due to noncardiac drugs. Most patients have easily identifiable risk factors. *Medicine* (2003) 82, 282–90.
2. Benoit SR, Mendelsohn AB, Nourjah P, Staffa JA, Graham DJ. Risk factors for prolonged QTc among US adults: Third National Health and Nutrition Survey. *Eur J Cardiovasc Prev Rehabil* (2005) 12, 363–8.
3. European Medicines Agency. Note for guidance on the clinical evaluation of QT/QTc interval prolongation and proarrhythmic potential for non-antiarrhythmic drugs. November 2005. Available at: http://www.ema.europa.eu/docs/en_GB/document_library/Scientific_guideline/2009/09/WC500002879.pdf (accessed 21/08/15).
4. US Food and Drug Administration. Guidance for Industry: E14 Clinical evaluation of QT/QTc interval prolongation and proarrhythmic potential for non-antiarrhythmic drugs. October 2005. Available at: http://www.fda.gov/downloads/Drugs/GuidanceComplianceRegulatoryInformation/Guidances/ucm073153.pdf (accessed 21/08/15).
5. Shaffer D, Singer S, Korvick J, Honig P. Concomitant risk factors in reports of torsades de pointes associated with macrolide use: review of the United States Food and Drug Administration Adverse Event Reporting System. *Clin Infect Dis* (2002) 35, 197–200.
6. Committee on Safety of Medicines/Medicines Control Agency. Drug-induced prolongation of the QT interval. *Current Problems* (1996) 22, 2.
7. Thomas SHL. Drugs, QT interval abnormalities and ventricular arrhythmias. *Adverse Drug React Toxicol Rev* (1994) 13, 77–102.
8. De Ponti F, Poluzzi E, Montanaro N. QT-interval prolongation by non-cardiac drugs: lessons to be learned from recent experience. *Eur J Clin Pharmacol* (2000) 56, 1–18.
9. Haverkamp W, Breithardt G, Camm AJ, Janse MJ, Rosen MR, Antzelevitch C, Escande D, Franz M, Malik M, Moss A, Shah R. The potential for QT prolongation and pro-arrhythmia by non-anti-arrhythmic drugs: clinical and regulatory implications. Report on a policy conference of the European Society of Cardiology. *Cardiovasc Res* (2000) 47, 219–33.
10. Bednar MM, Harrigan EP, Anziano RJ, Camm AJ, Ruskin JN. The QT interval. *Prog Cardiovasc Dis* (2001) 43 (Suppl 1): 1–45.
11. Kao LW, Furbee RB. Drug-induced Q–T prolongation. *Med Clin North Am* (2005) 89, 1125–44.
12. Glassman AH, Bigger JT. Antipsychotic drugs: prolonged QTc interval, torsade de pointes, and sudden death. *Am J Psychiatry* (2001) 158, 1774–82.
13. Stöllberger C, Huber JO, Finsterer J. Antipsychotic drugs and QT prolongation. *Int Clin Psychopharmacol* (2005) 20, 243–51.
14. Committee on Safety of Medicines/Medicines Control Agency. Risk of QT interval prolongation with methadone. *Current Problems* (2006) 31, 6.
15. Committee on Safety of Medicines/Medicines Control Agency. Cardiac arrhythmias associated with antipsychotic drugs. *Current Problems* (2006) 31, 9.

Flecainide + Amiodarone

Serum flecainide concentrations are increased by amiodarone. An isolated report describes a patient taking amiodarone who developed torsade de pointes when given flecainide.

Clinical evidence

In a study, amiodarone (1.2 g daily for 10 to 14 days then 600 mg daily) was given to 7 patients taking oral flecainide 200 to 500 mg daily. Amiodarone increased the trough plasma concentrations of flecainide by about 50%, and the flecainide dose needed to be reduced by one-third (an average reduction from 325 mg daily to 225 mg daily) to keep the flecainide levels constant. Observations in two patients suggested that the interaction begins soon after the amiodarone is started and takes 2 weeks or more to develop fully.[1] Other authors have also reported this interaction.[2-5] Another study found that amiodarone raised steady-state flecainide plasma levels by 37% in CYP2D6 extensive metabolisers (that is, those with normal levels of this isoenzyme), and by 55% in CYP2D6 poor metabolisers (that is, those lacking this isoenzyme).[6] However, in a later report of this study, the authors concluded that these differences were not clinically important, and that CYP2D6 phenotype does not affect the extent of the interaction between flecainide and amiodarone.[7]

An isolated report describes a patient taking amiodarone who developed torsade de pointes when also given flecainide.[8]

Mechanism

Amiodarone inhibits CYP2D6 by which flecainide is metabolised, resulting in raised flecainide levels. Other mechanisms might also be involved.[7]

Importance and management

The interaction between flecainide and amiodarone is established. The flecainide dose should be reduced by one-third to one-half if amiodarone is added.[1-5,7] Monitor patients closely for flecainide adverse effects (dizziness, nausea, and tremor) and, where possible, consider monitoring flecainide levels. Remember that any interaction could take 2 weeks or more to develop fully, and as amiodarone is cleared from the body slowly, this interaction is likely to persist for some weeks after it has been withdrawn.

1. Shea P, Lal R, Kim SS, Schechtman K, Ruffy R. Flecainide and amiodarone interaction. *J Am Coll Cardiol* (1986) 7, 1127–30.
2. Leclercq JF, Coumel P. La flécaïnide: un nouvel antiarythmique. *Arch Mal Coeur* (1983) 76, 1218–29.
3. Fontaine G, Frank R, Tonet JL. Association amiodarone-flécaïnide dans le traitement des troubles du rythme ventriculaires graves. *Arch Mal Coeur* (1984) 77, 1421.
4. Leclercq JF, Coumel P. Association amiodarone-flécaïnide dans le traitement des troubles du rythme ventriculaires graves. Résponse. *Arch Mal Coeur* (1984) 77, 1421–2.
5. Leclercq JF, Denjoy I, Mentré F, Coumel P. Flecainide acetate dose-concentration relationship in cardiac arrhythmias: influence of heart failure and amiodarone. *Cardiovasc Drugs Ther* (1990) 4, 1161–65.
6. Funck-Brentano C, Kroemer HK, Becquemont L, Bühl K, Eichelbaum M, Jaillon P. The interaction between amiodarone and flecainide is genetically determined. *Circulation* (1992) 86, (Suppl I), I–720.
7. Funck-Brentano C, Becquemont L, Kroemer HK, Bühl K, Knebel NG, Eichelbaum M, Jaillon P. Variable disposition kinetics and electrocardiographic effects of flecainide during repeated dosing in humans: contribution of genetic factors, dose-dependent clearance, and interaction with amiodarone. *Clin Pharmacol Ther* (1994) 55, 256–69.
8. Andrivet P, Beaslay V, Canh VD. Torsades de pointe with flecainide-amiodarone therapy. *Intensive Care Med* (1990) 16, 342–3.

Flecainide + Antiepileptics; Enzyme-inducing

Limited evidence suggests that carbamazepine, phenytoin or phenobarbital might slightly increase flecainide clearance.

Clinical evidence, mechanism, importance and management

Preliminary findings of a controlled study in 6 patients with epilepsy taking **phenytoin** or **phenobarbital** found that the pharmacokinetics of a single 2-mg/kg intravenous dose of flecainide were not generally different from those in a group of 7 healthy subjects not taking these antiepileptics. However, a 25 to 30% shorter flecainide half-life and lower urinary clearance of unchanged drug were noted in the group taking the antiepileptics.[1] The UK manufacturer of flecainide notes there is limited data indicating similar changes in flecainide elimination associated with **carbamazepine**.[2]

These changes are slight and the authors of the first study suggest that an adjustment of the flecainide dose is unlikely to be required in those also taking **phenytoin** or **phenobarbital**. These findings probably also apply to **primidone**, which is, in part, metabolised to phenobarbital, and **fosphenytoin**, a prodrug of phenytoin.

1. Pentikäinen PJ, Halinen MO, Hiepakorpi S, Chang SF, Conard GJ, McQuinn RL. Pharmacokinetics of flecainide in patients receiving enzyme inducers. *Acta Pharmacol Toxicol (Copenh)* (1986) 59 (Suppl 5), 91.
2. Tambocor 50 mg Tablets (Flecainide acetate). Meda Pharmaceuticals. UK Summary of product characteristics, July 2010.

Flecainide + Benziodarone

An isolated case report describes ECG changes in a patient taking flecainide with benziodarone.

Clinical evidence, mechanism, importance and management

A 71-year-old woman who had undergone kidney transplantation 7 years earlier and who was taking many drugs, including ciclosporin, cyclophosphamide and insulin was also taking flecainide, which controlled her paroxysmal atrial fibrillation. Atorvastatin was then restarted for hypercholesterolaemia and benziodarone 100 mg daily (because of intolerance to allopurinol) was added to treat hyperuricaemia. Three days later she presented with asthenia and poor overall condition, and later an ECG showed a number of changes including QTc interval prolongation of 482 milliseconds (22% increase) and PR interval prolongation of 203 milliseconds (18% increase). Creatinine concentrations were about 127 micromol/L, creatine phosphokinase concentrations were 354 units/L and urea concentrations were 155 mg/dL. Atorvastatin was stopped because of mild rhabdomyolysis and flecainide and benziodarone were both discontinued because an interaction was suspected. Symptoms resolved within 48 hours, with the ECG then becoming similar to baseline. Flecainide was restarted and the dose gradually increased to 100 mg daily.[1]

It was suggested that benziodarone might inhibit CYP2D6, which is partly involved in the metabolism of flecainide.[1] Note that benziodarone is chemically related to amiodarone, which has a similar effect, see 'Flecainide + Amiodarone', above. Mild renal impairment in the patient could also have contributed to the reduced flecainide elimination.

This is an isolated case and more study is needed to establish an interaction. Nevertheless, because of its similarities to the effects seen with the chemically related drug amiodarone, it would seem prudent to monitor cardiac effects if flecainide and benziodarone are given concurrently.

1. Gormaz CL, Page JCG, Fuentes FL. Pharmacological interaction between flecainide and benziodarone. *Rev Esp Cardiol* (2003) 56, 631–2.

Flecainide + Cimetidine

Cimetidine increases flecainide plasma concentrations.

Clinical evidence

In a study in 8 healthy subjects, cimetidine 1 g daily for one week increased the AUC of a single 200-mg dose of flecainide by 28%. The fraction of flecainide excreted unchanged in the urine was increased by 20%, but the total renal clearance was not altered.[1] In another study, in 11 patients, cimetidine 1 g daily for 5 days almost doubled the plasma concentrations of flecainide 200 mg daily measured 2 hours after the morning dose.[2]

Mechanism

Uncertain, but the raised flecainide concentrations seen probably occurred because cimetidine, a well-known, non-specific enzyme inhibitor, reduced the metabolism of flecainide (probably by CYP2D6) resulting in its accumulation.

Importance and management

The interaction between flecainide and cimetidine is established, although it is not extensively documented and the clinical outcome does not appear to have been assessed. Nevertheless, it would seem prudent to monitor for flecainide adverse effects (such as dizziness, nausea, and tremor) in patients given cimetidine, and consider the need to reduce the flecainide dose if appropriate. Note that additional caution is recommended in patients with renal impairment, as the interaction is likely to be enhanced.[1]

1. Tjandra-Maga TB, Van Hecken A, Van Melle P, Verbesselt R, De Schepper PJ. Altered pharmacokinetics of oral flecainide by cimetidine. *Br J Clin Pharmacol* (1986) 22, 108–110.
2. Nitsch J, Köhler U, Neyses L, Lüderitz B. Flecainid-Plasmakonzentraionen bei Hemmung des hepatischen Metabolismus durch Cimetidin. *Klin Wochenschr* (1987) 65 (Suppl IX), 250.

Flecainide + Colestyramine

An isolated report describes reduced plasma flecainide concentrations in a patient given colestyramine. However, small studies have not found an interaction.

Clinical evidence, mechanism, importance and management

A patient taking flecainide 100 mg twice daily had unusually low trough plasma concentrations (100 nanograms/mL) while taking colestyramine 4 g three times daily. When he stopped taking the colestyramine his plasma flecainide concentrations rose. However, a later study in 3 healthy subjects given flecainide 100 mg daily and colestyramine 4 g three times daily, found little or no evidence of an interaction: steady-state flecainide levels were 63.1 nanograms/mL and 59.1 nanograms/mL without and with colestyramine, respectively. *In vitro* studies also did not find any binding interaction between flecainide and colestyramine that might result in its reduced absorption from the gut.[1] The authors however suggest that the citric acid contained in the colestyramine formulation might have altered the urinary pH, which could have increased the renal clearance of the flecainide.[1]

Information on a possible interaction between flecainide and colestyramine seems to be limited to this preliminary report. Its general importance seems to be minor. Nevertheless it is generally recommended that other drugs should be given one hour before or 4 to 6 hours after colestyramine and, as the available evidence is so limited, it would seem prudent to continue to follow this recommendation.

1. Stein H, Hoppe U. Is there an interaction between flecainide and cholestyramine? *Naunyn Schmiedebergs Arch Pharmacol* (1989) 339 (Suppl), R114.

Flecainide + Food

The absorption of flecainide is not altered if it is taken with food in adults, but it might be reduced by milk in infants.

Clinical evidence, mechanism, importance and management

In a study in healthy adult subjects, food had no effect on the rate or extent of absorption of a single 200-mg dose of flecainide.[1] A premature baby being treated for refractory atrio-ventricular tachycardia with high doses of flecainide (40 mg/kg daily or 25 mg every 6 hours) developed flecainide toxicity (seen as ventricular tachycardia) when his **milk** feed was replaced by dextrose 5%. His serum flecainide concentrations approximately doubled. It was concluded that the **milk** had reduced flecainide absorption.[2]

Adult patients can take flecainide without regard to meals. **Milk**-fed infants might need their flecainide dose adjusting if **milk** intake is altered, but more study is needed to establish an interaction. Nevertheless, until more is known, it would seem prudent to monitor the effects of altering **milk** intake in infants given flecainide.

1. Tjandra-Maga TB, Verbesselt R, Van Hecken A, Mullie A, De Schepper PJ. Flecainide: single and multiple oral dose kinetics, absolute bioavailability and effect of food and antacid in man. *Br J Clin Pharmacol* (1986) 22, 309–16.
2. Russell GAB, Martin RP. Flecainide toxicity. *Arch Dis Child* (1989) 64, 860–2.

Flecainide + HIV-protease inhibitors

Ritonavir and tipranavir might increase flecainide concentrations. HIV-protease inhibitors boosted with ritonavir are predicted to interact similarly.

Clinical evidence

Direct evidence (from case reports or clinical studies) of an interaction between flecainide and the HIV-protease inhibitors is lacking; however, a review of HIV-protease inhibitor interactions reports that flecainide concentrations might be increased by **ritonavir**.[1]

Mechanism

Flecainide is metabolised by CYP2D6, of which ritonavir is a moderate inhibitor at high doses (500 mg twice daily) and a weak inhibitor at low doses (100 mg twice daily). Ritonavir could therefore increase flecainide concentrations, which might increase the risk of arrhythmias and other adverse effects. *In vitro* **tipranavir** has also been shown to be a CYP2D6 inhibitor,[2] and might also increase flecainide concentrations.

Importance and management

Evidence for an interaction between **ritonavir** and flecainide is limited, but what is predicted to occur is in line with the known pharmacokinetics of these drugs. As a result the manufacturers of ritonavir contraindicate its use with flecainide.[3,4] Similarly, the manufacturers of **tipranavir** contraindicate concurrent use.[2,5]

Other HIV-protease inhibitors are not known to affect CYP2D6. However, ritonavir is commonly used to boost the activity of other HIV-protease inhibitors, and at these low doses might cause small increases flecainide concentrations, the clinical relevance of which is unknown. Until more is known, a cautious approach would be to avoid the concurrent use of flecainide and HIV-protease inhibitors boosted with ritonavir. However, if concurrent use is necessary, monitor patients for an increase in flecainide adverse effects (such as dizziness, nausea, and tremor), adjusting the flecainide dose as necessary. Note that the manufacturers of **fosamprenavir**,[6,7] and **saquinavir**,[8,9] which should both be given with ritonavir, contraindicate the concurrent use of flecainide. Similarly, the UK manufacturer of **indinavir** contraindicates the concurrent use of flecainide, when indinavir is used in combination with ritonavir.[10]

1. Burger DM, Hoetelmans RMW, Koopmans PP, Meenhorst PL, Mulder JW, Hekster YA, Beijnen JH. Clinically relevant drug interactions with antiretroviral agents. *Antivir Ther* (1997) 2, 149–65.
2. Aptivus Soft Capsules (Tipranavir). Boehringer Ingelheim Ltd. UK Summary of product characteristics, December 2011.
3. Norvir Tablets (Ritonavir). AbbVie Ltd. UK Summary of product characteristics, September 2012.
4. Norvir Capsules (Ritonavir). Abbott Laboratories. US Prescribing information, March 2012.
5. Aptivus (Tipranavir). Boehringer Ingelheim Pharmaceuticals, Inc. US Prescribing information, April 2012.
6. Telzir (Fosamprenavir calcium). ViiV Healthcare UK Ltd. UK Summary of product characteristics, May 2011.
7. Lexiva (Fosamprenavir calcium). ViiV Healthcare. US Prescribing information, April 2013.
8. Invirase (Saquinavir mesilate). Roche Products Ltd. UK Summary of product characteristics, October 2013.
9. Invirase (Saquinavir mesylate). Genentech, Inc. US Prescribing information, February 2012.
10. Crixivan (Indinavir sulphate). Merck Sharp & Dohme Ltd. UK Summary of product characteristics, February 2012.

Flecainide + Quinidine or Quinine

Quinidine slightly increases the exposure to flecainide, whereas quinine very slightly increases the exposure to flecainide.

Clinical evidence

(a) Quinidine

In a single-dose study in 6 healthy subjects, a 50-mg oral dose of quinidine given the night before a 150-mg intravenous dose of flecainide decreased the clearance of flecainide by 23%, increased its AUC by 28% and prolonged its half-life by 22%.[1] In another study, 5 patients who were CYP2D6 extensive metabolisers (that is, those with normal amounts of this isoenzyme) taking long-term flecainide were given quinidine 50 mg every 6 hours for 5 days. The plasma concentration and clearance of *S*-(+)-flecainide were unchanged, but the plasma concentrations of *R*-(−)-flecainide increased by about 15% and its clearance was reduced by 15%. The effects of flecainide were increased, but the change was small and not statistically significant.[2]

(b) Quinine

In a study, 10 healthy subjects were given three 500-mg doses of quinine over 24 hours then a single 150-mg intravenous infusion of flecainide (given over 30 minutes). Quinine increased the AUC of flecainide by 21% and reduced its systemic clearance by 17%, whereas its renal clearance remained unchanged. The increases in the PR and QRS intervals caused by flecainide were increased by quinine, but the change was small and not statistically significant.[3]

Mechanism

Quinidine is known to be a potent inhibitor of CYP2D6, an isoenzyme by which flecainide is partly metabolised, resulting in a decrease in flecainide metabolism and a slight increase in its exposure. The study with quinidine suggests that quinine reduces the metabolism of flecainide, possibly by inhibiting CYP2D6.

Importance and management

The clinical importance of the pharmacokinetic interaction between flecainide and quinidine is uncertain, but it is probably small. However, flecainide blocks sodium channels, and the UK manufacturers do not recommend the concurrent use of other drugs that block sodium channels: one specifically names quinidine.[4]

The clinical importance of the interaction between flecainide and quinine does not appear to have been studied but it is probably small.

1. Munafo A, Buclin T, Tuto D, Biollaz J. The effect of a low dose of quinidine on the disposition of flecainide in healthy volunteers. *Eur J Clin Pharmacol* (1992) 43, 441–3.
2. Birgersdotter UM, Wong W, Turgeon J, Roden DM. Stereoselective genetically-determined interaction between chronic flecainide and quinidine in patients with arrhythmias. *Br J Clin Pharmacol* (1992) 33, 275–80.
3. Munafo A, Reymond-Michel G, Biollaz J. Altered flecainide disposition in healthy volunteers taking quinine. *Eur J Clin Pharmacol* (1990) 38, 269–73.
4. Flecainide acetate. Zentiva. UK Summary of product characteristics, February 2011.

Flecainide + SSRIs

Paroxetine slightly increases the exposure to flecainide and an isolated case report describes raised flecainide concentrations and adverse effects in a patient taking paroxetine. Fluoxetine would be expected to interact similarly. Other SSRIs have also been predicted to increase flecainide exposure.

Clinical evidence

In a study, 21 healthy Korean subjects with differing amounts of CYP2D6 were given **paroxetine** 20 mg daily for 7 days with a single 200-mg dose of flecainide on day 15. Paroxetine slightly increased the AUC of flecainide, by 29%, in the extensive metabolisers (that is, those with normal amounts of CYP2D6), and by 17% in the intermediate metabolisers (those with reduced amounts of CYP2D6), but did not affect the AUC in poor metabolisers (that is, those deficient in CYP2D6), when compared with a single dose of flecainide alone. The pharmacokinetics of flecainide alone did not differ between the different metaboliser groups.[1] A follow-on study by the same authors, found that the mean increase in QTcF interval (Fridericia's correction) resulting from flecainide alone, was further increased by **paroxetine**, but only in the extensive and intermediate metabolisers (by 6.5 milliseconds and 6.7 milliseconds, respectively). No serious adverse effects occurred during this study.[2]

A case report describes a 69-year-old patient who had been stable taking **paroxetine** 40 mg daily for at least 5 years, who developed confusion and paranoia about 2 weeks after starting to take flecainide 100 mg twice daily. On admission she had a flecainide plasma concentration of 1360 micrograms/L (therapeutic range 200 to 1000 micrograms/L). The symptoms resolved 3 days after paroxetine was stopped and the flecainide dose was reduced to 50 mg twice daily.[3]

Mechanism

Flecainide is metabolised by CYP2D6. This route of metabolism can be inhibited by paroxetine, a potent inhibitor of CYP2D6, resulting in an increased exposure to flecainide. CYP2D6 shows genetic polymorphism (see *Genetic factors in drug metabolism*, under 'Drug metabolism interactions', p.4, for further information). This interaction is therefore not apparent in poor metabolisers who are deficient in CYP2D6, but can occur in those with functional amounts of this isoenzyme.

Importance and management

The limited evidence available suggests that a pharmacokinetic interaction occurs between flecainide and **paroxetine**. The slight increase in flecainide exposure would not generally be expected to be of clinical relevance; however, any interaction might be of clinical importance in some patients, such as those with renal impairment. It would seem prudent to be alert for an increase in flecainide adverse effects (such as dizziness, nausea, and tremor) if paroxetine is also given, and consider a flecainide dose reduction, if necessary.

There appears to be no direct evidence for an interaction between flecainide and other SSRIs. **Fluoxetine** also inhibits CYP2D6 and so might be expected to interact in the same way as paroxetine. It would therefore seem prudent to apply similar caution.

Other SSRIs are weaker inhibitors of CYP2D6 than paroxetine (see 'Tricyclic and related antidepressants + SSRIs', p.1515, for the effects of these SSRIs on desipramine, a probe substrate for CYP2D6), and so a clinically relevant pharmacokinetic interaction with flecainide would seem unlikely to occur. Nevertheless, because flecainide has a narrow therapeutic window, until more is known bear the possibility of an interaction in mind should any otherwise unexplained flecainide adverse effects (such as dizziness, nausea, and tremor) occur in patients taking these SSRIs. Consider a flecainide dose reduction, if necessary.

1. Lim KS, Cho J-Y, Jang I-J, Kim B-H, Kim J, Jeon JY, Tae Y-M, Yi S, Eum S, Shin S-G, Yu K-S. Pharmacokinetic interaction of flecainide and paroxetine in relation to the CYP2D6*10 allele in healthy Korean subjects. *Br J Clin Pharmacol* (2008) 66, 660–6.
2. Lim KS, Jang I-J, Kim B-H, Kim J, Jeon J-Y, Tae Y-M, Yi S, Eum S, Cho J-Y, Shin S-G, Yu K-S. Changes in the QTc interval after administration of flecainide acetate, with and without coadministered paroxetine, in relation to cytochrome P450 2D6 genotype: data from an open-label, two-period, single-sequence crossover study in healthy Korean male subjects. *Clin Ther* (2010) 32, 659–66.
3. Tsao YY, Gugger JJ. Delirium in a patient with toxic flecainide plasma concentrations: the role of a pharmacokinetic drug interaction with paroxetine. *Ann Pharmacother* (2009) 43, 1366–9.

Flecainide + Thiazide diuretics

An isolated report describes cardiotoxicity in a patient taking flecainide, which was associated with an electrolyte imbalance caused by bendroflumethiazide.

Clinical evidence, mechanism, importance and management

A patient taking **bendroflumethiazide** developed syncope, weakness and fatigue 2 months after starting flecainide. He also had ECG changes (marked QRS widening) and gross hyponatraemia and hypokalaemia, which were consistent with flecainide cardiotoxicity exacerbated by electrolyte disturbances. The symptoms resolved when the electrolyte balance was corrected.[1]

Flecainide acts by a use-dependent block of sodium channels and hypertonic sodium salts have been used to reverse flecainide toxicity. Data in *animals* suggest flecainide might reduce salt absorption in the bowel.[1] This case report suggests hyponatraemia as well as hypokalaemia could contribute to flecainide toxicity.

Although this appears to be the only report of an interaction, it serves as a reminder that electrolytes should be carefully controlled in patients taking flecainide, and this is particularly important when other drugs that can cause electrolyte disturbances, such as the thiazides, are given.

1. Khavandi A, Walker PR. Flecainide cardiotoxicity precipitated by electrolyte imbalance. Caution with thiazide diuretics. *Emerg Med J* (2007) 24, e26.

Flecainide + Tobacco

Tobacco smokers need larger doses of flecainide than non-smokers to achieve the same therapeutic effects.

Clinical evidence

The chance observation that smokers appeared to have a reduced pharmacodynamic response to flecainide than non-smokers, prompted a meta-analysis[1] of the findings of 7 pre-marketing pharmacokinetic studies and 5 multicentre efficacy studies in which flecainide had been studied and in which the smoking habits of the subjects or patients had been also been recorded. In the pharmacokinetic studies, the clearance of flecainide was found to be about 50% higher in smokers than in non-smokers. In the efficacy studies, average clinically effective flecainide doses were found to be 338 mg daily for smokers and 288 mg daily for non-smokers, while trough plasma concentrations of flecainide were 1.74 nanograms/mL and 2.18 nanograms/mL, per mg dose, for the smokers and non-smokers, respectively. This confirmed that smokers needed higher doses of flecainide to achieve the same steady-state serum levels.[1]

Mechanism

In vitro, CYP1A2 has been shown to be involved in the metabolism of flecainide.[2] Tobacco smoke is a known inducer of CYP1A2 activity, so it is possible that the effects seen are a result of increased flecainide metabolism by this route.

Importance and management

The interaction between flecainide and tobacco is established. Smokers are likely to need higher doses of flecainide than non-smokers, but the way in which this interaction was identified suggests that in practice no specific action needs to be taken to accommodate it. It might be most relevant if a patient taking flecainide abruptly stops smoking. In this situation be alert for flecainide adverse effects (such as dizziness, nausea, tremor), and be aware that it is likely that the dose of flecainide will need to be reduced.

1. Holtzman JL, Weeks CE, Kvam DC, Berry DA, Mottonen L, Ekholm BP, Chang SF, Conard GJ. Identification of drug interactions by meta-analysis of premarketing trials: the effect of smoking on the pharmacokinetic and dosage requirements for flecainide acetate. *Clin Pharmacol Ther* (1989) 46, 1–8.
2. Doki K, Homma M, Kiga K, Aonuma K, Kohda Y. Effects of CYP2D6 genotypes on age-related change of flecainide metabolism: involvement of CYP1A2-mediated metabolism. *Br J Clin Pharmacol* (2009) 68, 89–96.

Flecainide + Urinary acidifiers or alkalinisers

The excretion of flecainide is increased if the urine is made acidic (e.g. with ammonium chloride) and reduced if the urine is made alkaline (e.g. with sodium bicarbonate).

Clinical evidence

Six healthy subjects were given a single 300-mg oral dose of flecainide on two occasions. On the first occasion flecainide was taken after **ammonium chloride** 1 g orally every 3 hours, and 2 g at bedtime, for a total of 21 hours to make the urine acidic (pH range 4.4 to 5.4). On the second occasion flecainide was taken after **sodium bicarbonate** 4 g every 4 hours for a total of 21 hours (including night periods) to make the urine alkaline (pH range 7.4 to 8.3). Over the next 32 hours, 44.7% of unchanged flecainide appeared in the acidic urine, but only 7.4% in alkaline urine.[1] This compares with 25% found by other researchers when urinary pH was not controlled.[1] A later similar study from the same research group broadly confirmed these findings; the elimination half-life of the flecainide was 10.7 hours in acidic urine and 17.6 hours in alkaline urine.[2] Another study also confirmed the effect of urinary pH on the excretion of flecainide, and found that the fluid load and the urinary flow rate had little effect on flecainide excretion.[3]

In a study in healthy adult subjects, three 15-mL doses of *Aldrox* (280 mg of **aluminium hydroxide** per 5 mL) had no effect on the rate or extent of absorption of a single 200-mg dose of flecainide.[4]

Mechanism

In alkaline urine at pH 8, much of the flecainide exists in the renal tubules in the non-ionised form (non-ionised fraction 0.04), which is more readily reabsorbed. In acidic urine at pH 5 more exists in the ionised form (non-ionised fraction 0.0001), which is less readily reabsorbed and is therefore lost in the urine.[3]

Importance and management

The interaction between flecainide and urinary acidifiers or alkalinisers is established, but its clinical importance is uncertain. The effects of these changes on the subsequent control of arrhythmias by flecainide in patients seem not to have been studied, but the outcome should be well monitored if patients are given drugs that considerably alter urinary pH (such as ammonium chloride, sodium bicarbonate or **acetazolamide**).

Large doses of some antacids might interact in the same way but one study suggests that aluminium hydroxide possibly does not interact. For a list of antacids and their effect on urinary pH, see 'Quinidine + Antacids or Urinary alkalinisers', p.293.

1. Muhiddin KA, Johnston A, Turner P. The influence of urinary pH on flecainide excretion and its serum pharmacokinetics. *Br J Clin Pharmacol* (1984) 17, 447–51.
2. Johnston A, Warrington S, Turner P. Flecainide pharmacokinetics in healthy volunteers: the influence of urinary pH. *Br J Clin Pharmacol* (1985) 20, 333–8.
3. Hertrampf R, Gundert-Remy U, Beckmann J, Hoppe U, Elsäßer W, Stein H. Elimination of flecainide as a function of urinary flow rate and pH. *Eur J Clin Pharmacol* (1991) 41, 61–3.
4. Tjandra-Maga TB, Verbesselt R, Van Hecken A, Mullie A, De Schepper PJ. Flecainide: single and multiple oral dose kinetics, absolute bioavailability and effect of food and antacid in man. *Br J Clin Pharmacol* (1986) 22, 309–16.

Flecainide + Verapamil

Although flecainide and verapamil have been used together successfully, serious and potentially life-threatening cardiogenic shock and asystole have been seen in a few patients, because the cardiac depressant effects of the two drugs can be additive.

Clinical evidence

A man with triple coronary artery disease taking flecainide 200 mg daily for recurrent ventricular tachycardia, developed severe cardiogenic shock within 2 days of increasing the flecainide dose to 300 mg daily and within one day of starting verapamil 80 mg daily. His blood pressure fell to 60/40 mmHg and he had an idioventricular rhythm of 88 bpm.[1] Another patient with atrial flutter and fibrillation was given digitalis and verapamil 120 mg three times daily. He was also given flecainide 150 mg daily for 10 days, but 3 days after the dose was increased to 200 mg daily he fainted, and later developed severe bradycardia (15 bpm) and asystoles of up to 14 seconds. He later died.[1] A further report describes atrioventricular block when a patient with a pacemaker took digoxin, flecainide and verapamil.[2]

Two earlier studies in patients[3] and healthy subjects[4] had found that the pharmacokinetics of flecainide and verapamil were only minimally affected by concurrent use, but the PR interval was increased by both drugs. Furthermore, additive depressant effects were seen on heart contractility and AV conduction, although no serious adverse responses occurred.

Mechanism

Flecainide and verapamil have little or no effects on the pharmacokinetics of each other,[3,4] but they can have additive depressant effects on the heart (negative inotropic and chronotropic) in both patients and healthy subjects.[1,3,4] Verapamil alone[5,6] and flecainide alone[7,8] have been responsible for asystole and cardiogenic shock in a few patients. In the cases cited above[1-3] the cardiac depressant effects were particularly serious because the patients already had compromised cardiac function.

Importance and management

The interaction between flecainide and verapamil is established, but the incidence of serious adverse effects is probably not great. The additive cardiac depressant effects are probably of little importance in many patients, but could represent 'the last straw' in a few who have seriously compromised cardiac function. The authors of one of the reports cited[1] advise careful monitoring if both drugs are used and emphasise the potential hazards of combining **class Ic antiarrhythmics** and verapamil.

1. Buss J, Lasserre JJ, Heene DL. Asystole and cardiogenic shock due to combined treatment with verapamil and flecainide. *Lancet* (1992) 340, 546.
2. Tworek DA, Nazari J, Ezri M, Bauman JL. Interference by antiarrhythmic agents with function of electrical cardiac devices. *Clin Pharm* (1992) 11, 48–56.
3. Landau S, Hogan C, Butler B, Somberg J. The combined administration of verapamil and flecainide. *J Clin Pharmacol* (1988) 28, 909.
4. Holtzman JL, Finley D, Mottonen L, Berry DA, Ekholm BP, Kvam DC, McQuinn RL, Miller AM. The pharmacodynamic and pharmacokinetic interaction between single doses of flecainide acetate and verapamil: effects on cardiac function and drug clearance. *Clin Pharmacol Ther* (1989) 46, 26–32.
5. Perrot B, Danchin N, De La Chaise AT. Verapamil: a cause of sudden death in a patient with hypertrophic cardiomyopathy. *Br Heart J* (1984) 51, 532–4.
6. Cohen IL, Fein A, Nabi A. Reversal of cardiogenic shock and asystole in a septic patient with hypertrophic cardiomyopathy on verapamil. *Crit Care Med* (1990) 18, 775–6.
7. Forbes WP, Hee TT, Mohiuddin SM, Hillman DE. Flecainide-induced cardiogenic shock. *Chest* (1988) 94, 1121.
8. Echt DS, Liebson PR, Mitchell LB, Peters RW, Obias-Manno D, Barker AH, Arensberg D, Baker A, Friedman L, Greene HL, Huther ML, Richardson DW, CAST investigators. Mortality and morbidity in patients receiving encainide, flecainide or placebo. *N Engl J Med* (1991) 324, 781–8.

Ibutilide + Amiodarone

Two reports describe the successful use of ibutilide and amiodarone for cardioversion. Both ibutilide and amiodarone can prolong the QT interval, and concurrent use would be expected to result in additive effects.

Clinical evidence, mechanism, importance and management

Intravenous ibutilide 2 mg has been used for cardioversion of atrial fibrillation or flutter in 70 patients taking long-term amiodarone. The QT interval was further prolonged (from 371 to 479 milliseconds). Only one patient had an episode of non-sustained torsade de pointes. Ibutilide was effective within 30 minutes of infusion in 39% of patients with atrial flutter, and 54% of patients with fibrillation.[1] A further report also found the use of ibutilide in 46 patients receiving amiodarone for atrial flutter and fibrillation as effective and safe as use of ibutilide alone (in 28 patients).[2]

The authors of one report[1] suggest that ibutilide may be useful for cardioversion in those already taking amiodarone. However, it is generally recommended that the concurrent use of two drugs that prolong the QT interval should be avoided. The manufacturer of ibutilide specifically recommends that other class III antiarrhythmics should not be given within 4 hours of an ibutilide infusion, and that ibutilide should not be given within five half-lives of these antiarrhythmics.[3] The concern is that a prolongation of the QT interval is associated with an increased risk of torsade de pointes, which is potentially life-threatening. See 'Drugs that prolong the QT interval + Other drugs that prolong the QT interval', p.272.

1. Glatter K, Yang Y, Chatterjee K, Modin G, Cheng J, Kayser S, Scheinman MM. Chemical cardioversion of atrial fibrillation or flutter with ibutilide in patients receiving amiodarone therapy. *Circulation* (2001) 103, 253–7.
2. Fragakis N, Papadopoulos N, Papanastasiou S, Kozirakis M, Maligkos G, Tsaritsaniotis E, Katsaris G. Efficacy and safety of ibutilide for cardioversion of atrial flutter and fibrillation in patients receiving amiodarone or propafenone. *Pacing Clin Electrophysiol* (2005) 28, 954–61.
3. Corvert (Ibutilide fumarate). Pharmacia & Upjohn. US Prescribing information, February 2006.

Ibutilide + Calcium-channel blockers

Calcium-channel blockers (predominantly non-dihydropyridine type) have not altered the safety or efficacy of ibutilide in clinical studies.

Clinical evidence, mechanism, importance and management

Retrospective analysis of three clinical studies found that calcium-channel blockers did not alter the ECG effects (QT prolongation) or the efficacy of ibutilide. In these three studies, 68 of the 130 patients taking ibutilide were also taking calcium-channel blockers. The report did not specify which calcium-channel blockers were used, except to say that only 12 of the 68 (19%) were taking a dihydropyridine-type.[1]

In vitro studies have shown that **nifedipine** (a dihydropyridine) attenuated the effects of ibutilide.[2] The findings of the above report[1] suggest that this may not be clinically important. However, since so few patients were taking a dihydropyridine, an effect specific to dihydropyridines cannot be excluded. Further study is needed.

1. Wood MA, Gilligan DM, Brown-Mahoney C, Nematzadeh F, Stambler BS, Ellenbogen KA. Clinical and electrophysiologic effects of calcium channel blockers in patients receiving ibutilide. *Am Heart J* (2002) 143, 176–80.
2. Lee KS, Lee EW. Ionic mechanism of ibutilide in human atrium: evidence for a drug-induced Na^+ current through a nifedipine inhibited inward channel. *J Pharmacol Exp Ther* (1998) 286, 9–22.

Ibutilide + Class Ic antiarrhythmics

Some evidence suggests that patients taking ibutilide have a less marked increase in QT interval, without a change in efficacy, when they are also given propafenone or flecainide.

Clinical evidence, mechanism, importance and management

The increase in QTc interval after intravenous ibutilide 2 mg was less in patients taking **propafenone** (5 patients) or **flecainide** (1 patient) than in 85 other patients who had taken ibutilide alone (34 milliseconds versus 65 milliseconds). The effect appeared to be dose-related, with higher propafenone doses causing the largest attenuation in the ibutilide-induced QT prolongation. The efficacy of ibutilide was unaltered.[1] In another study, 71 patients with atrial fibrillation or atrial flutter receiving either **propafenone** 300 to 900 mg daily or **flecainide** 100 to 300 mg daily underwent cardioversion with a single intravenous dose of ibutilide 1 mg over 10 minutes, followed if necessary by a further dose after an interval of 10 minutes. Torsade de pointes occurred in one patient with profound sinus node suppression after cardioversion, but the mean increase in the QT interval in response to ibutilide was attenuated (20 ± 54 milliseconds compared to reported range of 47 to 90 milliseconds) without a decrease in efficacy. However, the authors note that the risk of sustained torsade de pointes in this study appears to be similar to that seen in other studies of ibutilide.[2] In a further study in 100 patients with atrial fibrillation, undergoing elective cardioversion with either intravenous ibutilide (1 mg with a further 1 mg if required), or oral **propafenone** 600 mg plus intravenous ibutilide, cardioversion was achieved in 41% of 51 patients given ibutilide alone and about 71% of 49 patients given ibutilide and **propafenone**. Increases in the QTc interval were similar in both groups, but one case of torsade de pointes requiring electrical cardioversion occurred in one patient given ibutilide and **propafenone**.[3] A further report also found that the use of ibutilide in 30 patients receiving **propafenone** for atrial flutter and fibrillation was as effective and safe as use of ibutilide alone (in 28 patients).[4]

Ibutilide, a class III antiarrhythmic, is known to increase the QT interval, so increasing the risk of torsade de pointes. Class Ic antiarrhythmics such as **propafenone** and **flecainide** generally shorten the QT interval. It is possible that class Ic antiarrhythmics may usefully attenuate the risk of torsade de pointes with ibutilide,[1] and ibutilide may be useful in restoring sinus rhythm in patients taking class Ic antiarrhythmics.[2,3] However, the cases of torsade de pointes add a note of caution, and further study is needed.

1. Reiffel JA, Blitzer M. The actions of ibutilide and class Ic drugs on the slow sodium channel: new insights regarding individual pharmacologic effects elucidated through combination therapies. *J Cardiovasc Pharmacol Ther* (2000) 5, 177–81.
2. Hongo RH, Themistoclakis S, Raviele A, Bonso A, Rossillo A, Glatter A, Yang Y, Scheinman MM. Use of ibutilide in cardioversion of patients with atrial fibrillation or atrial flutter treated with Class IC agents. *J Am Coll Cardiol* (2004) 44, 864–8.
3. Korantzopoulos P, Kolettis TM, Papathanasiou A, Naka KK, Kolios P, Leontaridis I, Draganigos A, Katsouras CS, Goudenvenos JA. Propafenone added to ibutilide increases conversion rates of persistent atrial fibrillation. *Heart* (2006) 92, 631–4.
4. Fragakis N, Papadopoulos N, Papanastasiou S, Kozirakis M, Maligkos G, Tsaritsaniotis E, Katsaris G. Efficacy and safety of ibutilide for cardioversion of atrial flutter and fibrillation in patients receiving amiodarone or propafenone. *Pacing Clin Electrophysiol* (2005) 28, 954–61.

Ibutilide + Miscellaneous

Ibutilide can prolong the QT interval, therefore caution has been advised about the concurrent use of other drugs that can do the same. Ibutilide is reported not to interact with beta blockers or digoxin.

Clinical evidence, mechanism, importance and management

No specific drug interaction studies appear to have been undertaken with ibutilide, which is a class III antiarrhythmic, but because it can prolong the QT interval it has been recommended that other drugs that can do the same should be administered with caution, because of the potential additive effects.[1] The manufacturer of ibutilide[2] specifically recommends that class Ia and other class III antiarrhythmics should not be given within 4 hours of an ibutilide infusion, and that ibutilide should not be given within five half-lives of these antiarrhythmics (but see also, 'Ibutilide + Amiodarone', p.278). The concern is that a prolongation of the QT interval is associated with an increased risk of torsade de pointes, which is potentially life-threatening. The manufacturer of ibutilide specifically names **phenothiazines**, **tricyclic** and **tetracyclic antidepressants**, and **antihistamines**.[2] For further discussion of QT prolongation, and for further examples of drugs that prolong the QT interval, see also 'Drugs that prolong the QT interval + Other drugs that prolong the QT interval', p.272.

The concurrent use of **beta blockers** and **digoxin** during clinical studies is reported not to affect the safety or efficacy of ibutilide;[1,2] however, note that **sotalol** is known to prolong the QT interval.

Ibutilide is said not to affect the cytochrome P450 isoenzymes CYP3A4 or CYP2D6 and so metabolic interactions with drugs affected by these enzymes would not be expected.[1]

1. Cropp JS, Antal EG, Talbert RL. Ibutilide: a new Class III antiarrhythmic agent. *Pharmacotherapy* (1997) 17, 1–9.
2. Corvert (Ibutilide fumarate). Pharmacia & Upjohn. US Prescribing information, February 2006.

Lidocaine + Amiodarone

One man receiving intravenous lidocaine had a seizure about two days after starting to take amiodarone. Another man with sick sinus syndrome taking amiodarone had a sinoatrial arrest during placement of a pacemaker under local anaesthesia with lidocaine. There is conflicting evidence as to whether or not amiodarone affects the pharmacokinetics of intravenous lidocaine.

Clinical evidence

An elderly man taking digoxin, enalapril, amitriptyline and temazepam was treated for monomorphic ventricular tachycardia, firstly with procainamide, later replaced by a 2 mg/minute infusion of lidocaine, to which oral amiodarone 600 mg twice daily was added. After 12 hours his lidocaine concentration was 5.4 mg/L (reference range 1.5 to 5 mg/L), but 53 hours later he developed a seizure and his lidocaine concentration was found to have risen to 12.6 mg/L. A tomography brain scan found no abnormalities that could have caused the seizure and it was therefore attributed to the toxic lidocaine concentrations.[1]

An elderly man with long standing brady-tachycardia was successfully treated for atrial flutter firstly with a temporary pacemaker (later withdrawn) and amiodarone 600 mg daily. Ten days later, and 25 minutes after a permanent pacemaker was inserted under local anaesthesia with 15 mL of 2% lidocaine, severe sinus bradycardia and long sinoatrial arrest developed. He was effectively treated with atropine and isoprenaline, and cardiac massage.[2]

Six patients with symptomatic cardiac arrhythmias took part in a two-phase study. Initially, lidocaine 1 mg/kg was given intravenously over 2 minutes. In phase I, loading doses of amiodarone 500 mg daily for 6 days were given, followed by the same lidocaine dose. After 19 to 21 days, when the total cumulative amiodarone dose was 13 g, the same lidocaine dose was given again (phase II). The lidocaine AUC increased by about 20% and its systemic clearance decreased by about 20%. The elimination half-life and distribution volume at steady-state were unchanged. The pharmacokinetic parameters of lidocaine in phase II were the same as those in phase I, indicating that the interaction occurs early in the loading phase of amiodarone use.[3] This is in contrast with an earlier study, in which the pharmacokinetics of a bolus dose of lidocaine 1 mg/kg over 2 minutes were not altered in 10 patients who had taken amiodarone 200 to 400 mg daily (following a loading dose of 800 or 1200 mg) for 4 to 5 weeks.[4]

Mechanism

An *in vitro* study found that amiodarone might competitively inhibit lidocaine metabolism and *vice versa*. As CYP3A4 is partially involved in the metabolism of lidocaine, the interaction *in vivo* could be due to inhibition of CYP3A4 by amiodarone and/or its main metabolite, desethylamiodarone.[4]

The authors of the report describing the sinoatrial arrest suggest that this occurred because of a synergistic depression of the sinus node by both drugs.

Importance and management

A pharmacokinetic interaction between lidocaine and amiodarone is not established. However, in the study that did find an interaction, the effects were small, and would not be expected to be clinically relevant. The two reports of adverse interactions and the study in patients with arrhythmias illustrate the importance of good monitoring if both drugs are used as there is the possibility of a pharmacodynamic interaction. Furthermore, the manufacturers of some topical lidocaine preparations state that although specific interaction studies of topical lidocaine with class III antiarrhythmics such as amiodarone have not been undertaken, caution and close monitoring is important.[5,6] This might be particularly relevant if large doses of lidocaine are applied.

1. Siegmund JB, Wilson JH, Imhoff TE. Amiodarone interaction with lidocaine. *J Cardiovasc Pharmacol* (1993) 21, 513–15.
2. Keidar S, Grenadier E, Palant A. Sinoatrial arrest due to lidocaine injection in sick sinus syndrome during amiodarone administration. *Am Heart J* (1982) 104, 1384–5.
3. Ha HR, Candinas R, Steiger B, Meyer UA, Follath F. Interactions between amiodarone and lidocaine. *J Cardiovasc Pharmacol* (1996) 28, 533–9.
4. Nattel S, Talajic M, Beaudoin D, Matthews C, Roy D. Absence of pharmacokinetic interaction between amiodarone and lidocaine. *Am J Cardiol* (1994) 73, 92–4.
5. Xylocaine Spray (Lidocaine). AstraZeneca UK Ltd. UK Summary of product characteristics, April 2012.
6. EMLA Cream (Lidocaine with Prilocaine). AstraZeneca UK Ltd. UK Summary of product characteristics, July 2011.

Lidocaine + Atropine

Atropine delays the absorption of lidocaine, reduces its peak plasma concentrations, but does not alter its overall bioavailability.

Clinical evidence, mechanism, importance and management

A study in 4 healthy subjects found that the absorption of a single 400-mg oral dose of lidocaine was delayed when it was given at the same time as intramuscular atropine 600 micrograms (time to maximum plasma concentrations increased from 0.5 hours to 1.5 hours). Peak plasma lidocaine concentrations were reduced by about 30% by atropine, but there was no change in the AUC. Atropine probably delayed lidocaine absorption by inhibition of gastric emptying.[1]

These pharmacokinetic changes are relatively minor, and atropine would not be expected to alter the clinical effects of lidocaine.

1. Adjepon-Yamoah KK, Scott DB, Prescott LF. The effect of atropine on the oral absorption of lidocaine in man. *Eur J Clin Pharmacol* (1974) 7, 397–400.

Lidocaine + Azoles

Itraconazole increases the exposure to *oral* lidocaine, but does not appear to alter the exposure to intravenous or inhaled lidocaine. Other azoles might interact similarly.

Clinical evidence

In a randomised, crossover study, 9 healthy subjects were given either itraconazole 200 mg daily or placebo for 4 days. Itraconazole increased the AUC and peak plasma concentration of a single 1-mg/kg oral dose of lidocaine by 75% and 55%, respectively. Itraconazole did not affect the concentration of the main metabolite of lidocaine, monoethylglycinexylidide (MEGX).[1] In similar studies, itraconazole had no effect on the AUC and peak plasma concentration of lidocaine or MEGX after 1.5-mg/kg intravenous[2] or nebulised[3] dose of lidocaine.

Mechanism

Itraconazole is a potent inhibitor of CYP3A4, which is partially involved in the metabolism of lidocaine. Itraconazole therefore reduces the first-pass metabolism of oral lidocaine so that its plasma concentrations rise.

Importance and management

Information about the pharmacokinetic interaction between itraconazole and lidocaine is limited, and although itraconazole is a potent CYP3A4 inhibitor its effect on *oral* lidocaine appears to be only moderate. In addition, as lidocaine is not usually given orally the practical importance of any interaction is likely to be small. However, lidocaine is used for oro-pharyngeal topical anaesthesia, and there have been cases of toxicity after accidental ingestion. There is also a possibility of accidental oral ingestion during inhalation of lidocaine. In patients taking itraconazole, the toxicity of oral or oro-pharyngeal lidocaine might be increased and so it would seem prudent to be alert for lidocaine adverse effects (such as bradycardia, hypotension, pins and needles). It is likely that other azoles that are also potent inhibitors of CYP3A4 (**ketoconazole** and **voriconazole**) will interact similarly or perhaps have a greater effect, and so similar caution would seem to be appropriate if these drugs are given with oral or oro-pharyngeal lidocaine. **Fluconazole** and **posaconazole** are moderate CYP3A4 inhibitors and therefore they would be expected to interact to a lesser extent, which might not be clinically relevant.

1. Isohanni MH, Neuvonen PJ, Olkkola KT. Effect of erythromycin and itraconazole on the pharmacokinetics of oral lignocaine. *Pharmacol Toxicol* (1999) 84, 143–6.
2. Isohanni MH, Neuvonen PJ, Palkama VJ, Olkkola KT. Effect of erythromycin and itraconazole on the pharmacokinetics of intravenous lignocaine. *Eur J Clin Pharmacol* (1998) 54, 561–5.
3. Isohanni MH, Neuvonen PJ, Olkkola KT. Effect of itraconazole on the pharmacokinetics of inhaled lidocaine. *Basic Clin Pharmacol Toxicol* (2004) 95, 120–3.

Lidocaine + Barbiturates

Plasma lidocaine concentrations following slow intravenous injection might be reduced by phenobarbital and other barbiturates.

Clinical evidence

In a study, 7 patients with epilepsy were given a single 2-mg/kg dose of lidocaine by slow intravenous injection (rate about 100 mg over 15 minutes), while taking their usual antiepileptic drugs and sedatives (including phenytoin, barbiturates, phenothiazines, benzodiazepines), and after taking only **phenobarbital** 300 mg daily for 4 weeks. The same lidocaine dose was also given to 6 control subjects who had not received any other drugs. Plasma lidocaine concentrations achieved during the **phenobarbital** phase were found to be 18% and 29% lower at 30 minutes and 60 minutes, respectively, when compared with those achieved in the control patients. When the patients took their standard antiepileptic treatment, plasma lidocaine concentrations were 27% and 43% lower at 30 minutes and 60 minutes, respectively, when compared with the levels in the 6 control subjects. This suggests that combined treatment caused a greater reduction in lidocaine concentrations than **phenobarbital** alone.[1]

Mechanism

Barbiturates are known inducers of the cytochrome P450 enzyme system and would therefore be expected to increase the rate of lidocaine metabolism, possibly by inducing CYP1A2 and CYP3A4.

Importance and management

Direct information regarding the interaction between lidocaine and the barbiturates is very limited. As the reduction in lidocaine concentrations is small, and as intravenous lidocaine is usually titrated to effect no particular action seems likely to be needed; however, the lidocaine dose required to achieve the desired therapeutic response in patients taking phenobarbital or other barbiturates might be somewhat higher than in subjects not taking barbiturates.

1. Heinonen J, Takki S, Jarho L. Plasma lidocaine levels in patients treated with potential inducers of microsomal enzymes. *Acta Anaesthesiol Scand* (1970) 14, 89–95.

Lidocaine + Beta blockers

The plasma concentrations of lidocaine after intravenous and possibly oral use can be increased by propranolol. Isolated cases of toxicity attributed to this interaction have been reported. Nadolol and penbutolol possibly interact similarly, but there is uncertainty about metoprolol. Atenolol and pindolol do not appear to interact.

Clinical evidence

(a) Atenolol

A study in 7 healthy subjects pretreated with oral atenolol 50 mg daily for one week found that it did not affect the clearance of lidocaine after oral or intravenous use.[1]

(b) Metoprolol

In a study in 6 healthy subjects, pretreatment with metoprolol 100 mg twice daily for 2 days did not affect the pharmacokinetics of a single intravenous dose of lidocaine.[2] Similarly, another study in 7 healthy subjects did not find any changes in the pharmacokinetics of a single oral or intravenous dose of lidocaine after pretreatment with metoprolol 100 mg every 12 hours for one week.[1] In contrast, another study found that the clearance of a single intravenous dose of lidocaine was reduced by 31% by pretreatment with metoprolol 50 mg every 6 hours for one day.[3]

(c) Nadolol

A study in 6 healthy subjects receiving 30-hour infusions of lidocaine at a rate of 2 mg/minute found that pretreatment with nadolol 160 mg daily for 3 days raised the steady-state plasma lidocaine levels by 28% (from 2.1 micrograms/mL to 2.7 micrograms/mL) and reduced its plasma clearance by 17%.[4]

(d) Penbutolol

In a study in 7 healthy subjects, pre-treatment with penbutolol 60 mg daily increased the volume of distribution of a single 100-mg intravenous dose of lidocaine, thus prolonging its elimination half-life. However, the clearance of lidocaine was not affected.[5]

(e) Pindolol

A study in 8 healthy subjects found that pretreatment with intravenous pindolol 23 micrograms/kg did not affect the clearance of intravenous lidocaine.[6]

(f) Propranolol

A study in 6 healthy subjects receiving 30-hour infusions of lidocaine at a rate of 2 mg/minute found that pretreatment with propranolol 80 mg every 8 hours for 3 days raised the steady-state plasma lidocaine concentrations by 19% (from 2.1 micrograms/mL to 2.5 micrograms/mL) and reduced its plasma clearance by 16%.[4] Other similar studies have found a 23 to 30% increase in steady-state serum lidocaine concentrations and a 15 to 46% reduction in its plasma clearance on the concurrent use of propranolol.[3,6,7] Two cases of lidocaine toxicity attributed to an interaction with propranolol[8] were revealed by a search of the adverse drug reaction file of the FDA in the US in 1981. A further case of lidocaine toxicity (seizures) has been described in a man taking propranolol after the accidental *oral* ingestion of lidocaine for oesophageal anaesthesia. High serum concentrations of lidocaine were detected.[9]

(g) Other beta blockers

A matched study in 51 cardiac patients taking a variety of beta blockers (including **propranolol, metoprolol, timolol, pindolol**) found no differences in either total or free concentrations of lidocaine during a lidocaine infusion, but there was a trend towards increased bradycardia with the concurrent use of a beta blocker.[10]

Mechanism

Not fully agreed. There is some debate about whether the increased serum lidocaine concentrations largely occur because of the decreased cardiac output caused by the beta blockers, which decreases the flow of blood through the liver thereby reducing the metabolism of the lidocaine,[4] or because of direct liver enzyme inhibition.[11] An *in vitro* study in *animal* tissue found that propranolol decreased the binding of lidocaine to liver tissue, so that concurrent use might increase the free fraction of lidocaine excreted by the liver. Further study of this *in vitro* model is required.[12] There could also be a pharmacodynamic interaction, with an increased risk of myocardial depression.[10]

Importance and management

The interaction between systemic lidocaine and propranolol is established and possibly of some clinical relevance. It would seem prudent to monitor the effects of concurrent use and be alert for the need to reduce the intravenous lidocaine dose to avoid toxicity; however, note that the UK manufacturer of propranolol states that concurrent use should be avoided.[13]

The situation with other beta blockers is less clear. Nadolol appears to interact with lidocaine in a similar way to propranolol, but it is uncertain whether metoprolol interacts with lidocaine or not. It has been suggested that a higher intravenous loading dose (but not a higher maintenance dose) of lidocaine might be needed if penbutolol is used.[5] Atenolol and pindolol are reported not to cause a pharmacokinetic interaction with lidocaine.

Aside from the pharmacokinetic interactions, a pharmacodynamic interaction between systemic lidocaine and beta blockers resulting in bradycardia and myocardial depressant effects is possible. It would therefore be prudent to monitor the effects of the concurrent use of systemic lidocaine with any beta blocker.

For information regarding the use of lidocaine as a local anaesthetic in patients taking beta blockers, see 'Anaesthetics, local + Beta blockers', p.115.

1. Miners JO, Wing LMH, Lillywhite KJ, Smith KJ. Failure of 'therapeutic' doses of β-adrenoceptor antagonists to alter the disposition of tolbutamide and lignocaine. *Br J Clin Pharmacol* (1984) 18, 853–60.
2. Jordö L, Johnsson G, Lundborg P, Regårdh C-G. Pharmacokinetics of lidocaine in healthy individuals pretreated with multiple dose of metoprolol. *Int J Clin Pharmacol Ther Toxicol* (1984) 22, 312–15.
3. Conrad KA, Byers JM, Finley PR, Burnham L. Lidocaine elimination: effects of metoprolol and of propranolol. *Clin Pharmacol Ther* (1983) 33, 133–8.
4. Schneck DW, Luderer JR, Davis D, Vary J. Effects of nadolol and propranolol on plasma lidocaine clearance. *Clin Pharmacol Ther* (1984) 36, 584–7.
5. Ochs HR, Skanderra D, Abernethy DR, Greenblatt DJ. Effect of penbutolol on lidocaine kinetics. *Arzneimittelforschung* (1983) 33, 1680–1.
6. Svendsen TL, Tangø M, Waldorff S, Steiness E, Trap-Jensen J. Effects of propranolol and pindolol on plasma lignocaine clearance in man. *Br J Clin Pharmacol* (1982) 13, 223S–226S.
7. Ochs HR, Carstens G, Greenblatt DJ. Reduction in lidocaine clearance during continuous infusion and by co administration of propranolol. *N Engl J Med* (1980) 303, 373–7.
8. Graham CF, Turner WM, Jones JK. Lidocaine-propranolol interactions. *N Engl J Med* (1981) 304, 1301.
9. Parish RC, Moore RT, Gotz VP. Seizures following oral lidocaine for esophageal anesthesia. *Drug Intell Clin Pharm* (1985) 19, 199–201.
10. Wyse DG, Kellen J, Tam Y, Rademaker AW. Increased efficacy and toxicity of lidocaine in patients on beta-blockers. *Int J Cardiol* (1988) 21, 59–70.
11. Bax NDS, Tucker GT, Lennard MS, Woods HF. The impairment of lignocaine clearance by propranolol—major contribution from enzyme inhibition. *Br J Clin Pharmacol* (1985) 19, 597–603.
12. Tesseromatis C, Kotsiou A, Tsagataki M, Tigka E, Vovou J, Alevizou A, Perisanidis C, Saranteas T, Karakitsos D, Karabinis A, Kostopanagiotou G. *In vitro* binding of lidocaine to liver tissue under the influence of propranolol: another mechanism of interaction? *Eur J Drug Metab Pharmacokinet* (2007) 32, 213–17.
13. Half-Inderal LA (Propranolol hydrochloride). AstraZeneca UK Ltd. UK Summary of product characteristics, January 2011.

Lidocaine + Ciprofloxacin

Ciprofloxacin appears to slightly increase lidocaine exposure.

Clinical evidence

In a randomised, crossover study, 9 healthy subjects were given ciprofloxacin 500 mg or placebo twice daily for 5 doses. On day 3, they were given intravenous lidocaine 1.5 mg/kg over a 60-minute period, starting 1-hour after the morning dose of ciprofloxacin or placebo. Ciprofloxacin increased the maximum plasma concentration and AUC of lidocaine by 12% and 27%, respectively. The AUCs of the active lidocaine metabolites, monoethylglycinexylidide and 3-hydroxylidocaine, were decreased by 21% and 14%, respectively.[1]

Mechanism

Ciprofloxacin is a moderate inhibitor of CYP1A2, by which lidocaine is partially metabolised. Concurrent use therefore increases lidocaine exposure.

Importance and management

Evidence for an interaction between ciprofloxacin and lidocaine is limited to one study which suggests that ciprofloxacin only slightly increases lidocaine exposure. The clinical relevance of this increase seems likely to be small

1. Isohanni MH, Ahonen J, Neuvonen PJ, Olkkola KT. Effect of ciprofloxacin on the pharmacokinetics of intravenous lidocaine. *Eur J Anaesthesiol* (2005) 22, 795–9.

Lidocaine + Cocaine

Limited evidence suggests intravenous lidocaine use in patients with cocaine-associated myocardial infarction is not associated with major toxicity.

Clinical evidence, mechanism, importance and management

A retrospective study, covering a 6-year period in 29 hospitals, identified 29 patients (27 available for review) who received lidocaine for prophylaxis or treatment of cocaine-associated myocardial infarction. No patients exhibited bradycardia, sustained ventricular tachycardia or ventricular fibrillation, and no patients died.[1]

Both lidocaine and cocaine exhibit class I antiarrhythmic effects and are proconvulsants. Lidocaine could potentiate the cardiac and CNS adverse effects of cocaine. Therefore the use of lidocaine for cocaine-associated myocardial infarction is controversial. The lack of adverse effects in this study might have been due to delays of more than 5 hours between last exposure to cocaine and the use of lidocaine. These authors[1] and others[2,3] consider that the cautious use of lidocaine does not appear to be contraindicated in patients with cocaine-associated myocardial infarction who require an antiarrhythmic. However, extra care should be taken in patients who receive lidocaine shortly after cocaine.[1]

1. Shih RD, Hollander JE, Burstein JL, Nelson LS, Hoffman RS, Quick AM. Clinical safety of lidocaine in patients with cocaine-associated myocardial infarction. *Ann Emerg Med* (1995) 26, 702–6.
2. Derlet RW. More on lidocaine use in cocaine toxicity. *J Emerg Nurs* (1998) 24, 303.
3. Friedman MB. Is lidocaine contraindicated with cocaine? *J Emerg Nurs* (1997) 23, 520.

Lidocaine + Dextromethorphan

Intravenous lidocaine does not affect the pharmacokinetics of dextromethorphan.

Clinical evidence, mechanism, importance and management

Although *in vitro* data suggested that lidocaine inhibited oxidative metabolism reactions mediated by CYP2D6, a later *in vivo* study in 16 patients found that, while being given an infusion of lidocaine (serum concentration in the range of 3.2 to 55.9 micromol/L), the metabolism of a single 30-mg dose of dextromethorphan remained unchanged. All of the patients were CYP2D6 extensive metabolisers (that is, those with normal amounts of this isoenzyme). Note that dextromethorphan can be used as a probe substrate to assess the activity of drugs on CYP2D6, and it was therefore concluded that lidocaine is unlikely to affect the metabolism of drugs that are extensively metabolised by this isoenzyme.[1]

1. Bartoli A, Gatt G, Chimienti M, Corbellini D, Perrucca E. Does lidocaine affect oxidative dextromethorphan metabolism *in vivo*? *G Ital Chim Clin* (1993/4) 18, 125–9.

Lidocaine + Disopyramide

***In vitro* studies suggest that disopyramide can increase the levels of unbound lidocaine, but it is not known whether their combined effects have a clinically important cardiac depressant effect in practice.**

Clinical evidence, mechanism, importance and management

An *in vitro* study using serum taken from 9 patients receiving intravenous lidocaine for severe ventricular arrhythmias found that there was an average 20% increase in the free (unbound) fraction of lidocaine when disopyramide in a concentration of 14.7 micromol/L was added.[1] This appears to occur because disopyramide can displace lidocaine from its binding sites on plasma proteins (alpha-1-acid glycoprotein).

The importance of this possible displacement interaction in clinical practice is uncertain. The suggestion made by the authors[1] is that, although lidocaine has only a minor cardiac depressant effect, a transient 20% increase in the concentrations of free and active lidocaine in association with the negative inotropic effects of disopyramide might possibly be hazardous in patients with reduced cardiac function.

1. Bonde J, Jensen NM, Burgaard P, Angelo HR, Graudal N, Kampmann JP, Pedersen LE. Displacement of lidocaine from human plasma proteins by disopyramide. *Pharmacol Toxicol* (1987) 60, 151–5.

Lidocaine + Fluvoxamine

Fluvoxamine slightly reduces the clearance of intravenous lidocaine. The bioavailability of oral lidocaine is modestly increased by fluvoxamine.

Clinical evidence

In a crossover study, 9 healthy subjects were given fluvoxamine 100 mg daily alone, or with erythromycin 500 mg three times daily for 5 days, with a single *intravenous* dose of lidocaine 1.5 mg/kg on day 6. The clearance of lidocaine was reduced by 41% with fluvoxamine alone, and by 53% with the concurrent use of fluvoxamine and erythromycin.[1] The same study was repeated in 8 healthy subjects, who were given a single *oral* dose of lidocaine 1 mg/kg on day 6. The AUC and peak levels of lidocaine were increased threefold and 2.2-fold, respectively, by fluvoxamine alone, and 3.6-fold and 2.5-fold, respectively, by concurrent fluvoxamine and erythromycin. The half-life of lidocaine was increased by fluvoxamine and fluvoxamine with erythromycin, from 2.4 hours, to 3.1 hours and 3.8 hours, respectively. Fluvoxamine alone and fluvoxamine with erythromycin decreased the peak levels of the main metabolite of lidocaine, monoethylglycinexylidide (MEGX), by 50% and 30%, respectively.[2]

Mechanism

Fluvoxamine is an inhibitor of CYP1A2, by which lidocaine is partially metabolised, and therefore concurrent use results in an increase in lidocaine exposure. Lidocaine is also metabolised by CYP3A4, and an *in vitro* study found that fluvoxamine (a CYP1A2 inhibitor) was a more potent inhibitor of lidocaine metabolism than erythromycin (a CYP3A4 inhibitor).[3] Therefore CYP1A2 inhibition has more of an effect on lidocaine metabolism than CYP3A4 inhibition, and the effects of erythromycin on lidocaine metabolism are additional to those of fluvoxamine.

Importance and management

Information regarding an interaction between *oral* lidocaine and fluvoxamine seems limited, and as lidocaine is not usually given orally, the practical importance is minor. However, lidocaine is used for oro-pharyngeal topical anaesthesia, and there have been cases of toxicity after accidental oral ingestion. Thus, in a patient taking fluvoxamine, the toxicity of lidocaine given or absorbed *orally* could be increased. It would seem prudent to bear the possibility of an interaction in mind should a patient taking fluvoxamine and given oral or oro-pharyngeal lidocaine develop evidence of lidocaine toxicity (such as bradycardia, hypotension, pins and needles).

The evidence for an interaction between *intravenous* lidocaine and fluvoxamine is also limited; however, what is known suggests that the exposure to intravenous lidocaine will only be slightly increased, and any resultant effects possibly not of clinical relevance. However, further study is required to assess the clinical importance of the decrease in the active MEGX metabolite during prolonged intravenous lidocaine infusions.

1. Olkkola KT, Isohanni MH, Hamunen K, Neuvonen PJ. The effect of erythromycin and fluvoxamine on the pharmacokinetics of intravenous lidocaine. *Anesth Analg* (2005) 100, 1352–6.
2. Isohanni MH, Neuvonen PJ, Olkkola KT. Effect of fluvoxamine and erythromycin on the pharmacokinetics of oral lidocaine. *Basic Clin Pharmacol Toxicol* (2006) 99, 168–72.
3. Wang JS, Backman JT, Wen X, Taavitsainen P, Neuvonen PJ, Kivisto KT. Fluvoxamine is a more potent inhibitor of lidocaine metabolism than ketoconazole and erythromycin in vitro. *Pharmacol Toxicol* (1999) 85, 201–5.

Lidocaine + HIV-protease inhibitors

Ritonavir appears to increase lidocaine concentrations more than threefold. Other HIV-protease inhibitors might interact similarly.

Clinical evidence

Direct evidence (from case reports or clinical studies) of an interaction between lidocaine and the HIV-protease inhibitors is lacking; however, a review of HIV-protease inhibitor interactions reported that the plasma concentrations of lidocaine might be increased more than threefold by **ritonavir**.[1] The same review also states that **indinavir**, **nelfinavir** and **saquinavir** might interact similarly.

Mechanism

Lidocaine is partially metabolised by CYP3A4, of which ritonavir is a potent inhibitor. Concurrent use would therefore be expected to raise lidocaine concentrations. All HIV-protease inhibitors are, to varying degrees, inhibitors of CYP3A4, and would therefore be expected to raise lidocaine concentrations.

Importance and management

Evidence for an interaction between lidocaine and HIV-protease inhibitors is limited, but a rise in lidocaine concentrations would be expected from the known pharmacology of these drugs. A threefold increase in lidocaine concentrations would be expected to increase the risk of lidocaine adverse effects, including arrhythmias. If the concurrent use of lidocaine and a HIV-protease inhibitor cannot be avoided, it would seem prudent to monitor the outcome of concurrent use closely for lidocaine adverse effects (such as bradycardia, hypotension, pins and needles), monitoring lidocaine concentrations if possible. Reduce the lidocaine dose as necessary. However, note that the manufacturers of **darunavir**[2] and **saquinavir**[3] contraindicate concurrent use with lidocaine. Similarly, although some manufacturers of **fosamprenavir**,[4] **indinavir**,[5] **nelfinavir**[6] and **tipranavir**[7,8] do not specifically mention lidocaine, they do contraindicate the concurrent use of drugs with a narrow therapeutic range that are metabolised by CYP3A4, which could reasonably be expected to include lidocaine.

1. Burger DM, Hoetelmans RMW, Koopmans PP, Meenhorst PL, Mulder JW, Hekster YA, Beijnen JH. Clinically relevant drug interactions with antiretroviral agents. *Antivir Ther* (1997) 2, 149–165.
2. Prezista (Darunavir ethanolate). Janssen-Cilag Ltd. UK Summary of product characteristics, June 2012.
3. Invirase (Saquinavir mesilate). Roche Products Ltd. UK Summary of product characteristics, October 2013.
4. Telzir (Fosamprenavir calcium). ViiV Healthcare UK Ltd. UK Summary of product characteristics, May 2011.
5. Crixivan (Indinavir sulphate). Merck Sharp & Dohme Ltd. UK Summary of product characteristics, February 2012.
6. Viracept (Nelfinavir mesilate). Roche Products Ltd. UK Summary of product characteristics, June 2012.
7. Aptivus Soft Capsules (Tipranavir). Boehringer Ingelheim Ltd. UK Summary of product characteristics, December 2011.
8. Aptivus (Tipranavir). Boehringer Ingelheim Pharmaceuticals, Inc. US Prescribing information, April 2012.

Lidocaine + H_2-receptor antagonists

Cimetidine slightly reduces the clearance of intravenous and possibly oral lidocaine, and raises its serum concentrations in some patients. Lidocaine toxicity has occurred in some patients. Ranitidine appears to have negligible effects on lidocaine clearance.

Clinical evidence

(a) Cimetidine

In a study, 15 patients were given a 1-mg/kg intravenous loading dose of lidocaine followed by a continuous infusion of 2 or 3 mg/minute over 26 hours. At 6 hours a 300 mg intravenous dose of cimetidine was given, followed by 300 mg orally every 6 hours for 3 doses. After 26 hours (20 hours after cimetidine was started) the serum concentrations of lidocaine were 30% higher (5.6 micrograms/mL) than in a control group of 6 patients (4.3 micrograms/mL). The most substantial rise in concentrations occurred in the first 6 hours after cimetidine was started. Six patients developed toxic serum lidocaine concentrations (over 5 micrograms/mL) and two (with levels of 10 micrograms/mL and 11 micrograms/mL) experienced lethargy and confusion attributed to lidocaine toxicity, which disappeared when the lidocaine was stopped.[1]

In another study, patients with suspected myocardial infarction were given a 2 mg/minute infusion of lidocaine, and then, 11 to 20 hours later, two 300-mg oral doses of cimetidine 4 hours apart. Serum lidocaine concentrations, taken 24 hours after the initial cimetidine dose, had risen by 28%, and unbound levels had risen by 18%. In three of these patients whose diagnosis of myocardial infarction was subsequently confirmed, rises in total and unbound lidocaine serum levels of 24% and 9% occurred.[2] In contrast, a study in 6 patients with suspected myocardial infarction given lidocaine infusions, followed later by a cimetidine infusion, did not show an increase in the plasma concentrations of lidocaine.[3]

Studies in healthy subjects[4,5] have similarly found that oral cimetidine 300 mg four times daily increases the maximum concentrations of intravenous lidocaine (by 50%) and/or decreases its clearance (by 30%), and adverse effects (light-headedness, paraesthesia) developed.[4] However, other studies in healthy subjects have found that cimetidine 300 mg four times daily has no effect on intravenous lidocaine clearance.[6,7]

Cimetidine pretreatment increased the *oral* bioavailability of lidocaine by 35% in healthy subjects, and reduced the apparent clearance by 42%.[8] Another study found that 2 days of cimetidine pretreatment increased the AUC of lidocaine by 52% after the aerosol application of lidocaine 120 mg (12 sprays of *Xylocaine* 10%) to the oropharynx.[9]

An 89-year-old man with congestive heart failure taking oral cimetidine had two seizures 10 to 15 minutes after accidental *oral* ingestion of lidocaine solution for oesophageal anaesthesia. He had a high serum lidocaine level of 7.8 micrograms/mL.[10]

(b) Ranitidine

In a study in 10 healthy subjects, ranitidine 150 mg twice daily for 5 days increased the clearance of an intravenous dose of lidocaine by 9%, but did not alter the clearance of an oral lidocaine dose.[11] In two other studies, ranitidine 150 mg twice daily for one to 2 days did not change the clearance of intravenous lidocaine.[6,12]

Mechanism

Not established. It has been suggested that blockade of H_2-receptors results in reduced blood flow to the liver and that this might partly explain the effect of cimetidine on lidocaine concentrations seen.[1] However, cimetidine is also a well-known non-specific enzyme inhibitor and it is therefore more likely that lidocaine metabolism was reduced by this mechanism, resulting in a reduced clearance and raised serum lidocaine concentrations.

Importance and management

The interaction between intravenous lidocaine and cimetidine is well studied and established, but the effects appear to be small. However, some studies report an increase in the adverse effects of lidocaine when cimetidine is also given. It would therefore seem prudent to monitor patients given lidocaine with cimetidine for evidence of lidocaine toxicity (e.g. bradycardia, hypotension, pins and needles) and, where possible, check lidocaine concentrations. A reduced lidocaine infusion rate might be needed. Ranitidine would appear to be a non-interacting alternative to cimetidine, which might be suitable in some patients. Note that the interaction might possibly be of less importance in patients following a myocardial infarction because of the increased amounts of alpha-1-acid glycoprotein, which alters the concentrations of bound and free lidocaine.[2]

For a discussion on the potential for an interaction between cimetidine and lidocaine, when lidocaine is used as a local anaesthetic, see 'Anaesthetics, local + H_2-receptor antagonists', p.117.

1. Knapp AB, Maguire W, Keren G, Karmen A, Levitt B, Miura DS, Somberg JC. The cimetidine-lidocaine interaction. *Ann Intern Med* (1983) 98, 174–7.
2. Berk SI, Gal P, Bauman JL, Douglas JB, McCue JD, Powell JR. The effect of oral cimetidine on total and unbound serum lidocaine concentrations in patients with suspected myocardial infarction. *Int J Cardiol* (1987) 14, 91–4.
3. Patterson JH, Foster J, Powell JR, Cross R, Wargin W, Clark JL. Influence of a continuous cimetidine infusion on lidocaine plasma concentrations in patients. *J Clin Pharmacol* (1985) 25, 607–9.
4. Feely J, Wilkinson GR, McAllister CB, Wood AJJ. Increased toxicity and reduced clearance of lidocaine by cimetidine. *Ann Intern Med* (1982) 96, 592–4.
5. Bauer LA, Edwards WAD, Randolph FP, Blouin RA. Cimetidine-induced decrease in lidocaine metabolism. *Am Heart J* (1984) 108, 413–15.
6. Jackson JE, Bentley JB, Glass SJ, Fukui T, Gandolfi AJ, Plachetka JR. Effects of histamine-2 receptor blockade on lidocaine kinetics. *Clin Pharmacol Ther* (1985) 37, 544–8.
7. Powell JR, Foster J, Patterson JH, Cross R, Wargin W. Effect of duration of lidocaine infusion and route of cimetidine administration on lidocaine pharmacokinetics. *Clin Pharm* (1986) 5, 993–8.
8. Wing LMH, Miners JO, Birkett DJ, Foenander T, Lillywhite K, Wanwimolruk S. Lidocaine disposition—sex differences and effects of cimetidine. *Clin Pharmacol Ther* (1984) 35, 695–701.
9. Parish RC, Gotz VP, Lopez LM, Mehta JL, Curry SH. Serum lidocaine concentrations following application to the oropharynx: effects of cimetidine. *Ther Drug Monit* (1987) 9, 292–7.
10. Parish RC, Moore RT, Gotz VP. Seizures following oral lidocaine for esophageal anesthesia. *Drug Intell Clin Pharm* (1985) 19, 199–201.
11. Robson RA, Wing LMH, Miners JO, Lillywhite KJ, Birkett DJ. The effect of ranitidine on the disposition of lignocaine. *Br J Clin Pharmacol* (1985) 20, 170–3.
12. Feely J, Guy E. Lack of effect of ranitidine on the disposition of lignocaine. *Br J Clin Pharmacol* (1983) 15, 378–9.

Lidocaine + Macrolides

Erythromycin (a CYP3A4 inhibitor) appears to increase the plasma concentrations of oral and intravenous lidocaine. Other macrolides that inhibit CYP3A4 might interact similarly.

Clinical evidence

In a randomised, crossover study, 9 healthy subjects were given erythromycin 500 mg three times daily or placebo daily for 4 days. Erythromycin increased the AUC and maximum plasma concentration of a single 1-mg/kg *oral* dose of lidocaine by 50% and 40%, respectively. Erythromycin also increased the AUC of the main metabolite of lidocaine, monoethylglycinexylidide (MEGX), by 60%.[1]

In a similar study,[2] erythromycin had no effect on the AUC or maximum plasma concentration of a single 1.5-mg/kg intravenous dose of lidocaine, but increased the AUC of MEGX by 70%. In yet another study, erythromycin ethylsuccinate 600 mg three times daily for 5 doses had a minor effect on the pharmacokinetics of a single 1-mg/kg *intravenous* dose of lidocaine, decreasing the clearance of lidocaine by 18% and increasing the AUC of MEGX by 33%. There was no difference in the results from the 10 healthy subjects and the 20 patients with biopsy proven cirrhosis who were entered into the study.[3]

In another study, 9 healthy subjects were given fluvoxamine 100 mg daily alone or with erythromycin 500 mg three times daily for 5 days, with a single intravenous dose of lidocaine 1.5 mg/kg on day 6. The clearance of lidocaine was reduced 41% by fluvoxamine alone and 53% by concurrent fluvoxamine and erythromycin.[4] The same study was repeated in 8 healthy subjects who were given a single *oral* dose of lidocaine 1 mg/kg on day 6. The AUC and peak levels of lidocaine were increased threefold and 2.2-fold by fluvoxamine and 3.6-fold and 2.5-fold by concurrent fluvoxamine and erythromycin. The half-life of lidocaine was increased by fluvoxamine and fluvoxamine with erythromycin from 2.4 hours, to 3.1 hours and 3.8 hours, respectively. Fluvoxamine alone and fluvoxamine with erythromycin decreased the peak levels of MEGX by 50% and 30%, respectively.[5]

Mechanism

Lidocaine is metabolised by CYP1A2 and CYP3A4. Erythromycin is a moderate inhibitor of CYP3A4, and therefore concurrent use results in a reduction in the first-pass metabolism of *oral* lidocaine and an increase in its plasma concentrations. The increase in the main metabolite monoethylglycinexylidide (MEGX) could be due to either an increase in the production of this metabolite, or inhibition of its further metabolism. From the data with fluvoxamine, given with or without erythromycin, it would appear that lidocaine metabolism is more dependent on CYP1A2 than on CYP3A4.

Importance and management

Information regarding an interaction between *oral* lidocaine and erythromycin seems limited, and as lidocaine is not usually given orally the practical importance is minor. However, lidocaine is used for oro-pharyngeal topical anaesthesia, and there have been cases of toxicity after accidental ingestion. Thus, in a patient taking erythromycin, the toxicity of lidocaine given or absorbed *orally* might be somewhat increased. It would seem prudent to bear the possibility of an interaction in mind should a patient taking erythromycin and given oral or oro-pharyngeal lidocaine develop otherwise unexplained lidocaine toxicity (such as bradycardia, hypotension, pins and needles).

There appears to be more evidence regarding the interaction between *intravenous* lidocaine and erythromycin; however, some studies suggest that no increase in exposure occurs, and in others, only slight pharmacokinetic changes were found. Therefore the increase in *intravenous* lidocaine concentrations would not be expected to be clinically relevant. However, further study is required to assess the clinical importance of the increase in MEGX during prolonged intravenous lidocaine infusions. Other macrolides that also inhibit CYP3A4 (e.g. **clarithromycin** and **telithromycin**) would be expected to interact similarly.

1. Isohanni MH, Neuvonen PJ, Olkkola KT. Effect of erythromycin and itraconazole on the pharmacokinetics of oral lignocaine. *Pharmacol Toxicol* (1999) 84, 143–6.
2. Isohanni MH, Neuvonen PJ, Palkama VJ, Olkkola KT. Effect of erythromycin and itraconazole on the pharmacokinetics of intravenous lignocaine. *Eur J Clin Pharmacol* (1998) 54, 561–5.
3. Orlando R, Piccoli P, De Martin S, Padrini R, Palatini P. Effect of the CYP3A4 inhibitor erythromycin on the pharmacokinetics of lignocaine and its pharmacologically active metabolites in subjects with normal and impaired liver function. *Br J Clin Pharmacol* (2003) 55, 86–93.
4. Olkkola KT, Isohanni MH, Hamunen K, Neuvonen PJ. The effect of erythromycin and fluvoxamine on the pharmacokinetics of intravenous lidocaine. *Anesth Analg* (2005) 100, 1352–6.
5. Isohanni MH, Neuvonen PJ, Olkkola KT. Effect of fluvoxamine and erythromycin on the pharmacokinetics of oral lidocaine. *Basic Clin Pharmacol Toxicol* (2006) 99, 168–72.

Lidocaine + Mexiletine

A case report suggests that mexiletine might increase the toxicity of lidocaine.

Clinical evidence, mechanism, importance and management

A patient with cardiomyopathy taking mexiletine 300 mg twice daily developed lidocaine CNS toxicity within one hour of receiving a total of 600 mg of oral lidocaine for oesophageal burning. Her lidocaine concentration was raised at 26.9 micrograms/mL.[1] Similarly, involuntary motion and muscular stiffness occurred in a man taking oral mexiletine after he received an intravenous infusion of lidocaine for one day.[2] Studies in *animals* have shown that the concurrent use of mexiletine and intravenous lidocaine results in a decrease in the total clearance of lidocaine and an increase in its plasma concentrations. It appeared that this was due to mexiletine displacing the tissue binding of lidocaine and reducing its distribution.[3] Mexiletine is an oral lidocaine analogue, so it is perhaps not surprising the two drugs interact. The combination should be used with caution, especially during the initial stages of treatment. Where possible, lidocaine concentrations should be closely monitored. Note that, when lidocaine is used topically, particularly in large doses, additive systemic toxicity might occur in patients also taking mexiletine and caution with this combination is therefore advised.[4-6]

1. Geraets DR, Scott SD, Ballew KA. Toxicity potential of oral lidocaine in a patient receiving mexiletine. *Ann Pharmacother* (1992) 26, 1380–1.
2. Christie JM, Valdes C, Markowsky SJ. Neurotoxicity of lidocaine combined with mexiletine. *Anesth Analg* (1993) 77, 1291–4.
3. Maeda Y, Funakoshi S, Nakamura M, Fukuzawa M, Kugaya Y, Yamasaki M, Tsukiai S, Murakami T, Takano M. Possible mechanism for pharmacokinetic interaction between lidocaine and mexiletine. *Clin Pharmacol Ther* (2002) 71, 389–97.
4. EMLA Cream (Lidocaine with Prilocaine). AstraZeneca UK Ltd. UK Summary of product characteristics, July 2011.
5. Grunenthal Ltd. UK Summary of product characteristics, December 2011.
6. Xylocaine Spray (Lidocaine). AstraZeneca UK Ltd. UK Summary of product characteristics, April 2012.

Lidocaine + Omeprazole

Omeprazole does not appear to alter the pharmacokinetics of intravenous lidocaine.

Clinical evidence, mechanism, importance and management

In a study in 10 healthy subjects, omeprazole 40 mg daily for one week did not affect the AUC or half-life of a single 1-mg/kg intravenous dose of lidocaine or those of its main metabolite monoethylglycinexylidide (MEGX).[1] This study suggests that no intravenous lidocaine dose adjustment is necessary on the concurrent use of omeprazole.

1. Noble DW, Bannister J, Lamont M, Andersson T, Scott DB. The effect of oral omeprazole on the disposition of lignocaine. *Anaesthesia* (1994) 49, 497–500.

Lidocaine + Opioids

Morphine, given as an intravenous bolus, does not alter the concentrations of lidocaine, given as a continuous intravenous infusion. A case of respiratory depression has been reported when intravenous lidocaine was given to a patient who had been receiving fentanyl and morphine.

Clinical evidence, mechanism, importance and management

A double-blind study in 10 patients who were given continuous lidocaine infusions during a suspected myocardial infarction found that a 10-mg intravenous bolus dose of **morphine sulfate** did not alter the steady-state serum concentrations of lidocaine.[1] However, in one case, respiratory depression occurred within 5 minutes of giving intravenous lidocaine for an episode of ventricular tachycardia in a patient who had been receiving spinal **fentanyl** and **morphine**: the last dose of opioid had been given 4 hours previously. Naloxone successfully reversed this effect.[2] This appears to be an isolated case, and its general relevance is unknown.

For information on the use of opioids with lidocaine given as a local anaesthetic, see 'Opioids + Anaesthetics, local', p.162.

1. Vacek JL, Wilson DB, Hurwitz A, Gollub SB, Dunn MI. The effect of morphine sulfate on serum lidocaine levels. *Clin Res* (1988) 36, 325A.
2. Jensen E, Nader ND. Potentiation of narcosis after intravenous lidocaine in a patient given spinal opioids. *Anesth Analg* (1999) 89, 758–9.

Lidocaine + Phenytoin

The incidence of central toxic adverse effects might be increased by the concurrent intravenous infusion of lidocaine and phenytoin. Sinoatrial arrest has been reported in one patient. Phenytoin might cause small reductions in the concentrations of intravenous lidocaine, but modestly reduce the concentrations of oral lidocaine.

Clinical evidence

A study in 5 patients with suspected myocardial infarction, given lidocaine 0.5 to 3 mg/minute intravenously for at least 24 hours, followed by additional intravenous injections or infusions of phenytoin, found that the plasma concentrations of both drugs remained unchanged but the incidence of adverse effects (vertigo, nausea, nystagmus, diplopia, impaired hearing) were unusually high.[1] However, in another study, lidocaine 2 mg/kg was given intravenously to 7 patients with epilepsy taking their usual antiepileptics (including phenytoin, barbiturates, phenothiazines, benzodiazepines), and to 6 control subjects. Plasma lidocaine concentrations were 27% and 43% lower in the patients at 30 minutes and 60 minutes, respectively.[2] Another study found that the clearance of intravenous lidocaine was slightly greater in patients taking antiepileptics than in healthy subjects (850 mL/minute compared with 770 mL/minute) but this difference was not statistically significant.[3]

Sinoatrial arrest occurred in a man with heart block following a suspected myocardial infarction, after he received intravenous lidocaine 1 mg/kg over one minute, followed 3 minutes later by phenytoin 250 mg given over 5 minutes. The patient lost consciousness and his blood pressure could not be measured, but he responded to a 200-microgram dose of isoprenaline (isoproterenol).[4]

Other studies in patients with epilepsy and healthy subjects have found that phenytoin halves the bioavailability of *oral* lidocaine.[3,5]

Mechanism

Phenytoin and lidocaine appear to have additive cardiac depressant actions. Phenytoin is also a known inducer of the cytochrome P450 enzyme system and could therefore increase the rate of lidocaine metabolism, possibly via CYP1A2 and CYP3A4, resulting in reduced lidocaine concentrations. In addition, patients taking antiepileptics including phenytoin had higher plasma concentrations of alpha-1-acid glycoprotein, which might result in a lower free fraction of lidocaine in the plasma.[6]

Importance and management

Information regarding an interaction between intravenous lidocaine and phenytoin is limited and its importance is not well established. However, the case of sinoatrial arrest emphasises the need to exercise caution when giving two drugs that have cardiac depressant actions.

The reduction in the serum concentrations of intravenous lidocaine in patients taking antiepileptics, including phenytoin, is small and does not appear to be of clinical importance. The reduction in the bioavailability of oral lidocaine is larger, but as lidocaine is not usually given orally, the practical importance of this interaction would also seem to be small.

Note that **fosphenytoin** is a prodrug of phenytoin and would be expected to interact with lidocaine in the same way as phenytoin.

1. Karlsson E, Collste P, Rawlins MD. Plasma levels of lidocaine during combined treatment with phenytoin and procainamide. *Eur J Clin Pharmacol* (1974) 7, 455–9.
2. Heinonen J, Takki S, Jarho L. Plasma lidocaine levels in patients treated with potential inducers of microsomal enzymes. *Acta Anaesthesiol Scand* (1970) 14, 89–95.
3. Perucca E, Richens A. Reduction of oral bioavailability of lignocaine by induction of first pass metabolism in epileptic patients. *Br J Clin Pharmacol* (1979) 8, 21–31.
4. Wood RA. Sinoatrial arrest: an interaction between phenytoin and lignocaine. *BMJ* (1971) i, 645.
5. Perucca E, Hedges A, Makki KA, Richens A. A comparative study of antipyrine and lignocaine disposition in normal subjects and in patients treated with enzyme-inducing drugs. *Br J Clin Pharmacol* (1980) 10, 491–7.
6. Routledge PA, Stargel WW, Finn AL, Barchowsky A, Shand DG. Lignocaine disposition in blood in epilepsy. *Br J Clin Pharmacol* (1981) 12, 663–6.

Lidocaine + Procainamide

An isolated case of delirium has been described in a patient given intravenous lidocaine with procainamide.

Clinical evidence, mechanism, importance and management

A man with paroxysmal tachycardia, taking oral procainamide 1 g every 5 hours and receiving increasing doses of lidocaine by intravenous infusion (550 mg within 3.5 hours), became restless, noisy and delirious when given a further 250 mg intravenous dose of procainamide.[1] The symptoms disappeared within 20 minutes of discontinuing the lidocaine. The reason for this reaction is not understood but the symptoms suggest that the neurotoxic effects of the two drugs might be additive. Other studies in patients have found that lidocaine plasma concentrations are unaffected by intravenous or oral procainamide.[2] If both drugs are given it would be prudent to be alert for CNS adverse effects, and, where possible, consider stopping one of the drugs if these become troublesome.

1. Ilyas M, Owens D, Kvasnicka G. Delirium induced by a combination of anti-arrhythmic drugs. *Lancet* (1969) ii, 1368–9.
2. Karlsson E, Collste P, Rawlins MD. Plasma levels of lidocaine during combined treatment with phenytoin and procainamide. *Eur J Clin Pharmacol* (1974) 7, 455–9.

Lidocaine + Propafenone

Propafenone has negligible effects on the pharmacokinetics of intravenous lidocaine, but the severity and duration of the CNS adverse effects of lidocaine are increased by propafenone.

Clinical evidence, mechanism, importance and management

Twelve healthy subjects, who had been taking propafenone 225 mg every 8 hours for 4 days, were given a continuous infusion of lidocaine 2 mg/kg per hour for 22 hours. Propafenone increased the AUC of lidocaine by 7% and reduced its clearance by 7%. One poor metaboliser of propafenone (that is, a subject lacking CYP2D6) had an increase in lidocaine clearance. Increases in the PR and QRS intervals of 10 to 20% were also seen. Combined use increased the severity and duration of adverse effects (lightheadedness, dizziness, paraesthesia, lethargy, somnolence). One subject withdrew from the study as a result.[1] In another study, the concurrent use of lidocaine (100 mg bolus then a 2 mg/minute infusion) and propafenone (1 or 2 mg/kg infusion) produced a minor additional negative inotropic effect (which was not statistically significant) and reversed the prolongation in atrial and ventricular refractoriness produced by propafenone alone.[2]

There would therefore appear to be no clinically relevant pharmacokinetic interaction between these two drugs, but the increased CNS adverse effects might be poorly tolerated by some individuals, and cardiac depressant effects could also be additive.

1. Ujhelyi MR, O'Rangers EA, Fan C, Kluger J, Pharand C, Chow MSS. The pharmacokinetic and pharmacodynamic interaction between propafenone and lidocaine. *Clin Pharmacol Ther* (1993) 53, 38–48.
2. Feld GK, Nademanee K, Singh BN, Kirsten E. Hemodynamic and electrophysiologic effects of combined infusion of lidocaine and propafenone in humans. *J Clin Pharmacol* (1987) 27, 52–9.

Lidocaine + Rifampicin (Rifampin)

Rifampicin causes a very slight increase in the clearance of intravenous lidocaine.

Clinical evidence, mechanism, importance and management

In a study in 10 healthy subjects, rifampicin 600 mg daily for 6 days increased the clearance of a single 50-mg intravenous dose of lidocaine by 15%. In addition, plasma concentrations of the main metabolite of lidocaine, monoethylglycinexylidide (MEGX), increased by 34%, although this did not reach statistical significance.[1] Using cultured human hepatocytes it was found that rifampicin increases the metabolism of lidocaine, probably because it induces CYP3A4, which is partially concerned with the metabolism of lidocaine to MEGX.[2] These small changes in lidocaine pharmacokinetics are unlikely to be of much clinical importance, particularly as the intravenous lidocaine dose is usually titrated to effect.

1. Reichel C, Skodra T, Nacke A, Spengler U, Sauerbruch T. The lignocaine metabolite (MEGX) liver function test and P-450 induction in humans. *Br J Clin Pharmacol* (1998) 46, 535–9.
2. Li AP, Rasmussen A, Xu L, Kaminski DL. Rifampicin induction of lidocaine metabolism in cultured human hepatocytes. *J Pharmacol Exp Ther* (1995) 274, 673–7.

Lidocaine + Tobacco

Tobacco smoking reduces the bioavailability of oral, but not intravenous, lidocaine.

Clinical evidence, mechanism, importance and management

A study in 9 subjects found that the AUC of lidocaine when given orally, was almost 70% lower in the 4 smokers than in the 5 non-smokers. However, when lidocaine was given intravenously only small differences were seen.[1]

The reduced AUC of oral lidocaine in the smokers probably occurred because tobacco smoke is a known inducer of CYP1A2, the isoenzyme that is partially involved in the metabolism of lidocaine. Tobacco smoke therefore increased the rate of metabolism of lidocaine resulting in increased clearance and reduced exposure. In the case of intravenous lidocaine, the authors suggest that as first-pass metabolism is bypassed, the effect seen might be due to a smoking-related decrease in hepatic blood flow.[1]

In practical terms this interaction is unlikely to be of much clinical importance as lidocaine is not usually given orally.

1. Huet P-M, Lelorier J. Effects of smoking and chronic hepatitis B on lidocaine and indocyanine green kinetics. *Clin Pharmacol Ther* (1980) 28, 208–15.

Mexiletine + Amiodarone

Amiodarone does not affect the clearance of mexiletine.

Clinical evidence, mechanism, importance and management

In a study in 10 patients, the clearance of mexiletine was found to be unchanged when assessed after 1, 3 and 5 months of the concurrent use of amiodarone. In addition, the clearance of mexiletine did not differ between these patients and 155 other patients not taking amiodarone.[1]

Torsade de pointes has been described in a patient taking amiodarone and mexiletine,[2] but the manufacturer of mexiletine previously commented that this seemed to be an isolated case.[3] Note that the two drugs have been used together successfully.[4,5]

Class Ib antiarrhythmics, such as mexiletine, are usually associated with shortening of the QT interval, and could therefore be expected to reduce QT prolongation and the risk of torsade de pointes seen with amiodarone. This has been seen with quinidine (see 'Mexiletine + Quinidine', p.286).

1. Yonezawa E, Matsumoto K, Ueno K, Tachibana M, Hashimoto H, Komamura K, Kamakura S, Miyatake K, Tanaka K. Lack of interaction between amiodarone and mexiletine in cardiac arrhythmia patients. *J Clin Pharmacol* (2002) 42, 342–6.
2. Tartini R, Kappenberger L, Steinbrunn W. Gefährliche Interaktionen zwischen Amiodaron und Antiarrhythmika der Klasse I. *Schweiz Med Wochenschr* (1982) 112, 1585–7.
3. Boehringer Ingelheim. Personal Communication, July 1995.
4. Waleffe A, Mary-Rabine L, Legrand V, Demoulin JC, Kulbertus HE. Combined mexiletine and amiodarone treatment of refractory recurrent ventricular tachycardia. *Am Heart J* (1980) 100, 788–93.
5. Hoffmann A, Follath F, Burckhardt D. Safe treatment of resistant ventricular arrhythmias with a combination of amiodarone and quinidine or mexiletine. *Lancet* (1983) i, 704–5.

Mexiletine + Antacids

The rate of absorption of mexiletine is slowed by the antacid almasilate, but the extent of the absorption is unaltered. Other antacids might have similar effects.

Clinical evidence, mechanism, importance and management

In a study in healthy subjects, the antacid almasilate (*Gelusil*), given one hour before a single 400-mg dose of mexiletine, delayed mexiletine absorption (time to maximum concentration prolonged from 1.7 hours to 2.9 hours), but had no effect on the extent of its absorption.[1]

This slight delay in the absorption of mexiletine by almasilate would not be expected to be clinically relevant, as its overall absorption was unaffected. It seems likely that other antacids would also not affect the absorption of mexiletine by affecting gastric pH. However, note that some antacids (such as sodium bicarbonate) can affect *urinary* pH and might possibly affect mexiletine concentrations by this mechanism, see 'Mexiletine + Urinary acidifiers or alkalinisers', p.287.

1. Herzog P, Holtermüller KH, Kasper W, Meinertz T, Trenk D, Jähnchen E. Absorption of mexiletine after treatment with gastric antacids. *Br J Clin Pharmacol* (1982) 14, 746–7.

Mexiletine + Atropine or Metoclopramide

The rate of absorption of mexiletine is slowed by atropine and hastened by metoclopramide, but the extent of the absorption is unaltered.

Clinical evidence, mechanism, importance and management

A study in 8 healthy subjects found that a single 600-microgram dose of intravenous atropine reduced the rate of absorption of a single 400-mg oral dose of mexiletine (time to maximum concentration increased from 1.97 hours to 3.32 hours), but the AUC of mexiletine remained unaffected. Intravenous metoclopramide 10 mg increased the rate of absorption of mexiletine (time to maximum concentration reduced from 1.97 hours to 1.03 hours) but similarly did not affect the AUC of mexiletine.[1] This increased rate of absorption with metoclopramide appears to reverse the effect of diamorphine on mexiletine plasma concentrations, see 'Mexiletine + Opioids', p.285.

The achievement of steady-state mexiletine concentrations depends on the extent of its absorption, not on its rate, and therefore it seems very unlikely that atropine or metoclopramide will affect the antiarrhythmic effects of mexiletine during long-term use.[1] In general, no particular precautions would appear necessary on concurrent use of atropine or metoclopramide with mexiletine. However, these drugs might cause variations in the antiarrhythmic effects of initial oral mexiletine doses, which could be a problem if rapid control of the arrhythmia is essential.

1. Wing LMH, Meffin PJ, Grygiel JJ, Smith KJ, Birkett DJ. The effect of metoclopramide and atropine on the absorption of orally administered mexiletine. *Br J Clin Pharmacol* (1980) 9, 505–9.

Mexiletine + Beta blockers

The concurrent use of mexiletine and beta blockers can be clinically useful.

Clinical evidence, mechanism, importance and management

A study in 4 patients found that the concurrent use of mexiletine and **propranolol** 240 mg daily was more effective in blocking ventricular premature depolarisation (VPD) and ventricular tachycardia than mexiletine alone, and did not increase adverse effects. Plasma mexiletine concentrations were not altered by **propranolol**.[1] Similar efficacy was reported for **metoprolol** with mexiletine.[2] Success in decreasing VPDs was noted in 30% of 44 patients taking mexiletine and a beta blocker (unspecified) compared with only 14% of 185 subjects taking mexiletine alone.[3]

1. Leahey EB, Heissenbuttel RH, Giardina E-GV, Bigger JT. Combined mexiletine and propranolol treatment of refractory ventricular tachycardia. *BMJ* (1980) 281, 357–8.
2. Ravid S, Lampert S, Graboys TB. Effect of the combination of low-dose mexiletine and metoprolol on ventricular arrhythmia. *Clin Cardiol* (1991) 14, 951–5.
3. Bigger JT. The interaction of mexiletine with other cardiovascular drugs. *Am Heart J* (1984) 107, 1079–85.

Mexiletine + Fluconazole

Fluconazole does not affect the pharmacokinetics of mexiletine.

Clinical evidence, mechanism, importance and management

In a study, 6 healthy subjects were given a single 200-mg dose of mexiletine before and after taking fluconazole 200 mg daily for 7 days. Two of the subjects were given fluconazole 400 mg daily for a further 7 days. Fluconazole had no effect on the pharmacokinetics of mexiletine.[1] This study therefore suggests that mexiletine dose adjustments will not be necessary on the concurrent use of fluconazole.

1. Ueno K, Yamaguchi R, Tanaka K, Sakaguchi M, Morishima Y, Yamauchi K, Iwai A. Lack of a kinetic interaction between fluconazole and mexiletine. *Eur J Clin Pharmacol* (1996) 50, 129–31.

Mexiletine + HIV-protease inhibitors

Ritonavir appears to increase the concentrations of mexiletine. Tipranavir and any HIV-protease inhibitors boosted with ritonavir would be expected to interact similarly.

Clinical evidence, mechanism, importance and management

Direct evidence (from case reports or clinical studies) of an interaction between mexiletine and the HIV-protease inhibitors appears to be lacking; however, a review of HIV-protease inhibitor interactions reports that the plasma concentrations of mexiletine might be increased 1.5- to 3-fold by **ritonavir**.[1] Mexiletine is primarily metabolised by CYP2D6, of which **ritonavir** is an inhibitor, causing moderate inhibition at high doses (500 mg twice daily) and weak inhibition at low doses (100 mg twice daily). Concurrent use would therefore be expected to result in raised mexiletine concentrations, which might increase the risk of arrhythmias and other adverse effects. The manufacturer of ritonavir reports that cardiac adverse effects have been reported on concurrent use.[2] *In vitro* **tipranavir** has been shown to be a CYP2D6 inhibitor,[3] and so it might also interact with mexiletine in this way. The other HIV-protease inhibitors are not known to affect CYP2D6, and would not be expected to increase mexiletine concentrations when given alone. However, they are usually given with low-dose **ritonavir** as a pharmacokinetic enhancer and so small increases in mexiletine concentrations might occur on concurrent use, although the clinical relevance of this is unknown. Therefore, until more is known, it would seem prudent to monitor any patient taking mexiletine with **ritonavir**, **tipranavir** or any **HIV-protease inhibitor boosted with ritonavir** for an increase in mexiletine adverse effects (such as nausea, tremor, hypotension), and titrate the mexiletine dose slowly, according to clinical response.

1. Burger DM, Hoetelmans RMW, Koopmans PP, Meenhorst PL, Mulder JW, Hekster YA, Beijnen JH. Clinically relevant drug interactions with antiretroviral agents. *Antivir Ther* (1997) 2, 149–165.
2. Norvir Tablets (Ritonavir). AbbVie Ltd. UK Summary of product characteristics, September 2012.
3. Aptivus Soft Capsules (Tipranavir). Boehringer Ingelheim Ltd. UK Summary of product characteristics, December 2011.

Mexiletine + H_2-receptor antagonists

The pharmacokinetics of mexiletine are not altered by cimetidine or ranitidine. Cimetidine appears to reduce the gastric adverse effects of mexiletine.

Clinical evidence, mechanism, importance and management

In a study in 11 patients, the maximum and minimum plasma mexiletine concentrations were unaltered when **cimetidine** 300 mg four times daily was given for one week, and the frequency and severity of the ventricular arrhythmias for which they were being treated remained unchanged. Moreover the gastric adverse effects of mexiletine were reduced in half of the patients.[1] This study in patients confirms the findings of two other studies using **cimetidine** or **ranitidine** in healthy subjects.[2,3] There would seem to be no problems associated with giving these drugs concurrently, and some advantages.

1. Klein AL, Sami MH. Usefulness and safety of cimetidine in patients receiving mexiletine for ventricular arrhythmia. *Am Heart J* (1985) 109, 1281–6.
2. Klein A, Sami M, Selinger K. Mexiletine kinetics in healthy subjects taking cimetidine. *Clin Pharmacol Ther* (1985) 37, 669–73.
3. Brockmeyer NH, Breithaupt H, Ferdinand W, von Hattingberg M, Ohnhaus EE. Kinetics of oral and intravenous mexiletine: lack of effect of cimetidine and ranitidine. *Eur J Clin Pharmacol* (1989) 36, 375–8.

Mexiletine + Omeprazole

Omeprazole does not appear to affect the pharmacokinetics of mexiletine.

Clinical evidence, mechanism, importance and management

A crossover study in 9 healthy Japanese men found that when they were given mexiletine 200 mg after taking omeprazole 40 mg daily for 8 days, the serum concentration and AUC of mexiletine were unchanged. It was concluded that omeprazole does not affect the metabolism of mexiletine,[1] and no mexiletine dose adjustments would be expected to be necessary if these drugs are used concurrently.

1. Kusumoto M, Ueno K, Tanaka K, Takeda K, Mashimo K, Kameda T, Fujimura Y, Shibakawa M. Lack of pharmacokinetic interaction between mexiletine and omeprazole. *Ann Pharmacother* (1998) 32, 182–4.

Mexiletine + Opioids

The absorption of mexiletine is reduced following myocardial infarction, and further reduced and delayed if diamorphine or morphine is used concurrently. Other opioids might interact similarly.

Clinical evidence

A pharmacokinetic study found that the mean plasma concentrations of mexiletine (400 mg orally followed by 200 mg 2 hours later) in the first 3 hours were more than 50% lower in 6 patients who had suffered a myocardial infarction and who had been given **diamorphine** 5 to 10 mg or **morphine** 10 to 15 mg than in 4 patients who had not been given opioids. In addition, the AUC_{0-8} was 39% lower in those who had received opioids.[1]

In a further study about the prophylactic use of mexiletine, the same authors found that plasma mexiletine concentrations 3 hours after the first oral dose were 31% lower in 10 patients who had received opioids than in 6 patients who had not received opioids. These patients were from a subset that were subsequently shown not to have had a myocardial infarction.[1] In another similar study of mexiletine in acute myocardial infarction, the use of **diamorphine** was associated with low plasma mexiletine concentrations at 3 hours, and a possible reduction in the efficacy of mexiletine. In this study, pretreatment with intravenous **metoclopramide** tended to reduce the effect of **diamorphine** on mexiletine absorption,[2] although this was not noted in the other report.[1]

Mechanism

The reduced absorption of mexiletine would seem to result from inhibition of gastric emptying by diamorphine and morphine. Other mechanisms probably contribute to the delayed clearance of mexiletine.

Importance and management

The interaction between mexiletine and morphine or diamorphine is established, although information is limited. The delay and reduction in the absorption of mexiletine would seem to limit the value of oral mexiletine during the first few hours after a myocardial infarction, particularly if morphine or diamorphine are used. Mexiletine is no longer widely available, but the UK manufacturer previously suggested that a higher loading dose of oral mexiletine might be preferable in this situation. Alternatively, an intravenous dose of mexiletine may be given. In addition, they noted that it might be necessary to titrate the dose against therapeutic and adverse effects.[3] There seems to be no information about other opioids, but if the mechanism of interaction is correct, then other opioids would be expected to interact similarly.

1. Pottage A, Campbell RWF, Achuff SC, Murray A, Julian DC, Prescott LF. The absorption of oral mexiletine in coronary care patients. *Eur J Clin Pharmacol* (1978) 13, 393–9.
2. Smyllie HC, Doar JW, Head CD, Leggett RJ. A trial of intravenous and oral mexiletine in acute myocardial infarction. *Eur J Clin Pharmacol* (1984) 26, 537–42.
3. Mexitil (Mexiletine). Boehringer Ingelheim Ltd. UK Summary of product characteristics, May 2003.

Mexiletine + Phenytoin

Mexiletine exposure is moderately reduced by phenytoin.

Clinical evidence

The observation that 3 patients had unusually low plasma mexiletine concentrations while taking phenytoin prompted a pharmacokinetic study in 6 healthy subjects. After taking phenytoin 300 mg daily for one week, the mean AUC and half-life of a single 400-mg dose of mexiletine were reduced by an average of about 50% (half-life reduced from 17.2 hours to 8.4 hours).[1]

Mechanism

Phenytoin is a known moderate inducer of CYP1A2, by which mexiletine is partially metabolised. It therefore seems likely that phenytoin increased the metabolism of mexiletine by this route, leading to reduced mexiletine exposure.

Importance and management

Information seems to be limited to this report but the interaction between mexiletine and phenytoin appears to be established. It seems likely that the moderate reduction in mexiletine exposure could be clinically important in some individuals. It would therefore seem prudent to monitor mexiletine efficacy in patients also given phenytoin, and, where possible, monitor mexiletine concentrations, increasing the mexiletine dose if necessary. There seems to be no information about **fosphenytoin**, but as it is a prodrug of phenytoin, it seems likely that it will interact with mexiletine in a similar way to phenytoin.

1. Begg EJ, Chinwah PM, Webb C, Day RO, Wade DN. Enhanced metabolism of mexiletine after phenytoin administration. *Br J Clin Pharmacol* (1982) 14, 219–23.

Mexiletine + Propafenone

Propafenone increases mexiletine concentrations in some patients. Mexiletine does not appear to affect propafenone pharmacokinetics.

Clinical evidence

In one study in healthy subjects, propafenone reduced mexiletine clearance and increased plasma mexiletine concentrations in CYP2D6 extensive metabolisers (that is, those with normal levels of this isoenzyme), but had no effect in CYP2D6 poor metabolisers (that is, those lacking this isoenzyme). Propafenone effectively turned the extensive metabolisers into poor metabolisers. Mexiletine did not affect propafenone pharmacokinetics. In this study, overall changes in ECG parameters were minor during the concurrent use of mexiletine and propafenone.[1]

Mechanism

Propafenone is a known moderate inhibitor of CYP2D6, and it is likely that the increased mexiletine concentrations and reduced clearance seen, occurred as a result of inhibition of the metabolism of mexiletine by this pathway.

Importance and management

Evidence for an interaction between mexiletine and propafenone is limited to this one study, but although the use of the combination was not associated with important ECG changes, the potentiation of drug effects could predispose to proarrhythmias in patients with ischaemic heart disease. The authors suggest that slow dose titration of the combination might decrease the risk of adverse effects.[1] If propafenone is given to a patient taking mexiletine it would seem prudent to monitor the outcome for mexiletine adverse effects (such as nausea, tremor, hypotension), and decrease the dose of mexiletine if necessary.

1. Labbé L, O'Hara G, Lefebvre M, Lessard É, Gilbert M, Adedoyin A, Champagne J, Hamelin B, Turgeon J. Pharmacokinetic and pharmacodynamic interaction between mexiletine and propafenone in human beings. *Clin Pharmacol Ther* (2000) 68, 44–57.

Mexiletine + Quinidine

Quinidine slightly reduces mexiletine clearance in most patients. Mexiletine appears to limit the quinidine-induced increase in the QT interval.

Clinical evidence

Two studies[1,2] in healthy subjects have found that quinidine reduces the metabolism and excretion of mexiletine in CYP2D6 extensive metabolisers (that is, those with normal amounts of this isoenzyme). The total clearance of mexiletine was reduced by 24%.[2] Quinidine had no effect on mexiletine metabolism in CYP2D6 poor metabolisers (that is, those lacking this isoenzyme).

The concurrent use of mexiletine and quinidine (in lower doses) was reported to be more effective than either drug alone,[3,4] and the incidence of adverse effects was reduced. Mexiletine limited the quinidine-induced increase in QT interval,[3] and might prevent ventricular tachycardias in response to quinidine, which could be due to a prolonged ventricular refractory period.[5]

Mechanism

Quinidine is a potent inhibitor of CYP2D6, which is involved in the metabolism of mexiletine, leading to a reduction in mexiletine clearance in extensive metabolisers (those with normal levels of CYP2D6), but has no effect in poor metabolisers as they lack CYP2D6 and therefore depend on other routes of metabolism for mexiletine.

Importance and management

Evidence for a pharmacokinetic interaction between mexiletine and quinidine is limited, but the effects seen are consistent with the known inhibitory effect of quinidine on CYP2D6. These changes appear to be slight and are unlikely to be clinically relevant in most patients. However, bear the possibility of an interaction in mind should any unexplained mexiletine adverse effects (such as nausea, tremor, hypotension) occur in a patient also given quinidine. Note also that the combination can be clinically useful and mexiletine appears to limit quinidine-induced QT interval prolongation.

1. Broly F, Vandamme N, Caron J, Libersa C, Lhermitte M. Single-dose quinidine treatment inhibits mexiletine oxidation in extensive metabolizers of debrisoquine. *Life Sci* (1991) 48, PL-123–128.
2. Turgeon J, Fiset C, Giguère R, Gilbert M, Moerike K, Rouleau JR, Kroemer HK, Eichelbaum M, Grech-Bélanger O, Bélanger PM. Influence of debrisoquine phenotype and of quinidine on mexiletine disposition in man. *J Pharmacol Exp Ther* (1991) 259, 789–98.
3. Duff HJ, Roden D, Primm RK, Oates JA, Woosley RL. Mexiletine in the treatment of resistant ventricular arrhythmias: enhancement of efficacy and reduction of dose-related side effects by combination with quinidine. *Circulation* (1983) 67, 1124–8.
4. Giardina E-GV, Wechsler ME. Low dose quinidine-mexiletine combination therapy versus quinidine monotherapy for treatment of ventricular arrhythmias. *J Am Coll Cardiol* (1990) 15, 1138–45.
5. Bonavita GJ, Pires LA, Wagshal AB, Cuello C, Mittleman RS, Greene TO, Huang SKS. Usefulness of oral quinidine-mexiletine combination therapy for sustained ventricular tachyarrhythmias as assessed by programmed electrical stimulation when quinidine monotherapy has failed. *Am Heart J* (1994) 127, 847–51.

Mexiletine + Quinolones

Ciprofloxacin slightly reduces the clearance of mexiletine. Mexiletine might reduce sparfloxacin-induced QT prolongation.

Clinical evidence, mechanism, importance and management

(a) Ciprofloxacin

A study in healthy subjects found that the oral clearance of a single dose of mexiletine was reduced by about 8 to 20% when it was given on day 3 of a 5-day course of ciprofloxacin 750 mg twice daily. This was due to a decrease in the metabolic clearance of mexiletine, which presumably occurred because ciprofloxacin inhibits CYP1A2, which is involved in the metabolism of mexiletine.[1] It is unlikely that changes of this magnitude would be clinically relevant, and so no mexiletine dose adjustment appears to be necessary on the concurrent use of ciprofloxacin.

(b) Other quinolones

An *animal* study found that mexiletine might reduce the QT-prolonging effect of **sparfloxacin.**[2] This is in line with the known effects of mexiletine, and this effect would be expected to be replicated clinically, both with **sparfloxacin**, and other quinolones that prolong the QT interval (e.g. **gatifloxacin** and **moxifloxacin**).

1. Labbé L, Robitaille NM, Lefez C, Potvin D, Gilbert M, O'Hara G, Turgeon J. Effects of ciprofloxacin on the stereoselective disposition of mexiletine in man. *Ther Drug Monit* (2004) 26, 492–8.
2. Takahara A, Sugiyama A, Satoh Y, Hashimoto K. Effects of mexiletine on the canine model of sparfloxacin-induced long QT syndrome. *Eur J Pharmacol* (2003) 476, 115–22.

Mexiletine + Rifampicin (Rifampin)

Rifampicin reduces the exposure to mexiletine.

Clinical evidence

In a study in 8 healthy subjects, rifampicin 600 mg daily for 10 days reduced the AUC and half-life of a single 400-mg dose of mexiletine by about 40% and increased its clearance by about 50%.[1]

Mechanism

The probable reason for these pharmacokinetics changes is that rifampicin, a well-known, non-specific enzyme-inducer, increases the metabolism and clearance of mexiletine.

Importance and management

Evidence for an interaction between mexiletine and rifampicin is limited to this study, but an interaction would appear to be established. The slight changes in mexiletine exposure could be clinically important in some individuals. It would therefore seem prudent to monitor mexiletine efficacy in patients also given rifampicin, and, where possible, monitor mexiletine concentrations, increasing the mexiletine dose if necessary.

1. Pentikäinen PJ, Koivula IH, Hiltunen HA. Effect of rifampicin treatment on the kinetics of mexiletine. *Eur J Clin Pharmacol* (1982) 23, 261–6.

Mexiletine + SSRIs

Fluvoxamine slightly increases the exposure to mexiletine. Fluoxetine and paroxetine are predicted to inhibit the metabolism of mexiletine, but sertraline seems unlikely to interact.

Clinical evidence, mechanism, importance and management

(a) Fluvoxamine

In a study in 6 healthy subjects, **fluvoxamine** 50 mg twice daily for 7 days increased the AUC of a single 200-mg dose of mexiletine by 55%, and decreased its clearance by 37%.[1] It is likely that **fluvoxamine** increases the AUC of mexiletine by inhibiting CYP1A2, which is partially responsible for the metabolism of mexiletine.[1] These changes in mexiletine pharmacokinetics are only slight and unlikely to be clinically important in most patients. However, as many of the adverse effects of mexiletine are dose-related, it might be prudent to bear the possibility of an interaction in mind if mexiletine adverse effects (such as nausea, tremor, hypotension) occur in a patient also taking fluvoxamine.

(b) Other SSRIs

An *in vitro* study using human liver microsomes found that **paroxetine**, **fluoxetine**, and **sertraline** extensively inhibited the metabolism of mexiletine. Using a model to predict *in vivo* interactions, it was suggested that both **fluoxetine** and **paroxetine** might interact with mexiletine to a clinically relevant extent, whereas **sertraline** is less likely to interact.[2] It is important to note that such *in vitro* findings and related predictions for *in vivo* effects are not always reliable. However, this *in vitro* finding is consistent with the established inhibitory effect of these particular SSRIs on CYP2D6. Quinidine, a potent CYP2D6 inhibitor, has only slight effects on mexiletine metabolism (see 'Mexiletine + Quinidine', above), and therefore **fluoxetine** and **paroxetine**, which are also moderate to potent CYP2D6 inhibitors seem unlikely to interact to a clinically relevant extent. However, until more is known, it might be prudent to bear the possibility of an interaction in mind should any unexplained mexiletine adverse effects (such as nausea, tremor, hypotension) occur in a patient given **fluoxetine** or **paroxetine. Sertraline** is known to only be a weak CYP2D6 inhibitor and so would be unlikely to interact with mexiletine to a clinically relevant extent.

1. Kusumoto M, Ueno K, Oda A, Takeda K, Mashimo K, Takaya K, Fujimura Y, Nishihori T, Tanaka K. Effect of fluvoxamine on the pharmacokinetics of mexiletine in healthy Japanese men. *Clin Pharmacol Ther* (2001) 69, 104–7.
2. Hara Y, Nakajima M, Miyamoto K-I, Yokoi T. Inhibitory effects of psychotropic drugs on mexiletine metabolism in human liver microsomes: prediction of *in vivo* drug interactions. *Xenobiotica* (2005) 35, 549–60.

Mexiletine + Tobacco

Tobacco smoking reduces the elimination half-life of mexiletine but does not affect its absorption and distribution.

Clinical evidence, mechanism, importance and management

A study in 14 healthy subjects (6 smokers and 8 non-smokers) found that cigarette smoking had no effect on the absorption or distribution of a single 200-mg dose of mexiletine. However, smoking reduced the elimination half-life of mexiletine from 11.1 hours to 7.2 hours. Cigarette smoking was also found to induce the conjugation of mexiletine with glucuronic acid and the hydroxylation of mexiletine to hydroxymethylmexiletine but had no effect on the formation of *p*-hydroxymexiletine.[1]

Tobacco smoke is a known inducer of CYP1A2, which is involved in the metabolism of mexiletine, and so it seems likely that the effects seen are a result of increased mexiletine metabolism by this route. The clinical importance of this effect is not known, but as mexiletine is titrated to effect it would seem that any interaction would automatically be accounted for in smokers. If a patient taking mexiletine stops smoking, it would seem prudent to be alert for mexiletine adverse effects (such as nausea, tremor, hypotension), and decrease the dose of mexiletine, according to clinical response.

1. Grech-Bélanger O, Gilbert M, Turgeon J, LeBlanc P-P. Effects of cigarette smoking on mexiletine kinetics. *Clin Pharmacol Ther* (1985) 37, 638–43.

Mexiletine + Urinary acidifiers or alkalinisers

Large changes in urinary pH caused by acidifying or alkalinising drugs can have a large effect on the plasma concentrations of mexiletine in some patients.

Clinical evidence

In 4 healthy subjects, a single 200-mg intravenous dose of mexiletine was given, once when the urine was acidic (pH 5) after administration of **ammonium chloride**, and once when the urine was alkaline (pH 8) after administration of **sodium bicarbonate**. The plasma elimination half-life was shorter when the urine was acidic (2.8 hours) compared with when it was alkaline (8.6 hours). In addition, the percentage of mexiletine excreted unchanged in the urine was 58% in acidic urine and less than 1% in alkaline urine.[1] Similar results were found in another study.[2] A further study in patients with uncontrolled urinary pHs (range 5.04 to 7.86) given mexiletine orally for 5 days found that the plasma concentration of mexiletine correlated with urine pH. In addition, it was predicted that a normal variation in pH could cause more than a 50% variation in plasma mexiletine concentrations.[3] A later comprehensive pharmacokinetic study in 5 healthy subjects found that the renal clearance of mexiletine was 4 mL/minute in alkaline urine (pH 8) compared with 168 mL/minute in acidic urine (pH 5.2). In two subjects, this resulted in an increase in mexiletine plasma concentrations of 61% and 96%, respectively, but in the other three subjects the increase was less than 20%. Non-renal clearance (metabolic clearance) increased in the three subjects with little change in plasma concentrations, but was unaffected in the two subjects with large changes in plasma concentrations.[4]

Mechanism

Mexiletine is a basic drug, which undergoes greater reabsorption by the kidneys when in the non-ionised form in alkaline urine. Mexiletine is also extensively cleared by hepatic metabolism and only about 10% is excreted unchanged in the urine at physiological pH, although this is variable. Any changes in the renal clearance of mexiletine that occur as a result of urinary pH changes might therefore be expected to be compensated for by an increase in metabolic clearance, but this does not seem to occur in all patients.[4]

Importance and management

Although changes in urinary pH can affect the amount of mexiletine lost in the urine, the effect of diet or the concurrent use of alkalinisers (such as sodium bicarbonate, **acetazolamide**) or acidifiers (such as ammonium chloride) on the plasma concentrations of mexiletine does not appear to be predictable. There appear to be no reports of adverse interactions but concurrent use should be monitored. Mexiletine is no longer widely available, but the UK manufacturer previously recommended that the concurrent use of drugs that markedly acidify or alkalinise the urine should be avoided.[5] Drugs that might be implicated include ammonium chloride, sodium bicarbonate or acetazolamide. See also 'Quinidine + Antacids or Urinary alkalinisers', p.293, for a list of antacids and their effect on urinary pH.

1. Kiddie MA, Kaye CM, Turner P, Shaw TRD. The influence of urinary pH on the elimination of mexiletine. *Br J Clin Pharmacol* (1974) 1, 229–32.
2. Beckett AH, Chidomere EC. The distribution, metabolism and excretion of mexiletine in man. *Postgrad Med J* (1977) 53 (Suppl 1), 60–6.
3. Johnston A, Burgess CD, Warrington SJ, Wadsworth J, Hamer NAJ. The effect of spontaneous changes in urinary pH on mexiletine plasma concentrations and excretion during chronic administration to healthy volunteers. *Br J Clin Pharmacol* (1979) 8, 349–52.
4. Mitchell BG, Clements JA, Pottage A, Prescott LF. Mexiletine disposition: individual variation in response to urine acidification and alkalinisation. *Br J Clin Pharmacol* (1983) 16, 281–4.
5. Mexitil (Mexiletine). Boehringer Ingelheim Ltd. UK Summary of product characteristics, May 2003.

Procainamide + Amiodarone

When procainamide and amiodarone are used together the QT interval prolonging effects are increased. Serum procainamide levels are increased by about 60% and procainamide metabolite levels are increased by about 30% by amiodarone.

Clinical evidence

In a study, 12 patients were stabilised taking procainamide (2 to 6 g daily, or about 900 mg every 6 hours). When amiodarone (600 mg loading dose every 12 hours for 5 to 7 days, then 600 mg daily) was also given their mean serum procainamide levels rose by 57% (from 6.8 to 10.6 micrograms/mL) and their serum levels of the metabolite *N*-acetylprocainamide (NAPA) rose by 32% (from 6.9 to 9.1 micrograms/mL). Procainamide levels increased by more than 3 micrograms/mL in 6 of the patients. The increases usually occurred within 24 hours, but in other patients they occurred as late as 4 or 5 days. Toxicity was seen in 2 patients. Despite lowering the procainamide doses by 20%, serum procainamide levels were still higher (at 7.7 micrograms/mL) than before the amiodarone was started.[1]

In another study, intravenous procainamide was given once before (at a mean dose of 13 mg/kg), and once during (at a 30% reduced dose: mean 9.2 mg/kg) the use of amiodarone 1.6 g daily for 7 to 14 days. Amiodarone decreased the clearance of procainamide by 23% and increased its elimination half-life by 38%. Both drugs prolonged the QRS and QTc intervals, and the extent of prolongation was significantly greater with the combination than with either drug alone.[2]

Mechanism

The mechanism behind the pharmacokinetic interaction is not understood. The QT prolonging effects of the two drugs appear to be additive.

Importance and management

Information about an interaction between procainamide and amiodarone appears to be limited to these studies, but the interaction would seem to be established and clinically important. The authors of the pharmacokinetic studies, suggest that the dose of procainamide may need to be reduced by 20 to 50%. They also suggest that serum levels should be monitored and patients observed for adverse effects.[1,2] Remember that the interaction can develop within 24 hours.

Note that the concurrent use of two drugs that prolong the QT interval, such as amiodarone and procainamide, should generally be avoided. For further discussion, see also 'Drugs that prolong the QT interval + Other drugs that prolong the QT interval', p.272.

1. Saal AK, Werner JA, Greene HL, Sears GK, Graham EL. Effect of amiodarone on serum quinidine and procainamide levels. *Am J Cardiol* (1984) 53, 1264–7.
2. Windle J, Prystowsky EN, Miles WM, Heger JJ. Pharmacokinetic and electrophysiologic interactions of amiodarone and procainamide. *Clin Pharmacol Ther* (1987) 41, 603–10.

Procainamide + Antacids or Antidiarrhoeals

There is some inconclusive evidence that aluminium phosphate may possibly cause a small reduction in the absorption of procainamide. Kaolin-pectin appears to modestly reduce the bioavailability of procainamide.

Clinical evidence, mechanism, importance and management

A single 11-g dose of an **aluminium phosphate** antacid modestly reduced the AUC of a single 750-mg oral dose of procainamide by about 15%.[1] The clinical importance of this interaction is uncertain, but probably small.

In a study in 4 healthy subjects, **kaolin-pectin** was found to reduce the peak saliva concentrations and AUC of a single 250-mg dose of procainamide by about 30%. **Kaolin-pectin** and **magnesium trisilicate** absorbed procainamide *in vitro*.[2] The clinical importance of this is also uncertain, but the effects appear to be relatively modest. The same *in vitro* study found that *Simeco* (**co-dried aluminium hydroxide/ magnesium carbonate** with **magnesium hydroxide** and **simeticone**) and *Pepto-Bismol* (**bismuth salicylate**) did not adsorb procainamide[2] which suggests that they are unlikely to interact, but this needs confirmation.

1. Albin H, Vincon G, Bertolaso D, Dangoumau J. Influence du phosphate d'aluminium sur la biodisponibilité de la procaïnamide et du disopyramide. *Therapie* (1981) 36, 541–6.
2. Al-Shora HI, Moustafa MA, Niazy EM, Gaber M, Gouda MW. Interactions of procainamide, verapamil, guanethidine and hydralazine with adsorbent antacids and antidiarrhoeal mixtures. *Int J Pharmaceutics* (1988) 47, 209–13.

Procainamide + Beta blockers

The pharmacokinetics of procainamide are only slightly altered by propranolol and metoprolol. Both sotalol and procainamide have QT-interval prolonging effects, which may be additive if they are used together.

Clinical evidence, mechanism, importance and management

Preliminary results of a study in 6 healthy subjects found that long-term treatment with **propranolol** (period and dose not stated) increased the procainamide half-life from 1.71 to 2.66 hours and reduced the plasma clearance by 16%.[1] A later study in 8 healthy subjects found that the pharmacokinetics of a single 500-mg dose of procainamide were only slightly altered by **propranolol** 80 mg three times daily or **metoprolol** 100 mg twice daily. The procainamide half-life of 1.9 hours increased to 2.2 hours with **propranolol**, and to 2.3 hours with **metoprolol**, but no significant changes in total clearance occurred. No changes in the AUC of the metabolite *N*-acetylprocainamide were seen.[2] It seems unlikely that a clinically important adverse pharmacokinetic interaction normally occurs between these drugs.

A clinical study describes the successful use of procainamide with **sotalol**.[3] However, both **sotalol** and procainamide can prolong the QT interval, and there may be an increased risk of torsade de pointes arrhythmias if they are used together, see 'Drugs that prolong the QT interval + Other drugs that prolong the QT interval', p.272.

1. Weidler DJ, Garg DC, Jallad NS, McFarland MA. The effect of long-term propranolol administration on the pharmacokinetics of procainamide in humans. *Clin Pharmacol Ther* (1981) 29, 289.
2. Ochs HR, Carstens G, Roberts G-M, Greenblatt DJ. Metoprolol or propranolol does not alter the kinetics of procainamide. *J Cardiovasc Pharmacol* (1983) 5, 392–5.
3. Dorian P, Newman D, Berman N, Hardy J, Mitchell J. Sotalol and type IA drugs in combination prevent recurrence of sustained ventricular tachycardia. *J Am Coll Cardiol* (1993) 22, 106–13.

Procainamide + H_2-receptor antagonists

Serum procainamide levels can be increased by cimetidine and toxicity may develop, particularly in those who have a reduced renal clearance,

such as the elderly. Ranitidine and famotidine appear to interact with procainamide only minimally or not at all.

Clinical evidence

(a) Cimetidine

In one study, 36 elderly patients (aged 65 to 90 years) taking sustained-release oral procainamide every 6 hours had rises in mean steady-state serum levels of procainamide and its metabolite *N*-acetylprocainamide of 55% and 36%, respectively, after taking cimetidine 300 mg every 6 hours for 3 days. This was tolerated in 24 patients with serum procainamide and *N*-acetylprocainamide levels of less than 12 mg/L and less than 15 mg/L, respectively, without adverse effects. However, 9 patients had some mild adverse effects (nausea, weakness, malaise, PR interval increases of less than 20%), with serum procainamide and *N*-acetylprocainamide levels between 10 and 15 mg/L and 10 and 20 mg/L, respectively. Three patients experienced severe procainamide toxicity (e.g. ventricular rate above 150 bpm for between 30 seconds and 5 minutes) with serum procainamide and *N*-acetylprocainamide levels greater than 14 mg/L and 16 mg/L, respectively. These adverse effects were dealt with by stopping one or both drugs and symptoms resolved within 12 to 24 hours.[1] Another report describes an elderly man who developed procainamide toxicity after taking cimetidine 1.2 g daily. His procainamide dose was roughly halved (from 937.5 mg every 6 hours to 500 mg every 6 hours) to bring his serum procainamide and *N*-acetylprocainamide levels into the accepted therapeutic range.[2]

Four studies in healthy subjects have found that cimetidine increases the AUC of procainamide by 24 to 43%, and decreases its renal clearance by 31 to 40%,[3-6] these changes occurring even with single doses of cimetidine.[5] An increase in the steady-state levels of procainamide of 43% has been seen when cimetidine 1.2 g daily was also given.[6]

(b) Famotidine

In a study in 8 healthy subjects, famotidine 40 mg daily for 5 days did not affect the pharmacokinetics or pharmacodynamics of a single 5-mg/kg intravenous dose of procainamide.[7]

(c) Ranitidine

One study[8] found that ranitidine 150 mg twice daily for one day reduced the absorption of procainamide from the gut by 10% and reduced its renal excretion by 19%, increasing the procainamide and *N*-acetylprocainamide AUC by about 14%. Another study found no change in the steady-state pharmacokinetics of procainamide when ranitidine 150 mg twice daily was also given, except that ranitidine delayed the time to maximum plasma concentration (from 1.4 to 2.7 hours).[6] In a further study, in 13 healthy subjects, ranitidine 150 mg twice daily for 4 days caused no significant changes in the mean pharmacokinetics of oral procainamide 1 g. However, it appeared that subjects had either a modest 20% increase or decrease in procainamide clearance, with the direction of change related to their baseline procainamide clearance: the higher the baseline clearance the greater the decrease caused by ranitidine.[9]

Mechanism

Procainamide levels are increased because cimetidine reduces its renal excretion by about one-third or more, but the precise mechanism for this is uncertain. One suggestion is that it interferes with the active secretion of procainamide by the kidney tubules.[3,4]

Importance and management

The interaction between procainamide and cimetidine is established. Concurrent use should be undertaken with care because the safety margin of procainamide is low. Reduce the procainamide dosage as necessary. This is particularly important in the elderly because they have a reduced ability to clear both drugs. Ranitidine and famotidine appear not to interact to a clinically important extent, but it should be appreciated that what is known is based on studies in healthy subjects rather than patients.

1. Bauer LA, Black D, Gensler A. Procainamide-cimetidine drug interaction in elderly male patients. *J Am Geriatr Soc* (1990) 38, 467–9.
2. Higbee MD, Wood JS, Mead RA. Case report. Procainamide-cimetidine interaction. A potential toxic interaction in the elderly. *J Am Geriatr Soc* (1984) 32, 162–4.
3. Somogyi A, McLean A, Heinzow B. Cimetidine-procainamide pharmacokinetic interaction in man: evidence of competition for tubular secretion of basic drugs. *Eur J Clin Pharmacol* (1983) 25, 339–45.
4. Christian CD, Meredith CG, Speeg KV. Cimetidine inhibits renal procainamide clearance. *Clin Pharmacol Ther* (1984) 36, 221–7.
5. Lai MY, Jiang FM, Chung CH, Chen HC, Chao PDL. Dose dependent effect of cimetidine on procainamide disposition in man. *Int J Clin Pharmacol Ther Toxicol* (1988) 26, 118–21.
6. Rodvold KA, Paloucek FP, Jung D, Gallastegui J. Interaction of steady-state procainamide with H_2-receptor antagonists cimetidine and ranitidine. *Ther Drug Monit* (1987) 9, 378–83.
7. Klotz U, Arvela P, Rosenkranz B. Famotidine, a new H_2-receptor antagonist, does not affect hepatic elimination of diazepam or tubular secretion of procainamide. *Eur J Clin Pharmacol* (1985) 28, 671–5.
8. Somogyi A, Bochner F. Dose and concentration dependent effect of ranitidine on procainamide disposition and renal clearance in man. *Br J Clin Pharmacol* (1984) 18, 175–81.
9. Rocci ML, Kosoglou T, Ferguson RK, Vlasses PH. Ranitidine-induced changes in the renal and hepatic clearances of procainamide are correlated. *J Pharmacol Exp Ther* (1989) 248, 923–8.

Procainamide + Para-aminobenzoic acid (PABA)

A single case report found that para-aminobenzoic acid (PABA) increased the serum levels of procainamide and reduced the serum levels of the procainamide metabolite *N*-acetylprocainamide. In contrast, a later pharmacokinetic study in healthy subjects found that PABA had no effect on serum procainamide levels, and increased serum *N*-acetylprocainamide levels.

Clinical evidence, mechanism, importance and management

A 61-year-old man who had sustained ventricular tachycardia, which did not respond adequately to oral procainamide, was found to be a fast acetylator of procainamide, which resulted in particularly high serum levels of the procainamide metabolite (*N*-acetylprocainamide) in relation to his procainamide levels. When he was also given para-aminobenzoic acid (PABA) 1.5 g every 6 hours for 30 hours, to suppress the production of this metabolite, the serum level of procainamide increased, that of *N*-acetylprocainamide decreased, and control of his arrhythmia improved.[1] However, a later study in 10 healthy subjects, who were also fast acetylators of procainamide, found that PABA did not significantly affect the pharmacokinetics of procainamide. In addition, although PABA inhibited the production of *N*-acetylprocainamide, it also inhibited its renal excretion, so that the AUC and elimination half-life were increased. This suggests that PABA may in fact not be useful for increasing the efficacy and safety of procainamide.[2]

These contradictory findings are difficult to explain, but neither report suggests that concurrent use need be avoided.

1. Nylen ES, Cohen AI, Wish MH, Lima JL, Finkelstein JD. Reduced acetylation of procainamide by para-aminobenzoic acid. *J Am Coll Cardiol* (1986) 7, 185–7.
2. Tisdale JE, Rudis MI, Padhi ID, Svensson CK, Webb CR, Borzak S, Ware JA, Krepostman A, Zarowitz BJ. Inhibition of N-acetylation of procainamide by para-aminobenzoic acid in humans. *J Clin Pharmacol* (1995) 35, 902–10.

Procainamide + Probenecid

In a study in 6 healthy subjects, the pharmacokinetics of a single 750-mg intravenous dose of procainamide and its effects on the QT interval were not altered by pretreatment with probenecid 2 g.[1] No special precautions appear to be necessary on concurrent use.

1. Lam YWF, Boyd RA, Chin SK, Chang D, Giacomini KM. Effect of probenecid on the pharmacokinetics and pharmacodynamics of procainamide. *J Clin Pharmacol* (1991) 31, 429–32.

Procainamide + Quinidine

A single case report describes a patient who developed a marked increase in his procainamide levels when he was also given quinidine. The combination prolongs the QT interval, and should generally be avoided because of the increased risk of torsade de pointes.

Clinical evidence

A man with sustained ventricular tachycardia taking high-dose intravenous procainamide 2 g every 8 hours had a 70% increase in his steady-state plasma procainamide levels, from 9.1 nanograms/mL to 15.4 nanograms/mL, when he also took quinidine gluconate 324 mg every 8 hours. The procainamide half-life increased from 3.7 hours to 7.2 hours and its clearance fell from 27 L/hour to 16 L/hour. His QTc interval increased by 30 milliseconds, to 678 milliseconds.[1] In another study in patients with ventricular arrhythmias, quinidine was given with procainamide. The doses were adjusted, based in part on the QT interval. The QTc interval was longer when both drugs were given (499 milliseconds) than with each drug alone (quinidine 470 milliseconds, procainamide 460 milliseconds) despite reducing the doses when both drugs were given (mean quinidine dose reduced by 28%; mean procainamide dose reduced by 32%).[2]

Mechanism

It has been suggested that the quinidine interferes with one or more of the renal pathways by which procainamide is cleared from the body.[1]

Importance and management

Information on the possible pharmacokinetic interaction between procainamide and quinidine seems to be limited to this report. Both quinidine and procainamide are class Ia antiarrhythmics and prolong the QT interval, an effect that is increased by concurrent use. Such combinations should generally be avoided because of the increased risk of torsade de pointes. For further discussion of this effect, see 'Drugs that prolong the QT interval + Other drugs that prolong the QT interval', p.272.

1. Hughes B, Dyer JE, Schwartz AB. Increased procainamide plasma concentrations caused by quinidine: a new drug interaction. *Am Heart J* (1987) 114, 908–9.
2. Kim SG, Seiden SW, Matos JA, Waspe LE, Fisher JD. Combination of procainamide and quinidine for better tolerance and additive effects for ventricular arrhythmias. *Am J Cardiol* (1985) 56, 84–8.

Procainamide + Quinolones

Ofloxacin and levofloxacin cause moderate increases in the serum levels of procainamide, whereas ciprofloxacin has a lesser effect. However, the ECG appears to be unaltered in studies in healthy subjects given these quinolones with procainamide. An increased risk of torsade de pointes

would be expected if procainamide is used with gatifloxacin, moxifloxacin, or sparfloxacin, and possibly levofloxacin.

Clinical evidence

Nine healthy subjects were given a single 1-g oral dose of procainamide alone, then again with the fifth dose of **ofloxacin** (400 mg twice daily for five doses). **Ofloxacin** increased the AUC of procainamide by 27%, increased its maximum plasma levels by 21% (from 4.8 to 5.8 micrograms/mL) and reduced its total clearance by 22%, whereas the pharmacokinetics of the active metabolite of procainamide, *N*-acetylprocainamide, were not significantly altered.[1] In another study, 10 healthy subjects were given **levofloxacin** 500 mg daily or **ciprofloxacin** 500 mg twice daily, with a single 15-mg/kg intravenous dose of procainamide on day 5. **Levofloxacin** increased the AUC of procainamide by 21% and prolonged its half-life by about 19% (from 2.7 to 3.2 hours). The clearance of procainamide was reduced by 17% (range 4 to 46%) with renal clearance reduced by 26% (range 11 to 58%). The pharmacokinetics of *N*-acetylprocainamide were similarly affected. **Ciprofloxacin** caused only minor changes in procainamide and *N*-acetylprocainamide pharmacokinetics, although the renal clearance of procainamide was reduced by 15% (range 3 to 26%).[2]

Despite these pharmacokinetic changes, no ECG changes were detected. However, these studies[1,2] involved only single doses of procainamide with average maximum serum levels (about 4 to 6 micrograms/mL) at the lower end of the therapeutic range for procainamide, although in one study individual levels of up to 8.5 micrograms/mL were found.[1]

The QTc interval in an elderly patient with atrial fibrillation increased from 450 to 464 milliseconds 3 days after she was given a single intravenous dose of procainamide and also started taking **levofloxacin** 500 mg daily. Procainamide levels on day 3 were subtherapeutic (1.8 micrograms/mL). On day 4 the QTc interval had increased to 568 milliseconds, she developed polymorphic ventricular tachycardia, and by the evening the QTc interval had further increased to 577 milliseconds. **Levofloxacin** was discontinued on day 5 and the QTc interval returned to normal within 48 hours.[3] This effect was attributed to **levofloxacin**, and an interaction with procainamide was not considered.

An analysis of the Adverse Events Reporting System database of the FDA in the US looked at cases of torsade de pointes associated with quinolones reported up until May 2001. The quinolones included in the analysis were **ciprofloxacin, ofloxacin, levofloxacin, gatifloxacin,** and **moxifloxacin**, and in total there were 37 cases identified, of which 19 occurred in patients also taking other drugs known to prolong the QT interval. One of these 19 cases was noted in a patient taking procainamide with a quinolone [unspecified].[4]

Mechanism

The probable reason for the pharmacokinetic interaction is that levofloxacin, ofloxacin and to a lesser extent ciprofloxacin, inhibit the secretion of unchanged procainamide by the kidney tubules via renal drug transporters. Levofloxacin also appears to inhibit the secretion of *N*-acetylprocainamide. Some quinolones can prolong the QT interval, and these effects may be additive with the QT-prolonging effects of procainamide.

Importance and management

These results suggest that ofloxacin and levofloxacin affect the pharmacokinetics of procainamide to a modest extent; ciprofloxacin has lesser effects. The large interpatient variation found in these studies suggests it is possible that many patients will not experience a clinically significant interaction. However, in slow acetylators of procainamide, in whom renal clearance contributes to a larger fraction of total clearance, and those receiving higher doses of procainamide (serum levels greater than 10 micrograms/mL), the use of ofloxacin or levofloxacin could result in a clinically relevant effect. Therefore, it would be prudent to monitor the outcome if procainamide is given with these quinolones.

Evidence for an interaction between QT-prolonging quinolones and procainamide is limited but note that the concurrent use of two drugs that prolong the QT interval should generally be avoided, or undertaken with caution. For a further discussion of QT prolongation, see 'Drugs that prolong the QT interval + Other drugs that prolong the QT interval', p.272.

1. Martin DE, Shen J, Griener J, Raasch R, Patterson JH, Cascio W. Effects of ofloxacin on the pharmacokinetics and pharmacodynamics of procainamide. *J Clin Pharmacol* (1996) 36, 85–91.
2. Bauer LA, Black DJ, Lill JS, Garrison J, Raisys VA, Hooton TM. Levofloxacin and ciprofloxacin decrease procainamide and *N*-acetylprocainamide renal clearances. *Antimicrob Agents Chemother* (2005) 49, 1649–51.
3. Samaha FF. QTc interval prolongation and polymorphic ventricular tachycardia in association with levofloxacin. *Am J Med* (1999) 107, 528–9.
4. Frothingham R. Rates of torsades de pointes associated with ciprofloxacin, ofloxacin, levofloxacin, gatifloxacin, and moxifloxacin. *Pharmacotherapy* (2001) 21, 1468–72.

Procainamide + Sucralfate

Sucralfate does not appear to affect the absorption of procainamide.

Clinical evidence, mechanism, importance and management

In 4 healthy subjects, sucralfate 1 g taken 30 minutes before a single 250-mg dose of procainamide reduced the mean maximum salivary level of procainamide by 5.3%, but did not significantly affect either the AUC or the rate of absorption.[1] These results suggest that a clinically significant interaction between sucralfate and procainamide is unlikely.

1. Turkistani AAA, Gaber M, Al-Meshal MA, Al-Shora HI, Gouda MW. Effect of sucralfate on procainamide absorption. *Int J Pharmaceutics* (1990) 59, R1–R3.

Procainamide + Trimethoprim

Trimethoprim causes a marked increase in the plasma levels of procainamide and its active metabolite, *N*-acetylprocainamide.

Clinical evidence

Eight healthy subjects were given procainamide 500 mg every 6 hours for 3 days. The concurrent use of trimethoprim 200 mg daily increased the AUC_{0-12} of procainamide and its active metabolite, *N*-acetylprocainamide (NAPA), by 63% and 51%, respectively. The renal clearance of procainamide and NAPA decreased by 47% and 13%, respectively. The QTc prolonging effects of procainamide were increased to a significant, but slight, extent by trimethoprim.[1] Another study found that trimethoprim 200 mg daily reduced the renal clearance of a single 1-g dose of procainamide and NAPA by 45% and 26%, respectively. The QTc interval was increased by 30 milliseconds to 430 milliseconds.[2]

Mechanism

Trimethoprim decreases the renal clearance of both procainamide and its active metabolite by competing for active tubular secretion. It may also cause a small increase in the conversion of procainamide to *N*-acetylprocainamide.[1]

Importance and management

An established interaction but its documentation is limited. The need to reduce the procainamide dose should be anticipated if trimethoprim is given to patients already taking stable doses of procainamide. In practice the effects may be greater than those found in the studies cited because the renal excretion of procainamide is slower in the elderly than in young healthy subjects. Remember too that the daily dose of trimethoprim in **co-trimoxazole** (trimethoprim 160 mg with sulfamethoxazole 800 mg) may equal or exceed the doses used in the studies cited.

1. Kosoglou T, Rocci ML, Vlasses PH. Trimethoprim alters the disposition of procainamide and N-acetylprocainamide. *Clin Pharmacol Ther* (1988) 44, 467–77.
2. Vlasses PH, Kosoglou T, Chase SL, Greenspon AJ, Lottes S, Andress E, Ferguson RK, Rocci ML. Trimethoprim inhibition of the renal clearance of procainamide and N-acetylprocainamide. *Arch Intern Med* (1989) 149, 1350–3.

Propafenone + Azoles

Limited evidence suggests that ketoconazole might inhibit the metabolism of propafenone in some patients. Other azoles would be expected to interact similarly. An isolated case report describes a man taking propafenone who had a seizure two days after taking ketoconazole.

Clinical evidence

The preliminary results of a study in 12 healthy subjects given a single 300-mg dose of propafenone with or without **ketoconazole** 200 mg found that the increase in the AUC of propafenone with **ketoconazole** was greater in CYP2D6 poor metabolisers (that is, those lacking this isoenzyme) than in CYP2D6 extensive metabolisers (that is, those with normal amounts of this isoenzyme).[1]

A man who had been taking captopril and hydrochlorothiazide for 6 years and propafenone 300 mg daily for 4 years, without problems, and without any history of convulsive episodes, experienced a tonic-clonic seizure while watching television. It was later found that he had started to take **ketoconazole** 2 days previously for the treatment of a candidal infection.[2]

Mechanism

Propafenone is principally metabolised by CYP2D6, with CYP3A4 and CYP1A2 also involved. Ketoconazole is a potent inhibitor of CYP3A4. It therefore increases propafenone concentrations to some extent in CYP2D6 extensive metabolisers, but has a greater effect in CYP2D6 poor metabolisers, for whom routes other than CYP2D6 are more important in propafenone metabolism. For further comments on propafenone metabolism, see *Propafenone metabolism*, under 'Antiarrhythmics', p.260.

The authors of the case report postulate that the ketoconazole might have inhibited the metabolism of the propafenone so that this patient, in effect, developed an overdose.[2] However, convulsions with propafenone, even in overdose, are extremely rare.[3]

Importance and management

Evidence for an interaction between propafenone and the azoles appears to be limited and the general importance of this interaction is uncertain. As of 2006, there had been no other cases of an interaction reported to the manufacturer of propafenone.[4] As the available data suggest that a clinically relevant pharmacokinetic interaction could be possible in some patients (that is, those lacking CYP2D6, which is unlikely to be known in clinical practice), it would seem prudent to keep this interaction in mind, particularly if any unexplained propafenone adverse effects (such as hypotension, bradycardia, dizziness, dry mouth) occur in patients also given ketoconazole. If adverse effects become troublesome, adjust the propafenone dose, according to clinical need. The effect of other azoles does not appear to have been studied, but as they can all inhibit CYP3A4 (to a greater or lesser extent, see 'Table 1.9', p.11) it would seem prudent to consider the possibility of an interaction if any unexplained propafenone adverse effects occur on concurrent use, and follow the same advice.

1. Munoz CE, Ito S, Bend JR, Tesoro A, Freeman D, Spence JD, Bailey DG. Propafenone interaction with CYP3A4 inhibitors in man. *Clin Pharmacol Ther* (1997) 61, 154.
2. Duvelleroy Hommet C, Jonville-Bera AP, Autret A, Saudeau D, Autret E, Fauchier JP. Une crise convulsive chez un patient traité par propafénone et kétoconazole. *Therapie* (1995) 50, 164–5.
3. Arythmol (Propafenone hydrochloride). Abbott Laboratories Ltd. UK Summary of product characteristics, November 2012.
4. Abbott Laboratories. Personal communication, April 2006.

Propafenone + Barbiturates

Phenobarbital increases the metabolism of propafenone and reduces its exposure. Other barbiturates might interact similarly.

Clinical evidence, mechanism, importance and management

In a preliminary report of a study in 7 non-smoking subjects, **phenobarbital** 100 mg daily for 3 weeks reduced the concentrations of a single 300-mg dose of propafenone by 26 to 87% and reduced its AUC by 10 to 89%. The intrinsic clearance of propafenone was increased by 11 to 84%. The results in a further 4 heavy smokers were similar.[1]

Barbiturates are known inducers of the cytochrome P450 enzyme system and would therefore be expected to increase the rate of propafenone metabolism, possibly by inducing CYP1A2 and CYP3A4. For further comments on propafenone metabolism, see *Propafenone metabolism*, under 'Antiarrhythmics', p.260.

The clinical importance of this interaction awaits assessment, but until more is known, it would seem prudent to monitor concurrent use to ensure that propafenone remains effective if **phenobarbital** is started: the increases seen suggest that it may be ineffective in some patients. Other barbiturates would be expected to interact similarly.

1. Chan GL-Y, Axelson JE, Kerr CR. The effect of phenobarbital on the pharmacokinetics of propafenone in man. *Pharm Res* (1988) 5, S153.

Propafenone + Cimetidine

Cimetidine appears to interact minimally with propafenone.

Clinical evidence

A study in 12 healthy subjects given propafenone 225 mg every 8 hours for 5 days found that the concurrent use of cimetidine 400 mg every 8 hours, also given for 5 days, increased the mean maximum and steady-state plasma propafenone concentrations by 24% and 22%, respectively. However, there was wide intersubject variability and so these changes did not reach statistical significance. A slight increase in the QRS interval also occurred.[1]

Mechanism

Propafenone is principally metabolised by CYP2D6, with CYP3A4 and CYP1A2 also involved. Cimetidine is a well-known non-specific enzyme inhibitor, and is a weak inhibitor of both CYP3A4 and CYP1A2, and therefore has only small effects on propafenone metabolism. For further comments on propafenone metabolism, see *Propafenone metabolism*, under 'Antiarrhythmics', p.260.

Importance and management

Evidence for a pharmacokinetic interaction between propafenone and cimetidine is limited to this study in which none of the changes were considered clinically important.[1] However, the UK manufacturer of propafenone advises that all patients are closely monitored and the dose adjusted accordingly on concurrent use with CYP3A4 inhibitors, and they name cimetidine.[2] This is possibly because some patients lack CYP2D6, and this is unlikely to be known in clinical practice. In these patients the contribution of CYP3A4 is likely to be more important in propafenone metabolism, which creates the potential for a greater interaction with CYP3A4 inhibitors. Therefore, until more is known, it would seem prudent to monitor all patients for an increase in propafenone adverse effects (such as hypotension, bradycardia, dizziness, dry mouth), and adjust the propafenone dose if necessary.

1. Pritchett ELC, Smith WM, Kirsten EB. Pharmacokinetic and pharmacodynamic interactions of propafenone and cimetidine. *J Clin Pharmacol* (1988) 28, 619–24.
2. Arythmol (Propafenone hydrochloride). Abbott Laboratories Ltd. UK Summary of product characteristics, November 2012.

Propafenone + Grapefruit juice

Limited evidence suggests that grapefruit juice might inhibit the metabolism of propafenone in some patients.

Clinical evidence

Preliminary results of a study in 12 healthy subjects given a single 300-mg dose of propafenone with or without 250 mL of grapefruit juice found that the increase in the AUC of propafenone with grapefruit juice was greater in CYP2D6 poor metabolisers (that is, those lacking this isoenzyme) than in CYP2D6 extensive metabolisers (that is, those with normal amounts of this isoenzyme).[1]

Mechanism

Propafenone is principally metabolised by CYP2D6, with CYP3A4 and CYP1A2 also involved. Grapefruit juice can inhibit CYP3A4. It therefore increases propafenone concentrations to some extent in CYP2D6 extensive metabolisers, but has a greater effect in CYP2D6 poor metabolisers, for whom routes other than CYP2D6 are more important in propafenone metabolism. For further comments on propafenone metabolism, see *Propafenone metabolism*, under 'Antiarrhythmics', p.260.

Importance and management

Evidence for a pharmacokinetic interaction between propafenone and grapefruit juice appears to be limited to this study. The clinical importance of the finding is not certain, but it suggests that grapefruit juice might raise propafenone concentrations in some patients, that is, those lacking CYP2D6, although note that this is rarely known in clinical practice..As the effect of grapefruit juice could be variable between batches of juice and the effect could only be controlled by dose adjustments if patients consumed grapefruit juice consistently, it would seem prudent to initially monitor for propafenone adverse effects (such as hypotension, bradycardia, dizziness, dry mouth) and advise patients to avoid grapefruit juice if these become troublesome. If arrhythmias have been particularly difficult to control, a cautious approach would be to advise avoiding grapefruit juice altogether.

1. Munoz CE, Ito S, Bend JR, Tesoro A, Freeman D, Spence JD, Bailey DG. Propafenone interaction with CYP3A4 inhibitors in man. *Clin Pharmacol Ther* (1997) 61, 154.

Propafenone + HIV-protease inhibitors

Ritonavir might increase the concentrations of propafenone. Other HIV-protease inhibitors alone or boosted with ritonavir might interact similarly.

Clinical evidence

Direct evidence (from case reports or clinical studies) of an interaction between propafenone and the HIV-protease inhibitors appears to be lacking; however, a review of HIV-protease inhibitor interactions reports that the plasma concentrations of propafenone may be increased by **ritonavir**.[1] The review also states that **indinavir**, **nelfinavir** and **saquinavir** might increase plasma concentrations of propafenone.[1]

Mechanism

Propafenone is primarily metabolised by CYP2D6, with CYP1A2 and CYP3A4 also involved. Ritonavir is an inhibitor of both CYP2D6 and CYP3A4; having moderate effects on CYP2D6 at high doses (500 mg twice daily) and weak effects at low doses (100 mg twice daily), and potent effects on CYP3A4 both alone and when used as a pharmacokinetic enhancer (i.e. at high and low doses). The concurrent use of ritonavir would therefore be expected to increase propafenone concentrations. Of the other HIV-protease inhibitors, only tipranavir has been shown to inhibit CYP2D6 (*in vitro*).[2] All HIV-protease inhibitors are, to varying degrees, inhibitors of CYP3A4, and might only affect propafenone concentrations under certain circumstances, see 'Table 1.9', p.11, for further details.

Importance and management

Evidence for an interaction between **ritonavir** and propafenone is limited, but what is reported is in line with the known pharmacokinetics of these drugs. At high doses, ritonavir would be expected to increase propafenone concentrations in all patients. **Tipranavir** seems likely to interact similarly (see under *Mechanism*, above). As there is a risk of serious adverse effects, the manufacturers of ritonavir[3,4] and tipranavir[2,5] contraindicate the concurrent use of propafenone. The clinical relevance of an interaction with ritonavir given as a pharmacokinetic enhancer is less certain, as it will have less potent effects on propafenone metabolism at this lower dose. Nevertheless, a number of the HIV-protease inhibitors are contraindicated with propafenone, when ritonavir is also given, and, until more information is available, this seems a sensibly cautious approach with all HIV-protease inhibitors boosted with ritonavir. If concurrent use is considered to be unavoidable, it would be advisable to monitor propafenone concentrations wherever possible, and monitor closely for an increase in propafenone adverse effects (such as hypotension, bradycardia, dizziness, dry mouth).

Unlike tipranavir and ritonavir, other HIV-protease inhibitors do not inhibit CYP2D6, and they would therefore not be expected to interact with propafenone in all patients, when given unboosted. However, in poor metabolisers where propafenone metabolism is more dependent on CY3A4, these HIV-protease inhibitors could cause a clinically relevant interaction (see *Propafenone metabolism*, under 'Antiarrhythmics', p.260, for an explanation). It would therefore seem prudent to monitor the use of unboosted HIV-protease inhibitors and propafenone for an increase in propafenone adverse effects (such as hypotension, bradycardia, dizziness, dry mouth).

It is important to note, that metaboliser status is rarely known in clinical practice and therefore any cautions and contraindications apply to all patients, but may be more relevant in some than in others.

1. Burger DM, Hoetelmans RMW, Koopmans PP, Meenhorst PL, Mulder JW, Hekster YA, Beijnen JH. Clinically relevant drug interactions with antiretroviral agents. *Antivir Ther* (1997) 2, 149–165.
2. Aptivus Soft Capsules (Tipranavir). Boehringer Ingelheim Ltd. UK Summary of product characteristics, December 2011.
3. Norvir Tablets (Ritonavir). AbbVie Ltd. UK Summary of product characteristics, September 2012.
4. Norvir Capsules (Ritonavir). Abbott Laboratories. US Prescribing information, March 2012.
5. Aptivus (Tipranavir). Boehringer Ingelheim Pharmaceuticals, Inc. US Prescribing information, April 2012.

Propafenone + Macrolides

Limited evidence suggests that erythromycin (a CYP3A4 inhibitor) might inhibit the metabolism of propafenone in some patients. Other macrolides that inhibit CYP3A4 would be expected to interact similarly.

Clinical evidence

The preliminary results of a study in 12 healthy subjects given a single 300-mg dose of propafenone with or without erythromycin 250 mg found that the increase in the AUC of propafenone with erythromycin was greater in CYP2D6 poor metabolisers (that is, those lacking this isoenzyme) than in CYP2D6 extensive metabolisers (that is, those with normal amounts of this isoenzyme).[1]

Mechanism

Propafenone is principally metabolised by CYP2D6, with CYP3A4 and CYP1A2 also involved. Erythromycin is a moderate inhibitor of CYP3A4. It therefore increases propafenone concentrations to some extent in CYP2D6 extensive metabolisers, but has a greater effect in CYP2D6 poor metabolisers, for whom routes other than CYP2D6 are more important in propafenone metabolism. For further comments on propafenone metabolism, see *Propafenone metabolism*, under 'Antiarrhythmics', p.260.

Importance and management

Evidence for a pharmacokinetic interaction between propafenone and erythromycin appears to be limited to this study and its clinical importance is not certain. As the available data suggest that a clinically relevant pharmacokinetic interaction could be possible in some patients (that is, those lacking CYP2D6, which is unlikely to be known in clinical practice), it would seem prudent to bear this interaction in mind, particularly if any unexplained propafenone adverse effects (such as hypotension, bradycardia, dizziness, dry mouth) occur in patients also given erythromycin If adverse effects become troublesome, adjust the propafenone dose, according to clinical need. Other macrolides that inhibit CYP3A4, such as **clarithromycin** and **telithromycin**, would be expected to interact similarly.

1. Munoz CE, Ito S, Bend JR, Tesoro A, Freeman D, Spence JD, Bailey DG. Propafenone interaction with CYP3A4 inhibitors in man. *Clin Pharmacol Ther* (1997) 61, 154.

Propafenone + Mirtazapine

A case report describes seizures and cardiovascular toxicity in a patient taking propafenone after mirtazapine was added.

Clinical evidence, mechanism, importance and management

A case report describes seizures, bradycardia, plus prolonged QRS and QT intervals in a 69-year-old man taking propafenone 325 mg twice daily, aspirin, and multivitamins, when he took mirtazapine 15 mg at night for insomnia. The patient experienced a seizure approximately 12 hours after the first dose of mirtazapine, then two further seizures en route to hospital where he was noted to be hypotensive and bradycardic, and an ECG showed atrial fibrillation, right bundle branch block, a prolonged QRS interval, and a corrected QT interval of 500 milliseconds. The patient was intubated, sedated, and given fluid resuscitation, and 6 hours after admission an ECG showed sinus bradycardia with less prolonged QRS and QT intervals. Another ECG, 36 hours after admission, showed sinus rhythm, a normal QT interval, and a narrow QRS complex.

Propafenone is a substrate of CYP2D6, and the authors suggest that mirtazapine might have led to inhibition of CYP2D6 resulting in an increase in propafenone concentrations,[1] although clinical evidence of CYP2D6 inhibition by mirtazapine appears to be lacking, and the speed of the effect seen is possibly unlikely to be due to inhibition of isoenzymes. The authors also suggest that the patient might have been a CYP2D6 poor metaboliser (that is, those with a lower than normal activity of CYP2D6), and as such could already have had a higher propafenone concentration than an extensive metaboliser (that is, those with normal CYP2D6 activity), which was further exacerbated by mirtazapine.[1] Neither metaboliser status, or propafenone concentrations were assessed. Note that as with other antidepressants, the use of mirtazapine can be associated with an increased risk of seizures and this case could perhaps just be due to an adverse effect of mirtazapine. Prolongation of the QT interval has also been reported with mirtazapine, although usually with high doses and in association with other drugs that also prolong the QT interval.[2] The suggestion that the effects seen are due to a drug interaction between propafenone and mirtazapine is questionable, and therefore the general clinical relevance of this case is unclear.

1. Rajpurohit N, Aryal SR, Khan MA, Stys AT, Stys TP. Propafenone associated severe central nervous system and cardiovascular toxicity due to mirtazapine: a case of severe drug interaction. *S D Med* (2014) 67, 137–9.
2. Zispin SolTab (Mirtazapine). Merck Sharp & Dohme Ltd. UK Summary of product characteristics, February 2015.

Propafenone + Quinidine

Quinidine doubles the plasma concentrations of propafenone and halves the concentrations of its active metabolite in some patients.

Clinical evidence

Nine patients taking propafenone for frequent isolated ventricular ectopic beats, firstly had their dose reduced to 150 mg every 8 hours and then 4 days later the steady-state pharmacokinetics of propafenone were determined at this new dose. Quinidine was then added at a dose of 50 mg every 8 hours, and after a further 4 days the steady-state plasma propafenone concentrations in 7 CYP2D6 extensive metabolisers (that is, those with normal amounts of this isoenzyme) had more than doubled from 408 nanograms/mL to 1100 nanograms/mL, and the concentrations of the metabolite 5-hydroxypropafenone had approximately halved. However, the ECG intervals and arrhythmia frequency were unaltered. The steady-state plasma propafenone concentrations remained unchanged in the other 2 patients with reduced amounts of CYP2D6 (poor metabolisers).[1]

The same research group conducted a similar study in healthy subjects, which confirmed that quinidine increased the plasma concentration of propafenone in CYP2D6 extensive but not poor metabolisers. In addition, it was found that quinidine increased the extent of the beta-blockade caused by propafenone in extensive metabolisers to approach that seen in poor metabolisers.[2] CYP2D6 shows pronounced interethnic differences in expression, and another study found that the inhibition of propafenone metabolism by low-dose quinidine also occurs in Chinese as well as Caucasian patients.[3] A further study found that combining low-dose quinidine (150 mg daily) with standard doses of propafenone in patients with atrial fibrillation resulted in a similar control of the arrhythmia as increasing the propafenone dose, but caused less gastrointestinal adverse effects.[4]

Mechanism

Quinidine is a potent inhibitor of CYP2D6, which is responsible for the 5-hydroxylation of propafenone, resulting in a reduced rate of metabolism in CYP2D6 extensive metabolisers, but not in poor metabolisers, who lack this isoenzyme and therefore depend on other routes for propafenone metabolism. So, in extensive metabolisers, plasma propafenone concentrations are doubled, but the overall antiarrhythmic effects remain unchanged, possibly because the production of its active metabolite (5-hydroxypropafenone) is simultaneously halved.[1] Quinidine increases the beta-blocking effects of propafenone in extensive metabolisers because only the parent drug, and not the metabolites, has beta-blocking activity.[2]

Importance and management

Quinidine appears to increase propafenone concentrations in patients who are CYP2D6 extensive metabolisers, and might also affect the beta-blocking properties of propafenone in these patients. In one study the concurrent use of propafenone and quinidine was said to have an effect similar to increasing the propafenone dose.[4] Note that CYP2D6 metaboliser status is usually unknown in routine clinical practice, therefore it would seem prudent to monitor all patients taking propafenone and quinidine for an increase in propafenone adverse effects (such as hypotension, bradycardia, dizziness, dry mouth), and adjust the propafenone dose as necessary.

1. Funck-Brentano C, Kroemer HK, Pavlou H, Woosley RL, Roden DM. Genetically-determined interaction between propafenone and low dose quinidine: role of active metabolites in modulating net drug effect. *Br J Clin Pharmacol* (1989) 27, 435–44.
2. Mörike K, Roden D. Quinidine-enhanced β-blockade during treatment with propafenone in extensive metabolizer human subjects. *Clin Pharmacol Ther* (1994) 55, 28–34.
3. Fan C, Tang M, Lau C-P, Chow M. The effect of quinidine on propafenone metabolism in Chinese patients. *Clin Invest Med* (1998) (Suppl) S12.
4. Lau C-P, Chow MSS, Tse H-F, Tang M-O, Fan C. Control of paroxysmal atrial fibrillation recurrence using combined administration of propafenone and quinidine. *Am J Cardiol* (2000) 86, 1327–32.

Propafenone + Rifampicin (Rifampin)

Propafenone serum concentrations and therapeutic effects can be greatly reduced by rifampicin.

Clinical evidence

A man with ventricular arrhythmias successfully treated with propafenone had a large reduction in his plasma propafenone concentrations, from 993 nanograms/mL to 176 nanograms/mL, within 12 days of starting to take rifampicin 450 mg twice daily. Concentrations of the two active metabolites of propafenone were also altered, with 5-hydroxypropafenone concentrations reduced from 195 nanograms/mL to 64 nanograms/mL, and *N*-depropylpropafenone levels increased from 110 nanograms/mL to 192 nanograms/mL. His arrhythmias returned, but 2 weeks after stopping rifampicin his arrhythmias had disappeared and propafenone and its 5-hydroxy and *N*-depropyl metabolites had returned to acceptable concentrations (1411 nanograms/mL, 78 nanograms/mL and 158 nanograms/mL, respectively).[1]

In a study in young healthy subjects, rifampicin 600 mg daily for 9 days reduced the bioavailability of a single 300-mg oral dose of propafenone from 30% to 10% in CYP2D6 extensive metabolisers (that is, those with normal amounts of this isoenzyme), and from 81% to 48% in those lacking CYP2D6 (poor metabolisers). QRS prolongation decreased during enzyme induction. In contrast, in this study, rifampicin had no substantial effect on the pharmacokinetics of propafenone given intravenously.[2] Similar findings were reported in a further study by the same research group, in healthy elderly subjects.[3]

One report describes the use of rifampicin 600 mg daily to increase the metabolism of propafenone (as well as digoxin and warfarin) in a case of multiple drug overdose in a 16-year-old female. She had ingested 15 tablets each containing propafenone 300 mg (equivalent to 90 mg/kg) but concentrations of propafenone were not obtained. Other treatments including gastric lavage, activated charcoal, cardiac pacing and plasma exchange were also used so the contribution of rifampicin treatment to the patient's recovery is not known.[4]

Mechanism

Propafenone is principally metabolised by CYP2D6, although CYP1A2 and CYP3A4 are also involved. Rifampicin is a well-known non-specific enzyme inducer, which has the potential to increase the metabolism of propafenone by any of the isoenzymes involved in its metabolism. Rifampicin is also known to induce glucuronidation and might also increase the phase II glucuronidation of propafenone. The effect of rifampicin on gastrointestinal clearance of propafenone was greater than that of its hepatic clearance.[2,3]

Importance and management

The interaction between propafenone and rifampicin is established and clinically relevant. It would seem prudent to monitor concurrent use closely for a reduction in propafenone efficacy in patients also given rifampicin: the dose of oral propafenone is likely to need increasing.[3] Alternatively, the authors of the case report[1] advise the use of another antibacterial, where possible, because of the probable difficulty in adjusting the propafenone dose.

1. Castel JM, Cappiello E, Leopaldi D, Latini R. Rifampicin lowers plasma concentrations of propafenone and its antiarrhythmic effect. *Br J Clin Pharmacol* (1990) 30, 155–6.
2. Dilger K, Greiner B, Fromm MF, Hofmann U, Kroemer HK, Eichelbaum M. Consequences of rifampicin treatment on propafenone disposition in extensive and poor metabolizers of CYP2D6. *Pharmacogenetics* (1999) 9, 551–9.
3. Dilger K, Hofmann U, Klotz U. Enzyme induction in the elderly: Effect of rifampin on the pharmacokinetics and pharmacodynamics of propafenone. *Clin Pharmacol Ther* (2000) 67, 512–20.
4. Unal S, Bayrakci B, Yasar U, Karagoz T. Successful treatment of propafenone, digoxin and warfarin overdosage with plasma exchange therapy and rifampicin. *Clin Drug Invest* (2007) 27, 505–8.

Propafenone + SSRIs

In general, the SSRIs would be expected to inhibit the metabolism of propafenone, but the extent of this interaction varies by drug: fluoxetine and paroxetine would be expected to have the greatest effect, although fluvoxamine might also have an important effect in some patients.

Clinical evidence

In a study in healthy subjects, **fluoxetine** 20 mg daily for 10 days decreased the oral clearance of a single 400-mg dose of propafenone by 34% for both the *R*- and *S*-enantiomers. The maximum plasma concentrations were increased by 39% for *S*-propafenone and by 71% for *R*-propafenone. However, there were no differences in the changes to the PR and QRS intervals.[1]

A case report describes an elderly woman who had been taking propafenone 900 mg daily for more than 10 years for paroxysmal atrial fibrillation, who experienced chest tightness and dizziness 3 months after starting to take **citalopram** 10 mg daily, increased after one month to 20 mg daily. The episodes became more frequent in the following months and she had several falls but no acute coronary event was diagnosed. She was given amlodipine, glyceryl trinitrate patches and warfarin, but after a fall she became delirious. Amlodipine and glyceryl trinitrate were discontinued and her dose of propafenone was reduced to 450 mg daily and **citalopram** was continued at 20 mg daily. The patient recovered without any further symptoms during a one-year follow-up.[2]

Mechanism

Fluoxetine is an inhibitor of CYP2D6, which is responsible for the metabolism of propafenone to its primary active metabolite, 5-hydroxypropafenone. *In vitro* data have shown that, of the SSRIs, fluoxetine is the most potent inhibitor of propafenone 5-hydroxylation, followed by **paroxetine**. **Sertraline** and **fluvoxamine** have less effect on propafenone 5-hydroxylation, and citalopram has slight or no effects.[3] Although **fluvoxamine** only moderately inhibited propafenone 5-hydroxylation it did inhibit propafenone *N*-dealkylation[3] by inhibiting CYP1A2. This isoenzyme has only a minor role in the metabolism of propafenone, but it might assume greater importance in patients lacking CYP2D6 (poor metabolisers).[3] For further comments on propafenone metabolism, see *Propafenone metabolism*, under 'Antiarrhythmics', p.260.

Importance and management

Evidence for an interaction between **fluoxetine** and propafenone is limited. The study suggests that fluoxetine increases the maximum propafenone concentrations without affecting the ECG, but as the overall propafenone exposure was not assessed, and it was only a single-dose study, it is difficult to assess the clinical relevance of the interaction on the long-term concurrent use of both drugs. As with quinidine (see 'Propafenone + Quinidine', p.291), inhibition of 5-hydroxylation would be expected to increase the beta-blocking effects of propafenone, although note that fluoxetine is a less potent inhibitor of CYP2D6 than quinidine, and therefore its effects would be expected to be smaller. Until more is known, it would be prudent to use caution when giving fluoxetine with propafenone, monitoring for an increase in propafenone adverse effects (such as hypotension, bradycardia, dizziness, dry mouth) and consider decreasing the dose of propafenone if these become troublesome.

Evidence regarding an interaction with the other SSRIs is even more sparse. **Paroxetine** generally interacts in the same way as fluoxetine, and therefore similar precautions to those given for fluoxetine would be appropriate.

Fluvoxamine would not generally be expected to interact, except in patients who lack CYP2D6 (poor metabolisers), when other routes of propafenone metabolism become more important. As it is unlikely that the metaboliser status of patients will be known, it would seem prudent to monitor concurrent use in the same way as for fluoxetine.

The *in vitro* study with propafenone suggests that the other SSRIs, **citalopram** (and therefore probably **escitalopram**) and **sertraline**, have more minor, if any, effects on CYP2D6, and this is supported by the known clinical effects of these drugs on other CYP2D6 substrates (see 'Beta blockers + SSRIs', p.1022). Nevertheless, a small increase in propafenone concentrations is possible, and the case report with citalopram reinforces this. Therefore, if propafenone adverse effects (such as hypotension, bradycardia, dizziness, dry mouth) develop in a patient taking one of these SSRIs, it would be prudent to consider an interaction as a possible cause.

1. Cai WM, Chen B, Zhou Y, Zhang YD. Fluoxetine impairs the CYP2D6-mediated metabolism of propafenone enantiomers in healthy Chinese volunteers. *Clin Pharmacol Ther* (1999) 66, 516–21.
2. Garcia A. Adverse effects of propafenone after long-term therapy with the addition of citalopram. *Am J Geriatr Pharmacother* (2008) 6, 96–9.
3. Hemeryck A, De Vriendt C, Belpaire FM. Effect of selective serotonin reuptake inhibitors on the oxidative metabolism of propafenone: *in vitro* studies using human liver microsomes. *J Clin Psychopharmacol* (2000) 20, 428–34.

Quinidine + Amiloride

A single study found that the antiarrhythmic activity of quinidine can be opposed by amiloride.

Clinical evidence

A study in 10 patients with inducible sustained ventricular tachycardia was carried out to see whether a beneficial interaction occurred between quinidine and amiloride. Patients were given oral quinidine until their trough serum levels reached 10 micromol/L, or the maximum well-tolerated dose was reached. After electrophysiological studies, oral amiloride 5 mg twice daily was started, and increased up to 10 mg twice daily (if serum potassium levels remained normal) for 3 days. The electrophysiological studies were then repeated. Unexpectedly, 7 of the 10 patients demonstrated adverse responses while taking both drugs. Three developed sustained ventricular tachycardia and 3 others had somatic adverse effects (hypotension, nausea, diarrhoea), which prevented further studies being undertaken. One patient had 12 episodes of sustained ventricular tachycardia while taking both drugs. Amiloride had no effect on quinidine levels.[1]

Mechanism

Not understood. The combination of quinidine and amiloride increased the QRS interval, but did not prolong the QT interval more than quinidine alone.

Importance and management

So far the evidence seems to be limited to this single study but it suggests that amiloride can oppose the antiarrhythmic activity of quinidine. The full clinical implications of this interaction are not known, but it would clearly be prudent to consider monitoring to confirm that the quinidine continues to be effective if amiloride is given.

1. Wang L, Sheldon RS, Mitchell B, Wyse DG, Gillis AM, Chiamvimonvat N, Duff HJ. Amiloride-quinidine interaction: adverse outcomes. *Clin Pharmacol Ther* (1994) 56, 659–67.

Quinidine + Amiodarone

The QT interval prolonging effects of quinidine and amiodarone are increased when they are used together, and torsade de pointes has occurred. Amiodarone increases quinidine levels.

Clinical evidence

In a study, 11 patients were stabilised taking quinidine in daily doses of 1.2 to 4.2 g. When they were also given amiodarone (600 mg every 12 hours for 5 to 7 days, then 600 mg daily) their mean serum quinidine levels rose by an average of 32%, from 4.4 to 5.8 micrograms/mL and 3 of them had a substantial increase of 2 micrograms/mL. Signs of toxicity (diarrhoea, nausea, vomiting, hypotension) were seen in some patients, and the quinidine dose was reduced in 9 patients, by an average of 37%. Despite the dose reduction, the quinidine serum levels were still higher at 5.2 micrograms/mL than before the amiodarone was started.[1]

A test in a healthy subject found that 3 days after amiodarone 600 mg was added to quinidine 1.2 g daily, the serum quinidine levels doubled and the relative QT interval was prolonged from 1 (no drugs) to 1.2 (quinidine alone) to 1.4 (quinidine plus amiodarone).[2] This report also described 2 patients with minor cardiac arrhythmias who developed QT prolongation and torsade de pointes when given both drugs.[2] A Russian study of the use of the combination in atrial fibrillation reported that one of 52 patients had a 50% increase in the QT interval resulting in torsade de pointes and subsequently ventricular fibrillation, which required repeated defibrillation over 6 hours.[3] A 76-year-old man taking quinidine and amiodarone had a number of episodes of loss of consciousness, and subsequently QT prolongation and torsade de pointes, which stopped when the quinidine was discontinued.[4]

Successful and uneventful concurrent use has been described in a report of 4 patients taking quinidine (dose not stated) and amiodarone 200 mg five times weekly.[5] Another report describes the successful use of a short course of quinidine to convert chronic atrial fibrillation to sinus rhythm in 9 of 15 patients taking long-term amiodarone. Patients were hospitalised and continuously monitored. No proarrhythmias occurred and the QT interval remained within acceptable limits.[6]

Mechanism

The mechanism behind the pharmacokinetic interaction is not understood. The QT prolonging effects of the two drugs would be expected to be additive.

Importance and management

An established and clinically important pharmacokinetic and pharmacodynamic interaction. The pharmacokinetic component appears to occur in most patients, and to develop rapidly. The study suggests that the dose of quinidine may need to be reduced by 30 to 50% or more to keep quinidine at its pre-amiodarone level. Where possible, quinidine levels should be monitored.

The use of amiodarone with quinidine further prolongs the QT interval and increases the risk of torsade de pointes. The concurrent use of two drugs that prolong the QT interval should generally be avoided. For further discussion, see 'Drugs that prolong the QT interval + Other drugs that prolong the QT interval', p.272.

1. Saal AK, Werner JA, Greene HL, Sears GK, Graham EL. Effect of amiodarone on serum quinidine and procainamide levels. *Am J Cardiol* (1984) 53, 1265–7.
2. Tartini R, Kappenberger L, Steinbrunn W, Meyer UA. Dangerous interaction between amiodarone and quinidine. *Lancet* (1982) i, 1327–9.
3. Lipnitsky TN, Dorogan AV, Randin AG, Kotsuta GI. Clinical efficacy and potential hazards from combined kordarone-and-quinidine therapy in patients with atrial fibrillation (in Russian). *Klin Med (Mosk)* (1992) 70, 31–4.
4. Nattel S, Ranger S, Talajic M, Lemery R, Roy D. Erythromycin-induced long QT syndrome: concordance with quinidine and underlying cellular electrophysiologic mechanism. *Am J Med* (1990) 89, 235–8.
5. Hoffmann A, Follath F, Burckhardt D. Safe treatment of resistant ventricular arrhythmias with a combination of amiodarone and quinidine or mexiletine. *Lancet* (1983) i, 704–5.
6. Kerin NZ, Ansari-Leesar M, Faitel K, Narala C, Frumin H, Cohen A. The effectiveness and safety of the simultaneous administration of quinidine and amiodarone in the conversion of chronic atrial fibrillation. *Am Heart J* (1993) 125, 1017–21.

Quinidine + Antacids or Urinary alkalinisers

Large rises in urinary pH due to the concurrent use of some antacids, diuretics or alkaline salts can cause quinidine retention, which could lead to quinidine toxicity, but there seems to be only one case on record of an adverse interaction (with an aluminium/magnesium hydroxide antacid). Aluminium hydroxide alone appears not to interact with quinidine.

Clinical evidence

In a study in 4 subjects, the renal clearance of oral quinidine 200 mg every 6 hours was reduced by an average of 50% (from 53 to 26 mL/minute) when their urine was made alkaline (i.e. changed from pH 6 to 7, up to pH 7 to 8) with **sodium bicarbonate** and **acetazolamide** 500 mg twice daily. Below pH 6 their urinary quinidine level averaged 115 mg/L, whereas when urinary pH values rose above 7.5 the average urinary quinidine level was only 13 mg/L. The quinidine urinary excretion rate decreased from 103 micrograms/minute to 31 micrograms/minute. In 6 other subjects the rise in serum quinidine levels was reflected in a prolongation of the QT interval. Raising the urinary pH from about 6 to 7.5 in one individual increased serum quinidine levels from about 1.6 micrograms/mL to 2.6 micrograms/mL.[1]

A patient taking quinidine who took eight *Mylanta* tablets daily (**aluminium hydroxide** gel 200 mg, **magnesium hydroxide** 200 mg and simeticone 20 mg) for a week, with a little over one litre of fruit juice (orange and grapefruit) each day developed a threefold increase in serum quinidine levels (from 8 mg/L to 25 mg/L) and toxicity. However, note that the grapefruit juice (see 'Quinidine + Grapefruit juice', p.296) may have contributed. In 6 healthy subjects, this dose of *Mylanta* for 3 days produced consistently alkaline urine in 4 subjects; the addition of fruit juice produced consistently alkaline urine in a further subject.[2]

In 4 healthy subjects, 30 mL of **aluminium hydroxide** gel *(Amphogel)* given with, and one hour after, a single 200-mg dose of quinidine sulphate had no effect on serum quinidine levels, AUC or excretion (urine pH ranged from 5 to 6.2).[3] Two similar single-dose studies in healthy subjects found that the absorption and elimination of 400 mg of quinidine sulfate[4] or 648 mg of quinidine gluconate[5] was unaffected by 30 mL **aluminium hydroxide** gel, although the change in quinidine AUC did vary from a decrease of 18% to an increase of 35% in one study.[5] Urinary pH was unaffected in both studies.[4,5]

Mechanism

Quinidine is excreted unchanged in the urine. In acid urine much of the quinidine excreted by the renal tubules is in the ionised (lipid-insoluble) form, which is unable to diffuse freely back into the cells and so is lost in the urine. In alkaline urine more of the quinidine is in the non-ionised (lipid-soluble) form, which freely diffuses back into the cells and is retained. In this way the pH of the urine determines how much quinidine is lost or retained and thereby governs the serum levels. *In vitro* data suggest that changes in pH and adsorption effects within the gut due to antacids could also affect the absorption of quinidine.[6,7]

Importance and management

An established interaction, but with the exception of the one isolated case cited,[2] there seem to be no reports of problems in patients given quinidine and antacids or urinary alkalinisers. However, in the case quinidine was given with grapefruit juice, which may potentially have had an effect of its own, see 'Quinidine + Grapefruit juice', p.296. Nevertheless it would be prudent to monitor the effects if drugs that can markedly change urinary pH are started or stopped. Avoid concurrent use, or reduce the quinidine dose as necessary.

It is difficult to predict which antacids, if any, are likely to increase the serum levels of quinidine. As noted above, aluminium hydroxide gel and magnesium hydroxide (*Mylanta*) alkalinises urine and may interact. Similarly, magnesium and aluminium hydroxide (*Maalox*) can raise the urinary pH by about 0.9 and could possibly interact.[8] Magnesium hydroxide (*Milk of magnesia*) and **calcium carbonate-glycine** (*Titralac*) raise the urinary pH by about 0.5, so that a smaller effect is likely.[8] Aluminium hydroxide gel (*Amphogel*) and **dihydroxyaluminium glycinate** (*Robalate*) are reported to have no effect on urinary pH,[8] and the studies above confirm aluminium hydroxide gel does not generally interact.

1. Gerhardt RE, Knouss RF, Thyrum PT, Luchi RJ, Morris JJ. Quinidine excretion in aciduria and alkaluria. *Ann Intern Med* (1969) 71, 927–33.
2. Zinn MB. Quinidine intoxication from alkali ingestion. *Tex Med* (1970) 66, 64–6.
3. Romankiewicz JA, Reidenberg M, Drayer D, Franklin JE. The noninterference of aluminium hydroxide gel with quinidine sulfate absorption: an approach to control quinidine-induced diarrhea. *Am Heart J* (1978) 96, 518–20.
4. Ace LN, Jaffe JM, Kunka RL. Effect of food and antacid on quinidine bioavailability. *Biopharm Drug Dispos* (1983) 4, 183–90.
5. Mauro VF, Mauro LS, Fraker TD, Temesy-Armos PN, Somani P. Effect of aluminium hydroxide gel on quinidine gluconate absorption. *Ann Pharmacother* (1990) 24, 252–4.
6. Remon JP, Van Severen R, Braeckman P. Interaction entre antiarythmiques, antiacides et antidiarrhéiques. III. Influence d'antiacides et d'antidiarrhéiques sur la réabsorption in vitro de sels de quinidine. *Pharm Acta Helv* (1979) 54, 19–22.
7. Moustafa MA, Al-Shora HI, Gaber M, Gouda MW. Decreased bioavailability of quinidine sulphate due to interactions with adsorbent antacids and antidiarrhoeal mixtures. *Int J Pharmaceutics* (1987) 34, 207–11.
8. Gibaldi M, Grundhofer B, Levy G. Effect of antacids on pH of urine. *Clin Pharmacol Ther* (1974) 16, 520–5.

Quinidine + Antiepileptics

Serum quinidine levels can be reduced by phenytoin, phenobarbital or primidone. Fosphenytoin would be expected to interact similarly. Quinidine does not affect the metabolism of mephenytoin.

Clinical evidence

A man taking long-term **primidone** 500 mg daily was given quinidine sulfate 300 mg every 4 hours, but only attained a plasma quinidine level of 0.8 micrograms/mL with an estimated half-life of 5 hours. When **primidone** was discontinued, his quinidine level rose to 2.4 micrograms/mL and the half-life was 12 hours. **Phenobarbital** 90 mg daily was then started, and the quinidine level fell to 1.6 micrograms/mL with a half-life of 7.6 hours.

In another case, a woman required doses of quinidine sulfate of up to 800 mg every 4 hours to achieve therapeutic levels while taking **phenytoin**. When the **phenytoin** was stopped, quinidine toxicity occurred, and the dose was eventually halved. Further study was then undertaken in 4 healthy subjects. After taking either **phenytoin** (in doses adjusted to give levels of 10 to 20 micrograms/mL) or **phenobarbital** for 4 weeks the elimination half-life of a single 300-mg dose of quinidine sulfate was reduced by about 50% and the total AUC was reduced by about 60%.[1] Similar results were found with **phenytoin** in another study in 3 healthy subjects.[2] Other cases have also been reported with **phenytoin**, **primidone**, **pentobarbital** and **phenobarbital**.[3-6] In one case, when **phenytoin** was given with quinidine to a patient with recurrent ventricular tachycardia the quinidine levels fell by 44%.[3] In another report quinidine levels increased from a mean of 0.8 micrograms.mL to 2.2 micrograms/mL, 15 days after **pentobarbital** was discontinued.[4] Interestingly, in this case the patient was also taking digoxin, and stopping phenobarbital precipitated digoxin toxicity by causing an increase in quinidine levels.

A 3-year-old child taking both **phenobarbital** and **phenytoin** needed to take quinidine 300 mg every 4 hours to achieve therapeutic serum quinidine levels, and had an estimated quinidine half-life of only 1.4 hours.[5] Difficulty in achieving adequate serum quinidine levels was also reported in a woman taking **phenytoin** and **primidone**. Her quinidine half-life was 2.7 hours, about half that usually seen in adults.[6]

In a study in 10 healthy subjects, quinidine 200 mg had no effect on the metabolism (4-hydroxylation) of **mephenytoin** 100 mg.[7]

Mechanism

The evidence suggests that phenytoin, primidone or phenobarbital (all known enzyme-inducers) increase the hepatic metabolism of quinidine and thereby reduce its levels.[2]

Importance and management

Established interactions of clinical importance although the documentation is limited. The concurrent use of phenytoin (and therefore probably the prodrug, **fosphenytoin**), primidone, phenobarbital or any other barbiturate need not be avoided, but be alert for the need to increase the quinidine dose. If the antiepileptics are withdrawn the quinidine dose may need to be reduced to avoid quinidine toxicity. Where possible, quinidine serum levels should be monitored.

1. Data JL, Wilkinson GR, Nies AS. Interaction of quinidine with anticonvulsant drugs. *N Engl J Med* (1976) 294, 699–702.
2. Russo ME, Russo J, Smith RA, Pershing LK. The effect of phenytoin on quinidine pharmacokinetics. *Drug Intell Clin Pharm* (1982) 16, 480.
3. Urbano AM. Phenytoin-quinidine interaction in a patient with recurrent ventricular tachyarrhythmias. *N Engl J Med* (1983) 308, 225.
4. Chapron DJ, Mumford D, Pitegoff GI. Apparent quinidine-induced digoxin toxicity after withdrawal of pentobarbital. A case of sequential drug interactions. *Arch Intern Med* (1979) 139, 363–5.
5. Rodgers GC, Blackman MS. Quinidine interaction with anticonvulsants. *Drug Intell Clin Pharm* (1983) 17, 819–20.
6. Kroboth FJ, Kroboth PD, Logan T. Phenytoin-theophylline-quinidine interaction. *N Engl J Med* (1983) 308, 725.
7. Schellens JHM, Ghabrial H, van der Wart HHF, Bakker EN, Wilkinson GR, Breimer DD. Differential effects of quinidine on the disposition of nifedipine, sparteine and mephenytoin in humans. *Clin Pharmacol Ther* (1991) 50, 520–8.

Quinidine + Aspirin

A patient and two healthy subjects given quinidine and aspirin had a two- to threefold increase in bleeding times. The patient developed petechiae and gastrointestinal bleeding.

Clinical evidence, mechanism, importance and management

A patient with a prolonged history of paroxysmal atrial tachycardia was given quinidine 800 mg daily and aspirin 325 mg twice daily. After a week he developed generalised petechiae and blood in his faeces. His prothrombin and partial prothrombin times were normal but the template bleeding time was more than 35 minutes (reference range 2 to 10 minutes). Further study in 2 healthy subjects found that quinidine 975 mg daily given alone for 5 days and aspirin 650 mg three times daily given alone for 5 days prolonged bleeding times by 125% and 163% respectively; given together for 5 days the bleeding times were prolonged by 288%.[1] The underlying mechanism for this increase in bleeding time is not totally understood but it is believed to be the outcome of the additive effects of the two drugs, both of which can reduce platelet aggregation,[1] although with quinidine this antiplatelet effect usually only occurs as the result of a hypersensitivity reaction.

This seems to be the only study of this adverse interaction, and its general importance is uncertain.

1. Lawson D, Mehta J, Mehta P, Lipman BC, Imperi GA. Cumulative effects of quinidine and aspirin on bleeding time and platelet α_2-adrenoceptors: potential mechanism of bleeding diathesis in patients receiving this combination. *J Lab Clin Med* (1986) 108, 581–6.

Quinidine + Azoles

Itraconazole increases the plasma levels of quinidine, and a case report suggests that ketoconazole may also raise quinidine levels. Other azoles are predicted to interact similarly. An isolated report describes QT prolongation in a patient taking hydroquinidine and itraconazole.

Clinical evidence

(a) Itraconazole

In a randomised, crossover study, 9 healthy subjects were given a single 100-mg dose of quinidine sulfate on the final day of a 4-day course of either itraconazole 200 mg daily or placebo. Itraconazole caused a 60% increase in the peak plasma quinidine levels, a 2.4-fold increase in its AUC, a 60% increase in its elimination half-life and a 50% decrease in its renal clearance.[1] Similarly, another study in 6 healthy subjects found that itraconazole 100 mg daily for 6 days reduced the total clearance of a single 200-mg dose of quinidine sulfate by 61%, increased its elimination half-life by 35%, and decreased its renal clearance by 60%.[2]

An isolated report describes QT prolongation after itraconazole was given to an elderly patient taking **hydroquinidine**. The QT interval returned to normal after hydroquinidine was withdrawn.[3]

(b) Ketoconazole

An elderly man with chronic atrial fibrillation, taking quinidine sulfate 300 mg four times daily, was also given ketoconazole 200 mg daily, for candidal oesophagitis after antineoplastic therapy. Within 7 days his plasma quinidine levels had risen from a range of 1.4 to 2.7 mg/L up to 6.9 mg/L (reference range 2 to 5 mg/L) but there was no evidence of toxicity. The elimination half-life of quinidine was found to be 25 hours (reference range in healthy subjects 6 to 7 hours). The quinidine dose was reduced to 200 mg twice daily, but it needed to be increased to the former dose by the end of a month, even though ketoconazole was continued at the same dose.[4]

Mechanism

The most likely explanation for the rises in quinidine levels is that itraconazole and ketoconazole inhibit the metabolism of quinidine by the cytochrome P450 isoenzyme CYP3A4 in the gut wall and liver. Itraconazole may also inhibit the active secretion of quinidine by the renal tubules.[1,2] In the case with ketoconazole, it is unclear why the quinidine dose was subsequently returned to normal. Hydroquinidine is structurally related to quinidine and may interact similarly.

Importance and management

Direct information regarding an interaction between itraconazole and quinidine appears to be limited to these studies, but what is known suggests that this interaction is clinically important. The authors of one report advise that concurrent use of these drugs should therefore be well monitored and the dose of quinidine reduced accordingly.[1]

The isolated case with ketoconazole suggests that it may interact similarly, and other azoles (including **voriconazole**, **posaconazole** and possibly **fluconazole**) would also be expected to raise quinidine levels. Because of the risk of torsade de pointes with raised quinidine levels, the concurrent use of these azoles is generally contraindicated. Note that, a large proportion of **miconazole** oral gel (both prescription and non-prescription doses) may be swallowed, and therefore adequate systemic absorption may occur to produce an interaction.

1. Kaukonen K-M, Olkkola KT, Neuvonen PJ. Itraconazole increases plasma concentrations of quinidine. *Clin Pharmacol Ther* (1997) 62, 510–17.
2. Damkier P, Hansen LL, Brøsen K. Effect of diclofenac, disulfiram, itraconazole, grapefruit juice and erythromycin on the pharmacokinetics of quinidine. *Br J Clin Pharmacol* (1999) 48, 829–38.
3. Cruccu V, Pedretti D, Confalonieri F. Un caso di aspergillosi polmonare trattato efficacemente con itraconazolo. Possibile interferenza dell'antimicotico con la idrochinidina. *Clin Ter* (1995) 146, 383–9.
4. McNulty RM, Lazor JA, Sketch M. Transient increase in plasma quinidine concentrations during ketoconazole-quinidine therapy. *Clin Pharm* (1989) 8, 222–5.

Quinidine + Calcium-channel blockers

A few patients have had increases in their quinidine levels when stopping nifedipine, but in others no interaction has occurred. In contrast, one study suggests that quinidine serum levels may be slightly raised by nifedipine. Nifedipine levels may be modestly raised by quinidine.

Verapamil reduces the clearance of quinidine and in one patient the quinidine levels doubled and quinidine toxicity developed. Acute hypotension has also been seen in three patients taking quinidine when they were given verapamil intravenously. Felodipine and nisoldipine appear not to interact, and the situation with diltiazem is unclear.

Clinical evidence

(a) Diltiazem

A study in 10 healthy subjects given quinidine 600 mg twice daily and diltiazem 120 mg daily for 7 days found that concurrent use did not affect the pharmacokinetics of either drug.[1] These findings contrast with a crossover study in 12 healthy subjects. In this study, a single 60-mg dose of diltiazem was given before and after quinidine 100 mg twice daily for 5 doses, and a single 200-mg dose of quinidine was given before and after diltiazem 90 mg twice daily for 5 doses. The pharmacokinetics of diltiazem were unaffected by quinidine, but the AUC of quinidine was increased by 51% by diltiazem.[2] When quinidine was given after diltiazem pretreatment, there were significant increases in QTc and PR intervals, and a significant decrease in heart rate and diastolic blood pressure. Pretreatment with quinidine did not significantly alter the effects of diltiazem.[2]

(b) Felodipine

In a study in 12 healthy subjects, felodipine 10 mg daily for 3 days was found to have no clinically significant effect on the pharmacokinetics or haemodynamic and ECG effects of a single 400-mg dose of quinidine. Felodipine did cause a modest 22% decrease in the AUC of the quinidine metabolite 3-hydroxyquinidine.[3]

(c) Nifedipine

1. Nifedipine serum levels. In a study in 10 healthy subjects quinidine sulfate 200 mg every 8 hours increased the AUC of nifedipine by 37%, and heart rates were significantly increased. Quinidine levels were unchanged.[4] Another study found that quinidine had a modest inhibitory effect on the metabolism of nifedipine (half-life prolonged by 40%).[5] A further study in 12 healthy subjects found that the AUC of a single 20-mg dose of nifedipine was increased 16% by quinidine 200 mg and its clearance was reduced by 17%, but these modest changes were not considered clinically relevant.[6]

2. Quinidine serum levels. The quinidine serum levels of 2 patients taking quinidine sulfate 300 or 400 mg every 6 hours and nifedipine 10 or 20 mg every 6 or 8 hours doubled (from a range of 2 to 2.5 micrograms/mL up to 4.6 micrograms/mL and from 1.6 to 1.8 micrograms/mL up to 3.5 micrograms/mL, respectively) when the nifedipine was withdrawn. The increased serum quinidine levels were reflected in a prolongation of the QTc interval. However, in the first patient there had been no change in quinidine levels when nifedipine was initially added. Further, 4 other patients did not develop this interaction.[7] Two other reports[8,9] describe a similar response: the quinidine serum level doubled in one patient when the nifedipine was stopped,[8] and in the other it was found difficult to achieve adequate serum quinidine levels when nifedipine was added, even when the quinidine dosage was increased threefold. When the nifedipine was withdrawn, the quinidine levels rose once again.[9]

A study in 12 patients found no significant change in serum quinidine levels in the group as a whole when nifedipine was given, but one patient had a 41% decrease in quinidine levels.[10] Two other studies in healthy subjects found that the quinidine AUC was unchanged by nifedipine.[3,4]

A further study in 12 healthy subjects found that the AUC of a single 200-mg oral dose of quinidine sulfate was increased by 16% by nifedipine 20 mg. The quinidine clearance was reduced by 14% and the maximum serum level was raised by almost 20%. These modest changes were not considered clinically relevant.[6]

(d) Nisoldipine

An open, crossover study in 20 healthy subjects found that nisoldipine 20 mg had no effect on the bioavailability of quinidine gluconate 648 mg.[11]

(e) Verapamil

In a study in 6 healthy subjects, verapamil 80 mg three times daily for 3 days, decreased the clearance of a single 400-mg dose of quinidine sulfate by 32% and increased the half-life was by 35% (from 6.87 to 9.29 hours).[12]

A patient given quinidine gluconate 648 mg every 6 hours had an increase in serum quinidine levels from 2.6 micrograms/mL to 5.7 micrograms/mL after taking verapamil 80 mg every 8 hours for a week. He became dizzy and had blurred vision and was found to have atrioventricular block (heart rate 38 bpm) and a systolic blood pressure of 50 mmHg. In a subsequent study in this patient it was found that verapamil halved quinidine clearance and almost doubled its serum half-life.[13]

Three other patients given quinidine orally developed marked hypotension when given intravenous verapamil 2.5 or 5 mg (blood pressure reduced from 130/70 mmHg to 80/50 mmHg, systolic pressure reduced from 140 mmHg to 85 mmHg, and mean arterial pressure reduced from 100 mmHg to 60 mmHg, in the 3 patients respectively). In two of the patients, after quinidine was discontinued, the same dose of verapamil did not cause a reduction in blood pressure.[14]

Mechanism

Suggestions for how nifedipine could alter quinidine levels include changes in cardiovascular haemodynamics,[7] and effects on metabolism.[10] Quinidine possibly inhibits the metabolism of nifedipine by competing for metabolism by the cytochrome P450 isoenzyme CYP3A4.[5] The interaction with verapamil is probably due to an inhibitory effect of verapamil on the metabolism of quinidine (inhibition of cytochrome P450 isoenzyme CYP3A).[12,15] The marked hypotension observed may be related to the antagonistic effects of the two drugs on catecholamine-induced alpha-receptor induced vasoconstriction.[14]

Importance and management

The results of studies of the interaction between quinidine and **nifedipine** are somewhat contradictory, so that the outcome of concurrent use is uncertain. However, the increase in QTc interval seen in some patients suggests that some caution would be prudent. The increases in quinidine levels seen in the studies are generally modest, but the case reports suggest that greater increases may occur in some patients. Monitor concurrent use for quinidine adverse effects (e.g. nausea, diarrhoea, tinnitus) and decrease the dose accordingly. The increases in nifedipine levels are also modest, nevertheless, it would seem prudent to monitor for nifedipine adverse effects (e.g. greater than desired reductions in blood pressure, flushing, oedema) and reduce the nifedipine dose as necessary.

What is known about the interaction between quinidine and **verapamil** suggests that a reduction in the dose of the quinidine may be needed to avoid toxicity. If the verapamil is given intravenously, use with caution and be alert for evidence of acute hypotension. Monitor the effects of concurrent use closely. There is actually a fixed dose preparation containing verapamil and quinidine *(Cordichin)* available in Germany, which is used for the management of atrial fibrillation.

No interaction apparently occurs between quinidine and **felodipine** or **nisoldipine**. The situation with **diltiazem** is as yet uncertain but be alert for the need to reduce the quinidine dose.

1. Matera MG, De Santis D, Vacca C, Fici F, Romano AR, Marrazzo R, Marmo E. Quinidine-diltiazem: pharmacokinetic interaction in humans. *Curr Ther Res* (1986) 40, 653–6.
2. Laganière S, Davies RF, Carignan G, Foris K, Goernert L, Carrier K, Pereira C, McGilveray I. Pharmacokinetic and pharmacodynamic interactions between diltiazem and quinidine. *Clin Pharmacol Ther* (1996) 60, 255–64.
3. Bailey DG, Freeman DJ, Melendez LJ, Kreeft JH, Edgar B, Carruthers SG. Quinidine interaction with nifedipine and felodipine: pharmacokinetic and pharmacodynamic evaluation. *Clin Pharmacol Ther* (1993) 53, 354–9.
4. Bowles SK, Reeves RA, Cardozo L, Edwards DJ. Evaluation of the pharmacokinetic and pharmacodynamic interaction between quinidine and nifedipine. *J Clin Pharmacol* (1993) 33, 727–31.
5. Schellens JHM, Ghabrial H, van der Wart HHF, Bakker EN, Wilkinson GR, Breimer DD. Differential effects of quinidine on the disposition of nifedipine, sparteine and mephenytoin in humans. *Clin Pharmacol Ther* (1991) 50, 520–8.
6. Hippius M, Henschel L, Sigusch H, Tepper J, Brendel E. Hoffmann A. Pharmacokinetic interactions of nifedipine and quinidine. *Pharmazie* (1995) 50 613–16.
7. Farringer JA, Green JA, O'Rourke RA, Linn WA, Clementi WA. Nifedipine-induced alterations in serum quinidine concentrations. *Am Heart J* (1984) 108, 1570–2.
8. Van Lith RM, Appleby DH. Quinidine-nifedipine interaction. *Drug Intell Clin Pharm* (1985) 19, 829–31.
9. Green JA, Clementi WA, Porter C, Stigelman W. Nifedipine-quinidine interaction. *Clin Pharm* (1983) 2, 461–5.
10. Munger MA, Jarvis RC, Nair R, Kasmer RJ, Nara AR, Urbancic A, Green JA. Elucidation of the nifedipine-quinidine interaction. *Clin Pharmacol Ther* (1989) 45, 411–16.
11. Schall R, Müller FO, Groenewoud G, Hundt HKL, Luus HG, Van Dyk M, Van Schalkwyk AMC. Investigation of a possible pharmacokinetic interaction between nisoldipine and quinidine in healthy volunteers. *Drug Invest* (1994) 8, 162–170.
12. Edwards DJ, Lavoie R, Beckman H, Blevins R, Rubenfire M. The effect of coadministration of verapamil on the pharmacokinetics and metabolism of quinidine. *Clin Pharmacol Ther* (1987) 41, 68–73.
13. Trohman RG, Estes DM, Castellanos A, Palomo AR, Myerburg RJ, Kessler KM. Increased quinidine plasma concentrations during administration of verapamil; a new quinidine-verapamil interaction. *Am J Cardiol* (1986) 57, 706–7.
14. Maisel AS, Motulsky HJ, Insel PA. Hypotension after quinidine plus verapamil. Possible additive competition at alpha-adrenergic receptors. *N Engl J Med* (1985) 312, 167–70.
15. Kroemer HK, Gautier J-C, Beaune P, Henderson C, Wolf CR, Eichelbaum M. Identification of P450 enzymes involved in metabolism of verapamil in humans. *Naunyn Schmiedebergs Arch Pharmacol* (1993) 348, 332–7.

Quinidine + Colesevelam

In a study in 25 subjects, a single 4.5-g dose of colesevelam had no significant effect on the pharmacokinetics of a single 324-mg dose of quinidine [gluconate].[1] This suggests that colesevelam does not reduce the absorption of quinidine. No special precautions appear to be needed during concurrent use.

1. Donovan JM, Stypinski D, Stiles MR, Olson TA, Burke SK. Drug interactions with colesevelam hydrochloride, a novel, potent lipid-lowering agent. *Cardiovasc Drugs Ther* (2000) 14, 681–90.

Quinidine + Co-phenotrope (Atropine with Diphenoxylate)

Co-phenotrope slightly reduced the rate, but not the extent, of absorption of a single dose of quinidine.

Clinical evidence, mechanism, importance and management

In one study, 8 healthy subjects were given a single 300-mg dose of quinidine sulfate alone and after taking two tablets of co-phenotrope (atropine sulfate 25 micrograms, diphenoxylate 2.5 mg; *Lomotil*) at midnight on the evening before and another two tablets the next morning an hour before the quinidine.[1] It was found that the maximum plasma quinidine levels were reduced by 21% (from 2.1 to 1.65 micrograms/mL) by the co-phenotrope, the time to maximum level was prolonged from 0.89 hours to 1.21 hours, and there was a slight increase in elimination half-life from 5.7 hours to 6.8 hours. While these results were statistically significant, the changes were relatively small and it seems doubtful if they are clinically relevant, particularly as the extent of absorption was unchanged. However it needs to be emphasised that because the quinidine formulation used was an immediate-release preparation, these results may not necessarily apply to sustained-release preparations, and also may not apply if multiple doses of quinidine are used.

1. Ponzillo JJ, Scavone JM, Paone RP, Lewis GP, Rayment CM, Fitzsimmons WE. Effect of diphenoxylate with atropine sulfate on the bioavailability of quinidine sulfate in healthy subjects. *Clin Pharm* (1988) 7, 139–42.

Quinidine + Diazepam

A single-dose study suggests that diazepam does not affect the pharmacokinetics of quinidine.

Clinical evidence, mechanism, importance and management

A comparative study in 8 healthy subjects found that the pharmacokinetics of a single 250-mg dose of quinidine sulfate was unaltered by a single 10-mg dose of diazepam.[1] This suggests that no dose adjustment of quinidine is likely to be needed in patients given diazepam, but this ideally needs confirmation by further studies using multiple doses of both drugs.

1. Rao BR, Rambhau D. Absence of a pharmacokinetic interaction between quinidine and diazepam. *Drug Metabol Drug Interact* (1995) 12, 45–51.

Quinidine + Diclofenac

Diclofenac inhibits the metabolism (*N*-oxidation) of quinidine but does not affect other pharmacokinetic parameters.

Clinical evidence, mechanism, importance and management

In an open study, 6 healthy subjects were given a single 200-mg dose of quinidine sulfate before and on day 5 of a 6-day course of diclofenac 100 mg daily. Diclofenac reduced the *N*-oxidation of quinidine by 33%, but no other pharmacokinetic changes were found.[1] Diclofenac is a substrate for, and therefore a possible competitive inhibitor of the cytochrome P450 isoenzyme CYP2C9. These results suggest that CYP2C9 does not appear to have a major role in quinidine metabolism,[1] and so clinically relevant changes in quinidine pharmacokinetics with diclofenac would seem unlikely.

1. Damkier P, Hansen LL, Brøsen K. Effect of diclofenac, disulfiram, itraconazole, grapefruit juice and erythromycin on the pharmacokinetics of quinidine. *Br J Clin Pharmacol* (1999) 48, 829–38.

Quinidine + Disulfiram

Disulfiram does not affect the pharmacokinetics of quinidine.

Clinical evidence, mechanism, importance and management

In an open study, 6 healthy subjects were given a single 200-mg dose of quinidine sulfate before and on day 5 of a 6-day course of disulfiram 200 mg daily. There were no changes in quinidine pharmacokinetics during disulfiram use.[1] Disulfiram is thought to be an inhibitor of the cytochrome P450 isoenzyme CYP2E1, but this isoenzyme does not appear to have a major role in quinidine metabolism.[1] Disulfiram therefore seems unlikely to have a clinically relevant effect on the pharmacokinetics of quinidine.

1. Damkier P, Hansen LL, Brøsen K. Effect of diclofenac, disulfiram, itraconazole, grapefruit juice and erythromycin on the pharmacokinetics of quinidine. *Br J Clin Pharmacol* (1999) 48, 829–38.

Quinidine + Erythromycin

Erythromycin can increase quinidine levels and cause a small further increase in the QTc interval.

Clinical evidence

Preliminary results of a randomised, placebo-controlled study in 12 subjects found that when a single 400-mg dose of quinidine was given after oral erythromycin 500 mg three times daily for 5 days, the AUC of the QTc interval was prolonged by about 6%.[1] In a parallel study by the same group, peak levels of quinidine were increased by 39% (from 587 nanograms/mL to 816 nanograms/mL), and the AUC was increased by 62% by day 5 of the erythromycin phase. Peak levels of the main metabolite of quinidine, 3-hydroxyquinidine, were significantly reduced.[2] Another study in 6 healthy subjects found that oral erythromycin 250 mg four times daily for 6 days reduced the total clearance of a single 200-mg dose of quinidine sulfate by 34% and increased its maximum serum concentration by 39%.[3]

A 74-year-old man with a history of cardiac disease (coronary artery bypass graft surgery, ventricular tachycardia) taking quinidine sulfate 200 mg every 6 hours and several other drugs, including mexiletine, was hospitalised with suspected infection of his implantable cardioverter defibrillator. Within 2 days of starting erythromycin lactobionate 500 mg every 6 hours and ceftriaxone 1 g daily, both intravenously, his trough serum quinidine levels had risen by about 50% from about 2.8 mg/L to 4.2 mg/L. On day 7, metronidazole 500 mg every 8 hours was added and the erythromycin dosage was doubled, and the patient experienced an episode of torsade de pointes. By day 12 his serum quinidine levels had further risen to 5.8 mg/L, whereupon the quinidine dosage was reduced by 25%. Because an interaction between quinidine and erythromycin had by then been suspected, the antibacterials were replaced by doxycycline and ciprofloxacin. By day 21, the quinidine serum levels had fallen to their former levels. The patient had a prolonged QTc interval of 504 milliseconds on admission, and this did not change.[4]

A 95-year-old man developed QT interval prolongation, torsade de pointes, with a subsequent cardiac arrest when given quinidine and erythromycin, both orally.[5]

Mechanism

Not fully understood, but erythromycin inhibits the metabolism of quinidine,[2] possibly by inhibition of the cytochrome P450 isoenzyme CYP3A4,[3] thereby reducing its clearance from the body and increasing its effects. There are also a number of cases on record of prolongation of the QT interval and torsade de pointes associated with the use of intravenous erythromycin alone.[6] Therefore, quinidine and erythromycin may have additive effects on the QT interval in addition to the pharmacokinetic interaction.

Importance and management

Information about this interaction appears to be limited to these reports, but it would appear to be established. If erythromycin is essential in a patient taking quinidine, the effects of concurrent use should be well monitored, being alert for the development of raised plasma quinidine levels. Monitor for quinidine adverse effects (e.g. nausea, diarrhoea, tinnitus). The concurrent use of two drugs that prolong the QT interval should usually be undertaken with great caution. For further discussion, see 'Drugs that prolong the QT interval + Other drugs that prolong the QT interval', p.272).

1. Stanford RH, Geraets DR, Lee H-C, Min DI. Effect of oral erythromycin on quinidine pharmacodynamics in healthy volunteers. *Pharmacotherapy* (1997) 17, 1111.
2. Stanford RH, Park JM, Geraets Dr, Min DI, Lee H-C. Effect of oral erythromycin on quinidine pharmacokinetics in healthy volunteers. *Pharmacotherapy* (1998) 18, 426–7.
3. Damkier P, Hansen LL, Brøsen K. Effect of diclofenac, disulfiram, itraconazole, grapefruit juice and erythromycin on the pharmacokinetics of quinidine. *Br J Clin Pharmacol* (1999) 48, 829–38.
4. Spinler SA, Cheng JWM, Kindwall KE, Charland SL. Possible inhibition of hepatic metabolism of quinidine by erythromycin. *Clin Pharmacol Ther* (1995) 57, 89–94.
5. Lin JC, Quasny HA. QT prolongation and development of torsades de pointes with the concomitant administration of oral erythromycin base and quinidine. *Pharmacotherapy* (1997) 17, 626–30.
6. Gitler B, Berger LS, Buffa SD. Torsades de pointes induced by erythromycin. *Chest* (1994) 105, 368–72.

Quinidine + Fluvoxamine

Fluvoxamine appears to inhibit the metabolism and clearance of quinidine.

Clinical evidence, mechanism, importance and management

In a study, 6 healthy subjects were given a single 200-mg dose of quinidine sulfate before and on day 5 of a 6-day course of fluvoxamine 100 mg daily. The total apparent oral clearance of quinidine was reduced by 29%, and *N*-oxidation and 3-hydroxylation were reduced by 33% and 44%, respectively. The renal clearance and elimination half-life of quinidine were unchanged.[1] It was concluded that fluvoxamine inhibited the metabolism of quinidine by the cytochrome P450 isoenzyme CYP3A4, although a role for CYP1A2 and CYP2C19 was not excluded. The clinical relevance of these findings is unclear. However, it would seem prudent to monitor concurrent use for quinidine adverse effects (e.g. nausea, diarrhoea, tinnitus). More study is needed to assess the effect of multiple dosing and to establish the clinical significance of this interaction.

1. Damkier P, Hansen LL, Brøsen K. Effect of fluvoxamine on the pharmacokinetics of quinidine. *Eur J Clin Pharmacol* (1999) 55, 451–6.

Quinidine + Grapefruit juice

Grapefruit juice delays the absorption of quinidine and reduces its metabolism to some extent, but no clinically relevant adverse interaction seems to occur.

Clinical evidence, mechanism, importance and management

In one study, 12 healthy subjects were given quinidine sulfate 400 mg orally on two occasions, once with 240 mL of water and once with grapefruit juice. The pharmacokinetics of the quinidine were unchanged, except that its absorption was delayed (the time to reach maximum plasma concentrations was doubled from 1.6 hours to 3.3 hours) by grapefruit juice for reasons that are not understood. The AUC of the quinidine metabolite, 3-hydroxyquinidine was decreased by one-third, suggesting that grapefruit juice inhibits the metabolism of quinidine. No important changes in the QTc interval were seen.[1]

Similarly, another study in 6 healthy subjects found the total clearance of a single 200-mg dose of quinidine sulfate was reduced by 15% by 250 mL of grapefruit juice, with no change in its maximum level. There was a small reduction in metabolite formation suggesting only minor inhibition of metabolism.[2]

Grapefruit is known to inhibit the cytochrome P450 isoenzyme CYP3A4, which is involved with the metabolism of quinidine, so it seems likely that any interaction would occur via this pathway.[1,2] The effects of grapefruit juice appear to be modest, and these studies suggest that it is not usually necessary for patients on quinidine to avoid grapefruit juice. However, grapefruit juice may have contributed to raised quinidine levels and toxicity in a woman who took an antacid and one litre of fruit juice daily for a week, see 'Quinidine + Antacids or Urinary alkalinisers', p.293. It may therefore be prudent to be alert for an increase in quinidine adverse effects (e.g. nausea, diarrhoea, tinnitus), and consider avoiding grapefruit if these become troublesome.

1. Min DI, Ku Y-M, Geraets DR, Lee H-C. Effect of grapefruit juice on the pharmacokinetics and pharmacodynamics of quinidine in healthy volunteers. *J Clin Pharmacol* (1996) 36, 469–76.
2. Damkier P, Hansen LL, Brøsen K. Effect of diclofenac, disulfiram, itraconazole, grapefruit juice and erythromycin on the pharmacokinetics of quinidine. *Br J Clin Pharmacol* (1999) 48, 829–38.

Quinidine + HIV-protease inhibitors

In theory, the HIV-protease inhibitors will increase the concentrations of quinidine. Quinidine does not affect indinavir concentrations.

Clinical evidence

In a study in which quinidine sulphate 200 mg was given to 10 healthy subjects, followed one hour later by a single 400-mg dose of **indinavir**, the pharmacokinetics of **indinavir** were not notably affected.[1]

Direct evidence (from case reports or clinical studies) of an interaction between quinidine and the other HIV-protease inhibitors appears to be lacking; however, a review of HIV-protease inhibitor interactions reports that the plasma concentrations of quinidine might be increased by **ritonavir**. The same review states that **nelfinavir** and **saquinavir** might interact similarly.[2]

Mechanism

Quinidine is metabolised by CYP3A4, of which nelfinavir, ritonavir and saquinavir are all inhibitors. Note that the HIV-protease inhibitors are all inhibitors of CYP3A4, to varying degrees, and therefore would be expected to interact similarly.

Importance and management

Clinical evidence of an interaction between quinidine and the HIV-protease inhibitors is lacking; however, in theory, all HIV-protease inhibitors could raise quinidine concentrations. Raised concentrations of quinidine will increase the risk of arrhythmias and other adverse effects. The manufacturers of **ritonavir** contraindicate concurrent use with quinidine,[3,4] and for this reason, many of the manufacturers contraindicate the concurrent use of HIV-protease inhibitors boosted with ritonavir and quinidine. However, the UK manufacturer of **lopinavir**[5] states that caution is warranted on the concurrent use of quinidine and recommends monitoring quinidine concentrations, where possible. Note that quinidine adverse effects include nausea, diarrhoea, and tinnitus. In the US, most manufacturers advise caution and close monitoring of quinidine concentrations, with the exception of the manufacturers of **nelfinavir**,[6] **saquinavir**[7] and **tipranavir**,[8] who contraindicate the concurrent use of quinidine.

No dose adjustment of **indinavir** appears to be needed if the concurrent use of quinidine is necessary.

1. McCrea J, Woolf E, Sterrett A, Matthews C, Deutsch, Yeh KC, Waldman S, Bjornsson T. Effects of ketoconazole and other p-450 inhibitors on the pharmacokinetics of indinavir. *Pharm Res* (1996) 13 (9 Suppl), S485.
2. Burger DM, Hoetelmans RMW, Koopmans PP, Meenhorst PL, Mulder JW, Hekster YA, Beijnen JH. Clinically relevant drug interactions with antiretroviral agents. *Antivir Ther* (1997) 2, 149–165.
3. Norvir Tablets (Ritonavir). AbbVie Ltd. UK Summary of product characteristics, September 2012.
4. Norvir Capsules (Ritonavir). Abbott Laboratories. US Prescribing information, March 2012.
5. Kaletra Tablets (Lopinavir with Ritonavir). AbbVie Ltd. UK Summary of product characteristics, August 2012.
6. Viracept (Nelfinavir mesylate). Agouron Pharmaceuticals, Inc. US Prescribing information, May 2013.
7. Invirase (Saquinavir mesylate). Genentech, Inc. US Prescribing information, February 2012.
8. Aptivus (Tipranavir). Boehringer Ingelheim Pharmaceuticals, Inc. US Prescribing information, April 2012.

Quinidine + H_2-receptor antagonists

Quinidine serum levels can rise and toxicity may develop in some patients when they take cimetidine. An isolated case of ventricular bigeminy (a form of arrhythmia) occurred in a patient taking quinidine and ranitidine.

Clinical evidence

In a study in 6 healthy subjects, **cimetidine** 300 mg four times daily for 7 days prolonged the elimination half-life of a single 400-mg dose of quinidine sulfate by 55%, from 5.8 to 9 hours, and decreased its clearance by 37%. Peak plasma levels were raised by 21%. These changes were reflected in ECG changes, with 51% and 28% increases in the mean areas under the QT and QTc time curves, respectively, but these were not considered to be statistically significant.[1]

A later study in healthy subjects, prompted by the observation of 2 patients who developed toxic quinidine levels when given **cimetidine**, found essentially the same effects. The AUC and half-life of quinidine were increased by 15% and 23%, respectively, and the clearance was decreased by 25% by **cimetidine** 300 mg four times daily.[2] A further study in 4 healthy subjects found that **cimetidine** 300 mg four times daily for 5 days prolonged the elimination half-life of quinidine by 54% and decreased its total clearance by 36%.[3,4] In one study, the addition of **cimetidine** prolonged the QT interval by 30% more than the effect of quinidine alone.[4] A case report describes marked increases in both quinidine and digitoxin concentrations in a woman also given **cimetidine**.[5] Similarly, quinidine levels increased by up to 50%, without causing any adverse effects, when a man taking quinidine was given **cimetidine**.[6]

Ventricular bigeminy (a form of arrhythmia) occurred when a man taking quinidine was given **ranitidine**. His serum quinidine levels remained unchanged.[7]

Mechanism

It was originally suggested that the cimetidine inhibits the metabolism of the quinidine by the liver so that it is cleared more slowly.[2] However, further data suggest that cimetidine successfully competes with quinidine for its excretion by the kidneys.[8]

Importance and management

The interaction between quinidine and cimetidine is established and of clinical importance. The incidence is unknown. Be alert for changes in the response to quinidine if cimetidine is started or stopped. Ideally the quinidine serum levels should be monitored (consider monitoring in response to adverse effects such as hypotension, tinnitus and diarrhoea) and reduce the quinidine dose as necessary. Reductions of 25% (oral) and 35% (intravenous) have been suggested.[3] Those at greatest risk are likely to be patients with impaired renal function, patients with impaired liver function, the elderly, and those with serum quinidine levels already at the top end of the therapeutic range.[2] The situation with ranitidine is uncertain.

1. Hardy BG, Zador IT, Golden L, Lalka D, Schentag JJ. Effect of cimetidine on the pharmacokinetics and pharmacodynamics of quinidine. *Am J Cardiol* (1983) 52, 172–5.
2. Kolb KW, Garnett WR, Small RE, Vetrovec GW, Kline BJ, Fox T. Effect of cimetidine on quinidine clearance. *Ther Drug Monit* (1984) 6, 306–12.
3. MacKichan JJ, Boudoulas H, Schaal SF. Effect of cimetidine on quinidine bioavailability. *Biopharm Drug Dispos* (1989) 10, 121–5.
4. Boudoulas H, MacKichan JJ, Schaal SF. Effect of cimetidine on the pharmacodynamics of quinidine. *Med Sci Res* (1988) 16, 713–14.
5. Polish LB, Branch RA, Fitzgerald GA. Digitoxin-quinidine interaction: potentiation during administration of cimetidine. *South Med J* (1981) 74, 633–4.
6. Farringer JA, McWay-Hess K, Clementi WA. Cimetidine–quinidine interaction. *Clin Pharm* (1984) 3, 81–3.
7. Iliopoulou A, Kontogiannis D, Tsoutsos D, Moulopoulos S. Quinidine-ranitidine adverse reaction. *Eur Heart J* (1986) 7, 360.
8. Hardy BG, Schentag JJ. Lack of effect of cimetidine on the metabolism of quinidine: effect on renal clearance. *Int J Clin Pharmacol Ther Toxicol* (1988) 26, 388–91.

Quinidine + Kaolin-pectin

There is some evidence that kaolin-pectin can reduce the absorption of quinidine and lower its serum levels.

Clinical evidence, mechanism, importance and management

When 4 healthy subjects were given 30 mL of kaolin-pectin (*Kaopectate*), after a single 100-mg dose of oral quinidine sulfate, the maximal salivary quinidine concentration was reduced by 54% and its AUC was reduced by 58%, without any effect on the rate of absorption.[1] There is a correlation between salivary and serum concentrations after single (but not repeated) doses of quinidine.[2] This is consistent with *in vitro* data showing that quinidine is adsorbed onto kaolin and pectin.[1,3] Documentation appears to be limited to these two studies, but be alert for the need to increase the quinidine dose if kaolin-pectin is used concurrently.

1. Moustafa MA, Al-Shora HI, Gaber M, Gouda MW. Decreased bioavailability of quinidine sulphate due to interactions with adsorbent antacids and antidiarrhoeal mixtures. *Int J Pharmaceutics* (1987) 34, 207–11.
2. Narang PK, Carliner NH, Fisher ML, Crouthamel WG. Quinidine saliva concentrations: absence of correlation with serum concentrations at steady state. *Clin Pharmacol Ther* (1983) 34, 695–702.
3. Bucci AJ, Myre SA, Tan HSI, Shenouda LS. In vitro interaction of quinidine with kaolin and pectin. *J Pharm Sci* (1981) 70, 999–1002.

Quinidine + Laxatives

Quinidine plasma levels can be reduced by the anthraquinone laxative senna.

Clinical evidence, mechanism, importance and management

In a study in 7 patients with cardiac arrhythmias taking sustained-release quinidine bisulfate 500 mg every 12 hours, **senna** reduced plasma quinidine levels, measured 12 hours after the last dose of quinidine, by about 25%.[1] The modest reduction in quinidine levels might be of clinical importance in patients whose plasma levels are barely adequate to control their arrhythmia.

1. Guckenbiehl W, Gilfrich HJ, Just H. Einfluß von Laxantien und Metoclopramid auf die Chindin-Plasmakonzentration während Langzeittherapie bei Patienten mit Herzrhythmusstörugen. *Med Welt* (1976) 27, 1273–6.

Quinidine + Lidocaine

A single case report describes a man taking quinidine who had sinoatrial arrest when he was given intravenous lidocaine.

Clinical evidence, mechanism, importance and management

A man with Parkinson's disease was given quinidine 300 mg every 6 hours for the control of ventricular ectopic beats. After receiving two doses he was given lidocaine as well, initially as a bolus of 80 mg, followed by an infusion of 4 mg/minute because persistent premature ventricular beats developed. Within 2.5 hours the patient complained of dizziness and weakness, and was found to have sinus bradycardia, sinoatrial arrest and an atrioventricular escape rhythm. Normal sinus rhythm resumed when the lidocaine was stopped. Whether quinidine was a contributing factor in this reaction is uncertain.[1] However, this case emphasises the need to exercise caution when giving two drugs that have cardiac depressant actions.

1. Jeresaty RM, Kahn AH, Landry AB. Sinoatrial arrest due to lidocaine in a patient receiving quinidine. *Chest* (1972) 61, 683–5.

Quinidine + Metoclopramide

Metoclopramide has been seen to both modestly increase quinidine levels and modestly decrease quinidine exposure.

Clinical evidence

A study of a possible interaction between quinidine and metoclopramide was prompted by the case of a patient who was taking sustained-release quinidine (*Quinidex*) and whose arrhythmia became uncontrolled when metoclopramide was added. In a crossover study, 9 healthy subjects were given metoclopramide 10 mg every 6 hours, for 24 hours before and 48 hours after a single 600- or 900-mg oral dose of quinidine sulfate or quinidine alone. It was found that metoclopramide caused a mean 10% decrease in the AUC of quinidine, although two subjects had decreases of 23% and 28%, respectively. The elimination rate constant was unaffected.[1]

Another study, in patients taking sustained-release quinidine bisulfate 500 mg every 12 hours, found that metoclopramide 10 mg three times daily increased the mean plasma levels measured 3.5 hours after the last dose of quinidine by almost 20%, from 1.6 to 1.9 micrograms/mL, and increased the levels at 12 hours by about 16%, from 2.4 to 2.8 micrograms/mL.[2]

Mechanism

Not understood. Metoclopramide alters both the gastric emptying time and gastrointestinal motility, which can affect quinidine absorption.

Importance and management

Direct information seems to be limited to these studies using different quinidine preparations. The outcome of concurrent use is uncertain, but any effect generally seems small in most patients.

1. Yuen GJ, Hansten PD, Collins J. Effect of metoclopramide on the absorption of an oral sustained-release quinidine product. *Clin Pharm* (1987) 6, 722–5.
2. Guckenbiehl W, Gilfrich HJ, Just H. Einfluß von Laxantien und Metoclopramid auf die Chindin-Plasmakonzentration während Langzeittherapie bei Patienten mit Herzrhythmusstörugen. *Med Welt* (1976) 27, 1273–6.

Quinidine + Omeprazole

Omeprazole does not appear to alter the pharmacokinetics or QT-interval prolonging effects of quinidine.

Clinical evidence, mechanism, importance and management

In a study in 8 healthy subjects, omeprazole 40 mg daily for one week had no effect on the pharmacokinetics of a single 400-mg dose of quinidine sulfate. In addition, the corrected QT interval was not significantly changed.[1] There would not appear to be the need for any special precautions during concurrent use.

1. Ching MS, Elliott SL, Stead CK, Murdoch RT, Devenish-Meares S, Morgan DJ, Smallwood RA. Quinidine single dose pharmacokinetics and pharmacodynamics are unaltered by omeprazole. *Aliment Pharmacol Ther* (1991) 5, 523–31.

Quinidine + Quinolones

Ciprofloxacin does not normally appear to interact with quinidine to a clinically relevant extent. An increased risk of torsade de pointes might be expected if quinidine is used with gatifloxacin, moxifloxacin, or sparfloxacin.

Clinical evidence, mechanism, importance and management

In a study in 7 healthy subjects, **ciprofloxacin** 750 mg daily for 6 days did not significantly affect the pharmacokinetics of a single 400-mg oral dose of quinidine sulfate, and QRS and QTc prolongation were not significantly changed. The decrease in clearance ranged from a decrease of 10% to an increase of 20%, with a mean 1% increase, which is unlikely to be clinically relevant.[1] However an isolated case report describes a woman who started taking quinidine gluconate 324 mg every 8 hours while she was taking **ciprofloxacin** and metronidazole. Her first trough serum quinidine level was 6.3 micrograms/mL, which was slightly above the reference range of 2 to 5 micrograms/mL, but she had no evidence of toxicity. Quinidine was continued unchanged, and her next trough serum quinidine level was only 2.3 micrograms/mL, 3 days after finishing the course of antibacterials. This effect was tentatively attributed to the possible enzyme inhibitory effects of **ciprofloxacin** and metronidazole. This case is far from clear and so no firm conclusions can be reached.[2] There would seem to be little reason for avoiding concurrent use.

Some quinolones can prolong the QT interval, and would be expected to increase the risk of torsade de pointes when used with quinidine. Of the quinolones used clinically, **gatifloxacin**, **moxifloxacin**, and **sparfloxacin** are known to prolong the QT interval (see 'Table 9.2', p.273). The concurrent use of two drugs that prolong the QT interval should usually be avoided, or undertaken with great caution. For further discussion, see also 'Drugs that prolong the QT interval + Other drugs that prolong the QT interval', p.272.

1. Bleske BE, Carver PL, Annesley TM, Bleske JRM, Morady F. The effect of ciprofloxacin on the pharmacokinetic and ECG parameters of quinidine. *J Clin Pharmacol* (1990) 30, 911–15.
2. Cooke CE, Sklar GE, Nappi JM. Possible pharmacokinetic interaction with quinidine: ciprofloxacin or metronidazole? *Ann Pharmacother* (1996) 30, 364–6.

Quinidine + Rifamycins

The serum levels and therapeutic effects of quinidine can be markedly reduced by rifampicin.

Clinical evidence

It was noted that the control of ventricular arrhythmia deteriorated in a patient taking quinidine sulfate 800 mg daily within a week of **rifampicin** 600 mg daily being started. His serum quinidine level fell from 4 micrograms/mL to 0.5 micrograms/mL, and remained low despite doubling the quinidine dose to 1.6 g daily. The **rifampicin** was discontinued, and quinidine levels gradually increased over a week. Some signs of quinidine toxicity then occurred, and the quinidine dose was reduced back to 800 mg daily.[1] Further study in 4 healthy subjects found that **rifampicin** 600 mg daily for 7 days reduced the mean half-life of a single 6-mg/kg oral dose of quinidine sulfate by about 62% (from 6.1 hours to 2.3 hours) and reduced the AUC by 83%.[2] Similar findings were reported in 4 other subjects receiving the same dose of quinidine intravenously.[2]

Another case report describes a patient taking **rifampicin** who did not achieve adequate serum quinidine levels despite daily doses of quinidine of up to 3.2 g. When the **rifampicin** was stopped, ultimately, a reduced quinidine dose of 1.8 g daily achieved a serum level of 2 micrograms/mL, reflecting a 44% decrease in dose and a 43% increase in level.[3] In a further case, a patient taking quinidine and digoxin was given **rifampicin**: the quinidine levels fell, resulting in a fall in digoxin levels.[4]

Mechanism

Rifampicin is a potent enzyme-inducer, which markedly increases the metabolism of the quinidine by 3-hydroxylation and *N*-oxidation, thereby reducing its levels and effects.[5] It has been suggested that two of the quinidine metabolites (3-hydroxyquinidine and 2-oxoquinidinone) may be active, which might, to some extent, offset the effects of this interaction.[4]

Importance and management

An established and clinically important interaction, although documentation is limited. The dose of quinidine will need to be increased if rifampicin is given concurrently. Monitor the serum levels. Doubling the dose may not be sufficient.[2,4] An equivalent dosage reduction will be needed if the rifampicin is stopped. There does not seem to be any information regarding the other rifamycins, **rifabutin** (a weak enzyme inducer) and **rifapentine** (a moderate enzyme inducer). However, the manufacturers and the CSM in the UK warn that **rifabutin** may possibly reduce the effects of a number of drugs, including quinidine.[6,7]

1. Ahmad D, Mathur P, Ahuja S, Henderson R, Carruthers G. Rifampicin-quinidine interaction. *Br J Dis Chest* (1979) 73, 409–11.
2. Twum-Barima Y, Carruthers SG. Quinidine-rifampin interaction. *N Engl J Med* (1981) 304, 1466–9.
3. Schwartz A, Brown JR. Quinidine-rifampin interaction. *Am Heart J* (1984) 107, 789–90.
4. Bussey HI, Merritt GJ, Hill EG. The influence of rifampin on quinidine and digoxin. *Arch Intern Med* (1984) 144, 1021–3.
5. Damkier P, Hansen LL, Brøsen K. Rifampicin treatment greatly increases the apparent oral clearance of quinidine. *Pharmacol Toxicol* (1999) 85, 257–62.
6. Mycobutin (Rifabutin). Pfizer Ltd. UK Summary of product characteristics, December 2013.
7. Committee on the Safety of Medicines/Medicines Control Agency. Revised indication and drug interactions of rifabutin. *Current Problems* (1997) 23, 14.

Quinidine + Sucralfate

An isolated report describes a marked reduction in serum quinidine levels, which was attributed to the concurrent use of sucralfate.

Clinical evidence, mechanism, importance and management

An elderly woman was found to have subtherapeutic levels of warfarin, digoxin and sustained-release quinidine (serum quinidine level 0.31 micromol/L), even though they were given 2 hours apart from sucralfate. On hospitalisation, a variety of other medications were then started for chest pain (glyceryl trinitrate, diltiazem, pethidine (meperidine), promethazine), and on day 4 the sucralfate was stopped. On day 5, her serum quinidine level was 5.55 micromol/L.[1] The patient denied non-compliance, and the suggestion was that sucralfate can bind with quinidine within the gut and reduce its absorption. This isolated case appears to be the only report of an interaction between quinidine and sucralfate and its general importance is unclear.

1. Rey AM, Gums JG. Altered absorption of digoxin, sustained-release quinidine, and warfarin with sucralfate administration. *DICP Ann Pharmacother* (1991) 25, 745–6.

10

Antibacterials

This section deals with interactions where the effects of the antibacterial drugs are altered. In many cases the antibacterial drugs interact by affecting other drugs, and these interactions are dealt with elsewhere in this publication.

The antibacterials covered in this section are listed in 'Table 10.1', p.300.

Many of the interactions covered in this section concern absorption interactions, such as the ability of the tetracyclines and quinolones to chelate with divalent cations. More information on the mechanism of these interactions can be found in 'Drug absorption interactions', p.3.

Many monographs concern the use of multiple antibacterials. One of the great difficulties with these interactions is the often poor correlation between *in vitro* and *in vivo* studies, so it is difficult to get a thoroughly reliable indication of how the antibacterials will behave together in clinical practice. For example, two antibacterials might actually be less effective than one on its own, because, in theory, the effects of a bactericidal drug, which requires actively dividing cells for it to be effective, might be reduced by a bacteriostatic drug. However, in practice this seems to be less clinically important than might be expected and there are relatively few well-authenticated clinical examples.

(a) Macrolides

The most important clinical pharmacokinetic interactions caused by the macrolides are those resulting from inhibition of CYP3A4 and of P-glycoprotein.

- **Azithromycin** does not appear to inhibit CYP3A4, but might inhibit P-glycoprotein to a clinically relevant extent based on its effect on fexofenadine, (see 'Antihistamines + Macrolides', p.635).
- **Clarithromycin** is a potent inhibitor of CYP3A4. It is a clinically relevant inhibitor of P-glycoprotein, as demonstrated by its effects on digoxin (see 'Digoxin and related drugs + Macrolides', p.1100).
- **Erythromycin** is a moderate CYP3A4 inhibitor. It might also inhibit P-glycoprotein to a clinically relevant extent based on its effect on fexofenadine, (see 'Antihistamines + Macrolides', p.635).
- **Roxithromycin** is a weak inhibitor of CYP3A4 and **telithromycin** is a potent inhibitor of CYP3A4.

Azithromycin, clarithromycin, erythromycin, and telithromycin might prolong the QT interval, see 'Table 9.2', p.273 for further details.

(b) Quinolones

Some of the most important clinical interactions caused by the quinolones are those resulting from inhibition of CYP1A2 and from prolongation of the QT interval. **Enoxacin**, depending upon the dose, is a moderate to potent inhibitor of CYP1A2. **Ciprofloxacin** appears to moderately inhibit CYP1A2 while **norfloxacin** and **pefloxacin** are weak CYP1A2 inhibitors. **Gatifloxacin**, **moxifloxacin**, and **sparfloxacin** can prolong the QT interval (see 'Table 9.2', p.273).

(c) Rifamycins

Rifampicin (rifampin), a potent non-specific enzyme inducer, lowers the concentrations of many drugs. Rifampicin potently induces CYP3A4, moderately induces CYP2B6, CYP2C8, CYP2C9, and CYP2C19, weakly to moderately induces CYP1A2, and weakly induces CYP2D6. **Rifabutin** is potentially a weak CYP3A4 inducer, while **rifapentine**, though generally considered moderate, is potentially a potent inducer of CYP3A4.

Table 10.1 Antibacterials

Group	*Drugs*
Aminoglycosides	Amikacin, Astromicin, Dibekacin, Dihydrostreptomycin, Framycetin, Gentamicin, Isepamicin, Kanamycin, Micronomicin, Neomycin, Netilmicin, Paromomycin, Sisomicin, Streptomycin, Tobramycin
Antimycobacterials and related drugs	Aminosalicylic acid (PAS), Bedaquiline, Capreomycin, Clofazimine, Cycloserine, Dapsone, Ethambutol, Ethionamide, Isoniazid, Methaniazide, Protionamide, Pyrazinamide, Rifabutin, Rifampicin (Rifampin), Rifamycin, Rifapentine, Rifaximin
Carbapenems	Biapenem, Doripenem, Ertapenem, Faropenem, Imipenem, Meropenem, Panipenem
Cephalosporins	Cefaclor, Cefadroxil, Cefalexin, Cefaloglycin, Cefaloridine, Cefalotin, Cefamandole, Cefapirin, Cefatrizine, Cefazolin, Cefbuperazone, Cefcapene, Cefdinir, Cefditoren, Cefepime, Cefetamet, Cefixime, Cefmenoxime, Cefmetazole, Cefminox, Cefodizime, Cefonicid, Cefoperazone, Ceforanide, Cefotaxime, Cefotetan, Cefotiam, Cefoxitin, Cefpiramide, Cefpirome, Cefpodoxime, Cefprozil, Cefradine, Cefsulodin, Ceftaroline, Ceftazidime, Cefteram, Ceftezole, Ceftibuten, Ceftizoxime, Ceftobiprole, Ceftriaxone, Cefuroxime, Flomoxef, Latamoxef
Macrolides	Azithromycin, Clarithromycin, Dirithromycin, Erythromycin, Flurithromycin, Josamycin, Midecamycin, Rokitomycin, Roxithromycin, Spiramycin, Telithromycin, Troleandomycin
Penicillins	Amoxicillin, Ampicillin, Azidocillin, Azlocillin, Bacampicillin, Benzylpenicillin (Penicillin G), Carbenicillin, Carindacillin, Ciclacillin, Clometocillin, Cloxacillin, Dicloxacillin, Flucloxacillin, Mecillinam, Meticillin, Mezlocillin, Nafcillin, Oxacillin, Phenethicillin, Phenoxymethylpenicillin (Penicillin V), Piperacillin, Pivampicillin, Pivmecillinam, Procaine benzylpenicillin (Procaine penicillin), Propicillin, Sulbenicillin, Temocillin, Ticarcillin
Polypeptides	Bacitracin, Colistimethate sodium, Colistin, Dalbavancin, Oritavancin, Polymyxin B, Teicoplanin, Telavancin, Vancomycin
Quinolones	Cinoxacin, Ciprofloxacin, Enoxacin, Fleroxacin, Flumequine, Gatifloxacin, Gemifloxacin, Grepafloxacin, Levofloxacin, Lomefloxacin, Moxifloxacin, Nadifloxacin, Nalidixic acid, Norfloxacin, Ofloxacin, Oxolinic Acid, Pazufloxacin, Pefloxacin, Pipemidic Acid, Rosoxacin, Rufloxacin, Sparfloxacin, Temafloxacin, Tosufloxacin, Trovafloxacin
Sulfonamides	Co-trimoxazole, Phthalylsulfathiazole, Sulfadiazine, Sulfadimidine (Sulfamethazine), Sulfafurazole (Sulfisoxazole), Sulfaguanidine, Sulfamerazine, Sulfamethizole, Sulfamethoxazole, Sulfametopyrazine, Sulfametrole
Tetracyclines	Chlortetracyline, Demeclocycline, Doxycycline, Lymecycline, Methacycline, Minocycline, Oxytetracycline, Rolitetracycline, Tetracycline, Tigecycline
Miscellaneous	Aztreonam, Carumonam, Chloramphenicol, Cilastatin, Clindamycin, Daptomycin, Delamanid, Fosfomycin, Fusidic acid, Lincomycin, Linezolid, Loracarbef, Methenamine, Metronidazole, Mupirocin, Nitrofurantoin, Novobiocin, Pristinamycin, Quinupristin/Dalfopristin, Retapamulin, Spectinomycin, Trimethoprim

Aminoglycosides + Amphotericin B

One study in children suggested that amphotericin B decreased the clearance of amikacin and gentamicin. The concurrent use of aminoglycosides and amphotericin B can result in nephrotoxicity.

Clinical evidence, mechanism, importance and management

A study found that **amikacin** or **gentamicin** clearance was impaired in 12 of 17 children given amphotericin B. Serum creatinine increased by 50% or more in 3 of the children, but there was no significant increase in creatinine levels in 7 others. As a result, the aminoglycoside dose was decreased or the dose interval lengthened in 7 children.[1]

The renal function of 4 patients receiving moderate doses of **gentamicin** deteriorated when they were given amphotericin B. Both drugs are known to be nephrotoxic and it is suggested, on the basis of what was seen, that combined use may have had additive nephrotoxic effects.[2] A further retrospective analysis found that the use of **amikacin** tended to increase amphotericin B-related nephrotoxicity.[3]

A study assessing the risk factors for nephrotoxicity with aminoglycosides (**tobramycin** and **gentamicin**) enrolled 1489 patients, 157 of whom developed clinical nephrotoxicity. Of these patients 118 had no immediately identifiable cause (such as acute renal failure) and further evaluation of other risk factors found that the concurrent use of amphotericin B significantly increased the risk of nephrotoxicity.[4]

The nephrotoxicity of various combinations of antibiotics was assessed in 171 patients with cancer (139 given a combination of aminoglycoside with penicillin or cephalosporin; 32 given amphotericin B or vancomycin with other antibacterials). The highest nephrotoxicity (based on changes in urea and electrolytes) was found in patients receiving amphotericin B with an aminoglycoside and a cephalosporin.[5]

Two other studies did not find that aminoglycosides increased the risk of amphotericin B-associated toxicity (defined as a 100% or greater increase in serum creatinine),[6,7] although in one of the studies[7] the frequency of concurrent aminoglycoside use may have been too low to identify any evidence of increased nephrotoxic risk.

A case report describes hypomagnesaemic tetany, which developed in a patient who had received **gentamicin** for 9 days, followed immediately by an 8-day course of amphotericin B. Intravenous magnesium replacement resulted in immediate resolution of the tetany. The authors suggested that the hypomagnesaemia had occurred due to the additive magnesium-lowering effects of **gentamicin** and amphotericin B.[8]

Aminoglycosides are generally considered to be nephrotoxic, and therefore it is generally recommended that other nephrotoxic drugs (such as amphotericin B) should be avoided. However, concurrent use may be essential. Renal function and drug levels should be routinely monitored during the use of an aminoglycoside, and it may be prudent to increase the frequency of such monitoring in the presence of amphotericin B. Lipid formulations of amphotericin B are less nephrotoxic than the conventional formulation.[9] One manufacturer notes there was significantly less nephrotoxicity in patients receiving an aminoglycoside with liposomal amphotericin B (*Ambisome*) compared with aminoglycosides and conventional amphotericin B.[10]

1. Goren MP, Viar MJ, Shenep JL, Wright RK, Baker DK, Kalwinsky DK. Monitoring serum aminoglycoside concentrations in children with amphotericin B nephrotoxicity. *Pediatr Infect Dis J* (1988) 7, 698–703.
2. Churchill DN, Seely J. Nephrotoxicity associated with combined gentamicin-amphotericin B therapy. *Nephron* (1977) 19, 176–181.
3. Harbath S, Pestotnik SL, Lloyd JF, Burke JP, Samore MH. The epidemiology of nephrotoxicity associated with conventional amphotericin B therapy. *Am J Med* (2001) 111, 528–34.
4. Bertino JS, Booker LA, Franck PA, Jenkins PL, Franck KR, Nafziger AN. Incidence of and significant risk factors for aminoglycoside-associated nephrotoxicity in patients dosed by using individualized pharmacokinetic monitoring. *J Infect Dis* (1993) 167, 173–9.
5. Krčméry V, Fuchsberger P, Gočár M, Šalát T, Bodnárová J, Sobota R, Koza I, Švec J. Nephrotoxicity of aminoglycosides, polypeptides and cephalosporins in cancer patients. *Chemotherapy* (1991) 37, 287–91.
6. Fisher MA, Talbot GH, Maislin G, McKeon BP, Tynan KP, Strom BL. Risk factors for amphotericin B-associated nephrotoxicity. *Am J Med* (1989) 87, 547–52.
7. Zager RA, O'Quigley J, Zager BK, Alpers CE, Shulman HM, Gamelin LM, Stewart P, Thomas ED. Acute renal failure following bone marrow transplantation: a retrospective study of 272 patients. *Am J Kidney Dis* (1989) 13, 210–16.
8. Davies SV, Murray JA. Amphotericin B, aminoglycosides and hypomagnesaemic [sic] tetany. *BMJ* (1986) 292, 1395–6.
9. Dupont B. Overview of the lipid formulations of amphotericin B. *J Antimicrob Chemother* (2002) 49, (Suppl S1) 31–6.
10. AmBisome (Liposomal Amphotericin B). Gilead Sciences Ltd. UK Summary of product characteristics, January 2009.

Aminoglycosides + Carbapenems

No pharmacokinetic interaction of importance appears to occur between the aminoglycosides and the carbapenems.

Clinical evidence, mechanism, importance and management

The suspicion that low **tobramycin** levels in one patient might have been due to an interaction with **imipenem** with **cilastatin** was not confirmed in a later *in vitro* study.[1] It has also been suggested that the nephrotoxic effects of **imipenem** and the **aminoglycosides** might possibly be additive.[2] However, a study in healthy subjects given single intravenous doses of **imipenem** and **amikacin** found there was a transient increase in **imipenem** levels but no effects on other pharmacokinetic parameters of either drug.[3] In a study in 12 healthy subjects the concurrent use of **tobramycin** and **biapenem** did not alter the pharmacokinetics of either drug.[4] There would seem to be no reason for avoiding concurrent use.

1. Ariano RE, Kassum DA, Meatherall RC, Patrick WD. Lack of in vitro inactivation of tobramycin by imipenem/cilastatin. *Ann Pharmacother* (1992) 26, 1075–7.
2. Albrecht LM, Rybak MJ. Combination imipenem-aminoglycoside therapy. *Drug Intell Clin Pharm* (1986) 20, 506.
3. Adamis G, Papaionnou MG, Giamarellos-Bourboulis EJ, Gargalianos P, Kosmidis J, Giamarellou H. Pharmacokinetic interactions of ceftazidime, imipenem and aztreonam with amikacin in healthy volunteers. *Int J Antimicrob Agents* (2004) 23, 144–9.
4. Muralidharan G, Buice R, Depuis E, Carver A, Friederici D, Kinchelow T, Kinzig M, Kuye O, Sorgel F, Yacobi A, Mayer P. Pharmacokinetics of biapenem with and without tobramycin in healthy volunteers. *Pharm Res* (1993) 10 (10 Suppl), S-396.

Aminoglycosides + Cephalosporins

The nephrotoxic effects of gentamicin and tobramycin can be increased by cefalotin. Nephrotoxicity may also occur when other aminoglycosides are given with cephalosporins.

Clinical evidence

(a) Cefaloridine

Acute renal failure has been reported in a patient given **gentamicin** and cefaloridine.[1] One study reported an increase in the incidence of nephrotoxicity when cefaloridine was given with **gentamicin** (or other unnamed aminoglycosides), although other factors such as excessive dose or pre-existing renal impairment were also associated with the increase in cephalosporin nephrotoxicity in most cases.[2]

(b) Cefalotin

A randomised, double-blind study[3] in patients with sepsis found the following incidence of definite nephrotoxicity;

- **gentamicin** with **cefalotin** 30.4% (7 of 23 patients),
- **tobramycin** with **cefalotin** 20.8% (5 of 24),
- **gentamicin** with methicillin 10% (2 of 20),
- **tobramycin** with methicillin 4.3% (1 of 23).

A very considerable number of studies and case reports confirm an increase in the incidence of nephrotoxicity when **gentamicin**[2,4-14] or **tobramycin**[15,16] are used with **cefalotin**. However, some other studies have found no increase in nephrotoxicity with the combination.[17-20]

(c) Other cephalosporins

The nephrotoxicity of various combinations of antibacterials was assessed in 171 patients with cancer. In those receiving an aminoglycoside with a third generation cephalosporin, the most nephrotoxic combinations were found to be **gentamicin** with **cefotaxime** (although another study did not find this combination to be nephrotoxic[21]) and **amikacin** with **ceftriaxone**, where 5 of 20 and 5 of 13 patients, respectively, had increased serum creatinine. The following combinations were found to be safer: **amikacin** with **cefoxitin** or **ceftazidime**; **gentamicin** with **cefoxitin**; and **netilmicin** with **cefotaxime**.[22]

Another study assessing the risk factors for nephrotoxicity with aminoglycosides (**tobramycin** and **gentamicin**) enrolled 1489 patients, 157 of whom developed clinical nephrotoxicity. Of these patients 118 had no immediately identifiable cause (such as acute renal failure) and further evaluation of other risk factors found that the concurrent use of cephalosporins (including **cefazolin**, **cefotaxime**, **cefoxitin**, **cefamandole**, **cefuroxime**, **ceftriaxone**, and **ceftazidime**) significantly increased the risk of nephrotoxicity.[23]

Other adverse effects have also been reported. Hypokalaemia has also been described in patients taking cytotoxic drugs for leukaemia when they were given **gentamicin** and **cefalexin**,[24] and a study in healthy subjects found that **ceftazidime** may increase the levels of **amikacin**.[25]

In contrast, some studies have reported no adverse interactions between;

- **amikacin** and **cefepime**[26]
- **gentamicin** and **cefuroxime**,[27] or **cefazolin**,[20]
- **tobramycin** and **cefuroxime**,[28] **cefotaxime**,[29] **ceftazidime**[30] or **cefazolin**.[20]

Mechanism

Uncertain. The nephrotoxic effects of gentamicin and tobramycin are well documented, and some (mostly older) cephalosporins are known to be nephrotoxic, especially in high dose. However, it appears that doses that are well tolerated separately can become nephrotoxic when given together.[11]

Importance and management

The interaction between gentamicin and cefalotin is very well documented and potentially serious: there is less information about tobramycin with cefalotin, but they appear to interact similarly. The risk of nephrotoxicity is probably greatest if high doses of cefalotin are used in those with some existing renal impairment. One study suggests that short courses of treatment are sometimes justified,[12] but renal function should be very closely monitored and doses kept to a minimum. The combination of any aminoglycoside and cefalotin is probably best avoided in high-risk patients wherever possible.

The interaction between other aminoglycosides or cephalosporins is less well documented, but what is known suggests that they can, on occasion, interact similarly. Risk factors for this interaction are said to include raised aminoglycoside trough levels, decreased albumin, male gender, advanced age, increased length of treatment, liver disease or ascites, and some other diseases, including leukaemia,[23,31] although their significance in practice has been questioned.[23] It seems likely that the routine monitoring of renal function that is advised with aminoglycosides should be adequate to detect any interaction, but if renal impairment develops the contribution of an interaction should be considered.

1. Zazgornik J, Schmidt P, Lugscheider R, Kopsa H. Akutes Nierenversagen bei kombinierter Cephaloridin-Gentamycin-Therapie. *Wien Klin Wochenschr* (1973) 85, 839–41.
2. Foord RD. Cephaloridine, cephalothin and the kidney. *J Antimicrob Chemother* (1975) 1(suppl) 119–33.
3. Wade JC, Smith CR, Petty BG, Lipsky JJ, Conrad G, Ellner J, Lietman PS. Cephalothin plus an aminoglycoside is more nephrotoxic than methicillin plus an aminoglycoside. *Lancet* (1978) ii, 604–6.
4. Opitz A, Herrmann I, von Harrath D, Schaefer K. Akute niereninsuffizienz nach Gentamycin-Cephalosporin-Kombinationstherapie. *Med Welt* (1971) 22, 434–8.
5. Plager JE. Association of renal injury with combined cephalothin-gentamicin therapy among patients severely ill with malignant disease. *Cancer* (1976) 37, 1937–43.
6. The EORTC International Antimicrobial Therapy Project Group. Three antibiotic regimens in the treatment of infection in febrile granulocytopenic patients with cancer. *J Infect Dis* (1978) 137, 14–29.
7. Kleinknecht D, Ganeval D, Droz D. Acute renal failure after high doses of gentamicin and cephalothin. *Lancet* (1973) i, 1129.
8. Bobrow SN, Jaffe E, Young RC. Anuria and acute tubular necrosis associated with gentamicin and cephalothin. *JAMA* (1972) 222, 1546–7.
9. Fillastre JP, Laumonier R, Humbert G, Dubois D, Metayer J, Delpech A, Leroy J, Robert M. Acute renal failure associated with combined gentamicin and cephalothin therapy. *BMJ* (1973) 2, 396–7.
10. Cabanillas F, Burgos RC, Rodríguez RC, Baldizón C. Nephrotoxicity of combined cephalothin-gentamicin regimen. *Arch Intern Med* (1975) 135, 850–52.
11. Tvedegaard E. Interaction between gentamicin and cephalothin as cause of acute renal failure. *Lancet* (1976) ii, 581.
12. Hansen MM, Kaaber K. Nephrotoxicity in combined cephalothin and gentamicin therapy. *Acta Med Scand* (1977) 201, 463–7.
13. Schwartz JH, Schein P. Fanconi syndrome associated with cephalothin and gentamicin therapy. *Cancer* (1978) 41, 769–72.
14. Bailey RR. Renal failure in combined gentamicin and cephalothin therapy. *BMJ* (1973) 2, 776–7.
15. Tobias JS, Whitehouse JM, Wrigley PFM. Severe renal dysfunction after tobramycin/cephalothin therapy. *Lancet* (1976) i, 425.
16. Klastersky J, Hensgens C, Debusscher L. Empiric therapy for cancer patients: comparative study of ticarcillin-tobramycin, ticarcillin-cephalothin, and cephalothin-tobramycin. *Antimicrob Agents Chemother* (1975) 7, 640–45.
17. Fanning WL, Gump D, Jick H. Gentamicin- and cephalothin-associated rises in blood urea nitrogen. *Antimicrob Agents Chemother* (1976) 10, 80–82.
18. Stille W, Arndt I. Argumente gegen eine Nephrotoxizität von cephalothin und gentamycin. *Med Welt* (1972) 23, 1603–5.
19. Wellwood JM, Simpson PM, Tighe JR, Thompson AE. Evidence of gentamicin nephrotoxicity in patients with renal allografts. *BMJ* (1975) 3, 278–81.
20. Schentag JJ, Cerra FB, Plaut ME. Clinical and pharmacokinetic characteristics of aminoglycoside nephrotoxicity in 201 critically ill patients. *Antimicrob Agents Chemother* (1982) 21, 721–6.
21. Bethke RO, v. Gablenz E, Malerczyk V, Seidel G. Nierenverträglichkeit der kombinierten Behandlung mit Cefotaxim und Gentamicin. *Dtsch Med Wochenschr* (1981) 106, 334–6.
22. Krčméry V, Fuchsberger P, Gočár M, Šalát T, Bodnárová J, Sobota R, Koza I, Švec J. Nephrotoxicity of aminoglycosides, polypeptides and cephalosporins in cancer patients. *Chemotherapy* (1991) 37, 287–91.
23. Bertino JS, Booker LA, Franck PA, Jenkins PL, Franck KR, Nafziger AN. Incidence of and significant risk factors for aminoglycoside-associated nephrotoxicity in patients dosed by using individualized pharmacokinetic monitoring. *J Infect Dis* (1993) 167, 173–9.
24. Young GP, Sullivan J, Hurley A. Hypokalæmia due to gentamicin/cephalexin in leukaemia. *Lancet* (1973) ii, 855.
25. Adamis G, Papaioannou MG, Giamarellos-Bourboulis EJ, Gargalianos P, Kosmidis J, Giamarellou H. Pharmacokinetic interactions of ceftazidime, imipenem and aztreonam with amikacin in healthy volunteers. *Int J Antimicrob Agents* (2004) 23, 144–9.
26. Barbhaiya RH, Knupp CA, Pfeffer M, Pittman KA. Lack of pharmacokinetic interaction between cefepime and amikacin in humans. *Antimicrob Agents Chemother* (1992) 36, 1382–6.
27. Cockram CS, Richards P, Bax RP. The safety of cefuroxime and gentamicin in patients with reduced renal function. *Curr Med Res Opin* (1980) 6, 398–403.
28. Trollfors B, Alestig K, Rödjer S, Sandberg T, Westin J. Renal function in patients treated with tobramycin-cefuroxime or tobramycin-penicillin G. *J Antimicrob Chemother* (1983) 12, 641–5.
29. Kuhlmann J, Seidel G, Richter E, Grötsch H. Tobramycin nephrotoxicity: failure of cefotaxime to potentiate injury in patient. *Naunyn Schmiedebergs Arch Pharmacol* (1981) 316 (Suppl), R80.
30. Aronoff GR, Brier RA, Sloan RS, Brier ME. Interactions of ceftazidime and tobramycin in patients with normal and impaired renal function. *Antimicrob Agents Chemother* (1990) 34, 1139–42.
31. Streetman DS, Nafziger AN, Destache CJ, Bertino JS. Individualized pharmacokinetic monitoring results in less aminoglycoside-associated nephrotoxicity and fewer associated costs. *Pharmacotherapy* (2001) 21, 443–51.

Aminoglycosides + Clindamycin

Three cases of acute renal failure have been tentatively attributed to the use of gentamicin with clindamycin, and another report identified the combination as a risk factor for nephrotoxicity. However, other reports note no increased risk of nephrotoxicity when gentamicin or tobramycin was given with clindamycin.

Clinical evidence, mechanism, importance and management

Acute renal failure has been reported in 3 patients with normal renal function when they were given **gentamicin** 3.9 to 4.9 mg/kg daily and clindamycin 0.9 to 1.8 mg/kg daily for 13 to 18 days. They recovered within 3 to 5 days of discontinuing the antibacterials[1] but in one patient acute renal failure only developed after the clindamycin was stopped. The reasons for the renal failure are not known, but given the long courses of **gentamicin** involved, the possibility that renal impairment occurred as an adverse effect of the aminoglycoside alone cannot be excluded. However, one report identified the concurrent use of clindamycin as one of several factors that increased the risk of aminoglycoside-associated nephrotoxicity.[2]

The use of clindamycin with an aminoglycoside seems to be a fairly commonly used combination, especially following abdominal trauma. A study assessing the risk factors for nephrotoxicity with aminoglycosides (**tobramycin** and **gentamicin**) enrolled 1489 patients, 157 of whom developed clinical nephrotoxicity. Of these patients 118 had no immediately identifiable cause (such as acute renal failure) and further evaluation of other risk factors found that the concurrent use of clindamycin was not significantly associated with increased risk of nephrotoxicity.[3] This suggests that treatment with the combination is without nephrotoxic risk above and beyond that seen with an aminoglycoside alone. A short report has also indicated that the combination of **tobramycin** and clindamycin is not nephrotoxic.[4]

As renal function should be routinely monitored during the use of aminoglycosides, no additional precautions would be expected to be necessary if clindamycin is also given.

1. Butkus DE, de Torrente A, Terman DS. Renal failure following gentamicin in combination with clindamycin. Gentamicin nephrotoxicity. *Nephron* (1976) 17, 307–13.
2. Streetman DS, Nafziger AN, Destache CJ, Bertino JS. Individualized pharmacokinetic monitoring results in less aminoglycoside-associated nephrotoxicity and fewer associated costs. *Pharmacotherapy* (2001) 21, 443–51.
3. Bertino JS, Booker LA, Franck PA, Jenkins PL, Franck KR, Nafziger AN. Incidence of and significant risk factors for aminoglycoside-associated nephrotoxicity in patients dosed by using individualized pharmacokinetic monitoring. *J Infect Dis* (1993) 167, 173–9.
4. Gillett P, Wise R, Melikian V, Falk R. Tobramycin/cephalothin nephrotoxicity. *Lancet* (1976) i, 547.

Aminoglycosides + Loop diuretics

The concurrent use of aminoglycosides and etacrynic acid should be avoided because their damaging actions on the ear can be additive. Even sequential use may not be safe. Bumetanide and piretanide have been shown to interact similarly in *animals*. Although some patients have developed nephrotoxicity and/or ototoxicity while taking furosemide and an aminoglycoside, it has not been established that this was as a result of an interaction.

Clinical evidence

(a) Bumetanide

There seem to be no clinical reports of an interaction between aminoglycosides and bumetanide, but ototoxicity has been described in *animals* given **kanamycin** and bumetanide.[1,2]

(b) Etacrynic acid

Four patients with renal impairment became permanently deaf after they were given intramuscular **kanamycin** 1 to 1.5 g and intravenous etacrynic acid 50 to 150 mg. One patient also received **streptomycin**, and another also received oral **neomycin**. Deafness took between 30 minutes and almost 2 weeks to develop. In some cases deafness developed despite the doses being given on separate days, and in all cases it appeared irreversible.[3] A patient receiving **gentamicin** rapidly developed deafness when furosemide was replaced by intravenous etacrynic acid.[4]

There are other reports describing temporary, partial or total permanent deafness as a result of giving intravenous etacrynic acid with **gentamicin**,[5] intramuscular **kanamycin**,[5-7] oral **neomycin**,[8] or **streptomycin**.[6,9]

(c) Furosemide

An analysis of three, controlled, randomised, studies found that furosemide did not increase either aminoglycoside-induced nephrotoxicity, or ototoxicity: the aminoglycosides used were **amikacin**, **gentamicin**, and **tobramycin**. Nephrotoxicity developed in 20% (10 of 50 patients) given furosemide and 17% (38 of 222) not given furosemide. Auditory toxicity developed in 22% (5 of 23) given furosemide and 24% (28 of 119) not given furosemide.[4] Other clinical studies similarly suggest that furosemide does not increase aminoglycoside-associated renal damage.[10,11]

In contrast, a study assessing the risk factors for nephrotoxicity with aminoglycosides (**tobramycin** and **gentamicin**) enrolled 1489 patients, 157 of whom developed clinical nephrotoxicity. Of these patients 118 had no immediately identifiable cause (such as acute renal failure) and further evaluation of other risk factors found that the concurrent use of furosemide increased the risk of nephrotoxicity.[12] A clinical study evaluating a possible interaction also found that furosemide increased aminoglycoside-induced renal damage,[13] and there are clinical reports claiming that concurrent use results in ototoxicity, but usually only small numbers of patients were involved and control groups were not included.[14-18] A retrospective study of neonates suggested the possibility of increased ototoxicity but no firm conclusions could be drawn.[19]

Studies in patients and healthy subjects have found that furosemide reduces the renal clearance of **gentamicin**[20,21] and can cause a rise in both serum **gentamicin**[21] and **tobramycin** levels.[22] In contrast, a study in 6 healthy subjects found that although the AUC of a single parenteral 1-mg/kg dose of **gentamicin** was not affected by the administration of a single 0.25-mg/kg dose of furosemide, its clearance was increased during the first 3 hours The authors suggest that the observed increased clearance may reduce the nephrotoxic potential of this combination in patients with normal renal function.[23]

Ototoxicity has been described in *animals* given **kanamycin** and furosemide.[1,2]

(d) Piretanide

A study in 6 healthy subjects found that although the AUC of a single parenteral 1-mg/kg dose of **gentamicin** was not affected by the use of a single 0.1-mg/kg dose of piretanide, its clearance was increased during the first 3 hours. The authors suggest that the observed increased clearance may reduce the nephrotoxic potential of this combination in patients with normal renal function.[23]

Ototoxicity has been described in *animals* given **kanamycin** and piretanide.[24]

Mechanism

Aminoglycosides or etacrynic acid alone can damage the ear and cause deafness, the site of action of the aminoglycosides being the hair cell and that of etacrynic acid the stria vascularis. It appears that the effects of concurrent use are additive. Other loop diuretics can similarly damage hearing. *Animal* studies have shown that intramuscular neomycin can cause a fivefold increase in the concentration of etacrynate in cochlear tissues, and it is possible that the aminoglycoside has some effect on the tissues, which allows the etacrynic acid to penetrate more easily.[25] Similar results have been found with gentamicin.[26]

Importance and management

The interaction between etacrynic acid and the aminoglycosides is well established and well documented. The concurrent or sequential use of etacrynic acid with parenteral aminoglycosides should be avoided because permanent deafness may result. Patients with renal impairment seem to be particularly at risk, most likely because the drugs are less rapidly cleared. Most of the reports describe deafness after intravenous use, but it has also been seen when etacrynic acid is given orally alone.[9] If it is deemed absolutely necessary to use etacrynic acid and an intravenous aminoglycoside, minimal doses should be used and the effects on hearing should be monitored continuously. Not every aminoglycoside has been implicated, but their ototoxicity is clearly established and they may be expected to interact in a similar way. For this reason the same precautions should be used.

Although there is ample evidence of an adverse interaction between furosemide and aminoglycosides in *animals*,[2,27] the weight of clinical evidence suggests that furosemide does not normally increase either the nephrotoxicity or ototoxicity of the aminoglycosides. Nevertheless as there is still some uncertainty about the safety of concurrent use it would be prudent to monitor for any evidence of changes in aminoglycoside serum levels, and renal or hearing impairment. The authors of the major study cited[4] suggest that an interaction may possibly occur if high dose infusions of furosemide are used. The same precautions would seem to be appropriate with bumetanide and piretanide. Note that it is generally advised that aminoglycosides should not be used with other drugs that may cause ototoxicity or nephrotoxicity, such as etacrynic acid and furosemide, but in some cases concurrent use may be unavoidable.

1. Ohtani I, Ohtsuki K, Omata T, Ouchi J, Saito T. Interaction of bumetanide and kanamycin. *ORL J Otorhinolaryngol Relat Spec* (1978) 40, 216–25.
2. Brummett RE, Bendrick T, Himes D. Comparative ototoxicity of bumetanide and furosemide when used in combination with kanamycin. *J Clin Pharmacol* (1981) 21, 628–36.
3. Johnson AH, Hamilton CH. Kanamycin ototoxicity — possible potentiation by other drugs. *South Med J* (1970) 63, 511–13.
4. Smith CR, Lietman PS. Effect of furosemide on aminoglycoside-induced nephrotoxicity and auditory toxicity in humans. *Antimicrob Agents Chemother* (1983) 23, 133–7.
5. Meriwether WD, Mangi RJ, Serpick AA. Deafness following standard intravenous dose of ethacrynic acid. *JAMA* (1971) 216, 795–8.
6. Mathog RH, Klein WJ. Ototoxicity of ethacrynic acid and aminoglycoside antibiotics in uremia. *N Engl J Med* (1969) 280, 1223–4.
7. Ng PSY, Conley CE, Ing TS. Deafness after ethacrynic acid. *Lancet* (1969) i, 673–4.
8. Matz GJ, Beal DD, Krames L. Ototoxicity of ethacrynic acid. Demonstrated in a human temporal bone. *Arch Otolaryngol* (1969) 90, 152–5.
9. Schneider WJ, Becker EL. Acute transient hearing loss after ethacrynic acid therapy. *Arch Intern Med* (1966) 117, 715–17.
10. Bygbjerg IC, Møller R. Gentamicin-induced nephropathy. *Scand J Infect Dis* (1976) 8, 203–8.
11. Smith CR, Maxwell RR, Edwards CQ, Rogers JF, Lietman PS. Nephrotoxicity induced by gentamicin and amikacin. *Johns Hopkins Med J* (1978) 142, 85–90.
12. Bertino JS, Booker LA, Franck PA, Jenkins PL, Franck KR, Nafziger AN. Incidence of and significant risk factors for aminoglycoside-associated nephrotoxicity in patients dosed by using individualized pharmacokinetic monitoring. *J Infect Dis* (1993) 167, 173–9.
13. Prince RA, Ling MH, Hepler CD, Rainville EC, Kealey GP, Donta ST, LeFrock JL, Kowalsky SF. Factors associated with creatinine clearance changes following gentamicin therapy. *Am J Hosp Pharm* (1980) 37, 1489–95.
14. Gallagher KL, Jones JK. Furosemide-induced ototoxicity. *Ann Intern Med* (1979) 91, 744–5.
15. Noël P, Levy V-G. Toxicité rénale de l'association gentamicine-furosémide. Une observation. *Nouv Presse Med* (1978) 7, 351–3.
16. Brown CB, Ogg CS, Cameron JS, Bewick M. High dose frusemide in acute reversible intrinsic renal failure. A preliminary communication. *Scott Med J* (1974) 19, 35–9.
17. Thomsen J, Bech P, Szpirt W. Otological symptoms in chronic renal failure. The possible role of aminoglycoside-furosemide interaction. *Arch Otorhinolaryngol* (1976) 214, 71–9.
18. Bates DE, Beaumont SJ, Baylis BW. Ototoxicity induced by gentamicin and furosemide. *Ann Pharmacother* (2002) 36, 446–51.
19. Salamy A, Eldredge L, Tooley WH. Neonatal status and hearing loss in high-risk infants. *J Pediatr* (1989) 114, 847–52.
20. Lawson DH, Tilstone WJ, Semple PF. Furosemide interactions: studies in normal volunteers. *Clin Res* (1976) 24, 3.
21. Lawson DH, Tilstone WJ, Gray JMB, Srivastava PK. Effect of furosemide on the pharmacokinetics of gentamicin in patients. *J Clin Pharmacol* (1982) 22, 254–8.
22. Kaka JS, Lyman C, Kilarski DJ. Tobramycin-furosemide interaction. *Drug Intell Clin Pharm* (1984) 18, 235–8.
23. Whiting PH, Barber HE, Petersen J. The effect of frusemide and piretanide on the renal clearance of gentamicin in man. *Br J Clin Pharmacol* (1981) 12, 795–9.
24. Brummett RE. Ototoxicity resulting from the combined administration of potent diuretics and other agents. *Scand Audiol* (1981) (Suppl 14), 215–24.
25. Orsulakova A, Schacht J. A biochemical mechanism of the ototoxic interaction between neomycin and ethacrynic acid. *Acta Otolaryngol* (1982) 93, 43–8.
26. Tran Ba Huy P, Meulemans A, Manuel C, Sterkers O, Wassef M. Critical appraisal of the experimental studies on the ototoxic interaction between ethacrynic acid and aminoglycoside antibiotics. A pharmacokinetical standpoint. *Scand Audiol* (1981) (Suppl 14), 225–32.
27. Ohtani I, Ohtsuki K, Omata T, Ouchi J, Saito T. Potentiation and its mechanism of cochlear damage resulting from furosemide and aminoglycoside antibiotics. *ORL J Otorhinolaryngol Relat Spec* (1978) 40, 53–63.

Aminoglycosides + Magnesium compounds

A neonate with elevated serum magnesium levels had a respiratory arrest when given gentamicin.

Clinical evidence

An infant born to a woman whose pre-eclampsia had been treated with magnesium sulfate was found to have muscle weakness and a serum magnesium concentration of 1.77 mmol/L. The neonate was given ampicillin 100 mg/kg intravenously and **gentamicin** 2.5 mg/kg intramuscularly every 12 hours, starting 12 hours after birth. Soon after the second dose of **gentamicin** she stopped breathing and needed intubation. The **gentamicin** was stopped and the child improved.[1] *Animal* studies support this interaction.[1]

Mechanism

Magnesium ions and the aminoglycosides have neuromuscular blocking activity, which can be additive (see also 'Neuromuscular blockers + Magnesium compounds', p.129 and 'Neuromuscular blockers + Aminoglycosides', p.119). In the case cited here it seems that it was enough to block the actions of the respiratory muscles.

Importance and management

Direct information about this interaction is very limited, but it is well supported by the recognised pharmacological actions of magnesium and the aminoglycosides, and their interactions with conventional neuromuscular blockers. The aminoglycosides as a group should be avoided in hypermagnesaemic infants needing antibacterial treatment. If this is not possible, the effects on respiration should be closely monitored.

1. L'Hommedieu CS, Nicholas D, Armes DA, Jones P, Nelson T, Pickering LK. Potentiation of magnesium sulfate-induced neuromuscular weakness by gentamicin, tobramycin and amikacin. *J Pediatr* (1983) 102, 629–31.

Aminoglycosides + Miconazole

A report describes a reduction in tobramycin levels, which was attributed to the use of miconazole.

Clinical evidence, mechanism, importance and management

In 9 patients undergoing bone marrow transplantation intravenous miconazole significantly lowered the peak serum **tobramycin** levels, from 9.1 micrograms/mL to 6.7 micrograms/mL. Six patients needed **tobramycin** dose adjustments.[1] Miconazole was stopped in 4 patients, and **tobramycin** pharmacokinetic parameters returned to normal 4 to 8 days later. The reasons for this interaction are not understood. Although the use of **tobramycin** should be well monitored it would be prudent to increase the frequency in patients also given systemic miconazole (note that miconazole oral gel can have significant systemic absorption). There does not appear to be any information about other aminoglycosides and azole antifungals.

1. Hatfield SM, Crane LR, Duman K, Karanes C, Kiel RJ. Miconazole-induced alteration in tobramycin pharmacokinetics. *Clin Pharm* (1986) 5, 415–19.

Aminoglycosides + NSAIDs

There are conflicting reports as to whether or not serum gentamicin and amikacin levels are raised by indometacin or ibuprofen in premature infants.

Clinical evidence

(a) Amikacin

A study in 10 preterm infants with gestational ages ranging from 25 to 34 weeks, who were given amikacin, found that the use of **indometacin** 200 micrograms/kg every 8 hours, for up to 3 doses, caused a rise in the serum levels of amikacin. Trough and peak levels of amikacin were raised by 28% and 17%, respectively.[1]

In another study, preterm infants were given amikacin 20 mg/kg every 36 hours (gestational age less than 30 weeks) or every 24 hours (gestational age 30 to 31 weeks) with either **ibuprofen lysine** 10 mg/kg within 6 hours of birth, then a further 5 mg/kg dose 24 and 48 hours later, or placebo. The half-life of amikacin was increased from 12.4 hours to 16.4 hours and its clearance was reduced by 40% in infants who also received intravenous **ibuprofen lysine**.[2] Reductions in amikacin clearance, independent of gestational age were found by the same authors in another study in which preterm infants with gestational ages of between 24 and 34 weeks were given amikacin and **ibuprofen**.[3]

In contrast, another study in preterm infants given amikacin found no changes in its pharmacokinetics when **ibuprofen** or **indometacin** were given.[4]

(b) Gentamicin

A study in 10 preterm infants with gestational ages ranging from 25 to 34 weeks, who were given gentamicin, found that the use of **indometacin** 200 micrograms/kg every 8 hours, for up to 3 doses, caused a rise in the serum levels of gentamicin. Trough and peak levels of gentamicin were raised by 48% and 33%, respectively.[1] A later study[5] confirmed that **indometacin** (200 micrograms/kg given intravenously at 0 hours, then 100 micrograms/kg given at 12 hours and then 36 hours) decreased the clearance of 3-mg/kg daily doses of gentamicin by 23% in preterm infants weighing less than 1250 g.

In contrast, 8 out of 13 infants had no increase in their serum gentamicin levels when they were given **indometacin** 200 to 250 micrograms/kg every 12 hours for 3 doses. Of the remaining 5, slight to moderate rises occurred in 4, and a substantial rise occurred in just one.[6] In another study no significant changes in serum gentamicin levels were seen in 31 preterm newborns given parenteral **indometacin** 200 micrograms/kg every 12 hours for 3 doses.[7]

Mechanism

Aminoglycosides are excreted by renal filtration, which can be inhibited by indometacin or ibuprofen. This may result in the retention of the aminoglycoside.

Importance and management

Information seems to be limited to these conflicting studies, although supporting evidence for indometacin comes from the fact that it also causes the retention of digoxin in premature infants. The authors of one of the studies[6] suggest that the different results may be because aminoglycoside serum levels were lower in their study before the indometacin was given, and also because they measured the new steady-state levels after 40 to 60 hours instead of 24 hours. Whatever the explanation, concurrent use should be very closely monitored because toxicity is associated with raised aminoglycoside serum levels. It has been suggested that the aminoglycoside dose should be reduced before giving indometacin and aminoglycoside levels and renal function should be well monitored during concurrent use.[1] It has also been suggested that the dose interval of amikacin should be increased by at least 6 to 8 hours if ibuprofen lysine is also given during the first days of life.[2] Other aminoglycosides possibly behave similarly. This interaction does not seem to have been studied in adults.

1. Zarfin Y, Koren G, Maresky D, Perlman M, MacLeod S. Possible indomethacin-aminoglycoside interaction in preterm infants. *J Pediatr* (1985) 106, 511–13.
2. Allegaert K, Cossey V, Langhendries JP, Naulaers G, Vanhole C, Devlieger H, Van Overmeire B. Effects of co-administration of ibuprofen-lysine on the pharmacokinetics of amikacin in preterm infants during the first days of life. *Biol Neonate* (2004) 86, 207–11.
3. Allegaert K, Cossey V, Debeer A, Langhendries JP, Van Overmeire B, de Hoon J, Devlieger H. The impact of ibuprofen on renal clearance in preterm infants is independent of the gestational age. *Pediatr Nephrol* (2005) 20, 740–3.
4. Cuesta Grueso C, Gimeno Navarro A, Marqués Miñana MR, Peris Ribera JE, Morcillo Sopena F, Poveda Andrés JL. Efecto de la administración concomitante de indometacina o ibuprofeno en la farmacocinética de amikacina en neonatos prematuros. *Farm Hosp* (2006) 30, 149–53.
5. Dean RP, Domanico RS, Covert RF. Prophylactic indomethacin alters gentamicin pharmacokinetics in preterm infants <1250 grams. *Pediatr Res* (1994) 35, 83A.
6. Jerome M, Davis JC. The effects of indomethacin on gentamicin serum levels. *Proc West Pharmacol Soc* (1987) 30, 85–7.
7. Grylack LJ, Scanlon JW. Interaction of indomethacin (I) and gentamicin (G) in preterm newborns. *Pediatr Res* (1988) 23, 409A.

Aminoglycosides + Penicillins

The use of piperacillin is reported to be a risk factor for aminoglycoside-associated nephrotoxicity. A reduction in serum aminoglycoside levels can occur if aminoglycosides and penicillins are given to patients with severe renal impairment. No pharmacokinetic interaction of importance appears to occur with intravenous aminoglycosides and penicillins in those with normal renal function.

The serum levels of oral phenoxymethylpenicillin can be halved by oral neomycin.

Clinical evidence

A. Intravenous or intramuscular aminoglycosides

(a) Patients with normal renal function

A patient with normal renal function was given **gentamicin** 80 mg intravenously, with and without **carbenicillin** 4 g. The serum **gentamicin** concentration profiles in both cases were very similar.[1] No interaction was seen in 10 patients given **tobramycin** with **piperacillin**,[2] or in another 10 healthy subjects given daily **gentamicin** and **piperacillin** with **tazobactam**.[3] Only minimal pharmacokinetic changes were seen in 9 healthy subjects given **tobramycin** and **piperacillin** with **tazobactam**,[4] and 18 patients with cystic fibrosis (adults and children) given **tobramycin** with **ticarcillin**.[5] However, a study assessing the risk factors for nephrotoxicity with aminoglycosides (**tobramycin** and **gentamicin**) enrolled 1489 patients, 157 of whom developed clinical nephrotoxicity. Of these patients 118 had no immediately identifiable cause (such as acute renal failure) and further evaluation of other risk factors found that the concurrent use of **piperacillin**, but not **ticarcillin** or **carbenicillin** increased the risk of nephrotoxicity.[6]

(b) Patients with renal impairment

A study in 6 patients with renal failure requiring dialysis, who were receiving intravenous **carbenicillin** 8 to 15 g daily in 3 to 6 divided doses, found that in the presence of the penicillin, serum **gentamicin** levels did not exceed 4 micrograms/mL. When the **carbenicillin** was stopped, serum **gentamicin** levels rose.[7]

Other reports similarly describe unusually low **gentamicin** levels in patients with impaired renal function, given **carbenicillin**,[1,8-10] **piperacillin**,[11] or **ticarcillin**.[8,10,12] The half-life of **gentamicin** has been reported to be reduced by **carbenicillin** or **piperacillin** by about one-half or one-third.[8,11,13] Similarly, unusually low **tobramycin** levels have been reported in patients with impaired renal function, who were given **carbenicillin**,[7] **piperacillin**[14] or **ticarcillin**.[12]

In 3 patients receiving long-term haemodialysis, **piperacillin** doubled the clearance of **tobramycin** 2 mg/kg, and reduced its half-life from 73 hours to 22 hours.[15] In one patient, the half-life of **tobramycin** was reduced from an expected 70 hours to 10.5 hours, and the serum level of **tobramycin** was unexpectedly low, when **piperacillin** was given.[14]

In contrast one study found that **piperacillin** or **piperacillin** with **tazobactam** did not affect the pharmacokinetics of **tobramycin** in subjects with renal impairment.[16] Similarly, **piperacillin** 4 g every 12 hours did not affect the pharmacokinetics of **netilmicin** 2 mg/kg in 3 patients receiving long-term haemodialysis.[15]

B. Oral aminoglycosides

In 5 healthy subjects the serum concentrations of a 250-mg oral dose of **phenoxymethylpenicillin** were reduced by more than 50% after they took **neomycin** 3 g four times daily for 7 days. Normal penicillin pharmacokinetics were not seen until 6 days after the **neomycin** was withdrawn.[17]

Mechanism

The nephrotoxic effects of gentamicin and tobramycin are well documented. The reason why piperacillin but not carbenicillin or ticarcillin appears to increase the risk of nephrotoxicity in patients with normal renal function is not clear. One suggestion is that sodium loading may protect the kidney from tobramycin toxicity and piperacillin has only 40% as much sodium as ticarcillin.[6]

In vitro, the amino groups on the aminoglycosides and the beta-lactam ring on the penicillins interact chemically to form biologically inactive amides.[18] It has been suggested that this reaction may also occur in the plasma, causing a drop in the levels of active antibacterial.[13] The interaction occurs in those with poor renal function as the drugs persist in the plasma for longer, allowing a greater time for inactivation. This therefore means that the drug is lost more rapidly than has been accounted for by the renal function, and consequently lower than expected levels of the antibacterial result. However, the lack of interaction found in one study led to the conclusion that reported interactions in renal impairment may be due to *in vitro* inactivation after sample collection.[16]

In the case of phenoxymethylpenicillin, the levels are probably lowered because oral neomycin can cause a reversible malabsorption syndrome (histologically similar to nontropical sprue).

Importance and management

The concurrent use of piperacillin and aminoglycosides is reported to be a risk factor for nephrotoxicity in patients with normal renal function.[6,19] The nephrotoxic effects of gentamicin and tobramycin are well documented. Risk factors for nephrotoxicity include raised aminoglycoside trough levels, decreased albumin, male gender, advanced age, increased length of treatment, liver disease or ascites, and some other diseases, including leukaemia,[6,19] although their significance in practice has been questioned.[6] Renal function should be monitored if an aminoglycoside is given, but it may be prudent to increase the frequency of this monitoring if piperacillin is also given.

Other reports suggest that a pharmacokinetic interaction between parenteral aminoglycosides and piperacillin or other penicillins, resulting in reduced levels of the aminoglycoside, seems to occur in patients with renal impairment. In those cases where concurrent use is thought necessary, it has been recommended that the serum levels of both antibacterials are closely monitored.[7] However, note that antibacterial inactivation can continue in the assay sample, and one author[20] suggests that rapid assay is necessary, while others[16] note the importance of protecting samples against further inactivation. There would seem to be no reason for avoiding concurrent use in patients with normal renal function because no significant *in vivo* inactivation appears to occur. Moreover there is good clinical evidence that concurrent use is valuable, especially in the treatment of Pseudomonas infections.[1,21]

Evidence for an interaction between oral neomycin and penicillins seems limited to the report about phenoxymethylpenicillin, and its clinical significance is unclear. It seems possible that oral **kanamycin** and **paromomycin** might interact similarly, but this needs confirmation.

1. Eykyn S, Phillips I, Ridley M. Gentamicin plus carbenicillin. *Lancet* (1971) i, 545–6.
2. Lau A, Lee M, Flascha S, Prasad R, Sharifi R. Effect of piperacillin on tobramycin pharmacokinetics in patients with normal renal function. *Antimicrob Agents Chemother* (1983) 24, 533–7.
3. Hitt CM, Patel KB, Nicolau DP, Zhu Z, Nightingale CH. Influence of piperacillin-tazobactam on pharmacokinetics of gentamicin given once daily. *Am J Health-Syst Pharm* (1997) 54, 2704–8.
4. Lathia C, Sia L, Lanc R, Greene D, Kuye O, Batra V, Yacobi A, Faulkner R. Pharmacokinetics of piperacillin/tazobactam IV with and without tobramycin IV in healthy adult male volunteers. *Pharm Res* (1991) 8, (10 Suppl), S-303.
5. Roberts GW, Nation RL, Jarvinen AO, Martin AJ. An *in vivo* assessment of the tobramycin/ticarcillin interaction in cystic fibrosis patients. *Br J Clin Pharmacol* (1993) 36, 372–5.
6. Bertino JS, Booker LA, Franck PA, Jenkins PL, Franck KR, Nafziger AN. Incidence of and significant risk factors for aminoglycoside-associated nephrotoxicity in patients dosed by using individualized pharmacokinetic monitoring. *J Infect Dis* (1993) 167, 173–9.
7. Weibert R, Keane W, Shapiro F. Carbenicillin inactivation of aminoglycosides in patients with severe renal failure. *Trans Am Soc Artif Intern Organs* (1976) 22, 439–43.
8. Davies M, Morgan JR, Anand C. Interactions of carbenicillin and ticarcillin with gentamicin. *Antimicrob Agents Chemother* (1975) 7, 431–4.
9. Weibert RT, Keane WF. Carbenicillin-gentamicin interaction in acute renal failure. *Am J Hosp Pharm* (1977) 34, 1137–9.
10. Kradjan WA, Burger R. In vivo inactivation of gentamicin by carbenicillin and ticarcillin. *Arch Intern Med* (1980) 140, 1668–70.
11. Thompson MIB, Russo ME, Saxon BJ, Atkin-Thor E, Matsen JM. Gentamicin inactivation by piperacillin or carbenicillin in patients with end-stage renal disease. *Antimicrob Agents Chemother* (1982) 21, 268–73.
12. Chow MSS, Quintiliani R, Nightingale CH. In vivo inactivation of tobramycin by ticarcillin. A case report. *JAMA* (1982) 247, 658–9.
13. Riff LJ, Jackson GG. Laboratory and clinical conditions for gentamicin inactivation by carbenicillin. *Arch Intern Med* (1972) 130, 887–91.
14. Uber WE, Brundage RC, White RL, Brundage DM, Bromley HR. In vivo inactivation of tobramycin by piperacillin. *Ann Pharmacother* (1991) 25, 357–9.
15. Matzke GR, Halstenson CE, Heim KL, Abraham PA, Keane WF. Netilmicin disposition is not altered by concomitant piperacillin administration. *Clin Pharmacol Ther* (1985) 41, 210.
16. Dowell JA, Korth-Bradley J, Milisci M, Tantillo K, Amorusi P, Tse S. Evaluating possible pharmacokinetic interactions between tobramycin, piperacillin, and a combination of piperacillin and tazobactam in patients with various degrees of renal impairment. *J Clin Pharmacol* (2001) 41, 979–86.
17. Cheng SH, White A. Effect of orally administered neomycin on the absorption of penicillin V. *N Engl J Med* (1962) 267, 1296–7.
18. Perényi T, Graber H, Arr M. Über die Wechselwirkung der Penizilline und Aminoglykosid-Antibiotika. *Int J Clin Pharmacol Ther Toxicol* (1974) 10, 50–5.
19. Streetman DS, Nafziger AN, Destache CJ, Bertino JS. Individualized pharmacokinetic monitoring results in less aminoglycoside-associated nephrotoxicity and fewer associated costs. *Pharmacotherapy* (2001) 21, 443–51.
20. Russo ME. Penicillin-aminoglycoside inactivation: another possible mechanism of interaction. *Am J Hosp Pharm* (1980) 37, 702–4.
21. Kluge RM, Standiford HC, Tatem B, Young VM, Schimpff SC, Greene WH, Calia FM, Hornick RB. The carbenicillin-gentamicin combination against *Pseudomonas aeruginosa*. Correlation of effect with gentamicin sensitivity. *Ann Intern Med* (1974) 81, 584–7.

Aminoglycosides + Polygeline (*Haemaccel*)

The incidence of acute renal failure appears to be increased in cardiac surgical patients given polygeline (*Haemaccel*) with gentamicin.

Clinical evidence

The observation of a differing incidence of acute renal failure in patients undergoing coronary artery bypass surgery in two similar units, prompted a retrospective review of patient records. This showed that the only management differences were related to antibacterial prophylaxis and the bypass prime content (i.e. the solution used to prime the cardiopulmonary bypass circuit). Acute renal failure was defined as a more than 50% rise in serum creatinine on the first postoperative day in those patients whose creatinine was also greater than 120 micromol/L. Four groups of patients were identified, and the incidence of renal failure was as follows:

Group A: (polygeline plus **gentamicin** and flucloxacillin) 31% (28 of 91 patients);
Group B: (polygeline plus cefalotin)12% (9 of 72 patients);
Group C: (crystalloid plus **gentamicin** and flucloxacillin) 7% (4 of 57 patients);
Group D: (crystalloid plus cefalotin) 2% (1 of 47 patients).

Polygeline (*Haemaccel*) 1 litre, which is a urea linked gelatin colloid with a calcium concentration of 6.25 micromol/L, was used for groups A and B, with crystalloid-Hartmann's solution or Ringer's injection (calcium concentration 2 mmol/L) to make up the rest of the prime volume of 2 litres. Groups C and D received only crystalloid (no polygeline) in the prime. Albumin 100 mL was used in groups B and D.[1] However, the study has been criticised because other drugs that affect renal function (such as ACE inhibitors, cimetidine, NSAIDs or clonidine), which may have been taken by the patients were not considered.[2] This criticism has been refuted because of the large sample size involved.[3]

Mechanism

Not fully understood. It is thought that the relatively high calcium content of the polygeline may have potentiated gentamicin-associated nephrotoxicity. Hypercalcaemia has been shown in *animals* to increase aminoglycoside-induced nephrotoxicity.[4]

Importance and management

Information appears to be limited to this clinical study and *animal* studies, but the evidence available suggests that a clinically important adverse interaction occurs between these drugs. The incidence of acute renal failure in cardiac surgery patients is normally about 3 to 5%[5] which is low compared with the 31% shown by those given polygeline and gentamicin. The authors of the study advise avoidance of these two drugs. More study is needed.

1. Schneider M, Valentine S, Clarke GM, Newman MAJ, Peakcock J. Acute renal failure in cardiac surgical patients potentiated by gentamicin and calcium. *Anaesth Intensive Care* (1996) 24, 647–50.
2. Bolsin S, Jones S. Acute renal failure potentiated by gentamicin and calcium. *Anaesth Intensive Care* (1997) 25, 431–2.
3. Schneider M, Clarke GM, Valentine SJ, Peakcock J. Acute renal failure potentiated by gentamicin and calcium; reply. *Anaesth Intensive Care* (1997) 25, 432.
4. Elliott WC, Patchin DS, Jones DB. Effect of parathyroid hormone activity on gentamicin nephrotoxicity. *J Lab Clin Med* (1987) 109, 48–54.
5. Hilberman M, Myers BD, Carrie BJ, Derby G, Jamison RL, Stinson EB. Acute renal failure following cardiac surgery. *J Thorac Cardiovasc Surg* (1979) 77, 880–8.

Aminoglycosides + Vancomycin

The nephrotoxicity of the aminoglycosides appears to be potentiated by vancomycin.

Clinical evidence, mechanism, importance and management

A retrospective review of 105 patients who had received an aminoglycoside with vancomycin for at least 5 days found that nephrotoxicity occurred in 27% of the patients. Of these, 6 had no other identifiable cause for nephrotoxicity.[1] A study assessing the risks factors for nephrotoxicity with aminoglycosides (**tobramycin** and **gentamicin**) enrolled 1489 patients, 157 of whom developed clinical nephrotoxicity. Of these patients 118 had no immediately identifiable cause (such as acute renal failure) and further evaluation of other risk factors found that the concurrent use of vancomycin increased the risk of nephrotoxicity.[2]

A number of other studies,[3-9] including those where patients have had individualised pharmacokinetic monitoring,[3] and those using both once daily and multiple daily dosing,[4] have all found that vancomycin independently increases the risk of nephrotoxicity in patients receiving aminoglycosides. In one meta-analysis of 8 studies, the incidence of nephrotoxicity with the combination was 4.3% greater than with aminoglycosides alone and 13.3% greater than with vancomycin alone.[8]

Risk factors are said to include vancomycin peak and trough levels,[1,6] aminoglycoside trough levels,[1,3,6] decreased albumin concentrations,[2] male gender,[1-3] advanced age,[1-3] increased length of treatment,[1-3] liver disease or ascites,[1,2] as well as a large number of other disease states (such as leukaemia,[2] peritonitis[1] or neutropenia),[1] although their significance in practice has been questioned.[2]

The concurrent use of these antibacterials is therapeutically useful, but the risk of increased nephrotoxicity should be borne in mind. Therapeutic drug monitoring and regular assessment of renal function is warranted, as is recommended with the use of either drug alone.

1. Pauly DJ, Musa DM, Lestico MR, Lindstrom MJ, Hetsko CM. Risk of nephrotoxicity with combination vancomycin-aminoglycoside antibiotic therapy. *Pharmacotherapy* (1990) 10, 378–82.
2. Bertino JS, Booker LA, Franck PA, Jenkins PL, Franck KR, Nafziger AN. Incidence of and significant risk factors for aminoglycoside-associated nephrotoxicity in patients dosed by using individualized pharmacokinetic monitoring. *J Infect Dis* (1993) 167, 173–9.
3. Streetman DS, Nafziger AN, Destache CJ, Bertino JS. Individualized pharmacokinetic monitoring results in less aminoglycoside-associated nephrotoxicity and fewer associated costs. *Pharmacotherapy* (2001) 21, 443–51.
4. Rybak MJ, Abate BJ, Kang SL, Ruffing MJ, Lerner SA, Drusano GL. Prospective evaluation on the effect of an aminoglycoside dosing regimen on rates of observed nephrotoxicity and ototoxicity. *Antimicrob Agents Chemother* (1999) 43, 1549–55.
5. Farber BF, Moellering RC. Retrospective study of the toxicity of preparations of vancomycin from 1974 to 1981. *Antimicrob Agents Chemother* (1983) 23, 138–41.
6. Cimino MA, Rotstein C, Slaughter RL, Emrich LJ. Relationship of serum antibiotic concentrations to nephrotoxicity in cancer patients receiving concurrent aminoglycoside and vancomycin therapy. *Am J Med* (1987) 83, 1091–7.
7. Rybak MJ, Frankowski JJ, Edwards DJ, Albrecht LM. Alanine aminopeptidase and β_2-microglobulin excretion in patients receiving vancomycin and gentamicin. *Antimicrob Agents Chemother* (1987) 31, 1461–4.
8. Goetz MB, Sayers J. Nephrotoxicity of vancomycin and aminoglycoside therapy separately and in combination. *J Antimicrob Chemother* (1993) 32, 325–34.
9. Rybak MJ, Albrecht LM, Boike SC, Chandrasekar PH. Nephrotoxicity of vancomycin, alone and with an aminoglycoside. *J Antimicrob Chemother* (1990) 25, 679–87.

Aminoglycosides + Verapamil

Verapamil appears to protect the kidney from damage caused by gentamicin.

Clinical evidence, mechanism, importance and management

In a comparative study, 9 healthy subjects were given **gentamicin** alone (2 mg/kg loading dose, followed by doses every 8 hours to achieve a peak concentration of 5.5 mg/L and a trough concentration of 0.5 mg/L), and 6 other subjects were given the same dose of **gentamicin** with sustained-release verapamil 180 mg twice daily. The **gentamicin** AUCs of the two groups were virtually the same but the 24-hour urinary excretion of alanine aminopeptidase (AAP) was modestly reduced, by 18%, in the group given verapamil. The reduction in AAP excretion was particularly marked during the first 6 days.[1] The significance of urinary AAP is that this enzyme is found primarily in the brush border membranes of the proximal renal tubules, and its excretion is an early and sensitive marker of renal damage. Thus it seems that verapamil may modestly protect the kidneys from damage by **gentamicin**, but using a drug as potentially toxic as verapamil to provide this protection, when the risks of renal toxicity can be minimised by carefully controlling the **gentamicin** dose, is unwarranted. Information about other aminoglycosides and other calcium-channel blockers seems to be lacking.

1. Kazierad DJ, Wojcik GJ, Nix DE, Goldfarb AL, Schentag JJ. The effect of verapamil on the nephrotoxic potential of gentamicin as measured by urinary enzyme excretion in healthy volunteers. *J Clin Pharmacol* (1995) 35, 196–201.

Aminoglycosides; Amikacin + Dopamine

Dopamine probably does not alter the clearance of amikacin in premature infants.

Clinical evidence, mechanism, importance and management

A retrospective review of the amikacin levels achieved in 240 premature infants found that the median amikacin clearance in infants given dopamine was lower than in infants who did not receive dopamine. However, when the birth weight, gestational age, or use of non-selective COX inhibitors was considered, the change in clearance caused by dopamine was no longer significant.[1] The requirement for dopamine may indicate other medical issues that also have an impact on the clearance of amikacin, and it is therefore essential that doses of amikacin for such infants are individualised.

1. Allegaert K, Debeer A, Cossey V, Rayyan M, Devlieger H. Dopamine is not an independent risk factor for reduced amikacin clearance in extremely low-birth-weight infants. *Pediatr Crit Care Med* (2006) 7, 143–6.

Aminoglycosides; Tobramycin + Sucralfate

An *in vitro* study with tobramycin found that it became markedly and irreversibly bound to sucralfate at the pH values found in the gut. This suggests that the efficacy of tobramycin in gut decontamination might be decreased.

Clinical evidence, mechanism, importance and management

To simulate what might happen in the gut, tobramycin 50 mg/mL was mixed with sucralfate 500 mg in 40 mL of water at pH 3.5 and allowed to stand for 90 minutes at 25°C. Analysis of the solution showed that the tobramycin concentration fell rapidly and progressively over 90 minutes to about 1%. When the pH of the mixture was then raised to 6.5 to 7 for 90 minutes, there was no change in the concentration of tobramycin, suggesting that the interaction was irreversible.[1] The reason for this change is not known, but the authors of the study suggest that sucralfate forms insoluble chelates with tobramycin.[1]

It is not known how important this interaction is likely to be in practice, but the efficacy of tobramycin in gut decontamination may be decreased. Separating the doses of tobramycin and sucralfate might not be effective in some postoperative patients because their gastric function may not return to normal for up to 5 days, and some sucralfate might still be present when the next dose is given.[1] More study is needed to find out whether this interaction is clinically important, but in the meanwhile it would seem prudent to monitor concurrent use carefully, being alert for any evidence of reduced effects.

1. Feron B, Adair CG, Gorman SP, McClurg B. Interaction of sucralfate with antibiotics used for selective decontamination of the gastrointestinal tract. *Am J Hosp Pharm* (1993) 50, 2550–3.

Aminosalicylic acid + Antacids

An aluminium/magnesium hydroxide antacid had no significant effect on the pharmacokinetics of aminosalicylic acid in one study.

Clinical evidence, mechanism, importance and management

In a study, 12 healthy subjects were given a single 6-g dose of aminosalicylic acid with cycloserine, ethionamide and clofazimine, after an overnight fast, or with 15 mL of maximum strength ***Mylanta***, containing **aluminium/magnesium hydroxide** 400/400 mg and **simeticone** 40 mg/5 mL. The antacid had no significant effect on the pharmacokinetics of aminosalicylic acid.[1] No adjustments to the timing of dosing would therefore appear to be necessary if both drugs are given.

1. Peloquin CA, Zhu M, Adam RD, Singleton MD, Nix DE. Pharmacokinetics of para-aminosalicylic acid granules under four dosing conditions. *Ann Pharmacother* (2001) 35, 1332–8.

Aminosalicylic acid + Diphenhydramine

Diphenhydramine can cause a small reduction in the absorption of aminosalicylic acid from the gut.

Clinical evidence, mechanism, importance and management

A study in 9 healthy subjects[1] found that diphenhydramine 50 mg given intramuscularly 10 minutes before a 2-g oral dose of aminosalicylic acid, reduced the mean peak serum aminosalicylic acid levels by about 15%. This effect may occur because diphenhydramine reduces peristalsis in the gut, which in some way reduces aminosalicylic acid absorption. The extent to which diphenhydramine or any other anticholinergic drug diminishes the therapeutic response to long-term treatment with aminosalicylic acid is uncertain, but it is probably small.

1. Lavigne J-G, Marchand C. Inhibition of the gastrointestinal absorption of p-aminosalicylate (PAS) in rats and humans by diphenhydramine. *Clin Pharmacol Ther* (1973) 14, 404–12.

Aminosalicylic acid + Food

A high-fat meal increases the extent of absorption of aminosalicylic acid. Orange juice appears to have no significant effect on the pharmacokinetics of aminosalicylic acid.

Clinical evidence, mechanism, importance and management

In a study, 12 healthy subjects were given a single 6-g dose of aminosalicylic acid with cycloserine, ethionamide and clofazimine, after an overnight fast, with **orange juice** or a high-fat meal. The high-fat meal increased the maximum aminosalicylic acid plasma level and AUC by 50% and 70%, respectively, when compared with an overnight fast, although there was wide inter-individual variation in the effects of the meal. **Orange juice** had no significant effect on the pharmacokinetics of aminosalicylic acid.[1]

1. Peloquin CA, Zhu M, Adam RD, Singleton MD, Nix DE. Pharmacokinetics of para-aminosalicylic acid granules under four dosing conditions. *Ann Pharmacother* (2001) 35, 1332–8.

Aminosalicylic acid + Probenecid

The plasma levels of aminosalicylic acid can be raised up to fourfold by probenecid.

Clinical evidence, mechanism, importance and management

In a study in 7 patients, probenecid 500 mg every 6 hours increased the plasma levels of aminosalicylic acid 4 g by as much as fourfold.[1] Similar results are described in three other reports.[2-4]

The reasons for this effect are uncertain but it seems probable that probenecid successfully competes with aminosalicylic acid for active excretion by the kidney tubules, which results in the increased aminosalicylic acid levels.

The documentation of this interaction is old but it appears to be established. Such large increases in plasma aminosalicylic acid levels would be expected to lead to toxicity. It also seems possible that the dose of aminosalicylic acid could be reduced without losing the required therapeutic response, but this needs confirmation. Monitoring aminosalicylic acid levels, where possible, would probably be useful. Concurrent use should be undertaken with caution.

1. Boger WP, Pitts FW. Influence of *p*-(Di-*n*-propylsulfamyl)-benzoic acid, 'Benemid' on para-aminosalicylic acid (PAS) plasma concentrations. *Am Rev Tuberc* (1950) 61, 862–7.
2. Carr DT, Karlson AG, Bridge EV. Concentration of PAS and tuberculostatic potency of serum after administration of PAS with and without Benemid. *Proc Staff Meet Mayo Clin* (1952) 27, 209–15.
3. Breitenbucher RB, Amatuzio DS, Falk A. The effect of probenecid (Benemid) in enhancing para-aminosalicylic acid concentrations in the blood. *Am Rev Tuberc* (1952) 66, 228–32.
4. McLeod JA, Turnbull FWA, Crofton JW. The use of Benemid to enhance blood-levels of sodium para-aminosalicylate (PAS). *Tubercle* (1953) 34, 152–5.

Antibacterials + Immunoglobulins

One *animal* study found that for severe infections antibacterials were less effective in the presence of high-dose immunoglobulin, but this was not seen in less severe infections.

Clinical evidence, mechanism, importance and management

A study in an *animal* model of severe group B streptococcal infection found the following mortalities: 51% with **benzylpenicillin** 200 mg/kg alone, 88% with immunoglobulin and benzylpenicillin, and 100% with immunoglobulin 2 g/kg alone. A smaller dose of immunoglobulin 0.5 g/kg was not associated with an increase in mortality.[1] Roughly similar results were found when the penicillin was replaced by **ceftriaxone**.[1] In another study using a 1000-fold smaller inoculum of group B streptococci, there was no difference in mortality between **benzylpenicillin** 200 mg/kg daily alone and **benzylpenicillin** with immunoglobulin 0.25 to 2 g/kg, and there was some evidence of a lower incidence of bacteraemia with the combination.[1,2]

Immunoglobulins are used with antibacterials in the successful prevention of infections in clinical practice, and no special precautions appear to be needed in this situation. However, their clinical use for treating established infection is unclear, and the above findings suggest that some caution is warranted.

1. Kim KS. High-dose intravenous immune globulin impairs antibacterial activity of antibiotics. *J Allergy Clin Immunol* (1989) 84, 579–88.
2. Kim KS. Efficacy of human immunoglobulin and penicillin G in treatment of experimental group B streptococcal infection. *Pediatr Res* (1987) 21, 289–92.

Aztreonam + Other antibacterials

There appear to be no clinically significant pharmacokinetic interactions between aztreonam and amikacin, cefradine, clindamycin, gentamicin, metronidazole or nafcillin.

Clinical evidence, mechanism, importance and management

A study in healthy subjects given a single 1-g intravenous dose of aztreonam found that its maximum levels were reduced by 13% and 10% when it was given with **gentamicin** 80 mg and **metronidazole** 500 mg, respectively. Serum bound aztreonam fell by 5% when it was given with **nafcillin** 500 mg and increased by 5% when it was given with **cefradine** 1 g. When aztreonam 1 g and **clindamycin** 600 mg were given together, their renal excretion was increased by 5% and 11%, respectively. None of these changes was statistically significant.[1] Another study in healthy subjects found that the AUC of a 1-g intravenous dose of aztreonam was reduced by 22% by **amikacin** 500 mg, and the AUC of **amikacin** was increased by 27% by aztreonam.[2] These changes are modest and unlikely to be clinically significant in most patients.

1. Creasey WA, Adamovics J, Dhruv R, Platt TB, Sugerman AA. Pharmacokinetic interaction of aztreonam with other antibiotics. *J Clin Pharmacol* (1984) 24, 174–80.
2. Adamis G, Papaioannou MG, Giamarellos-Bourboulis EJ, Gargalianos P, Kosmidis J, Giamarellou H. Pharmacokinetic interactions of ceftazidime, imipenem and aztreonam with amikacin in healthy volunteers. *Int J Antimicrob Agents* (2004) 23, 144–9.

Bedaquiline + Miscellaneous

Ketoconazole and lopinavir boosted with ritonavir very slightly increase bedaquiline exposure; other potent CYP3A4 inhibitors would be expected to interact similarly. Additive QT-interval prolongation appears to occur when bedaquiline is given with clofazimine. Food increases the bioavailability of bedaquiline.

Isoniazid and pyrazinamide do not alter bedaquiline exposure and bedaquiline does not appear to alter the pharmacokinetics of ethambutol, kanamycin, pyrazinamide, ofloxacin, or cycloserine.

Clinical evidence, mechanism, importance and management

(a) Antibacterials

A study in healthy subjects found that the concurrent use of bedaquiline 400 mg daily, **isoniazid** 300 mg daily, and **pyrazinamide** 1 g daily for 5 days did not result in a clinically relevant change in the exposure to any of the drugs.[1] Similarly, in a placebo-controlled study in patients with multi-drug resistant tuberculosis , the use of bedaquiline did not affect the pharmacokinetics of **ethambutol**, **kanamycin**, **pyrazinamide**, **ofloxacin**, or **cycloserine**.[1,2] Dose adjustments of these drugs would therefore not be expected to be necessary on their concurrent use. See also *Clofazimine*, below.

(b) Clofazimine

In phase IIb studies, 17 patients taking clofazimine concurrently with bedaquiline for 24 weeks, had larger increases in QT-interval prolongation (mean QTcF increase 31.9 milliseconds) than those not taking clofazimine (mean QTcF increase 12.3 milliseconds).[2] Bedaquiline has some risk of prolonging the QT interval and can have an additive effect when used with other drugs that increase the QT interval, which would include, according to the manufacturers of bedaquiline, clofazimine.[1,2] See 'Drugs that prolong the QT interval + Other drugs that prolong the QT interval', p.272 for further information.

(c) Food

The UK and US manufacturers briefly note that the bioavailability of bedaquiline was increased about 2-fold when given with a standard meal, compared to the fasted state, and consequently they recommend taking bedaquiline with food.[1,2]

(d) Ketoconazole and other potent CYP3A4 inhibitors

A study in healthy subjects found that ketoconazole 400 mg daily for 4 days increased the exposure to bedaquiline 400 mg daily by 22%.[1] A study in healthy subjects found that **lopinavir boosted with ritonavir** 400/100 mg twice daily for 24 days increased the exposure to a single 400-mg dose of bedaquiline by 22%.[1]

Bedaquiline is metabolised by CYP3A4, of which ketoconazole and the HIV-protease inhibitors boosted with ritonavir are potent inhibitors. Concurrent use therefore increases the exposure to bedaquiline. These studies suggest that even the most potent CYP3A4 inhibitors result in only a very slight increase in bedaquiline exposure. Nevertheless, the UK manufacturer predicts that more prolonged use might have a greater effect, and advises that of the concurrent use of bedaquiline and moderate or potent CYP3A4 inhibitors for more than 14 days should be avoided.[2] The US manufacturer advises that potent CYP3A4 inhibitors for more than 14 days should be avoided unless the benefits of treatment outweigh the risk.[1] For a list of known, clinically relevant CYP3A4 inhibitors see 'Table 1.9', p.11. In addition to the drugs listed in this table, the UK manufacturer also names ciprofloxacin, although this is not known to be a clinically relevant inhibitor of CYP3A4. If concurrent use cannot be avoided, more frequent monitoring (such as ECG and liver transaminase monitoring) for bedaquiline adverse effects is recommended.

1. Sirturo (Bedaquiline). Janssen Therapeutics. US Prescribing information, May 2015.
2. Sirturo (Bedaquiline). Janssen-Cilag Ltd. UK Summary of product characteristics, April 2015.

Bedaquiline + NNRTIs

Nevirapine does not affect, and efavirenz has only a very slight effect on, bedaquiline exposure.

Clinical evidence

In a crossover study in 33 healthy subjects, **efavirenz** 600 mg daily for 14 days very slightly reduced the exposure to a single 400-mg dose of bedaquiline.[1]

The US manufacturer briefly notes that a study in HIV-positive patients found that **nevirapine** 200 mg twice daily for 4 weeks did not result in a clinically relevant change in the exposure to a single 400-mg dose of bedaquiline.[2]

Mechanism

Efavirenz is a moderate inducer of CYP3A4, by which bedaquiline is metabolised, and concurrent use decreases bedaquiline exposure.

Importance and management

Information for an interaction between bedaquiline and the NNRTIs is limited to two studies with efavirenz and nevirapine. The very slight decrease in bedaquiline exposure seen on concurrent use with **efavirenz** is unlikely to be clinically relevant, nevertheless, the UK and US manufacturers of bedaquiline advise that efavirenz, or other moderate inducers of CYP3A4, be avoided during treatment with bedaquiline.[2,3] For a list of moderate CYP3A4 inducers see 'Table 1.9', p.11. In addition to the drugs listed in this table, the UK manufacturer also names **etravirine**, although this is not generally considered to be a clinically relevant inhibitor of CYP3A4.

No bedaquiline dose adjustments are expected to be necessary on concurrent use with **nevirapine**.

1. Dooley KE, Park J-G, Swindells S, Allen R, Haas DW, Cramer Y, Aweeka F, Wiggins I, Gupta A, Lizak P, Qasba S, van Heeswijk R, Flexner C; ACTG 5267 Study Team. Safety, tolerability, and pharmacokinetic interactions of the antituberculous agent TMC207 (bedaquiline) with efavirenz in healthy volunteers: AIDS Clinical Trials Group Study A5267. *J Acquir Immune Defic Syndr* (2012) 59, 455–62.
2. Sirturo (Bedaquiline). Janssen Therapeutics. US Prescribing information, May 2015.
3. Sirturo (Bedaquiline). Janssen-Cilag Ltd. UK Summary of product characteristics, April 2015.

Bedaquiline + Rifamycins

Rifampicin and rifapentine moderately decrease bedaquiline exposure; other potent CYP3A4 inducers are predicted to interact similarly. Rifabutin is also predicted to decrease bedaquiline exposure.

Clinical evidence

A study in healthy subjects found that bedaquiline 300 mg daily and **rifampicin** 600 mg daily for 21 days reduced bedaquiline exposure by 52%.[1] Similarly, in another study in healthy subjects, **rifampicin** 600 mg daily given for 9 days before a single 400-mg dose of bedaquiline, was found to decrease the AUC and maximum concentration of bedaquiline by 53% and 40%, respectively. In the same study, **rifapentine** 600 mg daily given for 9 days before a single 400-mg dose of bedaquiline also decreased the AUC and maximum concentration of bedaquiline by 55% and 38%, respectively.[2]

Mechanism

Bedaquiline is metabolised by CYP3A4, of which both rifampicin and rifapentine are inducers. Concurrent use therefore reduces the exposure to bedaquiline.

Importance and management

The interaction between bedaquiline and **rifampicin** and **rifapentine** appears to be established but its clinical relevance is yet to be confirmed. The UK and US manufacturers advise that use of **rifampicin**, **rifapentine**, **rifabutin**, or other potent or moderate inducers of CYP3A4, be avoided during treatment with bedaquiline.[1,3] This would seem prudent given the risk that treatment failure would pose in a patient being treated with bedaquiline for multi-drug resistant tuberculosis. For a list of known, clinically relevant CYP3A4 inducers see 'Table 1.9', p.11.

1. Sirturo (Bedaquiline). Janssen Therapeutics. US Prescribing information, May 2015.
2. Winter H, Egizi E, Murray S, Erondu N, Ginsberg A, Rouse DJ, Severynse-Stevens D, Pauli E. Evaluation of the pharmacokinetic interaction between repeated doses of rifapentine or rifampin and a single dose of bedaquiline in healthy adult subjects. *Antimicrob Agents Chemother* (2015) 59, 1219–24
3. Sirturo (Bedaquiline). Janssen-Cilag Ltd. UK Summary of product characteristics, April 2015.

Carbapenems + Probenecid

Probenecid increases the AUC of doripenem and meropenem, but does not appear to interact with ertapenem to a clinically relevant extent.

Clinical evidence, mechanism, importance and management

(a) Doripenem

Probenecid increased the AUC of doripenem by 75% and prolonged its plasma elimination half-life by 53%. The manufacturer does not recommend the concurrent use of doripenem with probenecid.[1]

(b) Ertapenem

The use of probenecid with ertapenem is reported to decrease the renal clearance of unbound ertapenem by about 50%, probably because probenecid inhibits the renal tubular secretion of ertapenem. Probenecid slightly increased the elimination half-life and AUC of ertapenem and therefore concurrent use is considered unlikely to increase the effects of ertapenem.[2]

(c) Meropenem

In 6 healthy subjects probenecid 1 g given orally 2 hours before meropenem and 500 mg given orally 1.5 hours after meropenem, increased the AUC of meropenem 500 mg by 43%.[3] Another study in 6 healthy subjects found that probenecid 1.5 g in divided doses the day before meropenem and 500 mg one hour before meropenem increased the AUC of meropenem 1 g by up to 55% and increased its half-life by 33% (from 0.98 to 1.3 hours).[4] In both studies the serum levels of meropenem were modestly increased. This is possibly because meropenem and probenecid compete for active kidney tubular secretion.[5,6] The manufacturers say that because the potency and duration of meropenem are adequate without probenecid, they do not recommend concurrent use.[5,6]

1. Doribax (Doripenem). Ortho-McNeil Pharmaceuticals Inc. US Prescribing information, May 2009.
2. Nix DE, Majumdar AK, DiNubile MJ. Pharmacokinetics and pharmacodynamics of ertapenem: an overview for clinicians. *J Antimicrob Chemother* (2004) 53 (Suppl S2), ii23–ii28.
3. Ishida Y, Matsumoto F, Sakai O, Yoshida M, Shiba K. The pharmacokinetic study of meropenem: effect of probenecid and hemodialysis. *J Chemother* (1993) 5 (Suppl 1), 124–6.
4. Bax RP, Bastain W, Featherstone A, Wilkinson DM, Hutchison M, Haworth SJ. The pharmacokinetics of meropenem in volunteers. *J Antimicrob Chemother* (1989) 24 (Suppl A), 311–20.
5. Meronem (Meropenem). AstraZeneca UK Ltd. UK Summary of product characteristics, July 2007.
6. Merrem (Meropenem). AstraZeneca. US Prescribing information, July 2009.

Cephalosporins + Acetylcysteine

Acetylcysteine does not alter the pharmacokinetics of cefpodoxime or cefadroxil.

Clinical evidence, mechanism, importance and management

The pharmacokinetics of a single 200-mg dose of **cefpodoxime proxetil** are minimally affected by a single 200-mg dose of acetylcysteine.[1] Similarly, the pharmacokinetics of a single 1-g dose of **cefadroxil** are not significantly altered by acetylcysteine.[2] These interactions are unlikely to be of clinical importance.

1. Kees F, Wellenhofer M, Bröhl K, Grobecker H. Bioavailability of cefpodoxime proxetil with co-administered acetylcysteine. *Arzneimittelforschung* (1996) 46, 435–8.
2. Barkworth MF, Mangold B, Rehm KD, Schmieder G, Töberich H, Vinchenzo A, Weber J, Rübartsch C. Ermittlung der bioverfügbarkeit von cefadroxil bei gleichzeitiger gabe von N-acetylcystein. *Arzneimittelforschung* (1991) 41, 839–43.

Cephalosporins + Antacids

No clinically significant interactions appear to occur between an aluminium/magnesium hydroxide antacid and cefaclor AF, cefalexin, cefetamet pivoxil, cefixime or cefprozil; between *Alka-Seltzer* and cefixime; or between ceftibuten and *Mylanta*. In contrast, antacids reduce the bioavailability of cefpodoxime proxetil.

Clinical evidence, mechanism, importance and management

(a) Cefaclor

A study with cefaclor AF (a formulation with a slow rate of release) found that an **aluminium/magnesium hydroxide** antacid (*Maalox*) given one hour after the cefaclor AF to fed subjects reduced the AUC by 18%.[1] This reduction is small and unlikely to be clinically important.

(b) Cefalexin

An **aluminium/magnesium hydroxide** antacid (*Maalox*) given as 8 doses of 10 mL on day one and 2 doses of 10 mL on day 2, had only small and therapeutically unimportant effects on the pharmacokinetics of cefalexin 1 g.[2]

(c) Cefetamet pivoxil

Cefetamet pivoxil 1 g was given to 18 healthy subjects after breakfast with or without 80 mL of an **aluminium/magnesium hydroxide** antacid (*Maalox 70*) given the evening before, 2 hours before, and after breakfast. The pharmacokinetics of the cefetamet were unaffected by the antacid.[3]

(d) Cefixime

An **aluminium/magnesium hydroxide** antacid (*Maalox*) and ***Alka-Seltzer*** (aspirin, calcium phosphate, citric acid and **sodium bicarbonate**) do not significantly affect the absorption of cefixime.[4,5]

(e) Cefpodoxime proxetil

A study in 10 healthy subjects found that 10 mL of an **aluminium/magnesium hydroxide** antacid (*Maalox*) reduced the bioavailability of cefpodoxime proxetil by about 40%. This was considered to be due to reduced dissolution at increased gastric pH values.[6] These results confirm the findings of a previous study with **sodium bicarbonate** and **aluminium hydroxide**.[7] It has been recommended that cefpodoxime is given at least 2 hours after antacids.[6]

(f) Cefprozil

An **aluminium/magnesium hydroxide** antacid (*Maalox*) does not affect the bioavailability of cefprozil.[8]

(g) Ceftibuten

In 18 healthy subjects, 60 mL of an antacid containing **aluminium/magnesium hydroxide** plus **simeticone** (*Mylanta II*) was found not to affect the pharmacokinetics of ceftibuten 400 mg.[9]

1. Satterwhite JH, Cerimele BJ, Coleman DL, Hatcher BL, Kisicki J, DeSante KA. Pharmacokinetics of cefaclor AF: effects of age, antacids and H_2-receptor antagonists. *Postgrad Med J* (1992) 68 (Suppl 3), S3–S9.
2. Deppermann K-M, Lode H, Höffken G, Tschink G, Kalz C, Koeppe P. Influence of ranitidine, pirenzepine, and aluminum magnesium hydroxide on the bioavailability of various antibiotics, including amoxicillin, cephalexin, doxycycline and amoxicillin-clavulanic acid. *Antimicrob Agents Chemother* (1989) 33, 1901–1907.
3. Blouin RA, Kneer J, Ambros RJ, Stoeckel K. Influence of antacid and ranitidine on the pharmacokinetics of oral cefetamet pivoxil. *Antimicrob Agents Chemother* (1990) 34, 1744–8.
4. Petitjean O, Brion N, Tod M, Montagne A, Nicolas P. Étude de l'interaction pharmacocinétique entre le céfixime et deux antiacides. Résultats préliminaires. *Presse Med* (1989) 18, 1596–8.
5. Healy DP, Sahai JV, Sterling LP, Racht EM. Influence of an antacid containing aluminum and magnesium on the pharmacokinetics of cefixime. *Antimicrob Agents Chemother* (1989) 33, 1994–7.
6. Saathoff N, Lode H, Neider K, Depperman KM, Borner K, Koeppe P. Pharmacokinetics of cefpodoxime proxetil and interactions with an antacid and an H_2 receptor antagonist. *Antimicrob Agents Chemother* (1992) 36, 796–800.
7. Hughes GS, Heald DL, Barker KB, Patel RK, Spillers CR, Watts KC, Batts DH, Euler AR. The effects of gastric pH and food on the pharmacokinetics of a new oral cephalosporin, cefpodoxime proxetil. *Clin Pharmacol Ther* (1989) 46, 674–85.
8. Shyu WC, Wilber RB, Pittman KA, Barbhaiya RH. Effect of antacid on the bioavailability of cefprozil. *Antimicrob Agents Chemother* (1992) 36, 962–5.
9. Radwanski E, Nomeir A, Cutler D, Affrime M, Lin C-C. Pharmacokinetic drug interaction study: administration of ceftibuten concurrently with the antacid Mylanta double-strength liquid or with ranitidine. *Am J Ther* (1998) 5, 67–72.

Cephalosporins + Calcium-channel blockers

Nifedipine increases the levels of cefixime. The pharmacokinetics of cefpodoxime proxetil are not affected by nifedipine or diltiazem.

Clinical evidence, mechanism, importance and management

In 8 healthy subjects the AUC and peak serum levels of a single 200-mg dose of **cefixime** were increased by about 70% and 50%, respectively, when **cefixime** was taken 30 minutes after a 20-mg dose of **nifedipine**. The rate of absorption was also increased. One suggested reason for this interaction is that the **nifedipine** increases the absorption of the **cefixime** by affecting the carrier system across the epithelial wall of the gut.[1] It seems doubtful if this increased **cefixime** bioavailability is clinically important (the combination was well-tolerated) and no particular precautions would seem to be necessary on concurrent use.

In 12 healthy subjects, the pharmacokinetics of a single 200-mg dose of **cefpodoxime proxetil** were found to be unchanged by single doses of either **diltiazem** 60 mg or **nifedipine** 20 mg.[2] No special precautions would seem necessary during concurrent use.

Information about other cephalosporins and calcium-channel blockers seems to be lacking, but there seems to be no particular reason to suspect an interaction.

1. Duverne C, Bouten A, Deslandes A, Westphal J-F, Trouvin J-H, Farinotti R, Carbon C. Modification of cefixime bioavailability by nifedipine in humans: involvement of the dipeptide carrier system. *Antimicrob Agents Chemother* (1992) 36, 2462–7.
2. Deslandes A, Camus F, Lacroix C, Carbon C, Farinotti R. Effects of nifedipine and diltiazem on pharmacokinetics of cefpodoxime following its oral administration. *Antimicrob Agents Chemother* (1996) 40, 2879–81.

Cephalosporins + Colestyramine

Colestyramine binds with cefadroxil and cefalexin in the gut, which delays their absorption.

Clinical evidence

In 4 subjects, the peak serum levels of a 500-mg oral dose of **cefadroxil** were reduced and delayed when it was taken with 10 g of colestyramine, but the total amount absorbed was not affected.[1] Similar results were found in a study involving **cefalexin** and colestyramine.[2]

Mechanism

Colestyramine is an ion-exchange resin, which binds with these two cephalosporins in the gut. This prevents the early and rapid absorption of the antibacterial, but as the colestyramine/cephalosporin complex passes along the gastrointestinal tract, the antibacterial is progressively released and eventually virtually all of it becomes available for absorption.[1]

Importance and management

Direct information seems to be limited to the studies cited. The clinical significance is uncertain, but as the total amount of antibacterial absorbed is not reduced this interaction is probably of little importance. Information about other cephalosporins seems to be lacking.

1. Marino EL, Vicente MT and Dominguez-Gil A. Influence of cholestyramine on the pharmacokinetic parameters of cefadroxil after simultaneous administration. *Int J Pharmaceutics* (1983) 16, 23–30.
2. Parsons RL, Paddock GM. Absorption of two antibacterial drugs, cephalexin and co-trimoxazole, in malabsorption syndromes. *J Antimicrob Chemother* (1975) 1 (Suppl), 59–67.

Cephalosporins + Food

The bioavailabilities of cefadroxil, cefalexin, cefdinir, cefixime, cefprozil, and cefradine are not affected by food. Cefaclor may be given without regard to food but absorption of an extended-release preparation may be increased by food. The bioavailabilities of cefetamet pivoxil and cefuroxime axetil may be increased by food.

Clinical evidence, mechanism, importance and management

(a) Cefaclor

A study in 18 healthy subjects, the bioavailability and AUC of a single 250-mg capsule of cefaclor was unchanged when it was given after an overnight fast or within 30 minutes of different meals. The rate of absorption and its maximum plasma levels were decreased: a low-fat vegetarian diet produced the smallest decrease in maximum plasma levels (26%) and a high-fat non-vegetarian diet produced the largest decrease (47%), when compared with the levels achieved after an overnight fast. However, therapeutic efficacy (measured by time levels were above MIC_{50}) was not significantly altered.[1] In a further study, healthy subjects were given a single 500-mg dose of cefaclor as an extended-release tablet. The rate of absorption was decreased by food but compared with the fasting state, the maximum levels were increased; by 52% for rice-based diets, by 33% for low-fat-vegetarian food, by 29% for high-fat non-vegetarian food, by 13% for high-fat-vegetarian food, and by 7% for low-fat non-vegetarian food. Compared with the fasting state, all the diets increased the time above MIC_{90}, with a significant increase of almost 42% with low-fat vegetarian (wheat-based) food.[2] The manufacturer of immediate-release cefaclor capsules states that total absorption is the same whether the drug is given with or without food,[3] but for the extended-release preparation, as absorption is enhanced by food, the manufacturer recommends that this preparation should be taken with meals.[4]

(b) Cefadroxil

The manufacturers of cefadroxil state that the bioavailability of cefadroxil is unaffected by food so it may be taken either with meals or on an empty stomach.[5]

(c) Cefalexin

The manufacturers of cefalexin state that it is acid stable and may be given without regard to meals.[6]

(d) Cefdinir

In 6 healthy subjects, the pharmacokinetics of a single 100-mg dose of cefdinir were unaltered by a normal-protein diet, a high-protein diet, or a normal-protein diet supplemented with L-phenylalanine 7.5 g/day for 12 days.[7]

(e) Cefetamet pivoxil

A study found that the bioavailability of cefetamet pivoxil was up to 25% higher when it was given 10 minutes after a standard breakfast rather than in the fasting state.[8,9] In another study, healthy subjects were given oral cefetamet pivoxil hydrochloride 1 g (equivalent to 693 mg of cefetamet free acid) either: 1 hour before food with 200 mL of water; with a standard breakfast and a cup of tea or coffee; or one hour after breakfast with 200 mL of water. The cefetamet maximum plasma levels were 5.5 micrograms/mL, 5.47 micrograms/mL and 6.57 micrograms/mL, respectively, and the AUCs, compared to the fasting state were decreased by 6% when taken with breakfast and increased by 13% when taken one hour after breakfast. The time to reach maximum plasma levels was increased from 3.3 hours when given before food to 4.3 hours when given with food, and to 4.1 hours when given one hour after food.[10] It was thought possible that the amount of fluid taken with cefetamet may have affected absorption, but a study in which cefetamet 1 g was given under fasting conditions with either 250 or 450 mL of water found that increasing fluid intake did not affect absorption. Further, the absorption when taken with food, with or without 200 mL of water was similar. These changes are modest. Nevertheless, the authors recommended that cefetamet pivoxil should be taken within an hour of a meal to improve absorption. The delay in absorption was not considered to be of significance.[10]

(f) Cefixime

A study in healthy subjects given a single 400-mg dose of cefixime, either in the fasting state or immediately after a standard breakfast found that the time to peak serum levels was increased from about 3.8 hours to 4.8 hours when cefixime was given with food, probably because of delayed gastric emptying. The cefixime serum levels, AUC and 24-hour urinary recovery were similar for fasted and fed states.[11] Cefixime may be given without regard to meals.[11,12]

(g) Cefpodoxime proxetil

In a study in healthy subjects, cefpodoxime proxetil 400 mg tablets were given with 180 mL of water after an overnight fast, or either one hour before, with, or 2 hours after the start of a high-fat meal. Dosing one hour before the meal was similar to dosing in the fasting state. However, when cefpodoxime was taken with, or 2 hours after the meal its peak plasma levels were increased by about 45% and 46%, respectively, when compared with the peak levels achieved in the fasting state. The AUC was also increased, by 40%. The rate of cefpodoxime absorption was not greatly affected by food.[13] Studies with a 200-mg dose of cefpodoxime have also found that food increases the extent, but not the rate, of cefpodoxime absorption.[14] However, the extent of the food effect appears to be greater with the 400 mg dose. This is possibly because the bioavailability of the 400-mg tablets is less than that of the 200-mg tablets, so food may have a greater effect on the higher strength preparation.[13] In another study by the same authors the AUC and urinary excretion of cefpodoxime proxetil 200 mg given as a suspension were higher (11% and 14%, respectively) when taken with a high-fat meal rather than in the fasting state. Maximum plasma levels were not affected by a high-fat meal but the time to achieve maximum levels was prolonged.[15]

The manufacturers state that the bioavailability of cefpodoxime proxetil 100 mg tablets and suspension is increased by food.[16,17] The studies[13-15] suggest the increased bioavailability of the tablets, but possibly not that of the suspension, when given with food may be clinically significant.

(h) Cefprozil

A study in healthy subjects found that, although food caused slight changes in the rate of absorption of a 1-g dose of cefprozil its pharmacokinetics (including total absorption) were not significantly affected.[18]

(i) Cefradine

A study in healthy subjects given cefradine 500 mg in the fasting state or immediately after a meal found the time to peak levels was increased from 0.8 hours to 2 hours by food. Peak serum levels of cefradine were reduced by 45% when it was given after food. However, the half-life and AUC were not affected.[19] The manufacturer states that cefradine may be given without regard to meals.[20]

(j) Cefuroxime axetil

A study in healthy subjects given cefuroxime axetil 500 mg intravenously or oral doses of 125 mg to 1 g with or without food found that 36% and 52% of a 500-mg oral dose was absorbed in the fasting and fed states respectively.[21] In another study in healthy subjects, a single 1-g dose of cefuroxime axetil was given 2 hours before or 35 minutes after a standard cooked breakfast. The bioavailability of cefuroxime was markedly enhanced by food.[22] The manufacturer notes that optimum absorption of cefuroxime axetil occurs when it is given after a meal.[23] This is probably because of delayed gastric emptying and transit which allowed more complete dissolution and absorption.[22]

1. Karim S, Ahmed T, Monif T, Saha N, Sharma PL. The effect of four different types of food on the bioavailability of cefaclor. *Eur J Drug Metab Pharmacokinet* (2003), 28, 185–90.
2. Khan BAH, Ahmed T, Karim S, Monif T, Saha N. Comparative effect of different types of food on the bioavailability of cefaclor extended release tablet. *Eur J Drug Metab Pharmacokinet* (2004) 29, 125–32.
3. Distaclor (Cefaclor monohydrate). Flynn Pharma Ltd. UK Summary of product characteristics, November 2005.
4. Distaclor MR (Cefaclor monohydrate). Flynn Pharma Ltd. UK Summary of product characteristics, December 2006.
5. Baxan (Cefadroxil monohydrate). Bristol-Myers Pharmaceuticals. UK Summary of product characteristics, July 2005.
6. Keflex (Cefalexin monohydrate). Flynn Pharma Ltd. UK Summary of product characteristics, September 2005.
7. Fujita T, Nakamura K, Yamazaki A, Ozaki M, Sahashi K, Shichijo K, Nomura K, Maeda M, Nakamura T, Fujita T, Yokota S, Kuroyama S, Kumagai Y, Majima M, Ohtani Y. Effect of L-phenylalanine supplementation and a high-protein diet on pharmacokinetics of cefdinir in healthy volunteers: an exploratory study. *J Clin Pharm Ther* (2007) 32, 277–85.
8. Blouin RA, Kneer J, Stoeckel K. Pharmacokinetics of intravenous cefetamet (Ro 15-8074) and oral cefetamet pivoxil (R0-8075) in young and elderly subjects. *Antimicrob Agents Chemother* (1989) 33, 291–6.
9. Koup JR, Dubach UC, Brandt R, Wyss R, Stoeckel K. Pharmacokinetics of cefetamet (Ro 15-8074) and cefetamet pivoxil (Ro 15-8075) after intravenous and oral doses in humans. *Antimicrob Agents Chemother* (1988) 32, 573–9.
10. Tam YK, Kneer J, Dubach UC, Stoeckel K. Effects of timing of food and fluid volume on cefetamet pivoxil absorption in healthy normal volunteers. *Antimicrob Agents Chemother* (1990) 34, 1556–9.
11. Faulkner RD, Bohaychuk W, Haynes JD, Desjardins RE, Yacobi A, Silber BM. The pharmacokinetics of cefixime in the fasted and fed state. *Eur J Clin Pharmacol* (1988) 34, 525–8.
12. Suprax Tablets (Cefixime). Sanofi-Aventis. UK Summary of product characteristics, July 2008.
13. Borin MT, Driver MR, Forbes KK. Effect of timing of food on absorption of cefpodoxime proxetil. *J Clin Pharmacol* (1995) 35, 505–9.
14. Hughes GS, Heald DL, Barker KB, Patel RK, Spillers CR, Watts KC, Batts DH, Euler AR. The effects of gastric pH and food on the pharmacokinetics of a new oral cephalosporin, cefpodoxime proxetil. *Clin Pharmacol Ther* (1989) 46, 674–85.
15. Borin MT, Forbes KK. Effect of food on absorption of cefpodoxime proxetil oral suspension in adults. *Antimicrob Agents Chemother* (1995) 39, 273–5.
16. Orelox Tablets (Cefpodoxime proxetil). Sanofi-Aventis. UK Summary of product characteristics, December 2006.
17. Orelox Paediatric Granules for Oral Suspension (Cefpodoxime proxetil). Sanofi-Aventis. UK Summary of product characteristics, December 2006.
18. Shukla UA, Pittman KA, Barbhaiya RH. Pharmacokinetic interactions of cefprozil with food, propantheline, metoclopramide, and probenecid in healthy volunteers. *J Clin Pharmacol* (1992) 32, 725–31.
19. Mischler TW, Sugerman AA, Willard DA, Brannick LJ, Neiss ES. Influence of probenecid and food on the bioavailability of cephradine in normal male subjects. *J Clin Pharmacol* (1974) 14, 604–11.
20. Velosef (Cefradine). ER Squibb & Sons Ltd. UK Summary of product characteristics, June 2005.
21. Finn A, Straughn A, Meyer M, Chubb J. Effect of dose and food on the bioavailability of cefuroxime axetil. *Biopharm Drug Dispos* (1987) 8, 519–26.
22. Sommers DK, Van Wyk M, Moncrieff J, Schoeman HS. Influence of food and reduced gastric acidity on the bioavailability of bacampicillin and cefuroxime axetil. *Br J Clin Pharmacol* (1984) 18, 535–9.
23. Zinnat Tablets (Cefuroxime axetil). GlaxoSmithKline UK. UK Summary of product characteristics, July 2008.

Cephalosporins + H_2-receptor antagonists

Ranitidine and famotidine reduce the bioavailability of cefpodoxime proxetil. Ranitidine with sodium bicarbonate reduces the bioavailability of cefuroxime axetil. No clinically significant pharmacokinetic interactions appear to occur between cefaclor AF and cimetidine, or between cefetamet pivoxil, cefalexin or ceftibuten and ranitidine.

Clinical evidence

(a) Cefaclor

A study using cefaclor AF (a formulation with a slow rate of release) found that **cimetidine** 800 mg taken the previous night reduced its maximum plasma concentration by 12%.[1]

(b) Cefalexin

Ranitidine 150 mg for 3 doses had only small and therapeutically unimportant effects on the pharmacokinetics of cefalexin 1 g.[2] In another study in healthy subjects, **ranitidine** 150 mg for 3 doses prolonged the time to attain peak serum levels of a single 500-mg dose of cefalexin from 1.19 hours to 1.48 hours. Other pharmacokinetic parameters were not significantly affected. Similar results were found when **omeprazole** was given instead of ranitidine.[3]

(c) Cefetamet pivoxil

In 18 healthy subjects, **ranitidine** 150 mg twice daily for 4 days did not affect the pharmacokinetics of cefetamet pivoxil 1 g given after breakfast.[4]

(d) Cefpodoxime proxetil

A study in 10 healthy fasted subjects found that **famotidine** 40 mg reduced the bioavailability of cefpodoxime proxetil by about 40%.[5] This confirms the findings of a previous study with **ranitidine**.[6]

(e) Ceftibuten

In 18 healthy subjects **ranitidine** 150 mg every 12 hours for 3 days raised the maximum plasma levels and AUC of ceftibuten by 23% and 16%, respectively. However these values lie within the normal ranges seen in healthy subjects.[7]

(f) Cefuroxime axetil

Ranitidine 300 mg with sodium bicarbonate 4 g reduced the AUC of cefuroxime axetil 1 g by 43% when the combination was given to fasted subjects. However, when cefuroxime was given after food, its bioavailability was higher, and minimally affected by **ranitidine** plus sodium bicarbonate (10% reduction in AUC).[8]

Mechanism

The reduction in the bioavailability of some of the cephalosporins is thought to be due to reduced dissolution at increased gastric pH values.[5]

Importance and management

In most cases the interactions between the cephalosporins and H_2-receptor antagonists are not clinically significant. The clinical importance of the interaction with cefpodoxime has not been studied, but the manufacturer recommends that cefpodoxime is given at least 2 hours before H_2-receptor antagonists.[9] As it is thought that a change in gastric pH is responsible for this interaction it would seem likely that **proton pump inhibitors** will interact similarly.

As long as cefuroxime is taken with food (as is recommended[10]), any interaction is minimal. The bioavailability of cefetamet pivoxil,[4] and cefpodoxime proxetil,[5,6] are also enhanced by food so it is probable that any interaction with drugs that raise gastric pH may be similarly minimised.

1. Satterwhite JH, Cerimele BJ, Coleman DL, Hatcher BL, Kisicki J, DeSante KA. Pharmacokinetics of cefaclor AF: effects of age, antacids and H_2-receptor antagonists. *Postgrad Med J* (1992) 68 (Suppl 3), S3–S9.
2. Deppermann K-M, Lode H, Höffken G, Tschink G, Kalz C, Koeppe P. Influence of ranitidine, pirenzepine, and aluminum magnesium hydroxide on the bioavailability of various antibiotics, including amoxicillin, cephalexin, doxycycline and amoxicillin-clavulanic acid. *Antimicrob Agents Chemother* (1989) 33, 1901–1907.
3. Madaras-Kelly K, Michas P, George M, May MP, Adejare A. A randomized crossover study investigating the influence of ranitidine or omeprazole on the pharmacokinetics of cephalexin monohydrate. *J Clin Pharmacol* (2004) 44, 1391–7.

4. Blouin RA, Kneer J, Ambros RJ, Stoeckel K. Influence of antacid and ranitidine on the pharmacokinetics of oral cefetamet pivoxil. *Antimicrob Agents Chemother* (1990) 34, 1744–8.
5. Saathoff N, Lode H, Neider K, Depperman KM, Borner K, Koeppe P. Pharmacokinetics of cefpodoxime proxetil and interactions with an antacid and an H_2 receptor antagonist. *Antimicrob Agents Chemother* (1992) 36, 796–800.
6. Hughes GS, Heald DL, Barker KB, Patel RK, Spillers CR, Watts KC, Batts DH, Euler AR. The effects of gastric pH and food on the pharmacokinetics of a new oral cephalosporin, cefpodoxime proxetil. *Clin Pharmacol Ther* (1989) 46, 674–85.
7. Radwanski E, Nomeir A, Cutler D, Affrime M, Lin C-C. Pharmacokinetic drug interaction study: administration of ceftibuten concurrently with the antacid Mylanta double-strength liquid or with ranitidine. *Am J Ther* (1998) 5, 67–72.
8. Sommers De K, Van Wyk M, Moncrieff J, Schoeman HS. Influence of food and reduced gastric acidity on the bioavailability of bacampicillin and cefuroxime axetil. *Br J Clin Pharmacol* (1984) 18, 535–9.
9. Orelox Tablets (Cefpodoxime proxetil). Sanofi-Aventis. UK Summary of product characteristics, December 2006.
10. Zinnat Tablets (Cefuroxime axetil). GlaxoSmithKline UK. UK Summary of product characteristics, July 2008.

Cephalosporins + Loop diuretics

The nephrotoxic effects of cefaloridine and possibly cefalotin or cefacetrile appear to be increased by furosemide. Cefradine brain levels are reduced by furosemide. No important interactions appear to occur between furosemide and cefoxitin, ceftazidime, ceftriaxone, or cefuroxime.

Clinical evidence

(a) Nephrotoxicity

Nine out of 36 patients who developed acute renal failure while taking **cefaloridine** had also been taking a diuretic: furosemide was used in 7 cases. Other factors such as patient age and drug dose may also have been involved. The authors of this report related their observations to previous *animal* studies, which showed that potent diuretics such as furosemide and etacrynic acid enhanced the incidence and extent of tubular necrosis.[1] Several other reports describe nephrotoxicity in patients given both **cefaloridine** and furosemide.[2-4] There is a possibility that this effect also occurs with **cefalotin** and **cefacetrile** because *animal* studies found an increase in nephrotoxicity,[5,6] and there is a single report describing nephrotoxicity in one patient taking **cefalotin** with furosemide.[2] **Cefoxitin** seems to be relatively free of nephrotoxicity alone or with furosemide.[7]

(b) Changes in serum levels and clearance

A clinical study[8] found that furosemide 80 mg increased the serum half-life of **cefaloridine** by 25%, and in another study **cefaloridine** clearance was reduced by furosemide.[9] A further study found that brain concentrations of **cefradine** are markedly reduced by furosemide.[10] In a study in 6 healthy subjects, furosemide 40 mg, given one hour before a 1-g intramuscular dose of **ceftazidime**, raised the serum **ceftazidime** levels by about 20 to 40% over 8 hours and increased its AUC by 28%. Furosemide given 3 hours before **ceftazidime** had much smaller effects.[11] The serum half-lives of intravenous **cefoxitin** and **cefuroxime** were not affected by oral furosemide.[12] **Ceftriaxone** does not appear to interfere with the diuretic effects of furosemide.[13]

Mechanism

Cefaloridine is nephrotoxic, but why this should be increased by furosemide is not understood. It may possibly be related to a reduction in its clearance.[9]

Importance and management

The interaction between cefaloridine and furosemide is not well-established, but there is enough evidence to suggest that concurrent use should be undertaken with care. Age and/or renal impairment may possibly be predisposing factors. Renal function should be checked frequently if both drugs are given. A pharmacokinetic study suggests that the development of this adverse interaction may possibly depend on the time relationship of drug use, and it has been recommended that furosemide should be avoided for 3 or 4 hours before the cefaloridine.[14] There seems to be no evidence about other loop diuretics, but it seems possible that they will interact similarly.

Although the interaction between ceftazidime and furosemide does not appear to be clinically important, the UK manufacturer of ceftazidime states that the concurrent use of high doses of cephalosporins with other nephrotoxic drugs might adversely affect renal function.[15] The rest of the information about other cephalosporins and furosemide is fairly sparse. Most appear not to interact adversely, with a few possible exceptions, namely cefalotin (nephrotoxicity in a single case[2] and *animal* studies[5]) and cefacetrile (nephrotoxicity in *animal* studies[6]). Care is clearly prudent with these two cephalosporins.

1. Dodds MG, Foord RD. Enhancement by potent diuretics of renal tubular necrosis induced by cephaloridine. *Br J Pharmacol* (1970) 4, 227–36.
2. Simpson IJ. Nephrotoxicity and acute renal failure associated with cephalothin and cephaloridine. *N Z Med J* (1971) 74, 312–15.
3. Kleinknecht D, Jungers P, Fillastre J-P. Nephrotoxicity of cephaloridine. *Ann Intern Med* (1974) 80, 421–2.
4. Lawson DH, Macadam RF, Singh H, Gavras H, Linton AL. The nephrotoxicity of cephaloridine. *Postgrad Med J* (1970) 46 (Suppl), 36–9.
5. Lawson DH, Macadam RF, Singh H, Gavras H, Hartz S, Turnbull D, Linton AL. Effect of furosemide on antibiotic-induced renal damage in rats. *J Infect Dis* (1972) 126, 593–600.
6. Luscombe DK, Nichols PJ. Possible interaction between cephacetrile and frusemide in rabbits and rats. *J Antimicrob Chemother* (1975) 1, 67–77.
7. Trollfors B, Norrby R, Kristianson K, Nilsson NJ. Effects on renal function of treatment with cefoxitin alone or in combination with furosemide. *Scand J Infect Dis* (1978) (Suppl), 13, 73–7.
8. Norrby R, Stenqvist K, Elgefors B. Interaction between cephaloridine and furosemide in man. *Scand J Infect Dis* (1976) 8, 209–212.
9. Tilstone WJ, Semple PF, Lawson DH, Boyle JA. Effects of furosemide on glomerular filtration rate and clearance of practolol, digoxin, cephaloridine and gentamicin. *Clin Pharmacol Ther* (1977) 22, 389–94.
10. Adam D, Jacoby W, Raff WK. Beeinflussung der Antibiotika-Konzentration im Gewebe durch ein Saluretikum. *Klin Wochenschr* (1978) 56, 247–51.
11. Chrysos G, Gargalianos P, Lelekis M, Stefanou J, Kosmidis J. Pharmacokinetic interactions of ceftazidime and frusemide. *J Chemother* (1995) 7 (Suppl 4), 107–10.
12. Trollfors B, Norrby R. Effect of frusemide on the elimination of cefuroxime and cefoxitin. *J Antimicrob Chemother* (1989) 6, 405–7.
13. Korn A, Eichler HG, Gasic S. A drug interaction study of ceftriaxone and frusemide in healthy volunteers. *Int J Clin Pharmacol Ther Toxicol* (1986) 24, 262–4.
14. Kosmidis J, Polyzos A, Daikos GK. Pharmacokinetic interactions between cephalosporins and furosemide are influenced by administration time relationships. 11th International Congress of Chemotherapy, 1980. 673–5.
15. Fortum Injection (Ceftazidime pentahydrate). GlaxoSmithKline UK. UK Summary of product characteristics, June 2013.

Cephalosporins + Metoclopramide or Propantheline

The pharmacokinetics of cefprozil and cefpodoxime proxetil are minimally affected by propantheline and metoclopramide.

Clinical evidence, mechanism, importance and management

(a) Cefpodoxime

In 12 healthy subjects, the pharmacokinetics of a single 200-mg dose of cefpodoxime proxetil were not significantly altered when it was given 30 minutes after a single dose of metoclopramide 10 mg or propantheline 30 mg.[1]

(b) Cefprozil

A study in 15 healthy subjects who received a single 30-mg dose of metoclopramide or a single 30-mg dose of propantheline 30 minutes before a single 1 g dose of cefprozil, found that the pharmacokinetics of cefprozil were only minimally affected by these drugs.[2]

1. Hughes GS, Heald DL, Patel R, Spillers CR, Batts DH, Euler AR. Gastric emptying and the pharmacokinetics of the cephalosporin antibiotic, cefpodoxime proxetil. *Methods Find Exp Clin Pharmacol* (1990) 12, 197–204.
2. Shukla UA, Pittman KA, Barbhaiya RH. Pharmacokinetic interactions of cefprozil with food, propantheline, metoclopramide, and probenecid in healthy volunteers. *J Clin Pharmacol* (1992) 32, 725–31.

Cephalosporins + NSAIDs

The biliary excretion of ceftriaxone is increased by diclofenac. The clearance of ceftazidime is significantly reduced by indometacin in neonates Cefadroxil does not alter the pharmacokinetics of diclofenac.

Clinical evidence, mechanism, importance and management

(a) Diclofenac

The pharmacokinetics of diclofenac 100 mg daily were unaffected by either **cefadroxil** 2 g daily (8 patients) or doxycycline 100 mg daily (7 patients) for one week.[1] No special precautions are needed while taking either of these drugs and diclofenac.

A pharmacokinetic study in 8 patients who had undergone cholecystectomy and who had a T-drain in the common bile duct, found that diclofenac 50 mg every 12 hours increased the excretion of intravenous **ceftriaxone** 2 g in the bile by about fourfold and roughly halved the urinary excretion.[2] The clinical importance of this is uncertain, but probably small.

(b) Indometacin

A study found that the prenatal use of indometacin reduced the clearance of **ceftazidime** 25 mg/kg by 18% in 12 premature neonates (born at about 29 weeks) who were 10 days old. Further, in similar neonates who had not received indometacin, the clearance of **ceftazidime** increased over the first 10 days of life, but this was not seen when indometacin had been given.[3] A further study by the same authors intended to establish an appropriate dose of **ceftazidime** for premature neonates. This study found that in 25 subjects who had received indometacin prenatally, the clearance of **ceftazidime** was reduced by 31% and therefore the authors suggest that additional dose reductions are required. However, note that the effect of indometacin was cancelled out in neonates who had also received betamethasone prenatally.[4] *Animal* studies have shown that indometacin reduces **ceftazidime** excretion by decreasing its glomerular filtered load.[5]

The dose of **ceftazidime** in preterm infants in the first week of life is normally based on chronological age and glomerular filtration rate, although some have suggested that the gestational age should be taken into account.[4] Additional dose adjustments are recommended in preterm infants who are also given indometacin.[3,4]

1. Schumacher A, Geissler HE, Mutschler E, Osterburg M. Untersuchungen potentieller Interaktionen von Diclofenac-Natrium (Voltaren) mit Antibiotika. *Z Rheumatol* (1983) 42, 25–7.
2. Merle-Melet M, Bresler L, Lokiec F, Dopff C, Boissel P, Dureux JB. Effects of diclofenac on ceftriaxone pharmacokinetics in humans. *Antimicrob Agents Chemother* (1992) 36, 2331–3.
3. van den Anker JN, Hop WCJ, Schoemaker RC, Van der Heijden BJ, Neijens HJ, De Groot R. Ceftazidime pharmacokinetics in preterm infants: effect of postnatal age and postnatal exposure to indomethacin. *Br J Clin Pharmacol* (1995) 40, 439–43.
4. van den Anker JN, Schoemaker RC, Hop WCJ, van der Heijden BJ, Weber A, Sauer PJJ, Neijens HJ, de Groot R. Ceftazidime pharmacokinetics in preterm infants: effects of renal function and gestational age. *Clin Pharmacol Ther* (1995) 58, 650–9.
5. Carbon C, Dromer F, Brion N, Cremieux A-C, Contrepois A. Renal disposition of ceftazidime illustrated by interferences by probenecid, furosemide and indomethacin in rabbits. *Antimicrob Agents Chemother* (1984) 26, 373–7.

Cephalosporins + Probenecid

The serum levels of many cephalosporins are raised by probenecid. Possible exceptions include ceforanide, ceftazidime, ceftriaxone and latamoxef. The rise in serum levels may possibly increase the risk of nephrotoxicity with some cephalosporins such as cefaloridine and cefalotin.

Clinical evidence

Ten healthy subjects given a single 500-mg oral dose of **cefradine** or **cefaclor** developed markedly raised serum antibacterial concentrations when they were also given probenecid (500 mg doses taken 25, 13 and 2 hours before the antibacterial). Peak serum levels of the antibacterial were very roughly doubled.[1] Similar results were obtained in another study in healthy subjects given **cefradine** orally or intramuscularly.[2]

Although some cephalosporins do not appear to interact with probenecid, in general, most have their clearance reduced, their serum levels raised and sometimes their half-lives prolonged by probenecid, see 'Table 10.2', p.312.

Mechanism

Probenecid inhibits the excretion of most cephalosporins by the renal tubules by successfully competing for the excretory mechanisms. A fuller explanation of this mechanism is set out in 'Drug excretion interactions', p.11. Thus the cephalosporin is retained in the body and its serum levels rise. The extent of the rise cannot always be fully accounted for by this mechanism alone and it is suggested that some change in tissue distribution may sometimes have a part to play.[1]

Importance and management

An extremely well-documented interaction. The serum levels of many (but not all) cephalosporins will be higher if probenecid is given, but no special precautions are normally needed. The interaction has been used clinically; however, elevated serum levels of some cephalosporins, in particular cefaloridine and cefalotin, might possibly increase the risk of nephrotoxicity.

1. Welling PG, Dean S, Selen A, Kendall MJ, Wise R. Probenecid: an unexplained effect on cephalosporin pharmacology. *Br J Clin Pharmacol* (1979) 8, 491–5.
2. Mischler TW, Sugerman AA, Willard DA, Brannick LJ, Neiss ES. Influence of probenecid and food on the bioavailability of cephradine in normal male subjects. *J Clin Pharmacol* (1974) 14, 604–11.

Cephalosporins; Cefaclor + Cranberry juice

Cranberry juice does not appear to affect the pharmacokinetics of cefaclor.

Clinical evidence, mechanism, importance and management

In a study in 18 healthy subjects, 12 oz (about 350 mL) of cranberry juice taken twice daily for 2 days, then taken at the same time as a single 500-mg dose of cefaclor on day 3, had no effect on the pharmacokinetics of cefaclor. In this study, the cranberry juice used was *Ocean Spray* cranberry juice cocktail from concentrate containing 27% cranberry juice.[1]

Although the evidence is limited to this particular study, there appears to be no need for any special precautions when taking cranberry juice with cefaclor.

1. Li M, Andrew MA, Wang J, Salinger DH, Vicini P, Grady RW, Phillips B, Shen DD, Anderson GD. Effects of cranberry juice on pharmacokinetics of beta-lactam antibiotics following oral administration. *Antimicrob Agents Chemother* (2009) 53, 2725–32.

Cephalosporins; Cefalexin + Pirenzepine

Pirenzepine (50 mg for 4 doses) had only small and therapeutically unimportant effects on the pharmacokinetics of a 1-g dose of cefalexin.[1]

1. Deppermann K-M, Lode H, Höffken G, Tschink G, Kalz C, Koeppe P. Influence of ranitidine, pirenzepine, and aluminum magnesium hydroxide on the bioavailability of various antibiotics, including amoxicillin, cephalexin, doxycycline and amoxicillin-clavulanic acid. *Antimicrob Agents Chemother* (1989) 33, 1901–1907.

Cephalosporins; Cefalexin + Zinc compounds

Zinc sulphate appears to decrease the exposure to cephalexin when given at the same time, but not when it is given 3 hours after cefalexin.

Clinical evidence

In a randomised, crossover study in 12 healthy subjects, when **zinc sulfate** 250 mg (equivalent to 56 mg of elemental zinc) was given at the same time as cefalexin 500 mg, the AUC and plasma concentration of cefalexin were decreased by 27% and 31%, respectively, compared with when cefalexin was given alone. When zinc was given 3 hours before cefalexin, the AUC and plasma concentration of cefalexin were decreased by 18% and 11%, respectively. However, when zinc was given 3 hours after cefalexin, the pharmacokinetics of cefalexin were not notably altered.[1]

Mechanism

Unknown. The authors of the study speculate that zinc might interfere with intestinal drug transporters, or that zinc chelates with cefalexin (in a similar manner to the interactions with quinolones and tetracyclines).

Importance and management

Although evidence for an interaction appears to be limited to the one study, zinc sulphate appears to decrease exposure to cefalexin when given at the same time. The clinical relevance of the modest decrease in exposure to cefalexin is unknown, but it would seem prudent to bear this in mind if a patient is not responding as expected, and to separate the doses of zinc and cefalexin by at least 3 hours where possible. Other zinc compounds might interact similarly.

1. Ding Y, Jia YY, Li F, Liu WX, Lu CT, Zhu YR, Yang J, Ding LK, Yang L, Wen AD. The effect of staggered administration of zinc sulfate on the pharmacokinetics of oral cephalexin. *Br J Clin Pharmacol* (2012) 73, 422–7.

Cephalosporins; Cefalotin + Colistin

Renal failure has been attributed to the concurrent use of cefalotin and colistin.

Clinical evidence, mechanism, importance and management

Four patients developed acute renal failure, which appeared to be reversible, during treatment with colistin. Three were given cefalotin concurrently and the fourth had previously been taking this antibacterial.[1] An increase in renal toxicity associated with the concurrent use of these drugs has been described in another report.[2] The reason for this reaction is not known. What is known suggests that renal function should be closely monitored if these drugs are given concurrently or sequentially.

1. Adler S, Segal DP. Nonoliguric renal failure secondary to sodium colistimethate: a report of four cases. *Am J Med Sci* (1971) 262, 109–14.
2. Koch-Weser J, Sidel VW, Federman EB, Kanarek P, Finer DC, Eaton AE. Adverse effects of sodium colistimethate. Manifestations and specific reaction rates during 317 courses of therapy. *Ann Intern Med* (1970) 72, 857–68.

Cephalosporins; Cefdinir + Iron compounds

Ferrous sulfate markedly reduces the absorption of cefdinir.

Clinical evidence

When 6 healthy subjects were given **ferrous sulfate** (1050 mg of *Fero-Gradumet*, sustained release, equivalent to 210 mg of elemental iron) with cefdinir 200 mg the AUC of cefdinir was reduced by 93%. When **ferrous sulfate** was taken 3 hours after cefdinir, the absorption of cefdinir remained unchanged for 3 hours and then rapidly fell, the total AUC over 12 hours being reduced by 36%.[1] There have been a small number of reported cases of maroon or red stools in children who have taken cefdinir with iron supplements.[2,3] One of these cases occurred in a child who was receiving an iron-containing infant formula.[3]

Mechanism

It is believed that iron compounds chelate with cefdinir in the gut to produce a poorly absorbed complex, which may discolour the stools.

Importance and management

An established interaction of clinical importance. Avoid ferrous sulfate and other iron compounds while taking cefdinir. The manufacturer advises separating the administration of cefdinir and iron preparations by at least 2 hours, but notes that although iron-containing vitamin supplements may interact, iron-fortified infant formula may be taken with cefdinir.[4] Parents should be advised about the potential discoloration of the stools. There is no information to suggest that other cephalosporins interact in this way.

1. Ueno K, Tanaka K, Tsujimura K, Morishima Y, Iwashige H, Yamazaki K, Nakata I. Impairment of cefdinir absorption by iron ion. *Clin Pharmacol Ther* (1993) 54, 473–5.
2. Graves R, Weaver SP. Cefdinir-associated "bloody stools" in an infant. *J Am Board Fam Med* (2008) 21, 246–8.
3. Lancaster J, Sylvia LM, Schainker E. Nonbloody, red stools from coadministration of cefdinir and iron-supplemented infant formulas. *Pharmacotherapy* (2008) 28, 678–81.
4. Omnicef (Cefdinir). Abbott Laboratories. US Prescribing information, July 2007.

Cephalosporins; Cefotaxime + Penicillins

Azlocillin and mezlocillin may reduce the clearance of cefotaxime.

Clinical evidence, mechanism, importance and management

A patient with renal failure developed encephalopathy with focal motor status and generalised convulsions when given cefotaxime 2 g every 8 hours and **azlocillin** 5 g every 8 hours (high-dose).[1] In a study in subjects with either normal or impaired renal function, the clearance of a single dose of cefotaxime was reduced by 40 to 50% by **azlocillin** regardless of renal function.[2]

When 8 healthy subjects were given intravenous cefotaxime 30 mg/kg and **mezlocillin** 50 mg/kg together over 30 minutes the pharmacokinetics of the **mezlocillin**

Table 10.2 Effect of probenecid on the pharmacokinetics of the cephalosporins

Drug	*Route*	*Effect of probenecid*	*Refs*
Cefacetrile	Intramuscular	Mean serum half-life increased from 52 minutes to 90 minutes	1
Cefaclor	Oral	Serum level approximately doubled; renal excretion inhibited; renal excretion after 4 hours reduced by 61%	2,3
Cefadroxil	Oral	Probenecid 500 mg every 8 hours for 5 doses increased the half-life of cefadroxil from 1.13 hours to 1.63 hours and reduced its renal excretion by 58%; probenecid slightly increased and prolonged cefadroxil serum levels	4
Cefalexin	Oral	Reduced clearance	5
Cefaloglycin	Oral	Increased peak serum levels and duration of antibacterial activity	6
Cefaloridine	Intramuscular/Intravenous	Plasma levels increased by 20%. Clearance reduced by 24% (intravenous); increased serum levels; prolonged antibacterial activity (intramuscular)	7,8
Cefalotin	Intravenous	Plasma levels increased by 70%. Clearance reduced by 59%	7
Cefamandole	Intramuscular	Peak serum levels almost doubled; half-life prolonged from 1.1 hours to 2 hours	9
Cefazedone	Intravenous	AUC increased more than threefold; elimination half-life increased from 1.58 hours to 4.44 hours; total clearance reduced by 68%	10
Cefazolin	Intramuscular/Intravenous	At 6 hours serum levels of intramuscular dose doubled; after intravenous dose elimination half-life increased from 1.6 hours to 2.7 hours and mean serum level after 24 hours was increased from 1.1 mg/L to 2 mg/L; therapeutic levels at steady-state maintained by once daily rather than three times daily dose regimen	11-13
Cefditoren	Oral	Increased plasma half-life; decreased excretion and renal clearance	14
Cefmenoxime	Intravenous	Renal clearance of cefmenoxime reduced from 159 mL/minute to 66 mL/minute; AUC almost doubled	15
Cefmetazole	Intravenous	Mean AUC increased by about 58%; clearance reduced by about 36%; half-life increased from 1.5 hours to 2.27 hours	16
Cefonicid	Intramuscular	Probenecid 1 g increased the maximum levels of cefonicid 500 mg by 52%, increased the AUC twofold, increased the half-life from 3.5 hours to 7.5 hours, reduced elimination rates and decreased renal clearance	17
Ceforanide	Intramuscular	No significant effect	18
Cefotaxime	Intramuscular/Intravenous	Oral probenecid 500 mg every 6 hours for 24 hours before, and 1 g 30 minutes before, intravenous cefotaxime 1 g reduced renal clearance by about half and almost doubled its AUC. Delayed excretion and increased plasma levels due to effects on renal tubular transfer. Clearance of cefotaxime and also its metabolites decreased by probenecid	19-21
Cefoxitin	Intramuscular/Intravenous	Serum half-life increased from 39 minutes to 129 minutes and clearance halved (intravenous); greater increase in AUC when probenecid given 1 hour before rather than with cefoxitin (intravenous); increasing dose of probenecid from 1 to 2 g increased AUC of cefoxitin (intramuscular)	21-23
Cefprozil	Oral	Significant increase in half-life and maximum levels, AUC approximately doubled, and clearance decreased by about 60%	24
Cefradine	Oral/Intramuscular	Serum levels approximately doubled. Peak levels delayed (from 1 to 2 hours oral and from 1 to 1.5 hours intramuscular); half-lives prolonged	2,25
Ceftazidime	Intravenous	Probenecid 500 mg every 6 hours for 24 hours before and 1 g immediately before a single intravenous dose of ceftazidime 1 g did not significantly affect ceftazidime clearance. Pharmacokinetics of single 50-mg/kg dose of ceftazidime in patients with cystic fibrosis not affected by pre-treatment with probenecid 2 g	19,26
Ceftizoxime	Intramuscular/Intravenous	AUC increased by 49% (both routes); half-life increased from 1.7 hours to 2.3 hours (intravenous) and 1.9 hours to 2.8 hours (intramuscular)	27
Ceftriaxone	Intravenous	No significant effect	28
Cefuroxime	Intravenous	AUC increased by 44 to 50%; half-life prolonged by 63%; clearance decreased by 29%	29
Latamoxef	Intravenous	Probenecid 500 mg every 6 hours for 24 hours before and 1 g immediately before a single 1-g intravenous dose of latamoxef did not significantly affect latamoxef clearance	19

1. Wise R, Reeves DS. Pharmacological studies on cephacetrile in human volunteers. *Curr Med Res Opin* (1974) 2, 249–55.
2. Welling PG, Dean S, Selen A, Kendall MJ, Wise R. Probenecid: an unexplained effect on cephalosporin pharmacology. *Br J Clin Pharmacol* (1979) 8, 491–5.
3. Santoro J, Agarwal BN, Martinelli R, Wenger N, Levison ME. Pharmacology of cefaclor in normal volunteers and patients with renal failure. *Antimicrob Agents Chemother* (1978) 13, 951–4.
4. Mariño EL, Dominguez-Gil A. The pharmacokinetics of cefadroxil associated with probenecid. *Int J Clin Pharmacol Ther Toxicol* (1981) 19, 506–8.
5. Taylor WA, Holloway WJ. Cephalexin in the treatment of gonorrhea. *Int J Clin Pharmacol Ther Toxicol* (1972) 6, 7–9.
6. Applestein JM, Crosby EB, Johnson WD, Kaye D. In-vitro antimicrobial activity and human pharmacology of cephaloglycin. *Appl Microbiol* (1968) 16, 1006–10.

Continued

Table 10.2 Effect of probenecid on the pharmacokinetics of the cephalosporins (continued)

7. Tuano SB, Brodie JL, Kirby WMM. Cephaloridine versus cephalothin: relation of the kidney to blood level differences after parenteral administration. *Antimicrob Agents Chemother* (1966) 6, 101–6.
8. Kaplan KS, Reisberg BE, Weinstein L. Cephaloridine: antimicrobial activity and pharmacologic behaviour. *Am J Med Sci* (1967) 253, 667–74.
9. Griffith RS, Black HR, Brier GL, Wolny JD. Effect of probenecid on the blood levels and urinary excretion of cefamandole. *Antimicrob Agents Chemother* (1977) 11, 809–12.
10. Ungethüm W, Pabst J, Dingeldein E, Leopold G. Clinical pharmacology phase I of cefazedone, a new cephalosporin, in healthy volunteers; III. Investigations of the mechanism of renal elimination. *Arzneimittelforschung* (1979) 29, 443–8.
11. Duncan WC. Treatment of gonorrhea with cefazolin plus probenecid. *J Infect Dis* (1974) 130, 398–401.
12. Brown G, Zemcov SJV, Clarke AM. Effect of probenecid on cefazolin serum concentrations. *J Antimicrob Chemother* (1993) 31, 1009–1011.
13. Spina SP, Dillon EC. Effect of chronic probenecid therapy on cefazolin serum concentrations. *Ann Pharmacother* (2003) 37, 621–4.
14. Mayer M, Mulford D, Witt G. Effect of probenecid on the pharmacokinetics of cefditoren. 41st Annual Meeting of the Interscience Conference on Antimicrobial Agents and Chemotherapy, Chicago, Illinois. (2001) 41, Abstract 23.
15. Sennello LT, Quinn D, Rollins DE, Tolman KG, Sonders RC. Effect of probenecid on the pharmacokinetics of cefmenoxime. *Antimicrob Agents Chemother* (1983) 23, 803–7.
16. Ko H, Cathcart KS, Griffith DL, Peters GR, Adams WJ. Pharmacokinetics of intravenously administered cefmetazole and cefoxitin and effects of probenecid on cefmetazole elimination. *Antimicrob Agents Chemother* (1989) 33, 356–61.
17. Pitkin D, Dubb J, Actor P, Alexander F, Ehrlich S, Familiar R, Stote R. Kinetics and renal handling of cefonicid. *Clin Pharmacol Ther* (1981) 30, 587–93.
18. Jovanovich JF, Saravolatz LD, Burch K, Pohlod DJ. Failure of probenecid to alter the pharmacokinetics of ceforanide. *Antimicrob Agents Chemother* (1981) 20, 530–2.
19. Lüthy R, Blaser J, Bonetti A, Simmen H, Wise R, Siegenthaler W. Comparative multiple-dose pharmacokinetics of cefotaxime, moxalactam, and ceftazidime. *Antimicrob Agents Chemother* (1981) 20, 567–75.
20. Ings RMJ, Reeves DS, White LO, Bax RP, Bywater MJ, Holt HA. The human pharmacokinetics of cefotaxime and its metabolites and the role of renal tubular secretion on their elimination. *J Pharmacokinet Biopharm* (1985) 13, 121–42.
21. Bint AJ, Reeves DS, Holt HA. Effect of probenecid on serum cefoxitin concentrations. *J Antimicrob Chemother* (1977) 3, 627–8.
22. Reeves DS, Bullock DW, Bywater MJ, Holt HA, White LO, Thornhill DP. The effect of probenecid on the pharmacokinetics and distribution of cefoxitin in healthy volunteers. *Br J Clin Pharmacol* (1981) 11, 353–9.
23. Vlasses PH, Holbrook AM, Schrogie JJ, Rogers JD, Ferguson RK, Abrams WB. Effect of orally administered probenecid on the pharmacokinetics of cefoxitin. *Antimicrob Agents Chemother* (1980) 17, 847–55.
24. Shukla UA, Pittman KA, Barbhaiya RH. Pharmacokinetic interactions of cefprozil with food, propantheline, metoclopramide, and probenecid in healthy volunteers. *J Clin Pharmacol* (1992) 32, 725–31.
25. Mischler TW, Sugerman AA, Willard DA, Brannick LJ, Neiss ES. Influence of probenecid and food on the bioavailability of cephradine in normal male subjects. *J Clin Pharmacol* (1974) 14, 604–11.
26. Kercsmar CM, Stern RC, Reed MD, Myers CM, Murdell D, Blumer JL. Ceftazidime in cystic fibrosis: pharmacokinetics and therapeutic response. *J Antimicrob Chemother* (1983) 12 (Suppl. A) 289–95.
27. LeBel M, Paone RP, Lewis GP. Effect of probenecid on the pharmacokinetics of ceftizoxime. *J Antimicrob Chemother* (1983) 12, 147–55.
28. Stoeckel K, Trueb V, Dubach UC, McNamara PJ. Effect of probenecid on the elimination and protein binding of ceftriaxone. *Eur J Clin Pharmacol* (1988) 34, 151–6.
29. Garton AM, Rennie RP, Gilpin J, Marrelli M, Shafran SD. Comparison of dose doubling with probenecid for sustaining serum cefuroxime levels. *J Antimicrob Chemother* (1997) 40, 903–6.

were unchanged but the clearance of the cefotaxime was reduced by about 40%. However, in a series of 5 patients with end-stage renal disease no significant decrease in cefotaxime clearance was seen when **mezlocillin** was given.[3]

Doses of cefotaxime may need to be reduced in the presence of either **azlocillin** or **mezlocillin**. One report suggests a dose reduction of cefotaxime is advisable if the glomerular filtration rate is 20 to 40 mL/minute and **azlocillin** is also given.[2]

There seems to be no information about other penicillins.

1. Wroe SJ, Ellershaw JE, Whittaker JA, Richens A. Focal motor status epilepticus following treatment with azlocillin and cefotaxime. *Med Toxicol* (1987) 2, 233–4.
2. Kampf D, Borner K, Möller M, Kessel M. Kinetic interactions between azlocillin, cefotaxime, and cefotaxime metabolites in normal and impaired renal function. *Clin Pharmacol Ther* (1984) 35, 214–20.
3. Rodondi LC, Flaherty JF, Schoenfeld P, Barriere SL, Gambertoglio JG. Influence of coadministration on the pharmacokinetics of mezlocillin and cefotaxime in healthy volunteers and in patients with renal failure. *Clin Pharmacol Ther* (1989) 45, 527–34.

Cephalosporins; Cefotaxime + Phenobarbital

A 30-month study noted a very marked increase in drug-induced reactions in children in intensive care who were given high-dose phenobarbital and beta-lactam antibacterials (mainly cefotaxime). Twenty-four out of 49 children developed drug-induced reactions, which were mainly exanthematous skin reactions.[1] The reasons for this reaction are not known. It would seem prudent to consider this interaction in patients who develop skin reactions while taking both drugs.

1. Harder S, Schneider W, Bae ZU, Bock U, Zielen S. Unerwünschte Arzneimittelreaktionen bei gleichzeitiger Gabe von hochdosiertem Phenobarbital und Betalaktam-Antibiotika. *Klin Padiatr* (1990) 202, 404–7.

Cephalosporins; Ceftobiprole + Miscellaneous

Ceftobiprole is predicted to increase the exposure to some statins and glibenclamide.

Clinical evidence, mechanism, importance and management

(a) Glibenclamide (Glyburide)

The UK manufacturer of ceftobiprole states that *in vitro* studies indicated that ceftobiprole inhibits the organic anion transporting polypeptide, OATP1B1,[1] which is involved in the hepatic uptake of glibenclamide. They therefore predict that ceftobiprole might increase the exposure to glibenclamide.[1] However note that *in vitro* inhibitory activity does not always translate into a clinically relevant effect *in vivo*.

(b) Statins

The UK manufacturer of ceftobiprole states that in-vitro studies indicated that ceftobiprole inhibits the organic anion transporting polypeptides, OATP1B1 and OATP1B3,[1] which are involved in the hepatic uptake of statins. They therefore predict that ceftobiprole might increase the exposure to **pitavastatin**, **pravastatin**, and **rosuvastatin**.[1] However note that *in vitro* inhibitory activity does not always translate into a clinically relevant effect *in vivo*.

1. Zevtera (Ceftobiprole). Basilea Pharmaceutica. UK Summary of product characteristics, November 2013.

Cephalosporins; Ceftriaxone + Calcium compounds

Cases of cardio-respiratory arrest have been reported in neonates given intravenous ceftriaxone and calcium-containing fluids. Limited data suggests that adults given intravenous calcium chloride and intravenous ceftriaxone do not appear to have an increased risk of adverse effects.

Clinical evidence

(a) Adults

A retrospective cohort-study of patients undergoing continuous renal replacement therapy from January 2003 to December 2008 identified 142 patients given a continuous infusion of intravenous calcium chloride 8 mg/mL on the same day as receiving intravenous ceftriaxone. No statistically significant increase in the risk of adverse outcomes (such as respiratory events or hospital mortality) was found on concurrent use, when compared with patients not given ceftriaxone. However, the authors noted that the study was limited by low numbers of patients.[1]

(b) Neonates

In an analysis of post-marketing reports submitted to the FDA in the US between 1984 and 2007, cardio-respiratory arrest occurred in 7 neonates (3 weeks of age or younger, some of whom were pre-term) given ceftriaxone and calcium-containing fluids: 6 of these neonates died. A white crystalline precipitate was found in the renal, pulmonary and/or hepatic vasculature of 3 of these cases on autopsy. In all cases, ceftriaxone was given intravenously: one patient was given a bolus injection of 50 mg/kg over 2 minutes, while some were given high-dose intravenous infusions (doses ranging from 80 to 200 mg/kg/day). Calcium was given as intravenous calcium gluconate (either through the same line, through a Y-set, or in one case, by different intravenous lines) in 5 of the cases, whereas one was given intravenous calcium as part of parenteral nutrition.[2]

Mechanism

In vitro studies in adult plasma, and neonatal plasma from umbilical cord blood,[3] have shown that intravascular ceftriaxone-calcium precipitates are more likely to form in neonates than in other age groups.[4] Precipitates of ceftriaxone and calcium can also occur when ceftriaxone is mixed with calcium-containing solutions in the same intravenous line.[3] It has also been suggested that giving high doses of ceftriaxone by intravenous bolus injection (as occurred in some of the reported cases) rather than as an infusion might also increase the risk of precipitation due to transiently higher ceftriaxone concentrations.[2]

Importance and management

Evidence for an interaction between ceftriaxone and calcium compounds is limited, but the available information would appear to suggest that there is a possible increased risk of precipitation leading to serious, and in some cases fatal, adverse effects in neonates. In 2009, the FDA[3] in the US and the MHRA[5] in the UK recommended that intravenous ceftriaxone and intravenous calcium-containing solutions should not be given simultaneously because of a risk of calcium-ceftriaxone salt precipitation in all age groups. They further advised that the concurrent use of ceftriaxone and intravenous calcium-containing products is contraindicated in neonates (up to 28 days old). In patients aged 28 days or older, ceftriaxone and calcium-containing fluids can be infused sequentially, but only if the infusion lines are flushed thoroughly between infusions with a compatible solution[3,5] or if they are given through different infusion lines at different sites.[5]

For calcium-containing parenteral nutrition, the MHRA in the UK advises giving an alternative antibacterial to ceftriaxone; however, if this is not possible, parenteral nutrition and calcium-containing fluids can be given simultaneously but only if they are given through different infusion lines at different sites.[5]

There appears to be no data regarding a possible interaction with intramuscular ceftriaxone, or with oral calcium-containing products.[3]

Although strictly speaking this is a drug compatibility effect, rather than a drug interaction, it has been included in this publication because of the severity of the outcome.

1. Dalton BR, Zuege DJ, Shahpori R, Laupland KB. Concomitant ceftriaxone and high-concentration intravenous calcium therapy in adult critical care patients: a matched cohort study. *Ann Pharmacother* (2010) 44, 1158–63.
2. Bradley JS, Wassel RT, Lee L, Nambiar S. Intravenous ceftriaxone and calcium in the neonate: assessing the risk for cardiopulmonary adverse events. *Pediatrics* (2009), e609–e613.
3. FDA Information for healthcare professionals: ceftriaxone (marketed as Rocephin and generics). April 21st 2009. Available at: http://www.fda.gov/Drugs/DrugSafety/PostmarketDrugSafetyInformationforPatientsandProviders/DrugSafetyInformationforHeathcareProfessionals/ucm084263.htm (accessed 20/10/15).
4. Rocephin (Hydrated disodium ceftriaxone). Roche Products Ltd. UK Summary of product characteristics, July 2010.
5. Medicines and Healthcare Products Regulatory Agency and the Commission on Human Medicines. Ceftriaxone: incompatibility with calcium-containing solutions. *Drug Safety Update* (2009) 3, 2–3. Available at: https://www.gov.uk/drug-safety-update/ceftriaxone-rocephin-incompatible-with-solutions-containing-calcium (accessed 20/10/15).

Cephalosporins; Cefuroxime + Disulfiram

An isolated case report describes a disulfiram-like reaction when cefuroxime axetil was given to a patient taking disulfiram.

Clinical evidence

A patient taking disulfiram 125 mg daily for 18 months without problem, developed nausea, vomiting and stomach cramps one hour after taking one dose of cefuroxime axetil 250 mg. The symptoms lasted for about 9 hours, and the patient was not rechallenged.[1]

Mechanism

The authors[1] suggest that the reaction seen was due to the accumulation of acetaldehyde (produced when the axetil salt of cefuroxime is metabolised[2]), as a result of disulfiram inhibiting acetaldehyde dehydrogenase. The accumulation of acetaldehyde is generally thought to be responsible for most of the symptoms of the disulfiram reaction, see *Mechanism* under 'Alcohol + Disulfiram', p.67.

Importance and management

Information about an interaction between cefuroxime and disulfiram is limited to this isolated case report and it is unclear whether the amount of axetil-salt present in cefuroxime axetil preparations would be sufficient to produce acetaldehyde in such quantities that if accumulation occurred, a disulfiram reaction might result. However, note that very small amounts of alcohol have been reported to cause this reaction when taken with disulfiram, see 'Alcohol + Disulfiram', p.67. No specific precautions would seem necessary on concurrent use, but bear the interaction in mind in the case of symptoms relating to the disulfiram reaction.

1. Mattes JA. Antabuse reaction with ceftin. *Am J Psychiatry* (2006) 163, 2019–20.
2. Ceftin (Cefuroxime axetil). GlaxoSmithKline. US Prescribing information, January 2010.

Chloramphenicol + Cimetidine

Isolated reports describe fatal aplastic anaemia in two patients given intravenous chloramphenicol and cimetidine.

Clinical evidence, mechanism, importance and management

Pancytopenia and aplastic anaemia developed in a man taking cimetidine 1.2 g daily, within 18 days of being given intravenous chloramphenicol 1 g every 6 hours. It proved to be fatal.[1] Another patient, similarly treated, developed fatal aplastic anaemia after 19 days.[2] A drug interaction with cimetidine was suspected because the onset of pancytopenia was more rapid than in previous cases where chloramphenicol alone induced aplastic anaemia. This effect may occur because the bone marrow depressant effects of the two drugs are additive. There are at least 8 other cases of aplastic anaemia following the use of parenteral chloramphenicol in the absence of cimetidine.[2] The general importance of these observations is uncertain, but the authors of one of the reports suggest that these drugs should be used together with caution.

1. Farber BF, Brody JP. Rapid development of aplastic anemia after intravenous chloramphenicol and cimetidine therapy. *South Med J* (1981) 74, 1257–8.
2. West BC, DeVault GA, Clement JC, Williams DM. Aplastic anemia associated with parenteral chloramphenicol: review of 10 cases, including the second case of possible increased risk with cimetidine. *Rev Infect Dis* (1988) 10, 1048–51.

Chloramphenicol + Dapsone

Dapsone does not significantly affect the pharmacokinetics of oral chloramphenicol.

Clinical evidence, mechanism, importance and management

A comparison of the pharmacokinetics of oral chloramphenicol in 8 healthy subjects and 8 patients with uncomplicated lepromatous leprosy found that the half-life of a single 500-mg dose of chloramphenicol was prolonged from 4.3 hours to 6.4 hours in patients with leprosy, possibly due to changes in liver function. The elimination half-life of chloramphenicol was further increased, to about 8 hours, when the subjects were also given dapsone 100 mg daily for 8 days. However, this latter increase was not statistically significant. Although there was no clinically significant interaction between dapsone and chloramphenicol, the disposition of chloramphenicol may be altered in leprosy.[1]

1. Garg SK, Kumar B, Shukla VK, Bakaya V, Lal R, Kaur S. Pharmacokinetics of aspirin and chloramphenicol in normal and leprotic patients before and after dapsone therapy. *Int J Clin Pharmacol* (1988) 26, 204–5.

Chloramphenicol + Other antibacterials

An old report suggests that the use of chloramphenicol may antagonise the effects of ampicillin in bacterial meningitis. In contrast, no antagonism and even additive antibacterial effects have been described in other infections. Chloramphenicol levels have been markedly lowered by rifampicin (rifampin) in a small number of children.

Clinical evidence

(a) Antibacterial antagonism

A study in 264 patients (adults, and children over 2 months old) with acute bacterial meningitis found that when they were given **ampicillin** 150 mg/kg daily alone, the case-fatality ratio was 4.3% compared with 10.5% in comparable subjects given a combination of **ampicillin**, chloramphenicol 100 mg/kg daily (up to 4 g), and **streptomycin** 40 mg/kg daily (up to 2 g). The neurological sequelae (hemiparesis, deafness, cranial nerve palsies) were also markedly increased by the combined use of these drugs.[1] Antibacterial antagonism was clearly seen in a 10-week-old infant with *Salmonella enteritidis* meningitis, who was given chloramphenicol and **ceftazidime**.[2]

However, in contrast a report claims that antibacterial antagonism was not seen in 65 of 66 patients given chloramphenicol and **benzylpenicillin** for bronchitis or bronchopneumonia.[3] **Ampicillin** with chloramphenicol is more effective than chloramphenicol alone in the treatment of typhoid,[4] and in a study of 700 patients, **procaine benzylpenicillin** with chloramphenicol was shown to be more effective than chloramphenicol alone in the treatment of gonorrhoea (failure rates of 1.8% compared with 8.5%).[5]

(b) Pharmacokinetic interactions

In a study in premature and full-term neonates, infants and small children, it was found that the presence of **penicillin** markedly raised chloramphenicol levels.[6]

Two children, aged 2 and 5 years, with *Haemophilus influenzae* meningitis, were given chloramphenicol 100 mg/kg daily in four divided doses by infusion over 30 minutes. Within 3 days of starting **rifampicin (rifampin)** 20 mg/kg daily their peak serum chloramphenicol levels were reduced by 86% and 64%, respectively, and only returned to the therapeutic range when the chloramphenicol dose was increased to 125 mg/kg daily.[7]

Two other children, of 5 and 18 months, with *Haemophilus influenzae* infections, are also reported to have shown reductions of 75% and 94%, respectively, in serum chloramphenicol levels when given **rifampicin** 20 mg/kg daily for 4 days. These reductions occurred despite 20 to 25% increases in the chloramphenicol dose.[8]

Mechanism

By no means fully understood. Chloramphenicol inhibits bacterial protein synthesis and can change an actively growing bacterial colony into a static one. Thus the effects of a bactericide, such as penicillin, which interferes with cell wall synthesis, are blunted, and the death of the organism occurs more slowly. This would seem to explain the antagonism seen with some organisms.

It is thought that rifampicin (rifampin), a potent enzyme inducer, markedly increases the metabolism of chloramphenicol by the liver, thereby lowering its serum levels.[7,8]

Importance and management

Proven cases of antibacterial antagonism of chloramphenicol by penicillins in patients seem to be few in number, and there is insufficient evidence to impose a general prohibition, because, depending on the organism, penicillins and chloramphenicol have been used together with clear advantage.

So far only four cases of an interaction between rifampicin (rifampin) and chloramphenicol appear to have been reported. However, the evidence is of good quality and in line with the way rifampicin interacts with other drugs, so this interaction should be taken seriously. There is a risk that chloramphenicol levels will become subtherapeutic. The authors of the second report point out that raising the chloramphenicol dose may possibly expose the patient to a greater risk of bone marrow aplasia. They suggest delaying rifampicin prophylaxis in patients with invasive *Haemophilus influenzae* infections until the end of chloramphenicol treatment.

1. Mathies AW, Leedom JM, Ivler D, Wehrle PF, Portnoy B. Antibiotic antagonism in bacterial meningitis. *Antimicrob Agents Chemother* (1967) 7, 218–24.
2. French GL, Ling TKW, Davies DP, Leung DTY. Antagonism of ceftazidime by chloramphenicol in vitro and in vivo during treatment of gram negative meningitis. *BMJ* (1985) 291, 636–7.
3. Ardalan P. Zur Frage des Antagonismus von Penicillin und Chloramphenicolus klinischer Sicht. *Prax Pneumol* (1969) 23, 772–6.
4. De Ritis R, Giammanco G, Manzillo G. Chloramphenicol combined with ampicillin in treatment of typhoid. *BMJ* (1972) 4, 17–18.
5. Gjessing HC, Ödegaard K. Oral chloramphenicol alone and with intramuscular procaine penicillin in the treatment of gonorrhoea. *Br J Vener Dis* (1967) 43, 133–6.
6. Windorfer A, Pringsheim W. Studies on the concentrations of chloramphenicol in the serum and cerebrospinal fluid of neonates, infants and small children. *Eur J Pediatr* (1977) 124, 129–38.
7. Prober CG. Effect of rifampin on chloramphenicol levels. *N Engl J Med* (1985) 312, 788–9.
8. Kelly HW, Couch RC, Davis RL, Cushing AH, Knott R. Interaction of chloramphenicol and rifampin. *J Pediatr* (1988) 112, 817–20.

Chloramphenicol + Paracetamol (Acetaminophen)

Although there is limited evidence to suggest that paracetamol may affect chloramphenicol pharmacokinetics its validity has been criticised.

Clinical evidence, mechanism, importance and management

Three studies report alterations in the pharmacokinetics of chloramphenicol by paracetamol. The first was conducted in 6 adults in intensive care after an observation that the half-life of chloramphenicol was prolonged by paracetamol in children with kwashiorkor. The addition of 100 mg of intravenous paracetamol increased the half-life of chloramphenicol in the adults from 3.25 hours to 15 hours.[1] However, this study has been criticised because of potential errors in the method used to calculate the half-life,[2] the unusual doses used,[2,3] and because the pharmacokinetics of the chloramphenicol with and without paracetamol were calculated at different times after the administration of chloramphenicol.[4] It has also been pointed out that malnutrition (e.g. kwashiorkor) can increase the elimination rate and AUC of chloramphenicol independently of paracetamol.[2]

The second study demonstrated a different interaction, in that the clearance of chloramphenicol was *increased* and the half-life *reduced* by paracetamol.[5] This study has also been criticised as it does not account for the fact that chloramphenicol clearance increases over the duration of a treatment course, which suggests that the changes seen in the pharmacokinetics of chloramphenicol may be independent of the paracetamol.[6] The authors later admit this as a possibility.[7] The third study found no differences in the pharmacokinetics of chloramphenicol after the first dose, but at steady state, the AUC and peak serum levels of chloramphenicol were lower in children who also received paracetamol.[8]

Three other studies do not support the existence of a pharmacokinetic interaction between chloramphenicol and paracetamol.[2-4]

The clinical significance of these reports is unclear, and clinical evidence of toxicity or treatment failure of chloramphenicol appears to be lacking. It would seem prudent to remain aware of the potential for interaction, especially in malnourished patients, but routine monitoring would appear unnecessary without further evidence.

1. Buchanan N, Moodley GP. Interaction between chloramphenicol and paracetamol. *BMJ* (1979) 2, 307–308.
2. Kearns GL, Bocchini JA, Brown RD, Cotter DL, Wilson JT. Absence of a pharmacokinetic interaction between chloramphenicol and acetaminophen in children. *J Pediatr* (1985) 107, 134–9.
3. Rajpurohit R, Krishnaswamy K. Lack of effect of paracetamol on the pharmacokinetics of chloramphenicol in adult human subjects. *Indian J Pharm* (1984) 16, 124–8.
4. Stein CM, Thornhill DP, Neill P, Nyazema NZ. Lack of effect of paracetamol on the pharmacokinetics of chloramphenicol. *Br J Clin Pharmacol* (1989) 27, 262–4.
5. Spika JS, Davis DJ, Martin SR, Beharry K, Rex J, Aranda JV. Interaction between chloramphenicol and acetaminophen. *Arch Dis Child* (1986) 61, 1121–4.
6. Choonara IA. Interaction between chloramphenicol and acetaminophen. *Arch Dis Child* (1987) 62, 319.
7. Spika JS, Aranda JV. Interaction between chloramphenicol and acetaminophen. *Arch Dis Child* (1987) 62, 1087–8.
8. Bravo ME, Horwitz I, Contreras C, Olea I, Arancibia A. Influencia del paracetamol en la farmacocinética del cloramfenicol en pacientes con fiebre tifoídea. *Rev Chil Pediatr* (1987) 58, 117–20.

Chloramphenicol + Phenobarbital

Studies in children have found that phenobarbital can markedly reduce serum chloramphenicol levels. There is a single report, in one adult, of markedly increased serum phenobarbital levels caused by chloramphenicol.

Clinical evidence

(a) Effects on chloramphenicol

A study in a group of infants and children (aged one month to 12 years) given chloramphenicol 25 mg/kg every 6 hours found that 6 of them, also taking phenobarbital, had reduced serum chloramphenicol levels, when compared with 17 control patients. The peak levels were lowered by 34%, from 25.3 to 16.6 micrograms/mL, and the trough levels were lowered by 44%, from 13.4 to 7.5 micrograms/mL.[1] Two children aged 3 and 7 months were given chloramphenicol 100 mg/kg daily, initially intravenously, and later orally for *Haemophilus influenzae* meningitis. The chloramphenicol levels halved over the first 2 days of treatment, while the children were receiving phenobarbital 10 mg/kg daily to prevent convulsions. One child had serum chloramphenicol levels of only 5 micrograms/mL even though the initial doses used were expected to give levels of 15 to 25 micrograms/mL.[2]

Another study confirmed that this interaction occurred in 20 neonates, but no statistically significant effect was found in 40 infants.[3] Decreased chloramphenicol levels have been described in a single case report of a child who was also taking phenytoin and phenobarbital. The serum chloramphenicol levels were 35.1 micrograms/mL before the antiepileptics were started, 19.1 micrograms/mL after 2 days of phenytoin, and 13.2 micrograms/mL a month after the addition of phenobarbital.[4] For more information on the interaction of chloramphenicol with phenytoin see 'Phenytoin + Chloramphenicol', p.598.

(b) Effects on phenobarbital

A man admitted to hospital on numerous occasions for pulmonary complications associated with cystic fibrosis, had average serum phenobarbital levels of 33 micrograms/mL while taking phenobarbital 200 mg daily and oral chloramphenicol 600 mg every 6 hours. One week after the antibacterial was withdrawn, his serum phenobarbital levels were 24 micrograms/mL even though the phenobarbital dose was increased from 200 to 300 mg daily.[5]

Mechanism

Phenobarbital is a potent liver enzyme inducer, which can increase the metabolism and clearance of chloramphenicol (clearly demonstrated in *rats*[6]), so that its serum levels fall and its effects are reduced. Chloramphenicol inhibits the metabolism of the phenobarbital (also demonstrated in *animals*[7]) so that the effects of the barbiturate are increased.

Importance and management

This interaction appears to be established. The documentation is limited but what happened is consistent with the recognised enzyme-inducing actions of phenobarbital and the inhibitory actions of chloramphenicol. Concurrent use should be well monitored to ensure that chloramphenicol serum levels are adequate, and that phenobarbital levels do not become too high (indicators of toxicity include drowsiness, ataxia or dysarthria). Make appropriate dose adjustments as necessary.

1. Krasinski K, Kusmiesz H, Nelson JD. Pharmacologic interactions among chloramphenicol, phenytoin and phenobarbital. *Pediatr Infect Dis* (1982) 1, 232–5.
2. Bloxham RA, Durbin GM, Johnson T, Winterborn MH. Chloramphenicol and phenobarbitone—a drug interaction. *Arch Dis Child* (1979) 54, 76–7.
3. Windorfer A, Pringsheim W. Studies on the concentrations of chloramphenicol in the serum and cerebrospinal fluid of neonates, infants, and small children. *Eur J Pediatr* (1977) 124, 129–38.
4. Powell DA, Nahata MC, Durrell DC, Glazer JP, Hilty MD. Interactions among chloramphenicol, phenytoin, and phenobarbital in a pediatric patient. *J Pediatr* (1981) 98, 1001–1003.
5. Koup JR, Gibaldi M, McNamara P, Hilligoss DM, Colburn WA, Bruck E. Interaction of chloramphenicol with phenytoin and phenobarbital. Case report. *Clin Pharmacol Ther* (1978) 24, 571–5.
6. Bella DD, Ferrari V, Marca G,Bonanomi L. Chloramphenicol metabolism in the phenobarbital-induced rat. Comparison with thiamphenicol. *Biochem Pharmacol* (1968) 17, 2381–90.
7. Adams HR. Prolonged barbiturate anesthesia by chloramphenicol in laboratory animals. *J Am Vet Med Assoc* (1970) 157, 1908–13.

Clindamycin or Lincomycin + Food

The serum levels of lincomycin are markedly reduced (by up to two-thirds) if taken in the presence of food, but clindamycin is not significantly affected. Cyclamate sweeteners can also reduce the absorption of lincomycin.

Clinical evidence

In a study in 10 healthy subjects the mean peak serum levels of a single 500-mg oral dose of lincomycin were about 3 micrograms/mL when taken 4 hours before **breakfast**, 2 micrograms/mL when taken 1 hour before breakfast, and less than 1 microgram/mL when taken after breakfast. The mean total amounts of lincomycin recovered from the urine were 40.4 mg, 23.8 mg, and 8.9 mg, respectively.[1]

Reduced serum lincomycin levels due to the presence of **food** have been described in other reports,[2,3] but the absorption of clindamycin is not affected.[3,4]

Sodium cyclamate, an artificial sweetener found in diet foods, drinks and some pharmaceuticals, can also markedly reduce the absorption of lincomycin. The AUC of lincomycin 500 mg was reduced by about 75% by 1 Molar equivalent of **sodium cyclamate** (said to be an amount equal to only part of a bottle of diet drink, but exact quantity not stated).[5]

Mechanism

Not understood.

Importance and management

The food interaction with lincomycin is well established and of clinical importance. Lincomycin should not be taken with food or within several hours of eating a meal if adequate serum levels are to be achieved. An alternative is clindamycin, a synthetic derivative of lincomycin, which has the same antibacterial spectrum but is not affected by food.

1. McCall CE, Steigbigel NH, Finland M. Lincomycin: activity *in vitro* and absorption and excretion in normal young men. *Am J Med Sci* (1967) 254, 144–55.

2. Kaplan K, Chew WH, Weinstein L. Microbiological, pharmacological and clinical studies of lincomycin. *Am J Med Sci* (1965) 250, 137–46.
3. McGehee RF, Smith CB, Wilcox C, Finland M. Comparative studies of antibacterial activity in vitro and absorption and excretion of lincomycin and clinimycin. *Am J Med Sci* (1968) 256, 279–92.
4. Wagner JG, Novak E, Patel NC, Chidester CG, Lummis WL. Absorption, excretion and half-life of clinimycin in normal adult males. *Am J Med Sci* (1968) 256, 25–37.
5. Wagner JG. Aspects of pharmacokinetics and biopharmaceutics in relation to drug activity. *Am J Pharm Sci Support Public Health* (1969) 141, 5–20.

Clindamycin or Lincomycin + Kaolin

Kaolin-pectin can markedly reduce the absorption of lincomycin. The rate but not the extent of clindamycin absorption is altered by kaolin.

Clinical evidence

In 8 healthy subjects about 85 mL of *Kaopectate* (kaolin-pectin) reduced the absorption of lincomycin 500 mg by about 90%. Giving the *Kaopectate* 2 hours before the antibacterial had little or no effect on its absorption, whereas when *Kaopectate* was given 2 hours after lincomycin, the absorption was reduced by about 50%. The absorption rate of clindamycin is markedly prolonged by kaolin, but the extent of its absorption remains unaffected.[1]

Mechanism

It seems probable that the lincomycin becomes adsorbed onto the kaolin, thereby reducing its bioavailability. The kaolin also coats the lining of the gut and acts as a physical barrier to absorption.[2]

Importance and management

Information seems to be limited to this study, but the interaction between lincomycin and kaolin appears to be established and of clinical importance. For good absorption and a good antibacterial response separate their administration as much as possible, ideally giving the kaolin at least 2 hours before the antibacterial. Clindamycin appears to be a suitable alternative to lincomycin. However, note that marked diarrhoea is an indication that lincomycin or clindamycin should be stopped immediately. This is because it may be a sign of pseudomembranous colitis, which can be fatal.

1. Albert KS, DeSante KA, Welch RD, DiSanto AR. Pharmacokinetic evaluation of a drug interaction between kaolin-pectin and clindamycin. *J Pharm Sci* (1978) 67, 1579–82.
2. Wagner JG. Design and data analysis of biopharmaceutical studies in man. *Can J Pharm Sci* (1966) 1, 55–68.

Clofazimine + Miscellaneous

The bioavailability of a single dose of clofazimine is increased by a high-fat meal, and slightly decreased by orange juice and an aluminium/magnesium hydroxide antacid.

Clinical evidence, mechanism, importance and management

In a randomised, crossover study healthy subjects received a single 200-mg dose of clofazimine after a 12 hour fast (13 subjects), with 240 mL of **orange juice** (15 subjects), with a high-fat meal (15 subjects) or with 15 mL of an **aluminium/magnesium hydroxide** and **simeticone**-containing antacid given 9 hours before the clofazimine, at the time of dosing, and four times daily for the subsequent day. The high-fat meal increased the AUC and maximum plasma levels of clofazimine by 98% and 146%, respectively. The **orange juice** reduced the AUC and maximum plasma levels of clofazimine by 13% and 7%, respectively, and the **antacid** reduced the AUC and maximum plasma levels of clofazimine by 16% and 35%, respectively. There was wide inter-individual variation in each of the study groups.[1]

The clinical significance of the findings of this single-dose study with food is unclear; clofazimine has a half-life after repeated doses of about 70 days. The manufacturer advises that clofazimine is taken with meals.[2] The changes in clofazimine levels caused by the **antacid** and **orange juice** are small, and unlikely to be clinically relevant.

1. Nix DE, Adam RD, Auclair B, Krueger TS, Godo PG, Peloquin CA. Pharmacokinetics and relative bioavailability of clofazimine in relation to food, orange juice and antacid. *Tuberculosis (Edinb)* (2004) 84, 365–73.
2. Lamprene (Clofazimine). Novartis Pharmaceuticals Corporation. US Prescribing information, September 1998.

Colistin + Sucralfate

An *in vitro* study with colistin sulfate found that it became markedly and irreversibly bound to sucralfate at the pH values found in the gut.

Clinical evidence, mechanism, importance and management

To simulate what might happen in the gut, colistin sulfate 50 mg/L was mixed with sucralfate 500 mg in 40 mL of water at pH 3.5 and allowed to stand for 90 minutes at 25°C. Analysis of the solution showed that the colistin concentration fell rapidly and progressively over 90 minutes to about 40%. When the pH of the mixture was then raised to 6.5 to 7 for 90 minutes, there was no change in the concentration of colistin, suggesting that the interaction was irreversible.[1] The reason for this change is not known, but the suggestion is that sucralfate forms insoluble chelates with colistin.[1]

It is not known how important this interaction is likely to be in practice, but the efficacy of colistin in gut decontamination and gut infections may be decreased. Separating the doses might not be effective in some postoperative patients because their gastric function may not return to normal for up to 5 days, and some sucralfate might still be present when the next dose is given.[1] More study is needed to find out whether this interaction is clinically important, but in the meanwhile it would seem prudent to monitor concurrent use carefully, being alert for any evidence of reduced effects.

1. Feron B, Adair CG, Gorman SP, McClurg B. Interaction of sucralfate with antibiotics used for selective decontamination of the gastrointestinal tract. *Am J Hosp Pharm* (1993) 50, 2550–3.

Co-trimoxazole + Azithromycin

Azithromycin does not alter the pharmacokinetics of co-trimoxazole.

Clinical evidence, mechanism, importance and management

A study in 12 healthy subjects given co-trimoxazole (trimethoprim and sulfamethoxazole) 960 mg daily for 7 days found that a single 1.2-g dose of azithromycin given on day 7 did not alter the pharmacokinetics of either trimethoprim or sulfamethoxazole to a clinically relevant extent.[1]

1. Amsden GW, Foulds G, Thakker K. Pharmacokinetic study of azithromycin with fluconazole and cotrimoxazole (trimethoprim-sulfamethoxazole) in healthy volunteers. *Clin Drug Invest* (2000) 20, 135–42.

Co-trimoxazole + Azoles

Fluconazole, but not ketoconazole inhibits the metabolism of sulfamethoxazole to its hydroxylamine metabolite.

Clinical evidence, mechanism, importance and management

Ten healthy subjects were given co-trimoxazole (sulfamethoxazole 800 mg with trimethoprim 160 mg) either alone or one hour after either **fluconazole** 150 mg or **ketoconazole** 200 mg. **Ketoconazole** had no effect on the urinary recovery of sulfamethoxazole or its metabolites. However, **fluconazole** significantly inhibited the formation of sulfamethoxazole hydroxylamine and also inhibited the oxidation of sulfamethoxazole to its 5-methylhydroxy- and 5-methylhydroxy acetate metabolites. The amount of unchanged sulfamethoxazole or its *N*-acetyl or glucuronide metabolites were not affected by **fluconazole**.[1] Another study in HIV-positive patients given co-trimoxazole (sulfamethoxazole 800 mg with trimethoprim 160 mg daily) found that **fluconazole** 200 mg daily decreased the AUC, urinary recovery, and formation clearance of sulfamethoxazole hydroxylamine by 37%, 53% and 61% respectively.[2] As the hydroxylamine metabolite is possibly one of the causes of sulfamethoxazole toxicity, the concurrent use of **fluconazole** may be associated with reduced rates of sulfamethoxazole toxicity.[1,2]

Evidence about other azoles appears to be lacking, but they would, in general, be expected to interact similarly.

1. Gill HJ, Maggs JL, Madden S, Pirmohamed M, Park BK. The effect of fluconazole and ketoconazole on the metabolism of sulphamethoxazole. *Br J Clin Pharmacol* (1996) 42, 347–53.
2. Winter HR, Trapnell CB, Slattery JT, Jacobson M, Greenspan DL, Hooton TM, Unadkat JD. The effect of clarithromycin, fluconazole, and rifabutin on sulfamethoxazole hydroxylamine formation in individuals with human immunodeficiency virus infection (AATG 283). *Clin Pharmacol Ther* (2004) 76, 313–22.

Co-trimoxazole + Cimetidine

Cimetidine has no significant effect on the pharmacokinetics of co-trimoxazole.

Clinical evidence, mechanism, importance and management

In a placebo-controlled study, 6 healthy subjects were given cimetidine 400 mg every 6 hours for 6 days, with a single 960-mg dose of co-trimoxazole (trimethoprim with sulfamethoxazole) on day 6. Although trimethoprim levels were consistently higher in the presence of cimetidine, the slight difference was not statistically significant. Cimetidine had no effect on the pharmacokinetics of sulfamethoxazole.[1]

1. Rogers HJ, James CA, Morrison PJ, Bradbrook ID. Effect of cimetidine on oral absorption of ampicillin and co-trimoxazole. *J Antimicrob Chemother* (1980) 6, 297–300.

Co-trimoxazole + Kaolin-pectin

Kaolin-pectin can cause a small but probably clinically unimportant reduction in trimethoprim levels, and has no effect on sulfamethoxazole pharmacokinetics.

Clinical evidence, mechanism, importance and management

Co-trimoxazole suspension (trimethoprim 160 mg with sulfamethoxazole 800 mg) was given to 8 healthy subjects, with and without 20 mL of kaolin-pectin suspension. Kaolin-pectin reduced the AUC and the maximum serum levels of trimethoprim by about 12% and 20%, respectively. Changes in the sulfamethoxazole pharmacokinetics were not statistically significant.[1] The probable reason for this reduction in the trimethoprim AUC is that trimethoprim is adsorbed onto the kaolin-pectin, which reduces the amount available for absorption. However, the reduction is small and unlikely to be clinically relevant.

1. Gupta KC, Desai NK, Satoskar RS, Gupta C, Goswami SN. Effect of pectin and kaolin on bioavailability of co-trimoxazole suspension. *Int J Clin Pharmacol Ther Toxicol* (1987) 25, 320–1.

Co-trimoxazole + Prilocaine with Lidocaine

Methaemoglobinaemia developed in a baby treated with co-trimoxazole when *Emla* (prilocaine with lidocaine) cream was applied to his skin. Other drugs that cause methaemoglobinaemia are predicted to have similar effects.

Clinical evidence, mechanism, importance and management

A 12-week-old child, given co-trimoxazole for 2 months for pyelitis, was given 5 g of *Emla* cream (prilocaine 25 mg and lidocaine 25 mg per gram) applied to the back of his hands and the cubital regions. Unfortunately his operation was delayed, and 5 hours later, just before the operation began, his skin was noted to be pale and his lips had a brownish cyanotic colour. This was found to be due to the presence of 28% methaemoglobin (reference range less than 3%).[1] The authors of the report suggest that prilocaine together with sulfamethoxazole (both known to cause methaemoglobin formation) suppressed the activity of two enzymes (NADH-dehydrogenase and NADP-diaphorase), which normally keep blood levels of methaemoglobin to a minimum.[1] A study in 20 children[2] confirmed that *Emla* cream can increase methaemoglobin levels, although levels *decreased* in 6 of them. However, the maximum increase was 1.2% (from 0.7 to 1.9%), and the highest value was 2%, which was still within the reference range. Another study found similar small increases in methaemoglobin levels, and found that these remained elevated after 24 hours. The authors concluded that daily application of prilocaine with lidocaine may lead to accumulation, and a greater risk of toxicity.[3]

The case report appears to be unusual, but it has been suggested that there may be a special risk of methaemoglobinaemia with *Emla* in children with pre-existing anaemia, reduced renal excretion of the metabolites of prilocaine, or the concurrent use of sulfonamides.[3] It would seem prudent to keep *Emla* contact time to a minimum in these patients. Note that the UK and US manufacturers advise that *Emla* should not be applied to the skin of infants who are under the age of 12 months who are receiving treatment with methaemoglobin-inducing drugs. They specifically name the **sulfonamides**.[4] In addition, the manufacturers name a number of other drugs that they suggest may cause methaemoglobinaemia. This includes **aminosalicylic acid, benzocaine, chloroquine, dapsone, metoclopramide, nitrates, nitrofurantoin, nitroprusside, paracetamol (acetaminophen), phenacetin, phenobarbital, phenytoin**, and **primaquine**.[4,5]

1. Jakobson B, Nilsson A. Methemoglobinemia associated with a prilocaine-lidocaine cream and trimetho-prim-sulphamethoxazole. A case report. *Acta Anaesthesiol Scand* (1985) 29, 453–55.
2. Engberg G, Danielson K, Henneberg S, Nilsson A. Plasma concentrations of prilocaine and lidocaine and methaemoglobin formation in infants after epicutaneous application of a 5% lidocaine-prilocaine cream (Emla). *Acta Anaesthesiol Scand* (1987) 31, 624–8.
3. Frayling IM, Addison GM, Chattergee K, Meakin G. Methaemoglobinaemia in children treated with prilocaine-lignocaine cream. *BMJ* (1990) 301, 153–4.
4. EMLA Cream (Lidocaine with Prilocaine). AstraZeneca. US Prescribing information, May 2005.
5. EMLA Cream (Lidocaine with Prilocaine). AstraZeneca UK Ltd. UK Summary of product characteristics, July 2011.

Co-trimoxazole or Trimethoprim + Rifamycins

The pharmacokinetics of trimethoprim are not significantly affected by rifabutin, and probably not by rifampicin (rifampin). Trimethoprim does not affect the pharmacokinetics of rifampicin.

Rifabutin does not affect the pharmacokinetics of sulfamethoxazole, but significantly increases exposure to its hydroxylamine metabolite and as a result may increase adverse reactions to sulfamethoxazole in HIV-positive patients.

A significant reduction in co-trimoxazole levels and a decrease in prophylactic efficacy has been seen in HIV-positive patients taking rifampicin. Limited evidence suggests that co-trimoxazole can increase rifampicin levels.

Clinical evidence, mechanism, importance and management

(a) Rifabutin

Twelve HIV-positive patients taking co-trimoxazole (sulfamethoxazole and trimethoprim; strength not stated) twice daily for 7 days were also given rifabutin 300 mg daily for a further 14 days. The sulfamethoxazole component remained unaffected by rifabutin but the trimethoprim AUC was decreased by 22%. This small reduction is not expected to be clinically significant.[1] However, another study in HIV-positive patients given co-trimoxazole (sulfamethoxazole 800 mg with trimethoprim 160 mg daily) found that although rifabutin 300 mg daily had minimal effects on the disposition of sulfamethoxazole and its acetylated metabolite, it significantly increased the AUC, urinary recovery and formation clearance of its hydroxylamine metabolite by about 50%. As the hydroxylamine metabolite may be one of the factors associated with adverse reactions to sulfamethoxazole in HIV-positive patients, concurrent rifabutin may increase the rate of adverse reactions.[2]

(b) Rifampicin (Rifampin)

No significant pharmacokinetic interaction seems to occur when healthy subjects are given trimethoprim 240 mg daily with rifampicin 900 mg daily (both in divided doses). After 4 to 5 days, less trimethoprim is recovered in the urine, as more is metabolised before excretion due to the enzyme-inducing effects of rifampicin, but this does not appear to be of clinical importance.[3,4] Another study also notes that no clinically significant pharmacokinetic interaction occurs between trimethoprim and rifampicin.[5]

However, a case-control study of the efficacy of co-trimoxazole in preventing toxoplasmosis in HIV-positive patients found a link between rifampicin use and co-trimoxazole failure,[6] which prompted the authors to conduct a pharmacokinetic study. When rifampicin 600 mg daily was given to 10 HIV-positive patients with co-trimoxazole 960 mg daily, it was found that the AUCs of trimethoprim and sulfamethoxazole were reduced by 56% and 28%, respectively. These changes are sufficient to reduce the efficacy of co-trimoxazole treatment.[7] It would therefore seem prudent to consider this interaction when giving rifampicin to HIV-positive patients taking co-trimoxazole prophylaxis.

In one study, 15 patients with tuberculosis, who had taken rifampicin 450 mg daily for at least 15 days, were given co-trimoxazole (trimethoprim 320 mg and sulfamethoxazole 800 mg every 12 hours) for 5 to 10 days. Rifampicin levels were measured at five time points over 6 hours before and during co-trimoxazole treatment. At 4 and 6 hours, rifampicin levels were significantly higher (27% and 56%, respectively) during co-trimoxazole use, but peak levels were only increased by about 18%. Concurrent use did not result in any increase in adverse effects.[8]

1. Lee BL, Lampiris H, Colborn DC, Lewis RC, Narang PK, Sullam P. The effect of rifabutin (RBT) on the pharmacokinetics (PK) of trimethoprim-sulfamethoxazole (TMP-SMX) in HIV-infected patients. *Intersci Conf Antimicrob Agents Chemother* (1995) 35, 7.
2. Winter HR, Trapnell CB, Slattery JT, Jacobson M, Greenspan DL, Hooton TM, Unadkat JD. The effect of clarithromycin, fluconazole, and rifabutin on sulfamethoxazole hydroxylamine formation in individuals with human immunodeficiency virus infection (AACTG 283). *Clin Pharmacol Ther* (2004) 76, 313–22.
3. Buniva G, Palminteri R, Berti M. Kinetics of a rifampicin-trimethoprim combination. *Int J Clin Pharmacol Biopharm* (1979) 17, 256–9.
4. Emmerson AM, Grüneberg RN, Johnson ES. The pharmacokinetics in man of a combination of rifampicin and trimethoprim. *J Antimicrob Chemother* (1978) 4, 523–31.
5. Acocella G, Scotti R. Kinetic studies on the combination rifampicin-trimethoprim in man. *J Antimicrob Chemother* (1976) 2, 271–77.
6. Ribera E, Fernandez-Sola A, Juste C, Rovira A, Romero FJ, Armandas-Gil L, Ruiz I, Ocaña I, Pahissa A. Comparison of high and low doses of trimethoprim-sulfamethoxazole for primary prevention of toxoplasmic encephalitis in human immunodeficiency virus-infected patients. *Clin Infect Dis* (1999) 29, 1461–6.
7. Ribera E, Pou L, Fernandez-Sola A, Campos F, Lopez RM, Ocaña I, Ruiz I, Pahissa A. Rifampin reduces concentrations of trimethoprim and sulfamethoxazole in serum in human immunodeficiency virus infected patients. *Antimicrob Agents Chemother* (2001) 45, 3238–41.
8. Bhatia RS, Uppal R, Malhi R, Behera D, Jindal SK. Drug interaction between rifampicin and co-trimoxazole in patients with tuberculosis. *Hum Exp Toxicol* (1991) 10, 419–21.

Co-trimoxazole + Salbutamol (Albuterol)

Salbutamol reduces the rate but increases the extent of sulfamethoxazole absorption.

Clinical evidence, mechanism, importance and management

In 6 healthy subjects, oral salbutamol 4 mg four times daily for 2 weeks had no effect on the pharmacokinetics of a single 400-mg oral dose of sulfamethoxazole (given as co-trimoxazole), although the absorption rate constant was reduced by about 40% and the extent of absorption over 72 hours was increased by 23%.[1] A possible reason for these effects is that salbutamol stimulates the beta receptors in the gut, causing relaxation, which allows an increased contact time, and therefore increased absorption of sulfamethoxazole.[1] The clinical significance of this interaction is unknown, but it seems unlikely to be of importance. No interaction would be expected with inhaled salbutamol.

1. Adebayo GI, Ogundipe TO. Effects of salbutamol on the absorption and disposition of sulphamethoxazole in adult volunteers. *Eur J Drug Metab Pharmacokinet* (1989) 14, 57–60.

Cycloserine + Ethionamide

Neurotoxic adverse effects may be potentiated by the concurrent use of cycloserine and ethionamide.

Clinical evidence, mechanism, importance and management

Three cases of encephalopathy have been reported in patients taking antimycobacterial regimens that included ethionamide (and in 2 cases, isoniazid): in one case symptoms occurred during the concurrent use of ethionamide and cycloserine. All 3 patients recovered after the withdrawal of either ethionamide (and isoniazid) or cycloserine, and treatment with nicotinamide and other vitamin B compounds.[1] The manufacturers note that the concurrent use of ethionamide can potentiate the neurotoxic adverse effects of cycloserine.[2,3] The US manufacturer of ethionamide notes that convulsions have been reported in patients also taking cycloserine and they recommend special care with treatment regimens that include both drugs.[4]

1. Swash M, Roberts AH, Murnaghan DJ. Reversible pellagra-like encephalopathy with ethionamide and cycloserine. *Tubercle* (1972) 53, 132–6.
2. Cycloserine. King Pharmaceuticals Ltd. UK Summary of product characteristics, March 2007.
3. Seromycin (Cycloserine). Eli Lilly and Company. US Prescribing information, April 2005.
4. Trecator (Ethionamide). Wyeth Pharmaceuticals Inc. US Prescribing information, November 2007.

Cycloserine + Isoniazid

The adverse CNS effects of cycloserine are increased by isoniazid.

Clinical evidence, mechanism, importance and management

A report describes both an increase and a decrease in serum cycloserine levels in some subjects, which were apparently caused by isoniazid; however, the mean level of cycloserine was not significantly changed. Only one out of 11 patients taking cycloserine alone developed adverse effects (drowsiness, dizziness, unstable gait), but when isoniazid was added, 9 of the 11 developed these effects.[1] The manufacturers recommend monitoring for these adverse effects if both drugs are given and adjusting the doses as necessary to manage them.[2,3]

1. Mattila MJ, Nieminen E, Tiitinen H. Serum levels, urinary excretion, and side-effects of cycloserine in the presence of isoniazid and p-aminosalicylic acid. *Scand J Respir Dis* (1969) 50, 291–300.
2. Cycloserine. King Pharmaceuticals Ltd. UK Summary of product characteristics, March 2007.
3. Seromycin (Cycloserine). Eli Lilly and Company. US Prescribing information, April 2005.

Cycloserine + Miscellaneous

Orange juice and an aluminium/magnesium hydroxide-containing antacid do not affect the pharmacokinetics of cycloserine, but a high-fat meal delays its absorption.

Clinical evidence, mechanism, importance and management

(a) Antacids

A study in 12 healthy subjects found that the bioavailability of a single 500-mg dose of cycloserine was not affected by 15 mL of an antacid containing **aluminium/magnesium hydroxide** and **simeticone** (*Mylanta*) was given 9 hours before the cycloserine, at the same time as the cycloserine, immediately after meals, and at bedtime on both the dosing day and the following day.[1]

(b) Food

A study in 12 healthy subjects found that the bioavailability of a single 500-mg dose of cycloserine was not significantly affected by 240 mL of **orange juice**.[1] When cycloserine 500 mg was given 15 minutes after the start of a high-fat meal, which was completed within 30 minutes, its AUC was not affected, but its maximum serum levels were reduced by about 16% and the time to maximum levels was increased from 45 minutes to 3.5 hours. The authors suggest that, in patients with relatively low plasma levels or patients receiving once rather than twice daily doses, it is possible that the delay in absorption could result in increased periods of sub-inhibitory levels.[1] However, there is no evidence to suggest that this is clinically significant.

1. Zhu M, Nix DE, Adam RD, Childs JM, Peloquin CA. Pharmacokinetics of cycloserine under fasting conditions and with high-fat meal, orange juice, and antacids. *Pharmacotherapy* (2001) 21, 891–7.

Dapsone + Antacids

The absorption of dapsone is unaltered by an antacid containing aluminium/magnesium hydroxide and/or simeticone.

Clinical evidence, mechanism, importance and management

A study to see whether changes in gastric pH might affect the absorption of dapsone found that when a single 100-mg dose of dapsone was taken with the second of 11 doses of **aluminium/magnesium hydroxide** and **simeticone** (*Mylanta II*), given every hour, the absorption of the dapsone remained unchanged. The mean gastric pH rose from 2.3 before using the antacid, to 4.5 or higher while taking dapsone and the antacid.[1] In another study, 8 subjects were given a single 100-mg dose of dapsone as a liquid oral preparation followed immediately by 12.5 mL of an **aluminium/magnesium hydroxide** antacid (*Maalox TC*). The peak plasma levels of dapsone were increased by about 11% and the time to peak levels was reduced from 1.9 hours to 1.3 hours. However, the dapsone AUC and elimination rate were not affected.[2] No special precautions would therefore seem to be needed if *Mylanta II*, *Maalox TC* or any other similar antacid is used with dapsone. See also 'NRTIs + Dapsone', p.971, for a discussion of the effects of the buffer in didanosine tablets on dapsone absorption.

1. Breen GA, Brocavich JM, Etzel JV, Shah V, Schaefer P, Forlenza S. Evaluation of effects of altered gastric pH on absorption of dapsone in healthy volunteers. *Antimicrob Agents Chemother* (1994) 38, 2227–9.
2. Mirochnick M, Breña A, McNamara ER, Clarke D, Pelton S. Effect of antacid on dapsone absorption. *Pediatr AIDS HIV Infect* (1993) 4, 13–16.

Dalbavancin + Miscellaneous

Dalbavancin pharmacokinetics are not affected by aztreonam, fentanyl, furosemide, metronidazole, midazolam, paracetamol (acetaminophen), simvastatin, or the proton pump inhibitors, esomeprazole, lansoprazole, omeprazole, or pantoprazole. Dalbavancin is not expected to alter the pharmacokinetics of drugs that are substrates of cytochrome P450 isoenzymes.

Clinical evidence, mechanism, importance and management

The US manufacturer of dalbavancin notes that dalbavancin is not a substrate of cytochrome P450 isoenzymes *in vitro*,[1] and therefore drugs that are inhibitors or inducers of these isoenzymes would not expected to alter the pharmacokinetics of dalbavancin by this mechanism. Dalbavancin pharmacokinetics were not altered by **aztreonam**, **fentanyl**, **furosemide**, **metronidazole**, **midazolam**, **paracetamol (acetaminophen)**, some proton pump inhibitors (namely **esomeprazole**, **lansoprazole**, **omeprazole**, or **pantoprazole**), and **simvastatin** in a population pharmacokinetic analysis.[1]

The US manufacturer also briefly notes that dalbavancin is not an inducer or an inhibitor of cytochrome P450 isoenzymes *in vitro*,[1] and it would therefore not be expected to alter the pharmacokinetics of drugs that are substrates of these isoenzymes by this mechanism.

1. Dalvance (Dalbavancin). Durata Therapeutics Inc. US Prescribing information, May 2014.

Dapsone + Clarithromycin

Clarithromycin does not alter the metabolism of dapsone.

Clinical evidence, mechanism, importance and management

A study in 12 healthy subjects given single 100-mg doses of dapsone before and after taking clarithromycin 1 g twice daily for 10 days, found that the clearance of dapsone was unchanged. Of equal importance was finding that the AUC of the *N*-hydroxylation metabolite of dapsone, which appears to be responsible for its haematological toxicity (methaemoglobinaemia), was also unchanged.[1]

In another study, 11 HIV-positive patients were given dapsone 100 mg daily then clarithromycin 500 mg twice daily for 2 weeks. Clarithromycin had no effect on dapsone clearance or on the production of the hydroxylamine metabolite of dapsone.[2] These results suggest that the cytochrome P450 isoenzyme CYP3A4, which is inhibited by clarithromycin, is not involved in dapsone metabolism.[2]

Clarithromycin would not be expected to alter the toxicity of dapsone, and no special precautions are required during concurrent use.

1. Occhipinti DJ, Choi A, Deyo K, Danziger LH, Fischer JH. Influence of rifampin and clarithromycin on dapsone (D) disposition and methemoglobin concentrations. *Clin Pharmacol Ther* (1995) 57, 163.
2. Winter HR, Trapnell CB, Slattery JT, Jacobson M, Greenspan DL, Hooton TM, Unadkat JD. The effect of clarithromycin, fluconazole, and rifabutin on dapsone hydroxylamine formation in individuals with human immunodeficiency virus infection (AACTG 283). *Clin Pharmacol Ther* (2004) 76, 579–87.

Dapsone + Clofazimine

Dapsone can reduce the anti-inflammatory effects of clofazimine. Clofazimine does not affect the pharmacokinetics of dapsone.

Clinical evidence, mechanism, importance and management

Fourteen out of 16 patients with severe recurrent erythema nodosum leprosum (ENL) did not respond adequately when given dapsone and clofazimine and needed additional treatment with corticosteroids. When the dapsone was stopped the patients responded to clofazimine alone, and in some instances the ENL was controlled by smaller doses.[1] Further evidence of this interaction comes from a laboratory study, which suggests that the actions of clofazimine may be related to its ability to inhibit neutrophil migration (resulting in decreased numbers of neutrophils in areas of inflammation), whereas dapsone can have the opposite effect.[1] Although the information is very limited, it would seem prudent to avoid the concurrent use of dapsone and clofazimine in the treatment of ENL. The authors of this report[1] are at great pains to emphasise that what they describe only relates to the effects of dapsone on the anti-inflammatory effects of clofazimine, and not to the beneficial effects of concurrent use when treating drug-resistant *Mycobacterium leprae*.

A study in patients taking clofazimine and dapsone[2] and 4 other studies in patients also taking isoniazid or rifampicin suggest that clofazimine does not affect the pharmacokinetics of dapsone.[3-6] However, one earlier study[7] found that clofazimine transiently increased the renal excretion of dapsone in 9 of 17 patients with leprosy who had recently discontinued dapsone.

1. Imkamp FMJH, Anderson R, Gatner EMS. Possible incompatibility of dapsone with clofazimine in the treatment of patients with erythema nodosum leprosum. *Lepr Rev* (1982) 53, 148–9.
2. George J, Balakrishnan S, Bhatia VN. Drug interaction during multidrug regimens for treatment of leprosy. *Indian J Med Res* (1988) 87, 151–6.
3. Venkatesan K, Mathur A, Girdhar BK, Bharadwaj VP. The effect of clofazimine on the pharmacokinetics of rifampicin and dapsone in leprosy. *J Antimicrob Chemother* (1986) 18, 715–18.
4. Pieters FAJM, Woonink F, Zuidema J. Influence of once-monthly rifampicin and daily clofazimine on the pharmacokinetics of dapsone in leprosy patients in Nigeria. *Eur J Clin Pharmacol* (1988) 34, 73–6.
5. Venkatesan K, Bharadwaj VP, Ramu R, Desikan KV. Study on drug interactions. *Lepr India* (1980) 52, 229–35.
6. Balakrishnan S, Seshadri PS. Drug interactions— the influence of rifampicin and clofazimine on the urinary excretion of DDS. *Lepr India* (1981) 53, 17–22.
7. Grabosz JAJ, Wheate HW. Effect of clofazimine on the urinary excretion of DDS (Dapsone). *Int J Lepr* (1975) 43, 61–2.

Dapsone + Drugs that affect gastric pH

Cimetidine raises serum dapsone levels, and may reduce methaemoglobinaemia due to the hydroxylamine metabolite of dapsone. Cimetidine, ranitidine and omeprazole do not appear to affect the outcome of dapsone prophylaxis against pneumocystis pneumonia. The absorption of dapsone does not appear to be altered by nizatidine-induced increases in gastric pH.

Clinical evidence, mechanism, importance and management

In 7 healthy subjects **cimetidine** 400 mg three times daily for 3 days increased the AUC of a single 100-mg dose of dapsone by 40%.[1] The probable reason for this effect is that the **cimetidine** (a known non-specific enzyme inhibitor) inhibits the metabolism of the dapsone by the liver. Although this might be expected to increase the risk of haematological adverse effects of dapsone by raising its serum levels, **cimetidine** also apparently markedly reduces the production of the hydroxylamine metabolite of dapsone (the AUC fell by more than half). Dapsone hydroxylamine appears to be responsible for the methaemoglobinaemia and haemolysis that may occur with dapsone.[1] These findings were later confirmed in 6 patients taking long-term dapsone 75 to 350 mg daily who were given **cimetidine** 1.2 g daily for 2 weeks. Steady-state serum dapsone levels rose by about 47%, accompanied by a fall in serum methaemoglobin levels from 7.1% to 5.2% (reference range less than 2%) in the first week.[2] Similar findings were reported in a further 3-month study in 8 patients.[3] However, a sustained decrease in methaemoglobin was not seen, with levels returning to baseline at week 12, despite the continued use of **cimetidine**.[3] Another report based on a small number of patients, comparing those given **cimetidine**, **ranitidine** or **omeprazole** with those not taking acid suppression, found no difference in the outcome of dapsone prophylaxis for pneumocystis pneumonia in HIV-positive patients.[4] A study in healthy subjects found that the increase in pH produced by **nizatidine** did not result in any clinically significant changes in the rate or extent of dapsone absorption.[5] It would therefore seem that no additional precautions are needed if H_2-receptor antagonists or proton pump inhibitors are given to patients taking dapsone. Consider also 'Dapsone + Antacids', p.318.

1. Coleman MD, Scott AK, Breckenridge AM, Park BK. The use of cimetidine as a selective inhibitor of dapsone *N*-hydroxylation in man. *Br J Clin Pharmacol* (1990) 30, 761–7.
2. Coleman MD, Rhodes LE, Scott AK, Verbov JL, Friedmann PS, Breckenridge AM, Park BK. The use of cimetidine to reduce dapsone-dependent methaemoglobinaemia in dermatitis herpetiformis patients. *Br J Clin Pharmacol* (1992) 34, 244–9.
3. Rhodes LE, Tingle MD, Park BK, Chu P, Verbov JL, Friedmann PS. Cimetidine improves the therapeutic/toxic ratio of dapsone in patients on chronic dapsone therapy. *Br J Dermatol* (1995) 132, 257–62.
4. Huengsberg M, Castelino S, Sherrard J, O'Farrell N, Bingham J. Does drug interaction cause failure of PCP prophylaxis with dapsone? *Lancet* (1993) 341, 48.
5. Itokazu GA, Fischer JH, Manitpisitkul P, Hariharan R, Danziger LH. Lack of effect of nizatidine-induced elevation of gastric pH on the oral bioavailability of dapsone in healthy volunteers. *Pharmacotherapy* (2002) 22, 1420–5.

Dapsone + Fluconazole

Fluconazole decreases the production of the toxic metabolite of dapsone, and might therefore reduce the incidence of adverse reactions to dapsone.

Clinical evidence, mechanism, importance and management

Twelve HIV-positive patients were given dapsone 100 mg daily for 2 weeks and then in random order either fluconazole 200 mg daily, rifabutin 300 mg daily or fluconazole with rifabutin, each for 2 weeks. Dapsone pharmacokinetics were unaffected by fluconazole. However, fluconazole inhibited the production of the *N*-hydroxylamine metabolite of dapsone (AUC, urinary recovery, and formation clearance reduced by about 50%).[1]

Hydroxylamine is assumed to be responsible for the haematological toxicity of dapsone (methaemoglobinaemia). The findings of this study suggest that the production of this metabolite is mediated by the cytochrome P450 isoenzyme CYP2C9, which fluconazole inhibits.

On the basis of these results, fluconazole would not be expected to alter the efficacy of dapsone, but might reduce its toxicity. Further study is needed to assess this potential.

1. Winter HR, Trapnell CB, Slattery JT, Jacobson M, Greenspan DL, Hooton TM, Unadkat JD. The effect of clarithromycin, fluconazole, and rifabutin on dapsone hydroxylamine formation in individuals with human immunodeficiency virus infection (AACTG 283). *Clin Pharmacol Ther* (2004) 76, 579–87.

Dapsone + Probenecid

The serum levels of dapsone can be markedly raised by probenecid.

Clinical evidence

Twelve patients with quiescent tuberculoid leprosy were given dapsone 300 mg with probenecid 500 mg, and 5 hours later another 300-mg dose of dapsone. At 4 hours, the dapsone serum levels were raised by about 50%. The urinary excretion of dapsone and its metabolites were reduced.[1]

Mechanism

Not fully examined. It seems probable that the probenecid inhibits the renal excretion of dapsone by the kidney.

Importance and management

The documentation is very limited. It is likely that the probenecid will raise the serum levels of dapsone given long-term. The importance of this is uncertain, but the extent of the rise and evidence that the haematological toxicity of dapsone may be related to dapsone levels[2] suggests that it may well have some clinical importance. It would therefore seem prudent to monitor for dapsone adverse effects if probenecid is also given.

1. Goodwin CS, Sparell G. Inhibition of dapsone excretion by probenecid. *Lancet* (1969) ii, 884–5.
2. Ellard GA, Gammon PT, Savin JA, Tan RS-H. Dapsone acetylation in dermatitis herpetiformis. *Br J Dermatol* (1974) 90, 441–4.

Dapsone + Proguanil

No pharmacokinetic interaction appears to occur between dapsone and proguanil, and they have been successfully used together for malaria prophylaxis.

Clinical evidence, mechanism, importance and management

A study in 6 healthy subjects found that proguanil 200 mg daily had no effect on the pharmacokinetics of dapsone 10 mg daily, nor on its principal metabolite, monoacetyldapsone. The authors of this report are extremely cautious because, despite this lack of a pharmacokinetic interaction at these doses, they say that increased dapsone toxicity cannot be ruled out.[1] However, dapsone 25 mg was successfully used with proguanil 200 mg daily for malaria prophylaxis in the Vietnam war,[2] and the same regimen, but with the dapsone dose every third day was successful as prophylaxis against proguanil-resistant falciparum malaria in Papua New Guinea.[1] Moreover, a different dose (dapsone 4 or 12.5 mg with proguanil 200 mg daily), was well tolerated over a period of 80 days when used as malaria prophylaxis in Thailand.[3]

1. Edstein MD, Rieckmann KH. Lack of effect of proguanil on the pharmacokinetics of dapsone in healthy volunteers. *Chemotherapy* (1993) 39, 235–41.
2. Black RH. Malaria in the Australian army in South Vietnam. Successful use of a proguanil-dapsone combination for chemoprophylaxis of chloroquine-resistant falciparum malaria. *Med J Aust* (1973) 1, 1265–70.
3. Shanks GD, Edstein MD, Suriyamongkol V, Timsaad S, Webster HK. Malaria prophylaxis using proguanil/dapsone combinations on the Thai-Cambodian border. *Am J Trop Med Hyg* (1992) 46, 643–8.

Dapsone + Pyrimethamine

Pyrimethamine does not significantly affect the pharmacokinetics of dapsone.

Clinical evidence, mechanism, importance and management

A study in 7 healthy subjects given single doses of dapsone 100 mg, pyrimethamine 25 mg, or both drugs together found that the peak plasma levels of dapsone fell by 17%, its half-life was unchanged, and the apparent volume of distribution was increased by 26% (from 1.53 to 1.93 L/kg). The pharmacokinetics of pyrimethamine were not affected by dapsone.[1] In another study HIV-positive patients were given dapsone 200 mg weekly (the maximum tolerated dose) either alone or with pyrimethamine 25 mg weekly. In contrast to the earlier study, there was a *decrease* in the volume of distribution of dapsone when it was given with pyrimethamine, although dapsone levels were not significantly altered.[2] Furthermore, the tolerability of once-weekly dapsone with pyrimethamine was found to be similar to that of once-weekly dapsone alone.[2]

1. Ahmad RA, Rogers HJ. Pharmacokinetics and protein binding interactions of dapsone and pyrimethamine. *Br J Clin Pharmacol* (1980) 10, 519–24.
2. Falloon J, Lavelle J, Ogata-Arakaki D, Byrne A, Graziani A, Morgan A, Amantea MA, Ownby K, Polis M, Davey RT, Kovacs JA, Lane HC, Masur H, MacGregor RR. Pharmacokinetics and safety of weekly dapsone and dapsone plus pyrimethamine for prevention of pneumocystis pneumonia. *Antimicrob Agents Chemother* (1994) 38, 1580–7.

Dapsone + Rifamycins

Rifampicin (rifampin) increases the urinary excretion of dapsone, lowers its serum levels and increases the risk of toxicity (methaemoglobinaemia). Similarly, rifabutin increases the clearance of dapsone, and may also increase its toxicity.

Clinical evidence

(a) Rifabutin

Twelve HIV-positive patients were given dapsone 100 mg daily for 2 weeks and then, in random order, either rifabutin 300 mg daily, fluconazole 200 mg daily, or fluconazole with rifabutin, each for 2 weeks. Rifabutin alone increased the clearance of dapsone by 67%. When combined with fluconazole, rifabutin increased the clearance of dapsone by 38%, which shows that fluconazole (a known enzyme inhibitor) partially attenuates the enzyme-inducing effects of rifabutin. Rifabutin increased the formation clearance of dapsone by 92%, which was again attenuated by fluconazole. Rifabutin did not affect the AUC of the hydroxylamine metabolite of dapsone, which is thought to be associated with dapsone toxicity.[1]

Similarly, in a population analysis of 60 HIV-positive children, 7 of whom were also receiving rifabutin, factors associated with increased dapsone clearance included rifabutin use. It was suggested that dapsone clearance was increased by 38 to 50% in these children.[2]

(b) Rifampicin (Rifampin)

A study in 7 patients with leprosy given single doses of dapsone 100 mg and rifampicin 600 mg, alone or together, found that while the pharmacokinetics of rifampicin were not significantly changed, the half-life of dapsone was roughly halved and the AUC was reduced by about 20%.[3] Other studies in patients given both drugs for several days, similarly found reduced dapsone serum levels and an increased urinary excretion.[4-8] Likewise, a study in HIV-positive adults also found lowered dapsone levels in the presence of rifampicin.[9] Another study in 12 healthy subjects given a single 100-mg dose of dapsone before and after taking rifampicin 600 mg daily for 10 days, found that the clearance of dapsone was increased more than 3.5-fold (from 2.01 to 7.17 L/hour). Of equal importance was the finding that the production of the hydroxylamine metabolite of dapsone, which appears to be responsible for the haematological toxicity (methaemoglobinaemia), was markedly increased. The 24-hour AUC of methaemoglobin was increased by more than 60%,[10] suggesting that this interaction increases dapsone toxicity.

Mechanism

Rifampicin and rifabutin increase the metabolism and clearance of dapsone. Rifampicin also increases the blood levels of the toxic hydroxylamine metabolite of dapsone. Similarly, rifabutin increased the formation of this metabolite, although increases in the AUC were not seen.

Importance and management

The interaction between dapsone and rifampicin is established but of uncertain clinical importance. Concurrent use should be well monitored to confirm that treatment is effective. It may be necessary to raise the dose of dapsone. It has been pointed out that there is the risk of treatment failures for pneumocystis pneumonia as well as for leprosy.[11] Also be alert for any evidence of methaemoglobinaemia.

Although there is less information, rifabutin appears to interact similarly to rifampicin. When dapsone is given with rifabutin, the dose of dapsone may need to be increased, but this may increase exposure to the potentially toxic hydroxylamine metabolite.[1]

1. Winter HR, Trapnell CB, Slattery JT, Jacobson M, Greenspan DL, Hooton TM, Unadkat JD. The effect of clarithromycin, fluconazole, and rifabutin on dapsone hydroxylamine formation in individuals with human immunodeficiency virus infection (AACTG 283). *Clin Pharmacol Ther* (2004) 76, 579–87.
2. Mirochnick M, Cooper E, Capparelli E, McIntosh K, Lindsey J, Xu J, Jacobus D, Mofenson L, Bonagura VR, Nachman S, Yogev R, Sullivan JL, Spector SA. Population pharmacokinetics of dapsone in children with human immunodeficiency virus infection. *Clin Pharmacol Ther* (2001) 70, 24–32.
3. Krishna DR, Appa Rao AVN, Ramanakar TV, Prabhakar MC. Pharmacokinetic interaction between dapsone and rifampicin in leprosy patients. *Drug Dev Ind Pharm* (1986) 12, 443–59.
4. Balakrishnan S, Seshadri PS. Drug interactions – the influence of rifampicin and clofazimine on the urinary excretion of DDS. *Lepr India* (1981) 53, 17–22.
5. Peters JH, Murray JF, Gordon GR, Gelber RH, Laing ABG, Waters MFR. Effect of rifampin on the disposition of dapsone in Malaysian leprosy patients. *Fedn Proc* (1977) 36, 996.
6. George J, Balakrishnan S, Bhatia VN. Drug interaction during multidrug regimens for treatment of leprosy. *Indian J Med Res* (1988) 87, 151–6.
7. Pieters FAJM, Woonink F, Zuidema J. Influence of once-monthly rifampicin and daily clofazimine on the pharmacokinetics of dapsone in leprosy patients in Nigeria. *Eur J Clin Pharmacol* (1988) 34, 73–6.
8. Venkatesan K, Bharadwaj VP, Ramu G, Desikan KV. Study on drug interactions. *Lepr India* (1980) 52, 229–35.
9. Gatti G, Merighi M, Hossein J, Travaini S, Casazza R, Karlsson M, Cruciani M, Bassetti D. Population pharmacokinetics of dapsone administered biweekly to human immunodeficiency virus-infected patients. *Antimicrob Agents Chemother* (1996) 40, 2743–8.
10. Occhipinti DJ, Choi A, Deyo K, Danziger LH, Fischer JH. Influence of rifampin and clarithromycin on dapsone (D) disposition and methemoglobin concentrations. *Clin Pharmacol Ther* (1995) 57, 163.
11. Jorde UP, Horowitz HW, Wormser GP. Significance of drug interactions with rifampin in *Pneumocystis carinii* pneumonia prophylaxis. *Arch Intern Med* (1992) 152, 2348.

Dapsone + Trimethoprim

The serum levels of both dapsone and trimethoprim are possibly raised by concurrent oral use. Both increased efficacy and dapsone toxicity have been seen. Topical dapsone levels are also raised by trimethoprim given as co-trimoxazole.

Clinical evidence

Eighteen patients with AIDS, treated for pneumocystis pneumonia and taking dapsone 100 mg daily, were compared with 30 other patients taking dapsone with trimethoprim 20 mg/kg daily. Trimethoprim raised dapsone levels by 40% (from 1.5 to 2.1 micrograms/mL), at 7 days (steady-state). Dapsone toxicity (methaemoglobinaemia) was also increased.[1] Trimethoprim plasma levels were 48% higher in the 30 patients also taking dapsone when compared with another group of 30 patients given co-trimoxazole (trimethoprim with sulfamethoxazole), but the incidence of toxicity was higher in the co-trimoxazole group.[1] However, a later study by the same authors in 8 asymptomatic HIV-positive patients given dapsone 100 mg daily and trimethoprim 200 mg every 12 hours found that the steady-state pharmacokinetics of each drug was unaffected by the other, although the single dose pharmacokinetics indicated higher serum levels than at steady state for both drugs.[2]

A study in 17 patients with acne vulgaris who applied dapsone 5% gel topically, and took co-trimoxazole (trimethoprim with sulfamethoxazole) 960 mg twice daily, found no significant change in the pharmacokinetics of either trimethoprim or sulfamethoxazole. In contrast, the AUC and maximum plasma level of dapsone were increased by 45% and 39%, respectively. Further, the AUC and maximum plasma level of dapsone hydroxylamine, the metabolite responsible for the haematological adverse effects, were increased by 145% and 113%, respectively. However, these parameters were still lower than would be expected after an oral dose of dapsone 100 mg.[3]

Mechanism

Not understood. Dapsone and trimethoprim appear to have mutually inhibitory effects on clearance.

Importance and management

Information is limited. The difference between the results of the two studies using oral dapsone may be because the first was in patients with AIDS and pneumocystis pneumonia and the second was in asymptomatic HIV-positive patients whose drug metabolism may possibly be different. Concurrent use appears to be an effective form of treatment, but be alert for evidence of increased dapsone toxicity (methaemoglobinaemia). No adverse effects would be expected if topical dapsone is given with oral trimethoprim or co-trimoxazole.

1. Lee BL, Medina I, Benowitz NL, Jacob P, Wofsy CB, Mills J. Dapsone, trimethoprim, and sulfamethoxazole plasma levels during treatment of pneumocystis pneumonia in patients with acquired immunodeficiency syndrome (AIDS). *Ann Intern Med* (1989) 110, 606–11.
2. Lee BL, Safrin S, Makrides V, Gambertoglio JG. Zidovudine, trimethoprim, and dapsone pharmacokinetic interactions in patients with human immunodeficiency virus infection. *Antimicrob Agents Chemother* (1996) 40, 1231–6.
3. Thiboutot DM, Willmer J, Sharata H, Halder R, Garrett S. Pharmacokinetics of dapsone gel, 5% for the treatment of acne vulgaris. *Clin Pharmacokinet* (2007) 46, 697–712.

Dapsone + Ursodeoxycholic acid (Ursodiol)

A single case suggests that the effectiveness of dapsone in the treatment of dermatitis herpetiformis may be reduced by ursodeoxycholic acid.

Clinical evidence, mechanism, importance and management

A 61-year-old man taking dapsone 50 mg daily for dermatitis herpetiformis started taking ursodeoxycholic acid 450 mg twice daily for cholecystitis. Two weeks later the dermatitis herpetiformis worsened and the dose of dapsone was increased to 150 mg daily. However, his condition did not improve, so ursodeoxycholic acid was stopped and, as his condition improved, the dapsone dose was reduced to 100 mg, and then 50 mg daily. Two months later ursodeoxycholic acid was restarted and there was again an exacerbation of the dermatitis herpetiformis.[1] This case appears to have also been published elsewhere.[2] The general importance of this isolated report is unknown, but consider the possibility of reduced dapsone effects if ursodeoxycholic acid is also given.

1. Stroubou E, Dawn G, Forsyth A. Ursodeoxycholic acid causing exacerbation of dermatitis herpetiformis. *J Am Acad Dermatol* (2001) 45, 319–20.
2. Schmutz J-L, Barbaud A, Trechot PH. Interaction acide ursodéoxycholique-dapsone. *Ann Dermatol Venereol* (2003) 130, 391.

Daptomycin + Aminoglycosides

The pharmacokinetics of daptomycin are not altered by gentamicin or tobramycin. The pharmacokinetics of tobramycin are not altered by daptomycin.

Clinical evidence, mechanism, importance and management

(a) Gentamicin

In a crossover study in 11 healthy subjects who were given intravenous daptomycin 6 mg/kg daily for 3 days with 1 mg/kg gentamicin given every 8 hours starting after the second dose of daptomycin, there were no clinically significant changes in the pharmacokinetics of daptomycin.[1] No daptomycin dose adjustment therefore seems necessary on concurrent use.

(b) Tobramycin

In a crossover study, 6 healthy subjects were given daptomycin 2 mg/kg, tobramycin 1 mg/kg, or both drugs together. There was no change in the pharmacokinetics of either drug.[2] No dose adjustment of either drug would be expected to be necessary on concurrent use.

1. DeRyke CA, Sutherland C, Zhang B, Nicolau DP, Kuti JL. Serum bactericidal activities of high-dose daptomycin with and without coadministration of gentamicin against isolates of *Staphylococcus aureus* and *Enterococcus* species. *Antimicrob Agents Chemother* (2006) 50, 3529–3534.
2. Woodworth JR, Nyhart EH, Wolny JD, Brier GL, Black HR. Tobramycin and daptomycin disposition when co-administered to healthy volunteers. *J Antimicrob Chemother* (1994) 33, 655–9.

Daptomycin + Miscellaneous

The use of statins, probably fibrates and possibly ciclosporin with daptomycin may increase the risk of muscle toxicity. Daptomycin does not appear to interact with warfarin, but its use may result in falsely elevated prothrombin times. NSAIDs may reduce daptomycin excretion and concurrent use may increase the risks of renal impairment. Probenecid and aztreonam do not appear to affect the pharmacokinetics of daptomycin.

Clinical evidence, mechanism, importance and management

(a) Drugs causing myopathy

The US manufacturers describe a study in 20 healthy subjects taking **simvastatin** 40 mg daily, in which the addition of daptomycin 4 mg/kg per day for 14 days did not result in an increase in adverse effects, when compared with subjects given placebo. In contrast, in a phase III study of patients with bacteraemia, 5 out of 22 patients who were currently, or had recently, been taking a **statin** developed raised creatinine phosphokinase levels.[1] Furthermore, a case report describes a patient who was given daptomycin 6.5 mg/kg daily, who developed muscle pain and a raised creatinine phosphokinase level (20 771 units/L). He had been taking **simvastatin**, but this had been discontinued when the daptomycin was started.[2] It is difficult to know whether this was a result of an interaction as another case of rhabdomyolysis (creatinine phosphokinase 21 243 units/L) was attributed to the use of daptomycin alone: the patient was taking no other drugs known to cause myopathy (fibrates and statins specifically mentioned).[3] A review of patients with Gram-positive complicated skin and skin structure infections found that musculoskeletal pain or myalgia occurred in up to 0.4% of patients. In patients with similar infections treated with daptomycin the incidence of myopathy was slightly higher, at 0.2 to 0.9%,[4] suggesting that daptomycin may modestly increase the risk of muscle toxicity.

The manufacturers note that experience of the concurrent use of daptomycin with statins is limited, and therefore the use of a statin should be suspended if daptomycin is given,[1,5] unless the benefits of concurrent use outweigh the risks, in which case the patient's creatine kinase should be monitored more frequently than weekly.[5] See also *Muscle and liver toxicity*, under 'Lipid regulating drugs', p.1309, for further guidance on monitoring for statin-associated myopathy, and risk factors for muscle toxicity. The UK manufacturers give the same guidance for **fibrates** and **ciclosporin**, both of which have been associated with myopathy.[1]

(b) NSAIDs

The UK manufacturers note that NSAIDs (including coxibs) may reduce the renal excretion of daptomycin and have additive detrimental effects on renal function if used with daptomycin.[5] They advise caution on concurrent use, which in practice probably means keeping a close eye on renal function and monitoring for possible daptomycin adverse effects.

(c) Warfarin

The US manufacturers describe a study in 16 healthy subjects in which daptomycin 6 mg/kg daily for 5 days did not affect either the pharmacokinetics or the INR in response to a single 25-mg dose of warfarin. The pharmacokinetics of daptomycin were also unchanged.[1] However, as experience is limited the manufacturers advise monitoring the INR for the first few days of concurrent use. Note that daptomycin causes a concentration-dependent false prolongation of the prothrombin time.[1,5] This only appears to occur with recombinant thromboplastin reagents. Blood for INR testing should therefore be drawn during the daptomycin trough (i.e. immediately before the next dose). If a raised INR is found it is recommended that the INR should be re-tested, and alternative methods of monitoring should be considered.[1]

(d) Miscellaneous

The US manufacturers[1] briefly mention a small study in which daptomycin was given with **aztreonam** without any significant change in the pharmacokinetics of either drug. They also mention a study in which **probenecid** did not alter the pharmacokinetics of daptomycin.

1. Cubicin (Daptomycin). Cubist Pharmaceuticals, Inc. US Prescribing information, August 2008.
2. Echevarria K, Datta P, Cadena J, Lewis JS. Severe myopathy and possible hepatotoxicity related to daptomycin. *J Antimicrob Chemother* (2005) 55, 599–600.
3. Kazory A, Dibadj, K, Weiner ID. Rhabdomyolysis and acute renal failure in a patient treated with daptomycin. *J Antimicrob Chemother* (2006) 57, 578–9.
4. Fenton C, Keating GM, Curran MP. Daptomycin. *Drugs* (2004) 64, 445–55.
5. Cubicin (Daptomycin). Novartis Pharmaceuticals UK Ltd. UK Summary of product characteristics, July 2009.

Delamanid + Miscellaneous

Rifampicin appears to slightly decrease the exposure to delamanid. Other potent CYP3A4 inducers might interact similarly. Lopinavir boosted with ritonavir appears to slightly increase the exposure to a major metabolite of delamanid. Other potent CYP3A4 inhibitors might be expected to interact similarly. Food appears to greatly increase the absorption of delamanid. Delamanid does not appear to alter the exposure to rifampicin, lopinavir, ritonavir, isoniazid, or pyrazinamide, but might increase the plasma concentration of ethambutol. There appears to be no pharmacokinetic interaction between delamanid and efavirenz or tenofovir.

Clinical evidence, mechanism, importance and management

(a) CYP3A4 inducers

The UK manufacturer briefly reports that, in studies in healthy subjects, the exposure to delamanid 200 mg daily was decreased up to 45% by **rifampicin (rifampin)** 300 mg daily for 15 days (when given with isoniazid and pyrazinamide).[1] CYP3A4 appears to have a minor role in the metabolism of delamanid, and rifampicin is a well-known potent enzyme inducer. It can therefore induce CYP3A4 and decrease the exposure of delamanid, albeit only slightly. Despite such a small decrease in exposure, the UK manufacturer contraindicates the use of potent inducers of CYP3A4 with delamanid.[1] For a list of known, clinically relevant CYP3A4 inducers see 'Table 1.9', p.11. No clinically relevant decrease in delamanid exposure was observed with the moderate CYP3A4 inducer **efavirenz** when administered at a dose of 600 mg daily for 10 days in combination with delamanid 100 mg twice daily.[1] Note also, that the exposure of **rifampicin** and **efavirenz** in these studies, was not altered.[1]

(b) CYP3A4 inhibitors

The UK manufacturer briefly reports that, **lopinavir** boosted with **ritonavir** 400/100 mg twice daily increased the AUC of the delamanid metabolite, DM-6705, by 30% when it was given with delamanid 100 mg twice daily.[1] DM-6705 is metabolised by CYP3A4 and as it has been associated with QT interval prolongation (see 'Drugs that prolong the QT interval + Other drugs that prolong the QT interval', p.272), the UK manufacturer recommends that if concurrent use of delamanid with a potent inhibitor of CYP3A4 is necessary, very frequent ECG monitoring should be undertaken throughout the full delamanid treatment period.[1] For a list of known, clinically relevant CYP3A4 inhibitors, see 'Table 1.9', p.11. Note also, that the exposure of **lopinavir** and **ritonavir** in this study was not altered.[1]

(c) Food

The UK manufacturer briefly reports that a standard meal increased the bioavailability of delamanid about 2.7-fold, when compared with the fasted state. Delamanid should therefore be given with food.[1]

(d) Other drugs

The UK manufacturer briefly reports that in studies in healthy subjects, exposure to delamanid 100 mg twice daily was not altered by **tenofovir** 300 mg daily for 14 days, and the exposure to tenofovir was also not altered. In another study, delamanid 200 mg daily increased steady-state plasma concentrations of **ethambutol** 1100 mg daily by about 25%, but had no effect on the exposure of **isoniazid** 720 mg daily or of **pyrazinamide** 1800 mg daily (when also given with rifampicin). The clinical relevance of this increase in ethambutol concentration is unknown,[1] but given that it is only minor it might not be expected to be important.

1. Deltyba (Delamanid). Otsuka Novel Products GmbH. UK Summary of product characteristics, July 2014.

Ethambutol + Antacids

Aluminium hydroxide and aluminium/magnesium hydroxide can cause a small reduction in the absorption of ethambutol in some patients.

Clinical evidence, mechanism, importance and management

A study in 13 patients with tuberculosis, given a single 50-mg/kg dose of ethambutol, found that when they were also given three 1.5-g doses of **aluminium hydroxide gel** (at the same time and 15 and 30 minutes later) their peak serum ethambutol levels were delayed and reduced. The average urinary excretion of ethambutol over a 10-hour period was reduced by about 15%, but there were marked variations between individual patients. In some patients there was no interaction, and the absorption of ethambutol was even increased in others.[1] No interaction was seen in 6 healthy subjects similarly treated.[1] A further study in 14 healthy subjects found that 30 mL of an **aluminium/magnesium hydroxide** antacid decreased the AUC and maximum serum levels of a 25-mg/kg dose of ethambutol by 10% and 29%, respectively.[2]

The reason for this interaction is not understood, but **aluminium hydroxide** can affect gastric emptying. The reduction in absorption is generally small and variable, and it seems doubtful if it will have a significant effect on the treatment of tuberculosis. However, the authors of the second study suggest avoiding giving antacids at the same time as ethambutol,[2] and the US manufacturer states that **aluminium hydroxide**-containing antacids should not be taken until 4 hours after a dose of ethambutol.[3]

1. Mattila MJ, Linnoila M, Seppälä T, Koskinen R. Effect of aluminium hydroxide and glycopyrrhonium on the absorption of ethambutol and alcohol in man. *Br J Clin Pharmacol* (1978) 5, 161–6.
2. Peloquin CA, Bulpitt AE, Jaresko GS, Jelliffe RW, Childs JM, Nix DE. Pharmacokinetics of ethambutol under fasting conditions, with food, and with antacids. *Antimicrob Agents Chemother* (1999) 43, 568–72.
3. Myambutol (Ethambutol). X-Gen Pharmaceuticals Inc. US Prescribing information, April 2012.

Ethambutol + Food

The pharmacokinetics of ethambutol given with a high-fat breakfast were only slightly different to its pharmacokinetics when it is given in the fasting state.[1] Therefore ethambutol may be given without regard to meals.

1. Peloquin CA, Bulpitt AE, Jaresko GS, Jelliffe RW, Childs JM, Nix DE. Pharmacokinetics of ethambutol under fasting conditions, with food, and with antacids. *Antimicrob Agents Chemother* (1999) 43, 568–72.

Ethambutol + Rifabutin

Rifabutin does not appear to affect the pharmacokinetics of ethambutol.

Clinical evidence, mechanism, importance and management

Ten healthy subjects were given a single 1.2-g dose of ethambutol before and after taking rifabutin 300 mg daily for a week. No clinically relevant changes in the pharmacokinetics of ethambutol were seen.[1] Although 5 of the subjects experienced moderate to severe chills, and one had transient thrombocytopenia, these reactions are unlikely to have been due to an interaction. No special precautions would appear to be necessary during concurrent use.

1. Breda M, Benedetti MS, Bani M, Pellizzoni C, Poggesi I, Brianceschi G, Rocchetti M, Dolfi L, Sassella D, Rimoldi R. Effect of rifabutin on ethambutol pharmacokinetics in healthy volunteers. *Pharmacol Res* (1999) 40, 351–6.

Ethionamide + Isoniazid

Isoniazid may contribute to acute psychotic reactions associated with ethionamide, but evidence for this is limited.

Clinical evidence, mechanism, importance and management

Acute psychotic reactions occurring during treatment with either isoniazid or ethionamide are reported to be uncommon.[1] Acute mania occurred in a patient taking streptomycin, isoniazid and prednisolone for 4 months, and ethionamide and pyrazinamide for 27 days. It was thought that ethionamide was probably responsible for the psychotic reaction but that isoniazid and prednisolone may have potentiated the reaction.[2] In another patient, ethionamide was considered to be responsible for psychological changes, which resolved when the drug was stopped. However, the contribution of alcohol and other concurrent drugs such as isoniazid was not ruled out.[3] One study in patients found that ethionamide 750 mg increased the serum levels of a single 10-mg/kg dose of isoniazid at 4 hours but not at one or 10 hours, but this was not considered to be of therapeutic significance[4] and the toxic symptoms reported with the combination[5,6] were considered not to be due to increased isoniazid levels.[4]

A clinically significant interaction therefore seems unlikely, but as both drugs can, rarely, cause psychotic reactions these tentative reports cannot entirely be dismissed.

1. Sharma GS, Gupta PK, Jain NK, Shanker A, Nanawati V. Toxic psychosis to isoniazid and ethionamide in a patient with pulmonary tuberculosis. *Tubercle* (1979) 60, 171–2.
2. Narang RK. Acute psychotic reaction probably caused by ethionamide. *Tubercle* (1972) 137–8.
3. Lansdown FS, Beran M, Litwak T. Psychotoxic reaction during ethionamide therapy. *Am Rev Respir Dis* (1967) 95,1053–5.
4. Tiitinen H. Isoniazid and ethionamide serum levels and inactivation in Finnish subjects. *Scand J Respir Dis* (1969) 50, 110–24.
5. Brouet G, Marche J, Rist N, Chevallier J, LeMeur G. Observations on the antituberculous effectiveness of alpha-ethyl-thioisonicotinamide in tuberculosis in humans. *Am Rev Tuberc* (1959) 79, 6–18.
6. Trendelenburg F. Antibakterielle chemotherapie der tuberkulose. *Fortschr Arzneimittelforsch* (1964) 7, 193–303.

Ethionamide + Miscellaneous

A study in 12 healthy subjects found that the bioavailability of a single 500-mg dose of ethionamide was not significantly affected by food, orange juice or antacids, when compared with ethionamide bioavailability under fasting conditions. It was suggested that ethionamide may be given with food if tolerance is a problem.[1] The US manufacturer of ethionamide advises that it may be taken without regard to meals.[2]

1. Auclair B, Nix DE, Adam RD, James GT, Peloquin CA. Pharmacokinetics of ethionamide administered under fasting conditions or with orange juice, food, or antacids. *Antimicrob Agents Chemother* (2001) 45, 810–4.
2. Trecator (Ethionamide). Wyeth Pharmaceuticals Inc. US Prescribing information, November 2007.

Fidaxomicin + Miscellaneous

Ciclosporin increases the exposure to fidaxomicin, and other P-glycoprotein inhibitors might interact similarly. Food does not affect the absorption of fidaxomicin. Fidaxomicin has no effect on the pharmacokinetics of midazolam, omeprazole, or warfarin, and is predicted not to affect the pharmacokinetics of other substrates of CYP3A4, CYP2C19, or CYP2C9. Fidaxomicin has no effect on the pharmacokinetics of digoxin, but might possibly affect the exposure to dabigatran.

Clinical evidence, mechanism, importance and management

Note that fidaxomicin has minimal systemic absorption following oral administration and has a local action in the gut.[1,2]

(a) Ciclosporin

The UK and US manufacturers of fidaxomicin briefly report that, in a single-dose study in 14 healthy subjects, ciclosporin 200 mg given one hour before fidaxomicin 200 mg increased the AUC and maximum plasma concentration of fidaxomicin 4-fold and 2-fold, respectively. The AUC and maximum plasma concentration of the principle, active metabolite of fidaxomicin, OP-1118, were increased 9.5-fold and 4-fold, respectively.[1,2] Fidaxomicin and its active metabolite, OP-1118, are substrates of the drug transporter protein P-glycoprotein, which is inhibited by ciclosporin, concurrent use therefore results in an increase in their exposure. The US manufacturer comments that there was no attributable effect on safety or treatment outcomes after the concurrent use of a P-glycoprotein inhibitor use in controlled clinical studies, and therefore fidaxomicin can be given with P-glycoprotein inhibitors, without adjusting the dose.[1] In contrast, the UK manufacturer states that the clinical relevance of the increases in exposure is not known, and as such the concurrent use of fidaxomicin and potent inhibitors of P-glycoprotein is not recommended, and they name **amiodarone**, **ciclosporin**, **dronedarone**, **ketoconazole**, the macrolides **erythromycin** and **clarithromycin**, and **verapamil**.[2] For a list of P-glycoprotein inhibitors, see 'Table 1.12', p.14.

(b) Food

The UK and US manufacturers briefly report that, in a study in 28 healthy subjects, giving fidaxomicin with a high-fat meal resulted in decreases in the maximum plasma concentration of fidaxomicin and its active metabolite, OP-1118, of 22% and 33%, respectively, when compared with the fasting state, but had no effect on their AUCs and no clinically relevant effect on their maximum plasma concentrations. Fidaxomicin can therefore be given with or without food.[1,2]

(c) Other drugs

The US manufacturer briefly reports that, in clinical studies, **digoxin**, **midazolam**, **omeprazole**, and **warfarin** were given with fidaxomicin to assess the effect of fidaxomicin on P-glycoprotein, CYP3A4, CYP2C19, and CYP2C9, respectively. Fidaxomicin had no effect on the pharmacokinetics of any of these substrates, and so they state that no dose adjustment is necessary if fidaxomicin is administered with substrates of P-glycoprotein, CYP3A4, CYP2C19, or CYP2C9.[1]

The UK manufacturer notes that, although fidaxomicin 200 mg twice daily had a small, but not clinically relevant effect, on the exposure to digoxin, a known probe substrate for P-glycoprotein, a larger effect on other P-glycoprotein substrates with lower bioavailability more sensitive to intestinal P-glycoprotein inhibition (they name **dabigatran**) cannot be excluded.[2]

1. Dificid (Fidaxomicin). Optimer Pharmaceuticals Inc. US Prescribing information, May 2011.
2. Dificlir (Fidaxomicin). Astellas Pharma Ltd. UK Summary of product characteristics, March 2012.

Fosfomycin + Cimetidine

In a study in 9 healthy subjects, the pharmacokinetics of a 50-mg dose of fosfomycin were not significantly altered by two 400 mg doses of cimetidine, given the night before and 30 minutes before the fosfomycin.[1]

1. Bergan T, Mastropaolo G, Di Mario F, Naccarato R. Pharmacokinetics of fosfomycin and influence of cimetidine and metoclopramide on the bioavailability of fosfomycin trometamol. New Trends in Urinary Tract Infections (eds Neu and Williams) Int Symp Rome 1987, p 157–66. Published in 1988.

Fosfomycin + Metoclopramide

Metoclopramide reduces fosfomycin bioavailability.

Clinical evidence, mechanism, importance and management

Metoclopramide 20 mg given to 9 healthy subjects 30 minutes before fosfomycin 50 mg/kg reduced the peak serum levels of fosfomycin by 42% and reduced the AUC by 27%. These changes appear to occur because metoclopramide speeds the transit through the gut, so that less time is available for good absorption. However, despite these reductions, the urinary concentrations of fosfomycin remained above the minimum levels required for common urinary pathogens for at least 36 hours after the dose.[1] This suggests that the interaction is unlikely to be clinically important.

1. Bergan T, Mastropaolo G, Di Mario F, Naccarato R. Pharmacokinetics of fosfomycin and influence of cimetidine and metoclopramide on the bioavailability of fosfomycin trometamol. New Trends in Urinary Tract Infections (eds Neu and Williams) Int Symp Rome 1987, p 157–66. Published in 1988.

Fusidic acid + Colestyramine

***In vitro* studies have shown that colestyramine can bind with sodium fusidate in the gut, thereby reducing its activity,[1] and *in vivo animal* studies have shown peak fusidate levels are decreased by 33 to 77% by colestyramine,[2] but whether this also occurs clinically has not been confirmed. It is generally recommended that other drugs are given one hour before or 4 to 6 hours after colestyramine.**

1. Johns WH, Bates TR. Drug-cholestyramine interactions. I: Physicochemical factors affecting *in vitro* binding of sodium fusidate to cholestyramine. *J Pharm Sci* (1972) 61, 730–5.
2. Johns WH, Bates TR. Drug-cholestyramine interactions. II: Influence of cholestyramine on GI absorption of sodium fusidate. *J Pharm Sci* (1972) 61, 735–9.

Isoniazid + Aminosalicylic acid

Isoniazid levels are raised by aminosalicylic acid.

Clinical evidence, mechanism, importance and management

A study found that aminosalicylic acid significantly increased the plasma levels of isoniazid at 4 and 6 hours after administration by 32% and 114%, respectively in fast acetylators of isoniazid, and by 21% and 39%, respectively in slow acetylators of isoniazid. The half-life of isoniazid was increased from 1.32 hours to 2.89 hours in the fast acetylators and from 3.05 hours to 4.27 hours in the slow acetylators (see 'Genetic factors in drug metabolism', p.8, for more information about acetylator status). The effects were probably due to the inhibition of isoniazid metabolism by aminosalicylic acid.[1] There seem to be no reports of isoniazid toxicity arising from this interaction, but the manufacturers of isoniazid warn that adverse effects are more likely in the presence of aminosalicylic acid.[2]

1. Hanngren Å, Borgå O, Sjöqvist F. Inactivation of isoniazid (INH) in Swedish tuberculous patients before and during treatment with para-aminosalicylic acid (PAS). *Scand J Respir Dis* (1970) 51, 61–9.
2. Isoniazid Tablets. UCB Pharma Ltd. UK Summary of product characteristics, July 2009.

Isoniazid + Antacids

The absorption of isoniazid from the gut is modestly reduced by aluminium hydroxide, slightly reduced by magaldrate, and not affected by aluminium/magnesium hydroxide tablets or didanosine chewable tablets.

Clinical evidence

Aluminium hydroxide (*Amphojel*) 45 mL was given to 10 patients with tuberculosis at 6 am, 7 am and 8 am, followed immediately by isoniazid and any other medication they were receiving. The plasma isoniazid levels at one hour were decreased, and peak plasma levels occurring between one and 2 hours after the dose were reduced by about 25%, when adjusted for different doses.[1] The effect of **magaldrate** (hydrated magnesium aluminate) was smaller,[1] and in another well-controlled study **aluminium/magnesium hydroxide** (*Mylanta*) had no effect on isoniazid plasma levels.[2]

Didanosine chewable tablets contain antacids (**aluminium/magnesium hydroxide**) in the formulation, but it has been shown that they do not affect the bioavailability of isoniazid.[3]

Mechanism

Aluminium hydroxide delays gastric emptying,[4,5] causing retention of the isoniazid in the stomach. As isoniazid is largely absorbed from the intestine, this explains the slight decrease in plasma isoniazid concentrations. Aluminium hydroxide also appears to inhibit the absorption of isoniazid.

Importance and management

Information on this interaction is limited, and it is not established. The clinical importance of the modest reductions in isoniazid levels with aluminium hydroxide in one study is uncertain, but likely to be small. Aluminium/magnesium hydroxide did not interact, and neither did didanosine chewable tablets.

1. Hurwitz A, Schlozman DL. Effects of antacids on gastrointestinal absorption of isoniazid in rat and man. *Am Rev Respir Dis* (1974) 109, 41–7.
2. Peloquin CA, Namdar S, Dodge AA, Nix DE. Pharmacokinetics of isoniazid under fasting conditions, with food, and with antacids. *Int J Tuberc Lung Dis* (1999) 3, 703–710.
3. Gallicano K, Sahai J, Zaror-Behrens G, Pakuts A. Effect of antacids in didanosine tablet on bioavailability of isoniazid. *Antimicrob Agents Chemother* (1994) 38, 894–7.
4. Vats TS, Hurwitz A, Robinson RG, Herrin W. Effects of antacids on gastric emptying in children. *Pediatr Res* (1973) 7, 340.
5. Hava M, Hurwitz A. The relaxing effect of aluminium and lanthanum on rat and human gastric smooth muscle in vitro. *Eur J Pharmacol* (1973) 22, 156–61.

Isoniazid + Chlorpromazine

A study in 11 patients found that the half-life of isoniazid was increased by 41% when a single 300-mg dose of chlorpromazine was given one hour before a single 5 mg/kg intravenous dose of isoniazid.[1] The clinical relevance of this finding is unclear.

1. Matilla MJ, Takki S. Half-lives of isoniazid and salicylic acid in serum and their modification by different drugs in psychiatric patients. *Ann Med Exp Biol Fenn* (1969) 47, 124–8.

Isoniazid + Disulfiram

In most patients the concurrent use of isoniazid and disulfiram is uneventful, but difficulties in co-ordination, with changes in mental status, behaviour, and drowsiness have been reported in a small number of patients.

Clinical evidence

Seven patients with tuberculosis who had been taking isoniazid for at least 30 days, without problems, experienced adverse reactions within 2 to 8 days of starting to take disulfiram 500 mg daily. Among the symptoms were dizziness, disorientation, a staggering gait, insomnia, irritability and querulous behaviour, listlessness, and lethargy. One patient became hypomanic. Most of the patients were also taking chlordiazepoxide, and other drugs included aminosalicylic acid, streptomycin and phenobarbital. The adverse reactions decreased or disappeared when the disulfiram was either reduced to 250 or 125 mg daily, or withdrawn. These 7 patients represented less than one-third of those who received both drugs.[1] As disulfiram is known to inhibit the metabolism of chlordiazepoxide,[2] another 4 patients were given only isoniazid and disulfiram. Although their reaction was not as severe, all 4 developed drowsiness and depression.[1]

In contrast, another report describes the concurrent use of both drugs, without problems, in 200 patients.[3] A retrospective study in patients taking isoniazid-containing regimens for tuberculosis found no difference in the rate of toxicity in 13 patients taking disulfiram, when compared with a large group of patients not taking disulfiram. However, the small number of patients taking disulfiram in this study limits the strength of the negative finding.[4] Another patient taking disulfiram with isoniazid and rifampicin (rifampin) also did not experience any problems.[5]

Mechanism

Not understood. One idea is that some kind of synergy occurs between the two drugs because both can produce similar adverse effects if given in high doses. The authors of one report[1] speculate that isoniazid and disulfiram together inhibit two of three biochemical pathways concerned with the metabolism of dopamine. This leaves a third pathway open, catalysed by COMT (catechol-*O*-methyl transferase), which produces a number of methylated products of dopamine. These methylated products may possibly have been responsible for the mental and physical reactions seen.

Importance and management

Information about this interaction appears to be limited to the reports cited. Its incidence is uncertain but apparently quite small. Two-thirds of the patients in one study, and at least 200 other patients did not experience an interaction. It would therefore seem that concurrent use need not be avoided, but the response should be monitored. If marked changes in mental status occur, or there is unsteady gait, the manufacturers recommend that the disulfiram should be withdrawn.[6]

1. Whittington HG, Grey L. Possible interaction between disulfiram and isoniazid. *Am J Psychiatry* (1969) 125, 1725–9.
2. Antabuse (Disulfiram). Actavis UK Ltd. UK Summary of product characteristics, December 2011.
3. McNichol RW, Ewing JA, Faiman MD, eds. Disulfiram (Antabuse), a unique medical aid to sobriety: history, pharmacology, research, clinical use. Springfield Ill: Thomas; 1987 p. 47–90.
4. Burman WJ, Terra M, Breese P, Cohn D, Reves R. Lack of toxicity from concomitant directly observed disulfiram and isoniazid-containing therapy for active tuberculosis. *Int J Tuberc Lung Dis* (2002) 6, 839–42.
5. Rothstein E. Rifampin with disulfiram. *JAMA* (1972) 219, 1216.
6. Antabuse (Disulfiram). Odyssey Pharmaceuticals, Inc. US Prescribing information, December 2003.

Isoniazid + Etanercept

A case report describes a patient who developed optic neuritis while taking isoniazid and etanercept.

Clinical evidence, mechanism, importance and management

A case report describes a patient with rheumatoid arthritis who developed latent tuberculosis, and was given isoniazid and pyridoxine. Five days after starting to take these drugs, he also started treatment with subcutaneous etanercept twice weekly. Approximately 2 months later he experienced a reduction in visual acuity, which was attributed to optic neuritis. After stopping treatment with etanercept and isoniazid, and starting a corticosteroid, his condition improved. The authors of the case report considered that the combination of isoniazid and etanercept were causative factors in his optic neuritis, although either drug alone may have caused this adverse effect.[1] No particular precautions are warranted on the basis of this isolated case.

1. Noguera-Pons R, Borrás-Blasco J, Romero-Crespo I, Antón-Torres R, Navarro-Ruiz A, González-Ferrandez JA. Optic neuritis with concurrent etanercept and isoniazid therapy. *Ann Pharmacother* (2005) 39, 2131–5.

Isoniazid + Ethambutol

Ethambutol does not appear to affect isoniazid levels. However, it seems that the optic neuropathy caused by ethambutol may be increased by isoniazid.

Clinical evidence, mechanism, importance and management

In 10 patients with tuberculosis, the mean serum levels of a 300-mg dose of isoniazid were not significantly changed by a single 20-mg/kg dose of ethambutol.[1] The possible effects of concurrent use over a period of time were not studied. However, there is some evidence that the optic neuropathy caused by ethambutol may be increased by isoniazid, and any effects resolve more slowly after the use of isoniazid.[2-5] One group of authors recommends that both ethambutol and isoniazid should be stopped immediately if severe optic neuritis occurs. They further recommend that isoniazid should be stopped if less severe optic neuritis does not improve within 6 weeks after stopping ethambutol.[6]

1. Singhal KC, Varshney DP, Rathi R, Kishore K, Varshney SC. Serum concentration of isoniazid administered with and without ethambutol in pulmonary tuberculosis patients. *Indian J Med Res* (1986) 83, 360–2.
2. Renard G, Morax PV. Nevrite optique au cours des traitements antituberculeux. *Ann Ocul (Paris)* (1977) 210, 53–61.
3. Karmon G, Savir H, Zevin D, Levi J. Bilateral optic neuropathy due to combined ethambutol and isoniazid treatment. *Ann Ophthalmol* (1979) 11, 1013–17.
4. Garret CR. Optic neuritis in a patient on ethambutol and isoniazid evaluated by visual evoked potentials: Case report. *Mil Med* (1985) 150, 43–6.
5. Jimenez-Lucho VE, del Busto R, Odel J. Isoniazid and ethambutol as a cause of optic neuropathy. *Eur J Respir Dis* (1987) 71, 42–5.
6. Sivakumaran P, Harrison AC, Marschner J, Martin P. Ocular toxicity from ethambutol: a review of four cases and recommended precautions. *N Z Med J* (1998) 111, 428–30.

Isoniazid + Fluconazole

A double-blind, crossover study in 16 healthy subjects (8 fast and 8 slow acetylators of isoniazid) found that fluconazole 400 mg daily for a week had no clinically significant effect on the pharmacokinetics of isoniazid.[1] No special precautions would appear necessary during concurrent use.

1. Buss DC, Routledge PA, Hutchings A, Brammer KW, Thorpe JE. The effect of fluconazole on the acetylation of isoniazid. *Hum Exp Toxicol* (1991) 10, 85–6.

Isoniazid + Food

The absorption of isoniazid is reduced by food. See also 'Isoniazid + Food; Cheese or Fish', p.324 for toxic reactions between isoniazid and specific foods.

Clinical evidence

In 9 healthy subjects the mean peak serum levels of isoniazid 10 mg/kg were delayed, and reduced by 79%,when isoniazid was given with breakfast rather than when fasting. The AUC was reduced by 43%.[1] In another study in 14 healthy subjects given isoniazid with a full fat breakfast, the maximum serum levels of isoniazid were decreased by 51%, its absorption was delayed, and its AUC was decreased by 12%.[2] Similar results have been found in other studies.[3,4]

Mechanism

Uncertain. Food delays gastric emptying so that absorption further along the gut is also delayed, but the reduction in absorption is not understood.

Importance and management

Information is limited but the interaction seems to be established. For maximum absorption isoniazid should be taken without food, hence the manufacturer's guidance to take it at least 30 minutes before or 2 hours after food.[5]

1. Melander A, Danielson K, Hanson A, Jansson L, Rerup C, Scherstén B, Thulin T, Wåhlin E. Reduction of isoniazid bioavailability in normal men by concomitant intake of food. *Acta Med Scand* (1976) 200, 93–7.
2. Peloquin CA, Namdar S, Dodge AA, Nix DE. Pharmacokinetics of isoniazid under fasting conditions, with food, and with antacids. *Int J Tuberc Lung Dis* (1999) 3, 703–710.
3. Männistо P, Mäntylä R, Klinge R, Nykänen S, Koponen A, Lamminsivu U. Influence of various diets on the bioavailability of isoniazid. *J Antimicrob Chemother* (1982) 10, 427–34.
4. Zwolska Z, Niemirowska-Mikulska H, Augustynowicz-Kopeć E. Wpływ pożywienia na biologiczną dostępność izoniazydu (INH) u zdrowych ochotników. *Pneumonol Alergol Pol* (1998) 66, 412–21.
5. Isoniazid Tablets. UCB Pharma Ltd. UK Summary of product characteristics, July 2009.

Isoniazid + Food; Cheese or Fish

Patients taking isoniazid who eat some foods, particularly fish from the scombroid family (tuna, mackerel, salmon) that are not fresh, may experience an exaggerated histamine poisoning reaction. Cheese has also been implicated in this reaction, but the adverse effects may be due to the weak MAOI effects of isoniazid rather than histamine poisoning.

Clinical evidence

Three months after starting to take isoniazid 300 mg daily, a woman experienced a series of unpleasant reactions 10 to 30 minutes after eating cheese. These reactions included chills, headache (sometimes severe), itching of the face and scalp, slight diarrhoea, flushing of the face (and on one occasion the whole body), variable and mild tachycardia, and a bursting sensation in the head. Blood pressure measurements showed only a modest rise (from her normal blood pressure of 95/65 mmHg to 110/80 mmHg). No physical or biochemical abnormalities were found.[1]

Headache, dizziness, blurred vision, tachycardia, flushing and itching of the skin, redness of the eyes, burning sensation of the body, difficulty in breathing, abdominal colic, diarrhoea, vomiting, sweating and wheezing have all been described after other patients taking isoniazid ate cheese.[2-6] Certain tropical fish, including **tuna (skipjack** or **bonito**; ***Katsuwanus pelamis***),[7-11] ***Sardinella (Amblygaster) sirm***,[12] ***Rastrigella kanagurta***,[13] **saury (skipper** or **bill-fish)**[14] and others[15] are also implicated. There are a few hundred cases of this reaction on record.

Mechanism

The reaction appears to be an exaggeration of the histamine poisoning that can occur after eating some foods, such as members of the scombroid family of fish (tuna, mackerel, salmon, etc), if they are not fresh and adequately refrigerated. These fish (and some cheeses) have a high histidine content and under poor storage circumstances the histidine is decarboxylated by bacteria to produce unusually large amounts of histamine. Normally this is inactivated by histaminase in the body, but isoniazid is a potent inhibitor of this enzyme, which means that the histamine is absorbed largely unchanged and histamine poisoning develops.[16] Histamine survives all but very prolonged cooking. Tuna fish can contain 180 to 500 mg histamine per 100 g, other types of fish may contain as little as 0.5 to 7.5 mg.[10]

Alternatively, it has been suggested that the cases of reactions to cheese are caused by tyramine content and the weak MAOI properties of isoniazid. See 'MAOIs or RIMAs + Food; Tyramine-containing', p.1389, for more details of the mechanism of this interaction.

Importance and management

An established interaction of clinical importance. With the exception of one patient who appeared to have had a cerebrovascular accident,[9] the reactions experienced by the others were unpleasant and alarming but usually not serious or life-threatening. They required little or no treatment, although 'scombroid poisoning' in the absence of isoniazid is sometimes more serious. Two reports say that treatment with antihistamines can be effective.[10,15] Isoniazid has been in use since 1956 and there is little need to now introduce any general dietary restrictions, but if any of these reactions are experienced, examine the patient's diet and advise the avoidance of any probable offending foodstuffs. Very mature cheese and fish of the scombroid family (tuna, mackerel, salmon and other varieties of dark meat fish) that are not fresh are to be treated with suspicion, but the likely histamine or tyramine content of food cannot be assessed without undertaking a detailed analysis. See 'Table 32.2', p.1390, and 'Table 32.3', p.1390, for a list of tyramine-rich foods and drinks.

1. Smith CK, Durack DT. Isoniazid and reaction to cheese. *Ann Intern Med* (1978) 88, 520–1.
2. Uragoda CG, Lodha SC. Histamine intoxication in a tuberculous patient after ingestion of cheese. *Tubercle* (1979) 60, 59–61.
3. Lejonc JL, Gusmini D, Brochard P. Isoniazid and reaction to cheese. *Ann Intern Med* (1979) 91, 793.
4. Hauser MJ, Baier H. Interactions of isoniazid with foods. *Drug Intell Clin Pharm* (1982) 16, 617–18.
5. Toutoungi M, Carroll R, Dick P. Isoniazide (INH) and tyramine-rich food. *Chest* (1986) 89 (Suppl 6), 540S.
6. Carvalho ACC, Manfrin M, Gore RP, Capone S, Scalvini A, Armellini A, Giovine T, Carosi G, Matteelli A. Reaction to cheese during TB treatment. *Thorax* (2004) 59, 635.
7. Uragoda CG, Kottegoda SR. Adverse reactions to isoniazid on ingestion of fish with a high histamine content. *Tubercle* (1977) 58, 83–9.
8. Uragoda CG. Histamine poisoning in tuberculous patients after ingestion of tuna fish. *Am Rev Respir Dis* (1980) 121, 157–9.
9. Senanayake N, Vyravanathan S, Kanagasuriyam S. Cerebrovascular accident after a 'skipjack' reaction in a patient taking isoniazid. *BMJ* (1978) 2, 1127–8.
10. Senanayake N, Vyravanathan S. Histamine reactions due to ingestion of tuna fish (*Thunnus argentivittatus*) in patients on antituberculosis therapy. *Toxicon* (1981) 19, 184–5.
11. Morinaga S, Kawasaki A, Hirata H, Suzuki S, Mizushima Y. Histamine poisoning after ingestion of spoiled raw tuna in a patient taking isoniazid. *Intern Med* (1997) 36, 198–200.
12. Uragoda CG. Histamine poisoning in tuberculous patients on ingestion of tropical fish. *J Trop Med Hyg* (1978) 81, 243–5.
13. Uragoda CG. Histamine intoxication with isoniazid and a species of fish. *Ceylon Med J* (1978) 23, 109–10.
14. Miki M, Ishikawa T, Okayama H. An outbreak of histamine poisoning after ingestion of the ground saury paste in eight patients taking isoniazid in a tuberculous ward. *Intern Med* (2005) 44, 1133–6.
15. Diao Y *et al.* Histamine like reaction in tuberculosis patients taking fishes containing much of histamine under treatment with isoniazid in 277 cases. *Zhonghua Jie He He Hu Xi Xi Ji Bing Za Zhi* (1986) 9, 267–9, 317–18.
16. O'Sullivan TL. Drug-food interaction with isoniazid resembling anaphylaxis. *Ann Pharmacother* (1997) 31, 928–9.

Isoniazid + H_2-receptor antagonists

Cimetidine and ranitidine do not appear to affect the pharmacokinetics of isoniazid.

Clinical evidence, mechanism, importance and management

In 13 healthy subjects, **cimetidine** 400 mg or **ranitidine** 300 mg, three times daily, for 3 days had no effect on the pharmacokinetics of a single 10-mg/kg dose of isoniazid. The absorption and the metabolism of isoniazid were both unchanged.[1] No special precautions would appear to be necessary on concurrent use. Although data about other H_2-receptor antagonists appears to be lacking, based on this study, they would not be expected to interact with isoniazid.

1. Paulsen O, Höglund P, Nilsson L-G, Gredeby H. No interaction between H_2 blockers and isoniazid. *Eur J Respir Dis* (1986) 68, 286–90.

Isoniazid + Laxatives

Sodium sulfate and castor oil used as laxatives can cause a modest reduction in isoniazid absorption.

Clinical evidence, mechanism, importance and management

In an experimental study of the possible effects of laxatives on isoniazid absorption, healthy subjects were given 10 to 20 g of oral **sodium sulfate** or 20 g of **castor oil** (doses sufficient to provoke diarrhoea). Absorption, measured by the amount of isoniazid excreted in the urine, was decreased by 50% with **castor oil** and by 41% with **sodium sulfate** at 4 hours. However, serum levels of isoniazid were relatively unchanged. The overall picture was that while these laxatives can alter the pattern of absorption, they do not seriously impair the total amount of drug absorbed.[1]

1. Mattila MJ, Takki S, Jussila J. Effect of sodium sulphate and castor oil on drug absorption from the human intestine. *Ann Clin Res* (1974) 6, 19–24.

Isoniazid + Pethidine (Meperidine)

An isolated case report describes hypotension and lethargy in a patient after he took isoniazid with pethidine.

Clinical evidence, mechanism, importance and management

A patient became lethargic and his blood pressure fell from 124/68 mmHg to 84/50 mmHg within 20 minutes of being given pethidine 75 mg intramuscularly. An hour before, he had been given isoniazid. There was no evidence of fever or cardiac arrhythmias, and his serum electrolytes, glucose levels and blood gases were normal. His blood pressure returned to normal over the next 3 hours. He had previously had both pethidine and isoniazid separately without incident. He was subsequently uneventfully given intravenous morphine sulfate 4 mg every 2 to 4 hours.[1] The authors of the report attribute this reaction to the MAO-inhibitory properties of the isoniazid and equate it with the severe and potentially fatal interaction between MAOIs and pethidine (see 'MAOIs or RIMAs + Opioids; Pethidine (Meperidine)', p.1399), but in reality this reaction was mild and lacked many of the characteristics of the more serious reaction. Moreover, isoniazid possesses only mild MAO-inhibitory properties and does not normally interact to the same extent as the non-selective MAOIs.

There is too little evidence to advise against concurrent use, but bear this interaction in mind in case of an unexpected response to treatment.

1. Gannon R, Pearsall W, Rowley R. Isoniazid, meperidine, and hypotension. *Ann Intern Med* (1983) 99, 415.

Isoniazid + Prednisolone

Prednisolone can lower isoniazid levels.

Clinical evidence, mechanism, importance and management

Isoniazid 10 mg/kg daily was given to 26 patients with tuberculosis. The 13 slow acetylators of isoniazid had a 23% fall in plasma isoniazid levels when they were given

prednisolone 20 mg, while the 13 fast acetylators had a 38% fall over 8.5 hours (see 'Genetic factors in drug metabolism', p.8, for an explanation of acetylator status). The reasons for these changes are not understood but changes in the metabolism, and/or the excretion of the isoniazid by the kidney, are possibilities. Despite these changes the response to treatment was excellent.[1] In another group of 49 patients (including both slow and fast acetylators of isoniazid), rifampicin 12 mg/kg largely counteracted the isoniazid-lowering effects of **prednisolone**.[1]

None of these interactions were of clinical importance, but the authors point out that if the dose of isoniazid had been lower, its effects might have been reduced. Be aware of the possibility of a reduced response during concurrent use, and raise the isoniazid dose if necessary. There seems to be no information about other corticosteroids.

1. Sarma GR, Kailasam S, Nair NGK, Narayana ASL, Tripathy SP. Effect of prednisolone and rifampin on isoniazid metabolism in slow and rapid inactivators of isoniazid. *Antimicrob Agents Chemother* (1980) 18, 661–6.

Isoniazid + Propranolol

Propranolol causes a small reduction in the clearance of isoniazid.

Clinical evidence, mechanism, importance and management

In 6 healthy subjects, the clearance of a single 600-mg intravenous dose of isoniazid was reduced by 21%, from 16.4 to 13 L/hour, by propranolol 40 mg three times daily for 3 days.[1] It is suggested that propranolol reduces the clearance of isoniazid by inhibiting its metabolism (acetylation) by the liver.[1] However, as the increase in isoniazid levels is likely to be only modest this interaction is probably of little clinical importance.

1. Santoso B. Impairment of isoniazid clearance by propranolol. *Int J Clin Pharmacol Ther Toxicol* (1985) 23, 134–6.

Isoniazid + Pyrazinamide

A study in 19 patients with tuberculosis found that pyrazinamide did not affect serum levels of isoniazid.[1]

1. Levy D, Duysak S, Zylberberg B, Haapanen J, Russell WF, Middlebrook G. Effect of pyrazinamide on antimicrobially active serum isoniazid. *Dis Chest* (1960) 38, 148–51.

Isoniazid + Quinolones

Ciprofloxacin may cause a slight increase in the bioavailability of isoniazid, and pefloxacin may increase both the absorption and excretion of isoniazid.

Clinical evidence, mechanism, importance and management

(a) Ciprofloxacin

In a single-dose study, ciprofloxacin 500 mg was found to increase the absorption of isoniazid 300 mg by about 15%. The time to reach maximum plasma levels was increased from 3 hours to 4 hours. The rate of elimination and plasma half-life of isoniazid were not significantly affected.[1] In a very similar study, measurement of the salivary and urinary levels of isoniazid also found that ciprofloxacin increased the absorption of isoniazid, although the time to reach maximum salivary levels of isoniazid was shortened from 4 hours to 3 hours.[2] The urinary excretion was also increased by 38% in the presence of ciprofloxacin. The effects on isoniazid absorption may be due to inhibition of gastric motility and emptying by ciprofloxacin.[1] However, these effects are modest and unlikely to be clinically significant.

(b) Pefloxacin

In a study in 6 healthy subjects a single 400-mg dose of pefloxacin increased the maximum salivary levels and AUC of a single 300-mg dose of isoniazid almost twofold, indicating increased absorption. The time to reach maximum saliva concentrations was reduced from 5 hours to 4 hours. The excretion of isoniazid was also increased by 38%, as measured by an increased recovery from the urine.[3] The clinical relevance of the increased salivary levels of isoniazid is unclear. The authors suggest that concurrent use may lead to increased isoniazid toxicity. Therefore, until more is known, if patients develop isoniazid adverse effects (e.g. nausea, vomiting, constipation), while taking pefloxacin, consider this interaction as a possible cause.

1. Ofoefule SI, Obodo CE, Orisakwe OE, Ilondu NA, Afonne OJ, Maduka SO, Anusiem CA, Agbasi PU. Some plasma pharmacokinetic parameters of isoniazid in the presence of a fluoroquinolone antibacterial agent. *Am J Ther* (2001) 8, 243–6.
2. Ofoefule SI, Obodo CE, Orisakwe OE, Afonne JO, Ilondu NA, Agbasi PU, Anusiem CA, Maduka SO, Ilo CE. Salivary and urinary excretion and plasma-saliva concentration ratios of isoniazid in the presence of co-administered ciprofloxacin. *Am J Ther* (2002) 9, 15–18.
3. Ofoefule SI, Onyeagba OE, Orisakwe OE. Effects of pefloxacin on urinary and salivary concentrations of isoniazid in six healthy female volunteers. *Am J Ther* (2000) 7, 313–16.

Isoniazid + Rifamycins

The concurrent use of a rifamycin and isoniazid is common and therapeutically valuable, but there is evidence that the incidence of hepatotoxicity may be increased, particularly in slow acetylators of isoniazid. One study suggests the bioavailability of rifampicin may be reduced by isoniazid but other studies found no pharmacokinetic interaction. Rifabutin and rifampicin do not alter the pharmacokinetics of isoniazid.

Clinical evidence, mechanism, importance and management

(a) Rifabutin

In 6 healthy subjects, rifabutin 300 mg daily for 7 days had no significant effect on the pharmacokinetics of a single 300-mg dose of isoniazid or its metabolite acetylisoniazid.[1] Two of the 6 subjects were rapid acetylators of isoniazid (see 'Genetic factors in drug metabolism', p.8, for more information about acetylator status).

Although both drugs have been effectively used together in the treatment of tuberculosis, it is not clear whether concurrent use increases the incidence of hepatotoxicity, as occurs with isoniazid and rifampicin (see below). However, as regular monitoring of liver function is required for both isoniazid and rifabutin, no additional monitoring seems necessary on concurrent use. The manufacturer of rifabutin notes that haematological reactions of rifabutin could be increased by isoniazid, but, again, as regular monitoring of white blood cell and platelet counts is advised,[2] no additional monitoring seems necessary.

(b) Rifampicin (Rifampin)

Most studies have shown that the serum levels and half-lives of isoniazid and rifampicin are not significantly affected by concurrent use,[3-6] even in those with hepatic impairment.[6] There was also no difference[4] between rapid and slow acetylators of isoniazid, (see 'Genetic factors in drug metabolism', p.8, for more information about acetylator status). One single-dose study in healthy subjects found that isoniazid 12 mg/kg reduced the AUC of rifampicin 10 mg/kg by about 25%.[7] There is some evidence that the incidence and severity of hepatotoxicity rises if both drugs are given together.[8] Reports from India suggest that the incidence can be as high as 8 to 10%, while much lower figures of 2 to 3% are reported in the US.[9] There is one case report that appears to prove that hepatotoxicity can arise rapidly from the use of both drugs. The patient tolerated both drugs individually, but hepatotoxicity reappeared on concurrent use.[10]

The reasons for the hepatotoxicity are not fully understood but rifampicin or isoniazid alone can cause liver damage by their own toxic action. One suggestion is that the rifampicin alters the metabolism of isoniazid, resulting in the formation of hydrazine, which has proven to be hepatotoxic.[9-11] Higher plasma levels of hydrazine are said to occur in slow acetylators of isoniazid,[9] but this effects was not found in one study.[12] There has been at least one fatality caused by this combination.[13] The manufacturers of rifampicin advise that caution is particularly needed in patients with impaired liver function, the elderly, malnourished patients, and children under 2 years of age. In patients with normal pre-treatment liver function, after baseline LFTs, further tests are only needed if fever, vomiting, or jaundice occur, or if the patient deteriorates.[14] However, one of the manufacturers of isoniazid suggests that liver function tests should be reviewed monthly in patients receiving both drugs.[15]

1. Breda M, Painezzola E, Benedetti MS, Efthymiopoulos C, Carpentieri M, Sassella D, Rimoldi R. A study of the effects of rifabutin on isoniazid pharmacokinetics and metabolism in healthy volunteers. *Drug Metabol Drug Interact* (1993) 10, 323–40.
2. Mycobutin (Rifabutin). Pfizer Ltd. UK Summary of product characteristics, December 2013.
3. Boman G. Serum concentration and half-life of rifampicin after simultaneous oral administration of aminosalicylic acid or isoniazid. *Eur J Clin Pharmacol* (1974) 7, 217–25.
4. Sarma GR, Kailasam S, Nair NGK, Narayana ASL, Tripathy SP. Effect of prednisolone and rifampin on isoniazid metabolism in slow and rapid inactivators of isoniazid. *Antimicrob Agents Chemother* (1980) 18, 661–6.
5. Venho VMK, Koskinen R. The effect of pyrazinamide, rifampicin and cycloserine on the blood levels and urinary excretion of isoniazid. *Ann Clin Res* (1971) 3, 277–80.
6. Acocella G, Bonollo L, Garimoldi M, Mainardi M, Tenconi LT. Kinetics of rifampicin and isoniazid administered alone and in combination to normal subjects and patients with liver disease. *Gut* (1972) 13, 47–53.
7. Immanuel C, Gurumurthy P, Ramachandran G, Venkatesan P, Chandrasekaran V, Prabhakar R. Bioavailability of rifampicin following concomitant administration of ethambutol or isoniazid or pyrazinamide or a combination of the three drugs. *Indian J Med Res* (2003) 118, 109–14.
8. Steele MA, Burk RF, DesPrez RM. Toxic hepatitis with isoniazid and rifampin. A meta-analysis. *Chest* (1991) 99, 465–71.
9. Gangadharam PRJ. Isoniazid, rifampin and hepatotoxicity. *Am Rev Respir Dis* (1986) 133, 963–5.
10. Askgaard DS, Wilcke T, Døssing M. Hepatotoxicity caused by the combined action of isoniazid and rifampicin. *Thorax* (1995) 50, 213–14.
11. Pessayre D, Bentata M, Degott C, Nouel O, Miguet J-P, Rueff B, Benhamou J-P. Isoniazid-rifampin fulminant hepatitis. A possible consequence of the enhancement of isoniazid hepatotoxicity by enzyme induction. *Gastroenterology* (1977) 72, 284–9.
12. Jenner PJ, Ellard GA. Isoniazid-related hepatotoxicity: a study of the effect of rifampicin administration on the metabolism of acetylisoniazid in man. *Tubercle* (1989) 70, 93–101.
13. Lenders JWM, Bartelink AKM, van Herwaarden CLA, van Haelst UJGM, van Tongeren JHM. Dodelijke levercelnecrose na kort durende toediening van isoniazide en rifampicine aan een patiënt die reeds werd behandeld met anti-epileptica. *Ned Tijdschr Geneeskd* (1983) 127, 420–3.
14. Rifadin for Infusion (Rifampicin). Sanofi-Aventis. UK Summary of product characteristics, March 2009.
15. Isoniazid Ampoules. Cambridge Laboratories. UK Summary of product characteristics, April 2002.

Isoniazid + Salicylates

Isoniazid prolongs the half-life of salicylate in patients given aspirin.

Clinical evidence, mechanism, importance and management

In 8 patients it was found that the half-life of isoniazid was reduced by 14% when a single 2-g dose of sodium salicylate was given one hour before a single 5 mg/kg intravenous dose of isoniazid. This is unlikely to be clinically relevant. Further analysis in 10 patients found that the half-life of salicylate was almost doubled when a 2 g dose of aspirin was given with isoniazid 600 mg. A further dose of isoniazid was given 4 hours later.[1] The clinical relevance of this increase in the half-life of salicylate is unclear, but it seems likely to be small, particularly with antiplatelet doses of aspirin.

1. Matilla MJ, Takki S. Half-lives of isoniazid and salicylic acid in serum and their modification by different drugs in psychiatric patients. *Ann Med Exp Biol Fenn* (1969) 47, 124–8.

Isoniazid + SSRIs and related antidepressants

A few reports suggest that no important interaction occurs between isoniazid and the SSRIs or nefazodone. However, adverse reactions have been seen during concurrent use and one report found an increased discontinuation rate in patients taking an SSRI with isoniazid.

Clinical evidence

Two HIV-positive patients taking **fluoxetine** 20 mg daily were also given isoniazid. One of them tolerated the use of both drugs, but the other developed vomiting and diarrhoea, and after 10 days the **fluoxetine** was stopped.[1]

A woman who had been hospitalised for serious depression was given **nefazodone** 300 mg daily. A few days later she began to take isoniazid 300 mg daily, and was later discharged on an increased **nefazodone** dose of 400 mg daily. She was reported to have had no problems while taking both drugs over a 5-month period.[2]

A woman with tuberculosis taking isoniazid 300 mg daily presented with depression, and was given **sertraline** 50 mg daily, later raised to 150 mg daily, without problems. She responded well and was reported to have taken both drugs together for 8 months without problems.[2]

A retrospective review of HIV-positive patients who were taking either an SSRI, isoniazid, or both, found that the rate of discontinuation of the SSRI was higher in those also taking isoniazid (7 of 10 patients) than in the group of patients taking an SSRI alone (2 of 14). It is unclear why this rate was increased; little mention is made of the influence of other drugs or medical conditions.[3]

Mechanism

In theory isoniazid could interact with the SSRIs[4] because it has some weak MAO inhibitory activity. However, isoniazid rarely interacts like the non-selective MAOIs. This is because isoniazid seems to lack activity on mitochondrial MAO even though it has activity on plasma MAO. Therefore no adverse interaction would usually be expected.

Importance and management

Direct information about the concurrent use of isoniazid and SSRIs seems to be limited, but the case reports cited here[1,2,4] would suggest that the concurrent use of isoniazid and these SSRIs is normally without problems. However, also be aware that one report suggests the possibility of an increase in adverse effects with the combination of SSRIs and isoniazid.[3]

1. Judd FK, Mijch AM, Cockram A, Norman TR. Isoniazid and antidepressants: is there cause for concern? *Int Clin Psychopharmacol* (1994) 9, 123–5.
2. Malek-Ahmadi P, Chavez M, Contreras SA. Coadministration of isoniazid and antidepressant drugs. *J Clin Psychiatry* (1996) 57, 550.
3. Doyle ME, Hicks D, Aronson NE. Selective serotonin reuptake inhibitors and isoniazid: evidence of a potential adverse interaction. *Mil Med* (2001) 166, 1054–6.
4. Evans ME, Kortas KJ. Potential interaction between isoniazid and selective serotonin-reuptake inhibitors. *Am J Health-Syst Pharm* (1995) 52, 2135–6.

Linezolid + Antacids

A study in healthy subjects found that *Maalox 70mVal* suspension 10 mL (aluminium/magnesium hydroxide) did not affect the pharmacokinetics of a single 600-mg dose of linezolid.[1]

1. Grunder G, Zysset-Aschmann Y, Vollenweider F, Maier T, Krähenbühl S, Drewe J. Lack of pharmacokinetic interaction between linezolid and antacid in healthy volunteers. *Antimicrob Agents Chemother* (2006) 50, 68–72.

Linezolid + Aztreonam

In a single-dose study in healthy subjects, the pharmacokinetics of intravenous aztreonam 1 g and intravenous linezolid 375 mg were not affected by concurrent use. Therefore dose alterations are unlikely to be needed if both drugs are given.[1]

1. Sisson TL, Jungbluth GL, Hopkins NK. A pharmacokinetic evaluation of concomitant administration of linezolid and aztreonam. *J Clin Pharmacol* (1999) 39, 1277–82.

Linezolid + Clarithromycin

A case report describes increased exposure to linezolid on the concurrent use of clarithromycin.

Clinical evidence, mechanism, importance and management

A case report describes a 42-year-old man receiving linezolid 300 mg twice daily for resistant TB, whose linezolid AUC increased about 3.7-fold when clarithromycin 1 g daily was started. His liver and renal function were unchanged. Based on serum linezolid concentrations, his dose was reduced to 150 mg twice daily. After 6 months his sputum cultures and smear microscopy were negative and remained so up to 18 months post follow-up. The authors suggest that the increased linezolid exposure was due to inhibition of P-glycoprotein by clarithromycin.[1]

This is an isolated case and as such its general clinical relevance is not known. However, given the considerable increase in linezolid exposure seen and the potential for linezolid toxicity, it might be prudent to monitor linezolid concentrations on concurrent use with clarithromycin, considering the need to reduce the linezolid dose.

1. Bolhuis MS, van Altena R, Uges DRA, van der Werf TS, Kosterink JGW, Alffenaar J-WC. Clarithromycin significantly increases linezolid serum concentrations. *Antimicrob Agents Chemother* (2010) 54, 5418–9.

Linezolid + Dextromethorphan

There is no clinically important pharmacokinetic interaction between linezolid and dextromethorphan, but one case of concurrent use resulted in serotonin syndrome.

Clinical evidence, mechanism, importance and management

In a study in 14 healthy subjects, two 20-mg doses of dextromethorphan given 4 hours apart, before and during the use of linezolid 600 mg every 12 hours, had no effect on linezolid pharmacokinetics. The AUC and maximum concentration of the dextromethorphan metabolite, dextrorphan was decreased by 30%, but this was not considered sufficient to warrant any dosing alterations. There was no evidence of serotonin syndrome, as measured by changes in body temperature, alertness, and mental performance.[1] However, the manufacturer describes one case where the concurrent use of linezolid and dextromethorphan resulted in serotonin syndrome.[2] Linezolid has mild reversible MAOI activity, and serotonin syndrome has been described when dextromethorphan was taken by patients also taking antidepressant MAOIs, see 'MAOIs or RIMAs + Dextromethorphan and related cough suppressants', p.1387. If the concurrent use of linezolid and dextromethorphan is considered necessary, it would seem prudent to monitor for symptoms of serotonin syndrome. For more information on serotonin syndrome and its management, see 'Drugs that cause serotonin syndrome + Other drugs that cause serotonin syndrome', p.1471.

1. Hendershot PE, Antal EJ, Welshman IR, Batts DH, Hopkins NK. Linezolid: pharmacokinetic and pharmacodynamic evaluation of coadministration with pseudoephedrine HCl, phenylpropanolamine HCl, and dextromethorphan HBr. *J Clin Pharmacol* (2001) 41, 563–72.
2. Zyvox (Linezolid). Pharmacia Ltd. UK Summary of product characteristics, September 2014.

Linezolid + Diphenhydramine

A single case report describes delirium in a patient receiving linezolid and diphenhydramine.

Clinical evidence

A case report describes a patient taking linezolid 600 mg twice daily, with metronidazole, aztreonam and diphenhydramine to treat a rash caused by previous antibacterials. The patient developed delirium, with aggression and hallucinations 2 days after starting to take the diphenhydramine. The symptoms of delirium resolved 2 to 3 days after the diphenhydramine was withdrawn. Metronidazole was also stopped at the same time.[1]

Mechanism

There are several factors that could account for the delirium seen in this patient. Linezolid may have enhanced the antimuscarinic action of diphenhydramine resulting in the symptoms seen. In addition, psychotic disorders including hallucinations are a very rare adverse effect of metronidazole,[2] and can also occur due to sepsis.

Importance and management

Evidence for an interaction between diphenhydramine and linezolid appears to be limited to this isolated case, the reasons for which are not established. As such, no general recommendations can be made.

1. Serio RN. Acute delirium associated with combined diphenhydramine and linezolid use. *Ann Pharmacother* (2004) 38, 62–5.
2. Flagyl Tablets (Metronidazole). Zentiva. UK Summary of product characteristics, May 2011.

Linezolid + Food

Linezolid modestly increases the blood pressure response to oral tyramine. The bioavailability of linezolid is not affected by enteral feeds or food.

Clinical evidence, mechanism, importance and management

(a) Enteral feeds

In a study, 9 patients receiving enteral feeds were given a single 600-mg dose of linezolid as a suspension via a nasogastric tube or gastric tube. The rate and extent of linezolid absorption was not significantly different from that found in another 6 patients not receiving enteral feeds. No dose adjustments are therefore thought to be required if linezolid is given with enteral feeds.[1]

(b) Food

A study in healthy subjects found that the plasma levels following a single 375-mg oral dose of a linezolid tablet were 23% higher when given to fasted subjects than when it was taken immediately after a high-fat meal. However, the AUCs were not significantly different, indicating that the extent of absorption was not affected by food.[2] Another study in healthy subjects found that food delayed the rate but not the extent of absorption and distribution of linezolid into tissues.[3] The manufacturer of linezolid states that both the oral suspension and the film-coated tablets may be taken with or without food.[4]

(c) Tyramine-rich food

In a pharmacodynamic study in healthy subjects, the dose of oral tyramine required to raise the systolic blood pressure by 30 mmHg was decreased by a factor of about 3.5 (from a range of 300 to 600 mg without linezolid to 100 to 200 mg with linezolid) when the subjects were pretreated with linezolid 625 mg twice daily for 4 to 7 days. This increase in the pressor response to tyramine was similar to that seen with moclobemide 150 mg three times daily.[5] Further, another placebo-controlled study in healthy subjects found that single doses of linezolid 600 mg and moclobemide 300 mg also caused similar increases in the pressor response to intravenous tyramine, as measured by amount of tyramine required to raise the systolic blood pressure by 30 mmHg.[6]

Linezolid is a weak, non-selective inhibitor of MAO. As a consequence, it can inhibit the breakdown of tyramine by MAO in the gut, and can also potentiate the effect of tyramine at nerve endings, therefore causing an increase in blood pressure (see *Mechanism*, under 'MAOIs or RIMAs + Food; Tyramine-containing', p.1389). However, the extent of this rise was similar to that for moclobemide, which is much less than that seen with antidepressant MAOIs.

The manufacturers of linezolid recommend that patients should avoid large amounts of tyramine-rich foods and drinks[4,7] and should not consume more than 100 mg of tyramine per meal.[7] For a list of the possible tyramine-content of various foods and drinks, see 'Table 32.2', p.1390, 'Table 32.3', p.1390 and 'Table 32.4', p.1391, but note that these amounts are only a guide. The manufacturers advice is in line with the dietary restrictions recommended for RIMAs rather than the more stringent dietary recommendations required in patients taking non-selective MAOIs.

1. Nguyen M, Beringer P, Wong-Beringer A, Louie S, Gill M, Gurevitch A. Effect of continuous enteral feedings (TF) on oral bioavailability (F) of linezolid (LZD) in hospitalized patients. Abstracts of the 43rd Annual Interscience Conference on Antimicrobial Agents and Chemotherapy, Chicago, Il, 2003, 43, 36.
2. Welshman IR, Sisson TA, Jungbluth GL, Stalker D, Hopkins NK. Linezolid absolute bioavailability and the effect of food on oral bioavailability. *Biopharm Drug Dispos* (2001) 22, 91–7.
3. Islinger F, Dehghanyar P, Sauermann R, Burger C, Kloft C, Muller M, Joukhader C. The effect of food on plasma and tissue concentrations of linezolid after multiple doses. *Int J Antimicrob Agents* (2006) 27, 108–12.
4. Zyvox (Linezolid). Pharmacia Ltd. UK Summary of product characteristics, September 2015.
5. Antal EJ, Hendershot PE, Batts DH, Sheu W-P, Hopkins NK, Donaldson KM. Linezolid, a novel oxazolidinone antibiotic: assessment of monoamine oxidase inhibition using pressor response to oral tyramine. *J Clin Pharmacol* (2001) 41, 552–62.
6. Cantarini MV, Painter CJ, Gilmore EM, Bolger C, Watkins CL, Hughes AM. Effect of oral linezolid on the pressor response to intravenous tyramine. *Br J Clin Pharmacol* (2004) 58, 470–5.
7. Zyvox (Linezolid). Pfizer Inc. US Prescribing information, June 2015.

Linezolid + Mirtazapine

Serotonin syndrome might occur in patients taking linezolid with mirtazapine.

Clinical evidence

A patient taking linezolid 600 mg twice daily developed delirium, confusion and visual hallucinations (symptoms similar to those of the serotonin syndrome) 2 weeks after starting to take mirtazapine 15 or 30 mg daily and gabapentin 300 mg at night. Gabapentin was stopped and the delirium resolved. About 4 weeks later the delirium recurred and then resolved when the patient discontinued mirtazapine. Mirtazapine was restarted without recurrence of delirium. The patient subsequently took mirtazapine 15 mg daily with linezolid 600 mg twice daily without adverse effects.[1] See 'Linezolid + SSRIs', p.328, for mention of a case of serotonin syndrome in a patient taking mirtazapine, citalopram and linezolid.

Mechanism

Not fully understood. Linezolid has weak MAOI effects, and serotonin syndrome is known to occur when MAOIs are given with tricyclics (see 'MAOIs or RIMAs + Tricyclic and related antidepressants', p.1403), and SSRIs (see 'MAOIs or RIMAs + SSRIs', p.1401), which are related to mirtazapine.

Importance and management

Information on the interaction between linezolid and mirtazapine appears to be limited, but it is in line with the way both drugs are known to interact. The manufacturer of linezolid contraindicates the concurrent use of serotonergic drugs (which would include mirtazapine), unless it is essential.[2,3] If linezolid is given with mirtazapine, it would seem prudent to monitor closely for symptoms of serotonin syndrome (such as agitation, fever, hyperreflexia, incoordination, and tremor), which can take several weeks to manifest. For more information on serotonin syndrome and its management, see 'Drugs that cause serotonin syndrome + Other drugs that cause serotonin syndrome', p.1471.

1. Aga VM, Barklage NE, Jefferson JW. Linezolid, a monoamine oxidase inhibiting antibiotic, and antidepressants. *J Clin Psychiatry* (2003) 64, 609–11.
2. Zyvox (Linezolid). Pharmacia Ltd. UK Summary of product characteristics, September 2014.
3. Zyvox (Linezolid). Pfizer Inc. US Prescribing information, June 2015.

Linezolid + Miscellaneous

Linezolid is predicted to interact with a number of drugs (e.g. salbutamol, buspirone, inotropes and vasopressors, triptans) in the same way as the MAOIs. The concurrent use of linezolid and gentamicin does not affect the pharmacokinetics of either drug.

Clinical evidence, mechanism, importance and management

Linezolid is a weak, reversible, non-selective inhibitor of MAO. It is therefore expected to share the interactions of the antidepressant MAOIs, although the magnitude of any interaction is likely to be smaller. The UK manufacturer of linezolid[1] contraindicates its use with a number of drugs, unless facilities are available for close observation and monitoring of blood pressure. Similarly, the US manufacturer advises that patients should only receive linezolid with these drugs if they are observed for signs of serotonin syndrome.[2]

The drugs mentioned include:

- Beta agonist bronchodilators; consider 'MAOIs or RIMAs + Beta-agonist bronchodilators', p.1386.
- Buspirone; consider 'MAOIs + Buspirone', p.1387.
- Inotropes and vasopressors (e.g. adrenaline (epinephrine), noradrenaline (norepinephrine), dopamine, dobutamine); consider 'MAOIs or RIMAs + Inotropes and Vasopressors', p.1392.
- Triptans; consider 'Triptans + MAOIs', p.646.

For more information on serotonin syndrome and its management, see 'Drugs that cause serotonin syndrome + Other drugs that cause serotonin syndrome', p.1471.

The manufacturers also contraindicate the concurrent use of linezolid with or within 2 weeks of taking any other drug that inhibits MAO-A or MAO-B.[1] They specifically name the non-selective MAOIs **isocarboxazid** and **phenelzine**.[1,2] The UK manufacturer includes the RIMA, **moclobemide**, and the MAO-B inhibitor, **selegiline**.[1] See 'MAOIs + MAOIs or RIMAs', p.1394), and see 'MAO-B inhibitors + MAOIs or RIMAs', p.771.

The US manufacturer of linezolid notes that the pharmacokinetics of neither linezolid or gentamicin are altered when the two drugs are given together.[2]

1. Zyvox (Linezolid). Pharmacia Ltd. UK Summary of product characteristics, September 2014.
2. Zyvox (Linezolid). Pfizer Inc. US Prescribing information, June 2015.

Linezolid + Nasal decongestants

In one study the use of linezolid with phenylpropanolamine or pseudoephedrine resulted in additive hypertensive effects.

Clinical evidence

In a placebo-controlled study, 14 healthy patients were given two 60-mg doses of **pseudoephedrine** or two 25-mg doses of **phenylpropanolamine** 4 hours apart, with and without linezolid. The mean maximum blood pressure rise was 11 mmHg with placebo, 15 mmHg with linezolid, 18 mmHg with **pseudoephedrine** and 14 mmHg with **phenylpropanolamine**. When the subjects were given linezolid with **pseudoephedrine** the rise was 32 mmHg, which was similar to the 38 mmHg rise seen with linezolid plus **phenylpropanolamine**. However, these rises were transient, resolving in about 2 hours. No effects were seen on linezolid pharmacokinetics.[1]

Mechanism

Linezolid acts as a weak MAO-inhibitor, which allows the accumulation of some noradrenaline at adrenergic nerve endings associated with arterial blood vessels. Pseudoephedrine and phenylpropanolamine, both indirectly-acting sympathomimetics, can release these above-normal amounts of noradrenaline resulting in blood vessel constriction and a rise in blood pressure.

Importance and management

Evidence for an interaction between linezolid and phenylpropanolamine or pseudoephedrine appears to be limited to this report, but given what is known about the way non-selective MAOIs interact with these drugs (see 'MAOIs or RIMAs + Nasal decongestants and related drugs', p.1396) an interaction appears to be established. However, it should be said that the evidence available indicates that blood pressure rises are unlikely to be of the proportions seen with the antidepressant MAOIs, which result in hypertensive crises. The manufacturers of linezolid contraindicate the use of pseudoephedrine[2,3] and phenylpropanolamine[2] with linezolid unless there are facilities available for close observation of the patient and monitoring of blood pressure. The UK manufacturer additionally advises careful dose titration if concurrent use is undertaken.

Pseudoephedrine and phenylpropanolamine are present in some cough and cold remedies, which can be bought without prescription. Patients should be told to avoid these preparations while taking linezolid. There appears to be no direct information about **ephedrine**, but it would be expected to interact similarly.

1. Hendershot PE, Antal EJ, Welshman IR, Batts DH, Hopkins NK. Linezolid: pharmacokinetic and pharmacodynamic evaluation of coadministration with pseudoephedrine HCl, phenylpropanolamine HCl, and dextromethorphan HBr. *J Clin Pharmacol* (2001) 41, 563–72.
2. Zyvox (Linezolid). Pharmacia Ltd. UK Summary of product characteristics, September 2014.
3. Zyvox (Linezolid). Pfizer Inc. US Prescribing information, June 2015.

Linezolid + Pethidine (Meperidine)

A single case report describes serotonin syndrome, which developed when a patient was given pethidine and linezolid.

Clinical evidence, mechanism, importance and management

A case report describes a 27-year-old man who developed serotonin syndrome after receiving linezolid and pethidine. He developed myoclonus and paranoid ideations, with an elevated temperature, respiratory rate, heart rate and blood pressure 2 hours after receiving the third dose of linezolid, and half an hour after receiving pethidine for amphotericin-associated rigors. His neuropsychiatric symptoms resolved within 2 hours of stopping the pethidine.[1]

The UK manufacturer of linezolid[2] (a drug with weak, reversible, non-selective MAOI activity) contraindicates its use with pethidine, unless facilities are available for close observation and monitoring of blood pressure, because of the possibility of serious reactions, similar to those that have occurred with antidepressant MAOIs and pethidine, see 'MAOIs or RIMAs + Opioids; Pethidine (Meperidine)', p.1399. Similarly, the US manufacturer[3] advises that patients should only receive linezolid with pethidine if they are observed for signs of serotonin syndrome. For more information on serotonin syndrome and its management, see 'Drugs that cause serotonin syndrome + Other drugs that cause serotonin syndrome', p.1471.

1. Das PK, Warkentin DI, Hewko R, Forrest DL. Serotonin syndrome after concomitant treatment with linezolid and meperidine. *Clin Infect Dis* (2008) 46, 264–5.
2. Zyvox (Linezolid). Pharmacia Ltd. UK Summary of product characteristics, September 2014.
3. Zyvox (Linezolid). Pfizer Inc. US Prescribing information, June 2015.

Linezolid + Rifampicin (Rifampin)

Rifampicin reduces the exposure to linezolid.

Clinical evidence

In a crossover study in 16 healthy subjects given rifampicin 600 mg daily for 8 days with oral linezolid 600 mg twice daily for the last 5 doses, rifampicin decreased the AUC and maximum plasma concentration of linezolid by 32% and 21% respectively, compared with linezolid given alone.[1] In an earlier study, healthy subjects were given a single 600-mg dose of intravenous linezolid either alone or with a single 600-mg dose of intravenous rifampicin. This study also found that rifampicin reduced the serum concentrations of linezolid, by 10%, 20%, and 35% at 6 hours, 9 hours, and 12 hours, respectively.[2]

A retrospective analysis of results from routine therapeutic drug monitoring found that linezolid exposure was lower in 45 patients taking long-term oral linezolid with rifampicin (mostly for bone and joint infections). The linezolid AUC and minimum plasma concentration were 42% and 63% lower respectively in those taking linezolid with rifampicin compared with those taking linezolid alone. Patients taking rifampicin concurrently were also much less likely to experience thrombocytopenia, a dose-related adverse effect of linezolid, or to require linezolid dose reduction.[3]

A 31-year-old woman was given intravenous rifampicin 300 mg every 8 hours and linezolid 600 mg every 12 hours for an MRSA infection. During rifampicin treatment her linezolid maximum and minimum concentrations were 7.29 micrograms/mL and 2.04 micrograms/mL, respectively. However, when the rifampicin was stopped the linezolid maximum and minimum concentrations were higher, at 12.46 micrograms/mL and 5.03 micrograms/mL, respectively.[4] There are other case reports of this interaction between oral linezolid and rifampicin, including two cases in patients with orthopaedic implant infections, whose linezolid concentrations increased when rifampicin was stopped,[5] and a case where the effect of rifampicin on linezolid concentrations persisted for 2 to 3 weeks after rifampicin was stopped.[6]

Mechanism

Linezolid is only minimally metabolised by the cytochrome P450 enzyme system, so the reduction in concentrations seems unlikely to be due to increased metabolism associated with rifampicin enzyme induction. However, *in vitro* studies[1] suggest even this minimal metabolism might, in the presence of the potent enzyme inducer rifampicin, increase sufficiently to lower linezolid concentrations. It has been suggested that the reduction in linezolid plasma concentrations might be due to the induction of P-glycoprotein by rifampicin, resulting in increased excretion of linezolid;[2,4] however, others dispute that linezolid is a substrate for P-glycoprotein.[1] Further study is needed to establish the mechanism of this interaction.

Importance and management

A pharmacokinetic interaction between rifampicin and linezolid seems to be established, although the clinical significance of this interaction is not yet established. However, case reports suggest that treatment failure could result from subtherapeutic concentrations of linezolid. The available evidence suggests that, where possible, linezolid concentrations should be monitored if both drugs are given. If this is not possible it would seem prudent to monitor concurrent use closely to ensure that the antibacterial treatment is effective. Note that the effect of rifampicin on linezolid might persist for 2 to 3 weeks after rifampicin is stopped.

1. Gandelman K, Zhu T, Fahmi OA, Glue P, Lian K, Obach RS, Damle B. Unexpected effect of rifampin on the pharmacokinetics of linezolid: in silico and in vitro approaches to explain its mechanism. *J Clin Pharmacol* (2011) 51, 229–36.
2. Egle H, Trittler R, Kümmerer K, Lemmen SW. Linezolid and rifampicin: drug interaction contrary to expectations? *Clin Pharmacol Ther* (2005) 77,451–3.
3. Pea F, Viale P, Cojutti P, Del Pin B, Zamparini E, Furlanut M. Therapeutic drug monitoring may improve safety outcomes of long-term treatment with linezolid in adult patients. *J Antimicrob Chemother* (2012) 67, 2034–42.
4. Gebhart BC, Barker BC, Markewitz BA. Decreased serum linezolid levels in a critically ill patient receiving concomitant linezolid and rifampin. *Pharmacotherapy* (2007) 27, 476–9.
5. Hoyo I, Martínez-Pastor J, Garcia-Ramiro S, Climent C, Brunet M, Cuesta M, Mensa J, Soriano A. Decreased serum linezolid concentrations in two patients receiving linezolid and rifampicin due to bone infections. *Scand J Infect Dis* (2012) 44, 548–50.
6. Gervasoni C, Simonetti FR, Resnati C, Charbe N, Clementi E, Cattaneo D. Prolonged inductive effect of rifampicin on linezolid exposure. *Eur J Clin Pharmacol* (2015) 71, 643–4.

Linezolid + SNRIs

Serotonin syndrome has been reported in patients taking linezolid with venlafaxine or duloxetine. Other SNRIs might be predicted to be associated with the same risk.

Clinical evidence

(a) Duloxetine

A case report describes a 55-year-old woman taking duloxetine 60 mg daily who developed confusion, restlessness, and abnormal movements, 3 hours after receiving linezolid 600 mg. She also developed tachycardia, low grade fever, hyperreflexia, and was unable to stay awake. Serotonin syndrome was suspected, and her symptoms improved 12 hours after withholding duloxetine.[1]

(b) Venlafaxine

An 85-year-old man taking venlafaxine 150 mg daily was given ciprofloxacin, rifampicin, and linezolid 600 mg twice daily for a hip prosthesis infection. After 20 days he was found to be confused and disorientated, and 4 days later he was also drowsy, and suffering myoclonic jerks. Linezolid and venlafaxine were stopped and the symptoms resolved over 2 days.[2] Other cases of serotonin syndrome in patients taking venlafaxine and linezolid have also been reported,[3-6] including a case in which the patient continued to take venlafaxine, but at half the original dose,[3] and a case that also involved imipramine and lithium.[6] A further case report describes a 7-year-old boy taking venlafaxine and methylphenidate who was given linezolid for osteomyelitis. He took all three drugs (doses not stated) for several days without any alterations in vital signs or evidence of serotonin syndrome.[7]

Mechanism

Linezolid has weak MAOI effects, and serotonin syndrome is known to occur when MAOIs are given with venlafaxine, see 'MAOIs or RIMAs + SNRIs', p.1401.

Importance and management

Information about an interaction between linezolid and the SNRIs is limited to cases with duloxetine and venlafaxine, but it is consistent with the way both drugs are known to interact. The manufacturers of linezolid contraindicate the concurrent use of serotonergic drugs (which would include the SNRIs),[8,9] unless concurrent use is essential, when the UK manufacturer advises that patients should be closely monitored for signs and symptoms of serotonin syndrome. If such signs or symptoms occur, consideration should be given to stopping one or both drugs.[8] The US manufacturer advises that if a serotonergic antidepressant is already being taken, where there is no suitable alternative to linezolid, and the benefits of linezolid are considered to outweigh the risk of serotonin syndrome, then the antidepressant should be stopped, linezolid given, and the patient closely monitored for symptoms of serotonin syndrome for 2 weeks, or until 24 hours after the last linezolid dose, whichever comes first.[9] For more information on serotonin syndrome and its management, see 'Drugs that cause serotonin syndrome + Other drugs that cause serotonin syndrome', p.1471.

1. Strouse TB, Kerrihard TN, Forscher CA, Zakowski P. Serotonin syndrome precipitated by linezolid in a medically ill patient on duloxetine. *J Clin Psychopharmacol* (2006) 26, 681–3.
2. Jones SL, Athan E, O'Brien D. Serotonin syndrome due to co-administration of linezolid and venlafaxine. *J Antimicrob Chemother* (2004) 54, 289–90.
3. Bergeron L, Boulé M, Perreault S. Serotonin toxicity associated with concomitant use of linezolid. *Ann Pharmacother* (2005) 39, 956–61.
4. Packer S, Berman SA, Serotonin syndrome precipitated by the monoamine oxidase inhibitor linezolid. *Am J Psychiatry* (2007) 164, 346–7.
5. Mason LW, Randhawa KS, Carpenter EC. Serotonin toxicity as a consequence of linezolid use in revision hip arthroplasty. *Orthopedics* (2008) 31, 1140.
6. Miller DG, Lovell EO. Antibiotic-induced serotonin syndrome. *J Emerg Med* (2011) 40, 25–7.
7. Hammerness P, Parada H, Abrams A. Linezolid: MAOI activity and potential drug interactions. *Psychosomatics* (2002) 43, 248–9.
8. Zyvox (Linezolid). Pharmacia Ltd. UK Summary of product characteristics, September 2014
9. Zyvox (Linezolid). Pfizer Inc. US Prescribing information, June 2015.

Linezolid + SSRIs

Serotonin syndrome has been reported in patients taking linezolid with SSRIs.

Clinical evidence

In an analysis of phase III studies, changes in vital signs did not differ between patients given linezolid and comparator drugs (i.e. antibacterials) when either were used with drugs known to interact with MAOIs, including unnamed SSRIs.[1,2] However, a number of case reports describe serotonin syndrome in patients given linezolid and an SSRI. These are described in the sections below.

(a) Citalopram

A case report describes an 85-year-old woman taking citalopram who developed tremor, confusion, dysarthria, hyperreflexia, agitation, and restlessness after linezolid was started. Citalopram was stopped and the symptoms resolved over 72 hours.[3] There are several other similar case reports of this interaction between linezolid and citalopram,[4-9] including one patient who was given citalopram 40 mg daily and mirtazapine 30 mg daily, whose symptoms resolved 2 days after stopping linezolid,[6] and one patient who received citalopram 40 mg daily and continued to show signs of serotonin syndrome 10 days after the end of a 12-day course of linezolid, which were partially resolved by cyproheptadine.[8]

(b) Escitalopram

A patient taking escitalopram 10 mg daily was also given intravenous linezolid 600 mg twice daily. After 3 days of concurrent therapy, she experienced two seizures. She also demonstrated mental status changes, agitation, and diarrhoea. Other causes of the seizures could not be ruled out, but the authors consider this case was highly suggestive of serotonin syndrome.[8]

(c) Fluoxetine

One patient taking fluoxetine had a transient episode of asymptomatic hypertension after one dose of linezolid, but as this patient had no other symptoms of serotonin syndrome, it was not considered an interaction.[2] However, a 4-year-old girl given fluoxetine 5 mg daily developed symptoms of serotonin syndrome 2 days after starting linezolid 140 mg every 12 hours, and after a procedure for which she was given fentanyl 200 micrograms. Fentanyl might have been a contributing factor.[10]

A further case report describes a 23-year old patient who received 6 doses of linezolid 600 mg whilst also taking fluoxetine 80 mg daily and developed abdominal pain, and unsteady gait. His symptoms were attributed to serotonin syndrome, and improved after the linezolid was stopped.[11] Similarly, a 77-year-old man who had recently started taking fluoxetine developed agitation and confusion 48 hours after also starting linezolid. He worsened over the next 72 hours and developed clonus, hypertonicity, and weakness, and was diagnosed with serotonin syndrome. Both drugs were stopped and he subsequently recovered.[12] A woman who was given linezolid 18 days after stopping fluoxetine developed serotonin syndrome, and required treatment with cyproheptadine.[13]

(d) Paroxetine

Paroxetine has been implicated in the development of serotonin syndrome.[14,15] In one case paroxetine was stopped 3 days before linezolid was started.[14] In the other case, an elderly patient was given linezolid 600 mg every 12 hours, 21 days after amitriptyline 10 mg daily, paroxetine 20 mg daily, and alprazolam 500 micrograms daily were started.[15]

(e) Sertraline

A woman taking sertraline 100 mg daily developed serotonin syndrome (incoordination, confusion, and hypertension) 4 days after starting to take linezolid 600 mg twice daily. Her symptoms subsided 4 days after linezolid was withdrawn. She then required a further course of linezolid, and, despite stopping sertraline on day one, she again exhibited symptoms likely to be those of serotonin syndrome on day 9. The linezolid was stopped and cyproheptadine was given, and her symptoms resolved.[16] Other cases have also been published:[5,17,18] in one case symptoms resolved within one day of discontinuing linezolid and sertraline.[5]

Mechanism

Linezolid has weak MAOI effects, and serotonin syndrome is known to occur when MAOIs are given with SSRIs (see 'MAOIs or RIMAs + SSRIs', p.1401). In the case of the patient taking linezolid with amitriptyline and paroxetine, it is possible that an interaction between amitriptyline and paroxetine contributed to the development of serotonin syndrome.

Importance and management

Information on the interaction between linezolid and the SSRIs, appears to be limited, but what is known suggests that the interaction is probably rare. The manufacturers of linezolid contraindicate or recommend avoiding the concurrent use of SSRIs unless patients are closely observed[19] (for serotonin syndrome[20]) and have their blood pressure monitored.[19] If linezolid is used with a drug with serotonergic actions it would seem prudent to monitor for symptoms of serotonin syndrome, which can take several weeks to manifest. Note that in some cases, serotonin syndrome has occurred several days after stopping the SSRI. Consideration should be given to allowing a washout period after stopping the SSRI if clinically appropriate. For more information on serotonin syndrome and its management, see 'Drugs that cause serotonin syndrome + Other drugs that cause serotonin syndrome', p.1471.

1. Hartman CS, Leach TS, Todd WM, Hafkin B. Lack of drug-interaction with combination of linezolid and monoamine oxidase inhibitor-interacting medications. *Pharmacotherapy* (2000) 20, 1230.
2. Rubinstein E, Isturiz R, Standiford HC, Smith LG, Oliphant TH, Cammarata S, Hafkin B, Le V, Remington J. Worldwide assessment of linezolid's clinical safety and tolerability: comparator-controlled phase III studies. *Antimicrob Agents Chemother* (2003) 47, 1824–31.
3. Tahir N. Serotonin syndrome as a consequence of drug-resistant infections: an interaction between linezolid and citalopram. *J Am Med Dir Assoc* (2004) 5, 111–13.
4. Bernard L, Stern R, Lew D, Hoffmeyer P. Serotonin syndrome after concomitant treatment with linezolid and citalopram. *Clin Infect Dis* (2003) 36, 1197.
5. Hachem RY, Hicks K, Huen A, Raad I. Myelosuppression and serotonin syndrome associated with concurrent use of linezolid and selective serotonin reuptake inhibitors in bone marrow transplant recipients. *Clin Infect Dis* (2003) 37, 37: e8–e11.
6. DeBellis RJ, Schaefer OP, Liquori M, Volturo GA. Linezolid-associated serotonin syndrome after concomitant treatment with citalopram and mirtazepine [sic] in a critically ill bone marrow transplant recipient. *J Intensive Care Med* (2005) 20, 351–3.
7. Bergeron L, Boulé M, Perreault S. Serotonin toxicity associated with concomitant use of linezolid. *Ann Pharmacother* (2005) 39, 956–61.
8. Lorenz RA, Vandenberg AM, Canepa EA. Serotonergic antidepressants and linezolid: a retrospective chart review and presentation of cases. *Int J Psychiatry Med* (2008) 38, 81–90.
9. McClean M, Walsh JC, Condon F. Serotonin syndrome in an orthopaedic patient secondary to linezolid therapy for MRSA infection. *Isr J Med Sci* (2011) 180, 285–6.
10. Thomas CR, Rosenberg M, Blythe V, Meyer WJ. Serotonin syndrome and linezolid. *J Am Acad Child Adolesc Psychiatry* (2004) 43, 790.
11. Steinberg M, Morin AK. Mild serotonin syndrome associated with concurrent linezolid and fluoxetine. *Am J Health-Syst Pharm* (2007) 64, 59–62.
12. Shaikh ZS, Krueper S, Malins TJ. Serotonin syndrome: take a closer look at the unwell surgical patient. *Ann R Coll Surg Engl* (2011) 93, 569–72.
13. Morales N, Vermette H. Serotonin syndrome associated with linezolid treatment after discontinuation of fluoxetine. *Psychosomatics* (2005) 46, 274–5.
14. Wigen CL, Goetz MB. Serotonin syndrome and linezolid. *Clin Infect Dis* (2002) 34, 1651–2.
15. Morales-Molina JA, Mateu-de Antonio J, Grau Cerrato S, Marín-Casino M. Probable síndrome serotoninérgico por interacción entre amitriptilina, paroxetina y linezolid. *Farm Hosp* (2005) 29, 1–2.
16. Clark DB, Andrus MR, Byrd DC. Drug interactions between linezolid and selective serotonin reuptake inhibitors: case report involving sertraline and review of the literature. *Pharmacotherapy* (2006) 26, 269–76.
17. Lavery S, Ravi H, McDaniel WW, Pushkin YR. Linezolid and serotonin syndrome. *Psychosomatics* (2001) 42, 432–4.
18. Sola CL, Bostwick JM, Hart DA, Lineberry TW. Anticipating potential linezolid-SSRI interactions in the general hospital setting: an MAOI in disguise. *Mayo Clin Proc* (2006) 81, 330–4.
19. Zyvox (Linezolid). Pharmacia Ltd. UK Summary of product characteristics, September 2014.
20. Zyvox (Linezolid). Pfizer Inc. US Prescribing information, June 2015.

Linezolid + Tricyclic antidepressants

Serotonin syndrome has been reported in a patient taking linezolid with amitriptyline and paroxetine and is also predicted to occur if linezolid is given with any tricyclic antidepressant.

Clinical evidence, mechanism, importance and management

In an analysis of phase III studies, changes in vital signs did not differ between patients given linezolid and comparator drugs (i.e. antibacterials) when either were used with drugs known to interact with MAOIs, including unnamed cyclic antidepressants.[1,2] A case report describes serotonin syndrome in an elderly patient taking linezolid 600 mg every 12 hours, 21 days after amitriptyline 10 mg daily, paroxetine 20 mg daily and alprazolam 500 micrograms daily were started.[3] However, it seems possible that an interaction between amitriptyline and paroxetine, or between paroxetine and linezolid contributed to the development of serotonin syndrome in this case.

Information on an interaction between linezolid and the tricyclics is limited and inconclusive. However, both drugs have caused serotonin syndrome when given with other serotonergic drugs. The manufacturers of linezolid contraindicate or recommend avoiding the concurrent use of tricyclic antidepressants unless patients are closely observed[4] (for serotonin syndrome[5]) and have their blood pressure monitored.[4] If linezolid is used with a drug with serotonergic actions it would seem prudent to monitor for symptoms of serotonin syndrome, which may take several weeks to manifest. For more information on serotonin syndrome and its management, see 'Drugs that cause serotonin syndrome + Other drugs that cause serotonin syndrome', p.1471.

1. Hartman CS, Leach TS, Todd WM, Hafkin B. Lack of drug-interaction with combination of linezolid and monoamine oxidase inhibitor-interacting medications. *Pharmacotherapy* (2000) 20, 1230.
2. Rubinstein E, Isturiz R, Standiford HC, Smith LG, Oliphant TH, Cammarata S, Hafkin B, Le V, Remington J. Worldwide assessment of linezolid's clinical safety and tolerability: comparator-controlled phase III studies. *Antimicrob Agents Chemother* (2003) 47, 1824–31.
3. Morales-Molina JA, Mateu-de Antonio J, Grau Cerrato S, Marín-Casino M. Probable síndrome serotoninérgico por interacción entre amitriptilina, paroxetina y linezolid. *Farm Hosp* (2005) 29, 1–2.
4. Zyvox (Linezolid). Pharmacia Ltd. UK Summary of product characteristics, September 2014.
5. Zyvox (Linezolid). Pfizer Inc. US Prescribing information, June 2015.

Linezolid + Vitamins

The pharmacokinetics of linezolid are not affected by either vitamin C or vitamin E.

Clinical evidence, mechanism, importance and management

In a study, healthy subjects were given vitamin C 1 g daily or vitamin E 800 units daily for 8 days with a single 600-mg dose of linezolid on day 6. As *in vitro* studies have indicated that endogenous reactive oxygen species (ROS) may affect linezolid clearance, it was considered possible that antioxidant supplements may affect the balance of ROS and linezolid clearance. However, the study found that antioxidants (vitamins C and E) given in doses far higher than the recommended daily intake did not affect linezolid pharmacokinetics. Therefore no dose adjustments are considered necessary during concurrent use.[1]

1. Gordi T, Tan LH, Hong C, Hopkins NJ, Francom SF, Slatter JG, Antal EJ. The pharmacokinetics of linezolid are not affected by concomitant intake of the antioxidant vitamins C and E. *J Clin Pharmacol* (2003) 43, 1161–7.

Loracarbef + Acetylcysteine

A study in healthy subjects found that acetylcysteine 200 mg had no effect on the absorption of loracarbef 400 mg.[1]

1. Roller S, Lode H, Stelzer I, Deppermann KM, Boeckh M, Koeppe P. Pharmacokinetics of loracarbef and interaction with acetylcysteine. *Eur J Clin Microbiol Infect Dis* (1992) 11, 851–5.

Loracarbef + Food

Food reduces the maximum plasma levels of loracarbef, but does not alter its bioavailability.

Clinical evidence, mechanism, importance and management

Loracarbef 400 mg was given to 12 healthy subjects either in a fasting state or following a standard breakfast. Food slowed the rate of absorption, but not the total bioavailability of loracarbef.[1] In another study, food was found to decrease the maximum plasma levels of a single 200-mg dose of loracarbef and increase the time to achieve maximum levels but the AUC of loracarbef was not significantly affected by food.[2] In a crossover study 24 healthy subjects received a single 200-mg dose of loracarbef after an overnight fast, a vegetarian low-fat breakfast, a vegetarian high-fat breakfast, a non-vegetarian low-fat breakfast, and a non-vegetarian high-fat breakfast. There was no significant difference between the pharmacokinetics of loracarbef observed after each of the four different meals. There was, however, a significant decrease in the maximum plasma level of loracarbef between the fed state and the fasted state, ranging from a 43% decrease with a high-fat vegetarian meal, to a 59% decrease with a low-fat non-vegetarian meal.[3] Loracarbef should be taken one hour before or 2 hours after food.[4]

1. Roller S, Lode H, Stelzer I, Deppermann KM, Boeckh M, Koeppe P. Pharmacokinetics of loracarbef and interaction with acetylcysteine. *Eur J Clin Microbiol Infect Dis* (1992) 11, 851–5.
2. DeSante KA, Zeckel ML. Pharmacokinetic profile of loracarbef. *Am J Med* (1992) 92 (Suppl 6A), 16S–19S.
3. Bapujee AT, Singh T, Ahmed T, Monif T, Saha N, Sharma PL. The effect of four different types of diet on the bioavailability of loracarbef. *Eur J Drug Metab Pharmacokinet* (2007) 32, 205–11.
4. Lorabid (Loracarbef). Monarch Pharmaceuticals, Inc. US Prescribing information, September 2002.

Loracarbef + Probenecid

Probenecid increases the half-life of loracarbef by about 50% but the clinical importance of this is unknown.[1]

1. Force RW, Nahata MC. Loracarbef: a new orally administered carbacephem antibiotic. *Ann Pharmacother* (1993) 27, 321–9.

Macrolides + Antacids

Aluminium/magnesium hydroxide antacids may reduce the peak levels of azithromycin, and aluminium/magnesium hydroxide (with simeticone) can prolong the absorption of erythromycin. Aluminium/magnesium hydroxide antacids do not appear to significantly alter the pharmacokinetics of clarithromycin, roxithromycin or telithromycin.

Clinical evidence, mechanism, importance and management

In 10 healthy subjects the peak serum levels, but not the total absorption, of **azithromycin** was reduced by 30 mL of *Maalox* (**aluminium/magnesium hydroxide**).[1] It is suggested therefore that **azithromycin** should not be given at the same time as antacids,[2,3] but should be taken at least one hour before or 2 hours after.[2]

In 8 healthy subjects 30 mL of *Mylanta* (**aluminium/magnesium hydroxide** and [**simeticone**]) had no significant effect on the AUC, peak serum concentration, or time to peak serum concentration of **erythromycin stearate** 500 mg, but the mean elimination rate constant was more than doubled. It was suggested that the effect on elimination may be due to a possible prolonging of absorption, although the reason for this effect is unclear.[4] However, an *in vitro* study has suggested that the release and absorption of **erythromycin stearate** may be slowed in the presence of some antacids, including **aluminium** and **magnesium hydroxides**, **aluminium** and **magnesium trisilicates**, and **simeticone** because of adsorption of **erythromycin** by the antacids.[5] The clinical relevance of this is uncertain, but likely to be small.

Aluminium/magnesium hydroxide antacids are reported not to affect the pharmacokinetics of **clarithromycin**,[6] **roxithromycin**,[7] or **telithromycin**.[8,9]

1. Foulds G, Hilligoss DM, Henry EB, Gerber N. The effects of an antacid or cimetidine on the serum concentrations of azithromycin. *J Clin Pharmacol* (1991) 31, 164–7.
2. Hopkins S. Clinical toleration and safety of azithromycin. *Am J Med* (1991) 91 (Suppl 3A), 40S–45S.
3. Zithromax (Azithromycin). Pfizer Ltd. UK Summary of product characteristics, January 2015.
4. Yamreudeewong W, Scavone JM, Paone RP, Lewis GP. Effect of antacid coadministration on the bioavailability of erythromycin stearate. *Clin Pharm* (1989) 8, 352–4.
5. Arayne MS, Sultana N. Erythromycin-antacid interaction. *Pharmazie* (1993) 48, 599–602.
6. Zündorf H, Wischmann L, Fassenbender M, Lode H, Borner K, Koeppe P. Pharmacokinetics of clarithromycin and possible interaction with H_2 blockers and antacids. *Intersci Conf Antimicrob Agents Chemother* (1991) 31, 185.
7. Boeckh M, Lode H, Höffken G, Daeschlein S, Koeppe P. Pharmacokinetics of roxithromycin and influence of H_2-blockers and antacids on gastrointestinal absorption. *Eur J Clin Microbiol Infect Dis* (1992) 11, 465–8.
8. Ketek (Telithromycin). Sanofi-Aventis. US Prescribing information, January 2015.
9. Ketek (Telithromycin). Sanofi. UK Summary of product characteristics, November 2012.

Macrolides + Azoles

Moderate pharmacokinetic interactions appear to occur between several of the azoles and macrolides but many of these are unlikely to be of clinical significance. However, clarithromycin may almost double itraconazole levels, and ketoconazole may almost double telithromycin levels.

Clinical evidence, mechanism, importance and management

(a) Azithromycin

1. Fluconazole. Single doses of fluconazole 800 mg and azithromycin 1.2 g were given to 18 healthy subjects alone and together without any significant change in the pharmacokinetics of either drug.[1]

2. Voriconazole. In healthy subjects, azithromycin 500 mg daily for 3 days had no significant effect on the AUC and maximum plasma levels of voriconazole 200 mg twice daily.[2]

(b) Clarithromycin

1. Fluconazole. Twenty healthy subjects were given clarithromycin 500 mg twice daily for 8 days. Fluconazole 400 mg daily was added on day 5, followed by 200 mg daily on days 6 to 8. The fluconazole increased the minimum plasma levels of the clarithromycin by 33% and the AUC_{0-12} by 18%.[3] These relatively small changes in the pharmacokinetics of clarithromycin are almost certainly of little or no clinical importance.

2. Itraconazole. A study in 8 patients with AIDS, taking itraconazole 200 mg daily, found that when clarithromycin 500 mg twice daily for 14 days was also given, the maximum serum levels and the AUC of the itraconazole were increased by 90% and 92%, respectively.[4] A report of 3 patients who took clarithromycin with itraconazole describes clarithromycin and itraconazole levels above the expected values in each of the patients. In one patient the clarithromycin plasma level was more than double the expected upper level, and the itraconazole level was almost ninefold the expected level.[5] The first report does not comment on the outcome of this almost twofold increase in itraconazole levels, but none of the three patients in the second report experienced signs or symptoms of either clarithromycin or itraconazole toxicity.[5] However, it would seem prudent to be alert for the need to reduce its dosage. More study is needed.

3. Posaconazole. The manufacturer of posaconazole notes that it is metabolised by UDP glucuronidation, and is a substrate for P-glycoprotein, and suggests that inhibitors of these pathways, (they name clarithromycin) may increase posaconazole plasma levels.[6] The clinical relevance of any interaction has not been established.

(c) Erythromycin

1. Itraconazole. The manufacturer of itraconazole notes that the peak plasma levels and AUC of a single 200-mg dose of itraconazole were increased by 44% and 36%, respectively, by a single 1-g dose of erythromycin ethyl succinate.[7] However, no dose adjustments are recommended.

2. Posaconazole. The manufacturer of posaconazole notes that it is metabolised by glucuronidation, and is a substrate for P-glycoprotein, and suggests that inhibitors of these pathways, (they name erythromycin) may increase posaconazole plasma levels.[6] The clinical relevance of any interaction has not been established.

3. Voriconazole. In healthy subjects, erythromycin 1 g twice daily for 7 days had no significant effect on the AUC and maximum plasma levels of voriconazole 200 mg twice daily.[2]

(d) Telithromycin

In a study in which healthy subjects were given either telithromycin 800 mg daily, **ketoconazole** 800 mg daily or both drugs together, it was found that the AUC and peak plasma levels of telithromycin were increased by 95% and 51%, respectively. It may be prudent to monitor for telithromycin adverse effects on concurrent use. In a further related study, healthy subjects were given **itraconazole** 200 mg daily, telithromycin 800 mg daily, or both drugs together. **Itraconazole** was found to increase the AUC and peak plasma levels of telithromycin by 54% and 22%, respectively. No serious adverse effects were reported in either study and telithromycin did not increase the QTc intervals observed with either **ketoconazole** or **itraconazole** alone.[8,9] Another study[10] by the same authors, in subjects aged 60 years or older and with a creatinine clearance of 30 mL/minute or more, found that, when **ketoconazole** was given, levels of telithromycin were increased but were only slightly higher than those found in younger healthy subjects[8] in the earlier study.

1. Amsden GW, Foulds G, Thakker K. Pharmacokinetic study of azithromycin with fluconazole and cotrimoxazole (trimethoprim-sulfamethoxazole) in healthy volunteers. *Clin Drug Invest* (2000) 20, 135–42.
2. Purkins L, Wood N, Ghahramani P, Kleinermans D, Layton G, Nichols D. No clinically significant effect of erythromycin or azithromycin on the pharmacokinetics of voriconazole in healthy male volunteers. *Br J Clin Pharmacol* (2003) 56, 30–6.
3. Gustavson LE, Shi H, Palmer RN, Siepman NC, Craft JC. Drug interaction between clarithromycin and fluconazole in healthy subjects. *Clin Pharmacol Ther* (1996) 59, 185.
4. Hardin TC, Summers KS, Rinaldi MG, Sharkey PK. Evaluation of the pharmacokinetic interaction between itraconazole and clarithromycin following chronic oral dosing in HIV-infected patients. *Pharmacotherapy* (1997) 17, 195.
5. Auclair B, Berning SE, Huitt GA, Peloquin CA. Potential interaction between itraconazole and clarithromycin. *Pharmacotherapy* (1999) 19, 1439–44.
6. Noxafil (Posaconazole). Merck Sharp & Dohme Ltd. UK summary of product characteristics, December 2011.
7. Sporanox Capsules (Itraconazole). Ortho-McNeill-Janssen Pharmaceuticals, Inc. US Prescribing information, June 2011.
8. Shi J, Montay G, Leroy B, Bhargava V. Effects of ketoconazole and itraconazole on the pharmacokinetics of telithromycin, a new ketolide antibiotic. *Intersci Conf Antimicrob Agents Chemother* (2002) 42, 28.
9. Shi J, Montay G, Leroy B, Bhargava VO. Effects of itraconazole or grapefruit juice on the pharmacokinetics of telithromycin. *Pharmacotherapy* (2005) 25, 42–51.
10. Shi J, Chapel S, Montay G, Hardy P, Barrett JS, Sica D, Swan SK, Noveck R, Leroy B, Bhargava VO. Effect of ketoconazole on the pharmacokinetics and safety of telithromycin and clarithromycin in older subjects with renal impairment. *Int J Clin Pharmacol Ther* (2005) 43, 123–33.

Macrolides + Food

Food appears to halve the absorption of azithromycin from the capsule formulation, but does not alter the AUC of azithromycin tablets or suspension. The pharmacokinetics of telithromycin are not altered by food.

Clinical evidence, mechanism, importance and management

(a) Azithromycin

A review by the manufacturers briefly mentions that food reduced the absorption of azithromycin by about half.[1] It is suggested therefore that azithromycin *capsules* should not be given at the same time as food, but should be taken at least one hour before or 2 hours after a meal.[1,2] However, the US manufacturers note that a high-fat meal increased the maximum levels of azithromycin *tablets* by 23%, and had no effect on the AUC.[3] Similarly, food increased the maximum levels of azithromycin *suspension* by 56%, without altering the AUC.[3] Azithromycin suspension[2,3] and tablets[3] may therefore be taken without regard to food.

(b) Telithromycin

In a crossover study, 18 healthy subjects were given a single 800-mg dose of telithromycin after an overnight fast, or at the end of a high-fat breakfast. There was no clinically significant change in the pharmacokinetics of telithromycin when taken with food.[4] Telithromycin can therefore be taken alone, or with food.[5]

1. Hopkins S. Clinical toleration and safety of azithromycin. *Am J Med* (1991) 91 (Suppl 3A), 40S–45S.
2. Zithromax (Azithromycin). Pfizer Ltd. UK Summary of product characteristics, January 2015.
3. Zithromax (Azithromycin). Pfizer Inc. US Prescribing information, June 2012.
4. Bhargava V, Lenfant B, Perret C, Pascual M-H, Sultan E, Montay G. Lack of effect of food on the bioavailability of a new ketolide antibacterial, telithromycin. *Scand J Infect Dis* (2002) 34, 823–6.
5. Ketek (Telithromycin). Sanofi. UK Summary of product characteristics, November 2012.

Macrolides + Grapefruit juice

Grapefruit juice modestly increases the bioavailability of erythromycin, but does not affect the bioavailability of clarithromycin or telithromycin.

Clinical evidence

(a) Clarithromycin

In a study, 12 healthy subjects were given a single 500-mg dose of clarithromycin and 240 mL of either water or freshly squeezed grapefruit juice with and 2 hours after clarithromycin. Grapefruit juice increased the time to peak levels of both clarithromycin and its metabolite, 14-hydroxyclarithromycin, from about 82 minutes to 148 minutes and from about 85 minutes to 172 minutes, respectively, but it did not affect the extent of clarithromycin absorption and had no significant effects on any other pharmacokinetic parameters.[1]

(b) Erythromycin

A study in 6 healthy subjects given a single 400-mg dose of erythromycin with either water or grapefruit juice found that grapefruit juice increased the AUC and maximum plasma level of erythromycin by about 49% and 52%, respectively. The time to achieve maximum levels and the half-life of erythromycin were not affected.[2]

(c) Telithromycin

A study in 16 healthy subjects given telithromycin 800 mg daily found that grapefruit juice did not affect telithromycin pharmacokinetics.[3]

Mechanism

Some components of grapefruit juice, possibly flavonoids such as naringenin, or a psoralen, dihydroxybergamottin, may inhibit the activity of the cytochrome P450 isoenzyme CYP3A4 in the gut.[1] The levels of drugs metabolised by CYP3A4, such as the macrolides, may therefore be raised by grapefruit juice. Erythromycin levels, but not those of clarithromycin or telithromycin appear to be affected by grapefruit juice. It has been suggested that a drug with low or variable bioavailability may be more likely to have its levels increased by grapefruit juice and it has been suggested that this may partly explain why the pharmacokinetics of clarithromycin (bioavailability of about 55%) and telithromycin (bioavailability of about 60%) are not significantly affected.[1]

Importance and management

Information is very limited but it would appear that there is unlikely to be a clinically significant interaction between grapefruit juice and either clarithromycin or telithromycin. The increased bioavailability of erythromycin was found in a single-dose study and it has been suggested that more prolonged administration of erythromycin with grapefruit juice could increase levels further and potentially increase the risk of adverse effects.[4] More study is needed to establish this.

1. Cheng KL, Nafziger AN, Peloquin CA, Amsden GW. Effect of grapefruit juice on clarithromycin pharmacokinetics. *Antimicrob Agents Chemother* (1998) 42, 927–9.
2. Kanazawa S, Ohkubo T, Sugawara K. The effects of grapefruit juice on the pharmacokinetics of erythromycin. *Eur J Clin Pharmacol* (2001) 56, 799–803.
3. Shi J, Montay G, Leroy B, Bhargava VO. Effects of itraconazole or grapefruit juice on the pharmacokinetics of telithromycin. *Pharmacotherapy* (2005) 25, 42–51.
4. Amory JK, Amory DW. Oral erythromycin and the risk of sudden death. *N Engl J Med* (2005) 352, 302–3.

Macrolides + H_2-receptor antagonists

Cimetidine doubled the levels of erythromycin in one single-dose study, and a single case report describes reversible deafness, which was attributed to this interaction. No clinically significant interaction appears to occur when cimetidine is given with azithromycin or clarithromycin, or when ranitidine is given with clarithromycin, roxithromycin, or telithromycin.

Clinical evidence

(a) Cimetidine

A 64-year-old woman was admitted to hospital with cough, dyspnoea and pleuritic pain and was found to have an atypical pneumonia and renal impairment. All her antihypertensive treatment (methyldopa, propranolol, co-amilofruse) was stopped, due to hypotension, and her treatment for duodenal ulcer was changed from ranitidine 150 mg twice daily to cimetidine 400 mg at night. She was then given amoxicillin 500 mg three times daily and **erythromycin** stearate 1 g four times daily. Two days later she complained of 'fuzzy hearing' and audiometry showed a bilateral hearing loss. The **erythromycin** was stopped and her hearing returned to normal after 5 days.[1] This prompted a study of this possible interaction in 8 healthy subjects, which found that cimetidine 400 mg twice daily increased the AUC of a single 250-mg dose of **erythromycin** by 73%. Maximum serum **erythromycin** levels were doubled.[1]

The pharmacokinetics of **azithromycin** were not affected by a single 800-mg dose of cimetidine in one study,[2] and although cimetidine prolongs the absorption of **clarithromycin**, this is unlikely to be of clinical significance.[3]

(b) Ranitidine

The pharmacokinetics of **clarithromycin**,[4] **roxithromycin**[5] and **telithromycin**[6,7] are reported to be unaffected by ranitidine.

Mechanism

Cimetidine is known to inhibit the *N*-demethylation of erythromycin so that it is metabolised and cleared from the body more slowly and its serum levels rise. Deafness is known to be one of the adverse effects of erythromycin,[1] which usually occurs with high-doses or intravenous use, and was probably exacerbated by renal impairment[4] in the patient described above.

Importance and management

Clinical information about an interaction between cimetidine and erythromycin seems to be limited to this case and the associated single-dose study. The manufacturers note that, with erythromycin alone, reversible hearing loss has been reported, usually in patients with renal impairment and those receiving high doses[8] (greater than 4 g daily[9]) and usually when given by the intravenous route.[9] If deafness were to occur, the management would seem to be similar (withdraw the erythromycin) regardless of whether or not cimetidine was present, so no additional precautions seem necessary.

There is evidence that azithromycin and clarithromycin do not interact with cimetidine, and ranitidine does not interact with clarithromycin, roxithromycin or telithromycin. No interaction would be expected between the macrolides and other non-enzyme inducing H_2-receptor antagonists.

1. Mogford N, Pallett A, George C. Erythromycin deafness and cimetidine treatment. *BMJ* (1994) 309, 1620.
2. Foulds G, Hilligoss DM, Henry EB, Gerber N. The effects of an antacid or cimetidine on the serum concentrations of azithromycin. *J Clin Pharmacol* (1991) 31, 164–7.
3. Amsden GW, Cheng KL, Peloquin CA, Nafziger AN. Oral cimetidine prolongs clarithromycin absorption. *Antimicrob Agents Chemother* (1998) 42, 1578–80.
4. Zündorf H, Wischmann L, Fassenbender M, Lode H, Borner K, Koeppe P. Pharmacokinetics of clarithromycin and possible interaction with H_2 blockers and antacids. *Intersci Conf Antimicrob Agents Chemother* (1991) 31, 185.
5. Boeckh M, Lode H, Höffken G, Daeschlein S, Koeppe P. Pharmacokinetics of roxithromycin and influence of H_2-blockers and antacids on gastrointestinal absorption. *Eur J Clin Microbiol Infect Dis* (1992) 11, 465–8.
6. Ketek (Telithromycin). Sanofi-Aventis. US Prescribing information, January 2015.
7. Ketek (Telithromycin). Sanofi. UK Summary of product characteristics, November 2012.
8. PCE (Erythromycin particles in tablets). Abbott Laboratories. US Prescribing information, November 2008.
9. Erymax Capsules (Erythromycin). Cephalon Ltd. UK Summary of product characteristics, January 2009.

Macrolides + Penicillins

Although there is *in vitro* evidence of antagonism between erythromycin and penicillins, this combination has been used successfully to treat community-acquired pneumonia.

Clinical evidence, mechanism, importance and management

Some *in vitro* evidence suggests that antagonism may occur between erythromycin (a bacteriostatic drug) and penicillins (bactericidal drugs) when they are used against staphylococci[1] and *Streptococcus pneumoniae*.[2] However, another study has suggested that this *in vitro* antagonism against *S. pneumoniae* between 'penicillin' and erythromycin is minimal and dependent on the interpretative criteria applied.[3] Clinical evidence for this interaction is apparently lacking, and the combination is generally used successfully for pneumonia.[4] In the UK, the combination of amoxicillin and erythromycin or another macrolide (e.g. azithromycin or clarithromycin) has been recommended by the British Thoracic Society (BTS) for adult patients with non-severe community-acquired pneumonia who require hospital admission.[5] In addition, the

BTS has recommended an intravenous combination of a beta-lactamase stable antibacterial such as co-amoxiclav (amoxicillin with clavulanic acid) with a macrolide (erythromycin or clarithromycin) for severe community-acquired pneumonia in hospitalised patients.[5]

1. Manten A. Synergism and antagonism between antibiotic mixtures containing erythromycin. *Antibiot Chemother* (1954) 4, 1228–33.
2. Johansen HK, Jensen TG, Dessau RB, Lundgren B, Frimodt-Møller N. Antagonism between penicillin and erythromycin against Streptococcus pneumoniae in vitro and in vivo. *J Antimicrob Chemother* (2000) 46, 973–80.
3. Deshpande LM, Jones RN. Antagonism between penicillin and erythromycin against Streptococcus pneumoniae: Does it exist? *Diagn Microbiol Infect Dis* (2003) 46, 223–5.
4. Feldman C. Clinical relevance of antimicrobial resistance in the management of pneumococcal community-acquired pneumonia. *J Lab Clin Med* (2004) 143, 269–83.
5. British Thoracic Society. BTS Guidelines for the management of community acquired pneumonia in adults. *Thorax* (2001) 56 (suppl IV) iv1–iv64.
6. British Thoracic Society. BTS Guidelines for the management of community acquired pneumonia in adults – 2009 update. Available at https://www.brit-thoracic.org.uk/document-library/clinical-information/pneumonia/adult-pneumonia/bts-guidelines-for-the-management-of-community-acquired-pneumonia-in-adults-2009-update/ (accessed 21/10/15)

Macrolides + Rifamycins

Both rifabutin and rifampicin greatly reduce clarithromycin concentrations. Clarithromycin increases the concentrations of rifabutin and the combination is associated with an increased risk of uveitis and neutropenia. Rifampicin (rifampin) greatly reduces telithromycin concentrations. In one study, the concurrent use of rifabutin and azithromycin did not appear to affect the concentrations of either drug, but in a retrospective analysis there was a small increase in azithromycin exposure; a very high incidence of neutropenia was seen in one study of the combination.

Clinical evidence

(a) Rifabutin

1. Neutropenia. A study in 12 healthy subjects was designed to investigate the safety and possible interactions between rifabutin 300 mg daily, and **azithromycin** 250 mg daily or **clarithromycin** 500 mg twice daily, over 14 days. The subjects were matched against 18 healthy controls who received either of the macrolides or rifabutin alone. The study had to be abandoned after 10 days because 14 patients developed neutropenia; 2 taking rifabutin alone, and all 12 of those taking rifabutin with a macrolide. Eight subjects developed a fever, 5 required colony simulating factors, and 3 required hospitalisation.[1]

2. Pharmacokinetics. In a randomised study[2] investigating a possible regimen for the prophylaxis of *Mycobacterium avium* complex (MAC) disease, 12 HIV-positive patients were given **clarithromycin** 500 mg daily, to which rifabutin 300 mg daily was added on day 15. By day 42 the **clarithromycin** AUC had decreased by 44%, and the concentrations of the metabolite, 14-hydroxyclarithromycin, had increased by 57%. A further 14 patients were given rifabutin 300 mg daily with **clarithromycin** 500 mg every 12 hours from day 15. After 28 days the AUC of the rifabutin had increased by 99%, and the AUC of the active metabolite, 25-*O*-desacetyl-rifabutin, had increased by 375%. Another group of patients with MAC lung disease were given **clarithromycin** 500 mg twice daily. When rifabutin 600 mg was added the **clarithromycin** concentrations decreased by 63% (from 5.4 to 2 micrograms/mL).[3] Limited information from a randomised study in healthy subjects suggested similar results.[1] Fluconazole appears to further increase the effects of clarithromycin on rifabutin.[4]

In a retrospective study in patients with MAC lung disease, 10 patients taking **clarithromycin** with rifabutin had lower plasma concentrations of clarithromycin (1.8 micrograms/mL) than 60 controls (patients with *Mycobacterium absessus* complex lung disease) who took clarithromycin but not rifamycins (3.8 micrograms/mL). The effect of rifabutin on clarithromycin concentrations was smaller than that of rifampicin in the same study (see under Rifampicin, below).[5] In another retrospective study in patents with MAC lung disease, in those taking rifabutin, the AUC and maximum concentration of **azithromycin** (34 patients) was 35% and 49% higher respectively, while the AUC and maximum concentration of **clarithromycin** (5 patients) did not differ, when compared with those not taking a rifamycin.[6] One study suggests that there is no pharmacokinetic interaction between **azithromycin** and rifabutin.[1]

3. Uveitis or arthralgias. Uveitis, and in some cases pseudojaundice, aphthous stomatitis, and an arthralgia syndrome have been described in patients taking both **clarithromycin** 1 to 2 g daily and rifabutin 300 to 600 mg daily.[7-10] The authors of a study in which patients with pulmonary *Mycobacterium avium* complex disease were given rifabutin 600 mg daily with clarithromycin 500 mg twice daily (15 patients) or azithromycin 600 mg daily (11 patients) considered that overall there was a high incidence of adverse events, which included 2 patients in the clarithromycin group who developed uveitis requiring discontinuation of both drugs.[11]

Reports suggest that uveitis develops between 27 to 370 days after taking the combination.[8,9] The reaction appears to be dose-dependent. In patients taking rifabutin 600 mg with clarithromycin the incidence of uveitis was 14% in patients weighing more than 65 kg, 45% in those weighing between 55 and 65 kg and 64% in those weighing less than 55 kg. The risk of developing uveitis was reduced from a mean of 43% to 13% when the dose of rifabutin was reduced to 300 mg daily.[12] The presence of fluconazole does not appear to affect the development of uveitis in patients taking clarithromycin with rifabutin,[8,9,12] but it has been suggested that this was because only small doses (50 mg) were used.[9]

Uveitis did not develop in 8 patients taking rifabutin and **azithromycin** 500 mg daily,[9] although cases of uveitis have been reported in patients taking rifabutin, fluconazole, and **azithromycin** 1.2 g weekly but they have been attributed to an interaction between rifabutin and fluconazole.[13] See 'Azoles + Rifabutin', p.239.

(b) Rifampicin (Rifampin)

Patients with lung disease due to *Mycobacterium avium* complex (MAC) were given **clarithromycin** 500 mg twice daily. When rifampicin 600 mg daily was added, the mean serum concentrations of **clarithromycin** decreased by almost 90% (from 5.4 to 0.7 micrograms/mL).[3] Similar results are reported in two further studies.[14,15] In a retrospective study in patents with MAC lung disease, in those taking rifampicin, the AUC and maximum concentration of **clarithromycin** (39 patients) was 73% and 68% lower, respectively, while the AUC and maximum concentration of **azithromycin** (272 patients) was 24% and 23% lower, respectively, than in those not taking a rifamycin.[6] In another retrospective study in 120 patients with MAC lung disease, patients taking **clarithromycin** with rifampicin had much lower clarithromycin plasma concentrations (0.3 micrograms/mL) than 60 controls (patients with *Mycobacterium absessus* complex lung disease) who took clarithromycin but not rifamycins (3.8 micrograms/mL). Over 97% of the patients with MAC lung disease had clarithromycin concentrations below the target range (2 micrograms/mL), however, there was no association between low clarithromycin concentrations and treatment outcomes in this study.[5]

The UK manufacturer of **telithromycin** notes that rifampicin reduces its AUC and maximum serum concentration by 86% and 79%, respectively.[16]

Two cases of cholestatic jaundice have been reported in patients taking rifampicin with **troleandomycin**.[17,18]

Mechanism

Both rifabutin and rifampicin (rifampin) are known enzyme inducers, which can increase the metabolism of other drugs by the liver, thereby reducing their serum concentrations. Rifampicin is recognised as being the more potent inducer. Rifabutin is also a substrate for CYP3A4. Both clarithromycin and fluconazole are inhibitors of CYP3A4 and it is probable that clarithromycin and fluconazole exert additive effects resulting in greater inhibition of rifabutin metabolism than occurs with either drug alone.[4]

The mechanism behind the increase in azithromycin exposure by rifabutin is unknown. The reason for the uveitis is not known, but based on *animal* studies it has been suggested that it is associated with effective treatment of MAC and is due to release of a mycobacterial protein, rather than a toxic effect of the drugs.[19] It has been suggested that lower body-weight and concurrent clarithromycin might result in toxic rifabutin serum concentrations, although concurrent fluconazole, which increases rifabutin concentrations, does not appear to be a factor.[12] The hepatotoxicity seen with rifampicin and troleandomycin is probably due to additive effects as both drugs are known to be hepatotoxic.

Importance and management

Rifabutin and Rifampicin: Pharmacokinetics

Direct information appears to be limited to the reports cited but the interactions would appear to be established. What is not entirely clear is whether these interactions result in treatment failures because of the potentially subtherapeutic clarithromycin or azithromycin serum concentrations. Moreover, serum concentrations might not reflect bactericidal efficacy in the tissues. Because of the lack of information, be alert for evidence of reduced efficacy if clarithromycin or azithromycin and rifampicin are used.

Although rifabutin can lower clarithromycin concentrations, the efficacy of this combination for MAC infection is established, although not without risk, see *Uveitis*, below. Clarithromycin increases rifabutin concentrations and therefore increases the risks of adverse effects. Concurrent use might therefore be desirable, but monitoring for adverse effects is necessary.

Due to a pharmacokinetic interaction the UK manufacturers recommend that telithromycin should not be given during and for 2 weeks after the use of rifampicin.[16]

Rifabutin: Neutropenia

Information regarding neutropenia with macrolides and rifamycins is very limited but what is known suggests that white cell counts should be monitored closely if rifabutin is given with azithromycin or clarithromycin. Rifabutin is known to cause polyarthritis on rare occasions, but in conjunction with clarithromycin it appears to happen at much lower doses.[10] Careful monitoring is necessary.

Rifabutin: Uveitis

The CSM in the UK has warned about the need to be aware of the increased risk of uveitis with clarithromycin and rifabutin. If uveitis occurs they recommend that rifabutin should be stopped and the patient should be referred to an ophthalmologist. Because of the increased risk of uveitis they also state that consideration should be given to reducing the dose of rifabutin to 300 mg daily in the presence of macrolides.[20] A review and a case-control study also suggest that this dose is associated with a reduced risk of uveitis and maintains efficacy.[12,21] A similar suggestion has been made by others.[11]

1. Apseloff G, Foulds G, LaBoy-Goral L, Willavize S, Vincent J. Comparison of azithromycin and clarithromycin in their interactions with rifabutin in healthy volunteers. *J Clin Pharmacol* (1998) 38, 830–5.
2. Hafner R, Bethel J, Power M, Landry B, Banach M, Mole L, Standiford HC, Follansbee S, Kumar P, Raasch R, Cohn D, Mushatt D, Drusano G. Tolerance and pharmacokinetic interactions of rifabutin and clarithromycin in human immunodeficiency virus-infected volunteers. *Antimicrob Agents Chemother* (1998) 42, 631–9.

3. Wallace RJ, Brown BA, Griffith DE, Girard W, Tanaka K. Reduced serum levels of clarithromycin in patients treated with multidrug regimens including rifampin or rifabutin for *Mycobacterium avium-M. intracellulare* infection. *J Infect Dis* (1995) 171, 747–50.
4. Jordan MK, Polis MA, Kelly G, Narang PK, Masur H, Piscitelli SC. Effects of fluconazole and clarithromycin on rifabutin and 25-O-desacetylrifabutin pharmacokinetics. *Antimicrob Agents Chemother* (2000) 44, 2170–2.
5. Koh WJ, Jeong BH, Jeon K, Lee SY, Shin SJ. Therapeutic drug monitoring in the treatment of *Mycobacterium avium* complex lung disease. *Am J Respir Crit Care Med* (2012)186, 797–802.
6. van Ingen J, Egelund EF, Levin A, Totten SE, Boeree MJ, Mouton JW, Aarnoutse RE, Heifets LB, Peloquin CA, Daley CL. The pharmacokinetics and pharmacodynamics of pulmonary *Mycobacterium avium* complex disease treatment. *Am J Respir Crit Care Med* (2012) 186, 559–65.
7. Shafran SD, Deschênes J, Miller M, Phillips P, Toma E. Uveitis and pseudojaundice during a regimen of clarithromycin, rifabutin, and ethambutol. *N Engl J Med* (1994) 330, 438–9.
8. Becker K, Schimkat M, Jablonowski H, Häussinger D. Anterior uveitis associated with rifabutin medication in AIDS patients. *Infection* (1996) 24, 34–6.
9. Kelleher P, Helbert M, Sweeney J, Anderson J, Parkin J, Pinching A. Uveitis associated with rifabutin and macrolide therapy for *Mycobacterium avium intracellulare* infections in AIDS patients. *Genitourin Med* (1996) 72, 419–21.
10. Le Gars L, Collon T, Picard O, Kaplan G, Berenbaum F. Polyarthralgia-arthritis syndrome induced by low doses of rifabutin. *J Rheumatol* (1999) 26, 1201–2.
11. Griffith DE, Brown BA, Girard WM, Wallace RJ. Adverse events associated with high-dose rifabutin in macrolide-containing regimens for the treatment of *Mycobacterium avium* complex lung disease. *Clin Infect Dis* (1995) 21, 594–8.
12. Shafran SD, Singer J, Zarowny DP, Deschênes J, Phillips P, Turgeon F, Aoki FY, Toma E, Miller M, Duperval R, Lemieux C, Schlech WF, for the Canadian HIV Trials Network Protocol 010 Study Group. Determinants of rifabutin-associated uveitis in patients treated with rifabutin, clarithromycin, and ethambutol for *Mycobacterium avium* complex bacteremia: a multivariate analysis. *J Infect Dis* (1998) 177, 252–5.
13. Havlir D, Torriani F, Dubé M. Uveitis associated with rifabutin prophylaxis. *Ann Intern Med* (1994) 121, 510–12.
14. Yamamoto F, Harada S, Mitsuyama T, Harada Y, Kitahara Y, Yoshida M, Nakanishi Y. Concentration of clarithromycin and 14-R-hydroxyclarithromycin in plasma of patients with *Mycobacterium avium* complex infection, before and after the addition of rifampicin. *Jpn J Antibiot* (2004) 57, 124–33.
15. Taki H, Ogawa K, Nakagawa T, Kashima K, Tarumi O, Saitou Y, Yamada N, Tano M, Nikai T. Clinical analysis of drug interaction between rifampicin and clarithromycin which are used for treating pulmonary *Mycobacterium avium* complex infection. *Kekkaku* (2007) 82, 641–6.
16. Ketek (Telithromycin). Sanofi. UK Summary of product characteristics, November 2012.
17. Piette F, Peyrard P. Ictère bénin médicamenteux lors d'un traitement associant rifampicine-triacétyloléandomycine. *Nouv Presse Med* (1979) 8, 368–9.
18. Givaudan JF, Gamby T, Privat Y. Ictère cholestatique après association rifampicine-troléandomycine: une nouvelle observation. *Nouv Presse Med* (1979) 8, 2357.
19. Opremcak EM, Cynamon M. Uveitogenic activity of rifabutin and clarithromycin in the *Mycobacterium avium*-infected beige mice. Am Soc Microbiol 2nd Nat Conf. Human retroviruses and related infections. Washington DC, Jan 29—Feb 2 1995, 74.
20. Committee on Safety of Medicines. Rifabutin (Mycobutin) – uveitis. *Current Problems* (1994) 20, 4.
21. Committee on Safety of Medicines/Medicines Control Agency. Revised indications and drug interactions of rifabutin. *Current Problems* (1997) 23, 14.

Macrolides; Azithromycin + Ceftriaxone

A study in healthy subjects found that there did not appear to be a pharmacokinetic interaction between steady-state intravenous azithromycin and ceftriaxone: the combination was well-tolerated.[1]

1. Chiu LM, Menhinick AM, Johnson PW, Amsden GW. Pharmacokinetics of intravenous azithromycin and ceftriaxone when administered alone and concurrently to healthy volunteers. *J Antimicrob Chemother* (2002) 50, 1075–9.

Macrolides; Azithromycin + Chloroquine

A study in which healthy subjects were given azithromycin 1 g daily for 3 days either alone or with chloroquine base 600 mg daily on days 1 and 2, and 300 mg on day 3, found no pharmacokinetic interaction.[1]

1. Cook JA, Randinitis EJ, Bramson CR, Wesche DL. Lack of a pharmacokinetic interaction between azithromycin and chloroquine. *Am J Trop Med Hyg* (2006) 74, 407–12.

Macrolides; Clarithromycin + Disulfiram

Fatal toxic epidermal necrolysis and fulminant hepatitis occurred in a patient taking disulfiram and clarithromycin.

Clinical evidence, mechanism, importance and management

A 47-year-old man who had taken disulfiram 250 mg daily for about a month, with clarithromycin 500 mg twice daily and paracetamol 500 mg three times daily for one week, developed fatal toxic epidermal necrolysis and fulminant hepatitis. He had not drunk alcohol for several weeks and although he was taking paracetamol, the dose was below the toxic range and therefore an interaction between disulfiram and clarithromycin was considered probable.[1]

Disulfiram alone may cause hepatic toxicity, possibly as the result of hypersensitivity or toxic metabolites. It was suggested that inhibition of the cytochrome P450 isoenzyme CYP3A4 by clarithromycin could have resulted in the accumulation of toxic metabolites of disulfiram. Hepatocellular damage is uncommon in patients receiving clarithromycin alone, but may occur in patients with underlying disease. Both clarithromycin and disulfiram alone may cause adverse skin reactions, but neither has been reported to cause toxic epidermal necrolysis. The reason why this should occur on concurrent use is not understood.[1] Information seems to be limited to this single report, so no general conclusions can be drawn.

1. Masiá M, Gulierrez F, Jimeno A, Navarro A, Borrás J, Matarredona J, Martin-Hidalgo A. Fulminant hepatitis and fatal toxic epidermal necrolysis (Lyell disease) coincident with clarithromycin administration in an alcoholic patient receiving disulfiram therapy. *Arch Intern Med* (2002) 162, 474–6.

Macrolides; Erythromycin + Carbimazole

An isolated case describes torsade de pointes in an elderly patient taking carbimazole and oral erythromycin.

Clinical evidence

A 75-year-old woman with known mild mitral stenosis taking digoxin, furosemide, warfarin and carbimazole was given oral erythromycin 250 mg four times daily for a urinary tract infection. Three days later she experienced presyncopal episodes, and 4 days later she was admitted to hospital with syncope and self-terminating episodes of torsade de pointes. She completed the 7-day course of erythromycin on the day before admission. Five days after admission, when the QT interval was back to normal, she was inadvertently rechallenged with erythromycin, given as prophylaxis before permanent pacemaker insertion. After two doses of erythromycin 500 mg given at an interval of 6 hours, she developed torsade de pointes associated with a prolonged QT interval (QTc 612 milliseconds). The QT interval returned to normal 4 days after erythromycin was discontinued.[1]

Mechanism

QT prolongation and torsade de pointes are rare with oral erythromycin. Carbimazole is rapidly metabolised to thiamazole which is the active form of the drug. Thiamazole inhibits cytochrome P450 isoenzymes including CYP3A4 and it may therefore have inhibited the metabolism of erythromycin resulting in higher than normal levels. In addition, hypothyroidism can cause torsade de pointes, and therefore mild hypothyroidism induced by carbimazole could have contributed.[1] Furthermore, bradycardia (heart rate less than 60 bpm) may also have contributed to the development of torsade de pointes.

Importance and management

It was suggested that the combination of oral erythromycin and carbimazole could lead to torsade de pointes in susceptible individuals. In this case, female sex, presence of valvular heart disease, bradycardia, hypokalaemia, and hypothyroidism may all have been contributory factors.[1] See also, 'Drugs that prolong the QT interval + Other drugs that prolong the QT interval', p.272.

1. Koh TW. Risk of torsades de pointes from oral erythromycin with concomitant carbimazole (methimazole) administration. *PACE* (2001) 24, 1575–6.

Macrolides; Erythromycin + Sucralfate

Sucralfate does not appear to affect the pharmacokinetics of erythromycin.

Clinical evidence, mechanism, importance and management

In 6 healthy subjects the pharmacokinetics (elimination rate constant, half-life, AUC) of a single 400-mg dose of erythromycin ethylsuccinate were not significantly altered by a single 1-g dose of sucralfate. It was concluded that the therapeutic effects of erythromycin are unlikely to be affected by concurrent use.[1]

1. Miller LG, Prichard JG, White CA, Vytla B, Feldman S, Bowman RC. Effect of concurrent sucralfate administration on the absorption of erythromycin. *J Clin Pharmacol* (1990) 30, 39–44.

Macrolides; Erythromycin + Urinary acidifiers or alkalinisers

In the treatment of urinary tract infections, the antibacterial activity of erythromycin is maximal in alkaline urine and minimal in acidic urine.

Clinical evidence

Urine taken from 7 subjects receiving erythromycin 1 g every 8 hours, was tested against 5 genera of Gram-negative bacilli (*Escherichia coli*, *Klebsiella pneumoniae*, *Proteus mirabilis*, *Pseudomonas aeruginosa* and *Serratia* sp.) both before and after treatment with **acetazolamide** or **sodium bicarbonate**, given to alkalinise the urine. A direct correlation was found between the activity of the antibacterial and the pH of the urine. In general, acidic urine had little or no antibacterial activity, whereas alkalinised urine had activity.[1]

Clinical studies have confirmed the increased antibacterial effectiveness of erythromycin in the treatment of bacteriuria when the urine is made alkaline.[2,3]

Mechanism

The pH of the urine does not apparently affect the way the kidney handles erythromycin (most of it is excreted actively rather than passively) but it does have a direct influence on the way the antibacterial affects the micro-organisms. Mechanisms suggested include effects on bacterial cell receptors, the induction of active transport mechanisms on bacterial cell walls, and changes in ionisation of the antibacterial, which enables it to enter the bacterial cell more effectively.

Importance and management

An established interaction, which can be exploited. Should erythromycin be used to treat urinary tract infections its efficacy can be maximised by making the urine alkaline (for example with acetazolamide or sodium bicarbonate). Treatment with urinary acidifiers will minimise the activity of the erythromycin for urinary tract infections and should be avoided. There is no evidence that the efficacy of erythromycin in other infections is affected by urinary acidifiers or alkalinisers.

1. Sabath LD, Gerstein DA, Loder PB, Finland M. Excretion of erythromycin and its enhanced activity in urine against gram-negative bacilli with alkalinization. *J Lab Clin Med* (1968) 72, 916–23.
2. Zinner SH, Sabath LD, Casey JI, Finland M. Erythromycin and alkalinisation of the urine in the treatment of urinary-tract infections due to gram-negative bacilli. *Lancet* (1971) i, 1267–8.
3. Zinner SH, Sabath LD, Casey JI, Finland M. Erythromycin plus alkalinization in treatment of urinary infections. *Antimicrob Agents Chemother* (1969) 9, 413–16.

Methenamine + Urinary acidifiers or alkalinisers

Urinary alkalinisers (e.g. potassium or sodium citrate) and those antacids that can raise the urinary pH above 5.5 inhibit its activation of methenamine.

Clinical evidence, mechanism, importance and management

Methenamine and methenamine mandelate are only effective as urinary antiseptics if the pH is about 5.5 or lower, when formaldehyde is released. This is normally achieved by giving urinary acidifiers such as ammonium chloride, ascorbic acid,[1,2] or sodium acid phosphate. In the case of methenamine hippurate, the acidification of the urine is achieved by the presence of hippuric acid. The concurrent use of substances that raise the urinary pH such as **acetazolamide, sodium bicarbonate, potassium** or **sodium citrate** is clearly contraindicated. **Potassium citrate mixture BPC** has been shown to raise the pH by more than 1 at normal therapeutic doses, thereby making the urine sufficiently alkaline to interfere with the activation of methenamine to formaldehyde.[3] Some **antacids** (containing magnesium, aluminium or calcium as well as sodium bicarbonate, as mentioned above) can also cause a significant rise in the pH of the urine.[4]

1. Strom JG, Jun HW. Effect of urine pH and ascorbic acid on the rate of conversion of methenamine to formaldehyde. *Biopharm Drug Dispos* (1993) 14, 61–9.
2. Nahata MC, Cummins BA, McLeod DC, Schondelmeyer SW, Butler R. Effect of urinary acidifiers on formaldehyde concentration and efficacy with methenamine therapy. *Eur J Clin Pharmacol* (1982) 22, 281–4.
3. Lipton JH. Incompatibility between sulfamethizole and methenamine mandelate. *N Engl J Med* (1963) 268, 92.
4. Blondheim SH, Alkan WJ, Brunner D, eds. Frontiers of Internal Medicine. 1974. Basel: Karger; 1975 p. 404–8.

Metronidazole + Barbiturates

Phenobarbital markedly increases the metabolism of metronidazole and treatment failure has been reported in both adults and children.

Clinical evidence

A woman with vaginal trichomoniasis was given metronidazole on several occasions over the course of a year, but the infection flared up again as soon as it was stopped. When it was realised that she was also taking **phenobarbital** 100 mg daily, the metronidazole dose was doubled to 500 mg three times daily, and she was cured after a 7-day course.[1] A pharmacokinetic study found that the clearance of metronidazole was increased by **phenobarbital** (half-life 3.5 hours compared with the normal half-life of 8 to 9 hours).[1]

A retrospective study in children who had not responded to metronidazole for giardiasis or amoebiasis found that 80% of them had been taking long-term **phenobarbital**. In a prospective study in 36 children the normal recommended metronidazole dose had to be increased about threefold to 60 mg/kg to achieve a cure. The half-life of metronidazole in 15 other children taking **phenobarbital** was found to be 3.5 hours, compared with the normal half-life of 8 to 9 hours.[2]

Other studies in patients with Crohn's disease and healthy subjects have found that **phenobarbital** reduces the AUC of metronidazole by about one-third,[3] and increases the clearance of metronidazole by 50%.[4]

Mechanism

Phenobarbital is a known, potent liver-enzyme inducer, which increases the metabolism and clearance of metronidazole from the body.

Importance and management

An established and clinically important interaction. Monitor the effects of concurrent use and anticipate the need to increase the metronidazole dose two to threefold if phenobarbital is given. All of the barbiturates are potent liver enzyme inducers and would therefore be expected to interact similarly.

1. Mead PB, Gibson M, Schentag JJ, Ziemniak JA. Possible alteration of metronidazole metabolism by phenobarbital. *N Engl J Med* (1982) 306, 1490.
2. Gupte S. Phenobarbital and metabolism of metronidazole. *N Engl J Med* (1983) 308, 529.
3. Eradiri O, Jamali F, Thomson ABR. Interaction of metronidazole with phenobarbital, cimetidine, prednisone, and sulfasalazine in Crohn's disease. *Biopharm Drug Dispos* (1988) 9, 219–27.
4. Loft S, Sonne J, Poulsen HE, Petersen KT, Jørgensen BG, Døssing M. Inhibition and induction of metronidazole and antipyrine metabolism. *Eur J Clin Pharmacol* (1987) 32, 35–41.

Metronidazole + Chloroquine

An isolated report describes acute dystonia in one patient, which was attributed to an interaction between metronidazole and chloroquine.

Clinical evidence, mechanism, importance and management

A patient was given a 7-day course of metronidazole and ampicillin, following a laparoscopic investigation. She developed acute dystonic reactions (facial grimacing, coarse tremors, and an inability to maintain posture) on day 6, within 10 minutes of being given chloroquine phosphate (equivalent to 200 mg of base) and intramuscular promethazine 25 mg. The dystonic symptoms started to subside within 15 minutes of being given diazepam 5 mg intravenously, and had completely resolved within 2 hours.[1]

The authors of the report attribute the dystonia to an interaction between metronidazole and chloroquine as she had taken both drugs alone without adverse effect. However, they do not fully assess the possible contribution of **promethazine**, which is known to cause dystonias. It is therefore possible that the reaction seen was an adverse effect of the **promethazine**, or perhaps even an interaction between **promethazine** and chloroquine, which, very rarely, has been associated with movement disorders. No general recommendations can therefore be made from this single report.

1. Achumba JI, Ette EI, Thomas WOA, Essien EE. Chloroquine-induced acute dystonic reactions in the presence of metronidazole. *Drug Intell Clin Pharm* (1988) 22, 308–10.

Metronidazole and related drugs + Cimetidine

Cimetidine reduces the metabolism of tinidazole, and possibly also metronidazole.

Clinical evidence

(a) Metronidazole

In 6 healthy subjects, the half-life of a 400-mg intravenous dose of metronidazole was increased from 6.2 hours to 7.9 hours by cimetidine 400 mg twice daily for 6 days. The total plasma clearance of metronidazole was reduced by almost 30%.[1] However, in another study in 6 patients with Crohn's disease, cimetidine 600 mg twice daily for 7 days was found not to affect either the AUC or the half-life of metronidazole,[2] and no evidence of an interaction was found in a further study in 6 healthy subjects.[3]

(b) Tinidazole

In a study in 6 healthy subjects, cimetidine 400 mg twice daily for 7 days raised the peak serum levels of a single 600-mg dose of tinidazole by 21%, increased the 24-hour AUC by 40% and increased the half-life by 47%, from 7.66 to 11.23 hours.[4]

Mechanism

Cimetidine is a well known enzyme inhibitor, which probably inhibits the metabolism of the metronidazole and tinidazole by the liver.

Importance and management

Evidence for an interaction between metronidazole or tinidazole and cimetidine appears to be limited to these studies. With metronidazole, only one study found an interaction, but the effects were modest, and unlikely to be clinically relevant. Similarly the effects of cimetidine on tinidazole are small, and probably not of any clinical importance.

1. Gugler R, Jensen JC. Interaction between cimetidine and metronidazole. *N Engl J Med* (1983) 309, 1518–19.
2. Eradiri O, Jamali F, Thomson ABR. Interaction of metronidazole with phenobarbital, cimetidine, prednisone, and sulfasalazine in Crohn's disease. *Biopharm Drug Dispos* (1988) 9, 219–27.
3. Loft S, Døssing M, Sonne J, Dalhof K, Bjerrum K, Poulsen HE. Lack of effect of cimetidine on the pharmacokinetics and metabolism of a single oral dose of metronidazole. *Eur J Clin Pharmacol* (1988) 35, 65–8.
4. Patel RB, Shah GF, Raval JD, Gandhi TP, Gilbert RN. The effect of cimetidine and rifampicin on tinidazole kinetics in healthy human volunteers. *Indian Drugs* (1986) 23, 338–41.

Metronidazole + Corticosteroids

Prednisone slightly decreases metronidazole exposure. No pharmacokinetic interaction appears to occur between oral budesonide and metronidazole.

Clinical evidence, mechanism, importance and management

(a) Budesonide

In a study investigating the pharmacokinetics of budesonide in children with Crohn's disease, the absorption of oral budesonide 3 mg, taken as a single dose on day one followed by three times daily until the morning of day 8, was found to be delayed in a 15-year-old boy with Crohn's disease who took a 12-day course of metronidazole 1.2 g daily until the evening before the budesonide was started. It was suggested that this might have been due to altered intraluminal pH, or delayed gastric emptying or intestinal transit. However, the possibility of a pharmacokinetic interaction between budesonide and metronidazole prompted further investigation.[1] In a study in 12 healthy adult subjects, giving metronidazole 750 mg twice daily for 8 days, with a single 3-mg dose of budesonide on day 8, had no effect on the pharmacokinetics of either drug.[2] This would suggest that the delayed absorption seen in the case report was not due to a pharmacokinetic interaction between oral budesonide and metronidazole. No dose adjustment of either drug appears to be necessary on concurrent use.

(b) Prednisone

In a study in 6 patients with Crohn's disease, prednisone 10 mg twice daily for 6 days reduced the AUC of metronidazole 250 mg twice daily by 31%. It was suggested that this occurred because prednisone induces the metabolism of metronidazole by liver enzymes.[3] Information appears to be limited to this report and the interaction is probably of only limited clinical importance because the reduction in metronidazole exposure was slight.

1. Dilger K, Alberer M, Busch A, Enninger A, Behrens R, Koletzko S, Stern M, Beckmann C, Gleiter CH. Pharmacokinetics and pharmacodynamic action of budesonide in children with Crohn's disease. *Aliment Pharmacol Ther* (2006) 23, 387–95.
2. Dilger K, Fux R, Röck D, Mörike K, Gleiter CH. Effect of high-dose metronidazole on pharmacokinetics of oral budesonide and vice versa: a double drug interaction study. *J Clin Pharmacol* (2007) 47, 1532–9.
3. Eradiri O, Jamali F, Thomson ABR. Interaction of metronidazole with phenobarbital, cimetidine, prednisone, and sulfasalazine in Crohn's disease. *Biopharm Drug Dispos* (1988) 9, 219–27.

Metronidazole + Diosmin

Diosmin reduces the metabolism of metronidazole to some extent.

Clinical evidence, mechanism, importance and management

A single 800-mg dose of metronidazole was given to 12 healthy subjects following 9 days of treatment with diosmin 500 mg daily. The metronidazole AUC and maximum plasma concentrations were raised by 27% and 25%, respectively.[1] This interaction is thought to occur because of an inhibitory effect of diosmin on metronidazole metabolism by hepatic enzymes, and inhibition of P-glycoprotein. The increase in metronidazole levels is similar to that seen with other drugs (such as cimetidine, see 'Metronidazole and related drugs + Cimetidine', p.334), and are not considered to be clinically significant. Therefore no clinically significant pharmacokinetic interaction is likely to occur if metronidazole is given with diosmin.

1. Rajnarayana K, Reddy MS, Krishna DR. Diosmin pretreatment affects bioavailability of metronidazole. *Eur J Clin Pharmacol* (2003) 58, 803–807.

Metronidazole + Disulfiram

Acute psychoses and confusion can be caused by the concurrent use of metronidazole and disulfiram.

Clinical evidence, mechanism, importance and management

In a double-blind study in 58 hospitalised chronic alcoholics taking disulfiram, 29 patients were also given metronidazole 750 mg daily for a month, then 250 mg daily thereafter. Six of the 29 subjects in the group receiving metronidazole developed acute psychoses or confusion. Five of the 6 had paranoid delusions and in 3 visual and auditory hallucinations were also seen. The symptoms persisted for 2 to 3 days after the drugs were withdrawn, but had disappeared after about 2 weeks and did not reappear when disulfiram alone was restarted.[1] Similar reactions have been described in two other reports.[2,3]

The reason for this interaction is not understood, but it appears to be established. Concurrent use should be avoided or very well monitored. Withdrawing the drugs appears to resolve any adverse effects.

1. Rothstein E, Clancy DD. Toxicity of disulfiram combined with metronidazole. *N Engl J Med* (1969) 280, 1006–7.
2. Goodhue WW. Disulfiram-metronidazole (well-identified) toxicity. *N Engl J Med* (1969) 280, 1482–3.
3. Scher JM. Psychotic reaction to disulfiram. *JAMA* (1967) 201,1051.

Metronidazole + Mebendazole

A case-control study identified the concurrent use of metronidazole and mebendazole as a risk factor in an outbreak of Stevens-Johnson syndrome/toxic epidermal necrolysis.

Clinical evidence, mechanism, importance and management

A case control study was conducted in an attempt to identify risk factors associated with an outbreak of Stevens-Johnson syndrome/toxic epidermal necrolysis that occurred amongst Filipino workers in Taiwan. The risk of developing this serious condition was significantly higher in workers who had taken both metronidazole and mebendazole sometime in the preceding 6 weeks (odds ratio of 9.5). In addition, there was an increase in risk with higher doses of metronidazole.[1]

The information is limited to this report, which does not establish an interaction. However, Stevens-Johnson syndrome/toxic epidermal necrolysis is a serious condition, and therefore, the manufacturer of mebendazole states that the concurrent use of mebendazole and metronidazole should be avoided.[2] Caution would certainly seem appropriate if both drugs are considered essential.

1. Chen K-T, Twu S-J, Chang H-J, Lin R-S. Outbreak of Stevens-Johnson syndrome/toxic epidermal necrolysis associated with mebendazole and metronidazole use among Filipino laborers in Taiwan. *Am J Public Health* (2003) 93, 489–92.
2. Vermox (Mebendazole). Janssen-Cilag Ltd. UK Summary of product characteristics, May 2009.

Metronidazole + Miscellaneous

The absorption of metronidazole is unaffected by kaolin-pectin, but it is slightly reduced by an aluminium hydroxide antacid and colestyramine.

Clinical evidence, mechanism, importance and management

In 5 healthy subjects, the bioavailability of a single 500-mg dose of metronidazole was not significantly changed by 30 mL of a **kaolin-pectin** antidiarrhoeal mixture. However, a 15% reduction in metronidazole bioavailability occurred with 30 mL of an **aluminium hydroxide/simeticone** suspension, and a 21% reduction occurred with a single 4-g dose of **colestyramine**.[1] The clinical importance of these reductions is small, and no special precautions seem necessary on concurrent use.

1. Molokhia AM, Al-Rahman S. Effect of concomitant oral administration of some adsorbing drugs on the bioavailability of metronidazole. *Drug Dev Ind Pharm* (1987) 13, 1229–37.

Metronidazole + Omeprazole

Omeprazole has no clinically significant effect on the pharmacokinetics of oral or intravenous metronidazole.

Clinical evidence, mechanism, importance and management

In 14 healthy subjects the plasma pharmacokinetics of a single oral dose of metronidazole were unaffected by 5 days of pre-treatment with omeprazole 20 mg twice daily.[1] Similar results were found in other studies with oral and intravenous metronidazole.[2,3] However, when the pharmacokinetics of metronidazole were studied in the gastric juice of 8 healthy subjects it was found that the transfer of metronidazole into the gastric juice after an intravenous dose was reduced by omeprazole (from 15.5% to 2.6%).[2] In another study, omeprazole 20 mg daily for 7 days reduced the AUC in gastric juice of a single 500-mg intravenous dose of metronidazole by 32%, but this was seen only in *H. pylori* infected individuals and not those without the infection.[3] In a third study, in 24 healthy subjects, omeprazole 40 mg twice daily for 5 days reduced the AUC_{0-4} in gastric juice of a single 400-mg intravenous dose of metronidazole by 75%.[4] However, the levels of metronidazole in gastric juice still exceeded the MIC for *H. pylori*.[4]

The clinical relevance of these findings is unclear, but they seem likely to be limited.

See also 'Proton pump inhibitors + Penicillins', p.1154, for case reports of glossitis, stomatitis and a black tongue with lansoprazole and antibacterial regimens including metronidazole.

1. David FL, Da Silva CMF, Mendes FD, Ferraz JGP, Muscara MN, Moreno H, De Nucci G, Pedrazzoli J. Acid suppression by omeprazole does not affect orally administered metronidazole bioavailability and metabolism in healthy male volunteers. *Aliment Pharmacol Ther* (1998) 12, 349–54.
2. Jessa MJ, Goddard AF, Barrett DA, Shaw PN, Spiller RC. The effect of omeprazole on the pharmacokinetics of metronidazole and hydroxymetronidazole in human plasma, saliva and gastric juice. *Br J Clin Pharmacol* (1997) 44, 245–53.
3. Calafatti SA, dos Santos A, da Silva CMF, Deguer M, Carvalho AF, Mendes FD, Ferraz JGP, Bento AP, Pereira AA, Piovesana H, de Nucci G, Lerner F, Pedrazzoli J. Transfer of metronidazole to gastric juice: impact of *Helicobacter pylori* infection and omeprazole. *Scand J Gastroenterol* (2000) 35, 699–704.
4. Goddard AF, Jessa MJ, Barrett DA, Shaw PN, Idström J-P, Cederberg C, Spiller RC. Effect of omeprazole on the distribution of metronidazole, amoxicillin, and clarithromycin in human gastric juice. *Gastroenterology* (1996) 111, 358–67.

Metronidazole and related drugs + Rifampicin (Rifampin)

Rifampicin slightly decreases the exposure to metronidazole, ornidazole and tinidazole.

Clinical evidence

(a) Metronidazole

Intravenous metronidazole 500 mg or 1 g was given to 10 healthy subjects before and after they took rifampicin 450 mg daily for 7 days. Rifampicin slightly reduced the AUC of metronidazole by 33% and increased its clearance by 44%. Results were the same with both metronidazole doses.[1]

(b) Ornidazole

In a study in 8 healthy subjects, rifampicin 600 mg daily for 6 days slightly reduced the AUC of a single 500-mg dose of ornidazole by 21%.[2]

(c) Tinidazole

In a study in 6 healthy subjects, rifampicin 600 mg daily for 7 days reduced the maximum serum concentration of a single 600-mg dose of tinidazole by 22%, slightly reduced its AUC_{0-24} by 30% and reduced its half-life by 27% (from 7.66 to 5.6 hours).[3]

Mechanism

Rifampicin (a well-recognised and potent enzyme inducer) probably increases the metabolism of metronidazole, ornidazole, and tinidazole, but the specific mechanism is unknown.

Importance and management

These pharmacokinetic interactions would appear to be established. However, a 30% reduction in metronidazole exposure would not be expected to be of much clinical relevance and there do not appear to be any reports of an interaction in practice. The effect of rifampicin on ornidazole and tinidazole is smaller, and a clinically relevant reduction in the effects of these drugs is unlikely.

1. Djojosaputro M, Mustofa SS, Donatus IA, Santoso B. The effects of doses and pre-treatment with rifampicin on the elimination kinetics of metronidazole. *Eur J Pharmacol* (1990) 183, 1870–1.
2. Kumar YS, Ramesh S, Rao YM, Paradkar AR. Effect of rifampicin pretreatment on the transport across rat intestine and oral pharmacokinetics of ornidazole in healthy human volunteers. *Drug Metabol Drug Interact* (2007) 22, 151–63.
3. Patel RB, Shah GF, Raval JD, Gandhi TP, Gilbert RN. The effect of cimetidine and rifampicin on tinidazole kinetics in healthy human volunteers. *Indian Drugs* (1986) 23, 338–41.

Metronidazole + Sucralfate

Sucralfate does not alter the pharmacokinetics of metronidazole.

Clinical evidence, mechanism, importance and management

Because oral triple therapy to eradicate *Helicobacter pylori* using sucralfate instead of bismuth has yielded inconsistent results, a 5-day study was undertaken in 14 healthy subjects to investigate whether sucralfate interacts with metronidazole. It was found that sucralfate 2 g twice daily had no effect on the pharmacokinetics of a single 400-mg dose of metronidazole.[1] Sucralfate would therefore not be expected to alter the effects of metronidazole.

1. Amaral Moraes ME, De Almeida Pierossi M, Moraes MO, Bezerra FF, Ferreira De Silva CM, Dias HB, Muscará MN, De Nucci G, Pedrazzoli J. Short-term sucralfate administration does not alter the absorption of metronidazole in healthy male volunteers. *Int J Clin Pharmacol Ther* (1996) 34, 433–7.

Nitrofurantoin + Antacids

Magnesium trisilicate reduces the absorption of nitrofurantoin. Aluminium hydroxide is reported not to interact with nitrofurantoin. Whether other antacids interact adversely is uncertain.

Clinical evidence

In 6 healthy subjects, **magnesium trisilicate** 5 g in 150 mL of water reduced the absorption of a single 100-mg oral dose of nitrofurantoin by more than 50%. The time during which the concentration of nitrofurantoin in the urine was at, or above 32 micrograms/mL (a level stated to be the minimum inhibitory concentration) was also reduced.[1] The amounts of nitrofurantoin adsorbed by other antacids during *in vitro* tests were as follows: **magnesium trisilicate** and **charcoal** 99%, **bismuth subcarbonate** and **talc** 50 to 53%, **kaolin** 31%, **magnesium oxide** 27%, **aluminium hydroxide** 2.5% and **calcium carbonate** 0%.[1]

A crossover study in 6 healthy subjects confirmed that **aluminium hydroxide gel** does not affect the absorption of nitrofurantoin from the gut (as measured by its excretion into the urine).[2] Another study, in 10 healthy subjects, found that an antacid containing **aluminium/magnesium hydroxide** and **magnesium carbonate** reduced the absorption of nitrofurantoin by 22%.[3]

Mechanism

Antacids can, to a greater or lesser extent, adsorb nitrofurantoin onto their surfaces, as a result less is available for absorption by the gut and for excretion into the urine.

Importance and management

Information appears to be limited to these reports. There seems to be nothing in the literature confirming that a clinically important interaction occurs between nitrofurantoin and antacids. One reviewer offers the opinion that common antacid preparations are unlikely to interact with nitrofurantoin.[4]

It is not yet known whether magnesium trisilicate significantly reduces the antibacterial effectiveness of nitrofurantoin but the response should be monitored. While it is known that the antibacterial action of nitrofurantoin is increased by drugs that acidify the urine (so that reduced actions would be expected if the urine were made more alkaline by antacids) this again does not seem to have been confirmed. The results of the *in vitro* studies suggest that the possible effects of the other antacids are quite small, and aluminium hydroxide is reported not to interact.

1. Naggar VF, Khalil SA. Effect of magnesium trisilicate on nitrofurantoin absorption. *Clin Pharmacol Ther* (1979) 25, 857–63.
2. Jaffe JM, Hamilton B, Jeffers S. Nitrofurantoin-antacid interaction. *Drug Intell Clin Pharm* (1976) 10, 419–20.
3. Männistö P. The effect of crystal size, gastric content and emptying rate on the absorption of nitrofurantoin in healthy human volunteers. *Int J Clin Pharmacol Biopharm* (1978) 16, 223–8.
4. D'Arcy PF. Nitrofurantoin. *Drug Intell Clin Pharm* (1985) 19, 540–7.

Nitrofurantoin + Antigout drugs

On theoretical grounds the toxicity of nitrofurantoin may possibly be increased, and its efficacy in urinary tract infections decreased, by probenecid and sulfinpyrazone.

Clinical evidence, mechanism, importance and management

A study of the way the kidneys handle nitrofurantoin found that intravenous **sulfinpyrazone** 2.5 mg/kg reduced the secretion of nitrofurantoin by the renal tubules by about 50%.[1] This reduction would be expected to reduce its urinary antibacterial efficacy, and the higher serum levels might lead to increased systemic toxicity, but there do not seem to be any reports suggesting that this represents a real problem in practice. The same situation would also seem likely with **probenecid**, but there do not appear to be any reports confirming this interaction.

The clinical importance of both of these interactions is therefore uncertain, but it would seem prudent to be alert for any evidence of reduced antibacterial efficacy and increased systemic toxicity if either **sulfinpyrazone** or **probenecid** is used with nitrofurantoin.

1. Schirmeister J, Stefani F, Willmann H, Hallauer W. Renal handling of nitrofurantoin in man. *Antimicrob Agents Chemother* (1965) 5, 223–6.

Nitrofurantoin + Antimuscarinics or Diphenoxylate

Diphenoxylate and antimuscarinic drugs such as propantheline can double the absorption of nitrofurantoin in some patients.

Clinical evidence, mechanism, importance and management

In 6 healthy subjects **propantheline** 30 mg given 45 minutes before nitrofurantoin approximately doubled the absorption of nitrofurantoin 100 mg (as measured by the urinary excretion).[1] In another study, **diphenoxylate** 200 mg daily for 3 days nearly doubled nitrofurantoin absorption in 2 out of 6 men.[2] **Atropine** 500 micrograms given subcutaneously 30 minutes before a single 100-mg dose of nitrofurantoin had little effect on the bioavailability of nitrofurantoin, but the absorption and excretion into the urine was delayed.[3]

It was suggested that the reduced gut motility caused by these drugs allows the nitrofurantoin to dissolve more completely so that it is absorbed by the gut more easily. Whether this is of any clinical importance is uncertain but it could possibly increase the incidence of dose-related adverse reactions. So far there appear to be no reports of any problems arising from concurrent use.

1. Jaffe JM. Effect of propantheline on nitrofurantoin absorption. *J Pharm Sci* (1975) 64, 1729–30.
2. Callahan M, Bullock FJ, Braun J, Yesair DW. Pharmacodynamics of drug interactions with diphenoxylate (Lomotil®). *Fedn Proc* (1974) 33, 513.
3. Männistö P. The effect of crystal size, gastric content and emptying rate on the absorption of nitrofurantoin in healthy human volunteers. *Int J Clin Pharmacol Biopharm* (1978) 16, 223–8.

Nitrofurantoin + Azoles

In an isolated case hepatic and pulmonary toxicity occurred when nitrofurantoin was given with fluconazole, but not with itraconazole.

Clinical evidence, mechanism, importance and management

A 73-year-old man who had taken nitrofurantoin 50 mg daily for 5 years was given **fluconazole** 150 mg weekly for onychomycosis. At the start of treatment with **fluconazole** his hepatic enzyme levels were slightly raised, and 3 weeks later they were increased more than twofold. Two months after starting **fluconazole** the patient's hepatic enzyme levels had increased fivefold and he had fatigue, dyspnoea on exertion, pleuritic pain, burning tracheal pain, and a cough. Bilateral pulmonary disease was confirmed by chest X-rays, and pulmonary function tests suggested nitrofurantoin toxicity. Both **fluconazole** and nitrofurantoin were discontinued, and hepatic and lung function gradually improved.[1]

Either **fluconazole** or nitrofurantoin could have caused the liver toxicity. However, it was considered that both the lung and liver toxicity may have been due to an interaction between nitrofurantoin and **fluconazole**, possibly due to increased nitrofurantoin concentrations resulting from competition with **fluconazole** for renal tubular secretion.

Some 2 years earlier the patient had received pulse **itraconazole** (less than 1% excreted in the urine as active drug) with nitrofurantoin without raised liver enzymes or any other adverse effects.[1]

Information appears to be limited to this report, but bear it in mind in the event of increased nitrofurantoin adverse effects. More study is needed.

1. Linnebur SA, Parnes BL. Pulmonary and hepatic toxicity due to nitrofurantoin and fluconazole treatment. *Ann Pharmacother* (2004) 38, 612–16.

Nitrofurantoin + Metoclopramide

Metoclopramide reduces the absorption of nitrofurantoin.

Clinical evidence, mechanism, importance and management

In 10 healthy subjects the urinary excretion of a 100-mg dose of nitrofurantoin was approximately halved by pretreatment with a 10-mg intramuscular dose of metoclopramide and a 10-mg oral dose of metoclopramide given 30 minutes before the nitrofurantoin.[1]

It is thought that metoclopramide increases the gastric emptying rate, thus decreasing nitrofurantoin absorption. The practical importance of this is uncertain, and there seem to be no reports of an interaction in practice.

1. Männistö P. The effect of crystal size, gastric content and emptying rate on the absorption of nitrofurantoin in healthy human volunteers. *Int J Clin Pharmacol Biopharm* (1978) 16, 223–8.

Nitrofurantoin + Pyridoxine (Vitamin B_6)

Paraesthesias occurred in an elderly woman who had taken pyridoxine for several years and several courses of nitrofurantoin over a 10-year period.

Clinical evidence, mechanism, importance and management

A 73-year-old woman with a 10-year history of recurrent urinary-tract infections treated with nitrofurantoin 100 mg twice daily for 3 to 10 days, two to three times each year and who also took conjugated oestrogens, calcium and magnesium, and a vitamin B complex (including pyridoxine 100 mg for 5 years), reported tingling and burning sensation of the distal lower extremity and alternate sensations of hot and cold in both feet 3 weeks after taking a 6-day course of nitrofurantoin. She also had abdominal discomfort. Her pyridoxine levels were 88.6 nanograms/mL (reference range 2 to 26 nanograms/mL). No evidence of peripheral sensory motor neuropathy, lower motor neurone dysfunction, myopathic dysfunction, or abdominal problems was found, but one year after symptoms developed she still had paraesthesias of the distal lower extremity.[1]

Nitrofurantoin may cause neuropathy after both short- or long-term treatment and occurs more frequently in women and the elderly. Pyridoxine, particularly in high doses may cause sensory neuropathy. Either drug could have caused the paraesthesias. However, it has been suggested that concurrent use of nitrofurantoin with other neurotoxic medications may increase the potential for neurotoxicity. The reason for the elevated pyridoxine levels is unclear, but they may have contributed to the neuropathy.

Information appears to be limited to this report, but bear it in mind in the event of unexpected toxicity.

1. Lacerna RA, Chien C. Paresthesias developing in an elderly patient after chronic usage of nitrofurantoin and vitamin B_6. *J Am Geriatr Soc* (2003) 51, 1822–3.

Nitroxoline + Antacids

The antibacterial effects of nitroxoline have been found to be reduced *in vitro* by magnesium and calcium ions because they form chelates with the nitroxoline.[1] In the absence of any direct clinical information it would seem prudent to monitor concurrent use for any evidence that its antibacterial effects are reduced. In many interactions with antacids, separating administration by 2 to 3 hours is effective in minimising the extent of the effects.

1. Pelletier C, Prognon P, Bourlioux P. Roles of divalent cations and pH in mechanism of action of nitroxoline against *Escherichia coli* strains. *Antimicrob Agents Chemother* (1995) 707–13.

Novobiocin + Rifampicin (Rifampin)

Rifampicin reduces the half-life of novobiocin.

Clinical evidence, mechanism, importance and management

When 10 healthy subjects were given novobiocin 1 g daily for 13 days with rifampicin 600 mg daily, the novobiocin half-life was reduced from 5.85 hours to 2.66 hours and its AUC was reduced by almost 50%. There were no significant changes to the half-life or AUC of rifampicin. The serum novobiocin and rifampicin levels were not significantly altered and the trough serum levels of both antibacterials when given alone or concurrently remained in excess of the MIC for 90% of the strains of MRSA tested.[1] No special precautions would therefore seem to be necessary during concurrent use.

1. Drusano GL, Townsend RJ, Walsh TJ, Forrest A, Antal EJ, Standiford HC. Steady-state serum pharmacokinetics of novobiocin and rifampin alone and in combination. *Antimicrob Agents Chemother* (1986) 30, 42–5.

Ornidazole + Ketoconazole

Ketoconazole slightly increases the exposure to ornidazole.

Clinical evidence, mechanism, importance and management

In a study in 8 healthy subjects, ketoconazole 200 mg daily for 7 days slightly increased the AUC of a single 500-mg dose of ornidazole (given on day 7, one hour after the last dose of ketoconazole) by 31%.[1] *In vitro* study indicates that this effect was probably due to inhibition of P-glycoprotein by ketoconazole leading to increased ornidazole exposure, although a role for CYP3A4 inhibition was not ruled out.[1] The slight increase in ornidazole exposure seen in this study is not clinically important.

1. Ramesh S, Kumar YS, Rao YM. Effect of ketoconazole on the pharmacokinetics of ornidazole–a possible role of p-glycoprotein and CYP3A. *Drug Metabol Drug Interact* (2006) 22, 67–77.

Oritavancin + Miscellaneous

Oritavancin appears to slightly increase warfarin exposure, and is predicted to interact with other CYP2C9 substrates similarly. Oritavancin affects some coagulation tests (namely aPTT, INR, and prothrombin time), and can affect coagulation monitoring of other anticoagulants, such as heparin. Oritavancin appears to slightly decrease dextromethorphan exposure, and is predicted to interact with other CYP2D6 substrates similarly. Oritavancin does not appear to have a clinically relevant effect on caffeine, omeprazole, or midazolam exposure.

Clinical evidence, mechanism, importance and management

(a) Anticoagulants

The US manufacturer of oritavancin notes that in a study in 16 healthy subjects, a single 1.2-g dose of oritavancin increased the AUC of **warfarin** by 31%.[1] Warfarin can be used as a probe substrate to assess the activity of drugs on CYP2C9, and this slight increase in its exposure suggests that oritavancin is a weak inhibitor of CYP2C9. Oritavancin might be expected to increase the exposure to other CYP2C9 substrates, but this is not expected to be clinically relevant. However, the US manufacturer advises close monitoring for adverse effects when CYP2C9 substrates with a narrow therapeutic range are used concurrently with oritavancin.[1]

The US manufacturer also notes that oritavancin might falsely elevate aPTT for about 48 hours, and artificially prolong the prothrombin time and INR for up to 24 hours, after it is given by binding to the phospholipid reagents used to precipitate coagulation in some coagulation tests and preventing them from working. They predict that oritavancin will also interfere with the test for activated clotting time because it also relies on phospholipid reagents to initiate coagulation.[1] Many **anticoagulant drugs** require coagulation monitoring, and the manufacturer advises that if aPTT monitoring is necessary in a patient taking oritavancin, a coagulation test which does not use phospholipid reagents, such as a Factor Xa (chromogenic) assay should be used, or an alternative anticoagulant not requiring aPTT monitoring should be considered. They also specifically advise that the use of **unfractionated heparin** should be avoided for 48 hours after oritavancin is given.[1] For more information on coagulation tests, see 'Coagulation tests', p.371.

(b) CYP1A2 substrates

The US manufacturer of oritavancin notes that in a study in 16 healthy subjects, a single 1.2-g dose of oritavancin given with **caffeine** increased the urinary ratio of caffeine metabolites by 18%, but there was no change in the mean exposure to the caffeine metabolites.[1] Caffeine can be used as a probe substrate to assess the activity of drugs on CYP1A2, and this study shows that caffeine is not metabolised to a clinically relevant extent by oritavancin. It would suggest that a clinically relevant interaction between oritavancin and other CYP1A2 substrates is unlikely to occur via this mechanism. However note that, a multiple-dose study is needed fully to rule out an interaction and therefore further research is needed.

(c) CYP2C19 substrates

The US manufacturer of oritavancin notes that in a study in 16 healthy subjects, a single 1.2-g dose of oritavancin given with **omeprazole** (dose not stated), increased the ratio of omeprazole to 5-hydroxyomeprazole plasma concentrations by 15%.[1] This increase is unlikely to be clinically relevant. Omeprazole can be used as a probe substrate to assess the activity of drugs on CYP2C19, and this study suggests that a clinically relevant interaction between oritavancin and other CYP2C19 substrates via this mechanism is unlikely.

(d) CYP2D6 substrates

The US manufacturer of oritavancin notes that in a study in 16 healthy subjects, when given with **dextromethorphan** (dose not stated), a single 1.2-g dose of oritavancin decreased the ratio of dextromethorphan to dextrorphan concentrations in urine by 31%.[1] Dextromethorphan can be used as a probe substrate to assess the activity of drugs on CYP2D6, and this study shows that oritavancin is a weak inducer of this isoenzyme. Oritavancin might be expected to decrease the exposure to other CYP2D6 substrates, but this is not expected to be clinically relevant. However, the US manufacturer advises close monitoring for adverse effects when CYP2D6 substrates with a narrow therapeutic range are used concurrently with oritavancin.[1] For a list of CYP2D6 substrates, see 'Table 1.7', p.9.

(e) CYP3A4 substrates

The US manufacturer of oritavancin notes that in a study in 16 healthy subjects, a single 1.2-g dose of oritavancin decreased the AUC of **midazolam** by 18%.[1] Midazolam can be used as a probe substrate to assess the activity of drugs on CYP3A4. This study therefore suggests that oritavancin is not a clinically relevant inducer of CYP3A4. However, a multiple-dose study is needed to fully predict the extent of enzyme induction, therefore the possibility of a clinically relevant interaction between oritavancin and any CYP3A4 substrate cannot be ruled out. On this basis, the US manufacturer advises caution when oritavancin is given with drugs with a narrow therapeutic range which are metabolised by CYP3A4.[1] For a list of CYP3A4 substrates, see 'Table 1.10', p.12.

(f) P-glycoprotein inhibitors and substrates

The US manufacturer of oritavancin notes that *in vitro* studies suggest that oritavancin is not an inhibitor or substrate of P-glycoprotein.[1]

1. Orbactiv (Oritavancin). The Medicines Company. US Prescribing information, September 2014.

Penicillins + Acacia or Guar gum

The absorption of amoxicillin may be significantly reduced when given with or 2 hours after acacia. Guar gum causes a small reduction in the absorption of phenoxymethylpenicillin.

Clinical evidence, mechanism, importance and management

(a) Acacia

In healthy subjects the maximum serum levels and AUC of a single 500-mg dose of **amoxicillin** were reduced by 73% and 79%, respectively, when given with acacia (gum arabic: amount not stated) and by 56% and 49%, respectively, when given 2 hours after acacia. The pharmacokinetics of **amoxicillin** were not significantly affected when it was given 4 hours after acacia. Acacia is used in pharmaceutical preparations as a suspending, demulcent and emulsifying agent. Concurrent administration with **amoxicillin** could result in subtherapeutic levels of the antibacterial, but whether or not this would occur with the amount of acacia in a dose of a preparation containing it as an excipient is not known. In some countries acacia is given to patients with chronic renal failure. The authors suggest that if **amoxicillin** is used to treat urinary tract infections in patients also treated with acacia, it should be given 4 hours before or after the acacia.[1]

(b) Guar gum

In 10 healthy subjects, guar gum 5 g (*Guarem*, 95% guar gum) reduced the absorption of a single 1980-mg dose of **phenoxymethylpenicillin** (penicillin V). Peak serum penicillin levels were reduced by 25% and the AUC_{0-6} was reduced by 28%.[2] The reasons are not understood. The clinical significance of this interaction is uncertain, but the reduction in serum levels is only small. It would clearly only be important if the reduced amount of penicillin absorbed was inadequate to control infection The effect of guar gum on other penicillins seems not to have been studied.

1. Eltayeb IB, Awad AI, Elderbi MA, Shadad SA. Effect of gum arabic on the absorption of a single oral dose of amoxicillin in healthy Sudanese volunteers. *J Antimicrob Chemother* (2004) 54, 577–8.
2. Huupponen R, Seppälä P, Iisalo E. Effect of guar gum, a fibre preparation, on digoxin and penicillin absorption in man. *Eur J Clin Pharmacol* (1984) 26, 279–81.

Penicillins + Allopurinol

The incidence of skin rashes in patients taking either ampicillin or amoxicillin is increased by allopurinol.

Clinical evidence

A retrospective search through the records of 1324 patients, 67 of whom were taking allopurinol and **ampicillin**, found that 15 of them (22%) developed a skin rash compared with 94 (8%) of the patients not taking allopurinol.[1] The types of rash were not defined. Another study found that 35 out of 252 patients (14%) taking allopurinol and **ampicillin** developed a rash, compared with 251 out of 4434 (6%) taking **ampicillin** alone.[2] A parallel study revealed that 8 out of 36 patients (22%) taking **amoxicillin** and allopurinol developed a rash, whereas only 52 out of 887 (6%) did so when taking **amoxicillin** alone.[2]

A case report describes a patient who developed erythema multiforme shortly after starting **amoxicillin** and allopurinol and who was found to have both allopurinol hypersensitivity and type IV amoxicillin hypersensitivity.[3]

In contrast, one study did not find that the incidence of penicillin-related rashes was increased by allopurinol, and the authors suggested that this contrasting finding may be because exposure to penicillins was shorter in their study.[4]

Mechanism

Not understood. One suggestion is that the hyperuricaemia was responsible.[1] Another is that hyperuricaemic individuals may possibly have an altered immunological reactivity.[5]

Importance and management

An established interaction of limited importance. There would seem to be no strong reason for avoiding concurrent use, but prescribers should recognise that the development of a rash is by no means unusual. Whether this also occurs with penicillins other than ampicillin or amoxicillin is uncertain, and does not seem to have been reported.

1. Boston Collaborative Drug Surveillance Programme. Excess of ampicillin rashes associated with allopurinol or hyperuricemia. *N Engl J Med* (1972) 286, 505–7.
2. Jick H, Porter JB. Potentiation of ampicillin skin reactions by allopurinol or hyperuricemia. *J Clin Pharmacol* (1981) 21, 456–8.
3. Pérez A, Cabrerizo S, de Barrio M, Díaz MP, Herrero T, Tornero P, Baeza ML. Erythema-multiforme-like eruption from amoxicillin and allopurinol. *Contact Dermatitis* (2001) 44, 113–14.
4. Sonntag MR, Zoppi M, Fritschy D, Maibach R, Stocker F, Sollberger J, Buchli W, Hess T, Hoigné R. Exantheme unter haufig angewandten Antibiotika und antibakteriellen Chemotherepeutika (Penicilline, speziell Aminopenicilline, Cephalosporine und Cotrimoxazol) sowie Allopurinol. *Schweiz Med Wochenschr* (1986) 116, 142–5.
5. Fessel WJ. Immunologic reactivity in hyperuricemia. *N Engl J Med* (1972) 286, 1218.

Penicillins + Antacids

Aluminium/magnesium hydroxide and aluminium hydroxide do not significantly affect the bioavailability of amoxicillin or amoxicillin with clavulanic acid (co-amoxiclav). Antacids may reduce the absorption of the hydrochloride salt of pivampicillin.

Clinical evidence, mechanism, importance and management

(a) Amoxicillin or Co-amoxiclav

The pharmacokinetics of amoxicillin 1 g, and both amoxicillin and clavulanic acid (given as co-amoxiclav 625 mg), were not significantly altered by 10 doses of **aluminium/magnesium hydroxide** (*Maalox*) 10 mL, with the last dose given 30 minutes before amoxicillin.[1] Another study found that four 40-mg doses of **aluminium hydroxide** (*Aludrox*) given at 20 minute intervals had no effect on the pharmacokinetics of either amoxicillin or clavulanic acid (given as co-amoxiclav 750 mg with the second dose of antacid).[2]

There would seem to be no reason for avoiding the concurrent use of antacids and amoxicillin or co-amoxiclav.

(b) Pivampicillin

The UK manufacturers of pivampicillin[3] used to recommend that, because antacids may decrease pivampicillin absorption, concurrent use should be avoided. This warning relates to a hydrochloride salt formulation, which needs acidic conditions for optimal absorption, whereas the basic salt formulation should not be affected by any pH change.[4]

1. Deppermann K-M, Lode H, Höffken G, Tschink G, Kalz C, Koeppe P. Influence of ranitidine, pirenzepine, and aluminium magnesium hydroxide on the bioavailability of various antibacterials, including amoxicillin, cephalexin, doxycycline, and amoxicillin-clavulanic acid. *Antimicrob Agents Chemother* (1989) 33, 1901–7.
2. Staniforth DH, Clarke HL, Horton R, Jackson D, Lau D. Augmentin bioavailability following cimetidine, aluminum hydroxide and milk. *Int J Clin Pharmacol Ther Toxicol* (1985) 23, 145–7.
3. Pondocillin (Pivampicillin). Leo Laboratories Ltd. ABPI Compendium of Datasheets and Summaries of Product Characteristics, 1998–99, 625–6.
4. Leo Laboratories Limited. Personal communication, March 1995.

Penicillins + Catha (Khat)

Chewing khat reduces the absorption of ampicillin and, to a lesser extent, amoxicillin, but the effects are minimal 2 hours after khat chewing stops.

Clinical evidence, mechanism, importance and management

A study in 8 healthy Yemeni male subjects found that chewing khat reduced the absorption of oral **ampicillin** from the gut.[1] When **ampicillin** 500 mg was taken with 250 mL water 2 hours before, just before khat chewing started, or midway through a 4-hour chewing session, the amounts of unchanged **ampicillin** in the urine fell by 46%, 41% and 49%, respectively. Even when **ampicillin** was taken 2 hours after a chewing session had stopped, the amount of drug excreted unchanged in the urine fell by 12%. A parallel series of studies with **amoxicillin** 500 mg found much smaller reductions. The equivalent reductions were 14%, 9%, 22% and 13%. A similar study found that chewing khat resulted in variable reduction in the bioavailability of **amoxicillin** 500 mg, which was maximal (22%) when it was given midway during the 4-hour chewing period.[2]

The reasons for this interaction are not known, but the authors of the reports suggest that tannins from the khat might form insoluble and non-absorbable complexes with these penicillins, and possibly also directly reduce the way the gut absorbs them.[1]

Khat (the leaves and stem tips of *Catha edulis*) is chewed in some African and Arabian countries for its stimulatory properties. The authors of one of the studies concluded that both **ampicillin** and **amoxicillin** should be taken 2 hours after khat chewing to ensure that maximum absorption occurs.[1]

1. Attef OA, Ali A-AA, Ali HM. Effect of Khat chewing on the bioavailability of ampicillin and amoxycillin. *J Antimicrob Chemother* (1997) 39, 523–5.
2. Abdel Ghani YM, Etman MA, Nada AH. Effect of khat chewing on the absorption of orally administered amoxycillin. *Acta Pharm* (1999) 49, 43–50.

Penicillins + Chloroquine

Chloroquine reduces the absorption of ampicillin, but does not affect the absorption of ampicillin from bacampicillin.

Clinical evidence

In 7 healthy subjects, chloroquine 1 g reduced the absorption (as measured by excretion in the urine) of a single 1-g dose of oral **ampicillin** by about one-third (from 29 to 19%).[1] Another study by the same author demonstrated that the absorption of **ampicillin** from **bacampicillin** tablets was unaffected by chloroquine.[2]

Mechanism

A possible reason for the reduction in absorption is that the chloroquine irritates the gut so that the ampicillin is moved through more quickly, thereby reducing the time for absorption.

Importance and management

Information appears to be limited to the studies cited, which used large doses of chloroquine (1 g) when compared with those usually used for malarial prophylaxis (300 mg base weekly) or for rheumatic diseases (150 mg daily). The reduction in the ampicillin absorption is also only moderate. The general clinical importance of this interaction therefore seems likely to be small. However, one report suggests separating the dosing by not less than 2 hours.[1] An alternative would be to use bacampicillin (an ampicillin pro-drug), which does not appear to interact with chloroquine.[2] More study is needed to confirm and evaluate the importance of this interaction.

1. Ali HM. Reduced ampicillin bioavailability following oral coadministration with chloroquine. *J Antimicrob Chemother* (1985) 15, 781–4.
2. Ali HM. The effect of Sudanese food and chloroquine on the bioavailability of ampicillin from bacampicillin tablets. *Int J Pharmaceutics* (1981) 9, 185–90.

Penicillins + Food

The absorption of many penicillins is not significantly affected by food. The exceptions are ampicillin (food may reduce its levels by up to 50%), cloxacillin, and possibly pivampicillin and phenoxymethylpenicillin.

Clinical evidence, mechanism, importance and management

(a) Dietary fibre

In 10 healthy subjects the AUC of a single 500-mg oral dose of **amoxicillin** was found to be 12.17 micrograms/mL per hour when the subjects consumed a low-fibre diet (7.8 g of insoluble fibre daily) but only 9.65 micrograms/mL per hour when the subjects consumed a high-fibre diet (36.2 g of insoluble fibre daily); a difference of about 20%. Peak serum levels were the same and occurred at 3 hours.[1] The clinical relevance of these changes is likely to be minimal.

(b) Enteral and parenteral feeds

A single 250-mg intravenous dose of **ampicillin** was given to 7 healthy subjects 2 hours into a 12-hour infusion of parenteral nutrition or 4 hours after an enteral meal. The parenteral nutrition was of two types, one with and one without amino acids, calcium and phosphorus, both without lipids, and of similar calorific content and volume to the enteral feed. None of the three regimens altered the pharmacokinetics of intravenous **ampicillin**.[2] Note that the **ampicillin** was given in a separate limb to the parenteral nutrition.

(c) Food

1. Amoxicillin and Co-amoxiclav. When amoxicillin was taken after food, its serum levels were reduced by about 50% and its urinary excretion was reduced, when compared with the fasted state.[3] However, in another study in 16 healthy subjects, a standard breakfast had no effect on the AUC of a single 500-mg dose of amoxicillin.[4] Similarly, a crossover study in 18 healthy subjects given co-amoxiclav (amoxicillin 500 mg with **clavulanic acid** 250 mg), either 2 hours before or with a fried breakfast, found that the breakfast had no significant effect on the pharmacokinetics of amoxicillin or **clavulanic acid**. Moreover, a further study in 43 healthy subjects found that taking co-amoxiclav with food tended to minimise the incidence (but not the severity) of gastrointestinal adverse effects (watery stools, nausea and vomiting).[5] It would therefore be beneficial to take co-amoxiclav with a meal.

2. Ampicillin. When a single 500-mg dose of ampicillin was taken immediately after food, its serum levels were reduced by about 50% and its urinary excretion was reduced.[3] In 16 healthy subjects, a standard breakfast reduced the AUC of a single 500-mg dose of ampicillin by 31%.[4] Another study found ampicillin absorption was delayed and the total absorption reduced when it was taken with food. Urinary excretion of ampicillin was about 30% of a dose when given on an empty stomach and about 20% when given with food.[6] It is recommended that ampicillin is taken one hour before food or on an empty stomach to optimise absorption.

3. Bacampicillin. When 6 healthy subjects took a 1.6-g dose of bacampicillin either 35 minutes after breakfast or 2 hours before breakfast, its AUC was 26% lower with the post-breakfast dose, but this difference was not statistically significant.[7] On the basis of other work that also suggests that no important interaction occurs with food,[8,9] the manufacturers say that bacampicillin can be given without regard to the time of food intake.

4. Flucloxacillin. A study in children given flucloxacillin 12.5 mg/kg as either tablets or mixture found that while the absorption depended on both the formulation and age of the child, there was no difference in levels achieved when given to a subject when fasting or with a breakfast.[10] However, it is recommended that flucloxacillin is taken one hour before food or on an empty stomach to optimise absorption. The presence of food is reported to reduce the rate and extent of absorption of the related drug **cloxacillin**,[11] and therefore it may be prudent to follow the advice given for flucloxacillin.

5. Pivampicillin. A study in healthy subjects found the absorption of pivampicillin was delayed when it was given with food, but the amount absorbed was not affected. The urinary excretion of ampicillin following pivampicillin was about 60% of the dose when taken with or without food.[6] However, another study in which pivampicillin 350 mg was given in the fasting state or with a standardised cooked breakfast found that food both delayed and reduced the absorption of pivampicillin by almost 50%.[12]

6. Pivmecillinam. The manufacturer of pivmecillinam states that the tablets should preferably be taken with or immediately after a meal.[13]

(d) Milk

The peak levels and the AUCs of oral **phenoxymethylpenicillin** and *oral* **benzylpenicillin** were reduced by 40 to 60% in infants and children when they were given with milk.[14] It is recommended that **phenoxymethylpenicillin** is taken one hour before food or on an empty stomach to optimise absorption.

Co-amoxiclav (**amoxicillin** 500 mg with **clavulanic acid** 250 mg) was given to 16 healthy subjects at the same time as the second of four 200-mL glasses of milk (taken at 20 minute intervals). Although the bioavailability of the **amoxicillin** and **clavulanic acid** tended to be decreased, and the time to peak levels delayed, the changes did not reach statistical significance.[15] No special precautions would seem to be necessary.

1. Lutz M, Espinoza J, Arancibia A, Araya M, Pacheco I, Brunser O. Effect of structured dietary fiber on bioavailability of amoxicillin. *Clin Pharmacol Ther* (1987) 42, 220–4.
2. Koo WWK, Ke J, Tam YK, Finegan BA, Marriage B. Pharmacokinetics of ampicillin during parenteral nutrition. *J Parenter Enteral Nutr* (1990) 14, 279–82.
3. Welling PG, Huang H, Koch PA, Craig WA, Madsen PO. Bioavailability of ampicillin and amoxicillin in fasted and nonfasted subjects. *J Pharm Sci* (1977) 66, 549–52.
4. Eshelman FN, Spyker DA. Pharmacokinetics of amoxicillin and ampicillin: crossover study of the effect of food. *Antimicrob Agents Chemother* (1978) 14, 539–43.
5. Staniforth DH, Lillystone RJ, Jackson D. Effect of food on the bioavailability and tolerance of clavulanic acid/amoxycillin combination. *J Antimicrob Chemother* (1982) 10, 131–9.
6. Neuvonen PJ, Elonen E, Pentikainen PJ. Comparative effect of food on absorption of ampicillin and pivampicillin. *J Int Med Res* (1977) 5, 71–6.
7. Sommers DK, van Wyk M, Moncrieff J, Schoeman HS. Influence of food and reduced gastric acidity on the bioavailability of bacampicillin and cefuroxime axetil. *Br J Clin Pharmacol* (1984) 18, 535–9.
8. Magni L, Sjöberg B, Sjövall J, Wessman J. Clinical pharmacological studies with bacampicillin. *Chemotherapy* (1976) 5, 109–114.
9. Ali HM. The effect of Sudanese food and chloroquine on the bioavailability of ampicillin from bacampicillin tablets. *Int J Pharmaceutics* (1981) 9, 185–90.
10. Bergdahl S, Eriksson M, Finkel Y, Lännergren K. Oral absorption of flucloxacillin in infants and young children. *Acta Pharmacol Toxicol (Copenh)* (1986) 58, 255–8.
11. Babalola CP, Iwheye GB, Olaniyi AA. Effect of proguanil interaction on bioavailability of cloxacillin. *J Clin Pharm Ther* (2002) 27, 461–4.
12. Fernandez CA, Menezes JP, Ximenes J. The effect of food on the absorption of pivampicillin and a comparison with the absorption of ampicillin potassium. *J Int Med Res* (1973) 1, 530–3.
13. Selexid (Pivmecillinam hydrochloride). Leo Laboratories Ltd. UK Summary of product characteristics, January 2008.
14. McCracken GH, Ginsburg CM, Clahsen JC, Thomas ML. Pharmacologic evaluation of orally administered antibiotics in infants and children: effect of feeding on bioavailability. *Pediatrics* (1978) 62, 738–43.
15. Staniforth DH, Clarke HL, Horton R, Jackson D, Lau D. Augmentin bioavailability following cimetidine, aluminium hydroxide and milk. *Int J Clin Pharmacol Ther Toxicol* (1985) 23, 154–7.

Penicillins + H_2-receptor antagonists

Cimetidine does not adversely affect the bioavailability of ampicillin or co-amoxiclav, but the bioavailability of oral benzylpenicillin may be increased in some subjects. Ranitidine does not affect the pharmacokinetics of amoxicillin, but may possibly reduce the bioavailability of bacampicillin.

Clinical evidence, mechanism, importance and management

(a) Amoxicillin and Co-amoxiclav

Cimetidine 200 mg, given three times daily the day before and with a single 200-mg dose of co-amoxiclav (amoxicillin with clavulanic acid), had no significant effect on the bioavailability of amoxicillin or clavulanic acid.[1] Another study found that **ranitidine** (300 mg given the day before and 150 mg given with the antibacterial) had no effect on the pharmacokinetics of a single 1-g dose of amoxicillin.[2]

(b) Ampicillin

In a placebo-controlled study in 6 healthy subjects, **cimetidine** 400 mg every 6 hours for 6 days had no effect on the pharmacokinetics of a single 500-mg dose of ampicillin given on day 6.[3]

(c) Bacampicillin

One small study suggested that when bacampicillin was given with **ranitidine** 300 mg and **sodium bicarbonate** 4 g, the AUC was reduced by 78% when the drugs were given with breakfast and by 55% when the drugs were given without food.[4] However, these results have been criticised because the study only included 6 subjects and because of differences in methodology between the compared groups.[5] The findings remain unconfirmed, and their clinical significance is uncertain.

(d) Benzylpenicillin

A study using a 600-mg *oral* dose of benzylpenicillin found that **cimetidine** raised the benzylpenicillin serum levels by about threefold in one subject, but did not significantly affect benzylpenicillin levels in another 4 subjects.[5] The clinical significance of these findings is unclear, especially as benzylpenicillin is more usually given parenterally.

1. Staniforth DH, Clarke HL, Horton R, Jackson D, Lau D. Augmentin bioavailability following cimetidine, aluminum hydroxide and milk. *Int J Clin Pharmacol Ther Toxicol* (1985) 23, 145–7.
2. Deppermann K-M, Lode H, Höffken G, Tschink G, Kalz C, Koeppe P. Influence of ranitidine, pirenzepine, and aluminium magnesium hydroxide on the bioavailability of various antibiotics, including amoxicillin, cephalexin, doxycycline, and amoxicillin-clavulanic acid. *Antimicrob Agents Chemother* (1989) 33, 1901–7.
3. Rogers HJ, James CA, Morrison PJ and Bradbrook ID. Effect of cimetidine on oral absorption of ampicillin and cotrimoxazole. *J Antimicrob Chemother* (1980) 6, 297–300.
4. Sommers DK, van Wyk M, Moncrieff J, Schoeman HS. Influence of food and reduced gastric acidity on the bioavailability of bacampicillin and cefuroxime axetil. *Br J Clin Pharmacol* (1984) 18, 535–9.
5. Fairfax AJ, Adam J and Pagan FS. Effect of cimetidine on absorption of oral benzylpenicillin. *BMJ* (1977) 2, 820.

Penicillins + Miscellaneous

Aspirin, indometacin, phenylbutazone, sulfaphenazole and sulfinpyrazone prolong the half-life of benzylpenicillin. Some sulfonamides reduce oxacillin blood levels. Pirenzepine does not affect the pharmacokinetics of amoxicillin, and chlorothiazide, sulfamethizole and sulfamethoxypyridazine do not affect the half-life of benzylpenicillin.

Clinical evidence, mechanism, importance and management

Studies in patients given different drugs for 5 to 7 days showed the following increases in the half-life of **benzylpenicillin**: **aspirin** 63%, **indometacin** 22%, **phenylbutazone** 139%, **sulfaphenazole** 44% and **sulfinpyrazone** 65%. It seems likely that competition between these drugs and **benzylpenicillin** for excretion by the kidney tubules caused these increases.[1] Changes in the half-life of benzylpenicillin with **chlorothiazide**, **sulfamethizole** and **sulfamethoxypyridazine** were not significant.[1]

In healthy subjects, **sulfamethoxypyridazine** 3 g given 8 hours before a 1-g dose of oral **oxacillin** reduced the 6-hour urinary recovery by 55%. **Sulfaethidole** 3.9 g given 3 hours before the **oxacillin** reduced the 6-hour urinary recovery by 42%.[2]

Pirenzepine 50 mg given three times daily on the day before and with a single 1-g dose of **amoxicillin** had no significant effect on the pharmacokinetics of the antibacterial.[3]

None of the interactions listed appears to be adverse, and no particular precautions would seem necessary during concurrent use of these drugs and the penicillins. The importance of the interaction between **oxacillin** and the sulfonamides is uncertain, but it can easily be avoided by choosing alternative drugs.

1. Kampmann J, Hansen JM, Siersboek-Nielsen K, Laursen H. Effect of some drugs on penicillin half-life in blood. *Clin Pharmacol Ther* (1972) 13, 516–19.

2. Kunin CM. Clinical pharmacology of the new penicillins. II. Effect of drugs which interfere with binding to serum proteins. *Clin Pharmacol Ther* (1966) 7, 180–88.
3. Deppermann K-M, Lode H, Höffken G, Tschink G, Kalz C, Koeppe P. Influence of ranitidine, pirenzepine, and aluminium magnesium hydroxide on the bioavailability of various antibiotics, including amoxicillin, cephalexin, doxycycline, and amoxicillin-clavulanic acid. *Antimicrob Agents Chemother* (1989) 33, 1901–7.

Penicillins + Nifedipine

Nifedipine increases the absorption of amoxicillin from the gut. Nafcillin increases the clearance of nifedipine.

Clinical evidence, mechanism, importance and management

(a) Amoxicillin

In 8 healthy subjects when amoxicillin 1 g was given 30 minutes after a 20-mg nifedipine capsule, the peak serum amoxicillin levels were raised by 33%, the bioavailability was raised by 21% and the absorption rate was raised by 70%.[1] The authors speculate that the uptake of amoxicillin through the gut wall is increased by nifedipine in some way.[1] There would seem to be no good reason for avoiding concurrent use as overall the bioavailability was not significantly altered.

(b) Nafcillin

In a randomised, placebo-controlled study, 9 healthy subjects were given a single 10-mg nifedipine capsule after a 5-day course of nafcillin 500 mg four times daily. The nifedipine AUC was decreased by 63% and its clearance was increased by 145%, but the effect of these changes on nifedipine pharmacodynamics was not assessed. It was suggested that nafcillin is an inducer of cytochrome P450 isoenzymes, and increased the metabolism of nifedipine.[2] The clinical significance of these changes is unclear, but it may be prudent to be alert for any decrease in the efficacy of nifedipine.

1. Westphal J-F, Trouvin J-H, Deslandes A, Carbon C. Nifedipine enhances amoxicillin absorption kinetics and bioavailability in humans. *J Pharmacol Exp Ther* (1990) 255, 312–17.
2. Lang CC, Jamal SK, Mohamed Z, Mustafa MR, Mustafa AM, Lee TC. Evidence of an interaction between nifedipine and nafcillin in humans. *Br J Clin Pharmacol* (2003) 55, 588–90.

Penicillins + Probenecid

Probenecid reduces the excretion of the penicillins.

Clinical evidence

(a) Amoxicillin

In 10 healthy subjects a single 3-g dose of amoxicillin was given with or without probenecid 1 g. Two hours after administration, the serum levels of amoxicillin taken with probenecid were 55% higher than those with amoxicillin alone, and they remained higher for up to 18 hours.[1] Similar results were found in another study.[2] Amoxicillin 3 g twice daily plus placebo, amoxicillin 1 g twice daily plus probenecid 1 g twice daily, and amoxicillin 1 g twice daily plus probenecid 500 mg four times daily were given to 6 patients to treat bronchiectasis. The maximum serum concentration and half-life of both high- and low-dose amoxicillin were similar, but in the regimens containing probenecid the clearance of amoxicillin was reduced by two-thirds, when compared with amoxicillin given alone.[3]

(b) Amoxicillin with clavulanic acid

A crossover study in 16 healthy subjects found that probenecid, 1 g given 12 hours and one hour before a single 500-mg dose of amoxicillin, with or without 250 mg of clavulanic acid, had no significant effects on the pharmacokinetics of clavulanic acid. However, the AUC of amoxicillin was increased by 89% and 77% when given with clavulanic acid and alone, respectively, and the maximum plasma level of amoxicillin was increased by 54% and 29% when given with clavulanic acid and alone, respectively.[4]

(c) Benzylpenicillin

Four healthy subjects were given infusions of benzylpenicillin at three different rates, either alone or with probenecid (as a separate infusion), at rates to provide low and high plasma levels. An infusion rate of probenecid 83 mg/hour, corresponding to a daily dose of 2 g was found to produce about 90% inhibition of the tubular excretion of benzylpenicillin (at plasma levels of 25 mg/L). Doses of probenecid above 2 g daily did not have a significantly greater effect.[5]

(d) Mezlocillin

A study in healthy subjects found that probenecid 1 g, given one hour before an intramuscular injection of mezlocillin, increased the peak serum levels and AUC of mezlocillin by 65% and decreased the total clearance, renal clearance and apparent volume of distribution by 38%, 52%, and 35%, respectively.[6]

(e) Nafcillin

A study in 5 healthy subjects given 500 mg of intravenous nafcillin sodium with probenecid, 1 g given orally the previous night and 2 hours before the antibacterial, found that the urinary recovery of nafcillin was reduced from 30% to 17%, and its AUC was approximately doubled.[7]

(f) Piperacillin with Tazobactam

In 10 healthy subjects probenecid 1 g given one hour before a single infusion of piperacillin 3 g with tazobactam 375 mg caused a decrease of about 25% in the clearance of both components. The half-life of tazobactam was increased by 72%.[8] A study in 8 healthy subjects found that oral probenecid 1 g, given one hour before an intramuscular injection of piperacillin 1 g, increased both the peak plasma level and terminal half-life of piperacillin by 30% and increased its AUC by 60%. The apparent volume of distribution of piperacillin was reduced by 20% and renal clearance was reduced by 40%.[9]

(g) Pivampicillin

In a crossover study, healthy subjects were given either pivampicillin 350 mg every 8 hours or a tablet of MK-356 (approximately 350 mg of pivampicillin with 200 mg of probenecid). Peak ampicillin levels of 4 to 5 micrograms/mL were found about one hour after administration of the first and last dose of both treatments suggesting that probenecid did not affect the elimination of the ampicillin metabolite of pivampicillin. Administration of MK-356 (pivampicillin 700 mg with probenecid 400 mg) twice daily indicated that peak serum levels of ampicillin were increased and elimination rate slowed following successive doses.[10]

(h) Procaine benzylpenicillin

A study in patients given intramuscular procaine benzylpenicillin 2.4 or 4.8 g with or without probenecid 2 g found the peak serum levels were higher in patients given probenecid, but because of wide interpatient variation, possibly associated with differences in the release of penicillin from the injection sites; the exact potentiating effect of probenecid could not be determined.[11] However, another study in men and women given procaine benzylpenicillin 2.4 g and 4.8 g, respectively (for uncomplicated gonorrhoea), found treatment failure after one week in 15.4% of men and 10.4% of women. Failure rates were reduced to 1.8% and 3.7%, respectively, when oral probenecid 1 g was given with the penicillin.[12]

(i) Ticarcillin

Probenecid, either 500 mg twice daily, 1 g daily, or 2 g daily was added to ticarcillin 3 g every 4 hours, which was being given to treat infections in adult cystic fibrosis patients. In all cases the clearance of ticarcillin was reduced: by about 27% with the 500-mg dose regimen, by about 32% with the 1-g dose regimen and by about 43% with the 2-g dose regimen.[13]

Mechanism

In each case the penicillin competes with the probenecid for excretion by the renal tubules, although with nafcillin, non-renal clearance may also play a part.

Importance and management

In the case of amoxicillin, benzylpenicillin, nafcillin and ticarcillin the effects of probenecid are of clinical significance. The presence of clavulanic acid does not alter the interaction of amoxicillin with probenecid. In the case of the ticarcillin study the authors suggest that a 12-hourly dosing regimen could be used if probenecid is given concurrently, which has implications for home treatment. When piperacillin with tazobactam is given with probenecid the changes are not thought to provide any benefit in terms of dose reduction or alteration of the dose interval. Note that this is generally considered to be a beneficial interaction, but bear in mind that, in some cases, such as in renal impairment, the increase in penicillin levels may be undesirably large.

1. Shanson DC, McNabb R, Hajipieris P. The effect of probenecid on serum amoxycillin concentrations up to 18 hours after a single 3 g oral dose of amoxycillin: possible implications for preventing endocarditis. *J Antimicrob Chemother* (1984) 13, 629–32.
2. Barbhaiya R, Thin RN, Turner P, Wadsworth J. Clinical pharmacological studies of amoxycillin: effect of probenecid. *Br J Vener Dis* (1979) 55, 211–13.
3. Allen MB, Fitzpatrick RW, Barratt A, Cole RB. The use of probenecid to increase the serum amoxycillin levels in patients with bronchiectasis. *Respir Med* (1990) 84, 143–6.
4. Staniforth DH, Jackson D, Clarke HL, Horton R. Amoxycillin/clavulanic acid: the effect of probenecid. *J Antimicrob Chemother* (1983) 12, 273–5.
5. Overbosch D, Van Gulpen C, Hermans J, Mattie H. The effect of probenecid on the renal tubular excretion of benzylpenicillin. *Br J Clin Pharmacol* (1988) 25, 51–8.
6. Verbist L, Tjandramaga TB, Verbesselt R, De Schepper PJ. Pharmacocinétique de la mezlocilline. Comparaison avec l'ampicilline et influence du probénécide. *Nouv Presse Med* (1982) 11, 347–52.
7. Waller ES, Sharanevych MA, Yakatan GJ. The effect of probenecid on nafcillin disposition. *J Clin Pharmacol* (1982) 22, 482–9.
8. Ganes D, Batra V, Faulkner R, Greene D, Haynes J, Kuye O, Ruffner A, Shin K, Tonelli A, Yacobi A. Effect of probenecid on the pharmacokinetics of piperacillin and tazobactam in healthy volunteers. *Pharm Res* (1991) 8 (10 Suppl), S-299.
9. Tjandramaga TB, Mullie A, Verbesselt R, De Schepper PJ, Verbist L. Piperacillin: human pharmacokinetics after intravenous and intramuscular administration. *Antimicrob Agents Chemother* (1978) 14, 829–37.
10. Kampffmeyer HG, Hartmann I, Metz H, Breault GO, Skeggs HR, Till AE, Weidner L. Serum concentrations of ampicillin and probenecid and ampicillin excretion after repeated oral administration of a pivampicillin-probenecid salt (MK-356). *Eur J Clin Pharmacol* (1975) 9, 125–9.
11. Cornelius CE, Schroeter AL, Lester A, Martin JE. Variations in serum concentrations of penicillin after injections of aqueous procaine penicillin G with and without oral probenecid. *Br J Vener Dis* (1971) 47, 359–63.
12. Holmes KK, Karney WW, Harnisch JP, Wiesner PJ, Turck M, Pedersen AHB. Single-dose aqueous procaine penicillin G therapy for gonorrhea: use of probenecid and cause of treatment failure. *J Infect Dis* (1973) 127, 455–60.
13. Corvaia L, Li SC, Ioannides-Demos LL, Bowes G, Spicer WJ, Spelman DW, Tong N, McLean AJ. A prospective study of the effects of oral probenecid on the pharmacokinetics of intravenous ticarcillin in patients with cystic fibrosis. *J Antimicrob Chemother* (1992) 30, 875–8.

Penicillins + Tetracyclines

Data from the 1950s suggested that the tetracyclines can reduce the effectiveness of penicillins in the treatment of pneumococcal meningitis and probably scarlet fever. It is uncertain whether a similar interaction

occurs with other infections. This interaction may possibly be important only with those infections where a rapid kill is essential.

Clinical evidence

When **chlortetracycline** originally became available it was tested as a potential treatment for meningitis. In patients with pneumococcal meningitis it was found that intramuscular **benzylpenicillin** 600 mg every 2 hours was more effective than the same regimen of penicillin with intravenous **chlortetracycline** 500 mg every 6 hours. Out of 43 patients given penicillin alone, 70% recovered, compared with only 20% in another group of 14 essentially similar patients who had received both antibacterials.[1]

Another report about the treatment of pneumococcal meningitis with intramuscular or intravenous **penicillin** and intravenous tetracyclines (**chlortetracycline, oxytetracycline, tetracycline**) confirmed that the mortality was much lower in those given only penicillin, rather than the combination of penicillin and a tetracycline.[2] In the treatment of scarlet fever (Group A beta-haemolytic streptococci), no difference was seen in the initial response to treatment with penicillin (oral **procaine benzylpenicillin**) and **chlortetracycline** or the penicillin alone, but spontaneous re-infection occurred more frequently in those who had received both antibacterials.[3]

Mechanism

The generally accepted explanation is that bactericides such as the penicillins, which inhibit bacterial cell wall synthesis, require cells to be actively growing and dividing to be maximally effective, a situation that will not occur in the presence of bacteriostatic antibacterials, such as the tetracyclines.

Importance and management

Documentation is limited, but this is an apparently important interaction when treating pneumococcal meningitis and probably scarlet fever. However, the use of these antibacterials for such severe infections has largely been superseded. It has not been shown to occur when treating pneumococcal pneumonia.[4] It has been suggested that antagonism, if it occurs, may only be significant when it is essential to kill bacteria rapidly,[4] i.e. in serious infections such as meningitis or in neutropenic patients. Any penicillin and any tetracycline would be expected to behave in this way. The manufacturers of some tetracyclines (including doxycycline and oxytetracycline) advise that their use with penicillins should be avoided.[5-7]

Note that, the macrolides, which are also bacteriostatic would be expected to attenuate the action of penicillins, but this does not seem to occur in practice. See 'Macrolides + Penicillins', p.331.

1. Lepper MH, Dowling HF. Treatment of pneumococcic meningitis with penicillin compared with penicillin plus aureomycin: studies including observations on an apparent antagonism between penicillin and aureomycin. *Arch Intern Med* (1951) 88, 489–94.
2. Olsson RA, Kirby JC, Romansky MJ. Pneumococcal meningitis in the adult. Clinical, therapeutic and prognostic aspects in forty-three patients. *Ann Intern Med* (1961) 55, 545–9.
3. Strom J. The question of antagonism between penicillin and chlortetracycline, illustrated by therapeutical experiments in Scarlatina. *Antibiotic Med* (1955) 1,6–12.
4. Ahern JJ, Kirby WMM. Lack of interference of aureomycin with penicillin in treatment of pneumococcic pneumonia. *Arch Intern Med* (1953) 91, 197–203.
5. Vibramycin (Doxycycline hyclate). Pfizer Ltd. UK Summary of product characteristics, May 2008.
6. Oxytetracycline (Oxytetracycline dihydrate). Actavis UK Ltd. UK Summary of product characteristics, June 2007.
7. Tetracycline (Tetracycline hydrochloride). Actavis UK Ltd. UK Summary of product characteristics, March 2007.

Penicillins + Valproate

An isolated report describes hyperammonaemic encephalopathy in an elderly patient during treatment with valproate and pivmecillinam.

Clinical evidence, mechanism, importance and management

There is a report of hyperammonaemic encephalopathy which developed in a 72-year-old woman taking valproate monotherapy for partial epilepsy after she started treatment with **pivmecillinam** 600 mg daily. She recovered after discontinuation of valproate and use of cefuroxime instead of **pivmecillinam**.[1] Valproate may reduce serum carnitine,[1] for reasons that are not well understood.[2] Valproate-induced hyperammonaemic encephalopathy may be due to reduced carnitine levels.[1]

Pivmecillinam and **pivampicillin** are hydrolysed to release mecillinam or ampicillin, respectively, as well as pivalic acid and formaldehyde. One of the potential problems of these drugs is that the pivalic acid can react with carnitine to form pivaloyl-carnitine, which is excreted in the urine, and so the body can become depleted of carnitine. Carnitine deficiency also manifests as muscle weakness and cardiomyopathy.

The risks of carnitine deficiency due to **pivmecillinam** or **pivampicillin** seem to be small in healthy adults, but the manufacturer of **pivmecillinam** issues a warning about long-term or frequently repeated treatment.[3]

The authors of the report advise caution if **pivmecillinam** is added to treatment with valproate.[1] Although this appears to be the only report of an adverse effect due to the combined effects of **pivmecillinam** and valproate on carnitine levels, the manufacturer of **pivmecillinam** advises its avoidance with valproic acid or valproate.[3] **Pivampicillin** is likely to have a similar effect and should therefore probably also be avoided.

1. Lokrantz C-M, Eriksson B, Rosén I, Asztely F. Hyperammonemic encephalopathy induced by a combination of valproate and pivmecillinam. *Acta Neurol Scand* (2004) 109, 297–301.
2. Melegh B, Kerner J, Jaszai V, Bieber LL. Differential excretion of xenobiotic acyl-esters of carnitine due to administration of pivampicillin and valproate. *Biochem Med Metab Biol* (1990) 43, 30–8.
3. Selexid (Pivmecillinam hydrochloride). Leo Laboratories Ltd. UK Summary of product characteristics, January 2008.

Penicillins; Amoxicillin + Amiloride

Amiloride can cause a small reduction in the absorption of amoxicillin.

Clinical evidence, mechanism, importance and management

When 8 healthy subjects were given amiloride 10 mg followed 2 hours later by a single 1-g oral dose of amoxicillin, the bioavailability and maximum serum levels of amoxicillin were reduced by 27% and 25%, respectively, and the time to reach maximum levels was delayed from 1 hour to 1.56 hours. When amoxicillin was given intravenously its bioavailability was unchanged by amiloride.[1] A second study in which amiloride and amoxicillin were delivered directly to the jejunum found that amiloride had no effect on the jejunal permeability of amoxicillin.[2]

It is thought that the absorption of beta lactams like amoxicillin depends on a dipeptide carrier system in the cells lining the intestine (brush border membrane). This system depends on the existence of a pH gradient between the outside and inside of the cells, which is maintained by a Na-H exchanger. As this exchanger is inhibited by amiloride the reduced absorption seen in the first study would seem to be explained.

This reported reduction in the absorption of the amoxicillin is only small and unlikely to have very much clinical relevance. There seems to be no information about other penicillins.

1. Westphal JF, Jehl F, Brogard JM, Carbon C. Amoxicillin intestinal absorption reduction by amiloride: possible role of the Na(+)-H(+) exchanger. *Clin Pharmacol Ther* (1995) 57, 257–64.
2. Lennernäs H, Knutson L, Knutson T, Hussain A, Lesko L, Salmonson T, Amidon GL. The effect of amiloride on the in vivo effective permeability of amoxicillin in human jejunum: experience from a regional perfusion technique. *Eur J Pharm Sci* (2002) 15, 271–7.

Penicillins; Amoxicillin + Cranberry juice

Cranberry juice does not appear to affect the pharmacokinetics of amoxicillin.

Clinical evidence, mechanism, importance and management

In a crossover study in 18 healthy subjects, 8 oz (about 240 mL) of cranberry juice taken twice daily for 2 days, then taken at the same time as a single 2-g or 500-mg dose of oral amoxicillin on day 3, had no effect on the pharmacokinetics of amoxicillin. In this study, the cranberry juice used was *Ocean Spray* cranberry juice cocktail from concentrate containing 27% cranberry juice.[1]

Although the evidence is limited to this particular study, there appears to be no need for any special precautions when taking cranberry juice with amoxicillin.

1. Li M, Andrew MA, Wang J, Salinger DH, Vicini P, Grady RW, Phillips B, Shen DD, Anderson GD. Effects of cranberry juice on pharmacokinetics of beta-lactam antibiotics following oral administration. *Antimicrob Agents Chemother* (2009) 53, 2725–32.

Penicillins; Cloxacillin + Proguanil

Proguanil may reduce the bioavailability of cloxacillin.

Clinical evidence, mechanism, importance and management

A pharmacokinetic study in healthy subjects given cloxacillin 500 mg with or without proguanil 200 mg found that the total amount of cloxacillin excreted in the urine over 12 hours was reduced by up to 48% by proguanil. The time to maximum excretion and the half-life of cloxacillin were increased by 23% and 34%, respectively. The reasons why cloxacillin absorption is reduced by proguanil are not known, but it has been suggested that it may be due to adsorption of cloxacillin on to proguanil in the gut, formation of a drug-complex, increased gastric motility or increased beta-lactam ring hydrolysis leading to reduced cloxacillin bioavailability.[1] The clinical implications of the interaction are unknown.

1. Babalola CP, Iwheye GB, Olaniyi AA. Effect of proguanil interaction on bioavailability of cloxacillin. *J Clin Pharm Ther* (2002) 27, 461–4.

Penicillins; Dicloxacillin + Rifampicin (Rifampin)

Rifampicin increases the oral clearance of dicloxacillin and reduces its plasma levels.

Clinical evidence, mechanism, importance and management

A study in 18 healthy subjects found that rifampicin 600 mg daily for 10 days decreased the maximum plasma level of a single 1-g dose of dicloxacillin by 27% and increased its mean oral clearance by 26%. The mean absorption time increased from 0.71 hours to 1.34 hours. Rifampicin increased the formation clearance, maximum level and AUC of the 5-hydroxymetabolite of dicloxacillin by 135%, 119%, and 59%, respectively. Dicloxacillin is a substrate of P-glycoprotein and it was suggested that the effects of rifampicin on dicloxacillin were due to induction of both intestinal P-glycoprotein and dicloxacillin metabolism.[1] The changes in the levels of dicloxacillin are modest, and unlikely to be clinically relevant.

1. Putnam WS, Woo JM, Huang Y, Benet LZ. Effect of the *MDR1* C3435T variant and P-glycoprotein induction on dicloxacillin pharmacokinetics. *J Clin Pharmacol* (2005) 45, 411–21.

Penicillins; Flucloxacillin + Paracetamol (Acetaminophen)

A case report describes severe acidosis in a critically ill patient receiving paracetamol and flucloxacillin.

Clinical evidence, mechanism, importance and management

A case report describes a patient with sepsis and renal impairment who was admitted to an intensive care unit with a high anion gap (42 mmol/L) metabolic acidosis which was tentatively attributed to treatment with flucloxacillin and paracetamol. He had received 8 g of paracetamol and 16 g of flucloxacillin over the 4 days before admission. The patient was diagnosed with pyroglutamic acidaemia, which is defined as a high anion gap acidosis resulting from excess production of 5-oxoproline. It was suggested that the depletion of glutathione by paracetamol, and further inhibition of the production of glutathione from 5-oxoproline by flucloxacillin had contributed to this patients condition. Note that this patient was also receiving carbamazepine, phenobarbital and phenytoin, which the authors suggest may also have reduced glutathione stores.[1]

This is not an unusual combination of drugs, and the clinical significance of this case, in a patient with serious medical problems, to other patients is unclear.

1. Peter JV, Rogers N, Murty S, Gerace R, Mackay R, Peake SL. An unusual cause of severe metabolic acidosis. *Med J Aust* (2006) 185, 223–5.

Penicillins; Piperacillin with Tazobactam + Vancomycin

Vancomycin does not interact to a clinically relevant extent with piperacillin and tazobactam

Clinical evidence, mechanism, importance and management

A randomised, crossover study in 9 healthy subjects found that infusions of vancomycin 500 mg and piperacillin 3 g with tazobactam 375 mg had little or no effect on the pharmacokinetics of any of the antibacterials, except that the piperacillin AUC was slightly raised, by about 7%. It was concluded that no dose adjustments are needed if these drugs are given together.[1]

1. Vechlekar D, Sia L, Lanc R, Kuye O, Yacobi A, Faulkner R. Pharmacokinetics of piperacillin/tazobactam (Pip/Taz) IV with and without vancomycin IV in healthy adult male volunteers. *Pharm Res* (1992) 9 (10 Suppl), S-322.

Protionamide + Other antimycobacterials

Protionamide appears to be very hepatotoxic and this effect is possibly increased by the concurrent use of rifampicin (rifampin) or rifandin. Protionamide does not affect the pharmacokinetics of either dapsone or rifampicin.

Clinical evidence

In a study of 39 patients with leprosy, 39% became jaundiced after treatment for 24 to 120 days with **dapsone** 100 mg daily, protionamide 300 mg daily and **rifandin** [isopiperazinylrifamycin SV] 300 to 600 mg monthly. Laboratory evidence of liver damage occurred in 56% of patients, and despite the withdrawal of the drugs from all the patients, 2 of them died.[1] All the patients except two had previously taken **dapsone** alone for 3 to 227 months without reported problems.[1] In another group of patients with leprosy, 22% (11 of 50) had liver damage after treatment with **dapsone** 100 mg and protionamide 300 mg given daily, and **rifampicin** (rifampin) 900 mg, protionamide 500 mg and **clofazimine** 300 mg given monthly over a period of 30 to 50 days. One patient died.[1] Most of the patients recovered within 30 to 60 days after withdrawing the treatment. Jaundice, liver damage and deaths have occurred in other patients with leprosy given **rifampicin** and protionamide or **ethionamide**.[2-4]

Protionamide does not affect the pharmacokinetics of either **dapsone** or **rifampicin**.[5]

Mechanism

Although not certain, it seems probable that the liver damage was primarily caused by the protionamide, and possibly exacerbated by the rifampicin (rifampin) or the rifandin.

Importance and management

This serious and potentially life-threatening hepatotoxic reaction to protionamide is established, but the part played by the other drugs, particularly the rifampicin (rifampin), is uncertain. Strictly speaking this may not be an interaction. If protionamide is given the liver function should be very closely monitored in order to detect toxicity as soon as possible. This monitoring is probably sufficient to detect any adverse interaction.

1. Baohong J, Jiakun C, Chenmin W, Guang X. Hepatotoxicity of combined therapy with rifampicin and daily prothionamide for leprosy. *Lepr Rev* (1984) 55, 283–9.
2. Lesobre R, Ruffino J, Teyssier L, Achard F, Brefort G. Les ictères au cours du traitement par la rifampicine. *Rev Tuberc Pneumol (Paris)* (1969) 33, 393–403.
3. Report of the Third Meeting of the Scientific Working Group on Chemotherapy of Leprosy (THELEP) of the UNDP/World Bank/WHO Special Programme for Research and Training in Tropical Diseases. *Int J Lepr* (1981) 49, 431–6.
4. Cartel J-L, Millan J, Guelpa-Lauras C-C, Grosset JH. Hepatitis in leprosy patients treated by a daily combination of dapsone, rifampin, and a thioamide. *Int J Lepr* (1983) 51, 461–5.
5. Mathur A, Venkatesan K, Girdhar BK, Bharadwaj VP, Girdhar A, Bagga AK. A study of drug interactions in leprosy — 1. Effect of simultaneous administration of prothionamide on metabolic disposition of rifampicin and dapsone. *Lepr Rev* (1986) 57, 33–7.

Pyrazinamide + Antacids

In 14 healthy subjects, 30 mL of *Mylanta* (aluminium/magnesium hydroxide) given 9 hours before, with, and after a single 30-mg/kg dose of pyrazinamide decreased the time to peak absorption by 17%, but had no effect on other pharmacokinetic parameters.[1] This change is not clinically important.

1. Peloquin CA, Bulpitt AE, Jaresko GS, Jelliffe RW, James GT, Nix DE. Pharmacokinetics of pyrazinamide under fasting conditions, with food, and with antacids. *Pharmacotherapy* (1998) 18, 1205–11.

Pyrazinamide + Antigout drugs

Pyrazinamide commonly causes hyperuricaemia and may therefore reduce the uricosuric effect of benzbromarone and probenecid, however benzbromarone may have modest efficacy in reducing the hyperuricaemia caused by pyrazinamide. Allopurinol is unlikely to be effective against pyrazinamide-induced hyperuricaemia, and may exacerbate the situation.

Clinical evidence and mechanism

(a) Allopurinol

It is thought that pyrazinamide is hydrolysed in the body to pyrazinoic acid, which appears to be responsible for its hyperuricaemic effect. Pyrazinoic acid is oxidised by the enzyme xanthine oxidase to 5-hydroxypyrazoic acid.[1] As allopurinol is an inhibitor of xanthine oxidase, its presence increases pyrazinoic acid concentrations[2] thereby probably worsening pyrazinamide-induced hyperuricaemia.[3]

(b) Benzbromarone

In 5 subjects with hyperuricaemia and gout a single dose of pyrazinamide completely abolished the uricosuric effect of a single 160-mg dose of benzbromarone.[4] Other authors also briefly mention the same finding.[5] However in another study, when 10 patients taking pyrazinamide 35 mg/kg daily for tuberculosis were given benzbromarone 50 mg daily for 8 to 10 days, uric acid levels were reduced by an average of 24%, and returned to normal in 4 patients.[6] It is unclear from these studies whether or not pyrazinamide abolishes the uricosuric effects of benzbromarone.

(c) Probenecid

The interactions of probenecid and pyrazinamide and their effects on the excretion of uric acid are complex and intertwined. Probenecid increases the secretion of uric acid into the urine, apparently by inhibiting its reabsorption from the kidney tubules.[7] Pyrazinamide on the other hand decreases the secretion of uric acid into the urine by one-third to one-half,[8] resulting in a rise in the serum levels of urate in the blood, thereby causing hyperuricaemia.[8,9] The result of using probenecid and pyrazinamide together is not however merely the simple sum of these two effects. This is because pyrazinamide additionally decreases the metabolism of the probenecid and prolongs its uricosuric effects, and the effect of pyrazinamide is reduced. Also, probenecid inhibits the secretion of pyrazinamide, increasing its effects.[10]

Importance and management

Pyrazinamide commonly causes hyperuricaemia, and would be expected to antagonise the effects of uricosuric drugs such as benzbromarone. Benzbromarone may have modest efficacy in reducing hyperuricaemia caused by pyrazinamide, but further study is necessary to establish this.

If probenecid were to be used to treat the hyperuricaemia caused by pyrazinamide, the normal uricosuric effects of probenecid would be diminished, and larger doses would be required. Allopurinol would appear to be unsuitable for treating pyrazinamide-induced hyperuricaemia as it potentially exacerbates the situation.

Note that pyrazinamide should be used with caution[11] or is contraindicated[12] in patients with a history of gout. Baseline serum uric acid levels should be established in all patients given pyrazinamide.[12] If hyperuricaemia accompanied by gouty arthritis occurs (without liver dysfunction[12]), pyrazinamide should be stopped.[11,12]

1. Weiner IM, Tinker JP. Pharmacology of pyrazinamide: metabolic and renal function studies related to the mechanism of drug-induced urate retention. *J Pharmacol Exp Ther* (1972) 180, 411–34.
2. Lacroix C, Guyonnaud C, Chaou M, Duwoos H, Lafont O. Interaction between allopurinol and pyrazinamide. *Eur Respir J* (1988) 807–11.
3. Urban T, Maquarre E, Housset C, Chouaid C, Devin E, Lebeau B. Hypersensibilité à l'allopurinol. Une cause possible d'hépatite et d'éruption cutanéo-muqueuse chez un patient sous antituberculeux. *Rev Mal Respir* (1995) 12, 314–16.
4. Sinclair DS, Fox IH. The pharmacology of hypouricemic effect of benzbromarone. *J Rheumatol* (1975) 2, 437–45.
5. Sorensen LB, Levinson DJ. Clinical evaluation of benzbromarone. *Arthritis Rheum* (1976) 19, 183–90.
6. Kropp R. Zur urikosurischen Wirkung von Benzbromaronum an Modell der pyrizinamidbedingten Hyperurikämie. *Med Klin* (1970) 65, 1448–50.
7. Meisel AD, Diamond HS. Mechanism of probenecid-induced uricosuria: inhibition of reabsorption of secreted urate. *Arthritis Rheum* (1977) 20, 128.
8. Cullen JH, LeVine M, Fiore JM. Studies of hyperuricemia produced by pyrazinamide. *Am J Med* (1957) 23, 587–95.
9. Shapiro M, Hyde L. Hyperuricemia due to pyrazinamide. *Am J Med* (1957) 23, 596–9.
10. Yü T-F, Perel J, Berger L, Roboz J, Israili ZH, Dayton PG. The effect of the interaction of pyrazinamide and probenecid on urinary uric acid excretion in man. *Am J Med* (1977) 63, 723–8.
11. Rifater Tablets (Rifampicin, Isoniazid and Pyrazinamide). Sanofi-Aventis. UK Summary of product characteristics, March 2009.
12. Rifater (Rifampin, Isoniazid and Pyrazinamide). Sanofi-Aventis. US Prescribing information, April 2008.

Pyrazinamide + Food

In 14 subjects a high-fat breakfast approximately doubled the time to peak absorption of a single 30-mg/kg dose of pyrazinamide but had no effect on other pharmacokinetic parameters.[1] It would therefore seem that pyrazinamide may be taken without regard to meals.

1. Peloquin CA, Bulpitt AE, Jaresko GS, Jelliffe RW, James GT, Nix DE. Pharmacokinetics of pyrazinamide under fasting conditions, with food, and with antacids. *Pharmacotherapy* (1998) 18, 1205–11.

Quinolones + Antacids or Calcium compounds

The serum levels of many of the quinolone antibacterials can be reduced by aluminium and magnesium antacids. Calcium compounds interact to a lesser extent, and bismuth compounds interact only minimally.

Clinical evidence

There is a wealth of information about the interaction between quinolones and antacids and for simplicity this is summarised in 'Table 10.3', p.344. This table shows what happens to the maximum serum levels (C_{max}) and the relative bioavailabilities (%) when the quinolones listed have been given at the same time as antacids, and when separated by time intervals (e.g. −2 h; two hours before the antacid).

Mechanism

It is believed that certain of the quinolone functional groups (3-carboxyl and 4-oxo) form insoluble chelates with aluminium and magnesium ions within the gut, which reduces their absorption.[1-3] The stability of the chelate formed seems to be an important factor in determining the degree of interaction.[3] It has been suggested from *animal* studies that adsorption of quinolones by aluminium hydroxide re-precipitated in the small intestine may be a factor in the reduced bioavailability of quinolones.[4] See also 'Quinolones + Iron or Zinc compounds', p.350.

Importance and management

The interactions between quinolones and antacids are generally well documented, well established and, depending on the particular quinolone and antacid concerned, of clinical importance. The risk is that the serum levels of the antibacterial may fall below minimum inhibitory concentrations (i.e. become subtherapeutic, particularly against organisms such as staphylococci and *Pseudomonas aeruginosa*[5]), resulting in treatment failures.[6] From a review of the use of levofloxacin, it has been suggested that the low levels of quinolones which occur as a result of this interaction may contribute to the development of resistance.[7] The overall picture is that the aluminium/magnesium antacids interact to a greater extent than the calcium compounds, and bismuth compounds hardly at all.

Possible alternatives to the antacids, which do not appear to interact with the quinolones, include the H_2-receptor antagonists and omeprazole (see 'Quinolones + H_2-receptor antagonists', p.349, and 'Quinolones + Omeprazole', p.351, respectively).

Aluminium/magnesium antacids

'Table 10.3', p.344 shows that the aluminium/magnesium antacids can greatly reduce the bioavailabilities of the quinolones. Separating their administration to reduce the admixture of the two drugs in the gut minimises the interaction, a very broad rule-of-thumb being that the quinolones should be taken at least 2 hours before and not less than 4 to 6 hours after the antacid.[1,8-14] The only obvious exception is **fleroxacin**, which appears to interact minimally.

Bismuth compounds

As can be seen from 'Table 10.3', p.344, bismuth compounds have little or no effect on the bioavailability of **ciprofloxacin**. Information about other quinolones appears to be lacking. However, using **ciprofloxacin** as a guide it would seem that any interaction is likely only to be of minimal clinical importance, and no action appears to be necessary.

Calcium compounds

Information about the interactions with calcium carbonate is more limited than with the aluminium/magnesium antacids, but 'Table 10.3', p.344 shows that the bioavailabilities of **ciprofloxacin**, **norfloxacin**, and to a lesser extent **gemifloxacin**, can be reduced. Other calcium compounds, for example those used as phosphate binders, are likely to interact similarly. These reductions are less than those seen with the aluminium/magnesium antacids, but using **ciprofloxacin** as a guide a very broad rule-of-thumb would be to separate the drug administration by about 2 hours to minimise this interaction.[15,16] This is clearly not necessary with **levofloxacin**,[17] **lomefloxacin**,[18] **moxifloxacin**[19] or **ofloxacin**,[20] nor probably with some of the other quinolones that have yet to be studied, but in the absence of direct information a 2-hour separation errs on the side of caution.

Sodium antacids

Sodium bicarbonate does not interact significantly with **norfloxacin**[21] but information about other quinolones appears to be lacking. However, bear in mind that in the case of **ciprofloxacin** an excessive rise in urinary pH (which can be caused by antacids like sodium bicarbonate) may possibly result in urinary crystalluria and kidney damage.[22]

1. Nix DE, Watson WA, Lener ME, Frost RW, Krol G, Goldstein H, Lettieri J, Schentag JJ. Effects of aluminum and magnesium antacids and ranitidine on the absorption of ciprofloxacin. *Clin Pharmacol Ther* (1989) 46, 700–705.
2. Shimada J, Shiba K, Oguma T, Miwa H, Yoshimura Y, Nishikawa T, Okabayashi Y, Kitagawa T, Yamamoto S. Effect of antacid on absorption of the quinolone lomefloxacin. *Antimicrob Agents Chemother* (1992) 36, 1219–24.
3. Mizuki Y, Fujiwara I, Yamaguchi T. Pharmacokinetic interactions related to the chemical structures of fluoroquinolones. *J Antimicrob Chemother* (1996) 37 (Suppl), A41–A55.
4. Tanaka M, Kurata T, Fujisawa C, Ohshima Y, Aoki H, Okazaki O, Hakusui H. Mechanistic study of inhibition of levofloxacin absorption by aluminium hydroxide. *Antimicrob Agents Chemother* (1993) 37, 2173–8.
5. Preheim LC, Cuevas TA, Roccaforte JS, Mellencamp MA, Bittner MJ. Ciprofloxacin and antacids. *Lancet* (1986) ii, 48.
6. Noyes M, Polk RE. Norfloxacin and absorption of magnesium-aluminium. *Ann Intern Med* (1988) 109, 168–9.
7. Cohen KA, Lautenbach E, Weiner MG, Synnestvedt M, Gasink LB. Coadministration of oral levofloxacin with agents that impair absorption: impact on antibiotic resistance. *Infect Control Hosp Epidemiol* (2008) 29, 975–7.
8. Grasela TH, Schentag JJ, Sedman AJ, Wilton JH, Thomas DJ, Schultz RW, Lebsack ME, Kinkel AW. Inhibition of enoxacin absorption by antacids or ranitidine. *Antimicrob Agents Chemother* (1989) 33, 615–17.
9. Nix DE, Wilton JH, Ronald B, Distlerath L, Williams VC, Norman A. Inhibition of norfloxacin absorption by antacids. *Antimicrob Agents Chemother* (1990) 34, 432–5.
10. Forster T, Blouin R. The effect of antacid timing on lomefloxacin bioavailability. *Intersci Conf Antimicrob Agents Chemother* (1989) 29, 318.
11. Johnson RD, Dorr MB, Talbot GH, Caille G. Effect of Maalox on the oral absorption of sparfloxacin. *Clin Ther* (1998) 20, 1149–58.
12. Lober S, Ziege S, Rau M, Schreiber G, Mignot A, Koeppe P, Lode H. Pharmacokinetics of gatifloxacin and interaction with an antacid containing aluminum and magnesium. *Antimicrob Agents Chemother* (1999) 43, 1067–71.
13. Misiak P, Toothaker R, Lebsack M, Sedman A, Colburn W. The effect of dosing-time intervals on the potential pharmacokinetic interaction between oral enoxacin and oral antacid. *Intersci Conf Antimicrob Agents Chemother* (1988) 28, 367.
14. Miyata K, Ohtani H, Tsujimoto M, Sawada Y. Antacid interaction with new quinolones: dose regimen recommendations based on pharmacokinetic modelling of clinical data for ciprofloxacin, gatifloxacin and norfloxacin and metal cations. *Int J Clin Pharmacol Ther* (2007) 45, 63–70.
15. Lomaestro BM, Bailie GR. Effect of staggered dose of calcium on the bioavailability of ciprofloxacin. *Antimicrob Agents Chemother* (1991) 35, 1004–1007.
16. Lomaestro BM, Bailie GR. Effect of multiple staggered doses of calcium on the bioavailability of ciprofloxacin. *Ann Pharmacother* (1993) 27, 1325–8.
17. Shiba K, Sakai O, Shimada J, Okazaki O, Aoki H, Hakusui H. Effects of antacids, ferrous sulfate, and ranitidine on absorption of DR-3355 in humans. *Antimicrob Agents Chemother* (1992) 36, 2270–4.
18. Lehto P, Kivistö KT. Different effects of products containing metal ions on the absorption of lomefloxacin. *Clin Pharmacol Ther* (1994) 56, 477–82.
19. Stass H, Kubitza D. Profile of moxifloxacin drug interactions. *Clin Infect Dis* (2001) 32, (Suppl 1), S47–S50.
20. Sánchez Navarro A, Martínez Cabarga M, Dominguez-Gil Hurlé A. Comparative study of the influence of Ca^{2+} on absorption parameters of ciprofloxacin and ofloxacin. *J Antimicrob Chemother* (1994) 34, 119–25.
21. Okhamafe AO, Akerele JO, Chukuka CS. Pharmacokinetic interactions of norfloxacin with some metallic medicinal agents. *Int J Pharmaceutics* (1991) 68, 11–18.
22. Ciproxin Tablets (Ciprofloxacin hydrochloride). Bayer plc. UK Summary of product characteristics, November 2008.

Quinolones + Antineoplastics

The absorption of ciprofloxacin and ofloxacin can be reduced by some cytotoxic antineoplastics. Production of the active metabolite of cyclophosphamide may be reduced by ciprofloxacin.

Clinical evidence

(a) Ciprofloxacin

Six patients with newly diagnosed haematological malignancies (5 with acute myeloid leukaemia and one with non-Hodgkin's lymphoma) were given ciprofloxacin 500 mg twice daily to control possible neutropenic infections. It was found that, after 13 days of chemotherapy, their mean maximum serum ciprofloxacin levels had fallen by 46% (from 3.7 to 2 mg/L) and the AUC_{0-4} was reduced by 47%. There were large individual differences between the patients. The antineoplastics used were **cyclophosphamide**, **cytarabine**, **daunorubicin**, **doxorubicin**, **mitoxantrone** and **vincristine**.[1]

A study in 8 patients who received a course of CHOP (**cyclophosphamide**, **doxorubicin**, prednisolone and **vincristine**) found that oral ciprofloxacin, 1 g given in the evening and 500 mg given on the morning before intravenous **cyclophosphamide** was given, reduced the AUC of the active metabolite of **cyclophosphamide** by 32%.[2]

For mention that methotrexate toxicity has occurred in 2 patients during treatment with ciprofloxacin, see 'Methotrexate + Antibacterials; Ciprofloxacin', p.693.

(b) Ofloxacin

Ten patients with non-Hodgkin's lymphoma, hairy cell leukaemia or acute myeloid leukaemia were given ofloxacin 400 mg at breakfast time for antibacterial prophylaxis during neutropenia. Blood samples were taken 3 days before chemotherapy began and then at 2 to 3 days, 5 to 7 days, and 8 to 10 days. The maximum serum ofloxacin levels were reduced by 18% two to three days after the chemotherapy but none of the other pharmacokinetic measurements were changed by the antineoplastic treatment. The serum levels had returned to normal by 5 to 7 days. At all times serum levels exceeded the expected MICs of the gram-negative potential pathogens. The antineoplastics used were **cyclophosphamide**, **cytarabine**, **doxorubicin**, **etoposide**, **ifosfamide** (with mesna), **vincristine**.[3]

Mechanism

Uncertain. The reduction in serum levels seems to result from a reduction in the absorption of the quinolones by the small intestine, possibly related to the damaging effect cytotoxic antineoplastics have on the rapidly dividing cells of the intestinal mucosa. It was suggested that the production of the active metabolite of cyclophosphamide may have been inhibited by ciprofloxacin.

Table 10.3 The effect of antacids on the pharmacokinetics of quinolone antibacterials

Quinolone (mg:time)*	*Antacid or other coadministered drug*	*Maximum level (micrograms/mL)*		*Relative bioavailability (%)†*	*Refs*
		alone	*with*		
Ciprofloxacin					
250	$Mg(OH)_2 + Al(OH)_3$	3.69	less than 1.25	NR	1
500	$Mg(OH)_2 + Al(OH)_3$	2.6	0.88	NR	2
500: +24 h	$Mg(OH)_2 + Al(OH)_3$	1.7	0.1	NR	3
500: +24 h	$Mg(OH)_2 + Al(OH)_3$	1.9	0.13	9.5	4
750: -2 h	$Mg(OH)_2 + Al(OH)_3$	3.01	3.96	107	5
+0.08 h		3.42	0.68	15.1	
+2 h		3.42	0.88	23.2	
+4 h		3.01	2.62	70	
+6 h		2.63	2.64	108.5	
750: +0.08 h	$Al(OH)_3$	3.2	0.6	15.4	6
750	$Al(OH)_3$	2.3	0.8	NR	7
200	$Al(OH)_3$	1.3	0.2	12	8
250	$CaCO_3$	3.69	3.42 (ns)	NR	1
500	$CaCO_3$	1.53	1.37 (ns)	94 (ns)	9
500	$CaCO_3$	2.9	1.8	58.8	10
750: +0.08 h	$CaCO_3$	3.2	1.7	64.5	6
500: +2 h	$CaCO_3$	1.25	1.44	102.4	11
500	Mg citrate	2.4	0.6	21	12
500	Bismuth salicylate (subsalicylate)	3.8	2.9	83.8	13
750	Bismuth salicylate (subsalicylate)	2.95	2.57	87	14
500	Tripotassium dicitratobismuthate			100	12
400	Polycarbophil calcium	2.66	0.95	48	15
750	Calcium acetate	3.77	1.9	0.49	16
Enoxacin					
200	$Al(OH)_3$	2.26	0.46	15.4	17
400: +0.5 h	$Mg(OH)_2 + Al(OH)_3$	3.17	0.95	26.8	18
+2 h		3.17	1.95	52.3	
+8 h		3.17	2.88	82.7	
200	$Al(OH)_3$	2.3	0.5	15.8	8
Fleroxacin					
200	$Al(OH)_3$	2.4	1.8	82.8	8
Garenoxacin					
600	$Mg(OH)_2 + Al(OH)_3$	9.3	3.8	42	19
+4 h		9.3	7.9	84	
+2 h		9.3	7.7	78	
-2 h		9.3	11		
-4 h		9.3	9.4 (ns)	ns	
Gatifloxacin					
200	$Al(OH)_3$	1.71	0.75	45.9	20
400	$Mg(OH)_2 + Al(OH)_3$	3.8	1.2	35.6	21
400: -2 h		3.8	2.1	57.9	
+2 h		3.4	3.3	82.5	
+4 h		3.4	3.5 (ns)	100 (ns)	
Gemifloxacin					
320: +3 h	$Mg(OH)_2 + Al(OH)_3$	0.91	0.75	85.9	22
-0.17 h		0.91	0.13	16.8	
-2 h		0.91	0.99	101.2	
320	$CaCO_3$	1.13	0.9	77	23
320: -2 h		1.13	1.13	93	
+2 h		1.11	1.01	90	
Grepafloxacin					
200	$Al(OH)_3$	NR	NR	60	24
Levofloxacin					
100	$Al(OH)_3$	1.82	0.64	56.3	25, 26
100	$Al(OH)_3$	1.8	0.6	54.8	8
100	MgO	1.82	1.13	78.2	25, 26
100	$CaCO_3$	1.45	1.12	96.7	25, 26
750: -2 h	$CaCO_3$	9.7	8.8	ns	27

*Time interval between intake of quinolone and the other drug: – and + indicate that the quinolone was administered before and after, respectively, intake of the other drug.
†Calculated from AUC data.
NR = not reported; h = hour; ns = not significant.

Continued

Table 10.3 The effect of antacids on the pharmacokinetics of quinolone antibacterials (continued)

Quinolone (mg:time[*])*	*Antacid or other coadministered drug*	*Maximum level (micrograms/mL) alone*	*with*	*Relative bioavailability (%)*[†]	*Refs*
Lomefloxacin					
200	$Mg(OH)_2$ + $Al(OH)_3$	1.91	1.03	59.2	28
200	$Al(OH)_3$	2.2	1	65.2	8
NR: +2 h	$Mg(OH)_2$ + $Al(OH)_3$	2.85	2.67 (ns)	88.2	29
–2 h		2.85	2.16	80.4	
–4 h		2.85	2.67 (ns)	90.1	
400	$Mg(OH)_2$ + $Al(OH)_3$	3.25	1.31	52.1	30
400: +12 h		3.25	3.66 (ns)		
–4 h		3.25	3.69 (ns)		
400	$CaCO_3$	4.72	4.08	97.9 (ns)	31
Moxifloxacin					
400	$Mg(OH)_2$ + $Al(OH)_3$	2.57	1	74	32
400	Calcium lactate gluconate + $CaCO_3$	2.71	2.29	97.6	33
Norfloxacin					
200	$Al(OH)_3$	1.45	less than 0.01	2.7	17
400: +0.08 h	$Mg(OH)_2$ + $Al(OH)_3$	1.64	0.08	9 (based on urinary recovery)	34
–2 h		1.64	1.25	81.3	
200	$Al(OH)_3$	1.5	less than 0.1	3	8
400	$Al(OH)_3$	1.51	1.09	71.2 (from saliva)	35
400	Mg trisilicate	1.51	0.43	19.3 (from saliva)	35
400	$CaCO_3$	1.64	0.56	37.5	34
400	$CaCO_3$	1.51	1.08	52.8 (from saliva)	35
400	Bismuth salicylate (subsalicylate)			89.7 (ns)	36
400	Sodium bicarbonate	1.4	1.47	104.9 (ns)	35
Ofloxacin					
200	$Al(OH)_3$	3.23	1.31	52.1	17
200	$Al(PO_4)$			93.1 (ns)	37
200	MgO + $Al(OH)_3$	1.97	1.1	62	38
200: +24 h	$Mg(OH)_2$ + $Al(OH)_3$	2.6	0.7	30.8	4
400: +2 h	$Mg(OH)_2$ + $Al(OH)_3$	3.7	2.6	79.2	39
–2 h		3.7	3.8 (ns)	101.9 (ns)	
+24 h		3.7	3.5 (ns)	95.3 (ns)	
600	$Mg(OH)_2$ + $Al(OH)_3$	8.11	6.13	NR	40
200	$Al(OH)_3$	3.2	1.3	52.1	8
400: +2 h	$CaCO_3$	3.2	3.3 (ns)	103.6 (ns)	39
–2 h		3.2	3.3 (ns)	97.9 (ns)	
+24 h		3.2	3.5 (ns)	95.9 (ns)	
Pefloxacin					
400	$Mg(OH)_2$ + $Al(OH)_3$	5.14	1.95	44.2	41
400	$Mg(OH)_2$ + $Al(OH)_3$	3.95	1.25	NR	42
400	$Mg(OH)_2$ + $Al(OH)_3$	5.1	2	45.7	43
Rufloxacin					
400: +0.08 h	$Mg(OH)_2$ + $Al(OH)_3$	3.74	2.12	59.7	44
–4 h		3.74	3.97 (ns)	84.7	
Sparfloxacin					
400: –2 h	$Mg(OH)_2$ + $Al(OH)_3$	1.09	0.94	82.8	45
+2 h		1.09	0.77	77.2	
–4 h		1.09	1.17	93.4	
200	$Al(OH)_3$	1.09	1.17	94.7	8, 46
Tosufloxacin					
150	$Al(OH)_3$	0.3	0.1	29.2	8
300	$Al(OH)_3$	0.88	0.52	68	47
Trovafloxacin					
300: –2 h	$Mg(OH)_2$ + $Al(OH)_3$	2.8	2.5	71.7	48
+0.5 h		2.8	1.1	33.7	

[*]Time interval between intake of quinolone and the other drug: – and + indicate that the quinolone was administered before and after, respectively, intake of the other drug.
[†]Calculated from AUC data.
NR = not reported; h = hour; ns = not significant.

1. Fleming LW, Moreland TA, Stewart WK, Scott AC. Ciprofloxacin and antacids. *Lancet* (1986) ii, 294.
2. Preheim LC, Cuevas TA, Roccaforte JS, Mellencamp MA, Bittner MJ. Ciprofloxacin and antacids. *Lancet* (1986) ii, 48.
3. Höffken G, Borner K, Glatzel PD, Koeppe P, Lode H. Reduced enteral absorption of ciprofloxacin in the presence of antacids. *Eur J Clin Microbiol* (1985) 4, 345.
4. Höffken G, Lode H, Wiley R, Glatzel TD, Sievers D, Olschewski T, Borner K, Koeppe T. Pharmacokinetics and bioavailability of ciprofloxacin and ofloxacin: effect of food and antacid intake. *Rev Infect Dis* (1988) 10 (Suppl 1), S138–S139.
5. Nix DE, Watson WA, Lener ME, Frost RW, Krol G, Goldstein H, Lettieri J, Schentag JJ. Effects of aluminum and magnesium antacids and ranitidine on the absorption of ciprofloxacin. *Clin Pharmacol Ther* (1989) 46, 700–705.

Continued

Table 10.3 The effect of antacids on the pharmacokinetics of quinolone antibacterials (continued)

6. Frost RW, Lasseter KC, Noe AJ, Shamblen EC, Lettieri JT. Effects of aluminum hydroxide and calcium carbonate antacids on the bioavailability of ciprofloxacin. *Antimicrob Agents Chemother* (1992) 36, 830–2.
7. Golper TA, Hartstein AI, Morthland VH, Christensen JM. Effects of antacids and dialysate dwell times on multiple-dose pharmacokinetics of oral ciprofloxacin in patients on continuous ambulatory peritoneal dialysis. *Antimicrob Agents Chemother* (1987) 31, 1787–90.
8. Shiba K, Sakamoto M, Nakazawa Y, Sakai O. Effect of antacid on absorption and excretion of new quinolones. *Drugs* (1995) 49 (Suppl 2), 360–1.
9. Lomaestro BM, Bailie GR. Effect of multiple staggered doses of calcium on the bioavailability of ciprofloxacin. *Ann Pharmacother* (1993) 27, 1325–8.
10. Sahai J, Healey DP, Stotka J, Polk RE. The influence of chronic administration of calcium carbonate on the bioavailability of oral ciprofloxacin. *Br J Clin Pharmacol* (1993) 35, 302–4.
11. Lomaestro BM, Bailie GR. Effect of staggered dose of calcium on the bioavailability of ciprofloxacin. *Antimicrob Agents Chemother* (1991) 35, 1004–1007.
12. Brouwers JRBJ, van der Kam HJ, Sijtsma J, Proost JH. Important reduction of ciprofloxacin absorption by sucralfate and magnesium citrate solution. *Drug Invest* (1990) 2, 197–9.
13. Sahai J, Oliveras L, Garber G. Effect of bismuth subsalicylate (Peptobismol. PB) on ciprofloxacin (C) absorption: a preliminary investigation. *17th Int Congr Chemother*, June 1991, Berlin, Abstract 414.
14. Rambout L, Sahai J, Gallicano K, Oliveras L, Garber G. Effect of bismuth subsalicylate on ciprofloxacin bioavailability. *Antimicrob Agents Chemother* (1994) 38, 2187–90.
15. Kato R, Ueno K, Imano H, Kawai M, Kuwahara , Tsuchishita Y, Yonezawa E, Tanaka K. Impairment of ciprofloxacin absorption by calcium polycarbophil. *J Clin Pharmacol* (2002) 42, 806–11.
16. Kays MB, Overholser BR, Mueller BA, Moe SM, Sowinski KM. Effects of sevelamer hydrochloride and calcium acetate on the oral bioavailability of ciprofloxacin. *Am J Kidney Dis* (2003) 42, 1253–9.
17. Shiba K, Saito A, Miyahara T, Tachizawa H, Fujimoto T. Effect of aluminium hydroxide, an antacid, on the pharmacokinetics of new quinolones in humans. *Proc 15th Int Congr Chemother*, Istanbul 1987, 168–9.
18. Grasela TH, Schentag JJ, Sedman AJ, Wilton JH, Thomas DJ, Schultz RW, Lebsack ME, Kinkel AW. Inhibition of enoxacin absorption by antacids or ranitidine. *Antimicrob Agents Chemother* (1989) 33, 615–17.
19. Krishna G, Kisicki JC, Olsen S, Grasela DM, Wang Z. Effect of an aluminium- and magnesium-containing antacid on the bioavailability of garenoxacin in healthy volunteers. *Pharmacotherapy* (2007) 27, 963–9.
20. Shiba K, Kusajima H, Momo K. The effects of aluminium hydroxide, cimetidine, ferrous sulfate, green tea and milk on pharmacokinetics of gatifloxacin in healthy humans. *J Antimicrob Chemother* (1999) 44 (Suppl A), 141.
21. Lober S, Ziege S, Rau M, Schreiber G, Mignot A, Koeppe P, Lode H. Pharmacokinetics of gatifloxacin and interaction with an antacid containing aluminum and magnesium. *Antimicrob Agents Chemother* (1999) 43, 1067–71.
22. Allen A, Vousden M, Porter A, Lewis A. Effect of Maalox® on the bioavailability of oral gemifloxacin in healthy volunteers. *Chemotherapy* (1999) 45, 504–11.
23. Pletz MW, Petzold P, Allen A, Burkhardt O, Lode H. Effect of calcium carbonate on bioavailability of orally administered gemifloxacin. *Antimicrob Agents Chemother* (2003) 47, 2158–60.
24. Koneru B, Bramer S, Bricmont P, Maroli A, Shiba K. Effect of food, gastric pH and co-administration of antacid, cimetidine and probenecid on the oral pharmacokinetics of the broad spectrum antimicrobial agent grepafloxacin. *Pharm Res* (1996) 13 (9 Suppl), S414.
25. Shiba K, Sakai O, Shimada J, Okazaki O, Aoki H, Hakusui H. Effects of antacids, ferrous sulfate, and ranitidine on absorption of DR-3355 in humans. *Antimicrob Agents Chemother* (1992) 36, 2270–4.
26. Shiba K , Okazaki O, Aoki H, Shimada J, Sakai O. Influence of antacids and ranitidine on the absorption of levofloxacin in men. *Drugs* (1993) 45 (Suppl 3) 299–300.
27. Pai MP, Allen SE, Amsden GW. Altered steady state pharmacokinetics of levofloxacin in adult cystic fibrosis patients receiving calcium carbonate. *J Cyst Fibros* (2006) 5, 153–7.
28. Shimada J, Shiba K, Oguma T, Miwa H, Yoshimura Y, Nishikawa T, Okabayashi Y, Kitagawa T, Yamamoto S. Effect of antacid on absorption of the quinolone lomefloxacin. *Antimicrob Agents Chemother* (1992) 36, 1219–24.
29. Foster T, Blouin R. The effect of antacid timing on lomefloxacin bioavailability. *Intersci Conf Antimicrob Agents Chemother* (1989) 29, 318.
30. Kunka RL, Wong YY, Lyon JL. Effect of antacid on the pharmacokinetics of lemofloxacin. *Pharm Res* (1988) 5 (Suppl), S–165.
31. Lehto P, Kivistö KT. Different effects of products containing metal ions on the absorption of lomefloxacin. *Clin Pharmacol Ther* (1994) 56, 477–82.
32. Stass H, Böttcher M-F, Ochmann K. Evaluation of the influence of antacids and H_2 antagonists on the absorption of moxifloxacin after oral administration of a 400-mg dose to healthy volunteers. *Clin Pharmacokinet* (2001) 40 (Suppl 1), 39–48.
33. Stass H, Wandel C, Delesen H, Möller J-G. Effect of calcium supplements on the oral bioavailability of moxifloxacin in healthy male volunteers. *Clin Pharmacokinet* (2001) 40 (Suppl 1), 27–32.
34. Nix DE, Wilton JH, Ronald B, Distlerath L, Williams VC, Norman A. Inhibition of norfloxacin absorption by antacids. *Antimicrob Agents Chemother* (1990) 34, 432–5.
35. Okhamafe AO, Akerele JO, Chukuka CS. Pharmacokinetic interactions of norfloxacin with some metallic medicinal agents. *Int J Pharmaceutics* (1991) 68, 11–18.
36. Campbell NRC, Kara M, Hasinoff BB, Haddara WM, McKay DW. Norfloxacin interaction with antacids and minerals. *Br J Clin Pharmacol* (1992) 33, 115–16.
37. Martínez Carbaga M, Sánchez Navarro A, Colino Gandarillas CI, Domínguez-Gil A. Effects of two cations on gastrointestinal absorption of ofloxacin. *Antimicrob Agents Chemother* (1991) 35, 2102–5.
38. Shiba K, Yoshida M, Kachi M, Shimada J, Saito A, Sakai N. Effects of peptic ulcer-healing drugs on the pharmacokinetics of new quinolone (OFLX). *17th Int Congr Chemother*, June 1991, Berlin, Abstract 415.
39. Flor S, Guay DRP, Opsahl JA, Tack K, Matzke GR. Effects of magnesium-aluminum hydroxide and calcium carbonate antacids on bioavailability of ofloxacin. *Antimicrob Agents Chemother* (1990) 34, 2436–8.
40. Maesen FPV, Davies BI, Geraedts WH, Sumajow CA. Ofloxacin and antacids. *J Antimicrob Chemother* (1987) 19, 848–50.
41. Metz R, Jaehde U, Sörgel F, Wiesemann H, Gottschalk B, Stephan U, Schunack W. Pharmacokinetic interactions and non-interactions of pefloxacin. *Proc 15th Int Congr Chemother*, Istanbul, 1987, 997–9.
42. Vinceneux P, Weber P, Gaudin H, Boussougant Y. Diminution de l'absorption de la péfloxacine par les pansements gastriques. *Presse Med* (1986) 15, 1826.
43. Jaehde U, Sörgel F, Stephan U, Schunack W. Effect of an antacid containing magnesium and aluminum on absorption, metabolism and mechanism of renal elimination of pefloxacin in humans. *Antimicrob Agents Chemother* (1994) 38, 1129–33.
44. Lazzaroni M, Imbimbo BP, Bargiggia S, Sangaletti O, Dal Bo L, Broccali G, Bianchi Porro G. Effects of magnesium-aluminum hydroxide antacid on absorption of rufloxacin. *Antimicrob Agents Chemother* (1993) 37, 2212–16.
45. Johnson RD, Dorr MB, Talbot GH, Caille G. Effect of Maalox on the oral absorption of sparfloxacin. *Clin Ther* (1998) 20, 1149–58.
46. Shimada J, Saito A, Shiba K, Hojo T, Kaji M, Hori S, Yoshida M, Sakai O. Pharmacokinetics and clinical studies on sparfloxacin. *Chemotherapy (Tokyo)* (1991) 39 (Suppl 4), 234–44.
47. Minami R, Nakamura C, Inotsume N, Nakano M, Effects of aluminium hydroxide and famotidine on bioavailability of tosufloxacin in healthy volunteers. *Antimicrob Agents Chemother* (1998) 42, 453–5.
48. Teng R, Dogolo LC, Willavize SA, Freidman HL, Vincent J. Effect of Maalox and omeprazole on the bioavailability of trovafloxacin. *J Antimicrob Chemother* (1997) 39 (Suppl B), 93–7.

Importance and management

Direct information is limited, but the reports of reduced serum levels are consistent with the way cytotoxic antineoplastics can reduce the absorption of some other drugs; however, the authors suggest that these changes are probably clinically unimportant, because the serum levels achieved are likely to be sufficient to treat most infections. If the suggested mechanism of interaction is correct, no interaction should occur if quinolones are given parenterally. Nothing appears to be documented about any of the other quinolones.

The significance of the reduction in the active metabolite of cyclophosphamide seen in one study is unclear; however the authors suggest that a reduction in the therapeutic efficacy of cyclophosphamide may result and this combination should therefore be avoided. It has also been suggested that this interaction was a high-risk factor for relapse in patients undergoing bone marrow transplantation when ciprofloxacin was given as prophylaxis during cyclophosphamide use.[4]

1. Johnson EJ, MacGowan AP, Potter MN, Stockley RJ, White LO, Slade RR, Reeves DS. Reduced absorption of oral ciprofloxacin after chemotherapy for haematological malignancy. *J Antimicrob Chemother* (1990) 25, 837–42.
2. Afsharian P, Möllgård L, Hassan Z, Xie H, Kimby E, Hassan M. The effect of ciprofloxacin on cyclophosphamide pharmacokinetics in patients with non-Hodgkin lymphoma. *Eur J Haematol* (2005) 75, 206–211.
3. Brown NM, White LO, Blundell EL, Chown SR, Slade RR, MacGowan AP, Reeves DS. Absorption of oral ofloxacin after cytotoxic chemotherapy for haematological malignancy. *J Antimicrob Chemother* (1993) 32, 117–22.
4. Carlens S, Ringdén O, Aschan J, Hägglund H, Ljungman P, Mattsson J, Remberger M. Risk factors in bone marrow transplant recipients with leukaemia. Increased relapse risk in patients treated with ciprofloxacin for gut decontamination. *Clin Transplant* (1998) 12, 84–92.

Quinolones + Chinese herbal medicines

Sho-saiko-to, Rikkunshi-to and Sairei-to do not interact with ofloxacin, and Hotyu-ekki-to, Rikkunshi-to and Juzen-taiho-to do not interact with levofloxacin.

Clinical evidence, mechanism, importance and management

The bioavailability and urinary recovery of a single 200-mg oral dose of **ofloxacin** were not significantly altered in 7 healthy subjects by three Chinese herbal medicines (**Sho-saiko-to, Rikkunshi-to** or **Sairei-to**).[1] The bioavailability and renal excretion of a single 200-mg oral dose of **levofloxacin** was not affected in 8 healthy subjects given single 2.5-g doses of **Hotyu-ekki-to, Rikkunshi-to** or **Juzen-taiho-to**.[2] There would

Table 10.4 Herbs contained in some Chinese herbal remedies[1,2]

Herb (plant part)	*Amounts of herbs in the medicines (mg/2.5 g)*				
	Hotyu-ekki-to	**Rikkunshi-to**	**Juzen-taiho-to**	**Sho-saiko-to**	**Sairei-to**
Atractylodis lanceae (rhizome)	278	248	175		125
Ginseng (root)	278	248	175	188	125
Glycyrrhizae (root)	104	662	688	125	83
Aurantii nobilis (pericarp)	139	124			
Zizyphi (fruit)	139	124		188	125
Zingiberis (rhizome)	635	631		63	42
Astragali (root)	278		175		
Angelicae (root)	208		175		
Bupleuri (root)	139			438	292
Cimicifugae (rhizome)	669				
Hoelen		248	175		125
Pinelliae (tuber)		248		313	208
Cinnamomi (cortex)			175		83
Rehmanniae (root)			175		
Paeoniae (root)			175		
Cnidii (rhizome)			175		
Scutellariae (root)				188	125
Alismatis (rhizome)					208
Polyporus					125

1. Hasegawa T, Yamaki K, Nadai M, Muraoka I, Wang L, Takagi K, Nabeshima T. Lack of effect of Chinese medicines on bioavailability of ofloxacin in healthy volunteers. *Int J Clin Pharmacol Ther* (1994) 32, 57-61.
2. Hasegawa T, Yamaki K-I, Muraoka I, Nadai M, Takagi K, Nabeshima T. Effects of traditional Chinese medicines on pharmacokinetics of levofloxacin. *Antimicrob Agents Chemother* (1995) 39, 2135-7.

therefore seem to be no reason for avoiding concurrent use. Information about other quinolones is lacking. The ingredients of these herbal medicines are detailed in 'Table 10.4', above.

1. Hasegawa T, Yamaki K, Nadai M, Muraoka I, Wang L, Takagi K, Nabeshima T. Lack of effect of Chinese medicines on bioavailability of ofloxacin in healthy volunteers. *Int J Clin Pharmacol Ther* (1994) 32, 57–61.
2. Hasegawa T, Yamaki K-I, Muraoka I, Nadai M, Takagi K, Nabeshima T. Effects of traditional Chinese medicines on pharmacokinetics of levofloxacin. *Antimicrob Agents Chemother* (1995) 39, 2135–7.

Quinolones + Dairy products

Dairy products reduce the bioavailability of ciprofloxacin and norfloxacin, and to a minor extent, gatifloxacin, but not enoxacin, lomefloxacin, moxifloxacin, ofloxacin and probably not fleroxacin.

Clinical evidence

(a) Ciprofloxacin

A study in 7 healthy subjects found that 300 mL of **milk** or **yoghurt** reduced the peak plasma levels of a single 500-mg dose of ciprofloxacin by 36% and 47%, respectively, and reduced its AUC by 33% and 36%, respectively.[1] In another study 300 mL of **milk** reduced the AUC of ciprofloxacin 500 mg by about 30%.[2]

(b) Enoxacin

A study found that **milk** and a standard breakfast had no effect on enoxacin absorption.[3]

(c) Fleroxacin

In a study, a fat and liquid calcium meal had no clinically significant effect on the pharmacokinetics of fleroxacin.[4] In another study, **milk** had no effect on fleroxacin pharmacokinetics.[2]

(d) Gatifloxacin

In one study 200 mL of **milk** reduced the AUC of gatifloxacin 200 mg by about 15%.[5]

(e) Lomefloxacin

Milk had no effect on the pharmacokinetics of lomefloxacin.[6]

(f) Moxifloxacin

A study found that the rate of absorption of a single 400-mg dose of moxifloxacin was slightly delayed by 250 g of **yoghurt**. The maximum plasma level of moxifloxacin was reduced by about 15%, but its bioavailability was unaffected.[7]

(g) Norfloxacin

A study found that 300 mL of **milk** or **yoghurt** reduced the absorption and the peak plasma levels of a single 200-mg dose of norfloxacin by roughly 50%.[8]

(h) Ofloxacin

A study in 21 healthy subjects found that 8 oz (about 250 mL) of **milk** had no clinically significant effects on the absorption of 300 mg of ofloxacin.[9] Another study confirmed the lack of a significant interaction between ofloxacin and both **milk** and **yoghurt**.[10]

Mechanism

The proposed reason for these changes is that the calcium in milk and yoghurt or other dairy products combines with the ciprofloxacin and norfloxacin to produce insoluble chelates. Compare also 'Quinolones + Antacids or Calcium compounds', p.343.

Importance and management

The effect of these changes to ciprofloxacin and norfloxacin pharmacokinetics on the control of infection is uncertain but until the situation is clear patients should be advised not to take these dairy products within one to 2 hours of either ciprofloxacin or norfloxacin to prevent admixture in the gut. The slight reduction in gatifloxacin levels is probably not clinically relevant.

Enoxacin, lomefloxacin, moxifloxacin, ofloxacin and probably fleroxacin do not appear to interact with dairy products to a clinically relevant extent, and they may therefore provide a useful alternative to the interacting quinolones.

1. Neuvonen PJ, Kivistö KT, Lehto P. Interference of dairy products with the absorption of ciprofloxacin. *Clin Pharmacol Ther* (1991) 50, 498–502.
2. Hoogkamer JFW, Kleinbloesem CH. The effect of milk consumption on the pharmacokinetics of fleroxacin and ciprofloxacin in healthy volunteers. *Drugs* (1995) 49 (Suppl 2), 346–8.
3. Lehto P, Kivistö KT. Effects of milk and food on the absorption of enoxacin. *Br J Clin Pharmacol* (1995) 39, 194–6.
4. Bertino JS, Nafziger AN, Wong M, Stragand L, Puleo C. Effects of a fat- and calcium-rich breakfast on pharmacokinetics of fleroxacin administered in single and multiple doses. *Antimicrob Agents Chemother* (1994) 38, 499–503.
5. Shiba K, Kusajima H, Momo K. The effects of aluminium hydroxide, cimetidine, ferrous sulfate, green tea and milk on pharmacokinetics of gatifloxacin in healthy humans. *J Antimicrob Chemother* (1999) 44 (Suppl A), 141.
6. Lehto PL, Kivistö KT. Different effects of products containing metal ions on the absorption of lomefloxacin. *Clin Pharmacol Ther* (1994) 56, 477–82.
7. Stass H, Kubitza D. Effects of dairy products on the oral bioavailability of moxifloxacin, a novel 8-methoxyfluoroquinolone, in healthy volunteers. *Clin Pharmacokinet* (2001) 40 (Suppl 1) 33–8.
8. Kivistö KT, Ojala-Karlsson P, Neuvonen PJ. Inhibition of norfloxacin absorption by dairy products. *Antimicrob Agents Chemother* (1992) 36, 489–91.
9. Dudley MN, Marchbanks CR, Flor SC, Beals B. The effect of food or milk on the absorption kinetics of ofloxacin. *Eur J Clin Pharmacol* (1991) 41, 569–71.
10. Neuvonen PJ, Kivistö KT. Milk and yoghurt do not impair the absorption of ofloxacin. *Br J Clin Pharmacol* (1992) 33, 346–8.

Quinolones + Didanosine

An extremely marked reduction in the serum levels of ciprofloxacin occurs if it is given at the same time as didanosine tablets, because of an interaction with the antacid buffers in the didanosine formulation. Other quinolones are expected to interact similarly. Didanosine enteric-coated capsules do not interact with ciprofloxacin.

Clinical evidence

When 12 healthy subjects were given **ciprofloxacin** 750 mg with two didanosine placebo tablets (i.e. all of the antacid additives but no didanosine), the **ciprofloxacin** AUC and maximum serum levels were reduced by 98% and 93%, respectively.[1] The antacids in this formulation were dihydroxyaluminium sodium carbonate and magnesium hydroxide.

Other studies have looked at whether separating administration affects this interaction. When 16 HIV-positive patients were given **ciprofloxacin** 1.5 g daily 2 hours before didanosine tablets, the AUC of **ciprofloxacin** was reduced by only 26%.[2] Another study in just one subject found that when **ciprofloxacin** 500 mg was given 2 hours after taking two didanosine placebo tablets the **ciprofloxacin** serum levels were reduced below minimal inhibitory concentrations, but giving the **ciprofloxacin** 2 hours before the didanosine placebo tablets resulted in normal blood levels.[3]

The enteric-coated capsule formulation of didanosine (which does not contain antacids) does not interact with **ciprofloxacin.**[4]

Mechanism

Didanosine is extremely acid labile at pH values below 3, so one of the formulations contains buffering agents (dihydroxyaluminium sodium carbonate and magnesium hydroxide) to keep the pH as high as possible to minimise the acid-induced hydrolysis. Ciprofloxacin forms insoluble non-absorbable chelates with these metallic ions in the buffer so that its bioavailability is markedly reduced. See also 'Quinolones + Antacids or Calcium compounds', p.343.

Importance and management

Direct information is limited to these reports but the interaction between buffered didanosine and ciprofloxacin appears to be clinically important. Such drastic reductions in serum ciprofloxacin levels mean that minimal inhibitory concentrations are unlikely to be achieved. Ciprofloxacin should be given at least 2 hours before or 6 hours after didanosine tablets (see 'Quinolones + Antacids or Calcium compounds', p.343). Other quinolone antibacterials that interact with antacids are also expected to interact with didanosine tablets, but so far reports are lacking. Didanosine enteric-coated capsules do not interact.

1. Sahai J, Gallicano K, Oliveras L, Khaliq S, Hawley-Foss N, Garber G. Cations in the didanosine tablet reduce ciprofloxacin bioavailability. *Clin Pharmacol Ther* (1993) 53, 292–7.
2. Knupp CA, Barbhaiya RH. A multiple-dose pharmacokinetic interaction study between didanosine (Videx®) and ciprofloxacin (Cipro®) in male subjects seropositive for HIV but asymptomatic. *Biopharm Drug Dispos* (1997) 18, 65–77.
3. Sahai J. Avoiding the ciprofloxacin-didanosine interaction. *Ann Intern Med* (1995) 123, 394–5.
4. Damle BD, Mummaneni V, Kaul S, Knupp C. Lack of effect of simultaneously administered didanosine encapsulated enteric bead formulation (Videx EC) on oral absorption of indinavir, ketoconazole, or ciprofloxacin. *Antimicrob Agents Chemother* (2002) 46, 385–91.

Quinolones + Enteral feeds or Food

The absorption of ciprofloxacin can be reduced by enteral feeds. Moxifloxacin and ofloxacin are similarly affected, but the extent of the interaction is smaller. No interaction is seen with garenoxacin or gatifloxacin and enteral feeds.

Apart from dairy products most foods delay but do not reduce the absorption of ciprofloxacin, enoxacin, gemifloxacin, lomefloxacin, ofloxacin or sparfloxacin. A high-fat/high-calcium breakfast did not reduce ciprofloxacin levels. Calcium-fortified orange juice significantly reduces the absorption of ciprofloxacin, but not gatifloxacin or levofloxacin.

Clinical evidence

A. Enteral feeds

(a) Ciprofloxacin

When ciprofloxacin 750 mg was given to 13 fasted subjects with *Ensure* its oral bioavailability was reduced by 28% and its mean maximum serum levels were reduced by 48%. In this study the subjects were given 120 mL of the study liquid (*Ensure* or water) and this was repeated at 30-minute intervals for 5 doses. The ciprofloxacin was crushed and mixed with the second dose of the study liquid and the cup rinsed with another 60 mL of the study liquid.[1]

Other enteral feeds given orally (*Osmolite*, *Pulmocare*, and *Resource*) similarly reduced the bioavailability and maximum serum levels of ciprofloxacin by about one-quarter to one-third in two other studies.[2,3] One comparative study found that *Ensure* reduced the AUC of ciprofloxacin by 40% in men but by only 15% in women.[4]

In a study of 26 hospitalised patients, ciprofloxacin bioavailability was reduced by 53% and 67% by *Jevity* or *Sustacal*, respectively, when given via gastrostomy or jejunostomy tubes. Despite this, the serum levels achieved with gastrostomy tubes were roughly equivalent to those seen in subjects taking tablets orally.[5] In another study in patients given *Jevity* or *Osmolite*, the 4 patients with a nasoduodenal tube achieved a ciprofloxacin AUC that was about double that seen in the 3 patients with a nasogastric tube or a gastrostomy tube.[6] In contrast, in another study in healthy subjects, there was no difference in the bioavailability of ciprofloxacin when it was given alone or when it was given with *Osmolite* via a nasogastric tube.[7]

The bioavailability of ciprofloxacin 750 mg every 12 hours in 5 patients with severe gram-negative intra-abdominal infections was reduced by 47% when it was added to enteral feeding with *Nutrison* or *Nutrison E+* and given via nasogastric or nasoduodenal tubes. The serum levels were similar to those found in another 7 patients given ciprofloxacin with these enteral feeds and also to those found when the 5 original patients were given intravenous ciprofloxacin 400 mg every 12 hours.[8] In another study, in 12 intensive care patients, the AUC of ciprofloxacin 400 mg given by intravenous infusion was similar to that found after a dose of 750 mg given via nasogastric tube during enteral feeding with *Normo-Réal fibres*.[9]

(b) Garenoxacin

In a randomised crossover study, 18 healthy subjects received a single 600-mg dose of garenoxacin via a nasogastric tube, alone or 2 hours after the start of a 6-hour nasogastric feed of *Osmolite*. The pharmacokinetics of garenoxacin were not altered by the enteral feed.[10]

(c) Gatifloxacin

In a crossover study, 12 healthy subjects were given a single 400-mg dose of gatifloxacin alone, or with *Ensure* 120 mL given every 30 minutes for 5 doses, starting 30 minutes before the gatifloxacin. The AUC and maximum plasma levels of gatifloxacin were reduced by 26% and 45%, respectively, in the presence of *Ensure*.[11]

A randomised study in critically ill patients found no significant difference in the bioavailability of gatifloxacin given as a single 400-mg dose either nasogastrically or intravenously with two enteral feed schedules. Seven patients received continuous enteral feeds, and 8 patients received feeds interrupted for 2 hours before and after the administration of the gatifloxacin. In this study 5 different enteral feeds were given (*Glucerna, Impact, Jevity, Promote, and Pulmocare*) at rates ranging from 30 mL/hour to 75 mL/hour. There was significant variation in the bioavailability of gatifloxacin, most likely due to the critical illnesses of the patients.[12]

(d) Moxifloxacin

In a study in 12 healthy subjects, the oral bioavailability of a single 400-mg dose of moxifloxacin was decreased by 9% when it was given to as a suspension of a crushed tablet via a nasogastric tube with either water or *Isosource Energy*. This decrease was in comparison with oral administration of an uncrushed tablet with water. Maximum plasma levels were decreased by 5% and 12% after nasogastric administration with water and *Isosource Energy*, respectively.[13]

(e) Ofloxacin

The oral bioavailability of ofloxacin 400 mg was reduced by 10% when it was given to 13 healthy subjects with *Ensure*. The mean maximum serum ofloxacin levels were reduced by 36%. In this study the subjects were given 120 mL of the study liquid (*Ensure* or water) and this was repeated at 30-minute intervals for 5 doses. The ofloxacin was crushed and mixed with the second dose of the study liquid and the cup rinsed with another 60 mL of the study liquid.[1] Only small reductions in the AUCs of ofloxacin were seen in another study (11% in men, 13% in women) with *Ensure*.[4]

B. Food

Food delayed the absorption of **ciprofloxacin** and **ofloxacin** in 10 subjects, but their bioavailabilities remained unchanged.[14] A study in 12 healthy subjects found that standard or high-fat breakfasts did not affect the absorption of **ciprofloxacin.**[15] Another study in healthy subjects found that a standard breakfast reduced the bioavailability of a single 300-mg dose of **ofloxacin** by about 18%, but this was not considered clinically significant.[16] Other studies suggest that food delays the absorption of **ofloxacin**[17] and **lomefloxacin**[18] but the bioavailability is unchanged. Food also has no effect on the absorption of **enoxacin**, but high-carbohydrate meals delayed the peak serum levels by almost an hour.[19] The pharmacokinetics of **gemifloxacin** 320 mg or 640 mg[20] or **sparfloxacin** 200 mg[21] were not significantly affected when they were given to healthy subjects with high-fat or standard meals, although the absorption of **sparfloxacin** was slightly delayed.

C. Calcium-fortified foods

Calcium-fortified orange juice decreased the AUC of **ciprofloxacin** by 38% and decreased its maximum plasma level by 41%, when compared with water.[22] However, in another study, a high-fat/high-calcium breakfast did not affect the absorption of **ciprofloxacin.**[15]

The AUC of **gatifloxacin** was reduced by only 12% by calcium-fortified orange juice.[23] Similarly, in two studies, orange juice, calcium-fortified orange juice,[24] or a breakfast of calcium-fortified orange juice and cereal with or without milk[25] were found to decrease the bioavailability of **levofloxacin**. However, the **levofloxacin** AUC was decreased by less than 16%, an amount that rarely proves to be clinically significant.

Mechanism

Not fully understood. The quinolone antibacterials can form insoluble chelates with divalent ions, which reduces their absorption from the gut. Enteral feeds such as those used above contain at least two divalent ions, calcium and magnesium. However, an *in vitro* study found no evidence of chelate formation with ciprofloxacin, **levofloxacin** or ofloxacin and calcium or magnesium, and therefore suggested that either other divalent cations may be involved, or that the quinolones may be adsorbed onto other metal ions, proteins or fat in the enteral feed.[26]

It has also been suggested that alteration in pH as well as the presence of cations are required to form chelates with ciprofloxacin and while this helps explain the lack of effect of high calcium in a high-fat breakfast,[15] it does not explain the significant effect with enteral feeds or calcium-fortified orange juice. The differences seen in men and women are possibly due to a slower gastric emptying rate in men, which increases the exposure of the quinolone to the enteral feed.[4]

Importance and management

The interaction between ciprofloxacin and enteral feeds is established. No treatment failures have been reported but it may be clinically important. For example, if patients receiving enteral feeds were to be switched from parenteral to oral ciprofloxacin, there could be a significant reduction in serum ciprofloxacin levels. The authors of one study recommend that in patients with severe infections, such a switch from parenteral to nasogastric administration of ciprofloxacin should be restricted to those whose plasma ciprofloxacin levels can be routinely monitored. However, some have found the reduced levels with enteral feeding still provide adequate antibacterial levels,[8,27] but be alert for any evidence that ciprofloxacin is less effective and raise the dose as necessary. Use of enteral feeds with lower concentrations of divalent ions or even stopping tube feeding for a short period of time have been suggested as methods to try to improve ciprofloxacin absorption.[27] The authors of one *in vitro* study suggest that *Ensure* should be given at least 2 hours before or after fluoroquinolones.[26]

The interaction between ofloxacin or moxifloxacin and enteral feeds is much smaller and probably not clinically important but this needs confirmation. Garenoxacin and gatifloxacin appear not to interact. There are no specific reports about other quinolones but be alert for this interaction with any of them.

Apart from dairy products (see 'Quinolones + Dairy products', p.347), quinolones can be given with food without any decrease in levels. However, calcium-fortified foods may cause significant interactions with ciprofloxacin.

1. Mueller BA, Brierton DG, Abel SR, Bowman L. Effect of enteral feeding with *Ensure* on oral bioavailabilities of ofloxacin and ciprofloxacin. *Antimicrob Agents Chemother* (1994) 38, 2101–5.
2. Noer BL, Angaran DM. The effect of enteral feedings on ciprofloxacin pharmacokinetics. *Pharmacotherapy* (1990) 10, 254.
3. Piccolo ML, Toossi Z, Goldman M. Effect of coadministration of a nutritional supplement on ciprofloxacin absorption. *Am J Hosp Pharm* (1994) 51, 2697–9.
4. Sowinski KM, Abel SR, Clark WR, Mueller BA. Effect of gender on relative oral bioavailability of ciprofloxacin and ofloxacin when administered with an enteral feeding product. *Pharmacotherapy* (1997) 17, 1112.
5. Healy DP, Brodbeck MC, Clendening CE. Ciprofloxacin absorption is impaired in patients given enteral feedings orally and via gastrostomy and jejunostomy tubes. *Antimicrob Agents Chemother* (1996) 40, 6–10.
6. Yuk JH, Nightingale CH, Quintiliani R, Yeston NS, Orlando R, Dobkin ED, Kambe JC, Sweeney KR, Buonpane EA. Absorption of ciprofloxacin administered through a nasogastric tube or a nasoduodenal tube in volunteers and patients receiving enteral nutrition. *Diagn Microbiol Infect Dis* (1990) 13, 99–102.
7. Yuk JH, Nightingale CH, Sweeney KR, Quintiliani R, Lettieri JT, Frost RW. Relative bioavailability in healthy volunteers of ciprofloxacin administered through a nasogastric tube with and without enteral feeding. *Antimicrob Agents Chemother* (1989) 33, 1118–20.
8. de Marie S, VandenBergh MFQ, Buijk SLCE, Bruining HA, van Vliet A, Kluytmans JAJW, Mouton JW. Bioavailability of ciprofloxacin after multiple enteral and intravenous doses in ICU patients with severe gram-negative intra-abdominal infections. *Intensive Care Med* (1998) 24, 343–6.
9. Mimoz O, Binter V, Jacolot A, Edouard A, Tod M, Petitjean O, Samii K. Pharmacokinetics and absolute bioavailability of ciprofloxacin administered through a nasogastric tube with continuous enteral feeding to critically ill patients. *Intensive Care Med* (1998) 24, 1047–51.
10. Krishna G, Noveck R, Vargas R, Grasela D, Wang Z. Nasogastric administration of garenoxacin as crushed tablets with and without concomitant enteral feeding in healthy subjects. *Drugs R D* (2007) 8, 43–50.
11. Kays MB, Overholser BR, Lagvankar S, Goldman M, Sowinski KM. Effect of Ensure on the oral bioavailability of gatifloxacin in healthy volunteers. *Pharmacotherapy* (2005) 25, 1530–5.
12. Kanji S, McKinnon PS, Barletta JF, Kruse JA, Devlin JW. Bioavailability of gatifloxacin by gastric tube administration with and without concomitant enteral feeding in critically ill patients. *Crit Care Med* (2003) 31, 1347–52.
13. Burkhardt O, Stass H, Thuss U, Borner K, Welte T. Effects of enteral feeding on the oral bioavailability of moxifloxacin in healthy volunteers. *Clin Pharmacokinet* (2005) 44, 969–76.
14. Höffken G, Lode H, Wiley R, Glatzel TD, Sievers D, Olschewski T, Borner K, Koeppe T. Pharmacokinetics and bioavailability of ciprofloxacin and ofloxacin: effect of food and antacid intake. *Rev Infect Dis* (1988) 10 (Suppl 1), S138–S139.
15. Frost RW, Carlson JD, Dietz AJ, Heyd A, Lettieri JT. Ciprofloxacin pharmacokinetics after a standard or high-fat/high-calcium breakfast. *J Clin Pharmacol* (1989) 29, 953–5.
16. Verho M, Malerczyk V, Dagrosa E, Korn A. The effect of food on the pharmacokinetics of ofloxacin. *Curr Med Res Opin* (1986) 10, 166–71.
17. Dudley MN, Marchbanks CR, Flor SC, Beals B. The effect of food or milk on the absorption kinetics of ofloxacin. *Eur J Clin Pharmacol* (1991) 41, 569–71.
18. Hooper WD, Dickinson RG, Eadie MJ. Effect of food on absorption of lomefloxacin. *Antimicrob Agents Chemother* (1990) 34, 1797–9.
19. Somogyi AA, Bochner F, Keal JA, Rolan PE, Smith M. Effect of food on enoxacin absorption. *Antimicrob Agents Chemother* (1987) 31, 638–9.
20. Allen A, Bygate E, Clark D, Lewis A, Pay V. The effect of food on the bioavailability of oral gemifloxacin in healthy volunteers. *Int J Antimicrob Agents* (2000) 16, 45–50.
21. Johnson RD, Dorr MB, Hunt TL, Jensen BK, Talbot GH. Effects of food on the pharmacokinetics of sparfloxacin. *Clin Ther* (1999) 21, 982–91.
22. Neuhofel AL, Wilton JH, Victory JM, Hejmanowski LG, Amsden GW. Lack of bioequivalence of ciprofloxacin when administered with calcium-fortified orange juice: a new twist on an old interaction. *J Clin Pharmacol* (2002) 42, 461–6.
23. Wallace AW, Victory JM, Amsden GW. Lack of bioequivalence of gatifloxacin when coadministered with calcium-fortified orange juice in healthy volunteers. *J Clin Pharmacol* (2003) 43, 92–6.
24. Wallace AW, Victory JM, Amsden GW. Lack of bioequivalence when levofloxacin and calcium-fortified orange juice are coadministered to healthy volunteers. *J Clin Pharmacol* (2003) 43, 539–44.
25. Amsden GW, Whitaker A-M. Johnson PW. Lack of bioequivalence of levofloxacin when coadministered with a mineral-fortified breakfast of juice and cereal. *J Clin Pharmacol* (2003) 43, 990–95.
26. Wright DH, Pietz SL, Konstantinides FN, Rotschafer JC. Decreased *in vitro* fluoroquinolone concentrations after admixture with an enteral feeding formulation. *J Parenter Enteral Nutr* (2000) 24, 42–8.
27. Cohn SM, Sawyer MD, Burns GA, Tolomeo C, Milner KA. Enteric absorption of ciprofloxacin during tube feeding in the critically ill. *J Antimicrob Chemother* (1996) 38, 871–6.

Quinolones + H_2-receptor antagonists

Cimetidine can increase the serum levels of some quinolones (intravenous enoxacin or fleroxacin and oral clinafloxacin or pefloxacin). Famotidine can reduce the serum levels of norfloxacin, and ranitidine can reduce the absorption of enoxacin.

Clinical evidence and mechanism

(a) Ciprofloxacin

Neither **cimetidine**[1,2] nor **ranitidine**[3,4] appear to have a clinically important effect on the pharmacokinetics of ciprofloxacin.

(b) Clinafloxacin

Cimetidine 300 mg four times daily for 4 days increased the maximum serum levels of clinafloxacin by 15% and increased its AUC by 44%.[5]

(c) Enoxacin

The plasma levels of a 400-mg intravenous dose of enoxacin were higher when **cimetidine** 300 mg four times daily was given concurrently. Renal clearance and systemic clearance were reduced by 26% and 20%, respectively, and the elimination half-life was increased by 30%.[6]

In one study, **ranitidine** 150 mg twice daily did not affect the pharmacokinetics of a single 400-mg intravenous dose of enoxacin.[6] However, in another study, **ranitidine** 50 mg given intravenously 2 hours before a single 400-mg oral dose of enoxacin reduced the absorption of the enoxacin by 26 to 40%,[7,8] which seemed to be related to changes in gastric pH caused by **ranitidine**.[8]

(d) Fleroxacin

Cimetidine decreases the total clearance of fleroxacin by about 25%, without much effect on renal clearance, and increases its elimination half-life by 32%.[9]

(e) Gatifloxacin

Cimetidine does not alter the pharmacokinetics of gatifloxacin.[10]

(f) Levofloxacin

Cimetidine reduces the clearance of levofloxacin by about 25% and increased its AUC by almost 30%,[11] whereas **ranitidine** does not affect the pharmacokinetics of levofloxacin.[12]

(g) Lomefloxacin

Ranitidine does not affect the pharmacokinetics of lomefloxacin.[13,14]

(h) Moxifloxacin

Ranitidine does not affect the pharmacokinetics of moxifloxacin.[15]

(i) Norfloxacin

Famotidine given 8 hours before norfloxacin significantly reduced its maximum serum concentrations in 6 healthy subjects, but the AUC and urinary recovery rate were unchanged.[16]

(j) Ofloxacin

Cimetidine does not alter the pharmacokinetics of ofloxacin.[17]

(k) Pefloxacin

Cimetidine increases the AUC of intravenous pefloxacin by about 40%. It increases the half-life from 10.3 hours to 15.3 hours and the clearance of pefloxacin was reduced by almost 30%.[18]

(l) Sparfloxacin

Cimetidine does not alter the pharmacokinetics of sparfloxacin.[19]

(m) Tosufloxacin

Famotidine does not alter the pharmacokinetics of tosufloxacin.[20]

(n) Trovafloxacin

Cimetidine does not alter the pharmacokinetics of trovafloxacin.[21]

Importance and management

Although the pharmacokinetic changes seen in some of these studies are moderate, none has been shown to affect the outcome of treatment and they are probably only of minor clinical relevance.

1. Ludwig E, Graber H, Székely É, Csiba A. Metabolic interactions of ciprofloxacin. *Diagn Microbiol Infect Dis* (1990) 13, 135–41.
2. Prince RA, Liou W-S, Kasik JE. Effect of cimetidine on ciprofloxacin pharmacokinetics. *Pharmacotherapy* (1990) 10, 233.
3. Höffken G, Lode H, Wiley R, Glatzel TD, Sievers D, Olschewski T, Borner K, Koeppe T. Pharmacokinetics and bioavailability of ciprofloxacin and ofloxacin: effect of food and antacid intake. *Rev Infect Dis* (1988) 10 (Suppl 1), S138–9.
4. Nix DE, Watson WA, Lener ME, Frost RW, Krol G, Goldstein H, Letterei J, Schentag JJ. Effects of aluminum and magnesium antacids and ranitidine on the absorption of ciprofloxacin. *Clin Pharmacol Ther* (1989) 46, 700–5.
5. Randinitis EJ, Koup JR, Bron NJ, Hounslow NJ, Rausch G, Abel R, Vassos AB, Sedman AJ. Drug interaction studies with clinafloxacin and probenecid, cimetidine, phenytoin and warfarin. *Drugs* (1999) 58 (Suppl 2), 254–5.
6. Misiak PM, Eldon MA, Toothaker RD, Sedman AJ. Effects of oral cimetidine or ranitidine on the pharmacokinetics of intravenous enoxacin. *J Clin Pharmacol* (1993) 33, 53–6.

7. Grasela TH, Schentag JJ, Sedman AJ, Wilton JH, Thomas DJ, Schultz RW, Lebsack ME, Kinkel AW. Inhibition of enoxacin absorption by antacids or ranitidine. *Antimicrob Agents Chemother* (1989) 33, 615–17.
8. Lebsack ME, Nix D, Ryerson B, Toothaker RD, Welage L, Norman AM, Schentag JJ, Sedman AJ. Effect of gastric acidity on enoxacin absorption. *Clin Pharmacol Ther* (1992) 52, 252–6.
9. Portmann R. Influence of cimetidine on fleroxacin pharmacokinetics. *Drugs* (1993) 45 (Suppl 3), 471.
10. Shiba K, Kusajima H, Momo K. The effects of aluminium hydroxide, cimetidine, ferrous sulfate, green tea and milk on pharmacokinetics of gatifloxacin in healthy humans. *J Antimicrob Chemother* (1999) 44 (Suppl A), 141.
11. Gaitonde MD, Mendes P, House ESA, Lehr KH. The effects of cimetidine and probenecid on the pharmacokinetics of levofloxacin (LFLX). *Intersci Conf Antimicrob Agents Chemother* (1995) 35, 8.
12. Shiba K, Sakai O, Shimada J, Okazaki O, Aoki H, Hakusui H. Effects of antacids, ferrous sulphate, and ranitidine on absorption of DR-3355 in humans. *Antimicrob Agents Chemother* (1992) 36, 2270–4.
13. Nix D, Schentag J. Lomefloxacin (L) absorption kinetics when administered with ranitidine (R) and sucralfate (S). *Intersci Conf Antimicrob Agents Chemother* (1989) 29, 317.
14. Sudoh T, Fujimura A, Harada K, Sunaga K, Ohmori M, Sakamoto K. Effect of ranitidine on renal clearance of lomefloxacin. *Eur J Clin Pharmacol* (1996) 51, 95–8.
15. Stass H, Böttcher M-F, Ochmann K. Evaluation of the influence of antacids and H_2 antagonists on the absorption of moxifloxacin after oral administration of a 400-mg dose to healthy volunteers. *Clin Pharmacokinet* (2001) 40 (Suppl 1), 39–48.
16. Shimada J, Hori S. Effect of antiulcer drugs on gastrointestinal absorption of norfloxacin. *Chemotherapy (Tokyo)* (1992) 40, 1141–7.
17. Shiba K, Yoshida M, Kachi M, Shimada J, Saito A, Sakai N. Effects of peptic ulcer-healing drugs on the pharmacokinetics of new quinolone (OFLX). 17th International Congress on Chemotherapy, Berlin, June 1991. Abstract 415.
18. Sörgel F, Mahr G, Koch HU, Stephan U, Wiesemann HG, Malter U. Effects of cimetidine on the pharmacokinetics of pefloxacin in healthy volunteers. *Rev Infect Dis* (1988) 10 (Suppl 1), S137.
19. Gries JM, Honorato J, Taburet AM, Alvarez MP, Sadaba B, Azanza JR, Singlas E. Cimetidine does not alter sparfloxacin pharmacokinetics. *Int J Clin Pharmacol Ther* (1995) 33, 585–7.
20. Minami R, Nakamura C, Inotsume N, Nakano M. Effects of aluminium hydroxide and famotidine on bioavailability of tosufloxacin in healthy volunteers. *Antimicrob Agents Chemother* (1998) 42, 453–5.
21. Purkins L, Oliver SD, Willavize SA. An open, controlled, crossover study on the effects of cimetidine on the steady-state pharmacokinetics of trovafloxacin. *Eur J Clin Microbiol Infect Dis* (1998) 17, 431–3.

Quinolones + Iron or Zinc compounds

Ferrous fumarate, ferrous gluconate, ferrous sulfate and other iron compounds can reduce the absorption of ciprofloxacin, gatifloxacin, levofloxacin, moxifloxacin, norfloxacin, ofloxacin, sparfloxacin from the gut. Serum levels of the antibacterial may become subtherapeutic as a result. Limited evidence suggests that fleroxacin is not affected, lomefloxacin is only minimally affected and gemifloxacin is not affected when dosing is separated. Zinc appears to interact like the iron compounds. No interaction appears to occur with iron-ovotransferrin.

Clinical evidence

(a) Ciprofloxacin

The absorption of ciprofloxacin is markedly reduced by iron and zinc compounds. Several studies have clearly demonstrated reductions in the AUC and maximum serum levels of 30 to 90% with **ferrous fumarate**,[1] **ferrous gluconate**,[2] **ferrous sulfate**,[2-5] **iron-glycine sulfate**,[6] ***Centrum Forte***[2] (a multi-mineral preparation containing iron, magnesium, zinc, calcium, copper and manganese) and with ***Stresstabs 600-with-zinc***[4] (a multivitamin-with-zinc preparation). However **iron-ovotransferrin** has been found to have no significant effect on the absorption of ciprofloxacin.[7]

(b) Fleroxacin

A study in 12 subjects found that **ferrous sulfate** (equivalent to 100 mg of elemental iron) had no significant effect on the pharmacokinetics of fleroxacin.[8]

(c) Gatifloxacin

A study in 6 healthy subjects found that **ferrous sulfate** 160 mg given with gatifloxacin 200 mg decreased the maximum serum levels and AUC of gatifloxacin by 49% and 29%, respectively.[9]

A case report describes a woman who did not respond to treatment with gatifloxacin for hospital acquired pneumonia when it was given at the same time as a multivitamin preparation containing iron, magnesium and **zinc**. When administration was separated by 6 hours her clinical signs improved.[10]

(d) Gemifloxacin

In a study in 27 healthy subjects, gemifloxacin 320 mg was given either 3 hours before or 2 hours after **ferrous sulfate** 325 mg. The pharmacokinetics of gemifloxacin were not significantly altered in either case.[11]

(e) Levofloxacin

Ferrous sulfate has been found to reduce the bioavailability of levofloxacin by 79%.[12]

(f) Lomefloxacin

When lomefloxacin 400 mg was given with **ferrous sulfate** (equivalent to 100 mg of elemental iron), the lomefloxacin maximum serum levels were reduced by about 28% and the AUC was reduced by about 14%.[13]

(g) Moxifloxacin

In 12 healthy subjects **ferrous sulfate** (equivalent to 100 mg of elemental iron) reduced the AUC and maximum plasma levels of a single 400-mg dose of moxifloxacin by 39% and 59%, respectively. The rate of absorption was reduced (time to maximum plasma level increased from a mean of one hour to 2.79 hours).[14]

(h) Norfloxacin

In 8 healthy subjects **ferrous sulfate** reduced the AUC and maximum serum levels of a single 400-mg dose of norfloxacin by 73% and 75%, respectively.[5] **Ferrous sulfate** caused a 51% reduction in the AUC of norfloxacin in another study,[15,16] and a 97% reduction in bioavailability in a further single-dose study.[17] The same authors also found that both **ferrous sulfate** and **zinc sulfate** reduced the urinary recovery of norfloxacin by 55% and 56%, respectively.[18]

(i) Ofloxacin

In 8 healthy subjects **ferrous sulfate** (equivalent to 100 mg of elemental iron) reduced the AUC and maximum serum levels of a single 400-mg dose of ofloxacin by 25% and 36%, respectively.[5] In 9 healthy subjects **ferrous sulfate** 1050 mg decreased the absorption of ofloxacin 200 mg by 11%.[19] In 12 healthy subjects elemental iron 200 mg (in the form of an **iron-glycine-sulfate** complex) reduced the bioavailability of ofloxacin 400 mg by 36%.[6]

(j) Sparfloxacin

In a single-dose study in 6 subjects, **ferrous sulfate** 525 mg (equivalent to 170 mg of elemental iron) reduced the AUC of sparfloxacin 200 mg by 27%.[15,16]

Mechanism

It is believed that the quinolones form a complex with iron and zinc (by chelation between the metal ion and the 4-oxo and adjacent carboxyl groups), which is less easily absorbed by the gut. However, a study in *rats* using oral iron and intravenous ciprofloxacin suggested that the interaction may not be entirely confined to the gut.[20] This needs further study. Iron-ovotransferrin differs from other iron preparations in being able to combine directly with the transferrin receptors of intestinal cells, and appears to release little iron into the gut to interact with the quinolones.

Importance and management

The interactions between the quinolones and iron compounds are established and would appear to be of clinical importance because the serum antibacterial levels can become subtherapeutic. In descending order the extent of the interaction appears to be: norfloxacin, levofloxacin, ciprofloxacin, moxifloxacin, gatifloxacin, ofloxacin/sparfloxacin, then least affected, lomefloxacin.

None of these quinolones should be taken at the same time as any iron preparation that contains substantial amounts of iron (e.g. ferrous sulfate, ferrous gluconate, ferrous fumarate, iron-glycine sulfate). As the quinolones are rapidly absorbed, taking them 2 hours before the iron should minimise the risk of admixture in the gut and largely avoid this interaction. Information about other quinolones seems to be lacking but the same precautions should be taken with all of them except fleroxacin, which appears not to interact, and lomefloxacin, which seems to interact only minimally.

Iron-ovotransferrin does not interact with ciprofloxacin and is not expected to interact with any of the quinolones (see 'Mechanism') but this awaits confirmation.

There seems to be very little data about the interactions between zinc compounds and quinolones, but zinc appears to interact like iron and therefore the same precautions suggested for iron should be followed.

1. Brouwers JRBJ, Van der Kam HJ, Sijtsma J, Proost JH. Decreased ciprofloxacin absorption with concomitant administration of ferrous fumarate. *Pharm Weekbl (Sci)* (1990) 12, 182–3.
2. Kara M, Hasinoff BB, McKay DW, Campbell NRC. Clinical and chemical interactions between iron preparations and ciprofloxacin. *Br J Clin Pharmacol* (1991) 31, 257–61.
3. Le Pennec MP, Kitzis MD, Terdjman M, Foubard S, Garbarz E, Hanania G. Possible interaction of ciprofloxacin with ferrous sulphate. *J Antimicrob Chemother* (1990) 25, 184–5.
4. Polk RE, Healy DP, Sahai J, Drwal L, Racht E. Effect of ferrous sulfate and multivitamins with zinc on absorption of ciprofloxacin in normal volunteers. *Antimicrob Agents Chemother* (1989) 33, 1841–4.
5. Lehto P, Kivistö KT, Neuvonen PJ. The effect of ferrous sulphate on the absorption of norfloxacin, ciprofloxacin and ofloxacin. *Br J Clin Pharmacol* (1994) 37, 82–5.
6. Lode H, Stuhlert P, Deppermann KH, Mainz D, Borner K, Kotvas K, Koeppe P. Pharmacokinetic interactions between oral ciprofloxacin (CIP)/ofloxacin (OFL) and ferro-salts. *Intersci Conf Antimicrob Agents Chemother* (1989) 29,136.
7. Pazzucconi F, Barbi S, Baldassarre D, Colombo N, Dorigotti F, Sirtori CR. Iron-ovotransferrin preparation does not interfere with ciprofloxacin absorption. *Clin Pharmacol Ther* (1996) 59, 418–22.
8. Sörgel F, Naber KG, Kinzig M, Frank A, Birner B. Effect of ferrous sulfate on fleroxacin analyzed by the confidence interval (CI) approach. *Pharm Res* (1995) 12 (9 Suppl), S-422.
9. Shiba K, Kusajima H, Momo K. The effects of aluminium hydroxide, cimetidine, ferrous sulfate, green tea and milk on pharmacokinetics of gatifloxacin in healthy humans. *J Antimicrob Chemother* (1999) 44 (Suppl A), 141.
10. Mallet L, Huang A, Coadministration of gatifloxacin and multivitamin preparation containing minerals: potential treatment failure in an elderly patient. *Ann Pharmacother* (2005) 39, 150–2.
11. Allen A, Bygate E, Faessel H, Isaac L, Lewis A. The effect of ferrous sulphate and sucralfate on the bioavailability of oral gemifloxacin in healthy volunteers. *Int J Antimicrob Agents* (2000) 15, 283–9.
12. Shiba K, Okazaki O, Aoki H, Sakai O, Shimada J. Inhibition of DR-3355 absorption by metal ions. *Intersci Conf Antimicrob Agents Chemother* (1991) 31, 198.
13. Lehto P, Kivistö KT. Different effects of products containing metal ions on the absorption of lomefloxacin. *Clin Pharmacol Ther* (1994) 56, 477–82.
14. Stass H, Kubitza D. Effects of iron supplements on the oral bioavailability of moxifloxacin, a novel 8-methoxyfluoroquinolone, in humans. *Clin Pharmacokinet* (2001) 40 (Suppl 1), 57–62.
15. Kanemitsu K, Hori S, Yanagawa A, Shimada J. Effect of ferrous sulfate on the pharmacokinetics of sparfloxacin. *Chemotherapy* (1994) 42, 6–13.
16. Kanemitsu K, Hori S, Yanagawa A, Shimada J. Effect of ferrous sulfate on the absorption of sparfloxacin in healthy volunteers and rats. *Drugs* (1995) 49 (Suppl 2), 352–6.
17. Okhamafe AO, Akerele JO, Chukuka CS. Pharmacokinetic interactions of norfloxacin with some metallic medicinal agents. *Int J Pharmaceutics* (1991) 68, 11–18.
18. Campbell NRC, Kara M, Hasinoff BB, Haddara WM, McKay DW. Norfloxacin interaction with antacids and minerals. *Br J Clin Pharmacol* (1992) 33, 115–16.
19. Martínez Cabarga M, Sánchez Navarro A, Colino Gandarillas CI, Domínguez-Gil A. Effects of two cations on gastrointestinal absorption of ofloxacin. *Antimicrob Agents Chemother* (1991) 35, 2102–5.
20. Wong PY, Zhu M, Li RC. Pharmacokinetic and pharmacodynamic interactions between intravenous ciprofloxacin and oral ferrous sulfate. *J Chemother* (2000) 12, 286–93.

Quinolones + NSAIDs

Diclofenac appears to increase the exposure to a single-dose ciprofloxacin. A number of cases of convulsions have been seen in Japanese

patients given fenbufen with enoxacin, and there is also one possible case involving ofloxacin. Generally no interaction seems to occur with most quinolones and NSAIDs, except where there is a predisposition to convulsive episodes. Isolated cases of convulsions, other neurological toxicity or skin eruptions have been seen when ciprofloxacin was given with indometacin, mefenamic acid, or naproxen. These appear to be very rare events.

Clinical evidence

(a) Ciprofloxacin

As of 1995 the manufacturer of ciprofloxacin had, on record, two confirmed spontaneous reports of convulsions in patients taking ciprofloxacin and an NSAID; one with **mefenamic acid** and the other with **naproxen**.[1] These appear to be the only medically validated reports of an interaction between ciprofloxacin and an NSAID by 1995.[1]

A woman taking chloroquine 250 mg and **naproxen** 1 g daily developed dizziness, anxiety and tremors within a week of starting to take ciprofloxacin 1 g daily. The symptoms largely resolved when the chloroquine was stopped; it was not known if she also stopped the naproxen. Two months after chloroquine was discontinued, and while she was still taking ciprofloxacin, **indometacin** was started. This time she developed pain in her feet and became extremely tired. The pain partially subsided and the fatigue vanished when the ciprofloxacin was stopped. Later she was found to have some axonal demyelination, compatible with drug-induced polyneuropathy.[2]

A crossover study in 12 healthy subjects found that concurrent use of a single 50-mg dose of **diclofenac** with a single 500-mg dose of ciprofloxacin increased the AUC and the maximum plasma concentration of ciprofloxacin by 46% and 58%, respectively, when compared with ciprofloxacin given alone.[3] A study in 8 healthy subjects found that the pharmacokinetics of ciprofloxacin were unaffected by treatment with **fenbufen** for 3 days.[4] Another study, in 12 healthy subjects, found that the concurrent use of single doses of ciprofloxacin and **fenbufen** produced no evidence, using EEG recordings, of increased CNS excitatory effects.[5]

(b) Enoxacin

A total of 17 Japanese patients have been identified, with apparently no previous history of seizures, who in the 1986 to 1987 period developed convulsions when given **fenbufen** 400 mg to 1.2 g daily with enoxacin 200 to 800 mg.[6] Two case reports of this interaction have been published.[7,8] An 87-year-old Japanese woman taking enoxacin 200 mg also had convulsions after receiving a single 50-mg intravenous dose of **flurbiprofen**.[9]

(c) Levofloxacin

A study in 24 healthy subjects found plasma levels of single 125-mg and 500-mg doses of levofloxacin were increased by about 13%, 6.5 hours after they were given **fenbufen** 600 mg. No changes in CNS activity were found.[10]

(d) Ofloxacin

One patient taking **fenbufen** 800 mg had involuntary movements of the neck and upper extremities after taking ofloxacin 600 mg.[6] In 10 healthy subjects the pharmacokinetics of ofloxacin 200 mg twice daily were unchanged by **ketoprofen** 100 mg daily for 3 days.[11] The incidence of psychotic adverse effects (euphoria, hysteria, psychosis) in 151 patients taking ofloxacin were not increased by the concurrent use of NSAIDs (**aspirin**, **diclofenac**, **indometacin**, **dipyrone**).[12]

(e) Pefloxacin

In 10 healthy subjects the pharmacokinetics of pefloxacin 400 mg twice daily were not affected by **ketoprofen** 100 mg daily for 3 days.[11]

(f) Sparfloxacin

A 62-year-old woman developed drug eruptions (erythematous papules), which were attributed to sparfloxacin hypersensitivity induced by **mefenamic acid**.[13]

Mechanism

Not fully understood. Convulsions have occurred in a few patients taking quinolones alone, some of whom had epilepsy and some of whom did not, see 'Antiepileptics + Quinolones', p.566. Experiments in *mice* have shown that quinolones competitively inhibit the binding of GABA to its receptors.[14] GABA is an inhibitory transmitter in the CNS, which is believed to be involved in the control of convulsive activity. Enoxacin and fenbufen are known to affect the GABA receptor site in the hippocampus and frontal cortex of *mice*, which is associated with convulsive activity.[15] It could be that, if and when an interaction occurs, the NSAID simply lowers the amount of quinolone needed to precipitate convulsions in already susceptible individuals.

The mechanism behind the increase in exposure to ciprofloxacin when given with diclofenac is unclear. The authors of the study[3] note that diclofenac increased the extent of absorption, and decreased the clearance of ciprofloxacin; further research is needed.

Importance and management

The interaction between enoxacin and fenbufen is established, but it seems to be uncommon. Nevertheless, it would seem prudent to avoid the concurrent use of fenbufen with enoxacin; there are very many alternatives.

The evidence for an interaction between diclofenac and ciprofloxacin seems to be limited to one small single-dose study. Diclofenac appears to increase the exposure to, and maximum plasma concentrations of single-dose ciprofloxacin. The clinical relevance of these increases is unclear, but might be of more consequence in patients with renal impairment and in those with epilepsy. Until more is known, it might be prudent to consider the use of an alternative NSAID. Reports of adverse interactions between other quinolones and NSAIDs are extremely rare. The general warning about convulsions with quinolones and NSAIDs issued by the CSM in the UK[16] seems to be an extrapolation from the interaction between enoxacin and fenbufen, and from some *animal* experiments. In addition to the data cited above, an epidemiological study of 856 users of quinolones (ciprofloxacin, enoxacin, nalidixic acid) and a range of NSAIDs found no cases of convulsions.[17] The overall picture would therefore seem to be that although a potential for interaction exists, the risk is very small indeed and normally there would seem to be little reason for most patients taking quinolones to avoid NSAIDs. Patients with epilepsy are a possible exception and it would seem prudent to avoid quinolones and NSAIDs wherever possible in these patients.

1. Bomford J. Ciprofloxacin. *Pharm J* (1995) 255, 674.
2. Rollof J, Vinge E. Neurological adverse effects during concomitant treatment with ciprofloxacin, NSAIDS, and chloroquine: possible drug interaction. *Ann Pharmacother* (1993) 27, 1058–9.
3. Iqbal Z, Khan A, Naz A, Khan JA, Khan GS. Pharmacokinetic interaction of ciprofloxacin with diclofenac: a single-dose, two-period crossover study in healthy adult volunteers. *Clin Drug Investig* (2009) 29, 275–81.
4. Kamali F. Lack of a pharmacokinetic interaction between ciprofloxacin and fenbufen. *J Clin Pharm Ther* (1994) 19, 257–9.
5. Kamali F, Ashton CH, Marsh VR, Cox J. Is there a pharmacodynamic interaction between ciprofloxacin and fenbufen? *Br J Clin Pharmacol* (1997) 43, 545P–546P.
6. Lederle. Data on file. December 1995.
7. Takeo G, Shibuya N, Motomura M, Kanazawa H, Shishido H. A new DNA gyrase inhibitor induces convulsions: a case report and animal experiments. *Chemotherapy (Tokyo)* (1989) 37, 1154–9.
8. Morita H, Maemura K, Sakai Y, Kaneda Y. A case with convulsion, loss of consciousness and subsequent acute renal failure caused by enoxacin and fenbufen. *Nippon Naika Gakkai Zasshi* (1988) 77, 744–5.
9. Mizuno J, Takumi Z, Kaneko A, Tsutsui T, Tsutsui T, Zushi N, Machida K. Convulsion following the combination of single preoperative oral administration of enoxacine and single postoperative intravenous administration of flurbiprofen axetil. *Jpn J Anesthesiol* (2001) 50, 425–8.
10. Hoechst Marion Roussel Ltd. Data on file. Personal communication, January 1999.
11. Fillastre JP, Leroy A, Borsa-Lebas F, Etienne I, Gy C, Humbert G. Effects of ketoprofen (NSAID) on the pharmacokinetics of pefloxacin and ofloxacin in healthy volunteers. *Drugs Exp Clin Res* (1992) 18, 487–92.
12. Jüngst G, Weidmann E, Breitstadt A, Huppertz E. Does ofloxacin interact with NSAIDs to cause psychotic side effects? 17th International Congress on Chemotherapy, Berlin, June 23–8, 1991. Abstract 412.
13. Oiso N, Taniguchi S, Goto Y, Hisa T, Mizuno N, Mochida K, Hamada T, Yorifuji T. A case of drug eruption due to sparfloxacin (SPFX) and mefenamic acid. *Skin Res* (1995) 37, 321–7.
14. Hori S, Shimada J, Saito A, Matsuda M, Miyahara T. Comparison of the inhibitory effects of new quinolones on γ-aminobutyric acid receptor binding in the presence of antiinflammatory drugs. *Rev Infect Dis* (1989) 11 (Suppl 5), S1397–S1398.
15. Motomura M, Kataoka Y, Takeo G, Shibayama K, Ohishi K, Nakamura T, Niwa M, Tsujihata M, Nagataki S. Hippocampus and frontal cortex are the potential mediatory sites for convulsions induced by new quinolones and non-steroidal anti-inflammatory drugs. *Int J Clin Pharmacol Ther Toxicol* (1991) 29, 223–7.
16. Committee on Safety of Medicines. Convulsions due to quinolone antimicrobial agents. *Current Problems* (1991) 32, 2.
17. Mannino S, Garcia-Rodriguez LA, Jick SS. NSAIDs, quinolones and convulsions: an epidemiological approach. *Post Marketing Surveillance* (1992) 6, 119–28.

Quinolones + Omeprazole

Omeprazole has no clinically important effect on the pharmacokinetics of ciprofloxacin, garenoxacin, gemifloxacin, lomefloxacin, ofloxacin or trovafloxacin.

Clinical evidence, mechanism, importance and management

A single-dose study found that omeprazole 20 or 80 mg had no significant effect on the pharmacokinetics of single doses of **ofloxacin** 400 mg, **ciprofloxacin** 500 mg or **lomefloxacin** 250 or 400 mg.[1] Another study in 27 subjects found that omeprazole 40 mg daily for 3 days did not affect the pharmacokinetics of a single 1-g dose of an extended-release formulation of **ciprofloxacin** (*Depomed*).[2] Omeprazole 40 mg caused an 18% reduction in the AUC of a single 300-mg dose of **trovafloxacin** and a 32% reduction in the maximum serum levels, but this was considered not to be of clinical significance.[3] A randomised, crossover study in 12 healthy subjects found that the maximum serum levels and AUC of a single 320-mg dose of **gemifloxacin** were increased by 11% and 10%, respectively, by omeprazole 40 mg daily for 4 days. The confidence intervals indicated that the respective increases were unlikely to exceed 36% and 43%, and it was concluded that these two drugs could be given together without any need for dose adjustments.[4] In a study in 12 healthy subjects, slow-release omeprazole 40 mg daily did not affect the pharmacokinetics of a single 600-mg dose of **garenoxacin** and concurrent use did not increase adverse effects.[5]

1. Stuht H, Lode H, Koeppe P, Rost KL, Schaberg T. Interaction study of lomefloxacin and ciprofloxacin with omeprazole and comparative pharmacokinetics. *Antimicrob Agents Chemother* (1995) 39, 1045–9.
2. Washington C, Hou E, Hughes N, Berner B. Effect of omeprazole on bioavailability of an oral extended-release formulation of ciprofloxacin. *Am J Health-Syst Pharm* (2006) 63, 653–6.
3. Teng R, Dogolo LC, Willavize SA, Friedman HL, Vincent J. Effect of Maalox and omeprazole on the bioavailability of trovafloxacin. *J Antimicrob Chemother* (1997) 39 (Suppl B), 93–7.
4. Allen A, Vousden M, Lewis A. Effect of omeprazole on the pharmacokinetics of oral gemifloxacin in healthy volunteers. *Chemotherapy* (1999) 45, 496–503.
5. Krishna G, Kisicki JC, Olsen S, Grasela DM, Wang Z. The effect of omeprazole on the bioavailability and safety of garenoxacin in healthy volunteers. *J Clin Pharmacol* (2007) 47, 628–32.

Quinolones + Opioids

Morphine modestly reduces the AUC of trovafloxacin, but this is not considered to be clinically significant. Trovafloxacin did not alter the effects or pharmacokinetics of morphine. Oxycodone does not appear to significantly affect the pharmacokinetics of either levofloxacin or gati-

floxacin. It has been suggested that opiates decrease oral ciprofloxacin levels, but good evidence for this appears to be lacking.

Clinical evidence, mechanism, importance and management

(a) Ciprofloxacin

In one non-randomised study[1] the levels of oral ciprofloxacin were only 1.3 mg/L in the presence of intramuscular **papaveretum**, compared to 3.22 mg/L in a control group not receiving **papaveretum**. The authors say that this means the peak ciprofloxacin levels in the **papaveretum** group would not reach the MIC of a number of gut pathogens. They name *Bacteroides fragilis* (but it should be noted that the levels of the control group also did not reach the MIC of this organism), and *Enterococcus faecalis*, many strains of which are only moderately susceptible to ciprofloxacin anyway. Further, the **papaveretum** group in this study had only 4 patients, and, as the authors note, the control group was not matched.[1] Based on this rather slim evidence, some have suggested that the concurrent use of opioids and ciprofloxacin as pre-medication should be avoided.[2-4]

(b) Gatifloxacin

In 12 healthy subjects, the pharmacokinetics of gatifloxacin 400 mg were not significantly altered by **oxycodone** 5 mg every 4 hours.[5]

(c) Levofloxacin

In 8 healthy subjects, the pharmacokinetics of oral levofloxacin 500 mg were not significantly altered by **oxycodone** 5 mg every 4 hours.[6]

(d) Trovafloxacin

An intravenous infusion of **morphine** 150 micrograms/kg given with oral trovafloxacin 200 mg to 18 healthy subjects caused a 36% reduction in the trovafloxacin AUC and a 46% reduction in the maximum serum levels. These levels were considered sufficient for prophylaxis of infection, and remained above the MICs of the most likely organisms to cause post-surgical infections. The bioavailability and effects of **morphine** were not significantly changed by trovafloxacin.[7]

1. Morran C, McArdle C, Petitt L, Sleigh D, Gemmell C, Hichens M, Felmingham D, Tillotson G. Brief report: pharmacokinetics of orally administered ciprofloxacin in abdominal surgery. *Am J Med* (1989) 87, (Suppl 5A), 86S–88S.
2. Celltech Pharmaceutical Ltd. Personal Communication, August 2003.
3. Morphine Sulphate Injection. Wockhardt UK Ltd. UK Summary of product characteristics, September 2007.
4. Ciprofloxacin Solution for Infusion. Hospira UK Ltd. UK Summary of product characteristics, January 2008.
5. Grant EM, Nicolau DP, Nightingale C, Quintiliani R. Minimal interaction between gatifloxacin and oxycodone. *J Clin Pharmacol* (2002) 42, 928–32.
6. Grant EM, Zhong MK, Fitzgerald JF, Nicolau DP, Nightingale C, Quintiliani R. Lack of interaction between levofloxacin and oxycodone: pharmacokinetics and drug disposition. *J Clin Pharmacol* (2001) 41, 206–9.
7. Vincent J, Hunt T, Teng R, Robarge L, Willavize SA, Friedman HL. The pharmacokinetic effects of coadministration of morphine and trovafloxacin in healthy subjects. *Am J Surg* (1998) 176 (Suppl 6A), 32S–38S.

Quinolones + Opioids; Methadone

An isolated case describes sedation, confusion and respiratory depression, which was attributed to the inhibition of methadone metabolism by ciprofloxacin.

Clinical evidence

A woman taking methadone 140 mg daily for 6 years, to manage pain due to chronic intestinal pseudo-obstruction, was admitted to hospital because of a urinary tract infection and given ciprofloxacin 750 mg twice daily. Two days later she became sedated and confused. Ciprofloxacin was replaced with co-trimoxazole and the patient recovered within 48 hours. She was treated with ciprofloxacin for recurrent urinary-tract infections a further three times and on each occasion the patient became sedated, with her normal alertness regained on discontinuing ciprofloxacin. On the last occasion, when the venlafaxine that she had also been taking was replaced by fluoxetine, she also developed respiratory depression, which was reversed with naloxone.[1]

Mechanism

The cytochrome P450 isoenzymes CYP1A2, CYP2D6 and CYP3A4 are involved in the metabolism of methadone. Ciprofloxacin is a potent inhibitor of CYP1A2 and possibly has some effect on CYP3A4. It is therefore probable that the confusion and sedation seen in the patient were due to the inhibition of methadone metabolism. The use of fluoxetine (a known CYP2D6 inhibitor) may also have contributed.

Importance and management

This seems to be the only report of this interaction but it would appear to be of clinical importance. Care is needed if ciprofloxacin and methadone are given concurrently, especially if there are other factors present, such as smoking or the use of other enzyme inhibitors, which may also contribute to the interaction. Be alert for the need to change the methadone dose. Consider also 'Quinolones + Opioids', p.351.

1. Herrlin K, Segerdahl M, Gustafsson LL, Kalso E. Methadone, ciprofloxacin, and adverse drug reactions. *Lancet* (2000) 356, 2069–70.

Quinolones + Other antibacterials

There appear to be few documented cases of clinically relevant interactions between the quinolones and other antibacterials. However, note that clindamycin may antagonise the effects of ciprofloxacin on *Staphylococcus aureus*. Further, *in vitro* studies have demonstrated antagonistic antibacterial effects when nitrofurantoin and nalidixic acid are used together, and other quinolones are also said to antagonise the effects of nitrofurantoin.

Clinical evidence, mechanism, importance and management

(a) Aminoglycosides

A study found that a single 100-mg intravenous dose of **tobramycin** had no effect on the pharmacokinetics of **pefloxacin**, and **pefloxacin** did not affect the pharmacokinetics of **tobramycin**.[1] Similarly no pharmacokinetic interaction was found between **pefloxacin** and **amikacin**.[2]

(b) Cephalosporins

A study found that a single 2-g intravenous dose of **ceftazidime** had no effect on the pharmacokinetics of **pefloxacin**, and **pefloxacin** did not affect the pharmacokinetics of **ceftazidime**.[1]

In a study in 11 healthy subjects, the pharmacokinetics of **cefotaxime** and **ofloxacin** were similar, whether given alone or in combination, and the antimicrobial effect of the combination was additive for *Staphylococcus aureus*, *Streptococcus pneumoniae*, *Enterobacter cloacae* and *Klebsiella pneumoniae*, but not for *Pseudomonas aeruginosa*.[3]

(c) Clindamycin

One study found that the pharmacokinetics of intravenous **ciprofloxacin** 200 mg were not affected by intravenous clindamycin 600 mg and there is evidence that combined use may possibly enhance the antibacterial activity, particularly against *Staphylococcus aureus* and *Streptococcus pneumoniae*.[4] However, another study found that the serum bactericidal activity of **ciprofloxacin** against *Staphylococcus aureus* was completely antagonised by clindamycin, if the strains were susceptible to the latter.[5]

(d) Macrolides

A study designed to assess the potential interaction between **trovafloxacin** and **azithromycin** found no significant alteration in the pharmacokinetics of either drug.[6]

(e) Metronidazole

A study found that a single 400-mg oral dose of metronidazole had no effect on the pharmacokinetics of **pefloxacin**, and similarly **pefloxacin** did not affect the pharmacokinetics of metronidazole.[1] In other studies no interaction was found between **ciprofloxacin** or **ofloxacin** (both 200 mg intravenously) and metronidazole 500 mg intravenously;[7] and metronidazole with **ciprofloxacin** orally.[8]

A further study, investigating the use of metronidazole 500 mg intravenously and **ciprofloxacin** 200 mg intravenously, also did not find any significant pharmacokinetic changes, although metronidazole reduced the **ciprofloxacin** volume of distribution by 20%.[4] This is not expected to be clinically significant.

(f) Nitrofurantoin

The antibacterial activity of **nalidixic acid** can be attenuated by sub-inhibitory concentrations of nitrofurantoin. In 44 out of 53 strains of *Escherichia coli*, *Salmonella* and *Proteus*, antagonism was shown.[9] Another study confirmed these findings.[10] Whether this similarly occurs if both antibacterials are given to patients is uncertain, but the advice that concurrent use should be avoided when treating urinary tract infections seems sound.[9] Active division of bacteria is required for the bactericidal activity of quinolones such as nalidixic acid, and the presence of a bacteriostatic drug such as nitrofurantoin may inhibit its action.[11] Other quinolone antibacterials (not named) and nitrofurantoin have been found to be antagonistic *in vitro*, although the clinical significance of this is unknown.[12,13]

(g) Penicillins

A single-dose study in 6 healthy subjects found that intravenous **azlocillin** 60 mg/kg reduced the clearance of intravenous **ciprofloxacin** 4 mg/kg by 35%. The pharmacokinetics of **azlocillin** were not affected.[14] Another study found that when a single 4-g intravenous dose of **piperacillin** was given with **pefloxacin** 400 mg the pharmacokinetics of both drugs were unchanged.[1] In 6 healthy subjects the absorption of **ofloxacin** 400 mg was not altered by **amoxicillin** 3 g.[15]

In another study, in 12 healthy subjects, the serum bacterial activity of **ciprofloxacin** with **piperacillin** against a variety of organisms was found to be additive, rather than antagonistic or synergistic despite the fact that the clearance of **ciprofloxacin** was reduced by 24%.[16]

(h) Rifampicin (Rifampin)

1. Ciprofloxacin. A single-dose study in 5 healthy subjects found that ciprofloxacin 500 mg decreased the peak serum levels of rifampicin 600 mg by 12%, and prolonged its half-life from 3.5 hours to 3.8 hours.[17] In a further study, ciprofloxacin did not affect the percentage of rifampicin recovered in the urine, but it did increase its initial rate of excretion.[18] In 12 elderly patients (aged 67 to 95 years), ciprofloxacin 750 mg and rifampicin 300 mg, both given every 12 hours for 2 weeks, did not significantly affect the pharmacokinetics of either drug.[19] This is confirmed by other pharmacokinetic studies, one of which also reported that combined use provided excellent serum bactericidal activity against *Staphylococcus aureus* strains, although activity was modestly lower than rifampicin alone.[5,20,21] No special precautions would seem necessary if rifampicin is given with ciprofloxacin.

2. Fleroxacin. A study in 13 healthy subjects found that rifampicin 600 mg daily for a week increased the clearance of fleroxacin 400 mg daily by 15%. However, the fleroxacin levels remained above the MIC_{90} of methicillin-sensitive strains of *Staphylococcus aureus* and *Staphylococcus epidermidis* for at least 24 hours.[22]

3. Gatifloxacin. A study in 22 healthy subjects who took a single 400-mg dose of gatifloxacin alone, or with a combined preparation containing rifampicin 400 mg, isoniazid 300 mg and pyrazinamide 1.6 g, found that the AUC of gatifloxacin was increased by 10% when taken with the combined preparation. In addition, the AUC and maximum plasma concentration of rifampicin were reduced by 14% and 27%, respectively, by gatifloxacin.[23] The effect of these changes on the efficacy of treatment is unclear, but it seems likely to be small.

4. Moxifloxacin. A study in 19 patients who were nearing the end of treatment for tuberculosis with rifampicin 450 mg daily and isoniazid 600 mg daily found that the maximum plasma levels and AUC of moxifloxacin 400 mg daily for 5 days were reduced by 32% and 31%, respectively, when it was taken with the antimycobacterials, compared with when it was taken alone. It was also noted that the MIC of moxifloxacin against fast growing bacilli was achieved in only one patient taking moxifloxacin with the antimycobacterials, compared with 9 of 19 patients taking moxifloxacin alone.[24]Another study in healthy subjects found that the AUC of moxifloxacin 400 mg daily, given for 4 days alone, and then with rifampicin 600 mg daily for 10 days was reduced by 27% by rifampicin. There was no significant difference between the maximum plasma moxifloxacin levels achieved in each treatment period.[25] The clinical significance of these findings is unclear, but it seems likely to be small.

5. Pefloxacin. A study in 8 healthy subjects found that rifampicin 900 mg daily for 10 days decreased the half-life and AUC_{0-12} of pefloxacin 400 mg twice daily by about 30%, due to a 35% increase in total plasma clearance.[26] Despite these changes the serum pefloxacin levels still remained well above the MIC (0.5 mg/L) for 90% of strains of methicillin-sensitive *Staphylococcus aureus* and *Staphylococcus epidermidis*.[26] A single-dose study in 5 healthy subjects found that pefloxacin 500 mg increased the AUC of a single 600-mg dose of rifampicin about twofold.[27] In a further study the urinary recovery of rifampicin was increased from 16% of the dose to 20% by pefloxacin.[28] No special precautions would seem necessary if rifampicin is given with pefloxacin.

1. Metz R, Jaehde U, Wiesemann H, Gottschalk B, Stephan U, Schunack W. Pharmacokinetic interactions and non-interactions of pefloxacin. Proc 15th Int Congr Chemother, Istanbul, 1987, 997–9.
2. Sultan E, Richard C, Pezzano M, Auzepy P, Singlas E. Pharmacokinetics of pefloxacin and amikacin administered simultaneously to intensive care patients. *Eur J Clin Pharmacol* (1988) 34, 637–43.
3. Nix DE, Wilton JH, Hyatt J, Thomas J, Strenkoski-Nix LC, Forrest A, Schentag JJ. Pharmacodynamic modeling of the in vivo interaction between cefotaxime and ofloxacin by using serum ultrafiltrate inhibitory titers. *Antimicrob Agents Chemother* (1997) 41, 1108–14.
4. Deppermann K-M, Boeckh M, Grineisen S, Shokry F, Borner K, Koeppe P, Krasemann C, Wagner J, Lode H. Brief report: combination effects of ciprofloxacin, clindamycin, and metronidazole intravenously in volunteers. *Am J Med* (1989) 87 (Suppl 5A), 46S–48S.
5. Weinstein MP, Deeter RG, Swanson KA, Gross JS. Crossover assessment of serum bactericidal activity and pharmacokinetics of ciprofloxacin alone and in combination in healthy elderly volunteers. *Antimicrob Agents Chemother* (1991) 35, 2352–8.
6. Foulds G, Cohen MJ, Geffken A, Willavize S, Hunt T. Coadministration of azithromycin 1-g packet does not affect the bioavailability of trovafloxacin. *Intersci Conf Antimicrob Agents Chemother* (1998) 38, 31.
7. Boeckh M, Grineisen S, Shokry F, Koeppe P, Borner K, Krasemann C, Lode H. Pharmacokinetics and serum bactericidal activity (SBA) of ciprofloxacin (CIP) and ofloxacin (OFL) alone and in combination with metronidazole (METRO) or clindamycin (CLINDA). *Intersci Conf Antimicrob Agents Chemother* (1988) 28, 246.
8. Ludwig E, Graber H, Székely É, Csiba A. Metabolic interactions of ciprofloxacin. *Diagn Microbiol Infect Dis* (1990) 13, 135–41.
9. Stille W, Ostner KH. Antagonismus Nitrofurantoin-Nalidixinsaure. *Klin Wochenschr* (1966) 44, 155–6.
10. Piguet JD. L'action inhibitrice de la nitrofurantoïne sur le pouvoir bactériostatique *in vitro* de l'acide nalidixique. *Ann Inst Pasteur (Paris)* (1969) 116, 43–8.
11. NegGram (Nalidixic acid). Sanofi-Synthelabo Inc. US Prescribing information, April 2007.
12. Macrobid (Nitrofurantoin monohydrate/macrocrystals). Proctor & Gamble Pharmaceuticals, US Prescribing information, January 2009.
13. Macrodantin (Nitrofurantoin macrocrystals). Proctor & Gamble Pharmaceuticals, US Prescribing information, January 2009.
14. Barriere SL, Catlin DH, Orlando PL, Noe A, Frost RW. Alteration in the pharmacokinetic disposition of ciprofloxacin by simultaneous administration of azlocillin. *Antimicrob Agents Chemother* (1990) 34, 823–6.
15. Paintaud G, Alván G, Hellgren U, Nilsson-Ehle I. Lack of effect of amoxycillin on the absorption of ofloxacin. *Eur J Clin Pharmacol* (1993) 44, 207–9.
16. Strenkoski-Nix LC, Forrest A, Schentag JJ, Nix DE. Pharmacodynamic interactions of ciprofloxacin, piperacillin, and piperacillin/tazobactam in healthy volunteers. *J Clin Pharmacol* (1998) 38, 1063–71.
17. Orisakwe OE, Agbasi PU, Afonne OJ, Ofoefule SI, Obi E, Orish CN. Rifampicin pharmacokinetics with and without ciprofloxacin. *Am J Ther* (2001) 8, 151–3.
18. Orisakwe OE, Afonne OJ, Agbasi PU, Ofoefule SI. Urinary excretion of rifampicin in the presence of ciprofloxacin. *Am J Ther* (2004) 11, 171–4.
19. Chandler MHH, Toler SM, Rapp RP, Muder RR, Korvick JA. Multiple-dose pharmacokinetics of concurrent oral ciprofloxacin and rifampin therapy in elderly patients. *Antimicrob Agents Chemother* (1990) 34, 442–7.
20. Polk RE. Drug-drug interactions with ciprofloxacin and other fluoroquinolones. *Am J Med* (1989) 87 (Suppl 5A), 76S–81S.
21. Jhaj R, Roy A, Uppal R, Behera D. Influence of ciprofloxacin on pharmacokinetics of rifampin. *Curr Ther Res* (1997) 58, 260–5.
22. Schrenzel J, Dayer P, Leemann T, Weidekamm E, Portmann R, Lew DP. Influence of rifampin on fleroxacin pharmacokinetics. *Antimicrob Agents Chemother* (1993) 37, 2132–8.
23. McIlleron H, Norman J, Kanyok TP, Fourie PB, Horton J, Smith PJ. Elevated gatifloxacin and reduced rifampicin concentrations in a single-dose interaction study amongst healthy volunteers. *J Antimicrob Chemother* (2007) 60, 1398–1401.
24. Nijland HMJ, Ruslami R, Juwono Suroto A, Burger DM, Alisjahbana B, van Crevel R, Aarnoutse RE. Rifampicin reduces plasma concentrations of moxifloxacin in patients with tuberculosis. *Clin Infect Dis* (2007) 45, 1001–7.
25. Weiner M, Burman W, Luo C-C, Peloquin CA, Engle M, Goldberg S, Agarwal V, Vernon A. Effects of rifampin and multidrug resistance gene polymorphism on concentrations of moxifloxacin. *Antimicrob Agents Chemother* (2007) 51, 2861–6.
26. Humbert G, Brumpt I, Montay G, Le Liboux A, Frydman A, Borsa-Lebas F, Moore N. Influence of rifampin on the pharmacokinetics of pefloxacin. *Clin Pharmacol Ther* (1991) 50, 682–7.
27. Orisakwe OE, Akunyili DN, Agbasi PU, Ezejiofor NA. Some plasma and saliva pharmacokinetic parameters of rifampicin in the presence of pefloxacin. *Am J Ther* (2004) 11, 283–7.
28. Orisakwe OE, Agbasi PU, Ofoefule SI, Ilondu NA, Afonne OJ, Anusiem CA, Ilo CE, Maduka SO. Effect of pefloxacin on the urinary excretion of rifampicin. *Am J Ther* (2004) 11, 13–16.

Quinolones + Phosphate binders

The bioavailability of ciprofloxacin is markedly reduced by lanthanum. Other quinolones are likely to interact similarly. Sevelamer reduced the bioavailability of ciprofloxacin by 48% in one study.

Clinical evidence, mechanism, importance and management

(a) Lanthanum

In a randomised, crossover study, 12 healthy subjects received a single 750-mg dose of oral **ciprofloxacin** alone, or on the second day of a 2-day course of lanthanum 1 g three times daily. Lanthanum reduced the AUC and maximum plasma levels of **ciprofloxacin** by 54% and 56%, respectively.[1] It seems likely that **ciprofloxacin** forms an insoluble chelate with lanthanum within the gut, which reduces its absorption. Such a reduction in bioavailability may lead to subtherapeutic levels and hence reduced efficacy. It is therefore recommended that quinolones are not taken for 2 hours before or 4 hours after lanthanum.[2]

(b) Sevelamer

In a crossover study in 15 healthy subjects, the AUC of **ciprofloxacin** was reduced by 39% and its relative oral bioavailability was reduced by 48% when a single 750-mg dose of **ciprofloxacin** was taken with sevelamer 2.8 g. The reduction was variable.[3] The mechanism of the interaction is unknown. Based on the results of this study, sevelamer should not be given at the same time as **ciprofloxacin** because the efficacy of **ciprofloxacin** might be reduced in some patients. Note that the manufacturers of sevelamer suggest that, when giving any other oral drug for which a reduction in the bioavailability could have a clinically significant effect on safety or efficacy, the drug should be given at least one hour before or 3 hours after sevelamer.[4,5] Until more is known it would seem prudent to apply this advice to all quinolones.

1. How PP, Fischer JH, Arruda JA, Lau AH. Effects of lanthanum carbonate on the absorption and oral bioavailability of ciprofloxacin. *Clin J Am Soc Nephrol* (2007) 2, 1235–40.
2. Fosrenol (Lanthanum carbonate hydrate). Shire Pharmaceuticals Ltd. UK Summary of product characteristics, March 2013.
3. Kays MB, Overholser BR, Mueller BA, Moe SM, Sowinski KM. Effects of sevelamer hydrochloride and calcium acetate on the oral bioavailability of ciprofloxacin. *Am J Kidney Dis* (2003) 42, 1253–9.
4. Renagel (Sevelamer hydrochloride). Sanofi. UK Summary of product characteristics, February 2015.
5. Renvela (Sevelamer carbonate). Genzyme. US Prescribing information, May 2011.

Quinolones + Pirenzepine

In 10 healthy subjects, four doses of pirenzepine 50 mg delayed the absorption of ciprofloxacin and ofloxacin, but their bioavailabilities remained unchanged.[1] The delayed absorption is unlikely to be of clinical significance.

1. Höffken G, Lode H, Wiley R, Glatzel TD, Sievers D, Olschewski T, Borner K, Koeppe T. Pharmacokinetics and bioavailability of ciprofloxacin and ofloxacin: effect of food and antacid intake. *Rev Infect Dis* (1988) 10 (Suppl 1), S138–S139.

Quinolones + Probenecid

Probenecid increases the serum concentrations and/or decreases the urinary excretion of cinoxacin, ciprofloxacin, clinafloxacin, enoxacin, fleroxacin, gatifloxacin, gemifloxacin, levofloxacin, nalidixic acid and norfloxacin. Moxifloxacin, sparfloxacin, and probably ofloxacin, do not appear to interact with probenecid.

Clinical evidence

(a) Cinoxacin

A study in 6 healthy subjects found that probenecid 500 mg three times daily roughly doubled the serum concentration of a 3-hour intravenous infusion of cinoxacin. The renal clearance of cinoxacin was also reduced from 68% to 46%, both during and for the 4 hours after the infusion.[1]

(b) Ciprofloxacin

In one study, probenecid 1 g, given 30 minutes before ciprofloxacin 500 mg, was found to reduce the renal clearance of ciprofloxacin by up to 50%. Other pharmacokinetic parameters (maximum serum concentration, AUC) were unchanged and no accumulation of ciprofloxacin appeared to occur, probably due to an increase in extra-renal elimination.[2]

Another study found that the renal clearance of ciprofloxacin was reduced by 64% by probenecid. However, in contrast to the other study cited, the AUC of ciprofloxacin was increased by 74% and the AUC of its 2-aminoethylamino metabolite was increased by 234%. As a consequence, the concentration of ciprofloxacin in tears, sweat and saliva was also increased, but probenecid had no direct effect on ciprofloxacin distribution into these fluids.[3]

(c) Clinafloxacin

Probenecid 1 g, given one hour before a single 400-mg dose of clinafloxacin, reduced the total clearance and renal clearance of clinafloxacin by 24% and 36%, respectively, increased its AUC by 32%, and increased its elimination half-life from 6.3 hours to 7 hours.[4]

(d) Enoxacin

In one subject, the renal clearance of enoxacin 600 mg was approximately halved, and the half-life increased from 3.5 hours to 4.5 hours by a single 2.5-g dose of probenecid.[5]

(e) Fleroxacin

A study in 6 healthy subjects given a single 200-mg dose of fleroxacin, followed by 500 mg of probenecid 30 minutes, 12 hours, 24 hours and 36 hours later, found that the AUC of fleroxacin was increased by 37% and its urinary excretion was decreased by 22%.[6] Another study found that probenecid increased the AUC of fleroxacin 400 mg by 26% (not statistically significant), and had no effect on fleroxacin urinary excretion.[7]

(f) Gatifloxacin

A study in 6 healthy subjects found that probenecid 500 mg given one hour before and 12 and 24 hours after a single 200-mg oral dose of gatifloxacin increased the AUC of gatifloxacin by 42%, decreased its renal clearance by 38% and increased its elimination half-life from 7.1 hours to 10.2 hours.[8]

(g) Gemifloxacin

In a crossover study, 17 healthy subjects were given probenecid 4.5 g in divided doses over a 70-hour period with a single 320-mg dose of gemifloxacin given 10 hours after probenecid was started. Probenecid decreased the median total clearance and median renal clearance of gemifloxacin by 31% and 51%, respectively, and its elimination half-life was increased from 8.9 hours to 9.5 hours.[9]

(h) Levofloxacin

A study in 12 healthy subjects found that although probenecid reduced the renal clearance of a single 500-mg oral dose of levofloxacin by about one-third, and increased its AUC and half-life by similar amounts, the 72-hour urinary excretion of levofloxacin was unaltered.[10]

(i) Moxifloxacin

A study in 12 healthy subjects found that probenecid had no clinically significant effect on the pharmacokinetics of a single 400-mg dose of moxifloxacin.[11]

(j) Nalidixic acid

Two subjects, acting as their own controls, took nalidixic acid 500 mg with and without probenecid 500 mg. The maximum serum concentration of nalidixic acid were unaffected at 2 hours, but at 8 hours the concentration was increased 3-fold by probenecid.[12]

Another study, in 5 women with urinary tract infections treated with nalidixic acid, found that probenecid increased the maximum serum concentration and AUC of nalidixic acid by 43% and 74%, respectively.[13]

(k) Norfloxacin

In 5 subjects the mean 12-hour urinary recovery of norfloxacin 200 mg was reduced by about half when they were given probenecid 1 g. Norfloxacin serum concentrations were unaffected.[14]

(l) Ofloxacin

A study in 8 healthy subjects found that probenecid 500 mg increased the AUC of a single 200-mg dose of ofloxacin by 16% and decreased its total body clearance by 14%. Other pharmacokinetic parameters were not affected.[15]

(m) Sparfloxacin

In 6 healthy subjects, probenecid 1.5 g did not affect the clearance, the AUC or the half-life of sparfloxacin 200 mg to a statistically significant extent.[16]

Mechanism

The likely explanation for this interaction is that probenecid successfully competes with some quinolones for tubular excretion, so that their renal elimination is reduced. Some quinolones are more dependent on glomerular filtration than tubular excretion for elimination, and thus are unaffected by competition for tubular excretion.[7]

Importance and management

The interactions between the quinolones and probenecid are established, but their clinical importance seems not to have been assessed. The increased concentration and decreased renal excretion of clinafloxacin caused by probenecid are not considered large enough to warrant dose adjustment,[4] and most of the changes seen with the other quinolones were of a similar or lesser magnitude. However, caution has been advised if probenecid is given with a quinolone to patients with impaired renal function, or in the presence of other drugs that might also compete for renal excretion (such as some penicillins or cephalosporins).[3,4] Moxifloxacin and sparfloxacin appear not to interact, and so could be useful alternatives in some situations.

1. Rodriguez N, Madsen PO, Welling PG. Influence of probenecid on serum levels and urinary excretion of cinoxacin. *Antimicrob Agents Chemother* (1979) 15, 465–69.
2. Wingender W, Beerman D, Förster D, Graefe K-H, Kuhlmann J. Interactions of ciprofloxacin with food intake and drugs. *Curr Clin Pract Ser* (1986) 34, 136–40.
3. Jaehde U, Sörgel F, Reiter A, Sigl G, Naber KG, Schunack W. Effect of probenecid on the distribution and elimination of ciprofloxacin in humans. *Clin Pharmacol Ther* (1995) 58, 532–41.
4. Randinitis EJ, Koup JR, Bron NJ, Hounslow NJ, Rausch G, Abel R, Vassos AB, Sedman AJ. Drug interaction studies with clinafloxacin and probenecid, cimetidine, phenytoin and warfarin. *Drugs* (1999) 58 (Suppl 2), 254–5.
5. Wijnands WJA, Vree TB, Baars AM, van Herwaarden CLA. Pharmacokinetics of enoxacin and its penetration into bronchial secretions and lung tissue. *J Antimicrob Chemother* (1988) 21 (Suppl B), 67–77.
6. Shiba K, Saito A, Shimada J, Hori S, Kaji M, Miyahara T, Kusajima H, Kaneko S, Saito S, Uchida H. Interactions of fleroxacin with dried aluminium hydroxide gel and probenecid. *Rev Infect Dis* (1989) 11 (Suppl 5), S1097–S1098.
7. Weidekamm E, Portmann R, Suter K, Partos C, Dell D, Lücker PW. Single- and multiple dose pharmacokinetics of fleroxacin, a trifluorinated quinolone, in humans. *Antimicrob Agents Chemother* (1987) 31, 1909–14.
8. Nakashima M, Uematsu T, Kosuge K, Kusajima H, Ooie T, Masuda Y, Ishida R, Uchida H. Single- and multiple-dose pharmacokinetics of AM-1155, a new 6-fluoro-8-methoxy quinolone, in humans. *Antimicrob Agents Chemother* (1995) 39, 2635–40.
9. Landersdorfer CB, Kirkpatrick CMJ, Kinzig M, Bulitta JB, Holzgrabe U, Drusano GL, Sörgel F. Competitive inhibition of renal tubular secretion of gemifloxacin by probenecid. *Antimicrob Agents Chemother* (2009) 53, 3902–7.
10. Gaitonde MD, Mendes P, House ESA, Lehr KH. The effects of cimetidine and probenecid on the pharmacokinetics of levofloxacin (LVFX). *Intersci Conf Antimicrob Agents Chemother* (1995) 35, 8.
11. Stass H, Sachse R. Effect of probenecid on the kinetics of a single oral 400-mg dose of moxifloxacin in healthy male volunteers. *Clin Pharmacokinet* (2001) 40 (Suppl 1), 71–76.
12. Dash H, Mills J. Severe metabolic acidosis associated with nalidixic acid overdose. *Ann Intern Med* (1976) 84, 570–1.
13. Ferry N, Cuisinaud G, Pozet N, Zech PY, Sassard J. Influence du probénécide sur la pharmacocinétique de l'acide nalidixique. *Therapie* (1982) 37, 645–9.
14. Shimada J, Yamaji T, Ueda Y, Uchida H, Kusajima H, Irikura T. Mechanism of renal excretion of AM-715, a new quinolonecarboxylic acid derivative, in rabbits, dogs, and humans. *Antimicrob Agents Chemother* (1983) 23, 1–7.
15. Nataraj B, Rao Mamidi NVS, Krishna DR. Probenecid affects the pharmacokinetics of ofloxacin in healthy volunteers. *Clin Drug Invest* (1998) 16, 259–62.
16. Shimada J, Saito A, Shiba K, Hojo T, Kaji M, Hori S, Yoshida M, Sakai O. Pharmacokinetics and clinical studies of sparfloxacin. *Chemotherapy (Tokyo)* (1991) 39 (Suppl 4), 234–44.

Quinolones + Sucralfate

Sucralfate causes a marked reduction in the absorption of ciprofloxacin, enoxacin, gemifloxacin, lomefloxacin, moxifloxacin, ofloxacin, norfloxacin and sparfloxacin, but causes only a modest reduction in fleroxacin levels.

Clinical evidence

(a) Ciprofloxacin

In a study in 8 healthy subjects sucralfate 1 g four times daily reduced the AUC and maximum serum concentration of ciprofloxacin 500 mg by 88% and 90%, respectively.[1] A study in 12 healthy subjects found that a 1-g dose of sucralfate given 6 hours and 2 hours before a single 750-mg dose of ciprofloxacin, reduced the ciprofloxacin AUC by about 30%. In 3 subjects there were little or no changes in the AUC of ciprofloxacin but a decrease of more than 50% was seen in 4 others.[2] A related study in 12 healthy subjects found that the bioavailability of ciprofloxacin 750 mg was reduced by 7%, 20%, and 95%, respectively, when sucralfate was given 6 hours before, 2 hours before, or at the same time as, the ciprofloxacin.[3]

A patient given sucralfate 1 g four times daily had serum ciprofloxacin levels that were 85 to 90% lower than 5 other patients who were not taking sucralfate.[4] A single dose study found a 96% reduction in the AUC of ciprofloxacin following a 2-g dose of sucralfate.[5] Oral sucralfate does not alter the effects of ciprofloxacin on aerobic bacteria in the gut.[6]

(b) Enoxacin

In 8 healthy subjects when sucralfate 1 g was given 2 hours before or with enoxacin 400 mg the bioavailability of the enoxacin was reduced by 54% and 88%, respectively,. When sucralfate was given 2 hours after enoxacin its bioavailability was not affected.[7]

(c) Fleroxacin

In 20 healthy subjects, sucralfate 1 g every 6 hours reduced the bioavailability of fleroxacin 400 mg by 24%.[8]

(d) Gemifloxacin

In a study in 27 healthy subjects, gemifloxacin 320 mg was given either 3 hours before or 2 hours after sucralfate 2 g. The pharmacokinetics of gemifloxacin were not significantly altered when sucralfate was given after the gemifloxacin, probably due to its rapid absorption. However, when sucralfate was given 3 hours before gemifloxacin, its AUC and maximum plasma levels were decreased by 53% and 69%, respectively.[9]

(e) Levofloxacin

The pharmacokinetics of levofloxacin are unaffected by sucralfate taken 2 hours after the quinolone.[10]

(f) Lomefloxacin

A study in 12 subjects found that when lomefloxacin 400 mg was given 2 hours after sucralfate 1 g the lomefloxacin AUC and maximum serum concentration were reduced by about 25% and 30%, respectively.[11] Another study in 8 healthy subjects found that when lomefloxacin 400 mg was given with sucralfate 1 g, the lomefloxacin AUC was reduced by 51%.[12]

(g) Moxifloxacin

In 12 healthy subjects, a total of five doses of sucralfate 1 g, given at the same time as a single 400-mg dose of moxifloxacin and then 5, 10, 15, and 24 hours after the dose, reduced the AUC and maximum serum concentration of moxifloxacin by 40% and 29%, respectively.[13]

(h) Norfloxacin

A study in 8 healthy subjects found that sucralfate 1 g four times daily reduced the AUC of a single 400-mg dose of norfloxacin by 98%, when taken with the sucralfate, and by 42% when taken 2 hours after the sucralfate.[14] Another study found a reduction of 91% in the AUC of norfloxacin 400 mg when it was taken with sucralfate 1 g, but no reduction when norfloxacin was taken 2 hours before sucralfate.[15]

(i) Ofloxacin

A single-dose study found that sucralfate (dose not stated) reduced the maximum serum levels and AUC of a single 200-mg dose of ofloxacin by about two-thirds.[16] Another study found a reduction in the maximum serum levels and the AUC of ofloxacin of 70% and 61%, respectively, when ofloxacin 400 mg was taken with sucralfate 1 g, but no reduction when the ofloxacin was taken 2 hours before sucralfate.[15] Food reduced the extent of the interaction but it was still marked.[17]

(j) Sparfloxacin

In a study in 15 healthy subjects, sucralfate 1 g four times daily reduced the maximum serum levels, the AUC and the relative bioavailability of sparfloxacin 400 mg daily by 39%, 47%, and 44%, respectively.[18] In a study assessing staggered dosing of sucralfate 1.5 g on the pharmacokinetics of sparfloxacin 300 mg, the AUC of sparfloxacin was unaffected when sucralfate was given 4 hours after the quinolone, but was decreased by 34% when sucralfate was given 2 hours after the quinolone, and by 51% when sucralfate was given at the same time as the quinolone.[19]

Mechanism

The aluminium hydroxide component of sucralfate (about 200 mg in each gram) forms an insoluble chelate between the cation and the 4-keto and 3-carboxyl groups of the quinolone, which reduces its absorption. See 'Quinolones + Antacids or Calcium compounds', p.343, for more on this mechanism.

Importance and management

Established and clinically important interactions. Because it seems probable that serum ciprofloxacin, enoxacin, gemifloxacin, levofloxacin, lomefloxacin, moxifloxacin, ofloxacin, norfloxacin and sparfloxacin levels will be reduced to subtherapeutic concentrations if given with sucralfate, separate the doses as much as possible (by 2 hours or more), giving the quinolone first. The manufacturer of ciprofloxacin advises that it should be given one to 2 hours before, or 4 hours after, sucralfate.[20] The study with moxifloxacin suggested that sucralfate should not be given for 2 hours before or 4 hours after the quinolone, but more study is needed to confirm both these findings and the effectiveness of separating the doses; however, the UK manufacturer of moxifloxacin advises separating administration by 6 hours,[21] whereas the US manufacturer of moxifloxacin recommends that it is taken at least 4 hours before or 8 hours after sucralfate.[22] The interaction with fleroxacin is only modest (bioavailability reduced by 24%) and probably not clinically important, but some separation of the doses may reduce the interaction further. This needs confirmation. **Pefloxacin** interacts with antacids containing aluminium hydroxide (see 'Quinolones + Antacids or Calcium compounds', p.343) and is therefore likely to interact with sucralfate.

The H_2-receptor antagonists and (see 'Quinolones + H_2-receptor antagonists', p.349, and 'Quinolones + Omeprazole', p.351, respectively) do not interact with the quinolones and may therefore be alternatives to sucralfate in some situations.

1. Garrelts JC, Godley PJ, Peterie JD, Gerlach EH, Yakshe CC. Sucralfate significantly reduces ciprofloxacin concentrations in serum. *Antimicrob Agents Chemother* (1990) 34, 931–3.
2. Nix DE, Watson WA, Handy L, Frost RW, Rescott DL, Goldstein HR. The effect of sucralfate pretreatment on the pharmacokinetics of ciprofloxacin. *Pharmacotherapy* (1989) 9, 377–80.
3. Van Slooten AD, Nix DE, Wilton JH, Love JH, Spivey JM, Goldstein HR. Combined use of ciprofloxacin and sucralfate. *DICP Ann Pharmacother* (1991) 25, 578–82.
4. Yuk JH, Nightingale CN, Quintiliani R. Ciprofloxacin levels when receiving sucralfate. *JAMA* (1989) 262, 901.
5. Brouwers JRBJ, Van Der Kam HJ, Sijtsma J, Proost JH. Important reduction of ciprofloxacin absorption by sucralfate and magnesium citrate solution. *Drug Invest* (1990) 2, 197–9.
6. Krueger WA, Ruckdeschel G, Unertl K. Influence of intravenously administered ciprofloxacin on aerobic intestinal microflora and fecal drug levels when administered simultaneously with sucralfate. *Antimicrob Agents Chemother* (1997) 41, 1725–30.
7. Ryerson B, Toothaker R, Schleyer I, Sedman A, Colburn W. Effect of sucralfate on enoxacin pharmacokinetics. *Intersci Conf Antimicrob Agents Chemother* (1989) 29, 136.
8. Lubowski TJ, Nightingale CH, Sweeney K, Quintiliani R. Effect of sucralfate on pharmacokinetics of fleroxacin in healthy volunteers. *Antimicrob Agents Chemother* (1992) 36, 2758–60.
9. Allen A, Bygate E, Faessel H, Isaac L, Lewis A. The effect of ferrous sulphate and sucralfate on the bioavailability of oral gemifloxacin in healthy volunteers. *Int J Antimicrob Agents* (2000) 15, 283–9.
10. Lee L-J, Hafkin B, Lee I-D, Hoh J, Dix R. Effect of food and sucralfate on a single oral dose of 500 milligrams of levofloxacin in healthy subjects. *Antimicrob Agents Chemother* (1997) 41, 2196–2200.
11. Nix D, Schentag J. Lomefloxacin (L) absorption kinetics when administered with ranitidine (R) and sucralfate (S). *Intersci Conf Antimicrob Agents Chemother* (1989) 29, 317.
12. Lehto P, Kivistö KT. Different effects of products containing metal ions on the absorption of lomefloxacin. *Clin Pharmacol Ther* (1994) 56, 477–82.
13. Stass H, Schühly U, Möller J-G, Delesen H. Effects of sucralfate on the oral bioavailability of moxifloxacin, a novel 8-methoxyfluoroquinolone, in healthy volunteers. *Clin Pharmacokinet* (2001) 40 (Suppl 1), 49–55.
14. Parpia SH, Nix DE, Hejmanowski LG, Goldstein HR, Witton JH, Schentag JJ. Sucralfate reduces the gastrointestinal absorption of norfloxacin. *Antimicrob Agents Chemother* (1989) 33, 99–102.
15. Lehto P, Kivistö KT. Effect of sucralfate on absorption of norfloxacin and ofloxacin. *Antimicrob Agents Chemother* (1994) 38, 248–51.
16. Shiba K, Yoshida M, Kachi M, Shimada J, Saito A, Sakai N. Effects of peptic ulcer-healing drugs on the pharmacokinetics of new quinolone (OFLX). 17th Int Congr Chemother, June 1991, Berlin, Abstract 415.
17. Kawakami J, Matsuse T, Kotaki H, Seino T, Fukuchi Y, Orimo H, Sawada Y, Iga T. The effect of food on the interaction of ofloxacin with sucralfate in healthy volunteers. *Eur J Clin Pharmacol* (1994) 47, 67–9.
18. Zix JA, Geerdes-Fenge HF, Rau M, Vöckler J, Borner K, Koeppe P, Lode H. Pharmacokinetics of sparfloxacin and interaction with cisapride and sucralfate. *Antimicrob Agents Chemother* (1997) 41, 1668–1672.
19. Kamberi M, Nakashima H, Ogawa K, Oda N, Nakano S. The effect of staggered dosing of sucralfate on oral bioavailability of sparfloxacin. *Br J Clin Pharmacol* (2000) 49, 98–103.
20. Ciproxin Tablets (Ciprofloxacin hydrochloride). Bayer plc. UK Summary of product characteristics, November 2008.
21. Avelox (Moxifloxacin hydrochloride). Bayer plc. UK Summary of product characteristics, May 2012.
22. Avelox (Moxifloxacin hydrochloride). Bayer HealthCare Pharmaceuticals. US Prescribing information, December 2008.

Quinolones; Ciprofloxacin + Chloroquine

Chloroquine may modestly reduce ciprofloxacin levels.

Clinical evidence, mechanism, importance and management

A study in 5 healthy subjects who were given a single 500-mg dose of ciprofloxacin alone, or with a single 600-mg dose of chloroquine found that the maximum plasma level of ciprofloxacin was reduced by 18% by chloroquine, and was below the minimum inhibitory concentration for *Plasmodium falciparum*.[1] The same or a very similar study is reported elsewhere.[2] The authors of these reports suggest that the reduction in ciprofloxacin bioavailability may have implications for the management of infections resistant to chloroquine. More study is needed to establish the clinical relevance of this small decrease in ciprofloxacin levels.

For details of a possible interaction between a NSAID and ciprofloxacin in a patient also taking chloroquine, see 'Quinolones + NSAIDs', p.350.

1. Ilo EC, Orisakwe OE, Ilondu NA, Okwoli N, Brown SA, Elo-Ilo J, Agbasi PU. Effect of chloroquine on the bioavailability of ciprofloxacin in man. J Control Release. (2006) 116, e109–10.
2. Ilo CE, Ezejiofor NA, Agbakoba N, Brown SA, Maduagwuna CA, Agbasi PU, Orisakwe OE. Effect of chloroquine on the urinary excretion of ciprofloxacin. *Am J Ther* (2008) 15, 419–22.

Quinolones; Ciprofloxacin + Pancreatic enzymes

The pharmacokinetics of ciprofloxacin are not affected by pancreatic enzyme supplements.

Clinical evidence, mechanism, importance and management

Six patients with cystic fibrosis, chronically infected with *Pseudomonas aeruginosa* and who had received a range of drugs including ceftazidime, tobramycin, ticarcillin and salbutamol, demonstrated no significant changes in the pharmacokinetics of a single 250-mg dose of ciprofloxacin when it was given with standard doses of pancreatic enzymes (seven *Pancrease* capsules).[1] Another study in 12 patients with cystic fibrosis found that giving pancreatic enzyme supplements 30 minutes before a single 750-mg dose of ciprofloxacin did not alter the pharmacokinetics of ciprofloxacin.[2] No special precautions would seem to be necessary during concurrent use.

1. Mack G, Cooper PJ, Buchanan N. Effects of enzyme supplementation on oral absorption of ciprofloxacin in patients with cystic fibrosis. *Antimicrob Agents Chemother* (1991) 35, 1484–5.
2. Reed MD, Stern RC, Myers CM, Yamashita TS, Blumer JL. Lack of unique pharmacokinetic characteristics in patients with cystic fibrosis. *J Clin Pharmacol* (1988) 28, 691–9.

Quinolones; Ciprofloxacin + Phenazopyridine

Phenazopyridine appears to increase the bioavailability of ciprofloxacin.

Clinical evidence, mechanism, importance and management

A study in 23 healthy subjects given a single 500-mg dose of ciprofloxacin either alone or with phenazopyridine 200 mg found that phenazopyridine increased the AUC and mean residence time of ciprofloxacin by about 30%. The time to achieve maximum plasma levels was increased from 1 hours to 1.5 hours.[1] If anything, this seems likely to be a beneficial, rather than adverse, interaction.

1. Marcelín-Jiménez G, Ángeles AP, Martínez-Rossier L, Fernández A. Ciprofloxacin bioavailability is enhanced by oral co-administration with phenazopyridine: a pharmacokinetic study in a Mexican population. *Clin Drug Invest* (2006) 26, 323–8.

Quinolones; Ciprofloxacin + Ursodeoxycholic acid (Ursodiol)

An isolated report describes a reduction in serum ciprofloxacin levels in a patient taking ursodeoxycholic acid.

Clinical evidence, mechanism, importance and management

A man with metastatic colon cancer had unusually low serum levels of ciprofloxacin following oral dosing; his only other medication was ursodeoxycholic acid 300 mg twice daily for gallstones. Despite the low antibacterial serum levels the bacteraemia cleared. Several months later, when he was readmitted to hospital, both drugs were again given, initially staggered, and then later together. When taken together the AUC of ciprofloxacin was reduced by 50% by ursodeoxycholic acid.[1] The reason for this interaction is not understood.

This seems to be the first and only report of an interaction between a quinolone and ursodeoxycholic acid and its importance is uncertain. More study is needed to establish this interaction, its importance, and its mechanism.

1. Belliveau PP, Nightingale CH, Quintiliani R, Maderazo EG. Reduction in serum concentrations of ciprofloxacin after administration of ursodiol to a patient with hepatobiliary disease. *Clin Infect Dis* (1994) 19, 354–5.

Quinolones; Levofloxacin + Antiretrovirals

There appears to be no clinically important pharmacokinetic interaction between levofloxacin and efavirenz, nelfinavir or zidovudine.

Clinical evidence, mechanism, importance and management

A study in HIV-positive patients who were taking zidovudine and lamivudine with either **efavirenz** or **nelfinavir**, found that levofloxacin 500 mg daily for 4 days did not affect the steady-state pharmacokinetics of either **efavirenz** 600 mg daily or **nelfinavir** 750 mg three times daily. The pharmacokinetics of levofloxacin during the concurrent use of **efavirenz** or **nelfinavir** were unaffected, except for the time to reach maximum levels, which was increased from a range of 0.9 to 1.7 hours in control subjects, to 3.3 hours with **efavirenz**. This may have occurred as a result of delayed gastric emptying caused by the **efavirenz**. A clinically important interaction between levofloxacin and either **efavirenz** or **nelfinavir** is unlikely.[1]

A double-blind study in 16 HIV-positive patients taking **zidovudine** with levofloxacin 350 mg every 8 hours or placebo, did not find any changes in the pharmacokinetics of either drug.[2] No dose adjustments would therefore be expected to be necessary if both drugs are given.

1. Villani P, Viale P, Signorini L, Cadeo B, Marchetti F, Villani A, Fiocchi C, Regazzi MB, Carosi G. Pharmacokinetic evaluation of oral levofloxacin in human immunodeficiency virus-infected subjects receiving concomitant antiretroviral therapy. *Antimicrob Agents Chemother* (2001) 45, 2160–2.
2. Chien SC, Chow AT, Rogge MC, Williams RR, Hendrix CW. Pharmacokinetics and safety of oral levofloxacin in human immunodeficiency virus-infected individuals receiving concomitant zidovudine. *Antimicrob Agents Chemother* (1997) 41, 1765–9.

Quinolones; Lomefloxacin + Furosemide

Furosemide causes a small rise in the serum levels of lomefloxacin. The pharmacokinetics and diuretic effects of furosemide are not changed by lomefloxacin.

Clinical evidence, mechanism, importance and management

A study in 8 healthy subjects found that when a single 200-mg dose of lomefloxacin was taken with furosemide 40 mg, the AUC of lomefloxacin was increased by 12%. The maximum serum levels and the half-life of lomefloxacin were also increased, but not to a statistically significant extent.[1] The suggested reason for the interaction is that there is some competition between the two drugs for excretion by the renal tubules. No significant changes were seen in the pharmacokinetics of furosemide nor in its diuretic effects.[1] The small rise in the serum levels of lomefloxacin is almost certainly too small to be important and there would seem to be no reason for avoiding concurrent use. Information about other quinolone antibacterials appears to be lacking.

1. Sudoh T, Fujimura A, Shiga T, Sasaki M, Harada K, Tateishi T, Ohashi K, Ebihara A. Renal clearance of lomefloxacin is decreased by furosemide. *Eur J Clin Pharmacol* (1994) 46, 267–9.

Quinolones; Moxifloxacin + Itraconazole

A study in healthy subjects found that itraconazole 200 mg daily for 9 days did not affect the pharmacokinetics of a single 200-mg dose of moxifloxacin given on day 7. No clinically relevant changes were found in the pharmacokinetics of itraconazole.[1] No dose adjustments would seem to be necessary during concurrent use.

1. Stass H, Nagelschmitz J, Moeller J-G, Delesen. Pharmacokinetics of moxifloxacin are not influenced by a 7-day pre-treatment with 200 mg oral itraconazole given once a day in healthy subjects. *Int J Clin Pharmacol Ther* (2004) 42, 23–9.

Quinolones; Ofloxacin + Cetraxate

A single-dose study found that cetraxate (dose not stated) did not affect the pharmacokinetics of a single 200-mg dose of ofloxacin.[1] No dose adjustments would seem to be necessary on concurrent use.

1. Shiba K, Yoshida M, Kachi M, Shimada J, Saito A, Sakai N. Effects of peptic ulcer-healing drugs on the pharmacokinetics of new quinolone (OFLX). 17th Int Congr Chemother, June 1991, Berlin, Abstract 415.

Quinupristin with Dalfopristin + Miscellaneous

Quinupristin with dalfopristin modestly increases the levels of intravenous midazolam, a substrate for CYP3A4. The manufacturers therefore predict that quinupristin with dalfopristin will raise the levels of a number of other CYP3A4 substrates.

Clinical evidence, mechanism, importance and management

The manufacturers report a study in which quinupristin with dalfopristin raised the levels of an intravenous bolus dose of midazolam by 33 to 38%.[1,2] These effects are relatively modest, but oral doses of midazolam may be increased to a greater extent. Be alert for increased and/or prolonged sedation when both drugs are given. This study also suggests that quinupristin with dalfopristin is a moderate inhibitor of the cytochrome P450 isoenzyme CYP3A4, and this is supported by other studies in which the levels of CYP3A4 substrates were raised by quinupristin with dalfopristin (consider also 'Calcium-channel blockers + Quinupristin with Dalfopristin', p.1044). The manufacturers therefore predict that quinupristin with dalfopristin will raise the levels of other drugs metabolised by CYP3A4, including some antiarrhythmics (**disopyramide, lidocaine, quinidine**), antiretrovirals (such as **delavirdine, indinavir, nevirapine, ritonavir**), **carbamazepine, cisapride, methylprednisolone, paclitaxel,** and **vinca alkaloids** (the US manufacturer specifically mentions **vinblastine**).[1] It would therefore be prudent to be alert for increased adverse effects when these drugs are given to patients taking quinupristin with dalfopristin. However, the manufacturers also advise that the concurrent use of quinupristin with dalfopristin in patients taking drugs that are metabolised by CYP3A4 and which may prolong the QTc interval should be avoided.[1,2] This would be expected to include **cisapride**.

The manufacturers also name **diazepam** and the **statins** (the US manufacturer specifically mentions **lovastatin**) in their list of drugs that may have their levels raised by quinupristin with dalfopristin.[1,2] However, note that diazepam is not usually affected by CYP3A4 inhibitors, and the statins are not all metabolised by this route, see 'Lipid regulating drugs', p.1309. For a further list of CYP3A4 substrates, see 'Table 1.10', p.12.

The manufacturers also note that when healthy subjects were given **rifampicin** and quinupristin with dalfopristin the pharmacokinetics of both drugs were unchanged. However, the AUC of the sum of quinupristin and its active metabolites was increased by 43%.[2] The clinical relevance of this finding is unclear.

1. Synercid (Quinupristin/Dalfopristin). Pfizer Injectables. US Prescribing information, October 2013.
2. Synercid (Quinupristin/Dalfopristin). Monarch Pharmaceuticals Ireland Ltd. UK Summary of product characteristics, March 2005.

Retapamulin + Azoles

Ketoconazole increases the plasma levels and AUC of topical retapamulin. Other azoles may interact similarly.

Clinical evidence, mechanism, importance and management

The manufacturers note that the AUC and maximum plasma level of topical retapamulin ointment 1% applied to the abraded skin of healthy subjects was increased by 81% when they also took ketoconazole 200 mg twice daily.[1,2] However, this interaction is not expected to be clinically significant, and no dose adjustment of retapamulin is recommended due to its low systemic exposure following topical application.[1,2] Other azoles would be expected to interact similarly, or to a lesser extent.

1. Altargo (Retapamulin). GlaxoSmithKline UK. UK Summary of product characteristics, May 2007.
2. Altabax (Retapamulin). GlaxoSmithKline. US Prescribing information, May 2009.

Rifabutin + Cobicistat

Cobicistat markedly increases the exposure to the active 25-*O*-desacetyl metabolite of rifabutin.

Clinical evidence

The US manufacturer briefly reports that, in a study in 12 healthy subjects given rifabutin 150 mg every other day with cobicistat 150 mg once daily (as a pharmacokinetic enhancer with elvitegravir 150 mg once daily), the pharmacokinetics of rifabutin were the same as that for rifabutin 300 mg once daily alone. However, the AUC and maximum plasma concentration of the active 25-*O*-desacetyl metabolite of rifabutin were 6.3-fold and 4.8-fold higher, respectively.[1] The UK manufacturer adds that the AUC and the maximum concentration of cobicistat were not affected, but the minimum concentration was decreased by 66%.[2]

Mechanism

Rifabutin itself is partially metabolised by CYP3A4 whereas its active metabolite, 25-*O*-desacetyl rifabutin, is completely metabolised by CYP3A4. Therefore inhibition of CYP3A4 by cobicistat increases the plasma concentration of rifabutin and greatly increases the plasma concentration of its 25-*O*-desacetyl metabolite.

Importance and management

A pharmacokinetic interaction between rifabutin and cobicistat would appear to be established based on the known disposition of rifabutin and the potent inhibitory effects of cobicistat. The marked increase in the exposure to the active metabolite of rifabutin is likely to be clinically important. As such, the UK manufacturer of cobicistat does not recommend concurrent use with rifabutin.[2] However, if the combination is necessary, it advises that rifabutin should be given at a dose of 150 mg three times a week on set days,[2] and the US manufacturer advises giving the same dose every other day.[1] Both advise increased monitoring for rifabutin adverse effects, such as neutropenia and uveitis.[1,2] This would seem prudent given the known effects of the similarly potent CYP3A4 inhibitor ritonavir, see 'HIV-protease inhibitors + Rifamycins; Rifabutin', p.939.

1. Tybost (Cobicistat). Gilead Sciences, Inc. US Prescribing information, September 2014.
2. Tybost (Cobicistat). Gilead Sciences Ltd. UK Summary of product characteristics, October 2014.

Rifampicin (Rifampin) + Aminosalicylic acid

The serum levels of rifampicin are approximately halved if aminosalicylic acid granules containing bentonite are given.

Clinical evidence

In 30 patients with tuberculosis, the serum levels of rifampicin 10 mg/kg were reduced by more than 50% at 2 hours (from 6.06 to 2.91 micrograms/mL) by aminosalicylate.[1,2] Later studies in 6 healthy subjects found that this interaction was not due to the aminosalicylic acid itself but to the **bentonite**, which was the main excipient of the granules.[3] The rifampicin AUC was statistically unchanged in the presence of sodium aminosalicylate tablets (no **bentonite**), whereas it was reduced by more than 37% in the presence of **bentonite** from aminosalicylate granules.[3]

Other studies confirm this marked reduction in serum rifampicin levels in the presence of **bentonite** in aminosalicylic acid granules.[4]

Mechanism

The bentonite excipient in the aminosalicylic acid granules adsorbs the rifampicin onto its surface so that much less is available for absorption, which results in reduced serum levels.[3] Bentonite is a naturally occurring mineral (montmorillonite) consisting largely of hydrate aluminium silicate, and is similar to kaolin.

Importance and management

A well documented and clinically important interaction. Separating the administration of the two drugs by 8 to 12 hours to prevent their mixing in the gut has been suggested as an effective way to prevent this interaction.[1] Based on this interaction with rifampicin, one UK manufacturer of **rifabutin** gives the same administration advice.[5] An alternative is to give aminosalicylic acid preparations that do not contain bentonite.

1. Boman G, Hanngren Å, Malmborg A-S, Borgå O, Sjöqvist F. Drug Interaction: decreased serum concentrations of rifampicin when given with P.A.S. *Lancet* (1971) i, 800.
2. Boman G, Borgå O, Hanngren Å, Malmborg A-S and Sjöqvist F. Pharmacokinetic interactions between the tuberculostatics rifampicin, para-aminosalicylic acid and isoniazid. *Acta Pharmacol Toxicol (Copenh)* (1970) 28 (Suppl 1), 15.
3. Boman G, Lundgren P, Stjernström G. Mechanism of the inhibitory effect of PAS granules on the absorption of rifampicin: adsorption of rifampicin by an excipient, bentonite. *Eur J Clin Pharmacol* (1975) 8, 293–9.
4. Boman G. Serum concentration and half-life of rifampicin after simultaneous oral administration of aminosalicylic acid or isoniazid. *Eur J Clin Pharmacol* (1974) 7, 217–25.
5. Mycobutin (Rifabutin). Pfizer Ltd. UK Summary of product characteristics, December 2013.

Rifampicin (Rifampin) + Antacids

The absorption of rifampicin can be reduced by up to about one-third by antacids.

Clinical evidence

When 5 healthy subjects took a single 600-mg dose of rifampicin with various antacids the absorption of rifampicin was reduced. The antacids caused a fall in the urinary excretion of rifampicin as follows:

- 15 or 30 mL of **aluminium hydroxide gel** 29 to 31%;
- 2 or 4 g of **magnesium trisilicate** 31 to 36%;
- 2 g of **sodium bicarbonate** 21%.[1]

Three groups of 15 patients with tuberculosis were given a single oral dose of rifampicin 10 to 12 mg/kg, isoniazid 300 mg and ethambutol 20 mg/kg either alone or with about 20 mL of antacid. A 'significant number' of patients had peak rifampicin concentrations below 6.5 micrograms/mL (serum level quoted as necessary to achieve adequate lung concentrations) in the group receiving *Aludrox* (**aluminium hydroxide**), but no significant effect was noted in the group receiving *Gelusil* (**aluminium hydroxide** with **magnesium trisilicate**).[2] However, in a further study in 14 healthy subjects, 30 mL of *Mylanta* (**aluminium/magnesium hydroxide**) given 9 hours before, with and after rifampicin had no effect on rifampicin pharmacokinetics.[3]

Mechanism

It has been suggested that the rise in stomach pH caused by these antacids reduces the dissolution of the rifampicin and thereby inhibits its absorption. In addition, aluminium ions may form less soluble chelates with rifampicin, and magnesium trisilicate can adsorb rifampicin, both of which would also be expected to reduce bioavailability.[1]

Importance and management

Direct information seems to be limited to these reports. The effects of 20 to 35% reductions in rifampicin absorption do not appear to have been assessed, but if antacids are given it would be prudent to be alert for any evidence that treatment is less effective than expected. The US manufacturers of rifampicin advise giving rifampicin one hour before antacids.[4]

1. Khalil SAH, El-Khordagui LK, El-Gholmy ZA. Effect of antacids on oral absorption of rifampicin. *Int J Pharmaceutics* (1984) 20, 99–106.
2. Gupta PR, Mehta YR, Gupta ML, Sharma TN, Jain D, Gupta RB. Rifampicin-aluminium antacid interaction. *J Assoc Physicians India* (1988) 36, 363–4.
3. Peloquin CA, Namdar R, Singleton MD, Nix DE. Pharmacokinetics of rifampin under fasting conditions, with food, and with antacids. *Chest* (1999) 115, 12–18.
4. Rifadin (Rifampicin). Sanofi-Aventis US LLC. US Prescribing information, March 2007.

Rifampicin (Rifampin) + Barbiturates

Phenobarbital possibly modestly increases the clearance of rifampicin. The effect of rifampicin on phenobarbital levels is unknown, but rifampicin markedly increases the clearance of another barbiturate hexobarbital.

Clinical evidence, mechanism, importance and management

In one study, the serum levels of rifampicin were reduced by 20 to 40% in 12 of 15 patients taking **phenobarbital** 100 mg daily.[1] In another study, although **phenobarbital** 100 mg daily for 7 days reduced the mean half-life of a single 600-mg dose of rifampicin by 15%, this was not statistically significant. However, in a further 5 patients with cirrhosis of the liver, **phenobarbital** reduced the half-life of rifampicin by a mean of 2.2 hours.[2]

The effect of rifampicin on **phenobarbital** levels does not appear to have been studied, but rifampicin markedly increased the clearance of another barbiturate **hexobarbital**, which is used as a marker of drug metabolism.[3-6]

The evidence for an interaction between rifampicin and the barbiturates is limited. Both rifampicin and the barbiturates are potent liver enzyme inducers. The outcome of their effects when combined is not clear from the available data, but a reduction in the levels of both drugs seems possible. Concurrent use need not be avoided, but be alert for a reduced response to both the barbiturate and rifampicin.

1. de Rautlin de la Roy Y, Beauchant G, Breuil K, Patte F. Diminution du taux sérique de rifampicine par le phénobarbital. *Presse Med* (1971) 79, 350.
2. Acocella G, Bonollo L, Mainardi M, Margaroli P, Nicolis FB. Kinetic studies on rifampicin. III. Effect of phenobarbital on the half-life of the antibiotic. *Tijdschr Gastroenterol* (1974) 17, 151–8.
3. Breimer DD, Zilly W, Richter E. Influence of rifampicin on drug metabolism: differences between hexobarbital and antipyrine. *Clin Pharmacol Ther* (1977) 21, 470–81.
4. Zilly W, Breimer DD, Richter E. Induction of drug metabolism in man after rifampicin treatment measured by increased hexobarbital and tolbutamide clearance. *Eur J Clin Pharmacol* (1975) 9, 219–27.
5. Zilly W, Breimer DD, Richter E. Stimulation of drug metabolism by rifampicin in patients with cirrhosis or cholestasis measured by increased hexobarbital and tolbutamide clearance. *Eur J Clin Pharmacol* (1977) 11, 287–93.
6. Smith DA, Chandler MHH, Shedlofsky SI, Wedlund PJ, Blouin RA. Age-dependent stereoselective increase in the oral clearance of hexobarbitone isomers caused by rifampicin. *Br J Clin Pharmacol* (1991) 32, 735–9.

Rifampicin (Rifampin) + Clofazimine

Clofazimine does not affect the pharmacokinetics of rifampicin and rifampicin does not affect the bioavailability of clofazimine.

Clinical evidence, mechanism, importance and management

Clofazimine 100 mg daily, given to 15 patients with leprosy taking rifampicin 600 mg daily and dapsone 100 mg daily, had no effect on the pharmacokinetics of rifampicin.[1] A single-dose study found that the bioavailability of clofazimine remained unaltered when rifampicin was given, although a reduction in the rate of absorption was seen.[2] No special precautions would seem to be necessary on concurrent use.

1. Venkatesan K, Mathur A, Girdhar BK, Bharadwaj VP. The effect of clofazimine on the pharmacokinetics of rifampicin and dapsone in leprosy. *J Antimicrob Chemother* (1986) 18, 715–18.
2. Mehta J, Gandhi IS, Sane SB, Wamburkar MN. Effect of clofazimine and dapsone on rifampicin (Lositril) pharmacokinetics in multibacillary and paucibacillary leprosy cases. *Indian J Lepr* (1985) 57, 297–310.

Rifampicin (Rifampin) + Food

Food delays and reduces the absorption of rifampicin from the gut.

Clinical evidence

The absorption of a single 10-mg/kg dose of rifampicin was reduced when it was given to 6 healthy subjects with a standard Indian breakfast (125 g wheat, 10 g visible fat, 350 g vegetables). The AUC after 8 hours was reduced by 26% and the peak plasma levels were delayed, and reduced by about 30% (from 11.84 micrograms/mL at 2 hours to 8.35 micrograms/mL at 4 hours).[1] In another study, a high-fat breakfast reduced the maximum serum level of rifampicin 600 mg by 36% and delayed the absorption, but the AUC was not significantly altered.[2]

Mechanism

Not understood.

Importance and management

An established interaction. Rifampicin should be taken on an empty stomach (at least 30 minutes before a meal, or 2 hours after a meal) to ensure rapid and complete absorption.

1. Polasa K, Krishnaswamy K. Effect of food on bioavailability of rifampicin. *J Clin Pharmacol* (1983) 23, 433–7.
2. Peloquin CA, Namdar R, Singleton MD, Nix DE. Pharmacokinetics of rifampin under fasting conditions, with food, and with antacids. *Chest* (1999) 155, 12–18.

Rifampicin (Rifampin) + Probenecid

Probenecid increased rifampicin levels in one study, but not in another.

Clinical evidence, mechanism, importance and management

A study in 6 healthy subjects given probenecid 2 g, before and after a single 300-mg dose of rifampicin, found that probenecid increased the mean peak serum rifampicin levels by 86%. At 4, 6, and 9 hours after the dose the increases were 118%, 90%, and 102%, respectively.[1] However, subsequent studies in patients taking either rifampicin 600 mg daily, or rifampicin 300 mg daily given 30 minutes after a 2-g dose of probenecid, found that the probenecid group achieved serum rifampicin levels that were only about half of those achieved in patients taking rifampicin 600 mg alone, suggesting that no interaction occurred.[2] The reasons for these discordant results are not understood, although it has been suggested that erratic rifampicin absorption may have played a part.[2] The interaction is not proven, but it seems possible that some patients will experience a rise in rifampicin levels. Consider this interaction as a possible cause if rifampicin adverse effects are troublesome.

1. Kenwright S, Levi AJ. Impairment of hepatic uptake of rifamycin antibiotics by probenecid, and its therapeutic implications. *Lancet* (1973) ii, 1401–5.
2. Fallon RJ, Lees AW, Allan GW, Smith J, Tyrrell WF. Probenecid and rifampicin serum levels. *Lancet* (1975) ii, 792–4.

Rifapentine + Food

Food increases the bioavailability of rifapentine.

Clinical evidence, mechanism, importance and management

In a randomised, crossover study, 34 healthy subjects were given a single 900-mg dose of rifapentine, either in the fasted state, or 30 minutes after 4 different meals. When compared with the fasted state, food increased the oral bioavailability of rifapentine by 33 to 86% depending on the type of meal (high-fat breakfast 86%; low-fat, high-fluid breakfast 49%; high-fat, bulky breakfast 46%; low-fat, bulky breakfast 33%).[1] The US manufacturer briefly reports that in a study in asymptomatic HIV-infected subjects, the AUC and maximum concentration of rifapentine were increased by 51% and 53%, respectively, by the presence of food when compared with the fasted state. It is recommended that rifapentine is given with food.[2] This advice seems prudent given the possible consequences of reduced rifapentine absorption on the treatment of tuberculosis.

1. Zvada SP, Van Der Walt JS, Smith PJ, Fourie PB, Roscigno G, Mitchison D, Simonsson US, McIlleron HM. Effects of four different meal types on the population pharmacokinetics of single-dose rifapentine in healthy male volunteers. *Antimicrob Agents Chemother* (2010) 54, 3390–4.
2. Priftin (Rifapentine). Sanofi-Aventis US LLC. US Prescribing information, December 2014.

Rifaximin + Food

The exposure to rifaximin is increased by food.

Clinical evidence, mechanism, importance and management

The US manufacturer briefly reports that, in a study in 12 healthy subjects, the AUC of a single 550-mg dose of rifaximin, given 30 minutes after a high-fat meal, was increased 2-fold, and the time to maximum concentration was delayed, from 45 minutes to 90 minutes.[1] This is not expected to be clinically relevant, so the manufacturers therefore advise that rifaximin can be taken with or without food.[1,2]

1. Xifaxan (Rifaximin). Salix Pharmaceuticals, Inc. US Prescribing information, October 2011.
2. Xifaxanta (Rifaximin). Norgine Ltd. UK Summary of product characteristics, June 2011.

Sulfonamides + Anaesthetics, local

Para-aminobenzoic acid, derived from certain local anaesthetics, can reduce the effects of the sulfonamides and allow the development of local and even generalised infections. However, it should be noted that the limited evidence for this interaction is from the 1940s.

Clinical evidence

Four patients taking sulfonamides developed local infections in areas where **procaine** had been injected before diagnostic taps for meningitis, or draining procedures in empyema. Extensive cellulitis of the lumbar region occurred in one case, and abscesses appeared at the puncture sites in another. However, it should be noted that lumbar punctures were being done at least daily and up to four times a day in the 3 patients with meningitis.[1]

An *in vitro* study demonstrated that the amount of **procaine** in the pleural fluid after anaesthesia for thoracentesis was sufficient to inhibit the antibacterial activity of 0.005% **sulfapyridine** against type III pneumococci.[2] Another *in vitro* study found that some local anaesthetics derived from para-aminobenzoic acid (PABA) inhibited the bacteriostatic activity of **sulfapyridine** and **sulfathiazole** but some other local anaesthetics not derived from PABA did not affect the antibacterial activity of these sulfonamides.[3] Other studies in *animals* confirm that both *in vitro*[4-6] and *in vivo*[7] antagonism can occur between sulfonamides and local anaesthetics that are hydrolysed to **PABA**.

Mechanism

The ester type of local anaesthetic is hydrolysed within the body to produce para-aminobenzoic acid (PABA). Sulfonamides work by inhibiting bacterial DNA synthesis by competitively inhibiting folate production. The PABA competes with the sulfonamides, so higher PABA concentrations effectively dilute the effects of the sulfonamides.

Importance and management

Clinical examples of this interaction seem to be few and of poor quality (note that the patients were given repeated lumbar punctures, up to four times daily in some instances). It should also be noted that the supporting evidence (human, *animal* and *in vitro* studies) dates back to the mid-1940s with nothing more recent apparently on record. Local anaesthetics of the ester type that are hydrolysed to para-aminobenzoic acid (e.g. tetracaine, procaine, benzocaine) present the greatest risk of a reaction, whereas those of the amide type (bupivacaine, cinchocaine, lidocaine, mepivacaine and prilocaine) would not be expected to interact adversely. The evidence seems to be too slim to preclude concurrent use of these drugs, but it is perhaps worth considering this interaction if high or repeated doses of the local anaesthetic are used. However, note that high doses or prolonged use of these ester-type anaesthetics are best avoided given their toxicity when used in this manner.

1. Peterson OL, Finland M. Sulfonamide inhibiting action of procaine. *Am J Med Sci* (1944) 207, 166–75.
2. Boroff DA, Cooper A, Bullowa JGM. Inhibition of sulfapyridine by procaine in chest fluids after procaine anesthesia. *Proc Soc Exp Biol Med* (1941) 47,182–3.
3. Keltch AK, Baker LA, Krahl ME, Clowes GHA. Anti-sulfapyridine and anti-sulfathiazole effect of local anaesthetics derived from p-aminobenzoic acid. *Proc Soc Exp Biol Med* (1941) 47, 533–8.
4. Casten D, Fried JJ, Hallman FA. Inhibitory effect of procaine on the bacteriostatic activity of sulfathiazole. *Surg Gynecol Obstet* (1943) 76, 726–8.
5. Powell HM, Krahl ME, Clowes GHA. Inhibition of chemotherapeutic action of sulfapyridine by local anesthetics. *J Indiana State Med Assoc* (1942) 35, 62–3.
6. Walker BS, Derow MA. The antagonism of local anesthetics against the sulfonamides. *Am J Med Sci* (1945) 210, 585–8.
7. Pfeiffer CC, Grant CW. The procaine-sulfonamide antagonism: an evaluation of local anesthetics for use with sulfonamide therapy. *Anesthesiology* (1944) 5, 605–14.

Sulfonamides; Sulfafurazole (Sulfisoxazole) + Laxatives

Sodium sulfate and castor oil used as laxatives can cause a modest reduction in sulfafurazole absorption.

Clinical evidence, mechanism, importance and management

In an experimental study of the possible effects of laxatives on the absorption of sulfafurazole, healthy subjects were given 10 to 20 g of oral **sodium sulfate** or 20 g of **castor oil** (doses sufficient to provoke diarrhoea). Absorption, measured by the amount of sulfafurazole excreted in the urine, was decreased by 50% with **castor oil**, and by 33% with **sodium sulfate** at 4 hours. However, serum levels of the drugs were relatively unchanged. The overall picture was that while these laxatives can alter the pattern of absorption, they do not seriously impair the total amount of drug absorbed.[1]

1. Mattila MJ, Takki S, Jussila J. Effect of sodium sulphate and castor oil on drug absorption from the human intestine. *Ann Clin Res* (1974) 6, 19–24.

Telavancin + Miscellaneous

Telavancin can cause nephrotoxicity and ototoxicity, and the effects might be additive with nephrotoxic or ototoxic drugs. Concurrent administration of telavancin and midazolam did not alter the pharmacokinetics of either drug. Telavancin can interfere with some coagulation tests.

Clinical evidence, mechanism, importance and management

(a) CYP3A4 substrates

The US manufacturer of telavancin notes that in a study in 16 healthy subjects who were given a single 10-mg/kg dose of telavancin and a single 1-mg dose of intravenous **midazolam**, the pharmacokinetics of both telavancin and midazolam were unaffected.[1] The UK manufacturer briefly notes that in a clinical study in which multiple doses of telavancin were given with intravenous midazolam, telavancin pharmacokinetics were unaffected.[2] Midazolam can be used as a probe to assess the activity of drugs on CYP3A4. These studies therefore suggest that telavancin is not an inducer or inhibitor of CYP3A4, and a clinically relevant interaction with other CYP3A4 substrates is unlikely to occur by this mechanism.

(b) Drugs that affect coagulation

The UK and US manufacturers state that although it does not affect coagulation, telavancin can interfere with some coagulation tests (including activated clotting time, aPTT, coagulation based factor Xa activity assays, INR, and prothrombin time) if performed with blood drawn up to 18 hours after telavancin is given.[1,2] This occurs because telavancin binds to the phospholipid reagents used to precipitate coagulation in these tests, preventing them from working. Many **anticoagulant drugs** require coagulation monitoring, and the UK and US manufacturers advise that blood samples for coagulation tests should be taken as close as possible before the next dose of telavancin. Alternatively, if aPTT monitoring is necessary in a patient taking telavancin, a coagulation test which does not use phospholipid reagents, such as a Factor Xa (chromogenic) assay should be used, or an alternative anticoagulant not requiring aPTT monitoring should be considered.[1,2] The US manufacturer also specifically advises that the use of intravenous **unfractionated heparin** should be avoided with telavancin.[1] For more information on coagulation tests, see 'Coagulation tests', p.371.

(c) Nephrotoxic drugs

The US manufacturer of telavancin briefly notes that adverse renal effects occurred more often in patients taking telavancin with other drugs which affect renal function (they name **ACE inhibitors**, **loop diuretics**, and **NSAIDs**).[1] Telavancin is known to cause nephrotoxicity,[1,2] and therefore if given with other nephrotoxic drugs, the effects might be additive. The UK manufacturer recommends that telavancin should be used with caution in patients given nephrotoxic drugs.[2]

(d) Ototoxic drugs

Telavancin has been reported to cause ototoxicity (rarely deafness and uncommonly tinnitus)[2] and therefore if given with other ototoxic drugs (such as **aminoglycosides**, **NSAIDs**, **loop diuretics**, and platinum-based chemotherapy agents, such as **carboplatin** and **cisplatin**), the effects might be additive. The UK manufacturer of telavancin advises that if it is used with, or after, other ototoxic drugs, the patient's hearing should be closely monitored, and if hearing deteriorates the benefit of telavancin should be re-evaluated.[2]

1. Vibativ (Telavancin). Theravance Inc. US Prescribing information, December 2014.
2. Vibativ (Telavancin hydrochloride). Clinigen Healthcare Ltd. UK Summary of product information, September 2014.

Telavancin + Other antibacterials

Telavancin appears not to alter the pharmacokinetics of aztreonam or piperacillin with tazobactam, and the pharmacokinetics of telavancin appear not to be affected by aztreonam or piperacillin with tazobactam. No interaction is predicted to occur between telavancin and the beta lactams, clindamycin, the fluoroquinolones, or metronidazole.

Clinical evidence, mechanism, importance and management

A randomised crossover study, in which 11 healthy subjects were given either a single 10-mg/kg dose of telavancin alone, a single 2-g dose of **aztreonam**, or a combination of both drugs, found that concurrent use did not alter the pharmacokinetics of either drug. Another study by the same authors in 12 healthy subjects, given either a single 10-mg/kg dose of telavancin alone, a single 4.5-g dose of **piperacillin with tazobactam**, or both telavancin and piperacillin with tazobactam, found that concurrent use did not alter the pharmacokinetics of any of the three drugs.[1] Evidence from these single-dose studies suggests that no clinically relevant pharmacokinetic interaction occurs between telavancin and either aztreonam or piperacillin with tazobactam, and that no dose adjustments would appear necessary on concurrent use. However, note that a multiple-dose study is required to completely exclude such an interaction.

The UK manufacturer of telavancin briefly notes that no interaction is predicted to occur between telavancin and the **beta lactams**, **clindamycin**, the **fluoroquinolones**, or **metronidazole**, based on their pharmacokinetics.[2]

1. Wong SL Sörgel F, Kinzig M, Goldberg MR, Kitt MM, Barriere SL. Lack of pharmacokinetic drug interactions following concomitant administration of telavancin with aztreonam or piperacillin/tazobactam in healthy participants. *J Clin Pharmacol* (2009) 49, 816–23.
2. Vibativ (Telavancin hydrochloride). Clinigen Healthcare Ltd. UK Summary of product information, September 2014.

Tetracyclines + Antacids

The serum levels and therefore the therapeutic effectiveness of the tetracyclines can be markedly reduced or even abolished by antacids containing aluminium, bismuth, calcium or magnesium. Other antacids, such as sodium bicarbonate, may also reduce the bioavailability of some tetracyclines. Even intravenous doxycycline levels can be reduced by antacids.

Clinical evidence

(a) Aluminium-containing antacids

A study in 5 patients and 6 healthy subjects found that within 48 hours of starting to take about 10 mL of aluminium hydroxide gel (*Amphogel*) every 6 hours with **chlortetracycline** 500 mg the serum levels of the antibacterial were reduced by 80 to 90%. One patient had a recurrence of her urinary tract infection, which only subsided when the antacid was withdrawn, and one patient maintained **chlortetracycline** levels despite antacid use.[1] Similar results were obtained in other studies.[2,3]

Further studies have found similar interactions with other tetracyclines:

- 30 mL of aluminium hydroxide reduced **oxytetracycline** serum levels by more than 50%,[3]
- 20 mL of aluminium hydroxide caused a 75% reduction in **demeclocycline** serum levels,[4]
- 15 mL of aluminium hydroxide caused a 100% reduction in serum **doxycycline** levels,[5,6]
- 30 mL of aluminium/magnesium hydroxide (*Maalox*) caused a 90% reduction in **tetracycline** serum levels.[7]

Intravenous doxycycline also appears to be affected. The mean serum levels of an intravenous dose of **doxycycline** were found to be reduced by 36% when 30 mL of aluminium hydroxide was taken four times daily, for 2 days before and after the antibacterial.[8]

(b) Bismuth-containing antacids

Bismuth subsalicylate reduces the absorption of **tetracycline** by 34%[9] and reduces the maximum serum levels of **doxycycline** by 50%.[10] It has been suggested the excipient *Veegum* (magnesium aluminium silicate) in some bismuth subsalicylate formulations enhances this effect.[11] Bismuth carbonate similarly interacts with the tetracyclines *in vitro*.[12] An observation that patients given metronidazole, with bismuth and **tetracycline** taken at the same time, experienced a *Helicobacter pylori* eradication rate greater than that achieved with metronidazole and bismuth has led to the suggestion that the reduced absorption of **tetracycline** may not be as clinically relevant in the treatment of this disorder.[13]

(c) Calcium-containing antacids

There seem to be no direct clinical studies with calcium-containing antacids, but a clinically important interaction seems almost a certainty, based on *in vitro* studies with calcium carbonate,[12] calcium in milk, (see 'Tetracyclines + Food', p.360), dicalcium phosphate,[14] and calcium as an excipient in tetracycline capsules.[15]

(d) Magnesium-containing antacids

Magnesium sulfate certainly interacts with **tetracycline**, but in the only clinical study available[16] the amount of magnesium was much higher than would normally be found in the usual dose of antacid. It has been suggested the excipient *Veegum* (magnesium aluminium silicate) enhances the effect of some bismuth subsalicylate formulations on **tetracycline** absorption,[11] and in one study, 30 mL of aluminium/magnesium hydroxide (*Maalox*) caused a 90% reduction in **tetracycline** serum levels.[7]

(e) Sodium-containing antacids

In 8 subjects, sodium bicarbonate 2 g reduced the absorption of a 250-mg capsule of **tetracycline** by 50%. However, if the **tetracycline** was dissolved before administration, the absorption was unaffected by sodium bicarbonate.[17] Another study stated that sodium bicarbonate 2 g had an insignificant effect on **tetracycline** absorption.[7]

Mechanism

The tetracyclines bind with aluminium, bismuth, calcium, magnesium and other metallic ions to form compounds (chelates), which are much less soluble and therefore much less readily absorbed by the gut.[18] Because doxycycline undergoes enterohepatic recirculation, even intravenous doxycycline is affected, although less so than oral. It has also been suggested that the antacids reduce gastric acidity and thereby decrease the absorption of tetracyclines,[17] but studies demonstrating the lack of a significant interaction with H_2-receptor antagonists (see 'Tetracyclines + H_2-receptor antagonists', p.361), suggest that this is not the case. The reduced absorption with bismuth compounds may be because they adsorb tetracyclines.[9] The interaction of some tetracycline preparations with sodium bicarbonate is unexplained.

Importance and management

Extremely well-documented, and well-established interactions. Their clinical importance depends on how much the serum tetracycline levels are lowered, but with normal antacid doses the reductions cited above (50 to 100%) are large enough to mean that many organisms will not be exposed to minimum inhibitory concentrations (MIC) of antibacterial. As a general rule none of the aluminium, bismuth, calcium or magnesium-containing antacids should be given at the same time as the tetracycline antibacterials. If they must be used, separate the doses by 2 to 3 hours or more to prevent their admixture in the gut. This also applies to **quinapril** formulations containing substantial quantities of magnesium (such as *Accupro*), although the interaction is less pronounced (see 'Tetracyclines + Quinapril', p.362), and to **didanosine** tablets that are formulated with antacid.[19] The enteric-coated capsule formulation (which does not contain antacids) is not expected to interact.[20]

Patients should be warned about taking any antacids and indigestion preparations at the same time as tetracyclines. Instead of using antacids to minimise the gastric irritant effects of the tetracyclines it is usually recommended that tetracyclines are taken after food; however, it is not entirely clear how much this affects their absorption (see 'Tetracyclines + Food', p.360). H_2-receptor antagonists may be suitable non-interacting alternatives to antacids in some situations, see 'Tetracyclines + H_2-receptor antagonists', p.361.

1. Waisbren BA, Hueckel JS. Reduced absorption of aureomycin caused by aluminum hydroxide gel (*Amphojel*). *Proc Soc Exp Biol Med* (1950) 73, 73–4.
2. Seed JC, Wilson CE. The effect of aluminum hydroxide on serum aureomycin concentrations after simultaneous oral administration. *Bull Johns Hopkins Hosp* (1950) 86, 415–8.
3. Michel JC, Sayer RJ, Kirby WMM. Effect of food and antacids on blood levels of aureomycin and terramycin. *J Lab Clin Med* (1950) 36, 632–4.
4. Scheiner J, Altemeier WA. Experimental study of factors inhibiting absorption and effective therapeutic levels of declomycin. *Surg Gynecol Obstet* (1962) 114, 9–14.
5. Rosenblatt JE, Barrett JE, Brodie JL, Kirby WMM. Comparison of in vitro activity and clinical pharmacology of doxycycline with other tetracyclines. *Antimicrob Agents Chemother* (1966) 6, 134–41.
6. Deppermann K-M, Lode H, Höffken G, Tschink G, Kalz C, Koeppe P. Influence of ranitidine, pirenzepine, and aluminum magnesium hydroxide on the bioavailability of various antibiotics, including amoxicillin, cephalexin, doxycycline, and amoxicillin-clavulanic acid. *Antimicrob Agents Chemother* (1989) 33, 1901–7.
7. Garty M, Hurwitz A. Effect of cimetidine and antacids on gastrointestinal absorption of tetracycline. *Clin Pharmacol Ther* (1980) 28, 203–7.
8. Nguyen VX, Nix DE, Gillikin S, Schentag JJ. Effect of oral antacid administration on the pharmacokinetics of intravenous doxycycline. *Antimicrob Agents Chemother* (1989) 33, 434–6.
9. Albert KS, Welch RD, De Sante KA, Disanto AR. Decreased tetracycline bioavailability caused by a bismuth subsalicylate antidiarrheal mixture. *J Pharm Sci* (1979) 68, 586–8.

10. Ericsson CD, Feldman S, Pickering LK, Cleary TG. Influence of subsalicylate bismuth on absorption of doxycycline. *JAMA* (1982) 247, 2266–7.
11. Healy DP, Dansereau RJ, Dunn AB, Clendening CE, Mounts AW, Deepe GS. Reduced tetracycline bioavailability caused by magnesium aluminum silicate in liquid formulations of bismuth subsalicylate. *Ann Pharmacother* (1997) 31, 1460–4.
12. Christensen EKJ, Kerckhoffs HPM, Huizinga T. De invloed van antacida op de afgifte in vitro van tetracycline hydrochloride. *Pharm Weekbl* (1967) 102, 463–73.
13. Tkach CL, Ariano RE. Significance of a tetracycline and Pepto-Bismol interaction in the management of *Helicobacter pylori*-induced peptic ulcer disease. *Ann Pharmacother* (1998) 32, 387.
14. Boger WP, Gavin JJ. An evaluation of tetracycline preparations. *N Engl J Med* (1959) 261, 827–32.
15. Sweeney WM, Hardy SM, Dornbush AC, Ruegsegger JM. Absorption of tetracycline in human beings as affected by certain excipients. *Antibiotic Med Clin Ther* (1957) 4, 642–56.
16. Harcourt RS, Hamburger M. The effect of magnesium sulfate in lowering tetracycline blood levels. *J Lab Clin Med* (1957) 50, 464–8.
17. Barr WH, Adir J, Garrettson L. Decrease of tetracycline absorption in man by sodium bicarbonate. *Clin Pharmacol Ther* (1971) 12, 779–84.
18. Albert A, Rees CW. Avidity of the tetracyclines for the cations of metals. *Nature* (1956) 177, 433–4.
19. Videx Tablets (Didanosine). Bristol-Myers Squibb Pharmaceuticals Ltd. UK Summary of product characteristics, June 2009.
20. Videx EC (Didanosine). Bristol-Myers Squibb Pharmaceuticals Ltd. UK Summary of product characteristics, July 2009.

Tetracyclines + Antiepileptics; Enzyme-inducing

The serum levels of doxycycline are reduced and may fall below the accepted minimum inhibitory concentration in patients receiving long-term treatment with barbiturates, phenytoin or carbamazepine. Other tetracyclines do not appear to be affected.

Clinical evidence

A study in 14 patients taking **phenytoin** 200 to 500 mg daily, **carbamazepine** 300 mg to 1 g daily, or both, found that the half-life of **doxycycline** was approximately halved from 15.1 hours in patients not taking antiepileptics, to 7.2 hours in patients taking **phenytoin**, 8.4 hours in patients taking **carbamazepine**, and 7.4 hours in patients taking both drugs.[1]

Similar results were found in 16 other patients taking various combinations of **phenytoin, carbamazepine, primidone** or **phenobarbital**. The serum **doxycycline** levels of almost all of them fell below 0.5 micrograms/mL during the 12- to 24-hour period following their last dose of **doxycycline** 100 mg.[2] Other studies confirm this interaction between some **barbiturates (amobarbital, pentobarbital, phenobarbital)** and **doxycycline.**[3,4]

Tetracycline, methacycline, oxytetracycline, demeclocycline and **chlortetracycline** levels were not significantly affected by various combinations of **phenytoin, carbamazepine, primidone** or **phenobarbital**.[2]

Mechanism

Uncertain. These antiepileptics and barbiturates are known enzyme inducers and it seems probable that they increase the metabolism of the doxycycline by the liver, thereby increasing its clearance from the body.

Importance and management

The interactions between doxycycline and the enzyme-inducing antiepileptics are established, but the clinical significance of the reduction in levels does not seem to have been studied. Serum doxycycline levels below 0.5 micrograms/mL are less than the minimum inhibitory concentration (MIC) quoted by the authors, so that it seems likely that the antibacterial will be less effective. To accommodate this potential problem it has been suggested that the doxycycline dose could be doubled.[2] Alternatively any of the tetracyclines that are reported not to be affected by these antiepileptics (tetracycline, methacycline, oxytetracycline, demeclocycline and chlortetracycline) may provide a suitable alternative.[2]

1. Penttilä O, Neuvonen PJ, Aho K, Lehtovaara R. Interaction between doxycycline and some antiepileptic drugs. *BMJ* (1974) 2, 470–2.
2. Neuvonen PJ, Penttilä O, Lehtovaara R, Aho K. Effect of antiepileptic drugs on the elimination of various tetracycline derivatives. *Eur J Clin Pharmacol* (1975) 9, 147–54.
3. Neuvonen PJ, Penttilä O. Interaction between doxycycline and barbiturates. *BMJ* (1974) 1, 535–6.
4. Alestig K. Studies on the intestinal excretion of doxycycline. *Scand J Infect Dis* (1974) 6, 265–71.

Tetracyclines + Colestipol

Colestipol can reduce the absorption of tetracycline by about a half. Information about other tetracyclines is lacking but it seems likely that they will interact similarly.

Clinical evidence

In 9 healthy subjects, colestipol 30 g taken either in 180 mL of water or orange juice reduced the absorption of a single 500-mg dose of oral **tetracycline** by about 55%, as measured by recovery in the urine.[1]

Mechanism

Colestipol binds to bile acids in the gut and can also bind with some drugs, thereby reducing their availability for absorption. An *in vitro* study found a 30% binding with tetracycline.[2] The presence of citrate ions in the orange juice, which can also bind to colestipol, appears not to have a marked effect on the binding of the tetracycline.

Importance and management

An established interaction. Direct information seems to be limited to the report cited, but it is consistent with the way colestipol interacts with other drugs. In practice up to 30 g of colestipol is given daily in single or twice daily, in divided doses, and tetracycline 250 to 500-mg is given every 6 hours. As other drugs need to be given one hour before or 4 hours after colestipol it may be difficult to avoid some mixing in the gut. It seems very probable that a clinically important interaction will occur, but the extent to which the efficacy of tetracycline is affected seems not to have been determined. Advise patients to separate the doses as much as possible. Monitor the outcome well. Information about other tetracyclines is lacking but it also seems likely that they will interact similarly, but those that can be given less often may prove easier to administer, although note that doxycycline undergoes enterohepatic recirculation and therefore separating doses may not be completely effective.

1. Friedman H, Greenblatt DJ, LeDuc BW. Impaired absorption of tetracycline by colestipol is not reversed by orange juice. *J Clin Pharmacol* (1989) 29, 748–51.
2. Ko H, Royer ME. *In vitro* binding of drugs to colestipol hydrochloride. *J Pharm Sci* (1974) 63, 1914–20.

Tetracyclines + Diuretics

It has been recommended by some that the concurrent use of tetracyclines and diuretics should be avoided because of their association with rises in blood urea nitrogen levels.

Clinical evidence, mechanism, importance and management

A retrospective study of patient records as part of the Boston Collaborative Drug Surveillance Program showed that an association existed between tetracycline use with diuretics (not named) and rises in blood urea nitrogen (BUN) levels.[1] It was suggested that tetracyclines should be avoided in patients taking diuretics when alternative antibacterials could be substituted.[1] However, the results of this study have been much criticised as the authors could not exclude physician bias,[1,2] they did not define what was meant by 'clinically significant rise in BUN',[2] they did not state whether or not this rise affected patient outcomes,[2] they did not measure creatinine levels,[3] they did not specify which diuretics were involved,[2] and they did not adequately consider the fact that diuretics are known to cause rises in BUN.[4] The patients most affected also had the highest levels of BUN before starting tetracyclines. Tetracyclines alone are known to cause rises in BUN, especially where a degree of renal impairment exists, although it has been suggested that **doxycycline** is less prone to this effect.[4] It would seem that tetracyclines and diuretics may be used together safely, although it would be wise to give thought to the patient's renal function.

1. Boston Collaborative Drug Surveillance Program. Tetracycline and drug-attributed rises in blood urea nitrogen. *JAMA* (1972) 220, 377–9.
2. Tannenberg AM. Tetracyclines and rises in urea nitrogen. *JAMA* (1972) 221, 713.
3. Dijkhuis HJPM, van Meurs AJ. Tetracycline and BUN level. *JAMA* (1973) 223, 441.
4. Alexander MR. Tetracyclines and rises in urea nitrogen. *JAMA* (1972) 221, 713–14.

Tetracyclines + Food

The calcium in food can complex with tetracycline to reduce its absorption. This is particularly notable with dairy products, which can reduce the absorption of the tetracyclines by up to 80%, thereby reducing or even abolishing their therapeutic effects. Doxycycline and minocycline are less affected by dairy products (25 to 30% reduction) and lymecycline is not affected by milk. Orange juice and coffee do not interact with tetracycline.

Clinical evidence

(a) Dairy products

1. Demeclocycline. In 4 subjects given dairy products the serum levels of a 300-mg dose of demeclocycline were 70 to 80% lower, when compared with subjects who took demeclocycline with a meal containing no dairy products. The dairy products used were either 8 oz (about 250 mL) of **fresh pasteurized milk**, 8 oz of **buttermilk** or 4 oz of **cottage cheese**.[1]

2. Doxycycline. The plasma doxycycline levels were reduced by 20%, from 1.79 micrograms/mL to 1.45 micrograms/mL, 2 hours after a single 100-mg oral dose was taken with 240 mL of **milk**.[2] Another study, in 9 healthy subjects, found a 30% reduction in the absorption of doxycycline 200 mg, and a 24% reduction in its peak serum levels when it was taken with 300 mL of **fresh milk**.[3] However, two other studies suggest that the absorption of doxycycline 200 mg is unaffected by milk,[4,5] although in one study the half-life was almost halved and its clearance increased.[5]

3. Lymecycline. In 10 healthy subjects the absorption of lymecycline 300 mg twice daily has not been shown to be significantly affected by 300 g of **milk**.[6]

4. Methacycline. In one study 300 mL of **milk** reduced the absorption of methacycline 300 mg by about 63%.[4]

5. Minocycline. In one study about 180 mL (6 oz) of **homogenised milk** reduced the absorption of minocycline 100 mg by 27%.[7]

6. Oxytetracycline. In one study 300 mL of **milk** reduced the absorption of oxytetracycline 500 mg by about 64%.[4]

7. Tetracycline. In one study about 180 mL (6 oz) of **homogenised milk** reduced the absorption of tetracycline hydrochloride 250 mg by 65%.[7] In another study the absorption of tetracycline 500 mg was reduced by about 50% by 300 mL of **milk**.[4] The addition of 16 mL **evaporated milk** to tea and coffee reduced the bioavailability of a single 250-mg dose of tetracycline by about 40 to 50%.[8]

(b) Other calcium-containing foods or drinks

A study in 9 healthy subjects found that 200 mL of **orange juice** or **coffee** (milk content, if any, unstated) did not significantly affect the bioavailability of a single 250-mg dose of **tetracycline**. This is despite the fact that **orange juice** contains 35 to 70 mg calcium per 100 mL.[9]

Tetracycline 250 mg was given to 9 healthy subjects with 200 mL of water on an empty stomach. The **tetracycline** bioavailability was compared with its administration after a standard meal (two slices of bread, ham, tomato, and water, containing 145 mg calcium) and a Mexican meal (two tortillas, beans, two eggs, tomato and water, containing 235 mg calcium). The cumulative amounts of tetracycline excreted in the urine at 72 hours were about 151 mg (fasting), 90 mg (standard meal) and 68 mg (Mexican meal).[10] Another study in 23 healthy subjects also found a reduction in the maximum **tetracycline** plasma levels and AUC when it was taken with food.[11] A brief report describes a 14% reduction in the bioavailability of **minocycline** when 12 healthy subjects took **minocycline** with a standard meal, although there was wide inter-individual variation in the findings.[12] The absorption of a 300-mg dose of **demeclocycline** was not affected when it was given with a meal not containing dairy products,[1] and **doxycycline** seems to be minimally affected by food not containing dairy products.[2]

Mechanism

The tetracyclines have a strong affinity for the calcium ions that are found in abundance in dairy products and some foodstuffs. The tetracycline/calcium chelates formed are much less readily absorbed from the gastrointestinal tract and as a result the serum tetracycline levels achieved are much lower. Some tetracyclines have a lesser tendency to form chelates, which explains why their serum levels are reduced to a smaller extent.[13]

Orange juice appears not to interact, despite its calcium content, because at the relevant pH values in the gut, the calcium is bound to components within the orange juice (citric, tartaric and ascorbic acids) and is not free to combine with the tetracycline.[9]

Importance and management

Well documented and very well established interactions of clinical importance. Reductions in serum tetracycline levels of 50 to 80% caused by calcium-rich foods are sufficiently large to reduce or even abolish their antibacterial effects. For this reason tetracyclines should not be taken with milk or dairy products such as yoghurt or cheese. Separate the ingestion of these foods and tetracycline as much as possible. In the case of iron, which interacts by the same mechanism, 2 to 3 hours is enough. Doxycycline[3,14] and minocycline[7] are not affected as much by dairy products (reductions of about 25 to 30%), and lymecycline appears unaffected, and in this respect they may have some advantages over the other tetracyclines.

It is usual to recommend that tetracyclines are taken one hour before or 2 hours after food (which would be expected to contain at least some calcium), to minimise admixture in the gut and thereby reduce the effects of the interaction. The separation is something of a compromise, because food can help to minimise the gastric irritant effects of the tetracyclines.

1. Scheiner J, Altemeier WA. Experimental study of factors inhibiting absorption and effective therapeutic levels of declomycin. *Surg Gynecol Obstet* (1962) 114, 9–14.
2. Rosenblatt JE, Barrett JE, Brodie JL, Kirby WMM. Comparison of in vitro activity and clinical pharmacology of doxycycline with other tetracyclines. *Antimicrob Agents Chemother* (1966) 6, 134–41.
3. Meyer FP, Specht H, Quednow B, Walther H. Influence of milk on bioavailability of doxycycline — new aspects. *Infection* (1989) 17, 245–6.
4. Mattila MJ, Neuvonen PJ, Gothoni G, Hackman CR. Interference of iron preparations and milk with the absorption of tetracyclines. *Int Congr Ser* (1972) 254, 128–33.
5. Saux M-C, Mosser J, Pontagnier H, Leng B. Pharmacokinetic study of doxycycline polyphosphate after simultaneous ingestion of milk. *Eur J Drug Metab Pharmacokinet* (1983) 8, 43–9.
6. Ericson S, Gnarpe H. Lymecycline and concurrent ingestion of milk. *J Int Med Res* (1979) 7, 471–2.
7. Leyden JJ. Absorption of minocycline hydrochloride and tetracycline hydrochloride. Effect of food, milk, and iron. *J Am Acad Dermatol* (1985) 12, 308–12.
8. Jung H, Peregrina AA, Rodriguez JM, Moreno-Esparza R. The influence of coffee with milk and tea with milk on the bioavailability of tetracycline. *Biopharm Drug Dispos* (1997) 18, 459–63.
9. Jung H, Rivera O, Reguero MT, Rodríguez JM, Moreno-Esparza R. Influence of liquids (coffee and orange juice) on the bioavailability of tetracycline. *Biopharm Drug Dispos* (1990) 11, 729–34.
10. Cook HJ, Mundo CR, Fonseca L, Gasque L, Moreno-Esparza R. Influence of the diet on bioavailability of tetracycline. *Biopharm Drug Dispos* (1993) 14, 549–53.
11. Spénard J, Aumais C, Massicotte J, Brunet J-S, Tremblay C, Grace M, Lefebvre M. Effects of food and formulation on the relative bioavailability of bismuth biskalcitrate, metronidazole, and tetracycline given for *Helicobacter pylori* eradication. *Br J Clin Pharmacol* (2005) 60, 374–7.
12. Meyer FP. Minocycline for acne. Food reduces minocycline's bioavailability. *BMJ* (1996) 312, 1101.
13. Albert A, Rees CW. Avidity of the tetracyclines for the cations of metals. *Nature* (1956) 177, 433–4.
14. Siewert M, Blume H, Stenzhorn G, Kieferndorf U, Lenhard G. Zur Qualitätsbeurteilung von doxycyclinhaltigen ertigarzneimitteln. 3. Mitteilung: Vergleichende Bioverfügbarkeitsstudie unter Berücksichtigung einer Einnahme mit Milch. *Pharm Ztg* (1990) 3, 96–102.

Tetracyclines + H_2-receptor antagonists

Cimetidine reduces the absorption of tetracycline but does not appear to affect its serum levels. Ranitidine does not appear to affect the bioavailability of doxycycline. Information about other tetracyclines and H_2-receptor antagonists is lacking, but there would seem to be no reason to suspect that they will interact.

Clinical evidence, mechanism, importance and management

A study in 5 subjects found that **cimetidine** 200 mg three times daily and 400 mg at bedtime for 3 days reduced the absorption of a single 500-mg dose of a **tetracycline** capsule by about 30%, but had no effect on absorption when the **tetracycline** was given as a solution.[1] However, when **tetracycline** as either a tablet or a suspension was given to 6 subjects with **cimetidine** 1.6 g daily for 6 days, no changes in the plasma levels of **tetracycline** were seen.[2] Similar results were found in another study.[3]

In 10 healthy subjects, the bioavailability of **doxycycline** 200 mg was not altered by three 150-mg doses of **ranitidine**.[4]

No special precautions would seem necessary with either combination. Information about other tetracyclines seems to be lacking, but there would seem to be no reason to suspect that they will interact.

1. Cole JJ, Charles BG, Ravenscroft PJ. Interaction of cimetidine with tetracycline absorption. *Lancet* (1980) ii, 536.
2. Fisher P, House F, Inns P, Morrison PJ, Rogers HJ, Bradbrook ID. Effect of cimetidine on the absorption of orally administered tetracycline. *Br J Clin Pharmacol* (1980) 9, 153–8.
3. Garty M, Hurwitz A. Effect of cimetidine and antacids on gastrointestinal absorption of tetracycline. *Clin Pharmacol Ther* (1980) 28, 203–7.
4. Deppermann K-M, Lode H, Höffken G, Tschink G, Kalz C, Koeppe P. Influence of ranitidine, pirenzepine, and aluminum magnesium hydroxide on the bioavailability of various antibiotics, including amoxicillin, cephalexin, doxycycline, and amoxicillin-clavulanic acid. *Antimicrob Agents Chemother* (1989) 33, 1901–7.

Tetracyclines + Iron compounds

The absorption of both the tetracyclines and iron compounds is greatly reduced by concurrent use, leading to reduced serum concentrations of the tetracyclines. The therapeutic effectiveness of both might be reduced or even abolished.

Clinical evidence

(a) Effect on tetracyclines

An investigation in 10 healthy subjects given single oral doses of tetracyclines found that **ferrous sulfate** 200 mg decreased the serum antibacterial concentrations as follows: **doxycycline** 200 mg, 80 to 90%; **methacycline** 300 mg, 80 to 85%; **oxytetracycline** 500 mg, 50 to 60%; and **tetracycline** 500 mg, 40 to 50%.[1] Another study in two groups of 8 healthy subjects found that **ferrous sulfate** 300 mg reduced the absorption of **tetracycline** and **minocycline** by 81% and 77%, respectively.[2] Other studies found that in some instances iron caused the tetracycline serum concentrations to fall below minimum bacterial inhibitory concentrations.[3,4] If the iron was given 3 hours before or 2 hours after most tetracyclines, the serum concentrations were not notably reduced.[3-5] However, even when the iron was given up to 11 hours after **doxycycline**, serum concentrations were still lowered by 20 to 45%.[5] In contrast to this, another study found that four doses of **ferrous sulfate** (each equivalent to 80 mg of elemental iron) starting 11.5 hours after doxycycline did not affect the absorption of a 200-mg dose of **doxycycline**, and only reduced the AUC of a 100-mg dose of **doxycycline** by 17%.[6]

In 22 patients, an **iron polymaltose** complex, equivalent to 100 mg elemental iron, had no clinically relevant effect on the pharmacokinetics of a single 500-mg dose of **tetracycline**.[7]

A case report describes a 38-year-old HIV-positive man with a relapse of toxoplasmic encephalitis despite maintenance treatment with **minocycline** and clarithromycin. The patient was found to have a subtherapeutic plasma concentration of minocycline (0.3 mg/L, range 3 to 4 mg/L), thought to be the result of a drug interaction between **minocycline** and **ferrous oxalate**, a constituent of the *Disulone* tablets (also containing dapsone) he was taking for pneumocystis pneumonia prophylaxis.[8]

(b) Effect on iron

When **ferrous sulfate** 250 mg (equivalent to 50 mg of elemental iron) was given with **tetracycline** 500 mg, the absorption of iron was reduced by up to 78% in healthy subjects, and up to 65% in those with depleted iron stores.[9,10]

There was no change in the iron uptake into erythrocytes in 22 patients when an **iron polymaltose** complex, equivalent to 100 mg elemental iron, was given with a single 500-mg dose of **tetracycline**.[11]

Mechanism

The tetracyclines have a strong affinity for iron and form poorly soluble tetracycline/iron chelates, which are much less readily absorbed by the gut, and as a result the serum tetracycline concentrations achieved are much lower.[12,13] There is also less free iron available for absorption. Separating the administration of the two prevents their admixture.[3,4] However, doxycycline undergoes enterohepatic recycling, which could affect any attempt to keep the iron and antibacterial apart, although the importance of the enterohepatic recycling has been said to be minimal.[6] Even when given intravenously the half-life of doxycycline is reduced.[5] The different extent to which iron compounds interact with the tetracyclines appears to be a reflection of their ability to liberate ferrous and ferric ions, which are free to combine with the tetracycline.[14]

Importance and management

The interactions between the tetracyclines and iron compounds are well-documented, well-established, and of clinical importance. The 30 to 90% reductions in serum tetracycline concentrations that are caused by iron are so large that tetracycline concentrations might fall below the MIC,[4] possibly leading to treatment failure as in the case report. However, the extent of the reductions depends on a number of factors:

- *the particular tetracycline used:* tetracycline and oxytetracycline in the study cited above were the least affected;[1]

- *the time-interval between the administration of the two drugs:* giving the iron 3 hours before or 2 to 3 hours after the antibacterial is satisfactory with tetracycline itself,[3] but one study found that even 11 hours was inadequate for doxycycline;
- *the particular iron preparation used:* with tetracycline the reduction in serum concentrations with ferrous sulfate was 80 to 90%, with **ferrous fumarate, succinate,** and **gluconate,** 70 to 80%; with **ferrous tartrate,** 50%; and with **ferrous sodium edetate,** 30%. This was with doses containing equivalent amounts of elemental iron.[14] The small studies with **iron polymaltose** indicate that this preparation might have minimal interaction with tetracycline.

The interaction can therefore be accommodated by separating the doses as much as possible. It would also seem logical to choose one of the iron preparations causing minimal interference, but it seems unlikely that there will be a clinically relevant difference between those that are commonly available (i.e. sulfate, fumarate, and gluconate).

Only tetracycline, oxytetracycline, methacycline, minocycline, and doxycycline have been shown to interact with iron, but it seems reasonable to expect that the other tetracyclines will behave in a similar way.

1. Neuvonen PJ, Gothoni G, Hackman R, Björksten K. Interference of iron with the absorption of tetracyclines in man. *BMJ* (1970) 4, 532–4.
2. Leyden JJ. Absorption of minocycline hydrochloride and tetracycline hydrochloride. Effect of food, milk, and iron. *J Am Acad Dermatol* (1985) 12, 308–12.
3. Mattila MJ, Neuvonen PJ, Gothoni G, Hackman CR. Interference of iron preparations and milk with the absorption of tetracyclines. *Int Congr Ser* (1972) 254, 128–33.
4. Gothoni G, Neuvonen PJ, Mattila M, Hackman R. Iron-tetracycline interaction: effect of time interval between the drugs. *Acta Med Scand* (1972) 191, 409–11.
5. Neuvonen PJ, Penttilä O. Effect of oral ferrous sulphate on the half-life of doxycycline in man. *Eur J Clin Pharmacol* (1974) 7, 361–3.
6. Venho VMK, Salonen RO, Mattila MJ. Modification of the pharmacokinetics of doxycycline in man by ferrous sulphate or charcoal. *Eur J Clin Pharmacol* (1978) 14, 277–80.
7. Potgieter MA, Pretorius SG, Jacobs YL, Venter C, Venter JL, Geisser P. Effect of an oral iron(III)-hydroxide polymaltose complex on tetracycline pharmacokinetics in patients with iron deficiency anaemia. *Arzneimittelforschung* (2007) 57, 385–91.
8. Gallien S, Bigé N, Kitzis MD, Longuet P, Gervais A, Leport C. Drug-to-drug interaction between dapsone and minocycline: an unusual cause of relapse of toxoplasmic encephalitis in an HIV-infected patient. *Scand J Infect Dis* (2009) 41, 700–2.
9. Heinrich HC, Oppitz KH, Gabbe EE. Hemmung der Eisenabsorption beim Menschen durch Tetracyclin. *Klin Wochenschr* (1974) 52, 493–8.
10. Heinrich HC, Oppitz KH. Tetracycline inhibits iron absorption in man. *Naturwissenschaften* (1973) 60, 524–5.
11. Potgieter MA, Potgieter JH, Venter C, Venter JL, Geisser P. Effect of oral tetracycline on iron absorption from iron(III)-hydroxide polymaltose complex in patients with iron deficiency anaemia. *Arzneimittelforschung* (2007) 57, 376–84.
12. Albert A, Rees CW. Avidity of the tetracyclines for the cations of metals. *Nature* (1956) 177, 433–4.
13. Albert A, Rees C. Incompatibility of aluminium hydroxide and certain antibiotics. *BMJ* (1955) 2, 1027–8.
14. Neuvonen PJ, Turakka H. Inhibitory effect of various iron salts on the absorption of tetracycline in man. *Eur J Clin Pharmacol* (1974) 7, 357–60.

Tetracyclines + Kaolin-pectin

Kaolin-pectin reduces the absorption of tetracycline by about 50%.

Clinical evidence, mechanism, importance and management

Healthy subjects were given **tetracycline** 250 mg as a solution or as a capsule, with and without 30 mL of kaolin-pectin (*Kaopectate*). The absorption of both formulations was reduced by about 50% by the kaolin-pectin. Even when the kaolin-pectin was given 2 hours before or after the **tetracycline**, the drug absorption was still reduced by about 20%.[1] The likely reason for this interaction is that **tetracycline** becomes adsorbed onto the kaolin-pectin so that less is available for absorption.

If these two drugs are given together, consider separating the doses by at least 2 hours to minimise admixture in the gut. It may even then be necessary to increase the **tetracycline** dose. Information about other tetracyclines is lacking, but be aware that they may interact similarly.

1. Gouda MW. Effect of an antidiarrhoeal mixture on the bioavailability of tetracycline. *Int J Pharmaceutics* (1993) 89, 75–7.

Tetracyclines + Lanthanum

The bioavailability of tetracyclines is expected to be reduced by lanthanum, as concurrent use may result in the formation of insoluble chelates (as with other polyvalent cations). As a result, it is recommended that tetracyclines (the manufacturer names tetracycline and doxycycline) are not taken within 2 hours of a dose of lanthanum.[1]

1. Fosrenol (Lanthanum carbonate hydrate). Shire Pharmaceuticals Ltd. UK Summary of product characteristics, March 2013.

Tetracyclines + Metoclopramide

In 4 patients, metoclopramide 20 mg was found to double the rate of absorption and slightly reduce the maximum serum levels of a single 500-mg dose of tetracycline.[1] This appears to be of little clinical importance.

1. Nimmo J. The influence of metoclopramide on drug absorption. *Postgrad Med J* (1973) 49 (July Suppl), 25–8.

Tetracyclines + Quinapril

The absorption of tetracycline is reduced by the magnesium carbonate excipient in some quinapril formulations.

Clinical evidence

Quinapril, formulated as *Accupro*, contains **magnesium carbonate** as an excipient (250 mg in a 40 mg quinapril capsule, 47 mg in a 5 mg capsule). A pharmacokinetic study in 12 healthy subjects investigating the potential interaction between the **magnesium carbonate** in these capsules and **tetracycline** found that single doses of both strengths of *Accupro* capsules markedly reduced the absorption of **tetracycline**. The 5 mg and 40 mg *Accupro* capsules reduced the **tetracycline** AUC by 28% and 37%, respectively, and the maximum serum levels were reduced by 25% and 34%, respectively.[1]

Mechanism

The reason for these reductions in tetracycline levels is that the magnesium carbonate and the tetracycline form a less soluble chelate in the gut which is less well absorbed (see 'Tetracyclines + Antacids', p.359).

Importance and management

An established interaction but the extent of the reduction is only moderate and its clinical importance is uncertain. However, the authors of the study and the manufacturers[2] recommend that the concurrent use of *Accupro* and tetracycline should be avoided.[1] Other tetracyclines would be expected to behave similarly. One possible way to accommodate this interaction (as with the antacid interaction) is to separate the doses as much as possible (by about 2 to 3 hours) to minimise admixture in the gut.

Quinapril, formulated as *Quinil* tablets, contains **magnesium oxide**, and, based on the interaction with magnesium carbonate, the manufacturer advises that *Quinil* tablets should not be taken with tetracycline.[3]

1. Parke Davis Ltd. Data on file. Effect of magnesium-containing quinapril tablets on the single-dose pharmacokinetics of tetracycline in healthy volunteers; protocol 906–237, report RR 764–00872.
2. Accupro (Quinapril hydrochloride). Pfizer Ltd. UK Summary of product characteristics, June 2009.
3. Quinil (Quinapril hydrochloride). Tillomed Laboratories Ltd. UK Summary of product characteristics, May 2004.

Tetracyclines + Sucralfate

On theoretical grounds the absorption of tetracycline may possibly be reduced by sucralfate, but clinical confirmation of this appears to be lacking.

Clinical evidence, mechanism, importance and management

The manufacturers of sucralfate point out that it may reduce the bioavailability of **tetracycline**, probably because the two become bound together in the gut, thereby reducing absorption. It is suggested that they should be given 2 hours apart to minimise their admixture in the gut.[1] There do not appear to be any clinical reports in the literature confirming this potential interaction.

However, the formation of a **tetracycline**-sucralfate acid complex has been investigated in *animal* and *in vitro* studies and this indicates that the interaction may be clinically useful for *Helicobacter pylori* eradication because of direct delivery of **tetracycline** to the gastric mucosa for extended periods of time.[2-5]

1. Antepsin Suspension (Sucralfate). Chugai Pharma UK Ltd. UK Summary of product characteristics, September 2013.
2. Higo S, Ori K, Takeuchi H, Yamamoto H, Hino T, Kawashima Y. A novel evaluation method of gastric mucoadhesive property *in vitro* and the mucoadhesive mechanism of tetracycline-sucralfate acidic complex for eradication of *Helicobacter pylori*. *Pharm Res* (2004) 21, 413–9.
3. Higo S, Takeuchi H, Yamamoto H, Hino T, Kawashima Y. The acidic complexation of tetracycline with sucralfate for its mucoadhesive preparation. *Drug Dev Ind Pharm* (2004) 30, 715–24.
4. Yokel RA, Dickey KM, Goldberg AH. Selective adherence of a sucralfate-tetracycline complex to gastric ulcers: implications for the treatment of *Helicobacter pylori*. *Biopharm Drug Dispos* (1995) 16, 475–9.
5. Higo S, Takeuchi H, Yamamoto H, Hino T, Kawashima Y. Slow release of tetracycline from a mucoadhesive complex with sucralfate for eradication of *Helicobacter pylori*. *Chem Pharm Bull (Tokyo)* (2008) 56, 1412–16.

Tetracyclines + Thiomersal

Patients taking tetracyclines who use contact lens solutions containing thiomersal may experience an inflammatory ocular reaction.

Clinical evidence, mechanism, importance and management

The observation that 2 patients had ocular reactions (red eye, irritation, blepharitis) when they used a 0.004% thiomersal-containing contact lens solution while taking a tetracycline, prompted further study of this interaction. A questionnaire revealed another 9 similar cases that suddenly began shortly after patients who had used thiomersal-containing solutions for 6 months without problem started to take a tetracycline. In each case the reaction cleared when the thiomersal or the tetracycline was stopped. The same reaction was also clearly demonstrated in *rabbits*.[1] The reasons are not understood. It would seem prudent to avoid the concurrent use of these compounds.

1. Crook TG, Freeman JJ. Reactions induced by the concurrent use of thimerosal and tetracycline. *Am J Optom Physiol Opt* (1983) 60, 759–61.

Tetracyclines + Zinc compounds

The absorption of tetracycline can be reduced by as much as 50% by zinc sulphate. Doxycycline interacts minimally with zinc.

Clinical evidence

When **tetracycline** 500 mg was given to 7 subjects either alone or with zinc sulfate 200 mg (equivalent to 45 mg of elemental zinc) the **tetracycline** serum concentrations and AUC were reduced by about 30 to 40%.[1] This study was repeated with **doxycycline** 200 mg and zinc, but **doxycycline** absorption was not affected.[1] A reduction in **tetracycline** absorption of more than 50% has been seen in other studies when zinc was given concurrently.[2,3]

Tetracycline appears to cause minimal reductions in zinc concentrations.[2]

Mechanism

Zinc (like iron, calcium, magnesium and aluminium) forms a relatively stable and poorly absorbed chelate with tetracycline in the gut, which results in a reduction in the amount of antibacterial available for absorption.[4,5]

Importance and management

An established and moderately well documented interaction of clinical importance. Separate the administration of tetracycline and zinc compounds as much as possible to minimise admixture in the gut. In the case of iron (see 'Tetracyclines + Iron compounds', p.361), which interacts by the same mechanism, 2 to 3 hours is usually enough. Alternatively it would seem that doxycycline is less affected, so it may be a useful alternative.[1] Other tetracyclines would be expected to interact like tetracycline itself, but this needs confirmation. The small reduction in serum zinc concentrations is likely to be of little practical importance.[2]

1. Penttilä O, Hurme H, Neuvonen PJ. Effect of zinc sulphate on the absorption of tetracycline and doxycycline in man. *Eur J Clin Pharmacol* (1975) 9, 131–4.
2. Andersson K-E, Bratt L, Dencker H, Kamme C, Lanner E. Inhibition of tetracycline absorption by zinc. *Eur J Clin Pharmacol* (1976) 10, 59–62.
3. Mapp RK, McCarthy TJ. The effect of zinc sulphate and of bicitropeptide on tetracycline absorption. *S Afr Med J* (1976) 50, 1829–30.
4. Albert A, Rees CW. Avidity of the tetracyclines for the cations of metals. *Nature* (1956) 177, 433–4.
5. Doluisio JT, Martin AN. Metal complexation of the tetracycline hydrochlorides. *J Med Chem* (1963) 16, 16.

Tetracyclines; Doxycycline + Rifampicin (Rifampin)

Rifampicin may cause a marked reduction in doxycycline levels, which has led to treatment failures in some cases.

Clinical evidence

In 7 patients, rifampicin 10 mg/kg daily caused a considerable reduction in the serum levels of doxycycline 200 mg daily. The reduction was very marked in 4 patients but not significant in the other 3 patients. The AUC of doxycycline was reduced by 54%, its clearance was approximately doubled, and its half-life was reduced from about 14 hours to 9 hours.[1,2]

Five patients with brucellosis taking doxycycline 200 mg daily had a reduction in the doxycycline half-life from about 14.5 hours to 8 hours when they took rifampicin 200 mg daily.[3] Another study, in 20 patients treated for brucellosis, found that the mean AUC of doxycycline was nearly 60% lower in the presence of rifampicin, when compared with streptomycin. There were no treatment failures in the patients taking doxycycline and streptomycin, but two treatment failures occurred in the 10 patients taking doxycycline and rifampicin.[4]

A meta-analysis of 6 studies involving 544 patients with brucellosis found a significantly higher numbers of relapses and lower numbers of initial cures if doxycycline was given with rifampicin rather than streptomycin.[5]

Mechanism

Not established, but it seems almost certain that the rifampicin (a known potent enzyme inducer) increases the metabolism of the doxycycline thereby reducing its levels.

Importance and management

The interaction between doxycycline and rifampicin is established and of clinical importance. Monitor the effects of concurrent use and increase the doxycycline dose as necessary. No clinically important adverse interaction appears to occur between doxycycline and streptomycin.

1. Garraffo R, Dellamonica P, Fournier JP, Lapalus P, Bernard E, Beziau H, Chichmanian RM. Effet de la rifampicine sur la pharmacocinétique de la doxycycline. *Pathol Biol (Paris)* (1987) 35, 746–9.
2. Garraffo R, Dellamonica P, Fournier JP, Lapalus P, Bernard E. The effect of rifampicin on the pharmacokinetics of doxycycline. *Infection* (1988) 16, 297–8.
3. Bessard G, Stahl JP, Dubois F, Gaillat J, Micoud M. Modification de la pharmacocinetique de la doxycycline par l'administration de rifampicine chez l'homme. *Med Mal Infect* (1983) 13, 138–41.
4. Colmenero JD, Fernández-Gallardo LC, Agúndez JAG, Sedeño J, Benítez J, Valverde E. Possible implications of doxycycline-rifampin interaction for the treatment of brucellosis. *Antimicrob Agents Chemother* (1994) 38, 2798–2802.
5. Solera J, Martínez-Alfaro E, Sáez L. Metaanálisis sobre la eficacia de la combinación de rifampicina y doxiciclina en el tratamiento de la brucelosis humana. *Med Clin (Barc)* (1994) 102, 731–8.

Tetracyclines; Doxycycline + Simeticone

A study in 8 healthy subjects found that [simeticone] 2.25 g did not alter the bioavailability of a single 200-mg dose of doxycycline.[1]

1. Bistue C, Perez P, Becquart D, Vinçon G, Albin H. Effet du diméticone sur la biodisponibilité de la doxycycline. *Therapie* (1987) 42, 13–16.

Tetracyclines; Minocycline + Ethinylestradiol

There is some evidence that ethinylestradiol may accentuate the facial pigmentation that can be caused by minocycline.

Clinical evidence

Two teenage sisters with severe acne vulgaris, taking minocycline 50 mg four times daily for 14 days then 50 mg twice daily thereafter, developed dark-brown pigmentation in their acne scars when they took *Dianette* (cyproterone acetate and ethinylestradiol) for about 15 months.[1] The type of pigmentation was not identified because they both declined to have a biopsy, but in other cases it has been found to consist of haemosiderin, iron, melanin and a metabolic degradation product of minocycline.[1] Two other reports describe facial pigmentation in patients taking minocycline, two of whom were taking oral hormonal contraceptives containing ethinylestradiol.[2,3] Other young women who have developed minocycline pigmentation may also have been taking oral hormonal contraceptives because they fall into the right age-group, but this is not specifically stated in any of the reports.

Mechanism

Not understood. It seems possible that the facial pigmentation (melasma, chloasma) that can occur with hormonal contraceptives may have been additive with the effects of the minocycline.[1]

Importance and management

Evidence is very limited but it has been suggested that all patients given long-term minocycline treatment should be well screened for the development of pigmentation, particularly if they are taking other drugs such as the hormonal contraceptives that are known to induce hyperpigmentation.[1] Note that although isolated cases of contraceptive failure have been associated with the concurrent use of combined hormonal contraceptives and minocycline and other tetracyclines, no additional contraceptive precautions are necessary on concurrent use, see 'Combined hormonal contraceptives + Antibacterials', p.1162.

1. Eedy DJ, Burrows D. Minocycline-induced pigmentation occurring in two sisters. *Clin Exp Dermatol* (1991) 16, 55–7.
2. Ridgeway HA, Sonnex TS, Kennedy CTC, Millard PR, Henderson WJ, Gold SC. Hyperpigmentation associated with oral minocycline. *Br J Dermatol* (1982) 107, 95–102.
3. Prigent F, Cavelier-Balloy B, Tollenaere C, Civatte J. Pigmentation cutanée induite par la minocycline: deux cas. *Ann Dermatol Venereol* (1986) 113, 227–33.

Tetracyclines; Minocycline + Phenothiazines

An isolated report describes black galactorrhoea, which was attributed to an interaction between minocycline and perphenazine.

Clinical evidence, mechanism, importance and management

A woman taking minocycline 100 mg twice daily for 4 years to control pustulocystic acne, and also taking **perphenazine**, amitriptyline and diphenhydramine, developed irregular darkly pigmented macules in the areas of acne scarring and later began to produce droplets of darkly coloured milk. The milk was found to contain macrophages filled with positive iron-staining particles, assumed to be haemosiderin. The situation resolved when the drugs were withdrawn: the galactorrhoea within a week and the skin staining over 6 months.[1] Galactorrhoea is a known adverse effect of the phenothiazines and is due to an elevation of serum prolactin levels caused by the blockade of dopamine receptors in the hypothalamus. The dark colour appeared to be an adverse effect of the **minocycline**, which can cause haemosiderin to be deposited in cells, and in this instance to be scavenged by the macrophages that were then secreted in the milk. The general significance of this isolated case is unknown, but it seems likely to be small.

1. Basler RSW, Lynch PJ. Black galactorrhea as a consequence of minocycline and phenothiazine therapy. *Arch Dermatol* (1985) 121, 417–18.

Tetracyclines; Oxytetracycline + Pyridostigmine

When oxytetracycline 500 mg every 8 hours was given with pyridostigmine 30 mg every 8 hours the pharmacokinetics of both drugs were unchanged. There was an increase in erythrocyte cholinesterase activity when pyridostigmine was given with oxytetracycline, but the clinical significance of this finding is unclear.[1] It would appear that no dose adjustments are necessary on concurrent use.

1. Johnston A, Hedges A, Turner P. A study of the interaction between oxytetracycline and pyridostigmine. *Hum Toxicol* (1988) 7, 263–6.

Trimethoprim + Food or Guar gum

Guar gum and food can modestly reduce the absorption of trimethoprim suspension.

Clinical evidence, mechanism, importance and management

In a study over a 24-hour period, 12 healthy subjects were given a single 3-mg/kg oral dose of a trimethoprim suspension with food, with or without guar gum. The mean peak serum levels were reduced by food and by food given with 5 g of guar gum by 21% and 15%, respectively. Food, both with guar gum and alone, reduced the AUC of trimethoprim by about 22%.[1] The greatest individual reductions in peak serum levels and AUC were 44% and 36%, respectively with food, and 48% and 38%, respectively, with food and guar gum.[1] The reasons are not understood but it may be due to adsorption of the trimethoprim onto the food and guar gum.

The clinical importance of this interaction is uncertain but a modest reduction in absorption can occur in some individuals. However, trimethoprim is generally taken without regard to food, so this interaction would not appear to be significant in most patients.

1. Hoppu K, Tuomisto J, Koskimies O and Simell O. Food and guar decrease absorption of trimethoprim. *Eur J Clin Pharmacol* (1987) 32, 427–9.

Vancomycin + Colestyramine

Colestyramine may bind with vancomycin in the gut.

Clinical evidence, mechanism, importance and management

Colestyramine binds with vancomycin within the gut, thereby reducing its biological activity (about tenfold according to *in vitro* studies). The combination of vancomycin and colestyramine used to be used in antibacterial-associated colitis (now no longer recommended) and to overcome this interaction it was suggested that a vancomycin dose of 2 g daily should be used, and that administration of vancomycin and colestyramine should be separated as much as possible to minimise their admixture in the gut.[1] It is usually recommended that other drugs should be taken one hour before or 4 to 6 hours after colestyramine.

1. Taylor NS, Bartlett JG. Binding of *Clostridium difficile* cytotoxin and vancomycin by anion-exchange resins. *J Infect Dis* (1980) 141, 92–7.

Vancomycin + Indometacin

Indometacin reduces the renal clearance of vancomycin in premature neonates. This interaction does not appear to have been studied in adults.

Clinical evidence, mechanism, importance and management

In 6 premature neonates with patent ductus arteriosus given indometacin, the half-life of vancomycin 15 to 20 mg/kg given intravenously over one hour was found to be 24.6 hours, compared with only 7 hours in 5 other premature neonates without patent ductus arteriosus who were not given indometacin.[1] A second study, which included 4 premature infants who received vancomycin within 2 weeks of receiving indometacin for patent ductus arteriosus, suggested that only one of these infants had reduced vancomycin clearance as a result of indometacin use. This infant had received indometacin 4 days before starting vancomycin, and a 36-hour interval was required between doses to attain target vancomycin levels.[2] The reason for this effect is uncertain but it seems possible that the indometacin reduces the renal clearance of vancomycin. The authors of the first report suggest that the usual vancomycin maintenance dose should be halved if indometacin is also being used. If vancomycin therapeutic drug monitoring is possible it would be advisable to take levels and adjust the vancomycin dose and/or dosing interval accordingly. It is not known whether indometacin has the same effect on vancomycin in adults.

1. Spivey JM, Gal P. Vancomycin pharmacokinetics in neonates. *Am J Dis Child* (1986) 140, 859.
2. Asbury WH, Darsey EH, Rose WB, Murphy JE, Buffington DE, Capers CC. Vancomycin pharmacokinetics in neonates and infants: a retrospective evaluation. *Ann Pharmacother* (1993) 27, 490–6.

Vancomycin + Miscellaneous

The risk of nephrotoxicity and ototoxicity with vancomycin may possibly be increased if it is given with other drugs with similar toxic effects. There is some evidence to suggest that dobutamine, dopamine and furosemide can markedly reduce vancomycin serum levels following cardiac surgery.

Clinical evidence, mechanism, importance and management

A retrospective evaluation of the records of 18 critically ill patients in intensive care units following cardiac surgery, suggested that drugs with important haemodynamic effects (**dopamine**, **dobutamine**, **furosemide**) may lower the serum levels of vancomycin. It was noted that withdrawal of the interacting drugs was followed by an increase in the minimum steady-state serum levels of vancomycin, from 8.79 mg/L to 13.3 mg/L, despite no major changes in body-weight or estimated renal clearance. This resulted in a mean dose reduction of 4.26 mg/kg per day.

It is suggested that this interaction occurs because these drugs increase cardiac output, which increases the renal clearance of vancomycin, and therefore reduces its serum levels.[1] The clinical implication is that in this particular situation creatinine clearance is not as good a predictor of vancomycin clearance and consequently dose. Good therapeutic drug monitoring is needed to ensure that serum vancomycin levels are optimal. More confirmatory study is needed.

In addition, vancomycin is both potentially nephrotoxic and ototoxic, and its manufacturer therefore advises that it should be avoided with other drugs that have nephrotoxic potential, because the effects could be additive. They list **amphotericin B**, **aminoglycosides**, **bacitracin**, **colistin**, **polymyxin B** and **cisplatin**. They also list **etacrynic acid** and **furosemide** as potentially aggravating ototoxicity.[2] However, a review of 494 patients receiving **amphotericin B**, 57% of whom also received treatment with vancomycin, did not identify this combination as a risk factor for the development of nephrotoxicity.[3] In contrast, there is some evidence to suggest that additive nephrotoxicity can occur with the **aminoglycosides** (see 'Aminoglycosides + Vancomycin', p.305). The general warning issued by the manufacturers to monitor carefully therefore seems a reasonable precaution.

1. Pea F, Porreca L, Baraldo M, Furlanut M. High vancomycin dosage regimens required by intensive care unit patients cotreated with drugs to improve haemodynamics following cardiac surgical procedures. *J Antimicrob Chemother* (2000) 45, 329–35.
2. Vancomycin hydrochloride. Hospira UK Ltd. UK Summary of product characteristics, January 2008.
3. Harbarth S, Pestotnik SL, Lloyd JF, Burke JP, Samore MH. The epidemiology of nephrotoxicity associated with conventional amphotericin B therapy. *Am J Med* (2001) 111, 528–34.

Vancomycin + Theophylline

Theophylline appears not to interact with vancomycin in premature infants.

Clinical evidence, mechanism, importance and management

Five premature infants (mean gestational age of 25 weeks and weighing 1.1 kg) were given theophylline (serum levels of 6.6 mg/L) for apnoea of prematurity. It was found that the pharmacokinetics of vancomycin 20 mg/kg given every 12 to 18 hours for suspected sepsis were unchanged by the presence of the theophylline, when compared with previously published data on the pharmacokinetics of vancomycin in neonates.[1] There seems to be no other clinical reports about vancomycin with theophylline or aminophylline (which is metabolised to theophylline), and nothing to suggest that vancomycin has any effect on the serum levels of theophylline.

1. Ilagan NB, MacDonald JL, Liang K-C, Womack SJ. Vancomycin pharmacokinetics in low birth weight preterm neonates on therapeutic doses of theophylline. *Pediatr Res* (1996) 39, 74A.

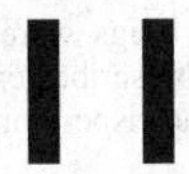

Anticholinesterases

The anticholinesterase drugs (or cholinesterase inhibitors) can be classified as **centrally-acting, reversible inhibitors** such as donepezil (used in the treatment of Alzheimer's disease), **reversible inhibitors with poor CNS penetration**, such as neostigmine (used in the treatment of myasthenia gravis), or **irreversible inhibitors**, such as ecothiopate and metrifonate. Note that organophosphorus insecticides are also potent cholinesterase inhibitors.

The centrally-acting anticholinesterases and the reversible anticholinesterases form the basis of this section, and these are listed in 'Table 11.1', below. Interactions where the anticholinesterases are affecting other drugs are covered elsewhere in the publication.

Centrally-acting anticholinesterases share a number of common pharmacodynamic interactions. The effects of anticholinesterases are expected to be additive with other cholinergic drugs or depolarising neuromuscular blockers, such as suxamethonium (succinylcholine), and antagonistic with antimuscarinic drugs or competitive (non-depolarising) neuromuscular blockers, such as tubocurarine (see 'Anticholinesterases; Centrally acting + Other drugs that affect acetylcholine', p.369). The concurrent use of anticholinesterases and drugs that slow the heart rate, such as beta blockers, some calcium-channel blockers, and some antiarrhythmics, might increase the risk of bradycardia, arrhythmias, or syncope. Anticholinesterases might have the potential to exacerbate or induce extrapyramidal symptoms, and so possibly increase the risk of adverse effects with antipsychotics (see 'Anticholinesterases; Centrally acting + Antipsychotics', p.366).

Due to their differing pharmacokinetic characteristics, the centrally-acting anticholinesterases have slightly different interaction profiles. Donepezil and galantamine are metabolised by CYP3A4 and CYP2D6, and so they might interact with ketoconazole (see "Anticholinesterases; Centrally acting + Quinidine', p.369), respectively. Rivastigmine, which is metabolised by conjugation, seems relatively free of *pharmacokinetic* interactions. Consideration of concurrent drug use would therefore seem to be an important factor in the choice of a centrally-acting anticholinesterase.

Table 11.1 Anticholinesterase drugs; reversible

Centrally-acting inhibitors used principally for Alzheimer's disease	*Inhibitors with poor CNS penetration used principally for myasthenia gravis*
Donepezil	Ambenonium
Galantamine	Distigmine
Rivastigmine	Edrophonium (mainly used diagnostically)
	Neostigmine
	Physostigmine
	Pyridostigmine (also used for glaucoma)

Anticholinesterases + Miscellaneous

A number of drugs can affect myasthenia gravis, often by increasing muscular weakness. This is, strictly speaking, a drug-disease interaction, but such effects might be expected to oppose the actions of the drugs used to treat myasthenia gravis. A number of drugs (e.g. chlorpromazine, methocarbamol, and propafenone) are clearly contraindicated in patients with myasthenia, and, as this is not strictly a drug interaction, they are not dealt with here. A number of case reports (see 'Table 11.2', p.367) describe the worsening or unmasking of myasthenia gravis with a range of different drugs. The evidence for many of these interactions is very sparse indeed, and in some instances they are simply rare and isolated cases. It would therefore be wrong to exaggerate their importance, but it would nevertheless be prudent to be alert for any evidence of worsening myasthenia if any of the drugs listed are added to established treatment.

Anticholinesterases + Ranitidine

In 10 patients with myasthenia gravis receiving long-term pyridostigmine, ranitidine 150 mg slightly reduced the renal clearance of pyridostigmine, but this was not statistically significant. Pyridostigmine plasma concentrations were unchanged.[1]

1. Eiermann, Sommer N, Winne D, Schumm F, Maier U, Breyer-Pfaff U. Renal clearance of pyridostigmine in myasthenic patients and volunteers under the influence of ranitidine and pirenzepine. *Xenobiotica* (1993) 23, 1263–75.

Anticholinesterases; Centrally acting + Amiodarone

The risk of adverse effects, including bradycardia, might be increased if a centrally-acting anticholinesterase is given with amiodarone.

Clinical evidence, mechanism, importance and management

An analysis of the French Pharmacovigilance Database for adverse drug reactions involving centrally-acting cholinesterases (**donepezil**, **galantamine**, and **rivastigmine**) up to March 2006 found 45 potential drug interactions between centrally-acting anticholinesterases and amiodarone. Eleven of these interactions were thought to have caused adverse reactions [probably bradycardia]. Inhibitors of CYP3A4, such as amiodarone, were also involved in pharmacokinetic interactions with **donepezil** and **galantamine**, which are substrates of this isoenzyme. However, the extent to which the plasma concentrations of donepezil and galantamine were increased is unknown.[1]

It would appear that the effects of these centrally-acting anticholinesterases on heart rate can be additive with those of amiodarone. Be alert for bradycardia if amiodarone is given with **donepezil**, **galantamine** or **rivastigmine**.

1. Tavassoli N, Sommet A, Lapeyre-Mestre M, Bagheri H, Montrastruc J-L. Drug interactions with cholinesterase inhibitors: an analysis of the French Pharmacovigilance Database and a comparison of two national drug formularies (Vidal, British National Formulary). *Drug Safety* (2007) 30, 1063–71.

Anticholinesterases; Centrally acting + Antipsychotics

No clinically relevant pharmacokinetic interaction appears to occur between risperidone and donepezil or galantamine, and the pharmacokinetics of thioridazine are not affected by donepezil. However, adverse effects such as movement disorders and neuroleptic malignant syndrome have occurred in patients given centrally-acting anticholinesterases with antipsychotics.

Clinical evidence

(a) Donepezil

1. Olanzapine. A 78-year-old man who had been taking olanzapine for 10 years experienced fatigue, progressive weakness, confusion, lethargy, and severe muscle stiffness within a week of starting to take donepezil. He was diagnosed as having a variant of neuroleptic malignant syndrome secondary to an interaction between the two drugs.[1]

2. Risperidone. In a randomised, crossover study, 24 healthy subjects were given risperidone 500 micrograms twice daily with donepezil 5 mg daily. Although donepezil caused slight changes in the exposure to risperidone and its metabolite, 9-hydroxyrisperidone, these were not considered clinically relevant. Concurrent use did not increase adverse effects.[2] In one study, 16 patients with schizophrenia taking risperidone were given donepezil 5 mg daily for 7 days without any alteration in their risperidone and 9-hydroxyrisperidone exposure. The pharmacokinetics of donepezil were similar in the risperidone-treated patients and healthy controls taking donepezil alone.[3] However, a case report describes the emergence of parkinsonian symptoms in an 80-year-old woman after she was given donepezil 5 mg daily, with risperidone 1 mg daily added 12 days later. Risperidone was discontinued and she recovered without treatment.[4] Similarly, another case report describes the onset of parkinsonian symptoms in a 69-year-old man taking risperidone 2 mg daily after he was given donepezil 10 mg daily for 4 weeks. Both drugs were stopped and the symptoms resolved after several days.[5] Another report describes extrapyramidal adverse effects in a 79-year-old woman taking donepezil and risperidone.[6]

3. Thioridazine. In a crossover study, 11 healthy subjects were given donepezil 5 mg daily for 16 days, with a single 50-mg dose of thioridazine on the final day. Although donepezil did not affect the pharmacokinetics of thioridazine or its effects on the QT interval, thioridazine, either alone or in combination with donepezil, was poorly tolerated, and resulted in postural hypotension and increases in heart rate.[7]

4. Tiapride. Severe parkinsonism developed in a 79-year-old woman taking tiapride 25 mg twice daily and donepezil 3 mg daily, after the dose of donepezil was increased to 5 mg daily. Both tiapride and donepezil were discontinued and, on the following day, her gait disturbance began to improve: in 10 days, she could walk without assistance and the rigidity had disappeared.[8]

(b) Galantamine

In a randomised, crossover study, 16 patients over 60 years of age were given a 14-day dose escalation of galantamine, after which they were given galantamine 12 mg twice daily with **risperidone** 500 micrograms twice daily, both for 13 doses. Although galantamine caused slight changes in the exposure to **risperidone** and its metabolite, 9-hydroxyrisperidone, their combined exposure (the active moiety) was unchanged. The combination was well tolerated.[9]

(c) Rivastigmine

A 58-year-old man receiving low-dose **olanzapine** and rivastigmine developed neuroleptic malignant syndrome 4 months after starting olanzapine and 6 weeks after his dose of rivastigmine was doubled to 6 mg twice daily. The patient fully recovered once the **olanzapine** was discontinued. **Olanzapine** was considered to be the probable cause of the patient's neuroleptic malignant syndrome, but it was suggested that rivastigmine might have contributed, possibly due to an acetylcholine/dopamine imbalance.[10]

In a study in 65 patients with Alzheimer's disease, 10 vascular dementia patients, and 15 mixed dementia patients, the patients were randomised to receive rivastigmine, **risperidone**, or both drugs together, for 20 weeks. No significant adverse events were reported on concurrent use.[11] However, a patient taking multiple drugs including **quetiapine**, **risperidone**, and rivastigmine experienced acute dystonia, which resolved over the next 48 hours after rivastigmine was discontinued and benzatropine given. Three days later, rivastigmine was restarted and the dystonia-like symptoms returned within 2 hours of her morning dose.[12]

Mechanism

Both antipsychotics and centrally-acting anticholinesterases can cause movement disorders and neuroleptic malignant syndrome when used alone, and these effects might be additive on concurrent use. In the case of donepezil and tiapride, it was suggested that the two drugs had caused an acetylcholine/dopamine imbalance in the striatum resulting in the symptoms seen.[8]

Importance and Management

Evidence for pharmacokinetic interactions between the centrally-acting anticholinesterases and antipsychotics is limited to the studies above. No clinically relevant pharmacokinetic interaction appears to occur between donepezil or galantamine and risperidone, and the pharmacokinetics of thioridazine are not affected by donepezil. However case reports have shown that adverse effects, such as movement disorders and neuroleptic malignant syndrome, can occur when centrally-acting anticholinesterases and antipsychotics are used together. Their concurrent use can be useful, and so need not be avoided, however patients given a centrally-acting anticholinesterase and any antipsychotic should be well monitored for antipsychotic adverse effects (such as extrapyramidal effects) and particularly for signs of neuroleptic malignant syndrome. It would seem prudent to use an alternative antipsychotic wherever possible if combinations are poorly tolerated, such as in the study above, when thioridazine was given with donepezil.

1. Warwick TC, Moningi V, Jami P, Lucas K, Molokwu O, Moningi S. Neuroleptic malignant syndrome variant in a patient receiving donepezil and olanzapine. *Nat Clin Pract Neurol* (2008) 4, 170–4.
2. Zhao Q, Xie C, Pesco-Koplowitz L, Jia X, Parier J-L. Pharmacokinetic and safety assessments of concurrent administration of risperidone and donepezil. *J Clin Pharmacol* (2003) 43, 180–6.
3. Reyes JF, Preskorn SH, Khan A, Kumar D, Cullen EI, Perdomo CA, Pratt RD. Concurrent administration of donepezil HCl and risperidone in patients with schizophrenia: assessment of pharmacokinetic changes and safety following multiple oral doses. *Br J Clin Pharmacol* (2004) 58, 50–7.
4. Liu H-C, Lin S-K, Sung S-M. Extrapyramidal side-effect due to drug combination of risperidone and donepezil. *Psychiatry Clin Neurosci* (2002) 54, 479.
5. Kang SH, Kim D-K. Drug induced parkinsonism caused by the concurrent use of donepezil and risperidone in a patient with traumatic brain injuries. *Ann Rehabil Med* (2013) 37,147–50.
6. Magnuson TM, Keller BK, Burke WJ. Extrapyramidal side effects in a patient treated with risperidone plus donepezil. *Am J Psychiatry* (1998) 155, 1458–9.
7. Ravic M, Warrington S, Boyce M, Dunn K, Johnston A. Repeated dosing with donepezil does not affect the safety, tolerability or pharmacokinetics of single-dose thioridazine in young volunteers. *Br J Clin Pharmacol* (2004) 58 (Suppl 1), 34–40.
8. Arai M. Parkinsonism onset in a patient concurrently using tiapride and donepezil. *Intern Med* (2000) 39, 863.
9. Huang F, Lasseter KC, Janssens L, Verhaeghe T, Lau H, Zhao Q. Pharmacokinetic and safety assessments of galantamine and risperidone after the two drugs are administered alone and together. *J Clin Pharmacol* (2002) 42, 1341–51.
10. Stevens DL, Lee MR, Padua Y. Olanzapine-associated neuroleptic malignant syndrome in a patient receiving concomitant rivastigmine therapy. *Pharmacotherapy* (2008) 28, 403–5.
11. Weiser M, Rotmensch HH, Korczyn AD, Hartman R, Cicin-Sain A, Anand R, and the Rivastigmine-Risperidone Study Group. A pilot, randomized, open-label trial assessing safety and pharmacokinetic parameters of co-administration of rivastigmine with risperidone in dementia patients with behavioral disturbances. *Int J Geriatr Psychiatry* (2002) 17, 343–6.
12. Pavlis CJ, Kutscher EC, Carnahan RM, Kennedy WK, Van Gerpen S, Schlenker E. Rivastigmine-induced dystonia. *Am J Health-Syst Pharm* (2007) 64, 2468–70.

Table 11.2 Case reports of drugs aggravating or unmasking myasthenia gravis

Drug	*Effect seen*	*Refs*
Acetazolamide 500 mg intravenously	Aggravation of muscular weakness in patients with myasthenia gravis taking unnamed anticholinesterases.	1
Ampicillin up to 1.5 g daily	Aggravation of myasthenic symptoms in 2 patients taking pyridostigmine.	2
Aspirin	Mild aggravation of myasthenic symptoms in a patient taking neostigmine.	3
Beta blockers	Deterioration in muscle strength in 2 patients taking pyridostigmine who were given timolol eye drops. Myasthenic symptoms in 3 patients (two taking propranolol and one taking oxprenolol). Fatal fulminant myasthenia gravis in a patient given acebutolol. In contrast 10 myasthenic patients with mild to moderate symptoms given intravenous propranolol 100 micrograms/kg without a worsening of neuromuscular transmission despite pyridostigmine dose reductions in 8 of those with mild symptoms.	4-8
Chloroquine	Persisting myasthenic symptoms, including muscular weakness, attributed to prior chloroquine use. Development of myasthenic symptoms in 3 patients, one who took chloroquine in overdose.	9-12
Ciprofloxacin	Aggravation of myasthenic symptoms in a patient taking pyridostigmine, and unmasking of myasthenia in one patient.	13,14
Dipyridamole* 75 mg three times daily	Aggravation of myasthenic symptoms in a patient taking distigmine.	15
Erythromycin 500 mg intravenously	Precipitation of a myasthenic crisis in an undiagnosed 15-year-old girl.	16
Imipenem/cilastatin 500 mg four times daily	Aggravation of myasthenic symptoms in a patient taking pyridostigmine.	17
Interferons	Development of myasthenia gravis in patients given interferon-alfa (5 patients), interferon-beta (2 patients) and peginterferon-alfa 2a (1 patient), and aggravation of myasthenic symptoms in 1 patient given interferon-beta.	18-25
Ketoprofen 50 mg daily	Aggravation of myasthenic symptoms in a patient taking neostigmine.	3
Lithium carbonate 600 mg daily	Unmasking of myasthenia in one patient.	26
Norfloxacin*	Aggravation of myasthenic symptoms in a patient taking pyridostigmine.	27
Oxytetracycline	Transient aggravation of myasthenic symptoms in one patient taking pyridostigmine.	28,29
Penicillamine	Aggravation of myasthenic symptoms in numerous patients taking anticholinesterases. Amitriptyline and imipramine also implicated in 2 cases.	30-33
Phenytoin 100 mg three times daily	Aggravation of myasthenic symptoms in an untreated patient.	34
Procainamide* 250 mg	Serious aggravation of myasthenic symptoms in a patient taking pyridostigmine. Two other less severe cases also reported.	35,36
Quinidine* up to 970 mg daily	Mild aggravation of myasthenic symptoms in one patient taking pyridostigmine and another taking neostigmine. Development of myasthenic symptoms in 2 undiagnosed patients.	36-38
Rolitetracycline	Aggravation of myasthenic symptoms in 4 patients, two patients taking various anticholinesterases (cases originally reported elsewhere).	28,29,39

*Drugs that should be used with caution in myasthenia gravis.

1. Carmignani M, Scoppetta C, Ranelletti OF, Tonali P. Adverse interaction between acetazolamide and anticholinesterase drugs at the normal and myasthenic neuromuscular junction level. *Int J Clin Pharmacol Ther Toxicol* (1984) 22, 140–4.
2. Argov Z, Brenner T, Abramsky O. Ampicillin may aggravate clinical and experimental myasthenia gravis. *Arch Neurol* (1986) 43, 255–6.
3. McDowell IFW, McConnell JB. Cholinergic crisis in myasthenia gravis precipitated by ketoprofen. *BMJ* (1985) 291, 1094.
4. Herishanu Y, Rosenberg P. Beta-blockers and myasthenia gravis. *Ann Intern Med* (1975) 83, 834–5.
5. Confavreux C, Charles N, Aimard G. Fulminant myasthenia gravis soon after initiation of acebutolol therapy. *Eur Neurol* (1990) 30, 279–81.
6. Verkijk A. Worsening of myasthenia gravis with timolol maleate eyedrops. *Ann Neurol* (1985) 17, 211–12.
7. Shaivitz SA. Timolol and myasthenia gravis. *JAMA* (1979) 242, 1611–12.
8. Jonkers I, Swerup C, Pirskanen R, Bjelak S, Matell G. Acute effects of intravenous injection of beta-adrenoreceptor- and calcium channel antagonists and agonists in myasthenia gravis. *Muscle Nerve* (1996) 19, 959–65.
9. De Bleecker J, De Reuck J, Quatacker J, Meire F. Persisting chloroquine-induced myasthenia? *Acta Clin Belg* (1991) 46, 401–6.
10. Robberecht W, Bednarik J, Bourgeois P, van Hees J, Carton H. Myasthenic syndrome caused by direct effect of chloroquine on neuromuscular junction. *Arch Neurol* (1989) 46, 464–8.
11. Sghirlanzoni A, Mantegazza R, Mora M, Pareyson D, Cornelio F. Chloroquine myopathy and myasthenia-like syndrome. *Muscle Nerve* (1988) 11, 114–19.
12. Pichon P, Soichot P, Loche D, Chapelon M. Syndrome myasthenique induit par une intoxication a la choroquine: une forme clinique inhabituelle confirmee par une atteinte oculaire. *Bull Soc Ophtalmol Fr* (1984) 84, 219–22.
13. Moore B, Safani M, Keesey J. Possible exacerbation of myasthenia gravis by ciprofloxacin. *Lancet* (1988) 1, 882.
14. Mumford CJ, Ginsberg L. Ciprofloxacin and myasthenia gravis. *BMJ* (1990) 301, 818.
15. Haddad M, Zelikovski A, Reiss R. Dipyridamole counteracting distigmine in a myasthenic patient. *IRCS Med Sci* (1986) 14, 297.
16. Absher JR, Bale JF. Aggravation of myasthenia gravis by erythromycin. *J Pediatr* (1991) 119, 155–6.
17. O'Riordan J, Javed M, Doherty C, Hutchinson M. Worsening of myasthenia gravis on treatment with imipenem/cilastatin. *J Neurol Neurosurg Psychiatry* (1994) 57, 383.
18. Batocchi AP, Evoli A, Servidei S, Palmisani MT, Apollo F, Tonali P. Myasthenia gravis during interferon alfa therapy. *Neurology* (1995) 45, 382–3.
19. Piccolo G, Franciotta D, Versino M, Alfonsi E, Lombardi M, Poma G. Myasthenia gravis in a patient with chronic active hepatitis C during interferon-α treatment. *J Neurol Neurosurg Psychiatry* (1996) 60, 348.
20. Mase G, Zorzon M, Biasutti E, Vitrani B, Cazzato G, Urban F, Frezza M. Development of myasthenia gravis during interferon-α treatment for anti-HCV positive chronic hepatitis. *J Neurol Neurosurg Psychiatry* (1996) 60, 348–9.
21. Oishi A, Miyamoto K, Kashii S, Yoshimura N. Retinopathy is not the only ocular symptom: myasthenia gravis in association with interferon therapy. *Br J Ophthalmol* (2005) 89, 1542–3.
22. Reffet A, Oddes B, Terrier F, Chauveau E, Casassus-Buihle D, Fraudin A. Survenue d'une crise myasthénique au cours du traitement par interféron d'une hépatite virale C. *Gastroenterol Clin Biol* (2007) 31, 1085–7.
23. Harada H, Tamaoka A, Kohno Y, Mochizuki A, Shoji S. Exacerbation of myasthenia gravis in a patient after interferon-β treatment for chronic active hepatitis C. *J Neurol Sci* (1999) 165, 182–3.
24. Dionisiotis J, Zoukos Y, Thomaides T. Development of myasthenia gravis in two patients with multiple sclerosis following interferon β treatment. *J Neurol Neurosurg Psychiatry* (2004) 75, 1079.
25. Borgia G, Reynaud L, Gentile I, Cerini R, Ciampi R, Dello Russo M, Piazza M. Myasthenia gravis during low-dose IFN-alpha therapy for chronic hepatitis C. *J Interferon Cytokine Res* (2001) 21, 469–70.
26. Neil JF, Himmelhoch JM, Licata SM. Emergence of myasthenia gravis during treatment with lithium carbonate. *Arch Gen Psychiatry* (1976) 33, 1090–2.
27. Rauser EH, Ariano RE, Anderson BA. Exacerbation of myasthenia gravis by norfloxacin. *DICP Ann Pharmacother* (1990) 24, 207–8.
28. Pittinger CB, Eryasa Y, Adamson R. Antibiotic-induced paralysis. *Anesth Analg* (1970) 49, 487–501.
29. Wullen F, Kast G, Bruck A. Über Nebenwirkungen bei Tetracyclin-Verabreichung an Myastheniker. *Dtsch Med Wochenschr* (1967) 92, 667–9.

Continued

Table 11.2 Case reports of drugs aggravating or unmasking myasthenia gravis (continued)

30. Vincent A, Newsom-Davis J, Martin V. Anti-acetylcholine receptor antibodies in D-penicillamine-associated myasthenia gravis. *Lancet* (1978) i, 1254.
31. Masters CL, Dawkins RL, Zilko PJ, Simpson JA, Leedman RJ, Lindstrom J. Penicillamine-associated myasthenia gravis, antiacetylcholine receptor and antistriational antibodies. *Am J Med* (1977) 63, 689–94.
32. Ferro J, Susano R, Gómez C, de Quirós FB. Miastenia inducida por penicilamina: ¿existe interacción con los antidepresivos tricíclicos? *Rev Clin Esp* (1993) 192, 358–9.
33. Russell AS, Linstrom JM. Penicillamine-induced myasthenia gravis associated with antibodies to acetylcholine receptor. *Neurology* (1978) 28, 847–9.
34. Brumlik J, Jacobs RS. Myasthenia gravis associated with diphenylhydantoin therapy for epilepsy. *Can J Neurol Sci* (1974) 1, 127–9.
35. Drachman DA, Skom JH. Procainamide - a hazard in myasthenia gravis. *Arch Neurol* (1965) 13, 316–20.
36. Kornfeld P, Horowitz SH, Genkins G, Papatestas AE. Myasthenia gravis unmasked by antiarrhythmic agents. *Mt Sinai J Med* (1976) 43, 10–14.
37. Stoffer SS, Chandler JH. Quinidine-induced exacerbation of myasthenia gravis in patient with Graves' disease. *Arch Intern Med* (1980) 140, 283–4.
38. Weisman SJ. Masked myasthenia gravis. *JAMA* (1949) 141, 917–18.
39. Gibbels E. Weitere Beobachtungen zur Nebenwirkung intravenöser Reverin-Gaben bei Myasthenia gravis pseudoparalytica. *Dtsch Med Wochenschr* (1967) 92, 1153–4.

Anticholinesterases; Centrally acting + Calcium-channel blockers

The risk of adverse effects, including bradycardia, might be increased if donepezil, galantamine, or rivastigmine are given concurrently with calcium-channel blockers.

Clinical evidence, mechanism, importance and management

An analysis of the French Pharmacovigilance Database for adverse drug reactions involving centrally-acting anticholinesterases (**donepezil**, **galantamine**, and **rivastigmine**) up to March 2006 found 40 potential drug interactions between centrally-acting anticholinesterases and calcium-channel blockers. Fifteen of these were thought to have caused adverse reactions [probably bradycardia]. CYP3A4 inhibitors such as **diltiazem** and **verapamil** were also involved in pharmacokinetic drug interactions with **donepezil** and **galantamine**, which are substrates of this isoenzyme. The extent to which the plasma concentrations of donepezil and galantamine were increased is unknown.[1] However, as the effects of the potent CYP3A4 inhibitor ketoconazole was only modest (see 'Anticholinesterases; Centrally acting + Ketoconazole or other CYP3A4 inhibitors', below), the effects of the moderate CYP3A4 inhibitors **diltiazem** and **verapamil** would not be expected to be clinically relevant.

It would appear that the effects of these centrally-acting anticholinesterases on heart rate can be additive with those of the calcium-channel blockers. Although not stated in the report, only the calcium-channel blockers that have effects on heart rate (that is, **diltiazem** and **verapamil**) would be expected to be implicated. However, in a case-control study of 161 patients taking cholinesterase inhibitors (mainly **donepezil**) admitted to hospital with a diagnosis of bradycardia, there was no increased risk in those who were also taking other drugs that slow the heart rate including beta blockers, digoxin, **diltiazem**, and **verapamil**. The odds ratio for hospitalisation for bradycardia was 2.13 for patients that had recently started a cholinesterase inhibitor and 2.34 in those also receiving other drugs that slow the heart rate.[2] Nevertheless, given that, rarely, case reports have described bradycardia, and that bradycardia is a known adverse effect of both the centrally-acting anticholinesterases and **diltiazem** and **verapamil**, it would be prudent to assume that some patients might be affected. Therefore, be alert for bradycardia on the concurrent use of these drugs and adjust treatment if necessary.

1. Tavassoli N, Sommet A, Lapeyre-Mestre M, Bagheri H, Montrastruc J-L. Drug interactions with cholinesterase inhibitors: an analysis of the French Pharmacovigilance Database and a comparison of two national drug formularies (Vidal, British National Formulary). *Drug Safety* (2007) 30, 1063–71.
2. Park-Wyllie LY, Mamdani MM, Li P, Gill SS, Laupacis A, Juurlink DN. Cholinesterase inhibitors and hospitalisation for bradycardia: a population-based study. *PLoS Med* (2009) 6, e1000157.

Anticholinesterases; Centrally acting + CYP3A4 inducers

Inducers of CYP3A4 might decrease donepezil plasma concentrations.

Clinical evidence, mechanism, importance and management

As **donepezil** is metabolised by CYP3A4, and its exposure is increased by the CYP3A4 inhibitor ketoconazole (see 'Anticholinesterases; Centrally acting + Ketoconazole or other CYP3A4 inhibitors', below), the UK and US manufacturers suggest that inducers of CYP3A4 might decrease **donepezil** exposure.[1,2] As the magnitude of the effect on donepezil exposure is unknown, such drug combinations should be used with care.[1] Bear the possibility of an interaction in mind if a reduced response to donepezil occurs on concurrent use. See 'Table 1.9', p.11 for a list of clinically relevant CYP3A4 inducers. Note that the manufacturers include dexamethasone as a CYP3A4 inducer, but dexamethasone does not usually cause clinically relevant interactions as a result of this effect.

1. Aricept (Donepezil hydrochloride). Eisai Ltd. UK Summary of product characteristics, January 2013.
2. Aricept (Donepezil hydrochloride). Eisai Inc. US Prescribing information, August 2013.

Anticholinesterases; Centrally acting + H_2-receptor antagonists

Cimetidine does not appear to affect the pharmacokinetics of donepezil or galantamine to a clinically relevant extent, and ranitidine does not affect the bioavailability of galantamine.

Clinical evidence, mechanism, importance and management

Centrally-acting anticholinesterases might be expected to increase gastric acid secretion due to increased cholinergic activity, but it is not clear whether this would oppose the actions of the H_2-receptor antagonists.

(a) Donepezil

In a crossover study, donepezil 5 mg daily was given to 18 healthy subjects with **cimetidine** 800 mg daily. It was found that after one week of concurrent use the maximum plasma concentration and AUC of donepezil were increased by 13% and 10%, respectively. Donepezil had no effect on the pharmacokinetics of **cimetidine**.[1] The changes in the pharmacokinetics of donepezil were not considered to be clinically relevant.[1]

(b) Galantamine

When a single 4-mg dose of galantamine was given on day 2 of a 3-day course of **cimetidine** 800 mg daily, the bioavailability of galantamine was increased by about 16%,[2] which would not be expected to be clinically relevant. **Ranitidine** 300 mg daily had no effect on galantamine bioavailability.[2]

1. Tiseo PJ, Perdomo CA, Friedhoff LT. Concurrent administration of donepezil HCl and cimetidine: assessment of pharmacokinetic changes following single and multiple doses. *Br J Clin Pharmacol* (1998) 46 (Suppl 1), 25–29.
2. Razadyne ER (Galantamine hydrobromide). Ortho-McNeil-Janssen Pharmaceuticals, Inc. US Prescribing information, July 2013.

Anticholinesterases; Centrally acting + HRT

Limited evidence suggests that oestrogens do not affect rivastigmine pharmacokinetics.

Clinical evidence, mechanism, importance and management

HRT did not enhance the response to **rivastigmine** in menopausal women with Alzheimer's disease.[1] **Rivastigmine** metabolism is minimally affected by the major cytochrome P450 isoenzymes, and analysis of population data from 70 subjects found that oestrogens did not affect **rivastigmine** pharmacokinetics.[2]

1. Rigaud AS, AndrÈ G, Vellas B, Touchon J, Pere JJ; French Study Group. No additional benefit of HRT on response to rivastigmine in menopausal women with AD. *Neurology* (2003) 60, 148–50.
2. Exelon (Rivastigmine tartrate). Novartis Pharmaceuticals Corp. US Prescribing information, July 2013.

Anticholinesterases; Centrally acting + Ketoconazole or other CYP3A4 inhibitors

Ketoconazole slightly increases the exposure to donepezil; other inhibitors of CYP3A4 might interact similarly. Galantamine exposure is increased by ketoconazole and is predicted to be increased by other potent CYP3A4 inhibitors. Erythromycin did not have a clinically relevant effect on the exposure to galantamine.

Clinical evidence, mechanism, importance and management

(a) Donepezil

Donepezil 5 mg daily was given to 18 healthy subjects with **ketoconazole** 200 mg daily, which is a specific and potent inhibitor of CYP3A4. After one week of concurrent use, the maximum plasma concentration and AUC of donepezil were increased by about 36%. Donepezil had no effect on the pharmacokinetics of **ketoconazole**.[1] None of the increases in donepezil exposure were considered to be clinically relevant, and the authors suggest that no dose modifications will be required on concurrent use with **ketoconazole** or other CYP3A4 inhibitors.[1] Despite this, the UK manufacturer recommends that donepezil should be used with care with CYP3A4 inhibitors[2] (see 'Table 1.9', p.11 for a list of clinically relevant CYP3A4 inhibitors).

(b) Galantamine

The UK and US manufacturers of galantamine note that **ketoconazole** increased the AUC of galantamine by 30%, probably by inhibiting CYP3A4, by which galantamine is metabolised.[3,4] The UK manufacturer therefore predicts that **ketoconazole** might increase the incidence of nausea and vomiting with galantamine, and suggests that, based on tolerability, a decrease in the maintenance dose can be considered.[3] Other potent CYP3A4 inhibitors would also be expected to increase the exposure to galantamine (see 'Table 1.9', p.11 for a list). Until the extent of the interaction with other potent CYP3A4 inhibitors is known, similar precautions as for ketoconazole seem prudent. **Erythromycin**, a moderate CYP3A4 inhibitor, only increased the AUC of galantamine by about 10%,[3,4] and so a clinically relevant interaction would not be expected on concurrent use. Other moderate CYP3A4 inhibitors (see 'Table 1.9', p.11

for a list) would not be expected to have a clinically relevant effect on the pharmacokinetics of galantamine, by this mechanism.

1. Tiseo PJ, Perdomo CA, Friedhoff LT. Concurrent administration of donepezil HCl and ketoconazole: assessment of pharmacokinetic changes following single and multiple doses. *Br J Clin Pharmacol* (1998) 46 (Suppl 1), 30–34.
2. Aricept (Donepezil hydrochloride). Eisai Ltd. UK Summary of product characteristics, January 2013.
3. Reminyl Tablets (Galantamine hydrobromide). Shire Pharmaceuticals Ltd. UK Summary of product characteristics, August 2013.
4. Razadyne ER (Galantamine hydrobromide). Ortho-McNeil-Janssen Pharmaceuticals, Inc. US Prescribing information, July 2013.

Anticholinesterases; Centrally acting + Memantine

Memantine does not appear to attenuate the anticholinesterase effects, nor affect the pharmacokinetics, of donepezil, galantamine, or rivastigmine. A case report describes PR-interval prolongation attributed to the concurrent use of donepezil and memantine.

Clinical evidence, mechanism, importance and management

(a) Donepezil

In a study, 19 healthy subjects were given memantine 10 mg before and on the last day of taking donepezil (5 mg daily for 7 days then 10 mg daily for 22 days). The pharmacokinetics of both drugs were not significantly affected by concurrent use, and the effects of donepezil on anticholinesterase were also unaffected.[1] Furthermore, a one-year efficacy and safety study reported that the combination is well tolerated and beneficial.[2]

A case report describes a 77-year-old woman with Alzheimer's disease who was started on a titrating dose of donepezil 10 mg daily. She developed PR-interval prolongation (of 240 milliseconds) after 30 days, which increased further (by 45 milliseconds) after being given memantine 5 mg daily on day 33. The memantine was stopped 3 days later, and on day 39 her PR-interval had decreased to 237 milliseconds. On day 75 her PR-interval had reduced to 208 milliseconds, but she was bradycardic so her donepezil dose was reduced to 5 mg daily. There was no change in the pharmacokinetics of either drug.[3] Donepezil and memantine are not known to cause PR-interval prolongation alone, however the authors state that the PR-interval prolongation seen might be due to combination of memantine with the donepezil dose increase.[3] Further study is required.

(b) Galantamine

A study in 15 healthy subjects found that the concurrent use of extended-release galantamine 16 mg daily with memantine 10 mg twice daily for 12 days did not affect the pharmacokinetics of galantamine and generally did not increase the incidence of adverse effects, although dizziness might have been more common.[4] Furthermore, a review of efficacy studies suggested that the effects of galantamine on anticholinesterase are unaffected by memantine, and that the combination is safe and generally well tolerated.[5]

(c) Rivastigmine

In vitro and *in vivo* studies demonstrate that the inhibition of cholinesterase by rivastigmine is not affected by the concurrent use of memantine.[6] A study in 16 patients with mild to moderate Alzheimer's disease taking rivastigmine 1.5 to 6 mg twice daily for 2 months or more found that memantine, increased in a gradual step-up approach to 10 mg twice daily, did not affect the pharmacokinetics of rivastigmine. The combination was well tolerated with adverse events being mild to moderate.[7]

1. Periclou AP, Ventura D, Sherman T, Rao N, Abramowitz WT. Lack of pharmacokinetic or pharmacodynamic interaction between memantine and donepezil. *Ann Pharmacother* (2004) 38, 1389–94.
2. Tariot PN, Farlow MR, Grossberg GT, Graham SM, McDonald S, Gergel I, for the Memantine Study Group. Memantine treatment in patients with moderate to severe Alzheimer Disease already receiving donepezil: a randomized controlled trial. *JAMA* (2004) 291, 317–24.
3. Igeta H, Suzuki Y, Motegi T, Sasaki A, Yokoyama Y, Someya T. Deterioration in donepezil-induced PR prolongation after a coadministration of memantine in a patient with Alzheimer's disease. *Gen Hosp Psychiatry* (2013) Epub.
4. Yao C, Raoufinia A, Gold M, Nye JS, Ramael S, Padmanabhan M, Walschap Y, Verhaeghe T, Zhao Q. Steady-state pharmacokinetics of galantamine are not affected by addition of memantine in healthy subjects. *J Clin Pharmacol* (2005) 45, 519–28.
5. Grossberg GT, Edwards KR, Zhao Q. Rationale for combination therapy with galantamine and memantine in Alzheimer's disease. *J Clin Pharmacol* (2006) 46, 17S–26S.
6. Exelon (Rivastigmine tartrate). Novartis Pharmaceuticals Corp. US Prescribing information, July 2013.
7. Shua-Haim J, Smith J, Picard F, Sedek G, Athalye S, Pommier F, Lefèvre G. Steady-state pharmacokinetics of rivastigmine in patients with mild to moderate Alzheimer's disease not affected by co-administration of memantine: an open-label, crossover, single-centre study. *Clin Drug Investig* (2008) 28, 361–74.

Anticholinesterases; Centrally acting + Other drugs that affect acetylcholine

The effects of centrally-acting anticholinesterases (e.g. donepezil) are expected to be additive with those of other anticholinesterases (e.g. neostigmine) and cholinergics (e.g. pilocarpine). The effects of centrally-acting anticholinesterases and drugs with antimuscarinic effects are expected to be antagonistic, but case reports have described the opposite effect.

Clinical evidence, mechanism, importance and management

Anticholinesterases increase acetylcholine concentrations: some are more selective for increasing acetylcholine concentrations in the brain (e.g. **donepezil**), whereas others (e.g. **neostigmine**, **pyridostigmine**) have a more generalised effect, see 'Table 11.1', p.365. Therefore, if both drugs are given together their effects might be expected to be additive. Similarly, additive effects might be expected if anticholinesterases are given with cholinergic drugs, such as **bethanechol** or **pilocarpine**, which mimic the effects of acetylcholine, and depolarising neuromuscular blockers such as **suxamethonium (succinylcholine)**, which act like acetylcholine to cause depolarisation. In contrast, competitive (non-depolarising) neuromuscular blockers (e.g. **tubocurarine**) compete with acetylcholine for receptors on the motor endplate of the neuromuscular junction and anticholinesterases such as neostigmine can oppose or reverse this blockade. See 'Neuromuscular blockers + Anticholinesterases', p.121, for reports of these interactions.

Drugs with **antimuscarinic** (anticholinergic) effects, which block the actions of acetylcholine, such as **atropine**, would be expected to oppose the actions of the anticholinesterases, and the findings of one long-term study suggested that concurrent use of these centrally-acting anticholinesterases and antimuscarinics might cause a greater rate of decline in cognitive function in patients with Alzheimer's disease.[1] Similar effects were found in another study in which urinary antimuscarinics (**oxybutynin**, **tolterodine**) were taken with **donepezil**, **rivastigmine**, or **galantamine**, although those with the lowest initial functional ability did not demonstrate any decline.[2] In another study, no decline in mental status was seen in patients taking centrally-acting anticholinesterases and antimuscarinics.[3]

In addition, an analysis of the French Pharmacovigilance Database for adverse drug reactions involving centrally-acting anticholinesterases (**donepezil**, **galantamine**, and **rivastigmine**) up to March 2006 found 118 potential drug-drug interactions with antimuscarinic drugs. Of these, 24 were thought to have caused adverse drug reactions,[4] although the exact nature of the adverse effects due to antimuscarinic drugs was not stated.

Case reports also describe an interaction between centrally-acting anticholinesterases and antimuscarinics. Two patients taking **donepezil** and one taking **rivastigmine** were given **tolterodine** (a urinary antimuscarinic). One patient (taking **donepezil**) developed confusion, while the other two developed delusional states. This is the opposite effect to the predicted interaction (where the anticholinesterase might be expected to oppose the antimuscarinic effects of **tolterodine**). The authors suggest that the combination causes 'cholinergic neurogenic hypersensitivity' similar to that seen as a withdrawal reaction to anticholinesterases.[5] In contrast, a case report describes the successful use of **tolterodine** 6 mg daily in a patient taking **donepezil** 10 mg daily. The authors of this report suggest that, despite the predictions of an interaction, a trial of an **antimuscarinic** for urinary incontinence might be worthwhile in patients taking centrally-acting anticholinesterases.[6]

Seizures have occurred in 2 patients taking the irreversible anticholinesterase, **metrifonate**, after antimuscarinics were started and then abruptly discontinued. One patient took **hyoscyamine** for about 10 days and then experienced a generalised tonic-clonic seizure approximately 36 hours after the hyoscyamine was stopped. Another patient taking metrifonate 60 mg daily for 6 weeks experienced seizures after she was prescribed **doxepin** cream for pruritus, which was applied liberally for 5 days.[7]

The authors suggested that, in both cases, excess cholinergic stimulation resulting in seizures was due to the abrupt discontinuation of the antimuscarinic and continued use of metrifonate.[7] It would therefore appear that the outcome of concurrent use is uncertain, but it would certainly be prudent to monitor the concurrent use of **donepezil**, **galantamine**, or **rivastigmine** and any cholinergic or antimuscarinic drug.

1. Lu C, Tune LE. Chronic exposure to anticholinergic medications adversely affects the course of Alzheimer disease. *Am J Geriatr Psychiatry* (2003) 11, 458–61.
2. Sink KM, Thomas J, Xu H, Craig B, Kritchevsky S, Sands LP. Dual use of bladder anticholinergics and cholinesterase inhibitors: long-term functional and cognitive outcomes. *J Am Geriatr Soc* (2008) 56, 847–53.
3. Bottiggi KA, Salazar JC, Yu L, Caban-Holt AM, Ryan M, Schmitt FA. Concomitant use of medications with anticholinergic properties and acetylcholinesterase inhibitors: impact on cognitive and physical functioning in Alzheimer disease. *Am J Geriatr Psychiatry* (2007) 15, 357–9.
4. Tavassoli N, Sommet A, Lapeyre-Mestre M, Bagheri H, Montrastruc J-L. Drug interactions with cholinesterase inhibitors: an analysis of the French Pharmacovigilance Database and a comparison of two national drug formularies (Vidal, British National Formulary). *Drug Safety* (2007) 30, 1063–71.
5. Edwards KR, O'Connor JT. Risk of delirium with concomitant use of tolterodine and acetylcholinesterase inhibitors. *J Am Geriatr Soc* (2002) 50, 1165–6.
6. Siegler EL, Reidenberg M. Treatment of urinary incontinence with anticholinergics in patients taking cholinesterase inhibitors for dementia. *Clin Pharmacol Ther* (2004) 75, 484–8.
7. Piecoro LT, Wermeling DP, Schmitt FA, Ashford JW. Seizures in patients receiving concomitant antimuscarinics and acetylcholinesterase inhibitor. *Pharmacotherapy* (1998) 18, 1129–32.

Anticholinesterases; Centrally acting + Quinidine

Quinidine inhibits the metabolism of galantamine, and is predicted to inhibit the metabolism of donepezil.

Clinical evidence, mechanism, importance and management

(a) Donepezil

In vitro study has shown that quinidine (an inhibitor of CYP2D6) inhibits donepezil metabolism[1,2] and, as no clinical information is available, the UK manufacturer suggests care with the combination:[1] increased donepezil concentrations and adverse effects are theoretically possible.

(b) Galantamine

A study in 8 healthy subjects given a single 10-mg dose of galantamine found that almost 20% of a dose of galantamine is excreted in the urine as *O*-demethylgalantamine glucuronide. Four of the 8 subjects were then given quinidine 250 mg twice daily for 2 days, with a single 15-mg dose of galantamine on day 2. Quinidine abolished the excretion of *O*-demethylgalantamine glucuronide in 3 subjects, and substantially reduced it in the fourth. The cumulative urinary recovery of unchanged galantamine increased by 60% in the presence of quinidine.[3] Quinidine is a known potent inhibitor of CYP2D6, by which galantamine is metabolised. Concurrent use therefore decreases the metabolism of galantamine. This would be expected to result in increased plasma concentrations of galantamine, but this does not appear to have been assessed in this study. A population pharmacokinetic analysis of a database of 852 patients with Alzheimer's disease, showed that the clearance of galantamine was decreased by about 25 to 33% by CYP2D6 inhibitors, including 7 patients receiving quinidine.[4] Consequently the UK manufacturer of galantamine suggests that the concurrent use of quinidine might result in increased adverse effects (mainly nausea and vomiting), and, if this occurs, a reduction in the maintenance dose of galantamine should be considered.[5] This seems prudent.

1. Aricept (Donepezil hydrochloride). Eisai Ltd. UK Summary of product characteristics, January 2013.
2. Aricept (Donepezil hydrochloride). Eisai Inc. US Prescribing information, August 2013.
3. Bachus R, Bickel U, Thomsen T, Roots I, Kewitz H. The *O*-demethylation of the antidementia drug galanthamine is catalysed by cytochrome P450 2D6. *Pharmacogenetics* (1999) 9, 661–8.
4. Razadyne ER (Galantamine hydrobromide). Ortho-McNeil-Janssen Pharmaceuticals, Inc. US Prescribing information, July 2013.
5. Reminyl Tablets (Galantamine hydrobromide). Shire Pharmaceuticals Ltd. UK Summary of product characteristics, August 2013.

Anticholinesterases; Centrally acting + SSRIs

Paroxetine and fluoxetine might increase donepezil and galantamine exposure. Sertraline does not appear to have a pharmacokinetic interaction with donepezil; concurrent use seems generally well tolerated, although there might be an increase in gastrointestinal adverse effects, and one report describes hepatotoxicity. No pharmacokinetic interaction occurs between rivastigmine and fluoxetine.

Clinical evidence, mechanism, importance and management

(a) Donepezil

Two case reports suggest that donepezil and **paroxetine** might interact, in one case with an increase in gastrointestinal adverse effects, and the other with increased CNS effects. These adverse effects were thought to occur because **paroxetine** might inhibit donepezil metabolism by CYP2D6.[1] A further report describes a patient taking **paroxetine** for 6 months who developed hypertonic limbs and severe gait disorders when donepezil 5 to 10 mg daily was also given.[2] The UK manufacturer of donepezil logically predicts that **fluoxetine** (a potent CYP2D6 inhibitor) could also inhibit the metabolism of donepezil, and until more information is available, they suggest care should be taken on the concurrent use of donepezil and CYP2D6 inhibitors[3] (see 'Table 1.7', p.9 for a list).

In a crossover study, 16 healthy subjects were given **sertraline** (50 mg daily increasing after 5 days to 100 mg daily) with donepezil 5 mg daily for 15 days. The pharmacokinetics of both drugs were not notably altered by concurrent use, and, although there was some indication that gastrointestinal adverse effects might have been increased, overall adverse effects were not changed.[4] Another study similarly found that the concurrent use of donepezil and **sertraline** was well tolerated with a relatively low incidence of adverse effects, although diarrhoea was noticeably more common with concurrent use than with donepezil alone.[5] A case report describes an 83-year-old woman taking **sertraline** 200 mg daily, who developed drug-induced cholestatic jaundice within 10 days of starting donepezil 5 mg daily. The authors suggest that although this reaction could have been in response to either drug, it might also have been precipitated by their concurrent use. The general significance of this report is unclear.[6]

(b) Galantamine

The UK and US manufacturers[7,8] note that an interaction study found that **paroxetine** 20 mg daily for 16 days increased the bioavailability of galantamine by about 40%, by inhibiting galantamine metabolism by CYP2D6. The UK manufacturer warns about the increased risk of galantamine adverse effects (in particular nausea and vomiting) if **paroxetine** is added, and suggests a reduction in the galantamine dose, based on tolerability.[7] They also predict that other SSRIs that are potent inhibitors of CYP2D6 might interact similarly[7] (see 'Table 1.7', p.9 for a list).

A population pharmacokinetic analysis of a database of 852 patients with Alzheimer's disease showed that the clearance of galantamine was decreased by about 25 to 33% by the concurrent use of several drugs, including **fluoxetine** (48 patients) and **fluvoxamine** (14 patients),[8] although it should be noted that **fluvoxamine** is not an inhibitor of CYP2D6. So far there appear to be no reports of adverse reactions with any of these drugs.

(c) Rivastigmine

The UK and US manufacturers of rivastigmine report that in studies in healthy subjects no pharmacokinetic interaction was seen between rivastigmine and **fluoxetine**.[9,10] No dose adjustment of either drug would appear necessary with concurrent use.

1. Carrier L. Donepezil and paroxetine: possible drug interaction. *J Am Geriatr Soc* (1999) 47, 1037.
2. Carcenac D, Martin-Hunyadi C, Kiesmann M, Demuynck-Roegel C, Alt M, Kuntzmann F. Syndrome extrapyramidal sous donepezil. *Presse Med* (2000) 29, 992–3.
3. Aricept (Donepezil hydrochloride). Eisai Ltd. UK Summary of product characteristics, January 2013.
4. Nagy CF, Kumar D, Perdomo CA, Wason S, Cullen EI, Pratt RD. Concurrent administration of donepezil HCl and sertraline HCl in healthy volunteers: assessment of pharmacokinetic changes and safety following single and multiple oral doses. *Br J Clin Pharmacol* (2004) 58 (Suppl 1), 25–33.
5. Finkel SI, Mintzer JE, Dysken M, Krishnan KRR, Burt T, McRae T. A randomized, placebo-controlled study of the efficacy and safety of sertraline in the treatment of the behavioral manifestations of Alzheimer's disease in outpatients treated with donepezil. *Int J Geriatr Psychiatry* (2004) 19, 9–18.
6. Verrico MM, Nace DA, Towers AL. Fulminant chemical hepatitis possibly associated with donepezil and sertraline therapy. *J Am Geriatr Soc* (2000) 48, 1659–63.
7. Reminyl Tablets (Galantamine hydrobromide). Shire Pharmaceuticals Ltd. UK Summary of product characteristics, August 2013.
8. Razadyne ER (Galantamine hydrobromide). Ortho-McNeil-Janssen Pharmaceuticals, Inc. US Prescribing information, July 2013.
9. Exelon (Rivastigmine hydrogen tartrate). Novartis Pharmaceuticals UK Ltd. UK Summary of product characteristics, April 2013.
10. Exelon (Rivastigmine tartrate). Novartis Pharmaceuticals Corp. US Prescribing information, July 2013.

Anticholinesterases; Centrally acting + Tobacco

Smoking tobacco increases the clearance of rivastigmine.

Clinical evidence, mechanism, importance and management

The US manufacturer[1] notes that population pharmacokinetic analysis (75 smokers and 549 non-smokers) showed that nicotine use increases **rivastigmine** clearance by 23%. Tobacco smoke contains aromatic hydrocarbons that are inducers of CYP1A2, but as rivastigmine is not metabolised by this isoenzyme, other mechanisms might have a part to play. **Donepezil** and **galantamine** are also not metabolised by CYP1A2, and therefore are not expected to interact with tobacco smoke by this mechanism.

One observational study has suggested that patients with Alzheimer's disease who are smokers might be more likely to have an improved response to the digit symbol substitution test (a psychomotor test) when taking centrally-acting anticholinesterases than non-smokers; however, this was not associated with improved functional ability.[2] Furthermore, smoking might also increase the risk of dementia and cognitive decline.[3]

1. Exelon (Rivastigmine tartrate). Novartis Pharmaceuticals Corp. US Prescribing information, July 2013.
2. Connelly PJ, Prentice NP. Current smoking and response to cholinesterase inhibitor therapy in Alzheimer's disease. *Dementia Geriatr Cogn Disord* (2005) 19, 11–14.
3. Duron E, Hanon O. Vascular risk factors, cognitive decline, and dementia. *Vasc Health Risk Manag* (2008) 4, 363–81.

Anticholinesterases; Centrally acting + Tricyclic antidepressants

Amitriptyline reduces the clearance of galantamine. The antimuscarinic effects of tricyclics might be additive with those of the centrally-acting anticholinesterases.

Clinical evidence, mechanism, importance and management

A population pharmacokinetic analysis of a database of 852 patients with Alzheimer's disease found that the clearance of **galantamine** was decreased by about 25 to 33% by the concurrent use of inhibitors of CYP2D6, which was said to include 17 patients receiving **amitriptyline**.[1] However, note that amitriptyline is more usually considered a substrate, rather than an inhibitor of this isoenzyme. Further, the effects of a reduction in clearance of galantamine of this magnitude do not appear to have been studied.

Also, note that amitriptyline and other tricyclic antidepressants have antimuscarinic adverse effects, which might affect the actions of the centrally-acting anticholinesterases, see 'Anticholinesterases; Centrally acting + Other drugs that affect acetylcholine', p.369.

1. Razadyne ER (Galantamine hydrobromide). Ortho-McNeil-Janssen Pharmaceuticals, Inc. US Prescribing information, July 2013.

Donepezil + Ginkgo (*Ginkgo biloba*)

Ginkgo does not appear to affect the pharmacokinetics or effects of donepezil.

Clinical evidence, mechanism, importance and management

In a pharmacokinetic study, 14 elderly patients with Alzheimer's disease were given donepezil 5 mg daily for at least 20 weeks, after which ginkgo extract 90 mg daily was also given for a further 30 days. Concurrent use did not affect the pharmacokinetics or cholinesterase activity of donepezil, and cognitive function appeared to be unchanged.[1] Therefore, over the course of 30 days, concurrent use appears neither beneficial nor detrimental.

1. Yasui-Furukori N, Furukori H, Kaneda A, Kaneko S, Tateishi T. The effects of *Ginkgo biloba* extracts on the pharmacokinetics and pharmacodynamics of donepezil. *J Clin Pharmacol* (2004) 44, 538–42.

Rivastigmine + Diazepam

Rivastigmine does not appear to affect the pharmacokinetics of diazepam.

Clinical evidence, mechanism, importance and management

The UK and US manufacturers of rivastigmine state that no pharmacokinetic interaction has been seen with diazepam in healthy subjects.[1,2] No diazepam dose adjustments would seem necessary if rivastigmine is also given.

1. Exelon (Rivastigmine hydrogen tartrate). Novartis Pharmaceuticals UK Ltd. UK Summary of product characteristics, April 2013.
2. Exelon (Rivastigmine tartrate). Novartis Pharmaceuticals Corp. US Prescribing information, July 2013.

12 Anticoagulants

The blood clotting process

When blood is lost or clotting is initiated in some other way, a complex cascade of biochemical reactions is set in motion, which ends in the formation of a network or clot of insoluble protein threads enmeshing the blood cells. These threads are produced by the polymerisation of the molecules of fibrinogen (a soluble protein present in the plasma) into threads of insoluble fibrin. The penultimate step in the chain of reactions requires the presence of an enzyme, thrombin, which is produced from its precursor prothrombin, already present in the plasma. This is initiated by factor III (tissue thromboplastin), and subsequently involves various factors including activated factor VII, IX, X, XI, and XII, and is inhibited by antithrombin III. Platelets are also involved in the coagulation process. Fibrinolysis is the mechanism of dissolution of fibrin clots, which can be promoted with thrombolytics. For further information on platelet aggregation and clot dissolution, see 'Antiplatelet drugs and Thrombolytics', p.776.

Mode of action of the anticoagulants

Anticoagulants can be divided into direct anticoagulants, which have an immediate effect, and the indirect anticoagulants, which inhibit the formation of coagulation factors, so have a delayed effect as they do not inactivate coagulation factors already formed. See 'Table 12.1', below, for a list.

(a) Direct anticoagulants

The direct anticoagulants include **heparin**, which principally enhances the effect of antithrombin III, thereby inhibiting the effect of thrombin (factor IIa) and activated factor X (factor Xa). **Low-molecular-weight heparins** are salts of fragments of heparin and act similarly, except that they have a greater effect on factor Xa than factor IIa. They have a longer duration of action than heparin and usually require less monitoring. The **heparinoids** (such as **danaparoid**) are similar.

A more recent introduction is the activated factor X inhibitors, the first of which was the synthetic polysaccharide **fondaparinux**, which is given subcutaneously. The oral activated factor X inhibitors **apixaban**, **edoxaban**, and **rivaroxaban** are structurally different to fondaparinux, but essentially act in a similar way.

The other group of direct anticoagulants are the **thrombin inhibitors**, which bind to the active thrombin site. These include recombinant forms or synthetic analogues of **hirudin**, such as **bivalirudin** and **lepirudin**. They also include **argatroban**, which is given intravenously, and the oral thrombin inhibitor, **dabigatran etexilate**, the prodrug of **dabigatran**. **Melagatran**, and its oral prodrug **ximelagatran**, act similarly, but have been withdrawn because of liver toxicity.

(b) Indirect anticoagulants

The indirect anticoagulants inhibit the vitamin K-dependent synthesis of factors VII, IX, X and II (prothrombin) in the liver, and are also referred to as **vitamin K antagonists**. The most commonly used are the **coumarins**, principally warfarin, but also acenocoumarol and phenprocoumon. Their target site of action is vitamin K epoxide reductase complex subunit 1 (VKORC1), and increasing evidence suggests that genetic polymorphisms in VKORC1 affect dose-requirements. The **indanediones**, such as phenindione, are now less frequently used. For many decades, the indirect anticoagulants have had the advantage over direct anticoagulants as they are orally active. They are often therefore referred to as **oral anticoagulants**, but this term has become misleading with the development of direct-acting oral anticoagulants, such as apixaban, dabigatran, edoxaban, and rivaroxaban, which have different monitoring requirements and interactions.

Coagulation tests

During anticoagulant therapy the aim is to give protection against intravascular clotting, without too great a risk of bleeding. To achieve this, doses of heparin and oral anticoagulants should be individually titrated until the desired response is attained. With the coumarin and indanedione oral anticoagulants, this procedure normally takes several days because they do not

Table 12.1 Anticoagulants

Class	*Drugs*
Parenteral anticoagulants	
Activated Factor X inhibitor	Fondaparinux sodium
Heparins	
Heparin	Heparin calcium, Heparin sodium
Low-molecular weight heparins	Bemiparin, Certoparin, Dalteparin, Enoxaparin, Nadroparin, Parnoparin, Reviparin, Tinzaparin
Heparinoids	Danaparoid, Dermatan sulphate, Pentosan polysulfate, Suleparoid, Sulodexide
Thrombin inhibitors, direct	
Hirudin analogues and recombinant hirudins	Bivalirudin, Desirudin, Lepirudin
Synthetic thrombin inhibitors	Argatroban
Oral anticoagulants	
Activated Factor X inhibitors	Apixaban, Edoxaban, Rivaroxaban
Thrombin inhibitors, direct	Dabigatran etexilate
Vitamin K antagonists	
Coumarins	Acenocoumarol, Dicoumarol, Ethyl biscoumacetate, Phenprocoumon, Warfarin
Indanediones	Fluindione, Phenindione

act directly on the blood clotting factors already in circulation, but on the rate of synthesis of new factors by the liver. The successful titration is determined by one of a number of different but closely related laboratory tests, see 'Table 12.2', below, and under the subsections below. Note that routine monitoring of the anticoagulant effect is not required for low-molecular weight heparins or heparinoids, except in patients at increased risk of bleeding such as those with renal impairment; or those who are overweight. Also, note that these tests cannot be used to monitor the anticoagulant effect of fondaparinux or the direct thrombin inhibitors, but these drugs do not require routine anticoagulant monitoring.

(a) Prothrombin time

The prothrombin time test (PT, Pro-Time, tissue factor induced coagulation time) is the most common coagulation test employed in clinical situations. It measures the time taken for a fibrin clot to form in a citrated plasma sample containing calcium ions and tissue thromboplastin. The PT is usually reported as the International Normalised Ratio (INR).

1. International normalised ratio (INR). The INR was adopted by the WHO in 1982 to standardise (using the International Sensitivity Index) oral anticoagulant therapy to take into account the sensitivities of the different thromboplastins used in laboratories across the world. The formula for calculating the INR is as follows:

INR = (patient's prothrombin time in seconds/mean normal prothrombin time in seconds)^{ISI}

The PT values obtained from the patient's sample are compared to a control, and this gives the INR. The higher the INR, the higher the PT value so if the patient's ratio is 2, this means the PT (and therefore clotting) is twice as long as the normal plasma. The British Corrected Ratio is essentially the same, but was calculated to a standard British thromboplastin.

2. Quick Value. The Quick Value (also called Quick time) is expressed as a percentage; the lower the value, the longer the blood takes to coagulate. Therefore as the Quick Value increases, the corresponding INR value gets smaller and vice versa.

(b) Activated partial thromboplastin time

The activated partial thromboplastin time (aPTT) is the second most common method for monitoring anticoagulant therapy, measuring all the clotting factors in the intrinsic pathway as opposed to the PT test, which measures the extrinsic pathway.

(c) Other methods of assessing clotting

Other tests used, which in some instances offer more sensitivity to specific aspects of therapy, include the prothrombin-proconvertin ratio (PP), the thrombotest, the thrombin clotting time test (TCT) the activated clotting time (ACT or activated coagulation time), the platelet count and the bleeding time test. The use of the most appropriate test will depend on the situation and the desired result.

Anticoagulant interactions

Stable oral anticoagulant therapy is difficult to achieve even during close monitoring. For example, in one controlled study in patients with atrial fibrillation, only 61% of INR values were within the target range of 2 to 3, despite monitoring the INR monthly and adjusting the warfarin dose appropriately.[1] A large number of factors can influence levels of coagulation, including diet, disease (fever, diarrhoea, heart failure, thyroid dysfunction), and the use of other drugs. It must therefore be remembered that it is particularly difficult to ascribe a change in INR specifically to a drug interaction in a single case report, and single case reports or a few isolated reports for widely used drugs do not prove that an interaction occurs. Nevertheless, either the addition or the withdrawal of drugs may upset the balance in a patient already well stabilised on an anticoagulant. Some drugs are well known to increase the activity of the anticoagulants and can cause bleeding if the dose of the anticoagulant is not reduced appropriately. Others reduce the activity and return the prothrombin time to normal. Both situations are serious and may be fatal, although excessive hypoprothrombinaemia manifests itself more obviously and immediately as bleeding and is usually regarded as the more serious. The interaction mechanism may be pharmacodynamic or pharmacokinetic: pharmacokinetic mechanisms are particularly well established and important for coumarin anticoagulants.

(a) Metabolism of the coumarins

The coumarins, warfarin, phenprocoumon and acenocoumarol, are racemic mixtures of *S*- and *R*-enantiomers. The *S*-enantiomers of these coumarins have several times more anticoagulant activity than the *R*-enantiomers. Reports suggest for example, that *S*-warfarin is three to five times more potent a vitamin K antagonist than *R*-warfarin. The *S*-enantiomer of warfarin is metabolised primarily by the cytochrome P450 isoenzyme CYP2C9. The metabolism of *R*-warfarin is more complex, but this enantiomer is primarily metabolised by CYP1A2, CYP3A4, CYP2C19 and CYP2C8. *S*-warfarin is eliminated in the bile and *R*-warfarin is excreted in the urine as inactive metabolites. There is much more known about the metabolism of warfarin compared with other anticoagulants, but it is established that *S*-phenprocoumon and *S*-acenocoumarol are also substrates for CYP2C9 and that they differ from warfarin in their hepatic metabolism, and stereospecific potency.[2]

It makes sense to assume therefore, that an inhibitor of CYP2C9 (e.g. fluconazole, see 'Coumarins + Azoles; Fluconazole', p.408) is likely to increase the concentration of the coumarin and enhance the anticoagulant effect. Drugs that induce CYP2C9 (e.g. rifampicin, see 'Coumarins + Antibacterials; Rifamycins', p.397) reduce plasma levels of the coumarins by increasing their clearance, and reduce the anticoagulant effect.

Genetic differences in the genes for these cytochrome P450 isoenzymes may have an important influence on drug metabolism of the coumarins. For example, different versions of the gene encoding CYP2C9 exist and the enzymatic activity of the most clinically important CYP2C9 variants, CYP2C9*2 and CYP2C9*3, is significantly reduced. Studies have suggested an association between patients possessing one or more of these variants and a low-dose requirement of warfarin. Similar observations have been made with the CYP2C9*3 variant and acenocoumarol.

While the metabolism of the coumarins, especially warfarin, are well known, the numerous interaction pathways and the variability in patient responses makes the clinical consequences of affecting their metabolism less accurate to predict than with other drugs.

(b) Other mechanisms for anticoagulant interactions

Some drugs, such as colestyramine (see 'Coumarins and related drugs + Bile-acid binding resins', p.414) may prevent the absorption of the coumarins and reduce their bioavailability. See also 'Drug absorption interactions', p.3. An increased risk of bleeding can occur if anticoagulants are given with other drugs that also impair coagulation by other mechanisms such as those drugs with an antiplatelet effect (see 'Coumarins and related drugs + Clopidogrel', p.417. Coumarins and indanediones act as vitamin K antagonists, and so dietary intake of vitamin K can also reduce or abolish their effects. Protein-binding displacement is another possible drug interaction mechanism but this usually plays a minor role compared with other mechanisms.[3] Consider also 'Protein-binding interactions', p.3.

Bleeding and its treatment

When prothrombin times become excessive, bleeding can occur. In order of decreasing frequency the bleeding shows itself as ecchymoses, blood in the

Table 12.2 Coagulation tests

Test	*Normal range*	*Therapeutic/diagnostic range*
Activated partial thromboplastin time	20 to 39 seconds after reagents added	1.5 to 2.5 x control
Bleeding time	1 to 9 minutes depending on method used	Critical value greater than 15 minutes
International normalised ratio	0.9 to 1.2	2 to 4 depending on indication for anticoagulation
Plasma thrombin time test	10 to 15 seconds	Greater than 15 seconds
Prothrombin-proconvertin ratio	70 to 130%	10 to 30%
Prothrombin time	10 to 15 seconds	1 to 2 x control
Quick value	70 to 130%	10 to 20%
Thrombin clotting time	70 to 120 seconds	150 to 600 seconds depending on indication for anticoagulation
Thrombotest	100%	10 to 20%

urine, uterine bleeding, black faeces, bruising, nose-bleeding, haematoma, gum bleeding, coughing and vomiting blood.

Vitamin K is an antagonist of the coumarin and indanedione oral anticoagulants. The British Society for Haematology has given advice on the appropriate course of action if bleeding occurs in patients taking warfarin, and this is readily available in summarised form in the British National Formulary.

If the effects of heparin are excessive it is usually sufficient just to stop the heparin, but protamine sulfate is a specific antidote if a rapid effect is required. Protamine sulfate only partially reverses the effect of low-molecular-weight heparins.

There is currently no known specific antidote for fondaparinux, or for the direct thrombin inhibitors.

1. Stroke Prevention in Atrial Fibrillation Investigators. Adjusted-dose warfarin versus low-intensity, fixed dose warfarin plus aspirin for high-risk patients with atrial fibrillation: Stroke Prevention in Atrial Fibrillation III randomised clinical trial. *Lancet* (1996) 348, 633–8.
2. Ufer M. Comparative pharmacokinetics of vitamin-K antagonists. Warfarin, phenprocoumon and acenocoumarol. *Clin Pharmacokinet* (2005) 44, 1227–46.
3. Sands CD, Chan ES, Welty TE. Revisiting the significance of warfarin protein-binding displacement interactions. *Ann Pharmacother* (2002) 36, 1642–4.

Activated factor X inhibitors + Antiplatelet drugs or NSAIDs

The pharmacokinetics and pharmacodynamics of apixaban are not altered by aspirin, but there is an increased risk of bleeding on concurrent use with aspirin and/or clopidogrel. Naproxen appears to increase the exposure to, and the pharmacodynamic effects of, apixaban. Neither aspirin, clopidogrel, nor naproxen alter the pharmacokinetics of rivaroxaban, or change the anticoagulant effects of rivaroxaban. However, there might be a minor increase in bleeding time during concurrent use. Edoxaban pharmacokinetics are not altered by naproxen or low doses of aspirin, but higher doses of aspirin slightly increase edoxaban exposure. Both aspirin and naproxen increase the bleeding time during concurrent use with edoxaban. Note that all NSAIDs and antiplatelets increase the risk of bleeding, and concurrent use with apixaban, edoxaban, or rivaroxaban might increase this risk.

Clinical evidence

(a) Aspirin

1. Apixaban. The UK manufacturer briefly notes that, no pharmacokinetic or pharmacodynamic interactions were seen when apixaban was given with aspirin 325 mg daily.[1] However, in a clinical trial in patients with atrial fibrillation, the concurrent use of aspirin (dose not stated) with apixaban, increased the risk of major bleeding from 1.8% per year to 3.4% per year.[1,2] In the APPRAISE-2 trial, in high-risk, post-acute coronary syndrome patients, the use of aspirin with apixaban was associated with a risk of major bleeding of 2.8% per year, compared with 0.6% per year for aspirin alone.[2] Note that this study was terminated early due to the increased risk of bleeding. See also *clopidogrel* below.

2. Edoxaban. A series of randomised, crossover studies in healthy subjects assessed the pharmacokinetic and pharmacodynamic effects of edoxaban 60 mg daily with low-dose (100 mg daily) and high-dose (325 mg daily) aspirin, for 5 days. The pharmacokinetics of edoxaban were not altered by low-dose aspirin, but high-dose aspirin increased the edoxaban AUC and maximum concentration by 30% and 35%, respectively. Low-dose aspirin with edoxaban increased bleeding times by about 2-fold compared with either aspirin or edoxaban given alone. A similar increase in bleeding time was found when high-dose aspirin was given with edoxaban. Edoxaban did not alter the effect of either dose of aspirin on platelet aggregation, and both doses of aspirin did not alter the effects of edoxaban on clotting parameters (inhibition of factor Xa activity, prolongation of prothrombin time, aPTT, or INR).[3] The UK manufacturer of edoxaban briefly notes that, in clinical studies, patients taking low dose aspirin (100 mg daily or less) or other antiplatelet drugs had a 2-fold increased risk of major bleeding compared to those not taking antiplatelet drugs. They also note that this same dose of aspirin did not alter the AUC or maximum concentration of edoxaban after a single-dose or at steady state.[4]

3. Rivaroxaban. In a controlled study in 13 healthy subjects, aspirin 500 mg on day one then 100 mg on day 2 had no effect on the pharmacokinetics of a single 15-mg dose of oral rivaroxaban given at the same time as aspirin on day 2. Concurrent use resulted in an increase in the bleeding time of 2.28 minutes compared with aspirin alone. Rivaroxaban did not alter the effect of aspirin on platelet aggregation and aspirin did not alter the effects of rivaroxaban on clotting parameters (inhibition of factor Xa activity, prolongation of prothrombin time, aPTT, and HepTest).[5] In a prospective analysis of patients treated with rivaroxaban for acute venous thromboembolism, the risk of clinically relevant bleeding (such as that requiring medical intervention) was increased in those also taking aspirin, compared with those not taking aspirin (hazard ratio 1.8). Note that this was similar to the increase seen with enoxaparin and aspirin.[6] In another analysis of patients taking rivaroxaban after total hip or knee arthroplasty, the risk of major or clinically relevant bleeding was increased in those taking aspirin or other antiplatelet drugs, compared with those not taking these drugs (relative risk 1.11). Note that this risk was not statistically significant and was similar to that seen with enoxaparin and aspirin or other antiplatelet drugs.[7]

(b) Clopidogrel or prasugrel

1. Apixaban. The UK manufacturer briefly notes that, in a phase I study, there was no increase in bleeding time or further inhibition of platelet aggregation, when **clopidogrel** 75 mg daily (alone or in combination with aspirin 162 mg daily) or **prasugrel** (60 mg followed by 10 mg daily) was given with apixaban, when compared with administration without apixaban.[1] However, in the APPRAISE-2 trial in high-risk, post-acute coronary syndrome patients, the use of aspirin and **clopidogrel** with apixaban was associated with a risk of major bleeding of 5.9% per year, compared with 2.5% per year for the antiplatelets alone.[2] Note that this study was terminated early due to the increased risk of bleeding. See also *aspirin* above.

2. Rivaroxaban. The UK manufacturer of rivaroxaban reports that no pharmacokinetic interaction occurred in patients given rivaroxaban with **clopidogrel** 300 mg as a single dose followed by 75 mg daily. However, an increase in bleeding times was reported in some patients.[8]

(c) NSAIDs

1. Apixaban. In a study in 21 healthy subjects, a single 500-mg dose of **naproxen** increased the AUC and maximum plasma concentration of a single 10-mg dose of apixaban by 54% and 61%, respectively. Clotting tests were also increased in-line with the increases in apixaban plasma concentration, but no changes in platelet aggregation, and no clinically relevant increase in bleeding time was seen. Also, the AUC and maximum plasma concentration of the **naproxen** were not affected by apixaban.[9]

2. Edoxaban. In a randomised, crossover study in 31 healthy subjects, **naproxen** 500 mg daily for 2 days did not alter the pharmacokinetics of edoxaban 60 mg given on day 2. However, bleeding times were increased about 2-fold with the combination, compared with either naproxen or edoxaban given alone. Edoxaban did not alter the effect of naproxen on platelet aggregation, and naproxen did not alter the effects of edoxaban on clotting parameters (inhibition of factor Xa activity, prolongation of prothrombin time, aPTT, or INR).[3] The UK manufacturer of edoxaban briefly notes that, in clinical studies, patients concurrently taking NSAIDs had an increased risk of clinically relevant bleeding.[4]

3. Rivaroxaban. In a controlled study in 11 healthy subjects, **naproxen** 500 mg daily on two consecutive days was given with a single 15-mg dose of oral rivaroxaban on the second day. Concurrent use increased bleeding time by a mean of 3.43 minutes compared with naproxen alone, and one subject had a greater increase. **Naproxen** increased the rivaroxaban AUC by 10%, but this was not statistically significant. Naproxen did not have any clinically relevant effect on the pharmacodynamics of rivaroxaban (prolongation of aPTT, prothrombin time, and HepTest, and inhibition of factor Xa activity).[10] In a prospective analysis of patients treated with rivaroxaban for acute venous thromboembolism, the risks of clinically relevant and major bleeding were increased in those also taking NSAIDs (unspecified), compared with those not taking NSAIDs (hazard ratios 1.90 and 2.56, respectively). Note that these increases were similar to those seen with enoxaparin and NSAIDs.[6] In another analysis of patients taking rivaroxaban after total hip or knee arthroplasty, the risk of major or clinically relevant bleeding was increased in those taking NSAIDs (unspecified), compared with those not taking NSAIDs (relative risk 1.28).[7]

Mechanism

Antiplatelet drugs and many NSAIDs increase the bleeding time. Rivaroxaban alone does not increase the bleeding time, but it appears to increase this effect when given with aspirin and NSAIDs, and possibly also clopidogrel. Concurrent use of apixaban with antiplatelet drugs or NSAIDs, does not appear to increase the bleeding time, however, apixaban with antiplatelet drugs does appear to increase the risk of bleeding. Edoxaban increases bleeding time, and concurrent use of aspirin (low- or high-dose) or naproxen with edoxaban increases the bleeding time compared with these drugs given alone. Naproxen increased the exposure to apixaban in a study,[9] but the mechanism behind this effect is not known; the authors suggest involvement of P-glycoprotein on the basis of *in vitro* investigation, but clinically, naproxen is not generally considered to be an inhibitor of P-glycoprotein.

Importance and management

Although the pharmacological studies described show that the pharmacokinetics of **apixaban** are not changed by aspirin, apixaban does appear to be associated with a higher risk of bleeding when combined with aspirin and/or clopidogrel. While naproxen appears to increase clotting tests and exposure to apixaban, no clinically relevant bleeding was noted and no changes in platelet aggregation were seen. The pharmacokinetics of **rivaroxaban** are not notably changed by aspirin, clopidogrel, or naproxen, however, a minor increase in bleeding time was seen when they were taken concurrently. **Edoxaban** appears to be associated with a higher risk of bleeding when combined with aspirin or NSAIDs, but no pharmacokinetic interactions occur. In general, it would be prudent to use NSAIDs and antiplatelet drugs, such as aspirin and clopidogrel, and these activated factor X inhibitors with caution because of the possible increased risk of haemorrhage.[1,8] Additional care should also be taken in those patients given combination antiplatelet therapies. The UK manufacturer of edoxaban advises against the concurrent use of aspirin at doses above 325 mg daily, and that doses above 100 mg daily should be under medical supervision. In addition, they advise against the concurrent use of other antiplatelet drugs, and the chronic use of NSAIDs.[4] The US manufacturer advises careful monitoring [presumably for signs and symptoms of bleeding] on concurrent use with low-dose aspirin and/or NSAIDs.[11] Note also that although aspirin and naproxen did not affect the clotting parameters used to monitor the effects of edoxaban and rivaroxaban in clinical studies, these parameters are not used in clinical practice to monitor the effects of these drugs due to lack of reliability.

1. Eliquis (Apixaban). Bristol-Myers Squibb-Pfizer. UK Summary of product characteristics, July 2014.
2. Eliquis (Apixaban). Bristol-Myers Squibb Co. US Prescribing information, June 2015.
3. Mendell J, Lee F, Chen S, Worland V, Shi M, Samama MM. The effects of the antiplatelet agents, aspirin and naproxen, on pharmacokinetics and pharmacodynamics of the anticoagulant edoxaban, a direct factor Xa inhibitor. *J Cardiovasc Pharmacol* (2013) 62, 212–21.
4. Lixiana (Edoxaban tosilate). Daiichi Sankyo UK Ltd. UK Summary of product characteristics, June 2015.
5. Kubitza D, Becka M, Mueck W, Zuehlsdorf M. Safety, tolerability, pharmacodynamics, and pharmacokinetics of rivaroxaban—an oral, direct factor Xa inhibitor—are not affected by aspirin. *J Clin Pharmacol* (2006) 46, 981–90.
6. Davidson BL, Verheijen S, Lensing AW, Gebel M, Brighton TA, Lyons RM, Rehm J, Prins MH. Bleeding risk of patients with acute venous thromboembolism taking nonsteroidal anti-inflammatory drugs or aspirin. *JAMA Intern Med* (2014) 174, 947–53.
7. Eriksson BI, Rosencher N, Friedman RJ, Homering M, Dahl OE. Concomitant use of medication with antiplatelet effects in patients receiving either rivaroxaban or enoxaparin after total hip or knee arthroplasty. *Thromb Res* (2012) 130, 147–51.
8. Xarelto (Rivaroxaban). Bayer plc. UK Summary of product characteristics, May 2015.
9. Frost C, Shenker A, Gandhi MD, Pursley J, Barrett YC, Wang J, Zhang D, Byon W, Boyd RA, LaCreta F. Evaluation of the effect of naproxen on the pharmacokinetics and pharmacodynamics of apixaban. *Br J Clin Pharmacol* (2014) 78, 877–85.
10. Kubitza D, Becka M, Mueck W, Zuehlsdorf M. Rivaroxaban (BAY 59-7939) – an oral, direct Factor Xa inhibitor – has no clinically relevant interaction with naproxen. *Br J Clin Pharmacol* (2007) 63, 469–76.
11. Savaysa (Edoxaban tosylate monohydrate). Daiichi Sankyo Inc. US Prescribing information, January 2015.

Activated factor X inhibitors + Drugs that induce CYP3A4 and/or P-glycoprotein

Rifampicin (rifampin) moderately decreases the exposure to apixaban and rivaroxaban. Other drugs that are both potent CYP3A4 inducers and P-glycoprotein inducers might interact similarly. Rifampicin slightly decreases the exposure to edoxaban, and other P-glycoprotein inducers might interact similarly.

Clinical evidence

(a) Apixaban

A preliminary report of a study in 20 healthy subjects states that **rifampicin (rifampin)** 600 mg once daily for 11 days decreased the AUC and maximum plasma concentration of a single 10-mg dose of oral apixaban by 54% and 42%, respectively.[1]

(b) Edoxaban

In a crossover study in 32 healthy subjects, **rifampicin (rifampin)** 600 mg once daily for 7 days decreased the AUC of a single 60-mg dose of oral edoxaban by 34% and increased its clearance by 33%. Rifampicin also increased the AUC of the active metabolites of edoxaban (M4 and M6) almost 3-fold.[2]

(c) Rivaroxaban

The UK and US manufacturers of rivaroxaban briefly report that in a study, **rifampicin (rifampin)** titrated up to 600 mg daily, decreased the AUC and maximum plasma concentration of rivaroxaban by about 50% and 22%, respectively, with an associated reduction in its anticoagulant effects.[3,4]

Mechanism

Rivaroxaban and apixaban are metabolised by CYP3A4 and are also substrates for P-glycoprotein. Rifampicin is a well-known inducer of cytochrome P450 isoenzymes, including CYP3A4, and it also induces P-glycoprotein. Concurrent use therefore results in decreased exposure to apixaban and rivaroxaban. Edoxaban is only minimally metabolised by CYP3A4, but it is a substrate for P-glycoprotein, and rifampicin probably decreases its exposure mainly by inducing P-glycoprotein.

Importance and management

A pharmacokinetic interaction between apixaban, edoxaban, or rivaroxaban, and rifampicin would seem to be established, and is likely to be clinically important. Therefore the US manufacturers of apixaban[5] and rivaroxaban[4] advise avoiding their concurrent use with drugs that are both P-glycoprotein inducers and potent CYP3A4 inducers (see 'Table 1.12', p.14 and 'Table 1.9', p.11, respectively, for lists). However, the UK manufacturer of apixaban[6] only contraindicates its concurrent use with drugs that are both P-glycoprotein inducers and potent CYP3A4 inducers when given for the treatment of deep vein thrombosis or pulmonary embolism. The UK manufacturer of rivaroxaban[3] recommends avoiding concurrent use with potent CYP3A4 inducers unless the patient is closely observed for signs and symptoms of thrombosis. Note that they name **St John's wort** as a potent CYP3A4 inducer, but St John's wort generally behaves as a moderate inducer. The US manufacturer of edoxaban[7] advises avoiding concurrent use with rifampicin, whereas the UK manufacturer[8] advises caution with drugs that are P-glycoprotein inducers (see 'Table 1.12', p.14 for a list). Note that they also name **phenytoin** and **phenobarbital** as P-glycoprotein inducers, but clinical evidence for such an effect with these drugs is lacking. Given the likely clinical risk of the reduced apixaban, edoxaban, and rivaroxaban efficacy that could result from decreased exposure on concurrent use with potent CYP3A4 inducers and/or P-glycoprotein inducers, it would seem prudent to consider using an alternative drug with these activated factor X inhibitors. However, if this is not possible, consideration should be given to switching to an alternative anticoagulant for which monitoring is available to ensure adequate anticoagulation is maintained.

1. Vakkalagadda B, Frost C, Wang J, Nepal S, Schuster A, Zhang D, Dias C, Yu Z, Shenker A, LaCreta F. Effect of rifampin on the pharmacokinetics of apixaban, an oral direct inhibitor of factor Xa [abstract no. 143]. *J Clin Pharmacol* (2009) 49, 1124.
2. Mendell J, Chen S, He L, Desai M, Parasramupria DA. The effect of rifampin on the pharmacokinetics of edoxaban in healthy adults. *Clin Drug Investig* (2015) 35, 447–53.
3. Xarelto (Rivaroxaban). Bayer plc. UK Summary of product characteristics, May 2015.
4. Xarelto (Rivaroxaban). Janssen Pharmaceuticals, Inc. US Prescribing information, January 2015.
5. Eliquis (Apixaban). Bristol-Myers Squibb Co. US Prescribing information, June 2015.
6. Eliquis (Apixaban). Bristol-Myers Squibb-Pfizer. UK Summary of product characteristics, July 2014.
7. Savaysa (Edoxaban tosylate monohydrate). Daiichi Sankyo Inc. US Prescribing information, January 2015.
8. Lixiana (Edoxaban tosilate). Daiichi Sankyo UK Ltd. UK Summary of product characteristics, June 2015.

Activated factor X inhibitors; Apixaban + Drugs that inhibit CYP3A4 and/or P-glycoprotein

Ketoconazole moderately increases apixaban exposure. Other drugs that are both potent CYP3A4 inhibitors and P-glycoprotein inhibitors might interact similarly. Diltiazem slightly increases apixaban exposure.

Clinical evidence

(a) Azoles

In a crossover study in 18 healthy subjects, **ketoconazole** 400 mg once daily for 6 days, increased the AUC and maximum plasma concentration of a single 10-mg dose of apixaban given on day 4, almost 2-fold and by 62%, respectively.[1]

(b) Diltiazem

In a crossover study in 18 healthy subjects, diltiazem 360 mg once daily for 10 days, increased the AUC and maximum plasma concentration of a single 10-mg dose of apixaban given on day 8, by 40% and 31%, respectively.[1]

Mechanism

Apixaban is metabolised by CYP3A4 and is also a substrate for P-glycoprotein. Ketoconazole is an inhibitor of CYP3A4 and P-glycoprotein, and therefore concurrent use increases apixaban exposure. Exposure to apixaban is also increased to a smaller extent by the concurrent use of diltiazem, which is an inhibitor of CYP3A4 only.

Importance and management

The interaction between apixaban and drugs that inhibit both CYP3A4 and P-glycoprotein seems to be established; however, the clinical relevance of the interaction appears to depend on the degree to which the interacting drug inhibits CYP3A4 and P-glycoprotein. **Ketoconazole** is a potent inhibitor of CYP3A4 and it inhibits P-glycoprotein, so that concurrent use with apixaban results in a moderate increase in its exposure. Therefore, for drugs that are both P-glycoprotein inhibitors and potent CYP3A4 inhibitors (see 'Table 1.12', p.14' and 'Table 1.9', p.11, respectively, for lists), the UK manufacturer of apixaban, does not recommend concurrent use.[2] However, the US manufacturer of apixaban only advises against concurrent use in patients already taking the low 2.5 mg twice daily dose of apixaban; and in other patients, advises reducing the dose by 50% if concurrent use is required.[3]

Diltiazem, a moderate CYP3A4 inhibitor, had a smaller effect than ketoconazole on apixaban, causing only a slight increase in its exposure. Such an increase is not considered clinically relevant, and no additional precautions are necessary on concurrent use of less potent CYP3A4 inhibitors or P-glycoprotein inhibitors with apixaban.

1. Frost CE, Byon W, Song Y, Wang J, Schuster AE, Boyd RA, Zhang D, Yu Z, Dias C, Shenker A, LaCreta F. Effect of ketoconazole and diltiazem on the pharmacokinetics of apixaban, an oral direct factor Xa inhibitor. *Br J Clin Pharmacol* (2015) 79, 838–46.
2. Eliquis (Apixaban). Bristol-Myers Squibb-Pfizer. UK Summary of product characteristics, July 2014.
3. Eliquis (Apixaban). Bristol-Myers Squibb Co. US Prescribing information, June 2015.

Activated factor X inhibitors; Apixaban + Food

Food does not affect the pharmacokinetics or pharmacodynamics of apixaban.

Clinical evidence, mechanism, importance and management

In a randomised, crossover study in 21 healthy subjects, the pharmacokinetics of a single 10-mg dose of apixaban were no different when given 5 minutes after a standardised high-fat, high-calorie breakfast, than when given after a 10 hour fast. The time to maximum concentration was prolonged by 1 hour when given with food. The pharmacodynamics of apixaban were similarly unaffected by food.[1] Apixaban can therefore be administered with or without food.

1. Frost C, Wang J, Nepal S, Schuster A, Barrett YC, Mosqueda-Garcia R, Reeves RA, LaCreta F. Apixaban, an oral, direct factor Xa inhibitor: single dose safety, pharmacokinetics, pharmacodynamics and food effect in healthy subjects. *Br J Clin Pharmacol* (2012) 75, 476–87.

Activated factor X inhibitors; Apixaban + LMWHs

Enoxaparin does not affect the pharmacokinetics of apixaban but concurrent use results in an additive effect on anti-Xa activity.

Clinical evidence, mechanism, importance and management

In a randomised, crossover study in 18 healthy subjects, the pharmacokinetics of a single 5-mg dose of apixaban were not affected by **enoxaparin** 40 mg given subcutaneously. However, on concurrent administration, peak anti-Xa activity was 42% higher than with apixaban alone. When **enoxaparin** was administered 6 hours after the apixaban was given, the peak anti-Xa activity was 15% higher than with apixaban alone.[1] Because of the risk of major bleeding, the MHRA in the UK contraindicates the concurrent use of apixaban with low-molecular-weight heparins, unless the patient is being switched to, or from, treatment with apixaban, in which case the switch should be conducted at the next scheduled dose.[2] It would seem prudent to monitor patients for signs of excessive bleeding on concurrent use.

1. Barrett YC, Wang J, Song Y, Pursley J, Wastall P, Wright R, Lacreta F, Frost C. A randomised assessment of the pharmacokinetic, pharmacodynamic and safety interaction between apixaban and enoxaparin in healthy subjects. *Thromb Haemost* (2012) 107, 916–24.
2. Medicines and Healthcare Products Regulatory Agency. New oral anticoagulants apixaban (Eliquis), dabigatran (Pradaxa) and rivaroxaban (Xarelto). *Drug Safety Update* (2013) 3, A1. Available at: https://www.gov.uk/drug-safety-update/new-oral-anticoagulants-apixaban-eliquis-dabigatran-pradaxa-and-rivaroxaban-xarelto (accessed 25/03/15).

Activated factor X inhibitors; Apixaban + Miscellaneous

The use of apixaban and warfarin increases the risk of bleeding. The use of apixaban with other anticoagulants, and drugs that affect bleeding would be expected to increase the risk of bleeding. There is no pharma-

cokinetic interaction between apixaban and atenolol. Famotidine does not alter the pharmacokinetics of apixaban.

Clinical evidence, mechanism, importance and management

(a) Anticoagulants

The UK and US manufacturers of apixaban briefly report that, in a clinical study in patients with atrial fibrillation, the use of apixaban with **warfarin** increased the risk of bleeding from 2.7% per year to 4.6% per year.[1,2] As such, the use of apixaban with anticoagulants is contraindicated by the MHRA in the UK, unless the patient is being switched to, or from, apixaban.[3] When switching from **warfarin** to apixaban, warfarin should be discontinued, and when the INR is less than 2, apixaban can be started.[1,2] When switching from apixaban to **warfarin**, the UK manufacturer advises continuing apixaban for 2 days after warfarin has been started, at which point the INR should be checked prior to the next dose of apixaban. Once the INR is equal or greater than 2, apixaban can be discontinued.[1] In contrast, the US manufacturer advises that because apixaban affects INR, such measurements made during combined treatment would not be reliable. Instead, they advise that apixaban is discontinued, and a parenteral anticoagulant with warfarin is started at the time the next scheduled apixaban dose would have been due. The parenteral anticoagulant can be stopped when the INR is within the acceptable range.[2] For discussion of the interaction between enoxaparin and apixaban, see 'Activated factor X inhibitors; Apixaban + LMWHs', p.375.

(b) Atenolol

The UK manufacturer briefly reports that, in a study the AUC and maximum plasma concentration of a single 10-mg dose of apixaban were only 15 and 18% lower, respectively, when administered with atenolol 100 mg, then when apixaban was administered alone. The pharmacokinetics of atenolol were not affected.[1] No dose adjustments would seem necessary on concurrent use.

(c) Famotidine

The UK manufacturer briefly reports that, in a study the pharmacokinetics of a single 10-mg dose of apixaban were not altered by administration with famotidine 40 mg.[1] No apixaban dose adjustment would seem necessary on concurrent use.

(d) Other drugs

The UK manufacturer specifically advises that concurrent use with **thrombolytics, GPIIb/IIIa receptor antagonists, thienopyridines, dipyridamole, dextran**, and **sulfinpyrazone** is not recommended.[1] See also 'Activated factor X inhibitors + Antiplatelet drugs or NSAIDs', p.374.

1. Eliquis (Apixaban). Bristol-Myers Squibb-Pfizer. UK Summary of product characteristics, July 2014.
2. Eliquis (Apixaban). Bristol-Myers Squibb Co. US Prescribing information, June 2015.
3. Medicines and Healthcare Products Regulatory Agency. New oral anticoagulants apixaban (Eliquis), dabigatran (Pradaxa) and rivaroxaban (Xarelto). *Drug Safety Update* (2013) 3, A1. Available at: https://www.gov.uk/drug-safety-update/new-oral-anticoagulants-apixaban-eliquis-dabigatran-pradaxa-and-rivaroxaban-xarelto (accessed 23/10/15).

Activated factor X inhibitors; Edoxaban + Drugs that inhibit P-glycoprotein

Amiodarone, dronedarone, quinidine, and verapamil slightly increase edoxaban exposure. Ciclosporin, erythromycin, and ketoconazole also appear to slightly increase edoxaban exposure. Other P-glycoprotein inhibitors might interact similarly. Atorvastatin has no effect on edoxaban exposure.

Clinical evidence

(a) Amiodarone

In a study in 28 healthy subjects, amiodarone 400 mg daily for 4 days increased the AUC and maximum plasma concentration of a single 60-mg dose of edoxaban given on day 4 by 40% and 66%, respectively.[1]

(b) Atorvastatin

In a crossover study in 29 healthy subjects, atorvastatin 80 mg daily for 8 days had no effect on the AUC of a single 60-mg dose of edoxaban given on day 7, but decreased the maximum plasma concentration of edoxaban by 14%.[1]

(c) Ciclosporin

The UK manufacturer of edoxaban briefly reports that, in a study, a single 500-mg dose of ciclosporin increased the AUC and maximum plasma concentration of a single 60-mg dose of edoxaban by 73% and 74%, respectively.[2]

(d) Dronedarone

In a crossover study in 31 healthy subjects, dronedarone 400 mg twice daily for 7 days, increased the AUC and maximum plasma concentration of a single 60-mg dose of edoxaban given on day 5 by 85% and 46%, respectively.[1]

(e) Erythromycin

The UK manufacturer of edoxaban briefly reports that, in a study, erythromycin 500 mg four times daily for 8 days, increased the AUC and maximum plasma concentration of a single 60-mg dose of edoxaban given on day 7 by 85% and 68%, respectively.[2]

(f) Ketoconazole

The UK manufacturer of edoxaban briefly reports that, in a study, ketoconazole 400 mg daily for 7 days, increased the AUC and maximum plasma concentration of a single 60-mg dose of edoxaban given on day 4 by 87% and 89%, respectively.[2]

(g) Quinidine

In a crossover study in 29 healthy subjects, quinidine 300 mg daily on day 1, 300 mg three times daily on days 2 to 3, and 300 mg daily on day 4, increased the AUC and maximum plasma concentration of a single 60-mg dose of edoxaban given on day 3 by 77% and 85%, respectively.[1] The UK and US manufacturers briefly report that, in a study, edoxaban had no effect on the AUC and maximum plasma concentration of quinidine.[2,3]

(h) Verapamil

In a crossover study in 30 healthy subjects, sustained-release verapamil 240 mg daily for 11 days increased the AUC and maximum plasma concentration of a single 60-mg dose of edoxaban given on day 10 by 53%.[1] The UK and US manufacturers briefly report that, in a study, edoxaban decreased the AUC and maximum plasma concentration of verapamil by 14% and 16%, respectively.[2,3]

Mechanism

Edoxaban is a substrate for P-glycoprotein. Amiodarone, ciclosporin, dronedarone, erythromycin, ketoconazole, quinidine and verapamil inhibit P-glycoprotein, so that concurrent use increases the exposure to edoxaban. Note that erythromycin, ketoconazole, and verapamil also inhibit CYP3A4 (albeit to varying extents), but the interaction is unlikely to be due to CYP3A4 inhibition because edoxaban is only minimally metabolised by this isoenzyme.

Importance and management

Evidence for an interaction between edoxaban and P-glycoprotein inhibitors is from controlled studies, and a pharmacokinetic interaction is established. Although the clinical relevance of the slight increases in exposure seen are not known, an increased risk of bleeding cannot be ruled out. On the basis of data from clinical studies in patients with atrial fibrillation that showed an increased risk of stroke with reduced edoxaban doses in patients also taking dronedarone, quinidine, or verapamil (despite a reduced risk of bleeding), the US manufacturer does not recommend reducing the dose of edoxaban when it is given for stroke prophylaxis in patients with atrial fibrillation who are also taking P-glycoprotein inhibitors.[3] However, they do recommend a dose reduction, to 30 mg daily, when edoxaban is given for the treatment of deep vein thrombosis or pulmonary embolism if patients are taking quinidine or verapamil, or during a short course of **azithromycin**, clarithromycin, erythromycin, oral **itraconazole**, or oral ketoconazole (the dose can be increased again after the course).[3] In contrast, the UK manufacturer recommends reducing the edoxaban dose to 30 mg daily with concurrent ciclosporin, dronedarone, erythromycin, or ketoconazole, regardless of the indication for the edoxaban. No dose reduction is recommended for concurrent amiodarone, quinidine, or verapamil.[2]

It is possible that any inhibitor of P-glycoprotein might interact similarly (for a list, see 'Table 1.12', p.14), and it would be prudent to be alert for signs of bleeding or anaemia on concurrent use with edoxaban, as with any anticoagulant. Note that edoxaban is used without routine coagulation monitoring.

No particular precautions are necessary with the concurrent use of atorvastatin and edoxaban. The clinical relevance of the small decrease in verapamil exposure with edoxaban is not known, but is unlikely to be important.

1. Mendell J, Zahir H, Matsushima N, Noveck R, Lee F, Chen S, Zhang G, Shi M. Drug-drug interaction studies of cardiovascular drugs involving P-glycoprotein, an efflux transporter, on the pharmacokinetics of edoxaban, an oral factor Xa inhibitor. *Am J Cardiovasc Drugs* (2013) 13, 331–42.
2. Lixiana (Edoxaban tosilate). Daiichi Sankyo UK Ltd. UK Summary of product characteristics, June 2015..
3. Savaysa (Edoxaban tosylate monohydrate). Daiichi Sankyo Inc. US Prescribing information, January 2015.

Activated factor X inhibitors; Edoxaban + Food

Food does not have a clinically relevant effect on the pharmacokinetics of edoxaban

Clinical evidence, mechanism, importance and management

In a randomised, crossover study, 32 healthy subjects were given a single 60-mg dose of edoxaban, either in the fasted state, or immediately after a high-fat meal. When compared with the fasted state, food had no clinically relevant effect on the pharmacokinetics of edoxaban.[1] Similarly, a study in 10 healthy subjects found that a high-fat meal had no clinically relevant effects on the pharmacokinetics of a single dose of edoxaban 60 mg.[2] Therefore, edoxaban can be taken without regard to meals.

1. Mendell J, Tachibana M, Shi M, Kunitada S. Effects of food on the pharmacokinetics of edoxaban, an oral direct factor Xa inhibitor, in healthy volunteers. *J Clin Pharmacol* (2011) 51, 687–94.
2. Ogata K, Mendell-Harary J, Tachibana M, Masumoto H, Oguma T, Kojima M, Kunitada S. Clinical safety, tolerability, pharmacokinetics, and pharmacodynamics of the novel factor Xa inhibitor edoxaban in healthy volunteers. *J Clin Pharm* (2010) 50, 743–53.

Activated factor X inhibitors; Edoxaban + LMWHs

Enoxaparin does not affect the pharmacokinetics of edoxaban, but concurrent use results in an additive effect on anti-Xa activity.

Clinical evidence, mechanism, importance and management

In a randomised, crossover study in 38 healthy subjects, the pharmacokinetics of a single 60-mg dose of edoxaban were not affected by **enoxaparin** 1 mg/kg given subcutaneously, compared with edoxaban given alone, whether they were given concurrently or 12 hours apart. However, on concurrent administration, maximum anti-Xa activity was 25% higher than with edoxaban alone. When edoxaban was administered 12 hours after the enoxaparin was given, the maximum anti-Xa activity was 12% higher than with edoxaban alone.[1] Because of the risk of major bleeding, the UK manufacturer[2] contraindicates the concurrent use of edoxaban with low-molecular-weight heparins, and the US manufacturer[3] does not recommend it, unless the patient is being switched to, or from, treatment with edoxaban, in which case the switch should be conducted at the next scheduled dose. It would seem prudent to monitor patients for signs of excessive bleeding on concurrent use.

1. Zahir H, Matsushima N, Halim AB, He L, Zhang G, Lee F, Worland V, Mendell. Edoxaban administration following enoxaparin: a pharmacodynamic, pharmacokinetic, and tolerability assessment in human subjects. *Thromb Haemost* (2012) 108, 166–75.
2. Lixiana (Edoxaban tosilate). Daiichi Sankyo UK Ltd. UK Summary of product characteristics, June 2015..
3. Savaysa (Edoxaban tosylate monohydrate). Daiichi Sankyo Inc. US Prescribing information, January 2015.

Activated factor X inhibitors; Edoxaban + Miscellaneous

The use of edoxaban with other anticoagulants, and drugs that affect bleeding, would be expected to increase the risk of bleeding. Esomeprazole does not appear to affect edoxaban exposure.

Clinical evidence, mechanism, importance and management

(a) Anticoagulants

Because of the risk of major bleeding, the UK manufacturer[1] contraindicates the concurrent use of edoxaban with other anticoagulants (including **unfractionated heparin**, heparin derivatives such as **fondaparinux**, and **oral anticoagulants**) and the US manufacturer[2] does not recommend it, unless the patient is being switched to, or from, treatment with edoxaban, in which case the switch should be conducted at the next scheduled dose. It would seem prudent to monitor patients for signs of excessive bleeding on concurrent use.

For discussion of the interaction between enoxaparin and edoxaban, see 'Activated factor X inhibitors; Edoxaban + LMWHs', p.376.

(b) Esomeprazole

The US manufacturer briefly notes that in a study, esomeprazole decreased the AUC of edoxaban by less than 10%.[2] The UK manufacturer briefly reports that **proton pump inhibitors** had no relevant effect on edoxaban exposure.[1] No special precautions would seem necessary on concurrent use.

(c) Other drugs

The UK and US manufacturers advise that concurrent use with **thrombolytics** or **fibrinolytics** might increase the risk of bleeding if used concurrently with edoxaban.[1,2] See also 'Activated factor X inhibitors + Antiplatelet drugs or NSAIDs', p.374.

1. Lixiana (Edoxaban tosilate). Daiichi Sankyo UK Ltd. UK Summary of product characteristics, June 2015..
2. Savaysa (Edoxaban tosylate monohydrate). Daiichi Sankyo Inc. US Prescribing information, January 2015.

Activated factor X inhibitors; Rivaroxaban + Atorvastatin

Atorvastatin does not alter the pharmacokinetics or pharmacodynamic effects of rivaroxaban, and rivaroxaban does not alter the pharmacokinetics of atorvastatin.

Clinical evidence, mechanism, importance and management

In a randomised crossover study, in 19 healthy subjects given atorvastatin 10 mg daily for three days, followed by atorvastatin 20 mg daily for four days (to achieve steady state), a single 20 mg dose of rivaroxaban did not affect the pharmacokinetics of steady state atorvastatin. In addition, atorvastatin (at steady state) did not affect the pharmacokinetics or pharmacodynamics of the single dose of rivaroxaban.[1] No dose adjustments are therefore necessary if these drugs are given together.

1. Kubitza D, Becka M, Roth A, Mueck W. Absence of clinically relevant interactions between rivaroxaban—an oral, direct Factor Xa inhibitor—and digoxin or atorvastatin in healthy subjects. J Int Med Res 2012 (40), 1688–1707.

Activated factor X inhibitors; Rivaroxaban + Drugs that affect gastric pH

Antacids, ranitidine, and omeprazole do not appear to affect the pharmacokinetics or pharmacodynamics of rivaroxaban. Other H_2-receptor antagonists or proton pump inhibitors would also not be expected to interact.

Clinical evidence

(a) Antacids

In a controlled study in fasted healthy subjects, simultaneous administration of a single 10-mL dose of an **aluminium/magnesium hydroxide** antacid (*Maalox*) had no effect on the pharmacokinetics or pharmacodynamics of a single 30-mg dose of oral rivaroxaban.[1]

(b) H_2-receptor antagonists

In a study in 12 healthy subjects, pretreatment with **ranitidine** 150 mg twice daily for 3 days did not alter the pharmacokinetics or pharmacodynamics of a single 30-mg dose of rivaroxaban.[1]

(c) Proton pump inhibitors

In a randomised, crossover study in 22 healthy subjects, pretreatment with **omeprazole** 40 mg daily for 5 days did not alter the pharmacokinetics or pharmacodynamics of a single 20-mg dose of rivaroxaban.[2]

Mechanism

Alteration of the gastric pH by antacids, ranitidine, and omeprazole does not affect rivaroxaban absorption.

Importance and management

Evidence for an interaction between rivaroxaban and antacids, ranitidine, or omeprazole is limited, but on the basis of these studies, no interaction would be expected. Other H_2-receptor antagonists and proton pump inhibitors do not appear to have been studied, but these would also not be expected to interact.

1. Kubitza D, Becka M, Zuehlsdorf M, Mueck W. Effect of food, an antacid, and the H_2 antagonist ranitidine on the absorption of BAY 59-7939 (rivaroxaban), an oral, direct factor Xa inhibitor, in healthy subjects. *J Clin Pharmacol* (2006) 46, 549–58.
2. Moore KT, Plotnikov AN, Thyssen A, Vaccaro N, Ariyawansa J, Burton PB. Effect of multiple doses of omeprazole on the pharmacokinetics, pharmacodynamics, and safety of a single dose of rivaroxaban. *J Cardiovasc Pharmacol* (2011) 58, 581–8.

Activated factor X inhibitors; Rivaroxaban + Drugs that inhibit CYP3A4 and/or P-glycoprotein

Ketoconazole and ritonavir moderately increase rivaroxaban exposure. Other drugs that are both potent CYP3A4 inhibitors and P-glycoprotein inhibitors might interact similarly. Clarithromycin, erythromycin, and fluconazole only slightly increase rivaroxaban exposure. Ciclosporin might increase rivaroxaban concentrations.

Clinical evidence

(a) Azoles

A crossover study found that, in 12 healthy subjects, giving **ketoconazole** 200 mg daily with a single 10 mg dose of rivaroxaban on day 4, resulted in an increase in the AUC and maximum concentration of rivaroxaban of 82% and 53%, respectively, when compared with rivaroxaban alone. Similarly, in 20 healthy subjects given rivaroxaban 10 mg daily alone for 5 days and then with **ketoconazole** 400 mg daily for a further 5 days, ketoconazole increased the AUC and maximum concentrations of rivaroxaban 2.6-fold and by 72%, respectively. While in another group of 13 healthy subjects given either a single 20 mg dose of rivaroxaban alone, or **fluconazole** 400 mg daily for 6 days, with rivaroxaban 20 mg on day 5, fluconazole increased the AUC and maximum concentration of rivaroxaban by 42% and 28%, respectively.[1]

(b) Ciclosporin

A retrospective review of 5 liver transplant patients taking ciclosporin and given rivaroxaban for various reasons (atrial fibrillation, pulmonary embolism, venous thrombosis, or hepatic artery thrombosis), found that the mean minimum rivaroxaban concentration (measured by anti-Xa activity assay) was 131.7 nanograms/mL (reference range 7 to 65 nanograms/mL). In 4 other patients taking tacrolimus, the mean minimum concentration was 20.3 nanograms/mL. Rivaroxaban doses had been adjusted according to renal function, but a dose reduction was necessary in 3 of the 5 patients taking ciclosporin (compared with none of those taking tacrolimus). During the following 19 months, 3 of the patients taking ciclosporin reported bleeding complications, 2 of whom were found to have rivaroxaban concentrations above the reference range. This compared with only 1 patient in the tacrolimus group, but whose rivaroxaban concentration was within the therapeutic range.[2]

(c) HIV-protease inhibitors

An interaction study found that, in 12 healthy subjects given a single 10-mg dose of rivaroxaban on day 1, **ritonavir** 600 mg twice daily on days 3 to 7, and a single-dose of both drugs on the morning of day 8, ritonavir increased the AUC and maximum concentration of rivaroxaban 2.5-fold and by 55%, respectively, when compared with rivaroxaban alone.[1] A case report describes a 52-year-old, HIV-positive man taking **darunavir boosted with ritonavir** 600/100 mg twice daily, who was started on rivaroxaban 10 mg daily for 6 weeks following an orthopaedic operation. The rivaroxaban concentration was measured after 2 weeks and the dose was halved because the concentration was about twice that predicted from population pharmacokinetic analyses. A few weeks later, while travelling in Mexico, the patient experienced acute bloody diarrhoea, which resolved after stopping rivaroxaban and with ciprofloxacin treatment. The bleeding was attributed to a drug interaction between rivaroxaban and **darunavir boosted with ritonavir**, and the diarrhoea was attributed to traveller's diarrhoea (salmonellosis, shigellosis, and *campylobacter* infections were excluded).[3]

(d) Macrolides

In a crossover study, 15 healthy subjects were given either a single 10 mg dose of rivaroxaban alone, or **clarithromycin** 500 mg twice daily for 4 days followed by both drugs on day 5. Clarithromycin increased the AUC and maximum concentration of rivaroxaban by 54% and 40%, respectively, when compared with rivaroxaban alone. In another group of 15 healthy subjects given either a single 10 mg dose of rivaroxaban alone, or **erythromycin** 500 mg three times daily for 4 days followed by a single 10 mg dose of rivaroxaban and a single 500 mg-dose of **erythromycin** on day 5, erythromycin increased the AUC and maximum concentration of rivaroxaban by 34% and 38%, respectively, compared with rivaroxaban alone.[1] Similarly, in a study in 8 subjects with normal renal function, **erythromycin** 500 mg three times daily for 6 days increased the AUC and maximum concentration of a single 10-mg dose of rivaroxaban given on day 5 by 38% and 40%, respectively. In the same study, subjects with mild (8 subjects) or moderate (8 subjects) renal impairment were also given the same treatments. When the pharmacokinetics of rivaroxaban in these subjects were compared with those of a single 10-mg dose given alone in the 8 subjects with normal renal function, the AUC and maximum plasma concentration were 80% and 56% higher, respectively, in those with mild renal impairment, and almost 2-fold and 77% higher, respectively in those with moderate renal impairment.[4]

Mechanism

Rivaroxaban is metabolised by CYP3A4 and is also a substrate for P-glycoprotein. Ritonavir (high-dose) and ketoconazole are inhibitors of CYP3A4, and are also inhibitors of P-glycoprotein, and therefore concurrent use increases rivaroxaban exposure. Clarithromycin and erythromycin also inhibit CYP3A4 (albeit to different extents) and P-glycoprotein, and appear to have a smaller effect on rivaroxaban exposure. Similarly, fluconazole is an inhibitor of CYP3A4, and appears to have a small effect on rivaroxaban exposure.

Importance and management

The interaction between rivaroxaban and drugs that inhibit both CYP3A4 and P-glycoprotein seems to be established; however, the clinical relevance of the interaction appears to depend on the degree to which the interacting drug inhibits CYP3A4 and P-glycoprotein. Both ritonavir and ketoconazole are potent CYP3A4 inhibitors and they inhibit P-glycoprotein, and concurrent use with rivaroxaban resulted in moderate increases in rivaroxaban exposure. Therefore, for drugs that are both P-glycoprotein inhibitors and potent CYP3A4 inhibitors (see 'Table 1.12', p.14 and 'Table 1.9', p.11, respectively, for lists), the UK and US manufacturers of rivaroxaban do not recommend concurrent use.[5,6] Note also, that although **clarithromycin** is considered a potent CYP3A4 inhibitor, as well as being a P-glycoprotein inhibitor, it does not appear to cause the same magnitude of effect on rivaroxaban exposure as ketoconazole and ritonavir; thus the increase in rivaroxaban exposure seen is not considered clinically relevant, and so clarithromycin is excluded from the above advice.

Erythromycin and **fluconazole**, are moderate inhibitors of CYP3A4 (and erythromycin also inhibits P-glycoprotein), so had a smaller effect on rivaroxaban exposure than ketoconazole and ritonavir. These effects are not considered clinically relevant, and no additional precautions are necessary on concurrent use with rivaroxaban, except perhaps in those with renal impairment.

Although **dronedarone** is an inhibitor of P-glycoprotein only, its use is not recommended by the UK manufacturer of rivaroxaban, because of a lack of clinical data.[5] Similarly, **ciclosporin** is an inhibitor of P-glycoprotein but not of CYP3A4, and more study is required to establish the clinical relevance of this interaction, if any.

1. Mueck W, Kubitza D, Becka M. Co-administration of rivaroxaban with drugs that share its elimination pathways: pharmacokinetic effects in healthy subjects. *Br J Clin Pharmacol* (2013) 76, 455–66.
2. Wannhoff A, Weiss KH, Schemmer P, Stremmel W, Gotthardt DN. Increased levels of rivaroxaban in patients after liver transplantation treated with cyclosporine A. *Transplantation* (2014) 98, e12–13.
3. Lakatos B, Stoeckle M, Elzi L, Battegay M, Marzolini C. Gastrointestinal bleeding associated with rivaroxaban administration in a treated patient infected with human immunodeficiency virus. *Swiss Med Wkly* (2014) Epub.
4. Moore KT, Vaidyanathan S, Natarajan J, Ariyawansa J, Haskell L, Turner KC. An open-label study to estimate the effect of steady-state erythromycin on the pharmacokinetics, pharmacodynamics, and safety of a single dose of rivaroxaban in subjects with renal impairment and normal renal function. *J Clin Pharmacol* (2014) 54, 1407–20.
5. Xarelto (Rivaroxaban). Bayer plc. UK Summary of product characteristics, May 2015.
6. Xarelto (Rivaroxaban). Janssen Pharmaceuticals, Inc. US Prescribing information, January 2015.

Activated factor X inhibitors; Rivaroxaban + Food

Food can increase the absorption of rivaroxaban, but this appears to be dose dependent.

Clinical evidence, mechanism, importance and management

In controlled studies in healthy subjects, the absorption of a single 10- or 20-mg dose of rivaroxaban was increased and delayed when it was given within 30 minutes of a standardised high-fat, high-calorie meal, when compared with the fasted state, as reflected by an increase in the AUC of about 25% and an increase in the time to maximum concentration from 2.75 hours to 4 hours. The increase in inhibition of factor Xa activity mirrored the increase in absorption (26% increase). Further study did not find any difference between the effect of a high-carbohydrate meal and a high-fat meal.[1] In randomised crossover studies, healthy subjects were given either oral rivaroxaban as a 10 mg tablet (24 subjects) or 20 mg tablet (22 subjects) after a 10-hour fast or with a standardised high fat, high calorie breakfast. In the 10-mg group there was no difference in exposure to rivaroxaban in the fed or fasted state, whereas in the 20-mg group there was an increase in the AUC and maximum concentrations of rivaroxaban of 39% and 76 %, respectively, when administered with food.[2] Similarly, in another randomised crossover study, in which 16 healthy subjects were given rivaroxaban 20 mg as a suspension, under fed and fasted conditions, the AUC and maximum concentrations of rivaroxaban were increased by 47% and 104%, respectively, in the fed as compared with the fasted state.[2] As a result, the UK and US manufacturers state that rivaroxaban can be taken with or without food when given at a dose of 2.5 mg or 10 mg,[3,4] but must be taken with food when given at a dose of 15 or 20 mg.[3,4]

In clinical studies in elective surgery, rivaroxaban has been given within one to 2 hours of food before surgery, and in the fasting state in the postoperative period. The authors of this report speculate that the smaller maximum concentrations of rivaroxaban in the fasted state might be somewhat beneficial for wound haemostasis in the postoperative period.[1]

1. Kubitza D, Becka M, Zuehlsdorf M, Mueck W. Effect of food, an antacid, and the H_2 antagonist ranitidine on the absorption of BAY 59-7939 (rivaroxaban), an oral, direct factor Xa inhibitor, in healthy subjects. *J Clin Pharmacol* (2006) 46, 549–58.
2. Stampfuss J, Kubitza D, Becka M, Mueck W. The effect of food on the absorption and pharmacokinetics of rivaroxaban. *Int J Clin Pharmacol Ther* (2013) 51, 549–61.
3. Xarelto (Rivaroxaban). Bayer plc. UK Summary of product characteristics, May 2015.
4. Xarelto (Rivaroxaban). Janssen Pharmaceuticals, Inc. US Prescribing information, January 2015.

Activated factor X inhibitors; Rivaroxaban + Midazolam

Rivaroxaban does not alter the pharmacokinetics of midazolam.

Clinical evidence, mechanism, importance and management

In a study in 12 healthy subjects, the concurrent use of a single 7.5-mg dose of midazolam and a single 20-mg dose of rivaroxaban had no effect on the pharmacokinetics of rivaroxaban, midazolam, or the metabolite of midazolam, α-hydroxymidazolam.[1]

No dose adjustments are therefore necessary if these drugs are given together.

Note that midazolam can be used as a probe substrate to assess the activity of drugs on CYP3A4. This study therefore suggests that rivaroxaban has no effect on CYP3A4 activity, and therefore is not expected to affect the exposure to other substrates of CYP3A4 via this mechanism.

1. Mueck W, Kubitza D, Becka M. Co-administration of rivaroxaban with drugs that share its elimination pathways: pharmacokinetic effects in healthy subjects. *Br J Clin Pharmacol* (2013) 76, 455–66.

Activated factor X inhibitors; Rivaroxaban + Other anticoagulants

Enoxaparin and warfarin do not affect the pharmacokinetics of rivaroxaban, but could have additive bleeding effects. The use of rivaroxaban with other anticoagulants would be expected to increase the risk of bleeding.

Clinical evidence, mechanism, importance and management

The UK and US manufacturers of rivaroxaban report that **enoxaparin**[1,2] and **warfarin**[2] do not affect the pharmacokinetics of rivaroxaban; however, the concurrent use of single doses of rivaroxaban 10 mg and 5 mg with enoxaparin 40 mg or warfarin 15 mg, respectively, had an additive effect on anti-factor Xa concentrations, with no additional effects on either prothrombin time or the aPTT. The US manufacturer[2] advises avoiding the use of rivaroxaban in patients taking other anticoagulants (not specified), due to the increased risk of additive bleeding effects, unless the benefit outweighs the risk; whereas the MHRA in the UK[3] contraindicates the use of rivaroxaban with any other anticoagulants except when changing treatment to or from rivaroxaban, or when using heparin to keep a central venous or arterial catheter open. It would seem prudent to monitor patients for signs of excessive bleeding if rivaroxaban is given with an anticoagulant.

1. Xarelto (Rivaroxaban). Bayer plc. UK Summary of product characteristics, May 2015.
2. Xarelto (Rivaroxaban). Janssen Pharmaceuticals, Inc. US Prescribing information, January 2015.
3. Medicines and Healthcare Products Regulatory Agency. New oral anticoagulants apixaban (Eliquis), dabigatran (Pradaxa) and rivaroxaban (Xarelto). *Drug Safety Update* (2013) 3, A1. Available at: https://www.gov.uk/drug-safety-update/new-oral-anticoagulants-apixaban-eliquis-dabigatran-pradaxa-and-rivaroxaban-xarelto (accessed 28/10/15).

Coumarins + ACE inhibitors

There is a single, isolated and unexplained case of melaena attributed to an interaction between acenocoumarol and fosinopril. No other ACE inhibitor studied has so far been shown to interact to a clinically relevant extent with the coumarins.

Clinical evidence

(a) Benazepril

In healthy subjects benazepril 20 mg daily for 7 days did not affect the steady-state plasma levels of either **warfarin** or **acenocoumarol**. The anticoagulant activity of **acenocoumarol** was not altered. The effects of **warfarin** were slightly reduced, as demonstrated by a mean reduction in PT of about 4%, but this is not enough to be clinically important.[1]

(b) Cilazapril

In 26 patients taking long-term **acenocoumarol** or **phenprocoumon**, cilazapril 2.5 mg daily for 3 weeks had no effect on the thrombotest times or coagulation factors II, VII and X.[2]

(c) Enalapril

Enalapril 20 mg for 5 days did not affect the anticoagulant effects of **warfarin** 2.5 to 7.5 mg daily, according to a brief summary of unpublished data cited in a review.[3]

(d) Fosinopril

A 74-year-old patient stabilised on **acenocoumarol**, **enalapril**, piretanide, and digoxin had the piretanide and **enalapril** switched to furosemide and fosinopril. Eleven days later, he presented with dark faeces (melaena) and had a low haemoglobin level. Fosinopril and acenocoumarol were stopped, and then **enalapril** and acenocoumarol were restarted. On gastrointestinal endoscopy, no explanation for the melaena was found, and his haemoglobin level had returned to normal 15 days later. This case was attributed to possible potentiation of the effect of acenocoumarol by fosinopril.[4]

(e) Moexipril

In 10 healthy subjects, the pharmacokinetics and pharmacodynamics of a single 50-mg dose of **warfarin** were not altered when it was given with the first dose of moexipril 15 mg daily for 6 days.[5]

(f) Ramipril

In 8 healthy subjects, ramipril 5 mg daily for 7 days had no effect on the steady-state pharmacokinetics or anticoagulant effects of **phenprocoumon**.[6] Similarly, ramipril 5 mg daily for 3 weeks did not alter the anticoagulant effects of **acenocoumarol** or **phenprocoumon** in patients stabilised on these anticoagulants, when compared with placebo.[7]

(g) Temocapril

In 24 healthy subjects, temocapril 20 mg daily for 2 weeks had no effect on the steady-state pharmacokinetics or pharmacodynamics of **warfarin**.[8] The absence of an interaction between **warfarin** and temocapril was also shown in another study.[9]

(h) Trandolapril

In a study in 19 healthy subjects,[10] **trandolapril** 2 mg daily for 13 days did not affect the pharmacodynamics of a single 25-mg dose of **warfarin** given on day 8.

Mechanism, importance and management

No important pharmacokinetic or pharmacodynamic interaction has been demonstrated for any ACE inhibitor and coumarin anticoagulant. Contrasting with all this evidence, there is a single, unexplained and isolated case of melaena attributed to an interaction between acenocoumarol and fosinopril. There seems to be no other evidence that fosinopril normally interacts with the oral anticoagulants and so this case report is unlikely to be of general significance. No special precautions would therefore seem necessary if any of these coumarin anticoagulants and ACE inhibitors are used concurrently.

1. Van Hecken A, De Lepeleire I, Verbesselt R, Arnout J, Angehrn J, Youngberg C, De Schepper PJ. Effect of benazepril, a converting enzyme inhibitor, on plasma levels and activity of acenocoumarol and warfarin. *Int J Clin Pharmacol Res* (1988) 8, 315–19.
2. Boeijinga JK, Breimer DD, Kraay CJ, Kleinbloesem CH. Absence of interaction between the ACE inhibitor cilazapril and coumarin derivatives in elderly patients on long term oral anticoagulants. *Br J Clin Pharmacol* (1992) 33, 553P.
3. Gomez HJ, Cirillo VJ, Irvin JD. Enalapril: a review of human pharmacology. *Drugs* (1985) 30 (Suppl 1), 13–24.
4. de Tomás ME, Sáez L, Beltrán S, Gato A. Probable interacción farmacológica entre fosinopril y acenocumarol. *Med Clin (Barc)* (1997) 108, 757.
5. Van Hecken A, Verbesselt R, Depré M, Tjandramaga TB, Angehrn J, Cawello W, De Schepper PJ. Moexipril does not alter the pharmacokinetics or pharmacodynamics of warfarin. *Eur J Clin Pharmacol* (1993) 45, 291–3.
6. Verho M, Malerczyk V, Grötsch H, Zenbil I. Absence of interaction between ramipril, a new ACE-inhibitor, and phenprocoumon, an anticoagulant agent. *Pharmatherapeutica* (1989) 5, 392–9.
7. Boeijinga JK, Matroos AW, van Maarschalkerweerd MW, Jeletich-Bastiaanse A, Breimer DD. No interaction shown between ramipril and coumarine derivatives. *Curr Ther Res* (1988) 44, 902–8.
8. Siepmann M, Kirch W, Kleinbloesem CH. Non-interaction of temocapril, an ACE-inhibitor, with warfarin. *Clin Pharmacol Ther* (1996) 59, 214.
9. Lankhaar G, Eckenberger P, Ouwerkerk MJA, Dingemanse J. Pharmacokinetic-pharmacodynamic investigation of a possible interaction between steady-state temocapril and warfarin in healthy subjects. *Clin Drug Invest* (1999) 17, 399–405.
10. Meyer BH, Muller FO, Badenhorst PN, Luus HG, De La Rey N. Multiple doses of trandolapril do not affect warfarin pharmacodynamics. *S Afr Med J* (1995) 85, 768–70.

Coumarins and related drugs + Alcohol

The effects of the coumarins are unlikely to be changed in those with normal liver function who drink small or moderate amounts of alcoholic beverages such as wine or spirits. A non-significant trend has been reported of an increased risk of serious bleeding in patients taking warfarin with a history of binge drinking.

Clinical evidence

(a) Patients and subjects free from liver disease

In a study in 8 healthy subjects anticoagulated with **warfarin**, the daily consumption of one pint (about 560 mL) of Californian white table wine for a 3-week period at meal times had no significant effects on either the serum **warfarin** levels or the anticoagulant response.[1]

Other studies in both patients[2,3] and healthy subjects[4,5] taking either **warfarin**[2,3,5] or **phenprocoumon**[4] have very clearly confirmed the absence of an interaction with wine,[3,5] gin,[4] or alcohol 40%.[2] In one of these studies the subjects were given almost 600 mL of a table wine (alcohol 12%) or 300 mL of a fortified wine (alcohol 20%) without adverse effects on coagulation.[5] Moreover, in men randomised to receive low-dose **warfarin** in a post-coronary artery bypass graft study, there was no significant difference in the incidence of an INR above 2 between 323 non-drinkers, 181 light drinkers (one to 6 drinks weekly), 75 moderate drinkers (7 to 13 drinks weekly) and 46 heavy drinkers (14 drinks or more weekly).[6]

In contrast to the above studies, a 58-year-old man stabilised on **warfarin** experienced a sharp rise in his INR to 8 when he started to drink half a can of light beer (5.35 g of alcohol) every other day. In the previous 5 months he had an INR in the range of 1.9 to 2.5 with a stable **warfarin** dose, and no other explanation for the change in INR was found. He stopped taking the alcohol, and was eventually restabilised on the original dose of **warfarin**.[7] In a prospective, longitudinal study of patients taking **warfarin**, there was a slight statistically significant increased risk of self-reported bleeding events in patients who had increased their alcohol consumption in the previous week (35 bleeds in 245 weeks, none of which were major; odds ratio 1.24).[8]

In a case-control study of risk factors for excessive anticoagulation, self-reported alcohol use (ranging from one drink every other day to 2 drinks daily) was actually associated with an 80% *lower* risk of an INR greater than 6 with **warfarin**.[9]

(b) Chronic alcoholics or those with liver disease

In one study, 15 alcoholics who had been drinking heavily (250 g of ethanol or more daily) for at least 3 months and 11 control subjects (minimal social drinkers or non-drinkers) were given a single 40-mg dose of **warfarin**. The half-life of **warfarin** was lower in the alcoholics (26.5 hours versus 41.1 hours), but a comparison of the prothrombin times with those of healthy subjects found no differences.[10]

One patient with liver cirrhosis had marked fluctuations in prothrombin times and **warfarin** levels associated with weekend binge drinking of vodka.[2] Another patient with abnormal liver function had a fall in plasma **warfarin** levels and effect when he stopped drinking 50 mL of whiskey daily. When rechallenged with alcohol, **warfarin** levels and effect rose, and he had a nosebleed.[11] In contrast, a large retrospective cohort study did not find a significantly increased risk of serious bleeding in 140 patients with a history of alcoholic binge drinking who were taking **warfarin**. The relative risk was 1.3 (0.8 to 1.9) compared with patients who had no record of alcohol abuse.[12]

Mechanism

It seems probable that, as in *rats*,[13] continuous heavy drinking stimulates the hepatic enzymes concerned with the metabolism of warfarin, leading to more rapid elimination.[10,14] The fluctuations in prothrombin times in those with liver impairment[2,11] may possibly occur because sudden large amounts of alcohol exacerbate the general dysfunction of the liver and this might affect the way it metabolises warfarin. Alcohol may also change the ability of the liver to synthesise clotting factors.[15] Constituents of beer other than alcohol may affect warfarin metabolism.[7]

Importance and management

The absence of an interaction between warfarin or phenprocoumon and alcohol in those free from liver disease is well documented and well established. It appears to be quite safe for patients taking oral anticoagulants to drink small or moderate amounts of wine or spirits (e.g. drinking within the generally accepted healthy daily limits). Even much less conservative amounts (up to 8 oz/250 mL of spirits[4] or a pint of wine (about 560 mL) daily[1]) do not create problems with anticoagulant control, so that there appears to be a good margin of safety even for the less than abstemious. Only warfarin and phenprocoumon appear to have been investigated, but other coumarin anticoagulants would be expected to behave similarly. The single case of increased INR in a patient who started to drink beer is unexplained, and therefore, further study with beer is needed to throw light on this possible interaction.

On the other hand, those who drink heavily may possibly need above-average doses of the coumarin, while limited evidence suggests that those with liver damage who binge drink may experience marked fluctuations in their prothrombin times. It might be prudent to avoid anticoagulation in this type of patient unless they can abstain from drinking. Nevertheless, although one cohort study in patients taking warfarin found a slight trend towards serious bleeding events in patients with a history of binge drinking, this was not significant, and other risk factors for bleeding were more important (highly variable prothrombin time ratio, or prothrombin time ratio greater than 2).[12]

Some sources also say that the indanedione **phenindione** may interact with alcohol, but there seems no direct evidence available to support this prediction.

1. O'Reilly RA. Lack of effect of mealtime wine on the hypoprothrombinemia of oral anticoagulants. *Am J Med Sci* (1979) 277, 189–94.
2. Udall JA. Drug interference with warfarin therapy. *Clin Med* (1970) 77, 20–25.
3. Karlson B, Leijd B, Hellström A. On the influence of vitamin K-rich vegetables and wine on the effectiveness of warfarin treatment. *Acta Med Scand* (1986) 220, 347–50.
4. Waris E. Effect of ethyl alcohol on some coagulation factors in man during anticoagulant therapy. *Ann Med Exp Biol Fenn* (1963) 41, 45–53.
5. O'Reilly RA. Lack of effect of fortified wine ingested during fasting and anticoagulant therapy. *Arch Intern Med* (1981) 141, 458–9.
6. Mukamal KJ, Smith CC, Karlamangla AS, Moore AA. Moderate alcohol consumption and safety of lovastatin and warfarin among men: the post-coronary artery bypass graft trial. *Am J Med* (2006) 119, 434–40.
7. Havrda DE, Mai T, Chonlahan J. Enhanced antithrombotic effect of warfarin associated with low-dose alcohol consumption. *Pharmacotherapy* (2005) 25, 303–7.
8. Shalansky S, Lynd L, Richardson K, Ingaszewski A, Kerr C. Risk of warfarin-related bleeding events and supratherapeutic international normalized ratios associated with complementary and alternative medicine: a longitudinal analysis. *Pharmacotherapy* (2007) 27, 1237–47.
9. Hylek EM, Heiman H, Skates SJ, Sheehan MA, Singer DE. Acetaminophen and other risk factors for excessive warfarin anticoagulation. *JAMA* (1998) 279, 657–62.
10. Kater RMH, Roggin G, Tobon F, Zieve P, Iber FL. Increased rate of clearance of drugs from the circulation of alcoholics. *Am J Med Sci* (1969) 258, 35–9.
11. Breckenridge A, Orme M. Clinical implications of enzyme induction. *Ann N Y Acad Sci* (1971) 179, 421–31.
12. Fihn SD, McDonell M, Martin D, Henikoff J, Vermes D, Kent D, White RH, for the Warfarin Optimized Oupatient Follow-up Study Group. Risk factors for complications of chronic anticoagulation: a multi-center study. *Ann Intern Med* (1993) 118, 511–20.
13. Rubin E, Hutterer F, Lieber CS. Ethanol increases hepatic smooth endoplasmic reticulum and drug-metabolizing enzymes. *Science* (1968) 159, 1469–70.

14. Kater RMH, Carruli N, Iber FL. Differences in the rate of ethanol metabolism in recently drinking alcoholic and nondrinking subjects. *Am J Clin Nutr* (1969) 22, 1608–17.
15. Riedler G. Einfluß des Alkohols auf die Antikoagulantientherapie. *Thromb Diath Haemorrh* (1966) 16, 613–35.

Coumarins + Aliskiren

Aliskiren did not alter the pharmacodynamics or pharmacokinetics of a single dose of acenocoumarol, nor does it appear to interact with warfarin. Warfarin does not increase the levels of aliskiren.

Clinical evidence, mechanism, importance and management

(a) Acenocoumarol

In a well-controlled study in 18 healthy subjects, aliskiren 300 mg daily for 10 days did not alter the anticoagulant effect of a single 10-mg dose of acenocoumarol given on day 8. No significant changes in the pharmacokinetics of either *R*- and *S*-acenocoumarol were reported.[1] This study suggests that no acenocoumarol dose adjustment or additional monitoring would be expected to be needed if aliskiren is used in patients taking acenocoumarol.

(b) Warfarin

In a placebo-controlled, crossover study in 15 healthy subjects, aliskiren 150 mg daily for 11 days did not alter the pharmacodynamics of a single dose of warfarin given on day 8. In addition, there was no change in the AUC or half-life of *R*- and *S*-warfarin.[2] However, the manufacturer says that there were technical difficulties with this study, which was considered deficient.[3] They therefore state in their product information that the effects of aliskiren on warfarin pharmacokinetics have not been evaluated.[4] Nevertheless, aliskiren did not interact with acenocoumarol, which has very similar metabolism to warfarin; therefore no interaction with warfarin would be anticipated.

The US manufacturers state that warfarin does not increase the levels of aliskiren.[5]

1. Huang H-LA, Vaidyanathan S, Yeh C-M, Bizot M-N, Dieterich HA, Dole WP, Howard D. Effect of aliskiren, an oral direct renin inhibitor, on the pharmacokinetics and pharmacodynamics of a single dose of acenocoumarol in healthy volunteers. *Curr Med Res Opin* (2008) 24, 2449–56.
2. Dieterle W, Corynen S, Mann J. Effect of the oral renin inhibitor aliskiren on the pharmacokinetics and pharmacodynamics of a single dose of warfarin in healthy subjects. *Br J Clin Pharmacol* (2004) 58, 433–6.
3. Personal communication. Novartis, October 2008.
4. Rasilez 300 mg Tablets (Aliskiren hemifumarate). Novartis Pharmaceuticals UK Ltd. UK Summary of product characteristics, August 2012.
5. Tekturna (Aliskiren hemifumarate). Novartis. US Prescribing information, September 2012.

Coumarins + Allopurinol

A number of studies and case reports suggest that allopurinol does not alter the pharmacokinetics or pharmacodynamics of warfarin. Nevertheless, a few case reports suggest that allopurinol might have increased the effect of warfarin, and similar cases have been reported with phenprocoumon. Allopurinol increased the half-life of dicoumarol in some healthy subjects, but there do not appear to be any reports of a clinically significant interaction.

Clinical evidence

(a) Dicoumarol

In 6 healthy subjects, allopurinol 2.5 mg/kg twice daily for 14 days increased the mean half-life of a single 4-mg/kg dose of dicoumarol from 51 hours to 153 hours, with large inter-individual variation.[1] In another similar study, only one of 3 healthy subjects had an increase in their dicoumarol half-life (from 13 hours to 17 hours) when they were also given allopurinol.[2]

(b) Phenprocoumon

Two patients, who had been stabilised on phenprocoumon for a few weeks, developed prolonged bleeding times, with haematuria in one of them, within 4 to 5 weeks of starting to take allopurinol 300 mg daily.[3]

(c) Warfarin

In a study in 8 healthy subjects, the half-life of a single 25-mg dose of warfarin was not altered by pretreatment with allopurinol 100 mg twice daily for 10 days.[2] Similarly, in 6 subjects, the elimination of a single 50-mg dose of warfarin was not altered by allopurinol 100 mg three times daily for 2 to 4 weeks, although one subject had a 30% reduction in the elimination of warfarin after 4 weeks.[4] No change was seen in the prothrombin ratios of 2 patients taking warfarin who took allopurinol 100 mg three times daily for 3 weeks.[4] In contrast, one patient stabilised on warfarin had a 42% increase in his prothrombin ratio after taking allopurinol 100 mg daily for 2 days.[5]

In a retrospective study[6] of the adverse effects of allopurinol in 1835 patients, 3 patients were identified who had developed excessive anticoagulation while taking warfarin and allopurinol. One of them developed extensive intrapulmonary haemorrhage and had a prothrombin time of 71 seconds. An increase in prothrombin time to 42 seconds was reported in an 82-year-old woman who had started taking warfarin 11 days previously, when she was also started on both allopurinol 300 mg daily and indometacin (which could have contributed, see 'Coumarins + NSAIDs; Indometacin and related drugs', p.453). The precise role of the allopurinol in this case is unclear.[7]

Mechanism

It has been suggested that, as in *rats*, allopurinol inhibits the metabolism of the anticoagulants by the liver, thereby prolonging their effects and half-lives.[1,2,5] There is a wide individual variability in the effects of allopurinol on drug metabolism,[4] so that only a few individuals are affected.

Importance and management

Documentation for an interaction between allopurinol and the coumarins is poor, and a pharmacokinetic interaction is not established. There appear to be few case reports of any important interaction. Nevertheless, consider increased monitoring of the anticoagulant effect in any patient taking a coumarin with allopurinol.

1. Vesell ES, Passananti GT, Greene FE. Impairment of drug metabolism in man by allopurinol and nortriptyline. *N Engl J Med* (1970) 283, 1484–8.
2. Pond SM, Graham GG, Wade DN, Sudlow G. The effects of allopurinol and clofibrate on the elimination of coumarin anticoagulants in man. *Aust N Z J Med* (1975) 5, 324–8.
3. Jähnchen E, Meinertz T, Gilfrich HJ. Interaction of allopurinol with phenprocoumon in man. *Klin Wochenschr* (1977) 55, 759–61.
4. Rawlins MD, Smith SE. Influence of allopurinol on drug metabolism in man. *Br J Pharmacol* (1973) 48, 693–8.
5. Barry M, Feeley J. Allopurinol influences aminophenazone elimination. *Clin Pharmacokinet* (1990) 19, 167–9.
6. McInnes GT, Lawson DH, Jick H. Acute adverse reactions attributed to allopurinol in hospitalised patients. *Ann Rheum Dis* (1981) 40, 245–9.
7. Self TH, Evans WE, Ferguson T. Drug enhancement of warfarin activity. *Lancet* (1975) ii, 557–8.

Coumarins + Alpha blockers

Tamsulosin does not appear to alter the pharmacokinetics or anticoagulant effect of acenocoumarol, and alfuzosin, doxazosin and terazosin do not appear to affect the response to warfarin.

Clinical evidence, mechanism, importance and management

(a) Alfuzosin

The UK manufacturer of alfuzosin reports that no pharmacodynamic or pharmacokinetic interaction was seen in healthy subjects given alfuzosin with **warfarin**.[1] The US manufacturer reports that in 6 healthy subjects, alfuzosin 5 mg twice daily for 6 days did not affect the pharmacological response to a single 25-mg dose of **warfarin**.[2] No warfarin dose adjustment would be expected to be needed on concurrent use.

(b) Doxazosin

The manufacturer of doxazosin reports that doxazosin has no effect on the protein binding of **warfarin** *in vitro*, and that no adverse effects have been reported with anticoagulants (unspecified).[3] No warfarin dose adjustment would be expected to be needed on concurrent use.

(c) Tamsulosin

In a double-blind, placebo-controlled, crossover study in 12 healthy subjects, tamsulosin 400 micrograms daily for 9 days had no effect on the pharmacokinetics or anticoagulant effects of a single 10-mg dose of **acenocoumarol** given on day five.[4] However, the UK manufacturer of tamsulosin states that **warfarin** might increase the elimination rate of tamsulosin.[5] The US manufacturer states that the findings of an *in vitro* metabolic interaction study between tamsulosin and **warfarin** were equivocal, and that they have not done a definitive drug interaction study; they therefore recommend caution with concurrent use.[6] Nevertheless, there do not appear to be any published cases of problems with the concurrent use of tamsulosin and **warfarin**, and the clinical study with **acenocoumarol**, which is metabolised in a similar way to **warfarin**, suggests that an interaction is unlikely.

(d) Terazosin

In a retrospective study of 26 men stabilised on **warfarin**, starting terazosin had no effect on their INRs. The patients had stable INRs for a least 2 consecutive measurements before receiving terazosin, and an INR taken within 14 days (9 patients) or 30 days (17 patients) of starting the terazosin.[7] Another study in 29 patients taking **warfarin** found that starting terazosin did not have a significant effect on anticoagulation.[8] Terazosin was used as a control comparator drug in these studies because of its lack of interaction with **warfarin**.[7,8] No warfarin dose adjustment would be expected to be needed on concurrent use.

1. Xatral (Alfuzosin hydrochloride). Sanofi. UK Summary of product characteristics, September 2013.
2. Uroxatral (Alfuzosin hydrochloride extended-release tablets). Sanofi-Aventis US LLC. US Prescribing information, October 2011.
3. Cardura (Doxazosin mesilate). Pfizer Ltd. UK Summary of product characteristics, August 2009.
4. Rolan P, Terpstra IJ, Clarke C, Mullins F, Visser JN. A placebo-controlled pharmacodynamic and pharmacokinetic interaction study between tamsulosin and acenocoumarol. *Br J Clin Pharmacol* (2003) 55, 314–16.
5. Tabphyn (Tamsulosin hydrochloride). ProStrakan. UK Summary of product characteristics, August 2008.
6. Flomax (Tamsulosin hydrochloride). Astellas Pharma Inc. US Prescribing information, May 2012.
7. Beckey NP, Parra D, Colon A. Retrospective evaluation of a potential interaction between azithromycin and warfarin in patients stabilized on warfarin. *Pharmacotherapy* (2000) 20, 1055–9.
8. Glasheen JJ, Fugit RV, Prochazka AV. The risk of overanticoagulation with antibiotic use in outpatients on stable warfarin regimens. *J Gen Intern Med* (2005) 20, 653–6.

Coumarins + 5-Alpha reductase inhibitors

Dutasteride and finasteride have no clinically significant effect on the pharmacokinetics or pharmacodynamics of warfarin.

Clinical evidence, mechanism, importance and management

In a study in 23 healthy subjects, dutasteride 500 micrograms daily taken with **warfarin** for 3 weeks had no effect on the pharmacokinetics of *S*- or *R*-warfarin, and the prothrombin time was unaffected by dutasteride.[1]

Similarly, the manufacturer of finasteride briefly notes that no clinically meaningful interaction was seen with **warfarin**.[2,3]

Therefore, no warfarin dose adjustment would be expected to be necessary on concurrent use of these 5-alpha reductase inhibitors.

1. Avodart (Dutasteride). GlaxoSmithKline. US Prescribing information, October 2012.
2. Proscar (Finasteride). Merck Sharp & Dohme Ltd. UK Summary of product characteristics, March 2008.
3. Proscar (Finasteride). Merck & Co., Inc. US Prescribing information, August 2010.

Coumarins + 5-Aminosalicylates

A single case report describes reduced warfarin effects in a patient given mesalazine. Another single case report describes a marked reduction in the response to warfarin when mesalazine was switched to sulfasalazine.

Clinical evidence

A woman stabilised on **warfarin** 5 mg daily, with INRs between 2 and 3, started taking **mesalazine** 800 mg three times daily for the treatment of a caecal ulcer. Four weeks later she presented to hospital with left leg pain, which was diagnosed as an acute popliteal vein thrombosis, and at the same time it was found that her prothrombin time and INR had fallen to 11.3 seconds and 0.9, respectively. The patient was treated with intravenous heparin. Over the next 10 days INRs of up to 1.7 were achieved by increasing the doses of **warfarin** up to 10 mg daily, but a satisfactory INR of 2.1 was only reached when the **mesalazine** was stopped. The report says that serum **warfarin** levels were not detectable during the use of **mesalazine**.[1] A 37-year-old woman taking **warfarin** 30 mg weekly with stable INRs between 2 and 3 in the previous 2 years (and also taking beclometasone, salbutamol, aspirin, azathioprine,and ethinyloestradiol with norgestrel), had her treatment for arthritis and ulcerative colitis changed from **mesalazine** to **sulfasalazine** 1 g four times daily. The day after the change her INR was found to be subtherapeutic (1.5) and she needed numerous increases in the **warfarin** doses over the next 6 weeks, eventually needing **warfarin** 75 mg weekly before acceptable INRs were achieved. During this period she developed a new deep vein thrombosis. When the **sulfasalazine** was later stopped and the **mesalazine** restarted, her **warfarin** dose was only 45 mg weekly.[2]

Mechanism

Not understood. Sulfasalazine is broken down in the colon to a sulfonamide, sulfapyridine, and 5-aminosalicylic acid (mesalazine). Some sulfonamides (see 'Coumarins and related drugs + Antibacterials; Sulfonamides and/or Trimethoprim', p.398) are known inhibitors of warfarin metabolism, and increase the effects of warfarin. In contrast, in the case with sulfasalazine, a marked decrease was noted.

Importance and management

Not established. The case of a reduction in effect of warfarin on starting mesalazine appears to be the first and only report of an interaction, which suggests that it is unlikely to be of general importance. Similarly, the case when mesalazine was switched to sulfasalazine is an unexplained and isolated case, and its validity has been debated.[3,4] There are no other reports in the literature and this possible interaction also seems unlikely to be of general importance. Consider these cases in the event of an unexpected response to treatment.

1. Marinella MA. Mesalamine and warfarin therapy resulting in decreased warfarin effect. *Ann Pharmacother* (1998) 32, 841–2.
2. Teefy AM, Martin JE, Kovacs MJ. Warfarin resistance due to sulfasalazine. *Ann Pharmacother* (2000) 34, 1265–8.
3. Sherman JJ. Comment: other factors should be considered in a possible warfarin and sulfasalazine interaction. *Ann Pharmacother* (2001) 35, 506.
4. Kovacs MJ, Teefy AM. Comment: other factors should be considered in a possible warfarin and sulfasalazine interaction. Author's reply. *Ann Pharmacother* (2001) 35, 506.

Coumarins and related drugs + Amiodarone

The anticoagulant effects of warfarin, phenprocoumon, and acenocoumarol are increased by amiodarone and bleeding might occur. The interaction can be maximal in 2 to 7 weeks, and could persist long after the amiodarone has been withdrawn. Amiodarone-induced thyrotoxicosis might also alter the INR in patients taking warfarin.

Clinical evidence

A. Inhibition of coumarin metabolism

(a) Acenocoumarol

A number of retrospective studies[1-4] have found that patients stabilised on acenocoumarol require a dose reduction when they are given amiodarone, the combined range in these studies being 4 to 69%. In a prospective study, 10 patients stabilised on acenocoumarol were given amiodarone 600 mg daily for a week, then 400 mg daily. Eight of the 10 patients had a decrease in prothrombin activity after a mean of 4 days of amiodarone. Six patients required a decrease in their acenocoumarol dose of 60% while taking amiodarone 600 mg daily, but by the third week of taking amiodarone 400 mg daily the effects had diminished, and only a 33% reduction in dose was necessary.[5] A couple of case reports of the interaction have also been published.[6,7]

(b) Phenprocoumon

Amiodarone appears to increase the effects of phenprocoumon, with one case series in 7 patients reporting that a 9 to 59% phenprocoumon dose reduction was required within 1 to 3 weeks of starting amiodarone.[8] Conversely, an early study in 12 patients stabilised on phenprocoumon and given amiodarone 400 mg to 1 g daily did not find any interaction.[9]

(c) Warfarin

In the one of the first reports of an interaction between amiodarone and warfarin, 5 out of 9 patients who were stabilised on warfarin developed signs of bleeding (4 had microscopic haematuria and one had diffuse ecchymoses) within 3 to 4 weeks of starting to take amiodarone (dose not stated). All 9 had increases in their prothrombin times averaging 21 seconds. It was necessary to decrease the warfarin dose by an average of one-third (range 16 to 45%) to return their prothrombin times to the therapeutic range. The effects of amiodarone persisted for 6 to 16 weeks in 4 of the patients from whom it was withdrawn.[10]

Since then numerous other case reports have described a prolongation in prothrombin times and/or bleeding in patients taking warfarin and also given amiodarone (maintenance doses of 100 to 800 mg daily, sometimes with initial higher loading doses).[11-20] One patient died of haemorrhage.[15] Warfarin dose reductions varied between about 25 to 60%,[13,15,17,20] with only a few patients not needing a reduction.[13] In one retrospective study, the required dose of warfarin was related to the amiodarone maintenance dose, leading to the recommendation that the warfarin dose should be reduced by 40% for a daily maintenance dose of amiodarone of 400 mg, by 35% for 300 mg, by 30% for 200 mg and by 25% for 100 mg.[20] Other studies have also found that amiodarone use was associated with a lower required warfarin dose[21-24] and this effect was seen within the first 5 days when amiodarone and warfarin were started simultaneously in 18 patients with atrial fibrillation.[23] One 80-week study reported that a clinically important interaction defined as an INR above 5 was most likely in the first 12 weeks of concurrent use, and was minimal thereafter.[25] Conversely, one large cohort study found no important increased risk of haemorrhage with the concurrent use of warfarin and amiodarone,[26] but it is possible that the patients were on stable therapy, or that the interaction was anticipated and managed accordingly.

A few pharmacokinetic studies have shown that amiodarone decreased the clearance of warfarin by 44 to 55% in patients,[16,27] and by 20 to 37% in healthy subjects given a single dose of warfarin after taking amiodarone for 3 to 4 days.[28,29] In the two studies in healthy subjects, amiodarone caused a similar decrease in the clearance of both *R*- and *S*-warfarin.[28,29] However, a recent study in patients concluded that amiodarone had a much greater effect on *S*-warfarin than on *R*-warfarin.[30]

B. Thyrotoxicosis (Hyperthyroidism)

The INR of a patient stabilised on **warfarin** and amiodarone was noted to increase from about 2 to 5.5 after he developed amiodarone-induced thyrotoxicosis.[31] Another three well-described cases of this potential interaction have been reported.[32]

Mechanism

Amiodarone inhibits the metabolism of warfarin, probably because it, and/or its metabolite desethylamiodarone,[33] inhibit CYP2C9, CYP3A4, and CYP1A2, which are all involved in the metabolism of warfarin.

Thyrotoxicosis, which can be caused by amiodarone, potentiates the effect of warfarin, see 'Coumarins and related drugs + Thyroid hormones and Antithyroid drugs', p.477. As a result less warfarin would be required to prolong the prothrombin time.[31,32]

Importance and management

The potentiating effect of amiodarone on coumarin anticoagulants is a well documented, established, and clinically important interaction. It appears to occur in most patients.[10,13,17] It would seem prudent to adjust the doses of the coumarin anticoagulants based on INR measurements. Some recommend that the dose of warfarin should initially be reduced by 25%[17] or 50%[13] when amiodarone is added to established anticoagulant treatment, with increased INR monitoring until a new steady-state is achieved. The potentiation of coumarins starts within a few days and is usually maximal by 2 to 7 weeks.[17,20,23,30] The final reduction in warfarin dose required might depend on the amiodarone maintenance dose: average warfarin dose reductions of 25% have been required for amiodarone 100 mg daily, 30 to 35% for amiodarone 200 mg daily, 35% for amiodarone 300 mg daily, 40 to 50% for amiodarone 400 mg daily, and 65% for amiodarone 600 mg daily.[16,20] These suggested reductions are broad generalisations and individual patients might need more or less.[4,34] If established amiodarone therapy is withdrawn in a patient taking warfarin, it is likely that the dose of warfarin will need increasing gradually over the first few months after amiodarone is stopped. This is because amiodarone has such a long half-life. If warfarin is required in a patient on established amiodarone therapy, a lower initial dose of warfarin should be used.

Similar advice applies to acenocoumarol and phenprocoumon, and probably also other coumarins. Some recommend an initial reduction in acenocoumarol dose of 50% when amiodarone is added,[1] whereas others recommend that the INR should be closely monitored, and the dose of acenocoumarol only reduced in response to an increase in INR.[34]

In patients stabilised on a coumarin and amiodarone, the possibility of amiodarone-induced thyroid dysfunction should be considered if an abrupt increase in INR occurs,[31,32] see 'Coumarins and related drugs + Thyroid hormones and Antithyroid drugs', p.477.

Some sources say that the metabolism of the indanedione, **phenindione**, is inhibited by amiodarone, but this appears to be an extrapolation from the known interaction with warfarin. There seems to be no clinical evidence available to support this prediction.

1. Caraco Y, Chajek-Shaul T. The incidence and clinical significance of amiodarone and acenocoumarol interaction. *Thromb Haemost* (1989) 62, 906–8.
2. Arboix M, Frati ME, Laporte J-R. The potentiation of acenocoumarol anticoagulant effect by amiodarone. *Br J Clin Pharmacol* (1984) 18, 355–60.

3. Pini M, Manotti C, Quintavalla R. Interaction between amiodarone and acenocoumarin. *Thromb Haemost* (1985) 54, 549.
4. Fondevila C, Meschengieser S, Lazzari MA. Amiodarone potentiates acenocoumarin. *Thromb Res* (1988) 53, 203–8.
5. Richard C, Riou B, Berdeaux A, Forunier C, Khayat D, Rimailho A, Giudicelli JF, Auzépy P. Prospective study of the potentiation of acenocoumarol by amiodarone. *Eur J Clin Pharmacol* (1985) 28, 625–9.
6. El Allaf D, Sprynger M, Carlier J. Potentiation of the action of oral anticoagulants by amiodarone. *Acta Clin Belg* (1984) 39, 306–8.
7. Bharat V, Mohanty B. Bleeding complication during coumarin therapy due to amiodarone and azithromycin. *J Assoc Physicians India* (2000) 48, 746–7.
8. Broekmans AW, Meyboom RHB. Bijwerkingen van geneesmiddelen. Potentiëring van het cumarine-effect door amiodaron (Cordarone). *Ned Tijdschr Geneeskd* (1982) 126, 1415–17.
9. Verstraete M, Vermylen J, Claeys H. Dissimilar effect of two anti-anginal drugs belonging to the benzofuran group on the action of coumarin derivatives. *Arch Int Pharmacodyn Ther* (1968) 176, 33–41.
10. Martinowitz U, Rabinovici J, Goldfarb D, Many A, Bank H. Interaction between warfarin sodium and amiodarone. *N Engl J Med* (1981) 304, 671–2.
11. Rees A, Dalal JJ, Reid PG, Henderson AH, Lewis MJ. Dangers of amiodarone and anticoagulant treatment. *BMJ* (1981) 282, 1756–7.
12. Serlin MJ, Sibeon RG, Green GJ. Dangers of amiodarone and anticoagulant treatment. *BMJ* (1981) 283, 58.
13. Hamer A, Peter T, Mandel WJ, Scheinman MM, Weiss D. The potentiation of warfarin anticoagulation by amiodarone. *Circulation* (1982) 65, 1025–29.
14. McGovern B, Garan H, Kelly E, Ruskin JN. Adverse reactions during treatment with amiodarone hydrochloride. *BMJ* (1983) 287, 175–80.
15. Raeder EA, Podrid PJ, Lown B. Side effects and complications of amiodarone therapy. *Am Heart J* (1985) 109, 975–83.
16. Almog S, Shafran N, Halkin H, Weiss P, Farfel Z, Martinowitz U, Bank H. Mechanism of warfarin potentiation by amiodarone: dose- and concentration-dependent inhibition of warfarin elimination. *Eur J Clin Pharmacol* (1985) 28, 257–61.
17. Kerin NZ, Blevins RD, Goldman L, Faitel K, Rubenfire M. The incidence, magnitude, and time course of the amiodarone-warfarin interaction. *Arch Intern Med* (1988) 148, 1779–81.
18. Cheung B, Lam FM, Kumana CR. Insidiously evolving, occult drug interaction involving warfarin and amiodarone. *BMJ* (1996) 312, 107–8.
19. Chan TYK. Drug interactions as a cause of over-anticoagulation and bleedings in Chinese patients receiving warfarin. *Int J Clin Pharmacol Ther* (1998) 36, 403–5.
20. Sanoski CA, Bauman JL. Clinical observations with the amiodarone/warfarin interaction: dosing relationships with long-term therapy. *Chest* (2002) 121, 19–23.
21. Whitley HP, Fermo JD, Chumney ECG, Brzezinski WA. Effect of patient-specific factors on weekly warfarin dose. *Ther Clin Risk Manag* (2007) 3, 499–504.
22. Gage BF, Eby C, Johnson JA, Deych E, Rieder MJ, Ridker PM, Milligan PE, Grice G, Lenzini P, Rettie AE, Aquilante CL, Grosso L, Marsh S, Langaee T, Farnett LE, Voora D, Veenstra DL, Glynn RJ, Barrett A, McLeod HL. Use of Pharmacogenetic and Clinical Factors to Predict the Therapeutic Dose of Warfarin. *Clin Pharmacol Ther* (2008).
23. Edwin SB, Jennings DL, Kalus JS. An evaluation of the early pharmacodynamic response after simultaneous initiation of warfarin and amiodarone. *J Clin Pharmacol* (2010) 50, 693–8.
24. McDonald MG, Au NT, Wittkowsky AK, Rettie AE. Warfarin-amiodarone drug-drug interactions: determination of $[I]_u/K_{I,u}$ for amiodarone and its plasma metabolites. *Clin Pharmacol Ther* (2012) 91, 709–17.
25. Lu Y, Won KA, Nelson BJ, Qi D, Rausch DJ, Asinger RW. Characteristics of the amiodarone-warfarin interaction during long-term follow-up. *Am J Health-Syst Pharm* (2008) 65, 947–52.
26. Zhang K, Young C, Berger J. Administrative claims analysis of the relationship between warfarin use and risk of hemorrhage including drug-drug and drug-disease interactions. *J Manag Care Pharm* (2006)12, 640–8.
27. Watt AH, Stephens MR, Buss DC, Routledge PA. Amiodarone reduces plasma warfarin clearance in man. *Br J Clin Pharmacol* (1985) 20, 707–9.
28. Heimark LD, Wienkers L, Kunze K, Gibaldi M, Eddy AC, Trager WF, O'Reilly RA, Goulart DA. The mechanism of the interaction between amiodarone and warfarin in humans. *Clin Pharmacol Ther* (1992) 51, 398–407.
29. O'Reilly RA, Trager WF, Rettie AE, Goulart DA. Interaction of amiodarone with racemic warfarin and its separate enantiomorphs in humans. *Clin Pharmacol Ther* (1987) 42, 290–4.
30. Matsumoto K, Ueno K, Nakabayashi T, Komamura K, Kamakura S, Miyatake K. Amiodarone interaction time differences with warfarin and digoxin. *J Pharm Technol* (2003) 19, 83–90.
31. Woeber KA, Warner I. Potentiation of warfarin sodium by amiodarone-induced thyrotoxicosis. *West J Med* (1999) 170, 49–51.
32. Kurnik D, Loebstein R, Farfel Z, Ezra D, Halkin H, Olchovsky D. Complex drug-drug-disease interactions between amiodarone, warfarin, and the thyroid gland. *Medicine* (2004) 83, 107–13.
33. Naganuma M, Shiga T, Nishikata K, Tsuchiya T, Kasaniki H, Fujii E. Role of desethylamiodarone in the anticoagulant effect of concurrent amiodarone and warfarin therapy. *J Cardiovasc Pharmacol Ther* (2001) 6, 363–7.
34. Fondevila C, Meschengieser S, Lazzari M. Amiodarone-acenocoumarin interaction. *Thromb Haemost* (1991) 65, 328.

Coumarins and related drugs + Anabolic steroids or Androgens

Increased anticoagulant effects and bleeding have been seen in patients taking a coumarin or the indanedione, phenindione, and an anabolic steroid or testosterone.

Clinical evidence

(a) Anabolic steroids

Six patients stabilised on **warfarin** or **phenindione** were given **oxymetholone** 15 mg daily. One patient developed extensive subcutaneous bleeding and another had haematuria. After 15 to 30 days all 6 patients had thrombotests of less than 5%, which returned to the therapeutic range within a few days of **oxymetholone** being withdrawn.[1] Other similar cases have been reported with **oxymetholone** and **warfarin**,[2-4] or **acenocoumarol**.[5] In 3 of the reports[1,3,4] the interaction was severe enough to discontinue the **oxymetholone**. In one patient[2] the **warfarin** dose was reduced by 59%, and in another[5] the **acenocoumarol** dose was reduced by 66 to 75%. Similarly increased anticoagulant effects and bleeding have been described in studies and case reports involving:

- **dicoumarol** with **norethandrolone**,[6]
- **dicoumarol** with **stanozolol**,[7]
- **phenindione** with **methandienone**,[8]
- **phenindione** with **ethylestrenol**,[9]
- **warfarin** with **methandienone**[2,8,10,11] (62% to 73% decrease in dose required in 3 cases[2] and 38% in 7 others[8]),
- **warfarin** with **stanozolol**[12-15] (40% and 64% decrease in dose required in 2 patients and about a 70% increase required after stopping stanozolol[12]).

In a pharmacokinetic study in 15 healthy subjects, the concurrent use of **warfarin** and **oxandrolone** 5 or 10 mg twice daily increased the *S*-warfarin AUC by 2.65-fold and doubled its half-life, and had similar effects on *R*-warfarin.[16] Microscopic haematuria occurred in 9 subjects and gingival bleeding in one. An 80 to 85% decrease in the dose of **warfarin** was necessary to maintain a target INR of 1.5.

(b) Androgens

A 58-year-old man receiving **methyltestosterone** replacement therapy 37.5 mg daily required a maintenance dose of **phenprocoumon** of just 0.94 mg daily compared with control subjects who required 2.62 mg daily.[17] One report notes that 3 patients receiving **warfarin** and *Sustanon* (containing four combined esters of **testosterone**) had no changes in their anticoagulant requirements,[4] whereas another report describes a woman who had a 78% and a 65% increase in prothrombin times on two occasions when using a 2% **testosterone propionate** vaginal ointment twice daily. She needed a 25% reduction in her **warfarin** dose.[18]

Mechanism

Not understood. One study found that norethandrolone did not alter the metabolism of dicoumarol, and did not alter the plasma levels of vitamin-K dependent clotting factors.[6] However, a more recent study of oxandrolone and warfarin suggests a pharmacokinetic basis for this interaction.[16]

Importance and management

The interactions between warfarin and the anabolic steroids are well documented, well established and clinically important. The effect develops rapidly, possibly within 2 to 3 days. Most, if not all, patients are affected.[1,6] If concurrent use cannot be avoided, the dose of the anticoagulant should be appropriately reduced. In a few cases, where patients have been able to be stabilised on the combination, up to 75% reductions in anticoagulant dose have been required, and the study with oxandrolone[16] suggests that an 85% reduction in the dose of warfarin might be necessary. After withdrawal of the interacting drug the anticoagulant dose will need to be increased.

It seems probable that all the coumarin and indanedione anticoagulants will interact with any 17-alkyl substituted anabolic steroid; effects have been seen on acenocoumarol, dicoumarol and phenindione. The situation with testosterone and other non 17-alkylated steroids is not clear as there are only case reports, which are conflicting. Until more is known it would seem prudent to increase the frequency of INR monitoring if these drugs are given with coumarins or indanediones.

1. Longridge RGM, Gillam PMS, Barton GMG. Decreased anticoagulant tolerance with oxymetholone. *Lancet* (1971) ii, 90.
2. Murakami M, Odake K, Matsuda T, Onchi K, Umeda T, Nishino T. Effects of anabolic steroids on anticoagulant requirements. *Jpn Circ J* (1965) 29, 243–50.
3. Robinson BHB, Hawkins JB, Ellis JE, Moore-Robinson M. Decreased anticoagulant tolerance with oxymetholone. *Lancet* (1971) i, 1356.
4. Edwards MS, Curtis JR. Decreased anticoagulant tolerance with oxymetholone. *Lancet* (1971) ii, 221.
5. de Oya JC, del Río A, Noya M, Villeneuva A. Decreased anticoagulant tolerance with oxymetholone in paroxysmal nocturnal hæmoglobinuria. *Lancet* (1971) ii, 259.
6. Schrogie JJ, Solomon HM. The anticoagulant response to bishydroxycoumarin. II. The effect of d-thyroxine, clofibrate, and norethandrolone. *Clin Pharmacol Ther* (1967) 8, 70–7.
7. Howard CW, Hanson SG, Wahed MA. Anabolic steroids and anticoagulants. *BMJ* (1977) 1, 1659–60.
8. Pyörälä K, Kekki M. Decreased anticoagulant tolerance during methandrostenolone therapy. *Scand J Clin Lab Invest* (1963) 15, 367–74.
9. Vere DW, Fearnley GR. Suspected interaction between phenindione and ethylœstrenol. *Lancet* (1968) ii, 281.
10. Dresdale FC, Hayes JC. Potential dangers in the combined use of methandrostenolone and sodium warfarin. *J Med Soc New Jers* (1967) 64, 609–12.
11. McLaughlin GE, McCarty DJ, Segal BL. Hemarthrosis complicating anticoagulant therapy. Report of three cases. *JAMA* (1966) 196, 1020–1.
12. Acomb C, Shaw PW. A significant interaction between warfarin and stanozolol. *Pharm J* (1985) 234, 73–4.
13. Cleverly CR. Personal communication, March 1987.
14. Shaw PW, Smith AM. Possible interaction of warfarin and stanozolol. *Clin Pharm* (1987) 6, 500–2.
15. Elwin C-E, Törngren M. Samtidigt intag av warfarin och stanozolol orsak till blödningar hos patienten. *Lakartidningen* (1988) 85, 3290.
16. Oxandrin (Oxandrolone). Savient Pharmaceuticals Inc. US Prescribing information, January 2006.
17. Husted S, Andreasen F, Foged L. Increased sensitivity to phenprocoumon during methyltestosterone therapy. *Eur J Clin Pharmacol* (1976) 10, 209–16.
18. Lorentz SM, Weibert RT. Potentiation of warfarin anticoagulation by topical testosterone ointment. *Clin Pharm* (1985) 4, 332–4.

Coumarins + Angiotensin II receptor antagonists

None of the angiotensin II receptor antagonists appear to interact with warfarin to a clinically relevant extent.

Clinical evidence

(a) Candesartan

In healthy subjects stabilised on individualised doses of **warfarin**, candesartan cilexetil 16 mg daily for 10 days reduced the trough serum levels of **warfarin** by 7%, but this had no effect on prothrombin times.[1]

(b) Eprosartan

No clinically relevant changes in anticoagulation occurred in 18 healthy subjects stabilised on **warfarin** with INRs between 1.3 and 1.6 when they were given eprosartan 300 mg twice daily for 7 days.[2]

(c) Irbesartan

Warfarin 2.5 to 10 mg daily was given to 16 healthy subjects for 2 weeks, with irbesartan 300 mg or a placebo daily for a further week. There was no evidence that irbesartan affected the pharmacokinetics or pharmacodynamics of **warfarin.**[3]

(d) Losartan

In a placebo-controlled, randomised, crossover study, 10 healthy subjects were given losartan 100 mg daily for 13 days with a single 30-mg dose of **warfarin** on day 7. The pharmacokinetics of **warfarin** (both *R*- and *S*-enantiomers) and its anticoagulant effects were not altered. Losartan, given alone for one week, also had no effect on prothrombin times.[4]

(e) Olmesartan

In a study in 24 healthy subjects given **warfarin** titrated to a Quick value of between 1.4 and 1.8 for 2 weeks, the addition of olmesartan 40 mg daily for a further 7 days had no effect on the pharmacokinetics of either *R*- or *S*-warfarin. There was also no change in Quick value or partial prothrombin time.[5]

(f) Telmisartan

Telmisartan 120 mg daily for 10 days was given to 12 healthy subjects stabilised on **warfarin**, with INRs of between 1.2 and 1.8. A small 11% decrease in the mean trough plasma **warfarin** concentration occurred, but the anticoagulation effect remained unchanged.[6]

(g) Valsartan

In a study in 12 healthy subjects, valsartan 160 mg daily was given for 7 days with **warfarin** 10 mg daily for the first 3 days. **Warfarin** had no effect on the pharmacokinetics of valsartan. Valsartan caused a small increase in prothrombin time of about 12%, which was not considered clinically important. **Warfarin** pharmacokinetics were not assessed.[7,8]

Mechanism

In vitro, various angiotensin II antagonists have some cytochrome P450 isoenzyme CYP2C9 inhibitory activity,[9] and it is therefore possible that they might reduce warfarin metabolism.

Importance and management

Despite the reported *in vitro* inhibitory effects on CYP2C9 reported for some angiotensin II antagonists, the available pharmacokinetic and pharmacodynamic studies show that the angiotensin II receptor antagonists (candesartan, eprosartan, irbesartan, losartan, olmesartan, telmisartan, valsartan) do not interact with warfarin to a clinically relevant extent. The lack of any published evidence to the contrary suggests that no warfarin dose adjustments should be needed if these drugs are given together.

1. Jonkman JHG, van Lier JJ, van Heiningen PNM, Lins R, Sennewald R, Högemann A. Pharmacokinetic drug interaction studies with candesartan cilexetil. *J Hum Hypertens* (1997) 11 (Suppl 2), S31–S35.
2. Kazierad DJ, Martin DE, Ilson B, Boike S, Zariffa N, Forrest A, Jorkasky DK. Eprosartan does not affect the pharmacodynamics of warfarin. *J Clin Pharmacol* (1998) 38, 649–53.
3. Mangold B, Gielsdorf W, Marino MR. Irbesartan does not affect the steady-state pharmacodynamics and pharmacokinetics of warfarin. *Eur J Clin Pharmacol* (1999) 55, 593–8.
4. Kong A-N T, Tomasko P, Waldman SA, Osborne B, Deutsch PJ, Goldberg MR, Bjornsson TD. Losartan does not affect the pharmacokinetics and pharmacodynamics of warfarin. *J Clin Pharmacol* (1995) 35, 1008–15.
5. Laeis P, Püchler K, Kirch W. The pharmacokinetic and metabolic profile of olmesartan medoxomil limits the risk of clinically relevant drug interaction. *J Hypertens* (2001) 19 (Suppl.), S21–S32.
6. Stangier J, Su C-APF, Hendriks MGC, van Lier JJ, Sollie FAE, Oosterhuis B, Jonkman JHG. Steady-state pharmacodynamics and pharmacokinetics of warfarin in the presence and absence of telmisartan in healthy male volunteers. *J Clin Pharmacol* (2000) 40, 1331–7.
7. Novartis Pharmaceuticals Ltd. Data on file. Protocol 40.
8. Knight H, Flesch G, Prasad P, Lloyd P, Douglas J. Lack of pharmacokinetic and pharmacodynamic interaction between valsartan and warfarin. *J Hypertens* (2000) 18 (Suppl 4), S89.
9. Kamiyama E, Yoshigae Y, Kasuya A, Takei M, Kurihara A, Ikeda T. Inhibitory effects of angiotensin receptor blockers on CYP2C9 activity in human liver microsomes. *Drug Metab Pharmacokinet* (2007) 22, 267–75.

Coumarins + Antacids

There is some evidence that the absorption of dicoumarol may be increased by magnesium hydroxide. Aluminium hydroxide does not interact with either warfarin or dicoumarol, and magnesium hydroxide does not interact with warfarin.

Clinical evidence

(a) Dicoumarol

In a study in 6 healthy subjects, **magnesium hydroxide** (*Milk of Magnesia*) 15 mL, taken with and 3 hours after a single dose of dicoumarol, was found to raise the peak plasma levels and AUC of dicoumarol by 75% and 50%, respectively. Conversely, **aluminium hydroxide** (*Amphogel*) 30 mL did not alter dicoumarol levels.[1]

(b) Warfarin

In a study in 6 healthy subjects, **aluminium/magnesium hydroxide** (*Maalox*) 30 mL, given with and for four 2-hourly doses after warfarin, had no effect on the plasma warfarin levels or on the anticoagulant response.[2] Similarly, neither **aluminium hydroxide** (*Amphogel*) 30 mL nor **magnesium hydroxide** (*Milk of Magnesia*) 15 mL, taken with and 3 hours after a single 75-mg dose of warfarin, had any effect on warfarin peak levels or AUC.[1]

Mechanism

It is suggested that dicoumarol forms a more readily absorbed chelate with magnesium so that its effects are increased.[1,3] An *in vitro* study suggested that the absorption of warfarin may be decreased by **magnesium trisilicate**,[4] where as another *in vitro* study found no effect.[5]

Importance and management

No special precautions need be taken if aluminium or magnesium hydroxide antacids are given to patients taking warfarin, or if aluminium hydroxide is given to those taking dicoumarol. Despite the evidence of increased absorption of dicoumarol with magnesium hydroxide, there seems to be no direct clinical evidence of any important adverse interaction for this combination, or indeed between any coumarin and an antacid.

1. Ambre JJ, Fischer LJ. Effect of coadministration of aluminum and magnesium hydroxides on absorption of anticoagulants in man. *Clin Pharmacol Ther* (1973) 14, 231–7.
2. Robinson DS, Benjamin DM, McCormack JJ. Interaction of warfarin and nonsystemic gastrointestinal drugs. *Clin Pharmacol Ther* (1971) 12, 491–5.
3. Akers MJ, Lach JL, Fischer LJ. Alterations in the absorption of dicoumarol by various excipient materials. *J Pharm Sci* (1973) 62, 391–5.
4. McElnay JC, Harron DWG, D'Arcy PF, Collier PS. Interaction of warfarin with antacid constituents. *BMJ* (1978) 2, 1166.
5. Khalil SA, Naggar VF, Zaghloul IA, Ismail AA. In vitro anticoagulant–antacid interactions. *Int J Pharmaceutics* (1984) 19, 307–21.

Coumarins + Antibacterials

Altered (usually enhanced) response to anticoagulation with a coumarin has been reported with virtually every class of antibacterial. While some such as sulfamethoxazole, clearly have a pharmacokinetic interaction, for others there is no clear explanation for why an interaction might be expected. Theoretical mechanisms include reduced intestinal bacterial production of vitamin K_2 substances, or reduced enterohepatic recycling. Possible confounding mechanisms include a reduction in dietary vitamin K_1 intake because of illness, or the effect of fever or infection on coagulation or drug metabolism.

Clinical evidence and mechanism

Various studies have implicated antibacterials in general as being a risk factor for over-anticoagulation. For example, in a large prospective cohort study, INR levels of greater than 7 were recorded in 31 patients. When compared with 100 patients with stable INRs, these 31 patients were more likely to have been treated with an antibacterial (not specified) in the previous 4 weeks (odds ratio 6.2), and more likely to have an intercurrent illness (odds ratio 4.48).[1] Various mechanisms may be responsible for these findings, and these are discussed below.

(a) Confounding effects relating to the infection

1. Dietary factors. Patients taking coumarins and related drugs are advised to maintain a constant dietary intake of vitamin K_1 as sustained changes in intake of vitamin K_1-rich foods, such as green leafy vegetables, causes clinically relevant changes in anticoagulation. See 'Coumarins and related drugs + Food; Vitamin K_1-rich', p.432. It is therefore possible that patients who stop eating for more than a day or so could develop over-anticoagulation. The same could happen with a reduced appetite leading to a sustained reduction in intake of vitamin K_1-rich foods.

2. Fever. Fever might possibly be a confounding factor in reports of interactions between antibacterials and warfarin, because it might increase the catabolism of vitamin K-dependent coagulation factors by producing a hypermetabolic state. However, in one cohort study, there was no difference in the frequency of fever between patients who developed over-anticoagulation (INR greater than 6) while taking antibacterials and those who did not develop over-anticoagulation while taking antibacterials.[2]

3. Reduced metabolism. There is some evidence from *animal* studies that infection can down regulate cytochrome P450 isoenzymes, which might result in reduced drug metabolism.[3] Whether the metabolism of warfarin is different during an acute infection does not appear to have been studied.

(b) Effects relating to the antibacterial

1. Direct anticoagulant effects. Cephalosporins and related beta lactams with an *N*-methylthiotetrazole or similar side-chain can occasionally cause enough hypoprothrombinaemia for bleeding to occur when they are used alone, and this effect might therefore be additive with coumarins, although there is not that much evidence to support this, see 'Coumarins and related drugs + Antibacterials; Cephalosporins and related drugs', p.385.

2. Intestinal production of vitamin K_2 substances by bacteria. The activity of intestinal microflora produces menaquinones (vitamin K_2 substances). Suppression of the microflora might therefore result in reduced vitamin K_2, and hence reduced synthesis of vitamin-K dependent clotting factors. There is some evidence from studies in healthy subjects receiving vitamin-K_1 restricted diets and taking warfarin that giving menaquinones (an extract of bacterially synthesised material) decreases the response to warfarin.[4] In addition, natto, a fermented soya bean product which is a rich source of bacterially-derived menaquinones, markedly inhibits the effect of warfarin (see 'Coumarins + Food; Soya bean products', p.431). It is therefore possible that antibacterials that decimate gut microflora might increase the effect of warfarin by reducing vitamin K_2 levels. However, this effect might be important only if vitamin-K_1 intake from dietary sources is also reduced.

3. Protein-binding displacement. Many drugs can displace warfarin from protein-binding sites leading to an increase in unbound (active) concentrations of warfarin. However, any effect is transient, as the unbound warfarin is quickly metabolised. The exception to this is if the metabolism of warfarin is markedly inhibited at the same time. On rare example of a drug that is known to interact by both these mechanisms is phenylbutazone, see 'Coumarins and related drugs + NSAIDs; Phenylbutazone and related drugs', p.455. Altered protein binding has not clearly been shown to be an important mechanism in any interaction between warfarin and an antibacterial, but it is often suggested as one.

4. Reduced or increased metabolism. Sulfamethoxazole clearly inhibits the metabolism of warfarin by the cytochrome P450 isoenzyme CYP2C9, so enhancing its effect. Some macrolides such as erythromycin inhibit CYP3A4, and therefore have a minor inhibitory effect on *R*-warfarin, which would, on its own, be unlikely to be of any clinical relevance. Conversely, rifampicin (rifampin), see 'Coumarins + Antibacterials; Rifamycins', p.397, is a well established inducer of drug metabolism, and clearly reduces the effect of warfarin. Nafcillin (see 'Coumarins + Antibacterials; Penicillins', p.391) also appears to markedly reduce the effects of warfarin. Most other antibacterial classes have no clinically relevant effect on warfarin pharmacokinetics.

Importance and management

All these factors in their own right might affect the intensity of anticoagulation. Therefore, a few case reports of an enhanced response to warfarin on starting a specific antibacterial does not necessarily imply that the antibacterial has a direct interaction with warfarin. Conversely, demonstration of a lack of a specific interaction between an antibacterial and warfarin in a controlled study does not mean that a patient prescribed that drug for an infection will not have a change in coagulation status. Therefore, if a patient is unwell enough to require an antibacterial, it may be prudent to increase monitoring of coagulation status even if no specific drug interaction is expected. Monitor within 3 days of starting the antibacterial. The expectation of an interaction should not exclude the use of an antibacterial if it is considered clinically appropriate.

1. Panneerselvam S, Baglin C, Lefort W, Baglin T. Analysis of risk factors for over-anticoagulation in patient receiving long-term warfarin. *Br J Haematol* (1998) 103, 422–4.
2. Visser LE, Penning-van Beest FJA, Kasbergen AAH, De Smet PAGM, Vulto AG, Hofman A, Stricker BHC. Overanticoagulation associated with combined use of antibacterial drugs and acenocoumarol or phenprocoumon anticoagulants. *Thromb Haemost* (2002) 88, 705–10.
3. Eschenauer G, Collins CD, Regal RE. Azithromycin-warfarin interaction: are we fishing with a red herring? *Pharmacotherapy* (2005) 25, 630–1.
4. Conly JM, Stein K, Worobetz L, Rutledge-Harding S. The contribution of vitamin K2 (menaquinones) produced by the intestinal microflora to human nutritional requirements for vitamin K. *Am J Gastroenterol* (1994) 89, 915–23.

Coumarins and related drugs + Antibacterials; Aminoglycosides

Limited data suggest that no clinically significant interaction occurs between dicoumarol or warfarin and oral neomycin or paromomycin in most patients. However, individual patients have shown some alteration in anticoagulant effect (usually increases) when given oral neomycin and parenteral streptomycin, and a marked increased risk of hospitalisation for bleeding has been reported in patients taking acenocoumarol and phenprocoumon and given neomycin.

Clinical evidence

(a) Neomycin

Six out of 10 patients taking **warfarin** who were given oral neomycin (2 g daily[1] or 4 g daily[2]) over a 3-week period had a gradual increase in their prothrombin times averaging 5.6 seconds.[1,2] Similarly, in patients taking an unnamed anticoagulant, 2 of 5 given oral neomycin with bacitracin had a fall in their prothrombin-proconvertin concentration from a range of 10 to 30% to less than 6%. This suggests an *increase* in anticoagulant effect.

Five of 7 patients taking unnamed anticoagulants had no change in their mean daily dose of anticoagulant when given oral **neomycin** 1 to 2 g daily for 18 weeks. Of the remaining two, one required an increase of about 100%, and one required a small 27% decrease.[3]

In a retrospective cohort study,[4] the relative risk of hospitalisation for bleeding in patients taking **acenocoumarol** or **phenprocoumon** and given neomycin was very high (relative risk 43). However, as the incidence of concurrent use was low (only 25 patients), the confidence interval was very broad (range 6 to 308).

(b) Paromomycin

The concurrent use of oral **paromomycin** 2 g daily with **dicoumarol** or **warfarin** did not alter anticoagulant requirements in 2 subjects.[5]

(c) Streptomycin

One of 3 patients given parenteral **streptomycin** 500 mg twice daily, and 2 patients given parenteral **streptomycin** 500 mg twice daily with 1 million units of penicillin daily had a fall in their prothrombin-proconvertin concentration from a range of 10 to 30% down to 6 to 9%. This suggests an *increase* in anticoagulant effect.[6]

Mechanism

Not understood. One idea is that these antibacterials increase the effects of these coumarins by diminishing the bacterial population in the gut, thereby reducing their production of vitamin K_2 substances, see 'Coumarins + Antibacterials', p.383. Another suggestion is that these antibacterials decrease the vitamin K_1 absorption as part of a general antibacterial-induced malabsorption syndrome.[7]

Importance and management

A sparsely documented interaction. The data implies that, rarely, an increased risk of bleeding may occur if aminoglycosides are given with coumarins but common experience seems to confirm that normally no interaction of any significance occurs. The data relating to acenocoumarol and phenprocoumon and neomycin need confirming.

One manufacturer of **gentamicin** suggests that concurrent use with oral anticoagulants may decrease thrombin levels,[8] which would be expected to increase the risk of bleeding, but there appears to be little evidence to suggest that this usually occurs. However, occasionally vitamin K deficiency and/or spontaneous bleeding is seen after the prolonged use of broad-spectrum antibacterials in association with a totally inadequate diet, starvation or some other condition in which the intake of vitamin K is very limited.[9,10] Under these circumstances the effects of the vitamin-K antagonist anticoagulants (both coumarins and **indanediones**) would be expected to be significantly increased and appropriate precautions should be taken.

1. Udall JA. Drug interference with warfarin therapy. *Clin Med* (1970) 77, 20–25.
2. Udall JA. Human sources and absorption of vitamin K in relation to anticoagulation stability. *JAMA* (1965) 194, 107–9.
3. Schade RWB, van't Laar A, Majoor CLH, Jansen AP. A comparative study of the effects of cholestyramine and neomycin in the treatment of type II hyperlipoproteinaemia. *Acta Med Scand* (1976) 199, 175–80.
4. Penning-van Beest FJA, Koerselman J, Herings RMC. Risk of major bleeding during concomitant use of antibiotic drugs and coumarin anticoagulants. *J Thromb Haemost* (2008) 6, 284–90.
5. Messinger WJ, Samet CM. The effect of a bowel sterilizing antibiotic on blood coagulation mechanisms. The anti-cholesterol effect of paromomycin. *Angiology* (1965) 16, 29–36.
6. Magid E. Tolerance to anticoagulants during antibiotic therapy. *Scand J Clin Lab Invest* (1962) 14, 565–6.
7. Faloon WW, Paes IC, Woolfolk D, Nankin H, Wallace K, Haro EN. Effect of neomycin and kanamycin upon intestinal absorption. *Ann N Y Acad Sci* (1966) 132, 879–87.
8. Gentamicin Paediatric Solution for Injection. Winthrop Pharmaceuticals UK Ltd. UK Summary of product characteristics, November 2006.
9. Haden HT. Vitamin K deficiency associated with prolonged antibiotic administration. *Arch Intern Med* (1957) 100, 986–8.
10. Frick PG, Riedler G, Brögli H. Dose response and minimal daily requirement for vitamin K in man. *J Appl Physiol* (1967) 23, 387–9.

Coumarins + Antibacterials; Aminosalicylic acid and/or Isoniazid

A report attributes bleeding in a patient taking warfarin to the concurrent use of isoniazid. Another report describes a markedly increased anticoagulant response in a patient taking warfarin when the dose was doubled and aminosalicylic acid and isoniazid were started.

Clinical evidence

A man who had recently started to take **warfarin** 10 mg daily and isoniazid 300 mg daily began to bleed (haematuria, bleeding gums) within 10 days of accidentally doubling his dose of isoniazid. His prothrombin time had increased from about 26 seconds to 53 seconds.[1] Another patient taking digoxin, potassium chloride, docusate, diazepam and **warfarin** 2.5 mg daily, was also given aminosalicylic acid 12 g, isoniazid 300 mg and pyridoxine 100 mg daily, and at the same time the warfarin dose was doubled to 5 mg daily. His prothrombin time increased from 18 seconds to 130 seconds over 20 days but no signs of bleeding were seen.[2]

Mechanism

Not understood. It seems possible that isoniazid may inhibit the metabolism of the coumarin anticoagulants, because *in vitro* study in human liver microsomes has shown that it inhibits *S*-warfarin 7-hydroxylation by the cytochrome P450 isoenzyme CYP2C9,[3] but this needs confirmation *in vivo*. Isoniazid increased the anticoagulant effects of dicoumarol in *dogs*[4] but not of warfarin in *rabbits*.[5] Two patients taking isoniazid, aminosalicylic acid and streptomycin (but not taking anticoagulants) developed haemorrhage, which was attributed to the effects of isoniazid alone.[6]

Importance and management

These two isolated cases of possible interactions are far from conclusive, and the interactions of warfarin with isoniazid and aminosalicylic acid are not established. Nevertheless, given that the *in vitro* data suggest that isoniazid might inhibit warfarin metabolism, some caution might be appropriate. If this is the case, similar caution may also need to be extended to other coumarins that are metabolised in the same way as warfarin, such as **acenocoumarol**. Further study is needed.

1. Rosenthal AR, Self TH, Baker ED, Linden RA. Interaction of isoniazid and warfarin. *JAMA* (1977) 238, 2177.
2. Self TH. Interaction of warfarin and aminosalicylic acid. *JAMA* (1973) 223, 1285.
3. Nishimura Y, Kurata N, Sakurai E, Yasuhara H. Inhibitory effect of antituberculosis drugs on human cytochrome P450-mediated activities. *J Pharmacol Sci* (2004) 96, 293–300.
4. Eade NR, McLeod PJ, MacLeod SM. Potentiation of bishydroxycoumarin in dogs by isoniazid and p-aminosalicylic acid. *Am Rev Respir Dis* (1971) 103, 792–9.
5. Kiblawi SS, Jay SJ, Bang NU, Rowe HM. Influence of isoniazid on the anticoagulant effect of warfarin. *Clin Ther* (1979) 2, 235–9.
6. Castell FA. Accion anticoagulante de la isoniazida. *Enferm Torax* (1969) 18, 153–62.

Coumarins and related drugs + Antibacterials; Cephalosporins and related drugs

Cephalosporins and related beta lactams with an *N*-methylthiotetrazole or similar side-chain can occasionally cause bleeding when they are used alone. These effects could therefore be additive with those of the coumarins. Some studies and cases of increased INRs and bleeding have been reported with both warfarin and acenocoumarol.

Of the cephalosporins not having an *N*-methylthiotetrazole or related side-chain, a few cases of over-anticoagulation have been reported for cefixime and cefaclor with coumarins and phenindione, an increased risk of haemorrhage has been reported in patients taking coumarins with cefuroxime and cefradine, and there is a report of an increased INR with warfarin and ceftaroline. Cefalexin does not appear to interact.

Clinical evidence

(a) Cephalosporins with N-methylthiotetrazole or similar side-chains

Note that cephalosporins with N-methylthiotetrazole or similar side-chains can cause bleeding alone. For example, serious bleeding following the use of **cefamandole** (in the absence of an anticoagulant) has been described in 3 out of 37 patients in one report,[1] and a further report highlights a further 16 cases.[2] Other similar cephalosporins and related beta lactams that have been reported to cause hypoprothrombinaemia when used alone include **cefoperazone,**[3-7] **cefotetan,**[8] **ceftriaxone,**[9] **cefalotin,**[10] **cefazolin,**[11-13] and **latamoxef.**[14,15] The incidence is very variable: in some instances only isolated cases have been reported whereas a 15% bleeding rate was found in one study[15] with **latamoxef** alone, 22% in another[14], but only 8% with **cefoxitin** alone.[14] These cephalosporins might therefore worsen the risk of bleeding by simple addition if given with coumarin or **indanedione** anticoagulants. In addition, some of them might also inhibit platelet function.[16]

1. Cefamandole or cefazolin. Two patients who had received prophylactic cefamandole before cardiac valve replacement developed unusually high prothrombin times, with bleeding in one case, within 48 hours of an initial dose of **warfarin** 10 mg. Because of this, the records of a total of 60 other patients who had undergone heart valve replacement surgery were reviewed. They had been given prophylactic antibacterials before the chest incision was made, and every 6 hours thereafter for about 72 hours. The 44 patients given cefamandole 2 g showed a much greater anticoagulant response than the 16 patients given vancomycin 500 mg. Fourteen of the cefamandole group had a prothrombin time greater than 32 seconds after the initial **warfarin** dose, compared with only one of the vancomycin group.[17] In a later randomised study by the same workers, the prothrombin times as a percentage of activity after 3 days of concurrent use with **warfarin** were cefamandole 29%, cefazolin 38%, and vancomycin 51%. This suggests that cefamandole had a much greater effect on anticoagulant response than vancomycin.[18]

2. Cefonicid. In a study in 9 patients stabilised on **warfarin**, there was no change in prothrombin times when they were given intravenous cefonicid 2 g daily for 7 days.[19] In contrast, a later study identified 9 patients taking **acenocoumarol** who had increased INRs within 3 to 8 days of being given cefonicid. They needed a reduction in the anticoagulant dose of about one-third to one-half.[20] Another patient stabilised on **acenocoumarol**, with a prothrombin index of 28% bled 2 days after starting cefonicid 1 g daily and had a prothrombin index of less than 5%.[21]

3. Cefotiam. Severe haemorrhage has been reported in 3 patients taking **acenocoumarol** with cefotiam. One developed an abdominal haematoma and an INR of 10.4 within 2 days. Another had gastrointestinal bleeding and melaena after one day of concurrent use. The third died from intracranial haemorrhage on the day she started cefotiam.[22]

4. Ceftriaxone. A case report describes a 67-year-old woman stabilised on **warfarin** for about 8 years, who experienced a greatly increased INR (10.74 compared with 1.9 to 3 previously) 4 days after receiving a single 1-g intramuscular dose of ceftriaxone. Phytomenadione was given and warfarin withheld for 1 day, after which her INR was 3.4 (within her target range). Her INR values remained stable for 4 to 5 weeks, when she again required a single 1-g intramuscular dose of ceftriaxone. At this time, she was also prescribed cefuroxime 500 mg twice daily for 7 days and phenazopyridine if needed. Four days after this second dose of ceftriaxone, her INR was again increased, this time to 16.99 (compared with 2.8 a week earlier). Phytomenadione was again administered and warfarin was withheld but her INR remained high at 4.6. After withholding warfarin for a further day, her INR returned to range at 2.1. She resumed her 7.5 mg daily warfarin dose and 1 week later her INR remained within range.[23]

(b) Cephalosporins without N-methylthiotetrazole or similar side-chains

1. Cefaclor. Over the period 1979 to 1997, the CSM in the UK had received reports of 3 cases of increased INRs, with or without clinical bleeding, in patients taking cefaclor with **acenocoumarol, warfarin**, or an unknown anticoagulant.[24] No cases seem to have been published.

2. Cefalexin. In a retrospective case-control study in patients taking **warfarin**, there was a small but statistically significant increase in the risk of hospitalisation for gastrointestinal haemorrhage in those who had received cefalexin 6 to 10 days before admission. However, the risk was similar to that 0 to 5 days before admission (during which time it is unlikely that any pharmacokinetic interaction would have occurred).[25]

3. Cefixime. Cefixime has also been implicated in a handful of cases of bleeding and/or increased INRs in patients taking **warfarin** or the indanedione **phenindione**, but the evidence is inconclusive.[26] No cases seem to have been published.

4. Cefradine. In a retrospective cohort study, the relative risk of hospitalisation for bleeding in patients taking **acenocoumarol** or **phenprocoumon** and also taking cefradine was very high (relative risk 43). This equated to 1 major bleed per 100 cefradine prescriptions during coumarin use.[27]

5. Ceftaroline. An 85-year-old woman with a therapeutic INR while receiving **warfarin** experienced an increased INR after receiving a course of ceftaroline for cellulitis.[28]

6. Cefuroxime. In a retrospective case-control study,[29] there was a modest increased risk of hospitalisation for haemorrhage in acutely ill elderly patients taking warfarin who had received cefuroxime prior to admission (odds ratio 1.62). A retrospective review of the effect of antibacterials on INR in children taking **warfarin** mentions that a 2-and-a-half-year-old child had an INR of 6.7 five days after starting oral cefuroxime.[30]

(c) Unnamed cephalosporins

In a prospective study of the effect of antibacterials on anticoagulation, none of the 36 patients taking **warfarin** and prescribed an oral cephalosporin (not named) experienced a change in their INR.[31] Conversely, a mean INR increase of 1.2 was reported in 12 children taking **warfarin** and receiving cephalosporins.[30] In a large analysis of claims data, use of cephalosporins (unnamed) with **warfarin** was associated with a very small increase in the risk of haemorrhage of 1.16, which was statistically significant.[32] Similarly, a prospective case-control study using health insurance data found that use of cephalosporins) with **warfarin** (36 patients) was associated with an increased risk of hospitalisation due to bleeding (odds ratio 2.45; range 1.52 to 3.95). Antibacterial and antifungal use in general was associated with an overall increased risk of 2.01 (range 1.62 to 2.5), with the greatest risk being associated with use during the 60 days prior to the bleed occurring.[33] A case-control study[34] in 2 553 patients taking **phenprocoumon** found that the risk of hospitalisation due to bleeding appeared to be increased in the 20 patients taking cephalosporins (drugs not stated).

Mechanism

Cephalosporins with an *N*-methylthiotetrazole side-chain can, like the oral anticoagulants, act as vitamin K antagonists to reduce the production of some blood clotting factors. They can therefore cause bleeding on their own, which would be expected to be additive when used with an anticoagulant. Some of these cephalosporins might also inhibit platelet function.[16]

Ceftriaxone seems to act similarly although it has an *N*-methylthio*triazine* ring instead, as does cefazolin, which has an *N*-methylthiadiazolethiol side-chain. **Aztreonam** can also increase the prothrombin time.[35-38]

Importance and management

Most cephalosporins and related beta lactams do not normally cause bleeding so would not be expected to have an additive interaction with the oral anticoagulants. In contrast, cephalosporins with the *N*-methylthiotetrazole or similar side-chains appear to increase the risk of bleeding, and might therefore interact. Both **cefamandole** and to a lesser extent **cefazolin** have been shown to increase the response to warfarin, and cases of over-anticoagulation have been reported for **cefonicid** and **cefotiam**. All other cephalosporins and related beta-lactams with the *N*-methylthiotetrazole or similar side-chains might be expected to interact similarly, but have not so far been reported to specifically interact with anticoagulants. These include **cefalotin, cefmenoxime, cefmetazole, cefminox, cefoperazone, ceforanide, cefotetan, cefpiramide**, and **latamoxef**. **Aztreonam** has also been predicted to interact similarly, although, again there are no reports. Patients most at risk seem to be those whose intake of vitamin K is restricted (such as poor diet or malabsorption syndromes) and those with renal impairment. The use of an anticoagulant represents just another factor that could precipitate bleeding.

A possible solution to the problem is to use a non-interacting cephalosporin. Alternatively the outcome should be closely monitored, particularly in the early stages of treatment, adjusting the anticoagulant dose if necessary. Excessive hypoprothrombinaemia can be controlled with vitamin K. Although they do not have an *N*-methylthiotetrazole side-chain, the manufacturers of **cefixime** and **cefaclor** have a few cases of over-anticoagulation on record, an increased risk of haemorrhage has been reported for **cefradine** and **cefuroxime**, and a case of an increased INR has been reported for **ceftaroline**. **Cefalexin** does not appear to interact.

Even with non-interacting cephalosporins, if a patient is unwell enough to require an antibacterial, it would be prudent to increase monitoring of coagulation status, bearing in mind that factors relating to acute infection rather than the antibacterial used to treat it could also be responsible for increased INRs or bleeding events (see also 'Coumarins + Antibacterials', p.383). Monitor within 3 days of starting the antibacterial.

1. Hooper CA, Haney BB, Stone HH. Gastrointestinal bleeding due to vitamin K deficiency in patients on parenteral cefamandole. *Lancet* (1980) i, 39–40.
2. Rymer W, Greenlaw CW. Hypoprothrombinemia associated with cefamandole. *Drug Intell Clin Pharm* (1980) 14, 780–3.
3. Meisel S. Hypoprothrombinemia due to cefoperazone. *Drug Intell Clin Pharm* (1984) 18, 316.
4. Cristiano P. Hypoprothrombinemia associated with cefoperazone treatment. *Drug Intell Clin Pharm* (1984) 18, 314–16.
5. Osborne JC. Hypoprothrombinemia and bleeding due to cefoperazone. *Ann Intern Med* (1985) 102, 721–2.
6. Freedy HR, Cetnarowski AB, Lumish RM, Schafer FJ. Cefoperazone-induced coagulopathy. *Drug Intell Clin Pharm* (1986) 20, 281–3.
7. Andrassy K, Koderisch J, Fritz S, Bechtold H, Sonntag H. Alteration of hemostasis associated with cefoperazone treatment. *Infection* (1986) 14, 27–31.

8. Conjura A, Bell W, Lipsky JJ. Cefotetan and hypoprothrombinemia. *Ann Intern Med* (1988) 108, 643.
9. Haubenstock A, Schmidt P, Zazgornik J, Balcke P, Kopsa H. Hypoprothrombinaemic bleeding associated with ceftriaxone. *Lancet* (1983) i, 1215–16.
10. Natelson EA, Brown CH, Bradshaw MW, Alfrey CP, Williams TW. Influence of cephalosporin antibiotics on blood coagulation and platelet function. *Antimicrob Agents Chemother* (1976) 9, 91–3.
11. Lerner PI, Lubin A. Coagulopathy with cefazolin in uremia. *N Engl J Med* (1974) 290, 1324.
12. Khaleeli M, Giorgio AJ. Defective platelet function after cephalosporin administration. *Blood* (1976) 48, 971.
13. Dupuis LL, Paton TW, Suttie JW, Thiessen JJ, Rachlis A. Cefazolin-induced coagulopathy. *Clin Pharmacol Ther* (1984) 35, 237.
14. Brown RB, Klar J, Lemeshow S, Teres D, Pastides H, Sands M. Enhanced bleeding with cefoxitin or moxalactam. Statistical analysis within a defined population of 1493 patients. *Arch Intern Med* (1986) 146, 2159–64.
15. Morris DL, Fabricius PJ, Ambrose NS, Scammell B, Burdon DW, Keighley MRB. A high incidence of bleeding is observed in a trial to determine whether addition of metronidazole is neeeded with latamoxef for prophylaxis in colorectal surgery. *J Hosp Infect* (1984) 5, 398–408.
16. Bang NU, Tessler SS, Heidenreich RO, Marks CA, Mattler LE. Effects of moxalactam on blood coagulation and platelet function. *Rev Infect Dis* (1982) 4 (Suppl), S546–S554.
17. Angaran DM, Dias VC, Arom KV, Northrup WF, Kersten TE, Lindsay WG, Nicoloff DM. The influence of prophylactic antibiotics on the warfarin anticoagulation response in the postoperative prosthetic cardiac valve patient. *Ann Surg* (1984) 199, 107–111.
18. Angaran DM, Dias VC, Arom KV, Northrup WF, Kersten TG, Lindsay WG, Nicoloff DM. The comparative influence of prophylactic antibiotics on the prothrombin response to warfarin in the post-operative prosthetic cardiac valve patient. *Ann Surg* (1987) 206, 155–61.
19. Angaran DM, Tschida VH, Copa AK. Effect of cefonicid (CN) on prothrombin time (PT) in outpatients (OP) receiving warfarin (W) therapy. *Pharmacotherapy* (1988) 8, 120.
20. Puente Garcia M, Bécares Martínez FJ, Merlo Arroyo J, García Sánchez G, García Díaz B, Cervero Jiménez M. Potenciación del efecto anticoagulante del acenocoumarol por cefonicid. *Rev Clin Esp* (1999) 199, 620–1.
21. Riancho JA, Olmos JM, Sedano C. Life-threatening bleeding in a patient being treated with cefonicid. *Ann Intern Med* (1995) 123, 472–3.
22. Gras-Champel V, Sauvé L, Perault MC, Laine P, Gouello JP, Decocq G, Masson H, Touzard M, Andréjak M. Association cefotiam et acenocoumarol: a propos de 3 cas d'hémorragies. *Therapie* (1998) 53, 191.
23. Clark TR, Burns S. Elevated international normalized ratio values associated with concomitant use of warfarin and ceftriaxone. *Am J Health-Syst Pharm* (2011) 68, 1603–5.
24. Eli Lilly and Company Limited. Personal communication, December 1997.
25. Schelleman H, Bilker WB, Brensinger CM, Han X, Kimmel SE, Hennessy S. Warfarin with fluoroquinolones, sulfonamides or azole antifungals: interactions and the risk of hospitalization for gastrointestinal bleeding. *Clin Pharmacol Ther* (2008) 84, 581–8.
26. Lederle Laboratories. Personal communication, December 1995.
27. Penning-van Beest FJA, Koerselman J, Herings RMC. Risk of major bleeding during concomitant use of antibiotic drugs and coumarin anticoagulants. *J Thromb Haemost* (2008) 6, 284–90.
28. Bohm NM, Crosby B. Hemarthrosis in a patient on warfarin receiving ceftaroline: a case report and brief review of cephalosporin interactions with warfarin. *Ann Pharmacother* (2012) 46, e19.
29. Stroud LF, Mamdami MM, Kopp A, Bell CM. The safety of levofloxacin in elderly patients on warfarin. *Am J Med* (2005) 118, 1417.
30. Johnson MC, Wood M, Vaughn V, Cowan L, Sharkey AM. Interaction of antibiotics and warfarin in pediatric cardiology patients. *Pediatr Cardiol* (2005) 26, 589–92.
31. Pharmacy Anticoagulant Clinic Study Group. A multicentre survey of antibiotics on the INR of anti-coagulated patients. *Pharm J* (1996) 257 (Pharmacy Practice Suppl), R30.
32. Zhang K, Young C, Berger J. Administrative claims analysis of the relationship between warfarin use and risk of hemorrhage including drug-drug and drug-disease interactions. *J Manag Care Pharm* (2006) 12, 640–8.
33. Baillargeon J, Holmes HM, Lin YL, Raji MA, Sharma G, Kuo YF. Concurrent use of warfarin and antibiotics and the risk of bleeding in older adults. *Am J Med* (2012) 125, 183–9.
34. Jobski K, Behr S, Garbe E. Drug interactions with phenprocoumon and the risk of serious haemorrhage: a nested case-control study in a large population-based German database. *Eur J Clin Pharmacol* (2011) 67, 941–51.
35. Bodey G, Reuben A, Elting L, Kantarjian H, Keating M, Hagemeister F, Koller C, Velasquez W, Papadopoulos N. Comparison of two schedules of cefoperazone plus aztreonam in the treatment of neutropenic patients with fever. *Eur J Clin Microbiol Infect Dis* (1991) 10, 551–8.
36. Rusconi F, Assael BM, Boccazzi A, Colombo R, Crossignani RM, Garlaschi L, Rancilio L. Aztreonam in the treatment of severe urinary tract infections in pediatric patients. *Antimicrob Agents Chemother* (1986) 30, 310–14.
37. Giamarellou H, Galanakis N, Dendrinos CH, Kanellakopoulou K, Petrikkos G, Koratzanis G, Daikos GK. Clinical experience with aztreonam in a variety of gram-negative infections. *Chemioterapia* (1985) 4 (Suppl 1), 75–80.
38. Giamerellou H, Koratzanis G, Kanellakopoulou K, Galanakis N, Papoulias G, El Messidi M, Daikos G. Aztreonam versus cefamandole in the treatment of urinary tract infections. *Chemioterapia* (1984) 3, 127–31.

Coumarins + Antibacterials; Chloramphenicol

There is some limited evidence to suggest that the anticoagulant effects of acenocoumarol and dicoumarol can be increased by oral chloramphenicol. An isolated report attributes a marked rise in the INR of a patient taking warfarin to the use of chloramphenicol eye drops.

Clinical evidence

A study in 4 patients found that the half-life of **dicoumarol** was increased on average from 8 hours to 25 hours when they were given oral chloramphenicol 2 g daily for 5 to 8 days.[1]

Three out of 9 patients taking an unnamed anticoagulant had a fall in their prothrombin-proconvertin values from a range of 10 to 30% down to less than 6% (suggesting an increased anticoagulant effect) when given oral chloramphenicol 1 to 2 g daily for 4 to 6 days. One patient had a smaller reduction.[2] In early clinical experience with **acenocoumarol**, one of 3 patients taking chloramphenicol had greater sensitivity to the anticoagulant.[3]

An isolated report describes an 83-year-old woman stabilised on **warfarin** who had a rise in her INR to about 8.9 from her normal range of 1.9 to 2.8 within 2 weeks of starting to use eye drops containing chloramphenicol 5 mg/mL, dexamethasone sodium phosphate 1 mg/mL and tetrahydrozoline hydrochloride 0.25 mg/mL. She used one drop in each eye four times daily.[4] Hypoprothrombinaemia and bleeding have also been described in patients given intramuscular,[5] intravenous,[5] or oral[6] chloramphenicol in the absence of an anticoagulant.

Mechanism

Uncertain. One suggestion is that the chloramphenicol inhibits the liver enzymes concerned with the metabolism of the anticoagulants so that their effects are prolonged and increased.[4] An *in vitro* study with human liver microsomes found that chloramphenicol did not inhibit the hydroxylation of *S*-warfarin, but it did inhibit *R*-warfarin metabolism, probably by the cytochrome P450 isoenzyme CYP3A4.[7] Another suggestion is that the antibacterial diminishes the gut bacteria thereby decreasing a source of vitamin K, but it is doubtful if these bacteria are normally an important source of the vitamin except in exceptional cases where dietary levels are very inadequate.[8] A third suggestion is that chloramphenicol blocks the production of prothrombin by the liver.[5] See also 'Coumarins + Antibacterials', p.383.

Importance and management

The documentation for the interaction between anticoagulants and oral chloramphenicol is very sparse and poor (the best being the pharmacokinetic report about dicoumarol) so that this interaction is by no means adequately established. There would therefore appear to be little reason for avoiding concurrent use, but it would seem prudent to monitor prothrombin times if oral chloramphenicol is started in patients taking a coumarin, being alert for the need to reduce the anticoagulant dose.

The report about an apparent interaction between warfarin and topical chloramphenicol is surprising because the amount of chloramphenicol absorbed from eye drops is relatively small and because, despite the very widespread use of warfarin and chloramphenicol for very many years, this report appears to be the only one. This suggests that any such interaction is very unlikely indeed.

1. Christensen LK, Skovsted L. Inhibition of drug metabolism by chloramphenicol. *Lancet* (1969) ii, 1397–9.
2. Magid E. Tolerance to anticoagulants during antibiotic therapy. *Scand J Clin Lab Invest* (1962) 14, 565–6.
3. Johnson R, David A, Chartier Y. Clinical experience with G-23350 (Sintrom). *Can Med Assoc J* (1957) 77, 756–61.
4. Leone R, Ghiotto E, Conforti A, Velo G. Potential interaction between warfarin and ocular chloramphenicol. *Ann Pharmacother* (1999) 33, 114.
5. Klippel AP, Pitsinger B. Hypoprothrombinemia secondary to antibiotic therapy and manifested by massive gastrointestinal hemorrhage. *Arch Surg* (1968) 96, 266–8.
6. Matsaniotis N, Messaritakis J, Vlachou C. Hypoprothrombinaemic bleeding in infants associated with diarrhoea and antibiotics. *Arch Dis Child* (1970) 45, 586–7.
7. Park J-Y, Kim K-A, Kim S-L. Chloramphenicol is a potent inhibitor of cytochrome P450 isoforms CYP2C19 and CYP3A4 in human liver microsomes. *Antimicrob Agents Chemother* (2003) 47, 3464–9.
8. Udall JA. Human sources and absorption of vitamin K in relation to anticoagulation stability. *JAMA* (1965), 194, 107–9.

Coumarins + Antibacterials; Clindamycin

Two isolated cases of a marked increase in INR and/or bleeding have been attributed to an interaction with clindamycin. However, a report found no cases of a serious increase in INR in patients taking acenocoumarol or phenprocoumon with clindamycin.

Clinical evidence, mechanism, importance and management

A 47-year-old woman with multiple medical problems stabilised on **warfarin** (and also taking azathioprine, captopril, furosemide, insulin, prednisone, levothyroxine, valproic acid and zolpidem) had all her teeth removed under general anaesthetic. Sixteen days later she needed a dental abscess drained and was given oral clindamycin 300 mg four times daily with ibuprofen 600 mg for any discomfort. On day 17 she needed a suture to stop some bleeding and her INR was found to be 3.5. By day 20 she had developed more severe oral bleeding, which needed emergency room treatment. Her INR was found to have risen to 13 and her haematocrit decreased to 18%. She was treated successfully with a blood transfusion and vitamin K.[1]

A retrospective review of the effect of antibacterials on INR in children taking **warfarin** mentions that an INR of 8.5 was noted in a 4-year-old child, 6 days after clindamycin was started.[2]

These appear to be isolated cases, from which no general conclusions should be drawn because the whole picture is so uncertain. Note that in a cohort study, none of 37 patients stabilised on **acenocoumarol** or **phenprocoumon** developed over-anticoagulation (an INR greater than 6) when they were given clindamycin.[3] However, if a patient is unwell enough to require an antibacterial, it may be prudent to increase monitoring of coagulation status even if no specific drug interaction is expected. Monitor within 3 days of starting the antibacterial (see also 'Coumarins + Antibacterials', p.383).

1. Aldous JA, Olson CJ. Managing patients on warfarin therapy: a case report. *Spec Care Dentist* (2001) 21, 109–112.
2. Johnson MC, Wood M, Vaughn V, Cowan L, Sharkey AM. Interaction of antibiotics and warfarin in pediatric cardiology patients. *Pediatr Cardiol* (2005) 26, 589–92.
3. Visser LE, Penning-van Beest FJA, Kasbergen AAH, De Smet PAGM, Vulto AG, Hofman A, Stricker BHC. Overanticoagulation associated with combined use of antibacterial drugs and acenocoumarol or phenprocoumon anticoagulants. *Thromb Haemost* (2002) 88, 705–10.

Coumarins + Antibacterials; Linezolid

Linezolid had only minor effects on the pharmacokinetics and anticoagulant activity of single-dose warfarin in one study.

Clinical evidence, mechanism, importance and management

Linezolid 600 mg twice daily was given to 13 healthy subjects for 5 days followed by a single 25-mg dose of **warfarin**. The pharmacokinetics of **warfarin** with linezolid were within 20% of those seen with **warfarin** alone, and the INR was minimally affected (about a 10% increase in maximal INR).[1] These effects were not considered to be clinically relevant.

However, if a patient is unwell enough to require an antibacterial, it may be prudent to increase monitoring of coagulation status even if no specific drug interaction is expected. Monitor within 3 days of starting the antibacterial. See also 'Coumarins + Antibacterials', p.383.

1. Azie NE, Stalker DJ, Jungbluth GL, Sisson T, Adams G. Effect of linezolid on CYP2C9 using racemic warfarin (W) as a probe. *Clin Pharmacol Ther* (2001) 69, 21.

Coumarins + Antibacterials; Macrolides

Most controlled studies suggest that macrolides do not cause clinically relevant changes in the pharmacokinetics or anticoagulant effects of warfarin. There is less information about other anticoagulants, but two retrospective studies of acenocoumarol and phenprocoumon have variously shown an increased risk (with azithromycin, clarithromycin, and erythromycin, though for erythromycin this was not statistically significant), and no increased risk of bleeding (with clarithromycin, erythromycin, and roxithromycin). Furthermore, a number of case reports describe large increases in INRs and/or bleeding in patients taking coumarins and macrolides.

Clinical evidence

(a) Azithromycin

The UK manufacturer of azithromycin notes that, in a pharmacokinetic study in healthy volunteers, azithromycin did not alter the anticoagulant effect of a single 15-mg dose of warfarin, but that post-marketing reports have suggested azithromycin might increase the anticoagulant effect when given with coumarin anticoagulants.[1] Several studies (including phase II and III studies) also suggest that no interaction occurs with warfarin. However, other studies and published case reports suggest an interaction may occur with coumarins. These are summarised in 'Table 12.3', p.388.

In addition, the manufacturers[2] stated that, as of December 1998, they had received 47 reports (40 in the US, 7 elsewhere in the world, including 2 in the UK) of possible interactions between azithromycin and warfarin. A 2004 report from the Australian Adverse Drug Reactions Advisory Committee said they had received 3 reports of interactions between warfarin and azithromycin,[3] which presumably includes the 2 published cases cited in the table.[4]

(b) Clarithromycin

There are no studies of the effect of clarithromycin on the pharmacokinetics of coumarins. However, there are numerous cases of increased INRs in published reports, and one cohort study suggesting that the use of clarithromycin is associated with an increased risk of bleeding in patients taking coumarins. Conversely, in an earlier cohort study by the same research group, the increased risk was small and not statistically significant. These are summarised in 'Table 12.3', p.388.

(c) Dirithromycin

In a study in 15 healthy subjects the pharmacokinetics and pharmacodynamics of a single 0.5-mg/kg dose of **warfarin** were not altered when it was given on day 10 of a 14-day course of dirithromycin 500 mg daily.[5]

(d) Erythromycin

A study in 12 healthy subjects found that the clearance of a single 1-mg/kg dose of **warfarin** was reduced by an average of 14% (range 0 to about 30%) when taken on day 5 of an 8-day course of erythromycin 250 mg every 6 hours. This change was greatest in those subjects with relatively slow warfarin clearance rates.[6] In another similar study, **warfarin** 0.5 mg/kg, given on day 10 of a 14-day course of erythromycin 250 mg four times daily increased the AUC of *S*-warfarin by 11% and of *R*-warfarin by 12%. The INR increased by 10%.[5] Similar effects were seen in another study in 8 patients stabilised on **warfarin** and who did not have infections. In these patients, erythromycin 333 mg three times daily for 7 days caused a mean 10% increase in the prothrombin time ratio, which was maximal by day 2 to 5. There was also a mean 9% increase in the total plasma warfarin concentration, which was similar for the *S*- and *R*-enantiomers, and was maximal by day 7. No patient had a prothrombin time ratio above the therapeutic range and none required a reduction in warfarin dose.[7]

In contrast to the modest effects in the above studies, various case reports have demonstrated a large increase in INR. These are summarised in 'Table 12.3', p.388.

(e) Midecamycin diacetate

The pharmacokinetics of a single 8-mg oral dose of **acenocoumarol** were not changed when it was taken on day 4 of a 9-day course of midecamycin diacetate 800 mg twice daily.[8]

(f) Roxithromycin

In a study in which **warfarin** was given at a daily dose sufficient to maintain the thrombotest percentages at 10 to 20%, there was no difference in warfarin dose or AUC between 10 subjects given roxithromycin 150 mg twice daily for 2 weeks and 11 subjects given placebo. The dose of **warfarin** and the AUC of warfarin increased by about 10% in both the roxithromycin group and the placebo group, which was taken as indicating that steady state had not been achieved. Serum roxithromycin concentrations were unchanged by warfarin.[9]

In contrast, there are case reports of an interaction with warfarin and other coumarins. These are summarised in 'Table 12.3', p.388.

(g) Telithromycin

In a placebo-controlled, crossover study in healthy subjects, telithromycin 800 mg daily for 7 days did not alter the pharmacodynamics of a single-dose of **warfarin** 25 mg given on day 4. There was a small 20% increase in the AUC of *R*-warfarin, and a 5% increase in the AUC of *S*-warfarin,[10] effects which the manufacturer does not consider to be clinically relevant.[11]

Conversely, there are a few reports of an interaction with warfarin and with acenocoumarol, see 'Table 12.3', p.388 for details.

(h) Unspecified macrolides

Details of studies assessing the effect of unspecified macrolides are summarised in 'Table 12.3', p.388.

Mechanism

Erythromycin, clarithromycin, and telithromycin are known inhibitors of CYP3A4. However, this isoenzyme has only a minor role in the metabolism of warfarin, specifically the less active *R*-isomer of warfarin. Consequently, only minor increases in the concentrations of warfarin have been seen in pharmacokinetic studies, which would generally not be expected to be clinically relevant. However, it is possible that even these small changes could be important in a very few patients, particularly those with a low prothrombin complex activity.[6] Other macrolides (azithromycin, dirithromycin, roxithromycin) have much less effect on CYP3A4 than erythromycin, clarithromycin, or telithromycin, and consequently would be expected to have even less effect on the pharmacokinetics of warfarin or acenocoumarol, which is borne out in the few studies available. Nevertheless, cases of interactions have been reported for nearly all these macrolides. Moreover, one cohort study found that clarithromycin increased the risk of an interaction and erythromycin did not. It is possible that there is some other, as yet unidentified, mechanism involved. Alternatively, it is equally possible that the relatively few cases just represent idiosyncratic effects attributable to other factors, such as those secondary to being acutely ill, and not to any interaction (see also 'Coumarins + Antibacterials', p.383).

Importance and management

A minor pharmacokinetic interaction between erythromycin and warfarin is established, but would not generally be expected to be clinically relevant. This is borne out by the relatively few published reports of an interaction see 'Table 12.3', p.388 for details. Other macrolides would be even less likely to inhibit the metabolism of warfarin or acenocoumarol than erythromycin, and this is borne out by studies with dirithromycin, midecamycin, and roxithromycin. Nevertheless, cases of important interactions have been reported for most of the other macrolides (azithromycin, clarithromycin, roxithromycin, and telithromycin). Moreover, one cohort study found an increased risk of over-anticoagulation with clarithromycin but not with erythromycin. Taken together, the available evidence suggests that, occasionally and unpredictably the effects of warfarin, acenocoumarol, or phenprocoumon might be considerably increased by the macrolides. It would therefore be prudent to increase monitoring in all patients when they are first given any macrolide antibacterial. There is some evidence that this may be particularly important in those who clear warfarin and other anticoagulants slowly and who therefore only need low doses. The elderly in particular would seem to fall into this higher risk category. With azithromycin, bear in mind that, because of its long half-life, the interaction might not become apparent until a couple of days after a short course of azithromycin has been stopped.

If a patient is unwell enough to require an antibacterial, it might be prudent to increase monitoring of coagulation status even if no specific drug interaction is expected, see also 'Coumarins + Antibacterials', p.383. Monitor within 3 days of starting the antibacterial.

1. Zithromax (Azithromycin). Pfizer Ltd. UK Summary of product characteristics, January 2015.
2. Pfizer Limited. Personal Communication, December 1998.
3. ADRAC. Macrolides and warfarin interaction. *Aust Adverse Drug React Bull* (2004) 23, 7.
4. Wiese MD, Cosh DG. Raised INR with concurrent warfarin and azithromycin. *Aust J Hosp Pharm* (1999) 29, 159–161.
5. Ellsworth A, Horn JR, Wilkinson W, Black DJ, Church L, Sides GD, Harris J, Cullen PD. An evaluation of the effect of dirithromycin (D) and erythromycin (E) on the pharmacokinetics and pharmacodynamics of warfarin (W). *Intersci Conf Antimicrob Agents Chemother* (1995) 35, 9.
6. Bachmann K, Schwartz JI, Forney R, Frogameni A, Jauregui LE. The effect of erythromycin on the disposition kinetics of warfarin. *Pharmacology* (1984) 28, 171–6.
7. Weibert RT, Lorentz SM, Townsend RJ, Cook CE, Klauber MR, Jagger PI. Effect of erythromycin in patients receiving long-term warfarin therapy. *Clin Pharm* (1989) 8, 210–14.
8. Couet W, Istin B, Decourt JP, Ingrand I, Girault J, Fourtillan JB. Lack of effect of ponsinomycin on the pharmacokinetics of nicoumalone enantiomers. *Br J Clin Pharmacol* (1990) 30, 616–20.
9. Paulsen O, Nilsson L-G, Saint-Salvi B, Manuel C, Lunell E. No effect of roxithromycin on pharmacokinetic or pharmacodynamic properties of warfarin and its enantiomers. *Pharmacol Toxicol* (1988) 63, 215–20.
10. Scholtz HE, Pretorius SG, Wessels DH, Mogilmicka EM, Van Niekerk N, Sultan E. HMR 3647, a new ketolide antimicrobial does not affect the pharmacodynamics or pharmacokinetics of warfarin in healthy adult males. Abstracts of the IDSA 37th Annual Meeting p. 976.
11. Ketek (Telithromycin). Sanofi. UK Summary of product characteristics, November 2012.

Coumarins + Antibacterials; Metronidazole and related drugs

Limited evidence suggests that metronidazole might cause a notable increase in INR, without bleeding, and increase the risk of haemorrhage in patients also taking warfarin. A few case reports support these findings. One early study found that metronidazole increased the half-life of a single dose of warfarin by one-third and increased its effects. A case-control study suggests that metronidazole greatly increases the risk

Table 12.3 Summary of the pharmacological evidence for and against an interaction between macrolides and coumarins

Study type (year)	*Group*	*Coumarin*	*Macrolide*	*Outcome*	*Refs*
Studies showing no interaction					
Phase II and III studies	Patients (number not stated)	Warfarin, single dose	Azithromycin, 500 mg on day 1 then 250 mg daily for 4 days	No effect on prothrombin time response	1
Retrospective (2000)	26 stable patients	Warfarin	Azithromycin	No evidence of effect on INR, measured within 14 days (9 patients) or 30 days (17 patients) of starting azithromycin*	2
Retrospective (2004)	17 patients	Warfarin	Azithromycin	No effect on INR*	3
Prospective (2013)	18 dental patients	Warfarin	Azithromycin, single 2-g dose	No effect on INR	4
Retrospective cohort (2008)	2907 Patients	Acenocoumarol or phenprocoumon	Clarithromycin	RR for hospitalisation for bleeding = 1.8 (range 0.4 to 7)	5
Cohort (2002)	78 patients	Acenocoumarol or phenprocoumon	Erythromycin	No cases of overanticoagulation (INR >6)	6
Retrospective cohort (2008)	645 Patients	Acenocoumarol or phenprocoumon	Erythromycin	RR for hospitalisation for bleeding = 4.2 (range 0.6 to 30)	5
Cohort (2002)	14 patients	Acenocoumarol or phenprocoumon	Roxithromycin	No cases of overanticoagulation (INR >6)	6
Studies showing an interaction					
Retrospective cohort (2008)	1947 Patients	Acenocoumarol or phenprocoumon	Azithromycin	RR for hospitalisation for bleeding = 4.1 (range 1 to 16.2) Equivalent to 1 major bleed per 1250 azithromycin prescription	5
Retrospective (2005)	32 stable patients	Warfarin	Azithromycin	Mean increase in INR of 0.51 after starting azithromycin; 5 patients had an INR >4 and one patient had an INR >5. INR was measured within 3 to 15 days of starting azithromycin	7
Retrospective (2013)	100 elderly patients	Warfarin	Azithromycin	Increased INR with mean weekly warfarin dose decreased from 30 mg to 29.2 mg	8
Cohort (2002)	Patients	Acenocoumarol or phenprocoumon	Clarithromycin	RR for over-anticoagulation (INR >6) = 11.7 (range 3.6 to 37.8). Risk highest within first 3 days of concurrent use	6
Prospective (1996)	35 patients	Warfarin	Unspecified macrolides	INR increased by an estimated 0.319	9
Retrospective review (2005)	18 children	Warfarin	Unspecified macrolides	Mean INR was increased by 0.9, but 2 children had large increases with azithromycin and erythromycin	10
Prospective case-control (2012)	24 Patients	Warfarin	Unspecified macrolides	Odds ratio for hospitalisation due to bleeding = 1.86 (range 1.08 to 3.21), compared with 2.01 for use of any antibacterial or antifungal	11
Case reports of an interaction					
Case report (2004)	57-year-old	Warfarin	Azithromycin, 500 mg on day 1 then 250 mg daily for 4 days	Two days after stopping azithromycin her INR increased to 8.32 (from a range of 1.75 to 3.03 prior to azithromycin). No signs or symptoms of bleeding, but did have fever on second day and she reduced her smoking, which may have been a factor (see Coumarins + Tobacco, p.479)	12
Case reports (1996 to 2004)	Patients	Warfarin	Azithromycin	Increased INR of 40% to 6-fold within 1 to 7 days of starting azithromycin≈	13-18
				Three patients had bleeding complications	14, 15, 17
				Four patients required vitamin K	14-17
Case report (1996)	75-year-old	Acenocoumarol	Clarithromycin, 250 mg twice daily	INR increased from 2.1 to 9 within a week of starting clarithromycin	19
Case report (1997)	5 stable patients	Acenocoumarol	Clarithromycin	Mean increase in INR from about 2.5 to 5.5; largest increase was from 1.95 to 7.01	20
Case report (1996)	70-year-old	Phenprocoumon	Clarithromycin, 500 mg daily	Increase in prothrombin time from a range of 140 to 180 seconds up to 304 seconds, but with no bleeding, within 4 days of starting clarithromycin. Phenoprocoumon was stopped and phytomenadine given. Patient restabilised on original phenprocoumon dose after clarithromycin stopped	21

* A major disadvantage of this study is the small numbers of patients who had an INR measurement within 7 days of starting azithromycin.
≈ Most patients had possible confounding factors, such as recent increases in warfarin dose,[15,16] other concurrent antibacterials,[16,18] fever and decreased appetite,[13,17] or complex disease states and heart failure.[14-17]
† Possible confounding factor of other concurrent antibacterials.[40]

Continued

Table 12.3 Summary of the pharmacological evidence for and against an interaction between macrolides and coumarins (continued)

Study type (year)	*Group*	*Coumarin*	*Macrolide*	*Outcome*	*Refs*
Case report (1992)	56-year-old	Warfarin	Clarithromycin	INR >10, resulting in fatal cerebrovascular bleed 3 days after starting clarithromycin	22
Case report (2001)	62-year-old	Warfarin	Clarithromycin, 250 mg twice daily	INR 8.2 with suprachoroidal haemorrhage and permanent vision loss 7 days after starting clarithromycin. Three days before starting the clarithromycin her INR was 2.3, and 3 days into treatment her INR was 2.9	23
Case reports (1997 to 1999)		Warfarin	Clarithromycin	INRs ranging from 5.6 to 90.3 within 4 to 12 days of starting, or 5 to 14 days of finishing a course of clarithromycin. No bleeding complications were noted	24-27
Case reports (2004)	6 patients	Warfarin	Clarithromycin	Median INR of 7.6, two patients were symptomatic	28
Case report (1986)	44-year-old	Acenocoumarol	Erythromycin, 14-day course	Haematuria on last day of course	29
Case report (1999)	68-year-old	Acenocoumarol	Erythromycin ethylsuccinate, 1.5 g daily	INR increased from a range of 3 to 4.5 to 15 one week after starting erythromycin, but no bleeding was seen	30
Case report (1980)	77-year-old	Warfarin	Erythromycin stearate, 500 mg four times daily	In the previous month the patient started digoxin, diuretics, and quinidine for AF. Her digoxin dose was decreased at that point and then increased by her GP after discharge. Two weeks later she received erythromycin for a chest infection and, within a week, her prothrombin time increased to 64 seconds; haematuria and bruising developed	31
Case reports (1982 to 2010)	At least 10 patients	Warfarin	Erythromycin as the base, ethylsuccinate, stearate or lactobionate	Bleeding and/or an increase in prothrombin time or INR[†]	32-40
Case reports (up to 2004)	19 patients	Warfarin	Erythromycin	Median INR of 9.7, four patients were symptomatic	28
Case report (2010)	77-year-old	Warfarin	Erythromycin 5% *ophthalmic ointment*	INR increased from a range of 1.8 to 2.5 up to 8.5 three weeks after starting the ointment. Her INR decreased when the ointment was stopped, but increased again when it was restarted	41
Case report (1992)	52-year-old	Warfarin	Erythromycin stearate 2 g daily	Sulfonamide-induced bullous haemorrhagic eruption occurred while also taking co-trimoxazole. The authors considered that an interaction between warfarin and erythromycin might have contributed to the haemorrhagic component. Note that co-trimoxazole could also interact, see Coumarins and related drugs + Antibacterials; Sulfonamides and/or Trimethoprim, p.398	42
Case report (1998)	79-year-old	Acenocoumarol	Roxithromycin, 150 mg twice daily	Abdominal wall haematoma developed 2 days after starting roxithromycin. On admission to hospital six days later, his INR was 5.9	43
Case report (1996)	75-year-old	Phenprocoumon	Roxithromycin, 300 mg daily for 5 days	Large increase in prothrombin time with no bleeding. Phenprocoumon was stopped and phytomenadione given. Patient restabilised on original phenprocoumon dose after roxithromycin stopped	21
Case reports (2004)	56 patients	Warfarin	Roxithromycin	Increased warfarin effects: median INR of 8.8 and median time to onset of 6 days. 27 patients were symptomatic, and there was 1 fatality due to widespread bleeding (INR of 11.6 by day 8)	28
Case report (2004)	73-year-old	Warfarin	Telithromycin, 800 mg daily for 5 days	Haemoptysis on last day of treatment, with an INR of 11. His INR 10 days before treatment was 3.1. Telithromycin was stopped and he was restabilised on his usual warfarin dose	44
Case reports (May 2003-Sept 2004)	7 patients	Warfarin (6 patients); unspecified (1 patient)	Telithromycin	Increased INR in 6 reports, but decreased INR in the seventh	45
Case report (2006)	84-year-old	Acenocoumarol	Telithromycin, 800 mg daily	Rectus sheath haematoma with an INR increase to 6, after 6 days of telithromycin	46

* A major disadvantage of this study is the small numbers of patients who had an INR measurement within 7 days of starting azithromycin.

≈ Most patients had possible confounding factors, such as recent increases in warfarin dose,[15,16] other concurrent antibacterials,[16,18] fever and decreased appetite,[13,17] or complex disease states and heart failure.[14-17]

† Possible confounding factor of other concurrent antibacterials.[40]

1. Hopkins S. Clinical toleration and safety of azithromycin. *Am J Med* (1991) 91 (Suppl 3A), 40S–45S.
2. Beckey NP, Parra D, Colon A. Retrospective evaluation of a potential interaction between azithromycin and warfarin in patients stabilized on warfarin. *Pharmacotherapy* (2000) 20, 1055–9.
3. McCall KL, Anderson HG, Jones AD. Determination of the lack of a drug interaction between azithromycin and warfarin. *Pharmacotherapy* (2004) 24, 188–94.

Continued

Table 12.3 Summary of the pharmacological evidence for and against an interaction between macrolides and coumarins (continued)

4. Kusafuka Y, Kurita H, Sakurai S, Suzuki S, Nakanishi Y, Katsuyama Y, Ohmori S. Effect of single-dose extended-release oral azithromycin on anticoagulation status in warfarinized patients. *Oral Surg Oral Med Oral Pathol Oral Radiol* (2013) 115, 148–51.
5. Penning-van Beest FJA, Koerselman J, Herings RMC. Risk of major bleeding during concomitant use of antibiotic drugs and coumarin anticoagulants. *J Thromb Haemost* (2008) 6, 284–90.
6. Visser LE, Penning-van Beest FJA, Kasbergen AAH, De Smet PAGM, Vulto AG, Hofman A, Stricker BHC. Overanticoagulation associated with combined use of antibacterial drugs and acenocoumarol or phenprocoumon anticoagulants. *Thromb Haemost* (2002) 88, 705–10.
7. Glasheen JJ, Fugit RV, Prochazka AV. The risk of overanticoagulation with antibiotic use in outpatients on stable warfarin regimens. *J Gen Intern Med* (2005) 20, 653–6.
8. Mergenhagen KA, Olbrych PM, Mattappallil A, Krajewski MP, Ott MC. Effect of azithromycin on anticoagulation-related outcomes in geriatric patients receiving warfarin. *Clin Ther* (2013) 35, 425–30.
9. Pharmacy Anticoagulant Clinic Study Group. A multicentre survey of the effect of antibiotics on the INR of anticoagulated patients. *Pharm J* (1996) 257 (Pharmacy Practice Suppl), R30.
10. Johnson MC, Wood M, Vaughn V, Cowan L, Sharkey AM. Interaction of antibiotics and warfarin in pediatric cardiology patients. *Pediatr Cardiol* (2005) 26, 589–92.
11. Baillargeon J, Holmes HM, Lin YL, Raji MA, Sharma G, Kuo YF. Concurrent use of warfarin and antibiotics and the risk of bleeding in older adults. *Am J Med* (2012) 125, 183–9.
12. Shrader SP, Fermo JD, Dzikowski AL. Azithromycin and warfarin interaction. *Pharmacotherapy* (2004) 24, 945–9.
13. Lane G. Increased hypoprothrombinemic effect of warfarin possibly induced by azithromycin. *Ann Pharmacother* (1996) 30, 884–5.
14. Woldtveldt BR, Cahoon CL, Bradley LA, Miller SJ. Possible increased anticoagulation effect of warfarin induced by azithromycin. *Ann Pharmacother* (1998) 32, 269–70.
15. Foster DR, Milan NL. Potential interaction between azithromycin and warfarin. *Pharmacotherapy* (1999) 19, 902–8.
16. Wiese MD, Cosh DG. Raised INR with concurrent warfarin and azithromycin. *Aust J Hosp Pharm* (1999) 29, 159–161.
17. Williams D, Ponte CD. Warfarin associated hypoprothrombinemia: an unusual presentation. *Am J Health-Syst Pharm* (2003) 60, 274–8.
18. Rao KB, Pallaki M, Tolbert SR, Hornick TR. Enhanced hypoprothrombinemia with warfarin due to azithromycin. *Ann Pharmacother* (2004) 38, 982–5.
19. Grau E, Real E, Pastor E. Interaction between clarithromycin and oral anticoagulants. *Ann Pharmacother* (1996) 30, 1495–6.
20. Sánchez B, Muruzábal MJ, Peralta G, Santiago G, Castilla A, Aguilera JP, Arjona R. Clarithromycin-oral anticoagulants interaction. Report of five cases. *Clin Drug Invest* (1997) 13, 220–2.
21. Meyboom RHB, Heere FJ, Egberts ACG, Lastdrager CJ. Vermoedelijke potentiëring van fenprocoumon door claritromycine en roxitromycine. *Ned Tijdschr Geneeskd* (1996) 140, 375–7.
22. Committee on Safety of Medicines. Reminders: interaction between macrolide antibiotics and warfarin. *Current Problems* (1992) 35, 4.
23. Dandekar SS, Laidlaw DAH. Suprachoroidal haemorrhage after addition of clarithromycin. *J R Soc Med* (2001) 94, 583–4.
24. Oberg KC. Delayed elevation of international normalized ratio with concurrent clarithromycin and warfarin therapy. *Pharmacotherapy* (1998) 18, 386–91.
25. Recker MW, Kier KL. Potential interaction between clarithromycin and warfarin. *Ann Pharmacother* (1997) 31, 996–8.
26. Gooderham MJ, Bolli P, Fernandez PG. Concomitant digoxin toxicity and warfarin interaction in a patient receiving clarithromycin. *Ann Pharmacother* (1999) 33, 796–9.
27. Byers M. Clarithromycin–warfarin interaction resulting in an elevated INR. *Can J Hosp Pharm* (1997) 50, 285–7.
28. ADRAC. Macrolides and warfarin interaction. Aust Adverse Drug React Bull (2004) 23, 7.
29. Grau E, Fontcuberta J, Félez J. Erythromycin-oral anticoagulants interaction. *Arch Intern Med* (1986) 146, 1639.
30. Grau E, Real E, Pastor E. Macrolides and oral anticoagulants: a dangerous association. *Acta Haematol* (1999) 102, 113–14.
31. Bartle WR. Possible warfarin-erythromycin interaction. *Arch Intern Med* (1980) 140, 985–7.
32. Husserl FE. Erythromycin-warfarin interaction. *Arch Intern Med* (1983) 143, 1831, 1836.
33. Sato RI, Gray DR, Brown SE. Warfarin interaction with erythromycin. *Arch Intern Med* (1984) 144, 2413–14.
34. Friedman HS, Bonventre MV. Erythromycin-induced digoxin toxicity. *Chest* (1982) 82, 202.
35. Hassell D, Utt JK. Suspected interaction: warfarin and erythromycin. *South Med J* (1985) 78, 1015–16.
36. Bussey HI, Knodel LC, Boyle DA. Warfarin-erythromycin interaction. *Arch Intern Med* (1985) 145, 1736–7.
37. O'Donnell D. Antibiotic-induced potentiation of oral anticoagulant agents. *Med J Aust* (1989) 150, 163–4.
38. Schwartz J, Bachmann K, Perigo E. Interaction between warfarin and erythromycin. *South Med J* (1983) 76, 91–3.
39. Wood GD, Deeble T. Warfarin: dangers with antibiotics. *Dent Update* (1993) 20, 350, 352–3.
40. Trivedi D, Newton JD, Mitra A, Puri P. A serious drug interaction leading to a spontaneous total hyphema. *J Postgrad Med* (2010) 56, 46–7.
41. Parker DL, Hoffmann TK, Tucker MA, Gerschutz GP, Malone PM. Elevated international normalized ratio associated with concurrent use of ophthalmic erythromycin and warfarin. *Am J Health-Syst Pharm* (2010) 67, 38–41.
42. Wolf R, Elman M, Brenner S. Sulfonamide-induced bullous hemorrhagic eruption in a patient with low prothrombin time. *Isr J Med Sci* (1992), 28, 882–4.
43. Chassany O, Logeart I, Choulika S, Caulin C. Hématome pariétal abdominal lors d'un traitement associant acénocoumarol et roxithromycine. *Presse Med* (1998) 27, 1103.
44. Kolilekas L, Anagnostopoulos GK, Lampaditis I, Eleftheriadis I. Potential interaction between telithromycin and warfarin. *Ann Pharmacother* (2004) 38, 1424–7.
45. Health Canada. Telithromycin (Ketek) and warfarin: suspected interaction. *Can Adverse React News* (2005) 15, 1.
46. García-Fuster MJ, Domínguez E, Martínez F, Forner MJ. Telitromicina, un posible nuevo potenciador del acenocumarol. *Med Clin (Barc)* (2006) 126, 797–8.

of bleeding in patients taking phenprocoumon. Two case reports describe increased INRs in patients taking nimorazole and phenprocoumon. Tinidazole might interact with the coumarins similarly.

Clinical evidence

(a) Metronidazole

In 8 healthy subjects, metronidazole 250 mg three times daily for one week increased the half-life of a single 1.5-mg/kg dose of **warfarin** by about one-third (from 35 hours to 46 hours), and increased the prothrombin time from a mean of 100 seconds to 142 seconds. When the warfarin enantiomers were given separately, the anticoagulant effects of *S*-warfarin were virtually doubled and the half-life increased by 60%, but the response to *R*-warfarin was only affected in one subject.[1] In a retrospective cohort study, 32 patients taking **warfarin** had an INR reading before and during concurrent metronidazole use. In these patients, the mean INR increased from 2.2 to a maximum of 4.3 by day 8. Fourteen of the 32 patients had an INR above 4, but no bleeding events were recorded.[2] In a large analysis of claims data, the use of metronidazole with **warfarin** was associated with an increased risk of haemorrhage (odds ratio of 1.6).[3] In another retrospective study in 20 patients receiving **warfarin** and started on metronidazole, 7 had a pre-emptive warfarin dose reduction (mean 34.6%) which resulted in an increase in INR of 0.19 when compared with an increase of 1.47 in the 13 patients who did not have a pre-emptive dose reduction. Furthermore, none of the patients who had a pre-emptive warfarin dose reduction had an INR of more than 4, while in those who had no pre-emptive dose reduction, 6 patients had an INR of greater than 4, and 2 patients had minor bleeding complications.[4]

Bleeding has been seen in 2 patients taking **warfarin** and metronidazole.[5,6] One patient had severe pain in one leg, ecchymoses, and haemorrhage of both legs, and an increase in her prothrombin time from 17 to 19 seconds, up to 147 seconds within 17 days of starting metronidazole.[5] A further report describes 3 elderly patients taking **warfarin**, who developed increased INRs after being given intravenous metronidazole.[7] In the first patient, the INR on admission was 4.6, and so warfarin was stopped. The next day metronidazole was given for about 24 hours, and on day 4 the INR had reached 10.3. In the second patient the INR on admission was 4.9 and so the warfarin was stopped. Later that day metronidazole was started, and the INR was reduced to 1.7 with fresh frozen plasma. Nevertheless by day 5 the INR had reached 6 (metronidazole had been stopped on day 2). In the third patient the INR on admission was 4 and so the warfarin was stopped. Later that day metronidazole was given, and the INR was reduced to 2.1 with fresh frozen plasma. Nevertheless by day 5 (while still receiving metronidazole) the INR had reached 10. In another case, an elderly woman taking **warfarin** developed a profuse nosebleed after a fall, with an INR of 8, nine days after starting metronidazole and levofloxacin (which can also interact, see 'Coumarins + Antibacterials; Quinolones', p.393). She was found to have an intracerebral haemorrhage.[8] An increased INR (from 3 to 4.2) was also seen in a patient taking **warfarin**,[9] after receiving metronidazole 400 mg three times daily with ciprofloxacin, and after erythromycin, both of which can also interact (see 'Coumarins + Antibacterials; Macrolides', p.387 and 'Coumarins + Antibacterials; Quinolones', p.393). A cohort study describes one patient taking **warfarin** who had severe bleeding and was found to have an INR of 4.5 two days after starting metronidazole.[10]

A case-control study[11] in 2 553 patients taking **phenprocoumon** found that the risk of hospitalisation due to bleeding appeared to be greatly increased with metronidazole use: odds ratio 9.49; range 2.44 to 37. However, note that only 6 patients were given metronidazole and there were only 4 patients in the control group.

(b) Nimorazole

A 66-year-old man who had been taking **phenprocoumon** for 15 years with an INR around 2.5 was diagnosed with carcinoma of the glottis. He received radiotherapy 6 times a week with nimorazole 2.5 g given 1.5 hours before the radiotherapy as a radiosensitiser. At the 16th dose he had haemoptysis, on the 17th dose continuous haematuria, and then on the 22nd dose his INR was found to be 7.5. Fluconazole had been started 4 days before the 22nd dose. When the patient had recovered and restarted **phenprocoumon**, he was rechallenged with nimorazole before his last 5 days of radiotherapy, with an INR increase from 3.7 to 5.3.[12,13]

Another report describes an 80-year-old woman with hypopharyngeal cancer who was treated with radiotherapy 6 times a week and given nimorazole 1.5 g before each dose. After her fourth dose of radiotherapy, she restarted **phenprocoumon** 1.5 mg three times a week. A few days later, there was an increase in her INR, and at the 13th radiotherapy dose she had an INR of 5.6 with gastrointestinal bleeding and haematemesis. She was also taking diclofenac and fluconazole,[13] both of which might interact with warfarin, see 'Coumarins + Azoles; Fluconazole', p.408 and 'Coumarins + NSAIDs; Diclofenac', p.451.

Mechanism

In the early study, it was suggested that metronidazole probably inhibits the activity of the enzymes responsible for the metabolism (ring oxidation) of the more potent isomer *S*-warfarin, but not *R*-warfarin.[1] Reduction of protein binding coupled with reduced metabolism was suggested by other authors.[7] Nimorazole potentially acts similarly. Note also that infection can affect coagulation status, see 'Coumarins + Antibacterials', p.383.

Importance and management

The interaction between **metronidazole** and warfarin appears to be established and clinically important, although the documentation is limited. Monitor the INR when both drugs are used, and adjust the warfarin dose accordingly. A pre-emptive dose reduction of warfarin by 30 to 35% has been suggested.[4] Due to the lack of control patients in the case-control study in patients given **phenprocoumon**, no conclusions can be drawn. Nothing seems to be documented about other anticoagulants, but it would be prudent to expect other coumarins to behave similarly to warfarin. The two case reports with **nimorazole** suggest that caution might also be warranted with this drug, and therefore probably all 5-nitroimidazoles, including **tinidazole**. Note that, if a patient is unwell enough to require an antibacterial, it would be prudent to increase monitoring of coagulation status even if no specific drug interaction is expected, see also 'Coumarins + Antibacterials', p.383. Monitor within 3 days of starting the antibacterial.

1. O'Reilly RA. The stereoselective interaction of warfarin and metronidazole in man. *N Engl J Med* (1976) 295, 354–7.
2. Laine K, Forsström J, Grönroos P, Irjala K, Kailajärvi M, Scheinin M.. Frequency and clinical outcome of potentially harmful drug metabolic interactions in patients hospitalized on internal and pulmonary medicine wards: focus on warfarin and cisapride. *Ther Drug Monit* (2000) 22, 503–9.
3. Zhang K, Young C, Berger J. Administrative claims analysis of the relationship between warfarin use and risk of hemorrhage including drug-drug and drug-disease interactions. *J Manag Care Pharm* (2006) 12, 640–8.
4. Holt RK, Anderson EA, Cantrell MA, Shaw RF, Egge JA. Preemptive dose reduction of warfarin in patients initiating metronidazole. *Drug Metabol Drug Interact* (2010) 25, 35–9.
5. Kazmier FJ. A significant interaction between metronidazole and warfarin. *Mayo Clin Proc* (1976) 51, 782–4.
6. Dean RP, Talbert RL. Bleeding associated with concurrent warfarin and metronidazole therapy. *Drug Intell Clin Pharm* (1980) 14, 864–6.
7. Tonna AP, Scott D, Keeling D, Tonna I. Metronidazole causes an unexpected rise in INR in anticoagulated patients even after warfarin has been stopped. *Hosp Pharm* (2007) 14, 65–7.
8. Howard-Thompson A, Hurdle AC, Arnold LB, Finch CK, Sands C, Self TH. Intracerebral hemorrhage secondary to a warfarin-metronidazole interaction. *Am J Geriatr Pharmacother* (2008) 6, 33–6.
9. Trivedi D, Newton JD, Mitra A, Puri P. A serious drug interaction leading to spontaneous total hyphema. *J Postgrad Med* (2010) 56, 46–7.
10. Gasse C, Hollowell J, Meier CR, Haefeli WE. Drug interactions and risk of acute bleeding leading to hospitalisation or death in patients with chronic atrial fibrillation treated with warfarin. *Thromb Haemost* (2005) 94, 537–43.
11. Jobski K, Behr S, Garbe E. Drug interactions with phenprocoumon and the risk of serious haemorrhage: a nested case-control study in a large population-based German database. *Eur J Clin Pharmacol* (2011) 67, 941–51.
12. Bjarnason NH, Specht L, Dalhoff K. Nimorazole may increase the effect of phenprocoumon. *Radiother Oncol* (2005) 74, 345.
13. Bjarnason NH, Christiansen M, Specht L. The nimorazole regimen in patients with head and neck cancer can increase the effect of vitamin K antagonists. *Acta Oncol* (2008) 47, 150–1.

Coumarins + Antibacterials; Nitrofurantoin

One retrospective study suggests that nitrofurantoin does not increase the risk of gastrointestinal bleeding in patients taking warfarin.

Clinical evidence, mechanism, importance and management

In a retrospective, case-control study, in patients aged 66 years or older taking **warfarin**, the risk of hospitalisation for upper gastrointestinal tract haemorrhage was not increased if nitrofurantoin had been taken in the 14 days before admission.[1] The limitations of this type of study mean that the clinical relevance of this finding is unclear. However, as with other antibacterials, if a patient is unwell enough to require an antibacterial, it might be prudent to increase monitoring of coagulation status even if no specific drug interaction is expected. Monitor within 3 days of starting the antibacterial. See also 'Coumarins + Antibacterials', p.383.

1. Fischer HD, Juurlink DN, Mamdani MM, Kopp A, Laupacis A. Hemorrhage during warfarin therapy associated with cotrimoxazole and other urinary tract anti-infective agents: a population-based study. *Arch Intern Med* (2010) 170, 617–21.

Coumarins + Antibacterials; Penicillins

Increased prothrombin times and/or bleeding in patients taking coumarins have been seen in some patients given amoxicillin (with or without clavulanic acid), intravenous benzylpenicillin, or pheneticillin. There is also some evidence that phenoxymethylpenicillin (penicillin V) does not increase the risk of bleeding in patients taking coumarins. In contrast, several cases of greatly *reduced* warfarin effects have been seen with nafcillin. Similarly, dicloxacillin might cause a modest reduction in warfarin effects, and an isolated case of thrombosis has been reported. A few case reports describe difficulties in achieving a therapeutic INR, despite increases in the dose of warfarin, when given with cloxacillin or flucloxacillin.

Clinical evidence

(a) Amoxicillin ± Clavulanic acid

An 81-year-old woman taking **acenocoumarol** 3 mg daily (INR 2.5 to 4) developed bruising and an increased INR of 7.1 within a week of starting amoxicillin 500 mg every 8 hours.[1] In another case, a man stabilised on **warfarin** (INR 2 to 3) had an INR of 5.7 and developed a rectus sheath haematoma 3 days after completing a 7-day-course of co-amoxiclav (amoxicillin with clavulanic acid).[2] In one case, an 85-year-old woman taking **warfarin** was found collapsed at home one week after completing a course of co-amoxiclav. She had an INR of greater than 10 and widespread haemorrhage, and died shortly afterwards.[3] Two cases of increased INRs have been reported in patients who took prophylactic single 3-g doses of amoxicillin before dental treatment.[3] Other possible cases of an interaction between **warfarin** and amoxicillin[4,5] and amoxicillin with clavulanic acid[5,6] have been reported.

A case-control study in 2 553 patients taking **phenprocoumon** found that the risk of hospitalisation due to bleeding appeared to be greater in the 12 patients taking co-amoxiclav than in the 28 patients taking amoxicillin alone (odds ratio 1.56; range 1.01 to 2.40, and 2.99; range 1.39 to 6.42, respectively).[7] Similarly, in another case-control study,[8] use of co-amoxiclav was found to be associated with an increased risk of an INR of greater than 6 (odds ratio 4.1; range 0.9 to 19.2) in patients stabilised on either **acenocoumarol** or **phenprocoumon**. Amoxicillin alone was associated with a smaller increased risk (odds ratio 1.7; range 0.6 to 4.7). Conversely, in a population-based cohort study,[9] conducted by the same research group in similar patients, the risk of over-anticoagulation (INR greater than or equal to 6) in patients taking either **acenocoumarol** or **phenprocoumon** was greater for amoxicillin alone than amoxicillin plus an enzyme inhibitor. The relative risk for amoxicillin alone was 10.5 (range 5.1 to 21.7) and for amoxicillin plus an enzyme inhibitor was 5.1 (range 1.9 to 13.9). The increased risk was observed in the early stages of concurrent use but was greater after 4 or more days of treatment.[9] In two further cohort studies by this same research group, the relative risk of hospitalisation for bleeding in patients taking **acenocoumarol** or **phenprocoumon** and given co-amoxiclav was 7 and 4.4, respectively,[10,11] and 3.1 for amoxicillin alone.[11] Nevertheless, they estimated that the individual risk of major bleeding was low at 1 per 1000 co-amoxiclav prescriptions.[11] In another retrospective study of paediatric patients taking **warfarin**, the mean INR increased by 0.8 in 20 children given amoxicillin and in 25 children given co-amoxiclav.[5]

In contrast to these reports of increased anticoagulation, a randomised, placebo-controlled, crossover study in 12 patients stabilised on **warfarin** but with no ongoing infection, found that the mean maximum increase in INR from baseline to day 10 was not affected by co-amoxiclav 1 g twice daily for 7 days.[12] Similarly, a retrospective case-control study in patients aged 66 years or older taking **warfarin**, found that the risk of hospitalisation due to gastrointestinal haemorrhage was not increased by administration of amoxicillin or **ampicillin** in the 14 days before admission.[13] A very brief report of an audit of an anticoagulant clinic, states that 5 patients who had taken amoxicillin had an unspecified decrease in prothrombin time.[14]

A pharmacokinetic study in 8 healthy subjects found that amoxicillin with clavulanic acid increased the AUC of a single 8-mg dose of **acenocoumarol** by about 20%. A subsequent population pharmacokinetic model found that the clearance of **acenocoumarol** was decreased by 15% by amoxicillin with clavulanic acid.[15] However, the authors note that this study had a number of limitations that may have affected the results (such as small size, large acenocoumarol dose).

(b) Benzylpenicillin

One patient stabilised on **warfarin** (prothrombin time 20 seconds) was found to have an increased prothrombin time of 32 seconds 8 days after starting intravenous benzylpenicillin [14.4 g] daily for subacute bacterial endocarditis. The benzylpenicillin was continued, and the warfarin dose reduced for 18 days. However, the prothrombin time decreased below the therapeutic range, and the warfarin dose was increased back to the original dose, still with continuation of the benzylpenicillin for a further 3 weeks.[16]

In a retrospective cohort study,[11] the relative risk of hospitalisation for bleeding in patients taking **acenocoumarol** or **phenprocoumon** and given benzathine benzylpenicillin was 5.8, but it was not statistically significant (range 0.8 to 41.5).

(c) Cloxacillin

A series of case reports describes 3 patients who experienced reduced anticoagulation on warfarin after undergoing valve replacement surgery and who were also given standard doses of intravenous antibacterial drugs (cloxacillin, ampicillin, and gentamicin in 2 patients, and cloxacillin only in the third) for the treatment of endocarditis. In all 3 patients, the INR began to decrease when cloxacillin was started (despite an increase in warfarin dose) and remained subtherapeutic for about 21 to 25 days after cloxacillin was stopped. All 3 patients subsequently achieved a therapeutic INR on the same, or a lower, warfarin dose than when they were given cloxacillin.[17] Similarly, a 40-year-old woman given a standard dose of intravenous cloxacillin for 4 weeks, followed by oral cloxacillin for 2 weeks, for the treatment of endocarditis, had difficulty in achieving a therapeutic INR (1.4 to 2.9) despite her warfarin dose being increased to 30 mg daily and being given intravenous heparin. Her INR stabilised 8 days after cloxacillin was stopped, and she was discharged on warfarin 8 mg daily.[18]

In contrast, a 70-year-old man stabilised on **warfarin** was started on cloxacillin (dose not stated) and 2 days later his INR had increased from 1.9 to 4.6. There were no signs of haemorrhage, and his warfarin was discontinued. His INR remained high (between about 3.5 and 5) for the remaining 8 days of the cloxacillin course. Three days after the cloxacillin was stopped his INR had decreased to 1.8 and warfarin was restarted at his previous dose.[19]

(d) Dicloxacillin

In a controlled study in 7 patients stabilised on **warfarin** and without infections, dicloxacillin 500 mg four times daily for 7 days reduced the mean prothrombin time by 1.9 seconds. One patient had a 5.6 second reduction.[20] This study was conducted because the authors had noted a case of a patient receiving **warfarin** who had a decrease in prothrombin time when dicloxacillin was started.[20] Another patient stabilised on **warfarin** had a 17% decrease in prothrombin times within 4 to 5 days of starting dicloxacillin 500 mg four times daily, with a documented 20 to 25% reduction in both *S*- and *R*-warfarin concentrations.[21] In a retrospective review, 7 other patients similarly treated were also identified as having a 17% reduction in prothrombin times.[21] In yet another case, a patient who had previously required **warfarin** 10 mg daily subsequently needed an increased dose of 15 mg daily while taking dicloxacillin 4 g daily long-term.[22] However, another case report[23] suggested a greater effect of dicloxacillin: a patient taking dicloxacillin 500 mg every 6 hours required an increase in **warfarin** dose from a range of 35 to 40 mg weekly up to 50 to 60 mg weekly, with INRs still being subtherapeutic (about 1.5). Moreover, when a woman taking **warfarin** was given dicloxacillin 500 mg four times daily she developed a heart valve thrombosis, suggesting inadequate anticoagulation. Her INR was 1.4, and an increased **warfarin** dose was required for 3 weeks after she stopped dicloxacillin.[24]

(e) Flucloxacillin

In one cohort study in patients taking **acenocoumarol** or **phenprocoumon**, no cases of over-anticoagulation (INR greater than 6) occurred in patients taking flucloxacillin (25 patients received this antibacterial).[9] Note that this study found an increased risk of over-anticoagulation for *amoxicillin*, see above. In another cohort study[11] by the same research group, the relative risk of hospitalisation for bleeding in patients taking **acenocoumarol** or **phenprocoumon** and given flucloxacillin was increased at 2.2 but this was not statistically significant (range 0.7 to 6.9).

Conversely, a case report describes a 68-year-old woman stabilised on **warfarin**, whose INR decreased from 3.5 to 1.4 and was hospitalised for an ischaemic stroke, 17 days after starting a course of flucloxacillin 500 mg and **phenoxymethylpenicillin** 999 mg, both four times daily, for a soft tissue infection. The patient had also taken the same combination of drugs previously and an INR of 1.8 was recorded 5 days after completing the course.[25] Another similar case report describes a 58-year-old man stabilised on warfarin (3 mg and 4 mg on alternate days) for 6 months prior to an elective joint fusion. Following surgery the patient was recommenced on his usual warfarin dose. On day 12 after surgery oral flucloxacillin (dose not stated) was started. On day 14 his INR was 2.9, but by day 16 his INR had decreased to 1.1 and his warfarin dose was increased to 8 mg. On day 17 his INR was 0.9, so the flucloxacillin was stopped and amoxicillin with clavulanic acid started; the patient was also given 5 mg warfarin and the following morning his INR had increased to 2.7.[26] A decrease in INR has also been reported in a 64-year-old man who was started on warfarin after mitral valve replacement surgery and was also given intravenous flucloxacillin for the treatment of infective endocarditis. For the first 4 weeks he received intravenous flucloxacillin 2 g every 6 hours and had difficulty in achieving a therapeutic INR despite warfarin doses between 5 and 10 mg daily. When the dose of flucloxacillin was increased to 2 g every 4 hours he experienced a further decrease in his INR despite an increase in warfarin dose to 25 mg daily. When flucloxacillin was discontinued, the patient's INR increased and his warfarin dose was reduced.[27]

(f) Nafcillin

The prothrombin time of a 29-year-old patient stabilised on **warfarin** decreased from a range of 20 to 25 seconds down to 16 seconds five days after intravenous nafcillin 2 g every 4 hours was started for endocarditis. Over the next 2 weeks the prothrombin time ranged between 14 and 17 seconds despite an eventual doubling of the **warfarin** dose, and heparin was substituted. In this patient the half-life of a single 30-mg dose of **warfarin** was 11 hours when nafcillin was taken, 17 hours four days after stopping nafcillin, and 44 hours eight months after the nafcillin was discontinued.[28] A case report describes a 39-year-old man taking warfarin 32 mg weekly, who required an eventual 2.75-fold dose increase to 88 mg weekly when his antibacterial for septic arthritis was changed from intravenous cefazolin to intravenous nafcillin 2 g every 4 hours. When the nafcillin was discontinued, he was eventually stabilised on **warfarin** 42 to 48 mg weekly.[29] At least 10 other cases of this **warfarin** resistance have been reported with high-dose nafcillin.[22,30-34]

(g) Pheneticillin

In one cohort study[9] in patients taking **acenocoumarol** or **phenprocoumon**, one case of over-anticoagulation (INR greater than 6) occurred in a group of 219 patients taking pheneticillin, giving a calculated relative risk of 0.9. In a further cohort study by the same research group,[11] the relative risk of hospitalisation for bleeding in patients taking **acenocoumarol** or **phenprocoumon** and given pheneticillin was 4.6.

(h) Phenoxymethylpenicillin (Penicillin V)

When 10 patients taking an unnamed anticoagulant were given intravenous phenoxymethylpenicillin calcium [187.5 mg] four times daily for 4 days, none had a change in their prothrombin-proconvertin value.[35] For mention that, in another study no patients taking penicillins including phenoxymethylpenicillin had an increase in INR see under *Unspecified penicillins*, below. However, in a retrospective cohort study,[11] the relative risk of hospitalisation for bleeding in patients taking **acenocoumarol** or **phenprocoumon** and given phenoxymethylpenicillin was 4.7, but it was not statistically significant (range 0.7 to 33.2).

For a description of a patient experiencing acute left hemiparesis and a decrease in INR while taking phenoxymethylpenicillin and **flucloxacillin**, see under *Flucloxacillin*, above.

(i) Unspecified penicillins

In one analysis of patients taking **warfarin** with antibacterials, there was no association between use of penicillins (**phenoxymethylpenicillin (penicillin V)** and broad-spectrum penicillins) and an increase in INR. The estimated change in INR was 0.117 in 109 patients given the combination.[36] In contrast, a prospective case-control study using health insurance data found that use of penicillins with **warfarin** was associated with an increased risk of bleeding (odds ratio 1.92, range 1.21 to 2.07). Antibacterial and antifungal use in general was associated with an overall increased risk of 2.01 (range 1.62 to 2.5), with the greatest risk being associated with use during the 60 days prior to the bleed occurring.[37]

Mechanism

Not understood. The interaction between nafcillin and warfarin is possibly due to increases in the metabolism of warfarin by the liver. Dicloxacillin also possibly reduces serum warfarin concentrations.[21] Other penicillins (ampicillin,[38] benzylpenicillin,[38,39] carbenicillin,[40-45] methicillin,[38] ticarcillin[46]) have caused increased bleeding times when given alone, principally due to platelet inhibition,[38-40] which may be additive with the effects of the anticoagulants. Broad-spectrum antibacterials might decrease the gut flora and thereby possibly decrease production of vitamin K. Other factors relating to the disease might be important, see 'Coumarins + Antibacterials', p.383.

Importance and management

The reduced effect of warfarin with **dicloxacillin** and **nafcillin** appears to be established. If these penicillins are used, increase monitoring of the INR and anticipate the need to increase the warfarin dose during concurrent use and decrease it on discontinuation of the penicillin. Some patients taking nafcillin have been warfarin resistant, and needed heparin treatment. A small number of case reports describe difficulty achieving a therapeutic INR with warfarin, both during treatment with cloxacillin or flucloxacillin, and for up to 25 days after discontinuation of cloxacillin. Until further evidence is available it would seem prudent to be aware of the possibility of an interaction and to monitor the patient's INR, and if necessary manage as advised for dicloxacillin and nafcillin (above).

Documented reports of interactions between the coumarins and other penicillins are relatively rare, bearing in mind how frequently these drugs are used, so that the broad picture is that no clinically relevant interaction normally occurs with most other penicillins. This lack of interaction was supported by one clinical study.[36] However, in one case-control study, co-amoxiclav increased the risk of bleeding, and the authors recommended avoiding this combination,[8] although a later cohort study by the same authors just recommended increased monitoring with amoxicillin or co-amoxiclav.[9] In yet another study, they estimated that the individual risk of major bleeding was low at 1 per 1000 co-amoxiclav prescriptions.[11]

Although there appear to be no reports of an interaction, if the mechanism of the interaction is correct, the **indanediones** are also likely to be affected. However, these interactions may be due to a number of different factors, and these are discussed in detail in 'Coumarins + Antibacterials', p.383. Therefore concurrent use should be monitored, so that the very occasional and unpredictable cases (increases or decreases in the anticoagulant effects) can be identified and managed accordingly.

1. Soto J, Sacristan JA, Alsar MJ, Fernandez-Viadero C, Verduga R. Probable acenocoumarol-amoxycillin interaction. *Acta Haematol (Basel)* (1993) 90, 195–7.
2. Kelly M, Moran J, Byrne S. Formation of rectus sheath hematoma with antibiotic use and warfarin therapy: a case report. *Am J Geriatr Pharmacother* (2005) 3, 266–9.
3. Wood GD, Deeble T. Warfarin: dangers with antibiotics. *Dent Update* (1993) 20, 350, 352–3.
4. Bandrowsky T, Vorono AA, Borris TJ, Marcantoni HW. Amoxicillin-related postextraction bleeding in an anticoagulated patient with tranexamic acid rinse. *Oral Surg Oral Med Oral Pathol Oral Radiol Endod* (1996) 82, 610–12.
5. Johnson MC, Wood M, Vaughn V, Cowan L, Sharkey AM. Interaction of antibiotics and warfarin in pediatric cardiology patients. *Pediatr Cardiol* (2005) 26, 589–92.
6. Davydov L, Yermolnik M, Cuni LJ. Warfarin and amoxicillin/clavulanate drug interaction. *Ann Pharmacother* (2003) 37, 367–70.
7. Jobski K, Behr S, Garbe E. Drug interactions with phenprocoumon and the risk of serious haemorrhage: a nested case-control study in a large population-based German database. *Eur J Clin Pharmacol* (2011) 67, 941–51.
8. Penning-van Beest FJA, van Meegen E, Rosendaal FR, Stricker BH. Drug interactions as a cause of overanticoagulation on phenprocoumon or acenocoumarol predominantly concern antibacterial drugs. *Clin Pharmacol Ther* (2001) 69, 451–57.
9. Visser LE, Penning-van Beest FJA, Kasbergen AAH, De Smet PAGM, Vulto AG, Hofman A, Stricker BHC. Overanticoagulation associated with combined use of antibacterial drugs and acenocoumarol or phenprocoumon anticoagulants. *Thromb Haemost* (2002) 88, 705–10.
10. Penning-van Beest F, Erkens J, Petersen K-U, Koelz HR, Herings R. Main comedications associated with major bleeding during anticoagulant therapy with coumarins. *Eur J Clin Pharmacol* (2005) 61, 439–44.
11. Penning-van Beest FJA, Koerselman J, Herings RMC. Risk of major bleeding during concomitant use of antibiotic drugs and coumarin anticoagulants. *J Thromb Haemost* (2008) 6, 284–90.
12. Zhang Q, Simoneau G, Verstuyft C, Drouet L, Bal dit Sollier C, Alvarez JC, Rizzo-Padoin N, Bergmann JF, Becquemont L, Mouly S. Amoxicillin/clavulanic acid-warfarin drug interaction: a randomized controlled trial. *Br J Clin Pharmacol* (2011) 71, 232–6.
13. Fischer HD, Juurlink DN, Mamdani MM, Kopp A, Laupacis A. Hemorrhage during warfarin therapy associated with cotrimoxazole and other urinary tract anti-infective agents: a population-based study. *Arch Intern Med* (2010) 170, 617–21
14. Radley AS, Hall J. Interactions. *Pharm J* (1992) 249, 81.
15. Delavenne X, Laporte S, Demasles S, Mallouk N, Basset T, Tod M, Girard P, Mismetti P. Investigation of PK-PD drug-drug interaction between acenocoumarol and amoxicillin plus clavulanic acid. *Fundam Clin Pharmacol* (2009) 23, 127–35.
16. Brown MA, Korchinski ED, Miller DR. Interaction of penicillin-G and warfarin? *Can J Hosp Pharm* (1979) 32, 18–19.
17. Khalili H, Nikvarz N, Najmeddin F, Dashti-Khavidaki S. A probable clinically significant interaction between warfarin and cloxacillin: three case reports. *Eur J Clin Pharmacol* (2013) 69, 721–4.
18. Ibrahim OM, Allam A. Warfarin resistance in a patient with prosthetic valve endocarditis treated with cloxacillin. *Saudi Pharm J* (1996) 4, 56–9.
19. Marusic S, Gojo-Tomic N, Bacic-Vrca V, Franic M. Enhanced anticoagulant effect of warfarin in a patient treated with cloxacillin. *Int J Clin Pharmacol Ther* (2012) 50, 431–3.
20. Krstenansky PM, Jones WN, Garewal HS. Effect of dicloxacillin sodium on the hypoprothrombinemic response to warfarin sodium. *Clin Pharm* (1987) 6, 804–6.
21. Mailloux AT, Gidal BE, Sorkness CA. Potential interaction between warfarin and dicloxacillin. *Ann Pharmacother* (1996) 30, 1402–7.
22. Taylor AT, Pritchard DC, Goldstein AO, Fletcher JL. Continuation of warfarin-nafcillin interaction during dicloxacillin therapy. *J Fam Pract* (1994) 39, 182–5.
23. Lacey CS. Interaction of dicloxacillin with warfarin. *Ann Pharmacother* (2004) 38, 898.
24. Halvorsen S, Husebye T, Arnesen H. Prosthetic heart valve thrombosis during dicloxacillin therapy. *Scand Cardiovasc J* (1999) 33, 366–8.
25. Merwick A, Hannon N, Kelly PJ, O'Rourke K. Warfarin-flucloxacillin interaction presenting as cardioembolic ischemic stroke. *Eur J Clin Pharmacol* (2010) 66, 643–4.
26. Garg A, Mohammed M. Decreased INR response secondary to warfarin-flucloxacillin interaction. *Ann Pharmacother* (2009) 43, 1374–5.

27. Choi PY, Phillips KL, Rae I. High-dose intravenous flucloxacillin may affect warfarin therapy. *Med J Aust* (2011) 194, 613.
28. Qureshi GD, Reinders TP, Somori GJ, Evans HJ. Warfarin resistance with nafcillin therapy. *Ann Intern Med* (1984) 100, 527–9.
29. Kim KY, Frey RJ, Epplen K, Foruhari F. Interaction between warfarin and nafcillin: case report and review of the literature. *Pharmacotherapy* (2007) 27, 1467–70.
30. Fraser GL, Miller M, Kane K. Warfarin resistance associated with nafcillin therapy. *Am J Med* (1989) 87, 237–8.
31. Davis RL, Berman W, Wernly JA, Kelly HW. Warfarin-nafcillin interaction. *J Pediatr* (1991) 118, 300–3.
32. Shovick VA, Rihn TL. Decreased hypoprothrombinemic response to warfarin secondary to the warfarin-nafcillin interaction. *DICP Ann Pharmacother* (1991) 25, 598–9.
33. Heilker GM, Fowler JW, Self TH. Possible nafcillin-warfarin interaction. *Arch Intern Med* (1994) 154, 822–4.
34. Baciewicz AM, Heugel AM, Rose PG. Probable nafcillin-warfarin interaction. *J Pharm Technol* (1999) 15, 5–7.
35. Magid E. [Tolerance to anticoagulants during antibiotic therapy]. *Scand J Clin Lab Invest* (1962) 14, 565–6.
36. Pharmacy Anticoagulant Clinic Study Group. A multicentre survey of antibiotics on the INR of anti-coagulated patients. *Pharm J* (1996) 257 (Pharmacy Practice Suppl), R30.
37. Baillargeon J, Holmes HM, Lin YL, Raji MA, Sharma G, Kuo YF. Concurrent use of warfarin and antibiotics and the risk of bleeding in older adults. *Am J Med* (2012) 125, 183–9.
38. Brown CH, Bradshaw MW, Natelson EA, Alfrey CP, Williams TW. Defective platelet function following the administration of penicillin compounds. *Blood* (1976) 47, 949–56.
39. Roberts PL. High-dose penicillin and bleeding. *Ann Intern Med* (1974) 81, 267–8.
40. Brown CH, Natelson EA, Bradshaw MW, Williams TW, Alfrey CP. The hemostatic defect produced by carbenicillin. *N Engl J Med* (1974) 291, 265–70.
41. McClure PD, Casserly JG, Monsier C, Crozier D. Carbenicillin-induced bleeding disorder. *Lancet* (1970) ii, 1307–8.
42. Waisbren BA, Evani SV, Ziebert AP. Carbenicillin and bleeding. *JAMA* (1971) 217, 1243.
43. Yudis M, Mahood WH, Maxwell R. Bleeding problems with carbenicillin. *Lancet* (1972) ii, 599.
44. Lurie A, Ogilvie M, Townsend R, Gold C, Meyers AM, Goldberg B. Carbenicillin-induced coagulopathy. *Lancet* (1970) i, 1114–15.
45. Andrassy K, Ritz E, Weisschedel E. Bleeding after carbenicillin administration. *N Engl J Med* (1975) 292, 109.
46. Brown CH, Natelson EA, Bradshaw MW, Alfrey CP, Williams TW. Study of the effects of ticarcillin on blood coagulation and platelet function. *Antimicrob Agents Chemother* (1975) 7, 652–7.

Coumarins + Antibacterials; Quinolones

Quinolones have at most, a small effect on the pharmacokinetics and pharmacodynamics of warfarin. However, isolated cases of increased effects and even bleeding have been reported in patients taking a coumarin with a quinolone, and retrospective studies suggest that there might be an increased risk of over-anticoagulation in patients taking acenocoumarol or phenprocoumon with norfloxacin and ciprofloxacin, and warfarin with gatifloxacin or levofloxacin.

Clinical evidence

(a) Ciprofloxacin

In a randomised, placebo-controlled study in 32 patients stabilised on **warfarin** and without infections, ciprofloxacin 750 mg twice daily for 12 days had no effect on *S*-warfarin concentrations, but did increase *R*-warfarin concentrations by 14.7%.[1] There are studies showing no effect of ciprofloxacin on the anticoagulant effects of coumarins, but there are also studies and case reports showing that an interaction might occur. These are summarised in 'Table 12.4', p.394.

(b) Clinafloxacin

Clinafloxacin 200 mg twice daily for 14 days had no effect on the steady-state concentrations of *S*-warfarin in healthy subjects, but the concentrations of the less active enantiomer *R*-warfarin were increased by 32% and the mean INR was increased by 13%.[2]

(c) Enoxacin

When a single 25-mg dose of **warfarin** was given to 6 healthy subjects on day 8 of a 14-day course of enoxacin 400 mg twice daily, the pharmacokinetics of *S*-warfarin were not altered, but the clearance of *R*-warfarin was decreased by 32% and its elimination half-life was prolonged from 36.8 hours to 52.2 hours. The overall anticoagulant response to the **warfarin** was unaltered.[3] A case report supports this finding, see 'Table 12.4', p.394.

(d) Fleroxacin

The pharmacokinetics of *R*- and *S*-warfarin, the prothrombin time and factor VII clotting time were unaffected when 12 healthy subjects were given a single 25-mg dose of **warfarin** on day 4 of a 9-day course of fleroxacin 400 mg daily.[4]

(e) Gatifloxacin

Gatifloxacin 400 mg daily for 11 days had no effect on the pharmacokinetics of a single 25-mg dose of **warfarin**, nor was the prothrombin time altered.[5] Other studies showing no effect on the anticoagulant effects of warfarin as well as studies and case reports suggesting an interaction might occur, are summarised in 'Table 12.4', p.394.

(f) Gemifloxacin

There is a study showing no effect of gemifloxacin on the anticoagulant effects of coumarins. This is summarised in 'Table 12.4', p.394.

(g) Levofloxacin

In a study[6] in 15 healthy subjects given a single 30-mg dose of **warfarin** on day 4, levofloxacin 500 mg twice daily for 9 days had no effect on the pharmacokinetics or pharmacodynamics of *R*- and *S*-warfarin. Several other studies found similar results, but in contrast there are also studies and case reports suggesting an interaction may occur. See 'Table 12.4', p.394 for a summary.

In addition to the studies summarised in the table, another study assessed the impact of pre-emptively reducing the **warfarin** dose by 10 to 20% in patients starting levofloxacin. In 10 patients who had a **warfarin** dose reduction, there was no change in mean INR before and after levofloxacin. However, 4 patients developed a *sub-therapeutic* INR, including two with borderline low INR values beforehand. In 13 patients who had no pre-emptive **warfarin** dose reduction, the INR increased from a mean of about 2.5 to about 4. Note that most of the patients had little change in their INR, but one patient had a marked increase in INR requiring oral vitamin K.[7]

(h) Moxifloxacin

The pharmacokinetics of *R*- and *S*-warfarin were not altered when a single 25-mg dose of **warfarin** was given on day 5 of an 8-day course of moxifloxacin 400 mg daily in healthy subjects. The prothrombin time increased by 3% (0 to 6%), which is not clinically relevant.[8]

In contrast, there are a number of case reports suggesting an interaction; these are summarised in 'Table 12.4', p.394.

(i) Nalidixic acid

There are case reports showing that nalidixic acid might interact with coumarins. These are summarised in 'Table 12.4', p.394.

(j) Norfloxacin

In a study[9] in 10 healthy subjects, norfloxacin 400 mg twice daily for 9 days was found not to alter either the pharmacokinetics or anticoagulant effects of a single 30-mg dose of **warfarin** given on day 4. A similar result was seen in a retrospective study, but conflicting case reports have been published. Similarly, contrasting effects have been seen with **acenocoumarol** and **phenprocoumon**. These are summarised in 'Table 12.4', p.394.

(k) Ofloxacin

In general, there does not seem to be an interaction between ofloxacin and acenocoumarol or phenprocoumon, as demonstrated by the majority of studies showing no effect, see 'Table 12.4', p.394 for details. Furthermore, for the period December 1990 to January 2004, Health Canada had not received any reports of suspected coagulation disorders associated with ofloxacin and **warfarin**.[10] However, there are 2 case reports of increased warfarin effects, which are summarised in 'Table 12.4', p.394.

(l) Pefloxacin

There is a case report showing that pefloxacin might interact with coumarins. This is summarised in 'Table 12.4', p.394.

Mechanism

Uncertain. It is not clear what other factors might have been responsible in those cases where the effects of the anticoagulants were increased. Factors relating to acute infection rather than the antibacterial used to treat it might be responsible for increased INRs, see also 'Coumarins + Antibacterials', p.383. However, one study that controlled for severity of infection indicated this was not the case and that an interaction between the quinolone and anticoagulant probably occurs.[11] *In vitro* experiments[12,13] have shown that nalidixic acid can displace warfarin from its binding sites on human plasma albumin, but this mechanism on its own is almost certainly not the full explanation. In a single-dose study enoxacin was shown to inhibit the metabolism of the less potent *R*-warfarin isomer, without affecting the anticoagulant response.[3] This effect may become important if accumulation of the *R*-warfarin isomer (which is cleared slowly) occurred during prolonged dosing.[14] Other quinolones might have similar effects. It has also been suggested that fluoroquinolones might suppress vitamin K-producing gut bacteria with resultant potentiation of anticoagulant effects,[15] see also 'Coumarins + Antibacterials', p.383.

Importance and management

The minor pharmacokinetic interaction between ciprofloxacin and warfarin would appear to be established, but unlikely to be clinically relevant. Similarly, no other quinolone has been shown to have a clinically important interaction with warfarin in a controlled prospective study. Despite this, there are numerous published case reports of marked over-anticoagulation with many of the quinolones, and other known unpublished cases reported to regulatory authorities. In addition, for levofloxacin there is some information from uncontrolled studies supporting an interaction in some patients. Nevertheless, given the widespread use of warfarin and quinolones, these interactions would appear to be rare.

The overall picture is that no adverse interaction normally occurs between the quinolones and coumarins, but rarely and unpredictably increased anticoagulant effects and even bleeding can occur with some of them. There is no need to avoid using any of the quinolones with the coumarins, and, in one study, pre-emptive warfarin dose reduction resulted in subtherapeutic INRs in some patients given levofloxacin, and was considered unnecessary.[7] Monitoring the INR within 3 to 5 days of starting the quinolone was considered reasonable. Note that, if a patient is unwell enough to require an antibacterial, it might be prudent to increase monitoring of coagulation status even if no specific drug interaction is expected, see also 'Coumarins + Antibacterials', p.383.

1. Israel DS, Stotka J, Rock W, Sintek CD, Kamada AK, Klein C, Swaim WR, Pluhar RE, Toscano JP, Lettieri JT, Heller AH, Polk RE. Effect of ciprofloxacin on the pharmacokinetics and pharmacodynamics of warfarin. *Clin Infect Dis* (1996) 22, 251–6.
2. Randinitis EJ, Koup JR, Bron NJ, Hounslow NJ, Rausch G, Abel R, Vassos AB, Sedman AJ. Drug interaction studies with clinafloxacin and probenecid, cimetidine, phenytoin and warfarin. *Drugs* (1999) 58 (Suppl 2), 254–5.

Table 12.4 Summary of the pharmacodynamic evidence for and against an interaction between quinolones and coumarins or indanediones

Study type (year)	*Group*	*Coumarin*	*Quinolone*	*Outcome*	*Refs*
Studies showing no interaction					
Randomised, placebo-controlled crossover (1996)	32 stable patients (without infection)	Warfarin	Ciprofloxacin 750 mg twice daily for 12 days	No clinically relevant effect on prothrombin time ratio with a mean increase of just 3% (range 0 to 6%)	1
Clinical (1991)	9 stable patients (without infection)	Warfarin	Ciprofloxacin 500 mg twice daily for 7 days	No difference in mean prothrombin time before and during treatment with ciprofloxacin	2
Randomised placebo-controlled (1992)	16 stable patients (without infection)	Warfarin	Ciprofloxacin 500 mg twice daily for 10 days (n=7)	No difference in INR was observed between or within treatment groups, nor in individual patients during treatment	3
Single-dose (2007)	18 healthy subjects	Warfarin 7.5 mg (single-dose)	Ciprofloxacin 500 mg controlled release tablet (single-dose)	No clinically relevant effect on anticoagulation	4
Retrospective, nested case-control crossover (2008)	Patients	Warfarin	Ciprofloxacin	Risk of hospitalisation for gastrointestinal bleeding no greater in patients who had taken ciprofloxacin in the 6 to 10 days before hospitalisation than in those who had taken cefalexin*	5
Population-based cohort study (2002)	19 patients	Acenocoumarol or phenprocoumon	Ciprofloxacin	No cases of overanticoagulation (INR >6)	6
Retrospective, nested case-control crossover (2008)	Patients	Warfarin	Gatifloxacin	Risk of hospitalisation for gastrointestinal bleeding no greater in patients who had taken gatifloxacin in the 6 to 10 days before hospitalisation than in those who had taken cefalexin*	5
Randomised, placebo-controlled (1999)	35 healthy subjects	Warfarin, fixed dose	Gemifloxacin, 320 mg daily for 7 days	INRs in range 1.3 to 1.8 did not increase when given gemifloxacin	7
Retrospective analysis (2006)	54 patients	Warfarin	Levofloxacin	Only 1 patient had an INR >4	8
Retrospective analysis (2005)	22 patients	Warfarin	Levofloxacin	No interaction detected, mean INR change 0.31, (p = 0.65)	9
Retrospective case-control (2005)	Acutely ill elderly patients	Warfarin	Levofloxacin	No increased risk of hospitalisation associated with use of levofloxacin prior to admission	10
Retrospective, nested case-control crossover (2008)	Patients	Warfarin	Levofloxacin	Risk of hospitalisation for gastrointestinal bleeding no greater in patients who had taken levofloxacin in the 6 to 10 days before hospitalisation than in those who had taken cefalexin*	5
Retrospective, nested case-control (2010)	Patients aged 66-years or older	Warfarin	Norfloxacin	Risk of hospitalisation for upper gastrointestinal tract haemorrhage no different in those who had taken norfloxacin in the preceding 14 days compared with controls (odds ratio 0.38)	11
Retrospective cohort (2008)	59 987 patients	Acenocoumarol or phenprocoumon	Norfloxacin (n=2714)	Relative risk of hospitalisation for bleeding = 2.2 (range 0.7 to 6.7)	12
Clinical (1987)	7 healthy subjects	Phenprocoumon	Ofloxacin, 200 mg daily for 7 days	No effect on prothrombin times	13
Population-based cohort study (2002)	33 patients	Acenocoumarol or phenprocoumon	Ofloxacin	No cases of overanticoagulation (INR >6)	6
Retrospective cohort (2008)	59 987 patients	Acenocoumarol or phenprocoumon	Ofloxacin (n=1395)	Relative risk of hospitalisation for bleeding = 2.8 (range 0.7 to 11.3)	12
Studies showing an interaction					
Retrospective, nested case-control (2010)	Patients aged 66-years or older	Warfarin	Ciprofloxacin	Risk of hospitalisation for upper gastrointestinal tract haemorrhage 2-fold higher in those that had taken ciprofloxacin in the preceding 14 days than in controls (odds ratio 1.94)	11
Retrospective cohort (2008)	59 987 patients	Acenocoumarol or phenprocoumon	Ciprofloxacin (n=2992)	Relative risk of hospitalisation for bleeding increased (RR = 3.9, range 1.8 to 8.2)	12
Case-control (2011)	Patients	Phenprocoumon	Ciprofloxacin	Risk of hospitalisation for bleeding increased (OR = 2.74, range 1.8 to 4.18)	14

* Cefalexin was used as a reference point to exclude the possibility that being ill and requiring an antibacterial could, in itself, affect coagulation.

≈ See Coagulation tests, p.371.

Continued

Table 12.4 Summary of the pharmacodynamic evidence for and against an interaction between quinolones and coumarins or indanediones (continued)

Study type (year)	*Group*	*Coumarin*	*Quinolone*	*Outcome*	*Refs*
Retrospective review (2002)	40 patients	Warfarin	Gatifloxacin	22 patients (55%) had an INR>3 during or within 48 hours after stopping gatifloxacin, compared with 37% of those taking ceftriaxone and/or azithromycin. Warfarin dose adjustments were needed in 38% of the gatifloxacin group, compared with 18% in patients taking other antibacterials. Infection severity did not differ between the groups	15
Retrospective analysis (2006)	38 patients	Warfarin	Gatifloxacin	8 patients had an INR>4, and 4 patients were treated with vitamin K	8
Uncontrolled, prospective (2003)	18 stable patients	Warfarin	Levofloxacin	No difference in mean INR before levofloxacin and the first INR taken a median of 5 days afterwards (2.61 versus 2.74), however, 4 patients had increased INR (to a range of 3.89 to 4.2) and 3 had decreased INR (to a range of 1.39 to 1.84) and required warfarin dose adjustments. Only 7 patients had therapeutic INRs (range 2 to 3) throughout the study and did not require warfarin dose adjustment	16
Retrospective cohort analysis (2005)	27 patients	Warfarin	Levofloxacin	Mean increase in INR of 0.85 and increased incidence of over-anticoagulation	17
Case-control (2011)	Patients	Phenprocoumon	Levofloxacin	Risk of hospitalisation for bleeding increased (OR = 4.4, range 2.45 to 7.89)	14
Case-control (2011)	Patients	Phenprocoumon	Moxifloxacin	Risk of hospitalisation for bleeding increased (OR = 3.51, range 1.77 to 6.96)	14
Population-based cohort (2002)	Patients	Acenocoumarol or phenprocoumon	Norfloxacin	RR of over-anticoagulation (INR >6) = 9.8. Risk greatest within first 3 days of treatment	6
Cohort (2005)	Patients	Acenocoumarol or phenprocoumon	Norfloxacin	RR of hospitalisation for bleeding = 5.9	18
Case-control (2011)	Patients	Phenprocoumon	Ofloxacin	Risk of hospitalisation for bleeding increased (OR = 3.6, range 1.3 to 10)	14
Prospective case-control (2012)	Patients	Warfarin	Unspecified quinolones	Odds ratio for bleeding risk = 1.69 (range 1.09 to 2.62), compared with 2.01 for use of an antibacterial or antifungal	19
Case reports of no interaction					
Case report (1988)	23-year-old	Warfarin 3 mg daily	Enoxacin 400 mg twice daily for 7 days	No effect on prothrombin time ratio	20
Case reports of an interaction					
Case reports (1989 to 2006)	About 100 patients	Warfarin	Ciprofloxacin	Modest to large increases in prothrombin times and/or bleeding	21-31
				Data, mainly from the FDA in the US, suggests that the median prothrombin time increase was 38 seconds, the INR 10, and the median time to detection after starting ciprofloxacin was 5.5 days. Hospitalisation was reported in 15 cases and bleeding in 25 cases	28
				At least 3 fatalities reported	28, 29, 31
Case report (2010)	70-year-old	Warfarin	Ciprofloxacin, 750 mg twice daily	Increase in INR from 3 to 4.2. However, the patient also received several other antibacterials which may also have been implicated	32
Case reports (2004)	13 patients	Warfarin	Gatifloxacin	Suspected coagulation disorders, all were considered serious and 2 were fatal	29
Case report (2006)	88-year-old	Warfarin	Gatifloxacin, 400 mg daily	INR too high to be determined. Patient was taking numerous drugs which included warfarin and gatifloxacin	33
Case report (2001)	2 patients	Warfarin	Levofloxacin, 500 mg daily	Increased INRs of 5.7 and 7.9 on routine testing shortly after stopping levofloxacin	34
Case reports (2001 to 2007)	9 patients	Warfarin	Levofloxacin, 500 mg daily for 5 to 10 days (or unstated)	Modest to large increases in INR	35-37
				Bleeding complications (epistaxis, haemopericardium) occurred in some	36, 37
				One case was fatal	37

* Cefalexin was used as a reference point to exclude the possibility that being ill and requiring an antibacterial could, in itself, affect coagulation.
≈ See Coagulation tests, p.371.

Continued

Table 12.4 Summary of the pharmacodynamic evidence for and against an interaction between quinolones and coumarins or indanediones (continued)

Study type (year)	*Group*	*Coumarin*	*Quinolone*	*Outcome*	*Refs*
Case reports over an 8-year period (2004)	16 patients	Warfarin	Levofloxacin	Suspected coagulation disorders, 14 were considered serious and 1 was fatal	29
Case reports (2003 to 2008)	12 patients	Warfarin	Moxifloxacin	Increased INRs	38-41
				5 patients had INRs increased to 5.7 to 12.8 within 4 to 12 days of starting moxifloxacin and one patient had a haemorrhage	40
				INR increased to 12 after 5 days of moxifloxacin with gross haematuria and diffuse ecchymosis	41
Case reports over a 3-year period (2004)	12 patients	Warfarin	Moxifloxacin	Suspected coagulation disorders, 11 were considered serious	29
Case report (2006)	1 patient	Warfarin	Moxifloxacin	INR increased from about 2 to >10, after 4 days of moxifloxacin	30
Case report (2011)	89-year-old	Warfarin	Moxifloxacin, single 400-mg dose	INR increased on 2 occasions (5.8 and 6.7) after taking moxifloxacin on day of BCG bladder instillations. On 2 other occasions INR increases were averted by precautionary measures. Note that the patient also received prophylactic doses of paracetamol (acetaminophen) with each bladder instillation, which has been reported to interact (see Coumarins and related drugs + Paracetamol (Acetaminophen), p.459)	42
Case report (1974)	55-year-old	Warfarin	Nalidixic acid, 500 mg four times daily	Increased prothrombin ratio from 2 to 3.6, with purpuric rash and bruising within 6 days of starting nalidixic acid	43
Case report (1987)	71-year-old	Warfarin	Nalidixic acid, 1 g three times daily	Prothrombin time of 60 seconds, 10 days after starting nalidixic acid	44
Case report (1996)	84-year-old	Warfarin	Nalidixic acid	INR increased from 1.9 to 9.6	45
Case report (1980)	65-year-old	Acenocoumarol	Nalidixic acid, 1 g daily	Hypoprothrombinaemia after taking nalidixic acid	46
Case report (1989)	91-year-old	Warfarin	Norfloxacin (dose not stated)	Brain haemorrhage within 11 days of starting norfloxacin. Her prothrombin time had increased from 21.6 to 36.5 seconds	47
Case reports over a 17-year period (2004)	6 patients	Warfarin	Norfloxacin	Suspected coagulation disorders, 4 were considered serious	29
Case reports (2006)	11 patients	Warfarin	Norfloxacin	Suspected interaction	30
Case report (1988)	40-year-old	Warfarin, 5 mg daily	Ofloxacin, 200 mg three times daily	INR increased from 2.5 to 4.4 within 2 days of starting ofloxacin, and increased to 5.8 after a further 2 days	48
Case report (1993)	73-year-old	Warfarin	Ofloxacin, 400 mg twice daily	Prothrombin time of 78 seconds and gross haematuria 5 days after starting ofloxacin	49
Case report (1986)	64-year-old	Acenocoumarol	Pefloxacin, 800 mg daily	Quick time≈ decreased from 26% to less than 5% within 5 days of starting pefloxacin and rifampicin 1.2 g daily. Note that rifampicin is an enzyme inducer, which normally causes a decrease in the effects of acenocoumarol (see Coumarins + Antibacterials; Rifamycins, p.397)	50

* Cefalexin was used as a reference point to exclude the possibility that being ill and requiring an antibacterial could, in itself, affect coagulation.

≈ See Coagulation tests, p.371.

1. Israel DS, Stotka J, Rock W, Sintek CD, Kamada AK, Klein C, Swaim WR, Pluhar RE, Toscano JP, Lettieri JT, Heller AH, Polk RE. Effect of ciprofloxacin on the pharmacokinetics and pharmacodynamics of warfarin. *Clin Infect Dis* (1996) 22, 251–6.
2. Rindone JP, Keuey CL, Jones WN, Garewal HS. Hypoprothrombinemic effect of warfarin not influenced by ciprofloxacin. *Clin Pharm* (1991) 10, 136–8. Erratum ibid, 429 [name].
3. Bianco TM, Bussey HI, Farnett LE, Linn WD, Roush MK, Wong YWJ. Potential warfarin-ciprofloxacin interaction in patients receiving long-term anticoagulation. *Pharmacotherapy* (1992) 12, 435–9.
4. Washington C, Hou SYE, Hughes NC, Campanella C, Berner B. Ciprofloxacin prolonged-release tablets do not affect warfarin pharmacokinetics and pharmacodynamics. *J Clin Pharmacol* (2007) 47, 1320–6.
5. Schelleman H, Bilker WB, Brensinger CM, Han X, Kimmel SE, Hennessy S. Warfarin with fluoroquinolones, sulfonamides or azole antifungals: interactions and the risk of hospitalization for gastrointestinal bleeding. *Clin Pharmacol Ther* (2008) 84, 581–8.
6. Visser LE, Penning-van Beest FJA, Kasbergen AAH, De Smet PAGM, Vulto AG, Hofman A, Stricker BHC. Overanticoagulation associated with combined use of antibacterial drugs and acenocoumarol or phenprocoumon anticoagulants. *Thromb Haemost* (2002) 88, 705–10.
7. Davy M, Bird N, Rost KL, Fuder H. Lack of effect of gemifloxacin on the steady-state pharmacodynamics of warfarin in healthy volunteers. *Chemotherapy* (1999) 45, 491–5.
8. Mathews S, Cole J, Ryono RA. Anticoagulation-related outcomes in patients receiving warfarin after starting levofloxacin or gatifloxacin. *Pharmacotherapy* (2006) 26, 1446–52.
9. McCall KL, Scott JC, Anderson HG. Retrospective evaluation of a possible interaction between warfarin and levofloxacin. *Pharmacotherapy* (2005) 25, 67–73.
10. Stroud LF, Mamdami MM, Kopp A, Bell CM. The safety of levofloxacin in elderly patients on warfarin. *Am J Med* (2005) 118, 1417.
11. Fischer HD, Juurlink DN, Mamdani MM, Kopp A, Laupacis A. Hemorrhage during warfarin therapy associated with cotrimoxazole and other urinary tract anti-infective agents: a population-based study. *Arch Intern Med* (2010) 170, 617–21.
12. Penning-van Beest FJ, Koerselman J, Herings RM. Risk of major bleeding during concomitant use of antibiotic drugs and coumarin anticoagulants. *J Thromb Haemost* (2008) 6, 284–90.
13. Verho M, Malerczyk V, Rosenkranz B, Grötsch H. Absence of interaction between ofloxacin and phenprocoumon. *Curr Med Res Opin* (1987) 10, 474–9.
14. Jobski K, Behr S, Garbe E. Drug interactions with phenprocoumon and the risk of serious haemorrhage: a nested case-control study in a large population-based German database. *Eur J Clin Pharmacol* (2011) 67, 941–51.
15. Artymowicz RJ, Cino BJ, Rossi JG, Walker JL, Moore S. Possible interaction between gatifloxacin and warfarin. *Am J Health-Syst Pharm* (2002) 59 1205–6.

Continued

Table 12.4 Summary of the pharmacodynamic evidence for and against an interaction between quinolones and coumarins or indanediones (continued)

16. Yamreudeewong W, Lower DL, Kilpatrick DM, Enlow AM, Burrows MM, Greenwood MC. Effect of levofloxacin coadministration on the international normalized ratios during warfarin therapy. *Pharmacotherapy* (2003) 23, 333–8.
17. Glasheen JJ, Fugit RV, Prochazka AV. The risk of overanticoagulation with antibiotic use in outpatients on stable warfarin regimens. *J Gen Intern Med* (2005) 20, 653–6.
18. Penning-van Beest F, Erkens J, Petersen KU, Koelz HR, Herings R. Main comedications associated with major bleeding during anticoagulant therapy with coumarins. *Eur J Clin Pharmacol* (2005) 61, 439–44.
19. Baillargeon J, Holmes HM, Lin YL, Raji MA, Sharma G, Kuo YF. Concurrent use of warfarin and antibiotics and the risk of bleeding in older adults. *Am J Med* (2012) 125, 183–9.
20. McLeod AD, Burgess C. Drug interaction between warfarin and enoxacin. *N Z Med J* (1988) 101, 216.
21. Mott FE, Murphy S, Hunt V. Ciprofloxacin and warfarin. *Ann Intern Med* (1989) 111, 542–3.
22. Linville D, Emory C, Graves L. Ciprofloxacin and warfarin interaction. *Am J Med* (1991) 90, 765.
23. Kamada AK. Possible interaction between ciprofloxacin and warfarin. *DICP Ann Pharmacother* (1990) 24, 27–8.
24. Johnson KC, Joe RH, Self TH. Drug interaction. J Fam Pract (1991) 33, 338.
25. Renzi R, Finkbeiner S. Ciprofloxacin interaction with warfarin: a potentially dangerous side-effect. *Am J Emerg Med* (1991) 9, 551–2.
26. Dugoni-Kramer BM. Ciprofloxacin-warfarin interaction. *DICP Ann Pharmacother* (1991) 25, 1397.
27. Jolson HM, Tanner A, Green L, Grasela TH. Adverse reaction reporting of interaction between warfarin and fluoroquinolones. *Arch Intern Med* (1991) 151, 1003–4.
28. Ellis RJ, Mayo MS, Bodensteiner DM. Ciprofloxacin-warfarin coagulopathy: a case series. *Am J Hematol* (2000) 63, 28–31.
29. Health Canada. Fluoroquinolones and warfarin: suspected interaction. *Can Adverse React News* (2004) 14, 1–2.
30. ADRAC. Fluoroquinolone antibiotics: interactions with warfarin. *Aust Adverse Drug React Bull* (2006) 25; 2.
31. Byrd DC, Gaskins SE, Parrish AM, Freeman LB. Warfarin and ciprofloxacin interaction: case report and controversy. *J Am Board Fam Pract* (1999) 12, 486–8.
32. Trivedi D, Newton JD, Mitra A, Puri P. A serious drug interaction leading to a spontaneous total hyphema. *J Postgrad Med* (2010) 56, 46–7.
33. Chock AWY, Stading JA. Indeterminable international normalized ratio with concurrent use of warfarin and gatifloxacin. *Am J Health-Syst Pharm* (2006) 63, 1539–42.
34. Ravnan SL, Locke C. Levofloxacin and warfarin interaction. *Pharmacotherapy* (2001) 21, 884–5.
35. Gheno G, Cinetto L. Levofloxacin-warfarin interaction. *Eur J Clin Pharmacol* (2001) 57, 427.
36. Jones CB, Fugate SE. Levofloxacin and warfarin interaction. *Ann Pharmacother* (2002) 36, 1554–7.
37. Vadlamudi RS, Smalligan RD, Ismail HM. Interaction between warfarin and levofloxacin: case series. *South Med J* (2007) 100, 720–4.
38. O'Connor KA, O'Mahony D. The interaction of moxifloxacin and warfarin in three elderly patients. *Eur J Intern Med* (2003) 14, 255–7.
39. Arnold LM, Nissen LR, Ng TMH. Moxifloxacin and warfarin: additional evidence for a clinically relevant interaction. *Pharmacotherapy* (2005) 25, 904–7.
40. Elbe DHT, Chang SW. Moxifloxacin-warfarin interaction: a series of five case reports. *Ann Pharmacother* (2005) 39, 361–4.
41. Yildiz F, Kurtaran B, Çayli M, Candevir A, Sümbül Z. A significant interaction between moxifloxacin and warfarin in a patient with a mitral bioprosthetic valve. *Heart Vessels* (2008) 4, 286–8.
42. Lee R, Wen A, Berube C. Moxifloxacin-acetaminophen-warfarin interaction during bacille Calmette-Guérin treatment for bladder cancer. *Am J Health-Syst Pharm* (2011) 68, 814–7.
43. Hoffbrand BI. Interaction of nalidixic acid and warfarin. *BMJ* (1974) 2, 666.
44. Leor J, Levartowsky D, Sharon C. Interaction between nalidixic acid and warfarin. *Ann Intern Med* (1987) 107, 601.
45. Gulløv AL, Koefoed BG, Petersen P. Interaktion mellem warfarin og nalidixinsyre. *Ugeskr Laeger* (1996) 158, 5174–5.
46. Potasman I, Bassan H. Nicoumalone and nalidixic acid interaction. *Ann Intern Med* (1980) 92, 571.
47. Linville T, Matanin D. Norfloxacin and warfarin. *Ann Intern Med* (1989) 110, 751–2.
48. Leor J, Matetzki S. Ofloxacin and warfarin. *Ann Intern Med* (1988) 109, 761. 49. Baciewicz AM, Ashar BH, Locke TW. Interaction of ofloxacin and warfarin. *Ann Intern Med* (1993) 119, 1223.
50. Pertek JP, Helmer J, Vivin P, Kipper R. Potentialisation d'une antivitamine K par l'association péfloxacine-rifampicine. *Ann Fr Anesth Reanim* (1986) 5, 320–1.

3. Toon S, Hopkins KJ, Garstang FM, Aarons L, Sedman A, Rowland M. Enoxacin-warfarin interaction: pharmacokinetic and stereochemical aspects. *Clin Pharmacol Ther* (1987) 42, 33–41.
4. Holazo AA, Soni PP, Kachevsky V, Min BH, Townsend L, Patel IH. Fleroxacin-warfarin interaction in humans. *Intersci Conf Antimicrob Agents Chemother* (1990) 30, 253.
5. Tequin (Gatifloxacin). Bristol-Myers Squibb Company. US Prescribing information, January 2006.
6. Liao S, Palmer M, Fowler C, Nayak RK. Absence of an effect of levofloxacin on warfarin pharmacokinetics and anticoagulation in male volunteers. *J Clin Pharmacol* (1996) 36, 1072–7.
7. Ahmed A, Stephens JC, Kaus CA, Fay WP. Impact of preemptive warfarin dose reduction on anticoagulation after initiation of trimethoprim-sulfamethoxazole or levofloxacin. *J Thromb Thrombolysis* (2008) 26, 44–8.
8. Müller FO, Hundt HKL, Muir AR, Potgieter MA, Terblanché J, Toerien CJ, Stass H. Study to investigate the influence of 400 mg BAY 12-8039 (M) given once daily to healthy volunteers on PK and PD of warfarin (W). *Intersci Conf Antimicrob Agents Chemother* (1998) 18, A-13.
9. Rocci ML, Vlasses PH, Distlerath LM, Gregg MH, Wheeler SC, Zing W, Bjornsson TD. Norfloxacin does not alter warfarin's disposition or anticoagulant effect. *J Clin Pharmacol* (1990) 30, 728–32.
10. Health Canada. Fluoroquinolones and warfarin: suspected interaction. *Can Adverse React News* (2004) 14, 1–2.
11. Artymowicz RJ, Cino BJ, Rossi JG, Walker JL, Moore S. Possible interaction between gatifloxacin and warfarin. *Am J Health-Syst Pharm* (2002) 59 1205–6.
12. Sellers EM, Koch-Weser J. Kinetics and clinical importance of displacement of warfarin from albumin by acidic drugs. *Ann N Y Acad Sci* (1971) 179, 213–25.
13. Sellers EM, Koch-Weser J. Displacement of warfarin from human albumin by diazoxide and ethacrynic, mefenamic, and nalidixic acids. *Clin Pharmacol Ther* (1970) 11, 524–9.
14. Bianco TM, Bussey HI, Farnett LE, Linn WD, Roush MK, Wong YWJ. Potential warfarin-ciprofloxacin interaction in patients receiving long-term anticoagulation. *Pharmacotherapy* (1992) 12, 435–9.
15. Leor J, Matetzki S. Ofloxacin and warfarin. *Ann Intern Med* (1988) 109, 761.

Coumarins + Antibacterials; Rifamycins

The anticoagulant effects of warfarin are considerably reduced by rifampicin (rifampin). Acenocoumarol and phenprocoumon are similarly affected. An isolated case describes reduced warfarin anticoagulant effects on the concurrent use of rifaximin.

Clinical evidence

(a) Acenocoumarol

The dose of acenocoumarol needed to be greatly increased in 18 patients who were given **rifampicin** 450 mg twice daily for 7 days to maintain the Quick value within the therapeutic range. The effect was apparent 5 to 8 days after starting the rifampicin, and had not reached a maximum at 14 days, at which point a mean 76% increase in the acenocoumarol dose was needed.[1] In another study, the Quick time of a single dose of acenocoumarol, measured 35 hours after the dose, was reduced by 44% when **rifampicin** 10 mg/kg daily was given for 2 weeks.[2] In one 73-year-old, a 6-fold increase in the dose of acenocoumarol was insufficient to maintain a therapeutic INR after starting **rifampicin** for endocarditis.[3]

(b) Phenprocoumon

In a study in healthy subjects, **rifampicin** 600 mg daily for 14 days increased the clearance of a single dose of phenprocoumon 2.2-fold.[4] Similarly, 2 patients stabilised on phenprocoumon required the dose to be doubled while taking **rifampicin** 600 mg daily (and isoniazid with or without ethambutol). In one case, the patient developed severe gross haematuria 3 months after **rifampicin** had been discontinued because the phenprocoumon dose had not been reduced.[5]

(c) Warfarin

1. Rifampicin (Rifampin). In one controlled study in 8 healthy subjects, rifampicin 600 mg daily for 21 days reduced the steady-state warfarin plasma concentrations by 85% (range 64% to 100%). In addition, rifampicin abolished the anticoagulant effect of warfarin (the prothrombin time averaged 27% of normal during warfarin alone, and 85% of normal when rifampicin was taken).[6] Similar findings were seen in two other single-dose studies with warfarin.[7,8] One of these measured the isomers of warfarin separately and found that rifampicin increased the clearance of *R*-warfarin 3-fold and *S*-warfarin 2-fold.[8] This interaction has also been described in a number of case reports.[9-14] In these reports the dose of warfarin was doubled[9,11] or even tripled[11] to accommodate this interaction, and reduced by an equivalent amount over two[10] to three weeks[12] after rifampicin was stopped. In one well-described case, a 3-fold increase in warfarin dose, from 5 to 15 mg daily over 4 months, did not achieve a therapeutic INR during the long-term use of rifampicin, and eventually a 5-fold increase in dose (25 mg daily) attained an INR of 1.7 and 1.9. A gradual 70% dose reduction over 4 to 5 weeks was required when the rifampicin was stopped.[14] In yet another case, a 5- to 6-fold increase in warfarin dose was not sufficient to maintain the INR in the therapeutic range, and enoxaparin was used instead of warfarin.[15]

A retrospective study[16] similarly found that the concurrent use of enzyme inducers (including rifampicin) greatly influenced the total weekly warfarin dose; further analysis found that the average additional amount of warfarin required in patients taking these drugs was 17.2 mg weekly.

2. Rifaximin. A 49-year-old woman whose INR had been stable between 2 and 3.5 while taking warfarin 7.5 mg daily for antiphospholipid syndrome, was diagnosed with small intestine bacterial overgrowth and given rifaximin 400 mg three times daily for 10 days, then 400 mg twice daily for 25 days. Within a few days of starting to take rifaximin, her INR had fallen to 1.2, and was only 1.4 about 4 weeks later, despite a gradual 50% increase in her warfarin dose. Twelve days after stopping rifaximin, her INR was 4.2, and her warfarin dose was reduced accordingly. About 5 weeks later she was restarted on rifaximin at the same dose for a 10-day course for another episode of small intestine bacterial overgrowth, and her INR fell from 1.9 to 1.5, despite a 50% increase in her warfarin dose.[17]

Mechanism

Rifampicin (rifampin) is a non-specific liver enzyme inducer with potent effects on CYP3A4, which increases the metabolism and clearance of the coumarins, thereby reducing their effects.[8] Other mechanisms might also be involved.[12] See also 'Coumarins + Antibacterials', p.383.

Rifaximin has been reported to induce CYP3A4 *in vitro*, but due to its low systemic bioavailability (less than 1%), and its lack of effect on the CYP3A4 probe substrate, midazolam (see 'Benzodiazepines + Rifaximin', p.837), the manufacturers consider the risk of systemic drug interactions to be low.[18] However, the authors of the case report,[17] suggest that rifaximin absorption was increased as a result of increased intestinal permeability caused by the small intestine bacterial overgrowth, and that this led to an increase in rifaximin systemic exposure sufficient to cause CYP3A4 induction.[17]

Importance and management

The interaction between **rifampicin (rifampin)** and the coumarins is very well documented, clinically important, and occurs in most patients. A sizeable reduction in anticoagulant effects is to be expected within one week of starting the rifampicin, and this is likely to persist for about 2 to 5 weeks after the rifampicin has been withdrawn. With warfarin there is evidence that the dose might need to be greatly increased (2- to 5-fold) over a number of weeks to accommodate this interaction, and reduced slowly by an equivalent amount following withdrawal of the rifampicin. Warfarin dose titrations should be carried out with close monitoring. Bridging therapy with heparin or a low-molecular-weight heparin might be appropriate until the warfarin dose is restabilised.

The general relevance of the isolated case report of decreased warfarin anticoagulation with **rifaximin** is unclear, as the patient's clinical condition could have increased rifaximin systemic exposure, and therefore contributed to the interaction. Nevertheless, until more is known, it would seem prudent to bear the possibility of an interaction in mind and consider increasing INR monitoring if rifaximin is started or stopped in a patient also taking warfarin.

There does not seem to be any information regarding the other rifamycins, **rifabutin** and **rifapentine** which are both enzyme inducers, although they possess less potent effects than rifampicin. However, the manufacturers and the CSM in the UK warn that rifabutin might reduce the effects of a number of drugs, including oral anticoagulants.[19,20]

1. Michot F, Bürgi M, Büttner J. Rimactan (Rifampizin) und Antikoagulantientherapie. *Schweiz Med Wochenschr* (1970) 100, 583–4.
2. Sennwald G. Etude de l'influence de la rifampicine sur l'effet anticoagulant de l'acénocoumarol. *Rev Med Suisse Romande* (1974) 94, 945–54.
3. Harmsze AM, Deneer VHM, Wiltink EH. Langdurig verminderd effect van cumarinederivaten na gebruik van rifampicine. *Ned Tijdschr Geneeskd* (2007) 151, 1945–9.
4. Ohnhaus EE, Kampschulte J, Mönig H. Effect of propranolol and rifampicin on liver blood flow and phenprocoumon elimination. *Acta Pharmacol Toxicol (Copenh)* (1986) 59 (Suppl 4), 92.
5. Boekhout-Mussert RJ, Bieger R, van Brummelen A, Lemkes HHPJ. Inhibition by rifampin of the anticoagulant effect of phenprocoumon. *JAMA* (1974) 229, 1903–4.
6. O'Reilly RA. Interaction of chronic daily warfarin therapy and rifampin. *Ann Intern Med* (1975) 83, 506–8.
7. O'Reilly RA. Interaction of sodium warfarin and rifampin. Studies in man. *Ann Intern Med* (1974) 81, 337–40.
8. Heimark LD, Gibaldi M, Trager WF, O'Reilly RA, Goulart DA. The mechanism of the warfarin-rifampicin drug interaction in humans. *Clin Pharmacol Ther* (1987) 42, 388–94.
9. Romankiewicz JA, Ehrman M. Rifampin and warfarin: a drug interaction. *Ann Intern Med* (1975) 82, 224–5.
10. Self TH, Mann RB. Interaction of rifampicin and warfarin. *Chest* (1975) 67, 490–1.
11. Fox P. Warfarin-rifampicin interaction. *Med J Aust* (1982) 1, 60.
12. Almog S, Martinowitz U, Halkin H, Bank HZ, Farfel Z. Complex interaction of rifampin and warfarin. *South Med J* (1988) 81, 1304–6.
13. Casner PR. Inability to attain oral anticoagulation: warfarin-rifampin interaction revisited. *South Med J* (1996) 89, 1200–3
14. Lee CR, Thrasher KA. Difficulties in anticoagulation management during coadministration of warfarin and rifampin. *Pharmacotherapy* (2001) 21, 1240–6.
15. Kim KY, Epplen K, Foruhari F, Alexandropoulos H. Update on the interaction of rifampin and warfarin. *Prog Cardiovasc Nurs* (2007) 22, 97–100.
16. Whitley HP, Fermo JD, Chumney ECG, Brzezinski WA. Effect of patient-specific factors on weekly warfarin dose. *Ther Clin Risk Manag* (2007) 3, 499–504.
17. Hoffman JT, Hartig C, Sonbol E, Lang M. Probable interaction between warfarin and rifaximin in a patient treated for small intestine bacterial overgrowth. *Ann Pharmacother* (2011) 45, e25.
18. Xifaxanta (Rifaximin). Norgine Ltd. UK Summary of product characteristics, June 2011.
19. Mycobutin (Rifabutin). Pfizer Ltd. UK Summary of product characteristics, December 2013.
20. Committee on the Safety of Medicines/Medicines Control Agency. Revised indication and drug interactions of rifabutin. *Current Problems* (1997) 23, 14.

Coumarins and related drugs + Antibacterials; Sulfonamides and/or Trimethoprim

Co-trimoxazole (sulfamethoxazole with trimethoprim) inhibits the metabolism of *S*-warfarin, and a number of case reports show that the anticoagulant effects of the coumarins can be increased. Case reports suggest that sulfafurazole, sulfadoxine, and sulfamethizole may have similar effects. Two cohort studies have suggested that trimethoprim alone may be associated with an increased risk of over-anticoagulation. Anecdotal evidence suggests that phenindione might not interact with co-trimoxazole, but sulfaphenazole has been reported to increase the effects of phenindione.

Clinical evidence

(a) Co-trimoxazole (Sulfamethoxazole with Trimethoprim)

1. Coumarins. Six out of 20 patients taking **warfarin** had an increase in their prothrombin ratios (to about 4 to 6) within 2 to 6 days of starting to take co-trimoxazole 960 mg twice daily.[1] One patient had a gastrointestinal haemorrhage and needed to be given vitamin K. The **warfarin** was temporarily withdrawn from 5 patients and the dose was reduced in one patient to control excessive hypoprothrombinaemia.[1]

Similarly, an increase in the effects of **warfarin**, with or without bleeding complications, in patients given co-trimoxazole has been described in a number of other case reports.[2-17] In a retrospective study of 16 patients stabilised on **warfarin**, there was a mean increase in INR of 1.75 after starting co-trimoxazole (7 patients had an INR greater than 4, and 5 patients had an INR greater than 5). The patients had stable INRs for a least two consecutive measurements before receiving co-trimoxazole, and an INR was taken within 3 to 15 days of starting the co-trimoxazole.[18] In one study in healthy subjects, co-trimoxazole 480 mg four times daily for 8 days increased the prothrombin time after a single dose of **warfarin** by 50%, but no change in the half-life of **warfarin** was seen.[19] However, in a later similar study by the same research group, in which **warfarin** was given as its separate isomers, co-trimoxazole increased the AUC of *S*-warfarin by 22% and caused a 5% decrease in AUC of *R*-warfarin.[20] A retrospective case-control study in patients aged 66 years or older taking **warfarin** found that the risk of hospitalisation for upper gastrointestinal tract hemorrhage was increased almost fourfold if co-trimoxazole had been taken in the preceding 14 days.[21] Another similar study in patients taking **warfarin** found that the risk of hospitalisation for gastrointestinal bleeding was higher in those patients who had taken co-trimoxazole in the 6 to 10 days before admission, than in those who had received cefalexin (adjusted odds ratio 1.68). In this study, cefalexin was used as a reference point to exclude the possibility that being ill and requiring an antibacterial could, in itself, affect coagulation.[22]

In a population based cohort study[23] in patients taking **acenocoumarol** or **phenprocoumon**, co-trimoxazole was associated with an increased risk of over-anticoagulation (INR greater than or equal to 6); the adjusted relative risk of over-anticoagulation was noted to be 20.1 (range 10.7 to 37.9). The risk was increased in the first 3 days of use (relative risk 16.6), but was greatest after 4 days of concurrent use (relative risk 23.2). In two other cohort studies by this same research group, the relative risk of hospitalisation for bleeding in patients taking **acenocoumarol** or **phenprocoumon** and given co-trimoxazole was lower at 6.2 and 5.1, respectively.[24,25]

In a study looking at management of the interaction, the risk of both moderate and severe over-anticoagulation with co-trimoxazole was markedly lower in patients who had their dose of anticoagulant reduced before receiving the antibacterials (preventive dose reduction) compared with those who did not (mean dose reduction 15% for **acenocoumarol** and 18% for **phenprocoumon**). Nevertheless, all patients who had taken co-trimoxazole spent considerably more time with subtherapeutic INRs in the 6 weeks after the antibacterial, although this tended to be less in patients who had a preventive dose reduction, and less if the preventive dose reduction was less than 20%.[26] In another study of preventive **warfarin** dose reduction (10 to 20%) in patients also taking co-trimoxazole,[27] none of 8 patients had a subtherapeutic INR and none had an INR of greater than 6, although 2 patients had a INR between 4 and 6. However, in the control group with no preventive dose reduction, 4 out of 9 patients had an INR greater than 6, with values ranging from 7.1 to 17.4.

2. Indanediones. In one anecdotal report, the author noted that in several years experience of the use of **phenindione** in an anticoagulant clinic serving 1 000 patients, he had not come across a clinically important case of anticoagulant potentiation with co-trimoxazole.[28] Nothing else seems to have been published on the combination, but note that another sulphonamide, sulfaphenazole, potentiated the effect of **phenindione**, see *Sulfaphenazole*, below.

(b) Sulfadoxine

A 19-year-old with a valve replacement and taking **warfarin** presented with melaena and coughing up blood about a week after self-medicating with *Fansidar* (sulfadoxine with pyrimethamine). He had not had his anticoagulant control monitored.[29]

(c) Sulfafurazole (Sulfisoxazole)

A man taking digitalis, diuretics, antacids and **warfarin** was later given sulfafurazole 500 mg every 6 hours. After 9 days, his prothrombin time had risen from 20 seconds to 28 seconds, and after 14 days he bled (haematuria, haemoptysis, gum bleeding). His prothrombin time had risen to 60 seconds.[30]

Another patient who had recently started taking **warfarin** developed haematuria and had a prolonged prothrombin time 7 days after also starting sulfafurazole.[31]

(d) Sulfamethizole

The half-life of **warfarin** was increased by over 40% (from 65 to 93 hours) in 2 patients taking sulfamethizole 1 g four times daily for a week.[32]

(e) Sulfaphenazole

Sixteen patients given single oral doses of **phenindione** and sulfaphenazole 500 mg had prothrombin time increases after 24 hours of 16.8 seconds, compared with 10.3 seconds in 12 other patients who took **phenindione** alone.[33]

(f) Trimethoprim

Trimethoprim with sulfamethoxazole (co-trimoxazole) is known to interact with coumarins, see *Co-trimoxazole*, above. However, there appear to be no controlled studies of the effect of trimethoprim alone on these drugs, and no case reports of any interaction. In one cohort study,12 patients taking **warfarin** had a small INR increase of about 0.36 when given trimethoprim, but this was not statistically significant.[34] In another cohort study in patients taking **acenocoumarol** or **phenprocoumon**, the use of trimethoprim was associated with an increased risk of over-anticoagulation (INR greater than or equal to 6). The adjusted relative risk of over-anticoagulation was noted to be 5.6 (range 1.3 to 23.1), and the greatest risk was in the first 3 days of concurrent use. The risk from trimethoprim alone in this study was less than that for co-trimoxazole.[23] However, in a further cohort study by this same research group, the relative risk of hospitalisation for bleeding in patients taking **acenocoumarol** or **phenprocoumon** and given trimethoprim was just 1.3, and it was not statistically significant (0.3 to 5.4).[25]

Mechanism

Not fully understood. Sulfamethoxazole is a known inhibitor of CYP2C9, by which *S*-warfarin in predominantly metabolised. The finding that co-trimoxazole (sulfamethoxazole with trimethoprim) caused a modest 22% increase in *S*-warfarin levels supports this mechanism.[20,35] Acenocoumarol and phenprocoumon are also metabolised by CYP2C9 and might be expected to be similarly affected. Plasma protein binding displacement has been suggested as a mechanism,[36,37] but on its own it does not provide an adequate explanation because the interaction is sustained.[23,35] Sulfonamides can drastically reduce the intestinal bacterial synthesis of vitamin K, but this is not normally an essential source of the vitamin unless dietary sources are exceptionally low,[35,38] see also 'Coumarins + Antibacterials', p.383.

Importance and management

The interaction between co-trimoxazole and the coumarins is well documented and well established. The incidence appears to be high. If bleeding is to be avoided the INR should be well monitored and the warfarin, acenocoumarol, or phenprocoumon dose should be reduced. Some consider that a pre-emptive warfarin dose reduction of about 10 to 20% reduces the risk of over-anticoagulation without increasing the risk of subtherapeutic INRs.[27] However, others suggest that co-trimoxazole should be avoided in patients taking coumarins, because they found that management of the interaction (either preventive or reactive dose reduction) resulted in an increased period of under-anticoagulation after the antibacterial. They suggest that an alternative antibacterial to co-trimoxazole is always available.[26]

Anecdotal evidence suggests that co-trimoxazole may not interact with phenindione, but note that sulfaphenazole did, so some caution is still appropriate.

The other interactions are poorly documented. However, it would seem prudent to follow the precautions suggested for co-trimoxazole if any sulfonamide is given with a coumarin or indanedione.

The relative silence in the literature for trimethoprim alone would suggest that, in practice, any interaction, if it occurs, is of only minor importance, and the anticoagulant dose probably needs little or no adjustment. However, note that two cohort studies have shown some increased risk when trimethoprim was given with warfarin, acenocoumarol or phenprocoumon so an interaction cannot entirely be dismissed.

1. Hassall C, Feetam CL, Leach RH, Meynell MJ. Potentiation of warfarin by co-trimoxazole. *Lancet* (1975) ii, 1155–6.
2. Barnett DB, Hancock BW. Anticoagulant resistance: an unusual case. *BMJ* (1975) 1, 608–9.
3. Tilstone WJ, Gray JMB, Nimmo-Smith RH, Lawson DH. Interaction between warfarin and sulphamethoxazole. *Postgrad Med J* (1977) 53, 388–90.
4. Errick JK, Keys PW. Co-trimoxazole and warfarin: case report of an interaction. *Am J Hosp Pharm* (1979) 35, 1399–1401.
5. Greenlaw CW. Drug interaction between co-trimoxazole and warfarin. *Am J Hosp Pharm* (1979) 36, 1155.
6. Keys PW. Drug interaction between co-trimoxazole and warfarin. *Am J Hosp Pharm* (1979) 36, 1155–6.
7. Kaufman JM, Fauver HE. Potentiation of warfarin by trimethoprim-sulfamethoxazole. *Urology* (1980) 16, 601–3.
8. Perkash A. Experience with the management of deep vein thrombosis in patients with spinal cord injury. Part II: a critical evaluation of the anticoagulant therapy. *Paraplegia* (1980) 18, 2–14.
9. Brooks BJ Jr, Mocklin KE. Retropharyngeal hematoma as a complication of warfarin therapy. *J La State Med Soc* (1981) 133, 156–7.
10. McQueen EG. New Zealand Committee on Adverse Drug Reactions. 17th Annual Report 1982. *N Z Med J* (1983) 96, 95–9.
11. O'Donnell D. Antibiotic-induced potentiation of oral anticoagulant agents. *Med J Aust* (1989) 150, 163–4.
12. Wolf R, Elman M, Brenner S. Sulfonamide-induced bullous hemorrhagic eruption in a patient with low prothrombin time. *Isr J Med Sci* (1992) 28, 882–4.
13. Erichsen C, Sondenaa K, Soreide JA, Andersen E, Tysvær A. Spontaneous liver hematomas induced by anti-coagulation therapy. A case report and review of the literature. *Hepatogastroenterology* (1993) 40, 402–6.
14. Cook DE, Ponte CD. Suspected trimethoprim/sulfamethoxazole-induced hypoprothrombinemia. *J Fam Pract* (1994) 39, 589–91.
15. Chafin CC, Ritter BA, James A, Self TH. Hospital admission due to warfarin potentiation by TMP-SMX. *Nurse Pract* (2000) 25, 73–75.
16. Saghbini S, Gynn TN. Unusual presentation of infected retroperitoneal hematoma induced from warfarin and sulfa antibiotics interaction (abstract 3879). *Blood* (2002) 100, 100b.
17. Weinberg AD, Altman JS, Pals JK. Quality improvement case study: warfarin sodium interactions. *J Am Med Dir Assoc* (2006) 7, 315–18.
18. Glasheen JJ, Fugit RV, Prochazka AV. The risk of overanticoagulation with antibiotic use in outpatients on stable warfarin regimens. *J Gen Intern Med* (2005) 20, 653–6.
19. O'Reilly RA, Motley CH. Racemic warfarin and trimethoprim-sulfamethoxazole interaction in humans. *Ann Intern Med* (1979) 91, 34–6.
20. O'Reilly RA. Stereoselective interaction of trimethoprim-sulfamethoxazole with the separated enantiomorphs of racemic warfarin in man. *N Engl J Med* (1980) 302, 33–5.
21. Fischer HD, Juurlink DN, Mamdani MM, Kopp A, Laupacis A. Hemorrhage during warfarin therapy associated with cotrimoxazole and other urinary tract anti-infective agents: a population-based study. *Arch Intern Med* (2010) 170, 617–21
22. Schelleman H, Bilker WB, Brensinger CM, Han X, Kimmel SE, Hennessy S. Warfarin with fluoroquinolones, sulfonamides or azole antifungals: interactions and the risk of hospitalization for gastrointestinal bleeding. *Clin Pharmacol Ther* (2008) 84, 581–8.
23. Visser LE, Penning-van Beest FJA, Kasbergen AAH, De Smet PAGM, Vulto AG, Hofman A, Stricker BHC. Overanticoagulation associated with combined use of antibacterial drugs and acenocoumarol or phenprocoumon anticoagulants. *Thromb Haemost* (2002) 88, 705–10.
24. Penning-van Beest F, Erkens J, Petersen KU, Koelz HR, Herings R. Main comedications associated with major bleeding during anticoagulant therapy with coumarins. *Eur J Clin Pharmacol* (2005) 61, 439–44.
25. Penning-van Beest FJA, Koerselman J, Herings RMC. Risk of major bleeding during concomitant use of antibiotic drugs and coumarin anticoagulants. *J Thromb Haemost* (2008) 6, 284–90.
26. Schalekamp T, van Geest-Daalderop JH, Kramer MH, van Holten-Verzantvoort AT, de Boer A. Coumarin anticoagulants and co-trimoxazole: avoid the combination rather than manage the interaction. *Eur J Clin Pharmacol* (2007) 63, 335–43.
27. Ahmed A, Stephens JC, Kaus CA, Fay WP. Impact of preemptive warfarin dose reduction on anticoagulation after initiation of trimethoprim-sulfamethoxazole or levofloxacin.*J Thromb Thrombolysis* (2008) 26, 44–8.
28. De Swiet J. Potentiation of warfarin by co-trimoxazole. *BMJ* (1975) 3, 491.
29. Obasohan AO, Ukoh V, Ajuyah CO. Prosthetic valve dysfunction in a Nigerian. *Trop Geogr Med* (1993) 45, 183–5.
30. Self TH, Evans W, Ferguson T. Interaction of sulfisoxazole and warfarin. *Circulation* (1975) 52, 528.
31. Sioris LJ, Weibert RT, Pentel PR. Potentiation of warfarin anticoagulation by sulfisoxazole. *Arch Intern Med* (1980) 140, 546–7.
32. Lumholtz B, Siersbaek-Nielsen K, Skovsted L, Kampmann J, Hansen JM. Sulphamethizole-induced inhibition of diphenylhydantoin, tolbutamide and warfarin metabolism. *Clin Pharmacol Ther* (1975) 17, 731.
33. Varma DR, Gupta RK, Gupta S, Sharma KK. Prothrombin response to phenindione during hypoalbuminaemia. *Br J Clin Pharmacol* (1975) 2, 467–8.
34. Pharmacy Anticoagulant Clinic Study Group. A multicentre survey of antibiotics on the INR of anticoagulated patients. *Pharm J* (1996) 257 (Pharmacy Practice Suppl), R30.
35. Fredricks DA. Comment: TMP/SMX—warfarin interaction. *DICP Ann Pharmacother* (1989) 23, 619–20.
36. Seiler K, Duckert F. Properties of 3-(1-phenyl-propyl)-4-oxycoumarin (Marcoumar®) in the plasma when tested in normal cases and under the influence of drugs. *Thromb Diath Haemorrh* (1968) 19, 389–96.
37. Solomon HM, Schrogie JJ. The effect of various drugs on the binding of warfarin-^{14}C to human albumin. *Biochem Pharmacol* (1967) 16, 1219–26.
38. Udall JA. Human sources and absorption of vitamin K in relation to anticoagulation stability. *JAMA* (1965) 194, 107–9.

Coumarins + Antibacterials; Teicoplanin or Vancomycin

An isolated case report describes a marked reduction in the effects of warfarin, which was attributed to the use of teicoplanin, although this could equally be explained by rifampicin treatment. Vancomycin possibly causes a small increase in the effects of warfarin, and may increase the risk of over-anticoagulation with acenocoumarol or phenprocoumon.

Clinical evidence, mechanism, importance and management

(a) Teicoplanin

A 60-year-old woman taking digoxin, furosemide and **warfarin** (INR 3.5 to 5) developed a fever after mitral valve replacement surgery and was given rifampicin 450 mg twice daily and teicoplanin 400 mg twice daily. Within 3 days her INR began to fall and by day 6 the anticoagulant effect was completely lost. Despite progressive **warfarin** increases to 10, 15, and then 20 mg daily, her INR stayed between 1.2 and 1.6, even when rifampicin was stopped, and remained low for a further 20 days, at which point the teicoplanin was also stopped.[1] Some of this resistance to **warfarin** was undoubtedly due to the rifampicin (a known and potent inducer of **warfarin** metabolism) but as the INRs remained depressed for a further 20 days after rifampicin was withdrawn the authors suggested that the teicoplanin had its own part to play. However, rifampicin has been shown is several cases to decrease the effects of warfarin for three or more weeks after its withdrawal (see 'Coumarins + Antibacterials; Rifamycins', p.397), so an interaction with teicoplanin would seem doubtful.

(b) Vancomycin

In a retrospective review of 60 patients undergoing heart valve replacement surgery and receiving prophylactic antibacterials, 44 patients given cefamandole had a much greater anticoagulant response to their first dose of **warfarin** than 16 patients given **vancomycin**.[2] In a later prospective study by the same workers, in patients taking warfarin with an antibacterial, after 3 days the prothrombin times as a percentage of activity were as follows: cefamandole 29%, cefazolin 38%, and **vancomycin** 51%, suggesting that cefamandole had a much greater effect on the anticoagulant response than **vancomycin**.[3]

In a cohort study, the use of **vancomycin** was associated with an increased risk of over-anticoagulation (an INR greater than 6) in patients stabilised on **acenocoumarol** or **phenprocoumon**. The relative risk was 13.6; however, the confidence interval was very large (1.7 to 107), so it is not possible to draw any firm conclusions from this.[4]

If a patient is unwell enough to require antibacterial therapy, it may be prudent to increase the monitoring of coagulation status even if no specific drug interaction is expected, see also 'Coumarins + Antibacterials', p.383.

1. Agosta FG, Liberato NL, Chiofalo F. Warfarin resistance induced by teicoplanin. *Haematologica* (1997) 82, 637–40.
2. Angaran DM, Dias VC, Arom KV, Northrup WF, Kersten TE, Lindsay WG, Nicoloff DM. The influence of prophylactic antibiotics on the warfarin anticoagulation response in the postoperative prosthetic cardiac valve patient. *Ann Surg* (1984) 199, 107–111.
3. Angaran DM, Dias VC, Arom KV, Northrup WF, Kersten TG, Lindsay WG, Nicoloff DM. The comparative influence of prophylactic antibiotics on the prothrombin response to warfarin in the postoperative prosthetic cardiac valve patient. *Ann Surg* (1987) 206, 155–61.
4. Visser LE, Penning-van Beest FJA, Kasbergen AAH, De Smet PAGM, Vulto AG, Hofman A, Stricker BHC. Overanticoagulation associated with combined use of antibacterial drugs and acenocoumarol or phenprocoumon anticoagulants. *Thromb Haemost* (2002) 88, 705–10.

Coumarins and related drugs + Antibacterials; Tetracyclines

Isolated cases suggest that doxycycline and tetracycline can increase the effects of coumarins. Similarly, some small studies (none controlled) suggest that chlortetracycline (alone or with oxytetracycline), doxycycline, or the tetracyclines as a class may increase the risks of over-anticoagulation, but there appear to be no studies of the effect of tetracyclines on the pharmacokinetics of coumarins. However, the related antibacterial, tigecycline, increased the AUC of warfarin, and has been found to increase the prothrombin time when given alone.

Clinical evidence

There are no controlled studies of the effect of any tetracycline on the pharmacokinetics or pharmacodynamics of warfarin or other coumarins, although there are data for tigecycline, a new glycylcycline antibacterial structurally related to the tetracyclines.

(a) Chlortetracycline

Six out of 9 patients taking an unnamed anticoagulant had a fall in their prothrombin-proconvertin concentration from a range of 10 to 30% to less than 6% when given chlortetracycline 250 mg four times a day for 4 days. Although the anticoagulant effects were increased, there was no evidence of bleeding.[1] In one early study of **dicoumarol** and **ethyl biscoumacetate**, the authors briefly comment that 4 cases of the concurrent use of chlortetracycline and oxytetracycline increased the prothrombin response.[2]

(b) Doxycycline

A woman stabilised on **warfarin** developed menorrhagia after taking doxycycline 100 mg twice daily for 10 days, and her prothrombin time ratio had increased from about 2 to 4.4.[3] Two other patients stabilised on **acenocoumarol** or **warfarin** developed markedly increased prothrombin ratios (3.82 and 4.09, respectively) with bruising, haematomas and bleeding when they took doxycycline.[4] Another patient with multiple medical problems, taking **warfarin** developed peritoneal bleeding and an INR of 7.2 (previously 2.6) 6 days after starting doxycycline 100 mg twice daily.[5] Yet another patient taking **warfarin** had an INR increase from 2.3 to 6.5 with prominent bruising when given doxycycline.[6]

In a population-based cohort study in patients taking **acenocoumarol** or **phenprocoumon**, doxycycline was found to increase the risk of over-anticoagulation (INR greater than or equal to 6) with an adjusted relative risk of 4.3 (range 1.8 to 10.4). The risks were greatest after 4 or more days of concurrent use.[7] In two other cohort studies by this same research group, the relative risk of hospitalisation for bleeding in patients taking **acenocoumarol** or **phenprocoumon** and given doxycycline was 4.2 and 2.4, respectively.[8,9] Nevertheless, they estimated that the individual risk of major bleeding was low at one per 2000 doxycycline dispensings.[9]

(c) Oxytetracycline

In one early study of **dicoumarol** and **ethyl biscoumacetate**, the authors briefly comment that 4 cases of the concurrent use of chlortetracycline and **oxytetracycline** increased the prothrombin response.[2]

(d) Tetracycline

In one analysis of haemorrhagic events in patients taking **dicoumarol** and antibacterials, one patient out of 20 who received tetracycline had a bleeding event.[10] A patient stabilised on **warfarin** had a marked increase in INR (from about 2 to 7.7) 6 weeks after starting to take tetracycline 250 mg four times daily. Warfarin was withheld for a few days, and then restarted at a 40% lower dose. The INR decreased over the following months, broadly in parallel with decreases in the tetracycline dose.[11] A patient taking **warfarin** bled (right temporal lobe haematoma) and had an extended prothrombin time a week after starting to take tetracycline and nystatin.[12] Another patient taking **warfarin** also bled (epistaxis, haematemesis, melaena) 3 weeks after starting to take tetracycline and nystatin.[12]

In a retrospective cohort study, the relative risk of hospitalisation for bleeding in patients taking **acenocoumarol** or **phenprocoumon** and given tetracycline was 8.7. However, the incidence of concurrent use was low so the confidence interval was very broad (range 1.2 to 62).[9]

(e) Tigecycline

The manufacturer notes that, in healthy subjects, intravenous tigecycline 100 mg then 50 mg every 12 hours decreased the clearance of *R*-warfarin by 40% and *S*-warfarin by 23% after a single 25-mg dose of **warfarin**. The AUCs of *R*- and *S*-warfarin were increased by 68% and 29%, respectively. However, the INR was not affected.[13,14]

(f) Unnamed tetracyclines

In a prospective study of the effect of antibacterials on anticoagulation, there was an estimated 0.53 increase in the INR in 9 patients taking warfarin and a tetracycline (unnamed). The effect with tetracyclines was greater than the effect of other antibacterials studied (penicillins, cephalosporins, macrolides).[15]

Mechanism

Not understood. Tetracyclines, in the absence of anticoagulants, can reduce prothrombin activity,[16] and both hypoprothrombinaemia and bleeding have been described.[17,18] It seems possible that very occasionally the anticoagulant and the tetracycline have additive hypoprothrombinaemic effects. In clinical studies, tigecycline alone has commonly caused a prolonged prothrombin time (incidence 1 to 10%) or uncommonly caused an increased INR (incidence 0.1 to 1%).[13] It is also possible that antibacterials can diminish the intestinal flora of the gut thereby depleting the body of vitamin K_2, although this might be clinically important only where normal dietary intake of vitamin K_1 is extremely low, see 'Coumarins + Antibacterials', p.383. There appear to be no data on the effect of tetracyclines on the pharmacokinetics of coumarins. Although tigecycline decreased the clearance of warfarin, the mechanism for this is unclear, and is not thought to be as a result of decreased cytochrome P450 metabolism.[13,14]

Importance and management

A relatively sparsely documented interaction, bearing in mind that the tetracyclines have been in very widespread use for many years. It can therefore reasonably be concluded that normally any changes are of little clinical relevance. As a few patients have unpredictably had increased anticoagulant effects and even bleeding, bear the possibility of an interaction in mind when a tetracycline is first added to established anticoagulant treatment with a coumarin. Moreover, if a patient is unwell enough to require an antibacterial, it may be prudent to increase monitoring of coagulation status even if no specific drug interaction is expected, see also 'Coumarins + Antibacterials', p.383. Monitor within 3 days of starting the antibacterial.

The increase in warfarin exposure by tigecycline did not alter its anticoagulant effects; however, as tigecycline alone can cause an increase in INR, it is recommended that the INR be closely monitored if patients taking warfarin are given tigecycline.[13,14] Similar precaution would seem prudent in patients taking other coumarins and given tigecycline.

There appears to be no information about the **indanediones**, but if the mechanism suggested is correct they may also interact like the coumarins.

1. Magid E. Tolerance to anticoagulants during antibiotic therapy. *Scand J Clin Lab Invest* (1962) 14, 565–6.
2. Scarrone LA, Beck DF, Wright IS. A comparative evaluation of Tromexan and dicumarol in the treatment of thromboembolic conditions — based on experience with 514 patients. *Circulation* (1952) 6, 489–514.
3. Westfall LK, Mintzer DL, Wiser TH. Potentiation of warfarin by tetracycline. *Am J Hosp Pharm* (1980) 37, 1620, 1625.
4. Caraco Y, Rubinow A. Enhanced anticoagulant effect of coumarin derivatives induced by doxycycline coadministration. *Ann Pharmacother* (1992) 26, 1084–6.
5. Baciewicz AM, Bal BS. Bleeding associated with doxycycline and warfarin treatment. *Arch Intern Med* (2001) 161, 1231.
6. Hasan SA. Interaction of doxycycline and warfarin: an enhanced anticoagulant effect. *Cornea* (2007) 26, 742–3.
7. Visser LE, Penning-van Beest FJA, Kasbergen AAH, De Smet PAGM, Vulto AG, Hofman A, Stricker BHC. Overanticoagulation associated with combined use of antibacterial drugs and acenocoumarol or phenprocoumon anticoagulants. *Thromb Haemost* (2002) 88, 705–10.
8. Penning-van Beest F, Erkens J, Petersen KU, Koelz HR, Herings R. Main comedications associated with major bleeding during anticoagulant therapy with coumarins. *Eur J Clin Pharmacol* (2005) 61, 439–44.
9. Penning-van Beest FJA, Koerselman J, Herings RMC. Risk of major bleeding during concomitant use of antibiotic drugs and coumarin anticoagulants. *J Thromb Haemost* (2008) 6, 284–90.
10. Chiavazza F, Merialdi A. Sulle interferenze fra dicumarolo e antibiotici. *Minerva Ginecol* (1973) 25, 630–1.
11. Danos EA. Apparent potentiation of warfarin activity by tetracycline. *Clin Pharm* (1992) 11, 806–8.
12. O'Donnell D. Antibiotic-induced potentiation of oral anticoagulant agents. *Med J Aust* (1989) 150, 163–4.
13. Tygacil (Tigecycline). Pfizer Ltd. UK Summary of product characteristics, December 2013.
14. Tygacil (Tigecycline). Wyeth Pharmaceuticals Inc. US Prescribing information, September 2009.
15. Pharmacy Anticoagulant Clinic Study Group. A multicentre survey of antibiotics on the INR of anti-coagulated patients. *Pharm J* (1996) 257 (Pharmacy Practice Suppl), R30.
16. Searcy RL, Simms NM, Foreman JA, Bergquist LM. Evaluation of the blood-clotting mechanism in tetracycline-treated patients. *Antimicrob Agents Chemother* (1964) 4, 179–83.
17. Rios JF. Hemorrhagic diathesis induced by antimicrobials. *JAMA* (1968) 205, 142.
18. Klippel AP, Pitsinger B. Hypoprothrombinemia secondary to antibiotic therapy and manifested by massive gastrointestinal hemorrhage. *Arch Surg* (1968) 96, 266–8.

Coumarins + Anticholinesterases; Centrally acting

Donepezil, galantamine, rivastigmine and tacrine do not appear to alter the pharmacokinetics or effects of warfarin.

Clinical evidence, mechanism, importance and management

(a) Donepezil

In an open-label, crossover study, 12 healthy men were given donepezil 10 mg daily for 19 days with a single 25-mg dose of **warfarin** on day 14. The pharmacokinetics of *R*- and *S*-warfarin and the prothrombin times were unchanged by the presence of the donepezil, and vital signs, ECG and laboratory tests were unaltered.[1] Therefore, no special precautions are needed on concurrent use.

(b) Galantamine

The manufacturers say that galantamine 24 mg daily had no effect on the pharmacokinetics of *R*- and *S*-warfarin after a single 25-mg dose of **warfarin**. In addition, galantamine did not alter the prothrombin time.[2,3] Therefore, no special precautions are needed on concurrent use.

(c) Rivastigmine

The manufacturers of rivastigmine[4,5] say that no pharmacokinetic interaction has been noted between rivastigmine and **warfarin** in healthy subjects. In addition, rivastigmine did not affect the increase in prothrombin time seen with **warfarin**. Therefore, no special precautions are needed on concurrent use.

(d) Tacrine

In a study in 10 patients stabilised on **warfarin,** the addition of tacrine 20 mg four times daily for 5 days had no significant effect on prothrombin times.[6] Therefore, no special precautions are needed on concurrent use.

1. Tiseo PJ, Foley K, Friedhoff LT. The effect of multiple doses of donepezil hydrochloride on the pharmacokinetic and pharmacodynamic profile of warfarin. *Br J Clin Pharmacol* (1998) 46 (Suppl 1), 45–50.
2. Reminyl Tablets (Galantamine hydrobromide). Shire Pharmaceuticals Ltd. UK Summary of product characteristics, August 2013.
3. Razadyne ER (Galantamine hydrobromide). Ortho-McNeil-Janssen Pharmaceuticals, Inc. US Prescribing information, July 2013.
4. Exelon (Rivastigmine hydrogen tartrate). Novartis Pharmaceuticals UK Ltd. UK Summary of product characteristics, April 2013.
5. Exelon (Rivastigmine tartrate). Novartis Pharmaceuticals Corp. US Prescribing information, July 2013.
6. Reece PA, Garnett WR, Rock WL, Taylor JR, Underwood B, Sedman AJ, Rajagopalan R. Lack of effect of tacrine administration on the anticoagulant activity of warfarin. *J Clin Pharmacol* (1995) 35, 526–8.

Coumarins + Antidiabetics; Alpha-glucosidase inhibitors

Miglitol and voglibose do not appear to alter the pharmacokinetics or effects of warfarin. There are isolated cases of reduced or increased INRs in patients given warfarin and acarbose.

Clinical evidence, mechanism, importance and management

(a) Acarbose

A 66-year-old man taking fosinopril, hydrochlorothiazide, diphenhydramine, insulin, glipizide and **warfarin** started taking acarbose to improve the control of his diabetes. Four days before starting acarbose his INR was 3.09, but after 2 weeks (25 mg acarbose daily for week one and then 50 mg daily for week 2) his INR had *risen* to 4.85. The **warfarin** was temporarily stopped, then it was reintroduced at a lower dose, and finally the acarbose was withdrawn, resulting in an INR of 2.84. No bleeding was seen.[1] In contrast, in 1997, the manufacturer had on record 2 other cases of patients taking **warfarin** whose INRs were *reduced* when acarbose was added. One of them stopped taking the acarbose, whereupon her INR returned to its previous value. The other patient needed an increased **warfarin** dose.[2]

These appear to be the only cases on record, and therefore the general picture is that usually no interaction occurs, but in isolated cases some changes in **warfarin** requirements occur. Bear this potential interaction in mind if anticoagulant control alters in a patient taking acarbose.

(b) Miglitol

In a double-blind, randomised, placebo-controlled study, 24 healthy subjects were given miglitol 100 mg three times daily for 7 days, with a single 25-mg oral dose of **warfarin** on day 4. Neither the pharmacokinetics nor the pharmacodynamics of *R*- or *S*-warfarin were affected by the miglitol.[3] No special precautions would therefore appear to be needed if these two drugs are used concurrently.

(c) Voglibose

Twelve healthy male subjects were given individually adjusted doses of **warfarin** to give Quick values of 30 to 40%, and then from day 11 to 15 they were also given voglibose 5 mg three times daily. It was found that the voglibose had no effect on the pharmacokinetics of **warfarin** nor on its anticoagulant effects.[4] No special precautions would therefore appear to be needed if these two drugs are used concurrently.

1. Morreale AP, Janetzky K. Probable interaction of warfarin and acarbose. *Am J Health-Syst Pharm* (1997) 54, 1551–2.
2. Bayer. Personal communication, December 1997.
3. Schall R, Müller FO, Hundt HKL, Duursema L, Groenewoud G, Middle MV. Study of the effect of miglitol on the pharmacokinetics and pharmacodynamics of warfarin in healthy males. *Arzneimittel-forschung* (1996) 46, 41–6.
4. Fuder H, Kleist P, Birkel M, Ehrlich A, Emeklibas S, Maslak W, Stridde E, Wetzelsberger N, Wieckhorst G, Lücker PW. The α-glucosidase inhibitor voglibose (AO-128) does not change pharmacodynamics or pharmacokinetics of warfarin. *Eur J Clin Pharmacol* (1997) 53, 153–7.

Coumarins + Antidiabetics; Dipeptidylpeptidase-4 inhibitors

Alogliptin, linagliptin, sitagliptin, and vildagliptin do not appear to alter the pharmacokinetics or anticoagulant effect of warfarin.

Clinical evidence, mechanism, importance and management

(a) Alogliptin

The US manufacturer of alogliptin briefly notes that, in clinical studies, when alogliptin 25 mg daily was given with *R*- or *S*-warfarin (at stable doses between 1 mg and 10 mg daily) for 7 days, no meaningful changes to the pharmacokinetics of warfarin were seen. In addition, no clinically relevant change in the prothrombin time or INR occurred.[1] No warfarin dose adjustment is expected to be necessary on concurrent use.

(b) Linagliptin

In a study in 18 healthy subjects, linagliptin 5 mg daily for 12 days had no effect on the pharmacokinetics of *R*- and *S*-warfarin when a single 10-mg dose of warfarin was given on day 6. Similarly, the anticoagulant effect of **warfarin** (prothrombin time and INR) was not altered by linagliptin.[2] No warfarin dosing adjustments would therefore be expected to be necessary on concurrent use.

(c) Sitagliptin

In a study in 11 healthy subjects, sitagliptin 200 mg for 11 days had no effect on the pharmacokinetics of *R*- and *S*-warfarin when a single 30-mg dose of warfarin was given on day 5. Similarly, the anticoagulant effect of **warfarin** (assessed by INR) was not altered by sitagliptin.[3] No warfarin dosing adjustments would therefore be expected to be necessary on concurrent use.

(d) Vildagliptin

In a controlled study in 15 healthy subjects, vildagliptin 100 mg daily for 6 days had no effect on the pharmacokinetics of *R*- and *S*-warfarin when a single 25-mg dose of **warfarin** was given on day 2. Similarly, the anticoagulant effect of **warfarin** (prothrombin time and INR) was not altered by vildagliptin.[4] No warfarin dosing adjustments would therefore be expected to be necessary on concurrent use.

1. Nesina (Alogliptin). Takeda Pharmaceuticals America, Inc. US Prescribing information, January 2013.
2. Graefe-Mody EU, Brand T, Ring A, Withopf B, Stangier J, Iovino M, Woerle H-J. Effect of linagliptin on the pharmacokinetics and pharmacodynamics of warfarin in healthy volunteers. *Int J Clin Pharmacol Ther* (2011) 49, 300–10.
3. Wright DH, Herman GA, Maes A, Liu Q, Johnson-Levonas AO, Wagner JA. Multiple doses of sitagliptin, a selective DPP-4 inhibitor, do not meaningfully alter pharmacokinetics and pharmacodynamics of warfarin. *J Clin Pharmacol* (2009) 49, 1157–67.
4. He Y-L, Sabo R, Riviere G-J, Sunkara G, Leon S, Ligueros-Saylan M, Rosenberg M, Dole WP, Howard D. Effect of the novel oral dipeptidyl peptidase IV inhibitor vildagliptin on the pharmacokinetics and pharmacodynamics of warfarin in healthy subjects. *Curr Med Res Opin* (2007) 23, 1131–8.

Coumarins + Antidiabetics; Glucagon-like peptide-1 receptor agonists

Albiglutide has no effect on the pharmacokinetics of, or response to, warfarin. Exenatide does not affect the pharmacokinetics of warfarin, but might alter the INR. Dulaglutide and lixisenatide do not appear to affect the pharmacokinetics of, or response to, warfarin, and liraglutide is predicted not to have any effect.

Clinical evidence, mechanism, importance and management

(a) Albiglutide

In a study in 15 healthy subjects, albiglutide 50 mg weekly had no effect on the AUC or maximum concentration of *R*- or *S*-warfarin after a single 25-mg dose of **warfarin** was given 3 days after the last dose of albiglutide, but did increase the median time to maximum concentration by 30 minutes. There was also no effect on INR.[1] No warfarin dose adjustment would seem necessary on concurrent use.

(b) Dulaglutide

The UK and US manufacturers briefly report that, in a study, dulaglutide had no effect on the AUC and maximum concentration of *R*-**warfarin**, or the AUC of *S*-**warfarin**, but did decrease the maximum concentration of *S*-warfarin by 22%. Time to maximum concentration of *R*- and *S*-warfarin was delayed by 6 and 4 hours, respectively, and this resulted in a similar delay in the time to maximum INR. These effects were not considered clinically relevant and no warfarin dose adjustment is advised on concurrent use.[2,3]

(c) Exenatide

In a controlled study in 15 healthy subjects, subcutaneous exenatide 5 micrograms twice daily for 2 days then 10 micrograms twice daily for 9 days had no effect on the pharmacokinetics of a single 25-mg dose of **warfarin** given on day 4. There was a 12% decrease in the maximum INR (1.72 versus 1.95).[4] Given the lack of a pharmacokinetic interaction, and minor decrease in anticoagulant effect, no **warfarin** dose adjustments are likely to be needed when exenatide is started. However, note that there are post-marketing reports of increased INR in patients receiving exenatide and warfarin, some associated with bleeding, and so close monitoring of the INR is recommended when exenatide is started or the dose increased,[5] with warfarin dose adjustment if necessary.

(d) Liraglutide

No interaction study has been conducted, but on the basis of data from other studies showing a lack of effect on the extent of absorption of paracetamol (acetaminophen) (see 'Paracetamol (Acetaminophen) + Antidiabetics', p.202), liraglutide would not be expected to alter the absorption of **warfarin**. In addition, liraglutide does not affect cytochrome P450, by which **warfarin** is principally metabolised. No interaction would therefore be expected. However, the UK manufacturer of liraglutide states that a clinically relevant interaction with active substances with a narrow therapeutic index such as **warfarin** cannot be excluded. They therefore recommend more frequent monitoring of the INR if patients taking **warfarin** are started on liraglutide.[6] As there is little clinical experience with liraglutide this might be prudent.

(e) Lixisenatide

The preliminary report of a randomised, crossover study in 16 healthy subjects, notes that lixisenatide 10 micrograms daily for 7 days, then 20 micrograms daily for 10 days, did not alter the AUC of a single 25-mg dose of **warfarin** given on day 11. The INR was also unaltered, but the warfarin maximum concentration was decreased by 19% and the time to maximum concentration was delayed by 7 hours.[7] No **warfarin** dose adjustment would seem necessary on concurrent use, but close monitoring of the INR on starting or stopping lixisenatide is recommended.[8]

1. Bush M, Scott R, Watanalumlerd P, Zhi H, Lewis E. Effects of multiple doses of albiglutide on the pharmacokinetics, pharmacodynamics, and safety of digoxin, warfarin, or a low-dose oral contraceptive. *Postgrad Med* (2012) 124, 55–72.
2. Trulicity (Dulaglutide). Eli Lilly and Company Ltd. UK Summary of product characteristics, November 2014.
3. Trulicity (Dulaglutide). Eli Lilly and Company. US Prescribing information, March 2015.
4. Soon D, Kothare PA, Linnebjerg H, Park S, Yuen E, Mace KF, Wise SD. Effect of exenatide on the pharmacokinetics and pharmacodynamics of warfarin in healthy Asian men. *J Clin Pharmacol* (2006) 46, 1179–87.
5. Byetta (Exenatide). AstraZeneca UK Ltd. UK Summary of product characteristics, January 2015.
6. Victoza (Liraglutide). Novo Nordisk Ltd. UK Summary of product characteristics, March 2015.
7. Liu Y, Ruus P, Steinstraesser A, Teichert L. Effect of the GLP-1 agonist lixisenatide on the pharmacokinetics of warfarin. *Diabetes* (2010) 59 (Suppl 1), 2128-PO.
8. Lyxumia (Lixisenatide). Sanofi. UK Summary of product characteristics, October 2014.

Coumarins + Antidiabetics; Nateglinide or Repaglinide

Nateglinide and repaglinide do not appear to interact with warfarin, and nateglinide does not interact with acenocoumarol.

Clinical evidence, mechanism, importance and management

(a) Nateglinide

In a randomised, double-blind study, 11 healthy subjects were given nateglinide 120 mg three times daily for 5 days, with a single 10-mg dose of **acenocoumarol** on day 3. Nateglinide had no effect on the tolerability, pharmacokinetics or anti-coagulant activity of **acenocoumarol**.[1]

In another study,12 healthy subjects were given nateglinide 120 mg three times daily for 4 days with a single 30-mg dose of **warfarin** on day 2. No pharmacokinetic or pharmacodynamic interaction was noted.[2] No dose adjustments would therefore be expected to be necessary if nateglinide is taken with either acenocoumarol or warfarin.

(b) Repaglinide

In a double-blind, placebo-controlled study in 28 healthy subjects who were stabilised on **warfarin**, repaglinide did not alter the anticoagulant effects of **warfarin** or the steady-state warfarin pharmacokinetics.[3] Therefore, no **warfarin** dose adjustment would be expected to be necessary on concurrent use.

1. Sunkara G, Bigler H, Wang Y, Smith H, Prasad P, McLeod J, Ligueros-Saylan M. The effect of nateglinide on the pharmacokinetics and pharmacodynamics of acenocoumarol. *Curr Med Res Opin* (2004) 20, 41–8.
2. Anderson DM, Shelley S, Crick N, Buraglio M. No effect of the novel antidiabetic agent nateglinide on the pharmacokinetics and anticoagulant properties of warfarin in healthy volunteers. *J Clin Pharmacol* (2002) 42, 1358–65.
3. Rosenberg M, Strange P, Cohen A. Assessment of pharmacokinetic (PK) and pharmacodynamic (PD) interaction between warfarin and repaglinide. *Diabetes* (1999) 48 (Suppl 1), A356.

Coumarins and related drugs + Antidiabetics; Sulfonylureas

Dicoumarol inhibits the metabolism of tolbutamide and increases its effects; cases of hypoglycaemic coma have been reported. Chlorpropamide may be similarly affected. Although isolated cases of interactions (raised prothrombin times, bleeding or hypoglycaemia) have been seen in patients taking other sulfonylureas and other coumarins, in general, no important interaction appears to occur. There also appears to be no interaction between phenindione and tolbutamide.

Clinical evidence

A. Coumarins

(a) Chlorpropamide

1. Acenocoumarol. A woman with normal renal function had an increase in the half-life of chlorpropamide to 88 hours (normally about 36 hours) when she took acenocoumarol.[1]

2. Dicoumarol. A 67-year-old non-diabetic man taking chlorpropamide for Parkinson's disease developed severe hypoglycaemia about 3 months after starting dicoumarol. He had high chlorpropamide levels with a half-life of 80 to 90 hours. Dicoumarol was withdrawn, and 3 weeks later his chlorpropamide half-life was 30 hours.[2] This observation prompted further study in 3 other patients and 2 non-diabetics. Dicoumarol doubled the serum chlorpropamide levels within 3 to 4 days and also more than doubled the half-life.[2]

(b) Glibenclamide (Glyburide)

1. Phenprocoumon. A small study in 4 subjects reported that the pharmacokinetics of glibenclamide were unchanged by phenprocoumon.[3] Similarly, the plasma levels and half-life of single doses of phenprocoumon did not differ between patients with type 2 diabetes managed by diet alone (12 patients) and those taking glibenclamide (9 patients).[4]

2. Warfarin. There do not appear to be any controlled studies on the effect of glibenclamide on the pharmacokinetics of warfarin, although *in vitro* data suggest that an effect is possible because glibenclamide inhibited *S*-warfarin hydroxylation (a 7 to 37% *in vivo* inhibition was predicted).[5] Moreover, an isolated report describes increased warfarin effects (INR increased from 2.3 to 6.6 with haematomas) in a patient given glibenclamide.[6]

(c) Glibornuride

Phenprocoumon, given to 3 subjects for 4 days, slightly increased the half-life of a single 25-mg dose of glibornuride by 29%.[7] The plasma levels and half-life of a single dose of **phenprocoumon** did not differ between patients with type 2 diabetes managed by diet alone (12 patients) and those taking glibornuride (12 patients).[4]

(d) Glimepiride

In healthy subjects, glimepiride 4 mg daily caused only minor, clinically unimportant changes in the prothrombin times (about 10% decrease in mean maximum prothrombin time) in response to single 25-mg doses of **warfarin**. In addition, glimepiride had no effect on the pharmacokinetics of *R*- and *S*-warfarin.[8]

(e) Tolbutamide

1. Dicoumarol. Dicoumarol has been found to increase the serum levels of tolbutamide, prolong its half-life (more than threefold), and reduce blood-glucose levels in both diabetics[9,10] and healthy subjects.[9-12] This may become excessive in a few patients and hypoglycaemic coma has been described in 3 diabetics,[9,13,14] and one non-diabetic.[15]

Two patients taking dicoumarol had marked increases in prothrombin times (a rise from 33 to 60 seconds) within 2 days of starting to take tolbutamide, but no bleeding occurred. However, no increases were seen in 3 other patients taking dicoumarol when they started tolbutamide.[16] Conversely, the half-life of dicoumarol was approximately halved in 2 out of 4 healthy subjects given tolbutamide, but the hypoprothrombinaemic effects were unchanged.[12] However, in a retrospective study there was no difference in the initial or average dose of dicoumarol between 15 patients taking tolbutamide and 24 control subjects taking insulin.[17]

2. Phenprocoumon. In 3 subjects, phenprocoumon, given for one week, did not alter the half-life of a single intravenous dose of tolbutamide 1 g.[10] Similarly, there was no difference in monthly tolbutamide levels, taken over a year, between 7 patients taking tolbutamide alone and 2 patients also taking phenprocoumon.[18]

The plasma levels and half-life of single doses of phenprocoumon did not differ between patients with type 2 diabetes managed by diet alone (12 patients) and those taking tolbutamide (10 patients).[4]

3. Warfarin. Giving warfarin for one week did not alter the half-life of a single intravenous dose of tolbutamide 1 g in 2 subjects.[10] Similarly, giving warfarin for a week did not alter serum tolbutamide levels in 2 patients with diabetes.[10] In a retrospective study, there was no difference in the initial or average dose of warfarin between 42 patients taking tolbutamide and 54 control subjects taking insulin.[17]

(f) Unspecified sulfonylureas

In a retrospective study, the initial rate of warfarin anticoagulation was faster (threefold faster rise in INR) in 6 patients also taking sulfonylurea antidiabetics than in 160 control patients and 16 patients with diabetes not taking sulfonylureas.[19] The findings of this study require confirmation in a controlled, prospective study.

B. Indanediones

In early studies, phenindione given for 6 days did not affect the half-life of a single dose of **tolbutamide** in a few subjects.[9,10] Similarly, the average plasma levels of **tolbutamide** in 3 patients taking phenindione were not different from 4 patients not taking phenindione.[9]

Mechanism

Dicoumarol appears to increase the effects of tolbutamide by inhibiting its metabolism by the liver.[9,11] This may also be true for chlorpropamide.[2] The increase in the anticoagulant effects of dicoumarol by tolbutamide may, in part, be due to a plasma protein binding interaction. In the case of phenprocoumon there seem to be several different mutually opposing processes going on, which cancel each other out.[12] There is no clear explanation for most of the isolated cases.

Importance and management

Information is patchy and very incomplete. The effect of dicoumarol on tolbutamide has been the most thoroughly investigated, and the interaction is clinically important. Increased blood-glucose lowering effects may be expected if dicoumarol is given to patients taking tolbutamide, and there is a risk of hypoglycaemic coma. Whether tolbutamide alters the anticoagulant response to dicoumarol is unclear. Avoid concurrent use unless the outcome can be well monitored and dose adjustments made. The same precautions should be taken with dicoumarol and chlorpropamide, but information is limited to one study.

Information on other interactions is limited to isolated cases, and these are therefore of doubtful general significance.

1. Petitpierre B, Perrin L, Rudhardt M, Herrera A, Fabre J. Behaviour of chlorpropamide in renal insufficiency and under the effect of associated drug therapy. *Int J Clin Pharmacol* (1972) 6, 120–4.
2. Kristensen M, Hansen JM. Accumulation of chlorpropamide caused by dicoumarol. *Acta Med Scand* (1968) 183, 83–6.
3. Schulz E, Schmidt FH. Über den Einfluß von Sulphaphenazol, Phenylbutazon und Phenprocumarol auf die Elimination von Glibenclamid beim Menschen. *Verh Dtsch Ges Inn Med* (1970) 76, 435–8.
4. Heine P, Kewitz H, Wiegboldt K-A. The influence of hypoglycaemic sulphonylureas on elimination and efficacy of phenprocoumon following a single oral dose in diabetic patients. *Eur J Clin Pharmacol* (1976) 10, 31–6.
5. Kim K-A, Park J-Y. Inhibitory effect of glyburide on human cytochrome P450 isoforms in human liver microsomes. *Drug Metab Dispos* (2003) 3, 1090–2.
6. Jassal SV. Drug points. *BMJ* (1991) 303, 789.
7. Eckhardt W, Rudolph R, Sauer H, Schubert WR, Undeutsch D. Zur pharmakologischen Interferenz von Glibornurid mit Sulfaphenazol, Phenylbutazon und phenprocoumon beim Menschen. *Arzneimittelforschung* (1972) 22, 2212–19.
8. Schaaf LJ, Sisson TA, Dietz AJ, Viveash DM, Oliver LK, Knuth DW, Carel BJ. Influence of multiple dose glimepiride on the pharmacokinetics and pharmacodynamics of racemic warfarin in healthy volunteers. *Pharm Res* (1994) 11 (10 Suppl), S-359.
9. Kristensen M, Hansen JM. Potentiation of the tolbutamide effect by dicoumarol. *Diabetes* (1967) 16, 211–14.
10. Skovsted L, Kristensen M, Hansen M, Siersbæk-Nielsen K. The effect of different oral anticoagulants on diphenylhydantoin (DPH) and tolbutamide metabolism. *Acta Med Scand* (1976) 199, 513–15.
11. Solomon HM, Schrogie JJ. Effect of phenyramidol and bishydroxycoumarin on the metabolism of tolbutamide in human subjects. *Metabolism* (1967) 16, 1029–33.
12. Jähnchen E, Meinertz T, Gilfrich H-J, Groth U. Pharmacokinetic analysis of the interaction between dicoumarol and tolbutamide in man. *Eur J Clin Pharmacol* (1976) 10, 349–56.
13. Spurny OM, Wolf JW, Devins GS. Protracted tolbutamide-induced hypoglycemia. *Arch Intern Med* (1965) 115, 53–6.
14. Fontana G, Addarii F, Peta G. Su di un caso di coma ipoglicemico in corso di terapia con tolbutamide e dicumarolici. *G Clin Med* (1968) 49, 849–58.
15. Schwartz JF. Tolbutamide-induced hypoglycemia in Parkinson's disease. A case report. *JAMA* (1961) 176, 106–9.
16. Chaplin H, Cassell M. Studies on the possible relationship of tolbutamide to dicumarol in anticoagulant therapy. *Am J Med Sci* (1958) 235, 706–15.
17. Poucher RL, Vecchio TJ. Absence of tolbutamide effect on anticoagulant therapy. *JAMA* (1966) 197, 1069–70.
18. Kolenda K-D, Grille W, Johnsen K. Arzneimittelwechselwirkungen bei der therapie mit tolbutamid. *Med Klin* (1979) 74, 1914–22.
19. Wilke RA, Berg RL, Vidaillet HJ, Caldwell MD, Burmester JK, Hillman MA. Impact of age, CYP2C9 genotype and concomitant medication on the rate of rise for prothrombin time during the first 30 days of warfarin therapy. *Clin Med Res* (2005) 3, 207–13.

Coumarins + Antidiabetics; Thiazolidinediones

Pioglitazone does not appear to alter the pharmacokinetics or anticoagulant effect of warfarin or phenprocoumon, and rosiglitazone does not affect the pharmacokinetics of warfarin. However, there is one

isolated report of two patients who required markedly increased warfarin doses after starting to take pioglitazone or rosiglitazone.

Clinical evidence

(a) Pioglitazone

In a study, pioglitazone 45 mg daily for 7 days did not alter the steady-state pharmacokinetics of **warfarin** and there was no significant change in prothrombin time.[1,2] Similar results were noted with **phenprocoumon**.[2] The US manufacturer also briefly mentions that pioglitazone had no effect on prothrombin time when it was given to patients stabilised on **warfarin**.[1]

However, there is an isolated report of an 84-year old woman (who had been on a stable maintenance dose of **warfarin** for the previous year) who, 12 weeks after starting to take pioglitazone 15 mg daily, had a subtherapeutic INR of 1.2. The patient denied any recent changes in diet or medication, including non-prescription and herbal medicines. An INR of 2.3 was eventually reached after her **warfarin** dose was increased by 88% from 8.5 mg to 16 mg weekly. A therapeutic INR was subsequently maintained at a similar dose over the following 18 months.[3]

(b) Rosiglitazone

The manufacturer briefly notes that rosiglitazone has been found to have no clinically relevant effect on the steady-state pharmacokinetics of **warfarin**.[4]

However, there is an isolated report of a 76-year-old man (who had been taking a stable dose of **warfarin** for the previous 18 months) who, 4 weeks after starting to take rosiglitazone 4 mg daily, had a subtherapeutic INR of 1.1. The patient denied any recent changes in diet or medication, including non-prescription and herbal medicines. An INR of 1.9 was eventually reached after increasing the **warfarin** dose by 75% from 24 mg weekly to 42 mg weekly. A therapeutic INR was subsequently maintained at a similar dose over the following 12 months.[3]

Mechanism

In vitro, troglitazone (the first thiazolidinedione, which has now been withdrawn) significantly inhibited the metabolism (7-hydroxylation) of *S*-warfarin by the cytochrome P450 isoenzyme CYP2C9; however, pioglitazone and rosiglitazone only slightly inhibited this activity.[5] Any inhibitory activity would be expected to increase warfarin effects, whereas the two cases suggest reduced effects. The authors suggest that the weak CYP3A4-inducing effect of pioglitazone might explain the interaction.[3] However, as CYP3A4 is only a minor enzyme in warfarin metabolism, and controlled pharmacokinetic studies have not shown an effect on warfarin pharmacokinetics, this explanation is unlikely.

Importance and management

Controlled studies have found no interaction between pioglitazone and warfarin or phenprocoumon, or between rosiglitazone and warfarin. This suggests that coumarin dose adjustments are unlikely to be needed when these antidiabetics are also given. Nevertheless, one report describes two patients who required increases in warfarin doses 4 to 12 weeks after starting pioglitazone or rosiglitazone. The general relevance of these two cases is uncertain, and such effects are likely to be picked up by routine INR monitoring.

1. Actos (Pioglitazone hydrochloride). Takeda Pharmaceutical Company Ltd. US Prescribing information, November 2013.
2. Kortboyer JM, Eckland DJA. Pioglitazone has low potential for drug interactions. *Diabetologia* (1999) 42 (Suppl 1), A228.
3. Hoffmann TK, Parker DL, Buch HA, Balusu P. Suspected suppression of the INR by thiazolidinediones: interaction between warfarin and TZDs. *Ann Pharmacother* (2006) 40, 994–6.
4. Avandia (Rosiglitazone maleate). GlaxoSmithKline. US Prescribing information, September 2013.
5. Yamazaki H, Suzuki M, Tane K, Shimada N, Nakajima M, Yokoi T. *In vitro* inhibitory effects of troglitazone and its metabolites on drug oxidation activities of human cytochrome P450 enzymes: comparison with pioglitazone and rosiglitazone. *Xenobiotica* (2000) 30, 61–70.

Coumarins + Antihistamines

Findings from a retrospective review suggest that the anticoagulant effects of acenocoumarol may be reduced by loratadine, ebastine, or cetirizine. Conversely, an isolated report describes bleeding and a markedly raised INR in an elderly man taking acenocoumarol and cetirizine.

Clinical evidence, mechanism, importance and management

A retrospective review of patients taking **acenocoumarol** with **loratadine**, **ebastine**, or **cetirizine** found that INRs were decreased during concurrent use, but no thromboembolic event was noted. The authors consider that temporary increases in the anticoagulant dose might be required in patients taking both drugs.[1]

In contrast, there is a case report of an 88-year-old man taking **acenocoumarol** for a deep vein thrombosis who developed acute and severe epistaxis after a fall. He had started to take **cetirizine** 10 mg daily for allergic rhinitis 3 days before the fall.[2] His INR was found to have risen from 1.5 to 14. The **cetirizine** concentration was found to be particularly high, possibly because of some degree of renal impairment, and it was thought that these high levels may have displaced **acenocoumarol** from its plasma protein binding sites. However, this mechanism on its own is now largely discredited as an explanation for interactions between anticoagulants and highly protein-bound drugs.

Information is limited, and given the widespread use of these drugs, any consistent clinically significant interaction might have been expected to have come to light by now. No specific precautions seem necessary if these drugs are given in combination, but bear the interaction in mind in the case of an unexpected response to treatment.

1. García Callejo FJ, Velert Vila MM, Marco Sanz M, Fernández Julián EN. Empleo simultáneo de antihistamínicos H_1 y anticoagulantes orales. *Acta Otorrinolaringol Esp* (2001) 52, 442–5.
2. Berod T, Mathiot I. Probable interaction between cetirizine and acenocoumarol. *Ann Pharmacother* (1997) 31, 122.

Coumarins + Antineoplastics; Cytotoxic

A number of case reports describe an increase in the effects of warfarin, accompanied by bleeding in some cases, caused by antineoplastic regimens including carboplatin, cisplatin, chlormethine, cyclophosphamide, high-dose cytarabine, doxorubicin, etoposide, ifosfamide with mesna, irinotecan, methotrexate, paclitaxel, procarbazine, vincristine or vindesine, and gemcitabine alone and with docetaxel and capecitabine. Conversely, a decrease in the effects of warfarin has been seen in individual cases with cyclophosphamide alone and mitotane alone, and no change in warfarin effect has been seen in one patient while receiving busulfan, cyclophosphamide, cytarabine, and melphalan each given alone.

Clinical evidence

(a) Busulfan

A man stabilised on **warfarin** had no change in his anticoagulant response while taking busulfan for 6 weeks.[1]

(b) Carboplatin

The INR of a man taking **warfarin** increased from a baseline range of 1.15 to 2.11 up to 12.6 within 16 days of a first course of chemotherapy with carboplatin and etoposide.[2]

(c) Cisplatin

A 50-year-old woman taking warfarin 3.25 mg daily for 3 weeks with a stable INR of 2.19 to 2.58, had an increase in her INR to 3.43 on day 3 of the first cycle of **irinotecan** with cisplatin. The warfarin was withheld for one day and restarted, with the dose adjusted to achieve a target INR. Before her second cycle of irinotecan with cisplatin her warfarin dose was 3.75 mg daily and her INR was 2.31; however, her INR rose again on day 3 of the chemotherapy cycle. Irinotecan and cisplatin were stopped because of a poor therapeutic response. Similar increases in INR were also seen in another patient taking warfarin on day 3 of each cycle of **irinotecan** with cisplatin chemotherapy. In both cases, dexamethasone (see 'Coumarins and related drugs + Corticosteroids or Corticotropin', p.419) and aprepitant (see 'Coumarins + Aprepitant', p.404), which could also have affected the anticoagulant response to warfarin, were given during each chemotherapy cycle, although the authors ruled these out as a cause of the increases in INR.[3] Another patient had an increase in the anticoagulant effect of **warfarin** while taking a combination regimen containing cisplatin, see *R-ESHAP*, below.

(d) Cyclophosphamide

A woman taking **warfarin** had a notable increase in her prothrombin time when her treatment with cyclophosphamide was withdrawn, suggesting that cyclophosphamide reduced the anticoagulant response.[4] Another patient had an increase in the anticoagulant effect of **warfarin** while taking a combination regimen containing cyclophosphamide, see *ProMace-Mopp*, below. In contrast, a man well stabilised on **warfarin** had no change in anticoagulant response while taking cyclophosphamide for 6 weeks.[1]

(e) Cytarabine

A man well stabilised on **warfarin** had no change in anticoagulant response while taking cytarabine for 6 weeks.[1]

(f) Etoposide

The INR of a man taking **warfarin** increased from a baseline range of 1.15 to 2.11 up to 12.6 within 16 days of a first course of chemotherapy with carboplatin and etoposide.[2] Another elderly man taking **warfarin** had a notable increase in prothrombin times (prolongation of 8 to 15 seconds) on two occasions when he took etoposide 500 mg and **vindesine** 5 mg.[5] Another patient had an increase in the anticoagulant effect of **warfarin** while taking a combination regimen containing etoposide, see *ProMace-Mopp*, below.

(g) Gemcitabine

A 63-year-old man needed a reduction in his weekly **warfarin** dose from 59.23 mg to 50.75 mg in order to keep his INR at about 2.5 during 2 cycles of gemcitabine. When the gemcitabine was stopped his **warfarin** dose had to be increased again.[6] Another case report describes a difficult to manage INR in a 70-year-old patient with pancreatic cancer given gemcitabine (as part of a regimen of gemcitabine, docetaxel, and capecitabine, and as monotherapy) after previously being stabilised on warfarin.[7] For discussion of the effect of capecitabine see 'Coumarins + Fluorouracil and related prodrugs', p.428. The UK manufacturers have information on 4 cases of suspected interactions between gemcitabine and **warfarin**, and one with **phenprocoumon** (reported by December 2000). Based on 724 reports of the concurrent use of gemcitabine and **anticoagulants**, this represents an incidence of the suspected interaction of 0.8%, which is low if there were a specific interaction.[8]

(h) Hydroxycarbamide

A man well stabilised on **warfarin** had no change in anticoagulant response while taking hydroxycarbamide for 6 weeks.[1]

(i) Ifosfamide

Three patients taking **warfarin** had a notable and very rapid increase in their INRs when given ifosfamide; with **mesna** and **cisplatin** with **etoposide**; or **doxorubicin**; or **doxorubicin** with **vincristine**.[9]

(j) Melphalan

A man well stabilised on **warfarin** had no change in anticoagulant response while taking melphalan for 6 weeks.[1]

(k) Mitotane

A patient who started to take mitotane 4 g [daily] for adrenal carcinoma was also given warfarin (5 mg and 2.5 mg on alternate days) 2 days later for a deep vein thrombosis. This patient required several increases in her warfarin dose (to 12.5 mg daily) over a 4-month period to maintain a therapeutic prothrombin time of about 22 seconds. A few weeks later she was found to have an increase in her prothrombin time to 27.1 seconds, so her warfarin dose was decreased to 10 mg daily. However, 3 months later she was admitted to hospital with haematemesis and gingival bleeding, and her prothrombin time was found to be 74.6 seconds. She was found to have a haemorrhage of a tumour in the right posterior fossa, and she died that day.[10]

(l) Paclitaxel

A woman who had been stable on **warfarin** for 2 months had an INR increase from 3 to 5.2 on the day after receiving paclitaxel and **carboplatin**. An increase in INR occurred after each subsequent cycle of chemotherapy.[11]

(m) ProMace-Mopp

The prothrombin times of an elderly man given **warfarin** increased by 50 to 100% in the middle of three cycles of treatment with ProMace-Mopp (**cyclophosphamide**, **doxorubicin**, **etoposide**, **chlormethine**, **vincristine**, **procarbazine**, **methotrexate**, and prednisone), and he developed a subconjunctival haemorrhage during the first cycle.[12]

(n) R-ESHAP

A 49-year-old man receiving R-ESHAP (rituximab, **etoposide**, **cisplatin**, high-dose **cytarabine**, and methylprednisolone) for lymphoma, was started on **warfarin** for the secondary prevention of pulmonary embolism with deep venous thrombosis, after the first course. After warfarin dose titration, he received a second course of R-ESHAP and his INR increased (from 1 to 5.28). After further warfarin dose adjustments to stabilise his INR, he received a third course of R-ESHAP and his INR increased again (from 2.44 to 4.71) but decreased to within the normal range (1.05, range 0.81 to 1.09) 5 days after the chemotherapy was completed.[13] Note that high doses of methylprednisolone increase the INR of patients taking coumarins (see 'Coumarins and related drugs + Corticosteroids or Corticotropin', p.419).

Mechanism

Not well understood. Coagulation control can be altered by many factors in severely ill patients with cancer, including altered diet due to lack of appetite and nausea and vomiting caused by antineoplastics. Antineoplastics that cause gastrointestinal toxicity might also alter the absorption of warfarin. The authors of the case report of an interaction with paclitaxel[11] and with cisplatin[3] suggest that the likely mechanism of action is displacement of warfarin from protein binding sites by paclitaxel and cisplatin. However, altered protein binding has not clearly been shown to be an important mechanism in warfarin interactions, as any effect is usually transient.

Importance and management

These are isolated cases, and no specific drug interaction is established for any of the cytotoxic antineoplastics covered here. Nevertheless, other factors due to the disease or patient might alter the response to anticoagulants. Therefore, the anticoagulant doses might need adjustment. Note that, from a disease perspective, when treating venous thromboembolic disease in patients with cancer, warfarin is generally inferior (higher risk of major bleeds and recurrent thrombosis) to low-molecular-weight heparins.[14]

Note that some cytotoxic antineoplastics do have specific interactions with coumarins, see 'Coumarins + Azathioprine or Mercaptopurine', p.407, and 'Coumarins + Fluorouracil and related prodrugs', p.428.

1. Spiers ASD, Mibashan RS. Increased warfarin requirement during mercaptopurine therapy: a new drug interaction. *Lancet* (1974) ii, 221–2.
2. Le AT, Hasson NK, Lum BL. Enhancement of warfarin response in a patient receiving etoposide and carboplatin chemotherapy. *Ann Pharmacother* (1997) 31, 1006–8.
3. Yano R, Kurokawa T, Tsuyoshi h, Shinagawa A, Sawamura Y, Matsunaga A, Nakamura T, Yoshida Y, Yoneda M, Kotsuji F, Masada M. Transient elevation of international normalized ratio during cisplatin-based chemotherapy in patients who are taking warfarin. *Ann Pharmacother* (2011) 45, e55.
4. Tashima CK. Cyclophosphamide effect on coumarin anticoagulation. *South Med J* (1979) 72, 633–4.
5. Ward K, Bitran JD. Warfarin, etoposide, and vindesine interactions. *Cancer Treat Rep* (1984) 68, 817–18.
6. Kinikar SA, Kolesar JM. Identification of a gemcitabine-warfarin interaction. *Pharmacotherapy* (1999) 19, 1331–3.
7. Saif MW, Wasif N. Interaction between capecitabine and gemcitabine with warfarin in a patient with pancreatic cancer. *JOP* (2008) 9, 739–43.
8. Kilgour-Christie J, Czarnecki A. Gemcitabine and the interaction with anticoagulants. *Lancet Oncol* (2002) 3, 460.
9. Hall G, Lind MJ, Huang M, Moore A, Gane A, Roberts JT, Cantwell BMJ. Intravenous infusions of ifosfamide/mesna and perturbation of warfarin anticoagulant control. *Postgrad Med J* (1990) 66, 860–1.
10. Cuddy PG, Loftus LS. Influence of mitotane on the hypoprothrombinemic effect of warfarin. *South Med J* (1986) 79, 387–8.
11. Thompson ME, Highley MS. Interaction between paclitaxel and warfarin. *Ann Oncol* (2003) 14, 500.
12. Seifter EJ, Brooks BJ, Urba WJ. Possible interactions between warfarin and antineoplastic drugs. *Cancer Treat Rep* (1985) 69, 244–5.
13. Suzuki T, Koga H, Yamazaki S, Saeki H, Tanaka H, Nishimura M, Nakaseko C, Nakasa H, Nakamura H, Ariyoshi N, Kitada M. Probable interaction between warfarin and antitumor agents used in R-ESHAP chemotherapy. *Clin Ther* (2008) 30, 1155–9.
14. Baglin TP, Keeling DM, Watson HG, for the British Committee for Standards in Haematology. Guidelines on oral anticoagulation (warfarin): third edition – 2005 update. *Br J Haematol* (2005) 132, 277–85.

Coumarins + Aprepitant

Aprepitant modestly reduces warfarin levels and slightly decreases the INR in healthy subjects. It is expected to interact similarly with acenocoumarol. Fosaprepitant, a prodrug of aprepitant, would be expected to interact similarly.

Clinical evidence, mechanism, importance and management

In a double-blind study, healthy subjects were stabilised on **warfarin** and then given either aprepitant (125 mg on day one, then 80 mg daily on days 2 and 3) or placebo. On day 3, there was no change in **warfarin** levels. However, by day 8 (5 days after stopping aprepitant) there was a 34% decrease in trough *S*-warfarin levels, and a 14% decrease in INR in the aprepitant group.[1]

Aprepitant is a moderate inducer of the cytochrome P450 isoenzyme CYP2C9, by which *S*-warfarin is metabolised. The manufacturer recommends that, in patients taking **warfarin**, the INR should be monitored closely for 2 weeks, particularly at 7 to 10 days,[2] after each 3-day course of aprepitant for chemotherapy,[2,3] or after each single 40-mg dose when given for the prevention of post-operative nausea and vomiting.[2] This seems a prudent precaution. The UK manufacturer[3] similarly recommends caution with **acenocoumarol**, which is also metabolised by CYP2C9. **Fosaprepitant**, a prodrug of aprepitant, would be expected to interact similarly, and therefore the same precautions would be appropriate if it is given to a patient taking a coumarin.

1. Depré M, Van Hecken A, Oeyen M, De Lepeleire I, Laethem T, Rothenberg P, Petty KJ, Majumdar A, Crumley T, Panebianco D, Bergman A, de Hoon JN. Effect of aprepitant on the pharmacokinetics and pharmacodynamics of warfarin. *Eur J Clin Pharmacol* (2005) 61, 341–6.
2. EMEND Capsules (Aprepitant). Merck & Co., Inc. US Prescribing information, August 2014.
3. EMEND (Aprepitant). Merck Sharp & Dohme Ltd. UK Summary of product characteristics, December 2013.

Coumarins + Aromatase inhibitors

The anticoagulant effects of warfarin and acenocoumarol can be markedly reduced by aminoglutethimide. An isolated case of thromboembolism has been loosely attributed to an interaction between letrozole and warfarin. However, anastrozole and letrozole do not affect the pharmacokinetics of warfarin, and exemestane would not be expected to interact.

Clinical evidence

(a) Aminoglutethimide

In a study in 9 patients being treated for breast cancer, aminoglutethimide 125 mg twice daily increased the clearance of a single-dose of *R*- or *S*-warfarin by 41% with marked variability between individuals (range 15 to 103%). Aminoglutethimide 250 mg four times daily increased the clearance of **warfarin** by 91%. The effects of the interaction had developed fully by 14 days. Both enantiomers of **warfarin** were equally affected.[1]

One 79-year-old woman taking aminoglutethimide 250 mg four times daily was resistant to **warfarin** requiring a dose of 17.5 to 20 mg daily. Two weeks after the aminoglutethimide was stopped, the required dose of **warfarin** gradually declined, eventually reaching a level of 3.75 and 5 mg on alternate days (about a fourfold reduction).[2] Another patient stabilised on **warfarin** gradually needed about a threefold increase in the **warfarin** dose after starting aminoglutethimide 250 mg four times a day.[2] The increased requirement persisted for 2 weeks after the aminoglutethimide was stopped, and then declined. A study briefly mentions a patient who needed greatly increased doses of **warfarin** after starting aminoglutethimide.[3] Three patients taking **acenocoumarol** needed a doubled dose to maintain adequate anticoagulation when they took aminoglutethimide 250 mg four times daily for 3 to 4 weeks.[4]

(b) Anastrozole

In a well-controlled study in 16 healthy men,[5] anastrozole (7 mg loading dose followed by 1 mg daily for a further 10 days) had no effect on the pharmacokinetics or pharmacodynamics of a single dose of **warfarin** given on day 3.

(c) Letrozole

The manufacturers report that letrozole had no clinically relevant effect on the pharmacokinetics of **warfarin**.[6,7]

A 72-year-old woman with breast cancer developed deep vein thrombosis while taking tamoxifen. **Warfarin** was started and the tamoxifen was switched to letrozole. Five months later she developed a pulmonary thromboembolism, and her INR was noted to be subtherapeutic. The authors suggested that the low INR may be due to an interaction between **warfarin** and letrozole; however, they also note that many other factors may have contributed to this patient developing a pulmonary embolism, such as a possible adverse effect of letrozole, obesity and related immobility, and therefore the exact cause is unknown.[8]

Mechanism

Uncertain. The most likely explanation is that aminoglutethimide, like glutethimide, stimulates the activity of the liver enzymes concerned with the metabolism of the coumarin anticoagulants, thereby reducing their levels and efficacy. Alternatively, it has been suggested that aminoglutethimide may affect blood steroid levels, which in turn might affect coagulation.[2] Letrozole is not reported to be an inducer of the cytochrome P450 isoenzymes CYP2C9 or CYP3A4, which are involved in the metabolism of coumarin anticoagulants.

Importance and management

The interaction of warfarin and acenocoumarol with aminoglutethimide is established and clinically important. Monitor the effects of adding aminoglutethimide to patients already taking these drugs and increase the anticoagulant dose as necessary. Up to four times the dose may be needed. The extent of the effects would appear to be related to the dose of aminoglutethimide used. Monitor the INR and reduce the anticoagulant dose accordingly if aminoglutethimide is withdrawn. Information about other coumarins is lacking but it would be prudent to apply the same precautions with any of them.

Conversely, controlled studies have shown no interaction between anastrozole or letrozole and warfarin, and the isolated case report does not firmly implicate an interaction with warfarin. Overall, this suggests that coumarin dose adjustments are unlikely to be needed when these aromatase inhibitors are used. There appears to be no published information of an interaction with **exemestane**. The US manufacturers state that it does not inhibit CYP2C9 or CYP3A4, therefore it is unlikely to have any significant pharmacokinetic interaction with warfarin.[9]

Note that tamoxifen also interacts with warfarin and possibly other coumarin anticoagulants in some patients, see 'Coumarins + Tamoxifen or Toremifene', p.476, for further information.

Consider also that, from a disease perspective, when treating venous thromboembolic disease in patients with cancer, warfarin is generally inferior (higher risk of major bleeds and recurrent thrombosis) to low-molecular-weight heparins.[10]

1. Lønning PE, Ueland PM, Kvinnsland S. The influence of a graded dose schedule of aminoglutethimide on the disposition of the optical enantiomers of warfarin in patients with breast cancer. *Cancer Chemother Pharmacol* (1986) 17, 177–81.
2. Lønning PE, Kvinnsland S, Jahren G. Aminoglutethimide and warfarin. A new important drug interaction. *Cancer Chemother Pharmacol* (1984) 12, 10–12.
3. Murray RML, Pitt P, Jerums G. Medical adrenalectomy with aminoglutethimide in the management of advanced breast cancer. *Med J Aust* (1981) 1, 179–81.
4. Bruning PF, Bonfrèr JGM. Aminoglutethimide and oral anticoagulant therapy. *Lancet* (1983) ii, 582.
5. Yates RA, Wong J, Seiberling M, Merz M, März W, Nauck M. The effect of anastrozole on the single-dose pharmacokinetics and anticoagulant activity of warfarin in healthy volunteers. *Br J Clin Pharmacol* (2001) 51, 429–35.
6. Femara (Letrozole). Novartis Pharmaceuticals UK Ltd. UK Summary of product characteristics, March 2009.
7. Femara (Letrozole). Novartis Pharmaceuticals. US Prescribing information, January 2009.
8. Oyan B, Altundag K, Ozisik Y. Does letrozole have any place in adjuvant setting in breast cancer patients with documented hypercoagulability? *Am J Clin Oncol* (2004) 27, 210–1.
9. Aromasin (Exemestane). Pfizer. US Prescribing information, October 2008.
10. Baglin TP, Keeling DM, Watson HG, for the British Committee for Standards in Haematology. Guidelines on oral anticoagulation (warfarin): third edition – 2005 update. *Br J Haematol* (2005) 132, 277–85.

Coumarins + Ascorbic acid (Vitamin C)

Although a few cases have been reported in which the effects of warfarin were reduced by ascorbic acid, four prospective studies have not found any interaction.

Clinical evidence

In a woman recently stabilised on **warfarin** 7.5 mg daily, who began to simultaneously take ascorbic acid (dose not stated) with her warfarin, the prothrombin time fell steadily from 23 seconds, to 19, 17, and then 14 seconds, with no response to an increase in the dose of **warfarin** to 10 mg, 15 mg, and finally 20 mg daily. The prothrombin time returned to 28 seconds within 2 days of stopping the ascorbic acid.[1] Another woman recently stabilised on warfarin 5 mg daily had a recurrence of acute thrombophlebitis with a prothrombin time of 12 seconds. She was unusually resistant to the actions of **warfarin** and required 25 mg daily before a notable increase in prothrombin times was achieved. On questioning, she had been taking massive amounts of ascorbic acid (about 16 g daily) for several weeks. She was eventually stabilised on warfarin 10 mg daily.[2] In another case, a 65-year-old man was started on warfarin but his INR remained below target range even at a **warfarin** dose of 20 mg daily. After known potential contributory factors were ruled out, his usual ascorbic acid dose (500 mg twice daily) was discontinued on day 8. Within 24 hours his INR had increased from 1.1 to 2.8, and the following day it had increased further to 15.4. Phytomenadione was administered and warfarin withheld for 2 days, after which his INR was 2.7 and he was eventually stabilised on 5 mg daily. Three months later his INR was found to be stable on 3.5 mg warfarin daily.[3]

In contrast, in prospective studies, no changes in the effects of **warfarin** were seen:

- in 5 patients given ascorbic acid 1 g daily for a fortnight,[4]
- in 11 patients (some taking **dicoumarol**) given ascorbic acid 4 g daily for 2 weeks,[5]
- in 14 patients given ascorbic acid 3 g then 5 g daily for one week or 5 patients given 10 g daily for one week:[6] a mean fall of 18% in total plasma **warfarin** concentrations was seen at all doses,
- in a 10-week study, where the proportion of patients requiring a change in **warfarin** dose did not differ between 84 patients given ascorbic acid (dose unstated) and 96 control patients (31 patients versus 18 patients required a dose reduction, and 7 versus 13 required a dose increase, respectively).[7]

Mechanism

Not understood. One *animal* study has demonstrated this interaction[8] and others have not,[9,10] but none of them has provided any definite clues about why it ever occurs. One suggestion is that high doses of ascorbic acid can cause diarrhoea, which might prevent adequate absorption of the anticoagulant.

Importance and management

Four clinical studies in patients stabilised on warfarin have not found that ascorbic acid alters the anticoagulant effect of warfarin, even using very large doses of ascorbic acid (up to 10 g daily), even though there are a few reports of reduced warfarin efficacy. Coumarin dose adjustments would therefore seem unlikely to be needed when ascorbic acid is also used.

1. Rosenthal G. Interaction of ascorbic acid and warfarin. *JAMA* (1971) 215, 1671.
2. Smith EC, Skalski RJ, Johnson GC, Rossi GV. Interaction of ascorbic acid and warfarin. *JAMA* (1972) 221, 1166.
3. Sattar A, Willman JE, Kolluri R. Possible warfarin resistance due to interaction with ascorbic acid: case report and literature review. *Am J Health-Syst Pharm* (2013) 70, 782–6.
4. Hume R, Johnstone JMS, Weyers E. Interaction of ascorbic acid and warfarin. *JAMA* (1972) 219, 1479.
5. Blakely JA. Interaction of warfarin and ascorbic acid. 1st Florence Conference on Haemostasis and Thrombosis, May 1977. Abstracts p 99.
6. Feetam CL, Leach RH, Meynell MJ. Lack of a clinically important interaction between warfarin and ascorbic acid. *Toxicol Appl Pharmacol* (1975) 31, 544–7.
7. Dedichen J. The effect of ascorbic acid given to patients on chronic anticoagulant therapy. *Boll Soc Ital Cardiol* (1973) 18, 690–2.
8. Sigell LT, Flessa HC. Drug interactions with anticoagulants. *JAMA* (1970) 214, 2035–8.
9. Weintraub M, Griner PF. Warfarin and ascorbic acid: lack of evidence for a drug interaction. *Toxicol Appl Pharmacol* (1974) 28, 53–6.
10. Deckert FW. Ascorbic acid and warfarin. *JAMA* (1973) 223, 440.

Coumarins and related drugs + Aspirin or other Salicylates

Antiplatelet doses of aspirin (75 to 325 mg daily) increase the risk of bleeding when given with warfarin, although, in most studies the absolute risks have been small. In addition to increased bleeding, high doses of aspirin (4 g daily or more) can increase prothrombin times.

Clinical evidence

A. Analgesic-dose aspirin

In a pharmacological study in patients stabilised on **acenocoumarol**, aspirin 2.4 g daily for one week increased faecal blood loss from an average of 1.1 mL to 4.7 mL. While taking aspirin, 11 of 17 patients required a 29% reduction in their **acenocoumarol** dose from a mean of 3.1 mg to 2.2 mg. One patient required a small increase of 0.5 mg, and the remaining 5 required a dose reduction of less than 0.5 mg.[1]

In another study in healthy subjects, aspirin 1.95 g daily for 11 days had no effect on the prothrombin time response to a single dose of **warfarin** given on day 4. When 11 healthy subjects were stabilised on **dicoumarol** or **warfarin** and given aspirin 1.95 g daily, 7 had no important change in prothrombin time activity, and 4 had a small reduction (of 5 to 10%). Two subjects had signs of bleeding, but neither had a reduction in prothrombin time activity. A further 4 subjects stabilised on **warfarin** received a higher dose of aspirin (3.9 g daily), and all 4 had a reduction in prothrombin time activity of 6 to 12% and signs of bleeding occurred. The bleeding time was considerably prolonged by the combination of aspirin 1.95 g daily and **warfarin** when compared with **warfarin** alone (10.3 minutes versus 4 minutes).[2] In a study in 12 healthy subjects stabilised on **warfarin**, aspirin 2.6 g daily for one week reduced the mean prothrombin concentrations by about 2.75%.[3] In two further studies in healthy subjects, aspirin 6 g daily modestly prolonged prothrombin times,[4,5] and in one study this effect tended to be reversed by vitamin K.[4]

In contrast, in another study in 10 patients, adding aspirin 3 g daily to **warfarin** for 2 weeks had no effect on prothrombin times (20.9 seconds versus 21.2 seconds).[6]

B. Antiplatelet-dose aspirin

In a study in healthy subjects, low-dose aspirin 75 mg daily doubled the normal blood loss from the gastric mucosa. However, concurrent **warfarin** (dose individualised to achieve an INR of 1.4 to 1.6) did not increase the gastric mucosal bleeding any further.[7]

In a large population-based, retrospective case control-study using records from the UK General Practice Research Database from 2000 to 2005, the use of **warfarin** with aspirin was associated with a greater increased risk of gastrointestinal bleeding when compared with either drug alone (rate ratio of 6.48 for concurrent use compared with 1.94 for **warfarin** and 1.39 for aspirin).[8] This study did not specify the indication for concurrent use. In a similar retrospective cohort study from the Netherlands, the use of **acenocoumarol** or **phenprocoumon** with antithrombotic salicylates (not specified) was associated with an increased risk of major bleeding (relative risk 3).[9]

(a) Atrial fibrillation

In a large study in patients with atrial fibrillation, the cumulative incidence of bleeding events after 3 years was no different in those receiving fixed low-dose **warfarin** 1.25 mg daily with aspirin 300 mg daily (24.4%) than with fixed low-dose **warfarin** alone (24.7%) or aspirin 300 mg daily alone (30%).[10] This study also contained an adjusted-dose **warfarin**-only group, which proved more effective than the other group, so the study was terminated early. Other studies have found similar results.[11] However, in a large, retrospective, cohort study in Denmark from 1997 to 2006, patients who were discharged from hospital with a diagnosis of atrial fibrillation and were taking warfarin and aspirin were found to have an increased risk of admission to hospital with bleeding, when compared with warfarin alone (adjusted hazard ratio 1.83). The authors note that they had no information on the patients' INR.[12] Similarly, in another large cohort study in the UK, patients newly diagnosed with atrial fibrillation between 1993 and 2008 and prescribed warfarin and aspirin were found to have an increased risk of experiencing a bleeding event (minor or major) when compared with those who received either aspirin or warfarin alone (adjusted hazard ratio 2.87 compared with 1.25 and 2.08, respectively).[13] In another study, the combination of adjusted dose **fluindione** (INR 2 to 2.6) with aspirin 100 mg daily was associated with a much higher incidence of haemorrhagic complications than **fluindione** alone (13.1% versus 1.2%). The overall balance of benefit to risk could not be assessed because of the low incidence of the primary endpoint (ischaemic events).[14]

(b) Myocardial infarction

1. Primary prevention. In a large primary prevention study in men at high risk of ischaemic heart disease, the incidence of haematuria was 2-fold higher in those receiving both low-dose aspirin 75 mg daily and low-intensity **warfarin** (INR 1.5) than in those receiving low-dose aspirin alone, or low-intensity **warfarin** alone. Similarly, the incidence of minor episodes of bleeding (nose bleeds, bruising, rectal bleeding, pink/red urine) was 1.27-fold higher in those receiving the combination than in those receiving low-dose aspirin alone, or low-intensity **warfarin** alone (49% versus 38% and 39%, respectively), although the difference was not statistically significant. There was no difference in incidence of major and intermediate episodes of bleeding.[15]

2. Secondary prevention. In a meta-analysis of randomised, controlled studies in patients following myocardial infarction or acute coronary syndrome, intensive **warfarin** (INR greater than 2) with aspirin 80 to 325 mg daily was associated with a 2.5-fold increased risk of major bleeding, when compared with aspirin alone, although the actual incidence was low (1.5% versus 0.6%).[16] This analysis excluded studies of coronary stenting. In another similar meta-analysis, the concurrent use of aspirin and **warfarin** (INR 2 to 3) was associated with an odds ratio of 2.3 for a major bleed, when compared with aspirin alone.[17] The number needed to treat to cause one major bleed was 100. This compared with a number needed to treat to avoid one major adverse event (death, myocardial infarction or stroke) of 33.

Similarly, in an observational cohort study of elderly survivors of acute myocardial infarction, the rate of bleeding was higher in patients receiving **warfarin** with aspirin (0.08 per patient-year), than in patients receiving aspirin alone (0.03 per patient-year).[18] Using lower intensity **warfarin** with the low-dose aspirin was still associated with more major bleeding than aspirin alone (1.77 in one study, although this is less than higher intensity **warfarin**; 2.3 as mentioned above). Nevertheless, low-intensity **warfarin** with low-dose aspirin does not appear to be any more effective than aspirin alone.[17,19]

(c) Peripheral arterial disease

In a meta-analysis of studies of patients with peripheral arterial disease, the concurrent use of **oral anticoagulants** with aspirin increased the risk of major bleeding about 2-fold when compared with aspirin alone, and appeared to be associated with increased mortality.[20]

In one open-label, randomised, clinical study, patients with peripheral arterial disease were assigned to take an antiplatelet alone (1081 patients taking aspirin, clopidogrel, or ticlopidine) or to take an antiplatelet with **warfarin** or **acenocoumarol** (1080 patients, target INR of 2 to 3). The risk of life-threatening bleeding was 3.4-fold higher with the concurrent use of an anticoagulant and an antiplatelet than with the antiplatelet alone (4% versus 1.2%), and moderate and minor bleeding were also increased (relative risk of 2.8 and 3.6, respectively).[21]

(d) Prosthetic heart valves

In one randomised study in patients with artificial heart valves, the risk of bleeding episodes requiring blood transfusion or hospitalisation was much higher among those taking aspirin 500 mg daily and **warfarin** (14%), when compared with those taking **warfarin** and dipyridamole 400 mg daily (4%), and compared with a non-randomised control group taking **warfarin** alone (5%). Bleeding was mainly gastrointestinal or cerebral. All of those with intracerebral bleeding died.[22]

A further study found that aspirin 1 g daily, given with **unnamed anticoagulants**, was associated with a 3-fold higher incidence of bleeding episodes than those taking anticoagulants alone (13.9 per 100 patients per year versus 4.7 per 100 patients per year).[23,24] However, in another study there was no difference in haemorrhagic risk between patients receiving aspirin 500 mg daily and **acenocoumarol** or **acenocoumarol** alone.[25]

More recent studies have used lower doses of aspirin. In one study in patients stabilised on **warfarin** with a target INR of 3.0 to 4.5, the addition of aspirin 100 mg daily increased the risk of any bleeding 1.55-fold, when compared with placebo (35% versus 22% per year), mainly due to an increase in minor haematuria, nosebleeds, and bruising. However, the risk was more than offset by the overall reduction in mortality.[26]

The preliminary report of a meta-analysis of these four studies, concluded that the concurrent use of **oral anticoagulants** and aspirin (100 mg to 1 g daily) reduced mortality and embolic complications in patients with prosthetic heart valves, with an estimated increased odds ratio of major bleeds of 1.7 and of total bleeds of 1.98. Nevertheless the overall picture was that the benefits possibly outweighed the problems.[27] In a subsequent meta-analysis,[28] which excluded one non-randomised study,[22] but included two other randomised controlled studies, the risk of major bleeding for the combination of **warfarin** and aspirin was 1.53. For the two studies using low-dose aspirin (100 mg daily), there did not appear to be an excess risk of major bleeding.[28] Another analysis of these studies provided essentially the same risk of increased major bleeding with the combination.[29]

Mechanism

Aspirin has a direct irritant effect on the stomach lining and can cause gastrointestinal bleeding, even in doses as low as 75 mg daily.[30] It also decreases platelet aggregation and prolongs bleeding times. At low doses of aspirin, this increases the risk of haemorrhage with warfarin without elevating the INR. In addition, large doses of aspirin (4 g daily or more) alone are known to have a direct hypoprothrombinaemic effect, which is reversible by vitamin K.[4,5] This effect of aspirin can be additive with the effects of the anticoagulant.

Importance and management

The interaction of high-dose aspirin and warfarin is not well documented, but is clinically important. It is usual to avoid normal analgesic and anti-inflammatory doses of aspirin while taking any coumarin anticoagulant, although only dicoumarol, acenocoumarol, and warfarin appear to have been investigated. Patients should be told that many non-prescription analgesic, antipyretic, cold, and influenza preparations contain substantial amounts of aspirin. Warn them that it could be listed as acetylsalicylic acid. Paracetamol is a safer analgesic substitute (but not entirely without problems, see 'Coumarins and related drugs + Paracetamol (Acetaminophen)', p.459).

The effect of low-dose aspirin, used for its antiplatelet effects, with warfarin has been far more extensively studied. Overall, the evidence shows that the combination is still associated with an increased risk of bleeding over either drug alone, and, from controlled studies, this is in the region of 1.5- to 2.5-fold, although two population studies have suggested that the risk may be greater in the primary care setting.[8,9] Nevertheless, the absolute risk is small. A 2-fold increased risk of haematuria and a small increased risk of minor bleeding of 1.27 was still seen in the study using the lowest dose of warfarin (INR 1.5) with just 75 mg of aspirin a day.[15] In certain patient groups the benefits of concurrent use have been clearly shown to outweigh this increased risk of bleeding, such as in patients with prosthetic heart valves at high risk of thromboembolism. In these patients, those who are at risk of gastrointestinal bleeding should additionally receive gastroprotection such as proton pump inhibitors. In addition, in the long-term, aspirin doses should be limited to no more than 81 mg daily.[31]

For a review of the risk of bleeding when using warfarin with dual, or triple, antiplatelet therapy, such as low-dose aspirin and/or clopidogrel, see 'Coumarins and related drugs + Clopidogrel', p.417.

Note that cases of increased INRs and/or bleeding have been reported in patients taking warfarin who have used *topical* salicylates, see 'Coumarins + Salicylates; Topical', p.468.

1. Watson RM, Pierson RN. Effect of anticoagulant therapy upon aspirin-induced gastrointestinal bleeding. *Circulation* (1961) 24, 613–16.
2. O'Reilly RA, Sahud MA, Aggeler PM. Impact of aspirin and chlorthalidone on the pharmacodynamics of oral anticoagulant drugs in man. *Ann N Y Acad Sci* (1971) 179, 173–86.
3. Holmes EL. Pharmacology of the fenamates: IV. Toleration by normal human subjects. *Ann Phys Med* (1966) 9 (Suppl), 36–49.
4. Shapiro S. Studies on prothrombin. VI. The effect of synthetic vitamin K on the prothrombinopenia induced by salicylate in man. *JAMA* (1944) 125, 546–8.
5. Quick AJ, Clesceri L. Influence of acetylsalicylic acid and salicylamide on the coagulation of blood. *J Pharmacol Exp Ther* (1960) 128, 95–8.
6. Udall JA. Drug interference with warfarin therapy. *Clin Med* (1970) 77, 20–5.
7. Prichard PJ, Kitchingman GK, Walt RP, Daneshmend TK, Hawkey CJ. Human gastric mucosal bleeding induced by low dose aspirin, but not warfarin. *BMJ* (1989) 298, 493–6.
8. Delaney JA, Opatrny L, Brophy JM, Suissa S. Drug–drug interactions between antithrombotic medications and the risk of gastrointestinal bleeding. *CMAJ* (2007) 177, 347–51.
9. Penning-van Beest F, Erkens J, Petersen K-U, Koelz HR, Herings R. Main comedications associated with major bleeding during anticoagulant therapy with coumarins. *Eur J Clin Pharmacol* (2005) 61, 439–44.
10. Gulløv AL, Koefoed BG, Petersen P, Pedersen TS, Andersen ED, Godtfredsen J, Boysen G. Fixed minidose warfarin and aspirin alone and in combination vs adjusted-dose warfarin for stroke prevention in atrial fibrillation. Second Copenhagen atrial fibrillation, aspirin, and anticoagulant study. *Arch Intern Med* (1998) 158, 1513–21.
11. Stroke Prevention in Atrial Fibrillation Investigators. Adjusted-dose warfarin versus low-intensity, fixed-dose warfarin plus aspirin for high-risk patients with atrial fibrillation: Stroke Prevention in Atrial Fibrillation III randomised clinical trial. *Lancet* (1996) 348, 633–38.
12. Hansen ML, Sørensen R, Clausen MT, Fog-Petersen ML, Raunsø J, Gadsbøll N, Gislason GH, Folke F, Andersen SS, Schramm TK, Abildstrøm SZ, Poulsen HE, Køber L, Torp-Pedersen C. Risk of bleeding with single, dual, or triple therapy with warfarin, aspirin, and clopidogrel in patients with atrial fibrillation. *Arch Intern Med* (2010) 170, 143341.
13. Azoulay L, Dell'Aniello S, Simon T, Renoux C, Suissa S. The concurrent use of antithrombotic therapies and the risk of bleeding in patients with atrial fibrillation. *Thromb Haemost* (2013) 109, 431–39.
14. Lechat P, Lardoux H, Mallet A, Sanchez P, Derumeaux G, Lecompte T, Maillard L, Mas JL, Mentre F, Pousset F, Lacomblez L, Pisica G, Solbes-Latourette S, Raynaud P, Chaumet-Riffaud P for the FFAACS Investigators. Anticoagulant (fluindione)-aspirin combination in patients with high-risk atrial fibrillation. A randomized trial. *Cerebrovasc Dis* (2001) 12, 245–52.
15. The Medical Research Council's General Practice Research Framework. Thrombosis prevention trial: randomised trial of low-intensity oral anticoagulation with warfarin and low-dose aspirin in the primary prevention of ischaemic heart disease in men at increased risk. *Lancet* (1998) 351, 233–41.
16. Rothberg MB, Celestin C, Fiore LD, Lawler E, Cook JR. Warfarin plus aspirin after myocardial infarction or the acute coronary syndrome: meta-analysis with estimates of risk and benefit. *Ann Intern Med* (2005) 143, 241–50.
17. Andreotti F, Testa L, Biondi-Zoccai GG, Crea F. Aspirin plus warfarin compared to aspirin alone after acute coronary syndromes: an updated and comprehensive meta-analysis of 25,307 patients. *Eur Heart J* (2006) 27, 519–26.
18. Buresly K, Eisenberg MJ, Zhang X, Pilote L. Bleeding complications associated with combinations of aspirin, thienopyridine derivatives, and warfarin in elderly patients following acute myocardial infarction. *Arch Intern Med* (2005) 165, 784–9.
19. Fiore LD, Ezekowitz MD, Brophy MT, Lu D, Sacco J, Peduzzi P. Department of Veterans Affairs Cooperative Studies Program clinical trial comparing combined warfarin and aspirin with aspirin alone in survivors of acute myocardial infarction: primary results of the CHAMP study. *Circulation* (2002) 105, 557–63.
20. WAVE investigators. The effects of oral anticoagulants in patients with peripheral arterial disease: rationale, design, and baseline characteristics of the Warfarin and Antiplatelet Vascular Evaluation (WAVE) trial, including a meta-analysis of trials. *Am Heart J* (2006) 151, 1–9.
21. Anand S, Yusuf S, Xie C, Pogue J, Eikelboom J, Budaj A, Sussex B, Liu L, Guzman R, Cina C, Crowell R, Keltai M, Gosselin G, for the Warfarin Antiplatelet Vascular Evaluation Trial Investigators. Oral anticoagulant and antiplatelet therapy and peripheral arterial disease. *N Engl J Med* (2007) 357, 217–27.
22. Chesebro JH, Fuster V, Elveback LR, McGoon DC, Pluth JR, Puga FJ, Wallace RB, Danielson GK, Orszulak TA, Piehler JM, Schaff HV. Trial of combined warfarin plus dipyridamole or aspirin therapy in prosthetic heart valve replacement: danger of aspirin compared with dipyridamole. *Am J Cardiol* (1983) 51, 1537–41.

23. Dale J, Myhre E, Storstein O, Stormorken H, Efskind L. Prevention of arterial thromboembolism with acetylsalicylic acid. A controlled clinical study in patients with aortic ball valves. *Am Heart J* (1977) 94, 101–111.
24. Dale J, Myhre E, Loew D. Bleeding during acetylsalicylic acid and anticoagulant therapy in patients with reduced platelet reactivity after aortic valve replacement. *Am Heart J* (1980) 99, 746–52.
25. Altman R, Boullon F, Rouvier J, Rada R, de la Fuente L, Favaloro R. Aspirin and prophylaxis of thromboembolic complications in patients with substitute heart valves. *J Thorac Cardiovasc Surg* (1976) 72, 127–9.
26. Turpie AGG, Gent M, Laupacis A, Latour Y, Gunstensen J, Basile F, Klimek M, Hirsh J. A comparison of aspirin with placebo in patients treated with warfarin after heart-valve replacement. *N Engl J Med* (1993) 329, 524–9.
27. Fiore L, Brophy M, Deykin D, Cappelleri J, Lau J. The efficacy and safety of the addition of aspirin in patients treated with oral anticoagulants after heart valve replacement: a meta-analysis. *Blood* (1993) 82 (10 Suppl 1), 409a.
28. Little SH, Massel DR. Antiplatelet and anticoagulation for patients with prosthetic heart valves. Available in The Cochrane Database of Systematic Reviews; Issue 4. Chichester: John Wiley; 2006 (accessed 20070606).
29. Larson RJ, Fischer ES. Should aspirin be continued in patients started on warfarin? A systematic review and meta-analysis. *J Gen Intern Med* (2004) 19, 879–86.
30. Weil J, Colin-Jones D, Langman M, Lawson D, Logan R, Murphy M, Rawlins M, Vessey M, Wainwright P. Prophylactic aspirin and risk of peptic ulcer bleeding. *BMJ* (1995) 310: 827–30.
31. Bhatt DL, Scheiman J, Abraham NS, Antman EM, Chan FKL, Furberg CD, Johnson DA, Mahaffey KW, Quigley EM. ACCF/ACG/AHA 2008 Expert Consensus Document on Reducing the Gastrointestinal Risks of Antiplatelet Therapy and NSAID Use. A Report of the American College of Cardiology Foundation Task Force on Clinical Expert Consensus Documents. *Circulation* (2008) 118, 1894–909.

Coumarins + Atovaquone

An isolated report describes a raised INR, which developed in a patient taking warfarin, after atovaquone was started.

Clinical evidence

A single case report describes a 53-year-old HIV-positive man taking atovaquone 1.5 g daily for prophylaxis of pneumocystis pneumonia, and warfarin for the treatment of pulmonary and venous emboli, whose INR rose from 2.3 to 3.5 after 7 days of concurrent use. His INR remained high (reaching 4.2) despite several decreases in his warfarin dose, but he did not report any adverse effects or signs of haemorrhage during this time. Approximately one month later the atovaquone was stopped, and the following day his INR fell to 1.7.[1]

Mechanism

Both warfarin and atovaquone are highly protein bound and the authors suggest that atovaquone may have displaced warfarin from its plasma protein binding site,[1] thereby increasing the concentration of free and active warfarin. However, protein-binding displacement is considered to only play a minor role in coumarin drug interactions (see *Anticoagulant interactions*, under 'Anticoagulants', p.371).

Importance and management

Information regarding an interaction between atovaquone and warfarin is limited to this single case report and other confounding factors were possibly involved (such as poor compliance, health status including alcohol and illicit drug consumption, and a lack of good historical INR data), making the general importance of this report unclear. Based on the available information, no specific precautions would seem necessary if atovaquone is given to patients taking warfarin, but bear the interaction in mind in the case of an unexpected response to treatment.

1. Hidalgo K, Lyles A, Dean SR. A potential interaction between warfarin and atovaquone. *Ann Pharmacother* (2011) 45, e3.

Coumarins + Azathioprine or Mercaptopurine

Large decreases in the effects of warfarin have been seen with concurrent use of azathioprine and mercaptopurine. A decrease in the effects of acenocoumarol has also been seen with mercaptopurine, and a decrease in the effects of phenprocoumon has been seen with azathioprine.

Clinical evidence

(a) Azathioprine

In a survey of 103 patients with antiphospholipid syndrome taking **warfarin**, the use of azathioprine appeared to increase **warfarin** requirements. Twelve of 26 patients (46%) requiring more than 10 mg of **warfarin** daily were taking azathioprine when compared with 15 of 77 patients (19%) requiring less than 10 mg **warfarin** daily.[1] There are a number of case reports of an interaction between coumarins and azathioprine. In one case, a woman who was resistant to **warfarin**, needing 14 to 17 mg daily while taking azathioprine, began to bleed (epistaxis, haematemesis) when the azathioprine was stopped. She was restabilised on **warfarin** 5 mg daily.[2] Reduced **warfarin** effects were seen in 2 other patients taking azathioprine,[3,4] one of whom had a sizeable fall in serum **warfarin** concentrations while taking azathioprine.[4] Two women with systemic lupus erythematosus taking **phenprocoumon**[5] and a third taking **warfarin**[6] had sizeable decreases in their INRs during treatment with azathioprine. Another woman needed an almost 4-fold increase in the dose of **warfarin** when she was given azathioprine.[7] In a retrospective analysis of patients with antiphospholipid syndrome admitted to hospital with serious bleeding, 3 patients taking azathioprine had a serious bleed, and in two of these cases the bleed occurred when their azathioprine dose was reduced.[8] In another case, a patient required about double the **warfarin** dose when her azathioprine dose was increased from 150 mg daily to 200 mg daily. Four weeks after the azathioprine was stopped abruptly because of suspected liver toxicity, her INR had increased from 1.8 to 14, and she had bruising and mild epistaxis.[9] A further case has been reported where a patient required a **warfarin** dose increase from 37.5 mg weekly to 112 mg weekly when azathioprine 150 mg daily was started in order to maintain an INR of 2.5.[10] In two other cases, sizeable warfarin dose increases were needed in patients given azathioprine.[11]

(b) Mercaptopurine

A man well stabilised on **warfarin** had a notable reduction in his anticoagulant response on two occasions while taking mercaptopurine 100 to 150 mg daily: the anticoagulant response returned when mercaptopurine was stopped. He had previously had no changes in anticoagulant response when receiving 6-week courses of single drugs, including **busulfan**, **cyclophosphamide**, **cytarabine**, **hydroxycarbamide**, **mitobronitol**, **demecolcine**, and **melphalan**.[12] A woman needed a large increase in her dose of **acenocoumarol**, from 21 mg weekly to 70 mg weekly, when she was given mercaptopurine 100 mg daily.[13] Another patient had a reduction in INR, from 3 to 1.1, two weeks after starting mercaptopurine and methotrexate. His **warfarin** requirements varied up to about 3-fold over 3 cycles of this chemotherapy, increasing during the mercaptopurine cycle and decreasing when in between cycles of treatment.[14]

Mechanism

Not well understood. From early studies in *rats*, it was concluded that mercaptopurine possibly increases the synthesis or activation of prothrombin, and that it does not alter the half-life, volume of distribution, or clearance of warfarin.[15] The authors of one case report noted a lower plasma warfarin concentration during the use of azathioprine in one patient.[4] Azathioprine is metabolised to mercaptopurine, and would therefore be expected to interact similarly.

Importance and management

Although the evidence is limited, it seems that mercaptopurine and azathioprine can greatly decrease the anticoagulant response to coumarins, and that the anticoagulant doses might need to be considerably increased to achieve adequate anticoagulation. It would therefore be prudent to closely monitor concurrent use.

Note that, from a disease perspective, when treating venous thromboembolic disease in patients with cancer, warfarin is generally inferior (higher risk of major bleeds and recurrent thrombosis) to low-molecular-weight heparins.

1. Khamashta MA, Cuadrado MJ, Mujic F, Taub N, Hunt BJ, Hughes GRV. Effect of azathioprine on the anticoagulant activity of warfarin in patients with the antiphospholipid syndrome. *Lupus* (1998) 7 (Suppl 2), S227.
2. Singleton JD, Conyers L. Warfarin and azathioprine: an important drug interaction. *Am J Med* (1992) 92, 217.
3. Rivier G, Khamashta MA, Hughes GRV. Warfarin and azathioprine: a drug interaction does exist. *Am J Med* (1993) 95, 342.
4. Rotenberg M, Levy Y, Shoenfeld Y, Almog S, Ezra D. Effect of azathioprine on the anticoagulant activity of warfarin. *Ann Pharmacother* (2000) 34, 120–2.
5. Jeppesen U, Rasmussen JM, Brøsen K. Clinically important interaction between azathioprine (Imurel) and phenprocoumon (Marcoumar). *Eur J Clin Pharmacol* (1997) 52, 503–4.
6. Walker J, Mendelson H, McClure A Smith MD. Warfarin and azathioprine: clinically significant drug interaction. *J Rheumatol* (2002) 29, 398–9.
7. Havrda DE, Rathbun S, Scheid D. A case report of warfarin resistance due to azathioprine and review of the literature. *Pharmacotherapy* (2001) 21, 355–7.
8. Castellino G, Cuadrado MJ, Godfrey T, Khamashta MA, Hughes GRV. Characteristics of patients with antiphospholipid syndrome with major bleeding after oral anticoagulant treatment. *Ann Rheum Dis* (2001) 60, 527–30.
9. Ng HJ, Crowther MA. Azathioprine and inhibition of the anticoagulant effect of warfarin: evidence from a case report and a literature review. *Am J Geriatr Pharmacother* (2006) 4, 75–7.
10. Vazquez SR, Rondina MT, Pendleton RC. Azathioprine-induced warfarin resistance. *Ann Pharmacother* (2008) 42, 1118–23.
11. Amato M, Mantha S, Corneau R, Sherry P, Tsapatsaris N. Azathioprine induced warfarin resistance: case reports and potential interaction mechanism. *J Thromb Thrombolysis* (2008) 25, 111.
12. Spiers ASD, Mibashan RS. Increased warfarin requirement during mercaptopurine therapy: a new drug interaction. *Lancet* (1974) ii, 221–2.
13. Fernández MA, Regadera A, Aznar J. Acenocoumarol and 6-mercaptopurine: an important drug interaction. *Haematologica* (1999) 84, 664–5.
14. Martin LA, Mehta SD. Diminished anticoagulant effects of warfarin with concomitant mercaptopurine therapy. *Pharmacotherapy* (2003) 23, 260–4.
15. Martini A, Jähnchen E. Studies in rats on the mechanisms by which 6-mercaptopurine inhibits the anticoagulant effect of warfarin. *J Pharmacol Exp Ther* (1977) 201, 547–53.

Coumarins + Azoles; Bifonazole or Econazole

Several case reports describe a raised INR and bleeding in patients taking warfarin and using topical econazole. One case report describes a raised INR in a patient taking warfarin and using bifonazole lotion. Two case reports describe markedly raised INRs in patients taking acenocoumarol and using econazole lotion.

Clinical evidence

(a) Bifonazole

An 85-year-old woman taking **warfarin** 4 mg daily was found to have an increased INR (greater than 5) within two days of starting to apply bifonazole cream 1% to her buttocks.[1]

(b) Econazole

A 79-year-old man, taking long-term **warfarin**, was given econazole cream for a fungal groin infection. Within one week of starting to apply the cream, he noticed bruising, including a large area on his hip, resulting from a trivial injury, and prolonged bleeding from a small cut.[2] His INR was found to have increased from 2.2 to 12. He was also taking glucosamine with chondroitin, which seems unlikely to have been responsible as this was not a new medication. Another report describes raised INRs (greater than 5) in 4 patients taking warfarin, which developed within a few days of starting to use topical econazole 1% (as a cream or lotion). In all four cases the econazole was applied to a fairly large area, and in two cases the area was occluded.[1]

An 84-year-old woman who had been stabilised on **acenocoumarol** for 10 years, was admitted to hospital with life-threatening laryngeal, sublingual and epiglottal haematomas 17 days after starting to use topical econazole lotion 1% three times daily for a dermatitis affecting 12% of her body surface. Her aPTT was found to be greater than 120 seconds and her INR exceeded laboratory limits. Prothrombin complex concentrate and vitamin K were given and her coagulation tests returned to normal after 36 hours. The acenocoumarol was substituted with aspirin and she was discharged 10 days later with no further problems.[3] A case report describes an 85-year-old woman taking **acenocoumarol** 1.25 mg daily who developed a raised INR following application of econazole 1% lotion and powder to the vulva and groin under occlusion. Oral vitamin K was given but her INR increased to above 14, until the econazole was stopped.[1]

Mechanism

Econazole is structurally similar to miconazole, an inhibitor of CYP2C9 and CYP3A4, which have major and minor roles, respectively, in warfarin metabolism. It seems likely that sufficient econazole was absorbed through the infected (and in some cases, occluded) skin to inhibit warfarin metabolism, leading to raised levels, and the increase in INR seen.

Importance and management

Evidence for an interaction between the coumarins and topical econazole and bifonazole is limited. The manufacturer notes that econazole normally has very low systemic bioavailability after topical application, and therefore clinically relevant interactions are rare.[4,5] Nevertheless, they advise increasing the frequency of monitoring in patients taking warfarin or acenocoumarol and given topical econazole. The French manufacturer of bifonazole states that only 1% of bifonazole is absorbed under occlusion when it is applied to healthy skin, but that this can be 4 to 5 times higher if the skin is inflamed.[6] In general, it would seem prudent to consider closer monitoring of the anticoagulant effects in any patient taking a coumarin if they need to use large amounts of econazole or bifonazole, especially on broken, damaged or occluded skin.

1. Alexandra J-F, Pautas E, Gouin-Thibault I, Siguret V, Loriet M-A. Overanticoagulation with coumarin and cutaneous azole therapy. *Ann Intern Med* (2008) 8, 633–5.
2. Lang PG, LeClercq AH. Increase in anticoagulant effect of warfarin in a patient using econazole cream. *J Am Acad Dermatol* (2006) 55, S117–S119.
3. Wey P-F, Petitjeans F, Lions C, Ould-Ahmed M, Escarment J. Laryngeal dyspnea in relation to an interaction between acenocoumarol and topical econazole lotion. *Am J Geriatr Pharmacother* (2008) 6, 173–7.
4. Pevaryl Topical Cream (Econazole nitrate). Janssen-Cilag Ltd. UK Summary of product characteristics, February 2011.
5. Gyno-Pevaryl Vaginal Pessaries (Econazole nitrate). Janssen-Cilag Ltd. UK Summary of product characteristics, March 2011.
6. Amycor (Bifonazole). Merck Serono. French Prescribing information, April 2011.

Coumarins + Azoles; Fluconazole

Fluconazole causes a dose-related reduction in the metabolism of warfarin, and increases its anticoagulant effect. Cases of minor to major bleeding have been reported, and one study found an increased risk of hospitalisation due to gastrointestinal bleeding in patients who had also taken fluconazole. There is one similar case report with acenocoumarol and fluconazole.

Clinical evidence

(a) Acenocoumarol

A patient stabilised on acenocoumarol suffered an intracranial haemorrhage (prothrombin time 170 seconds) 5 days after starting to take fluconazole 200 mg daily for the management of relapsed prosthetic valve candidal endocarditis.[1]

(b) Warfarin

1. Multiple-dose fluconazole. In a well-designed study in healthy subjects, fluconazole was given at three dose levels (100 mg, 200 mg, and 400 mg daily) for 14 days with a single dose of warfarin given both before fluconazole and on day 7. In this study, fluconazole potentiated the anticoagulant effect of warfarin in a dose-related manner. The duration of anticoagulant effect was 4 to 7 days for the single dose of warfarin alone, 5 to 9 days with fluconazole 100 mg daily, 6 to 11 days with fluconazole 200 mg daily, and 8 to 15 days with fluconazole 400 mg daily. Fluconazole increased the exposure of both *R*- and *S*-warfarin. With fluconazole 100 mg, 200 mg, and 400 mg, the AUC of *R*-warfarin was increased by 28%, 63%, and 70%, respectively, and that of *S*-warfarin by 35%, 86%, and 100%, respectively.[2] Two other studies in healthy subjects have found broadly similar results.[3-5]

The clinical importance of this interaction was shown in an earlier study, which found that when fluconazole 100 mg daily was given to 7 patients stabilised on warfarin, the prothrombin time increased from 15.8 seconds on day one, to 18.9 seconds on day 5, and 21.9 seconds on day 8. Fluconazole was stopped early in 3 of the patients due to high prothrombin times, but none exceeded an increase of more than 9.7 seconds, and no bleeding occurred.[6] In addition a retrospective case-control study in patients taking warfarin found that the risk of hospitalisation for gastrointestinal haemorrhage was increased in patients who had been given fluconazole 11 to 15 days before admission, when compared with those who had received cefalexin (adjusted odds ratio 2.09). In this study, cefalexin was used as a reference point to exclude the effect that illness requiring drug treatment could have on coagulation.[7] Similarly, a prospective case-control study using health insurance data found that use of azoles (including fluconazole) with **warfarin** was associated with an increased risk of bleeding (odds ratio 4.57, range 1.9 to 11.03). Antibacterial and antifungal use in general was associated with an overall increased risk of 2.01 (range 1.62 to 2.5), with the greatest risk being associated with use during the 60 days prior to the bleed occurring.[8]

At least 6 reports have described increased prothrombin times or INRs in patients stabilised on warfarin who took fluconazole in doses of 50 to 400 mg daily.[9-15] Several patients had haemorrhagic effects (gastrointestinal bleeding, melaena, ocular haemorrhage, spinal epidural haematoma).[9,11,13-15]

2. Single-dose fluconazole. Six women taking stable doses of warfarin with an INR between 2 and 3 were given a single 150-mg dose of fluconazole, and their prothrombin time measured on days 2, 5 and 8. The prothrombin time increased by 11% on day 2, by 34% on day 5, and by 2% on day 8: none of these differences was statistically significant. However, three of the women had an increase in INR to above 4 or had bleeding.[16]

Mechanism

In vitro studies using human liver microsomes clearly demonstrate that fluconazole inhibits the metabolism (7-hydroxylation) of *S*-warfarin by CYP2C9 and the metabolism of *R*-warfarin by CYP3A4, and possibly other isoenzymes involved in the metabolism of warfarin.[17] *In vivo*, this results in the accumulation of warfarin and in an increase in its effects, possibly leading to bleeding.[5]

Importance and management

An established and clinically important interaction. If fluconazole is given to patients taking warfarin or acenocoumarol the prothrombin times should be very well monitored and the anticoagulant dose reduced as necessary. On the basis of pharmacokinetic studies it has been predicted that the warfarin dose may need to be reduced, but the size of the reduction depends on the fluconazole dose being used. A reduction of about 20% may be required when using fluconazole 50 mg daily, whereas a reduction of about 70% may be required when using fluconazole 600 mg daily. These larger reductions should be made gradually over 5 days or so.[18] However, remember that individual variations between patients can be considerable and factors such as infection can also affect coagulation (see 'Coumarins + Antibacterials', p.383). Most of the available data relate to multiple-dose fluconazole, with just one small study with a single-dose of fluconazole 150 mg. Although the effect in this study was not as great as that for multiple-dose fluconazole, it suggests that careful monitoring of prothrombin times is still required.[16]

Ketoconazole (see 'Coumarins + Azoles; Ketoconazole', p.409) and itraconazole (see 'Coumarins + Azoles; Itraconazole', below), appear less likely to interact.

1. Isalska BJ, Stanbridge TN. Fluconazole in the treatment of candidal prosthetic valve endocarditis. *BMJ* (1988) 297, 178–9.
2. Neal JM, Kunze KL, Levy RH, O'Reilly RA, Trager WF. K_iIV, an in vivo parameter for predicting the magnitude of a drug interaction arising from competitive enzyme inhibition. *Drug Metab Dispos* (2003) 31, 1043–8.
3. Lazar JD, Wilner KD. Drug interactions with fluconazole. *Rev Infect Dis* (1990) 12 (Suppl 3), S327–S333.
4. Rieth H, Sauerbrey N. Interaktionsstudien mit Fluconazol, einem neuen Triazolantimykotikum. *Wien Med Wochenschr* (1989) 139, 370–4.
5. Black DJ, Kunze KL, Wienkers LC, Gidal BE, Seaton TL, McDonnell ND, Evans JS, Bauwens JE, Trager WF. Warfarin-fluconazole II. A metabolically based drug interaction: *in vivo* studies. *Drug Metab Dispos* (1996) 24, 422–8.
6. Crussell-Porter LL, Rindone JP, Ford MA, Jaskar DW. Low-dose fluconazole therapy potentiates the hypoprothrombinemic response of warfarin sodium. *Arch Intern Med* (1993) 153, 102–4.
7. Schelleman H, Bilker WB, Brensinger CM, Han X, Kimmel SE, Hennessy S. Warfarin with fluoroquinolones, sulfonamides or azole antifungals: interactions and the risk of hospitalization for gastrointestinal bleeding. *Clin Pharmacol Ther* (2008) 84, 581–8.
8. Baillargeon J, Holmes HM, Lin YL, Raji MA, Sharma G, Kuo YK. Concurrent use of warfarin and antibiotics and the risk of bleeding in older adults. *Am J Med* (2012) 125, 183–9.
9. Seaton TL, Celum CL, Black DJ. Possible potentiation of warfarin by fluconazole. *DICP Ann Pharmacother* (1990) 24, 1177–8.
10. Tett S, Carey D, Lee H-S. Drug interactions with fluconazole. *Med J Aust* (1992) 156, 365.
11. Kerr HD. Case report: potentiation of warfarin by fluconazole. *Am J Med Sci* (1993) 305, 164–5.
12. Gericke KR. Possible interaction between warfarin and fluconazole. *Pharmacotherapy* (1993) 13, 508–9.
13. Baciewicz AM, Menke JJ, Bokar JA, Baud EB. Fluconazole-warfarin interaction. *Ann Pharmacother* (1994) 28, 1111.
14. Mootha VV, Schluter ML, Das A. Intraocular hemorrhages due to warfarin-fluconazole drug interaction in a patient with presumed *Candida* endophthalmitis. *Arch Ophthalmol* (2002) 120, 94–5.
15. Allison EJ, McKinney TJ, Langenberg JN. Spinal epidural haematoma as a result of warfarin/fluconazole drug interaction. *Eur J Emerg Med* (2002) 9, 175–7.
16. Turrentine MA. Single dose fluconazole for vulvovaginal candidiasis; impact on prothrombin time in women taking warfarin. *Obstet Gynecol* (2006) 107, 310–3.
17. Kunze KL, Wienkers LC, Thummel KE, Trager WF. Warfarin-fluconazole I. Inhibition of the human cytochrome P450-dependent metablism of warfarin by fluconazole: *in vitro* studies. *Drug Metab Dispos* (1996) 24, 414–21.
18. Kunze KL, Trager WF. Warfarin-fluconazole III. A rational approach to management of a metabolically based drug interaction. *Drug Metab Dispos* (1996) 24, 429–35.

Coumarins + Azoles; Itraconazole

An isolated report describes a very large increase in the anticoagulant effects of warfarin, accompanied by bruising and bleeding, in a patient given itraconazole. One case suggests that itraconazole might increase the risk of over-anticoagulation with acenocoumarol or phenprocoumon.

Clinical evidence

A woman stabilised on **warfarin** 5 mg daily and also taking ipratropium bromide, salbutamol, budesonide, quinine sulfate, and omeprazole, was given itraconazole 200 mg twice daily for oral candidiasis caused by the inhaled steroid. Within

4 days she developed generalised bleeding and recurrent nosebleeds. Her INR had increased to more than 8. The **warfarin** and itraconazole were stopped, but the next day she had to be admitted to hospital for intractable bleeding and increased bruising, for which she was treated with fresh frozen plasma. Two days later, when the bleeding had stopped and her INR had returned to 2.4, she was restarted on **warfarin** and later restabilised on her original dose.[1] A prospective case-control study using health insurance data found that use of azoles (including itraconazole) with **warfarin** was associated with an increased risk of bleeding (odds ratio 4.57, range 1.9 to 11.03). Antibacterial and antifungal use in general was associated with an overall increased risk of 2.01 (range 1.62 to 2.5), with the greatest risk being associated with use during the 60 days prior to the bleed occurring.[2]

In one cohort study in patients taking **acenocoumarol** or **phenprocoumon**, itraconazole considerably increased the risk of over-anticoagulation (INR greater than 6: relative risk of 13.9, range 1.7 to 115). However, the authors say this figure should be interpreted cautiously since it was based on just one case.[3]

Mechanism

Itraconazole is a known inhibitor of CYP3A4, but this isoenzyme is involved only in the metabolism of the less potent *R*-warfarin, and therefore inhibition would not be expected to have an important effect on warfarin metabolism. However, there appear to be no pharmacological studies to confirm this. Omeprazole (see 'Coumarins + Proton pump inhibitors', p.464), might also have had some minor part to play in the case described.[1]

Importance and management

A minor to modest pharmacokinetic interaction would be predicted between itraconazole and the coumarins, but as yet there appear to be no studies to confirm this. The case report and cohort study suggest that this interaction might be clinically important in some individuals. However, the general importance of this interaction, if it occurs, is not clear. As such it would seem prudent to bear it in mind in cases of otherwise unexplained increase in INR, or signs of over-anticoagulation (bleeding, bruising) and manage accordingly. Further study is needed.

1. Yeh J, Soo S-C, Summerton C, Richardson C. Potentiation of action of warfarin by itraconazole. *BMJ* (1990) 301, 669.
2. Baillargeon J, Holmes HM, Lin YL, Raji MA, Sharma G, Kuo YF. Concurrent use of warfarin and antibiotics and the risk of bleeding in older adults. *Am J Med* (2012) 125, 183–9.
3. Visser LE, Penning-van Beest FJA, Kasbergen AAH, De Smet PAGM, Vulto AG, Hofman A, Stricker BHC. Overanticoagulation associated with combined use of antifungal agents and coumarin anticoagulants. *Clin Pharmacol Ther* (2002) 71, 496–502.

Coumarins + Azoles; Ketoconazole

Limited evidence suggests that the anticoagulant effect of warfarin is unchanged by ketoconazole. However, there are four isolated cases of an increase in the anticoagulant effects of warfarin with ketoconazole. Topical ketoconazole does not appear to interact with acenocoumarol or phenprocoumon.

Clinical evidence

(a) Systemic ketoconazole

Two healthy subjects had no changes in their anticoagulant response to **warfarin** when they were given ketoconazole 200 mg daily over a 3-week period.[1,2] However, an elderly woman, stabilised on **warfarin** for 3 years, complained of spontaneous bruising 3 weeks after starting a course of ketoconazole 200 mg twice daily. Her British Comparative Ratio was found to have risen from 1.9 to 5.4. Her liver function was normal. She was restabilised on her previous **warfarin** dose 3 weeks after the ketoconazole was withdrawn.[3] In 1984, the CSM in the UK had one report of an 84-year-old man taking **warfarin** whose British Comparative Ratio rose to 4.8 when he was given ketoconazole, and fell to 1.4 when it was withdrawn.[3] In 1986, the manufacturers of ketoconazole had one other report of an elderly man taking **warfarin** whose prothrombin time rose from a range of 34 to 39 seconds to over 60 seconds when he was given ketoconazole 400 mg daily.[4] Another case describes a 59-year-old man stabilised on **warfarin** 52.5 mg weekly, who was started on high-dose ketoconazole (400 mg three times daily) for prostate cancer. Upon initiation, his warfarin dose was reduced by 35% to avoid over-anticoagulation. However, on day 9 his INR was 3.82 and so his warfarin dose was reduced further to 30 mg weekly (a 43% reduction from baseline). On day 20 his INR was 3.16 and subsequently his INR was restabilised at target levels.[5] A prospective case-control study using health insurance data found that use of azoles (including ketoconazole) with **warfarin** was associated with an increased risk of bleeding (odds ratio 4.57, range 1.9 to 11.03). Antibacterial and antifungal use in general was associated with an overall increased risk of 2.01 (range 1.62 to 2.5), with the greatest risk being associated with use during the 60 days prior to the bleed occurring.[6]

(b) Topical ketoconazole

In one cohort study in patients taking **acenocoumarol** or **phenprocoumon**, topical ketoconazole did not increase the relative risk of over-anticoagulation (INR greater than 6; relative risk 1.1, range 0.3 to 4.3). However, this figure should be interpreted cautiously as it was based on just two patients.[7]

Mechanism

In a study in *rats*,[8] ketoconazole potentiated the anticoagulant effect of acenocoumarol, but at much higher doses than miconazole (which is known to interact, see 'Coumarins and related drugs + Azoles; Miconazole', below). It is now well-known that ketoconazole is an inhibitor of CYP3A4, but this isoenzyme has only a minor role in the metabolism of warfarin, specifically the less active *R*-isomer.

Importance and management

Information about this interaction seems to be limited to the reports cited. Its general importance and incidence is therefore uncertain, but it is probably quite small. However, it would seem prudent to bear the possibility of an interaction in mind should any unexplained increase in the coumarin anticoagulant effects occur in a patient given both drugs.

1. Brass C, Galgiani JN, Blaschke TF, Defelice R, O'Reilly RA, Stevens DA. Disposition of ketoconazole, an oral antifungal, in humans. *Antimicrob Agents Chemother* (1982) 21, 151–8.
2. Stevens DA, Stiller RL, Williams PL, Sugar AM. Experience with ketoconazole in three major manifestations of progressive coccidioidomycosis. *Am J Med* (1983) 74, 58–63.
3. Smith AG. Potentiation of oral anticoagulants by ketoconazole. *BMJ* (1984) 288, 188–9.
4. Janssen Pharmaceutical Limited. Personal communication, April 1986.
5. Jackevicius CA, Ton MN. Enhanced interaction between warfarin and high-dose keotoconazole: a case report. *Case Report Med* (2009) Epub.
6. Baillargeon J, Holmes HM, Lin YL, Raji MA, Sharma G, Kuo YF. Concurrent use of warfarin and antibiotics and the risk of bleeding in older adults. *Am J Med* (2012) 125, 183–9.
7. Visser LE, Penning-van Beest FJA, Kasbergen AAH, De Smet PAGM, Vulto AG, Hofman A, Stricker BHC. Overanticoagulation associated with combined use of antifungal agents and coumarin anticoagulants. *Clin Pharmacol Ther* (2002) 71, 496–502.
8. Niemegeers CJE, Levron JC, Awouters F, Janssen PAJ. Inhibition and induction of microsomal enzymes in the rat. A comparative study of four antimycotics: miconazole, econazole, clotrimazole and ketoconazole. *Arch Int Pharmacodyn Ther* (1981) 251, 26–38.

Coumarins and related drugs + Azoles; Miconazole

The anticoagulant effects of acenocoumarol, phenprocoumon, and warfarin can be greatly increased if miconazole is given orally as an oral (buccal) gel, and bleeding can occur. Oral miconazole has also been reported to interact with ethyl biscoumacetate, fluindione, phenindione, and tioclomarol in a few reports. The interaction has also rarely been seen in some women using intravaginal miconazole, and in those using a miconazole cream on the skin.

Clinical evidence

(a) Oral gel

In one early report, a patient with a prosthetic heart valve and stabilised on **warfarin** developed blood blisters and bruised easily 12 days after starting miconazole gel 250 mg four times a day for a presumed fungal mouth infection. Her prothrombin time ratio had increased from less than 3 to about 16. She was subsequently restabilised in the absence of miconazole on her former dose of **warfarin**.[1]

Numerous other cases of this interaction with **warfarin** have been reported, and, where stated, often involved the use of 5 mL (125 mg) of the gel four times daily for oral candidiasis.[2-14] However, cases have occurred with lower doses; one case of an increase in INR to 11.4 with frank haematuria and spontaneous bruising was reported in a woman who had used 30 g of non-prescription miconazole (*Daktarin*) over 8 days (estimated daily dose of 75 mg),[7] and three other cases have occurred with non-prescription miconazole.[13-15] In another case, the interaction occurred with use of the miconazole gel locally around the corners of the lips for angular cheilitis.[11]

In 1996, the New Zealand Centre for Adverse Reactions Monitoring reported 5 patients taking **warfarin** whose INRs increased from normal values to between 7.5 and 18 within 7 to 15 days of starting to use miconazole oral gel.[5] In 2002, the Australian Adverse Drug Reactions Advisory Committee (ADRAC) stated that they had received 18 reports of this interaction. In the 17 cases for which it was documented, the INR was above 7.5. Eight of the cases had bleeding complications, 9 required vitamin K, and 5 required fresh frozen plasma.[16] A small retrospective report found that in 32 patients stable taking warfarin and given miconazole oral gel the INR was increased from a mean of 2.44 (range of 1.92 to 3.18) to 8.8 (range of 4.9 to 16.9). The mean warfarin dose required by these patients was reduced (from 15.7 mg before to 10.8 mg after miconazole oral gel was started). Bleeding was reported in 15 patients.[17]

A few similar cases have also been reported for **acenocoumarol**[18-20] with miconazole oral gel. In addition, in one cohort study in patients taking **acenocoumarol** or **phenprocoumon**, the use of oral miconazole (form and doses not stated) greatly increased the risk of over-anticoagulation (INR greater than 6: adjusted relative risk 36.6; range 12.4 to 108). When analysed separately, the adjusted relative risk was higher for **acenocoumarol** than **phenprocoumon** (35.1 versus 16.5).[21]

A case has also been reported with the indanedione, **fluindione**.[22]

(b) Skin creams

An 80-year-old man stabilised on **warfarin** with an INR of 2.2 to 3.1 was found to have an INR of 21.4 at a routine check 2 weeks after starting to use miconazole cream for a fungal infection in his groin. He showed no evidence of bruising or bleeding.[23] In 2001, Health Canada reported that they had on record a case of an 80-year-old man taking **warfarin** and using topical miconazole who had a cerebral vascular accident, although this case was complicated by multiple medical conditions and medications.[24] In 2002, the Australian Adverse Drug Reactions Advisory Committee stated that they had received one report of an interaction involving topical miconazole cream.[16] Between April 2001 and July 2010, the Netherlands Pharmacovigilance Foundation (Lareb) received four case reports of patients (aged 59 to 80 years old) using topical miconazole who developed an increased INR. Two patients were taking **acenocoumarol**, and two were taking **phenprocoumon**.[25]

In one cohort study in patients taking **acenocoumarol** or **phenprocoumon**, the use of topical miconazole was associated with a small increased risk of over-anticoagulation (INR greater than 6: adjusted relative risk 1.4) but this was not statistically significant. Note that this was much lower than the increased risk seen with oral miconazole (relative risk 36.6).[21]

(c) Tablets

In a study in 6 healthy subjects, miconazole 125 mg daily for 18 days (in the form of *tablets*) caused a 5-fold increase in the prothrombin time response to a single dose of **warfarin** given on day 3. In addition, there was a 3-fold increase in the AUC of warfarin, with *S*-warfarin most affected (4-fold), and *R*-warfarin increased 1.7-fold.[26] In one early case report with warfarin, one patient with a prosthetic heart valve and stabilised on **warfarin** was found to have a prothrombin time ratio of 23.4 within 10 days of starting miconazole tablets 250 mg four times a day for a suspected fungal diarrhoea. He developed two haematomas soon after both drugs were withdrawn, and was subsequently restabilised, in the absence of miconazole, on his former dose of **warfarin**.[1]

The Centres de Pharmacovigilance Hospitalière in Bordeaux have on record 5 cases where miconazole (oral doses of 500 mg daily, where stated; form not mentioned) was responsible for a large increase in prothrombin times and/or bleeding (haematomas, haematuria, gastrointestinal bleeding) in patients taking the coumarins **acenocoumarol** (2 cases), **ethyl biscoumacetate** (1 case), and **tioclomarol** (1 case), and the indanedione **phenindione** (1 case).[27] Other cases and reports of this interaction involving **acenocoumarol** have been described elsewhere.[28-30]

(d) Vaginal dose forms

In 1999, the Netherlands Pharmacovigilance Foundation (Lareb) reported two elderly women patients taking **acenocoumarol** whose INRs increased sharply and rapidly when they were given miconazole pessaries 400 mg daily for 3 days.[31] Another report describes the development of bruising and an INR of almost 10 in a 55-year-old woman taking **warfarin** on the third day of using 200-mg miconazole pessaries. For a subsequent course of intravaginal miconazole 100 mg daily for 7 days, the dose of warfarin was decreased by 28%, and her INR was 3.27.[32] Yet another report describes haemorrhage of the kidney in a 52-year old woman taking **warfarin** after she used vaginal miconazole for 12 days.[24] An asymptomatic increase in INR (from 2 to 5) was seen in 50-year-old woman stabilised on **warfarin**, after she had used non-prescription vaginal miconazole cream for 5 days. Her INR returned to baseline after stopping the miconazole.[33] In one cohort study in patients taking **acenocoumarol** or **phenprocoumon**, the use of vaginal miconazole was associated with a small increased risk of over-anticoagulation (INR greater than 6: adjusted relative risk 4.3) but this was not statistically significant. Note that this was much lower than the increased risk seen with oral miconazole (relative risk 36.6).[21] A small retrospective case study found that in 3 patients stable taking warfarin and given intravaginal miconazole pessaries, the INR was increased from a mean of 3 to 4.9. The mean warfarin dose required by these patients was reduced (from 14.5 mg before, to 12 mg after, intravaginal miconazole was used).[17]

(e) Unspecified route

A prospective case-control study using health insurance data found that use of azoles (including miconazole) with **warfarin** was associated with an increased risk of bleeding (odds ratio 4.57, range 1.9 to 11.03). Antibacterial and antifungal use in general was associated with an overall increased risk of 2.01 (range 1.62 to 2.5), with the greatest risk being associated with use during the 60 days prior to the bleed occurring.[34]

Mechanism

Miconazole is an inhibitor of CYP2C9 by which *S*-warfarin is metabolised, and, to a lesser extent, it also inhibits the metabolism of *R*-warfarin, probably by inhibiting CYP3A4. Even low oral doses of miconazole (125 mg daily) greatly inhibit warfarin metabolism, so it is not surprising that prescription doses of miconazole oral gel (480 to 960 mg daily) interact, as the gel is swallowed after retaining in the mouth. Very unusually, the low absorption of miconazole from the vagina and even exceptionally through the skin, can result in increased anticoagulant effects. Acenocoumarol would be expected to be similarly affected.

Importance and management

The interaction of **miconazole oral gel** and **miconazole tablets** with the coumarins is a very well established and potentially serious interaction. Most of the reports are about warfarin or acenocoumarol, but many other coumarins and indanediones, have been implicated. In some cases the bleeding has taken 7 to 15 days to develop,[1,3,27] whereas others have bled within only 3 days.[29,32] Increased INRs have been seen even sooner. Given the extent of the interaction, usual prescription doses of miconazole oral gel (5 to 10 mL (120 to 240 mg) four times daily) should generally be avoided in patients taking any oral anticoagulant. Should concurrent use be necessary, prothrombin times should be closely monitored and suitable dose reductions made. The interaction has also been seen with non-prescription miconazole (one 30 g tube given over 8 days, or about 75 mg daily), which is not surprising in the context of the pharmacokinetic study, and suggests that patients taking coumarins and indanediones should also avoid using non-prescription miconazole. Nevertheless, the UK patient information leaflet for non-prescription *Daktarin* oral gel simply advises patients taking oral anticoagulants to talk to their doctor, and does not advise avoiding the product.[35] Nystatin and amphotericin are possible alternative antifungals to miconazole for mouth infections. However, note that one report suggests that nystatin might also interact with warfarin, see 'Coumarins + Nystatin', p.456.

An interaction with **intravaginal miconazole** would not normally be expected because its systemic absorption is usually very low (less than 2%) in healthy women of child-bearing age.[36] However, the reports cited above show that sufficient absorption to provoke an interaction can apparently occur in a few patients, particularly in those with conditions that allow increased absorption to occur (for example, in postmenopausal women with inflamed vaginal tissue). Appropriate monitoring is therefore needed even with this route of administration in potentially at-risk women taking coumarins.

Topical (cutaneous) miconazole would also not be expected to interact, but the case reports cited shows that some caution could be warranted, especially if applied to a large surface area, close to mucous membranes, to broken skin, and/or to skin under occlusion.

1. Watson PG, Lochan RG, Redding VJ. Drug interaction with coumarin derivative anticoagulants. *BMJ* (1982) 285, 1044–5.
2. Colquhoun MC, Daly M, Stewart P, Beeley L. Interaction between warfarin and miconazole oral gel. *Lancet* (1987) i, 695–6.
3. Bailey GM, Magee P, Hickey FM, Beeley L. Miconazole and warfarin interaction. *Pharm J* (1989) 242, 183.
4. Shenfield GM, Page M. Potentiation of warfarin action by miconazole oral gel. *Aust N Z J Med* (1991) 21, 928.
5. Pillans P, Woods DJ. Interaction between miconazole oral gel (Daktarin) and warfarin. *N Z Med J* (1996) 109, 346.
6. Ariyaratnam S, Thakker NS, Sloan P, Thornhill MH. Potentiation of warfarin anticoagulant activity by miconazole oral gel. *BMJ* (1997) 314, 349.
7. Evans J, Orme DS, Sedgwick ML, Youngs GR. Treating oral candidiasis: potentially fatal. *Br Dent J* (1997) 182, 452.
8. Marco M, Guy AJ. Retroperitoneal haematoma and small bowel intramural haematoma caused by warfarin and miconazole interaction. *Int J Oral Maxillofac Surg* (1997) 27, 485.
9. Pemberton MN, Sloan P, Ariyaratnam S, Thakker NS, Thornhill MH. Derangement of warfarin anticoagulation by miconazole oral gel. *Br Dent J* (1998) 184, 68–9.
10. Øgard CG, Vestergaad H. Interaktion mellem warfarin og oral miconazol-gel. *Ugeskr Laeger* (2000) 162, 5511.
11. Ezsiás A, Wojnarowska F, Juniper R. Topical use of miconazole antifungal oral gel on warfarinized patients: a word of caution. *Dent Update* (1997) 24, 421–2.
12. Silingardi M, Ghirarduzzi A, Tincani E, Iorio A, Iori I. Miconazole oral gel potentiates warfarin anticoagulant activity. *Thromb Haemost* (2000) 83, 794–5.
13. Pemberton MN, Oliver RJ, Theaker ED. Miconazole oral gel and drug interactions. *Br Dent J* (2004) 196, 529–31.
14. Baker S. Miconazole oral gel and warfarin. *Pharm J* (2008) 280, 308.
15. Spence C. Protect patients from harm. *Pharm J* (2008) 280, 656.
16. ADRAC. Miconazole oral gel elevates INR –a reminder. *Aust Adverse Drug React Bull* (2002) 21; 14–15.
17. Kovac M, Mitic G, Kovac Z. Miconazole and nystatin used as topical antifungal drugs interact equally strongly with warfarin. *J Clin Pharm Ther* (2012) 37, 45–8.
18. Marotel C, Cerisay D, Vasseur P, Rouvier B, Chabanne JP. Potentialisation des effets de l'acénocoumarol par le gel buccal de miconazole. *Presse Med* (1986) 15, 1684–5.
19. Ducroix JP, Smail A, Sevenet F, Andrejak M, Baillet J. Hématome oesophagien secondaire à une potentialisation des effets de l'acénocoumarol par le gel buccal de miconazole. *Rev Med Interne* (1989) 10, 557–9.
20. Ortín M, Olalla JI, Muruzábal MJ, Peralta FG, Gutiérrez MA. Miconazole oral gel enhances acenocoumarol anticoagulant activity: a report of three cases. *Ann Pharmacother* (1999) 33, 175–77.
21. Visser LE, Penning-van Beest FJA, Kasbergen AAH, De Smet PAGM, Vulto AG, Hofman A, Stricker BHC. Overanticoagulation associated with combined use of antifungal agents and coumarin anticoagulants. *Clin Pharmacol Ther* (2002) 71, 496–502.
22. Ponge T, Rapp MJ, Fruneau P, Ponge A, Wassen-Hove L, Larousse C, Cottin S. Interaction médicamenteuse impliquant le miconazole en gel et la fluindione. *Therapie* (1987) 42, 412–13.
23. Devaraj A, O'Beirne JP, Veasey R, Dunk AA. Interaction between warfarin and topical miconazole cream. *BMJ* (2002) 325, 77.
24. Anon. Miconazole-warfarin interaction: increased INR. *Can Med Assoc J* (2001) 165, 81.
25. Broos N, van Puijenbroek EP. Interactions between topical miconazole and coumarins. *Eur J Clin Pharmacol* (2010) 66, 1171–2.
26. O'Reilly RA, Goulart DA, Kunze KL, Neal J, Gibaldi M, Eddy AC, Trager WF. Mechanisms of the stereoselective interaction between miconazole and racemic warfarin in human subjects. *Clin Pharmacol Ther* (1992) 51, 656–67.
27. Loupi E, Descotes J, Lery N, Evreux J C. Interactions médicamenteuses et miconazole. *Therapie* (1982) 37, 437–41.
28. Anon. New possibilities in the treatment of systemic mycoses. Reports on the experimental and clinical evaluation of miconazole. Round table discussion and Chairman's summing up. *Proc R Soc Med* (1977), 70 (Suppl l), 51–4.
29. Ponge T, Barrier J, Spreux A, Guillou B, Larousse C, Grolleau JY. Potentialisation des effets de l'acénocoumarol par le miconazole. *Therapie* (1982) 37, 221–2.
30. Goenen M, Reynaert M, Jaumin P, Chalant CH, Tremouroux J. A case of candida albicans endocarditis three years after an aortic valve replacement. *J Cardiovasc Surg* (1977) 18, 391–6.
31. Lansdorp D, Bressers HPHM, Dekens-Konter JAM, Meyboom RHB. Potentiation of acenocoumarol during vaginal administration of miconazole. *Br J Clin Pharmacol* (1999) 47, 225–6.
32. Thirion DJ, Zanetti LAF. Potentiation of warfarin's hypoprothrombinemic effect with miconazole vaginal suppositories. *Pharmacotherapy* (2000) 20, 98–9.
33. Thomas JL, Dunn D, Pelletier A, Franks AS. Hyperprothrombinemia as a result of a possible warfarin and intravaginal miconazole interaction. *South Med J* (2010) 103, 1063–5.
34. Baillargeon J, Holmes HM, Lin YL, Raji MA, Sharma G, Kuo YF. Concurrent use of warfarin and antibiotics and the risk of bleeding in older adults. *Am J Med* (2012) 125, 183–9.
35. Daktarin Oral Gel (Miconazole). Janssen-Cilag Ltd. UK Patient information leaflet, July 2013.
36. Daneshmend TK. Systemic absorption of miconazole from the vagina. *J Antimicrob Chemother* (1986) 18, 507–11.

Coumarins + Azoles; Voriconazole

In one pharmacodynamic study, voriconazole approximately doubled the prothrombin time in response to warfarin.

Clinical evidence

In a placebo-controlled, crossover study, when 16 healthy subjects were given voriconazole 300 mg twice daily for 12 days, with a single 30-mg dose of **warfarin** on day 7, the maximal increase in prothrombin time was about doubled.[1] The increase in prothrombin time was still present 6 days after the **warfarin** dose when given with voriconazole, but had returned to baseline 6 days after the **warfarin** was given alone. Two subjects were withdrawn from the study because of an unacceptable increased prothrombin time.[1] A prospective case-control study using health insurance data found that use of azoles (including voriconazole) with **warfarin** was associated with an increased risk of bleeding (odds ratio 4.57, range 1.9 to 11.03). Antibacterial and antifungal use in general was associated with an overall increased risk of 2.01 (range 1.62 to 2.5), with the greatest risk being associated with use during the 60 days prior to the bleed occurring.[2]

Mechanism

Voriconazole is a known inhibitor of CYP2C9 and CYP3A4, by which the coumarins are metabolised, which results in an enhanced anticoagulant effect.

Importance and management

Evidence is limited to the one study, but given the magnitude of the effects seen, and the known inhibitory effects of voriconazole on the isoenzymes involved in the metabolism of the coumarins, the interaction is likely to be clinically important. If voriconazole is added to treatment with any coumarin, the prothrombin times should be more frequently monitored and the anticoagulant dose reduced as necessary.

1. Purkins L, Wood N, Kleinermans D, Nichols D. Voriconazole potentiates warfarin-induced prothrombin time prolongation. *Br J Clin Pharmacol* (2003) 56 (Suppl 1), 24–9.
2. Baillargeon J, Holmes HM, Lin YL, Raji MA, Sharma G, Kuo YK. Concurrent use of warfarin and antibiotics and the risk of bleeding in older adults. *Am J Med* (2012) 125, 183–9.

Coumarins + Barbiturates

The effects of the coumarins are substantially reduced by the barbiturates. Primidone is metabolised to phenobarbital and is expected to interact similarly.

Clinical evidence

(a) Phenobarbital

A study in 16 patients stabilised on **warfarin** found that when they were also given phenobarbital 2 mg/kg their average daily **warfarin** requirements rose over a 4-week period by 25% (from 5.7 to 7.1 mg daily).[1] In another study in patients stabilised on **warfarin**, phenobarbital 100 mg at night for 4 weeks reduced the mean prothrombin time by 13%.[2] In a prospective cohort study in children, the use of phenobarbital or carbamazepine was associated with a higher dose of **warfarin** to maintain the target INR (0.24 mg/kg versus 0.15 mg/kg).[3]

Other studies have found that phenobarbital causes a 29% or 46% reduction in the half-life of **warfarin**,[4,5] and that the reduction was similar for both *R*- and *S*-warfarin.[6] A retrospective analysis in patients taking **warfarin** revealed that the use of phenobarbital was associated with more erratic anticoagulation control, and that discontinuation of phenobarbital in a patient taking **warfarin** resulted in severe hypoprothrombinaemia and haematuria 2 weeks later.[7]

A reduced anticoagulant response has also been described in studies with phenobarbital and **dicoumarol**,[8-10] and 2 cases have been reported with phenobarbital and **ethyl biscoumacetate**.[11] One retrospective study[12] found that the concurrent use of enzyme inducers (including phenobarbital and **primidone**) significantly influenced the total weekly **warfarin** dose; further analysis found that an average additional amount of **warfarin** required in patients taking these drugs was 17.2 mg weekly.

In contrast, there is one isolated report of a woman stabilised on **warfarin** who developed haematuria 3 days after starting to take phenobarbital 60 mg four times daily.[13]

(b) Other barbiturates

An investigation in 12 patients taking either **warfarin** or **phenprocoumon** found that **secbutabarbital sodium**, 15 mg four times daily for the first week and 30 mg four times daily for the next 2 weeks, increased their anticoagulant requirements by 35 to 60%, reaching a maximum after 4 to 5 weeks.[14]

This interaction has also been described in pharmacological studies between:

- **acenocoumarol** and **pentobarbital**,[15] or **heptabarb**;[16]
- **dicoumarol** and **aprobarbitone**,[17] **heptabarb**,[16,18] or **vinbarbital**;[17]
- **ethyl biscoumacetate** and **heptabarb**;[16]
- **warfarin** and **amobarbital**,[19-21] **heptabarb**,[22] **secobarbital**,[2,19-21,23-25] or **secbutobarbital**.[14]

Cases have been described in patients taking **ethyl biscoumacetate** who were taking **amobarbital**, **heptabarb**, or **secobarbital**.[11] Cases have also been described of apparent resistance to coumarins in patients taking barbiturates,[17,26] and of bleeding in patients who were stabilised on a coumarin and a barbiturate when they stopped taking the barbiturate.[17,26,27]

Mechanism

Pharmacokinetic studies in man and *animals*[4,5,20-22,24] clearly show that the barbiturates are potent liver enzyme inducers, which increase the metabolism and clearance of the coumarins. The effect is similar on both *R*- and *S*-warfarin.[6,25] Barbiturates may also reduce the absorption of dicoumarol from the gut.[18]

Importance and management

The interactions between the coumarins and barbiturates are clinically important and very well documented. The reduced anticoagulant effects expose the patient to the risk of thrombus formation if the dose is not increased appropriately. A very large number of coumarin and barbiturate pairs have been found to interact and the others may be expected to behave similarly. The reduction in the anticoagulant effects begins within one week, sometimes within 2 to 4 days, reaching a maximum after about 3 weeks, and it may still be evident up to 6 weeks after stopping the barbiturate.[14] Patients' responses can vary considerably. Stable anticoagulant control can be re-established[28] in the presence of the barbiturate by increasing the anticoagulant dose by about 30 to 60%.[1,7,10,14] Care must be taken not to withdraw the barbiturate without also reducing the anticoagulant dose, otherwise over-anticoagulation will occur. Alternative non-interacting drugs, such as the benzodiazepines (see 'Coumarins + Benzodiazepines and related drugs', p.412), are now considered more appropriate sedatives than the barbiturates.

Primidone is metabolised to phenobarbital and is therefore expected to have a similar effect to phenobarbital. This is suggested by the findings of the retrospective study, and therefore, it would be prudent to be alert for reduced anticoagulant effects if primidone is given concurrently with a coumarin.

1. Robinson DS, MacDonald MG. The effect of phenobarbital administration on the control of coagulation achieved during warfarin therapy in man. *J Pharmacol Exp Ther* (1966) 153, 250–3.
2. Udall JA. Clinical implications of warfarin interactions with five sedatives. *Am J Cardiol* (1975) 35, 67–71.
3. Streif W, Marzinotto AV, Massicotte P, Chan AKC, Julian JA, Mitchell L. Analysis of warfarin therapy in pediatric patients: a prospective cohort study of 319 patients. *Blood* (1999) 94, 3007–14.
4. Corn M. Effect of phenobarbital and glutethimide on biological half-life of warfarin. *Thromb Diath Haemorrh* (1966) 16, 606–12.
5. MacDonald MG, Robinson DS, Sylwester D, Jaffe JJ. The effects of phenobarbital, chloral betaine, and glutethimide administration on warfarin plasma levels and hypoprothrombinemic responses in man. *Clin Pharmacol Ther* (1969) 10, 80–4.
6. Orme M, Breckenridge A. Enantiomers of warfarin and phenobarbital. *N Engl J Med* (1976) 295, 1482.
7. MacDonald MG, Robinson DS. Clinical observations of possible barbiturate interference with anticoagulation. *JAMA* (1968) 204, 97–100.
8. Corn M, Rockett JF. Inhibition of bishydroxycoumarin activity by phenobarbital. *Med Ann Dist Columbia* (1965) 34, 578–9, 588.
9. Cucinell SA, Conney AH, Sansur M, Burns JJ. Drug interactions in man. I. Lowering effect of phenobarbital on plasma levels of bishydroxycoumarin (Dicumarol) and diphenylhydantoin (Dilantin). *Clin Pharmacol Ther* (1965) 6, 420–9.
10. Goss JE, Dickhaus DW. Increased bishydroxycoumarin requirements in patients receiving phenobarbital. *N Engl J Med* (1965) 273, 1094–5.
11. Avellaneda M. Interferencia de los barbituricos en la accion del Tromexan. *Medicina (B Aires)* (1955) 15, 109–15.
12. Whitley HP, Fermo JD, Chumney ECG, Brzezinski WA. Effect of patient-specific factors on weekly warfarin dose. *Ther Clin Risk Manag* (2007) 3, 499–504.
13. Taylor PJ. Hemorrhage while on anticoagulant therapy precipitated by drug interaction. *Ariz Med* (1967) 24, 697–9.
14. Antlitz AM, Tolentino M, Kosai MF. Effect of butabarbital on orally administered anticoagulants. *Curr Ther Res* (1968) 10, 70–3.
15. Kroon C, de Boer A, Hoogkamer JFW, Schoemaker HC, vd Meer FJM, Edelbroek PM, Cohen AF. Detection of drug interactions with single dose acenocoumarol: new screening method? *Int J Clin Pharmacol Ther Toxicol* (1990) 28, 355–60.
16. Dayton PG, Tarcan Y, Chenkin T, Weiner M. The influence of barbiturates on coumarin plasma levels and prothrombin response. *J Clin Invest* (1961) 40, 1797–1802.
17. Johansson S-A. Apparent resistance to oral anticoagulant therapy and influence of hypnotics on some coagulation factors. *Acta Med Scand* (1968) 184, 297–300.
18. Aggeler PM, O'Reilly RA. Effect of heptabarbital on the response to bishydroxycoumarin in man. *J Lab Clin Med* (1969) 74, 229–38.
19. Breckenridge A, Orme M. Clinical implications of enzyme induction. *Ann N Y Acad Sci* (1971) 179, 421–31.
20. Robinson DS, Sylwester D. Interaction of commonly prescribed drugs and warfarin. *Ann Intern Med* (1970) 72, 853–6.
21. Whitfield JB, Moss DW, Neale G, Orme M, Breckenridge A. Changes in plasma γ-glutamyl transpeptidase activity associated with alterations in drug metabolism in man. *BMJ* (1973) 1, 316–18.
22. Levy G, O'Reilly RA, Aggeler PM, Keech GM. Pharmacokinetic analysis of the effect of barbiturate on the anticoagulant action of warfarin in man. *Clin Pharmacol Ther* (1970) 11, 372–7.
23. Feuer DJ, Wilson WR, Ambre JJ. Duration of effect of secobarbital on the anticoagulant effect and metabolism of warfarin. *Pharmacologist* (1974) 16, 195.
24. Breckenridge A, Orme ML'E, Davies L, Thorgeirsson SS, Davies DS. Dose-dependent enzyme induction. *Clin Pharmacol Ther* (1973) 14, 514–20.
25. O'Reilly RA, Trager WF, Motley CH, Howald W. Interaction of secobarbital with warfarin pseudoracemates. *Clin Pharmacol Ther* (1980) 28, 187–95.
26. Reverchon F, Sapir M. Constatation clinique d'un antagonisme entre barbituriques et anticoagulants. *Presse Med* (1961) 69, 1570–1.
27. Macgregor AG, Petrie JC and Wood RA. Therapeutic conferences. Drug interaction. *BMJ* (1971) 1, 389–91.
28. Williams JRB, Griffin JP, Parkins A. Effect of concomitantly administered drugs on the control of long term anticoagulant therapy. *Q J Med* (1976) 45, 63–73.

Coumarins + Benfluorex

Benfluorex does not alter the anticoagulant effects of phenprocoumon.

Clinical evidence, mechanism, importance and management

No significant changes occurred in the prothrombin times of 22 patients stabilised on **phenprocoumon** when they were given benfluorex 150 mg three times daily for 9 weeks, when compared with equivalent periods before and after taking benfluorex.[1]

1. De Witte P, Brems HM. Co-administration of benfluorex with oral anticoagulant therapy. *Curr Med Res Opin* (1980) 6, 478–80.

Coumarins and related drugs + Benzbromarone or Benziodarone

The anticoagulant effects of warfarin are increased by benzbromarone and bleeding has been seen. Similarly, the anticoagulant effects of acenocoumarol, ethyl biscoumacetate, diphenadione and warfarin are increased by benziodarone. Clorindione, dicoumarol and phenindione were not affected by benziodarone in one study. Phenprocoumon was not affected by benziodarone in one study, but was in another.

Clinical evidence

(a) Benzbromarone

The observation that 2 patients bled (haematuria, gastrointestinal bleeding) when given **warfarin** and benzbromarone, prompted a more detailed study in 7 other patients who were stabilised on both drugs. The thrombotest values of these 7 averaged 24.7% while taking both **warfarin** and benzbromarone (average dosage 57.1 mg daily), but when the benzbromarone was stopped for a week they rose to 47.3%. On restarting the benzbromarone the thrombotest values decreased to 30.3% (indicating an enhanced anticoagulant effect). The Factor II activity paralleled the thrombotest values. The total plasma **warfarin** levels were reduced during the period that benzbromarone was stopped.[1] Another later study found that the **warfarin** requirements of 13 patients given benzbromarone 50 mg daily were 36% lower than in 18 other patients given **warfarin** alone (3.9 versus 2.5 mg daily). The oral clearance of *S*-warfarin was 54% lower in the benzbromarone recipients, but the clearance of *R*-warfarin did not differ between the groups.[2] These two studies confirm observations in other patients with prosthetic valve replacements who had haemorrhagic tendencies when given both drugs.[1]

Early information about benzbromarone noted that no increase in the anticoagulant effects of the coumarins **acenocoumarol** and **ethyl biscoumacetate** or the indanedione **phenindione** had been seen in a few patients also given benzbromarone.[3]

(b) Benziodarone

Benziodarone 200 mg three times daily for 2 days then 100 mg three times daily thereafter was given to 90 patients taking various anticoagulants. To maintain constant prothrombin-proconvertin percentages the coumarin anticoagulant doses were reduced as follows: **ethyl biscoumacetate** 17% (9 patients), **acenocoumarol** 25% (7) and **warfarin** 46% (15). No changes in dose were needed in patients taking **dicoumarol** (9) or **phenprocoumon** (8). For the indanedione anticoagulants, a dose reduction of 42% was required in 8 patients taking **diphenadione**, but no changes were needed in those taking **clorindione** (5 patients) or **phenindione** (10 patients).[4] A parallel study in healthy subjects also found that benziodarone 300 mg or 600 mg daily increased the effects of a single dose of **warfarin**.[4]

In another study, benziodarone 300 to 600 mg daily increased the anticoagulant effects of **phenprocoumon** in just 9 out of 29 patients.[5] Plasma levels of **ethyl biscoumacetate** after a single intravenous dose were increased by pre-treatment with benziodarone 600 mg daily for 6 days.[5]

Mechanism

Benzbromarone selectively inhibits the metabolism of *S*-warfarin by the cytochrome P450 isoenzyme CYP2C9 so that its effects are increased. The metabolism of the *R*-warfarin remains unchanged.[2] Acenocoumarol and phenprocoumon are also known to be metabolised by CYP2C9, and would therefore be expected to interact similarly. Benziodarone is another benzofuran derivative with a similar structure to benzbromarone, and therefore probably interacts by a similar mechanism.

Importance and management

The interaction between warfarin and benzbromarone or benziodarone is established and clinically important. If benzbromarone is given to a patient taking warfarin, monitor prothrombin times and be alert for the need to reduce the dosage by about one-third to prevent over-anticoagulation. Information about other coumarins is limited, but what is known about the mechanism of action suggests that acenocoumarol and phenprocoumon would also be predicted to interact, and this has been shown for benziodarone and acenocoumarol or phenprocoumon, in a few patients. The limited evidence suggesting an interaction with some indanediones also suggests that some caution is appropriate with these drugs as well.

1. Shimodaira H, Takahashi K, Kano K, Matsumoto Y, Uchida Y, Kudo T. Enhancement of anticoagulant action by warfarin-benzbromarone interaction. *J Clin Pharmacol* (1996) 36, 168–74.
2. Takahashi H, Sato T, Shimoyama Y, Shioda N, Shimizu T, Kubo S, Tamura N, Tainaka H, Yasumori T, Echizen H. Potentiation of anticoagulant effect of warfarin caused by enantioselective metabolic inhibition by the uricosuric agent benzbromarone. *Clin Pharmacol Ther* (1999) 66, 569–81.
3. Masbernard A. Quoted as personal communication (1977) by Heel RC, Brogden RN, Speight TM, Avery GS. Benzbromarone: a review of its pharmacological properties and therapeutic use in gout and hyperuricaemia. *Drugs* (1977) 14, 349–66.
4. Pyörälä K, Ikkala E, Siltanen P. Benziodarone (Amplivix®) and anticoagulant therapy. *Acta Med Scand* (1963) 173, 385–9.
5. Verstraete M, Vermylen J, Claeys H. Dissimilar effect of two anti-anginal drugs belonging to the benzofuran group on the action of coumarin derivatives. *Arch Int Pharmacodyn Ther* (1968) 176, 33–41.

Coumarins + Benzethonium chloride

A rise in INR occurred in a couple who took a grapefruit seed extract product containing considerable amounts of the preservative benzethonium chloride for three days, and one of them developed a minor haematoma.

Clinical evidence

A couple, both well stabilised on warfarin, took some drops of a grapefruit seed extract product (*Estratto di Semillas di Pompelmo*, Lakshmi, Italy) for 3 days. No more was taken, but after a further 3 days the woman developed a minor subcutaneous haematoma, and her INR was found to be 7.9. The man was found to have an INR of 5.1, with no evidence of bleeding.[1]

Mechanism

The product used was stated to contain grapefruit seed extract, glycerol and water. However, chemical analysis of this product revealed that it also contained considerable amounts (77 mg/mL) of the preservative, benzethonium chloride, and did not contain any significant amount of natural substances from grapefruit seeds. The constituents of two other commercial grapefruit seed products were similar on analysis (*Citroseed* and *Citricidal*).

Further, *in vitro* analysis found that benzethonium chloride, and the three products, were potent inhibitors of the cytochrome P450 isoenzyme CYP2C9, suggesting that they could inhibit the metabolism of warfarin.

Importance and management

Data presented in this report, and other papers (one of which is cited as an example[2]), suggests that the primary constituent of many grapefruit seed extract products appears to be the preservative benzethonium chloride. The evidence from the two cases, backed by *in vitro* data, suggests that this has the potential to interact with warfarin. On this basis, it would probably be prudent for patients taking warfarin to avoid grapefruit seed extract products, or for concurrent use to be monitored closely. Some caution might also be appropriate with other pharmaceutical preparations containing benzethonium chloride.

1. Brandin H, Myrberg O, Rundlöf T, Arvidsson AK, Brenning G. Adverse effects by artificial grapefruit seed extract products in patients on warfarin therapy. *Eur J Clin Pharmacol* (2007) 63, 565–70.
2. Takeoka G, Dao L, Wong RY, Lundin R, Mahoney N. Identification of benzethonium chloride in commercial grapefruit seed extracts. *J Agric Food Chem* (2001) 49, 3316–20.

Coumarins + Benzodiazepines and related drugs

A large number of combinations of coumarins and benzodiazepines have been studied, without finding any evidence of an adverse interaction. An interaction between any coumarin and a benzodiazepine is therefore unlikely, but there are three unexplained and unconfirmed cases of increased or decreased anticoagulant responses, which were attributed to an interaction.

Clinical evidence

A. Benzodiazepines

(a) Chlordiazepoxide

In a placebo-controlled study in 7 patients stabilised on **warfarin**, chlordiazepoxide 10 mg three times daily for 2 weeks had no effect on anticoagulant control.[1] Other studies in healthy subjects[2,3] and patients[4] have similarly found that chlordiazepoxide does not alter the anticoagulant effect or the half-life of **warfarin**. Similarly, chlordiazepoxide 10 mg three times daily for 10 days had no effect on the half-life of a single intravenous dose of **ethyl biscoumacetate** in healthy subjects.[5] However, one patient stabilised on warfarin had a small 18% fall in mean plasma **warfarin** levels with a corresponding change in the anticoagulant response when given chlordiazepoxide 15 mg daily.[6]

(b) Diazepam

In 4 patients stabilised on **warfarin**, diazepam 5 mg three times daily for 30 days had no effect on anticoagulant control (thrombotest). In one of the patients, the half-life of **warfarin** was measured, and this was not changed by diazepam.[4] Similarly, diazepam 5 mg daily did not alter the anticoagulant response or the half-life of a single dose of **warfarin** in healthy subjects.[3]

However, there are two discordant reports. A patient stabilised on **dicoumarol** developed multiple ecchymoses and a prothrombin time of 53 seconds within 2 weeks of starting to take **diazepam** 5 mg four times daily.[7] The New Zealand Committee on Adverse Drug Reactions has received one report of an increased anticoagulant effect in a patient taking **warfarin** with **diazepam**.[8] It is by no means certain that these responses were due to an interaction.

(c) Flurazepam

In healthy subjects, flurazepam 30 mg at bedtime for 28 days had no effect on the half-life of a single dose of **warfarin** given on days 14 and 28, but there was a slight statistically significant reduction in prothrombin time. In a further placebo-controlled study in 12 patients stabilised on **warfarin**, flurazepam 30 mg at night for 28 days had no effect on prothrombin time or plasma warfarin concentrations.[9]

(d) Midazolam

In a pharmacokinetic study in 12 healthy subjects, **warfarin** and midazolam were given together as probe substrates for the cytochrome P450 isoenzymes CYP2C9 and CYP3A4, respectively. The *S*-warfarin AUC and midazolam plasma clearance were not altered by concurrent use.[10]

(e) Nitrazepam

In two reports by the same researchers, nitrazepam 10 mg at night for 30 days had no effect on steady-state **warfarin** levels or anticoagulant control in a few patients stabilised on **warfarin**.[4,6] In a placebo-controlled study in 22 patients stabilised on **phenprocoumon**, nitrazepam 5 mg at night for 2 weeks had no effect on thrombotest times.[11]

(f) Oxazepam

Oxazepam 10 mg in the morning and 10 to 20 mg in the evening for 3 weeks had no effect on anticoagulant response in 21 patients stabilised on **phenprocoumon**.[12]

B. Non-benzodiazepine hypnotics

(a) Eszopiclone

In a study in healthy subjects, eszopiclone 3 mg daily for 5 days had no effect on the AUC of *S*- or *R*-warfarin after a single 25-mg dose of **warfarin** and there was no change in the INR.[13]

(b) Zaleplon

In a study in healthy subjects, zaleplon 20 mg daily for 12 days had no effect on the AUC of *S*- or *R*-warfarin after a single 25-mg dose of **warfarin**. There was a minor 17% increase in the maximum serum levels of *S*-warfarin. However, zaleplon did not alter the prothrombin time response to **warfarin**.[14,15]

(c) Zolpidem

The prothrombin times of 8 healthy subjects given **warfarin** were unaffected by zolpidem 20 mg daily for 4 days.[16]

Mechanism

The three discordant reports describing an interaction are not understood. Enzyme induction is a possible explanation in one case with chlordiazepoxide,[6] because increases in the urinary excretion of 6-beta-hydroxycortisol (a marker of enzyme induction) have been described during chlordiazepoxide use.[4,6]

Importance and management

The weight of evidence and common experience shows that the benzodiazepines do not interact with the coumarins. Not all of the coumarins and benzodiazepines have been examined, but none of the possible pairs would be expected to interact. Similarly, based on pharmacodynamic studies, no interaction would be anticipated with the newer non-benzodiazepine hypnotics eszopiclone, zaleplon or zolpidem. As eszopiclone is metabolised to **zopiclone**, an interaction between zopiclone and warfarin would also not be expected, although there is no published data to confirm this.

1. Lackner H, Hunt VE. The effect of Librium on hemostasis. *Am J Med Sci* (1968) 256, 368–72.
2. Robinson DS, Sylwester D. Interaction of commonly prescribed drugs and warfarin. *Ann Intern Med* (1970) 72, 853–6.
3. Solomon HM, Barakat MJ, Ashley CJ. Mechanisms of drug interaction. *JAMA* (1971) 216, 1997–9.
4. Orme M, Breckenridge A, Brooks RV. Interactions of benzodiazepines with warfarin. *BMJ* (1972) 3, 611–14.
5. van Dam FE, Gribnau-Overkamp MJH. The effect of some sedatives (phenobarbital, gluthetimide, chlordiazepoxide, chloral hydrate) on the rate of disappearance of ethyl biscoumacetate from the plasma. *Folia Med Neerl* (1967) 10, 141–5.
6. Breckenridge A, Orme M. Clinical implications of enzyme induction. *Ann N Y Acad Sci* (1971) 179, 421–31.
7. Taylor PJ. Hemorrhage while on anticoagulant therapy precipitated by drug interaction. *Ariz Med* (1967) 24, 697–9.
8. McQueen EG. New Zealand Committee on Adverse Drug Reactions: Ninth Annual Report 1974. *N Z Med J* (1974) 80, 305–11.
9. Robinson DS, Amidon EL. Interaction of benzodiazepines with warfarin in man. In: Garattini S, Mussini E, Randall LO, eds. The Benzodiazepines. New York: Raven Press, 1973. p. 641–6.
10. Chainuvati S, Nafziger AN, Leeder JS, Gaedigk A, Kearns GL, Sellers E, Zhang Y, Kashuba AD, Rowland E, Bertino JS. Combined phenotypic assessment of cytochrome p450 1A2, 2C9, 2C19, 2D6, and 3A, N-acetyltransferase-2, and xanthine oxidase activities with the "Cooperstown 5+1 cocktail". *Clin Pharmacol Ther* (2003) 74, 437–47.
11. Bieger R, De Jonge H, Loeliger EA. Influence of nitrazepam on oral anticoagulation with phenprocoumon. *Clin Pharmacol Ther* (1972) 13, 361–5.
12. Schneider J, Kamm G. Beeinflußt Oxazepam (Adumbran®) die Antikoagulanzientherapie mit Phenprocoumon? *Med Klin* (1978) 73, 153–6.
13. Maier G, Roach J, Rubens R. Evaluation of pharmacokinetic and pharmacodynamic interactions between eszopiclone and warfarin. *Sleep* (2004) 27 (Suppl), A56.
14. Darwish M. Overview of drug interaction studies with zaleplon. Poster presented at 13th Annual Meeting of Associated Professional Sleep Studies (APSS), Orlando, Florida, June 23rd, 1999.
15. Darwish M. Analysis of potential drug interactions with zaleplon. *J Am Geriatr Soc* (1999) 47, S62.
16. Sauvanet JP, Langer SZ, Morselli PL, eds. Imidazopyridines in Sleep Disorders. New York: Raven Press; 1988 p. 165–73.

Coumarins and related drugs + Beta blockers

The effects of the coumarins are not normally altered by any beta blocker. However, propranolol has caused small increases in warfarin levels in a couple of studies, and an isolated case described an increased INR in a patient taking warfarin and propranolol.

Clinical evidence

(a) Acenocoumarol

In a study in 4 patients stabilised on acenocoumarol there was no difference in anticoagulation tests when **atenolol** 100 mg daily, **metoprolol** 100 mg twice daily, or placebo, was given for 3 weeks.[1]

(b) Phenindione

In one early clinical study, haemorrhagic tendencies without any changes in Quick value or any other impairment of coagulation were described in three patients stabilised on phenindione within 6 weeks of starting **propranolol**.[2]

(c) Phenprocoumon

In healthy subjects, a single dose of **atenolol** 100 mg or **metoprolol** 100 mg did not affect the AUC of a single dose of phenprocoumon, although phenprocoumon levels were slightly higher at 4 and 6 hours after the **metoprolol** dose. Nevertheless, neither beta blocker altered the prothrombin time response.[3]

In healthy subjects, **carvedilol** 25 mg daily for 7 days had no effect on the pharmacokinetics of a single 15-mg dose of phenprocoumon given on day 5 phenprocoumon.[4]

In 12 patients stabilised on phenprocoumon, there was no difference in Quick time between those randomised to receive **pindolol** 5 mg three times daily for 6 weeks and those who received placebo.[5]

(d) Warfarin

In 6 patients stabilised on warfarin, **acebutolol** 300 mg three times daily for 3 days had no effect on prothrombin time response.[6] Similarly, in one patient taking warfarin, neither **atenolol** 100 mg daily nor **metoprolol** 100 mg twice daily for 3 weeks had any effect on prothrombin time.[1] Similarly, in studies in healthy subjects the following beta blockers had no clinically relevant effects on the pharmacokinetics and/or anticoagulant response to warfarin; **atenolol** 100 mg daily,[7] **betaxolol** 20 mg daily,[8] **bisoprolol** 10 mg daily,[9] **esmolol**,[10] **metoprolol** 100 mg twice daily[7] or **nebivolol** 10 mg daily.[11]

In contrast, the minimum steady-state plasma **warfarin** levels of 6 healthy subjects rose by 15% when they took **propranolol** 80 mg twice daily in one study.[12] Similarly, in another study in 6 healthy subjects given **propranolol** 80 mg twice daily for 7 days with a single dose of warfarin on day 4, the AUC of warfarin was increased by about 16% and the in maximum serum level was increased by 23%, but there was no change in the prothrombin time.[7] A patient stabilised on **warfarin** had a rise in his British Corrected Ratio from a low of 1.3 up to 2.5 while taking **propranolol** 80 mg twice daily.[13]

Mechanism

None known.

Importance and management

Overall, the findings of these pharmacological studies in patients and healthy subjects confirm the general clinical experience that the effects of the coumarins are not normally altered by the beta blockers. No special precautions are needed on concurrent use. The only uncertainty is with propranolol, which has caused a small rise in warfarin levels in two studies, and for which there is one case report describing an increased INR with warfarin. Even so, a clinically significant interaction would seem to be extremely rare.

1. Mantero F, Procidano M, Vicariotto MA , Girolami A. Effect of atenolol and metoprolol on the anticoagulant activity of acenocoumarin. *Br J Clin Pharmacol* (1984) 17 (Suppl), 94S–96S.
2. Neilson GH, Seldon WA. Propranolol in angina pectoris. *Med J Aust* (1969) 1, 856–57.
3. Spahn H, Kirch W, Mutschler E, Ohnhaus EE, Kitteringham NR, Lögering HJ, Paar D. Pharmacokinetic and pharmacodynamic interactions between phenprocoumon and atenolol or metoprolol. *Br J Clin Pharmacol* (1984) 17, 97S–102S.
4. Harder S, Brei R, Caspary S, Merz PG. Lack of a pharmacokinetic interaction between carvedilol and digitoxin or phenprocoumon. *Eur J Clin Pharmacol* (1993) 44, 583–6.
5. Vinazzer H. Effect of the beta-receptor blocking agent Visken® on the action of coumarin. *Int J Clin Pharmacol* (1975) 12, 458–60.
6. Ryan JR. Clinical pharmacology of acebutolol. *Am Heart J* (1985) 109, 1131–6.
7. Bax NDS, Lennard MS, Tucker GT, Woods HF, Porter NR, Malia RG, Preston FE. The effect of β-adrenoceptor antagonists on the pharmacokinetics and pharmacodynamics of warfarin after a single dose. *Br J Clin Pharmacol* (1984) 17, 553–7.
8. Thiercelin JF, Warrington SJ, Thenot JP, Orofiamma B. Lack of interaction of betaxolol on warfarin induced hypocoagulability. In: Aiache JM, Hirtz J, eds. Proc 2nd Eur Cong Biopharm Pharmacokinet Vol III: Clinical Pharmacokinetics. Paris: Imprimerie de l'Université de Clermont Ferrand; 1984. pp 73–80.
9. Warrington SJ, Johnston A, Lewis Y, Murphy M. Bisoprolol: studies of potential interactions with theophylline and warfarin in healthy volunteers. *J Cardiovasc Pharmacol* (1990) 16 (Suppl 5), S164–S168.
10. Lowenthal DT, Porter RS, Saris SD, Bies CM, Slegowski MB, Staudacher A. Clinical pharmacology, pharmacodynamics and interactions with esmolol. *Am J Cardiol* (1985) 56, 14F–17F.
11. Lawrence TE, Liu S, Bland TM, Chervenick SW, Huang MY, Rackley RJ. Single-dose pharmacokinetics and anticoagulant activity of warfarin is unaffected by nebivolol in healthy volunteers. *Clin Pharmacol Ther* (2005) 77, P39.
12. Scott AK, Park BK, Breckenridge AM. Interaction between warfarin and propranolol. *Br J Clin Pharmacol* (1984) 17, 559–64.
13. Bax NDS, Lennard MS, Al-Asady S, Deacon CS, Tucker GT, Woods HF. Inhibition of drug metabolism by β-adrenoceptor antagonists. *Drugs* (1983) 25 (Suppl 2), 121–6.

Coumarins + Bicalutamide, Flutamide, or Nilutamide

A few cases have been reported of flutamide possibly increasing the anticoagulant effects of warfarin. Based on limited *in vitro* evidence, it has been predicted that bicalutamide and nilutamide might interact with coumarins.

Clinical evidence and mechanism

(a) Bicalutamide

The manufacturers say that *in vitro* studies show that bicalutamide can displace **warfarin** from its protein binding sites.[1,2] It used to be thought that the displacement of **warfarin** from its protein binding sites by other drugs normally resulted in clinically important interactions, but that is now known to rarely be true (see 'Protein-binding interactions', p.3). In 1995, the manufacturers said that they did not know of any reports of an interaction between **warfarin** and bicalutamide, apart from an isolated case of a raised INR in one patient taking **warfarin** with bicalutamide 150 mg, but no causal link with bicalutamide was established.[3] In a clinical study of bicalutamide and finasteride, it was briefly stated that one patient developed a prolonged prothrombin time while also taking **warfarin**.[4] To date, there appear to be no other published cases of an interaction.

(b) Flutamide

In 1990, the manufacturer had 5 cases on record of patients with prostatic cancer receiving **warfarin** whose prothrombin times had increased when they were given flutamide. For example, one patient needed reductions in his **warfarin** dose from 35 mg weekly to 22.5 mg weekly over a 2-month period. Another had a prothrombin time rise from 15 seconds to 37 seconds within 4 days of starting flutamide 750 mg daily.[5] There appears to be no published information about this interaction.

(c) Nilutamide

The manufacturer notes that, *in vitro*, nilutamide has been shown to inhibit cytochrome P450 isoenzymes (specific isoenzymes not stated). Because of this, they suggest that nilutamide might increase the toxicity of drugs with a low therapeutic margin such as the vitamin K antagonists (i.e. **coumarins** and **indanediones**). There appears to be no published information about this interaction.

Importance and management

No interaction is established, and had there been any interaction, it might have been expected to come to light by now. The lack of any published case reports suggests that there is little reason to believe that these non-steroidal anti-androgens specifically interact with warfarin. Despite this, the manufacturers of bicalutamide, flutamide and nilutamide recommend that the prothrombin time be carefully monitored when these drugs are given with coumarins, adjusting the dose when necessary.[1,2,6,7]

Consider also that, from a disease perspective, when treating venous thromboembolic disease in patients with cancer, warfarin is generally inferior (higher risk of major bleeds and recurrent thrombosis) to low-molecular-weight heparins.[8]

1. Casodex 50 mg Film-coated Tablets (Bicalutamide). AstraZeneca UK Ltd. UK Summary of product characteristics, January 2011.
2. Casodex (Bicalutamide). AstraZeneca. US Prescribing information, November 2009.
3. Zeneca. Personal Communication, October 1995.
4. Tay M-H, Kaufman DS, Regan MM, Leibowitz SB, George DJ, Febbo PG, Manola J, Smith MR, Kaplan ID, Kantoff PW, Oh WK. Finasteride and bicalutamide as primary hormonal therapy in patients with advanced adenocarcinoma of the prostate. *Ann Oncol* (2004) 15, 974–8.
5. Schering-Plough Ltd. Personal communication, March 1990.
6. Drogenil (Flutamide). Schering-Plough Ltd. UK Summary of product characteristics, August 2007.
7. Nilandron (Nilutamide). Sanofi-Aventis US LLC. US Prescribing information, June 2006.
8. Baglin TP, Keeling DM, Watson HG, for the British Committee for Standards in Haematology. Guidelines on oral anticoagulation (warfarin): third edition – 2005 update. *Br J Haematol* (2005) 132, 277–85.

Coumarins and related drugs + Bile-acid binding resins

The anticoagulant effects of phenprocoumon and warfarin can be reduced by colestyramine. Conversely, an isolated report describes unexpected sensitivity to warfarin in a patient taking colestyramine, which was attributed to a possible reduction in vitamin K absorption with colestyramine. Colestipol does not alter the absorption or effect of phenprocoumon or warfarin, and colesevelam does not alter the pharmacokinetics of warfarin.

Clinical evidence

(a) Colesevelam

In a single-dose study in 24 healthy subjects, colesevelam 4.5 g had no effect on the pharmacokinetics of **warfarin** 10 mg.[1]

(b) Colestipol

In a placebo-controlled, single-dose study in 4 healthy subjects, **phenprocoumon** plasma levels and the prothrombin response were unaffected by colestipol 8 g given at the same time as **phenprocoumon** 12 mg.[2] Similarly, in a study in healthy subjects quoted in a review,[3] the concurrent use of colestipol 10 g did not cause any changes in the absorption of a single 10-mg dose of **warfarin**.

The long-term use of colestipol might have the potential to decrease fat soluble vitamins such as vitamin K, which result in a prolonged prothrombin time,[4] and thereby increase the effect of warfarin. However, the manufacturers report that in a study, the use of colestipol resulted in a prolonged prothrombin time in only one patient.[4]

(c) Colestyramine

1. Phenprocoumon. It was noted that establishing effective anticoagulation was difficult in patients taking phenprocoumon with colestyramine, in spite of doubling the dose of phenprocoumon. This prompted a study in healthy subjects in which it was found that concurrent single doses of phenprocoumon and colestyramine markedly reduced the plasma levels and effect of phenprocoumon.[5] In another study using *intravenous* phenprocoumon, colestyramine reduced the effect of the anticoagulant by this route, presumably by reducing enterohepatic recycling.[6] This fact has been used clinically to enhance the elimination of phenprocoumon after phenprocoumon overdose. In one case, the half-life of phenprocoumon was measured as 6.8 days without colestyramine, and 3.5 days with colestyramine 4 g three times daily.[7]

A patient stabilised on phenprocoumon developed a fatal valve thrombosis after starting colestyramine, despite separation of doses in accordance with the manufacturer's instructions.[8]

2. Warfarin. In a study, 10 subjects were given warfarin alone or with colestyramine, for one-week periods. When warfarin was taken 30 minutes after colestyramine, peak warfarin levels were reduced by 52% and the prolongation in prothrombin times was reduced by 27%, compared with warfarin alone. However, when warfarin was taken 6 hours after colestyramine, peak warfarin levels were reduced by only 16%, and the prolongation in prothrombin times was the same as with warfarin alone.[9]

Comparable results were found in another similar study; simultaneous administration of warfarin and colestyramine reduced the prothrombin time response by 21%, and separation by 3 hours still caused an 11% reduction in the prothrombin time response.[10] Another study using *intravenous* warfarin has shown that colestyramine also reduces the effect of warfarin by this route, presumably by reducing enterohepatic recycling.[11] Note that colestyramine has been used to speed up the elimination of warfarin in cases of over-anticoagulation.[12,13]

Another report describes a patient taking colestyramine 4 g three times daily who was successfully stabilised on warfarin with alternating doses of 5 mg and 7.5 mg daily. The warfarin was given at 8 am, then the colestyramine at 12 noon with lunch, with dinner, and with an evening snack.[14]

In contrast, an isolated report describes a 77-year-old patient taking multiple medications including colestyramine who was found to have a very high prothrombin time of 78.9 seconds and microscopic haematuria 6 weeks after starting warfarin 5 mg daily. Four days after starting the warfarin her prothrombin time was 17.1 seconds, and it had not been checked again.[15] However, as it is not certain that this patient was properly stabilised on warfarin this may simply have been an effect of the warfarin alone.

Mechanism

Colestyramine binds to coumarins in the gut, thereby preventing their absorption.[5,10,16,17] Data with *intravenous* warfarin and phenprocoumon show that they undergo enterohepatic recycling, and that colestyramine can reduce this as well.[6,11] The long-term use of colestyramine also reduces the absorption of fat-soluble vitamins such as vitamin K so that it can have some direct hypoprothrombinaemic effects of its own.[18,19] This may to some extent offset the full effects of its interaction with anticoagulants. Colestipol on the other hand appears not to bind to any great extent at the pH values in the gut,[2] although, in the same way as colestyramine, it might reduce absorption of vitamin K and prolong the prothrombin time.[4] The paradoxical increase in the effects of warfarin in the isolated case cited above was attributed to the effect of colestyramine on vitamin K.[15]

Importance and management

The interaction of colestyramine with phenprocoumon and warfarin is established, and can be clinically important. If concurrent use is thought necessary, prothrombin times should be monitored and the dose of the anticoagulant increased appropriately. Giving the colestyramine 4 to 6 hours after the anticoagulant has been shown to minimise the effects of this interaction,[9,14] and it is a standard recommendation that other drugs should be given one hour before or 4 to 6 hours after colestyramine. However, despite adequate separation of doses, one patient taking phenprocoumon developed fatal valve thrombosis when given colestyramine, leading the authors to suggest that colestyramine should not be used in patients taking oral anticoagulants.[8] Information about other anticoagulants is lacking but as colestyramine interacts with dicoumarol and ethyl biscoumacetate in *animals*[17] it would be prudent to expect all coumarins to interact similarly. Bear in mind that long-term colestyramine can reduce vitamin K absorption and can cause hypoprothrombinaemia. This might result in an increased effect of warfarin, as has been suggested in one unconfirmed case report, but there seems to be no other evidence to suggest that this is clinically relevant.

No special precautions appear to be necessary if warfarin or phenprocoumon and colestipol or colesevelam are given concurrently. But, as with colestyramine, bear in mind that the long-term use of colestipol might reduce vitamin K absorption and cause hypoprothrombinaemia. This might result in an increased effect of warfarin.

There appear to be no reports of an interaction with the **indanediones**, however, should long-term use of a bile-acid binding resin result in reduced vitamin K absorption and subsequent hypoprothrombinaemia, this would be expected to be additive with the anticoagulant effects of these drugs.

1. Donovan JM, Stypinski D, Stiles MR, Olson TA, Burke SK. Drug interactions with colesevelam hydrochloride, a novel, potent lipid-lowering agent. *Cardiovasc Drugs Ther* (2000) 14, 681–90.
2. Harvengt C, Desager JP. Effects of colestipol, a new bile acid sequestrant, on the absorption of phenprocoumon in man. *Eur J Clin Pharmacol* (1973) 6, 19–21.
3. Heel RC, Brogden RN, Pakes GE, Speight TM, Avery GS. Colestipol: a review of its pharmacological properties and therapeutic effects in patients with hypercholesterolaemia. *Drugs* (1980) 19, 161–80.
4. Colestid (Colestipol). Pharmacia Ltd. UK Summary of product characteristics, June 2007.
5. Hahn KJ, Eiden W, Schettle M, Hahn M, Walter E, Weber E. Effect of cholestyramine on the gastro-intestinal absorption of phenprocoumon and acetylosalicylic acid in man. *Eur J Clin Pharmacol* (1972) 4, 142–5.
6. Meinertz T, Gilfrich H-J, Groth U, Jonen HG, Jähnchen E. Interruption of the enterohepatic circulation of phenprocoumon by cholestyramine. *Clin Pharmacol Ther* (1977) 21, 731–5.
7. Meinertz T, Gilfrich H-J, Bork R, Jähnchen E. Treatment of phenprocoumon intoxication with cholestyramine. *BMJ* (1977) 2, 439.
8. Balmelli N, Domine F, Pfisterer M, Krähenbühl S, Marsch S. Fatal drug interaction between colestyramine and phenprocoumon. *Eur J Intern Med* (2002) 13, 210–11.
9. Kuentzel WP, Brunk SF. Cholestyramine-warfarin interaction in man. *Clin Res* (1970) 18, 594.
10. Robinson DS, Benjamin DM, McCormack JJ. Interaction of warfarin and nonsystemic gastrointestinal drugs. *Clin Pharmacol Ther* (1971) 12, 491–5.
11. Jähnchen E, Meinertz T, Gilfrich H-J, Kersting F, Groth U. Enhanced elimination of warfarin during treatment with cholestyramine. *Br J Clin Pharmacol* (1978) 5, 437–40.
12. Roberge RJ, Rao P, Miske GR, Riley TJ. Diarrhea-associated over-anticoagulation in a patient taking warfarin: therapeutic role of cholestyramine. *Vet Hum Toxicol* (2000) 42, 351–3.
13. Renowden S, Westmoreland D, White JP, Routledge PA. Oral cholestyramine increases elimination of warfarin after overdose. *Br Med J (Clin Res Ed)* (1985) 291, 513–14.
14. Cali TJ. Combined therapy with cholestyramine and warfarin. *Am J Pharm Sci Support Public Health* (1975) 147, 166–9.
15. Lawlor DP, Hyers TM. Extreme prolongation of the prothrombin time in a patient receiving warfarin and cholestyramine. *Cardiovasc Rev Rep* (1993) April, 72–4.
16. Gallo DG, Bailey KR, Sheffner AL. The interaction between cholestyramine and drugs. *Proc Soc Exp Biol Med* (1965) 120, 60–5.
17. Tembo AV, Bates TR. Impairment by cholestyramine of dicumarol and tromexan absorption in rats: a potential drug interaction. *J Pharmacol Exp Ther* (1974) 191, 53–9.
18. Casdorph HR. Safe uses of cholestyramine. *Ann Intern Med* (1970) 72, 759.
19. Gross L, Brotman M. Hypoprothrombinemia and hemorrhage associated with cholestyramine therapy. *Ann Intern Med* (1970) 72, 95–6.

Coumarins + Boldo or Fenugreek

A report describes a woman taking warfarin whose INR rose modestly when she began to take boldo and fenugreek.

Clinical evidence

A woman taking **warfarin** for atrial fibrillation whose INR was normally within the range 2 to 3 had a modest rise in her INR to 3.4, apparently due to the use of 10 drops of boldo after meals and one capsule of fenugreek before meals. A week after stopping these two herbal medicines her INR had fallen to 2.6. When she restarted them, her INR rose to 3.1 after a week, and to 3.4 after 2 weeks. Her INR was later restabilised in her normal range while continuing to take these two herbs by reducing the **warfarin** dose by 15%.[1] The patient had no undesirable reactions (e.g. bruising or bleeding).

Mechanism

The mechanism of this apparent interaction remains unknown, and it is not known whether both herbs or just one was responsible for what happened. Both boldo and fenugreek have been reported to contain natural coumarins, but it is unclear whether they have any anticoagulant activity. Consider also, 'Coumarins + Herbal medicines; Miscellaneous', p.439.

Importance and management

Evidence is limited to one isolated case. Because of the many other factors influencing anticoagulant control, it is not possible to reliably ascribe a change in INR specifically to a drug interaction in a single case report without other supporting evidence. It may be better to advise patients to discuss the use of any herbal products they wish to try, and to increase monitoring if this is thought advisable. Cases of uneventful use should be reported, as they are as useful as possible cases of adverse effects.

1. Lambert JP, Cormier A. Potential interaction between warfarin and boldo-fenugreek. *Pharmacotherapy* (2001) 21, 509–12.

Coumarins + Broxuridine

A case report describes an increase in the effects of warfarin in a patient taking broxuridine.

Clinical evidence, mechanism, importance and management

A man taking **warfarin** and with grade III anaplastic astrocytoma was given intravenous broxuridine as a radiosensitiser. His prothrombin times were unaffected by the first course of broxuridine 1.4 g daily for 4 days, but became more prolonged with successive courses, and after the fourth course his prothrombin time reached about 45 seconds. This was managed with 10 mg of vitamin K. Warfarin was stopped after a significant increase in his prothrombin time also took place with a fifth cycle of broxuridine 990 mg daily.[1] The clinical relevance of this single case is uncertain.

1. Oster SE, Lawrence HJ. Potentiation of anticoagulant effect of coumadin by 5-bromo-2´-deoxyuridine (BUDR). *Cancer Chemother Pharmacol* (1988) 22, 181.

Coumarins + Buflomedil

Buflomedil does not alter the anticoagulant effect of acenocoumarol.

Clinical evidence, mechanism, importance and management

In a randomised study in patients with severe or recurrent venous thrombosis, there was no difference in dose of **acenocoumarol** necessary to reach an INR of 2.5 to 3.5 between 100 patients taking **acenocoumarol** with buflomedil 600 mg daily and 100 patients taking **acenocoumarol** alone. No patients had severe bleeding, and 3 to 4% of patients in both groups had moderate bleeding (haematomas, haematuria).[1] This suggests that no **acenocoumarol** dose adjustments are likely to be needed when it is used with buflomedil.

1. Moriau M, Lavenne-Pardonge E, Crasborn L, von Frenckell R, Col-Debeys C. The treatment of severe or recurrent deep venous thrombosis. Beneficial effect of the co-administration of antiplatelet agents with or without rheological effects, and anticoagulants. *Thromb Res* (1995) 78, 469–82.

Coumarins and related drugs + Calcium-channel blockers

Amlodipine and felodipine do not affect the anticoagulant effects of warfarin. Diltiazem, and possibly verapamil, may cause a minor decrease in warfarin metabolism, but the anticoagulant effect of warfarin is unlikely to be affected. Verapamil does not appear to alter the anticoagulant effects of phenindione.

Clinical evidence

(a) Dihydropyridine calcium-channel blockers

The manufacturers say that **amlodipine** did not significantly alter the effect of **warfarin** on prothrombin times in healthy subjects.[1,2]

In healthy subjects given **warfarin** until steady state, **felodipine** 10 mg daily for 14 days did not alter the dose of **warfarin** required to maintain a stable INR, or affect the pharmacokinetics of *S*- or *R*-warfarin.[3] Because **felodipine** does not interact with **warfarin** it has been used as a control drug in retrospective cohort studies assessing **warfarin** drug interactions.[4,5]

(b) Diltiazem

In a study, 11 healthy men were given racemic **warfarin**, and 8 were given *R*-warfarin, both as a single 1.5-mg/kg intravenous dose. Another 10 subjects were given *S*-warfarin as a single 0.75-mg/kg intravenous dose. After taking diltiazem 120 mg three times daily (for 4 days before and 9 days after the dose of **warfarin**) the clearance of *R*-warfarin was decreased by about 20% but the more potent *S*-warfarin remained unaffected. The total anticoagulant response remained unchanged.[6] Similarly, in another study in 20 healthy subjects, diltiazem 30 mg three times daily for one week caused no clinically relevant changes in the anticoagulant effects of a single dose of **warfarin**. There was a small 13% decrease in **warfarin** clearance and an 8% increase in its AUC in the presence of diltiazem, but these changes were not statistically significant.[7]

However, one report describes a patient stabilised on **warfarin** with an INR in the range of 2.5 to 3 who was found to have an INR of 4.2 two weeks after starting diltiazem 180 mg daily.[8]

(c) Verapamil

In a small study in 20 patients to investigate the effectiveness of verapamil 80 mg three times daily for 2 weeks for angina, 10 of these patients were also taking **phenindione** during the study. Although not specifically studied, the authors of this study reported that there was no significant change in the sensitivity of these 10 patients to **phenindione** during the use of verapamil.[9]

Mechanism

Diltiazem is a known inhibitor of the cytochrome P450 isoenzyme CYP3A4. However, this isoenzyme has only a minor role in the metabolism of warfarin, specifically in the metabolism of the less active *R*-isomer of warfarin. Consequently, only minor increases in the levels of warfarin have been seen in pharmacokinetic studies, which would generally not be expected to be clinically relevant. Verapamil is also an inhibitor of CYP3A4, but the dihydropyridine calcium-channel blockers are not.

Importance and management

No special precautions would seem to be necessary during the concurrent use of warfarin and dihydropyridine calcium-channel blockers. Although the minor pharmacokinetic interaction between diltiazem and warfarin would appear to be established, in the studies cited this did not change anticoagulant control, and is therefore unlikely to be of clinical importance. Verapamil would be expected to cause a similar, minor pharmacokinetic interaction to diltiazem, which would be unlikely to result in clinically significant effects, although the only available data to confirm this appears to be the small study reported above. The absence of adverse reports about these very widely used drugs suggests that concurrent use is normally uneventful.

1. Istin (Amlodipine besilate). Pfizer Ltd. UK Summary of product characteristics, July 2007.
2. Norvasc (Amlodipine besylate). Pfizer Inc. US Prescribing information, August 2006.
3. Grind M, Murphy M, Warrington S, Åberg J. Method for studying drug-warfarin interactions. *Clin Pharmacol Ther* (1993) 54, 381–7.
4. McCall KL, Anderson HG, Jones AD. Determination of the lack of a drug interaction between azithromycin and warfarin. *Pharmacotherapy* (2004) 24, 188–94.
5. McCall KL, Scott JC, Anderson HG. Retrospective evaluation of a possible interaction between warfarin and levofloxacin. *Pharmacotherapy* (2005) 25, 67–73.
6. Abernethy DR, Kaminsky LS, Dickinson TH. Selective inhibition of warfarin metabolism by diltiazem in humans. *J Pharmacol Exp Ther* (1991) 257, 411–15.
7. Stoysich AM, Lucas BD, Mohiuddin SM, Hilleman DE. Further elucidation of pharmacokinetic interaction between diltiazem and warfarin. *Int J Clin Pharmacol Ther* (1996) 34, 56–60.
8. Böttiger Y. Interagerar cardizem och waran? *Lakartidningen* (2008) 105, 373.
9. Phear DN. Verapamil in angina: a double-blind trial. *BMJ* (1968) 2, 740–1.

Coumarins + Carbamazepine and related drugs

The anticoagulant effects of warfarin can be greatly reduced by carbamazepine. Two case reports suggest phenprocoumon is similarly affected, and one case has been described with acenocoumarol. A small study suggests that oxcarbazepine might not interact with warfarin; however, it did reduce the anticoagulant effects of warfarin in one case. Eslicarbazepine appears to cause a small decrease in exposure to *S*-warfarin but not *R*-warfarin.

Clinical evidence

(a) Carbamazepine

1. Acenocoumarol. A man taking stable doses of acenocoumarol and carbamazepine 200 mg daily started coughing up blood about 4 weeks after carbamazepine was stopped, and he was found to be over-anticoagulated. The acenocoumarol was stopped for 48 hours and he was given vitamin K.[1]

2. Phenprocoumon. A man in his mid-twenties developed multiple thrombotic episodes due to hereditary resistance to activated protein C. Because of cerebral embolic strokes, he developed epileptic seizures and was given carbamazepine 400 mg daily, followed 6 days later by phenprocoumon. It was found that relatively large doses of phenprocoumon (8 mg daily) had to be given without achieving adequate anticoagulation (Quick value 50 to 60%; target 10 to 20%) until the carbamazepine was withdrawn, whereupon the phenprocoumon dose could be reduced to 1.5 mg daily with a Quick value of 30 to 40%.[2] Similarly, another patient stabilised on phenprocoumon was found to have a greatly reduced anticoagulant effect (a dramatic increase in his Quick value), 21 days after he started taking carbamazepine 400 mg daily. The values returned to normal when the carbamazepine was stopped.[3]

3. Warfarin. In one study, 2 patients taking warfarin with carbamazepine (200 mg daily for the first week, 400 mg daily for the second, and 600 mg for the third) had a decrease of about 50% in their serum warfarin concentrations, and sharp increases in their prothrombin-proconvertin percentages.[4] The half-life of a single intravenous dose of warfarin in 3 other patients fell by about 11%, 53%, and 60%, respectively, when they were similarly treated.[4] In another analysis, warfarin dose requirements were 2.3-fold higher in 5 patients stabilised on warfarin and carbamazepine than in 54 patients taking warfarin without any interacting drugs (median 9 mg daily versus 3.86 mg daily). The 5 patients taking carbamazepine had higher clearances of both *R*- and *S*-warfarin, and had about 11-fold higher plasma concentrations of the 10-hydroxymetabolite of warfarin.[5] In a prospective cohort study in children, the use of phenobarbital or carbamazepine was associated with a higher dose of warfarin to maintain the target INR (0.24 mg/kg versus 0.15 mg/kg).[6] A retrospective study similarly found that the concurrent use of enzyme inducers (including carbamazepine) considerably influenced the total weekly warfarin dose; further analysis found that an average additional amount of warfarin required in patients taking these drugs was 17.2 mg weekly.[7]

An interaction between warfarin and carbamazepine has been described in 5 case reports.[8-12] One of these reports describes a patient stabilised on warfarin and carbamazepine who developed widespread dermal ecchymoses and a prothrombin time of 70 seconds, one week after stopping carbamazepine. She was restabilised on approximately half the dose of warfarin in the absence of carbamazepine.[11]

(b) Eslicarbazepine

In a study in 13 healthy subjects given **warfarin** until their INR was stabilised between 1.3 and 1.8, eslicarbazepine 1.2 g for 7 days caused a 23% reduction in the AUC, and a 20% reduction in the maximum plasma concentration of *S*-warfarin. The pharmacokinetics of *R*-warfarin were not altered by eslicarbazepine. There was also a 4% increase in the INR during concurrent use, but this was below the threshold set for clinical importance.[13]

(c) Oxcarbazepine

In a study in 7 healthy subjects given **warfarin** until steady-state, oxcarbazepine 450 mg twice daily for one week increased the mean Quick values from 36.6% to only 38.1%, which was not statistically significant.[14] In contrast, a case report describes a 16-year-old man whose INR was stabilised within the range of 2 to 3 with warfarin 10 mg daily. Six months after starting oxcarbazepine (dose unknown) his INR started to decrease and after one year of concurrent use, his INR had decreased to 1.23. His INR could still not be stabilised after oxcarbazepine was stopped, despite warfarin dose increases (time scale unknown). As a result, the warfarin was discontinued and treatment changed. The patient was found to be a CYP2C9 poor metaboliser, and this case was further complicated by the presence of another genotype (related to vitamin K epoxide reductase) capable of affecting warfarin dosing, making its implications difficult to assess.[15]

Mechanism

The metabolism of *S*-warfarin occurs principally via CYP2C9 and as such, *S*-warfarin is used as a probe substrate for assessing CYP2C9 activity. The metabolism of *R*-warfarin involves CYP3A4. Carbamazepine is a potent CYP3A4 inducer and, from the evidence cited above, it appears to have some effect on CYP2C9, resulting in increased warfarin metabolism. Acenocoumarol and phenprocoumon are also metabolised via CYP2C9. The extent of the interactions between coumarins and carbamazepine might be related to the CYP2C9 genotype (see *Genetic factors in drug metabolism* in 'Drug metabolism interactions', p.4), when the metabolism of warfarin by CYP3A4 is likely to be more important, but this requires further study.

Oxcarbazepine is not known to affect the metabolism of drugs by CYP2C9, but it does induce CYP3A4. The reason for the effect on *S*-warfarin seen with eslicarbazepine is not known; the authors[13] suggest a possible very weak inductive effect on CYP2C9, but this requires further study. Eslicarbazepine is also an inducer of CYP3A4.

Importance and management

The interaction between warfarin and **carbamazepine** is fairly well documented, established, and clinically important, although the incidence is uncertain and it might be more important in poor metabolisers (those with low CYP2C9 activity) than extensive metabolisers (those with normal CYP2C9 activity). Because metaboliser status is generally unknown in practice, the following advice should be applied to all patients. Monitor the anticoagulant response more closely if carbamazepine is added to established treatment with warfarin and anticipate the need to increase the dose. **Oxcarbazepine** might interact with warfarin, but not to the same extent as carbamazepine; be aware that it might have an important effect in poor metabolisers and warfarin dose adjustments might be necessary. The concurrent use of **eslicarbazepine** and warfarin would not seem to warrant additional INR monitoring; however, given the small study size and inter-individual variability associated with warfarin response, increased monitoring of INR when starting or stopping eslicarbazepine, would seem prudent and is recommended by the UK manufacturer of eslicarbazepine.[16]

Information about an interaction between phenprocoumon or acenocoumarol and carbamazepine seems to be limited to the three reports cited. Nevertheless it would be prudent to monitor concurrent use in any patient, being alert for the need to increase the coumarin dose. Evidence for an interaction between oxcarbazepine or eslicarbazepine and phenprocoumon or acenocoumarol is lacking, but they might be expected to interact similarly to carbamazepine.

1. Rivière I, Barjhoux C, Mallaret M. Hémoptysie sous acénocoumarol: rôle de L'arrêt d'un inducteur enzymatique (carbamazépine). *Therapie* (1994) 49, 142–3.
2. Böttcher T, Buchmann J, Zettl U-K, Benecke R. Carbamazepine-phenprocoumon interaction. *Eur Neurol* (1997) 38, 132–3.
3. Schlienger R, Kurmann M, Drewe J, Müller-Spahn F, Seifritz E. Inhibition of phenprocoumon anticoagulation by carbamazepine. *Eur Neuropsychopharmacol* (2000) 10, 219–21.
4. Hansen JM, Siersbæk-Nielsen K, Skovsted L. Carbamazepine-induced acceleration of diphenylhydantoin and warfarin metabolism in man. *Clin Pharmacol Ther* (1971) 12, 539–43.
5. Herman D, Locatelli I, Grabnar I, Peternel P, Stegnar M, Lainščak M, Mrhar A, Breskvar K, Dolžan V. The influence of co-treatment with carbamazepine, amiodarone and statins on warfarin metabolism and maintenance dose. *Eur J Clin Pharmacol* (2006) 62, 291–6.
6. Streif W, Marzinotto AV, Massicotte P, Chan AKC, Julian JA, Mitchell L. Analysis of warfarin therapy in pediatric patients: a prospective cohort study of 319 patients. *Blood* (1999) 94, 3007–14.
7. Whitley HP, Fermo JD, Chumney ECG, Brzezinski WA. Effect of patient-specific factors on weekly warfarin dose. *Ther Clin Risk Manag* (2007) 3, 499–504.
8. Ross JRY, Beeley L. Interaction between carbamazepine and warfarin. *BMJ* (1980) 1, 1415–16.
9. Kendall AG, Boivin M. Warfarin-carbamazepine interaction. *Ann Intern Med* (1981) 94, 280.
10. Massey EW. Effect of carbamazepine on Coumadin metabolism. *Ann Neurol* (1983) 13, 691–2.
11. Denbow CE, Fraser HS. Clinically significant hemorrhage due to warfarin-carbamazepine interaction. *South Med J* (1990) 83, 981.
12. Parrish RH, Pazdur DE, O'Donnell PJ. Effect of carbamazepine initiation and discontinuation on antithrombotic control in a patient receiving warfarin: case report and review of the literature. *Pharmacotherapy* (2006) 26, 1650–3.
13. Vaz-da-Silva M, Almeida L, Falcão A, Soares E, Maia J, Nunes T, Soares-da-Silva P. Effect of eslicarbazepine acetate on the steady-state pharmacokinetics and pharmacodynamics of warfarin in healthy subjects during a three-stage, open-label, multiple-dose, single-period study. *Clin Ther* (2010) 32, 179–92.
14. Krämer G, Tettenborn B, Klosterkov Jensen P, Menge GP, Stoll KD. Oxcarbazepine does not affect the anticoagulant activity of warfarin. *Epilepsia* (1992) 33, 1145–8.
15. Nevruz O, Baysan O, Yokuşoğlu M. Warfarin resistance induced by oxcarbazepine. *Anadolu Kardiyol Derg* (2009) 9, 358–9.
16. Zebinix (Eslicarbazepine acetate). Eisai Ltd. UK Summary of product characteristics, August 2012.

Coumarins + Carbon tetrachloride

A single case report describes an increase in the anticoagulant effects of dicoumarol in a patient who accidentally drank some cleaning liquid containing carbon tetrachloride.

Clinical evidence, mechanism, importance and management

A patient, well stabilised on **dicoumarol**, accidentally drank a small amount of cleaning liquid later estimated to contain just 0.1 mL of carbon tetrachloride. The next day his prothrombin time had risen to 41 seconds. This value was about the same after another day even though the **dicoumarol** had been withdrawn, and marked hypoprothrombinaemia persisted for another 5 days.[1]

The probable reason for this reaction is that carbon tetrachloride is very toxic to the liver, the changed anticoagulant response being a manifestation of this. Carbon tetrachloride, once used as an anthelmintic in man, is no longer used in human medicine, but is still employed as an industrial solvent and degreasing agent. On theoretical grounds it would seem possible for anticoagulated patients exposed to substantial amounts of the vapour to experience this interaction, but this has not been reported.

1. Luton EF. Carbon tetrachloride exposure during anticoagulant therapy. Dangerous enhancement of hypoprothrombinemic effect. *JAMA* (1965) 194, 1386–7.

Coumarins + Chamomile

A single case report describes a woman stabilised on warfarin who developed a marked increase in her INR with bleeding complications five days after she started using two chamomile products.

Clinical evidence

A 70-year-old woman stabilised on **warfarin** with an INR of 3.6 started drinking 4 to 5 cups of chamomile tea (an infusion of *Matricaria chamomilla*) daily for chest congestion, and using a chamomile-based skin lotion 4 to 5 times daily for foot oedema. About 5 days later she developed ecchymoses and was found to have an INR of 7.9, a retroperitoneal haematoma and other internal haemorrhages.[1]

Mechanism

German chamomile contains the natural coumarin compounds, umbelliferone and herniarin. However, these compounds do not possess the minimum structural requirements (a C-4 hydroxyl substituent and a C-3 non-polar carbon substituent) required for anticoagulant activity. German chamomile essential oil extracts do not appear to significantly affect the cytochrome P450 isoenzyme CYP2C9, the main isoenzyme involved in the metabolism of warfarin, but the effects of chamomile tea do not appear to have been studied.

Importance and management

This appears to be the first report of an interaction between warfarin and German chamomile. There seem to be no reports of German chamomile alone causing anticoagulation, and the natural coumarin constituents of German chamomile do not appear to possess anticoagulant activity, which might suggest that the risk of an additive effect is small. Furthermore, a pharmacokinetic basis for this interaction has not been established. Because of the many other factors influencing anticoagulant control, it is not possible to reliably ascribe a change in INR specifically to a drug interaction in a single case report without other supporting evidence. It may be better to advise patients to discuss the use of any herbal products they wish to try, and to increase monitoring if this is thought advisable. Cases of uneventful use should be reported, as they are as useful as possible cases of adverse effects.

1. Segal R, Pilote L. Warfarin interaction with *Matricaria chamomilla*. *Can Med Assoc J* (2006) 174, 1281–2.

Coumarins + Chinese angelica (*Angelica sinensis*)

Two case reports describe a very marked increase in the anticoagulant effects of warfarin when Chinese angelica was given.

Clinical evidence

A 46-year-old African-American woman with atrial fibrillation taking **warfarin** had a greater than twofold increase in her prothrombin time and INR after taking Chinese angelica for 4 weeks. The prothrombin time and INR were back to normal 4 weeks after stopping Chinese angelica.[1] In another case, a woman who had been taking **warfarin** for 10 years developed widespread bruising and an INR of 10, a month after starting to take Chinese angelica.[2]

Mechanism

The reasons for this interaction are not fully understood but Chinese angelica is known to contain natural coumarin derivatives, which may possibly have anticoagulant properties: these could be additive with those of warfarin. The data suggest that alteration of warfarin levels is not involved, but other studies suggest that the herb may inhibit the cytochrome P450 isoenzyme CYP2C9, which is the main route of warfarin metabolism.

Importance and management

Clinical evidence for an interaction between Chinese angelica and warfarin appears to be limited to the case reports cited, and an interaction is not fully established. Nevertheless, it would seem prudent to warn patients taking warfarin, and possibly other coumarin anticoagulants, of the potential risks of also taking Chinese angelica. For safety, the use of Chinese angelica should be avoided unless the effects on anticoagulation can be monitored. More study is needed.

1. Page RL, Lawrence JD. Potentiation of warfarin by dong quai. *Pharmacotherapy* (1999) 19, 870–6.
2. Ellis GR, Stephens MR. Untitled report. *BMJ* (1999) 319, 650.

Coumarins and related drugs + Chitosan

An isolated report describes an increase in the INR of an elderly man taking warfarin when he also took chitosan.

Clinical evidence

A case report describes an 83-year-old man, with type 2 diabetes who was receiving **warfarin** (2.5 mg daily for one year, with an INR of between 2 and 3) for atrial fibrillation. At a routine blood test his INR was found to be about 3.7, and, although the dose of **warfarin** was halved, 3 days later his INR was more than 9. On discussion, it was established that he had recently started taking chitosan 1.2 g twice daily. He was advised to stop this supplement and was subsequently restabilised on **warfarin**. About one month later, the patient restarted the chitosan, which again resulted in a raised INR.[1]

Mechanism

Chitosan sulfate has been reported to have anticoagulant activity, but this has not been found with chitosan. The authors therefore suggest that chitosan impaired the absorption of fat soluble vitamins, including vitamin K. Warfarin is a vitamin-K antagonist and a reduction in vitamin K would be expected to enhance its effects.

Importance and management

Evidence is limited to this case, and the mechanism is largely speculative; however an interaction seems probable. The evidence is too slim to forbid patients taking warfarin from also taking chitosan, but it would seem prudent to discuss the possible outcome and advise an increase in the frequency of anticoagulant monitoring; measuring the INR after a few days of concurrent use seems reasonable. There appears to be no evidence regarding other anticoagulants, but if the mechanism is correct, all vitamin K antagonists (coumarins and **indanediones**) would be expected to be similarly affected.

1. Huang S-S, Sung S-H, Chiang C-E. Chitosan potentiation of warfarin effect. *Ann Pharmacother* (2007) 41, 1912–14.

Coumarins + Chlorpromazine

Chlorpromazine probably does not interact significantly with the coumarins.

Clinical evidence, mechanism, importance and management

Although in one early report, chlorpromazine 40 to 100 mg daily was said to have 'slightly sensitised' 2 out of 8 patients to the effects of **acenocoumarol**[1] and in another was reported to increase its anticoagulant effects in *animals*,[2] there appears to be nothing else published to suggest that an interaction occurs. *In vitro* study in human liver microsomes[3] found that chlorpromazine did not inhibit CYP2C9, the cytochrome P450 isoenzyme predominantly involved in the metabolism of **warfarin** and other coumarins. No coumarin dose adjustments would therefore be expected to be needed on concurrent use.

1. Johnson R, David A, Chartier Y. Clinical experience with G-23350 (Sintrom). *Can Med Assoc J* (1957) 77, 756–61.
2. Weiner M. Effect of centrally active drugs on the action of coumarin anticoagulants. *Nature* (1966) 212, 1599–1600.
3. Shin J-G, Soukhova N, Flockhart DA. Effect of antipsychotic drugs on human liver cytochrome P-450 (CYP) isoforms in vitro: preferential inhibition of CYP2D6. *Drug Metab Dispos* (1999) 27, 1078–84.

Coumarins and related drugs + Cilostazol

Cilostazol does not appear to have a clinically relevant effect on the pharmacokinetics or pharmacodynamics of warfarin. Nevertheless, as with other antiplatelet drugs, concurrent use might increase the bleeding risk.

Clinical evidence, mechanism, importance and management

In a crossover study in 15 healthy subjects, cilostazol 100 mg twice daily for 13 days did not alter the pharmacokinetics of a single 25-mg dose of warfarin given on day 7. Also, prothrombin times, aPTT, and bleeding time were unaffected.[1]

No specific interaction would be expected during concurrent use. Nevertheless, because cilostazol is an antiplatelet drug, and the effects of antiplatelet drugs can be additive with those of anticoagulants, the UK manufacturer advises caution with the concurrent use of anticoagulants, and more frequent monitoring to reduce the possibility of bleeding. Further, note that use of cilostazol in patients receiving two or more additional antiplatelet drugs or anticoagulants is contraindicated.[2] For discussion of the increased bleeding risk associated with combining other antiplatelet drugs and anticoagulants, see 'Coumarins and related drugs + Aspirin or other Salicylates', p.405.

1. Mallikaarjun S, Bramer SL. Effect of cilostazol on the pharmacokinetics and pharmacodynamics of warfarin. *Clin Pharmacokinet* (1999) 37 (Suppl 2), 79–86.
2. Pletal (Cilostazol). Otsuka Pharmaceuticals (UK) Ltd. UK Summary of product characteristics, October 2013.

Coumarins + Cinacalcet

Cinacalcet does not appear to affect the pharmacokinetics or anticoagulant effects of warfarin.

Clinical evidence, mechanism, importance and management

In a placebo-controlled study, 21 healthy subjects were given cinacalcet 30 mg twice daily for 15 doses, with a single 25-mg dose of warfarin on day 5. Cinacalcet did not affect the pharmacokinetics of warfarin or its effects on prothrombin time.[1] This study suggests that the dose of warfarin is unlikely to need adjusting in patients given cinacalcet.

1. Padhi D, Sullivan JT. Cinacalcet does not affect the pharmacokinetics or pharmacodynamics of warfarin. *Drugs R D* (2007) 8, 79–87.

Coumarins and related drugs + Clopidogrel

Clopidogrel does not appear to have a clinically relevant effect on the pharmacokinetics or pharmacodynamics of warfarin. Nevertheless, the concurrent use of clopidogrel, either with warfarin or with warfarin and aspirin, increases the risk of bleeding. Limited data suggests that phenprocoumon reduces the antiplatelet effects of clopidogrel.

Clinical evidence

(a) Clopidogrel and Warfarin

In a well-controlled study involving 43 patients who had been taking warfarin for at least 2 months, the addition of clopidogrel 75 mg daily for 8 days had no effect on warfarin plasma concentrations or INRs. No bleeding occurred with clopidogrel and no serious adverse events were reported.[1]

In a large, retrospective, cohort study in Denmark from 1997 to 2006, patients who were discharged from hospital with a diagnosis of atrial fibrillation taking warfarin and clopidogrel were found to have an increased risk of admission to hospital with bleeding, when compared with clopidogrel or warfarin alone (adjusted hazard ratio 3.08, compared with 1.06 and 1, respectively).[2] Similarly, in another large cohort study in the UK, patients newly diagnosed with atrial fibrillation between 1993 and 2008 and prescribed warfarin and clopidogrel were found to have an increased risk of experiencing a bleeding event (minor or major) when compared to those who received clopidogrel or warfarin alone (adjusted hazard ratio 2.74 compared with 1.57 and 2.08, respectively).[3] In an open study of 50 patients who underwent endovascular treatment for peripheral arterial disease, and were randomised to receive either clopidogrel alone or in combination with warfarin, 21% of patients in the combination group and 7% in the clopidogrel group had a bleeding event, however this was not a statistically significant difference.[4]

(b) Triple therapy

Dual antiplatelet therapy (usually low-dose aspirin with clopidogrel) is increasingly used in acute coronary syndromes in situations where the benefits have been shown to outweigh the small increased risk of bleeding with the combination (see 'Aspirin + Clopidogrel and related drugs', p.782). Some patients also require anticoagulants for additional indications, for example, for atrial fibrillation or mechanical valves. However, there are limited clinical study data on the benefits and risks of dual antiplatelet therapy plus an anticoagulant (triple therapy).

In a 2008 review of 12 studies (mostly retrospective cohort studies),[5] the increased risk of bleeding events for triple therapy versus dual therapy was 3- to 6-fold in 8 of the studies, with 4 of the studies reporting no increased risk of major bleeding events. In one of these studies, patients who had been taking **warfarin** long-term and who underwent stent implantation and were subsequently discharged taking aspirin, clopidogrel, and **warfarin**, had a higher risk of bleeding compared with those taking dual therapy: the incidence of major bleeding was 6.6% and the incidence of minor bleeding was 14.9% in those taking triple therapy, compared with 0% and 3.8% for major and minor bleeding, respectively, in patients taking dual therapy with no

warfarin.[6] In 2011, a further meta analysis of 9 studies (from 2005 to 2008) found that triple therapy with **warfarin**, aspirin, and clopidogrel after percutaneous stent implantation increased the risk of major bleeding (odds ratio 2.12), when compared with dual antiplatelet therapy, but had no statistically significant increased risk of minor bleeding.[7] Similar outcomes were found in another 2011 meta-analysis, which included some of the same studies.[8] A further meta-analysis reports an incidence of bleeding of 9.2% in patients who had undergone stent placement and received **warfarin**, aspirin, and clopidogrel.[9] In an observational cohort study of elderly survivors of acute myocardial infarction, the rate of bleeding was higher in patients receiving **warfarin** with aspirin (0.08 per patient year), or the triple drug combination of **warfarin** and aspirin with either clopidogrel or ticlopidine (0.09 per patient year), than in patients receiving aspirin alone (0.03 per patient year).[10] In a large, retrospective, cohort study in Denmark from 1997 to 2006, patients who were discharged from hospital with a diagnosis of atrial fibrillation taking **warfarin**, aspirin, and clopidogrel were found to have a higher risk of admission to hospital with bleeding, when compared to dual therapy with **warfarin** and aspirin (adjusted hazard ratio 3.7 compared with 1.83). In addition the risk of gastrointestinal and airways bleeding was even higher (adjusted hazard ratio 5.38 and 4.94, respectively).[2] Similarly, in another large cohort study in the UK, patients newly diagnosed with atrial fibrillation between 1993 and 2008 and prescribed **warfarin**, aspirin, and clopidogrel were found to have an increased risk of experiencing a bleeding event (minor or major) when compared to those who received dual therapy with **warfarin** and aspirin (adjusted hazard ratio 3.75 compared with 2.87).[3]

In an observational study in 1 223 patients taking aspirin and clopidogrel, patients also taking **phenprocoumon** (124 patients) were found to have about 35% higher platelet aggregation than those not taking phenprocoumon, with about one-third of these patients classified as clopidogrel low-responders. However, the clinical relevance of this was not studied.[11]

Mechanism

As with other antiplatelet drugs (see 'Coumarins and related drugs + Aspirin or other Salicylates', p.405), the concurrent use of clopidogrel and oral anticoagulants can increase the risk or intensity of bleeding.

The authors of the study with phenprocoumon suggest that it might compete with clopidogrel for metabolism by CYP2C9 and CYP3A4, reducing the metabolism of clopidogrel to its active metabolite, leading to a reduction in its antiplatelet effect.[11] However, note that interactions by substrate competition are rarely clinically relevant.

Importance and management

The concurrent use of **warfarin** and clopidogrel (with or without aspirin) increases the risk of bleeding. These combinations should therefore be used only when there is a clear indication for using both an anticoagulant and antiplatelet, and the expected benefits are likely to outweigh the increased risks of bleeding. The American College of Cardiology and American Heart Association 2012 joint guidelines for the management of patients with acute coronary syndromes[12] recommend that if warfarin is added to dual antiplatelet therapy, it might be reasonable to target an INR of 2 to 2.5. In addition, a 2010 guideline on the use of proton pump inhibitors and thienopyridines recommends that a proton pump inhibitor should be considered for gastroprotection in patients who require antiplatelet therapy and have multiple risk factors for gastrointestinal bleeding, such as the use of an anticoagulant. The guideline also suggests that the benefit of using a proton pump inhibitor in these patients may outweigh any potential reduction in the cardiovascular efficacy of the antiplatelet drug because of a drug-drug interaction.[13] Note that the use of clopidogrel with a proton pump inhibitor is controversial (see 'Clopidogrel + Proton pump inhibitors and other CYP2C19 inhibitors', p.788). The European 2010 guidelines for atrial fibrillation recommend that, following coronary artery stenting in patients with atrial fibrillation requiring oral anticoagulation, triple therapy with warfarin, aspirin, and clopidogrel can be given temporarily (duration dependent on risk of haemorrhage, clinical setting, and type of stent), followed by warfarin (INR 2 to 2.5) and clopidogrel, or alternatively aspirin, for up to 12 months post-stent, followed by lifelong warfarin (INR 2 to 3). Gastric protection with a proton pump inhibitor is also recommended, where necessary.[14] However, note that, in the UK, the manufacturers of clopidogrel actually state that the concurrent use of warfarin is not recommended,[15] whereas the US manufacturers just recommend caution.[16]

The US manufacturer[16] notes that *in vitro* clopidogrel has been reported to inhibit CYP2C9. However, no relevant increase in warfarin concentrations was found in the study[1] reported above, and the UK manufacturer notes that no clinically relevant interaction was reported in patients taking phenytoin or tolbutamide, which are also metabolised by CYP2C9, during the CAPRIE study. Also, no clinically relevant interaction occurs between clopidogrel and *fluvastatin* (see 'Clopidogrel + Statins', p.792), another substrate of CYP2C9. Therefore a pharmacokinetic interaction between clopidogrel and warfarin seems unlikely.

The clinical relevance of the increase in platelet aggregation in patients taking aspirin and clopidogrel plus **phenprocoumon** is unknown, although the authors[11] suggest that this reduction in antiplatelet effects may be offset by the anticoagulant effects of phenprocoumon. Further study is needed.

1. Lidell C, Svedberg L-E, Lindell P, Bandh S, Job B, Wallentin L. Clopidogrel and warfarin: absence of interaction in patients receiving long-term anticoagulant therapy for non-valvular atrial fibrillation. *Thromb Haemost* (2003) 89, 842–6.
2. Hansen ML, Sørensen R, Clausen MT, Fog-Petersen ML, Raunsø J, Gadsbøll N, Gislason GH, Folke F, Andersen SS, Schramm TK, Abildstrøm SZ, Poulsen HE, Køber L, Torp-Pedersen C. Risk of bleeding with single, dual, or triple therapy with warfarin, aspirin, and clopidogrel in patients with atrial fibrillation. *Arch Intern Med* (2010) 170, 1433–41.
3. Azoulay L, Dell'Aniello S, Simon T, Renoux C, Suissa S. The concurrent use of antithrombotic therapies and the risk of bleeding in patients with atrial fibrillation. *Thromb Haemost* (2013) 109, 431–39.
4. Li H, Zhang F, Liang G, Luo X, Zhang C, Feng Y, Guo M. A prospective randomised controlled clinical trial on clopidogrel combined with warfarin versus clopidogrel alone in the prevention of restenosis after endovascular treatment of the femoropopliteal artery. *Ann Vasc Surg* (2013) 27, 627–33.
5. Hermosillo AJ, Spinler SA. Aspirin, clopidogrel, and warfarin: is the combination appropriate and effective or inappropriate and too dangerous? *Ann Pharmacother* (2008) 42, 790–805.
6. Khurram Z, Chou E, Minutello R, Bergman G, Parikh M, Naidu S, Wong SC, Hong MK. Combination therapy with aspirin, clopidogrel and warfarin following coronary stenting is associated with a significant risk of bleeding. *J Invasive Cardiol* (2006) 18, 162–4.
7. Zhao H-J, Zheng Z-T, Wang Z-H, Li S-H, Zhang Y, Zhong M, Zhang W. "Triple therapy" rather than "triple threat". A meta-analysis of the two antithrombotic regimens after stent implantation in patients receiving long-term oral anticoagulant treatment. *Chest* (2011) 139, 260–70.
8. Gao F, Zhou YJ, Wang ZJ, Yang SW, Nie B, Liu XL, Jia DA, Yan ZX. Meta-analysis of the combination of warfarin and dual antiplatelet therapy after coronary stenting in patients with indications for chronic oral anticoagulation. *Int J Cardiol* (2011) 148, 96–101.
9. Orford JL, Fasseas P, Melby S, Burger K, Steinhubl SR, Holmes DR, Berger PB. Safety and efficacy of aspirin, clopidogrel, and warfarin after coronary stent placement in patients with an indication for anticoagulation. *Am Heart J* (2004) 147, 463–7.
10. Buresly K, Eisenberg MJ, Zhang X, Pilote L. Bleeding complications associated with combinations of aspirin, thienopyridine derivatives, and warfarin in elderly patients following acute myocardial infarction. *Arch Intern Med* (2005) 165, 784–9.
11. Sibbing D, von Beckerath N, Morath T, Stegherr J, Mehilli J, Sarafoff N, Braun S, Schulz S, Schömig A, Kastrati A. Oral anticoagulation with coumarin derivatives and antiplatelet effects of clopidogrel. *Eur Heart J* (2010) 31, 1205–11.
12. Jneid H, Anderson JL, Wright RS, Adams CD, Bridges CR, Casey DE, Ettinger SM, Fesmire FM, Ganiats TG, Lincoff AM, Peterson ED, Philippides GJ, Theroux P, Wenger NK, Zidar JP. 2012 ACCF/AHA focused update of the guideline for the management of patients with unstable angina/non-ST-elevation myocardial infarction (updating the 2007 guideline and replacing the 2011 focused update). A Report of the American College of Cardiology Foundation/American Heart Association Task Force on Practice Guidelines. *J Am Coll Cardiol* (2012) 60, 645.
13. Abraham NS, Hlatky MA, Antman EM, Bhatt DL, Bjorkman DJ, Clark CB, Furberg CD, Johnson DA, Kahi CJ, Laine L, Mahaffey KW, Quigley EM, Scheiman J, Sperling LS, Tomaselli GF. ACCF/ACG/AHA 2010 Expert Consensus Document on the concomitant use of proton pump inhibitors and thienopyridines: a focused update of the ACCF/ACG/AHA 2008 Expert Consensus Document on Reducing the Gastrointestinal Risks of Antiplatelet Therapy and NSAID Use. A Report of the American College of Cardiology Foundation Task Force on Expert Consensus Documents. *Circulation* (2010) 122, 2619–33.
14. Camm AJ, Kirchhof P, Lip GYH, Schotten U, Savalieva I, Ernst S, Van Gelder IC, Al-Attar N, Hindricks G, Prendergast B, Heidbuchal H, Alfieri O, Angelini A, Atar D, Colonna P, De Caterina R, De Sutter J, Goette A, Gorenek B, Heldal M, Hohloser SH, Kolh P, Le Heuzey J-Y, Ponikowski P, Rutten FH. Guidelines for the management of atrial fibrillation. The Task Force for the management of atrial fibrillation of the European Society of Cardiology (ESC). Eur Heart J (2010) 31, 2369–429. Erratum *ibid* (2011) 32, 1172.
15. Plavix (Clopidogrel hydrogen sulphate). Sanofi-aventis. UK Summary of product characteristics, January 2014.
16. Plavix (Clopidogrel bisulfate). Bristol-Myers Squibb/Sanofi Pharmaceuticals Partnership. US Prescribing information, December 2011.

Coumarins + Cloral hydrate and related drugs

The anticoagulant effects of warfarin are increased in the first few days of cloral hydrate use, but this is normally of little or no clinical importance. Cloral betaine and triclofos may be expected to behave similarly.

Clinical evidence

In a retrospective study in patients just starting **warfarin**, the same loading doses of **warfarin** were given to 32 patients taking **cloral hydrate** daily and 67 patient who did not receive cloral hydrate. The **warfarin** requirements of the **cloral** group during the first 4 days fell by about one-third, but rose again to control requirements by the fifth day.[1]

In a study in 8 subjects, the concurrent use of **warfarin** (loading dose 25 mg then 5 mg daily for 5 days) and **cloral hydrate** 1 g each night resulted in potentiation of the effect of **warfarin**, when compared with placebo (increase in prothrombin time of about 3 to 4 seconds). However, in a longer term study, the addition of **cloral hydrate** 500 mg at night for 4 weeks to subjects stabilised on **warfarin** did not alter the average prothrombin time before, during, and after the use of **cloral** (18.9 seconds, 19.3 seconds, and 19.2 seconds, respectively).[2,3] Similar results have been described in other studies in patients taking **warfarin** and **cloral hydrate**[4-8] or **triclofos**.[9] **Cloral betaine** appears to behave similarly.[10] An isolated and by no means fully explained case of fatal hypoprothrombinaemia occurred in a patient taking **dicoumarol** who was given **cloral hydrate** for 10 days, later replaced by secobarbital.[11] Another patient taking **dicoumarol** had a reduction in prothrombin times when given **cloral hydrate**.[11]

Mechanism

Cloral hydrate is mainly metabolised to trichloroacetic acid, which then successfully competes with warfarin for its binding sites on plasma proteins.[6] As a result, free and active molecules of warfarin are displaced into the plasma water and the effects of the warfarin are increased. However, this effect is only short-lived because the warfarin molecules become exposed to metabolism by the liver, so the warfarin level is reduced.

Importance and management

The interaction between warfarin and cloral hydrate is well documented and well understood, but normally of little or no clinical importance. There is very good evidence that concurrent use need not be avoided.[1-8] However, it may be prudent to keep an eye on the anticoagulant response during the first 4 to 5 days, just to make sure it does not become excessive. It is not certain whether other anticoagulants behave in the same way because the evidence is sparse, indirect and inconclusive,[11,12] but what is known suggests that the coumarins probably do. Triclofos and cloral betaine appear to behave like cloral hydrate. Dichloralphenazone on the other hand interacts quite differently (see 'Coumarins + Dichloralphenazone', p.422).

1. Boston Collaborative Drug Surveillance Program. Interaction between chloral hydrate and warfarin. *N Engl J Med* (1972) 286, 53–5.

2. Udall JA. Warfarin-chloral hydrate interaction. Pharmacological activity and significance. *Ann Intern Med* (1974) 81, 341–4.
3. Udall JA. Warfarin interactions with chloral hydrate and glutethimide. *Curr Ther Res* (1975) 17, 67–74.
4. Griner PF, Raisz LG, Rickles FR, Wiesner PJ, Odoroff CL. Chloral hydrate and warfarin interaction: clinical significance? *Ann Intern Med* (1971) 74, 540–3.
5. Udall JA. Clinical implications of warfarin interactions with five sedatives. *Am J Cardiol* (1975) 35, 67–71.
6. Sellers EM, Koch-Weser J. Kinetics and clinical importance of displacement of warfarin from albumin by acidic drugs. *Ann N Y Acad Sci* (1971) 179, 213–25.
7. Breckenridge A, Orme ML'E, Thorgeirsson S, Davies DS, Brooks RV. Drug interactions with warfarin: studies with dichloralphenazone, chloral hydrate and phenazone (antipyrine). *Clin Sci* (1971) 40, 351–64.
8. Breckenridge A, Orme M. Clinical implications of enzyme induction. *Ann N Y Acad Sci* (1971) 179, 421–31.
9. Sellers EM, Lang M, Koch-Weser J, Colman RW. Enhancement of warfarin-induced hypoprothrombinemia by triclofos. *Clin Pharmacol Ther* (1972) 13, 911–15.
10. MacDonald MG, Robinson DS, Sylwester D, Jaffe JJ. The effects of phenobarbital, chloral betaine, and glutethimide administration on warfarin plasma levels and hypoprothrombinemic responses in man. *Clin Pharmacol Ther* (1969) 10, 80–4.
11. Cucinell SA, Odessky L, Weiss M, Dayton PG. The effect of chloral hydrate on bishydroxycoumarin metabolism. A fatal outcome. *JAMA* (1966) 197, 144–6.
12. van Dam FE, Gribnau-Overkamp MJH. The effect of some sedatives (phenobarbital, gluthetimide, chlordiazepoxide, chloral hydrate) on the rate of disappearance of ethyl biscoumacetate from the plasma. *Folia Med Neerl* (1967) 10, 141–5.

Coumarins + Coenzyme Q_{10} (Ubidecarenone)

Ubidecarenone did not alter the INR or required warfarin dose in a controlled study in patients stabilised on warfarin. However, two reports describe reduced anticoagulant effects of warfarin in four patients taking ubidecarenone. A transient increase in INR has been reported in one patient taking ubidecarenone and warfarin. A 4-month prospective, longitudinal study describes an increased risk of self-reported bleeding events in patients taking coenzyme Q_{10} with warfarin.

Clinical evidence

In a randomised, crossover study in 21 patients stabilised on **warfarin**, coenzyme Q_{10} 100 mg daily (*Bio-Quinone*) for 4 weeks did not alter the INR or the required dose of **warfarin**, when compared with placebo.[1] Similarly, 2 patients taking coenzyme Q_{10} to treat alopecia caused by **warfarin** treatment did not have any notable changes in INR, except that one had a transient INR *increase* when coenzyme Q_{10} was started.[2]

In a 4-month prospective, longitudinal study of 78 patients taking **warfarin** and a herbal product or dietary supplement, there was a statistically significant *increased* risk of self-reported bleeding events in 14 patients taking **warfarin** and coenzyme Q_{10} (57 bleeding events, none major, in a total of 181 weeks of concurrent use for an odds ratio of 3.7).[3] There were 4 elevated INRs (specific values not given) for 55 weeks of concurrent use, but this was not a statistically significant increase in risk. Note that the coenzyme Q_{10} products used were not mentioned and some patients were taking more than one potentially interacting supplement. The authors acknowledge that their finding might be due to chance and not a true interaction.

In contrast, another report describes 3 patients taking **warfarin** who had a reduction in their INR while taking coenzyme Q_{10}. In two of these patients, INR reductions from about 2.5 to 1.4 occurred when they took coenzyme Q_{10} 30 mg daily for 2 weeks. The INRs rapidly returned to normal when the coenzyme Q_{10} was stopped.[4] In two other cases, patients appeared to have a reduced response to **warfarin** while taking coenzyme Q_{10}, and responded normally when it was stopped.[5,6]

Mechanism

Not known. Coenzyme Q_{10} may have some vitamin K-like activity, which would explain the decrease in INR. In a study in *rats*, coenzyme Q_{10} reduced the anticoagulant effect of warfarin and increased the clearance of both enantiomers of warfarin.[7] Explanations for the increase in bleeding or INRs are unknown.

Importance and management

The well-controlled study suggests that coenzyme Q_{10} does not interact with warfarin, and that no warfarin dose adjustment would be expected to be necessary in patients who take this substance. However, the contrasting findings of a *decrease* in warfarin effect in the case reports, and an *increase* in bleeding events in the epidemiological study, introduce a note of caution. Moreover, the authors of the controlled study do recommend close monitoring of the INR if a patient decides to use coenzyme Q_{10}, because the underlying health problem resulting in them choosing to take this substance may alter their response to warfarin.[1] Until more is known it would seem prudent to increase the frequency of INR monitoring in patients taking warfarin if coenzyme Q_{10} is started.

1. Engelsen J, Nielsen JD, Winther K. Effect of coenzyme Q_{10} and ginkgo biloba on warfarin dosage in stable, long-term warfarin treated outpatients. A randomised, double blind, placebo-crossover trial. *Thromb Haemost* (2002) 87, 1075–6.
2. Nagao T, Ibayashi S, Fujii K, Sugimori H, Sadoshima S, Fujishima M. Treatment of warfarin-induced hair loss with ubidecarenone. *Lancet* (1995) 346, 1104–5.
3. Shalansky S, Lynd L, Richardson K, Ingaszewski A, Kerr C. Risk of warfarin-related bleeding events and supratherapeutic international normalized ratios associated with complementary and alternative medicine: a longitudinal analysis. *Pharmacotherapy* (2007) 27, 1237–47.
4. Spigset O. Reduced effect of warfarin caused by ubidecarenone. *Lancet* (1994) 344, 1372–3.
5. Landbo C, Almdal TP. Interaction mellem warfarin og coenzym Q10. *Ugeskr Laeger* (1998) 160, 3226–7.
6. Porterfield LM. Why did the response to warfarin change? *RN* (2000) 63, 107.
7. Zhou S, Chan E. Effect of ubidecarenone on warfarin anticoagulation and pharmacokinetics of warfarin enantiomers in rats. *Drug Metabol Drug Interact* (2001) 18, 99–122.

Coumarins and related drugs + Colchicine

Five cases of a possible marked increase in the effect of fluindione caused by colchicine have been reported.

Clinical evidence, mechanism, importance and management

The national pharmacovigilance system in France has reported 5 cases where colchicine appeared to increase the anticoagulant effect of the indanedione **fluindione**. All 5 patients were stabilised on **fluindione** and were given short-term colchicine 1 to 6 mg daily for an acute attack of gout. All 5 patients had markedly raised INRs (6.5 to in excess of 18), but only one had clinical bleeding (haemorrhoidal bleeding).[1] The authors[1] consider that colchicine may have been a factor in a case of raised INR with **warfarin**,[2] which was attributed solely to fluvoxamine (consider also 'Coumarins and related drugs + SSRIs', p.469).

The mechanism of this interaction is unknown, although the authors rule out protein binding or P-glycoprotein alterations. They suggest that it may occur because colchicine decreases the expression of various cytochrome P450 isoenzymes, so decreasing the metabolism of **fluindione**.[1]

This appears to be the only evidence of an interaction of coumarins or indanediones with colchicine, and is insufficient to justify increased monitoring in all patients.

1. Gras-Champel V, Ohlmann P, Polard E, Wiesel M-L, Imbs J-L, Andréjak M. Can colchicine potentiate the anticoagulant effect of fluindione? *Eur J Clin Pharmacol* (2005) 61, 555–6.
2. Yap KB, Low ST. Interaction of fluvoxamine with warfarin in an elderly woman. *Singapore Med J* (1999) 40, 480–2.

Coumarins + COMT inhibitors

Entacapone slightly increases *R*-warfarin levels and causes a slight increase in INR. Tolcapone is not expected to alter the pharmacokinetics of *S*-warfarin.

Clinical evidence

In a double-blind, crossover study in 12 healthy subjects given individualised **warfarin** doses to achieve an INR of between 1.4 and 1.8, **entacapone** 200 mg four times daily slightly increased the INR by 13%. The AUC of *R*-warfarin was increased by 18%, with no change in the AUC of the more potent *S*-warfarin.[1]

Mechanism

Not known. Based on *in vitro* data, both entacapone and tolcapone were thought to potentially interfere with the metabolism of drugs by the cytochrome P450 isoenzyme CYP2C9, such as *S*-warfarin.[2-4] However, the above study found that entacapone does not alter *S*-warfarin pharmacokinetics, and tolcapone is also not expected to interact by this mechanism because it does not interact with tolbutamide, another CYP2C9 substrate. Consider also 'Sulfonylureas; Tolbutamide + Tolcapone', p.554.

Importance and management

The minor pharmacokinetic interaction between entacapone and warfarin would appear to be established, but its clinical relevance is uncertain. Changes of this magnitude would not generally be expected to be clinically relevant, and there do not appear to be any published case reports of problems. Nevertheless, it is possible that some patients might show a greater effect, and the manufacturer in the UK recommends that the INR be monitored when entacapone is started in patients taking warfarin.[2]

Similarly, although the manufacturers do not predict a pharmacokinetic interaction between **tolcapone** and warfarin, they still recommend monitoring because of the limited clinical information on the combination.[3,4]

1. Dingemanse J, Meyerhoff C, Schadrack J. Effect of the catechol-*O*-methyltransferase inhibitor entacapone on the steady-state pharmacokinetics and pharmacodynamics of warfarin. *Br J Clin Pharmacol* (2002) 53, 485–91.
2. Comtess (Entacapone). Orion Pharma (UK) Ltd. UK Summary of product characteristics, September 2008.
3. Tasmar (Tolcapone). Meda Pharmaceuticals. UK Summary of product characteristics, January 2009.
4. Tasmar (Tolcapone). Valeant Pharmaceuticals North America. US Prescribing information, June 2009.

Coumarins and related drugs + Corticosteroids or Corticotropin

In general, high doses of corticosteroids and corticotrophin increase the INR in patients taking coumarins or fluindione: this has resulted in bleeding in some patients. However, one study found that prednisone opposes the effect of dicoumarol, and case reports describe a reduction in the effects of ethyl biscoumacetate in patients given corticotrophin or cortisone.

Clinical evidence

(a) Corticotropin

Ten out of 14 patients receiving long-term treatment with either **dicoumarol** or **phenindione** had a small but definite increase in their anticoagulant responses when they were given intramuscular or intravenous corticotropin for 4 to 9 days.[1] A patient stable on **ethyl biscoumacetate** developed frank melaena and microscopic haematuria within 3 days of starting treatment with intravenous corticotropin 10 mg twice daily.[2]

In contrast, a decrease in the anticoagulant effects of **ethyl biscoumacetate** was described in one patient given corticotropin and one patient given **cortisone**.[3]

(b) Dexamethasone

The INR and plasma anticoagulant concentrations were studied in 9 patients stabilised on anticoagulants (8 taking **fluindione** and one taking **warfarin**) during a total of 10 cycles of dexamethasone (40 mg/day for 4 days every 28 days) alone (4 patients) or with melphalan (5 patients). The INR increased in all patients from a mean of 2.75 at baseline to 5.22 within 3 to 6 days of starting dexamethasone. No major bleeding occurred, although 2 cases of minor bleeding were reported. Oral anticoagulants were temporarily withheld during 8 out of 10 cycles, and oral vitamin K 1 mg was taken by 2 patients during 2 cycles. An increase in the plasma concentration of fluindione of about 37% was noted (4 patients monitored), and the only patient taking warfarin had an increase in the warfarin plasma concentration (of about 28%), although neither of these results was statistically significant.[4]

(c) Methylprednisolone

A sharp increase in the INR of a patient with antiphospholipid syndrome occurred after methylprednisolone was added to treatment with an unnamed oral anticoagulant.[5,6] This prompted a controlled study in 10 patients stabilised on anticoagulants (8 taking **fluindione** and 2 taking **acenocoumarol**) and 5 patients not taking an anticoagulant. It was found that pulse high-dose intravenous methylprednisolone (500 mg or 1 g) increased the mean INR of those patients taking an anticoagulant from a baseline of 2.75 to 8.04, but had no effect on the prothrombin time in those taking methylprednisolone alone.[5,6] Two patients stabilised on **warfarin** are also reported to have had significant prolongations in their prothrombin times when given high-dose methylprednisolone (960 mg or 1 g, followed by **dexamethasone** 60 mg three times daily for 3 days in one case) for the treatment of multiple sclerosis.[7]

Moreover, in a retrospective study, short-term oral corticosteroid use (methylprednisolone or prednisone) was associated with an increase in INR in patients taking **warfarin**, see under *Prednisone*, below.

(d) Prednisone

An early study in 24 patients anticoagulated for several days with **dicoumarol** found that 2 hours after receiving prednisone 10 mg their silicone coagulation time had decreased from 28 minutes to 24 minutes, and 2 hours later had further decreased to 22 minutes, suggesting that prednisone opposes the effect of dicoumarol.[8]

In contrast, in a retrospective analysis of 24 patients stabilised on **warfarin**, short-term oral corticosteroid use (prednisone in 12 patients and **methylprednisolone** in 12 patients for between 5 and 30 days, doses not specified) increased the INR on 29 of 32 occasions, decreased it on 2 occasions, and did not change it on one occasion. The mean INR increased from 2.33 to 3.57 (measured at a mean of 6.7 days after starting the corticosteroid). Warfarin dose adjustments (reduction and/or withheld dose) were required on 16 occasions. On 5 occasions the INR was elevated to greater than 5 (three times with prednisone and twice with **methylprednisolone**).[9] Similarly, in a study of children with acute leukaemia receiving high-dose prednisone 60 mg/m^2 daily with low-dose **warfarin** for the prevention of central line-associated thrombosis, the warfarin requirement while they were taking the steroid was about half that required during periods without it (0.057 mg/kg versus 0.12 mg/kg daily).[10] Moreover, there is case report of a man taking **warfarin** and prednisone whose INR fluctuations appeared to correlate with when he stopped (subtherapeutic) or re-started (supratherapeutic) prednisone.[11]

In a study to investigate the effects of reducing the **warfarin** dose in anticipation of an interaction with **prednisone**, patients stable taking warfarin were either given a pre-emptive 10 to 20% warfarin dose reduction before starting prednisone (20 patients) or the warfarin dose was adjusted in response to INR changes after starting prednisone (control group, 17 patients). Patients in the control group had a trend towards a higher risk of an INR greater than one point above the upper limit than those whose warfarin dose was pre-emptively reduced, although this was not statistically significant. However, patients whose warfarin dose was initially reduced when prednisone was started had a greater risk of having a subtherapeutic INR, when compared with the control group. The median prednisone dose in both groups was 40 mg daily for at least 5 days[12]

(e) Unspecified corticosteroids

An analysis of a cohort of children receiving **warfarin** found that there was no difference in the dose of **warfarin** required to achieve and maintain the target INR between **warfarin** courses if corticosteroids were given (38 courses) and courses where corticosteroids were not given (314 courses). However, courses with corticosteroids were associated with a higher percentage of INR measurements greater than the target (21% versus 14%).[13]

Mechanism

Not understood. Corticotropin, cortisone, and prednisone can increase the coagulability of the blood in the absence of anticoagulants, and might therefore antagonise their effects.[14,15] Conversely, it has been suggested that methylprednisolone and prednisone might inhibit the metabolism of anticoagulants increasing their effects.[6] However, note that, if anything, corticosteroids, particularly dexamethasone, are usually considered to be inducers of cytochrome P450 isoenzymes.

Importance and management

The interaction of low to moderate doses of corticosteroids with coumarins is by no means established. There are a few reports from the 1950s and 60s, with very little appearing to have been published until more recently. Nevertheless, in two of the more recent retrospective analyses, the use of corticosteroids appeared to be associated with a higher incidence of INRs over the target range or lower warfarin requirements. The most constructive thing that can be said is that if corticotropin (corticotrophin, ACTH) or any low-dose corticosteroid is given to patients taking anticoagulants, be aware that a modest change in coagulation requirements might occur.

Although the evidence is limited, marked INR increases have been reported with high-dose dexamethasone, prednisone, or methylprednisolone, and INRs should be closely monitored (daily has been recommended[6]) if these, or other high-dose corticosteroids, are added to established treatment with any coumarin or indanedione oral anticoagulant; the anticoagulant dose should be adjusted if necessary. Although one study suggests that a pre-emptive reduction in the warfarin dose might possibly reduce the risk of over-anticoagulation, this could result in an increased risk of a subtherapeutic INR. Also note that corticosteroids are associated with a weak increase in peptic ulceration and gastrointestinal bleeding, and the risk of this could theoretically be increased if over-anticoagulation occurs.

1. Hellem AJ, Solem JH. The influence of ACTH on prothrombin-proconvertin values in blood during treatment with dicumarol and phenylindanedione. *Acta Med Scand* (1954) 150, 389–93.
2. van Cauwenberge H, Jacques LB. Haemorrhagic effect of ACTH with anticoagulants. *Can Med Assoc J* (1958) 79, 536–40.
3. Chatterjea JB, Salomon L. Antagonistic effects of A.C.T.H. and cortisone on the anticoagulant activity of ethyl biscoumacetate. *BMJ* (1954) 2, 790–2.
4. Sellam J, Costedoat-Chalumeau N, Amoura Z, Aymard G, Choquet S, Trad S, Vignes BL, Hulot J-S, Berenbaum F, Lechat P, Cacoub P, Ankri A, Mariette X, Leblond V, Piette J-C. Potentiation of fluindione or warfarin by dexamethasone in multiple myeloma and AL amyloidosis. *Joint Bone Spine* (2007) 74, 446–52.
5. Costedoat-Chalumeau N, Amoura Z, Wechsler B, Ankri A, Piette J-C. Implications of interaction between vitamin K antagonists and high-dose intravenous methylprednisolone in the APS. *J Autoimmun* (2000) 15, A22.
6. Costedoat-Chalumeau N, Amoura Z, Aymard G, Sevin O, Wechsler B, Cacoub P, Huong Du, Le Th, Diquet B, Ankri A, Piette J-C. Potentiation of vitamin K antagonists by high-dose intravenous methylprednisolone. *Ann Intern Med* (2000) 132, 631–5.
7. Kaufman M. Treatment of multiple sclerosis with high-dose corticosteroids may prolong the prothrombin time to dangerous levels in patients taking warfarin. *Multiple Sclerosis* (1997) 3, 248–9.
8. Menczel J, Dreyfuss F. Effect of prednisone on blood coagulation time in patients on dicumarol therapy. *J Lab Clin Med* (1960) 56, 14–20.
9. Hazlewood KA, Fugate SE, Harrison DL. Effect of oral corticosteroids on chronic warfarin therapy. *Ann Pharmacother* (2006) 40, 2101–6.
10. Ruud E, Holmstrøm H, Bergan S, Wesenberg F. Oral anticoagulation with warfarin is significantly influenced by steroids and CYP2C9 polymorphisms in children with cancer. *Pediatr Blood Cancer* (2008) 50, 710–13.
11. Stading JA, Chock A, Faulkner MA, Skrabal MZ. Effects of prednisone on the International Normalized Ratio. *Am J Health-Syst Pharm* (2006) 63, 2354–6. Erratum: *ibid.* (2007) 64, 130 authors added.
12. Dowd MB, Vavra KA, Witt DM, Delate T, Martinez K. Empiric warfarin dose adjustment with prednisone therapy. A randomized, controlled trial. *J Thromb Thrombolysis* (2011) 31, 472–7.
13. Streif W, Marzinotto AV, Massicotte P, Chan AKC, Julian JA, Mitchell L. Analysis of warfarin therapy in pediatric patients: a prospective cohort study of 319 patients. *Blood* (1999) 94, 3007–14.
14. Cosgriff SW, Diefenbach AF, Vogt W. Hypercoagulability of the blood associated with ACTH and cortisone therapy. *Am J Med* (1950) 9, 752–6.
15. Ozsoylu S, Strauss HS, Diamond LK. Effects of corticosteroids on coagulation of the blood. *Nature* (1962) 195, 1214–15.

Coumarins + Cranberry products

A number of case reports suggest that cranberry juice can increase the INR of patients taking warfarin, and one patient has died as a result of this interaction. Other patients have developed unstable INRs, or, in one isolated case, a *reduced* INR. However, in five controlled studies, cranberry juice did not alter the anticoagulant effect of warfarin, or had only very minor effects on the INR. Neither cranberry juice nor the extract altered warfarin pharmacokinetics. An isolated report describes raised INR in a patient taking warfarin, after consumption of large amounts of cranberry sauce.

Clinical evidence

(a) Case reports

1. Cranberry juice. In September 2003, the MHRA/CSM in the UK noted that they had received 5 reports suggesting an interaction between **warfarin** and cranberry juice since 1999 (3 cases of INR increases, one case of unstable INR and one case of a decrease in INR).[1] By October 2004, the MHRA/CSM reported that they had now received 12 reports of a suspected interaction, including 5 additional cases of bleeding episodes and two additional cases of unstable INRs in patients drinking cranberry juice while taking warfarin.[2] The most serious case involved a man taking **warfarin** whose INR markedly increased (INR greater than 50) 6 weeks after starting to drink cranberry juice. He died from gastrointestinal and pericardial haemorrhages.[1,3,4] Further details of this case included that he had recently been taking cefalexin (not known to interact) for a chest infection, and had been eating virtually nothing for at least 2 weeks,[3] a fact that would have contributed to the increase in anticoagulation.

In a further published case report, a patient stabilised on **warfarin** was found to have INRs of 10 to 12 before a surgical procedure, although he had no previous record of an INR greater than 4. Vitamin K was given, and heparin was substituted for warfarin. When warfarin was restarted postoperatively, the INR quickly rose to 8 and then to 11 with haematuria, and postoperative bleeding. The patient was drinking almost 2 litres of cranberry juice daily, because of recurrent urinary tract infections, and was advised to stop drinking this. Three days later the INR had stabilised at 3 with no further intervention.[5] Another report describes a patient stabilised on **warfarin** whose INR rose from an average of about 2 to 4.6 after drinking about 1420 mL of cranberry juice cocktail (cranberry fruit juice 18%) daily for 2 days. A few months later, her INR rose again, from an average of about 2 to 6.5 after drinking about

1893 mL of the same juice, daily for 3 or 4 days.[6] Similarly, a case of fluctuating INR (between 1 and 10) in a patient taking **warfarin** has been attributed to cranberry juice.[7]

In the US, a case of major bleeding and a high INR has been reported in a man taking **warfarin**, which occurred shortly after cranberry juice 710 mL daily was started.[8] Another case, describes an increase in the INR of a patient receiving **warfarin**, from below 3 to 6.45, without bleeding, after the patient drank about 2 litres of cranberry/apple juice over the last week. Of note, the patient was subsequently restabilised on a lower dose of warfarin and may have taken an extra dose of warfarin in the week before the raised INR was measured.[9]

2. Cranberry sauce. A single case report describes a patient stabilised on **warfarin**, whose INR rose from between 2 and 3 up to 4.8, after consuming about 113 g of cranberry sauce daily for 7 days. Warfarin was stopped for 2 days, after which the dose was reduced, and 7 days after the cranberry sauce was discontinued the patient's INR returned to previous levels.[10]

(b) Controlled studies

1. Cranberry juice. In a placebo-controlled study, 30 patients on stable doses of **warfarin** drank 240 mL of cranberry juice or placebo once daily for 2 weeks. Mean INR values were not found to be different between the two groups during, or one week after the study period. Maximum plasma levels of both *R*- and *S*-warfarin were also no different between the two groups.[11] The preliminary findings of this study have been reported elsewhere.[12] Another study in 7 male patients, also found that 250 mL of cranberry juice for 7 days had no effect on INR values.[13] Similarly, an open-label study in 9 male patients taking stable doses of **warfarin** found that 240 mL of cranberry juice *twice* daily for 7 days did not change mean prothrombin times from baseline values during, or one day after the study.[14]

However, note that the daily volume of cranberry juice in these studies was lower than the daily volume in the couple of case reports where cranberry juice intake is known. Nevertheless, in another controlled study in 10 healthy subjects, a higher volume of cranberry juice (200 mL *three* times daily) for 10 days did not alter the effect of a single 10-mg dose of **warfarin** (given on day 5) on the maximum thromboplastin time or AUC of the thromboplastin time.[15] In addition, cranberry juice had no effect on warfarin pharmacokinetics, except that there was a slight, but not statistically significant, 7% *decrease* in the AUC of *S*-warfarin.

2. Cranberry concentrate. A study in 12 healthy subjects found that cranberry juice concentrate, given as 2 capsules three times daily for 21 days (equivalent to 57 g of fruit daily), had no effect on the maximum INR after a single 25-mg dose of **warfarin** given on day 15 (2.8 versus 2.6). However, the AUC of the INR was slightly increased by 28%, which was statistically significant, but the clinical relevance of this measure is uncertain. The cranberry concentrate had no effect on platelet aggregation, and had no effect on the pharmacokinetics of either *R*- or *S*-warfarin.[16]

Mechanism

Not known. It was originally suggested that one or more of the constituents of cranberry juice might inhibit the metabolism of warfarin by CYP2C9, thereby reducing its clearance from the body and increasing its effects.[1] However, five studies have shown that cranberry juice or cranberry extracts do not alter the pharmacokinetics of warfarin, and cranberry juice had no effect on flurbiprofen pharmacokinetics, a drug used as a surrogate index of CYP2C9 activity.[17] An interaction might therefore be via a pharmacodynamic mechanism. For example, the salicylate constituent of commercial cranberry juice might cause hypoprothrombinaemia.[18]

Importance and management

An interaction is not established. Controlled studies have not found a pharmacokinetic interaction, and only one of five studies found any evidence for an increase in warfarin effect. Moreover, the clinical relevance of the finding of this study of a 0.2 increase in INR and 28% increase in AUC of the INR is likely to be slight at most, and does not fit with the sometimes marked increase in INR seen in some case reports. This might be explained if the interaction is dose dependent (in one of the cases where cranberry intake was mentioned a quantity of 2 litres daily was being consumed), or if it is product dependent (i.e. due to a constituent present in the cranberry juice that is not standardised for and varies widely). However, it could also be that there is no specific interaction, and that the case reports just represent idiosyncratic reactions in which other unknown factors (e.g. altered diet) were more important.

In 2004, on the basis of the then available case reports and lack of controlled studies, the CSM/MHRA in the UK advised that patients taking warfarin should avoid drinking cranberry juice unless the health benefits are considered to outweigh any risks. They recommended increased INR monitoring for any patient taking warfarin and who has a regular intake of cranberry juice.[2] They also advised similar precautions with other cranberry products (such as capsules or concentrates).[2] These might still be prudent precautions, although the controlled studies now available do provide some reassurance that, in otherwise healthy individuals, moderate doses of cranberry juice are unlikely to have an important impact on anticoagulation control.

The report of raised INR after consumption of large amounts of cranberry sauce is an isolated one and the amount of cranberry sauce consumed was unusually large. As such its general importance is unclear. Nevertheless it would seem unnecessary to extend the warning about other cranberry products to include cranberry sauce on the basis of this one report.

1. Committee on Safety of Medicines/Medicines and Healthcare products Regulatory Agency. Possible interaction between warfarin and cranberry juice. *Current Problems* (2003) 29, 8.
2. Committee on Safety of Medicines/Medicines and Healthcare products Regulatory Agency. Interaction between warfarin and cranberry juice: new advice. *Current Problems* (2004) 30, 10.
3. Suvarna R, Pirmohamed M, Henderson L. Possible interaction between warfarin and cranberry juice. *BMJ* (2003) 327, 1454.
4. Griffiths AP, Beddall A, Pegler S. Fatal haemopericardium and gastrointestinal haemorrhage due to possible interaction of cranberry juice with warfarin. *J R Soc Promot Health* (2008) 128, 324–6.
5. Grant P. Warfarin and cranberry juice: an interaction? *J Heart Valve Dis* (2004) 13, 25–6.
6. Hamann GL, Campbell JD, George CM. Warfarin-cranberry juice interaction. *Ann Pharmacother* (2011) 45, e17 [Epub].
7. Walsh KM. Getting to yes. *J Am Geriatr Soc* (2005) 53, 1072.
8. Rindone JP, Murphy TW. Warfarin-cranberry juice interaction resulting in profound hypoprothrombinemia and bleeding. *Am J Ther* (2006) 13, 283–4.
9. Paeng CH, Sprague M, Jackevicius CA. Interaction between warfarin and cranberry juice. *Clin Ther* (2007) 29, 1730–5.
10. Mergenhagen KA, Sherman O. Elevated international normalized ratio after concurrent ingestion of cranberry sauce and warfarin. *Am J Health-Syst Pharm* (2008) 65, 2113–16.
11. Ansell J, McDonough M, Zhao Y, Harmatz JS, Greenblatt DJ. The absence of an interaction between warfarin and cranberry juice: a randomized double-blind trial. *J Clin Pharmacol* (2009) 49, 824–30.
12. Ansell J, McDonough M, Harmatz JS, Greenblatt DJ. A randomized, double-blind trial of the interaction between cranberry juice and warfarin. *J Thromb Thrombolysis* (2008) 25, 112.
13. Li Z, Seeram NP, Carpenter CL, Thames G, Minutti C, Bowerman S. Cranberry does not affect prothrombin time in male subjects on warfarin. *J Am Diet Assoc* (2006) 106, 2057–61.
14. Mellen CK, Ford M, Rindone J. Effect of high-dose cranberry juice on the pharmacodynamics of warfarin in patients. *Br J Clin Pharmacol* (2010) 70, 139–42.
15. Lilja JJ, Backman JT, Neuvonen PJ. Effects of daily ingestion of cranberry juice on the pharmacokinetics of warfarin, tizanidine, and midazolam—probes of CYP2C9, CYP1A2, and CYP3A4. *Clin Pharmacol Ther* (2007) 81, 833–9.
16. Mohammed Abdul MI, Jiang X, Williams KM, Day RO, Roufogalis BD, Liauw WS, Xu H, McLachlan AJ. Pharmacodynamic interaction of warfarin with cranberry but not with garlic in healthy subjects. *Br J Pharmacol* (2008) 154, 1691–1700.
17. Greenblatt DJ, von Moltke LL, Perloff ES, Luo Y, Harmatz JS, Zinny MA. Interaction of flurbiprofen with cranberry juice, grape juice, tea, and fluconazole: in vitro and clinical studies. *Clin Pharmacol Ther* (2006) 79, 125–33.
18. Isele H. Tödliche Blutung unter Warfarin plus Preiselbeersaft. Liegt's an der Salizylsäure? *MMW Fortschr Med* (2004) 146, 13.

Coumarins + *Curbicin*

The INR of one patient taking warfarin modestly increased after he took *Curbicin* (saw palmetto, cucurbita, and vitamin E). This product has also been associated with an increased INR in a patient not taking anticoagulants. Excessive bleeding during surgery has been reported in another patient who had been taking saw palmetto.

Clinical evidence

A 61-year-old man taking **warfarin** and simvastatin, with a stable INR of around 2.4, had an increase in his INR to 3.4 within 6 days of starting to take 5 tablets of *Curbicin* daily. Within a week of stopping the *Curbicin*, his INR had fallen to its previous value. Another elderly man who was not taking any anticoagulants and was taking 3 tablets of *Curbicin* daily was found to have an INR of 2.1 (normal 0.9 to 1.2). His INR decreased (1.3 to 1.4) when he was given vitamin K, but did not normalise until a week after the *Curbicin* was stopped. *Curbicin* is a herbal remedy used for micturition problems, and contains extracts from the fruit of *Serenoa repens* (**saw palmetto**) and the seed of *Cucurbita pepo*.[1]

In addition, saw palmetto has been attributed to excessive bleeding in a 53-year-old man undergoing a surgical procedure to remove a brain tumour. An estimated 2 litres of blood was lost during surgery and bleeding time did not return to normal for 5 days. The patient denied taking NSAIDs pre-operatively but admitted to taking saw palmetto for benign prostatic hypertrophy.[2]

Mechanism

The authors of the first report suggest that what happened was possibly due to the presence of vitamin E in the *Curbicin* preparation (each tablet contains 10 mg), but vitamin E does not normally affect INRs. Experimental evidence suggests that saw palmetto may inhibit the cytochrome P450 isoenzyme CYP2C9, which is an important route of warfarin metabolism.

Importance and management

Evidence appears to be limited to case reports and an experimental study of unknown clinical relevance. Because of the many other factors influencing anticoagulant control, it is not possible to reliably ascribe a change in INR specifically to a drug interaction in a single case report without other supporting evidence. It may be better to advise patients to discuss the use of any herbal products they wish to try, and to increase monitoring if this is thought advisable. Cases of uneventful use should be reported, as they are as useful as possible cases of adverse effects.

1. Yue, Q-Y, Jansson K. Herbal drug Curbicin and anticoagulant effect with and without warfarin: possibly related to the vitamin E component. *J Am Geriatr Soc* (2001) 49, 838.
2. Cheema P, El-Mefty O, Jazieh AR. Intraoperative haemorrhage associated with the use of extract of Saw Palmetto herb: a case report and review of literature. *J Intern Med* (2001) 250, 167–9.

Coumarins + Danazol or Gestrinone

Increased anticoagulant effects and bleeding have been seen in a few patients taking warfarin with danazol. A case describes similar effects in a patient taking warfarin and gestrinone.

Clinical evidence

(a) Danazol

A 40-year-old woman stabilised on **warfarin** 6 mg daily with a prothrombin ratio of 2.3 presented after vomiting blood. She was found to have a prothrombin ratio of 14, and required fresh frozen plasma and 2 litres of blood. Three weeks previously she had been prescribed danazol 200 mg twice daily.[1] Four other similar cases of this interaction with danazol have been reported.[2-4] In two of the cases the patients were subsequently stabilised on **warfarin** and danazol, but with 50 to 70% lower **warfarin** doses.[3,4]

(b) Gestrinone

A bulletin includes a brief mention of an increased INR with vaginal bleeding and multiple bruising in a woman taking **warfarin** and gestrinone.[5]

Mechanism

The reason for this interaction is unknown, but both danazol and gestrinone have androgenic properties, and anabolic steroids (see 'Coumarins and related drugs + Anabolic steroids or Androgens', p.382), are known to increase the effects of warfarin.

Importance and management

Although data are limited, the interaction with danazol would appear to be established, and close monitoring of the INR is advisable if danazol is added to established treatment with a coumarin. Some suggest that the initial dose of the anticoagulant should be halved when danazol is started.[2] However, others note that this may not be appropriate in patients at high thrombogenic risk, such as those with mechanical valves. In these patients, they recommend a cautious reduction in dose with weekly monitoring of the INR until it becomes stable (several weeks).[4] Gestrinone might be expected to interact similarly, and some caution is therefore appropriate.

1. Goulbourne IA, Macleod DAD. An interaction between danazol and warfarin. Case report. *Br J Obstet Gynaecol* (1981) 88, 950–1.
2. Small M, Peterkin M, Lowe GDO, McCune G, Thomson JA. Danazol and oral anticoagulants. *Scott Med J* (1982) 27, 331–2.
3. Meeks ML, Mahaffey KW, Katz MD. Danazol increases the anticoagulant effect of warfarin. *Ann Pharmacother* (1992) 26, 641–2.
4. Booth CD. A drug interaction between danazol and warfarin. *Pharm J* (1993) 250, 439.
5. Beeley L, Cunningham H, Carmichael A, Brennan A. *Adverse Drug React Bull* (1992) 35, 18.

Coumarins and related drugs + Danshen (*Salvia miltiorrhiza*)

Three case reports indicate that danshen may increase the effects of warfarin, resulting in bleeding.

Clinical evidence

A woman taking **warfarin**, furosemide and digoxin, who began to take danshen on alternate days, was hospitalised a month later with anaemia and bleeding (prothrombin time greater than 60 seconds, INR greater than 5.62). The anaemia was attributed to occult gastrointestinal bleeding and the over-anticoagulation to an interaction with the danshen. She was later restabilised on warfarin in the absence of the danshen with an INR of 2.5, and within 4 months her haemoglobin levels were normal.[1]

A man taking **warfarin**, digoxin, captopril and furosemide with an INR of about 3, developed chest pain and breathlessness about 2 weeks after starting to take danshen. He was found to have a massive pleural effusion, and an INR of more than 8.4. He was later discharged on his usual dose of warfarin with an INR stable at 3, in the absence of the danshen.[2]

Over-anticoagulation was investigated in Chinese patients admitted to a medical unit during a 9-month period in 1994/1995. An interaction with **warfarin** was reported in a patient using a medicated oil product that contained methyl salicylate 15%, and an analgesic balm that contained danshen, methyl salicylate 50% and diclofenac.[3]

Mechanism

Danshen has antiplatelet actions, which may be additive with the anticoagulant effect of warfarin. The mechanism for the increase in warfarin levels is unknown, because the studies suggest that the usual extracts of danshen do not inhibit the cytochrome P450 isoenzyme CYP2C9, the main route of warfarin metabolism.

Importance and management

Evidence appears to be limited to three case studies, which alone would be insufficient to establish an interaction. Further, one of these cases included the use of methyl salicylate, which has been shown to interact with warfarin. The pharmacokinetic effects of the usual extracts of danshen seem to suggest that an interaction resulting in raised warfarin levels is unlikely in most patients. However, because danshen may have antiplatelet effects, an interaction between warfarin and danshen, resulting in increased bleeding, is possible. Clinically the use of an antiplatelet drug with an anticoagulant should generally be avoided in the absence of a specific indication. It may therefore be prudent to advise against concurrent use. However, if concurrent use is felt desirable it would seem sensible to warn patients to be alert for any signs of bruising or bleeding, and report these immediately, should they occur.

1. Yu CM, Chan JCN, Sanderson JE. Chinese herbs and warfarin potentiation by 'Danshen'. *J Intern Med* (1997) 241, 337–9.
2. Izzat MB, Yim APC, El-Zufari MH. A taste of Chinese medicine. *Ann Thorac Surg* (1998) 66, 941–2.
3. Chan TYK. Drug interactions as a cause of overanticoagulation and bleedings in Chinese patients receiving warfarin. *Int J Clin Pharmacol Ther* (1998) 36, 403–5.

Coumarins + Dichloralphenazone

The anticoagulant effects of warfarin are reduced by dichloralphenazone.

Clinical evidence

Five patients stabilised taking **warfarin** long-term and given dichloralphenazone 1.3 g each night for 30 days had a reduction of about 50% (range 20 to 69%) in plasma **warfarin** levels and a fall in the anticoagulant response during the last 14 days of concurrent use. Another patient given dichloralphenazone 1.3 g nightly for one month had a 70% fall in plasma **warfarin** levels and a thrombotest percentage rise from 9% to 55% (indicating a reduced anticoagulant effect). These values returned to normal when the hypnotic was withdrawn.[1,2]

Mechanism

The phenazone component of dichloralphenazone is a potent liver enzyme inducer (see 'Coumarins + NSAIDs; Phenazone (Antipyrine)', p.455), which increases the metabolism and clearance of the warfarin, thereby reducing its effects.[1,2] The effects of the cloral hydrate component (see 'Coumarins + Cloral hydrate and related drugs', p.418) appear to be minimal.

Importance and management

Information is limited, but the interaction between warfarin and dichloralphenazone appears to be established and clinically important, probably affecting most patients. The dose of warfarin will need to be increased to accommodate this interaction. If the effect of warfarin has been reduced by using dichloralphenazone, it may take up to a month for it to restabilise. There does not appear to be any information about other anticoagulants, but other coumarins would be expected to be similarly affected. The benzodiazepines (see 'Coumarins + Benzodiazepines and related drugs', p.412) are generally preferred hypnotics, and do not interact.

1. Breckenridge A, Orme ML'E, Thorgeirsson S, Davies DS, Brooks RV. Drug interaction with warfarin: studies with dichloralphenazone, chloral hydrate and phenazone (antipyrine). *Clin Sci* (1971) 40, 351–64.
2. Breckenridge A, Orme M. Clinical implications of enzyme induction. *Ann N Y Acad Sci* (1971) 179, 421–31.

Coumarins and related drugs + Dipyridamole

The concurrent use of dipyridamole and a coumarin does not alter the prothrombin time, but it might cause an increased risk of serious bleeding. There is some evidence that the risk of bleeding may be lower, without a reduction in efficacy, if the INR is maintained within a lower range.

Clinical evidence

(a) Prosthetic heart valves

In a short-term study in 6 patients stabilised on **warfarin**, the addition of dipyridamole 75 mg three times daily did not alter prothrombin time ratios measured 8 times over 17 days.[1]

A meta-analysis of 6 randomised, controlled studies of the combined use of an oral anticoagulant [presumably a coumarin or indanedione] and dipyridamole compared with an oral anticoagulant alone, found no increased risk of *any* bleeding events when dipyridamole was given (odds ratio 1.001).[2] In contrast, in a later meta-analysis of the same studies, the risk of *major* bleeding with the addition of dipyridamole was increased (odds ratio 2.22). In addition to the difference in classification of bleeding events, the authors of the second analysis stated that they had used published data from two studies, which showed a slightly higher bleeding risk, whereas the earlier meta-analysis had used unpublished data from these studies, showing a lower bleeding risk.[3]

In one randomised study, the risk of excessive bleeding was 4% in patients taking **warfarin** and dipyridamole 400 mg daily, compared with 14% in patients taking **warfarin** and aspirin 500 mg daily. When compared with a non-randomised control group taking **warfarin** alone, the risk of excessive bleeding was not increased by dipyridamole (4% with both drugs versus 5% with **warfarin** alone).[4]

In another randomised study, the risk of bleeding was lower (1% versus 3.7%) in patients receiving dipyridamole 225 mg daily with **phenindione** at a target INR of 2 to 2.5 than in patients receiving **phenindione** alone with a target INR of 2.5 to 3.5, and the combination was more effective.[5] Similarly, the risk of bleeding was lower with a lower target INR of 2 to 3 than with a target INR of 3 to 4.5 (3.9% versus 20.8%) in patients taking **acenocoumarol**, aspirin 330 mg twice daily and dipyridamole 75 mg twice daily.[6]

(b) Other conditions

In a randomised study in patients with severe or recurrent venous thrombosis, there was no difference in dose of **acenocoumarol** necessary to reach an INR of 2.5 to 3.5 between 100 patients taking **acenocoumarol** with dipyridamole 400 mg daily and 100 patients taking **acenocoumarol** alone. None of the patients had severe bleeding, and 3 to 4% of patients in both groups had moderate bleeding (haematomas, haematuria).[7]

Thirty patients with glomerulonephritis stabilised on either **warfarin** (28 patients) or **phenindione** (2 patients) with a prothrombin activity of between 20 to 30% of control had no significant changes in prothrombin times when they were given dipyridamole in doses increased from 100 mg daily up to a maximum of 400 mg daily over about a month. Twelve to 19 days after starting dipyridamole, 3 patients with normal renal function developed mild bleeding (epistaxis, bruising, haematuria), which resolved when either drug was withdrawn or the dose reduced.[8]

In a retrospective, cohort study in patients taking oral anticoagulants with or without antiplatelet drugs, including dipyridamole, the concurrent use of an antiplatelet drug was found to significantly increase the risk of bleeding compared with an oral anticoagulant alone: 4.2% of patients receiving an anticoagulant and an antiplatelet drug had a bleeding event compared with 2% of the patients taking an oral anticoagulant alone. No additional beneficial reduction in the risk of thromboembolism was found.[9]

Mechanism

Dipyridamole reduces platelet adhesiveness or aggregation, which prolongs bleeding time. This may increase the risk or severity of bleeding if over-anticoagulation occurs.

Importance and management

There is clearly some uncertainty regarding the increased risk of bleeding with the combination of warfarin and dipyridamole, with one analysis finding no increased risk,[2] and a second finding about a doubling of risk of serious bleeding.[3] The authors of the second analysis consider that their results represent a more conservative estimate of bleeding risk.[3] There is some evidence that maintaining anticoagulant control at the lower end of the therapeutic range minimises possible bleeding complications and it would therefore seem prudent to consider this wherever possible.

1. Donaldson DR, Sreeharan N, Crow MJ, Rajah SM. Assessment of the interaction of warfarin with aspirin and dipyridamole. *Thromb Haemost* (1982) 47, 77.
2. Pouleur H, Buyse M. Effects of dipyridamole in combination with anticoagulant therapy on survival and thromboembolic events in patients with prosthetic heart valves. A meta-analysis of the randomized trials. *J Thorac Cardiovasc Surg* (1995) 110, 463–72.
3. Little SH, Massel DR. Antiplatelet and anticoagulation for patients with prosthetic heart valves. Available in The Cochrane Database of Systematic Reviews; Issue 4. Chichester: John Wiley; 2003 (accessed 06/06/07).
4. Chesebro JH, Fuster V, Elveback LR, McGoon DC, Pluth JR, Puga FJ, Wallace RB, Danielson GK, Orszulak TA, Piehler JM, Schaff HV. Trial of combined warfarin plus dipyridamole or aspirin therapy in prosthetic heart valve replacement: danger of aspirin compared with dipyridamole. *Am J Cardiol* (1983) 51, 1537–41.
5. Hassouna A, Allam H, Awad A, Hassaballah F. Standard versus low-level anticoagulation combined to low-dose dipyridamole after mitral valve replacement. *Cardiovasc Surg* (2000) 8, 491–8.
6. Altman R, Rouvier J, Gurfinkel E, D'Ortencio O, Manzanel R, de La Fuente L, Favaloro RG. Comparison of two levels of anticoagulant therapy in patients with substitute heart valves. *J Thorac Cardiovasc Surg* (1991) 101, 427–31.
7. Moriau M, Lavenne-Pardonge E, Crasborn L, von Frenckell R, Col-Debeys C. The treatment of severe or recurrent deep venous thrombosis. Beneficial effect of the co-administration of antiplatelet agents with or without rheological effects, and anticoagulants.*Thromb Res* (1995) 78, 469–82.
8. Kalowski S, Kincaid-Smith P. Interaction of dipyridamole with anticoagulants in the treatment of glomerulonephritis. *Med J Aust* (1973) 2, 164–6.
9. Johnson SG, Rogers K, Delate T, Witt DM. Outcomes associated with combined antiplatelet and anticoagulant therapy. *Chest* (2008) 133, 948–54.

Coumarins + Disopyramide

In two small uncontrolled studies, the anticoagulant effects of warfarin were slightly reduced by disopyramide. In contrast, there is an isolated report of a patient who needed his warfarin dose to be doubled after *stopping* disopyramide.

Clinical evidence

In a preliminary report of a study in 10 patients with recent atrial fibrillation taking **warfarin** and with a British Corrected Ratio of 2 to 3, disopyramide (dose not stated) increased the clearance of **warfarin** by 21%.[1] Similarly, another study found that 2 out of 3 patients needed a slight **warfarin** dose increase of about 10% after cardioversion and after starting disopyramide 200 mg three times daily for atrial fibrillation.[2]

In contrast, another report describes a patient who, following a myocardial infarction, was given **warfarin** 3 mg daily and disopyramide 100 mg every 6 hours with digoxin, furosemide and potassium supplements. When the disopyramide was withdrawn his **warfarin** requirements doubled over a 9-day period.[3,4]

Mechanism

Unknown. One idea is that when the disopyramide controls fibrillation, changes occur in cardiac output and in the flow of blood through the liver, which might have an effect on the synthesis of the blood clotting factors.[2,5] But the discordant response in the isolated case remains unexplained.

Importance and management

The interaction between disopyramide and warfarin is very poorly documented and not established. Limited data suggest only a minor interaction occurs (a slight reduction in anticoagulant effect), but an isolated case suggests a greater and opposite effect. Bear the possibility of an interaction in mind in the case of an unexpected response to warfarin in a patient starting or stopping disopyramide.

1. Woo KS, Chan K, Pun CO. The mechanisms of warfarin-disopyramide interaction. *Circulation* (1987) 76 (Suppl 4), IV-520.
2. Sylvén C, Anderson P. Evidence that disopyramide does not interact with warfarin. *BMJ* (1983) 286, 1181.
3. Haworth E, Burroughs AK. Disopyramide and warfarin interaction. *BMJ* (1977) 2, 866–7.
4. Marshall J. Personal communication, 1987.
5. Ryll C, Davis LJ. Warfarin-disopyramide interaction? *Drug Intell Clin Pharm* (1979) 13, 260.

Coumarins + Disulfiram

The anticoagulant effects of warfarin were increased by disulfiram in two studies, and two cases showing this effect have also been reported.

Clinical evidence

In one study in 7 healthy subjects, **warfarin** (adjusted to maintain a prothrombin activity of 40%) was given alone for 21 days, then given with disulfiram 500 mg daily for 21 days. The plasma **warfarin** levels of 5 of the 7 subjects rose by an average of 20% and their prothrombin activity fell from about 34% to 24% of normal (suggesting an increased anticoagulant effect); one of the subjects had little change, and the other had the opposite effect.[1] Other experiments with single doses of **warfarin** confirm these results.[1] However, a further study found that, although disulfiram potentiated the effect of *S*-warfarin, it did not change the plasma levels of either *R*- or *S*-warfarin.[2]

An alcoholic patient stabilised on **warfarin** had an increase in his prothrombin time associated with gross haematuria when disulfiram 250 mg daily was given. Two subsequent attempts to introduce disulfiram 250 mg on alternate days also had a similar effect. He was eventually stabilised on a 43% lower daily dose of warfarin and disulfiram 250 mg daily.[3] Another case of increased prothrombin time and the need for a reduced warfarin dose has been reported.[4]

Mechanism

Not fully understood. The suggestion[1] that disulfiram inhibits the liver enzymes concerned with the metabolism of warfarin has not been confirmed by later studies.[2] It has instead been suggested[2] that disulfiram may chelate with the metal ions necessary for the production of active thrombin from prothrombin, thereby augmenting the actions of warfarin.

Importance and management

An interaction appears to be established, although direct information about patients is very limited. What is known suggests that most individuals will demonstrate this interaction. If concurrent use is thought appropriate, the effects of warfarin should be monitored and suitable dose adjustments made when adding or withdrawing disulfiram. Care should be taken when starting warfarin in patients already taking disulfiram, and consideration should be given to using a smaller loading dose.

1. O'Reilly RA. Interaction of sodium warfarin and disulfiram (Antabuse®) in man. *Ann Intern Med* (1973) 78, 73–6.
2. O'Reilly RA. Dynamic interaction between disulfiram and separated enantiomorphs of racemic warfarin. *Clin Pharmacol Ther* (1981) 29, 332–6.
3. Rothstein E. Warfarin effect enhanced by disulfiram. *JAMA* (1968) 206, 1574–5.
4. Rothstein E. Warfarin effect enhanced by disulfiram (Antabuse). *JAMA* (1972) 221, 1052–3.

Coumarins and related drugs + Ditazole

Ditazole does not alter the anticoagulant effects of acenocoumarol. Nevertheless, as with other antiplatelet drugs, concurrent use might increase bleeding risk.

Clinical evidence, mechanism, importance and management

Fifty patients with artificial heart valves taking **acenocoumarol** had no changes in their prothrombin times while taking ditazole 800 mg daily.[1] Nevertheless, as with other antiplatelet drugs, such as aspirin (see 'Coumarins and related drugs + Aspirin or other Salicylates', p.405), concurrent use with oral anticoagulants might increase the risk or intensity of bleeding. Some caution is therefore appropriate on concurrent use.

1. Jacovella G, Milazzotto F. Ricerca di interazioni fra ditazolo e anticoagulanti in portatori di protesi valvolari intracardiache. *Clin Ter* (1977) 80, 425–31.

Coumarins and related drugs + Diuretics

Although cases of an interaction have been reported, in general, the loop diuretics, bumetanide, furosemide, and torasemide, the potassium-sparing diuretic spironolactone, and the thiazides, chlortalidone and chlorothiazide, have been found either not to interact with, or to cause only a small reduction in the effects of, the coumarin anticoagulants. The exceptions are tienilic acid, which has a pharmacokinetic interaction with warfarin and increases its effects, and possibly etacrynic acid, which on rare occasions has caused a large increase in the effects of warfarin. An isolated case of increased effects of warfarin with potassium canrenoate has also been reported.

Clinical evidence

A. Loop diuretics

(a) Bumetanide

In 10 healthy subjects, bumetanide 1 mg daily for 14 days did not alter the anticoagulant effect of a single-dose of **warfarin** given on day 8, and did not alter serum **warfarin** concentrations.[1] This confirms findings of a previous study in 5 healthy subjects given single-dose **warfarin** after bumetanide 2 mg daily for 5 days.[2]

(b) Etacrynic acid

A case report describes a large increase in the anticoagulant effects of **warfarin** in a woman with hypoalbuminaemia on two occasions when she was given etacrynic acid 150 mg to 300 mg daily.[3] In a preliminary report of a cohort study, it was stated that a therapeutically important interaction between **warfarin** and etacrynic acid was documented, but no details are given.[4]

(c) Furosemide

In 6 healthy subjects, plasma concentrations, half-lives, and prothrombin times were not altered when a single 50-mg dose of **warfarin** was given after furosemide 80 mg daily for 5 days.[2] However, a 28% decrease in the INR of one patient taking **warfarin** was seen when furosemide was taken on a regular basis. This was attributed to volume depletion caused by the diuretic, although interpretation of this case is complicated by the patient's admission of previous non-compliance and abuse of alcohol and cocaine.[5] In a pharmacokinetic study in 17 healthy subjects, furosemide 40 mg twice daily had no effect on the pharmacokinetics of a single 0.22-mg/kg dose of **phenprocoumon**.[6] In another study in 22 patients with congestive heart failure stabilised on **phenprocoumon**, furosemide 40 mg daily for 8 days did not alter the anticoagulant effects or required dose of **phenprocoumon**.[7]

(d) Tienilic acid (Ticrynafen)

In 6 healthy subjects, tienilic acid 250 mg daily for about 14 days caused a mean 3.6-fold increase in the anticoagulant effect of a single 1.5-mg/kg dose of **warfarin** given on day 4. Analysis showed the interaction was stereoselective, with the AUC of *S*-warfarin increased by 2.9-fold, and the AUC for *R*-warfarin increased by only 8%.[8] Two patients taking **ethyl biscoumacetate** began to bleed spontaneously (haematuria, ecchymoses of the legs, and gastrointestinal bleeding) when they started to take tienilic acid 250 mg daily. The thrombotest percentage of one of them was found to have fallen by 10%.[9] Increased anticoagulant effects and/or bleeding, which began within a few days, have been described in a number of other case reports in patients given tienilic acid while taking **ethyl biscoumacetate**,[10,11] **acenocoumarol**,[12] or **warfarin**.[10,13]

(e) Torasemide

In a study in 24 patients with congestive heart failure stabilised on **phenprocoumon**, torasemide 20 mg daily for 8 days did not alter the anticoagulant effects or required dose of **phenprocoumon**.[7]

A 43-year-old woman taking **warfarin** 7.5 mg daily had an increase in her INR from 3.1 to 6.2 within one week of stopping furosemide and starting to take torasemide 40 mg in the morning and 20 mg in the afternoon. The patient had no other changes to her medication, diet, alcohol intake, or other factors that are known to affect the anticoagulant effects of warfarin. Her warfarin dose was withheld and then restarted to eventually stabilise at a dose of 7.5 mg daily (except for 5 mg daily on Tuesdays and Fridays), with torasemide continued at the same dose. Note that in the 10 months before starting torasemide, the patient's weekly warfarin dose had been between 47.5 mg and 52.5 mg, with an INR ranging between 1.3 and 5.1, which had been attributed to other causes such as changes in diet.[14]

B. Potassium-sparing diuretics

In a study in 9 healthy subjects, **spironolactone** 50 mg four times daily for about 16 days reduced the prothrombin time response to a single-dose of warfarin given on day 8 by 24%, when compared with **warfarin** alone. Plasma **warfarin** concentrations remained unchanged.[15]

A case report describes a 77-year-old woman stabilised on **warfarin** 35 mg weekly for the previous 5 years (INR about 2), who developed an extensive haematoma 2 weeks after **potassium canrenoate** 50 mg daily was added to her existing medication (furosemide, bisoprolol, ramipril). Her INR was measured as 10.8, her **warfarin** was stopped, and she was given vitamin K. When her INR was 1.0, warfarin was retitrated, and stabilised, within the range of 2 to 3, on a dose of 22.5 mg weekly (while still taking the potassium canrenoate).[16]

C. Thiazides

(a) Chlortalidone

Six healthy subjects given a single 1.5-mg/kg dose of **warfarin** had reduced hypoprothrombinaemia (prothrombin activity reduced from 77 to 58 units) when they were also given chlortalidone 100 mg daily for 7 days with the **warfarin** given on the first day, although the plasma **warfarin** concentrations remained unaltered.[17] Similarly, reduced anticoagulant effects have been described when chlortalidone was given with **phenprocoumon**, but no important effects were seen when chlortalidone was given with **acenocoumarol**.[18]

(b) Chlorothiazide

A study in 8 healthy subjects given single 40- to 60-mg doses of **warfarin** before and after chlorothiazide 1 g daily for 21 days found that the mean half-life of the anticoagulant was increased from 39 hours to 44 hours, but the prothrombin time was only decreased by 0.3 seconds.[19]

(c) Unspecified thiazides

In contrast to the studies described above, a retrospective analysis of 551 patients taking **phenindione**, **phenprocoumon**, or **warfarin**, found that concurrent use of a thiazide (drugs not specified) increased the risk of a major bleed (defined as bleeding that required hospitalisation) by 5.2%.[20] However, note that this study was conducted during the 1980's and the finding does not appear to have been confirmed subsequently.

D. Unspecified diuretics

A retrospective study in 123 patients stabilised on **warfarin**, found no change in the INR within 30 days of giving patients a diuretic or increasing their diuretic dose, when compared with the INR within the previous 30 days before the diuretic was started or increased.[21]

Mechanism

It has been suggested that the diuresis induced by chlortalidone, furosemide, and spironolactone reduces plasma water, which leads to a concentration of the blood clotting factors.[5,15,17] Etacrynic acid can displace warfarin from its plasma protein binding sites,[22] and it was originally thought that other diuretics also interacted by drug displacement.[9,23,24] Only 3% of total plasma warfarin is in the free active form, thus a small displacement could result in marked enhancement of activity,[3] but it is almost certain that this, on its own, does not explain the interaction described.[4] Tienilic acid (ticrynafen), a loop diuretic which is structurally related to etacrynic acid, reduces the metabolism of *S*-warfarin (but not *R*-warfarin) thereby prolonging its stay in the body and increasing its effects.[8] It is possible that etacrynic acid interacts by a similar mechanism. Displacement of warfarin from protein-binding sites by torasemide, was one of the suggestions as to the reason for the case report of an increased INR on concurrent use,[14] and this was similarly implicated in the case of an increased INR with potassium canrenoate and warfarin.[16] The authors also suggested that this effect might only be clinically relevant in patients with a genetic polymorphism in vitamin K epoxide reductase complex subunit 1 (VKORC1), as was the case with their patient, which results in a lower dose of warfarin being required.[16]

Note that, in general protein-binding displacement is considered to only play a minor role in coumarin drug interactions (see *Anticoagulant interactions*, under 'Anticoagulants', p.371).

Importance and management

The documentation relating to diuretics in general (other than tienilic acid) is limited and seems to be confined to the reports cited here, most of which are single-dose pharmacological studies. The evidence suggests that, in general, these diuretics either do not interact at all with the coumarins, or interact only to an extent which is of little clinical relevance. This seems to be supported by the limited number of case reports of problems with these combinations, and is in general agreement with common experience. No precautions normally seem to be necessary, except possibly with etacrynic acid where it might be prudent to monitor the outcome, particularly in those with hypoalbuminaemia or renal impairment. The proposed increased risk of major bleeding with the concurrent use of thiazides has not subsequently been confirmed.

The interaction between the coumarins and tienilic acid is established and of clinical importance, but the incidence is uncertain. Concurrent use should be avoided. If that is not possible, prothrombin times should be closely monitored and the anticoagulant dose reduced as necessary. Note that tienilic acid has been withdrawn in many countries because of its hepatotoxicity.

1. Nipper H, Kirby S, Iber FL. The effect of bumetanide on the serum disappearance of warfarin sodium. *J Clin Pharmacol* (1981) 21, 654–6.
2. Nilsson CM, Horton ES, Robinson DS. The effect of furosemide and bumetanide on warfarin metabolism and anticoagulant response. *J Clin Pharmacol* (1978) 18, 91–4.
3. Petrick RJ, Kronacher N, Alcena V. Interaction between warfarin and ethacrynic acid. *JAMA* (1975) 231, 843–4.
4. Koch-Weser J. Hemorrhagic reactions and drug interactions in 500 warfarin-treated patients. *Clin Pharmacol Ther* (1973) 14, 139.
5. Laizure SC, Madlock L, Cyr M, Self T. Decreased hypoprothrombinemic effect of warfarin associated with furosemide. *Ther Drug Monit* (1997) 19, 361–3.
6. Mönig H, Böhm M, Ohnhaus EE, Kirch W. The effects of frusemide and probenecid on the pharmacokinetics of phenprocoumon. *Eur J Clin Pharmacol* (1990) 39, 261–5.
7. Piesche L, Bölke T. Comparative clinical trial investigating possible interactions of torasemide (20 mg o. d.) or furosemide (40 mg o.d.) with phenprocoumon in patients with congestive heart failure. *Int Congr Ser* (1993) 1023, 267–70.
8. O'Reilly RA. Ticrynafen-racemic warfarin interaction: hepatotoxic or stereoselective? *Clin Pharmacol Ther* (1982) 32, 356–61.
9. Detilleux M, Caquet R, Laroche C. Potentialisation de l'effet des anticoagulants coumariniques par un nouveau diurétique, l'acide tiénilique. *Nouv Presse Med* (1976) 5, 2395.
10. Prandota J, Pankow-Prandota L. Kliniczne znamienna interakcja nowego leku moczopednego kwasu tienylowego z lekami przeciwzakrzepowymi pochodnymi kumaryny. *Przegl Lek* (1982) 39, 385–8.
11. Portier H, Destaing F, Chauve L. Potentialisation de l'effet des anticoagulants coumariniques par l'acide tiénilique: une nouvelle observation. *Nouv Presse Med* (1977) 6, 468.
12. Grand A, Drouin B, Arche G-J. Potentialisation de l'action anticoagulante des anti-vitamines K par l'acide tiénilique. *Nouv Presse Med* (1977) 6, 2691.
13. McLain DA, Garriga FJ, Kantor OS. Adverse reactions associated with ticrynafen use. *JAMA* (1980) 243, 763–4.
14. Bird J, Carmona C. Probable interaction between warfarin and torsemide. *Ann Pharmacother* (2008) 42, 1893–8.
15. O'Reilly RA. Spironolactone and warfarin interaction. *Clin Pharmacol Ther* (1980) 27, 198–201.
16. Maggini V, Pugi A, Coletta D, Vietri M, Giusti B, Prisco D, Mugelli A, Lapi F, Vannacci A. A severe case of warfarin-canrenoate interaction: a role for genetic predisposition? *Br J Haematol* (2010) 150, 482–3.
17. O'Reilly RA, Sahud MA, Aggeler PM. Impact of aspirin and chlorthalidone on the pharmacodynamics of oral anticoagulant drugs in man. *Ann N Y Acad Sci* (1971) 179, 173–86.
18. Vinazzer H. Die Beeinflussung der Antikoagulantientherapie durch ein Diuretikum. *Wien Z Inn Med* (1963) 44, 323–7.
19. Robinson DS, Sylwester D. Interaction of commonly prescribed drugs and warfarin. *Ann Intern Med* (1970) 72, 853–6.
20. Launbjerg J, Egeblad H, Heaf J, Nielsen NH, Fugleholm AM, Ladefoged K. Bleeding complications to oral anticoagulant therapy: multivariate analysis of 1010 treatment years in 551 outpatients. *J Intern Med* (1991) 229, 351–5.
21. Edwards HD, Webb RD, Conway SE. Effect of oral diuretics on chronic warfarin therapy: a retrospective study. *Expert Opin Drug Safety* (2012) 11, 375–80.
22. Sellers EM, Koch-Weser J. Kinetics and clinical importance of displacement of warfarin from albumin by acidic drugs. *Ann N Y Acad Sci* (1971) 179, 213–25.
23. Slattery JT, Levy G. Ticrynafen effect on warfarin protein binding in human serum. *J Pharm Sci* (1979) 68, 393.
24. Prandota J, Albengres E, Tillement JP. Effect of tienilic acid (Diflurex) on the binding of warfarin ^{14}C to human plasma proteins. *Int J Clin Pharmacol Ther Toxicol* (1980) 18, 158–62.

Coumarins + Dofetilide

Dofetilide did not alter the anticoagulant effect of warfarin in one study.

Clinical evidence, mechanism, importance and management

In a placebo-controlled study in 14 healthy subjects, dofetilide 750 micrograms twice daily for 8 days had no effect on the prothrombin time in response to a single 40-mg dose of **warfarin** given on day 5.[1] No dose adjustment of **warfarin** would be anticipated to be needed on concurrent use.

1. Nichols DJ, Dalrymple I, Newgreen MW, Kleinermans D. The effect of dofetilide on pharmacodynamics of warfarin and pharmacokinetics of digoxin. *Eur Heart J* (1999) 20 (Abstr Suppl), 586.

Coumarins + Dronedarone

Studies suggest that dronedarone has very slight effects on warfarin exposure, but a number of case reports link increased INRs to the concurrent use of dronedarone.

Clinical evidence

The exposure to *S*-warfarin was very slightly increased by 20% when healthy subjects were also given dronedarone 600 mg twice daily (note this is higher than the recommended dose of 400 mg twice daily). The exposure to *R*-warfarin was unaffected and there was no clinically significant increase in INR.[1,2] However, the US manufacturer states that, when compared with placebo, more patients taking oral anticoagulants (not specified) had INRs of 5 or more, which was not associated with an increased risk of bleeding, after taking dronedarone in the ATHENA study. In most cases, the INR rose within one week of starting dronedarone.[1] Furthermore, a letter describes 3 patients taking **warfarin** who had increases in their INR of 50 to 100% after dronedarone was added.[3] In addition, a case report describes a 72-year-old woman who had been stable taking **warfarin** 25 mg/week and sotalol had her antiarrhythmic drug changed to dronedarone 400 mg twice daily. About 10 days later, she was seen in clinic and found to have an INR of 4.8, the **warfarin** dose was decreased by 5 mg/week, and 2 weeks later her INR had reduced to 2.7. Follow up over the next 11 months found a stable INR at the lower **warfarin** dose.[4]

Mechanism

Unclear. Dronedarone is known to inhibit CYP3A4, but in the study, it did not affect the pharmacokinetics of *R*-warfarin, which is metabolised, in part, by this isoenzyme. Dronedarone is not an established inhibitor of CYP2C9, by which *S*-warfarin is metabolised. In both the case reports, the patients had diarrhoea, but in one patient at least, the warfarin dose remained stable after the diarrhoea had resolved, so what part the diarrhoea had to play is unclear.

Importance and management

Evidence for an interaction between warfarin and dronedarone is somewhat conflicting, with one pharmacokinetic study finding only a slight effect on warfarin, whereas data from a study into the effect of dronedarone on hospitalisation, and a few unconfirmed case reports, finding an increased tendency to raised INRs after dronedarone is started. Until more is known it would seem prudent to increase the frequency of INR monitoring after dronedarone is first started and adjust the dose of warfarin accordingly. There does not appear to be any information about other coumarins, but it might be prudent to consider similar monitoring to that suggested for warfarin on the concurrent use of dronedarone.

1. Multaq (Dronedarone). Sanofi-Aventis U.S. LLC. US Prescribing information, March 2014.
2. Multaq (Dronedarone hydrochloride). Sanofi. UK Summary of product characteristics, November 2013.
3. Reiffel JA. An important drug interaction between dronedarone and warfarin that may be extrapolated to other drugs that can alter gastrointestinal function. *Am Heart J* (2011) 161, e5.
4. Pogge EK, Haber SL. Elevated international normalized ratio associated with use of dronedarone and warfarin. *Ann Pharmacother* (2011) 45, e46.

Coumarins + Endothelin receptor antagonists

Bosentan appears to cause a slight reduction in warfarin exposure, which might result in an increase in warfarin requirements in some patients. Ambrisentan and macitentan did not alter warfarin pharmacokinetics or pharmacodynamics in studies in healthy subjects.

Clinical evidence

(a) Ambrisentan

In a crossover study, 22 healthy subjects were given ambrisentan 10 mg daily for 8 days with a single 25-mg dose of **warfarin** on day 8. There was a 5% increase in the AUC of *R*-warfarin, and an 8% and 10% decrease in the maximum concentrations of *R*- and *S*-warfarin, respectively. The maximum prothrombin time was decreased by about 14%.[1] The UK manufacturer notes that, in patients, ambrisentan did not alter the weekly **warfarin** dose, prothrombin time, or INR. The pharmacokinetics of ambrisentan are also not affected by warfarin.[2]

(b) Bosentan

In a well-controlled study, 12 healthy subjects were given bosentan 500 mg twice daily or placebo for 10 days, with a single 26-mg dose of **warfarin** on day 6. Bosentan reduced the AUC of *R*-warfarin by 38% and reduced the AUC of *S*-warfarin by 29%. A decrease in the anticoagulant effects of **warfarin** was also noted, with a 23% reduction in prothrombin time occurring with bosentan.[3]

A few case reports highlight the clinical importance of this interaction. A 35-year-old woman taking **warfarin** with a stable INR of 2 to 3 over three months started taking bosentan 62.5 mg twice daily. After 10 days her INR was 1.7, and remained at this level over the next 4 weeks, despite an increase in her weekly **warfarin** dose from 27.5 mg to 40 mg. The bosentan dose was then increased to the maintenance dose of 125 mg twice daily, and two further weekly increases in **warfarin** dose were made. The INR was then high (3.2 to 4.1) for 3 weeks, before she was finally stabilised on **warfarin** 45 mg each week.[4] In a second case, the INR decreased to 1.5 on starting bosentan, necessitating an increase in **warfarin** dose from 30 mg weekly to 40 mg weekly. However, when the bosentan dose was later decreased from 250 mg daily to 125 mg daily, the INR increased to 4.6, and the warfarin dose was reduced to 35 mg weekly.[5] In another case, a 52-year-old woman with a stable INR while taking 52.5 mg warfarin weekly, required a 14% increase in her warfarin dose (to 60 mg weekly) three weeks after starting bosentan 125 mg daily. About 5 weeks after her bosentan dose was increased to 250 mg daily, her warfarin dose needed to be increased further to 65 mg weekly. For personal reasons, the patient discontinued both drugs for 7 days, after which the warfarin and bosentan doses were retitrated, and she then required 75 mg warfarin weekly (a 43% increase from her original dose).[6]

The UK manufacturer of bosentan notes that, in clinical experience, the use of bosentan with **warfarin** did not result in clinically relevant changes in the INR or **warfarin** dose. There was no difference in the frequency of **warfarin** dose changes (due to INR changes or adverse effects) between bosentan or placebo recipients.[7] However, in the STRIDE-2 study, where 52 patients with pulmonary arterial hypertension took bosentan at usual prescribed doses, daily warfarin dose requirements were 5.1 mg daily, compared with 3.7 mg in 51 patients given placebo. The average number of patients with an INR greater than 3.5 during this study was 20% lower than in the placebo group, but this did not reach statistical significance.[8]

(c) Macitentan

The UK and US manufacturers briefly report that, in a study, the maximum concentrations of *R*- and *S*-warfarin were not altered after a single 25-mg dose of warfarin was given with macitentan 10 mg daily, and there was no effect on the INR. The pharmacokinetics of macitentan, and its active metabolite, were also unaffected.[9,10]

Mechanism

Bosentan induces both CYP3A4 and CYP2C9, which are involved in the metabolism of *R*-warfarin and *S*-warfarin, respectively.[3] Therefore, the use of bosentan increases the metabolism of warfarin, leading to reduced anticoagulant effects. Ambrisentan and macitentan have been shown not to induce or inhibit CYP3A4 or CYP2C9 *in vitro*,[2,9] and so they would be expected to have no effect on warfarin metabolism.

Importance and management

Both the studies and the case reports suggest that a clinically relevant reduction in the effects of warfarin might occur in some patients taking **bosentan**, although exactly how frequently this might occur is unclear. The UK manufacturer of bosentan states that the INR should be closely monitored in any patient taking warfarin when bosentan is started and during dose titration.[7] Given the higher dose requirements reported in the STRIDE-2 study, this seems a prudent precaution. Other coumarins should be similarly monitored on concurrent use with bosentan.

Available evidence suggests that no clinically relevant interaction occurs between warfarin and **ambrisentan** or **macitentan**, therefore no special precautions are necessary on concurrent use.

1. Walker G, Mandagere A, Dufton C, Venitz J. The pharmacokinetics and pharmacodynamics of warfarin in combination with ambrisentan in healthy volunteers. *Br J Clin Pharmacol* (2009) 67, 527–34.
2. Volibris (Ambrisentan). GlaxoSmithKline UK. UK Summary of product characteristics, September 2014.
3. Weber C, Banken L, Birnboeck H, Schulz R. Effect of the endothelin-receptor antagonist bosentan on the pharmacokinetics and pharmacodynamics of warfarin. *J Clin Pharmacol* (1999) 39, 847–54.
4. Murphey LM, Hood EH. Bosentan and warfarin interaction. *Ann Pharmacother* (2003) 37, 1028–31.
5. Holm L, Jansson Å, Noher H. Warfarin och bosentan interagerar. *Lakartidningen* (2007) 104, 2248.
6. Spangler ML, Saxena S. Warfarin and bosentan interaction in a patient with pulmonary hypertension secondary to bilateral pulmonary emboli. *Clin Ther* (2010) 32, 53–6.
7. Tracleer (Bosentan monohydrate). Actelion Pharmaceuticals UK Ltd. UK Summary of product characteristics, September 2013.
8. Barst RJ, Langleben D, Badesch D, Frost A, Lawrence EC, Shapiro S, Naeije R, Galie N, on behalf of the STRIDE-2 study group. Treatment of pulmonary arterial hypertension with the selective endothelin-A receptor antagonist sitaxsentan. *J Am Coll Cardiol* (2006) 47, 2049–56.
9. Opsumit (Macitentan). Actelion Pharmaceuticals UK Ltd. UK Summary of product characteristics, May 2014.
10. Opsumit (Macitentan). Actelion Pharmaceuticals US, Inc. US Prescribing information, October 2013.

Coumarins + Etanercept

Etanercept did not alter the pharmacodynamics or pharmacokinetics of a single dose of warfarin in one study.

Clinical evidence, mechanism, importance and management

In a study in 12 healthy subjects, subcutaneous etanercept 25 mg twice weekly for 7 doses did not alter the pharmacodynamics (INR) of a single dose of **warfarin** given with the last dose of etanercept. In addition, there was no change in the AUC of *R*- and *S*-warfarin.[1]

This study suggests that no **warfarin** dose adjustments would be expected to be needed if etanercept is used in patients taking **warfarin**.

1. Zhou H, Patat A, Parks V, Buckwalter M, Metzger D, Korth-Bradley J. Absence of a pharmacokinetic interaction between etanercept and warfarin. *J Clin Pharmacol* (2004) 44, 543–50.

Coumarins + Ethchlorvynol

The anticoagulant effects of dicoumarol and warfarin are reduced by ethchlorvynol.

Clinical evidence

Six patients who had recently started taking **dicoumarol** had a rise in their Quick index from 38% to 55% (indicating a reduction in anticoagulant effect) while taking ethchlorvynol 1 g daily over an 18-day period. Another patient stabilised on **dicoumarol** became over-anticoagulated and developed haematuria on two occasions when ethchlorvynol was withdrawn for periods of 6 days and 4 days.[1] A marked reduction in the anticoagulant effects of **warfarin** occurred in another patient given ethchlorvynol.[2]

Mechanism

Uncertain. The idea that ethchlorvynol increases the metabolism of the anticoagulants by the liver has not been confirmed by studies in *dogs* and *rats*.[3]

Importance and management

Information is very sparse and limited to dicoumarol and warfarin, but the interaction seems to be established. Be alert for other coumarins to behave similarly. Anticipate the need to alter the anticoagulant dose if ethchlorvynol is started or stopped. The benzodiazepines may be a useful non-interacting alternative to ethchlorvynol, see 'Coumarins + Benzodiazepines and related drugs', p.412.

1. Johansson S-A. Apparent resistance to oral anticoagulant therapy and influence of hypnotics on some coagulation factors. *Acta Med Scand* (1968) 184, 297–300.
2. Cullen SI and Catalano PM. Griseofulvin-warfarin antagonism. *JAMA* (1967) 199, 582–3.
3. Martin YC. The effect of ethchlorvynol on the drug-metabolizing enzymes of rats and dogs. *Biochem Pharmacol* (1967) 16, 2041–4.

Coumarins and related drugs + Ezetimibe

No clinically significant interaction occurred between ezetimibe and warfarin in one study. However, there have been post-marketing reports of raised INRs in patients taking warfarin or fluindione after they were also given ezetimibe.

Clinical evidence, mechanism, importance and management

In a two-way, crossover study, 12 healthy subjects were given ezetimibe 10 mg or placebo daily for 11 days, with a single 25-mg dose of **warfarin** on day 7. The pharmacokinetics and pharmacodynamics (prothrombin time) of **warfarin** were not significantly altered by ezetimibe. In addition, the pharmacokinetics of ezetimibe were similar to those previously seen with the drug alone.[1]

However, the UK manufacturers of ezetimibe state that there have been post-marketing reports of raised INRs in patients taking **warfarin** or **fluindione** after they were also given ezetimibe. They therefore advise that the INR should be monitored if ezetimibe is given with any coumarin or **fluindione**[2] (this is probably a prudent precaution for any **indanedione**), and the US manufacturer states the same for **warfarin**.[3] Nevertheless, there do not appear to be any published case reports, or other evidence, which suggests that any interaction is not established, and probably rare.

1. Bauer KS, Kosoglou T, Statkevich P, Calzetta A, Maxwell SE, Patrick JE, Batra V. Ezetimibe does not affect the pharmacokinetics or pharmacodynamics of warfarin. *Clin Pharmacol Ther* (2001) 69, P5.
2. Ezetrol (Ezetimibe). MSD-SP Ltd. UK Summary of product characteristics, September 2010.
3. Zetia (Ezetimibe). Merck/Schering-Plough Pharmaceuticals. US Prescribing information, August 2013.

Coumarins + Felbamate

An isolated case report describes a marked increase in the effect of warfarin, which was attributed to starting felbamate, although stopping carbamazepine and phenobarbital could have been the cause.

Clinical evidence, mechanism, importance and management

A 62-year-old man with a seizure disorder who was receiving **warfarin** had his antiepileptic treatment with carbamazepine, phenobarbital and sodium valproate discontinued and replaced by felbamate 2.4 g daily and later 3.2 g daily. Within 14 days his INR had risen from his usual range of 2.5 to 3.5 up to 7.8. After stopping and later restarting **warfarin** his INR rose within about 14 days to 18.2. He was eventually restabilised on about half his former **warfarin** dose. The authors of the report suggest that the withdrawal of the carbamazepine and phenobarbital was an unlikely reason for this reaction because no increases in **warfarin** dose had been needed when they were started.[1] Suspicion therefore fell on the felbamate, but it is clearly difficult to be sure that the withdrawal of the enzyme-inducing antiepileptics did not have some part to play. A letter commenting on this report[2] favours the idea that what occurred was in fact due to the withdrawal of the carbamazepine (see 'Coumarins + Carbamazepine and related drugs', p.415), and phenobarbital (see 'Coumarins + Barbiturates', p.411).

The general importance of this interaction (if such it is) is uncertain, and this appears to be the only case. Bear it in mind in the event of an unexpected response to **warfarin**.

1. Tisdel KA, Israel DS, Kolb KW. Warfarin-felbamate interaction: first report. *Ann Pharmacother* (1994) 28, 805.
2. Glue P, Banfield CR, Colucci RD, Perhach JL. Comment: warfarin-felbamate interaction. *Ann Pharmacother* (1994) 28, 1412–13.

Coumarins and related drugs + Fibrates

Bezafibrate, clofibrate, ciprofibrate, and fenofibrate increase the effects of the coumarins, and clofibrate also interacts with phenindione. These interactions have been fatal in a few cases. Gemfibrozil did not interact with warfarin in a controlled study, although a retrospective study and several cases describing bleeding have been reported.

Clinical evidence

(a) Bezafibrate

In a study in patients with hyperlipidaemia, stabilised on **phenprocoumon**, it was necessary to reduce the anticoagulant dose by about 20% when bezafibrate 450 mg daily was given to 10 patients for 4 weeks, and by 33% when bezafibrate 600 mg daily was given to 5 patients.[1] In another study in 22 patients taking bezafibrate 400 mg daily, the dose of **acenocoumarol** had to be reduced by 20% to maintain a constant INR.[2]

A patient (with hypoalbuminaemia due to nephrotic syndrome and chronic renal failure) stabilised on **acenocoumarol** developed severe haematemesis with an INR of 25.9, two weeks after starting to take bezafibrate 800 mg daily.[3] A woman stabilised on **warfarin** and bezafibrate 400 mg daily had an increase in her INR to 5.29 after being given an incorrect double dose of bezafibrate for a few days, and a man had a reduced response to **warfarin** (INR 1.5) when he stopped taking bezafibrate for one week.[4]

(b) Ciprofibrate

In a well-controlled study, 12 young healthy men were given a single 25-mg dose of **warfarin** on day 21 of a 26-day course of ciprofibrate 100 mg daily. The ciprofibrate increased the anticoagulant response to **warfarin** by 50% and caused a 28% decrease in the apparent intrinsic clearance of *S*-warfarin, which is the more active enantiomer.[5]

(c) Clofibrate

1. Coumarins. In a study including 11 patients stabilised on **warfarin**, clofibrate with androsterone (*Atromid*), given for 5 to 7 months, reduced the weekly **warfarin** dose requirement in all patients by a mean of 32%, with variability between patients.[6,7] This interaction has been confirmed in a number of other similar studies in patients stabilised on **warfarin** and given clofibrate,[8,9] or clofibrate with androsterone,[10] with only 2 of 10 patients affected in one study[8] but all 13 patients affected in another study.[10] One fatal case of haemorrhage has been reported in a man stabilised on **warfarin** who was given clofibrate 500 mg four times daily for one week.[11]

The interaction has been studied in 4 healthy subjects given the enantiomers of **warfarin** separately. In this study, clofibrate increased the effect of *S*-warfarin without altering its clearance, whereas there was no alteration of the effect of *R*-warfarin and an increase in its clearance.[12] In another study in 10 healthy subjects, clofibrate 500 mg four times daily for 18 days increased the anticoagulant effect of a single dose of **dicoumarol** given on day 14 without altering the half-life or plasma **dicoumarol** concentrations.[13]

2. Indanediones. Ten out of 15 patients stabilised on **phenindione** needed a 33% reduction in **phenindione** dose and 5 of them bled (haematuria or haematoma) when they were given clofibrate, or clofibrate with androsterone (*Atromid*).[7] In another series, of 13 patients stabilised on **phenindione** and given clofibrate with androsterone (*Atromid*) there were 5 cases of haemorrhagic episodes, two of which were not associated with a prolonged prothrombin time, and one of which was fatal.[14,15] In yet another study, clofibrate with androsterone appeared to be less effective in reducing serum cholesterol in patients taking **phenindione** than in 12 other patients taking clofibrate alone.[16]

(d) Fenofibrate

In an early clinical study of fenofibrate, 2 patients stabilised on **acenocoumarol** needed a 30% reduction in their dose to maintain the same prothrombin time when they were given long-term fenofibrate 200 mg in the morning and 100 mg in the evening.[17] In other similar studies, reductions in the dose of unnamed **coumarins** of 12% (range 0 to 21%)[18] or about one-third[19] were needed when fenofibrate was given. One patient developed haematuria.[20]

A number of case reports of this interaction have subsequently been published, as follows:

- A patient taking **warfarin** had an increase in his INR to 8.5 (from a previous range of 2 to 2.5) within one week of starting to take fenofibrate 200 mg daily. His INR later restabilised when the **warfarin** dose was reduced by 27%.[21]
- A patient taking **warfarin** had a large increase in INR from a range of 2.8 to 3.5 up to 5.6 within 10 days of starting to take fenofibrate (dose not stated).[21]
- A patient taking **warfarin** bled, and was found to have an INR of 18 when his gemfibrozil was replaced by fenofibrate.[22]

- In 2 cases, 30 to 40% reductions in the **warfarin** dose were required when fenofibrate was given.[23]

(e) Gemfibrozil

In a well-controlled study, gemfibrozil 600 mg twice daily for 8 days did not alter the anticoagulant effect of a single dose of **warfarin** given on day 3. In addition, gemfibrozil unexpectedly slightly decreased the AUC of both *R*- and *S*-warfarin (by 6% and 11%, respectively).[24] In contrast, a large retrospective, case-control study in patients taking **warfarin**, and who were hospitalised for a gastrointestinal bleed, found that initiation of gemfibrozil was associated with an increased risk of bleeding (odds ratio 1.96). Long-term use of warfarin (for more than 3 months) did not increase this risk (odds ratio 1.88).[25] Several cases support this finding: A brief report describes bleeding ('menstrual cycle prolonged and lots of blood clots') and much higher prothrombin times (values not given) 2 weeks after a woman stabilised on **warfarin** started to take gemfibrozil 1.2 g daily in divided doses. Halving the **warfarin** dose resolved the problem.[26] Another patient stabilised on **warfarin** developed severe hypoprothrombinaemia (INR 43) and bleeding (melaena, bruising) 4 weeks after starting to take gemfibrozil 1.2 g daily.[27] A further case describes an increase in INR (5.8), in the absence of bleeding, in a 62-year-old man stabilised on **warfarin** 45 mg weekly, 3 weeks after starting gemfibrozil 600 mg twice daily. Gradual reduction of his warfarin dose to 35 to 37.5 mg weekly returned his INR to within the range of 2 to 3. Four months later the gemfibrozil was stopped due to myalgia, and his warfarin dose was increased to his previous dose.[28]

Mechanism

Uncertain. Clofibrate can displace warfarin from its plasma protein binding sites,[5,29-31] but this does not adequately explain the interaction. Another suggestion is that the fibrates have an additive pharmacodynamic effect with these anticoagulants.[1,12] Altered metabolism might also account for the interaction with ciprofibrate, because it decreased the clearance of *S*-warfarin.[5] However, this did not occur with clofibrate[12,13] or gemfibrozil.[24]

Importance and management

The interactions of clofibrate with dicoumarol, warfarin, and phenindione are established, clinically important, and potentially serious. Severe bleeding (fatal in some instances) has been seen. The incidence of the interaction is reported to be between 20% and 100%, but it would be prudent to assume that all patients will be affected. Coumarin dose reductions of one-third to one-half might be needed to avoid the risk of bleeding. Monitor the INR and adjust the dose accordingly. Information about other coumarins and indanediones is lacking but it would be prudent to assume that they will interact with clofibrate in a similar way.

Bezafibrate, ciprofibrate, and fenofibrate have interacted similarly with coumarins. Therefore, the same precautions suggested for clofibrate should be followed if any of these fibrates are given with any oral anticoagulant.

Gemfibrozil did not interact with warfarin in a pharmacological study, but a large retrospective study suggests an increased risk (almost 2-fold) of bleeding in warfarin users started on gemfibrozil and 3 cases of an increased effect of warfarin have been reported, so it would seem prudent to apply the same precautions on its concurrent use with any coumarin.

1. Zimmermann R, Ehlers W, Walter E, Hoffrichter A, Lang PD, Andrassy K, Schlierf G. The effect of bezafibrate on the fibrinolytic enzyme system and the drug interaction with racemic phenprocoumon. *Atherosclerosis* (1978) 29, 477–85.
2. Manotti C, Quintavalla R, Pini M, Tomasini G, Vargiu G, Dettori AG. Interazione farmacologica tra bezafibrato in formulazione retard ed acenocumarolo. Studio clinico. *G Arterioscler* (1991) 16, 49–52.
3. Blum A, Seligmann H, Livneh A, Ezra D. Severe gastrointestinal bleeding induced by a probable hydroxycoumarin-bezafibrate interaction. *Isr J Med Sci* (1992) 28, 47–9.
4. Beringer TRO. Warfarin potentiation with bezafibrate. *Postgrad Med J* (1997) 73, 657–8.
5. Sanofi Withrop Ltd. Personal communication, December 1997.
6. Roberts SD, Pantridge JF. Effect of Atromid on requirements of warfarin. *J Atheroscler Res* (1963) 3, 655–7.
7. Oliver MF, Roberts SD, Hayes D, Pantridge JF, Suzman MM, Bersohn I. Effect of Atromid and ethyl chlorophenoxyisobutyrate on anticoagulant requirements. *Lancet* (1963) i, 143–4.
8. Udall JA. Drug interference with warfarin therapy. *Clin Med* (1970) 77, 20–5.
9. Eastham RD. Warfarin dosage, clofibrate, and age of patient. *BMJ* (1973) ii, 554.
10. Counihan TB, Keelan P. Atromid in high cholesterol states. *J Atheroscler Res* (1963) 3, 580–3.
11. Solomon RB, Rosner F. Massive hemorrhage and death during treatment with clofibrate and warfarin. *N Y State J Med* (1973) 73, 2002.
12. Bjornsson TD, Meffin PJ, Blaschke TF. Interaction of clofibrate with the optical enantiomorphs of warfarin. *Pharmacologist* (1976) 18, 207.
13. Schrogie JJ, Solomon HM. The anticoagulant response to bishydroxycoumarin. II. The effect of d-thyroxine, clofibrate, and norethandrolone. *Clin Pharmacol Ther* (1967) 8, 70–7.
14. Rogen AS, Ferguson JC. Clinical observations on patients treated with Atromid and anticoagulants. *J Atheroscler Res* (1963) 3, 671–6.
15. Rogen AS, Ferguson JC. Effect of Atromid on anticoagulant requirements. *Lancet* (1963) i, 272.
16. Williams GEO, Meynell MJ, Gaddie R. Atromid and anticoagulant therapy. *J Atheroscler Res* (1963) 3, 658–70.
17. Harvengt C, Heller F, Desager JP. Hypolipidemic and hypouricemic action of fenofibrate in various types of hyperlipoproteinemias. *Artery* (1980) 7, 73–82.
18. Stähelin HB, Seiler W, Pult N. Erfahrungen mit dem Lipidsenker Procetofen (Lipanthyl®). *Schweiz Rundsch Med Prax* (1979) 68, 24–8.
19. Raynaud P. Un nouvel hypolipidemiant: le procetofene. *Rev Med Tours* (1977) 11, 325–30.
20. Lauwers PL. Effect of procetofene on blood lipids of subjects with essential hyperlipidaemia. *Curr Ther Res* (1979) 26, 30–8.
21. Ascah KJ, Rock GA, Wells PS. Interaction between fenofibrate and warfarin. *Ann Pharmacother* (1998) 32, 765–8.
22. Aldridge MA, Ito MK. Fenofibrate and warfarin interaction. *Pharmacotherapy* (2001) 21, 886–9.
23. Kim KY, Mancano MA. Fenofibrate potentiates warfarin effects. *Ann Pharmacother* (2003) 37, 212–15.
24. Lilja JJ, Backman JT, Neuvonen PJ. Effect of gemfibrozil on the pharmacokinetics and pharmacodynamics of racemic warfarin in healthy subjects. *Br J Clin Pharmacol* (2005) 59, 433–9.
25. Schelleman H, Bilker WB, Brensinger CM, Wan F, Yang YX, Hennessy S. Fibrate/statin initiation in warfarin users and gastrointestinal bleeding risk. *Am J Med* (2010) 123, 151–7.
26. Ahmad S. Gemfibrozil interaction with warfarin sodium (Coumadin). *Chest* (1990) 98, 1041–2.
27. Rindone JP, Keng HC. Gemfibrozil-warfarin interaction resulting in profound hypoprothrombinemia. *Chest* (1998) 114, 641–2.
28. Dixon DL, Williams VG. Interaction between gemfibrozil and warfarin: case report and review of the literature. *Pharmacotherapy* (2009) 29, 744–8.
29. Solomon HM, Schrogie JJ, Williams D. The displacement of phenylbutazone-C^{14} and warfarin-C^{14} from human albumin by various drugs and fatty acids. *Biochem Pharmacol* (1968) 17, 143–51.
30. Solomon HM, Schrogie JJ. The effect of various drugs on the binding of warfarin-^{14}C to human albumin. *Biochem Pharmacol* (1967) 16, 1219–26.
31. Bjornsson TD, Meffin PJ, Swezey S, Blaschke TF. Clofibrate displaces warfarin from plasma proteins in man: an example of a pure displacement interaction. *J Pharmacol Exp Ther* (1979) 210, 316–21.

Coumarins + Fish oils

The concurrent use of fish oils does not appear to alter warfarin efficacy, nor the incidence of bleeding episodes. However, there are a couple of reports of an increased INR in patients taking warfarin and fish oils, and one of a life-threatening bleed without an increase in INR in a patient taking high-dose fish oils with aspirin and warfarin.

Clinical evidence

In one early study, 40 patients took 4 g of a fish oil preparation daily for 4 weeks, and 18 of these patients were taking **warfarin**. In the group as a whole (40 patients), the bleeding time was prolonged from 240 seconds to 270 seconds. In the subset of patients taking **warfarin** who had stable anticoagulant control in the preceding 3 months (15 patients), the thrombotest was shortened from 114 seconds to 90 seconds, although no changes in **warfarin** dose were made. One patient taking **warfarin** had a minor nosebleed.[1] In a large randomised study of the effect of fish oils or placebo, taken with either aspirin or **warfarin** over 9 months, there was no difference in the frequency of bleeding episodes between 132 patients taking **warfarin** and fish oil 4 g daily and 154 patients taking **warfarin** alone (17 versus 14, respectively).[2] In yet another small controlled study in 6 patients, the use of fish oils 3 g or 6 g daily for 4 weeks did not alter the INR in patients receiving stable **warfarin** therapy.[3]

Two cases of a possible interaction with an increase in INR have been reported. In one, a woman had INRs in the range of 2 to 3 for five months while taking **warfarin** 1.5 mg and 1 mg on alternate days. During this time, she started taking 1 g of a fish oil preparation daily with no change in her INR. Her **warfarin** was then increased to 1.5 mg daily, with stable INRs for about 5 months. A routine INR was then found to be 4.3 (increased from 2.8 one month earlier). One week previously, she had started to take fish oils 2 g daily (double the previous dose). The dose of **warfarin** was reduced to 1.5 mg and 1 mg on alternate days, and she was asked to reduce the fish oils back to 1 g daily. Eight days later her INR was 1.6, and the **warfarin** was increased back to 1.5 mg daily.[4] In another case, an increase in INR from between 2 and 3 up to 6, without bleeding complications, occurred 2 weeks after a patient started taking fish oils 2 g daily and trazodone 50 mg daily.[5]

In yet another report, a subdural haematoma developed after a minor fall in an elderly patient stabilised on **warfarin** and low-dose aspirin who had been taking omega-3 fatty acids 6 g daily for a year. His INR was only minimally elevated at the time (3.2 compared with 2.8 previously).[6] Note that use of low-dose aspirin with **warfarin** increases the risk of bleeding, see 'Coumarins and related drugs + Aspirin or other Salicylates', p.405.

Mechanism

Fish oils contain omega-3 fatty acids particularly **eicosapentaenoic acid** and **docosahexaenoic acid**. These are considered to have some antiplatelet activity, and might prolong the bleeding time. In addition, they might reduce concentrations of some coagulation factors. They can therefore increase the risk of bleeding when used with warfarin, similarly to antiplatelet doses of aspirin (see 'Coumarins and related drugs + Aspirin or other Salicylates', p.405), but this would not be expected to alter the INR.

Importance and management

An interaction between warfarin and fish oils is not established. One large study found no increase in bleeding episodes in over 150 patients taking warfarin and fish oils, suggesting that most patients do not develop an interaction. Nevertheless, a much larger study would be needed to quantify any excess risk in the order of that seen with antiplatelet doses of aspirin. Based on the possible modest increase in bleeding times with high-dose fish oils, the manufacturers of one product, *Omacor* (omega-3-acid ethyl esters), state that although there have been no reports of haemorrhage with concurrent use, patients receiving anticoagulants should be monitored, and the dose of anticoagulant adjusted as necessary.[7] However, monitoring the INR would not pick up a pharmacodynamic interaction.

1. Smith P, Arnesen H, Opstad T, Dahl KH, Eristsland J. Influence of highly concentrated N-3 fatty acids on serum lipids and hemostatic variables in survivors of myocardial infarction receiving either oral anticoagulants or matching placebo. *Thromb Res* (1989) 53, 467–74.
2. Eritsland J, Arnesen H, Seljeflot I, Kierulf P. Long-term effects of *n*-3 polyunsaturated fatty acids on haemostatic variables and bleeding episodes in patients with coronary artery disease. *Blood Coag Fibrinol* (1995) 6, 17–22.
3. Bender NK, Kraynak MA, Chiquette E, Linn WD, Clark GM, Bussey HI. Effects of marine fish oils on the anticoagulation status of patients receiving chronic warfarin therapy. *J Thromb Thrombolysis* (1998) 5, 257–261.
4. Buckley MS, Goff AD, Knapp WE. Fish oil interaction with warfarin. *Ann Pharmacother* (2004) 38, 50–3.
5. Jalili M, Dehpour AR. Extremely prolonged INR associated with warfarin in combination with both trazodone and omega-3 fatty acids. *Arch Med Res* (2007) 38, 901–4.
6. McClaskey EM, Michalets EL. Subdural haematoma after a fall in an elderly patient taking high-dose omega-3 fatty acids with warfarin and aspirin: case report and review of the literature. *Pharmacotherapy* (2007) 27, 152–60.
7. Omacor (Omega-3-acid ethyl esters 90). Abbott Healthcare Products Ltd. UK Summary of product characteristics, April 2013.

Coumarins + Fluorouracil and related prodrugs

Fluorouracil greatly increases the anticoagulant effects of warfarin, and cases of serious bleeding have been reported. The fluorouracil prodrugs, capecitabine and tegafur, appear to interact similarly.

Clinical evidence

(a) Capecitabine

In an open study, 4 patients with breast or colorectal cancer received a single 20-mg dose of **warfarin** 8 days before starting oral capecitabine (3 cycles of capecitabine 1250 mg/m^2 twice daily for 14 days, then 7 days rest) and again on day 12 of the third cycle of capecitabine. Capecitabine increased the AUC of *S*-warfarin by 57% and increased its elimination half-life by 51%, without any changes to *R*-warfarin. The maximum INR was increased by 90% and the AUC of the INR increased 2.8-fold. Three of the patients required vitamin K. Because of the clear, statistically significant findings in these 4 patients, the study was terminated early.[1]

Various cases of this interaction have been reported.[2-8] In one of these reports, 2 patients starting **warfarin** developed gastrointestinal bleeding with an INR of greater than 10, after 2 cycles of capecitabine.[2] In another case, a patient who had been taking long-term **warfarin** required a gradual 85% reduction in the warfarin dose to 0.78 mg daily over 3 cycles of capecitabine and **irinotecan**, and required an increase to 4 mg daily over the 3 weeks after stopping chemotherapy.[4] Another patient required a 50% reduction in the **warfarin** dose while taking capecitabine.[6] An almost 3-fold increase in INR was seen in a patient previously stabilised on **warfarin** after a regimen containing capecitabine (with gemcitabine and docetaxel) was started, but the INR returned to near baseline after the capecitabine was stopped.[7] A 4-fold increase in INR was seen in a patient receiving **warfarin** 1 mg daily as prophylaxis for catheter-associated thrombosis, 21 days after starting capecitabine.[8] In addition, in a retrospective analysis of 21 patients who received **warfarin** with capecitabine, 6 patients required a warfarin dose reduction, and there were 4 episodes of major bleeding.[9] Another retrospective analysis of 6 patients receiving **warfarin** and capecitabine found that the mean change in INR from baseline was 5.11, with a maximum of 7.13 (range 2.67 to 16.71). An INR of greater than 9 was recorded in one patient and 4 patients required a warfarin dose reduction of 41%.[10] Conversely, in another analysis, there was not that much difference in the rates of bleeding events and elevated INRs between patients receiving warfarin with capecitabine and those receiving warfarin alone, although the authors concluded that this might just reflect appropriate management of the interaction.[11]

The manufacturers of **capecitabine** also report that this interaction has occurred with other coumarins including **phenprocoumon**,[12,13] and that some cases have been fatal.[13]

(b) Fluorouracil and fluorouracil-based regimens

In an early clinical study, 25 patients with colon cancer were given bolus fluorouracil 15 to 20 mg/kg weekly and **warfarin** daily, titrated to maintain the prothrombin time in the 20 to 30% range, and modified weekly as necessary. Three patients developed blood loss from the gut, which was controlled by giving a transfusion (type unnamed) and stopping the **warfarin**. This study did not report the required dose of warfarin, or how often it needed adjusting in these patients.[14] A retrospective analysis of 9 patients receiving **warfarin** and 5-fluorouracil found that the mean change in INR from baseline was 4.62 with a maximum of 6.3 (range 2 to 19.1). An INR of greater than 9 was recorded in 2 patients and 4 patients required a warfarin dose reduction of 38%.[10]

Various case reports have described clinically important over-anticoagulation with the concurrent use of dose-adjusted **warfarin** (for treatment of deep vein thrombosis, or in patients with prosthetic heart valves) and fluorouracil, either alone,[15,16] with folinic acid (leucovorin),[17-20] or levamisole.[18,21,22] In one well-described case, an elderly man taking **warfarin** long-term was found to have an INR of almost 40 (usual INR 3) four weeks after he started taking fluorouracil (450 mg/m^2 daily for 5 days then once weekly) and **levamisole** (50 mg every 8 hours for 3 days every other week). He required a two-thirds reduction in his **warfarin** dose. Later, when the chemotherapy was withheld for 5 weeks, his INR became subtherapeutic, and then increased again when the chemotherapy was re-started.[21] In another retrospective case series, 4 patients taking **warfarin** long-term (target INR 2 to 3) required an 18 to 74% reduction in their **warfarin** dose during the use of fluorouracil and **folinic acid** or **levamisole**. The maximum INR in 3 of these patients was 3.66 to 8.15, and the other patient had a maximum INR of 23.7 and a retroperitoneal bleed.[18]

Other cases of over-anticoagulation have been reported with **warfarin** and fluorouracil-based regimens including CMF (**cyclophosphamide**, **methotrexate**, and fluorouracil);[18,23,24] CMF plus **vincristine** and prednisone;[25] fluorouracil, **cisplatin**, and **etoposide**;[26] and fluorouracil, **cisplatin**, and **mitomycin**.[16]

A case has also been reported with the use of fixed-dose **warfarin** (1 mg daily) for prophylaxis of venous catheter-associated thrombosis in a patient receiving fluorouracil with **vinblastine**.[27] Similarly, in a large retrospective analysis of fixed dose **warfarin**, 31 of 95 patients given regimens based on continuous infusions of **fluorouracil** had INR elevations above 1.5, and, of these, 18 had an INR of 3 to 4.9 and seven had an INR of more than 5. Epistaxis and haematuria occurred in 8 of the patients. The regimens used were fluorouracil with **folinic acid**; folinic acid, fluorouracil, and **oxaliplatin** (FOLFOX); and folinic acid, fluorouracil, and **irinotecan** (FOLFIRI).[28] In a further analysis of the use of fixed dose **warfarin** with the FOLFOX regimen, 25 of 50 patients had an INR greater than 1.5 (range 1.55 to 9.4). Two of these developed haematuria and one had a nosebleed.[29]

(c) Tegafur

Increased INRs and bleeding (haemoptysis) were seen in a patient taking **warfarin** when *Orzel* (uracil with tegafur in a 4:1 molar ratio) was given, and a 63% reduction in the warfarin dose was needed.[30] The manufacturers of *Uftoral* (tegafur with uracil) also say that sizeable elevations in prothrombin times and INRs have been reported in patients taking **warfarin** when *Uftoral* was given concurrently.[31] Similarly, a number of case reports attribute greatly increased INRs in patients receiving **warfarin** to an interaction with a combination preparation of tegafur, gimeracil, and oteracil potassium.[32-34] In all 9 patients in one report, a raised INR was seen within the 3-week course and in 5 of these patients, reduction in dose, or cessation, of warfarin was necessary.[32] In 3 other patients, the INR was increased by about 50% within 8 to 17 days of concurrent use, and warfarin dose adjustments were necessary.[33]

Mechanism

Uncertain. However, in a pharmacokinetic study in *rats*, fluorouracil greatly reduced the total clearance of *S*-warfarin by inhibiting its metabolism.[35] In addition, in a small clinical study, fluorouracil inhibited the metabolism of losartan, used as a probe substrate for CYP2C9 (see 'Angiotensin II receptor antagonists; Losartan + Fluorouracil', p.49). This suggests that fluorouracil possibly inhibits warfarin metabolism via CYP2C9 resulting in increased anticoagulant effects. Fluorouracil prodrugs such as capecitabine and tegafur would be expected to interact by the same mechanism.

Importance and management

The interactions between warfarin and fluorouracil and its prodrugs are fairly well-documented and are established interactions of clinical importance. Prothrombin times should be more frequently monitored in patients taking warfarin or other **coumarins**, and requiring fluorouracil, capecitabine, tegafur, or other fluorouracil prodrugs, anticipating the need to reduce the warfarin dose. Note that, from a disease perspective, when treating venous thromboembolic disease in patients with cancer, warfarin is generally inferior (higher risk of major bleeds and recurrent thrombosis) to low-molecular-weight heparins.[36]

1. Camidge R, Reigner B, Cassidy J, Grange S, Abt M, Weidekamm, Jodrell D. Significant effect of capecitabine on the pharmacokinetics and pharmacodynamics of warfarin in patients with cancer. *J Clin Oncol* (2005) 23, 4719–25.
2. Copur MS, Ledakis P, Bolton M, Morse AK, Werner T, Norvell M, Muhvic J, Chu E. An adverse interaction between warfarin and capecitabine: a case report and review of the literature. *Clin Colorectal Cancer* (2001) 3, 182–4.
3. Buyck HCE, Buckley N, Leslie MD, Plowman PN. Capecitabine-induced potentiation of warfarin. *Clin Oncol* (2003) 15, 297.
4. Janney LM, Waterbury NV. Capecitabine–warfarin interaction. *Ann Pharmacother* (2005) 39, 1546–51.
5. Issacs K, Haim N. Adverse interaction between capecitabine and warfarin resulting in altered coagulation parameters and bleeding: case report and review of the literature. *J Chemother* (2005) 17, 339–42.
6. Yildirim Y, Ozyilkan O, Akcali Z, Basturk B. Drug interaction between capecitabine and warfarin: a case report and review of the literature. *Int J Clin Pharmacol Ther* (2006) 44, 80–2.
7. Saif MW, Wasif N. Interaction between capecitabine and gemcitabine with warfarin in a patient with pancreatic cancer. *JOP* (2008) 9, 739–43.
8. Giunta G. Adverse interaction between capecitabine and warfarin resulting in altered coagulation parameters: a review of the literature starting from a case report. *Case Report Med* (2010) Epub.
9. Shah HR, Ledbetter L, Diasio R, Saif MW. A retrospective study of coagulation abnormalities in patients receiving concomitant capecitabine and warfarin. *Clin Colorectal Cancer* (2006) 5, 354–8.
10. Shah SR, Martin R, Dowell JE, Gressett Ussery SM. Comparison of the 5-fluorouracil-warfarin and capecitabine-warfarin drug interactions. *Pharmacotherapy* (2010) 30, 1259–65.
11. Yood MU, Quesenberry CP, Alford SH, Tsai A-L, Wells KE, Yood SM, Ackermann Shiff SP. An observational study examining the impact of capecitabine on warfarin antithrombotic activity and bleeding complications. *Curr Med Res Opin* (2006) 22, 307–14.
12. Xeloda (Capecitabine). Roche Products Ltd. UK Summary of product characteristics, June 2011.
13. Xeloda (Capecitabine). Roche Laboratories Inc. US Prescribing information, February 2011.
14. Chlebowski RT, Gota CH, Chann KK, Weiner JM, Block JB, Batemen JR. Clinical and pharmacokinetic effects of combined warfarin and 5-fluorouracil in advanced colon cancer. *Cancer Res* (1982) 42, 4827–30.
15. Wajima T, Mukhopadhyay P. Possible interactions between warfarin and 5-fluorouracil. *Am J Hematol* (1992) 40, 238.
16. Morita N, Kashihara K, Tagashira H, Otsuka H, Yoneda K, Murase T, Tsujikawa T, Furutani S, Furutani K, Minato M, Nishitani H. Two cases of retroperitoneal hematoma caused by combination of anticoagulant therapy and 5-fluorouracil. *J Med Invest* (2005) 52, 114–17.
17. Brown MC. Multisite mucous membrane bleeding due to a possible interaction between warfarin and 5-fluorouracil. *Pharmacotherapy* (1997) 17, 631–3.
18. Kolesar JM, Johnson CL, Freeberg BL, Berlin JD, Schiller JH. Warfarin-5-FU interaction – a consecutive case series. *Pharmacotherapy* (1999) 19, 1445–9.
19. Carabino J, Wang F. International normalized ratio fluctuation with warfarin-fluorouracil therapy. *Am J Health-Syst Pharm* (2002), 59, 875.
20. Davis DA, Fugate SE. Increasing warfarin dosage reductions associated with concurrent warfarin and repeated cycles of 5-fluorouracil therapy. *Pharmacotherapy* (2005) 25, 442–7.
21. Scarfe MA, Israel MK. Possible drug interaction between warfarin and combination of levamisole and fluorouracil. *Ann Pharmacother* (1994) 28, 464–7.
22. Wehbe TW, Warth JA. A case of bleeding requiring hospitalisation that was likely caused by an interaction between warfarin and levamisole. *Clin Pharmacol Ther* (1996) 59, 360–2. Erratum *ibid.* 60, 137.
23. Seifter EJ, Brooks BJ, Urba WJ. Possible interactions between warfarin and antineoplastic drugs. *Cancer Treat Rep* (1985) 69, 244–5.
24. Malacarne P, Maestri A. Possible interactions between antiblastic agents and warfarin inducing prothrombin time abnormalities. *Recenti Prog Med* (1996) 87, 135.
25. Booth BW, Weiss RB. Venous thrombosis during adjuvant chemotherapy. *N Engl J Med* (1981) 305, 170.
26. Aki Z, Kotiloğlu G, Özyilkan Ö. A patient with a prolonged prothrombin time due to an adverse interaction between 5-fluorouracil and warfarin. *Am J Gastroenterol* (2000) 95, 1093–4.
27. Brown MC. An adverse interaction between warfarin and 5-fluorouracil; a case report and review of the literature. *Chemotherapy* (1999) 45, 392–5.
28. Masci G, Magagnoli M, Zucali PA, Castagna L, Carnaghi C, Sarina B, Pedicini V, Fallini M, Santoro A. Minidose warfarin prophylaxis for catheter-associated thrombosis in cancer patients: can it be safely associated with fluorouracil-based chemotherapy? *J Clin Oncol* (2003) 21, 736–9.
29. Magagnoli M, Masci G, Carnagi C, Zucali PA, Castagna L, Morenghi E, Santoro A. Minidose warfarin is associated with a high incidence of international normalized ratio elevation during chemotherapy with FOLFOX regimen. *Ann Oncol* (2003) 14, 959–60.
30. Karwal MW, Schlueter AJ, Arnold MM, Davis RT. Presumed drug interaction between Orzel® and warfarin. *Blood* (1999) 94 (10 Suppl 1, part 2), 106b.
31. Uftoral (Tegafur and uracil). Merck Serono. UK Summary of product characteristics, April 2011.
32. Yamada T, Watanabe H, Yano T, Nonaka T, Takada A, Sonoda M, Kubota T. The timing of expression of blood coagulation abnormality in patients treated with warfarin and S-1 concomitantly. *Yakugaku Zasshi* (2010) 130, 955–60.

33. Yamamuro F, Miki A, Kondo G, Maeda T, Satoh H, Hori S, Sawada Y. Individual differences in prothrombin time-international normalized ratio variation following coadministration of the anticancer agents S-1and warfarin: 3 case reports. *Int J Clin Pharmacol Ther* (2011) 49, 700–4.
34. Marutaka M, Kubota Y, Yoshida R, Orita Y. Difficult management of warfarin anticoagulant therapy due to S-1 administration for gastric cancer – report of a case. *Gan To Kagaku Ryoho* (2009) 36, 1561–3.
35. Zhou Q, Chan E. Effect of 5-fluorouracil on the anticoagulant activity and the pharmacokinetics of warfarin enantiomers in rats. *Eur J Pharm Sci* (2002) 17, 73–80.
36. Baglin TP, Keeling DM, Watson HG, for the British Committee for Standards in Haematology. Guidelines on oral anticoagulation (warfarin): third edition – 2005 update. *Br J Haematol* (2006) 132, 277–85.

Coumarins + Flupirtine

Flupirtine does not appear to interact with phenprocoumon.

Clinical evidence, mechanism, importance and management

Twelve healthy subjects had no significant changes in their plasma levels of **phenprocoumon** 1.5 mg daily when they were given flupirtine 100 mg three times daily for 14 days. The prothrombin times were also not significantly changed.[1] Therefore, **phenprocoumon** dose adjustments would not be expected to be needed if these drugs are given concurrently.

1. Harder S, Thürmann P, Hermann R, Weller S, Mayer M. Effects of flupirtine coadministration on phenprocoumon plasma concentrations and prothrombin time. *Int J Clin Pharmacol Ther* (1994) 32, 577–581.

Coumarins + Folic acid

Folic acid increases the metabolism of *S*-7-hydroxywarfarin, a metabolite of *S*-warfarin, but this does not appear to affect the anticoagulant activity of warfarin.

Clinical evidence

In a prospective study, 24 patients stabilised on warfarin were given folic acid 5 mg daily for 30 to 60 days. There was a 47% increase in the metabolic clearance of *S*-7-hydroxywarfarin, a metabolite of *S*-warfarin, whereas the pharmacokinetics of *R*-warfarin, *S*-warfarin and *R*-7-hydroxy-warfarin were unaffected. No statistically significant differences were found in the dose of warfarin needed, or the INR of patients during the study, when compared with before folic acid supplementation.[1]

Mechanism

S-warfarin is mainly metabolised by CYP2C9, whereas *R*-warfarin is metabolised by a number of isoenzymes, with very little metabolised by CYP2C9. The authors suggested that the effect of folic acid on the clearance of *S*-7-hydroxywarfarin (a metabolite of *S*-warfarin), and the lack of effect on the *R*-isomer, might be attributed to folic acid inducing CYP2C9.[1] However, a statistically significant difference in the clearance of *S*-warfarin would be expected if folic acid was a clinically relevant inhibitor of CYP2C9.

Importance and management

Evidence for an interaction between warfarin and folic acid appears to be limited to this one study, which found that the small changes in the pharmacokinetics of *S*-7-hydroxywarfarin did not result in any clinically relevant changes in INR. Based on the available evidence, no increase in monitoring or dose adjustment seems necessary on concurrent use.

1. Muszkat M, Bialer O, Blotnick S, Adar L, Xie H-G, Ufer M, Cascorbi I, Caraco Y. Effects of folic acid supplementation on the pharmacokinetics and anticoagulant effect of warfarin: an open-label, prospective study of long-term administration in adults. *Clin Ther* (2010) 32, 347–56.

Coumarins + Fondaparinux

Warfarin does not alter the pharmacokinetics of fondaparinux, and fondaparinux does not alter the effect of warfarin on prothrombin time.

Clinical evidence, mechanism, importance and management

In a placebo-controlled study, 12 healthy subjects were given subcutaneous fondaparinux 4 mg daily for 5 days, with warfarin 15 mg given on day 4 and 10 mg on day 5. Warfarin had no effect on fondaparinux pharmacokinetics. In addition, the effect of warfarin on prothrombin time was not altered by fondaparinux.[1]

Fondaparinux is an anticoagulant that is an indirect inhibitor of activated factor Xa, and it is sometimes used as a 'bridge' to oral anticoagulation. The findings of this study show that the prothrombin time (INR) can still be used to monitor the effect of coumarin anticoagulants during the switch from fondaparinux to oral anticoagulants.

1. Faaij RA, Burggraaf J, Schoemaker RC, van Amsterdam RGM, Cohen AF. Absence of an interaction between the synthetic pentasaccharide fondaparinux and oral warfarin. *Br J Clin Pharmacol* (2002) 54, 304–8.

Coumarins + Food

The rate of absorption of dicoumarol can be increased by food. Three patients had modest increases in warfarin requirements after starting high-protein, low-carbohydrate diets. The rate of absorption of phenprocoumon can be decreased by wheat bran.

Clinical evidence and mechanism

(a) Dicoumarol

A study in 10 healthy subjects found that the peak serum concentrations of a single 250-mg dose of dicoumarol, were increased on average by 85% by food. Two subjects had increases of 242% and 206%, respectively.[1] Food might cause prolonged retention of dicoumarol in the upper part of the gut, leading to increased tablet dissolution and increased absorption.

(b) Phenprocoumon

A pharmacokinetic study in 7 healthy subjects found that the rate of absorption of a single 0.23-mg/kg dose of phenprocoumon was decreased by 35 g of wheat bran taken immediately before phenprocoumon, but the maximum plasma concentration was not altered. There was also a decrease in the total body clearance and clearance of free phenprocoumon (18% and 25% respectively). The mechanism for the reduced clearance is unknown, but the authors' suggestions include inhibition of the glucuronidation of phenprocoumon by wheat bran and an effect on bile salts.[2] The clinical relevance of this finding is unknown, but seems likely to be small.

(c) Warfarin

One report describes 2 patients who had well-documented decreases in INR values with modest increases in warfarin requirements (22% and 30%) after switching to high-protein, low-carbohydrate diets (the *Atkins* diet and the *South Beach* diet). On stopping these diets, both patients were eventually restabilised on their original warfarin doses.[3] Another similar case of a 16% increase in warfarin requirement with a high-protein diet has been reported.[4]

The mechanism for these cases is unknown, but suggested reasons include an increase in albumin with increased protein intake (leading to increased warfarin binding), an induction of cytochrome P450 isoenzymes with increased protein intake (increasing warfarin clearance), or increased intake of dietary vitamin-K, or a combination of these mechanisms.[5]

Importance and management

None of these interactions are very well documented, and their clinical relevance is unclear. Nevertheless, any big changes in diet have the potential to alter the effects of warfarin on the INR, and it would therefore be prudent to increase monitoring in patients wishing to start a diet. Note that vitamin K in food commonly interacts with warfarin, and these interactions are discussed in 'Coumarins and related drugs + Food; Vitamin K_1-rich', p.432.

Other food substances are discussed in their own monographs. Consider also:

- 'Coumarins + Cranberry products', p.420,
- 'Coumarins and related drugs + Food; Enteral and parenteral nutrition', below,
- 'Coumarins + Grapefruit juice', p.436,
- 'Coumarins + Food; Ice cream', p.431,
- 'Coumarins + Food; Mango fruit', p.431,
- 'Coumarins + Quinine', p.466, for tonic water,
- 'Coumarins + Food; Soya bean products', p.431,
- 'Coumarins + Sucrose polyesters', p.475, for additives in potato crisps.

1. Melander A, Wåhlin E. Enhancement of dicoumarol bioavailability by concomitant food intake. *Eur J Clin Pharmacol* (1978) 14, 441–4.
2. Kitteringham NR, Mineshita S, Ohnhaus EE. The effect of wheat bran on the pharmacokinetics of phenprocoumon in normal volunteers. *Klin Wochenschr* (1985) 63, 537–9.
3. Beatty SJ, Mehta BH, Rodis JL. Decreased warfarin effect after initiation of high-protein, low-carbohydrate diets. *Ann Pharmacother* (2005) 39, 744–7.
4. Hornsby LB, Hester EK, Donaldson AR. Potential interaction between warfarin and high dietary protein intake. *Pharmacotherapy* (2008) 28, 536–9.
5. Rodis JL, Beatty SJ, Mehta BH. Comment: Decreased warfarin effect after initiation of high-protein, low-carbohydrate diets. *Ann Pharmacother* (2005) 39, 1371–2; author reply 1372.

Coumarins and related drugs + Food; Enteral and parenteral nutrition

A number of early case reports described warfarin resistance in patients taking enteral feeds that contained large amounts of added vitamin K_1. However, products with a lower vitamin K_1 content have also been reported to interact. Lipid emulsions containing soya oil might contain sufficient natural vitamin K_1 to alter warfarin requirements. Parenteral multivitamin preparations might also contain vitamin K_1.

Clinical evidence

A. Enteral feeds

Case reports from the early 1980s described patients stabilised on **warfarin** who experienced a reversal of the anticoagulant effect when they started taking the liquid dietary supplements *Ensure*,[1,2] or *Osmolite*.[3] Other patients who were resistant to **warfarin** were found to be taking *Ensure*[4] or *Ensure Plus*.[5,6] At this time, these products contained large amounts of vitamin K_1 (240 to 380 micrograms per 240 or

250 mL, an amount equivalent to approximately 1 mg of vitamin K_1 for every 1 000 calories). Two of the patients were successfully anticoagulated with **warfarin** when their enteral nutrition was switched to *Compleat B* (vitamin K_1 16.6 micrograms/250 mL)[6] or *Meritene* (trace of vitamin K_1).[4] In response to these reports, *Ensure*, *Ensure-Plus*, and *Osmolite* were reformulated to reduce the vitamin K_1 content to 50 micrograms in 240 mL (140 micrograms per 1000 calories).[4] However, further case reports for *Ensure Plus*[7] and *Osmolite*[8] suggested that this lower vitamin K content might still be sufficient to cause an interaction. The vitamin K_1 content of these products was reduced further to 36 to 37 micrograms per 1000 calories,[9] but even then a case of increased **warfarin** requirement was reported with *Ensure*.[10] In another case, a patient taking *Osmolite* and intermittent *Ensure Plus* (total mean vitamin K_1 dose 81 micrograms daily) only achieved satisfactory anticoagulation with **warfarin** when the *Osmolite* was stopped, which reduced the vitamin K_1 intake to 36 micrograms daily.[11] Another patient given *Osmolite* (vitamin K_1 68.4 micrograms daily), only achieved satisfactory anticoagulation with **warfarin** when the dose was given separately from the *Osmolite*.[12]

A further case report describes a patient in whom *Isocal* 3550 mL daily (equivalent to 460 micrograms of vitamin K_1) caused an increase in **warfarin** requirement from 8 mg daily to 13 mg daily.[13] Another patient had a decrease in anticoagulant response requiring an increase in **warfarin** dose when she started a weight-reducing diet consisting solely of *Nutrilite 330* (vitamin K content unknown),[14] and one patient required twice the dose of **acenocoumarol** during a period of enteral feeding (vitamin K_1 200 micrograms daily).[15]

Isocal and *Sustacal* have also been implicated in two cases of **warfarin** resistance in a further report.[16] A study in 6 patients found a small increase in INR of 0.74 when continuous enteral feeding was withheld for one hour before and after warfarin administration, although the mean daily dose of **warfarin** did not differ. However, note that there was also a small difference in vitamin K intake of 25 micrograms daily less during the period of separation of administration.[17] This same feeding schedule resulted in achievement of a therapeutic INR in a 56-year-old man taking warfarin who had a previously unstable INR, although a change in feed to one with a lower vitamin K content (103 micrograms daily versus 204 micrograms daily) was instigated at the same time as the change to feeding schedule.[18]

In a prospective cohort study in 319 children, the use of enteral nutrition (mostly vitamin K supplemented formula, and some vitamin K supplemented tube feeds) was associated with a higher dose of **warfarin** to achieve a target INR (0.28 versus 0.16 mg/kg) and similarly a higher dose of **warfarin** was needed to maintain the INR (0.26 versus 0.11 mg/kg).[19]

B. Parenteral nutrition

(a) Intravenous lipids

Warfarin resistance was seen in a patient who was given a constant intravenous infusion of **soya oil emulsion** (*Intralipid*). In this case intravenous **warfarin** up to 15 mg daily only slightly prolonged the prothrombin time.[20] In another patient, an emulsified infusion of **propofol** containing 10% **soya oil** antagonised the effect of **warfarin**; anticoagulation was not achieved until the **propofol** was discontinued despite an increase in the **warfarin** dose to 30 mg daily. The dose of propofol given was estimated to provide about 154 to 231 micrograms of vitamin K_1 daily. The same effect was later seen when the patient was given parenteral nutrition supplemented with 20% *Liposyn II*, which also contains **soya oil**, and was estimated to provide 53 micrograms of vitamin K_1 daily.[21]

(b) Multivitamins

The FDA in the US requires that multivitamin products for inclusion in total parenteral nutrition contain 150 micrograms of vitamin K_1. The aim of this is to provide a daily physiological amount of the vitamin, rather than the previous practice of giving a large single weekly dose. Previously, patients taking anticoagulants were not given this single large weekly dose, therefore it is anticipated that with this multivitamin preparation, **warfarin** doses for anticoagulation might be higher than previously needed. What effect this amount of vitamin K_1 will have on the fixed-dose **warfarin** used for prophylaxis of catheter-associated thrombosis is not known.[22] In the UK, *Vitlipid N* contains vitamin K_1 (phytomenadione) 15 micrograms/mL for adults and 20 micrograms/mL for children under 11 years.

Mechanism

The coumarin and **indanedione** anticoagulants are vitamin K antagonists, and consequently giving vitamin K_1 reduces their effects. The dose at which this might become clinically important is not firmly established, but in one controlled study 150 micrograms of vitamin K_1 daily produced a clinically relevant effect in 25% of subjects (see 'Coumarins + Vitamin K_1-containing dietary supplements', p.484). There is also some evidence that a physicochemical interaction (possibly binding to protein) might occur between warfarin and enteral feeds.[12,16] See also 'Coumarins + Food', p.429, for mention that high-protein diets appear to increase warfarin requirements.

Lipid emulsions given as part of parenteral nutrition often contain soya oil, which has a moderate amount of vitamin K (see 'Table 12.5', below). These preparations might also have direct coagulation effects.[21] Parenteral nutrition can also be supplemented with vitamin K.

Importance and management

The interactions between the vitamin K content of enteral or parenteral nutrition and coumarins or indanediones are established and of clinical importance. Be aware that enteral feeds might contain sufficient vitamin K to alter coagulation status, so starting, stopping or changing between these feeds might affect dose requirements of these vitamin K antagonists. It is also possible that there is a local interaction, as in one case separating the administration of the warfarin and an enteral feed by 3 hours or more was effective,[12] and in another study[17] withholding the enteral feed for one hour before and after warfarin administration reduced the effect of the interaction. It would therefore seem prudent to separate administration of warfarin doses and enteral feed where possible, by stopping the feed (perhaps for one hour) either side of the warfarin dose. It should be remembered that the rate of feeding should be adjusted accordingly to accommodate this break while maintaining the same daily intake. Patients should also be advised not to add or substitute dietary supplements such as *Ensure* without increased monitoring of their coagulation status.

Fat emulsions used for parenteral use containing soya oil might contain sufficient vitamin K_1 for daily needs. Parenteral multivitamin preparations might also contain sufficient vitamin K_1 to provoke an interaction. It would be advisable to keep the vitamin K_1 intake constant in any patient taking a coumarin or indanedione who requires long-term supplemental or total parenteral nutrition. If the amount of lipid and/or multivitamins is altered, anticipate a change in warfarin requirement.

Table 12.5 Foods with a moderate to high content of Vitamin K_1 (phytomenadione)

Foods	*Vitamin K_1 content (micrograms/100 g)*
Vegetables	
Asparagus	51 to 80
Beet greens	484
Broccoli	101 to 156
Brussels sprouts	122 to 289
Cabbage	50 to 98
Collards (non-heading cabbage)	440 to 623
Endive	231
Kale	817 to 882
Kelp seaweed	66
Lettuce (iceberg to green leaf)	24 to 174
Parsley (fresh or dried)	360 to 1640
Spinach	270 to 575
Spring onions	207
Turnip greens	367 to 519
Fats and oils	
Soya oil	25 to 145
Rapeseed oil	112 to 150
Olive oil	30 to 60
Margarines	40 to 110
Fruit and nuts	
Avocado	14 to 20
Cashew nuts	19 to 64
Kiwi fruit	25 to 40
Pine nuts	33 to 74
Prunes, dried	1.4 to 68

Data from:

1. Booth SL, Sadowski JA, Pennington JAT. Phylloquinone (vitamin K1) content of foods in the U.S. Food and Drug Administration's Total Diet Study. *J Agric Food Chem* (1995) 43, 1574–9.
2. Piironen V, Koivu T, Tammisalo O, Mattila P. Determination of phylloquinone in oils, margarines and butter by high-performance liquid chromatography with electrochemical detection. *Food Chem* (1997) 59, 473–80.
3. Koivu TJ, Pirronen VI, Henttonen SK, Mattila PH. Determination of phylloquinone in vegetables, fruits and berries by high-performance liquid chromatography with electrochemical detection. *J Agric Food Chem* (1997) 45, 4644–49.
4. Bolton-Smith C, Price RJG, Fenton ST, Harrington DJ, Shearer MJ. Compilation of a provisional UK database for the phylloquinone (vitamin K1) content of foods. *Br J Nutr* (2000) 83, 389–99.
5. USDA National Nutrient Database for Standard Reference, Release 28. Vitamin K (phylloquinone) (μg) Content of selected foods per 100 g. Available at: http://ndb.nal.usda.gov/ndb/nutrients/index, p. (accessed 21/10/2015).
6. Dismore ML, Haytowitz DB, Gebhardt SE, Peterson JW, Booth SL. Vitamin K content of nuts and fruits in the US diet. *J Am Diet Assoc* (2003) 103, 1650–2.
7. Schurgers LJ, Vermeer C. Determination of phylloquinone and menaquinones in food. Effect of food matrix on circulating vitamin K concentrations. *Haemostasis* (2000) 30, 298–307.

Although there is only a single case, bear in mind that propofol could interact because it is formulated with soya oil, which contains vitamin K_1.

1. O'Reilly RA, Rytand DA. 'Resistance' to warfarin due to unrecognized vitamin K supplementation. *N Engl J Med* (1980) 303, 160–1.
2. Westfall LK. An unrecognized cause of warfarin resistance. *Drug Intell Clin Pharm* (1981) 15, 131.
3. Lader EW, Yang L, Clarke A. Warfarin dosage and vitamin K in Osmolite. *Ann Intern Med* (1980) 93, 373–4.
4. Lee M, Schwartz RN, Sharifi R. Warfarin resistance and vitamin K. *Ann Intern Med* (1981) 94, 140–1.
5. Michaelson R, Kempin SJ, Navia B, Gold JWM. Inhibition of the hypoprothrombinemic effect of warfarin (Coumadin®) by Ensure-Plus, a dietary supplement. *Clin Bull* (1980) 10, 171–2.
6. Zallman JA, Lee DP, Jeffrey PL. Liquid nutrition as a cause of warfarin resistance. *Am J Hosp Pharm* (1981) 38, 1174.
7. Griffith LD, Olvey SE, Triplett WC, Stotter Cuddy ML. Increasing prothrombin times in a warfarin-treated patient upon withdrawal of Ensure Plus. *Crit Care Med* (1982) 10, 799–800.
8. Parr MD, Record KE, Griffith GL, Zeok JV, Todd EP. Effect of enteral nutrition on warfarin therapy. *Clin Pharm* (1982) 1, 274–6.
9. Kutsop JJ. Update on vitamin K_1 content of enteral products. *Am J Hosp Pharm* (1984) 41, 1762.
10. Howard PA, Hannaman KN. Warfarin resistance linked to enteral nutrition products. *J Am Diet Assoc* (1985) 85, 713–15.
11. Martin JE, Lutomski DM. Warfarin resistance and enteral feedings. *J Parenter Enteral Nutr* (1989) 13, 206–8.
12. Petretich DA. Reversal of Osmolite-warfarin interaction by changing warfarin administration time. *Clin Pharm* (1990) 9, 93.
13. Watson AJM, Pegg M, Green JRB. Enteral feeds may antagonise warfarin. *BMJ* (1984) 288, 557.
14. Oren B, Shvartzman P. Unsuspected source of vitamin K in patients treated with anticoagulants: a case report. *Fam Pract* (1989) 6, 151–2.
15. Van Iersel MB, Blenke AAM, Kremer HPH, Hekster YA. Een patiënt met verminderde gevoeligheid voor acenocoumarol tijdens gebruik van sondevoeding. *Ned Tijdschr Geneeskd* (2004) 148, 1155–6.
16. Penrod LE, Allen JB, Cabacungan LR. Warfarin resistance and enteral feedings: 2 case reports and a supporting in vitro study. *Arch Phys Med Rehabil* (2001) 82, 1270–3.
17. Dickerson RN, Garmon WM, Kuhl DA, Minard G, Brown RO. Vitamin K-independent warfarin resistance after concurrent administration of warfarin and continuous enteral nutrition. *Pharmacotherapy* (2008) 28, 308–13.
18. Krajewski KC, Butterfoss K. Achievement of therapeutic international normalized ratio following adjustment of tube feeds. *J Clin Pharmacol* (2011) 51, 440–3.
19. Streif W, Marzinotto AV, Massicotte P, Chan AKC, Julian JA, Mitchell L. Analysis of warfarin therapy in pediatric patients: a prospective cohort study of 319 patients. *Blood* (1999) 94, 3007–14.
20. Lutomski DM, Palascak JE, Bower RH. Warfarin resistance associated with intravenous lipid administration. *J Parenter Enteral Nutr* (1987) 11, 316–18.
21. MacLaren R, Wachsman BA, Swift DK, Kuhl DA. Warfarin resistance associated with intravenous lipid administration: discussion of propofol and review of the literature. *Pharmacotherapy* (1997) 17, 1331–7.
22. Helphingstine CJ, Bistrian BR. New Food and Drug Administration requirements for inclusion of vitamin K in adult parenteral multivitamins. *J Parenter Enteral Nutr* (2003) 27, 220–4.

Coumarins + Food; Ice cream

Two isolated reports describe antagonism of the effects of warfarin by ice cream.

Clinical evidence, mechanism, importance and management

A woman taking **warfarin** 22.5 mg daily did not have the expected prolongation of her prothrombin time. It was then discovered that she took the **warfarin** in the evening and she always ate ice cream before going to bed. When the **warfarin** was taken in the mornings, the prothrombin time increased.[1] Another patient's **warfarin** requirements almost doubled when she started to eat very large quantities of ice cream (one litre each evening). She took the **warfarin** at 6 pm and ate the ice cream at about 10 pm.[2] The effect was not seen when she ate normal amounts of ice cream (3 or 4 normal size portions weekly).

The reason for these isolated cases is unknown. Vitamin K in food commonly interacts with warfarin (see 'Coumarins and related drugs + Food; Vitamin K_1-rich', p.432), but ice cream does not contain important amounts of this vitamin. Given the rarity of reports, it would appear very unlikely that eating ice cream as part of a normal diet will have any effect on INR. However, be aware that any big changes in diet have the potential to alter the INR in response to **warfarin**. Consider also 'Coumarins + Food', p.429.

1. Simon LS, Likes KE. Hypoprothrombinemic response due to ice cream. *Drug Intell Clin Pharm* (1978) 12, 121–2.
2. Blackshaw CA, Watson VA. Interaction between warfarin and ice cream. *Pharm J* (1990) 244, 318.

Coumarins + Food; Mango fruit

A daily intake of one to six mangoes was considered the reason for a moderate increase in the anticoagulant effects of warfarin in one report. None of the patients in whom this interaction was seen showed any evidence of bleeding.

Clinical evidence, mechanism, importance and management

In 13 patients taking **warfarin**, eating mango fruit appeared to increase their INRs by an average of 38% (from 2.79 to 3.85), but no bleeding occurred. No other explanation for the increased INRs could be identified. The patients were reported to have eaten one to 6 mangoes daily for 2 days to one month before attending the anticoagulant clinic. When mango was identified as a possible cause for their increased INRs, the patients were told to stop eating mango, whereupon their mean INR fell within 2 weeks, by almost 18%. When two of the patients whose mean INRs had originally risen by 13% were later rechallenged with mango (rather less than before), their mean INR rose by 9%.[1]

The reason for this apparent interaction is not known, but the authors of the report speculate about the possible role of vitamin A (reported to be 8061 units in an average sized mango of 130 g, without seed). In practical terms this increase in INR would not seem to represent a serious problem, although note that one patient's INR rose to 5.1 (a 54% increase).

There appear to be no other reports in the literature of an interaction between mango and **warfarin**, nor of interactions between mango and any other oral anticoagulant. More study of this interaction is needed, but at the present time there is insufficient reason to suggest that patients taking **warfarin** should avoid mango fruit.

1. Monterrey-Rodriguez J, Feliú JF, Rivera-Miranda GC. Interaction between warfarin and mango fruit. *Ann Pharmacother* (2002) 36, 940–1.

Coumarins + Food; Pomegranate juice

Case reports suggest that pomegranate juice increases the INR in response to warfarin. Other coumarins could potentially interact similarly.

Clinical evidence

A 64-year-old woman, who had been stable taking a number of drugs, including warfarin, was referred to an anticoagulation clinic because of fluctuating INRs. It was discovered that over the last few months the patient had been drinking pomegranate juice two to three times each week. The patient was advised to stop drinking pomegranate juice, and when her INR was measured 2 weeks later it was found to have fallen, from 2.2 to 1.7. She was subsequently stabilised on a new warfarin regimen while not drinking pomegranate juice, although subsequently she was found to have a further reduction in INR, which this time was unexplained.[1]

In another case, a 34-year-old woman stable taking warfarin following a mitral valve replacement developed a large haematoma in her thigh, and was found to have an INR of 14. On questioning, it was discovered that she had consumed about 3 litres of pomegranate juice over the previous week. She was subsequently restabilised after being advised to stop drinking the pomegranate juice.[2]

Mechanism

In vitro,[3] pomegranate juice has been shown to be an inhibitor of the cytochrome P450 isoenzyme CYP2C9, the main isoenzyme involved in the metabolism of the more active *S*-isomer of warfarin. It therefore seems possible that pomegranate juice decreases warfarin metabolism, leading to raised levels and an increase in its anticoagulant effects.

Importance and management

Evidence for an interaction between pomegranate and warfarin is limited to these case reports; however, the *in vitro* findings of a possible metabolic basis for this interaction (see *Mechanism*, above) give further weight to the suggestion of an interaction. Nevertheless, controlled studies are ideally required to establish an interaction. There is currently insufficient evidence to suggest that patients taking warfarin should avoid pomegranate juice, but it may be prudent to consider pomegranate juice consumption in a patient with otherwise unexplained fluctuations in INR, or unexpectedly raised INRs.

Evidence regarding other coumarins is lacking, but all are metabolised, at least in part, by CYP2C9 and it therefore seems possible that they may interact in the same way as warfarin.

1. Komperda KE. Potential interaction between pomegranate juice and warfarin. *Pharmacotherapy* (2009) 29, 1002–1006.
2. Jarvis S, Li C, Bogle RG. Possible interaction between pomegranate juice and warfarin. *Emerg Med J* (2010) 27, 74–5.
3. Nagata M, Hidaka M, Sekiya H, Kawano Y, Yamasaki K, Okumura M, Arimori K. Effects of pomegranate juice on human cytochrome P450 2C9 and tolbutamide pharmacokinetics in rats. *Drug Metab Dispos* (2007) 35, 302–307.

Coumarins + Food; Soya bean products

Natto, a Japanese food made from fermented soya bean, can reduce the effects of warfarin and acenocoumarol, because of the high levels of vitamin K_2 substance produced in the fermentation process. In one study, soya bean protein also reduced the effects of warfarin, and a similar case has been reported with soy milk. Two cases of 'warfarin resistance' have been seen in patients given intravenous soya oil emulsions.

Clinical evidence

(a) Fermented soya bean products (natto)

In a controlled study in 12 healthy subjects stabilised on **acenocoumarol**, a single meal containing 100 g of natto decreased the mean INR from 2.1 to 1.5 after 24 hours, and the INR had still not returned to the original level after 7 days (INR 1.75 one week later). The effect was considered clinically important in 6 of the 12 subjects.[1] Similarly, in an earlier retrospective study in 10 patients taking **warfarin**, eating natto caused the thrombotest values to rise from a range of 12 to 29% up to a range of 33 to 100%. The extent of the rise appeared to be related to the amount of natto eaten. The thrombotest values fell again when the natto was stopped. A healthy subject taking **warfarin**, with a thrombotest value of 40%, ate 100 g of natto. Five hours later the thrombotest value was unchanged, but 24 hours later it was 86%, and after 48 hours it was 90% (suggesting that the anticoagulant effect was decreased).[2]

(b) Soya milk

In a 70-year-old man stabilised on **warfarin** 3 mg daily, consumption of soya milk 480 mL daily (240 mL of both *Sun Soy* and *8th Continent* mixed together) decreased the INR from 2.5 to 1.6 after about 4 weeks.[3] One week after stopping the soya milk, his INR was 1.9, and 4 weeks after it was 2.5.

(c) Soya oil

Soya oil is an important source of dietary vitamin K, see 'Table 12.5', p.430.

In a study in 115 Brazilian patients with vascular disease, consumption of soybean oil (median 11.4 g per day) contributed about 29% of the vitamin K_1 intake, as estimated by 24-hour diet recall. Recent vitamin K_1 consumption was associated with a reduced INR and prothrombin time. The other major contributor to recent vitamin K_1 consumption was kidney beans, which although low in vitamin K themselves, are traditionally prepared in Brazil in soybean oil.[4]

For two cases of 'warfarin resistance' with intravenous soya oil emulsions, see 'Coumarins and related drugs + Food; Enteral and parenteral nutrition', p.429.

(d) Soya protein

In a study in 10 patients with hypercholesterolaemia who were stabilised on **warfarin**, substitution of all animal protein for textured **soya protein** for 4 weeks caused a marked reduction (Quick value approximately doubled) in the anticoagulant effects of warfarin by the second week.[5]

Mechanism

Soya beans are a moderate source of vitamin K_1 (19 micrograms per 100 g),[6] and soya oil and products derived from it are an important dietary source of vitamin K. However, the soy milk brand taken in the case report did not contain vitamin K,[3] and another reference source lists soya milk as containing just 7.5 micrograms vitamin K per 250 mL,[6] which would not be expected to cause an interaction. Why this product decreased the effect of warfarin is therefore open to speculation.

The vitamin K content of textured soya protein is unknown. Note that **soy sauce** made from soya and wheat is reported to contain no vitamin K, and soft **tofu** made from the curds by coagulating soya milk contains only low levels (2 micrograms per 100 g).[6] In contrast, fermented soya bean products such as natto contain very high levels of a particular vitamin K_2 substance (MK-7)[7], because of the fermentation process with *Bacillus natto*. In addition, the bacteria might continue to act in the gut to increase the synthesis and subsequent absorption of vitamin K_2.[2] Although the role of vitamin K_2 in anticoagulation is less well established than vitamin K_1, it appears that this also opposes the actions of coumarins and indanediones, which are vitamin K antagonists.

Importance and management

The interaction between warfarin and fermented soya bean products is established and likely to be clinically relevant in all patients. Patients taking coumarin and probably **indanedione** anticoagulants should probably be advised to avoid natto, unless they want to consume a regular, constant amount.

Although information is limited, it appears that soya protein might also modestly reduce the effect of warfarin. In particular, complete substitution of animal protein for soya protein appears to reduce the effect of warfarin. A single report suggests that soy milk might also interact, and similarly, case reports suggest that soya milk and soya oil might also interact, and therefore some caution would be prudent with these products. On the basis of known vitamin K-content, **whole soya beans** could potentially reduce the effect of warfarin, whereas **soy sauce** should not.[6] Note that patients taking coumarins and **indanediones** are advised to have their INR checked if they markedly change their diet. This would seem particularly important if they decide to change their intake of soya-related products.

1. Schurgers LJ, Shearer MJ, Hamulyák K, Stöcklin E, Vermeer C. Effect of vitamin K intake on the stability of oral anticoagulant treatment: dose-response relationships in healthy subjects. *Blood* (2004) 104, 2682–9.
2. Kudo T. Warfarin antagonism of natto and increase in serum vitamin K by intake of natto. *Artery* (1990) 17, 189–201.
3. Cambria-Kiely JA. Effect of soy milk on warfarin efficacy. *Ann Pharmacother* (2002) 36, 1893–6.
4. Custódio das Dôres SM, Booth SL, Martini LA, de Carvalho Gouvêa VH, Padovani CR, de Abreu Maffei FH, Campana ÁO, Rupp de Paiva SA. Relationship between diet and anticoagulant response to warfarin: a factor analysis. *Eur J Nutr* (2007) 46, 147–54.
5. Gaddi A, Sangiorgi Z, Ciarrocchi A, Braiato A, Descovich GC. Hypocholesterolemic soy protein diet and resistance to warfarin therapy. *Curr Ther Res* (1989) 45, 1006–10.
6. USDA National Nutrient Database for Standard Reference, Release 28. Vitamin K (phylloquinone) (µg) Content of selected foods per 100 g. Available at: http://ndb.nal.usda.gov/ndb/nutrients/index (accessed 21/10/15).
7. Schurgers LJ, Vermeer C. Determination of phylloquinone and menaquinones in food. Effect of food matrix on circulating vitamin K concentrations. *Haemostasis* (2000) 30, 298–307.

Coumarins and related drugs + Food; Vitamin K_1-rich

Unintentional and unwanted antagonism of warfarin has occurred in patients who ate exceptionally large amounts of some green vegetables, which can contain considerable amounts of vitamin K_1. Isolated cases have also been reported with avocado, green tea (very large quantities), liver, and seaweed sushi. Large amounts of kidney beans might also have a similar effect. Foods containing high amounts of vitamin K_2 substances such as fermented soya beans might also interact.

Clinical evidence and mechanism

The coumarin and indanedione oral anticoagulants are vitamin K antagonists, which inhibit the enzyme vitamin K epoxide reductase so reducing the synthesis of vitamin K-dependent blood clotting factors by the liver. If the intake of dietary vitamin K_1 increases, the synthesis of the blood clotting factors begins to return to normal. As a result the prothrombin time also begins to fall to its normal value. Naturally occurring vitamin K_1 (phytomenadione) is found only in plants.

A. Individual foodstuffs

(a) Avocado

Two women taking **warfarin** had a reduction in their INRs (from 2.5 to 1.7 and from 2.7 to 1.6, respectively) when they started to eat avocado 100 g daily, or 200 g of avocado on two consecutive days. Their INRs climbed again when the avocado was stopped.[1] Avocado contains a small to moderate amount of vitamin K_1, see 'Table 12.5', p.430, so might occasionally reduce the efficacy of **warfarin** if eaten in these quantities.

(b) Green tea

A patient taking **warfarin** had a reduction in his INR from a range of 3.2 to 3.79 down to 1.37, which was attributed to the ingestion of very large quantities of green tea (about 2 to 4 litres each day for a week). This interaction was attributed to the vitamin-K content of the tea.[2] However, although dried tea, including green tea, is very high in vitamin-K_1, the brewed liquid made from the tea contains inconsequential amounts of vitamin K_1 (which is a fat-soluble vitamin),[1,3] and is therefore not considered to contribute any vitamin K_1 to the diet.[3] The reason for this interaction is therefore unclear, unless the patient was eating some of the brewed tea leaves. A pharmacokinetic interaction also appears unlikely, because, although black tea inhibited CYP2C9 *in vitro*, brewed tea had no effect on the CYP2C9 substrate flurbiprofen in healthy subjects.[4] CYP2C9 is important in the metabolism of the more potent *S*-warfarin. For discussion of a case where a patient had an increase in INR after stopping taking a herbal preparation of which green tea leaves were one of 25 ingredients, see 'Coumarins + Vitamin K_1-rich herbal medicines', p.485.

(c) Green vegetables

In a formal study in patients stabilised on **warfarin**, one day of a high intake of vitamin K_1-rich vegetables (**brussels sprouts** 400 g, **broccoli** 400 g, **lettuce** 750 g, or **spinach** 300 g, estimated to contain 1 mg of vitamin K_1 daily) decreased anticoagulant effects: the thrombotest values rose above the normal range of 10 to 25% in 2 of 5 patients in 2 to 3 days. Two days of a high intake of the same vegetable caused values above the therapeutic range in 3 of 7 patients, and 7 days intake did the same in 9 of 13 patients.[5] In another similar study, intake of **spinach** 250 g or **broccoli** 250 g daily for 7 days increased the mean thrombotest values to above the therapeutic limit of 15%, and the effect was similar to that of a supplement containing phytomenadione 250 micrograms daily. A reduction in the anticoagulant effect of **warfarin** was also seen in one healthy subject who ate about 450 g **spinach** daily.[6,7]

In a pharmacokinetic study in healthy subjects, a daily intake of 400 g of **brussels sprouts** for 2 weeks slightly decreased the AUC of **warfarin** by 16% and increased its metabolic clearance by 27%.[8] This is probably because **brussels sprouts** induce CYP1A2, which has a role in the metabolism of warfarin (see *Metabolism of the coumarins*, under 'Anticoagulants', p.371).

A few cases of this interaction (often described as warfarin resistance) have been reported in patients taking **dicoumarol**,[9] or **warfarin**[10-13] when consuming large amounts of green vegetables (about 300 to 700 g daily),[11,12] such as **spinach**,[9,14] **broccoli**,[11,12] or a weight-loss diet consisting of **lettuce**, **turnip greens**, and **broccoli**.[13] The dietary vitamin K was estimated to be 1.3 g daily in one case,[10] and 6 g daily in another.[13] In two cases, patients suffered a serious thromboembolic event.[12,13] For discussion of a case where a patient had an increase in INR after stopping a herbal preparation, of which spinach, broccoli and cabbage were 3 of 25 ingredients, see 'Coumarins + Vitamin K_1-rich herbal medicines', p.485.

Conversely, a single intake of **spinach** 250 g or **broccoli** 250 g had no effect on thrombotest values over 7 days.[14] Similarly, in another study in healthy subjects stabilised on **acenocoumarol**, a single meal containing either **spinach** 400 g or **broccoli** 400 g with corn oil caused just 0.27 and 0.41 reductions in the mean INR, an effect that was not considered clinically relevant. These reductions were equivalent to that seen with about 200 micrograms of vitamin K_1.[15]

(d) Liver

A patient taking **acenocoumarol** had a soft tissue bleed, and was found to have a very low thrombotest value of about 3%. She had always consumed about 142 g daily of green vegetables, but about 4 months previously had been advised to stop eating liver (750 g weekly) as part of a low-fat diet.[16] In another case, a man taking **warfarin** 5 mg daily had diffuse bruising and an INR of 5.6 two weeks after he was advised to stop eating pork liver[12] (1 kg per week). He was eventually restabilised on just 1.5 mg of warfarin daily. Early studies found that liver contained high levels of vitamin K, but more recent studies using more specific detection techniques have shown that liver generally contains very low levels of vitamin K_1 (4 and 7 micrograms in 100 g).[17] However, liver might contain vitamin K_2 substances in sufficient levels to be of possible nutritional relevance.[17,18] The precise role of vitamin K_2 substances in anticoagulation control is less clear, but natto, which is a rich source of these, clearly reduces the effects of coumarins. See 'Coumarins + Food; Soya bean products', p.431.

(e) Seaweed

A patient taking **warfarin** had, on two occasions, reduced INRs of 1.6 and 1.8 (usual range 2 to 3) within 24 hours of eating sushi with seaweed (*asakusa-nori*). It was estimated that she had consumed only about 45 micrograms of vitamin K_1, which would not usually interact. However, if her vitamin K stores were low, this amount could have accounted for a large percentage of her vitamin K intake or stores, and might therefore have interacted.[19] Note that **kelp** is a moderate source of vitamin K, see 'Table 12.5', p.430.

(f) Other foodstuffs

In a study in 115 Brazilian patients with vascular disease, consumption of large amounts of **kidney beans** (median 90 g per day) contributed about 11% of the vitamin K_1 intake, as estimated by 24-hour diet recall. Recent vitamin K_1 consumption was associated with reduced INR and prothrombin time. Kidney beans were identified as an important factor in anticoagulation response.[20] However, note that the vitamin K_1 content of kidney beans is low, and they are usually prepared in Brazil with soybean oil which is a rich source of vitamin K[20] (see also 'Coumarins + Food; Soya bean products', p.431). In an early report, a Japanese man recently stabilised on **warfarin** developed bleeding episodes on two occasions shortly after resuming his usual diet of Japanese food (specific foods not mentioned), suggesting increased warfarin effects. However, ingestion of three similar Japanese meals in a 24-hour period had no effect on the prothrombin time in 6 Caucasian patients taking **warfarin**.[21]

B. Overall dietary vitamin K intake

(a) Correlation with INR

Some evidence suggests that the average dietary vitamin K_1 intake is correlated with the efficacy of **warfarin**. In one study, patients consuming a diet containing more than 250 micrograms daily of vitamin K_1 had a lower INR five days after starting **warfarin** than patients consuming less dietary vitamin K_1 (median INR 1.9 versus 3). Also, the high-vitamin K_1 group needed a higher maintenance **warfarin** dose (5.7 mg daily versus 3.5 mg daily).[22] In another study, multiple regression analysis indicated that, in patients taking warfarin, the INR was altered by 1, by a weekly change in the intake of vitamin K of 714 micrograms.[23] Similarly, for each increase in daily dietary vitamin K_1 intake of 100 micrograms, the INR decreased by just 0.2 in another study.[24]

In a randomised, crossover study in patients taking **warfarin** or **phenprocoumon**, increasing the dietary intake of vitamin K_1 by 500% relative to the baseline value (from 118 to 591 micrograms daily) for 4 days only modestly decreased the INR from 3.1 to 2.8 on day 4. Decreasing the dietary intake of vitamin K_1 by 80% (from 118 to 26 micrograms daily) for 4 days increased the INR from just 2.6 to 3.3 on day 7.[25]

In a prospective observational study of 5 817 patient visits to anticoagulant clinics,[26] a change in dietary vitamin K intake was found to be the second most prevalent predictor of non-therapeutic INR (after change in health status) with an odds ratio of 6.4.

(b) Stability of anticoagulant control

A number of studies have found that patients with a very low dietary vitamin K_1 intake are more sensitive to alterations in vitamin K_1 intake, and have less stable anticoagulant control. A prospective, cohort study found that the risk of subtherapeutic INR was increased (hazard ratio 1.33) in those patients with a low usual intake of vitamin K (less than 100 micrograms per day), when compared with patients with a normal usual intake (100 to 300 micrograms per day), but the risk was decreased (hazard ratio 0.8) in those with a high usual intake (greater than 300 micrograms per day). Further, in those patients with low usual vitamin K intake there was a threefold increased risk of subtherapeutic INR if their recent daily intake was equivalent to normal levels. This was not the case in patients whose usual intake was normal or high.[27] In a study in 26 patients with unstable control of anticoagulation, dietary intake of vitamin $K_1$was much lower than in 26 matched patients with stable anticoagulant control (29 micrograms daily versus 76 micrograms daily).[28] Similarly, in another study, high dietary vitamin K intake (greater than 195 micrograms daily) was associated with greater stability of the long-term anticoagulant effect of **warfarin**.[29] In another study in 10 patients with poorly controlled anticoagulation taking **acenocoumarol**, a diet with a low, controlled vitamin K_1 content of 20 to 40 micrograms daily increased the percentage of INR values within the therapeutic range, when compared with a control group of 10 patients not subjected to any dietary restrictions.[30] Supplementation of the diet with small doses of vitamin K_1 has had a similar effect, see 'Coumarins + Vitamin K_1-containing dietary supplements', p.484.

Importance and management

A very well established, well documented and clinically important drug-food interaction, expected to occur with every coumarin or indanedione anticoagulant because they have a common mode of action. The evidence suggests that, in patients with normal vitamin K_1 status, in general, clinically relevant changes in coagulation status require large continued changes in intake of vitamin K_1 from foods. However, there is some evidence to suggest that patients with low dietary vitamin K_1 intake might be sensitive to smaller changes in dietary vitamin K_1, and that higher intake could lessen the impact of incidental intake of vitamin-K_1 rich foods.[27] There is also some evidence that patients with high dietary intake of vitamin K_1 show a lower variability in vitamin K intake than those with low dietary intake.[31] This suggests that patients taking anticoagulants should be advised to eat a normal balanced diet, maintaining a relatively consistent amount of vitamin-K_1 rich foods. They should be told to avoid making major changes to their diet, including starting a weight-loss diet, without increased monitoring of their INR. It is estimated that a normal Western diet contains 300 to 500 micrograms of vitamin K_1 daily. The minimum daily requirement is about 1 micrograms/kg and, in the US, an adequate intake has been determined to be 120 micrograms for adult men and 90 micrograms daily for adult women. 'Table 12.5', p.430, gives the vitamin K_1 content of some vitamin-K_1 rich foods; however, it is important to note that these are not the bioavailable contents, which could be much lower for green vegetables, particularly if they are eaten in the absence of fat.[18,32] Nevertheless, green leafy vegetables usually contribute 40 to 50% of the total intake, followed by certain vegetable oils and margarines made from these oils.[33] Also, processed foods can have moderate to high vitamin K_1 levels if they contain fats with high vitamin K_1 levels. Note that some foods that have a low vitamin K_1 content can contribute considerably to total intake because of how often they are eaten. Cooking and freezing do not alter the vitamin K_1 content, but vitamin K_1 in oils is degraded by exposure to light.[34] In the US, a chart has been devised to help patients and researchers determine the daily intake of vitamin K_1.[35]

For the effect of multivitamins containing vitamin K_1, see 'Coumarins + Vitamin K_1-containing dietary supplements', p.484, and for the effect of supplements in enteral and parenteral feeds, see 'Coumarins and related drugs + Food; Enteral and parenteral nutrition', p.429.

There is growing evidence that vitamin K_2 substances (menaquinones) might also be important, and in one analysis rich dietary sources of these included goose liver paste, hard and soft cheeses, egg yolk,[18] and natto, the effect of which is already established, see 'Coumarins + Food; Soya bean products', p.431.

1. Blickstein D, Shaklai M, Inbal A. Warfarin antagonism by avocado. *Lancet* (1991) 337, 914–15.
2. Taylor JR, Wilt VM. Probable antagonism of warfarin by green tea. *Ann Pharmacother* (1999) 33, 426–8.
3. Booth SL, Madabushi HT, Davidson KW, Sadowski JA. Tea and coffee brews are not dietary sources of vitamin K-1 (phylloquinone). *J Am Diet Assoc* (1995) 95, 82–3.
4. Greenblatt DJ, von Moltke LL, Perloff ES, Luo Y, Harmatz JS, Zinny MA. Interaction of flurbiprofen with cranberry juice, grape juice, tea, and fluconazole: in vitro and clinical studies. *Clin Pharmacol Ther* (2006) 79, 125–33.
5. Pedersen FM, Hamberg O, Hess K, Ovesen L. The effect of dietary vitamin K on warfarin-induced anticoagulation. *J Intern Med* (1991) 229, 517–20.
6. Udall JA, Krock LB. A modified method of anticoagulant therapy. *Curr Ther Res* (1968) 10, 207–11.
7. Udall JA. Human sources and absorption of vitamin K in relation to anticoagulation stability. *JAMA* (1965) 194, 127–9.
8. Ovesen L, Lyduch S, Idorn ML. The effect of a diet rich in brussels sprouts on warfarin pharmacokinetics. *Eur J Clin Pharmacol* (1988) 33, 521–3.
9. Anon. Leafy vegetables in diet alter prothrombin time in patients taking anticoagulant drugs. *JAMA* (1964) 187, 27.
10. Qureshi GD, Reinders P, Swint JJ, Slate MB. Acquired warfarin resistance and weight-reducing diet. *Arch Intern Med* (1981) 141, 507–9.
11. Kempin SJ. Warfarin resistance caused by broccoli. *N Engl J Med* (1983) 308, 1229–30.
12. Chow WH, Chow TC, Tse TM, Tai YT, Lee WT. Anticoagulation instability with life-threatening complication after dietary modification. *Postgrad Med J* (1990) 66, 855–7.
13. Walker FB. Myocardial infarction after diet-induced warfarin resistance. *Arch Intern Med* (1984) 144, 2089–90.
14. Karlson B, Leijd B, Hellström A. On the influence of vitamin K-rich vegetables and wine on the effectiveness of warfarin treatment. *Acta Med Scand* (1986) 220, 347–50.
15. Schurgers LJ, Shearer MJ, HamulyâK K, Stöcklin E, Vermeer C. Effect of vitamin K intake on the stability of oral anticoagulant treatment: dose-response relationships in healthy subjects. *Blood* (2004) 104, 2682–9.
16. Kalra PA, Cooklin M, Wood G, O'Shea GM, Holmes AM. Dietary modification as a cause of anticoagulation instability. *Lancet* (1988) ii, 803.
17. Shearer MJ, Bach A, Kohlmeier M. Chemistry, nutritional sources, tissue distribution and metabolism of vitamin K with special reference to bone health. *J Nutr* (1996) 126, 1181S–1186S.
18. Schurgers LJ, Vermeer C. Determination of phylloquinone and menaquinones in food. Effect of food matrix on circulating vitamin K concentrations. *Haemostasis* (2000) 30, 298–307.
19. Bartle WR, Madorin P, Ferland G. Seaweed, vitamin K, and warfarin. *Am J Health-Syst Pharm* (2001) 58, 2300.
20. Custódio das Dôres SM, Booth SL, Martini LA, de Carvalho Gouvêa VH, Padovani CR, de Abreu Maffei FH, Campana ÁO, Rupp de Paiva SA. Relationship between diet and anticoagulant response to warfarin: a factor analysis. *Eur J Nutr* (2007) 46, 147–54.
21. Flannery EP, MacDonald BS, O'Leary DS, McGinty JM. Japanese-restaurant syndrome. *N Engl J Med* (1971) 285, 414.
22. Lubetsky A, Dekel-Stern E, Chetrit A, Lubin F, Halkin H. Vitamin K intake and sensitivity to warfarin in patients consuming regular diets. *Thromb Haemost* (1999) 81, 396–9.
23. Couris R, Tataronis G, McCloskey W, Oertel L, Dallal G, Dwyer J, Blumberg JB. Dietary vitamin K variability affects International normalized ratio (INR) coagulation indices. *Int J Vitam Nutr Res* (2006) 76, 65–74.
24. Khan T, Wynne H, Wood P, Torrance A, Hankey C, Avery P, Kesteven P, Kamali F. Dietary vitamin K influences intra-individual variability in anticoagulant response to warfarin. *Br J Haematol* (2004) 124, 348–54.
25. Franco V, Polanczyk CA, Clausell N, Rohde LE. Role of dietary vitamin K intake in chronic oral anticoagulation: prospective evidence from observational and randomized protocols. *Am J Med* (2004) 116, 651–6.
26. Cryder B, Felczak M, Janociak J, Dela Pena L, Allen S, Gutierrez P. Prevalent aetiologies of non-therapeutic warfarin anticoagulation in a network of pharmacist-managed anticoagulation clinics. *J Clin Pharm Ther* (2011) 36, 64–70.
27. Rombouts EK, Rosendaal FR, van der Meer FJM. Influence of dietary vitamin K intake on subtherapeutic oral anticoagulant therapy. *Br J Haematol* (2010) 149, 598–605.
28. Sconce E, Khan T, Mason J, Noble F, Wynne H, Kamali F. Patients with unstable control have a poorer dietary intake of vitamin K compared to patients with stable control of anticoagulation. *Thromb Haemost* (2005) 93, 872–5.
29. Kim KH, Choi WS, Lee JH, Lee H, Yang DH, Chae SC. Relationship between dietary vitamin K intake and the stability of anticoagulation effect in patients taking long-term warfarin. *Thromb Haemost* (2010) 104, 755–9.
30. Sorano GG, Biondi G, Conti M, Mameli G, Licheri D, Marongiu F. Controlled vitamin K content diet for improving the management of poorly controlled anticoagulated patients: a clinical practice proposal. *Haemostasis* (1993) 23, 77–82.
31. Presse N, Kergoat M-J, Ferland G. High usual dietary vitamin K intake is associated with low relative variability in vitamin K intake: implications for anticoagulant therapy. *Br J Haematol* (2011) 153, 129–30.
32. Gijsbers BLMG, Jie K-SG, Vermeer C. Effect of food composition on vitamin K absorption in human volunteers. *Br J Nutr* (1996) 76, 223–9.
33. Booth SL, Suttie JW. Dietary intake and adequacy of vitamin K. *J Nutr* (1998) 128, 785–8.
34. Booth SL, Centurelli MA. Vitamin K: a practical guide to the dietary management of patients on warfarin. *Nutr Rev* (1999) 57, 288–96.
35. Couris RR, Tataronis GR, Booth SL, Dallal GE, Blumberg JB, Dwyer JT. Development of a self-assessment instrument to determine daily intake and variability of dietary vitamin K. *J Am Coll Nutr* (2000) 19, 801–6.

Coumarins and related drugs + Garlic

An isolated report described increases in the anticoagulant effects of warfarin in two patients taking garlic supplements. Another report described a decrease in anticoagulant effects of fluindione in a patient taking garlic tablets. Garlic supplements alone have also rarely been associated with bleeding. However, in one study, aged garlic extract did not increase the INR or risk of bleeding in patients taking warfarin.

Clinical evidence

(a) Fluindione

In an 82-year-old man stabilised on fluindione 5 mg (dosage frequency not stated) for chronic atrial fibrillation, the INR dropped to below its usual range (2 to 3) when garlic tablets 600 mg daily were taken, and remained below 2 for 12 consecutive days despite an increase in fluindione dose to 10 mg. The INR returned to normal, with an associated reduction in fluindione dose, when the garlic tablets were stopped. He was also taking enalapril 20 mg, furosemide 40 mg and pravastatin 20 mg (dose frequency not stated).[1]

(b) Warfarin

The INR of a patient stabilised on warfarin more than doubled and haematuria occurred 8 weeks after the patient started to take three *Höfels garlic pearles* daily. The situation resolved when the garlic was stopped. The INR rose on a later occasion while the patient was taking two *Kwai* garlic tablets daily. The INR of another patient was also more than doubled by six *Kwai* garlic tablets daily.[2,3]

In contrast, in a placebo-controlled study in 48 patients stabilised on warfarin, there was no change in INR or evidence of increased bleeding in those receiving 5 mL of aged garlic extract (*Kyolic*) twice daily for 12 weeks.[4] Similarly, in a preliminary report of the use of alternative and complementary medicines in 156 patients taking warfarin, there was no apparent increased risk of bleeding or raised INRs in 57 patients taking potentially interacting complementary medicines (garlic in 10%), compared with 84 who did not.[5]

Mechanism

Garlic has been associated with decreased platelet aggregation, which has on at least two documented occasions led to spontaneous bleeding in the absence of an anticoagulant.[6,7] These effects might therefore increase the risk of bleeding with anticoagulants, see also 'Coumarins + Herbal medicines; Miscellaneous', p.439.

Importance and management

Information about an adverse interaction between warfarin and garlic seems to be limited to two cases from one author. Similarly, the data regarding indanediones is sparse, with just one case reported. Bearing in mind the wide-spread use of garlic and garlic products, and the limited information from the review,[5] and study with aged garlic extract,[4] it seems most unlikely that garlic usually has any generally important interaction with these anticoagulants. Nevertheless, bear the possibility in mind in the event of an unexpected response to treatment.

In addition, garlic may have some antiplatelet effects, and although there appear to be no clinical reports of an adverse interaction between garlic and antiplatelet drugs, it may be prudent to consider the potential for an increase in the severity of bleeding if garlic is given with anticoagulants.

1. Pathak A, Léger P, Bagheri H, Senard J-M, Boccalon H, Montastruc J-L. Garlic interaction with fluindione: a case report. *Therapie* (2003) 58, 380–81.
2. Sunter W. Warfarin and garlic. *Pharm J* (1991) 246, 722.
3. Sunter W. Personal communication, July 1991.
4. Macan H, Uykimpang R, Alconcel M, Takasu J, Razon R, Amagase H, Niihara Y. Aged garlic extract may be safe for patients on warfarin therapy. *J Nutr* (2006) 136 (3 Suppl), 793S–795S.
5. Shalansky S, Neall E, Lo M, Abd-Elmessih E, Vickars L, Lynd L. The impact of complementary and alternative medicine use on warfarin-related adverse outcomes. *Pharmacotherapy* (2002) 22, 1345.
6. German K, Kumar U, Blackford HN. Garlic and the risk of TURP bleeding. *Br J Urol* (1995) 76, 518.
7. Rose KD, Croissant PD, Parliament CF, Levin MP. Spontaneous spinal epidural hematoma with associated platelet dysfunction from excessive garlic ingestion: a case report. *Neurosurgery* (1990) 26, 880–2.

Coumarins + Ginger

Evidence from pharmacological studies suggests that ginger does not increase the anticoagulant effect of warfarin, neither does it alter coagulation or platelet aggregation on its own. However, two case reports describe markedly raised INRs with phenprocoumon and warfarin, which were associated with eating dried ginger and drinking ginger tea. A prospective, longitudinal study also reports of an increased risk of self-reported bleeding events in patients taking warfarin and ginger.

Clinical evidence

In a randomised, crossover study in 12 healthy subjects, 3 ginger capsules taken three times daily for 2 weeks did not affect either the pharmacokinetics or pharmacodynamics (INR) of a single 25-mg dose of **warfarin** taken on day 7. The brand of ginger used was *Blackmores Travel Calm Ginger*, each capsule containing an extract equivalent to 400 mg of ginger rhizome powder. Moreover, ginger alone did not affect the INR or platelet aggregation.[1]

However, a case report describes a rise in INR to greater than 10, with epistaxis, in a woman stabilised on **phenprocoumon** several weeks after she started to eat ginger regularly in the form of pieces of dried ginger and tea from ginger powder. She was eventually restabilised on the original dose of **phenprocoumon**, and was advised to stop taking ginger.[2] Another very similar case has been described in a woman taking **warfarin**.[3]

Moreover, in a prospective, longitudinal study of patients taking **warfarin** and a herbal product or dietary supplement, there was a statistically significant increased risk of self-reported bleeding events in patients taking **warfarin** and ginger (7 bleeds in 25 weeks, none of which were major: odds ratio 3.2).[4] No elevated INRs were reported for the combination. Note that the number of patients taking ginger was not reported, except to say it was less than 5% of 171; so it was less than 8 patients. Also, the ginger products used were not mentioned and some patients were taking more than one potentially interacting supplement.

Mechanism

Ginger (*Zingiber officinale*) has sometimes been listed as a herb that interacts with warfarin[5,6] on the basis that *in vitro* it inhibits platelet aggregation. However, this antiplatelet effect has generally not been demonstrated in controlled clinical studies (three of which have been reviewed[7]). Consider also 'Coumarins + Herbal medicines; Miscellaneous', p.439.

Importance and management

Evidence from a controlled study suggests that ginger does not increase the anticoagulant effect of warfarin. Despite it being cited as a herb that inhibits platelet aggregation, there is limited evidence that it increases bleeding when given alone or with warfarin, and there are just two case reports of markedly raised INRs with phenprocoumon and warfarin, which were associated with ginger root and ginger tea. Because of the many other factors influencing anticoagulant control, it is not possible to reliably ascribe a change in INR specifically to a drug interaction in a single case report without other supporting evidence. It may be better to advise patients to discuss the use of any herbal products they wish to try, and to increase monitoring if this is thought advisable. Cases of uneventful use should be reported, as they are as useful as possible cases of adverse effects.

1. Jiang X, Williams KM, Liauw WS, Ammit AJ, Roufogalis BD, Duke CC, Day RO, McLachlan AJ. Effect of ginkgo and ginger on the pharmacokinetics and pharmacodynamics of warfarin in healthy subjects. *Br J Clin Pharmacol* (2005) 59, 425–32.
2. Krüth P, Brosi E, Fux R, Mörike K, Gleiter CH. Ginger-associated overanticoagulation by phenprocoumon. *Ann Pharmacother* (2004) 38, 257–60.
3. Lesho EP, Saullo L, Udvari-Nagy S. A 76-year-old woman with erratic anticoagulation. *Cleve Clin J Med* (2004) 71, 651–6.
4. Shalansky S, Lynd L, Richardson K, Ingaszewski A, Kerr C. Risk of warfarin-related bleeding events and supratherapeutic international normalized ratios associated with complementary and alternative medicine: a longitudinal analysis. *Pharmacotherapy* (2007) 27, 1237–47.
5. Argento A, Tiraferri E, Marzaloni M. Anticoagulanti orali e piante medicinali. Una interazione emergente. *Ann Ital Med Int* (2000) 15, 139–43.
6. Braun L. Herb-drug interaction guide. *Aust Fam Physician* (2001) 30, 473–6.
7. Vaes LPJ, Chyka PA. Interactions of warfarin with garlic, ginger, ginkgo, or ginseng: nature of the evidence. *Ann Pharmacother* (2000) 34, 1478–82.

Coumarins + Ginkgo (*Ginkgo biloba*)

Evidence from pharmacological studies in patients and healthy subjects suggests that ginkgo extracts do not interact with warfarin. However, an isolated report describes intracerebral haemorrhage associated with the use of ginkgo and warfarin, and there are a few reports of bleeding associated with the use of ginkgo alone.

Clinical evidence

In a randomised, crossover study in 21 patients stabilised on **warfarin**, ginkgo extract 100 mg daily (*Bio-Biloba*) for 4 weeks did not alter the INR or the required dose of **warfarin**, when compared with placebo.[1] Similarly, in another study in healthy subjects,[2] *Tavonin* (containing standardised dry extract EGb 761 of ginkgo equivalent to 2 g of leaf) 2 tablets three times daily for 2 weeks did not affect either the pharmacokinetics or pharmacodynamics (INR) of a single dose of **warfarin** given on day 7. Moreover, a retrospective review of 21 clinical cases involving the concurrent use of ginkgo and **warfarin** also found no evidence of altered INRs.[3] Similarly, a retrospective review of claims data found that the risk of haemorrhage in 60 patients taking ginkgo and antiplatelet drugs or anticoagulants (warfarin) was not increased, however note that this was based on only 3 patients experiencing a haemorrhage.[4]

Conversely, a report describes an intracerebral haemorrhage in an elderly woman within 2 months of her starting to take ginkgo. Her prothrombin time was found to be 16.9 seconds and her partial thromboplastin time was 35.5 seconds. She had been taking **warfarin** uneventfully for 5 years.[5] The author of the report speculated that ginkgo may have contributed towards the haemorrhage.

Mechanism

Uncertain. Isolated cases of bleeding have been reported with ginkgo alone: in a review,[6] and a retrospective study.[4] The study also suggested that the risk of bleeding in elderly patients (65 years or older) who were prescribed ginkgo alone was 3.8 (range 2.8 to 5.2), however, the background risk of bleeding was not identified. In pharmacological studies, ginkgo extract alone did not alter coagulation parameters or platelet aggregation.[2,3] However, in *animal* studies it was found that the AUC of warfarin was decreased by 23% during EGb 761 administration, and the prothrombin time was also reduced by EGb 761, which would suggest that ginkgo should *reduce* the effects of warfarin.[3] In healthy subjects, ginkgo extract had no effect on diclofenac or tolbutamide, which were used as marker substrates for CYP2C9, suggesting that it will not alter the metabolism of *S*-warfarin.[7]

Importance and management

There is good evidence from pharmacological studies in patients and healthy subjects that ginkgo extract would not be expected to interact with warfarin. However, there is one case report of over-anticoagulation, and a few reports of bleeding with ginkgo alone. This is insufficient evidence to justify telling patients taking warfarin to avoid ginkgo, but they should be told to monitor for early signs of bruising or bleeding and seek informed professional advice if any bleeding problems arise.

1. Engelsen J, Nielsen JD, Winther K. Effect of coenzyme Q_{10} and ginkgo biloba on warfarin dosage in stable, long-term warfarin treated outpatients. A randomised, double blind, placebo-crossover trial. *Thromb Haemost* (2002) 87, 1075–6.
2. Jiang X, Williams KM, Liauw WS, Ammit AJ, Roufogalis BD, Duke CC, Day RO, McLachlan AJ. Effect of ginkgo and ginger on the pharmacokinetics and pharmacodynamics of warfarin in healthy subjects. *Br J Clin Pharmacol* (2005) 59, 425–32.
3. Lai C-F, Chang C-C, Fu C-H, Chen C-M. Evaluation of the interaction between warfarin and ginkgo biloba extract. *Pharmacotherapy* (2002) 22, 1326.

4. Chan ALF, Leung HWC, Wu JW, Chien TW. Risk of hemorrhage with co-prescriptions for *Ginkgo biloba* and antiplatelet or anticoagulant drugs. *J Altern Complement Med* (2011) 17, 513–7.
5. Matthews MK. Association of *Ginkgo biloba* with intracerebral hemorrhage. *Neurology* (1998) 50, 1933.
6. Vaes LPJ, Chyka PA. Interactions of warfarin with garlic, ginger, ginkgo, or ginseng: nature of the evidence. *Ann Pharmacother* (2000) 34, 1478–82.
7. Mohutsky MA, Anderson GA, Miller JW, Elmer GW. *Ginkgo biloba:* evaluation of CYP2C9 drug interactions in vitro and in vivo. *Am J Ther* (2006) 13, 24–31.

Coumarins + Ginseng

One pharmacological study found that *Panax quinquefolius* (American ginseng) modestly decreased the effect of warfarin, whereas another study found that *Panax ginseng* (Asian ginseng) did not alter the pharmacokinetics or the effect of a single dose of warfarin. Two other studies suggest that *Panax ginseng* does not affect the INR in patients taking warfarin. Two case reports describe decreased warfarin effects, one with thrombosis, attributed to the use of ginseng (probably *Panax ginseng*), while 3 possible cases of increased warfarin effects have been reported in patients after use of a product containing *Panax ginseng*, one requiring hospitalisation.

Clinical evidence

In a placebo-controlled study in 20 healthy subjects, 12 were given **warfarin** 5 mg daily for 3 days alone then again on days 15 to 17 of a 3-week course of *Panax quinquefolius* (American ginseng) 1 g twice daily. In those given ginseng, the maximum INR was modestly reduced by 0.16, compared with a minor reduction of 0.02 in the 8 subjects given placebo. There was also a modest reduction in the AUC of **warfarin**. In this study, *Panax quinquefolius* root was ground and capsulated.[1]

Evidence from two earlier case reports supports a reduction in warfarin effect. A man taking **warfarin** long-term, and also diltiazem, glyceryl trinitrate, and salsalate, had a decrease in his INR from 3.1 to 1.5 within 2 weeks of starting to take ginseng capsules (*Ginsana*) three times daily. This preparation contains 100 mg of standardised concentrated ginseng [probably *Panax ginseng* (Asian ginseng)] in each capsule. Within 2 weeks of stopping the ginseng his INR had increased again to 3.3.[2] Another patient taking **warfarin** was found to have thrombosis of a prosthetic aortic valve, with a subtherapeutic INR of 1.4. Three months before this episode his INR had become persistently subtherapeutic, requiring a progressive increment in his **warfarin** dose. It was suggested that this might have been because he had begun using a ginseng product (not identified).[3]

In contrast, in a randomised, crossover study, 31 patients stabilised on **warfarin** were given 1 g of *Panax ginseng* (as Korean red ginseng extract) and **warfarin** for 6 weeks. The INR was reduced on concurrent use of the Korean red ginseng extract, compared with placebo.[4] In another randomised, crossover study in 12 healthy subjects, ginseng capsules 1 g three times daily for 2 weeks did not affect either the pharmacokinetics or pharmacodynamics (INR) of a single 25-mg dose of **warfarin** taken on day 7. The brand of ginseng used was *Golden Glow*, each capsule containing an extract equivalent to 0.5 g of *Panax ginseng* (Asian ginseng) root.[5] Similarly in a randomised controlled study in 25 patients, where one group received *Panax ginseng* (Asian ginseng) and **warfarin**, and the other group received **warfarin** alone , there appeared to be no statistically significant difference in the effect on INR between the 2 groups.[6] However, a case report describes how a 71-year-old man taking **warfarin** with an INR within the range of 1.8 to 2.2, was admitted to intensive care with an intracerebral haematoma which required surgery, 7 days after starting the Chinese herbal product *shengmai-yin*, which contains *Panax ginseng* (Asian ginseng). His INR was 5.08, which was reduced to 1.67 after stopping the warfarin and the herbal product, and giving vitamin K.[7] Two other possible cases of increased INR have been reported in patients taking **warfarin** after use of a product containing *Panax ginseng* (Asian ginseng).[8]

Mechanism

It is unclear why ginseng might reduce the efficacy of warfarin, particularly as no pharmacokinetic interaction occurs. The authors of one study[4] suggest that an interaction might occur due to the vitamin K content of Korean red ginseng. They also note that the ginsenosides are steroidal saponins and as such could induce the metabolism of warfarin, but this seems unlikely, see 'Coumarins and related drugs + Corticosteroids or Corticotropin', p.419.

In vitro experiments have found that *Panax ginseng* contains antiplatelet components that inhibit platelet aggregation and thromboxane formation,[9] although antiplatelet activity was not demonstrated in a study in healthy subjects.[10] If an antiplatelet effect were confirmed, this might suggest the possibility of an *increased* risk of bleeding with the combination of ginseng and warfarin; three possible cases exist[7,8]. There are a few reports of vaginal bleeding in women using ginseng preparations (unspecified) in the absence of an anticoagulant,[11-13] but these are probably due to a possible hormonal effect of ginseng.

Importance and management

The available evidence suggests that *Panax quinquefolius* (American ginseng) might *decrease* the effect of warfarin, however this is based on one small study. There is some evidence to suggest that *Panax ginseng* (Asian ginseng) does not interact with warfarin. However, there are conflicting case reports; two cases report decreased warfarin effects attributed to the use of ginseng (probably *Panax ginseng*) whereas three others report an increase in INR after use of a product containing *Panax ginseng*.

There has been criticism of the design of some studies, with the suggestion that in a well-designed study patients should be stabilised on warfarin before giving ginseng.[14]

Until further information becomes available it would seem prudent to be alert for decreased effects of warfarin and related drugs in patients using ginseng, particularly *Panax quinquefolius*. However, the possibility of an increased risk of bleeding due to the antiplatelet component of *Panax ginseng* cannot entirely be ruled out, and was possibly seen in three patients, although studies suggest that this is unlikely.

1. Yuan C-S, Wei G, Dey L, Karrison T, Nahlik L, Maleckar S, Kasza K, Ang-Lee M, Moss J. Brief communication: American ginseng reduces warfarin's effect in healthy patients. *Ann Intern Med* (2004) 141, 23–27.
2. Janetzky K, Morreale AP. Probable interaction between warfarin and ginseng. *Am J Health-Syst Pharm* (1997) 54, 692–3.
3. Rosado MF. Thrombosis of a prosthetic aortic valve disclosing a hazardous interaction between warfarin and a commercial ginseng product. *Cardiology* (2003) 99, 111.
4. Lee YH, Lee BK, Choi YJ, Yoon IK, Chang BC, Gwak HS. Interaction between warfarin and Korean red ginseng in patients with cardiac valve replacement. *Int J Cardiol* (2010) 145, 275–6.
5. Jiang X, Williams KM, Liauw WS, Ammit AJ, Roufogalis BD, Duke CC, Day RO, McLachlan AJ. Effect of St John's wort and ginseng on the pharmacokinetics and pharmacodynamics of warfarin in healthy subjects. *Br J Clin Pharmacol* (2004) 57, 592–99.
6. Lee SH, Ahn YM, Ahn SY, Doo HK, Lee BC. Interaction between warfarin and Panax ginseng in ischemic stroke patients. *J Altern Complement Med* (2008) 14, 715–21.
7. Su Q, Li Y. Interaction between warfarin and the herbal product Shengmai-yin: a case report of intracerebral hematoma. *Yonsei Med J* (2010) 51, 793–6.
8. Turfan M, Tasal A, Ergun F, Ergelen M. A sudden rise in INR due to combination of Tribulus terrestris, Avena sativa, and Panax ginseng (Clavis Panax). *Turk Kardiyol Dern Ars* (2012) 40, 259–61.
9. Kuo S-C, Teng C-M, Leed J-C, Ko F-N, Chen S-C, Wu T-S. Antiplatelet components in Panax ginseng. *Planta Med* (1990) 56, 164–7.
10. Beckert BW, Concannon MJ, Henry SL, Smith DS, Puckett CL. The effect of herbal medicines on platelet function: an in vivo experiment and review of the literature. *Plast Reconstr Surg* (2007) 120, 2044–50.
11. Hopkins MP, Androff L, Benninghoff AS. Ginseng face cream and unexplained vaginal bleeding. *Am J Obstet Gynecol* (1988) 159, 1121–2.
12. Greenspan EM. Ginseng and vaginal bleeding. *JAMA* (1983) 249, 2018.
13. Kabalak AA, Soyal OB, Urfalioglu A, Saracoglu F, Gogus N. Menometrorrhagia and tachyarrhythmia after using oral and topical ginseng. *J Womens Health (Larchmt)* (2004) 13, 830–833.
14. Shao J, Jia L. Potential serious interactions between nutraceutical ginseng and warfarin in patients with ischemic stroke. *Trends Pharmacol Sci* (2013) 34, 85–6.

Coumarins + Glucagon

In one early analysis, the anticoagulant effects of warfarin were markedly increased by very large doses of glucagon (total dose exceeding 50 mg over 2 days), but not by doses of less than 30 mg over one to 2 days.

Clinical evidence

In an analysis of 24 patients taking **warfarin** who were given glucagon for inadequate cardiac contractility, no potentiation of the action of **warfarin** was noted in 11 patients given a total of less than 30 mg of glucagon over one to 2 days. However, 8 out of 9 patients had a marked increase in anticoagulant effects (prothrombin times of 30 to 50 seconds or more) when they were given higher doses of glucagon (62 to 362 mg over 3 to 8 days). Three of them bled. The interaction was not able to be assessed in 4 patients.[1]

Mechanism

Unknown. Changes in the production of blood clotting factors and an increase in the affinity of warfarin for its site of action have been proposed.[1] A study in *guinea pigs* using **acenocoumarol** suggested that changes in warfarin metabolism or its absorption from the gut are *not* responsible.[2]

Importance and management

Direct information is limited to the report cited,[1] which relates to doses far in excess of those used clinically for hypoglycaemia (1 mg) or in the management of beta blocker overdose (2 to 10 mg then 50 micrograms/kg per hour). As such, its findings are probably of no general relevance. Its authors recommend that if glucagon 25 mg per day or more is given for two or more days, the dose of warfarin should be reduced in anticipation of the interaction, and prothrombin time closely monitored.[1]

1. Koch-Weser J. Potentiation by glucagon of the hypoprothrombinemic action of warfarin. *Ann Intern Med* (1970) 72, 331–5.
2. Weiner M, Moses D. The effect of glucagon and insulin on the prothrombin response to coumarin anticoagulants. *Proc Soc Exp Biol Med* (1968) 127, 761–3.

Coumarins + Glucosamine ± Chondroitin

A few reports suggest that glucosamine with or without chondroitin might increase the INR in patients taking warfarin. In contrast, one case of a decreased INR has been reported when glucosamine was given with acenocoumarol.

Clinical evidence

The first indication of a possible interaction between **warfarin** and glucosamine was in 2001, when the Canadian Adverse Drug Reaction Monitoring Program briefly reported that an increase in INR had been noted when glucosamine was given to patients taking **warfarin**, and that INR values decreased when glucosamine was stopped.[1] In 2004, a full case report was published. In this case, a 69-year-old man stabilised on **warfarin** 47.5 mg weekly had an increase in his INR from 2.58 to 4.52 four weeks after starting to take 6 capsules of *Cosamin DS* (glucosamine hydrochloride 500 mg, sodium chondroitin sulfate 400 mg, manganese ascorbate per capsule) daily. His **warfarin** dose was reduced to 40 mg weekly, and his INR returned to the target range of 2 to 3 (INR 2.15) with continued *Cosamin DS* therapy.[2] A comment on this report noted that this is twice the usual dose of glucosamine.[3] Since then, one other similar case of a modest rise in INR has been published. A man taking **warfarin** and glucosamine hydrochloride 500 mg with chondroitin sulfate 400 mg twice daily had a gradual increase in his INR (from 2.3 to 4.7 over 5 weeks) when he trebled the dose of the glucosamine supplement.[4]

Analysis of regulatory authority data has revealed other unpublished reports. In 2006 the CHM in the UK reported that they had received 7 reports of an increase in INR in patients taking **warfarin** after they started taking glucosamine supplements.[5] In 2007, a search of the FDA database identified 20 possible cases,[4] and a search of the WHO database identified 22 possible case reports of an increase in **warfarin** effect with glucosamine, which originated from Australia, Canada, Denmark, Sweden, the UK, and the USA.[6] In two of the WHO cases, chondroitin was used, but the other cases were with glucosamine alone. Of 15 reports giving details of time to onset, the increased INR was noted within 3 days (in a 99-year-old) and up to 6 months; most commonly the interaction took several weeks to manifest.[6]

In contrast, a 71-year-old man stabilised on **acenocoumarol** 15 mg weekly had a *decrease* in his INR to 1.6 after taking glucosamine sulfate (*Xicil*) 1.5 g daily for 10 days. The glucosamine was stopped and the INR reached 2.1. When the glucosamine was restarted, with an increase in **acenocoumarol** dose to 17 mg weekly, the INR only reached 1.9. The glucosamine was eventually stopped.[7] Similarly, the WHO database contained one report of a *decreased* effect of **warfarin** with glucosamine.[6] The Australian Adverse Drug Reactions Advisory Committee have also identified 12 cases of alterations in INR in patients taking **warfarin**. Nine of these cases are included in the WHO report.[8]

There do not appear to have been any controlled studies of the effects of glucosamine supplements on the pharmacodynamics or pharmacokinetics of oral anticoagulants.

Mechanism

Unknown. Evidence from a phenotyping study in healthy subjects, suggests that glucosamine does not inhibit CYP2C9, which is involved in the metabolism of warfarin, to a clinically relevant extent.[9] This requires confirmation, but would appear to support the general lack of pharmacokinetic interaction.

Importance and management

Glucosamine is a widely used supplement, particularly in the middle-aged and elderly, who are also the group most likely to be using warfarin or similar anticoagulants. Despite this, there are just three published reports of a possible interaction, two describing moderate increases in INR and one a decrease. Even taking into account the possible cases reported to regulatory authorities, the interaction would seem to be quite rare. Nevertheless, the cases described suggest it would be prudent to monitor the INR more closely if glucosamine is started or stopped. Also, if a patient shows an unexpected change in INR, bear in mind the possibility of self-medication with supplements such as glucosamine.

Note that in 2006 the CHM in the UK recommended that patients taking warfarin do not take glucosamine,[5] but subsequent UK-approved labelling for the prescription-only glucosamine product *Dolenio* recommends close monitoring when a patient taking a coumarin anticoagulant starts or stops glucosamine.[10]

1. Canadian Adverse Drug Reaction Monitoring Programme (CADRMP). Communiqué. Warfarin and glucosamine: interaction. *Can Adverse Drug React News* (2001) 11, 8.
2. Rozenfeld V, Crain JL, Callahan AK. Possible augmentation of warfarin effect by glucosamine-chondroitin. *Am J Health-Syst Pharm* (2004) 61, 306–7.
3. Scott GN. Interaction of warfarin with glucosamine—chondroitin. *Am J Health-Syst Pharm* (2004) 61, 1186.
4. Knudsen JF, Sokol GH. Potential glucosamine-warfarin interaction resulting in increased international normalized ratio: case report and review of the literature and MedWatch database. *Pharmacotherapy* (2008) 28, 540–48.
5. Commission on Human Medicines/Medicines and Healthcare Products Regulatory Agency. Glucosamine adverse reactions and interactions. *Current Problems* (2006) 31, 8. Available at: https://assets.digital.cabinet-office.gov.uk/media/547307e5e5274a1301000030/con2023860.pdf (accessed 20/10/15).
6. Yue Q-Y, Strandell J, Myrberg O. Concomitant use of glucosamine potentiates the effect of warfarin. The Uppsala Monitoring Centre. Available at: http://www.who-umc.org/graphics/25284.pdf (accessed 20/10/15).
7. Garrote García M, Iglesias Piñeiro MJ, Martín Álvarez R, Pérez González J. Interacción farmacológica del sulfato de glucosamina con acenocumarol. *Aten Primaria* (2004) 33, 162–4.
8. Adverse Drug Reactions Advisory Committee (ADRAC). Interaction between glucosamine and warfarin. *Aust Adverse Drug React Bull* (2008) 27, 3.
9. Rosenborg S, Stenberg M, Otto S, Ostervall J, Masquelier M, Yue Q-Y, Bertilsson L, Eliasson E. Clinically significant CYP2C inhibition by noscapine but not by glucosamine. *Clin Pharmacol Ther* (2010) 88, 343–46.
10. Dolenio (Glucosamine sulphate). Blue Bio Pharmaceuticals Ltd. UK Summary of product characteristics, March 2012.

Coumarins and related drugs + Glycoprotein IIb/IIIa-receptor antagonists

Warfarin has been reported not to increase bleeding with eptifibatide, whereas it does increase bleeding with tirofiban. Nevertheless, an increased risk of bleeding is generally anticipated if glycoprotein IIb/IIIa-receptor antagonists (abciximab, eptifibatide or tirofiban) are given with any coumarins or indanediones.

Clinical evidence

The UK manufacturer of **eptifibatide** briefly reports that concurrent use with **warfarin** did not appear to increase the risk of major and minor bleeding. They also note that, in a population pharmacokinetic study, there was no evidence of a pharmacokinetic interaction between **eptifibatide** and warfarin.[1]

Conversely, the UK manufacturer of **tirofiban** briefly notes that the concurrent use of **warfarin** with tirofiban and heparin increased the risk of bleeding.[2]

Mechanism

Glycoprotein IIb/IIIa-receptor antagonists have antiplatelet effects, which may be additive with other drugs that affect haemostasis resulting in an increased risk of bleeding.

Importance and management

Glycoprotein IIb/IIIa-receptor antagonists are generally used together with low-dose aspirin and heparin, see also 'Glycoprotein IIb/IIIa-receptor antagonists + Heparin or LMWHs', p.796. The manufacturers of **abciximab**, eptifibatide and tirofiban generally advise caution on their concurrent use with other drugs that affect haemostasis because of the likely further increased risk of bleeding.[1-6] They specifically name oral anticoagulants[1-6] (such as warfarin). Note that the US manufacturer of abciximab contraindicates the use of oral anticoagulants within 7 days of treatment with abciximab unless the INR is 1.2 or less.[4] The UK manufacturer[2] of tirofiban also contraindicates the use of tirofiban in patients with an INR greater than 1.5.

1. Integrilin (Eptifibatide). GlaxoSmithKline UK. UK Summary of product characteristics, April 2011.
2. Aggrastat (Tirofiban hydrochloride monohydrate). Iroko Cardio GmbH. UK Summary of product characteristics, September 2010.
3. ReoPro (Abciximab). Eli Lilly and Company Ltd. UK Summary of product characteristics, March 2011.
4. ReoPro (Abciximab). Centocor. US Prescribing information, November 2005.
5. Integrilin (Eptifibatide). Schering-Plough. US Prescribing information, March 2011.
6. Aggrastat (Tirofiban hydrochloride). Medicure Pharma, Inc. US Prescribing information, July 2008.

Coumarins + Grapefruit juice

Grapefruit juice may cause a modest rise in the INR some patients taking warfarin and one case report describes a marked rise in INR, which was attributed to grapefruit juice. However, other studies have suggested that grapefruit juice does not interact with warfarin or acenocoumarol.

Clinical evidence

(a) Acenocoumarol

In the preliminary report of a single-dose, placebo-controlled study in 12 healthy subjects, 150 mL of grapefruit juice did not alter the maximum INR of a 10-mg dose of acenocoumarol, and the AUCs of *S*- and *R*-acenocoumarol were not altered.[1,2]

(b) Warfarin

In a study in 9 patients stabilised on warfarin, consumption of grapefruit juice 240 mL three times daily for one week had no effect on the INR or prothrombin times.[3] Similarly, in the preliminary report of a two-way crossover study in 24 patients stabilised on warfarin, the frequency of the **warfarin** dosage adjustments needed by the group as a whole, when taking 250 mL grapefruit juice daily for 4 weeks was the same as when taking a placebo (orange juice). However, 4 individuals had a clinically significant, progressive and sustained 12 to 25% decrease in the warfarin dose to INR ratio when taking grapefruit juice, but not orange juice.[4] A 64-year-old man stabilised on warfarin was found to have an INR of 6.29 on routine testing 10 days after starting to drink about 1.5 litres of grapefruit juice daily. However, when the author took warfarin to achieve an INR of 2 to 3 and then drank 1.5 litres of grapefruit juice daily there was no clinically relevant change in his INR.[5]

Mechanism

It was suggested that the patients who showed some evidence of an interaction between grapefruit juice and warfarin may possibly have had an increased susceptibility to the inhibitory effects of grapefruit juice on the activity of the cytochrome P450 isoenzyme CYP3A4 in the gut.[4] Note that CYP3A4 has a minor role in the metabolism of *R*-warfarin, which is a much less potent anticoagulant than *S*-warfarin.

Importance and management

Information is limited. One study with warfarin suggests that some patients might require a slight reduction in dose if they regularly consume grapefruit juice, but further study is needed. Current evidence suggests that routine testing should be sufficient to detect any interaction.

For discussion of the interaction of warfarin with grapefruit seed extract, thought to be due to the preservative benzethonium chloride, see 'Coumarins + Benzethonium chloride', p.412.

1. Van Rooij J, van der Meer FJM, Schoemaker HC, Cohen AF. Comparison of the effect of grapefruit juice and cimetidine on pharmacokinetics and anticoagulant effect of a single dose of acenocoumarol. *Br J Clin Pharmacol* (1993) 35, 548P.
2. van der Meer FJM. Personal communication, April 1994.
3. Sullivan DM, Ford MA, Boyden TW. Grapefruit juice and the response to warfarin. *Am J Health-Syst Pharm* (1998) 55, 1581–3.
4. Dresser GK, Munoz C, Cruikshank M, Kovacs M, Spence JD. Grapefruit juice-warfarin interaction in anticoagulated patients. *Clin Pharmacol Ther* (1999) 65, 193.
5. Bartle WR. Grapefruit juice might still be factor in warfarin response. *Am J Health-Syst Pharm* (1999) 56, 676.

Coumarins + Griseofulvin

The anticoagulant effects of warfarin may be reduced by griseofulvin in some patients.

Clinical evidence

The anticoagulant effects of **warfarin** were modestly and markedly reduced in 2 patients, respectively, stabilised on **warfarin** when they were given griseofulvin 1 g daily in divided doses. Griseofulvin 1 g daily had no effect on the prothrombin time in one healthy subject given **warfarin**, whereas 2 g daily caused a marked reduction in the prothrombin time. Another healthy subject had no interaction, even when the griseofulvin dose was raised to 4 g daily for 2 weeks.[1]

In another study there was no change in the mean prothrombin time in 10 patients stabilised on **warfarin** when they were given griseofulvin 1 g daily in divided doses for 2 weeks. Four of the patients had an equivocal average reduction in prothrombin time of 4.2 seconds.[2] One case report describes decreased anticoagulant effects in a man stabilised on **warfarin** when he took griseofulvin 250 mg twice daily, which took 12 weeks to develop fully.[3] He eventually needed a 41% increase in his daily dose of **warfarin**. Another report very briefly mentions a case of a coagulation defect in a patient taking **warfarin** and griseofulvin.[4]

Mechanism

Not understood. It has been suggested that the griseofulvin acts as a liver enzyme inducer, which increases the metabolism of the warfarin, thereby reducing its effects.[1,3]

Importance and management

The interaction between warfarin and griseofulvin is poorly documented and not well established. However, it possibly results in a clinically significant interaction in some patients. Because of the uncertainty, and the known enzyme-inducing effects of griseofulvin, the prothrombin times of all patients taking warfarin who are given griseofulvin should be monitored, and suitable warfarin dose increases made as necessary.

1. Cullen SI, Catalano PM. Griseofulvin-warfarin antagonism. *JAMA* (1967) 199, 582–3.
2. Udall JA. Drug interference with warfarin therapy. *Clin Med* (1970) 77, 20–5.
3. Okino K, Weibert RT. Warfarin-griseofulvin interaction. *Drug Intell Clin Pharm* (1986) 20, 291–3.
4. McQueen EG. New Zealand Committee on Adverse Drug Reactions: 14th Annual Report 1979. *N Z Med J* (1980) 91, 226–9.

Coumarins and related drugs + H_2-receptor antagonists

The anticoagulant effects of warfarin can be increased by cimetidine. Acenocoumarol interacts similarly, but phenprocoumon appears not to be affected. In one patient the effects of phenindione were modestly increased by cimetidine. Famotidine, nizatidine, ranitidine and roxatidine normally do not appear to interact with the coumarins, although isolated cases of bleeding have been reported.

Clinical evidence

(a) Cimetidine

A brief report in 1978, published as a letter by the manufacturers of cimetidine, stated that preliminary details of a study in healthy subjects indicated that cimetidine 1 g daily could cause a prothrombin time rise of about 20% in patients stabilised on **warfarin**. At that time, they were aware of 17 cases worldwide, most of moderate rises in prothrombin times.[1]

A number of studies[2,3] and case reports[4-8] have confirmed this interaction with **warfarin**. In the studies, plasma **warfarin** levels were reported to rise by 25% and 80%, and prothrombin times were increased by 18% and 20% by cimetidine 1.2 g daily. In the case reports, severe bleeding (haematuria, internal haemorrhages) and very prolonged prothrombin times have been seen in a few patients given cimetidine 900 mg or 1.2 g daily.[4,6-8]

In another study, 7 out of 14 patients stabilised on **warfarin** had a greater than 30 second increase in their prothrombin time, whereas the other 7 had no prolongation or only a minor prolongation in their prothrombin time when they were given cimetidine 1.2 g daily for 10 days.[9] A study in 27 patients found that, although the AUC of **warfarin** was increased by 21 to 39% and its clearance fell by 22 to 28%, prothrombin times only increased by 2 to 2.6 seconds by cimetidine 800 mg or 1.2 g daily.[10] A pharmacokinetic study in 6 healthy subjects found that cimetidine did not affect *S*-warfarin but increased the trough plasma levels of *R*-warfarin by 28%, with minimal effect on prothrombin times.[11] Other pharmacokinetic studies have confirmed that the interaction affects only *R*-warfarin.[12-15] In one analysis of the concurrent use of **warfarin** and an H_2-receptor antagonist in hospitalised patients, there was no difference in the intensity of prothrombin time monitoring, and no difference in bleeding rates between 35 patients receiving cimetidine, 38 patients receiving ranitidine, or 36 patients receiving famotidine. Two patients in the cimetidine group had a bleed after they had taken both drugs for one or two days but neither had abnormally high prothrombin times.[16]

In three studies, the AUC of single-dose **acenocoumarol** was increased by cimetidine, and the prothrombin time prolonged,[17-19] with the effect greatest for *R*-acenocoumarol.[19] However, another study found no interaction.[20] Data from one patient taking **acenocoumarol** and one taking **phenindione** showed that cimetidine increased their anticoagulant effects.[2] In one study in patients stabilised on **phenprocoumon**, cimetidine 400 mg twice daily did not alter the pharmacokinetics of **phenprocoumon** or its anticoagulant effect.[21]

(b) Famotidine

In a study in 8 healthy subjects taking doses of **warfarin** titrated to prolong the prothrombin time by 2 to 5 seconds (mean dose 4 mg daily), famotidine 40 mg daily for 7 days did not affect prothrombin times, thrombotest coagulation times or steady-state plasma **warfarin** levels.[22] No changes in prothrombin times were seen in 3 patients stabilised on **acenocoumarol** or **fluindione** when they were given famotidine.[23] However, in another report 2 patients taking **warfarin** are said to have had prolonged prothrombin times and bled when they took famotidine.[24]

(c) Nizatidine

In 7 healthy subjects taking **warfarin**, nizatidine 300 mg daily for 2 weeks had no significant effect on the prothrombin times, kaolin-cephalin clotting times, the activity of factors II, VII, XI and X, or on steady-state serum **warfarin** levels.[25] A lack of a pharmacokinetic interaction was also reported in the preliminary results of another study.[26] An isolated case of gastrointestinal bleeding, associated with markedly prolonged prothrombin times, occurred after a 78-year-old took six doses of nizatidine 300 mg.[24]

(d) Ranitidine

In a study in 5 healthy subjects, ranitidine 200 mg twice daily for 2 weeks had no effect on **warfarin** concentrations or prothrombin times.[27] In another study in 11 healthy subjects, ranitidine 150 mg twice daily for 3 days had no effect on the pharmacodynamics or pharmacokinetics of a single dose of **warfarin**.[3] The same finding was reported in another similar study.[15] In contrast, in a fourth study in 5 subjects, ranitidine 150 mg twice daily for a week reduced the clearance of a single dose of **warfarin** by almost 30%, but the half-life was not significantly changed and prothrombin times were not measured.[28] Ranitidine 750 mg daily given to 2 subjects reduced the **warfarin** clearance by more than 50%.[28] In an isolated case, a patient stabilised on ranitidine 150 mg twice daily and **warfarin** vomited blood one week after her ranitidine dose was doubled to 300 mg twice daily. Her prothrombin time had risen from 17.6 seconds to 36.7 seconds. She was subsequently restabilised on ranitidine 150 mg twice daily and the original dose of **warfarin** with a prothrombin time between 19 and 20 seconds.[29]

In one study in 10 patients stabilised on **phenprocoumon**, ranitidine 150 mg twice daily for 14 days had no effect on anticoagulation or on phenprocoumon plasma levels.[30]

(e) Roxatidine

In a study in 12 healthy subjects, roxatidine 150 mg daily for 4 days had no effect on the steady-state pharmacokinetics of **warfarin** or the prothrombin ratio.[31]

Mechanism

Cimetidine binds with the cytochrome P450 isoenzymes and inhibits oxidative metabolism in the liver. Although cimetidine is considered to be a general inhibitor, it exhibits a degree of specificity for certain isoenzymes such as CYP1A2 and CYP2C19. These isoenzymes are principally involved in the metabolism of *R*-warfarin and not *S*-warfarin. Thus, the interaction between warfarin and cimetidine has been found to be stereoselective (i.e. cimetidine interacts with the *R*-isomer but not with the *S*-isomer).[11-14] As *R*-warfarin is the less active isomer, and the pharmacokinetic interaction is not marked, the interaction is generally modest. The other H_2-receptor antagonists normally do not act as enzyme inhibitors.

Importance and management

The interaction between warfarin and cimetidine is well documented, well established and potentially clinically important. Its effects are generally modest, but rarely, patients have shown a marked interaction. Because of this unpredictability, and to avoid bleeding, the response should be closely monitored in every patient when cimetidine is first added, being alert for the need to reduce the warfarin dose. The onset of the interaction appears rapid and its effects have been seen within days,[4,7] and even as early as 24 hours.[9] The effect of low non-prescription doses of cimetidine on warfarin do not appear to have been studied. Acenocoumarol is reported to interact similarly, and there is one case of phenindione being affected. Expect other coumarins and indanediones to behave in the same way, with the possible exception of phenprocoumon, which was not affected in one study.

Famotidine, nizatidine, ranitidine and roxatidine normally appear not to interact with the coumarins although note that, in rare cases, increases in prothrombin times and bleeding have been seen.

1. Flind AC. Cimetidine and oral anticoagulants. *Lancet* (1978) ii, 1054.
2. Serlin MJ, Sibeon RG, Mossman S, Breckenridge AM, Williams JRB, Atwood JL, Willoughby JMT. Cimetidine: interaction with oral anticoagulants in man. *Lancet* (1979) ii, 317–19.
3. O'Reilly RA. Comparative interaction of cimetidine and ranitidine with racemic warfarin in man. *Arch Intern Med* (1984) 144, 989–91.
4. Silver BA, Bell WR. Cimetidine potentiation of the hypoprothrombinemic effect of warfarin. *Ann Intern Med* (1979) 90, 348–9.
5. Hetzel D, Birkett D, Miners J. Cimetidine interaction with warfarin. *Lancet* (1979) ii, 639.
6. Wallin BA, Jacknowitz A, Raich PC. Cimetidine and effect of warfarin. *Ann Intern Med* (1979) 90, 993.
7. Kerley B, Ali M. Cimetidine potentiation of warfarin action. *Can Med Assoc J* (1982) 126, 116.
8. Devanesen S. Prolongation of prothrombin time with cimetidine. *Med J Aust* (1981) 1, 537.
9. Bell WR, Anderson KC, Noe DA, Silver BA. Reduction in the plasma clearance rate of warfarin induced by cimetidine. *Arch Intern Med* (1986) 146, 2325–8.
10. Sax MJ, Randolph WC, Peace KE, Chretien S, Frank WO, Braverman AJ, Gray DR, McCree LC, Wyle F, Jackson BJ, Beg MA, Young MD. Effect of two cimetidine regimens on prothrombin time and warfarin pharmacokinetics during long-term warfarin therapy. *Clin Pharm* (1987) 6, 492–5.
11. Niopas I, Toon S, Aarons L, Rowland M. The effect of cimetidine on the steady-state pharmacokinetics and pharmacodynamics of warfarin in humans. *Eur J Clin Pharmacol* (1999) 55, 399–404.

12. Choonara IA, Cholerton S, Haynes BP, Breckenridge AM, Park BK. Stereoselective interaction between the R enantiomer of warfarin and cimetidine. *Br J Clin Pharmacol* (1986) 21, 271–77.
13. Toon S, Hopkins KJ, Garstang FM, Diquet B, Gill TS, Rowland M. The warfarin-cimetidine interaction: stereochemical considerations. *Br J Clin Pharmacol* (1986) 21, 245–6.
14. Niopas I, Toon S, Rowland M. Further insight into the stereoselective interaction between warfarin and cimetidine in man. *Br J Clin Pharmacol* (1991) 32, 508–11.
15. Toon S, Hopkins KJ, Garstang FM, Rowland M. Comparative effects of ranitidine and cimetidine on the pharmacokinetics and pharmacodynamics of warfarin in man. *Eur J Clin Pharmacol* (1987) 32, 165–72.
16. Greaney JJ, Souney PF, Scavone JM. A review of monitoring intensity and bleeding complications in hospitalized patients receiving concurrent warfarin and histamine$_2$ antagonist therapy. *J Pharmacoepidemiol* (1994) 3, 27–45.
17. van Rooij J, van der Meer FJM, Schoemaker HC, Cohen AF. Comparison of the effect of grapefruit juice and cimetidine on pharmacokinetics and anticoagulant effect of a single dose of acenocoumarol. *Br J Clin Pharmacol* (1993) 35, 548P.
18. Kroon C, de Boer A, Hoogkamer JFW, Schoemaker HC, vd Meer FJM, Edelbroek PM, Cohen AF. Detection of drug interactions with single dose acenocoumarol: new screening method? *Int J Clin Pharmacol Ther Toxicol* (1990) 28, 355–60.
19. Gill TA, Hopkins KJ, Bottomley J, Gupta SK, Rowland M. Cimetidine-nicoumalone interaction in man: stereochemical considerations. *Br J Clin Pharmacol* (1989) 27, 469–74.
20. Thijssen HHW, Janssen GMJ, Baars LGM. Lack of effect of cimetidine on pharmacodynamics and kinetics of single oral doses of R- and S-acenocoumarol. *Eur J Clin Pharmacol* (1986) 30, 619–23.
21. Harenberg J, Staiger C, de Vries JX, Walter E, Weber E, Zimmermann R. Cimetidine does not increase the anticoagulant effect of phenprocoumon. *Br J Clin Pharmacol* (1982) 14, 292–3.
22. De Lepeleire I, van Hecken A, Verbesselt R, Tjandra-Maga TB, Buntinx A, Distlerath L, De Schepper PJ. Lack of interaction between famotidine and warfarin. *Int J Clin Pharmacol Res* (1990) 10, 167–71.
23. Chichmanian RM, Mignot G, Spreux A, Jean-Girard C, Hofliger P. Tolérance de la famotidine. Étude du réseau médecins sentinelles en pharmacovigilance. *Therapie* (1992) 47, 239–43.
24. Shinn AF. Unrecognized drug interactions with famotidine and nizatidine. *Arch Intern Med* (1991) 151, 814.
25. Cournot A, Berlin I, Sallord JC, Singlas E. Lack of interaction between nizatidine and warfarin during chronic administration. *J Clin Pharmacol* (1988) 28, 1120–2.
26. Callaghan JT, Nyhart EH. Drug interactions between H$_2$-blockers and theophylline (T) or warfarin (W). *Pharmacologist* (1988) 30, A14.
27. Serlin MJ, Sibeon RG, Breckenridge AM. Lack of effect of ranitidine on warfarin action. *Br J Clin Pharmacol* (1981) 12, 791–4.
28. Desmond PV, Mashford ML, Harman PJ, Morphett BJ, Breen KJ, Wang YM. Decreased oral warfarin clearance after ranitidine and cimetidine. *Clin Pharmacol Ther* (1984) 35, 338–41.
29. Baciewicz AM, Morgan PJ. Ranitidine-warfarin interaction. *Ann Intern Med* (1990) 112, 76–7.
30. Harenberg J, Zimmermann R, Kommerell B, Weber E. Interaktion von Ranitidin mit oralen Antikoagulantien. *Dtsch Med Wochenschr* (1983) 108, 1536.
31. Bender W, Brockmeier D. Pharmacokinetic characteristics of roxatidine. *J Clin Gastroenterol* (1989) 11 (Suppl 1), S6–S19.

Coumarins + HCV-Protease inhibitors

A case report describes changes in INR in a patient taking warfarin, after telaprevir was started. Boceprevir is predicted to interact similarly. Paritaprevir (in a fixed-dose combination) and simeprevir do not appear to alter the pharmacokinetics of warfarin.

Clinical evidence

(a) Boceprevir

The US manufacturer predicts that boceprevir could increase or decrease the plasma concentration of warfarin, which might alter its anticoagulant effects.[1]

(b) Paritaprevir

The UK manufacturer briefly reports that, in a study in healthy subjects given a single 5-mg dose of warfarin with paritaprevir 150 mg daily (in a fixed-dose combination with ombitasvir and ritonavir, and given with and without dasabuvir), there were no effects on the pharmacokinetics of *R*- and *S*-warfarin or paritaprevir.[2]

(c) Simeprevir

The UK and US manufacturers briefly report that, in a study in 16 healthy subjects given a single 10-mg dose of warfarin with simeprevir 150 mg daily for 11 days, the AUC and maximum concentration of *S*-warfarin were unaffected.[3,4]

(d) Telaprevir

The UK and US manufacturers of telaprevir predict that it might increase or decrease the plasma concentration of warfarin.[5,6] A case report describes a 45-year-old man, stable taking warfarin 6 mg daily with an INR within the target range of 2.5 to 3.5 for 8 months, whose INR increased to 6, 2 days after telaprevir 750 mg three times daily was started as part of triple therapy for hepatitis C. The patient was instructed to stop warfarin for 2 days and then restart at a dose of 5 mg daily, and to be alert for signs of bruising or bleeding. The patient decided to stop the warfarin for 5 days, after which his INR was only 1.1. Over the following 6 weeks his warfarin dose was increased to 9 mg daily and he achieved an INR of 2.5 at this dose. However, during the remaining weeks of his telaprevir course, and for several weeks after it was completed, his INR fluctuated and was mostly higher than the top of the target range, despite warfarin dose changes, but was eventually near its original level.[7]

Mechanism

The HCV-protease inhibitors are inhibitors of CYP3A4 (albeit to varying extents), but this isoenzyme is involved only in the metabolism of the less potent *R*-warfarin, and therefore inhibition would not be expected to have a notable effect on warfarin metabolism. In addition, boceprevir[1] and telaprevir[5,6] do not inhibit CYP2C9 *in vitro*, the main isoenzyme involved in the metabolism of the more potent *S*-warfarin (see Metabolism of the coumarins, under 'Anticoagulants', p.371). The studies with paritaprevir (in a fixed-dose combination) and simeprevir suggests that they do not affect CYP2C9 *in vivo*.

Importance and management

Evidence for an interaction between the HCV-protease inhibitors and warfarin is limited to a case report with telaprevir. Based on the known disposition and interactions of boceprevir, telaprevir, and warfarin, it would seem unlikely that a clinically important pharmacokinetic interaction would occur. However, a small effect on warfarin metabolism cannot be ruled out, but this needs confirmation. The US manufacturer of boceprevir,[1] and the UK and US manufacturers of telaprevir,[5,6] advise monitoring the INR on concurrent use and, until more is known, this would seem prudent. The studies with paritaprevir (in a fixed dose combination) and with simeprevir suggest that they do not alter warfarin metabolism and that no dose adjustment is necessary on concurrent use. However, note that the UK manufacturers of paritaprevir (in a fixed dose combination) and of simeprevir advise monitoring of the INR if given with warfarin.[2,3] This would seem a sensible precaution.

1. Victrelis (Boceprevir). Merck & Co., Inc. US Prescribing information, July 2014.
2. Viekirax (Ombitasvir, paritaprevir, ritonavir). AbbVie Ltd. UK Summary of product characteristics, January 2015.
3. Olysio (Simeprevir sodium). Janssen-Cilag Ltd. UK Summary of product characteristics, May 2014.
4. Olysio (Simeprevir sodium). Janssen Products, LP. US Prescribing information, November 2014.
5. Incivo (Telaprevir). Janssen-Cilag Ltd. UK Summary of product characteristics, July 2014.
6. Incivek (Telaprevir). Vertex Pharmaceuticals, Inc. US Prescribing information, October 2013.
7. Gatti DC, Cha A. Apparent interaction between telaprevir and warfarin in a patient with chronic hepatitis C viral infection. *Am J Health-Syst Pharm* (2012) 69, 2062–5.

Coumarins + Heparin

Heparin may prolong the prothrombin time, and increase the risk of bleeding with warfarin.

Clinical evidence, mechanism, importance and management

Heparin may prolong the one-stage prothrombin time.[1] The US manufacturer notes that, if a valid prothrombin time is to be obtained in a patient starting **warfarin** or other coumarins, a period of a least 5 hours after the last intravenous heparin dose or 24 hours after the last subcutaneous dose should be left before measuring the prothrombin time.[2] Note that it is usual clinical practice to start heparin and a coumarin at the same time to ensure the patient is anticoagulated until warfarin reaches steady-state, and to discontinue the heparin when the INR is stable.

1. Lutomski DM, Djuric PE, Draeger RW. Warfarin therapy: the effect of heparin on prothrombin times. *Arch Intern Med* (1987) 147, 432–3.
2. Heparin Sodium Injection. Pharmacia & Upjohn. US Prescribing information, December 2000.

Coumarins and related drugs + Heparinoids

Some of the normal tests of anticoagulation (prothrombin time, thrombotest) are unreliable for a few hours after giving intravenous danaparoid to patients taking coumarins. Oral pentosan polysulfate sodium did not alter the pharmacokinetics or pharmacodynamics of warfarin in healthy subjects, but note that this heparinoid is associated with rectal bleeding. An isolated case report describes bleeding in a patient taking acenocoumarol after a heparinoid-impregnated bandage was applied.

In general, the use of heparinoids with coumarins or indanediones would be expected to increase the risk of bleeding.

Clinical evidence, mechanism, importance and management

(a) Intravenous danaparoid

A study in 6 healthy subjects taking **acenocoumarol** (steady-state thrombotest values of 10 to 15%), found that a single intravenous bolus injection of 3250 anti-Xa units of danaparoid prolonged the prothrombin time and thrombotest for up to one hour and 5 hours, respectively, which was more than would have been expected by the simple addition of the effects of both drugs. However, no significant differences were seen in bleeding time, and danaparoid did not alter **acenocoumarol** pharmacokinetics.[1] The authors concluded that when monitoring the anticoagulant effects of **acenocoumarol**, the prothrombin time and the thrombotest may therefore be unreliable for at least one hour and 5 hours, respectively, after intravenous danaparoid has been given. This advice would apply equally to other coumarins and other drugs monitored using these tests, such as the indanediones.

(b) Pentosan polysulfate sodium

In a placebo-controlled, crossover study in 24 healthy subjects stabilised on **warfarin**, oral pentosan polysulfate sodium 100 mg every 8 hours for 7 days did not alter the anticoagulant effect of **warfarin** or the pharmacokinetics of *R*- or *S*-warfarin.[2] The authors consider it appears that, unlike intravenous administration, oral pentosan polysulfate sodium has no anticoagulant activity. However, the manufacturer notes that rectal haemorrhage was reported as an adverse effect in 6.3% of patients receiving pentosan polysulfate sodium at a dose of 300 mg daily.[3] On the basis of the pharmacological study, the authors considered that it seems unnecessary to make changes in the warfarin dose or the oral pentosan polysulfate sodium dose when the two drugs are used together. However, they do recommend careful monitoring on starting concurrent use.[2] Logic would suggest that, if bleeding occurs, this could be more severe in anticoagulated patients. The patient information provided by the manufacturer states that concurrent use of pentosan polysulfate and warfarin should be avoided until they have spoken with their doctor.[3] See also *Topical heparinoid*, below.

(c) Topical heparinoid

A man who was well stabilised on **acenocoumarol** and also taking metoprolol, dipyridamole and isosorbide dinitrate began to bleed within about 3 days of starting to use a medicated bandage on an inflamed lesion on his hand, probably caused by a mosquito bite. His prothrombin percentage was found to have fallen to less than 10%. The bandage was impregnated with a semi-synthetic heparinoid compound based on **xylane acid polysulfate** [possibly **pentosan polysulfate**].[4] It would appear that enough of the heparinoid had been absorbed through his skin to increase his anticoagulation to the point where he began to bleed. This case is unusual but it illustrates the need to keep a close watch on patients who are given several drugs that can potentially cause bleeding.

1. Stiekema JCJ, de Boer A, Danhof M, Kroon C, Broekmans AW, van Dinther TG, Voerman J, Breimer DD. Interaction of the combined medication with the new low-molecular-weight heparinoid Lomoparan® (Org 10172) and acenocoumarol. *Haemostasis* (1990) 20,136–46.
2. Modi NB, Kell S, Simon M, Vargas R. Pharmacokinetics and pharmacodynamics of warfarin when coadministered with pentosan polysulfate sodium. *J Clin Pharmacol* (2005) 45, 919–26.
3. Elmiron (Pentosan polysulfate sodium). Ortho-McNeil Pharmaceutical, Inc. US Prescribing information, December 2008.
4. Potel G, Maulaz B, Pabœuf C, Touze MD, Baron D. Potentialisation de l'acénocoumarol après application cutanée d'un héparinoïde semi-synthétique. *Therapie* (1989) 44, 67–8.

Coumarins + Herbal medicines; Miscellaneous

Many of the interactions of herbal medicines (health foods, dietary supplements) with warfarin in the published literature are solely hypothetical based on the postulated pharmacological effects of known chemical constituents of the plants. These mechanisms are discussed further below. Where specific clinical data on a herbal medicine interaction with warfarin are available, this is covered in a separate monograph.

All patients should be encouraged to report their use of herbal medicines and food supplements and cases of uneventful concurrent use should be published as well as cases of possible interactions to increase the clinical information available.

Clinical evidence and mechanism

(a) Antiplatelet effects

Antiplatelet doses of aspirin (see 'Coumarins and related drugs + Aspirin or other Salicylates', p.405), do not alter the anticoagulant efficacy of warfarin (INR); however, these doses of aspirin by themselves increase the risk of gastrointestinal bleeding, and the risk of this is higher in patients taking warfarin. On this basis, many herbs with antiplatelet activity *in vitro* are suggested to interact with warfarin. To establish the increased risk with antiplatelet doses of aspirin with warfarin, very large studies were needed because the absolute risks are small (about 1 in 100 in one study). Studies of this size are very unlikely to be conducted with herbal medicines. One way might be to compare the *in vivo* antiplatelet activity of the herbal product with that of aspirin 75 mg, and then to extrapolate to the likely increased risk of bleeding.

(b) Coumarin constituents

There is a misconception that if a plant contains natural coumarins it will have anticoagulant properties. More than 3 400 coumarins occur naturally throughout at least 160 plant families. Of these, just 13 have been tested for antithrombotic or anticoagulant activity, and only about half (7) were found to be active.[1] There are no established interactions between warfarin and herbal medicines that have been attributed to the coumarin content of the herb. Even in the classic case of hemorrhagic death of livestock that led to the discovery of dicoumarol, it was the action of the mould on the coumarin in the sweet clover that led to the production of the anticoagulant, so consumption of a spoiled product would seem to be necessary for this interaction to occur. This suggests that the occurrence of coumarins in dietary supplements or herbal medicines should not trigger immediate concern.[1]

(c) Vitamin K content

Vitamin K is found in highest levels in green leafy vegetables, which, if ingested in sufficient quantities, can markedly reduce the effects of warfarin and related drugs (see 'Coumarins and related drugs + Food; Vitamin K_1-rich', p.432). It would therefore not be surprising if many herbal medicines derived from dark green leaves contain vitamin K. However, whether enough of these herbs could be taken to cause an interaction seems less likely than with foods. Nevertheless, two case reports of altered coagulation status attributed to the vitamin K content of herbal preparations have been reported, see 'Coumarins + Vitamin K_1-rich herbal medicines', p.485.

Importance and management

There are many reviews of the effect of various herbal medicines on warfarin. Most of these include interactions based on theoretical data, based on the knowledge that a plant has been shown to contain antiplatelet substances or coumarins. The problem with these lists is that a suggested interaction might never be clinically relevant if, for example, the coumarins present are found not to be anticoagulants, or the substances are found in such small quantities and the herb cannot be ingested in sufficient amounts to cause an interaction. With natural substances, there is also the problem of chemical variations between batches of product if they are not standardised. Moreover, even isolated reports of an interaction between a herbal medicine and warfarin cannot definitively establish that such an interaction exists (see also *Anticoagulant interactions*, under 'Anticoagulants', p.371).

Because of the potential for interactions, some consider that patients taking warfarin would be well advised to avoid all herbal medications. However, this approach may not be practical: there are many papers showing that patients taking warfarin do use a number of herbal medicines and dietary supplements (19.2% in a UK survey;[2] 26% in a Hong Kong survey[3]). If patients have been told to avoid all herbal products, they may be less likely to admit to their use, and become less cautious in the future if they discover that the use of one product is uneventful. It may be better to advise patients to discuss the use of any products they wish to try, and to increase monitoring if this is thought necessary. Cases of uneventful use should be reported, as they are as useful as possible cases of adverse use.

1. Booth NL, Nikolic D, van Breemen RB, Geller SE, Banuvar S, Shulman LP, Farnsworth NR. Confusion regarding anticoagulant coumarins in dietary supplements. *Clin Pharmacol Ther* (2004) 76, 511–16.
2. Simth L, Ernst E, Ewings P, Myers P, Smith C. Co-ingestion of herbal medicines and warfarin. *Br J Gen Pract* (2004) 54, 439–41.
3. Wong RSM, Cheng G, Chan TYK. Use of herbal medicines by patients receiving warfarin. *Drug Safety* (2003) 26, 585–8.

Coumarins + Herbicides

An isolated report describes a marked increase in the anticoagulant effects of acenocoumarol, with bleeding, caused by the use of a herbicide containing thiocarbamates.

Clinical evidence, mechanism, importance and management

A 55-year-old patient with mitral and aortic prostheses, stabilised on **acenocoumarol** 2 mg daily and with an INR of 3.6 to 4.2 was hospitalised because of severe and uncontrollable gum bleeding. He responded when given a transfusion of fresh plasma. The cause of the marked increase in the anticoagulant effects of the **acenocoumarol** was eventually identified as almost certainly being due to the use of a herbicide (*SATURN-S*) containing **thiobencarb** and **molinate** (two thiocarbamates), which the patient was using to spray his rice crop. The **thiobencarb** can be absorbed through the skin and the **molinate** by inhalation. Just how these two compounds interact with **acenocoumarol** is not known but the authors of the report suggest that these herbicides may possibly have inhibited the metabolism of the anticoagulant, thereby increasing its effects. The patient was later restabilised on his former dose of **acenocoumarol**.[1]

This seems to be the first and only report of this interaction but it highlights one of the possible risks of using chemical sprays that have never been formally tested for their potential to interact with drugs. A similar problem has been seen with insecticides, see 'Coumarins + Insecticides', p.441.

1. Fernández MA, Aznar J. Potenciación del efecto anticoagulante del acenocumarol por un herbicida. *Rev Iberoamer Tromb Hemostasia* (1988) 1, 40–1.

Coumarins + HIV-protease inhibitors

In pharmacokinetic studies, ritonavir did not affect the exposure to *S*-warfarin but slightly decreased the exposure to *R*-warfarin, while lopinavir boosted with ritonavir slightly decreased the exposure to both *R*- and *S*-warfarin. Darunavir boosted with ritonavir also slightly reduced the exposure to *S*-warfarin. A number of case reports describe an interaction with HIV-protease inhibitors, most of which show a decrease in warfarin or acenocoumarol effects, although some show an increase in warfarin effects.

Clinical evidence

(a) Acenocoumarol

A 46-year-old HIV-positive man, with mitraortic valve replacements, stabilised on acenocoumarol (INR 2.5 to 3.5) for 5 years and taking zidovudine and didanosine for 17 months, was found to have a dramatic decrease in his INR when his drug regimen was changed to stavudine, lamivudine, and **ritonavir** 600 mg twice daily. Increasing the acenocoumarol dose over 5 days from an average of 24 mg to more than 70 mg did not increase the INR to within the target range. The INR returned to baseline within 4 days of stopping **ritonavir**, and the acenocoumarol dose could be reduced to 3 mg daily. The patient was subsequently given **nelfinavir** and a similar, though less dramatic interaction occurred: while taking **nelfinavir** an INR of 2.5 was achieved with a 210% increase in the acenocoumarol dose.[1] Another case describes a 51-year-old HIV-positive man, with poorly controlled INR, who had a further decrease in his INR after **atazanavir** boosted with ritonavir 300/100 mg daily was started. An acenocoumarol dose increase from 6.7 mg daily (INR about 2) to 8.3 mg daily did not achieve adequate INR control.[2]

(b) Warfarin

1. Darunavir. The US manufacturer of darunavir reports that, in a study in 12 subjects, darunavir boosted with ritonavir 600/100 mg daily reduced the AUC and maximum plasma concentration of a single 10-mg dose of *S*-warfarin by 21% and 8%, respectively. In addition, darunavir boosted with ritonavir increased the AUC and maximum plasma concentration of the 7-hydroxy metabolite of *S*-warfarin by 23% and 42%, respectively.[3]

2. Fosamprenavir. A 60-year-old HIV-positive man, stabilised on warfarin (mean daily dose 3 mg) required no warfarin dose modification after he was started on abacavir, lamivudine, and fosamprenavir 1400 mg twice daily. The authors also describe two other cases where warfarin was added to antiretroviral therapy. A 49-year-old man taking abacavir, lamivudine, and fosamprenavir 1400 mg twice daily, who was started on warfarin following a mechanical valve replacement, required only a minor warfarin dose adjustment (from 2 to 2.5 mg daily to 2.5 mg daily) to achieve the desired INR. A

33-year-old man whose antiretroviral treatment was changed to abacavir, lamivudine, and fosamprenavir 1400 mg twice daily because of poor INR control while taking abacavir, lamivudine, and *lopinavir boosted with ritonavir* (see below), required a warfarin dose reduction from 9 mg daily to 4.25 to 5 mg daily. This lower dose maintained his INR within the desired range.[4]

3. Indinavir. A 50-year-old HIV-positive man, stabilised on warfarin (prothrombin complex activity (PCA) range of 20 to 35%), started taking indinavir 800 mg every 8 hours, but it had to be withdrawn after 12 days because of a generalised skin rash. It was then found that the indinavir had caused a moderate reduction in his level of anticoagulation: 10 and 25 days after indinavir was stopped his PCA was 53% and 43%, respectively. The warfarin dose was increased to 6.25 and 7.5 mg on alternate days for one week, during which time a PCA of 34% was achieved, and he was then given warfarin 6.25 mg daily.[5] This patient subsequently needed an increase in warfarin dose when given *ritonavir*, see below. Another patient had a modest rise in INR to 4.5 when his dose of ritonavir was reduced from 600 mg twice daily to 200 mg twice daily and indinavir 800 mg twice daily added. This case suggests that any effect of high-dose ritonavir was greater than that of indinavir boosted with ritonavir.[6]

4. Lopinavir. In a pharmacokinetic study in healthy subjects,[7] lopinavir boosted with ritonavir 400/100 mg twice daily for 10 days slightly decreased the AUCs of *R*- and *S*-warfarin by 37% and 29%, respectively, after a single 10-mg dose of warfarin and vitamin K were given on day 7. The effect of this reduction on the anticoagulant activity of warfarin was not assessed, since vitamin K was given to inhibit the pharmacological effect of warfarin without affecting its pharmacokinetics.

However, there are several case reports suggesting a marked reduction in warfarin effects with lopinavir boosted with ritonavir. In one case, a man taking warfarin required a progressive daily dose increase from between 3.75 to 5 mg up to 10 mg after restarting an antiretroviral regimen including lopinavir with ritonavir. When the HIV-protease inhibitors were later stopped, the warfarin dose needed to be reduced again.[8] A 33-year-old man taking abacavir, lamivudine, and lopinavir boosted with ritonavir, was started on warfarin 7 mg daily for a DVT followed by pulmonary embolism, but after several months his INR could not be maintained within the desired range even at a dose of 9 mg daily. He similarly required a dose reduction when the lopinavir boosted with ritonavir was switched to *fosamprenavir* (see above).[4] In another case, a man was eventually stabilised on warfarin 13 mg daily while taking lopinavir boosted with ritonavir, which was over twice his original dose of 5.5 mg daily.[9] Yet another describes a man who required a 40% warfarin dose increase from 12.5 to 17.5 mg daily when switched from nelfinavir to lopinavir boosted with ritonavir.[10]

5. Nelfinavir. A man taking abacavir, tenofovir, and nelfinavir needed an increase in his warfarin dose from 45 mg weekly to 70 mg weekly to achieve a therapeutic INR.[10] Of the other drugs he was taking, ribavirin has been reported to increase warfarin requirements (see 'Coumarins + Ribavirin', p.467). Another patient required a high warfarin dose of 12.5 mg daily while taking a nelfinavir-containing regimen,[10] but this was less than that required while he was taking lopinavir boosted with ritonavir (17.5 mg daily) or nevirapine (20 mg daily). Consider also 'Coumarins + NNRTIs', p.448.

6. Ritonavir. The US manufacturer reports that, in 12 healthy subjects given ritonavir 400 mg every 12 hours for 12 days, there was a 9% increase (not statistically significant) in the AUC of *S*-warfarin, while the AUC of *R*-warfarin was slightly decreased (by 33%), after a single 5-mg dose of warfarin.[11] The effect of these changes on prothrombin time was not mentioned, but potentially could result in an increased warfarin effect due to the more potent *S*-warfarin, or a decreased effect due to the *R*-warfarin. Both of these outcomes have been reported in individual cases. An increase in warfarin effect was seen in a man taking warfarin 10 mg daily (INRs 2.4 to 3) when his treatment for HIV was changed from efavirenz and abacavir to ritonavir, nelfinavir, and *Combivir* (zidovudine with lamivudine). Within 5 days his INR had increased to 10.4, without any sign of bleeding. It proved difficult to achieve acceptable and steady INRs both while in hospital and after discharge, but eventually it was discovered that the patient could not tolerate liquid ritonavir because of nausea and vomiting, so he had sometimes skipped or lowered the ritonavir dose, or even refused to take it. On the occasions where no ritonavir or low-dose ritonavir was taken, the INRs had been low, whereas when he took the full dose of ritonavir the INRs were high.[12]

In contrast, the INR of a 27-year-old HIV-positive woman taking warfarin decreased when she was given ritonavir, clarithromycin, and zidovudine. It was necessary almost to double the warfarin dose to maintain satisfactory INRs. Three months later when the ritonavir was withdrawn, her INR more than tripled within a week. Her final warfarin maintenance dose was half of that needed before the ritonavir was started, and a quarter of the dose needed just before she stopped the ritonavir. This case was complicated by the use or withdrawal of a number of other drugs (co-trimoxazole, rifabutin, an oral hormonal contraceptive, megestrol), which can also interact with warfarin.[13] Similarly, in another patient taking warfarin 6.25 mg daily with a prothrombin activity complex (PCA) of about 34%, a decrease in warfarin effects (PCA increase to 62%) was noted 20 days after starting ritonavir (escalating doses up to 600 mg every 12 hours). The warfarin dose was then increased to 8.75 mg daily and 24 days later a satisfactory PCA of 33% was achieved.[5] This patient had previously had a decrease in warfarin effects while taking *indinavir*, see above. A patient stabilised on warfarin was found to have a subtherapeutic INR of 1 and required a 62% increase in warfarin dose when his HIV-protease inhibitor was switched from saquinavir to ritonavir 600 mg twice daily. Another patient taking ritonavir and saquinavir needed a very high warfarin dose to achieve a therapeutic INR.[6]

7. Saquinavir. A 73-year-old man who was HIV-positive and who had been taking warfarin, co-trimoxazole, nizatidine, stavudine, and lamivudine for 7 months started taking saquinavir 600 mg three times daily. His INR, which had been stable at around 2 for five months, increased to about 2.5 after 4 weeks, and to about 4.2 after 8 weeks, which the author of the report attributed to an interaction with the saquinavir. The situation was solved by reducing the warfarin dose by 20%.[14]

8. Tipranavir. The UK manufacturer of tipranavir briefly reports that in a pharmacokinetic study, at steady state, tipranavir boosted with ritonavir reduced the AUC of *S*-warfarin by 12%.[15]

Mechanism

HIV-protease inhibitors are well known to alter the metabolism of many drugs by inhibition, but sometimes by induction of cytochrome P450 isoenzymes, see 'Table 21.2', p.894, so it is not surprising that they alter the effects of warfarin, although the precise mechanism is unclear. The findings of the two pharmacokinetic studies suggest that, with warfarin, induction predominates, and that the anticoagulant effects are likely to be decreased. However, the modest reductions in concentrations seen do not explain the sometimes dramatic reduction in anticoagulant effects.

Importance and management

Pharmacokinetic studies have suggested that ritonavir, darunavir boosted with ritonavir, and lopinavir boosted with ritonavir slightly reduce the exposure to warfarin. Clinical information on an interaction between coumarins and HIV-protease inhibitors is limited to the case reports cited, most of which show a decrease in warfarin or acenocoumarol effects (with indinavir, lopinavir boosted with ritonavir, nelfinavir, ritonavir, saquinavir boosted with ritonavir, or atazanavir boosted with ritonavir), although a couple show an increase in warfarin effects (nelfinavir boosted with ritonavir or saquinavir). These cases show it would be prudent to monitor the prothrombin times and INRs in any patient if a HIV-protease inhibitor is added or changed, being alert for the need to modify the coumarin dose. Similarly, in any patient taking a HIV-protease inhibitor who requires warfarin, the INR may be more difficult to maintain and dose adjustments might be necessary. A few cases suggest that fosamprenavir does not interact with warfarin in the same way and might be an alternative in hard to manage patients, but this requires further study.

1. Libre JM, Romeu J, López E, Sirera G. Severe interaction between ritonavir and acenocoumarol. *Ann Pharmacother* (2002) 36, 621–3.
2. Welzen MEB, van den Berk GEL, Hamers RL, Burger DM. Interaction between antiretroviral drugs and acenocoumarol. *Antivir Ther* (2011) 16, 249–52.
3. Prezista (Darunavir ethanolate). Janssen Pharmaceuticals, Inc. US Prescribing information, May 2012.
4. Honda H, Gatanaga H, Matsumura J, Kamimura M, Goto K, Tsukada K, Honda M, Teruya K, Kikuchi Y, Oka S. Favourable use of non-boosted fosamprenavir in patients treated with warfarin. *Int J STD AIDS* (2009) 20, 441.
5. Gatti G, Alessandrini A, Camera M, Di Biagnio A, Bassetti M, Rizzo F. Influence of indinavir and ritonavir on warfarin anticoagulant activity. *AIDS* (1998) 12, 825–6.
6. Flamm JA, King J, Cohen S. Increased warfarin requirements in HIV(+) patients with deep venous thrombosis on HIV protease inhibitors. *Clin Infect Dis* (1999) 29, 1004.
7. Yeh RF, Gaver VE, Patterson KB, Rezk NL, Baxter-Meheux F, Blake MJ, Eron JJ, Klein CE, Rublein JC, Kashuba ADM. Lopinavir/ritonavir induces the hepatic activity of cytochrome P450 enzymes CYP2C9, CYP2C19, and CYP1A2 but inhibits the hepatic and intestinal activity of CYP3A as measured by a phenotyping drug cocktail in healthy volunteers. *J Acquir Immune Defic Syndr* (2006) 42, 52–60.
8. Bonora S, Lanzafame M, D'Avolio A, Trentini L, Lattuada E, Concia E, Di Perri G. Drug interactions between warfarin and efavirenz or lopinavir-ritonavir in clinical treatment. *Clin Infect Dis* (2008) 46, 146–7.
9. Hughes CA, Freitas A, Miedzinski LJ. Interaction between lopinavir/ritonavir and warfarin. *CMAJ* (2007) 177, 357–9.
10. Fulco PP, Zingone MM, Higginson RT. Possible antiretroviral therapy–warfarin drug interaction. *Pharmacotherapy* (2008) 28, 945–9.
11. Norvir Capsules (Ritonavir). Abbott Laboratories. US Prescribing information, March 2012.
12. Newshan G, Tsang P. Ritonavir and warfarin interaction. *AIDS* (1999) 13, 1788–9.
13. Knoell KR, Young TM, Cousins ES. Potential interaction involving warfarin and ritonavir. *Ann Pharmacother* (1998) 32, 1299–1302.
14. Darlington MR. Hypoprothrombinemia during concomitant therapy with warfarin and saquinavir. *Ann Pharmacother* (1997) 31, 647.
15. Aptivus Soft Capsules (Tipranavir). Boehringer Ingelheim Ltd. UK Summary of product characteristics, December 2011.

Coumarins + Hormonal contraceptives or HRT

Acenocoumarol dose requirements appear to be about 20% lower during the use of a combined hormonal contraceptive. An isolated report describes a marked increase in the INR of a woman taking warfarin when she was given emergency contraception with levonorgestrel. In contrast, the anticoagulant effects of dicoumarol and phenprocoumon were slightly decreased by oral contraceptives. Ethinylestradiol with norgestimate did not appear to have much effect on the clearance of warfarin.

There is conflicting data on whether or not the use of HRT (oral or topical) affects warfarin or phenindione dosing. In one case, the acenocoumarol dose was increased by 75% when oral conjugated oestrogens were changed to transdermal estradiol.

Clinical evidence

A. Hormonal contraceptives

(a) Acenocoumarol

The anticoagulant requirements of 12 patients taking acenocoumarol were about 20% lower while they were taking a combined hormonal contraceptive (average 19 months) than when they were not taking a contraceptive (average 12 months). Even then, they were anticoagulated to a higher degree while taking the contraceptive (prothrombin ratio of 1.67 compared with 1.5) than with the anticoagulant alone. The contraceptives used were *Neogynona*, *Microgynon*, *Eugynon* (**ethinylestradiol** with **levonorgestrel**) or *Topasel* (intramuscular **estradiol enantate** with **algestone**).[1]

(b) Dicoumarol

A study in 4 healthy subjects given single 150- or 200-mg doses of dicoumarol on day 17 of a 20-day course of *Enovid* (**noretynodrel** and **mestranol**) found that the anticoagulant effects were decreased in 3 of the 4 subjects, although the dicoumarol half-life remained unaltered.[2]

(c) Phenprocoumon

In a controlled study in 14 healthy women, the clearance of a single 0.22-mg/kg dose of phenprocoumon was increased by 20% in the 7 subjects taking oral combined hormonal contraceptives, compared with the 7 control subjects not taking hormonal contraceptives.[3]

(d) Warfarin

In a pharmacokinetic study, a single dose of warfarin 10 mg (given with vitamin K 10 mg to prevent anticoagulant effects) was given to 10 women before and while they were taking an oral combined hormonal contraceptive (**ethinylestradiol** 35 micrograms with **norgestimate** 180 micrograms to 250 micrograms for 3 weeks). The mean clearance of *S*-warfarin was not significantly changed, although there was wide variability with 5 subjects having an increase in clearance, 3 having a decrease, and 2 having little change.[4]

A 39-year-old woman with familial type 1 antithrombin deficiency and a history of extensive deep vein thrombosis and pulmonary embolism, taking warfarin, was given **levonorgestrel** for emergency contraception. Within 3 days her INR had risen from 2.1 to 8.1. No bleeding occurred. Her INR returned to normal after stopping the warfarin for 2 days.[5]

B. HRT

In a retrospective analysis, 18 women were identified who had started HRT while taking **warfarin** (16 patients) or **phenindione** (2 patients). A wide variety of HRT preparations were being used, including topical and oral preparations, oestrogens with or without progestogens, and progestogens alone. Half of the women taking **warfarin** had no change in their warfarin dose requirement after starting HRT. Five required a less than 10% increase or decrease in average **warfarin** dose, and 3 required a 13%, 22%, and 28% increase in their average **warfarin** dose, the latter two of these being the only 2 women taking oestrogen-only oral HRT. Of the 2 women taking **phenindione**, one needed no change in dose, and the other a 4.6% increase in dose.[6]

In one case, a postmenopausal 53-year-old woman needed an increase in her daily dose of **acenocoumarol** from 2 to 3.5 mg when her HRT was changed from **oral conjugated oestrogens** 0.625 mg daily to **transdermal estradiol** 50 micrograms daily. When the oral HRT was restarted, her **acenocoumarol** requirements returned to their former levels.[7]

Mechanism

Not understood. The oral contraceptives are known to be associated with a small increased risk of venous thromboembolism in otherwise healthy women, and are therefore contraindicated in women who have had thrombosis. HRT also increases the risk of venous thromboembolism. Oestrogens can apparently increase the metabolism (glucuronidation) of phenprocoumon.[3] The authors of the report about levonorgestrel suggest that it might have displaced the warfarin from its binding sites thereby increasing its activity,[5] although this mechanism is now generally discounted.

Ethinylestradiol with norgestimate did not appear to have an important effect on the activity of the cytochrome P450 isoenzyme CYP2C9, as assessed by the clearance of *S*-warfarin.[4]

Importance and management

Direct information seems to be limited to these reports. Combined hormonal contraceptives (both oral and patch) are normally contraindicated in those with thromboembolic disorders but if they must be used, be alert for any changes in the anticoagulant response if a hormonal contraceptive is started or stopped. The report about the apparent interaction between warfarin and postcoital levonorgestrel seems to be isolated and therefore its general importance is unknown. Note that intrauterine levonorgestrel has been used for menorrhagia in women taking warfarin.[8]

There is very limited published information available on the concurrent use of warfarin and HRT. The retrospective study suggests that usually HRT causes no or only minor changes in warfarin or phenindione requirements.

Note that, because of the increased risk of developing venous thromboembolism with HRT, the use of HRT in women already taking an anticoagulant requires careful consideration of the risks and benefits.

1. de Teresa E, Vera A, Ortigosa J, Alonso Pulpon L, Puente Arus A, de Artaza M. Interaction between anticoagulants and contraceptives: an unsuspected finding. *BMJ* (1979) 2, 1260–1.
2. Schrogie JJ, Solomon HM, Zieve PD. Effect of oral contraceptives on vitamin K-dependent clotting activity. *Clin Pharmacol Ther* (1967) 8, 670–5.
3. Mönig H, Baese C, Heidemann HT, Ohnhaus EE, Schulte HM. Effect of oral contraceptive steroids on the pharmacokinetics of phenprocoumon. *Br J Clin Pharmacol* (1990) 30, 115–18.
4. Shelepova T, Nafziger AN, Victory J, Kashuba AD, Rowland E, Zhang Y, Sellers E, Kearns G, Leeder JS, Gaedigk A, Bertino JS. Effect of a triphasic oral contraceptive on drug-metabolizing enzyme activity as measured by the validated Cooperstown 5+1 cocktail. *J Clin Pharmacol* (2005) 45, 1413–21.
5. Ellison J, Thomson AJ, Greer IA, Walker ID. Apparent interaction between warfarin and levonorgestrel used for emergency contraception. *BMJ* (2000) 321, 1382.
6. McLintock LA, Dykes A, Tait RC, Walker ID. Interaction between hormone replacement therapy preparations and oral anticoagulant therapy. *Br J Obstet Gynaecol* (2003) 110, 777–9.
7. Interference with oral anticoagulant treatment by oestrogen - influence of oestrogen administration route. *Thromb Haemost* (1999) 81, 471–2.
8. Pisoni CN, Cuadrado MJ, Khamashta MA, Hunt BJ. Treatment of menorrhagia associated with oral anticoagulation: efficacy and safety of the levonorgestrel releasing intrauterine device (Mirena coil). *Lupus* (2006) 15, 877–80.

Coumarins + Insecticides

A patient had a marked increase in his response to acenocoumarol when exposed to insecticides containing ivermectin and methidathion. Another patient was resistant to the effects of warfarin after very heavy exposure to a toxaphene and lindane-containing insecticide.

Clinical evidence

(a) Acenocoumarol

A farmer in Spain, normally well stabilised on acenocoumarol and amiodarone, had marked rises in his INR, from 3.5 up to 7.9, requiring a reduction in his anticoagulant dose (from 12 to 8 mg weekly), which occurred during the summer months. No bleeding occurred. It was then discovered that he was using insecticides containing **ivermectin** and an organophosphate **methidathion** on his trees without any protective clothing.[1]

(b) Warfarin

A rancher in the US, who was taking warfarin, had a very marked reduction in his anticoagulant response after dusting his sheep with an insecticide containing 5% **toxaphene (camphechlor)** and 1% **lindane (gamma-benzene hexachloride)**. Over a 2-year period he had periods of considerable warfarin resistance, which were linked to the use of this insecticide. Normally warfarin 7.5 mg daily maintained his prothrombin time in the therapeutic range, but after exposure to the insecticide even 15 mg daily failed to have any effect.[2] The dusting was done by putting the insecticide in a sack and hitting the sheep with it in an enclosed barn.[2]

Mechanism

The interaction between acenocoumarol and ivermectin with methidathion is not understood. When used on its own, ivermectin used for onchocerciasis normally has no effect on prothrombin times,[3,4] but two unexplained cases of prolonged prothrombin times associated with the development of haematomas have been reported.[5] Methidathion is an organophosphate. Lindane and other chlorinated hydrocarbon insecticides are known liver enzyme inducers,[6] which increase the metabolism and clearance of the warfarin, thereby reducing or even abolishing its effects.

Importance and management

Information about these interactions appears to be limited to these isolated case reports. Neither interaction is well established or of general clinical importance. The chlorinated hydrocarbon insecticides have been withdrawn from general use in most countries so that the possibility of an interaction with any anticoagulant is now very small. No other cases of an interaction between an anticoagulant and ivermectin, whether used as an insecticide or for the treatment of onchocerciasis, appear to have been reported.

As a general rule, farm workers and others should use proper protection (gloves, masks, protective clothing) if they are exposed to substantial amounts of any insecticide, because these can be both directly toxic and can also apparently interact with some prescribed drugs, including the anticoagulants, even if only very rarely.

1. Fernandéz MA, Ballasteros S, Aznar J. Oral anticoagulants and insecticides. *Thromb Haemost* (1998) 80, 724.
2. Jeffery WH, Ahlin TA, Goren C, Hardy WR. Loss of warfarin effect after occupational insecticide exposure. *JAMA* (1976) 236, 2881–2.
3. Richards FO, McNeeley MB, Bryan RT, Eberhard ML, McNeeley DF, Lammie PJ, Spencer HC. Ivermectin and prothrombin time. *Lancet* (1989) i, 1139–40.
4. Pacque MC, Munoz B, White AT, Williams PN, Greene BM, Taylor HR. Ivermectin and prothrombin time. *Lancet* (1989) i, 1140.
5. Homeida MMA, Bagi IA, Ghalib HW, El Sheikh H, Ismail A, Yousif MA, Sulieman S, Ali HM, Bennett JL, Williams J. Prolongation of prothrombin time with ivermectin. *Lancet* (1988) i, 1346–7.
6. Kolmodin B, Azarnoff DL, Sjöqvist F. Effect of environmental factors on drug metabolism: Decreased plasma half-life of antipyrine in workers exposed to chlorinated hydrocarbon insecticides. *Clin Pharmacol Ther* (1969) 10, 638–42.

Coumarins + Interferons

Two isolated reports indicate that the effects of acenocoumarol and warfarin may be increased by interferons. Conversely, there is evidence that suggests that peginterferon alfa-2b might modestly increase the metabolism of warfarin and other coumarins.

Clinical evidence

The manufacturer of **peginterferon alfa-2b** notes that, in a pharmacokinetic probe study in patients with chronic hepatitis C, **peginterferon alfa-2b** increased the activity of cytochrome P450 isoenzyme CYP2C8/9 by 28%, as assessed by tolbutamide pharmacokinetics.[1,2] This suggests that this interferon might increase the metabolism of *S*-warfarin, the more potent isomer, and therefore decrease the effects of **warfarin**. However, in a similar study in healthy subjects, **peginterferon alfa-2a** had no effect on tolbutamide pharmacokinetics.[3]

However, a woman stabilised on long-term **warfarin** 2.5 to 3.5 mg daily had a prothrombin time rise from 16.7 seconds to 20.4 seconds after receiving 6 million units of **interferon-alfa** daily for 10 days, then three times a week, for chronic hepatitis C. Her serum **warfarin** levels rose from about 0.8 micrograms/mL to 5.2 micrograms/mL. She responded to a reduction in the **warfarin** dose to 2 mg daily. The authors of the report also say that they have seen 4 other patients taking **warfarin** who needed a dose reduction when given interferon, two of them while taking **interferon beta** and the other two while taking **interferon alfa-2b**.[4]

Similarly, a woman taking **acenocoumarol** 1 mg and 2 mg on alternate days had gingival bleeding and a thrombotest change from 35% to 19% (indicating an increased anticoagulant effect) within 6 weeks of starting treatment with 3 million units of **interferon-alfa 2b** three times weekly for chronic hepatitis C. Her thrombotest percentages stabilised between 25 and 40% when the **acenocoumarol** dose was reduced to 1 mg daily. A later reduction in the interferon dose caused a decrease in the anticoagulant effects of **acenocoumarol**.[5]

Mechanism

Not understood. The authors of both reports suggest that interferon reduces the metabolism of the anticoagulants by the liver, thereby reducing their clearance and increasing their effects.[4,5] Some early *in vitro* studies did show that interferons might inhibit some drug metabolising enzymes.[6] Conversely, data for peginterferon alfa-2b suggest that it might modestly increase the metabolism of warfarin by the cytochrome P450 isoenzyme CYP2C9, which would reduce its anticoagulant effects. The manufacturer suggests that this might be because of the improvement in liver function seen when peginterferon is used in chronic hepatitis,[2] rather than any direct effect of peginterferon. However, the effect was not seen for all cytochrome P450 isoenzymes, and the opposite was seen in the two case reports described when other interferons were used for chronic hepatitis.

Importance and management

These two reports seem to be the only ones to describe an increased effect of the coumarins with an interferon, so the interaction is by no means established. Conversely, the data for peginterferon alfa-2b suggest that there might be a modest increase in activity of CYP2C9. Whether this is sufficient to cause a relevant decrease in the effect of warfarin remains to be seen. Nevertheless, the manufacturer advises caution with warfarin.[1,2] It would seem prudent to consider increased monitoring if any of these interferons is given to patients taking coumarins. For a case of decreased warfarin effects in a patient given interferon alfa-2b and ribavirin, see 'Coumarins + Ribavirin', p.467.

1. PegIntron (Peginterferon alfa-2b). Schering Corp. US Prescribing information, August 2009.
2. ViraferonPeg (Peginterferon alfa-2b). Schering-Plough Ltd. UK Summary of product characteristics, November 2009.
3. Pegasys (Peginterferon alfa-2a). Roche Products Ltd. UK Summary of product characteristics, October 2013.
4. Adachi Y, Yokoyama Y, Nanno T, Yamamoto T. Potentation of warfarin by interferon. *BMJ* (1995) 311, 292.
5. Serratrice J, Durand J-M, Morange S. Interferon-alpha 2b interaction with acenocoumarol. *Am J Hematol* (1998) 57, 89–92.
6. Okuno H, Kitao Y, Takasu M, Kano H, Kunieda K, Seki T, Shiozaki Y, Sameshima Y. Depression of drug metabolizing activity in the human liver by interferon-α. *Eur J Clin Pharmacol* (1990) 39, 365–7.

Coumarins + Ispaghula (Psyllium)

Ispaghula (psyllium) did not affect either the absorption or the anticoagulant effects of warfarin in one study. A cohort study also found no evidence of an interaction in patients taking acenocoumarol or phenprocoumon and ispaghula.

Clinical evidence, mechanism, importance and management

In a study in 6 healthy subjects, ispaghula (given as a 14-g dose of colloid (*Metamucil*) in a small amount of water with a single 40-mg dose of **warfarin**, and three further doses of ispaghula every 2 hours thereafter) did not affect either the absorption or the anticoagulant effects of the **warfarin**.[1] Similarly, in a population-based cohort study in patients taking **acenocoumarol** or **phenprocoumon**, there was no increased risk of over-anticoagulation (INR greater than 6) associated with the use of ispaghula (psyllium seeds), although the number of people treated was small.[2] No alteration of the anticoagulant response would therefore be expected on concurrent use.

1. Robinson DS, Benjamin DM, McCormack JJ. Interaction of warfarin and nonsystemic gastrointestinal drugs. *Clin Pharmacol Ther* (1971) 12, 491–5.
2. Visser LE, Penning-van Beest FJA, Wilson JHP, Vulto AG, Kasbergen AAH, De Smet PAGM, Hofman A, Stricker BHC. Overanticoagulation associated with combined use of lactulose and acenocoumarol or phenprocoumon. *Br J Clin Pharmacol* (2003) 57, 522–4.

Coumarins + Lanthanum

Lanthanum does not appear to alter the pharmacokinetics of a single dose of warfarin.

Clinical evidence, mechanism, importance and management

In a pharmacokinetic study in healthy subjects, lanthanum carbonate (3 doses of 1 g the day before **warfarin**, then 1 g thirty minutes before **warfarin**) had no effect on the pharmacokinetics of a single dose of **warfarin**.[1]

Lanthanum carbonate is a phosphate-binding drug, and does not appear to alter **warfarin** absorption. This suggests that no **warfarin** dose adjustments would be expected to be needed on concurrent use. However, note that the pharmacodynamics of **warfarin** (e.g. the effects on INR) were not assessed in this study.

1. Fiddler G. Fosrenol (lanthanum carbonate) does not affect the pharmacokinetics of concomitant treatment with warfarin. *J Am Soc Nephrol* (2002) 13, 749A–750A.

Coumarins + Laropiprant

Laropiprant has no clinically relevant effect on the pharmacokinetics or anticoagulant effect of warfarin.

Clinical evidence

In a randomised, crossover study, 12 healthy subjects were given laropiprant 40 mg daily for 12 days with a single 30-mg dose of warfarin on day 6. Laropiprant had no effect on the AUC of either enantiomers of warfarin, but negligibly increased their maximum level (by 11% and 13%), which just reached statistical significance for the *R*-enantiomer. However, laropiprant did not alter the AUC of the INR.[1]

Mechanism

Warfarin is principally metabolised by CYP2C9, and the data here suggest that laropiprant has no clinically relevant effect on this isoenzyme.

Importance and management

Laropiprant does not alter warfarin exposure and does not affect the INR in response to warfarin (the possible tiny increase in maximum warfarin levels is not clinically relevant). Therefore, on a pharmacokinetic basis, it is unlikely that concurrent use would require warfarin dose adjustments. However, note that laropiprant is available only in a combination product with nicotinic acid, which might alter the response to warfarin and other oral anticoagulants, see 'Coumarins and related drugs + Nicotinic acid (Niacin)', p.448.

1. Schwartz JI, Liu F, Stroh M, Gipson A, Johnson-Levonas AO, Lasseter KC, Lai E, Wagner JA. Influence of laropiprant, a selective prostaglandin D_2 receptor 1 antagonist, on the pharmacokinetics and pharmacodynamics of warfarin. *Am J Ther* (2009) 16, 215–23.

Coumarins + Lasofoxifene

In a study, lasofoxifene caused a minor decrease in the prothrombin time in response to warfarin without changing warfarin pharmacokinetics.

Clinical evidence, mechanism, importance and management

In 12 healthy postmenopausal women, lasofoxifene 4 mg on day one then 500 micrograms daily for 13 days had no effect on the pharmacokinetics of *R*- or *S*-warfarin when a single 20-mg dose of **warfarin** was given on day 8. However, the maximum prothrombin time was decreased by 16%, with a similar decrease in the maximum INR, which was reduced from 1.9 to 1.6.[1]

Because this slight decrease in **warfarin** effects has been seen with raloxifene (see 'Coumarins + Raloxifene', p.467), the authors suggested that it might be because oestrogenic compounds increase plasma concentrations of vitamin K-dependent clotting factors.[1]

The authors suggest that the small decrease in **warfarin** effect with lasofoxifene may not be clinically relevant. Nevertheless, they say that until more data are available on longer-term concurrent use, it is recommended that prothrombin times should be monitored (presumably with any coumarin) when starting or stopping lasofoxifene.[1] This seems a sensible precaution.

1. Ouellet D, Bramson C, Carvajal-Gonzalez S, Roman D, Randinitis E, Remmers A, Gardner MJ. Effects of lasofoxifene on the pharmacokinetics and pharmacodynamics of single-dose warfarin. *Br J Clin Pharmacol* (2006) 61, 741–5.

Coumarins + Laxatives

In one cohort study, the long-term use of lactulose appeared to be associated with an increased risk of over-anticoagulation. Limited evidence suggested no interaction occurred with liquid paraffin or colocynth.

Clinical evidence

In a population-based cohort study in patients taking **acenocoumarol** or **phenprocoumon**, lactulose significantly increased the risk of over-anticoagulation (INR greater than 6) with a relative risk of 3.4 (range 2.2 to 5.3). When analysed by duration of use, less than 27 days use of **lactulose** actually decreased the risk of over-anticoagulation, whereas longer use was associated with an increased risk. In this study, neither **liquid paraffin** nor **colocynth** preparations were associated with an increased risk of over-anticoagulation, but the numbers of patients taking these drugs was small.[1]

Mechanism

In theory, drugs that shorten gastrointestinal transit time such as laxatives and liquid paraffin (mineral oil) might be expected to decrease the absorption of both vitamin K and the coumarins or indanediones. Decreasing the absorption of vitamin K would be expected to increase the effect of these anticoagulants, which could be offset by the decrease in absorption of the anticoagulant. In the case of short-term lactulose use, it was suggested that decreasing the colonic pH might have increased the absorption of vitamin K, thereby reducing the effect of the coumarin. On longer term use, it was postulated that lactulose might reduce faecal flora that produce vitamin K, so increasing the risk of over-anticoagulation.[1] Liquid paraffin might also be expected to impair the absorption of vitamin K.

Importance and management

The cohort study cited appears to be the first and only evidence of a possible interaction with laxatives, and it suggests that the long-term use of lactulose may increase the effect of coumarins. This finding requires confirmation in a controlled pharmacological study. Until further data are available, it may be prudent to consider the possibility of an interaction in any patient taking lactulose long-term. Limited evidence suggests that no interaction occurs with liquid paraffin or colocynth but this needs confirmation. Clinical evidence for an interaction with other laxatives is lacking, despite the theoretical considerations.

1. Visser LE, Penning-van Beest FJA, Wilson JHP, Vulto AG, Kasbergen AAH, De Smet PAGM, Hofman A, Stricker BHC. Overanticoagulation associated with combined use of lactulose and acenocoumarol or phenprocoumon. *Br J Clin Pharmacol* (2003) 57, 522–4.

Coumarins + Leflunomide or Teriflunomide

There are a few reports of increased INRs, some with bleeding complications, in patients taking warfarin with leflunomide. Teriflunomide might decrease the INR in patients taking warfarin.

Clinical evidence

(a) Leflunomide

A short report describes a patient taking **warfarin** whose INR increased from 2.5 to over 6, resulting in a hospital admission, shortly after she started taking leflunomide (3 days of 100 mg daily).[1]

Another report describes a patient taking **warfarin** who developed haematuria after taking leflunomide 100 mg daily for 2 days. His INR was found to have increased from 3.4 to over 11, and **warfarin** was discontinued. The haematuria spontaneously resolved, but as the INR remained elevated for the next 2 days he was given 1 mg of vitamin K, which brought his INR down to 1.9. He was later stabilised on **warfarin** 1 mg daily with a leflunomide maintenance dose of 20 mg daily.[2] The authors of this report stated that at that time (2002) the CSM in the UK had received over 300 reports of leflunomide increasing the INRs of patients taking **warfarin**;[2] however, this was an error, and the report should have read that of 300 reports of increased INRs with **warfarin** and another drug, *four* reports related to leflunomide.[3] An additional case describes a patient who required a 22% decrease in her weekly **warfarin** dose after starting leflunomide.[4]

(b) Teriflunomide

The UK and US manufacturers of teriflunomide briefly note that, a 25% *lower* INR was seen when warfarin was given with teriflunomide, when compared with warfarin alone.[5,6]

Mechanism

Uncertain, as teriflunomide (the major active metabolite of leflunomide) has been shown not to affect the pharmacokinetics of *S*-warfarin[5,6] (the more active isomer of warfarin), which is metabolised by CYP2C9. Furthermore, the lower INR reported with teriflunomide, is the opposite of that seen with leflunomide. The mechanism(s) behind the effects on INR seen is therefore not known, and requires further study.

Importance and management

Evidence for an interaction between the coumarins and leflunomide is based only on case reports with warfarin, nevertheless given the increased INRs and episodes of bleeding reported, it would seem prudent to closely monitor the INR of any patient taking warfarin, or another coumarin, with leflunomide.

Teriflunomide might be expected to interact similarly. However, the evidence for an interaction with the coumarins is much more limited, and it suggests that the INR might be *lower* than expected on concurrent use. Close INR monitoring would be prudent on concurrent use of teriflunomide and any coumarin.

1. Mason JP. Warfarin and leflunomide. *Pharm J* (2000) 265, 267.
2. Lim V, Pande I. Leflunomide can potentiate the anticoagulant effect of warfarin. *BMJ* (2002) 325, 1333. Erratum *ibid.* (2003) 326, 432.
3. Anonymous. Corrections and clarifications: drug points. *BMJ* (2003) 326, 432.
4. Chonlahan J, Halloran MA, Hammonds A. Leflunomide and warfarin interaction: case report and review of the literature. *Pharmacotherapy* (2006) 26, 868–71.
5. Aubagio (Teriflunomide). Genzyme Therapeutics. UK Summary of product characteristics, September 2014.
6. Aubagio (Teriflunomide). Genzyme Corp. US Prescribing information, October 2014.

Coumarins + Leukotriene antagonists

Zafirlukast increases the anticoagulant effects of warfarin and bleeding has been seen. Pranlukast is predicted to interact similarly. In contrast, montelukast did not alter the pharmacokinetics or anticoagulant effects of single-dose warfarin.

Clinical evidence

(a) Montelukast

In a placebo-controlled, randomised study, 12 healthy subjects were given oral montelukast 10 mg daily for 12 days and a single 30-mg dose of **warfarin** on day 7. It was found that the pharmacokinetics of the **warfarin** were virtually unchanged by the montelukast, and prothrombin times and INRs were not significantly altered.[1]

(b) Zafirlukast

In a placebo-controlled study, 16 healthy subjects taking zafirlukast 80 mg twice daily for 10 days were given a single 25-mg dose of **warfarin** on day 5. The mean AUC of *S*-warfarin was increased by 63% and the half-life by 36%, but the pharmacokinetics of *R*-warfarin were not significantly changed. The mean prothrombin time increased by 35%.[2]

An 85-year-old woman taking **warfarin**, salbutamol (albuterol), diltiazem, digoxin, furosemide and potassium was admitted to hospital with various cardiac-related problems and bleeding (epistaxis, melaena, multiple bruising), which was attributed to the use of zafirlukast 20 mg twice daily. Her INR had risen from 1.1 (measured 6 months previously) to 4.5. The report does not say how long she had been taking the both drugs together.[3]

Mechanism

The reason for the interaction is thought to be that the zafirlukast inhibits the cytochrome P450 isoenzyme CYP2C9, which metabolises *S*-warfarin.[2,4] *In vitro* studies suggest that **pranlukast** has a similar effect.[5]

Importance and management

Information appears to be limited to these reports but the interaction with zafirlukast would seem to be established. If zafirlukast is given to patients stabilised on warfarin, monitor prothrombin times well and be alert for the need to reduce the warfarin dose to avoid over-anticoagulation. Other coumarins might be expected to be affected similarly. Pranlukast is also predicted to interact with the coumarins, as it is also an inhibitor of CYP2C9. In contrast, montelukast does not appear to interact with warfarin, and no warfarin dose adjustments are predicted to be needed on concurrent use.

1. Van Hecken A, Depre M, Verbesselt R, Wynants K, De Lepeleire I, Arnoudt J, Wong PH, Freeman A, Holland S, Gertz B, De Schepper PJ. Effect of montelukast on the pharmacokinetics and pharmacodynamics of warfarin in healthy subjects. *J Clin Pharmacol* (1999) 39, 495–500.
2. Suttle AB, Vargo DL, Wilkinson LA, Birmingham BK, Lasseter K. Effect of zafirlukast on the pharmacokinetics of R- and S-warfarin in healthy men. *Clin Pharmacol Ther* (1997) 61, 186.
3. Morkunas A, Graeme K. Zafirlukast-warfarin drug interaction with gastrointestinal bleeding. *J Toxicol Clin Toxicol* (1997) 35, 501.
4. Accolate (Zafirlukast). AstraZeneca UK Ltd. UK Summary of product characteristics, February 2011.
5. Liu KH, Lee YM, Shon JH, Kim MJ, Lee SS, Yoon YR, Cha IJ, Shin JG. Potential of pranlukast and zafirlukast in the inhibition of human liver cytochrome P450 enzymes. *Xenobiotica* (2004) 34, 429–38.

Coumarins + Levetiracetam

In a controlled study, levetiracetam did not alter the pharmacokinetics or pharmacodynamics of warfarin.

Clinical evidence, mechanism, importance and management

In a randomised, double-blind, placebo-controlled study in 42 healthy subjects stabilised on **warfarin**, levetiracetam 1 g twice daily for 7 days had no significant effect on the pharmacokinetics of *R*- or *S*-warfarin and the INRs were not significantly altered.[1] No **warfarin** dose adjustments would therefore be expected to be needed on concurrent use.

1. Ragueneau-Majlessi I, Levy RH, Meyerhoff C. Lack of effect of repeated administration of levetiracetam on the pharmacodynamic and pharmacokinetic profiles of warfarin. *Epilepsy Res* (2001) 47, 55–63.

Coumarins + Levocarnitine

Two isolated reports describe a marked increase in the anticoagulant effects of acenocoumarol in patients taking levocarnitine, one of which was associated with melaena.

Clinical evidence, mechanism, importance and management

A woman who had taken **acenocoumarol** for 17 years because of aortic and mitral prosthetic valves, was admitted to hospital with melaena within 5 days of starting to take levocarnitine 1 g daily, which she was prescribed for congestive heart failure. Her INR had risen from 2.1 to 7. Endoscopy and colonoscopy revealed diffuse bleeding from superficial erosions in the gut. She was discharged 10 days later with the same dose of **acenocoumarol** and an INR of 2.1 without the levocarnitine.[1] A similar case has been described in a man stabilised on **acenocoumarol** (INR 1.99 to 2.94) who had a rise in INR to 4.65 despite a dose correction. The increases in INR occurred when he was using levocarnitine 1 g daily for 10 weeks in the form of a drink (*Maximize*) promoted for bodybuilding and fitness training. When this product was discontinued, the INR returned to the therapeutic range.[2]

The reason for this apparent interaction is not known. These seem to the only recorded cases of an interaction between a coumarin and levocarnitine, but it may be prudent to bear this interaction in mind if levocarnitine is taken with acenocoumarol, or possibly any coumarin, being alert for an increased response.

1. Martinez E, Domingo P, Roca-Cusachs A. Potentiation of acenocoumarol action by L-carnitine. *J Intern Med* (1993) 233, 94.
2. Bachmann HU, Hoffmann A. Interaction of food supplement L-carnitine with oral anticoagulant acenocoumarol. *Swiss Med Wkly* (2004) 134, 385.

Coumarins + Levosimendan

Levosimendan does not alter the effects of warfarin. There is no pharmacokinetic interaction between levosimendan and warfarin.

Clinical evidence, mechanism, importance and management

In an open, randomised, crossover study, 10 healthy subjects were given a single 25-mg oral dose of **warfarin** both before and on day 4 of a 9-day course of oral levosimendan 500 micrograms four times daily. No clinically relevant changes in the anticoagulant effects of the **warfarin** were seen, and levosimendan alone had no effect on blood coagulation. In addition, there was no important pharmacokinetic interaction between **warfarin** and levosimendan. No interactions would therefore be expected if both drugs are used concurrently.[1]

1. Antila S, Jarvinen A, Honkanen T, Lehtonen L. Pharmacokinetic and pharmacodynamic interactions between the new calcium sensitiser levosimendan and warfarin. *Eur J Clin Pharmacol* (2000) 56, 705–10.

Coumarins + Lycium (*Lycium barbarum*)

A case report suggests that lycium may enhance the effects of warfarin.

Clinical evidence

A 61-year-old Chinese woman stabilised on **warfarin** (INRs normally 2 to 3) had an unexpected rise in her INR to 4.1, which was identified during a routine monthly check. No bleeding was seen. She was also taking atenolol, benazepril, digoxin and fluvastatin. It was found that 4 days before visiting the clinic she had started to take one glass (about 170 mL) 3 or 4 times daily of a Chinese herbal tea made from the fruits of lycium to treat blurred vision caused by a sore eye. When the herbal treatment was stopped, her INRs rapidly returned to normal.

Mechanism

Warfarin is metabolised by a number of isoenzymes, the most important being the cytochrome P450 isoenzyme CYP2C9. Inhibition of this isoenzyme may therefore lead to increased warfarin levels and effects. The authors also carried out an *in vitro* study and concluded that although lycium is a weak inhibitor of CYP2C9, this is insufficient to cause an interaction. However, they note that other mechanisms cannot be ruled out.[1]

Importance and management

Although the authors suggest avoiding the concurrent use of lycium and warfarin,[1] because of the many other factors influencing anticoagulant control, it is not possible to reliably ascribe a change in INR specifically to a drug interaction in a single case report without other supporting evidence. It may be better to advise patients to discuss the use of any herbal products they wish to try, and to increase monitoring if this is thought advisable. Cases of uneventful use should be reported, as they are as useful as possible cases of adverse effects. It should be noted that lycium berries are also used as an ingredient in Chinese foods.

1. Lam AY, Elmer GW, Mohutsky M. Possible interaction between warfarin and *Lycium barbarum*. *Ann Pharmacother* (2001) 35, 1199–1201.

Coumarins + MAOIs or RIMAs

Although some *animal* data show that the non-selective MAOIs increase the effects of some oral anticoagulants, there appears to be no clinical evidence of an interaction. Moclobemide did not interact with phenprocoumon in a pharmacological study, and limited data suggests that it does not interact with warfarin.

Clinical evidence, mechanism, importance and management

(a) MAOIs

A number of studies in *animals*[1-4] have shown that some of the non-selective MAOIs can increase the effects of some oral anticoagulants. However, there appear to be no clinical studies or case reports of this interaction and therefore no particular precautions seem to be necessary on concurrent use.

(b) Moclobemide

A study in healthy subjects found that moclobemide 200 mg three times daily for 7 days did not alter the anticoagulant effects of steady-state **phenprocoumon**.[5] No **phenprocoumon** dose adjustments would be expected to be needed on concurrent use.

There appears to be just one review that mentions the possible interaction of moclobemide with **warfarin**.[6] This review reports that (in 1996), the manufacturer had on file six possible cases of anticoagulation problems in patients taking **warfarin** and moclobemide. On the basis that moclobemide is an inhibitor of CYP2C19 and possibly also CYP1A2, the reviewers considered that moclobemide could theoretically increase the plasma concentration of *S*-warfarin, and so stated that an interaction with **warfarin** was likely. However, CYP2C19 and CYP1A2 are just two of a number of isoenzymes involved in metabolism of *R*-warfarin, which is the less pharmacologically active isomer of **warfarin**. Other CYP2C19 inhibitors, such as omeprazole (see 'Coumarins + Proton pump inhibitors', p.464), and ticlopidine (see 'Coumarins + Ticlopidine', p.478), usually have no clinically relevant effect on the plasma concentration of **warfarin**. In addition, in a retrospective study in patients taking warfarin, the concurrent use of moclobemide was not associated with an increased risk of bleeding, when compared with patients taking warfarin alone.[7]

This, and the absence of published reports of problems, suggests that moclobemide is unlikely to interact with **warfarin**. There appears to be no evidence about other coumarins, but there seems to be no reason to suspect that they might interact.

1. Fumarola D, De Rinaldis P. Ricerche sperimentali sugli inibitori della mono-aminossidasi. Influenza della nialamide sulla attività degli anticoagulanti indiretti. (1964) 49, 1248–66.
2. Reber K, Studer A. Beeinflussung der Wirkung einiger indirekter Antikoagulantien durch Monoaminoxydase-Hemmer. *Thromb Diath Haemorrh* (1965) 14, 83–7.
3. de Nicola P, Fumarola D, de Rinaldis P. Beeinflussung der gerinnungshemmenden Wirkung der indirekten Antikoagulantien durch die MAO-Inhibitoren. *Thromb Diath Haemorrh* (1964) 12 (Suppl), 125–7.
4. Hrdina P, Rusnáková M, Kovalčík V. Changes of hypoprothrombinaemic activity of indirect anticoagulants after MAO inhibitors and reserpine. *Biochem Pharmacol* (1953) 12 (Suppl), 241.
5. Amrein R, Güntert TW, Dingemanse J, Lorscheid T, Stabl M, Schmid-Burgk W. Interactions of moclobemide with concomitantly administered medication: evidence from pharmacological and clinical studies. *Psychopharmacology (Berl)* (1992) 106, S24–S31.
6. Duncan D, Sayal K, McConnell H, Taylor D. Antidepressant interactions with warfarin. *Int Clin Psychopharmacol* (1998) 13, 87–94.
7. Hauta-Aho M, Tirkkonen T, Vahlberg T, Laine K. The effect of drug interactions on bleeding risk associated with warfarin therapy in hospitalized patients. *Ann Med* (2009) 41, 619–28.

Coumarins + Medroxyprogesterone or Megestrol

High-dose medroxyprogesterone acetate and megestrol prolonged the half-life of single-dose warfarin in one small study in patients with advanced breast cancer.

Clinical evidence, mechanism, importance and management

In a study in patients with advanced breast cancer, a single 0.3-mg/kg dose of **warfarin** was given to 2 patients before and after oral medroxyprogesterone acetate 500 mg twice daily for 5 weeks and to 2 patients before and after megestrol 160 mg daily for 5 weeks. The half-life of **warfarin** was increased by 71% and the clearance decreased by 35%.[1] Although the evidence is limited, what is known suggests that it would be prudent to monitor prothrombin times in patients taking **warfarin** who are given high-dose medroxyprogesterone acetate or megestrol, being alert for any increased warfarin effects.

1. Lundgren S, Kvinnsland S, Utaaker E, Bakke O, Ueland PM. Effect of oral high-dose progestins on the disposition of antipyrine, digitoxin, and warfarin in patients with advanced breast cancer. *Cancer Chemother Pharmacol* (1986) 18, 270–5.

Coumarins + Mefloquine

The effects of warfarin and an unnamed coumarin were increased in two patients who took mefloquine.

Clinical evidence, mechanism, importance and management

A 66-year-old man taking **warfarin** and various other drugs presented to an emergency department unwell with a distended abdomen while travelling in Kenya. His prothrombin time was grossly prolonged and the distension was found to be due to bleeding. One week before travel he had started mefloquine 250 mg weekly without a check of his prothrombin time. He was given subcutaneous enoxaparin instead of **warfarin** while continuing the mefloquine. Another patient taking a coumarin and oral antidiabetics presented with hypoglycaemia and a large haematoma of the right leg after taking 3 doses of mefloquine 250 mg weekly. His INR was 6.4.[1]

The author considered that mefloquine may have caused the increased anticoagulation in these two cases, and suggested that mefloquine should be started several weeks before travel to allow for monitoring of any changes in anticoagulant effects.[1] The manufacturers of mefloquine also recommend that, before departure, travellers also taking anticoagulants should be checked for any alteration in anticoagulant effect.[2] This is probably prudent, although patients should be advised that many other factors associated with travel, such as altered diet, could contribute to a change in anticoagulant control.

1. Loefler I. Mefloquine and anticoagulant interaction. *J Travel Med* (2003) 10, 194–5.
2. Lariam (Mefloquine hydrochloride). Roche Products Ltd. UK Summary of product characteristics, November 2011.

Coumarins + Melatonin

Case reports suggest that melatonin may raise or lower the INR in response to warfarin.

Clinical evidence

Six case reports of a suspected interaction between melatonin and **warfarin** have been documented by the WHO Uppsala Monitoring Centre, and have been briefly summarised in a review of melatonin.[1] In three cases, the prothrombin time was increased, with bleeding events in two (nosebleed, eye haemorrhage, bruising) occurring up to 8 days after starting to take melatonin. The other three cases reports describe a prothrombin time decrease.[1]

Mechanism

Unknown. Melatonin did not inhibit the cytochrome P450 isoenzyme CYP2C9 *in vitro*,[2] and would not therefore be expected to alter warfarin metabolism by this mechanism.

Importance and management

These appear to be the only reports in the literature of a possible interaction between melatonin and warfarin. They are difficult to interpret, because they include both increased and decreased warfarin effects, and it is possible that they are just idiosyncratic cases. Because of these cases, a study designed to exclude a pharmacokinetic and/or pharmacodynamic interaction would be useful. Until more is known, bear these cases in mind in the event of an unexpected change in coagulation status in patients also taking melatonin supplements.

1. Herxheimer A, Petrie KKJ. Melatonin for the prevention and treatment of jet lag. Available in the Cochrane Database of Systematic Reviews; Issue 1. Chichester: John Wiley; 2009.
2. Yeleswaram K, Vachharajani N, Santone K. Involvement of cytochrome P-450 isozymes in melatonin metabolism and clinical implications. *J Pineal Res* (1999) 26, 190–1.

Coumarins + Melilot (*Melilotus officinalis*)

The INR of a patient taking acenocoumarol was increased after she used a melilot-containing topical cream, and a woman who had been drinking large quantities of a herbal tea containing melilot developed a prolonged prothrombin time.

Clinical evidence

A 66-year-old taking **acenocoumarol**, levothyroxine and prazepam had an increase in her INR after massaging a proprietary topical cream (*Cyclo 3*) containing melilot and butcher's broom on her legs three times daily. On the first occasion her INR rose from about 2 to 5.8 after 7 days of use, and on a later occasion it rose to 4.6 after 10 days of use.[1] In another report, a woman with unexplained abnormal menstrual bleeding was found to have a prothrombin time of 53 seconds, and laboratory tests showed that her blood clotting factors were abnormally low. When given parenteral vitamin K her prothrombin time rapidly returned to normal (suggesting that she was taking a vitamin K antagonist of some kind). She strongly denied taking any anticoagulant drugs, but it was eventually discovered that she had been drinking large quantities of a herbal tea containing among other ingredients tonka beans, melilot and sweet woodruff, all of which might contain natural coumarins.[2]

Mechanism

Unknown. Melilot is known to contain natural coumarins, which can be turned into dicoumarol by moulds, see 'Coumarins + Herbal medicines; Miscellaneous', p.439.

Importance and management

Evidence appears to be limited to these isolated cases, which are not established. Many factors influence anticoagulant control, and therefore it is not possible to reliably ascribe a change in INR specifically to a drug interaction in a single case report without other supporting evidence. It may be better to advise patients to discuss the use of any herbal products they wish to try, and to increase monitoring if this is thought advisable. Cases of uneventful use should be reported, as they are as useful as possible cases of adverse effects.

1. Chiffoleau A, Huguenin H, Veyrac G, Argaiz V, Dupe D, Kayser M, Bourin M, Jolliet P. Interaction entre mélilot et acénocoumarol ? (mélilot-*ruscus aculeatus*). *Therapie* (2001) 56, 321–7.
2. Hogan RP. Hemorrhagic diathesis caused by drinking an herbal tea. *JAMA* (1983) 249, 2679–80.

Coumarins + Menthol

Two case reports describe a reduction in the effects of warfarin, which were attributed to the use of menthol cough lozenges.

Clinical evidence, mechanism, importance and management

A 57-year-old man taking **warfarin** 49 mg weekly with an INR in the range of 2.3 to 2.7 for the previous 3 weeks was found to have an INR of 1.45. He had been unwell with a flu-like illness over the past week, for which he had been taking about 6 *Halls* menthol cough lozenges (cough drops) per day for 4 days. He said he had not changed his diet or missed any warfarin doses. The **warfarin** dose was increased to 53 mg weekly for a week with an INR rise to 2.2, then the **warfarin** dose was decreased to 52 mg weekly with an INR of 3.06, so the previous dose of 49 mg weekly was resumed with an INR of 2.92.[1]

In a second case, a 46-year-old man taking warfarin 50 mg weekly had a reduction in his INR from 2.6 to 1.6 after taking 8 to 10 menthol cough drops daily, due to dry conditions in his work place. Despite increases in his warfarin dose over a period of 3 weeks his INR remained at 1.6. Five days after stopping the cough drops his INR increased, and he was subsequently re-stabilised on a warfarin dose of 40 mg weekly.[2]

Whether these cases represent an interaction with the menthol lozenges is uncertain. Further study is needed.

1. Kassebaum PJ, Shaw DL, Tomich DJ. Possible warfarin interaction with menthol cough drops. *Ann Pharmacother* (2005) 39, 365–7.
2. Coderre K, Faria C, Dyer E. Probable warfarin interaction with menthol cough drops. *Pharmacotherapy* (2010) 30, 110.

Coumarins + Meprobamate

The anticoagulant effects of warfarin are not altered to a clinically relevant extent by meprobamate.

Clinical evidence, mechanism, importance and management

In a study, 9 patients stabilised on **warfarin** were given meprobamate 400 mg four times daily for 2 weeks. Three patients had a small increase in their prothrombin time, five had a small decrease and one patients remained unaffected: all the changes were considered to fall within the range of variations normally seen in clinical practice.[1] Moreover, in a later placebo-controlled study in 17 patients taking **warfarin**, the 8 patients who were also given meprobamate 2.4 g daily for 4 weeks had only a small clinically unimportant reduction in their prothrombin time.[2] Similar results were found in another study.[3] No **warfarin** dose adjustments would therefore seem to be needed if meprobamate is added to established treatment with **warfarin**.

1. Udall JA. Warfarin therapy not influenced by meprobamate. A controlled study in nine men. *Curr Ther Res* (1970) 12, 724–8.
2. Gould L, Michael A, Fisch S, Gomprecht RF. Prothrombin levels maintained with meprobamate and warfarin. A controlled study. *JAMA* (1972) 220, 1460–2.
3. deCarolis PP, Gelfand ML. Effect of tranquilizers on prothrombin time response to coumarin. *J Clin Pharmacol* (1975) 15, 557.

Coumarins + Metformin

One patient had a notable increase in the effects of phenprocoumon when she stopped taking metformin for a short period, and there is some evidence that metformin increases the metabolism of phenprocoumon. Another patient developed metformin-induced lactic acidosis after warfarin-induced bleeding caused renal obstruction.

Clinical evidence

(a) Phenprocoumon

The Quick value of a 58-year-old woman stabilised on **metformin** 1.7 g twice daily and phenprocoumon 3 to 4.5 mg daily decreased from a range of 20 to 30% down to 0% when she stopped taking the **metformin** while on holiday. Despite the increased anticoagulant effect no signs of bleeding were observed, and she was eventually restabilised on the original doses of both drugs.[1] This case prompted a further observational study in 13 patients with type 2 diabetes. It was found that the 7 patients taking **metformin** 1.1 to 3 g daily were less well anticoagulated than those taking only 400 mg to 1 g of **metformin**, even though the mean phenprocoumon dose was slightly higher in those taking the higher **metformin** dose (2.57 mg daily versus 2.27 mg daily).[1] In another study, the half-life of phenprocoumon was reduced by about one-third (from 123 to 85 hours) by **metformin** 1.7 g daily.[1]

(b) Warfarin

An elderly woman taking warfarin 5 mg daily and **metformin** 1 g twice daily developed fatigue, epistaxis, haematuria, and gingival bleeding, with an INR of 16.9, which was treated with vitamin K. The following morning, she was given **metformin**, then she was found to have a retroperitoneal haematoma and bilateral perinephric blood with obstruction of both renal collecting systems. Over the next 8 hours, she developed progressive metabolic acidosis and suffered a cardiopulmonary arrest. Her serum **metformin** concentration was 7.3 micrograms/mL (therapeutic range 1 to 2 micrograms/mL). It was suggested that **metformin** accumulation occurred because of renal impairment caused by the site of renal bleeding secondary to the excessive effects of warfarin. This then resulted in metabolic acidosis.[2]

Mechanism

Metformin possibly reduces the effects of phenprocoumon by altering blood flow to the liver and interfering with enterohepatic circulation.

Importance and management

The information about an interaction with metformin and warfarin appears to be limited to these isolated reports, none of which definitively suggest that the metformin altered anticoagulant effects. In general no interaction would be expected between metformin and warfarin.

There is some evidence that a small increase in the dose of phenprocoumon might be necessary if metformin is given, but it seems likely that this can be managed with routine anticoagulant monitoring.

1. Ohnhaus EE, Berger W, Duckert F, Oesch F. The influence of dimethylbiguanide on phenprocoumon elimination and its mode of action. *Klin Wochenschr* (1983) 61, 851–8.
2. Schier JG, Hoffman RS, Nelson LS. Metformin-induced acidosis due to a warfarin adverse drug event. *Ann Pharmacother* (2003) 37, 1145.

Coumarins + Methylphenidate

Methylphenidate appears not to interact with ethyl biscoumacetate.

Clinical evidence, mechanism, importance and management

In one study in 4 healthy subjects, the half-life of a single dose of **ethyl biscoumacetate** was approximately doubled after they took methylphenidate 20 mg daily for 3 to 5 days.[1] However, a later double-blind, placebo-controlled study did not find an interaction: the half-life of **ethyl biscoumacetate** was not altered by methylphenidate

20 mg daily for 4 days in 4 healthy subjects, and was not different to that seen in 4 subjects given placebo.[2] The first authors suggested that methylphenidate inhibits the metabolism of **ethyl biscoumacetate**, but this seems unlikely given the findings of the second study.

Although the findings of these two studies are at odds with each other, the better-controlled study and the lack of reports of problems in the literature suggest that an interaction is unlikely. There does not seem to be any information about other coumarins. Nevertheless, the manufacturers recommend caution and suggest that patients taking coumarins should have their INR monitored if methylphenidate is started or stopped.[3,4] This seems over-cautious. Similarly, the manufacturer of **dexmethylphenidate**, the d-isomer of methylphenidate, notes the possibility of an interaction between methylphenidate and the coumarins.[5] Although they make no direct recommendation for the use of **dexmethylphenidate** with coumarins, until more is known, it may be prudent to follow the same precautions given for methylphenidate.

1. Garrettson LK, Perel JM, Dayton PG. Methylphenidate interaction with both anticonvulsants and ethyl biscoumacetate. *JAMA* (1969) 207, 2053–6.
2. Hague DE, Smith ME, Ryan JR, McMahon FG. The effect of methylphenidate and prolintane on the metabolism of ethyl biscoumacetate. *Clin Pharmacol Ther* (1971) 12, 259–62.
3. Ritalin (Methylphenidate hydrochloride). Novartis Pharmaceuticals UK Ltd. UK Summary of product characteristics, May 2011.
4. Ritalin (Methylphenidate hydrochloride). Novartis. US Prescribing information, December 2010.
5. Focalin XR (Dexmethylphenidate hydrochloride). Novartis. US Prescribing information, December 2013.

Coumarins + Metoclopramide

Metoclopramide caused a minor decrease in the AUC of phenprocoumon, without altering its anticoagulant effects. There is one case report of an interaction between phenprocoumon and metoclopramide.

Clinical evidence, mechanism, importance and management

An elderly woman taking **phenprocoumon** and metoclopramide developed a renal bleed and a low Quick time shortly after stopping metoclopramide.[1] This prompted a study in 12 healthy subjects, in which metoclopramide 30 mg daily for 10 days slightly reduced the AUC of a single dose of **phenprocoumon** given on day 4 by 16%, but no significant changes were seen in the anticoagulant effects.[2] The study findings suggests that no **phenprocoumon** dose adjustment would be expected to be necessary if these two drugs are given together. There seems to be no published information about a possible interaction with any other coumarins, and given the widespread use of both metoclopramide and **warfarin**, an interaction appears to be unlikely.

1. Bruhn HD, Kirch W, Ohnhaus EE. Arzneimittelinteraktionen. Metoclopramid-phenprocoumon. *Dtsch Med Wochenschr* (1987) 112, 742.
2. Wesermeyer D, Mönig H, Gaska T, Masuch S, Seiler KU, Huss H, Bruhn HD. Der Einfluß von Cisaprid und Metoclopramid auf die Bioverfügbarkeit von Phenprocoumon. *Hamostaseologie* (1991) 11, 95–102.

Coumarins + Metrifonate

Metrifonate did not interact with single-dose warfarin in one study.

Clinical evidence, mechanism, importance and management

A double-blind, placebo-controlled, crossover study in 14 healthy subjects found that metrifonate 50 mg daily for 8 days did not change the pharmacokinetics and pharmacodynamics of a single 25-mg dose of **warfarin** given on day 4. Plasma **warfarin** levels and prothrombin times remained unchanged.[1] This suggests that no **warfarin** dose adjustments are likely to be needed if these two drugs are used concurrently.

1. Heinig R, Kitchin N, Rolan P. Disposition of a single dose of warfarin in healthy individuals after pretreatment with metrifonate. *Clin Drug Invest* (1999) 18, 151–9.

Coumarins + Mirtazapine

In one study, mirtazapine slightly increased the INR in subjects given warfarin. One retrospective study found no increased risk of bleeding in patients taking mirtazapine and warfarin whereas another found an increased risk on concurrent use.

Clinical evidence, mechanism, importance and management

In a study in 16 healthy subjects stabilised on individual doses of **warfarin**,[1] mirtazapine 15 mg for 2 days then 30 mg daily for 5 days increased the mean INR from 1.6 to 1.8. This small increase was not considered clinically relevant.[1] In a retrospective study in patients taking warfarin, the concurrent use of mirtazapine was not associated with an increased risk of bleeding, when compared with patients taking warfarin alone.[2] However, another retrospective case-control study in patients taking **warfarin** who were given their first 30-day prescription for mirtazapine, found that concurrent use increased the risk of hospitalisation for gastrointestinal bleeding (adjusted odds ratio 1.75). However, no increased risk of gastrointestinal bleeding was found with subsequent prescriptions. Note that, in this study, mirtazapine was used as a non-interacting reference when studying the interaction of SSRIs and warfarin (see 'Coumarins and related drugs + SSRIs', p.469), and the authors suggested that the unexpected increased risk of bleeding might have been due to other confounding factors not controlled by the analysis.[3] Further study is therefore needed to clarify this reported effect. Based on the small change reported in the first study, the UK and US manufacturers state that a more pronounced effect cannot be excluded at higher doses of mirtazapine. For this reason, they very cautiously advise that the INR should be monitored if mirtazapine is given with warfarin.[4,5] However, there do not appear to be any published reports of alterations in INR with this combination.

1. Spaans E, van den Heuvel MW, Chin-Kon-Sung UG, Colbers EPH, Peeters PAM, Sitsen JMA . The effect of mirtazapine on steady state prothrombin time during warfarin therapy. *Pharmacol Toxicol* (2001) 89 (Suppl 1), 80.
2. Hauta-Aho M, Tirkkonen T, Vahlberg T, Laine K. The effect of drug interactions on bleeding risk associated with warfarin therapy in hospitalized patients. *Ann Med* (2009) 41, 61928.
3. Schelleman H, Brensinger CM, Bilker WB, Hennessy S. Antidepressant-warfarin interaction and associated gastrointestinal bleeding risk in a case-control study. *PLoS One* (2011) 6, e21447.
4. Zispin SolTab (Mirtazapine). Merck Sharp & Dohme Ltd. UK Summary of product characteristics, February 2015.
5. Remeron (Mirtazapine). Merck Sharp & Dohme Corp. US Prescribing information, January 2014.

Coumarins + Misoprostol

An isolated report describes a reduction in the anticoagulant effects of acenocoumarol, which was attributed to the use of misoprostol.

Clinical evidence, mechanism, importance and management

A 39-year-old woman taking **acenocoumarol**, celiprolol, triamterene, cyclothiazide, pravastatin and diosmin had a rise in her prothrombin levels from 0.3 to 1 within 8 days of starting to take diclofenac and misoprostol 400 micrograms daily. A day after these two drugs had been withdrawn her prothrombin level had fallen to 0.67, and after another 3 days to 0.32.[1] The reasons for this reaction are not known, but suspicion falls on the misoprostol because diclofenac, if and when it interacts with coumarins, increases rather than reduces their effects (see 'Coumarins + NSAIDs; Diclofenac', p.451). However, just why misoprostol should cause these changes is not clear.

This is an isolated case, complicated by the presence of a number of other drugs, which suggests that it is unlikely to be of general importance. More study is needed.

1. Martin MP, Jonville-Bera AP, Bera F, Caillard X, Autret E. Interaction entre le misoprostol et l'acénocoumarol. *Presse Med* (1995) 24, 195.

Coumarins + Modafinil

Modafinil does not alter the pharmacokinetics or effect of single-dose warfarin.

Clinical evidence, mechanism, importance and management

In a placebo-controlled study, when 14 healthy subjects taking modafinil 200 to 400 mg daily long-term were given a single 5-mg dose of warfarin, there were no changes in the pharmacokinetics of *R*- and *S*-warfarin. In addition, there was no change in clotting time.[1]

This study was conducted because, *in vitro*, modafinil was shown to be an inhibitor of the cytochrome P450 isoenzyme CYP2C9, and warfarin is an accepted probe substrate of this isoenzyme. It is well recognised that *in vitro* findings do not always predict what will happen *in vivo*, and the findings of the study show that modafinil is not a clinically relevant inhibitor of CYP2C9. Nevertheless, on the basis that this was a single-dose study, the authors suggest some caution.[1] The manufacturers recommend that prothrombin times should be monitored more frequently[2] particularly during the first 2 months of concurrent use and after changes in modafinil dose.[3] This is a cautious interpretation, and a pharmacokinetic interaction seems unlikely.

There appears to be no information regarding the possibility of an interaction between **armodafinil** (the *R*-isomer of modafinil) and warfarin. As modafinil did not affect the pharmacokinetics of a single dose of warfarin a pharmacokinetic interaction between armodafinil and warfarin seems unlikely. However, as the manufacturer of armodafinil states that a pharmacodynamic interaction cannot be ruled out, they advise more frequent monitoring of the prothrombin time or INR if armodafinil is given to patients taking warfarin.[4]

1. Robertson P, Hellriegel ET, Arora S, Nelson M. Effect of modafinil at steady state on the single-dose pharmacokinetic profile of warfarin in healthy volunteers. *J Clin Pharmacol* (2002) 42, 205–14.
2. Provigil (Modafinil). Cephalon, Inc. US Prescribing information, October 2010.
3. Provigil (Modafinil). Cephalon (UK) Ltd. UK Summary of product characteristics, August 2013.
4. Nuvigil (Armodafinil). Cephalon, Inc. US Prescribing information, June 2013.

Coumarins + Monoclonal antibodies

An isolated report describes an increase in the effects of warfarin in two women taking trastuzumab. An increase in INR was seen in a patient receiving a regimen containing rituximab. Bevacizumab and ranibizumab might theoretically increase the risk of bleeding in patients taking anticoagulants.

Clinical evidence

(a) Bevacizumab

The UK manufacturer notes that treatment with bevacizumab is associated with an increased risk of haemorrhage, especially tumour-associated haemorrhage, and they advise caution in patients already taking full-dose anticoagulants.[1] An analysis of data from 3 clinical studies found that in patients who developed a venous thrombosis while receiving bevacizumab, the use of **warfarin** did not appear to increase the risk of severe bleeding.[2] Further, a retrospective review of 12 patients taking **warfarin** who were subsequently started on bevacizumab, found that 2 of these patients developed asymptomatic haemorrhage compared with 7 of 244 patients treated with bevacizumab who were not receiving any anticoagulants. The authors concluded that anticoagulation did not lead to any major haemorrhages and is not a contraindication to starting bevacizumab.[3] In contrast, in a retrospective review of 282 patients treated with bevacizumab, 64 received concurrent anticoagulants and of these, 13 received **warfarin**. The rate of serious haemorrhage (grade 3 or above) was higher in those patients who received anticoagulants than in those who did not, but the type of anticoagulant (low-molecular weight heparin versus warfarin) was not associated with the risk of haemorrhage. Due to a small number of patients taking warfarin, it was not possible to assess the haemorrhage risk based on anticoagulant taken.[4]

A retrospective case series in 104 patients receiving *intravitreal* injections of either bevacizumab or **ranibizumab** (number of injections not specified), whilst also taking **warfarin**, found no bleeding complications.[5]

(b) Ranibizumab

A retrospective study of 50 patients undergoing intravitreal injections (149 injections) of ranibizumab 0.5 mg and instructed to continue with their normal anticoagulant dosing with coumarins (specific drugs not stated), found no serious bleeding complications. Minor subconjunctival bleeding occurred after 17.4% of injections and was associated with an average INR of 2.6, compared with 2.3 without bleeding.[6] Another retrospective case series, found no bleeding complications in 104 patients taking **warfarin** and also receiving intravitreal injections of either **bevacizumab** or ranibizumab (number of injections not specified).[5]

(c) Rituximab

A 49-year-old man receiving R-ESHAP (rituximab, etoposide, cisplatin, high-dose cytarabine, and methylprednisolone) for lymphoma, was started on **warfarin** for the secondary prevention of pulmonary embolism with deep venous thrombosis, after the first course. After warfarin dose titration, he received a second course of R-ESHAP and his INR increased (from 1 to 5.28). After further warfarin dose adjustments to stabilise his INR, he received a third course of R-ESHAP and his INR increased again (from 2.44 to 4.71) but was within the normal range (1.05, range 0.81 to 1.09) 5 days after the chemotherapy was completed.[7] Note that etoposide has been seen to increase the effects of warfarin (see 'Coumarins + Antineoplastics; Cytotoxic', p.403) and high doses of methylprednisolone increase the INR of patients taking coumarins (see 'Coumarins and related drugs + Corticosteroids or Corticotropin', p.419), therefore an interaction with rituximab is by no means established.

(d) Trastuzumab

Two women stabilised on **warfarin** developed nosebleeds after 10 and 8 doses of trastuzumab (one dose given each week), and were found to have INRs of 6 and 5.8, respectively.[8] However, the US manufacturer notes that, in an analysis of clinical study data, the rate of bleeding events was similar for patients receiving or not receiving trastuzumab, with or without anticoagulants.[9]

Mechanism

The reason for the increased INRs seen with trastuzumab or rituximab and warfarin is not known. Theoretically, bevacizumab and ranibizumab could have additive effects with anticoagulants because they are associated with an increased risk of haemorrhage, although in the case of ranibizumab the incidence in clinical studies was generally low and showed no consistent pattern.[10]

Importance and management

Evidence for an interaction between rituximab or trastuzumab and warfarin is limited to case reports and so their general relevance is uncertain, but bear them in mind in the event of an unexpected response to treatment. Note that factors related to illness, such as decreased appetite, can alter warfarin requirements. A pharmacodynamic interaction between bevacizumab or ranibizumab and warfarin with an increased risk of bleeding is theoretically possible, although some limited evidence suggests that this might not be the case. Nevertheless, it would seem prudent to monitor patients for signs of bleeding with concurrent use.

Note too, that from a disease perspective, when treating venous thromboembolic disease in patients with cancer, warfarin is generally inferior (higher risk of major bleeds and recurrent thrombosis) to low-molecular-weight heparins.[11]

1. Avastin (Bevacizumab). Roche Products Ltd. UK Summary of product characteristics, February 2014.
2. Leighl NB, Bennouna J, Yi J, Moore N, Hambleton J, Hurwitz H. Bleeding events in bevacizumab-treated cancer patients who received full-dose anticoagulation and remained on study. *Br J Cancer* (2011) 104, 413–8.
3. Nghiemphu P, Green RM, Pope WB, Lai A, Cloughesy TF. Safety of anticoagulation use and bevacizumab in patients with glioma. *Neuro Oncol* (2008) 10, 355–60.
4. Norden AD, Bartolomeo J, Tanaka S, Drappatz J, Ciampa AS, Doherty LM, LaFrankie DC, Ruland S, Quant EC, Beroukhim R, Wen PY. Safety of concurrent bevacizumab therapy and anticoagulation in glioma patients. *J Neurooncol* (2012) 106, 121–5.
5. Mason JO, Frederick PA, Neimkin MG, White MF, Feist RM, Thomley ML, Albert MA. Incidence of hemorrhagic complications after intravitreal bevacizumab (avastin) or ranibizumab (lucentis) injections on systemically anticoagulated patients. *Retina* (2010) 1386–9.
6. Loukopoulos V, Meier C, Gerding H. Hemorrhagic complications after intravitreal injections of ranibizumab in patients under coumarin-type anticoagulation. *Klin Monbl Augenheilkd* (2010) 227, 289–91.
7. Suzuki T, Koga H, Yamazaki S, Saeki H, Tanaka H, Nishimura M, Nakaseko C, Nakasa H, Nakamura H, Ariyoshi N, Kitada M. Probable interaction between warfarin and antitumor agents used in R-ESHAP chemotherapy. *Clin Ther* (2008) 30, 1155–9.
8. Nissenblatt MJ, Karp GI. Bleeding risk with trastuzumab (Herceptin) treatment. *JAMA* (1999) 282, 2299–2300.
9. Stewart SJ. Bleeding risk with trastuzumab (Herceptin) treatment. In reply. *JAMA* (1999) 282, 2300–1.
10. Lucentis (Ranibizumab). Novartis Pharmaceuticals UK Ltd. UK Summary of product characteristics, July 2013.
11. Baglin TP, Keeling DM, Watson HG, for the British Committee for Standards in Haematology. Guidelines on oral anticoagulation (warfarin): third edition – 2005 update. *Br J Haematol* (2005) 132, 277–85.

Coumarins + Moracizine

Moracizine did not alter the pharmacodynamics of single-dose warfarin, and had no clinically relevant effect on warfarin pharmacokinetics. However, an isolated report describes bleeding in a patient taking warfarin with moracizine.

Clinical evidence

In a study in 12 healthy subjects, moracizine 250 mg every 8 hours for 21 days caused little or no change in the pharmacokinetics of a single 25-mg dose of **warfarin** given on day 14. There was only a slight decrease in the **warfarin** elimination half-life, from 37.6 hours to 34.2 hours, and no change in prothrombin times.[1,2] The manufacturer also noted that clinical experience in 34 patients suggests that no significant changes in **warfarin** dose requirements are needed after moracizine is started.[1]

However, in one case report the prothrombin time of a woman taking **warfarin**, digoxin, captopril and prednisone rose from a range of 15 to 20 seconds up to 41 seconds within 4 days of starting moracizine 300 mg three times daily. She bled (haematemesis, haematuria), but responded rapidly to withdrawal of the **warfarin** and moracizine, and phytomenadione.[3]

Mechanism

Not understood.

Importance and management

Information appears to be limited to these reports. The study and early clinical experience suggest that no interaction occurs. The case of an increased effect seems to be an isolated report, and therefore unlikely to be of general importance.

1. Siddoway LA, Schwartz SL, Barbey JT, Woosley RL. Clinical pharmacokinetics of moricizine. *Am J Cardiol* (1990) 65, 21D–25D.
2. Benedek IH, King S-YP, Powell RJ, Agra AM, Schary WL, Pieniaszek HJ. Effect of moricizine on the pharmacokinetics and pharmacodynamics of warfarin in healthy volunteers. *J Clin Pharmacol* (1992) 32, 558–63.
3. Serpa MD, Cossolias J, McGreevy MJ. Moricizine-warfarin: a possible interaction. *Ann Pharmacother* (1992) 26, 127.

Coumarins + Nefazodone or Trazodone

A handful of case reports describe a moderate reduction in the anticoagulant effects of warfarin caused by trazodone, and another case report describes a rise in INR. In one study, nefazodone slightly decreased the level of *S*-warfarin and did not alter the prothrombin ratio.

Clinical evidence

(a) Nefazodone

In one study, 17 healthy subjects given **warfarin** to achieve a prothrombin ratio of 1.2 to 1.5 for 14 days were then given nefazodone 200 mg or placebo every 12 hours for a further 7 days. The only pharmacokinetic changes were a 12% decrease in the AUC and maximum serum levels of *S*-warfarin. No changes occurred in the prothrombin ratios.[1]

(b) Trazodone

In an early case series, a patient stabilised on **warfarin** was given trazodone 75 mg daily for 8 days without any significant changes in the prothrombin time. Similarly, the same dose of trazodone had no obvious effect on the prothrombin time of a patient who had recently started taking **phenprocoumon** or another patient who had recently started taking **ethyl biscoumacetate**.[2]

However, in another report, a woman needed a small increase in her **warfarin** dose, from 6.4 mg daily to 7.5 mg daily, when she was given trazodone 300 mg daily, in order to maintain her prothrombin time at 20 seconds. Her **warfarin** requirements fell when the trazodone was later withdrawn.[3] A retrospective review from June 1998 to June 1999 identified 75 patients taking both trazodone and **warfarin**. Of the patients who had started trazodone during this period (number not stated), at least 3 had a probable interaction. One had a decrease in INR from 2.79 to 1.07 six days after starting trazodone, and needed a 25% increase in the dose of **warfarin**. Another patient had an increase in INR when he ran out of trazodone, and a decrease in INR on restarting the trazodone. A third required a 39% increase in **warfarin** dose after starting trazodone.[4] Conversely, there is a report of a rise in INR from between 2 and 3 up to 6, without bleeding complications, that occurred in a patient 2 weeks after trazodone 50 mg daily and fish oil 2 g daily were started.[5] The manufacturer in the US notes that there have been reports of both increased and decreased prothrombin times in patients taking warfarin with trazodone.[6]

Mechanism

Unknown.

Importance and management

The limited evidence available suggests that some patients might require a moderate increase in warfarin dose when starting trazodone, and, conversely, there is one possible case of an increase in INR. Therefore, it might be prudent to monitor the INR in all patients taking warfarin if trazodone is started or stopped, adjusting the warfarin dose if necessary. The clinical relevance of the 12% decrease in *S*-warfarin levels see with nefazodone is likely to be minor. The authors of the study concluded that no change in warfarin dose is likely to be required on concurrent use.[1]

1. Salazar DE, Dockens RC, Milbrath RL, Raymond RH, Fulmor IE, Chaikin PC, Uderman HD. Pharmacokinetic and pharmacodynamic evaluation of warfarin and nefazodone coadministration in healthy subjects. *J Clin Pharmacol* (1995) 35, 730–8.
2. Cozzolino G, Pazzaglia I, De Gaetano V, Macri M. Clinical investigation on the possible interaction between anti-coagulants and a new psychotropic drug (Trazodone). *Clin Eur* (1972) 11, 593–607.
3. Hardy J-L, Sirois A. Reduction of prothrombin and partial thromboplastin times with trazodone. *Can Med Assoc J* (1986) 135, 1372.
4. Small NL, Giamonna KA. Interaction between warfarin and trazodone. *Ann Pharmacother* (2000) 34, 734–6.
5. Jalili M, Dehpour AR. Extremely prolonged INR associated with warfarin in combination with both trazodone and omega-3 fatty acids. *Arch Med Res* (2007) 38, 901–4.
6. Desyrel (Trazodone hydrochloride). Bristol-Myers Squibb Company. US Prescribing information, February 2009.

Coumarins and related drugs + Nicotinic acid (Niacin)

Nicotinic acid might affect the anticoagulant response to coumarins and indanediones.

Clinical evidence, mechanism, importance and management

In a case report,[1] a 69-year-old patient stable whilst taking **warfarin** 2.5 mg daily for 18 months was given extended-release nicotinic acid 500 mg daily, with no subsequent change in her INR. However, one week after her nicotinic acid dose was increased to 1 g daily, her INR increased to greater than 12.3. Nicotinic acid was stopped and by day 2 her INR had reduced to 4.8. This appears to be the only published case report of an interaction; however, the US manufacturer states that nicotinic acid has been associated with a small (4%) increase in the prothrombin time, which could be additive with the effects of anticoagulants, such as the coumarins and indanediones. Nicotinic acid has also been associated with an 11% reduction in the platelet count. The manufacturer therefore advises caution on the concurrent use of anticoagulants and nicotinic acid, and states that the prothrombin time and platelet counts should be monitored.[2]

1. Christopher A. Critically elevated INR in a patient on warfarin after increase in extended-release niacin dose. *Ann Pharmacother* (2011) 45, e58.
2. Niaspan (Niacin). Abbott Laboratories. US Prescribing information, April 2015.

Coumarins + Nitazoxanide

Nitazoxanide does not alter the pharmacokinetics or pharmacodynamics of warfarin.

Clinical evidence, mechanism, importance and management

In a phase I crossover study in healthy subjects, nitazoxanide 500 mg twice daily for 6 days did not alter the pharmacokinetics of a single 25-mg dose of **warfarin** given on day 1.The pharmacodynamics of **warfarin** were similarly unaffected.[1] The US manufacturer warns that the nitazoxanide metabolite, tizoxanide, is highly protein-bound and advises caution with other highly protein-bound drugs with a narrow therapeutic index (they name **warfarin**) as competition for binding sites might occur.[2] However, protein-binding displacement is considered to only play a minor role in coumarin drug interactions (see *Anticoagulant interactions*, under 'Anticoagulants', p.371), and the results of the study suggest that no interaction occurs.

1. Vets E, Rossignol JF, Jackson AS. Effects of nitazoxanide on pharmacokinetics and pharmacodynamics of a single dose of warfarin. *Am J Health-Syst Pharm* (2009) 66, 838–42.
2. Alinia (Nitazoxanide). Romark Laboratories, LC. US Prescribing information, October 2007.

Coumarins + NNRTIs

Two reports suggest that warfarin requirements are markedly increased by nevirapine. There is one case report of an unusually low warfarin dose requirement in a patient taking an efavirenz-based regimen; however, a single case report with acenocoumarol and efavirenz found an increased acenocoumarol dose requirement. The effect of other NNRTIs is unclear.

Clinical evidence

(a) Efavirenz

A woman taking efavirenz, didanosine and lamivudine was started on **warfarin** for a deep vein thrombosis. After 12 days she was discharged with an INR between 2 and 3 on a mean daily dose of warfarin of 5 mg. About one week later her INR was 2.7, but then 3 days later she had blood in the urine and an INR of 7. She was eventually stabilised on a much lower mean dose of warfarin of 1.25 mg daily.[1] In another case report, a 51-year-old man receiving **acenocoumarol** 4.2 mg daily required a dose increase to 6.7 mg daily in order to achieve a target INR of between 2.5 and 3.5 but this could not be maintained and his antiretroviral regimen was changed.[2]

(b) Etravirine

In a study, 12 healthy subjects were given a single 10-mg dose of **warfarin** on day one and day 14 of a 14-day course of etravirine 200 mg twice daily. Etravirine increased the ratio of the AUC of *S*-warfarin to 7-hydroxy-*S*-warfarin by 63%.[3]

(c) Nevirapine

A man taking **warfarin** 2.5 mg daily (INR 2.1 to 2.4) needed a doubled **warfarin** dose when his treatment with zidovudine and didanosine was replaced by stavudine, lamivudine and nevirapine. A few days later, when his treatment was again changed to stavudine, lamivudine and saquinavir, his original **warfarin** dose was found to be adequate. Another patient was resistant to doses of **warfarin** of up to 17 mg daily while taking zidovudine, lamivudine and nevirapine, but he responded to **warfarin** 5 mg daily when the nevirapine was withdrawn. The warfarin dose had to be raised to 12 mg daily when nevirapine was restarted. Yet another patient showed resistance to **warfarin** while taking nevirapine.[4] Similarly, in another report, a patient taking lamivudine 150 mg twice daily, zidovudine 300 mg twice daily and nevirapine 200 mg twice daily required a high **warfarin** dose of 20 mg daily to maintain a therapeutic INR. When his antiretroviral regimen was changed to nelfinavir, didanosine and tenofovir, a reduction in his warfarin dose to 12.5 mg daily was required.[5] Note that nelfinavir may also interact with warfarin, see 'Coumarins + HIV-protease inhibitors', p.439.

Mechanism

The finding of greatly increased warfarin requirements with nevirapine was not predicted from *in vitro* studies,[6] in which nevirapine did not inhibit CYP2C9, by which the more potent *S*-warfarin is metabolised, and had mixed (induction and inhibition) effects on CYP3A4, which partly metabolises *R*-warfarin. Although induction of CYP3A4 might reduce *R*-warfarin concentrations, the clinical effect of this would be expected to be modest.

In vitro efavirenz inhibits CYP2C9 and induces CYP3A4,[7] and its effects on the clinical pharmacokinetics of warfarin are unknown. In one case, the authors suggested that efavirenz inhibited warfarin metabolism,[1] but it is unclear why this became suddenly apparent 3 weeks after starting concurrent use. The authors of the case involving acenocoumarol suggest that efavirenz induces acenocoumarol metabolism, resulting in the need for higher anticoagulant doses.[2]

Importance and management

Information on **nevirapine** seems to be limited to these four cases, but it would be prudent to monitor prothrombin times and INRs in any patient if warfarin and nevirapine are used concurrently, being alert for the need to increase the warfarin dose (possibly twofold). Information about other coumarins seems to be lacking, but if the suggested mechanism is correct, all coumarins would be expected to interact to some extent.

Increased monitoring on the concurrent use of **efavirenz** and warfarin or acenocoumarol would also seem advisable, but note; the only case available involving warfarin appears to suggest a decreased warfarin requirement, while the case involving acenocoumarol suggests an increased acenocoumarol requirement. Until more is known, it would seem prudent to monitor all coumarins and adjust the dose accordingly.

Etravirine has weak effects on both CYP3A4 and CYP2C9, the isoenzymes involved in the metabolism of warfarin and could therefore have some modest effects on warfarin metabolism. Until the clinical relevance of this is known it might be prudent to be alert for increased warfarin effects.

Delavirdine inhibits CYP3A4, but the effect of this alone on warfarin concentrations is probably modest. Nevertheless, the US manufacturer of delavirdine advises monitoring the INR of patients also given warfarin.[8]

1. Bonora S, Lanzafame M, D'Avolio A, Trentini L, Lattuada E, Concia E, Di Perri G. Drug interactions between warfarin and efavirenz or lopinavir-ritonavir in clinical treatment. *Clin Infect Dis* (2008) 46, 146–7.
2. Welzen MEB, van den Berk GEL, Hamers RL, Burger DM. Interaction between antiretroviral drugs and acenocoumarol. *Antivir Ther* (2011) 16, 249–52.
3. Schöller-Gyüre M, Kakuda TN, Stevens T, Aharchi F, De Smedt G, Peeters M, Hoetelmans RMW. Effect of etravirine on cytochrome P450 isoenzymes assessed by the Cooperstown 5+1 cocktail. 48th Annual ICAAC/ IDSA 46th General Meeting, Washington DC, 25th–28th October 2008.
4. Dionisio D, Mininni S, Bartolozzi D, Esperti F, Vivarelli A, Leoncini F. Need for increased dose of warfarin in HIV patients taking nevirapine. *AIDS* (2001) 15, 277–8.
5. Fulco PP, Zingone MM, Higginson RT. Possible antiretroviral therapy-warfarin drug interaction. *Pharmacotherapy* (2008) 28, 945–9.
6. Viramune (Nevirapine). Boehringer Ingelheim Pharmaceuticals, Inc. US Prescribing information, November 2011.
7. Sustiva (Efavirenz). Bristol-Myers Squibb Company. US Prescribing information, August 2012.
8. Rescriptor (Delavirdine mesylate). Pfizer Inc. US prescribing information, May 2008.

Coumarins + Noscapine

Noscapine appears to increase the INR in response to warfarin, and bleeding has been seen. Other coumarins might interact similarly.

Clinical evidence

A number of letters[1-3] describe cases of increased INRs, which have been attributed to an interaction between noscapine and warfarin; in total 16 cases appear to have been described, with the highest INR being greater than 8. Bleeding appears to have been reported in only one case.[2] One of these reports describes 4 patients who developed increased INRs (of 4.4 to greater than 6) after the addition of noscapine 50 mg three times daily. No bleeding events occurred in any of the 4 patients, and all were restabilised on their original dose of warfarin after the noscapine was stopped.[1]

Mechanism

An *in vitro* study[4] and a phenotyping study in healthy subjects,[5] suggest that noscapine might cause clinically relevant inhibition of CYP2C9, which is involved in the metabolism of warfarin. Noscapine[5] might also cause clinically relevant inhibition of CYP2C19, and to a lesser extent,[4] CYP3A4; both these enzymes are also involved in the metabolism of warfarin. It therefore appears that concurrent use decreases warfarin metabolism, resulting in increased warfarin effects.

Importance and management

Evidence appears to be limited to case reports and *in vitro* study; however, an interaction appears to be established, although ideally a controlled pharmacokinetic study is needed to confirm this. Many commentators suggest that the concurrent use of noscapine and warfarin should be avoided, and where possible, this seems prudent. If concurrent use is considered desirable, it would seem prudent to increase the frequency of INR monitoring. Increased INRs have been reported as early as 3 days after concurrent use.

Information about other coumarins appears to be lacking, but all are metabolised, at least in part, by CYP2C9 and it therefore seems possible that they might interact in the same way as warfarin.

1. Scordo MG, Melhus H, Stjernberg E, Edvardsson AM, Wadelius M. Warfarin-noscapine interaction: a series of four case reports. *Ann Pharmacother* (2008) 42, 448–50.
2. Ohlsson S, Holm L, Myrberg O, Sundström A, Yue Q-Y. Noscapine may increase the effect of warfarin. *Br J Clin Pharmacol* (2007) 65, 277–8.
3. Mhyr K. Noskapin og warfarin – en potensielt farlig interaksjon. *Tidsskr Nor Laegeforen* (2009) 129, 540.
4. Fang Z-Z, Zhang Y-Y, Ge G-B, Huo H, Liang S-C, Yang L. Time dependent inhibition (TDI) of CYP3A4 and CYP2C9 by noscapine potentially explains clinical noscapine-warfarin interaction. *Br J Clin Pharmacol* (2010) 69, 193–9.
5. Rosenborg S, Stenberg M, Otto S, Östervall J, Masquelier M, Yue Q-Y, Bertilsson L, Eliasson E. Clinically significant CYP2C inhibition by noscapine but not by glucosamine. *Clin Pharmacol Ther* (2010) 88, 343–46.

Coumarins and related drugs + NSAIDs

The concurrent use of NSAIDs and coumarin anticoagulants increases the risk of gastrointestinal haemorrhage and, to a lesser extent, non-gastrointestinal bleeds. Care is needed with the combination. Some individual NSAIDs also alter the pharmacokinetics and/or pharmacodynamics of warfarin, and these effects are covered in specific monographs.

Clinical evidence

(a) Bleeding

In a retrospective cohort study of patients hospitalised for peptic ulcer disease, the current use of both oral anticoagulants and NSAIDs was associated with a large increase in the risk of haemorrhagic peptic ulcer disease of 12.7 (95% confidence interval 6.3 to 25.7). This was much higher than the risk associated with NSAIDs alone or oral anticoagulants alone (both about a 4-fold increased risk). In this study, about 10% of the hospitalisations for haemorrhagic peptic ulcer disease in patients taking anticoagulants were attributed to the concurrent use of NSAIDs. The oral anticoagulants used were the coumarins **warfarin**, **phenprocoumon**, and **acenocoumarol**, and the indanediones **phenindione** and **anisindione**. The NSAIDs used were non-acetylated salicylates, **ibuprofen**, **indometacin**, **sulindac**, **naproxen**, **fenoprofen**, **piroxicam**, **tolmetin**, and **meclofenamate**.[1]

Several case-control studies have assessed the risk of bleeding in patients taking **warfarin** and NSAIDs. In one, patients taking **warfarin** who were admitted to hospital with upper gastrointestinal haemorrhage were considerably more likely to be taking non-selective NSAIDs (odds ratio 1.9). A similar increased risk was seen with the coxibs **celecoxib** and **rofecoxib**.[2] In another study, non-selective NSAID and coxib use was associated with an increased risk of bleeding of all diagnoses (odds ratio 2.57 and 3.10, respectively), but when analysed according to bleeding diagnosis, only NSAIDs were associated with an increased risk of lower gastrointestinal bleeding to a statistically significant degree (odds ratio 3.96).[3] Further, in a large population-based, retrospective case control-study using records from the UK General Practice Research Database from 2000 to 2005, the use of **warfarin** with NSAIDs was associated with an increased risk of gastrointestinal bleeding when compared with either drug alone (rate ratio of 4.79 for concurrent use compared with 1.94 for warfarin and 1.78 for NSAIDs). A very similar increased risk (rate ratio 4.62) was seen with the coxibs, **celecoxib** and **rofecoxib**.[4] Consider also, 'Coumarins and related drugs + NSAIDs; Coxibs', p.450. The most commonly used NSAIDs were **diclofenac**, **ibuprofen**, and **naproxen**, and the full list of NSAIDs considered was **aclofenac** (sic), **dexibuprofen**, **dexketoprofen**, **diclofenac**, **diflunisal**, **etodolac**, **fenoprofen**, **ibuprofen**, **indomethacin**, **ketoprofen**, **ketorolac**, **lornoxicam**, **mefenamic acid**, **meloxicam**, **nabumetone**, **naproxen**, **nimesulide**, **piroxicam**, **sulindac**, **tenoxicam**, **tolfenamic acid**, and **tiaprofenic acid**.[3,4] A retrospective case-control study in 98 patients receiving warfarin and started on a NSAID (**aceclofenac**, **celecoxib**, **fenoprofen**, **ibuprofen**, **meloxicam**, **naproxen**, **rofecoxib**, or **zaltoprofen**), found that the INR was increased by at least 15% in 39.8% of the patients. The only NSAID associated with a statistically significant increased risk was **meloxicam** (odds ratio 4.88).[5] Consider also, 'Coumarins + NSAIDs; Oxicam derivatives', p.454.

In another case-control study, the use of NSAIDs with the coumarins **acenocoumarol** or **phenprocoumon** was associated with an increased risk of hospitalisation for gastrointestinal bleeding (odds ratio 4.6) and, to a lesser extent, non-gastrointestinal bleeding (odds ratio 1.7).[6] Similarly, a case-control study[7] in 2 553 **phenprocoumon** users found that the risk of hospitalisation due to bleeding (including gastrointestinal bleeding) was increased with NSAID use, with the following specific odds ratios: **diclofenac** OR 1.60, **ibuprofen** OR 1.63, **ketoprofen** OR 8.06, and **naproxen** OR 4.29. Likewise, in a questionnaire-based study, 12.2% of patients taking **acenocoumarol** or **phenprocoumon** who had a bleeding complication were found to have used an NSAID in the previous month compared with only 2.5% of coumarin users who did not have a bleed (an increased relative risk of bleeding of 5.8).[8]

In contrast, in a large analysis of claims data, use of NSAIDs (unnamed) with **warfarin** was, unexpectedly, not associated with an increased risk of haemorrhage.[9]

(b) Pharmacokinetic interactions

In one cohort study in patients taking **acenocoumarol** or **phenprocoumon**, the use of NSAIDs that are known substrates of CYP2C9 (**celecoxib**, **diclofenac**, **flurbiprofen**, **ibuprofen**, **indometacin**, **ketoprofen**, **meloxicam**, **naproxen**, and **piroxicam**) increased the risk of over-anticoagulation (INR greater than 6) to varying degrees depending on the patient's CYP2C9 metaboliser status. In patients who were CYP2C9 extensive metabolisers (that is, those with normal CYP2C9 activity), the relative risk was 1.69. However, the relative risk was greater (2.28) in patients who were CYP2C9 intermediate metabolisers (those with reduced activity of this isoenzyme), and particularly high (10.8) in those who were CYP2C9 poor metabolisers (those with little or no activity of this isoenzyme).[10] In another smaller retrospective cohort study, giving the CYP2C9 substrates **diclofenac**, **naproxen**, or **ibuprofen** increased the INR above the therapeutic range in 52 of 112 patients taking **acenocoumarol**. However, in this study CYP2C9 genotype did not influence the interaction between **acenocoumarol** and **diclofenac**, **naproxen**, and **ibuprofen**.[11] In a prospective study in 100 patients started on **acenocoumarol** after total hip replacement surgery, those who were CYP2C9 intermediate or poor metabolisers were at a higher risk of increased INRs (over 4.9) following concurrent use of an NSAID. Of the 35 patients who were CYP2C9 intermediate or poor metabolisers, 20 were also taking NSAIDs and 7 had an INR of greater than 4.9. The 65 patients who were CYP2C9 extensive metabolisers had a similar mean INR irrespective of whether they were taking NSAIDs.[12]

For more general information about the genetic variations in cytochrome P450 isoenzymes, see 'Genetic factors in drug metabolism', p.8.

(c) Other effects

In a prospective study, the concurrent use of musculoskeletal drugs (said to be mainly NSAIDs, with none specified) was associated with an apparent risk of INR instability (odds ratio 1.68) in 125 hospitalised patients starting **acenocoumarol**.[13] Instability was defined as not having two consecutive INRs within the range of 2 to 3. However, most of the patients defined as unstable had INRs below the therapeutic range, and it was suggested that this might have just reflected conservative dosing of the anticoagulant in patients already taking NSAIDs because of the possible interaction. This would result in these patients taking longer to reach the therapeutic range, and is not therefore an interaction as such.

Mechanism

NSAIDs, to a greater or lesser extent irritate the stomach lining, which can result in gastrointestinal bleeding, which will be more severe in anticoagulated patients. Many also have antiplatelet activity, which can prolong bleeding times, and contribute to the increased bleeding risk.

Phenylbutazone and related drugs (see 'Coumarins and related drugs + NSAIDs; Phenylbutazone and related drugs', p.455) are well known to inhibit the metabolism of warfarin by CYP2C9. *S*-phenprocoumon and *S*-acenocoumarol are also substrates for CYP2C9. Few other NSAIDs are known CYP2C9 inhibitors; however; many are CYP2C9 substrates. People who are CYP2C9 poor metabolisers (that is, those with little or no activity of this isoenzyme (about 5 to 11% of Caucasians)) have a lower metabolising capacity for warfarin, acenocoumarol, and phenprocoumon and are therefore likely to require much lower maintenance doses. Some believe that concurrent use of an NSAID that is a CYP2C9 substrate might result in reduced metabolism of these anticoagulants, however, note that interactions by substrate competition are rarely clinically relevant.

Importance and management

The available data indicate that the risk of bleeding is increased if NSAIDs are used in patients taking coumarin or **indanedione** anticoagulants. For this reason, it would be prudent to avoid the unnecessary concurrent use of NSAIDs when simple analgesics are adequate. When concurrent use is necessary, extra caution would be appropriate. It would be advisable to avoid NSAIDs with higher risks of inducing gastrointestinal bleeds, and possibly also to consider prophylactic mucosal protection. Note that patients at higher risk of NSAID-induced gastrointestinal bleeding and those prone to warfarin-related bleeding are likely to be at increased risk. Further study is required to ascertain whether people who are CYP2C9 intermediate or poor metabolisers are at increased risk of an interaction when given NSAIDs.

1. Shorr RI, Ray WA, Daugherty JR, Griffin MR. Concurrent use of nonsteroidal anti-inflammatory drugs and oral anticoagulants places elderly persons at high risk for hemorrhagic peptic ulcer disease. *Arch Intern Med* (1993) 153, 1665–70.
2. Battistella M, Mamdami MM, Juurlink DN, Rabeneck L, Laupacis A. Risk of upper gastrointestinal hemorrhage in warfarin users treated with nonselective NSAIDs or COX-2 inhibitors. *Arch Intern Med* (2005) 165, 189–92.
3. Hauta-Aho M, Tirkkonen T, Vahlberg T, Laine K. The effect of drug interactions on bleeding risk associated with warfarin therapy in hospitalized patients. *Ann Med* (2009) 41, 619–28.
4. Delaney JA, Opatrny L, Brophy JM, Suissa S. Drug–drug interactions between antithrombotic medications and the risk of gastrointestinal bleeding. *CMAJ* (2007) 177, 347–51.
5. Choi KH, Kim AJ, Son IJ, Kim KH, Kim KB, Ahn H, Lee EB. Risk factors of drug interaction between warfarin and nonsteroidal anti-inflammatory drugs in practical setting. *J Korean Med Sci* (2010) 25, 337–41.
6. Schalekamp T, Klungel OH, Souverein PC, de Boer A. Increased bleeding risk with concurrent use of selective serotonin reuptake inhibitors and coumarins. *Arch Intern Med* (2008) 168, 180–5.

7. Jobski K, Behr S, Garbe E. Drug interactions with phenprocoumon and the risk of serious haemorrhage: a nested case-control study in a large population-based German database. *Eur J Clin Pharmacol* (2011) 67, 941–51.
8. Knijff-Dutmer EAJ, Schut GA, van de Laar MAFJ. Concomitant coumarin-NSAID therapy and risk for bleeding. *Ann Pharmacother* (2003) 37, 12–16.
9. Zhang K, Young C, Berger J. Administrative claims analysis of the relationship between warfarin use and risk of hemorrhage including drug-drug and drug-disease interactions. *J Manag Care Pharm* (2006) 12, 640–8.
10. Visser LE, van Schaik RH, van Vliet M, Trienekens PH, De Smet PAGM, Vulto AG, Hofman A, van Duijn CM, Stricker BHC. Allelic variants of cytochrome P450 2C9 modify the interaction between nonsteroidal anti-inflammatory drugs and coumarin anticoagulants. *Clin Pharmacol Ther* (2005) 77, 479–85.
11. van Dijk KN, Plat AW, van Dijk AAC, Piersma-Wichers M, de Vries-Bots AMB, Slomp J, de Jong-van den Berg LTW, Brouwers JRBJ. Potential interaction between acenocoumarol and diclofenac, naproxen and ibuprofen and role of CYP2C9 genotype. *Thromb Haemost* (2004) 91, 95–101.
12. Beinema MJ, de Jong PH, Salden HJM, van Wijnen M, van der Meer J, Brouwers JRBJ. The influence of NSAIDs on coumarin sensitivity in patients with CYP2C9 polymorphism after total hip replacement surgery. *Mol Diagn Ther* (2007) 11, 123–8.
13. Van den Bemt PMLA, Joosten P, Risselada A, van den Boogaart MHA, Egberts ACG, Brouwers JRBJ. Stabilization of oral anticoagulant therapy in hospitalized patients and characteristics associated with lack of stabilization. *Pharm World Sci* (2000) 22, 147–51.

Coumarins + NSAIDs; Benzydamine

Oral benzydamine did not alter the anticoagulant effects of phenprocoumon. Topical formulations of benzydamine (mouthwash and spray) would not be expected to interact.

Clinical evidence, mechanism, importance and management

In 10 patients stabilised on **phenprocoumon**, the anticoagulant response was not significantly changed by benzydamine 50 mg three times daily for 2 weeks, although there was some evidence of an increase in blood levels of the anticoagulant.[1] This suggests that no **phenprocoumon** dose adjustments are likely to be needed on concurrent use. Note that benzydamine tends to be used as a topical mouthwash or spray. Neither of these topical formulations would be expected to interact.

1. Duckert F, Widmer LK, Madar G. Gleichzeitige Behandlung mit oralen Antikoagulantien und Benzydamin. *Schweiz Med Wochenschr* (1974) 104, 1069–71.

Coumarins + NSAIDs; Clonixin

Clonixin lysine did not appear to alter the anticoagulant effects of phenprocoumon in a pharmacological study. However, note that all NSAIDs increase the risk of bleeding, and an increased risk is seen when they are combined with anticoagulants.

Clinical evidence, mechanism, importance and management

In a randomised, crossover study in 12 healthy men, the pharmacokinetics and the anticoagulant activity of a single 18-mg dose of **phenprocoumon** were unchanged by clonixin lysine 125 mg five times daily, given for 3 days before and for 13 days after the **phenprocoumon**.[1]

On the basis of this study, no adjustment in coumarin dose would be expected to be needed when clonixin is used. However, care is still needed with every NSAID, because, to a greater or lesser extent, they irritate the stomach lining, which can result in gastrointestinal bleeding, which will be more severe in anticoagulated patients. Consider also, 'Coumarins and related drugs + NSAIDs', p.449.

1. Russmann S, Dilger K, Trenk D, Nagyivanyi P, Jänchen E. Effect of lysine clonixinate on the pharmacokinetics and anticoagulant activity of phenprocoumon. *Arzneimittelforschung* (2001) 51, 891–895.

Coumarins and related drugs + NSAIDs; Coxibs

Etoricoxib, lumiracoxib and rofecoxib cause a slight increase in the INR in response to warfarin, whereas celecoxib and parecoxib have no effect. However, raised INRs accompanied by bleeding, particularly in the elderly, have been attributed to the use of warfarin and celecoxib or rofecoxib. In addition, the use of celecoxib or rofecoxib is associated with an increased risk of hospitalisation for upper gastrointestinal haemorrhage, which was of a similar magnitude to that seen with non-selective NSAIDs.

Clinical evidence

(a) Celecoxib

In a placebo-controlled study, **warfarin** 2 to 5 mg daily was given to 24 healthy subjects to maintain a stable prothrombin time of 1.2 to 1.7 times their pretreatment values for at least 3 consecutive days. They were then given placebo or celecoxib 200 mg twice daily for a week. It was found that the steady-state pharmacokinetics of both *S*- and *R*-warfarin and the prothrombin times were unchanged by the presence of the celecoxib.[1]

Similarly, in a crossover study in 15 osteoarthritic patients stabilised on **warfarin**, celecoxib 200 mg daily for 5 weeks did not alter the mean INR when compared with codeine (see 'Coumarins + Opioids; Codeine', p.457). One patient had an INR of 4.9 when taking celecoxib.[2] However, in 16 patients stabilised on **warfarin** and given celecoxib 200 mg daily for 3 weeks, the INR increased by 13%, 6% and 5% at week one, 2 and 3, respectively, the change at week one being statistically significant.[3] Furthermore, in another analysis of 28 patients taking **warfarin** who were prescribed either celecoxib or rofecoxib, 13 had increases in their INR, of which 7 (5 taking celecoxib) had no other explanation for the INR increase other than the use of the coxib. The average increase in INR in these 7 patients was 1.5, and one patient had bruising and epistaxis and required treatment with phytomenadione.[4]

Case reports of an interaction have also been published.[5-10] In one report, an 88-year-old woman stabilised on **warfarin** had a rise in her INR from 3.1 to 5.8 when celecoxib 200 mg daily was substituted for diclofenac. After several **warfarin** dose adjustments she was later restabilised on a 25% lower **warfarin** dose.[5] There is a similar case report of a 77-year old patient who required a 10% decrease in her **warfarin** dose to maintain her target INR when celecoxib 100 mg twice daily was also given.[8] In another case, the patient was shown to have a variant of CYP2C9, with lower metabolising capacity, which was thought to explain the interaction,[10] see also *Mechanism*, below. The manufacturers also noted that bleeding events have been reported with this combination, predominantly in the elderly, which led to a change in the product labelling.[11] A 2001 report from the Australian Adverse Drug Reactions Advisory Committee noted they had received 21 reports of increases in the INR in patients taking **warfarin** with celecoxib since the introduction of celecoxib in October 1999. Six of these cases reported bleeding complications. In addition, they had 11 cases of bleeding in patients taking the combination, with no reference to INR, or with an unchanged INR in one case.[12] A review of adverse effects of coxibs mentioned 2 patients taking **warfarin** who had increases in their INR while taking celecoxib.[13]

Moreover, in a case-control study, patients taking **warfarin** and admitted to hospital with upper gastrointestinal haemorrhage were significantly more likely to be also taking celecoxib (odds ratio 1.7). A similar increased risk was seen with rofecoxib and non-selective NSAIDs[14] (see 'Coumarins and related drugs + NSAIDs', p.449). The same findings were reported in another study for celecoxib and rofecoxib considered together.[15] In a retrospective analysis, the relative risk of all bleeding complications was slightly increased (1.34) in 123 patients taking celecoxib with **warfarin** when compared with 1022 control patients taking **warfarin** alone.[16]

(b) Etoricoxib

In a controlled study in 14 healthy subjects stabilised on **warfarin**, etoricoxib 120 mg daily for 21 days increased the INR by about 13%. There was no change in the pharmacokinetics of *S*-warfarin, and the AUC of *R*-warfarin showed a minor 10% increase.[17]

(c) Lumiracoxib

The manufacturer noted that in healthy subjects stabilised on **warfarin**, lumiracoxib 400 mg daily increased the INR by about 15%.[18] Lumiracoxib has been withdrawn from a number of countries because of reports of liver toxicity.

(d) Parecoxib

In a randomised study in healthy subjects given **warfarin**, the use of intravenous parecoxib 10 mg twice daily for 7 days had no significant effects on prothrombin times when compared with placebo. Parecoxib did not affect the pharmacokinetics of *S*- or *R*-warfarin.[19]

(e) Rofecoxib

In a study in 12 healthy subjects,[20] rofecoxib 50 mg daily for 12 days increased the maximum INR after a single 30-mg dose of **warfarin** given on day 7 by about 14%. In a steady-state study, 15 healthy subjects were given **warfarin** 5 mg daily to produce a stable prothrombin time of 1.4 to 1.7 for at least 3 consecutive days. They were then additionally given rofecoxib 25 mg or placebo daily for 3 weeks. It was found that the 24-hour average INR was increased by 9% by rofecoxib. Rofecoxib had no effect on the pharmacokinetics of the more potent *S*-warfarin enantiomer, but the AUC of *R*-warfarin was increased by about 40% in both the single dose and steady-state studies.[20] Moreover, in 16 patients stabilised on **warfarin** and given rofecoxib 25 mg daily for 3 weeks, the INR increased by 5%, 9%, and 5% at week one, 2, and 3, respectively, the change at week 2 being statistically significant.[3]

In one case report, an increase in INR was seen in two elderly patients taking **warfarin** and rofecoxib. The INRs were raised, in one case from less than 3 to 4.1 within a month of starting rofecoxib 12.5 mg daily, and in the other case from 3.2 to 4.6 within 2 days of starting rofecoxib. The INRs decreased when the **warfarin** dose was reduced.[4] In another case, this time in a patient taking **acenocoumarol**, the INR rose from the range of 2 to 3 up to over 8 two weeks after starting rofecoxib 50 mg daily.[21] A further possible case with **acenocoumarol** has been reported.[22] A 2002 report from the Australian Adverse Drug Reactions Advisory Committee noted that they had received 8 reports of increases in the INR of patients taking **warfarin** with rofecoxib since the introduction of rofecoxib in late 2000. Two of these cases reported bleeding complications. A further patient died of a cerebral haemorrhage, although the INR was stable.[23] A review of the adverse effects of coxibs included 5 patients taking **warfarin** who had increases in their INR while taking rofecoxib and **warfarin**.[13] Moreover, in a case-control study, patients taking **warfarin** and admitted to hospital with an upper gastrointestinal haemorrhage were significantly more likely to be also taking rofecoxib (odds ratio 2.4).[14] The same findings were reported in another study for celecoxib and rofecoxib considered together.[15] Note that rofecoxib has generally been withdrawn because of adverse cardiovascular effects.

Mechanism

Non-selective NSAIDs (see 'Coumarins and related drugs + NSAIDs', p.449), inhibit platelet aggregation and cause gastrointestinal toxicity, which can result in bleeding, the risk of which is increased in patients taking anticoagulants. Although coxibs are generally considered to be associated with a lower risk of gastrointestinal haemorrhage than non-selective NSAIDs, the only available comparative epidemiological studies found a similar increased risk of bleeding when coxibs were given with warfarin.

There is also possibly a pharmacokinetic interaction. Both warfarin and celecoxib are substrates of the cytochrome P450 isoenzyme CYP2C9, and it is possible that people with variants of CYP2C9 with lower metabolising capacity may develop an interaction if given the combination. See 'Coumarins and related drugs + NSAIDs', p.449, for further discussion on this, and for more general information, see 'Genetic factors in drug metabolism', p.8.

Rofecoxib possibly inhibits the metabolism of the less active *R*-warfarin by inhibition of CYP1A2,[20] and the active *R*-acenocoumarol by the same isoenzyme and CYP2C19.[21] It is unclear how etoricoxib increased R-warfarin levels as it has no known inhibitory effects on cytochrome P450, and the minor rise in warfarin levels is unlikely to completely account for the modest increase in INR.[17]

Importance and management

The interaction of the coumarins with these coxibs leading to raised INRs can be clinically significant, but is apparently rare. For example, of the 4 million prescriptions for celecoxib dispensed over the 18-month period from December 1998, about 1% were estimated to be for patients who would have been taking warfarin,[11] and only a handful of cases of an interaction had been reported. However, the manufacturers recommend that anticoagulant activity should be monitored in patients taking warfarin, other coumarins, or indanediones, particularly in the first few days after initiating or changing the dose of a coxib. Others recommend increased monitoring for 3 weeks.[3] Moreover, remember that all NSAIDS, including coxibs, can irritate the gastrointestinal tract and cause bleeding, the risk of which is increased with anticoagulants. Consider also, 'Coumarins and related drugs + NSAIDs', p.449.

1. Karim A, Tolbert D, Piergies A, Hubbard RC, Harper K, Wallemark C-B, Slater M, Geis GS. Celecoxib does not significantly alter the pharmacokinetics or hypoprothrombinemic effect of warfarin in healthy subjects. *J Clin Pharmacol* (2000) 40, 655–63.
2. Dentali F, Douketis JD, Woods K, Thabane L, Foster G, Holbrook A, Crowther M. Does celecoxib potentiate the anticoagulant effect of warfarin? A randomized, double-blind, controlled trial. *Ann Pharmacother* (2006) 40, 1241–7.
3. Schaefer MG, Plowman BK, Morreale AP, Egan M. Interaction of rofecoxib and celecoxib with warfarin. *Am J Health-Syst Pharm* (2003) 60, 1319–23.
4. Stading JA, Skrabal MZ, Faulkner MA. Seven cases of interaction between warfarin and cyclooxygenase-2 inhibitors. *Am J Health-Syst Pharm* (2001) 58, 2076–80.
5. Haase KK, Rojas-Fernandez CH, Lane L, Frank DA. Potential interaction between celecoxib and warfarin. *Ann Pharmacother* (2000) 34, 666–7.
6. Linder JD, Mönkemüller KE, Davis JV, Wilcox CM. Cyclooxygenase-2 inhibitor celecoxib: a possible cause of gastropathy and hypoprothrombinemia. *South Med J* (2000) 93, 930–2.
7. Mersfelder TL, Stewart LR. Warfarin and celecoxib interaction. *Ann Pharmacother* (2000) 34, 325–7.
8. O'Donnell DC, Hooper JS. Increased international normalized ratio in a patient taking warfarin and celecoxib. *J Pharm Technol* (2001), 17, 3–5.
9. Stoner SC, Lea JW, Dubisar BM, Farrar C. Possible international normalized ratio elevation associated with celecoxib and warfarin in an elderly psychiatric patient. *J Am Geriatr Soc* (2003) 51, 728–9.
10. Malhi H, Atac B, Daly AK, Gupta S. Warfarin and celecoxib interaction in the setting of cytochrome P450 (CYP2C9) polymorphism with bleeding complication. *Postgrad Med J* (2004) 80, 107–9.
11. FDA MedWatch Program, May 1999. Available at: http://www.fda.gov/Safety/MedWatch/default.htm (accessed 22/10/15).
12. ADRAC. Interaction of celecoxib and warfarin. *Aust Adverse Drug React Bull* (2001) 20, 2.
13. Verrico MM, Weber RJ, McKaveney TP, Ansani NT, Towers AL. Adverse drug events involving COX-2 inhibitors. *Ann Pharmacother* (2003) 37, 1203–13.
14. Battistella M, Mamdami MM, Juurlink DN, Rabeneck L, Laupacis A. Risk of upper gastrointestinal hemorrhage in warfarin users treated with nonselective NSAIDs or COX-2 inhibitors. *Arch Intern Med* (2005) 165, 189–92.
15. Delaney JA, Opatrny L, Brophy JM, Suissa S. Drug–drug interactions between antithrombotic medications and the risk of gastrointestinal bleeding. *CMAJ* (2007) 177, 347–51.
16. Chung L, Chakravarty EF, Kearns P, Wang C, Bush TM. Bleeding complications in patients on celecoxib and warfarin. *J Clin Pharm Ther* (2005) 30, 471–7.
17. Schwartz JI, Agrawal NGB, Hartford AH, Cote J, Hunt TL, Verbesselt R, Eckols DR, Gottesdiener KM. The effect of etoricoxib on the pharmacodynamics and pharmacokinetics of warfarin. *J Clin Pharmacol* (2007) 47, 620–7.
18. Prexige (Lumiracoxib). Novartis Pharmaceuticals UK Ltd. UK Summary of product characteristics, February 2007.
19. Karim A, Bradford D, Qian J, Hubbard R. The COX-2-specific inhibitor parecoxib sodium does not affect warfarin pharmacokinetic and pharmacodynamic parameters. American College of Emergency Physicians. Scientific Assembly, Chicago, Illinois, 15-18 October 2001. Abstract 130.
20. Schwartz JI, Bugianesi KJ, Ebel DL, De Smet M, Haesen R, Larson PJ, Ko A, Verbesselt R, Hunt TL, Lins R, Lens S, Porras AG, Dieck J, Keymeulen B, Gertz BJ. The effect of rofecoxib on the pharmacodynamics and pharmacokinetics of warfarin. *Clin Pharmacol Ther* (2000) 68, 626–36.
21. Girardin F, Siegenthaler M, de Moerloose P, Desmeules J. Rofecoxib interaction with oral anticoagulant acenocoumarol. *Eur J Clin Pharmacol* (2003) 59, 489–90.
22. Tewari P, Nath SS, Mazumdar G. Increased prothrombin time and lactic acidosis: rofecoxib drug interaction with acenocoumarin and metformin. *Ann Card Anaesth* (2007) 10, 58–60.
23. ADRAC. Interaction of rofecoxib with warfarin. *Aust Adverse Drug React Bull* (2002) 21, 3.

Coumarins + NSAIDs; Diclofenac

Diclofenac does not appear to alter the anticoagulant effect of acenocoumarol, phenprocoumon or warfarin. However, isolated cases of raised INRs have been reported. Note that all NSAIDs increase the risk of bleeding, and an increased risk is seen when they are given with anticoagulants.

Clinical evidence

In a crossover study in 29 patients stabilised on **acenocoumarol**, diclofenac 25 mg four times daily for one week did not alter the anticoagulant effect (prothrombin value) of **acenocoumarol**, when compared with placebo.[1] Other studies similarly confirm that diclofenac does not alter the anticoagulant effect of either **phenprocoumon**[2] or **warfarin**.[3]

However, a patient taking **acenocoumarol** developed a pulmonary haemorrhage associated with a very prolonged prothrombin time within 10 days of starting to take diclofenac.[4] Another report mentions a Chinese patient taking **warfarin** who developed an INR of 4 within 4 days of using a 1% diclofenac topical gel for joint pain.[5]

In a retrospective cohort study of patients taking **acenocoumarol** or **phenprocoumon**, diclofenac was associated with a 2.6-fold increased risk of hospitalisation for bleeding.[6] For a discussion of other studies, including one assessing the effect of CYP2C9 substrates such as diclofenac, on the risk of bleeding when used with **warfarin**, see 'Coumarins and related drugs + NSAIDs', p.449.

There is a report of the rare adverse effect, coumarin necrosis, occurring in an elderly man taking **acenocoumarol**, in which acute renal impairment aggravated by diclofenac was considered a contributory factor.[7]

Mechanism

See 'Coumarins and related drugs + NSAIDs', p.449.

Importance and management

On the basis of the pharmacological studies, no adjustment in coumarin dose would be anticipated to be needed when diclofenac is used. The isolated cases of raised INRs are unexplained. However, care is still needed with every NSAID because, to a greater or lesser extent, they irritate the stomach lining, which can result in gastrointestinal bleeding, which will be more severe in anticoagulated patients. For more information about this and potential CYP2C9-mediated interactions, see 'Coumarins and related drugs + NSAIDs', p.449.

1. Michot F, Ajdacic K, Glaus L. A double-blind clinical trial to determine if an interaction exists between diclofenac sodium and the oral anticoagulant acenocoumarol (nicoumalone). *J Int Med Res* (1975) 3, 153–7.
2. Krzywanek HJ, Breddin K. Beeinflußt Diclofenac die orale Antikoagulantientherapie und die Plättchenaggregation? *Med Welt* (1977) 28, 1843–5.
3. Fitzgerald DE, Russell JG. Voltarol and warfarin, an interaction? In: Chiswell RJ, Birdwood GFB, eds. Current Themes in Rheumatology: Cambridge: Cambridge Medical Publications :p 26–7.
4. Cuadrado Gómez LM, Palau Beato E, Pérez Venegas J, Pérez Moro E. Hemorragia pulmonar debido a la interacción de acenocumarina y diclofenac sódico. *Rev Clin Esp* (1987) 181, 227–8.
5. Chan TYK. Drug interactions as a cause of overanticoagulation and bleedings in Chinese patients receiving warfarin. *Int J Clin Pharmacol Ther* (1998) 36, 403–5.
6. Penning-van Beest F, Erkens J, Petersen K-U, Koelz HR, Herings R. Main comedications associated with bleeding during anticoagulant therapy with coumarins. *Eur J Clin Pharmacol* (2005) 61, 439–44.
7. Muniesa C, Marcoval J, Moreno A, Giménez S, Sánchez J, Ferreres JR, Peyrí J. Coumarin necrosis induced by renal insufficiency. *Br J Dermatol* (2004) 151, 502–4.

Coumarins + NSAIDs; Diflunisal

There is limited evidence to suggest that diflunisal might increase the anticoagulant effects of acenocoumarol and possibly warfarin, but apparently not phenprocoumon. All NSAIDs increase the risk of bleeding, and should be used with care in patients taking oral anticoagulants.

Clinical evidence

The total plasma **warfarin** levels of 5 healthy subjects fell by about one-third (from 741 to 533 nanograms/mL) when they were given diflunisal 500 mg twice daily for 2 weeks. Also, unbound **warfarin** increased from 1.02% to 1.34%, but the anticoagulant response was unaffected. When the diflunisal was withdrawn the anticoagulant response was reduced.[1]

A brief report states that 3 out of 6 subjects taking **acenocoumarol** had significant increases in prothrombin times, but no interaction was seen in 2 subjects taking **phenprocoumon**, when they were given diflunisal 750 mg daily.[2]

Mechanism

Uncertain. Diflunisal can displace warfarin from its plasma protein binding sites, but this on its own is almost certainly not the full explanation.[1] The fall in anticoagulant response when diflunisal was stopped is possibly linked to a difference in the rates that total and unbound plasma warfarin returned to their original levels.[1]

Importance and management

This interaction is neither well defined nor well documented and its importance is uncertain. However, the reports cited suggest that an increased anticoagulant effect should be looked for if diflunisal is added to established treatment with any anticoagulant. A decreased effect might be expected if diflunisal is withdrawn. Note that care is needed with every NSAID because, to a greater or lesser extent, they irritate the stomach lining, which can result in gastrointestinal bleeding, which will be more severe in anticoagulated patients. Consider also 'Coumarins and related drugs + NSAIDs', p.449.

1. Serlin MJ, Mossman S, Sibeon RG, Tempero KF, Breckenridge AM. Interaction between diflunisal and warfarin. *Clin Pharmacol Ther* (1980) 28, 493–8.
2. Tempero KF, Cirillo VJ, Steelman SL. Diflunisal: a review of pharmacokinetic and pharmacodynamic properties, drug interactions, and special tolerability studies in humans. *Br J Clin Pharmacol* (1977) 4, 31S–36S.

Coumarins + NSAIDs; Dipyrone (Metamizole sodium)

One report claims that dipyrone does not interact with phenprocoumon or ethyl biscoumacetate, whereas another describes a rapid but transient increase in the effects of ethyl biscoumacetate with dipyrone. All NSAIDs

increase the risk of bleeding, and an increased risk is seen when they are given with anticoagulants.

Clinical evidence, mechanism, importance and management

A single 1-g dose of dipyrone did not alter the steady-state anticoagulant effects of either **phenprocoumon** (5 subjects) or **ethyl biscoumacetate** (6 subjects).[1] Conversely, another report describes a short-lived but rapid increase (within 4 hours) in the effects of **ethyl biscoumacetate** caused by single 1-g dose metamizole sodium.[2] The reasons are not understood. However, care is still needed with every NSAID because, to a greater or lesser extent, they irritate the stomach lining, which can result in gastrointestinal bleeding, which will be more severe in anticoagulated patients. Consider also 'Coumarins and related drugs + NSAIDs', p.449.

1. Badian M, Le Normand Y, Rupp W, Zapf R. There is no interaction between dipyrone (metamizol) and the anticoagulants, phenprocoumon and ethylbiscoumacetate, in normal caucasian subjects. *Int J Pharmaceutics* (1984) 18, 9–15.
2. Mehvar SR, Jamali F. Dipyrone-ethylbiscoumacetate interaction in man. *Indian J Pharm* (1981) 7, 293–9.

Coumarins + NSAIDs; Etodolac

In a pharmacological study, etodolac did not interact significantly with warfarin. Note that all NSAIDs increase the risk of bleeding, and an increased risk is seen when they are combined with anticoagulants.

Clinical evidence, mechanism, importance and management

In a three-period, crossover study, each period lasting 2.5 days, 18 healthy subjects were given **warfarin** 20 mg on day one, 10 mg on days 2 and 3 and etodolac 200 mg every 12 hours. Although the median peak serum levels of the **warfarin** fell by 19% and the median total clearance rose by 13% in the presence of etodolac, the prothrombin time response remained unchanged.[1,2] On the basis of this study, no adjustment in coumarin dose would be expected to be needed when etodolac is used. However, care is still needed with every NSAID, because, to a greater or lesser extent, they irritate the stomach lining, which can result in gastrointestinal bleeding, which will be more severe in anticoagulated patients. Consider also 'Coumarins and related drugs + NSAIDs', p.449.

1. Ermer JC, Hicks DR, Wheeler SC, Kraml M, Jusko WJ. Concomitant etodolac affects neither the unbound clearance nor the pharmacologic effect of warfarin. *Clin Pharmacol Ther* (1994) 55, 305–16.
2. Zvaifler N. A review of the antiarthritic efficacy and safety of etodolac. *Clin Rheumatol* (1989) 8 (Suppl 1), 43–53.

Coumarins and related drugs + NSAIDs; Fenamates

The anticoagulant effects of acenocoumarol, phenprocoumon and warfarin may be increased by floctafenine, glafenine, meclofenamic acid, and mefenamic acid. Tolfenamic acid is expected to interact similarly. However, limited evidence from one small study found glafenine did not alter the response to acenocoumarol, or ethyl biscoumacetate. Note also that all NSAIDs increase the risk of bleeding, and an increased risk is seen when they are given with anticoagulants.

Clinical evidence

(a) Floctafenine

In a double-blind study in 20 patients stabilised on **acenocoumarol** or **phenprocoumon** and given either floctafenine 200 mg or placebo four times daily for 3 weeks, floctafenine prolonged their thrombotest times by an average of about one-third, even though the anticoagulant dose of some of the patients was reduced.[1]

(b) Glafenine

In a double-blind study in 20 patients stabilised on **phenprocoumon** and given either glafenine 200 mg or placebo three times daily it was noted that within a week of starting glafenine there was a significant increase in thrombotest times.[2] In another report, 5 out of 7 patients needed a **phenprocoumon** dose reduction while taking glafenine.[3] Conversely, in another study, 10 patients taking **acenocoumarol**, **ethyl biscoumacetate** or **'indanedione'** had no changes in their anticoagulant response when given glafenine 800 mg daily over a 4-week period.[4]

(c) Meclofenamic acid

After taking sodium meclofenamate 200 to 300 mg daily for 7 days, the average dose of **warfarin** required by 7 patients fell from 6.5 to 4.25 mg daily, and by the end of 4 weeks it was 5.5 mg (a 16% reduction with a 0 to 25% range).[5]

(d) Mefenamic acid

After taking mefenamic acid 500 mg four times daily for a week, the mean prothrombin concentrations of 12 healthy subjects stabilised on **warfarin** fell by about 3.5%. Microscopic haematuria was seen in 3 of them, but no overt haemorrhage occurred. Their prothrombin concentrations were 15 to 25% of normal, well within the accepted anticoagulant range.[6]

Mechanism

Uncertain. Mefenamic acid can displace warfarin from its plasma protein binding sites,[7-9] and *in vitro* studies have shown that therapeutic concentrations (equivalent to 4 g daily) can increase the unbound and active warfarin concentrations by 140 to 340%,[7,8] but this interaction mechanism alone is only likely to have a transient effect. See also 'Coumarins and related drugs + NSAIDs', p.449.

Importance and management

The pharmacological studies cited suggest that all the fenamates can cause a small to modest increase in the effects of the coumarins. If both drugs are given, increase monitoring and anticipate the need for a small reduction in the coumarin dose. Although there are no data regarding concurrent use with the fenamate **tolfenamic acid**, the manufacturer similarly recommends close monitoring of coagulation.[10] Also note that, all NSAIDs, to a greater or lesser extent irritate the stomach lining, which can result in gastrointestinal bleeding, which will be more severe in anticoagulated patients. Consider also 'Coumarins and related drugs + NSAIDs', p.449.

1. Boeijinga JK, van de Broeke RN, Jochemsen R, Breimer DD, Hoogslag MA, Jeletich-Bastiaanse A. De invloed van floctafenine (Idalon) op antistollingsbehandeling met coumarinederivaten. *Ned Tijdschr Geneeskd* (1981) 125, 1931–5.
2. Boeijinga JK, van der Vijgh WJF. Double blind study of the effect of glafenine (Glifanan®) on oral anticoagulant therapy with phenprocoumon (Marcumar®). *Eur J Clin Pharmacol* (1977) 12, 291–6.
3. Boeijinga JK, Bing GT, van der Meer J. De invloed van glafenine (Glifanan) op antistollingsbehandeling met coumarinederivaten. *Ned Tijdschr Geneeskd* (1974) 118, 1895–8.
4. Raby C. Recherches sur une éventuelle potentialisation de l'action des anticoagulants de synthèse par la glafénine. *Therapie* (1977) 32, 293–9.
5. Baragar FD, Smith TC. Drug interaction studies with sodium meclofenamate (Meclomen®). *Curr Ther Res* (1978) 23 (April Suppl), S51–S59.
6. Holmes EL. Pharmacology of the fenamates: IV. Toleration by normal human subjects. *Ann Phys Med* (1966) 9 (Suppl), 36–49.
7. Sellers EM, Koch-Weser J. Displacement of warfarin from human albumin by diazoxide and ethacrynic, mefenamic and nalidixic acids. *Clin Pharmacol Ther* (1970) 11, 524–9.
8. Sellers EM, Koch-Weser J. Kinetics and clinical importance of displacement of warfarin from albumin by acidic drugs. *Ann N Y Acad Sci* (1971) 179, 213–25.
9. McElnay JC, D'Arcy PFD. Displacement of albumin-bound warfarin by anti-inflammatory agents *in vitro*. *J Pharm Pharmacol* (1980) 32, 709–11.
10. Clotam Rapid (Tolfenamic acid). Galen Ltd. UK Summary of product characteristics, February 2009.

Coumarins + NSAIDs; Ibuprofen and related drugs

Ibuprofen, indoprofen, ketoprofen, naproxen and oxaprozin do not appear to alter the anticoagulant effect of coumarins. However, isolated cases of raised INRs have been described with ibuprofen and ketoprofen, and an increased risk of bleeding has been reported with naproxen. A slight increase in anticoagulant effect has been seen with fenbufen, flurbiprofen and tiaprofenic acid. Note also that all NSAIDs increase the risk of bleeding, and an increased risk is seen when they are given with anticoagulants.

Clinical evidence

(a) Fenbufen

In a study in 10 healthy subjects who were stabilised on **warfarin** and then given either fenbufen 400 mg twice daily or placebo for one week, the prothrombin times were increased by 1.9 seconds within 2 days in the fenbufen recipients, and the serum **warfarin** levels fell by 14%.[1]

(b) Flurbiprofen

In a study in 19 patients stable taking **phenprocoumon** and given flurbiprofen 50 mg three times daily for 2 weeks, a small but significant fall in the Quick value occurred (from 25.05% to 20.68%). Two patients bled (haematuria, epistaxis, haemorrhoidal bleeding) and the prothrombin times of 3 patients fell below the therapeutic range.[2] A case report describes 2 patients taking **acenocoumarol** who had a rise in thrombotest times and bled (haematuria, melaena, haematomas) within 2 to 3 days of starting to take flurbiprofen 150 to 300 mg daily.[3]

(c) Ibuprofen

Ibuprofen 600 mg to 2.4 g daily for 7 to 14 days did not alter the effects of coumarins in studies in patients stabilised on **phenprocoumon**;[4-6] healthy subjects[7,8] or patients[8] stabilised on **warfarin**; or patients stabilised on **dicoumarol**.[9] In one study in 20 patients taking **warfarin**, ibuprofen 600 mg three times daily for one week had no effect on prothrombin time; however, it did prolong bleeding time (4 cases above the therapeutic range) and microscopic haematuria and haematoma were seen.[10] Note that, this finding is probably more of a function of the effect of ibuprofen than an interaction *per se*,[11] although it does explain why the combination of an anticoagulant and an NSAID has an increased risk of haemorrhage.

An isolated case report describes subclinical bleeding with a raised INR in a 74-year-old woman with multiple medical problems taking **warfarin** when she was given ibuprofen.[12]

In a retrospective cohort study of patients taking **acenocoumarol** or **phenprocoumon**, ibuprofen was associated with a 2.2-fold increased risk of hospitalisation for bleeding. The study specifically looked at potentially interacting drugs taken by at least 50 patients, and there were at least 5 cases of bleeding with ibuprofen.[13] A case report describes a woman taking **warfarin**, with an INR of 2.1 on admission, who had a fatal gastrointestinal bleed after taking ibuprofen (dose unknown) for foot pain in the previous week.[14] For other studies, including one assessing the effect of CYP2C9 substrates, such as ibuprofen, on the risk of bleeding with warfarin, see 'Coumarins and related drugs + NSAIDs', p.449.

(d) Indoprofen

In a placebo-controlled study in 18 patients stabilised on **warfarin** and given indoprofen 600 mg daily for 7 days, found no changes occurred in any of the blood coagulation measurements made.[15]

(e) Ketoprofen

In a study in 15 healthy subjects stabilised on **warfarin**, ketoprofen 100 mg twice daily for 7 days had no effect on prothrombin times or coagulation cascade parameters, and there was no evidence of bleeding.[16] This contrasts with an isolated case of bleeding in a patient taking **warfarin** (prothrombin time increased from 18 seconds to 41 seconds) one week after starting ketoprofen 25 mg three times daily.[17]

(f) Naproxen

In a study in 10 healthy subjects, naproxen 375 mg twice daily for 17 days did not alter the pharmacokinetics of a single dose of **warfarin** given on day 10, or alter its anticoagulant effects.[18] Similar results were found in a study of **warfarin** at steady state.[19] A further study in patients taking **phenprocoumon** found that naproxen 250 mg twice daily transiently increased the anticoagulant effects and caused an unimportant change in primary bleeding time.[20]

In a retrospective cohort study of patients taking **acenocoumarol** or **phenprocoumon**, naproxen was associated with a 6.5-fold increased risk of hospitalisation for bleeding. The study specifically looked at potentially interacting drugs taken by at least 50 patients, and there were at least 9 cases of bleeding for naproxen.[13] For other studies, including one assessing the effect of CYP2C9 substrates, such as naproxen, on the risk of bleeding with warfarin, see 'Coumarins and related drugs + NSAIDs', p.449.

(g) Oxaprozin

In a study in 10 healthy subjects stabilised on **warfarin** for an average of 15 days, oxaprozin 1.2 g daily for 7 days did not significantly alter prothrombin times.[21]

(h) Tiaprofenic acid

In a study in 6 healthy subjects, the anticoagulant effects and the pharmacokinetic profile of **phenprocoumon** remained unchanged when they took tiaprofenic acid daily for 2 days.[22] This study is also published elsewhere.[23] No significant interaction occurred in 9 patients stabilised on **acenocoumarol** and given tiaprofenic acid 200 mg three times daily for 2 weeks, but in 4 patients a 'rebound' rise in prothrombin percentages occurred following the withdrawal of the NSAID.[24] However, an elderly man taking **acenocoumarol** had severe epistaxis and bruising 4 to 6 weeks after starting to take tiaprofenic acid 300 mg twice daily. His prothrombin time had risen to 129 seconds.[25]

Mechanism

When given alone, ibuprofen and related drugs can prolong bleeding times because of their antiplatelet effects.[11] They may also cause gastrointestinal toxicity. Because of these effects, the risk of bleeding is increased in patients taking anticoagulants by the concurrent use of NSAIDs. Most of the propionic acid derivatives can displace the anticoagulants from plasma protein binding sites to some extent, but this mechanism on its own is rarely, if ever, responsible for clinically important drug interactions.

Importance and management

It is well established that ibuprofen does not alter the anticoagulant effect of warfarin or other coumarins, (although isolated and unexplained cases of bleeding or raised INRs have occurred, but only very rarely). On the basis of these studies, no adjustment in coumarin dose would be anticipated to be needed when ibuprofen is used. Pharmacological studies also show no interaction for related propionic acid derivatives including indoprofen, ketoprofen, naproxen and oxaprozin, although the documentation is more limited. A slight increase in anticoagulant effects has been seen with fenbufen, flurbiprofen, and possibly tiaprofenic acid, although this is probably of limited clinical relevance. However, note that care is still needed with every NSAID, because, to a greater or lesser extent, they irritate the stomach lining, which can result in gastrointestinal bleeding, which will be more severe in anticoagulated patients. For more information about this, and potential CYP2C9-mediated interactions, see 'Coumarins and related drugs + NSAIDs', p.449.

1. Savitsky JP, Terzakis T, Bina P, Chiccarelli F, Haynes J. Fenbufen-warfarin interaction in healthy volunteers. *Clin Pharmacol Ther* (1980) 27, 284.
2. Marbet GA, Duckert F, Walter M, Six P, Airenne H. Interaction study between phenprocoumon and flurbiprofen. *Curr Med Res Opin* (1977) 5, 26–31.
3. Stricker BHC, Delhez JL. Interaction between flurbiprofen and coumarins. *BMJ* (1982) 285, 812–13.
4. Thilo D, Nyman F, Duckert F. A study of the effects of the anti-rheumatic drug ibuprofen (Brufen) on patients being treated with the oral anti-coagulant phenprocoumon (Marcoumar). *J Int Med Res* (1974) 2, 276–8.
5. Duckert F. The absence of effect of the antirheumatic drug ibuprofen on oral anticoagulation with phenprocoumon. *Curr Med Res Opin* (1975) 3, 556–7.
6. Boekhout-Mussert MJ, Loeliger EA. Influence of ibuprofen on oral anti-coagulation with phenprocoumon. *J Int Med Res* (1974) 2, 279–83.
7. Penner JA, Abbrecht PH. Lack of interaction between ibuprofen and warfarin. *Curr Ther Res* (1975) 18, 862–71.
8. Goncalves L. Influence of ibuprofen on haemostasis in patients on anticoagulant therapy. *J Int Med Res* (1973) 1, 180–3.
9. Marini U, Cecchi A, Venturino M. Mancanza di interazione tra ibuprofen lisinato e anticoagulanti orali. *Clin Ter* (1985) 112, 25–9.
10. Schulman S, Henriksson K. Interaction of ibuprofen and warfarin on primary haemostasis. *Br J Rheumatol* (1989) 28, 46–9.
11. Pullar T. Interaction of ibuprofen and warfarin on primary haemostasis. *Br J Rheumatol* (1989) 28, 265–6.
12. Ernst ME, Buys LM. Reevaluating the safety of concurrent warfarin and ibuprofen. *J Pharm Technol* (1997) 13, 244–7.
13. Penning-van Beest F, Erkens J, Petersen K-U, Koelz HR, Herings R. Main comedications associated with bleeding during anticoagulant therapy with coumarins. *Eur J Clin Pharmacol* (2005) 61, 439–44.
14. Gabb GM. Fatal outcome of interaction between warfarin and a non-steroidal anti-inflammatory drug. *Med J Aust* (1996) 164, 700–1.
15. Jacono A, Caso P, Gualtieri S, Raucci D, Bianchi A, Vigorito C, Bergamini N, Iadevaia V. Clinical study of the possible interactions between indoprofen and oral anticoagulants. *Eur J Rheumatol Inflamm* (1981) 4, 32–5.
16. Mieszczak C, Winther K. Lack of interaction of ketoprofen with warfarin. *Eur J Clin Pharmacol* (1993) 44, 205–6.
17. Flessner MF, Knight H. Prolongation of prothrombin time and severe gastrointestinal bleeding associated with combined use of warfarin and ketoprofen. *JAMA* (1988) 259, 353.
18. Slattery JT, Levy G, Jain A, McMahon FG. Effect of naproxen on the kinetics of elimination and anticoagulant activity of a single dose of warfarin. *Clin Pharmacol Ther* (1979) 25, 51–60.
19. Jain A, McMahon FG, Slattery JT, Levy G. Effect of naproxen on the steady-state serum concentration and anticoagulant activity of warfarin. *Clin Pharmacol Ther* (1979) 25, 61–6.
20. Angelkort B. Zum einfluß von Naproxen auf die thrombozytäre Blutstillung und die Antikoagulantien-Behandlung mit Phenprocoumon. *Fortschr Med* (1978) 96, 1249–52.
21. Davis LJ, Kayser SR, Hubscher J, Williams RL. Effect of oxaprozin on the steady-state anticoagulant activity of warfarin. *Clin Pharm* (1984) 3, 295–7.
22. Dürr J, Pfeiffer MH, Wetzelsberger K, Lücker PW. Untersuchung zur Frage einer Interaktion von Tiaprofensäure und Phenprocoumon. *Arzneimittelforschung* (1981) 31, 2163–7.
23. Lücker PW, Penth B, Wetzelsberger K. Pharmacokinetic interaction between tiaprofenic acid and several other compounds for chronic use. *Rheumatology (Oxford)* (1982) 7, 99–106.
24. Meurice J. Interaction of tiaprofenic acid and acenocoumarol. *Rheumatology (Oxford)* (1982) 7, 111–17.
25. Whittaker SJ, Jackson CW, Whorwell PJ. A severe, potentially fatal, interaction between tiaprofenic acid and nicoumalone. *Br J Clin Pract* (1986) 40, 440.

Coumarins + NSAIDs; Indometacin and related drugs

The anticoagulant effects of acenocoumarol, phenprocoumon and warfarin are not affected by indometacin, and the anticoagulant effects of phenprocoumon are not affected by acemetacin. However, isolated cases of raised INRs and bleeding complications have been reported. Also, note that, like all NSAIDs, indometacin increases the risk of bleeding, the risk of which is further increased in patients taking anticoagulants.

Clinical evidence

(a) Acemetacin

In a placebo-controlled study in 20 patients stabilised on **phenprocoumon**, acemetacin 60 mg three times daily for 3 weeks did not alter the thromboplastin value.[1]

(b) Indometacin

In a placebo-controlled, double-blind study in 8 healthy subjects, indometacin 100 mg daily for 5 days had no effect on the anticoagulant effects of steady-state **warfarin**.[2] Similarly, when 19 healthy subjects took either indometacin 25 mg four times daily or placebo for 11 days, the anticoagulant effects and the half-life of single doses of **warfarin** were not affected.[2]

Other studies in healthy subjects and patients anticoagulated with **acenocoumarol**[3] or **phenprocoumon**[4-6] similarly found that the anticoagulant effects were not changed by indometacin.

However, isolated cases of possible interactions in patients taking **warfarin** have been reported.[7-9] One patient had a rise in INR from 2 to 5.3,[8] and another had a rise from 2.75 to 3.42, then to 3.6 despite a reduction in **warfarin** dose.[9] However, there are other possible interpretations of this case.[10] In another report a patient taking indometacin appeared to have an enhanced response to **warfarin**, which subsequently improved when ibuprofen was substituted for indometacin.[7] The preliminary report of an analysis of possible drug interactions with **warfarin** stated that indometacin was found to have a clinically relevant effect on the anticoagulant action of warfarin.[11] One patient taking **warfarin** and indometacin died from acute peptic ulceration.[12] In another report, a patient who was very sensitive to **acenocoumarol** was found to have melaena and an INR of greater than 10 one week after starting indometacin and tetrazepam. He was found to have low levels of the cytochrome P450 isoenzyme CYP2C9 (poor metaboliser phenotype of CYP2C9 variant *3).[13]

For studies, including one assessing the effect of CYP2C9 substrates, such as indometacin, on the risk of bleeding with warfarin, see 'Coumarins and related drugs + NSAIDs', p.449.

Mechanism

None. Indometacin reduces platelet aggregation and thereby prolongs bleeding when it occurs. Acemetacin would act similarly since it is a glycolic acid ester of indometacin and indometacin is the major metabolite.

Importance and management

In pharmacological studies it is well established that indometacin does not normally alter the anticoagulant effects acenocoumarol, phenprocoumon or warfarin. No coumarin dose adjustments would therefore expected to be needed during concurrent use. However, caution is still appropriate, because indometacin, like other NSAIDs, can cause gastrointestinal irritation, ulceration and bleeding, which will be more severe in anticoagulated patients. For more information about this and potential CYP2C9-mediated interactions, see 'Coumarins and related drugs + NSAIDs', p.449.

1. Hess H, Koeppen R. Kontrollierte Doppelblindestudie zur Frage einer möglichen Interferenz von Acemetacin mit einer laufenden Antikoagulanzien-Therapie. *Arzneimittelforschung* (1980) 30, 1421–3.
2. Vesell ES, Passananti GT, Johnson AO. Failure of indomethacin and warfarin to interact in normal human volunteers. *J Clin Pharmacol* (1975) 15, 486–95.
3. Gáspárdy G, Bálint G, Gáspárdy G. Wirkung der Kombination Indomethacin und Syncumar (Acenocumarol) auf den Prothrombinspiegel im Blutplasma. *Z Rheumaforsch* (1967) 26, 332–5.
4. Müller G, Zollinger W. The influence of indomethacin on blood coagulation, particularly with regard to the interference with anticoagulant treatment. In: Heister R, Hofmann HF eds. International Symposium on Inflammation. Munich: Urban and Schwarzenburg, 1966: 1–12.
5. Frost H, Hess H. Concomitant administration of indomethacin and anticoagulants. In: Heister R, Hofmann HF eds. International Symposium on Inflammation. Munich: Urban and Schwarzenburg, 1966: 1–3.

6. Muller KH, Herrmann K. Is simultaneous therapy with anticoagulants and indomethacin feasible? *Med Welt* (1966) 17, 1553–4.
7. Self TH, Soloway MS, Vaughn D. Possible interaction of indomethacin and warfarin. *Drug Intell Clin Pharm* (1978) 12, 580–1.
8. Chan TYK. Prolongation of prothrombin time with the use of indomethacin and warfarin. *Br J Clin Pract* (1997) 51, 177–8.
9. Chan TYK, Lui SF, Chung SY, Luk S, Critchley JAJH. Adverse interaction between warfarin and indomethacin. *Drug Safety* (1994) 10, 267–9.
10. Day R, Quinn D. Adverse interaction between warfarin and indomethacin. *Drug Safety* (1994) 11, 213–14.
11. Koch-Weser J. Haemorrhagic reactions and drug interactions in 500 warfarin-treated patients. *Clin Pharmacol Ther* (1973) 14, 139.
12. McQueen EG. New Zealand Committee on Adverse Reactions: fourteenth annual report 1979. *N Z Med J* (1980) 91, 226–9.
13. Zarza J, Hermida J, Montes R, Páramo JA, Rocha E. Major bleeding during combined treatment with indomethacin and low doses of acenocoumarol in a homozygous patient for 2C9*3 variant of cytochrome P-450 CYP2C9. *Thromb Haemost* (2003) 90, 161–2.

Coumarins and related drugs + NSAIDs; Ketorolac

Ketorolac does not alter the pharmacokinetics of, or prothrombin time response to, warfarin. However, ketorolac has been associated with serious gastrointestinal bleeding.

Clinical evidence, mechanism, importance and management

In a placebo-controlled, crossover study[1] in 10 healthy subjects, ketorolac 10 mg four times daily for 12 days caused no major changes in the pharmacokinetics of *R*- or *S*-warfarin, nor in the prothrombin time after a single 25-mg dose of **warfarin** given on day 6. This suggests that ketorolac is normally unlikely to affect the anticoagulant response of patients taking **warfarin** long-term, and that no warfarin dose adjustments would be expected to be necessary on concurrent use. However, in 1993 the CSM in the UK reported on an analysis of adverse reactions associated with ketorolac: they had received 5 reports of postoperative haemorrhage and four reports of gastrointestinal haemorrhage (one fatal) in patients taking ketorolac.[2] As result of this analysis, the use of ketorolac with anticoagulants was contraindicated in the UK.[2,3] In the US, the manufacturers stated that patients taking anticoagulants have an increased risk of bleeding complications if they are also given ketorolac, and therefore they should be used together extremely cautiously. They noted that, in particular, there is an increased risk of intramuscular haematoma from intramuscular ketorolac in patients taking anticoagulants.[4] This advice is prudent, because it is now established that use of any NSAID increases the risk of gastrointestinal bleeding when used with anticoagulants, see 'Coumarins and related drugs + NSAIDs', p.449, and it would therefore be wise to avoid the concurrent use of NSAIDs that have a higher risk of gastrointestinal toxicity such as ketorolac.

1. Toon S, Holt BL, Mullins FGP, Bullingham R, Aarons L, Rowland M. Investigations into the potential effects of multiple dose ketorolac on the pharmacokinetics and pharmacodynamics of racemic warfarin. *Br J Clin Pharmacol* (1990) 30, 743–50.
2. Committee on the Safety of Medicines/Medicines Control Agency. Ketorolac: new restrictions on dose and duration of treatment. *Current Problems* (1993) 19, 5–6.
3. Toradol (Ketorolac trometamol). Roche Products Ltd. UK Summary of product characteristics, July 2009.
4. Toradol (Ketorolac tromethamine). Roche Pharmaceuticals. US Prescribing information, September 2002.

Coumarins + NSAIDs; Nabumetone

Nabumetone does not appear to alter the anticoagulant effects of acenocoumarol or warfarin. However, an isolated report describes a raised INR and haemarthrosis in one patient taking warfarin, which was attributed to an interaction with nabumetone. Note that all NSAIDs increase the risk of bleeding, and an increased risk is seen when they are given with anticoagulants.

Clinical evidence, mechanism, importance and management

In a study in 12 healthy subjects, nabumetone 2 g daily for 2 weeks did not significantly alter the anticoagulant effects of steady-state **warfarin**.[1] Similarly, nabumetone 1 to 2 g daily for 6 weeks had no effect on the INR in 58 patients stabilised on **warfarin**.[2] Another clinical study in osteoarthritis patients also found that there was no difference in the proportion of patients with no INR change and no change in **acenocoumarol** dose in 27 patients given nabumetone 1 to 2 g daily for 4 weeks and 29 patients given placebo.[3] Moreover, nabumetone does not appear to affect bleeding time, platelet aggregation or prothrombin times in the absence of an anticoagulant.[4] However, an isolated and unexplained report describes an increase in INR from 2 to 3.7 and haemarthrosis in a patient taking **warfarin** a week after nabumetone 750 mg twice daily was added.[5]

On the basis of the above studies, no coumarin dose adjustment would be expected to be needed with nabumetone. However, care is still needed with every NSAID because, to a greater or lesser extent, they irritate the stomach lining, which can result in gastrointestinal bleeding, which will be more severe in anticoagulated patients. Consider also 'Coumarins and related drugs + NSAIDs', p.449.

1. Fitzgerald DE. Double-blind study to establish whether there is any interaction between nabumetone and warfarin in healthy adult male volunteers. In: Panayi GS, Price JD, Rotman H, eds. Nabumetone: a novel anti-inflammatory. *Roy Soc Med Int Congr Symp* (1984) 69, 47–53.
2. Hilleman DE, Mohiuddin SM, Lucas BD. Hypoprothrombinemic effect of nabumetone in warfarin-treated patients. *Pharmacotherapy* (1993) 13, 270–1.
3. Pardo A, García-Losa M, Fernández-Pavón A, del Castillo S, Pascual-García T, García-Méndez E, Dal-Ré R. A placebo-controlled study of interaction between nabumetone and acenocoumarol. *Br J Clin Pharmacol* (1999) 47, 441–4.
4. Al Balla S, Al Momen AK, Al Arfaj H, Al Sugair S, Gader AMA. Interaction between nabumetone — a new non-steroidal anti-inflammatory drug — and the haemostatic system ex vivo. *Haemostasis* (1990) 20, 270–5.
5. Dennis VC, Thomas BK, Hanlon JE. Potentiation of oral anticoagulation and hemarthrosis associated with nabumetone. *Pharmacotherapy* (2000) 20, 234–9.

Coumarins + NSAIDs; Nimesulide

In pharmacological studies, nimesulide did not alter the effects of acenocoumarol or warfarin. Note that all NSAIDs increase the risk of bleeding, and an increased risk is seen when they are given with anticoagulants.

Clinical evidence, mechanism, importance and management

In a pilot study in 6 patients stabilised on **acenocoumarol**, a single 100-mg dose of nimesulide did not affect the clotting mechanisms, although the platelet aggregating response to adenosine diphosphate, adrenaline (epinephrine) and collagen was reduced for 2 to 4 hours.[1] Ten patients stabilised on **warfarin** 5 mg daily had no significant changes in their prothrombin times, partial thromboplastin time or bleeding times when they were given nimesulide 100 mg twice daily for a week.[2] However, a few patients had some increase in anticoagulant activity.[1]

These studies suggest that no coumarin dose adjustments are expected to be needed when nimesulide is used. However, care is still needed with every NSAID because, to a greater or lesser extent, they irritate the stomach lining, which can result in gastrointestinal bleeding, which will be more severe in anticoagulated patients. Consider also 'Coumarins and related drugs + NSAIDs', p.449.

1. Perucca E. Drug interactions with nimesulide. *Drugs* (1993) 46 (Suppl 1), 79–82.
2. Auteri A, Bruni F, Blardi P, Di Renzo M, Pasqui AL, Saletti M, Verzuri MS, Scaricabarozzi I, Vargiu G, Di Perri T. Clinical study on pharmacological interaction between nimesulide and warfarin. *Int J Clin Pharmacol Res* (1991) 11, 267–70.

Coumarins + NSAIDs; Oxicam derivatives

Piroxicam increases plasma levels of *R*-acenocoumarol, and a few cases of raised INRs and bleeding have been reported when it was given with acenocoumarol or warfarin. In pharmacological studies, lornoxicam modestly increased the anticoagulant effects of warfarin, and possibly decreased the effect of phenprocoumon, but it did not interact with acenocoumarol. Studies have indicated that meloxicam does not interact with warfarin, and that tenoxicam does not interact with warfarin or phenprocoumon. Note that all NSAIDs increase the risk of bleeding, and an increased risk is seen when they are given with anticoagulants.

Clinical evidence

(a) Lornoxicam

In an open, crossover study in 6 healthy subjects, lornoxicam 8 mg twice daily for 7 days had no effect on the pharmacokinetics or the anticoagulant activity of a single 10-mg dose of **acenocoumarol** given on day 4.[1]

In an open, crossover study in 6 healthy subjects, lornoxicam 8 mg twice daily for 21 days increased the bioavailabilities of *S*- and *R*-phenprocoumon by 14% and 6%, respectively, and decreased their clearances by 15% and 6%, respectively, after a single 9-mg dose of **phenprocoumon** given on day 4. Despite the minor pharmacokinetic changes, statistically significant reductions in the activities of factors II and VII were seen.[2]

Lornoxicam 4 mg twice daily was given to 12 healthy subjects for 5 days, and then **warfarin** was added until a stable prothrombin time, averaging about 23.6 seconds, was achieved. The period to achieve this varied from 9 to 24 days, depending on the subject. The **warfarin** was then continued and the lornoxicam withdrawn, whereupon the mean prothrombin time fell to 19.5 seconds, the INR fell from 1.48 to 1.23 and the serum **warfarin** levels fell by 25%.[3]

(b) Meloxicam

In a group of 13 healthy subjects stabilised with INRs of 1.2 to 1.8, meloxicam 15 mg daily for 7 days did not significantly affect the pharmacokinetics of **warfarin** or INR values[4].

(c) Piroxicam

1. Acenocoumarol. In a single-dose study in healthy subjects, when piroxicam 40 mg was given with acenocoumarol 4 mg the AUC of the less active *R*-isomer was increased by 47% and its maximum plasma level was increased by 28%.[5]

In patients stabilised on acenocoumarol, piroxicam 20 mg daily for 2 weeks increased the effects of acenocoumarol in 4 out of 11 patients: the effect was considered mild in 3 patients, and significant in the fourth, although no specific values were given.[6] A further patient taking acenocoumarol developed gastrointestinal bleeding 3 days after starting to take piroxicam 20 mg daily. His INR rose from 2.2 to 6.5.[7]

2. Warfarin. A man stabilised on warfarin had a fall in his prothrombin time from a range of 1.7 to 1.9 times his control value to 1.3 when he stopped taking piroxicam 20 mg daily. The prothrombin times rose and fell when he re-started and then stopped the piroxicam.[8] Another patient taking warfarin had an increase in her prothrombin time (from a range of 16.5 to 18.1 seconds, up to 24.9 seconds) when piroxicam

20 mg daily was started, and a decrease when it was then stopped.[9] The INR of two Chinese patients rose to 4.5 and 4.2 after they were given piroxicam 20 mg daily and 0.5% topical piroxicam gel. One of them had bruises over the legs within 3 days.[10]

A woman who spread **warfarin** rat poison with her bare hands developed intracerebral bleeding, possibly exacerbated by piroxicam, which she took occasionally.[11]

(d) Tenoxicam

In single-dose and steady-state studies in a total of 16 healthy subjects, tenoxicam 20 mg daily for 14 days had no significant effect on the anticoagulant effects of **warfarin** or on bleeding times.[12] This report also mentions case studies in a small number of patients and healthy subjects, which similarly found that tenoxicam had no significant effect on the anticoagulant effects of **phenprocoumon**.[12]

Mechanism

Piroxicam inhibits the metabolism of *R*-acenocoumarol, but its effect on the metabolism of warfarin is unknown. Lornoxicam inhibited the metabolism of warfarin, but not acenocoumarol, *in vitro*.[13] In addition NSAIDs have antiplatelet effects, which can prolong bleeding if it occurs. They may also cause gastrointestinal toxicity. Because of these effects, in patients taking anticoagulants, the risk of bleeding is increased by NSAIDs.

Importance and management

The interaction of piroxicam with acenocoumarol would appear to be established, and case reports suggest that warfarin might be similarly affected. The UK manufacturer of piroxicam[14] contraindicates the concurrent use of anticoagulants, such as warfarin. This seems overly cautious; nevertheless, if piroxicam is given with a coumarin, it would be prudent to monitor the outcome well and anticipate the need to reduce the anticoagulant dose. Lornoxicam appears to have a similar effect with warfarin, although no cases of an interaction have been reported. Meloxicam and tenoxicam appear not to interact. However, care is still needed with every NSAID because, to a greater or lesser extent, they irritate the stomach lining, which can result in gastrointestinal bleeding, which will be more severe in anticoagulated patients. Consider also 'Coumarins and related drugs + NSAIDs', p.449.

1. Masche UP, Rentsch KM, von Felten A, Meier PJ, Fattinger KE. No clinically relevant effect of lornoxicam intake on acenocoumarol pharmacokinetics and pharmacodynamics. *Eur J Clin Pharmacol* (1999) 54, 865–8.
2. Masche UP, Rentsch KM, von Felten A, Meier PJ, Fattinger KE. Opposite effects of lornoxicam co-administration on phenprocoumon pharmacokinetics and pharmacodynamics. *Eur J Clin Pharmacol* (1999) 54, 857–64.
3. Ravic M, Johnston A, Turner P, Ferber HP. A study of the interaction between lornoxicam and warfarin in healthy volunteers. *Hum Exp Toxicol* (1990) 9, 413–14.
4. Türck D, Su CAPF, Heinzel G, Busch U, Bluhmki E, Hoffmann J. Lack of interaction between meloxicam and warfarin in healthy volunteers. *Eur J Clin Pharmacol* (1997) 51, 421–5.
5. Bonnabry P, Desmeules J, Rudaz S, Leemann T, Veuthey J-L, Dayer P. Stereoselective interaction between piroxicam and acenocoumarol. *Br J Clin Pharmacol* (1996) 41, 525–30.
6. Jacotot B. Interaction of piroxicam with oral anticoagulants. 9th European Congress of Rheumatology, Wiesbaden, September 1979, pp 46–47.
7. Desprez D, Blanc P, Larrey D, Michel H. Hémorragie digestive favorisée par une hypocoagulation excessive due à une interaction médicamenteuse piroxicam — antagoniste de la vitamine K. *Gastroenterol Clin Biol* (1992) 16, 906–7.
8. Rhodes RS, Rhodes PJ, Klein C, Sintek CD. A warfarin-piroxicam drug interaction. *Drug Intell Clin Pharm* (1985) 19, 556–8.
9. Mallet L, Cooper JW. Prolongation of prothrombin time with the use of piroxicam and warfarin. *Can J Hosp Pharm* (1991) 44, 93–4.
10. Chan TYK. Drug interactions as a cause of overanticoagulation and bleedings in Chinese patients receiving warfarin. *Int J Clin Pharmacol Ther* (1998) 36, 403–5.
11. Abell TL, Merigian KS, Lee JM, Holbert JM, McCall JW. Cutaneous exposure to warfarin-like anticoagulant causing an intracerebral hemorrhage: a case report. *Clin Toxicol* (1994) 32, 69–73.
12. Eichler H-G, Jung M, Kyrle PA, Rotter M, Korn A. Absence of interaction between tenoxicam and warfarin. *Eur J Clin Pharmacol* (1992) 42, 227–9.
13. Kohl C, Steinkellner M. Prediction of pharmacokinetic drug/drug interactions from in vitro data: interactions of the nonsteroidal anti-inflammatory drug lornoxicam with oral anticoagulants. *Drug Metab Dispos* (2000) 28, 161–8.
14. Feldene (Piroxicam). Pfizer Ltd. UK Summary of product characteristics, July 2009.

Coumarins + NSAIDs; Phenazone (Antipyrine)

The anticoagulant effects of warfarin are reduced by phenazone.

Clinical evidence

The plasma **warfarin** concentrations were halved (from 2.93 to 1.41 micrograms/mL) and the anticoagulant effects reduced accordingly after 5 patients took phenazone 600 mg daily for 50 days.[1] The thrombotest percentage of one patient rose from 5% to 50%. In an associated study it was found that phenazone 600 mg daily for 30 days caused a reduction in the **warfarin** half-life from 47 hours to 27 hours and from 69 hours to 39 hours, respectively, in 2 patients.[1,2]

Mechanism

Phenazone is an enzyme inducer, which increases the metabolism and clearance of warfarin, thereby reducing its effects.[1,2]

Importance and management

An established interaction. The effects of concurrent use should be monitored and the dose of warfarin increased appropriately. However, note that phenazone is little used clinically, and an alternative NSAID that does not alter the metabolism of coumarins would be more appropriate (see 'Coumarins and related drugs + NSAIDs', p.449). Other coumarins might be expected to be similarly affected.

1. Breckenridge A, Orme M. Clinical implications of enzyme induction. *Ann N Y Acad Sci* (1971) 179, 421–31.
2. Breckenridge A, Orme ML'E, Thorgeirsson S, Davies DS, Brooks RV. Drug interactions with warfarin: studies with dichloralphenazone, chloral hydrate and phenazone (antipyrine). *Clin Sci* (1971) 40, 351–64.

Coumarins and related drugs + NSAIDs; Phenylbutazone and related drugs

The anticoagulant effects of warfarin are markedly increased by azapropazone, oxyphenbutazone and phenylbutazone. Feprazone appears to interact similarly.

Bleeding has also been seen in patients taking phenindione or phenprocoumon when given phenylbutazone, but successful concurrent use has been achieved with both phenprocoumon and acenocoumarol. Note also that all NSAIDs increase the risk of bleeding, and an increased risk is seen when they are given with anticoagulants.

Clinical evidence

(a) Azapropazone

A woman taking digoxin, furosemide, spironolactone, allopurinol, and **warfarin** (prothrombin ratio 2.8) developed haematemesis within 4 days of starting to take azapropazone 300 mg four times a day. Her prothrombin ratio was found to have risen to 15.7. Subsequent gastroscopic examination revealed a benign ulcer, the presumed site of the bleeding.[1]

Several other patients are reported to have developed this interaction. Bruising or bleeding (melaena, epistaxis, haematuria) and prolonged prothrombin times have occurred within a few days of starting azapropazone.[2-4] Two patients died.[3,4]

(b) Feprazone

Five patients stabilised on **warfarin** had a mean prothrombin time rise from 29 seconds to 38 seconds after taking feprazone 200 mg twice daily for 5 days, despite a 40% reduction in the **warfarin** dose (from 5 to 3 mg daily). Four days after feprazone was stopped, their prothrombin times were almost back to usual. The interaction with feprazone was less marked than that with phenylbutazone.[5]

(c) Oxyphenbutazone

A man stabilised on **warfarin** developed gross haematuria within 9 days of starting to take oxyphenbutazone 400 mg daily. His prothrombin time had increased to 68 seconds.[6] Two similar cases have been described elsewhere.[7,8] A clinical study has found that oxyphenbutazone slows the clearance of **dicoumarol**.[9]

(d) Phenylbutazone

In a study in 3 subjects and one patient, phenylbutazone 200 mg three times daily and twice daily, respectively, given for 11 to 19 days before and 11 days after a single dose of **warfarin**, markedly increased the prothrombin time, but *decreased* the half-life of **warfarin**, and the **warfarin** AUC.[10] In another study that gave the enantiomers of **warfarin** separately, it was found that phenylbutazone inhibited the clearance of *S*-warfarin, but increased the clearance of *R*-warfarin.[11] This was confirmed in other studies, where the AUC of *R*-warfarin was decreased by 41% and the AUC of *S*-warfarin increased by 18%.[12]

A number of other studies have found markedly increased prothrombin times in patients[5,13] or healthy subjects[14] taking **warfarin** and given phenylbutazone. Moreover, there are a number of case reports demonstrating the clinical importance of this interaction.[10,15-19] In one, a man stabilised on **warfarin** following mitral valve replacement was later given phenylbutazone for back pain by his general practitioner. On admission to hospital a week later he had epistaxis, and his face, legs and arms had begun to swell. He had extensive bruising of the jaw, elbow and calves, some evidence of gastrointestinal bleeding, and a prothrombin time of 89 seconds. Two similar cases have also been reported.[18] A similar interaction occurs between phenylbutazone and **phenprocoumon**. In one study in healthy subjects, phenylbutazone 300 mg daily for 14 days doubled the prothrombin time response to a single dose of phenprocoumon given on day 4, while decreasing the phenprocoumon AUC by 31%.[20] Cases of a clinically important interaction have also been reported for **phenprocoumon**.[21] In one early report, the required dose of **acenocoumarol** was 25% lower in patients taking phenylbutazone.[22] A single unconfirmed report describes this interaction in two patients taking **phenindione**.[23]

Mechanism

Phenylbutazone very effectively displaces the coumarins and indanediones from their plasma protein binding sites, thereby increasing the concentrations of free and active anticoagulant (an effect easily demonstrated *in vitro*[10,24-28]). By itself, the importance of this mechanism is usually small, since any displaced drug is then available to be cleared, so any effect is usually transient (see 'Protein-binding interactions', p.3). However, phenylbutazone also inhibits the metabolism of *S*-warfarin (the more potent of the two warfarin enantiomers) so its effects are increased and prolonged.[11,12,29] In studies, the unbound clearance of *S*-warfarin was decreased about three- to four-fold.[29,30] In contrast, the unbound clearance of *R*-warfarin is not altered, so the total clearance of *R*-warfarin is increased due to displacement.[29] Thus, overall, it appears that phenylbutazone decreases total plasma warfarin levels, while increasing its effect. Azapropazone[31-33] and oxyphenbutazone (the major metabolite of phenylbutazone) probably act similarly.

Importance and management

The pharmacokinetic interaction between warfarin and azapropazone or phenylbutazone is very well established and clinically important. Serious bleeding can result and concurrent use should be avoided. Feprazone and oxyphenbutazone appear to interact similarly. Much less is known about phenindione with phenylbutazone, but they probably interact similarly.[23] Direct evidence of a serious interaction with phenprocoumon seems to be limited to two reports, and there is some evidence (from one paper published in 1957) that successful and apparently uneventful concurrent use is possible, presumably because in the case cited the response and the anticoagulant doses were carefully controlled.[34] However, the practicalities of such close monitoring outside of a study are unclear. One study found that 25% less acenocoumarol was needed in patients given phenylbutazone.[22] Remember too that phenylbutazone and related drugs affect platelet aggregation and can cause gastrointestinal bleeding, and the risk of this is increased in patients taking an anticoagulant. It would seem advisable to use an alternative NSAID that interacts to a lesser extent, such as ibuprofen or naproxen, although it should be noted that no NSAID is entirely free from interactions with anticoagulants. Consider also 'Coumarins and related drugs + NSAIDs', p.449.

1. Powell-Jackson PR. Interaction between azapropazone and warfarin. *BMJ* (1977) 1, 1193–4.
2. Green AE, Hort JF, Korn HET, Leach H. Potentiation of warfarin by azapropazone. *BMJ* (1977) 1, 1532.
3. Anon. Interactions. Doctors warned on warfarin dangers. *Pharm J* (1983) 230, 676.
4. Win N, Mitchell DC, Jones PAE, French EA. Azapropazone and warfarin. *BMJ* (1991) 302, 969–70.
5. Chierichetti S, Bianchi G, Cerri B. Comparison of feprazone and phenylbutazone interaction with warfarin in man. *Curr Ther Res* (1975) 18, 568–72.
6. Taylor PJ. Hemorrhage while on anticoagulant therapy precipitated by drug interaction. *Ariz Med* (1967) 24, 697–9.
7. Hobbs CB, Miller AL, Thornley JH. Potentiation of anticoagulant therapy by oxyphenylbutazone (a probable case). *Postgrad Med J* (1965) 41, 563–5.
8. Fox SL. Potentiation of anticoagulants caused by pyrazole compounds. *JAMA* (1964) 188, 320–1.
9. Weiner M, Siddiqui AA, Bostanci N, Dayton PG. Drug interactions: the effect of combined administration on the half-life of coumarin and pyrazolone drugs in man. *Fedn Proc* (1965) 24, 153.
10. Aggeler PM, O'Reilly RA, Leong I, Kowitz PE. Potentiation of anticoagulant effect of warfarin by phenylbutazone. *N Engl J Med* (1967) 276, 496–501.
11. Lewis RJ, Trager WF, Chan KK, Breckenridge A, Orme M, Rowland M, Schary W. Warfarin. Stereochemical aspects of its metabolism and the interaction with phenylbutazone. *J Clin Invest* (1974) 53, 1607–17.
12. O'Reilly RA, Trager WF, Motley CH, Howald W. Stereoselective interaction of phenylbutazone with [$^{12}C/^{13}C$] warfarin pseudoracemates in man. *J Clin Invest* (1980) 65, 746–53.
13. Udall JA. Drug interference with warfarin therapy. *Clin Med* (1970) 77, 20–5.
14. Schary WL, Lewis RJ, Rowland M. Warfarin-phenylbutazone interaction in man: a long-term multiple-dose study. *Res Commun Chem Pathol Pharmacol* (1975) 10, 663–72.
15. Eisen MJ. Combined effect of sodium warfarin and phenylbutazone. *JAMA* (1964) 189, 64–5.
16. McLaughlin GE, McCarty DJ, Segal BL. Hemarthrosis complicating anticoagulant therapy. Report of three cases. *JAMA* (1966) 196, 1020–1.
17. Hoffbrand BI, Kininmonth DA. Potentiation of anticoagulants. *BMJ* (1967) 2, 838–9.
18. Bull J, Mackinnon J. Phenylbutazone and anticoagulant control. *Practitioner* (1975) 215, 767–9.
19. Robinson DS. The application of basic principles of drug interaction to clinical practice. *J Urol (Baltimore)* (1975) 113, 100–7.
20. O'Reilly RA. Phenylbutazone and sulfinpyrazone interaction with oral anticoagulant phenprocoumon. *Arch Intern Med* (1982) 142, 1634–7.
21. Sigg A, Pestalozzi H, Clauss A, Koller F. Verstärkung der Antikoagulantienwirkung durch Butazolidin. *Schweiz Med Wochenschr* (1956) 42, 1194–5.
22. Guggisberg W, Montigel C. Erfahrungen mit kombinierter Butazolidin-Sintrom-Prophylaxe und Butazolidin-prophylaxe thromboembolischer Erkrangungen. *Ther Umsch* (1958) 15, 227.
23. Kindermann A. Vaskuläres Allergid nach Butalidon und Gefahren kombinierter Anwendung mit Athrombon (Phenylindandion). *Dermatol Wochenschr* (1961) 143, 172–8.
24. O'Reilly RA. The binding of sodium warfarin to plasma albumin and its displacement by phenylbutazone. *Ann N Y Acad Sci* (1973) 226, 293–308.
25. Seiler K, Duckert F. Properties of 3-(1-phenyl-propyl)-4-oxycoumarin (Marcoumar®) in the plasma when tested in normal cases under the influence of drugs. *Thromb Diath Haemorrh* (1968) 19, 389–96.
26. Tillement J-P, Zini R, Mattei C, Singlas E. Effect of phenylbutazone on the binding of vitamin K antagonists to albumin. *Eur J Clin Pharmacol* (1973) 6, 15–18.
27. Solomon HM, Schrogie JJ. The effect of various drugs on the binding of warfarin-^{14}C to human albumin. *Biochem Pharmacol* (1967) 16, 1219–26.
28. O'Reilly RA. Interaction of several coumarin compounds with human and canine plasma albumin. *Mol Pharmacol* (1971) 7, 209–18.
29. Banfield C, O'Reilly R, Chan E, Rowland M. Phenylbutazone-warfarin interaction in man: further stereochemical and metabolic considerations. *Br J Clin Pharmacol* (1983) 16, 669–75.
30. Chan E, McLachlan A, O'Reilly R, Rowland M. Stereochemical aspects of warfarin drug interactions: use of a combined pharmacokinetic-pharmacodynamic model. *Clin Pharmacol Ther* (1994) 56, 286–94.
31. McElnay JC, D'Arcy PF. Interaction between azapropazone and warfarin. *BMJ* (1977) 2, 773–4.
32. McElnay JC, D'Arcy PF. The effect of azapropazone on the binding of warfarin to human serum proteins. *J Pharm Pharmacol* (1978) 30 (Suppl), 73P.
33. McElnay JC, D'Arcy PF. Interaction between azapropazone and warfarin. *Experientia* (1978) 34, 1320–1.
34. Kaufmann P. Vergleich zwischen einer Thromboembolieprophylaxe mit Antikoagulantien und mit Butazolidin. *Schweiz Med Wochenschr* (1957) 87 (Suppl 24), 755–9.

Coumarins + NSAIDs; Sulindac

Sulindac does not usually appear to significantly alter the anticoagulant effect of warfarin or phenprocoumon; however, isolated cases of a modest to marked increase in the anticoagulant effects of warfarin have been reported. Note that all NSAIDs increase the risk of bleeding, and an increased risk is seen when they are given with anticoagulants.

Clinical evidence

In a study in healthy subjects stabilised on **warfarin**, sulindac 200 mg twice daily for 7 days did not significantly alter the prothrombin time, when compared with placebo, although the prothrombin time was slightly higher in the sulindac group.[1] Similarly, in 20 patients stabilised on **phenprocoumon**, sulindac 200 to 400 mg daily for 4 weeks did not alter measures of coagulation or bleeding time.[2]

However, a patient stabilised on **warfarin**, ferrous sulfate, phenobarbital and sulfasalazine had a marked increase in his prothrombin time ratio from about 3.2 to 10 after taking sulindac 100 mg twice daily for 5 days.[3-5] There are 5 similar cases of this interaction on record.[1,5-8] One of the patients had a gastrointestinal bleed after taking only three 100-mg doses of sulindac, although this patient was also taking flurbiprofen.[5] Another patient was stabilised on about a 40% lower dose of **warfarin** with continuation of the sulindac.[6] Another patient had a potassium-losing renal tubular defect, which was thought to contribute to the interaction.[1] In one of these cases, the patient, who was also taking a corticosteroid, developed a retropharyngeal haematoma.[8]

Mechanism

Not understood. In one patient, renal impairment may have caused sulindac accumulation, which in turn may have affected warfarin pharmacokinetics.[1] See also 'Coumarins and related drugs + NSAIDs', p.449.

Importance and management

The pharmacological studies cited suggest that usually no coumarin dose adjustment would be needed in patients given sulindac. However, the isolated cases of an interaction suggest that, rarely, some patients may be affected. Also note that all NSAIDs can irritate the gastric mucosa, affect platelet activity and cause gastrointestinal bleeding, which will be more severe in anticoagulated patients. Consider also 'Coumarins and related drugs + NSAIDs', p.449.

1. Loftin JP, Vesell ES. Interaction between sulindac and warfarin: different results in normal subjects and in an unusual patient with a potassium-losing renal tubular defect. *J Clin Pharmacol* (1979) 19, 733–42.
2. Schenk H, Klein G, Haralambus J, Goebel R. Coumarintherapie unter dem antirheumaticum sulindac. *Z Rheumatol* (1980) 39, 102–8.
3. Beeley L. *Adverse Drug React Bull* (1978) No. 6.
4. Beeley L, Baker S. Personal communication, 1978.
5. Ross JRY, Beeley L. Sulindac, prothrombin time, and anticoagulants. *Lancet* (1979) ii, 1075.
6. Carter SA. Potential effect of sulindac on response of prothrombin-time to oral anticoagulants. *Lancet* (1979) ii, 698–9.
7. McQueen EG. New Zealand Committee on Adverse Drug Reactions. 17th Annual Report 1982. *N Z Med J* (1983) 96, 95–9.
8. Thatcher J, George D. Retropharyngeal hematoma as a new cause of acute upper airway obstruction in rheumatoid arthritis. *J Rheumatol* (1987) 14, 1172–3.

Coumarins + NSAIDs; Tolmetin

In pharmacological studies, tolmetin did not alter the anticoagulant effect of the coumarins; however, isolated cases of raised INRs have been described. Note that all NSAIDs increase the risk of bleeding, and an increased risk is seen when they are given with anticoagulants.

Clinical evidence

In a placebo-controlled study, no changes in prothrombin times occurred in 15 healthy subjects stabilised on **warfarin** when they took tolmetin 400 mg three times daily for 14 days.[1] Similarly, no changes in prothrombin times occurred in 15 patients taking **phenprocoumon** when they were given tolmetin 200 mg four times daily for 10 days.[2] Bleeding times were reported to be slightly prolonged, though not to a clinically relevant extent.[2] Bleeding times were not significantly altered in healthy subjects given **acenocoumarol** and tolmetin 400 mg twice daily, or patients taking **acenocoumarol** and tolmetin.[3] However, there is a single published case report of a diabetic patient stabilised on **warfarin**, insulin, digoxin, theophylline, ferrous sulfate, furosemide and sodium polystyrene sulfonate who had a nosebleed after taking three 400-mg doses of tolmetin. His prothrombin time had risen from a range of 15 to 22 seconds up to 70 seconds.[4] The manufacturers of tolmetin and the FDA in the US also have 10 other cases on record involving tolmetin and warfarin,[4,5] received over a 10-year period.[5]

Mechanism

See 'Coumarins and related drugs + NSAIDs', p.449.

Importance and management

The pharmacological studies cited suggest that usually no coumarin dose adjustment would be needed in patients given tolmetin. The isolated cases of an interaction are unexplained. However, care is needed with every NSAID because, to a greater or lesser extent, they irritate the stomach lining, which can result in gastrointestinal bleeding, which will be more severe in anticoagulated patients. Consider also 'Coumarins and related drugs + NSAIDs', p.449.

1. Whitsett TL, Barry JP, Czerwinski AW, Hall WH, Hampton JW. Tolmetin and warfarin: a clinical investigation to determine if interaction exists. In 'Tolmetin, A New Non-steroidal Anti-Inflammatory Agent.' Ward JR (ed). Proceedings of a Symposium, Washington DC, April 1975, Excerpta Medica, Amsterdam, New York, p. 160–7.
2. Rüst O, Biland L, Thilo D, Nyman D, Duckert F. Prüfung des Antirheumatikums Tolmetin auf Interaktionen mit oralen Antikoagulantien. *Schweiz Med Wochenschr* (1975) 105, 752–3.
3. Malbach E. Über die Beeinflussung der Blutungszeit durch Tolectin. *Schweiz Rundsch Med Prax* (1978) 67, 161–3.
4. Koren JF, Cochran DL, Janes RL. Tolmetin-warfarin interaction. *Am J Med* (1987) 82, 1278–9.
5. Santopolo AC. Tolmetin-warfarin interaction. *Am J Med* (1987) 82, 1279–80.

Coumarins + Nystatin

A case series reported raised INRs and bleeding in patients stable taking warfarin and given nystatin oral suspension.

Clinical evidence

A retrospective case series identified patients who had been stable taking warfarin between 2002 and 2010 and who had also been given topical antifungals, including nystatin oral solution. Eight patients given nystatin oral solution for at least one week had raised INRs: the INR was increased from a mean of 2.5 (range 1.99 to 3.5) to 10.6 (range 4.5 to 19.3). The mean warfarin dose required by patients using nystatin was reduced, from 14.5 mg before nystatin was started to 9 mg after nystatin was started. Bleeding occurred in 4 of the 8 patients, resulting in haematuria (2 patients), haematoma (one patient) and rectal bleeding with haematoma (one patient): 2 of these patients needed treating with frozen fresh plasma infusions. The authors state that none of the patients were recorded as having any dietary changes, altered alcohol intake or taking other potentially interacting drugs.[1]

Mechanism

Unknown. Nystatin is not known to affect cytochrome P450 and would therefore not be expected to interact with warfarin by this mechanism.

Importance and management

An interaction between warfarin and nystatin is not yet established. This case series appears to be the only published report of an interaction between warfarin and nystatin and given its nature, a definitive conclusion cannot be drawn from its findings. Further study is needed to establish if an interaction occurs, and if so, its underlying mechanism. Nevertheless, until more is known, it would seem prudent to bear this report in mind should any otherwise unexplained change in anticoagulation control occur in patients taking warfarin and given nystatin.

1. Kovac M, Mitic G, Kovac Z. Miconazole and nystatin used as topical antifungal drugs interact equally strongly with warfarin. *J Clin Pharm Ther* (2012) 37, 45.

Coumarins + Olanzapine

A single dose of olanzapine did not alter the pharmacokinetics or anticoagulant effect of a single dose of warfarin.

Clinical evidence, mechanism, importance and management

In a three-way, randomised, crossover study, 15 healthy subjects were given olanzapine 10 mg, **warfarin** 20 mg or both drugs together as single doses. No significant changes were seen in the pharmacokinetics of either drug, and the adverse effects of the olanzapine and the anticoagulant effects of the **warfarin** were unchanged.[1] Similarly, a 71-year-old woman stabilised on **warfarin** 15 mg/week with an INR of 2.6 had no significant change in her INR after taking olanzapine 20 mg daily for 6 weeks (INR 2.6 when taking 15 mg/week and 2 while taking 12.5 mg/week).[2] This evidence suggests that no **warfarin** dose adjustments are expected to be needed on concurrent use with olanzapine.

1. Maya JF, Callaghan JT, Bergstrom RF, Cerimele BJ, Kassahun K, Nyhart EH, Brater DC. Olanzapine and warfarin drug interaction. *Clin Pharmacol Ther* (1997) 61, 182.
2. Rogers T, de Leon J, Atcher D. Possible interaction between warfarin and quetiapine. *J Clin Psychopharmacol* (1999) 19, 382–3.

Coumarins + Opioids; Codeine

Codeine does not alter the anticoagulant effect of warfarin.

Clinical evidence, mechanism, importance and management

In a crossover study in 15 patients stabilised on **warfarin** and with osteoarthritis pain, codeine phosphate 7 to 15 mg three or four times daily for 5 weeks did not alter the mean INR when compared with celecoxib[1] (see 'Coumarins and related drugs + NSAIDs; Coxibs', p.450).

Codeine was used as a control analgesic in this study because it does not interact with **warfarin**, although this appears to be based on the absence of any evidence of an interaction, and the fact that it is unlikely to alter **warfarin** metabolism, rather than any direct evidence. Nevertheless, the lack of an interaction in this study suggests that codeine is not expected to alter **warfarin** dosing requirements.

1. Dentali F, Douketis JD, Woods K, Thabane L, Foster G, Holbrook A, Crowther M. Does celecoxib potentiate the anticoagulant effect of warfarin? A randomized, double-blind, controlled trial. *Ann Pharmacother* (2006) 40, 1241–7.

Coumarins + Opioids; Dextropropoxyphene (Propoxyphene)

In one study, dextropropoxyphene did not alter the prothrombin time in patients taking unspecified coumarins. There are isolated cases of patients taking warfarin who have had a marked increase in their prothrombin time and/or bleeding when given co-proxamol (dextropropoxyphene with paracetamol (acetaminophen)).

Clinical evidence

(a) Dextropropoxyphene

A double-blind study in 23 patients anticoagulated with un-named coumarins and given dextropropoxyphene 450 mg daily for 15 days or ibuprofen did not find any change in prothrombin times with either drug.[1]

(b) Dextropropoxyphene with Paracetamol (Acetaminophen)

A man taking **warfarin** developed marked haematuria within 6 days of starting to take two tablets of co-proxamol three times daily. Thirteen days previously his **warfarin** dose had been increased from 6 mg to 7 mg daily (thrombotest 16%), and then 9 days previously it had been reduced back to 6 mg daily (thrombotest 5%). His plasma **warfarin** levels had risen by one-third (from 1.8 to 2.4 micrograms/mL) despite the reduction in **warfarin** dose.[2] A woman, stable for 6 weeks on **warfarin**, developed gross haematuria 11 hours after starting co-proxamol. She had taken 6 tablets of co-proxamol over a 6-hour period. Her prothrombin time increased from about 30 to 40 seconds up to 130 seconds.[2]

This interaction has been reported in several other patients taking **warfarin**.[3-6] The prothrombin time of one of them rose from 28 to 44 seconds up to 80 seconds within 3 days of substituting paracetamol with two tablets of co-proxamol four times daily.[4] Another developed a prothrombin time of more than 50 seconds after taking 30 tablets of *Darvocet-N 100* (dextropropoxyphene 100 mg, paracetamol 650 mg) and possibly an unknown amount of ibuprofen over a 3-day period.[5]

Mechanism

Not understood. The effect dextropropoxyphene has on the metabolism of the warfarin enantiomers does not appear to have been studied. Dextropropoxyphene does not interact with other cytochrome P450 isoenzyme CYP2C9 substrates such as tolbutamide (see 'Antidiabetics + Dextropropoxyphene (Propoxyphene)', p.507), although it does interact with the CYP3A4 substrate carbamazepine (see 'Carbamazepine and related drugs + Dextropropoxyphene (Propoxyphene)', p.570). There is also the possibility that the paracetamol component had some part to play (see also 'Coumarins and related drugs + Paracetamol (Acetaminophen)', p.459). Alternatively, these cases may just represent idiosyncratic reactions.

Importance and management

Information about this interaction is very sparse and seems to be limited to the reports cited. The cases cited could just be idiosyncratic reactions. Bear them in mind in the event of an unexpected response to treatment.

1. Franchimont P, Heynen G. Comparative study of ibuprofen and dextropropoxyphene in scapulo-humeral periarthritis following myocardial infarction. 13th International Congress of Rheumatol, Kyoto, Japan. 30th Sept–6th Oct 1973.
2. Orme M, Breckenridge A, Cook P. Warfarin and Distalgesic interaction. *BMJ* (1976) i, 200.
3. Jones RV. Warfarin and Distalgesic interaction. *BMJ* (1976) i, 460.
4. Smith R, Prudden D, Hawkes C. Propoxyphene and warfarin interaction. *Drug Intell Clin Pharm* (1984) 18, 822.
5. Justice JL, Kline SS. Analgesics and warfarin. A case that brings up questions and cautions. *Postgrad Med* (1988) 83, 217-8, 220.
6. Pilszek FH, Moloney D, Sewell JR. Case report: increased anticoagulant effect of warfarin in patient taking a small dose of co-proxamol. Personal communication, 1994.

Coumarins + Opioids; Hydrocodone

In an isolated report, the anticoagulant effects of warfarin were increased by hydrocodone in one patient and in one healthy subject.

Clinical evidence, mechanism, importance and management

A patient, stabilised on **warfarin** (and also taking digoxin, propranolol, clofibrate and spironolactone) had a rise in his prothrombin time of about 2 to 3 times his control value when he began to take *Tussionex* (hydrocodone with phenyltoloxamine) for a chronic cough. When the cough syrup was discontinued, his prothrombin time fell again. In a subsequent study in one healthy subject the equivalent dose of hydrocodone increased the elimination half-life of **warfarin** from 30 hours to 42 hours.[1] The reason for this interaction is not known, and this early report appears to be the only information available. Any interaction is not therefore established.

1. Azarnoff DL. Drug interactions: the potential for adverse effects. *Drug Inf J* (1972) 6, 19–25.

Coumarins + Opioids; Meptazinol

The anticoagulant effects of warfarin were not altered by meptazinol in one study.

Clinical evidence, mechanism, importance and management

Meptazinol 200 mg four times daily for 7 days had no significant effect on the prothrombin indexes of 6 elderly patients stabilised on **warfarin**, nor on the required **warfarin** dose.[1] No **warfarin** dose adjustments would be expected to be needed on concurrent use.

1. Ryd-Kjellen E, Alm A. Effect of meptazinol on chronic anticoagulant therapy. *Hum Toxicol* (1986) 5, 101–2.

Coumarins and related drugs + Opioids; Tramadol

In one study tramadol did not change the mean INR in response to phenprocoumon, although two patients had INR increases. Isolated cases of an increase in anticoagulant effects of warfarin, acenocoumarol, phenprocoumon and fluindione have been reported in patients given tramadol. One retrospective cohort study also found an increased risk of

bleeding when acenocoumarol or phenprocoumon was given with tramadol.

Clinical evidence

In a double-blind, placebo-controlled, crossover study the mean INR of 19 patients anticoagulated with **phenprocoumon** was unchanged when they were given tramadol 50 mg three times daily for one week.[1,2] Although the mean difference was not changed, one patient had an INR rise from 4 to 7.3, and another had an INR rise from just under 5 to 6, while taking tramadol, but not while taking placebo.

A brief report describes 5 elderly patients (aged 71 to 84 years), anticoagulated with **warfarin** or **phenprocoumon** and taking a range of other drugs, who had clinically important rises in INRs (up to threefold) shortly after starting to take tramadol. One of the patients had gastrointestinal bleeding. Three of the patients were able to continue the tramadol with a reduced anticoagulant dose.[3]

In another report, a 61-year old woman with a mitral valve replacement stabilised on **warfarin** developed ecchymoses about 2 weeks after starting tramadol 50 mg every 6 hours. Her prothrombin time was found to have risen to 39.6 seconds and her INR was 10.6. These values returned to normal when the tramadol was withdrawn and **warfarin** was temporarily stopped.[4] Other cases have been reported with **warfarin**[5,6] and **phenprocoumon**.[7] In 2004, the Australian Adverse Drug Reactions Advisory Committee said they had received 11 reports of increases in INR or a haemorrhagic event in patients taking **warfarin** and given tramadol. Two patients died of haemorrhagic stroke. They note that this number of cases suggests that the interaction is an uncommon event.[8] Up until March 2003, the Swedish Adverse Drug Reactions Advisory Committee had received reports of 17 cases of a suspected interaction between tramadol and **warfarin** resulting in increases in the INR (to 3.4 to 8.5) and bleeding complications in 35% of patients. One patient who continued tramadol needed the **warfarin** dose to be almost halved.[9] The French regulatory authority has received 2 possible cases with **warfarin** and with the indanedione, **fluindione**, and one possible case with **acenocoumarol**; they note however, that other factors could have contributed to the cases reported.[10] The New Zealand regulatory authority has also commented on 4 possible cases with **warfarin**, two of which they considered were likely due to an interaction.[11]

In a retrospective cohort study of patients taking **acenocoumarol** or **phenprocoumon**, tramadol was associated with a threefold increased risk of hospitalisation for bleeding. The study specifically looked at potentially interacting drugs taken by at least 50 patients and with at least 5 cases of bleeding.[12]

Mechanism

Unknown. It has been suggested that the interaction might be related to a variation in a cytochrome P450 isoenzyme genotype. Seven of 10 patients from the 17 suspected cases of interaction in Sweden had defective CYP2D6 alleles. The authors suggested that as this isoenzyme metabolises tramadol, these patients might have changes in tramadol metabolism that could increase the risk of an interaction with warfarin by CYP3A4. However, CYP3A4 only has a role in the metabolism of *R*-warfarin and inhibition of CYP3A4 usually results in no more than a modest increase in INR. Moreover, defective CYP2D6 alleles have a population prevalence of 42.2%, so if this were the mechanism, many more cases would be expected. Because of the rarity of reports, it could just be that it is not really an interaction, and that there were unknown confounding factors in the suspected cases. Possible confounding factors include age, renal impairment, dehydration, under-nourishment, and other medications.[10]

Importance and management

An interaction between tramadol and coumarins or indanediones is not established. One pharmacological study did not show a clear interaction for phenprocoumon and tramadol, although data from 2 patients suggested the possibility. Moreover, isolated cases of an interaction with warfarin, acenocoumarol, phenprocoumon and fluindione have been published or reported to regulatory authorities, but the incidence seems to be low. Because of the uncertainty, it would be prudent to consider monitoring prothrombin times in any patient taking coumarins or indanediones when tramadol is first added, being aware that a small proportion of patients may need a reduction in the anticoagulant dose. Consider using an alternative, non-interacting opioid such as codeine, if appropriate. Further study is needed.

1. Boeijinga JK, van Meegen E, van den Ende R, Schook CE, Cohen AF. Lack of interaction between tramadol and coumarins. *J Clin Pharmacol* (1998) 38, 966–70.
2. Boeijinga JK, van Meegen E, van den Ende R, Schook CE, Cohen AF. Is there interaction between tramadol and phenprocoumon? *Lancet* (1997) 350, 1552.
3. Jensen K. Interaktion mellem tramadol og orale antikoagulantia. *Ugeskr Laeger* (1997) 159, 785–6.
4. Sabbe JR, Sims PJ, Sims MH. Tramadol-warfarin interaction. *Pharmacotherapy* (1998) 18, 871–3.
5. Scher ML, Huntington NH, Vitillo JA. Potential interaction between tramadol and warfarin. *Ann Pharmacother* (1997) 31, 646–7.
6. Dumo PA, Kielbasa LA. Successful anticoagulation and continuation of tramadol therapy in the setting of a tramadol-warfarin interaction. *Pharmacotherapy* (2006) 26, 1654–7.
7. Madsen H, Rasmussen JM, Brøsen K. Interaction between tramadol and phenprocoumon. *Lancet* (1997) 350, 637.
8. ADRAC. Tramadol-warfarin interaction. *Aust Adverse Drug React Bull* (2004) 23, 16.
9. Hedenmalm K, Lindh JD, Säwe J, Rane A. Increased liability of tramadol-warfarin interaction in individuals with mutations in the cytochrome *P450* 2D6 gene. *Eur J Clin Pharmacol* (2004) 60, 369–72.
10. Chiffoleau A, Veyrac G, Dudouet D, Miremont G, Merle L, David-Laroche M, Bourin M, Jolliet P. Tramadol et anticoagulants oraux: interaction ou facteurs confondants? *Therapie* (2003) 58, 471–4.
11. Savage R. Evidence for tramadol-warfarin interaction. *Prescriber Update* (2006) 27, 23–4.
12. Penning-van Beest F, Erkens J, Petersen K-U, Koelz HR, Herings R. Main comedications associated with bleeding during anticoagulant therapy with coumarins. *Eur J Clin Pharmacol* (2005) 61, 439–44.

Coumarins and related drugs + Orlistat

Orlistat had no effect on the pharmacodynamics or pharmacokinetics of single-dose warfarin in a study in healthy subjects. However, orlistat reduces fat absorption, and might therefore reduce vitamin K absorption. There is a published report of a patient taking warfarin who developed a modest increase in INR after taking orlistat. Similar cases have been reported to regulatory authorities.

Clinical evidence

In a placebo-controlled, randomised, crossover study, 12 healthy subjects were given orlistat 120 mg three times daily for 16 days, with a single 30-mg dose of **warfarin** on day 11. The pharmacokinetics and pharmacodynamics of the **warfarin** were not altered by the orlistat, and markers of vitamin K nutritional status were not affected.[1] However, regarding this study, the manufacturers US prescribing information states that vitamin K levels did tend to decline in subjects taking orlistat.[2] It is also noted that increased INRs and changes in the anticoagulant response have been reported in patients taking orlistat and anticoagulants.[2] In addition, in 2001 the Canadian regulatory authorities reported that unexpected increases in INR were noted after orlistat was given to patients taking either **warfarin** or **acenocoumarol**. These were managed by dose adjustments of the coumarin or discontinuing orlistat.[3]

In a published report, a 66-year-old man stabilised on **warfarin** for 2.5 years who started taking orlistat 120 mg three times daily for weight reduction had a modest increase in his INR, from less than 3, to 4.7 within 18 days. **Warfarin** was withheld and he was later restabilised on approximately two-thirds of the previous dose while continuing the orlistat.[4]

Mechanism

Orlistat may reduce the absorption of fat soluble vitamins including vitamin K,[4,5] and a change to a lower fat diet associated with the use of orlistat may also contribute to changes in the balance between vitamin K and **warfarin**.[4]

Importance and management

The manufacturers say that patients stabilised on anticoagulants [coumarins and **indanediones**] and given orlistat should be closely monitored for changes in coagulation parameters.[2,5] Given the reports of changes in INRs, and the fact that changes in dietary vitamin K (see 'Coumarins and related drugs + Food; Vitamin K_1-rich', p.432), are known to affect warfarin efficacy, this seems prudent in patients taking any coumarin or indanedione.

1. Zhi J, Melia AT, Guerciolini R, Koss-Twardy SG, Passe SM, Rakhit A, Sadowski JA. The effect of orlistat on the pharmacokinetics and pharmacodynamics of warfarin in healthy volunteers. *J Clin Pharmacol* (1996) 36, 659–666.
2. Xenical (Orlistat). Roche Pharmaceuticals. US Prescribing information, December 2013 .
3. Canadian Adverse Drug Reaction Monitoring Program. Communiqué. Orlistat (Xenical) interaction with coumarin derivatives: increased INR. *Can Adverse Drug React News* (2001) 11 (Jul), 7.
4. MacWalter RS, Fraser HW, Armstrong KM. Orlistat enhances warfarin effect. *Ann Pharmacother* (2003) 37, 510–12.
5. Xenical (Orlistat). Roche Products Ltd. UK Summary of product characteristics, April 2014.

Coumarins + Oseltamivir

No pharmacokinetic interaction occurs between oseltamivir and warfarin. However isolated cases of increased INRs have been reported.

Clinical evidence

In a randomised, crossover study, 20 patients taking warfarin, with a stable INR in the range 2 to 3.5 for at least 2 weeks before the study, were given oseltamivir 75 mg twice daily for 4.5 days or warfarin alone. Oseltamivir did not affect the pharmacokinetics of warfarin and had no clinically relevant effect on the INR. The pharmacokinetics of oseltamivir were no different to historical controls.[1] In contrast, a retrospective review of patients taking warfarin and oseltamivir between September 2009 and February 2010, found that of 15 patients whose INR had previously been stable and who had their INR measured with 10 days of starting oseltamivir, 7 had an increase in INR after oseltamivir was started (mean INR 2.08 prior to oseltamivir compared with 5.15 after). The INR of the other 8 patients remained stable. Bleeding events occurred in 3 of the patients whose INR was increased, and within 5 days of stopping warfarin their INRs returned to normal.[2]

Both the MHRA in the UK and Health Canada have received reports of an increase in clotting time when patients taking warfarin were given oseltamivir.[3,4] Between January 1999 and November 2005, Health Canada received 19 reports (11 submitted by the same source) of an increase in the INR in patients taking warfarin and given oseltamivir. However, in 3 of these cases the warfarin dose had been increased after starting oseltamivir, and in 2 cases the patients were taking other drugs known to interact with warfarin. Three cases of a *decrease* in the INR were also reported. On this basis, a causative relationship could not be established.[4] Anticoagulant control can be affected by influenza and its associated symptoms (such as fever and decreased appetite), and in 2009 the MHRA in the UK stated that there is no strong evidence to suggest that a drug interaction exists between oseltamivir and warfarin.[3]

Mechanism

Uncertain. Oseltamivir is not known to have an important effect on cytochrome P450 (by which warfarin is predominantly metabolised), and the study[1] supports the lack of a pharmacokinetic interaction.

Importance and management

Evidence for an interaction is limited and conflicting. No pharmacokinetic interaction occurs between warfarin and oseltamivir, but case reports of increased INR exist.

However, it is difficult to establish whether the cases reported represent a true drug interaction or an effect related to the patients underlying infection. On balance, it would seem unlikely that the effects seen are due to an interaction. However, until further data is available to confirm a lack of an interaction, it would be prudent to bear the case reports in mind if a patient taking warfarin develops an unexpected alteration in bleeding times after starting oseltamivir.

1. Davies, BE, Aceves Baldó P, Lennon-Chrimes S, Brewster M. Effect of oseltamivir treatment on anticoagulation: a cross-over study in warfarinized patients. *Br J Clin Pharmacol* (2010) 70, 834–43.
2. Lee SH, Kang HR, Jung JW, Kwon JW, Hong KS, Yu KS, Cho SH. Effect of oseltamivir on bleeding risk associated with warfarin therapy: a retrospective review. *Clin Drug Investig* (2012) 32, 131–7.
3. Medicines and Healthcare Products Regulatory Agency. UK Suspected Adverse Drug Reaction (ADR) Analysis: influenza antivirals – oseltamivir (Tamiflu) and zanamivir (Relenza), November 2009. Available at: http://webarchive.nationalarchives.gov.uk/20141205150130/http://www.mhra.gov.uk/home/groups/pl-p/documents/websiteresources/con062634.pdf (accessed 21/10/15).
4. Health Canada. Oseltamivir (Tamiflu) and warfarin: suspected increase in INR. *Can Adverse React News* (2006) 16, 1–2.

Coumarins + Oxolamine

Oxolamine markedly increases the effect of warfarin.

Clinical evidence, mechanism, importance and management

In a retrospective study, 11 patients were identified who had been receiving stable doses of **warfarin** and were then given oxolamine in doses of 100 to 600 mg daily for 3 to 10 days. Of six patients who did not have their **warfarin** dose adjusted, the INR increased by 70 to 190% from a range of 1.51 to 2.82 up to a range of 3.24 to 6.45. One patient had a **warfarin** dose reduction of 14%, with an INR increase from 2.29 to 9.11. Four patients had their **warfarin** dose reduced by 30 to 36%, but one of these still had an INR increase from 2.14 to 4.01. Two of the 11 patients developed a haematoma.[1] In a further prospective study, 6 patients receiving stable doses of **warfarin** were given oxolamine 300 to 600 mg daily for 4 to 7 days, and the **warfarin** dose was reduced by 50% on starting oxolamine. Three patients had no change in INR, one had a 24% increase and two had a 6% and 17% decrease.[1]

The mechanism of this interaction is unknown. Although published information is limited to this study, an interaction seems to be established. If any patient taking **warfarin** requires oxolamine, anticipate the need to roughly halve the **warfarin** dose.

1. Min KA, Zhu X, Oh JM, Shin WG. Effect of oxolamine on anticoagulant effect of warfarin. *Am J Health-Syst Pharm* (2006) 63, 153–6.

Coumarins and related drugs + Paracetamol (Acetaminophen)

A number of studies have found an increase in the anticoagulant effect of coumarins but fewer have reported no effect. The size of the increased effect seems to be only minor to modest. One retrospective cohort study reported that concurrent use tends to increase the incidence of upper gastrointestinal bleeding. There are isolated case reports of an increase in anticoagulant effects in patients taking warfarin, acenocoumarol, or fluindione with paracetamol.

Clinical evidence

Over 15 published studies have investigated whether or not paracetamol alters the effect of the coumarins, with fewer finding no effect than finding an increased effect, see 'Table 12.6', p.460. Nevertheless, all the randomised, controlled studies finding an interaction have demonstrated only a minor to modest effect (e.g. average increase in INR of 1.2 in one well-controlled study[1,2]). The only study to show a much greater effect (an increased odds ratio of an INR above 6 ranging from 3.5 to 10 for different doses of paracetamol alone or combined with an opioid) was a retrospective case-control study,[3,4] which has the limitations of being non-randomised with all the attendant problems of controlling for possible confounding variables.[5-7] Excluding this study, there appears to be no obvious explanation for the disparate findings between the studies finding an interaction and those not, either by study group, coumarin used, or dose of paracetamol.

There are only 7 published case reports of a possible interaction between paracetamol without opioids and a coumarin (**warfarin** or **acenocoumarol**), and two case reports of a possible interaction with the indanedione, **fluindione**, which are summarised in 'Table 12.6', p.460. In addition, there are two reports of a possible interaction with paracetamol combined with codeine or dihydrocodeine listed in 'Table 12.6', p.460, and 7 others with paracetamol combined with dextropropoxyphene (propoxyphene), see 'Coumarins + Opioids; Dextropropoxyphene (Propoxyphene)', p.457. Note that this incidence is very rare, given the widespread use of paracetamol, and the fact that it is generally considered safe for use with warfarin. Moreover, in response to one case-control study[3] other clinicians running outpatient anticoagulant clinics have contended that they have not seen an interaction with paracetamol in their experience.[6,7]

Mechanism

Not understood. It is possible that paracetamol or one of its metabolites inhibits the enzymes in the vitamin K cycle, and so has additive effects with anticoagulants.[2,8]

A pharmacokinetic interaction has been proposed, but this seems unlikely. Paracetamol does not inhibit CYP2C9, which is the major isoenzyme involved in the metabolism of *S*-warfarin.[9] Paracetamol is mainly metabolised by glucuronidation and sulfation,[10,11] but CYP1A2, CYP3A4, and CYP2E1 metabolise up to 15% of paracetamol under normal conditions.[10] *R*-warfarin is mainly metabolised by CYP3A4 and CYP1A2.[10,11] It has been suggested that in conditions such as ageing, hypoxia, or hypertension, the isoenzymes play a more important part in paracetamol metabolism. Consequently paracetamol might then theoretically compete with the metabolism of *R*-warfarin to a sufficient degree to provoke an interaction,[11] however, evidence to suggest that competition for metabolism by the same isoenzyme results in clinically relevant interactions is generally lacking. In addition, as the *S*-enantiomer has considerably greater anticoagulant activity than the *R*-enantiomer, interactions with *R*-warfarin are considered by some to be of questionable importance.[7] Moreover, this explanation might explain rare case reports, but not the small increases in INR seen in some studies in otherwise healthy subjects and patients.

Yet another idea is that it is the indications for paracetamol use such as pain or fever that cause the interaction, rather than paracetamol *per se*,[12] but this does not explain why an interaction has been found in otherwise healthy patients or subjects given paracetamol in controlled studies.

Importance and management

Despite the number of studies, an interaction between paracetamol and the coumarins is not firmly established, and the importance of the findings remain controversial. Some consider that the dose of paracetamol and its duration of use should be minimised in patients taking coumarins.[10,13] However, in randomised controlled studies, even maximum daily doses of paracetamol (4 g daily) for 2 weeks, had, at most, a modest effect, see 'Table 12.6', p.460. A dose-related effect has been suggested in a case-controlled study,[3] but a more recent randomised controlled study did not find a dose-response (i.e. there was a small change in INR of 0.5 with both 1.5 g daily and 3 g daily).[12] Further evidence is therefore required on the possible dose-response effect, and whether there is any value in minimising the dose. Moreover, on the basis of the studies suggesting an interaction, many have advocated increased monitoring in patients starting regular paracetamol. However, others consider that an increase in monitoring is unnecessary, or that increased monitoring during paracetamol use is not necessary unless the underlying illness (e.g. fever) requires increased monitoring. On the basis of the available data, it is not possible to firmly recommend increased monitoring, or dismiss its advisability. Further study is clearly needed.

Paracetamol is still considered to be safer than aspirin (see 'Coumarins and related drugs + Aspirin or other Salicylates', p.405) or NSAIDs (see 'Coumarins and related drugs + NSAIDs', p.449) as an analgesic in the presence of an anticoagulant because it does not affect platelets or cause gastric bleeding.

1. Mahé I, Bertrand N, Drouet L, Simoneau G, Mazoyer E, Bal dit Sollier C, Caulin C, Bergmann JF. Paracetamol: a haemorrhagic risk factor in patients on warfarin. *Br J Clin Pharmacol* (2005) 59, 371–4.
2. Mahé I, Bertrand N, Drouet L, Bal Dit Sollier C, Simoneau G, Mazoyer E, Caulin C, Bergmann J-F. Interaction between paracetamol and warfarin in patients: a double-blind, placebo-controlled, randomized study. *Haematologica* (2006) 91, 1621–7.
3. Hylek EM, Heiman H, Skates SJ, Sheehan MA, Singer DE. Acetaminophen and other risk factors for excessive warfarin anticoagulation. *JAMA* (1998) 279, 657–62.
4. Hylek EM. Acetaminophen and risk factors for excess anticoagulation with warfarin. *JAMA* (1998) 280, 697.
5. Gray CD. Acetaminophen and risk factors for excess anticoagulation with warfarin. *JAMA* (1998) 280, 695.
6. Amato MG, Bussey H, Farnett L, Lyons R. Acetaminophen and risk factors for excess anticoagulation with warfarin. *JAMA* (1998) 280, 695–6.
7. Riser J, Gilroy C, Hudson P, McCay L, Willis TA. Acetaminophen and risk factors for excess anticoagulation with warfarin. *JAMA* (1998) 280, 696.
8. Thijssen HH, Soute BA, Vervoort LM, Claessens JG. Paracetamol (acetaminophen) warfarin interaction: NAPQI, the toxic metabolite of paracetamol, is an inhibitor of enzymes in the vitamin K cycle. *Thromb Haemost* (2004) 92, 797–802.
9. Takigawa T, Tainaka H, Mihara K, Ogata H. Inhibition of S-warfarin metabolism by nonsteroidal antiinflammatory drugs in human liver microsomes *in vitro*. *Biol Pharm Bull* (1998) 21, 541–3.
10. Shek KLA, Chan L-N, Nutescu E. Warfarin-acetaminophen drug interaction revisited. *Pharmacotherapy* (1999) 19, 1153–8.
11. Lehmann DF. Enzymatic shunting: resolving the acetaminophen-warfarin controversy. *Pharmacotherapy* (2000) 20, 1464–8.
12. Gadisseur APA, van der Meer FJM, Rosendaal FR. Sustained intake of paracetamol (acetaminophen) during oral anticoagulant therapy with coumarins does not cause clinically important INR changes: a randomized double-blind clinical trial. *J Thromb Haemost* (2003) 1: 714–17.
13. Bell WR. Acetaminophen and warfarin: an undesirable synergy. *JAMA* (1998) 279, 702–3.

Coumarins + Pentoxifylline

Some studies have found that pentoxifylline does not alter the anticoagulant effects of phenprocoumon or acenocoumarol; however, one study suggests that there might be an increased risk of serious bleeding if pentoxifylline is given with acenocoumarol. Pentoxifylline alone has rarely been associated with bleeding.

Clinical evidence

The anticoagulant effects of **phenprocoumon** were not altered by pentoxifylline 400 mg four times daily for 27 days in 10 patients stabilised on **phenprocoumon**. Two patients had a slight increase in platelet aggregation.[1]

In a randomised study in patients with recurrent venous thrombosis, there was no difference in the dose of **acenocoumarol** necessary to reach an INR of 2.5 to 3.5 between 100 patients taking **acenocoumarol** with pentoxifylline 1.2 g daily and 100 patients taking **acenocoumarol** alone. No patients had severe bleeding, and 3% to 4% of patients in both groups had moderate bleeding (haematomas, haematuria).[2] However, in another placebo-controlled study of either pentoxifylline 400 mg three times daily, **acenocoumarol** (adjusted to maintain an INR of 2 to 4.5), or both drugs together, three major haemorrhagic problems (2 fatal cerebral, one gastrointestinal) occurred in the 36 patients taking both drugs. In the 36 patients taking **acenocoumarol** alone, one case of cerebral haemorrhage (resulting in hemiplegia) and another of

Table 12.6 Summary of the evidence for and against an interaction between paracetamol (acetaminophen) and coumarins or indanediones

Study type (year)	*Group*	*Coumarin*	*Paracetamol*	*Outcome*	*Refs*
Studies showing no interaction					
Randomised, crossover (1999)	20 healthy subjects	Warfarin, single-dose	1 g four times daily for one day, and 22 days	No change in warfarin pharmacokinetics or anticoagulant effect with either 1 day or 22 days	1
Clinical (1970)	10 patients	Stable warfarin	3.25 g daily for 2 weeks	No change in average prothrombin time	2
Randomised, placebo-controlled (1969)	20 patients	Phenprocoumon (19 patients) Warfarin (1 patient)	Two doses of 650 mg four hours apart	No change in average prothrombin time over 3 days	3
Randomised, placebo-controlled (2003)	31 patients	Phenprocoumon	Placebo (10 patients), 500 mg three times daily (11 patients), or 1 g three times daily (10 patients) for 2 weeks	Mean rise in INR of 0.46 at day 8 for both doses, which was not considered clinically relevant	4
Cohort (2002)	54 patients taking paracetamol and 180 others not taking paracetamol	Phenprocoumon	2 to 2.5 g per day for 3 days preceding INR determination	No change in anticoagulant effect	5
Cohort (recently started) (2002)	54 patients and 20 controls not given paracetamol	Acenocoumarol or phenprocoumon	Mean of 2.1 g daily	No difference in changes in INR between groups	6
Studies showing an interaction					
Randomised, placebo-controlled, crossover (1968)	50 patients	Stable warfarin, dicoumarol, anisindione,* phenprocoumon	650 mg four times daily for 2 weeks	Average increase in prothrombin time of 3.6 seconds	7
Randomised, placebo-controlled (1982, 1983)	20 patients	Stable acenocoumarol (8 patients) or phenprocoumon (12 patients)	500 mg four times daily for 3 weeks (10 patients); placebo (10 patients)	Average increase in thrombotest value of about 20 seconds (14% increase), which necessitated a reduction in coumarin dose in 5 patients	8,9
Randomised, placebo-controlled, crossover (1984)	15 healthy subjects	Stable warfarin	4 g daily for 2 weeks	7 of 15 subjects had a prothrombin ratio rise of more than 20% while taking paracetamol compared with 1 of 15 taking placebo	10
Randomised, placebo-controlled, crossover (2005, 2006)	19 patients	Stable warfarin	4 g daily for 2 weeks	INR increased by a mean of 1.20 to a mean maximum of 3.45 in patients taking paracetamol, but did not change with placebo	11,12
Case-control (1998)	93 cases with INR greater than 6 and 196 controls (INR 1.7 to 3.3)	Warfarin	325 mg each week to greater than 1.3 g daily	52 cases (56%) and 70 controls (36%) reported using paracetamol in the preceding week.† The increased risk (3.5 to 10-fold) was related to paracetamol dose	13
Cohort (2001)	4204 patients	Warfarin and/or Phenprocoumon		Standardised incidence ratio of hospitalisation for upper GI bleeding was higher with combined use of paracetamol (4.4) than oral anticoagulants alone (2.8)	14
Cohort (2007)	171 patients	Warfarin		Statistically significant increased risk of self-reported bleeding events (142 bleeds in 697 weeks, none of which were serious, for an odds ratio of 1.41)	15
Randomised, placebo-controlled (2007)	36 patients	Warfarin	1 g four times daily (12 patients), or 1 g twice daily with placebo twice daily (12 patients) or placebo four times daily (12 patients), for four weeks	Statistically significant increase in mean INR between placebo and both paracetamol groups (maximum mean increase in INR of 1 in the paracetamol 4 g group at week 3)	16
Case-control (2010)	53 patients with matched controls	Warfarin		Post-mortem analysis suggested that in patients taking warfarin with paracetamol the prevalence of a fatal bleed was 4.6 times higher when compared with paracetamol alone, and 2.7 times higher when compared with warfarin alone	17

*Note that this is an indanedione
†Including 11 cases and 6 controls who reported taking a preparation of paracetamol in combination with an opioid, mostly codeine and oxycodone
‡There are also cases reported with dextropropoxyphene/paracetamol., p.457

Continued

Table 12.6 Summary of the evidence for and against an interaction between paracetamol (acetaminophen) and coumarins or indanediones (continued)

Study type (year)	*Group*	*Coumarin*	*Paracetamol*	*Outcome*	*Refs*
Randomised, placebo-controlled (2011)	45 patients	Stable warfarin	2 g daily (18 patients), or 3 g daily (18 patients) or placebo (9 patients), for 10 days	Mean maximum INR increase of 0.7 and 0.67 for 2 g and 3 g paracetamol doses, respectively	18
Case reports of an interaction: paracetamol					
Case report (1999)	72-year-old	Acenocoumarol	1 to 2 g daily long-term	13 days after stopping paracetamol, the INR decreased from a range of 2.5 to 3 down to 1.62. INR gradually increased on restarting paracetamol	19
Case report (2004)	77-year-old	Acenocoumarol	2 to 2.5 g daily for a few weeks	INR 5.4 then 9.1 one week later. Patient restabilised on same acenocoumarol dose and asked not to take more paracetamol than 2 g daily for more than 3 days	20
Case report (2005)	72-year-old	Fluindione	4 g daily for 10 days for knee pain	INR of 8 with skin haematomas and gingival bleeding. Two weeks previously the INR had been 2.3	21
Case report (2006)	46-year-old	Fluindione	2 to 3 g daily for 10 days for phlebitis-related pain	INR of 4.46 decreased to 2.68 within 1 day of stopping paracetamol	22
Case report (2002)	62-year-old	Warfarin	4 to 5 g (duration not stated)	INR of 7.5, with retroperitoneal haematoma. One month previously the INR had been 2.5	23
Case report (2003)	74-year-old	Warfarin	a. 1 g twice daily for 3 days b. 1 g four times daily for 3 days	a. INR of 3.4 then 4 b. INR increased from 2.3 to 6.4	24
Case report (2004)	76-year-old	Warfarin	Patient recently taking more paracetamol for a flare of arthritis	INR increase from 2.1 to 7, with haematuria and gingival bleeding	25
Case report (2011)	89-year-old	Warfarin	3 to 4 g for one day	INR increased (up to 6.7) after taking paracetamol on day of BCG bladder instillations on 2 occasions. On 2 other occasions INR increases were averted by precautionary measures. Note that the patient also received single prophylactic doses of moxifloxacin with each bladder instillation, which has (rarely) been reported to interact (see Coumarins + Antibacterials; Quinolones, p.393)	26
Case report (2007)	81-year-old	Warfarin	4 g daily for 3 days then as required for 4 days (total dose not stated)	INR of 16.39 with gastrointestinal bleeding. INR fell to below 2 within 48 hours of treatment	27
Paracetamol in combination with opioids‡					
Case report (1991)	66-year-old	Warfarin	Paracetamol/codeine; about 1.6 g daily of paracetamol over 10 days	Increase in prothrombin time from range of 15 to 19 up to 96 seconds. Haematuria and gingival bleeding	28
Case report (1997)	63-year-old	Warfarin	a. Paracetamol/dihydrocodeine 500 mg/10 mg, four daily for 7 days b. Paracetamol/codeine 500 mg/30 mg, three daily for 8 days	a. Increase in INR to 9.6 then 12, with gingival bleeding b. Increase in INR to 8.5	29

*Note that this is an indanedione
†Including 11 cases and 6 controls who reported taking a preparation of paracetamol in combination with an opioid, mostly codeine and oxycodone
‡There are also cases reported with dextropropoxyphene/paracetamol., p.457

1. Kwan D, Bartle WR, Walker SE. The effects of acetaminophen on pharmacokinetics and pharmacodynamics of warfarin. *J Clin Pharmacol* (1999) 39, 68–75.
2. Udall JA. Drug interference with warfarin therapy. *Clin Med* (1970) 77, 20–5.
3. Antlitz AM, Awalt LF. A double blind study of acetaminophen used in conjunction with oral anticoagulant therapy. *Curr Ther Res* (1969) 11, 360–1.
4. Gadisseur APA, van der Meer FJM, Rosendaal FR. Sustained intake of paracetamol (acetaminophen) during oral anticoagulant therapy with coumarins does not cause clinically important INR changes: a randomized double-blind clinical trial. *J Thromb Haemost* (2003) 1, 714–17.
5. Fattinger K, Frisullo R, Masche U, Braunschweig S, Meier PJ, Roos M. No clinically relevant drug interaction between paracetamol and phenprocoumon based on a pharmacoepidemiological cohort study in medical inpatients. *Eur J Clin Pharmacol* (2002) 57, 863–7.
6. van den Bemt PMLA, Geven LM, Kuitert NA, Risselada A, Brouwers JRBJ. The potential interaction between oral anticoagulants and acetaminophen in everyday practice. *Pharm World Sci* (2002) 24, 201–4.
7. Antlitz AM, Mead JA ,Tolentino MA. Potentiation of oral anticoagulant therapy by acetaminophen. *Curr Ther Res* (1968) 10, 501–7.
8. Boeijinga J, Boerstra EE, Ris P, Breimer DD, Jeletich-Bastiaanse A. Interaction between paracetamol and coumarin anticoagulants. *Lancet* (1982) 1, 506.
9. Boeijinga JK, Boerstra EE, Ris P, Breimer DD, Jeletich-Bastiaanse A. De invloed van paracetamol op antistollingsbehandeling met coumarinederivaten. *Pharm Weekbl* (1983) 118, 209–12.
10. Rubin RN, Mentzer RL, Budzynski AZ. Potentiation of anticoagulant effect of warfarin by acetaminophen (TylenolR). *Clin Res* (1984) 32, 698A.

Continued

Table 12.6 Summary of the evidence for and against an interaction between paracetamol (acetaminophen) and coumarins or indanediones (continued)

11. Mahé I, Bertrand N, Drouet L, Simoneau G, Mazoyer E, Bal dit Sollier C, Caulin C, Bergmann JF. Paracetamol: a haemorrhagic risk factor in patients on warfarin. *Br J Clin Pharmacol* (2005) 59, 371–4.
12. Mahé I, Bertrand N, Drouet L, Bal Dit Sollier C, Simoneau G, Mazoyer E, Caulin C, Bergmann J-F. Interaction between paracetamol and warfarin in patients: a double-blind, placebo-controlled, randomized study. *Haematologica* (2006) 91, 1621–7.
13. Hylek EM, Heiman H, Skates SJ, Sheehan MA, Singer DE. Acetaminophen and other risk factors for excessive warfarin anticoagulation. *JAMA* (1998) 279, 657–62.
14. Johnsen SP, Sorensen HT, Mellemkjoer L, Blot WJ, Nielsen GL, McLaughlin JK, Olsen JH. Hospitalisation for upper gastrointestinal bleeding associated with the use of oral anticoagulants. *Thromb Haemost* (2001) 86, 563–8.
15. Shalansky S, Lynd L, Richardson K, Ingaszewski A, Kerr C. Risk of warfarin-related bleeding events and supratherapeutic international normalized ratios associated with complementary and alternative medicine: a longitudinal analysis. *Pharmacotherapy* (2007) 27, 1237–47.
16. Parra D, Beckey NP, Stevens GR. The effect of acetaminophen on the international normalized ratio in patients stabilized on warfarin therapy. *Pharmacotherapy* (2007) 27, 675–83.
17. Launiainen T, Sajantila A, Rasanen I, Vuori E, Ojanperä I. Adverse interaction of warfarin and paracetamol: evidence from a post-mortem study. *Eur J Clin Pharmacol* (2010) 66, 97–103.
18. Zhang Q, Bal-dit-Sollier C, Drouet L, Simoneau G, Alvarez JC, Pruvot S, Aubourg R, Berge N, Bergmann JF, Mouly S, Mahé I. Interaction between acetaminophen and warfarin in adults receiving long-term oral anticoagulants: a randomized controlled trial. *Eur J Clin Pharmacol* (2011) 67, 309–14.
19. Bagheri H, Bernhard NB, Montastruc JL. Potentiation of acenocoumarol anticoagulant effect by acetaminophen. *Ann Pharmacother* (1999) 33, 506.
20. Thijssen HH, Soute BA, Vervoort LM, Claessens JG. Paracetamol (acetaminophen) warfarin interaction: NAPQI, the toxic metabolite of paracetamol, is an inhibitor of enzymes in the vitamin K cycle. *Thromb Haemost* (2004) 92, 797–802.
21. Ornetti P, Ciappuccini R, Tavernier C, Maillefert JF. Interaction between paracetamol and oral anticoagulants. *Rheumatology* (Oxford) (2005) 44, 1584–5.
22. Wilouin F, Baune B, Lidove O, Papo T, Farinott R. Interaction entre le paracétamol et la fluindione: à propos d'un cas. *Thérapie* (2006) 61, 75–7. Correction. *ibid.*, (268).
23. Andrews FJ. Retroperitoneal haematoma after paracetamol increased anticoagulation. *Emerg Med J* (2002) 19. 84–5.
24. Gebauer MG, Nyfort-Hansen K, Henschke PJ, Gallus AS. Warfarin and acetaminophen interaction. *Pharmacotherapy* (2003) 23, 109–112.
25. Lesho EP, Saullo L, Udvari-Nagy S. A 76-year-old woman with erratic anticoagulation. *Cleve Clin J Med* (2004) 71, 651–56.
26. Lee R, Wen A, Berube C. Moxifloxacin-acetaminophen-warfarin interaction during bacille Calmette-Guérin treatment for bladder cancer. *Am J Health-Syst Pharm* (2011) 68, 814–7.
27. Dharmarajan L, Sajjad W. Potentially lethal acetaminophen-warfarin interaction in an older adult: an under-recognized phenomenon? *J Am Med Dir Assoc* (2007) 8, 545–7.
28. Bartle WR, Blakely JA. Potentiation of warfarin anticoagulation by acetaminophen. *JAMA* (1991) 265, 1260.
29. Fitzmaurice DA, Murray JA. Potentiation of anticoagulant effect of warfarin. *Postgrad Med J* (1997) 73, 439–40.

haematuria with epistaxis occurred. This difference was not statistically significant, but the authors considered that the risk of bleeding was probably increased by the combination.[3] In this study, 69% of patients had an INR within desired range, and 7% had an INR above 4.5.

Mechanism

Pentoxifylline alone has rarely been associated with bleeding,[4] which could potentially be more severe in patients taking anticoagulants. Nevertheless, the manufacturers say that a causal relationship between pentoxifylline and bleeding has not been established.[5,6]

Importance and management

Information is limited, and an interaction is not established. In the US, the manufacturer recommends that patients taking **warfarin** should have more frequent monitoring of coagulation parameters when given pentoxifylline,[6] and this might be a prudent precaution with this and any other coumarin.

1. Ingerslev J, Mouritzen C, Stenbjerg S. Pentoxifylline does not interfere with stable coumarin anticoagulant therapy: a clinical study. *Pharmatherapeutica* (1986) 4, 595–600.
2. Moriau M, Lavenne-Pardonge E, Crasborn L, von Frenckell R, Col-Debeys C. The treatment of severe or recurrent deep venous thrombosis. Beneficial effect of the co-administration of antiplatelet agents with or without rheological effects, and anticoagulants. *Thromb Res* (1995) 78, 469–82.
3. Dettori AG, Pini M, Moratti A, Paolicelli M, Basevi P, Qintavalla R, Manotti C, Di Lecce C and The APIC Study Group. Acenocoumarol and pentoxifylline in intermittent claudication. A controlled clinical study. *Angiology* (1989) 40, 237–48.
4. Oren R, Yishar U, Lysy J, Livshitz T, Ligumsky M. Pentoxifylline-induced gastrointestinal bleeding. *DICP Ann Pharmacother* (1991) 25, 315–16.
5. Trental 400 (Pentoxifylline). Sanofi-Aventis. UK Summary of product characteristics, October 2006.
6. Trental (Pentoxifylline). Sanofi-Aventis US LLC. US Prescribing information, October 2007.

Coumarins + Phosphodiesterase type-5 inhibitors

In pharmacological studies, sildenafil did not interact with warfarin or acenocoumarol. However, in patients with pulmonary hypertension, there is some evidence of an increased risk of bleeding with concurrent use, even though nosebleeds were a common adverse effect of sildenafil alone. Two possible cases of increased INRs have been reported in patients taking acenocoumarol or warfarin, and sildenafil. Studies suggest that avanafil, tadalafil, and vardenafil do not interact with warfarin.

Clinical evidence

(a) Avanafil

The US manufacturer briefly reports that, in a crossover study, 24 healthy subjects were given avanafil 200 mg daily for 9 days with a single 25-mg dose of **warfarin** on day 3. The AUC of *S*-warfarin was increased by about 1.6%, but its maximum concentration was decreased by 5.2%. Prothrombin times and INR were unchanged.[1]

(b) Sildenafil

The UK and US manufacturers of sildenafil note that no interaction occurred when sildenafil 50 mg was given with **warfarin** 40 mg,[2-5] or when sildenafil 100 mg was given with **acenocoumarol**.[4] However, in studies in patients with pulmonary hypertension, nosebleeds were a common adverse effect (9%), and the concurrent use of vitamin K antagonists and sildenafil resulted in a greater incidence of reports of bleeding (primarily nosebleeds; 9% compared with 2%) than placebo.[5]

A 68-year-old man taking **acenocoumarol** and enalapril had an increase in his INR from 3.05 to 7.7 without bleeding complications after taking sildenafil. The patient continued to take sildenafil once a week, and the daily dose of **acenocoumarol** was split into two, with a return to stable therapeutic INR values. Another patient taking **warfarin**, ranitidine, and pravastatin had an increase in INR on three occasions after taking sildenafil once a week, omitting the dose of ranitidine when he took the sildenafil. On one of these occasions, he had bleeding gums. This increase in INR no longer occurred when he started taking the ranitidine with the sildenafil.[6]

(c) Tadalafil

A double-blind, randomised, crossover study in which a single dose of **warfarin** was given on day 7 of 12 consecutive days of treatment with either tadalafil 10 mg or placebo found that tadalafil did not affect the AUCs of either *S*-warfarin or *R*-warfarin, and prothrombin times were unchanged.[7]

(d) Vardenafil

The UK and US manufacturers note that no pharmacokinetic interaction was observed when vardenafil was given with **warfarin**,[8,9] and the prothrombin time and other pharmacodynamic parameters were unchanged.[9]

Mechanism

An interaction as a result of altered coumarin metabolism is unlikely with any of these phosphodiesterase type-5 inhibitors. The two cases of interactions with sildenafil are unexplained. It is not obvious why dividing the acenocoumarol dose, or using ranitidine, would have reversed an interaction.

Sildenafil alone appears to commonly cause nosebleeds in patients with pulmonary hypertension. The reason for this is unknown, but studies with human platelets indicate that sildenafil potentiates the antiaggregatory effect of sodium nitroprusside *in vitro*.[2-5]

Importance and management

There is no established pharmacokinetic or pharmacodynamic interaction between the phosphodiesterase type-5 inhibitors and warfarin, and no warfarin dose adjustment would therefore be expected to be needed on concurrent use. However, in pulmonary hypertension, **sildenafil** appears to increase the risk of nosebleeds, and this might be greater in patients taking coumarins. Similarly, the two possible cases with acenocoumarol and warfarin, although not conclusive, do introduce a note of caution.

1. Stendra (Avanafil). Vivus, Inc. US Prescribing information, January 2015.
2. Viagra (Sildenafil citrate). Pfizer Ltd. UK Summary of product characteristics, June 2015.
3. Viagra (Sildenafil citrate). Pfizer Inc. US Prescribing information, March 2015.
4. Revatio Tablets (Sildenafil citrate). Pfizer Ltd. UK Summary of product characteristics, April 2015.
5. Revatio (Sildenafil citrate). Pfizer Inc. US Prescribing information, April 2015.
6. Fernández MA, Romá E. International normalized ratio increase in patients taking oral anticoagulant therapy and using sildenafil (Viagra®). *Haematologica* (2003) 88, ELT34.
7. Eli Lilly and Company. Personal communication, March 2003.
8. Levitra (Vardenafil hydrochloride). Bayer plc. UK Summary of product characteristics, April 2014.
9. Levitra (Vardenafil hydrochloride). Bayer Healthcare Pharmaceuticals Inc. US Prescribing information, April 2014.

Coumarins + Picotamide

Picotamide did not alter the anticoagulant effects of warfarin. Nevertheless, as with other antiplatelet drugs, concurrent use might increase the bleeding risk.

Clinical evidence, mechanism, importance and management

Picotamide 300 mg three times daily for 10 days did not alter the anticoagulant effects of established **warfarin** therapy in 10 patients with aortic or mitral valve prostheses.[1] No **warfarin** dose adjustments would therefore be expected to be needed on concurrent use. Nevertheless, as with other antiplatelet drugs, such as aspirin (see 'Coumarins and related drugs + Aspirin or other Salicylates', p.405), the concurrent use of oral anticoagulants might increase the risk or intensity of bleeding. Some caution is therefore appropriate on concurrent use.

1. Parise P, Gresele P, Viola E, Ruina A, Migliacci R, Nenci GG. La picotamide non interferisce con l'attività anticoagulante del warfarin in pazienti portatori di protesi valvolari cardiache. *Clin Ter* (1990) 135, 479–82.

Coumarins + Piracetam

Piracetam does not appear to affect the dose of acenocoumarol required to produce a given INR. A single case report describes a woman stabilised on warfarin who began to bleed within one month of starting to take piracetam.

Clinical evidence, mechanism, importance and management

In a randomised study in patients with severe or recurrent venous thrombosis, there was no difference in the dose of **acenocoumarol** necessary to reach an INR of 2.5 to 3.5 between 100 patients taking **acenocoumarol** with high-dose piracetam 9.6 g daily and 100 patients taking **acenocoumarol** alone. No patients had severe bleeding, and 3 to 4% of patients in both groups had moderate bleeding (haematomas, haematuria). The addition of piracetam decreased platelet aggregation, levels of fibrinogen, and blood viscosity.[1]

A woman taking **warfarin**, insulin, levothyroxine and digoxin complained of menorrhagia at a routine follow up. Investigations revealed that her British Corrected Ratio had risen to 4.1 (from a range of 2.3 to 2.8), and that one month previously she had started to take low-dose piracetam 200 mg three times daily. Within 2 days of withdrawing both the **warfarin** and piracetam her British Corrected Ratio had fallen to 2.07, and the original dose of warfarin was restarted.[2]

Piracetam alone is known to decrease platelet aggregation,[1] and might therefore be expected to increase the risk of bleeding with anticoagulants, similar to other drugs with antiplatelet activity such as aspirin (see 'Coumarins and related drugs + Aspirin or other Salicylates', p.405). The early case appears to be the only report of a possible interaction, but some caution might be prudent on concurrent use.

1. Moriau M, Lavenne-Pardonge E, Crasborn L, von Frenckell R, Col-Debeys C. The treatment of severe or recurrent deep venous thrombosis. Beneficial effect of the co-administration of antiplatelet agents with or without rheological effects, and anticoagulants. *Thromb Res* (1995) 78, 469–82.
2. Pan HYM, Ng RP. The effect of Nootropil in a patient on warfarin. *Eur J Clin Pharmacol* (1983) 24, 711.

Coumarins + Pirmenol

The anticoagulant effects of warfarin are not altered by pirmenol.

Clinical evidence, mechanism, importance and management

The prothrombin time response to a single 25-mg dose of **warfarin** was slightly reduced (reductions ranged from 0.2 to 1.3 seconds) in most of the 12 healthy subjects who had taken pirmenol 150 mg twice daily for 14 days, with warfarin taken on day 8.[1] This suggested that some changes in the dose of **warfarin** might be required in practice, but a later placebo-controlled study found that the prothrombin times of 10 patients stabilised on **warfarin** were not significantly changed when they were given oral pirmenol 150 mg twice daily for 14 days.[2] No **warfarin** dose adjustments would therefore be expected to be required on concurrent use.

1. Janiczek N, Bockbrader HN, Lebsack ME, Sedman AJ, Chang T. Effect of pirmenol (CI-845) on prothrombin (PT) time following concomitant administration of pirmenol and warfarin to healthy volunteers. *Pharm Res* (1988) 5, S-155.
2. Stringer KA, Switzer DF, Abadier R, Lebsack ME, Sedman A, Chrymko M. The effect of pirmenol administration on the anti-coagulant activity of warfarin. *J Clin Pharmacol* (1991) 31, 607–10.

Coumarins and related drugs + Prasugrel

The use of prasugrel with coumarins and indanediones may increase the risk of bleeding. Prasugrel does not affect the pharmacokinetics of S-warfarin.

Clinical evidence, mechanism, importance and management

The UK manufacturer reports that prasugrel has no effect on the metabolism of S-warfarin by CYP2C9.[1] The US manufacturer briefly reports that the concurrent use of prasugrel with **warfarin** 15 mg significantly prolonged bleeding times (amount not stated).[2] The concurrent use of prasugrel in patients taking other coumarins has not been studied.[1]

The UK manufacturer of prasugrel advises caution on the concurrent use of coumarins because of the theoretical possibility of an increased risk of bleeding.[1] If concurrent use is necessary, the patient should be monitored for signs of increased bleeding, and told to report any unexplained bruising or bleeding.[1]

Due to the actions of both drugs there is a possible increased risk of bleeding on the concurrent use of prasugrel and an **indanedione**. If prasugrel is given with an indanedione it would seem prudent to follow the same precautions advised for the coumarins.

1. Efient (Prasugrel hydrochloride). Eli Lilly and Company Ltd. UK Summary of product characteristics, December 2013.
2. Effient (Prasugrel). Eli Lilly and Company. US Prescribing information, November 2013.

Coumarins + Probenecid

In healthy subjects, probenecid increased the clearance of single-dose phenprocoumon without altering its anticoagulant effect. The anticoagulant effects of multiple-dose phenprocoumon might be expected to be decreased by probenecid, but this requires confirmation.

Clinical evidence, mechanism, importance and management

In 9 healthy subjects probenecid 500 mg four times daily for 7 days reduced the AUC of a single 0.22-mg/kg dose of **phenprocoumon** given on day one by 47% and reduced the elimination half-life by about one-third. Nevertheless, the reduction in prothrombin time by **phenprocoumon** was not altered by probenecid.[1]

The reasons for this interaction are not understood, but one possibility is that, while probenecid inhibits the glucuronidation of **phenprocoumon** (its normal route of metabolism), it may also increase the formation of hydroxylated metabolites so that its overall loss is increased.[1]

Although the anticoagulant effect of single-dose **phenprocoumon** was not altered in this study, its findings suggests that, in the presence of probenecid, the dose of phenprocoumon might need to be increased, but this awaits formal clinical confirmation in a multiple-dose study. Nevertheless, bear the possibility in mind. Nothing further seems to have been published on this potential interaction and there seems to be nothing documented about other coumarins.

1. Mönig H, Böhm M, Ohnhaus EE, Kirch W. The effects of frusemide and probenecid on the pharmacokinetics of phenprocoumon. *Eur J Clin Pharmacol* (1990) 39, 261–5.

Coumarins + Proguanil

An isolated report describes bleeding in a patient stabilised on warfarin after she took proguanil for about five weeks.

Clinical evidence

A woman stabilised on **warfarin** developed haematuria, bruising, and abdominal and flank discomfort about 5 weeks after starting to take proguanil 200 mg daily. Her prothrombin ratio was found to be 8.6. Within 12 hours of being given fresh frozen plasma and vitamin K her prothrombin ratio had fallen to 2.3. During the 5 weeks she had travelled from Britain to Thailand, Bali, Australia and then New Zealand, and her prothrombin ratio had not been checked during this time.[1]

Mechanism

If this case report does represent an interaction, the mechanism is unknown. The manufacturer speculates that proguanil possibly interferes with the metabolic pathway of warfarin and related anticoagulants.[2] However, this seems unlikely as there is no evidence that proguanil inhibits CYP2C9, the principal isoenzyme involved in the metabolism of warfarin.

Importance and management

The general importance of the isolated case describing an increased prothrombin ratio in a patient taking warfarin and proguanil seems limited, especially as factors related to travel (such as a changing diet and changing dose times in different time zones) might have had a part to play (see *Anticoagulant interactions*, under 'Anticoagulants', p.371, for a discussion of the fact that isolated cases of interactions with warfarin do not prove that an interaction occurs). Nevertheless, the manufacturer states that proguanil can potentiate the anticoagulant effect of warfarin and related anticoagulants, and they therefore advise caution when starting or stopping proguanil in a patient taking anticoagulants.[2] However, given the lack of evidence for a pharmacokinetic interaction coupled with an isolated unproven case report, it seems unlikely that any caution is required in patients taking a coumarin and given proguanil. Note that patients taking warfarin or a related anticoagulant and arranging travel should plan their anticoagulant therapy carefully (e.g. timing of doses).

1. Armstrong G, Beg MF, Scahill S. Warfarin potentiated by proguanil. *BMJ* (1991) 303, 789.
2. Paludrine (Proguanil hydrochloride). AstraZeneca UK Ltd. Summary of product characteristics, December 2009.

Coumarins + Prolintane

The anticoagulant effects of ethyl biscoumacetate are not affected by prolintane.

Clinical evidence, mechanism, importance and management

The response to a single 20-mg/kg dose of **ethyl biscoumacetate** was studied in 4 healthy subjects given prolintane 20 mg daily for 4 days. Assessments were made before prolintane, on day one of prolintane, and 8 days after prolintane was stopped. The mean half-life of the anticoagulant and prothrombin times remained unchanged.[1] No **ethyl biscoumacetate** dose adjustments would appear to be required on concurrent use.

1. Hague DE, Smith ME, Ryan JR, McMahon FG. The effect of methylphenidate and prolintane on the metabolism of ethyl biscoumacetate. *Clin Pharmacol Ther* (1971) 12, 259–62.

Coumarins and related drugs + Propafenone

The anticoagulant effects of warfarin, and possibly fluindione and phenprocoumon, are increased by propafenone.

Clinical evidence

The mean steady-state plasma levels of 8 healthy subjects taking **warfarin** 5 mg daily rose by 38% after they took propafenone 225 mg three times daily for a week. Five of the 8 had a distinct prothrombin time increase. The average rise in prothrombin time of the whole group was about 7 seconds, which was considered to be clinically significant.[1] Two case reports describe marked increases in the anticoagulant effects of **fluindione** and **phenprocoumon** in 2 patients taking propafenone.[2,3]

Mechanism

Propafenone may reduce the metabolism of these anticoagulants, thereby increasing their effects. From *in vitro* data, it was concluded that propafenone would affect only *R*-warfarin, whereas both *R*- and *S*-acenocoumarol were affected.[4]

Importance and management

Information seems to be limited to these reports but they suggest that anticoagulant control should be well monitored if propafenone is given to patients taking warfarin, and probably also phenprocoumon and the indanedione fluindione. The anticoagulant dose should be reduced where necessary. It would be prudent to apply the same precautions with any other coumarin or indanedione.

1. Kates RE, Yee Y-G, Kirsten EB. Interaction between warfarin and propafenone in healthy volunteer subjects. *Clin Pharmacol Ther* (1987) 42, 305–11.
2. Körst HA, Brandes J-W, Littmann K-P. Cave: Propafenon potenziert Wirkung von oralen Antikoagulantien. *Med Klin* (1981) 76, 349–50.
3. Welsch M, Heitz C, Stephan D, Imbs JL. Potentialisation de l'effet anticoagulant de la fluindione par la propafénone. *Therapie* (1991) 46, 254–5.
4. Hermans JJR, Thijssen HHW. Human liver microsomal metabolism of the enantiomers of warfarin and acenocoumarol: P450 isozyme diversity determines the differences in their pharmacokinetics. *Br J Pharmacol* (1993) 110, 482–90.

Coumarins and related drugs + Prostaglandins

The concurrent use of high-dose, intravenous epoprostenol and warfarin may increase the risk of pulmonary haemorrhage. Treprostinil does not appear to alter the pharmacokinetics or the anticoagulant effects of warfarin, and also did not appear to increase the risk of bleeding when used with warfarin in clinical studies. Beraprost did not alter the pharmacokinetics of fluindione. Inhaled iloprost did not appear to increase the incidence of bleeding in clinical studies in patients using anticoagulants. Because these prostaglandins inhibit platelet aggregation, some caution is appropriate on the concurrent use of anticoagulants.

Clinical evidence

(a) Beraprost

In a controlled study in 12 healthy subjects, oral beraprost sodium 40 micrograms three times daily for 3 days did not alter the pharmacokinetics of a single 20-mg dose of **fluindione** given on day 3. This dose of fluindione had only a marginal effect on the INR, and this effect was not altered by beraprost.[1]

(b) Epoprostenol

In a small retrospective review of 31 patients with primary pulmonary hypertension receiving **warfarin** and continuous intravenous epoprostenol, 9 patients were identified who experienced 11 bleeding episodes (9 cases of pulmonary haemorrhage, 2 of nasal bleeding). Of the 9 cases of pulmonary haemorrhage, 8 were identified clinically by persistent haemoptysis, and 2 cases were associated with severe respiratory distress. Of the 7 patients with an INR available at the time of the first bleeding episode, 6 had an INR under 2 and one had an INR of 3.1. The dose of epoprostenol in patients with bleeds ranged from 28.1 to 164 nanograms/kg per minute, and no patient receiving less than 28 nanograms/kg per minute had a bleed. There was no significant difference in survival in patients with a bleeding episode and those without.[2] In contrast, the manufacturer states that, in clinical studies, there was no evidence of increased bleeding in patients taking anticoagulants and receiving infusions of epoprostenol.[3]

(c) Iloprost

The manufacturer of iloprost notes that there was no difference in the incidence of bleeding between patients receiving inhaled iloprost and those given placebo in clinical studies in which a high proportion of patients were taking anticoagulants (unnamed). However, they note that bleeding events (mostly haematomas) were common.[4]

(d) Treprostinil

In a crossover study in 15 healthy subjects, continuous subcutaneous treprostinil 5 then 10 nanograms/kg every minute for 9 days did not alter the pharmacodynamics (INR) of a single 25-mg oral dose of **warfarin** given on day 3. In addition, there was no change in the pharmacokinetics of *R*- and *S*-warfarin.[5] In the discussion of this study, the authors mention an unpublished retrospective review of data from placebo-controlled clinical studies in patients with pulmonary artery hypertension. From this there was no evidence to suggest that the concurrent use of **warfarin** and treprostinil (155 patients) was associated with increased bleeding or coagulation-related events, when compared with warfarin and placebo (156 patients).[5]

Mechanism

Epoprostenol (prostacyclin) and its analogues beraprost, iloprost and treprostinil are vasodilators that also inhibit platelet aggregation. As such, it is anticipated that they might increase the potential for bleeding when given with anticoagulants.

Importance and management

Anticoagulants such as warfarin are commonly used in patients with pulmonary artery hypertension, a condition for which the prostaglandins beraprost, epoprostenol, iloprost and treprostinil are indicated, so the combination is likely to be used frequently. Because these prostaglandins are potent inhibitors of platelet aggregation, they might increase the risk of bleeding with anticoagulants (including coumarins and **indanediones**), although the manufacturers say that there was no evidence of increased bleeding in clinical studies using epoprostenol,[3] or treprostinil.[5] Nevertheless, limited evidence from the small survey in Japanese patients given epoprostenol suggests that this may be the case with high-dose epoprostenol. In this study, the authors commented that they no longer use anticoagulants in patients receiving high-dose epoprostenol.[2] However, the manufacturer states that in clinical studies of epoprostenol almost all patients with pulmonary hypertension were receiving oral anticoagulants, and, unless contraindicated, they recommend concurrent oral anticoagulation in those patients with either primary pulmonary hypertension or pulmonary hypertension secondary to scleroderma to reduce the risk of thromboembolism.[3] Some caution would be appropriate if any of these prostaglandins is given with a coumarin or **indanedione**.

Some prostaglandins, such as epoprostenol, may also be used for other indications, such as maintaining renal dialysis catheter patency or for treating peripheral ischaemia: similar caution should be used if these patients are taking anticoagulants.[6]

1. Warot D, Berlin I, Aymard G, Ankri A, Fabry C, Besse B, Lechat P, Diquet B. Beraprost sodium-fluindione combination in healthy subjects: pharmacokinetic and pharmacodynamic aspects. *Fundam Clin Pharmacol* (2000) 14, 231–6.
2. Ogawa A, Matsubara H, Fujio H, Miyaji K, Nakamura K, Morita H, Saito H, Fukushima Kusano K, Emori T, Date H, Ohe T. Risk of alveolar hemorrhage in patients with primary pulmonary hypertension: anticoagulation and epoprostenol therapy. *Circ J* (2005) 69, 216–20.
3. Flolan (Epoprostenol sodium). GlaxoSmithKline. US Prescribing information, January 2008.
4. Ventavis (Iloprost trometamol). Bayer plc. UK Summary of product characteristics, July 2011.
5. Wade M, Hunt TL, Lai AA. Effect of continuous subcutaneous treprostinil therapy on the pharmacodynamics and pharmacokinetics of warfarin. *J Cardiovasc Pharmacol* (2003) 41, 908–15.
6. Flolan (Epoprostenol). GlaxoSmithKline UK. UK Summary of product characteristics, September 2006.

Coumarins + Proton pump inhibitors

Omeprazole causes a minor increase in *R*-warfarin concentrations and might enhance the anticoagulant effect of warfarin. Conversely, in studies, dexlansoprazole, lansoprazole, pantoprazole, and rabeprazole did not alter warfarin pharmacokinetics or its anticoagulant effect, and esomeprazole did not increase the anticoagulant effect of warfarin to a clinically relevant extent, although cases of an enhanced effect have been reported with all these combinations. A study in patients taking warfarin post-heart surgery appears to suggest that rabeprazole has less effect on INR and bleeding complications than lansoprazole. Esomeprazole and lansoprazole appear to increase the risk of over-anticoagulation with acenocoumarol, but omeprazole, pantoprazole, and rabeprazole do not, although a case of an enhanced effect has been reported with acenocoumarol and omeprazole. Esomeprazole and omeprazole appear to enhance the anticoagulant effect of phenprocoumon, but pantoprazole does not appear to have the same effect.

Clinical evidence

(a) Dexlansoprazole

In a pharmacokinetic study in 18 healthy subjects, dexlansoprazole MR 90 mg for 11 days, did not affect the pharmacokinetics of *R*- or *S*-warfarin after a single 25-mg dose of **warfarin** was given on day 6. Similarly no effect on INR was seen.[1]

(b) Esomeprazole

1. Acenocoumarol. A prospective cohort study in 2 755 patients who had been taking acenocoumarol for at least 6 weeks, found that the concurrent use of esomeprazole was associated with an almost 2-fold increased risk (hazard ratio 1.99) of over-anticoagulation (defined as INR greater than or equal to 6).[2]

2. Phenprocoumon. In a retrospective analysis of 597 patients taking phenprocoumon, and who achieved a stable dose within 1 year of starting, the mean phenprocoumon dose in 18 patients also taking esomeprazole was 1.88 mg daily compared with 2.27 mg daily in those not taking esomeprazole (or **omeprazole**).[3]

3.Warfarin. The UK and US manufacturers state that esomeprazole 40 mg daily did not cause any clinically relevant effects on anticoagulant times in patients stabilised on warfarin, but a few isolated cases of increased INRs have been reported post-marketing.[4,5]

(c) Lansoprazole

1. Acenocoumarol. A prospective cohort study in 2 755 patients who had been taking acenocoumarol for at least 6 weeks, found that the concurrent use of lansoprazole was associated with a increased risk (hazard ratio 1.49) of over-anticoagulation (defined as INR greater than or equal to 6).[2]

2. Warfarin. A study in 24 healthy subjects stabilised on warfarin found that lansoprazole 60 mg daily for 9 days had no effect on the pharmacokinetics of either *S*- or *R*-warfarin, and did not alter the effect of warfarin on prothrombin times.[6] However, in a retrospective analysis of 240 patients who underwent open heart surgery and were given a proton pump inhibitor and warfarin (3 mg daily), the mean INR on day 4 in the 126 patients taking lansoprazole 15 mg daily was 2.06 compared with an INR of 1.66 in the 114 patients taking **rabeprazole** 10 mg daily, Furthermore, 7 patients taking lansoprazole had delayed bleeding complications compared with none in those patients taking **rabeprazole**.[7] In 1998 the manufacturers of lansoprazole had on record two reports of possible interactions. An elderly patient taking warfarin developed an INR of 7 when lansoprazole was added. Despite a warfarin dose adjustment he had a gastrointestinal haemorrhage, a myocardial infarction and died after 3 weeks. Another man taking warfarin (as well as amiodarone, furosemide and lisinopril) became confused, had hallucinations and developed an increased INR (value not known) when given lansoprazole. The lansoprazole was stopped after 4 days, and he then recovered. However, it is uncertain whether this was an interaction or whether he had taken an incorrect warfarin dose because of his confusion.[8]

(d) Omeprazole

1. Acenocoumarol. In a placebo-controlled study in 8 healthy subjects, omeprazole 40 mg daily for 3 days had no effect on the pharmacokinetics of *R*- or *S*-acenocoumarol when a single 10-mg dose of acenocoumarol was given on day 2. In addition, omeprazole did not alter the anticoagulant effects of acenocoumarol.[9] Similarly, there was no evidence of an interaction in a retrospective study of 118 patients given acenocoumarol with omeprazole and 299 patients taking acenocoumarol without omeprazole (matched for age and sex).[10] Furthermore, in a retrospective cohort study of patients taking acenocoumarol, omeprazole was not associated with an increased risk of hospitalisation for bleeding;[11] nor was it associated with an increased risk of over-anticoagulation (defined as INR greater than or equal to 6) in a prospective cohort study in 2 755 patients taking acenocoumarol for at least 6 weeks.[2] However, an isolated case report describes a 78-year-old woman who had been taking acenocoumarol for 60 days and who developed gross haematuria within 5 days of starting omeprazole 20 mg daily. Her INR had increased from a range of 2.5 to 3 up to 5.7, and when the omeprazole was stopped, her INR decreased.[12]

2. Phenprocoumon. In a retrospective cohort study of patients taking phenprocoumon, omeprazole was not associated with an increased risk of hospitalisation for bleeding.[11] However, in a retrospective analysis of 597 patients taking phenprocoumon, and who achieved a stable dose within 1 year of starting, the mean phenprocoumon dose in 46 patients also taking omeprazole was 1.78 mg daily compared with 2.27 mg daily in those not taking omeprazole (or **esomeprazole**),[3] There is also a report of two possible cases of an interaction.[13] One patient who was given phenprocoumon (loading dose 12 mg on day one, 9 mg on day 2, 3 mg on day 3, and further as required) and omeprazole 20 mg daily concurrently, had an INR of 3.28 by the fourth day. The phenprocoumon was withheld, but the INR remained high for 9 days, when the omeprazole was stopped. Four days later the INR was 1.5 and phenprocoumon was restarted at 16.5 mg per week, and stabilised at 9 to 10.5 mg per week. She subsequently had a similar loading dose without problems, in the absence of omeprazole, after phenprocoumon had been stopped for 3 weeks before surgery.[13] Another patient stabilised on phenprocoumon 18 mg per week required a slight reduction in dose to 16.5 mg per week after starting omeprazole 20 mg daily.[13]

3. Warfarin. In 21 healthy subjects who had been stabilised on warfarin, omeprazole 20 mg daily for 2 weeks caused a small but statistically significant decrease in the mean thrombotest percentage, from 21.1% to 18.7%. *S*-warfarin serum concentrations remained unchanged, but a small 12% increase in *R*-warfarin concentrations was seen.[14] In a further study, no changes in coagulation times or thrombotest values occurred in 28 patients anticoagulated with warfarin and given omeprazole 20 mg daily for 3 weeks. *S*-warfarin concentrations were unchanged, while a 9.5% increase in *R*-warfarin concentrations occurred.[15] A study in 7 patients who were CYP2C19 poor metabolisers and 10 patients who were CYP2C19 extensive metabolisers (that is, those with little or no activity of this isoenzyme and those with normal activity of this isoenzyme, respectively) specifically looked at the effect of different CYP2C19 genotypes on the metabolism of warfarin, and also the influence of omeprazole on this interaction. The AUC of *R*-warfarin (from a single 10-mg dose of racemic warfarin) was found to be 24% higher in poor metabolisers than in extensive metabolisers. Omeprazole 20 mg daily taken for 11 days increased the AUC of *R*-warfarin (taken on day 7) in the extensive metabolisers to a level comparable with that in the poor metabolisers. Omeprazole had no effect on *S*-warfarin, and no effect on anticoagulant activity in any subject.[16] However, a man stabilised on warfarin 5 mg daily developed widespread bruising and haematuria 2 weeks after starting to take omeprazole 20 mg daily. His prothrombin time was found to have increased to 48 seconds. He was later restabilised on omeprazole 20 mg daily with the warfarin dose reduced to 2 mg daily.[17]

(e) Pantoprazole

1. Acenocoumarol. A prospective cohort study in 2 755 patients who had been taking acenocoumarol for at least 6 weeks, found that the concurrent use of pantoprazole was not associated with an increased risk of over-anticoagulation (defined as INR greater than or equal to 6).[2]

2. Phenprocoumon. The prothrombin time ratio in 16 healthy subjects taking individualised maintenance phenprocoumon doses was not changed when they were given pantoprazole 40 mg daily for 5 days, nor was there any change in the pharmacokinetics of *R*- and *S*-phenprocoumon.[18]

3. Warfarin. In 26 healthy subjects, pantoprazole 40 mg daily for 8 days caused no change in the response to a single 25-mg dose of warfarin given on day 2. The pharmacokinetics of *R*- and *S*-warfarin were unaltered, and no changes in the pharmacodynamics of the warfarin (prothrombin time, factor VII) were seen.[19] However, the manufacturer notes that there have been post-marketing reports of increased INR and prothrombin time in patients taking pantoprazole and warfarin.[20]

(f) Rabeprazole

1. Acenocoumarol. A prospective cohort study in 2 755 patients who had been taking acenocoumarol for at least 6 weeks, found that the concurrent use of rabeprazole was not associated with an increased risk of over-anticoagulation (defined as INR greater than or equal to 6).[2]

2. Warfarin. In a placebo-controlled study, a single 0.75-mg/kg dose of warfarin was given to 21 patients before and after rabeprazole 20 mg daily for 7 days. No changes in prothrombin times or in the pharmacokinetics of *R*- or *S*-warfarin were seen.[21] However, the manufacturer notes that there have been reports of increased INR and prothrombin time in patients receiving rabeprazole and warfarin.[22]

For mention of a retrospective analysis of patients taking warfarin with rabeprazole or lansoprazole, see under *Lansoprazole*, above.

Mechanism

Studies have shown that omeprazole partially inhibits the metabolism of *R*-warfarin, but not *S*-warfarin,[23,24] which is consistent with the findings in the pharmacokinetic studies above, the known involvement of CYP2C19 in the metabolism of *R*-warfarin, and the CYP2C19 inhibitory effects of omeprazole. It also partially inhibits the metabolism of acenocoumarol.[23] It has been suggested that the interaction might occur only in patients who are CYP2C19 poor metabolisers (seen in about 5% of Caucasians), and who have 5- to 10-fold higher concentrations of omeprazole than extensive metabolisers.[9] However, in the one study addressing this, the effect of CYP2C19 genotype was not clinically relevant.[16] For further discussion of the effect of genetics on drug metabolism, see 'Genetic factors in drug metabolism', p.8. Other proton pump inhibitors are generally considered to have less potential for pharmacokinetic interactions than omeprazole, but even with these, isolated cases of anticoagulant interactions have been reported.

Importance and management

The very minor pharmacokinetic interaction between omeprazole and warfarin, resulting in a less than 15% increase in *R*-warfarin concentrations (the less active isomer), is established, but probably of limited clinical relevance. This is borne out by the fact there is only one published case report of an interaction between these commonly prescribed drugs. No pharmacokinetic or pharmacodynamic interaction occurred between warfarin and dexlansoprazole, lansoprazole, pantoprazole, or rabeprazole in clinical studies. However the retrospective analysis of patients receiving warfarin with either lansoprazole or rabeprazole in patients post-heart surgery appears to suggest that lansoprazole might increase INR and bleeding complications, and that rabeprazole might be the safer choice in this group of patients.

One study suggested that esomeprazole and lansoprazole are associated with an increased risk of over-anticoagulation when taken with acenocoumarol and isolated cases of increased INRs have been reported for esomeprazole, lansoprazole, pantoprazole, omeprazole, and rabeprazole with acenocoumarol (one published), phenprocoumon (2 published), and warfarin. It is possible that the isolated cases of interactions with proton pump inhibitors just represent idiosyncratic effects attributable to other factors, and not to any interaction. An analysis of data from the FDA database for adverse events and drug interactions, found a low frequency (about 0.1 per million packages) of drug interactions between omeprazole, lansoprazole, or pantoprazole and vitamin K antagonists (drugs not stated).[25]

Nevertheless, when prescribing proton pump inhibitors to patients taking coumarins it would seem prudent to bear in mind that rarely bleeding can occur. Note that the US prescribing information for every proton pump inhibitor states that patients taking a proton pump inhibitor and warfarin might need to be monitored for increases in INR and prothrombin time. The advice in the UK varies from recommending monitoring with warfarin or coumarin derivatives on starting or stopping esomeprazole,[4] recommending monitoring with coumarins after starting or stopping pantoprazole, or during irregular use,[26] to no advice with lansoprazole,[27] omeprazole,[28] or rabeprazole.[29]

1. Vakily M, Lee RD, Wu J, Gunawardhana L, Mulford D. Drug interaction studies with dexlansoprazole modified release (TAK-390MR), a proton pump inhibitor with a dual delayed-release formulation: results of four randomized, double-blind, crossover, placebo-controlled, single-centre studies. *Clin Drug Invest* (2009) 29, 35–50.
2. Teichert M, van Noord C, Uitterlinden AG, Hofman A, Buhre PN, De Smet PAGM, Straus S, Stricker BH, Visser LE. Proton pump inhibitors and the risk of overanticoagulation during acenocoumarol maintenance treatment. *Br J Haematol* (2011) 153, 379–85.
3. Verhoef TI, Zuurhout MJL, van Schie RMF, Redekop WK, van der Meer FJM, le Cessie S, Schalekamp T, de Boer A, Maitland-van der Zee AH. The effect of omeprazole and esomeprazole on the maintenance dose of phenprocoumon. *Br J Clin Pharmacol* (2012) 74, 1068–9.
4. Nexium Tablets (Esomeprazole magnesium trihydrate). AstraZeneca UK Ltd. UK Summary of product characteristics, August 2013.
5. Nexium (Esomeprazole magnesium). AstraZeneca Pharmaceuticals LP. US Prescribing information, November 2012.
6. Cavanaugh JH, Winters EP, Cohen A, Locke CS, Braeckman R. Lack of effect of lansoprazole on steady state warfarin metabolism. *Gastroenterology* (1991) 100, A40.
7. Hata M, Hayasaka M, Sezal A, Nilno T, Yoda M, Unosawa S, Taoka M, Osaka S, Furukawa N, Kimura H, Minami K. Proton pump inhibitors may increase the risk of delayed bleeding complications after open heart surgery if used concomitantly with warfarin. *Thorac Cardiovasc Surg* (2008) 56, 274–7.
8. Wyeth. Personal communication, January 1998.

9. de Hoon JNJM, Thijssen HHW, Beysens AJMM, Van Bortel LMAB. No effect of short-term omeprazole intake on acenocoumarol pharmacokinetics and pharmacodynamics. *Br J Clin Pharmacol* (1997) 44, 399–401.
10. Vreeburg EM, De Vlaam-Schluter GM, Trienekens PH, Snel P, Tytgat GNJ. Lack of effect of omeprazole on oral acenocoumarol anticoagulant therapy. *Scand J Gastroenterol* (1997) 32, 991–4.
11. Penning-van Beest F, Erkens J, Petersen K-U, Koelz HR, Herings R. Main comedications associated with bleeding during anticoagulant therapy with coumarins. *Eur J Clin Pharmacol* (2005) 61, 439–44.
12. García B, Lacambra C, Garrote F, García-Plaza I, Solis J. Possible potentiation of anticoagulant effect of acenocoumarol by omeprazole. *Pharm World Sci* (1994) 16, 231–2.
13. Enderle C, Müller W, Grass U. Drug interaction: omeprazole and phenprocoumon. *BMC Gastroenterol* (2001) 1, 2.
14. Sutfin T, Balmer K, Boström H, Eriksson S, Höglund P, Paulsen O. Stereoselective interaction of omeprazole with warfarin in healthy men. *Ther Drug Monit* (1989) 11, 176–84.
15. Unge P, Svedberg L-E, Nordgren A, Blom H, Andersson T, Lagerström P-O, Idström J-P. A study of the interaction of omeprazole and warfarin in anticoagulated patients. *Br J Clin Pharmacol* (1992) 34, 509–12.
16. Uno T, Sugimoto K, Sugawara K, Tateishi T. The role of cytochrome P2C19 in R-warfarin pharmacokinetics and its interaction with omeprazole. *Ther Drug Monit* (2008) 30, 276–81.
17. Ahmad S. Omeprazole-warfarin interaction. *South Med J* (1991) 84, 674–5.
18. Ehrlich A, Fuder H, Hartmann M, Wieckhorst G, Timmer W, Huber R, Birkel M, Bliesath H, Steinijans VW, Wurst W, Lücker PW. Lack of pharmacokinetic and pharmacodynamic interaction between pantoprazole and phenprocoumon in man. *Eur J Clin Pharmacol* (1996) 51, 277–281.
19. Duursema L, Müller FO, Schall R, Middle MV, Hundt HKL, Groenewoud G, Steinijans VW, Bliesath H. Lack of effect of pantoprazole on the pharmacodynamics and pharmacokinetics of warfarin. *Br J Clin Pharmacol* (1995) 39, 700–703.
20. Protonix (Pantoprazole sodium). Wyeth Pharmaceuticals Inc. US Prescribing information, December 2014.
21. Humphries TJ, Nardi RV, Spera AC, Lazar JD, Laurent AL, Spanyers SA. Coadministration of rabeprazole sodium (E3810) does not affect the pharmacokinetics of anhydrous theophylline or warfarin. *Gastroenterology* (1996) 110 (Suppl), A138.
22. Aciphex (Rabeprazole sodium). Eisai Inc. US Prescribing information, November 2013.
23. Hermans JJ, Thijssen HH. Human liver microsomal metabolism of the enantiomers of warfarin and acenocoumarol: P450 isozyme diversity determines the differences in their pharmacokinetics. *Br J Pharmacol* (1993) 111, 482–90.
24. Chainuvati S, Nafziger AN, Leeder JS, Gaedigk A, Kearns GL, Sellers E, Zhang Y, Kashuba ADM, Rowland E, Bertino JS. Combined phenotypic assessment of cytochrome P450 1A2, 2C9, 2C19, 2D6, and 3A, *N*-acetyltransferase-2, and xanthine oxidase activities with the "Cooperstown 5+1 cocktail". *Clin Pharmacol Ther* (2003) 74, 437–47.
25. Labenz J, Petersen KU, Rösch W, Koelz HR. A summary of Food and Drug Administration-reported adverse events and drug interactions occurring during therapy with omeprazole, lansoprazole and pantoprazole. *Aliment Pharmacol Ther* (2003) 17, 1015–19.
26. Pantoprazole Gastro-Resistant Tablets (Pantoprazole sodium sesquihydrate). Sandoz Ltd. UK Summary of product characteristics, September 2013.
27. Zoton (Lansoprazole). Pfizer Ltd. UK Summary of product characteristics, June 2012.
28. Losec Capsules (Omeprazole). AstraZeneca UK Ltd. UK Summary of product characteristics, May 2013.
29. Pariet (Rabeprazole sodium). Eisai Ltd. UK Summary of product characteristics, March 2013.

Coumarins + Quetiapine

A case report describes a woman taking warfarin who developed a raised INR when quetiapine was started.

Clinical evidence, mechanism, importance and management

A 71-year old woman receiving long-term treatment with **warfarin**, phenytoin, olanzapine and benztropine had her **warfarin** dose slightly reduced (from 20 to 19.5 mg weekly) because her INR was raised (from 1.6 to 2.6). Eight days later her treatment with olanzapine was changed to quetiapine 200 mg daily, and after 5 days her INR was 2.7. Two weeks later she was found to have an INR of 9.2. The quetiapine was stopped and she was given two doses of vitamin K by injection. The only clinical symptoms seen were a small amount of bleeding from the injection site and a bruise on her hand. She was eventually later restabilised taking phenytoin, olanzapine and **warfarin** 21 mg weekly with an INR of 1.6.

The reasons for this apparent interaction are not known, but the authors suggest that the quetiapine may have inhibited the metabolism of the **warfarin** (possibly by competitive inhibition of the cytochrome P450 isoenzymes CYP3A4 and CYP2C9), thereby increasing its effects. They also suggest that the phenytoin may have had some part to play.[1] This is only an isolated case and as such an interaction is not confirmed, but bear it in mind in the case of an unexpected response to concurrent use.

1. Rogers T, de Leon J, Atcher D. Possible interaction between warfarin and quetiapine. *J Clin Psychopharmacol* (1999) 19, 382–3.

Coumarins + Quilinggao

A single case report describes a man who had a marked increase in his INR with bleeding complications, nine days after he switched the brand of quilinggao he was using.

Clinical evidence

A 61-year-old man stabilised on **warfarin** with an INR in the range of 1.6 to 2.8 was found to have an INR greater than 6 and skin bruising, and complained of gum bleeding and epistaxis in the previous 3 days. For the past 3 years he had taken quilinggao, apparently without problems. However, 9 days previously he had started taking a different brand of quilinggao. He was eventually stabilised on the previous dose of **warfarin** with an INR of 2.5, but after discharge started taking a third brand of quilinggao, and 3 days later had an INR of 5.2.[1]

Mechanism

Quilinggao is a Chinese herbal product made from a mixture of herbs. The first brand did not contain any herbs suspected to have anticoagulant effects except one with possible antiplatelet activity, but the second brand contained Chinese peony (*Paeoniae rubra*), *Poncirus trifoliata* and a couple of other herbs known to contain substances with anticoagulant or antiplatelet effects *in vitro*, but see also 'Coumarins + Herbal medicines; Miscellaneous', p.439.

Importance and management

This appears to be the only case of a possible interaction, and as such the interaction is not established. Quilinggao did not affect anticoagulant control in this patient for a number of years, and then did after switching brands. Bear the possibility of an interaction in mind.

1. Wong ALN, Chan TYK. Interaction between warfarin and the herbal product *quilinggao*. *Ann Pharmacother* (2003) 37, 836–8.

Coumarins + Quinidine

Quinidine does not appear to alter the anticoagulant effect of warfarin; however, isolated reports of increased warfarin effects and bleeding, and also decreased dicoumarol and warfarin effects have been reported. Quinidine does not alter the half-life of phenprocoumon.

Clinical evidence

In a controlled study, 10 patients receiving long-term treatment with **warfarin** 2.5 to 12.5 mg daily had no significant alteration in their prothrombin times when they were given quinidine 200 mg four times daily for 2 weeks.[1,2] Similarly, in a retrospective analysis of 8 patients stabilised on **warfarin**, there was no change in anticoagulant control associated with starting or stopping quinidine (600 mg to 1.2 g daily as sulfate or 660 mg daily as gluconate).[3] In the preliminary report of another study in 5 healthy subjects, quinidine 100 mg daily, started 7 days after a single 12-mg dose of **phenprocoumon**, did not change the elimination half-life of **phenprocoumon**.[4]

In contrast, another report described 3 patients stabilised on **warfarin**, with Quick values within the range of 15 to 25%, who began to bleed within 7 to 10 days of starting to take quinidine 800 mg to 1.2 g daily. Their Quick values were found to have fallen to 6 to 8%. Bleeding ceased when the warfarin was withdrawn.[5] There is one other case report of haemorrhage associated with the concurrent use of **warfarin** and quinidine,[6] and in an analysis of haemorrhage in patients taking anticoagulants, it was reported that quinidine seemed partly responsible for some cases.[7]

In a further report, 4 patients taking **warfarin** or **dicoumarol** needed dose *increases* of 8 to 24% to maintain adequate anticoagulation after DC conversion for atrial fibrillation and starting quinidine 400 mg three times daily.[8]

Mechanism

Uncertain. The cases of increased warfarin effects were attributed to quinidine possibly having a direct hypoprothrombinaemic effect of its own.[5] The cases of a slight decrease in anticoagulant effect were attributed to changes in haemodynamic factors as a result of cardioversion.[8]

Importance and management

In one study and one retrospective analysis, quinidine had no effect on the anticoagulant control with warfarin in patients. Therefore, no interaction would normally be anticipated. However, a few isolated cases of increased anticoagulant effect with bleeding have been reported. Nevertheless, the literature is limited, and based almost solely on evidence from more than 40 years ago. The lack of reports of any further interactions in this time suggests that a clinically relevant interaction is unlikely. Limited evidence suggests that quinidine does not alter phenprocoumon pharmacokinetics.

1. Udall JA. Quinidine and hypoprothrombinemia. *Ann Intern Med* (1968) 69, 403–4.
2. Udall JA. Drug interference with warfarin therapy. *Clin Med* (1970) 77, 20–5.
3. Jones FL. More on quinidine-induced hypoprothrombinaemia. *Ann Intern Med* (1968) 69, 1074.
4. Iven H, Lerche L, Kaschube M. Influence of quinine and quinidine on the pharmacokinetics of phenprocoumon in rat and man. *Eur J Pharmacol* (1990) 183, 662.
5. Koch-Weser J. Quinidine-induced hypoprothrombinemic hemorrhage in patients on chronic warfarin therapy. *Ann Intern Med* (1968) 68, 511–17.
6. Gazzaniga AB, Stewart DR. Possible quinidine-induced hemorrhage in a patient on warfarin sodium. *N Engl J Med* (1969) 280, 711–12.
7. Beaumont JL, Tarrit A. Les accidents hémorrhagiques survenus au cours de 1500 traitements anticoagulants. *Sang* (1955) 26, 680–94.
8. Sylvén C, Anderson P. Evidence that disopyramide does not interact with warfarin. *BMJ* (1983) 286, 1181.

Coumarins + Quinine

Isolated reports describe increased anticoagulant effects in two women taking warfarin and a man taking phenprocoumon, which were attributed to the quinine content of tonic water. Limited evidence suggests that quinine does not alter the half-life of phenprocoumon.

Clinical evidence

In the preliminary report of a study in 5 healthy subjects, quinine 100 mg daily started 7 days after a single 12-mg dose of **phenprocoumon** did not change the elimination half-life of **phenprocoumon** in the following 7 days.[1]

However, a patient taking long-term **phenprocoumon** repeatedly developed extensive haematuria within 24 hours of drinking one litre of Indian tonic water containing 30 mg of quinine.[1]

A woman stabilised on **warfarin** needed a dose reduction from 6 mg to 4 mg daily when she started to drink up to 1.5 litres of tonic water containing quinine each day.

Her **warfarin** requirements rose again when the tonic water was stopped. Another woman needed a **warfarin** dose reduction from 4 mg to 2 mg daily when she started to drink over 2 litres of tonic water daily. These patients were probably taking about 80 to 180 mg of quinine daily.[2]

Mechanism

Not understood. Two studies[3,4] using the Page method (Russell viper venom)[5] to measure prothrombin times showed that marked increases of up to 12 seconds could occur when 330-mg doses of quinine were given in the absence of an anticoagulant, but other studies[4,6] using the Quick method found that the prothrombin times were only prolonged by up to 2.1 seconds. The changes in prothrombin times could be completely reversed by vitamin K (menadiol sodium diphosphate),[3,4] which suggests that quinine, like the **indanediones** and coumarins, is a competitive inhibitor of vitamin K.

Importance and management

The interaction between quinine and the coumarins is not established. The lack of reports relating to the therapeutic use of quinine suggest that no interaction of clinical importance occurs, and because the only reports relate to tonic water, it cannot be excluded that some other ingredient is responsible for the effect seen in these patients. Also, they may just represent idiosyncratic reactions. Nevertheless, because some isolated cases appear to suggest that very exceptionally decreased anticoagulant requirements and even bleeding can occur when large quantities of tonic water are ingested the possibility of a rare interaction cannot entirely be dismissed.

1. Iven H, Lerche L, Kaschube M. Influence of quinine and quinidine on the pharmacokinetics of phenprocoumon in rat and man. *Eur J Pharmacol* (1990) 183, 662.
2. Clark DJ. Clinical curio: warfarin and tonic water. *BMJ* (1983) 286, 1258.
3. Pirk LA, Engelberg R. Hypoprothrombinemic action of quinine sulfate. *JAMA* (1945) 128, 1093–5.
4. Pirk LA, Engelberg R. Hypoprothrombinemic action of quinine sulfate. *Am J Med Sci* (1947) 213, 593–7.
5. Page RC, de Beer EJ, Orr ML. Prothrombin studies using Russell viper venom. II. Relation of clotting time to prothrombin concentration in human plasma. *J Lab Clin Med* (1941) 27, 197–201.
6. Quick AJ. Effect of synthetic vitamin K and quinine sulfate on the prothrombin level. *J Lab Clin Med* (1946) 31, 79–84.

Coumarins + Raloxifene

Raloxifene may cause a minor increase in warfarin levels. However, a 10% decrease in prothrombin time may also occur. Other coumarins would be expected to be similarly affected.

Clinical evidence, mechanism, importance and management

In a study in 15 healthy postmenopausal women, raloxifene 120 mg daily for 15 days had minor effects on the pharmacokinetics and pharmacodynamics of a single 20-mg dose of **warfarin** given on day 11. The clearance of both *R*- and *S*-warfarin was slightly decreased (by 7% and 14%, respectively), with similar increases in AUC. Conversely, a 10% reduction in the maximum prothrombin time was reported.[1] As has been suggested for lasofoxifene (see 'Coumarins + Lasofoxifene', p.442), this might be because oestrogenic compounds increase plasma concentrations of vitamin K-dependent clotting factors, so antagonising the effect of **warfarin**.

The manufacturers recommend that because modest decreases in prothrombin times have been seen, which may develop over several weeks, prothrombin times should be monitored.[2,3] In the UK, they extend this recommendation to cover the use of other coumarins.[2]

1. Miller JW, Skerjanec A, Knadler MP, Ghosh A, Allerheiligen SRB. Divergent effects of raloxifene HCl on the pharmacokinetics and pharmacodynamics of warfarin. *Pharm Res* (2001) 18, 1024–8.
2. Evista (Raloxifene hydrochloride). Daiichi Sankyo UK Ltd. UK Summary of product characteristics, August 2003.
3. Evista (Raloxifene hydrochloride). Eli Lilly and Company. US Prescribing information, October 2008.

Coumarins + Retinoids

Two isolated case reports describe reduced warfarin effects in one patient given etretinate, and in one patient given isotretinoin. Acitretin did not significantly alter the anticoagulant effects of phenprocoumon in healthy subjects.

Clinical evidence

(a) Phenprocoumon

Acitretin 50 mg daily for 10 days slightly increased the Quick test of 10 healthy subjects stabilised on phenprocoumon, from 22% to 24%, and the corresponding INR value decreased from 2.91 to 2.71. However, these changes were not considered to be clinically significant.[1]

(b) Warfarin

1. Etretinate. A man with T-cell lymphoma who had recently been given chemotherapy (cyclophosphamide, doxorubicin, vincristine and prednisolone) was anticoagulated with warfarin after developing a pulmonary embolism. About three weeks later, he started etretinate 40 mg daily and it was found necessary to increase his warfarin dose from 7 to 10 mg daily. His liver function tests were normal.[2] This patient had also recently started taking 'co-proxamol', p.457, 'tolbutamide', p.402, and 'cimetidine', p.437, but all of these have been reported to only rarely *increase* the effect of warfarin.

2. Isotretinoin. A 61-year-old man stabilised on warfarin 2.5 mg daily for 2 to 3 years had a decrease in his INR to below 2.5 after starting oral cefpodoxime proxetil 200 mg twice daily and oral isotretinoin 30 mg daily for inflammatory lesions of the face. He required an increase in warfarin dose to 3.75 mg daily. The cefpodoxime was stopped after 10 days without a further change in his warfarin requirement. However, when the isotretinoin was discontinued after 40 days, the INR progressively increased and the warfarin dose was eventually reduced to the pre-isotretinoin dose of 2.5 mg daily.[3]

Mechanism

Not understood. It has been suggested that etretinate or isotretinoin may increase the rate of metabolism of warfarin.[2,3]

Importance and management

Information appears to be limited to these reports. The clinical relevance of the two case reports of a modest increase in warfarin requirements on starting etretinate or isotretinoin is uncertain. No definite conclusions can be drawn from these isolated cases. The study with acitretin suggests that no phenprocoumon dose adjustments are expected to be needed on starting acitretin.

1. Hartmann D, Mosberg H, Weber W. Lack of effect of acitretin on the hypoprothrombinemic action of phenprocoumon in healthy volunteers. *Dermatologica* (1989) 178, 33–6.
2. Ostlere LS, Langtry JAA, Jones S, Staughton RCD. Reduced therapeutic effect of warfarin caused by etretinate. *Br J Dermatol* (1991) 124, 505–10.
3. Fiallo P. Reduced therapeutic activity of warfarin during treatment with oral isotretinoin. *Br J Dermatol* (2004) 150, 164.

Coumarins + Ribavirin

Ribavirin appears to decrease the anticoagulant effects of warfarin.

Clinical evidence

A 61-year-old patient who had been taking **warfarin** for a number of years with an INR in the range of 1.8 to 2.7 required a progressive 40% increase in his **warfarin** dose (from 45 to 62.5 mg weekly) over the month after starting oral ribavirin 600 mg twice daily and subcutaneous interferon alfa-2b for active hepatitis C infection. During the following 11 months, the **warfarin** dose was stabilised at 57.5 mg weekly. Three weeks after discontinuation of the ribavirin and interferon, his INR had increased from 2.2 to 3.4 requiring a reduction in his **warfarin** dose to 47.5 mg weekly. One year later, when the patient was rechallenged with ribavirin alone (1 g daily for 4 weeks), his INR decreased from 2.6 to 1.8 and he required a weekly **warfarin** dose of 52.5 mg.[1]

For mention of another patient requiring a high **warfarin** dose (70 mg weekly), which was attributed to nelfinavir, but who was also receiving ribavirin, see 'Coumarins + HIV-protease inhibitors', p.439.

Mechanism

Unknown. The few cases with interferon (see 'Coumarins + Interferons', p.441) have suggested that interferon may *increase* the effect of warfarin. In this case, ribavirin seems to have decreased the effect of warfarin, and overridden any effect of interferon. However, ribavirin is not known to be an inhibitor or inducer of any cytochrome P450 isoenzyme.

Importance and management

This is the only case of this interaction, so it is not established, although the evidence on rechallenge with ribavirin alone lends weight to the effects potentially being due to an interaction. The authors recommended increased monitoring of anticoagulant effects in patients taking warfarin requiring ribavirin. Until more is known, this may be prudent.

1. Schulman S. Inhibition of warfarin activity by ribavirin. *Ann Pharmacother* (2002) 36, 72–4.

Coumarins + Riociguat

Riociguat does not appear to affect the pharmacokinetics or pharmacodynamics of warfarin and is not expected to alter the prothrombin time when given with other coumarins. Warfarin marginally decreased riociguat maximum concentrations.

Clinical evidence, mechanism, importance and management

A crossover study in 22 healthy subjects given riociguat 2.5 mg three times daily for 10 days, with a single 25-mg dose of warfarin on day 7, found that riociguat did not alter the pharmacodynamics of warfarin as assessed by the effects on prothrombin time and factor VII. The pharmacokinetics of *R*- and *S*-warfarin were not altered by riociguat. Warfarin did not affect the AUC of riociguat, but decreased the riociguat maximum concentration by 16%. This small decrease is unlikely to be clinically relevant,[1] and no dose adjustment of either drug would therefore seem necessary on concurrent use. The UK manufacturer of riociguat notes that riociguat is not expected to affect the prothrombin time when given with other coumarins.[2]

1. Frey R, Mück W, Kirschbaum N, Krätzschmar J, Weimann G, Wensing G. Riociguat (BAY 63-2521) and warfarin: a pharmacodynamic and pharmacokinetic interaction study. *J Clin Pharmacol* (2011) 51, 1051–60.
2. Adempas (Riociguat). Bayer plc. UK Summary of product characteristics, October 2014.

Coumarins + Roflumilast

There is no pharmacokinetic interaction between roflumilast and warfarin. Roflumilast does not alter the pharmacodynamics of warfarin.

Clinical evidence, mechanism, importance and management

In a placebo-controlled, crossover study in 21 healthy subjects, the pharmacokinetics and pharmacodynamics of a single 25-mg dose of **warfarin** given on day 8 were not altered by roflumilast 500 micrograms daily for 12 days. The pharmacokinetics of roflumilast were similarly unaffected.[1] No dose adjustments would seem necessary on concurrent use.

1. McCracken N, Lahu G, Bethke TD. Lack of pharmacokinetic and pharmacodynamic interactions of roflumilast with (*R, S*)-warfarin in healthy adult subjects. *Int J Clin Pharmacol Ther* (2011) 49, 388–96.

Coumarins + Ropinirole

A man stabilised on warfarin had an increase in his INR, necessitating a 25% decrease in his warfarin dose, while taking ropinirole.

Clinical evidence, mechanism, importance and management

A frail 63-year-old man taking levodopa with carbidopa daily and **warfarin** 4 mg daily with a stable INR ranging from 1.8 to 2.6 over the past 14 months was evaluated for possible progression of Parkinson's disease. He was then given ropinirole 250 micrograms three times daily with a 25% reduction in the dose of levodopa with carbidopa, and 9 days later his INR was noted to have increased to 4.6, but there were no apparent signs of bleeding. **Warfarin** was withheld for 4 days, and then restarted at 2 mg daily, and increased to 3 mg daily 19 days later when his INR was 1.2. After one month the ropinirole was discontinued because of adverse gastrointestinal effects, and 2 months later his INR was 1.4 necessitating an increase in the **warfarin** dose to the original dose of 4 mg daily.[1] The mechanism of this probable interaction is unknown, and it appears to be the first evidence of such an interaction. No definite conclusions can be drawn from this isolated case.

1. Bair JD, Oppelt TF. Warfarin and ropinirole interaction. *Ann Pharmacother* (2001) 35, 1202–4.

Coumarins + Royal jelly

An isolated report describes a patient taking warfarin, who developed a raised INR with haematuria one week after starting a royal jelly supplement.

Clinical evidence, mechanism, importance and management

An 87-year-old man stabilised on warfarin (INR 1.9 to 2.4) and a variety of other drugs presented with haematuria and was found to have an INR of 6.88. He reported starting to take a supplement containing just royal jelly one week earlier. The name of the supplement and the dose taken were not given in the report.[1]

Royal jelly is a substance secreted by worker honeybees (*Apis mellifera*) to feed their larvae. It is essentially a nutrient substance, and why it might interact with warfarin is unknown. This appears to be an isolated case, and its general relevance is therefore uncertain.

1. Lee NJ, Fermo JD. Warfarin and royal jelly interaction. *Pharmacotherapy* (2006) 26, 583–6.

Coumarins + Salicylates; Topical

Cases of increased warfarin effects have been reported with topical methyl salicylate or trolamine salicylate.

Clinical evidence

Methyl salicylate, in the form of gels, oil, or ointment applied to the skin, has been found to increase the effects of **warfarin**. Bleeding and bruising and/or increased INRs have been seen with both high[1-5] and low doses[6] of topical **methyl salicylate**. One report[7] described the possible additive effects of **methyl salicylate oil** (*Kwan Loong Medicated Oil*) and a decoction of *Danshen* (the root of *Salvia miltiorrhiza*) on the response to **warfarin** (see also 'Coumarins and related drugs + Danshen (*Salvia miltiorrhiza*)', p.422). An increased prothrombin time has also been reported with topical **trolamine salicylate.**[3]

Mechanism

Methyl and trolamine salicylates possibly interact like high-dose aspirin (see 'Coumarins and related drugs + Aspirin or other Salicylates', p.405), if they are absorbed through the skin. In one case report, the blood-salicylate concentration suggested significant percutaneous absorption.[1] However, in a study in healthy subjects, systemic absorption of salicylate was low after a single application of *Deep Heat* (local absorption was comparatively high).[8]

Importance and management

Although the evidence is limited, it appears that topical methyl salicylate and trolamine salicylate might be sufficiently absorbed in some circumstances to increase the effect of warfarin. Bear the potential for an interaction in mind should a patient have an otherwise unexplained increase in their INR or experience bleeding.

1. Chow WH, Cheung KL, Ling HM, See T. Potentiation of warfarin anticoagulation by topical methylsalicylate ointment. *J R Soc Med* (1989) 82, 501–2.
2. Yip ASB, Chow WH, Tai YT, Cheung KL. Adverse effect of topical methylsalicylate ointment on warfarin anticoagulation: an unrecognized potential hazard. *Postgrad Med J* (1990) 66, 367–9.
3. Littleton F. Warfarin and topical salicylates. *JAMA* (1990) 263, 2888.
4. Chan TY. Drug interactions as a cause of overanticoagulation and bleedings in Chinese patients receiving warfarin. *Int J Clin Pharmacol Ther* (1998) 36, 403–5.
5. Chan TYK. Life-threatening retroperitoneal bleeding due to warfarin-drug interactions. *Pharmacoepidemiol Drug Safety* (2009) 18, 420–2.
6. Joss JD, LeBlond RF. Potentiation of warfarin anticoagulation associated with topical methyl salicylate. *Ann Pharmacother* (2000) 34, 729–33.
7. Tam LS, Chan TYK, Leung WK, Critchley JAJH. Warfarin interactions with Chinese traditional medicines: danshen and methyl salicylate medicated oil. *Aust N Z J Med* (1995) 25, 258.
8. Collins AJ, Notarianni LJ, Ring EFJ, Seed MP. Some observations on the pharmacology of 'deep-heat', a topical rubifacient. *Ann Rheum Dis* (1984) 43, 411–15.

Coumarins + Sevelamer

Sevelamer does not alter the pharmacokinetics of warfarin.

Clinical evidence, mechanism, importance and management

In a study in healthy subjects, the pharmacokinetics of a single 30-mg oral dose of **warfarin** were not statistically changed by sevelamer 2.4 g (equivalent to 6 capsules). Five more doses of sevelamer were given with meals over 2 days to check whether it had any effect on the enterohepatic circulation of **warfarin**. No effect was seen.[1] Thus it appears that sevelamer does not bind to **warfarin** within the gut to reduce its absorption. No warfarin dose adjustment would be expected to be required on concurrent use.

1. Burke SK, Amin NS, Incerti C, Plone MA, Watson N. Sevelamer hydrochloride (Renagel®), a non-absorbed phosphate-binding polymer, does not interfere with digoxin or warfarin pharmacokinetics. *J Clin Pharmacol* (2001) 41, 193–8.

Coumarins + SNRIs

A study involving duloxetine and warfarin found no pharmacodynamic interaction; however, case reports with acenocoumarol and warfarin suggest that, occasionally, interactions might occur. A case of an increased INR requiring warfarin dose reduction has been reported in a patient taking milnacipran. Unpublished cases of bleeding and increased prothrombin times have been reported with venlafaxine and warfarin. Note that SNRIs alone have, rarely, been associated with bleeding, and there is the theoretical possibility that the risk might be increased when used with warfarin and related drugs.

Clinical evidence

(a) Duloxetine

In a study, healthy subjects stabilised on **warfarin** were given duloxetine 60 mg daily (15 subjects) or duloxetine 120 mg daily (14 subjects) for 9 to 14 days. There was no statistically significant change in the INR with either dose and the pharmacokinetics of warfarin were unchanged. However, the addition of duloxetine 60 mg led to a small 75-second increase in the bleeding time seen with warfarin alone, whereas the 120-mg dose had no statistically significant effect on bleeding time.[1] A woman taking **warfarin** with a stable INR (mean 2.2 over the previous year) developed petechiae and purpura 55 days after starting duloxetine 30 mg daily, and was found to have an INR of 5. Warfarin was stopped on day 58, but the INR continued to increase to greater than 19 on day 85, and she was given vitamin K. On day 94 the duloxetine was stopped. Warfarin was restarted on day 110 and by day 140 the INR was 2.2 with the warfarin dose stabilised at the original level.[2] A 44-year-old woman taking warfarin, had an INR within the range of 0.83 to 4.09 (mean 2.09). Six days after starting duloxetine 60 mg daily, her INR increased to 13.3. Duloxetine and warfarin were stopped, red blood cells and vitamin K were given, and the next day her INR decreased to 2.89. This case was complicated by the presence of altered liver function tests (which returned to baseline on day 13) and other drugs that can interact with warfarin (although no recent change in her drug regimen had occurred, except for the addition of duloxetine). An interaction is therefore not established in this case.[3] Conversely, a patient taking **acenocoumarol** had a decrease in INR (from about 2.6 to 1.5) after taking a single 60-mg dose of duloxetine, the effect of which persisted for 3 weeks.[4]

(b) Milnacipran

A report briefly describes a 53-year old man who had been stable taking **warfarin** 2 mg daily for several years whose INR increased to 3, about 24 days after starting milnacipran. His warfarin dose was initially reduced to 1.5 mg daily and adjusted over the course of the next few months. He was finally stabilised on milnacipran 150 mg daily and a reduced dose of warfarin 1.14 mg daily.[5]

(c) Venlafaxine

The possible interactions of **warfarin** or other anticoagulants with venlafaxine do not appear to have been studied, but in May 2000, the manufacturers of venlafaxine had on record 6 case reports of increased prothrombin times, increased INRs, and bleeding (haematuria, gastrointestinal bleeding, melaena, haemarthrosis) in patients taking **warfarin** with venlafaxine.[6] A case report describes a patient taking **warfarin** and fluvoxamine who had an increased INR which resolved when fluvoxamine was changed to venlafaxine, see 'Coumarins and related drugs + SSRIs', below.

In a cohort study, 6 of 14 patients taking **acenocoumarol** and also taking venlafaxine had an INR greater than 6 on at least one occasion in the study period (hazard ratio 2.19).[7]

Mechanism

The reasons for the bleeding events and increased INRs seen on the concurrent use of a coumarin and a SNRI are not understood, especially as no pharmacokinetic interaction appears to occur between warfarin and duloxetine, and none would be expected between venlafaxine or milnacipran and warfarin. Serotonin release by platelets plays an important role in haemostasis, and, as with all drugs that inhibit serotonin reuptake (see 'Coumarins and related drugs + SSRIs', below), SNRIs such as duloxetine, milnacipran, and venlafaxine can uncommonly cause ecchymosis, mucosal bleeding and, rarely, prolonged bleeding time and haemorrhage. This theoretically might result in an increased risk of bleeding when used with warfarin and related drugs, but would not explain the increased INRs. In a large case-control study, venlafaxine alone was associated with an increased risk of gastrointestinal haemorrhage (rate ratio 1.85), but the study was insufficiently powered to detect whether the concurrent use of warfarin increased this.[8] Note that there was no interaction effect between SSRIs and warfarin for gastrointestinal bleeds in this study.

Importance and management

Evidence for an interaction between the SNRIs and the coumarins is limited to case reports and so an interaction is not established. The general relevance of the unpublished cases with venlafaxine and the cases with duloxetine and milnacipran are therefore uncertain, particularly given that a controlled study found no interaction with duloxetine. However, the SNRIs are known to have effects on bleeding when used alone, and this would reasonably be expected to be worsened in the presence of an anticoagulant. Thus the manufacturers of **desvenlafaxine**[9] and **levomilnacipran**[10] also advise caution on their use in patients taking drugs that interfere with homeostasis, and both name warfarin and other anticoagulants. If one subscribes to the view that increased monitoring is necessary when any drug is started or stopped in a patient on warfarin or related drugs, then it would be prudent to monitor prothrombin times with venlafaxine, duloxetine, and milnacipran. Also bear in mind the possibility of increased bleeding risk in the absence of alterations in INR when any SNRI is used with warfarin.

1. Chappell J, Jingsong H, Knadler MP, Mitchell M, Lee D, Lobo E. Effects of duloxetine on the pharmacodynamics and pharmacokinetics of warfarin at steady state in healthy subjects. *J Clin Pharmacol* (2009) 49, 1456–66.
2. Glueck CJ, Khalil Q, Winiarska M, Wang P. Interaction of duloxetine and warfarin causing severe elevation of international normalized ratio. *JAMA* (2006) 295, 1517–18.
3. Gimenez C, Guce G, Lingisetty C, Bernhardt L. Severe INR elevation related to duloxetine use: a case report. *Psychosomatics* (2011) 52, 583–5.
4. Monastero R, Camarda R, Camarda C. Potential drug-drug interaction between duloxetine and acenocoumarol in a patient with Alzheimer's disease. *Clin Ther* (2007) 29, 2706–9.
5. Sawamura J, Kozaki K, Mochizuki S, Ishigooka J. Possible interaction between milnacipran and warfarin potassium. *J Clin Pharmacol* (2012) 52, 780–1.
6. Wyeth Laboratories. Personal communication, May 2000.
7. Teichert M, Visser LE, Uitterlinden AG, Hofman A, Buhre PJ, Straus S, De Smet PAGM, Stricker BH. Selective serotonin re-uptake inhibiting antidepressants and the risk of overanticoagulation during acenocoumarol maintenance treatment. *Br J Clin Pharmacol* (2011) 72, 798–805.
8. Opatrny L, Delaney JA, Suissa S. Gastro-intestinal haemorrhage risks of selective serotonin receptor antagonist therapy: a new look. *Br J Clin Pharmacol* (2008) 66, 76–81.
9. Pristiq (Desvenlafaxine succinate). Wyeth Pharmaceutical Inc. US Prescribing information, July 2014.
10. Fetzima (Levomilnacipran). Forest Pharmaceuticals Inc. US Prescribing information, July 2014.

Coumarins + Sodium-glucose co-transporter-2 inhibitors

Canagliflozin does not appear to alter the pharmacokinetics or anticoagulant effects of warfarin. Dapagliflozin did not alter the pharmacokinetics of warfarin, or affect the INR. The pharmacokinetics of empagliflozin and warfarin do not appear to be altered on concurrent use.

Clinical evidence, mechanism, importance and management

(a) Canagliflozin

In a randomised, crossover study, 13 healthy subjects were given canagliflozin 300 mg daily for 12 days with a single 30-mg dose of warfarin on day 6. The pharmacokinetics of *R*- or *S*-warfarin were unaffected, and there was no change in the INR, when compared with when warfarin was given alone.[1] No warfarin dose adjustment would seem necessary on concurrent use.

(b) Dapagliflozin

In a randomised, crossover study, 14 healthy subjects were given dapagliflozin 20 mg on day 1 followed by 10 mg daily for 7 days, with a single 25-mg dose of warfarin on day 2. The pharmacokinetics of *R*- or *S*-warfarin were unaffected and there was no change in the INR, when compared with when given alone.[2] No warfarin dose adjustment would seem necessary on concurrent use.

(c) Empagliflozin

In a crossover study, 18 healthy subjects were given empagliflozin 25 mg once daily for 12 days with a single dose of warfarin 25 mg given on day 6. The AUC and maximum plasma concentration of *R*- or *S*-warfarin were not affected, when compared with warfarin given alone, and there was no change in the AUC or maximum plasma concentration of empagliflozin. There was a small 13% change in the INR, but this was not considered to be clinically relevant.[3] No dose adjustment of either drug appears necessary on concurrent use.

1. Devineni D, Manitpisitkul P, Vaccaro N, Bernard A, Skee D, Mamidi RN, Tian H, Weiner S, Stieltjes H, Sha S, Rothenberg P. Effect of canagliflozin, a sodium glucose co-transporter 2 inhibitor, on the pharmacokinetics of oral contraceptives, warfarin, and digoxin in healthy participants. *Int J Clin Pharmacol Ther* (2015) 53, 41–53.
2. Kasichayanula S, Chang M, Liu X, Shyu W-C, Griffen SC, LaCreta FP, Boulton DW. Lack of pharmacokinetic interactions between dapagliflozin and simvastatin, valsartan, warfarin or digoxin. *Adv Therapy* (2012) 29, 163–77.
3. Macha S, Rose P, Mattheus M, Pinnetti S, Woerle HJ. Lack of drug-drug interaction between empagliflozin, a sodium glucose cotransporter 2 inhibitor, and warfarin in healthy volunteers. *Diabetes Obes Metab* (2013) 15, 316–23.

Coumarins + Sodium edetate

A man had a reduction in the effects of warfarin, which was attributed to intravenous chelation therapy that included sodium edetate.

Clinical evidence, mechanism, importance and management

A 64-year-old man who had been taking **warfarin** for 3 weeks, with a gradually increasing dose to 25 mg weekly, had an INR decrease from 2.6 to 1.6 the day after he received intravenous chelation therapy with sodium edetate. He was given a single 10-mg dose of **warfarin** that day, then continued on his 25 mg weekly dose, with an INR in the range of 2.3 to 2.8. The chelation therapy also contained high-dose vitamin C along with various other vitamins and electrolytes.[1] Whether this case represents an interaction with the chelation therapy is uncertain. Further study is needed.

1. Grebe HB, Gregory PJ. Inhibition of warfarin anticoagulation associated with chelation therapy. *Pharmacotherapy* (2002) 22, 1067–69.

Coumarins and related drugs + SSRIs

Fluvoxamine increases warfarin plasma concentrations, and increased INRs have been seen in several cases of the concurrent use of these drugs. In another study with warfarin and paroxetine, the majority of patients experienced no interaction, but a few had minor bleeding events. Other studies suggest that citalopram and sertraline do not significantly alter the pharmacokinetics or effects of warfarin. However, isolated reports describe bleeding in patients taking SSRIs and coumarins or fluindione. In addition, SSRIs alone have, rarely, been associated with bleeding, and some (but not all) retrospective studies suggest that the risk of bleeding might be increased when SSRIs are given with coumarins.

Clinical evidence

(a) Citalopram

In a study in 12 healthy subjects given a single 25-mg oral dose of **warfarin** either alone or on day 15 of a 21-day course of citalopram 40 mg daily, the pharmacokinetics of both *R*- and *S*-warfarin remained unchanged in the presence of the citalopram, but the maximum prothrombin time was increased by 6.4% (1.6 seconds). This was not considered to be clinically relevant.[1]

A retrospective case-control study in patients taking **warfarin** who were given their first 30-day prescription for citalopram found that the concurrent use of citalopram increased the risk of hospitalisation for gastrointestinal bleeding (adjusted odds ratio 1.73). However, no increased risk of gastrointestinal bleeding was found with subsequent prescriptions.[2] Another retrospective study found an increased risk of bleeding on the concurrent use of SSRIs (including citalopram) and warfarin, see under *Various SSRIs*, below.

A 63-year-old patient who had just started **acenocoumarol** 18 mg weekly developed spontaneous gingival haemorrhage 10 days after also starting citalopram 20 mg daily for depression. Her INR had increased from a value of 1.8 to greater than 15. She was treated with 2 units of blood and citalopram was withdrawn. Her INR decreased to 1.95 within 5 days and she was able to continue on **acenocoumarol** 18 mg weekly.[3]

(b) Fluoxetine

In a study in 3 healthy subjects, the half-life of a single 20-mg dose of **warfarin** was not altered by either a single 30-mg dose of fluoxetine given 3 hours before the **warfarin**, or by fluoxetine 30 mg daily for a week with the **warfarin** dose given 3 hours after the last dose of fluoxetine. In addition, fluoxetine had no effect on the warfarin-induced prolongation of prothrombin time.[4] In another study, 6 patients stabilised on **warfarin** had no clinically relevant changes in their prothrombin times or INRs while taking fluoxetine 20 mg daily for 21 days. The greatest change was a decrease in prothrombin time of 3.5% (15%) in one patient.[5]

However, there are few reports of increases in INR in patients taking **warfarin** with fluoxetine. In one report, the INR of a man stabilised on **warfarin**, amiodarone, furosemide, digoxin, ciprofloxacin, and levothyroxine increased sharply from a range of 1.8 to 2.3 up to 14.9 within 5 days of starting fluoxetine 30 mg daily.[6] The INR of another man with metastatic carcinoma taking **warfarin**, dexamethasone, bisacodyl, and lactulose rose from a range of 2.5 to 3.5 up to 15.5 within 2 weeks of starting fluoxetine 20 mg daily. He showed microscopic haematuria but no bleeding.[6] Other reports describe an abdominal haematoma,[6] cerebral haemorrhage,[7] severe bruising,[8] and increases in INRs[9] in patients taking fluoxetine and **warfarin**. In 1993, the CSM in the UK was also said to have 4 other similar cases on record.[9] In the preliminary report of one retrospective review of patients' records, all of 8 evaluable cases of concurrent use of fluoxetine and **warfarin** had an abnormally prolonged prothrombin time.[10]

In a case-control study in patients stabilised on **warfarin**, the increase in risk of hospitalisation for an upper gastrointestinal bleed after starting either fluvoxamine or fluoxetine was marginally higher than for other SSRIs (relative risk 1.2 versus 1.1), but neither risk was statistically significant.[11] Note that fluvoxamine and fluoxetine were not considered separately, and the number taking each one was not stated. However, another retrospective case-control study in patients taking **warfarin** who were given their first 30-day prescription for fluoxetine found that the concurrent use of fluoxetine increased the risk of hospitalisation for gastrointestinal bleeding (adjusted odds ratio 1.63). However, no increased risk of gastrointestinal bleeding was found with subsequent prescriptions.[2] Another retrospective study found an increased risk of bleeding on the concurrent use of SSRIs (including fluoxetine) and warfarin, see under *Various SSRIs*, below.

(c) Fluvoxamine

In a study in healthy subjects, fluvoxamine 50 mg three times daily for 12 days increased steady-state plasma **warfarin** concentrations by about 65% and increased prothrombin times by 28%.[12,13] A worldwide literature search by the manufacturers of fluvoxamine identified only 11 reported interactions between **warfarin** and fluvoxamine by 1995, all with clinical signs that included prolonged prothrombin times.[14] An 80-year-old woman who had recently started taking **warfarin**, digoxin, and colchicine (see 'Coumarins and related drugs + Colchicine', p.419) had an increase in her INR from 1.8 to about 10 within a week of starting to take fluvoxamine 25 mg daily. Both the **warfarin** and fluvoxamine were stopped, but her INR only stabilised on the original dose of **warfarin** after the colchicine was withdrawn.[15] Another report describes a 79-year-old woman admitted to hospital because of suicidal thoughts. She was taking **warfarin** (INR 1.6 to 1.8) and citalopram 10 mg at night and other medications including paracetamol with dextropropoxyphene. On the third day in hospital the citalopram dose was increased to 30 mg at bedtime; after 2 days it was stopped and fluvoxamine 50 mg daily was started to treat depression and possibly obsessive thoughts. Within 4 days the patient's INR had increased to 3.7. Fluvoxamine was replaced with venlafaxine and **warfarin** was omitted for one day. The INR gradually decreased to the normal range over about 7 days.[16]

A further isolated report describes a woman stabilised on **fluindione** whose INR rose to 7.13 (from a normal value of about 2.5) within 13 days of starting to take fluvoxamine 100 mg daily. She had received fluoxetine, dosulepin, and lorazepam for 15 days before fluvoxamine was started.[17]

In a case-control study in patients stabilised on **warfarin**, the increase in risk of hospitalisation for an upper gastrointestinal bleed after starting either fluvoxamine or fluoxetine was marginally higher than for other SSRIs (relative risk 1.2 versus 1.1), but neither risk was statistically significant.[11] Note that fluoxetine and fluvoxamine were not considered separately, and the number taking each one was not stated.

In a cohort study, patients taking **acenocoumarol** with fluvoxamine (8 of 36 patients) were found to have an increased risk of an INR greater than 6 (hazard ratio 2.46).[18]

(d) Paroxetine

In a study in healthy subjects, paroxetine 30 mg daily, given with **warfarin** 5 mg daily, did not increase mean prothrombin times to a clinically relevant extent, but mild, clinically relevant bleeding was seen in 5 out of 27 subjects given both drugs. Two withdrew from the study because of increased prothrombin times, and another because of haematuria. The pharmacokinetics of warfarin and paroxetine remained unchanged by concurrent use.[19] In a brief retrospective review, 4 patients taking **warfarin** were said to have had an increase in INR by an average of 3 points (increases of nearly 100% in some cases) associated with the use of paroxetine and sertraline.[20] A retrospective case-control study in patients taking **warfarin** who were given their first 30-day prescription for paroxetine found that the concurrent use of paroxetine increased the risk of hospitalisation for gastrointestinal bleeding (adjusted odds ratio 1.64). However, no increased risk of gastrointestinal bleeding was found with subsequent prescriptions.[2] Another retrospective study found an increased risk of bleeding on the concurrent use of SSRIs (including paroxetine) and warfarin, see under *Various SSRIs*, below.

A single case report[21] describes severe bleeding (abdominal haematoma) in a patient taking **acenocoumarol** and paroxetine when given phenytoin, but it is not clear whether the paroxetine had any part to play in what happened (see 'Phenytoin + Coumarins and related drugs', p.598).

(e) Sertraline

In a placebo-controlled study in healthy subjects, sertraline in increasing doses up to 200 mg daily for 22 days increased the prothrombin time AUC in response to a single 0.75-mg/kg dose of **warfarin** by 8%. This was statistically significant, but regarded as too small to be clinically relevant.[22]

In a brief retrospective review, 4 patients taking **warfarin** were said to have had an increase in INR by an average of 3 points (increases of nearly 100% in some cases) associated with the use of paroxetine and sertraline.[20] A retrospective case-control study in patients taking **warfarin** who were given their first 30-day prescription for sertraline found no increased risk of hospitalisation for gastrointestinal bleeding on concurrent use.[2] However, another retrospective study found an increased risk of bleeding on the concurrent use of SSRIs (including sertraline) and warfarin, see under *Various SSRIs*, below.

(f) Various SSRIs

In a large case-control study using data from the Netherlands, the concurrent use of coumarins (**acenocoumarol** and **phenprocoumon**) and SSRIs increased the risk of hospitalisation for non-gastrointestinal bleeding (odds ratio 1.7). However, the risk of hospitalisation for gastrointestinal bleeding was not increased (odds ratio 0.8).[23] Another case-control study using data from the UK General Practice Research Database, also found no increased risk of gastrointestinal haemorrhage with the concurrent use of **warfarin** and SSRIs compared with warfarin or an SSRI given alone (rate ratio 0.81).[24,25] In yet another analysis, **warfarin** alone was associated with an increased risk of haemorrhagic stroke (odds ratio 3), whereas SSRIs alone were not (odds ratio 0.8). The concurrent use of SSRIs and **warfarin** did not increase the risk compared with warfarin alone (odds ratios 4.7 versus 3).[26]

Other studies have found an increased risk of bleeding on the concurrent use of warfarin and an SSRI. In one retrospective study in patients taking **warfarin**, the concurrent use of any antidepressant (including SSRIs, some tricyclics, trazodone and bupropion) was not associated with an increased risk of bleeding. However, further analysis found that the concurrent use of an SSRI was associated with an increased risk of any bleeding, major bleeding and hospitalisation due to haemorrhage (odds ratio 2.6, 4.4 and 7, respectively), when compared with patients taking warfarin and not taking an SSRI. When these results were adjusted for factors associated with an increased risk of bleeding in the study (haematocrit and creatinine concentrations) and for patient factors that differed between both groups (such as female sex, history of stroke or gastrointestinal bleed), the risk of any bleed was still increased.[27] Similarly, in another retrospective study in patients taking **warfarin**, the concurrent use of an SSRI (**citalopram**, **fluoxetine**, **paroxetine**, and **sertraline**) was associated with an increased risk of bleeding (adjusted odds ratio 2.57), when compared with patients taking **warfarin** only. In particular, these patients had an increased risk of upper gastrointestinal bleeding, more so than lower gastrointestinal bleeding or intracranial haemorrhage (adjusted odds ratio 5.49, compared with 1.33 and 1.47, respectively). In this study, **clomipramine** was included with the SSRIs group and **fluvoxamine** was analysed separately as a CYP2C9 inhibitor; however, both drugs only represented a small percentage of the analysed data for each group.[28] Another retrospective cohort study[29] and a case-control study[2] also found similar results. However, in the case-control study mirtazapine was used as a non-interacting reference, and this was also found to increase the rate of hospitalisation for a gastrointestinal bleed in patients taking warfarin. The authors state that it is possible that other patient factors not controlled during the analysis affected the results and that this suggests that a drug-drug interaction between warfarin and the SSRIs might not be the cause of this adverse outcome.[29]

Mechanism

Pharmacokinetic interactions. Fluvoxamine is a weak inhibitor of CYP2C9, by which *S*-warfarin is metabolised, and is also a potent inhibitor of CYP1A2 and CYP2C19, by which the less active *R*-warfarin is partially metabolised. Consequently, fluvoxamine would be expected to increase warfarin effects. *In vitro*, fluoxetine, paroxetine, sertraline, and citalopram had little or no inhibitory effect on CYP2C9 mediated *S*-warfarin hydroxylation.[30] In addition, these SSRIs do not inhibit CYP1A2 or CYP2C19, therefore they would not be anticipated to increase warfarin concentrations.

Pharmacodynamic interactions. Serotonin release by platelets plays an important role in haemostasis, and epidemiological studies and case reports suggest that SSRIs alone are rarely associated with bleeding events.[23,31]

Importance and management

A pharmacokinetic interaction between fluvoxamine and warfarin that leads to increased anticoagulant effects is established. Therefore, the anticoagulant effects should be monitored when fluvoxamine is started, being alert for the need to decrease the coumarin dose.

None of the other SSRIs studied (citalopram, fluoxetine, paroxetine) have been shown to alter the pharmacokinetics of warfarin. Neither fluoxetine nor paroxetine increased the prothrombin time, but citalopram and sertraline caused a less than 10% increase in prothrombin time, and a few patients taking paroxetine with warfarin had bleeds. **Escitalopram** is the *S*-isomer of citalopram, and as such would be expected to interact in the same way as citalopram. However, in general, these effects would not be expected to be clinically relevant. Nevertheless, because SSRIs alone can rarely cause bleeding, some predict that this could result in additive effects with coumarins and indanediones, and recommend caution with all SSRIs. Some of the available retrospective data appears to support this prediction, as well as a possible excess risk of gastrointestinal bleeding, whereas other studies did not find this effect. The increased risk of bleeding might also be relevant for bleeds from other sites (e.g. intracranial). As there are case reports of interactions with warfarin for many of the SSRIs (citalopram, fluoxetine, paroxetine, sertraline), it would seem prudent to bear these in mind in a patient taking both drugs.

1. Priskorn M, Sidhu JS, Larsen F, Davis JD, Khan AZ, Rolan PE. Investigation of multiple dose citalopram on the pharmacokinetics and pharmacodynamics of racemic warfarin. *Br J Clin Pharmacol* (1997) 44, 199–202.
2. Schelleman H, Brensinger CM, Bilker WB, Hennessy S. Antidepressant-warfarin interaction and associated gastrointestinal bleeding risk in a case-control study. *PLoS One* (2011) 6, e21447.
3. Borrás-Blasco J, Marco-Garbayo JL, Bosca-Sanleon B, Navarro-Ruiz A. Probable interaction between citalopram and acenocoumarol. *Ann Pharmacother* (2002) 36, 345.
4. Rowe H, Carmichael R, Lemberger L. The effect of fluoxetine on warfarin metabolism in the rat and man. *Life Sci* (1978) 23, 807–12.
5. Ford MA, Anderson ML, Rindone JP, Jaskar DW. Lack of effect of fluoxetine on the hypoprothrombinemic response of warfarin. *J Clin Psychopharmacol* (1997) 17, 110–12.
6. Hanger HC, Thomas F. Fluoxetine and warfarin interactions. *N Z Med J* (1995), 108, 157.
7. Dent LA, Orrock MW. Warfarin-fluoxetine and diazepam-fluoxetine interaction. *Pharmacotherapy* (1997) 17, 170–2.
8. Claire RJ, Servis ME, Cram DL. Potential interaction between warfarin sodium and fluoxetine. *Am J Psychiatry* (1991) 148, 1604.
9. Woolfrey S, Gammack NS, Dewar MS, Brown PJE. Fluoxetine-warfarin interaction. *BMJ* (1993) 307, 241.
10. Wu J-R, Li P-YY, Yang Y-HK. Concurrent use of fluoxetine and warfarin prolongs prothrombin time: a retrospective survey. *Pharmacotherapy* (1997) 17, 1080.

11. Kurdyak PA, Juurlink DN, Kopp A, Herrmann N, Mamdani MM. Antidepressants, warfarin, and the risk of hemorrhage. *J Clin Psychopharmacol* (2005) 25, 561–4.
12. Benfield P, Ward A. Fluvoxamine. A review of its pharmacodynamic and pharmacokinetic properties, and therapeutic efficacy in depressive illness. *Drugs* (1986) 32, 313–34.
13. Solvay. Personal communication, December 2006.
14. Wagner W, Vause EW. Fluvoxamine. A review of global drug-drug interaction data. *Clin Pharmacokinet* (1995) 29 (Suppl 1), 26–32.
15. Yap KB, Low ST. Interaction of fluvoxamine with warfarin in an elderly woman. *Singapore Med J* (1999) 40, 480–2.
16. Limke KK, Shelton AR, Elliott ES. Fluvoxamine interaction with warfarin. *Ann Pharmacother* (2002) 36, 1890–2.
17. Nezelof S, Vandel P, Bonin B. Fluvoxamine interaction with fluindione: a case report. *Therapie* (1997) 52, 608–9.
18. Teichert M, Visser LE, Uitterlinden AG, Hofman A, Buhre PJ, Straus S, De Smet PAGM, Stricker BH. Selective serotonin re-uptake inhibiting antidepressants and the risk of overanticoagulation during acenocoumarol maintenance treatment. *Br J Clin Pharmacol* (2011) 72, 798–805.
19. Bannister SJ, Houser VP, Hulse JD, Kisicki JC, Rasmussen JGC. Evaluation of the potential for interactions of paroxetine with diazepam, cimetidine, warfarin, and digoxin. *Acta Psychiatr Scand* (1989) 80 (Suppl 350), 102–6.
20. Askinazi C. SSRI treatment of depression with comorbid cardiac disease. *Am J Psychiatry* (1996) 153, 135–6.
21. Abad-Santos F, Carcas AJ, Capitán CF, Frias J. Case report. Retroperitoneal haematoma in a patient treated with acenocoumarol, phenytoin and paroxetine. *Clin Lab Haematol* (1995) 17, 195–7.
22. Apseloff G, Wilner KD, Gerber N, Tremaine LM. Effect of sertraline on protein binding of warfarin. *Clin Pharmacokinet* (1997) 32 (Suppl 1), 37–42.
23. Schalekamp T, Klungel OH, Souverein PC, de Boer A. Increased bleeding risk with concurrent use of selective serotonin reuptake inhibitors and coumarins. *Arch Intern Med* (2008) 168, 180–5.
24. Opatrny L, Delaney JA, Suissa S. Gastro-intestinal haemorrhage risks of selective serotonin receptor antagonist therapy: a new look. *Br J Clin Pharmacol* (2008)66, 76–81.
25. Suissa S. Personal communication, September 2008.
26. Kharofa J, Sekar P, Haverbusch M, Moomaw C, Flaherty M, Kissela B, Broderick J, Woo D. Selective serotonin reuptake inhibitors and risk of hemorrhagic stroke. *Stroke* (2007) 38, 3049–51.
27. Cochran KA, Cavallari LH, Shapiro NL, Bishop JR. Bleeding incidence with concomitant use of antidepressants and warfarin. *Ther Drug Monit* (2011) 33, 433–8.
28. Hauta-Aho M, Tirkkonen T, Vahlberg T, Laine K. The effect of drug interactions on bleeding risk associated with warfarin therapy in hospitalized patients. *Ann Med* (2009) 41, 619–28.
29. Wallerstedt SM, Gleerup H, Sundström A, Stigendal L, Ny L. Risk of clinically relevant bleeding in warfarin-treated patients – influence of SSRI treatment. *Pharmacoepidemiol Drug Safety* (2009) 18, 412–6.
30. Hemeryck A, De Vriendt C, Belpaire FM. Inhibition of CYP2C9 by selective serotonin reuptake inhibitors: in vitro studies with tolbutamide and (S)-warfarin using human liver microsomes. *Eur J Clin Pharmacol* (1999) 54, 947–51.
31. Consumers' Association. Do SSRIs cause gastrointestinal bleeding? *Drug Ther Bull* (2004) 42, 17–18.

Coumarins + St John's wort (*Hypericum perforatum*)

St John's wort can reduce the anticoagulant effects of phenprocoumon and warfarin. An isolated report described an increased anticoagulant effect in response to warfarin on the concurrent use of St John's Wort.

Clinical evidence

(a) Phenprocoumon

In a randomised, placebo-controlled, crossover study in 10 healthy men,[1] St John's wort extract (*LI 160, Lichtwer Pharma*) 900 mg daily for 11 days negligibly reduced the AUC of a single 12-mg dose of phenprocoumon by 17%.

A case report describes a 75-year-old woman taking phenprocoumon who had a reduced anticoagulant response (a rise in the Quick value) 2 months after starting to take St John's wort.[2]

(b) Warfarin

In a randomised, crossover study in 12 healthy subjects, one tablet of St John's wort three times daily for 3 weeks slightly decreased the AUC of both *R*- and *S*-warfarin by about 25%. In this study, the brand of St John's wort used was *Bioglan* tablets, each tablet containing an extract equivalent to 1 g of *Hypericum perforatum* flowering herb top containing 825 micrograms of hypericin and 12.5 mg of hyperforin, and warfarin was given as a single 25-mg dose on day 14.[3]

Over the 1998 to 1999 period, the Swedish Medical Products Agency received 7 case reports of patients stabilised on warfarin whose INRs decreased when St John's wort was started. Their INRs fell from the normal therapeutic range of about 2 to 4, to about 1.5. Two patients needed warfarin dose increases of 6.6% and 15%, respectively, when St John's wort was added. The INRs of 4 of the patients returned to their former values when the St John's wort was stopped.[4] A retrospective study[5] similarly found that the concurrent use of enzyme inducers (including St John's wort) greatly influenced the total weekly warfarin dose; further analysis found that an average additional amount of warfarin of 17.2 mg weekly was required in patients taking these drugs.

In contrast, a case report describes an 85-year-old patient taking warfarin 5 mg daily for almost a year without problems, who developed upper gastrointestinal bleeding, requiring hospitalisation, one month after starting St John's wort. On admission his haemoglobin was 7.9 g/dL and his INR was 6.2. After supportive treatment, the bleeding ceased and endoscopy before discharge revealed no clinically important pathology.[6]

Mechanism

Uncertain, but it has been suggested that the St John's wort increases the metabolism and clearance of the coumarins,[1,3,4] possibly by induction of CYP3A4 and CYP2C9 as both *R*- and *S*-warfarin were affected.[3] However, note that St John's wort had no effect on the metabolism of tolbutamide, which is commonly used as a probe substrate for CYP2C9 activity (see 'Sulfonylureas + St John's wort (*Hypericum perforatum*)', p.552). Note also that St John's wort does not generally *inhibit* cytochrome P450 isoenzymes *in vivo*, as was suggested by the authors of the case report showing increased warfarin effects.[6]

Importance and management

Information seems to be limited to these reports, but a pharmacokinetic interaction between the coumarins and St John's wort would seem to be established, which might be clinically important in some patients. It would be prudent to monitor the INRs of patients taking phenprocoumon, warfarin, or any other coumarin, if they start taking St John's wort, being alert for the need to increase the anticoagulant dose accordingly. This interaction should also be borne in mind as a possible cause in cases where an otherwise unexplained decrease in INR occurs, and scrutiny of the patients other medications, particularly self medications, should be undertaken for the presence of St John's wort. Note that the CSM in the UK advise that St John's wort should not be used with warfarin. They state that the degree of induction of warfarin metabolism is likely to vary because amounts of active ingredients can vary between St John's wort preparations. If a patient is already taking warfarin and St John's wort, they advise checking the INR, stopping the St John's wort, and then monitoring the INR closely and adjusting the anticoagulant dose as necessary.[7]

Note that the case report of increased effect of warfarin,[6] is in stark contrast to the other evidence and is not in line with how St John's wort is understood to affect drug metabolism. It is therefore unlikely to be of any general importance.

1. Maurer A, Johne A, Bauer S, Brockmöller J, Donath F, Roots I, Langheinrich M, Hübner W-D. Interaction of St John's wort extract with phenprocoumon. *Eur J Clin Pharmacol* (1999) 55, A22.
2. Bon S, Hartmann, Kuhn M. Johanniskraut: Ein Enzyminduktor? *Schweiz Apothekerzeitung* (1999) 16, 535–6.
3. Jiang X, Williams KM, Liauw WS, Ammit AJ, Roufogalis BD, Duke CC, Day RO, McLachlan AJ. Effect of St John's wort and ginseng on the pharmacokinetics and pharmacodynamics of warfarin in healthy subjects. *Br J Clin Pharmacol* (2004) 57, 592–9.
4. Yue Q-Y, Bergquist C, Gerdén B. Safety of St John's wort *(Hypericum perforatum)*. *Lancet* (2000) 355, 576–7.
5. Whitley HP, Fermo JD, Chumney ECG, Brzezinski WA. Effect of patient-specific factors on weekly warfarin dose. *Ther Clin Risk Manag* (2007) 3, 499–504.
6. Uygur Bayramiçli O, Kalkay MN, Oskay Bozkaya E, Doğan Köse E, Iyigün Ö, Görük M, Sezgin G. St. John's wort (Hypericum perforatum) and warfarin: Dangerous liaisons. *Turk J Gastroenterol* (2011) 22, 115.
7. Committee on Safety of Medicines. Message from Professor A Breckenridge, Chairman, Committee on Safety of Medicines, and Fact Sheet for Health Care Professionals, February 2000. Available at http://webarchive.nationalarchives.gov.uk/20141205150130/http://www.mhra.gov.uk/Safetyinformation/Safetywarningsalertsandrecalls/Safetywarningsandmessagesformedicines/CON2015756 (accessed 21/10/15).

Coumarins and related drugs + Statins

Studies and case reports have suggested that fluvastatin can increase warfarin exposure and/or effects. Rosuvastatin can increase the anticoagulant effects of warfarin but does not alter warfarin pharmacokinetics. Other studies with atorvastatin, lovastatin, pravastatin, and simvastatin suggest that they do not usually alter the effects of warfarin, although isolated cases of bleeding have been seen when these statins were given with coumarins and fluindione. Pitavastatin does not appear to alter the effects or pharmacokinetics of warfarin.

Clinical evidence

Pharmacological studies of the effect of statins on **warfarin** are summarised in 'Table 12.7', p.472. These show that **rosuvastatin** increases **warfarin** effects without altering **warfarin** pharmacokinetics, and that **fluvastatin**, at high clinical doses, can increase *S*-warfarin exposure. Conversely, **atorvastatin**, **pravastatin**, **lovastatin**, and **simvastatin** appear to have little effect on the anticoagulant effects of **warfarin**. **Pitavastatin** appears to have no effect on **warfarin** effects or pharmacokinetics.[1] Nevertheless, isolated case reports of interactions with coumarins have been reported for all statins and these are summarised in 'Table 12.8', p.474.

Moreover, in one analysis of 42 patients taking warfarin and starting **fluvastatin** 20 mg daily,[2] three patients had a modest rise in INR (further details given in 'Table 12.8', p.474), 5 patients had possible elevations in INR, 17 patients had no change, and data were not available for 17.

An early report, from the first 7 months after **lovastatin** became available in the US, notes that the manufacturers had received 10 spontaneous reports of bleeding and/or increased prothrombin times in patients taking **warfarin** with lovastatin.[3,4] In an analysis of factors that might be useful to construct a warfarin-dosing algorithm, **warfarin** maintenance doses were found to be 12% lower in patients taking **simvastatin**.[5] In another similar analysis, there was a trend towards a lower **warfarin** dose with a lower plasma concentration of 10-hydroxywarfarin (a metabolite of *R*-warfarin) in 17 patients taking simvastatin or lovastatin.[6]

In the preliminary analysis of a large, retrospective, case-control study in patients taking warfarin, the use of statins in patients who were receiving **warfarin** did not decrease the risk for bleeding (odds ratio 0.91).[7] In contrast, another large retrospective case-control study in patients taking warfarin and who were hospitalised for a gastrointestinal bleed, found that initiation of **simvastatin** or **atorvastatin** was associated with an increased risk of bleeding (odds ratio 1.33 and 1.29, respectively) and this was further increased in patients who had taken warfarin for 3 months or more (odds ratio 1.46 and 1.39, respectively). **Pravastatin** was not associated with an increased risk of bleeding.[8]

Coumarins are not expected to alter statin pharmacokinetics or effects. However, an isolated report[9] describes rhabdomyolysis with acute renal failure in an 82-year-old man taking **simvastatin** 20 mg daily within 7 days of starting **warfarin** 5 mg daily; his INR was raised to 4.3.

Table 12.7 Summary of pharmacological studies of the effect of statins on warfarin

Study type	*Group*	*Warfarin*	*Statin dose*	*Findings*		*Refs*
				Pharmacokinetics	*Anticoagulant effects*	
Atorvastatin						
Prospective	12 patients	Stable therapy	80 mg daily for 14 days	NR	Prothrombin time decreased from 18.6 to 17 seconds on days 3 to 5, but was not changed on other days	1
Fluvastatin						
Placebo-controlled	Healthy subjects	Single 30-mg dose	40 mg daily for 8 days	No change in racemic warfarin levels	No change in prothrombin complex activity	2
Crossover	18 healthy subjects	Single 10-mg dose	40 mg twice daily for 18 days	Increase in AUC of *S*-warfarin of 42% in smokers and 26% in non-smokers	NR	3
Lovastatin						
NR	Patients	Stable therapy	NR	NR	No change in prothrombin time	4
Crossover, placebo-controlled	8 patients	Stable therapy	40 mg daily for 7 days	NR	INR increased from 2.6 to 3 (17%) by day 7	5
Pitavastatin						
Open-label, crossover	Healthy subjects	Stable therapy	4 mg daily for 9 days	No change in pharmacokinetics of *S*- or *R*-warfarin	No change in INR over the 8 days of concurrent use	6
Open-label	23 healthy subjects	Stable therapy	4 mg daily for 9 days	No change in pharmacokinetics of *S*- or *R*-warfarin	No change in INR over the 8 days of concurrent use	7
Pravastatin						
Prospective	Healthy subjects	5 mg daily	20 mg twice daily	17% increase in warfarin AUC*	No change in prothrombin time on concurrent use for 6 days	8
Crossover, placebo-controlled	8 patients	Stable therapy	20 mg daily for 7 days	NR	No change in INR over the 7 days	5
NR	Elderly healthy subjects	Stable therapy	40 mg	NR	No change in prothrombin time	9
Rosuvastatin						
Placebo-controlled, crossover	18 healthy subjects	Single 25-mg dose	40 mg daily for 10 days	No change in pharmacokinetics of *S*- or *R*-warfarin	INR AUC increased by 10%, and maximum INR increased by 19%	10
Prospective	7 patients	Stable therapy	10 mg daily for up to 14 days then 80 mg daily for up to 14 days	NR	With 10 mg daily, 2 patients had INR increases of 1.5 and 3.7 to values greater than 4. With 80 mg daily, 4 of 5 patients had increases of 1.5 to 2.6 to values greater than 4	10
Placebo-controlled, crossover	12 healthy subjects	5 mg daily for 14 days	40 mg daily for 7 days	NR	No change in steady-state warfarin pharmacodynamics	11
Open-label, crossover	Healthy subjects	Stable therapy	40 mg daily for 9 days	No change in pharmacokinetics of *S*- or *R*-warfarin	INR increased from a mean of 1.74 to 1.9 over the 8 days of concurrent use	6
Simvastatin						
Retrospective analysis of a placebo-controlled study	23 patients	NR	20 mg or 40 mg daily	NR	INR increased from a mean of 2.6 to 3.4 in the simvastatin group without changes in warfarin dose, compared with a decrease from 2.6 to 2.4 in the placebo group	12
NR	Healthy subjects	NR	20 mg or 40 mg daily	NR	INR increased from a mean of 1.7 to 1.8	13,14
Retrospective cohort	46 patients	Stable with no change	Switch from pravastatin to simvastatin	NR	Mean INR increased from 2.42 to 2.74. Eleven patients had a warfarin dose adjustment after the INR change, 7 a decrease and 4 an increase	15
Retrospective	29 patients	Stable therapy	NR	NR	Warfarin dose decreased from a mean of 4.2 mg daily before to 3.8 mg daily after, while INR increased from a mean of 2.5 to 3.15	16

NR = not reported.

*Attributed to warfarin being nearer steady state by the combined phase of this longitudinal study, in which there was no washout between phases, and sequence of phases was pravastatin alone for 3.5 days, warfarin alone for 6 days, and then both drugs for 6 days.

Continued

Table 12.7 Summary of pharmacological studies of the effect of statins on warfarin (continued)

Study type	*Group*	*Warfarin*	*Statin dose*	*Findings*		*Refs*
				Pharmacokinetics	*Anticoagulant effects*	
Historical control group taking warfarin alone	56 patients 56 controls	Stable therapy	20 mg daily (35 patients) or 40 mg daily (21 patients)	Median clearance of *S*-warfarin was 18%, and *R*-warfarin 23%, lower in patients than controls	Mean dose of warfarin was 3.3 mg daily in patients and 4 mg in controls	17

NR = not reported.
*Attributed to warfarin being nearer steady state by the combined phase of this longitudinal study, in which there was no washout between phases, and sequence of phases was pravastatin alone for 3.5 days, warfarin alone for 6 days, and then both drugs for 6 days.

1. Stern R, Abel R, Gibson GL, Besserer J. Atorvastatin does not alter the anticoagulant activity of warfarin. *J Clin Pharmacol* (1997) 37, 1062–4.
2. Lescol (Fluvastatin sodium). Novartis Pharmaceuticals Corp. US Prescribing information, October 2006.
3. Kim MJ, Nafzinger AN, Kashuba AD, Kirchheiner J, Bauer S, Gaedigk A, Bertino JS. Effects of fluvastatin and cigarette smoking on CYP2C9 activity measured using the probe S-warfarin. *Eur J Clin Pharmacol* (2006) 62, 431–6.
4. Mevacor (Lovastatin). Merck & Co., Inc. US Prescribing information, September 2008.
5. O'Rangers EA, Ford M, Hershey A. The effect of HMG-coA reductase inhibitors on the anticoagulant response to warfarin. *Pharmacotherapy* (1994) 14, 349.
6. Yu CY, Campbell SE, Zhu B, Knadler MP, Small DS, Sponseller CA, Hunt TL, Morgan RE. Effect of pitavastatin vs. rosuvastatin on international normalized ratio in healthy volunteers on steady-state warfarin. *Curr Med Res Opin* (2012) 28, 187-94.
7. Inagaki Y, Hunt T, Arana B, Gosho M, Morgan R. Drug-drug interaction study to assess the effects of multiple-dose pitavastatin on steady-state warfarin in healthy adult volunteers. *J Clin Pharmacol* (2011) 51, 1302-9.
8. ER Squibb. Data on file. A report on the pharmacokinetic and pharmacodynamic interaction of pravastatin and warfarin in healthy male volunteers (Protocol No 27, 201-59). 1988.
9. Pravachol (Pravastatin sodium). Bristol-Myers Squibb Co. US Prescribing information, March 2007.
10. Simonson SG, Martin PD, Mitchell PD, Lasseter K, Gibson G, Schneck DW. Effect of rosuvastatin on warfarin pharmacodynamics and pharmacokinetics. *J Clin Pharmacol* (2005) 45, 927–34.
11. Jindal D, Tandon M, Sharma S, Pillai KK. Pharmacodynamic evaluation of warfarin and rosuvastatin co-administration in healthy subjects. *Eur J Clin Pharmacol* (2005) 61, 621–25.
12. Keech A, Collins R, MacMahon S, Armitage J, Lawson A, Wallendszus K, Fatemian M, Kearney E, Lyon V, Mindell J, Mount J, Painter R, Parish S, Slavin B, Sleight P, Youngman L, Peto R for the Oxford Cholesterol Study Group. Three-year follow-up of the Oxford cholesterol study: assessment of the efficacy and safety of simvastatin in preparation for a large mortality study. *Eur Heart J* (1994) 15, 255–69.
13. Zocor (Simvastatin). Merck Sharp & Dohme Ltd. UK Summary of product characteristics, October 2009.
14. Zocor (Simvastatin). Merck & Co., Inc. US Prescribing information, June 2008.
15. Lin JC, Ito MK, Stolley SN, Morreale AP, Marcus DB. The effect of converting from pravastatin to simvastatin on the pharmacodynamics of warfarin. *J Clin Pharmacol* (1999) 39, 86–90.
16. Hickmott H, Wynne H, Kamali F. The effect of simvastatin co-medication on warfarin anticoagulation response and dose requirements. *Thromb Haemost* (2003) 89, 949–50.
17. Sconce EA, Khan TI, Daly AK, Wynne HA, Kamali F. The impact of simvastatin on warfarin disposition and dose requirements. *J Thromb Haemost* (2006) 4, 1422–4.

Mechanism

Fluvastatin is a weak inhibitor of CYP2C9, by which *S*-warfarin (which has greater anticoagulant activity than *R*-warfarin) is metabolised. Evidence from an interaction study with the CYP2C9 substrate diclofenac suggests that this interaction is most likely with higher and sustained fluvastatin concentrations,[10] which might explain why, with warfarin, it was demonstrated in healthy subjects with the maximum recommended daily dose of 80 mg daily, but not the more commonly encountered clinical dose of 40 mg daily, and why it has not been seen in all patients.

Lovastatin and simvastatin appear less likely to interact via CYP2C9,[11] although it is possible they might interact via other isoenzymes. In one analysis, patients taking these statins had lower plasma concentrations of 10-hydroxywarfarin, a metabolite of *R*-warfarin, but clearance of *R*-warfarin was not reduced.[6] It might be that because warfarin has multiple routes of metabolism, other isoenzymes can 'pick up' warfarin metabolism if competition for metabolism occurs. Interactions might therefore only occur if other confounding factors are present. Alternatively, the cases seen might just represent idiosyncratic reactions.

Rosuvastatin clearly shows a dose related increase in warfarin effects, but this was not due to an increase in *R*- or *S*-warfarin concentrations, and the mechanism for this effect is unknown.[12]

Bear in mind that patients starting a statin might also alter their dietary fat consumption. Vegetable fats are a good source of vitamin K (see 'Table 12.5', p.430), and a marked reduction in the consumption of foods rich in these fats could increase the sensitivity to warfarin.

Importance and management

Data are limited, which is surprising given the widespread use of statins and warfarin, and are sometimes contradictory, all of which complicates making firm recommendations. Some evidence suggests that a slight pharmacokinetic interaction occurs between **fluvastatin** and warfarin at high doses, and this would explain the case reports of an interaction with this statin. The clinical evidence suggests that only some patients develop an important interaction (3 of 25 evaluable patients in one analysis). Clearly, with **fluvastatin**, increased monitoring is required when starting or stopping the statin, or changing the dose. Similar advice also applies to **rosuvastatin**, which has the best pharmacological data on concurrent use in patients, clearly showing that clinically important increases in INR can occur. In contrast to fluvastatin, this interaction does not appear to have a pharmacokinetic basis.

Data for **simvastatin** appear to be limited to retrospective analyses, with only one poor quality study reporting pharmacokinetic data, which suggested a minor reduction in warfarin clearance with simvastatin. In general the studies show that simvastatin can cause a minor increase in warfarin effects. This would appear to be supported by the fact that there is only one fully published report of an interaction in a patient taking warfarin and one for acenocoumarol. Some consider that any interaction is of limited clinical importance, and that the statin could be switched to simvastatin without any additional monitoring over and above that usually practised for warfarin.[13] However, others,[14,15] including the manufacturers[16,17] recommend increased monitoring when starting or stopping the statin, or changing the dose, and this might be prudent. There are even less data for **lovastatin**, an analogue of simvastatin, but it appears to interact similarly to simvastatin, and the US manufacturer recommends the same increased monitoring as for simvastatin.[18] There appear to be no data on the effect of lovastatin on the pharmacokinetics of coumarins.

In one pharmacological study, **atorvastatin** did not interact with warfarin, and no cases of an interaction have been published. This suggests that with this statin, no increased monitoring is necessary. In the US, the manufacturer does not give any advice on monitoring,[19] but in the UK, the manufacturer recommends increased monitoring when starting or stopping atorvastatin, or changing the dose,[20] which seems over-cautious.

Limited data for **pravastatin** also suggest that no interaction occurs with warfarin, there being just one isolated case report with the indanedione, fluindione. No increased monitoring would appear to be necessary on concurrent use.

In a study in healthy subjects, **pitavastatin** did not appear to interact with warfarin, but the US manufacturer nevertheless advises that INR and prothrombin time should be monitored when pitavastatin is given with warfarin.[1]

1. Livalo (Pitavastatin). Kowa Pharmaceuticals America, Inc. US Prescribing information, October 2013.
2. Trilli LE, Kelley CL, Aspinall SL, Kroner BA. Potential interaction between warfarin and fluvastatin. *Ann Pharmacother* (1996) 30, 1399–1402.
3. Tobert JA, Shear CL, Chremos AN, Mantell GE. Clinical experience with lovastatin. *Am J Cardiol* (1990) 65, 23F–26F.
4. Tobert JA. Efficacy and long-term adverse effect pattern of lovastatin. *Am J Cardiol* (1988) 62, 28J–34J.
5. Gage BF, Eby C, Milligan PE, Banet GA, Duncan JR, McLeod HL. Use of pharmacogenetics and clinical factors to predict the maintenance dose of warfarin. *Thromb Haemost* (2004) 91, 87–94.
6. Herman D, Locatelli I, Grabnar I, Peternel P, Stegnar M, Lainščak M, Mrhar A, Breskvar K, Dolžan V. The influence of co-treatment with carbamazepine, amiodarone and statins on warfarin metabolism and maintenance dose. *Eur J Clin Pharmacol* (2006) 62, 291–6.
7. Douketis JD, Melo M, Bell CM, Mamdani MM. Does statin therapy decrease the risk for bleeding in patients who are receiving warfarin? *Am J Med* (2007) 120, 369.
8. Schelleman H, Bilker WB, Brensinger CM, Wan F, Yang YX, Hennessy S. Fibrate/statin initiation in warfarin users and gastrointestinal bleeding risk. *Am J Med* (2010) 123, 151–7.
9. Mogyorósi A, Bradley B, Showalter A, Schubert ML. Rhabdomyolysis and acute renal failure due to combination therapy with simvastatin and warfarin. *J Intern Med* (1999) 246, 599–602.
10. Transon C, Leemann T, Vogt N, Dayer P. In vivo inhibition profile of cytochrome P450TB (CYP2C9) by (±)-fluvastatin. *Clin Pharmacol Ther* (1995) 58, 412–17.
11. Transon C, Leemann T, Dayer P. In vitro comparative inhibition profiles of major human drug metabolising cytochrome P450 isozymes (CYP2C9, CYP2D6 and CYP3A4) by HMG-CoA reductase inhibitors. *Eur J Clin Pharmacol* (1996) 50, 209–15.
12. Simonson SG, Martin PD, Mitchell PD, Lasseter K, Gibson G, Schneck DW. Effect of rosuvastatin on warfarin pharmacodynamics and pharmacokinetics. *J Clin Pharmacol* (2005) 45, 927–34.
13. Lin JC, Ito MK, Stolley SN, Morreale AP, Marcus DB. The effect of converting from pravastatin to simvastatin on the pharmacodynamics of warfarin. *J Clin Pharmacol* (1999) 39, 86–90.
14. Hickmott H, Wynne H, Kamali F. The effect of simvastatin co-medication on warfarin anticoagulation response and dose requirements. *Thromb Haemost* (2003) 89, 949–50.
15. Westergren T, Johansson P, Molden E. Probable warfarin–simvastatin interaction. *Ann Pharmacother* (2007) 41, 1292–5.
16. Zocor (Simvastatin). Merck Sharp & Dohme Ltd. UK Summary of product characteristics, June 2015.
17. Zocor (Simvastatin). Merck & Co., Inc. US Prescribing information, March 2015.
18. Mevacor (Lovastatin). Merck & Co., Inc. US Prescribing information, February 2014.
19. Lipitor (Atorvastatin calcium). Pfizer Inc. US Prescribing information, March 2015.
20. Lipitor (Atorvastatin calcium trihydrate). Pfizer Ltd. UK Summary of product characteristics, March 2015.

Table 12.8 Summary of the case reports of statins interacting with coumarins

Year of study	Patient	Coumarin	Statin dose (duration before event)	INR or PT* before	INR or PT after	Bleeding complications	Longer-term management	Refs
Fluvastatin								
1996	68-year-old	Warfarin	20 mg daily (6 weeks)	3	4.8	None	Warfarin dose decreased by 14%	1
			40 mg daily (2 months)	2.9	3.81	None	Warfarin dose decreased by 12.5%	
	61-year-old	Warfarin	20 mg daily (4 weeks**)	2.29	3.54	None	Warfarin dose decreased by 10%	
	71-year-old	Warfarin	20 mg daily (3 weeks**)	2.92	4.45	None	Warfarin dose decreased by 14%	
1997	68-year-old	Warfarin	20 mg daily (2 weeks)	2.11 to 2.99	4.17	None	Warfarin dose decreased by 18%, then increased back again on withdrawal of fluvastatin	2
	83-year-old	Warfarin	20 mg daily (1 week)	1.84 to 2.73	3.47	None	Warfarin dose decreased by 36%, then increased back again on withdrawal of fluvastatin	
	51-year-old	Warfarin	20 mg daily (1 week)	1.95 to 3.4	4.2	Minor rectal bleeding	Warfarin dose decreased by 13%	
2004	67-year-old	Warfarin	80 mg daily (5 weeks†)	2 to 3	6.6	None	Fluvastatin switched back to atorvastatin, and warfarin restablised at a 14% lower dose	3
Lovastatin								
1990	48-year-old	Warfarin	20 mg daily (3 weeks)	PT 18 to 24 seconds	PT 48 seconds	Minor rectal bleeding	Warfarin dose decreased by 60%	4
	58-year-old	Warfarin	20 mg daily (10 days)	PT 19 to 22 seconds	PT 42 seconds	Epistaxis and haematuria	Warfarin dose decreased by 60%	
1992	85-year-old	Warfarin	20 mg daily (2 weeks)	PT 15 to 17 seconds	PT 24 seconds	None	Lovastatin discontinued	5
1995	78-year-old	Warfarin	40 mg daily (2 months)	1.9 to 3.1	12.3	Gross haematuria, haematoma	Lovastatin discontinued	6
Pravastatin								
1996	64-year-old	Fluindione‡	10 mg daily (5 days)	2.5 to 3.5	10.2	Haematuria	Not reported	7
Rosuvastatin								
2004	74-year-old	Warfarin	Not reported (4 weeks)	2	8	Bruising, haematuria	Not reported	8
2005	36-year-old	Acenocoumarol	10 mg daily (about 45 days)	2 to 3	5.8	Haematoma	Rosuvastatin discontinued	9
2005	56-year-old	Warfarin	20 mg daily (about 8 weeks)	Stable before and twice during	5.9	None	Rosuvastatin discontinued and atorvastatin started	10
Simvastatin								
1996	70-year-old	Acenocoumarol	20 mg daily (3 weeks)	2 to 3.5	9	Not reported	Simvastatin discontinued	11
2007	82-year-old	Warfarin	10 mg daily (4 weeks†)	2.6	>8	Cerebral haemorrhage	Fatal	12

*Prothrombin time
**Switched from lovastatin
†Switched from atorvastatin
‡Note that this is an indanedione

1. Trilli LE, Kelley CL, Aspinall SL, Kroner BA. Potential interaction between warfarin and fluvastatin. *Ann Pharmacother* (1996) 30, 1399–1402.
2. Kline SS, Harrell CC. Potential warfarin-fluvastatin interaction. *Ann Pharmacother* (1997) 31, 790.
3. Andrus MR. Oral anticoagulant drug interactions with statins: case report of fluvastatin and review of the literature. *Pharmacotherapy* (2004) 24, 285–90.
4. Ahmad S. Lovastatin. Warfarin interaction. *Arch Intern Med* (1990) 150, 2407.
5. Hoffman HS. The interaction of lovastatin and warfarin. *Conn Med* (1992) 56, 107.
6. Iliadis EA, Konwinski MF. Lovastatin during warfarin therapy resulting in bleeding. *PA Medicine* (1995) 98, 31.
7. Trenque T, Choisy H, Germain M-L. Pravastatin: interaction with oral anticoagulant? *BMJ* (1996) 312, 886.
8. Barry M. Rosuvastatin–warfarin drug interaction. *Lancet* (2004) 363, 328.
9. Mondillo S, Ballo P, Galderisi M. Rosuvastatin–acenocoumarol interaction. *Clin Ther* (2005) 27, 782–4.
10. Finsterer J, Stöllberger C. Myalgia, hyper-CK-aemia, and hypocoagulability in a patient under rosuvastatin and warfarin. *Eur J Neurol* (2005) 12, 660.
11. Grau E, Perella M, Pastor E. Simvastatin-oral anticoagulant interaction. *Lancet* (1996) 347, 405–6.
12. Westergren T, Johansson P, Molden E. Probable warfarin–simvastatin interaction. *Ann Pharmacother* (2007) 41, 1292–5.

Coumarins + Sucralfate

The simultaneous administration of warfarin and sucralfate did not alter the anticoagulant effect of warfarin in studies in patients on stable therapy. However, case reports describe a marked reduction in the effects of warfarin in four patients taking sucralfate.

Clinical evidence

In an open, crossover study in 8 elderly patients taking **warfarin**, their anticoagulant response (thromboplastin time) and plasma **warfarin** levels remained unchanged while taking sucralfate 1 g three times a day over a 2-week period.[1] Similarly, in a preliminary report of another study, sucralfate 1 g four times daily for 2 weeks had no effect on prothrombin time or plasma **warfarin** levels in 5 patients on stable **warfarin** therapy.[2] In both these studies, the daily **warfarin** dose was taken simultaneously with one of the sucralfate doses.[1,2]

However, there are four case reports of reduced **warfarin** effects with sucralfate. In one of these, a man taking several drugs (digoxin, furosemide, chlorpropamide, potassium chloride) had serum **warfarin** levels that were about two-thirds lower when he was given sucralfate (dose not stated). When the sucralfate was withdrawn, his serum **warfarin** levels rose to their former levels accompanied by a prolongation of prothrombin times.[3] Another patient taking sucralfate had subtherapeutic prothrombin times on starting **warfarin**, despite **warfarin** doses of up to 17.5 mg daily. When the sucralfate was stopped his prothrombin time rose to 1.5 times the control, even though the **warfarin** dose was reduced to 10 mg daily.[4] One other patient appeared to have reduced responses to **warfarin** while taking sucralfate, despite separation of administration.[5] However, another patient taking **warfarin** and sucralfate had a reduced response to **warfarin** only when it was taken simultaneously with sucralfate, but not when administration was separated.[6]

Mechanism

Unknown. It is suggested that the sucralfate may possibly adsorb the warfarin so that its bioavailability is reduced.[4]

Importance and management

The documentation regarding an interaction between warfarin and sucralfate appears to be limited to the reports cited. Any interaction would therefore seem to be uncommon. Concurrent use need not be avoided, but bear this interaction in mind if a patient has a reduced anticoagulant response to warfarin. Note that, although separating dosing has been suggested as a strategy for avoiding this interaction, one of the cases occurred despite this.

1. Neuvonen PJ, Jaakkola A, Tötterman J, Penttilä O. Clinically significant sucralfate-warfarin interaction is not likely. *Br J Clin Pharmacol* (1985) 20, 178–80.
2. Talbert RL, Dalmady-Israel C, Bussey HI, Crawford MH, Ludden TM. Effect of sucralfate on plasma warfarin concentration in patients requiring chronic warfarin therapy. *Drug Intell Clin Pharm* (1985) 19, 456–7.
3. Mungall D, Talbert RL, Phillips C, Jaffe D, Ludden TM. Sucralfate and warfarin. *Ann Intern Med* (1983) 98, 557.
4. Braverman SE, Marino MT. Sucralfate-warfarin interaction. *Drug Intell Clin Pharm* (1988) 22, 913.
5. Rey AM, Gums JG. Altered absorption of digoxin, sustained-release quinidine, and warfarin with sucralfate absorption. *DICP Ann Pharmacother* (1991) 25, 745–6.
6. Parrish RH, Waller B, Gondalia BG. Sucralfate-warfarin interaction. *Ann Pharmacother* (1992) 26, 1015–16.

Coumarins + Sucrose polyesters

Short-term, moderate consumption of potato crisps containing sucrose polyesters (*Olestra, Olean*), which include vitamin K_1, did not alter the INR in response to warfarin.

Clinical evidence

In a randomised, double-blind, placebo-controlled study in 36 patients stabilised on **warfarin**, sucrose polyester 12 g daily (as *Pringles Original Flavor Fat Free Potato Crisps with Olean* 42 g) for one week did not significantly alter the anticoagulant effects of **warfarin** (mean INR increase of 0.02, versus 0.17 for placebo). After one week, greater than expected numbers of patients from both the placebo and sucrose polyester groups had INRs outside the therapeutic range of 2 to 3 (3 sucrose polyester recipients and 3 placebo recipients had an INR above 3 (max 4.1) and 2 in the sucrose polyester group and one in the placebo group had an INR less than 2). Two of each group also withdrew because of diarrhoea: their INRs were therapeutic. Only 22 patients entered the second week of the study, and there was no important effect on INR in these patients after the second week.[1]

Mechanism

Sucrose polyesters are non-absorbable, non-calorific fat replacements. It has been concluded that sucrose polyesters are unlikely to reduce the absorption of oral drugs in general; however, they are known to reduce the absorption of some fat-soluble vitamins, and therefore might lower vitamin K stores.[2] Because of this, snacks containing *Olestra* are supplemented with vitamin K_1 at a level of 8 micrograms per gram of *Olestra*.[3] It is possible that this supplementation could be insufficient to offset the vitamin K-lowering effect and therefore increase patient sensitivity to warfarin, or it could be too much and result in an antagonism of warfarin.

Importance and management

No evidence was found in the above study to suggest that short-term moderate consumption of a snack containing sucrose polyesters (12 g daily, including 96 micrograms of vitamin K daily) altered the anticoagulant effect of warfarin. In 1996, the FDA in the US considered that the changes in dietary vitamin K intake attributable to eating vitamin-K compensated *Olestra* would likely be within the normal range of dietary variation.[3] However, an intake similar to this of a vitamin K_1 supplement has altered coagulation status in some subjects (see 'Coumarins + Vitamin K_1-containing dietary supplements', p.484), and pure vitamin K_1 is much more bioavailable than that from plant sources (see 'Coumarins and related drugs + Food; Vitamin K_1-rich', p.432). Some consider that the snacks may have an impact on serum vitamin K levels.[4] Given these concerns, further study is probably needed.

1. Beckey NP, Korman LB, Parra D. Effect of the moderate consumption of olestra in patients receiving long-term warfarin therapy. *Pharmacotherapy* (1999) 19, 1075–9.
2. Goldman P. Olestra: assessing its potential to interact with drugs in the gastrointestinal tract. *Clin Pharmacol Ther* (1997) 61, 613–18.
3. Department of Health and Human Services. Food and Drug Administration. Food additives permitted for direct addition to food for human consumption; Olestra. *Fed Regist* (1996) 61, 3118–73.
4. Harrell CC, Kline SS. Vitamin K–supplemented snacks containing olestra: implication for patients taking warfarin. *JAMA* (1999), 282, 1133–4.

Coumarins + Sulfinpyrazone

The anticoagulant effects of warfarin are markedly increased by sulfinpyrazone, and there are case reports of moderate to serious bleeding on concurrent use. Acenocoumarol is modestly affected. Phenprocoumon does not appear to be significantly affected. The antiplatelet effects of sulfinpyrazone might increase the risk of bleeding with coumarins.

Clinical evidence

(a) Acenocoumarol

In a placebo-controlled, crossover study in 22 patients taking acenocoumarol, sulfinpyrazone 800 mg daily for 2 weeks led to a drop in the mean prothrombin time requiring a reduction in the anticoagulant dose by an average of 20%. Four patients withdrew because of bleeding episodes, 3 patients while taking sulfinpyrazone and one while taking placebo.[1]

(b) Phenprocoumon

In a study in 6 healthy subjects, sulfinpyrazone 400 mg daily for 17 days had little effect on phenprocoumon levels after a single 0.6-mg/kg dose of phenprocoumon given on day 4. The AUC of prothrombin time increased in 4 subjects and decreased in 2, resulting in an overall non-significant mean increase of 16%.[2] Similar findings were reported in another study of similar design.[3]

(c) Warfarin

In a double-blind, placebo-controlled study in 11 patients stabilised on warfarin, sulfinpyrazone 200 mg four times daily for 6 to 12 months reduced the average warfarin dose requirement by 44% from 7.3 to 4.1 mg week, compared with no change in the placebo group. There were four episodes of bleeding (haematoma, epistaxis and bleeding gums) in 3 patients receiving sulfinpyrazone and one in the placebo group. The authors noted it was difficult to regulate anticoagulant control in the patients taking sulfinpyrazone.[4,5] Similarly, in another study, the prothrombin ratios of 5 patients taking warfarin rose rapidly over 2 to 3 days after sulfinpyrazone 200 mg every 6 hours was added. The average warfarin requirements fell by 46% and 2 patients needed vitamin K to combat the excessive hypoprothrombinaemia. When the sulfinpyrazone was withdrawn, the warfarin requirements returned to their former levels within one to 2 weeks.[6]

A number of case reports have described increased effects of warfarin in patients starting sulfinpyrazone,[7-12] or an exaggerated anticoagulant response in patients taking sulfinpyrazone and then starting warfarin.[13] Moderate to severe bleeding occurred in some instances.[8,10,11] An increased anticoagulant effect of warfarin in the first 15 days after starting sulfinpyrazone, followed by an unexplained progressive increased warfarin dose requirement has been described in one report.[14] However, this may have had other explanations, as a constant potentiation of warfarin is usually seen on long-term sulfinpyrazone use.[5]

In subsequent studies in healthy subjects, sulfinpyrazone 200 mg twice daily for 10 days was shown to augment the effect of warfarin (99% or 83% increase in the AUC of the prothrombin time) by inhibiting the clearance of *S*-warfarin (by 51% or 40%) when a single dose of warfarin was given on day 4. In contrast, sulfinpyrazone did not alter the effect of *R*-warfarin, and actually increased its clearance by 30% or 42%.[15,16]

Mechanism

Sulfinpyrazone inhibits the metabolism of the more potent *S*-isomer of warfarin, probably because its sulfide metabolite inhibits the cytochrome P450 isoenzyme CYP2C9.[17] It probably interacts by a similar mechanism with acenocoumarol. It could be speculated that sulfinpyrazone induces the metabolism of *R*-warfarin via CYP1A2, as it modestly induces the metabolism of theophylline (see 'Theophylline + Sulfinpyrazone', p.1460). Some early *in vitro* evidence[18] suggested that plasma protein binding displacement might explain this interaction, but a study in healthy subjects found that sulfinpyrazone did not alter the free fraction of either *R*- or *S*-warfarin.[19] Sulfinpyrazone also has antiplatelet effects, so might be expected to increase the risk or severity of bleeding should over-anticoagulation occur.

Importance and management

The increased effect of warfarin with sulfinpyrazone is a well established interaction of clinical importance. If sulfinpyrazone is added, the prothrombin time should be well monitored and suitable anticoagulant dose reductions made. Halving the dose of warfarin[4,6,20] has proven to be adequate in patients taking sulfinpyrazone 600 to 800 mg daily. The interaction with acenocoumarol[1] is less marked, and a 20% dose reduction appears adequate in patients taking sulfinpyrazone 600 to 800 mg daily. Phenprocoumon is reported not to have a pharmacokinetic interaction with sulfinpyrazone. Bear in mind that the antiplatelet effects of sulfinpyrazone might increase the risk of bleeding with coumarins.

1. Michot F, Holt NF, Fontanilles F. Über die Beeinflussung der gerinnungshemmenden Wirkung von Acenocoumarol durch Sulfinpyrazon. *Schweiz Med Wochenschr* (1981) 111, 255–60.
2. O'Reilly RA. Phenylbutazone and sulphinpyrazone interaction with oral anticoagulant phenprocoumon. *Arch Intern Med* (1982) 142, 1634–7.
3. Heimark LD, Toon S, Gibaldi M, Trager WF, O'Reilly RA, Goulart DA. The effect of sulfinpyrazone on the disposition of pseudoracemic phenprocoumon in humans. *Clin Pharmacol Ther* (1987) 42, 312–19.
4. Girolami A, Fabris F, Casonato A, Randi ML. Potentiation of anticoagulant response to warfarin by sulphinpyrazone: a double-blind study in patients with prosthetic heart valves. *Clin Lab Haematol* (1982) 4, 23–6.
5. Girolami A, Schivazappa L, Fabris F, Randi ML. Biphasic sulphinpyrazone-warfarin interaction. *BMJ* (1981) 283, 1338.
6. Miners JO, Foenander T, Wanwimolruk S, Gallus AS, Birkett DJ. Interaction of sulphinpyrazone with warfarin. *Eur J Clin Pharmacol* (1982) 22, 327–31.
7. Davis JW, Johns LE. Possible interaction of sulfinpyrazone with coumarins. *N Engl J Med* (1978) 299, 955.
8. Mattingly D, Bradley M, Selley PJ. Hazards of sulphinpyrazone. *BMJ* (1978) 2, 1786–9.
9. Weiss M. Potentiation of coumarin effect by sulfinpyrazone. *Lancet* (1979) i, 609.
10. Gallus A, Birkett D. Sulphinpyrazone and warfarin: a probable drug interaction. *Lancet* (1980) i, 535–6.
11. Thompson PL, Serjeant C. Potentially serious interaction of warfarin with sulphinpyrazone. *Med J Aust* (1981) 1, 41.
12. Jamil A, Reid JM, Messer M. Interaction between sulphinpyrazone and warfarin. *Chest* (1981) 79, 375.
13. Bailey RR, Reddy J. Potentiation of warfarin action by sulphinpyrazone. *Lancet* (1980) i, 254.
14. Nenci GG, Agnelli G, Berrettini M. Biphasic sulphinpyrazone-warfarin interaction. *BMJ* (1981) 282, 1361–2.
15. O'Reilly RA. Stereoselective interaction of sulfinpyrazone with racemic warfarin and its separated enantiomorphs in man. *Circulation* (1982) 65, 202–7.
16. Toon S, Low LK, Gibaldi M, Trager WF, O'Reilly RA, Motley CH, Goulart DA. The warfarin-sulfinpyrazone interaction: stereochemical considerations. *Clin Pharmacol Ther* (1986) 39, 15–24.
17. He M, Kunze KL, Trager WF. Inhibition of (*S*)-warfarin metabolism by sulfinpyrazone and its metabolites. *Drug Metab Dispos* (1995) 23, 659–63.
18. Seiler K, Duckert F. Properties of 3-(1-phenyl-propyl)-4-oxycoumarin (Marcoumar®) in the plasma when tested in normal cases and under the influence of drugs. *Thromb Diath Haemorrh* (1968) 19, 389–96.
19. O'Reilly RA, Goulart DA. Comparative interaction of sulfinpyrazone and phenylbutazone with racemic warfarin: alteration *in vivo* of free fraction of plasma albumin. *J Pharmacol Exp Ther* (1981) 219, 691–4.
20. Tulloch JA, Marr TCK. Sulphinpyrazone and warfarin after myocardial infarction. *BMJ* (1979) ii, 133.

Coumarins + Tamoxifen or Toremifene

Tamoxifen appears to increase the effects of warfarin and cases of serious bleeding, in one case fatal, have been reported. A case report describes a similar effect with acenocoumarol. It has been suggested that a similar interaction might occur with toremifene and the coumarins.

Clinical evidence

A woman who had been taking **warfarin** for 11 years after a heart valve replacement (prothrombin time of 23 to 34 seconds taking **warfarin** 27 to 28.5 mg weekly), was given tamoxifen 10 mg twice daily after mastectomy for early breast cancer. Three days later her prothrombin time was 39 seconds, and 3 weeks later it was 75.6 seconds, although this was attributed to a 5-day course of co-trimoxazole, and so the warfarin dose was unchanged. Six weeks later she developed haematemesis, abdominal pain, and haematuria, and her prothrombin time was found to be 206 seconds. She was restabilised on a little over half the **warfarin** dose (17.5 mg weekly) while continuing to take tamoxifen.[1] Another case report describes a significantly increased INR and rectal bleeding in a patient who had been taking tamoxifen 20 mg daily long-term and had recently started taking warfarin. The patient had an initial increase in the INR to about 10, which stabilised when omeprazole was stopped and the patient was discharged with an INR of 2.3. However, 7 days later, the patient was readmitted with an INR of 10.8 and rectal bleeding.[2] In another case, a 43-year-old woman was given **warfarin** for a deep vein thrombosis. Seven weeks later tamoxifen 40 mg daily was started, and her prothrombin time increased from 19 seconds to 38 seconds. A warfarin dose reduction from 5 to 1 mg daily was eventually needed to keep her prothrombin time within the range of 20 to 25 seconds. A subsequent retrospective study of the records of women with breast cancer who had been admitted to hospital for serious thromboembolism from 1981 to 1986 revealed 5 other patients taking tamoxifen when **warfarin** was started, and 13 patients not taking tamoxifen. Of the 5 patients taking tamoxifen, 2 had shown large increases in prothrombin times, and bleeding, shortly after receiving loading doses of **warfarin** (three daily doses of 10 mg, 10 mg and 5 mg). The other 3 patients needed daily **warfarin** doses of 2 mg, 2 mg and 3 mg, respectively, which were about one-third of those taken by the 13 other patients not taking tamoxifen (mean 6.25 mg).[3] In another retrospective analysis of hospital admissions from 1980 to 1988, 22 patients were identified who had been given tamoxifen with **warfarin**. Of these, 17 had no problems, but 2 developed grossly elevated British Comparative Ratios and 3 developed serious bleeding.[4] A retrospective analysis of patients diagnosed with cerebral haemorrhage due to warfarin or warfarin drug interactions reported an 84-year old patient stabilised on warfarin for at least one year for thromboembolism who had an increased INR of 3.7 while taking tamoxifen.[5]

A 53-year-old woman who had been taking **acenocoumarol** for 2 years after a heart valve replacement died after a massive brain haemorrhage about 3 weeks after starting to take tamoxifen 20 mg daily for a benign breast condition.[6]

Mechanism

The mechanism for this interaction is unclear. However, one study has reported that tamoxifen might inhibit the metabolism of losartan by CYP2C9, see 'Angiotensin II receptor antagonists; Losartan + Tamoxifen', p.49. CYP2C9 is the isoenzyme involved in the metabolism of the more potent isomer *S*-warfarin, and therefore concurrent use might lead to increased warfarin concentrations and effects.

Importance and management

Evidence for an interaction between **tamoxifen** and warfarin is limited to the above reports, but it appears that a clinically important interaction can occur, which apparently affects some but not all patients. Monitor the effects closely if tamoxifen is given to patients taking warfarin or acenocoumarol, and reduce the anticoagulant dose as necessary; the reports indicate a reduction of between one-half to two-thirds for warfarin. Consider also that, from a disease perspective, when treating venous thromboembolic disease in patients with cancer, warfarin is generally inferior (higher risk of major bleeds and recurrent thrombosis) to low-molecular-weight heparins.[7]

Because of the data with tamoxifen, the UK manufacturer[8] of **toremifene** recommends avoiding the concurrent use of coumarins, whereas the US manufacturer recommends careful monitoring of prothrombin time.[9] However, there appear to be no published reports of any interaction between toremifene and warfarin.

1. Lodwick R, McConkey B, Brown AM, Beeley L. Life threatening interaction between tamoxifen and warfarin. *BMJ* (1987) 295, 1141.
2. Mishra D, Paudel R, Kishore PV, Palaian S, Bista D, Mishra P. Interaction between warfarin and tamoxifen: a case report. *Kathmandu Univ Med J (KUMJ)* (2007) 5, 105–7.
3. Tenni P, Lalich DL, Byrne MJ. Life threatening interaction between tamoxifen and warfarin. *BMJ* (1989) 298, 93.
4. Ritchie LD, Grant SMT. Tamoxifen-warfarin interaction: the Aberdeen hospitals drug file. *BMJ* (1989) 298, 1253.
5. Jönsson AK, Spigset O, Jacobsson I, Hägg S. Cerebral haemorrhage induced by warfarin – the influence of drug-drug interactions. *Pharmacoepidemiol Drug Safety* (2007) 16, 309–15.
6. Gustovic P, Baldin B, Tricoire MJ, Chichmanian RM. Interaction tamoxifène-acénocoumarol. Une interaction potentiellement dangereuse. *Therapie* (1994) 49, 55–6.
7. Baglin TP, Keeling DM, Watson HG, for the British Committee for Standards in Haematology. Guidelines on oral anticoagulation (warfarin): third edition – 2005 update. *Br J Haematol* (2005) 132, 277–85.
8. Fareston (Toremifene citrate). Orion Pharma (UK) Ltd. UK Summary of product characteristics, January 2009.
9. Fareston (Toremifene citrate). GTx, Inc. US Prescribing information, March 2011.

Coumarins + Tegaserod

Tegaserod does not appear to alter the pharmacokinetics or pharmacodynamics of warfarin.

Clinical evidence, mechanism, importance and management

In a study in healthy subjects, tegaserod 6 mg twice daily for 7 days did not alter the pharmacokinetics of either *S*- or *R*-warfarin when a single 30-mg dose of **warfarin** was given on day 4. Similarly, tegaserod did not alter the prothrombin time response to warfarin. No warfarin dose adjustments are therefore recommended when tegaserod is given with **warfarin**.[1] Note that tegaserod has been associated with an excess risk of rare serious cardiovascular ischaemic events,[2] and it should generally not be used in patients with cardiac disease.

1. Ledford P, On N, Lingueros-Saylan M. Tegaserod does not significantly affect the pharmacokinetics and pharmacodynamics of warfarin in healthy subjects [abstract A1184]. Gastroenterology (200) 118, 5445.
2. Dear Dr Letter. Novartis Pharmaceuticals Corp. March 30, 2007.

Coumarins + Terbinafine

Terbinafine does not affect the pharmacokinetics or anticoagulant effects of warfarin. However, there is one isolated case of markedly reduced anticoagulation, and one case of markedly increased anticoagulation when terbinafine was given with warfarin. No increased risk of over-anticoagulation appears to occur when acenocoumarol or phenprocoumon are given with oral or topical terbinafine.

Clinical evidence

In a randomised, placebo-controlled, study in 16 healthy subjects, terbinafine 250 mg daily for 14 days did not alter the pharmacokinetics or anticoagulant effects of a single 30-mg oral dose of **warfarin** given on day 8.[1] In a post-marketing surveillance study of terbinafine, 26 patients were identified who were also taking **warfarin** and there was no evidence to suggest an interaction occurred in these patients.[2,3] In one cohort study in patients taking **acenocoumarol** or **phenprocoumon**, the concurrent use of oral terbinafine (49 patients) or cutaneous terbinafine (29 patients) was not associated with an increased risk of over-anticoagulation (INR greater than 6).[4]

However, an isolated report describes a 68-year-old woman taking long-term **warfarin** whose INR fell from 2.1 to 1.1 within one month of starting a 3-month course of terbinafine 250 mg daily for tinea unguium. It was necessary to raise her **warfarin** dose from 5.5 mg daily to a range of 7.5 mg to 8 mg daily while taking the terbinafine, and to reduce it stepwise to 5.5 mg over the 4 weeks after the terbinafine was stopped.[5] In contrast, another isolated case report describes an elderly woman stabilised on **warfarin** and cimetidine who developed gastrointestinal bleeding about one month after starting to take terbinafine 250 mg daily. Her INR had increased from 3.1 (about 4 weeks previously) to 11 on admission to hospital.[6]

Mechanism

The isolated cases are not understood, and have been questioned.[7] They may simply represent idiosyncratic reactions.

Importance and management

The available evidence suggests that no interaction usually occurs between the coumarins and terbinafine, and no coumarin dose adjustment is therefore predicted to be needed during concurrent use. The two isolated cases of opposite effects are rarities, and unexplained. There is insufficient evidence to recommend monitoring all patients; however, bear the isolated case reports in mind in the event of an unexpected response.

1. Guerret M, Francheteau P, Hubert M. Evaluation of effects of terbinafine on single oral dose pharmacokinetics and anticoagulant actions of warfarin in healthy volunteers. *Pharmacotherapy* (1997) 17, 767–73.
2. O'Sullivan DP, Needham CA, Bangs A, Atkin K, Kendall FD. Postmarketing surveillance of oral terbinafine in the UK; report of a large cohort study. *Br J Pharmacol* (1996) 42, 559–65.
3. Novartis. Personal communication, February 1998.
4. Visser LE, Penning-van Beest FJA, Kasbergen AAH, De Smet PAGM, Vulto AG, Hofman A, Stricker BHC. Overanticoagulation associated with combined use of antifungal agents and coumarin anticoagulants. *Clin Pharmacol Ther* (2002) 71, 496–502.
5. Warwick JA, Corrall RJ. Serious interaction between warfarin and oral terbinafine. *BMJ* (1998) 316, 440.
6. Gupta AK, Ross GS. Interaction between terbinafine and warfarin. *Dermatology* (1998) 196, 266–7.
7. Gantmacher J, Mills-Bomford J, Williams T. Interaction between warfarin and oral terbinafine. *BMJ* (1998) 317, 205.

Coumarins + Tetracyclic antidepressants

Maprotiline does not appear to alter the anticoagulant effect of acenocoumarol. Mianserin does not appear alter the anticoagulant effect of phenprocoumon, however, two isolated cases of an increased effect of warfarin and a decreased effect of acenocoumarol have been reported in patients taking mianserin.

Clinical evidence

(a) Maprotiline

In a study in 20 patients stabilised on **acenocoumarol**, the anticoagulant effects of **acenocoumarol** were not affected by maprotiline 50 mg three times daily for 2 weeks.[1]

(b) Mianserin

In a randomised, double-blind study in 60 patients taking **phenprocoumon** for 5 weeks, there was no difference in anticoagulant control and **phenprocoumon** dose between placebo recipients and those receiving mianserin, either up to 30 mg daily or up to 60 mg daily, for 20 days.[2]

A single case report describes a man stabilised on **warfarin** whose British standard ratio rose from 1.8 to 4.6 (prothrombin time rise from 20 to 25 seconds) after taking mianserin 10 mg daily for 7 days.[3] However, another patient taking **warfarin** received mianserin in varying doses of up to 120 mg daily for 22 weeks without any change in prothrombin ratio.[4] A further patient stabilised on **acenocoumarol** and amiodarone needed an *increase* in his **acenocoumarol** dose after starting mianserin, and a decrease when this drug was stopped.[5]

Mechanism

Not understood. The cases with mianserin might just represent idiosyncratic reactions.

Importance and management

Maprotiline does not interact with acenocoumarol and mianserin does not interact with phenprocoumon. The isolated cases of an increase in warfarin effects and a decrease in acenocoumarol effects with mianserin are unexplained, and probably of little general relevance.

1. Michot F, Glaus K, Jack DB, Theobald W. Antikoagulatorische Wirkung von Sintrom® und Konzentration von Ludiomil® im Blut bei gleichzeitiger Verabreichung beider Präparate. *Med Klin* (1975) 70, 626–9.
2. Kopera H, Schenk H, Stulemeijer S. Phenprocoumon requirement, whole blood coagulation time, bleeding time and plasma γ-GT in patients receiving mianserin. *Eur J Clin Pharmacol* (1978) 13, 351–6.
3. Warwick HMC, Mindham RHS. Concomitant administration of mianserin and warfarin. *Br J Psychiatry* (1983) 143, 308.
4. Shelly RK. Mianserin and warfarin. *Br J Psychiatry* (1984) 145, 97–8.
5. Baettig D, Tillement J-P, Baumann P. Interaction between mianserin and acenocoumarin: a single case study. *Int J Clin Pharmacol Ther* (1994) 32, 165–7.

Coumarins + Thalidomide

No pharmacokinetic interaction appears to occur between thalidomide and single-dose warfarin.

Clinical evidence, mechanism, importance and management

A preliminary report of a randomised, crossover study in 13 healthy men, states that thalidomide 200 mg daily for 4 days had no effect on the pharmacokinetics or anticoagulant effect of a single 25-mg dose of warfarin. Similarly, the pharmacokinetics of thalidomide were not affected by warfarin.[1] Nevertheless, because patients with cancer have an increased risk of thromboembolism, and the metabolism of warfarin might be increased by corticosteroids which are given with thalidomide regimens, the UK manufacturer of thalidomide recommends that the INR is closely monitored on concurrent use with warfarin, and for several weeks after thalidomide (with corticosteroids) is stopped.[2] However, note that some corticosteroids, particularly in high doses, have been reported to *increase* INRs in patients taking warfarin, see 'Coumarins and related drugs + Corticosteroids or Corticotropin', p.419.

1. Wu A, Shenounda M, Ayalasomayujula S, DeGroot B, Scheffler M. Thalomide (Thalidomide) does not affect the pharmacokinetics and pharmacodynamics of warfarin in healthy subjects. 34th Annual Meeting American College of Clinical Pharmacology, Rockville, Maryland, 2005. Abstract 41. *J Clin Pharmacol* (2005) 45, 1067–96.
2. Thalidomide Celgene (Thalidomide). Celgene Ltd. UK Summary of product characteristics, June 2014.

Coumarins and related drugs + Thyroid hormones and Antithyroid drugs

Hypothyroidism might decrease, and hyperthyroidism increases, the metabolism of the clotting factors. Correction of these disease states therefore alters anticoagulant requirements. Bleeding has been seen in patients given thyroid hormones without an adjustment of their anticoagulant dose, and increased coumarin requirements have been seen in patients given thiamazole or carbimazole.

Clinical evidence

(a) Hypothyroidism and Thyroid compounds

In a large retrospective case-control study in elderly patients stabilised on warfarin, the risk of hospitalisation due to bleeding, was no different between 10 532 patients who received **levothyroxine** during the 30 days preceding the bleed, and 40 693 matched control patients who did not experience bleeding.[1] However, in a study in 7 patients with myxoedema (hypothyroidism), the response to a single-dose of **warfarin** was increased after 3 months of treatment with **liothyronine** (when euthyroid), when compared with that before treatment, without a change in plasma warfarin concentrations.[2]

Various case reports describe similar effects.[3-6] In one report, brief mention is made of one patient who had an increased response to **warfarin** after an increase in the dose of thyroid replacement therapy, and of another patient taking long-term **warfarin** who had a bleeding episode when thyroid replacement therapy was started.[3] Another patient taking **warfarin** developed oral mucosal bleeding with an INR of greater than 11 when her hypothyroidism was overcorrected with **levothyroxine**, although she had no clinical signs of hyperthyroidism.[4] In another case, a subdural haematoma occurred in a child stabilised on **warfarin** when **levothyroxine** was started, and her dose of **warfarin** was eventually reduced from 7.5 mg daily to 5 mg daily.[5]

A patient with myxoedema required a gradual reduction in his dose of **phenindione** from 200 mg daily to 75 mg daily as his thyroid status was corrected by **liothyronine**.[6] A similar patient required a reduction in the dose of **acenocoumarol**, from 16 mg daily to 5 mg daily, when hypothyroidism was corrected with **liothyronine**.[6]

(b) Hyperthyroidism and Antithyroid compounds

In 5 patients with hyperthyroidism, the response to a single dose of **warfarin** was decreased (prothrombin ratio 1.35 versus 1.75) after treatment with **iodine-131** (when euthyroid), when compared with before treatment. Three of the 5 patients required a small increase in their warfarin dose of between 0.5 mg and 1 mg. There was no difference in the plasma half-life of **warfarin**.[7] Another similar study also reported a decreased sensitivity to **warfarin** after correction of hyperthyroidism, but found that the plasma half-life and plasma concentrations of **warfarin** were higher after treatment.[8]

Various case reports describe alterations in anticoagulant effects.[4,9-14] In one, a hyperthyroid patient taking **warfarin** had a large increase in his prothrombin times on two occasions when his treatment with **thiamazole (methimazole)** was stopped and he became hyperthyroid again.[9] Another similar case has been described where the required dose of **warfarin** increased from 35 mg weekly to 65 mg weekly as the patients hyperthyroid state was corrected with **thiamazole** 30 mg daily. However, the patient then became hypothyroid and required up to 85 mg of **warfarin** weekly. When the **thiamazole** dose was withheld for 5 days and then reduced to 5 mg daily, the patient rapidly developed an increased INR of 7 without bleeding complications.[10] Another hyperthyroid patient could not achieve a therapeutic INR with **warfarin** while receiving **thiamazole**, but after the thiamazole was switched to lithium she achieved an INR of 3 on warfarin 10 mg daily.[14] In another report, a patient required just 0.5 mg of **warfarin** daily while hyperthyroid.[4] Another case of possible enhanced response to **warfarin** in a hyperthyroid patient has been reported.[11,12] A woman taking **acenocoumarol**, required a dose reduction as she became hyperthyroid and the dose of **acenocoumarol** was increased again when she was treated with **carbimazole**.[13]

Mechanism

In hypothyroid patients the catabolism (destruction) of the blood clotting factors (II, VII, IX and X) is low and this tends to cancel, to some extent, the effects of the anticoagulants, which reduce blood clotting factor synthesis. Conversely, in hyperthyroid patients in whom the catabolism is increased, the net result is an increase in the effects of the anticoagulants.[15] In studies in healthy subjects, **dextrothyroxine** (which has weak thyroid activity compared with levothyroxine) potentiated the anticoagulant effect of **dicoumarol**[16] and warfarin[17] without altering the half-life and plasma concentrations of the anticoagulants, and without altering vitamin K-dependent clotting activity.[16] Because of this, it was suggested that the thyroid hormones might increase the affinity of the anticoagulants for its receptor sites.[16,17]

Importance and management

The interaction between oral anticoagulants and thyroid hormones is well documented and could be clinically important.

In hypothyroid patients taking an anticoagulant who are subsequently treated with thyroid hormones as replacement therapy the INR should be well monitored and a downward adjustment of the anticoagulant dose as treatment proceeds might be needed if excessive hypoprothrombinaemia and bleeding are to be avoided. The more recent case-control study indicates that the risk of bleeding in patients taking both warfarin and levothyroxine might not be as great as previously thought, however it would still be prudent to closely monitor the INR on concurrent use.

Conversely, as the thyroid status of hyperthyroid patients returns to normal with the use of antithyroid drugs (e.g. carbimazole, thiamazole, **propylthiouracil**) an increase in the anticoagulant requirements would be expected. As this is more of a drug-disease interaction than a direct drug-drug interaction, it is therefore likely to occur with any coumarin or indanedione given with any drug that affects thyroid function. Close anticoagulant monitoring and dose adjustment are required, particularly while thyroid hormone concentrations are being stabilised. Note that, in one case the authors commented that the magnitude and clinical complexity of the interaction between the drugs and disease state was unexpected.[10]

Also note that propylthiouracil in the absence of an anticoagulant, has very occasionally been reported to cause hypoprothrombinaemia and bleeding.[18,19]

Some drugs can alter thyroid status as an unwanted effect, and this will also alter the response to the oral anticoagulants. For example, amiodarone (see 'Coumarins and related drugs + Amiodarone', p.381), can cause thyrotoxicosis, which decreases warfarin requirements. Also, the use of **dextrothyroxine** for hypercholesterolaemia decreased the required dose of warfarin[20,21] and dicoumarol,[22] presumably because it has weak thyroid activity.

1. Pincus D, Gomes T, Hellings C, Zheng H, Paterson JM, Mamdani MM, Juurlink DN. A population-based assessment of the drug interaction between levothyroxine and warfarin. *Clin Pharmacol Ther* (2012) 92, 766–70.
2. Rice AJ, McIntosh TJ, Fouts JR, Brunk SF, Wilson WR. Decreased sensitivity to warfarin in patients with myxedema. *Am J Med Sci* (1971) 262, 211–15.
3. Hansten PD. Oral anticoagulants and drugs which alter thyroid function. *Drug Intell Clin Pharm* (1980) 14, 331–4.
4. Chute JP, Ryan CP, Sladek G, Shakir KMM. Exacerbation of warfarin-induced anticoagulation by hyperthyroidism. *Endocr Pract* (1997) 3, 77–9.
5. Costigan DC, Freedman MH, Ehrlich RM. Potentiation of oral anticoagulant effect by L-thyroxine. *Clin Pediatr (Phila)* (1984) 23, 172–4.
6. Walters MB. The relationship between thyroid function and anticoagulant therapy. *Am J Cardiol* (1963) 11, 112–14.
7. Kellett HA, Sawers JSA, Boulton FE, Cholerton S, Park BK, Toft AD. Problems of anticoagulation with warfarin in hyperthyroidism. *Q J Med* (1986) 58, 43–51.
8. McIntosh TJ, Brunk SF, Kölln I, Fouts JR, Wilson WR. Increased sensitivity to warfarin in thyrotoxicosis. *J Clin Invest* (1970) 49, 63a–64a.
9. Vagenakis AG, Cote R, Miller ME, Braverman LE, Stohlman F. Enhancement of warfarin-induced hypoprothrombinemia by thyrotoxicosis. *Johns Hopkins Med J* (1972) 131, 69–73.
10. Busenbark LA, Cushnie SA. Effect of Graves' disease and methimazole on warfarin anticoagulation. *Ann Pharmacother* (2006) 40, 1200–3.
11. Self TH, Straughn AB, Weisburst MR. Effect of hyperthyroidism on hypoprothrombinemic response to warfarin. *Am J Hosp Pharm* (1976) 33, 387–9.
12. Self T, Weisburst M, Wooton E, Straughn A, Oliver J. Warfarin-induced hypoprothrombinemia. Potentiation by hyperthyroidism. *JAMA* (1975) 231, 1165–6.
13. John GT, Punnoose E, Narasimhan G, Pulimood BM. Enhanced action of acenocoumarin in hyperthyroidism. *J Assoc Physicians India* (1994) 42, 575.
14. Akin F, Yaylali GF, Bastemir M, Yapar B. Effect of methimazole on warfarin anticoagulation in a case of Graves' disease. *Blood Coag Fibrinol* (2008) 19, 89–91.
15. Loeliger EA, van der Esch B, Mattern MJ, Hemker HC. The biological disappearance rate of prothrombin, factors VII, IX and X from plasma in hypothyroidism, hyperthyroidism and during fever. *Thromb Diath Haemorrh* (1964) 10, 267–77.
16. Schrogie JJ, Solomon HM. The anticoagulant response to bishydroxycoumarin. II. The effect of d-thyroxine, clofibrate and norethandrolone. *Clin Pharmacol Ther* (1967) 8, 70–7.
17. Solomon HM, Schrogie JJ. Change in receptor site affinity: a proposed explanation for the potentiating effect of d-thyroxine on the anticoagulant response to warfarin. *Clin Pharmacol Ther* (1967) 8, 797–9.
18. D'Angelo G, Le Gresley LP. Severe hypoprothrombinæmia after propylthiouracil therapy. *Can Med Assoc J* (1959) 81, 479–81.
19. Gotta AW, Sullivan CA, Seaman J, Jean-Gilles B. Prolonged intraoperative bleeding caused by propylthiouracil-induced hypoprothrombinemia. *Anesthesiology* (1972) 37, 562–3.
20. Owens JC, Neeley WB, Owen WR. Effect of sodium dextrothyroxine in patients receiving anticoagulants. *N Engl J Med* (1962) 266, 76–9.
21. Winters WL, Soloff LA. Observations on sodium d-thyroxine as a hypocholesterolemic agent in persons with hypercholesterolemia with and without ischemic heart disease. *Am J Med Sci* (1962) 243, 458–69.
22. Jones RJ, Cohen L. Sodium dextro-thyroxine in coronary disease and hypercholesterolemia. *Circulation* (1961) 24, 164–70.

Coumarins + Tiabendazole

An isolated case report describes a marked increase in the anticoagulant effects of acenocoumarol in a patient given tiabendazole.

Clinical evidence, mechanism, importance and management

An increase in the anticoagulant effects of **acenocoumarol** occurred in a patient with nephrotic syndrome undergoing dialysis, who was given tiabendazole 8 g daily for 2 days, on two occasions about 7 weeks apart.[1] On both occasions, his INR rose from 2.9 to more than 5 without any clinical consequence. The reasons for this effect are not understood, nor is the general importance of this interaction known. There seem to be no other reports.

1. Henri P, Mosquet B, Hurault de Ligny B, Lacotte J, Cardinau E, Moulin M, Ryckelinck JP. Imputation d'une hypocoagulabilité à l'interaction tiabendazole-acénocoumarol. *Therapie* (1993) 48, 500–501.

Coumarins and related drugs + Tibolone

Tibolone may increase the INR in some patients taking warfarin or phenindione.

Clinical evidence

In a well-controlled study in 16 postmenopausal women taking **warfarin**, the use of tibolone 2 mg daily for 21 days increased the mean INR by just 0.4. No clinically significant adverse effects occurred on concurrent use.[1] In a retrospective analysis, five women were identified who had started tibolone while taking **warfarin** or **phenindione**. All of the 5 patients had an increase in INR to a range of 4.6 to 9.5 after starting tibolone, and required reductions in their anticoagulant dose (range of 12 to 53% reductions in **warfarin** dose, and 56% for **phenindione**). One further patient who discontinued tibolone while taking **warfarin** required an increase in her **warfarin** dose from 6 to 7.5 mg daily.[2]

Mechanism

Not understood. Tibolone alone increases fibrinolytic activity without altering the prothrombin time,[3] and might therefore be expected to increase the risk of bleeding with anticoagulants. However, this would not result in raised INRs, and it was suggested that the effect on the INR might be because of the androgenic effect of tibolone causing a reduction in factor VIIa.[2]

Importance and management

There is very limited published information available on the concurrent use of warfarin and tibolone. The study suggests tibolone causes minor increases in INR; however, the retrospective analysis reported more clinically significant increases in the INR, and reduced warfarin and phenindione requirements of up to about 50%. Because of this, increased INR monitoring is advised when starting tibolone in patients stabilised on warfarin, other coumarins, or indanediones.

1. Elbers J, Hageluken C, Wadham A. Tibolone (Livial®) enhances warfarin-induced anticoagulation in postmenopausal women. *Maturitas* (2007) 56, 94–100.
2. McLintock LA, Dykes A, Tait RC, Walker ID. Interaction between hormone replacement therapy preparations and oral anticoagulant therapy. *Br J Obstet Gynaecol* (2003) 110, 777–9.
3. Cortes-Prieto J. Coagulation and fibrinolysis in post-menopausal women treated with Org OD 14. *Maturitas* (1987) Suppl 1, 67–72.

Coumarins + Ticlopidine

The anticoagulant effects of acenocoumarol may be modestly reduced by ticlopidine. However, the anticoagulant effects of warfarin are unchanged by ticlopidine. As with other antiplatelet drugs, concurrent use with coumarins might possibly increase bleeding risk. Cholestatic hepatitis has been reported in some patients given warfarin and ticlopidine.

Clinical evidence

(a) Acenocoumarol

A retrospective study of 36 patients with heart valve prostheses found that when they took ticlopidine 250 mg daily, 29 of them needed a mean 13% increase in their acenocoumarol dose from 15.5 to 17.5 mg weekly, accompanied by a small INR rise from 3.05 to 3.13. One patient needed a dose increase from 14 to 22 mg weekly. INR changes were detectable with a week of starting the ticlopidine.[1]

(b) Warfarin

Ticlopidine 250 mg twice daily for 2 weeks, given to 9 men taking warfarin long-term, increased the mean *R*-warfarin levels by 26% but did not change *S*-warfarin levels or their INRs.[2] *R*-warfarin is the much less active of the two enantiomers. In a Japanese study, 4 out of 132 patients (3%) given both warfarin and ticlopidine after cardiovascular surgery developed cholestatic hepatitis.[3]

Mechanism

It seems possible that ticlopidine inhibits the metabolism of *R*-warfarin, but the interaction with acenocoumarol is not understood. Ticlopidine alone can cause raised liver enzymes and cholestatic hepatitis,[4] and whether these cases with warfarin represent an interaction is unclear.

Importance and management

Information seems to be limited to the reports cited. A small to moderate increase in the acenocoumarol dose may be needed if ticlopidine is added, but none seems to be necessary with warfarin. However, as with other antiplatelet drugs, such as aspirin (see 'Coumarins and related drugs + Aspirin or other Salicylates', p.405), an increased risk of bleeding (a combination of anticoagulant and platelet anti-aggregant activity) might be anticipated on concurrent use. The manufacturer states that the long-term safety of concurrent use of ticlopidine with oral anticoagulants has not been established, and they recommend that if a patient is switched from an anticoagulant to ticlopidine, the anticoagulant should be discontinued before ticlopidine is given.[4] For discussion of the combined use of anticoagulants and dual antiplatelet therapy (aspirin plus a thienopyridine derivative such as ticlopidine), see under 'Coumarins and related drugs + Clopidogrel', p.417.

Whether the incidence of cholestatic hepatitis is higher with the concurrent use of warfarin and ticlopidine than with ticlopidine alone is unclear.

1. Salar A, Domenech P, Martinez F. Ticlopidine antagonizes acenocoumarol treatment. *Thromb Haemost* (1997) 77, 223–4.
2. Gidal BE, Sorkness CA, McGill KA, Larson R, Levine RR. Evaluation of a potential enantioselective interaction between ticlopidine and warfarin in chronically anticoagulated patients. *Ther Drug Monit* (1995) 27, 33–8.
3. Takase K, Fujioka H, Ogasawara M, Aonuma H, Tameda Y, Nakano T, Kosaka Y. Drug-induced hepatitis during combination therapy of warfarin potassium and ticlopidine hydrochloride. *Mie Med J* (1990) 40, 27–32.
4. Ticlid (Ticlopidine hydrochloride). Roche Laboratories Inc. US Prescribing information, March 2001.

Coumarins + Tobacco

Analysis of data from four studies suggests that warfarin dose requirements might be greater in smokers than non-smokers and two cases have been reported of patients who required warfarin dose reductions on stopping smoking. Smoking appears to cause a small increase in the clearance of warfarin and a minor reduction in warfarin levels.

One patient who stopped chewing tobacco had an increase in INR.

Clinical evidence

(a) Chewing tobacco

In a patient using smokeless tobacco (chewing tobacco) for greater than 85% of waking hours, the INR was found to have increased from 1.1 to 2.3 six days after discontinuation of tobacco use. This patient had usually had an INR of 1.1 to 1.9 since restarting warfarin 4 months earlier, despite gradually increasing the warfarin dose from 10 mg daily to 25 mg daily alternating with 30 mg daily. However, during this time, he did have two INR spikes of 2.5 and 4.2, which were attributed to dietary changes,[1] but see *Mechanism*, below.

(b) Smoking tobacco

An analysis of data from four cross-sectional studies including 2 133 patients, found that smoking was associated with a 13% increase in warfarin dose requirements compared with not smoking. All studies included in the analysis had adjusted for relevant clinical and pharmacogenomic factors (such as CYP2C9 polymorphisms), but did not show heterogeneity (that is, the studies did not conform to the same experimental protocols).[2] In a retrospective study of factors relating to **warfarin** dose, smoking status appeared to be a factor in **warfarin** dose requirements.[3] In contrast, in a retrospective study of patients who had undergone cardiac valve replacement, there was no statistically significant difference between the **warfarin** dose requirements of 117 non-smokers, 23 light smokers (20 or less cigarettes daily) or 34 heavy smokers (greater than 20 cigarettes daily).[4] The same finding had earlier been briefly reported by the Boston Collaborative Drug Surveillance Program.[5]

Pharmacokinetic studies lend some weight to the idea that warfarin requirements are greater in smokers. In a controlled study in 9 healthy subjects who normally smoked at least one pack of cigarettes daily (size unknown) and who were given **warfarin** to steady-state, smoking abstention for about 6 weeks increased the average steady-state **warfarin** levels by 13%, decreased **warfarin** clearance by 13% and increased the **warfarin** half-life by 23%, but no changes in the prothrombin time occurred.[6] A population pharmacokinetic analysis similarly found that smoking appeared to increase **warfarin** clearance by 10%.[7] However, note that smoking status had no effect on the AUC of *S*-warfarin used as a probe substrate for assessing CYP2C9 activity.[8]

Further, some case reports also support these findings. An 80-year-old man taking **warfarin** had a steady rise in his INR (from a range of 2 to 2.8 up to 3.7) over a 3-month period when he gave up smoking. No bleeding occurred. His dose of **warfarin** was reduced by 14%, and the INR stabilised at 2.3 to 2.8 over the next 9 months.[9] Similarly, another patient required a 23% reduction in **warfarin** dose after stopping smoking following recovery from bacterial meningitis.[10]

Mechanism

Some of the components of tobacco smoke act as cytochrome P450 isoenzyme inducers, which might cause a small increase in the metabolism of warfarin. When smoking stops and the enzymes are no longer stimulated, the metabolism of warfarin falls slightly and its effects are correspondingly slightly increased. Tobacco smoke is known to induce CYP1A2, which has a partial role in the metabolism of the less active *R*-warfarin enantiomer. The metabolism of *S*-warfarin is primarily by CYP2C9, and this does not appear to be affected by smoking.[8]

The possible case of an interaction with smokeless tobacco was attributed to the very high vitamin K content of tobacco resulting in relative warfarin resistance (consider also 'Coumarins and related drugs + Vitamin K substances', p.484). However, there were two previous INR spikes in this patient, which were attributed to dietary changes,[1] an explanation that seems unlikely if there was a high background vitamin K intake from the tobacco. The reasons for the effects in this case are therefore unclear.

Importance and management

Evidence is limited and in some instances conflicting, but the overall picture seems to be that smoking and giving up smoking do have a small to modest effect on the response to warfarin (decreased and increased respectively), and it is likely that only the occasional patient will need a small dose alteration. This should easily be detected in the course of routine INR checks; be alert for the potential need to alter warfarin doses in patients who have changed their smoking status. Note that tobacco smoking increases cardiovascular disease risk, and patients requiring anticoagulants should be encouraged and helped to stop smoking.

The isolated case with smokeless tobacco is unclear, further study is needed.

1. Kuykendall JR, Houle MD, Rhodes RS. Possible warfarin failure due to interaction with smokeless tobacco. *Ann Pharmacother* (2004) 38, 595–7.
2. Nathisuwan S, Dilokthornsakul P, Chaiyakunapruk N, Morarai T, Yodting T, Piriyachananusorn N. Assessing evidence of interaction between smoking and warfarin: a systematic review and meta-analysis. *Chest* (2011) 139, 1130–9.
3. Lee VWY, You JHS, Lee KKC, Chau TS, Waye MMY, Cheng G. Factors affecting the maintenance stable warfarin dosage in Hong Kong Chinese patients. *J Thromb Thrombolysis* (2005) 20, 33–8.
4. Weiner B, Faraci PA, Fayad R, Swanson L. Warfarin dosage following prosthetic valve replacement: effect of smoking history. *Drug Intell Clin Pharm* (1984) 18, 904–6.
5. Mitchell AA. Smoking and warfarin dosage. *N Engl J Med* (1972) 287, 1153–4.
6. Bachmann K, Shapiro R, Fulton R, Carroll FT, Sullivan TJ. Smoking and warfarin disposition. *Clin Pharmacol Ther* (1979) 25, 309–15.
7. Mungall DR, Ludden TM, Marshall J, Hawkins DW, Talbert RL, Crawford MH. Population pharmacokinetics of racemic warfarin in adult patients. *J Pharmacokinet Biopharm* (1985) 13, 213–27.
8. Kim MJ, Nafzinger AN, Kashuba AD, Kirchheiner J, Bauer S, Gaedigk A, Bertino JS. Effects of fluvastatin and cigarette smoking on CYP2C9 activity measured using the probe S-warfarin. *Eur J Clin Pharmacol* (2006) 62, 431–6.
9. Colucci VJ. Increase in international normalized ratio associated with smoking cessation. *Ann Pharmacother* (2001) 35, 385–6.
10. Evans M, Lewis GM. Increase in international normalized ratio after smoking cessation in a patient receiving warfarin. *Pharmacotherapy* (2005) 25, 1656–9.

Coumarins + Tricyclic antidepressants

Amitriptyline and nortriptyline do not appear to alter the half-life of warfarin, and probably do not alter that of dicoumarol. Limited evidence suggests that the use of tricyclics might be associated with greater variability in prothrombin times or an increased risk of bleeding. An isolated case of the potentiation of warfarin by lofepramine has been reported.

Clinical evidence

(a) Dicoumarol

A study in 6 healthy subjects given **nortriptyline** 200 micrograms/kg three times daily for 8 days, reported that it increased the mean half-life of dicoumarol from 35 hours to 106 hours. In a parallel group, the same dose of **nortriptyline** also increased the half-life of antipyrine.[1] However, in later identical studies by the same research group, **nortriptyline** decreased the half-life of antipyrine in one study, and had no effect in another.[2] The authors were unable to explain these disparate findings with antipyrine,[2] and they cast doubt on the results seen with dicoumarol. In a later study by another group, both **amitriptyline** 75 mg daily and **nortriptyline** 40 mg daily had no consistent effect on the half-life of a single dose of dicoumarol, although there was some evidence of increased dicoumarol plasma concentrations (about 24% with nortriptyline and 6% with **amitriptyline**).[3]

(b) Phenprocoumon

A retrospective analysis of 7 patients taking phenprocoumon and **amitriptyline** found unpredictable fluctuations in prothrombin times (said to be massive, both increases and decreases were seen); these were absent in a control group of 7 other patients not taking **amitriptyline**. Note that the **amitriptyline** dose was not stable. Anticoagulant control improved on stopping the **amitriptyline** in 5 of the patients.[4] The same authors reported another similar case in a patient taking phenprocoumon and **amitriptyline**.[5]

(c) Warfarin

In a study in 12 healthy subjects,[3] **amitriptyline** 75 mg daily or **nortriptyline** 40 mg daily for 13 days did not affected the plasma half-life of a single dose of warfarin given on day 9. However, in the preliminary report of an analysis of 500 patients taking warfarin, a statistically significant difference in the warfarin dose index (prothrombin time prolongation/cumulative warfarin dose) before, during and after therapy was detected for a number of unexpected drugs including **amitriptyline**. However, no further details were given.[6] In another analysis of the stability of anticoagulant control in 277 patients, the use of tricyclics (**imipramine**, **amitriptyline**, **nortriptyline**) in 16 patients was associated with an increased need for anticoagulant dose modifications (average 3.56 over 6 months). Most of the patients were taking warfarin.[7] In a retrospective study, **clomipramine** was associated with an increased risk of haemorrhage in patients taking warfarin; however, in this study it was grouped with the SSRIs which appear to increase the risk of bleeding, see 'Coumarins and related drugs + SSRIs', p.469.

A retrospective case-control study in patients taking warfarin who were given their first 30-day prescription for **amitriptyline** found that concurrent use increased the risk of hospitalisation for gastrointestinal bleeding (adjusted odds ratio 1.47). No statistically significant increased risk of gastrointestinal bleeding was found with the second 30-day prescription but an increased risk was found with the third or fourth 30-day prescription (adjusted odds ratio 1.61).[8] Further, a case-control study using data from the UK General Practice Research Database, found no increased risk of gastrointestinal haemorrhage with the concurrent use of warfarin and tricyclics compared with warfarin or tricyclics given alone.[9]

Mechanism

Not understood. One suggestion is that the tricyclic antidepressants inhibit the metabolism of the anticoagulant (seen in *animals* with nortriptyline or amitriptyline and warfarin,[10] but not with **desipramine** and **acenocoumarol**[11]). However, the tricyclics are not established inhibitors of the metabolism of any drug so this seems unlikely. Another suggestion is that the tricyclics slow gastrointestinal motility because of their antimuscarinic effects, thereby increasing the time available for the dissolution and absorption of dicoumarol.[3]

Importance and management

Information about interactions between the coumarins and tricyclic antidepressants is limited, patchy, and inconclusive. It appears that amitriptyline and nortriptyline do not alter the half-life of warfarin, and probably do not affect that of dicoumarol either. A greater fluctuation in anticoagulant control was noted in two analyses, one with warfarin and one with phenprocoumon. However, these were uncontrolled studies, and the findings need confirming in a randomised study. In addition, the data regarding a possible increased risk of bleeding on concurrent use is retrospective and conflicting. Moreover, there do not appear to be any published case reports of an interaction between tricyclics and warfarin. Thus, there is insufficient evidence to recommend any particular precautions in patients taking coumarins and requiring tricyclics. However, consider the possibility of an interaction if the INR is difficult to stabilise.

1. Vesell ES, Passananti GT, Greene FE. Impairment of drug metabolism in man by allopurinol and nortriptyline. *N Engl J Med* (1970) 283, 1484–8.
2. Vesell ES, Passananti GT, Aurori KC. Anomalous results of studies on drug interaction in man. *Pharmacology* (1975) 13, 101–111.
3. Pond SM, Graham GG, Birkett DJ, Wade DN. Effects of tricyclic antidepressants on drug metabolism. *Clin Pharmacol Ther* (1975) 18, 191–9.
4. Hampel H, Berger C, Kuss H-J, Müller-Spahn F. Unstable anticoagulation in the course of amitriptyline treatment. *Pharmacopsychiatry* (1996) 29, 33–7.
5. Hampel H, Berger C, Müller-Spahn F. Modified anticoagulant potency in an amitriptyline-treated patient? *Acta Haematol (Basel)* (1996) 96, 178–80.
6. Koch-Weser J. Hemorrhagic reactions and drug interactions in 500 warfarin-treated patients. *Clin Pharmacol Ther* (1973) 14, 139.
7. Williams JRB, Griffin JP, Parkins A. Effect of concomitantly administered drugs on the control of long term anticoagulant therapy. *Q J Med* (1976) 45, 63.
8. Schelleman H, Brensinger CM, Bilker WB, Hennessy S. Antidepressant-warfarin interaction and associated gastrointestinal bleeding risk in a case-control study. *PLoS One* (2011) 6, e21447.
9. Opatrny L, Delaney JA, Suissa S. Gastro-intestinal haemorrhage risks of selective serotonin receptor antagonist therapy: a new look. *Br J Clin Pharmacol* (2008) 66, 76–81.
10. Loomis CW, Racz WJ. Drug interactions of amitriptyline and nortriptyline with warfarin in the rat. *Res Commun Chem Pathol Pharmacol* (1980) 30, 41–58.
11. Weiner M. Effect of centrally active drugs on the action of coumarin anticoagulants. *Nature* (1966) 212, 1599–1600.

Coumarins and related drugs + Tyrosine kinase inhibitors

Isolated cases of increased INRs and bleeding have been reported in patients taking warfarin with erlotinib, gefitinib, imatinib, and sorafenib. In studies, regorafenib slightly increased warfarin exposure, but pazopanib and a single dose of nilotinib did not affect the pharmacokinetics of warfarin. Many tyrosine kinase inhibitors when given alone can cause bleeding, and the risk of this is likely to be increased in patients taking anticoagulants.

Clinical evidence

(a) Erlotinib

A case report describes a 47-year-old man stabilised on **warfarin** whose INR increased from 2.89 to 5.3 after 7 days of erlotinib 150 mg daily for lung cancer. Warfarin was discontinued for 2 days, but his INR increased further to 9.1 and he had a haematoma on his elbow, at which point erlotinib was stopped. Vitamin K was given, and the following day his INR was 2.4. Note that the patient experienced severe diarrhoea after starting erlotinib, and this might have resulted in reduced warfarin absorption.[1] The UK and US manufacturers briefly note that increased INRs and bleeding, including gastrointestinal bleeding, have been reported in patients taking erlotinib, some of whom were also taking **warfarin**, and some cases were fatal.[2,3]

(b) Gefitinib

A retrospective review of 12 patients with non-small cell lung cancer treated with gefitinib, and who were also receiving **warfarin**, found that the effects of warfarin were increased in 50% of these patients.[4] The cases of two of these patients are described in detail elsewhere; a woman stabilised on **warfarin** required a gradual decrease in her **warfarin** dose from 4 mg daily to 2.5 mg daily after starting gefitinib 250 mg/m^2 daily for lung cancer, whereas in the second patient, the effect of **warfarin** was not increased while taking gefitinib.[5] The UK manufacturer of gefitinib notes that increased INRs and bleeding have been reported in patients taking **warfarin** and gefitinib.[6] Note that gefitinib alone is associated with an increased risk of bleeding.[6]

(c) Imatinib

In 2001, the UK manufacturer of imatinib noted that they were aware of one patient taking **warfarin** who had altered prothrombin times while receiving imatinib in a clinical study.[7] An unacceptably high incidence of thromboembolic events was seen in a phase I study of imatinib given with estramustine and escalating doses of docetaxel, in which patients were given prophylactic doses of warfarin (2 mg daily). The study was stopped early, but the authors state that an interaction with warfarin is unlikely to be responsible for the thromboembolic events because, with docetaxel 70 mg/m^2, an *increased* prothrombin time was seen in 2 subjects.[8] A report describes 8 chronic myeloid leukaemia patients stabilised on **warfarin**, who also received imatinib at a standard dose of 400 mg daily. None of the patients required a reduced imatinib dose for haematological or non-haematological toxicity, and none had abnormal INR values. No bleeding or other thrombotic events were seen.[9] Imatinib alone is associated with thrombocytopenia and haemorrhage.[10,11]

(d) Nilotinib

In a single-dose study in 18 healthy subjects, nilotinib 800 mg had no effect on the pharmacokinetics of *R*- or *S*-warfarin after administration of **warfarin** 25 mg. The anticoagulant response was similarly unaffected.[12] Note, that a single-dose study is not long enough to adequately assess enzyme induction or inhibition and therefore, it is unclear what effect nilotinib might have at steady state. Note also that nilotinib alone can cause thrombocytopenia and haemorrhage.[13,14]

(e) Pazopanib

In a pharmacokinetic study in patients with cancer, pazopanib 800 mg once daily for 17 days had no effect on the pharmacokinetics of a single 10-mg dose of **warfarin**.[15] Note that pazopanib alone can cause haemorrhage.[16,17]

(f) Regorafenib

The US manufacturer briefly notes that in a study in patients with advanced solid tumours, regorafenib 160 mg daily for 14 days increased the AUC of a single 10-mg dose of **warfarin** by 25%.[18] Note that regorafenib alone can cause haemorrhage, which has resulted in fatalities in some cases.[18]

(g) Sorafenib

The UK manufacturer briefly notes, that in a study in patients given sorafenib and **warfarin**, the INR did not differ compared with placebo.[19] However, increased INRs and infrequent bleeding have been reported in patients taking **warfarin** with sorafenib. Note also, that sorafenib alone is associated with an increased risk of bleeding.[19,20]

During a study, a patient taking **warfarin** and sorafenib developed gastrointestinal bleeding with an INR of 5.8. After treatment interruption and warfarin adjustment to give an INR of 2 to 3, sorafenib was restarted, but the INR increased again to 4.3 with mild gastrointestinal bleeding. The report did not describe the time course of the events.[21] In another published case, a 70-year-old man who had been taking **warfarin** 36 mg weekly for about 5 months was started on sorafenib 200 mg daily for hepatocellular carcinoma. About 20 days later his INR was normal (2.9), but after a further 12 days he had lower extremity haemorrhage and an INR of 39.5. Sorafenib was stopped and he eventually resumed warfarin 36 mg weekly with therapeutic INRs. He then restarted sorafenib, and his INR increased to 4.7 after 16 days.[22] This case is difficult to interpret because the first INR change did not occur quickly enough to implicate altered metabolism of warfarin, and the second increase in INR was much less than the first. This patient had previously had subtherapeutic INRs due to occasionally forgetting doses.[22] A further case in a 60-year-old man with hepatocellular carcinoma and taking **warfarin**, similarly describes increased warfarin effects and a lower extremity haemorrhage, when the dose of sorafenib was increased to 600 mg daily (after 63 days).[23]

(h) Other tyrosine kinase inhibitors

Severe, and sometimes fatal, haemorrhages have occurred in patients when **axitinib**,[24,25] **cabozantinib**,[26] **dasatinib**,[27,28] **ponatinib**,[29,30] **sunitinib**,[31,32] or **vandetanib**[33,34] were given alone. **Bosutinib**[35,36] and **ruxolitinib**[37] have been associated with an increased risk of bleeding when given alone.

Mechanism

The metabolism of *S*-warfarin is principally via CYP2C9. A number of tyrosine kinase inhibitors have been found to be inhibitors of this isoenzyme *in vitro*, including imatinib,[10,11] nilotinib,[13,14] pazopanib,[16,17] regorafenib,[18] and sorafenib,[19,20] although note that imatinib was used at higher concentrations than those usually achieved clinically.[10] From the study cited above, regorafenib also appears to have an effect on CYP2C9 *in vivo*. However, the *in vitro* findings were not confirmed in studies with pazopanib or sorafenib which showed no effect on warfarin pharmacokinetics, and the true effect of nilotinib (that is, after repeated dosing) is not known.

The metabolism of *R*-warfarin involves CYP3A4, which is also inhibited by a number of tyrosine kinase inhibitors (see 'Table 1.9', p.11), but as *R*-warfarin is far less potent than *S*-warfarin, inhibition of this isoenzyme would not be expected to have an important effect on warfarin metabolism.

The effects of warfarin might be additive with the bleeding effects associated with many of the tyrosine kinase inhibitors.

Importance and management

The only established pharmacokinetic interaction between the tyrosine kinase inhibitors and warfarin is with regorafenib, which slightly increased warfarin exposure. Such an increase would be expected to be clinically important and increased monitoring of the INR would seem prudent on concurrent use. Consideration should also be given to the need for a reduction in warfarin dose. However, a pharmacodynamic interaction with the risk of increased bleeding is a theoretical possibility with many of the tyrosine kinase inhibitors, including axitinib, bosutinib, cabozantanib, **dasatinib**, gefitinib, erlotinib, imatinib, nilotinib, pazopanib, ponatinib, ruxolitinib, sorafenib, sunitinib, and vandetanib. Note also that factors related to illness such as decreased appetite can alter warfarin requirements. These factors, coupled with the fact that there have been several reports of altered INRs in patients given tyrosine kinase inhibitors, suggest that it would be prudent to increase the monitoring of warfarin and other coumarin or indanedione anticoagulant effects in patients also given a tyrosine kinase inhibitor. The UK and US manufacturers of imatinib specifically advise that patients should be given alternative anticoagulants to warfarin, such as heparin or low-molecular-weight heparins.[10,11]

Note that, from a disease perspective, when treating venous thromboembolic disease in patients with cancer, warfarin is generally inferior (higher risk of major bleeds and recurrent thrombosis) to low-molecular-weight heparins.[38]

Note also that warfarin can be used as a probe substrate to assess the activity of drugs on CYP2C9. The study with regorafenib therefore suggests that it is a weak inhibitor of CYP2C9. The studies with pazopanib and sorafenib suggest that they are not inhibitors of CYP2C9.

1. Thomas KS, Billingsley A, Amarshi N, Nair BA. Elevated international normalized ratio associated with concomitant warfarin and erlotinib. *Am J Health-Syst Pharm* (2010) 67, 1426–9.
2. Tarceva (Erlotinib hydrochloride). OSI Pharmaceuticals, LLC. US Prescribing information, May 2013.
3. Tarceva (Erlotinib hydrochloride). Roche Products Ltd. UK Summary of product characteristics, June 2013.
4. Arai S, Mitsufuji H, Nishii Y, Onoda S, Ryuge S, Wada M, Katono K, Iwasaki M, Takakura A, Otani S, Yamamoto M, Yanaihara T, Yokoba M, Kubota M, Katagiri M, Fukui T, Kobayashi H, Yanase N, Hataishi R, Masuda N. Effect of gefitinib on warfarin antithrombotic activity. *Int J Clin Oncol* (2009) 14, 332–6.
5. Onoda S, Mitsufuji H, Yanase N, Ryuge S, Kato E, Wada M, Ishii K, Hagiri S, Yamamoto M, Yokoba M, Yanaihara T, Kuboto M, Takada N, Katagiri M, Abe T, Tanaka M, Kobayashi H, Masuda N. Drug interaction between gefitinib and warfarin. *Jpn J Clin Oncol* (2005) 35, 478–82.
6. Iressa (Gefitinib monohydrate). AstraZeneca UK Ltd. UK Summary of product characteristics, June 2013.

7. Novartis Pharmaceuticals UK Limited. Personal communication, December 2001.
8. Lin AM, Rini BI, Derynck MK, Weinberg V, Park M, Ryan CJ, Rosenberg JE, Bubley G, Small EJ. A phase I trial of docetaxel/estramustine/imatinib in patients with hormone-refractory prostate cancer. *Clin Genitourin Cancer* (2007) 5, 323–8.
9. Breccia M, Santopietro M, Loglisci G, Stagno F, Cannella L, Carmosino I, Alimena G. Concomitant use of imatinib and warfarin in chronic phase chronic myeloid leukemia patients does not interfere with drug efficacy. *Leuk Res* (2010) 34, e224–e225.
10. Glivec (Imatinib mesilate). Novartis Pharmaceuticals UK Ltd. UK Summary of product characteristics, July 2013.
11. Gleevec (Imatinib mesylate). Novartis Pharmaceuticals Corp. US Prescribing information, February 2013.
12. Yin OQP, Gallagher N, Fischer D, Zhao L, Zhou W, Leroy E, Golor G, Schran H. Effects of nilotinib on single-dose warfarin pharmacokinetics and pharmacodynamics. *Clin Drug Investig* (2011) 31, 169–79.
13. Tasigna (Nilotinib hydrochloride monohydrate). Novartis Pharmaceuticals UK Ltd. UK Summary of product characteristics, June 2015.
14. Tasigna (Nilotinib hydrochloride monohydrate). Novartis Pharmaceuticals Corp. US Prescribing information, January 2015.
15. Goh BC, Reddy NJ, Dandamudi UB, Laubscher KH, Peckham T, Hodge JP, Suttle AB, Arumugham T, Xu Y, Xu C-F, Lager J, Dar MM, Lewis LD. An evaluation of the drug interaction potential of pazopanib, an oral vascular endothelial growth factor receptor tyrosine kinase inhibitor, using a modified Cooperstown 5 +1 cocktail in patients with advanced solid tumours. *Clin Pharmacol Ther* (2010) 88, 652–9.
16. Votrient (Pazopanib hydrochloride). GlaxoSmithKline UK. UK Summary of product characteristics, July 2015.
17. Votrient (Pazopanib hydrochloride). GlaxoSmithKline. US Prescribing information, April 2015.
18. Stivarga (Regorafenib). Bayer HealthCare Pharmaceuticals Inc. US Prescribing information, August 2013.
19. Nexavar (Sorafenib tosylate). Bayer plc. UK Summary of product characteristics, November 2014.
20. Nexavar (Sorafenib tosylate). Bayer HealthCare Pharmaceuticals Inc. US Prescribing information, November 2013.
21. Laber DA, Mushtaq M. Compassionate use of sorafenib in patients with advanced renal cell cancer. *Clin Genitourin Cancer* (2009) 7, 34–8.
22. Moretti LV, Montalvo RO. Elevated international normalized ratio associated with concurrent use of sorafenib and warfarin. *Am J Health-Syst Pharm* (2009) 66, 2123–5.
23. Shiozawa K, Watanabe M, Hirano N, Wakui N, Kikuchi Y, Hara F Ishii K, Iida K, Sumino Y. Gastrointestinal hemorrhage associated with concurrent use of sorafenib and warfarin for hepatocellular carcinoma. *Gan To Kagaku Ryoho* (2011) 38, 1713–15.
24. Inlyta (Axitinib). Pfizer Ltd. UK Summary of product characteristics, May 2015.
25. Inlyta (Axitinib). Pfizer Inc. US Prescribing information, August 2014.
26. Cometriq (Cabozantinib malate). Exelixis, Inc. US Prescribing information, November 2012
27. Sprycel (Dasatinib monohydrate). Bristol-Myers Squibb Pharmaceutical Ltd. UK Summary of product characteristics, July 2013.
28. Sprycel (Dasatinib monohydrate). Bristol-Myers Squibb Company. US Prescribing information, October 2011.
29. Iclusig (Ponatinib). ARIAD Pharmaceuticals, Inc. US Prescribing information, September 2014.
30. Iclusig (Ponatinib). ARIAD Pharma Ltd. UK Summary of product characteristics, April 2015.
31. Sutent (Sunitinib malate). Pfizer Ltd. UK Summary of product characteristics, June 2015.
32. Sutent (Sunitinib malate). Pfizer Inc. US Prescribing information, April 2015.
33. Caprelsa (Vandetanib). AstraZeneca UK Ltd. UK Summary of product characteristics, October 2014.
34. Caprelsa (Vandetanib). AstraZeneca Pharmaceuticals LP. US Prescribing information, June 2011.
35. Bosulif (Bosutinib monohydrate). Pfizer Ltd. UK Summary of product characteristics, July 2015.
36. Bosulif (Bosutinib monohydrate). Pfizer Inc. US Prescribing information, November 2014.
37. Jakavi (Ruxolitinib phosphate). Novartis Pharmaceuticals UK Ltd. UK Summary of product characteristics, April 2015.
38. Baglin TP, Keeling DM, Watson HG; British Committee for Standards in Haematology. Guidelines on oral anticoagulation (warfarin): third edition–2005 update. *Br J Haematol* (2006) 132, 277–85.

Coumarins + Urinary antimuscarinics

Fesoterodine, solifenacin, and tolterodine do not appear to alter the pharmacokinetics or anticoagulant effect of warfarin; however, isolated cases of increased INRs have been reported when patients taking warfarin also took tolterodine. Darifenacin does not alter the prothrombin time in response to warfarin.

Clinical evidence

(a) Darifenacin

The US manufacturer notes that steady-state darifenacin 30 mg daily did not alter the prothrombin time after a single 30-mg dose of **warfarin**.[1]

(b) Fesoterodine

In a crossover study in healthy subjects, fesoterodine 8 mg daily for 9 days had no effect on the pharmacokinetics or anticoagulant effects of a single 25-mg dose of warfarin, taken on day 3, when compared with warfarin alone.[2]

(c) Solifenacin

In a placebo-controlled, crossover study in healthy subjects, solifenacin 10 mg daily for 10 days had no effect on the pharmacokinetics of *S*- or *R*-warfarin after a single 25-mg dose of **warfarin** was given on day 10. In addition, solifenacin did not alter the prothrombin time.[3]

(d) Tolterodine

In a placebo-controlled study in healthy subjects, tolterodine 2 mg twice daily for 7 days did not affect the pharmacokinetics of *R*- or *S*-warfarin after a single 25-mg dose of **warfarin** given on day 4, nor were the pharmacokinetics of tolterodine altered by **warfarin**. In addition, the prothrombin time and factor VII activity were not altered by tolterodine.[4] However, a report describes 2 patients on stable **warfarin** doses who had elevated INRs shortly after tolterodine 2 mg daily was started and stopped: one patient had an INR of 6.1 one day after stopping tolterodine, which had been taken for 13 days, and the other patient had an INR of 7.4 two days after stopping tolterodine, which had been taken for 8 days. In both cases no bleeding occurred and **warfarin** was withheld for three doses and successfully reinstated at the original dose.[5] Another case report describes a patient who required a 15% reduction in her **warfarin** dose while taking tolterodine 4 mg daily. Her maximum INR had been 3.9. However, she had undergone several warfarin dose increases over the previous 2 months and her INR had been fluctuating.[6]

Mechanism

As the controlled study found no pharmacokinetic interaction between tolterodine and warfarin, the mechanism for the interaction in the case reports is unknown.

Importance and management

The controlled study with tolterodine suggests that no warfarin dose adjustment would be expected to be necessary when tolterodine is added to warfarin. However, the three cases introduce a note of caution. Although additional monitoring would seem over-cautious on the basis of these cases, bear them in mind in the case of an unexpected response to warfarin.

The studies above suggest that no pharmacokinetic or pharmacodynamic interaction occurs between warfarin and darifenacin, fesoterodine, or solifenacin, and so no warfarin dose adjustment or additional monitoring would be expected to be needed on concurrent use.

1. Enablex (Darifenacin hydrobromide). Novartis. US Prescribing information, January 2010.
2. Malhotra B, Alvey C, Gong J, Li X, Duczynski G, Gandelman K. Effects of fesoterodine on the pharmacokinetics and pharmacodynamics of warfarin in healthy volunteers. *Br J Clin Pharmacol* (2011) 72, 257–62.
3. Smulders RA, Kuipers ME, Krauwinkel WJJ. Multiple doses of the antimuscarinic agent solifenacin do not affect the pharmacodynamics or pharmacokinetics of warfarin or the steady-state pharmacokinetics of digoxin in healthy subjects. *Br J Clin Pharmacol* (2006) 62, 210–17.
4. Rahimy M, Hallén B, Narang P. Effect of tolterodine on the anticoagulant actions and pharmacokinetics of single-dose warfarin in healthy volunteers. *Arzneimittelforschung* (2002) 52, 890–5.
5. Colucci VJ, Rivey MP. Tolterodine-warfarin drug interaction. *Ann Pharmacother* (1999) 33, 1173–6.
6. Taylor JR. Probable interaction between tolterodine and warfarin. *Pharmacotherapy* (2006) 26, 719–21.

Coumarins and related drugs + Vaccines; Influenza

The concurrent use of warfarin and influenza vaccination is usually safe and uneventful, but there are reports of bleeding in a handful of patients (fatal in one case and life-threatening in another) attributed to an interaction. Acenocoumarol also does not normally interact with influenza vaccination.

Clinical evidence

(a) Effect on anticoagulant control

Seventeen studies on the effects of influenza vaccine on the anticoagulant effect of coumarins have been published, and these are summarised in 'Table 12.9', p.482. Most of these are non-controlled studies in small to moderate numbers of patients, and the majority did not demonstrate a significant change in prothrombin time or INR in patients taking coumarins, including the two randomised placebo-controlled studies, and one very large retrospective cohort study. Some studies found a slight change in anticoagulant effect (both slight increases and slight reductions), but they are probably of limited clinical relevance. However, in one large case-control study, a clear increase in INR from 2.64 to 3.85 was seen in about half of the 90 patients involved in the study, and 2 of these patients had bleeding episodes. The reasons for the clear difference between this study and the many others are not known.

There are also various brief case reports of a possible interaction. One case report describes a 64-year-old man taking warfarin whose INR had been relatively stable (roughly ranging between 1.4 and 4.7) over the previous 6 months. Four-and-a-half weeks after receiving an inactivated influenza vaccine, he experienced rectal bleeding followed by a fatal intracranial bleed at which time his INR was found to be greater than 15. As none of his other medication had been changed for at least 6 months, the authors attributed these effects to an interaction between warfarin and the influenza vaccine. However, the authors note that the patient had no observed complications with previous influenza vaccination while taking warfarin and they suggest that variations in vaccine preparation may influence this interaction.[1] A very brief report in a review paper describes a patient receiving **warfarin** who had serious bleeding, which was almost fatal, after receiving a 'flu shot'. No further details are given.[2] In a third case, an elderly man receiving **warfarin** developed bleeding (haematemesis and melaena) within 10 days of being given an influenza vaccination. His prothrombin time was found to be 36 seconds.[3]

(b) Route of injection of vaccine

In a randomised study in 26 patients stabilised on **warfarin**, there was no difference in injection site adverse events between intramuscular or subcutaneous injection of a standard trivalent influenza vaccine, and no patient had bruising or swelling. In addition, both routes of administration produced similar levels of antibody titres.[4] In another study that specifically assessed the local reactions to intramuscular influenza vaccination, there were no detectable local complications after intramuscular injection, including no change in arm circumference.[5]

Mechanism

Not understood. In a placebo-controlled study in healthy subjects, influenza vaccination did not alter the half-life of either *R*- or *S*-warfarin.[3] It has therefore been suggested that when an interaction occurs the synthesis of the blood clotting factors is altered.[3]

Importance and management

A well-investigated interaction, but with some contradictory data. The weight of evidence suggests that influenza vaccination in those taking warfarin is normally safe and uneventful; nevertheless, it would be prudent to be on the alert because very occasionally and unpredictably bleeding may occur. Acenocoumarol appears not to be affected. Limited evidence suggests that intramuscular administration of the vaccine is not associated with increased local complications, but also that subcutaneous admin-

Table 12.9 Summary of the evidence for and against an interaction between influenza vaccine and coumarins

Study type (year)	*Group*	*Coumarin*	*Influenza vaccine*	*Route*	*Notes*	*Refs*
Studies showing no interaction						
Prospective (1983)	33 patients and 15 controls	Warfarin	Not stated	Not stated	No evidence of an interaction (one vaccinated patient had haematuria 27 days later, and one control patient had epistaxis)	1
Prospective series (1984)	21 patients	Stable warfarin	Trivalent type A and B, Wyeth	Not stated	No change in average prothrombin time at 0, 3, 7, 10 and 14 days after vaccination	2
Randomised, placebo-controlled (1984)	25 patients vaccinated and 25 placebo	Stable warfarin	Trivalent type A and B (*Fluvirin*)	Deep subcutaneous	No change in mean ratio of prothrombin times at 0, 2, 7 and 21 days after vaccination	3
Prospective (1984)	4 healthy subjects	Low-dose warfarin	*Influvac*	Intramuscular	No change in average prothrombin time at 7, 11, 14, 16, 21 and 28 days after vaccination, and no change in warfarin levels	4
Prospective series (1985)	7 patients	Stable warfarin	Trivalent type A and B, Wyeth	Not stated	No change in prothrombin time at 4, 6, 10, 14 and 21 days after vaccination	5
Prospective series (1986)	26 patients	Stable warfarin	Trivalent (subvirion) type A and B (*Fluogen*)	Intramuscular	No change in mean INR at day 14 after vaccination	6
Prospective series (1986)	7 patients and 9 controls	Stable warfarin	Trivalent type A and B, Wyeth	Not stated	No change in prothrombin time at 1, 3 and 5 weeks after vaccination, or compared with controls	7
Prospective series (1990)	9 patients	Stable warfarin	Trivalent, split virion, A and B (*MFV-Ject*)	Not stated	No significant change in INR at 3, 6, 8, 10, 13, 22 and 30 days after vaccination (mean decrease of 4.8%)	8
Prospective series (1993)	43 patients	Stable acenocoumarol	Trivalent type A and B	Subcutaneous	No change in mean INR at 7, 15 and 30 days after vaccination. INR values increased in 3 patients and decreased in 6 patients requiring modification in acenocoumarol dose	9
Prospective series (1995)	41 patients	Stable warfarin	Not stated	Intramuscular	No significant change in prothrombin time at 3, 7 and 14 days after vaccination, and no local complications	10
Prospective series (2007)	78 patients	Stable warfarin	Not stated	Not stated	No apparent effect on INR within 10 days of vaccination	11
Retrospective cohort (2007)	4923 patients	Stable warfarin	Trivalent inactivated	Not stated	No change in mean INR in the 14 or 28 days after vaccination	12
Randomised, placebo-controlled (2010)	100 patients	Stable warfarin	Trivalent adjuvanted A and B (Fluad, Novartis)	Intramuscular	No change in mean INR or warfarin weekly doses at 7, 14 and 28 days after vaccination. No major bleeding or thrombotic events within 6 months of vaccination.	13
Studies showing an increase in effect						
Prospective series (1984)	8 patients	Stable warfarin	Trivalent type A and B	Not stated	All patients had an increase in prothrombin time to at least the upper limit of their range for the previous year (40% from baseline)*	14
Prospective series (1986)	10 patients	Stable warfarin	Trivalent (subvirion) type A and B (*Fluogen*)	Intramuscular	Slight maximal 7.6% increase in mean INR at day 14 after vaccination	6
Case-control (2003)	90 patients and 45 controls	Stable warfarin (98%) Acenocoumarol (2%)	*Inflexel V*, *Isiflu V*, *Fluad*, or *Agrippal*	Intramuscular	49 out of 90 patients had a clear increase in INR from a mean of 2.64 to 3.85, and 2 of these had bleeding episodes. In the remaining patients and controls there was no change in INR	15
Studies showing a decrease in effect						
Prospective series (1988)	24 patients	Stable warfarin	Trivalent type A and B	Not stated	A slight 8.3% decrease in prothrombin time occurred in the first 2 weeks after vaccination.	16
Prospective series (2002)	73 patients and 72 controls	Stable warfarin	Not stated	Subcutaneous	Overall, there was no change in anticoagulation, but the 34 vaccinated patients aged 70 or more had a slight reduction in INR in month after vaccination (mean 2.8 versus 2.99)	17

*Other researchers[5] state that their analysis of these data failed to show a statistical difference after vaccination.

1. Patriarca PA, Kendal AP, Stricof RL, Weber JA, Meissner MK, Dateno B. Influenza vaccination and warfarin or theophylline toxicity in nursing-home residents. *N Engl J Med* (1983) 308, 1601–2.
2. Lipsky BA, Pecoraro RE, Roben NJ, de Blaquiere P, Delaney CJ. Influenza vaccination and warfarin anticoagulation. *Ann Intern Med* (1984) 100, 835–7.
3. Farrow PR, Nicholson KG. Lack of effect of influenza and pneumococcal vaccines on anticoagulation by warfarin. *J Infect* (1984) 9, 157–60.

Continued

Table 12.9 Summary of the evidence for and against an interaction between influenza vaccine and coumarins (continued)

4. Scott AK, Cannon J, Breckenridge AM. Lack of effect of influenza vaccination on warfarin in healthy volunteers. *Br J Clin Pharmacol* (1984) 19, 144P–145P.
5. Gomolin IH, Chapron DJ, Luhan PA. Lack of effect of influenza vaccine on theophylline levels and warfarin anticoagulation in the elderly. *J Am Geriatr Soc* (1985) 33, 269–72.
6. Weibert RT, Lorentz SM, Norcross WA, Klauber MR, Jagger PI. Effect of influenza vaccine in patients receiving long-term warfarin therapy. *Clin Pharm* (1986) 5, 499–503.
7. Gomolin IH. Lack of effect of influenza vaccine on warfarin anticoagulation in the elderly. *Can Med Assoc J* (1986) 135, 39–41.
8. Arnold WSG, Mehta MK, Roberts JS. Influenza vaccine and anticoagulation control in patients receiving warfarin. *Br J Clin Pract* (1990) 44, 136–9.
9. Souto JC, Oliver A, Montserrat I, Mateo J, Sureda A, Fontcuberta J. Lack of effect of influenza vaccine on anticoagulation by acenocoumarol. *Ann Pharmacother* (1993) 27, 365–8.
10. Raj G, Kumar R, McKinney WP. Safety of intramuscular influenza immunization among patients receiving long-term warfarin anticoagulation therapy. *Arch Intern Med* (1995) 155, 1529–31.
11. MacCallum P, Madhani M, Mt-Isa S, Ashby D. Lack of effect of influenza immunisation on anticoagulant control in patients on long-term warfarin. *Pharmacoepidemiol Drug Saf* (2007) 16, 786–9.
12. Jackson ML, Nelson JC, Chen RT, Davis RL, Jackson LA; for the Vaccine Safety Datalink investigators. Vaccines and changes in coagulation parameters in adults on chronic warfarin therapy: a cohort study. *Pharmacoepidemiol Drug Saf* (2007) 16, 790–6.
13. Iorio A, Basileo M, Marcucci M, Guercini F, Camilloni B, Paccamiccio E, Vecchioli M, Iorio AM. Influenza vaccination and vitamin K antagonist treatment: a placebo-controlled, randomized, double-blind crossover study. *Arch Intern Med* (2010) 170, 609–16.
14. Kramer P, Tsuru M, Cook CE, McClain CJ, Holtzman JL. Effect of influenza vaccine on warfarin anticoagulation. *Clin Pharmacol Ther* (1984) 35, 416–18.
15. Paliani U, Filippucci E, Gresele P. Significant potentiation of anticoagulation by flu-vaccine during the season 2001-2002. *Haematologica* (2003) 88, 599–600.
16. Bussey HI, Saklad JJ. Effect of influenza vaccine on chronic warfarin therapy. *Drug Intell Clin Pharm* (1988) 22, 198–201.
17. Poli D, Chiarugi L, Capanni M, Antonucci E, Abbate R, Gensini GF, Prisco D. Need of more frequent international normalized ratio monitoring in elderly patients on long-term anticoagulant therapy after influenza vaccination. *Blood Coag Fibrinol* (2002) 13, 297–300.

istration is effective. Because of the theoretical risk of local muscle haematoma, it may be preferable to give influenza vaccines by deep subcutaneous injection in patients taking coumarins and related anticoagulants.

Pneumococcal, tetanus and hepatitis A vaccines do not appear to alter anticoagulant status, see 'Coumarins + Vaccines; Miscellaneous', p.483.

1. Carroll DN, Carroll DG. Fatal intracranial bleed potentially due to a warfarin and influenza vaccine interaction. *Ann Pharmacother* (2009) 43, 754–60.
2. Sumner HW, Holtzman JL, McClain CJ. Drug-induced liver disease. *Geriatrics* (1981) 36, 83–96.
3. Kramer P, Tsuru M, Cook CE, McClain CJ, Holtzman JL. Effect of influenza vaccine on warfarin anticoagulation. *Clin Pharmacol Ther* (1984) 35, 416–18.
4. Delafuente JC, Davis JA, Meuleman JR, Jones RA. Influenza vaccination and warfarin anticoagulation: a comparison of subcutaneous and intramuscular routes of administration in elderly men. *Pharmacotherapy* (1998) 18, 631–6.
5. Raj G, Kumar R, McKinney WP. Safety of intramuscular influenza immunization among patients receiving long-term warfarin anticoagulation therapy. *Arch Intern Med* (1995) 155, 1529–31.

Coumarins + Vaccines; Miscellaneous

Pneumococcal, tetanus with diphtheria toxoid, and hepatitis A vaccines do not appear to alter the response to warfarin.

Clinical evidence, mechanism, importance and management

In a large, retrospective, cohort study in patients stabilised on warfarin, there was no clinically relevant change in INR found between mean values in the 14 days or 28 days after vaccination with a 23-valent **pneumococcal polysaccharide** vaccine (1207 patients), **tetanus** plus **diphtheria toxoid** vaccine (1024 patients), or **hepatitis A** vaccine (121 patients) compared with mean values at other times. The change in mean INR was 0.01 to 0.03.[1] Similarly, in an earlier placebo-controlled study, a 14-valent **pneumococcal vaccine** (*Pneumovax*) did not have any effect on anticoagulant control at 2, 7 and 21 days after vaccination.[2] These studies suggest that no alteration in coagulation status would be anticipated after use of these vaccines.

For discussion of the numerous studies with influenza vaccine, see 'Coumarins and related drugs + Vaccines; Influenza', p.481.

1. Jackson ML, Nelson JC, Chen RT, Davis RL, Jackson LA; for the Vaccine Safety Datalink investigators. Vaccines and changes in coagulation parameters in adults on chronic warfarin therapy: a cohort study. *Pharmacoepidemiol Drug Safety* (2007) 16, 790–6.
2. Farrow PR, Nicholson KG. Lack of effect of influenza and pneumococcal vaccines on anticoagulation by warfarin. *J Infect* (1984) 9, 157–60.

Coumarins + Valproate

An isolated case describes a patient who had an increase in her INR the day after starting valproic acid, but was eventually restabilised on the original dose of warfarin while still taking the valproic acid. Valproic acid did not alter the anticoagulant effects of phenprocoumon in one patient. Note that valproate alone can cause altered bleeding time, bruising, haematoma, epistaxis, haemorrhage, and thrombocytopenia.

Clinical evidence

A woman was given **warfarin** for a deep vein thrombosis, and was stabilised on 5 mg alternating with 2.5 mg daily with an INR of between 1.8 and 2.6. Valproic acid 250 mg twice daily and fluphenazine 5 mg daily were then added. The morning after her first dose of valproic acid, the INR increased to 3.9, and **warfarin** dose was decreased to 2.5 mg daily. Four days later the valproic acid dose was doubled, and numerous **warfarin** dose adjustments were needed to keep the INR therapeutic. However, 3 weeks after starting the valproic acid she was discharged on the same **warfarin** dose as before the valproic acid was started.[1] In one patient taking **phenprocoumon**, valproic acid 500 mg to 1 g daily did not alter the prothrombin time ratio.[2]

Mechanism

There is *in vitro* evidence that the serum binding of warfarin is decreased by sodium valproate so that free warfarin levels rise,[1,3,4] by 32% according to one study.[1] The increase in free warfarin levels is transient until a new equilibrium is reached, but theoretically could result in a transient increase in INR, as is seen with cloral hydrate (see 'Coumarins + Cloral hydrate and related drugs', p.418).

Valproate inhibits the second stage of platelet aggregation, and a reversible prolongation of bleeding times and thrombocytopenia has been reported, usually with high doses, which can result in spontaneous bruising and bleeding.

Importance and management

Evidence for an interaction is limited. There seem to be no other reports of problems associated with the concurrent use of valproate and warfarin, nor any other direct evidence that an interaction of clinical importance normally occurs. It may be that any interaction occurs only transiently when valproate is added, and the situation rapidly restabilises without any real need to adjust the warfarin dose. Nevertheless, the manufacturers of sodium valproate and divalproex recommend closely monitoring the prothrombin time because of the possibility of warfarin protein binding displacement.[5-8] Note that valproate alone can cause thrombocytopenia and spontaneous bruising or bleeding, and if these effects occur, the manufacturers recommend withdrawing valproate pending investigations.[5-8] A reduction of the valproate dose or permanent withdrawal of valproate may be required.[6]

1. Guthrie SK, Stoysich AM, Bader G, Hilleman DE. Hypothesized interaction between valproic acid and warfarin. *J Clin Psychopharmacol* (1995) 15, 138–9.
2. Schlienger R, Kurmann M, Drewe J, Müller-Spahn F, Seifritz E. Inhibition of phenprocoumon anticoagulation by carbamazepine. *Eur Neuropsychopharmacol* (2000) 10, 219–21.
3. Urien S, Albengres E, Tillement J-P. Serum protein binding of valproic acid in healthy subjects and in patients with liver disease. *Int J Clin Pharmacol Ther Toxicol* (1981) 19, 319–25.
4. Panjehshahin MR, Bowmer CJ, Yates MS. Effect of valproic acid, its unsaturated metabolites and some structurally related fatty acids on the binding of warfarin and dansylsarcosine to human albumin. *Biochem Pharmacol* (1991) 41, 1227–33.
5. Epilim (Sodium valproate). Sanofi-Aventis. UK Summary of product characteristics, November 2008.
6. Depakote (Divalproex sodium). Abbott Laboratories. US Prescribing information, October 2006.
7. Depakote (Valproate semisodium). Sanofi-Aventis. UK Summary of product characteristics, November 2009.
8. Depakene (Valproic acid). Abbott Laboratories. US Prescribing information, January 2007.

Coumarins + Varenicline

Varenicline does not appear to alter the pharmacokinetics or anticoagulant effect of warfarin.

Clinical evidence, mechanism, importance and management

In a controlled study in 24 smokers, varenicline 1 mg twice daily for 13 days had no effect on the pharmacokinetics of a single 25-mg dose of warfarin given on day 8. There was no difference in warfarin pharmacodynamics (INR time curve).[1] The lack of pharmacokinetic interaction is consistent with *in vitro* findings.[1] No warfarin dose adjustments would be expected to be needed in patients taking varenicline. Nevertheless, bear in mind that smoking cessation (for which varenicline is used as an aid) can sometimes cause a minor to modest decrease in warfarin requirements, see 'Coumarins + Tobacco', p.479.

1. Burstein AH, Clark DJ, O'Gorman M, Willavize SA, Brayman TG, Grover GS, Walsky RL, Obach RS, Faessel HM. Lack of pharmacokinetic and pharmacodynamic interactions between a smoking cessation therapy, varenicline, and warfarin: an in vivo and in vitro study. *J Clin Pharmacol* (2007) 47, 1421–9.

Coumarins + Vinpocetine

In healthy subjects, the anticoagulant effect and the AUC of warfarin was slightly reduced by vinpocetine.

Clinical evidence, mechanism, importance and management

In a study in 18 healthy subjects taking vinpocetine 10 mg three times daily for 19 days, the anticoagulant effects and pharmacokinetics of a single 25-mg dose of **warfarin** were compared when given before vinpocetine was started, and on day 15.[1] A small 15% reduction in the mean prothrombin time occurred, and also an 8%

reduction in the AUC of **warfarin**. The clinical relevance of these changes is unclear; however, they are slight, and a clinically relevant interaction would not be expected.

1. Hitzenberger G, Sommer W, Grandt R. Influence of vinpocetine on warfarin-induced inhibition of coagulation. *Int J Clin Pharmacol Ther Toxicol* (1990) 28, 323–8.

Coumarins + Vitamin E substances

The anticoagulant effects of warfarin are usually unchanged by small to large doses of vitamin E, although one isolated case of bleeding has been attributed to concurrent use. The effects of dicoumarol may be slightly increased by vitamin E.

Clinical evidence

(a) Dicoumarol

A study in 3 healthy subjects found that 42 units of vitamin E daily for one month increased the response to a single dose of dicoumarol after 36 hours (decrease in prothrombin activity from 52% to 33%).[1]

(b) Warfarin

In a double-blind, placebo-controlled study in 25 patients stabilised on warfarin, moderate to large daily doses of vitamin E (800 or 1200 units) for one month caused no clinically relevant changes in prothrombin times and INRs.[2] Similarly, in another study in 12 patients taking warfarin, the anticoagulant effects of warfarin were unchanged by smaller daily doses of 100 or 400 units of vitamin E given for 4 weeks.[3]

However, in one case, a patient taking warfarin (and multiple other drugs) developed ecchymoses and haematuria, which was attributed to him taking 1 200 units of vitamin E daily over a 2-month period. His prothrombin time was found to be 36 seconds. A later study in this patient found that 800 units of vitamin E daily for 6 weeks reduced his blood clotting factor levels, increased the prothrombin time from about 21 seconds to 29 seconds, and caused ecchymoses.[4] In addition, a modest rise in the INR of one patients with *Curbicin* was considered to be possible due to the presence of vitamin E in the *Curbicin* preparation (each tablet contains 10 mg).[5] For further information, see 'Coumarins + *Curbicin*', p.421.

Moreover, in a population cohort study, the concurrent use of vitamin E and warfarin was associated with an increased risk of mortality (adjusted hazard ratio 3.7). The hazard ratio for warfarin alone was 1.6 and for vitamin E alone was 0.91. The findings of this observational data require confirmation.[6]

Mechanism

Not understood. The suggested explanation is that vitamin E interferes with the activity of vitamin K in producing the blood clotting factors,[4,7] and increases in the dietary requirements of vitamin K.[8,9]

Importance and management

Information is limited but the evidence suggests that most patients taking warfarin are unlikely to have changes in coagulation status if given even quite large daily doses (up to 1 200 units) of vitamin E. Nevertheless, the isolated case cited here suggests that occasionally and unpredictably the warfarin effects can be changed. It has been recommended that prothrombin times should be monitored when vitamin E is first given (within one to 2 weeks has been recommended).[2] The same precautions could be applied to dicoumarol as well. However, as only one case of bleeding has been reported this does seem somewhat over-cautious. However, the finding of higher mortality in the observation cohort introduces some caution about the value of vitamin E supplements in patients taking warfarin. This requires further study. Information about other oral anticoagulants is lacking.

1. Schrogie JJ. Coagulopathy and fat-soluble vitamins. *JAMA* (1975) 232, 19.
2. Kim JM, White RH. Effect of vitamin E on the anticoagulant response to warfarin. *Am J Cardiol* (1996) 77, 545–6.
3. Corrigan JJ, Ulfers LL. Effect of vitamin E on prothrombin levels in warfarin-induced vitamin K deficiency. *Am J Clin Nutr* (1981) 34, 1701–5.
4. Corrigan JJ, Marcus FI. Coagulopathy associated with vitamin E ingestion. *JAMA* (1974) 230, 1300–1.
5. Yue, Q-Y, Jansson K. Herbal drug Curbicin and anticoagulant effect with and without warfarin: possibly related to the vitamin E component. *J Am Geriatr Soc* (2001) 49, 838.
6. Hayden KM, Welsh-Bohmer KA, Wengreen HJ, Zandi PP, Lyketsos CG, Breitner JCS, for the Cache County Investigators. Risk of mortality with vitamin E supplements: the Cache County study. *Am J Med* (2007) 120, 180–4.
7. Booth SL, Golly I, Sacheck JM, Roubenoff R, Dallal GE, Hamada K, Blumberg JB. Effect of vitamin E supplementation on vitamin K status in adults with normal coagulation status. *Am J Clin Nutr* (2004) 80, 143–8.
8. Anon. Vitamin K, vitamin E and the coumarin drugs. *Nutr Rev* (1982) 40, 180–2.
9. Anon. Megavitamin E supplementation and vitamin K-dependent carboxylation. *Nutr Rev* (1983) 41, 268–70.

Coumarins and related drugs + Vitamin K substances

The effects of the coumarin and indanedione anticoagulants can be reduced or abolished by vitamin K_1 (phytomenadione). Unintentional and unwanted antagonism can occur in patients unknowingly taking vitamin K_1. There is also a case of antagonism of acenocoumarol in a patient using a proprietary chilblain product containing the vitamin K_4 substance acetomenaphthone.

Clinical evidence

A woman taking **acenocoumarol** had a fall in her British Corrected Ratio to 1.2 (normal range 1.8 to 3) within 2 days of starting to take a non-prescription chilblain preparation (*Gon*) containing **acetomenaphthone** 10 mg per tablet. She took a total of 50 mg of vitamin K_4 over 48 hours.[1]

Mechanism

The coumarin and indanedione oral anticoagulants are vitamin K antagonists, and probably inhibit the enzyme vitamin K epoxide reductase so reducing the synthesis of vitamin K-dependent blood clotting factors by the liver. If the intake of vitamin K_1 increases, the competition swings in favour of the vitamin and the synthesis of the blood clotting factors begins to return to normal. As a result the prothrombin time also begins to fall to its normal value. The role of other vitamin K substances, such as K_4 and K_2, in coagulation is less clear.

Importance and management

The interaction with vitamin K_1 is very well established and clinically important, and is expected to occur with every coumarin and indanedione oral anticoagulant because they have a common mode of action as vitamin K antagonists. Vitamin K treatment is used as an effective antidote for excessive oral anticoagulation. The drug intake and diet of any patient who shows warfarin resistance should be investigated for the possibility of this interaction. It can be accommodated either by increasing the anticoagulant dose, or by reducing the intake of vitamin K_1. For more information on specific situations, see 'Coumarins + Vitamin K_1-containing dietary supplements', below, 'Coumarins and related drugs + Food; Enteral and parenteral nutrition', p.429, and 'Coumarins and related drugs + Food; Vitamin K_1-rich', p.432.

However, the role of other vitamin K substances in coagulation is less clear. The case report with acetomenaphthone, a vitamin K_4 substance suggests that this can also antagonise the effect of vitamin K antagonists. It may be prudent for patients to avoid preparations containing this substance. Similarly, the antagonism of coumarins by fermented soya beans has been attributed to the vitamin K_2 content (see 'Coumarins + Food; Soya bean products', p.431).

1. Heald GE, Poller L. Anticoagulants and treatment for chilblains. *BMJ* (1974) 1, 455.

Coumarins + Vitamin K_1-containing dietary supplements

In patients with normal vitamin K status, multivitamin supplements containing small amounts of vitamin K_1 (phytomenadione) will generally have no clinically important effect on the INR or anticoagulant requirements. Larger doses of vitamin K are likely to require a dose adjustment in a proportion of patients. Conversely, in patients with poor vitamin K status, even low vitamin K doses may have an important effect.

Clinical evidence

In a controlled study in healthy subjects stabilised on individual doses of **acenocoumarol**, the dose of vitamin K_1 tablets required to cause a statistically significant reduction in INR was 150 micrograms daily (INR 1.59 versus 2.04). Each dose of vitamin K_1 was taken daily for a week, and in successive weeks the dose was increased in increments of 50 micrograms from 50 to 300 micrograms daily, then 500 micrograms daily for the final week. The authors noted that their usual clinical criteria requiring an adjustment in **acenocoumarol** dose would have been met in 3 of the 12 subjects at a dose of vitamin K_1 of 150 micrograms daily.[1]

However, in another study in 9 patients stabilised on **warfarin** with low vitamin K levels the median INR dropped by 0.51 requiring a **warfarin** dose increase of 5.3% after they took just one multivitamin tablet containing vitamin K_1 25 micrograms daily for 4 weeks. Conversely, in a control group with normal plasma vitamin K levels, the same multivitamin did not change the INR or warfarin requirement.[2] In a well-controlled study in patients with unstable control of anticoagulation, vitamin K_1 150 micrograms daily increased the **warfarin** requirement by 16% from a mean of 3.8 mg daily to 4.4 mg daily, but also improved stability of control.[3]

In another study in patients taking **phenprocoumon**, supplementation with vitamin K_1 50 micrograms daily for 3 weeks had little effect on the INR, and required just a 3% increase in **phenprocoumon** dose. A higher dose of vitamin K_1 of 100 micrograms daily resulted in a mean dose increase of 9%. On stopping the supplements, a mean 7% decrease in dose was needed. However, there was wide variation between patients.[4]

A patient who required **warfarin** 15 to 17.5 mg daily to maintain an INR of about 3 was found to be taking vitamin K (dose not stated) as part of a vitamin supplement. When he stopped taking the vitamin K, his **warfarin** dose requirement decreased to between 10.5 and 12.5 mg daily.[5] In another report, a woman required an increase in her **warfarin** dose from 45 mg to 60 mg weekly when she started taking a daily multivitamin containing vitamin K_1 25 micrograms (*Centrum Plus*). Two weeks after stopping the multivitamin, she had haematuria and flank pain and was found to have a haematoma of the kidney and an INR of 13.2. A second patient had an acute occlusion of an aorto-bifemoral graft, requiring emergency surgery, 4 weeks after starting *Centrum Plus*. His INR had fallen from a mean of 2.48 to 1.1. A third patient had a fall in INR from a mean of 2.54 to 1.65 after taking *Centrum Plus* for 2 weeks. It was suggested that all three patients had low levels of vitamin K.[6] Similarly, an 89-year-old woman admitted to hospital with an INR of 2 while taking 30 mg warfarin weekly, was commenced on a daily multivitamin containing vitamin K_1 36 micrograms (*Centrum*). Over the following 3 days her INR fell from 1.5 to 1.1, despite an increase in her warfarin dose (not stated). The *Centrum* was stopped and her INR rose to 2.5 over the following 3 days. The patient's vitamin K status was not defined, but she was described as having a reduced appetite resulting in a recent 4 kg weight loss.[7]

A further case report describes a 64-year-old man taking warfarin and vitamin K_1 at a dose of 100 micrograms daily to decrease INR variability. He was stabilised on warfarin 6.5 to 7.5 mg weekly and the vitamin K_1 supplement for 9 months, with a mean INR of 2.02. After discontinuing his vitamin K_1 for one week, his INR was 1.5 and he denied any missed doses of warfarin. The vitamin K_1 was discontinued and his warfarin dose increased to 8 mg weekly. Two weeks later, the patients INR had risen to 8.5 with no acute bleeding and he reported no changes medication or diet. A 2.5 mg dose of vitamin K_1 was given and warfarin was withheld for 2 days, after which his INR decreased to 2.9. Vitamin K_1 supplementation was restarted and warfarin was also restarted, at a dose of 7 mg weekly. Subsequently his INR remained relatively stable.[8]

Mechanism

Vitamin K_1 reduces the effect of vitamin K-antagonists (coumarins and **indanediones**). The dose of vitamin K_1 at which this becomes clinically important appears to depend on the vitamin K status of the individual.

Importance and management

The data from the controlled studies suggest that taking multivitamin supplements containing 10 to 50 micrograms of vitamin K_1 is probably acceptable in most patients taking coumarins or indanediones, and is likely to require no change or only small changes to the anticoagulant dose. However, in patients with poor vitamin K status, even these low levels of vitamin K may be sufficient to antagonise the effect of the anticoagulant. Note that a review of selected US supplements found that they contained 10 to 80 micrograms of vitamin K_1. Therefore, patients should be advised to *not* take a multivitamin preparation containing vitamin K_1 (phytomenadione) without increased monitoring when starting or stopping treatment. Because of this, and because of the increasing recognition of the importance of vitamin K in bone health, some consider that patients taking anticoagulants should be advised to consume sufficient vitamin K to meet the recommended adequate intakes.[9] Consider also *Importance and management* under 'Coumarins and related drugs + Food; Vitamin K_1-rich', p.432. Others have even suggested that a low and steady vitamin K supplement can reduce the risk of excessive anticoagulation without altering efficacy.[3,10] Note also, that vitamin K_1 supplementation can be used therapeutically as an adjunct to warfarin in patients with unstable anticoagulation.

1. Schurgers LJ, Shearer MJ, Hamulyák K, Stöcklin E, Vermeer C. Effect of vitamin K intake on the stability of oral anticoagulant treatment: dose-response relationships in healthy subjects. *Blood* (2004) 104, 2682–9.
2. Kurnik D, Loebstein R, Rabinovitz H, Austerweil N, Halkin H, Almog S. Over-the-counter vitamin K_1-containing multivitamin supplements disrupt warfarin anticoagulation in vitamin K_1-depleted patients. A prospective, controlled trial. *Thromb Haemost* (2004) 92, 1018–24.
3. Sconce E, Avery P, Wynne H, Kamali F. Vitamin K supplementation can improve stability of anticoagulation for patients with unexplained variability in response to warfarin. *Blood* (2007) 109, 2419–23.
4. Rombouts EK, Rosendaal FR, van der Meer FJM. The effect of vitamin K supplementation on anticoagulant treatment. *J Thromb Haemost* (2006) 4, 691–2.
5. Eliason BC, Larson W. Acetaminophen and risk factors for excess anticoagulation with warfarin. *JAMA* (1998) 280, 696–7.
6. Kurnik D, Lubetsky A, Almog S, Halkin H. Multivitamin supplements may affect warfarin anticoagulation in susceptible patients. *Ann Pharmacother* (2003) 37, 1603–6.
7. Ducharlet KN, Katz B, Leung S. Multivitamin supplement interaction with warfarin therapy. *Australas J Ageing* (2011) 30, 41–2.
8. Miesner AR, Sullivan TS. Elevated international normalized ratio from vitamin K supplement discontinuation. *Ann Pharmacother* (2011) 45, e2.
9. Johnson MA. Influence of vitamin K on anticoagulant therapy depends on vitamin K status and the source and chemical forms of vitamin K. Nutr Rev 2003; 63, 91–7
10. Oldenburg J. Vitamin K intake and stability of oral anticoagulant treatment. *Thromb Haemost* (2005) 93, 799–800.

Coumarins + Vitamin K_1-rich herbal medicines

A man had a modest rise in his INR after stopping taking a herbal nutritional supplement (*Nature's Life Greens*), which contained a number of plants known to be high in vitamin K_1. Another patient had a subtherapeutic INR after starting to drink a plant extract juice (called *Noni Juice*).

Clinical evidence, mechanism, importance and management

(a) Nature's Life Greens

A 72-year-old man stabilised on **warfarin** was found to have an INR of 4.43 at a routine clinic visit, which was increased from 3.07 six weeks previously. The patient had stopped taking a herbal product *Nature's Life Greens* that month because he did not have enough money to buy it. He had been taking it for the past 7 years as a vitamin supplement because he had previously been instructed to limit his intake of green leafy vegetables. He was eventually restabilised on **warfarin** and the same nutritional product.

The product label listed 25 vegetables without stating the amounts or concentrations,[1] but at least 5 of the listed ingredients are known to contain high levels of vitamin K_1 including **parsley**, **green tea leaves**, spinach, broccoli, and cabbage (see also 'Coumarins and related drugs + Food; Vitamin K_1-rich', p.432). It is therefore likely it contained sufficient vitamin K to antagonise the effect of the **warfarin** so that when it was stopped the warfarin requirements fell, and without an appropriate adjustment in dose, this resulted in an increased INR.

This case reinforces the view that all patients taking **warfarin** should seek advice when they want to stop or start any herbal medicine or nutritional supplement.

(b) Plant juices

A 41-year-old woman stabilised on **warfarin** was found to have an INR of 1.6 at a routine clinic visit. The only possible cause identified was that the patient had begun to drink one to two small glasses daily of *Noni Juice 4 Everything.* This was identified as a brown liquid that contains extracts and derivates from more than 115 components. The authors noted that many of the listed plants contained vitamin K and that vitamin K was listed as a separate component, indicating that the juice might have been fortified with vitamin K. The patient was given heparin and then discharged on her previous dose of **warfarin**, and advised to stop taking this brand of juice.[2]

The authors concluded that this case reinforces the view that all patients taking **warfarin** should seek advice when they want to stop or start any herbal medicine or nutritional supplement.

1. Bransgrove LL. Interaction between warfarin and a vitamin K-containing nutritional supplement: a case report. *J Herb Pharmacother* (2001) 1, 85–89.
2. Carr ME, Klotz J, Bergeron M. Coumadin resistance and the vitamin supplement "Noni". *Am J Hematol* (2004) 77, 103–4.

Coumarins + Zileuton

Zileuton slightly increases the anticoagulant effects of warfarin and slightly increases *R*-warfarin levels.

Clinical evidence

In a placebo-controlled study, zileuton 600 mg every 6 hours for 6 days or placebo was given to healthy subjects who had been stabilised on racemic **warfarin** to achieve prothrombin times of 14 to 18 seconds for one week. The zileuton had no effect on the pharmacokinetics of *S*-warfarin, but the *R*-warfarin AUC rose by 22%, and its clearance fell by 15%. The mean prothrombin times increased by 2.3 seconds (morning) and 2 seconds (evening) in the zileuton group. The corresponding increases in the placebo group were 0.7 and 0.2 seconds, respectively.[1]

Mechanism

It seems likely that zileuton inhibits the metabolism of *R*-warfarin, probably by the cytochrome P450 isoenzyme CYP1A2.[2]

Importance and management

Information seems to be limited to this study, but the pharmacokinetic interaction appears to be established. The clinical significance of a 2 second rise in prothrombin times is unclear, but it seems likely to be small. The lack of any published reports of problems with the combination would tend to support this.

1. Awni WM, Hussein Z, Granneman GR, Patterson KJ, Dube LM, Cavanaugh JH. Pharmacodynamic and stereoselective pharmacokinetic interactions between zileuton and warfarin in humans. *Clin Pharmacokinet* (1995) 29 (Suppl 2), 67–76.
2. Lu P, Schrag ML, Slaughter DE, Raab CE, Shou M, Rodrigues AD. Mechanism-based inhibition of human liver microsomal cytochrome P450 1A2 by zileuton, a 5-lipoxygenase inhibitor. *Drug Metab Dispos* (2003) 31, 1352–60.

Drotrecogin alfa + Other drugs that affect coagulation

The concurrent use of drotrecogin alfa and prophylactic doses of heparin causes a slight increased risk of non-serious bleeding. The manufacturers of drotrecogin alfa caution its use in patients taking or who have recently received therapeutic doses of heparin, hirudins, oral anticoagulants, antiplatelet drugs, NSAIDs, prostacyclins, and thrombolytics.

Clinical evidence, mechanism, importance and management

(a) Heparins

Heparins are frequently used for prophylaxis of venous thromboembolic events in patients with severe sepsis. Because drotrecogin alfa increases the risk of bleeding, there has been concern that its use with heparin would further increase bleeding risk. Nevertheless, in phase III studies of drotrecogin alfa, two-thirds of patients received prophylactic doses of heparin or low-molecular-weight heparin with no observed increase in the risk of serious bleeding events reported.[1,2] Moreover, in a more recent study in patients treated with drotrecogin and randomised to receive prophylactic heparins or placebo, no increased risk of serious bleeding or adverse effects was found.[3] Except for a slight increase in any bleeding event in the first 6 days (10.8% heparin, 8.1% placebo), there was no difference in serious bleeding events, central nervous system bleeding events, or fatal bleeds on concurrent use. The US manufacturer notes that, in this study, the clearance and steady-state level of drotrecogin alfa (24 micrograms/kg per hour for 96 hours) was not affected by prophylactic **enoxaparin** 40 mg every 24 hours, or **unfractionated sodium heparin** 5000 units every 12 hours (although this was not evaluated when heparin 5000 units was given every 8 hours).[4] It therefore appears that low-dose heparin may be given for the prophylaxis of venous thromboembolic events concurrently with drotrecogin alfa. No dose adjustments are required.[1]

There appear to be little data on using drotrecogin alfa with therapeutic doses of heparin. The US manufacturer states that the increased risk of bleeding should be carefully considered when deciding to use drotrecogin alfa with therapeutic doses of heparin for treating an active thromboembolic event.[4] In the UK, the manufacturers specifically contraindicate use with heparin at doses of 15 units/kg per hour or more.[1]

(b) Other drugs affecting coagulation

Because of the possible increased risk of bleeding, the manufacturers state that the risks of giving drotrecogin alfa should be weighed against the benefits in patients who have received **thrombolytics** within 3 days, **oral anticoagulants** within 7 days, or **aspirin** (US information specifies greater than 650 mg daily) or other **antiplatelet drugs** within 7 days.[1,4] Caution should be used when prescribing these drugs and other drugs that affect haemostasis, such as the **hirudins**, **prostacyclins** such as **iloprost**, and other drugs that adversely affect platelet function such as **NSAIDs**, in patients given drotrecogin alfa.[1]

1. Xigris (Drotrecogin alfa). Eli Lilly and Company Ltd. UK Summary of product characteristics, December 2008.
2. Meshaka P. Question de l'agence européenne du médicament (EMEA): interaction drotrécogine alfa (activée) et héparine à dose prophylactique. *Ann Fr Anesth Reanim* (2003) 22, 23–7.
3. Levi M, Levy M, Williams MD, Douglas I, Artigas A, Antonelli M, Wyncoll D, Janes J, Booth FV, Wang D, Sundin DP, Macias WL for the Xigris and Prophylactic HepaRin Evaluation in Severe Sepsis (XPRESS) Study Group. Prophylactic heparin in patients with severe sepsis treated with drotrecogin alfa (activated). *Am J Respir Crit Care Med* (2007) 176, 483–90.
4. Xigris (Drotrecogin alfa). Eli Lilly and Company. US Prescribing information, October 2008.

Fondaparinux + Antiplatelet drugs or NSAIDs

Neither aspirin nor piroxicam appear to alter the pharmacokinetics of fondaparinux, and no significant change in bleeding time has been reported with concurrent use. However, concurrent use may be expected to increase the risk of bleeding.

Clinical evidence

In a study in 16 healthy subjects, a single 975-mg dose of **aspirin** given on day 4 of an 8-day course of subcutaneous fondaparinux 10 mg daily had no effect on fondaparinux pharmacokinetics. The increase in bleeding time with fondaparinux and **aspirin** was greater than with **aspirin** alone, but this was not statistically significant. **Aspirin** had no effect on the small prolongation of aPTT seen with fondaparinux.[1]

In another study, **piroxicam** 20 mg daily for 10 days was given to 12 healthy subjects with fondaparinux 10 mg daily starting on day 7. Both drugs were also given alone. **Piroxicam** had no effect on fondaparinux pharmacokinetics, and had no effect on the small prolongation of aPTT seen with fondaparinux. There was no difference in bleeding time between the treatments.[1]

Mechanism

Fondaparinux commonly causes bleeding as a consequence of its action.[2] As antiplatelet drugs and NSAIDs also increase the risk of bleeding, the risk and severity of bleeding is likely to be increased with the combination.

Importance and management

The pharmacological studies described show that the pharmacokinetics of fondaparinux are not changed by aspirin and piroxicam, and that there is only a minor increase in bleeding time. Nevertheless, the manufacturers of fondaparinux say that antiplatelet drugs (**aspirin, dipyridamole, sulfinpyrazone, ticlopidine** or **clopidogrel**) and NSAIDs should be used with caution because of the possible increased risk of haemorrhage. They recommend that if concurrent use is essential, close monitoring is necessary.[2,3] This is considered particularly important in patients undergoing peridural or spinal anaesthesia or spinal puncture, in whom antiplatelet drugs, NSAIDs and fondaparinux are possible risk factors for epidural or spinal haematoma resulting in prolonged or permanent paralysis.[2,3]

1. Ollier C, Faaij RA, Santoni A, Duvauchelle T, van Haard PMM, Schoemaker RC, Cohen AF, de Greef R, Burggraaf J. Absence of interaction of fondaparinux sodium with aspirin and piroxicam in healthy male volunteers. *Clin Pharmacokinet* (2002) 41 (Suppl 2), 31–37.
2. Arixtra (Fondaparinux sodium). GlaxoSmithKline UK. UK Summary of product characteristics, March 2009.
3. Arixtra (Fondaparinux sodium). GlaxoSmithKline. US Prescribing information, October 2009.

Fondaparinux + Miscellaneous

In the UK, the manufacturer of fondaparinux recommends avoiding other drugs that may enhance the risk of haemorrhage. They specifically name, desirudin, fibrinolytics, glycoprotein IIb/IIIa-receptor antagonists, heparin, heparinoids and low-molecular-weight heparins.[1] Similarly, in the US, the manufacturer states that drugs that may enhance the risk of haemorrhage should be discontinued before starting fondaparinux. They say that if concurrent use is essential, close monitoring may be appropriate.[2] See also 'Coumarins + Fondaparinux', p.429, and 'Fondaparinux + Antiplatelet drugs or NSAIDs', above.

1. Arixtra (Fondaparinux sodium). GlaxoSmithKline UK. UK Summary of product characteristics, March 2009.
2. Arixtra (Fondaparinux sodium). GlaxoSmithKline. US Prescribing information, October 2009.

Heparin or LMWHs + Antiplatelet drugs; Aspirin

The concurrent use of aspirin with heparin or low-molecular-weight heparins slightly increases the risk of haemorrhage. Concurrent use may be a contributing factor to the very rare complication of epidural or spinal haematoma occurring after epidural anaesthesia.

Clinical evidence

(a) Heparin

Eight out of 12 patients with hip fractures developed serious bleeding when they were given heparin 5 000 units subcutaneously every 12 hours and aspirin 600 mg twice daily as perioperative prophylaxis for deep vein thrombosis. Haematomas of the hip and thigh occurred in 3 patients, bleeding through the wound in 4, and uterine bleeding in the other patient.[1] In a large, randomised, placebo-controlled study, aspirin 500 mg three times daily, subcutaneous heparin 5000 units twice daily, or the combination were compared for prophylaxis of deep vein thrombosis in 1 210 patients undergoing surgery. Haemorrhage severe enough to discontinue the prophylaxis occurred in significantly more patients in the combination group (11 of 402 patients versus 3 of 404 patients in the heparin and aspirin alone groups). In addition, minor haemorrhage occurred more frequently in the combination group (89 patients) compared with aspirin alone (41 patients) or heparin alone (30 patients).[2] In another randomised study in patients with acute unstable angina, the combination of aspirin 325 mg twice daily and an intravenous infusion of heparin 1 000 units/hour resulted in slightly greater incidence of serious bleeding than either drug alone (3.3% for concurrent use versus 1.7% for either drug alone).[3]

In an epidemiological study of hospitalised patients receiving heparin, the incidence of bleeding was almost 2.4 times higher in 302 patients also receiving aspirin than in 2354 patients not given aspirin (doses not stated). Surgical patients were excluded from this analysis, as were patients with a discharge diagnosis of cancer or haematological disease.[4]

(b) LMWHs

In a crossover study in 9 healthy subjects, the bleeding time was prolonged by the use of aspirin 300 mg daily and subcutaneous **reviparin** 6 300 units daily, when compared with either drug alone (9.6 minutes versus 5.5 minutes and 5 minutes, respectively). However, the affect of aspirin on platelet aggregation and the effect of **reviparin** on aPTT were not altered by concurrent use.[5] However, in a clinical study in patients undergoing surgery for total hip or knee replacement, there was no difference in risk of bleeding or other bleeding-related parameters (total blood loss, need for transfusion, mean change in haemoglobin levels) between patients receiving **enoxaparin** and aspirin (51 patients) and those receiving **enoxaparin** and no aspirin (394 patients). Aspirin use was low-dose (up to 500 mg daily).[6] In addition, in an analysis of risk factors for bleeding in patients receiving **enoxaparin** for treating acute coronary syndrome, the use of aspirin was not associated with an increased risk of any bleeding.[7]

During a 5-year period in one hospital, 3 elderly patients had presented with sudden severe abdominal pain after coughing, which was found to be due to a rectus muscle sheath haematoma. These patients had been receiving subcutaneous **enoxaparin** 40 mg daily for an average of 6 days with aspirin 100 mg daily.[8] Other cases of retroperitoneal haematoma have been reported with **enoxaparin** in which aspirin may have been one of various contributing factors.[9-12] Similarly, the use of aspirin may have been one of a number of contributing factors in a case of spinal epidural haematoma occurring with **enoxaparin.**[13]

Mechanism

Aspirin inhibits platelet aggregation and prolongs bleeding times, and increases the risk of upper gastrointestinal haemorrhage, even at doses of 300 mg daily and less.[14] This risk is likely to be higher in patients also taking anticoagulants. See also 'Coumarins and related drugs + Aspirin or other Salicylates', p.405.

Importance and management

The concurrent use of heparin or LMWHs with aspirin is indicated in specific situations such as the prophylaxis of ischaemic complications of unstable angina.[15] However, unless specifically indicated, it may be prudent to avoid the concurrent use of aspirin with these drugs, because of the likely increased risk of bleeding. If they are used together, some caution and consideration of increased monitoring would seem appropriate.

Heparin and some LMWHs have rarely caused epidural or spinal haematomas resulting in long-term or permanent paralysis when used for thromboprophylaxis in procedures involving spinal/epidural anaesthesia or spinal puncture. The risk of this may be increased if they are used concurrently with other drugs affecting haemostasis such as aspirin, and extreme caution is needed if concurrent use is considered appropriate in these situations.

1. Yett HS, Skillman JJ, Salzman EW. The hazards of aspirin plus heparin. *N Engl J Med* (1978) 298, 1092.
2. Vinazzer H, Loew D, Simma W, Brücke P. Prophylaxis of postoperative thromboembolism by low dose heparin and by acetylsalicylic acid given simultaneously. A double-blind study. *Thromb Res* (1980) 17, 177–84.
3. Théroux P, Ouimet H, McCans J, Latour J-G, Joly P, Lévy G, Pelletier E, Juneau M, Stasiak J, deGuise P, Pelletier GB, Rinzler D, Waters DD. Aspirin, heparin, or both to treat acute unstable angina. *N Engl J Med* (1988) 319, 1105–11.
4. Walker AM, Jick H. Predictors of bleeding during heparin therapy. *JAMA* (1980) 244, 1209–12.
5. Klinkhardt U, Breddin HK, Esslinger HU, Haas S, Kalatzis A, Harder S. Interaction between the LMWH reviparin and aspirin in healthy volunteers. *Br J Clin Pharmacol* (2000) 49, 337–41.
6. Dahl OE, Ögren M, Agnelli G, Eriksson BI, Cohen AT, Mouret P, Rosencher N, Bylock A, Panfilov S, Andersson M. Assessment of bleeding after concomitant administration of antiplatelet and anticoagulant agents in lower limb arthroplasty. *Pathophysiol Haemost Thromb* (2006) 35, 428–34.
7. Macie C, Forbes L, Foster GA, Douketis JD. Dosing practices and risk factors for bleeding in patients receiving enoxaparin for the treatment of an acute coronary syndrome. *Chest* (2004) 125, 1616–21.
8. Macías-Robles MD, Peliz MG, Gonzalez-Ordonez AJ. Prophylaxis with enoxaparin can produce a giant abdominal wall haematoma when associated with low doses of aspirin among elderly patients suffering cough attacks. *Blood Coag Fibrinol* (2005) 16, 217–19.
9. Melde SL. Enoxaparin-induced retroperitoneal hematoma. *Ann Pharmacother* (2003) 37, 822–4.
10. Kavanagh D, Hill ADK, Martin S, Power C, McDermott EW, O'Higgins N, Murphy K. Life threatening haemorrhagic events associated with the administration of low-molecular-weight-heparin. *Thromb Haemost* (2004) 91, 833–4.
11. Malik A, Capling R, Bastani B. Enoxaparin-associated retroperitoneal bleeding in two patients with renal insufficiency. *Pharmacotherapy* (2005) 25, 769–72.
12. Ernits M, Mohan PS, Fares LG, Hardy H. A retroperitoneal bleed induced by enoxaparin therapy. *Am Surg* (2005) 71, 430–3.
13. Chan L, Bailin MT. Spinal epidural hematoma following central neuraxial blockade and subcutaneous enoxaparin: a case report. *J Clin Anesth* (2004) 16, 382–5.

14. Weil J, Colin-Jones D, Langman M, Lawson D, Logan R, Murphy M, Rawlins M, Vessey M, Wainwright P. Prophylactic aspirin and risk of peptic ulcer bleeding. *BMJ* (1995) 310: 827–30.
15. Harrington RA, Becker RC, Cannon CP, Gutterman D, Lincoff AM, Popma JJ, Steg G, Guyatt GH, Goodman SG; American College of Chest Physicians. Antithrombotic therapy for non-ST-segment elevation acute coronary syndromes: American College of Chest Physicians Evidence-Based Clinical Practice Guidelines (8th Edition). *Chest* (2008) 133 (6 Suppl), 670S–707S.

Heparin or LMWHs + Antiplatelet drugs; Miscellaneous

The dose of heparin does not need adjusting when clopidogrel is also given. The antiplatelet effects of clopidogrel and ticagrelor are not altered by heparin. Nevertheless, the concurrent use of heparin or low-molecular-weight heparins with antiplatelet drugs increases the risk of bleeding.

Clinical evidence

(a) Clopidogrel

In a placebo-controlled study in 12 healthy subjects, the dose of heparin given over 4 days did not need modification when clopidogrel 75 mg daily was also given, and the inhibitory effects of clopidogrel on platelet aggregation were unchanged by concurrent use.[1] Moreover, the manufacturers of clopidogrel note that in various large clinical studies in patients with acute coronary syndrome or myocardial infarction, most patients received heparin or LMWHs without an obvious difference in the rate of bleeding or the incidence of major bleeding.[2,3] Nevertheless, in an analysis of risk factors for bleeding in 208 patients receiving **enoxaparin** for acute coronary syndrome, the use of clopidogrel was associated with an increased risk of any bleeding (odds ratio 2.49).[4]

In one case the use of **enoxaparin** with clopidogrel was considered to be a contributing factor in a case of spinal epidural haematoma occurring after spinal anaesthesia.[5] Another similar case occurred in a patient taking clopidogrel and given **dalteparin**,[6] and serious retroperitoneal bleeding occurred in a patient with acute coronary syndrome receiving **enoxaparin**, clopidogrel and aspirin.[7]

(b) Prasugrel

The manufacturer reports that heparin, given as a single intravenous bolus of 100 units/kg, had no significant effect on the antiplatelet effect of prasugrel. They also report that no clinically significant interaction was reported with the use of prasugrel and LMWHs in phase III clinical studies. However, they advise that concurrent use might increase the risk of bleeding.[8]

(c) Ticagrelor

The UK manufacturer of ticagrelor states that in the PLATO study, ticagrelor was given with heparin or LMWHs without and evidence of clinically significant adverse interactions. Additionally, they state that in clinical interaction studies, neither heparin nor enoxaparin had an effect on the pharmacokinetics of ticagrelor or its active metabolite. However, they advise that concurrent use might increase the risk of bleeding.[9]

(d) Ticlopidine

The manufacturer of ticlopidine notes that it has been used concurrently with heparin for about 12 hours in studies of cardiac stenting, but that longer-term safety has not been established.[10]

Mechanism

Antiplatelet drugs increase the risk of bleeding, and the risk is likely to be increased further in patients who are anticoagulated with heparin or LMWHs.

Importance and management

The concurrent use of heparin or LMWHs with antiplatelet drugs such as clopidogrel is indicated in specific conditions such as acute coronary syndrome. However, unless specifically indicated, the concurrent use of heparin or LMWHs with antiplatelet drugs should probably be avoided because of the likely increase in haemorrhagic risk. If they are used together, the manufacturers of the LMWHs (**bemiparin**, dalteparin, enoxaparin, **tinzaparin**) recommend caution or careful clinical and laboratory monitoring.

Heparin and some LMWHs have rarely caused epidural or spinal haematomas resulting in long-term or permanent paralysis when used for thromboprophylaxis in procedures involving spinal/epidural anaesthesia or spinal puncture. The risk of this might be increased if they are used concurrently with other drugs affecting haemostasis such as antiplatelet drugs, and extreme caution is needed if concurrent use is considered appropriate in these situations.

Consider also 'Heparin or LMWHs + Antiplatelet drugs; Aspirin', p.486, and 'Glycoprotein IIb/IIIa-receptor antagonists + Miscellaneous', p.797.

1. Caplain H, D'Honneur G, Cariou R. Prolonged heparin administration during clopidogrel treatment in healthy subjects. *Semin Thromb Hemost* (1999) 25 (Suppl 2), 61–4.
2. Plavix (Clopidogrel hydrogen sulphate). Sanofi-aventis. UK Summary of product characteristics, January 2014.
3. Plavix (Clopidogrel bisulfate). Bristol-Myers Squibb/Sanofi Pharmaceuticals Partnership. US Prescribing information, December 2011.
4. Macie C, Forbes L, Foster GA, Douketis JD. Dosing practices and risk factors for bleeding in patients receiving enoxaparin for the treatment of an acute coronary syndrome. *Chest* (2004) 125, 1616–21.
5. Litz RJ, Gottschlich B, Stehr SN. Spinal epidural hematoma after spinal anesthesia in a patient treated with clopidogrel and enoxaparin. *Anesthesiology* (2004) 101, 1467–70.
6. Tam NLK, Pac-Soo C, Pretorius PM. Epidural haematoma after a combined spinal-epidural anaesthetic in a patient treated with clopidogrel and dalteparin. *Br J Anaesth* (2006) 96, 262–5.
7. Ernits M, Mohan PS, Fares LG, Hardy H. A retroperitoneal bleed induced by enoxaparin therapy. *Am Surg* (2005) 71, 430–3.
8. Efient (Prasugrel hydrochloride). Eli Lilly and Company Ltd. UK Summary of product characteristics, December 2013.
9. Brilique (Ticagrelor). AstraZeneca UK Ltd. UK Summary of product characteristics, July 2015.
10. Ticlid (Ticlopidine hydrochloride). Roche Laboratories Inc. US Prescribing information, March 2001.

Heparin + Antibacterials; Cephalosporins

Although a number of cephalosporins have been associated with an increased risk of bleeding, in one study cefamandole did not appear to increase the anticoagulant effects of prophylactic doses of heparin.

Clinical evidence

In a randomised study of 24 patients undergoing hip replacement with prophylactic heparin, prolongation of prothrombin time, partial thromboplastin time, thrombin clotting time, platelet count, or bleeding time were no different when patients given cefamandole were compared with patients given oxacillin and gentamicin, and both groups of patients had similar changes in coagulation parameters to those seen in another group of patients given heparin alone,[1] implying that cefamandole did not affect the response to heparin.

In this study patients were given subcutaneous heparin 5 000 units every 12 hours, with intravenous antibacterial prophylaxis for 3 days, with either cefamandole 2 g three times daily, or the combination of oxacillin 1 g four times daily and gentamicin 80 mg three times daily.

Mechanism

For further information regarding the effects of cephalosporins on coagulation see 'Coumarins and related drugs + Antibacterials; Cephalosporins and related drugs', p.385.

Importance and management

A number of cephalosporins can affect coagulation parameters and the study cited was designed to assess if these effects altered the response to heparin. Although the study found no effect on coagulation parameters, it is possible that adverse effects are rare, and the study was not large enough to detect the occasional patient who might experience such a reaction. Indeed, most of the data regarding an adverse effect on the INR in patients taking a cephalosporin and warfarin comes from case studies. The evidence is insufficient to either recommend monitoring for all patients or to exclude the possibility of an interaction; however, with anticoagulant doses of heparin it seems likely that routine monitoring would be adequate to detect any adverse reaction.

Further details about the cephalosporins that might affect bleeding, and situations where patients might be more at risk of developing an interaction, are given under *Importance and Management* in 'Coumarins and related drugs + Antibacterials; Cephalosporins and related drugs', p.385.

1. Agnelli G, Guerciolini R, Boldrini F, Tonzani A, Della Torre P, Nenci GG, del Favero A. Effects of cefamandole on hemostasis in patients undergoing hip replacement with heparin prophylaxis. *Chemioterapia* (1988) 7, 396–9.

Heparin + Aprotinin

The activated clotting time (ACT) may not be a reliable method to monitor heparin when aprotinin is used concurrently. This is because aprotinin increases the ACT monitored by some methods, without actually increasing anticoagulation.

Clinical evidence, mechanism, importance and management

Aprotinin prolongs the activated clotting time (ACT) as measured by a celite surface activation method, although the kaolin ACT is much less affected.[1] Therefore, if the ACT is used to monitor the effectiveness of heparin anticoagulation during cardiopulmonary bypass incorporating aprotinin, this may lead to an overestimation of the degree of anticoagulation. This may result in patients not receiving additional necessary heparin during extended extracorporeal circulation, or receiving excess protamine to reverse the effects of heparin at the end of the procedure. The UK manufacturer of aprotinin noted that it is not necessary to adjust the usual regimen of heparin and protamine used in cardiopulmonary bypass procedures when aprotinin is also used.[2] The US manufacturer provided additional detailed information on appropriate methods to monitor heparin anticoagulation in the presence of aprotinin.[1] Note that aprotinin has generally been withdrawn because of a possible increased risk of death when it is used in cardiac surgery.

1. Trasylol (Aprotinin). Bayer HealthCare. US Prescribing information, December 2003.
2. Trasylol (Aprotinin). Bayer plc. UK Summary of product characteristics, September 2006.

Heparin + Dextrans

The concurrent use of heparin and dextrans can further prolong clotting time and increase the risk of bleeding.

Clinical evidence, mechanism, importance and management

A study in 9 patients with peripheral vascular disease given 500 mL of dextran found that the mean clotting time one hour after an infusion of 10 000 units of heparin was increased from 36 minutes to 69 minutes. Dextran alone had no effect, but the mean clotting time after 5000 units of heparin with dextran was almost the same as after 10 000 units of heparin alone.[1,2] This study would seem to support two other reports[3,4] of an increase in the incidence of bleeding in those given both heparin and dextran 70. Uneventful concurrent use[5,6] has been described with dextran 40.

Note that these findings are probably of little clinical significance if these drugs are given for their anticoagulant effects; however, increased anticoagulation may be undesirable if dextrans are used as volume expanders in patients already receiving heparin. In this situation some caution is warranted.

1. Atik M. Potentiation of heparin by dextran and its clinical implication. *Thromb Haemost* (1977) 38, 275.
2. Atik M. Personal communication, April 1980.
3. Bloom WL, Brewer SS. The independent yet synergistic effects of heparin and dextran. *Acta Chir Scand* (1968) 387 (Suppl), 53–7.
4. Morrison ND, Stephenson CBS, Maclean D, Stanhope JM. Deep vein thrombosis after femoropopliteal bypass grafting with observations on the incidence of complications following the use of dextran 70. *N Z Med J* (1976) 84, 233–6.
5. Schöndorf TH, Weber U. Prevention of deep vein thrombosis in orthopedic surgery with the combination of low dose heparin plus either dihydroergotamine or dextran. *Scand J Haematol* (1980) 36 (Suppl), 126–40.
6. Serjeant JCB. Mesenteric embolus treated with low-molecular weight dextran. *Lancet* (1965) i, 139–40.

Heparin + LMWHs; Enoxaparin

There is some evidence that patients receiving enoxaparin preoperatively require more heparin during surgery.

Clinical evidence, mechanism, importance and management

In a clinical study, 30 patients with unstable coronary disease treated preoperatively with enoxaparin needed more heparin to maintain an activated clotting time above 480 seconds during surgery than 31 stable control patients not treated with enoxaparin. In addition, the enoxaparin recipients had higher heparin levels and lower antithrombin values compared with control patients. All patients were taking low-dose aspirin until the day before surgery, and received tranexamic acid as a bolus dose before cardiopulmonary bypass.[1]

The reasons for these differences are unclear, and their clinical relevance is uncertain. Further study is needed.

1. Pleym H, Videm V, Wahba A, Åsberg A, Amundsen T, Bjella L, Dale O, Stenseth R. Heparin resistance and increased platelet activation in coronary surgery patients treated with enoxaparin preoperatively. *Eur J Cardiothorac Surg* (2006) 29, 933–40.

Heparin + Miscellaneous

Changes in the protein binding of diazepam, propranolol, quinidine and verapamil caused by heparin do not appear to be of clinical importance.

Clinical evidence, mechanism, importance and management

A number of studies have found that heparin reduces the plasma protein binding of several drugs including **diazepam**,[1,2] **propranolol**,[1] **quinidine**[3] and **verapamil**[4] in man and in *animals*. For example, 3 patients taking oral **propranolol** and 5 patients given intramuscular **diazepam** 10 mg were given 3000 units of heparin just before cardiac catheterisation. Five minutes after the heparin was given, the free fraction of **diazepam** was found to have risen fourfold (from 1.8 to 7.9%) while the free **diazepam** levels had similarly risen (from 2 to 8.4 nanograms/mL). The free fraction of the **propranolol** rose from 7.4% to 12.5% and the free levels rose from 1.7 nanograms/mL to 2.7 nanograms/mL.[1]

It was suggested that these changes occur because heparin displaces these drugs from their binding sites on the plasma albumin and that these changes in protein binding might possibly have some clinical consequences. For example, there could, theoretically, be sudden increases in sedation or respiratory depression because of the rapid increase in the active (free) fraction of **diazepam**.

However, these changes are unlikely to be of clinical importance (see 'Protein-binding interactions', p.3). One study even suggested that the heparin-induced protein binding changes are an artefact of the study methods used,[5] and this would seem to be supported by an experimental study, which found that heparin did not have any effect on the beta-blockade caused by **propranolol**.[6] Moreover, there seem to be no other reports confirming that these interactions are of real clinical importance. No special precautions would seem to be necessary.

1. Wood AJJ, Robertson D, Robertson RM, Wilkinson GR, Wood M. Elevated plasma free drug concentrations of propranolol and diazepam during cardiac catheterization. *Circulation* (1980) 62, 1119–22.
2. Routledge PA, Kitchell BB, Bjornsson TD, Skinnner T, Linnoila M, Shand DG. Diazepam and N-desmethyldiazepam redistribution after heparin. *Clin Pharmacol Ther* (1980) 27, 528–32.
3. Kessler KM, Leech RC, Spann JF. Blood collection techniques, heparin and quinidine protein binding. *Clin Pharmacol Ther* (1979) 25, 204–10.
4. Keefe DL, Yee Y-G, Kates RE. Verapamil protein binding in patients and normal subjects. *Clin Pharmacol Ther* (1981) 29, 21–6.
5. Brown JE, Kitchell BB, Bjornsson TD, Shand DG. The artifactual nature of heparin-induced drug protein-binding alterations. *Clin Pharmacol Ther* (1981) 30, 636–43.
6. DeLeve LD, Piafsky KM. Lack of heparin effect on propranolol-induced β-adrenoceptor blockade. *Clin Pharmacol Ther* (1982) 31, 216.

Heparin + Nitrates

The effects of heparin were reduced by an infusion of glyceryl trinitrate in some studies, but other studies have not confirmed this interaction. No interaction has been seen with heparin and isosorbide dinitrate or molsidomine.

Clinical evidence

(a) Glyceryl trinitrate (Nitroglycerin)

An interaction between heparin and glyceryl trinitrate was originally reported[1] in 1985. A lower aPTT value was found in patients receiving both intravenous glyceryl trinitrate and heparin, when compared with control patients receiving heparin alone. In a further study in healthy subjects, the same effect was seen with the propylene glycol diluent alone, so the interaction was attributed to the diluent.[1] However, in another study, the same interaction was noted in 2 patients receiving a glyceryl trinitrate preparation without propylene glycol. In this study, while receiving intravenous glyceryl trinitrate, 7 patients with coronary artery disease needed an increased dose of intravenous heparin to achieve satisfactory aPTT ratios of 1.5 to 2.5 on eight occasions. When the glyceryl trinitrate was stopped, in 6 out of 8 occasions there was a marked increase in aPTT values to 3.5. One patient had transient haematuria.[2]

Four other studies have also found a reduction in the effects of heparin in the presence of intravenous glyceryl trinitrate.[3-6] In one of these, the prothrombin time of 27 patients given heparin was more than halved (from 130 to about 60 seconds) when they were given intravenous glyceryl trinitrate 2 to 5 mg/hour. The prothrombin time rose again when the glyceryl trinitrate was stopped.[3] In one study, there was some evidence that the effect might occur only at higher doses of intravenous glyceryl trinitrate (above 350 micrograms/minute),[5] whereas in another, an effect was seen at low doses of 25 to 50 micrograms/minute.[6]

In contrast to the above studies, a total of 12 other studies have found no changes in aPTT in patients[7-16] or healthy subjects[17,18] given intravenous glyceryl trinitrate with heparin. In the randomised, placebo-controlled studies in healthy subjects, a 60-minute infusion of glyceryl trinitrate 5 mg had no effect on the aPTT or prothrombin time following a 5000 unit intravenous injection of heparin,[17] and a 100 micrograms/minute infusion of glyceryl trinitrate did not alter the anticoagulant effect of a 40 units/kg bolus of intravenous heparin in 7 healthy subjects.[18] Two randomised, placebo-controlled studies in patients have also not found any effect of intravenous glyceryl trinitrate on a heparin infusion titrated to a given effect,[12] or on an intravenous heparin bolus dose.[14] In the first of these studies, the glyceryl trinitrate preparation contained propylene glycol.[12]

(b) Isosorbide dinitrate

In a randomised, placebo-controlled study in 12 patients receiving a stable infusion of heparin, the use of isosorbide dinitrate 4.8 ± 0.8 mg/hour for 24 hours did not alter the AUC of the prothrombin time, when compared with placebo, nor was there any change in prothrombin time in the 5 hours after stopping the nitrate.[12] Similarly, other studies have not found any important change in anticoagulation when intravenous isosorbide dinitrate is given with heparin.[8,14,16]

(c) Molsidomine

In a study in 15 patients given intravenous heparin then intravenous molsidomine 2 mg/hour, molsidomine had no effect on the prothrombin time.[19]

Mechanism

Not understood. One study suggests that what occurs is related to a glyceryl trinitrate-induced antithrombin III abnormality, and is apparent at doses above 350 micrograms/minute.[5] One study found that heparin levels were lowered,[6] whereas another reported unchanged heparin levels.[3]

Importance and management

The discord between these reports for glyceryl trinitrate infusion is not understood. However, the best controlled studies in the largest number of patients have not found any evidence of an interaction. On balance therefore, it appears that a clinically relevant interaction is generally unlikely to be seen. Moreover, given that heparin is routinely monitored, it is likely that if any interaction occurs, it will be rapidly detected and compensated for. No special precautions would appear to be needed if heparin is given with molsidomine or isosorbide dinitrate.

1. Col J, Col-Debeys C, Lavenne-Pardonge E, Meert P, Hericks L, Broze MC, Moriau M. Propylene glycol-induced heparin resistance during nitroglycerin infusion. *Am Heart J* (1985) 110, 171–3.
2. Habbab MA, Haft JI. Heparin resistance induced by intravenous nitroglycerin. A word of caution when both drugs are used concomitantly. *Arch Intern Med* (1987) 147, 857–60.
3. Pizzulli L, Nitsch J, Lüderitz B. Hemmung der Heparinwirkung durch Glyceroltrinitrat. *Dtsch Med Wochenschr* (1988) 113, 1837–40.
4. Dascalov TN, Chaushev AG, Petrov AB, Stancheva LG, Stanachcova SD, Ivanov AA. Nitroglycerin inhibition of the heparin effect in acute myocardial infarction patients. *Eur Heart J* (1990) 11 (Abstract Suppl), 321.
5. Becker RC, Corrao JM, Bovill EG, Gore JM, Baker SP, Miller ML, Lucas FV, Alpert JA. Intravenous nitroglycerin-induced heparin resistance: a qualitative antithrombin III abnormality. *Am Heart J* (1990) 119, 1254–61.
6. Brack MJ, More RS, Hubner PJB, Gerschlick AH. The effect of low dose nitroglycerine on plasma heparin concentrations and activated partial thromboplastin times. *Blood Coag Fibrinol* (1993) 4, 183–6.
7. Lepor NE, Amin DK, Berberian L, Shah PK. Does nitroglycerin induce heparin resistance? *Clin Cardiol* (1989) 12, 432–4.
8. Pye M, Olroyd KG, Conkie J, Hutton I, Cobbe SM. A clinical and in vitro study on the possible interaction of intravenous nitrates with heparin anticoagulation. *Clin Cardiol* (1994) 17, 658–61.
9. Gonzalez ER, Jones HD, Graham S, Elswick RK. Assessment of the drug interaction between intravenous nitroglycerin and heparin. *Ann Pharmacother* (1992) 26, 1512–14.
10. Reich DL, Hammerschlag BC, Rand JH, Perucho-Powell MH, Thys DM. Modest doses of nitroglycerin do not interfere with beef lung heparin anticoagulation in patients taking nitrates. *J Cardiothorac Vasc Anesth* (1992) 6, 677–9.
11. Nottestad SY, Mascette AM. Nitroglycerin-induced resistance: absence of interaction at clinically relevant doses. *Mil Med* (1994) 159, 569–71.
12. Bechtold H, Kleist P, Landgraf K, Möser K. Einfluß einer niedrigdosierten intravenösen Nitrattherapie auf die antikoagulatorische Wirkung von Heparin. *Med Klin* (1994) 89, 360–6.

13. Berk SI, Grunwald A, Pal S, Bodenheimer MM. Effect of intravenous nitroglycerin on heparin dosage requirements in coronary artery disease. *Am J Cardiol* (1993) 72, 393–6.
14. Muikku O. Isosorbide dinitrate does not interfere with heparin anticoagulation: a placebo-controlled comparison with nitroglycerin in patients scheduled for coronary artery surgery. *Acta Anaesthesiol Scand* (1994) 38, 583–6.
15. Williams H, Langlosi PF, Kelly JL. The effect of simultaneous intravenous administration of nitroglycerin and heparin on partial thromboplastin time. *Mil Med* (1995) 160, 449–52.
16. Koh KK, Park GS, Song JH, Moon TH, In HH, Kim JJ, Lee HJ, Cho SK, Kim SS. Interaction of intravenous heparin and organic nitrates in acute ischemic syndromes. *Am J Cardiol* (1995) 76, 706–9.
17. Bode V, Welzel D, Franz G, Polensky U. Absence of drug interaction between heparin and nitroglycerin. *Arch Intern Med* (1990) 150, 2117–19.
18. Schoenenberger RA, Ménat L, Weiss P, Marbet GA, Ritz R. Absence of nitroglycerin-induced heparin resistance in healthy volunteers. *Eur Heart J* (1992) 13, 411–14.
19. Wiemer M, Pizzulli L, Reichert H, Lüderitz B. Gibt es eine Wechselwirkung zwischen Heparin und Moldisomin?. *Med Klin* (1994) 89, 45–6.

Heparin or LMWHs + NSAIDs

Some evidence suggests that the bleeding risk is increased when enoxaparin is used with NSAIDs, whereas other evidence suggests no increased bleeding risk with these drugs. The bleeding time was prolonged when ketorolac was given with dalteparin, but not when it was given with heparin. Parecoxib does not alter the effect of heparin on aPTT. Cases of spinal haematomas after epidural anaesthesia have been reported with the concurrent use of heparin or low-molecular-weight heparins and NSAIDs.

Clinical evidence

(a) Heparin

In a crossover, placebo-controlled study in healthy subjects, there was no evidence of an interaction between **ketorolac** and heparin in terms of prolongation of skin bleeding time, platelet aggregation, anti-factor Xa activity, or kaolin-cephalin clotting time. In this study, two doses of oral **ketorolac** were given (the previous evening, and in the morning), then two 10-mg intramuscular doses of ketorolac were given at 10 am and 2 pm, with simultaneous doses of subcutaneous heparin 5000 units.[1] Similarly, in an open-label, crossover study in 18 healthy subjects, giving heparin on day 5 of the use of intravenous **parecoxib** 40 mg twice daily for 6 days produced no clinically or statistically significant differences in coagulation parameters (prothrombin time, aPTT and platelet counts), when compared with heparin alone (bolus dose of heparin 4000 units then a 36-hour infusion of 10 to 14 units/kg). The use of these drugs together was well tolerated. However, prolongation of bleeding time was not assessed.[2]

Use of heparin and **ibuprofen** were considered to be contributing factors in a case of spinal haematoma occurring after epidural anaesthesia.[3]

(b) Low-molecular-weight heparins

In a placebo-controlled, crossover study in healthy subjects, giving **ketorolac** with **dalteparin** resulted in prolongation of the skin bleeding time, when compared with ketorolac alone (13.95 minutes versus 10.55 minutes). **Dalteparin** alone had no effect on the bleeding time when compared with placebo. In this study, two doses of oral **ketorolac** 30 mg were given the day before, and one dose an hour after a single 5000-unit subcutaneous dose of **dalteparin**. The combination did not have any greater effect on platelet aggregation, anti-factor Xa activity, or aPTT time than the individual drugs alone.[4] In an analysis of risk factors for bleeding in patients receiving **enoxaparin** for acute coronary syndrome, the use of NSAIDs was associated with an increased risk of any bleeding (odds ratio 3.44), but not major bleeding.[5] However, a study in hip replacement patients given subcutaneous **enoxaparin** 40 mg daily found that there were no significant differences in intra-operative blood loss, post-operative drainage, transfusion requirements, bruising, wound oozing, and leg swelling between 34 patients given intramuscular **ketorolac** 30 mg on induction of anaesthesia then daily for 4 days postoperatively and 26 patients given unnamed opioids. Patients in this study had any previous NSAID medication stopped 4 weeks before admission, and were not taking aspirin.[6] Similarly, in a large study in patients undergoing surgery for total hip or knee replacement, there was no difference in risk of bleeding or other bleeding-related parameters (total blood loss, need for transfusion, mean change in haemoglobin levels) between patients receiving **enoxaparin** and NSAIDs (830 patients) and those receiving **enoxaparin** and no NSAIDs (394 patients). NSAIDs permitted in this study were said to be short-acting (with a half-life up to 20 hours), but none were specifically named.[7]

The use of **enoxaparin, ketorolac**, and aspirin were considered to be contributing factors in a case of spinal haematoma occurring after lumbar puncture, which resulted in paraplegia.[8] Another case has also been briefly described.[9] In an analysis of reports from the FDA in the US, 16 of 43 patients who developed spinal or epidural haematoma after receiving **enoxaparin** had received concurrent drugs known to prolong bleeding, such as **ketorolac** or other NSAIDs.[10]

Mechanism

NSAIDs, to a greater or lesser extent, irritate the stomach lining. This can result in gastrointestinal bleeding, which will be more severe in anticoagulated patients. Many NSAIDs also have antiplatelet activity, which can prolong bleeding times. There are studies showing that use of NSAIDs increases the risk of perioperative bleeding (one is cited as an example[11]), and theoretically this might be greater in those also receiving heparins.

Importance and management

An interaction between NSAIDs and heparins (including low-molecular-weight heparins) is established. The CSM in the UK and the UK manufacturers say that ketorolac is contraindicated with anticoagulants, including low-dose **heparin**.[12,13] Conversely, the US manufacturers of ketorolac advise that physicians should carefully weigh the benefits against the risks and use concurrent heparin only extremely cautiously.[14]

If NSAIDs and LMWHs are used together, the manufacturers of the LMWHs (**bemiparin, dalteparin, enoxaparin, tinzaparin**) recommend caution or careful clinical and laboratory monitoring.

Heparin and some LMWHs have rarely caused epidural or spinal haematomas resulting in long-term or permanent paralysis when used for thromboprophylaxis in procedures involving spinal/epidural anaesthesia or spinal puncture. The risk of this may be increased if they are used concurrently with other drugs affecting haemostasis such as ketorolac or other NSAIDs, and extreme caution is needed if concurrent use is considered appropriate in these situations.

1. Spowart K, Greer IA, McLaren M, Lloyd J, Bullingham RES, Forbes CD. Haemostatic effects of ketorolac with and without concomitant heparin in normal volunteers. *Thromb Haemost* (1988) 60, 382–6.
2. Noveck RJ, Hubbard RC. Parecoxib sodium, an injectable COX-2 specific inhibitor, does not affect unfractionated heparin-regulated blood coagulation parameters. *J Clin Pharmacol* (2004) 44, 474–80.
3. Litz RJ, Hübler M, Koch T, Albrecht DM. Spinal-epidural hematoma following epidural anesthesia in the presence of antiplatelet and heparin therapy. *Anesthesiology* (2001) 95, 1031–3.
4. Greer IA, Gibson JL, Young A, Johnstone J, Walker ID. Effect of ketorolac and low-molecular-weight heparin individually and in combination on haemostasis. *Blood Coag Fibrinol* (1999) 10, 367–73.
5. Macie C, Forbes L, Foster GA, Douketis JD. Dosing practices and risk factors for bleeding in patients receiving enoxaparin for the treatment of an acute coronary syndrome. *Chest* (2004) 125, 1616–21.
6. Weale AE, Warwick DJ, Durant N, Prothero D. Is there a clinically significant interaction between low molecular weight heparin and non-steroidal analgesics after total hip replacement? *Ann R Coll Surg Engl* (1995) 77, 35–7.
7. Dahl OE, Ögren M, Agnelli G, Eriksson BI, Cohen AT, Mouret P, Rosencher N, Bylock A, Panfilov S, Andersson M. Assessment of bleeding after concomitant administration of antiplatelet and anticoagulant agents in lower limb arthroplasty. *Pathophysiol Haemost Thromb* (2006) 35, 428–34.
8. Chan L, Bailin MT. Spinal epidural hematoma following central neuraxial blockade and subcutaneous enoxaparin: a case report. *J Clin Anesth* (2004) 16, 382–5.
9. Price AJ, Obeid D. Is there a clinical interaction between low molecular weight heparin and non-steroidal analgesics after total hip replacement? *Ann R Coll Surg Engl* (1995) 77, 395.
10. Wysowski DK, Talarico L, Bacsanyi J, Botstein P. Spinal and epidural hematoma and low-molecular-weight heparin. *N Engl J Med* (1998) 338, 1774–5.
11. Slappendel R, Weber EWG, Benraad B, Dirksen R, Bugter MLT. Does ibuprofen increase perioperative blood loss during hip arthroplasty? *Eur J Anaesthesiol* (2002) 19, 829–31.
12. Committee on Safety of Medicines/Medicines Control Agency. Ketorolac: new restrictions on dose and duration of treatment. *Current Problems* (1993) 19, 5–6.
13. Toradol (Ketorolac trometamol). Roche Products Ltd. UK Summary of product characteristics, July 2009.
14. Toradol (Ketorolac tromethamine). Roche Pharmaceuticals. US Prescribing information, September 2002.

Heparin + Probenecid

An isolated case report from the 1950s suggests that the effects of heparin may be possibly increased by probenecid, and bleeding may occur.

Clinical evidence, mechanism, importance and management

In 1950 (but not reported until 1975) a woman with subacute bacterial endocarditis was given probenecid orally and penicillin by intravenous drip, which was kept open with minimal doses of heparin. After about 20 000 units of heparin had been given over a 3-week period, increasing epistaxis developed and the clotting time was found to be 24 minutes (reference range 5 to 6 minutes). This was controlled with protamine.[1] However, no reports of this interaction appear to have been made subsequently. This interaction seems unlikely to be of general significance.

1. Sanchez G. Enhancement of heparin effect by probenecid. *N Engl J Med* (1975) 292, 48.

Heparin or LMWHs + SSRIs

Severe bleeding was attributed to the use of tinzaparin in an elderly woman with renal impairment taking fluoxetine.

Clinical evidence, mechanism, importance and management

A 78-year-old woman taking **fluoxetine** was started on once-daily subcutaneous injections of weight-adjusted **tinzaparin** for a deep vein thrombosis. Five days later she suffered a massive intraperitoneal and parietal haematoma. Poor renal function in this patient could have led to accumulation of the low-molecular-weight heparin, but **fluoxetine** was also considered a contributing factor because SSRIs have antiplatelet effects and can contribute to bleeding.[1] Consider also 'Coumarins and related drugs + SSRIs', p.469. The general relevance of this isolated case is unclear.

1. de Maistre E, Allart C, Lecompte T, Bollaert P-E. Severe bleeding associated with use of low molecular weight heparin and selective serotonin reuptake inhibitors. *Am J Med* (2002) 113, 530–2.

Heparin or LMWHs + Tobacco

There is some evidence that the anticoagulant effects of heparin and dalteparin might be marginally reduced in smokers. In the short-term, enoxaparin might be more effective than heparin in smokers.

Clinical evidence, mechanism, importance and management

In a study of the factors affecting the sensitivity of individuals to heparin, the heparin half-life in smokers was 0.62 hours compared with 0.97 hours in non-smokers. Heparin dose requirements in the smokers were minimally increased (18.8 units/hour compared with 16 units/hour). However, when lean body-weight was taken into account, smoking status was no longer related to heparin clearance.[1]

In the Global Utilization of Streptokinase and tPA for Occluded Coronary Arteries (GUSTO-I) study, cigarette smokers had lower aPTT compared with non-smokers, even after adjusting for weight, age, and sex.[2] In a retrospective analysis of weight-based heparin dosing, smoking was predictive of a subtherapeutic aPTT response.[3]

In a sub-study of **dalteparin** for unstable coronary artery disease, high-dose weight-adjusted dalteparin was associated with lower anti-factor Xa activity and a lower risk of bleeding in smokers than non-smokers..[4] In contrast, a study in 294 patients given **enoxaparin** 1 mg/kg twice daily, found that supratherapeutic concentrations of anti-factor Xa (greater than 1.2 IU/mL) were more than twice as frequent in smokers than non-smokers (12.1% versus 4.9%, respectively).[5] Further, a post-hoc analysis of the data for current smokers, former smokers, and non-smokers from another study population (SYNERGY), found that the adjusted odds ratio for 30-day death or myocardial infarction in patients receiving **enoxaparin**, compared with those receiving unfractionated heparin, was 0.74 in current smokers, 1.03 in former smokers, and 1.07 in non-smokers. However, this benefit was not seen at 6 months or one year. The authors suggested that this effect might be related to the anti-factor Xa activity of enoxaparin, but this remains to be confirmed.[6]

The limited data provide some evidence that the anticoagulant effects of heparin and **dalteparin** might be reduced in smokers, whether or not this affects their efficacy does not appear to have been established. Other data suggest that, in the short-term at least, **enoxaparin** might be more effective than heparin in smokers. Nevertheless, smoking status is not usually a factor used in calculating the dose of heparins. Note that as unfractionated heparin is usually dose adjusted according to bleeding times, any minor interaction should be accounted for in this adjustment.

1. Cipolle RJ, Seifert RD, Neilan BA, Zaske DE, Haus E. Heparin kinetics: variables related to disposition and dosage. *Clin Pharmacol Ther* (1981) 29, 387–93.
2. Granger CB, Hirsh J, Califf RM, Col J, White HD, Betriu A, Woodlief LH, Lee KL, Bovill EG, Simes RJ, Topol EJ; for the GUSTO-I Investigators. Activated partial thromboplastin time and outcome after thrombolytic therapy for acute myocardial infarction: results from the GUSTO-I trial. *Circulation* (1996) 93, 870–8.
3. Lackie CL, Luzier AB, Donovan JA, Feras HI, Forrest A. Weight-based heparin dosing: clinical response and resource utilization. *Clin Ther* (1998) 20, 699–710.
4. Toss H, Wallentin L, Siegbahn A. Influence of sex and smoking habits on anticoagulant activity in low-molecular-weight heparin treatment of unstable coronary artery disease. *Am Heart J* (1999) 137, 72–8.
5. Saliba W, Nitzan O, Rock W, Ron G, Zalman L, Goldstein L, Lavi I, Elias M. Non-therapeutic anti-FXa levels are common among medical ward patients treated with enoxaparin. *Ann Hematol* (2011) 90, 1345–51.
6. Leung S, Gallup D, Mahaffey KW, Cohen M, Antman EM, Goodman SG, Harrington RA, Langer A, Aylward P, Ferguson JJ, Califf RM on behalf of the SYNERGY trial investigators. Smoking status and antithrombin therapy in patients with non-ST-segment elevation acute coronary syndrome. *Am Heart J* (2008) 156, 177–84.

Heparinoids; Danaparoid + Antiplatelet drugs or NSAIDs

No haemostatic interaction was noted between danaparoid and aspirin in healthy subjects. However, caution is recommended on concurrent use because of the possibility of increased bleeding risk.

Clinical evidence

In a randomised, crossover study in healthy subjects, there were no important alterations in coagulation tests and plasma anti-Xa activity when danaparoid (3250 anti-Xa units intravenous bolus followed by 750 units subcutaneously twice daily for 8 days) was given with **aspirin** 500 mg, 14 hours and 2 hours before the intravenous danaparoid. Similarly, danaparoid did not alter the effects of **aspirin** on platelet function, but the prolongation in bleeding time tended to be longer after the combination.[1]

Mechanism

The manufacturer notes that, in general, combination with antithrombotics that act by other mechanisms, such as aspirin, would be additive.[2]

Importance and management

Any effects in the study with aspirin where not considered to be clinically relevant.[1,2] The manufacturers note that danaparoid may be used with drugs that interfere with platelet function, such as aspirin and NSAIDs, but considers that caution remains necessary.[2,3] This is considered particularly important in patients undergoing peridural or spinal anaesthesia or spinal puncture, in whom the use of NSAIDs, and probably also danaparoid, are risk factors for epidural or spinal haematoma resulting in prolonged or permanent paralysis.[2,3]

1. de Boer A, Danhof M, Cohen AF, Magnani HN, Breimer DD. Interaction study between Org 10172, a low molecular weight heparinoid, and acetylsalicylic acid in healthy male volunteers. *Thromb Haemost* (1991) 66, 202–7.
2. Orgaran (Danaparoid sodium). Organon Canada Ltd. Canadian product monograph, June 2001.
3. Orgaran (Danaparoid sodium). Organon Laboratories Ltd. UK Summary of product characteristics, July 2003.

Heparinoids; Danaparoid + Diuretics

Chlortalidone had no clinically relevant effect on the anti-Xa activity of danaparoid in healthy subjects, but it caused an increase in the volume of distribution of antithrombin activity of uncertain relevance. Nevertheless, in clinical use danaparoid is frequently used with a number of other drugs including diuretics, and there is no evidence of an interaction.

Clinical evidence, mechanism, importance and management

In a randomised, crossover study in healthy subjects, a slight decrease in clearance (7%) and volume of distribution (19%) of the anti-Xa activity of danaparoid (3250 anti-Xa units intravenous bolus) occurred when it was given about 12 hours after a single 100-mg dose of chlortalidone. Conversely, the apparent volume of distribution of antithrombin activity was increased by 80%. However, chlortalidone did not change the effect of danaparoid on clotting tests, except for a 4% increase in prothrombin time, which was thought to be a spurious finding.[1] The reasons for these changes are uncertain.

The minor changes in anti-Xa activity are unlikely to be clinically relevant.[1,2] However, the authors considered that relevance of the change in antithrombin activity was uncertain.[1] Nevertheless, the manufacturer notes that, in clinical use, danaparoid has frequently been used with a variety of drugs, including diuretics, and that there is no evidence of any direct interaction with danaparoid.[2]

1. de Boer A, Stiekema JC, Danhof M, Breimer DD. Influence of chlorthalidone on the pharmacokinetics and pharmacodynamics of Org 10172 (Lomoparan®), a low molecular weight heparinoid, in healthy volunteers. *J Clin Pharmacol* (1991) 31, 611–17.
2. Organ (Danaparoid). Organon Canada Ltd. Canadian Prescribing information, June 2001.

Heparinoids; Danaparoid + Penicillins

Cloxacillin and ticarcillin caused an increase in elimination half-life of anti-Xa activity of danaparoid in one study. Ticarcillin had no effect on haemostasis, but cloxacillin appeared to have some pro-coagulant effects, which were not likely to be due to an interaction with danaparoid.

Clinical evidence

(a) Cloxacillin

In a randomised, crossover study in 6 healthy subjects, there was a 74% increase in the elimination half-life of the plasma anti-Xa activity of danaparoid (3250 anti-Xa units intravenous bolus) when it was given with oral cloxacillin 500 mg four times daily for 3 days beginning 24 hours before the danaparoid. Unexpectedly, there were slight decreased effects on thrombin time and bleeding time, and increased effects on aPTT with the combination, effects that were attributed to cloxacillin alone.[1]

(b) Ticarcillin

In a randomised, crossover study in 12 healthy subjects, there was a 56% increase in the elimination half-life of the plasma anti-Xa activity of danaparoid (3250 anti-Xa units intravenous bolus) when it was given with intravenous ticarcillin 4 g four times daily for 2 days beginning immediately before the danaparoid. There were no changes in haemostatic parameters when ticarcillin was given with danaparoid.[1]

Mechanism

Uncertain, but penicillins might compete with danaparoid for renal tubular secretion.[1]

Importance and management

The pharmacokinetic changes seen in the studies with cloxacillin and ticarcillin were not considered clinically relevant.[1,2] In addition, the haemostatic changes seen in the study with cloxacillin were unlikely to be due to an interaction.[1] The manufacturer notes that in clinical use danaparoid has frequently been used with a variety of drugs, including antibacterials, and that there is no evidence of any direct interaction with danaparoid.[2]

1. de Boer A, Stiekema JCJ, Danhof M, van Dinther TG, Boeijinga JK, Cohen AF, Breimer DD. Studies of interaction of a low-molecular-weight heparinoid (Org 10172), with cloxacillin and ticarcillin in healthy male volunteers. *Antimicrob Agents Chemother* (1991) 35, 2110–15.
2. Orgaran (Danaparoid). Organon Canada Ltd. Canadian product monograph, June 2001.

Indanediones + Haloperidol

A single case report describes a marked reduction in the anticoagulant effects of phenindione in a patient given haloperidol.

Clinical evidence, mechanism, importance and management

A man stabilised on **phenindione** 50 mg daily was given haloperidol by injection (5 mg every 8 hours for 24 hours) followed by 3 mg twice daily by mouth. Adequate anticoagulation was not achieved even when the **phenindione** dose was increased to 150 mg daily. When the haloperidol dose was halved, the necessary dose of anti-coagulant was reduced to 100 mg daily, and only when the haloperidol was withdrawn was it possible to achieve adequate anticoagulation with the original dose.[1] The reasons for this effect are not understood. This appears to be the only report of an interaction, and its general importance is therefore limited. Bear it in mind in the event of an unexpected response to treatment.

1. Oakley DP, Lautch H. Haloperidol and anticoagulant treatment. *Lancet* (1963) ii, 1231.

Indanediones + Oxaceprol

An isolated report describes a marked reduction in the response to fluindione in a patient given oxaceprol.

Clinical evidence, mechanism, importance and management

A 77-year-old woman with hypertension and atrial fibrillation, taking propafenone, furosemide, enalapril and **fluindione** 15 mg daily, started taking oxaceprol 300 mg daily. Within 2 days her Quick Time had risen from 26% to 57% and by the end of the week to 65%. When the oxaceprol was withdrawn, her Quick value returned to its previous range of 23 to 30%.[1] The mechanism for this effect is not understood. The general importance of this interaction is unclear, but bear it in mind when prescribing oxaceprol and **fluindione**. Be alert for the need to modify the anticoagulant dose.

1. Bannwarth B, Tréchot P, Mathieu J, Froment J, Netter P. Interaction oxacéprol-fluindione. *Therapie* (1990) 45, 162–3.

LMWHs; Dalteparin + Miscellaneous

The anticoagulant effects of dalteparin are predicted to be enhanced and reduced by various concurrent medications.

Clinical evidence, mechanism, importance and management

The UK manufacturer of dalteparin advises that the anticoagulant effect could be enhanced by other **anticoagulants**, **vitamin K antagonists** (i.e. coumarins and related drugs and indanediones), **dextran**, **thrombolytics**, **sulfinpyrazone** (see 'Heparin or LMWHs + Antiplatelet drugs; Miscellaneous', p.487), **probenecid** (see also 'Heparin + Probenecid', p.489for a case report), and **etacrynic acid**.[1] If concurrent use is essential, it would be prudent to monitor for signs of bleeding.

The manufacturer also advises that the anticoagulant effect might be reduced by **antihistamines**, **cardiac glycosides**, **tetracyclines**, and **ascorbic acid**.[1] Further, they state that because heparin has been shown to interact with intravenous **glyceryl trinitrate** (see 'Heparin + Nitrates', p.488), high-dose **penicillin**, and **quinine**, an interaction between these drugs and dalteparin cannot be ruled out.[1] The clinical relevance of these predications is unclear.

1. Fragmin (Dalteparin sodium). Pharmacia Ltd. UK Summary of product characteristics, February 2013.

Thrombin inhibitors + Antiplatelet drugs

Low-dose aspirin does not appear to alter the pharmacokinetics or pharmacodynamic effects of argatroban. Neither abciximab nor eptifibatide appear to alter argatroban pharmacokinetics. The concurrent use of aspirin and high-dose dabigatran slightly increased the risk of major haemorrhage. From clinical studies, no pharmacodynamic interaction appears to occur between bivalirudin and aspirin, ticlopidine, clopidogrel, prasugrel, abciximab, eptifibatide, or tirofiban.

Clinical evidence, mechanism, importance and management

A. Synthetic thrombin inhibitors

(a) Argatroban

In a study in healthy subjects, pretreatment with oral **aspirin** 162.5 mg, given 26 and 2 hours before argatroban 1 microgram/kg per minute over 4 hours, caused no changes in the pharmacokinetics or pharmacodynamic effects of the argatroban.[1]

In a large clinical study of the concurrent use of argatroban and a glycoprotein IIb/IIIa-receptor antagonist (**abciximab** or **eptifibatide**) in patients undergoing percutaneous coronary intervention, the pharmacokinetics of argatroban (using a population model assessment) were similar to those previously seen in healthy subjects. This suggests that neither **abciximab** nor **eptifibatide** alter argatroban pharmacokinetics.[2] Nevertheless, the manufacturer warns that the use of argatroban with antiplatelet drugs can increase the risk of bleeding.[3]

(b) Dabigatran

In a study in patients with atrial fibrillation given dabigatran 50 to 300 mg twice daily alone or with **aspirin** 81 mg or 325 mg daily, the risk of major haemorrhage was higher with concurrent use of **aspirin** and dabigatran 300 mg twice daily (4 of 64 patients) than with dabigatran 300 mg twice daily alone (0 of 105 patients). Three major haemorrhages occurred at the 325 mg **aspirin** dose and one at the 81 mg dose, and **aspirin** was subsequently stopped in all patients receiving the 300 mg twice daily dose of dabigatran. With the lower doses of dabigatran, the total number of bleeding events tended to be higher in the groups also receiving **aspirin** (about 22% versus 15% for the 150 mg twice daily dabigatran dose, and 9.5% versus 3.4% for the 50 mg twice daily dose).[4] Note that this is not a licensed indication for dabigatran, and the 600 mg daily dose is much higher than that recommended in elective orthopaedic surgery.

A study in patients undergoing total hip replacements and randomised to receive either dabigatran 150 mg or 220 mg daily or enoxaparin allowed patients to continue to take low-dose **aspirin** (less than 160 mg daily) during the study. The full paper gave no specific data on the distribution of **aspirin** use between the groups or specifically if **aspirin** use contributed to the risk of bleeding;[5] however, some data were given in a subsequent letter.[6] The authors stated that there was no significant difference in efficacy or safety outcomes among patients receiving low-dose **aspirin** and those not taking **aspirin**, although the proportion of patients taking **aspirin** with dabigatran was small (at about 4 to 5%).[6]

The manufacturer states that drugs that can enhance the risk of haemorrhage should not be given concurrently or should be given with caution with dabigatran. They specifically recommend avoiding the use of the antiplatelet drugs **clopidogrel**, **ticlopidine**, **glycoprotein IIb/IIIa-receptor antagonists**, and **sulfinpyrazone** and state that if concurrent use is essential, patients should be closely monitored for signs and symptoms of bleeding.[7] Although not specifically mentioned, it would be prudent to similarly monitor the concurrent use of antiplatelet doses of **aspirin**.

B. Hirudins

(a) Bivalirudin

The UK manufacturer states that no pharmacodynamic interactions were detected when bivalirudin was used with platelet inhibitors, including **aspirin**, **ticlopidine**, **clopidogrel**, **abciximab**, **eptifibatide**, and **tirofiban**.[8] Similarly, the manufacturer of **prasugrel** reports that, in phase III studies, no clinically significant interaction was noted with the concurrent use of bivalirudin.[9]

The US manufacturer states that bivalirudin is intended for use with **aspirin** 300 to 325 mg daily, and has been studied only in patients receiving **aspirin**.[10] Both manufacturers state that bivalirudin can be used with a glycoprotein IIb/IIIa-receptor antagonist[8,10] (e.g. **abciximab**, **eptifibatide**, **tirofiban**). Nevertheless, the US manufacturer states that in clinical studies, the concurrent use of bivalirudin with glycoprotein IIb/IIIa-receptor antagonists was associated with increased risks of major bleeding events compared to patients not receiving them.[10] The UK manufacturer recommends regular monitoring of haemostasis when bivalirudin is used with platelet inhibitors.[8]

In general, due to the actions of these drugs, concurrent use with bivalirudin may possibly increase the risk of bleeding.[8,10] Be aware of the potential for this interaction if bleeding occurs.

(b) Lepirudin

The manufacturers of lepirudin state that no formal interaction studies have been done but they reasonably warn about the increased risks of bleeding if antiplatelet drugs such as **clopidogrel**, **ticlopidine**, **abciximab**, **eptifibatide** or **tirofiban** are used concurrently.[11,12]

1. Clarke RJ, Mayo G, FitzGerald GA, Fitzgerald DJ. Combined administration of aspirin and a specific thrombin inhibitor in man. *Circulation* (1991) 83, 1510–8.
2. Cox DS, Kleiman NS, Boyle DA, Aluri J, Parchman G, Holdbrook F, Fossler MJ. Pharmacokinetics and pharmacodynamics of argatroban in combination with a platelet glycoprotein IIB/IIIA receptor antagonist in patients undergoing percutaneous coronary intervention. *J Clin Pharmacol* (2004) 44, 981–90.
3. Argatroban. GlaxoSmithKline. US Prescribing information, March 2009.
4. Ezekowitz MD, Reilly PA, Nehmiz G, Simmers TA, Nagarakanti R, Parcham-Azad K, Pedersen KE, Lionetti DA, Stangier J, Wallentin L. Dabigatran with or without concomitant aspirin compared with warfarin alone in patients with nonvalvular atrial fibrillation (PETRO study). *Am J Cardiol* (2007) 100, 1419–26.
5. Eriksson BI, Dahl OE, Rosencher N, Kurth AA, van Dijk CN, Frostick SP, Prins MH, Hettiarachchi R, Hantel S, Schnee J, Büller HR, for the RE-NOVATE study group. Dabigatran etexilate versus enoxaparin for prevention of venous thromboembolism after total hip replacement: a randomised, double-blind, non-inferiority trial. *Lancet* (2007) 370, 949–56.
6. Eriksson BI, Hantel. Dabigatran versus enoxaparin after total hip replacement. Authors' reply. *Lancet* (2007) 370, 2003.
7. Pradaxa 110 mg Capsules (Dabigatran etexilate mesilate). Boehringer Ingelheim Ltd. UK Summary of product characteristics, December 2014.
8. Angiox (Bivalirudin). The Medicines Company. UK Summary of product characteristics, November 2009.
9. Efient (Prasugrel hydrochloride). Eli Lilly and Company Ltd. UK Summary of product characteristics, December 2013.
10. Angiomax (Bivalirudin). The Medicines Company. US Prescribing information, December 2005.
11. Refludan (Lepirudin). Celgene Ltd. UK Summary of product characteristics, March 2007.
12. Refludan (Lepirudin). Bayer HealthCare Pharmaceuticals Inc. US Prescribing information, December 2006.

Thrombin inhibitors + Other drugs that affect coagulation

The use of argatroban with warfarin and related oral anticoagulants has an effect on the measurement of the INR, and the manufacturer provides equations to adjust for this. Argatroban does not alter warfarin pharmacokinetics. The manufacturers warn of the increased bleeding risks if argatroban, bivalirudin, dabigatran, or lepirudin are used with other anticoagulants.

Clinical evidence, mechanism, importance and management

A. Synthetic thrombin inhibitors

(a) Argatroban

In a study in 12 healthy subjects, argatroban 1.25 micrograms/kg per minute was given for 100 hours, with a single 7.5-mg dose of **warfarin** given at hour 4. Neither drug affected the pharmacokinetics of the other. The single dose of **warfarin** in this study did not add to the anticoagulant effect of argatroban.[1] However, a previous study found that the INR and prothrombin time were increased when **warfarin** (7.5 mg on day one, then 3 to 6 mg for 9 days) was used with argatroban (1 to 4 micrograms/kg per minute for 5 hours daily for 11 days), but without any additional effect on vitamin K-dependent factor Xa activity.[2] A similar finding was reported in a study using **acenocoumarol** or **phenprocoumon** and argatroban.[3]

This means that the INR reading needs to be corrected before it can be used as a clinical indicator of coagulation status when **warfarin** or other vitamin K antagonists (i.e. any coumarin or **indanedione**) are used with argatroban. The manufacturer provides detailed information on how this should be done while switching from argatroban to **warfarin**.[4]

Argatroban is currently licensed for use in patients with or at risk of heparin-induced thrombocytopenia, and the manufacturer states that if **heparin** is to be switched to argatroban, sufficient time for the effect of heparin on the aPTT to decrease should be allowed before starting argatroban. They recommend that all parenteral anticoagulants should be discontinued before starting argatroban.[4]

(b) Dabigatran

The UK manufacturer states that drugs that might enhance the risk of haemorrhage should not be given concurrently, or should be given with caution, to patients receiving dabigatran. They contraindicate the concurrent use of dabigatran and vitamin K antagonist anticoagulants[5] (i.e. **coumarins** and **indanediones**), **rivaroxaban**, **apixaban**, and parenteral anticoagulants such as **heparin**, heparin derivatives, **low-molecular-weight heparins**, **dextrans**, **desirudin** and **fondaparinux**, except when switching to, or from, dabigatran, or when **heparin** is given at doses necessary to maintain a patent central venous or arterial catheter. They recommend starting parenteral anticoagulants 12 hours (when given for atrial fibrillation) or 24 hours (when given for venous thromboembolism) after the last dose of dabigatran. They also state that when switching patients from a parenteral anticoagulant to dabigatran, dabigatran should be started at the same time as, or up to 2 hours before, the next scheduled dose of the parenteral anticoagulant would have been due, or at the time of discontinuation of the parenteral anticoagulant in case of continuous treatment. When switching from dabigatran to a vitamin K antagonist anticoagulant for atrial fibrillation, they state that the vitamin K antagonist anticoagulant should be started 3 days before stopping dabigatran in patients with a creatinine clearance greater than 50 mL/minute, or 2 days before stopping dabigatran in patients with a creatinine clearance of 30 to 50 mL/minute. When switching from a vitamin K antagonist anticoagulant to dabigatran for atrial fibrillation, the manufacturers state that dabigatran can be started when the patient's INR is less than 2.0.[5]

B. Hirudins

(a) Bivalirudin

In the US, the manufacturers state that the concurrent use of bivalirudin with **heparin** or **warfarin** was associated with increased risks of major bleeding events, when compared with patients not receiving these drugs concurrently.[6] In the UK, the manufacturers state that bivalirudin can be started 30 minutes after stopping intravenous **heparin**, but 8 hours should be left after stopping a **low-molecular-weight heparin** given subcutaneously.[7] They recommend regular monitoring of haemostasis when bivalirudin is used with other anticoagulants.[7]

(b) Lepirudin

The manufacturers of lepirudin say that no formal interaction studies have been done but they reasonably warn about the increased risks of bleeding if vitamin K antagonists (i.e. **coumarins** and **indanediones**) are used concurrently.[8,9] Their recommendation for changing from lepirudin to an oral anticoagulant is to reduce the lepirudin dose gradually to reach an aPTT ratio just above 1.5 before beginning the oral anticoagulant, which should be started at the intended maintenance dose without a loading dose. They suggest that parenteral anticoagulation should be continued for 4 to 5 days, and then stopped when the INR stabilises within the target range.[8,9]

1. Brown PM, Hursting MJ. Lack of pharmacokinetic interactions between argatroban and warfarin. *Am J Health-Syst Pharm* (2002) 59, 2078–83.
2. Sheth SB, DiCicco RA, Hursting MJ, Montague T, Jorkasky DK. Interpreting the international normalized ratio (INR) in individuals receiving argatroban and warfarin. *Thromb Haemost* (2001) 85, 435–40. Correction. ibid. 86, 727.
3. Harder S, Graff J, Klinkhardt U, von Hentig N, Walenga JM, Watanabe H, Osakabe M, Breddin HK. Transition from argatroban to oral anticoagulation with phenprocoumon or acenocoumarol: effects on prothrombin time, activated partial thromboplastin time, and Ecarin clotting time. *Thromb Haemost* (2004) 91, 1137–45.
4. Argatroban. GlaxoSmithKline. US Prescribing information, March 2009.
5. Pradaxa 110 mg Capsules (Dabigatran etexilate mesilate). Boehringer Ingelheim Ltd. UK Summary of product characteristics, December 2014.
6. Angiomax (Bivalirudin). The Medicines Company. US Prescribing information, December 2005.
7. Angiox (Bivalirudin). The Medicines Company. UK Summary of product characteristics, November 2009.
8. Refludan (Lepirudin). Celgene Ltd. UK Summary of product characteristics, March 2007.
9. Refludan (Lepirudin). Bayer HealthCare Pharmaceuticals Inc. US Prescribing information, December 2006.

Thrombin inhibitors + Thrombolytics

The risks of bleeding are expected to be increased if argatroban, bivalirudin, dabigatran or lepirudin are used with thrombolytics.

Clinical evidence, mechanism, importance and management

A. Synthetic thrombin inhibitors

(a) Argatroban

The manufacturer of argatroban notes that, in patients with acute myocardial infarction receiving both argatroban and a thrombolytic (**streptokinase** or **alteplase**), the incidence of intracranial bleeding was 1% (8 out of 810 patients).[1] They therefore state that the safety and effectiveness of argatroban with thrombolytics has not been established, and that concurrent use may increase the risk of bleeding.[1]

(b) Dabigatran

The UK manufacturer of dabigatran states that concurrent use of thrombolytics might increased risk of haemorrhage.[2]

B. Hirudins

(a) Bivalirudin

The US manufacturer of bivalirudin states that the concurrent use of thrombolytics was associated with increased risks of major bleeding events.[3]

(b) Lepirudin

The manufacturers of lepirudin say that no formal interaction studies have been undertaken but they reasonably warn that the concurrent use of lepirudin and thrombolytics (they name **alteplase** and **streptokinase**) may increase the risk of bleeding complications and considerably enhance the effect of lepirudin on the aPTT.[4,5] The UK manufacturers advise a dose reduction of lepirudin with concurrent use; however, they state that the optimal dose for concurrent use with a thrombolytic is not known.[4]

1. Argatroban. GlaxoSmithKline. US Prescribing information, March 2009.
2. Pradaxa 110 mg Capsules (Dabigatran etexilate mesilate). Boehringer Ingelheim Ltd. UK Summary of product characteristics, December 2014.
3. Angiomax (Bivalirudin). The Medicines Company. US Prescribing information, December 2005.
4. Refludan (Lepirudin). Celgene Ltd. UK Summary of product characteristics, March 2007.
5. Refludan (Lepirudin). Bayer HealthCare Pharmaceuticals Inc. US Prescribing information, December 2006.

Thrombin inhibitors; Argatroban + Erythromycin

Erythromycin has no effect on the pharmacokinetics or anticoagulant activity of argatroban.

Clinical evidence, mechanism, importance and management

In 10 healthy subjects, erythromycin 500 mg four times daily was given for 7 days with a 5-hour intravenous infusion of argatroban 1 microgram/kg per minute on day 6. Erythromycin had no effect on the pharmacokinetics of argatroban, and had no effect on the argatroban-induced prolongation of the aPTT.[1] No special precautions are likely to be required on the concurrent use of argatroban and erythromycin.

1. Tran JQ, Di Cicco RA, Sheth SB, Tucci M, Peng L, Jorkasky DK, Hursting MJ, Benincosa LJ. Assessment of the potential pharmacokinetic and pharmacodynamic interactions between erythromycin and argatroban. *J Clin Pharmacol* (1999) 39, 513–19.

Thrombin inhibitors; Argatroban + Lidocaine

No pharmacokinetic interaction occurs between argatroban and lidocaine, and lidocaine does not appear to alter the anticoagulant effects of argatroban.

Clinical evidence, mechanism, importance and management

In a study in 12 healthy subjects, lidocaine 2 mg/kg per hour was infused for 16 hours (after a loading dose of 1.5 mg/kg over 10 minutes) alone, then with intravenous argatroban 1.5 micrograms/kg per minute for 16 hours. Concurrent use did not affect the pharmacokinetics of either drug, and lidocaine did not alter the effect of argatroban on aPTT.[1] No special precautions appear likely to be necessary on concurrent use of lidocaine and argatroban.

1. Inglis AML, Sheth SB, Hursting MJ, Tenero DM, Graham AM, DiCicco RA. Investigation of the interaction between argatroban and acetaminophen, lidocaine, or digoxin. *Am J Health-Syst Pharm* (2002) 59, 1257–66.

Thrombin inhibitors; Argatroban + Paracetamol (Acetaminophen)

No pharmacokinetic interaction occurs between argatroban and paracetamol, and paracetamol does not alter the anticoagulant effects of argatroban.

Clinical evidence, mechanism, importance and management

In 11 healthy subjects, paracetamol 1 g every 6 hours for 5 doses had no effect on the pharmacokinetics of a 19-hour infusion of argatroban 1.5 micrograms/kg per minute, started with the second dose of paracetamol. In addition, argatroban had no effect on paracetamol pharmacokinetics. Paracetamol did not alter the effect of argatroban on the aPTT.[1] No special precautions appear necessary on the concurrent use of paracetamol and argatroban.

1. Inglis AML, Sheth SB, Hursting MJ, Tenero DM, Graham AM, DiCicco RA. Investigation of the interaction between argatroban and acetaminophen, lidocaine, or digoxin. *Am J Health-Syst Pharm* (2002) 59, 1257–66.

Thrombin inhibitors; Dabigatran + Amiodarone

Amiodarone increases the exposure to dabigatran.

Clinical evidence

In a population pharmacokinetic analysis of the RE-LY trial, concurrent use of amiodarone increased the AUC of dabigatran (110 mg or 150 mg twice daily) by 12%.[1] The UK and US manufacturers briefly note that, in a study, a single 600-mg dose of amiodarone increased the AUC and maximum concentration of dabigatran (dose not stated) by about 60% and 50%, respectively.[2,3] However, the US manufacturer also states that amiodarone increased the renal clearance of dabigatran by 65% which offset the increase in exposure.[3] Dabigatran did not affect the pharmacokinetics of amiodarone.[3]

A case report describes an 82-year-old female, taking carvedilol, simvastatin, furosemide, and amiodarone, who was switched from warfarin to dabigatran 150 mg twice daily one week before she presented with an INR of 7.25 and a PTT of 135 seconds. The dabigatran was stopped, and her bleeding disorder resolved over the next 4 days.[4]

Mechanism

Dabigatran etexilate, the prodrug for the active metabolite dabigatran, is a substrate for P-glycoprotein. Amiodarone inhibits P-glycoprotein, leading to an increase in the concentration of dabigatran. The bleeding disorder in the case report was attributed to the patient's decreased renal function and the concurrent use of amiodarone, resulting in an increase in dabigatran exposure.[4]

Importance and management

The interaction between dabigatran and amiodarone is established and might be of clinical importance, particularly in the elderly and those with, or at risk of, renal impairment. However, the evidence is difficult to interpret due to the large difference in exposure to dabigatran seen in the two studies. These differences could be accounted for by the increased renal excretion.

As dabigatran is licensed at different doses for different indications, the manufacturers give different guidance on the management of this interaction, depending on the clinical indication for dabigatran. For **venous thromboembolism prophylaxis**, the UK manufacturer recommends that the dose of dabigatran should be reduced to 150 mg daily (as two 75 mg capsules) taken at the same time as amiodarone.[2] Note that amiodarone has a long half-life and therefore the potential for an interaction with dabigatran could still exist for several weeks after stopping amiodarone. For **stroke prophylaxis**, no dabigatran dose adjustment is necessary.[2,3] In addition, close monitoring for signs of bleeding or anaemia is recommended on concurrent use, and dabigatran should be discontinued if bleeding occurs. Note that there have been reports of false positive INR elevations and that the INR is not a reliable test in patients receiving dabigatran.[2] Dabigatran is used without routine coagulation monitoring, but it can be monitored with aPTT and ecarin clotting time (ECT).[2,3] ECT is the more sensitive and accurate measure, but is not widely available. Note that the UK manufacturer suggests that the aPTT might not be suitable for precise measurement of the anticoagulant effects of dabigatran at high plasma concentrations, and they advise caution when interpreting high aPPT measurements.[2]

1. Liesenfeld KH, Lehr T, Dansirikul C, Reilly PA, Connolly SJ, Ezekowitz MD, Yusuf S, Wallentin L, Haertter S, Staab A. Population pharmacokinetic analysis of the oral thrombin inhibitor dabigatran etexilate in patients with non-valvular atrial fibrillation from the RE-LY trial. *J Thromb Haemost* (2011) 9, 2168–75.
2. Pradaxa 110 mg Capsules (Dabigatran etexilate mesilate). Boehringer Ingelheim Ltd. UK Summary of product characteristics, December 2014.
3. Pradaxa (Dabigatran etexilate mesylate). Boehringer Ingelheim Pharmaceuticals, Inc. US Prescribing information, September 2014.
4. Fountzilas C, George J, Levine R. Dabigatran overdose secondary to acute kidney injury and amiodarone use. *N Z Med J* (2013) 126, 110–12.

Thrombin inhibitors; Dabigatran + Miscellaneous

No significant pharmacokinetic interaction occurs between dabigatran and atorvastatin, or diclofenac. However, concurrent use with NSAIDs might increase the risk of haemorrhage, and should be well monitored. Ranitidine has no effect on the absorption of dabigatran. Pantoprazole modestly reduces the bioavailability of dabigatran but does not reduce its therapeutic efficacy.

Clinical evidence, mechanism, importance and management

(a) Atorvastatin

In a study in 22 healthy subjects, atorvastatin 80 mg daily for 4 days slightly reduced the overall exposure to dabigatran 150 g twice daily taken for 4 days by a minor 16%.[1] Atorvastatin is a substrate of the cytochrome P450 isoenzyme CYP3A4, and the results of this study suggest that dabigatran does not significantly affect CYP3A4. These findings confirmed *in vitro* interaction studies, which found that dabigatran does not inhibit or induce CYP3A4. Therefore no special precautions are necessary on the concurrent use of atorvastatin and dabigatran.

(b) Food

In a study in 18 healthy subjects, although food delayed the time to the peak plasma concentration of dabigatran by around 2 hours, it had no effect on the overall bioavailability (AUC) of dabigatran when compared with fasting conditions.[2] Therefore, the manufacturer states that it may be taken with or without food.[3]

(c) NSAIDs

No pharmacokinetic interaction occurred between dabigatran and **diclofenac** in a study in healthy subjects.[3] Diclofenac is a substrate of the cytochrome P450 isoenzyme CYP2C9, and the findings confirmed *in vitro* interaction studies, which found that dabigatran does not inhibit or induce CYP2C9. Nevertheless, drugs such as the NSAIDs may increase the risk of haemorrhage, and should be used cautiously with dabigatran. The manufacturers advise that patients taking NSAIDs with dabigatran should be closely monitored for signs of bleeding, particularly with NSAIDs that have a half-life of greater than 12 hours.[3] Caution would seem appropriate.

(d) Proton pump inhibitors

In a study in 18 healthy subjects, pre-treatment with **pantoprazole** 40 mg twice daily for 2 days reduced the AUC and maximum concentration of a single 150-mg dose of dabigatran by around 22% and 33%, respectively. However, high intersubject variability in these parameters was reported, which the authors suggested may have been due to the interindividual efficacy of pantoprazole.[2] Similarly, in another study in 35 healthy elderly subjects, **pantoprazole** 40 mg twice daily for 10 days, started 2 days before dabigatran 150 mg twice daily for 7 days, reduced the overall bioavailability of dabigatran by around 20 to 24%. However these decreases in bioavailability did not result in a significant reduction in the anticoagulant effect of dabigatran, as measured by the aPTT and ecarin clotting time (ECT). The pharmacokinetic interaction was slightly greater (29% reduction in bioavailability) when the 4 subjects who did not respond to pantoprazole were excluded, along with the one subject with hypoacidity.[4] This suggests that the effect of pantoprazole on dabigatran absorption might be due to reduced gastric acidity, but see also *Ranitidine*, below.

The effect of pantoprazole on dabigatran pharmacokinetics is modest, and probably unlikely to be clinically relevant. The manufacturer notes that the concurrent use of pantoprazole and other proton pump inhibitors with dabigatran in clinical studies did not result in a reduction in its efficacy and no effects on bleeding were seen.[3] Therefore no dabigatran dose alteration appears to be necessary if dabigatran is given with pantoprazole, and probably also other proton pump inhibitors.

(e) Ranitidine

The manufacturer of dabigatran briefly states that ranitidine had no clinically relevant effect on the extent of absorption of dabigatran.[3] No special precautions are therefore needed on the concurrent use of dabigatran and ranitidine.

1. Stangier J, Rathgen K, Stähle H, Reseski K, Körnicke T, Roth W. Coadministration of dabigatran etexilate and atorvastatin: assessment of potential impact on pharmacokinetics and pharmacodynamics. *Am J Cardiovasc Drugs* (2009) 9, 59–68.
2. Stangier J, Eriksson BI, Dahl OE, Ahnfelt L, Nehmiz G, Stähle H, Rathgen K, Svärd R. Pharmacokinetic profile of the oral direct thrombin inhibitor dabigatran etexilate in healthy volunteers and patients undergoing total hip replacement. *J Clin Pharmacol* (2005) 45, 555–63.
3. Pradaxa 110 mg Capsules (Dabigatran etexilate mesilate). Boehringer Ingelheim Ltd. UK Summary of product characteristics, December 2014.
4. Stangier J, Stähle H, Rathgen K, Fuhr R. Pharmacokinetics and pharmacodynamics of the direct oral thrombin inhibitor dabigatran in healthy elderly subjects. *Clin Pharmacokinet* (2008) 47, 47–59.

Thrombin inhibitors; Dabigatran + P-glycoprotein inducers

Rifampicin (rifampin) moderately decreases the exposure to single-dose dabigatran, which would be expected to decrease its anticoagulant effect. Other inducers of P-glycoprotein are predicted to interact similarly.

Clinical evidence, mechanism, importance and management

In a study in 24 healthy subjects, **rifampicin** (rifampin) 600 mg daily for 7 days decreased the AUC and maximum concentration of a single 150-mg dose of dabigatran by 67% and 65.5%, respectively. The exposure to dabigatran returned to about baseline values within 7 days of stopping rifampicin.[1]

Rifampicin is an inducer of P-glycoprotein, of which dabigatran etexilate (the prodrug for the active metabolite, dabigatran) is a substrate. The concurrent use of dabigatran and rifampicin, or other P-glycoprotein inducers, would therefore be best avoided. For a list of other P-glycoprotein inducers, see 'Table 1.12', p.14.[2] Note that the UK manufacturer additionally names **phenytoin**.[2]

1. Härtter S, Koenen-Bergmann M, Sharma A, Nehmiz G, Lemke U, Timmer W, Reilly PA. Decrease in the oral bioavailability of dabigatran etexilate after co-medication with rifampicin. *Br J Clin Pharmacol* (2012) 74, 490–500.
2. Pradaxa 110 mg Capsules (Dabigatran etexilate mesilate). Boehringer Ingelheim Ltd. UK Summary of product characteristics, December 2014.

Thrombin inhibitors; Dabigatran + P-glycoprotein inhibitors

Dronedarone, ketoconazole, quinidine, and ticagrelor (which are all P-glycoprotein inhibitors) increase the exposure to dabigatran. Other P-glycoprotein inhibitors are predicted to have a similar effect, although in one study clarithromycin did not affect the exposure to dabigatran to a clinically relevant extent.

Clinical evidence

(a) Amiodarone

For details of the interaction between dabigatran and amiodarone, see 'Thrombin inhibitors; Dabigatran + Amiodarone', p.492.

(b) Clarithromycin

The UK manufacturer briefly reports that, in a study, clarithromycin 500 mg twice daily increased the AUC and maximum concentration of dabigatran by 19% and 15%, respectively.[1]

(c) Dronedarone

The UK manufacturer briefly reports that, in a study, when dronedarone was given at the same time as dabigatran, the dabigatran AUC and maximum plasma concentration were increased about 2.4-fold and 2.3-fold, respectively, with dronedarone 400 mg twice daily, and about 2.1-fold and 1.9-fold, respectively, after a single 400-mg dose of dronedarone. When single and multiple doses of dronedarone were given 2 hours after the dabigatran, the dabigatran AUC was increased 1.3-fold and 1.6-fold, respectively.[1] The UK manufacturer of dronedarone briefly reports that, in a study, dronedarone 400 mg twice daily doubled the AUC_{0-24} of dabigatran 150 mg daily and increased its maximum concentration by 70%.[2]

(d) Ketoconazole

The UK and US manufacturers briefly report that, in a study, a single 400-mg dose of ketoconazole increased the AUC and maximum concentration of dabigatran 2.4-fold, and multiple doses of ketoconazole 400 mg daily increased the AUC and maximum concentration of dabigatran 2.5-fold.[1,3]

(e) Quinidine

The UK and US manufacturers briefly report that, in a study, when dabigatran (dose not specified) taken twice daily for 3 days was given with quinidine 200 mg, taken every 2 hours up to a total dose of 1 g, on day 3, the AUC and maximum concentration of dabigatran were increased by 53% and 56%, respectively.[1,3]

(f) Verapamil

For details of the interaction between dabigatran and verapamil, see 'Thrombin inhibitors; Dabigatran + Verapamil', below.

(g) Ticagrelor

The UK manufacturer briefly reports that, simultaneous administration of a single 75-mg dose of dabigatran with a 180-mg loading dose of ticagrelor resulted in a 1.7-fold and almost a 2-fold increase in the AUC and maximum plasma concentration of dabigatran, respectively. After multiple doses of ticagrelor 90 mg twice daily, the dabigatran AUC and maximum plasma concentration were increased 1.5-fold and 1.6-fold, respectively.[1]

Mechanism

Dabigatran etexilate, the prodrug for the active metabolite dabigatran, is a substrate for P-glycoprotein. Clarithromycin, dronedarone, ketoconazole, quinidine, and ticagrelor are thought to inhibit P-glycoprotein, leading to an increase in the concentration of dabigatran.

Importance and management

The interaction between dabigatran and P-glycoprotein inhibitors appears to be established, although the extent of the interaction appears to differ between the inhibitors. On the basis of the marked effects of **ketoconazole** and **dronedarone** on dabigatran exposure, the UK manufacturer of dabigatran contraindicates concurrent use with both of these drugs.[1] However, the US manufacturer only recommends avoiding concurrent use in patients with severe renal impairment, and further, states that in patients with moderate renal impairment, the dose of dabigatran should be reduced to 75 mg twice daily in patients also taking ketoconazole or dronedarone.[3] In contrast, the US manufacturer of dronedarone states that no dabigatran dose adjustment is necessary on concurrent use.[4]

The UK manufacturer predicts a number of other drugs will interact with dabigatran in the same way as ketoconazole, and so contraindicates their concurrent use. They name **itraconazole**, **ciclosporin (cyclosporine)**, and **tacrolimus**.[1] They also advise caution with the concurrent use of **posaconazole**.[1]

As dabigatran is licensed at different doses for different indications, the manufacturers give different guidance on the management of the interaction with other P-glycoprotein inhibitors, depending on the clinical indication for dabigatran, which is given in the sections below:

1. Clarithromycin. The very slight increase in dabigatran exposure seen in the study cited is unlikely to be clinically relevant, and suggests that no dabigatran dose adjustment would be necessary on the concurrent use of clarithromycin; however, the UK manufacturer states that a clinically relevant interaction in patients cannot be ruled out, and they advise close monitoring, particularly in patients with renal impairment.[1]

2. Quinidine. For **venous thromboembolism prophylaxis**, the UK manufacturer recommends that the dose of dabigatran should be reduced to 150 mg daily (as two 75 mg capsules) taken at the same time as quinidine,[1] and this seems a prudent precaution. For **stroke prophylaxis**, no dabigatran dose adjustment is necessary.[1,3]

3. Ticagrelor. As ticagrelor has antiplatelet activity and increases dabigatran exposure [although note this was only slight], concurrent use is cautioned due to the increased risk of bleeding.[1]

General advice

For all P-glycoprotein inhibitors (for a list, see 'Table 1.12', p.14), close monitoring for signs of bleeding or anaemia is advised on concurrent use, and dabigatran should be discontinued if severe bleeding occurs. Similar advice is given by the UK manufacturer of **telithromycin**, which states that it is a P-glycoprotein inhibitor and might therefore increase dabigatran concentrations.[5] However, on the basis of the interaction between clarithromycin and dabigatran, it would seem unlikely that a clinically relevant interaction will occur with telithromycin.

Note that dabigatran is used without routine coagulation monitoring, but it can be monitored with aPTT and ecarin clotting time (ECT).[1,3] ECT is the more sensitive and accurate measure, but is not widely available. Note that the UK manufacturer suggests that the aPTT might not be suitable for precise measurement of the anticoagulant effects of dabigatran at high plasma concentrations, and they advise caution when interpreting high aPPT measurements.[1]

1. Pradaxa 110 mg Capsules (Dabigatran etexilate mesilate). Boehringer Ingelheim Ltd. UK Summary of product characteristics, December 2014.
2. Multaq (Dronedarone hydrochloride). Sanofi. UK Summary of product characteristics, November 2013.
3. Pradaxa (Dabigatran etexilate mesylate). Boehringer Ingelheim Pharmaceuticals, Inc. US Prescribing information, September 2014.
4. Multaq (Dronedarone). Sanofi-Aventis U.S. LLC. US Prescribing information, March 2014.
5. Ketek (Telithromycin). Sanofi. UK Summary of product characteristics, November 2012.

Thrombin inhibitors; Dabigatran + Verapamil

Verapamil increases the exposure to dabigatran.

Clinical evidence

A population pharmacokinetic analysis of the RE-LY trial found that concurrent use of verapamil increased the AUC of dabigatran (110 mg or 150 mg twice daily) by 23%.[1] In a two-part, crossover study in healthy subjects the AUC and maximum concentration of a single dose of dabigatran 150 mg were increased 2.4-fold and 2.8-fold, respectively, by a single 120-mg dose of *immediate-release* verapamil given 1 hour before the dabigatran. A 240-mg dose of *extended-release* verapamil had a much smaller effect, resulting in increases in dabigatran AUC and maximum concentration of 71% and 91%, respectively. Twice-daily doses of *immediate-release* verapamil had a similar effect, increasing the AUC and maximum concentration of dabigatran by 54% and 63%, respectively. When *immediate-release* verapamil was given 2 hours after the dabigatran, the increase in dabigatran AUC and maximum concentration was less than 20%.[2]

Mechanism

Dabigatran etexilate, the prodrug for the active metabolite dabigatran, is a substrate for P-glycoprotein. Verapamil is an inhibitor of P-glycoprotein, and concurrent use results in increased exposure to dabigatran.

Importance and management

The interaction between dabigatran and verapamil is established and likely to be clinically important, although the timing of administration of the two drugs influences the size of the effect. As such, this is a factor in the advice for concurrent use of verapamil and dabigatran. As dabigatran is licensed at different doses for different indications, the manufacturers give different guidance on the management of this interaction, depending on the clinical indication for dabigatran. For **venous thromboembolism prophylaxis**, the UK manufacturer recommends that the dose of dabigatran should be reduced to 150 mg daily (as two 75 mg capsules) taken at the same time as verapamil, with a further dose reduction to 75 mg daily considered in those patients with moderate renal impairment.[3] For **stroke prophylaxis**, the UK manufacturer[3] advises that the dose of dabigatran should be reduced to 110 mg twice daily, taken at the same time as verapamil, whereas the US manufacturer states that no dose adjustment is necessary.[4]

In addition, close monitoring for signs of bleeding or anaemia is recommended on concurrent use, and dabigatran should be discontinued if bleeding occurs. Note that dabigatran is used without routine coagulation monitoring, but it can be monitored with aPTT and ecarin clotting time (ECT).[3,4] ECT is the more sensitive and accurate measure, but is not widely available. Note that the UK manufacturer suggests that the aPTT might not be suitable for precise measurement of the anticoagulant effects of dabigatran at high plasma concentrations, and they advise caution when interpreting high aPPT measurements.[3]

1. Liesenfield KH, Lehr T, Dansirikul C, Reilly PA, Connolly SJ, Ezekowitz MD, Yusuf S, Wallentin L, Haertter S, Staab A. Population pharmacokinetic analysis of the oral thrombin inhibitor dabigatran etexilate in patients with non-valvular atrial fibrillation from the RE-LY trial. *J Thromb Haemost* (2011) 9, 2168–75.
2. Härtter S, Sennewald R, Nehmiz G, Reilly P. Oral bioavailability of dabigatran etexilate (Pradaxa®) after co-medication with verapamil in healthy subjects. *Br J Clin Pharmacol* (2012) 75, 1053–62.
3. Pradaxa 110 mg Capsules (Dabigatran etexilate mesilate). Boehringer Ingelheim Ltd. UK Summary of product characteristics, December 2014.
4. Pradaxa (Dabigatran etexilate mesylate). Boehringer Ingelheim Pharmaceuticals, Inc. US Prescribing information, September 2014.

Thrombin inhibitors; Ximelagatran + Miscellaneous

Aspirin did not alter the pharmacokinetics of melagatran, the active metabolite of ximelagatran, or its effects on the aPTT, but the combination had additive effects on bleeding time. Erythromycin and azithromycin increase the AUC of melagatran, the active metabolite of ximelagatran, and cause a small additional effect on coagulation parameters. The concurrent use of amiodarone and ximelagatran caused a slight increase in the AUC of melagatran and a slight decrease in the AUC of amiodarone.

No pharmacokinetic interaction occurs between ximelagatran and atorvastatin or digoxin, and concurrent use does not change coagulation status. No pharmacokinetic interaction appears to occur between ximelagatran and diazepam, diclofenac or nifedipine. This suggests that ximelagatran has no clinically relevant effect on drugs that are substrates for the cytochrome P450 isoenzymes CYP2C9, CYP2C19, and CYP3A4.

Clinical evidence, mechanism, importance and management

(a) Amiodarone

In a placebo-controlled study in 26 healthy subjects, ximelagatran 36 mg was given every 12 hours for 8 days with a single 600-mg dose of amiodarone on day 4. Concurrent use resulted in a slight 21% increase in the AUC of melagatran (the active metabolite of ximelagatran), and a slight 15% decrease in the AUC of amiodarone. Amiodarone did not alter the effect of melagatran on aPTT.[1] The mechanism of this interaction is unknown. The pharmacokinetic changes seen were not considered to be clinically relevant.

(b) Antibacterials

In 16 healthy subjects, **erythromycin** 500 mg three times daily was given for 5 days with a single 36-mg oral dose of ximelagatran given before erythromycin, and on day 5. Erythromycin increased the AUC of melagatran (the active metabolite of ximelagatran) by 82%, and the maximum plasma level by 76%. This resulted in a small increase in peak aPTT from 41 seconds to 44 seconds.[2] In another study, healthy subjects were given a single 36-mg dose of ximelagatran on day 1 and 5 of a 5-day course of azithromycin (500 mg on day 1 followed by 250 mg on days 2 to 5). **Azithromycin** increased the AUC of melagatran by 60% and caused a minor 15% increase in the peak aPTT. **Cefuroxime** (250 mg twice daily for 9 doses) also caused a minor increase in the AUC of melagatran of 23%, without affecting the aPTT, and **amoxicillin**, **ciprofloxacin** and **doxycycline** did not interact.[3]

Ximelagatran is not metabolised by cytochrome P450 isoenzymes, so the known inhibitory effect of erythromycin on CYP3A4 is not thought to be the mechanism for this interaction. The mechanism may involve inhibition of transport proteins, possibly P-glycoprotein.[2,3]

Based on the findings of a pharmacokinetic interaction with a small pharmacodynamic effect it would certainly be prudent to be cautious if ximelagatran is used in patients taking azithromycin or erythromycin, although note that the pharmacodynamic effect was small and the combination of erythromycin and ximelagatran was well tolerated.[2]

(c) Aspirin

In young healthy subjects, aspirin 450 mg the day before, and 150 mg just before melagatran had no effect on the pharmacokinetics of intravenous melagatran 4.12 mg. In addition, aspirin did not alter the increases seen in aPTT or activated clotting time seen with melagatran. Both aspirin and melagatran increased bleeding time, and the increase with the combination was additive.[4]

(d) Atorvastatin

In 15 healthy subjects, ximelagatran 36 mg twice daily was given for 5 days with a single 40-mg dose of atorvastatin on day 4. There was no change in the pharmacokinetics of either drug or their active metabolites. Atorvastatin did not alter the effect of melagatran on aPTT.[5] No special precautions are expected to be needed if ximelagatran is used in patients taking atorvastatin.

(e) Diazepam

In 24 healthy subjects, ximelagatran 24 mg twice daily was given for 8 days with a single 100-microgram/kg intravenous dose of diazepam on day 3. There was no change in the pharmacokinetics of either drug or of *N*-desmethyl-diazepam.[6]

Metabolism of diazepam to *N*-desmethyl-diazepam occurs via the cytochrome P450 isoenzyme CYP2C19, and *in vitro* studies had shown that melagatran was a weak inhibitor of this isoenzyme.[6] However, the lack of a pharmacokinetic interaction with diazepam suggests that no clinically relevant interaction occurs, and is also unlikely with other CYP2C19 substrates[6] by this mechanism (for a list see 'Table 1.6', p.8).

(f) Diclofenac

In a single-dose study in 24 healthy subjects, simultaneous administration of ximelagatran 24 mg and enteric-coated diclofenac 50 mg caused no change in the pharmacokinetics of either drug. In this study, there was also no additional effect of the combination on activated partial thromboplastin time or capillary bleeding time, suggesting that no pharmacodynamic interaction occurs.[6]

Diclofenac is a substrate for the cytochrome P450 isoenzyme CYP2C9, and *in vitro* study has shown that ximelagatran and melagatran are weak inhibitors of this isoenzyme.[6] However, the lack of a pharmacokinetic interaction with diclofenac suggests that no clinically relevant interaction occurs, and is also unlikely with other CYP2C9 substrates[6] by this mechanism (for a list see 'Table 1.5', p.7).

(g) Digoxin

In a double-blind, crossover study, 16 healthy subjects were given oral ximelagatran 36 mg twice daily or placebo for 8 days and a single 500-microgram oral dose of digoxin on day 4. Ximelagatran had no effects on the pharmacokinetics of digoxin. Similarly, digoxin had no effects on the pharmacokinetics of melagatran (the active metabolite) when ximelagatran was given orally. The anticoagulant effect of melagatran (measured as aPTT prolongation) was not altered by digoxin.[7]

(h) Nifedipine

In a single-dose study in 34 healthy subjects, giving ximelagatran 24 mg four hours after slow-release nifedipine 60 mg caused no change in the pharmacokinetics of either drug.[6]

Nifedipine is a substrate for the cytochrome P450 isoenzyme CYP3A4, and *in vitro* studies had shown that ximelagatran metabolites might be weak inhibitors of this isoenzyme.[6] However, the lack of a pharmacokinetic interaction with nifedipine suggests that no clinically relevant interaction occurs, and is also unlikely with other CYP3A4 substrates[6] by this mechanism (for a list see 'Table 1.10', p.12).

1. Teng R, Sarich TC, Eriksson UG, Hamer JE, Gillette S, Schützer K-M, Carlson GF, Knowey PR. A pharmacokinetic study of the combined administration of amiodarone and ximelagatran, an oral direct thrombin inhibitor. *J Clin Pharmacol* (2004) 44, 1063–71.
2. Eriksson UG, Dorani H, Karlsson J, Fritsch H, Hoffmann K-J, Olsson L, Sarich TC, Wall U, Schützer K-M. Influence of erythromycin on the pharmacokinetics of ximelagatran may involve inhibition of P-glycoprotein-mediated excretion. *Drug Metab Dispos* (2006) 34, 775–82.
3. Dorani H, Schützer K-M, Sarich TC, Wall U, Logren U, Ohlsson L, Eriksson UG. Pharmacokinetics and pharmacodynamics of the oral direct thrombin inhibitor ximelagatran co-administered with different classes of antibiotics in healthy volunteers. *Eur J Clin Pharmacol* (2007) 63, 571–81.
4. Fager G, Cullberg M, Eriksson-Lepkowska M, Frison L, Eriksson UG. Pharmacokinetics and pharmacodynamics of melagatran, the active form of the oral direct thrombin inhibitor ximelagatran, are not influenced by acetylsalicylic acid. *Eur J Clin Pharmacol* (2003) 59, 283–9.
5. Sarich TC, Schützer K-M, Dorani H, Wall U, Kalies I, Ohlsson L, Eriksson UG. No pharmacokinetic or pharmacodynamic interaction between atorvastatin and the oral direct thrombin inhibitor ximelagatran. *J Clin Pharmacol* (2004) 44, 928–34.
6. Bredberg E, Andersson TB, Frison L, Thuresson A, Johansson S, Eriksson-Lepkowska M, Larsson M, Eriksson UG. Ximelagatran, an oral direct thrombin inhibitor, has a low potential for cytochrome P450-mediated drug-drug interactions. *Clin Pharmacokinet* (2003) 42, 765–77.
7. Sarich TC, Schützer K-M, Wollbratt M, Wall U, Kessler E, Eriksson UG. No pharmacokinetic or pharmacodynamic interaction between digoxin and the oral direct thrombin inhibitor ximelagatran in healthy volunteers. *J Clin Pharmacol* (2004) 44, 935–41.

13

Antidiabetics

The antidiabetics are used to control diabetes mellitus, a disease in which there is total or partial failure of the beta-cells within the pancreas to secrete enough insulin, one of the hormones concerned with the handling of glucose. There are two main types of diabetes: one develops early in life and occurs when the ability of the pancreas suddenly, and often almost totally, fails to produce insulin. This type is called type 1, juvenile, or insulin-dependent diabetes (IDDM), and requires insulin replacement therapy. The other form is type 2, maturity-onset, or non-insulin dependent diabetes mellitus (NIDDM), which is most often seen in those over 40 years of age. This occurs when the pancreas gradually loses the ability to produce insulin over a period of months or years and/or resistance to the action of insulin develops. It is often associated with being overweight and can sometimes be satisfactorily controlled simply by losing weight and adhering to an appropriate diet. This might then be augmented with oral antidiabetic drugs, and eventually insulin. A classification of the antidiabetics is given in 'Table 13.1', p.497.

Modes of action of the antidiabetics

A. Parenteral antidiabetics

(a) Amylin analogues

Pramlintide is a synthetic analogue of amylin, a pancreatic hormone involved in glucose homoeostasis. It slows the rate of gastric emptying and reduces appetite. It is given subcutaneously immediately before meals, and is used in patients already receiving insulin.

(b) Glucagon-like peptide-1 receptor agonists

Albiglutide, dulaglutide, exenatide, liraglutide, and lixisenatide are incretin mimetics that act as glucagon-like peptide-1 (GLP-1) receptor agonists, increasing insulin secretion when glucose concentrations are high. These drugs are given subcutaneously, as an adjunct, in patients with type 2 diabetes who are already receiving metformin, a sulfonylurea, or both.

(c) Insulin

Insulin extracted from the pancreatic tissue of pigs and cattle is so similar to human insulin that it can be used as a replacement. However, human insulin, manufactured by genetically engineered microorganisms, is more commonly used. Insulin is usually given by injection in order to bypass the enzymes of the gut, which would digest and destroy it like any other protein. The onset and duration of action of insulin can be prolonged by forming a complex with zinc or protamine. Various insulin analogues have been developed, which have specific pharmacokinetic profiles. Insulin aspart, glulisine, and lispro have a faster onset and shorter duration of action than soluble insulin. Insulin glargine and detemir both have a prolonged duration of action, as does insulin degludec, a human insulin analogue. An inhaled form of insulin for use in adult patients with diabetes mellitus was launched and subsequently discontinued (*Exubera*), but others are still in development.

B. Oral antidiabetics

(a) Aldose reductase inhibitors

Epalrestat inhibits the enzyme aldose reductase, which converts glucose to sorbitol. The accumulation of sorbitol might play a role in some diabetic complications.

(b) Alpha-glucosidase inhibitors

Acarbose, miglitol, and voglibose act against alpha glucosidases and specifically against sucrase in the gut to delay the digestion and absorption of monosaccharides from starch and sucrose.

(c) Biguanides

The mode of action of the biguanides, such as metformin, is unclear, but they do not stimulate the pancreas to release insulin like the sulfonylureas. Instead, they may delay the gastrointestinal absorption of glucose, increase insulin sensitivity and the uptake of glucose into cells, and inhibit gluconeogenesis. Their use is restricted to type 2 diabetes because they are not effective unless insulin is present.

(d) Dipeptidylpeptidase-4 inhibitors

Alogliptin, linagliptin, saxagliptin, sitagliptin, and vildagliptin increase the concentration of incretin hormones by reducing their degradation via the enzyme dipeptidylpeptidase-4, and so augment insulin secretion. They are principally used in type 2 diabetes in combination with metformin and/or a sulfonylurea.

(e) Meglitinides

Nateglinide and repaglinide act similarly to the sulfonylureas (see below) to increase endogenous insulin secretion, and so are used in type 2 diabetes.

(f) Sodium-glucose co-transporter-2 inhibitors

Canagliflozin, dapagliflozin and empagliflozin enhance the urinary excretion of glucose by suppressing the renal reabsorption of glucose. They are used in type 2 diabetes, as monotherapy or in combination with insulin or other antidiabetics.

(g) Sulfonylureas

The sulfonylurea and other sulfonamide-related compounds, such as chlorpropamide and tolbutamide, were the first synthetic compounds used in medicine as antidiabetics. Among their actions, they stimulate the remaining beta-cells of the pancreas to grow and secrete insulin which, with a restricted diet, controls blood glucose concentrations and permits normal metabolism to occur. Clearly they can only be effective in those patients with diabetes whose pancreas still has the capacity to produce some insulin, so their use is confined to type 2 diabetes.

(h) Thiazolidinediones

Pioglitazone and rosiglitazone decrease peripheral insulin resistance by acting as agonists and hence activating gamma-PPAR (peroxisome proliferator-activated receptor). They are used in type 2 diabetes. However, due to concerns about the cardiovascular safety of rosiglitazone, its use is heavily restricted and in some countries it has been withdrawn from use.

(i) Other oral antidiabetics

Outside orthodox Western medicine, there are herbal preparations which are used to treat diabetes and which can be given by mouth. Blueberries were traditionally used by the Alpine peasants, and bitter gourd, or karela (*Momordica charantia*), is an established part of herbal treatment in the Indian subcontinent and elsewhere. Traditional Chinese medicine also has herbal medicines for diabetes. As yet it is not known how these herbal medicines act and their efficacy awaits formal clinical evaluation.

Interactions

The most common interactions with antidiabetic drugs are those that result in an increase or decrease in blood glucose concentrations, thereby disturbing the control of diabetes. These are detailed in this section, and might be a result of pharmacodynamic or pharmacokinetic effects.

(a) Pharmacodynamic effects

Antidiabetic drugs with differing mechanisms of action are often used in combination in clinical practice to achieve better glycaemic control than

Table 13.1 Drugs used in the management of diabetes

Group		*Drugs*
Parenteral antidiabetics		
Amylin analogues		Pramlintide
Glucagon-like peptide-1 receptor agonists (Incretin mimetics)		Albiglutide, Dulaglutide, Exenatide, Liraglutide, Lixisenatide
Insulins	Short-acting	Soluble insulin
	Intermediate- and long-acting	Insulin zinc suspension, Isophane insulin, Protamine zinc insulin
	Short-acting analogues	Insulin aspart, Insulin glulisine, Insulin lispro
	Intermediate to long-acting analogues	Insulin aspart protamine, Insulin degludec, Insulin detemir, Insulin glargine, Insulin lispro protamine
Oral antidiabetics		
Aldose reductase inhibitors		Epalrestat
Alpha glucosidase inhibitors		Acarbose, Miglitol, Voglibose
Biguanides		Buformin, Metformin
Meglitinides		Nateglinide, Repaglinide
Dipeptidylpeptidase-4 inhibitors		Alogliptin, Linagliptin, Saxagliptin, Sitagliptin, Vildagliptin
Sodium-glucose co-transporter-2 inhibitors		Canagliflozin, Dapagliflozin, Empagliflozin
Sulfonylureas		Acetohexamide, Carbutamide, Chlorpropamide, Glibenclamide (Glyburide), Glibornuride, Gliclazide, Glimepiride, Glipizide, Gliquidone, Glisentide, Glisolamide, Glisoxepide, Glycyclamide, Tolazamide, Tolbutamide
Thiazolidinediones		Pioglitazone, Rosiglitazone
Other drugs		Guar gum

monotherapy. As a result their effects can be additive and the risk of hypoglycaemia can be increased, although this is not the case for all combinations. It is most common when the individual antidiabetics increase insulin secretion and are associated with hypoglycaemia when used alone (for example the sulfonylureas).

(b) Pharmacokinetic effects

The cytochrome P450 enzyme system is involved in the metabolism of a number of oral antidiabetics, as outlined below.

1. Dipeptidylpeptidase-4 inhibitors. Of the dipeptidylpeptidase-4 inhibitors, saxagliptin is extensively metabolised by CYP3A4 to its principal metabolite (which is about half as active as the parent compound) and its pharmacokinetics are thus affected by ketoconazole (see 'Dipeptidylpeptidase-4 inhibitors + Ketoconazole and other CYP3A4 inhibitors', p.523).

2. Meglitinides. Repaglinide is principally metabolised by CYP2C8, with some involvement of CYP3A4 (as demonstrated by the administration of gemfibrozil and itraconazole, see 'Meglitinides + Azoles; Itraconazole or Ketoconazole', p.528 and 'Meglitinides + Fibrates', p.528), and the organic anion transporter protein, OATP1B1. Nateglinide is principally metabolised by CYP2C9.

3. Sulfonylureas. The sulfonylureas are all mainly metabolised by CYP2C9, albeit to varying degrees (see 'Sulfonylureas + Azoles; Fluconazole', p.543). Tolbutamide can be used as a probe substrate to assess the activity of drugs on CYP2C9.

4. Thiazolidinediones. Rosiglitazone and pioglitazone are both metabolised by CYP2C8 (see 'Thiazolidinediones + Fibrates', p.555).

Other interactions where the antidiabetic drug is the affecting drug are described elsewhere.

Alpha-glucosidase inhibitors + Antacids

Antacids appear not to interact with acarbose or miglitol.

Clinical evidence, mechanism, importance and management

(a) Acarbose

A placebo-controlled study in 24 healthy subjects given a 75-g dose of sucrose, found that 10 mL of *Maalox 70* (**aluminium/magnesium hydroxide**) had no effect on the blood glucose- and insulin-lowering effects of acarbose 100 mg. It was concluded that no special precautions are needed if this, or similar antacids, are used with acarbose.[1]

(b) Miglitol

The US manufacturer briefly notes that, in 12 healthy subjects, concurrent use of an antacid (not specified) did not alter the pharmacokinetics of miglitol.[2] No miglitol dose adjustment would be expected to be necessary on concurrent use.

1. Höpfner M, Durani B, Spengler M, Fölsch UR. Effect of acarbose and simultaneous antacid therapy on blood glucose. *Arzneimittelforschung* (1997) 47, 1108–1111.
2. Glyset (Miglitol). Pfizer Inc. US Prescribing information, September 2012.

Alpha-glucosidase inhibitors + Charcoal or Digestive enzymes

The absorption of acarbose and miglitol is predicted to be reduced by charcoal or digestive enzyme preparations.

Clinical evidence, mechanism, importance and management

The manufacturers of acarbose[1,2] and miglitol[3] reasonably suggest that concurrent use of intestinal adsorbents (e.g. charcoal), or digestive enzyme preparations containing carbohydrate splitting enzymes (such as amylase or pancreatin), should be avoided because, theoretically, they would be expected to reduce the effects of these alpha-glucosidase inhibitors.

1. Glucobay (Acarbose). Bayer plc. UK Summary of product characteristics, July 2013.
2. Precose (Acarbose). Bayer HealthCare Pharmaceuticals Inc. US Prescribing information, March 2011.
3. Glyset (Miglitol). Pfizer Inc. US Prescribing information, September 2012.

Alpha-glucosidase inhibitors + Metformin

Some minor decreases in the plasma concentrations of metformin have been seen on concurrent use with acarbose or miglitol.

Clinical evidence

A study in 6 healthy subjects found that **acarbose** 50 to 100 mg three times daily reduced the maximum serum concentrations and the AUC_{0-9} of metformin 1 g by about 35%, but its 24-hour urinary excretion was unchanged.[1] Another study in 19 diabetic patients given **acarbose** 50 or 100 mg three times daily and metformin 500 mg twice daily, found that **acarbose** reduced the metformin AUC by 12 to 13%, and its maximum plasma concentration by 17 to 20%. Nevertheless, the drug combination reduced the postprandial glucose concentration at 3 hours by 15% more than when metformin was given alone.[2] There was no increased incidence of hypoglycaemia when **acarbose** was used with metformin.[3]

The US manufacturer briefly notes that, in a study in healthy subjects, **miglitol** 100 mg three times daily for 7 days reduced the AUC and maximum concentration of a single 1-g dose of metformin by 12% and 13%, respectively, although this difference was not statistically significant.[4]

Mechanism

The reason for the minor pharmacokinetic changes seen is uncertain.

Importance and management

Evidence for a pharmacokinetic interaction between alpha-glucosidase inhibitors and metformin is limited, but the pharmacokinetic changes seen are minor and unlikely to be clinically relevant. The UK manufacturer of acarbose states that while acarbose does not cause hypoglycaemia when given alone, it might increase the blood glucose-lowering effects of metformin.[5] It might therefore be necessary to reduce the dose of one or both antidiabetic drugs. No dose adjustment is recommended for miglitol when given with metformin.[4] However, it is prudent to monitor blood glucose concentrations when any change is made to the medication regimen of a patient with diabetes. There appears to be no information for an interaction between voglibose and metformin, but a similar precaution would seem prudent. Note, that if hypoglycaemia occurs, it should be treated with glucose (dextrose), not sucrose, because alpha-glucosidase inhibitors delay the digestion and absorption of disaccharides such as sucrose, but do not affect monosaccharides.[3-5]

1. Scheen AJ, Fierra Alves de Magalhaes AC, Salvatore T, Lefebrve PJ. Reduction of the acute bioavailability of metformin by the α-glucosidase inhibitor acarbose in normal man. *Eur J Clin Invest* (1994) 24 (Suppl 3), 50–4.
2. Lettieri J, Liu MC, Sullivan JT, Heller AH. Pharmacokinetic (PK) and pharmacodynamic (PD) interaction between acarbose (A) and metformin (M) in diabetic (NIDDM) patients. *Clin Pharmacol Ther* (1998) 63, 155.
3. Precose (Acarbose). Bayer HealthCare Pharmaceuticals Inc. US Prescribing information, March 2011.
4. Glyset (Miglitol). Pfizer Inc. US Prescribing information, September 2012.
5. Glucobay (Acarbose). Bayer plc. UK Summary of product characteristics, July 2013.

Alpha-glucosidase inhibitors + Miscellaneous

Neomycin might increase the efficacy and the gastrointestinal adverse effects of acarbose. Paralytic ileus has been reported in a Japanese patient given acarbose and promethazine. The pharmacokinetics of nifedipine do not appear to be altered by acarbose or miglitol. Acarbose did not alter ranitidine pharmacokinetics in one study, but miglitol decreased the exposure to ranitidine.

Clinical evidence, mechanism, importance and management

(a) Antimuscarinics

A 69-year-old man with a partial gastrectomy and type 2 diabetes, receiving insulin 24 units and **acarbose** 300 mg daily, was admitted to hospital with diabetic gangrene. After developing cold symptoms he was given *PL granules* (salicylamide, paracetamol, caffeine, and **promethazine** methylene disalicylate). The next day he experienced sudden abdominal pain, nausea, and vomiting, which was diagnosed as paralytic ileus. He was given intravenous fluids and piperacillin. Oral intake and **acarbose** were withheld and the ileus resolved after 2 days. The authors note that there are several reports of ileus developing in Japanese patients within 3 months of treatment with alpha-glucosidase inhibitors such as **acarbose**. The risk seems to be increased with increasing age, a history of abdominal surgery, and a Japanese diet (high in carbohydrates and fibre) rather than Western diet. However, in this case the patient had been taking **acarbose** for 15 months without problem, and it is possible that the antimuscarinic effects of **promethazine** may have contributed to the development of ileus.[1] The general clinical relevance of this case is uncertain. However, the authors consider that patients at risk should be monitored if they are given alpha-glucosidase inhibitors, especially if the dose is increased or if antimuscarinics are also given.[1]

(b) Neomycin

Neomycin alone has been reported to reduce postprandial blood glucose concentrations, and might enhance the reduction in postprandial glucose concentrations associated with **acarbose**.[2] In 7 healthy subjects, neomycin 1 g three times daily increased the unpleasant gastrointestinal adverse effects (flatulence, cramps, and diarrhoea) of **acarbose** 200 mg three times daily.[3] The UK manufacturer of acarbose suggests that if these adverse effects are severe, a temporary reduction in the dose of acarbose might be needed.[4]

(c) Nifedipine

The UK and US manufacturers of **acarbose** state that in a pilot study of a possible interaction with nifedipine, no significant or reproducible changes were seen in plasma nifedipine profiles.[4,5] Similarly, the US manufacturer of **miglitol** briefly notes that it had no effect on the pharmacokinetics and pharmacodynamics of nifedipine.[6] No nifedipine dose adjustment would seem necessary on concurrent use with acarbose or miglitol.

(d) Ranitidine

The US manufacturer of **acarbose** briefly notes that it had no effect on the pharmacokinetics or pharmacodynamics of ranitidine in healthy subjects.[5] The US manufacturer of **miglitol** notes that it reduced the bioavailability of ranitidine by 60%.[6] No ranitidine dose adjustment would seem necessary on concurrent use with acarbose. The clinical relevance of the reduction in ranitidine exposure with miglitol has not been assessed, but consider an interaction should any unexplained reduction in ranitidine efficacy occur.

1. Oba K, Kudo R, Yano M, Watanabe K, Ajiro Y, Okazaki K, Susuki T, Nakano H, Metori S. Ileus after administration of cold remedy in an elderly diabetic patient treated with acarbose. *J Nippon Med Sch* (2001) 68, 61–4.
2. Bayer, Personal Communication, June 1993.
3. Lembcke B, Caspary WF, Fölsch UR, Creutzfeldt W. Influence of neomycin on postprandial metabolic changes and side effects of an α-glucosidehydrolase inhibitor (BAY g 5421). I. Effects on intestinal hydrogen gas production and flatulence. In Frontiers of Hormone Research, vol 7. The Entero-Insular Axis. Satellite Symposium to Xth IDF-Meeting, September 7–8, Göttingen 1979, p 294–5.
4. Glucobay (Acarbose). Bayer plc. UK Summary of product characteristics, July 2013.
5. Precose (Acarbose). Bayer HealthCare Pharmaceuticals Inc. US Prescribing information, March 2011.
6. Glyset (Miglitol). Pfizer Inc. US Prescribing information, September 2012.

Alpha-glucosidase inhibitors + Sulfonylureas

Minor decreases in the plasma concentration of glibenclamide (glyburide) have been seen on concurrent use with acarbose or miglitol. Voglibose had no effect on glibenclamide pharmacokinetics in one study. Alpha-glucosidase inhibitors cause a moderate additional blood glucose-lowering effect when used with other antidiabetics, such as the sulfonylureas.

Clinical evidence

(a) Acarbose

A randomised, crossover study in 6 patients with type 2 diabetes, given acarbose 100 mg three times daily or placebo for 7 days with a single 5-mg dose of **glibenclamide** on day 7, found no effect on the pharmacokinetics of glibenclamide.[1]

(b) Miglitol

A randomised, placebo-controlled study in 28 patients with type 2 diabetes mellitus, given **glibenclamide** 2.5 mg twice daily with either miglitol 100 mg three times daily or placebo for 2 days, found that miglitol reduced the maximum plasma glibenclamide concentration and AUC by 16% and 19%, respectively. Nevertheless, the average blood glucose concentrations were reduced more by the drug combination than by glibenclamide alone: over 5 hours there was a 15% greater reduction, and over 10 hours a 9% greater reduction.[2] The US manufacturer of miglitol briefly reports several studies between miglitol and glibenclamide. In one study, 6 healthy subjects were given miglitol 50 mg three times daily for 4 days, followed by miglitol 100 mg three times daily for 2 days or placebo, and a single 5-mg dose of glibenclamide. The maximum glibenclamide concentration and AUC were 17% and 25% lower, respectively, when glibenclamide was given with miglitol than when it was given alone. In another study, diabetic patients taking glibenclamide 3.5 mg daily, received miglitol 100 mg three times daily for 7 days or placebo. The glibenclamide AUC was 18% lower in those patients receiving miglitol, but this did not reach statistical significance. A further study in diabetic patients receiving glibenclamide 10 mg daily, found that maximum glibenclamide concentrations were 16% and 8% lower at 6-months and 1-year, respectively, in those patients also receiving miglitol 100 mg three times daily than in those taking glibenclamide alone. This difference was also not statistically significant. There was no increased incidence of hypoglycaemia when miglitol was used with sulfonylureas in clinical studies, compared with that seen with sulfonylureas alone.[3]

(c) Voglibose

In a double-blind crossover study, 12 healthy male subjects were given either voglibose 5 mg, or placebo, three times daily for 8 days, and a single 1.75-mg dose of **glibenclamide** at the same time as the first dose of the voglibose or placebo on the morning of day 8. Voglibose had no effect on the pharmacokinetics of glibenclamide.[4]

Mechanism

The reason for the minor pharmacokinetic changes seen is uncertain.

Importance and management

Evidence for interactions between alpha-glucosidase inhibitors and the sulfonylureas appear to be limited to these studies with glibenclamide. The pharmacokinetic changes seen on the concurrent use of glibenclamide and acarbose, miglitol, or voglibose are minor and unlikely to be clinically relevant. The manufacturers state that while alpha-glucosidase inhibitors such as acarbose and miglitol do not cause hypoglycaemia when given alone, they might increase the blood glucose-lowering effects of the sulfonylureas, for which reason it might be necessary to reduce the sulfonylurea dose. Monitor the outcome on blood glucose concentrations when acarbose, miglitol, or voglibose is first given with a sulfonylurea. Any hypoglycaemic episodes should be treated with glucose (dextrose), not sucrose, because alpha-glucosidase inhibitors delay the digestion and absorption of disaccharides such as sucrose, but do not affect monosaccharides.[3,5,6] In general, it is prudent to monitor blood glucose concentrations when any change is made to the medication regimen of a patient with diabetes, and this should be sufficient to detect any interaction, should it occur.

1. Gerard J, Lefebvre PJ, Luyckx AS. Glibenclamide pharmacokinetics in acarbose-treated type 2 diabetics. *Eur J Clin Pharmacol* (1984) 27, 233–6.
2. Sullivan JT, Lettieri JT, Heller AH. Effects of miglitol on pharmacokinetics and pharmacodynamics of glyburide. *Clin Pharmacol Ther* (1998) 63, 155.
3. Glyset (Miglitol). Pfizer Inc. US Prescribing information, September 2012.
4. Kleist P, Ehrlich A, Suzuki Y, Timmer W, Wetzelsberger N, Lücker PW, Fuder H. Concomitant administration of the α-glucosidase inhibitor voglibose (AO-128) does not alter the pharmacokinetics of glibenclamide. *Eur J Clin Pharmacol* (1997) 53, 149–52.
5. Precose (Acarbose). Bayer HealthCare Pharmaceuticals Inc. US Prescribing information, March 2011.
6. Glucobay (Acarbose). Bayer plc. UK Summary of product characteristics, July 2013.

Alpha-glucosidase inhibitors; Acarbose + Colestyramine

Colestyramine might enhance the effect of acarbose, and insulin concentrations might rebound if both drugs are stopped at the same time.

Clinical evidence, mechanism, importance and management

Colestyramine 12 g daily for 6 days, given to 8 healthy subjects taking acarbose 100 mg three times daily, improved the reduction in postprandial insulin concentrations.[1] The mean serum insulin concentrations decreased by 23% while taking both drugs, but showed a rebound 31% increase above baseline when both drugs were stopped.[1] The clinical importance of the effects of colestyramine on acarbose in patients with diabetes is uncertain, although the UK manufacturer of acarbose notes that some enhancement of the effects of acarbose might occur, and they suggest care if both drugs are stopped at the same time because of the possible rebound phenomenon with respect to insulin concentrations.[2]

1. Bayer, Personal Communications, June-July 1993.
2. Glucobay (Acarbose). Bayer plc. UK Summary of product characteristics, July 2013.

Alpha-glucosidase inhibitors; Acarbose + Thiazolidinediones; Rosiglitazone

A minor decrease in rosiglitazone exposure has been seen on concurrent use with acarbose in one study.

Clinical evidence

A study in 16 healthy subjects found that acarbose 100 mg three times daily for one week reduced the AUC of a single 8-mg oral dose of rosiglitazone by 12%.[1]

Mechanism

The reason for the minor reduction in rosiglitazone exposure is uncertain.

Importance and management

Evidence for a pharmacokinetic interaction between acarbose and rosiglitazone is limited to one study. However, the reduction in rosiglitazone exposure seen is minor and unlikely to be clinically relevant. No dose adjustments would be expected to be necessary on concurrent use. However, it is prudent to monitor blood glucose concentrations when any change is made to the medication regimen of a patient with diabetes. Note that if hypoglycaemia occurs, it should be treated with glucose (dextrose), not sucrose, because alpha-glucosidase inhibitors delay the digestion and absorption of disaccharides such as sucrose, but do not affect monosaccharides.[2-4]

1. Miller AK, Inglis AM, Culkin KT, Jorkaksy DK, Freed MI. The effect of acarbose on the pharmacokinetics of rosiglitazone. *Eur J Clin Pharmacol* (2001) 57, 105–9.
2. Precose (Acarbose). Bayer HealthCare Pharmaceuticals Inc. US Prescribing information, March 2011.
3. Glyset (Miglitol). Pfizer Inc. US Prescribing information, September 2012.
4. Glucobay (Acarbose). Bayer plc. UK Summary of product characteristics, July 2013.

Antidiabetics + ACE inhibitors

The concurrent use of ACE inhibitors and antidiabetics normally appears to be uneventful but hypoglycaemia, marked in some instances, has occurred in a small number of patients with diabetes taking insulin or sulfonylureas with captopril, enalapril, lisinopril, or perindopril. This has been attributed, but not proved, to be due to an interaction.

Clinical evidence

Numerous case reports, small case-control studies, and a pharmacological study in healthy subjects suggest that ACE inhibitors increase the risk of hypoglycaemia when used with insulin or oral antidiabetics (mainly sulfonylureas where specified), and these are summarised in 'Table 13.2', p.500. Conversely several larger case-control studies and two randomised controlled studies have not found a notably increased risk of hypoglycaemia with ACE inhibitors in patients with diabetes, and these are also summarised in Table 13.2, p.500. It is worth highlighting that one of these, conducted by the United Kingdom Prospective Diabetes Study Group, found that the number of patients experiencing hypoglycaemic attacks did not differ between patients receiving **atenolol** 50 to 100 mg daily or **captopril** 25 to 50 mg twice daily for hypertension.[1] For more information about the use of beta blockers with antidiabetics, see 'Antidiabetics + Beta blockers', p.504 and 'Sulfonylureas; Glibenclamide (Glyburide) + Carvedilol', p.554.

Mechanism

The hypoglycaemia is not fully understood. An increase in glucose utilisation and increased insulin sensitivity have been suggested.[2,3] A review of studies in *rats* indicates that blockade of the renin angiotensin system might affect the pancreas, skeletal muscle, and adipose tissue leading to these effects;[4] further clinical study is required to established whether this is also the case in humans. Other possibilities (such as altered renal function) are discussed in a series of letters in *The Lancet*.[5-10] There is also an isolated report of persistent severe hypoglycaemia in a non-diabetic patient associated with both **captopril** and **ramipril**.[11] Conversely, high natural ACE activity has been associated with a higher risk of severe hypoglycaemia in patients with type 1 diabetes receiving insulin and not taking ACE inhibitors, leading to the hypothesis that ACE inhibitors might reduce the risk of hypoglycaemia in these individuals.[12]

Importance and management

The interaction between the antidiabetics and the ACE inhibitors is not well established, not understood, and remains the subject of considerable study and debate. However, some cases of severe hypoglycaemia have undoubtedly occurred in patients with diabetes managed with insulin or sulfonylureas as a result of the use of ACE inhibitors. Nevertheless, some authors consider the risk of severe hypoglycaemia in patients with diabetes taking ACE inhibitors to be very low, and inconsequential, when compared with the benefits of this class of drugs in diabetes.[13] Moreover, some evidence suggests that ACE inhibitors might have beneficial or neutral effects on insulin sensitivity and glycaemic control,[14-16] and a number of guidelines on the treatment of hypertension in diabetes, recommend that patients with diabetes and hypertension should be given an ACE inhibitor.[17,18] To be on the safe side, it might be prudent to warn all patients receiving insulin or sulfonylureas who are just starting any ACE inhibitor (although only captopril, enalapril, lisinopril, and perindopril have been implicated) that excessive hypoglycaemia has been seen very rarely and unpredictably. The problem has been resolved in some patients by reducing the sulfonylurea dose by 50 to 75%.[19,20]

Cases with other oral antidiabetics are lacking, but note that some manufacturers warn that ACE inhibitors might decrease blood glucose concentrations on concurrent use, and advise that antidiabetic dose adjustments might be necessary.

The pharmacokinetic interactions and/or other effects of antidiabetic drugs with ACE inhibitors are covered under the individual drug groups elsewhere in this chapter.

A false positive urine ketone test can also occur with captopril when using the alkaline-nitroprusside test (*Ketodiastix*), which might affect the monitoring of diabetic control.[21]

1. UK Prospective Diabetes Study Group. Efficacy of atenolol and captopril in reducing risk of macrovascular and microvascular complications in type 2 diabetes: UKPDS 39. *BMJ* (1998) 317, 713–20.

Table 13.2 Interactions between antidiabetics and ACE inhibitors

Patients	*ACE inhibitor*	*Antidiabetic*	*Notes*	*Refs*
Evidence for hypoglycaemia				
1 case	Captopril 50 mg/day	Glibenclamide (glyburide) 10.5 mg/day Metformin 1.7 g/day	Blood glucose 2.2 mmol/L 24 hours after the addition of captopril.	1
1 case	Captopril	Glibenclamide 10.5 mg/day Metformin 1.7 g/day	Blood glucose of 2.9 mmol/L 48 hours after starting captopril. Antidiabetic drugs stopped.	1
3 cases	Captopril	Glibenclamide	Hypoglycaemia reported to a Spanish Regional Pharmacosurveillance centre.	2
1 case	Captopril 12.5 mg/day	Glibenclamide 2.5 mg/day	Hypoglycaemia 7 hours after first dose, blood glucose 2.1 mmol/L, glibenclamide stopped.	3
1 case	Captopril	Unspecified oral antidiabetic	Hypoglycaemia, oral antidiabetic withdrawn.	4
5 cases	Captopril	Unspecified sulfonylureas	Hypoglycaemia reported to Centres Regionaux de Pharmacovigilance in France.	5
3 cases case control study	Captopril	Unspecified oral antidiabetics	Risk of hypoglycaemia increased 3.1-fold.	6
9 cases case control study	Captopril	Insulin	Risk of hypoglycaemia increased 3.7-fold.	6
4 cases	Captopril	Insulin	Hypoglycaemia reported to a Spanish Regional Pharmacosurveillance centre.	2
3 cases	Captopril	Insulin	Unexplained hypoglycaemia.	4
1 case	Enalapril 5 mg/day	Glibenclamide 5 mg/day	Hypoglycaemia, blood glucose 2.3 mmol/L. Dose of glibenclamide reduced to 2.5 mg/day.	3
2 cases	Enalapril 5 mg/day	Glibenclamide 5 mg/day	Hypoglycaemic attacks, glibenclamide reduced to 1.25 mg/day.	7
9 healthy subjects (double-blind, crossover study)	Enalapril 5 mg/day, then 10 mg/day	Glibenclamide 3.5 mg single dose	Hypoglycaemic effects of glibenclamide temporarily enhanced between 2 and 4 hours after enalapril was taken.	8
4 cases	Enalapril	Glibenclamide	Hypoglycaemia reported to a Spanish Regional Pharmacosurveillance centre.	2
1 case	Enalapril	Gliclazide 80 mg/day	Hypoglycaemia when enalapril dose increased from 5 to 10 mg/day.	9
4 cases	Enalapril	Unspecified sulfonylureas	Hypoglycaemia reported to Centres Regionaux de Pharmacovigilance in France.	5
1 case	Enalapril	Unspecified sulfonylurea	Recurrent hypoglycaemia, sulfonylurea withdrawn.	10
10 cases case control study	Enalapril	Unspecified sulfonylurea Insulin	2.4-fold increase in the risk of hypoglycaemia with sulfonylureas. However, no increased risk was seen in insulin users. In addition when all ACE inhibitors were considered together, no significant increase in risk was seen.	11
2 cases case control study	Enalapril	Unspecified oral antidiabetics	Non-significant 5.4-fold increase in the risk of hypoglycaemia.	6
3 cases case control study	Enalapril	Insulin	Non-significant 1.7-fold increase in the risk of hypoglycaemia.	6
1 case	Enalapril	Insulin	Reduced insulin requirements.	10
11 cases	Enalapril	Insulin	Hypoglycaemia reported to a Spanish Regional Pharmacosurveillance centre.	2
1 case	Lisinopril	Glibenclamide and metformin	Hypoglycaemia reported to a Spanish Regional Pharmacosurveillance centre.	2
1 case	Lisinopril 10 mg/day	Gliclazide	Hypoglycaemia resolved on stopping gliclazide.	9
1 case	Perindopril	Glibenclamide	Hypoglycaemia reported to a Spanish Regional Pharmacosurveillance centre.	2
1 case	Ramipril 2.5 mg/day	Glibenclamide 5 mg/day Metformin 1.7 g/day	Patient also on naproxen, renal function deteriorated causing hypoglycaemia due to accumulation of oral antidiabetics.	12
7 cases case control study	Unspecified ACE inhibitor	Insulin or oral antidiabetics	3.2-fold increase in the risk of hypoglycaemia leading to hospitalisation.	13

Continued

Table 13.2 Interactions between antidiabetics and ACE inhibitors (continued)

Patients	*ACE inhibitor*	*Antidiabetic*	*Notes*	*Refs*
Evidence of no interaction				
8 cases	Captopril 37.5 mg/day	Insulin	No change to daily insulin requirements. No evidence of symptomatic hypoglycaemia.	14
38 cases	Captopril 50 to 100 mg/day or Enalapril 20 to 40 mg/day	Insulin or oral antidiabetics	Antidiabetic treatment unaltered, no evidence of unusual or unexplained hypoglycaemia.	15
18 cases double blind controlled study	Enalapril 20 to 40 mg/day	Insulin	No change to daily insulin requirements. No evidence of unexplained hypoglycaemia.	15
428 patients randomised controlled study	Lisinopril 10 to 20 mg/day or placebo	Insulin	No difference in the number of hypoglycaemic episodes between lisinopril and placebo recipients.	16
22 cases case control study	Captopril or Enalapril	Insulin or oral antidiabetics	Data from Centres Regionaux de Pharmacovigilance in France used. No increased risk of hypoglycaemia detected.	17
598 cases of hypoglycaemia in a retrospective study	Captopril or Enalapril or other classes of antihypertensive	Insulin or oral antidiabetics	No statistically significant increase or decrease in the risk of serious hypoglycaemia among users of ACE inhibitors or any other class of antihypertensives compared with non users of antihypertensives.	18
758 patients randomised controlled study	Captopril 50 to 100 mg/day or atenolol	Insulin or oral antidiabetics or diet alone	The proportion of patients with hypoglycaemic attacks did not differ between the captopril and atenolol groups.	19
336 reports case control study	Captopril or Enalapril	Antidiabetics	Data from the French pharmacovigilance database used. No increased risk of hypoglycaemia detected when confounding by indication considered.	20

1. Rett K, Wicklmayr M, Dietz GJ. Hypoglycemia in hypertensive diabetic patients treated with sulfonylureas, biguanides and captopril. *N Engl J Med* (1988) 319, 1609.
2. Aguirre C, Ayani I, Rodriguez-Sasiain JM. Hypoglycaemia associated with angiotensin converting enzyme inhibitors. *Therapie* (1995) 50 (Suppl), 198.
3. Arauz-Pacheco C, Ramirez LC, Rios JM, Raskin P. Hypoglycemia induced by angiotensin-converting enzyme inhibitors in patients with non-insulin-dependent diabetes receiving sulfonylurea therapy. *Am J Med* (1990) 89, 811-13.
4. Ferriere M, Lachkar H, Richard J-L, Bringer J, Orsetti A, Mirouze J. Captopril and insulin sensitivity. *Ann Intern Med* (1985) 102, 134-5.
5. Girardin E, Vial T, Pham E, Evreux J-C. Hypoglycémies induites par les sulfamides hypoglycémiants. *Ann Med Interne (Paris)* (1992) 143, 11-17.
6. Herings RMC, de Boer A, Stricker BHC, Leufkens HGM, Porsius A. Hypoglycaemia associated with use of inhibitors of angiotensin converting enzyme. *Lancet* (1995) 345, 1195-8.
7. Ahmad S. Drug interaction induces hypoglycemia. *J Fam Pract* (1995) 40, 540-1.
8. Rave K, Flesch S, Kühn-Velten WN, Hompesch BC, Heinemann L, Heise T. Enhancement of blood glucose lowering effect of a sulfonylurea when coadministered with an ACE inhibitor: results of a glucose-clamp study. *Diabetes Metab Res Rev* (2005) 21, 459–64.
9. Veyre B, Ginon I, Vial T, Dragol F, Daumont M. Hypoglycémies par interférence entre un inhibiteur de l'enzyme de conversion et un sulfamide hypoglycémiant. *Presse Med* (1993) 22, 738.
10. McMurray J, Fraser DM. Captopril, enalapril and blood glucose. *Lancet* (1986) i, 1035.
11. Thamer M, Ray NF, Taylor T. Association between antihypertensive drug use and hypoglycemia: a case-control study of diabetic users of insulin or sulfonylureas. *Clin Ther* (1999) 21, 1387-1400.
12. Collin M, Mucklow JC. Drug interactions, renal impairment and hypoglycaemia in a patient with type II diabetes. *Br J Clin Pharmacol* (1999) 48, 134-7.
13. Morris AD, Boyle DIR, McMahon AD, Pearce H, Evans JMM, Newton RW, Jung RT, MacDonald TM, The DARTS/MEMO collaboration. ACE inhibitor use is associated with hospitalization for severe hypoglycaemia in patients with diabetes. *Diabetes Care* (1997) 20, 1363-7.
14. Winocour P, Waldek S, Anderson DC. Captopril and blood glucose. *Lancet* (1986) ii, 461.
15. Passa P, Marre M, Leblanc H. Enalapril, captopril and blood glucose. *Lancet* (1986) i, 1447.
16. The EUCLID study group. Randomised placebo-controlled trial of lisinopril in normotensive patients with insulin-dependent diabetes and normoalbuminuria or microalbuminuria. *Lancet* (1997) 349, 1787-92.
17. Moore N, Kreft-Jais C, Haramburu F, Noblet C, Andrejak M, Ollagnier M, Bégaud B. Reports of hypoglycaemia associated with the use of ACE inhibitors and other drugs: a case/non-case study in the French pharmacovigilance system database. *Br J Clin Pharmacol* (1997) 44, 513-8.
18. Shorr RI, Ray WA, Daugherty JR, Griffin MR. Antihypertensives and the risk of serious hypoglycemia in older persons using insulin or sulfonylureas. *JAMA* (1997) 278, 40–3.
19. UK Prospective Diabetes Study Group. Efficacy of atenolol and captopril in reducing risk of macrovascular and microvascular complications in type 2 diabetes: UKPDS 39. *BMJ* (1998) 317, 713–20.
20. Grégoire F, Pariente A, Fourrier-Reglat A, Haramburu F, Bégaud B, Moore N. A signal of increased risk of hypoglycaemia with angiotensin receptor blockers caused by confounding. *Br J Clin Pharmacol* (2008) 66, 142–5.

2. Ferriere M, Lachkar H, Richard J-L, Bringer J, Orsetti A, Mirouze J. Captopril and insulin sensitivity. *Ann Intern Med* (1985) 102, 134–5.
3. Girardin E, Vial T, Pham E, Evreux J-C. Hypoglycémies induites par les sulfamides hypoglycémiants. *Ann Med Interne (Paris)* (1992) 143, 11–17.
4. van der Zijl NJ, Moors CCM, Goossens GH, Blaak EE, Diamant M. Does interference with the renin-angiotensin system protect against diabetes? Evidence and mechanisms. *Diabetes Obes Metab* (2012) 14, 586–95.
5. van Haeften TW. ACE inhibitors and hypoglycaemia. *Lancet* (1995) 346, 125.
6. Kong N, Bates A, Ryder REJ. ACE inhibitors and hypoglycaemia. *Lancet* (1995) 346, 125.
7. Feher MD, Amiel S. ACE inhibitors and hypoglycaemia. *Lancet* (1995) 346, 125–6.
8. Davie AP. ACE inhibitors and hypoglycaemia. *Lancet* (1995) 346, 126.
9. Wildenborg IHM, Veenstra J, van der Voort PHJ, Verdegaal WP, Silberbusch J. ACE inhibitors and hypoglycaemia. *Lancet* (1995) 346, 126.
10. Herings RMC, de Boer A, Stricker BHC, Leufkens HGM, Porsius AJ. ACE inhibitors and hypoglycaemia. *Lancet* (1995) 346, 126–7.
11. Elorriaga-Sánchez F, Corrales-Bobadilla H, Sosa-Trinidad E, Domínguez-Quezada B. Hipoglucemia severa secundaria a inhibidores de la enzima convertidora de angiotensina en ausencia de diabetes mellitus. Reporte de un caso. *Gac Med Mex* (2001) 137, 249–52.
12. Pedersen-Bjergaard U, Agerholm-Larsen B, Pramming S, Hougaard P, Thorsteinsson B. Prediction of severe hypoglycaemia by angiotensin-converting enzyme activity and genotype in type 1 diabetes. *Diabetologia* (2003) 46, 89–96.
13. Scheen AJ. Drug interactions of clinical importance with antihyperglycaemic agents: an update. *Drug Safety* (2005) 28, 601–31.
14. Sarafidis PA, Bakris GL. Antihypertensive therapy and the risk of new-onset diabetes. *Diabetes Care* (2006) 29, 1167–9.
15. Sarafidis PA, McFarlane SI, Bakris GL. Antihypertensive agents, insulin sensitivity, and new-onset diabetes. *Curr Diab Rep* (2007) 7, 191–9.
16. DREAM Trial Investigators, Bosch J, Yusuf S, Gerstein HC, Pogue J, Sheridan P, Dagenais G, Diaz R, Avezum A, Lanas F, Probstfield J, Fodor G, Holman RR. Effect of ramipril on the incidence of diabetes. *N Engl J Med* (2006) 355, 1551–62.
17. National Institute for Clinical Excellence. Type 2 diabetes: the management of type 2 diabetes: partial update (issued March 2010). Available at: http://www.nice.org.uk/guidance/CG87 (accessed 21/10/15).
18. American Diabetes Association. Standards of medical care in diabetes—2011. *Diabetes Care* (2011) 34 (Suppl 1), S11–S61.
19. Arauz-Pacheco C, Ramirez LC, Rios JM, Raskin P. Hypoglycemia induced by angiotensin-converting enzyme inhibitors in patients with non-insulin-dependent diabetes receiving sulfonylurea therapy. *Am J Med* (1990) 89, 811–13.
20. Ahmad S. Drug interaction induces hypoglycemia. *J Fam Pract* (1995) 40, 540–1.
21. Warren SE. False-positive urine ketone test with captopril. *N Engl J Med* (1980) 303, 1003–4.

Antidiabetics + Alcohol

Patients with diabetes need not abstain from alcohol, but they should drink only in moderation and accompanied by food. Epidemiological evidence suggests that heart disease might be less common in patients

with diabetes who drink in moderation. However, alcohol makes the signs of hypoglycaemia less clear and delayed hypoglycaemia can occur. The CNS depressant effects of alcohol in conjunction with hypoglycaemia can make driving or the operation of dangerous machinery much more hazardous.

Clinical evidence

1. Effect on glucose concentrations. The effect of alcohol on the blood glucose concentrations of patients with diabetes is variable and has been the subject of much research. Blood glucose concentrations might be reduced, remain unchanged, or be increased by alcohol, depending on the amount drunk at one time, if it is drunk with food or not, and if use is chronic and excessive.[1]

Early studies showed both hypoglycaemic effects and no effect on blood glucose concentrations after alcohol consumption in patients with diabetes. For specific information about the effect of alcohol in patients receiving insulin, see 'Insulin + Alcohol', p.526, or tolbutamide, see 'Sulfonylureas + Alcohol', p.539'.

More recently, a cross-sectional study of 38 564 diabetic patients found that moderate alcohol consumption was associated with improved glycaemic control, assessed using HbA_{1c} concentrations, such that the highest HbA_{1c} concentrations were associated with minimal alcohol consumption or lifetime abstention, and the lowest HbA_{1c} concentrations with consumption of 2 to 2.9 drinks/day.[2] A review of six earlier studies drew similar conclusions.[3] However, 2 other much smaller studies found that regular alcohol intake (defined in one study as mean 45 g/day[4]) worsened glycaemic control.[4,5]

2. Effect on diabetic complications. A review of 4 epidemiological studies concluded that heart disease is less common in people with diabetes who drink moderate amounts of alcohol than in those who do not.[3]

Mechanism

The exacerbation of hypoglycaemia by alcohol is not fully understood. However, it is known that if hypoglycaemia occurs when liver glycogen stores are low, the liver turns to the formation of new glucose from amino acids (gluconeogenesis). This gluconeogenesis is inhibited by the presence of alcohol so that the decrease in blood glucose concentrations might not be prevented and a full-scale hypoglycaemic episode can result.

Importance and management

The documentation of the interactions between antidiabetic drugs and alcohol is surprisingly patchy (with the exception of chlorpropamide and alcohol, see 'Sulfonylureas + Alcohol', p.539), but they are of recognised clinical importance.

The following contains the main recommendations of the Diabetes UK nutrition guidelines and patient information:[6,7] most patients with diabetes need not avoid alcohol totally, but they are advised not to exceed 2 units (for women) or 3 units (for men) daily. A drink (or unit) is defined in 'Table 3.1', p.52. The intake of drinks with high-carbohydrate content (sweet sherries, sweet wines, most liqueurs, and low alcohol wines) should be limited. Patients with diabetes should not drink on an empty stomach and they should know that the warning signs of hypoglycaemia might possibly be obscured by the effects of the alcohol. Driving or handling dangerous machinery should be avoided because the CNS depressant effects of alcohol plus hypoglycaemia can be particularly hazardous. Warn patients of the risks of hypoglycaemia occurring several hours after drinking. Those with peripheral neuropathy should be told that alcohol could aggravate the condition and they should not have more than one drink daily. Provided drinking is restricted as suggested, and drinks containing a lot of carbohydrate are avoided, there is no need to include the drink in the dietary allowance. However, patients with diabetes on a weight-reducing diet should try to limit intake to the occasional drink and should include it in their daily calorie allowance.

The advice of the American Diabetes Association is similar: if individuals choose to drink alcohol, daily intake should be limited to one drink (for women) or 2 drinks (for men). To reduce the risk of hypoglycaemia in individuals using insulin or oral insulin secretagogues, alcohol should be consumed with food.[1]

There is some evidence that heart disease in patients with diabetes might be less common in patients who consume moderate amounts of alcohol, but this is currently not sufficient to recommend that patients who do not drink alcohol should begin to drink in moderation.[3]

1. American Diabetes Association. Nutrition recommendations and interventions for diabetes. *Diabetes Care* (2008) 31 (Suppl 1), S61–S78.
2. Ahmed AT, Karter AJ, Warton EM, Doan JU, Weisner CM. The relationship between alcohol consumption and glycemic control among patients with diabetes: the Kaiser Permanente Northern California Diabetes Registry. *J Gen Intern Med* (2008) 23, 275–82.
3. Howard AA, Arnsten JH, Gourevitch MN. Effect of alcohol consumption on diabetes mellitus: a systematic review. *Ann Intern Med* (2004) 140, 211–19.
4. Ben G, Gnudi L, Maran A, Gigante A, Duner E, Iori E, Tiengo A, Avogaro A. Effects of chronic alcohol intake on carbohydrate and lipid metabolism in subjects with type II (non-insulin dependent) diabetes. *Am J Med* (1991) 90, 70–6.
5. Tsai CS, Oke TO, Tam CW, Olubadewo JO, Ochillo RF. The effect of regular alcohol use on the management of non-insulin diabetes mellitus. *Cell Mol Biol (Noisy-le-grand)* (2003) 49, 1327–32.
6. Diabetes UK. Evidence-based nutrition guidelines for the prevention and management of diabetes (May 2011). Available at: http://www.diabetes.org.uk/Documents/Reports/Nutritional_guidelines200911.pdf (accessed 20/10/15).
7. Diabetes UK. Alcohol and Diabetes (May 2009). Available at: http://www.diabetes.org.uk/Documents/catalogue/Alcohol%20and%20diabetes%202009.pdf (accessed 20/10/15).

Antidiabetics + Anabolic steroids or Androgens

Nandrolone, methandienone, testosterone, and stanozolol can enhance the blood glucose-lowering effects of insulin, and testosterone might also improve glycaemic control in those taking oral antidiabetics.

Clinical evidence

(a) Insulin

In a study in 54 patients with diabetes taking **nandrolone phenylpropionate** 25 mg weekly, or **nandrolone decanoate** 50 mg given every 3 weeks by intramuscular injection, it was found necessary to reduce the **insulin** dose by an average of 36% (reduction of 4 to 56 units) in about one-third of the patients.[1] In another placebo-controlled study in hypogonadal men with type 2 diabetes, of 10 patients using **insulin**, 5 reduced their daily insulin dose (by a mean of 7 units) while receiving intramuscular **testosterone esters** (*Sustanon*) once every 2 weeks for 3 months.[2]

Other reports similarly describe an enhanced reduction in blood glucose concentrations in patients with diabetes receiving **insulin** and **nandrolone**,[3,4] **methandienone**,[5] **testosterone propionate**,[6] or **stanozolol**.[7] No changes were seen when **ethylestrenol** was used.[1,3]

(b) Oral antidiabetics

In a placebo-controlled study in hypogonadal men with type 2 diabetes, intramuscular **testosterone esters** (*Sustanon*) once every 2 weeks for 3 months reduced fasting glucose by a mean of 1.6 mmol/L and HbA_{1c} by 0.37% (from over 7.4% to about 7.1%) in the 14 who were taking oral antidiabetics (11 patients) or diet alone (3 patients). The oral antidiabetics being taken were **metformin** alone or with **gliclazide** and/or **rosiglitazone**.[2] However, a study in 11 men with normal testosterone concentrations and type 2 diabetes given intramuscular testosterone 100 mg every 3 weeks, for 3 months, found no effect on glucose tolerance or insulin sensitivity. The oral antidiabetics being taken were **glibenclamide (glyburide)**, **gliclazide**, and **glipizide** with or without **metformin**.[8]

Mechanism

Uncertain. Some evidence suggests that androgens improve insulin sensitivity, although androgens are often considered to impair glucose tolerance. A reduction in blood glucose concentrations has been seen in healthy subjects given testosterone propionate.[9] In contrast, another study in healthy subjects given testosterone supplementation for 2 years, found no effect on glucose tolerance or insulin sensitivity.[10]

Importance and management

The interactions between the anabolic steroids or androgens and antidiabetics are established, but the total picture is incomplete because not all of the anabolic steroids appear to have been studied and they might not necessarily behave identically. A reduction in the dose requirements of insulin (of an average of one-third[1]) might be expected in many patients with the steroids cited. Some improvement in glycaemic control might also occur in patients receiving oral antidiabetics. Given these results, and the fact that, conversely, anabolic steroids have also been shown to *impair* glucose tolerance it would seem prudent to closely monitor blood glucose concentrations on concurrent use with any antidiabetic drug.

1. Houtsmuller AJ. The therapeutic applications of anabolic steroids in ophthalmology: biochemical results. *Acta Endocrinol (Copenh)* (1961) 39 (Suppl 63), 154–74.
2. Kapoor D, Goodwin E, Channer KS, Jones TH. Testosterone replacement therapy improves insulin resistance, glycaemic control, visceral adiposity and hypercholesterolaemia in hypogonadal men with type 2 diabetes. *Eur J Endocrinol* (2006) 154, 899–906.
3. Dardenne U. The therapeutic applications of anabolic steroids in ophthalmology. *Acta Endocrinol (Copenh)* (1961) 39 (Suppl 63), 143–53.
4. Weissel W. Anaboles Hormon bei malignem oder kompliziertem Diabetes mellitus. *Wien Klin Wochenschr* (1962) 74, 234–6.
5. Landon J, Wynn V, Samols E, Bilkus D. The effect of anabolic steroids on blood sugar and plasma insulin levels in man. *Metabolism* (1963) 12, 924–35.
6. Veil WH, Lippross O. 'Unspezifische' wirkungen der Männlichen keimdrücenhormone. *Klin Wochenschr* (1938) 17, 655–8.
7. Pergola F. El estanozolol, nuevo anabolico. *Prensa Med Argent* (1962) 49, 274–90.
8. Lee CH, Kuo SW, Hung YJ, Hsieh CH, He CT, Yang TC, Lian WC, Chyi-Fan S, Pei D. The effect of testosterone supplement on insulin sensitivity, glucose effectiveness, and acute insulin response after glucose load in male type 2 diabetics. Endocr Res. (2005) 31, 139–48.
9. Talaat M, Habib YA, Habib M. The effect of testosterone on the carbohydrate metabolism in normal subjects. *Arch Int Pharmacodyn Ther* (1957) 111, 215–26.
10. Basu R, Dalla Man C, Campioni M, Basu A, Nair KS, Jensen MD, Khosla S, Klee G,Toffolo G, Cobelli C, Rizza RA. Effect of 2 years of testosterone replacement on insulin secretion, insulin action, glucose effectiveness, hepatic insulin clearance, and postprandial glucose turnover in elderly men. *Diabetes Care* (2007) 30, 1972–8.

Antidiabetics + Angiotensin II receptor antagonists

There is some experimental evidence that suggests that losartan and eprosartan possibly reduce awareness of hypoglycaemic symptoms, but no increased risk was seen in a large epidemiological study.

Clinical evidence

A study in 16 healthy subjects found that a single 600-microgram dose of **eprosartan** did not significantly affect adrenaline (epinephrine) release in response to **insulin**-induced hypoglycaemia, but the eprosartan tended to blunt some of the haemodynamic responses to hypoglycaemia.[1] Theoretically, therefore, hypoglycaemic symptoms could be reduced in some patients with diabetes. Three patients with type 1 diabetes spontaneously reported reduced awareness of hypoglycaemic symptoms (tremor, palpitations, nervousness) after **losartan** was started. A placebo-controlled study in 16 healthy subjects given **losartan** 50 mg daily for 8 days confirmed an attenuation of the symptomatic and hormonal responses to hypoglycaemia.[2] However, in contrast, an early similar study found no such effect.[3] The French pharmacovigilance database was examined for an association between angiotensin II receptor antagonists and reported hypoglycaemia. Although an association was found (odds ratio 2) this was confounded by an association between use of angiotensin II receptor antagonists and antidiabetic drugs. When looking specifically at patients taking antidiabetic drugs, there was no association between angiotensin II receptor antagonist use and hypoglycaemia, and in fact, a reduced risk of reporting hypoglycaemia (odds ratio 0.4). Angiotensin II receptor antagonists used in order of frequency included **losartan**, **irbesartan**, **valsartan**, **candesartan**, **telmisartan**, and **eprosartan**.[4]

Mechanism

It has been suggested that blocking angiotensin II will block the adrenaline (epinephrine) response to insulin-induced hypoglycaemia, and thereby reduce awareness of hypoglycaemia. However, early studies found that angiotensin II receptor antagonists of the AT1 subtype, such as losartan, were not able to do this on their own, and AT2 subtype blockers were needed as well.[3,5]

Importance and management

There is some experimental evidence that suggests that symptoms of hypoglycaemia might be reduced by losartan and possibly other angiotensin II receptor antagonists, although one epidemiological study provided some reassurance that this might not be clinically important. Bear the possibility in mind. Note that it is prudent to monitor blood glucose concentrations when any change is made to the medication regimen of a patient with diabetes, and this should be sufficient to detect any interaction, should it occur. Further clinical study is needed, but note that this is similar to the possible effect of ACE inhibitors, see 'Antidiabetics + ACE inhibitors', p.499.

The pharmacokinetic interactions of antidiabetic drugs with angiotensin II receptor antagonists are covered under the individual drug groups elsewhere in this chapter.

1. Christensen M, Ibsen H, Worck R. Effect of eprosartan on catecholamines and peripheral haemodynamics in subjects with insulin-induced hypoglycaemia. *Clin Sci* (2005) 108, 113–19.
2. Deininger E, Oltmanns KM, Wellhoener P, Fruehwald-Schultes B, Kern W, Heuer B, Dominiak P, Born J, Fehm HL, Peters A. Losartan attenuates symptomatic and hormonal responses to hypoglycemia in humans. *Clin Pharmacol Ther* (2001) 70, 362–9.
3. Worck RH, Ibsen H, Frandsen E, Dige-Petersen H. AT_1 receptor blockade and the sympathoadrenal response to insulin-induced hypoglycemia in humans. *Am J Physiol* (1997) 272, E415–E421.
4. Grégoire F, Pariente A, Fourrier-Reglat A, Haramburu F, Bégaud B, Moore N. A signal of increased risk of hypoglycaemia with angiotensin receptor blockers caused by confounding. *Br J Clin Pharmacol* (2008) 66, 142–5.
5. Worck RH, Frandsen E, Ibsen H, Petersen JS. AT_1 and AT_2 receptor blockade and epinephrine release during insulin-induced hypoglycemia. *Hypertension* (1998) 31, 384–90.

Antidiabetics + Antimalarials

Hydroxychloroquine can reduce insulin requirements, which has resulted in hypoglycaemia in patients with diabetes managed with insulin. Hydroxychloroquine has also improved glycaemic control in patients taking glibenclamide (glyburide) and rosiglitazone. Similarly, hypoglycaemia has occurred in a patient taking chloroquine and insulin, and quinine reduces blood glucose concentrations in patients taking gliclazide.

Clinical evidence

(a) Effect on diabetic control

1. Chloroquine. A case report describes a patient with type 1 diabetes, who had developed insulin resistance and was maintained on intravenous **insulin**, who showed a dramatic return of sensitivity to subcutaneous **insulin**, heralded by a series of hypoglycaemic attacks, within 15 days of starting to take chloroquine phosphate 200 mg every 8 hours.[1] Similarly, chloroquine phosphate (150 mg of chloroquine base) four times daily improved glucose tolerance in 5 out of 6 patients with type 2 diabetes controlled by diet, but had little effect in healthy subjects.[2]

2. Hydroxychloroquine. The effect of hydroxychloroquine on diabetic control with **insulin** or **glibenclamide (glyburide)** was investigated in a randomised, double-blind, placebo-controlled study in 38 patients with poorly controlled type 2 diabetes. The addition of hydroxychloroquine 200 mg three times daily to **insulin** caused a notable improvement in the glycaemic profile and the daily **insulin** dose had to be reduced by about 25%. Patients taking **glibenclamide** with hydroxychloroquine also had a notable improvement in their plasma glucose concentrations. One patient receiving **insulin** and hydroxychloroquine had severe hypoglycaemia after 2 months of concurrent use, and it was necessary to drastically reduce the daily dose of **insulin**.[3] In another similar study, 135 patients with poorly controlled type 2 diabetes taking **glibenclamide** 10 mg twice daily were randomised to receive placebo or hydroxychloroquine 300 mg daily, increased up to a maximum of 300 mg twice daily. Fewer patients stopped hydroxychloroquine than placebo because of a lack of effect on improving blood glucose control (54% versus 82%). In addition, hydroxychloroquine reduced HbA_{1c} by 0.96% more than placebo.[4]

A case report describes a 77-year old man receiving a stable dose of **insulin** of 16 units twice daily who was diagnosed with rheumatoid arthritis. He was started on prednisolone 5 mg daily and hydroxychloroquine 400 mg daily, with an increase in insulin dose of 4 units daily in anticipation of prednisolone-induced impairment of glucose control. However he continued to have nightly hypoglycaemic episodes, and, one week later he had a hypoglycaemic attack requiring intravenous dextrose. His insulin dose was reduced back to the original dose, and over 6 weeks was gradually reduced to 10 units twice daily with good glycaemic control.[5] Similarly, a 49-year old woman with type 2 diabetes and systemic lupus erythematosus (SLE) stabilised on **rosiglitazone** 8 mg daily and **insulin** 25 units daily, reported episodes of hypoglycaemia immediately after starting hydroxychloroquine 200 mg twice daily. The patient herself stopped the insulin but continued with the hydroxychloroquine, rosiglitazone, and other stable medications (methotrexate, prednisone, aspirin, hydrochlorthiazide/triamterene, and folic acid). Her blood glucose concentrations normalised within 2 days of her making this change, and 2 months later her HbA_{1c} was 5.7% (compared with 6.2% before starting the hydroxychloroquine). Six months later the rosiglitazone was switched to **pioglitazone**, and her HbA_{1c} remained stable at 5.8%.[6]

3. Quinine. A study in 12 patients (age 51 to 79 years) with type 2 diabetes taking **gliclazide**, and 10 similar, non-diabetic subjects, found that a single 600-mg dose of **quinine sulphate** at night reduced serum glucose concentrations in both groups, without affecting serum insulin concentrations.[7] Profound and persistent hypoglycaemia was seen in one patient with type 2 diabetes and severe falciparum malaria treated with **quinine**, but the hypoglycaemia evolved before the use of **quinine** and resolved as the parasitaemia was successfully eradicated, despite continuation of the **quinine**. Subsequently, as she had discontinued antidiabetic medication (**chlorpropamide**) before hospital admission, hyperglycaemia developed (blood glucose ranging from 7.5 to 16 mmol/L) despite continuing to take **quinine**.[8]

Mechanism

Quinine has been shown in experimental studies to stimulate insulin release, whereas this was not shown for chloroquine, mefloquine, amodiaquine, and halofantrine.[9] A later study in patients with diabetes found that chloroquine both inhibits insulin degradation and increases insulin secretion.[10] A study in obese non-diabetic subjects suggests that hydroxychloroquine can improve insulin sensitivity.[11]

Importance and management

An interaction between antidiabetics and antimalarials is not well established, but it appears that hydroxychloroquine can cause a modest reduction in blood glucose concentrations, which is additive with antidiabetic treatment, such as insulin, glibenclamide (glyburide), and rosiglitazone or pioglitazone. Bear this in mind if hydroxychloroquine is required in a patient with diabetes. Note that it is prudent to monitor blood glucose concentrations when any change is made to the medication regimen of a patient with diabetes, and this would seem to be sufficient to detect any interaction with hydroxychloroquine, should it occur. Chloroquine appears to act similarly. Mefloquine and quinine have also been reported to reduce blood glucose concentrations. Some evidence is complicated by the use of quinine in malaria, as malaria can also cause hypoglycaemia.

1. Rees RG, Smith MJ. Effect of chloroquine on insulin and glucose homoeostasis in normal subjects and patients with non-insulin dependent diabetes mellitus. *BMJ* (1987) 294, 900–1.
2. Smith GD, Amos TAS, Mahler R, Peters TJ. Effect of chloroquine on insulin and glucose homoeostasis in normal subjects and patients with non-insulin-dependent diabetes mellitus. *BMJ* (1987) 294, 465–7.
3. Quatraro A, Consoli G, Magno M, Caretta F, Nardozza A, Ceriello A, Giugliano D. Hydroxychloroquine in decompensated, treatment-refractory noninsulin-dependent diabetes mellitus. A new job for an old drug? *Ann Intern Med* (1990) 112, 678–81.
4. Gerstein HC, Thorpe KE, Taylor DW, Haynes RB. The effectiveness of hydroxychloroquine in patients with type 2 diabetes mellitus who are refractory to sulfonylureas–a randomized trial. *Diabetes Res Clin Pract* (2002) 55, 209–19.
5. Shojania K, Koehler BE, Elliott T. Hypoglycemia induced by hydroxychloroquine in a type II diabetic treated for polyarthritis. *J Rheumatol* (1999) 26, 195–6.
6. Kang L, Mikuls TR, O'Dell JR. Hydroxychloroquine: a diabetic drug in disguise? *BMJ Case Rep* (2009) Epub.
7. Dyer JR, Davis TME, Giele C, Annus T, Garcia-Webb P, Robson J. The pharmacokinetics and pharmacodynamics of quinine in the diabetic and non-diabetic elderly. *Br J Clin Pharmacol* (1994) 38, 205–12.
8. Shalev O, Tsur A, Rahav G. Falciparum malaria-induced hypoglycaemia in a diabetic patient. *Postgrad Med J* (1992) 68, 281–2.
9. Phillips RE, Looareesuwan S, White NJ, Chanthavanich P, Karbwang J, Supanaranond W, Turner RC, Warrell DA. Hypoglycaemia and antimalarial drugs: quinidine and release of insulin. *BMJ* (1986) 292, 1319–21.
10. Powrie JK, Smith GD, Shojaee-Moradie F, Sönksen PH, Jones RH. Mode of action of chloroquine in patients with non-insulin-dependent diabetes mellitus. *Am J Physiol* (1991) 260, E897–E904.
11. Mercer E, Rekedal L, Garg R, Lu B, Massarotti EM, Solomon DH. Hydroxychloroquine improves insulin sensitivity in obese non-diabetic individuals. *Arthritis Res Ther* (2012) 14, R135.

Antidiabetics + Antipsychotics

Chlorpromazine appears to increase blood glucose concentrations, particularly in daily doses of 100 mg or more, and other classical antipsychotics appear to act similarly. The atypical antipsychotics are also associated with an increased risk of glucose intolerance. One epidemiological study found classical antipsychotics (haloperidol, pipamperone, levomepromazine, and zuclopenthixol) to be associated with an increased risk of needing insulin. Another epidemiological study found that patients with diabetes were particularly at risk of hospitalisation for hyperglycaemia during their first month of treatment with both classical and atypical antipsychotics.

Clinical evidence

(a) Classical antipsychotics

Early in the use of classical antipsychotics it was shown that they were associated with new-onset diabetes and impaired glucose control. For example, one long-term study was undertaken over the period 1955 to 1966 in a large number of women treated for a year or longer with **chlorpromazine** 100 mg daily or more, or corresponding doses of **perphenazine**, **thioridazine**, or **trifluoperazine**. This found that about 25% developed hyperglycaemia accompanied by glycosuria, compared with less than 9% in a control group who were not taking phenothiazines. Of those given a phenothiazine, about a quarter had complete remission of the symptoms when the drug was withdrawn or the dose reduced.[1]

Other reports also describe this response to **chlorpromazine**.[2-11] However, in contrast one study in 850 patients suggests that **chlorpromazine** has no effect on blood glucose concentrations. Five patients developed diabetes, but this was believed to be due to factors other than the use of **chlorpromazine**.[12] **Chlorpromazine** 50 to 70 mg daily does not affect blood glucose concentrations significantly.[11] Further, a more recent analysis (discussed further under *Atypical antipsychotics*, below) did not find an increased risk of glucose intolerance with **chlorpromazine** or **haloperidol**, and notes that the number of reports of glucose intolerance with these drugs has remained small.[13]

Very much less appears to have been published about the effect of these antipsychotics on the control of existing diabetes. The large study above that found no effect of **chlorpromazine** on blood glucose concentrations included 22 patients with diabetes, who also had no significant changes in their blood glucose concentrations.[12] Nevertheless, in a large cohort study in 2 585 patients with type 2 diabetes who had been taking oral antidiabetics for at least 2 years, the use of antipsychotics was associated with a 2-fold increased risk of needing **insulin** at 2 years after diagnosis when compared with non-users of antipsychotics (18.4% versus 9.3%). In addition, more patients taking antipsychotics were switched to insulin alone rather than receiving oral antidiabetics with insulin. However, no difference in rates of initiation of insulin was found for later years after the diagnosis of diabetes (3, 4 or 5 years). The antipsychotics most frequently being used were **haloperidol**, **pipamperone**, **levomepromazine**, and **zuclopenthixol**. Too few patients were receiving an atypical antipsychotic for these results to be analysed separately.[14] Moreover, in a case-control study of older patients with diabetes hospitalised for hyperglycaemia, the concurrent use of a classical antipsychotic (not named) was associated with an increased risk of hyperglycaemia. This occurred irrespective of diabetes treatment. With **insulin** use the adjusted rate ratio was 1.27, with **oral antidiabetics** alone was 1.31, and with diet alone was 3.43. The risk appeared to be greater during initial use, with the adjusted rate ratio 8 to 15 times higher. Furthermore, of those patients who had taken an antipsychotic for up to one month, almost 70% of the episodes of hyperglycaemia occurred within the first 14 days of treatment.[15]

(b) Atypical antipsychotics

There are lots of reports on the increased risk of new-onset diabetes with atypical antipsychotic drugs, and they are not cited here. There is some evidence that the risk of new-onset diabetes might be higher with atypical antipsychotics than classical antipsychotics. For example, an analysis of reports of glucose intolerance in the adverse reaction database of the WHO Collaborating Centre for International Drug Monitoring found that **clozapine**, **olanzapine**, and **risperidone** were associated with an increased risk of glucose intolerance, whereas the classical antipsychotics chlorpromazine and haloperidol were not. It is uncertain whether this is a dose-related effect. Additional risk factors with these antipsychotics were an underlying diabetic condition, weight increase, male gender, or the concurrent use of valproic acid, SSRIs, or buspirone.[13] However, a recent meta-analysis of all the available evidence found that the atypical antipsychotics were associated with only a tentative small increased risk of diabetes when compared with classical antipsychotics (relative risk 1.32).[16]

Very much less appears to have been published about the effect of any antipsychotics on control of existing diabetes. In a case-control study of older patients with diabetes hospitalised for hyperglycaemia, current atypical antipsychotic treatment (**olanzapine**, **quetiapine**, or **risperidone**) was associated with an increased risk of hyperglycaemia, particularly during the first month of treatment. The adjusted relative risk of developing hyperglycaemia in patients taking an atypical antipsychotic and managed with insulin, oral hypoglycaemic drugs, or diet alone was 1.4, 1.37, and 2.37, respectively.[15]

Mechanism

Although some studies found that drugs such as chlorpromazine and haloperidol were not associated with glucose intolerance,[11,13] it seems that chlorpromazine can inhibit the release of insulin, and possibly cause adrenaline release from the adrenals, both of which could result in an increase in blood glucose concentrations. This might be a dose-related effect.[11] Further, chlorpromazine might cause aggregation and inactivation of insulin by reduction of disulfide bonds.[17] Clozapine might induce insulin resistance and a compensatory increase in insulin secretion. Patients might develop diabetes if this compensatory increase is not achieved. Alternatively or additionally, weight gain is a common adverse effect of antipsychotics, and might contribute to worsening of metabolic control.[13,14] Schizophrenia itself might be associated with an increased risk of hyperglycaemia.

Importance and management

A long-established reaction first recognised in the early 1950s. The incidence of hyperglycaemia with chlorpromazine in doses of 100 mg or more is about 25%. Increases in the dose requirements of the antidiabetic should be anticipated during concurrent use.[1] Smaller chlorpromazine doses, of 50 to 70 mg daily do not appear to cause hyperglycaemia. Other classical and atypical antipsychotics appear to act similarly. In patients with diabetes, one study found evidence of an association between antipsychotic drug use and worsening of metabolic control and another found an increased risk of hospitalisation for hyperglycaemia, especially in the first month of use of the antipsychotic. It would seem prudent to increase monitoring for glycaemic control, particularly when starting or stopping any classical or atypical antipsychotic in a patient with diabetes.

1. Thonnard-Neumann E. Phenothiazines and diabetes in hospitalized women. *Am J Psychiatry* (1968) 124, 978–82.
2. Hiles BW. Hyperglycaemia and glycosuria following chlorpromazine therapy. *JAMA* (1956) 162, 1651.
3. Dobkin AB, Lamoureux L, Letienne R, Gilbert RGB. Some studies with Largactil. *Can Med Assoc J* (1954) 70, 626–8.
4. Célice J, Porcher P, Plas F, Hélie J, Peltier A. Action de la chlorpromazine sur la vésicule biliare et le clon droit. *Therapie* (1955) 10, 30–38.
5. Charatan FBE, Bartlett NG. The effect of chlorpromazine ('Largactil') on glucose tolerance. *J Ment Sci* (1955) 101, 351–3.
6. Cooperberg AA, Eidlow S. Haemolytic anemia, jaundice and diabetes mellitus following chlorpromazine therapy. *Can Med Assoc J* (1956) 75, 746–9.
7. Blair D, Brady DM. Recent advances in the treatment of schizophrenia: group training and tranquillizers. *J Ment Sci* (1958) 104, 625–64.
8. Amidsen A. Diabetes mellitus as a side effect of treatment with tricyclic neuroleptics. *Acta Psychiatr Scand* (1964) 40 (Suppl 180), 411–14.
9. Arneson GA. Phenothiazine derivatives and glucose metabolism. *J Neuropsychiatr* (1964) 5, 181–5.
10. Korenyi C, Lowenstein B. Chlorpromazine induced diabetes. *Dis Nerv Syst* (1971) 29, 827–8.
11. Erle G, Basso M, Federspil G, Sicolo N, Scandellari C. Effect of chlorpromazine on blood glucose and plasma insulin in man. *Eur J Clin Pharmacol* (1977) 11, 15–18.
12. Schwarz L, Munoz R. Blood sugar levels in patients treated with chlorpromazine. *Am J Psychiatry* (1968) 125, 253–5.
13. Hedenmalm K, Hägg S, Ståhl M, Mortimer Ö, Spigset O. Glucose intolerance with atypical antipsychotics. *Drug Safety* (2002) 25, 1107–16.
14. Spoelstra JA, Stolk RP, Cohen D, Klungel OH, Erkens JA, Leufkens HGM, Grobbee DE. Antipsychotic drugs may worsen metabolic control in type 2 diabetes mellitus. *J Clin Psychiatry* (2004) 65, 674–8.
15. Lipscombe LL, Lévesque L, Gruneir A, Fischer HD, Juurlink DN, Gill SS, Herrmann N, Hux JE, Anderson GM, Rochon PA. Antipsychotic drugs and hyperglycemia in older patients with diabetes. *Arch Intern Med* (2009) 169, 1282–9.
16. Smith M, Hopkins D, Peveler RC, Holt RIG, Woodward M, Ismail K. First- v. second-generation antipsychotics and risk for diabetes in schizophrenia: systematic review and meta-analysis. *Br J Psychiatry* (2008) 192, 406–11.
17. Bhattacharyya J, Das KP. Aggregation of insulin by chlorpromazine. *Biochem Pharmacol* (2001) 62, 1293–7.

Antidiabetics + Beta blockers

In patients with diabetes using insulin, the normal recovery reaction (increase in blood sugar) if hypoglycaemia occurs might be impaired to some extent by propranolol, but serious and severe hypoglycaemia seems rare. Cardioselective beta blockers seem less likely to interact.

The blood glucose-lowering effects of the sulfonylureas might be reduced by the beta blockers. Whether insulin or oral antidiabetic drugs are given, patients should be made aware that some of the familiar warning signs of hypoglycaemia (tachycardia, tremor) might not occur, although sweating could be increased. Hypoglycaemia in patients taking beta blockers has been noted to result in increases in blood pressure and possibly bradycardia in some studies.

Clinical evidence

A. Effects on blood glucose.

(a) Insulin

Although **propranolol** has occasionally been associated with spontaneous episodes of hypoglycaemia in non-diabetics,[1] and a number of studies in patients with diabetes[2] and healthy subjects[3-6] have found that **propranolol** impairs the normal blood glucose rebound if blood glucose concentrations decrease, there appear to be few reports of severe hypoglycaemia or coma in patients with diabetes receiving insulin and **propranolol**. Marked hypoglycaemia and/or coma occurred in 5 patients with diabetes receiving insulin as a result of the use of **propranolol**,[1,7,8] **pindolol**,[8] or **timolol** eye drops.[9] Other contributory factors (fasting, haemodialysis, etc.) probably had some part to play.[8] **Metoprolol** interacts like **propranolol** but to a lesser extent,[3,5,10] whereas **acebutolol**,[2,5] **alprenolol**,[11] **atenolol**,[2,12,13] **oxprenolol**,[10] **penbutolol**,[6] and **pindolol**[14] have been found to interact minimally or not at all. Note that the conflicting reports with **pindolol** mean that the exact effect of this beta blocker is not clear. **Carvedilol** has been associated with the onset of diabetes mellitus in one patient.[15] **Propranolol** (a peripheral vasoconstrictor) has also been found to reduce the rate of absorption of subcutaneous insulin by almost 50%, but the importance of this is uncertain.[16] However, a large case-control study found no statistically significant increase or decrease in the risk of a serious hypoglycaemic episode in patients over 65 years of age receiving insulin and taking either cardioselective beta blockers (**atenolol** and **metoprolol**) or non-cardioselective beta blockers (**propranolol** and **nadolol**) when compared with patients taking no antihypertensive drugs. Overall, of the different antihypertensive drug classes, the risk of hypoglycaemia was lowest with cardioselective beta blockers and highest with non-cardioselective beta blockers, although none of the changes were statistically significant when controlled for demographic factors and markers of comorbidity.[17] Similarly, in two other case-control studies, there was no increase in the risk of hypoglycaemia in patients with diabetes receiving insulin and also taking a beta blocker.[18,19]

(b) Oral antidiabetics

The sulfonylurea-induced insulin release from the pancreas can be inhibited by beta blockers so that the blood glucose-lowering effects are opposed to some extent.

- **Acebutolol** appears to inhibit the effects of **glibenclamide (glyburide)**,[20] but has no effect on **tolbutamide**.[21] Also, two isolated cases of hypoglycaemia have been seen with acebutolol, in one patient taking **gliclazide** and one patient taking **chlorpropamide**.[22]
- **Betaxolol** had no effect on the response to **glibenclamide** or **metformin** in one study.[23]

- **Metoprolol** did not affect the insulin-response to **tolbutamide** in one study.[24]
- **Propranolol** inhibits the effects of **glibenclamide**,[20] and **chlorpropamide**[25] and reduced the insulin-response to **tolbutamide** in one study,[26] but not in another.[24] Also, an isolated report describes hyperosmolar non-ketotic coma in a patient taking **tolbutamide** and propranolol.[27]

It is worth noting that the United Kingdom Prospective Diabetes Study Group (UKPDS) used **atenolol** 50 to 100 mg daily or captopril 25 to 50 mg twice daily for hypertension in patients with diabetes taking a range of antidiabetic drugs. Those given **atenolol** had a slightly greater increase in HbA_{1c} concentrations, and gained slightly more weight (3.4 kg for the **atenolol** group compared with 1.6 kg for the captopril group over 9 years). However, both drugs were equally effective in reducing the risk of predefined clinical end points (e.g. diabetic complications, death related to diabetes, heart failure). The number of patients experiencing hypoglycaemic attacks did not differ between the two antihypertensives.[28] This would suggest that beta blockers are generally useful in the treatment of patients with diabetes. Another large case-control study found no statistically significant increase or decrease in the risk of a serious hypoglycaemic episode in elderly patients taking sulfonylureas with either cardioselective beta blockers (**atenolol** and **metoprolol**) or non-cardioselective beta blockers (**propranolol** and **nadolol**) when compared with patients taking no antihypertensive drugs.[17]

B. Hypertension.

Marked increases in blood pressure and bradycardia can develop if hypoglycaemia occurs in patients with diabetes receiving **insulin** and a beta blocker.[29] In one study in patients with diabetes, insulin-induced hypoglycaemia resulted in blood pressure increases of 38.8/14.3 mmHg in those taking **propranolol** 80 mg twice daily, 27.9/0 mmHg in those taking **atenolol** 100 mg daily, and in those taking placebo the systolic blood pressure rose by 15.2 mmHg whereas the diastolic blood pressure decreased by 9.9 mmHg.[30] In another study, **insulin**-induced hypoglycaemia resulted in increases in blood pressure of 27/14 mmHg in those taking **alprenolol** 200 to 800 mg daily, but no increase occurred in those taking **metoprolol** 100 to 400 mg daily.[31] A report describes an increase in blood pressure to 258/144 mmHg in a patient having a hypoglycaemic episode within 2 days of starting **propranolol**.[7] Another patient taking **metoprolol** 50 mg twice daily experienced an increase in blood pressure from 190/96 mmHg to 230/112 mmHg during a hypoglycaemic episode.[29]

Mechanism

One of the normal physiological responses to a decrease in blood glucose concentrations is the mobilisation of glucose from the liver under the stimulation of adrenaline from the adrenals. This mobilisation is blocked by non-cardioselective beta blockers (such as propranolol) so that recovery from hypoglycaemia is delayed and might even proceed into a full-scale episode in a patient with diabetes who is prone to hypoglycaemia. Normally the adrenaline would also increase the heart rate, but with the beta-receptors in the heart already blocked this fails to occur. An increase in blood pressure occurs because the stimulant effects of adrenaline on the beta-2 receptors (vasodilation) are blocked leaving the alpha (vasoconstriction) effects unopposed.

Non-selective beta blockers can also block beta-2 receptors in the pancreas concerned with insulin-release, so that the effects of the sulfonylureas could be blocked.

Importance and management

Extremely well-studied interactions. Concurrent use can be uneventful but there are some risks. Patients with diabetes receiving insulin might have a prolonged or delayed recovery response to hypoglycaemia while taking a beta blocker, but very severe hypoglycaemia and/or coma is rare. If hypoglycaemia occurs it might be accompanied by a sharp increase in blood pressure. The risk is greatest with propranolol and possibly other non-cardioselective blockers and least with the cardioselective blockers. The cardioselectivity of a number of beta blockers is given in 'Table 22.1', p.999. Monitor the effects of concurrent use well, avoid the non-cardioselective beta blockers where possible, and check for any evidence that the insulin dose needs some adjustment. Warn all patients that some of the normal premonitory signs of a hypoglycaemic attack might not appear, in particular tachycardia and tremors, whereas the hunger, irritability, and nausea signs might be unaffected and sweating could even be increased.

Patients with diabetes taking oral sulfonylureas rarely seem to have serious hypoglycaemic episodes caused by beta blockers, and any reductions in the blood glucose-lowering effects of the sulfonylureas normally appear to be of little clinical importance. The cardioselective beta blockers are probably safer than those that are non-selective. Nevertheless, always monitor concurrent use to confirm that diabetic control is well maintained, adjusting the dose of antidiabetic as necessary, and warn all patients (as above) that some of the premonitory signs of hypoglycaemia might not occur.

One experimental study indicated that no interaction occurred between betaxolol and **metformin**,[23] but direct information about other beta blockers seems to be lacking.

There is also a hint from one report that the peripheral vasoconstrictive effects of non-cardioselective beta blockers and the poor peripheral circulation in patients with diabetes could be additive,[7] which is another possible reason for avoiding this type of beta blocker in diabetic patients.

Cases with other oral antidiabetics are lacking, but note that some manufacturers warn that beta blockers might alter their glycaemic effects and mask the premonitory signs of hypoglycaemia.

The pharmacokinetic interactions and/or other effects of antidiabetic drugs with beta blockers are covered under the relevant drug groups elsewhere in this chapter.

1. Kotler MN, Berman L, Rubenstein AH. Hypoglycaemia precipitated by propranolol. *Lancet* (1966) 2, 1389–90.
2. Deacon SP, Karunanayake A, Barnett D. Acebutolol, atenolol, and propranolol and metabolic responses to acute hypoglycaemia in diabetics. *BMJ* (1977) 2, 1255–7.
3. Davidson NM, Corrall RJM, Shaw TRD, French EB. Observations in man of hypoglycaemia during selective and non-selective beta-blockade. *Scott Med J* (1976) 22, 69–72.
4. Abramson EA, Arky RA, Woeber KA. Effects of propranolol on the hormonal and metabolic responses to insulin-induced hypoglycaemia. *Lancet* (1966) ii, 1386–9.
5. Newman RJ. Comparison of propranolol, metoprolol, and acebutolol on insulin-induced hypoglycaemia. *BMJ* (1976) 2, 447–9.
6. Sharma SD, Vakil BJ, Samuel MR, Chadha DR. Comparison of penbutolol and propranolol during insulin-induced hypoglycaemia. *Curr Ther Res* (1979) 26, 252–9.
7. McMurtry RJ. Propranolol, hypoglycemia, and hypertensive crisis. *Ann Intern Med* (1974) 80, 669–70.
8. Samii K, Ciancioni C, Rottembourg J, Bisseliches F, Jacobs C. Severe hypoglycaemia due to beta-blocking drugs in haemodialysis patients. *Lancet* (1976) i, 545–6.
9. Angelo-Nielsen K. Timolol topically and diabetes mellitus. *JAMA* (1980) 244, 2263.
10. Viberti GC, Keen H, Bloom SR. Beta blockade and diabetes mellitus: effect of oxprenolol and metoprolol on the metabolic, cardiovascular, and hormonal response to insulin-induced hypoglycemia in insulin-dependent diabetics. *Metabolism* (1980) 29, 873–9.
11. Eisalo A, Heino A, Munter J. The effect of alprenolol in elderly patients with raised blood pressure. *Acta Med Scand* (1974) (Suppl), 554, 23–31.
12. Deacon SP, Barnett D. Comparison of atenolol and propranolol during insulin-induced hypoglycaemia. *BMJ* (1976) 2, 272–3.
13. Waal-Manning HJ. Atenolol and three nonselective β-blockers in hypertension. *Clin Pharmacol Ther* (1979) 25, 8–18.
14. Patsch W, Patsch JR, Sailer S. Untersuchung zur Wirkung von Pindolol auf Kohlehydrat- und Fettstoffwechsel bei Diabetes Mellitus. *Int J Clin Pharmacol Biopharm* (1977) 15, 394–6.
15. Kobayakawa N, Sawaki D, Otani Y, Sekita G, Fukushima K, Takeuchi H, Aoyagi T. A case of severe diabetes mellitus occurred during management of heart failure with carvedilol and furosemide. *Cardiovasc Drugs Ther* (2003) 17, 295.
16. Veenstra J, van der Hulst JP, Wildenborg IH, Njoo SF, Verdegaal WP, Silberbusch J. Effect of antihypertensive drugs on insulin absorption. *Diabetes Care* (1991) 14, 1089–92.
17. Shorr RI, Ray WA, Daugherty JR, Griffin MR. Antihypertensives and the risk of serious hypoglycemia in older persons using insulin or sulfonylureas. *JAMA* (1997) 278, 40–3.
18. Thamer M, Ray NF, Taylor T. Association between antihypertensive drug use and hypoglycemia: a case-control study of diabetic users of insulin or sulfonylureas. *Clin Ther* (1999) 21, 1387–1400.
19. Herings RMC, de Boer A, Stricker BHC, Leufkens HGM, Porsius A. Hypoglycaemia associated with use of inhibitors of angiotensin converting enzyme. *Lancet* (1995) 345, 1195–8.
20. Zaman R, Kendall MJ, Biggs PI. The effect of acebutolol and propranolol on the hypoglycaemic action of glibenclamide. *Br J Clin Pharmacol* (1982) 13, 507–12.
21. Ryan JR. Clinical pharmacology of acebutolol. *Am Heart J* (1985) 109, 1131–6.
22. Girardin E, Vial T, Pham E, Evreux J-C. Hypoglycémies induites par les sulfamides hypoglycémiants. *Ann Med Interne (Paris)* (1992) 143, 11–17.
23. Sinclair AJ, Davies IB, Warrington SJ. Betaxolol and glucose-insulin relationships: studies in normal subjects taking glibenclamide or metformin. *Br J Clin Pharmacol* (1990) 30, 699–702.
24. Tötterman KJ, Groop LC. No effect of propranolol and metoprolol on the tolbutamide-stimulated insulin-secretion in hypertensive diabetic and non-diabetic patients. *Ann Clin Res* (1982) 14, 190–3.
25. Holt RJ, Gaskins JD. Hyperglycemia associated with propranolol and chlorpropamide coadministration. *Drug Intell Clin Pharm* (1981) 15, 599–600.
26. Massara F, Strumia E, Camanni F, Molinatti GM. Depressed tolbutamide-induced insulin response in subjects treated with propranolol. *Diabetologia* (1971) 7, 287–9.
27. Podolsky S, Pattavina CG. Hyperosmolar nonketotic diabetic coma: a complication of propranolol therapy. *Metabolism* (1973) 22, 685–93.
28. UK Prospective Diabetes Study Group. Efficacy of atenolol and captopril in reducing risk of macrovascular and microvascular complications in type 2 diabetes: UKPDS 39. *BMJ* (1998) 317, 713–20.
29. Shepherd AMM, Lin M-S, Keeton TK. Hypoglycemia-induced hypertension in a diabetic patient on metoprolol. *Ann Intern Med* (1981) 94, 357–8.
30. Ryan JR, LaCorte W, Jain A, McMahon FG. Hypertension in hypoglycemic diabetics treated with β-adrenergic antagonists. *Hypertension* (1985) 7, 443–6.
31. Östman J, Arner P, Haglund K, Juhlin-Dannfelt A, Nowak J, Wennlund A. Effect of metoprolol and alprenolol on the metabolic, hormonal, and haemodynamic response to insulin-induced hypoglycaemia in hypertensive, insulin-dependent diabetics. *Acta Med Scand* (1982) 211, 381–5.

Antidiabetics + Calcium-channel blockers

Calcium-channel blockers are known to have effects on insulin secretion and glucose regulation, but clinically important disturbances in the control of diabetes caused by these drugs appear to be rare. A report describes a patient whose diabetes worsened, requiring an increase in the dose of insulin, when diltiazem was given, and a similar case has occurred in a patient taking nifedipine. Deterioration in glucose tolerance has also occurred during nifedipine use. Hypoglycaemia occurred in a patient taking gliclazide and nicardipine.

Clinical evidence

(a) Dihydropyridines

A study in 20 patients with type 2 diabetes (5 taking **metformin** and 15 diet-controlled) found that both **nifedipine** 10 mg every 8 hours and **nicardipine** 30 mg every 8 hours for 4 weeks did not affect either glucose tolerance tests or the control of their diabetes, but both systolic and diastolic blood pressures were reduced by 4 to 7 mmHg.[1] No important changes in glucose metabolism occurred in 6 patients with type 2 diabetes taking **glibenclamide** (**glyburide**) when they were given **nifedipine** 20 to 60 mg daily for 12 to 25 weeks.[2] Similarly, other studies have found no important changes in glucose tolerance or the control of diabetes in patients taking **chlorpropamide**,[3] **glibenclamide**,[4] **gliclazide**,[5] **glipizide**,[3,6] or unspecified antidiabetics[7,8] while also taking **nifedipine**,[3,5-7] **nimodipine**,[4] or **nitrendipine**.[8] No change in **insulin** dose was needed in one patient taking **nicardipine**[9] and in 4 patients taking **nitrendipine**.[8] However, there are reports of a deterioration in glucose tolerance during the use of **nifedipine** in a total of 12 subjects with impaired glucose tolerance.[10,11] A further case report describes a 30% increase in the **insulin** requirements of a man with diabetes after he took **nifedipine** 60 mg daily.[12] An isolated case of hypoglycaemia has been described in a patient taking **gliclazide** when **nicardipine** was given.[13] However, a large case-control study found no statistically significant increase or decrease in the risk of a serious hypoglycaemic episode in patients over 65 years of age taking insulin or sulfonylureas, who were also taking calcium-channel blockers (**nifedipine** and **verapamil** were the most frequently used), when compared with patients not taking antihypertensive drugs.[14]

(b) Diltiazem

A patient with type 1 diabetes developed worsening and intractable hyperglycaemia (mean serum glucose concentrations above 13 mmol/L) when given diltiazem 90 mg every 6 hours. Her **insulin** requirements dropped when the diltiazem was withdrawn. When she started taking diltiazem 30 mg every 6 hours her blood glucose concentrations were still high, but she needed less **insulin** than when taking the higher diltiazem dose.[15]

A study in 12 healthy subjects found that diltiazem 60 mg three times daily had no effect on the secretion of **insulin** or glucagon, or on plasma glucose concentrations.[16] Similarly, diltiazem 120 mg three times daily for 3 days had no effect on **insulin** and glucose concentrations during an oral glucose tolerance test in 10 patients taking **gliclazide**.[5]

(c) Verapamil

A study in 23 patients with type 2 diabetes, 7 of whom were taking **glibenclamide (glyburide)**, found that verapamil improved the response to an oral glucose tolerance test but did not increase the blood glucose-lowering effects of the **glibenclamide**.[17] Two studies in patients with type 2 diabetes found that verapamil improved the response to glucose tolerance tests,[18,19] but in one of the studies, no alterations in the blood glucose-lowering effects of **glibenclamide** were found.[18] A large case-control study found no statistically significant increase or decrease in the risk of a serious hypoglycaemic episode in patients over 65 years of age taking insulin or sulfonylureas, who were also taking calcium-channel blockers (**nifedipine** and **verapamil** were the most frequently used), when compared with patients not taking antihypertensive drugs.[14]

Mechanism

The changes that occur are not fully understood. Suggestions include: inhibition of insulin secretion by the calcium-channel blockers and inhibition of glucagon secretion by glucose; changes in glucose uptake by the liver and other cells; increases in blood glucose following catecholamine release after vasodilation, and changes in glucose metabolism. In contrast, one study in non-diabetics suggested that long-acting nifedipine could improve insulin sensitivity.[20]

Importance and management

Very extensively studied, but many of the reports describe single-dose studies or multiple-dose studies in healthy subjects (only a few are cited here), which do not give a clear picture of what might be expected in patients with diabetes. Those studies that have concentrated on diabetic patients indicate that the control of diabetes is not usually adversely affected by calcium-channel blockers, although isolated cases with diltiazem, nicardipine, and nifedipine have been reported.[12,13,15] Therefore, in general, no particular precautions would normally seem necessary; although note that it is prudent to monitor blood glucose concentrations when any change is made to the medication regimen of a patient with diabetes. If an otherwise unexplained worsening of diabetic control occurs, consider the use of a calcium-channel blocker as a possible cause.

The pharmacokinetic interactions of antidiabetic drugs with calcium-channel blockers are covered under the individual drug groups elsewhere in this chapter.

1. Collins WCJ, Cullen MJ, Feely J. Calcium channel blocker drugs and diabetic control. *Clin Pharmacol Ther* (1987) 42, 420–3.
2. Kanatsuna T, Nakano K, Mori H, Kano Y, Nishioka H, Kajiyama S, Kitagawa Y, Yoshida T, Kondo M, Nakamura N, Aochi O. Effects of nifedipine on insulin secretion and glucose metabolism in rats and hypertensive type 2 (non-insulin dependent) diabetics. *Arzneimittelforschung* (1985) 35, 514–17.
3. Donnelly T, Harrower ADB. Effect of nifedipine on glucose tolerance and insulin secretion in diabetic and non-diabetic patients. *Curr Med Res Opin* (1980) 6, 690–3.
4. Mück W, Heine PR, Breuel H-P, Niklaus H, Horkulak J, Ahr G. The effect of multiple oral dosing of nimodipine on glibenclamide pharmacodynamics and pharmacokinetics in elderly patients with type-2 diabetes mellitus. *Int J Clin Pharmacol Ther* (1995) 33, 89–94.
5. Monges AM, Pisano P, Aujoulat P, Salducci D, Durand A, Panagides D, Bory M, Crevat A. ¹H nuclear magnetic resonance and clinical studies of interaction of calcium antagonists and hypoglycemic sulfonylureas. *Fundam Clin Pharmacol* (1991) 5, 527–38.
6. Connacher AA, El Debani AH, Isles TE, Stevenson IH. Disposition and hypoglycaemic action of glipizide in diabetic patients given a single dose of nifedipine. *Eur J Clin Pharmacol* (1987) 33, 81–3.
7. Abadie E, Passa P. Diabetogenic effects of nifedipine. *BMJ* (1984) 289, 438.
8. Trost BN, Weidmann P. 5 years of antihypertensive monotherapy with the calcium antagonist nitrendipine do not alter carbohydrate homeostasis in diabetic patients. *Diabetes Res Clin Pract* (1988) 5 (Suppl 1), S511.
9. Sakata S, Miura K. Effect of nicardipine in a hypertensive patient with diabetes mellitus. *Clin Ther* (1984) 6, 600–2.
10. Guigliano D, Torella R, Cacciapuoti F, Gentile S, Verza M, Varricchio M. Impairment of insulin secretion in man by nifedipine. *Eur J Clin Pharmacol* (1980) 18, 395–8.
11. Bhatnagar SK, Amin MMA, Al-Yusuf AR. Diabetogenic effects of nifedipine. *BMJ* (1984) 289, 19.
12. Heyman SN, Heyman A, Halperin I. Diabetogenic effect of nifedipine. *DICP Ann Pharmacother* (1989) 23, 236–7.
13. Girardin E, Vial T, Pham E, Evreux J-C. Hypoglycémies induites par les sulfamides hypoglycémiants. *Ann Med Interne (Paris)* (1992) 143, 11–17.
14. Shorr RI, Ray WA, Daugherty JR, Griffin MR. Antihypertensives and the risk of serious hypoglycemia in older persons using insulin or sulfonylureas. *JAMA* (1997) 278, 40–3.
15. Pershadsingh HA, Grant N, McDonald JM. Association of diltiazem therapy with increased insulin resistance in a patient with type I diabetes mellitus. *JAMA* (1987) 257, 930–1.
16. Segrestaa JM, Caulin C, Dahan R, Houlbert D, Thiercelin JF, Herman P, Sauvanet JP, Laurribaud J. Effect of diltiazem on plasma glucose, insulin and glucagon during an oral glucose tolerance test in healthy volunteers. *Eur J Clin Pharmacol* (1984) 26, 481–3.
17. Röjdmark S, Andersson DEH. Influence of verapamil on human glucose tolerance. *Am J Cardiol* (1986) 57, 39D–43D.
18. Röjdmark S, Andersson DEH. Influence of verapamil on glucose tolerance. *Acta Med Scand* (1984) (Suppl), 681, 37–42.
19. Andersson DEH, Röjdmark S. Improvement of glucose tolerance by verapamil in patients with non-insulin-dependent diabetes mellitus. *Acta Med Scand* (1981) 210, 27–33.
20. Koyama Y, Kodama K, Suzuki M, Harano Y. Improvement of insulin sensitivity by a long-acting nifedipine preparation (nifedipine-CR) in patients with essential hypertension. *Am J Hypertens* (2002) 15, 927–31.

Antidiabetics + Cibenzoline (Cifenline)

Hypoglycaemia has been seen in patients taking cibenzoline with antidiabetics.

Clinical evidence, mechanism, importance and management

A report describes an elderly patient with type 2 diabetes controlled by diet who developed hypoglycaemia and associated dementia-like symptoms while taking low-dose cibenzoline.[1] Hypoglycaemia also occurred in a 61-year-old patient with renal impairment taking **gliclazide** and cibenzoline.[2] In a study of reports of hypoglycaemia in the French pharmacovigilance database, cibenzoline was used as a positive control, and a very strong association between cibenzoline and hypoglycaemia was noted, both in reports including antidiabetic drugs (odds ratio 5) and in reports not including antidiabetic drugs (odds ratio 174). The odds ratio of hypoglycaemia compared with all reports for the study as a whole was 107 (78 to 148).[3]

The reasons for this effect are not understood. However, in a controlled study in patients with abnormal glucose tolerance and ventricular arrhythmias, cibenzoline exerted a hypoglycaemic effect by facilitating insulin secretion.[4]

This appears to be a drug-disease rather than a drug-drug interaction and diabetic patients do not seem to be more at risk than non-diabetics, but good monitoring is advisable if cibenzoline is given, particularly if risk factors such as increased age, renal impairment, malnutrition and high cibenzoline dose are present.

1. Sakane N, Onishi N, Katamura M, Sato H, Takamasu M, Yoshida T. Cifenline succinate and dementia in an elderly NIDDM patient. *Diabetes Care* (1998) 21, 320–1.
2. Girardin E, Vial T, Pham E, Evreux J-C. Hypoglycémies induites par les sulfamides hypoglycémiants. *Ann Med Interne (Paris)* (1992) 143, 11–17.
3. Grégoire F, Pariente A, Fourrier-Reglat A, Haramburu F, Bégaud B, Moore N. A signal of increased risk of hypoglycaemia with angiotensin receptor blockers caused by confounding. *Br J Clin Pharmacol* (2008) 66, 142–5.
4. Saikawa T, Arita M, Yamaguchi K, Ito M. Hypoglycemic effect of cibenzoline in patients with abnormal glucose tolerance and frequent ventricular arrhythmias. *Cardiovasc Drugs Ther* (2000) 14, 665–9.

Antidiabetics + Clonidine

Some evidence suggests that clonidine might suppress the signs and symptoms of hypoglycaemia in patients with diabetes. Marked hyperglycaemia occurred in a child using insulin when clonidine was given. However, the effect of clonidine on carbohydrate metabolism appears to be variable, as other reports have described both increases and decreases in blood glucose concentrations. Clonidine premedication might decrease or increase the hyperglycaemic response to surgery.

Clinical evidence

(a) Non-diabetics

Studies in healthy subjects and patients with hypertension found that their normal response to hypoglycaemia (tachycardia, palpitations, perspiration) caused by a 0.1 unit/kg dose of **insulin** was greatly reduced when they were taking clonidine 450 to 900 micrograms daily.[1,2] A study in healthy subjects and non-diabetic patients found that clonidine increases blood glucose concentrations, apparently by reducing insulin secretion,[3] whereas, in contrast, hypoglycaemia was associated with clonidine testing for growth hormone deficiency in 4 children.[4] Furthermore, in yet another study, clonidine 100 or 200 micrograms twice daily had no effect on fasting glucose concentrations or oral glucose tolerance testing.[5]

(b) Patients with diabetes

A 9-year-old girl with type 1 diabetes stabilised with **insulin** 4 units daily, developed substantial hyperglycaemia and needed up to 56 units of **insulin** daily when she began to take clonidine 50 micrograms daily for Tourette's syndrome. When the clonidine was stopped, she had numerous hypoglycaemic episodes, and within a few days it was possible to reduce her daily dose of **insulin** to 6 units.[6] A patient with type 2 diabetes and hypertension experienced elevated blood glucose concentrations and decreased insulin secretion when clonidine was given.[7] However, a study in 10 patients with diabetes and hypertension found that although clonidine impaired the response to an acute glucose challenge, it did not have a clinically relevant effect on diabetic control over a 10-week period.[8] Similarly, in 20 patients with type 2 diabetes and hypertension, clonidine 75 to 300 micrograms daily for 3 months had no effect on glucose control. The antidiabetic therapy (sulfonylureas (11 patients), metformin (2 patients), a combination (3 patients), or diet alone (4 patients)) was kept constant.[9]

In contrast, a placebo-controlled, crossover study in 20 patients with type 2 diabetes found that transdermal clonidine reduced mean fasting plasma glucose concentrations by 9%.[10]

(c) Hyperglycaemia during surgery

Forty patients with type 2 diabetes (controlled by diet alone, **sulfonylureas**, **biguanides**, or **insulin**), having eye surgery under general anaesthesia, were given either clonidine 225 to 375 micrograms or flunitrazepam as premedication. In patients with diabetes there is an increase in blood glucose during stress because of an increase in catecholamine release. Therefore the patients were also given a continuous infusion of **insulin** to maintain blood glucose at 5.5 to 11.1 mmol/L. Clonidine decreased the **insulin** requirement because of improved blood glucose control due to inhibition of catecholamine release.[11] Contrasting results were found in a study in 16 non-diabetic women undergoing abdominal hysterectomy. Eight were given intravenous clonidine 1 microgram/kg, and 8 control patients were given saline. Intraoperative plasma glucose concentrations were higher in the clonidine group and these patients also had lower insulin concentrations.[12]

Mechanism

The suggested reason for a reduced response to hypoglycaemia in healthy subjects is that clonidine depresses the output of the catecholamines (adrenaline (epinephrine), noradrenaline (norepinephrine)), which are secreted in an effort to increase blood glucose concentrations, and which are also responsible for the signs of a normal response to hypoglycaemia (tachycardia, palpitations, perspiration).[2] It seems possible that clonidine will similarly suppress the signs and symptoms of hypoglycaemia that can occur in patients with diabetes, but there seem to be no reports confirming this.

Importance and management

The effect of clonidine on carbohydrate metabolism in patients with diabetes appears to be variable and the general importance of these interactions is uncertain. In patients with diabetes there is an increase in blood glucose concentrations during stress because of an increase in catecholamine release. The influence of clonidine on the surgical stress response appears to vary depending on the dose of clonidine and the type of surgery.[12] Thus, clonidine at about 4 micrograms/kg might attenuate the hyperglycaemic response to neurosurgical and non-abdominal procedures, but low-dose clonidine accentuates the hyperglycaemic response to lower abdominal surgery, which results from a decrease in plasma insulin.[11,12] It would seem prudent to be aware of this interaction in patients with diabetes, and to act accordingly should an effect be seen. No additional monitoring, over and above that which would normally occur in patients with diabetes undergoing surgery or when any drug is added to antidiabetic treatment, would appear necessary.

1. Hedeland H, Dymling J-F, Hökfelt B. The effect of insulin induced hypoglycaemia on plasma renin activity and urinary catecholamines before and following clonidine (Catapresan) in man. *Acta Endocrinol (Copenh)* (1972) 71, 321–30.
2. Hedeland H, Dymling J-F, Hökfelt B. Pharmacological inhibition of adrenaline secretion following insulin induced hypoglycaemia in man: the effect of Catapresan. *Acta Endocrinol (Copenh)* (1971) 67, 97–103.
3. Metz SA, Halter JB, Robertson RP. Induction of defective insulin secretion and impaired glucose tolerance by clonidine. Selective stimulation of metabolic alpha-adrenergic pathways. *Diabetes* (1978) 27, 554–62.
4. Huang C, Banerjee K, Sochett E, Perlman K, Wherrett D, Daneman D. Hypoglycemia associated with clonidine testing for growth hormone deficiency. *J Pediatr* (2001) 139, 323–4.
5. Molitch ME, Hou SH, Gottesman S, Kapcala LP, Kopelman RI, Madias NE. Effects of antihypertensive medications on carbohydrate metabolism. *Curr Ther Res* (1986) 39, 398–407.
6. Mimouni-Bloch A, Mimouni M. Clonidine-induced hyperglycemia in a young diabetic girl. *Ann Pharmacother* (1993) 27, 980.
7. Okada S, Miyai Y, Sato K, Masaki Y, Higuchi T, Ogino Y, Ota Z. Effect of clonidine on insulin secretion: a case report. *J Int Med Res* (1986) 14, 299–302.
8. Guthrie GP, Miller RE, Kotchen TA, Koenig SH. Clonidine in patients with diabetes and mild hypertension. *Clin Pharmacol Ther* (1983) 34, 713–17.
9. Nilsson-Ehle P, Ekberg M, Fridström P, Ursing D, Lins L-E. Lipoproteins and metabolic control in hypertensive type II diabetics treated with clonidine. *Acta Med Scand* (1988) 224, 131–4.
10. Giugliano D, Acampora R, Marfella R, La Marca C, Marfella M, Nappo F, D'Onofrio F. Hemodynamic and metabolic effects of transdermal clonidine in patients with hypertension and non-insulin-dependent diabetes mellitus. *Am J Hypertens* (1998) 11, 184–9.
11. Belhoula M, Ciébiéra JP, De La Chapelle A, Boisseau N, Coeurveille D, Raucoules-Aimé M. Clonidine premedication improves metabolic control in type 2 diabetic patients during ophthalmic surgery. *Br J Anaesth* (2003) 90, 434–9.
12. Lattermann R, Schricker T, Georgieff M, Schreiber M. Low dose clonidine premedication accentuates the hyperglycemic response to surgery. *Can J Anesth* (2001) 48, 755–9.

Antidiabetics + Corticosteroids

The blood glucose-lowering effects of the antidiabetics are opposed by corticosteroids with glucocorticoid (hyperglycaemic) activity and clinically important hyperglycaemia has been seen with systemic corticosteroids. A report also describes deterioration in diabetic control with *inhaled* high-dose fluticasone, then high-dose budesonide, in a patient taking glibenclamide and metformin. High doses of high-potency corticosteroid creams might also, rarely, cause hyperglycaemia.

Clinical evidence, mechanism, importance and management

(a) Local corticosteroids

1. Inhaled. A 67-year-old man with diabetes taking **glibenclamide** 5 mg daily and **metformin** 1.7 g daily had a deterioration in diabetic control (glycosuria and an increase in HbA_{1c}) 3 weeks after starting inhaled **fluticasone** 2 mg daily, by metered dose inhaler with a spacer device, for asthma. The **fluticasone** dose was gradually decreased to 500 micrograms daily after about 3 months, with an improvement in diabetic control. Subsequently, the **fluticasone** dose was increased from 500 micrograms to 1 mg, and within a week he again developed glycosuria.[1] This same patient was later given inhaled high-dose **budesonide** 2 mg daily and he again developed glycosuria and increased HbA_{1c} concentrations, which improved as the dose was gradually decreased to 800 micrograms daily.[2] The adverse effects of *systemic* corticosteroids on glucose tolerance are well known. Although only one case appears to have been reported, it suggests that high-dose inhaled corticosteroids might have a similar effect. It might be prudent to increase monitoring of diabetic control in patients requiring high-dose corticosteroids and consider reducing the dose of the inhaled corticosteroid if possible, or adjusting the dose of the antidiabetic medication as necessary.

2. Topical. Two patients with an abnormal response to the glucose tolerance test, but without overt signs of diabetes mellitus, developed postprandial hyperglycaemia and one developed glycosuria when they used topical corticosteroids for severe psoriasis. These patients were given 15 g of **halcinonide** 0.1% or **betamethasone** 0.1% cream, applied every 12 hours for 15 days under occlusive dressings.[3] These cases appear to be rare, and were associated with high doses of potent or very potent corticosteroids, used under occlusive dressings, which increases systemic absorption. No additional special precautions would generally appear to be necessary in diabetics using moderate amounts of topical corticosteroids.

(b) Systemic corticosteroids

Systemic corticosteroids with glucocorticoid activity can increase blood glucose concentrations and induce diabetes.[4] This can oppose the blood glucose-lowering effects of the antidiabetics used in the treatment of diabetes mellitus. For example, a disturbance of the control of diabetes is very briefly described in a patient given **insulin** and **hydrocortisone**.[5] A study in 5 patients with type 2 diabetes taking **chlorpropamide** found that a single 200-mg dose of **cortisone** modified their glucose tolerance. The blood glucose concentrations of 4 of them increased (3 showed an initial reduction), whereas in a previous test with **chlorpropamide** alone the blood glucose concentrations of 4 of them had decreased.[6] This almost certainly reflects a direct antagonism between the pharmacological effects of the two drugs. Another glucocorticoid, **prednisone**, had no effect on the metabolism or clearance of **tolbutamide** in healthy subjects.[7]

There are very few studies of this interaction, probably because the hyperglycaemic activity of the **corticosteroids** has been known for such a long time that the outcome of concurrent use is self-evident. The effects of systemic corticosteroids in patients with diabetes should be closely monitored, and the dose of the antidiabetic increased as necessary. Antidiabetics are sometimes needed in non-diabetic patients taking **corticosteroids** to reduce blood glucose concentrations.

1. Faul JL, Tormey W, Tormey V, Burke C. High dose inhaled corticosteroids and dose dependent loss of diabetic control. *BMJ* (1998) 317, 1491.
2. Faul JL, Cormican LJ, Tormey VJ, Tormey WP, Burke CM. Deteriorating diabetic control associated with high-dose inhaled budesonide. *Eur Respir J* (1999) 14, 242–3.
3. Gomez EC, Frost P. Induction of glycosuria and hyperglycemia by topical corticosteroid therapy. *Arch Dermatol* (1976) 112, 1559–62.
4. David DS, Cheigh JS, Braun DW, Fotino M, Stenzel KH, Rubin AL. HLA-A28 and steroid-induced diabetes in renal transplant patients. *JAMA* (1980) 243, 532–3.
5. Manchon ND, Bercoff E, Lemarchand P, Chassagne P, Senant J, Bourreille J. Fréquence et gravité des interactions médicamenteuses dan une population âgée: étude prospective concernant 639 malades. *Rev Med Interne* (1989) 10, 521–5.
6. Danowski TS, Mateer FM, Moses C. Cortisone enhancement of peripheral utilization of glucose and the effects of chlorpropamide. *Ann N Y Acad Sci* (1959) 74, 988–96.
7. Breimer DD, Zilly W, Richter E. Influence of corticosteroid on hexobarbital and tolbutamide disposition. *Clin Pharmacol Ther* (1978) 24, 208–12.

Antidiabetics + Danazol

In theory, danazol would be expected to oppose the effects of antidiabetics.

Clinical evidence, mechanism, importance and management

A study in 14 non-diabetic subjects found that 3 months of treatment with danazol 600 mg daily caused a mild, but definite, deterioration in glucose tolerance, associated with high insulin concentrations. Insulin resistance was also seen in 5 subjects taking danazol when they were given intravenous **tolbutamide**.[1] Similarly, another study in 9 non-diabetic women found that danazol 600 mg daily increased insulin concentrations in response to glucose or intravenous **tolbutamide**.[2]

Danazol is known to cause insulin resistance and might therefore affect diabetic control, and some caution would therefore seem prudent if danazol is given to patients with diabetes. Danazol would be expected to oppose the actions of antidiabetics to some extent, but there do not appear to be any studies assessing the clinical relevance of this. If concurrent danazol is considered necessary, as when any change is made to the medication regimen of a patient with diabetes, it would be prudent to monitor blood glucose concentrations.

1. Wynn V. Metabolic effects of danazol. *J Int Med Res* (1977) 5 (Suppl 3), 25–35.
2. Goettenberg N, Schlienger J L, Becmeur F, Dellenbach P. Traitement de l'endométriose pelvienne par le danazol. Incidence sur le métabolisme glucidique. *Nouv Presse Med* (1982) 11, 3703–6.

Antidiabetics + Dextropropoxyphene (Propoxyphene)

Dextropropoxyphene does not appear to affect the pharmacokinetics of tolbutamide. Hypoglycaemia was seen in one patient taking an unnamed sulfonylurea with co-proxamol and in another with diet-controlled diabetes given dextropropoxyphene with paracetamol (acetaminophen). Hypoglycaemia has also been reported in non-diabetic patients given dextropropoxyphene alone.

Clinical evidence, mechanism, importance and management

After 6 healthy subjects took dextropropoxyphene 65 mg every 8 hours for 4 days, the clearance of a 500-mg intravenous dose of **tolbutamide** was not affected.[1] There is an isolated case of hypoglycaemia in a patient taking an unnamed **sulfonylurea** with **co-proxamol** (dextropropoxyphene with paracetamol (acetaminophen)).[2] A case report describes an 82-year-old woman with type 2 diabetes (controlled by diet alone) and end stage renal disease who developed recurrent hypoglycaemic episodes after starting dextropoxyphene 65 mg with **paracetamol** (**acetaminophen**) 650 mg (*Depain X*) four times daily. Drug-related hypoglycaemia was suspected, so the *Depain X* was stopped and the hypoglycaemia resolved.[3] In a study of reports of hypoglycaemia in the French pharmacovigilance database between 1997 and 2010, 72 cases of hypoglycaemia were associated with dextropropoxyphene use, which occurred after a median of 4 days. At least one risk factor for hypoglycaemia was found in 58% of these cases, with 32% having diabetes and 18% having renal insufficiency.[4] There are also several reports of hypoglycaemia in non-diabetic patients taking dextropropoxyphene alone,[5-10] sometimes associated with renal failure,[5,6,10] advanced age,[7] or with high doses or in overdose.[8]

The general importance of these isolated reports is uncertain, and bearing in mind the length of time these drugs have been available, there would normally seem to be little reason for avoiding the concurrent use of antidiabetics and dextropropoxyphene, or for taking particular precautions.

1. Robson RA, Miners JO, Whitehead AG, Birkett DJ. Specificity of the inhibitory effect of dextropropoxyphene on oxidative drug metabolism in man: effects on theophylline and tolbutamide disposition. *Br J Clin Pharmacol* (1987) 23, 772–5.
2. Girardin E, Vial T, Pham E, Evreux J-C. Hypoglycémies induites par les sulfamides hypoglycémiants. *Ann Med Interne (Paris)* (1992) 143, 11–17.
3. Lee HT, Tseng WC, Tarng DC. Recurrent hypoglycaemia in a hemodialysis patient related to propoxyphene treatment. *J Chin Med Assoc* (2007) 70, 286–8.
4. Bourne C, Gouraud A, Daveluy A, Grandvuillemin A, Auriche P, Descotes J, Vial T, the French Association of Pharmacovigilance Centres. Tramadol and hypoglycaemia: comparison with other step 2 analgesic drugs. *Br J Clin Pharmacol* (2012) 75, 1063–7.
5. Wiederholt IC, Genco M, Foley JM. Recurrent episodes of hypoglycemia induced by propoxyphene. *Neurology* (1967) 17, 703–6.
6. Almirall J, Montoliu J, Torras A, Revert L. Propoxyphene-induced hypoglycemia in a patient with chronic renal failure. *Nephron* (1989) 53, 273–5.
7. Laurent M, Gallinari C, Bonnin M, Soubrie C. Hypoglycémie sous dextropropoxyphène chez des grands vieillards: 7 observations. *Presse Med* (1991) 20, 1628.
8. Karunakara BP, Maiya PP, Hegde SR, Pradeep GCM. Accidental dextropropoxyphene poisoning. *Indian J Pediatr* (2003) 70, 357–8.
9. Santos Gil I, Junquera Crespo M, Sanz Sanz J, Lahulla Pastor F. Hipglucernia secundaria a ingestión de dextropropoxifeno en un paciente adicto a drogas. Med Clin (Barc) 1998, 110, 475–6.
10. Shah P, Aniszweski J, Service FJ. Propoxyphene-induced hypoglycaemia in renal failure. *Endocr Pract* (2006) 12, 170–3.

Antidiabetics + Disopyramide

Isolated reports describe severe hypoglycaemia when disopyramide was given to patients with diabetes taking gliclazide, glimepiride, or metformin and/or insulin.

Clinical evidence, mechanism, importance and management

Two case reports describe severe hypoglycaemia in patients with diabetes who were taking **gliclazide**[1] and **glimepiride**[2] after starting disopyramide 300 mg daily. A further case of hypoglycaemia associated with disopyramide occurred in a 70-year-old woman who had been taking **metformin** 500 mg twice daily and **insulin** 62 units daily. Within 3 months of starting disopyramide 250 mg twice daily her **insulin** dose was reduced to 24 units daily, she stopped taking **metformin**, and was eating 'substantial snacks' to avoid hypoglycaemia.[3] The **insulin** requirements of 2 other patients with type 2 diabetes were greatly reduced when disopyramide was started.[4,5]

Disopyramide has been associated with hypoglycaemia, and the UK and US manufacturers note that those particularly at risk are the elderly, the malnourished, and those with diabetes, and that impaired renal function and impaired cardiac function might be predisposing factors.[6,7] They advise close monitoring of blood glucose concentrations[6,7] and withdrawal of disopyramide if problems arise.[6] This is not simply a problem for patients with diabetes, but certainly within the context of diabetes the blood glucose-lowering effects of disopyramide could cause particular difficulties.

1. Wahl D, de Korwin JD, Paille F, Trechot P, Schmitt J. Hypoglycémie sévère probablement induite par le disopyramide chez un diabétique. *Therapie* (1988) 43, 321–2.
2. Negishi M, Shimomura K, Proks P, Mori M, Shimomura Y. Mechanism of disopyramide-induced hypoglycaemia in a patient with Type 2 diabetes. *Diabet Med* (2009) 26, 76–8.
3. Reynolds RM, Walker JD. Hypoglycaemia induced by disopyramide in a patient with type 2 diabetes mellitus. *Diabet Med* (2001) 18, 1009–10.
4. Onoda N, Kawagoe M, Shimizu M, Komori T, Takahashi C, Oomori Y, Hirata Y. A case of non-insulin dependent diabetes mellitus whose insulin requirement was markedly reduced after disopyramide treatment for arrhythmia. *Nippon Naika Gakkai Zasshi* (1989) 78, 820–5.
5. Taketa K, Yamamoto Y. Hypoglycemic effect of disopyramide in a case of diabetes mellitus under insulin treatment. *Acta Med Okayama* (1980) 34, 289–92.
6. Rythmodan Capsules (Disopyramide). Sanofi UK Summary of product characteristics, August 2013.
7. Norpace (Disopyramide). Pfizer Inc. US Prescribing information, September 2006.

Antidiabetics + Disulfiram

Disulfiram appears not to affect the control of diabetes mellitus. Disulfiram does not affect the pharmacokinetics of tolbutamide.

Clinical evidence, mechanism, importance and management

The UK manufacturer of disulfiram advises that caution should be exercised if it is used in patients with diabetes.[1] However, a review[2] of a clinician's experience with disulfiram in over 20 000 alcoholics, includes its use in several hundred patients with diabetes mellitus over 20 years without any apparent adverse effects, and concludes that any theoretical interaction is rarely, if ever, applicable to clinical practice. It would be reasonable to assume that many of these patients were also taking **insulin** or one of the older oral antidiabetics. There do not appear to be any reported cases in the literature of adverse interactions between disulfiram and any of the antidiabetics. In a study in 5 healthy subjects, disulfiram (400 mg three times daily for one day, then once daily for one day, then 200 mg daily for 2 days) had no effect on the half-life or clearance of intravenous **tolbutamide** 500 mg.[3] The conclusion to be drawn from all of this is that any reaction is very rare (if it ever occurs), and no special precautions would normally appear to be necessary on concurrent use of disulfiram and antidiabetic drugs.

1. Antabuse (Disulfiram). Actavis UK Ltd. UK Summary of product characteristics, December 2011.
2. McNichol RW, Ewing JA, Faiman MD, eds. Disulfiram (Antabuse): a unique medical aid to sobriety: history, pharmacology, research, clinical use. Springfield, Ill: Thomas; 1987. p. 47–90.
3. Svendsen TL, Kristensen MB, Hansen JM, Skovsted L. The influence of disulfiram on the half life and metabolic clearance rate of diphenylhydantoin and tolbutamide in man. *Eur J Clin Pharmacol* (1976) 9, 439–41.

Antidiabetics + Diuretics; Loop

The control of diabetes is not usually affected to a clinically relevant extent by etacrynic acid, furosemide, or torasemide. However, a few reports suggest that etacrynic acid and furosemide can, rarely, increase blood glucose concentrations.

Clinical evidence

(a) Etacrynic acid

A double-blind study in 24 hypertensive patients, 8 of whom had diabetes, found that etacrynic acid 200 mg daily for 6 weeks impaired the glucose tolerance and increased the blood glucose concentrations of the patients with diabetes to the same extent as **hydrochlorothiazide** 200 mg daily in both the patients with diabetes and non-diabetics.[1] However, in other studies no change in carbohydrate metabolism or glucose tolerance was seen in 6 patients with diabetes given etacrynic acid 150 mg daily for a week,[2] or in 10 patients described as pre-diabetic given etacrynic acid 50 mg for a week.[3]

(b) Furosemide

Although furosemide can elevate blood glucose concentrations,[4] worsen glucose tolerance,[5] and occasionally cause glycosuria or even acute diabetes in individual patients,[6,7] the general picture is that the control of diabetes is not usually affected by furosemide.[8] No change in glucose tolerance was seen in 10 patients described as pre-diabetic when they were given furosemide 40 mg daily for a week.[3] No clinically relevant changes in the control of diabetes were seen in a 3-month study of 29 patients with type 2 diabetes taking furosemide 40 mg daily and an average of 7 mg of **glibenclamide (glyburide)** daily.[9]

(c) Torasemide

A three-month study in 32 patients with congestive heart failure and type 2 diabetes mellitus taking **glibenclamide** found that torasemide 5 mg daily caused a small but clinically insignificant decrease in blood glucose concentrations.[9]

Mechanism

Uncertain.

Importance and management

Information is limited. Some impairment of glucose tolerance might occur, but there seems to be a lack of evidence in the literature to show that any loop diuretic has much effect on the control of diabetes in most patients.

1. Russell RP, Lindeman RD, Prescott LF. Metabolic and hypotensive effects of ethacrynic acid. Comparative study with hydrochlorothiazide. *JAMA* (1968) 205, 81–5.
2. Dige-Petersen H. Ethacrynic acid and carbohydrate metabolism. *Nord Med* (1966) 75, 123–5.
3. Káldor A, Gachályi B, Sebestyén K. Diabetogenic effect of oral diuretics in asymptomatic diabetes. *Int J Clin Pharmacol Biopharm* (1975) 11, 232–4.
4. Hutcheon DE, Leonard G. Diuretic and antihypertensive action of frusemide. *J Clin Pharmacol* (1967) 7, 26–33.
5. Breckenridge A, Welborn TA, Dollery CT, Fraser R. Glucose tolerance in hypertensive patients on long-term diuretic therapy. *Lancet* (1967) i, 61–4.
6. Toivonen S, Mustala O. Diabetogenic action of frusemide. *BMJ* (1966) i, 920–21.
7. Kobayakawa N, Sawaki D, Otani Y, Sekita G, Fukushima K, Takeuchi H, Aoyagi T. A case of severe diabetes mellitus occurred during management of heart failure with carvedilol and furosemide. *Cardiovasc Drugs Ther* (2003) 17, 295.
8. Bencomo L, Fyvolent J, Kahana S, Kahana L. Clinical experience with a new diuretic, furosemide. *Curr Ther Res* (1965) 7, 339–45.
9. Lehnert H, Schmitz H, Beyer J, Wilmbusse H, Piesche L. Controlled clinical trial investigating the influence of torasemide and furosemide on carbohydrate metabolism in patients with cardiac failure and concomitant type II diabetes. *Int Congr Ser* (1993) 1023, 271–4.

Antidiabetics + Diuretics; Thiazide and related or Potassium-sparing

By increasing blood glucose concentrations, the thiazide and related diuretics can reduce the effects of the antidiabetics and impair the control of diabetes. However, this effect appears to be dose-related, and is less frequent at the low doses now more commonly used for hypertension. Hyponatraemia has rarely been reported when chlorpropamide was given with a thiazide and potassium-sparing diuretic. An isolated report describes severe hypoglycaemia in a patient taking glibenclamide (glyburide) shortly after metolazone was started. Voglibose had no effect on the pharmacokinetics of hydrochlorothiazide, and hydrochlorothiazide did not appear to alter metformin pharmacokinetics. Triamterene is predicted to increase blood glucose concentrations.

Clinical evidence

(a) Effects on glucose control

Chlorothiazide, the first of the thiazide diuretics, was found within a year of its introduction in 1958 to have hyperglycaemic effects.[1] Since then a very large number of reports have described hyperglycaemia, the precipitation of diabetes in pre-diabetics, and the disturbance of blood glucose control in patients with diabetes taking thiazides. One example from many:

A long-term study in 53 patients with type 2 diabetes found that **chlorothiazide** 500 mg or 1 g daily or **trichlormethiazide** 4 or 8 mg daily caused a mean increase in blood glucose concentrations from about 6.7 mmol/L to 7.8 mmol/L. Only 7 patients needed a change in their treatment: 4 required more of their oral antidiabetic, 2 an increase in **insulin** dose, and one was transferred from **tolbutamide** to **insulin**. The oral antidiabetics used included **tolbutamide**, **chlorpropamide**, and **acetohexamide**.[2]

An increase in blood glucose concentrations has been observed with **bendroflumethiazide**,[3,4] **benzthiazide**,[5] **hydrochlorothiazide** 100 to 300 mg daily,[3] and **chlortalidone** 50 to 100 mg daily.[6] A study in hypertensive patients found that **chlortalidone** 50 mg daily increased glucose and insulin concentrations, but **hydrochlorothiazide** 50 mg daily alone or as part of a potassium and/or magnesium-sparing regimen did not.[7]

More recent data suggest that the effects of thiazides on blood glucose might be dose related. In a double-blind randomised study comparing the effects of 1.25 or 5 mg of **bendroflumethiazide** on blood glucose, the lower dose had no effects on insulin action, whereas when the higher dose was given, there was evidence of impaired glucose tolerance.[8] A review of the literature on **hydrochlorothiazide** similarly reports that low doses (6.25 to 12.5 mg) lack clinically important effects on blood glucose concentrations.[9]

A man with type 2 diabetes, stable taking **glibenclamide (glyburide)** 10 mg daily and hospitalised for congestive heart failure, became clinically hypoglycaemic (blood glucose concentrations unmeasurable by *Labstix*) within 40 hours of starting **metolazone** 5 mg daily. He was treated with intravenous glucose. Although both **glibenclamide (glyburide)** and **metolazone** were stopped, he had 4 further hypoglycaemic episodes over the next 30 hours.[10] The reasons are not understood. *In vitro* studies did not find any evidence that **metolazone** displaces **glibenclamide** from its protein binding sites, which might possibly have provided some explanation for what happened.[10]

The hypoglycaemic responses of 10 healthy subjects were studied following an intravenous infusion of **tolbutamide** 3 mg/kg, given 3 days before and one hour after the last dose of oral **cicletanine** 100 mg daily for a week.[11] No clinically relevant changes were seen. Note that, studies in *animals* and in non-diabetic hypertensive patients found that, at therapeutic doses, **cicletanine** did not affect glycoregulation.[12] The conclusion to be drawn is that **cicletanine** is unlikely to affect the control of diabetes in patients, but this needs confirmation from longer-term clinical studies.

(b) Hyponatraemia

A hospital report describes 8 cases of low serum sodium concentrations observed over a 5-year period in patients taking **chlorpropamide** and **hydrochlorothiazide** 50 mg with amiloride 5 mg.[13]

(c) Pharmacokinetics

A study in 12 healthy subjects given a single 25-mg dose of **hydrochlorothiazide** before and after taking **voglibose** 5 mg three times daily for 11 days found that **voglibose** increased the **hydrochlorothiazide** AUC and maximum plasma concentrations by 8% and 15%, respectively. These changes were not considered to be clinically relevant. The combination was well tolerated and adverse events were unchanged.[14]

In a study in 6 patients with diabetes taking **metformin**, adding **hydrochlorothiazide** for 2 weeks (4 patients), or stopping **hydrochlorothiazide** for 2 weeks (2 patients), had no effect on metformin AUC or clearance. This study was undertaken because of an earlier indication in 2 of these patients that hydrochlorothiazide might have increased metformin concentrations, but this was not confirmed.[15]

Mechanism

Not understood. One study suggested that the hyperglycaemia is due to the inhibition of insulin release by the pancreas.[16] Another suggestion is that the peripheral action of insulin is affected in some way.[5,17] There is also evidence that the effects might be related in part to potassium depletion.[18] The hyponatraemia appears to be due to the additive sodium-losing effects of chlorpropamide, the thiazide and amiloride. Obese patients might be more sensitive to the effects of hydrochlorothiazide on insulin metabolism.[7]

Importance and management

The reduction in the blood glucose-lowering effects of the antidiabetics on concurrent use with thiazides is extremely well documented (not all references are given here) but of only modest practical importance, particularly as much of the data relates to higher doses of thiazides than those now used clinically for hypertension. Low doses of thiazides have a lesser effect on plasma glucose, and UK guidelines on the treatment of hypertension in diabetes recommend the use of thiazides as add-on therapy if ACE inhibitors or angiotensin II receptor antagonists alone are not effective.[19] If higher doses are used, increased monitoring of diabetic control would seem prudent. There is evidence that the full effects could take many months to develop in some patients.[4] Most patients respond to a modest increase in the dose of their antidiabetics. This interaction might be expected to occur with all thiazides and possibly related diuretics, such as chlortalidone.

The US manufacturer of **triamterene** notes that it might increase blood glucose concentrations, and that dose adjustments of antidiabetics might be necessary on concurrent use.[20] The UK manufacturer of triamterene states that it should be used with caution in patients with diabetes.[21] However, there appears to be no evidence of potassium-sparing diuretics affecting glucose control. Note also, that they are rarely used alone (mostly being used in combination with a thiazide or loop diuretic), and are included as add-on treatment for hypertension in diabetes if ACE inhibitors or angiotensin II receptor antagonists with a thiazide are not effective.[19]

Hyponatraemia is a rare but recognised adverse effect of the thiazides and potassium-sparing diuretics, and no additional precautions would therefore seem necessary.

1. Wilkins RW. New drugs for the treatment of hypertension. *Ann Intern Med* (1959) 50, 1–10.
2. Kansal PC, Buse J, Buse MG. Thiazide diuretics and control of diabetes mellitus. *South Med J* (1969) 62, 1374–9.
3. Goldner MG, Zarowitz H, Akgun S. Hyperglycemia and glycosuria due to thiazide derivatives administered in diabetes mellitus. *N Engl J Med* (1960) 262, 403–5.
4. Lewis PJ, Kohner EM, Petrie A, Dollery CT. Deterioration of glucose tolerance in hypertensive patients on prolonged diuretic treatment. *Lancet* (1976) i, 564–6.
5. Runyan JW. Influence of thiazide diuretics on carbohydrate metabolism in patients with mild diabetes. *N Engl J Med* (1962) 267, 541–3.
6. Carliner NH, Schelling J-L, Russell RP, Okun R, Davis M. Thiazide- and phthalimidine-induced hyperglycemia in hypertensive patients. *JAMA* (1965) 191, 535–40.
7. Siegel D, Saliba P, Haffner S. Glucose and insulin levels during diuretic therapy in hypertensive men. *Hypertension* (1994) 23, 688–94.
8. Harper R, Ennis CN, Sheridan B, Atkinson AB, Johnston GD, Bell PM. Effects of low dose versus conventional dose thiazide diuretic on insulin action in essential hypertension. *BMJ* (1994) 309, 226–30.
9. Neutel JM. Metabolic manifestations of low-dose diuretics. *Am J Med* (1996) 101 (Suppl 3A), 71S–82S.
10. George S, McBurney A, Cole A. Possible protein binding displacement interaction between glibenclamide and metolazone. *Eur J Clin Pharmacol* (1990) 38, 93–5.
11. Bayés MC, Barbanoj MJ, Vallès J, Torrent J, Obach R, Jané F. A drug interaction study between cicletanine and tolbutamide in healthy volunteers. *Eur J Clin Pharmacol* (1996) 50, 381–4.
12. Mashori GR, Tariq AR, Shahimi MM, Suhaimi H. The effects of cicletanine, a new antihypertensive agent on insulin release in rat isolated pancreas by the perfusion technique. *Singapore Med J* (1996) 37, 278–81.
13. Zalin AM, Hutchinson CE, Jong M, Matthews K. Hyponatraemia during treatment with chlorpropamide and Moduretic (amiloride plus hydrochlorothiazide). *BMJ* (1984) 289, 659.
14. Kleist P, Suzuki Y, Thomsen T, Möller M, Römer A, Hucke HP, Kurowski M, Eckl KM. Voglibose has no effect on the pharmacokinetics of hydrochlorothiazide. *Eur J Clin Pharmacol* (1998) 54, 273–4.
15. Sung EYY, Moore MP, Lunt H, Doogue M, Zhang M, Begg EJ. Do thiazide diuretics alter the pharmacokinetics of metformin in patients with type 2 diabetes already established on metformin? *Br J Clin Pharmacol* (2009) 67, 130–1.
16. Fajans SS, Floyd JC, Knopf RF, Rull J, Guntsche EM, Conn JW. Benzothiadiazine suppression of insulin release from normal and abnormal islet tissue in man. *J Clin Invest* (1966) 45, 481–92.
17. Remenchik AP, Hoover C, Talso PJ. Insulin secretion by hypertensive patients receiving hydrochlorothiazide. *JAMA* (1970) 212, 869.
18. Rapoport MI, Hurd HF. Thiazide-induced glucose intolerance treated with potassium. *Arch Intern Med* (1964) 113, 405–8.
19. National Institute for Clinical Excellence. Type 2 diabetes: the management of type 2 diabetes: partial update (issued March 2010). Available at: http://www.nice.org.uk/nicemedia/pdf/CG87NICEGuideline.pdf (accessed 22/10/15)
20. Dyrenium (Triamterene). WellSpring Pharmaceutical Corp. US Prescribing information, March 2009.
21. Dytac (Triamterene). Mercury Pharma Group. UK Summary of product characteristics, September 2012.

Antidiabetics + Glucosamine ± Chondroitin

In a controlled study, glucosamine supplements with chondroitin had no effect on glycaemic control in patients taking oral antidiabetic drugs, but increases in blood glucose concentrations have occurred in patients with treated and untreated diabetes.

Clinical evidence, mechanism, importance and management

In 2000, the Canadian Adverse Drug Reaction Monitoring Programme (CADRMP) briefly reported that unexpected increases in blood glucose concentrations had occurred in patients with diabetes taking glucosamine sulfate, or glucosamine with chondroitin.[1] Similarly, increases in glucose concentrations were seen in 3 osteoarthritis patients with previously undiagnosed (and hence untreated) diabetes (2 patients) or glucose intolerance (1 patient) after taking glucosamine sulfate 1.5 g, but no effect on insulin concentrations was seen.[2] However, in a well controlled study, *Cosamin DS* (glucosamine hydrochloride 1.5 g plus chondroitin sulfate sodium 1.2 g) daily for 90 days had no effect on the control of diabetes (HbA_{1c}) in 22 patients with type 2 diabetes, 18 of whom were receiving oral antidiabetics (specific drugs not named) and 4 who were diet controlled.[3]

Endogenous glucosamine has a role in glucose metabolism, and might increase insulin resistance, which has led to concerns about its effects in diabetes. In one case, glucosamine reduced hypoglycaemic episodes in a patient with metastatic insulinoma.[4]

An interaction between antidiabetics and glucosamine is not established, and the results of the controlled study suggest that glucosamine supplements are unlikely to affect the control of diabetes. However, it has been suggested that the results might not be applicable to patients with later stages of diabetes[5] (i.e. those with type 2 diabetes who require, or are expected to require, insulin). Therefore, it might be prudent to increase monitoring of blood glucose concentrations in these patients if glucosamine supplements are taken. Also, if glucose control unexpectedly deteriorates, bear in mind the possibility of self-medication with supplements such as glucosamine.

1. Canadian Adverse Drug Reaction Monitoring Programme (CADRMP). Communiqué. Glucosamine sulfate: hyperglycemia. *Can Adverse Drug React News* (2000) 10 (Oct), 7.
2. Biggee BA, Blinn CM, Nuite M, Silbert JE, McAlindon TE. Effects of oral glucosamine sulphate on serum glucose and insulin during an oral glucose tolerance test of subjects with osteoarthritis. *Ann Rheum Dis* (2007) 66, 260–2.
3. Scroggie DA, Albright A, Harris MD. The effect of glucosamine-chondroitin supplementation on glycosylated hemoglobin levels in patients with type 2 diabetes mellitus: a placebo-controlled, double-blinded, randomized clinical trial. *Arch Intern Med* (2003) 163, 1587–90.
4. Chan NN, Baldeweg SE, Tan TMM, Hurel SJ. Glucosamine sulphate and osteoarthritis. *Lancet* (2001) 357, 1618–19.
5. Jain RK, McCormick JC. Can glucosamine supplements be applied for all patients with type 2 diabetes with osteoarthritis? *Arch Intern Med* (2004) 164, 807.

Antidiabetics + Guanethidine and related drugs

Limited evidence suggests that guanethidine has blood glucose-lowering activity, which might add to the effects of conventional antidiabetics. One

case report suggests soluble insulin might exaggerate the hypotensive effects of debrisoquine.

Clinical evidence

(a) Debrisoquine

An man with type 1 diabetes taking debrisoquine 20 mg twice daily developed severe postural hypotension within an hour of receiving 28 units of a short-acting **insulin** (soluble insulin) and 20 units of **isophane insulin**. He became dizzy and was found to have a standing blood pressure of 97/72 mmHg. The postural fall in systolic pressure was 65 mmHg. There was no evidence of hypoglycaemia and no hypotension when using 48 units of **isophane insulin** without the soluble insulin.[1] **Insulin** can cause hypotension but this is only seen in those with an impaired reflex control of blood pressure.[1]

(b) Guanethidine

A patient with diabetes needed an **insulin** dose increase from 70 to 94 units daily when guanethidine was withdrawn.[2] A later study in 3 patients with type 2 diabetes found that guanethidine 50 to 90 mg daily caused a notable improvement in their glucose tolerance.[3] Two other reports also suggest that guanethidine has blood glucose-lowering effects.[4,5]

Mechanism

It has been suggested that the interaction between insulin and guanethidine occurs because guanethidine can impair the homoeostatic mechanism concerned with increasing blood glucose concentrations, by affecting the release of catecholamines. The balance of the system thus impaired tends to be tipped in favour of a reduced blood glucose concentration, resulting in a reduced requirement for the antidiabetic drug. The interaction between debrisoquine and insulin is not understood.

Importance and management

Information about the interactions between guanethidine or debrisoquine and insulin is very limited, and their general importance is uncertain. Increase the frequency of blood glucose monitoring in patients taking antidiabetics if guanethidine or related drugs are started or stopped. Also monitor patients given debrisoquine (no longer generally available) and insulin, particularly if they are taking vasodilators, to ensure that excessive hypotension does not develop.

1. Hume L. Potentiation of hypotensive effect of debrisoquine by insulin. *Diabet Med* (1985) 2, 390–1.
2. Gupta KK, Lillicrap CA. Guanethidine and diabetes. *BMJ* (1968) 2, 697–8.
3. Gupta KK. The anti-diabetic action of guanethidine. *Postgrad Med J* (1969) 45, 455–6.
4. Kansal PC, Buse J, Durling FC, Buse MG. Effect of guanethidine and reserpine on glucose tolerance. *Curr Ther Res* (1971) 13, 517–22.
5. Woeber KA, Arky R, Braverman LE. Reversal by guanethidine of abnormal oral glucose tolerance in thyrotoxicosis. *Lancet* (1966) i, 895–8.

Antidiabetics + Hormonal contraceptives

The control of diabetes might be affected in some women while taking hormonal contraceptives, but it is unusual for it to be seriously disturbed. Irrespective of diabetic control, hormonal contraceptives should be used with caution in patients with diabetes because of the increased risk of arterial disease.

Clinical evidence

(a) Glucose tolerance

1. Healthy women. There are numerous reports of the effect of contraceptive steroids on glucose tolerance in non-diabetics. More recent reports from studies using low-dose oral combined hormonal contraceptives, support the suggestion that changes in glucose metabolism are minimal.[1,2] Problems with glucose metabolism seem very unlikely when the dose of oestrogen is less than 50 micrograms.[3] The progestogen in the hormonal contraceptive might also be important.[3-6] Progestogens with androgenic properties, such as **norgestrel**, **levonorgestrel**, and to a lesser extent **norethisterone (norethindrone)**, might affect carbohydrate metabolism. **Etynodiol (etynodrel)**, which has weak androgenic activity, was found to cause smaller reductions in glucose tolerance, and **noretynodrel** was found to have no effect.[3-5] Studies of healthy, non-diabetic women using oral combined hormonal contraceptives containing **ethinylestradiol** 20 to 40 micrograms with third generation progestogens (**gestodene**, **desogestrel**, or **norgestimate**) found no effect on carbohydrate metabolism in women using monophasic oral hormonal contraceptives, but impaired glucose tolerance developed in 10% of the women taking oral triphasic combined hormonal contraceptives. It was considered that the clinical consequences of impaired glucose tolerance and reduced **insulin** sensitivity induced by hormonal contraceptives are probably confined to risk groups, such as women with ovarian hyperandrogenism, obesity, previous gestational diabetes mellitus, perimenopausal women, or women with a family history of diabetes.[7]

2. Women with diabetes. In one study in 179 diabetic women, 34% needed an increase and 7% needed a decrease in their insulin dose when they were given an oral combined hormonal contraceptive.[8] However, there was no control group in this study so it is not possible to assess to what extent these changes were attributable to the contraceptives or to other factors. There are also a few scattered reports of individual patients with diabetes who experienced a marked disturbance of their diabetic control when given an oral hormonal contraceptive, some of which were low dose.[9-12] However, in a study of 38 patients with type 1 diabetes it was found that progestogen-only and oral combined hormonal contraceptives had little effect on the control of diabetes,[13] and another report[14] about women taking *Orthonovin* (**norethisterone** with **mestranol**) stated that no insulin dose changes were necessary. Similarly, no change in glycaemic control was found in 22 women with well-regulated type 1 diabetes who took a monophasic combination of **ethinylestradiol** with **gestodene** for one year.[7]

(b) Thromboembolic risk

A study in 11 patients with **insulin**-dependent diabetes, free of vascular complications, and taking low-dose oral hormonal contraceptives (**ethinylestradiol** 30 micrograms with **gestodene** 75 micrograms) found that although the plasma concentrations of most haemostatic variables were comparable to those of non-diabetics using the same contraceptive preparation, the rate of fibrin formation was increased and the fibrinolytic response attenuated. This suggests that women with diabetes can have a higher sensitivity to the thrombogenic effects of hormonal contraceptives.[7]

Mechanism

The reasons for changes in glucose metabolism are not understood. Many mechanisms have been considered including changes in cortisol secretion, alterations in tissue glucose utilisation, production of excessive amounts of growth hormone, and alterations in liver function.[15] Combined hormonal contraceptives have well known cardiovascular risks which are known to be increased in women with cardiovascular risk factors such as diabetes.

Importance and management

The effect of hormonal contraceptives on diabetic control is moderately well documented. Concurrent use need not be avoided in diabetes, but some patients might need a small adjustment in their dose of antidiabetic drug. However, it seems likely that routine blood glucose monitoring will identify any problems. Serious disturbances of diabetic control seem extremely rare. Of more concern in women with diabetes is the additive risk of vascular disease. Bear in mind that the lowest-strength oral combined hormonal contraceptive preparations (20 micrograms of oestrogen) are considered to be more appropriate for patients with risk factors for circulatory disease such as diabetics (provided a combined hormonal contraceptive is otherwise suitable), so the potential for interference with their diabetic control will also be minimised if this recommendation is followed. The choice of progestogen might also be important, with levonorgestrel appearing to have the most detrimental effect on glucose control, but less effect on thromboembolic risk. In women with diabetes and other vascular disease, combined hormonal contraceptives are generally not considered suitable, and oral progestogen-only contraceptives or implants are acceptable.[16]

The pharmacokinetic interactions of antidiabetic drugs with combined hormonal contraceptives are covered under the individual drugs or drug groups in the hormonal contraceptives section.

1. Miccoli R, Orlandi MC, Fruzzetti F, Giampietro O, Melis G, Ricci C, Bertolotto A, Fioretti P, Navalesi R, Masoni A. Metabolic effects of three new low-dose pills: a six-month experience. *Contraception* (1989) 39, 643–52.
2. Troisi RJ, Cowie CC, Harris MI. Oral contraceptive use and glucose metabolism in a national sample of women in the United States. *Am J Obstet Gynecol* (2000) 183, 389–95.
3. Spellacy WN. Carbohydrate metabolism during treatment with estrogen, progestogen, and low-dose oral contraceptives. *Am J Obstet Gynecol* (1982) 142, 732–4.
4. Perlman JA, Russell-Briefel R, Ezzati T, Lieberknecht G. Oral glucose tolerance and the potency of contraceptive progestins. *J Chron Dis* (1985) 38, 857–64.
5. Wynn V. Effect of duration of low-dose oral contraceptive administration on carbohydrate metabolism. *Am J Obstet Gynecol* (1982) 142, 739–46.
6. Knopp RH, Broyles FE, Cheung M, Moore K, Marcovina S, Chandler WL. Comparison of the lipoprotein, carbohydrate, and hemostatic effects of phasic oral contraceptives containing desogestrel or levonorgestrel. *Contraception* (2001) 63, 1–11.
7. Petersen KR. Pharmacodynamic effects of oral contraceptive steroids on biochemical markers for arterial thrombosis. Studies in non-diabetic women and in women with insulin-dependent diabetes mellitus. *Dan Med Bull* (2002) 49, 43–60.
8. Zeller WJ, Brehm H, Schöffling K, Melzer H. Verträglichkeit von hormonalen Ovulationshemmern bei Diabetikerinnen. *Arzneimittelforschung* (1974) 24, 351–7.
9. Kopera H, Dukes MNG, Ijzerman GL. Critical evaluation of clinical data on *Lyndiol*. *Int J Fertil* (1964) 9, 69–74.
10. Peterson WF, Steel MW, Coyne RV. Analysis of the effect of ovulatory suppressants on glucose tolerance. *Am J Obstet Gynecol* (1966) 95, 484–8.
11. Reder JA, Tulgan H. Impairment of diabetic control by norethynodrel with mestranol. *N Y State J Med* (1967) 67, 1073–4.
12. Rennie NJ. Hyperglycaemic episodes in a young woman after taking levonorgestrel-containing oral contraceptives. *N Z Med J* (1994) 107, 440–1.
13. Rådberg T, Gustafson A, Skryten A, Karlsson K. Oral contraception in diabetic women. Diabetes control, serum and high density lipoprotein lipids during low-dose progestogen, combined oestrogen/progestogen and non-hormonal contraception. *Acta Endocrinol (Copenh)* (1981) 98, 246–51.
14. Tyler ET, Olson HJ, Gotlib M, Levin M, Behne D. Long term usage of norethindrone with mestranol preparations in the control of human fertility. *Clin Med* (1964) 71, 997–1024.
15. Spellacy WN. A review of carbohydrate metabolism and the oral contraceptives. *Am J Obstet Gynecol* (1969) 104, 448–60.
16. Faculty of Sexual and Reproductive Healthcare. UK medical eligibility criteria for contraceptive use (UKMEC). 2009. Available at: http://www.fsrh.org/pdfs/UKMEC2009.pdf (accessed 21/10/15).

Antidiabetics + Isoniazid

Some reports suggest that isoniazid might affect the control of diabetes with insulin or tolbutamide.

Clinical evidence

A study in 6 patients with diabetes taking **insulin** found that isoniazid 300 to 400 mg daily increased their fasting blood glucose concentrations by 40% (from an average of about 14.2 mmol/L to 19.8 mmol/L), and their glucose tolerance curves increased and returned to normal range more slowly. After 6 days of treatment the average increase was only 20%. Two other patients needed an increased dose of **insulin** while taking

Table 13.3 Drugs commonly associated with effects that might alter blood-glucose control independent of a pharmacokinetic drug interaction*

Drug	*Comments*
ACE inhibitors	There is a strong association between ACE inhibitor use and the occurrence of hypoglycaemia, but this is not fully established, see 'Antidiabetics + ACE inhibitors', p.499.
Anabolic steroids (nandrolone, methandienone, and stanozolol)	Anabolic steroids have androgenic activity and might be expected to behave in the same way as testosterone (below).
Antipsychotics	There is evidence to indicate that both the classical and atypical antipsychotics can cause hyperglycaemia and might increase the incidence of new onset diabetes, see 'Antidiabetics + Antipsychotics', p.503.
Asparaginase	Asparaginase might induce temporary diabetes mellitus, which resolves when asparaginase is stopped.
Beta blockers (especially non-cardioselective)	Beta blockers can cause hypoglycaemia in non-diabetics and have been associated with prolonged or delayed recovery from hypoglycaemia as well as masking of hypoglycaemia symptoms in patients with diabetes. They can also oppose the effects of sulfonylureas. See 'Antidiabetics + Beta blockers', p.504.
Capecitabine	Control of diabetes is said to be affected by capecitabine.
Cibenzoline (Cifenline)	Cibenzoline has been strongly associated with causing hypoglycaemia, and this has been seen to affect the control of diabetes, see 'Antidiabetics + Cibenzoline (Cifenline)', p.506.
Corticosteroids	Corticosteroids impair carbohydrate tolerance and can unmask latent diabetes mellitus. These effects have resulted in impairment of diabetic control with a range of antidiabetics, see 'Antidiabetics + Corticosteroids', p.507.
Cyclophosphamide	Reported to alter carbohydrate metabolism.
Danazol	Reported to cause insulin resistance and this has affected the control of diabetes with antidiabetic drugs, see 'Antidiabetics + Danazol', p.507.
Disopyramide	Hypoglycaemia, sometimes severe, can occur with disopyramide and this can affect the control of diabetes, see 'Antidiabetics + Disopyramide', p.508. Patients at particular risk are the elderly, the malnourished, diabetics, and those with impaired renal and/or cardiac function.
Fenfluramine	Fenfluramine has established blood glucose-lowering effects.[1]
Isoniazid	Isoniazid is associated with hyperglycaemia, see 'Antidiabetics + Isoniazid', p.510.
Nicotinic acid (Niacin)	Impaired glucose tolerance.
Pentoxifylline	High doses of pentoxifylline given intravenously have, rarely, enhanced the blood glucose-lowering effects of insulin and oral antidiabetics. Oral pentoxifylline does not appear to have the same effect.
Quinine	Quinine can cause hypoglycaemia which is more common after intravenous use. This can affect the control of diabetes, see 'Antidiabetics + Antimalarials', p.503. Note that malaria itself can also cause hypoglycaemia.
SSRIs	There is an association between SSRI use and altered glycaemic control, including improved control as well as hypo- and hyper-glycaemia, but this is not fully established, see 'Antidiabetics + SSRIs', p.518.
Testosterone	Testosterone appears to improve insulin sensitivity, which has resulted in reduced insulin requirements in patients with diabetes, see 'Antidiabetics + Anabolic steroids or Androgens', p.502.

1. Turtle JR, Burgess JA. Hypoglycemic action of fenfluramine in diabetes mellitus. *Diabetes* (1973) 22, 858–67.
*This list is not exhaustive

isoniazid 200 mg daily, but this was reduced again when the isoniazid was withdrawn.[1]

Another study found that isoniazid had a hypoglycaemic effect in 6 out of 8 patients with diabetes.[2] A 500-mg dose of isoniazid caused an 18% (range 5 to 34%) reduction in blood glucose concentrations after 4 hours; 3 g of **tolbutamide** caused a 28% (19 to 43%) reduction, and together they caused a 35% (17 to 57%) reduction. However, one patient had a 10% increase in blood glucose concentrations after taking isoniazid, a 41% decrease after taking **tolbutamide**, and a 30% decrease after taking both drugs. The diabetic control of another patient was not affected by either drug.[2]

For mention of a case of increased insulin requirements in a patient taking isoniazid with rifampicin (rifampin), see 'Insulin + Rifampicin (Rifampin)', p.527.

Mechanism

Isoniazid is associated with hyperglycaemia and therefore the effects with insulin are not unexpected, whereas the effects with tolbutamide are unexplained.

Importance and management

Isoniazid is known to be associated with hyperglycaemia (see 'Table 13.3', above) and might therefore be expected to affect the control of diabetes. The finding with insulin is therefore expected, whereas the findings with tolbutamide are contrary to what might be expected. Nevertheless, given the effects of isoniazid alone on blood glucose, it would be prudent for patients with diabetes given isoniazid to be monitored for changes in diabetic control. Appropriate dose adjustments of the antidiabetic should be made where necessary.

1. Luntz GRWN, Smith SG. Effect of isoniazid on carbohydrate metabolism in controls and diabetics. *BMJ* (1953) i, 296–9.
2. Segarra FO, Sherman DS, Charif BS. Experiences with tolbutamide and chlorpropamide in tuberculous diabetic patients. *Ann N Y Acad Sci* (1959) 74, 656–61.

Antidiabetics + Karela (*Momordica charantia*)

The blood glucose-lowering effects of chlorpropamide and other antidiabetics can be increased by karela.

Clinical evidence

A report of a patient whose diabetes was poorly controlled on diet and **chlorpropamide**, but much better controlled when she ate curry containing karela, provides evidence that the blood glucose-lowering effects of karela and conventional oral antidiabetics can be additive.[1] Other small, non-controlled studies have subsequently shown that karela produces a notable improvement in glucose tolerance in patients with type 2 diabetes, both when they were taking **chlorpropamide**,[2] **tolbutamide**,[2] **glibenclamide**,[2,3] **glymidine**,[2] **metformin**,[3] or unspecified oral antidiabetics,[4] and when they were not taking antidiabetics.[5-7] In these studies, karela was given orally as a juice from the fruit,[2,5] dried powdered fruit,[6,7] fried fruits,[2] aqueous extract,[7] solvent extract from the fruit,[3] or as a suspension of fruit pulp.[4]

However, in a small randomised placebo-controlled study in 40 patients with type 2 diabetes given karela capsules (*Charantia*) taken three times daily after meals for 3 months, both karela and placebo had no statistically significant effect on HbA_{1c} (there was a very slight *increase* of 0.28% and 0.5%, respectively) and there was no change in mean fasting blood glucose concentrations (slight decrease with karela and increase with placebo). In this study, karela was taken in addition to standard **oral antidiabetics** (types not stated), and patients included both those newly diagnosed and those with established diabetes, with HbA_{1c} levels of 7 to 9%.[8]

A case report describes hypoglycaemic coma and seizures in two young non-diabetic children after they were given bitter melon (karela) tea.[9]

Mechanism

Karela (also known as bitter melon, bitter gourd, balsam pear, cundeamor) is the fruit of *Momordica charantia* which is indigenous to Asia and South America. The blood glucose-lowering effects of karela might be due to its content of polypeptide P, a blood glucose-lowering peptide,[10] also known as vegetable insulin (v-insulin).[11] This substance is effective when given subcutaneously,[11] but its oral activity is uncertain.[12] Other blood glucose-lowering compounds isolated from karela include charantin (sterol glucoside mixture in the fruit) and vicine a pyrimidine nucleoside found in the seeds). Karela fruit might have both insulin-like effects and stimulate insulin secretion.[12]

Importance and management

Karela is available in the UK and elsewhere, and is used to flavour foods such as curries, and also used as a herbal medicine for the treatment of diabetes mellitus. Its blood glucose-lowering activity appears to be established, although the best-controlled study so far found its effects to be minimal. Health professionals should therefore be aware that patients might possibly be using karela as well as more conventional drugs to control their diabetes. Irregular consumption of karela as part of the diet could possibly contribute to unexplained fluctuations in diabetic control.

1. Aslam M, Stockley IH. Interaction between curry ingredient (karela) and drug (chlorpropamide). *Lancet* (1979) i, 607.
2. Leatherdale BA, Panesar KR, Singh G, Atkins TW, Bailey CJ, Bignell AHC. Improvement in glucose tolerance due to Momordica charantia (karela). *BMJ* (1981) 282, 1823–4.
3. Tongia A, Tongia SK, Dave M. Phytochemical determination and extraction of Momordica charantia fruit and its hypoglycemic potentiation of oral hypoglycemic drugs in diabetes mellitus (NIDDM). *Indian J Physiol Pharmacol* (2004) 48, 241–44.
4. Ahmad N, Hassan MR, Halder H, Bennoor KS. Effect of *Momordica charantia* (Karolla) extracts on fasting and postprandial serum glucose levels in NIDDM patients. *Bangladesh Med Res Counc Bull* (1999) 25, 11–13.
5. Welihinda J, Karunanayake EH, Sheriff MHR, Jaysinghe KSA . Effect of *Momordica charantia* on the glucose tolerance in maturity onset diabetes. *J Ethnopharmacol* (1986) 17, 277–82.
6. Akhtar MS. Trial of Momordica Charantia Linn (Karela) powder in patients with maturity-onset diabetes. *J Pakistan Med Assoc* (1982) 32, 106–7.
7. Srivastava Y, Venkatakrishna-Bhatt H, Verma Y, Venkaiah K, Raval BH. Antidiabetic and adaptogenic properties of *Momordica charantia* extract: an experimental and clinical evaluation. *Phytother Res* (1993) 7, 285–9.
8. Dans AML, Villarruz MVC, Jimeno CA, Javelosa MAU, Chua J, Bautista R, Velez GGB. The effect of *Momordica charantia* capsule preparation on glycemic control in type 2 diabetes mellitus needs further studies. *J Clin Epidemiol* (2007) 60, 554–9.
9. Hulin A, Wavelet M, Desbordes JM. Intoxication aiguë par *Momordica charantia* (sorrossi). A propos de deux cas. *Sem Hop Paris* (1988) 64, 2847–8.
10. Khanna P, Jain SC, Panagariya A, Dixit VP. Hypoglycemic activity of polypeptide-p from a plant source. *J Nat Prod* (1981) 44, 648–55.
11. Baldwa VS, Bhandari CM, Pangaria A, Goyal RK. Clinical trial in patients with diabetes mellitus of an insulin-like compound obtained from plant source. *Ups J Med Sci* (1977) 82, 39–41.
12. Raman A, Lau C. Anti-diabetic properties and phytochemistry of *Momordica charantia* (Cucurbitaceae). *Phytomedicine* (1996) 2, 349–62.

Antidiabetics + Ketotifen

The concurrent use of biguanides and ketotifen resulted in a decrease in the number of platelets in one study in patients with diabetes.

Clinical evidence, mechanism, importance and management

A study in 30 hospitalised patients with diabetes (10 diet controlled, 10 taking unnamed **sulfonylureas**, 10 taking unnamed **biguanides**) found that the concurrent use of oral ketotifen 4 mg daily for 14 days was generally well tolerated (as assessed by an array of laboratory tests, including electrolytes, renal function, liver transaminases, haematology screen). However, those taking **biguanides** had a considerable decrease in platelet counts and 3 had a marked decrease on day 14 to slightly below 100×10^9/L, which returned to normal after a few days.[1] This finding underlies the precaution issued by the UK manufacturer of oral ketotifen,[2] that the concurrent use of oral antidiabetics and ketotifen should be avoided until this effect is explained. However, no other studies appear to have confirmed the decrease in platelet count, so that its general importance remains uncertain, but given the passage of time since this study was conducted, it would seem unlikely to be clinically relevant.

1. Doleček R. Ketotifen in the treatment of diabetics with various allergic conditions. *Pharmatherapeutica* (1981) 2, 568–74.
2. Zaditen tablets (Ketotifen hydrogen fumarate).Swedish Orphan Biovitrum Ltd. UK Summary of product characteristics, September 2011.

Antidiabetics + Linezolid

An isolated case report describes severe hypoglycaemia in a patient receiving insulin, glibenclamide (glyburide), and metformin after linezolid was started.

Clinical evidence, mechanism, importance and management

A 64-year-old man with type 2 diabetes, stabilised on **insulin** 55 units daily, **glibenclamide (glyburide)** 5 mg twice daily, and **metformin** 1 g twice daily, developed severe hypoglycaemia 7 days after starting linezolid 600 mg twice daily for a resistant wound infection. He decreased his insulin dose by 10 units daily and stopped the **glibenclamide**, but there was no improvement in his symptoms. Two days later he took no medication and increased his food intake, which led to some resolution of symptoms. He was admitted to hospital after further fluctuations in his blood glucose concentrations and recurring hypoglycaemic symptoms despite intravenous glucose treatment. The linezolid was stopped, all blood glucose-lowering medication was withheld, and during the following 48 hours he experienced no further hypoglycaemic events. Starting about two-and-a-half days post-admission, his **insulin**, **glibenclamide**, and **metformin** were reintroduced, and three weeks after admission he was discharged on insulin and metformin with **doxycycline**. At follow-up 9 months later, he was stabilised on **insulin** 65 units daily and **metformin** 1 g twice daily without any further episodes of hypoglycaemia. The patient had no previous history of hypoglycaemia of note and was considered to be compliant with medication, leading the authors to suggest that the addition of the linezolid precipitated this patient's hypoglycaemia.[1]

This is an isolated report and as such its general clinical relevance is not known. However, note that linezolid is a weak, reversible, non-selective inhibitor of MAO, and there are reports of hypoglycaemia occurring with the antidepressant MAOIs and other antidiabetics (see 'Antidiabetics + MAOIs or RIMAs', p.513).

1. Bodnar T, Starr K, Halter JB. Linezolid-associated hypoglycaemia in a 64-year-old man with type 2 diabetes. *Am J Geriatr Pharmacother* (2011) 9, 88–92.

Antidiabetics + Lithium

An isolated report describes a diabetic patient receiving insulin who developed hyperglycaemia when his lithium concentrations were high. Conversely, in another isolated case of a patient with type 2 diabetes, glucose control improved when lithium was started. Lithium use has been associated with increased blood glucose concentrations and the development of diabetes mellitus.

Clinical evidence

One patient with mania and diabetes developed hyperglycaemia, in the presence of a constant **insulin** dose, when his lithium serum concentrations were high (about 1.4 mmol/L), but reducing the lithium concentration to 1.1 mmol/L led to a lowering of the fasting blood glucose.[1] In contrast, a patient with type 2 diabetes managed with diet and insulin, had a reduction in blood glucose on starting lithium. Insulin was stopped, and at a one-year follow up she was said to have normal blood glucose concentrations without dietary restrictions or insulin.[2]

Mechanism

Uncertain. A study in 10 psychiatric patients found that lithium carbonate for 2 weeks increased their blood glucose concentrations and impaired their glucose tolerance.[3] There are also a few case reports of hyperglycaemia, impaired glucose tolerance, and diabetes mellitus in patients taking lithium.[4-6] However, a long-term investigation over a period of 6 years, involving 460 patients, found that the mean blood glucose concentrations remained the same before and after the use of lithium. One patient did develop diabetic ketoacidosis after 4 years of uneventful lithium use, but the authors concluded that the long-term use of lithium did not increase the risk of developing diabetes mellitus.[7] Further, in a study in 6 patients with type 2 diabetes controlled by diet alone, lithium, taken for one week, did not alter the metabolic response to a standard 50 g carbohydrate breakfast.[8] Conversely, there is an isolated case of a patient who developed temporary diabetes requiring insulin after the *withdrawal* of lithium.[9] Note that the incidence of diabetes tends to be higher in patients with manic depression than in the general population.[10]

Importance and management

There are only a couple of reports of disturbed diabetic control in patients taking lithium. The association between lithium and increased blood glucose concentrations and the development of diabetes mellitus is unclear, and there is little or no evidence that its use normally causes important changes in diabetic control. No special precautions would seem necessary on concurrent use, but if glycaemic control changes when lithium is started, bear this interaction in mind. Note that it is prudent to monitor blood glucose concentrations when any change is made to the medication regimen of a patient with diabetes.

1. Waziri R, Nelson J. Lithium in diabetes mellitus: a paradoxical response. *J Clin Psychiatry* (1978) 39, 623–5.
2. Saran AS. Antidiabetic effects of lithium. *J Clin Psychiatry* (1982) 43, 383–4.
3. Shopsin B, Stern S, Gershon S. Altered carbohydrate metabolism during treatment with lithium carbonate. *Arch Gen Psychiatry* (1972) 26, 566–71.
4. Craig J, Abu-Saleh M, Smith B, Evans I. Diabetes mellitus in patients on lithium. *Lancet* (1977) ii, 1028.
5. Johnston BB. Diabetes mellitus in patients on lithium. *Lancet* (1977) ii, 935.
6. Martinez-Maldonado M, Terrell J. Lithium carbonate-induced nephrogenic diabetes insipidus and glucose intolerance. *Arch Intern Med* (1973) 132, 881–4.
7. Vestergaard P, Schou M. Does long-term lithium treatment induce diabetes mellitus? *Neuropsychobiology* (1987) 17, 130–2.
8. Jones GR, Lazarus JH, Davies CJ, Greenwood RH. The effect of short term lithium carbonate in type II diabetes mellitus. *Horm Metab Res* (1983) 15, 422–4.
9. Okosieme OE, Campbell A, Patton K, Evans ML. Transient diabetes associated with withdrawal of lithium therapy. *Diabetes Care* (2006) 29, 1181.
10. Russell JD, Johnson GFS. Affective disorders, diabetes mellitus and lithium. *Aust N Z J Psychiatry* (1981) 15, 349–53.

Antidiabetics + Miscellaneous

The risk of hypoglycaemia is increased if pegvisomant is given with insulin or oral antidiabetics. The use of etanercept can result in hypoglycaemia in patients with diabetes taking antidiabetic drugs.

Clinical evidence, mechanism, importance and management

(a) Etanercept

The UK manufacturer states that, in patients with diabetes receiving medication [not stated], there have been cases of hypoglycaemia, and that doses of **antidiabetic** drugs might need to be reduced on concurrent use.[1]

(b) Pegvisomant

The UK manufacturer states that, in a study in patients with diabetes treated with **insulin** or **oral antidiabetics**, there was an increased risk of hypoglycaemia, and that a reduction in the dose of insulin or the antidiabetic might be necessary on concurrent use. This is as a result of altered insulin sensitivity by pegvisomant.[2]

1. Enbrel (Etanercept). Pfizer Ltd. UK Summary of product characteristics, October 2013
2. Somavert (Pegvisomant). Pfizer Ltd. UK Summary of product characteristics, December 2011.

Antidiabetics + MAOIs or RIMAs

The blood glucose-lowering effects of insulin and the oral antidiabetics can be increased by non-selective MAOIs. Moclobemide does not appear to interact with chlorpropamide, glibenclamide (glyburide), gliclazide, or metformin.

Clinical evidence

(a) Moclobemide

A study in healthy subjects given **glibenclamide (glyburide)** 2.5 mg daily found that moclobemide 200 mg three times daily for a week had no effect on glucose or insulin concentrations after oral glucose tolerance tests.[1] In clinical studies, 8 patients with diabetes taking **glibenclamide** , **gliclazide**, **metformin**, or **chlorpropamide** were given moclobemide, and there was no effect on blood glucose concentrations or any other evidence of an interaction.[1]

(b) Non-selective MAOIs

A patient with diabetes receiving **insulin** experienced postural syncope and hypoglycaemia, which required a reduction in **insulin** dose, when **mebanazine** was also taken.[2] Other reports in patients with diabetes indicate that **mebanazine** increases the blood glucose-lowering effects of **insulin**, **tolbutamide**, and **chlorpropamide,** and improves diabetic control.[3-6]

Mechanism

Not fully understood. Mebanazine,[4] iproniazid,[7] isocarboxazid,[8] phenelzine,[4] and tranylcypromine[9] have all been shown to reduce blood glucose concentrations in the absence of conventional antidiabetics, possibly due to some direct action on the pancreas, which causes the release of insulin.[9] It would seem that this can be additive with the effects of conventional antidiabetics.

Importance and management

The interaction between the non-selective MAOIs and antidiabetics is an established interaction of only modest clinical importance. It can benefit the control of diabetes in many patients, but some individuals might need a reduction in the dose of their antidiabetic to avoid excessive hypoglycaemia. The effects of concurrent use should be monitored. This interaction would seem possible with any combination of an antidiabetic drug and a non-selective MAOI.

No clinically important interaction seems to occur between chlorpropamide, glibenclamide, gliclazide, or metformin and moclobemide.

1. Amrein R, Güntert TW, Dingemanse J, Lorscheid T, Stabl M, Schmid-Burgk W. Interactions of moclobemide with concomitantly administered medication: evidence from pharmacological and clinical studies. *Psychopharmacology (Berl)* (1992) 106, S24–S31.
2. Cooper AJ, Keddie KMG. Hypotensive collapse and hypoglycaemia after mebanazine-a monoamine oxidase inhibitor. *Lancet* (1964) i, 1133–5.
3. Wickström L, Pettersson K. Treatment of diabetics with monoamine-oxidase inhibitors. *Lancet* (1964) ii, 995–7.
4. Adnitt PI. Hypoglycemic action of monoamineoxidase inhibitors (MAOI's). *Diabetes* (1968) 17, 628–33.
5. Cooper AJ. The action of mebanazine, a mono amine oxidase inhibitor antidepressant drug in diabetes-part II. *Int J Neuropsychiatry* (1966) 2, 342–5.
6. Adnitt PI, Oleesky S, Schnieden H. The hypoglycaemic action of monoamineoxidase inhibitors (MAOI's). *Diabetologia* (1968) 4, 379.
7. Weiss J, Weiss S, Weiss B. Effects of iproniazid and similar compounds on the gastrointestinal tract. *Ann N Y Acad Sci* (1959) 80, 854–9.
8. van Praag HM, Leijnse B. The influence of some antidepressives of the hydrazine type on the glucose metabolism in depressed patients. *Clin Chim Acta* (1963) 8, 466–75.
9. Bressler R, Vargas-Cordon M, Lebovitz HE. Tranylcypromine: a potent insulin secretagogue and hypoglycemic agent. *Diabetes* (1968) 17, 617–24.

Antidiabetics + Orlistat

Orlistat does not alter the pharmacokinetics of glibenclamide or metformin. Orlistat improved glycaemic control, which resulted in the need to reduce the dose of glibenclamide (glyburide) or glipizide in almost half the patients in one study. In other studies, orlistat also reduced the dose requirement for metformin and for insulin. Orlistat and cimetidine might have contributed to a case of metformin-associated lactic acidosis. An isolated case report describes acute pancreatitis after orlistat was added to sitagliptin.

Clinical evidence

(a) Acarbose

The UK manufacturer of orlistat states that in the absence of pharmacokinetic studies its concurrent use with acarbose should be avoided.[1]

(b) Insulin

In a randomised, placebo-controlled, double-blind study in patients with type 2 diabetes receiving insulin, with or without **metformin** or a **sulfonylurea**, orlistat 120 mg three times daily for one year, and a reduced-calorie diet improved glycaemic control and allowed a greater reduction in insulin dose (mean reduction of 8.1 units daily versus 1.6 units daily for placebo). Hypoglycaemic episodes occurred in about 17% of orlistat recipients and about 10% of placebo recipients: three orlistat recipients and one placebo recipient required medical intervention due to hypoglycaemia.[2] For discussion of a retrospective analysis of patients with type 2 diabetes taking metformin, a sulfonylurea, and/or insulin with orlistat, see under *Metformin*, below.

(c) Metformin

In a randomised, crossover study in 21 healthy subjects given metformin 500 mg daily for 6 days, orlistat 120 mg three times daily had no effect on the pharmacokinetics of metformin.[3] In a randomised, placebo-controlled, study in patients with type 2 diabetes taking metformin with or without a sulfonylurea (mainly **glibenclamide (glyburide)** or **glipizide**), orlistat 120 mg three times daily for one year improved glycaemic control and allowed a small reduction in the dose of metformin (mean daily reduction of 16 mg versus a mean increase of 49 mg for placebo). Twice as many patients in the orlistat group either reduced or discontinued one or more of their antidiabetics (17% versus 8% with placebo). Hypoglycaemic episodes (mild to moderate and not requiring treatment) occurred in 10% of orlistat recipients and 4% of placebo recipients.[4] Similarly, improvement in glycaemic control and a reduced requirement for oral antidiabetics was reported in another study.[5]

A 59-year-old woman with type 2 diabetes taking long-term metformin 500 mg three times daily, developed metformin-associated lactic acidosis with cardiovascular collapse and acute renal failure. Three months previously she had started orlistat 120 mg three times daily, which caused abdominal pain and chronic diarrhoea. During the 4 days before hospital admission, she was prescribed **cimetidine** 400 mg twice daily for her abdominal pain (presumed to be due to reactivation of a previously diagnosed duodenal ulcer). The metformin-associated lactic acidosis was considered to have been precipitated by the combination of orlistat and cimetidine.[6]

A retrospective analysis of 7 studies in obese patients with type 2 diabetes taking **metformin**, a **sulfonylurea** (type not stated), and/or **insulin**, found that orlistat 120 mg three times daily for 6 or 12 months reduced fasting blood glucose concentrations more than placebo by week 4. This reduction preceded most of the weight loss by these patients. Orlistat also appeared to improve glycaemic control more than was predicted due to weight loss alone.[7]

(d) Sitagliptin

A case report describes a 53-year-old woman with type 2 diabetes who had been taking sitagliptin 100 mg daily for 8 weeks, and who developed acute pancreatitis 4 weeks after orlistat was added. On admission the sitagliptin and orlistat were stopped, and over the following 5 days her abdominal pain improved and a normal diet was resumed without problems. **Metformin** and **gliclazide** were started and orlistat was added without problems, and the patient was discharged. The patient had no previous history of pancreatitis and had previously taken orlistat with metformin and gliclazide for 8 months without problems, and had tolerated sitagliptin alone for 8 weeks, also with no problems.[8]

(e) Sulfonylureas

A randomised, crossover study in 12 healthy subjects found that orlistat 80 mg three times daily for a little over 4 days had no effect on the pharmacokinetics of a single 5-mg oral dose of **glibenclamide (glyburide)** and the blood glucose lowering effects remained unchanged.[9] A later one-year, randomised, placebo-controlled, study in obese patients with type 2 diabetes, in which 139 patients took orlistat, found that orlistat reduced fasting blood glucose and HbA_{1c} concentrations. In addition, 43% of patients taking orlistat 120 mg three times daily were able to decrease their sulfonylurea dose (**glibenclamide** or **glipizide**), and 11.7% of them were able to discontinue the sulfonylurea. The average dose decrease was 23% compared with 9% in the placebo group.[10] For discussion of a retrospective analysis of patients with type 2 diabetes taking metformin, a sulfonylurea, and/or insulin with orlistat, see under *Metformin*, above.

Mechanism

The improved glycaemic control seen with orlistat in patients with diabetes might be partly due to the beneficial effects of weight reduction on glycaemic control, however in some studies the reduction in HbA_{1c} was not entirely dependent on the magnitude of weight loss.[2,7] The authors of the retrospective analysis suggest other mechanisms, including improvement of insulin sensitivity, might be involved, but this requires further study.[7]

Pancreatitis has been reported, post-marketing, for both sitagliptin and orlistat, and the case report is perhaps due to additive effects as both drugs had been taken previously without problems.

Importance and management

The majority of evidence regarding the use of orlistat in patients with diabetes, relates to a drug-disease interaction rather than a drug-drug interaction. That relating to drug-drug effects shows that there is no pharmacokinetic interaction between orlistat and metformin or glibenclamide (glyburide). The isolated report of pancreatitis with sitagliptin and orlistat is of unknown general clinical importance. Regarding drug-disease effects, the benefits of orlistat on glycaemic control in overweight or obese patients with diabetes are established. Diabetic control should be more closely monitored in patients taking orlistat, and the doses of antidiabetic drugs adjusted as necessary.

1. Xenical (Orlistat). Roche Products Ltd. UK Summary of product characteristics, April 2014.
2. Kelly DE, Bray GA, Pi-Sunyer FX, Klein S, Hill J, Miles J, Hollander P. Clinical efficacy of orlistat therapy in overweight and obese patients with insulin-treated type 2 diabetes. A 1-year randomized controlled trial. *Diabetes Care* (2002) 25, 1033–41. Correction. ibid., 2119 and ibid. (2003) 26, 971.
3. Zhi J, Moore R, Kanitra L, Mulligan TE. Pharmacokinetic evaluation of the possible interaction between selected concomitant medications and orlistat at steady state in healthy subjects. *J Clin Pharmacol* (2002) 42, 1011–19.
4. Miles JM, Leiter L, Hollander P, Wadden T, Anderson JW, Doyle M, Foreyt J, Aronne L, Klein S. Effect of orlistat in overweight and obese patients with type 2 diabetes treated with metformin. *Diabetes Care* (2002) 25, 1123–8.
5. Berne C; the Orlistat Swedish Type 2 diabetes Study Group. A randomized study of orlistat in combination with a weight management programme in obese patients with type 2 diabetes treated with metformin. *Diabet Med* (2005) 22, 612–18.
6. Dawson D, Conlon C. Case study: metformin-associated lactic acidosis. Could orlistat be relevant? *Diabetes Care* (2003) 26, 2471–2.
7. Jacob S, Rabbia M, Meier MK, Hauptman J. Orlistat 120 mg improves glycaemic control in type 2 diabetic patients with or without concurrent weight loss. *Diabetes Obes Metab* (2009) 11, 361–71.
8. Garg R, Hussey C, Ibrahim S. Pancreatitis associated with the use of sitagliptin and orlistat combination: a case report. *Diabet Med* (2010) 27, 485–6.
9. Zhi J, Melia AT, Koss-Twardy SG, Min B, Guerciolini R, Freundlich NL, Milla G, Patel IH. The influence of orlistat on the pharmacokinetics and pharmacodynamics of glyburide in healthy volunteers. *J Clin Pharmacol* (1995) 35, 521–5.
10. Hollander PA, Elbein SC, Hirsch IB, Kelley D, McGill J, Taylor T, Weiss SR, Crockett SE, Kaplan RA, Comstock J, Lucas CP, Lodewick PA, Canovatchel W, Chung J, Hauptman J. Role of orlistat in the treatment of obese patients with type 2 diabetes. A 1-year randomized double-blind study. *Diabetes Care* (1998) 21, 1288–94.

Antidiabetics + Other drugs that affect blood glucose concentrations

A number of drugs, such as pentoxifylline, can affect blood glucose concentrations, which can result in a disturbance of diabetic control in patients taking antidiabetic drugs.

Clinical evidence, mechanism, importance and management

If a drug has been reported to cause hypoglycaemia or hyperglycaemia, it could disturb the control of diabetes. As this effect could occur whether or not an antidiabetic drug is being taken, it is, strictly speaking, a drug-disease interaction or an adverse effect. Nevertheless, because this effect could be additive with, or antagonise the effects of, the antidiabetics it is included here for completeness. For some examples of drugs, other than the antidiabetics, that can affect blood glucose concentrations, see 'Table 13.3', p.511. Note that this table is not an exhaustive list of these drugs.

Interactions where a drug affects the exposure to an antidiabetic (a pharmacokinetic interaction), leading to an increase or reduction in its effects, or where other adverse effects have been reported, in addition to affecting blood glucose concentrations, are covered in individual, specific monographs.

Antidiabetics + Phosphodiesterase type-5 inhibitors

Sildenafil does not alter the pharmacokinetics of tolbutamide. Vardenafil does not alter the pharmacokinetics or pharmacodynamics of glibenclamide (glyburide). Avanafil does not appear to alter the pharmacokinetics of rosiglitazone.

Clinical evidence, mechanism, importance and management

(a) Avanafil

The US manufacturer briefly reports that, in a crossover study in 20 healthy male subjects, a single 200-mg dose of avanafil increased the AUC of a single 8-mg dose of **rosiglitazone** by just 2%.[1] Note that rosiglitazone can be used as a probe substrate to assess the activity of drugs on CYP2C8. This study therefore suggests that avanafil is not an inducer or inhibitor of this isoenzyme. No rosiglitazone dose adjustment would seem necessary on concurrent use, but it is prudent to monitor blood glucose concentrations when any change is made to the medication regimen of a patient with diabetes.

(b) Sildenafil

The UK and US manufacturers briefly report that, in a study, sildenafil 50 mg did not alter the pharmacokinetics of **tolbutamide** 250 mg,[2,3] probably because sildenafil is only a weak inhibitor of CYP2C9 by which **tolbutamide** is metabolised. This is consistent with the way other CYP2C9 substrates behave with sildenafil, see *Warfarin*, under 'Coumarins + Phosphodiesterase type-5 inhibitors', p.462. No tolbutamide dose adjustment would seem necessary on concurrent use, but it is prudent to monitor blood glucose concentrations when any change is made to the medication regimen of a patient with diabetes.

(c) Vardenafil

The UK manufacturers of vardenafil briefly report that the relative bioavailability of a 3.5 mg dose of **glibenclamide (glyburide)** was not affected by a single 20-mg dose of vardenafil,[4] and that vardenafil had no effect on **glibenclamide** pharmacodynamics (glucose and insulin concentrations).[5] They also state that **glibenclamide** had no effect on the pharmacokinetics of a 20-mg dose of vardenafil.[4]

Also, although no specific pharmacokinetic study has been conducted, the manufacturers state that population pharmacokinetic analysis suggests that **sulfonylureas** (not named) and **metformin** have no effect on vardenafil pharmacokinetics.[4] No dose adjustments seem necessary on concurrent use, but it is prudent to monitor blood glucose concentrations when any change is made to the medication regimen of a patient with diabetes.

1. Stendra (Avanafil). Vivus, Inc. US Prescribing information, January 2015.
2. Viagra (Sildenafil citrate). Pfizer Ltd. UK Summary of product characteristics, June 2015.
3. Viagra (Sildenafil citrate). Pfizer Inc. US Prescribing information, March 2015.
4. Levitra (Vardenafil hydrochloride). Bayer plc. UK Summary of product characteristics, April 2014.
5. Levitra (Vardenafil hydrochloride). Bayer HealthCare Pharmaceuticals Inc. US Prescribing information, April 2014.

Antidiabetics + Quinolones

A number of reports describe severe hypoglycaemia or hyperglycaemia in patients with diabetes taking gatifloxacin and various antidiabetics including insulin, metformin, pioglitazone, repaglinide, rosiglitazone, some sulfonylureas, or voglibose. There appears to be a much higher incidence of these effects with gatifloxacin than other quinolones. Levofloxacin does not affect the pharmacokinetics of glibenclamide (glyburide) and ciprofloxacin might slightly increase glibenclamide exposure, but neither drug appears to affect glucose concentrations. However, a retrospective study and isolated reports describe hypoglycaemia in diabetic patients taking glibenclamide, gliclazide, or glipizide, when ciprofloxacin, levofloxacin, or norfloxacin was given, and fatalities have occurred. The pharmacokinetics of rosiglitazone are not affected by ciprofloxacin.

Clinical evidence

(a) Effects on blood glucose control

Numerous case reports suggest that some quinolones are associated with hypoglycaemia or hyperglycaemia when used with insulin and oral antidiabetics, and these are summarised in 'Table 13.4', p.515. Analysis of FDA data, case-control studies and other small studies, support these reports and suggest that the risk of hypoglycaemia varies between individual drugs; details are provided below.

A search of the FDA database for adverse drug events associated with **gatifloxacin**, **ciprofloxacin**, **levofloxacin**, and **moxifloxacin** between November 1997 and September 2003 found 10 025 unique adverse events, including 568 involving glucose homoeostasis abnormalities, of which 25 were fatal. **Gatifloxacin** use was associated with 453 (80%) of the adverse events involving glucose homoeostasis, and 17 of these were fatal compared with 3, 5, and 0 fatalities with **ciprofloxacin**, **levofloxacin**, and **moxifloxacin**, respectively. Of all the adverse events associated with **gatifloxacin**, 24% involved glucose homoeostasis, compared with **ciprofloxacin** (1.3%), **levofloxacin** (1.6%), and **moxifloxacin** (1.3%). The risk of adverse events involving glucose homoeostasis was higher in older patients, in patients taking medications for diabetes (almost 70% of those taking **gatifloxacin** were also using **insulin** or **oral antidiabetics**), and in patients with renal impairment whose dose had not been appropriately adjusted.[1]

In another analysis, large case-control studies were conducted in a cohort of elderly patients from Ontario, Canada, who had taken broad-spectrum antibacterials and been treated in hospital for either hypoglycaemia or hyperglycaemia within 30 days of taking the antibacterial. **Gatifloxacin** was associated with a 4.3-fold increased risk of hypoglycaemia when compared with macrolides, and **levofloxacin** was associated with a 1.5-fold increased risk, whereas there was no increased risk with **moxifloxacin** or **ciprofloxacin**. Similarly, **gatifloxacin** was associated with a 16.7-fold increased risk of hyperglycaemia when compared with macrolides, whereas no other quinolones were associated with an increased risk. The risk of hypoglycaemia or hyperglycaemia with **gatifloxacin** was no different between those patients receiving treatment for diabetes and those who were not. Overall, 1.1% of courses of **gatifloxacin** were associated with hospital visits for dysglycaemia compared with 0.3% for **ciprofloxacin**, 0.3% for **levofloxacin**, 0.2% for **moxifloxacin**, and 0.1% for macrolides.[2] In a study in patients with type 2 diabetes controlled by diet and exercise alone, **gatifloxacin** 400 mg daily for 10 days had no clinically important effect on glucose tolerance or most aspects of glucose homoeostasis, but did cause a brief increase in the serum concentrations of insulin.[3]

In a further retrospective, case-control study, of 7 414 patients taking **glibenclamide (glyburide)**, and hospitalised or given emergency treatment for hypoglycaemia, 69 had recently received a course of **ciprofloxacin**, and 140 had received a course of **levofloxacin**. No statistically significant increased risk of hypoglycaemia was found in those who had been dispensed a prescription for **ciprofloxacin** from day one to 5 before the hypoglycaemia episode, relative to cefalexin (which was used as a non-interacting control). For **levofloxacin** for the same period, the adjusted odds ratio was 2.3. However, for those who had been dispensed a prescription for **ciprofloxacin** within days 6 to 10 of the hypoglycaemic episode, the adjusted odds ratio for the risk of developing hypoglycaemia on the concurrent use of **glibenclamide** was 2.1, relative to cefalexin (non-interacting control), and for **levofloxacin** for the same period, was 2.8. In the 5 559 patients taking **glipizide**, and hospitalised or given emergency treatment for hypoglycaemia, 33 had recently received a course of **ciprofloxacin** and 89 had received a course of **levofloxacin**. Ciprofloxacin use was not associated with a statistically significant increased risk of hypoglycaemia. However, for those who were dispensed **levofloxacin** within days 1 to 5, or days 6 to 10, of the diagnosis of hypoglycaemia, the adjusted odds ratio for the risk of an interaction was 2.1 and 1.8, respectively, relative to the non-interacting control cefalexin.[4]

A pooled analysis from clinical and post-marketing studies suggested that **moxifloxacin** had no clinically relevant effect on blood glucose homoeostasis, even in patients with diabetes mellitus.[5] The UK manufacturer of **norfloxacin**, briefly notes that concurrent use with **glibenclamide** has resulted in severe hypoglycaemia.[6]

Table 13.4 Interactions between antidiabetics and quinolones

Patients	*Quinolone (oral unless specified)*	*Antidiabetic*	*Notes*	*Refs*
1 case	Ciprofloxacin 500 mg/day	Glibenclamide (glyburide) 5 mg/day	Confusion, slurred speech, and diaphoresis within a week of starting ciprofloxacin. Glibenclamide serum concentrations several times greater than normally seen. Intravenous glucose required to correct hypoglycaemia.	1
2 cases	Ciprofloxacin 500 mg/day	Glibenclamide (glyburide) 2.5 mg/day and 10 mg/day	Hypoglycaemia developed after first or second dose of ciprofloxacin given for a wound infection and a urinary tract infection, although involvement of ciprofloxacin in the latter case is disputed.	2–4
1 case	Ciprofloxacin 500 mg/day	Glipizide 5 mg	Severe hypoglycaemia a few hours after first dose of ciprofloxacin. Due to a previous history with levofloxacin, octreotide was administered resulting in normal glucose concentrations within 2 hours.	5
70 patients (post-marketing study)	Gatifloxacin 400 mg/day for 14 days	Metformin with or without glibenclamide (glyburide)	Initial hypoglycaemia (within first 2 days) followed by hyperglycaemia from day 3 onwards.	6
1 case	Gatifloxacin 200 mg/day	Glibenclamide (glyburide) 5 mg/day Pioglitazone 30 mg/day	Severe, persistent hypoglycaemia within an hour of first gatifloxacin dose, which resolved on discontinuation of all 3 drugs and did not return when glibenclamide and pioglitazone restarted.	7
1 case	Gatifloxacin 400 mg/day (intravenous)	Glimepiride 3 mg/day	Severe hypoglycaemia 12 hours after first gatifloxacin dose, which resolved on discontinuation of both drugs and did not return on restarting the glimepiride.	7
1 case	Gatifloxacin 400 mg/day	Repaglinide 1.5 mg/day	Repaglinide discontinued 6 hours after first gatifloxacin dose due to lack of appetite, but 2 hours after second gatifloxacin dose, severe hypoglycaemia developed and the patient experienced a tonic-clonic seizure. Hypoglycaemia persisted for 32 hours after gatifloxacin discontinued. Repaglinide restarted after 4 days with no further problems.	7
1 case	Gatifloxacin 400 mg/day	Insulin 10 units/day Repaglinide 6 mg/day Voglibose 600 micrograms/day	Severe hypoglycaemia developed after first gatifloxacin dose and persisted for 2 days despite a reduction in insulin dose. On the third day, all antidiabetic drugs were discontinued and blood glucose concentrations returned to baseline within 2 days.	8
2 cases	Gatifloxacin 400 mg/day	Glibenclamide (glyburide) 1.25 mg/day and 5 mg/day	Hypoglycaemia requiring treatment with intravenous glucose.	9,10
3 cases	Gatifloxacin 400 mg/day	Glibenclamide (glyburide) 5 to 10 mg/day Metformin 1.7 to 2.5 g/day	Severe hypoglycaemia, including coma after first gatifloxcain dose.	11,12
1 case	Gatifloxacin 400 mg/day	Glibenclamide (glyburide) 15 mg/day Rosiglitazone 4 mg/day	Hypoglycaemic coma after first gatifloxacin dose.	10
1 case	Gatifloxacin 400 mg/day	Glipizide 5 mg/day Insulin 3 units (one dose)	Hypoglycaemia developed after first gatifloxacin dose and persisted for 12 hours despite intravenous glucose. Hypoglycaemia occurred again after second gatifloxacin dose and glucose concentrations returned to normal within 24 hours of stopping both drugs.	9
1 case	Gatifloxacin 200 mg/day	Glipizide 10 mg/day Metformin 2 g/day	Severe *hyperglycaemia* within 48 hours of starting gatifloxacin which resolved with low-dose intravenous insulin but returned the following day after another gatifloxacin dose while receiving subcutaneous insulin.	9
1 case	Gatifloxacin 400 mg/day	Glipizide 2.5 mg/day	Severe *hyperglycaemia* developed 9 days into a course of gatifloxacin. After receiving subcutaneous insulin, gatifloxacin dose was reduced to 200 mg/day but *hyperglycaemia* returned and only resolved after discontinuation of gatifloxacin and regular subcutaneous insulin.	13
2 cases	Gatifloxacin unknown dose and 400 mg/day	Nil	*Hyperglycaemia* in non-diabetic patients within 48 to 72 hours of starting gatifloxacin.	8,9

Continued

Table 13.4 Interactions between antidiabetics and quinolones (continued)

Patients	Quinolone (oral unless specified)	Antidiabetic	Notes	Refs
1 case	Levofloxacin 250 mg/day	Gliclazide 200 mg/day	Hypoglycaemia, experienced with glibenclamide and metformin after starting gatifloxacin, did not return after the patient was switched to gliclazide and levofloxacin.	11
1 case	Levofloxacin 250 mg/day (intravenous)	Glibenclamide (glyburide) 5 mg/day	Fatal hypoglycaemia occurred after glibenclamide was restarted during a course of levofloxacin.	14
1 case	Levofloxacin 500 mg/day	Glibenclamide (glyburide) 5 mg/day	Hypoglycaemia occurred 12 hours after first dose of levofloxacin, and hypoglycaemia-induced anoxic brain injury occurred 12 hours after second dose.	15
1 case	Levofloxacin 750 mg every 2 days	Glipizide 10 mg/day	Hypoglycaemia occurred in a malnourished man.	16
1 case	Levofloxacin 250 mg/day (intravenous)	Glipizide	First dose of levofloxacin given 8 hours after last dose of glipizide. Hypoglycaemia developed on day 2, and persisted for 72 hours. Levofloxacin stopped on day 4, and hypoglycaemia resolved 2 days later.	17
2 cases	Levofloxacin 500 mg/day	Glibenclamide (glyburide) 5 to 7.5 mg/day Metformin 800 mg to 1.2 g/day	Hypoglycaemic coma occurred 72 hours and 1 week after levofloxacin administration and resolved upon discontinuation of the levofloxacin.	18
1 case	Levofloxacin 500 mg/day	Insulin 34 units/day	Episodes of severe hypoglycaemia 3 days after starting levofloxacin, which continued despite stopping insulin. Hypoglycaemia resolved 3 days after levofloxacin was discontinued.	19
1 case	Levofloxacin	Insulin	Recurrent severe hypoglycaemia on days 6 to 8 of a course of levofloxacin, despite discontinuation of insulin on day 3. Hypoglycaemia resolved 24 hours after stopping levofloxacin, but was followed by central pontine myelinolysis and quadriplegia, which was attributed to the hypoglycaemia.	20
1 case	Levofloxacin 500 mg/day	Nil	Hypoglycaemia occurred in a patient with diet-controlled diabetes on days 2 and 3 of a course of levofloxacin. Intravenous glucose required to correct hypoglycaemia, which resolved on discontinuation of levofloxacin.	21

1. Roberge RJ, Kaplan R, Frank R, Fore C. Glyburide-ciprofloxacin interaction with resistant hypoglycaemia. *Ann Emerg Med* (2000) 36, 160–3.
2. Whitely MS, Worldling J, Patel S, Gibbs KB. Hypoglycaemia in a diabetic patient, associated with ciprofloxacin therapy. *Pract Diabetes* (1993) 10, 35.
3. Lin G, Hays DP, Spillane L. Refractory hypoglycemia from ciprofloxacin and glyburide interaction. *J Toxicol Clin Toxicol* (2004) 42, 295–7.
4. Roberge R. Comment on "refractory hypoglycemia from ciprofloxacin and glyburide interaction". *Clin Toxicol* (2005) 43, 213–14.
5. Kelesidis T, Canseco E. Quinolone-induced hypoglycemia: a life-threatening but potentially reversible side effect. *Am J Med* (2010) 123, e5–e6.
6. Tequin (Gatifloxacin). Bristol-Myers Squibb Company. US Prescribing information, January 2006.
7. Menzies DJ, Dorsainvil PA, Cunha BA, Johnson DH. Severe and persistent hypoglycemia due to gatifloxacin interaction with oral hypoglycemic agents. *Am J Med* (2002) 113, 232–4.
8. Khovidhunkit W, Sunthornyothin S. Hypoglycemia, hyperglycemia, and gatifloxacin. *Ann Intern Med* (2004) 141, 969.
9. Biggs WS. Hypoglycemia and hyperglycemia associated with gatifloxacin use in elderly patients. *J Am Board Fam Pract* (2003) 16, 455–7.
10. Bhasin R, Arce FC, Pasmantier R. Hypoglycemia associated with the use of gatifloxacin. *Am J Med Sci* (2005) 330, 250–3.
11. LeBlanc M, Bélanger C, Cossette P. Severe and resistant hypoglycemia associated with concomitant gatifloxacin and glyburide therapy. *Pharmacotherapy* (2004) 24, 926–31.
12. Baker SE, Hangii MC. Possible gatifloxacin-induced hypoglycemia. *Ann Pharmacother* (2002) 36, 1722–6.
13. Bobba RK, Arsura EL. Hyperglycemia in an elderly diabetic patient: drug-drug or drug-disease interaction? *South Med J* (2006) 99, 94–5.
14. Friedrich LV, Dougherty R. Fatal hypoglycemia associated with levofloxacin. *Pharmacotherapy* (2004) 24, 1807–12.
15. Lawrence KR, Adra M, Keir C. Hypoglycemia-induced anoxic brain injury possibly associated with levofloxacin. *J Infect* (2006) 52, e177–e180.
16. Garber SM, Pound MW, Miller SM. Hypoglycemia associated with the use of levofloxacin. *Am J Health-Syst Pharm* (2009) 66, 1014–19.
17. Kelesidis T, Canseco E. Levofloxacin-induced hypoglycemia: a rare but life-threatening side effect of a widely used antibiotic. *Am J Med* (2009) 122, e3–e4.
18. Micheli L, Sbrilli M, Nencini C. Severe hypoglycaemia associated with levofloxacin in Type 2 diabetic patients receiving polytherapy: two case reports. *Int J Clin Pharmacol Ther* (2012) 50, 302–6.
19. Gibert AE, Porto FS. Hypoglycemia and levofloxacin: a case report. *Clin Infect Dis* (2008) 46, 1126–27.
20. Vallurupalli S, Huesmann G, Gregory J, Jacoby MG. Levofloxacin-associated hypoglycaemia complicated by central pontine myelinolysis and quadripleigia. *Diabet Med* (2008) 25, 856–9.
21. Kanbay M, Aydogan T, Bozalan R, Isik A, Uz B, Kaya A, Akcay A. A rare but serious side effect of levofloxacin: hypoglycaemia in a geriatric patient. *Diabetes Care* (2006) 29, 1716–7.

(b) Pharmacokinetic studies

1. Ciprofloxacin. A study in 12 patients with type 2 diabetes taking **glibenclamide (glyburide)** 10 mg in the morning, plus in some instances 5 mg in the evening, found that ciprofloxacin 1 g daily for a week appeared to increase the maximum serum concentration of **glibenclamide** by 20 to 30%, and slightly increase its AUC by 25 to 36%. However, none of these changes were statistically significant, and, more importantly, blood glucose concentrations were not altered.[7] In a randomised, crossover study in 9 healthy subjects, a single 200-mg intravenous dose of ciprofloxacin had no effect on the pharmacokinetics of a single 1.25-mg oral dose of **glibenclamide** given 20 minutes later.[8]

In a randomised, crossover study in 24 healthy subjects, there was no change in the pharmacokinetics of a single 8-mg dose of **rosiglitazone** when given with a single 500-mg dose of ciprofloxacin. The effect on blood glucose concentrations was not assessed.[9]

2. Levofloxacin. A randomised, crossover study in 24 healthy subjects found that oral levofloxacin had no effect on the pharmacokinetics of a single oral dose of **glibenclamide** nor its effect on glucose concentrations.[10]

3. Moxifloxacin. The UK manufacturer notes that the concurrent use of moxifloxacin and **glibenclamide** resulted in an approximate 21% decrease in the maximum plasma concentration of **glibenclamide** in subjects with diabetes, but this did not alter blood glucose and endogenous insulin.[11]

4. Ofloxacin. The UK manufacturer of ofloxacin states that it might increase the serum concentration of glibenclamide: they state that this is based on unpublished case reports of an interaction and the possibility that the interaction is due to a class effect of the quinolones.[12,13]

Mechanism

Uncertain. However, it has been suggested that quinolones might increase insulin secretion,[14,15] in a similar manner to quinine (see 'Antidiabetics + Antimalarials', p.503). Gatifloxacin appears to increase insulin release initially, but then decrease insulin productivity or increase insulin disintegration.[16] Of the quinolones, the severe effects of gatifloxacin on glucose homoeostasis appear to be unique, with levofloxacin and ciprofloxacin having a very much smaller effect.[2,17]

The authors of one report suggest that ciprofloxacin might have inhibited the metabolism of glibenclamide, thereby increasing its serum concentrations.[18] This might possibly be exaggerated in elderly patients whose liver function could be reduced. Ciprofloxacin appears not to affect hepatic uptake of glibenclamide by the organic anion transporting polypeptide 2B1 (OATP2B1),[8] and is not known to be an inhibitor of CYP2C9, by which glibenclamide is metabolised.

Importance and management

Evidence for a pharmacokinetic interaction between the quinolones and antidiabetics is limited, but ciprofloxacin does not affect rosiglitazone pharmacokinetics and levofloxacin does not affect the pharmacokinetics of glibenclamide (glyburide). Ciprofloxacin might slightly increase glibenclamide exposure, but this is unlikely to be clinically important. There are numerous case reports of hypoglycaemia, sometimes severe or fatal, occurring with the concurrent use of most quinolones (although not moxifloxacin) and antidiabetics (largely glibenclamide). Gatifloxacin has been much more frequently associated with disturbances of blood glucose (hypo- and hyper-glycaemia) than other quinolones. When available for systemic use, the US manufacturer of gatifloxacin initially advised that the signs and symptoms of *hypo*glycaemia should be monitored, especially in the first 3 days of concurrent use, and signs and symptoms of *hyper*glycaemia should be monitored, especially with continued use beyond 3 days.[19] However, later they contraindicated its use in patients with diabetes,[20] and eventually withdrew the product.[21] Where still available for systemic use, these precautions would seem sensible. Note, that these concerns do not apply to gatifloxacin applied topically as eye drops.

The retrospective study with glipizide and glibenclamide (glyburide) suggests that the concurrent use of levofloxacin, and possibly ciprofloxacin might increase the risk of hypoglycaemia, although further study is needed to confirm this. Isolated cases of hypoglycaemia in patients with diabetes have also been reported for ciprofloxacin, levofloxacin, and norfloxacin. The general clinical relevance of these cases is uncertain, but the consequences have the potential to be severe and so should be kept in mind if concurrent use is necessary. When any change is made to the medication regimen of a patient with diabetes, it would be prudent to monitor blood glucose concentrations, and this would seem to be particularly important in the elderly, who appear to be more at risk.

1. Frothingham R. Glucose homeostasis abnormalities associated with use of gatifloxacin. *Clin Infect Dis* (2005) 41, 1269–76.
2. Park-Wyllie LY, Juurlink DN, Kopp A, Shah BR, Stukel TA, Stumpo C, Dresser L, Low DE, Mamdani MM. Outpatient gatifloxacin therapy and dysglycemia in older adults. *N Engl J Med* (2006) 354, 1352–61.
3. Gajjar DA, LaCreta FP, Kollia GD, Stolz RR, Berger S, Smith WB, Swingle M, Grasela DM. Effect of multiple-dose gatifloxacin or ciprofloxacin on glucose homeostasis and insulin production in patients with noninsulin-dependent diabetes mellitus maintained with diet and exercise. *Pharmacotherapy* (2000) 20, 76S–86S.
4. Schelleman H, Bilker WB, Brensinger CM, Wan F, Hennessy S. Anti-infectives and the risk of severe hypoglycemia in users of glipizide or glyburide. *Clin Pharmacol Ther* (2010) 88, 214
5. Gavin JR, Kubin R, Choudhri S, Kubitza D, Himmel H, Gross R, Meyer JM. Moxifloxacin and glucose homeostasis. A pooled-analysis of the evidence from clinical and postmarketing studies. *Drug Safety* (2004) 27, 671–86.
6. Utinor (Norfloxacin). Merck Sharp & Dohme Ltd. UK Summary of product characteristics, October 2009.
7. Ludwig E, Szekely E, Graber H, Csiba A. Study of interaction between oral ciprofloxacin and glibenclamide. *Eur J Clin Microbiol Infect Dis* (1991) 10 (Special issue) 378–9.
8. Zheng HX, Huang Y, Frassetto LA, Benet LZ. Elucidating rifampin's inducing and inhibiting effects on glyburide pharmacokinetics and blood glucose in healthy volunteers: unmasking the differential effects of enzyme induction and transporter inhibition for a drug and its primary metabolite. *Clin Pharmacol Ther* (2009) 85, 78–85.
9. Kumar JNS, Devi P, Narasu L, Mullangi R. Effect of ciprofloxacin and ibuprofen on the *in vitro* metabolism of rosiglitazone and oral pharmacokinetics of rosiglitazone in healthy human volunteers. *Eur J Drug Metab Pharmacokinet* (2008) 33, 237–42.
10. Hoechst Marion Roussel, Personal Communication, March 1999.
11. Avelox (Moxifloxacin hydrochloride). Bayer plc. UK Summary of product characteristics, May 2012.
12. Tarivid (Ofloxacin). Sanofi-Aventis. UK Summary of product characteristics, December 2013.
13. Sanofi-aventis. Personal communication, November 2009.
14. Lin G, Hays DP, Spillane L. Refractory hypoglycemia from ciprofloxacin and glyburide interaction. *J Toxicol Clin Toxicol* (2004) 42, 295–7.
15. Friedrich LV, Dougherty R. Fatal hypoglycemia associated with levofloxacin. *Pharmacotherapy* (2004) 24, 1807–12.
16. Tomita T, Onishi M, Sato E, Kimura Y, Kihira K. Gatifloxacin induces augmented insulin release and intracellular insulin depletion of pancreatic islet cells. *Biol Pharm Bull* (2007) 30, 644–7.
17. Menzies DJ, Dorsainvil PA, Cunha BA, Johnson DH. Severe and persistent hypoglycemia due to gatifloxacin interaction with oral hypoglycemic agents. *Am J Med* (2002) 113, 232–4.
18. Roberge RJ, Kaplan R, Frank R, Fore C. Glyburide-ciprofloxacin interaction with resistant hypoglycaemia. *Ann Emerg Med* (2000) 36, 160–3.
19. Tequin (Gatifloxacin). Bristol-Myers Squibb Company. US Prescribing information, January 2006.
20. Bristol-Myers Squibb. Dear Healthcare Provider letter. February 15, 2006. Available at: http://www.fda.gov/downloads/Safety/MedWatch/SafetyInformation/SafetyAlertsforHumanMedicalProducts/UCM153428.pdf (accessed 22/10/15).
21. FDA. Determination that Tequin (gatifloxacin) was withdrawn from sale for reasons of safety or effectiveness. *Fed Regist* (2008) 73, 52357–8.

Antidiabetics + Somatostatin analogues

Octreotide decreases insulin resistance and therefore might affect diabetic control, and in one patient, fatal diabetic ketoacidosis occurred when octreotide was withdrawn. Octreotide appears to have little effect in those with intact insulin reserves (type 2 diabetes) and it might reduce sulfonylurea-induced hypoglycaemia. Lanreotide can also affect glucose concentrations in patients with diabetes.

Clinical evidence

(a) Insulin

1. Type 1 diabetes. Seven patients with type 1 diabetes and poor metabolic control while using insulin, were given **octreotide** 50 micrograms subcutaneously three times daily (at 8, 15, and 23 hours) or by continuous subcutaneous infusion (62.5 or 112.5 micrograms over 24 hours). Their blood glucose concentrations were about 50% lower than when they were given insulin alone. The effects of **octreotide** on blood glucose concentrations were virtually the same regardless of route of administration or dose.[1] Another study in 6 patients with type 1 diabetes also found that **octreotide** 50 micrograms subcutaneously before meals reduced their daily insulin requirements by about 50%,[2] and other studies confirm that **octreotide** behaves in this way.[3,4] An isolated report describes clinical and biochemical improvement with **lanreotide** 30 mg intramuscularly every 10 days, in a man with diabetes and acromegaly whose glucose concentrations were poorly controlled with insulin. However, he experienced hypoglycaemia when the **lanreotide** was replaced with intramuscular **octreotide** 20 mg (depot preparation), and he had to reduce his insulin dose by 30 to 50% for the first week after each **octreotide** injection.[5] Another report describes deterioration in glucose tolerance leading to death from diabetic ketoacidosis when **octreotide** was stopped in a patient with acromegaly and insulin-resistant diabetes mellitus.[6]

2. Type 2 diabetes. Eight obese patients with type 2 diabetes that was not controlled with oral antidiabetics and who needed insulin, had no clinically important increases in blood glucose concentrations following a meal when they were given subcutaneous **octreotide** 25 micrograms.[7] **Octreotide** reduced insulin requirements in 6 patients with type 2 diabetes and chronic renal failure, but did not greatly affect the glycaemic profile of similar patients with diabetes and normal renal function. This effect was thought to be due to a greater reduction in glucagon concentrations, which are elevated in renal failure.[8]

(b) Oral antidiabetics

Octreotide does not appear to have a clinically relevant beneficial, or harmful effect on the blood glucose-lowering effects of oral antidiabetics such as **glibenclamide (glyburide)** in patients with type 2 diabetes, although some metabolic changes can occur, including suppression of postprandial serum insulin concentrations.[9,10] A retrospective study of 9 patients with hypoglycaemia occurring as a result of a sulfonylurea overdose (with **glibenclamide** or **glipizide**) found that there was a notable reduction in the number of episodes of hypoglycaemia after **octreotide** was given (29 episodes before, versus 2 episodes after, **octreotide**).[11]

Mechanism

Octreotide is an analogue of the natural hormone somatostatin, and similarly has blood glucose-lowering effects because it inhibits the actions of glucagon and growth hormone (which increase blood glucose concentrations), and because it also delays the absorption of carbohydrate from the gut. However, somatostatin is also diabetogenic, because it suppresses insulin release. In type 1 diabetes, because there is no endogenous insulin, the blood glucose-lowering effects predominate. In non-diabetics and patients with type 2 diabetes, the actions might cancel out, or there might be poorer glycaemic control. Octreotide is thought to cause less suppression of insulin release than somatostatin, but this could still be important in those with insulin-secreting reserves.

Lanreotide, like somatostatin and its analogues, might produce a transient inhibition of the secretion of insulin and glucagon,[12] but lanreotide might have less affinity for receptors found in the pancreas and so possibly produces a different response to that of octreotide.[5,13]

Sulfonylureas lower blood glucose concentrations primarily by facilitating preformed insulin release from pancreatic beta cells, and octreotide might oppose this by directly inhibiting insulin secretion from the pancreas.[11]

Importance and management

The interaction between insulin and octreotide in patients with type 1 diabetes is established, and hypoglycaemia has been reported. If both drugs are used, anticipate the need to reduce the insulin dose. The studies cited above[1,2] suggest that a reduction of about 50% is possibly required.

The UK manufacturer of octreotide states that in patients with type 2 diabetes with intact insulin reserves, octreotide might result in prandial *increases* in glycaemia,[14] but two clinical studies in patients with type 2 diabetes given glibenclamide (glyburide) did not show any deterioration (or benefit) in glycaemia.[9,10] However, octreotide has been reported to reduce sulfonylurea-induced hypoglycaemia. Octreotide appears to affect insulin secretion, and therefore glucose tolerance, and so it would certainly be prudent to monitor the effects of giving octreotide with any of the oral antidiabetics.

The UK manufacturer of lanreotide also recommends that blood glucose concentrations should be monitored in patients with diabetes to determine whether antidiabetic treatment needs to be adjusted,[12] which seems prudent.

1. Lunetta M, Di Mauro M, Le Moli R, Nicoletti F. Effect of octreotide on blood glucose and counter-regulatory hormones in insulin-dependent diabetic patients: the role of dose and route of administration. *Eur J Clin Pharmacol* (1996) 51, 139–44.
2. Rios MS, Navascues I, Saban J, Ordoñez A, Sevilla F, Del Pozo E. Somatostatin analog SMS 201–995 and insulin needs in insulin-dependent diabetic patients studied by means of an artificial pancreas. *J Clin Endocrinol Metab* (1986) 63, 1071–4.
3. Candrina R, Giustina G. Effect of a new long-acting somatostatin analogue (SMS 201–995) on glycemic and hormonal profiles in insulin-treated type II diabetic patients. *J Endocrinol Invest* (1988) 11, 501–7.
4. Hadjidakis DJ, Halvatsiotis PG, Ioannou YJ, Mavrokefalos PJ, Raptis SA. The effects of the somatostatin analogue SMS 201–995 on carbohydrate homeostasis of insulin-dependent diabetics as assessed by the artificial endocrine pancreas. *Diabetes Res Clin Pract* (1988) 5, 91–8.
5. Webb SM, Ortega E, Rodríguez-Espinosa J, Mato M-E, Corcoy R. Decreased insulin requirements after LAR-octreotide but not after lanreotide in an acromegalic patient. *Pituitary* (2001) 4, 275–8.
6. Abrahamson MJ. Death from diabetic ketoacidosis after cessation of octreotide in acromegaly. *Lancet* (1990) 336, 318–19.
7. Giustina A, Girelli A, Buffoli MG, Cimino A, Legati F, Valentini U, Giustina G. Low-dose octreotide is able to cause a maximal inhibition of the glycemic responses to a mixed meal in obese type 2 diabetic patients treated with insulin. *Diabetes Res Clin Pract* (1991) 14, 47–54.
8. Di Mauro M, Papalia G, Le Moli R, Nativo B, Nicoletti F, Lunetta M. Effect of octreotide on insulin requirement, hepatic glucose production, growth hormone, glucagon and c-peptide levels in type 2

diabetic patients with chronic renal failure or normal renal function. *Diabetes Res Clin Pract* (2001) 51, 45–50.
9. Davies RR, Miller M, Turner SJ, Watson M, McGill A, Ørskov H, Alberti KGMM, Johnston DG. Effects of somatostatin analogue SMS 201–995 in non-insulin-dependent diabetes. *Clin Endocrinol (Oxf)* (1986) 25, 739–47.
10. Williams G, Füessl HS, Burrin JM, Chilvers E, Bloom SR. Postprandial glycaemic effects of a long-acting somatostatin analogue (octreotide) in non-insulin dependent diabetes mellitus. *Horm Metab Res* (1988) 20, 168–170.
11. McLaughlin SA, Crandall CS, McKinney PE. Octreotide: an antidote for sulfonylurea-induced hypoglycemia. *Ann Emerg Med* (2000) 36, 133–8.
12. Somatuline Autogel (Lanreotide acetate). Ipsen Ltd. UK Summary of product characteristics, October 2013.
13. Baldelli R, Battista C, Leonetti F, Ghiggi M-R, Ribaudo M-C, Paoloni A, D'Amico E, Ferretti E, Baratta R, Liuzzi A, Trischitta V, Tamburrano G. Glucose homeostasis in acromegaly: effects of long-acting somatostatin analogues treatment. *Clin Endocrinol (Oxf)* (2003) 59, 492–9.
14. Sandostatin (Octreotide). Novartis Pharmaceuticals UK Ltd. UK Summary of product characteristics, June 2012.

Antidiabetics + SSRIs

In various clinical studies in patients with diabetes, SSRIs have generally caused minor improvements in glycaemic control. However, isolated cases of severe hypoglycaemia, hyperglycaemia, and hypoglycaemia unawareness have been reported.

Clinical evidence

One research group from the Netherlands has conducted a number of analyses to look at the association between antidepressants and dysglycaemia.[1-4] In one analysis of cases of patients hospitalised for hypoglycaemia, use of antidepressants (including SSRIs) was not associated with an increased risk. The authors suggested that there was a trend for an increased risk with SSRIs when compared with antidepressants not affecting serotonin uptake,[1] but there were too few cases to reasonably assess this. Conversely, in an analysis of spontaneous reports in the WHO adverse drug reaction database, use of antidepressants was associated with a small increased risk of both hyperglycaemia (odds ratio 1.5) and hypoglycaemia (odds ratio 1.8). SSRIs had a slightly greater risk of hypoglycaemia than hyperglycaemia (odds ratio 2 versus 1.4), which was not statistically significant.[2] In a further longitudinal study in 133 patients using **insulin** for at least 12 months before starting an antidepressant, and for at least 6 months with an antidepressant, the dose of insulin used did not change after starting the antidepressant. When analysed by type, the 85 SSRI users (individual SSRIs not named) had a small 13% decrease in dose of **insulin** while taking the antidepressant.[3] A small, open study found that mean **insulin** requirements in 4 patients (2 with type 2 diabetes and 2 with type 1) also taking an SSRI (**citalopram** in 1 patient, **sertraline** in 2 patients, and **paroxetine** in 1 patient), increased by 2.4% during 210 days of follow-up, compared with 18.3% in 8 patients (5 with type 2 diabetes and 3 with type 1) not receiving an SSRI. However, 1 patient not receiving an SSRI experienced an increased insulin requirement of 86.4%, which, when excluded, reduced the overall increase in this group to 8.5%. Mean HbA_{1c} concentrations were 7.2% lower in SSRI users compared with 0.5% in non-users. None of these differences reached statistical significance.[4]

(a) Citalopram

In a small uncontrolled study in 14 patients with diabetes (type 1 or 2 managed with **insulin** and/or **oral antidiabetics**) given citalopram (10 mg daily increased to 20 mg daily if needed for 16 weeks), there was a non-statistically significant modest improvement in measures of glycaemic control (HbA_{1c} decreased by 0.36%).[5] The fact that this study was small and not placebo-controlled limits its findings, but it does provide some indication that major effects of citalopram on glucose control are possibly uncommon.

(b) Fluoxetine

Various placebo-controlled clinical studies in patients with type 1 or 2 diabetes receiving **insulin** and/or **oral antidiabetics** have shown that fluoxetine can cause weight loss, reduce fasting plasma glucose concentrations, and improve glycaemic control (modest decrease in HbA_{1c} concentrations),[6-8] which in some cases were statistically significantly greater than with placebo. In one study in patients receiving **insulin**, a decrease in the daily **insulin** dose was required over the 24 weeks (44% reduction in dose compared with 20% for placebo).[9]

A patient with **insulin**-dependent diabetes experienced symptoms of hypoglycaemia (nausea, tremor, sweating, anxiety, lightheadedness) after starting to take fluoxetine 20 mg each night. The symptoms disappeared when the fluoxetine was stopped and reappeared when it was restarted. However, blood glucose concentrations were found to be normal (9 to 11 mmol/L), so it is likely that the effects were purely adverse effects of fluoxetine that were mistaken for symptoms of hypoglycaemia.[10] A further case report describes a patient who experienced symptoms of hypoglycaemia and whose blood glucose concentrations decreased on several occasions (lowest result, 2.36 mmol/L) while taking **glibenclamide (glyburide)** 20 mg daily and fluoxetine 20 mg daily.[11] In contrast, another patient with type 1 diabetes experienced a loss of hypoglycaemic awareness while taking fluoxetine 40 mg daily. Approximately one month after fluoxetine was started, he reported an increased incidence of hypoglycaemia, but these episodes were not accompanied by typical adrenergic symptoms (which he had previously experienced). After 3 grand mal seizures which occurred with blood glucose readings ranging from 1.9 to 2.2 mmol/L, the dose of fluoxetine was gradually decreased. Hypoglycaemic unawareness resolved when the fluoxetine dose was reduced to 10 mg every second day. Within weeks of discontinuing fluoxetine, blood glucose concentrations had increased considerably and hypoglycaemia did not recur.[12] These authors reported two very similar cases with **paroxetine** and **sertraline**.[13] However, in a placebo-controlled study in 18 patients with type 1 diabetes, fluoxetine 20 mg daily titrated to 80 mg daily over 6 weeks actually had no effect on hypoglycaemic symptoms experienced during induced hypoglycaemia (clamp study). Moreover, fluoxetine greatly increased the physiological counter-regulatory responses (e.g. adrenaline (epinephrine) release) to induced hypoglycaemia.[14]

The UK and US manufacturers of fluoxetine state that hypoglycaemia has occurred in patients with diabetes when they took fluoxetine alone, and hyperglycaemia has developed following discontinuation.[15,16]

(c) Fluvoxamine

Hyperglycaemia occurred in a 60-year-old woman with type 2 diabetes managed with **insulin**, 5 days after fluvoxamine was started. Blood glucose concentrations, which had approximately doubled, decreased when the fluvoxamine was stopped, but increased and then decreased again when the fluvoxamine was restarted and then stopped.[17]

(d) Paroxetine

In a small placebo-controlled study in 15 patients with type 2 diabetes given paroxetine 20 mg daily, there was a non-statistically significant modest improvement in measures of glycaemic control. HbA_{1c} decreased by 0.44% compared with 0.07% in the placebo group.[18] This study provides some indication that major effects of paroxetine on glucose control are possibly uncommon.

For mention of a case of reduced hypoglycaemic awareness in a patient with type 1 diabetes given paroxetine, see *Fluoxetine*, above.

(e) Sertraline

There is a report of a patient with schizoaffective disorder and type 2 diabetes who developed hypoglycaemia during treatment with sertraline, risperidone, and **glibenclamide**.[19] For mention of a case of reduced hypoglycaemic awareness in a patient with type 1 diabetes given sertraline, see *Fluoxetine*, above. In contrast, another report describes a patient with diet-controlled type 2 diabetes, whose glucose concentrations increased after initiation of sertraline treatment.[20]

Mechanism

The SSRIs themselves appear to be associated with some effects on glucose homeostasis. For example, in one pharmacodynamic study, fluoxetine improved insulin sensitivity in patients with type 2 diabetes managed with diet alone.[21]

Importance and management

Evidence for an effect of SSRIs on diabetic control is somewhat limited and not entirely conclusive. Studies seem to suggest that the use of SSRIs might result in some improvement in glycaemic control, perhaps by improving insulin sensitivity, but isolated cases of severe hypo- or hyper-glycaemia have been reported, including one case of reduced hypoglycaemic awareness. It is also important to note that this might be a drug-disease effect rather than a drug-drug interaction (see 'Sulfonylureas + SSRIs', p.551 and 'Thiazolidinediones; Rosiglitazone + SSRIs; Fluvoxamine', p.560, for details of a lack of pharmacokinetic interactions). Nevertheless, the dose requirements of insulin or oral antidiabetics might change on concurrent use with SSRIs and it would be prudent to increase the frequency of blood glucose monitoring if an SSRI is started or stopped.

The pharmacokinetic interactions of antidiabetic drugs with SSRIs are covered under the individual drugs or drug groups elsewhere in this chapter.

1. Derijks HJ, Heerdink ER, De Koning FH, Janknegt R, Klungel OH, Egberts AC. The association between antidepressant use and hypoglycaemia in diabetic patients: a nested case-control study. *Pharmacoepidemiol Drug Safety* (2008) 17, 336–44.
2. Derijks HJ, Meyboom RH, Heerdink ER, De Koning FHP, Janknegt R, Lindquist M, Egberts ACG. The association between antidepressant use and disturbances in glucose homeostasis: evidence from spontaneous reports. *Eur J Clin Pharmacol* (2008) 64, 531–8.
3. Knol MJ, Derijks HJ, Geerlings MI, Heerdink ER, Souverein PC, Gorter KJ, Grobbee DE, Egberts ACG. Influence of antidepressants on glycaemic control in patients with diabetes mellitus. *Pharmacoepidemiol Drug Safety* (2008) 17, 577–86.
4. Derijks HJ, Janknegt R, Heerdink ER, De Koning FHP, Krekels MM, Looij B-J, Egberts ACG. Influence of antidepressant use on glycemic control in patients with diabetes mellitus: an open-label comparative study. *J Clin Psychopharmacol* (2009) 29, 405–8.
5. Amsterdam JD, Shults J, Rutherford N, Schwartz S. Safety and efficacy of s-citalopram in patients with co-morbid major depression and diabetes mellitus. *Neuropsychobiology* (2006) 54, 208–14.
6. Breum L, Bjerre U, Bak JF, Jacobsen S, Astrup A. Long-term effects of fluoxetine on glycemic control in obese patients with non-insulin-dependent diabetes mellitus or glucose intolerance: influence on muscle glycogen synthase and insulin receptor kinase activity. *Metabolism* (1995) 44, 1570–6.
7. Daubresse J-C, Kolanowski J, Krzentowski G, Kutnowski M, Scheen A, Van Gaal L. Usefulness of fluoxetine in obese non-insulin-dependent diabetics: a multicenter study. *Obes Res* (1996) 4, 391–6.
8. Lustman PJ, Freedland KE, Griffith LS, Clouse RE. Fluoxetine for depression in diabetes: a randomized double-blind placebo-controlled trial. *Diabetes Care* (2000) 23, 618–23.
9. Gray DS, Fujioka K, Devine W, Bray GA. A randomized double-blind clinical trial of fluoxetine in obese diabetics. *Int J Obes* (1992) 16 (Suppl 4), S67–S72.
10. Lear J, Burden AC. Fluoxetine side-effects mimicking hypoglycaemia. *Lancet* (1992) 339, 1296.
11. Deeg MA, Lipkin EW. Hypoglycaemia associated with the use of fluoxetine. *West J Med* (1996) 164, 262–3.
12. Sawka AM, Burgart V, Zimmerman D. Loss of hypoglycemia awareness in an adolescent with type 1 diabetes mellitus during treatment with fluoxetine hydrochloride. *J Pediatr* (2000) 136, 394–6.
13. Sawka AM, Burgart V, Zimmerman D. Loss of awareness of hypoglycemia temporally associated with selective serotonin reuptake inhibitors. *Diabetes Care* (2001) 24, 1845–6..
14. Briscoe VJ, Ertl AC, Tate DB, Davis SN. Effects of the selective serotonin reuptake inhibitor fluoxetine on counterregulatory responses to hypoglycemia in individuals with type 1 diabetes. *Diabetes* (2008) 57, 3315–22.
15. Prozac (Fluoxetine hydrochloride). Eli Lilly and Company Ltd. UK Summary of product characteristics, October 2014.
16. Prozac (Fluoxetine hydrochloride). Eli Lilly and Company. US Prescribing information, July 2014.
17. Oswald P, Souery D, Mendlewicz J. Fluvoxamine-induced hyperglycaemia in a diabetic patient with comorbid depression. *Int J Neuropsychopharmacol* (2003) 6, 85–7.
18. Paile-Hyvärinen M, Wahlbeck K, Eriksson JG. Quality of life and metabolic status in mildly depressed women with type 2 diabetes treated with paroxetine: a single-blind randomised placebo controlled trial. *BMC Fam Pract* (2003) 4, 7.

19. Takhar J, Williamson P. Hypoglycemia associated with high doses of sertraline and sulphonylurea compound in a noninsulin-dependent diabetes mellitus patient. *Can J Clin Pharmacol* (1999) 6, 12–14.
20. Sansone RA, Sansone LA. Sertraline-induced hyperglycemia: case report. *Int J Psychiatry Med* (2003) 33, 103–5.
21. Maheux P, Ducros F, Bourque J, Garon J, Chiasson J-L. Fluoxetine improves insulin sensitivity in obese patients with non-insulin-dependent diabetes mellitus independently of weight loss. *Int J Obes Relat Metab Disord* (1997) 21, 97–102.

Antidiabetics + Sugar-containing pharmaceuticals

Some pharmaceutical preparations might contain sufficient amounts of sugar to affect the control of diabetes.

Clinical evidence, mechanism, importance and management

Pharmaceuticals, especially liquid formulations, might contain considerable amounts of sugar. The extent to which the use of preparations like these will affect the control of diabetes clearly depends upon the amounts taken, but the problem is by no means merely theoretical. One report describes the loss of diabetic control (glycosuria) in a woman with type 1 diabetes receiving insulin when given psyllium effervescent powder (*Metamucil* instant-mix), which contains sugar.[1]

The range of other sugar-containing preparations is far too extensive to be listed here. Because of concerns over sugar-containing medicines and dental caries, in children in particular, the number of sugar-free preparations has grown considerably over recent years. In the UK, the BNF and MIMS provide guidance as to which preparations are sugar-free. Patients with diabetes should be warned about sugar-containing medicines, and given guidance about the terminology used in labelling. Sweetening agents of note to diabetics include: **invert sugar** (dextrose and fructose), **invert syrup** (67% w/w invert sugar), **syrup BP** (66% w/w sucrose), **glucose liquid** (dextrose content 10 to 20%), **glucose syrup** (33.3% liquid glucose in syrup), and **honey** (70 to 80% glucose and fructose).[2]

1. Catellani J, Collins RJ. Drug labelling. *Lancet* (1978) ii, 98.
2. Greenwood J. Sugar content of liquid prescription medicines. *Pharm J* (1989) 243, 553–7.

Antidiabetics + Sulfinpyrazone

Sulfinpyrazone has no effect on the insulin requirements of patients with diabetes, nor does it affect the control of diabetes in patients taking glibenclamide (glyburide). Increased blood glucose-lowering effects might occur if sulfinpyrazone is given with tolbutamide, but there appear to be no case reports of this interaction. Sulfinpyrazone slightly increases nateglinide exposure.

Clinical evidence

(a) Insulin

A double-blind study in 41 adult patients with diabetes found that sulfinpyrazone 600 to 800 mg daily had no clinically relevant effects on insulin requirements over a 12-month period.[1]

(b) Nateglinide

In a crossover study in healthy subjects, sulfinpyrazone 200 mg twice daily for 7 days slightly increased the mean AUC of a single 120-mg dose of nateglinide by 28%, but did not change the mean maximum plasma concentration.[2]

(c) Sulfonylureas

A study in 19 patients with type 2 diabetes taking **glibenclamide (glyburide)** found that sulfinpyrazone 800 mg daily did not affect diabetic control.[3]

A detailed study of the pharmacokinetics of **tolbutamide** in 6 healthy subjects found that sulfinpyrazone 200 mg every 6 hours for a week, almost doubled the half-life of a 500-mg intravenous dose of **tolbutamide**, from 7.3 hours to 13.2 hours, and slightly reduced the clearance by 40%.[4]

Mechanism

Sulfinpyrazone is an inhibitor of CYP2C9, by which tolbutamide and nateglinide are metabolised, resulting in increased exposure and possibly increased effects. Other sulfonylureas are also metabolised by CYP2C9 and might be similarly affected.

Importance and management

Information about an interaction between tolbutamide and sulfinpyrazone appears to be limited to the study cited. There appear to be no reports of adverse interactions in patients, but the study suggests that increased blood glucose-lowering effects, and possibly hypoglycaemia, could occur if the dose of tolbutamide is not reduced. Such an interaction has been described with phenylbutazone, which has a close structural similarity to sulfinpyrazone (see 'Sulfonylureas + NSAIDs; Phenylbutazone and related drugs', p.549). As when any change is made to the medication regimen of a patient with diabetes, if sulfinpyrazone is added to established treatment with tolbutamide, it would be prudent to monitor blood glucose concentrations. It is also possible that other sulfonylureas metabolised similarly to tolbutamide might be affected in the same way, and similar monitoring would therefore seem sensible on concurrent use with sulfinpyrazone.

The effect of the slight increase in nateglinide exposure when given with sulfinpyrazone has not been assessed in patients with diabetes, but it seems unlikely that it would be clinically relevant. Nevertheless, as above it would be prudent to monitor blood glucose concentrations on concurrent use. There seems to be nothing documented about any other clinically important interactions between antidiabetics and sulfinpyrazone.

1. Pannebakker MAG, den Ottolander GJH, ten Pas JG. Insulin requirements in diabetic patients treated with sulphinpyrazone. *J Int Med Res* (1979) 7, 328–31.
2. Sabia H, Sunkara G, Ligueros-Saylan M, Wang Y, Smith H, McLeod J, Prasad P. Effect of a selective CYP2C9 inhibitor on the pharmacokinetics of nateglinide in healthy subjects. *Eur J Clin Pharmacol* (2004) 60, 407–12.
3. Kritz H, Najemnik C, Irsigler K. Interaktionsstudie mit Sulfinpyrazon (Anturan) und Glibenclamid (Euglucon) bei Typ-II-Diabetikern. *Wien Med Wochenschr* (1983) 133, 237–43.
4. Miners JO, Foenander T, Wanwimolruk S, Gallus AS, Birkett DJ. The effect of sulphinpyrazone on oxidative drug metabolism in man: inhibition of tolbutamide elimination. *Eur J Clin Pharmacol* (1982) 22, 321–6.

Antidiabetics + Terbinafine

Terbinafine is reported not to interact with tolbutamide, and did not affect glucose control in a study in patients receiving insulin or oral antidiabetics.

Clinical evidence

A large-scale post-marketing survey did not find any interaction in patients taking terbinafine with **tolbutamide** (number unknown),[1] and a subgroup analysis of this survey found no additional risk in 154 patients taking antidiabetics with terbinafine.[2] In a clinical study in 89 patients with diabetes and toenail fungal infections, oral terbinafine 250 mg daily for 12 weeks had no effect on blood glucose concentrations in 83% of patients. Eleven (12.4%) of the patients had an elevated blood glucose concentration at baseline, which was normal at the end of the study, and 4 patients had a normal baseline blood glucose concentration, which became elevated at the end of the study. No episodes of hypoglycaemia were reported. Patients in this study were receiving **insulin** or **oral antidiabetics** (not specified).[3]

Mechanism

On the basis of *in vitro* studies, terbinafine is unlikely to alter the metabolism of tolbutamide.[4]

Importance and management

Terbinafine does not appear to interact with tolbutamide or affect glucose control in patients receiving insulin or oral antidiabetics. No special precautions would seem necessary on concurrent use, however it is prudent to monitor blood glucose concentrations when any change is made to the medication regimen of a patient with diabetes.

1. Hall M, Monka C, Krupp P, O'Sullivan D. Safety of oral terbinafine. Results of a postmarketing surveillance study in 25 884 patients. *Arch Dermatol* (1997) 133, 1213–19.
2. O'Sullivan DP, Needham CA, Bangs A, Atkin K, Kendall FD. Postmarketing surveillance of oral terbinafine in the UK: report of a large cohort study. *Br J Clin Pharmacol* (1996) 42, 559–65.
3. Farkas B, Paul C, Dobozy A, Hunyadi J, Horváth A, Fekete G. Terbinafine (Lamisil®) treatment of toenail onychomycosis in patients with insulin-dependent and non-insulin-dependent diabetes mellitus: a multi-centre trial. *Br J Dermatol* (2002) 146, 254–60.
4. Back DJ, Stevenson P, Tjia JF. Comparative effects of two antimycotic agents, ketoconazole and terbinafine, on the metabolism of tolbutamide, ethinyloestradiol, cyclosporin and ethoxycoumarin by human liver microsomes *in vitro*. *Br J Clin Pharmacol* (1989) 28, 166–70.

Antidiabetics + Tetracyclines

The blood glucose-lowering effects of insulin and the sulfonylureas can sometimes be increased by oxytetracycline. There is also a case of hypoglycaemia involving insulin and doxycycline. Doxycycline might improve diabetic control in patients taking antidiabetics.

Clinical evidence

(a) Demeclocycline

A brief comment in a report suggests that demeclocycline might not affect **chlorpropamide** disposition.[1]

(b) Doxycycline

A study in patients with type 2 diabetes [treated with unspecified oral antidiabetics] and periodontal disease found that in those taking doxycycline 100 mg daily for 2 weeks (as an adjunct to topical treatment with water, chlorhexidine, or povidone-iodine), mean HbA_{1c} values were reduced by almost 10% from baseline, at 3 months.[2] In contrast, in another study in patients with diabetes (stable taking oral antidiabetics, including **glibenclamide (glyburide)** and/or **metformin**, or **insulin**) and periodontal disease, doxycycline 100 mg daily for 2 weeks (as an adjunct to sub-gingival debridement) did not result in a reduction in mean HbA_{1c} values at 3 months. However, in patients who received low-dose doxycycline 20 mg daily for 3 months, mean HbA_{1c} values were reduced by 0.9% units. This did not reach statistical significance but was statistically significantly different compared with the effect of the 100 mg dose. Note, that there were no changes in random plasma glucose concentrations in any group.[3] Another study in 132 patients with poorly controlled diabetes (HbA_{1c} greater than or equal to 8.5%) and periodontal disease, who received doxycycline 100 mg daily for 14 days, found no differences in mean HbA_{1c} values between groups.[4]

A report briefly lists a case of hypoglycaemia when a patient receiving **insulin** was given doxycycline,[5] and another case describes doxycycline-induced hypoglycaemia in an elderly patient with diabetes managed by diet alone.[6] The half-life of **glymidine** has been found to be prolonged from 4.6 hours to 7.6 hours by doxycycline,[7] whereas a brief comment in another report suggests that doxycycline might not affect **chlorpropamide** disposition.[1]

(c) Oxytetracycline

A patient with diabetes who had poorly controlled blood glucose concentrations needed a large reduction in his **insulin** dose, from 208 to 64 units daily, in order to control the hypoglycaemia that developed when oxytetracycline 250 mg four times daily was given. Hypoglycaemia was also seen when the same patient was given a second course of oxytetracycline, at the same dose, and in another patient given oxytetracycline 250 mg twice daily.[8] Marked hypoglycaemia occurred in an elderly patient taking **tolbutamide** when oxytetracycline was given,[9] and another study in patients with diabetes similarly found that oxytetracycline could reduce blood glucose concentrations.[10]

Mechanism

Not understood. Several mechanisms have been suggested including a prolongation of the half-life of insulin and interference with adrenaline-induced glycaemia.[6] The effect of doxycycline on HbA_{1c} values was suggested to be due to reduced protein glycation, which has been shown in *animal* and *in vitro* studies.[3] This requires further study.

Importance and management

Information about adverse interactions between the sulfonylureas or insulin and the tetracyclines is very limited indeed, and clinically important effects appear to be very uncommon. Concurrent use need not be avoided, however it is prudent to monitor blood glucose concentrations when any change is made to the medication regimen of a patient with diabetes. Some studies[2-4] suggest that periodontal use of doxycycline might improve HbA_{1c} values, although note that the studies have a number of limitations (including small sample size, short duration etc.), and so the general importance of this is yet to be established.

1. Petitpierre B, Perrin L, Rudhardt M, Herrera A, Fabre J. Behaviour of chlorpropamide in renal insufficiency and under the effect of associated drug therapy. *Int J Clin Pharmacol* (1972) 6, 120–24.
2. Grossi SG, Skrepcinski FB, DeCaro T, Robertson DC, Ho AW, Dunford RG, Genco RJ. Treatment of periodontal disease in diabetics reduces glycated hemoglobin. *J Periodontol* (1997) 68, 713–9.
3. Engebretson SP, Hey-Hadavi J. Sub-antimicrobial doxycycline for periodontitis reduces hemoglobin A1c in subjects with type 2 diabetes: a pilot study. *Pharmacol Res* (2011) 64, 624–9.
4. Jones JA, Miller DR, Wehler CJ, Rich SE, Krall-Kaye EA, McCoy LC, Christiansen CL, Rothendler JA, Garcia RI. Does periodontal care improve glycemic control? The department of veterans affairs dental diabetes study. *J Clin Periodontol* (2007) 34, 46–52.
5. New Zealand Committee on Adverse Drug Reactions. Ninth Annual Report. *N Z Dent J* (1975) 71, 28–32.
6. Odeh M, Oliven A. Doxycycline-induced hypoglycemia. *J Clin Pharmacol* (2000) 40, 1173–4.
7. Held H, Kaminski B, von Olderhausen HF. Die beeinflussung der Elimination von Glycodiazin durch Leber- und Nierenfunctionssorungen und durch eine Behandlung mit Phenylbutazon, Phenprocoumarol und Doxycyclin. *Diabetologia* (1970) 6, 386.
8. Miller JB. Hypoglycaemic effect of oxytetracycline. *BMJ* (1966) 2, 1007.
9. Hiatt N, Bonorris G. Insulin response in pancreatectomized dogs treated with oxytetracycline. *Diabetes* (1970) 19, 307–10.
10. Sen S, Mukerjee AB. Hypoglycaemic action of oxytetracycline. A preliminary study. *J Indian Med Assoc* (1969) 52, 366–9.

Antidiabetics + Thioctic acid

Thioctic acid is reported not to interact with acarbose, metformin, or glibenclamide (glyburide).

Clinical evidence, mechanism, importance and management

A crossover study in 24 healthy subjects given tablets containing thioctic acid 200 mg and **metformin** 500 mg found that the pharmacokinetics of **metformin** were unchanged by the presence of thioctic acid. The authors briefly comment that there was also no pharmacodynamic interaction,[1] but note that the report gives very few details. A further study in 24 healthy subjects found that a single 600-mg dose of thioctic acid given with **glibenclamide (glyburide)** 3.5 mg did not result in any clinically relevant pharmacokinetic interaction, and thioctic acid did not alter the effect of **glibenclamide** on glucose or insulin concentrations.[2] Similarly, there was no evidence of a change in thioctic acid pharmacokinetics or pharmacodynamics when it was given to healthy subjects with **acarbose** 50 mg.[2]

No special precautions seem to be required if thioctic acid is given to patients taking **acarbose**, **metformin**, or **glibenclamide**. However, it is prudent to monitor blood glucose concentrations when any change is made to the medication regimen of a patient with diabetes.

1. Schug BS, Schneider E, Elze M, Fieger-Büschges H, Larsimont V, Popescu G, Molz KH, Blume HH, Hermann R. Study of pharmacokinetic interaction of thioctic acid and metformin. *Eur J Clin Pharmacol* (1997) 52 (Suppl), A140.
2. Gleiter CH, Schreeb KH, Freudenthaler S, Thomas M, Elze M, Fieger-Büschges H, Potthast H, Schneider E, Schug BS, Blume HH, Hermann R. Lack of interaction between thioctic acid, glibenclamide and acarbose. *Br J Clin Pharmacol* (1999) 48, 819–25.

Antidiabetics + Tibolone

Tibolone might impair glucose tolerance and therefore possibly reduce the effects of the antidiabetics.

Clinical evidence, mechanism, importance and management

A metabolic study in 10 women with type 2 diabetes stabilised with diet and oral antidiabetics, and given tibolone 2.5 mg daily, found there were no changes in glycaemic control, as measured by HbA_{1c}.[1] Conversely, a longer 12-month study in 14 women with type 2 diabetes given tibolone found a slight deterioration in glycaemic control (as measured by serum fructosamine).[2] In 1994, the manufacturers of tibolone noted that on their adverse drug event database they had only 3 cases of aggravation of diabetes during the use of tibolone, which they considered a very low number in relation to the extent of tibolone use.[3]

Although apparently uncommon, it would appear that the control of diabetes might be affected in patients given tibolone. It would therefore seem prudent to increase the frequency of blood glucose monitoring if tibolone is started.

1. Feher MD, Cox A, Levy A, Mayne P, Lant AF. Short term blood pressure and metabolic effects of tibolone in postmenopausal women with non-insulin dependent diabetes. *Br J Obstet Gynaecol* (1996) 103, 281–3.
2. Prelevic GM, Beljic T, Balint-Peric L, Ginsburg J. Metabolic effects of tibolone in postmenopausal women with non-insulin dependent diabetes mellitus. *Maturitas* (1998) 28, 271–6.
3. Atsma WJ. Is Livial diabetogenic? *Maturitas* (1994) 19, 239–40.

Antidiabetics + Tobacco or Nicotine

Patients with diabetes who smoke tobacco might need more subcutaneous insulin than non-smokers. Smoking and, to a lesser extent, nicotine patches, can increase insulin resistance, and stopping smoking can improve glycaemic control in patients with both type 1 and type 2 diabetes. However, the effects of smoking on diabetes appear to be complex, as some studies have reported that smoking does not affect insulin sensitivity or glycaemic control. Preliminary evidence shows that smoking increases the absorption of inhaled insulin.

Clinical evidence and mechanism

(a) Insulin

A study in 163 patients with type 1 diabetes found that, on average, the 114 who smoked needed 15 to 20% more subcutaneous insulin than the non-smokers, and up to 30% more insulin if they smoked heavily.[1] Possible mechanisms include decreased absorption of insulin from the subcutaneous tissue because of peripheral vasoconstriction,[2] and a considerable increase (40 to 100%) in the concentrations of the hormones that oppose the actions of insulin.[3,4]

Serum insulin concentrations during the first 6 hours after inhaled insulin were 58% higher in smokers than in non-smokers, and maximum insulin concentrations were about 3-fold higher. Minor hypoglycaemia requiring a glucose infusion occurred in 12 smokers, but in only one non-smoker. The increased absorption was possibly due to cigarette smoke increasing the permeability of the alveolar-capillary barrier.[5] It should be noted that the first marketed inhaled insulin (*Exubera*, now withdrawn) was contraindicated in patients who smoked, or had smoked within the past 6 months.[6]

(b) Oral antidiabetics

In a double-blind, crossover study in 12 smokers with type 2 diabetes, stabilised with diet alone or with oral antidiabetics, the effect of smoking one cigarette every hour for 6 hours was compared with transdermal nicotine (30 cm^2 patch) or a placebo patch. Cigarette smoking and the nicotine patch did not affect endogenous insulin secretion, when compared with placebo, but smoking impaired peripheral insulin action, and resulted in lower rates of glucose utilisation and greater hepatic glucose production. The nicotine patch similarly impaired insulin action, but this was much less pronounced than after cigarette smoking, possibly due to the lower plasma concentrations of nicotine attained with the patch.[7]

In a study in patients with type 2 diabetes, stabilised with diet alone or diet and **sulfonylureas** (with or without **metformin**), insulin resistance was higher in the 28 smokers than the 12 non-smokers.[8]

Importance and management

The majority of evidence regarding smoking and diabetes, relates to a drug-disease interaction rather than a drug-drug interaction. That relating to drug-drug effects suggests that subcutaneous insulin requirements might be greater in smokers than non-smokers, and that insulin concentrations after inhalation might be greatly enhanced by smoking. Insulin resistance might also be higher in patients taking oral antidiabetics who are smokers, than in those who are non-smokers.

Regarding drug-disease effects, studies have reported that smoking in patients with diabetes is associated with poor glycaemic control,[9] microalbuminuria,[9] and impaired insulin clearance.[10] However, other studies have suggested that smoking does not affect insulin requirement in patients with type 1 diabetes[11] or have an important effect on glycaemic control in patients with type 1 or type 2 diabetes.[3,11,12] In contrast, another study found that glycaemic control (as measured by HbA_{1c}) was modestly improved in subjects with type 1 and type 2 diabetes, one year after they had stopped smoking. This improved control was considered clinically important.[13] There are numerous other studies on the relationship between smoking and diabetes or insulin resistance in non-diabetics, and only a few are cited here as examples. Some studies have indicated that smoking could increase the risk of type 2 diabetes (relative risk of 2.6) and that tobacco use is associated with a low insulin response.[14] However, other studies suggest that a causal relationship between smoking and insulin resistance is unlikely,[15,16] although in one of the studies[16] exposure to environmental tobacco smoke was associated with lower insulin sensitivity.

Glycaemic control is not the only factor of importance with smoking in patients with diabetes. Cigarette smoking can also accelerate progression of atherosclerosis, increase blood pressure, and increase macrovascular complications.[7,16,17] Patients with diabetes who smoke should be given all the help they need to stop smoking.[9,17]

1. Madsbad S, McNair P, Christensen MS, Christiansen C, Faber OK, Binder C, Transbøl I. Influence of smoking on insulin requirement and metabolic status in diabetes mellitus. *Diabetes Care* (1980) 3, 41–3.

2. Klemp P, Staberg B, Madsbad S, Kølendorf K. Smoking reduces insulin absorption from subcutaneous tissue. *BMJ* (1982) 284, 237.
3. Helve E, Yki-Järvinen H, Koivisto VA. Smoking and insulin sensitivity in type I diabetic patients. *Metabolism* (1986) 35, 874–7.
4. Chiodera P, Volpi R, Capretti L, Speroni G, Necchi-Ghiri S, Caffarri G, Colla R, Coiro V. Abnormal effect of cigarette smoking on pituitary hormone secretions in insulin-dependent diabetes mellitus. *Clin Endocrinol (Oxf)* (1997) 46, 351–7.
5. Himmelmann A, Jendle J, Mellén A, Petersen AH, Dahl UL, Wollmer P. The impact of smoking on inhaled insulin. *Diabetes Care* (2003) 26, 677–82.
6. Exubera (Insulin, human). Pfizer Ltd. UK Summary of product characteristics, April 2006.
7. Epifano L, Di Vincenzo A, Fanelli C, Porcellati F, Perriello G, De Feo P, Motolese M, Brunetti P, Bolli GB. Effect of cigarette smoking and of a transdermal nicotine delivery system on glucoregulation in type 2 diabetes mellitus. *Eur J Clin Pharmacol* (1992) 43, 257–63.
8. Targher G, Alberiche M, Zenere MB, Bonadonna RC, Muggeo M, Bonora E. Cigarette smoking and insulin resistance in patients with noninsulin-dependent diabetes mellitus. *J Clin Endocrinol Metab* (1997) 82, 3619–24.
9. Nilsson PM, Gudbjörnsdottir S, Eliasson B, Cederholm J, for the Steering Committee of the Swedish National Diabetes Register. Smoking is associated with increased HbA_{1c} values and microalbuminuria in patients with diabetes – data from the National Diabetes Register in Sweden. *Diabetes Metab* (2004) 30, 261–8.
10. Bott S, Shafagoj YA, Sawicki PT, Heise T. Impact of smoking on the metabolic action of subcutaneous regular insulin in type 2 diabetic patients. *Horm Metab Res* (2005) 37, 445–9.
11. Mathiesen ER, Søegaard U, Christiansen JS. Smoking and glycaemic control in male insulin dependent (type 1) diabetics. *Diabetes Res* (1984) 1, 155–7.
12. McCulloch P, Lee S, Higgins R, McCall K, Schade DS. Effect of smoking on hemoglobin A_{1c} and body mass index in patients with type 2 diabetes mellitus. *J Investig Med* (2002) 50, 284–7.
13. Gunton JE, Davies L, Wilmshurst E, Fulcher G, McElduff A. Cigarette smoking affects glycemic control in diabetes. *Diabetes Care* (2002) 25, 796–7.
14. Persson P-G, Carlsson S, Svanström L, Östenson C-G, Efendic S, Grill V. Cigarette smoking, oral moist snuff use and glucose intolerance. *J Intern Med* (2000) 248, 103–110.
15. Wareham NJ, Ness EM, Byrne CD, Cox BD, Day NE, Hales CN. Cigarette smoking is not associated with hyperinsulinemia: evidence against a causal relationship between smoking and insulin resistance. *Metabolism* (1996) 45, 1551–6.
16. Henkin L, Zaccaro D, Haffner S, Karter A, Rewers M, Sholinsky P, Wagenknecht L. Cigarette smoking, environmental tobacco smoke exposure and insulin sensitivity: the Insulin Resistance Atherosclerosis Study. *Ann Epidemiol* (1999) 9, 290–6.
17. American Diabetes Association. Smoking and diabetes. *Diabetes Care* (2004) 27 (Suppl 1), S74–S75.

Antidiabetics + Tricyclic and related antidepressants

Interactions between antidiabetics and tricyclic or tetracyclic antidepressants appear to be rare, but isolated cases of hypoglycaemia and one of altered insulin requirements have been reported.

Clinical evidence

(a) Retrospective evidence

One research group from the Netherlands has conducted a number of analyses to look at the association between antidepressants and dysglycaemia.[1-3] In one analysis of cases of patients hospitalised for hypoglycaemia, the use of antidepressants (including tricyclics and related drugs) was not associated with an increased risk. The authors suggested that there was a trend for an increased risk with amitriptyline, doxepin, and imipramine, as a group, when compared with maprotiline, nortriptyline, mianserin, and mirtazapine, as a group,[1] but there were too few cases to reasonably assess this. Conversely, in an analysis of spontaneous reports in the WHO adverse drug reaction database, the use of antidepressants was associated with a small increased risk of both hyperglycaemia (odds ratio 1.5) and hypoglycaemia (odds ratio 1.8). Tricyclics and related drugs had a slightly greater risk of hyperglycaemia than hypoglycaemia, but this was not statistically significant.[2] In a further longitudinal study in 133 patients using **insulin** for at least 12 months before starting an antidepressant, and for at least 6 months with an antidepressant, the dose of insulin used did not change after starting the antidepressant. When analysed by antidepressant type, no change in insulin requirement was seen with tricyclic antidepressants.[3]

(b) Prospective studies

A study in 4 patients suggested that **amitriptyline** 75 mg daily for 9 days did not affect the half-life of a single 500-mg dose of **tolbutamide**.[4] Although there is some evidence of a change in glucose metabolism during treatment with **mianserin**,[5-7] the alteration did not affect the control of diabetes in a study in 10 patients and there appear to be no reports of adverse effects caused by concurrent use.[6]

(c) Case reports

In contrast to the above data, there are five case reports describing alterations in glycaemic control:

- A patient taking **tolazamide** became hypoglycaemic 11 days after starting to take **doxepin** 250 mg daily. The patient was eventually stabilised on a daily dose of **tolazamide** that was only 10% of that used before the **doxepin** was given.[8]
- A patient taking **chlorpropamide** (initially 25 mg increased to 75 mg daily) developed marked hypoglycaemia 3 days after starting **nortriptyline** 125 mg daily. The **chlorpropamide** was stopped.[8]
- A patient receiving **insulin** developed violent and agitated behaviour (but no adrenergic symptoms) and hypoglycaemia when she started to take **amitriptyline** 25 mg at bedtime.[9]
- An elderly woman with diabetes taking **glibenclamide (glyburide)** and **phenformin** [now largely withdrawn] developed hypoglycaemia when given **maprotiline**. She was restabilised on half the dose of **glibenclamide** and **phenformin**.[10]
- A patient receiving **insulin** required a 17% increase in her dose when **imipramine** was increased from 25 mg once daily to 25 mg twice daily. She required a 51% decrease in her insulin dose when the imipramine was discontinued.[11]

Mechanism

The reason for the cases of hypoglycaemia and altered insulin requirements is unknown. Depression *per se*, might alter factors (e.g. weight gain or weight loss) that influence glucose homeostasis.

Importance and management

Apart from the isolated cases there seems to be very little evidence that the tricyclic or tetracyclic antidepressants can cause hypoglycaemia or alter insulin requirements in patients with diabetes. Bearing in mind the length of time these groups of drugs have been available, the risk of a clinically important interaction would seem to be very small. Therefore no particular precautions seem warranted on concurrent use.

1. Derijks HJ, Heerdink ER, De Koning FH, Janknegt R, Klungel OH, Egberts AC. The association between antidepressant use and hypoglycaemia in diabetic patients: a nested case-control study. *Pharmacoepidemiol Drug Safety* (2008) 17, 336–44.
2. Derijks HJ, Meyboom RHB, Heerdink ER, De Koning FHP, Janknegt R, Lindquist M, Egberts ACG. The association between antidepressant use and disturbances in glucose homeostasis: evidence from spontaneous reports. *Eur J Clin Pharmacol* (2008) 64, 531–8.
3. Knol MJ, Derijks HJ, Geerlings MI, Heerdink ER, Souverein PC, Gorter KJ, Grobbee DE, Egberts ACG. Influence of antidepressants on glycaemic control in patients with diabetes mellitus. *Pharmacoepidemiol Drug Safety* (2008) 17, 577–86.
4. Pond SM, Graham GG, Birkett DJ, Wade DN. Effects of tricyclic antidepressants on drug metabolism. *Clin Pharmacol Ther* (1975) 18, 191–9.
5. Fell PJ, Quantock DC, van der Burg WJ. The human pharmacology of GB94–a new psychotropic agent. *Eur J Clin Pharmacol* (1973) 5, 166–73.
6. Peet M, Behagel H. Mianserin: a decade of scientific development. *Br J Clin Pharmacol* (1978) 5, 5S–9S.
7. Brogden RN, Heel RC, Speight TM, Avery GS. Mianserin: a review of its pharmacological properties and therapeutic efficacy in depressive illness. *Drugs* (1978) 16, 273–301.
8. True BL, Perry PJ, Burns EA. Profound hypoglycemia with the addition of a tricyclic antidepressant to maintenance sulfonylurea therapy. *Am J Psychiatry* (1987) 144, 1220–1.
9. Sherman KE, Bornemann M. Amitriptyline and asymptomatic hypoglycemia. *Ann Intern Med* (1988) 109, 683–4.
10. Zogno MG, Tolfo L, Draghi E. Hypoglycemia caused by maprotiline in a patient taking oral antidiabetics. *Ann Pharmacother* (1994) 28, 406.
11. Derijks HJ, De Koning FH, Meyboom RH, Heerdink ER, Spooren PF, Egberts AC. Impaired glucose homeostasis after imipramine intake in a diabetic patient. *J Clin Psychopharmacol* (2005) 25, 621–3.

Antidiabetics + Tyrosine kinase inhibitors

An improvement in diabetic control with a reduction in dose of insulin or oral antidiabetics has been seen in a few reports of diabetics given imatinib for chronic myelogenous leukaemia, but one report found no benefit. In one case, an increased insulin dose was required with imatinib and then subsequently also with nilotinib, but a reduced insulin requirement then occurred with dasatinib. Tofacitinib appears to have no effect on the pharmacokinetics of metformin.

Clinical evidence

Use of **imatinib** 400 or 600 mg daily for the treatment of chronic myelogenous leukaemia (CML) was associated with improved glycaemic control in 6 of 7 patients with diabetes who had a clinical response to the drug. This allowed a reduction in **insulin** dose in 2 patients and a reduction in the dose of **oral antidiabetic** (not specified) in 4 patients.[1] The same research group described a further case, in a woman with type 2 diabetes managed with **insulin**, who had a sequential reduction in fasting blood glucose and HbA_{1c} over 18 weeks after starting **imatinib** 400 mg daily.[2] Another case report describes a 70-year-old woman with type 2 diabetes who needed a reduction in her **insulin** dose when she was given **imatinib** for CML. Later, while still taking imatinib, she was able to stop the insulin completely.[3] However, in a retrospective review of patients who had received **imatinib**, of 7 patients who had pre-existing type 2 diabetes, and 2 who developed diabetes during therapy, no effect of **imatinib** on glycaemic control was noted.[4]

In contrast, in another patient, the use of **imatinib** was associated with an increased **insulin** dose, and, the use of **nilotinib** (which proved ineffective for CML) for 3 months was associated with a further increased insulin requirement. However, the subsequent use of **dasatinib** resulted in two episodes of hypoglycaemia, and a reduced **insulin** requirement.[5]

The US manufacturer of **tofacitinib** briefly notes that, in a study, it had no clinically important effect on the pharmacokinetics of **metformin**.[6]

Mechanism

It was thought that imatinib and dasatinib might have a direct effect on glycaemic control,[1,3,5] rather than an indirect effect by improving the leukaemia.[1] It has also been suggested that imatinib might ameliorate fibrotic and amyloid damage to the islet cells of the pancreas which occurs in type 2 diabetes.[7] Nilotinib is reported to cause hyperglycaemia,[5,8] so it is perhaps not surprising that this drug caused an increase in insulin requirements.

Importance and management

These preliminary findings suggest that diabetic patients should be closely monitored if given tyrosine kinase inhibitors, such as dasatinib, imatinib, or nilotinib, because of the possibility of altered glucose metabolism. Further study is needed.

No metformin dose adjustments appear necessary on concurrent use with tofacitinib.

1. Breccia M, Muscaritoli M, Aversa Z, Mandelli F, Alimena G. Imatinib mesylate may improve fasting blood glucose in diabetic Ph+ chronic myelogenous leukemia patients responsive to treatment. *J Clin Oncol* (2004) 22, 4653–55.

2. Breccia M, Muscaritoli M, Alimena G. Reduction of glycosilated (sic) haemoglobin with stable plasma insulin level in a ph+ cml diabetic patient responsive to imatinib. *Haematologica* (2005) 90 (Suppl), ECR21.
3. Veneri D, Franchini M, Bonora E. Imatinib and regression of type 2 diabetes. *N Engl J Med* (2005) 352, 1049–50.
4. Dingli D, Wolf RC, Vella A. Imatinib and type 2 diabetes. *Endocr Pract* (2007) 13, 126–30.
5. Breccia M, Muscaritoli M, Cannella L, Stefanizzi C, Frustaci A, Alimena G. Fasting glucose improvement under dasatinib treatment in an accelerated phase chronic myeloid leukemia patient unresponsive to imatinib and nilotinib. *Leuk Res* (2008) 32, 1626–8.
6. Xeljanz (Tofacitinib citrate). Pfizer Inc. US Prescribing information, November 2012.
7. Welsh N. Does the small tyrosine kinase inhibitor imatinib mesylate counteract diabetes by affecting pancreatic islet cell amyloidosis and fibrosis? *Expert Opin Invest Drugs* (2012) 21, 1743–50.
8. Tasigna (Nilotinib hydrochloride monohydrate). Novartis Pharmaceuticals UK Ltd. UK Summary of product characteristics, December 2013.

Dipeptidylpeptidase-4 inhibitors + ACE inhibitors or Angiotensin II receptor antagonists

No clinically relevant pharmacokinetic interactions have been detected between vildagliptin and ramipril or valsartan. Sitagliptin appears to alter the hypotensive effects of enalapril.

Clinical evidence

(a) Sitagliptin

In a study in patients with metabolic syndrome, sitagliptin 100 mg daily for 5 days increased the hypotensive response to both **enalapril** 5 mg daily (8 patients) and placebo (9 patients), but reduced the hypotensive response to **enalapril** 10 mg daily (7 patients).[1]

(b) Vildagliptin

In a crossover study in 18 healthy subjects, the pharmacokinetics of vildagliptin, **ramipril**, and its active metabolite, ramiprilat, were not altered when vildagliptin 100 mg daily was given with **ramipril** 5 mg daily for 7 days, when compared with either drug alone.[2]

In another similar study in 28 healthy subjects, the pharmacokinetics of vildagliptin were not altered when vildagliptin 100 mg daily was given with **valsartan** 320 mg daily for 7 days, whereas vildagliptin negligibly increased the AUC of **valsartan** by 24%, when compared with either drug alone.[2] Note that the increase in valsartan exposure in one subject was considerably greater than in all other subjects.

Mechanism

The authors of the study of enalapril and sitagliptin suggest that maximal ACE inhibition together with inhibition of dipeptidylpeptidase-4 results in an increase in substance P, which stimulates the sympathetic nervous system, thereby reducing the hypotensive effects of the ACE inhibitor.[1]

Importance and management

These studies provide evidence that there is no clinically relevant pharmacokinetic interaction between vildagliptin and **ramipril** or **valsartan**. On this basis, no pharmacokinetic interaction would be anticipated with vildagliptin and any ACE inhibitor or angiotensin II receptor antagonist, and no dose adjustments would seem necessary. However, it is prudent to monitor blood glucose concentrations when any change is made to the medication regimen of a patient with diabetes.

The general relevance of the reported effect of sitagliptin on the blood pressure-lowering effects of ACE inhibitors requires further study. However, until more is known it would seem prudent to bear the possibility of an interaction in mind should any otherwise unexplained changes in blood pressure occur on concurrent use.

For conflicting data on the possible increased risk of hypoglycaemia when some antidiabetics are used with ACE inhibitors and angiotensin-II receptor antagonists, see 'Antidiabetics + ACE inhibitors', p.499 and 'Antidiabetics + Angiotensin II receptor antagonists', p.502.

1. Marney A, Kunchakarra S, Byrne L, Brown NJ. Interactive hemodynamic effects of dipeptidyl peptidase-IV inhibition and angiotensin-converting enzyme inhibition in humans. *Hypertension* (2010) 56, 728–33.
2. He Y-L, Ligueros-Saylan M, Sunkara G, Sabo R, Zhao C, Wang Y, Campestrini J, Pommier F, Dole K, Marion A, Dole WP, Howard D. Vildagliptin, a novel dipeptidyl peptidase IV inhibitor, has no pharmacokinetic interactions with the antihypertensive agents amlodipine, valsartan, and ramipril in healthy subjects. *J Clin Pharmacol* (2008) 48, 85–95.

Dipeptidylpeptidase-4 inhibitors + Calcium-channel blockers

Diltiazem moderately increases the exposure to saxagliptin, but slightly reduces that of its active metabolite. Verapamil is expected to interact similarly. No pharmacokinetic interaction occurs between vildagliptin and amlodipine.

Clinical evidence

(a) Amlodipine

In a crossover study in 19 healthy subjects, the pharmacokinetics of **vildagliptin** and amlodipine were not altered when **vildagliptin** 100 mg daily was given with amlodipine 5 mg daily for 10 days.[1]

(b) Diltiazem

In a study in 12 healthy subjects, modified-release diltiazem 360 mg daily for 8 days increased the maximum concentration of **saxagliptin** by 63% and increased the AUC 2.1-fold, when a single 10-mg dose of saxagliptin was given on day 8. In addition, there was a reduction of 36% in the AUC of the active metabolite of **saxagliptin** (which is about half as potent as saxagliptin). **Saxagliptin** had no effect on the pharmacokinetics of diltiazem.[2]

Mechanism

Diltiazem is a moderate inhibitor of CYP3A4, by which saxagliptin is metabolised to its principal metabolite (which is about half as active as the parent compound). This leads to an increase in saxagliptin exposure and possibly its effects.

Importance and management

The pharmacokinetic interaction between diltiazem and **saxagliptin** is established, but its clinical relevance has not yet been assessed. Until more is known, it would seem prudent to monitor concurrent use for an increase in the blood glucose-lowering effects of saxagliptin as well as its other adverse effects (such as headache, dizziness, and vomiting). **Verapamil**, also a moderate inhibitor of CYP3A4, would be predicted to interact similarly.

There is no clinically relevant pharmacokinetic interaction between **vildagliptin** and amlodipine, and no dose adjustments would seem necessary. However, it is prudent to monitor blood glucose concentrations when any change is made to the medication regimen of a patient with diabetes.

1. He Y-L, Ligueros-Saylan M, Sunkara G, Sabo R, Zhao C, Wang Y, Campestrini J, Pommier F, Dole K, Marion A, Dole WP, Howard D. Vildagliptin, a novel dipeptidyl peptidase IV inhibitor, has no pharmacokinetic interactions with the antihypertensive agents amlodipine, valsartan, and ramipril in healthy subjects. *J Clin Pharmacol* (2008) 48, 85–95.
2. Patel CG, Li L, Girgis S, Kornhauser DM, Frevert EU, Boulton DW. Two-way pharmacokinetic interaction studies between saxagliptin and cytochrome P450 substrates or inhibitors: simvastatin, diltiazem extended-release, and ketoconazole. *Clin Pharmacol* (2011) 2, 13

Dipeptidylpeptidase-4 inhibitors + Ciclosporin

Single-dose ciclosporin slightly increased sitagliptin exposure, but did not alter alogliptin pharmacokinetics.

Clinical evidence, mechanism, importance and management

(a) Alogliptin

The US manufacturer of alogliptin briefly notes that, in a clinical study, a single 600-mg dose of ciclosporin did not meaningfully alter the pharmacokinetics of a single 25-mg dose of alogliptin. No alogliptin dose adjustment is necessary on concurrent use.[1]

(b) Sitagliptin

A crossover study in 8 healthy subjects found that when a single 100-mg dose of sitagliptin was given with a single 600-mg dose of ciclosporin there was a 68% increase in the maximum plasma concentration of sitagliptin, with a slight increase in overall exposure to sitagliptin (AUC increased by 28%). There was no change in renal clearance of sitagliptin, or time to reach maximum concentrations.[2]

It is likely that ciclosporin enhances the absorption of sitagliptin by inhibiting P-glycoprotein. However, the changes seen were considered unlikely to be clinically meaningful, because of the apparent wide therapeutic index of sitagliptin.[2] Note that one of the rare adverse effects of ciclosporin is hyperglycaemia.

1. Nesina (Alogliptin). Takeda Pharmaceuticals America, Inc. US Prescribing information, January 2013.
2. Krishna R, Bergman A, Larson P, Cote J, Lasseter K, Dilzer S, Wang A, Zeng W, Chen L, Wagner J, Herman G. Effect of a single cyclosporine dose on the single-dose pharmacokinetics of sitagliptin (MK-0431), a dipeptidyl peptidase-4 inhibitor, in healthy male subjects. *J Clin Pharmacol* (2007) 47, 165–74.

Dipeptidylpeptidase-4 inhibitors + Drugs that affect gastric pH

The pharmacokinetics of saxagliptin are not altered by antacids, famotidine, or omeprazole. The pharmacokinetics of alogliptin and cimetidine were not altered when both drugs were given concurrently.

Clinical evidence, mechanism, importance and management

(a) Antacids

In a study in 15 healthy subjects, the AUC of **saxagliptin** was unchanged when a single 10-mg dose of saxagliptin was given at the same time as 30 mL of an antacid containing **aluminium/magnesium hydroxide** with simeticone.[1] The saxagliptin maximum concentration was decreased by 26%, but this is not expected to be clinically relevant. No saxagliptin dose adjustment is likely to be needed if antacids are also given.

(b) Cimetidine

In a randomised crossover study in 18 healthy subjects, the concurrent administration of **alogliptin** 100 mg daily with cimetidine 400 mg daily for 6 days did not alter the pharmacokinetics of either drug. No dose adjustments would seem necessary on concurrent use.[2]

(c) Famotidine

In a study in 15 healthy subjects, the AUC of **saxagliptin** was unchanged when a single 10-mg dose of saxagliptin was given 3 hours after a single 40-mg dose of famotidine.[1] No saxagliptin dose adjustment is likely to be needed if famotidine is also given.

(d) Omeprazole

In a study in 15 healthy subjects, there was no change in the pharmacokinetics of **saxagliptin** when a single 10-mg dose of saxagliptin was given on day 5 of omeprazole 40 mg daily for 5 days.[1] No saxagliptin dose adjustment is likely to be needed if omeprazole is also given.

1. Boulton DW, Adams D, Li L, Patel CG, Komoroski BJ, Whigan D, Frevert EU, Goyal A, Kornhauser DM. 36th Annual Meeting of the American College of Clinical Pharmacology, San Francisco, California, 2007.
2. Karim A, Covington P, Christopher R, Davenport M, Fleck P, Li X, Wann E, Mekki Q. Pharmacokinetics of alogliptin when administered with food, metformin, or cimetidine: a two-phase, crossover study in healthy subjects. *Int J Clin Pharmacol Ther* (2010) 48, 46–58.

Dipeptidylpeptidase-4 inhibitors + Food

Food does not affect the pharmacokinetics of alogliptin, linagliptin, saxagliptin, sitagliptin, or vildagliptin.

Clinical evidence, mechanism, importance and management

(a) Alogliptin

In a randomised, crossover study, 36 healthy subjects were given a single 100-mg dose of alogliptin immediately after a high-fat, high-calorie breakfast or after an overnight fast. The AUC of alogliptin was unaffected by food, but the maximum concentration was reduced by 14%. The time to maximum concentration was delayed by 30 minutes by food, but this was not statistically significant. As alogliptin has a wide therapeutic range, the minor reduction in maximum concentration was not considered clinically important.[1] Alogliptin can be given without regard to food.

(b) Linagliptin

In a randomised, crossover study, 32 healthy subjects were given a single 5-mg dose of linagliptin immediately after a high-fat, high-calorie (945 kcal) breakfast or after an overnight fast. The AUC of linagliptin was unaffected by food, but the maximum concentration was reduced by 15%. The time to maximum concentration was delayed by about 2 hours by food. The authors state that plasma linagliptin concentrations were still sufficient in the fed state, despite the minor reduction in maximum concentration, to achieve sufficient therapeutic inhibition of DPP-4, therefore this change was not clinically relevant.[2] Linagliptin can be given without regard to food.

(c) Saxagliptin

In a randomised, crossover study in 14 healthy subjects, administration of a single 10-mg dose of saxagliptin within 30 minutes of a high-fat meal resulted in a 27% increase in the AUC of saxagliptin, and an 18% reduction in the maximum concentration of its active metabolite, when compared with the fasted state. The time to maximum saxagliptin concentration was increased by food by about 30 minutes. None of the changes were statistically significant and were also not considered clinically relevant.[3] Saxagliptin can be given without regard to food.

(d) Sitagliptin

In a randomised, crossover study in 12 healthy subjects, administration of a single 100-mg dose of sitagliptin 5 minutes after a high-fat meal (about 57% fat) had no effect on its pharmacokinetics, when compared with the fasted state.[4] Sitagliptin can be given without regard to food.

(e) Vildagliptin

In a randomised, crossover study, 24 healthy subjects were given a single 100-mg dose of vildagliptin within 5 minutes of a high-fat, high-calorie (1000 kcal) breakfast or after an overnight fast. There was no change in the AUC of vildagliptin, and the maximum concentration was reduced by about 20%. The time to maximum concentration was increased by about 45 minutes by food. The authors state that plasma vildagliptin concentrations were still sufficient in the fed state, despite the minor reduction in maximum concentration, to achieve sufficient therapeutic inhibition of DPP-4, and therefore this change was not clinically relevant.[5] Another crossover study in 12 patients with type 2 diabetes, found that the pharmacokinetics and pharmacodynamics of vildagliptin 50 mg twice daily were unaffected when it was given 30 minutes, or immediately, before food.[6] Vildagliptin can be given without regard to food.

1. Karim A, Covington P, Christopher R, Davenport M, Fleck P, Li X, Wann E, Mekki Q. Pharmacokinetics of alogliptin when administered with food, metformin, or cimetidine: a two-phase, crossover study in healthy subjects. *Int J Clin Pharmacol Ther* (2010) 48, 46–58.
2. Graefe-Mody U, Giessmann T, Ring A, Iovino M, Woerle H-J. A randomized, open-label, crossover study evaluating the effect of food on the relative bioavailability of linagliptin in healthy subjects. *Clin Ther* (2011) 33, 1096–1103.
3. Patel CG, Zhang J, Li L, Gooding L, Croop R, Li T, Boulton DW. Effect of a high-fat meal on the pharmacokinetics of saxagliptin in healthy subjects. *J Clin Pharmacol* (2010) 50, 1211–16.
4. Bergman A, Ebel D, Liu F, Stone J, Wang A, Zeng W, Chen L, Dilzer S, Lasseter K, Herman G, Wagner J, Krishna R. Absolute bioavailability of sitagliptin, an oral dipeptidyl peptidase-4 inhibitor, in healthy subjects. *Biopharm Drug Dispos* (2007) 28, 315–22.
5. Sunkara G, Sabo R, Wang Y, He Y-L, Campestrini J, Rosenberg M, Howard D, Dole WP. Dose proportionality and the effect of food on vildagliptin, a novel dipeptidyl peptidase IV inhibitor, in healthy volunteers. *J Clin Pharmacol* (2007) 47, 1152–8.
6. He YL, Ito H, Yamaguchi M, Terao S, Shimada S, Irie S, Sekiguchi K. Effects of meal timing relative to dosing on the pharmacokinetics and pharmacodynamics of vildagliptin in Japanese patients with type 2 diabetes. *Int J Clin Pharmacol Ther* (2012) 50, 237–47.

Dipeptidylpeptidase-4 inhibitors + Ketoconazole and other CYP3A4 inhibitors

Ketoconazole, a potent CYP3A4 inhibitor, moderately increases the exposure to saxagliptin and very markedly reduces the exposure to its active metabolite. Other potent inhibitors of CYP3A4 would be expected to interact similarly. Ketoconazole did not alter the pharmacokinetics of alogliptin and ritonavir moderately increases the exposure to linagliptin; other potent CYP3A4 inhibitors would be expected to interact similarly.

Clinical evidence

(a) Alogliptin

The US manufacturer of alogliptin briefly reports that ketoconazole 400 mg daily for 7 days had no meaningful effect on the pharmacokinetics of a single 25-mg dose of alogliptin.[1]

(b) Linagliptin

The UK manufacturer of linagliptin briefly reports that, in a study, multiple doses of **ritonavir** 200 mg twice daily increased the AUC and maximum concentration of a single 5-mg dose of linagliptin 2-fold and 3-fold, respectively. The unbound concentration of linagliptin (usually less than 1% of linagliptin dose) was increased 4- to 5-fold. However, simulations of steady-state linagliptin suggested that this increase in exposure would not lead to an accumulation of linagliptin.[2]

(c) Saxagliptin

In a study in 15 healthy subjects, ketoconazole 200 mg every 12 hours for 9 days increased the AUC of a single 100-mg dose of saxagliptin, given on day 9, 2.5-fold, and increased its maximum concentration by 62%. In addition, ketoconazole reduced the AUC of the active metabolite of saxagliptin by 91% and reduced its maximum concentration by 95%.[3] Saxagliptin 100 mg caused a 13% decrease in the AUC of ketoconazole.[3]

The US manufacturer of saxagliptin also reports that ketoconazole 200 mg daily for 7 days increased the AUC of a single 20-mg dose of saxagliptin 3.7-fold and increased its maximum concentration 2.4-fold.[4]

Mechanism

Ketoconazole is a potent inhibitor of CYP3A4, by which saxagliptin is metabolised to its principal metabolite (which is about half as active as the parent compound), leading to an increase in saxagliptin exposure and a decrease in the exposure to its active metabolite. Metabolism by CYP3A4 is a minor route for linagliptin, however it is affected by the potent CYP3A4 inhibitor, ritonavir. Alogliptin is not extensively metabolised by cytochrome P450 isoenzymes, and so ketoconazole has no effect on its exposure. Linagliptin[2] and saxagliptin[4] are also P-glycoprotein substrates, but the exact role, if any, of this transporter in these interactions is unclear.

Importance and management

Ketoconazole moderately increases **saxagliptin** exposure, but any effect of this should be partially offset by the very marked reduction in the exposure to its active metabolite (which is about half as potent as saxagliptin) and therefore the clinical relevance of this interaction with use of lower daily doses of saxagliptin (such as 5 mg daily) is not known. Nevertheless, the US manufacturer[4] recommends that the saxagliptin dose be limited to 2.5 mg daily when used with ketoconazole or other potent inhibitors of CYP3A4. 'Table 1.9', p.11, includes a list of known, clinically relevant CYP3A4 inhibitors. In addition the manufacturer also names indinavir and nefazodone as potent inhibitors of CYP3A4; however, note that these drugs appear to be moderate CYP3A4 inhibitors, and so might be expected to behave more like diltiazem (see 'Dipeptidylpeptidase-4 inhibitors + Calcium-channel blockers', p.522).

The moderate increase in **linagliptin** exposure reported with ritonavir is not expected to be clinically relevant,[2] and so no linagliptin dose adjustment appears necessary on concurrent use with ritonavir or other potent inhibitors of CYP3A4 (see 'Table 1.9', p.11, for a list).

The lack of effect of ketoconazole on **alogliptin** means that no dose adjustment is necessary on concurrent use, and therefore no dose adjustment would appear to be necessary on the concurrent use of alogliptin with other potent inhibitors of CYP3A4 (see 'Table 1.9', p.11, for a list).

There appears to be no clinical data for the concurrent use of other dipeptidylpeptidase-4 inhibitors with potent CYP3A4 inhibitors. Nevertheless, the UK manufacturer of **sitagliptin** does not rule out the possibility of an interaction with potent CYP3A4 inhibitors (see 'Table 1.9', p.11, for a list) in patients with severe renal impairment or end-stage renal disease, in whom metabolism could play a more important role in elimination.[5] However, as the dose of sitagliptin should be adjusted based on renal function, any theoretical interaction with potent CYP3A4 inhibitors seems unlikely to be clinically relevant.

In general, it is prudent to monitor blood glucose concentrations when any change is made to the medication regimen of a patient with diabetes, and this should be sufficient to detect any interaction with these drugs should it occur.

1. Nesina (Alogliptin). Takeda Pharmaceuticals America, Inc. US Prescribing information, January 2013.
2. Trajenta (Linagliptin). Boehringer Ingelheim Ltd. UK Summary of product characteristics, August 2013.
3. Patel CG, Li L, Girgis S, Kornhauser DM, Frevert EU, Boulton DW. Two-way pharmacokinetic interaction studies between saxagliptin and cytochrome P450 substrates or inhibitors: simvastatin, diltiazem extended-release, and ketoconazole. *Clin Pharmacol* (2011) 3, 13–25.
4. Onglyza (Saxagliptin). Bristol-Myers Squibb. US Prescribing information, May 2013.
5. Januvia (Sitagliptin phosphate monohydrate). Merck Sharp & Dohme Ltd. UK Summary of product characteristics, December 2012.

Dipeptidylpeptidase-4 inhibitors + Metformin

No pharmacokinetic interactions have been detected between metformin and alogliptin, linagliptin, saxagliptin, sitagliptin, or vildagliptin.

Clinical evidence and mechanism

(a) Alogliptin

In a randomised, crossover study in 17 healthy subjects, the concurrent use of alogliptin 100 mg once daily and metformin 1 g twice daily for 6 days, had no effect on the pharmacokinetics of alogliptin. There was also no effect on the maximum concentrations of metformin, but there was a 19% increase in its AUC.[1]

(b) Linagliptin

In a randomised, crossover study in 14 healthy subjects, the concurrent use of linagliptin 10 mg daily and metformin 850 mg three times daily had no effect on the pharmacokinetics of metformin. In addition, there was no change in the pharmacokinetics of linagliptin, except for a 20% increase in its AUC.[2]

(c) Saxagliptin

In a crossover study in 16 healthy subjects, there was no change in the pharmacokinetics of a single 1-g dose of metformin when it was given with a single 100-mg dose of saxagliptin. In addition, there was no change in the AUC of saxagliptin, but there was a 21% decrease in the maximum saxagliptin concentration.[3]

(d) Sitagliptin

In a randomised, crossover study in 13 patients with type 2 diabetes, there were no changes in the pharmacokinetics of sitagliptin or metformin when sitagliptin 50 mg twice daily was given with metformin 1 g twice daily for 7 days.[4]

(e) Vildagliptin

In a randomised, crossover study in 17 patients with type 2 diabetes, when vildagliptin 100 mg daily was given with metformin 1 g daily, there was no change in AUC of vildagliptin, but there was a 15% increase in AUC of metformin. The maximum concentration of vildagliptin was decreased by 18%, but the maximum concentration of metformin was unaffected.[5]

Importance and management

The minor increase in the exposure to linagliptin, and the minor decreases in the maximum concentrations of saxagliptin and vildagliptin, when given with metformin were not considered to be clinically relevant.[2,3,5] Similarly the negligible increases in exposure to metformin seen on concurrent use with alogliptin and with vildagliptin were not considered to be a clinically important.[1,5] These combinations of drugs are used in the management of diabetes for their additive blood glucose lowering effects, and the studies show that there are no pharmacokinetic interactions that will complicate such use.

1. Karim A, Covington P, Christopher R, Davenport M, Fleck P, Li X, Wann E, Mekki Q. Pharmacokinetics of alogliptin when administered with food, metformin, or cimetidine: a two-phase, crossover study in healthy subjects. *Int J Clin Pharmacol* (2010) 48, 46–58.
2. Graefe-Mody EU, Padula S, Ring A, Withopf B, Dugi KA. Evaluation of the potential for steady-state pharmacokinetic and pharmacodynamic interactions between the DPP-4 inhibitor linagliptin and metformin in healthy subjects. *Curr Med Res Opin* (2009) 25, 1963–72.
3. Patel CG, Kornhauser D, Vachharajani N, Komoroski B, Brenner E, Handschuh del Corral M, Li L, Boulton DW. Saxagliptin, a potent, selective inhibitor of DPP-4, does not alter the pharmacokinetics of three oral antidiabetic drugs (metformin, glyburide or pioglitazone) in healthy subjects. *Diabetes Obes Metab* (2011) 13, 604–14.
4. Herman GA, Bergman A, Yi B, Kipnes M; Sitagliptin Study 012 Group. Tolerability and pharmacokinetics of metformin and the dipeptidyl peptidase-4 inhibitor sitagliptin when co-administered in patients with type 2 diabetes. *Curr Med Res Opin* (2006) 22, 1939–47.
5. He Y-L, Sabo R, Picard F, Wang Y, Herron J, Ligueros-Saylan M, Dole WP. Study of the pharmacokinetic interaction of vildagliptin and metformin in patients with type 2 diabetes. *Curr Med Res Opin* (2009) 25, 1265–72.

Dipeptidylpeptidase-4 inhibitors + Rifampicin (Rifampin) and other CYP3A4 inducers

Rifampicin, a potent CYP3A4 inducer, moderately reduces the exposure to saxagliptin but did not alter the exposure to its active metabolite. Rifampicin slightly reduces the exposure to linagliptin. Other potent inducers of CYP3A4 might be expected to interact similarly.

Clinical evidence

(a) Linagliptin

The UK and US manufacturers of linagliptin briefly report that, rifampicin 600 mg daily reduced the AUC of multiple-dose linagliptin 5 mg daily by about 40% and reduced the maximum concentration by 44%,[1,2] resulting in a 30% reduction in the minimum amount of dipeptidyl peptidase-4 inhibition.[1]

(b) Saxagliptin

In a study in healthy subjects, rifampicin 600 mg daily for 6 days reduced the AUC of a single 5-mg dose of saxagliptin by 76% and reduced the maximum concentration by 53%. There was no change in the pharmacokinetics of the active metabolite of saxagliptin. However, there was no overall change in the dipeptidylpeptidase-4 inhibitory activity of saxagliptin over 24 hours when given with rifampicin.[3]

Mechanism

Rifampicin is a potent inducer of CYP3A4 by which saxagliptin is metabolised to its principal metabolite (which is about half as active as the parent compound),[4] leading to a decrease in saxagliptin exposure, although there was no corresponding increase in exposure to its active metabolite. Metabolism by CYP3A4 is a minor route for linagliptin,[1] and it is therefore less affected than saxagliptin by rifampicin. Linagliptin[1] and saxagliptin[4] are also P-glycoprotein substrates, but the exact role, if any, of this transporter in these interactions is unclear.

Importance and management

Evidence for interactions between inducers of CYP3A4 and the dipeptidylpeptidase-4 inhibitors appears limited to the studies cited between rifampicin and linagliptin or saxagliptin. Rifampicin moderately reduces saxagliptin exposure, but there is no corresponding increase in exposure to the active metabolite (which is about half as potent as saxagliptin) to offset this. The clinical relevance of this has not been assessed, but no saxagliptin dose adjustment would seem necessary because dipeptidylpeptidase-4 inhibitory activity was not altered. Nevertheless, until more is known, it cannot be ruled out that rifampicin might reduce the blood glucose-lowering effect of saxagliptin, and monitoring of diabetic control on the concurrent use of potent inducers of CYP3A4 would seem prudent. 'Table 1.9', p.11 includes a list of known, clinically relevant CYP3A4 inducers. In addition to the drugs listed in this table, the UK manufacturer also names **dexamethasone**,[5] however, note that clinically important interactions with dexamethasone as a result of this mechanism is generally lacking. Further study is needed to establish the clinical relevance of these interactions.

The reduction in linagliptin exposure seen with rifampicin, and the overall dipeptidylpeptidase-4 inhibitory activity, might reduce its efficacy.[1,2] Although they have not been studied, other potent CYP3A4 inducers (see 'Table 1.9', p.11 for a list) would be expected to interact similarly. The advice of the US manufacturer[2] to consider alternatives to CYP3A4 inducers appears a overly cautious, but it would seem prudent to monitor concurrent use of linagliptin with potent CYP3A4 inducers to ensure linagliptin remains effective, adjusting the linagliptin dose if necessary.

In general, it is prudent to monitor blood glucose concentrations when any change is made to the medication regimen of a patient with diabetes, and this should be sufficient to detect any interaction with these drugs should it occur.

1. Trajenta (Linagliptin). Boehringer Ingelheim Ltd. UK Summary of product characteristics, August 2013.
2. Tradjenta (Linagliptin). Boehringer Ingelheim International GmbH. US Prescribing information, June 2013.
3. Upreti VV, Boulton DW, Li L, Ching A, Su H, LaCreta FP, Patel CG. Effect of rifampicin on the pharmacokinetics and pharmacodynamics of saxagliptin, a dipeptidyl peptidase-4 inhibitor, in healthy subjects. *Br J Clin Pharmacol* (2011) 72, 92–102.
4. Onglyza (Saxagliptin). Bristol-Myers Squibb. US Prescribing information, May 2013.
5. Onglyza (Saxagliptin). Bristol Myers Squibb-AstraZeneca EEIG. UK Summary of product characteristics, July 2013.

Dipeptidylpeptidase-4 inhibitors + Sulfonylureas or Insulin

No clinically relevant pharmacokinetic interactions appear to occur between alogliptin, linagliptin, saxagliptin, sitagliptin, or vildagliptin and glibenclamide (glyburide). Alogliptin appears not to alter the pharmacokinetics of tolbutamide. The risk of hypoglycaemia might be increased by the concurrent use of a dipeptidylpeptidase-4 inhibitor and a sulfonylurea or insulin.

Clinical evidence

(a) Alogliptin

In a randomised, crossover study in 24 healthy subjects, there was no change in the pharmacokinetics of **glibenclamide (glyburide)** when a single 5-mg dose was given before and on the last day of alogliptin 25 mg daily for 7 days, except for a minor 15% increase in the glibenclamide maximum concentration.[1] In a large placebo controlled study, where alogliptin 12.5 mg or 25 mg was given to patients with type 2 diabetes taking **glibenclamide**, the incidence of hypoglycaemia in patients taking alogliptin 25 mg was similar to placebo (9.6% v 11.1%). In those taking alogliptin 12.5 mg the incidence of hypoglycaemia was 15.8%.[2] The US manufacturer briefly notes that, in clinical studies, alogliptin 100 mg daily for 7 days did not meaningfully alter the systemic exposure to **tolbutamide**, when administered as a single 500-mg dose as part of a cocktail.[3] In a randomised, placebo-controlled study, patients with type 2 diabetes receiving **insulin**, or insulin with **metformin**, were given alogliptin 12.5 mg or 25 mg daily. There was no difference in the incidence of hypoglycaemia in those given alogliptin, compared with placebo.[4]

(b) Linagliptin

In a randomised, crossover study in 19 healthy subjects, a single 1.75-mg dose of **glibenclamide** given on day 6 of linagliptin 5 mg daily, had no effect on the pharmacokinetics of linagliptin. Linagliptin reduced the AUC and maximum concentration of glibenclamide by about 14%.[5]

(c) Saxagliptin

In a randomised crossover study in 30 healthy subjects, there was no change in the AUC of a single 5-mg dose of **glibenclamide** or a single 10-mg dose of saxagliptin when both drugs were given together, but there was a minor 16% increase in the glibenclamide maximum concentration and an 8% increase in the saxagliptin maximum concentration.[6]

In a large placebo-controlled study where saxagliptin 2.5 mg or 5 mg was given to patients with type 2 diabetes taking **glibenclamide**, the incidence of reports of hypoglycaemia in patients taking saxagliptin was a little higher (13.3% and 14.6%

for the two doses, respectively), than with placebo (10.1%), but did not reach statistical significance.[7] The manufacturer briefly notes that, when saxagliptin 5 mg was added to **insulin** (with or without metformin) the incidence of confirmed symptomatic hypoglycaemia was 5.3% compared with 3.3% with placebo.[8]

(d) Sitagliptin

In a randomised, crossover study in 8 healthy subjects, a single 1.25-mg dose of **glibenclamide** given on day 5 of sitagliptin 200 mg daily for 6 days, had no effect on the pharmacokinetics of glibenclamide.[9]

In a large (n=441) placebo-controlled study where sitagliptin 100 mg was given to patients with type 2 diabetes taking **glimepiride** or glimepiride and **metformin**, there appeared to be an increased incidence of hypoglycaemia in patients taking sitagliptin (12.2%) when compared with placebo (1.8%).[10] The manufacturer briefly notes that, when sitagliptin 100 mg was added to **insulin** (with or without metformin) the incidence of hypoglycaemia was 15.5% compared with 7.8% with placebo.[11]

(e) Vildagliptin

In a randomised, crossover study in 17 patients with type 2 diabetes, there were no changes in the pharmacokinetics of vildagliptin or **glibenclamide** when vildagliptin 100 mg twice daily was given with glibenclamide 10 mg daily. As expected, the combination had greater glucose lowering effects than either drug alone.[12]

In a large (n=515) placebo-controlled study, the incidence of hypoglycaemia when vildagliptin 50 mg or 100 mg daily was added to **glimepiride** was 1.2% and 3.6%, respectively, compared with 0.6% for placebo added to **glimepiride**.[13] The UK manufacturer briefly notes that, when vildagliptin 50 mg twice daily was added to **insulin** (with or without **metformin**) the incidence of hypoglycaemia was 8.4% compared with 7.2% with placebo.[14]

Mechanism

Sulfonylureas increase the risk of hypoglycaemia because they increase the secretion of insulin. Dipeptidylpeptidase-4 inhibitors might further increase this risk because they slow the inactivation of incretin hormones, which also increases the release of insulin.

Importance and management

Sulfonylureas and dipeptidylpeptidase-4 inhibitors are used concurrently in the management of diabetes for their additive blood glucose-lowering effects, and the studies show that there are no clinically relevant pharmacokinetic interactions that will complicate this use. Bear in mind that the risk of hypoglycaemia might be greater with the combination of a dipeptidylpeptidase-4 inhibitor and a sulfonylurea. Because of this, when starting the dipeptidylpeptidase-4 inhibitor in a patient already taking a sulfonylurea, consideration should be given to lowering the dose of the sulfonylurea. Some dipeptidylpeptidase-4 inhibitors have been shown to increase the incidence of hypoglycaemia when added to insulin (sitagliptin and saxagliptin) and for this reason their use in combination is cautioned and the dose of insulin might need to be reduced. The same advice is given for the use of most other dipeptidylpeptidase-4 inhibitors with insulin, with the exception of vildagliptin.

It is prudent to monitor blood glucose concentrations when any change is made to the medication regimen of a patient with diabetes, and this should be sufficient to detect any interaction between dipeptidylpeptidase-4 inhibitors and sulfonylureas or insulin, should it occur, and allow any necessary dose adjustments to be made.

Note that tolbutamide can be used as a probe substrate to assess the activity of drugs on CYP2C9. The study with alogliptin therefore suggests that alogliptin is not an inhibitor or inducer of CYP2C9.

1. Karim A, Laurent A, Munsaka M, Wann E, Fleck P, Mekki Q. Coadministration of pioglitazone or glyburide and alogliptin: pharmacokinetic drug interaction assessment in healthy participants. *J Clin Pharmacol* (2009) 49, 1210–19.
2. Pratley RE, Kipnes MS, Fleck PR, Wilson C, Mekki Q; Alogliptin Study 007 Group. Efficacy and safety of the dipeptidylpeptidase-4 inhibitor alogliptin in patients with type 2 diabetes inadequately controlled by glyburide monotherapy. *Diabetes Obes Metab* (2009) 11, 167–76.
3. Nesina (Alogliptin). Takeda Pharmaceuticals America, Inc. US Prescribing information, January 2013.
4. Rosenstock J, Rendell MS, Gross JL, Fleck PR, Wilson CA, Mekki Q. Alogliptin added to insulin therapy in patients with type 2 diabetes reduces HbA1c without causing weight gain or increased hypoglycaemia. *Diabetes Obes Metab* (2009) 11, 1145–52.
5. Graefe-Mody U, Rose P, Ring A, Zander K, Iovino M, Woerle H-J. Assessment of the pharmacokinetic interaction between the novel DPP-4 inhibitor linagliptin and a sulfonylurea, glyburide, in healthy subjects. *Drug Metab Pharmacokinet* (2011) 26, 123–9.
6. Patel CG, Kornhauser D, Vachharajani N, Komoroski B, Brenner E, Handschuh del Corral M, Li L, Boulton DW. Saxagliptin, a potent, selective inhibitor of DPP-4, does not alter the pharmacokinetics of three oral antidiabetic drugs (metformin, glyburide or pioglitazone) in healthy subjects. *Diabetes Obes Metab* (2011) 13, 604–14.
7. Chacra AR, Tan GH, Apanovitch A, Ravichandran S, List J, Chen R; CV181-040 Investigators. Saxagliptin added to a submaximal dose of sulphonylurea improves glycaemic control compared with uptitration of sulphonylurea in patients with type 2 diabetes: a randomised controlled trial. *Int J Clin Pract* (2009) 63, 1395–1406.
8. Onglyza (Saxagliptin). Bristol-Myers Squibb. US Prescribing information, May 2013
9. Mistry GC, Bergman AJ, Zheng W, Hreniuk D, Zinny MA, Gottesdiener KM, Wagner JA, Herman GA, Ruddy M. Sitagliptin, an dipeptidyl peptidase-4 inhibitor, does not alter the pharmacokinetics of the sulphonylurea, glyburide, in healthy subjects. *Br J Clin Pharmacol* (2008) 66, 36–42.
10. Hermansen K, Kipnes M, Luo E, Fanurik D, Khatami H, Stein P. Efficacy and safety of the dipeptidylpeptidase-4 inhibitor, sitagliptin, in patients with type 2 diabetes mellitus inadequately controlled on glimepiride alone or on glimepiride and metformin. *Diabetes Obes Metab* (2007) 9, 733–45.
11. Januvia (Sitagliptin). Merck & Co. Inc. US Prescribing information, February 2014
12. Serra D, He Y-L, Bullock J, Riviere G-J, Balez S, Schwartz S, Wang Y, Ligueros-Saylan M, Jarugula V, Dole WP. Evaluation of pharmacokinetic and pharmacodynamic interaction between the dipeptidyl peptidase IV inhibitor vildagliptin, glyburide and pioglitazone in patients with Type 2 diabetes. *Int J Clin Pharmacol Ther* (2008) 46, 349–64..
13. Garber AJ, Foley JE, Banerji MA, Ebeling P, Gudbjörnsdottir S, Camisasca R-P, Couturier A, Baron MA. Effects of vildagliptin on glucose control in patients with type 2 diabetes inadequately controlled with a sulfonylurea. *Diabetes Obes Metab* (2008) 10, 1047–56.
14. Galvus (Vildagliptin). Novartis Pharmaceuticals UK Ltd. UK Summary of product characteristics, July 2013.

Dipeptidylpeptidase-4 inhibitors + Thiazolidinediones

No clinically relevant pharmacokinetic interactions have been seen between sitagliptin and rosiglitazone, or between alogliptin, linagliptin, saxagliptin, or vildagliptin and pioglitazone. There might be an increased risk of peripheral oedema if saxagliptin is used with a thiazolidinedione.

Clinical evidence

(a) Alogliptin

In a crossover study in 27 healthy subjects, the concurrent use of alogliptin 25 mg daily and **pioglitazone** 45 mg daily for 12 days increased the AUC of alogliptin by 10% and caused no changes in the pharmacokinetics of pioglitazone or its active metabolites.[1] In a phase III clinical study, there was no difference in incidence of peripheral oedema when alogliptin was used with pioglitazone.[2]

(b) Linagliptin

In a randomised, crossover study in 20 healthy subjects, the concurrent use of **pioglitazone** 45 mg daily and linagliptin 10 mg daily for 7 days increased the AUC of linagliptin by 13% and increased its maximum concentration by 7%. The maximum concentration of pioglitazone was reduced by 14%.[3]

(c) Saxagliptin

In a study in 28 healthy subjects, when saxagliptin 10 mg daily and **pioglitazone** 45 mg daily were given together for 5 days, the pharmacokinetics of saxagliptin and pioglitazone were not appreciably affected when compared with either drug alone.[4] In a large placebo-controlled clinical study where saxagliptin 2.5 mg daily or 5 mg daily was added to the established use of **pioglitazone** or **rosiglitazone** in patients with type 2 diabetes, there was a higher incidence of peripheral oedema in those given saxagliptin 5 mg than those given saxagliptin 2.5 mg or placebo (8.1%, 3.1% and 4.3%, respectively).[5]

(d) Sitagliptin

In a randomised, crossover study in 12 healthy subjects, a single 4-mg dose of **rosiglitazone** given on day 5 of sitagliptin 200 mg daily for 5 days had no effect on the pharmacokinetics of rosiglitazone.[6]

(e) Vildagliptin

In a randomised, crossover study in 15 patients with type 2 diabetes, when vildagliptin 100 mg twice daily was given with **pioglitazone** 45 mg daily, the pharmacokinetics of vildagliptin and pioglitazone were not appreciably affected when compared with either drug alone. As expected, the combination had greater glucose lowering effects than either drug alone.[7] In a large, controlled clinical study in patients with type 2 diabetes, the combination of vildagliptin with **pioglitazone** in low doses (50 mg and 15 mg daily, respectively) was associated with the lowest occurrence of peripheral oedema (3.5%) compared with 5.2% for vildagliptin 100 mg daily, 6.1% for vildagliptin 100 mg with pioglitazone 30 mg daily, and 9.3% for pioglitazone 30 mg daily.[8]

Mechanism

Both groups of drugs lower blood glucose concentrations, and as might be expected, the effects are additive.

Importance and management

Dipeptidylpeptidase-4 inhibitors and thiazolidinediones are used in the management of diabetes for their additive blood glucose-lowering effects, and the studies show that there are no clinically relevant pharmacokinetic interactions that will complicate such use. Bear in mind the possibility of an increased risk of peripheral oedema if saxagliptin is given with a thiazolidinedione.

1. Karim A, Laurent A, Munsaka M, Wann E, Fleck P, Mekki Q. Coadministration of pioglitazone or glyburide and alogliptin: pharmacokinetic drug interaction assessment in healthy participants. *J Clin Pharmacol* (2009) 49, 1210–19.
2. Pratley RE, Reusch JE-B, Fleck PR, Wilson CA, Mekki Q; Alogliptin Study 009 Group. Efficacy and safety of the dipeptidyl peptidase-4 inhibitor alogliptin added to pioglitazone in patients with type 2 diabetes: a randomized, double-blind, placebo-controlled study. *Curr Med Res Opin* (2009) 25, 2361–71.
3. Graefe-Mody EU, Jungnik A, Ring A, Woerle HJ, Dugi KA. Evaluation of the pharmacokinetic interaction between the dipeptidyl peptidase-4 inhibitor linagliptin and pioglitazone in healthy volunteers. *Int J Clin Pharmacol Ther* (2010) 48, 652–61.
4. Patel CG, Kornhauser D, Vachharajani N, Komoroski B, Brenner E, Handschuh del Corral M, Li L, Boulton DW. Saxagliptin, a potent, selective inhibitor of DPP-4, does not alter the pharmacokinetics of three oral antidiabetic drugs (metformin, glyburide or pioglitazone) in healthy subjects. *Diabetes Obes Metab* (2011) 13, 604–14.
5. Hollander P, Li J, Allen E, Chen R. Saxagliptin added to a thiazolidinedione improves glycemic control in patients with type 2 diabetes and inadequate control on thiazolidinedione alone. *J Clin Endocrinol Metab* (2009) 94, 4810–9.
6. Mistry GC, Bergman AJ, Luo W-L, Cilissen C, Haazen W, Davies MJ, Gottesdiener KM, Wagner JA, Herman GA. Multiple-dose administration of sitagliptin, a dipeptidyl peptidase-4 inhibitor, does not alter the single-dose pharmacokinetics of rosiglitazone in healthy subjects. *J Clin Pharmacol* (2007) 47, 159–64.
7. Serra D, He Y-L, Bullock J, Riviere G-J, Balez S, Schwartz S, Wang Y, Ligueros-Saylan M, Jarugula V, Dole WP. Evaluation of pharmacokinetic and pharmacodynamic interaction between the dipeptidyl peptidase IV inhibitor vildagliptin, glyburide and pioglitazone in patients with Type 2 diabetes. *Int J Clin Pharmacol Ther* (2008) 46, 349–64..
8. Rosenstock J, Kim SW, Baron MA, Camisasca RP, Cressier F, Couturier A, Dejager S. Efficacy and tolerability of initial combination therapy with vildagliptin and pioglitazone compared with component monotherapy in patients with type 2 diabetes. *Diabetes Obes Metab* (2007) 9, 175–85.

Dipeptidylpeptidase-4 inhibitors; Alogliptin + Miscellaneous

Alogliptin does not appear to alter the pharmacokinetics of caffeine, dextromethorphan, fexofenadine, or midazolam. Fluconazole and gemfibrozil do not appear to alter the pharmacokinetics of alogliptin.

Clinical evidence, mechanism, importance and management

(a) Caffeine

The US manufacturer of alogliptin briefly notes that, in a clinical study, alogliptin 100 mg daily for 7 days did not meaningfully alter the systemic exposure to caffeine (a CYP1A2 probe substrate) when given as a single 200-mg dose as part of a cocktail.[1] This therefore suggests that alogliptin is not an inducer or inhibitor of CYP1A2.

(b) Dextromethorphan

The US manufacturer of alogliptin briefly notes that, in clinical studies, alogliptin 100 mg daily for 7 days did not meaningfully alter the pharmacokinetics of dextromethorphan (a CYP2D6 probe substrate) when given as a single 30-mg dose as part of a cocktail.[1] This therefore suggests that alogliptin is not an inducer or inhibitor of CYP2D6.

(c) Fexofenadine

The US manufacturer of alogliptin briefly notes that, in clinical studies, alogliptin 100 mg daily for 7 days did not meaningfully alter the pharmacokinetics of fexofenadine (a P-glycoprotein substrate) when given as a single 80-mg dose as part of a cocktail. No fexofenadine dose adjustment is necessary on concurrent use.[1] This therefore suggests that alogliptin is not an inducer or inhibitor of P-glycoprotein (see also 'Digoxin + Dipeptidylpeptidase-4 inhibitors', p.1093).

(d) Fluconazole

The US manufacturer of alogliptin briefly notes that, in a clinical study the CYP2C9 inhibitor fluconazole at a dose of 200 mg daily for 7 days, did not meaningfully alter the pharmacokinetics of a single 25-mg dose of alogliptin. No alogliptin dose adjustment is necessary on concurrent use.[1]

(e) Gemfibrozil

The US manufacturer of alogliptin briefly notes that, in a clinical study the CYP2C8 inhibitor gemfibrozil at a dose of 600 mg twice daily for 7 days, did not meaningfully alter the pharmacokinetics of a single 25-mg dose of alogliptin. No alogliptin dose adjustment is necessary on concurrent use.[1]

(f) Midazolam

The US manufacturer of alogliptin briefly notes that, in clinical studies, alogliptin 100 mg daily for 7 days did not meaningfully alter the pharmacokinetics of the CYP3A4 probe substrate midazolam, when administered as a single 4-mg dose as part of a cocktail.[1] This therefore suggests that alogliptin is not an inducer or inhibitor of CYP3A4.

1. Nesina (Alogliptin). Takeda Pharmaceuticals America, Inc. US Prescribing information, January 2013.

Glucagon-like peptide-1 receptor agonists + Other antidiabetics

The pharmacokinetics of liraglutide and insulin detemir were not altered by concurrent administration. Dulaglutide does not appear to alter the pharmacokinetics of metformin or sitagliptin, but the exposure to dulaglutide appears to be slightly increased by sitagliptin. The use of glucagon-like peptide-1 receptor agonists and sulfonylureas or insulin can increase the risk of hypoglycaemia.

Clinical evidence, mechanism, importance and management

(a) Albiglutide

The use of albuglutide in combination with **insulin** or a **sulfonylurea** might increase the risk of hypoglycaemia, but this risk might be reduced by reducing the dose of insulin or the sulfonylurea.[1]

(b) Dulaglutide

The UK and US manufacturers briefly report that, in a study, multiple doses of dulaglutide increased the AUC of steady-state **metformin** by up to 15%, and decreased the maximum concentration by 12%, but had no effect on time to maximum concentration.[2,3] In another study, single-dose dulaglutide did not alter **sitagliptin** exposure, but after two doses of dulaglutide, the sitagliptin AUC and maximum concentration were decreased by about 7% and 23%, respectively. Time to maximum concentration was increased by 30 minutes.[2] The AUC and maximum concentration of a single 1.5-mg dose of dulaglutide were increased by about 38% and 27%, respectively, by steady state sitagliptin 100 mg.[3] No **metformin**[2,3] or **sitagliptin**[3] dose adjustments are recommended on concurrent use, and the US manufacturer advises that the slight increase in dulaglutide exposure when given with sitagliptin is not clinically relevant.[3] However, the UK manufacturer advises that this increase might lead to a greater effect on blood glucose concentrations.[2] Furthermore, the use of dulaglutide in combination with **insulin** or a **sulfonylurea** might increase the risk of hypoglycaemia, but this risk might be reduced by reducing the dose of insulin or the sulfonylurea.[2,3]

(c) Exenatide

Exenatide is not expected to alter the pharmacokinetics of **metformin** or the **sulfonylureas** on concurrent use.[4] However, the concurrent use of exenatide and **sulfonylureas** in clinical trials, resulted in an increased risk of hypoglycaemia. A reduction in the dose of the sulfonylurea should be considered on concurrent use with exenatide to reduce the risk of hypoglycaemia.[4,5] Similarly, if exenatide is given with **insulin**, the dose of insulin should be evaluated and possibly reduced in patients at increased risk of hypoglycaemia.[4,5] The US manufacturer also states that exenatide should not be given with prandial insulin,[5] and the UK manufacturer notes that use with **alpha-glucosidase inhibitors**, **dipeptidylpeptidase-4 inhibitors**, **meglitinides**, and other glucagon-like peptide-1 receptor agonists has not been studied, and is not recommended.[5]

(d) Liraglutide

In a study in 32 patients with type 2 diabetes given a single 0.5 units/kg dose of **insulin detemir** with steady-state liraglutide 1.8 mg, there were no pharmacokinetic changes for either drug. The glucose lowering effect of the combination was about the sum of the effect of each drug when given alone.[6]

The use of liraglutide in combination with **insulin** or a **sulfonylurea** might increase the risk of hypoglycaemia, but this risk might be reduced by reducing the dose of insulin or the sulfonylurea.[7,8]

(e) Lixisenatide

The use of lixisenatide with basal **insulin** *or* a **sulfonylurea** increases the risk of hypoglycaemia and a reduction in the dose of the sulfonylurea or insulin should be considered in order to reduce the risk. The use of lixisenatide with basal insulin *and* a sulfonylurea is not recommended.[9]

1. Tanzeum (Albiglutide). GlaxoSmithKline LLC. US Prescribing information, May 2015.
2. Trulicity (Dulaglutide). Eli Lilly and Company Ltd. UK Summary of product characteristics, November 2014.
3. Trulicity (Dulaglutide). Eli Lilly and Company. US Prescribing information, March 2015.
4. Byetta (Exenatide). AstraZeneca UK Ltd. UK Summary of product characteristics, January 2015.
5. Byetta (Exenatide). AstraZeneca Pharmaceuticals LP. US Prescribing information, February 2015.
6. Morrow L, Hompesch M, Guthrie H, Chang D, Chatterjee DJ. Co-administration of lirgaglutide with insulin detemir demonstrates additive pharmacodynamic effects with no pharmacokinetic interaction. *Diabetes Obes Metab* (2011) 13, 75–80.
7. Victoza (Liraglutide). Novo Nordisk Inc. US Prescribing information, March 2015.
8. Victoza (Liraglutide). Novo Nordisk Ltd. UK Summary of product characteristics, March 2015.
9. Lyxumia (Lixisenatide). Sanofi. UK Summary of product characteristics, October 2014.

Insulin + Alcohol

Hypoglycaemia has been reported in small studies, after patients had consumed varying amounts of alcohol.

Clinical evidence, mechanism, importance and management

In one early study, 2 out of 7 patients with diabetes receiving insulin became severely hypoglycaemic after drinking the equivalent of about 3 measures of spirits.[1] In a hospital study over a 3-year period, five patients with type 1 diabetes were hospitalised with severe hypoglycaemia after binge-drinking. Two of them died without recovery from the initial coma, and the other 3 suffered permanent damage to the nervous system.[2] In another study it was found that alcohol was involved in about 4% of hypoglycaemic episodes requiring hospitalisation.[3] In contrast to these alcohol-induced hypoglycaemic episodes, it was found in another study[4] that dry wine had little effect on blood glucose concentrations.

For general advice about the consumption of alcohol in diabetes, see 'Antidiabetics + Alcohol', p.501.

1. Walsh CH, O'Sullivan DJ. Effect of moderate alcohol intake on control of diabetes. *Diabetes* (1974) 23, 440–2.
2. Arky RA, Veverbrants E, Abramson EA. Irreversible hypoglycemia. A complication of alcohol and insulin. *JAMA* (1968) 206, 575–8.
3. Potter J, Clarke P, Gale EAM, Dave SH, Tattersall RB. Insulin-induced hypoglycaemia in an accident and emergency department: the tip of an iceberg? *BMJ* (1982) 285, 1180–2.
4. Lolli G, Balboni C, Ballatore C, Risoldi L, Carletti D, Silvestri L, Pacifici De Tommaso G. Wine in the diets of diabetic patients. *Q J Stud Alcohol* (1963) 24, 412–6.

Insulin + Allopurinol

Allopurinol adversely affected glycaemic control in a patient with type 2 diabetes receiving insulin.

Clinical evidence, mechanism, importance and management

A case report describes improved glycaemic control in a patients with type 2 diabetes after allopurinol was stopped. Despite restricted food intake and an increasing dose of insulin, his glycaemic control was poor (fasting blood glucose 14.8 mmol/L) when he took allopurinol 100 mg twice daily. However, within a few days of stopping the allopurinol, an unexpected improvement in glycaemic control was observed (fasting blood glucose reduced to less than 11 mmol/L). He was later rechallenged with allopurinol, which resulted in reduced glucose tolerance, but increased insulin response, suggesting increased insulin resistance. Hyperuricaemia was later controlled with **probenecid**, which did not adversely affect glycaemic control.[1] This is an isolated report and as such, its general clinical relevance is uncertain.

1. Ohashi K, Ishibashi S, Yazaki Y, Yamada N. Improved glycemic control in a diabetic patient after discontinuation of allopurinol administration. *Diabetes Care* (1998) 21, 192–3.

Insulin + Azoles; Itraconazole

Itraconazole does not usually disturb the control of diabetes, although there are rare reports of hyperglycaemia or hypoglycaemia associated with its concurrent use with insulin.

Clinical evidence, mechanism, importance and management

Post-marketing surveillance of adverse event reports in patients receiving itraconazole with insulin over 10 years, indicated that, in most patients, diabetic control was not affected. However, of the 98 adverse events reported, there were 10 reports suggesting hyperglycaemia and 6 reports suggesting hypoglycaemia.[1] In clinical studies, only one of 189 patients with diabetes taking antidiabetic drugs, including insulin, experienced aggravated diabetes when given itraconazole.[1] The patient in question was also receiving ciclosporin for a kidney transplant. No special precautions would seem necessary, but it is prudent to monitor blood glucose concentrations when any change is made to the medication regimen of a patient with diabetes.

1. Verspeelt J, Marynissen G, Gupta AK, De Doncker P. Safety of itraconazole in diabetic patients. *Dermatology* (1999) 198, 382–4.

Insulin + Benzodiazepines

An isolated case of hyperglycaemia has been seen in an insulin-treated patient with type 2 diabetes while receiving chlordiazepoxide. The effects of lorazepam were found to be increased when patients were given beef or pork insulin compared with human insulin.

Clinical evidence, mechanism, importance and management

A woman with long-standing type 2 diabetes, which was stabilised with 45 units of isophane insulin suspension daily, had an increase in her mean fasting blood glucose from about 12 mmol/L to 21 mmol/L during a 3-week period while taking **chlordiazepoxide** 40 mg daily.[1] A preliminary report in 8 healthy patients with type 1 diabetes, given **lorazepam** 2 mg, suggested that while they were given human insulin they were more alert and less sedated than when given beef or pork insulin.[2]

There seems to be nothing in the literature to suggest that a clinically important adverse interaction normally takes place between insulin and the benzodiazepines. No special precautions would appear to be necessary.

1. Zumoff B, Hellman L. Aggravation of diabetic hyperglycemia by chlordiazepoxide. *JAMA* (1977) 237, 1960–1.
2. Dahlan AA, Vrbancic MI, Hogan TE, Woo D, Herman RI. Greater sedative response to lorazepam in patients with insulin-dependent diabetes mellitus while on treatment with beef/pork versus human insulin. *Clin Invest Med* (1993) 16 (4 Suppl), B18.

Insulin + Co-trimoxazole

There appear to be no reports of a serious adverse interaction between insulin and co-trimoxazole.

Clinical evidence, mechanism, importance and management

In one study, co-trimoxazole did not alter blood glucose or insulin concentrations in 8 patients receiving **insulin**.[1] However, note that co-trimoxazole alone can rarely cause hypoglycaemia (see *Mechanism* in 'Sulfonylureas + Antibacterials; Sulfonamides and/or Trimethoprim', p.542). It is prudent to monitor blood glucose concentrations when any change is made to the medication regimen of a diabetic patient.

1. Mihic M, Mautner LS, Feness JZ, Grant K. Effect of trimethoprim-sulfamethoxazole on blood insulin and glucose concentrations of diabetics. *Can Med Assoc J* (1975), 112, 80S–82S.

Insulin + Miscellaneous

The blood-glucose lowering effects of insulin might be increased by alpha-glucosidase inhibitors. Insulin does not affect the hypocholesterolaemic effects of colestipol.

Clinical evidence, mechanism, importance and management

(a) Alpha-glucosidase inhibitors

The manufacturers state that while alpha-glucosidase inhibitors, such as acarbose and miglitol, do not cause hypoglycaemia when given alone, they might increase the blood glucose-lowering effects of insulin, for which reason it might be necessary to reduce the insulin dose. Monitor the outcome when acarbose, miglitol, or voglibose is first given. Any hypoglycaemic episodes should be treated with glucose (dextrose), not sucrose, because alpha-glucosidase inhibitors delay the digestion and absorption of disaccharides such as sucrose, but do not affect monosaccharides.[1-3]

(b) Colestipol

In a randomised study in 12 patients with diabetes whose serum cholesterol concentrations were elevated, no antagonism of the hypocholesterolaemic effects of colestipol was seen in 2 patients receiving insulin. The control of diabetes was not affected by the colestipol.[4]

1. Precose (Acarbose). Bayer HealthCare Pharmaceuticals Inc. US Prescribing information, March 2011.
2. Glyset (Miglitol). Pfizer Inc. US Prescribing information, September 2012.
3. Glucobay (Acarbose). Bayer plc. UK Summary of product characteristics, July 2013.
4. Bandisode MS, Boshell BR. Hypocholesterolemic activity of colestipol in diabetes. *Curr Ther Res* (1975) 18, 276–84.

Insulin + Naltrexone

The insulin requirements of a patient increased when naltrexone was given.

Clinical evidence, mechanism, importance and management

A patient with type 1 diabetes was given naltrexone in an experimental study of the treatment of anorexia nervosa. During two periods of 5 days while taking the naltrexone (dose not stated), the blood glucose concentrations of the patient remained unchanged, but the insulin dose requirements increased from 52.8 and 61.4 units daily to 71.4 and 76 units daily (an increase of about 30%). The reason is not known, but the authors of this report point out that this apparent interaction must have been due to the actions of insulin, rather than on its release, because this patient had no endogenous insulin.[1]

The general clinical importance of this interaction is not known, but it would be prudent to be alert for any evidence of increased insulin requirements if naltrexone is used in any patient.

1. Marrazzi MA, Jacober S, Luby ED. A naltrexone-induced increase in insulin requirement. *J Clin Psychopharmacol* (1994) 14, 363–5.

Insulin + Nifedipine

Nifedipine increased the absorption of subcutaneous insulin in healthy subjects.

Clinical evidence, mechanism, importance and management

A study in 7 healthy subjects found that nifedipine 10 mg, given 30 minutes prior to a subcutaneous injection of insulin, increased the rate of insulin absorption by about 50%.[1] The general importance of this is uncertain.

For discussion of the general effects of calcium channel blockers on diabetes control, see 'Antidiabetics + Calcium-channel blockers', p.505.

1. Veenstra J, van der Hulst JP, Wildenborg IH, Njoo SF, Verdegaal WP, Silberbusch J. Effect of antihypertensive drugs on insulin absorption. *Diabetes Care* (1991) 14, 1089–92.

Insulin + Penicillamine

Two case reports describe hypoglycaemia in patients stabilised on insulin, after penicillamine was added.

Clinical evidence, mechanism, importance and management

A 60-year-old man stabilised on insulin for almost 30 years (40 units daily), with no history of hypoglycaemia, was started on penicillamine 250 mg daily for rheumatoid arthritis. After 8 weeks, he experienced symptoms of severe hypoglycaemia, including convulsions and mental confusion, over 3 consecutive nights. His insulin dose was reduced by 8 units and his symptoms resolved. Similarly, a 36-year-old woman stabilised on insulin (28 units in the morning and 16 units in the evening) was also prescribed penicillamine 250 mg daily then 500 mg daily, and 6 weeks later developed symptoms suggestive of hypoglycaemia over several nights. Her insulin dose was reduced by 10 units and symptoms resolved.[1] The reason for these effects is unclear, but an immunological mechanism has been suggested.[1,2] These are isolated cases and as such are unlikely to be of general clinical importance.

1. Elling P, Elling H. Penicillamine, captopril, and hypoglycaemia. *Ann Intern Med* (1985) 103, 644–5.
2. Becker RC, Martin RG. Penicillamine-induced insulin antibodies. *Ann Intern Med* (1985) 104, 127–8.

Insulin + Rifampicin (Rifampin)

An isolated report describes an increased insulin requirement in a patient with type 1 diabetes taking rifampicin and isoniazid.

Clinical evidence

A case report describes a 54-year-old woman with type 1 diabetes whose insulin requirements increased from 36 units daily to 48 units daily when she took rifampicin 300 mg and **isoniazid** 150 mg twice daily. Immediately on discontinuing her antimycobacterials, she developed frequent hypoglycaemic attacks, which persisted until her insulin dose was reduced back to 36 units daily.[1]

Mechanism

Unexplained, although there is a case of a patient who developed diabetes requiring insulin treatment while receiving rifampicin and ethambutol, which resolved when the antimycobacterials were stopped.[2] It is possible that rifampicin or tuberculosis *per se* might cause hyperglycaemia.[2] The authors of the case report state that isoniazid was not responsible for the change in the patient's insulin requirement, however note that isoniazid is associated with hyperglycaemia, see 'Antidiabetics + Isoniazid', p.510.

Importance and management

The isolated case of increased insulin requirement suggests that rifampicin might possibly affect the glycaemic control of patients with type 1 diabetes, but this needs further investigation. As isoniazid is known to be associated with hyperglycaemia, it is possible that it played a part in this case. Until more is known, it might be prudent for patients on insulin also given rifampicin (with or without isoniazid) to be monitored for changes in the control of their diabetes. Appropriate insulin dose adjustments should be made where necessary.

1. Atkin SL, Masson EA, Bodmer CW, Walker BA, White MC. Increased insulin requirement in a patient with type 1 diabetes on rifampicin. *Diabet Med* (1993) 10, 392.
2. Waterhouse M, Wilson C, White VLC, Chowdhury TA. Resolution of insulin-requiring diabetes after cessation of chemotherapy for tuberculosis. *J R Soc Med* (2005) 98, 270–1.

Insulin + Salicylates

Aspirin and other salicylates can lower blood glucose concentrations, but small analgesic doses do not normally have an adverse effect on diabetic control. Larger doses of salicylates might have a more important effect.

Clinical evidence

Twelve children with type 1 diabetes receiving insulin had a reduction in their blood glucose concentrations (from about 10.4 to 8.8 mmol/L) averaging 15% when they were given **aspirin** (patients under 27.2 kg given 1.2 g daily, patients over 27.2 kg given 2.4 g daily) for a week. No major changes in insulin doses were necessary.[1]

Eight patients receiving 12 to 48 units of insulin zinc suspension daily required no insulin when, for 2 to 3 weeks, they took **aspirin** in doses of 3.5 to 7.5 g daily, which were large enough to give maximum therapeutic serum salicylate concentrations of about 2.5 to 3.3 mmol/L. Six other patients were able to reduce their insulin requirements by about 20 to 65%.[2] In a randomised, placebo-controlled study in 40 obese, non-diabetic subjects given **salsalate** 3 g daily for 7 days, the fasting plasma glucose concentration after an oral glucose tolerance test was reduced by 4.7%, when compared with placebo. Serum insulin concentrations were increased.[3] Similar results were seen in another study in 28 obese, non-diabetic subjects given **triflusal** 600 or 900 mg daily for 4 weeks.[4]

Mechanism

It has been known for over 100 years that aspirin and salicylates have blood glucose-lowering properties and, in relatively large doses, can be used on their own in the treatment of diabetes.[5-9] The exact mechanism is unknown, but it has been suggested that the salicylates inhibit one of the chronic inflammatory pathways, resulting in a reduction in insulin resistance and an increase in insulin sensitivity.[10] Further study is required.

Importance and management

The interaction between insulin and the salicylates is established but of limited importance. Considering the extremely wide use of aspirin it might reasonably be expected that any generally serious interaction would have come to light by now. The data available, coupled with the common experience of patients with diabetes,[11] is that excessive and unwanted hypoglycaemia is very unlikely with small to moderate analgesic doses of salicylates. Some downward adjustment of the dose of insulin may be appropriate if large doses of salicylates are used.

1. Kaye R, Athreya BH, Kunzman EE, Baker L. Antipyretics in patients with juvenile diabetes mellitus. *Am J Dis Child* (1966) 112, 52–5.
2. Reid J, Lightbody TD. The insulin equivalence of salicylate. *BMJ* (1959) i, 897–900.
3. Koska J, Ortega E, Bunt JC, Gasser A, Impson J, Hanson RL, Forbes J, de Courten B, Krakoff J. The effect of salsalate on insulin action and glucose tolerance in obese non-diabetic patients: results of a randomised double-blind placebo-controlled study. *Diabetologia* (2009) 52, 385–93.
4. Fernandez-Real JM, Lopez-Bermejo A, Ropero AB, Piquer S, Nadal A, Bassols J, Casamitjana R, Gomis R, Arnaiz E, Perez I, Ricart W. Salicylates increase insulin secretion in healthy obese subjects. *J Clin Endocrinol Metab* (2008) 93, 2523–30.
5. Gilgore SG, Rupp JJ. The long-term response of diabetes mellitus to salicylate therapy. Report of a case. *JAMA* (1962) 180, 65–6.
6. Reid J, Macdougall AI, Andrews MM. Aspirin and diabetes mellitus. *BMJ* (1957) 2, 1071–4.
7. Ebstein W. Zur Therapie des Diabetes mellitus, insbesondere über die Anwendung des salicylsauren Natron bei demselben. Berl Klin Wschr (1876) 13, 337–40.
8. Bartels K. Ueber die therapeutische Verwerthung der Salizylsäure und ihres Nastronsalzes in der inneren Medicin. Dtsch Med Wschr (1878) 4, 423–5.
9. Cattaneo AG, Caviezel F, Pozza G. Pharmacological interaction between tolbutamide and acetylsalicylic acid: study on insulin secretion in man. *Int J Clin Pharmacol Ther Toxicol* (1990) 28, 229–34.
10. Rumore MM, Kim KS. Potential role of salicylates in type 2 diabetes. *Ann Pharmacother* (2010) 44, 1207–21.
11. Logie AW, Galloway DB, Petrie JC. Drug interactions and long-term antidiabetic therapy. *Br J Clin Pharmacol* (1976) 3, 1027–32.

Meglitinides + Azoles; Itraconazole or Ketoconazole

Itraconazole slightly increased repaglinide exposure, but very markedly increased repaglinide exposure when also given with gemfibrozil. Itraconazole slightly increased nateglinide exposure when given with gemfibrozil. Ketoconazole caused a negligible increase in repaglinide exposure.

Clinical evidence

(a) Itraconazole

In healthy subjects, itraconazole 200 mg then 100 mg twice daily for 3 days increased the AUC of a single 250-microgram dose of **repaglinide** by 40%. No change was noted in blood glucose concentrations, when compared with **repaglinide** alone.[1] However, itraconazole enhanced the pharmacokinetic interaction between gemfibrozil and **repaglinide**; itraconazole with gemfibrozil increased the AUC of **repaglinide** nearly 20-fold and considerably enhanced the blood glucose-lowering effect of **repaglinide**. In a similar study in healthy subjects, itraconazole with gemfibrozil increased the AUC of a single 30-mg dose of **nateglinide** by 47%, without causing any notable change in its blood glucose response.[2]

(b) Ketoconazole

In healthy subjects, ketoconazole 200 mg daily for 5 days increased the AUC of a single 2-mg dose of **repaglinide** by 15% and increased its maximum plasma concentration by 8%.[3]

Mechanism

Repaglinide is principally metabolised by CYP2C8, with some involvement of CYP3A4. Itraconazole and ketoconazole are potent inhibitors of CYP3A4, and are expected to increase repaglinide exposure, but. only minor changes in repaglinide pharmacokinetics were seen with these azoles, and this is likely a result of the compensatory capacity of the CYP2C8 pathway. However, when this pathway is also inhibited, as with gemfibrozil, the effect on repaglinide exposure is greatly enhanced (see 'Meglitinides + Fibrates', below).

The organic anion transporter protein OATP1B1 is involved in the hepatic uptake of repaglinide, and gemfibrozil has been shown to inhibit OATP1B1 *in vitro*, and this might also contribute to the increased exposure.[4]

Nateglinide is principally metabolised by CYP2C9, with some involvement of CYP3A4, and so concurrent use of itraconazole increases nateglinide exposure.

Importance and management

Evidence for a pharmacokinetic interaction between repaglinide and itraconazole or ketoconazole is limited, but in general the increase in exposure is minor and unlikely to be clinically relevant. It is prudent to monitor blood glucose concentrations when any change is made to the medication regimen of a patient with diabetes, and this would seem sensible when either itraconazole or ketoconazole are required in patients receiving repaglinide. Note that the effect of itraconazole, and possibly ketoconazole, on repaglinide could potentially be more important if a drug that inhibits CYP2C8, such as gemfibrozil, is also given, and increased monitoring of blood glucose concentrations is advisable (although note that the combination of gemfibrozil and repaglinide is contraindicated, see 'Meglitinides + Fibrates', below). See 'Table 1.4', p.6 for a list of clinically relevant CYP2C8 inhibitors.

The effect of itraconazole on nateglinide exposure was only slight, but note that this was in combination with gemfibrozil and so the exact effect of itraconazole is not known. There was no effect on blood glucose response, but the general advice to monitor blood glucose concentrations when any change is made to the medication regimen of a patient with diabetes would seem prudent on concurrent use.

1. Niemi M, Backman JT, Neuvonen M, Neuvonen PJ. Effects of gemfibrozil, itraconazole, and their combination on the pharmacokinetics and pharmacodynamics of repaglinide: potentially hazardous interaction between gemfibrozil and repaglinide. *Diabetologia* (2003) 46, 347–51.
2. Niemi M, Backman JT, Juntti-Patinen L, Neuvonen M, Neuvonen PJ. Coadministration of gemfibrozil and itraconazole has only a minor effect on the pharmacokinetics of the CYP2C9 and CYP3A4 substrate nateglinide. *Br J Clin Pharmacol* (2005) 60, 208–17.
3. Hatorp V, Hansen KT, Thomsen MS. Influence of drugs interacting with CYP3A4 on the pharmacokinetics, pharmacodynamics, and safety of the prandial glucose regulator repaglinide. *J Clin Pharmacol* (2003) 43, 649–60.
4. Kudo T, Hisaka A, Sugiyama Y, Ito K. Analysis of the repaglinide concentration increase produced by gemfibrozil and itraconazole based inhibition of the hepatic uptake transporter and metabolic enzymes. *Drug Metab Dispos* (2013) 41, 362–71.

Meglitinides + Fibrates

The combination of gemfibrozil and repaglinide results in a marked increase in repaglinide exposure and can cause serious hypoglycaemia. Nateglinide exposure is only slightly increased by gemfibrozil, when given with itraconazole. No pharmacokinetic interaction occurs between repaglinide and bezafibrate or fenofibrate, and the blood-glucose lowering effect of repaglinide was not altered.

Clinical evidence

A. Bezafibrate

In a randomised, crossover study in 12 healthy subjects bezafibrate 400 mg daily for 5 days had no effect on the pharmacokinetics of a single 250-microgram dose of **repaglinide**, and did not alter its blood glucose-lowering effect.[1]

B. Fenofibrate

In a randomised, crossover study in 12 healthy subjects, fenofibrate 200 mg daily for 5 days had no effect on the pharmacokinetics of a single 250-microgram dose of **repaglinide**, and did not alter its blood glucose-lowering effect.[1]

C. Gemfibrozil

(a) Nateglinide

In a randomised, crossover study, 9 healthy subjects were given gemfibrozil 600 mg daily and a 200-mg dose of itraconazole, followed by itraconazole 100 mg twice daily, for 3 days, with a single 30-mg dose of nateglinide given on day 3. The AUC of nateglinide was increased by 47%, but the blood glucose response was not altered.[2]

(b) Repaglinide

In a randomised, crossover study, 12 healthy subjects were given gemfibrozil 600 mg twice daily for 5 doses, with a 250-microgram dose of repaglinide one hour after the final gemfibrozil dose. Gemfibrozil increased the AUC of repaglinide 8-fold and increased its plasma concentration nearly 29-fold.[3] The repaglinide AUC was increased 5-fold even when the dose of repaglinide was taken 12 hours after the final dose of gemfibrozil.[4] Two other studies in healthy subjects evaluated the effects of increasing doses of gemfibrozil (30 mg, 100 mg, or 600 mg twice daily for 5 days,[5] and single 30-mg, 100-mg, 300-mg and 900-mg doses[6]) on the pharmacokinetics of a single 250-microgram dose of repaglinide. The AUC of repaglinide was increased in a dose-dependent manner with increases of 3.4-, 5.5-, and 7-fold, respectively,[5] and 1.8-, 4.5-, 6.7-, and 8.3-fold, respectively.[6]

When gemfibrozil and repaglinide were given with itraconazole these effects were further increased (see 'Meglitinides + Azoles; Itraconazole or Ketoconazole', p.528). In addition, the blood glucose-lowering effects of repaglinide were considerably enhanced and prolonged, both by gemfibrozil alone and in combination with itraconazole.[3] In 2003, the European Agency for the Evaluation of Medicinal Products (now the European Medicines Agency) had received five reports of serious hypoglycaemic episodes with gemfibrozil and repaglinide.[7]

Mechanism

It is thought that gemfibrozil inhibits the metabolism of repaglinide by CYP2C8, and that inhibition of CYP3A4 (repaglinide's other main route of metabolism) by itraconazole further blocks repaglinide metabolism,[3] leading to an increase in repaglinide exposure. According to one study, the organic anion transporting polypeptide 1B1 (OATP1B1) appears to have a limited role in the interaction of gemfibrozil with repaglinide, with genetic polymorphism determining the extent of the interaction.[8] An *in vitro* modelling study also showed involvement of OATP1B1 in this interaction, but in contrast, the authors suggest that this is an important contributory pathway.[9] The involvement of glucuronidation in the metabolism of repaglinide has also been studied *in vitro*, and it is suggested that inhibition of this pathway by gemfibrozil (via UGT1A1) contributes to the interaction.[10] It seems possible that any or all of these mechanisms might contribute towards enhanced hypoglycaemia. Further study is needed to determine the exact mechanisms involved.

Gemfibrozil might inhibit the CYP2C9-mediated metabolism of nateglinide, resulting in an increase in nateglinide exposure.[2]

Importance and management

A pharmacokinetic interaction between gemfibrozil and repaglinide is established and clinically important. Such that, on the basis of the marked increase in repaglinide exposure,[3] and following the five reports of serious hypoglycaemic episodes with gemfibrozil and repaglinide, the European Agency for the Evaluation of Medicinal Products contraindicated concurrent use.[7] No interaction occurs between bezafibrate or fenofibrate and repaglinide.

Only slight increases in nateglinide exposure have been seen with gemfibrozil, but note that this was in combination with itraconazole, which can also increase repaglinide exposure (see 'Meglitinides + Azoles; Itraconazole or Ketoconazole', p.528), and so the exact effect of gemfibrozil is not known. The blood glucose response was unaffected, but nevertheless, it is prudent to monitor blood glucose concentrations when any change is made to the medication regimen of a patient with diabetes, and this would seem sensible on concurrent use of nateglinide and gemfibrozil.

1. Kajosaari LI, Backman JT, Neuvonen M, Laitila J, Neuvonen PJ. Lack of effect of bezafibrate and fenofibrate on the pharmacokinetics and pharmacodynamics of repaglinide. *Br J Clin Pharmacol* (2004) 58, 390–6.
2. Niemi M, Backman JT, Juntti-Patinen L, Neuvonen M, Neuvonen PJ. Coadministration of gemfibrozil and itraconazole has only a minor effect on the pharmacokinetics of the CYP2C9 and CYP3A4 substrate nateglinide. *Br J Clin Pharmacol* (2005) 60, 208–17.
3. Niemi M, Backman JT, Neuvonen M, Neuvonen PJ. Effects of gemfibrozil, itraconazole, and their combination on the pharmacokinetics and pharmacodynamics of repaglinide: potentially hazardous interaction between gemfibrozil and repaglinide. *Diabetologia* (2003) 46, 347–51.
4. Tornio A, Niemi M, Neuvonen M, Laitila J, Kalliokoski A, Neuvonen PJ, Backman JT. The effect of gemfibrozil on repaglinide pharmacokinetics persists for at least 12 h after the dose: evidence for mechanism-based inhibition of CYP2C8 *in vivo*. *Clin Pharmacol Ther* (2008) 84, 403–11.
5. Honkalammi J, Niemi M, Neuvonen PJ, Backman JT. Gemfibrozil is a strong inactivator of CYP2C8 in very small multiple doses. *Clin Pharmacol Ther* (2012) 91, 846–55.
6. Honkalammi J, Niemi M, Neuvonen PJ, Backman JT. Dose-dependent interaction between gemfibrozil and repaglinide in humans: strong inhibition of CYP2C8 with subtherapeutic gemfibrozil doses. *Drug Metab Dispos* (2011) 39, 1977–86.
7. EMEA public statement on repaglinide (NovoNorm/Prandin): contraindication of concomitant use of repaglinide and gemfibrozil, 21 May 2003, London. Available at http://www.ema.europa.eu/ema/index.jsp?curl=pages/news_and_events/news/2010/08/news_detail_001082.jsp&mid=WC0b01ac058004d5c1 (accessed 21/10/15).
8. Kalliokoski A, Backman JT, Kurkinen KJ, Neuvonen PJ, Niemi M. Effects of gemfibrozil and atorvastatin on the pharmacokinetics of repaglinide in relation to *SLCO1B1* polymorphism. *Clin Pharmacol Ther* (2008) 84, 488–96.
9. Varma MVS, Lai Y, Kimoto E, Goosen TC, El-Kattan AF, Kumar V. Mechanistic modelling to predict the transporter-and enzyme-mediated drug-drug interactions of repaglinide. *Pharm Res* (2013) 30, 1188–99.
10. Gan J, Chen W, Shen H, Gao L, Hong Y, Tian Y, Li W, Zhang Y, Tang Y, Zhang H, Humphreys WG, Rodrigues AD. Repaglinide-gemfibrozil drug interaction: inhibition of repaglinide glucuronidation as a potential additional contributing mechanism. *Br J Clin Pharmacol* (2010) 70, 870–80.

Meglitinides + Food

The rate of absorption and maximum concentration of nateglinide are increased if it is taken before food. The rate of absorption of repaglinide is not affected when it is taken before food, but there is a minor decrease in its maximum concentration.

Clinical evidence, mechanism, importance and management

(a) Nateglinide

In a randomised, crossover study, 12 healthy subjects were given a single 60-mg dose of nateglinide 10 minutes before, and immediately after, a high-fat breakfast, and single 30-mg and 60-mg doses under fasting conditions. Compared with the fasted state, taking nateglinide 10 minutes before the meal resulted in a 12% increase in maximum concentration and a 52% decrease in time to maximum concentration without any effect on overall exposure (AUC). In contrast, when the nateglinide was given after the meal, the maximum concentration was decreased by 34% and the time to maximum concentration was increased by 22%, again, without any effect on overall exposure. Regardless of timing, nateglinide and food resulted in a larger increase in insulin concentrations than nateglinide alone. When nateglinide was taken prior to food, no meal-time increase in blood glucose concentrations occurred.[1] Other studies have similarly found a faster increase and higher maximum concentrations when nateglinide was given before food than after.[2,3] In one of these studies,[2] the composition of the meal (high in carbohydrate, fat or protein) did not alter these effects. Nateglinide is therefore best taken prior to meals.

(b) Repaglinide

In a study in 24 healthy subjects, taking a single 2-mg dose of repaglinide 15 minutes before a high-fat meal reduced its maximum concentration and AUC by 20% and 12%, respectively. There was no change in time to maximum concentration.[4] These small changes in repaglinide pharmacokinetics are unlikely to be clinically relevant, and repaglinide is recommended to be taken prior to meals.

1. Karara AH, Dunning BE, McLeod JF. The effects of food on the oral bioavailability and the pharmacodynamic actions of the insulinotropic agent nateglinide in healthy subjects. *J Clin Pharmacol* (1999) 39, 172–9.
2. Luzio SD, Anderson DM, Owens DR. Effects of timing of administration and meal composition on the pharmacokinetic and pharmacodynamic characteristics of the short-acting oral hypoglycaemic agent nateglinide in healthy subjects. *J Clin Endocrinol Metab* (2001) 86, 4874–80.
3. Anderson D, Shelley S, Kellett N, Marshall D, Nimmo W. The effect of nateglinide taken with food on gastric emptying rates in healthy subjects. *Clin Ther* (2003) 25, 1722–38.
4. Hatorp V, Bayer T. Repaglinide bioavailability in the fed or fasting state. *J Clin Pharmacol* (1997) 37, 875.

Meglitinides + Rifamycins and other enzyme inducers

Rifampicin slightly to moderately reduces repaglinide exposure, although the size of the effect might depend on whether they are given separately or simultaneously. Nateglinide exposure might also be reduced by concurrent use of rifampicin. Other inducers of CYP3A4 and CYP2C8 are predicted to interact similarly.

Clinical evidence

(a) Nateglinide

In a randomised, crossover study, 10 healthy subjects were given a single 60-mg dose of nateglinide the day after a 5-day course of **rifampicin** 600 mg daily. **Rifampicin** reduced the AUC_{0-7} of nateglinide by 24% (range 5 to 53%) and decreased the nateglinide half-life from 1.6 hours to 1.3 hours. Overall **rifampicin** did not decrease the blood glucose-lowering effects of nateglinide.[1] However, because of the high degree of intersubject variation, the authors suggest that the blood glucose-lowering effects of nateglinide might be reduced in some subjects.[1]

(b) Repaglinide

In a randomised, crossover study in 8 healthy subjects, a single 4-mg dose of repaglinide was given one hour after the final dose of **rifampicin** 600 mg daily for 7 days. **Rifampicin** decreased the AUC of repaglinide by 31% and the maximum plasma concentration by 26%, but the blood glucose-lowering effect of repaglinide was not affected.[2] In another similar study,[3] pretreatment with **rifampicin** 600 mg daily for 5 days decreased the AUC of a single 500-microgram dose of repaglinide given on day 6 by 57% and decreased the maximum concentration by 41%. In this study, **rifampicin** reduced the blood glucose-lowering effect of repaglinide by 35%. A third study, also of similar design, investigated the effect of **rifampicin** 600 mg daily for 7 days on a single 4-mg dose of repaglinide given at the same time as the last **rifampicin** dose on day 7, or 24 hours later. When **rifampicin** was given simultaneously, the median AUC of repaglinide was reduced by almost 50%, but when the repaglinide was given 24 hours after the last **rifampicin** dose, the median AUC was reduced by 80%.[4]

Mechanism

Rifampicin is a moderate inducer of CYP2C8 and CYP2C9, and a potent inducer of CYP3A4. Nateglinide is principally metabolised by CYP2C9, with some involvement of CYP3A4, and so concurrent use of rifampicin reduces nateglinide exposure. Repaglinide is principally metabolised by CYP2C8, with some involvement of CYP3A4, and rifampicin similarly reduces repaglinide exposure. However, rifampicin is also an inhibitor of the organic anion transporter protein OATP1B1, which is involved in the hepatic uptake of repaglinide and this might account for the differing size of effect between simultaneous and separate administration seen in the studies. When administered simultaneously, it appears that inhibition of OATP1B1 reduces the inductive effect of rifampicin resulting in only slight reductions in repaglinide exposure, but when administration is separated, the inductive effects of rifampicin predominate and a greater reduction in repaglinide exposure is seen. This has been demonstrated in *in vitro* studies,[5] and there is also evidence with atorvastatin, that the effect of OATP inhibition by rifampicin varies with simultaneous versus separated administration, and single versus multiple-dosing (see 'Statins + Rifampicin (Rifampin)', p.1355). *In vitro* studies with nateglinide suggest that OATP1B1 (and 1B3) might contribute to the hepatic uptake, but the possibility of drug-drug interactions via this route was considered to be low.[6]

Importance and management

A pharmacokinetic interaction between rifampicin and repaglinide is established and could be clinically important, especially if the doses are not given simultaneously. The UK manufacturer of repaglinide advises that dose adjustments might be needed and they should be based on careful monitoring of blood glucose concentrations on initiation, during repeated administration, and upon withdrawal of rifampicin, and for 2 weeks after discontinuation.[7] This would seem prudent, as would simultaneous administration to reduce the size of the effect. Although not studied with repaglinide, the effect of single-dose rifampicin might be different than that with multiple doses, as seen with atorvastatin (see 'Statins + Rifampicin (Rifampin)', p.1355). Careful monitoring of blood glucose concentrations if rifampicin is to be administered as very short courses or repeated single-doses, as is the case for meningococcal prophylaxis (2 days) or leprosy (once monthly), respectively, would seem prudent, as the inhibitory effects of rifampicin might be expected to predominate due to the inductive effects requiring several days to develop. Separating administration of repaglinide and rifampicin might reduce the size of the effect in these scenarios.

A possible interaction between repaglinide and other inducers of CYP2C8 or CYP3A4 cannot be excluded, see 'Table 1.4', p.6 and 'Table 1.9', p.11, respectively, for a list of clinically relevant inducers. For mention that high doses of **phenytoin** have rarely caused hyperglycaemia, see 'Phenytoin + Antidiabetics', p.592. In general, it is prudent to monitor blood glucose concentrations when any change is made to the medication regimen of a patient with diabetes, and this should be sufficient to detect any interaction with these drugs should it occur.

Information regarding an interaction between nateglinide and rifampicin is more limited, but might be clinically relevant interaction in some patients. Monitoring of blood glucose concentrations, as is prudent when any change is made to the medication regimen of patient with diabetes, should identify any interaction, and the dose of nateglinide can be adjusted if necessary.

There does not seem to be any information regarding an interaction between the meglitinides and **rifabutin** or **rifapentine**. However, as both drugs are probably moderate inducers of CYP3A4, the same advice as for other CYP3A4 inducers should be followed.

1. Niemi M, Backman JT, Neuvonen M, Neuvonen PJ. Effect of rifampicin on the pharmacokinetics and pharmacodynamics of nateglinide in healthy subjects. *Br J Clin Pharmacol* (2003) 56, 427–32.
2. Hatorp V, Hansen KT, Thomsen MS. Influence of drugs interacting with CYP3A4 on the pharmacokinetics, pharmacodynamics, and safety of the prandial glucose regulator repaglinide. *J Clin Pharmacol* (2003) 43, 649–60.
3. Niemi M, Backman JT, Neuvonen M, Neuvonen PJ, Kivistö KT. Rifampin decreases the plasma concentrations and effects of repaglinide. *Clin Pharmacol Ther* (2000) 68, 495–500.
4. Bidstrup TB, Stilling N, Damkier P, Scharling B, Thomsen MS, Brøsen K. Rifampicin seems to act as both an inducer and an inhibitor of the metabolism of repaglinide. *Eur J Clin Pharmacol* (2004) 60, 109–14.
5. Varma MV, Lin J, Bi YA, Rotter CJ, Fahmi OA, Lam J, El-Kattan AF, Goosen TC, Lai Y. Quantitative prediction of repaglinide-rifampicin complex drug interactions using dynamic and static mechanistic models: delineating differential CYP3A4 induction and OATP1B1 inhibition potential of rifampicin. *Drug Metab Dispos* (2013) 41, 966–74.
6. Takanohashi T, Kubo S, Arisaka H, Shinkai K, Ubukata K. Contribution of organic anion transporting polypeptide (OATP) 1B1 and OATP1B3 to hepatic uptake of nateglinide, and the prediction of drug-drug interactions via these transporters. *J Pharm Pharmacol* (2012) 64, 199–206.
7. Prandin (Repaglinide). Novo Nordisk Ltd. UK Summary of product characteristics, April 2012

Meglitinides + Statins

Simvastatin and atorvastatin had no clinically relevant effect on the pharmacokinetics of repaglinide, and fluvastatin had no clinically relevant effect on the pharmacokinetics of nateglinide.

Clinical evidence, mechanism, importance and management

(a) Nateglinide

In the preliminary report of a study in healthy subjects, **fluvastatin** 30 mg daily for 8 days caused a 18% increase in the AUC of a single 120-mg dose of nateglinide, with no change in blood glucose concentrations.[1] No nateglinide dose adjustment would seem necessary on concurrent use, but note that it is prudent to monitor blood glucose concentrations when any change to a diabetic patient's medication regimen is made.

(b) Repaglinide

In a three-period, crossover study in 12 healthy subjects, the concurrent use of **simvastatin** 20 mg daily and repaglinide 2 mg three times daily for 5 days increased the AUC of repaglinide by 8%, and increased its maximum concentration by 26%, although there was high variability in these findings. There was a higher incidence of adverse events (headache was most common, then hypoglycaemia) during concurrent use compared with either drug alone (45 events with both drugs, 23 events with repaglinide alone, and 13 events with **simvastatin** alone). However, these adverse events were mild or moderate, and were considered to be due to the additive effects of both drugs.[2] In another study in healthy subjects, **atorvastatin** 40 mg daily for 3 doses had little effect on the pharmacokinetics of a single 250-microgram dose of repaglinide given one hour after the final dose of atorvastatin. The only statistically significant changes (18% increase in AUC, and 41% increase in maximum concentration) were in the subset of subjects with a genetically reduced ability to clear repaglinide by the organic anion transporting polypeptide 1B1 (OATP1B1),[3] but these are unlikely to be clinically relevant. No repaglinide dose adjustment would seem necessary on its concurrent use with atorvastatin or simvastatin, but note that it is prudent to monitor blood glucose concentrations when any change is made to the medication regimen of a patient with diabetes.

1. Uchida S, Nishio S, Li XD, Ito T, Morita H, Nakamura H, Yamada H, Watanabe H, Ohashi K. Influences of CYP2C9 genotype and fluvastatin on pharmacokinetics and pharmacodynamics of nateglinide. *Clin Pharmacol Ther* (2005) 77, P74.
2. Hatorp V, Hansen KT, Thomsen MS. Influence of drugs interacting with CYP3A4 on the pharmacokinetics, pharmacodynamics, and safety of the prandial glucose regulator repaglinide. *J Clin Pharmacol* (2003) 43, 649–60.
3. Kalliokoski A, Backman JT, Kurkinen KJ, Neuvonen PJ, Niemi M. Effects of gemfibrozil and atorvastatin on the pharmacokinetics of repaglinide in relation to *SLCO1B1* polymorphism. *Clin Pharmacol Ther* (2008) 84, 488–96.

Meglitinides; Nateglinide + Azoles; Fluconazole or Miconazole

Fluconazole slightly increased nateglinide exposure, and miconazole is predicted to interact similarly.

Clinical evidence

In a randomised, crossover study, 10 healthy subjects were given a single 30-mg dose of nateglinide on the last day of a 4-day course of **fluconazole** (given as 400 mg on day one, then 200 mg daily). **Fluconazole** increased the AUC of nateglinide by 48% (range 20 to 73%) and increased the nateglinide half-life from 1.6 hours to 1.9 hours. Despite these pharmacokinetic changes **fluconazole** did not potentiate the blood glucose-lowering effects of nateglinide.[1]

Mechanism

Fluconazole is a weak to moderate inhibitor of CYP2C9 (depending on the dose given), by which nateglinide is predominantly metabolised, and so its exposure is increased, and its blood glucose-lowering effects would be predicted to be enhanced (although this was not seen in the study, see *Importance and management* below), on concurrent use. Fluconazole is also a moderate inhibitor of CYP3A4, which is involved in the metabolism of nateglinide, although to a lesser extent than CYP2C9.

Importance and management

Evidence for a pharmacokinetic interaction between fluconazole and nateglinide is limited to this one study, but the findings are consistent with the known effects of fluconazole and the known metabolism of nateglinide, and an interaction is established. However, note that a sub-therapeutic dose of nateglinide was used which might have resulted in a lower increase in nateglinide exposure (slight rather than moderate) than might have been expected given the known potency of fluconazole at the doses used , and no increase in the blood glucose-lowering effects of nateglinide was seen. In clinical practice, a greater increase in nateglinide exposure would be predicted and a greater blood glucose-lowering effect might possibly occur on concurrent use. The combination need not be avoided, but it would seem prudent to be aware of the potential for a greater than expected effect of nateglinide and to adjust the dose if necessary. The general advice to monitor blood glucose concentrations when any change is made to the medication regimen of a patient with diabetes should be sufficient to detect any interaction, should it occur.

Miconazole is also a moderate CYP2C9 inhibitor, when given orally, and has been predicted to interact similarly with nateglinide, but this requires confirmation. Although there are no specific data, a large proportion of miconazole oral gel (both prescription and non-prescription doses) could be swallowed and therefore adequate systemic absorption might occur to produce an interaction. It is therefore possible that oral miconazole gel might interact similarly. Intravaginal miconazole and miconazole topical creams are probably unlikely to interact, because absorption by these routes is minimal.

1. Niemi M, Neuvonen M, Juntti-Patinen L, Backman JT, Neuvonen PJ. Effect of fluconazole on the pharmacokinetics and pharmacodynamics of nateglinide. *Clin Pharmacol Ther* (2003) 74, 25–31.

Meglitinides; Nateglinide + Diclofenac

The pharmacokinetics of nateglinide and diclofenac are not altered by concurrent use.

Clinical evidence, mechanism, importance and management

In a randomised crossover study, 18 healthy subjects were given modified-release diclofenac 75 mg on the same day as two 120-mg doses of nateglinide, given 4 hours apart. The pharmacokinetics of both drugs were unaltered by concurrent use, and there was no difference in the blood glucose concentrations.[1] No dose adjustments would seem necessary on concurrent use, however it is prudent to monitor blood glucose concentrations when any change is made to the medication regimen of a patient with diabetes.

1. Anderson DM, Shelley S, Crick N, Buraglio M. A 3-way crossover study to evaluate the pharmacokinetic interaction between nateglinide and diclofenac in healthy volunteers. *Int J Clin Pharmacol Ther* (2002) 40, 457–64.

Meglitinides; Repaglinide + Antibacterials; Co-trimoxazole or Trimethoprim

Trimethoprim slightly increases repaglinide exposure. A case report describes hypoglycaemia in a patient, after co-trimoxazole was added to repaglinide.

Clinical evidence

In a randomised, crossover study in 9 healthy subjects, trimethoprim 160 mg twice daily for 3 days increased the AUC of a single 250-microgram dose of repaglinide by 61% and increased its maximum plasma concentration by 41%. However, the blood glucose-lowering effect of this small dose of repaglinide was unchanged.[1]

A case report describes a 76-year-old man with diabetes, stabilised on repaglinide 1 mg three times daily, who developed symptomatic hypoglycaemia 5 days after starting a course of **co-trimoxazole** 960 mg daily for a urinary tract infection. Both medications were stopped and his blood glucose concentrations returned to normal after intravenous glucose was given. Five days later, repaglinide was restarted with no further hypoglycaemia. Note that the patient had no previous history of hypoglycaemia but did have impaired renal function.[2]

Mechanism

Repaglinide, is principally metabolised by CYP2C8, which might be inhibited by trimethoprim, resulting in increased repaglinide exposure and possibly increased effects.

Importance and management

A pharmacokinetic interaction between trimethoprim and repaglinide is established. However, the clinical relevance of the pharmacokinetic changes has not been assessed. The case report of hypoglycaemia after the addition of co-trimoxazole to repaglinide suggests that the clinical effect could be important, but note that co-trimoxazole can (albeit rarely) cause hypoglycaemia when given alone. The authors note that **sulfamethoxazole** induced hypoglycaemia could not be ruled out.[2] A clinically important effect might therefore occur on concurrent use and, as such, the UK manufacturer of repaglinide[3] suggests that the concurrent use of trimethoprim should be avoided as the effect of larger doses of both drugs is unknown. The US manufacturer suggests caution, and advises that repaglinide dose adjustments might be necessary.[4] If trimethoprim is required in a patient taking repaglinide, it would seem prudent to increase the frequency of blood glucose monitoring. This would also seem sensible if co-trimoxazole is required.

1. Niemi M, Kajosaari LI, Neuvonen M, Backman JT, Neuvonen PJ. The CYP2C8 inhibitor trimethoprim increases the plasma concentrations of repaglinide in healthy subjects. *Br J Clin Pharmacol* (2003) 57, 441–7.
2. Roustit M, Blondel E, Villier C, Fonrose X, Mallaret MP. Symptomatic hypoglcemia associated with trimethoprim/sulfamethoxazole and repaglinide in a diabetic patient. *Ann Pharmacother* (2010) 44, 764–7.
3. Prandin (Repaglinide). Novo Nordisk Ltd. UK Summary of product characteristics, April 2012.
4. Prandin (Repaglinide). Novo Nordisk Inc. US Prescribing information, September 2011.

Meglitinides; Repaglinide + Cimetidine

Cimetidine does not alter the pharmacokinetics of repaglinide.

Clinical evidence, mechanism, importance and management

A crossover study in 14 healthy subjects found that cimetidine 400 mg twice daily had no effect on the pharmacokinetics of repaglinide 2 mg three times daily.[1] No repaglinide dose adjustment would seem necessary on concurrent use, but note that it is prudent to monitor blood glucose concentrations when any change is made to the medication regimen of a patient with diabetes.

1. Hatorp V, Thomsen MS. Drug interaction studies with repaglinide: repaglinide on digoxin or theophylline pharmacokinetics and cimetidine on repaglinide pharmacokinetics. *J Clin Pharmacol* (2000) 40, 184–92.

Meglitinides; Repaglinide + Colesevelam

The pharmacokinetics of repaglinide are not affected by colesevelam.

Clinical evidence, mechanism, importance and management

In a randomised, crossover study in 33 healthy subjects, colesevelam 3.75 g reduced the maximum concentration of repaglinide 2 mg by 19% when taken at the same time. The AUC of repaglinide was reduced by 7%, but this was not clinically relevant. No interaction was seen when repaglinide was taken one hour before colesevelam.[1] There would therefore appear to be no reason to separate administration of repaglinide and colesevelam, but note that it is prudent to monitor blood glucose concentrations when any change is made to the medication regimen of a patient with diabetes.

1. Brown KS, Armstrong IC, Wang A, Walker JR, Noveck RJ, Swearingen D, Allison M, Kissling JC, Kisicki J, Salazar DE. Effect of the bile acid sequestrant colesevelam on the pharmacokinetics of pioglitazone, repaglinide, estrogen estradiol, norethindrone, levothyroxine, and glyburide. *J Clin Pharmacol* (2010) 50, 554–65.

Meglitinides; Repaglinide + Grapefruit juice

Grapefruit juice caused a negligible increase in repaglinide exposure in one study.

Clinical evidence, mechanism, importance and management

In a study in 36 healthy subjects, drinking 300 mL of grapefruit juice with a single dose of repaglinide increased the AUC of repaglinide by 13% without any effect on blood glucose concentrations. The effect was more noticeable with a low 250 microgram dose of repaglinide than with the therapeutic dose of 2 mg.[1] Repaglinide is predominantly metabolised by CYP2C8, with some involvement of CYP3A4. Grapefruit juice is a known weak inhibitor of CYP3A4, and so the small increase in AUC of repaglinide in this study is most likely due to inhibition of intestinal CYP3A4 by grapefruit juice constituents. However, an increase of this size is not clinically relevant.

1. Bidstrup TB, Damkier P, Olsen AK, Ekblom M, Karlsson A, Brøsen K. The impact of CYP2C8 polymorphism and grapefruit juice on the pharmacokinetics of repaglinide. *Br J Clin Pharmacol* (2006) 61, 49–57.

Meglitinides; Repaglinide + HIV-protease inhibitors

Atazanavir monotherapy is predicted to increase repaglinide exposure. Other HIV-protease inhibitors boosted with ritonavir are also predicted to increase the exposure to repaglinide.

Clinical evidence, mechanism, importance and management

The US manufacturer of **atazanavir** briefly notes that it is a weak inhibitor of CYP2C8 and advises that caution should be used when it is used concurrently with drugs that are mainly metabolised by CYP2C8 and which have a narrow therapeutic range, such as repaglinide.[1] Repaglinide is also partially metabolised by CYP3A4, therefore as all **HIV-protease inhibitors** when boosted with ritonavir are potent inhibitors of this isoenzyme, they might also be expected to increase repaglinide exposure. Until more is known about the clinical outcome of concurrent use, it might be prudent to bear in mind the possibility of an interaction if an increase in repaglinide adverse effects (such as hypoglycaemia) occurs, and adjust the repaglinide dose as necessary.

1. Reyataz (Atazanavir sulfate). Bristol-Myers Squibb. US Prescribing information, August 2013.

Meglitinides; Repaglinide + Macrolides

Clarithromycin and telithromycin slightly increase repaglinide exposure. A case report describes severe hypoglycaemia in a patient taking repaglinide with clarithromycin.

Clinical evidence

(a) Clarithromycin

In a randomised, crossover study in 9 healthy subjects, pre-treatment with clarithromycin 250 mg twice daily for 4 days increased the AUC of a single 250-microgram dose of repaglinide, given on day 5, by 40% and increased its maximum plasma concentration by 67%. There was a similar corresponding increase in circulating insulin concentrations, but blood glucose concentrations were unchanged.[1]

An 80-year-old man with diabetes taking repaglinide 500 micrograms three times daily had a hypoglycaemic episode requiring intravenous glucose within 48 hours of starting clarithromycin 500 mg twice daily, and another similar episode 2 days later. Repaglinide was stopped, and no further hypoglycaemic episodes occurred.[2]

(b) Telithromycin

In a randomised, crossover study in 12 healthy subjects, pre-treatment with telithromycin 800 mg daily for 3 days increased the AUC of a single 250-microgram dose of repaglinide, given on day 3, by 77% and increased its maximum plasma concentration by 38%. In addition, it increased the blood glucose-lowering effect of repaglinide.[3]

Mechanism

Repaglinide is primarily metabolised by CYP2C8, with some involvement of CYP3A4. Clarithromycin and telithromycin are both potent inhibitors of CYP3A4 and so increase repaglinide exposure. However, the increases seen were only slight, and might be a result of the compensatory capacity of the CYP2C8 pathway. Further study is needed to determine the exact mechanisms involved.

Importance and management

A pharmacokinetic interaction between clarithromycin or telithromycin and repaglinide is established. The slight increase in repaglinide exposure is generally unlikely to be clinically important (especially as infections can increase blood glucose concentrations), although the doses of repaglinide used in these studies were lower than the doses that are used clinically. However, note that a case of severe hypoglycaemia in a patient has been reported after clarithromycin was started. It would, however, be prudent to monitor blood glucose concentrations on the concurrent use of these drugs, and to adjust the dose of repaglinide if necessary. Other macrolides that inhibit CYP3A4 (such as erythromycin) would be expected to interact in a similar manner.

1. Niemi M, Neuvonen PJ, Kivistö KT. The cytochrome P4503A4 inhibitor clarithromycin increases the plasma concentrations and effects of repaglinide. *Clin Pharmacol Ther* (2001) 70, 58–65.
2. Khamaisi M, Leitersdorf E. Severe hypoglycemia from clarithromycin-repaglinide drug interaction. *Pharmacotherapy* (2008) 28, 682–4.
3. Kajosaari LI, Niemi M, Backman JT, Neuvonen PJ. Telithromycin, but not montelukast, increases the plasma concentrations and effects of the cytochrome P450 3A4 and 2C8 substrate repaglinide. *Clin Pharmacol Ther* (2006) 79, 231–42.

Meglitinides; Repaglinide + Montelukast

Montelukast does not alter the pharmacokinetics of repaglinide.

Clinical evidence, mechanism, importance and management

In a randomised, crossover study in 12 healthy subjects given montelukast 10 mg daily for 3 days with a single 250-microgram dose of repaglinide on day 3, there was no change in the pharmacokinetics of repaglinide compared with when used alone.[1]

In vitro, montelukast inhibited CYP2C8, by which repaglinide is principally metabolised. As repaglinide is a sensitive CYP2C8 substrate, the lack of effect in this study provides evidence that montelukast does not inhibit CYP2C8 *in vivo*, and no interaction occurs with repaglinide. No repaglinide dose adjustment is therefore expected to be necessary if montelukast is also given. However, note that it is prudent to monitor blood glucose concentrations when any change is made to the medication regimen of a patient with diabetes.

1. Kajosaari LI, Niemi M, Backman JT, Neuvonen PJ. Telithromycin, but not montelukast, increases the plasma concentrations and effects of the cytochrome P450 3A4 and 2C8 substrate repaglinide. *Clin Pharmacol Ther* (2006) 79, 231–42.

Meglitinides; Repaglinide + Nifedipine

Nifedipine does not alter the pharmacokinetics of repaglinide.

Clinical evidence, mechanism, importance and management

A randomised, crossover study in healthy subjects found that nifedipine 10 mg daily for 5 days, decreased the maximum plasma concentration of repaglinide 2 mg three times daily for 5 days by 4.8% and decreased the AUC by 8%, but neither change was statistically significant.[1] No special precautions would seem necessary on concurrent use, but note that it is prudent to monitor blood glucose concentrations when any change is made to the medication regimen of a patient with diabetes.

For discussion of the general effects of calcium channel blockers on diabetes control, see 'Antidiabetics + Calcium-channel blockers', p.505.

1. Hatorp V, Hansen KT, Thomsen MS. Influence of drugs interacting with CYP3A4 on the pharmacokinetics, pharmacodynamics, and safety of the prandial glucose regulator repaglinide. *J Clin Pharmacol* (2003) 43, 649–60.

Meglitinides; Repaglinide + St John's wort (*Hypericum perforatum*)

St John's wort does not alter the pharmacokinetics of repaglinide.

Clinical evidence, mechanism, importance and management

In a randomised, crossover study in 15 healthy subjects, St John's wort 325 mg three times daily was given for 14 days with a single 1-mg dose of repaglinide and 75 g of glucose on day 15. St John's wort had no effect on the pharmacokinetics of repaglinide, or on its effects on blood glucose or insulin concentrations.[1]

Repaglinide is a sensitive substrate for CYP2C8 and so this study suggests that St John's wort does not alter the activity of this isoenzyme. No special precautions would seem necessary on concurrent use of repaglinide and St John's wort.

1. Fan L, Zhou G, Guo D, Liu Y-L, Chen W-Q, Liu Z-Q, Tan Z-R, Sheng D, Zhou H-H, Zhang W. The pregnane X receptor agonist St John's wort has no effects on the pharmacokinetics and pharmacodynamics of repaglinide. *Clin Pharmacokinet* (2011) 50, 605–11.

Meglitinides; Repaglinide + Thiazolidinediones; Pioglitazone

There is no pharmacokinetic interaction between repaglinide and pioglitazone.

Clinical evidence, mechanism, importance and management

In a randomised, crossover study, 12 healthy subjects were given pioglitazone 30 mg daily for 5 days, with a single 250-microgram dose of repaglinide on day 5. The pharmacokinetics of both drugs were unaffected by concurrent administration. Similarly, there was no change in the glycaemic effect of repaglinide when administered with pioglitazone.[1] This combination is used in the management of diabetes for its additive glucose lowering effects, and this study shows that there is no pharmacokinetic interaction that will complicate this use. Note, that the lack of increased glycaemic effect with combined use seen in this study, is most likely a result of the study design.

1. Kajosaari LI, Jakkola T, Neuvonen PJ, Backman JT. Pioglitazone, an in vitro inhibitor of CYP2C8 and CYP3A4, does not increase the plasma concentrations of the CYP2C8 and CYP3A4 substrate repaglinide. *Eur J Clin Pharmacol* (2006) 62, 217–23.

Metformin + Aliskiren

The concurrent use of metformin and aliskiren slightly reduced aliskiren exposure but did not alter metformin exposure in one study.

Clinical evidence, mechanism, importance and management

In a study in 19 healthy subjects, giving aliskiren 300 mg daily with metformin 1 g daily for 4 days reduced the AUC of aliskiren by 27% and reduced the AUC of metformin by 12%, when compared with either drug given alone.[1] The reason for these minor changes is unclear; however, they are not considered to be clinically relevant.

1. Vaidyanathan S, Maboudian M, Warren V, Yeh C-M, Dieterich HA, Howard D, Dole WP. A study of the pharmacokinetic interactions of the direct renin inhibitor aliskiren with metformin, pioglitazone and fenofibrate in healthy subjects. *Curr Med Res Opin* (2008) 24, 2313–26.

Metformin + Cefalexin

Cefalexin negligibly increased metformin exposure in a single-dose study.

Clinical evidence, mechanism, importance and management

In a randomised crossover study in 12 healthy subjects, a single 500-mg dose of cefalexin increased the AUC and maximum serum concentration of a single 500-mg dose of metformin by 24% and 34%, respectively. Cefalexin reduced the renal clearance of metformin by 14% by inhibiting metformin tubular secretion via the organic cation system.[1] The clinical relevance of these small changes is uncertain, but they could possibly be greater with longer-term use. The authors recommend that patients receiving metformin with cefalexin should have metformin concentrations monitored or an alternative antibacterial to cefalexin should be considered.[1] However, based on the available evidence this seems somewhat overcautious. Note that it is prudent to monitor blood glucose concentrations when any change is made to the medication regimen of a patient with diabetes, which should be sufficient to detect any interaction, should it occur.

1. Jayasagar G, Krishna Kumar M, Chandrasekhar K, Madhusudan Rao C, Madhusudan Rao Y. Effect of cephalexin on the pharmacokinetics of metformin in healthy human volunteers. *Drug Metabol Drug Interact* (2002) 19, 41–8.

Metformin + Cimetidine

Cimetidine appears to slightly increase the exposure to metformin by reducing its clearance, and might have contributed to two cases of metformin-associated lactic acidosis.

Clinical evidence

Cimetidine 800 mg daily for 5 days was found to reduce the renal clearance of metformin 250 mg daily in 7 healthy subjects by 27% and increase the AUC by about 50%.[1] A 59-year-old woman with type 2 diabetes taking long-term metformin 500 mg three times daily developed severe metabolic acidosis with cardiovascular collapse and acute renal failure. Three months previously she had started orlistat 120 mg three times daily, which caused chronic diarrhoea. During the 4 days before hospital admission, she was prescribed cimetidine 400 mg twice daily for her abdominal pain. The metformin-associated lactic acidosis was considered to have been precipitated by the orlistat and cimetidine.[2] Another case report describes a 59-year-old woman who developed lactic acidosis, renal failure, and acute pancreatitis 9 days after cimetidine (dose unknown) was added to her medication, which included metformin. After the cimetidine and metformin were discontinued, and she was dialysed for 24 hours, her laboratory results returned to normal and she was discharged within 72 hours without further problems.[3]

Mechanism

Cimetidine appears to inhibit the excretion of metformin by the kidneys,[1] and this might have contributed to the cases of metformin-associated lactic acidosis described.[2,3]

Importance and management

Evidence for an interaction between metformin and cimetidine is limited, and an interaction is not established. It has been suggested that the dose of metformin might need to be reduced if cimetidine is used, bearing in mind the possibility of lactic acidosis,[1] and there are two cases where cimetidine could have contributed to lactic acidosis. This should be taken into consideration if metformin and cimetidine are to be used concurrently. Note that it is prudent to monitor blood glucose concentrations when any change is made to the medication regimen of a patient with diabetes.

1. Somogyi A, Stockley C, Keal J, Rolan P, Bochner F. Reduction of metformin renal tubular secretion by cimetidine in man. *Br J Clin Pharmacol* (1987) 23, 545–51.
2. Dawson D, Conlon C. Case study: metformin-associated lactic acidosis. Could orlistat be relevant? *Diabetes Care* (2003) 26, 2471–2.
3. Boehm KM, Gunaga S. Cimetidine-induced lactic acidosis and acute pancreatitis. *South Med J* (2010) 103, 849.

Metformin + Eslicarbazepine

Eslicarbazepine did not alter the pharmacokinetics of metformin in one study.

Clinical evidence, mechanism, importance and management

In a randomised, crossover study in 19 healthy subjects given eslicarbazepine 1.2 g daily for 6 days with a single 850-mg dose of metformin on day 5, the pharmacokinetics of metformin were unchanged, compared with metformin given alone.[1] No metformin dose adjustment would be expected to be necessary on concurrent use with eslicarbazepine. However, note that it is prudent to monitor blood glucose concentrations when any change is made to the medication regimen of a patient with diabetes.

1. Rocha JF, Vaz-da-Silva M, Almeida L, Falcão A, Nunes T, Santos AT, Martins F, Fontes-Ribeiro C, Macedo T, Soares-da-Silva P. Effect of eslicarbazepine acetate on the pharmacokinetics of metformin in healthy subjects. *Int J Clin Pharmacol Ther* (2009) 47, 255–61.

Metformin + Ginkgo (*Ginkgo biloba*)

Ginkgo does not appear to alter the pharmacokinetics of metformin, and appears to have a small beneficial effect on glycaemic control.

Clinical evidence, mechanism, importance and management

In a small crossover study that included 10 patients with type 2 diabetes taking metformin, use of ginkgo (EGb 761) 120 mg daily for 3 months resulted in a small improvement in HbA_{1c} when compared with placebo (HbA_{1c} 7.2% versus 7.7%). The pharmacokinetics of metformin were assessed on one day at the end of the study, when the usual daily dose of metformin was taken with the daily dose of ginkgo. Ginkgo did not appear to have any effects on metformin pharmacokinetics.[1] In a further 10 healthy subjects, ginkgo 120 mg daily had no effect on the pharmacokinetics of a single 500-mg dose of metformin, except for a reduction in the time to reach the maximum plasma concentration.[1]

This study indicates that ginkgo is unlikely to alter the pharmacokinetics of metformin. In addition, it provides some limited evidence that it might have a small beneficial effect on glycaemic control, although this requires confirmation in a larger study.

1. Kudolo GB, Wang W, Javors M, Blodgett J. The effect of the ingestion of Ginkgo biloba extract (EGb 761) on the pharmacokinetics of metformin in non-diabetic and type 2 diabetic subjects–a double blind placebo-controlled, crossover study. *Clin Nutr* (2006) 25, 606–16.

Metformin + Guar gum

Guar gum slightly reduced metformin exposure in healthy subjects, but it enhanced its postprandial hypoglycaemic effect.

Clinical evidence, mechanism, importance and management

In a single-dose study, guar gum 10 g reduced the absorption rate of metformin 1.7 g and reduced the AUC by 39% in 6 healthy subjects, but the total reduction in postprandial blood glucose concentrations was increased.[1]

It seems doubtful that this minor pharmacokinetic interaction has much, if any, clinical relevance because guar gum can improve the metabolic control, and decrease serum lipids, in patients with type 2 diabetes.[2]

1. Gin H, Orgerie MB, Aubertin J. The influence of guar gum on absorption of metformin from the gut in healthy volunteers. *Horm Metab Res* (1989) 21, 81–3.
2. Uusitupa M, Södervik H, Silvasti M, Karttunen P. Effects of a gel forming dietary fiber, guar gum, on the absorption of glibenclamide and metabolic control and serum lipids in patients with non-insulin-dependent (type 2) diabetes. *Int J Clin Pharmacol Ther Toxicol* (1990) 28, 153–7.

Metformin + HIV-integrase inhibitors; Dolutegravir

Dolutegravir appears to increase the exposure to metformin.

Clinical evidence

In the preliminary report of a study, healthy subjects were given metformin 500 mg twice daily for 22 days, with dolutegravir 50 mg daily (14 subjects) or 50 mg twice daily (13 subjects) given from days 6 to 12. The AUC and maximum concentration of metformin were increased by 79% and 66%, respectively, when given with dolutegravir 50 mg daily, and 2.4- and 2.1-fold, respectively, when given with dolutegravir 50 mg twice daily.[1]

Mechanism

In vitro,[2] dolutegravir inhibits the organic cation transporter OCT-2, and the multidrug and toxin extrusion transporter protein, MATE-1. Metformin is a substrate for OCT-2, and it is thought that both OCT-2 and MATE-1 are involved in the renal transport of metformin. Concurrent use would therefore be expected to increase metformin exposure. Further study is required to confirm this.

Importance and management

A pharmacokinetic interaction between metformin and dolutegravir appears to occur, but it is not established. Metformin exposure is increased, and the possibility of increased effects cannot be ruled out. As it is prudent to monitor blood glucose concentrations when any change is made to the medication regimen of a patient with diabetes, any such effect should be identified and any related metformin dose adjustment should be made.

1. Zong J, Borland J, Jerva F, Wynne B, Choukour M, Song I. The effect of dolutegravir on the pharmacokinetics of metformin in healthy subjects. *J Int AIDS Soc* (2014) 17 (Suppl 3), Abstract 19584.
2. Tivicay (Dolutegravir sodium). ViiV Healthcare UK Ltd. UK Summary of product characteristics, September 2014.

Metformin + Iodinated contrast media

Parenteral administration of iodinated contrast media can cause renal failure, which could result in lactic acidosis in patients taking metformin.

Clinical evidence, mechanism, importance and management

Parenteral administration of iodinated contrast media to patients taking metformin might result in lactic acidosis. However, the problem is reported to occur only if the contrast media causes renal failure and metformin use is continued. This is because metformin is mainly excreted by the kidneys and in renal failure toxic concentrations may accumulate,[1] which might result in lactic acidosis. A literature search identified 18 cases of lactic acidosis after the use of contrast media in patients taking metformin.[2] Of these 18 cases, 14 or 15 were associated with pre-existing renal impairment and 2 cases with other contraindications to metformin (sepsis and cirrhosis). The remaining case was in an elderly woman with neurological disease. Note that diabetes-related renal impairment per se is an important risk factor for contrast-media associated renal failure.[2,3]

The UK and US manufacturers of metformin state that it should be stopped before, or at the time of giving, the contrast media and not restarted until 48 hours later, and then only after renal function has been re-checked and found to be normal.[4,5] Guidelines issued by the European Society of Urogenital Radiology[6] on iodine-based contrast media, suggest that there is no need to stop metformin before giving the contrast media in patients with normal renal function (estimated glomerular filtration rate of 60 mL/minute/1.73 m^2 or greater). In patients with an estimated glomerular filtration rate of 30 to 59 mL/minute/1.73 m^2, or an increased serum creatinine concentration, metformin should be withheld for 48 hours before and after the contrast media, and only restarted if creatinine concentrations are unchanged.[6] Metformin and/or contrast media are not usually recommended in patients with an estimated glomerular filtration rate of less than 30 mL/minute/1.73 m^2. In emergency cases where renal function is abnormal or unknown, alternative imaging should be used, if possible. If this is not possible, then the risks and benefits of using contrast media should be weighed carefully. If concurrent use is necessary, the metformin should be stopped, and special care taken with intravenous hydration and monitoring of renal function and lactic acidosis.[6] The American College of Radiology make similar recommendations, but additionally mention risk factors for lactic acidosis with metformin (e.g. liver impairment, alcohol abuse, myocardial ischaemia, sepsis), and recommend additional caution if these factors are also present. For example, patients with normal renal function and multiple risk factors should withhold from taking metformin for 48 hours after the administration of iodinated contrast media, and consideration should be given to measuring the serum creatinine before re-starting metformin.[7] They also note that elderly patients with reduced muscle mass might have an apparently 'normal' serum creatinine in the presence of marked renal impairment,[7] therefore the same precautions might also warranted.

Although these guidelines minimise the risk, some patients can still develop an adverse reaction. For example, in an analysis of 97 patients taking metformin who were given intravenous contrast media, 4 developed contrast media-associated nephropathy (all 4 had baseline normal renal function). These patients could have been at increased risk of metformin-associated lactic acidosis had the metformin not been stopped and withheld.[8] Furthermore, a fatal case of metformin-induced lactic acidosis occurred in a 47-year-old man with normal renal function who was admitted as an emergency for aneurysmal subarachnoid haemorrhage and who underwent two contrast procedures (CT scan and angiography) with ionic contrast iohexol.[9]

1. Rasuli P, Hammond DI. Metformin and contrast media: where is the conflict? *Can Assoc Radiol J* (1998) 49, 161–6.
2. Morcos SK, Thomsen HS. European Society of Urogenital Radiology guidelines on administering contrast media. *Abdom Imaging* (2003) 28, 187–190.
3. Thomsen HS, Morcos SK. Contrast media and the kidney: European Society of Urogenital Radiology (ESUR) guidelines. *Br J Radiol* (2003) 76, 513–8.
4. Glucophage (Metformin hydrochloride). Merck Serono. UK Summary of product characteristics, October 2010.
5. Glucophage (Metformin hydrochloride). Bristol-Myers Squibb Co. US Prescribing information, January 2009.
6. European Society of Urogenital Radiology. ESUR guidelines on contrast media version 8.1, May 2012. Available at: http://www.esur.org/esur-guidelines/contrast-media-81 (accessed 20/10/15).
7. American College of Radiology. Manual on contrast media, version 10.1, 2015. Available at: http://www.acr.org/quality-safety/resources/contrast-manual (accessed 20/10/15).

8. Parra D, Legreid AM, Beckey NP, Reyes S. Metformin monitoring and change in serum creatinine levels in patients undergoing radiologic procedures involving administration of intravenous contrast media. *Pharmacotherapy* (2004) 24, 987–93. Erratum ibid., 1489.
9. Jain V, Sharma D, Prabhakar H, Dash HH. Metformin-associated lactic acidosis following contrast media-induced nephrotoxicity. Eur J Anaesthesiol. (2008) 25, 166–7.

Metformin + Megilitinides; Nateglinide

No pharmacokinetic interaction occurs between metformin and nateglinide.

Clinical evidence, mechanism, importance and management

In a randomised, crossover study, 12 patients with type 2 diabetes taking metformin 500 mg three times daily were given nateglinide 120 mg three times daily for 1 day. There were no changes to the pharmacokinetics of either drug when given together, compared with when given alone. The post-prandial reduction in plasma glucose concentrations was greater after combined administration than with either drug alone.[1] This combination is used in the management of diabetes for its additive glucose lowering effects, and this study shows that there is no pharmacokinetic interaction that will complicate this use.

1. Hirschberg Y, Karara AH, Pietri AO, McLeod JF. Improved control of mealtime glucose excursions with coadministration of nateglinide and metformin. *Diabetes Care* (2000) 23, 349–53.

Metformin + Miscellaneous

An increased risk of lactic acidosis is predicted if metformin is taken with excessive alcohol. Nifedipine does not appear to affect the pharmacokinetics of metformin, and colesevelam is predicted not to affect the absorption of metformin.

Clinical evidence, mechanism, importance and management

(a) Alcohol

The UK manufacturers of metformin advise against its concurrent use with alcohol due to the increased risk of lactic acidosis in acute alcohol intoxication. Metformin should also not be given to alcoholic patients because of the risk of liver damage.[1] There appears to be a lack of information relating to normal alcohol consumption, and so it would seem unlikely that occasional consumption of one or two units of alcohol would pose a risk. Note also, the general advice for consumption of alcohol in diabetes in 'Antidiabetics + Alcohol', p.501.

(b) Colesevelam

The US manufacturers of colesevelam state that metformin did not bind with colesevelam during *in vitro* testing, so they consider a clinical interaction unlikely.[2] There would therefore appear to be no reason to separate administration of metformin and colesevelam, but note that it is prudent to monitor blood glucose concentrations when any change is made to the medication regimen of a patient with diabetes.

(c) Nifedipine

One US manufacturer of nifedipine noted that in a single-dose study in healthy subjects, nifedipine increased the AUC of metformin by 9%, and increased its maximum concentration by 20%.[3] No metformin dose adjustment would seem necessary on concurrent use, but note that it is prudent to monitor blood glucose concentrations when any change is made to the medication regimen of a patient with diabetes. For discussion of the general effects of calcium channel blockers on diabetes control, see 'Antidiabetics + Calcium-channel blockers', p.505.

1. Glucophage (Metformin hydrochloride). Merck Serono. UK Summary of product characteristics, October 2010.
2. Welchol (Colesevelam hydrochloride). Daiichi Sankyo, Inc. US Prescribing information, January 2014.
3. Adalat CC (Nifedipine). Bayer HealthCare. US Prescribing information, August 2005.

Metformin + NRTIs

Two cases of lactic acidosis, one of which was fatal, have been reported in patients taking metformin with NRTIs (didanosine, stavudine, tenofovir).

Clinical evidence, mechanism, importance and management

A patient taking **didanosine** 300 mg daily, **stavudine** 30 mg twice daily, **tenofovir** 300 mg daily, co-trimoxazole 160/800 mg daily, clarithromycin 500 mg twice daily, and ganciclovir 1 g three times daily developed severe lactic acidosis 7 days after starting to take metformin 500 mg twice daily. Two months before starting metformin he was found to have abnormal liver enzymes with signs of fatty changes in his liver and his lactic acid concentration was 1.8 mmol/L (normal range 0.2 to 1.8 mmol/L), however, his liver enzymes and lactic acid concentrations were found to have worsened on admission (lactic acid 14.6 mmol/L). The antiretrovirals and metformin were stopped, but he developed cardiac failure and died. The authors suggested that hepatic steatosis due to NRTI-induced mitochondrial damage reduced hepatic lactate clearance, which was exacerbated by the addition of metformin.[1]

Another case of lactic acidosis has been reported in a patient with coronary heart disease and diabetes stable taking metformin 850 mg three times daily when he started to take **tenofovir** 300 mg daily with emtricitabine and efavirenz (doses not stated). Ten days before admission his renal function had been normal but was found to have deteriorated on admission. He was treated with continuous haemofiltration and recovered.[2] However, one small, placebo-controlled clinical study found no increase in lactate concentrations in patients taking antiretrovirals including NRTIs who were also given low-dose metformin 500 mg twice daily for 3 months.[3] In a meta-analysis of randomised controlled studies evaluating the effects of antidiabetics in the treatment of HIV-associated lipodystrophy syndrome, 9 studies included the use of metformin (including that mentioned above). Where reported, the incidence of alterations in lactate concentrations was not statistically different between study arms (including metformin, placebo, and no treatment). There were 4 cases of elevated lactate concentrations which required treatment withdrawal or study discontinuation.[4]

Evidence for an increase in the risk of lactic acidosis on the concurrent use of metformin and NRTIs appears to be limited to the isolated case reports cited. Both NRTIs and metformin can themselves cause lactic acidosis, and so until more is known, it would seem prudent to bear the case reports in mind on concurrent use.

1. Worth L, Elliott J, Anderson J, Sasadeusz J, Street A, Lewin S. A cautionary tale: fatal lactic acidosis complicating nucleoside analogue and metformin therapy. *Clin Infect Dis* (2003) 37, 315–6.
2. Aperis G, Paliouras C, Zervos A, Arvanitis A, Alivanis P. Lactic acidosis after concomitant treatment with metformin and tenofovir in a patient with HIV infection. *J Ren Care* (2011) 37, 25–9.
3. Hadigan C, Corcoran C, Basgoz N, Davis B, Sax P, Grinspoon S. Metformin in the treatment of HIV lipodystrophy syndrome. A randomized controlled trial. *JAMA* (2000) 284, 472–77.
4. Sheth SH, Larson RJ. The efficacy and safety of insulin-sensitizing drugs in HIV-associated lipodystrophy syndrome: a meta-analysis of randomized trials. *BMC Infect Dis* (2010) 10, 183.

Metformin + NSAIDs; Coxibs

Rofecoxib and celecoxib might have been a precipitating factor in cases of acute renal failure and metformin-associated lactic acidosis.

Clinical evidence, mechanism, importance and management

A 58-year-old woman with longstanding type 2 diabetes taking metformin 500 mg twice daily, developed serious acute renal failure and lactic acidosis one month after starting **rofecoxib**. She made a full recovery. **Rofecoxib** could have precipitated acute renal failure, which would lead to the accumulation of metformin, and metformin-associated lactic acidosis.[1] Another similar case has been reported in a 61-year-old woman taking metformin and given **rofecoxib**.[2] Similarly, renal failure and metformin-associated lactic acidosis occurred in a 50-year-old woman taking metformin 2 months after starting **celecoxib**. In this case, hydrochlorothiazide and candesartan were thought to have contributed to the renal failure.[3] For cases of hypoglycaemia attributed to ramipril and **naproxen**-induced renal failure in a patient taking metformin and glibenclamide, and chlorpropamide and **fenclofenac** in a patient also taking metformin, see 'Sulfonylureas + NSAIDs', p.548.

Reports of adverse interactions between metformin and NSAIDs appear to be limited to those cited, and involved other precipitating factors, suggesting that in general no interaction would be expected and that routine monitoring of renal function would seem sufficient.

1. Price G. Metformin lactic acidosis, acute renal failure and rofecoxib. *Br J Anaesth* (2003) 91, 909–10.
2. Tewari P, Nath SS, Mazumdar G. Increased prothrombin time and lactic acidosis: rofecoxib drug interaction with acenocoumarin and metformin. *Ann Card Anaesth* (2007) 10, 58–60.
3. Audia P, Feinfeld DA, Dubrow A, Winchester JF. Metformin-induced lactic acidosis and acute pancreatitis precipitated by diuretic, celecoxib, and candesartan-associated acute kidney dysfunction. *Clin Toxicol* (2008) 46, 164–6.

Metformin + Pyrimethamine

In a single-dose study, pyrimethamine slightly increased metformin exposure.

Clinical evidence

In a crossover study, 8 healthy subjects were given a single 250-mg dose of metformin one hour after a single 50-mg dose of pyrimethamine. The renal clearance of metformin was reduced by 35% and the maximum concentration and AUC were increased by about 36%. Plasma lactate concentrations were unaffected, but plasma creatinine concentrations were increased.[1]

Mechanism

In vitro, pyrimethamine is an inhibitor of MATE (multidrug and toxin extrusion) transporter proteins that are thought to be involved in the urinary excretion of metformin.[1] This study suggests that pyrimethamine might also exert this effect *in vivo*. Further study is needed.

Importance and management

The changes in metformin pharmacokinetics with pyrimethamine are unlikely to be of general clinical importance. No special precautions or dose adjustment would seem necessary on concurrent use, but note that it is prudent to monitor blood glucose concentrations when any change is made to the medication regimen of a patient with diabetes.

1. Kusuhara H, Ito S, Kumagai Y, Jiang M, Shiroshita T, Moriyama Y, Inoue K, Yuasa H, Sugiyama Y. Effects of a MATE protein inhibitor, pyrimethamine, on the renal elimination of metformin at oral microdose and at therapeutic dose in healthy subjects. *Clin Pharmacol Ther* (2011) 89, 837–44.

Metformin + Rifamycins

Rifampicin appears to increase the absorption of metformin, leading to a negligible increase in its exposure.

Clinical evidence

In a study, 16 healthy subjects underwent oral glucose tolerance testing in the morning and were given two doses of metformin 1 g at 8pm on day one and 750 mg the following morning on day 2, and then on days 13 and 14, following a 10-day course of **rifampicin** 600 mg daily. **Rifampicin** increased the AUC of metformin by 13%. The blood glucose-lowering effects of metformin were increased by about 45% by **rifampicin** pre-treatment. **Rifampicin** pre-treatment also increased the renal tubular clearance of metformin.[1]

Mechanism

It is suggested that the increase in metformin exposure might be due to induction of organic cation transporters (OCT1 and OCT3) in the intestine by rifampicin, although further study is needed to confirm this. Other transporters might also have been involved.[1]

Importance and management

The interaction between **metformin** and rifampicin is not established. The limited data from one small study suggest that rifampicin does not have a clinically relevant effect on single-dose metformin exposure. However, as its blood glucose-lowering effects were increased, it would seem prudent to bear the possibility of an interaction in mind should any unexpected increase in metformin effects occur in patients also given rifampicin. As it is prudent to monitor blood glucose concentrations when any change is made to the medication regimen of a patient with diabetes, any such effect should be identified and any related metformin dose adjustment should be made.

There does not seem to be any information regarding an interaction between metformin and **rifabutin** or **rifapentine**. The UK manufacturer and the CSM in the UK warn that rifabutin might possibly reduce the effects of a number of drugs, including oral antidiabetics (not specified).[2,3] However, this warning is based on rifabutin's effects on CYP3A4, but as metformin is not metabolised by CYP3A4, no interaction is expected to occur between these two drugs via this route.

1. Cho SK, Yoon JS, Lee MG, Lee DH, Lim LA, Park K, Park MS, Chung J-Y. Rifampin enhances the glucose-lowering effect of metformin and increases OCT1 mRNA levels in healthy participants. *Clin Pharmacol Ther* (2011) 89, 416–21.
2. Mycobutin (Rifabutin). Pfizer Ltd. UK Summary of product characteristics, December 2013.
3. Committee on the Safety of Medicines/Medicines Control Agency. Revised indication and drug interactions of rifabutin. *Current Problems* (1997) 23, 14. Available at: http://webarchive.nationalarchives.gov.uk/20141205150130/http://www.mhra.gov.uk/home/groups/pl-p/documents/websiteresources/con2023238.pdf (accessed 21/10/15)

Sodium-glucose co-transporter-2 inhibitors + Dipeptidylpeptidase-4 inhibitors

The pharmacokinetics of dapagliflozin and sitagliptin were not affected by concurrent use in a single-dose study. The pharmacokinetics of empagliflozin and sitagliptin, and of empagliflozin and linagliptin, were not affected by concurrent use. Concurrent use might increase the risk of hypoglycaemia.

Clinical evidence, mechanism, importance and management

(a) Dapagliflozin

In a randomised, crossover study, 18 healthy subjects were given a single 20-mg dose of dapagliflozin with a single 100-mg dose of **sitagliptin**. There were no changes in the pharmacokinetics of either drug, compared with administration alone.[1] The pharmacodynamic effects were not studied, but on the basis of an increased incidence of hypoglycaemia with insulin or sulfonylureas and dapagliflozin, the UK and US manufacturers of dapagliflozin advise that the dose of insulin or insulin secretagogues (which would include the dipeptidylpeptidase-4 inhibitors) might need to be reduced on concurrent use with dapagliflozin.[2,3] No pharmacokinetic interaction occurs between dapagliflozin and **sitagliptin**, but monitoring of blood glucose concentrations if dapagliflozin is to be given concurrently with any dipeptidylpeptidase-4 inhibitor would be prudent.

(b) Empagliflozin

In a randomised, crossover study, 16 healthy subjects were given empagliflozin 50 mg once daily and **sitagliptin** 100 mg once daily for 5 days. There were no clinically relevant changes in the AUC or maximum plasma concentration of either drug, compared with when they were given alone.[4] In another randomised, crossover study, 16 healthy subjects were given empagliflozin 50 mg once a day and **linagliptin** 5 mg once a day for 7 days. There was no change in the AUC or maximum plasma concentration of either drug, compared with when they were given alone.[5]

No clinically relevant interaction occurs between empagliflozin and sitagliptin or linagliptin, but monitoring of blood glucose concentrations if empagliflozin is to be given concurrently with any dipeptidylpeptidase-4 inhibitor would be prudent. On the basis of an increased incidence of hypoglycaemia with insulin or sulfonylureas and empagliflozin, the UK and US manufacturers of empagliflozin advise that the dose of insulin or insulin secretagogues (which would include the dipeptidylpeptidase-4 inhibitors) might need to be reduced on concurrent use because of an increased risk of hypoglycaemia.[6,7]

1. Kasichayanula S, Liu X, Shyu WC, Zhang W, Pfister M, Griffen SC, Li T, LaCreta FP, Boulton DW. Lack of pharmacokinetic interaction between dapagliflozin, a novel sodium-glucose transporter 2 inhibitor, and metformin, pioglitazone, glimepiride or sitagliptin in healthy subjects. *Diabetes Obes Metab* (2011) 13, 47–54.
2. Forxiga (Dapagliflozin propanediol monohydrate). Bristol Myers Squibb-AstraZeneca EEIG. UK Summary of product characteristics, October 2014.
3. Farxiga (Dapagliflozin). AstraZeneca Pharmaceuticals LP. US Prescribing Information. March 2015.
4. Brand T, Macha S, Mattheus M, Pinnetti S, Woerle HJ. Pharmacokinetics of empagliflozin, a sodium glucose cotransporter-2 (SGLT-2) inhibitor, coadministered with sitagliptin in healthy volunteers. *Adv Therapy* (2012) 29, 889–99.
5. Friedrich C, Metzmann K, Rose P, Mattheus M, Pinnetti S, Woerle HJ. A randomised, open-label, crossover study to evaluate the pharmacokinetics of empagliflozin and linagliptin after coadministration in healthy male volunteers. *Clin Ther* (2013) 35, A33–42.
6. Jardiance (Empagliflozin). Boehringer Ingelheim Pharmaceuticals, Inc. US Prescribing information, June 2015.
7. Jardiance (Empagliflozin). Boehringer Ingelheim Ltd. UK Summary of product characteristics, January 2015.

Sodium-glucose co-transporter-2 inhibitors + Diuretics

Hydrochlorothiazide does not appear to affect the pharmacokinetics of canagliflozin to a clinically relevant extent. There appears to be no pharmacokinetic interaction between hydrochlorothiazide and dapagliflozin or empagliflozin, or between bumetanide and dapagliflozin. Diuretics are predicted to have additive effects with the sodium-glucose co-transporter-2 inhibitors, and might cause dehydration or hypotension.

Clinical evidence, mechanism, importance and management

(a) Pharmacokinetics

In a pharmacokinetic study, 28 healthy subjects were given **canagliflozin** 300 mg with **hydrochlorothiazide** 25 mg once daily, both for 7 days. The AUC and maximum concentration of canagliflozin were increased by 12% and 15%, respectively,[1] but these increases are not expected to be clinically relevant, and no canagliflozin dose adjustment would appear necessary on concurrent use.

Pharmacokinetic studies with **dapagliflozin** and **hydrochlorothiazide** or **bumetanide** found no effects on the pharmacokinetics of any of these drugs.[2]

The US manufacturer of **empagliflozin** briefly notes that, in a study, the pharmacokinetics of **hydrochlorothiazide** 25 mg once daily and empagliflozin 25 mg once daily were not altered when used concurrently. They also briefly note that, in a study, the pharmacokinetics of **torasemide** 5 mg once daily and a single 25mg dose of **empagliflozin** were not altered on concurrent use.[3]

(b) Pharmacodynamics

Due to their mechanism of action, **canagliflozin**, **dapagliflozin**, and **empagliflozin** all cause diuresis and can cause volume depletion and hypotension. As a result, their use with diuretics, especially **loop diuretics** and **thiazides**,[2-4] is cautioned. Additionally, **canagliflozin** might cause hyperkalaemia and it should also be used with caution with **potassium-sparing diuretics**.[4]

1. Devineni D, Vaccaro N, Polidori D, Rusch S, Wajs E. Effects of hydrochlorothiazide on the pharmacokinetics, pharmacodynamics, and tolerability of canagliflozin, a sodium glucose co-transporter 2 inhibitor, in healthy participants. *Clin Ther* (2014) 36, 698–710..
2. Forxiga (Dapagliflozin propanediol monohydrate). Bristol Myers Squibb-AstraZeneca EEIG. UK Summary of product characteristics, October 2014.
3. Jardiance (Empagliflozin). Boehringer Ingelheim Pharmaceuticals, Inc. US Prescribing information, June 2015.
4. Invokana (Canagliflozin). Janssen Pharmaceuticals, Inc. US Prescribing information, September 2015.

Sodium-glucose co-transporter-2 inhibitors + Food

Food does not affect the pharmacokinetics of canagliflozin, dapagliflozin, or empagliflozin.

Clinical evidence, mechanism, importance and management

(a) Canagliflozin

The US manufacturer briefly notes that, co-administration of a high-fat meal had no effect on the pharmacokinetics of canagliflozin. Canagliflozin can be taken without regard to meals, however, because it delays the intestinal absorption of glucose and this might reduce postprandial glucose excursions, it is recommend that it is taken before the first meal of the day.[1]

(b) Dapagliflozin

In a randomised, crossover study, 14 healthy subjects were given a single 10-mg dose of dapagliflozin after an overnight fast, or 5 minutes after finishing a high-fat meal (52% of calories from fat). The overall exposure (AUC) of dapagliflozin was not affected by food, but the maximum concentration was decreased by 31%. The time to maximum concentration was delayed by about 1 hour. These changes were not considered clinically important.[2] Dapagliflozin can be given without regard to food.

(c) Empagliflozin

In a randomised, crossover study 18 healthy subjects were given a single dose of empagliflozin 25 mg after an overnight fast, or 30 minutes after a high fat, high calorie meal. The AUC and maximum concentration of empagliflozin were decreased by 16% and 37%, respectively, when given with food. The time to maximum concentration was delayed by 1.5 hours. These changes were not considered to be clinically relevant,[3] therefore empagliflozin can be given with or without food.

1. Invokana (Canagliflozin). Janssen Pharmaceuticals, Inc. US Prescribing information, September 2015.
2. Kasichayanula S, Liu X, Zhang W, Pfister M, Reele SB, Aubry A-F, LaCreta FP, Boulton DW. Effect of a high-fat meal on the pharmacokinetics of dapagliflozin, a selective SGLT2 inhibitor, in healthy subjects. *Diabetes Obes Metab* (2011) 13, 770–3.
3. Macha S, Jungnik A, Hohl K, Hobson D, Salsali A, Woerle HJ. Effect of food on the pharmacokinetics of empagliflozin, a sodium glucose cotransporter 2 (SGLT2) inhibitor, and assessment of dose proportionality in health volunteers. *Int J Clin Pharmacol Ther* (2013) 51, 873–9.

Sodium-glucose co-transporter-2 inhibitors + Hormonal contraceptives

The pharmacokinetics of canagliflozin do not appear to be altered by ethinylestradiol or levonorgestrel. Canagliflozin does not appear to alter the exposure to ethinylestradiol or levonorgestrel. Empagliflozin does not affect pharmacokinetics of ethinylestradiol or levonorgestrel.

Clinical evidence, mechanism, importance and management

(a) Canagliflozin

In a pharmacokinetic study, 24 healthy women were given canagliflozin 200 mg daily for 6 days, with a single-dose of a combined hormonal contraceptive (**ethinylestradiol** 30 micrograms with **levonorgestrel** 150 micrograms) given on day 6. The overall exposure of **ethinylestradiol** and **levonorgestrel** were unaffected by canagliflozin, but the maximum concentrations of both drugs were increased by 24% and 28%, respectively.[1] The pharmacokinetics of canagliflozin were not affected upon concurrent use. No canagliflozin dose adjustment would appear necessary on concurrent use. As contraceptive exposure (the overall extent of absorption) is the clinically important factor for contraceptive steroids, and this was unchanged by canagliflozin, no special precautions would appear necessary on concurrent use.

(b) Empagliflozin

In a phase I study, 18 healthy women were given a combined hormonal contraceptive (containing **ethinylestradiol** 30 micrograms and **levonorgestrel** 150 micrograms) once daily for 21 days, with empagliflozin 25 mg once daily given on days 15 to 21. The pharmacokinetics of ethinylestradiol and levonorgestrel were unaffected by concurrent use.[2] No ethinylestradiol or levonorgestrel dose adjustment would therefore appear necessary on concurrent use with empagliflozin.

1. Devineni D, Manitpisitkul P, Vaccaro N, Bernard A, Skee D, Mamidi RN, Tian H, Weiner S, Stieltjes H, Sha S, Rothenberg P. Effect of canagliflozin, a sodium glucose co-transporter 2 inhibitor, on the pharmacokinetics of oral contraceptives, warfarin, and digoxin in healthy participants. *Int J Clin Pharmacol Ther* (2015) 53, 41–53.
2. Macha S, Mattheus M, Pinnetti S, Woerle HJ, Broedl UC. Effect of empagliflozin on the steady-state pharmacokinetics of ethinylestradiol and levonorgestrel in healthy female volunteers. *Clin Drug Investig* (2013) 33, 351–357.

Sodium-glucose co-transporter-2 inhibitors + Metformin

The pharmacokinetics of canagliflozin and metformin and empagliflozin and metformin do not appear to be affected by concurrent use. The pharmacokinetics of dapagliflozin and metformin were not affected by concurrent use in a single-dose study.

Clinical evidence, mechanism, importance and management

(a) Canagliflozin

The US manufacturer of canagliflozin briefly notes that, in a study, a single 2-g dose of metformin increased the AUC of canagliflozin 300 mg daily for 7 days by 10%. Its maximum concentration was unaffected. The AUC of metformin was increased by 20%, but its maximum concentration was unaffected.[1] These changes are not considered to be clinically relevant and no dose adjustments would appear necessary on concurrent use, but note that it is prudent to monitor blood glucose concentrations when any change is made to the medication regimen of a patient with diabetes.

(b) Dapagliflozin

In a randomised, crossover study, 18 healthy subjects were given a single 20-mg dose of dapagliflozin with a single 1-g dose of metformin. There were no changes in the pharmacokinetics of either drug, compared with when they were given alone.[2] No dose adjustments are necessary on concurrent use, but note that it is prudent to monitor blood glucose concentrations when any change is made to the medication regimen of a patient with diabetes.

(c) Empagliflozin

In a randomised, crossover study, 16 healthy subjects were given empagliflozin 50 mg once daily for 9 days, with metformin 1 g twice daily given on days 6 to 8 and metformin 1 g given on the morning of day 9. The pharmacokinetics of both drugs were not affected by concurrent use, compared with each drug given alone.[3] No dose adjustment is necessary upon concurrent use, but note that it is prudent to monitor blood glucose concentrations when any change is made to the medication regimen of a patient with diabetes.

1. Invokana (Canagliflozin). Janssen Pharmaceuticals, Inc. US Prescribing information, September 2015.
2. Kasichayanula S, Liu X, Shyu WC, Zhang W, Pfister M, Griffen SC, Li T, LaCreta FP, Boulton DW. Lack of pharmacokinetic interaction between dapagliflozin, a novel sodium-glucose transporter 2 inhibitor, and metformin, pioglitazone, glimepiride or sitagliptin in healthy subjects. *Diabetes Obes Metab* (2011) 13, 47–54.
3. Macha S, Dieterich S, Mattheus M, Seman LJ, Broedl UC, Woerle HJ. Pharmacokinetics of empagliflozin, a sodium glucose cotransporter-2 (SGLT2) inhibitor, and metformin following co-administration in healthy volunteers. *Clin Pharmacol Ther* (2013) 51, 132–40.

Sodium-glucose co-transporter-2 inhibitors + Miscellaneous

ACE inhibitors or angiotensin II receptor antagonists are predicted to have additive effects with the sodium-glucose co-transporter-2 inhibitors, and might cause dehydration or hypotension. Concurrent use of canagliflozin, dapagliflozin, or empagliflozin with meglitinides might increase the risk of hypoglycaemia.

Clinical evidence, mechanism, importance and management

(a) Drugs affecting the renin-angiotensin system

Due to their mechanism of action, **canagliflozin**, **dapagliflozin**, and **empagliflozin** all cause diuresis and can cause volume depletion and hypotension. As a result, the use of canagliflozin with drugs affecting the renin-angiotensin system, such as **ACE inhibitors** and **angiotensin II receptor antagonists**, is cautioned by the UK manufacturer.[1] Similar caution on the concurrent use of these drugs with dapagliflozin or empagliflozin might be prudent.

(b) Meglitinides

Due to the increased risk of hypoglycaemia seen with **sulfonylureas** in studies (see 'Sodium-glucose co-transporter-2 inhibitors + Sulfonylureas or Insulin', p.537), **insulin secretagogues** (which would include the meglitinides) should be given with caution with **canagliflozin**,[1] **dapagliflozin**,[2] and **empagliflozin**.[3,4] To reduce the risk of hypoglycaemia, consideration should be given to reducing the meglitinide dose.[1,2] Direct evidence for an increased risk of hypoglycaemia if **canagliflozin**, **dapagliflozin**, or **empagliflozin** are given concurrently with repaglinide or nateglinide is lacking, but note that it is prudent to monitor blood glucose concentrations when any change is made to the medication regimen of a patient with diabetes.

1. Invokana (Canagliflozin). Janssen Pharmaceuticals, Inc. US Prescribing information, September 2015.
2. Forxiga (Dapagliflozin propanediol monohydrate). Bristol Myers Squibb-AstraZeneca EEIG. UK Summary of product characteristics, October 2014.
3. Jardiance (Empagliflozin). Boehringer Ingelheim Pharmaceuticals, Inc. US Prescribing information, June 2015.
4. Jardiance (Empagliflozin). Boehringer Ingelheim Ltd. UK Summary of product characteristics, January 2015.

Sodium-glucose co-transporter-2 inhibitors + Pioglitazone

The pharmacokinetics of dapagliflozin and pioglitazone were not affected by concurrent use in a single-dose study. The pharmacokinetics of empagliflozin were increased by pioglitazone in one study, but not affected to a clinically relevant extent in another.

Clinical evidence, mechanism, importance and management

(a) Dapagliflozin

In a randomised, crossover study, 22 healthy subjects were given a single 50-mg dose of dapagliflozin with a single 45-mg dose of pioglitazone. There were no changes in the pharmacokinetics of dapagliflozin, compared with administration alone. The AUC of pioglitazone was unaltered, but the maximum concentration was reduced by 7%.[1] No dose adjustments are necessary on concurrent use, but note that it is prudent to monitor blood glucose concentrations when any change is made to the medication regimen of a patient with diabetes.

(b) Empagliflozin

In a randomised, crossover study, 16 healthy subjects were given empagliflozin 50 mg once daily for 12 days, with pioglitazone 45 mg once daily given on days 6 to 12. The pharmacokinetics of empagliflozin were not affected, but the AUC and maximum concentration of pioglitazone were increased by 50% and 70%, respectively, when compared to pioglitazone alone.[2] As the authors of the study did not expect to see an interaction (pioglitazone is a substrate of CYP2C8, but empagliflozin had no effect on cytochrome P450 isoenzymes *in vitro*), they carried out a second study using a similar crossover design. In the second study, 15 healthy subjects were given pioglitazone 45 mg once daily either alone or with empagliflozin 10 mg, 25 mg, or 50 mg once daily for 7 days. The pharmacokinetics of pioglitazone were not affected to a clinically relevant extent on concurrent use with empagliflozin. The authors state that the dose-adjusted minimum plasma concentrations of empagliflozin were comparable to those seen in the first study.[2]

The reason for the difference in the results between the two studies is not known, however the changes in pioglitazone exposure are unlikely to be clinically relevant, and no dose adjustments would be expected on concurrent use, but note that it is prudent to monitor blood glucose concentrations when any change is made to the medication regimen of a patient with diabetes.

1. Kasichayanula S, Liu X, Shyu WC, Zhang W, Pfister M, Griffen SC, Li T, LaCreta FP, Boulton DW. Lack of pharmacokinetic interaction between dapagliflozin, a novel sodium-glucose transporter 2 inhibitor, and metformin, pioglitazone, glimepiride or sitagliptin in healthy subjects. *Diabetes Obes Metab* (2011) 13, 47–54.
2. Macha S, Mattheus M, Pinnetti S, Broedl UC, Woerle HJ. Pharmacokinetics of empagliflozin and pioglitazone after coadministration in healthy volunteers. *Clin Ther* (2015) 37, 1503–16.

Sodium-glucose co-transporter-2 inhibitors + Probenecid

Probenecid caused a small increase in the exposure to empagliflozin and it negligibly increases the exposure to canagliflozin.

Clinical evidence, mechanism, importance and management

(a) Canagliflozin

In a pharmacokinetic study, 12 healthy subjects were given canagliflozin 300 mg once daily for 17 days with probenecid 500 mg twice daily on days 15 to 17. The AUC and maximum concentration of canagliflozin were increased by 20% and 15%, respectively, when compared with canagliflozin alone.[1] Canagliflozin is a substrate of UGT, and it has been suggested that the increase in canagliflozin exposure is due to possible inhibition of UGT by probenecid.[1] However, this small increase in canagliflozin exposure is not considered to be clinically relevant, and so no dose adjustment is necessary upon concurrent use.

(b) Empagliflozin

In a randomised, crossover study, 18 healthy subjects were given probenecid 500 mg twice daily for 4 days with a single dose of empagliflozin 10 mg on day 2. The AUC and maximum plasma concentration of empagliflozin were increased by 52% and 24%, respectively, when compared with empagliflozin given alone.[2]

Probenecid is an inhibitor of organic anion transporter 3 (OAT3) and possibly also an inhibitor of UGT. Empagliflozin is a substrate, of OAT3 and UGT and therefore the increase in exposure is likely due to one or both of these mechanisms. However, the authors do not consider the small increase in empagliflozin exposure to be clinically relevant, and state that no dose adjustment is necessary upon concurrent use.[2]

1. Devineni D, Vaccaro N, Murphy J, Curtin C, Mamidi RN, Weiner S, Wang SS, Ariyawansa J, Stieltjes H, Wajs E, Di Prospero NA, Rothenberg P. Effect of rifampin, cyclosporine A, and probenecid on the pharmacokinetic profile of canagliflozin, a sodium glucose co-transporter 2 inhibitor, in healthy participants. *Int J Clin Pharmacol Ther* (2015) 53, 115–28.
2. Macha S, Koenen R, Sennewald R, Schöne K, Hummel N, Riedmaier S, Woerle HJ, Salsali A, Broedl UC. Effect of gemfibrozil, rifampicin, or probenecid on the pharmacokinetics of the SGLT2 inhibitor empagliflozin in healthy volunteers. *Clin Ther* (2014) 36, 280–90.

Sodium-glucose co-transporter-2 inhibitors + Rifampicin (Rifampin)

Rifampicin causes a small reduction in dapagliflozin exposure and appears to modestly reduce canagliflozin exposure. Other inducers of glucuronidation might interact similarly. Rifampicin increases the exposure to empagliflozin.

Clinical evidence

(a) Canagliflozin

In a pharmacokinetic study, 14 healthy subjects were given rifampicin (rifampin) 600 mg daily for 9 days with a single 300-mg dose of canagliflozin on day 7. The AUC and maximum concentration were decreased by 51% and 30%, respectively.[1]

(b) Dapagliflozin

In a pharmacokinetic study, 14 healthy subjects were given rifampicin 600 mg daily for 10 days, with dapagliflozin 10 mg daily on days 6 to 8. The AUC of dapagliflozin was reduced by 22%. Only a minor (about 10%) decrease in urinary glucose excretion was seen.[2]

(c) Empagliflozin

In a randomised, crossover study, 18 healthy subjects were given a single dose of empagliflozin 10 mg with a single dose of rifampicin 600 mg. The AUC and maximum plasma concentration of empagliflozin were increased by 35% and 74%, respectively, compared with empagliflozin given alone. The time to maximum concentration was decreased by 30 minutes.[3]

Mechanism

Canagliflozin and dapagliflozin are both primarily metabolised via glucuronidation to inactive metabolites. The glucuronosyltransferase, UGT1A9, is the major enzyme responsible, with UGT2B4 also being involved in the metabolism of canagliflozin. It is suggested that rifampicin induces glucuronidation via these enzymes, resulting in reduced exposure.[1] With regards to the increase in empagliflozin exposure seen, the authors suggest that rifampicin inhibited the organic anion transporter proteins OATP1B1 and OATP1B3,[3] of which empagliflozin is a substrate *in vitro*. The US manufacturer of empagliflozin notes that the effect of induction of glucuronosyltransferases by rifampicin on empagliflozin exposure has not been evaluated.[4] Further study is needed.

Importance and management

A pharmacokinetic interaction appears to occur between rifampicin and canagliflozin, dapagliflozin, or empagliflozin, but might only be clinically important for canagliflozin. The pharmacodynamic effects of the moderate reduction in canagliflozin exposure were not studied, but a reduction in efficacy cannot be ruled out. As such, if concurrent use is unavoidable, and additional glycaemic control is required, consider increasing the canagliflozin dose to 300 mg once daily in patients tolerating canagliflozin 100 mg once daily and whose renal function is satisfactory.[5] Other inducers of glucuronidation might interact similarly; the authors of the canagliflozin study name **carbamazepine**, **efavirenz**, **phenytoin** (and therefore possibly **fosphenytoin**, a prodrug of phenytoin), **phenobarbital** (and therefore possibly **primidone**, which is metabolised to phenobarbital), **ritonavir**, and **St John's wort**.[1]

No dapagliflozin dose adjustment with concurrent rifampicin would appear necessary, and no interaction would be expected with other inducers of glucuronidation.

The increase in empagliflozin exposure is not expected to be clinically relevant, therefore no empagliflozin dose adjustment would appear necessary with the concurrent use of rifampicin.

Note that it is prudent to monitor blood glucose concentrations when any change is made to the medication regimen of a patient with diabetes.

1. Devineni D, Vaccaro N, Murphy J, Curtin C, Mamidi RN, Weiner S, Wang SS, Ariyawansa J, Stieltjes H, Wajs E, Di Prospero NA, Rothenberg P. Effect of rifampin, cyclosporine A, and probenecid on the pharmacokinetic profile of canagliflozin, a sodium glucose co-transporter 2 inhibitor, in healthy participants. *Int J Clin Pharmacol Ther* (2015) 53, 115–28.
2. Kasichayanula S, Liu X, Griffen SC, LaCreta FP, Boulton DW. Effects of rifampin and mefenamic acid on the pharmacokinetics and pharmacodynamics of dapagliflozin. *Diabetes Obes Metab* (2013) 15, 280–3.
3. Macha S, Koenen R, Sennewald R, Schöne K, Hummel N, Riedmaier S, Woerle HJ, Salsali A, Broedl UC. Effect of gemfibrozil, rifampicin, or probenecid on the pharmacokinetics of the SGLT2 inhibitor empagliflozin in healthy volunteers. *Clin Ther* (2014) 36, 280–90.
4. Jardiance (Empagliflozin). Boehringer Ingelheim Pharmaceuticals, Inc. US Prescribing information, June 2015.
5. Invokana (Canagliflozin). Janssen Pharmaceuticals, Inc. US Prescribing information, September 2015.

Sodium-glucose co-transporter-2 inhibitors + Simvastatin

Canagliflozin does not appear to alter the pharmacokinetics of simvastatin. The pharmacokinetics of dapagliflozin were unaffected by simvastatin, and there was a negligible increase in simvastatin exposure on concurrent use. In a single dose study, the pharmacokinetics of empagliflozin and simvastatin were unaffected by concurrent use.

Clinical evidence, mechanism, importance and management

(a) Canagliflozin

The US manufacturer of canagliflozin briefly notes that, in a study, the pharmacokinetics of a single 40-mg dose of simvastatin were unaffected by canagliflozin 300 mg daily for 7 days. The AUC and maximum concentration of simvastatin acid were increased by 18% and 26%, respectively.[1] No simvastatin dose adjustment would appear necessary on concurrent use.

(b) Dapagliflozin

In a randomised, crossover study, 23 healthy subjects were given a single 20-mg dose of dapagliflozin with a single 40-mg dose of simvastatin. The pharmacokinetics of dapagliflozin were unaffected by simvastatin. The AUCs of simvastatin and simvastatin acid were increased by 19% and 30%, respectively, but the maximum concentrations were unaffected.[2] No dapagliflozin dose adjustment appears necessary on concurrent use, but note that it is prudent to monitor blood glucose concentrations when any change is made to the medication regimen of a patient with diabetes. The negligible increase in simvastatin exposure would not indicate any dose adjustment is necessary on concurrent use.

(c) Empagliflozin

In a randomised, cross-over study, 17 healthy subjects were given a single dose of empagliflozin 25 mg with a single dose of simvastatin 40 mg. Simvastatin had no effect on the AUC or maximum concentration of empagliflozin, when compared with empagliflozin given alone. Empagliflozin had no effect on the AUC or maximum concentration of simvastatin or its metabolite, simvastatin acid, compared with simvastatin given alone.[3] No dose adjustment of either drug would appear necessary on concurrent use.

1. Invokana (Canagliflozin). Janssen Pharmaceuticals, Inc. US Prescribing information, September 2015.
2. Kasichayanula S, Chang M, Liu X, Shyu W-C, Griffen SC, LaCreta FP, Boulton DW. Lack of pharmacokinetic interactions between dapagliflozin and simvastatin, valsartan, warfarin or digoxin. *Adv Therapy* (2012) 29, 163–77.
3. Macha S, Lang B, Pinnetti S, Broedl UC. Pharmacokinetics of empagliflozin, a sodium glucose cotransporter-2 inhibitor, and simvastatin following co-administration in healthy volunteers. *Int J Clin Pharmacol* (2014) 52, 973–80.

Sodium-glucose co-transporter-2 inhibitors + Sulfonylureas or Insulin

Canagliflozin does not alter the pharmacokinetics of glibenclamide (glyburide). The pharmacokinetics of dapagliflozin or empagliflozin and glimepiride are not affected by concurrent use. The hypoglycaemic effect of insulin or sulfonylureas might be enhanced by canagliflozin, dapagliflozin, or empagliflozin.

Clinical evidence, mechanism, importance and management

A. Hypoglycaemia.

(a) Canagliflozin

In clinical studies, the incidence of hypoglycaemia was higher when canagliflozin was combined with **insulin** or a **sulfonylurea** than when used alone. As a result, the use of canagliflozin with these antidiabetics is cautioned and a lower dose of insulin or sulfonylurea might be required.[1]

(b) Dapagliflozin

In studies where dapagliflozin was added to a **sulfonylurea** or **insulin**, there were higher incidences of hypoglycaemia than when the sulfonylurea or insulin was used alone. For example, in a study with **glimepiride**, the incidence of minor hypoglycaemia in the group given dapagliflozin and glimepiride was 6%, and in the group given glimepiride alone the incidence was 2.1%. Similarly, in a study with **insulin**, the incidence of minor hypoglycaemia was 40.3% and 53.1% in the combination group and 34% and 41.6% in the insulin alone group after 24 weeks and 104 weeks of concurrent use, respectively. The dose of insulin or sulfonylurea might need to be reduced if used concurrently with dapagliflozin to reduce the risk of hypoglycaemia.[2]

(c) Empagliflozin

The US and UK manufacturers of empagliflozin briefly report that the risk of hypoglycaemia is increased when it is used with **insulin** or a **sulfonylurea**, and that a lower dose of insulin or sulfonylurea might be required to reduce this risk.[3,4]

B. Pharmacokinetics.

(a) Canagliflozin

The US manufacturer of canagliflozin briefly reports that, in a study the pharmacokinetics of a single 1.25-mg dose of **glibenclamide (glyburide)** were not altered by canagliflozin 200 mg daily for 6 days.[1] No pharmacokinetic interaction would appear to occur, but note that the hypoglycaemic effect of sulfonylureas might be enhanced if used concurrently with canagliflozin, see *Hypoglycaemia* above.

(b) Dapagliflozin

In a randomised, cross over study, 18 healthy subjects were given a single 20-mg dose of dapagliflozin with a single 4-mg dose of **glimepiride**. The pharmacokinetics of dapagliflozin were unaffected by **glimepiride**. The maximum concentration of **glimepiride** was unaffected by dapagliflozin and the AUC was not altered to a clinically relevant extent.[5] No clinically important pharmacokinetic interaction occurs between dapagliflozin and **glimepiride**, but note that the hypoglycaemic effect of sulfonylureas might be enhanced if used concurrently with dapagliflozin, see *Hypoglycaemia* above.

(c) Empagliflozin

The US manufacturer of empagliflozin briefly reports that, in a study, subjects were given a single dose of empagliflozin 50 mg with a single dose of **glimepiride** 1 mg. The pharmacokinetics of both drugs were unaffected.[3] No pharmacokinetic interaction would appear to occur on concurrent use, but note that the hypoglycaemic effect of sulfonylureas might be enhanced if used concurrently with empagliflozin, see *Hypoglycaemia* above.

1. Invokana (Canagliflozin). Janssen Pharmaceuticals, Inc. US Prescribing information, September 2015.
2. Forxiga (Dapagliflozin propanediol monohydrate). Bristol Myers Squibb-AstraZeneca EEIG. UK Summary of product characteristics, October 2014.
3. Jardiance (Empagliflozin). Boehringer Ingelheim Pharmaceuticals, Inc. US Prescribing information, June 2015.
4. Jardiance (Empagliflozin). Boehringer Ingelheim Ltd. UK Summary of product characteristics, January 2015.
5. Kasichayanula S, Liu X, Shyu WC, Zhang W, Pfister M, Griffen SC, Li T, LaCreta FP, Boulton DW. Lack of pharmacokinetic interaction between dapagliflozin, a novel sodium-glucose transporter 2 inhibitor, and metformin, pioglitazone, glimepiride or sitagliptin in healthy subjects. *Diabetes Obes Metab* (2011) 13, 47–54.

Sodium-glucose co-transporter-2 inhibitors; Canagliflozin + Ciclosporin

The pharmacokinetics of canagliflozin do not appear to be altered to a clinically relevant extent by ciclosporin.

Clinical evidence, mechanism, importance and management

In a pharmacokinetic study, 17 healthy subjects were given canagliflozin 300 mg daily for 8 days with a single 400-mg dose of ciclosporin on day 8. The AUC of canagliflozin was increased by 25%, but its maximum concentration was not affected.[1]

This increase is not expected to be clinically relevant, and no canagliflozin dose adjustment would appear necessary on concurrent use. However note that canagliflozin is a substrate of the drug transporter P-glycoprotein, which can be inhibited by ciclosporin, and a single-dose of ciclosporin might not be sufficient to exert this effect, such that the effect of repeated doses of ciclosporin might be different. It is prudent to monitor blood glucose concentrations when any change is made to the medication regimen of a patient with diabetes, and this should be sufficient to detect any interaction should it occur on repeated ciclosporin dosing. Further study is needed.

1. Devineni D, Vaccaro N, Murphy J, Curtin C, Mamidi RN, Weiner S, Wang SS, Ariyawansa J, Stieltjes H, Wajs E, Di Prospero NA, Rothenberg P. Effect of rifampin, cyclosporine A, and probenecid on the pharmacokinetic profile of canagliflozin, a sodium glucose co-transporter 2 inhibitor, in healthy participants. *Int J Clin Pharmacol Ther* (2015) 53, 115–28.

Sodium-glucose co-transporter-2 inhibitors; Canagliflozin + Paracetamol (Acetaminophen)

Canagliflozin does not appear to alter the pharmacokinetics of paracetamol (acetaminophen).

Clinical evidence, mechanism, importance and management

The US manufacturer of canagliflozin briefly notes that, in a study, the pharmacokinetics of a single 1-g dose of paracetamol (acetaminophen) were not altered by canagliflozin 300 mg twice daily for 25 days.[1] No dose adjustment would appear necessary on concurrent use.

1. Invokana (Canagliflozin). Janssen Pharmaceuticals, Inc. US Prescribing information, September 2015.

Sodium-glucose co-transporter-2 inhibitors; Dapagliflozin + Alpha-glucosidase inhibitors; Voglibose

The pharmacokinetics of dapagliflozin are not affected by voglibose.

Clinical evidence, mechanism, importance and management

In a study in 22 type 2 diabetics given a single 10-mg dose of dapagliflozin with voglibose 200 micrograms three times daily, the pharmacokinetics of dapagliflozin were unchanged, when compared with when it was given alone.[1] No dapagliflozin dose adjustment would seem necessary on concurrent use. However, note that it is prudent to monitor blood glucose concentrations when any change is made the medication regimen of a patient with diabetes.

1. Imamura A, Kusunoki M, Ueda S, Hayashi N, Imai Y. Impact of voglibose on the pharmacokinetics of dapagliflozin in Japanese patients with type 2 diabetes. *Diabetes Ther* (2013) 4, 41–9.

Sodium-glucose co-transporter-2 inhibitors; Dapagliflozin + Angiotensin II receptor antagonists; Valsartan

In a single-dose study, the pharmacokinetics of dapagliflozin and valsartan were not affected by concurrent use.

Clinical evidence, mechanism, importance and management

In a randomised, crossover study,[1] 23 healthy subjects were given a single 20-mg dose of dapagliflozin with a single 320-mg dose of valsartan. The maximum concentration of dapagliflozin was reduced by 12%, when compared with when given alone, but its AUC was unaffected. The valsartan AUC was increased by 6% and its maximum concentration was reduced by 6%. These changes were not considered clinically important and no dose adjustments would seem necessary on concurrent use. However, note that it is prudent to monitor blood glucose concentrations when any change is made to the medication regimen of a patient with diabetes.

1. Kasichayanula S, Chang M, Liu X, Shyu W-C, Griffen SC, LaCreta FP, Boulton DW. Lack of pharmacokinetic interactions between dapagliflozin and simvastatin, valsartan, warfarin or digoxin. *Adv Therapy* (2012) 29, 163–77.

Sodium-glucose co-transporter-2 inhibitors; Dapagliflozin + Mefenamic acid

Mefenamic acid modestly increases dapagliflozin exposure.

Clinical evidence

In a pharmacokinetic study, 16 healthy subjects were given mefenamic acid 250 mg with dapagliflozin 10 mg, followed by mefenamic acid 250 mg every 6 hours (11 doses), for 3 days. The AUC of dapagliflozin was increased by 51%, and there was an increase in urinary glucose excretion of about 18%.[1]

Mechanism

Dapagliflozin is primarily metabolised via glucuronidation to an inactive metabolite, with the glucuronyltransferase UGT1A9 being the major enzyme responsible. The authors[1] suggest that mefenamic acid inhibits UGT1A9, and hence increases dapagliflozin exposure. Further study is needed to confirm the action of mefenamic acid on UGT1A9.

Importance and management

The exposure to dapagliflozin is modestly increased by mefenamic acid, but this appears to be of no clinical importance. No dapagliflozin dose adjustment would appear necessary on concurrent use, but note that it is prudent to monitor blood glucose concentrations when any change is made to the medication regimen of a patient with diabetes.

1. Kasichayanula S, Liu X, Griffen SC, LaCreta FP, Boulton DW. Effects of rifampicin and mefenamic acid on the pharmacokinetics and pharmacodynamics of dapagliflozin. *Diabetes Obes Metab* (2013) 15, 280–3.

Sodium-glucose co-transporter-2 inhibitors; Empagliflozin + Gemfibrozil

The concurrent use of gemfibrozil and empagliflozin resulted in a small increase in empagliflozin exposure in one study.

Clinical evidence

In a randomised, crossover study, 18 healthy subjects were given gemfibrozil 600 mg twice a day for 5 days with a single-dose of empagliflozin 25 mg on day 3. The AUC and maximum concentration of empagliflozin were increased by 60% and 17%, respectively, when compared with empagliflozin alone.[1]

Mechanism

Gemfibrozil is an inhibitor of the organic anion transporting polypeptide, OATP1B1. Empagliflozin is a substrate of this transporter and concurrent use increases empagliflozin exposure.

Importance and management

Evidence of an interaction between empagliflozin and gemfibrozil is limited to one single-dose study. However, the increase in the exposure to empagliflozin seen does not appear to be clinically relevant, and the authors of the study suggest that no empagliflozin dose adjustment is necessary upon concurrent use.[1]

1. Macha S, Koenen R, Sennewald R, Schöne K, Hummel N, Riedmaier S, Woerle HJ, Salsali A, Broedl UC. Effect of gemfibrozil, rifampicin, or probenecid on the pharmacokinetics of the SGLT2 inhibitor empagliflozin in healthy volunteers. *Clin Ther* (2014) 36, 280–90.

Sodium-glucose co-transporter-2 inhibitors; Empagliflozin + Ramipril

Concurrent use of empagliflozin and ramipril negligibly increases the exposure to ramipril, but does not affect the exposure to empagliflozin.

Clinical evidence, mechanism, importance and management

In a randomised, crossover study, 22 healthy subjects were given empagliflozin 25 mg once daily with ramipril (2.5 mg on day one, then 5 mg once daily) for 5 days. The AUC and maximum concentration of ramipril were increased by 11% and 9%, respectively, however, the AUC and maximum concentration of ramiprilat, the active metabolite of ramipril, were not affected by concurrent use. The AUC and maximum concentration of empagliflozin were also not affected.[1] The increase in ramipril is not considered to be clinically relevant, therefore no dose adjustment is required upon concurrent use.

1. Macha S, Sennewald R, Rose P, Schoene K, Pinnetti S, Woerle HJ, Broedl UC. Lack of clinically relevant drug-drug interaction between empagliflozin, a sodium glucose cotransporter 2 inhibitor, and verapamil, ramipril, or digoxin in healthy volunteers. *Clin Ther* (2013) 35, 226–35.

Sodium-glucose co-transporter-2 inhibitors; Empagliflozin + Verapamil

The pharmacokinetics of empagliflozin were not altered by concurrent use of verapamil in a single-dose study.

Clinical evidence, mechanism, importance and management

In a randomised, crossover study, 16 healthy subjects were given a single 25-mg dose of empagliflozin followed by a single 120-mg dose of verapamil, one hour later. The AUC and maximum concentration of empagliflozin were not affected on concurrent use, compared with empagliflozin given alone.[1]

In vitro, empagliflozin has been shown to be a substrate of P-glycoprotein.[1] Verapamil is a P-glycoprotein inhibitor, but its apparent lack of effect on empagliflozin exposure suggests that empagliflozin is not a substrate for this transporter protein *in vivo*. No dose adjustment would appear to be required upon the concurrent use of verapamil and empagliflozin. Other drugs which are inducers or inhibitors of P-glycoprotein might not be expected to affect the exposure to empagliflozin by this mechanism (see 'Table 1.12', p.14 for a list).

1. Macha S, Sennewald R, Rose P, Schoene K, Pinnetti S, Woerle HJ, Broedl UC. Lack of clinically relevant drug-drug interaction between empagliflozin, a sodium glucose cotransporter 2 inhibitor, and verapamil, ramipril, or digoxin in healthy volunteers. *Clin Ther* (2013) 35, 226–35.

Sulfonylureas + ACE inhibitors

No pharmacokinetic interaction appears to occur between spirapril and glibenclamide. An isolated report describes pancytopenia after glipizide was started in a patient already taking enalapril.

Clinical evidence

(a) Glibenclamide (Glyburide)

A brief report states that **spirapril** did not have a pharmacokinetic interaction with glibenclamide (glyburide).[1]

(b) Glipizide

An isolated case report describes pancytopenia (possibly drug related) in a 72-year old man taking **enalapril**, an alpha blocker, and a calcium antagonist, shortly after he started to take glipizide 5 mg twice daily for diabetes.[2]

Mechanism

Blood dyscrasias are a rare adverse effect of ACE inhibitors used alone, and have also occurred with glipizide alone. Whether concurrent use could increase this risk is uncertain.

Importance and management

No pharmacokinetic interaction appears to occur between glibenclamide and spirapril. The isolated case of pancytopenia when glipizide was given with enalapril is probably of limited general relevance. For discussion of the potential hypoglycaemic effects of combining sulfonylureas and ACE inhibitors, see 'Antidiabetics + ACE inhibitors', p.499.

1. Grass P, Gerbeau C, Kutz K. Spirapril: pharmacokinetic properties and drug interactions. *Blood Press Suppl* (1994) 2, 7–13.
2. Ocaña J, Torres M, Gómez Navarro L, Chevarría JL. Pancitopenia como efecto indeseable de la asociación de enalapril y glipizida en la insuficiencia renal. *Nefrologia* (2007) 27, 655–6.

Sulfonylureas + Alcohol

A flushing reaction is common in patients taking chlorpropamide who drink alcohol, but is less common with other sulfonylureas. Limited evidence suggests that alcoholic patients might require above-average doses of tolbutamide.

Clinical evidence

(a) Effect on glucose concentrations

Alcohol has been reported to prolong, but not increase, the blood glucose-lowering effects of **glipizide**,[1] but wine had little effect on the blood glucose concentrations of patients taking tolbutamide.[2] Another study in 10 elderly patients (age range 60 to 75 years) with type 2 diabetes taking **glibenclamide** 20 mg daily found that intravenous infusion of ethanol (equivalent to one to 2 units of alcoholic drinks) greatly decreased the nadir plasma glucose concentration during a fast.[3]

(b) Flushing reaction

About one-third of patients taking **chlorpropamide** who drink alcohol, even in quite small amounts, experience a warm, tingling or burning sensation of the face, and sometimes the neck and arms as well. It might also involve the conjunctivae. This can begin within 5 to 20 minutes of drinking, reaching a peak within 30 to 40 minutes, and can persist for one to 2 hours. Very occasionally headache occurs, and light-headedness, palpitations, wheezing, and breathlessness have also been experienced.[4,5]

This disulfiram-like flushing reaction has been described in numerous reports (far too many to list here) involving large numbers of patients taking **chlorpropamide**. These reports have been extensively reviewed.[4,6-8] A similar reaction can occur, but much less frequently, with other sulfonylureas including **carbutamide**,[9] **glibenclamide (glyburide)**,[5,10] **gliclazide**,[11] **glipizide**,[5] **tolazamide**,[12] and **tolbutamide**,[13,14] especially when wine was consumed on an empty stomach.[2] In one crossover study, evident flushing phenomenon after an oral ethanol-loading test was seen in 6 of 10 patients taking **chlorpropamide**, 3 of 10 taking **tolbutamide**, 2 of 10 taking **glibenclamide**, one of 10 taking **glibornuride**, and none of 10 taking **glipizide**.[15]

(c) Pharmacokinetic effects

A study found that the mean half-life of **tolbutamide** in alcoholics was about one-third lower than in control subjects.[16]

Mechanism

The chlorpropamide-alcohol flush reaction, although extensively studied, is by no means fully understood. It seems to be related to the disulfiram-alcohol reaction, and is accompanied by an increase in blood-acetaldehyde concentrations (see also 'Alcohol + Disulfiram', p.67). It also appears to be genetically determined[5] and might involve both prostaglandins and endogenous opioids.[17] The decreased half-life of tolbutamide in alcoholics is probably due to the inducing effects of alcohol on liver microsomal enzymes.[16,18,19]

Importance and management

The **chlorpropamide**-alcohol interaction (flushing reaction) is very well documented, and while established, is of minimal importance. It is a nuisance and possibly socially embarrassing but normally requires no treatment. Patients should be warned about the reaction. The incidence is said to lie between 13 and 33%[20,21] although one study claims that it might be as low as 4%.[22] As it can be provoked by quite small amounts of alcohol (half a glass of sherry or wine) it is virtually impossible for sensitive patients to avoid it if they drink. Most manufacturers issue warnings about the possibility of this reaction with other sulfonylureas, but it is very rarely seen and can therefore almost always be avoided by replacing chlorpropamide with another sulfonylurea.

Alcoholic individuals might need above-average doses of tolbutamide.

For general advice about the consumption of alcohol in diabetes, see 'Antidiabetics + Alcohol', p.501.

1. Hartling SG, Faber OK, Wegmann M-L, Wahlin-Boll E and Melander A. Interaction of ethanol and glipizide in humans. *Diabetes Care* (1987) 10, 683–6.
2. Lolli G, Balboni C, Ballatore C, Risoldi L, Carletti D, Silvestri L, Pacifici De Tommaso G. Wine in the diets of diabetic patients. *Q J Stud Alcohol* (1963) 24, 412–6.
3. Burge MR, Zeise T-M, Sobhy TA, Rassam AG, Schade DS. Low-dose ethanol predisposes elderly fasted patients with type 2 diabetes to sulfonylurea-induced low blood glucose. *Diabetes Care* (1999) 22, 2037–43.
4. Johnston C, Wiles PG, Pyke DA. Chlorpropamide-alcohol flush: the case in favour. *Diabetologia* (1984) 26, 1–5.
5. Leslie RDG, Pyke DA. Chlorpropamide-alcohol flushing: a dominantly inherited trait associated with diabetes. *BMJ* (1978) 2, 1519–21.
6. Hillson RM, Hockaday TDR. Chlorpropamide-alcohol flush: a critical reappraisal. *Diabetologia* (1984) 26, 6–11.
7. Waldhäusl W. To flush or not to flush? Comments on the chlorpropamide-alcohol flush. *Diabetologia* (1984) 26, 12–14.
8. Groop L, Eriksson CJP, Huupponen R, Ylikarhi R, Pelkonen R. Roles of chlorpropamide, alcohol and acetaldehyde in determining the chlorpropamide-alcohol flush. *Diabetologia* (1984) 26, 34–38.
9. Signorelli S. Tolerance for alcohol in patients on chlorpropamide. *Ann N Y Acad Sci* (1959) 74, 900–903.
10. Stowers JM. Alcohol and glibenclamide. *BMJ* (1971) 3, 533.
11. Conget JI, Vendrell J, Esmatjes E, Halperin I. Gliclazide alcohol flush. *Diabetes Care* (1989) 12, 44.

12. McKendry JBR, Gfeller KF. Clinical experience with the oral antidiabetic compound tolazamide. *Can Med Assoc J* (1967) 96, 531–5.
13. Dolger H. Experience with the tolbutamide treatment of five hundred cases of diabetes on an ambulatory basis. *Ann N Y Acad Sci* (1957) 71, 275–9.
14. Büttner H. Äthanolunverträglichkeit beim Menschen nach Sulfonylharnstoffen. *Dtsch Arch Klin Med* (1961) 207, 1–18.
15. Lao B, Czyzyk A, Szutowski M, Szczepanik Z. Alcohol tolerance in patients with non-insulin-dependent (type 2) diabetes treated with sulphonylurea derivatives. *Arzneimittelforschung* (1994) 44, 727–34.
16. Carulli N, Manenti F, Gallo M, Salvioli GF. Alcohol-drugs interaction in man: alcohol and tolbutamide. *Eur J Clin Invest* (1971) 1, 421–4.
17. Johnston C, Wiles PG, Medbak S, Bowcock S, Cooke ED, Pyke DA, Rees LH. The role of endogenous opioids in the chlorpropamide alcohol flush. *Clin Endocrinol (Oxf)* (1984) 21, 489–97.
18. Kater RMH, Roggin G, Tobon F, Zieve P, Iber FL. Increased rate of clearance of drugs from the circulation of alcoholics. *Am J Med Sci* (1969) 258, 35–9.
19. Kater RMH, Tobon F, Iber FL. Increased rate of tolbutamide metabolism in alcoholic patients. *JAMA* (1969) 207, 363–5.
20. Fitzgerald MG, Gaddie R, Malins JM, O'Sullivan DJ. Alcohol sensitivity in diabetics receiving chlorpropamide. *Diabetes* (1962) 11, 40–3.
21. Daeppen JP, Hofstetter JR, Curchod B, Saudan Y. Traitment oral du diabete par un nouvel hypoglycemiant, le P 607 ou Diabinese. *Schweiz Med Wochenschr* (1959) 89, 817–19.
22. De Silva NE, Tunbridge WMG, Alberti KGMM. Low incidence of chlorpropamide-alcohol flushing in diet-treated, non-insulin-dependent diabetics. *Lancet* (1981) i, 128–31.

Sulfonylureas + Allopurinol

Severe hypoglycaemia and coma occurred in one patient taking gliclazide and allopurinol. The half-life of chlorpropamide was increased after the addition of allopurinol in 3 patients. Allopurinol caused a minor decrease in the half-life of tolbutamide in healthy subjects.

Clinical evidence

(a) Chlorpropamide

A brief report describes 6 patients taking chlorpropamide with allopurinol. The half-life of chlorpropamide in one patient with gout and normal renal function exceeded 200 hours (normally 36 hours) after allopurinol had been taken for 10 days, and in 2 other patients the half-life of chlorpropamide was extended to 44 hours and 55 hours. The other 3 patients were given allopurinol for only one or 2 days and the half-life of chlorpropamide remained unaltered.[1]

(b) Gliclazide

Severe hypoglycaemia (1.6 mmol/L) and coma occurred in a patient with renal impairment taking gliclazide and allopurinol.[2] Hypoglycaemia has been seen in another patient taking both drugs, but an interaction is less clear, as enalapril and ranitidine, which might also (rarely) interact were also involved.[2]

(c) Tolbutamide

In 10 healthy subjects, allopurinol 2.5 mg/kg twice daily for 15 days reduced the half-life of intravenous tolbutamide by 25% (from 360 to 267 minutes).[3,4]

Mechanism

Not understood. In the case of chlorpropamide it has been suggested that the interaction possibly involves some competition for renal tubular mechanisms.[1]

Importance and management

Information regarding interactions between the sulfonylureas and allopurinol is very limited. Only gliclazide has been implicated in severe hypoglycaemia with allopurinol and there seem to be no reports of either grossly enhanced hypoglycaemia with chlorpropamide and allopurinol, or a reduced effect with tolbutamide and allopurinol. Nevertheless, one UK manufacturer of glimepiride, predicts that allopurinol might potentiate its glucose-lowering effects, and warns that hypoglycaemia might occur on concurrent use.[5] More study is needed to find out whether any of these interactions have general clinical importance, but it seems unlikely.

1. Petitpierre B, Perrin L, Rudhardt M, Herrera A, Fabre J. Behaviour of chlorpropamide in renal insufficiency and under the effect of associated drug therapy. *Int J Clin Pharmacol* (1972) 6, 120–4.
2. Girardin E, Vial T, Pham E, Evreux J-C. Hypoglycémies induites par les sulfamides hypoglycémiants. *Ann Med Interne (Paris)* (1992) 143, 11–17.
3. Gentile S, Porcellini M, Loguercio C, Foglia F, Coltorti M. Modificazioni della depurazione plasmatica di tolbutamide e rifamicina-SV indotte dal trattamento con allopurinolo in volontari sono. *Progr Med (Napoli)* (1979) 35, 637–42.
4. Gentile S, Porcellini M, Foglia F, Loguercio C, Coltorti M. Influenza di allopurinolo sull'emivita plasmatica di tolbutamide e rifamicina-SV in soggetti sani. *Boll Soc Ital Biol Sper* (1979) 55, 345–8.
5. Amaryl (Glimepiride). Zentiva. UK Summary of product characteristics, October 2013.

Sulfonylureas + Angiotensin II receptor antagonists

Glibenclamide (glyburide) causes a small reduction in valsartan exposure. No pharmacokinetic interaction occurs between glibenclamide and candesartan or between tolbutamide and irbesartan. Eprosartan does not alter the efficacy of glibenclamide.

Clinical evidence and mechanism

(a) Candesartan

In a randomised, crossover study in 12 healthy male subjects, **glibenclamide (glyburide)** 3.5 mg daily did not alter the pharmacokinetics of candesartan 16 mg daily, both given for 7 days. The pharmacokinetics of glibenclamide were not altered by the candesartan.[1]

(b) Eprosartan

In a randomised, crossover study, 15 patients with type 2 diabetes stable taking **glibenclamide (glyburide)** 3.75 to 10 mg daily for at least 30 days, were given eprosartan 200 mg twice daily for 7 days or placebo. Eprosartan had no effect on their 24-hour plasma glucose concentrations. No pharmacokinetic data were reported.[2]

(c) Irbesartan

A study in 18 healthy subjects given irbesartan 300 mg daily and **tolbutamide** 1 g daily, either alone or in combination, found no difference in the pharmacokinetics of either drug.[3]

(d) Valsartan

In a randomised, crossover study, 12 healthy subjects were given single oral doses of valsartan 160 mg and **glibenclamide (glyburide)** 1.75 mg, alone and together.[4] Glibenclamide decreased the valsartan AUC by 16%, but the plasma concentrations of valsartan showed wide variations between subjects. The pharmacokinetics of glibenclamide were not affected.[4]

Importance and management

No pharmacokinetic interaction occurs between candesartan and glibenclamide or irbesartan and tolbutamide and no special precautions are necessary if given together. The slight increase in valsartan concentrations seen with glibenclamide is unlikely to be clinically important and no special precautions would seem necessary on concurrent use. Similarly, eprosartan did not alter the glycaemic effects of glibenclamide and concurrent use requires no special precautions. Nevertheless, it is prudent to monitor blood glucose concentrations when any change is made to the medication regimen of a patient with diabetes. For discussion of the potential hypoglycaemic effects of combining sulfonylureas and angiotensin II receptor antagonists, see 'Antidiabetics + Angiotensin II receptor antagonists', p.502.

1. Jonkman JHG, van Lier JJ, van Heiningen PNM, Lins R, Sennewald R, Högemann A. Pharmacokinetic drug interaction studies with candesartan cilexetil. *J Hum Hypertens* (1997) 11 (Suppl 2), S31–S35.
2. Martin DE, DeCherney GS, Ilson BE, Jones BA, Boike SC, Freed MI, Jorasky DK. Eprosartan, an angiotensin II receptor antagonist, does not affect the pharmacodynamics of glyburide in patients with type II diabetes mellitus. *J Clin Pharmacol* (1997) 37, 155–9.
3. Marino MR, Vachharajani NN. Drug interactions with irbesartan. *Clin Pharmacokinet* (2001) 40, 605–14.
4. Novartis Pharmaceuticals Ltd. Data on file. Protocol 52.

Sulfonylureas + Antacids

The rate of absorption of some sulfonylureas is increased by some antacids, but there appear to be no reports of adverse responses in diabetic patients as a result of any of these interactions.

Clinical evidence

(a) Chlorpropamide

Magnesium hydroxide 850 mg increased the rate of absorption of chlorpropamide 250 mg in healthy subjects, but the insulin and glucose responses were unaffected.[1]

(b) Glibenclamide (Glyburide)

A randomised, crossover, single-dose study in 7 healthy subjects found that **magnesium hydroxide** 850 mg had little effect on the rate or extent of absorption of a micronised glibenclamide preparation (*Semi-Euglucon*), but in a similar study in 6 healthy subjects it caused a 3-fold increase in the maximum plasma concentration and the bioavailability of a non-micronised preparation (*Gilemid*).[2] *Maalox* (**aluminium/magnesium hydroxide**) increased the AUC of glibenclamide (given as *Daonil*) by one-third, and increased its maximum serum concentration by 50%.[3]

Sodium bicarbonate 1 to 3 g considerably increased the early bioavailability of non-micronised glibenclamide in healthy subjects, but its overall exposure and the insulin and glucose responses remained unaltered.[4]

(c) Glipizide

Sodium bicarbonate 3 g greatly increased the absorption of glipizide 5 mg and enhanced its effects to some extent, but the total absorption was unaltered.[5] The 30 minute, 1-hour, and 2-hour AUCs, were increased 6-fold, 4-fold, and 2-fold, respectively, and the time to reach the maximum serum concentration decreased from 2.5 hours to one hour. **Aluminium hydroxide** 1 g did not appear to affect the absorption of glipizide 5 mg.[5] **Magnesium hydroxide** 850 mg considerably increased the rate of absorption of glipizide 5 mg: the 30-minute and one-hour AUCs being increased by 180% and 69%, respectively.[6]

(d) Tolbutamide

In 8 healthy subjects **magnesium hydroxide** 850 mg increased the 1-hour and 2-hour AUCs of a single 500-mg dose of tolbutamide 5-fold and 2.5-fold, respectively when compared to a control group not given magnesium hydroxide. The total AUC was unaffected. The maximum insulin response was increased 4-fold and occurred about an hour earlier, and the glucose responses were also larger, and occurred earlier.[1]

Mechanism

Uncertain. The small increase in gastric pH caused by these antacids possibly increases the solubility of these sulfonylureas and therefore increases their absorption.[7]

Importance and management

Although some interactions between antacids and sulfonylureas have occurred in studies, no reports of adverse reactions appear to have been published. However, note

Table 13.5 Interactions between sulfonylureas and sulfonamides

Drugs	*Information documented*	*Refs*
Chlorpropamide		
+ sulfafurazole (sulfisoxazole)	1 case of acute hypoglycaemia	1
+ sulfadimidine	1 case of acute hypoglycaemia	2
+ co-trimoxazole	2 cases of acute hypoglycaemia	3, 4
Glibenclamide		
+ co-trimoxazole	In a large review of glibenclamide-associated hypoglycaemia 6 of 57 patients were also taking co-trimoxazole 1 case of hypoglycaemia No pharmacokinetic interaction in 8 patients	5 6 7
Glibornuride		
+ sulfaphenazole	Half-life increased by 34% in 4 subjects (2 diabetic, 2 healthy)	8
Gliclazide		
+ co-trimoxazole	4 cases of acute hypoglycaemia	6
Glipizide		
+ co-trimoxazole	1 case of acute hypoglycaemia No pharmacokinetic interaction, or change in blood glucose-lowering effects in 8 healthy subjects	9 10
Tolbutamide		
+ co-trimoxazole	Clearance of intravenous tolbutamide reduced by 25%, half-life increased by 30% in 7 healthy subjects	12
+ sulfafurazole (sulfisoxazole)	3 cases of severe hypoglycaemia No pharmacokinetic interaction	13, 14 15, 16
+ sulfamethizole	Half-life of tolbutamide increased 60%. Metabolic clearance reduced by about 40%	17
+ sulfaphenazole	Two cases of severe hypoglycaemia Half-life of tolbutamide increased three to sixfold	16 15, 16, 18, 19, 20
+ sulfadiazine	Half-life of tolbutamide increased by about 57%	18
+ sulfadimethoxine	No pharmacokinetic interaction	15, 16
+ sulfamethoxazole	Clearance reduced 14%, half-life increased 20% after intravenous use Half-life increased by about 65%	12 15
+ sulfamethoxypyridazine	No pharmacokinetic interaction	16
Unnamed sulfonylurea		
+ co-trimoxazole	1 case of acute hypoglycaemia	11

1. Tucker HSG, Hirsch JI. Sulfonamide-sulfonylurea interaction. *N Engl J Med* (1972) 286, 110–11.
2. Dall JLC, Conway H, McAlpine SG. Hypoglycaemia due to chlorpropamide. *Scott Med J* (1967) 12, 403–4.
3. Ek I. Långvarigt klorpropamidutlöst hypoglykemitillstand Låkemedelsinteraktion? *Lakartidningen* (1974) 71, 2597–8.
4. Baciewicz AM, Swafford WB. Hypoglycemia induced by the interaction of chlorpropamide and co-trimoxazole. *Drug Intell Clin Pharm* (1984) 18, 309–10.
5. Asplund K, Wiholm B-E, Lithner F. Glibenclamide-associated hypoglycaemia: a report on 57 cases. *Diabetologia* (1983) 24, 412–7.
6. Girardin E, Vial T, Pham E, Evreux J-C. Hypoglycémies induites par les sulfamides hypoglycémiants. *Ann Med Interne* (Paris) (1992) 143, 11–17.
7. Sjöberg S, Wiholm BE, Gunnarsson R, Emilsson H, Thunberg E, Christenson I, Östman J. Lack of pharmacokinetic interaction between glibenclamide and trimethoprim-sulphamethoxazole. *Diabet Med* (1987) 4, 245–7.
8. Eckhardt W, Rudolph R, Sauer H, Schubert WR, Undeutsch D. Zur pharmakologischen Interferenz von Glibornurid mit Sulfaphenazol, Phenylbutazon und Phenprocoumon beim Menschen. *Arzneimittelforschung* (1972) 22, 2212–19.
9. Johnson JF, Dobmeier ME. Symptomatic hypoglycemia secondary to a glipizide-trimethoprim/sulfamethoxazole drug interaction. *DICP Ann Pharmacother* (1990) 24, 250–1.
10. Kradjan WA, Witt DM, Opheim KE, Wood FC. Lack of interaction between glipizide and co-trimoxazole. *J Clin Pharmacol* (1994) 34, 997–1002.
11. Mihic M, Mautner LS, Feness JZ, Grant K. Effect of trimethoprim-sulfamethoxazole on blood insulin and glucose concentrations of diabetics. *Can Med Assoc J* (1975), 112, 80S–82S.
12. Wing LMH, Miners JO. Cotrimoxazole as an inhibitor of oxidative drug metabolism: effects of trimethoprim and sulphamethoxazole separately and combined on tolbutamide disposition. *Br J Clin Pharmacol* (1985) 20, 482–5.
13. Soeldner JS, Steinke J. Hypoglycemia in tolbutamide-treated diabetes. *JAMA* (1965) 193, 148–9.
14. Robinson DS. The application of basic principles of drug interaction to clinical practice. *J Urol* (1975) 113, 100–107.
15. Dubach UC, Buckert A, Raaflaub J. Einfluss von Sulfonamiden auf die blutzuckersenkende Wirkung oraler Antidiabetica. *Schweiz Med Wochenschr* (1966) 96, 1483–6.
16. Christensen LK, Hansen JM, Kristensen M. Sulphaphenazole-induced hypoglycaemic attacks in tolbutamide-treated diabetics. *Lancet* (1963) ii, 1298–1301.
17. Lumholtz B, Siersbaek-Nielsen K, Skovsted L, Kampmann J, Hansen JM. Sulphamethizole-induced inhibition of diphenylhydantoin, tolbutamide, and warfarin metabolism. *Clin Pharmacol Ther* (1975) 17, 731–4.
18. Kristensen M, Christensen LK. Drug induced changes of the blood glucose lowering effect of oral hypoglycemic agents. *Acta Diabetol Lat* (1969) 6 (Suppl 1), 116–23.
19. Back DJ, Tjia J, Mönig H, Ohnhaus EE, Park BK. Selective inhibition of drug oxidation after simultaneous administration of two probe drugs, antipyrine and tolbutamide. *Eur J Clin Pharmacol* (1988) 34, 157–63.
20. Veronese ME, Miners JO, Randles D, Gregov D, Birkett DJ. Validation of the tolbutamide metabolic ratio for population screening with use of sulfaphenazole to produce model phenotypic poor metabolizers. *Clin Pharmacol Ther* (1990) 47, 403–11.

that patients taking glipizide with sodium bicarbonate or magnesium hydroxide, or tolbutamide with magnesium hydroxide might experience transient hypoglycaemia. Generally no action seems necessary, but if a problem does occur, separating the doses as much as possible would probably minimise any effects. Giving glibenclamide 30 minutes to one hour before the antacid has been suggested as a strategy to minimise any interaction.[3]

1. Kivistö KT, Neuvonen PJ. Effect of magnesium hydroxide on the absorption and efficacy of tolbutamide and chlorpropamide. *Eur J Clin Pharmacol* (1992) 42, 675–80.
2. Neuvonen PJ, Kivistö KT. The effects of magnesium hydroxide on the absorption and efficacy of two glibenclamide preparations. *Br J Clin Pharmacol* (1991) 32, 215–20.
3. Zuccaro P, Pacifici R, Pichini S, Avico U, Federzoni G, Pini LA, Sternieri E. Influence of antacids on the bioavailability of glibenclamide. *Drugs Exp Clin Res* (1989) 15, 165–9.
4. Kivistö KT, Lehto P, Neuvonen PJ. The effects of different doses of sodium bicarbonate on the absorption and activity of non-micronized glibenclamide. *Int J Clin Pharmacol Ther Toxicol* (1993) 31, 236–40.
5. Kivistö KT, Neuvonen PJ. Differential effects of sodium bicarbonate and aluminium hydroxide on the absorption and activity of glipizide. *Eur J Clin Pharmacol* (1991) 40, 383–6.
6. Kivistö KT, Neuvonen PJ. Enhancement of absorption and effect of glipizide by magnesium hydroxide. *Clin Pharmacol Ther* (1991) 49, 39–43.
7. Lehto P, Laine K, Kivistö K, Neuvonen PJ. The effect of pH on the *in vitro* dissolution of sulfonylurea preparations — a mechanism for the antacid-sulfonylurea interaction? *Therapie* (1995) 50 (Suppl), 413.

Sulfonylureas + Antibacterials; Sulfonamides and/or Trimethoprim

The blood glucose-lowering effects of some of the sulfonylureas are increased by some, but not all, sulfonamides. Occasionally and unpredictably acute hypoglycaemia has occurred in individual patients taking various combinations of sulfonamides and sulfonylureas. Trimethoprim negligibly reduces the clearance of tolbutamide. Co-trimoxazole alone can rarely cause hypoglycaemia.

Clinical evidence

Numerous case reports and studies of the effects of concurrent sulfonylurea and sulfonamide use exist, the details of which are summarised in 'Table 13.5', p.541.

(a) Co-trimoxazole

In a large, retrospective, case-control study, of 7 414 patients taking **glibenclamide (glyburide)**, and hospitalised or given emergency treatment for hypoglycaemia, 73 had recently received a course of **co-trimoxazole**. For those who took **co-trimoxazole** within days one to 5 or days 6 to 10 of the hypoglycaemic episode, the adjusted odds ratio for the risk of developing hypoglycaemia on the concurrent use of **glibenclamide** was 1.6 and 2.7, respectively, when compared with cefalexin (which was used a non-interacting control). Of the 5 559 patients who were taking **glipizide**, and hospitalised or given emergency treatment for hypoglycaemia, 73 had recently received a course of **co-trimoxazole**. For those who took **co-trimoxazole** within days one to 5 or days 6 to 10 of the diagnosis of hypoglycaemia, the adjusted odds ratio for the risk of an interaction was 2.4 and 3.1, respectively, when compared with cefalexin. Note that the concurrent use of **glibenclamide** or **glipizide** with cefalexin increased the risk of severe hypoglycaemia, which indicates that infection *per se* contributes to the increased risk of hypoglycaemia in patients also taking antibacterials.[1] Similarly, a 7-year, case-control study in elderly patients found that 909 patients taking **glibenclamide**, and admitted to hospital with hypoglycaemia, were over 6 times more likely to have also been taking co-trimoxazole (adjusted odds ratio, 6.6) in the previous week, compared with control patients receiving glibenclamide who were not admitted for hypoglycaemia. The concurrent use of glibenclamide with amoxicillin (used as a non-interacting control) was not associated with an increased risk of hypoglycaemia (adjusted odds ratio, 1.5).[2]

For a report of the concurrent use of co-trimoxazole and fluconazole causing hypoglycaemia when given with gliclazide, see 'Sulfonylureas + Azoles; Fluconazole', p.543.

(b) Trimethoprim

In a crossover study in 7 healthy subjects, trimethoprim 150 mg twice daily for 7 days reduced the clearance of a single intravenous 500-mg dose of tolbutamide by 11% and prolonged the elimination half-life by 19%.[3]

Mechanism

The sulfonamides might inhibit the metabolism of the sulfonylureas increasing their serum concentrations and blood glucose-lowering effects.[4-7] Many of the sulfonylureas are metabolised by CYP2C9 (see 'Table 1.5', p.7), and some of the sulfonamides are known to be inhibitors of this isoenzyme (although perhaps to varying extents, *see below*). Tolbutamide, is used as a probe substrate to assess the activity of drugs on CYP2C9.

Of the sulfonamides, *in vitro* data suggest that sulfaphenazole is a potent inhibitor of CYP2C9, with sulfadiazine, sulfamethizole, sulfafurazole (sulfisoxazole), and sulfamethoxazole being moderate to weak inhibitors, and sulfapyridine, sulfadimethoxine, and sulfamonomethoxine having little inhibitory activity.[8] Information from clinical studies to support this appears to be lacking.

CYP2C9 shows genetic polymorphism (see 'Genetic factors in drug metabolism', p.8), and therefore any interaction might only be clinically relevant in a subgroup of the population. There is also some evidence that the sulfonamides can displace the sulfonylureas from their protein binding sites,[7] however, note that the effect of displacement from plasma protein binding sites by itself, is usually transient as any displaced drug is then available to be cleared (see 'Protein-binding interactions', p.3).

Where some of the cases of hypoglycaemia cannot be predicted on pharmacokinetic grounds, it is worth noting that hypoglycaemia induced by co-trimoxazole, in the absence of a conventional antidiabetic,[9-14] and sometimes associated with renal failure,[11] high dose of sulfonamide,[9,13] advanced age,[10,12] or malnutrition,[9] has been described.

The reduced tolbutamide clearance with trimethoprim[3] suggests inhibition of CYP2C9, and the authors of an *in vitro* study also suggested the possibility of a slight inhibitory effect of trimethoprim on CYP2C9,[15] but other supporting data is lacking. Note that trimethoprim is considered a weak CYP2C8 inhibitor, but this isoenzyme has not been shown to be involved in the metabolism of tolbutamide *in vivo*.

Importance and management

Evidence for an interaction between the sulphonamides or co-trimoxazole and the sulfonylureas is limited. Most sulfonamides seem to have caused marked problems (acute hypoglycaemia), although in only a few patients and serious interactions are uncommon. However, the retrospective case-control studies suggest that patients taking glipizide or glibenclamide might have a clinically relevant increased risk of hypoglycaemia if taken with co-trimoxazole. On this basis, if concurrent co-trimoxazole is required in a patient established on a sulfonylurea, warn the patient that increased blood glucose-lowering effects, sometimes excessive, are a possibility, but that problems appear to be uncommon or rare. It is prudent to monitor blood glucose concentrations when any change is made to the medication regimen of a patient with diabetes, and this would therefore seem particularly relevant in this situation. Note also, that co-trimoxazole alone can rarely cause hypoglycaemia (see *Mechanism*, above). Advice concerning concurrent use of other sulfonamides is limited by the small volume of specific data, and no clinically relevant interaction would be expected between trimethoprim and tolbutamide, but the aforementioned general monitoring advice would appear to be sufficient to detect any relevant effects should they occur.

1. Schelleman H, Bilker WB, Brensinger CM, Wan F, Hennessy S. Anti-infectives and the risk of severe hypoglycemia in users of glipizide or glyburide. *Clin Pharmacol Ther* (2010) 88, 214
2. Juurlink DN, Mamdani M, Kopp A, Laupacis A, Redelmeier DA. Drug-drug interactions among elderly patients hospitalized for drug toxicity. *JAMA* (2003) 289, 1652–8.
3. Wing LMH, Miners JO. Cotrimoxazole as an inhibitor of oxidative drug metabolism: effects of trimethoprim and sulphamethoxazole separately and combined on tolbutamide disposition. *Br J Clin Pharmacol* (1985) 20, 482–5.
4. Lumholtz B, Siersbaek-Nielsen K, Skovsted L, Kampmann J, Hansen JM. Sulphamethizole-induced inhibition of diphenylhydantoin, tolbutamide, and warfarin metabolism. *Clin Pharmacol Ther* (1975) 17, 731–4.
5. Kristensen M, Christensen LK. Drug induced changes of the blood glucose lowering effect of oral hypoglycemic agents. *Acta Diabetol Lat* (1969) 6 (Suppl 1), 116–23.
6. Christensen LK, Hansen JM, Kristensen M. Sulphaphenazole-induced hypoglycaemic attacks in tolbutamide-treated diabetics. *Lancet* (1963) ii, 1298–1301.
7. Hellman B. Potentiating effects of drugs on the binding of glibenclamide to pancreatic beta cells. *Metabolism* (1974) 23, 839–46.
8. Komatsu K, Ito K, Nakajima Y, Kanamitsu S-I, Imaoka S, Funae Y, Green CE, Tyson CA, Shimada N, Sugiyama Y. Prediction of in vivo drug-drug interactions between tolbutamide and various sulfonamides in humans based on in vitro experiments. *Drug Metab Dispos* (2000) 28, 475–81.
9. Hekimsoy Z, Biberoğlu S, Çömleçki A, Tarhan O, Mermut C, Biberoğlu K. Trimethoprim-sulfamethoxazole-induced hypoglycemia in a malnourished patient with severe infection. *Eur J Endocrinol* (1997) 136, 304–6.
10. Mathews WA, Manint JE, Kleiss J. Trimethoprim-sulfamethoxazole-induced hypoglycemia as a cause of altered mental status in an elderly patient. *J Am Board Fam Pract* (2000) 13, 211–12.
11. Lee AJ, Maddix DS. Trimethoprim/sulfamethoxazole-induced hypoglycemia in a patient with acute renal failure. *Ann Pharmacother* (1997) 31, 727–32.
12. Rutschmann OT, Wicki J, Micheli P, Kondo Oestreicher M, Guillermin Spahr ML, Droz M. Co-trimoxazole administration: a rare cause of hypoglycemia in elderly persons. *Schweiz Med Wochenschr* (1998) 128, 1171–4.
13. Johnson JA, Kappel JE, Sharif MN. Hypoglycemia secondary to trimethoprim/sulfamethoxazole administration in a renal transplant patient. *Ann Pharmacother* (1993) 27, 304–6.
14. Nunnari G, Celesia BM, Bellissimo F, Tosto S, La Rocca M, Giarratana F, Benanti F, Caltabiano E, Russo R, Cacopardo B. Trimethoprim-sulfamethoxazole-associated severe hypoglycaemia: a sulfonylurea-like effect. *Eur Rev Med Pharmacol Sci* (2010) 14, 1015–8.
15. Wen X, Wang J-S, Backman JT, Laitila J, Neuvonen PJ. Trimethoprim and sulfamethoxazole are selective inhibitors of CYP2C8 and CYP2C9, respectively. *Drug Metab Dispos* (2002) 30, 631–5.

Sulfonylureas + Aprepitant

Aprepitant slightly reduces tolbutamide exposure. Other sulfonylureas might be similarly affected.

Clinical evidence

In a study in 12 healthy subjects, aprepitant (125 mg on day one, then 80 mg daily on days 2 and 3) decreased the AUC of a single 500-mg dose of tolbutamide by 23%, 28%, and 15%, when given on days 4, 8, and 15, respectively, when compared with 12 subjects not given aprepitant.[1] Even less effect was seen in another study[2] where a single 40-mg oral dose of aprepitant given on day one decreased the AUC of tolbutamide by 8% on day 2, by 16% on day 4, by 15% on day 8, and by 10% on day 15.

Mechanism

Aprepitant induces of CYP2C9 by which tolbutamide is metabolised. Concurrent use therefore increases tolbutamide metabolism, which leads to a reduction in tolbutamide exposure.

Importance and management

Evidence is limited, but what is known suggests that aprepitant increases the metabolism of tolbutamide. However, the clinical relevance of these small changes has not been assessed, but they are unlikely to be important. Nevertheless, the UK manufacturer recommends caution when tolbutamide is used with aprepitant (at the higher doses for chemotherapy induced nausea and vomiting).[3] No clinically relevant interaction is expected with the low single-dose of aprepitant used for post-operative nausea and vomiting.[2] Note that **fosaprepitant** is a prodrug of aprepitant, and it might therefore be expected to interact similarly. Other **sulfonylureas** which are also metabolised by CYP2C9 would be predicted to be similarly affected.

In general, it is prudent to monitor blood glucose concentrations when any change is made to the medication regimen of a patient with diabetes, and this should be sufficient to detect any interaction with these drugs should it occur.

Note that tolbutamide can be used as a probe substrate to assess the activity of drugs on CYP2C9. This study therefore suggests that aprepitant is a weak inducer of CYP2C9.

1. Shadle CR, Lee Y, Majumdar AK, Petty KJ, Gargano C, Bradstreet TE, Evans JK, Blum RA. Evaluation of potential inductive effects of aprepitant on cytochrome P450 3A4 and 2C9 activity. *J Clin Pharmacol* (2004) 44, 215–23.
2. EMEND Capsules (Aprepitant). Merck & Co., Inc. US Prescribing information, August 2014.
3. EMEND (Aprepitant). Merck Sharp & Dohme Ltd. UK Summary of product characteristics, December 2013.

Sulfonylureas + Azoles; Fluconazole

Fluconazole does not appear to affect the diabetic control of most patients taking sulfonylureas, but isolated reports describe severe hypoglycaemia in patients taking glipizide or gliclazide with fluconazole. Furthermore, some evidence suggests that the blood glucose-lowering effects and risk of hypoglycaemia with both glipizide and glibenclamide (glyburide) might be increased by fluconazole. The exposure to glimepiride is moderately increased by fluconazole, but only slight increases appear to occur with other sulfonylureas.

Clinical evidence

(a) Chlorpropamide

In a study, fluconazole increased the AUC of a single 250-mg dose of chlorpropamide by 28% in 18 healthy subjects given fluconazole 100 mg daily for 7 days, but the maximum plasma concentrations and blood glucose concentrations were unchanged. There was no evidence of hypoglycaemia.[1]

(b) Glibenclamide (Glyburide)

In a study, fluconazole increased the AUC of a single 5-mg dose of glibenclamide by 44%, and increased its maximum plasma concentrations by 19% in 20 healthy subjects given fluconazole 100 mg daily for 7 days. The change in blood glucose concentrations was not statistically significant but the number of subjects who had symptoms of hypoglycaemia increased.[2] In another study, a group of 14 postmenopausal women with diabetes and vulvovaginal candidiasis, taking either gliclazide or glibenclamide, were given fluconazole 50 mg daily for 14 days. None of the patients in this study developed symptoms of hypoglycaemia and their HbA_{1c} and fructosamine concentrations were unchanged. No pharmacokinetic data were reported.[3] In a large, retrospective, case-control study, of 7 414 patients taking glibenclamide, and hospitalised or given emergency treatment for hypoglycaemia, 11 had recently received a course of fluconazole. No statistically significant increased risk of hypoglycaemia occurred when fluconazole was dispensed one to 5 days before the episode of hypoglycaemia. However, for those who were given fluconazole within days 6 to 10 of the hypoglycaemic episode, the adjusted odds ratio for the risk of developing hypoglycaemia on the concurrent use of glibenclamide was 2.2, relative to cefalexin (which was given as a non-interacting control).[4] A retrospective, observational review of 3884 patients with type 2 diabetes taking sulphonylureas (glibenclamide, **glimepiride**, or **glipizide**) found that maximum fasting plasma glucose concentrations were lower in patients also taking a CYP2C9 inhibitor (including fluconazole), when compared to patients only taking a sulfonylurea.[5]

(c) Gliclazide

A group of 14 postmenopausal women with diabetes taking either gliclazide or glibenclamide, who developed vulvovaginal candidiasis, were given fluconazole 50 mg daily for 14 days. None of the patients developed symptoms of hypoglycaemia and their HbA_{1c} and fructosamine concentrations were unchanged. No pharmacokinetic data were reported.[3] However, a 56-year-old HIV-positive patient (antiretroviral treatment refused) with type 2 diabetes who had been taking gliclazide for 2 years was given fluconazole 50 mg daily for 2 weeks for oral candidiasis, and prophylactic co-trimoxazole (sulfamethoxazole 400 mg and trimethoprim 80 mg daily). One week after the re-introduction of fluconazole at a higher dose of 200 mg daily he was hospitalised because of weakness and aggressive behaviour. His blood glucose concentration was 2.2 mmol/L and gliclazide was stopped. He experienced a brief loss of consciousness 2 days later while driving his car, but his condition then improved and neurological symptoms did not recur during 3 months of follow-up without gliclazide treatment.[6] For the possible contribution of sulfamethoxazole to this interaction, see *Mechanism*, below.

(d) Glimepiride

A double-blind crossover study in 12 healthy subjects found that fluconazole 400 mg on day one, then 200 mg daily for a further 3 days, increased the AUC of a single 500-microgram dose of glimepiride about 2.5-fold, and increased the maximum plasma concentration by 50%. Fluconazole increased the mean elimination half-life of glimepiride from 2 hours to 3.3 hours. There were no statistically significant changes in blood glucose concentrations and no hypoglycaemia.[7] For mention of a retrospective, observational review which included the concurrent use of glimepiride and fluconazole, see *Glibenclamide* above.

(e) Glipizide

In a study, fluconazole increased the AUC of a single 2.5-mg dose of glipizide by 49%, and increase its maximum serum concentration by 17% in 13 healthy subjects given fluconazole 100 mg daily for 7 days. Although blood glucose concentrations were lowered, the change was not statistically significant. However, the number of subjects who had symptoms suggestive of hypoglycaemia increased.[8]

Of the 5 559 patients in a large, retrospective, case-control study, who were taking glipizide, and hospitalised or given emergency treatment for hypoglycaemia, 19 had recently received a course of fluconazole. For those who were given a prescription for fluconazole within days one to 5 or 6 to 10 of the diagnosis of hypoglycaemia, the adjusted odds ratio for the risk of an interaction was 2 and 2.5, respectively, relative to cefalexin (which was given as a non-interacting control).[4] A patient with diabetes taking glipizide 2.5 mg three times daily went into a hypoglycaemic coma within 4 days of starting to take fluconazole 200 mg daily. Her blood glucose concentrations had decreased to less than about 0.05 mmol/L. She rapidly recovered when given glucose.[9] For mention of a retrospective, observational review which included the concurrent use of glipizide and fluconazole, see *Glibenclamide* above.

(f) Tolbutamide

In a study, fluconazole increased the AUC of a single 500-mg dose of tolbutamide by about 50%, and increased its maximum plasma concentrations by about 11% in 13 healthy subjects given a single 150-mg dose of fluconazole, and then 6 doses of fluconazole 100 mg daily. The half-life of the tolbutamide was increased about 60%. Blood glucose concentrations remained unaltered and none of the subjects showed any evidence of hypoglycaemia.[10,11]

Mechanism

Fluconazole is a weak to moderate inhibitor of CYP2C9 (depending on the dose given), by which many of the sulfonylureas are metabolised. Inhibition of this isoenzyme leads to an accumulation of the sulfonylurea and an increase in its effects would be expected. The hypoglycaemia in the patient taking gliclazide and fluconazole might have been enhanced by sulfamethoxazole,[6] which also inhibits CYP2C9 (see also 'Sulfonylureas + Antibacterials; Sulfonamides and/or Trimethoprim', p.542).

Importance and management

Evidence for an interaction between fluconazole and the sulfonylureas seems to be restricted to case reports, with studies finding at worst moderate effects on sulfonylurea pharmacokinetics which did not lead to alterations in blood glucose concentrations. However, note that most studies were in healthy subjects and all used low, or subtherapeutic (in the case of glimepiride), doses of the sulfonylurea, so in clinical practice greater than expected blood glucose-lowering effects might be seen. Furthermore, the increased plasma concentrations of glipizide and glimepiride, and the single case of severe hypoglycaemia, as well as the hypoglycaemic symptoms shown by those taking glibenclamide (glyburide) or gliclazide suggest that patients taking these sulfonylureas in particular should be warned to be alert for any evidence of hypoglycaemia. It is prudent to monitor blood glucose concentrations when any change is made to the medication regimen of a patient with diabetes, and this should detect any interaction with fluconazole, should it occur, and allow any necessary sulfonylurea dose adjustments to be made.

1. Pfizer Ltd. Data on file. A volunteer-blind, placebo-controlled study to assess potential interaction between fluconazole and chlorpropamide in healthy male volunteers (Protocol 238).
2. Pfizer Ltd. Data on file. A volunteer-blind, placebo-controlled study to assess potential interaction between fluconazole and glibenclamide in healthy male volunteers. (Protocol 236).
3. Rowe BR, Thorpe J, Barnett A. Safety of fluconazole in women taking oral hypoglycaemic agents. *Lancet* (1992) 339, 255–6.
4. Schelleman H, Bilker WB, Brensinger CM, Wan F, Hennessy S. Anti-infectives and the risk of severe hypoglycemia in users of glipizide or glyburide. *Clin Pharmacol Ther* (2010) 88, 214
5. Tirkkonen T, Heikkilä P, Huupponen R, Laine K. Potential CYP2C9-mediated drug-drug interactions in hospitalized type 2 diabetes mellitus patients treated with the sulphonylureas glibenclamide, glimepiride or glipizide. *J Intern Med* (2010) 268, 359–66.
6. Abad S, Moachon L, Blanche P, Bavoux F, Sicard D, Salmon-Céron D. Possible interaction between gliclazide, fluconazole and sulfamethoxazole resulting in severe hypoglycaemia. *Br J Clin Pharmacol* (2001) 52, 456–7.
7. Niemi M, Backman JT, Neuvonen M, Laitila J, Neuvonen PJ, Kivistö KT. Effects of fluconazole and fluvoxamine on the pharmacokinetics and pharmacodynamics of glimepiride. *Clin Pharmacol Ther* (2001) 69, 194–200.
8. Pfizer Ltd. Data on file. A volunteer-blind, placebo-controlled study to assess potential interaction between fluconazole and glipizide in healthy male volunteers. (Protocol 237).
9. Fournier JP, Schneider S, Martinez P, Mahagne MH, Ducoeur S, Haffner M, Thiercelin D, Chichmanain RM, Bertrand F. Coma hypoglycémique chez une patiente traitée par glipizide et fluconazole: une possible interaction? *Therapie* (1992) 47, 446–7.
10. Lazar JD, Wilner KD. Drug interactions with fluconazole. *Rev Infect Dis* (1990) 12 (Suppl 3), S327–S333.
11. Pfizer Ltd. Data on file. A double-blind placebo-controlled study to assess the potential interaction between fluconazole and tolbutamide in healthy male volunteers.

Sulfonylureas+ Azoles; Itraconazole or Ketoconazole

Itraconazole appears not to affect diabetic control in most patients, but there are reports of hypoglycaemia or hyperglycaemia associated with its use in patients taking glibenclamide. Ketoconazole slightly increased tolbutamide exposure and increased its blood glucose-lowering effects.

Clinical evidence

(a) Itraconazole

Post-marketing surveillance of adverse event reports in patients receiving itraconazole with an oral antidiabetic (mostly a **sulfonylurea**) over 10 years, indicated that in most patients diabetic control was not affected. However, of the 74 adverse events reported, there were 5 reports suggesting hyperglycaemia (all 5 were in patients taking **gliben-**

clamide (glyburide)) and 3 reports suggesting hypoglycaemia (2 of which were in patients taking **glibenclamide**, the other patient was taking an unspecified sulfonylurea).[1] In clinical studies, only one of 189 patients with diabetes taking antidiabetics drugs, including sulfonylureas, experienced aggravated diabetes when given itraconazole.[1] The patient in question was also receiving ciclosporin for a kidney transplant.

(b) Ketoconazole

After an overnight fast and breakfast the next morning, 7 healthy subjects were given a single 500-mg dose of **tolbutamide** before and after taking ketoconazole 200 mg daily for a week. Ketoconazole increased the elimination half-life of **tolbutamide** more than 3-fold (from 3.7 to 12.3 hours) and increased its AUC by 77%. Ketoconazole increased the blood glucose-lowering effects of **tolbutamide** by about 10 to 15%, and 5 of the subjects experienced mild hypoglycaemic symptoms (weakness, sweating, and a reeling sensation) at about 2 hours after the dose.[2]

Mechanism

Tolbutamide and many of the other sulfonylureas are principally metabolised by CYP2C9. Ketoconazole is not known to be an inhibitor of CYP2C9 and so the reason for the slight increase in tolbutamide exposure seen is unclear.

Importance and management

Evidence for an interaction between the sulfonylureas and itraconazole or ketoconazole is limited. It appears that itraconazole does not usually disturb the control of diabetes, although there are rare reports of hyperglycaemia or hypoglycaemia associated with its use with glibenclamide.

Ketoconazole slightly increased tolbutamide exposure and its blood glucose-lowering effects in one study. In general, it is prudent to monitor blood glucose concentrations when any change is made to the medication regimen of a patient with diabetes, and this would seem to be sufficient to detect any interaction with itraconazole or ketoconazole, should one occur.

1. Verspeelt J, Marynissen G, Gupta AK, De Doneker P. Safety of itraconazole in diabetic patients. *Dermatology* (1999) 198, 382–4.
2. Krishnaiah YSR, Satyanarayana S, Visweswaram D. Interaction between tolbutamide and ketoconazole in healthy subjects. *Br J Clin Pharmacol* (1994) 37, 205–7.

Sulfonylureas + Azoles; Miscellaneous

Hypoglycaemia has been seen in a few diabetic patients taking tolbutamide, glibenclamide, or gliclazide when they were given miconazole tablets. Posaconazole slightly enhanced the blood glucose-lowering effects of glipizide in healthy subjects, but did not affect the metabolism of a single dose of tolbutamide. Voriconazole is predicted to increase the concentrations of the sulfonylureas, and a case report describes this effect in a patient given voriconazole and glimepiride. Clotrimazole used intravaginally appears not to interact with gliclazide or glibenclamide.

Clinical evidence

(a) Clotrimazole

A group of 15 postmenopausal diabetic women with vulvovaginal candidiasis taking either **gliclazide** or **glibenclamide (glyburide)** were treated with intravaginal clotrimazole 100 mg daily for 14 days. None of the patients developed symptoms of hypoglycaemia and their HbA_{1c} and fructosamine concentrations were unchanged. No pharmacokinetic data were reported.[1]

(b) Miconazole

A diabetic patient taking **tolbutamide** was hospitalised with severe hypoglycaemia about 10 days after starting to take miconazole tablets.[2] In 1983 the French Commission Nationale de Pharmacovigilance reported 6 cases of hypoglycaemia in diabetic patients taking sulfonylureas (5 with **gliclazide** and one with **glibenclamide (glyburide)**), which occurred within 2 to 6 days of miconazole being started.[2] The same organisation reported a further 8 cases in the 1985 to 1990 period.[3] Three other cases of hypoglycaemia (two with **gliclazide** and one with **glibenclamide**) are reported elsewhere, in patients given miconazole up to 750 mg daily.[4]

(c) Posaconazole

A study in 12 healthy subjects found that posaconazole 400 mg twice daily for 10 days had no effect on the steady-state pharmacokinetics of **glipizide** 10 mg daily, but there was a small decrease in blood glucose concentrations following concurrent use. **Glipizide** did not affect the pharmacokinetics of posaconazole.[5] In another study, posaconazole 200 mg daily for 10 days had no effect on **tolbutamide** metabolism.[6]

(d) Voriconazole

A diabetic patient taking **glimepiride** 1 mg daily developed acute myeloid leukemia with febrile neutropenia, for which he was given voriconazole 400 mg every 12 hours for one day, followed by 200 mg every 12 hours. On day 2, the patient developed excessive and pressurised speech, confusion, and delirium with a blood glucose concentration of 40 mg/dL. Despite initial stabilisation with a 25% dextrose infusion he dropped into unconsciousness 2 hours later with glucose concentrations of 38 mg/dL. He regained consciousness when given 25% dextrose after which both glimepiride and voriconazole were discontinued. The hypoglycaemia persisted for 48 hours following discontinuation of both drugs.[7]

Mechanism

Miconazole and voriconazole are inhibitors of CYP2C9, by which many of the sulfonylureas are metabolised. Inhibition of this isoenzyme would therefore be expected to lead to an accumulation of the sulfonylurea and therefore an increase in its effects, as seen with miconazole tablets. Clotrimazole is probably not absorbed in sufficient quantities to cause an interaction.

Importance and management

The interaction between miconazole tablets and the sulfonylureas is established and clinically important, but of uncertain incidence. Concurrent use need not be avoided, but it should be monitored, and the dose of the sulfonylurea reduced if necessary. Although there are no specific data, a large proportion of miconazole oral gel (both prescription and non-prescription doses) might be swallowed and therefore adequate systemic absorption could occur to produce an interaction. It is therefore possible that oral miconazole gel might interact similarly to miconazole tablets. Intravaginal miconazole and miconazole topical creams are probably unlikely to interact, because absorption by these routes is minimal.

Posaconazole slightly enhanced the blood glucose-lowering effects of glipizide in healthy subjects, but the clinical relevance of this is not known. Posaconazole does not appear to affect tolbutamide metabolism.

The UK and US manufacturers of voriconazole predict that it will increase the concentrations of the sulfonylureas and they advise increased blood glucose monitoring in patients taking sulfonylureas, with dose reductions if necessary.[8,9] The case report involving glimepiride suggests that this is probably prudent.

Information about intravaginal clotrimazole is very sparse, but it appears not to interact with gliclazide or glibenclamide, and probably not with any of the other oral antidiabetics, not least because its absorption from the vagina is very small.

1. Rowe BR, Thorpe J, Barnett A. Safety of fluconazole in women taking oral hypoglycaemic agents. *Lancet* (1992) 339, 255–6.
2. Meurice JC, Lecomte P, Renard JP, Girard JJ. Interaction miconazole et sulfamides hypoglycémiants. *Presse Med* (1983) 12, 1670.
3. Girardin E, Vial T, Pham E, Evreux J-C. Hypoglycémies induites par les sulfamides hypoglycémiants. *Ann Med Interne (Paris)* (1992) 143, 11–17.
4. Loupi E, Descotes J, Lery N, Evreux JC. Interactions médicamenteuses et miconazole. A propos de 10 observations. *Therapie* (1982) 37, 437–41.
5. Courtney R, Sansone A, Statkevich P, Martinho M, Laughlin M. Assessment of the pharmacokinetic (PK), pharmacodynamic (PD) interaction potential between posaconazole and glipizide in healthy volunteers. *Clin Pharmacol Ther* (2003) 73, P45.
6. Wexler D, Courtney R, Richards W, Banfield C, Lim J, Laughlin M. Effect of posaconazole on cytochrome P450 enzymes: a randomized, open-label, two-way crossover study. *Eur J Pharm Sci* (2004) 21, 645–53.
7. Shobha JC, Muppidi MR. Interaction between voriconazole and glimepiride. *J Postgrad Med* (2010) 56, 44–5.
8. VFEND (Voriconazole). Pfizer Ltd. UK Summary of product characteristics, October 2014.
9. VFEND (Voriconazole). Pfizer Inc. US Prescribing information, February 2014.

Sulfonylureas + Benzodiazepines

No adverse interaction was seen in two patients taking tolbutamide and chlordiazepoxide. In a study, the pharmacokinetics of chlorpropamide were not affected by diazepam.

Clinical evidence, mechanism, importance and management

Two patients with type 2 diabetes who were taking **tolbutamide** 500 mg and 2 g daily, had no changes in fasting blood glucose concentrations while taking **chlordiazepoxide** 40 mg daily for 20 to 25 days.[1] In another study **diazepam** did not change the half-life of **chlorpropamide**.[2] No dose adjustments would seem necessary on concurrent use.

1. Zumoff B, Hellman L. Aggravation of diabetic hyperglycemia by chlordiazepoxide. *JAMA* (1977) 237, 1960–1.
2. Petitpierre B, Perrin L, Rudhardt M, Herrera A, Fabre J. Behaviour of chlorpropamide in renal insufficiency and under the effect of associated drug therapy. *Int J Clin Pharmacol* (1972) 6, 120–4.

Sulfonylureas + Bile-acid binding resins

The absorption of glipizide might be reduced if it is taken at the same time as colestyramine, but tolbutamide does not appear to be affected. Colesevelam might reduce the absorption of glibenclamide if it is taken at the same time. Diabetic control in patients taking chlorpropamide, tolbutamide, or tolazamide was not affected by the addition of colestipol, but the hypocholesterolaemic effects of colestipol were inhibited in these patients.

Clinical evidence

(a) Colesevelam

In a randomised, crossover study in 18 healthy subjects, colesevelam 3.75 g reduced the AUC of **glibenclamide (glyburide)** 3 mg by 32% and reduced the maximum concentration by 47%, when taken at the same time. When the glibenclamide was taken one hour before colesevelam, the AUC and maximum concentration were still reduced, but to a lesser extent: by 20% and 15%, respectively. In a similar study in 33 healthy subjects, when glibenclamide was taken 4 hours before colesevelam, the AUC and maximum concentration were not affected.[1]

(b) Colestipol

In a randomised study in 12 diabetic patients with elevated serum cholesterol concentrations, the concurrent use of **chlorpropamide**, **tolbutamide**, or **tolazamide** with phenformin in 4 patients, inhibited the normal hypocholesterolaemic effects of colestipol 5 g three times daily. The control of diabetes was not affected by the colestipol.[2]

(c) Colestyramine

1. Glipizide. In 6 healthy subjects, colestyramine 8 g in 150 mL of water reduced the absorption of a single 5-mg dose of glipizide by a mean of 29%. One subject had a 41% reduction in glipizide concentrations. Maximum serum concentrations were reduced by 33%. The AUC_{0-10} was used to measure absorption.[3]

2. Tolbutamide. A single-dose study indicated that colestyramine 8 g, given 2 minutes before, and 6 and 12 hours after a 500-mg dose of tolbutamide, did not reduce the amount of tolbutamide absorbed, although the rate of absorption might have changed.[4]

Mechanism

Colestyramine, colestipol, and colesevelam are bile-acid binding resins, intended to bind to bile acids within the gut, but they can also bind with some acidic drugs thereby reducing the amount available for absorption.

Importance and management

Evidence for an interaction between the sulfonylureas and bile-acid binding resins is limited to specific drug combination studies, but is largely consistent with how bile-acid binding resins are known to interact, although the clinical importance of any interaction, where it occurs, is variable. Information about glipizide is limited to a single-dose study so that the clinical importance of the reduction in glipizide concentrations with colestyramine is unknown, but it would seem prudent to monitor the effects of concurrent use in patients. It has been suggested[3] that the glipizide should be taken one to 2 hours before the colestyramine to minimise admixture in the gut, but this might only be partially effective because it is believed that glipizide undergoes some entero-hepatic circulation (i.e. after absorption it is excreted in the bile and reabsorbed). The effect of colestyramine on other sulfonylureas is uncertain, with the exception of tolbutamide, which is reported not to interact.

Colesevelam appears to reduce the absorption of glibenclamide and this might have a modest clinically relevant effect. The US manufacturer recommends that glibenclamide should be taken at least 4 hours before colesevelam.[5]

The study with colestipol found no effect on the diabetic control of diabetics taking chlorpropamide, tolbutamide, or tolazamide (with phenformin, although note that phenformin has been withdrawn from many countries due to severe, often fatal, lactic acidosis), but did suggest that it might not be suitable for lowering the blood cholesterol concentrations in these patients. More study is needed to confirm these findings.

1. Brown KS, Armstrong IC, Wang A, Walker JR, Noveck RJ, Swearingen D, Allison M, Kissling JC, Kisicki J, Salazar DE. Effect of the bile acid sequestrant colesevelam on the pharmacokinetics of pioglitazone, repaglinide, estrogen estradiol, norethindrone, levothyroxine, and glyburide. *J Clin Pharmacol* (2010) 50, 554–65.
2. Bandisode MS, Boshell BR. Hypocholesterolemic activity of colestipol in diabetes. *Curr Ther Res* (1975) 18, 276–84.
3. Kivistö K T, Neuvonen P J. The effect of cholestyramine and activated charcoal on glipizide absorption. *Br J Clin Pharmacol* (1990) 30, 733–6.
4. Hunninghake D B, Pollack E. Effect of bile acid sequestering agents on the absorption of aspirin, tolbutamide and warfarin. *Fedn Proc* (1977) 35, 996.
5. Welchol (Colesevelam hydrochloride). Daiichi Sankyo, Inc. US Prescribing information, January 2014.

Sulfonylureas + Bosentan

There appears to be an increased risk of liver toxicity if bosentan is given with glibenclamide (glyburide). Glibenclamide slightly reduces bosentan exposure, and bosentan slightly reduces glibenclamide exposure. Bosentan is predicted to reduce the plasma concentrations, and possibly the effect, of other similarly metabolised sulfonylureas.

Clinical evidence

In clinical studies, bosentan was noted to be associated with dose-related asymptomatic elevations in liver enzymes in some patients, and these elevations were higher in patients also receiving **glibenclamide (glyburide)**.[1] Study in *rats* suggested that the concurrent use of bosentan and **glibenclamide** caused increases in serum bile salt concentrations that were greater than with either drug alone.[1] In addition, *in vitro* study showed that bosentan inhibits the bile salt export pump,[1] which is also inhibited by **glibenclamide**.

Because of the possibility that there might be a pharmacokinetic component to the interaction, the pharmacokinetics of both bosentan and **glibenclamide** were determined in a crossover study in 12 healthy subjects. However, **glibenclamide** actually reduced the maximum plasma concentration and AUC of bosentan by 24% and 29%, respectively, while bosentan reduced the maximum plasma concentration and AUC of **glibenclamide** by 22% and 40%, respectively. Two subjects had asymptomatic elevated liver enzyme concentrations while taking bosentan with **glibenclamide**.[2]

Mechanism

Bosentan is an inducer of CYP2C9 and CYP3A4. **Glibenclamide** is principally metabolised by CYP2C9, and this might explain the reduced **glibenclamide** concentrations seen.

Importance and management

Although limited, the available evidence for an increased risk of liver toxicity with bosentan and glibenclamide suggests that the combination would be best avoided and an alternative antidiabetic drug used. From a pharmacokinetic perspective, a 40% decrease in glibenclamide exposure might possibly reduce its blood glucose-lowering effects to a clinically relevant extent, and although there are no data, bosentan would be expected to reduce the plasma concentrations of other oral antidiabetics that are predominantly metabolised by CYP2C9 or CYP3A4. As many other **sulfonylureas** are principally metabolised by CYP2C9, they would be predicted to be similarly affected. If used concurrently, the possibility of worsened glucose control in patients using these drugs should be considered. The general advice to monitor blood glucose concentrations when any change is made to the medication regimen of a patient with diabetes, should be sufficient to detect any interaction with these drugs should it occur.

1. Fattinger K, Funk C, Pantze M, Weber C, Reichen J, Stieger B, Meier PJ. The endothelin antagonist bosentan inhibits the canalicular bile salt export pump: a potential mechanism for hepatic adverse reactions. *Clin Pharmacol Ther* (2001) 69, 223–31.
2. van Giersbergen PLM, Treiber A, Clozel M, Bodin F, Dingemanse J. In vivo and in vitro studies exploring the pharmacokinetic interaction between bosentan, a dual endothelin receptor antagonist, and glyburide. *Clin Pharmacol Ther* (2002) 71, 253–62.

Sulfonylureas + Calcium-channel blockers

The pharmacokinetics of glibenclamide do not appear to be altered by nimodipine or verapamil, and the pharmacokinetics of glipizide do not appear to be altered by nifedipine. There appears to be no pharmacokinetic interaction between tolbutamide and diltiazem.

Clinical evidence, mechanism, importance and management

For discussion of the general effects of calcium channel blockers on diabetes control, see 'Antidiabetics + Calcium-channel blockers', p.505

(a) Glibenclamide (Glyburide)

In an uncontrolled study in 11 diabetic patients stabilised on glibenclamide, there was no difference in the pharmacokinetics of glibenclamide after the addition of **nimodipine** 30 mg three times daily for 6 days when compared with glibenclamide alone.[1] A crossover study in 9 healthy subjects found that **verapamil** 120 mg increased the AUC of glibenclamide 5 mg by 26%, but plasma glucose concentrations were unchanged.[2] No special precautions would seem necessary if glibenclamide is to be given with verapamil or nimodipine, but note that it is prudent to monitor blood glucose concentrations when any change is made to the medication regimen of a patient with diabetes.

(b) Glipizide

A randomised, crossover study in 6 patients with type 2 diabetes taking glipizide 5 to 30 mg daily for the previous 2 months, found that a single 20-mg dose of **nifedipine** had no effect on the pharmacokinetics of glipizide.[3] No special precautions would seem necessary on concurrent use, but note that it is prudent to monitor blood glucose concentrations when any change is made to the medication regimen of a patient with diabetes.

(c) Tolbutamide

A randomised, crossover study in 8 healthy subjects found that a single 500-mg dose of tolbutamide had no effect on the serum concentrations of a single 60-mg dose of **diltiazem**. There was an increase of about 10% in the AUC_{0-24} and maximum serum concentrations of tolbutamide in the presence of **diltiazem**. The blood glucose-lowering effects of tolbutamide were not changed.[4] No special precautions would seem necessary on concurrent use, but note that it is prudent to monitor blood glucose concentrations when any change is made to the medication regimen of a patient with diabetes.

1. Mück W, Heine PR, Breuel H-P, Niklaus H, Horkulak J, Ahr G. The effect of multiple oral dosing of nimodipine on glibenclamide pharmacodynamics and pharmacokinetics in elderly patients with type-2 diabetes mellitus. *Int J Clin Pharmacol Ther* (1995) 33, 89–94.
2. Semple CG, Omile C, Buchanan KD, Beastall GH, Paterson KR. Effect of oral verapamil on glibenclamide stimulated insulin secretion. *Br J Clin Pharmacol* (1986) 22, 187–90.
3. Connacher AA, El Debani AH, Isles TE, Stevenson IH. Disposition and hypoglycaemic action of glipizide in diabetic patients given a single dose of nifedipine. *Eur J Clin Pharmacol* (1987) 33, 81–3.
4. Dixit AA, Rao YM. Pharmacokinetic interaction between diltiazem and tolbutamide. *Drug Metabol Drug Interact* (1999) 15, 269–77.

Sulfonylureas + Chloramphenicol

Chloramphenicol increases the plasma concentration of tolbutamide. The blood glucose-lowering effects of tolbutamide and chlorpropamide can be increased by chloramphenicol and acute hypoglycaemia can occur.

Clinical evidence

Studies in patients with diabetes have found that chloramphenicol 2 g daily can increase the serum concentration and half-life of **tolbutamide** 2- to 3-fold,[1,2] and reduce blood glucose concentrations by about 25 to 30%.[2,3] Three case reports also describe clinical effects. In one, a man taking chloramphenicol 2 g daily started taking **tolbutamide** 2 g daily. Three days later he had a typical hypoglycaemic collapse and was found to have serum **tolbutamide** concentrations 3- to 4-fold higher than expected.[1] Hypoglycaemia, acute in one case, also developed in two other patients taking **tolbutamide** with chloramphenicol.[4,5]

In another study chloramphenicol 1 to 2 g daily caused an average 2-fold increase in the half-life of **chlorpropamide**.[6]

Mechanism

Chloramphenicol inhibits the liver enzymes concerned with the metabolism of tolbutamide, and probably chlorpropamide as well, leading to their accumulation in the body. This is reflected in prolonged half-lives, reduced blood glucose concentrations, and occasionally acute hypoglycaemia.[1-4,6]

Importance and management

The interaction between tolbutamide and chloramphenicol is well established and of clinical importance. The incidence is uncertain, but increased blood glucose-lowering effects should be expected if both drugs are given. The interaction between chlorpropamide and chloramphenicol is less well documented. Nevertheless, monitor concurrent use carefully and reduce the dose of the sulfonylurea as necessary. Some patients might show a particularly exaggerated response. The manufacturers of other sulfonylureas often list chloramphenicol as an interacting drug, based on its interactions with tolbutamide and chlorpropamide, but direct information of an interaction does not appear to be available. No interaction would be expected with chloramphenicol eye drops, because the systemic absorption is likely to be small.

1. Christensen LK, Skovsted L. Inhibition of drug metabolism by chloramphenicol. *Lancet* (1969) ii, 1397–9.
2. Brunová E, Slabochová Z, Platilová H, Pavlík F, Grafnetterová J, Dvořáček K. Interaction of tolbutamide and chloramphenicol in diabetic patients. *Int J Clin Pharmacol Biopharm* (1977) 15, 7–12.
3. Brunová E, Slabochová Z, Platilová H. Influencing the effect of Dirastan (tolbutamide). Simultaneous administration of chloramphenicol in patients with diabetes and bacterial urinary tract inflammation. *Cas Lek Cesk* (1974) 113, 72–5.
4. Ziegelasch H-J. Extreme hypoglykämie unter kombinierter behandlung mit tolbutamid, n-1-butylbiguanidhydrochlorid und chloramphenikol. *Z Gesamte Inn Med* (1972) 27, 63–6.
5. Soeldner JS, Steinke J. Hypoglycemia in tolbutamide-treated diabetes. *JAMA* (1965) 193, 398–9.
6. Petitpierre B, Perrin L, Rudhardt M, Herrera A, Fabre J. Behaviour of chlorpropamide in renal insufficiency and under the effect of associated drug therapy. *Int J Clin Pharmacol* (1972) 6, 120–4.

Sulfonylureas + Echinacea

Echinacea negligibly increases tolbutamide exposure.

Clinical evidence

In a pharmacokinetic study, 12 healthy subjects were given *Echinacea purpurea* root 400 mg four times daily for 8 days with a single 500-mg dose of tolbutamide on day 6. The AUC of tolbutamide was increased by 14% and the time to maximum concentration was increased from 4 to 6 hours.[1] The oral clearance was decreased by a mean of 11%, although 2 subjects had a 25% or greater reduction.

Mechanism

Note that tolbutamide can be used as a probe substrate to assess the activity of drugs on CYP2C9. This study therefore suggests that echinacea is not a clinically relevant inhibitor of CYP2C9 and is unlikely to affect other CYP2C9 substrates (which would include other **sulfonylureas**) by this mechanism.

Importance and management

The available evidence is from one well-designed pharmacokinetic study. Although echinacea did have some effect on the pharmacokinetics of tolbutamide, the effect on exposure was negligible and would not be expected to be clinically relevant. Therefore no tolbutamide dose adjustments appear necessary if echinacea is also taken. Although evidence for other sulfonylureas is generally lacking, an interaction with Echinacea would not be expected, see under *Mechanism*, above.

1. Gorski JC, Huang S-M, Pinto A, Hamman MA, Hilligoss JK, Zaheer NA, Desai M, Miller M, Hall SD. The effect of echinacea (*Echinacea purpurea* root) on cytochrome P450 activity in vivo. *Clin Pharmacol Ther* (2004) 75, 89–100.

Sulfonylureas + Grapefruit juice

Grapefruit juice did not alter the pharmacokinetics of glibenclamide in one study.

Clinical evidence, mechanism, importance and management

In a study in healthy subjects, grapefruit juice 200 mL three times daily for 2 days, and then simultaneously with a single 875-microgram dose of **glibenclamide**, had no effect on the pharmacokinetics of **glibenclamide**.[1]

No pharmacokinetic interaction would therefore be expected on clinical use, either with glibenclamide, or other sulfonylureas that are similarly metabolised.

1. Lilja JJ, Niemi M, Fredrikson H, Neuvonen PJ. Effects of clarithromycin and grapefruit juice on the pharmacokinetics of glibenclamide. *Br J Clin Pharmacol* (2007) 63, 732–40.

Sulfonylureas + Guar gum or Glucomannan

Guar gum appears not to affect the absorption of glipizide or glibenclamide (glyburide). Glucomannan appears to reduce the initial absorption of glibenclamide, but also to enhance its hypoglycaemic effect.

Clinical evidence, mechanism, importance and management

(a) Glucomannan

Glucomannan 3.9 g reduced the plasma concentration of a single 2.5-mg dose of **glibenclamide (glyburide)** in 9 healthy subjects. Four samples taken over 30 to 150 minutes found that the plasma concentrations of **glibenclamide** were reduced by about 50%.[1] Despite this, plasma glucose concentrations were lower with the combination than with **glibenclamide** alone. Because plasma samples were not taken beyond 150 minutes, it is unclear what effect glucomannan has on the extent of **glibenclamide** absorption. The clinical relevance of these changes is unclear, but they seem unlikely to be important.

(b) Guar gum

In one study in 10 healthy subjects guar gum was found to have no effect on the AUC or maximum serum concentration of a single 2.5-mg dose of **glipizide**. In this study **glipizide** was given alone, or 30 minutes before breakfast, compared with guar gum granules (4.75 g guar gum) given either with the breakfast or with the **glipizide**.[2]

In one comparative study, guar gum was found to reduce the AUC of **glibenclamide (glyburide)** from one formulation (*Semi-Euglucon*) by about 30%, but not another formulation (*Semi-Euglucon-N*),[3] possibly because the latter preparation is more rapidly and completely absorbed. Similarly, in a crossover study in 9 patients with type 2 diabetes, guar gum granules 5 g three times daily with meals did not affect the AUC or maximum serum concentration of **glibenclamide** 3.5 mg twice daily from *Semi-Euglucon-N*. In addition, the combination slightly reduced fasting blood glucose when compared with baseline values.[4]

It seems doubtful that any of these modest pharmacokinetic interactions has much, if any, clinical relevance because guar gum can improve the metabolic control and decrease serum lipids in patients with type 2 diabetes.[4]

1. Shima K, Tanaka A, Ikegami H, Tabata M, Sawazaki N, Kumahara Y. Effect of dietary fiber, glucomannan, on absorption of sulfonylurea in man. *Horm Metab Res* (1983) 15, 1–3.
2. Huupponen R, Karhuvaara S, Seppälä P. Effect of guar gum on glipizide absorption in man. *Eur J Clin Pharmacol* (1985) 28, 717–9.
3. Neugebauer G, Akpan W, Abshagen U. Interaktion von Guar mit Glibenclamid und Bezafibrat. *Beitr Infusionther Klin Ernahr* (1983) 12, 40–7.
4. Uusitupa M, Södervik H, Silvasti M, Karttunen P. Effects of a gel forming dietary fiber, guar gum, on the absorption of glibenclamide and metabolic control and serum lipids in patients with non-insulin-dependent (type 2) diabetes. *Int J Clin Pharmacol Ther Toxicol* (1990) 28, 153–7.

Sulfonylureas + H_2-receptor antagonists

On the whole cimetidine and ranitidine do not appear to alter diabetic control on concurrent use with sulfonylureas, although cases of adverse effects have been seen when glibenclamide (glyburide) was given with ranitidine, and when gliclazide or glipizide were given with cimetidine.

Clinical evidence

(a) Chlorpropamide

Cimetidine had no effect on the pharmacokinetics of chlorpropamide in healthy subjects,[1] and in another study the blood glucose-lowering effects of chlorpropamide remained unaltered when **cimetidine** was given.[2]

(b) Glibenclamide (Glyburide)

A study in healthy subjects reported that the blood glucose-lowering effects of glibenclamide were marginally reduced by **cimetidine** and **ranitidine**. This occurred despite the fact that **cimetidine** increased the AUC of glibenclamide by 37% and ranitidine had no pharmacokinetic effect on glibenclamide.[3] Severe hypoglycaemia was seen in a patient taking glibenclamide 5 mg daily when **ranitidine** 150 mg twice daily was also taken.[4] Conversely, a study in healthy subjects found that the blood glucose-lowering effects of glibenclamide remained unaltered by **cimetidine**.[2]

(c) Gliclazide

An elderly patient with type 2 diabetes taking gliclazide 160 mg daily developed very low blood glucose concentrations (1 mmol/L) after starting to take **cimetidine** 800 mg daily.[5]

(d) Glimepiride

In a study in healthy subjects no effects on the pharmacokinetics or pharmacodynamics of glimepiride were seen when given with either **cimetidine** or **ranitidine**.[6]

(e) Glipizide

Six patients with type 2 diabetes were given **cimetidine** 400 mg one hour before taking a dose of glipizide (average dose 5.8 mg) and then 3 hours later they were given a standard meal with **cimetidine** 200 mg. The expected increase in blood glucose concentrations after the meal was reduced by 40%, and in two of the patients plasma glucose concentrations decreased to less than 3 mmol/L. Cimetidine increased the glipizide AUC by 23%.[7,8] However, a study in healthy subjects found that the hypoglycaemic activity of glipizide remained unaltered by **cimetidine**.[2] Two studies in patients with type 2 diabetes found that **ranitidine** 150 mg increased the AUC of glipizide by 29% and 34%,[8,9] and reduced the expected increase in blood sugar concentrations after a meal by 22%.[8] However, another study by the same research group reported that **ranitidine** 300 mg had no effects on either the pharmacokinetics or the effects of glipizide, except that the absorption was delayed.[10]

(f) Tolbutamide

The pharmacokinetics of tolbutamide 250 mg daily for 4 days were not changed in 7 healthy subjects when **cimetidine** 800 mg daily was added for a further 4 days.[11] Other studies also found no pharmacokinetic interaction between tolbutamide and **cimetidine**,[12,13] or between tolbutamide and **ranitidine**,[13] and the hypoglycaemic activity of tolbutamide remained unaltered by **cimetidine**.[2] In contrast, in another study in healthy subjects, the AUC of tolbutamide was found to be increased by 20% and the elimination half-life decreased by 17% by **cimetidine** 1.2 g daily, but plasma glucose concentrations were not changed. **Ranitidine** 300 mg had no effect.[14] A later study found effectively the same results.[15]

(g) Unnamed sulfonylureas

A report briefly describes hypoglycaemia when 2 patients taking unnamed sulfonylureas were given **cimetidine**.[16]

Mechanism

Where an interaction occurs[14] it might be because the cimetidine inhibits the metabolism of the sulfonylurea by the liver, thereby increasing its effects.

Importance and management

The many studies cited here show that cimetidine generally causes no important changes in the pharmacokinetics or pharmacodynamics of the sulfonylureas (chlorpropamide, glimepiride, and tolbutamide). Similarly, ranitidine did not interact with glimepiride or tolbutamide. Only a few isolated cases of hypoglycaemia have been reported with ranitidine or cimetidine and sulfonylureas (glibenclamide (glyburide), gliclazide, and unnamed), and only one research group has found a possible increase in the blood glucose-lowering effect of glipizide with cimetidine and ranitidine. In general, no dose adjustment or special precautions would seem necessary on concurrent use. However, it is generally considered prudent to monitor blood glucose concentrations when any change is made to the medication regimen of a patient with diabetes.

1. Shah GF, Ghandi TP, Patel PR, Patel MR, Gilbert RN, Shridhar PA. Tolbutamide and chlorpropamide kinetics in the presence of cimetidine in human volunteers. *Indian Drugs* (1985) 22, 455–8.
2. Shah GF, Ghandi TP, Patel PR, Patel MR, Gilbert RN, Shridhar PA. The effect of cimetidine on the hypoglycaemic activity of four commonly used sulphonylurea drugs. *Indian Drugs* (1985) 22, 570–2.
3. Kubacka RT, Antal EJ, Juhl RP. The paradoxical effect of cimetidine and ranitidine on glibenclamide pharmacokinetics and pharmacodynamics. *Br J Clin Pharmacol* (1987) 23, 743–51.
4. Lee K, Mize R, Lowenstein SR. Glyburide-induced hypoglycemia and ranitidine. *Ann Intern Med* (1987) 107, 261–2.
5. Archambeaud-Mouveroux F, Nouaille Y, Nadalon S, Treves R, Merle L. Interaction between gliclazide and cimetidine. *Eur J Clin Pharmacol* (1987) 31, 631.
6. Schaaf LJ, Welshman IR, Viveash DM, Carel BJ. The effects of cimetidine and ranitidine on glimepiride pharmacokinetics and pharmacodynamics in normal subjects. *Pharm Res* (1994) 11 (10 Suppl), S–360.
7. Feely J, Peden N. Enhanced sulphonylurea-induced hypoglycaemia with cimetidine. *Br J Clin Pharmacol* (1983) 15, 607P.
8. Feely J, Collins WCJ, Cullen M, El Debani AH, MacWalter RS, Peden NR, Stevenson IH. Potentiation of the hypoglycaemic response to glipizide in diabetic patients by histamine H_2–receptor antagonists. *Br J Clin Pharmacol* (1993) 35, 321–3.
9. MacWalter RS, El Debani AH, Feeley J, Stevenson IH. Potentiation by ranitidine of the hypoglycaemic response to glipizide in diabetic patients. *Br J Clin Pharmacol* (1985) 19, 121P–122P.
10. Stevenson IH, El Debani AH, MacWalter RS. Glipizide pharmacokinetics and effect in diabetic patients given ranitidine. *Acta Pharmacol Toxicol (Copenh)* (1986) 59 (Suppl 4), 97.
11. Stockley C, Keal J, Rolan P, Bochner F, Somogyi A. Lack of inhibition of tolbutamide hydroxylation by cimetidine in man. *Eur J Clin Pharmacol* (1986) 31, 235–7.
12. Dey NG, Castleden CM, Ward J, Cornhill J, McBurney A. The effect of cimetidine on tolbutamide kinetics. *Br J Clin Pharmacol* (1983) 16, 438–440.
13. Adebayo GI, Coker HAB. Lack of efficacy of cimetidine and ranitidine as inhibitors of tolbutamide metabolism. *Eur J Clin Pharmacol* (1988) 34, 653–6.
14. Cate EW, Rogers JF, Powell JR. Inhibition of tolbutamide elimination by cimetidine but not ranitidine. *J Clin Pharmacol* (1986) 26, 372–7.
15. Toon S, Holt BL, Mullins FGP, Khan A. Effects of cimetidine, ranitidine and omeprazole on tolbutamide pharmacokinetics. *J Pharm Pharmacol* (1995) 47, 85–88.
16. Girardin E, Vial T, Pham E, Evreux J-C. Hypoglycémies induites par les sulfamides hypoglycémiants. *Ann Med Interne (Paris)* (1992) 143, 11–17.

Sulfonylureas + Macrolides

A retrospective case-control study found an increased risk of hypoglycaemia in patients taking glibenclamide (glyburide) or glipizide with clarithromycin, and, in a pharmacokinetic study, clarithromycin slightly increased glibenclamide exposure. The same effect might occur with tolbutamide. An increased risk of hypoglycaemia was not found with azithromycin or erythromycin; however, isolated cases of hypoglycaemia have been described with erythromycin.

An isolated report describes severe liver damage with prolonged cholestasis in a patient taking chlorpropamide and erythromycin.

Clinical evidence

(a) Effects on blood glucose control

In a large, retrospective, case-control study of 7 414 patients taking **glibenclamide (glyburide)**, and hospitalised or given emergency treatment for hypoglycaemia, 74 patients had recently received a course of **clarithromycin**. For those who were dispensed a prescription for clarithromycin within days one to 5 of the hypoglycaemic episode, the adjusted odds ratio for the risk of developing hypoglycaemia on the concurrent use of glibenclamide was 5, when compared with cefalexin (which was given as a non-interacting control). The risk of hypoglycaemia in those who took **glibenclamide** with clarithromycin 6 to 10 days before the hypoglycaemia was not increased to a statistically significant extent. Of the 5 559 patients who were taking **glipizide**, and hospitalised or given emergency treatment for hypoglycaemia, 31 had recently received a course of **clarithromycin**. For those who took clarithromycin within days one to 5 of the hypoglycaemia, the adjusted odds ratio for the risk of developing hypoglycaemia was 2.9 relative to cefalexin. The risk of hypoglycaemia in those who took **glipizide** with clarithromycin 6 to 10 days could not be assessed due a low number of cases. No statistically significant increased risk was found on the concurrent use of **azithromycin** or **erythromycin** with **glibenclamide** or **glipizide**.[1] Two isolated cases of severe hypoglycaemia occurred in elderly patients with type 2 diabetes and renal impairment given **glibenclamide** or **glipizide** and **clarithromycin**.[2] A further case of hypoglycaemia occurred when an elderly patient, with diabetes and normal renal function taking **glibenclamide** 5 mg daily, also took **clarithromycin** 1 g daily as part of an *Helicobacter pylori* eradication regimen.[3] A case of hypoglycaemia was reported in a patient taking **glibenclamide** and **erythromycin**.[4]

In a placebo-controlled study involving 34 patients with type 2 diabetes (most of whom were taking **glibenclamide** or **glipizide**) found that oral **erythromycin** 400 mg three times daily for a week reduced fructosamine and fasting blood glucose concentrations and increased insulin secretion. Glycaemic control was also improved in a similar study using oral **erythromycin** 200 mg three times daily for 4 weeks.[5] A later study by the same research group found greater improvements in glucose control in patients with type 2 diabetes taking **glibenclamide** when given **erythromycin** 400 mg daily before sleep.[6] Further studies have shown that **erythromycin** increases gastric motility, which results in better control of blood glucose in patients with type 2 diabetes.[7,8]

(b) Effects on the liver

A man with type 2 diabetes taking **chlorpropamide** was given **erythromycin ethylsuccinate** 1 g daily for 3 weeks for a respiratory infection. Two weeks later he complained of increasing fatigue and fever. A short episode of pruriginous skin rash was followed by the appearance of dark urine, jaundice, and hepatomegaly. The picture over the next 2 years was that of profound cholestasis, complicated by steatorrhoea and marked hyperlipidaemia with disappearance of interlobular bile ducts. He died of ischaemic cardiomyopathy.[9]

(c) Pharmacokinetic studies

In a randomised, crossover study in 12 healthy subjects, **clarithromycin** 250 mg twice daily for 2 days increased the AUC of a single 875-microgram dose of **glibenclamide**, given on day 3, by 35% and increased the maximum plasma concentration by 25%.[10] A similar study in 12 patients with type 2 diabetes found that **erythromycin** base 333 mg three times daily for 4 days had no effect on the pharmacokinetics of a single 5-mg dose of **glibenclamide**, given on day 4, or on its blood glucose-lowering effects.[11] A single-dose study in 9 healthy subjects found that **clarithromycin** 250 mg increased the rate of absorption and maximum plasma concentrations of **tolbutamide** 500 mg by about 20% and increased the AUC by 26%. Hypoglycaemia, reported as uneasiness and giddiness, occurred on taking the combination.[12]

Mechanism

The reasons for the serious reaction with chlorpropamide and erythromycin are not understood, but the authors point out that liver damage occurs in a very small number of patients given sulfonylureas, such as chlorpropamide, and also with erythromycin. They suggest that there might have been an interaction between the two drugs. This case is also complicated by a history of long-term use of phenformin, which is known to be hepatotoxic.[9]

It is possible that clarithromycin increased glibenclamide exposure by inhibiting P-glycoprotein.[10] Further study is needed.

Importance and management

The pharmacokinetics of glibenclamide (glyburide) and tolbutamide are altered by clarithromycin and the glucose lowering effects might be enhanced (concurrent tolbutamide and clarithromycin resulted in hypoglycaemia[12]). Limited data from the retrospective study and case reports also suggests that hypoglycaemia can occur. Some caution would seem warranted on the concurrent use of clarithromycin and a sulfonylurea and, as is the case when any change is made to the medication regimen of a patient with diabetes, it would be prudent to monitor blood glucose concentrations, adjusting the dose of the sulfonylurea if necessary. Patients should be warned that increased blood glucose-lowering effects, sometimes excessive, might possibility occur.

An interaction between erythromycin and the sulfonylureas is not established, and from the retrospective, case-control study, no clinically relevant interaction appears to occur between azithromycin and glipizide or glibenclamide. However, it would be prudent to monitor blood glucose concentrations when any change is made to the medication regimen of a patient with diabetes.

No general conclusions can be drawn from the unusual case with chlorpropamide and erythromycin.

1. Schelleman H, Bilker WB, Brensinger CM, Wan F, Hennessy S. Anti-infectives and the risk of severe hypoglycemia in users of glipizide or glyburide. *Clin Pharmacol Ther* (2010) 88, 214
2. Bussing R, Gende A. Severe hypoglycemia from clarithromycin-sulfonylurea drug interaction. *Diabetes Care* (2002) 25, 1659–60.
3. Leiba A, Leibowitz A, Grossman E. An unusual case of hypoglycemia in a diabetic patient. *Ann Emerg Med* (2004) 44, 427–8.
4. Girardin E, Vial T, Pham E, Evreux J-C. Hypoglycémies induites par les sulfamides hypoglycémiants. *Ann Med Interne (Paris)* (1992) 143, 11–17.

5. Ueno N, Inui A, Asakawa A, Takao F, Tani S, Komatsu Y, Itoh Z, Kasuga M. Erythromycin improves glycaemic control in patients with type II diabetes mellitus. *Diabetologia* (2000) 43, 411–15.
6. Ueno N, Inui A, Asakawa A, Takao F, Ichibangase A, Komatsu Y, Kasuga M. Erythromycin administration before sleep is effective in decreasing fasting hyperglycemia in type 2 diabetic patients. *Diabetes Care* (2001) 24, 607.
7. Chang C-T, Shiau Y-C, Lin C-C, Li T-C, Lee C-C, Kao C-H. Improvement of esophageal and gastric motility after 2-week treatment of oral erythromycin in patients with non-insulin-dependent diabetes mellitus. *J Diabetes Complications* (2003) 17, 141–4.
8. Gonlachanvit S, Hsu C-W, Boden GH, Knight LC, Maurer AH, Fisher RS, Parkman HP. Effect of altering gastric emptying on postprandial plasma glucose concentrations following a physiologic meal in type-II diabetic patients. *Dig Dis Sci* (2003) 48, 488–97.
9. Geubel AP, Nakad A, Rahier J, Dive C. Prolonged cholestasis and disappearance of interlobular bile ducts following chlorpropamide and erythromycin ethylsuccinate. Case of drug interaction? *Liver* (1988) 8, 350–3.
10. Lilja JJ, Niemi M, Fredrikson H, Neuvonen PJ. Effects of clarithromycin and grapefruit juice on the pharmacokinetics of glibenclamide. *Br J Clin Pharmacol* (2007) 63, 732–40.
11. Fleishaker JC, Phillips JP. Evaluation of a potential interaction between erythromycin and glyburide in diabetic volunteers. *J Clin Pharmacol* (1991) 31, 259–62.
12. Jayasagar G, Dixit AA, Kirshan V, Rao YM. Effect of clarithromycin on the pharmacokinetics of tolbutamide. *Drug Metabol Drug Interact* (2000) 16, 207–15.

Sulfonylureas + Methylphenidate

A single case report describes reduced serum glucose concentrations when methylphenidate was given to a patient with type 2 diabetes taking glipizide. It seems possible that other sulfonylureas could interact similarly, although this needs confirmation.

Clinical evidence

A 38-year-old woman with type 2 diabetes and a complex medical history, taking **glipizide** 10 mg twice daily, **metformin** 500 mg twice daily, and **insulin**, started taking methylphenidate 10 mg twice daily as part of her rehabilitation after resection of a cerebellar tumour. After 4 days it was noted that her serum glucose concentration was decreasing, requiring a reduction in her **insulin** dose, although there appeared to be no changes in her diet. Overall, she had a 26% decrease in her mean blood glucose concentration.[1]

Mechanism

It is not clear how methylphenidate alone could cause changes in blood glucose concentrations, but one suggestion was that it had direct and/or indirect effects on pancreatic or hepatic function.[1] An interaction with **metformin** was considered unlikely as it is mainly excreted renally.[1] However, it was considered possible that methylphenidate might have inhibited the metabolism of **glipizide** by CYP2C9, resulting in increased glipizide concentrations, a prolongation of its half-life, and a more marked effect on serum glucose concentrations.[1] However, note that methylphenidate is not considered to be a clinically relevant inhibitor of CYP2C9.

Importance and management

Information is limited to this one case report, nevertheless, the authors suggest that if methylphenidate is given to patients with diabetes, close monitoring of glucose concentrations might be prudent.[1] Adjust the dose of the antidiabetics as necessary. If the suggested mechanism of interaction is correct, then other sulfonylureas, many of which are also CYP2C9 substrates, might be expected to interact similarly, but this needs confirmation.

1. Gontkovsky ST, Nevels R, McDonald NB, Winkelmann MH. Decreased serum glucose levels after initiation of methylphenidate in a patient status post-cerebellar tumour resection. A potential interaction with glipizide. *Clin Drug Invest* (2007) 27, 719–25.

Sulfonylureas + NSAIDs

No adverse interaction normally occurs between most NSAIDs and sulfonylureas. However, there are isolated cases of hypoglycaemia in patients given diflunisal with glibenclamide, fenclofenac with chlorpropamide and metformin, ibuprofen with glibenclamide, indometacin with chlorpropamide, and naproxen with glibenclamide and metformin.

Clinical evidence and mechanism

(a) Chlorpropamide

Ibuprofen 1.2 g daily for 4 weeks had no clinically important effect on the blood glucose concentrations of 10 patients with type 2 diabetes taking chlorpropamide 62.5 to 375 mg daily.[1]

A woman whose type 2 diabetes was well controlled with chlorpropamide 500 mg daily and **metformin** 1.7 g daily, developed hypoglycaemia within 2 days of changing her NSAIDs from **flurbiprofen** 150 mg daily and **indometacin** 150 mg daily to **fenclofenac** 1.2 g daily. The antidiabetic drugs were withdrawn the next day, but later in the evening she went into a hypoglycaemic coma. The reason for this is not understood, but it was attributed to a protein binding interaction between chlorpropamide and **fenclofenac**.[2]

(b) Glibenclamide (Glyburide)

1. Acemetacin. No changes in the control of diabetes were seen in 20 patients with type 2 diabetes taking glibenclamide when they were given acemetacin 60 mg three times daily.[3]

2. Bromfenac. The blood glucose concentrations of 12 patients with diabetes taking glibenclamide 10 mg daily were unchanged by bromfenac 50 mg three times daily for 3 days, and the pharmacokinetics of glibenclamide were also unaltered.[4]

3. Diclofenac. The blood glucose concentrations of 12 patients with diabetes and rheumatic diseases taking glibenclamide were unchanged by diclofenac 150 mg daily for 4 days.[5]

4. Diflunisal. An isolated case of hypoglycaemia has been reported in a patient taking glibenclamide with diflunisal.[6]

5. Etodolac. Etodolac does not appear to affect the pharmacokinetics of glibenclamide.[7]

6. Ibuprofen. A study in 16 healthy subjects found that ibuprofen did not affect the pharmacokinetics of glibenclamide. However, ibuprofen with glibenclamide caused a greater blood glucose-lowering effect than glibenclamide alone, but the clinical importance of this was uncertain.[8] A 72-year-old man with longstanding type 2 diabetes, well-controlled with glibenclamide 2.5 mg daily, took a single 150-mg dose of ibuprofen, and 30 minutes later experienced severe nausea, sweating, and palpitations, which were immediately relieved by taking sugar. The symptoms occurred again the next morning after a second dose of ibuprofen, and after a further dose in the afternoon he became unconscious and was given intravenous glucose. Ibuprofen was withdrawn and there were no further episodes of hypoglycaemia. It was also noted that hypoglycaemia had not occurred when he had previously taken aspirin, paracetamol, or diclofenac.[9]

7. Lornoxicam. In 15 healthy subjects, lornoxicam 4 mg twice daily for 6 days had no effect on the pharmacokinetics of a single 5-mg dose of glibenclamide. The pharmacokinetics of lornoxicam also remained unchanged. However, concurrent use increased plasma insulin concentrations, slightly increased the AUC (by 47%), and lowered serum glucose concentrations (by 8%), but this is probably not clinically important.[10]

8. Naproxen. A case of severe hypoglycaemia in a patient with diabetes was attributed to the accumulation of glibenclamide and **metformin** due to deterioration in renal function caused by the concurrent use of ramipril and naproxen.[11]

9. Nimesulide. Although a preliminary report suggested that nimesulide slightly increased the effects of glibenclamide,[12] a later study using various [unnamed] sulfonylureas did not find that it affected fasting blood glucose concentrations or the glucose tolerance of patients with diabetes.[12]

10. Parecoxib. The UK manufacturer of parecoxib (the prodrug of valdecoxib), briefly notes that coadministration with glibenclamide did not affect either the pharmacokinetics of glibenclamide or its effects on insulin or blood glucose concentrations.[13]

11. Piroxicam. Healthy subjects and patients with type 2 diabetes had an increased hypoglycaemic response to glibenclamide (blood glucose concentrations reduced by 13 to 15%) when they were given piroxicam 10 mg.[14]

12. Tenoxicam. Tenoxicam 20 mg daily was found not to affect the glycoregulation of 8 healthy subjects given glibenclamide 2.5 mg daily.[15]

13. Tolmetin. No changes were seen in the blood glucose concentrations of 40 patients with diabetes taking glibenclamide when they were given either tolmetin 1.2 g or placebo daily for 5 days.[16]

(c) Glibornuride

A study in healthy subjects found that **tenoxicam** 20 mg daily did not affect the pharmacokinetics of glibornuride or its effect on plasma insulin and blood glucose concentrations.[17]

(d) Glipizide

In a study in 6 healthy subjects, **indobufen** 200 mg twice daily for 5 days caused a 25% increase in the AUC of a single 5-mg dose of glipizide and a non-significant reduction in their blood glucose concentrations.[18] No important changes in blood glucose concentrations occurred in 24 patients with type 2 diabetes taking tolbutamide or glipizide when they took **indoprofen** 600 mg daily for 5 days.[19] A study in healthy subjects found that although **indoprofen** (200 mg on day one, then 600 mg daily on days 3 to 8) lowered the plasma concentrations of a single 5-mg dose of glipizide, the blood glucose concentrations remained unaffected.[20]

(e) Tolbutamide

Numerous studies in patients with type 2 diabetes, have found no effects on the pharmacokinetics of tolbutamide and/or blood glucose concentrations when given with **sulindac** 400 mg daily,[21] **naproxen** 375 mg every 12 hours for 3 days,[22] or **indoprofen** 600 mg daily for 5 days [patients took tolbutamide or glipizide].[19] In a study in 7 healthy subjects, the pharmacokinetics of a single 500-mg dose of tolbutamide were unaffected after they took **tenoxicam** 20 mg daily for 14 days, and blood glucose concentrations were not altered.[23] A report also briefly states that no changes in blood tolbutamide concentrations or in fasting blood glucose concentrations were seen in patients with diabetes given **diflunisal** 375 mg twice daily.[24] In contrast, in other patients taking tolbutamide it was found that **ibuprofen** lowered fasting blood glucose concentrations, but not below the lower limits of normal.[25]

Importance and management

The reports briefly cited here indicate that no adverse or clinically relevant interaction normally occurs between the sulfonylureas and the NSAIDs named. The general silence in the literature would seem to confirm this. Nevertheless, it is prudent to monitor blood glucose concentrations when any change is made to the medication regimen of a patient with diabetes. Adverse interactions can certainly occur between sulfonylureas and azapropazone, phenylbutazone, oxyphenbutazone, and the salicylates, see 'Sulfonylureas + NSAIDs; Phenylbutazone and related drugs', below, and 'Sulfonylureas + Salicylates', p.551.

1. Shah SJ, Bhandarkar SD, Satoskar RS. Drug interaction between chlorpropamide and non-steroidal anti-inflammatory drugs, ibuprofen and phenylbutazone. *Int J Clin Pharmacol Ther Toxicol* (1984) 22, 470–2.
2. Allen PA, Taylor RT. Fenclofenac and thyroid function tests. *BMJ* (1980) 281, 1642.
3. Haupt E, Hoppe FK, Rechziegler H, Zündorf P. Zur Frage der Interaktionen von nichtsteroidalen Antirheumatika mit oralen Antidiabetika: Acemetacin-Glibenclamid. *Z Rheumatol* (1987) 46, 170–3.
4. Boni JP, Cevallos WH, DeCleene S, Korth-Bradley JM. The influence of bromfenac on the pharmacokinetics and pharmacodynamic responses to glyburide in diabetic subjects. *Pharmacotherapy* (1997) 17, 783–90.
5. Chlud K. Untersuchungen zur Wechselwirkung von Diclofenac und Glibenclamid. *Z Rheumatol* (1976) 35, 377–82.
6. Girardin E, Vial T, Pham E, Evreux J-C. Hypoglycémies induites par les sulfamides hypoglycémiants. *Ann Med Interne (Paris)* (1992) 143, 11–17.
7. Zvaifler N. A review of the antiarthritic efficacy and safety of etodolac. *Clin Rheumatol* (1989) 8 (Suppl 1), 43–53.
8. Kubacka RT, Antal EJ, Juhl RP, Welshman IR. Effects of aspirin and ibuprofen on the pharmacokinetics and pharmacodynamics of glyburide in healthy subjects. *Ann Pharmacother* (1996) 30, 20–26.
9. Sone H, Takahashi A, Yamada N. Ibuprofen-related hypoglycemia in a patient receiving sulfonylurea. *Ann Intern Med* (2001) 134, 344.
10. Ravic M, Johnston A, Turner P. Clinical pharmacological studies of some possible interactions of lornoxicam with other drugs. *Postgrad Med J* (1990) 66 (Suppl 4), S30–S34.
11. Collin M, Mucklow JC. Drug interactions, renal impairment and hypoglycaemia in a patient with type II diabetes. *Br J Clin Pharmacol* (1999) 48, 134–7.
12. Perucca E. Drug interactions with nimesulide. *Drugs* (1993) 46 (Suppl 1), 79–82.
13. Dynastat (Parecoxib sodium). Pfizer Ltd. UK Summary of product characteristics, June 2013.
14. Diwan PV, Sastry MSP, Satyanarayana NV. Potentiation of hypoglycemic response of glibenclamide by piroxicam in rats and humans. *Indian J Exp Biol* (1992) 30, 317–9.
15. Hartmann D, Korn A, Komjati M, Heinz G, Haefelfinger P, Defoin R, Waldhäusl WK. Lack of effect of tenoxicam on dynamic responses to concurrent oral doses of glucose and glibenclamide. *Br J Clin Pharmacol* (1990) 30, 245–52.
16. Chlud K, Kaik B. Clinical studies of the interaction between tolmetin and glibenclamide. *Int J Clin Pharmacol Biopharm* (1977) 15, 409–10.
17. Stoeckel K, Trueb V, Dubach UC, Heintz RC, Ascalone V, Forgo I, Hennes U. Lack of effect of tenoxicam on glibornuride kinetics and response. *Br J Clin Pharmacol* (1985) 19, 249–54.
18. Elvander-Ståhl E, Melander A, Wåhlin-Boll E. Indobufen interacts with the sulphonylurea, glipizide, but not with the β-adrenergic receptor antagonists, propranolol and atenolol. *Br J Clin Pharmacol* (1984) 18, 773–8.
19. Pedrazzi F, Bommartini F, Freddo J, Emanueli A. A study of the possible interaction of indoprofen with hypoglycemic sulfonylureas in diabetic patients. *Eur J Rheumatol Inflamm* (1981) 4, 26–31.
20. Melander A, Wåhlin-Boll E. Interaction of glipizide and indoprofen. *Eur J Rheumatol Inflamm* (1981) 4, 22–5.
21. Ryan JR, Jain AK, McMahon FG, Vargas R. On the question of an interaction between sulindac and tolbutamide in the control of diabetes. *Clin Pharmacol Ther* (1977) 21, 231–3.
22. Whiting B, Williams RL, Lorenzi M, Varady JC, Robins DS. Effect of naproxen on glucose metabolism and tolbutamide kinetics and dynamics in maturity onset diabetics. *Br J Clin Pharmacol* (1981) 11, 295–302.
23. Day RO, Geisslinger G, Paull P, Williams KM. The effect of tenoxicam on tolbutamide pharmacokinetics and glucose concentrations in healthy volunteers. *Int J Clin Pharmacol Ther* (1995) 33, 308–10.
24. Tempero KF, Cirillo VJ, Steelman SL. Diflunisal: a review of the pharmacokinetic and pharmacodynamic properties, drug interactions, and special tolerability studies in humans. *Br J Clin Pharmacol* (1977) 4, 31S–36S.
25. Andersen LA. Ibuprofen and tolbutamide drug interaction study. *Br J Clin Pract* (1980) 34 (Suppl 6), 10–12.

Sulfonylureas + NSAIDs; Phenylbutazone and related drugs

The blood glucose-lowering effects of acetohexamide, carbutamide, chlorpropamide, glibenclamide (glyburide), glymidine, and tolbutamide can be increased by phenylbutazone. Severe hypoglycaemia has occurred in a few patients. Similarly, azapropazone can increase the effects of tolbutamide and cause severe hypoglycaemia. Oxyphenbutazone might be expected to behave similarly. Dipyrone and mofebutazone did not interact with glibenclamide.

Clinical evidence

(a) Azapropazone

A woman whose diabetes was well controlled for 3 years with **tolbutamide** 500 mg twice daily, became confused and semi-comatose 4 days after starting to take azapropazone 900 mg daily. She complained of having felt agitated since starting the azapropazone, so it was withdrawn on suspicion of causing hypoglycaemia. Later that evening she became semi-comatose and was found to have a plasma glucose concentration of 2 mmol/L.[1] A subsequent study in 3 healthy subjects found that azapropazone 900 mg daily increased the plasma half-life of **tolbutamide** 500 mg 3-fold (from 7.7 to 25.2 hours) and reduced its clearance accordingly.[1] Acute hypoglycaemia occurred in another patient taking **tolbutamide** 500 mg three times daily, 5.5 hours after a single 600-mg dose of azapropazone was taken.[2]

(b) Dipyrone (Metamizole)

One randomised, placebo-controlled, crossover study in 12 diabetic patients taking **glibenclamide (glyburide)** suggested that metamizole 1 g daily for 2 days did not interact with **glibenclamide**: no relevant alteration in blood glucose concentrations was found.[3]

(c) Mofebutazone

Mofebutazone 900 mg daily has not been found to cause any clinically important changes in blood glucose concentrations in patients taking **glibenclamide (glyburide)**.[4]

(d) Oxyphenbutazone

Oxyphenbutazone has been found to alter[5] or increase **glymidine** concentrations[6] and **tolbutamide** concentrations.[7,8]

(e) Phenylbutazone

A man with type 2 diabetes taking **tolbutamide** experienced an acute hypoglycaemic episode 4 days after starting phenylbutazone 200 mg three times daily, although there was no change in his diet or in the dose of **tolbutamide**. He was able to control the hypoglycaemia by eating a large bar of chocolate.[9]

There are numerous other case reports and studies of this interaction involving phenylbutazone with **acetohexamide**,[10] **carbutamide**,[11] **chlorpropamide**,[12-14] **glibenclamide (glyburide)**,[15] **glymidine**,[16] and **tolbutamide**,[13,17-23] some of which describe acute hypoglycaemic episodes.[10,12,13,18,20] Several of these interactions have been fatal.[13,23] There is a report suggesting that the interaction between **glibornuride** and phenylbutazone might not be clinically important.[24] In contrast to these reports, a single study describes a paradoxical *increase* in blood glucose concentrations in 3 African patients taking **tolbutamide** and phenylbutazone.[25] In addition to these reports there is some evidence that **tolbutamide** increases the metabolism of phenylbutazone by 42%,[22] but the extent to which this affects its therapeutic effects is uncertain.

Mechanism

Not fully resolved. Some evidence suggests that phenylbutazone can inhibit the renal excretion of glibenclamide (glyburide),[15] tolbutamide,[19] and the active metabolite of acetohexamide[10] so that they are retained in the body longer and their blood glucose-lowering effects are increased and prolonged. It has also been shown that phenylbutazone can inhibit the metabolism of the sulfonylureas[7,22] as well as causing their displacement from protein binding sites.[26] Azapropazone also possibly inhibits the metabolism of tolbutamide,[1] as well as maybe causing displacement from plasma protein binding sites.[2] However, note that the effect of displacement from plasma protein binding sites by itself, is usually transient as any displaced drug is then available to be cleared (see 'Protein-binding interactions', p.3).

Importance and management

The interactions between the sulfonylureas and phenylbutazone are well documented and potentially clinically important. Blood glucose concentrations can be lowered, but the number of reports of acute hypoglycaemic episodes seems to be small. Concurrent use should therefore be well monitored. A reduction in the dose of the sulfonylurea might be necessary if excessive hypoglycaemia is to be avoided. Not all sulfonylureas have been shown to interact (glibornuride probably does not do so) but it would be prudent to assume that they all interact until there is good evidence to suggest otherwise. Oxyphenbutazone might be expected to interact like phenylbutazone (it is a metabolite of phenylbutazone) but, unexpectedly, possibly not mofebutazone, although more study would be needed to confirm this.

The information regarding an interaction between azapropazone and the sulfonylureas seems to be limited to the cases and small study involving tolbutamide. Nevertheless, the manufacturer of azapropazone (when it was available) stated that the concurrent use of sulfonylureas was not recommended.[27]

1. Andreasen PB, Simonsen K, Brocks K, Dimo B, Bouchelouche P. Hypoglycaemia induced by azapropazone-tolbutamide interaction. *Br J Clin Pharmacol* (1981) 12, 581–3.
2. Waller DG, Waller D. Hypoglycaemia due to azapropazone-tolbutamide interaction. *Br J Rheumatol* (1984) 23, 24–5.
3. Haupt E, Hoppe FU, Bamberg E. Zur frage der Wechselwirkungen von Analgetika und oralen Antidiabetika. Metamizol – Glibenclamid. *Med Welt* (1989) 40, 681–3.
4. Speders S. Mofebutazon — Prufung einer moglichen Interaktion mit Glibenclamid. *Fortschr Med* (1993) 111, 366–8.
5. Held H, Scheible G. Interaktion von Phenylbutazon und Oxyphenbutazon mit glymidine. *Arzneimittelforschung* (1981) 31, 1036–8.
6. Held H, Scheible G, von Olderhausen HF. Über Stoffwechsel und Interferenz von Arzneimitteln bei Gesunden und Leberkranken. *Tag Deut Ges Inn Med (Wiesbaden)* (1970) 76, 1153–7.
7. Pond SM, Birkett DJ, Wade DN. Mechanisms of inhibition of tolbutamide metabolism: Phenylbutazone, oxyphenbutazone, sulfaphenazole. *Clin Pharmacol Ther* (1977) 22, 573–9.
8. Kristensen M, Christensen LK. Drug induced changes of the blood glucose lowering effect of oral hypoglycemic agents. *Acta Diabetol Lat* (1969) 6 (Suppl 1), 116–36.
9. Mahfouz M, Abdel-Maguid R, El-Dakhakhny M. Potentiation of the hypoglycaemic action of tolbutamide by different drugs. *Arzneimittelforschung* (1970) 20, 120–2.
10. Field JB, Ohta M, Boyle C, Remer A. Potentiation of acetohexamide hypoglycemia by phenylbutazone. *N Engl J Med* (1967) 277, 889–94.
11. Kaindl F, Kretschy A, Puxkandl H, Wutte J. Zur steigerung des Wirkundseffektes peroraler Antidiabetika durch Pyrazolonderivate. *Wien Klin Wochenschr* (1961) 73, 79–80.
12. Dalgas M, Christiansen I, Kjerulf K. Fenylbutazoninduceret hypoglykaemitilfaelde hos klorpropamidbehandlet diabetiker. *Ugeskr Laeger* (1965) 127, 834–6.
13. Schulz E. Schwere hypoglykämische Reaktionen nach den Sulfonylharnstoffen Tolbutamid, Carbutamid und Chlorpropamid. *Arch Klin Med* (1968) 214, 135–62.
14. Shah SJ, Bhandarkar SD, Satoskar RS. Drug interaction between chlorpropamide and non-steroidal anti-inflammatory drugs, ibuprofen and phenylbutazone. *Int J Clin Pharmacol Ther Toxicol* (1984) 22, 470–2.
15. Schulz E, Koch K, Schmidt FH. Ursachen der Potenzierung der hypoglykämischen Wirkung von Sulfonylharnstoff-derivaten durch Medikamente. II. Pharmakokinetik und Metabolismus von Glibenclamid (HN 419) in Gegenwart von Phenylbutazon. *Eur J Clin Pharmacol* (1971) 4, 32–7.
16. Held H, Kaminski B, von Olderhausen HF. Die beeinflussung der Elimination von Glycodiazin durch Leber-und Nierenfunktionsstorungen und durch eine Behandlung mit Phenylbutazon, Phenprocumarol und Doxycyclin. *Diabetologia* (1970) 6, 386–91.
17. Gulbrandsen R. Økt tolbutamid-effekt ved hjelp av fenylbutazon? *Tidsskr Nor Laegeforen* (1959) 79, 1127–8.
18. Tannenbaum H, Anderson LG, Soeldner JS. Phenylbutazone-tolbutamide drug interaction. *N Engl J Med* (1974) 290, 344.
19. Ober K-F. Mechanism of interaction of tolbutamide and phenylbutazone in diabetic patients. *Eur J Clin Pharmacol* (1974) 7, 291–4.
20. Dent LA, Jue SG. Tolbutamide-phenylbutazone interaction. *Drug Intell Clin Pharm* (1976) 10, 711.
21. Christensen LK, Hansen JM, Kristensen M. Sulphaphenazole-induced hypoglycaemic attacks in tolbutamide-treated diabetics. *Lancet* (1963) ii, 1298–1301.
22. Szita M, Gachályi B, Tornyossy M, Káldor A. Interaction of phenylbutazone and tolbutamide in man. *Int J Clin Pharmacol Ther Toxicol* (1990) 18, 378–80.

23. Slade IH, Iosefa RN. Fatal hypoglycemic coma from the use of tolbutamide in elderly patients: report of two cases. *J Am Geriatr Soc* (1967) 15, 948–50.
24. Eckhardt W, Rudolph R, Sauer H, Schubert WR, Undeutsch D. Zur pharmackologischen Interferenz von Glibornurid mit Sulfaphenazol, Phenylbutazon und Phenprocoumon beim Menschen. *Arzneimittelforschung* (1972) 22, 2212–19.
25. Owusu SK, Ocran K. Paradoxical behaviour of phenylbutazone in African diabetics. *Lancet* (1972) i, 440–41.
26. Hellman B. Potentiating effects of drugs on the binding of glibenclamide to pancreatic beta cells. *Metabolism* (1974) 23, 839–46.
27. Rheumox (Azapropazone dihydrate). Goldshield Pharmaceuticals Ltd. UK Summary of product characteristics, February 2000.

Sulfonylureas + Probenecid

The clearance of chlorpropamide is reduced by probenecid. Tolbutamide appears not to interact with probenecid.

Clinical evidence, mechanism, importance and management

A study in 6 patients given single oral doses of **chlorpropamide** found that probenecid 1 to 2 g daily increased the **chlorpropamide** half-life from about 36 hours to 50 hours.[1] It seems that the probenecid reduces the renal excretion of **chlorpropamide**. Another report in healthy subjects suggested that the half-life of **tolbutamide** was also prolonged by probenecid,[2] but this was not confirmed by a further controlled study.[3]

Information is very limited but it might be necessary to reduce the dose of **chlorpropamide** in the presence of probenecid. It seems unlikely that a clinically important interaction will occur with **tolbutamide**. Information about other sulfonylureas appears to be lacking, but note that one UK manufacturer of **glimepiride** predicts that probenecid might potentiate the glucose-lowering effects of glimepiride and warns that hypoglycaemia could occur on concurrent use.[4]

1. Petitpierre B, Perrin L, Rudhardt M, Herrera A, Fabre J. Behaviour of chlorpropamide in renal insufficiency and under the effect of associated drug therapy. *Int J Clin Pharmacol* (1972) 6, 120–4.
2. Stowers JM, Mahler RF, Hunter RB. Pharmacology and mode of action of the sulphonylureas in man. *Lancet* (1958) i, 278–83.
3. Brook R, Schrogie JJ, Solomon HM. Failure of probenecid to inhibit the rate of metabolism of tolbutamide in man. *Clin Pharmacol Ther* (1968) 9, 314–17.
4. Amaryl (Glimepiride). Zentiva. UK Summary of product characteristics, October 2013.

Sulfonylureas + Rifamycins

Rifampicin has also been shown to slightly to moderately reduce the exposure to glibenclamide (glyburide), however, conversely, a single intravenous dose of rifampicin given with glibenclamide moderately *increased* its exposure. Rifampicin (rifampin) moderately reduces the exposure to gliclazide and slightly reduces the exposure to glimepiride and glipizide. Limited evidence appears to show a similar effect on chlorpropamide, glymidine, and tolbutamide.

Clinical evidence

(a) Chlorpropamide

A single case report describes a man with type 2 diabetes who needed an increase in his dose of chlorpropamide from 250 to 400 mg daily when he was given **rifampicin** 600 mg daily. His chlorpropamide serum concentrations increased dramatically 12 months later when the **rifampicin** was withdrawn.[1]

(b) Glibenclamide (Glyburide)

A study in 29 patients with type 2 diabetes taking glibenclamide, found that when they were also given **rifampicin** 450 or 600 mg daily for 10 days, their blood glucose concentrations, both fasting and after meals, were increased. Glibenclamide dose changes were needed in 15 out of 17 patients in whom the diabetes became uncontrolled. Their blood glucose concentrations normalised 6 days after stopping **rifampicin**.[2] Another patient with type 2 diabetes taking glibenclamide had a deterioration in diabetic control over the 8 months after she started **rifampicin**, which required an increase in glibenclamide dose and the addition of insulin. On stopping **rifampicin**, her minimum serum glibenclamide concentrations increased, from 40 nanograms/mL to 200 nanograms/mL, but there was no appreciable change in blood glucose concentrations.[3]

A randomised, crossover study in 10 healthy subjects found that **rifampicin** 600 mg daily for 5 days decreased the AUC of a single 1.75-mg dose of glibenclamide given on day 6 by 39% and the maximum plasma concentration by 22%. The elimination half-life was shortened from 2 hours to 1.7 hours and the maximum reduction in blood glucose concentration was decreased by 36% by **rifampicin**.[4] However, in contrast, in a similar study in 9 healthy subjects, a single 600-mg intravenous dose of **rifampicin** given over 30 minutes immediately before a single 1.25-mg dose of glibenclamide, caused a (2.2-fold) *increase* in the AUC of glibenclamide, leading to a greater reduction in blood glucose concentrations and hypoglycaemia in one subject. When a single 600-mg intravenous dose of rifampicin was given on day 7 after 6 days of oral rifampicin 600 mg daily, there was a 28% reduction in the AUC of glibenclamide given immediately afterwards, which was considerably less than the 65% reduction seen 2 days later.[5]

(c) Gliclazide

A 65-year-old patient with type 2 diabetes taking gliclazide 80 mg daily for 2 years without problem was given **rifampicin** 450 mg daily, isoniazid, ethambutol, and clarithromycin for an atypical mycobacteriosis. Fasting blood glucose concentrations became increased requiring an increase in the dose of gliclazide to 120 mg daily then 160 mg daily. The plasma concentration of gliclazide on day 75 was 1.4 micrograms/mL, 2 hours after an 80-mg dose. When **rifampicin** was stopped the gliclazide concentration increased to 4.7 micrograms/mL and the dose was reduced back to 80 mg daily.[6] A study in 9 healthy subjects found that pre-treatment with **rifampicin** 600 mg for 6 days decreased the AUC of a single 80-mg dose of gliclazide given on day 7 by 70%. The mean elimination half-life of gliclazide was reduced from 9.5 hours to 3.3 hours and the gliclazide oral clearance was increased by about 4-fold. The blood glucose-lowering effects of gliclazide were reduced by **rifampicin** (blood glucose concentrations increased from 8 mmol/L to 9.4 mmol/L).[7]

(d) Glimepiride

A randomised, crossover study in 10 healthy subjects found that **rifampicin** 600 mg daily for 5 days decreased the AUC of a single 1-mg dose of glimepiride given on day 6 by 34%. **Rifampicin** reduced the elimination half-life of glimepiride by 25%. However, no statistically significant differences in blood glucose concentrations were found between the **rifampicin** and placebo regimens.[8]

(e) Glipizide

A randomised, crossover study in 10 healthy subjects found that **rifampicin** 600 mg daily for 5 days decreased the AUC of a single 2.5-mg dose of glipizide given on day 6 by 22%. The elimination half-life was shortened from 3 hours to 1.9 hours by **rifampicin**. However, no statistically significant differences in blood glucose concentrations were found.[4]

(f) Glymidine

In one study the half-life of glymidine was reduced by about one-third by the concurrent use of **rifampicin**.[9]

(g) Tolbutamide

After treatment for 4 weeks with **rifampicin** the half-life of tolbutamide in 9 patients with diabetes and tuberculosis was reduced by 43%, and its serum concentration measured at 6 hours was halved, when compared with other patients not taking **rifampicin**.[10] Similar results have been found in other studies in patients with cirrhosis or cholestasis[11] and in healthy subjects.[12] Where assessed, there was no difference in the effects of tolbutamide on blood glucose concentrations between treatments.[10]

Mechanism

Rifampicin is a well-known enzyme inducer, and moderately induces CYP2C9, which is involved in the metabolism of chlorpropamide, glibenclamide (glyburide), gliclazide, glimepiride, and glipizide, resulting in reduced exposure. Tolbutamide is also metabolised by CYP2C9 (it is used a probe substrate to assess the activity of drugs on this isoenzyme) and its concentrations are reduced by concurrent rifampicin. However, rifampicin is also an inhibitor of hepatic organic anion-transporting polypeptide 1B1 (OATP1B1), which is involved in the hepatic uptake of glibenclamide and this effect might explain the difference in the size of effect between simultaneous and separated administration, and the differing effects of single-dose and multiple-dose rifampicin. Acute administration of a single intravenous dose of rifampicin with glibenclamide inhibited glibenclamide uptake into the liver, and reduced its metabolism,[5] resulting in moderately increased exposure. However, when administration was separated, a moderate *reduction* in glibenclamide exposure was seen (due to CYP2C9 induction). When a single-dose of rifampicin was given simultaneously with glibenclamide after a multiple-dose rifampicin regimen, there was only a slight reduction in glibenclamide exposure, suggesting that the OATP1B1 inhibiting effects of rifampicin reduced the size of the CYP2C9 inducing effects. There is also evidence with repaglinide (see 'Meglitinides + Rifamycins and other enzyme inducers', p.529) and atorvastatin (see 'Statins + Rifampicin (Rifampin)', p.1355), that the effect of OATP inhibition by rifampicin varies in this way.

Importance and management

A pharmacokinetic interaction between glibenclamide (glyburide), gliclazide, glimepiride, or glipizide and rifampicin (rifampin) is established, but the clinical importance of this varies, as is the effect of rifampicin on the pharmacokinetic parameters measured in the tolbutamide studies. The effect of the reduced exposure seen with glibenclamide and gliclazide can be clinically important, and patients taking these sulfonylureas might need an increase in their sulfonylurea dose while taking rifampicin. It would be prudent to monitor blood glucose concentrations on concurrent use of rifampicin, adjusting the sulfonylurea dose accordingly, remembering that the effects of rifampicin can continue beyond stopping, and monitoring for 2 weeks after stopping is advisable. In the case of glibenclamide, the timing of administration might also be important, as could the duration of rifampicin. With multiple-dose rifampicin regimens, simultaneous administration might reduce the size of the effect. The study using a single intravenous dose of rifampicin suggested that the effect of oral glibenclamide given at a similar time might be increased. Whether this occurs with the first oral dose of rifampicin was not studied, but this has been seen with atorvastatin (see 'Statins + Rifampicin (Rifampin)', p.1355). On this basis, if rifampicin is to be given with glibenclamide, as very short courses or repeated single-doses, as is the case for meningococcal prophylaxis (2 days) or leprosy (once monthly), respectively, careful monitoring of blood glucose concentrations would seem prudent, as the inhibitory effects of rifampicin would be expected to predominate due to the inductive effects requiring several days to develop. Separated administration might reduce the size of the effect in these scenarios.

Caution might also be warranted for chlorpropamide, but the documentation for this interaction is very limited. The effect of rifampicin on the blood glucose-lowering effects of glimepiride, glipizide, or tolbutamide might be of only limited clinical importance. Nevertheless, it is prudent to monitor blood glucose concentrations when any change is made to the medication regimen of a patient with diabetes.

There does not seem to be any information regarding **rifabutin** and **rifapentine**; however, the UK manufacturer and the CSM in the UK warn that rifabutin might possibly reduce the effects of a number of drugs, including oral antidiabetics (not specified).[13,14]

1. Self TH, Morris T. Interaction of rifampin and chlorpropamide. *Chest* (1980) 77, 800–801.
2. Surekha V, Peter JV, Jeyaseelan L, Cherian AM. Drug interaction: rifampicin and glibenclamide. *Natl Med J India* (1997) 10, 11–12.
3. Self TH, Tsiu SJ, Fowler JW. Interaction of rifampin and glyburide. *Chest* (1989) 96, 1443–4.
4. Niemi M, Backman JT, Neuvonen M, Neuvonen PJ, Kivistö KT. Effects of rifampin on the pharmacokinetics and pharmacodynamics of glyburide and glipizide. *Clin Pharmacol Ther* (2001) 69, 400–6.
5. Zheng HX, Huang Y, Frassetto LA, Benet LZ. Elucidating rifampin's inducing and inhibiting effects on glyburide pharmacokinetics and blood glucose in healthy volunteers: unmasking the differential effects of enzyme induction and transporter inhibition for a drug and its primary metabolite. *Clin Pharmacol Ther* (2009) 85, 78–85.
6. Kihara Y, Otsuki M. Interaction of gliclazide and rifampicin. *Diabetes Care* (2000) 23, 1204–5.
7. Park J-Y, Kim K-A, Park P-W, Park C-W, Shin J-G. Effect of rifampin on the pharmacokinetics and pharmacodynamics of gliclazide. *Clin Pharmacol Ther* (2003) 74, 334–40.
8. Niemi M, Kivistö KT, Backman JT, Neuvonen PJ. Effect of rifampicin on the pharmacokinetics and pharmacodynamics of glimepiride. *Br J Clin Pharmacol* (2000) 50, 591–5.
9. Held H, Schoene B, Laar HJ, Fleischmann R. Die Aktivität der Benzpyrenhydroxylase im Leberpunktat des Menschen in vitro und ihre Beziehung zur Eliminations-geschwindigkeit von Glycodiazin in vivo. *Verh Dtsch Ges Inn Med* (1974) 80, 501–3.
10. Syvälahti E, Pihlajamäki K, Iisalo E. Effect of tuberculostatic agents on the response of serum growth hormone and immunoreactive insulin to intravenous tolbutamide, and on the half-life of tolbutamide. *Int J Clin Pharmacol Biopharm* (1976) 13, 83–9.
11. Zilly W, Breimer DD, Richter E. Stimulation of drug metabolism by rifampicin in patients with cirrhosis or cholestasis measured by increased hexobarbital and tolbutamide clearance. *Eur J Clin Pharmacol* (1977) 11, 287–93.
12. Zilly W, Breimer DD, Richter E. Induction of drug metabolism in man after rifampicin treatment measured by increased hexobarbital and tolbutamide clearance. *Eur J Clin Pharmacol* (1975) 9, 219–27.
13. Mycobutin (Rifabutin). Pfizer Ltd. UK Summary of product characteristics, December 2013.
14. Committee on the Safety of Medicines/Medicines Control Agency. Revised indication and drug interactions of rifabutin. *Current Problems* (1997) 23, 14. Available at: http://webarchive.nationalarchives.gov.uk/20141205150130/http://www.mhra.gov.uk/home/groups/pl-p/documents/websiteresources/con2023238.pdf (accessed 22/10/15)

Sulfonylureas + Salicylates

Aspirin and other salicylates can lower blood glucose concentrations, but small analgesic doses do not normally have an adverse effect on patients taking sulfonylureas. Larger doses of salicylates might have a more important effect.

Clinical evidence

(a) Chlorpropamide

In 5 healthy subjects the blood glucose-lowering effects of chlorpropamide and **sodium salicylate** were found to be additive. A further study in 6 healthy subjects found that chlorpropamide 100 mg given with **sodium salicylate** 1.5 g lowered blood glucose concentrations by the same amount as either chlorpropamide 200 mg or **sodium salicylate** 3 g alone.[1]

The blood glucose concentrations of a patient taking chlorpropamide 500 mg daily were lowered about two-thirds by **aspirin** in doses sufficient to give serum salicylate concentrations of about 1.9 mmol/L.[2]

(b) Glibenclamide (Glyburide)

In a study, 16 healthy subjects took a single 5-mg dose of glibenclamide both before and on the fourth day of taking **aspirin** 975 mg four times daily for 4 days. It was found that the **aspirin** reduced the AUC_{0-4} of the glibenclamide by 68% and reduced its mean maximum serum concentrations by 35%. The effects of these changes on glucose tolerance tests and insulin responses were difficult to interpret, but there was no clear evidence that any clinically relevant changes occurred.[3]

Mechanism

It has been known for over 100 years that aspirin and salicylates have blood glucose-lowering properties and in relatively large doses can be used on their own in the treatment of diabetes.[4-8] The simplest explanation for this interaction with sulfonylureas is that the blood glucose-lowering effects are additive,[1] but there is some evidence that other mechanisms might come into play.[8] In addition, aspirin can increase serum chlorpropamide concentrations, possibly by interfering with renal tubular excretion, and therefore the effects of chlorpropamide are enhanced.[2]

Importance and management

The interaction between the sulfonylureas and the salicylates is established but of limited importance. Considering the extremely wide use of aspirin it might reasonably be expected that any generally serious interaction would have come to light by now. The data available, coupled with the common experience of diabetic patients,[9] is that excessive and unwanted hypoglycaemia is very unlikely with small to moderate analgesic doses of salicylates. Some downward adjustment of the dose of the sulfonylurea might be appropriate if large doses of salicylates are used. Information about **other antidiabetics** and salicylates appears to be lacking, but they are expected to behave similarly.

1. Richardson T, Foster J, Mawer GE. Enhancement by sodium salicylate of the blood glucose lowering effect of chlorpropamide - drug interaction or summation of similar effects? *Br J Clin Pharmacol* (1986) 22, 43–48.
2. Stowers JM, Constable LW, Hunter RB. A clinical and pharmacological comparison of chlorpropamide and other sulfonylureas. *Ann N Y Acad Sci* (1959) 74, 689–95.
3. Kubacka RT, Antal EJ, Juhl RP, Welshman IR. Effects of aspirin and ibuprofen on the pharmacokinetics and pharmacodynamics of glyburide in healthy subjects. *Ann Pharmacother* (1996) 30, 20–6.
4. Gilgore SG, Rupp JJ. The long-term response of diabetes mellitus to salicylate therapy. Report of a case. *JAMA* (1962) 180, 65–6.
5. Reid J, Macdougall AI, Andrews MM. Aspirin and diabetes mellitus. *BMJ* (1957) 2, 1071–4.
6. Ebstein W. Zur Therapie des Diabetes mellitus, insbesondere über die Anwendung des salicylsauren Natron bei demselben. Berl Klin Wschr (1876) 13, 337–40.
7. Bartels K. Ueber die therapeutische Verwerthung der Salizylsäure und ihres Nastronsalzes in der inneren Medicin. Dtsch Med Wschr (1878) 4, 423–5.
8. Cattaneo AG, Caviezel F, Pozza G. Pharmacological interaction between tolbutamide and acetylsalicylic acid: study on insulin secretion in man. *Int J Clin Pharmacol Ther Toxicol* (1990) 28, 229–34.
9. Logie AW, Galloway DB, Petrie JC. Drug interactions and long-term antidiabetic therapy. *Br J Clin Pharmacol* (1976) 3, 1027–32.

Sulfonylureas + SSRIs

Fluvoxamine slightly reduces the clearance of tolbutamide and increases the maximum plasma concentrations of glimepiride. Fluoxetine did not alter the pharmacokinetics of tolbutamide, and sertraline does not appear to affect the pharmacokinetics of glibenclamide (glyburide) or tolbutamide.

Clinical evidence

(a) Fluoxetine

In a crossover study in healthy subjects, fluoxetine, given as a single 30-mg dose, or 30 mg daily for 8 days, did not affect the pharmacokinetics or the blood glucose-lowering effects of a single 1-g dose of **tolbutamide**.[1]

(b) Fluvoxamine

A randomised, crossover study in 14 healthy subjects given fluvoxamine 75 or 150 mg daily for 5 days, with a single 500-mg dose of **tolbutamide** on the third day, found that the clearance of **tolbutamide** was reduced by 19% by the 75 mg dose, and reduced by 33% by the 150 mg dose of fluvoxamine. The clearance of its metabolites (4-hydroxytolbutamide and carboxytolbutamide) was also decreased.[2]

A randomised, crossover study in 12 healthy subjects given fluvoxamine 100 mg or placebo daily for 4 days, with a single 500-microgram dose of **glimepiride** on the fourth day, found the AUC of **glimepiride** was not affected by fluvoxamine. Maximum plasma concentrations of **glimepiride** were increased by 43% and the elimination half-life was prolonged from 2 hours to 2.3 hours, but there was no notable change in the effects of **glimepiride** on blood glucose concentrations.[3]

(c) Sertraline

In a randomised study, sertraline 200 mg daily for 22 days appeared to decrease the clearance of a single 1-g intravenous dose of **tolbutamide** by 16% in 11 healthy subjects when compared with 12 other subjects taking placebo.[4] In another study, the pharmacokinetics of a single 5-mg dose of **glibenclamide (glyburide)** appeared to be unaffected by sertraline, taken in increasing doses up to 200 mg daily over 15 days in 11 healthy subjects when compared with 10 other subjects given placebo. Blood glucose concentrations were also no different.[5]

Mechanism

Fluvoxamine inhibits CYP2C9, by which tolbutamide is metabolised. Glimepiride is also metabolised by CYP2C9 and this mechanism might partly explain the increase in plasma concentrations of glimepiride. However, as the glimepiride AUC was not increased, and the half-life was only minimally increased, the increase in plasma concentrations might also be due to an increased rate of glimepiride absorption caused by the SSRI.[2,3]

Importance and management

Fluoxetine and fluvoxamine do not cause any clinically relevant pharmacokinetic interactions with tolbutamide or glimepiride, and sertraline does not appear to alter the pharmacokinetics of tolbutamide or glibenclamide. No dose adjustments would seem necessary. As other sulfonylureas are metabolised similarly, no dose adjustments with these would be expected to be necessary either on concurrent use with these SSRIs. Other SSRIs are not known to affect CYP2C9, and therefore no interaction would be expected between these and any sulfonylurea by this mechanism. Note that the concurrent use of SSRIs and antidiabetics has been associated with changes to glycaemic control (see 'Antidiabetics + SSRIs', p.518 for details), therefore it is prudent to monitor blood glucose concentrations on stopping or starting a SSRI, and also when any change is made to the medication regimen of a patient with diabetes.

Tolbutamide can be used as a probe substrate to assess the activity of drugs on CYP2C9. This study therefore suggests that fluvoxamine (at a dose of 150 mg daily) is a weak inhibitor of CYP2C9.

1. Lemberger L, Bergstrom RF, Wolen RL, Farid NA, Enas GG, Aronoff GR. Fluoxetine: clinical pharmacology and physiologic disposition. *J Clin Psychiatry* (1985) 46, 14–19.
2. Madsen H, Enggaard TP, Hansen LL, Klitgaard NA, Brøsen K. Fluvoxamine inhibits the CYP2C9 catalysed biotransformation of tolbutamide. *Clin Pharmacol Ther* (2001) 69, 41–7.
3. Niemi M, Backman JT, Neuvonen M, Laitila J, Neuvonen PJ, Kivistö KT. Effects of fluconazole and fluvoxamine on the pharmacokinetics of glimepiride. *Clin Pharmacol Ther* (2001) 69, 194–200.
4. Tremaine LM, Wilner KD, Preskorn SH. A study of the potential effect of sertraline on the pharmacokinetics and protein binding of tolbutamide. *Clin Pharmacokinet* (1997) 32 (Suppl 1), 31–6.
5. Invicta Pharmaceuticals. Data on file. A double blind placebo controlled, multiple dose study to assess potential interaction between oral sertraline (200 mg) and glibenclamide (5 mg) in healthy male volunteers (Study 223). 1991.

Sulfonylureas + St John's wort (*Hypericum perforatum*)

St John's wort slightly decreased gliclazide exposure, but did not affect the metabolism of tolbutamide.

Clinical evidence

(a) Gliclazide

In a crossover study in 21 healthy subjects, a 300-mg dose of a St John's wort preparation with a high hyperforin content (*LI 160, Lichtwer Pharma*) was given 3 times daily for 15 days. On the last day of treatment, a single 80-mg dose of gliclazide was given, followed 30 minutes later by glucose 75 g. St John's wort reduced AUC of gliclazide by 35% and reduced the maximum concentrations by 22%. The clearance was increased by 47%. No statistically significant changes were found in the $AUC_{0\text{-}4}$ or blood concentrations of glucose or insulin.[1]

(b) Tolbutamide

In a pharmacokinetic study, St John's wort 900 mg daily had no effect on the metabolism of a single dose of tolbutamide either after one day or after 2 weeks of use. The St John's wort product used provided about 33 mg of hyperforin daily.[2] Similarly, in a placebo-controlled study, a St John's wort preparation with low hyperforin content (*Esbericum*) at a dose of 240 mg daily (which provided about 3.5 mg of hyperforin daily) appeared to have no effect on tolbutamide metabolism in healthy subjects when compared with other subjects receiving placebo.[3]

Mechanism

Gliclazide is a substrate of CYP2C9 and the authors suggest that St John's wort induces this isoenzyme, thereby increasing the metabolism of gliclazide and reducing its exposure. The magnitude of this effect was not influenced by CYP2C9 genotype.[1] However, the fact that tolbutamide, which can be used as a probe substrate to assess the activity of drugs on CYP2C9 was unaffected by St John's wort, suggests that other factors could be involved.

Importance and management

There is evidence for a pharmacokinetic interaction between St John's wort and gliclazide, although the mechanism by which this occurs is unclear. The small reduction in gliclazide exposure does not appear to be clinically important as its blood-glucose-lowering effects were unaffected. No pharmacokinetic interaction occurs with St John's wort and tolbutamide and no special precautions appear to be necessary if these drugs are used together. However, it is generally considered prudent to monitor blood glucose concentrations when any change is made to the medication regimen of a patient with diabetes.

1. Xu H, Williams KM, Liauw WS, Murray M, Day RO, McLachlan AJ. Effects of St John's wort and CYP2C9 genotype on the pharmacokinetics and pharmacodynamics of gliclazide. *Br J Pharmacol* (2008) 153, 1579–86.
2. Wang Z, Gorski JC, Hamman MA, Huang S-M, Lesko LJ, Hall SD. The effects of St John's wort (*Hypericum perforatum*) on human cytochrome P450 activity. *Clin Pharmacol Ther* (2001) 70, 317–26.
3. Arold G, Donath F, Maurer A, Diefenbach K, Bauer S, Henneicke-von Zepelin H-H, Friede M, Roots I. No relevant interaction with alprazolam, caffeine, tolbutamide, and digoxin by treatment with a low-hyperforin St John's wort extract. *Planta Med* (2005) 71, 331–7.

Sulfonylureas + Statins

Lovastatin does not appear to alter the pharmacokinetics of chlorpropamide, and the pharmacokinetics of tolbutamide do not appear to be altered by fluvastatin or simvastatin. Glibenclamide (glyburide) exposure appears to be slightly increased by fluvastatin and simvastatin. No changes in diabetic control were seen for any combination.

Clinical evidence

(a) Chlorpropamide

A study in 7 patients with type 2 diabetes and hypercholesterolaemia, taking chlorpropamide 125 to 750 mg daily, found that **lovastatin** 20 mg twice daily for 6 weeks did not alter chlorpropamide plasma concentrations, and the diabetic control remained unaltered. The study also showed comparable reductions in low-density lipoprotein cholesterol (reduced by 28%) to those seen in non-diabetic patients.[1]

(b) Glibenclamide (Glyburide)

In a placebo-controlled study, two groups of 16 healthy subjects taking **fluvastatin** 40 mg or **simvastatin** 20 mg daily for 15 days were given a single 3.5-mg oral dose of glibenclamide on days one, 8, and 15. The maximum plasma concentration and the AUC of glibenclamide appeared to be increased by about 20% by the statins when compared with a group of 16 other healthy subjects given placebo. The blood glucose-lowering effects of glibenclamide remained virtually unchanged by both **fluvastatin** and **simvastatin** in these subjects, and also when **fluvastatin** was tested in a group of 32 patients with type 2 diabetes.[2] Nevertheless, the UK and US manufacturers of **fluvastatin** report a study in which a higher dose of **fluvastatin**, 40 mg twice daily for 14 days, was given to 32 patients with diabetes stable taking glibenclamide 5 to 20 mg daily. **Fluvastatin** increased the AUC of glibenclamide by about 70% and increased the maximum serum concentration by 50%, although there were no clinically important changes in blood glucose concentrations. Glibenclamide increased the AUC of fluvastatin by 44% and increased the maximum concentration by 51%.[3,4]

(c) Tolbutamide

In a placebo-controlled study, two groups of 16 healthy subjects taking **fluvastatin** 40 mg or **simvastatin** 20 mg daily for 15 days were given a single 1-g dose of oral tolbutamide on days one, 8, and 15. The pharmacokinetics of the tolbutamide appeared to be affected only to a very minor extent, and the blood glucose-lowering effects of the tolbutamide were no different, when compared with a group of 16 other healthy subjects given placebo.[2]

Mechanism

The changes in the pharmacokinetics of glibenclamide (glyburide) caused by fluvastatin and simvastatin are not understood.

Importance and management

There is little evidence to suggest that special precautions appear to be needed by patients with diabetes taking any of the pairs of sulfonylureas and statins cited here (chlorpropamide with lovastatin; or glibenclamide or tolbutamide with fluvastatin or simvastatin). Nevertheless, the UK and US manufacturers of fluvastatin recommend close monitoring on concurrent use if the fluvastatin dose is changed[4] or increased to 80 mg daily.[3]

It is prudent to monitor blood glucose concentrations when any change is made to the medication regimen of a patient with diabetes, and this should be sufficient to identify any changes to diabetic control should they occur after the introduction of a statin.

Note that a number of the large-scale studies of the use of lipid-regulating drugs in primary or secondary prevention of cardiovascular events included patients with diabetes. A review of these subgroups concluded that statins were the drug of choice for lipid-lowering therapy in patients with type 2 diabetes and known coronary artery disease or other cardiovascular risk factors. There was no evidence to recommend one statin over another.[5] NICE guidelines in the UK recommend use of a statin in patients with type 2 diabetes with relevant cardiovascular risks.[6]

1. Johnson BF, LaBelle P, Wilson J, Allan J, Zupkis RV, Ronca PD. Effects of lovastatin in diabetic patients treated with chlorpropamide. *Clin Pharmacol Ther* (1990) 48, 467–72.
2. Appel S, Rüfenacht T, Kalafsky G, Tetzloff W, Kallay Z, Hitzenberger G, Kutz K. Lack of interaction between fluvastatin and oral hypoglycemic agents in healthy subjects and in patients with non-insulin-dependent diabetes mellitus. *Am J Cardiol* (1995) 76, 29A–32A.
3. Lescol (Fluvastatin sodium). Novartis Pharmaceuticals UK Ltd. UK Summary of product characteristics, November 2013.
4. Lescol (Fluvastatin sodium). Novartis Pharmaceuticals Corp. US Prescribing information, October 2012.
5. Snow V, Aronson MD, Hornbake ER, Mottur-Pilson C, Weiss KB, for the Clinical Efficacy Assessment Subcommittee of the American College of Physicians. Lipid control in the management of type 2 diabetes mellitus: a clinical practice guideline from the American College of Physicians. *Ann Intern Med* (2004) 140, 644–9.
6. National Institute for Clinical Excellence. Type 2 diabetes: the management of type 2 diabetes: partial update (issued March 2010). Available at: http://www.nice.org.uk/nicemedia/pdf/CG87NICEGuideline.pdf (accessed 21/10/15)

Sulfonylureas or Insulin + Fibrates

A number of reports describe hypoglycaemia and/or an enhancement of the effects of antidiabetic drugs (mostly insulin and sulfonylureas) in patients given fibrates, but there is also some evidence of improved glycaemic control or no effect. The antidiuretic effects of clofibrate in the treatment of diabetes insipidus are opposed by glibenclamide (glyburide).

Clinical evidence

A. Bezafibrate

Three elderly patients with type 2 diabetes and mild renal impairment taking **glibenclamide (glyburide)** developed hypoglycaemia when they were given bezafibrate: one of them needed a 60% dose reduction, another was given **tolbutamide** instead, and the third was able to stop both **glibenclamide** and **buformin**.[1] During the period 1985 to 1990, the French Centres Régionaux de Pharmacovigilance recorded 7 cases of hypoglycaemia, which developed in patients taking unnamed sulfonylureas when they were given fibrates (one case with bezafibrate).[2] In contrast, a study conducted in patients with type 2 diabetes taking gliclazide or glibenclamide found that bezafibrate improved blood glucose control.[3]

B. Ciprofibrate

During the period 1985 to 1990, the French Centres Régionaux de Pharmacovigilance recorded 7 cases of hypoglycaemia, which developed in patients taking unnamed **sulfonylureas** when they were given fibrates (3 cases with ciprofibrate).[2] In contrast, in a randomised crossover study in patients with type 2 diabetes treated with diet and **sulfonylureas** (drugs not specified), the addition of ciprofibrate had no effect on glycaemic control.[4]

C. Clofibrate

(a) Hypoglycaemia

Over a 5-day period while taking clofibrate 2 g daily, the control of diabetes was improved in 6 out of 13 patients with type 2 diabetes taking various unnamed sulfonylureas. Hypoglycaemia (blood glucose concentrations of about 1.7 to 2.2 mmol/L) was seen in 4 patients.[5] Other studies confirm that in some, but not all, patients, blood glucose concentrations can decrease while taking clofibrate and the control of the diabetes can improve.[6-13] In one study the half-life of **chlorpropamide** ranged from 40 to 62 hours in 5 subjects taking clofibrate compared with a mean of about 36 hours in control subjects.[14]

(b) Reduced antidiuretic effects

Clofibrate 2 g daily reduced the volume of urine excreted by 2 patients with pituitary diabetes insipidus, but when **glibenclamide** was also given the volume increased once again. Without treatment they excreted 5.8 litres and 6.5 litres of urine daily, and this reduced to only 2.4 litres and 1.7 litres, respectively, while taking clofibrate, whereas with **glibenclamide** and clofibrate they excreted 3.6 litres and 3.7 litres daily, respectively.[15]

D. Fenofibrate

During the period 1985 to 1990, the French Centres Régionaux de Pharmacovigilance recorded 7 cases of hypoglycaemia, which developed in patients taking unnamed sulfonylureas when they were given fibrates (3 cases with fenofibrate).[2]

E. Gemfibrozil

Fasting blood glucose concentrations decreased in 10 patients with diabetes, and increased in 4 of 14 patients with diabetes receiving **insulin**, **acetohexamide**, **chlorpropamide**, or **glipizide** who were given gemfibrozil (800 mg daily initially, reduced later to 400 to 600 mg daily).[16] Another study found that of 20 patients, 9 required a slight increase in the dose of **insulin** or sulfonylurea (**glibenclamide** or **chlorpropamide**), and one a decreased dose, when they were given gemfibrozil 800 mg to 1.6 g daily.[17] A single report describes hypoglycaemia, which occurred in a diabetic taking **glibenclamide** when they were given gemfibrozil 1.2 g daily. The **glibenclamide** dose was reduced from 5 to 1.25 mg daily with satisfactory diabetic control. When the gemfibrozil was later stopped and restarted, the dose of the **glibenclamide** had to be increased and then reduced.[18] Similarly, a case report describes frequent hypoglycaemia and greatly reduced **insulin** requirements in a 76-year-old type 2 diabetic, after gemfibrozil 450 mg daily was added. His insulin dose needed to be reduced by more than 65% (from 148 units daily to 48 units daily) in order to maintain appropriate glucose concentrations.[19] A placebo-controlled study in 10 healthy subjects found that gemfibrozil 600 mg twice daily for 5 doses increased the AUC of a single 500-microgram dose of **glimepiride** by 23%, but there were no important changes in serum insulin or blood glucose.[20]

Mechanism

The suggested reasons for the alteration in diabetic control with fibrates include the displacement of the sulfonylureas from their plasma protein binding sites,[8] alterations in their renal excretion,[14] and a decrease in insulin resistance.[7,21] Clofibrate has also been shown to have a blood glucose-lowering action of its own, which improves the glucose tolerance of patients with diabetes.[13]

Gemfibrozil might inhibit the CYP2C9-mediated metabolism of glimepiride and other sulfonylureas such as glipizide, glibenclamide, or **gliclazide**.[20] It seems possible that any, or all, of these mechanisms might contribute towards enhanced hypoglycaemia.

Importance and management

The interaction between the sulfonylureas and clofibrate is established and well documented. The incidence is uncertain, but what is known suggests that between about one-third and one-half of patients could be affected. Alteration in diabetic control, most usually hypoglycaemia, has been seen in patients with diabetes taking sulfonylureas with bezafibrate, ciprofibrate, fenofibrate, and gemfibrozil, and the dose of the antidiabetic might need adjustment. Patients should be warned that excessive hypoglycaemia occurs occasionally and unpredictably. In general, it is prudent to monitor blood glucose concentrations when any change is made to the medication regimen of a patient with diabetes, and this would seem sufficient to detect and manage any interaction between sulfonylureas and fibrates should it occur.

Note that fibrates are recommended by NICE in the UK for the treatment of increased triglyceride concentrations in patients with type 2 diabetes when other causes have been addressed, and when cardiovascular risk is high (in addition to a statin).[22] The use of fibrates is also included in the recommendations of the American Heart Association and American Diabetes Association joint statement on the primary prevention of cardiovascular diseases in diabetes.[23]

Information about reduced diuretic effects is limited. It would seem prudent to avoid the concurrent use of drugs with actions that are antagonistic.

1. Ohsawa K, Koike N, Takamura T, Nagai Y, Kobayashi KI. Hypoglycaemic attacks after administration of bezafibrate in three cases of non-insulin dependent diabetes mellitus. *J Jpn Diabetes Soc* (1994) 37, 295–300.
2. Girardin E, Vial T, Pham E, Evreux J-C. Hypoglycémies induites par les sulfamides hypoglycémiants. Recensement par les Centres Régionaux de Pharmacovigilance français de 1985 à 1990. *Ann Med Interne (Paris)* (1992) 143, 11–17.
3. Ogawa S, Takeuchi K, Sugimura K, Fukuda M, Lee R, Ito S, Sato T. Bezafibrate reduces blood glucose in type 2 diabetes mellitus. *Metabolism* (2000) 49, 331–4.
4. Hernández-Mijares A, Lluch I, Vizcarra E, Martínez-Triguero ML, Ascaso JF, Carmena R. Ciprofibrate effects on carbohydrate and lipid metabolism in type 2 diabetes mellitus subjects. *Nutr Metab Cardiovasc Dis* (2000) 10, 1–6.
5. Daubresse J-C, Luyckx AS, Lefebvre PJ. Potentiation of hypoglycemic effect of sulfonylureas by clofibrate. *N Engl J Med* (1976) 294, 613.
6. Jain AK, Ryan JR, McMahon FG. Potentiation of hypoglycemic effect of sulfonylureas by halofenate. *N Engl J Med* (1975) 293, 1283–6.
7. Ferrari C, Frezzati S, Testori GP, Bertazzoni A. Potentiation of hypoglycemic response to intravenous tolbutamide by clofibrate. *N Engl J Med* (1976) 294, 1184.
8. Jain AK, Ryan JR, McMahon FG. Potentiation of hypoglycemic effect of sulfonylureas by clofibrate. *N Engl J Med* (1976) 294, 613.
9. Daubresse J-C, Daigneux D, Bruwier M, Luyckx A, Lefebvre PJ. Clofibrate and diabetes control in patients treated with oral hypoglycaemic agents. *Br J Clin Pharmacol* (1979) 7, 599–603.
10. Miller RD. *Atromid* in the treatment of post-climacteric diabetes. *J Atheroscler Res* (1963) 3, 694–700.
11. Csögör SI, Bornemisza P. The effect of clofibrate (Atromid) on intravenous tolbutamide, oral and intravenous glucose tolerance tests. *Clin Trials J* (1977) 14, 15–19.
12. Herriott SC, Percy-Robb IW, Strong JA, Thomson CG. The effect of Atromid on serum cholesterol and glucose tolerance in diabetes mellitus. *J Atheroscler Res* (1963) 3, 679–88.
13. Barnett D, Craig JG, Robinson DS, Rogers MP. Effect of clofibrate on glucose tolerance in maturity-onset diabetes. *Br J Clin Pharmacol* (1977) 4, 455–8.
14. Petitpierre B, Perrin L, Rudhardt M, Herrera A, Fabre J. Behaviour of chlorpropamide in renal insufficiency and under the effect of associated drug therapy. *Int J Clin Pharmacol* (1972) 6, 120–4.
15. Radó JP, Szende L, Marosi J, Juhos E, Sawinsky I, Takó J. Inhibition of the diuretic action of glibenclamide by clofibrate, carbamazepine and 1-deamino-8-D-arginine-vasopressin (DDAVP) in patients with pituitary diabetes insipidus. *Acta Diabetol Lat* (1974) 11, 179–97.
16. de Salcedo I, Gorringe JAL, Silva JL, Santos JA. Gemfibrozil in a group of diabetics. *Proc R Soc Med* (1976) 69 (Suppl 2), 64–70.
17. Konttinen A, Kuisma I, Ralli R, Pohjola S, Ojala K. The effect of gemfibrozil on serum lipids in diabetic patients. *Ann Clin Res* (1979) 11, 240–5.
18. Ahmad S. Gemfibrozil: interaction with glyburide. *South Med J* (1991) 84, 102.
19. Klein J, Ott V, Schütt M, Klein HH. Recurrent hypoglycaemic episodes in a patient with type 2 diabetes under fibrate therapy. *J Diabetes Complications* (2002) 16, 246–8.
20. Niemi M, Neuvonen PJ, Kivistö KT. Effect of gemfibrozil on the pharmacokinetics and pharmacodynamics of glimepiride. *Clin Pharmacol Ther* (2001) 70, 439–45.
21. Ferrari C, Frezzati S, Romussi M, Bertazzoni A, Testori GP, Antonini S, Paracchi A. Effects of short-term clofibrate administration on glucose tolerance and insulin secretion in patients with chemical diabetes or hypertriglyceridemia. *Metabolism* (1977) 26, 129–39.
22. National Institute for Clinical Excellence. Type 2 diabetes: the management of type 2 diabetes: partial update (issued March 2010). Available at: http://www.nice.org.uk/nicemedia/pdf/CG87NICEGuideline.pdf (accessed 22/10/15).
23. Buse JB, Ginsberg HN, Bakris GL, Clark NG, Costa F, Eckel R, Fonseca V, Gerstein HC, Grundy S, Nesto RW, Pignone MP, Plutzky J, Porte D, Redberg R, Stitzel KF, Stone NJ. Primary prevention of cardiovasular diseases in people with diabetes mellitus: A scientific statement from the American Heart Association and the American Diabetes Association. *Circulation* (2007) 115, 114–26.

Sulfonylureas; Chlorpropamide + Nevirapine

In a single-dose study, nevirapine did not alter the exposure to, or blood glucose-lowering effects of, chlorpropamide.

Clinical evidence, mechanism, importance and management

In a single-dose study in 6 fasting subjects, simultaneous administration of **nevirapine** 200 mg with **chlorpropamide** 250 mg had no effect on the AUC of chlorpropamide, when compared with chlorpropamide alone, and no effect on plasma glucose concentrations.[1]

This study provides some evidence that nevirapine might not alter the exposure to, or effect of chlorpropamide, but this needs confirming in a study with longer-term nevirapine use, as the enzyme-inducing effects of nevirapine would not be maximal with a simultaneous single dose. The general advice to monitor blood glucose concentrations when any change is made to the medication regimen of a patient with diabetes, should be sufficient to detect any interaction, should it occur.

1. Bakare-Odunola MT, Enemali I, Garba M, Obodozie OO, Mustapha KB. The influence of lamivudine, stavudine and nevirapine on the pharmacokinetics of chlorpropamide in human subjects. *Eur J Drug Metab Pharmacokinet* (2008) 33, 165–71.

Sulfonylureas; Chlorpropamide + NRTIs

In a single-dose study, lamivudine and stavudine slightly reduced chlorpropamide exposure, and thereby reduced its effects on blood glucose concentrations.

Clinical evidence, mechanism, importance and management

In a single-dose study in 6 fasting subjects, the simultaneous administration of **lamivudine** 150 mg with **chlorpropamide** 250 mg reduced the AUC of chlorpropamide by 42% when compared with chlorpropamide alone. A similar 41% reduction in the AUC of chlorpropamide was seen when **stavudine** 40 mg was given simultaneously. With both NRTIs, the plasma glucose concentrations were higher than with chlorpropamide alone.[1]

The finding of this study is surprising as NRTIs are not known to decrease the absorption or induce the metabolism of any other drugs. Further study is needed to confirm these findings, especially with multiple doses. Until such time, bear the possibility of an interaction in mind if chlorpropamide efficacy is poor in patients taking these NRTIs. The general advice to monitor blood glucose concentrations when any change is made to the medication regimen of a patient with diabetes should be sufficient to detect any interaction, should it occur.

1. Bakare-Odunola MT, Enemali I, Garba M, Obodozie OO, Mustapha KB. The influence of lamivudine, stavudine and nevirapine on the pharmacokinetics of chlorpropamide in human subjects. *Eur J Drug Metab Pharmacokinet* (2008) 33, 165–71.

Sulfonylureas; Chlorpropamide + Sucralfate

Sucralfate does not affect the pharmacokinetics of chlorpropamide.

Clinical evidence, mechanism, importance and management

A randomised, crossover study in 12 healthy subjects found that sucralfate 1 g four times daily, given one hour before meals, had no effect on the pharmacokinetics of a single 250-mg dose of chlorpropamide given at the same time as sucralfate.[1] No additional precautions would therefore seem to be necessary on concurrent use. However, it is prudent to monitor blood glucose concentrations when any change is made to the medication regimen of a patient with diabetes.

1. Letendre PW, Carlson JD, Siefert RD, Dietz AJ, Dimmit D. Effect of sucralfate on the absorption and pharmacokinetics of chlorpropamide. *J Clin Pharmacol* (1986) 26, 622–5.

Sulfonylureas; Chlorpropamide + Urinary acidifiers or alkalinisers

On theoretical grounds the response to chlorpropamide might be decreased if the urine is made alkaline, and increased if urine is acidified.

Clinical evidence, mechanism, importance and management

A study in 6 healthy subjects given a 250-mg oral dose of chlorpropamide found that when the urine was made alkaline (pH 7.1 to 8.2) with **sodium bicarbonate**, the half-life of the chlorpropamide was reduced from 50 hours to 13 hours, and the 72-hour clearance was increased 4-fold. In contrast, when the urine was acidified (pH 5.5 to 4.7) with **ammonium chloride**, the chlorpropamide half-life was increased from 50 hours to 69 hours and the 72-hour urinary clearance was decreased to 5%, and non-renal (i.e. metabolic) clearance predominated.[1] Another study[2] found that the renal clearance of chlorpropamide was almost 100 times greater at pH 7 than at pH 5. The reason for this effect is that changes in urinary pH affect the ionisation of chlorpropamide, and this affects the ability of the kidney to reabsorb it from the kidney filtrate (see more details under 'Drug excretion interactions', p.11). Thus, urinary pH determines the relative contribution of renal and metabolic clearance.

There appear to be no reports of adverse interactions between chlorpropamide and drugs that can alter urinary pH, but prescribers should be aware of the possibilities: a reduced response if the pH is considerably increased and renal clearance predominates (e.g. with **sodium bicarbonate**, **acetazolamide**, some **antacids**); an increased response if the pH is made more acidic than usual and metabolic clearance predominates (e.g. with **ammonium chloride**). Perhaps more importantly, the effects of drugs that alter the hepatic clearance of chlorpropamide are likely to be more important when its renal clearance is low (i.e. when the urine is acidic).[2]

1. Neuvonen PJ, Kärkkäinen S. Effects of charcoal, sodium bicarbonate, and ammonium chloride on chlorpropamide kinetics. *Clin Pharmacol Ther* (1983) 33, 386–93.
2. Neuvonen PJ, Kärkkäinen S, Lehtovaara R. Pharmacokinetics of chlorpropamide in epileptic patients: effects of enzyme induction and urine pH on chlorpropamide elimination. *Eur J Clin Pharmacol* (1987) 32, 297–301.

Sulfonylureas; Glibenclamide (Glyburide) + Carvedilol

No pharmacokinetic interaction appears to occur between glibenclamide (glyburide) and carvedilol.

Clinical evidence, mechanism, importance and management

No pharmacokinetic interaction was seen in a study in healthy subjects given a single 1.75-mg dose of glibenclamide (glyburide) with carvedilol 25 mg daily for 6 days.[1] No dose adjustments would seem necessary on concurrent use, but note that it is prudent to monitor blood glucose concentrations when any change is made to the medication regimen of a patient with diabetes.

For discussion of the potential glycaemic effects of combining sulfonylureas and beta-blockers, see 'Antidiabetics + Beta blockers', p.504, and for discussion of a theoretical pharmacokinetic interaction between tolbutamide and propranolol, see 'Beta blockers; Propranolol + Miscellaneous', p.1026.

1. Harder S, Merz PG, Rietbrock N. Lack of pharmacokinetic interaction between carvedilol and digitoxin, phenprocoumon or glibenclamide. *Cardiovasc Drugs Ther* (1993) 7 (Suppl 2), 447.

Sulfonylureas; Glibenclamide (Glyburide) + Pantoprazole

The concurrent use of glibenclamide (glyburide) and pantoprazole does not affect the pharmacokinetics of either drug, and pantoprazole does not alter the glucose-lowering effect of glibenclamide.

Clinical evidence, mechanism, importance and management

Pantoprazole 40 mg daily, or placebo, were given to 20 healthy subjects for 5 days. On day 5 the subjects were also given 3.5 mg of a micronised preparation of glibenclamide (glyburide). The pharmacokinetics of the glibenclamide and the pharmacodynamic profiles of glucose and insulin serum concentrations were not altered, and the pharmacokinetics of pantoprazole were not affected. It was concluded that dose changes of the micronised preparation of glibenclamide are not needed during treatment with pantoprazole.[1] Nevertheless, it is prudent to monitor blood glucose concentrations when any change is made to the medication regimen of a patient with diabetes.

1. Walter-Sack IE, Bliesath H, Stötzer F, Huber R, Steinijans VW, Ding R, Mascher H, Wurst W. Lack of pharmacokinetic and pharmacodynamic interaction between pantoprazole and glibenclamide in humans. *Clin Drug Invest* (1998) 15, 253–60.

Sulfonylureas; Glibenclamide (Glyburide) + Vinpocetine

Vinpocetine does not alter the pharmacokinetics or efficacy of glibenclamide.

Clinical evidence, mechanism, importance and management

A study in 18 elderly patients, with type 2 diabetes and symptoms of dementia, who were taking glibenclamide (glyburide), found that 4 days of treatment with vinpocetine 10 mg three times daily did not affect either the pharmacokinetics of the glibenclamide or the control of blood glucose concentrations.[1] There would seem to be no reason for avoiding concurrent use, nevertheless, it is prudent to monitor blood glucose concentrations when any change is made to the medication regimen of a patient with diabetes.

1. Grandt R, Braun W, Schulz H-U, Lührmann B, Frercks H-J. Glibenclamide steady-state plasma levels during concomitant vinpocetine administration in type II diabetic patients. *Arzneimittelforschung* (1989) 39, 1451–4.

Sulfonylureas; Glipizide + Ezetimibe

No pharmacokinetic interaction appears to occur between ezetimibe and glipizide. The glucose lowering effect of glipizide did not appear to be affected by ezetimibe.

Clinical evidence, mechanism, importance and management

In a study in 12 healthy subjects given ezetimibe 10 mg daily for 8 days, the pharmacokinetics and pharmacodynamics of a single 10-mg dose of glipizide given on day 8 were unaltered, when compared with glipizide alone.[1] In another similar study, the AUC and maximum concentration of total ezetimibe (ezetimibe plus its glucuronide metabolite) were unaltered by a single 10-mg dose of glipizide, when compared with ezetimibe alone.[2] This suggests that no interaction occurs, and no dose adjustments would seem necessary on concurrent use.

1. Statkevich P, Reyderman L, Kosoglou T et al. Ezetimibe does not affect the pharmacokinetics and pharmacodynamics of glipizide. *Clin Pharmacol Ther* (2001) 69, P67.
2. Kosoglou T, Statkevich P, Reyderman L, Pember LJC, Maxwell SE, Courtney R, Krishna G, Cutler DL. Effects of selected drugs on exposure to ezetimibe. *Eur Heart J* (2003) 24 (Suppl), 462.

Sulfonylureas; Glipizide + Heparin

An isolated report describes hypoglycaemia in a diabetic patient taking glipizide, which was attributed to the concurrent use of heparin.

Clinical evidence, mechanism, importance and management

A diabetic man taking glipizide 5 mg daily for 6 months, with fair control of his diabetes and no reports of hypoglycaemia, was hospitalised for the treatment of a foot ulcer. Over a period of 4 days he experienced recurring episodes of hypoglycaemia after taking his routine 5 mg daily dose of glipizide. It was suggested that this could possibly have been due to an interaction with subcutaneous heparin calcium 5000 units every 12 hours which might have displaced the glipizide from its protein binding sites.[1] No other information seems to be available. The general importance of this report is unknown, but seems likely to be small.

1. McKillop G, Fallon M, Slater SD. Possible interaction between heparin and a sulphonylurea a cause of prolonged hypoglycaemia? *BMJ* (1986) 293, 1073.

Sulfonylureas; Tolbutamide + Methysergide

An early study indicated that methysergide might enhance the insulin-secreting effects of tolbutamide without altering the glucose-lowering effect.

Clinical evidence, mechanism, importance and management

In 8 patients with type 2 diabetes, pretreatment with methysergide 2 mg every 6 hours for 2 days increased the amount of insulin secreted in response to a 1-g intravenous dose of tolbutamide by almost 40%, however, there was no effect on the glucose-lowering effect of tolbutamide.[1] This is an isolated study, and given the passing of a considerable amount of time since its publication with no further evidence coming to light, it is unlikely to be clinically relevant.

1. Baldridge JA, Quickel KE, Feldman JM and Lebovitz HE. Potentiation of tolbutamide-mediated insulin release in adult onset diabetics by methysergide maleate. *Diabetes* (1974) 23, 21–4.

Sulfonylureas; Tolbutamide + Tolcapone

In a single-dose study, tolcapone did not alter tolbutamide pharmacokinetics.

Clinical evidence, mechanism, importance and management

In a single-dose study in 12 healthy subjects, tolcapone 200 mg had no effect on the pharmacokinetics of tolbutamide 500 mg, and did not alter the glucose-lowering effect of tolbutamide.[1] This study was conducted because *in vitro* evidence had shown that tolcapone inhibits CYP2C9, by which tolbutamide is metabolised. However, these findings in healthy subjects suggest that no clinically relevant changes in the pharmacokinetics of tolbutamide are likely.

1. Jorga KM, Fotteler B, Gasser R, Banken L, Birnboeck H. Lack of interaction between tolcapone and tolbutamide in healthy volunteers. *J Clin Pharmacol* (2000) 40, 544–51.

Thiazolidinediones + Azoles; Itraconazole or Ketoconazole

Itraconazole had no effect on pioglitazone pharmacokinetics in healthy subjects. Ketoconazole slightly increased the AUC of rosiglitazone and pioglitazone in healthy subjects.

Clinical evidence

(a) Itraconazole

In a study in 12 healthy subjects, itraconazole 200 mg then 100 mg twice daily for 4 days did not alter the pharmacokinetics of a single 15-mg dose of **pioglitazone**.[1]

(b) Ketoconazole

In 10 healthy Korean subjects, ketoconazole 200 mg twice daily for 5 days increased the AUC of a single 8-mg dose of **rosiglitazone** by 47%.[2]

The US manufacturer briefly states that, in a 7-day study ketoconazole 200 mg twice daily increased the AUC of **pioglitazone** 45 mg daily by 34%.[3]

Mechanism

Unknown. Rosiglitazone is principally metabolised by CYP2C8, with some involvement of CYP2C9. Although it has been suggested that ketoconazole might inhibit the metabolism of rosiglitazone via both these pathways,[2] ketoconazole is normally only considered to be a clinically important inhibitor of CYP3A4.

Importance and management

Evidence for a pharmacokinetic interaction between pioglitazone or rosiglitazone and itraconazole or ketoconazole is limited. Itraconazole does not appear to alter the pharmacokinetics of pioglitazone, therefore no dose adjustments are expected to be necessary on concurrent use. The increased rosiglitazone and pioglitazone exposures seen with ketoconazole were minor and are unlikely to be clinically relevant. It is prudent to monitor blood glucose concentrations when any change is made to the medication regimen of a patient with diabetes, and this would seem sensible when either itraconazole or ketoconazole are given to patients taking rosiglitazone or pioglitazone.

1. Jaakkola T, Backman JT, Neuvonen M, Neuvonen PJ. Effects of gemfibrozil, itraconazole, and their combination on the pharmacokinetics of pioglitazone. *Clin Pharmacol Ther* (2005) 77, 404–14.
2. Park J-Y, Kim K-A, Shin J-G, Lee KY. Effect of ketoconazole on the pharmacokinetics of rosiglitazone in healthy subjects. *Br J Clin Pharmacol* (2004) 58, 397–402.
3. Actos (Pioglitazone hydrochloride). Takeda Pharmaceutical Company Ltd. US Prescribing information, November 2013.

Thiazolidinediones + Febuxostat

Febuxostat does not alter the pharmacokinetics of rosiglitazone, and is not expected to affect the pharmacokinetics of pioglitazone.

Clinical evidence, mechanism, importance and management

In a randomised, crossover study, 36 healthy subjects were given febuxostat 120 mg daily for 9 days with a single 4-mg dose of **rosiglitazone** on day 5. The pharmacokinetics of **rosiglitazone** were not altered by febuxostat.[1] No pharmacokinetic interaction would be expected on concurrent use, and no rosiglitazone dose adjustment would seem necessary. However, note that it is prudent to monitor blood glucose concentrations when any change is made to the medication regimen of a patient with diabetes.

Note that **rosiglitazone** can be used as a probe substrate to assess the activity of drugs on CYP2C8. This study therefore suggests that febuxostat is not an inhibitor or inducer of CYP2C8. No pharmacokinetic interaction would therefore be expected between febuxostat and **pioglitazone** by this mechanism.

1. Naik H, Wu JT, Palmer R, McLean L. The effects of febuxostat on the pharmacokinetic parameters of rosiglitazone, a CYP2C8 substrate. *Br J Clin Pharmacol* (2012) 74, 327–35.

Thiazolidinediones + Fibrates

Gemfibrozil markedly increases the exposure to pioglitazone and rosiglitazone. There are cases of paradoxical reductions in HDL-cholesterol with the combination of fibrates and thiazolidinediones.

Clinical evidence

(a) Bezafibrate or Fenofibrate

There are reports of paradoxical reductions in HDL-cholesterol concentrations in a few patients taking a fibrate (bezafibrate, fenofibrate) with a thiazolidinedione, and a few are cited as examples.[1-6] In one analysis, this was more likely with the combination than either a fibrate or **rosiglitazone** alone.[4] This has been confirmed in 2 patients who were prospectively followed and who both had reductions in HDL-cholesterol concentrations while receiving fenofibrate and **rosiglitazone**, but whose concentrations increased (to baseline or near baseline) when one of the drugs was stopped and decreased again after rechallenge.[6]

(b) Gemfibrozil

In a study in healthy subjects, gemfibrozil 600 mg twice daily for 4 days increased the AUC of a single 4-mg dose of **rosiglitazone** 2.3-fold, the maximum plasma concentration by 20%, and the 24-hour plasma concentration almost 10-fold.[7] In the same way, gemfibrozil increased the AUC of a single dose of **pioglitazone** 3.2-fold without altering its maximum concentration, but increased the 48-hour plasma concentration approximately 15-fold.[8] A similar increase in the AUC of **pioglitazone** was reported in another study.[9] In these studies, the effects of these pharmacokinetic changes on the pharmacodynamics of rosiglitazone or pioglitazone were not assessed.[7-9]

Mechanism

Gemfibrozil inhibits the CYP2C8-mediated metabolism of rosiglitazone and pioglitazone.[7,8]

Usually, fibrates, and also thiazolidinediones, increase HDL-cholesterol, but both thiazolidinediones and fibrates alone have caused paradoxical reductions in HDL-cholesterol. The reason for this is unknown.

Importance and management

A pharmacokinetic interaction between rosiglitazone or pioglitazone and gemfibrozil is established, and marked increases in the exposure to rosiglitazone and pioglitazone result, but the clinical relevance of these changes has not been assessed. Until further experience is gained, caution is warranted. Note that it is prudent to monitor blood glucose concentrations when any change is made to the medication regimen of a patient with diabetes, and this should be sufficient to detect any interaction should it occur.

The general relevance of the cases of paradoxical reductions in HDL-cholesterol in patients taking a fibrate with rosiglitazone or pioglitazone is unclear, but bear them in mind in the event of an unexpected response to treatment.

Note that rosiglitazone can be used as a probe substrate to assess the activity of drugs on CYP2C8. This study therefore suggests that gemfibrozil is a potent inhibitor of CYP2C8. For a list of CYP2C8 substrates see 'Table 1.4', p.6.

1. Normén L, Frohlich J, Montaner J, Harris M, Elliott T, Bondy G. Combination therapy with fenofibrate and rosiglitazone paradoxically lowers serum HDL cholesterol. *Diabetes Care* (2004) 27, 2241–2.
2. Senba H, Kawano M, Kawakami M. Severe decrease in serum HDL-cholesterol during combination therapy of bezafibrate and pioglitazone. *J Atheroscler Thromb* (2006) 13, 263–4.
3. Shetty C, Balasubramani M, Capps N, Milles J, Ramachandran S. Paradoxical HDL-C reduction during rosiglitazone and fibrate treatment. *Diabet Med* (2007) 24, 94–7.
4. Keidar S, Guttmann H, Stam T, Fishman I, Shapira C. High incidence of reduced plasma HDL cholesterol in diabetic patients treated with rosiglitazone and fibrate. *Pharmacoepidemiol Drug Safety* (2007) 16, 1192–4.
5. Venero CV, Thompson PD, Fernandez AB. Reduced high-density lipoprotein cholesterol in patients receiving rosiglitazone and fenofibrate. *Am J Med* (2008) 121, e3–e4.
6. Schwing W, Hustak L, Taylor HC. Paradoxical severe decrease in high-density lipoprotein cholesterol due to rosiglitazone-fenofibrate interaction. *Endocr Pract* (2010) 16, 382–8.
7. Niemi M, Backman JT, Granfors M, Laitila J, Neuvonen M, Neuvonen PJ. Gemfibrozil considerably increases the plasma concentrations of rosiglitazone. *Diabetologia* (2003) 46, 1319–23.
8. Jaakkola T, Backman JT, Neuvonen M, Neuvonen PJ. Effects of gemfibrozil, itraconazole, and their combination on the pharmacokinetics of pioglitazone. *Clin Pharmacol Ther* (2005) 77, 404–14.
9. Deng L-J, Wang F, Li H-D. Effect of gemfibrozil on the pharmacokinetics of pioglitazone. *Eur J Clin Pharmacol* (2005) 61, 831–6.

Thiazolidinediones + Ibuprofen

Ibuprofen does not appear to alter the pharmacokinetics of rosiglitazone. The risk of fluid retention with pioglitazone or rosiglitazone might be increased by the NSAIDs.

Clinical evidence, mechanism, importance and management

In a randomised, crossover study in 24 healthy subjects, there was no change in the pharmacokinetics of a single 8-mg dose of **rosiglitazone** when it was given with a single 400-mg dose of ibuprofen. The effect on blood glucose concentrations was not measured.[1]

There appears to be no pharmacokinetic interaction between rosiglitazone and ibuprofen. The effect on blood glucose concentrations is not known, but given the lack of effect on rosiglitazone pharmacokinetics, an effect on blood glucose concentrations would seem unlikely. Nevertheless, it is prudent to monitor blood glucose concentrations when any change is made to the medication regimen of a patient with diabetes.

The manufacturers of pioglitazone and rosiglitazone state that they can cause fluid retention, which might exacerbate or precipitate heart failure,[2,3] particularly in those with limited cardiac reserve.[2] As **NSAIDs** can cause fluid retention, some caution in this regard would be appropriate on the concurrent use of pioglitazone or rosiglitazone and NSAIDs.

1. Kumar JNS, Devi P, Narasu L, Mullangi R. Effect of ciprofloxacin and ibuprofen on the *in vitro* metabolism of rosiglitazone and oral pharmacokinetics of rosiglitazone in healthy human volunteers. *Eur J Drug Metab Pharmacokinet* (2008) 33, 237–42.
2. Actos (Pioglitazone hydrochloride). Takeda UK Ltd. UK Summary of product characteristics, November 2013.
3. Avandia (Rosiglitazone maleate). GlaxoSmithKline. US Prescribing information, September 2013.

Thiazolidinediones + Insulin

Pioglitazone and rosiglitazone can cause fluid retention and peripheral oedema, which can worsen or cause heart failure. There is evidence that the incidence of these effects is higher with the concurrent use of insulin. In addition, there might be an increased risk of myocardial ischaemia

when rosiglitazone is used with insulin. The incidence of hypoglycaemia might also be increased, and the required dose of insulin reduced.

Clinical evidence

(a) Pioglitazone

In one 16-week, randomised, placebo-controlled study,[1] pioglitazone 15 or 30 mg with insulin was compared with insulin alone in 566 patients with long-standing diabetes. Oedema was reported in 15.3% of the patients receiving pioglitazone with insulin (12.6% and 17.6% with pioglitazone 15 mg and 30 mg, respectively) compared with 7% when insulin was given alone. Four of the 379 patients given pioglitazone and insulin developed congestive heart failure compared with none of the 187 patients given insulin alone; all 4 had a history of cardiovascular disease.[2] In an analysis of 8 randomised controlled studies in which pioglitazone was given to patients already receiving insulin, concurrent use was associated with a tendency for more hypoglycaemic episodes (relative risk 1.27), a greater increase in weight (about 3 kg), a reduction in required insulin dose (about 12 units/day), and a more frequent incidence of peripheral oedema.[3]

One case report describes a 57-year-old obese man with type 2 diabetes, no history of heart failure and excellent exercise tolerance, who was given insulin and pioglitazone 30 mg daily. Over the first 4 weeks after starting pioglitazone he experienced considerable weight gain and subsequently developed heart failure and pulmonary oedema.[4]

(b) Rosiglitazone

A randomised, double-blind, placebo-controlled study in patients with poorly-controlled type 2 diabetes receiving insulin twice daily found that the addition of rosiglitazone 2 or 4 mg twice daily for 26 weeks improved the control of their blood glucose concentrations and they needed less insulin.[5] Mean total daily insulin reductions were 12% for the 4 mg dose, 5.6% for the 2 mg dose, and 0.6% for placebo. Symptoms consistent with hypoglycaemia also occurred more frequently with the combination; 67% with the 4 mg rosiglitazone dose, 53% with the 2 mg dose, and 38% with placebo. The incidence of oedema was about 3-fold higher in those patients given insulin and rosiglitazone; 16.2% with the 4 mg dose, and 13.1% with the 2 mg dose, compared with 4.7% in those given placebo. Congestive heart failure occurred in 4 of 209 patients receiving the combination compared with one of 104 receiving placebo. However, 2 of the patients receiving rosiglitazone had a history of coronary heart disease.[5] Other cases of peripheral oedema and congestive heart failure have been reported.[6-8]

From an analysis of the results of 7 placebo-controlled clinical studies, there was an incidence of heart failure of 1% with insulin monotherapy and 2.3% when combined with rosiglitazone. In addition, there was an increased risk of myocardial infarction (odds ratio of 5.6), MACE (a composite of myocardial infarction, cardiovascular death, or stroke; odds ratio of 2.14), and all-cause death (odds ratio of 2.19) when rosiglitazone is used with insulin.[9]

Mechanism

Pioglitazone or rosiglitazone alone might exacerbate or precipitate heart failure because they can cause fluid retention and weight gain.[2,9,10] The incidence appears to be greatly increased in patients who are also receiving insulin. An estimated 2 to 5% of patients receiving thiazolidinedione monotherapy and 5 to 15% receiving concurrent insulin experience peripheral oedema.[11] Fluid retention and tissue oedema appear to be part of a vascular 'leak' syndrome but, additionally, thiazolidinediones can potentiate the renal effects of insulin on sodium and water retention. It is conceivable that increased fluid retention caused by thiazolidinediones might alter the already precarious volume status in patients with underlying cardiac or renal impairment thus leading to congestive heart failure.[11] However, congestive heart failure has been estimated to occur in as many as 12% of patients who have type 2 diabetes[11] and whether the incidence of heart failure in patients given thiazolidinediones and insulin is simply a reflection of other factors that increase the risk in these patients, or due to some specific interaction with insulin, remains to be established.

Importance and management

The fact that rosiglitazone and pioglitazone can cause weight gain and peripheral oedema, and that the incidence of this is greater in patients who are also using insulin is well established. However, the relevance of this has been the subject of much debate. In addition, the relationship of rosiglitazone to myocardial ischaemia has been under close scrutiny, resulting in the European Medicines Agency withdrawing the drug from the market in 2010 having concluded that the safety restrictions put in place as a result of a review in 2007 had not led to a situation where the benefits of use outweighed the risks.[12] Similarly, in the US, the use of rosiglitazone is greatly restricted by the FDA, and use with insulin is not recommended.[9] Pioglitazone can be used in combination with insulin, but because of the risk of cardiac failure such use should be accompanied by close monitoring for signs and symptoms of heart failure, weight gain and oedema.[2,10] If oedema occurs in a patient taking a thiazolidinedione, the possible causes should be assessed,[13] and if symptoms and signs suggest congestive heart failure, they should be managed according to current guidelines.[2] The dose of the thiazolidinedione should be reduced or discontinued.[2,13]

Concurrent use of insulin and a thiazolidinedione increases the incidence of hypoglycaemia. It has been noted that in patients receiving insulin, the insulin dose may need to be reduced by 10 to 25% if pioglitazone 15 or 30 mg daily is given.[2]

1. Rosenstock J, Einhorn D, Hershon K, Glazer NB, Yu S; Pioglitazone 014 Study Group. Efficacy and safety of pioglitazone in type 2 diabetes: a randomised, placebo-controlled study in patients receiving stable insulin therapy. *Int J Clin Pract* (2002) 56, 251–7.
2. Actos (Pioglitazone hydrochloride). Takeda Pharmaceutical Company Ltd. US Prescribing information, November 2013.
3. Clar C, Royle P, Waugh N. Adding pioglitazone to insulin containing regimens in type 2 diabetes: systematic review and meta-analysis. *PLoS One* (2009) 4, e6112.
4. Cheng AYY, Fantus IG. Thiazolidinedione-induced congestive heart failure. *Ann Pharmacother* (2004) 38, 817–20.
5. Raskin P, Rendell M, Riddle MC, Dole JF, Freed MI, Rosenstock J; Rosiglitazone Clinical Trials Study Group. A randomized trial of rosiglitazone therapy in patients with inadequately controlled insulin-treated type 2 diabetes. *Diabetes Care* (2001) 24, 1226–32.
6. Buch HN, Baskar V, Barton DM, Kamalakannan D, Akarca C, Singh BM. Combination of insulin and thiazolidinedione therapy in massively obese patients with type 2 diabetes. *Diabet Med* (2002) 19, 572–4.
7. Singh N. Rosiglitazone and heart failure: long-term vigilance. *J Cardiovasc Pharmacol Ther* (2004) 9, 21–5.
8. Bell DSH. Unilateral edema due to a thiazolidinedione. *Diabetes Care* (2003) 26, 2700.
9. Avandia (Rosiglitazone maleate). GlaxoSmithKline. US Prescribing information, September 2013.
10. Actos (Pioglitazone hydrochloride). Takeda UK Ltd. UK Summary of product characteristics, November 2013.
11. Scheen AJ. Combined thiazolidinedione-insulin therapy. Should we be concerned about safety? *Drug Safety* (2004) 27, 841–56.
12. European Medicines Agency. Press release. European Medicines Agency recommends suspension of Avandia, Avandamet and Avaglim: Anti-diabetes medication to be taken off the market. London, 23 September 2010. Available at: http://www.ema.europa.eu/docs/en_GB/document_library/Press_release/2010/09/WC500096996.pdf (accessed 21/10/15).
13. Nesto RW, Bell D, Bonow RO, Fonseca V, Grundy SM, Horton ES, Le Winter M, Porte D, Semenkovich CF, Smith S, Young LH, Kahn R. Thiazolidinedione use, fluid retention, and congestive heart failure: a consensus statement from the American Heart Association and American Diabetes Association. *Circulation* (2003) 108, 2941–8.

Thiazolidinediones + Leukotriene antagonists

Montelukast and zafirlukast do not alter the pharmacokinetics of pioglitazone, and montelukast does not alter the pharmacokinetics of rosiglitazone.

Clinical evidence

In a controlled study in healthy subjects, both **montelukast** 10 mg daily for 6 days and **zafirlukast** 20 mg twice daily for 6 days did not affect either the AUC of a single 15-mg dose of **pioglitazone** given on day 3, or the metabolites of pioglitazone.[1] Similarly, **montelukast** 10 mg daily for 6 days had no effect on the AUC of a single 4-mg dose of **rosiglitazone** 4 mg given on day 5. In addition, there was no change in the AUC ratio of the *N*-desmethyl metabolite to rosiglitazone.[2]

Mechanism

In vitro, the leukotriene antagonists inhibited the metabolism of pioglitazone and rosiglitazone by CYP2C8.[3,4] However, the clinical studies provide conclusive evidence that this interaction does not occur *in vivo*, and this emphasises the fact that positive *in vitro* findings will not always directly translate to the clinical situation.

Importance and management

No pharmacokinetic interaction is expected if montelukast or zafirlukast are given with pioglitazone or rosiglitazone, and therefore dose adjustments of these antidiabetics are not expected to be necessary on concurrent use.

1. Jaakkola T, Backman JT, Neuvonen M, Niemi M, Neuvonen PJ. Montelukast and zafirlukast do not affect the pharmacokinetics of the CYP2C8 substrate pioglitazone. *Eur J Clin Pharmacol* (2006) 62, 503–9.
2. Kim K-A, Park P-W, Kim KR, Park J-Y. Effect of multiple doses of montelukast on the pharmacokinetics of rosiglitazone, a CYP2C8 substrate, in humans. *Br J Clin Pharmacol* (2007) 63, 339–45.
3. Walsky RL, Obach RS, Gaman EA, Gleeson J-PR, Proctor WR. Selective inhibition of human cytochrome P4502C8 by montelukast. *Drug Metab Dispos* (2005) 33, 413–18.
4. Jaakkola T, Laitila J, Neuvonen PJ, Backman JT. Pioglitazone is metabolised by CYP2C8 and CYP3A4 *in vitro*: potential for interactions with CYP2C8 inhibitors. *Basic Clin Pharmacol Toxicol* (2006) 99, 44–51.

Thiazolidinediones + Metformin

The pharmacokinetics of metformin are not altered by pioglitazone or rosiglitazone, and metformin does not alter the pharmacokinetics of rosiglitazone.

Clinical evidence, mechanism, importance and management

In healthy subjects, **pioglitazone** 45 mg daily for 7 days did not alter the pharmacokinetics of a single 1-g dose of metformin.[1,2]

The steady-state pharmacokinetics of metformin 500 mg twice daily and **rosiglitazone** 2 mg twice daily were not affected when they were given to healthy subjects for 4 days.[3]

The combination of a thiazolidinedione and metformin is used in the management of diabetes for additive blood glucose lowering effects, and the studies show that there are no pharmacokinetic interactions that will complicate their concurrent use. Because neither metformin nor thiazolidinediones increase the secretion of insulin, the risk of hypoglycaemia is not increased by the combination.

1. Actos (Pioglitazone hydrochloride). Takeda Pharmaceutical Company Ltd. US Prescribing information, November 2013
2. Kortboyer JM, Eckland DJA. Pioglitazone has low potential for drug interactions. *Diabetologia* (1999) 42 (Suppl 1), A228.
3. Di Cicco RA, Allen A, Carr A, Fowles S, Jorkasky DK, Freed MI. Rosiglitazone does not alter the pharmacokinetics of metformin. *J Clin Pharmacol* (2000) 40, 1280–5.

Thiazolidinediones + Nifedipine

Pioglitazone and rosiglitazone do not alter the pharmacokinetics of nifedipine. Nifedipine does not affect the pharmacokinetics of pioglitazone.

Clinical evidence, mechanism, importance and management

For discussion of the general effects of calcium channel blockers on diabetes control, see 'Antidiabetics + Calcium-channel blockers', p.505.

(a) Pioglitazone

The US manufacturer of pioglitazone briefly notes that, in a study in 24 healthy subjects, pioglitazone 45 mg daily for 4 days given with nifedipine extended-release 30 mg daily for 4 days resulted in a 13% decrease in the nifedipine AUC and a 17% decrease in the maximum concentration. Whereas in 23 healthy subjects given nifedipine extended-release 30 mg daily with pioglitazone 45 mg daily for 7 days, nifedipine had no effect on the AUC or maximum concentration of pioglitazone .[1] Such small changes in the pharmacokinetics of nifedipine are unlikely to be clinically important, and no special precautions on concurrent use would seem necessary.

(b) Rosiglitazone

In a randomised, crossover study in 26 healthy subjects, rosiglitazone 8 mg daily for 2 weeks was found to have no effect on the pharmacokinetics of a single 20-mg dose of nifedipine.[2] No special precautions on concurrent use would seem necessary.

1. Actos (Pioglitazone hydrochloride). Takeda Pharmaceutical Company Ltd. US Prescribing information, November 2013.
2. Harris RZ, Inglis AML, Miller AK, Thompson KA, Finnerty D, Patterson S, Jorkasky DK, Freed MI. Rosiglitazone has no clinically significant effect on nifedipine pharmacokinetics. *J Clin Pharmacol* (1999) 39, 1189–94.

Thiazolidinediones + Ranitidine

Ranitidine does not alter the pharmacokinetics of pioglitazone or rosiglitazone. Pioglitazone does not alter the pharmacokinetics of ranitidine.

Clinical evidence, mechanism, importance and management

(a) Pioglitazone

A crossover study in 23 healthy subjects found that when pioglitazone 45 mg daily was given with ranitidine 150 mg twice daily, the pharmacokinetics of both drugs were not affected.[1] No dose adjustments would seem necessary on concurrent use, but note that it is prudent to monitor blood glucose concentrations when any change is made to the medication regimen of a patient with diabetes.

(b) Rosiglitazone

A crossover study in 12 healthy subjects found that pre-treatment with ranitidine 150 mg twice daily for 4 days had no effect on the pharmacokinetics of either a single 4-mg oral dose, or a single 2-mg intravenous dose, of rosiglitazone.[2] No rosiglitazone dose adjustment would seem necessary on concurrent use, but note that it is prudent to monitor blood glucose concentrations when any change is made to the medication regimen of a patient with diabetes.

1. Glazer NB, Sanes-Miller C. Pharmacokinetics of coadministration of pioglitazone with ranitidine. *Diabetes* (2001) 50 (suppl 2) A114.
2. Miller AK, DiCicco RA, Freed MI. The effect of ranitidine on the pharmacokinetics of rosiglitazone in healthy adult male volunteers. *Clin Ther* (2002) 24, 1062–71.

Thiazolidinediones + Rifamycins

Rifampicin moderately reduces the exposure to pioglitazone and rosiglitazone.

Clinical evidence

(a) Pioglitazone

A randomised, crossover study in 10 healthy subjects found that **rifampicin** 600 mg daily for 6 days decreased the AUC of a single 30-mg dose of pioglitazone by 54%. In addition, **rifampicin** decreased the AUC of the active metabolites of pioglitazone by about 36%, and shortened the half-life by about 52%.[1]

(b) Rosiglitazone

In a randomised, crossover study in 10 healthy subjects, **rifampicin** 600 mg daily for 5 days reduced the AUC of a single 4-mg dose of rosiglitazone by 54% and reduced its maximum plasma concentration by 28%. **Rifampicin** increased the formation of the metabolite, *N*-desmethylrosiglitazone.[2] Very similar findings were reported in a study in healthy Korean subjects.[3]

Mechanism

Rifampicin is a moderate inducer of CYP2C8, by which rosiglitazone and pioglitazone are principally metabolised, and hence their exposure decreases on concurrent use with rifampicin. In the case of rosiglitazone, CYP2C9 is a minor pathway of metabolism (rifampicin is also a moderate inducer of this isoenzyme) and the authors of one study suggested that this might also play some part in this interaction.[3]

Importance and management

A pharmacokinetic interaction between rifampicin and pioglitazone or rosiglitazone is established, although the clinical relevance has not been assessed. The moderate reduction in the exposure to both antidiabetic drugs could reduce diabetic control and so it would be prudent to monitor blood glucose concentrations if rifampicin is also given, and to increase the dose of rosiglitazone or pioglitazone accordingly. Note that the effects of rifampicin can continue for up to 2 weeks after it has been stopped, and blood glucose monitoring should continue during this time, with pioglitazone or rosiglitazone doses being reduced accordingly to avoid hypoglycaemia.

There does not seem to be any information regarding an interaction between the thiazolidinediones and **rifabutin** or **rifapentine**; however, the UK manufacturer and the CSM in the UK warn that **rifabutin** might possibly reduce the effects of a number of drugs, including oral antidiabetics (not specified).[4,5]

1. Jaakkola T, Backman JT, Neuvonen M, Laitila J, Neuvonen PJ. Effect of rifampicin on the pharmacokinetics of pioglitazone. *Br J Clin Pharmacol* (2006) 61, 70–78.
2. Niemi M, Backman JT, Neuvonen PJ. Effects of trimethoprim and rifampin on the pharmacokinetics of the cytochrome P450 2C8 substrate rosiglitazone. *Clin Pharmacol Ther* (2004) 76, 239–49.
3. Park J-Y, Kim K-A, Kang M-H, Kim S-L, Shin J-G. Effect of rifampin on the pharmacokinetics of rosiglitazone in healthy subjects. *Clin Pharmacol Ther* (2004) 75, 157–62.
4. Mycobutin (Rifabutin). Pfizer Ltd. UK Summary of product characteristics, December 2013.
5. Committee on the Safety of Medicines/Medicines Control Agency. Revised indication and drug interactions of rifabutin. *Current Problems* (1997) 23, 14. Available at: http://webarchive.nationalarchives.gov.uk/20141205150130/http://www.mhra.gov.uk/home/groups/pl-p/documents/websiteresources/con2023238.pdf (accessed 21/10/15)

Thiazolidinediones + St John's wort (*Hypericum perforatum*)

St John's wort appears to slightly decrease rosiglitazone exposure.

Clinical evidence

A preliminary report of a pharmacokinetic study in healthy subjects, states that St John's wort 900 mg daily decreased the AUC of a single 8-mg dose of rosiglitazone by 26% and increased its clearance by 35%.[1]

Mechanism

Unknown. Rosiglitazone is metabolised principally by CYP2C8, and the authors of the above study concluded that St John's wort induces this isoenzyme. The magnitude of the effect of St John's wort was not influenced by CYP2C8 genotype.[1] However, note that repaglinide is a sensitive CYP2C8 substrate, and was not affected by St John's wort (see 'Meglitinides; Repaglinide + St John's wort (*Hypericum perforatum*)', p.532), casting some doubt on this suggested mechanism. Further study is required to determine the exact mechanism involved.

Importance and management

Evidence for a pharmacokinetic interaction between rosiglitazone and St John's wort is extremely limited and is not consistent with what is known about these two drugs. The clinical relevance of the slight reduction in rosiglitazone exposure has not been assessed, but it would seem unlikely to be important. However, the authors state that St John's wort use should be monitored when patients are given CYP2C8 substrates, but its lack of effect on the sensitive CYP2C8 substrate repaglinide, suggests that this might not be necessary. This would also be expected to be the case for the CYP2C8 substrate, **pioglitazone. Pioglitazone** is also a substrate for CYP3A4, of which St John's wort is an established inducer. However, a large decrease in **pioglitazone** concentrations on concurrent use with St John's wort would not be expected on the basis that rifampicin, a more potent enzyme inducer than St John's wort, only caused a moderate reduction in pioglitazone exposure (see 'Thiazolidinediones + Rifamycins', above).

Note that it is generally considered prudent to monitor blood glucose concentrations when any change is made to the medication regimen of a patient with diabetes.

1. Hruska MW, Cheong JA, Langaee TY, Frye RF. Effect of St John's wort administration on CYP2C8 mediated rosiglitazone metabolism. *Clin Pharmacol Ther* (2005) 77, P35.

Thiazolidinediones + Statins

Pioglitazone does not appear to alter the pharmacokinetics of atorvastatin or simvastatin in healthy subjects. Atorvastatin does not appear to alter the pharmacokinetics of pioglitazone in healthy subjects. Most studies have shown no increased incidence of adverse effects when pioglitazone or rosiglitazone were used with atorvastatin or simvastatin, but one study suggested a possible excess of hepatic adverse events in patients taking atorvastatin with these drugs.

Clinical evidence

(a) Adverse events

The adverse event reporting database of the FDA in the US was reviewed for reactions affecting muscle, liver, pancreas, or bone marrow where **simvastatin** or **atorvastatin** were implicated and where antidiabetic drugs also featured. Of the 3 767 events identified for **atorvastatin**, 40 also involved rosiglitazone and 20 also involved pioglitazone. Of the 3 651 events identified for **simvastatin**, 10 also involved rosiglitazone and 9 also involved pioglitazone. About half of these events involving pioglitazone or rosiglitazone resulted in hospitalisation or death. Although the data did not allow for an assessment of whether this rate was greater than that expected, the authors noted that if **simvastatin** is used as the control, the data suggest that the number of cases of adverse events with **atorvastatin** and a thiazolidinedione are greater than would be expected by chance alone.[1] A similar, earlier review by the same authors, had also suggested that patients receiving thiazolidinediones (95% taking **troglitazone**) were more likely to develop hepatotoxicity if taking **atorvastatin** than **simvastatin**.[2] However, note that **troglitazone** has now been withdrawn due to its hepatotoxic effects.

In contrast, information from clinical use does not appear to confirm this finding. For example, use of **rosiglitazone** with **atorvastatin** in 149 patients with type 2 diabetes for 16 weeks was well tolerated and more specifically, combination use was not associated with any hepatic adverse events, increases in hepatic enzymes, or evidence of musculoskeletal toxicity.[3] Similarly the clinical use of **rosiglitazone** or **pioglitazone** with **simvastatin** in 100 patients with type 2 diabetes was not associated with any difference in tolerability.[4] However, neither of these studies was powered to accurately assess adverse event rates and these comments are offered as observations.

(b) Pharmacokinetic studies

In a randomised, crossover study in 12 healthy subjects, **pioglitazone** 45 mg daily for 10 days, did not alter the pharmacokinetics of **simvastatin** 80 mg daily also given for 10 days.[5] Similarly, a preliminary report of another study in healthy subjects, reports that there was no pharmacokinetic interaction between **pioglitazone** 45 mg daily and **atorvastatin** 80 mg daily taken for up to 7 days.[6]

Mechanism

Simvastatin, and to some extent atorvastatin, are metabolised by CYP3A4. Pioglitazone might be a weak inducer of CYP3A4 (see 'Thiazolidinediones; Pioglitazone + Benzodiazepines', p.559), and rosiglitazone is not known to affect CYP3A4, so no change in simvastatin or atorvastatin exposure would be expected on concurrent use. Note that both the thiazolidinediones and the statins are associated with hepatic adverse effects when given alone.

Importance and management

Limited evidence from the studies that exist, and the known metabolic effects of the drugs, would suggest that no pharmacokinetic interaction would be expected to occur between the thiazolidinediones and statins. Most studies show no increased incidence of adverse effects when pioglitazone or rosiglitazone were used with atorvastatin or simvastatin. The clinical relevance of the apparent increased incidence of adverse muscle and liver effects with the use of pioglitazone or rosiglitazone together with atorvastatin is unclear. Further study is needed.

1. Alsheikh-Ali AA, Karas RH. Adverse events with concomitant use of simvastatin or atorvastatin and thiazolidinediones. *Am J Cardiol* (2004) 93, 1417–18.
2. Alsheikh-Ali AA, Abourjaily HM, Karas RH. Risk of adverse events with concomitant use of atorvastatin or simvastatin and glucose-lowering drugs (thiazolidinediones, metformin, sulfonylurea, insulin, acarbose). *Am J Cardiol* (2002) 89, 1308–10.
3. Freed MI, Ratner R, Marcovina SM, Kreider MM, Biswas N, Cohen BR, Brunzell JD; Rosiglitazone Study 108 Investigators. Effects of rosiglitazone alone and in combination with atorvastatin on the metabolic abnormalities in type 2 diabetes mellitus. *Am J Cardiol* (2002) 90, 947–52.
4. Lewin AJ, Kipnes MS, Meneghini LF, Plotkin DJ, Perevozskaya IT, Shah S, Maccubbin DL, Mitchel YB, Tobert JA; Simvastatin/Thiazolidinedione Study Group. Effects of simvastatin on the lipid profile and attainment of low-density lipoprotein cholesterol goals when added to thiazolidinedione therapy in patients with type 2 diabetes mellitus: a multicenter, randomized, double-blind, placebo-controlled trial. *Clin Ther* (2004) 26, 379–89.
5. Prueksaritanont T, Vega JM, Zhao J, Gagliano K, Kuznetsova O, Musser B, Amin RD, Liu L, Roadcap BA, Dilzer S, Lasseter KC, Rogers JD. Interactions between simvastatin and troglitazone or pioglitazone in healthy subjects. *J Clin Pharmacol* (2001) 41, 573–81.
6. Karim A, Schwartz L, Perez A, Chao C. Lack of clinically significant interaction in coadministration of pioglitazone and atorvastatin calcium. *Diabetes* (2003) 52 (suppl 1) A449.

Thiazolidinediones + Sulfonylureas

Pioglitazone does not alter glipizide pharmacokinetics. Rosiglitazone does not have a clinically important effect on glibenclamide (glyburide) pharmacokinetics, and does not alter glimepiride pharmacokinetics. The use of thiazolidinediones with sulfonylureas increases the risk of hypoglycaemia, and the concurrent use of rosiglitazone and sulfonylureas might be associated with a greater risk of fluid retention, particularly with higher rosiglitazone doses.

Clinical evidence

(a) Pioglitazone

In healthy subjects, pioglitazone 45 mg daily for 7 days did not alter the steady-state pharmacokinetics of **glipizide** 5 mg daily.[1,2] The UK and US manufacturers note that hypoglycaemia is more common when pioglitazone is given with a sulfonylurea.[1,3]

(b) Rosiglitazone

Rosiglitazone 2 mg twice daily for 7 days did not alter the mean steady-state 24-hour plasma glucose concentrations in diabetic patients taking **glibenclamide (glyburide)** 3.75 to 10 mg daily. However, rosiglitazone 8 mg daily for 8 days caused a decrease of about 30% in the AUC of **glibenclamide** in healthy Caucasian subjects, and a slight increase in the AUC of **glibenclamide** in Japanese subjects.[4] No pharmacokinetic interaction appears to occur between **glimepiride** and rosiglitazone.[4]

The US manufacturer notes that hypoglycaemia is more common when rosiglitazone is given with a sulfonylurea.[4] Furthermore, the combined use of rosiglitazone and a sulfonylurea leads to an increase in weight, which is greater than with rosiglitazone alone or with the concurrent use of metformin.[4] In addition, in clinical studies, the incidence of oedema was greater with rosiglitazone and sulfonylureas than with rosiglitazone and metformin.[4]

Mechanism

Thiazolidinediones increase insulin sensitivity, and therefore cause an increased incidence of hypoglycaemia when used with sulfonylureas. The reason for the increase in glibenclamide exposure on concurrent use with rosiglitazone is unknown as rosiglitazone is not known to be an enzyme inhibitor.

Importance and management

Evidence for a pharmacokinetic interaction between the thiazolidinediones and the sulfonylureas is limited, but based on that available, no dose changes appear to be needed if glipizide, glibenclamide, or glimepiride are used with the thiazolidinediones. The changes in glibenclamide exposure in Caucasian and Japanese patients were not considered clinically relevant.[4] Additive hypoglycaemia, weight gain, or oedema might occur on concurrent use of thiazolidinediones and sulfonylureas. In general, it is prudent to monitor blood glucose concentrations when any change is made to the medication regimen of a patient with diabetes, and this should be sufficient to identify any adverse effects should they occur; any relevant dose adjustments can then be made.

1. Actos (Pioglitazone hydrochloride). Takeda Pharmaceutical Company Ltd. US Prescribing information, November 2013.
2. Kortboyer JM, Eckland DJA. Pioglitazone has low potential for drug interactions. *Diabetologia* (1999) 42 (Suppl 1), A228.
3. Actos (Pioglitazone hydrochloride). Takeda UK Ltd. UK Summary of product characteristics, November 2013.
4. Avandia (Rosiglitazone maleate). GlaxoSmithKline. US Prescribing information, September 2013.

Thiazolidinediones + Trimethoprim

Trimethoprim slightly increases pioglitazone and rosiglitazone exposure.

Clinical evidence

(a) Pioglitazone

In a randomised, crossover study in 16 healthy subjects, trimethoprim 160 mg twice daily for 6 days increased the AUC of a single 15-mg dose of pioglitazone given on day 3 by 42%, without any change in the peak plasma concentration. The formation of various pioglitazone metabolites was slightly reduced.[1]

(b) Rosiglitazone

In a randomised, crossover study in 10 healthy subjects, trimethoprim 160 mg twice daily for 4 days increased the AUC of a single 4-mg dose of rosiglitazone given on day 3 by 37%. The half-life of rosiglitazone was increased by 26% but the maximum plasma concentration was only increased by 14%.[2] Similarly, in another study, trimethoprim 200 mg twice daily for 5 days increased the AUC of a single 8-mg dose of rosiglitazone by 31% and increased its half-life by 27%.[3]

Mechanism

Pioglitazone and rosiglitazone are principally metabolised by CYP2C8, which can be inhibited by trimethoprim, and hence pioglitazone and rosiglitazone exposure increases.

Importance and management

A pharmacokinetic interaction between trimethoprim and rosiglitazone or pioglitazone is established. However, the clinical relevance of the pharmacokinetic changes has not been assessed. The slight increase in the exposure to both antidiabetic drugs is unlikely to be clinically important, but it is prudent to monitor blood glucose concentrations when any change is made to the medication regimen of a patient with diabetes.

1. Tornio A, Niemi M, Neuvonen PJ, Backman JT. Trimethoprim and the *CYP2C8**3 allele have opposite effects on the pharmacokinetics of pioglitazone. *Drug Metab Dispos* (2008) 36, 73–80.
2. Niemi M, Backman JT, Neuvonen PJ. Effects of trimethoprim and rifampin on the pharmacokinetics of the cytochrome P450 2C8 substrate rosiglitazone. *Clin Pharmacol Ther* (2004) 76, 239–49.
3. Hruska MW, Amico JA, Langaee TY, Ferrell RE, Fitzgerald SM, Frye RF. The effect of trimethoprim on CYP2C8 mediated rosiglitazone metabolism in human liver microsomes and healthy subjects. *Br J Clin Pharmacol* (2005) 59, 70–9.

Thiazolidinediones; Pioglitazone + Aliskiren

There was no pharmacokinetic interaction between pioglitazone and aliskiren in one study.

Clinical evidence, mechanism, importance and management

In a study in 29 healthy subjects, the concurrent use of aliskiren 300 mg daily with pioglitazone 45 mg daily for 7 days had no effect on the AUC of aliskiren and reduced the AUC of pioglitazone by just 6%, when compared with either drug given alone. There was no change in the AUC of pioglitazone metabolites.[1] No dose adjustment of either drug would therefore be expected to be needed if aliskiren is given with pioglitazone.

1. Vaidyanathan S, Maboudian M, Warren V, Yeh C-M, Dieterich HA, Howard D, Dole WP. A study of the pharmacokinetic interactions of the direct renin inhibitor aliskiren with metformin, pioglitazone and fenofibrate in healthy subjects. *Curr Med Res Opin* (2008) 24, 2313–26.

Thiazolidinediones; Pioglitazone + Aspirin

Pioglitazone potentiates the effects of aspirin on platelet aggregation and function. Pioglitazone alone also appears to inhibit platelet function.

Clinical evidence, mechanism, importance and management

In a study, 20 healthy subjects and 20 diabetic patients each took single-doses of pioglitazone (30 mg) and **aspirin** (81 mg) alone, and together. Various methods were used to evaluate their effects on platelet aggregation and function. When aggregation was initiated with arachidonic acid, pioglitazone alone did not affect platelet aggregation, but when given with **aspirin** there was a greater reduction in platelet aggregation than with aspirin alone. In contrast, pioglitazone alone did inhibit platelet function, and when given with **aspirin**, it also potentiated the effect of aspirin alone on platelet function.[1]

It is suggested that pioglitazone exerts its antiplatelet effect through activation of PPARγ (peroxisome proliferator-activated receptor gamma).[1] Further study is needed to determine the clinical relevance of this interaction. Note that aspirin and other salicylates can lower blood glucose concentrations, see 'Sulfonylureas + Salicylates', p.551.

1. Mongan J, Mieszczanska HZ, Smith BH, Messing SP, Phipps RP, Francis CW. Pioglitazone inhibits platelet function and potentiates the effects of aspirin: a prospective observation study. *Thromb Res* (2012) 129, 760–4.

Thiazolidinediones; Pioglitazone + Benzodiazepines

Pioglitazone caused a slight decrease in the AUC of midazolam in healthy subjects.

Clinical evidence, mechanism, importance and management

The US manufacturer briefly notes that, in a study in 21 healthy subjects, pioglitazone 45 mg daily for 15 days reduced the AUC of a single 7.5-mg dose of **midazolam** by 26% and reduced the maximum concentration by 26%.[1]

Midazolam can be used as a probe substrate to assess the activity of drugs on CYP3A4. This study therefore suggests that pioglitazone might be a weak inducer of CYP3A4, but this requires confirmation. The clinical relevance of this small decrease in **midazolam** exposure has not been assessed, but it is likely to be minor. No midazolam dose adjustment would seem necessary on concurrent use with pioglitazone.

1. Actos (Pioglitazone hydrochloride). Takeda Pharmaceutical Company Ltd. US Prescribing information, November 2013.

Thiazolidinediones; Pioglitazone + Colesevelam

The pharmacokinetics of pioglitazone are not affected by colesevelam.

Clinical evidence, mechanism, importance and management

In a randomised, crossover study in 33 healthy subjects, colesevelam 3.75 g did not alter the pharmacokinetics of pioglitazone 30 mg when given at the same time or when pioglitazone was given 1 hour before the colesevelam.[1] There would therefore appear to be no reason to separate administration of pioglitazone and colesevelam, but note that it is prudent to monitor blood glucose concentrations when any change is made to the medication regimen of a patient with diabetes.

1. Brown KS, Armstrong IC, Wang A, Walker JR, Noveck RJ, Swearingen D, Allison M, Kissling JC, Kisicki J, Salazar DE. Effect of the bile acid sequestrant colesevelam on the pharmacokinetics of pioglitazone, repaglinide, estrogen estradiol, norethindrone, levothyroxine, and glyburide. *J Clin Pharmacol* (2010) 50, 554–65.

Thiazolidinediones; Pioglitazone + Fexofenadine

The pharmacokinetics of pioglitazone and fexofenadine do not appear to be affected by concurrent use.

Clinical evidence, mechanism, importance and management

A preliminary report of a study in healthy subjects indicated that the pharmacokinetics of pioglitazone 45 mg daily are not affected by fexofenadine 60 mg twice daily, and that pioglitazone does not affect the pharmacokinetics of fexofenadine.[1] No dose adjustments would seem necessary on concurrent use.

1. Robert M. Pharmacokinetics of coadministration of pioglitazone with fexofenadine. *Diabetes* (2001) 50 (Suppl 2), A443.

Thiazolidinediones; Rosiglitazone + Alcohol

Alcohol, taken with a meal, does not alter the glucose lowering effects of rosiglitazone.

Clinical evidence, mechanism, importance and management

An 8-week study in type 2 diabetics taking rosiglitazone 8 mg daily or placebo, found that 0.6 g/kg of alcohol taken with a meal did not have a clinically relevant effect on plasma glucose concentrations and no episodes of hypoglycaemia were seen.[1] No special precautions would be appear to be necessary on consumption of alcohol with rosiglitazone. However, adherence to the general advice about the consumption of alcohol in diabetes is necessary; see 'Antidiabetics + Alcohol', p.501 for details.

1. Culkin KT, Patterson SD, Jorkasky DK, Freed MI. Rosiglitazone (RSG) does not increase the risk of alcohol-induced hypoglycemia in diet-treated type 2 diabetics. *Diabetes* (1999) 48 (Suppl 1), A350.

Thiazolidinediones; Rosiglitazone + Food

Rosiglitazone exposure is not altered by food.

Clinical evidence, mechanism, importance and management

In a randomised, crossover study, 12 healthy subjects were given a single 2-mg dose of rosiglitazone after a high-fat breakfast or in the fasted state. The overall exposure (AUC) to rosiglitazone was not affected by food, but the maximum concentration was reduced by 20% and the time to maximum concentration increased by 1.75 hours, when compared with the fasted state.[1] The lack of effect on overall exposure to rosiglitazone means that it can be given without regard to food.

1. Freed MI, Allen A, Jorkasky DK, DiCicco RA. Systemic exposure to rosiglitazone is unaltered by food. *Eur J Clin Pharmacol* (1999) 55, 53–6.

Thiazolidinediones; Rosiglitazone + HIV-protease inhibitors

Atazanavir alone slightly increased the exposure to rosiglitazone, but atazanavir boosted with ritonavir negligibly decreased rosiglitazone exposure. Rosiglitazone appears to have no effect on the pharmacokinetics of lopinavir when boosted with ritonavir.

Clinical evidence

(a) Atazanavir

The US manufacturer notes that atazanavir 400 mg daily for 6 days increased the AUC of a single 4-mg dose of **rosiglitazone** given on day 6 by 35%. Conversely, atazanavir boosted with ritonavir 300/100 mg daily caused a 17% decrease in rosiglitazone AUC.[1]

(b) Lopinavir

In a study that included 4 patients taking lopinavir boosted with ritonavir 400/100 mg twice daily with NRTIs, **rosiglitazone** 4 mg daily for 28 days had no effect on the AUC, minimum concentrations, and maximum concentrations of lopinavir.[2]

Mechanism

The mechanism by which atazanavir increases rosiglitazone exposure is unclear, but might be the result of weak inhibition of CYP2C8 which is the principal route of rosiglitazone metabolism (although note that rosiglitazone is not a sensitive CYP2C8 substrate). Further study is needed. The finding that rosiglitazone appears not to affect lopinavir pharmacokinetics is not unexpected as rosiglitazone does not affect CYP3A4, by which lopinavir is metabolised.

Importance and management

The small changes in rosiglitazone pharmacokinetics seen with atazanavir alone and atazanavir boosted with ritonavir are probably unlikely to be clinically relevant.

Rosiglitazone appears not to affect lopinavir pharmacokinetics. The effect of lopinavir boosted with ritonavir on rosiglitazone pharmacokinetics does not appear to have been studied, but it might be expected to interact like atazanavir boosted with ritonavir, causing a minor decrease in the AUC of rosiglitazone. Therefore, it appears that a clinically relevant pharmacokinetic interaction is unlikely.

1. Reyataz (Atazanavir sulfate). Bristol-Myers Squibb. US Prescribing information, August 2013.
2. Oette M, Kurowski M, Feldt T, Kroidl A, Sagir A, Vogt C, Wettstein M, Häussinger D. Impact of rosiglitazone treatment on the bioavailability of antiretroviral compounds in HIV-positive patients. *J Antimicrob Chemother* (2005) 56, 416–19.

Thiazolidinediones; Rosiglitazone + Laropiprant

Laropiprant does not alter the pharmacokinetics of rosiglitazone.

Clinical evidence, mechanism, importance and management

In a randomised, crossover study in 12 healthy subjects, laropiprant 40 mg daily for 7 days was given with a single 4-mg dose of rosiglitazone on day 6. Laropiprant did not alter the pharmacokinetics of rosiglitazone.[1]

Rosiglitazone is known to be principally metabolised by CYP2C8, and laropiprant has been reported to be a moderate CYP2C8 inhibitor[1] *in vitro*. Nevertheless, the findings of this study indicate that laropiprant is unlikely to be a clinically relevant CYP2C8 inhibitor. Therefore, based on this pharmacokinetic study, no rosiglitazone dose adjustment would be expected to be needed in patients taking laropiprant. However, note that laropiprant is only available as a combination product with nicotinic acid, which might cause a deterioration in diabetic control, see 'Table 13.3', p.511.

The lack of a pharmacokinetic interaction in this study indicates that laropiprant is unlikely to interact with other drugs that are CYP2C8 substrates by this mechanism.

1. Schwartz JI, Stroh M, Gao B, Liu F, Rosko K, Zajic S, Meehan AJ, Ruckle J, Lai E, Wagner JA. Effects of laropiprant, a selective prostaglandin D(2) receptor 1 antagonist, on the pharmacokinetics of rosiglitazone. *Cardiovasc Ther* (2009) 27, 239–45.

Thiazolidinediones; Rosiglitazone + NNRTIs

Rosiglitazone appears to have no effect on the pharmacokinetics of efavirenz, but limited evidence suggests it might decrease nevirapine concentrations.

Clinical evidence, mechanism, importance and management

In a study which included 10 patients taking **efavirenz** 600 mg daily and four taking **nevirapine** 200 mg twice daily (both given with NRTIs), **rosiglitazone** 4 mg daily for 28 days had no effect on the AUC, minimum concentrations, or maximum concentrations of **efavirenz**, but the maximum concentration of **nevirapine** decreased by 44%. The AUC and minimum concentration of **nevirapine** also appeared to decrease, but these were not statistically significant.[1] A mechanism for this effect is not clear, as **rosiglitazone** is not known to be an enzyme inducer.

Because of the small number of patients taking **nevirapine**, the findings of this study require confirmation. Until more is known, it might be prudent to increase monitoring of antiretroviral efficacy and/or drug concentrations when **rosiglitazone** is used with **nevirapine**. **Rosiglitazone** appears not to alter the pharmacokinetics of **efavirenz**.

1. Oette M, Kurowski M, Feldt T, Kroidl A, Sagir A, Vogt C, Wettstein M, Häussinger D. Impact of rosiglitazone treatment on the bioavailability of antiretroviral compounds in HIV-positive patients. *J Antimicrob Chemother* (2005) 56, 416–19.

Thiazolidinediones; Rosiglitazone + SSRIs; Fluvoxamine

Fluvoxamine slightly increases rosiglitazone exposure.

Clinical evidence

In a crossover study in healthy subjects, fluvoxamine 50 mg daily for 4 days increased the AUC of **rosiglitazone** by 21% when a single 4-mg dose was given on day 4. There was no change in pharmacokinetics of the *N*-desmethyl metabolite.[1]

Mechanism

Fluvoxamine might have a weak inhibitory effect on CYP2C8, by which rosiglitazone is metabolised.[1]

Importance and management

Fluvoxamine slightly increases rosiglitazone exposure, but the clinical relevance of this was not assessed. Nevertheless, although it would seem unlikely such a small increase in exposure would affect diabetic control, it is prudent to monitor blood glucose concentrations when any change is made to the medication regimen of a patient with diabetes. Note also that the concurrent use of SSRIs and other antidiabetics has been associated with changes to glycaemic control, see 'Antidiabetics + SSRIs', p.518 for details.

1. Pedersen RS, Damkier P, Brosen K. The effects of human CYP2C8 genotype and fluvoxamine on the pharmacokinetics of rosiglitazone in healthy subjects. *Br J Clin Pharmacol* (2006) 62, 682–9.

Thiazolidinediones; Rosiglitazone + Sucralfate

Sucralfate does not affect the pharmacokinetics of rosiglitazone.

Clinical evidence, mechanism, importance and management

A randomised, crossover, single-dose study in 9 healthy subjects, found that sucralfate 2 g taken 45 minutes before rosiglitazone 8 mg had no effect on the pharmacokinetics of rosiglitazone. No special precautions are needed on concurrent use.[1] However, it is prudent to monitor blood glucose concentrations when any change is made to the medication regimen of a patient with diabetes.

1. Rao MNVS, Mullangi R, Katneni K, Ravikanth B, Babu AP, Rani UP, Naidu MUR, Srinivas NR, Rajagopalan R. Lack of effect of sucralfate on the absorption and pharmacokinetics of rosiglitazone. *J Clin Pharmacol* (2002) 42, 670–5.

14

Antiepileptics

The antiepileptic drugs find their major application in the treatment of various kinds of epilepsy, although some of them are also used for other conditions, such as pain management.

Drug interactions

The drugs used as antiepileptics are a disparate group, and their interactions need to be considered individually. Carbamazepine and phenytoin have established ranges of therapeutic plasma levels and these are typically fairly narrow. Modest changes in their plasma levels may therefore be clinically important.

(a) Carbamazepine and related drugs

1. Carbamazepine. Carbamazepine is extensively metabolised by CYP3A4 to the active metabolite, carbamazepine-10,11-epoxide, which is then further metabolised. The concurrent use of carbamazepine and CYP3A4 inhibitors or inducers can therefore lead to toxicity or reduced efficacy. However, importantly, carbamazepine induces CYP3A4 and also induces its own metabolism (autoinduction). Because of this, it is important that drug interaction studies are multiple dose and carried out at steady state. Autoinduction also means that moderate inducers of CYP3A4 might have less of an effect on steady-state carbamazepine concentrations than expected. Both carbamazepine and **oxcarbazepine** can act as inhibitors of CYP2C19, see 'Phenytoin + Carbamazepine and related drugs', p.597. There are also some differences in the effects of carbamazepine and oxcarbazepine, which as yet are not fully explained but might be a result of effects on different isoenzymes or different mechanisms of drug interaction. In particular, there is growing evidence for carbamazepine affecting other isoenzymes, such as a weak inducing effect on CYP2D6 and P-glycoprotein, which have not yet been shown for oxcarbazepine.

2. Oxcarbazepine. Oxcarbazepine is a derivative of carbamazepine and is extensively metabolised to its active metabolite, monohydroxyoxcarbazepine, which is then further metabolised to dihydroxyoxcarbazepine, which is inactive. Monohydroxyoxcarbazepine is principally responsible for the antiepileptic activity of oxcarbazepine. Originally, it was thought that oxcarbazepine did not interact in the same way as carbamazepine and other enzyme-inducing antiepileptics, but growing evidence is challenging this view. In particular, oxcarbazepine is a clinically important inducer of CYP3A4, with similar effects to carbamazepine in some cases (see 'Combined hormonal contraceptives + Carbamazepine and related drugs', p.1172, and 'Tyrosine kinase inhibitors + Antiepileptics; Enzyme-inducing', p.727). For a further mention of the similarities and differences to carbamazepine, see under *Carbamazepine*, above.

3. Eslicarbazepine. Eslicarbazepine is a derivative of carbamazepine, but perhaps more importantly is the *S*-isomer of the active metabolite of oxcarbazepine, monohydroxyoxcarbazepine. Eslicarbazepine is given as the acetate which is rapidly converted in the body to eslicarbazepine. Like carbamazepine and oxcarbazepine, eslicarbazepine induces CYP3A4 and inhibits CYP2C19.

(b) Phenobarbital

Phenobarbital is an inducer of a wide range of cytochrome P450 isoenzymes, and can increase the metabolism of a variety of drugs. It might, itself, also be affected by some enzyme inducers or inhibitors, although these interactions are less established.

(c) Phenytoin

Phenytoin is extensively metabolised by hydroxylation, principally by CYP2C9, although CYP2C19 also plays a role. These isoenzymes show genetic polymorphism (see 'Genetic factors in drug metabolism', p.8, for more information) and CYP2C19 might assume a greater role in individuals who have are CYP2C9 poor metabolisers (that is, patients lacking or deficient in this isoenzyme). The concurrent use of inhibitors of CYP2C9, and sometimes also CYP2C19, can lead to phenytoin toxicity. In addition, phenytoin metabolism is saturable (it shows non-linear pharmacokinetics), and therefore small changes in either the metabolism or the dose of phenytoin can result in large changes in its plasma concentrations. Moreover, phenytoin is highly protein bound, and drugs that alter its protein binding could alter its concentrations. Although protein binding interactions are usually not clinically relevant (unless metabolism is also inhibited, see 'Phenytoin + Valproate', p.609), they can be important in interpreting drug concentrations.

(d) Valproate

Valproate is a generic term that is applied in this section to cover valproic acid and its salts and esters. Valproate undergoes glucuronidation and β-oxidation, and possibly also some metabolism by CYP2C isoenzymes. It can therefore undergo drug interactions by a variety of mechanisms. It acts as an inhibitor of glucuronidation and so might affect other drugs that undergo glucuronidation. Valproate also has non-linear pharmacokinetics due to saturation of plasma protein binding, and so could interact with drugs that alter its protein binding. However, note that, although protein binding interactions are usually not clinically relevant unless metabolism is also inhibited, they can be important in interpreting drug concentrations.

(e) Other antiepileptics

Of the newer antiepileptics, both felbamate and topiramate are weak inducers of CYP3A4. They might also inhibit CYP2C19. They are also partially metabolised by the cytochrome P450 isoenzyme system, so can have their metabolism altered by other drugs such as the enzyme-inducing antiepileptics.

Gabapentin, lamotrigine, levetiracetam, tiagabine, vigabatrin, and zonisamide do not appear to act as inhibitors or inducers of cytochrome P450 isoenzymes, and so appear to cause less drug interactions than the older antiepileptics. Moreover, gabapentin, levetiracetam, and vigabatrin do not appear to be metabolised by the cytochrome P450 system, so appear to be little affected by drug interactions that result from this mechanism. Tiagabine and zonisamide are metabolised by the cytochrome P450 system, so might have their metabolism altered by other drugs such as the enzyme-inducing antiepileptics. Lamotrigine is metabolised by glucuronidation, and might be affected by inhibitors (e.g. valproate) or inducers (e.g. carbamazepine, phenytoin) of this process. Lamotrigine might also act as an inducer of glucuronidation, and could therefore affect the pharmacokinetics of valproate.

Rufinamide undergoes hydrolysis by carboxylesterases. It is not significantly metabolised by cytochrome P450 isoenzymes, but its plasma concentrations are slightly reduced by other antiepileptics such as phenytoin, phenobarbital and primidone. It does act as an inducer of CYP3A4, although clinically significant interactions by this mechanism are uncommon.

Stiripentol is metabolised by a number of isoenzymes but interactions as a result of this effect have yet to be established. Stiripentol inhibits CYP3A4, and might inhibit CYP1A2 and CYP2C19, but the clinical relevance of its effects on these latter two isoenzymes have not been established.

Antiepileptics; Enzyme-inducing + Acetazolamide

Severe osteomalacia and rickets have been seen in a few patients taking phenytoin, phenobarbital, or primidone with acetazolamide. A marked reduction in serum primidone levels with a loss in seizure control, rises in serum carbamazepine levels with toxicity, and rises in phenytoin levels have also been described in a very small number of patients given acetazolamide.

Clinical evidence

(a) Osteomalacia

Severe osteomalacia developed in 2 women taking **phenytoin** or **primidone** and **phenobarbital** when they were given acetazolamide 750 mg daily, despite a normal intake of calcium. When acetazolamide was withdrawn, the hyperchloraemic acidosis that had been seen in both patients abated and their high urinary excretion of calcium fell by 50%.[1,2]

Similar cases have been described in 3 children, who developed rickets after taking acetazolamide, **phenytoin** and **primidone**, with **phenobarbital** and/or metharbital.[3]

(b) Reduced serum primidone levels

A patient taking primidone had an increase in seizure-frequency and a virtual absence of primidone (or its metabolite, phenobarbital) in the serum while taking acetazolamide 250 mg daily. Primidone levels rose when the acetazolamide was withdrawn, probably due to improved absorption. A subsequent study in 2 other patients found that acetazolamide had a small effect on primidone absorption in one patient, and no effect in the other.[4]

(c) Increased serum carbamazepine levels

A 9-year-old girl and two teenage boys, all of them taking the highest doses of carbamazepine tolerable without adverse effects, developed signs of toxicity after taking acetazolamide 250 to 750 mg daily. Their serum carbamazepine levels were found to have increased by about 25 to 50%. In one instance toxicity appeared within 48 hours.[5]

The seizure control of 54 children with grand mal and temporal lobe epilepsy was improved when acetazolamide 10 mg/kg daily was given with carbamazepine. Serum carbamazepine levels rose by 1 to 6 mg/L in 60% of the 33 patients sampled. Adverse effects developed in 10 children, and in 8 children this was within 1 to 10 days of starting the acetazolamide. The adverse effects responded to a reduction in the carbamazepine dose.[6]

(d) Increased serum phenytoin levels

When acetazolamide was given with phenytoin to 6 children, 5 of them had an increase in their phenytoin level (range 20 to 132%, representing an increase of 3 to 12.5 mg/L), and one had a slight decrease (20% or 3 mg/L) [values estimated from figure].[7]

Mechanism

Uncertain. Mild osteomalacia induced by antiepileptics is a recognised phenomenon[8] (see also 'Vitamin D substances + Antiepileptics; Enzyme-inducing', p.1416). It seems that this is exaggerated by acetazolamide, which increases urinary calcium excretion, possibly by causing systemic acidosis, which results from the reduced absorption of bicarbonate by the kidney. The changes in the antiepileptic levels are not understood.

Importance and management

The documentation of all of these interactions is very limited, and their incidence is uncertain. Concurrent use should be monitored for the possible development of osteomalacia or altered antiepileptic levels (reduced primidone efficacy, and increased carbamazepine or phenytoin adverse effects) and steps taken to accommodate them. Withdraw the acetazolamide if necessary, or adjust the dose of the antiepileptic appropriately. In the case of the children with rickets[3] the acetazolamide was withdrawn and high doses of vitamin D was given. It seems possible that other carbonic anhydrase inhibitors may behave like acetazolamide.

1. Mallette LE. Anticonvulsants, acetazolamide and osteomalacia. *N Engl J Med* (1975) 293, 668.
2. Mallette LE. Acetazolamide-accelerated anticonvulsant osteomalacia. *Arch Intern Med* (1977) 137, 1013–17.
3. Matsuda I, Takekoshi Y, Shida N, Fujieda K, Nagai B, Arashima S, Anakura M, Oka Y. Renal tubular acidosis and skeletal demineralization in patients on long-term anticonvulsant therapy. *J Pediatr* (1975) 87, 202–5.
4. Syversen GB, Morgan JP, Weintraub M, Myers GJ. Acetazolamide-induced interference with primidone absorption. *Arch Neurol* (1977) 34, 80–4.
5. McBride MC. Serum carbamazepine levels are increased by acetazolamide. *Ann Neurol* (1984) 16, 393.
6. Forsythe WI, Owens JR, Toothill C. Effectiveness of acetazolamide in the treatment of carbamazepine-resistant epilepsy in children. *Dev Med Child Neurol* (1981) 23, 761–9.
7. Norell E, Lilienbeg G, Gamstorp I. Systematic determination of the serum phenytoin level as an aid in the management of children with epilepsy. *Eur Neurol* (1975) 13, 232–44.
8. Anast CS. Anticonvulsant drugs and calcium metabolism. *N Engl J Med* (1975) 292, 587–8.

Antiepileptics + Aciclovir

Isolated reports describe a marked reduction in phenytoin and valproate levels in two children given aciclovir. Seizure frequency increased.

Clinical evidence, mechanism, importance and management

A 7-year-old boy with epilepsy taking **phenytoin**, **valproate** and nitrazepam was given oral aciclovir 1 g daily for 6 days. After 4 days his trough plasma **phenytoin** levels had fallen from 17 micrograms/mL to 5 micrograms/mL, and his trough **valproate** levels similarly fell, from 32 micrograms/mL to 22 micrograms/mL. When the aciclovir was stopped the plasma levels of both antiepileptics rose over a period of 3 to 6 days. During the period when the antiepileptic levels were restabilising, the seizure frequency markedly increased and his EEG worsened.

The reason for this apparent interaction is not known, but the authors of the report suggest that aciclovir may possibly have reduced the absorption of these antiepileptics, in some way not understood.[1] Reduced **phenytoin** and **valproate** levels during treatment with aciclovir have been reported in another child.[2]

These cases appear to be the only reports of an interaction between aciclovir and valproate or phenytoin, and their general clinical importance is not known. More study is needed to establish an interaction.

1. Parmeggiani A, Riva R, Posar A, Rossi PG. Possible interaction between acyclovir and antiepileptic treatment. *Ther Drug Monit* (1995) 17, 312–15.
2. Iglesias Iglesias A-A, Ortega García MP, Guevara Serrano J. Disminución de la concentración sérica de antiepilépticos durante el tratamiento con aciclovir. *Med Clin (Barc)* (2005) 124, 355–6.

Antiepileptics + Antineoplastics; Cytotoxic

Carbamazepine, phenytoin, and valproate serum concentrations can be reduced by several antineoplastic drug regimens and seizures can occur if the antiepileptic doses are not raised appropriately. The effects of many antineoplastics are reduced or changed by enzyme-inducing antiepileptics. Increased haematological toxicity can occur if valproate is given with fotemustine and cisplatin.

Clinical evidence

(a) Antiepileptic concentrations reduced

There are a number of reports (mainly case reports) that implicate a variety of types of chemotherapy in reducing the concentrations of **carbamazepine**, **phenytoin**, and **valproate**. See 'Table 14.1', p.563, for details.

(b) Antineoplastic effects reduced or altered

A number of antiepileptic drugs affect the concentrations of various antineoplastics. These are discussed elsewhere. See:

- 'Anthracyclines; Doxorubicin + Barbiturates', p.655,
- 'Busulfan + Phenytoin', p.667,
- 'Cyclophosphamide or Ifosfamide + Barbiturates', p.670,
- 'Cyclophosphamide or Ifosfamide + Phenytoin', p.673,
- 'Etoposide + Antiepileptics; Enzyme-inducing', p.677,
- 'Tyrosine kinase inhibitors + Antiepileptics; Enzyme-inducing', p.727,
- 'Irinotecan + Antiepileptics', p.685,
- 'Methotrexate + Antiepileptics; Enzyme-inducing', p.696,
- 'Procarbazine + Antiepileptics; Enzyme-inducing', p.708,
- 'Streptozocin + Phenytoin', p.710,
- 'Taxanes + Rifampicin (Rifampin) and other enzyme inducers', p.717,
- 'Teniposide + Antiepileptics; Enzyme-inducing', p.719,
- 'Topotecan + Phenytoin', p.724,
- 'Toremifene + Antiepileptics; Enzyme-inducing', p.725.
- 'Vinca alkaloids + Antiepileptics; Enzyme-inducing', p.744.

(c) Miscellaneous

One report found that **valproate** increased haematological toxicity in patients taking **fotemustine** and **cisplatin**.[1]

Mechanism

Not fully understood, but a suggested reason for the reduction in serum antiepileptic concentrations is that these antineoplastics damage the intestinal wall, which reduces the absorption of the antiepileptic. Other mechanisms might also have some part to play.

Importance and management

Information about an interaction between the antiepileptics and the cytotoxic antineoplastics is scattered and incomplete. However, it appears that reduced antiepileptic concentrations can occur, possibly leading to loss of efficacy. Where possible, it would be prudent to avoid the concurrent use of enzyme-inducing antiepileptics and antineoplastics. If this is not possible, serum antiepileptic concentrations should be closely monitored during concurrent use with any of these antineoplastics, making dose adjustments as necessary. Note also, that phenytoin toxicity has been seen in patients taking phenytoin and fluorouracil or fluorouracil prodrugs, see 'Phenytoin + Fluorouracil and related prodrugs', p.600, for further details. Advice on the management of

Table 14.1 Reduced antiepileptic levels during antineoplastic therapy

Antiepileptic	*Antineoplastic*	*Malignancy*	*Outcome*	*Refs*
Phenytoin	Cisplatin Carmustine	Brain tumours	A retrospective study reviewed the effects of 3 or more cycles of 72 hours of carmustine and cisplatin chemotherapy in 19 patients who did not vomit. A phenytoin dose increase was required in three-quarters of patients, which was, on average, 40% of the original dose (range 20 to 100%). The effect on phenytoin levels persisted after the chemotherapy had finished, with levels returning to normal 2 to 3 weeks later.	1
Phenytoin	Cisplatin Vinblastine Bleomycin	Metastatic germ cell tumour	Estimated phenytoin level 15 micrograms/mL, but level only reached 2 micrograms/mL. Patient fitted.	2
Phenytoin Primidone	Cisplatin Vinblastine Bleomycin	Metastatic embryonal cell cancer	Phenytoin 800 mg daily gave a level of 15 micrograms/mL whilst receiving chemotherapy. After chemotherapy the same dose produced a toxic level of 42.8 micrograms/mL. Phenobarbital levels unaffected.	3
Phenytoin Phenobarbital	Vinblastine Carmustine Methotrexate	Lung cancer with brain metastases	Phenytoin levels fell from 9.4 micrograms/mL to 5.6 micrograms/mL 24 hours after vinblastine. Patient fitted. Phenytoin levels returned to normal 2 weeks after chemotherapy. Phenobarbital levels unaffected.	4
Phenytoin Carbamazepine Sodium valproate	Doxorubicin Cisplatin Cyclophosphamide Altretamine	Papillary adenocarcinoma of the ovaries	Seizures occurred 2 to 3 days after starting chemotherapy. All drug levels dropped to one-third or lower. Doses increased to compensate, which led to phenytoin toxicity when the chemotherapy finished.	5
Phenytoin	Carboplatin	Small cell lung cancer with brain metastases	Phenytoin level dropped from 9.7 micrograms/mL to 4.6 micrograms/mL 10 days into chemotherapy, resulting in seizures. Phenytoin dose had to be increased by 35% to achieve a level of 10.7 micrograms/mL.	6
Phenytoin	Dacarbazine Carmustine Cisplatin Tamoxifen	Malignant melanoma with brain metastases	Phenytoin level of only 2.5 micrograms/mL despite a loading 1-g dose and a daily dose of 500 mg phenytoin.	7
Phenytoin followed by Carbamazepine	Vincristine Cytarabine Hydroxycarbamide Daunorubicin Methotrexate Tioguanine Cyclophosphamide Carmustine	Stage IV T-cell lymphoma	Phenytoin failed to reach therapeutic levels and so was substituted with carbamazepine. Chemotherapy caused carbamazepine levels to drop below therapeutic levels resulting in seizures. Increasing the dose from 30 mg/kg to 50 mg/kg per day prevented subtherapeutic levels.	8
Phenytoin	Methotrexate Mercaptopurine Vincristine	Acute lymphoblastic leukaemia	Phenytoin levels dropped from 19.8 micrograms/mL on the day before chemotherapy to 3.6 micrograms/mL on the 6th day of chemotherapy.	9
Phenytoin	Cisplatin Carmustine Etoposide	CNS tumours	Dose of phenytoin had to be increased by 50 to 300% in 10 patients to maintain phenytoin levels in the therapeutic range.	10
Sodium valproate	Methotrexate (high dose)	Acute lymphoblastic leukaemia	A child had a seizure a few hours after methotrexate. Serum valproate levels reduced by 75%. The valproate dose was increased by 50% and clonazepam added.	11
Sodium valproate	Methotrexate Cytarabine Nimustine (by CSF perfusion)	Glioblastoma	CSF valproic acid levels reduced by 70% during the perfusion, but returned to normal levels within 7 hours.	12
Sodium valproate Phenytoin	Cisplatin Etoposide Bleomycin	Testicular cancer	Serum valproate levels reduced by 50% after the first cycle and generalised tonic-clonic seizures occurred. There was no effect on phenytoin levels.	13

1. Grossman SA, Sheidler VR, Gilbert MR. Decreased phenytoin levels in patients receiving chemotherapy. *Am J Med* (1989) 87, 505–10.
2. Sylvester RK, Lewis FB, Caldwell KC, Lobell M, Perri R, Sawchuk RA. Impaired phenytoin bioavailability secondary to cisplatinum, vinblastine, and bleomycin. *Ther Drug Monit* (1984) 6, 302-5.
3. Fincham RW, Schottelius DD. Case report. Decreased phenytoin levels in antineoplastic therapy. *Ther Drug Monit* (1979) 1, 277-83.
4. Bollini P, Riva R, Albani F, Ida N, Cacciari L, Bollini C, Baruzzi A. Decreased phenytoin level during antineoplastic therapy: a case report. *Epilepsia* (1983) 24, 75-8.
5. Neef C, de Voogd-van der Straaten I. An interaction between cytostatic and anticonvulsant drugs. *Clin Pharmacol Ther* (1988) 43, 372-5.
6. Dofferhoff ASM, Berensen HH, Naalt Jvd, Haaxma-Reiche H, Smit EF, Postmus PE. Decreased phenytoin level after carboplatin treatment. *Am J Med* (1990) 89, 247-8.
7. Gattis WA, May DB. Possible interaction involving phenytoin, dexamethasone, and antineoplastic agents: a case report and review. *Ann Pharmacother* (1996) 30, 520-6.
8. Nahum MP, Ben Arush MW, Robinson E. Reduced plasma carbamazepine level during chemotherapy in a child with malignant lymphoma. *Acta Paediatr Scand* (1990) 79, 873-5.
9. Jarosinski PF, Moscow JA, Alexander MS, Lesko LJ, Balis FM, Poplack DG. Altered phenytoin clearance during intensive treatment for acute lymphoblastic leukemia. *J Pediatr* (1988) 112, 996-9.
10. Ghosh C, Lazarus HM, Hewlett JS, Creger RJ. Fluctuation of serum phenytoin concentrations during autologous bone marrow transplant for primary central nervous system tumors. *J Neurooncol* (1992) 12, 25-32.
11. Schrøder H, Østergaard JR. Interference of high-dose methotrexate in the metabolism of valproate? *Pediatr Hematol Oncol* (1994) 11, 445-9.
12. Morikawa N, Mori T, Abe T, Kawashima H, Takeyama M, Hori S. Pharmacokinetics of cytosine arabinoside, methotrexate, nimustine and valproic acid in cerebrospinal fluid during cerebrospinal fluid perfusion chemotherapy. *Biol Pharm Bull* (2000) 23, 784-7.
13. Ikeda H, Murakami T, Takano M, Usui T, Kihira K. Pharmacokinetic interaction on valproic acid and recurrence of epileptic seizures during chemotherapy in an epileptic patient. *Br J Clin Pharmacol* (2005) 59, 593-7.

altered antineoplastic concentrations with antiepileptics is discussed in the individual monographs.

1. Bourg V, Lebrun C, Chichmanian RM, Thomas P, Frenay M. Nitroso-urea–cisplatin-based chemotherapy associated with valproate: increase of haematologic toxicity. *Ann Oncol* (2001) 12, 217–9.

Antiepileptics; Enzyme-inducing + Calcium carbimide or Disulfiram

Phenytoin levels are markedly and rapidly increased by disulfiram. Phenytoin toxicity can develop. There is evidence that phenobarbital and carbamazepine levels are not affected by disulfiram, and that phenytoin levels are not affected by calcium carbimide.

Clinical evidence

(a) Calcium carbimide

A study in 4 patients found that calcium carbimide 50 mg daily for a week followed by 100 mg daily for 2 weeks had no effect on serum **phenytoin** levels.[1]

(b) Disulfiram

The serum **phenytoin** levels of 4 patients rose by 100 to 500% over a 9-day period when they were given disulfiram 400 mg daily. **Phenytoin** levels were still rising even 3 to 4 days after the disulfiram was withdrawn, and had still not returned to normal after 14 days. Two patients developed signs of mild **phenytoin** toxicity.[2] In a follow-up study in two of the patients, one developed ataxia and both had a rise in serum **phenytoin** levels, of 25% and 50%, respectively, during 5 days of disulfiram treatment.[1] In 10 healthy subjects disulfiram increased the half-life of **phenytoin** from 11 hours to 19 hours.[3] There are also other case reports describing this interaction.[4-8]

Phenobarbital levels (from **primidone** in 3 patients and **phenobarbital** in one patient) fluctuated by about 10% (which is unlikely to be clinically significant) when disulfiram was given for 9 days.[1,2]

A case report suggested that **carbamazepine** did not interact with disulfiram,[6] and this has been confirmed in a study of 5 epileptic, non-alcoholic patients.[9]

Mechanism

Disulfiram inhibits the liver enzymes concerned with the metabolism of phenytoin (possibly the cytochrome P450 isoenzyme CYP2C9) thereby reducing its metabolism and resulting in a rise in its serum levels, to toxic concentrations in some instances. One study concluded that the inhibition was non-competitive.[7]

Importance and management

The interaction between phenytoin and disulfiram is established, moderately well documented, clinically important and potentially serious. It seems to occur in most patients and develops rapidly. Recovery may take 2 to 3 weeks after the disulfiram is withdrawn. It has been suggested that the dose of phenytoin could be reduced to accommodate the interaction, but it may be difficult to maintain the balance required. Monitor for phenytoin adverse effects (e.g. blurred vision, nystagmus, ataxia or drowsiness) and monitor phenytoin levels if both drugs are given.[1]

Carbamazepine and phenobarbital do not appear to interact with disulfiram, and calcium carbimide does not appear to interact with phenytoin.

1. Olesen OV. The influence of disulfiram and calcium carbimide on the serum diphenylhydantoin excretion of HPPH in the urine. *Arch Neurol* (1967) 16, 642–4.
2. Olesen OV. Disulfiramum (Antabuse®) as inhibitor of phenytoin metabolism. *Acta Pharmacol Toxicol (Copenh)* (1966) 24, 317–22.
3. Svendsen TL, Kristensen MB, Hansen JM, Skovsted L. The influence of disulfiram on the half-life and metabolic clearance rate of diphenylhydantoin and tolbutamide in man. *Eur J Clin Pharmacol* (1976) 9, 439–41.
4. Kiørboe E. Phenytoin intoxication during treatment with Antabuse® (Disulfiram). *Epilepsia* (1966) 7, 246–9.
5. Kiørboe E. Antabus som årsag til forgiftning med fenytoin. *Ugeskr Laeger* (1966) 128, 1531–6.
6. Dry J, Pradalier A. Intoxication par la phénytoïne au cours d'une association thérapeutique avec le disulfirame. *Therapie* (1973) 28, 799–802.
7. Taylor JW, Alexander B, Lyon LW. Mathematical analysis of a phenytoin-disulfiram interaction. *Am J Hosp Pharm* (1981) 38, 93–5.
8. Brown CG, Kaminsky MJ, Feroli ER, Gurley HT. Delirium with phenytoin and disulfiram administration. *Ann Emerg Med* (1983) 12, 310–13.
9. Krag B, Dam M, Angelo H, Christensen JM. Influence of disulfiram on the serum concentration of carbamazepine in patients with epilepsy. *Acta Neurol Scand* (1981) 63, 395–8.

Antiepileptics + Chinese herbal medicines

A study in patients with epilepsy found that Saiko-ka-ryukotsu-borei-to (TJ-12) enhanced the antiepileptic effects of carbamazepine. Paeoniae radix does not appear to affect the pharmacokinetics of valproic acid.

Clinical evidence

(a) Carbamazepine

A study in patients with epilepsy found the antiepileptic effects of carbamazepine were enhanced by concurrent **Saiko-ka-ryukotsu-borei-to (TJ-12)**;[1] patients experienced fewer seizures and had improved neurological symptoms.[2]

(b) Valproate

In 6 healthy subjects, the pharmacokinetics of a single 200-mg dose of valproic acid were unaffected by 1.2 g of a powder extract of **Paeoniae radix** taken daily for 7 days.[3]

Mechanism

Not fully understood. As a pharmacokinetic interaction has not been found between Saiko-ka-ryukotsu-borei-to and carbamazepine, the enhanced effects found in the patients with epilepsy may therefore have been due to a pharmacodynamic interaction.[2] Paeoniae radix (the dried root of *Paeonia lactiflora*[3]) is reported to reduce the rate of gastric emptying;[3] however, this does not appear to affect valproate absorption.

Importance and management

Evidence is limited, but there appears to be no evidence of an adverse effect when using Paeoniae radix with valproate, or Saiko-ka-ryukotsu-borei-to with carbamazepine. More study is needed to confirm all these findings. Note that adulteration of Chinese medicines with various antiepileptics may lead to unexpected toxicity.[4]

1. Senzaki A, Okubo Y, Matuura M, Kojima T, Toru M. Clinical studies on effects of Saiko-ka-ryukotsu-borei-to (TJ-12) for adult patients with symptomatic localization-related epilepsy. *Rinsho Seishin Igaku* (1993) 22, 641–6.
2. Ohnishi N, Nakasako S, Okada K, Umehara S, Takara K, Nagasawa K, Yoshioka M, Kuroda K, Yokoyama T. Studies on interactions between traditional herbal and Western medicines. IV: Lack of pharmacokinetic interactions between Saiko-ka-ryukotsu-borei-to and carbamazepine in rats. *Eur J Drug Metab Pharmacokinet* (2001) 26, 129–35.
3. Chen LC, Chou MH, Lin MF, Yang LL. Lack of pharmacokinetic interaction between valproic acid and a traditional Chinese medicine, Paeoniae Radix, in healthy volunteers. *J Clin Pharm Ther* (2000) 25, 453–9.
4. Lau KK, Lai CK, Chan AYM. Phenytoin poisoning after using Chinese proprietary medicines. *Hum Exp Toxicol* (2000) 19, 385–6.

Antiepileptics + Folinates

If folate supplements are given to treat folate deficiency, which can be caused by the use of antiepileptics (phenytoin, phenobarbital, primidone and possibly carbamazepine and pheneturide), the serum antiepileptic levels may fall, leading to decreased seizure control in some patients.

Clinical evidence

A study in 50 folate-deficient patients with epilepsy (taking **phenytoin**, **phenobarbital** and **primidone** in various combinations) found that after one month of treatment with folic acid 5 mg daily, the plasma **phenytoin** levels of one group of 10 patients had fallen from 20 micrograms/mL to 10 micrograms/mL. In another group of patients taking folic acid 15 mg daily, the levels of **phenytoin** fell from 14 micrograms/mL to 11 micrograms/mL. Only one patient (in the 5-mg folic acid group) had a marked increase in seizure frequency and severity. No alterations were seen in **phenobarbital** levels.[1]

Another long-term study in 26 patients with folic acid deficiency (serum folate less than 5 nanograms/mL) and taking two or more drugs (**phenytoin**, **phenobarbital**, **primidone**), found that the mental state of 22 patients (as shown by increased alertness, concentration, sociability etc.) improved to a variable degree when they were given folic acid 5 mg three times daily. However, the frequency and severity of seizures in 13 patients (50%) increased to such an extent that the folic acid had to be withdrawn from 9 of them.[2]

Similar results, both of increased seizure activity and decreased serum folate levels, have been described in other studies and reports in patients taking **phenytoin**, **phenobarbital**, **primidone** and **pheneturide**.[3-7]

Another report describes a lack of **phenytoin** efficacy in a patient receiving *UFT* (tegafur and uracil) with **folinic acid**, which was attributed to the effect of the **folinic acid** on **phenytoin** levels.[8]

Mechanism

Patients taking antiepileptics may have subnormal serum folic acid levels. Frequencies of 27 to 76% have been reported for phenobarbital, primidone, and phenytoin, alone or in various combinations.[9] There is conflicting information regarding **carbamazepine**[10-13] and **valproate**[10,11,13] causing reduced folic acid levels. **Zonisamide** has not been shown to reduce serum folate levels.[10] One possible explanation is that a reduction in folate occurs with enzyme-inducing antiepileptics, which make excessive demands on folate for the synthesis of the enzymes concerned with drug metabolism, but does not occur with valproate and zonisamide, which are not enzyme inducers. Ultimately the metabolism of the enzyme-inducing antiepileptics becomes limited by the lack of folate, and patients may also develop a reduction in their general mental health[2] and even frank megaloblastic anaemia.[9,14] If folic acid is then given to treat this deficiency, the metabolism of the antiepileptic increases,[15] resulting in a reduction in serum antiepileptic levels, which in some instances may become so low that seizure control is partially or totally lost.

Importance and management

A very well documented and clinically important interaction, which has been the subject of review.[16] Reductions in serum phenytoin levels of 16 to 50% have been described in patients taking 5 to 15 mg folic acid daily for 2 to 4 weeks.[1,3,17] One report suggests that folate doses as low as 1 mg daily may affect phenytoin levels and that even smaller doses may be advisable.[6]

If folic acid supplements are given to folate-deficient patients with epilepsy taking phenytoin, phenobarbital, primidone, and possibly pheneturide, their serum antiepileptic levels should be well monitored so that suitable dose increases can be made. Less information is available about primidone and phenobarbital, but similar precautions would seem prudent. An interaction with carbamazepine is not established, but as some evidence suggests that it may interact similarly some caution is warranted.

1. Baylis EM, Crowley JM, Preece JM, Sylvester PE, Marks V. Influence of folic acid on blood-phenytoin levels. *Lancet* (1971) i, 62–4.
2. Reynolds EH. Effects of folic acid on the mental state and fit-frequency of drug-treated epileptic patients. *Lancet* (1967) i, 1086–9.
3. Strauss RG, Bernstein R. Folic acid and Dilantin antagonism in pregnancy. *Obstet Gynecol* (1974) 44, 345–8.
4. Latham AN, Millbank L, Richens A, Rowe DJF. Liver enzyme induction by anticonvulsant drugs, and its relationship to disturbed calcium and folic acid metabolism. *J Clin Pharmacol* (1973) 13, 337–42.
5. Berg MJ, Fincham RW, Ebert BE, Schottelius DD. Phenytoin pharmacokinetics: before and after folic acid administration. *Epilepsia* (1992) 33, 712–20.
6. Seligmann H, Potasman I, Weller B, Schwartz M, Prokocimer M. Phenytoin-folic acid interaction: a lesson to be learned. *Clin Neuropharmacol* (1999) 5, 268–72.
7. Steinweg DL, Bentley ML. Seizures following reduction in phenytoin level after orally administered folic acid. *Neurology* (2005) 64, 1982.
8. Veldhorst-Janssen NML, Boersma HH, de Krom MCTFM, van Rijswijk REN. Oral tegafur/folinic acid chemotherapy decreases phenytoin efficacy. *Br J Cancer* (2004) 90, 745.
9. Davis RE, Woodliff HJ. Folic acid deficiency in patients receiving anticonvulsant drugs. *Med J Aust* (1971) 2, 1070–2.
10. Kishi T, Fujita N, Eguchi T, Ueda K. Mechanism for reduction of serum folate by antiepileptic drugs during prolonged therapy. *J Neurol Sci* (1997) 145, 109–12.
11. Karabiber H, Sonmezgoz E, Ozerol E, Yakinci C, Otlu B, Yologlu S. Effects of valproate and carbamazepine on serum levels of homocysteine, vitamin B12, and folic acid. *Brain Dev* (2003) 25, 113–5.
12. Deda G, Çaksen H, İçağasioğlu D. Effect of long-term carbamazepine therapy on serum lipids, vitamin B_{12} and folic acid levels in children. *J Pediatr Endocrinol Metab* (2003) 16, 193–6.
13. Sener U, Zorlu Y, Karaguzel O, Ozdamar O, Coker I, Topbas M. Effects of common anti-epileptic drug monotherapy on serum levels of homocysteine, vitamin B12, folic acid and vitamin B6. *Seizure* (2006) 15, 79–85.
14. Ryan GMS, Forshaw JWB. Megaloblastic anaemia due to phenytoin sodium. *BMJ* (1955) 11, 242–3.
15. Berg MJ, Fischer LJ, Rivey MP, Vern BA, Lantz RK, Schottelius DD. Phenytoin and folic acid interaction: a preliminary report. *Ther Drug Monit* (1983) 5, 389–94.
16. Lewis DP, Van Dyke DC, Willhite LA, Stumbo PJ, Berg MJ. Phenytoin-folic acid interaction. *Ann Pharmacother* (1995) 29, 726–35.
17. Furlanut M, Benetello P, Avogaro A, Dainese R. Effects of folic acid on phenytoin kinetics in healthy subjects. *Clin Pharmacol Ther* (1978) 24, 294–7.

Antiepileptics + Ginkgo (*Ginkgo biloba*)

Case reports describe seizures in three patients taking valproate, or valproate and phenytoin, when ginkgo was also taken.

Clinical evidence

A 55-year-old man taking **valproate** and **phenytoin** for a seizure disorder that developed following coronary artery bypass surgery, suffered a fatal breakthrough seizure while swimming a year later. Analysis of his medical history showed that he had unexplained subtherapeutic serum levels of **valproate** and **phenytoin** on three occasions over the previous year. It was later found that the patient had also been taking numerous vitamins, supplements and herbal medicines without the knowledge of his physician, of which a ginkgo extract was stated to be the most common ingredient.[1] The only other herbal medicines named in the report were ginseng and saw palmetto.

In another case, a 78-year-old man, whose epileptic seizures had been well controlled by **valproate** 1.2 g daily for 7 years, suffered a cluster of seizures after taking a ginkgo extract 120 mg daily for 2 weeks for the management of mild cognitive impairment. The ginkgo was stopped and the patient was reportedly seizure-free 8 months later. All other medications taken by the patient remained unchanged.[2]

An 84-year-old epileptic woman with severe dementia taking **valproate** 1.2 g daily had been seizure-free for 2 years. After taking a ginkgo extract 120 mg daily for 12 days prescribed by her psychiatrist, she suffered a cluster of seizures, which were treated with intravenous diazepam in the emergency department. The ginkgo extract was stopped on admission and the patient remained free of seizures 4 months later. All other medications taken by the patient were unchanged.[2]

Mechanism

Unknown. Ginkgo *seeds* (nuts) contain the neurotoxin 4-*O*-methoxypyridoxine (ginkgotoxin), which indirectly inhibits the activity of glutamate decarboxylase, which in turn results in seizure induction by lowering the levels of γ-amino-butyric acid (GABA). A large quantity of ginkgo nuts (about 70 to 80) alone have been reported to be the cause of seizures in a healthy 36-year-old woman.[3] However, leaf extracts would not generally be expected to contain sufficient levels of this neurotoxin to be a problem.

Another possible mechanism is induction of the cytochrome P450 isoenzyme CYP2C19 by ginkgo. Phenytoin is a substrate of CYP2C19 and therefore, in theory, ginkgo may increase the metabolism of phenytoin and thereby reduce its levels. Ginkgo has been seen to induce CYP2C19 in clinical studies. See 'Proton pump inhibitors + Ginkgo (*Ginkgo biloba*)', p.1152.

Importance and management

Evidence for an interaction between ginkgo and valproate and phenytoin appears to be limited to case reports. The only case that measured serum levels of these antiepileptics is complicated by the use of numerous other supplements. An interaction is therefore by no means established. Nevertheless, it may be prudent to consider the possibility of reduced effects if a patient taking phenytoin and/or valproate wishes to also take ginkgo.

1. Kupiec T, Raj V. Fatal seizures due to potential herb-drug interactions with Ginkgo biloba. *J Anal Toxicol* (2005) 29, 755–8.
2. Granger AS. Ginkgo biloba precipitating epileptic seizures. *Age Ageing* (2001) 30, 523–5.
3. Miwa H, Iijima M, Tanaka S, Mizuno Y. Generalised convulsions after consuming a large amount of ginkgo nuts. *Epilepsia* (2001) 42, 280–281.

Antiepileptics + Mefloquine

A woman whose epilepsy was controlled with valproic acid developed convulsions when she took mefloquine.

Clinical evidence, mechanism, importance and management

An isolated report describes a 20-year-old woman, with a 7-year history of epilepsy (bilateral myoclonus and generalised tonic-clonic seizures) controlled with **valproic acid** 1.3 g daily, who developed tonic-clonic seizures 8 hours after taking the second of 3 prophylactic doses of mefloquine 250 mg.[1] It is not clear whether this resulted from a drug-drug or a drug-disease interaction. The manufacturer of mefloquine advises its avoidance in those with a history of convulsions as it may increase the risk of convulsions. In these patients mefloquine should be used only for curative treatment if compelling reasons exist.[2]

1. Besser R, Krämer G. Verdacht auf anfallfördernde Wirkung von Mefloquin (Lariam®). *Nervenarzt* (1991) 62, 760–1.
2. Lariam (Mefloquine hydrochloride). Roche Products Ltd. UK Summary of product characteristics, November 2011.

Antiepileptics + Melatonin

Carbamazepine levels are not affected by melatonin. Melatonin levels are predicted to be reduced by carbamazepine.

Clinical evidence, mechanism, importance and management

In a placebo-controlled study on the effects of melatonin on antioxidant enzymes, melatonin 6 to 9 mg/kg daily for 14 days was given to children with epilepsy taking carbamazepine. The serum levels of carbamazepine and its metabolite carbamazepine-10,11-epoxide were not affected by melatonin. Melatonin appeared to antagonise the accumulation of reactive oxygen species (which can be damaging to cells in the body) caused by carbamazepine.[1]

One manufacturer predicts that carbamazepine may increase the metabolism of melatonin (by induction of the cytochrome P450 isoenzyme CYP1A2), thereby decreasing its levels.[2] However, note that carbamazepine is not a particularly potent inducer of this isoenzyme. Furthermore, when 22 children with epilepsy were given either **carbamazepine** or **valproate**, with a single 6- or 9-mg dose of melatonin, the serum levels of melatonin increased from 1.5 picograms/mL to 165 picograms/mL (range: 50 to 350 picograms/mL) in the **carbamazepine** group and from 1.3 picograms/mL to 78 picograms/mL (range 13 to 260 picograms/mL) in the **valproate** group. Although median levels of melatonin in the **carbamazepine** group were about twice those in the **valproate** group, the difference was not statistically significant because of the wide range of results.[3]

It appears that dose adjustments are unlikely to be needed on the concurrent use of melatonin and carbamazepine.

1. Gupta M, Gupta YK, Agarwal S, Aneja S, Kalaivani M, Kohli K. Effects of add-on melatonin administration on antioxidant enzymes in children with epilepsy taking carbamazepine monotherapy: a randomized, double-blind, placebo-controlled trial. *Epilepsia* (2004) 45, 1636–9.
2. Circadin (Melatonin). Flynn Pharma Ltd. UK Summary of product characteristics, August 2011.
3. Gupta M, Kohli K, Gupta YK. Modulation of serum concentrations of melatonin by carbamazepine and valproate. *Indian J Physiol Pharmacol* (2006) 50, 79–82.

Antiepileptics + Orlistat

Orlistat might reduce the absorption of lamotrigine. It is predicted to affect other antiepileptics similarly.

Clinical evidence, mechanism, importance and management

A patient with epilepsy taking **lamotrigine** 200 mg daily had an increase in seizure frequency from one each month to more than one each week after starting to take orlistat 120 mg three times daily. It was suggested that orlistat, which is known to affect the absorption of lipophilic drugs, might have reduced the absorption of lamotrigine which is considered to be highly lipophilic.[1]

This appears to be the only published report of an interaction between orlistat and any antiepileptic. However, the MHRA in the UK notes that loss of seizure control has been reported during concurrent use of orlistat and antiepileptic drugs such as lamotrigine and **valproate**. Further, they note that the absorption of antiepileptics might be reduced by orlistat resulting in loss of seizure control, and advise that patients should be monitored for changes in seizure frequency and severity on concurrent use, and they suggest separating administration of the antiepileptic and orlistat.[2]

For details of a lack of effect on the pharmacokinetics of phenytoin, see 'Phenytoin + Orlistat', p.604.

1. Bigham S, McGuigan C, MacDonald BK. Reduced absorption of lipophilic anti-epileptic medications when used concomitantly with the anti-obesity drug orlistat. *Epilepsia* (2006) 47, 2207.
2. Medicines and Healthcare Products Regulatory Agency and the Commission on Human Medicines. Orlistat safety update. *Drug Safety Update* (2010) 3, 4–5. Available at: http://webarchive.nationalarchives.gov.uk/20141205150130/http://www.mhra.gov.uk/home/groups/pl-p/documents/publication/con071086.pdf (accessed 21/10/15).

Antiepileptics; Enzyme-inducing + Quinine

Preliminary evidence suggests that the effects of carbamazepine and phenobarbital may be increased by quinine, possibly leading to toxicity. An isolated report suggests that phenytoin may reduce the levels of quinine but the levels of phenytoin do not appear to be affected by quinine.

Clinical evidence, mechanism, importance and management

Single doses of **carbamazepine** 200 mg, **phenobarbital** 120 mg or **phenytoin** 200 mg were given to 3 groups of 6 healthy subjects, with and without a single 600-mg dose of quinine sulfate. The AUC of **carbamazepine** and **phenobarbital** were increased by 104% and 57%, respectively, and the peak plasma levels were increased by 81% and 53%, respectively. **Phenytoin** was not significantly affected. The reasons for these effects are not known but the authors suggest that quinine inhibits the metabolism of **carbamazepine** and **phenobarbital** (but not **phenytoin**) by the liver, so that their levels become raised.[1]

In an earlier study in 2 healthy subjects, **phenobarbital** 125 mg daily for 4 days caused only a small reduction in the plasma half-life of quinine.[2]

Information seems to be limited to these studies. The importance of the interactions with **carbamazepine** and **phenobarbital** await assessment in a clinically realistic situation (i.e. in patients taking multiple doses) but in the meantime it would seem prudent to monitor for adverse effects of **carbamazepine** (e.g. nausea, vomiting, ataxia, drowsiness) or **phenobarbital** (e.g. hypotension, irritability, sedation) if quinine is also taken.

An isolated report describes a 22-month-old girl taking **phenytoin**, **sodium valproate** and **topiramate** for epilepsy, who was given quinine sulfate (initially intravenously, then orally) followed by a single dose of sulfadoxine with pyrimethamine for malaria. Her malaria film became negative after 4 days of the 7-day quinine course. About one month later she was found to have recrudescent falciparum malaria, and so she was given quinine sulfate and then atovaquone with proguanil. Although it is possible that quinine resistance may have occurred, the authors also considered that enzyme induction by **phenytoin** may have led to suboptimal quinine levels.[3]

Although quinine does not appear to affect **phenytoin** levels, the isolated case report suggests that levels of quinine may be reduced in the presence of **phenytoin**. Until more is known it would seem prudent to monitor concurrent use carefully.

1. Amabeoku GJ, Chikuni O, Akino C, Mutetwa S. Pharmacokinetic interaction of single doses of quinine and carbamazepine, phenobarbitone and phenytoin in healthy volunteers. *East Afr Med J* (1993) 70, 90–3.
2. Saggers VH, Hariratnajothi N, McLean AEM. The effect of diet and phenobarbitone on quinine metabolism in the rat and in man. *Biochem Pharmacol* (1970) 19, 499–503.
3. Fabre C, Criddle J, Nolder D, Klein JL. Recrudescence of imported falciparum malaria after quinine therapy: potential drug interaction with phenytoin. *Trans R Soc Trop Med Hyg* (2005) 99, 871–3.

Antiepileptics + Quinolones

Studies suggest that ciprofloxacin, clinafloxacin, and enoxacin do not usually have a clinically significant effect on phenytoin concentrations. However, case reports describe changes (both increases and decreases) in phenytoin concentrations in patients given ciprofloxacin. One single dose study suggests that ciprofloxacin might affect carbamazepine concentrations but this needs confirmation.

Clinical evidence

(a) Carbamazepine

In a single-dose pharmacokinetic study, 8 healthy subjects were given carbamazepine 200 mg, alone and with ciprofloxacin 500 mg. Ciprofloxacin increased the maximum plasma concentration and AUC of carbamazepine by 55% and 54%, respectively.[1]

(b) Phenytoin

1. Ciprofloxacin. In a study in 4 healthy subjects there was no difference in the pharmacokinetics of **phenytoin** 200 mg daily when it was given with ciprofloxacin 500 mg twice daily. However, one of the 4 subjects experienced a 30% decrease in the **phenytoin** maximum serum concentrations when ciprofloxacin was added.[2] Four case reports describe decreases of 50% or more in **phenytoin** serum concentrations when ciprofloxacin was added, accompanied by seizures in 3 instances.[3-6] Another report describes unexpectedly low **phenytoin** concentrations (measured after a loading dose) in a woman taking ciprofloxacin.[7]

Conversely, **phenytoin** concentrations increased in an elderly woman, possibly as a result of the ciprofloxacin she was taking.[8] In another study in 7 patients taking **phenytoin**, ciprofloxacin 500 mg twice daily for 10 days caused no statistically significant change in **phenytoin** concentrations, although there was a tendency for an increase (mean 24% rise).[9]

In one report, blood concentrations of **phenytoin** and **valproic acid** were not affected by ciprofloxacin although a seizure occurred on the fourth day of concurrent use.[10] Other cases describe seizures in patients taking **phenytoin** when given ciprofloxacin, but with little or no information on **phenytoin** concentrations.[11]

2. Clinafloxacin. In a study, **phenytoin** 300 mg daily was given to healthy subjects for 10 days, then clinafloxacin 400 mg twice daily was added for a further 2 weeks. The maximum serum **phenytoin** concentrations increased by 18% (from 6.74 to 7.95 mg/L), the AUC rose by 20% and the clearance decreased by 17%.[12]

3. Enoxacin. In a study in healthy subjects, enoxacin did not appear to alter **phenytoin** serum concentrations, nor were multiple-dose serum enoxacin concentrations significantly altered by **phenytoin**.[13]

Mechanism

Fluoroquinolones alone rarely cause convulsions both in patients with and without a history of seizures. The mechanism for the effect of ciprofloxacin on phenytoin concentrations is unknown, and is unlikely to be due to effects on hepatic metabolism or oral absorption.[14,15] However, ciprofloxacin decreased phenytoin concentrations in an *animal* study, and a suggested reason for this was increased urinary excretion.[16]

The authors of the study with ciprofloxacin and carbamazepine suggest a role for CYP1A2 and or CYP3A4, but this requires confirmation.

Importance and management

The known potential for quinolones to induce seizures suggests that these antibacterials should either be avoided in patients with epilepsy, or only used when the benefits of treatment outweigh the potential risks of seizures. Some of the reactions seem to be drug-disease interactions rather than drug-drug interactions, the usual outcome being that the control of epilepsy is worsened. However, it appears that ciprofloxacin might also alter (usually decrease) phenytoin concentrations, and if this combination is used it would be prudent to consider monitoring phenytoin concentrations. Enoxacin appears not to alter phenytoin concentrations.

Information regarding an interaction between ciprofloxacin and carbamazepine is limited to one small study. The authors suggest that, based on their findings, consideration should be given to monitoring carbamazepine concentrations in patients given ciprofloxacin. However, carbamazepine is known to induce its own metabolism on continued use and therefore this study needs repeating in a larger number of subjects with carbamazepine at steady state before any firm recommendations can be made.

1. Shahzadi A, Javed I, Aslam B, Muhammad F, Asi MR, Ashraf MY, Zia-Ur-Rhaman. Therapeutic effects of ciprofloxacin on the pharmacokinetics of carbamazepine in healthy adult male volunteers. *Pak J Pharm Sci* (2011) 24, 63–8.
2. Job ML, Arn SK, Strom JG, Jacobs NF, D'Souza MJ. Effect of ciprofloxacin on the pharmacokinetics of multiple-dose phenytoin serum concentrations. *Ther Drug Monit* (1994) 16, 427–31.
3. Dillard ML, Fink RM, Parkerson R. Ciprofloxacin-phenytoin interaction. *Ann Pharmacother* (1992) 26, 263.
4. Pollak PT, Slayter KL. Hazards of doubling phenytoin dose in the face of an unrecognized interaction with ciprofloxacin. *Ann Pharmacother* (1997) 31, 61–4.
5. Brouwers PJ, DeBoer LE, Guchelaar H-J. Ciprofloxacin-phenytoin interaction. *Ann Pharmacother* (1997) 31, 498.
6. Otero M-J, Morán D, Valverde M-P. Interaction between phenytoin and ciprofloxacin. *Ann Pharmacother* (1999) 33, 251–2.
7. McLeod R, Trinkle R. Comment: unexpectedly low phenytoin concentration in a patient receiving ciprofloxacin. *Ann Pharmacother* (1998) 32, 1110–11.
8. Hull RL. Possible phenytoin-ciprofloxacin interaction. *Ann Pharmacother* (1993) 27, 1283.
9. Schroeder D, Frye J, Alldredge B, Messing R, Flaherty J. Effect of ciprofloxacin on serum phenytoin concentrations in epileptic patients. *Pharmacotherapy* (1991) 11, 275.
10. Slavich IL, Gleffe R, Haas EJ. Grand mal epileptic seizures during ciprofloxacin therapy. *JAMA* (1989) 261, 558–9.
11. Anon. Risk of seizures from concomitant use of ciprofloxacin and phenytoin in patients with epilepsy. *Can Med Assoc J* (1998) 158, 104–5.
12. Randinitis EJ, Koup JR, Bron NJ, Hounslow NJ, Rausch G, Abel R, Vassos AB, Sedman AJ. Drug interaction studies with clinafloxacin and probenecid, cimetidine, phenytoin and warfarin. *Drugs* (1999) 58 (Suppl 2), 254–5.
13. Thomas D, Humphrey G, Kinkel A, Sedman A, Rowland M, Toon S, Aarons L, Hopkins K. A study to evaluate the potential pharmacokinetic interaction between oral enoxacin (ENX) and oral phenytoin (PHE). *Pharm Res* (1986) 3 (Suppl), 99S.
14. Pollak PT, Slayter KL. Comment: ciprofloxacin-phenytoin interaction. *Ann Pharmacother* (1997) 31, 1549–50.
15. Brouwers PJ, de Boer LE, Guchelaar H-J. Comment: ciprofloxacin-phenytoin interaction. *Ann Pharmacother* (1997) 31, 1550.
16. al-Humayyd MS. Ciprofloxacin decreases plasma phenytoin concentrations in the rat. *Eur J Drug Metab Pharmacokinet* (1997) 22, 35–9.

Antiepileptics + St John's wort (*Hypericum perforatum*)

St John's wort modestly increased the clearance of single-dose carbamazepine in one study, but had no effect on multiple-dose carbamazepine pharmacokinetics in another study. Carbamazepine does not appear to significantly affect the pharmacokinetics of hypericin or pseudohypericin (constituents of St John's wort). St John's wort increases the clearance of mephenytoin, and is predicted to reduce the blood levels of phenytoin and phenobarbital, but this awaits clinical confirmation.

Clinical evidence

In a multiple-dose study in 8 healthy subjects, St John's wort had no effect on the pharmacokinetics of **carbamazepine** or its active metabolite, carbamazepine-10,11-epoxide. In this study, subjects took **carbamazepine** 200 mg increased to 400 mg daily alone for 20 days, then with St John's wort 300 mg (standardised to 0.3% hypericin) three times daily for a further 14 days.[1] In contrast, the AUC of a single 400-mg dose of **carbamazepine** was reduced by 21% after St John's wort 300 mg was given three times daily for 14 days, and the AUC of the 10,11-epoxide metabolite was increased by 26%.[2]

A double-blind, placebo-controlled study in healthy subjects found that, apart from a modest 29% decrease in the AUC of pseudohypericin, **carbamazepine** did not significantly affect the pharmacokinetics of either hypericin or pseudohypericin, which are both constituents of St John's wort.[3]

In another placebo-controlled study in 6 extensive metabolisers of CYP2C19 (that is, those with normal levels of this isoenzyme), St John's wort 300 mg three times daily for 14 days increased the clearance of a single oral dose of **mephenytoin** 100 mg given on day 15, by about 3-fold. There were no significant effects when **mephenytoin** was given to 6 poor metabolisers of CYP2C19 (that is, those lacking this isoenzyme). Each St John's wort tablet contained 0.3% hypericin and 4% hyperforin.[4]

Mechanism

St John's wort is a known inducer of the cytochrome P450 isoenzyme CYP3A4, and the results with single-dose carbamazepine are as predicted. However, carbamazepine is also an inducer of CYP3A4, which induces its own metabolism (autoinduction). It is suggested that St John's wort is not sufficiently potent an inducer to further induce carbamazepine metabolism when autoinduction has occurred,[1] and therefore a small interaction is seen with single doses but no interaction is seen with multiple doses. However, the lack of effect seen in some of these studies may also be due to the different preparations used, and therefore differing levels of hyperforin.

Mephenytoin is a substrate of CYP2C19 and St John's wort appears to induce this isoenzyme.

Importance and management

The available evidence suggests that a clinically significant interaction between carbamazepine and St John's wort is unlikely. Before the publication of the above reports, the CSM in the UK had advised that patients taking a number of drugs including the antiepileptics carbamazepine, **phenytoin** and **phenobarbital** should not take St John's wort.[5] This advice was based on predicted pharmacokinetic interactions. In the light of the above studies, this advice may no longer apply to carbamazepine, although further study is needed. As the pharmacokinetic effects reported were modest, it may not be necessary for patients taking carbamazepine to avoid St John's wort; however, concurrent use should probably still be monitored to ensure adequate carbamazepine levels and efficacy.

Until more is known, it would probably be prudent to avoid the concurrent use of St John's wort in patients taking mephenytoin, **phenytoin** and **phenobarbital** (and therefore **primidone**), especially as **phenytoin** is also a substrate of CYP2C19, which St John's wort also appears to induce.

1. Burstein AH, Horton RL, Dunn T, Alfaro RM, Piscitelli SC, Theodore W. Lack of effect of St John's wort on carbamazepine pharmacokinetics in healthy volunteers. *Clin Pharmacol Ther* (2000) 68, 605–12.
2. Burstein AH, Piscitelli SC, Alfaro RM, Theodore W. Effect of St John's wort on carbamazepine single-dose pharmacokinetics. *Epilepsia* (2001) 42 (Suppl 7), 253.
3. Johne A, Perloff ES, Bauer S, Schmider J, Mai I, Brockmöller J, Roots I. Impact of cytochrome P-450 inhibition by cimetidine and induction by carbamazepine on the kinetics of hypericin and pseudohypericin in healthy volunteers. *Eur J Clin Pharmacol* (2004) 60, 617–22.
4. Wang L-S, Zhu B, El-Aty AMA, Zhou G, Li Z, Wu J, Chen G-L, Liu J, Tang ZR, An W, Li Q, Wang D, Zhou H-H. The influence of St. John's wort on CYP2C19 activity with respect to genotype. *J Clin Pharmacol* (2004) 44, 577–81.
5. Committee on the Safety of Medicines (UK). Message from Professor A Breckenridge (Chairman of CSM) and Fact Sheet for Health Care Professionals, 29th February 2000.

Antiepileptics + Terbinafine

A report describes the development of fatal toxic epidermal necrolysis shortly after a patient taking phenobarbital and carbamazepine started taking terbinafine. Another report describes elevated carbamazepine levels with symptoms of toxicity when a patient taking carbamazepine also took terbinafine.

Clinical evidence

A report describes a 26-year-old woman with cerebral palsy who had been taking **phenobarbital** 15 mg with **carbamazepine** 400 mg daily for 12 years to control epilepsy, and who developed fatal toxic epidermal necrolysis 2 weeks after starting oral terbinafine 250 mg daily for tinea corporis. The reasons are not understood, but the authors point out that all three drugs can cause adverse skin reactions (erythema multiforme) and suggest that some synergism may have occurred.[1] It is uncertain whether this was a true interaction or a terbinafine adverse effect.

A further report describes a 50-year-old man taking **carbamazepine** who developed symptoms of **carbamazepine** toxicity including gait ataxia, dizziness and falls and raised carbamazepine levels about 3 days after starting to take terbinafine 250 mg daily. These symptoms resolved on stopping the terbinafine, but recurred when treatment was restarted. It was suggested that terbinafine may have inhibited the metabolism of **carbamazepine**. A **carbamazepine** level of 17.2 micrograms/mL was recorded, which had only fallen to 2 micrograms/mL 10 days after stopping all treatment.[2]

Mechanism

The mechanism of this interaction is unclear, as terbinafine is thought to only affect the cytochrome P450 isoenzyme CYP2D6, which is not a major route of carbamazepine metabolism.

An antiepileptic drug hypersensitivity syndrome characterised by fever, skin rash (which may rarely be severe) and internal organ involvement (agranulocytosis, hepatitis, nephritis, and myositis) may occur 2 to 8 weeks after starting treatment with carbamazepine or phenytoin. As the patient in the first case report had been taking these drugs for several years, they are unlikely to be the cause, but this syndrome may also occur with other drugs including terbinafine.[3]

Importance and management

These appear to be isolated cases, and their general significance is unknown. If a patient taking terbinafine and carbamazepine experiences otherwise unexplained signs of carbamazepine toxicity (e.g. nausea, vomiting, ataxia and drowsiness) it may be prudent to suspect an interaction. Take carbamazepine levels and adjust the dose accordingly.

1. White SI, Bowen-Jones D. Toxic epidermal necrolysis induced by terbinafine in a patient on long-term anti-epileptics. *Br J Dermatol* (1996) 134, 188–9.
2. Baath NS, Hong J, Sattar SP. Possible carbamazepine toxicity with terbinafine. *Can J Clin Pharmacol* (2006) 13, e228–e231.
3. Schlienger RG, Shear NH. Antiepileptic drug hypersensitivity syndrome. *Epilepsia* (1998) 39 (Suppl 7), S3–S7.

Antiepileptics; Enzyme-inducing + Tobacco

Smoking tobacco appears to have no important effect on the serum levels of phenytoin, phenobarbital or carbamazepine.

Clinical evidence, mechanism, importance and management

A comparative study in 88 patients with epilepsy, taking **phenobarbital**, **phenytoin** and **carbamazepine** alone or in combination, found that although tobacco smoking had a tendency to lower the steady-state serum levels of these drugs, a statistically significant effect on the concentration-dose ratios was only found in the patients taking **phenobarbital**.[1] However, in another study in healthy subjects, there was no difference in the pharmacokinetics of a single 60-mg dose of **phenobarbital** in smokers and non-smokers.[2] In practical terms smoking appears to have only a negligible effect on the serum levels of these antiepileptic drugs and patients with epilepsy who smoke are unlikely to need higher doses than non-smokers.

1. Benetello P, Furlanut M, Pasqui L, Carmillo L, Perlotto N, Testa G. Absence of effect of cigarette smoking on serum concentrations of some anticonvulsants in epileptic patients. *Clin Pharmacokinet* (1987) 12, 302–4.
2. Mirfazaelian A, Jahanzad F, Tabatabaei-far M, Farsam H, Mahmoudian M. Effect of smoking on single dose pharmacokinetics of phenobarbital. *Biopharm Drug Dispos* (2001) 22, 403–6.

Antiepileptics; Enzyme-inducing + Vitamin B substances

High daily doses of pyridoxine can reduce phenytoin and phenobarbital levels in some patients. Some evidence suggests that high doses of nicotinamide reduce the conversion of primidone to phenobarbital, and increase carbamazepine levels.

Clinical evidence

(a) Nicotinamide

Nicotinamide 41 to 178 mg/kg daily increased the levels of **primidone** and decreased the levels of **primidone**-derived phenobarbital in 3 children. Although two of the children had refractory seizures, seizure frequency decreased while they were taking nicotinamide. Two of the children taking **carbamazepine** had increases in their **carbamazepine** levels.[1]

(b) Pyridoxine

Pyridoxine 200 mg daily for 4 weeks reduced the **phenobarbital** serum levels of 5 patients with epilepsy by about 50%. Reductions in serum **phenytoin** levels of about 35% (range 17 to 70%) were also seen when patients were given pyridoxine 80 to 400 mg daily for 2 to 4 weeks. However, no interaction occurred in a number of other patients taking these drugs.[2]

Mechanism

It is suggested that the pyridoxine increases and nicotinamide decreases the activity of the liver enzymes concerned with the metabolism of these antiepileptics.[1,2]

Importance and management

Information seems to be limited, but what is known suggests that the concurrent use of carbamazepine, phenytoin, phenobarbital or primidone should be monitored if large doses of pyridoxine or nicotinamide are used, being alert for the need to modify the antiepileptic dose. It seems unlikely that small doses (as in multivitamin preparations) will interact to any great extent.

1. Bourgeois BF, Dodson WE, Ferrendelli JA. Interactions between primidone, carbamazepine, and nicotinamide. *Neurology* (1982) 32, 1122–26.
2. Hansson O, Sillanpaa M. Pyridoxine and serum concentration of phenytoin and phenobarbitone. *Lancet* (1976) i, 256.

Carbamazepine + Allopurinol

There is some evidence to suggest that high-dose allopurinol (15 mg/kg or 600 mg daily) can gradually raise serum carbamazepine levels by about one-third. It appears that allopurinol 300 mg daily has no effect on carbamazepine levels.

Clinical evidence

In a 6-month study, 7 patients with epilepsy taking antiepileptics including carbamazepine, were also given allopurinol 100 mg three times daily for 3 months then 200 mg three times daily for 3 months. The mean trough steady-state serum carbamazepine levels of 6 of the patients rose by 30% or more and the carbamazepine clearance fell by 32% during the second 3-month period. A reduction in the carbamazepine dose was needed in 3 patients because of the symptoms that developed.[1] Similarly, in 11 patients taking antiepileptics including carbamazepine, allopurinol 10 mg/kg increased to 15 mg/kg daily for 12 weeks increased carbamazepine levels by 29%.[2] Conversely, in another study, allopurinol (150 mg daily in those less than 20 kg, and 300 mg daily for other patients) for 4 months had no effect on carbamazepine levels in 53 patients taking antiepileptics including carbamazepine.[3]

Mechanism

Uncertain. A possible explanation is that allopurinol can act as a liver enzyme inhibitor, which reduces the metabolism and clearance of carbamazepine.

Importance and management

Information is limited to these studies, but be alert for the need to reduce the dose of carbamazepine if high doses of allopurinol are used long-term. This interaction apparently takes several weeks or even months to develop fully. From one study, it appears that no interaction occurs between carbamazepine and low-dose allopurinol (such as that used for gout).

1. Mikati M, Erba G, Skouteli H, Gadia C. Pharmacokinetic study of allopurinol in resistant epilepsy: evidence for significant drug interactions. *Neurology* (1990) 40 (Suppl 1), 138.
2. Coppola G, Pascotto A. Double-blind, placebo-controlled, cross-over trial of allopurinol as add-on therapy in childhood refractory epilepsy. *Brain Dev* (1996) 18, 50–2.
3. Zagnoni PG, Bianchi A, Zolo P, Canger R, Cornaggia C, D'Alessandro P, DeMarco P, Pisani F, Gianelli M, Verzé L, Viani F, Zaccara G. Allopurinol as add-on therapy in refractory epilepsy: a double-blind placebo-controlled randomized study. *Epilepsia* (1994) 35, 107–12.

Carbamazepine + Amiodarone

Amiodarone does not appear to affect the pharmacokinetics of carbamazepine.

Clinical evidence, mechanism, importance and management

A single 400-mg dose of carbamazepine was given to 9 patients with cardiac disease (premature ventricular contractions, supraventricular tachycardia, sinus arrhythmia) before and after they took amiodarone 200 mg twice daily for a month. The pharmacokinetics of carbamazepine were found to be unchanged by amiodarone. This suggests that no clinically important interaction occurs, but it needs confirmation in patients who are given both drugs long term. Furthermore, the authors postulate that a higher amiodarone dose may inhibit the metabolism of the carbamazepine by the liver,[1] this also needs confirmation.

1. Leite SAO, Leite PJM, Rocha GA, Routledge PA, Bittencourt PRM. Carbamazepine kinetics in cardiac patients before and during amiodarone. *Arq Neuropsiquiatr* (1994) 52, 210–15.

Carbamazepine + Aspirin or NSAIDs

Carbamazepine levels are unaffected by aspirin or tolfenamic acid.

Clinical evidence, mechanism, importance and management

The carbamazepine levels of 10 patients were unaffected when they took aspirin 1.5 g daily for 3 days.[1] Similarly, the carbamazepine levels of 11 patients were not significantly affected by tolfenamic acid 300 mg, given for 3 days. It would appear that no carbamazepine dose adjustments are necessary in patients also given aspirin or tolfenamic acid.

1. Neuvonen PJ, Lehtovaara R, Bardy A, Elomaa E. Antipyretic analgesics in patients on anti-epileptic drug therapy. *Eur J Clin Pharmacol* (1979) 15, 263–8.

Carbamazepine + Azoles

Ketoconazole causes a small to moderate rise in serum carbamazepine concentrations. Case reports describe a large rise in carbamazepine concentrations in patients taking fluconazole; sometimes accompanied by toxicity. Adverse effects were seen in another patient when carbamazepine was given with miconazole. Carbamazepine can reduce the concentrations of itraconazole, and is predicted to lower the concentrations of posaconazole and voriconazole.

Clinical evidence

(a) Fluconazole

A 33-year-old man whose seizures were stabilised by carbamazepine became extremely lethargic after taking fluconazole 150 mg daily for 3 days. His carbamazepine concentration was found to have risen from 11.1 micrograms/mL to 24.5 micrograms/mL. Symptoms resolved when both drugs were stopped, and carbamazepine was later re-introduced without problem.[1] Another epileptic patient, treated with carbamazepine, lamotrigine and barbexaclone for many years, developed blurred vision and dizziness when she took fluconazole 150 mg with her morning dose of antiepileptics. The symptoms worsened over 11 days of fluconazole treatment during which she complained of severe diplopia, oscillopsia, nausea, vomiting and gait instability and her carbamazepine concentrations were found to have more than doubled. Twenty-four hours after fluconazole withdrawal, carbamazepine concentrations returned to normal and the symptoms resolved. Lamotrigine and **barbexaclone** concentrations were not notably affected by fluconazole.[2] A similar case describes a 40-year-old woman with bipolar disorder, stabilised having taken carbamazepine 600 mg daily for 10 years, who experienced double vision, nausea, vomiting and dizziness 2 days after starting fluconazole 150 mg daily. Over the following 2 days her symptoms worsened and on day 4 she was admitted to hospital where her carbamazepine concentration was found to be more than twofold higher than the previous level, taken 16 days before admission (18 [micrograms/mL] versus 7.3 micrograms/mL). Fluconazole was withdrawn and after one day her symptoms had resolved and her neurological examination was normal. Her carbamazepine concentration returned to 9 micrograms/mL, five days after the fluconazole was stopped.[3] Another well-documented case report describes a threefold increase in carbamazepine concentrations (without any signs of toxicity) 10 days after fluconazole 400 mg daily was started.[4]

(b) Itraconazole

A patient taking itraconazole 200 mg daily was noted to have low itraconazole concentrations (0.15 mg/L) about 14 days after starting carbamazepine 400 mg daily; about 2 months later itraconazole was undetectable. About 3 weeks after stopping carbamazepine, the itraconazole concentration had reached the reference range (0.36 mg/L).[5]

For mention of 2 patients taking carbamazepine with phenytoin, who had undetectable or very low itraconazole concentrations, and who relapsed or did not respond to itraconazole, see 'Phenytoin + Azoles', p.595.

(c) Ketoconazole

A study in 8 patients with epilepsy taking carbamazepine found that oral ketoconazole 200 mg daily for 10 days increased their serum carbamazepine concentrations by 29% (from 5.6 micrograms/mL to 7.2 micrograms/mL) without affecting carbamazepine-10,11-epoxide levels. When the ketoconazole was stopped the serum carbamazepine concentrations returned to their former levels.[6]

(d) Miconazole

A patient receiving long-term treatment with carbamazepine 400 mg daily developed malaise, myoclonia and tremor within 3 days of being given oral miconazole 1.125 g. The same reaction occurred on each subsequent occasion that miconazole was given. These toxic effects disappeared when miconazole was withdrawn.[7]

Mechanism

Carbamazepine concentrations are thought to rise because azoles inhibit CYP3A4, which is concerned with the metabolism of carbamazepine. Different azoles affect CYP3A4 to varying degrees, see *Azoles* in 'Anthelmintics, Antifungals, and Antiprotozoals', p.225. Carbamazepine is an enzyme inducer, and appears to decrease the concentrations of azoles by increasing their metabolism.

Importance and management

Evidence for these interactions between carbamazepine and the azoles is limited and in some cases the effects are only modest. Nevertheless, it would seem prudent to monitor the outcome of adding an azole to established carbamazepine treatment, being alert for any evidence of increased carbamazepine adverse effects (e.g. nausea, vomiting, ataxia and drowsiness).

Note also that carbamazepine can reduce the concentrations of azoles: a large reduction in itraconazole concentrations has been reported, and one manufacturer of itraconazole consequently states that the concurrent use of carbamazepine is not recommended.[8] Based on the interaction with phenytoin (see 'Phenytoin + Azoles', p.595), which results in reduced **posaconazole** concentrations, the manufacturer of posaconazole suggests that concurrent use of carbamazepine should be avoided, unless the benefits outweigh the risks.[9] If both drugs are given it would seem sensible to consider increasing the posaconazole dose, and increase monitoring of carbamazepine concentrations. Similarly, the manufacturers of **voriconazole** contraindicate the concurrent use of carbamazepine.[10,11]

1. Nair DR, Morris HH. Potential fluconazole-induced carbamazepine toxicity. *Ann Pharmacother* (1999) 33, 790–2.
2. Ulivelli M, Rubegni P, Nuti D, Bartalini S, Giannini F, Rossi S. Clinical evidence of fluconazole-induced carbamazepine toxicity. *J Neurol* (2004) 251, 622–3.
3. Tsouli S, Maranis S, Kyritsis AP. Fluconazole-carbamazepine interaction in a patient with bipolar disorder. *Psychiatry Clin Neurosci* (2011) 65, 112.
4. Finch CK, Green CA, Self TH. Fluconazole-carbamazepine interaction. *South Med J* (2002) 95, 1099–1100.
5. Bonay M, Jonville-Bera AP, Diot P, Lemarie E, Lavandier M, Autret E. Possible interaction between phenobarbital, carbamazepine and itraconazole. *Drug Safety* (1993) 9, 309–11.
6. Spina E, Arena D, Scordo MG, Fazio A, Pisani F, Perucca E. Elevation of plasma carbamazepine concentrations by ketoconazole in patients with epilepsy. *Ther Drug Monit* (1997) 19, 535–8.
7. Loupi E, Descotes J, Lery N, Evreux JC. Interactions médicamenteuses et miconazole. A propos de 10 observations. *Therapie* (1982) 37, 437–41.
8. Sporanox Capsules (Itraconazole). Janssen-Cilag Ltd. UK Summary of product characteristics, October 2011.
9. Noxafil (Posaconazole). Merck Sharp & Dohme Ltd. UK Summary of product characteristics, September 2014.
10. VFEND (Voriconazole). Pfizer Ltd. UK Summary of product characteristics, October 2014.
11. VFEND (Voriconazole). Pfizer Inc. US Prescribing information, February 2014.

Carbamazepine + Bile-acid binding resins

In a study in 6 healthy subjects, colestyramine 8 g did not affect the absorption of carbamazepine 400 mg, whereas colestipol 10 g reduced it by 10%. Both colestyramine and colestipol were given as a single dose

5 minutes after the carbamazepine.[1] This small reduction is unlikely to be clinically important.

1. Neuvonen PJ, Kivistö K, Hirvisalo EL. Effects of resins and activated charcoal on the absorption of digoxin, carbamazepine and frusemide. *Br J Clin Pharmacol* (1988) 25, 229–33.

Carbamazepine and related drugs + Calcium-channel blockers

Both diltiazem and verapamil can increase carbamazepine concentrations, causing toxicity. A single case report describes neurological toxicity in a patient taking phenytoin and carbamazepine with isradipine. Limited evidence suggests that amlodipine and nifedipine do not affect the plasma concentration of carbamazepine and that verapamil slightly reduces exposure to the active metabolite of oxcarbazepine.

The plasma concentrations of felodipine, nifedipine, nilvadipine, and nimodipine are reduced by carbamazepine. Felodipine concentrations are minimally reduced by oxcarbazepine.

Clinical evidence

(a) Diltiazem

A patient with epilepsy taking carbamazepine 400 mg in the morning and 600 mg in the evening developed symptoms of toxicity (dizziness, nausea, ataxia, and diplopia) within 2 days of starting to take diltiazem 60 mg three times daily. His carbamazepine serum concentration had increased by about 40% to 21 micrograms/mL, but decreased when diltiazem was stopped. No interaction occurred when diltiazem was replaced by **nifedipine** 20 mg three times daily.[1] Other case reports describe carbamazepine toxicity and an increase in its serum concentration of up to 4-fold in a total of 11 patients given diltiazem.[2-7] One patient required a 62% reduction in the carbamazepine dose.[2] Another patient had a modest decrease in the serum concentration of carbamazepine of 54% when diltiazem was *stopped*.[8]

For a further case report involving diltiazem, see *Nifedipine*, below.

(b) Felodipine

After taking felodipine 10 mg daily for 4 days, 10 patients with epilepsy (including 4 taking carbamazepine alone and 3 taking carbamazepine with phenytoin) had reduced felodipine plasma concentrations (maximum plasma concentration of 1.6 nanomol/L compared with 8.9 nanomol/L in 12 control subjects). The bioavailability of felodipine was reduced to 6.6% of the bioavailability in the control subjects.[9]

A study in 8 subjects found that the AUC of felodipine was reduced by 28% by oxcarbazepine 600 to 900 mg daily for a week.[10]

(c) Isradipine

A man taking carbamazepine and phenytoin developed neurological toxicity while taking isradipine, which was attributed to an interaction between phenytoin and isradipine.[11] However, although the plasma concentration of carbamazepine remained within the therapeutic range, a commentator suggested that an interaction between carbamazepine and isradipine was plausible.[12]

(d) Nifedipine

In 12 patients with epilepsy, nifedipine 20 mg twice daily for 2 weeks did not affect the steady-state plasma concentration of carbamazepine.[13] Similarly, a retrospective study of 5 patients suggested that nifedipine does not usually increase the plasma concentration of carbamazepine or cause toxicity.[4] However, one patient had a small increase in the serum concentration of carbamazepine when nifedipine was replaced by **diltiazem**. When **diltiazem** was replaced by **amlodipine**, his carbamazepine serum concentration returned to normal, suggesting that neither nifedipine nor **amlodipine** interacted with carbamazepine.[14] Another patient had no change in the plasma concentration of carbamazepine when also given nifedipine.[1]

A study in 12 patients with epilepsy, receiving long-term treatment with carbamazepine, found that the AUC of concurrent nifedipine 20 mg was only 22% of the values seen in 12 healthy subjects not taking carbamazepine.[13]

(e) Nilvadipine

A 59-year-old man taking nilvadipine 8 mg daily for hypertension and haloperidol for psychotic symptoms was given carbamazepine because haloperidol alone did not control symptoms of mania. The carbamazepine dose was gradually increased from 100 mg to 600 mg daily. Although the manic symptoms were improved, his blood pressure rose to 230/140 mmHg after 3 days of carbamazepine 600 mg daily. Blood pressure was temporarily controlled by **nifedipine** 10 mg sublingually. Retrospective analyses found that the plasma concentration of nilvadipine was reduced by carbamazepine 100 and 300 mg daily and undetectable when the carbamazepine dose was increased to 600 mg daily. The plasma concentration of nilvadipine increased after carbamazepine was discontinued and his blood pressure returned to normal after about 2 weeks.[15]

(f) Nimodipine

A study in 8 patients with epilepsy who had been taking antiepileptics long-term (including 2 taking carbamazepine with phenobarbital, one taking carbamazepine with clobazam, and one taking carbamazepine with phenytoin) found that the AUC of a single 60-mg oral dose of nimodipine was only about 15% of that achieved in a group of healthy subjects not taking antiepileptics,[16] suggesting that carbamazepine lowers nimodipine exposure.

(g) Verapamil

Carbamazepine toxicity developed in 6 patients with epilepsy within 36 to 96 hours of them starting to take verapamil 120 mg three times daily. The symptoms disappeared when verapamil was withdrawn. The total carbamazepine plasma concentration had increased by 46% (a 33% increase in the free carbamazepine plasma concentration). Rechallenge of two of the patients, who only experienced mild toxicity with a lower dose of verapamil 120 mg twice a day, caused a similar increase in the carbamazepine concentration, again with mild toxicity. This report also describes another patient who had an increased carbamazepine serum concentration while also taking verapamil.[17] Carbamazepine toxicity is described in 3 other patients, again caused by verapamil.[18,19] The verapamil was successfully replaced by **nifedipine** in one patient.[18]

In a study, 10 healthy subjects were given oxcarbazepine 450 mg twice daily and then also verapamil 120 mg twice daily for 5 days. The AUC of the monohydroxy derivative of oxcarbazepine (the active metabolite) decreased by about 20%, but the AUC of oxcarbazepine was unaltered.[20]

Mechanism

Diltiazem and verapamil are moderate inhibitors of CYP3A4, by which carbamazepine is metabolised, and concurrent use therefore increases its serum concentration. In contrast, carbamazepine is a potent inducer of CYP3A4, by which the majority of the calcium-channel blockers are metabolised, at least in part, resulting in a reduction in their exposure. Oxcarbazepine is also an inducer of CYP3A4, but only had a very small effect on felodipine suggesting that felodipine is not particularly dependent on this isoenzyme for its metabolism.

Importance and management

Information about the effects of calcium-channel blockers on **carbamazepine** pharmacokinetics is limited, but what is known indicates that if carbamazepine is given with verapamil or diltiazem, the carbamazepine dose might need to be reduced to avoid toxicity. A 50% reduction in the dose of carbamazepine has been suggested if diltiazem is to be used.[5] Other calcium-channel blockers are not CYP3A4 inhibitors and therefore would not be expected to interact.

Evidence from one small study suggests that the pharmacokinetics of **oxcarbazepine** are not affected to a clinically important extent by verapamil. Evidence with other calcium-channel blockers is lacking.

Carbamazepine has been shown to decrease the exposure to a number of calcium-channel blockers. The majority of the calcium-channel blockers would be expected to interact similarly, as most are also metabolised by CYP3A4. If a calcium-channel blocker is given to a patient taking carbamazepine, expect to need to use a larger dose. If carbamazepine is added to existing treatment with a calcium-channel blocker, monitor the blood pressure and expect to need to increase the dose. Note that the manufacturer of nimodipine[21] contraindicates its use with carbamazepine because of the possibility of a large reduction in its bioavailability. Evidence for an effect of oxcarbazepine on the pharmacokinetics of the calcium-channel blockers is limited to one small study, showing only a small effect on felodipine which is unlikely to be clinically important. Further study with other calcium-channel blockers, which are more dependent on CYP3A4 for their metabolism, is needed.

1. Brodie MJ, Macphee GJA. Carbamazepine neurotoxicity precipitated by diltiazem. *BMJ* (1986) 292, 1170–1.
2. Eimer M, Carter BL. Elevated serum carbamazepine concentrations following diltiazem initiation. *Drug Intell Clin Pharm* (1987) 21, 340–2.
3. Ahmad S. Diltiazem-carbamazepine interaction. *Am Heart J* (1990) 120, 1485–6.
4. Bahls FH, Ozuna J, Ritchie DE. Interactions between calcium channel blockers and the anticonvulsants carbamazepine and phenytoin. *Neurology* (1991) 41, 740–2.
5. Shaughnessy AF, Mosley MR. Elevated carbamazepine levels associated with diltiazem use. *Neurology* (1992) 42, 937–8.
6. Maoz E, Grossman E, Thaler M, Rosenthal T. Carbamazepine neurotoxic reaction after administration of diltiazem. *Arch Intern Med* (1992) 152, 2503–4.
7. Wijdicks EFM, Arendt C, Bazzell MC. Postoperative ophthalmoplegia and ataxia due to carbamazepine toxicity facilitated by diltiazem. *J Neuroophthalmol* (2004) 24, 95.
8. Gadde K, Calabrese JR. Diltiazem effect on carbamazepine levels in manic depression. *J Clin Psychopharmacol* (1990) 10, 378–9.
9. Capewell S, Freestone S, Critchley JAJH, Pottage A, Prescott LF. Reduced felodipine bioavailability in patients taking anticonvulsants. *Lancet* (1988) ii, 480–2.
10. Zaccara G, Gangemi PF, Bendoni L, Menge GP, Schwabe S, Monza GC. Influence of single and repeated doses of oxcarbazepine on the pharmacokinetic profile of felodipine. *Ther Drug Monit* (1993) 15, 39–42.
11. Cachat F, Tufro A. Phenytoin/isradipine interaction causing severe neurologic toxicity. *Ann Pharmacother* (2002) 36: 1399–1402.
12. Hauben M. Comment: phenytoin/isradipine interaction causing severe neurologic toxicity. *Ann Pharmacother* (2002) 36: 1974–5.
13. Routledge PA, Soryal I, Eve MD, Williams J, Richens A, Hall R. Reduced bioavailability of nifedipine in patients with epilepsy receiving anticonvulsants. *Br J Clin Pharmacol* (1998) 45, 196P.
14. Cuadrado A, Sánchez MB, Peralta G, González M, Verdejo A, Amat G, Bravo J, Fdez Cortizo MJ, Adín J, De Cos MA, Mediavilla A, Armijo JA. Carbamazepine-amlodipine: a free interaction association? *Methods Find Exp Clin Pharmacol* (1996) 18 (Suppl C), 65.
15. Yasui-Furukori N, Tateishi T. Carbamazepine decreases antihypertensive effect of nilvadipine. *J Clin Pharmacol* (2002) 42, 100–3.
16. Tartara A, Galimberti CA, Manni R, Parietti L, Zucca C, Baasch H, Caresia L, Mück W, Barzaghi N, Gatti G, Perucca E. Differential effects of valproic acid and enzyme-inducing anticonvulsants on nimodipine pharmacokinetics in epileptic patients. *Br J Clin Pharmacol* (1991) 32, 335–40.
17. Macphee GJA, McInnes GT, Thompson GG, Brodie MJ. Verapamil potentiates carbamazepine neurotoxicity: a clinically important inhibitory interaction. *Lancet* (1986) i, 700–3.
18. Beattie B, Biller J, Mehlhaus B, Murray M. Verapamil-induced carbamazepine neurotoxicity. *Eur Neurol* (1988) 28, 104–5.
19. Price WA, DiMarzio LR. Verapamil-carbamazepine neurotoxicity. *J Clin Psychiatry* (1988) 49, 80.
20. Krämer G, Tettenborn B, Flesch G. Oxcarbazepine-verapamil drug interaction in healthy volunteers. *Epilepsia* (1991) 32 (Suppl 1), 70–1.
21. Nimotop Tablets (Nimodipine). Bayer plc. UK Summary of product characteristics, October 2012.

Carbamazepine + Danazol

Serum carbamazepine levels can be doubled by danazol and carbamazepine toxicity may occur.

Clinical evidence

The serum carbamazepine levels of 6 patients with epilepsy approximately doubled within 7 to 30 days of taking danazol 400 to 600 mg daily. Acute carbamazepine toxicity (dizziness, drowsiness, blurred vision, ataxia, nausea) was experienced by 5 out of the 6 patients.[1]

Other reports similarly describe rises in serum carbamazepine levels of 50 to 100% (with toxicity seen in some instances) when danazol was given.[2-4]

Mechanism

Danazol inhibits the metabolism (by the epoxide-trans-diol pathway) of carbamazepine by the liver, thereby reducing its loss from the body.[2,5] During the use of danazol the clearance of carbamazepine has been found to be reduced by 60%.[2]

Importance and management

An established and clinically important interaction. If concurrent use is necessary carbamazepine serum levels should be monitored and the dose reduced as necessary.

1. Zeilinski JJ, Lichten EM, Haidukewych D. Clinically significant danazol-carbamazepine interaction. *Ther Drug Monit* (1987) 9, 24–7.
2. Krämer G, Theisohn M, von Unruh GE, Eichelbaum M. Carbamazepine-danazol drug interaction: its mechanism examined by a stable isotope technique. *Ther Drug Monit* (1986) 8, 387–92.
3. Hayden M, Buchanan N. Danazol-carbamazepine interaction. *Med J Aust* (1991) 155, 851.
4. Nelson MV. Interaction of danazol and carbamazepine. *Am J Psychiatry* (1988) 145, 768–9.
5. Krämer G, Besser R, Theisohn M, Eichelbaum M. Carbamazepine-danazol drug interaction: mechanism and therapeutic usefulness. *Acta Neurol Scand* (1984) 70, 249.

Carbamazepine + Dantrolene and Oxybutynin

Carbamazepine toxicity has been reported in a patient given oxybutynin and dantrolene.

Clinical evidence, mechanism, importance and management

A woman with incomplete tetraplegia who had taken carbamazepine 1 g daily for neuropathic pain for 2 years was given dantrolene in a gradually increasing dose and oxybutynin 5 mg twice daily. Two weeks after starting oxybutynin and while receiving dantrolene 125 mg daily, she experienced dizziness and vomiting, drowsiness, confusion, slurred speech, and nystagmus, and was found to have a raised carbamazepine level of 16 micrograms/mL. All drugs were stopped and the plasma carbamazepine level fell to 8.3 micrograms/mL (reference range 4 to 12 micrograms/mL). Because of pain, urinary frequency and spasticity, daily doses of carbamazepine 600 mg, oxybutynin 10 mg and dantrolene 100 mg were restarted, which resulted in a carbamazepine level of 9.2 micrograms/mL. The dantrolene dose was increased to 125 mg daily because of continuing spasticity, but after one day, symptoms of carbamazepine toxicity occurred and the carbamazepine plasma level was 29 micrograms/mL. Carbamazepine and oxybutynin were discontinued and the dantrolene dose was reduced to 25 mg. In order to relieve the patient's symptoms of pain and spasticity, carbamazepine 400 mg daily and dantrolene 25 mg daily were given (carbamazepine levels of 8.4 micrograms/mL at 7 days). The addition of oxybutynin 5 mg daily was associated with an increase in the carbamazepine level to 32 micrograms/mL and symptoms of toxicity. Carbamazepine was replaced by valproate 600 mg daily, which appeared to be beneficial and without an interaction with dantrolene or oxybutynin.[1]

Oxybutynin was being taken on each occasion when carbamazepine levels increased and therefore it was suggested that oxybutynin inhibited the metabolism of carbamazepine by the cytochrome P450 isoenzyme CYP3A4. Dantrolene was also being taken and the second episode of carbamazepine toxicity occurred after the dantrolene dose was increased. The exact mechanism of dantrolene metabolism is not known but it may decrease the activity of cytochrome P450 isoenzymes in a dose-dependent manner. However, there appears to be little evidence to suggest that these two drugs generally inhibit the metabolism of other drugs, and therefore the mechanism, and an interaction, is not established. The authors recommend careful monitoring and, if necessary, dose adjustments if carbamazepine is given with dantrolene and/or oxybutynin.[1]

1. Vander T, Odi H, Bluvstein , Ronen J, Catz A. Carbamazepine toxicity following oxybutynin and dantrolene administration; a case report. *Spinal Cord* (2005) 43, 252–5.

Carbamazepine + Dextromethorphan

Dextromethorphan appears not to affect the serum levels of carbamazepine.

Clinical evidence, mechanism, importance and management

A double-blind, crossover study in 5 patients with severe complex partial seizures found that dextromethorphan 120 mg daily in liquid form (*Delsym*) over 3 months had no effect on their serum carbamazepine levels. There was a non-significant alteration in the complex partial seizure and tonic-clonic seizure frequency.[1] No carbamazepine dose adjustment therefore appears necessary if dextromethorphan is also taken.

1. Fisher RS, Cysyk BJ, Lesser RP, Pontecorvo MJ, Ferkany JT, Schwerdt PR, Hart J, Gordon B. Dextromethorphan for treatment of complex partial seizures. *Neurology* (1990) 40, 547–9.

Carbamazepine and related drugs + Dextropropoxyphene (Propoxyphene)

Carbamazepine levels can be raised by dextropropoxyphene. Oxcarbazepine appears not to interact with dextropropoxyphene.

Clinical evidence

(a) Carbamazepine

The observation of toxicity (headache, dizziness, ataxia, nausea, tiredness) in patients taking both carbamazepine and dextropropoxyphene prompted further study. Five patients taking carbamazepine who were given dextropropoxyphene 65 mg three times daily had a mean rise in their serum carbamazepine levels of 65%, and 3 patients developed signs of carbamazepine toxicity. Carbamazepine levels were not taken in a further 2 patients because they withdrew from the study after 2 days of treatment due to adverse effects.[1,2] In a further study a 66% rise in carbamazepine levels was seen after 6 days of treatment with dextropropoxyphene.[3]

Carbamazepine toxicity due to this interaction has been reported elsewhere,[4-7] and rises in trough serum carbamazepine levels of 69% to 600% have been described.[8] A study in the elderly compared groups of patients taking either carbamazepine or dextropropoxyphene alone, with patients taking both drugs (21 subjects). The carbamazepine dose was about one- third lower in those taking both drugs, yet the mean serum carbamazepine levels were still 25% higher than in the patients not taking dextropropoxyphene. The prevalence of adverse effects was also higher in patients taking both drugs.[9]

(b) Oxcarbazepine

In a study in 7 patients with epilepsy or trigeminal neuralgia, dextropropoxyphene 65 mg three times daily for 7 days did not affect the steady-state levels of the active metabolite of oxcarbazepine.[10]

Mechanism

Uncertain. It is suggested that dextropropoxyphene inhibits the metabolism of carbamazepine by the liver, leading to its accumulation in the body.[1,2]

Importance and management

The interaction between carbamazepine and dextropropoxyphene is very well established and clinically important. If concurrent use is necessary reduce the dose of carbamazepine appropriately to prevent the development of toxicity. In many cases it may be simpler to use a non-interacting analgesic, although the occasional single dose of dextropropoxyphene probably does not matter. No special precautions seem necessary with oxcarbazepine.

1. Dam M, Christiansen J. Interaction of propoxyphene with carbamazepine. *Lancet* (1977) ii, 509.
2. Dam M, Kristensen CB, Hansen BS, Christiansen J. Interaction between carbamazepine and propoxyphene in man. *Acta Neurol Scand* (1977) 56, 603–7.
3. Hansen BS, Dam M, Brandt J, Hvidberg EF, Angelo H, Christensen JM, Lous P. Influence of dextropropoxyphene on steady state serum levels and protein binding of three anti-epileptic drugs in man. *Acta Neurol Scand* (1980) 61, 357–67.
4. Yu YL, Huang CY, Chin D, Woo E, Chang CM. Interaction between carbamazepine and dextropropoxyphene. *Postgrad Med J* (1986) 62, 231–3.
5. Kubacka RT, Ferrante JA. Carbamazepine-propoxyphene interaction. *Clin Pharm* (1983) 2, 104.
6. Risinger MW. Carbamazepine toxicity with concurrent use of propoxyphene: a report of five cases. *Neurology* (1987) 37 (Suppl 1), 87.
7. Allen S. Cerebellar dysfunction following dextropropoxyphene-induced carbamazepine toxicity. *Postgrad Med J* (1994) 70, 764.
8. Oles KS, Mirza W, Penry JK. Catastrophic neurologic signs due to drug interaction: Tegretol and Darvon. *Surg Neurol* (1989) 32, 144–51.
9. Bergendal L, Friberg A, Schaffrath AM, Holmdahl M, Landahl S. The clinical relevance of the interaction between carbamazepine and dextropropoxyphene in elderly patients in Gothenburg, Sweden. *Eur J Clin Pharmacol* (1997) 53, 203–6.
10. Mogensen PH, Jorgensen L, Boas J, Dam M, Vesterager A, Flesch G, Jensen PK. Effects of dextropropoxyphene on the steady-state kinetics of oxcarbazepine and its metabolites. *Acta Neurol Scand* (1992) 85, 14–17.

Carbamazepine and related drugs + Diuretics

Hyponatraemia has been reported in patients taking carbamazepine with furosemide, hydrochlorothiazide, or hydrochlorothiazide and paroxetine. Hyponatraemia occurred in another patient taking oxcarbazepine and furosemide.

Clinical evidence, mechanism, importance and management

Two patients with epilepsy taking carbamazepine developed symptomatic hyponatraemia while also taking **hydrochlorothiazide** or **furosemide**.[1] Another case has been described when a patient taking carbamazepine also took **hydrochlorothiazide** and paroxetine.[2] A further case describes a patient taking **hydrochlorothiazide** who developed hyponatraemia within 2 weeks of starting to take carbamazepine 200 mg twice daily. Carbamazepine was continued but **hydrochlorothiazide** was stopped and sodium levels returned to normal within one week indicating that in this patient each drug appeared to be well tolerated alone.[3]

Another report describes a patient with a 20-year history of complex partial seizures treated with oxcarbazepine 1800 mg daily (30 mg/kg daily) who developed confusion, auditory and visual hallucinations and delirium about one month after starting to take **furosemide** 25 mg daily for hypertension. Sodium levels were found to have decreased from 138 mmol/L to 115 mmol/L with concurrent **furosemide** and an EEG showed abnormal activity compared to baseline values before she started **furosemide**. Oxcarbazepine and **furosemide** were stopped and valproic acid and amlodipine started, and within 20 days the neurological symptoms had stopped, the EEG normalised to baseline, and sodium levels increased to within the reference range.[4]

The reasons for the interaction between carbamazepine or oxcarbazepine and diuretics are uncertain but all these drugs can cause sodium to be lost from the body. This seems to be an uncommon interaction, but be aware that it can occur.

1. Yassa R, Nastase C, Camille Y, Henderson M, Belzile L, Beland F. Carbamazepine, diuretics and hyponatremia: a possible interaction. *J Clin Psychiatry* (1987) 48, 281–3.
2. Kalksma R, Leemhuis MP. Hyponatriëmie bij gebruik van thiazidediuretica: let op combinaties van geneesmiddelen die dit effect versterken. *Ned Tijdschr Geneeskd* (2002) 146, 1521–5.
3. Ranta A, Wooten GF. Hyponatremia due to an additive effect of carbamazepine and thiazide diuretics. *Epilepsia* (2004) 45, 879.
4. Siniscalchi A, Mancuso F, Scornaienghi D, Ferreri G, De Saro G. Acute encephalopathy induced by oxcarbazepine and furosemide. *Ann Pharmacother* (2004) 38, 509–10.

Carbamazepine + Eslicarbazepine or Oxcarbazepine

Eslicarbazepine and oxcarbazepine appear to minimally affect the pharmacokinetics of carbamazepine. Carbamazepine appears to have only minor effects on the pharmacokinetics of oxcarbazepine and slightly reduces exposure to eslicarbazepine.

Clinical evidence

(a) Effects on carbamazepine

A study in 9 patients with epilepsy found that when oxcarbazepine 300 mg three times daily was given with carbamazepine, there were no clinically relevant changes in the pharmacokinetics of carbamazepine.[1] However, analysis of data from clinical studies found that oxcarbazepine decreased the plasma concentration of carbamazepine by about 15 to 22%.[2,3] The UK manufacturer of oxcarbazepine also briefly notes a 30% increase in the concentration of the carbamazepine metabolite, carbamazepine-10,11-epoxide, in the presence of oxcarbazepine.[2]

A population pharmacokinetic model using data from 641 patients enrolled in phase III eslicarbazepine studies, predicted that carbamazepine clearance was increased by up to 14% by eslicarbazepine.[4] However, the UK manufacturer of eslicarbazepine briefly notes that in a study in healthy subjects given eslicarbazepine 800 mg daily and carbamazepine 400 mg twice daily, there was no effect on exposure to carbamazepine or its metabolite, carbamazepine-10,11-epoxide.[5]

(b) Effects on eslicarbazepine

The UK manufacturer of eslicarbazepine briefly notes that a study in healthy subjects found that the concurrent use of eslicarbazepine 800 mg daily and carbamazepine 400 mg twice daily, resulted in a 32% decrease in eslicarbazepine exposure.[5] A population pharmacokinetic model using data from 641 patients enrolled in phase III eslicarbazepine studies, found that the concurrent use of carbamazepine (in 351 patients) increased the clearance of eslicarbazepine up to 2.5-fold.[4]

(c) Effects on oxcarbazepine

In a study in patients given oxcarbazepine 300 mg three times daily, the pharmacokinetics of oxcarbazepine were unaffected by the presence of carbamazepine, but the AUC of the active metabolite, monohydroxyoxcarbazepine, was 40% lower in the presence of carbamazepine.[1] In another study, the concentration of monohydroxyoxcarbazepine was statistically significantly lower (exact figure not stated) in patients taking carbamazepine than in patients not taking enzyme-inducing antiepileptics.[6] Similarly, in a study in children, carbamazepine was found to increase the apparent clearance of monohydroxyoxcarbazepine by 31 to 35%.[7]

Mechanism

Oxcarbazepine is an inducer of CYP3A4, of which carbamazepine is a metabolite and also an inducer. As a result, oxcarbazepine reduces the concentrations of carbamazepine and its active metabolite, carbamazepine-10,11-epoxide. Carbamazepine does not appear to affect the metabolism of oxcarbazepine, but does induce that of its active metabolite, monohydroxyoxcarbazepine. The decreased exposure to eslicarbazepine seen with carbamazepine might be due to induction of glucuronidation by carbamazepine.

Importance and management

Information on the interaction between carbamazepine and oxcarbazepine or eslicarbazepine is limited. The concentrations of both carbamazepine and its active metabolite, carbamazepine-10,11-epoxide, are reduced by **oxcarbazepine**, but this is probably not clinically relevant. It appears that oxcarbazepine concentrations are unaffected by carbamazepine, but concentrations of the active metabolite of oxcarbazepine, monohydroxyoxcarbazepine, are reduced. The clinical importance of this is unclear, but note that monohydroxyoxcarbazepine is principally responsible for the antiepileptic activity of oxcarbazepine. In addition, there is the theoretical risk that monohydroxyoxcarbazepine concentrations might increase and become toxic if carbamazepine is withdrawn.[1]

Evidence for an interaction between **eslicarbazepine** and carbamazepine is conflicting, but overall a clinically important effect would seem unlikely. However, carbamazepine seems to cause a slight reduction in exposure to eslicarbazepine, and the UK manufacturer of eslicarbazepine suggests that the dose might need to be increased, based on individual response, if given with carbamazepine.[5] They also note that the frequency of adverse effects (such as double vision, abnormal coordination, and dizziness) were between 2.5- and 5-fold higher in patients taking both eslicarbazepine and carbamazepine compared with those not taking carbamazepine.[5] It would seem prudent to be aware of such effects if both drugs are taken.

1. McKee PJW, Blacklaw J, Forrest G, Gillham RA, Walker SM, Connelly D, Brodie MJ. A double blind, placebo-controlled interaction study between oxcarbazepine and carbamazepine, sodium valproate and phenytoin in epileptic patients. *Br J Clin Pharmacol* (1994) 37, 27–32.
2. Trileptal (Oxcarbazepine). Novartis Pharmaceuticals UK Ltd. UK Summary of product characteristics. April 2012.
3. Hossain M, Sallas W, D'Souza J. Drug-drug interaction profile of oxcarbazepine in children and adults. *Neurology* (1999) 52 (Suppl 2), A525.
4. Falcão A, Fuseau E, Nunes T, Almeida L, Soares-da-Silva P. Pharmacokinetics, drug interactions and exposure-response relationship of eslicarbazepine acetate in adult patients with partial-onset seizures: population pharmacokinetic and pharmacokinetic/pharmacodynamic analyses. *CNS Drugs* (2012) 26, 79–91.
5. Zebinix (Eslicarbazepine acetate). Eisai Ltd. UK Summary of product characteristics, August 2012.
6. Barcs G, Walker EB, Elger CE, Scaramelli A, Stefan H, Sturm Y, Moore A, Flesch G, Kramer L, D'Souza J. Oxcarbazepine placebo-controlled, dose-ranging trial in refractory partial epilepsy. *Epilepsia* (2000) 41, 1597–1607.
7. Sallas WM, Milosavljev S, D'Souza J, Hossain M. Pharmacokinetic drug interactions in children taking oxcarbazepine. *Clin Pharmacol Ther* (2003) 74, 138–49.

Carbamazepine and related drugs + Felbamate

Felbamate modestly reduces carbamazepine serum concentrations but increases the concentrations of its active metabolite, carbamazepine-10,11-epoxide. Carbamazepine might reduce felbamate concentrations. Felbamate has no clinically relevant effect on the pharmacokinetics of oxcarbazepine, but concurrent use appears to increase the incidence of adverse effects.

Clinical evidence

(a) Carbamazepine

The carbamazepine serum concentrations of 22 patients, with doses adjusted to keep concentrations in the range of 4 to 12 micrograms/mL, were reduced by 25% (range 10 to 42%) when they were given felbamate 3 g daily. The reduction occurred within a week, reaching a plateau after 2 to 4 weeks, and returning to the original concentrations within 2 to 3 weeks of stopping felbamate.[1] Other studies in patients with epilepsy have found reductions in carbamazepine concentrations of between 18 and 31% when felbamate was given.[2-7] Some of these studies also found that the serum concentrations of the active carbamazepine metabolite, carbamazepine-10,11-epoxide, rose by 33 to 57%.[1,4,5]

Carbamazepine increases the clearance of felbamate by up to about 50%.[8-10]

(b) Oxcarbazepine

A double-blind, randomised study in 8 healthy subjects found that oxcarbazepine 300 to 600 mg every 12 hours, given with felbamate 600 to 1200 mg every 12 hours for 10 days, had no effect on the plasma concentrations of the major active metabolite of oxcarbazepine (monohydroxyoxcarbazepine). However, the concentrations of dihydroxyoxcarbazepine (a minor, inactive metabolite) were reduced, and the maximum serum concentrations of oxcarbazepine were reduced, by about 20%. Although these changes were not considered to be clinically relevant, the incidence of some adverse effects (dizziness, somnolence, nausea, diplopia) increased during concurrent use.[11]

Mechanism

Not established. It was suggested that felbamate does not induce the metabolism of carbamazepine by CYP3A4, but it does appear to alter the interaction of carbamazepine with CYP3A4.[12]

Importance and management

An interaction between carbamazepine and felbamate is established, but its clinical importance is uncertain because the modest reduction in carbamazepine serum concentrations would seem to be offset by the rise in the concentrations of its metabolite, carbamazepine-10,11-epoxide, which also has antiepileptic activity. However, be alert for any changes in antiepileptic control and consider monitoring carbamazepine concentrations, adjusting the dose as necessary. The importance of the increased felbamate clearance is uncertain. More study is needed.

The changes in oxcarbazepine pharmacokinetics seen with felbamate are unlikely to be clinically important, but it might be prudent to consider this interaction as a possible cause if oxcarbazepine adverse effects become troublesome in a patient also taking felbamate.

1. Albani F, Theodore WH, Washington P, Devinsky O, Bromfield E, Porter RJ, Nice FJ. Effect of Felbamate on plasma levels of carbamazepine and its metabolites. *Epilepsia* (1991) 32, 130–2.
2. Graves NM, Holmes GB, Fuerst RH, Leppik IE. Effect of felbamate on phenytoin and carbamazepine serum concentrations. *Epilepsia* (1989) 30, 225–9..
3. Fuerst RH, Graves NM, Leppik IE, Brundage RC, Holmes GB, Remmel RP. Felbamate increases phenytoin but decreases carbamazepine concentrations. *Epilepsia* (1988) 29, 488–91.
4. Howard JR, Dix RK, Shumaker RC, Perhach JL. The effect of felbamate on carbamazepine pharmacokinetics. *Epilepsia* (1992) 33 (Suppl 3), 84–5.
5. Wagner ML, Remmel RP, Graves NM, Leppik IE. Effect of felbamate on carbamazepine and its major metabolites. *Clin Pharmacol Ther* (1993) 53, 536–43.
6. Theodore WH, Raubertas RF, Porter RJ, Nice F, Devinsky O, Reeves P, Bromfield E, Ito B, Balish M. Felbamate: a clinical trial for complex partial seizures. *Epilepsia* (1991) 32, 392–7.
7. Leppik IE, Dreifuss FE, Pledger GW, Graves NM, Santilli N, Drury I, Tsay JY, Jacobs MP, Bertram E, Cereghino JJ, Cooper G, Sahlroot JT, Sheridan P, Ashworth M, Lee SI, Sierzant TL. Felbamate for partial seizures: results of a controlled clinical trial. *Neurology* (1991) 41, 1785–9.
8. Wagner ML, Graves NM, Marienau K, Holmes GB, Remmel RP, Leppik IE. Discontinuation of phenytoin and carbamazepine in patients receiving felbamate. *Epilepsia* (1991) 32, 398–406.
9. Kelley MT, Walson PD, Cox S, Dusci LJ. Population pharmacokinetics of felbamate in children. *Ther Drug Monit* (1997) 19, 29–36.

10. Banfield CR, Zhu G-RR, Jen JF, Jensen PK, Schumaker RC, Perhach JL Affrime MB, Glue P. The effect of age on the apparent clearance of felbamate: a retrospective analysis using nonlinear mixed-effects modeling. *Ther Drug Monit* (1996) 18, 19–29.
11. Hulsman JARJ, Rentmeester TW, Banfield CR, Reidenberg P, Colucci RD, Meehan JW, Radwanski E, Mojaverian P, Lin C-C, Nezamis J, Affrime MB, Glue P. Effects of felbamate on the pharmacokinetics of the monohydroxy and dihydroxy metabolites of oxcarbazepine. *Clin Pharmacol Ther* (1995) 58, 383–9.
12. Egnell A-C, Houston B, Boyer S. In vivo CYP3A4 heteroactivation is a possible mechanism for the drug interaction between felbamate and carbamazepine. *J Pharmacol Exp Ther* (2003) 305, 1251–62.

Carbamazepine + Gemfibrozil

Two patients had a rise in their carbamazepine levels after they took gemfibrozil.

Clinical evidence, mechanism, importance and management

Two patients, stable taking carbamazepine, had rises in their serum carbamazepine levels when they were given gemfibrozil for type IV hyperlipoproteinaemia. One patient had a rise of about 30% (from 8.8 micrograms/mL to 11.4 micrograms/mL) within 4 days of starting to take gemfibrozil 300 mg daily, and the other patient had a rise of 65% (from 8.3 micrograms/mL to 13.7 micrograms/mL) three months after gemfibrozil 300 mg twice daily was started.[1] It was suggested that the clearance of carbamazepine is increased in those with elevated cholesterol and total lipids. Thus, when the condition is treated with gemfibrozil, the clearance becomes more normal, which results in a rise in the serum carbamazepine levels.[2] These appear to be the only reports of an interaction, and their clinical importance is uncertain, but consider the possibility of an interaction if carbamazepine toxicity (nausea, vomiting, ataxia and drowsiness) develops in a patient given gemfibrozil.

1. Denio L, Drake ME, Pakalnis A. Gemfibrozil-carbamazepine interaction in epileptic patients. *Epilepsia* (1988) 29, 654.
2. Wichlinski LM, Sieradzki E, Gruchala M. Correlation between the total cholesterol serum concentration data and carbamazepine steady-state blood levels in humans. *Drug Intell Clin Pharm* (1983) 17, 812–14.

Carbamazepine + Grapefruit juice

Grapefruit juice increases carbamazepine levels. A case of possible carbamazepine toxicity has been seen when a man taking carbamazepine started to eat grapefruit.

Clinical evidence

A 58-year-old man, taking carbamazepine 1 g daily for epilepsy, developed visual disturbances with diplopia, and was found to have a carbamazepine level of 11 micrograms/mL (reference range 4 to 10 micrograms/mL). Previous levels had not exceeded 5.4 micrograms/mL. The patient said that one month previously he had started to eat one whole grapefruit each day. The levels restabilised at 5.1 micrograms/mL after the carbamazepine dose was reduced to 800 mg daily.[1]

A randomised, crossover study in 10 patients with epilepsy taking carbamazepine 200 mg three times daily found that a single 300-mL drink of grapefruit juice increased the plasma levels and AUC of carbamazepine by about 40%.[2]

Mechanism

The cytochrome P450 isoenzyme CYP3A4 is the main enzyme involved in the metabolism of carbamazepine. Components of whole grapefruit and grapefruit juice are known to inhibit CYP3A4, which could lead to a reduction in the metabolism of carbamazepine, and therefore an increase in its levels.[1-3]

Importance and management

Although the information is sparse, the interaction has been predicted, demonstrated in a study, and has also occurred in practice. The authors of the study[2] suggest that grapefruit juice should be avoided in patients taking carbamazepine. In the case report,[1] the patient continued to eat grapefruit, and this was successfully managed by a reduction in the carbamazepine dose. However, it should be noted that intake of a set amount of grapefruit would need to be maintained for this approach to have a chance of working, and even then, the natural variability in the constituents of grapefruit may make adequate control difficult. The manufacturers advise carbamazepine dose adjustment and monitoring of carbamazepine levels in patients taking substances that may raise carbamazepine levels, such as grapefruit juice.[4] If monitoring is not practical, or regular intake of grapefruit is not desired, it would seem prudent to avoid grapefruit and grapefruit juice.

1. Bonin B, Vandel P, Vandel S, Kantelip JP. Effect of grapefruit intake on carbamazepine bioavailability: a case report. *Therapie* (2001) 56, 69–71.
2. Garg SK, Kumar N, Bhargava VK, Prabhakar SK. Effect of grapefruit juice on carbamazepine bioavailability in patients with epilepsy. *Clin Pharmacol Ther* (1998) 64, 286–8.
3. Ameer B, Weintraub RA. Drug interactions with grapefruit juice. *Clin Pharmacokinet* (1997) 33, 103–21.
4. Tegretol Tablets (Carbamazepine). Novartis Pharmaceuticals UK Ltd. UK Summary of product characteristics, May 2012.

Carbamazepine and related drugs + H_2-receptor antagonists

The serum levels of those taking long-term carbamazepine may transiently increase, possibly accompanied by an increase in adverse effects, for the first few days after starting to take cimetidine, but these adverse effects rapidly disappear. Cimetidine does not appear to have this effect on oxcarbazepine levels. Ranitidine appears not to interact with carbamazepine.

Clinical evidence

(a) Carbamazepine

The steady-state carbamazepine levels of 8 healthy subjects taking carbamazepine 300 mg twice daily were increased by 17% within 2 days of them starting to take **cimetidine** 400 mg three times daily. Adverse effects occurred in 6 subjects, but after 7 days of treatment the carbamazepine levels had fallen again and the adverse effects disappeared.[1]

Conversely, the steady-state carbamazepine levels of 7 epileptic patients receiving long-term treatment remained unaltered when they were given **cimetidine** 1 g daily for a week.[2] Another study also found a lack of an interaction in 11 patients with epilepsy.[3] However, an 89-year-old woman taking carbamazepine 600 mg daily developed symptoms of carbamazepine toxicity within 2 days of starting to take **cimetidine** 400 mg daily, and had a rise in serum carbamazepine levels, which fell when the **cimetidine** was withdrawn.[4] The effects of **cimetidine** may be additive with those of isoniazid, see 'Carbamazepine + Isoniazid or Rifampicin (Rifampin)', p.573.

The results of these studies in patients and subjects taking carbamazepine long-term differ from single-dose studies and short-term studies in healthy subjects. For example, a 20% fall in clearance[5] and a 26% increase in the AUC[6] have been reported, which would indicate that there may be some potential for a clinically significant interaction (see 'Mechanism' below).

In 8 healthy subjects **ranitidine** 300 mg daily did not affect the pharmacokinetics of a single 600-mg dose of carbamazepine.[7]

(b) Oxcarbazepine

In 8 healthy subjects, **cimetidine** 400 mg twice daily for 7 days did not affect the pharmacokinetics of a single 600-mg oral dose of oxcarbazepine.[8]

Mechanism

Not fully understood. It is thought that cimetidine can inhibit the activity of the liver enzymes concerned with the metabolism of carbamazepine (such as the cytochrome P450 isoenzyme CYP3A4), resulting in its reduced clearance from the body. The autoinducing effects of carbamazepine oppose this, although one study suggests the autoinducing effects of carbamazepine are blocked by cimetidine.[9] However, autoinduction would possibly explain why the single-dose and short-term studies in healthy subjects suggest that a clinically important interaction could occur, but in practice the combination causes few problems in patients receiving long-term carbamazepine.

Importance and management

The interaction between carbamazepine and cimetidine is established but of minimal importance. Patients receiving long-term treatment with carbamazepine should be warned that for the first few days after starting to take cimetidine they may possibly experience some increase in carbamazepine adverse effects (nausea, headache, dizziness, fatigue, drowsiness, ataxia, an inability to concentrate, a bitter taste). However, because the serum levels are only transiently increased, these effects should subside and disappear by the end of a week. Ranitidine appears to be a non-interacting alternative to cimetidine.

1. Dalton MJ, Powell JR, Messenheimer JA, Clark J. Cimetidine and carbamazepine: a complex drug interaction. *Epilepsia* (1986) 27, 553–8.
2. Sonne J, Lühdorf K, Larsen NE and Andreasen PB. Lack of interaction between cimetidine and carbamazepine. *Acta Neurol Scand* (1983) 68, 253–6.
3. Levine M, Jones MW, Sheppard I. Differential effect of cimetidine on serum concentrations of carbamazepine and phenytoin. *Neurology* (1985) 35, 562–5.
4. Telerman-Topet N, Duret ME, Coërs C. Cimetidine interaction with carbamazepine. *Ann Intern Med* (1981) 94, 544.
5. Webster LK, Mihaly GW, Jones DB, Smallwood RA, Phillips JA, Vajda FJ. Effect of cimetidine and ranitidine on carbamazepine and sodium valproate pharmacokinetics. *Eur J Clin Pharmacol* (1984) 27, 341–3.
6. Dalton MJ, Powell JR, Messenheimer JA. The influence of cimetidine on single-dose carbamazepine pharmacokinetics. *Epilepsia* (1985) 26, 127–30.
7. Dalton MJ, Powell JR, Messenheimer JA. Ranitidine does not alter single-dose carbamazepine pharmacokinetics in healthy adults. *Drug Intell Clin Pharm* (1985) 19, 941–4.
8. Keränen T, Jolkkonen J, Klosterskov-Jensen P, Menge GP. Oxcarbazepine does not interact with cimetidine in healthy volunteers. *Acta Neurol Scand* (1992) 85, 239–42.
9. Macphee GJA, Thompson GG, Scobie G, Agnew E, Park BK, Murray T, McColl KEL, Brodie MJ. Effects of cimetidine on carbamazepine auto- and hetero-induction in man. *Br J Clin Pharmacol* (1984) 18, 411–19.

Carbamazepine + Influenza vaccines

Influenza vaccination appears to raise carbamazepine levels. In one case this resulted in carbamazepine toxicity.

Clinical evidence, mechanism, importance and management

The serum carbamazepine levels of 20 children rose by 47% from 6.17 micrograms/mL to 9.04 micrograms/mL 14 days after they were given 0.5 mL of influenza vaccine USP, types A and B, whole virus (Squibb). Levels remained elevated on day 28.[1] A teenager taking carbamazepine 400 mg in the morning and 600 mg at night with gabapentin 600 mg three times daily developed signs of carbamazepine toxicity (unsteady, lethargic, slurred speech) 13 days after she was given an influenza vaccination (*Fluzone*, Aventis Pasteur). Her serum carbamazepine level was 27.5 micrograms/mL (previous levels 8.2 to 12.4 micrograms/mL), and she required ventilation for 19 hours. A urine drug screen was positive for tricyclic antidepressants and cocaine, but it was eventually concluded that these were likely to represent false-positive results.[2]

It has been suggested that the vaccine inhibits the liver enzymes concerned with the metabolism of carbamazepine, and therefore raises its levels. The moderate increase in serum carbamazepine levels seen in the first study is unlikely to have much clinical relevance as the vaccine is usually given as a single dose and therefore levels will decline over time. However, the case report of markedly increased carbamazepine levels introduces a note of caution.

1. Jann MW, Fidone GS. Effect of influenza vaccine on serum anticonvulsant concentrations. *Clin Pharm* (1986) 5, 817–20.
2. Robertson WC. Carbamazepine toxicity after influenza vaccination. *Pediatr Neurol* (2002) 26, 61–3.

Carbamazepine + Isoniazid or Rifampicin (Rifampin)

Carbamazepine levels are markedly and very rapidly increased by isoniazid and toxicity can occur. Rifampicin has been reported both to augment and negate this interaction. There is evidence to suggest that carbamazepine may potentiate isoniazid hepatotoxicity.

Clinical evidence

Disorientation, listlessness, aggression, lethargy and, in one case, extreme drowsiness developed in 10 out of 13 patients taking carbamazepine when they were given isoniazid 200 mg daily. Serum carbamazepine levels were measured in 3 of the patients and they were found to have risen above the reference range (initial level not stated).[1]

Carbamazepine toxicity, associated with marked rises in serum carbamazepine levels, has been described in other reports.[2-5] Some of the patients were also taking sodium valproate, which does not seem to be implicated in the interaction, and in one case cimetidine (see also 'Carbamazepine and related drugs + H_2-receptor antagonists', p.572) was thought to have potentiated the interaction.[5]

One report describes carbamazepine toxicity in a patient given isoniazid, but only when rifampicin was present as well. Usually the enzyme-inducing effects of rifampicin would be expected to counteract any enzyme inhibition by isoniazid, so this report is somewhat inexplicable.[6] Conversely, a case report describes reduced carbamazepine levels in a woman given rifampicin and isoniazid, which resulted in reduced carbamazepine efficacy (symptoms of hypomania).[7]

Isoniazid-induced fulminant liver failure occurred in a 16-year-old girl taking carbamazepine and clonazepam, within 5 days of starting isoniazid, rifampicin and pyrazinamide. She recovered with supportive measures and later tolerated the antiepileptics with concurrent rifampicin and pyrazinamide.[8] Isoniazid hepatotoxicity has also occurred in a 74-year-old woman[9] and a 10-year-old boy[10] taking carbamazepine, shortly after treatment with isoniazid, rifampicin, and ethambutol, with or without pyrazinamide, was started.

Mechanism

Unknown. It has been suggested that isoniazid inhibits the activity of the cytochrome P450 isoenzyme CYP3A4, which is concerned with the metabolism of carbamazepine, causing it to accumulate in the body;[11] however, isoniazid does not usually cause clinically relevant interactions by this mechanism. Rifampicin is a potent enzyme inducer, and would be expected to negate the effects of isoniazid, and to induce the metabolism of carbamazepine. This is supported by one report, but not another.

Importance and management

The documentation is limited, but a clinically important and potentially serious interaction is established between isoniazid and carbamazepine. Toxicity can develop quickly (within 1 to 5 days) and also seems to disappear quickly if the isoniazid is withdrawn. Concurrent use should not be undertaken unless the effects can be closely monitored and suitable downward dose adjustments made (a carbamazepine dose reduction of between one-half and two-thirds was effective in 3 patients[1]). It seems probable that slow metabolisers of isoniazid may develop this interaction more quickly and to a greater extent than fast metabolisers.[2]

The effect of concurrent rifampicin on the interaction between isoniazid and carbamazepine is unclear. One report showed negation of the interaction, whereas another showed potential augmentation.

Limited evidence suggests that carbamazepine may potentiate isoniazid hepatotoxicity; routine isoniazid monitoring should be adequate to detect any interaction.

1. Valsalan VC, Cooper GL. Carbamazepine intoxication caused by interaction with isoniazid. *BMJ* (1982) 285, 261–2.
2. Wright JM, Stokes EF, Sweeney VP. Isoniazid-induced carbamazepine toxicity and vice versa: a double drug interaction. *N Engl J Med* (1982) 307, 1325–7.
3. Block SH. Carbamazepine-isoniazid interaction. *Pediatrics* (1982) 69, 494–5.
4. Poo Argüelles P, Samarra Riera JM, Gairí Tahull JM, Vernet Bori A. Interacción carbamacepina-tuberculostáticos. *Med Clin (Barc)* (1984) 83, 867–8.
5. García B, Zaborras E, Areas V, Obeso G, Jiménez I, de Juana P, Bermejo T. Interaction between isoniazid and carbamazepine potentiated by cimetidine. *Ann Pharmacother* (1992) 26, 841–2.
6. Fleenor ME, Harden JW, Curtis G. Interaction between carbamazepine and antituberculosis agents. *Chest* (1991) 99, 1554.
7. Zolezzi M, Antituberculosis agents and carbamazepine. *Am J Psychiatry* (2002) 159, 874.
8. Campos-Franco J, González-Quintela A, Alende-Sixto MR. Isoniazid-induced hyperacute liver failure in a young patient receiving carbamazepine. *Eur J Intern Med* (2004) 15, 396–7.
9. Barbare JC, Lallement PY, Vorhauer W, Veyssier P. Hépatotoxicité de l'isoniazide: influence de la carbamazépine? *Gastroenterol Clin Biol* (1986) 10, 523–4.
10. Berkowitz FE, Henderson SL, Fajman N, Schoen B, Naughton M. Acute liver failure caused by isoniazid in a child receiving carbamazepine. *Int J Tuberc Lung Dis* (1998) 2, 603–6.
11. Desta Z, Soukhova NV, Flockhart DA. Inhibition of cytochrome P450 (CYP450) isoforms by isoniazid: potent inhibition of CYP2C19 and CYP3A. *Antimicrob Agents Chemother* (2001) 45, 384–92.

Carbamazepine and related drugs + Lamotrigine

Most studies have found that lamotrigine has no effect on the pharmacokinetics of carbamazepine or its metabolite, carbamazepine-10,11-epoxide. However, some studies have found that lamotrigine raises the plasma concentration of carbamazepine-10,11-epoxide. Symptoms of toxicity have been seen irrespective of changes in concentration. Carbamazepine decreases lamotrigine concentrations. Lamotrigine did not appear to alter the pharmacokinetics of oxcarbazepine in one study, but did reduce oxcarbazepine metabolism in another study. Similarly conflicting effects on lamotrigine concentrations have been seen with concurrent use of oxcarbazepine, with symptoms of increased toxicity also reported.

The pharmacokinetics of eslicarbazepine are not altered by lamotrigine, but lamotrigine clearance might be minimally increased on concurrent use.

Clinical evidence

(a) Effects on carbamazepine

In 3 patients with epilepsy, the addition of lamotrigine increased the serum concentration of carbamazepine-10,11-epoxide, the active metabolite of carbamazepine, but the concentration of carbamazepine remained unchanged. One of the patients had a carbamazepine-10,11-epoxide serum concentration of 4.7 to 8.7 micrograms/mL while taking carbamazepine 1.1 g daily and lamotrigine. When the lamotrigine was stopped, her carbamazepine-10,11-epoxide concentration decreased to 2 to 2.2 micrograms/mL. Symptoms of toxicity occurred in 2 patients (dizziness, double vision, drowsiness, nausea).[1]

In another study in 9 patients, the addition of lamotrigine 200 mg increased the serum carbamazepine-10,11-epoxide concentration by 45%. Toxicity was seen in 4 patients (dizziness, double vision, nausea).[2] The addition of lamotrigine resulted in cerebellar toxicity (nausea, vertigo, nystagmus, ataxia) in 8 out of 9 patients taking subtoxic, and just-tolerated, doses of carbamazepine when lamotrigine was added. Analysis showed that in all 8 cases, one or more of the serum concentrations of carbamazepine, carbamazepine-10,11-epoxide, or lamotrigine had become unusually high.[3]

In contrast, other studies have found that the concurrent use of lamotrigine and carbamazepine does not result in any clinically important pharmacokinetic changes. Lamotrigine did not affect carbamazepine concentrations[4-8] or carbamazepine-10,11-epoxide concentrations in several studies[6,7,9] However, in one study, 9 of 47 subjects developed double vision or dizziness, predominantly in those whose carbamazepine concentration was already high before the lamotrigine was added.[6] In another study in 14 children, lamotrigine had no effect on the concentration of carbamazepine, and actually decreased the concentration of carbamazepine-10,11-epoxide by 23%. Two children developed double vision, which was unrelated to the drug concentrations, but responded to a reduction in the lamotrigine dose in one child, and a reduction in the carbamazepine dose in the other.[10]

(b) Effects on eslicarbazepine

A pharmacokinetic study in 14 healthy subjects given eslicarbazepine 600 mg daily on days one and 2, and then 1.2 g daily on days 3 to 27, found that the addition of lamotrigine (50 mg daily on days 9 and 10, increasing to 150 mg daily from day 11 to 27) did not alter the pharmacokinetics of eslicarbazepine.[11] Similarly, a population pharmacokinetic model using data from 641 patients enrolled in phase III eslicarbazepine studies, also found that the concurrent use of lamotrigine (in 148 patients) did not alter the pharmacokinetics of eslicarbazepine.[12]

(c) Effects on lamotrigine

1. Carbamazepine. In a retrospective study, the lamotrigine serum concentration-to-dose ratio was much lower in patients also taking carbamazepine than in those taking lamotrigine monotherapy (0.38 versus 0.84).[13] Other studies have reported similar findings.[14-16] In one of these studies, an increase in the concentration of lamotrigine of about 60% occurred in patients taking lamotrigine with carbamazepine when the carbamazepine was withdrawn.[16] Similarly, a case report describes a rapid increase in the concentration of lamotrigine when carbamazepine was withdrawn.[17] A review of patients taking antiepileptics found that carbamazepine increased the clearance of lamotrigine by 30 to 50%.[18]

2. Eslicarbazepine. In a pharmacokinetic study in 14 healthy subjects, eslicarbazepine (given as 600 mg daily on days 9 and 10, and 1.2 g daily on days 11 to 27) did not alter the pharmacokinetics of lamotrigine (give as 50 mg daily on days one and 2, and 150 mg daily on days 3 to 27).[11] A population pharmacokinetic model using data from 641 patients enrolled in phase III eslicarbazepine studies, found that lamotrigine clearance was increased by 12% by eslicarbazepine.[12]

3. Oxcarbazepine. In an analysis of a retrospective study, lamotrigine concentrations were about 34% lower in 14 patients also taking oxcarbazepine than in 64 patients taking lamotrigine alone, when corrected for dose. In this study, the effect of oxcarbazepine was less than that of carbamazepine (34% versus 47%).[15] Similarly, in another analysis, the addition of oxcarbazepine to lamotrigine reduced the concentrations of lamotrigine by 15 to 75%.[19] However, in contrast to these findings, one study in healthy subjects found that oxcarbazepine had no effect on the pharmacokinetics of lamotrigine, although adverse effects were reported to be more frequent and severe during concurrent use.[20] A report describes two cases of serious mouth ulcers (such that swallowing and eating were difficult) that developed after oxcarbazepine was withdrawn from patients also taking lamotrigine, and were attributed to gradually increasing lamotrigine concentrations once oxcarbazepine had been stopped. In the first patient, the ulcers developed 39 days after oxcarbazepine was stopped and resolved 4 days after lamotrigine was stopped, and in the second patient the ulcers appeared 22 days after the oxcarbazepine dose was reduced from 1200 mg daily to 600 mg daily and resolved after both oxcarbazepine and lamotrigine were stopped.[21]

(d) Effects on oxcarbazepine

A retrospective analysis found that monohydroxyoxcarbazepine-concentration to oxcarbazepine-dose ratios were higher in 7 patients also taking lamotrigine than in those taking oxcarbazepine alone.[22] However, in contrast to these findings, one study in healthy subjects found that lamotrigine had no effect on the pharmacokinetics of oxcarbazepine or its metabolite, monohydroxyoxcarbazepine, although adverse effects were reported to be more frequent and more severe during concurrent use.[20]

Mechanism

The reasons for the effects of lamotrigine on carbamazepine and oxcarbazepine pharmacokinetics are not clear. It has been suggested that a pharmacodynamic interaction between carbamazepine and lamotrigine might account for the toxic symptoms seen in some patients.[3,6] Evidence with oxcarbazepine is conflicting; in one study lamotrigine appeared to increase the metabolism of oxcarbazepine but another study found no pharmacokinetic interaction.

Lamotrigine is metabolised by glucuronidation, which might be induced by carbamazepine and possibly oxcarbazepine,[23] resulting in reduced lamotrigine concentrations.

Importance and management

Overall, lamotrigine does not appear to have a clinically relevant effect on **carbamazepine** concentrations. However, toxicity has occurred, and therefore patients should be well monitored if both drugs are given, with consideration given to decreasing the carbamazepine dose if CNS adverse effects occur. In one case, reducing the dose of lamotrigine was effective in resolving the adverse effects.

Carbamazepine induces the metabolism of lamotrigine, and the recommended starting dose and long-term maintenance dose of lamotrigine in patients already taking carbamazepine is twice that of patients taking lamotrigine monotherapy.[24,25] However, if patients are also taking valproate in addition to carbamazepine, the lamotrigine dose should be reduced.[24,25] Consider also, 'Lamotrigine + Valproate', p.587.

The situation with **oxcarbazepine** is less clear, with reports of both reduced lamotrigine concentrations (although perhaps to a lesser extent than with carbamazepine) and no effect on lamotrigine concentrations. The UK and US manufacturers of lamotrigine do not advise any lamotrigine dose adjustments on concurrent use with oxcarbazepine.[24,25] The UK manufacturer of oxcarbazepine notes that concurrent use with lamotrigine has been associated with an increased risk of adverse effects (such as nausea, drowsiness, dizziness, and headache) and that dose adjustments or monitoring of plasma concentration might be necessary, particularly in children.[26] The cases of mouth ulcers occurring some time after discontinuation, or dose reduction, of oxcarbazepine are isolated and, as such, their general clinical importance is uncertain, but bear them in mind in case of an unexpected response to treatment.

The pharmacokinetics of **eslicarbazepine** do not appear to be affected by lamotrigine, and the effect of eslicarbazepine on lamotrigine clearance is unlikely to be clinically important. It would therefore not seem necessary to adjust eslicarbazepine or lamotrigine doses on concurrent use.

1. Graves NM, Ritter FJ, Wagner ML, Floren KL, Alexander BJ, Campbell JI, Leppik IE. Effect of lamotrigine on carbamazepine epoxide concentrations. *Epilepsia* (1991) 32 (Suppl 3), 13.
2. Warner T, Patsalos PN, Prevett M, Elyas AA, Duncan JS. Lamotrigine-induced carbamazepine toxicity: an interaction with carbamazepine-10,11-epoxide. *Epilepsy Res* (1992) 11, 147–50.
3. Wolf P. Lamotrigine: preliminary clinical observations on pharmacokinetics and interactions with traditional antiepileptic drugs. *J Epilepsy* (1992) 5, 73–9.
4. Jawad S, Richens A, Goodwin G, Yuen WC. Controlled trial of lamotrigine (Lamictal) for refractory partial seizures. *Epilepsia* (1989) 30, 356–63.
5. Eriksson A-S, Hoppu K, Nergårdh A, Boreus L. Pharmacokinetic interactions between lamotrigine and other antiepileptic drugs in children with intractable epilepsy. *Epilepsia* (1996) 37, 769–73.
6. Besag FMC, Berry DJ, Pool F, Newbery JE, Subel B. Carbamazepine toxicity with lamotrigine: a pharmacokinetic or pharmacodynamic interaction? *Epilepsia* (1998) 39, 183–7.
7. Malminiemi K, Keränen T, Kerttula T, Moilanen E, Ylitalo P. Effects of short-term lamotrigine treatment on pharmacokinetics of carbamazepine. *Int J Clin Pharmacol Ther* (2000) 38, 540–5.
8. Pereira LRL, Velasco TR, Ceiki-Sakamoto A, de Carvalho D. Evaluación de la interacción medicamentosa de la carbamacepina y la lamotrigina en el tratamiento de los pacientes epilépticos refractarios. *Rev Neurol* (2006) 43, 74–7.
9. Pisani F, Xiao B, Fazio A, Spina E, Perucca E, Tomson T. Single dose pharmacokinetics of carbamazepine-10,11-epoxide in patients on lamotrigine monotherapy. *Epilepsy Res* (1994) 19, 245–8.
10. Eriksson A-S, Boreus LO. No increase in carbamazepine-10,11-epoxide during addition of lamotrigine treatment in children. *Ther Drug Monit* (1997) 19, 499–501.
11. Almeida L, Nunes T, Sicard E, Rocha J-F, Falcão A, Brunet J-S, Lefebvre M, Soares-da-Silva P. Pharmacokinetic interaction study between eslicarbazepine acetate and lamotrigine in healthy subjects. *Acta Neurol Scand* (2010) 121, 257–64.
12. Falcão A, Fuseau E, Nunes T, Almeida A, Soares-da-Silva P. Pharmacokinetics, drug interactions and exposure-response relationship of eslicarbazepine acetate in adult patients with partial-onset seizures: population pharmacokinetic and pharmacokinetic/pharmacodynamic analyses. *CNS Drugs* (2012) 26, 79–91.
13. Armijo JA, Bravo J, Cuadrado A, Herranz JL. Lamotrigine serum concentration-to-dose ratio: influence of age and concomitant antiepileptic drugs and dosage implications. *Ther Drug Monit* (1999) 21, 182–90.
14. Böttiger Y, Svensson J-O, Ståhle L. Lamotrigine drug interactions in a TDM material. *Ther Drug Monit* (1999) 21, 171–4.
15. May TW, Rambeck B, Jürgens U. Influence of oxcarbazepine and methsuximide on lamotrigine concentrations in epileptic patients with and without valproic acid comedication: results of a retrospective study. *Ther Drug Monit* (1999) 21, 175–81.
16. Anderson GD, Gidal BE, Messenheimer J, Gilliam FG. Time course of lamotrigine de-induction: impact of step-wise withdrawal of carbamazepine or phenytoin. *Epilepsy Res* (2002) 49, 211–17.
17. Koch HJ, Szecsey A, Vogel M. Clinically relevant reduction of lamotrigine concentrations by carbamazepine. *Eur Psychiatry* (2003) 18, 42.
18. Weintraub D, Buchsbaum R, Resor SR, Hirsch LJ. Effect of antiepileptic drug comedication on lamotrigine clearance. *Arch Neurol* (2005) 62, 1432–6.
19. Krämer G, Dorn T, Etter H. Oxcarbazepine: clinically relevant drug interaction with lamotrigine. *Epilepsia* (2003) 44 (Suppl 9), 95–6.
20. Theis JGW, Sidhu J, Palmer J, Job S, Bullman J, Ascher J. Lack of pharmacokinetic interaction between oxcarbazepine and lamotrigine. *Neuropsychopharmacology* (2005) 30, 2269–74.
21. O'Neill A, de Leon J. Two case reports of oral ulcers with lamotrigine several weeks after oxcarbazepine withdrawal. *Bipolar Disord* (2007) 9, 310–3.
22. Guénault N, Odou P, Robert H. Increase in dihydroxycarbamazepine serum levels in patients co-medicated with oxcarbazepine and lamotrigine. *Eur J Clin Pharmacol* (2003) 59, 781–2.
23. Trileptal (Oxcarbazepine). Novartis Pharmaceuticals Corp. US Prescribing information, March 2011.
24. Lamictal (Lamotrigine). GlaxoSmithKline UK. UK Summary of product characteristics, July 2012.
25. Lamictal (Lamotrigine). GlaxoSmithKline. US Prescribing information, November 2011.
26. Trileptal (Oxcarbazepine). Novartis Pharmaceuticals UK Ltd. UK Summary of product characteristics, April 2012.

Carbamazepine + Loxapine

An increase in the serum levels of the epoxide metabolite of carbamazepine has been reported in patients given loxapine.

Clinical evidence, mechanism, importance and management

One patient taking loxapine 500 mg daily developed toxicity (ataxia, nausea, anxiety) when given carbamazepine 600 mg daily, even though the serum carbamazepine level was low to normal.[1] In another case, neurotoxicity (ataxia, lethargy, visual disturbances) developed in a man given carbamazepine and loxapine.[2] In both cases, the toxicity appeared to be due to elevated carbamazepine-10,11-epoxide levels (the metabolite of carbamazepine).[1,2] The problem resolved when the carbamazepine doses were reduced. The reasons for these effects are not understood, and evidence appears to be limited to the two cases cited. The general significance of these reports is therefore unclear. Consider the possibility of an interaction if a patient taking carbamazepine and loxapine develops neurotoxic adverse effects.

1. Pitterle ME, Collins DM. Carbamazepine-10,11-epoxide evaluation associated with coadministration of loxitane or amoxapine. *Epilepsia* (1988) 29, 654.
2. Collins DM, Gidal BE, Pitterle ME. Potential interaction between carbamazepine and loxapine: case report and retrospective review. *Ann Pharmacother* (1993) 27, 1180–3.

Carbamazepine + Macrolides

Carbamazepine levels are markedly and rapidly increased by clarithromycin, erythromycin or troleandomycin, and toxicity can often develop within 1 to 5 days. Telithromycin is predicted to interact similarly. Studies suggest that azithromycin, flurithromycin, josamycin, midecamycin, and roxithromycin have no interaction, or no clinically significant interaction, with carbamazepine, but note that a case of carbamazepine toxicity has been reported in a patient given roxithromycin.

Clinical evidence

(a) Azithromycin

In a study in healthy subjects, azithromycin 500 mg daily for 3 days had no effect on the pharmacokinetics of carbamazepine 200 mg twice daily or its active metabolite, carbamazepine-10,11-epoxide.[1]

(b) Clarithromycin

A pharmacokinetic study[2] in healthy subjects found that clarithromycin 500 mg every 12 hours for 5 days increased the AUC of a single 400-mg dose of carbamazepine by 26%. A retrospective study of 5 patients with epilepsy found that when they were given clarithromycin (dose not stated) their serum carbamazepine levels rose by 20 to 50% within 3 to 5 days, despite 30 to 40% reductions in the carbamazepine dose in 4 of them. Carbamazepine levels in the toxic range were seen in 3 of them, and their carbamazepine doses were then even further reduced.[3] A number of case reports have described carbamazepine toxicity following the addition of clarithromycin in adults,[4-7] and children.[7-9] Two other patients with epilepsy had marked rises in serum carbamazepine levels when they were given clarithromycin 500 mg three times daily and omeprazole.[10] It is not clear whether the omeprazole also had some part to play.[11,12] See also 'Carbamazepine + Proton pump inhibitors', p.577. One case report describes a patient taking carbamazepine 200 mg twice daily who developed hyponatraemia 4 days after the addition of clarithromycin 500 mg twice daily: the hyponatraemia resolved when the clarithromycin was stopped.[13]

(c) Erythromycin

An 8-year-old girl taking phenobarbital 50 mg and carbamazepine 800 mg daily was given 500 mg, then later 1 g of erythromycin daily. Within 2 days she began to experience balancing difficulties and ataxia, which were eventually attributed to carbamazepine toxicity. Her serum carbamazepine levels were found to have risen from a little below 10 micrograms/mL to over 25 micrograms/mL (reference range 2 to 10 micrograms/mL). The levels rapidly returned to normal after carbamazepine was withheld for 24 hours and the erythromycin stopped.[14]

A study in 7 healthy subjects confirmed that erythromycin can cause significant increases in carbamazepine levels,[15] and a study in 8 healthy subjects found that the clearance of carbamazepine is reduced by an average of 20% (range 5 to 41%) by erythromycin 1 g daily for 5 days.[16] Another study, in healthy subjects given erythromycin 500 mg three times daily for 10 days, found that the clearance of a single dose of carbamazepine was reduced by about 20% and the maximum serum levels of carbamazepine-10,11-epoxide were reduced by about 40% by erythromycin.[17]

Marked rises in serum carbamazepine levels (up to fivefold in some cases) and/or toxicity (including cases of hepatorenal failure and AV block as well as more typical signs of carbamazepine toxicity) have been described in over 30 cases involving both children and adults. Symptoms commonly began within 24 to 72 hours of starting erythromycin, although in some cases it was as early as 8 hours. In most cases toxicity resolved within 3 to 5 days of stopping the erythromycin.[8,18-36]

(d) Flurithromycin

In a study in healthy subjects, flurithromycin 500 mg three times daily for a week increased the AUC of a single 400-mg dose of carbamazepine by about 20% and moderately reduced the production of carbamazepine-10,11-epoxide.[37]

(e) Josamycin

In studies in healthy subjects and in patients, josamycin 1 g twice daily for a week reduced the clearance of carbamazepine by about 20%.[38-40]

(f) Midecamycin acetate

A single-dose study in 14 subjects found that after taking midecamycin acetate 800 mg twice daily for 8 days the AUC of a single 200-mg dose of carbamazepine was increased by 15%, and the AUC of its active metabolite, carbamazepine-10,11-epoxide, was reduced by 26%.[41] Another study in patients taking carbamazepine found that the addition of midecamycin acetate 600 mg twice daily caused a small increase in the trough serum levels of carbamazepine, and only a 12% increase in its AUC.[42]

(g) Roxithromycin

In a study in healthy subjects, roxithromycin 150 mg twice daily for 8 days did not affect the pharmacokinetics of a single 200-mg dose of carbamazepine.[43] However, an isolated report describes carbamazepine toxicity (levels increased to 21.7 mg/L) in a patient taking carbamazepine and atorvastatin the day after she started to take roxithromycin 150 mg twice daily. Roxithromycin and atorvastatin were stopped and the carbamazepine level fell to 12.5 mg/L within a day. The increased carbamazepine levels were attributed to the concurrent use of roxithromycin.[44]

(h) Troleandomycin

In 8 patients with epilepsy, symptoms of carbamazepine toxicity (dizziness, nausea, vomiting, excessive drowsiness) developed within 24 hours of them also starting to take troleandomycin. The 2 patients available for examination had a sharp rise in serum carbamazepine levels, from about 5 micrograms/mL to 28 micrograms/mL over 3 days, and a rapid fall following withdrawal of the troleandomycin.[45,46]

Another report by the same authors describes a total of 17 similar cases of carbamazepine toxicity caused by troleandomycin.[18] Some of the patients had three or fourfold increases in serum carbamazepine levels. Another case has been described elsewhere.[14] In most instances the serum carbamazepine levels returned to normal within about 3 to 5 days of withdrawing the macrolide.[18]

Mechanism

It seems probable that clarithromycin, erythromycin and troleandomycin, and to a lesser extent some of the other macrolides, slow the rate of metabolism of the carbamazepine by the cytochrome P450 isoenzyme CYP3A4 so that the antiepileptic accumulates within the body.[47,48] Telithromycin is predicted to interact similarly.[49] It was suggested that the carbamazepine toxicity seen with roxithromycin may have been mediated by P-glycoprotein inhibition, which occurred as a result of an interaction between roxithromycin and atorvastatin; however, roxithromycin is a modest CYP3A4 inhibitor, and so it seems possible that it may have interacted by this mechanism.

Importance and management

The interaction between carbamazepine and troleandomycin is established, clinically important and potentially serious. The incidence is high. The rapidity of its development (within 24 hours in some cases) and the extent of the rise in serum carbamazepine levels suggest that it would be difficult to control carbamazepine levels by reducing the dose. Concurrent use should probably be avoided.

The interaction between carbamazepine and erythromycin is also very well documented, well established and of clinical importance. Concurrent use should be avoided unless the effects can be very closely monitored by measurement of serum carbamazepine levels and suitable dose reductions made. Toxic symptoms (ataxia, vertigo, drowsiness, lethargy, confusion, diplopia) can develop within 24 hours, but serum carbamazepine levels can return to normal within 8 to 12 hours of withdrawing the antibacterial.[38] Similar precautions would seem prudent if **telithromycin** is given with carbamazepine. However, the manufacturer of telithromycin advises avoidance of the combination, and suggests that telithromycin should not be used within 2 weeks of stopping carbamazepine. They also suggest that the levels of the antibacterial may be reduced.[49]

The interaction between carbamazepine and clarithromycin is also established, clinically important and potentially serious. It has been recommended that the carbamazepine dose should be reduced by 30 to 50% during treatment with clarithromycin, with monitoring within 3 to 5 days, and patients should be told to tell their doctor of any symptoms of toxicity (dizziness, diplopia, ataxia, mental confusion).

Analysis of the interactions between the macrolides and carbamazepine has shown that patients requiring high doses of carbamazepine to reach therapeutic levels are likely to have a greater rise in their carbamazepine levels.[50] The extent of the interactions is also correlated with the macrolide dose.[50]

Josamycin, flurithromycin, midecamycin acetate and roxithromycin appear to be safer alternatives to either clarithromycin, erythromycin, telithromycin or troleandomycin. Nevertheless a small or moderate reduction in the dose of carbamazepine may be needed, with subsequent good monitoring. Pharmacokinetic data suggest that azithromycin does not interact.

1. Rapeport WG, Dewland PM, Muirhead DC, Forster PL. Lack of an interaction between azithromycin and carbamazepine. *Br J Clin Pharmacol* (1992) 33, 551P.
2. Richens A, Chu S-Y, Sennello LT, Sonders RC. Effect of multiple doses of clarithromycin (C) on the pharmacokinetics (Pks) of carbamazepine (Carb). *Intersci Conf Antimicrob Agents Chemother* (1990) 30, 213.
3. O'Connor NK, Fris J. Clarithromycin-carbamazepine interaction in a clinical setting. *J Am Board Fam Pract* (1994) 7, 489–92.
4. Albani F, Riva R, Baruzzi A. Clarithromycin-carbamazepine interaction: a case report. *Epilepsia* (1993) 34, 161–2.
5. Yasui N, Otani K, Kaneko S, Shimoyama R, Ohkubo T, Sugawara K. Carbamazepine toxicity induced by clarithromycin coadministration in psychiatric patients. *Int Clin Psychopharmacol* (1997) 12, 225–9.
6. Tatum WO, Gonzalez MA. Carbamazepine toxicity in an epileptic induced by clarithromycin. *Hosp Pharm* (1994) 29, 45–6.
7. Gélisse P, Hillaire-Buys D, Halaili E, Jean-Pastor M-J, Vespignan H, Coubes P, Crespel A. Carbamazépine et clarithromycine: une interaction médicamenteuse cliniquement significative. *Rev Neurol (Paris)* (2007) 163, 1096–9.
8. Stafstrom CE, Nohria V, Loganbill H, Nahouraii R, Boustany R-M, DeLong GR. Erythromycin-induced carbamazepine toxicity: a continuing problem. *Arch Pediatr Adolesc Med* (1995) 149, 99–101.
9. Carmona Ibáñez G, Guevara Serrano J, Gisbert González S. Toxicidad de carbamacepina inducida por eritromicina. Un problema frencuente. *Farm Clin* (1996) 13, 698–700.
10. Metz DC, Getz HD. *Helicobacter pylori* gastritis therapy with omeprazole and clarithromycin increases serum carbamazepine levels. *Dig Dis Sci* (1995) 40, 912–15.
11. Dammann H-G. Therapy with omeprazole and clarithromycin increases serum carbamazepine levels in patients with *H.pylori* gastritis. *Dig Dis Sci* (1996) 41, 519.
12. Metz DC, Getz HD. Therapy with omeprazole and clarithromycin increases serum carbamazepine levels in patients with *H.pylori* gastritis. *Dig Dis Sci* (1996) 41, 519–20.
13. Kanbay M, Alkis M, Turgut F, Uz E, Bavbek N, Akcay A. Hyponatremia due to an additive effect of carbamazepine and clarithromycin. *South Med J* (2007) 100, 222.
14. Amedee-Manesme O, Rey E, Brussieux J, Goutieres F, Aicardi J. Antibiotiques à ne jamais associer à la carbamazépine. *Arch Fr Pediatr* (1982) 39, 126.
15. Miles MV, Tennison MB. Erythromycin effects on multiple-dose carbamazepine kinetics. *Ther Drug Monit* (1989) 11, 47–52.
16. Wong YY, Ludden TM, Bell RD. Effect of erythromycin on carbamazepine kinetics. *Clin Pharmacol Ther* (1983) 33, 460–4.
17. Barzaghi N, Gatti G, Crema F, Monteleone M, Amione C, Leone L, Perucca E. Inhibition by erythromycin of the conversion of carbamazepine to its active 10,11-epoxide metabolite. *Br J Clin Pharmacol* (1987) 24, 836–8.
18. Mesdjian E, Dravet C, Cenraud B, Roger J. Carbamazepine intoxication due to triacetyloleandomycin administration in epileptic patients. *Epilepsia* (1980) 21, 489–96.
19. Straughan J. Erythromycin-carbamazepine interaction? *S Afr Med J* (1982) 61, 420–1.
20. Vajda FJE, Bladin PF. Carbamazepine-erythromycin-base interaction. *Med J Aust* (1984) 140, 81.
21. Hedrick R, Williams F, Morin R, Lamb WA, Cate JC. Carbamazepine-erythromycin interaction leading to carbamazepine toxicity in four epileptic children. *Ther Drug Monit* (1983) 5, 405–7.
22. Miller SL. The association of carbamazepine intoxication and erythromycin use. *Ann Neurol* (1985) 18, 413.
23. Berrettini WH. A case of erythromycin-induced carbamazepine toxicity. *J Clin Psychiatry* (1986) 47, 147.
24. Carranco E, Kareus J, Co S, Peak V, Al-Rajeh S. Carbamazepine toxicity induced by concurrent erythromycin therapy. *Arch Neurol* (1985) 42, 187–8.
25. Goulden KJ, Camfield P, Dooley JM, Fraser A, Meek DC, Renton KW, Tibbles JAR. Severe carbamazepine intoxication after coadministration of erythromycin. *J Pediatr* (1986) 109, 135–8.
26. Wroblewski BA, Singer WD, Whyte J. Carbamazepine-erythromycin interaction. Case studies and clinical significance. *JAMA* (1986) 255, 1165–7.
27. Kessler JM. Erythromycin-carbamazepine interaction. *S Afr Med J* (1985) 67, 1038.
28. Jaster PJ, Abbas D. Erythromycin-carbamazepine interaction. *Neurology* (1986) 36, 594–5.
29. Loiseau P, Guyot M, Pautrizel B, Vincon G, Albin H. Intoxication par la carbamazépine due à l'interaction carbamazépine-érythromycine. *Presse Med* (1985) 14, 162.
30. Zitelli BJ, Howrie DL, Altman H, Marcon TJ. Erythromycin-induced drug interactions. *Clin Pediatr (Phila)* (1987) 26, 117–19.
31. Goldhoorn PB, Hofstee N. Een interactie tussen erytromycine en carbamazepine. *Ned Tijdschr Geneeskd* (1989) 133, 1944.
32. Mitsch RA. Carbamazepine toxicity precipitated by intravenous erythromycin. *DICP Ann Pharmacother* (1989) 23, 878–9.
33. Macnab AJ, Robinson JL, Adderly RJ, D'Orsogna L. Heart block secondary to erythromycin-induced carbamazepine toxicity. *Pediatrics* (1987) 80, 951–3.
34. Woody RC, Kearns GL, Bolyard KJ. Carbamazepine intoxication following the use of erythromycin in children. *Pediatr Infect Dis J* (1987) 6, 578–9.
35. Mota CR, Carvalho C, Mota C, Ferreira P, Vilarinho A, Pereira E. Severe carbamazepine toxicity induced by concurrent erythromycin therapy. *Eur J Pediatr* (1996) 155, 345–8.
36. Viani F, Claris-Appiani A, Rossi LN, Giani M, Romeo A. Severe hepatorenal failure in a child receiving carbamazepine and erythromycin. *Eur J Pediatr* (1992) 151, 715–16.
37. Barzaghi N, Gatti G, Crema F, Faja A, Monteleone M, Amione C, Leone L, Perucca E. Effect of flurithromycin, a new macrolide antibiotic, on carbamazepine disposition in normal subjects. *Int J Clin Pharmacol Res* (1988) 8, 101–5.
38. Albin H, Vinçon G, Pehourcq F, Dangoumau J. Influence de la josamycine sur la pharmacocinétique de la carbamazépine. *Therapie* (1982) 37, 151–6.
39. Vinçon G, Albin H, Demotes-Mainard F, Guyot M, Brachet-Liermain A, Loiseau P. Pharmacokinetic interaction between carbamazepine and josamycin. Proc Eur Congr Biopharmaceutics Pharmacokinetics vol III: Clinical Pharmacokinetics. Edited by Aiache JM and Hirtz J. Published by Imprimerie de l'Université de Clermont-Ferrand. (1984) pp 270–6.
40. Vinçon G, Albin H, Demotes-Mainard F, Guyot M, Bistue C, Loiseau P. Effects of josamycin on carbamazepine kinetics. *Eur J Clin Pharmacol* (1987) 32, 321–3.
41. Couet W, Istin B, Ingrand I, Girault J, Fourtillan J-B. Effect of ponsinomycin on single-dose kinetics and metabolism of carbamazepine. *Ther Drug Monit* (1990) 12, 144–9.
42. Zagnoni PG, DeLuca M, Casini A. Carbamazepine-miocamycin interaction. *Epilepsia* (1991) 32 (Suppl 1), 28.
43. Saint-Salvi B, Tremblay D, Surjus A, Lefebvre MA. A study of the interaction of roxithromycin with theophylline and carbamazepine. *J Antimicrob Chemother* (1987) 20 (Suppl B), 121–9.
44. Corbin C, Mosquet B, Lacotte J, Debruyne D, Denise P, Viader F, Coquerel A. Surdosage en carbamazépine après association à l'atorvastatine et à la roxithromycine. *Therapie* (2004) 59, 267–9.
45. Dravet C, Mesdjian E, Cenraud B, Roger J. Interaction between carbamazepine and triacetyloleandomycin. *Lancet* (1977) i, 810–11.
46. Dravet C, Mesdjian E, Cenraud B, Roger J. Interaction carbamazépine triacétyloléandomycine: une nouvelle interaction médicamenteuse? *Nouv Presse Med* (1977) 6, 467.
47. Pessayre D, Larrey D, Vitaux J, Breil P, Belghiti J, Benhamou J-P. Formation of an inactive cytochrome P-450 Fe(II)-metabolite complex after administration of troleandomycin in humans. *Biochem Pharmacol* (1982) 31, 1699–1704.
48. Levy RH, Johnson CM, Thummel KE, Kerr BM, Kroetz DL, Korzecwa KR, Gonzales FJ. Mechanism of the interaction between carbamazepine and erythromycin. *Epilepsia* (1993) 34 (Suppl 6), 37–8.
49. Ketek (Telithromycin). Sanofi. UK Summary of product characteristics, November 2012.
50. Pauwels O. Factors contributing to carbamazepine-macrolide interactions. *Pharmacol Res* (2002) 45, 291–8.

Carbamazepine and related drugs + MAOIs or RIMAs

Phenelzine and tranylcypromine do not appear to interact adversely with carbamazepine. The manufacturers predict that toxic reactions will develop if carbamazepine, eslicarbazepine, and oxcarbazepine are given with an MAOI.

Carbamazepine appears to slightly reduce the exposure to moclobemide. A tolerability study found no evidence of an interaction between carbamazepine and moclobemide.

Clinical evidence, mechanism, importance and management

(a) MAOIs

There appear to be no reports of adverse reactions during the concurrent use of MAOIs and carbamazepine, **eslicarbazepine**, or **oxcarbazepine**. However, the manufacturers of carbamazepine,[1] **eslicarbazepine**,[2] and **oxcarbazepine**[3] all suggest that an interaction is possible because of the close structural similarity between these drugs and the tricyclic antidepressants, which are known to interact adversely with the MAOIs, resulting in toxic reactions such as serotonin syndrome. The UK manufacturer of carbamazepine[1] does not recommend the concurrent use of MAOIs and suggests that MAOIs should be discontinued at least 2 weeks before carbamazepine is started. However, several reports describe the successful use of carbamazepine and MAOIs, namely **tranylcypromine**[4-6] and **phenelzine**.[6,7] Bearing in mind that the MAOIs and the tricyclics can be given together under certain well controlled conditions (see 'MAOIs or RIMAs + Tricyclic and related antidepressants', p.1403), the warning about the risks might possibly prove to be over-cautious.

Note that, rarely, the MAOIs have been seen to cause convulsions and they should therefore be used cautiously in patients with epilepsy.

(b) RIMAs

In a drug interaction study in patients with depression, moclobemide 150 mg three times daily was given alone (6 patients) or with carbamazepine 200 mg twice daily (7 patients) for 5 weeks. In the group taking carbamazepine, the AUC, maximum plasma concentration, and minimum plasma concentration of moclobemide were 35%, 28%, and 39% lower, respectively, on day 28 when compared with those receiving moclobemide alone. This was thought to be due to carbamazepine increasing the metabolism of moclobemide by CYP2C19.[8] Another study, which assessed tolerability, adverse effects, and vital signs in 3 patients given moclobemide with carbamazepine for 4 weeks, found no evidence of an interaction.[9]

The slight reduction in moclobemide exposure would not be expected to be of general relevance, as the study suggested that efficacy was not reduced and no clinically important changes in blood pressure or heart rate or other adverse effects occurred.[8] The available evidence therefore suggests that no particular precautions are necessary if moclobemide is given to patients taking carbamazepine.

1. Tegretol Tablets (Carbamazepine). Novartis Pharmaceuticals UK Ltd. UK Summary of product characteristics, May 2012.
2. Zebinix (Eslicarbazepine acetate). Eisai Ltd. UK Summary of product characteristics, August 2012.
3. Trileptal (Oxcarbazepine). Novartis Pharmaceuticals UK Ltd. UK Summary of product characteristics, April 2012.
4. Lydiard RB, White D, Harvey B, Taylor A. Lack of pharmacokinetic interaction between tranylcypromine and carbamazepine. *J Clin Psychopharmacol* (1987) 7, 360.
5. Joffe RT, Post RM, Uhde TW. Lack of pharmacokinetic interaction of carbamazepine with tranylcypromine. *Arch Gen Psychiatry* (1985) 42, 738.
6. Ketter TA, Post RM, Parekh PI, Worthington K. Addition of monoamine oxidase inhibitors to carbamazepine: preliminary evidence of safety and antidepressant efficacy in treatment-resistant depression. *J Clin Psychiatry* (1995) 56, 471–5.
7. Yatham LN, Barry S, Mobayed M, Dinan TG. Is the carbamazepine-phenelzine combination safe? *Am J Psychiatry* (1990) 147, 367.
8. Rakic Ignjatovic A, Milijkovic B, Todorovic D, Timotijevic I, Pokrajac M. Moclobemide monotherapy vs. Combined therapy with valproic acid or carbamazepine in depressive patients: a pharmacokinetic interaction study. *Br J Clin Pharmacol* (2008) 67, 199–208.
9. Amrein R, Güntert TW, Dingemanse J, Lorscheid T, Stabl M, Schmid-Burgk W. Interactions of moclobemide with concomitantly administered medication: evidence from pharmacological and clinical studies. *Psychopharmacology (Berl)* (1992) 106, S24–S31.

Carbamazepine + Metronidazole

Increased serum carbamazepine levels and toxicity have been seen in a patient given metronidazole.

Clinical evidence, mechanism, importance and management

A woman taking carbamazepine 1 g daily started taking co-trimoxazole twice daily and metronidazole 250 mg three times daily for diverticulitis. After 2 days the co-trimoxazole was stopped, she was changed to intravenous metronidazole 500 mg three times daily, and cefazolin 500 mg every 8 hours. After 2 days she complained of diplopia, dizziness and nausea, and her serum carbamazepine levels were found to have risen from 9 micrograms/mL to 14.3 micrograms/mL. A month later (presumably after the metronidazole had been withdrawn) her serum carbamazepine levels had fallen to 7.1 micrograms/mL. The reasons for this reaction are not understood.[1]

This appears to be the only report of an interaction between carbamazepine and metronidazole, so its general importance is uncertain.

1. Patterson BD. Possible interaction between metronidazole and carbamazepine. *Ann Pharmacother* (1994) 28, 1303–4.

Carbamazepine + Nefazodone

Five patients developed elevated serum carbamazepine levels and toxicity when nefazodone was given. A study in healthy subjects using lower carbamazepine doses found only modest increases in carbamazepine levels, and no evidence of toxicity when nefazodone was given. Carbamazepine markedly reduces nefazodone levels.

Clinical evidence

A patient taking carbamazepine 1 g daily developed evidence of toxicity (lightheadedness, ataxia) within 15 days of starting to take nefazodone (initially 100 mg twice daily increasing to 150 mg twice daily after a week). Her serum carbamazepine levels had risen from below 8.3 micrograms/mL up to 10.8 micrograms/mL. It was found necessary to reduce the carbamazepine dose to 600 mg daily to eliminate these adverse effects and to achieve a serum level of 7.4 micrograms/mL.[1] In 4 other patients taking carbamazepine 800 mg or 1 g daily the addition of nefazodone caused up to threefold rises in carbamazepine levels. The carbamazepine dose was reduced by 25 to 60%.[1,2] In a study in 12 healthy subjects, no evidence of toxicity was seen when carbamazepine 200 mg twice daily was given with nefazodone 200 mg twice daily for 5 days. However, the exposure to carbamazepine was slightly increased (23% increase in AUC) and the exposure to nefazodone markedly decreased (93% decrease in AUC). The authors suggest that there may be a greater effect with higher doses of carbamazepine.[3]

Mechanism

Both drugs are metabolised by the cytochrome P450 isoenzyme CYP3A4. Nefazodone is known to inhibit CYP3A4, whereas carbamazepine is a potent inducer of CYP3A4. Hence concurrent use reduces carbamazepine metabolism, leading to raised levels, and increases nefazodone metabolism, leading to lowered levels.

Importance and management

Information is limited, but it would seem prudent to monitor for signs of carbamazepine toxicity if nefazodone is added to established treatment, especially with doses of carbamazepine above 800 mg. The nefazodone dose may need to be increased in the presence of carbamazepine, so be alert for a reduced effect. Nefazodone has largely been withdrawn, but the US manufacturer of nefazodone did contraindicate its concurrent use with carbamazepine.[4]

1. Ashton AK, Wolin RE. Nefazodone-induced carbamazepine toxicity. *Am J Psychiatry* (1996) 153, 733.
2. Roth L, Bertschy G. Nefazodone may inhibit the metabolism of carbamazepine: three case reports. *Eur Psychiatry* (2001) 16, 320–1.
3. Laroudie C, Salazar DE, Cosson J-P, Cheuvart B, Istin B, Girault J, Ingrand I, Decourt J-P. Carbamazepine-nefazodone interaction in healthy subjects. *J Clin Psychopharmacol* (2000) 20, 46–53.
4. Nefazodone hydrochloride. Watson Laboratories Inc. US Prescribing information, June 2004.

Carbamazepine and related drugs + Phenobarbital

Carbamazepine concentrations are reduced to some extent by phenobarbital, whereas the concentrations of its active metabolite, carbamazepine-10,11-epoxide, are increased. In children, phenobarbital clearance is decreased by carbamazepine. Oxcarbazepine concentrations and those of its active metabolite, monohydroxyoxcarbazepine, are reduced by phenobarbital. Oxcarbazepine caused a minor increase in the concentrations of phenobarbital in one study. Eslicarbazepine does not appear to affect phenobarbital concentrations but barbiturates might increase eslicarbazepine clearance.

Clinical evidence

(a) Carbamazepine

A comparative study found that, on average, patients taking both carbamazepine and phenobarbital (44 patients) had carbamazepine serum concentrations that were 18% lower than those taking carbamazepine alone (43 patients).[1] Similar results were found in other studies in both adult and paediatric patients taking both drugs.[2-5] Concentrations of the active metabolite, carbamazepine-10,11-epoxide, were increased.[3-6] However, one study found that, after a single dose of carbamazepine, the clearance of the metabolite, carbamazepine-10,11-epoxide, was higher and its plasma half-life shorter in patients with epilepsy taking phenobarbital, when compared with healthy subjects not taking phenobarbital.[7]

In a prospective study, the clearance of phenobarbital in 222 patients receiving monotherapy was compared with that in 63 patients who were also taking carbamazepine. The clearance of carbamazepine was found to be decreased by phenobarbital. Further, the effects of carbamazepine on phenobarbital clearance were maximal in young children (about 54%) and minimal in adults.[8]

(b) Eslicarbazepine

A population pharmacokinetic model using data from 641 patients enrolled in phase III eslicarbazepine studies, found that the clearance of eslicarbazepine was increased by 60% by the concurrent use of phenytoin or a barbiturate (84 patients, but no breakdown for specific drugs). Eslicarbazepine was not found to alter the clearance of phenobarbital.[9]

(c) Oxcarbazepine

The AUCs of oxcarbazepine and its active metabolite, monohydroxyoxcarbazepine, were 43% and 25% lower, respectively, in 8 patients taking phenobarbital than in 8 control subjects. There were no other important effects on the pharmacokinetics of oxcarbazepine.[10] Similarly, in another study, concentrations of monohydroxyoxcarbazepine were statistically significantly lower (exact figure not stated) in patients taking phenobarbital than in those not taking enzyme-inducing antiepileptics.[11] In a study in children, phenobarbital was found to increase the apparent clearance of monohydroxyoxcarbazepine by 31 to 35%.[12] Another study found that the serum concentrations of monohydroxyoxcarbazepine were not affected by phenobarbital but its further conversion to dihydroxyoxcarbazepine was increased.[13]

An analysis of data from clinical studies found that oxcarbazepine increased phenobarbital concentrations by about 14%.[14,15]

Mechanism

Phenobarbital, carbamazepine, and oxcarbazepine are known enzyme inducers, and might therefore be expected to increase each other's metabolism (for details of the effects of carbamazepine and oxcarbazepine on each other see 'Carbamazepine + Eslicarbazepine or Oxcarbazepine', p.571). However, it appears that oxcarbazepine might actually inhibit the metabolism of phenobarbital, raising its concentrations, although the mechanism for this is not known. Phenobarbital might also induce the metabolism of the carbamazepine metabolite, carbamazepine-10,11-epoxide,[7] and the active metabolite of oxcarbazepine, monohydroxyoxcarbazepine.[13]

Importance and management

An interaction between **carbamazepine** and phenobarbital is established and important. It would be prudent to monitor phenobarbital concentrations in children also given carbamazepine, as changes in clearance might affect dose requirements. The small reduction in serum carbamazepine concentrations probably has little practical importance, especially as the metabolite carbamazepine-10,11-epoxide also has antiepileptic activity. Consider also 'Carbamazepine + Primidone', below.

The evidence with **oxcarbazepine** and phenobarbital suggests that an interaction occurs, but the clinical importance is perhaps limited. The increase in phenobarbital concentrations seen is small and unlikely to be clinically important. However, the decrease in the concentrations of the active oxcarbazepine metabolite, monohydroxyoxcarbazepine, which is principally responsible for the antiepileptic activity of oxcarbazepine, are unclear but could be clinically important and require further study. Until more is known, it might be prudent to monitor for the desired effect if both drugs are given concurrently. The increase in monohydroxyoxcarbazepine metabolism to dihydroxyoxcarbazepine is a minor step in the metabolism of monohydroxyoxcarbazepine, and so the overall antiepileptic action of oxcarbazepine is unlikely to be altered by this.

Information with **eslicarbazepine** and phenobarbital is limited, but no effect on phenobarbital concentrations appears to occur on concurrent use. Be aware of the possible need to increase the eslicarbazepine dose if phenobarbital or a barbiturate is also given.

1. Christiansen J, Dam M. Influence of phenobarbital and diphenylhydantoin on plasma carbamazepine levels in patients with epilepsy. *Acta Neurol Scand* (1973) 49, 543–6.
2. Cereghino JJ, Brock JT, Van Meter JC, Penry JK, Smith LD, White BG. The efficacy of carbamazepine combinations in epilepsy. *Clin Pharmacol Ther* (1975) 18, 733–41.
3. Rane A, Höjer B, Wilson JT. Kinetics of carbamazepine and its 10,11-epoxide metabolite in children. *Clin Pharmacol Ther* (1976) 19, 276–83.
4. Rambeck B, May T, Juergens U. Serum concentrations of carbamazepine and its epoxide and diol metabolites in epileptic patients: the influence of dose and comedication. *Ther Drug Monit* (1987) 9, 298–303.
5. Liu H, Delgado MR. Interactions of phenobarbital and phenytoin with carbamazepine and its metabolites' concentrations, concentration ratios, and level/dose ratios in epileptic children. *Epilepsia* (1995) 36, 249–54.
6. Dam M, Jensen A, Christiansen J. Plasma level and effect of carbamazepine in grand mal and psychomotor epilepsy. *Acta Neurol Scand* (1975) 75 (Suppl 51), 33–8.
7. Spina E, Martines C, Fazio A, Trio R, Pisani F, Tomson T. Effect of phenobarbital on the pharmacokinetics of carbamazepine-10,11-epoxide, an active metabolite of carbamazepine. *Ther Drug Monit* (1991) 13, 109–12.
8. Yukawa E, To H, Ohdo S, Higuchi S, Aoyama T. Detection of a drug-drug interaction on population-based phenobarbitone clearance using nonlinear mixed-effects modelling. *Eur J Clin Pharmacol* (1998) 54, 69–74.
9. Falcão A, Fuseau E, Nunes T, Almeida L, Soares-da-Silva P. Pharmacokinetics, drug interactions and exposure-response relationship of eslicarbazepine acetate in adult patients with partial-onset seizures: population pharmacokinetic and pharmacokinetic/pharmacodynamic analyses. *CNS Drugs* (2012) 26, 79–91.
10. Tartara A, Galimberti CA, Manni R, Morini R, Limido G, Gatti G, Bartoli A, Strad G, Perucca E. The pharmacokinetics of oxcarbazepine and its active metabolite 10-hydroxy-carbazepine in healthy subjects and in epileptic patients taking phenobarbitone or valproic acid. *Br J Clin Pharmacol* (1993) 36, 366–8.
11. Barcs G, Walker EB, Elger CE, Scaramelli A, Stefan H, Sturm Y, Moore A, Flesch G, Kramer L, D'Souza J. Oxcarbazepine placebo-controlled, dose-ranging trial in refractory partial epilepsy. *Epilepsia* (2000) 41, 1597–1607.
12. Sallas WM, Milosavljev S, D'Souza J, Hossain M. Pharmacokinetic drug interactions in children taking oxcarbazepine. *Clin Pharmacol Ther* (2003) 74, 138–49.
13. Kumps A, Wurth C. Oxcarbazepine disposition: preliminary observations in patients. *Biopharm Drug Dispos* (1990) 11, 365–70.
14. Trileptal (Oxcarbazepine). Novartis Pharmaceuticals UK Ltd. UK Summary of product characteristics. April 2012.
15. Hossain M, Sallas W, D'Souza J. Drug-drug interaction profile of oxcarbazepine in children and adults. *Neurology* (1999) 52 (Suppl 2), A525.

Carbamazepine + Primidone

A single case report suggests that primidone can reduce the effects of carbamazepine. Other evidence suggests that carbamazepine might reduce primidone serum concentrations and increase primidone-derived phenobarbital concentrations.

Clinical evidence

A 15-year-old boy had complex partial seizures that were not controlled despite treatment with primidone 12 mg/kg daily and carbamazepine 10 mg/kg daily, both in three divided doses. Even when the carbamazepine dose was increased to 20 mg/kg daily and then 30 mg/kg daily his carbamazepine serum concentrations only reached 4.8 micrograms/mL, and his seizures continued. When the primidone was gradually withdrawn, his carbamazepine serum concentrations increased to 12 micrograms/mL and his seizures completely disappeared.[1]

An analysis of the serum concentrations of antiepileptic drugs in children found that the serum concentrations of primidone tended to be lower in those also taking carbamazepine, but no details were given.[2] Another study found that the concentrations of phenobarbital derived from primidone were 42 micrograms/mL in patients taking primidone, carbamazepine and phenytoin, 24.7 micrograms/mL in patients taking phenytoin and primidone, and just 9.9 micrograms/mL in patients taking primidone alone.[3] A further study found that primidone concentrations were lower in patients also taking carbamazepine, but there were no notable changes in primidone-derived phenobarbital concentrations. The concentrations of carbamazepine-10,11-epoxide, a metabolite of carbamazepine, were increased by primidone.[4] In a retrospective study, the plasma concentrations-to-dose ratio for primidone was lower in patients also taking carbamazepine than in those taking primidone alone, and the primidone-derived phenobarbital concentrations were higher.[5]

Mechanism

When primidone was stopped in the single case cited, the clearance of carbamazepine decreased by about 60%.[1] This is consistent with the known enzyme-inducing effects of primidone (converted in the body to phenobarbital), which can increase the metabolism of other drugs by the liver. There is some evidence to suggest that carbamazepine might increase the metabolism of primidone to phenobarbital.

Importance and management

Direct evidence for the interaction between carbamazepine and primidone seems to be limited to these reports. It might be prudent to monitor concurrent use, and adjust the antiepileptic doses if necessary. Consider also 'Carbamazepine and related drugs + Phenobarbital', p.576.

1. Benetello P, Furlanut M. Primidone-carbamazepine interaction: clinical consequences. *Int J Clin Pharmacol Res* (1987) 7, 165–8.
2. Windorfer A, Sauer W. Drug interactions during anticonvulsant therapy in childhood: diphenylhydantoin, primidone, phenobarbitone, clonazepam, nitrazepam, carbamazepin and dipropylacetate. *Neuropadiatrie* (1977) 8, 29–41.
3. Callaghan N, Feeley M, Duggan F, O'Callaghan M, Seldrup J. The effect of anticonvulsant drugs which induce liver microsomal enzymes on derived and ingested phenobarbitone levels. *Acta Neurol Scand* (1977) 56, 1–6.
4. Callaghan N, Duggan B, O'Hare J, O'Driscoll D. Serum levels of phenobarbitone and phenylethylmalonamide with primidone used as a single drug and in combination with carbamazepine or phenytoin. In Johannessen SI et al. Antiepileptic Therapy: Advances in Drug Monitoring. New York: Raven Press; 1980, 307–13.
5. Battino D, Avanzini G, Bossi L, Croci D, Cusi C, Gomeni C, Moise A. Plasma levels of primidone and its metabolite phenobarbital: effect of age and associated therapy. *Ther Drug Monit* (1983) 5, 73–9.

Carbamazepine + Probenecid

Probenecid appears to increase the metabolism of carbamazepine to carbamazepine-10,11-epoxide.

Clinical evidence, mechanism, importance and management

In a placebo-controlled study, 10 healthy subjects were given probenecid 500 mg twice daily for 10 days with a single 200-mg dose of carbamazepine on day 6. The AUC of carbamazepine was decreased by about 19% and the AUC of carbamazepine-10,11-epoxide was increased by about 33%. Probenecid tended to decrease the formation of conjugated forms of both carbamazepine and its epoxide metabolite but this was not statistically significant. Probenecid increased the oral clearance of carbamazepine by 26%.

The increased metabolism of carbamazepine to carbamazepine-10,11-epoxide was thought to be due to induction of cytochrome P450 isoenzymes CYP3A4 and CYP2C8 by probenecid.[1] The clinical significance of the increase in levels of the active metabolite, carbamazepine-10,11-epoxide is unclear. This was a single-dose study, and it is known that following multiple doses, carbamazepine also induces its own metabolism by CYP3A4. The effect of carbamazepine on this isoenzyme would be expected to be much greater than any effect of probenecid, which does not usually cause clinically relevant interactions by this mechanism.

1. Kim K-A, Oh SO, Park P-W, Park J-Y. Effect of probenecid on the pharmacokinetics of carbamazepine in healthy subjects. *Eur J Clin Pharmacol* (2005) 61, 275–80.

Carbamazepine + Proton pump inhibitors

Omeprazole markedly raises the levels of a single dose of carbamazepine, but has no significant effect on the levels of carbamazepine taken long-term. Some anecdotal reports suggest that carbamazepine levels may

possibly be reduced by lansoprazole. Pantoprazole did not affect the pharmacokinetics of carbamazepine in one study.

Clinical evidence

(a) Lansoprazole

In 2001 the manufacturers of lansoprazole had on record 5 undetailed case reports of apparent interactions between lansoprazole and carbamazepine. One of them describes the development of carbamazepine toxicity when lansoprazole was added, but there is some doubt about this case because it is thought that the patient may have started to take higher doses of carbamazepine.

The other 4 cases are consistent, in that carbamazepine levels fell shortly after lansoprazole was added and/or the control of seizures suddenly worsened. One patient had a fall in carbamazepine serum levels from 11.5 mg/mL to 7.7 mg/L. The carbamazepine levels of another patient returned to normal when the lansoprazole was stopped.[1]

(b) Omeprazole

In a study in 7 patients, omeprazole 20 mg daily for 14 days was found to increase the AUC of a single 400-mg dose of carbamazepine by 75%. The clearance of carbamazepine was reduced by 40% and its elimination half-life was more than doubled (from 17.2 to 37.3 hours).[2] In a study in 10 healthy subjects, omeprazole 20 mg twice daily for 14 days increased the AUC, peak plasma level and elimination half-life of a single 400-mg dose of sustained-release carbamazepine (*Mazetol*) by about 90%, 31%, and 57%, respectively.[3] However, a retrospective study of the records of 10 patients who had been taking omeprazole 20 mg daily with long-term carbamazepine (rather than a single dose) found a non-significant reduction in carbamazepine serum levels.[4]

(c) Pantoprazole

In healthy subjects, pantoprazole 40 mg daily for 5 days had no effect on the AUC of carbamazepine or its metabolite, carbamazepine-10,11-epoxide, after a single 400-mg dose of carbamazepine.[5]

Mechanism

Omeprazole may inhibit the oxidative metabolism of single doses of carbamazepine. However, when carbamazepine is taken continuously it induces its own metabolism by the cytochrome P450 isoenzyme CYP3A4, thereby possibly opposing the effects of this interaction.[4]

Importance and management

It seems that in practice no clinically relevant interaction is likely to occur between omeprazole and carbamazepine. For lansoprazole, information seems to be limited to this handful of reports from which no broad general conclusions can be drawn. Pantoprazole appears not to affect the pharmacokinetics of carbamazepine.

1. Wyeth (UK). Personal communication, September 2001.
2. Naidu MUR, Shoba J, Dixit VK, Kumar A, Kumar TR, Sekhar KR, Sekhar EC. Effect of multiple dose omeprazole on the pharmacokinetics of carbamazepine. *Drug Invest* (1994) 7, 8–12.
3. Dixit RK, Chawla AB, Kumar N, Garg SK. Effect of omeprazole on the pharmacokinetics of sustained-release carbamazepine in healthy male volunteers. *Methods Find Exp Clin Pharmacol* (2001) 23, 37–9.
4. Böttiger Y, Bertilsson L. No effect on plasma carbamazepine concentration with concomitant omeprazole treatment. *Drug Invest* (1995) 9, 180–1.
5. Huber R, Bliesath H, Hartmann M, Steinijans VW, Koch H, Mascher H, Wurst W. Pantoprazole does not interact with the pharmacokinetics of carbamazepine. *Int J Clin Pharmacol Ther* (1998) 36, 521–4.

Carbamazepine + Retinoids

An isolated report describes a patient who did not respond to etretinate until the carbamazepine she was taking was withdrawn. A study in one patient found that isotretinoin modestly reduced the plasma levels of both carbamazepine and its active metabolite.

Clinical evidence, mechanism, importance and management

(a) Etretinate

A girl taking carbamazepine and valproate and with pityriasis rubra pilaris did not respond to etretinate for a period of 2 months and had none of its characteristic mucocutaneous adverse effects. When the carbamazepine was withdrawn and the valproate dose increased, she had a good response to etretinate within 6 weeks. It was suggested that carbamazepine may have reduced the bioavailability or increased the metabolism of etretinate.[1] Note that etretinate is extensively metabolised to acitretin, and that acitretin use is now preferred to etretinate. This appears to be an isolated case, and its general relevance to the use of etretinate or acitretin is unknown.

(b) Isotretinoin

The AUC of carbamazepine in a patient with epilepsy taking carbamazepine 600 mg daily was reduced by 11% when isotretinoin 500 micrograms/kg daily was taken, and by 24% when isotretinoin 1 mg/kg daily was taken. The AUC of carbamazepine-10,11-epoxide (the active metabolite of carbamazepine) was reduced by 21% and 44% by the small and large doses of isotretinoin, respectively. The patient had no adverse effects.[2] Although the author of the report suggests that monitoring may be necessary in patients given both drugs, changes of this magnitude, especially those seen with the lower dose of isotretinoin, are not usually clinically significant.

1. Mohammed KN. Unresponsiveness to etretinate during anticonvulsant therapy. *Dermatology* (1992)185, 79.
2. Marsden JR. Effect of isotretinoin on carbamazepine pharmacokinetics. *Br J Dermatol* (1988) 119, 403–4.

Carbamazepine + SNRIs

Carbamazepine does not appear to alter the pharmacokinetics of levomilnacipran or milnacipran, and these drugs do not appear to affect carbamazepine pharmacokinetics. The concurrent use of venlafaxine and carbamazepine led to hyponatraemia in one patient.

Clinical evidence, mechanism, importance and management

(a) Levomilnacipran

The US manufacturer of levomilnacipran briefly notes that in a study, carbamazepine (dose not specified) decreased the AUC and maximum concentration of levomilnacipran by about 25%, but the pharmacokinetics of carbamazepine were not affected.[1] The minor change in levomilnacipran exposure is not deemed clinically relevant, and no dose adjustments are recommended on concurrent use.[1]

(b) Milnacipran

The US manufacturer briefly notes that in a study, giving milnacipran 100 mg daily with carbamazepine 200 mg twice daily did not result in a clinically relevant change in the pharmacokinetics of milnacipran. No change in the pharmacokinetics of carbamazepine or its epoxide metabolite were seen.[2] No dose adjustments are necessary on concurrent use.

(c) Venlafaxine

A case report describes a woman taking carbamazepine 800 mg at breakfast, and 400 mg at lunch and dinner, lamotrigine 100 mg twice daily and phenobarbital 100 mg twice daily, who developed hyponatraemia following the addition of venlafaxine 150 mg daily and mirtazapine. Her sodium concentration decreased from 142.5 mmol/L at the time when venlafaxine was added, to 124.8 mmol/L 2 years later, at which point she experienced syncope. The authors attribute this to the syndrome of inappropriate secretion of antidiuretic hormone caused by the combination of carbamazepine, lamotrigine, and venlafaxine.[3] However, carbamazepine and venlafaxine are associated with this effect, whereas lamotrigine is not. Therefore an interaction between venlafaxine and carbamazepine seems a likely cause of the hyponatraemia. The clinical relevance of this case is unclear.

Note that venlafaxine can cause seizures and should therefore be used with caution in patients with epilepsy.

1. Fetzima (Levomilnacipran hydrochloride). Forest Pharmaceuticals, Inc. US Prescribing information, July 2014.
2. Savella (Milnacipran hydrochloride). Forest Pharmaceuticals, Inc. US prescribing information, January 2015.
3. Ruiz Ginés MA, García García S, Ruiz Ginés JA. Tze Kiong E, Fernández Rodríguez E. Hiponatremia sintomática secundaria a tratamiento conjunto antiocomicial y antidepresivo: ¿riesgo de muerte súbita en epilepsia? *An Med Interna* (2007) 24, 335–8.

Carbamazepine + SSRIs

Carbamazepine exposure can be increased by fluoxetine and fluvoxamine, resulting in toxicity. Citalopram, paroxetine, and sertraline do not appear to affect the pharmacokinetics of carbamazepine, but an increase in carbamazepine concentrations was seen in one case involving sertraline.

Citalopram, paroxetine, and sertraline concentrations might be reduced by carbamazepine. The use of carbamazepine with an SSRI has, rarely, led to effects such as hyponatraemia, serotonin syndrome, and parkinsonism.

Clinical evidence

(a) Citalopram

In a study in 12 healthy subjects, citalopram 40 mg daily for 2 weeks did not affect the pharmacokinetics of carbamazepine 400 mg daily.[1] An approximate 30% decrease in citalopram concentrations occurred in 6 patients taking citalopram 40 to 60 mg daily when they were given carbamazepine 200 to 400 mg daily for 4 weeks. Despite this decrease, concurrent use was considered clinically useful.[2] Similarly, two patients with epilepsy, major depression, and panic disorder had increased citalopram concentrations (one had an improved antidepressant response, but the other patient experienced tremor and increased anxiety) when carbamazepine was replaced with oxcarbazepine.[3]

(b) Fluoxetine

Two patients developed carbamazepine toxicity (including diplopia, blurred vision, tremor, vertigo, nausea, and tinnitus) within 7 and 10 days of starting to take fluoxetine 20 mg daily. Their serum carbamazepine concentrations were found to have increased by about 33% and 60%, respectively. The problem was resolved in one patient by reducing the carbamazepine dose from 1 g to 800 mg daily, and in the other by stopping fluoxetine.[4] The effects seen in these cases are supported by a study in 6 healthy patients, where adding fluoxetine 20 mg daily to steady-state carbamazepine caused an increase in the AUC of carbamazepine and carbamazepine-10,11-epoxide (its active metabolite) of about 25 to 50%.[5]

In contrast, in 8 patients with epilepsy taking stable doses of carbamazepine, fluoxetine 20 mg daily for 3 weeks was found to have no effect on the serum concentrations of carbamazepine or carbamazepine-10,11-epoxide.[6]

Aside from these pharmacokinetic changes two cases of parkinsonism developed within 3 and 9 days of adding fluoxetine to carbamazepine treatment. In both cases carbamazepine concentrations were unaffected.[7] A case of serotonin syndrome (including shivering, agitation, myoclonic-like leg contractions, and diaphoresis) has also been seen in a woman taking carbamazepine 200 mg daily and fluoxetine 20 mg daily.[8]

(c) Fluvoxamine

Increased serum concentrations and signs of carbamazepine toxicity (nausea, vomiting) were seen in 3 patients taking long-term carbamazepine when they were given fluvoxamine. In one patient, the carbamazepine concentration almost doubled within 10 days of starting fluvoxamine 50 to 100 mg daily. The interaction was accommodated by reducing the carbamazepine dose by 200 mg daily in all three (from 1 g to 800 mg in one patient, and from 800 to 600 mg daily in the other two).[9,10] An approximate doubling of carbamazepine concentrations has also been seen in other patients given fluvoxamine.[11-14]

In contrast, in 7 patients with epilepsy taking stable doses of carbamazepine, fluvoxamine 100 mg daily for 3 weeks was found to have no effect on the serum concentrations of carbamazepine or carbamazepine-10,11-epoxide.[6] Furthermore, a literature search[15] by the manufacturers of fluvoxamine only identified 8 cases of an interaction between fluvoxamine and carbamazepine up until 1995.

(d) Paroxetine

In patients with epilepsy, paroxetine 30 mg daily for 16 days did not affect the plasma concentration or therapeutic effects of carbamazepine. The steady-state paroxetine plasma concentration was lower in those taking carbamazepine (27 nanograms/mL) than in those taking sodium valproate (73 nanograms/mL).[16]

An elderly patient taking carbamazepine 200 mg daily then 400 mg daily for neuropathic pain associated with herpes zoster infection, was given paroxetine 20 mg daily for depression. He developed vertigo, bradycardia, and syncope and his plasma sodium was found to be low (120 mmol/L). Sodium concentrations returned to normal (135 mmol/L) over several weeks after carbamazepine was withdrawn.[17]

(e) Sertraline

A placebo-controlled study in 13 healthy subjects (7 taking sertraline, 6 taking placebo) found that sertraline 200 mg daily for 17 days had no effect on the pharmacokinetics of carbamazepine 200 mg twice daily or on its metabolite, carbamazepine-10,11-epoxide. In addition, sertraline did not potentiate the cognitive effects of carbamazepine.[18]

However, an isolated report describes a woman who had taken carbamazepine 600 mg and flecainide 100 mg daily for 2 years, who had a rise in her minimum serum carbamazepine concentration from 4.7 micrograms/mL to 8.5 micrograms/mL within 4 weeks of starting sertraline 100 mg daily. After 3 months of treatment, her carbamazepine concentration was 11.9 micrograms/mL. At the same time she developed pancytopenia (interpreted as a toxic bone marrow reaction to the increased carbamazepine concentration), which improved when both carbamazepine and sertraline were stopped.[19]

An isolated report describes a woman with a schizoaffective disorder, successfully treated for 3 years with haloperidol and carbamazepine, who was given sertraline 50 mg daily for depression. When she failed to respond, the sertraline dose was progressively increased to 300 mg daily but her sertraline plasma concentration remained low (about 17 to 25% of that predicted). Another patient taking carbamazepine similarly failed to respond to the addition of sertraline and had a low sertraline concentration.[20] In an analysis of plasma sertraline concentrations, the concentration-to-daily-dose ratio of sertraline was 68% lower in patients who had taken sertraline with carbamazepine compared with those who had taken sertraline without carbamazepine,[21] suggesting that carbamazepine lowered the concentration of sertraline.

Mechanism

The evidence suggests that fluoxetine and fluvoxamine inhibit the metabolism of carbamazepine by the liver (presumably by inhibiting CYP3A4) so that its loss from the body is reduced, leading to a rise in its serum concentration.[5,12] Fluoxetine and fluvoxamine both have some minor inhibitory effects on CYP3A4.

Citalopram, sertraline and paroxetine are all metabolised by CYP2D6, to varying degrees, with CYP3A4 also being involved in the metabolism of citalopram and sertraline (also to varying degrees). Carbamazepine is a potent inducer of CYP3A4 and a weak inducer of CYP2D6, which results in reduced exposure to these SSRIs. Carbamazepine and paroxetine might cause hyponatraemia so the reduced sodium concentrations seen could be due to the combined adverse effects of these drugs.[17,22]

Importance and management

Information on an interaction between carbamazepine and fluoxetine or fluvoxamine appears to be limited to these reports. Not all patients appear to be affected, but because it is not possible to identify which patients are at risk, it would seem prudent to be alert for an increase in the carbamazepine serum concentration and toxicity (such as nausea, vomiting, ataxia, and drowsiness) if fluoxetine or fluvoxamine is used concurrently. If toxicity is suspected, monitor the carbamazepine concentration, and reduce the dose as necessary. The manufacturers of fluoxetine suggest that carbamazepine should be started at or adjusted towards the lower end of the dose range in those taking fluoxetine. They additionally suggest caution if fluoxetine has been taken during the previous 5 weeks.[23]

There would seem to be no particular need to monitor the carbamazepine concentration in patients taking citalopram, paroxetine, or sertraline. However, be aware that these SSRIs might be less effective in the presence of carbamazepine. Consider increasing the dose if necessary.

Note that SSRIs can increase seizure frequency and should therefore be used with caution in patients with epilepsy, and avoided in those with unstable epilepsy.

1. Møller SE, Larsen F, Khan AZ, Rolan PE. Lack of effect of citalopram on the steady-state pharmacokinetics of carbamazepine in healthy male subjects. *J Clin Psychopharmacol* (2001) 21, 493–9.
2. Steinacher L, Vandel P, Zullino DF, Eap CB, Brawand-Amey M, Baumann P. Carbamazepine augmentation in depressive patients non-responding to citalopram: a pharmacokinetic and clinical pilot study. *Eur Neuropsychopharmacol* (2002) 12, 255–60.
3. Leinonen E, Lepola U, Koponen H. Substituting carbamazepine with oxcarbazepine increases citalopram levels. A report on two cases. *Pharmacopsychiatry* (1996) 29, 156–8.
4. Pearson HJ. Interaction of fluoxetine with carbamazepine. *J Clin Psychiatry* (1990) 51, 126.
5. Grimsley SR, Jann MW, Carter JG, D'Mello AP, D'Souza MJ. Increased carbamazepine plasma concentrations after fluoxetine coadministration. *Clin Pharmacol Ther* (1991) 50, 10–15.
6. Spina E, Avenoso A, Pollicino AM, Caputi AP, Fazio A, Pisani F. Carbamazepine coadministration with fluoxetine or fluvoxamine. *Ther Drug Monit* (1993) 15, 247–50.
7. Gernaat HBPE, van de Woude J, Touw DJ. Fluoxetine and parkinsonism in patients taking carbamazepine. *Am J Psychiatry* (1991) 148, 1604–5.
8. Dursun SM, Mathew VM, Reveley MA. Toxic serotonin syndrome after fluoxetine plus carbamazepine. *Lancet* (1993) 342, 442–3.
9. Fritze J, Unsorg B, Lanczik M. Interaction between carbamazepine and fluvoxamine. *Acta Psychiatr Scand* (1991) 84, 583–4.
10. Fritze J, Lanczik M. Pharmacokinetic interactions of carbamazepine and fluvoxamine. *Pharmacopsychiatry* (1993) 26, 153.
11. Bonnet P, Vandel S, Nezelof S, Sechter D, Bizouard P. Carbamazepine, fluvoxamine. Is there a pharmacokinetic interaction? *Therapie* (1992) 47, 165.
12. Martinelli V, Bocchetta A, Palmas AM, del Zompo M. An interaction between carbamazepine and fluvoxamine. *Br J Clin Pharmacol* (1993) 36, 615–16.
13. Debruille C, Robert H, Cottencin O, Regnaut N, Gignac C. Interaction carbamazépine/fluvoxamine: à propos de deux observations. *J Pharm Clin* (1994) 13, 128–30.
14. Cottencin O, Regnaut N, Thevenon Gignac C, Thomas P, Goudemand M, Debruille C, Robert H. Interaction carbamazepine-fluvoxamine sur le taux plasmatique de carbamazepine. *Encephale* (1995) 21, 141–5.
15. Wagner W, Vause EW. Fluvoxamine. A review of global drug-drug interaction data. *Clin Pharmacokinet* (1995) 29 (Suppl 1), 26–32.
16. Andersen BB, Mikkelsen M, Versterager A, Dam M, Kristensen HB, Pedersen B, Lund J, Mengel H. No influence of the antidepressant paroxetine on carbamazepine, valproate and phenytoin. *Epilepsy Res* (1991) 10, 201–4.
17. Sempere i Verdú E, Bel Reverter M, Palop Larrea V, Hidalgo Mora JJ. Hiponatremia por carbamazepina y paroxetina. *Aten Primaria* (2004) 33, 473.
18. Rapeport WG, Williams SA, Muirhead DC, Dewland PM, Tanner T, Wesnes K. Absence of a sertraline-mediated effect on the pharmacokinetics and pharmacodynamics of carbamazepine. *J Clin Psychiatry* (1996) 57 (Suppl 1), 20–3.
19. Joblin M, Ghose K. Possible interaction of sertraline with carbamazepine. *N Z Med J* (1994) 107, 43.
20. Khan A, Shad MU, Preskorn SH. Lack of sertraline efficacy probably due to an interaction with carbamazepine. *J Clin Psychiatry* (2000) 61, 526–7.
21. Pihlsgård M, Eliasson E.Significant reduction of sertraline plasma levels by carbamazepine and phenytoin. *Eur J Clin Pharmacol* (2002) 57, 915–16.
22. Ruiz Ginés MA, García García S, Ruiz Ginés JA. Tze Kiong E, Fernández Rodríguez E. Hiponatremia sintomática secundaria a tratamiento conjunto antiocomicial y antidepresivo: ¿riesgo de muerte súbita en epilepsia? *An Med Interna* (2007) 24, 335–8.
23. Prozac (Fluoxetine hydrochloride). Eli Lilly and Company Ltd. UK Summary of product characteristics, October 2014.

Carbamazepine + Ticlopidine

One case report suggests that ticlopidine may have increased carbamazepine levels, with associated toxicity.

Clinical evidence, mechanism, importance and management

A 67-year-old man taking carbamazepine 600 mg twice daily developed symptoms of carbamazepine toxicity (drowsiness, dizziness, ataxia) within a week of starting to take ticlopidine 250 mg twice daily. His carbamazepine level one week after starting the ticlopidine was 17.7 [micrograms/mL], but it had been only 10.1 [micrograms/mL] five weeks earlier. The carbamazepine dose was reduced to 500 mg twice daily, which resolved the symptoms, and resulted in a carbamazepine level of 12.5 [micrograms/mL] one week later. After stopping the ticlopidine, carbamazepine levels fell to 9.9 [micrograms/mL]. It was suggested that ticlopidine may interfere with carbamazepine metabolism.[1] However, carbamazepine is principally metabolised by the cytochrome P450 isoenzyme CYP3A4, and ticlopidine is not usually considered an inhibitor of this isoenzyme. This appears to be the only report of an interaction between carbamazepine and ticlopidine, and its general relevance is uncertain.

1. Brown RIG, Cooper TG. Ticlopidine-carbamazepine interaction in a coronary stent patient. *Can J Cardiol* (1997) 13, 853–4.

Carbamazepine + Trazodone

A single case report describes a moderate rise in carbamazepine levels in a patient given trazodone. Carbamazepine may moderately decrease trazodone levels.

Clinical evidence, mechanism, importance and management

A 53-year-old man who had been taking carbamazepine 700 mg daily for 7 months (serum levels 7.2 mg/L and 7.9 mg/L) started taking trazodone 100 mg daily. Two months later his serum carbamazepine levels were 10 mg/L and the concentration-to-dose ratio had increased by about 26%, but no signs or symptoms of carbamazepine toxicity were seen. The reasons for this interaction are not known but the authors suggest that it might occur because trazodone inhibits the cytochrome P450 isoenzyme CYP3A4, resulting in a reduction in the metabolism of carbamazepine.[1]

This seems to be the first and only report of raised carbamazepine levels with trazodone, and its general importance is unknown. The rise was only moderate and in this case was clinically irrelevant, but a carbamazepine serum rise of 26% might possibly be of importance in those patients with serum levels already near the top end of the therapeutic range. Therefore if carbamazepine adverse effects (e.g. nausea, vomiting, ataxia, drowsiness) develop in a patient taking trazodone, consider an interaction as a possible cause.

In 6 patients taking trazodone 150 or 300 mg daily, the addition of carbamazepine 400 mg daily for 4 weeks decreased the plasma levels of trazodone by 24%, and decreased the levels of the active metabolite of trazodone by 40%.[2] However, the combination was considered clinically useful in three of the cases.[2,3] In another study, when carbamazepine 400 mg daily was given with trazodone 100 to 300 mg daily, the plasma levels of trazodone and its active metabolite were reduced by 76% and 60%, respectively.[4,5] The FDA in the US and the manufacturers of trazodone recommend that patients should be closely monitored and trazodone doses increased if necessary when both drugs are given.[4-7]

1. Romero AS, Delgado RG, Peña MF. Interaction between trazodone and carbamazepine. *Ann Pharmacother* (1999) 33, 1370.
2. Otani K, Ishida M, Kaneko S, Mihara K, Ohkubo T, Osanai T, Sugawara K. Effects of carbamazepine coadministration on plasma concentrations of trazodone and its active metabolite, *m*-chlorophenylpiperazine. *Ther Drug Monit* (1996) 18, 164–7.
3. Otani K, Yasui N, Kaneko S, Ohkubo T, Osanai T, Sugawara K. Carbamazepine augmentation therapy in three patients with trazodone-resistant unipolar depression. *Int Clin Psychopharmacol* (1996) 11, 55–7.
4. Desyrel (Trazodone hydrochloride). Bristol-Myers Squibb Company. US Prescribing information, February 2009.
5. Trazodone hydrochloride. Apotex Inc. US Prescribing information, August 2014.
6. Molipaxin Tablets (Trazodone hydrochloride). Sanofi-Aventis. UK Summary of product characteristics, March 2008.
7. Lewis-Hall FC. Bristol-Myers Squibb Company. Letter to healthcare professionals, April 2004.

Carbamazepine + Valnoctamide

Carbamazepine toxicity may develop if valnoctamide is also taken.

Clinical evidence

A study in 6 patients with epilepsy taking carbamazepine 800 to 1200 mg daily found that valnoctamide 200 mg three times daily for 7 days caused a 1.5- to 6.5-fold increase in the serum levels of carbamazepine-10,11-epoxide (an active metabolite of carbamazepine). Clinical signs of carbamazepine toxicity (drowsiness, ataxia, nystagmus) were seen in 4 patients. Two patients were also taking phenobarbital or phenytoin, and the serum levels of these drugs were unaffected by valnoctamide.[1] A further study in 6 healthy subjects found that valnoctamide 600 mg daily for 8 days increased the half-life of carbamazepine-10,11-epoxide, after a single 100-mg dose of carbamazepine, threefold (from 6.7 to 19.7 hours) and decreased its oral clearance fourfold.[2]

Mechanism

Valnoctamide inhibits the enzyme epoxide hydrolase, which is concerned with the metabolism and elimination of carbamazepine and its active epoxide metabolite.[1,2]

Importance and management

Information is limited but the interaction between carbamazepine and valnoctamide appears to be established. Patients taking carbamazepine who also take valnoctamide could rapidly develop carbamazepine toxicity because the metabolism of its major metabolite, carbamazepine-10,11-epoxide, is inhibited. This interaction is very similar to the interaction that occurs between carbamazepine and valpromide (an isomer of valnoctamide), see 'Carbamazepine and related drugs + Valproate', below. Concurrent valnoctamide should be avoided unless the carbamazepine dose can be reduced appropriately.

1. Pisani F, Fazio A, Artesi C, Oteri G, Spina E, Tomson T, Perucca E. Impairment of carbamazepine-10,11-epoxide elimination by valnoctamide, a valpromide isomer, in healthy subjects. *Br J Clin Pharmacol* (1992) 34, 85–7.
2. Pisani F, Haj-Yehia A, Fazio A, Artesi C, Oteri G, Perucca E, Kroetz DL, Levy RH, Bialer M. Carbamazepine-valnoctamide interaction in epileptic patients: in vitro/in vivo correlation. *Epilepsia* (1993) 34, 954–9.

Carbamazepine and related drugs + Valproate

Carbamazepine concentrations are usually only minimally affected by sodium valproate, valproic acid or valpromide, but a larger rise in the concentrations of its active metabolite, carbamazepine-10,11-epoxide, might occur.

Carbamazepine might reduce the serum concentrations of valproate. Concurrent use might increase the incidence of sodium valproate-induced hepatotoxicity.

No pharmacokinetic interaction appears to occur between eslicarbazepine or oxcarbazepine and valproate. An isolated report describes valproate toxicity after oxcarbazepine was added. Concentrations of the active metabolite of oxcarbazepine, monohydroxyoxcarbazepine, might be reduced when oxcarbazepine is given with valproate. When carbamazepine is switched to oxcarbazepine, valproate concentrations might rise.

Clinical evidence

(a) Effects on carbamazepine

1. Sodium valproate or Valproic acid. A study in 7 adult patients with epilepsy who had been taking carbamazepine 8.3 to 13.3 mg/kg for more than 2 months found that their steady-state carbamazepine serum concentrations were reduced by an average of 24% (range 3 to 59%) over a 6-day period when they were given sodium valproate 1 g twice daily. The carbamazepine concentrations were reduced in 6 of the patients and remained unchanged in one. The concentrations of the active metabolite of carbamazepine, carbamazepine-10,11-epoxide, increased by a mean of 38%, with small decreases or no change in 4 patients and 24 to 150% increases in the remaining 3 patients.[1,2]

Other reports state that reductions,[3,4] no changes[3,5-7] and even a small increase[4] in carbamazepine concentrations have been seen in some patients also taking sodium valproate or valproic acid. The serum concentrations of carbamazepine-10,11-epoxide are reported to be increased by about 50 to 100%.[6,8-10] This active metabolite might cause the development of marked adverse effects such as blurred vision, dizziness, vomiting, tiredness and even nystagmus.[6-8,11] Acute psychosis, tentatively attributed to elevated epoxide concentrations, occurred when carbamazepine was given to a patient taking sodium valproate.[12]

2. Valpromide. Symptoms of carbamazepine toxicity, without increases in carbamazepine concentrations, developed in 5 out of 7 patients with epilepsy taking carbamazepine when concurrent treatment with sodium valproate was replaced by valpromide. The toxicity appeared to be connected with a 4-fold increase in the serum concentrations of the active metabolite of carbamazepine, carbamazepine-10,11-epoxide, which rose to 8.5 micrograms/mL.[13]

In another study in 6 patients with epilepsy the serum concentrations of carbamazepine-10,11-epoxide increased by 4.3-fold (range 2.1- to 9.6-fold) within a week of starting valpromide, and two of the patients developed confusion, dizziness and vomiting. The symptoms disappeared and carbamazepine-10,11-epoxide serum concentrations reduced when the valpromide dose was reduced by one-third.[6]

A study in healthy subjects given a single 100-mg oral dose of carbamazepine-10,11-epoxide confirmed that valpromide 300 mg twice daily for 8 days reduced carbamazepine-10,11-epoxide clearance by 73%, and increased its maximum concentrations by 62%.[14]

(b) Effects on eslicarbazepine

A population pharmacokinetic model using data from 641 patients enrolled in phase III eslicarbazepine studies found that the exposure to eslicarbazepine was not affected by the concurrent use of **valproic acid** (172 patients).[15]

(c) Effects on oxcarbazepine

A study in 35 patients with epilepsy found that when oxcarbazepine 300 mg three times daily was added to treatment with **sodium valproate** for 3 weeks there were no clinically relevant changes in the pharmacokinetics of oxcarbazepine.[16] In a study in children given oxcarbazepine, **valproic acid** had no effect on the clearance of the active metabolite of oxcarbazepine, monohydroxyoxcarbazepine.[17] Similarly, another study found no difference in the pharmacokinetics of oxcarbazepine or its active metabolite, monohydroxyoxcarbazepine, between 8 patients taking valproate and 8 controls.[18] In contrast, the manufacturers of oxcarbazepine, briefly note that **valproic acid** reduced the concentrations of monohydroxyoxcarbazepine by 18%.[19,20]

(d) Effects on valproate

A pharmacokinetic study in 6 healthy subjects found that carbamazepine 200 mg daily increased the valproic acid clearance over a 17-day period by 30%.[21]

Other reports have described reductions in serum valproate concentrations of 34 to 38% when carbamazepine was added,[22-24] and increases of 50 to 65% when carbamazepine was withdrawn.[25,26] The increase appears to reach a plateau after about 4 weeks.[26] A pharmacokinetic model has been devised to estimate valproate clearance when it is given with carbamazepine.[27]

A study in 35 patients with epilepsy found that when oxcarbazepine 300 mg three times daily was added to treatment with sodium valproate for 3 weeks there were no clinically relevant changes in the pharmacokinetics of valproate.[16]

A population pharmacokinetic model using data from 641 patients enrolled in phase III eslicarbazepine studies, found that the clearance of valproic acid was not affected by concurrent use.[15] A case report describes a 51-year-old woman taking valproate 1.5g twice daily who was started on oxcarbazepine titrated to 600 mg twice daily for persistent mania. Her valproate dose was reduced to 1 g twice daily but 4 weeks later, she developed symptoms attributed to catatonia (prolonged speech latency, thought blocking, hypoactivity and needed total assistance for meals, ambulation etc.). Valproate toxicity was suspected when her total valproate concentration was found to be 115.6 micrograms/mL (compared with 105 micrograms/mL on admission) and her free valproate concentration was more than double the top of the reference range (47.8 micrograms/mL, range 6 to 20 micrograms/mL). Oxcarbazepine was stopped and 5 days later her total and free valproate concentrations had more or less returned to normal. Oxcarbazepine was restarted at a dose of 300 mg twice daily and similar rises in valproate concentrations were seen 5 days later but returned to normal within 7 days of oxcarbazepine being stopped.[28]

(e) Effects of replacing carbamazepine with oxcarbazepine on valproate

A double-blind, crossover comparison of oxcarbazepine and carbamazepine in patients with epilepsy found that when carbamazepine was replaced by oxcarbazepine in 14 patients also taking valproate, the serum concentrations of valproate increased by 32%. In 18 patients taking carbamazepine, valproate and **phenytoin**, replacement of carbamazepine with oxcarbazepine caused an increase in the valproate serum concentrations of 21%. The study extended over 12 weeks to establish steady-state concentrations.[29] Another study in 4 patients with epilepsy (aged 13 to 17 years) found that the concentration-to-dose ratio of free valproate increased when the patients were switched from carbamazepine to oxcarbazepine, with an increase in valproate adverse effects, which resolved when the valproate dose was decreased.[30]

(f) Other effects

Evidence from epidemiological studies suggests that the risk of fatal hepatotoxicity is higher when valproate is given with other antiepileptics than when it is given alone, especially in infants.[31,32] A single case report describes hepatocellular and cholestatic jaundice and a reversible Parkinsonian syndrome in a woman taking sodium valproate and carbamazepine, which reversed when the carbamazepine was withdrawn. Concentrations of both drugs did not exceed the therapeutic range at any stage. The Parkinsonian syndrome was attributed to a drug interaction, whereas the hepatotoxicity was considered most likely to be due to carbamazepine, although valproate might have contributed.[33]

Mechanism

The evidence suggests that carbamazepine increases the metabolism of valproate, so that it is cleared from the body more quickly. Carbamazepine might also increase the formation of a minor but hepatotoxic metabolite of valproic acid (2-propyl-4-pentenoic acid or 4-ene-VPA).[34,35]

The latter stages of carbamazepine metabolism appear to be inhibited by both valproate and its amide derivative, valpromide.[36] The concentrations of the metabolite, carbamazepine-10,11-epoxide, increase during concurrent use, probably by inhibition of its metabolism to carbamazepine-10,11-trans-diol,[37-39] by epoxide hydrolase. Valpromide was found to be about 100 times more potent an inhibitor of this enzyme than valproic acid *in vitro*[40] and caused a 3-fold higher rise in epoxide concentrations than valproate in one study.[6] The carbamazepine-10,11-epoxide metabolite has antiepileptic activity, but it might also cause toxicity if its serum concentrations become excessive.[6,41]

It has also been suggested that valproate is not a selective inhibitor of epoxide hydrolase but that it inhibits all the steps of the epoxide-diol pathway.[42] The trans-diol metabolite is then further converted by glucuronidation, and it seems that this step is also inhibited.[39]

Importance and management

An interaction between **carbamazepine** and valproate is moderately well documented, and established. A small to modest reduction in carbamazepine concentrations might occur, but there could be a modest or greater rise in the active epoxide metabolite. Therefore, be alert for signs of toxicity, which could indicate high concentrations of carbamazepine-10,11-epoxide and a need to reduce the carbamazepine dose. Also be alert for reductions in the serum concentrations of valproate if carbamazepine is added. Sodium valproate has been associated with serious hepatotoxicity, especially in children aged less than 3 years, and this has been more common in those receiving other antiepileptics. Sodium valproate monotherapy is to be preferred in this group.

There is also some debate about whether the combination of valproate (especially valpromide) and carbamazepine should be avoided, not only because of the risk of toxicity but also because inhibition of epoxide hydrolase might be undesirable.[13] This enzyme is possibly important for the detoxification of a number of teratogenic, mutagenic and carcinogenic epoxides.[6,13] More study is needed.

Information about the concurrent use of **oxcarbazepine** and valproate is more limited than with carbamazepine, but no pharmacokinetic interaction appears to occur. The report[28] describing valproate toxicity after oxcarbazepine was started is isolated, and the general clinical importance of this is unclear. Concentrations of the active metabolite of oxcarbazepine, monohydroxyoxcarbazepine, might be reduced, but the clinical importance of this is not known. If oxcarbazepine is substituted for carbamazepine, be aware that the concentrations of valproate could increase.

The effects of concurrent use of **eslicarbazepine** and valproate are not well studied, but the limited evidence available suggests that an interaction does not occur.

1. Levy RH, Morselli PL, Bianchetti G, Guyot M, Brachet-Liermain A, Loiseau P. Interaction between valproic acid and carbamazepine in epileptic patients. In: RH Levy, (ed). Metabolism of Antiepileptic Drugs. New York: Raven Press, 1984: 45–51.
2. Levy RH, Moreland TA, Morselli PL, Guyot M, Brachet-Liermain A, Loiseau P. Carbamazepine/valproic acid interaction in man and rhesus monkey. *Epilepsia* (1984) 25, 338–45.
3. Wilder BJ, Willmore LJ, Bruni J, Villarreal HJ. Valproic acid: interaction with other anticonvulsant drugs. *Neurology* (1978) 28, 892–6.
4. Varma R, Michos GA, Varma RS, Hoshino AY. Clinical trials of Depakene (valproic acid) coadministered with other anticonvulsants in epileptic patients. *Res Commun Psychol Psychiatr Behav* (1980) 5, 265–73.
5. Fowler GW. Effects of dipropylacetate on serum levels of anticonvulsants in children. *Proc West Pharmacol Soc* (1978) 21, 37–40.
6. Pisani F, Fazio A, Oteri G, Ruello C, Gitto C, Russo R, Perucca E. Sodium valproate and valpromide: differential interactions with carbamazepine in epileptic patients. *Epilepsia* (1986) 27, 548–52.
7. Sunaoshi W, Miura H, Takanashi S, Shira H, Hosoda N. Influence of concurrent administration of sodium valproate on the plasma concentrations of carbamazepine and its epoxide and diol metabolites. *Jpn J Psychiatry Neurol* (1991) 45, 474–7.
8. Kutt H, Solomon G, Peterson H, Dhar A, Caronna J. Accumulation of carbamazepine epoxide caused by valproate contributing to intoxication syndromes. *Neurology* (1985) 35 (Suppl 1), 286.
9. Liu H, Delgado MR. Improved therapeutic monitoring of drug interactions in epileptic children using carbamazepine polytherapy. *Ther Drug Monit* (1994) 16, 132–8.
10. Macphee GJA, Mitchell JR, Wiseman L, McLellan AR, Park BK, McInnes GT, Brodie MJ. Effect of sodium valproate on carbamazepine disposition and psychomotor profile in man. *Br J Clin Pharmacol* (1988) 25, 59–66.
11. Rambeck B, Sälke-Treumann A, May T, Boenigk HE. Valproic acid-induced carbamazepine-10,11-epoxide toxicity in children and adolescents. *Eur Neurol* (1990) 30, 79–83.
12. McKee RJW, Larkin JG, Brodie MJ. Acute psychosis with carbamazepine and sodium valproate. *Lancet* (1989) i, 167.
13. Meijer JWA, Binnie CD, Debets RMChr, Van Parys JAP and de Beer-Pawlikowski NKB. Possible hazard of valpromide-carbamazepine combination therapy in epilepsy. *Lancet* (1984) i, 802.
14. Perucca E, Pisani F, Spina E, Oteri G, Fazio A, Bertilsson L. Effects of valpromide and viloxazine on the elimination of carbamazepine-10,11-epoxide, an active metabolite of carbamazepine. *Pharm Res* (1989) 21, 111–12.
15. Falcão A, Fuseau E, Nunes T, Almeida L, Soares-da-Silva P. Pharmacokinetics, drug interactions and exposure-response relationship of eslicarbazepine acetate in adult patients with partial-onset seizures: population pharmacokinetic and pharmacokinetic/pharmacodynamic analyses. *CNS Drugs* (2012) 26, 79–91.
16. McKee PJW, Blacklaw J, Forrest G, Gillham RA, Walker SM, Connelly D, Brodie MJ. A double blind, placebo-controlled interaction study between oxcarbazepine and carbamazepine, sodium valproate and phenytoin in epileptic patients. *Br J Clin Pharmacol* (1994) 37, 27–32.
17. Sallas WM, Milosavljev S, D'Souza J, Hossain M. Pharmacokinetic drug interactions in children taking oxcarbazepine. *Clin Pharmacol Ther* (2003) 74, 138–49.
18. Tartara A, Galimberti CA, Manni R, Morini R, Limido G, Gatti G, Bartoli A, Strada G, Perucca E. The pharmacokinetics of oxcarbazepine and its active metabolite 10-hydroxy-carbazepine in healthy subjects and in epileptic patients treated with phenobarbitone or valproic acid. *Br J Clin Pharmacol* (1993) 36, 366–8.
19. Trileptal (Oxcarbazepine). Novartis Pharmaceuticals UK Ltd. UK Summary of product characteristics, April 2012.
20. Trileptal (Oxcarbazepine). Novartis Pharmaceuticals Corp. US Prescribing information, March 2011.
21. Bowdle TA, Levy RH, Cutler RE. Effects of carbamazepine on valproic acid kinetics in normal subjects. *Clin Pharmacol Ther* (1979) 26, 629–34.
22. Reunanen MI, Luoma P, Myllylä VV, Hokkanen E. Low serum valproic acid concentrations in epileptic patients on combination therapy. *Curr Ther Res* (1980) 28, 456–62.
23. May T, Rambeck B. Serum concentrations of valproic acid: influence of dose and comedication. *Ther Drug Monit* (1985) 7, 387–90.
24. Panesar SK, Orr JM, Farrell K, Burton RW, Kassahun K, Abbott FS. The effect of carbamazepine on valproic acid disposition in adult volunteers. *Br J Clin Pharmacol* (1989) 27, 323–8.
25. Henriksen O, Johannessen SI. Clinical and pharmacokinetic observations on sodium valproate — a 5 year follow-up study in 100 children with epilepsy. *Acta Neurol Scand* (1982) 65, 504–23.
26. Jann MW, Fidone GS, Israel MK, Bonadero P. Increased valproate serum concentrations upon carbamazepine cessation. *Epilepsia* (1988) 29, 578–81.
27. Yukawa E, Honda T, Ohdo S, Higuchi S, Aoyama T. Detection of carbamazepine-induced changes in valproic acid relative clearance in man by simple pharmacokinetic screening. *J Pharm Pharmacol* (1997) 49, 751–6.
28. Xiong GL, Ferranti J, Leamon MH. Toxic interaction between valproate and oxcarbazepine: a case detected by the free valproate level. *J Clin Psychopharmacol* (2008) 28, 472–3.
29. Houtkooper MA, Lammertsma A, Meyer JWA, Goedhart DM, Meinardi H, van Oorschot CAEH, Blom GF, Höppener RJEA, Hulsman JARJ. Oxcarbazepine (GP 47.680): a possible alternative to carbamazepine? *Epilepsia* (1987) 28, 693–8.
30. Battino D, Croci D, Granata T, Bernadi G, Monza G. Changes in unbound and total valproic acid concentrations after replacement of carbamazepine with oxcarbazepine. *Ther Drug Monit* (1992) 14, 376–9.
31. Dreifuss FE, Santilli N, Langer DH, Sweeney KP, Moline KA, Menander KB. Valproic acid hepatic fatalities: a retrospective review. *Neurology* (1987) 37, 379–85.
32. Dreifuss FE, Langer DH, Moline KA, Maxwell DE. Valproic acid hepatic fatalities. II. US experience since 1984. *Neurology* (1989) 39, 201–7.
33. Froomes PR, Stewart MR. A reversible Parkinsonian syndrome and hepatotoxicity following addition of carbamazepine to sodium valproate. *Aust N Z J Med* (1994) 24, 413–14.
34. Levy RH, Rettenmeier AW, Anderson GD, Wilensky AJ, Friel PN, Baillie TA, Acheampong A, Tor J, Guyot M, Loiseau P. Effects of polytherapy with phenytoin, carbamazepine, and stiripentol on formation of 4-ene-valproate, a hepatotoxic metabolite of valproic acid. *Clin Pharmacol Ther* (1990) 48, 225–35.
35. Kondo T, Otani K, Hirano T, Kaneko S, Fukushima Y. The effects of phenytoin and carbamazepine on serum concentrations of mono-unsaturated metabolites of valproic acid. *Br J Clin Pharmacol* (1990) 29, 116–9.
36. Pisani F, Fazio A, Oteri G, Spina E, Perucca E and Bertilsson L. Effect of valpromide on the pharmacokinetics of carbamazepine-10,11-epoxide. *Br J Clin Pharmacol* (1988) 25, 611–13.
37. Pisani F, Caputo M, Fazio A, Oteri G, Russo M, Spina E, Perucca E, Bertilsson L. Interaction of carbamazepine-10,11-epoxide, an active metabolite of carbamazepine, with valproate: a pharmacokinetic study. *Epilepsia* (1990) 31, 339–42.
38. Robbins DK, Wedlund PJ, Kuhn R, Baumann RJ, Levy RH, Chang S-L. Inhibition of epoxide hydrolase by valproic acid in epileptic patients receiving carbamazepine. *Br J Clin Pharmacol* (1990) 29, 759–62.
39. Bernus I, Dickinson RG, Hooper WD, Eadie MJ. The mechanism of the carbamazepine-valproate interaction in humans. *Br J Clin Pharmacol* (1997) 44, 21–27.
40. Kerr BM, Rettie AE, Eddy AC, Loiseau P, Guyot M, Wilensky AJ, Levy RH. Inhibition of human liver microsomal epoxide hydrolase by valproate and valpromide: in vitro/in vivo correlation. *Clin Pharmacol Ther* (1989) 46, 82–93. Correction. ibid. 343.
41. Levy RH, Kerr BM, Loiseau P, Guyot M and Wilensky AJ. Inhibition of carbamazepine epoxide elimination by valpromide and valproic acid. *Epilepsia* (1986) 27, 592.
42. Svinarov DA, Pippenger CE. Valproic acid-carbamazepine interaction: is valproic acid a selective inhibitor of epoxide hydrolase? *Ther Drug Monit* (1995) 17, 217–20.

Carbamazepine + Vigabatrin

Vigabatrin does not normally alter carbamazepine levels, although one study has found a modest increase, and one a modest decrease, in carbamazepine levels when vigabatrin was given.

Clinical evidence

In an early clinical study in 12 patients, vigabatrin 2 to 3 g daily did not change the serum levels of carbamazepine.[1] Similarly, other studies found that carbamazepine levels were not significantly altered by the addition of vigabatrin.[2,3] However, in one study, in which 59 patients taking carbamazepine received vigabatrin, 34 patients had an increase in carbamazepine levels, 3 had no change, and 22 had a decrease in carbamazepine levels, resulting in a mean overall increase of 6%, which was not significant.[4] Similarly, in another study 46 out of 66 patients had an increase in carbamazepine level of at least 10% (mean increase about 24%), and in 24 of these patients the carbamazepine level exceeded the reference range.[5] In this study, the increase in carbamazepine level was greater the lower the initial carbamazepine level.[5] In contrast, one study in 15 patients reported a mean 18% *decrease* in carbamazepine levels when vigabatrin was added.[6]

Mechanism

Not understood.

Importance and management

The studies seem to suggest that any change in carbamazepine levels with vigabatrin is of borderline clinical significance and therefore the majority of patients will not be affected. Any change is likely to be more important in patients at the top of the therapeutic carbamazepine range. It would therefore seem prudent to be alert for any increase in carbamazepine adverse effects (such as nausea and vomiting, ataxia, and drowsiness) and consider taking carbamazepine levels and reducing the carbamazepine dose if these develop.

1. Tassinari CA, Michelucci R, Ambrosetto G, Salvi F. Double-blind study of vigabatrin in the treatment of drug-resistant epilepsy. *Arch Neurol* (1987) 44, 907–10.

2. Rimmer EM, Richens A. Interaction between vigabatrin and phenytoin. *Br J Clin Pharmacol* (1989) 27, 27S–33S.
3. Bernardina BD, Fontana E, Vigevano F, Fusco L, Torelli D, Galeone D, Buti D, Cianchetti C, Gnanasakthy A, Iudice A. Efficacy and tolerability of vigabatrin in children with refractory partial seizures: a single-blind dose-increasing study. *Epilepsia* (1995) 36, 687–91.
4. Browne TR, Mattson RH, Penry JK, Smith DB, Treiman DM, Wilder BJ, Ben-Menachem E, Napoliello MJ, Sherry KM, Szabo GK. Vigabatrin for refractory complex partial seizures: multicenter single-blind study with long-term follow up. *Neurology* (1987) 37, 184–9.
5. Jędrzejczak J, Dławichowska E, Owczarek K, Majkowski J. Effect of vigabatrin addition on carbamazepine blood serum levels in patients with epilepsy. *Epilepsy Res* (2000) 39, 115–20.
6. Sánchez-Alcaraz A, Quintana B, López E, Rodríguez I, Llopis P. Effect of vigabatrin on the pharmacokinetics of carbamazepine. *J Clin Pharm Ther* (2002) 27, 427–30.

Eslicarbazepine + Food

Food does not affect the pharmacokinetics of eslicarbazepine.

Clinical evidence, mechanism, importance and management

In a controlled, crossover study in 17 healthy subjects the pharmacokinetics of a single 800-mg dose of eslicarbazepine were no different when given after a standard meal or after a 10-hour fast.[1] Similarly, another controlled study in 12 healthy subjects found that the pharmacokinetics of a single 800-mg dose of eslicarbazepine were no different when given after a standard high-fat meal or after a 10-hour fast.[2] Eslicarbazepine can therefore be given without regard to food.

1. Fontes-Ribeiro C, Macedo T, Nunes T, Neta C, Vasconcelos T, Cerdeira R, Lima R, Rocha JF, Falcão A, Almeida L, Soares-da-Silva P. Dosage form proportionality and food effect of the final tablet formulation of eslicarbazepine acetate: randomized, open-label, crossover, single-centre study in healthy volunteers. *Drugs R D* (2008) 9, 447–54.
2. Maia J, Vaz-da-Silva M, Almeida L, Falcão A, Silveira P, Guimarães S, Graziela P, Soares-da-Silva P. Effect of food on the pharmacokinetic profile of eslicarbazepine acetate (BIA 2-093). *Drugs R D* (2005) 6, 201–6.

Ethosuximide + Isoniazid

A single report describes a patient who developed psychotic behaviour and signs of ethosuximide toxicity when isoniazid was also given.

Clinical evidence, mechanism, importance and management

An patient with epilepsy, who had been stable taking ethosuximide and sodium valproate for 2 years, developed persistent hiccuping, nausea, vomiting, anorexia and insomnia within a week of starting to take isoniazid 300 mg daily. Psychotic behaviour gradually developed over the next 5 weeks and so the isoniazid was stopped. The appearance of these symptoms appeared to be related to the sharp rise in serum ethosuximide levels (from about 50 micrograms/mL up to 198 micrograms/mL).[1] It is suggested that the isoniazid may have inhibited the metabolism of the ethosuximide, leading to accumulation and toxicity. The general importance of this case is uncertain. More study is needed to establish an interaction.

1. van Wieringen A, Vrijlandt CM. Ethosuximide intoxication caused by interaction with isoniazid. *Neurology* (1983) 33, 1227–8.

Ethosuximide + Other antiepileptics

Minor to modest falls in ethosuximide levels may occur if carbamazepine, primidone or phenytoin are also given, whereas methylphenobarbital or valproate may cause a rise in ethosuximide levels. Lamotrigine appears not to affect ethosuximide levels.

Ethosuximide is reported to have caused phenytoin toxicity in a few cases, and it appears that ethosuximide can reduce valproate levels.

Clinical evidence

(a) Barbiturates

In a retrospective analysis, the level-to-dose ratio of ethosuximide was 33% lower in 29 patients with epilepsy taking ethosuximide and **primidone** than in 39 patients taking ethosuximide alone,[1] suggesting that primidone reduces ethosuximide levels.

Similarly, in a study that compared the pharmacokinetics of a single dose of ethosuximide in 10 patients with epilepsy taking **phenobarbital**, phenytoin and/or carbamazepine with 12 healthy controls, the epileptic group had markedly shorter (about halved) ethosuximide half-lives.[2] Conversely, another report stated that ethosuximide levels tended to rise (amount not stated) when **methylphenobarbital** was given (the opposite effect to that which would be expected), but ethosuximide did not appear to be affected by **phenobarbital** or **primidone**.[3] Phenobarbital levels (derived from **primidone**) do not appear to be affected by ethosuximide.[4]

(b) Carbamazepine

A study in 6 healthy subjects taking ethosuximide 500 mg daily found that the mean plasma levels of ethosuximide were reduced by 17% (from 32 mg/mL to 27 mg/mL) by carbamazepine 200 mg daily for 18 days. One individual had a 35% reduction in ethosuximide levels.[5] Another study, which compared 10 patients with epilepsy taking enzyme-inducing antiepileptic drugs, including 4 taking carbamazepine, with 12 healthy controls found that the epileptic group had markedly shorter (about halved) ethosuximide half-lives.[2]

In contrast, the concurrent use of carbamazepine did not affect the correlation between ethosuximide dose and levels in another study.[3]

(c) Lamotrigine

Five children taking ethosuximide and various other antiepileptics had no change in their plasma ethosuximide levels when lamotrigine was also given.[6]

(d) Phenytoin

A study compared the pharmacokinetics of a single dose of ethosuximide in 10 patients with epilepsy taking phenobarbital, phenytoin and/or carbamazepine with 12 healthy controls. The epileptic group had markedly shorter (about halved) ethosuximide half-lives.[2] In contrast, the concurrent use of phenytoin did not affect the correlation between ethosuximide levels and dose in another study.[3]

Three cases have occurred in which ethosuximide appeared to have been responsible for increasing phenytoin levels,[7-9] leading to the development of phenytoin toxicity in 2 patients.[8,9]

(e) Valproate

Four out of 5 patients taking ethosuximide (average dose 27 mg/kg) had an increase in their serum levels of about 50% (from 73 micrograms/mL to 112 micrograms/mL), within 3 weeks of starting to take valproic acid (adjusted to the maximum tolerated dose). Sedation occurred and ethosuximide dose reductions were necessary.[10] In a single-dose study in 6 healthy subjects, the use of sodium valproate for 9 days was reported to have increased the ethosuximide half-life and reduced its clearance by 15%.[11] However, other studies have described no changes[12,13] or even lower serum ethosuximide levels (level to dose ratio reduced by 36%) when valproate was given.[1]

One study in 13 children found that ethosuximide can lower valproate serum levels. In the presence of ethosuximide the valproate levels were lower than with valproate alone (87 micrograms/mL versus 120 micrograms/mL). After stopping ethosuximide the valproate levels rose by about 40%.[14]

Mechanism

The most probable explanation for the fall in ethosuximide levels is that carbamazepine and the other enzyme-inducing antiepileptics increase the metabolism and clearance of ethosuximide, which is known to be metabolised by the cytochrome P450 subfamily CYP3A.[2]

Importance and management

The concurrent use of antiepileptics is common and often advantageous. Information on these interactions is sparse and even contradictory and their clinical importance is uncertain. Nevertheless, good monitoring would clearly be appropriate if these drugs are used with ethosuximide to monitor for potential toxicity and to ensure adequate seizure control.

1. Battino D, Cusi C, Franceschetti S, Moise A, Spina S, Avanzini G. Ethosuximide plasma concentrations: influence of age and associated concomitant therapy. *Clin Pharmacokinet* (1982) 7, 176–80.
2. Giaccone M, Bartoli A, Gatti G, Marchiselli R, Pisani F, Latella MA, Perucca E. Effect of enzyme inducing anticonvulsants on ethosuximide pharmacokinetics in epileptic patients. *Br J Clin Pharmacol* (1996) 41, 575–9.
3. Smith GA, McKauge L, Dubetz D, Tyrer JH, Eadie MJ. Factors influencing plasma concentrations of ethosuximide. *Clin Pharmacokinet* (1979) 4, 38–52.
4. Schmidt D. The effect of phenytoin and ethosuximide on primidone metabolism in patients with epilepsy. *J Neurol* (1975) 209, 115–23.
5. Warren JW, Benmaman JD, Wannamaker BB, Levy RH. Kinetics of a carbamazepine-ethosuximide interaction. *Clin Pharmacol Ther* (1980) 28, 646–51.
6. Eriksson A-S, Hoppu K, Nergårdh A, Boreus L. Pharmacokinetic interactions between lamotrigine and other antiepileptic drugs in children with intractable epilepsy. *Epilepsia* (1996) 37, 769–73.
7. Lander CM, Eadie MJ, Tyrer JH. Interactions between anticonvulsants. *Proc Aust Assoc Neurol* (1975) 12, 111–16.
8. Dawson GW, Brown HW, Clark BG. Serum phenytoin after ethosuximide. *Ann Neurol* (1978) 4, 583–4.
9. Frantzen E, Hansen JM, Hansen OE, Kristensen M. Phenytoin (Dilantin) intoxication. *Acta Neurol Scand* (1967) 43, 440–6.
10. Mattson RH, Cramer JA. Valproic acid and ethosuximide interaction. *Ann Neurol* (1980) 7, 583–4.
11. Pisani F, Narbone MC, Trunfio C, Fazio A, La Rosa G, Oteri G, Di Perri R. Valproic acid-ethosuximide interaction: a pharmacokinetic study. *Epilepsia* (1984) 25, 229–33.
12. Fowler GW. Effect of dipropylacetate on serum levels of anticonvulsants in children. *Proc West Pharmacol Soc* (1978) 21, 37–40.
13. Bauer LA, Harris C, Wilensky AJ, Raisys VA, Levy RH. Ethosuximide kinetics: possible interaction with valproic acid. *Clin Pharmacol Ther* (1982) 31, 741–5.
14. Sälke-Kellermann RA, May T, Boenigk HE. Influence of ethosuximide on valproic acid serum concentrations. *Epilepsy Res* (1997) 26, 345–349.

Ethosuximide + Ritonavir

Ritonavir is predicted to increase the plasma concentration of ethosuximide.

Clinical evidence, mechanism, importance and management

The US manufacturer of ritonavir states that it might increase the plasma concentration of ethosuximide, and that a dose reduction of ethosuximide might be needed with concurrent use. Monitoring of ethosuximide plasma concentration is recommended, if available.[1] However, the UK manufacturer[2] does not mention this interaction, and there appear to be no published clinical data regarding this.

1. Norvir Capsules (Ritonavir). Abbott Laboratories. US Prescribing information, March 2012.
2. Norvir Tablets (Ritonavir). AbbVie Ltd. UK Summary of product characteristics, September 2012.

Felbamate + Antacids

In one study, an aluminium/magnesium hydroxide-containing antacid had no effect on the absorption of felbamate.

Clinical evidence, mechanism, importance and management

Felbamate 2.4 g daily was given to 9 women with epilepsy for 2 weeks. For a third week the felbamate was taken with an antacid containing **aluminium/magnesium hydroxide** (*Maalox Plus*). No significant changes in the plasma levels or AUC of felbamate were seen.[1] No felbamate dose adjustments would seem to be needed if it is taken with this or any other similar antacid.

1. Sachdeo RC, Narang-Sachdeo SK, Howard JR, Dix RK, Shumaker RC, Perhach JL, Rosenberg A. Effect of antacid on the absorption of felbamate in subjects with epilepsy. *Epilepsia* (1993) 34 (Suppl 6), 79–80.

Felbamate + Erythromycin

Erythromycin does not alter the pharmacokinetics of felbamate.

Clinical evidence, mechanism, importance and management

In a randomised, crossover study, 12 patients with epilepsy were given felbamate 3 g or 3.6 g daily, either alone or with erythromycin 333 mg every 8 hours for 10 days. The pharmacokinetics of felbamate were unchanged by erythromycin.[1] There would therefore seem no need to adjust the dose of felbamate if erythromycin is given.

1. Sachdeo RJ, Narang-Sachdeo SK, Montgomery PA, Shumaker RC, Perhach JL, Lyness WH, Rosenberg A. Evaluation of the potential interaction between felbamate and erythromycin in patients with epilepsy. *J Clin Pharmacol* (1998) 38, 184–90.

Felbamate + Gabapentin

There is some evidence that the half-life of felbamate may be prolonged by gabapentin.

Clinical evidence, mechanism, importance and management

In a retrospective examination of clinical data from patients taking felbamate, its half-life was found to be 24 hours in 40 patients taking felbamate alone, whereas in 18 other patients also taking gabapentin (including 7 taking a third drug), the half-life of felbamate was extended to 32.7 hours.[1] The practical clinical importance of this effect is uncertain. More study is needed.

1. Hussein G, Troupin AS, Montouris G. Gabapentin interaction with felbamate. *Neurology* (1996) 47, 1106.

Fosphenytoin + Miscellaneous

Fosphenytoin is a prodrug of phenytoin, which is rapidly and completely hydrolysed to phenytoin in the body. It is predicted to interact with other drugs in the same way as phenytoin.[1,2] No drugs are known to interfere with the conversion of fosphenytoin to phenytoin.[2]

1. Fierro LS, Savulich DH, Benezra DA. Safety of fosphenytoin sodium. *Am J Health-Syst Pharm* (1996) 53, 2707–12.
2. Pro-Epanutin (Fosphenytoin sodium). Pfizer Ltd. UK Summary of product characteristics, December 2008.

Gabapentin + Antacids

Aluminium/magnesium hydroxide slightly reduces the absorption of gabapentin.

Clinical evidence, mechanism, importance and management

An **aluminium/magnesium hydroxide** antacid (*Maalox TC*) reduced the bioavailability of gabapentin 400 mg by about 20% when given either at the same time or 2 hours after gabapentin. When the antacid was given 2 hours before gabapentin, the bioavailability was reduced by about 10%.[1] These small changes are unlikely to be of clinical importance. Nevertheless, the manufacturers of gabapentin recommend that it is taken at least 2 hours after **aluminium/magnesium-containing antacids**.[2,3]

1. Busch JA, Radulovic LL, Bockbrader HN, Underwood BA, Sedman AJ, Chang T. Effect of Maalox TC® on single-dose pharmacokinetics of gabapentin capsules in healthy subjects. *Pharm Res* (1992) 9 (10 Suppl), S-315.
2. Neurontin (Gabapentin). Pfizer Ltd. UK Summary of product characteristics, April 2012.
3. Neurontin (Gabapentin). Pfizer Inc. US Prescribing information, July 2012.

Gabapentin + Cimetidine

Cimetidine increases the exposure to gabapentin and its prodrug, gabapentin enacarbil, and decreases gabapentin clearance.

Clinical evidence

In a study in 12 subjects, cimetidine 300 mg decreased the oral clearance of gabapentin by 14%, and creatinine clearance decreased by 10%, suggesting a decrease in renal excretion of gabapentin.[1]

In a pharmacokinetic study in 11 healthy subjects, the concurrent use of gabapentin enacarbil 1.2 g daily and cimetidine 400 mg four times daily for 4 days increased the gabapentin AUC by 24% but did not alter the AUC of cimetidine.[2]

Mechanism

Gabapentin is excreted renally by the organic cation transporter (OCT) OCTN1, which is inhibited by cimetidine. Concurrent use therefore results in a decrease in gabapentin clearance. Gabapentin enacarbil is a prodrug of gabapentin that is rapidly converted to gabapentin before reaching the systemic circulation.

Importance and management

The negligible effect of cimetidine on the exposure to gabapentin is not clinically important. No dose adjustment is needed on concurrent use

1. Neurontin (Gabapentin). Pfizer Inc. US Prescribing information, July 2012.
2. Lal R, Sukbuntherng J, Luo W, Vicente V, Blumenthal R, Ho J, Cundy KC. Clinical pharmacokinetic drug interaction studies of gabapentin enacarbil, a novel transported prodrug of gabapentin, with naproxen and cimetidine. *Br J Clin Pharmacol* (2010) 69, 498–507.

Gabapentin + Food

Food, including protein and enteral feeds, does not have a clinically important effect on the absorption of gabapentin.

Clinical evidence, mechanism, importance and management

A high-protein meal (80 g of total protein) increased the maximum serum levels of a single 800-mg dose of gabapentin by 36% in healthy subjects. The AUC was increased by 11%, which was not statistically significant. These findings were the opposite of those expected, because L-amino acids compete for gabapentin intestinal transport *in vitro*.[1] Another study also reported no significant differences in the pharmacokinetics of gabapentin when a single 400- or 800-mg dose was given after a high protein meal rather than in the fasting state.[2]

In another single-dose study, the absorption of gabapentin from capsules did not differ when given intact or opened and mixed with either apple sauce or orange juice, but tended to be higher (AUC increased by 26%) when opened and mixed with a protein-containing vehicle (chocolate pudding).[3] Similarly, no change in absorption was found when gabapentin syrup was mixed with tap water, grape juice, or an **enteral feed** (*Sustacal*), but a modest 31% increase in the AUC was seen when the gabapentin was mixed with **chocolate milk**.[4]

These small changes are unlikely to be of clinical importance, so it does not matter when gabapentin is taken in relation to food.

1. Gidal BE, Maly MM, Budde J, Lensmeyer GL, Pitterle ME, Jones JC. Effect of a high-protein meal on gabapentin pharmacokinetics. *Epilepsy Res* (1996) 23, 71–6.
2. Benetello P, Furlanut M, Fortunato M, Baraldo M, Pea F, Tognon A, Testa G. Oral gabapentin disposition in patients with epilepsy after a high-protein meal. *Epilepsia* (1997) 38, 1140–2.
3. Gidal BE, Maly MM, Kowalski JW, Rutecki PA, Pitterle ME, Cook DE. Gabapentin absorption: effect of mixing with foods of varying macronutrient composition. *Ann Pharmacother* (1998) 32, 405–9.
4. Parnell J, Sheth R, Limdi N, Gidal BE. Oral absorption of gabapentin syrup is not impaired by concomitant administration with various beverages or enteral nutrition supplement. *Epilepsia* (2001) 42 (Suppl 7), 91.

Gabapentin + Naproxen

Naproxen negligibly increases the exposure to gabapentin and its prodrug, gabapentin enacarbil.

Clinical evidence

The US manufacturer of gabapentin briefly notes that in a study in 18 subjects, the concurrent use of naproxen 250 mg with gabapentin 125 mg appeared to increase the absorption of gabapentin by 12% to 15%. Gabapentin had no effect on naproxen pharmacokinetics.[1]

In a pharmacokinetic study in 10 healthy subjects, the concurrent use of gabapentin enacarbil 1.2 g daily and naproxen 500 mg twice daily for 5 days increased the AUC of gabapentin by 13% but did not alter the AUC of naproxen.[2]

Mechanism

Gabapentin enacarbil is a prodrug of gabapentin that, unlike gabapentin, is actively absorbed in the gastrointestinal tract by high-capacity nutrient transporters including mono-carboxylate transporter-1 (MCT-1). Naproxen is also a substrate for MCT-1. The concurrent use of substrates of this transporter does not, therefore, appear to result in a clinically relevant effect.

Importance and management

The pharmacokinetic interaction seen when naproxen is given with gabapentin enacarbil is not clinically relevant, and no dose adjustment is required on concurrent use. Similarly, the pharmacokinetic interaction between naproxen and gabapentin is not clinically relevant. However, the US manufacturer of gabapentin states that the doses used were lower than those used clinically, and that the magnitude of the interaction with clinically used doses is unknown.[1] Nevertheless, the lack of interaction with gabapentin enacarbil, which is rapidly converted to gabapentin during absorption, suggests that no interaction will occur when naproxen is used with gabapentin at usual doses.

1. Neurontin (Gabapentin). Pfizer Inc. US Prescribing information, July 2012.
2. Lal R, Sukbuntherng J, Luo W, Vicente V, Blumenthal R, Ho J, Cundy KC. Clinical pharmacokinetic drug interaction studies of gabapentin enacarbil, a novel transported prodrug of gabapentin, with naproxen and cimetidine. *Br J Clin Pharmacol* (2010) 69, 498–507.

Gabapentin + Other antiepileptics

Gabapentin does not normally affect the pharmacokinetics of carbamazepine, eslicarbazepine, phenytoin, phenobarbital, or valproate, and these drugs do not normally affect the pharmacokinetics of gabapentin. However, isolated reports describe increased phenytoin serum concentrations and toxicity in two patients given gabapentin.

Clinical evidence, mechanism, importance and management

The pharmacokinetics of both **phenytoin** and gabapentin remained unchanged in 8 patients with epilepsy who were given gabapentin 400 mg three times daily for 8 days, in addition to **phenytoin**, which they had been taking for at least 2 months.[1] Other studies confirm that the steady-state pharmacokinetics of **phenytoin** are unaffected by gabapentin, and that the pharmacokinetics of gabapentin are similarly unaffected by **phenytoin**.[2,3] These reports contrast with an isolated report of a patient taking **phenytoin**, **carbamazepine**, and **clobazam** whose serum **phenytoin** concentrations increased 3- to 4-fold, with symptoms of toxicity, on two occasions when gabapentin 300 to 600 mg daily was given. **Carbamazepine** serum concentrations remained unchanged. The author suggests that this differing reaction might be because the patient was taking more than one antiepileptic, unlike previous studies where only single drugs had been used.[4] However, another case of **phenytoin** toxicity, possibly attributable to gabapentin, has been described in a patient who was not taking any other antiepileptics.[5]

Gabapentin does not affect the plasma concentration of **phenobarbital**, nor is it affected by **phenobarbital**.[2,3,6] Other studies confirm that the steady-state pharmacokinetics of **carbamazepine**, **eslicarbazepine**, and **valproate** are unaffected by gabapentin, and that the pharmacokinetics of gabapentin are similarly unaffected by these antiepileptics.[2,3,7,8]

It would seem therefore that no dose adjustments are normally needed if gabapentin is added to treatment with most of these antiepileptics. However, if gabapentin is added to **phenytoin** it would be wise to bear the possibility of an increase in **phenytoin** concentration in mind. Be alert for phenytoin adverse effects (e.g. blurred vision, nystagmus, ataxia, or drowsiness).

For mention that gabapentin might prolong the half-life of felbamate, see 'Felbamate + Gabapentin', p.583.

For mention of the lack of interaction between levetiracetam and gabapentin, see 'Levetiracetam + Other antiepileptics', p.588.

1. Anhut H, Leppik I, Schmidt B, Thomann P. Drug interaction study of the new anticonvulsant gabapentin with phenytoin in epileptic patients. *Naunyn Schmiedebergs Arch Pharmacol* (1988) 337 (Suppl), R127.
2. Brockbrader HN, Radulovic LL, Loewen G, Chang T, Welling PG, Reece PA, Underwood B, Sedman AJ. Lack of drug-drug interactions between Neurontin (gabapentin) and other antiepileptic drugs. 20th International Epilepsy Congress, Oslo, Norway. July 1993 (Abstract).
3. Richens A. Clinical pharmacokinetics of gabapentin. In: Chadwick D, ed. New Trends in Epilepsy Management: The Role of Gabapentin. International Congress and Symposium Series No 198, Royal Society of Medicine Services, London, NY 1993, 41–6.
4. Tyndel F. Interaction of gabapentin with other antiepileptics. *Lancet* (1994) 343, 1363–4.
5. Sánchez-Romero A, Durán-Quintana JA, García-Delgado R, Margariot-Rangel C, Proveda-Andrés JL. Posible interacción gabapentina-fenitoína. *Rev Neurol* (2002) 34, 952–3.
6. Hooper WD, Kavanagh MC, Herkes GK, Eadie MJ. Lack of a pharmacokinetic interaction between phenobarbitone and gabapentin. *Br J Clin Pharmacol* (1991) 31, 171–4.
7. Radulovic LL, Wilder BJ, Leppik IE, Bockbrader HN, Chang T, Posvar EL, Sedman AJ, Uthman BM, Erdman GR. Lack of interaction of gabapentin with carbamazepine or valproate. *Epilepsia* (1994) 35, 155–61.
8. Falcão A, Fuseau E, Nunes T, Almeida A, Soares-da-Silva P. Pharmacokinetics, drug interactions and exposure-response relationship of eslicarbazepine acetate in adult patients with partial-onset seizures: population pharmacokinetic and pharmacokinetic/pharmacodynamic analyses. *CNS Drugs* (2012) 26, 79–91.

Gabapentin + Probenecid

A brief report notes that probenecid had no effect on the renal clearance of gabapentin. No study details were given.[1]

1. Busch JA, Bockbrader HN, Randinitis EJ, Chang T, Welling PG, Reece PA, Underwood B, Sedman AJ, Vollmer KO, Türck D. Lack of clinically significant drug interactions with Neurontin (Gabapentin). 20th International Epilepsy Congress. Oslo, Norway, July 1993. Abstract 013958.

Lacosamide + Miscellaneous

No clinically relevant pharmacokinetic interactions occur between lacosamide and digoxin, metformin or omeprazole. Food does not affect the pharmacokinetics of lacosamide. Lacosamide does not affect the pharmacokinetics of midazolam to a clinically relevant extent. Potent enzyme inducers such as rifampicin (rifampin) are predicted to reduce the levels of lacosamide. Caution is required if class I antiarrhythmics are given with lacosamide because of the possibility of enhanced PR prolongation.

Clinical evidence, mechanism, importance and management

(a) Antiarrhythmics

Dose-dependent prolongation of the PR interval may occur with lacosamide.[1,2] The UK manufacturer advises that lacosamide should be used with caution in patients taking class I antiarrhythmics (see 'Table 9.1', p.260) or other drugs that prolong the PR interval. See also 'Lacosamide + Other antiepileptics', below.

(b) Enzyme inducers

The UK manufacturer notes that potent enzyme inducers (presumably CYP3A4 inducers as they name **rifampicin (rifampin)** and **St John's wort**) may moderately reduce the exposure to lacosamide and advises caution when starting or ending treatment with these drugs in patients taking lacosamide.[1] For a list of CYP3A4 inducers, see 'Table 1.9', p.11.

(c) Food

In a study, 24 healthy subjects were given a single 300-mg dose of lacosamide in the fasted state or after a high-fat meal. Food did not affect lacosamide pharmacokinetics,[3] and it may therefore be taken without regard to food.[1,2]

(d) Omeprazole

The US manufacturer notes that plasma levels of the (inactive[1]) *O*-desmethyl metabolite of lacosamide were decreased by about 60% in the presence of omeprazole,[2] possibly due to inhibition of lacosamide metabolism by cytochrome P450 isoenzyme CYP2C19.[1] This would not be expected to be clinically relevant. Lacosamide 300 mg twice daily did not affect the pharmacokinetics of a single 40-mg dose of omeprazole,[1,2] although the US manufacturer states that *in vitro* data suggest that lacosamide has the potential to inhibit CYP2C19.[2] However, one *in vitro* study suggests the interaction only occurs at levels 30-fold higher than therapeutic lacosamide plasma levels.[4]

(e) Other drugs

In studies in healthy subjects there were no pharmacokinetic interactions between lacosamide and **digoxin** or **metformin**.[1,2,5] Lacosamide increased the maximum level of **midazolam** in one study, but did not increase its AUC; this would not be expected to be clinically relevant.[1]

1. Vimpat (Lacosamide). UCB Pharma Ltd. UK Summary of product characteristics, July 2012.
2. Vimpat (Lacosamide). UCB, Inc. US Prescribing information, February 2012.
3. Horstmann R, Bonn R, Cawello W, Doty P, Rudd D. Basic clinical investigations of the new antiepileptic drug SPM 927. *Epilepsia* (2002) 43 (Suppl. 7) 188.
4. Beyreuther BK, Freitag J, Heers C, Krebsfänger N, Scharfenecker U, Stöhr T. Lacosamide: a review of preclinical properties. *CNS Drug Rev* (2007) 13, 21–42.
5. Thomas D, Scharfenecker U, Schiltmeyer B, Doty P, Cawello W, Horstmann R. Low potential for drug-drug-interaction of lacosamide [abstract no. 2.235]. *Epilepsia* (2006) 4, 200. Available at: http://onlinelibrary.wiley.com/doi/10.1111/j.1528-1167.2006.00001_6.x/epdf (accessed 21/10/15).

Lacosamide + Other antiepileptics

No significant pharmacokinetic interaction appears to occur between lacosamide and carbamazepine, lamotrigine, oxcarbazepine, or valproate. Lacosamide does not affect plasma levels of phenytoin or phenobarbital, clonazepam, gabapentin, levetiracetam, topiramate and zonisamide. However, limited evidence suggests that the enzyme-inducing antiepileptics may reduce lacosamide exposure.

Clinical evidence, mechanism, importance and management

(a) Carbamazepine or Oxcarbazepine

In a study in 19 healthy subjects given lacosamide 200 mg twice daily, modified-release carbamazepine 200 mg twice daily had no clinically significant effect on the pharmacokinetics of lacosamide.[1] In a further study in 18 healthy subjects given modified-release carbamazepine 200 mg twice daily with lacosamide 200 mg twice daily, there were no significant changes in the pharmacokinetics of carbamazepine.[1] In studies in patients with uncontrolled partial seizures taking one or two antiepileptic drugs, the addition of lacosamide 100 mg to 600 mg daily did not affect the plasma levels of carbamazepine and its 10,11-epoxide metabolite or oxcarbazepine.[2,3] In placebo-controlled clinical studies in patients with partial-onset seizures, the plasma levels of carbamazepine and carbamazepine-10,11-epoxide or the active metabolite of oxcarbazepine, monohydroxyoxcarbazepine, were unaffected by the concurrent use lacosamide.[4] The manufacturers of lacosamide note that, in a population pharmacokinetic analysis, the concurrent use of lacosamide with other antiepileptic drugs known to be enzyme inducers (carbamazepine, phenytoin, phenobarbital) decreased the exposure of lacosamide by 15 to 25%.[4,5] This finding is expected to be of limited clinical relevance, and it would appear that, in general, no dose adjustment of either carbamazepine or lacosamide is likely to be needed on concurrent use. However, the manufacturers advise caution if lacosamide is given with drugs known to be associated with PR prolongation, and they name carbamazepine.[4,5] However, the UK manufacturer states that a subgroup analysis of clinical study results did not find an increase in PR prolongation in patients given lacosamide and carbamazepine.[5]

(b) Lamotrigine

In studies in patients with uncontrolled partial seizures taking one or two antiepileptic drugs, the addition of lacosamide in doses of 100 mg to 600 mg daily did not affect plasma levels of lamotrigine.[2,3] The UK manufacturer advises caution if lacosamide is given with drugs known to be associated with PR prolongation, and they name lamotrigine; however, they state that subgroup analysis of clinical study results did not find an increase in PR prolongation in patients given lacosamide and lamotrigine.[5]

(c) Phenobarbital or Phenytoin

In studies in patients with uncontrolled partial seizures taking one or two antiepileptic drugs, the addition of lacosamide in doses of 100 mg to 600 mg daily did not affect the plasma levels of phenytoin.[2,3] In clinical studies, lacosamide did not affect the plasma levels of phenobarbital.[4] The manufacturer of lacosamide notes that, in a population pharmacokinetic analysis in patients with partial-onset seizures, the concurrent use of lacosamide with other antiepileptic drugs known to be enzyme inducers (carbamazepine, phenytoin, phenobarbital) decreased the exposure of lacosamide by 15 to 25%.[4,5] However, this would be expected to be of little clinical relevance, and no dose adjustments would be expected to be needed if lacosamide is given with phenytoin or phenobarbital.

(d) Pregabalin

The UK manufacturer of lacosamide advises caution if lacosamide is given with drugs known to be associated with PR prolongation, and they name pregabalin.[5]

(e) Valproate

Phase I studies in healthy subjects have found no pharmacokinetic interaction between lacosamide and valproate.[6] In studies in patients with uncontrolled partial seizures taking one or two antiepileptic drugs, the addition of lacosamide in doses of 100 mg to 600 mg daily did not affect the plasma levels of valproate.[2,3] Further, in clinical studies, the concurrent use of lacosamide did not affect the plasma levels of valproate.[4] No dose adjustment of lacosamide or valproate appears to be necessary on concurrent use.

(f) Other antiepileptics

In studies in patients with uncontrolled partial seizures taking one or two antiepileptic drugs, the addition of lacosamide in doses of 100 mg to 600 mg daily did not affect the plasma levels of **gabapentin**, **levetiracetam**, **topiramate**, or **zonisamide**.[2,3] In clinical studies, the concurrent use of lacosamide did not affect the steady-state levels of **clonazepam**.[4]

1. Cawello W, Nickel B, Eggert-Formella A. No pharmacokinetic interaction between lacosamide and carbamazepine in healthy volunteers. *J Clin Pharmacol* (2009) Oct 19.
2. Jatuzis D, Biton V, Ben-Menachem E, Abou-Khalil B, Doty P, Rudd GD. Evaluation of the effect of oral lacosamide on concomitant AED plasma concentrations in patients with partial seizures. *Epilepsia* (2005) 46 (Suppl 8), 170.
3. Fountain NB, Horstmann R, Cawello W, Doty P, Rudd GD. Absence of effect of adjunctive SPM927 on concomitant AED plasma concentrations in subjects with partial seizures. *Epilepsia* (2003) 44 (Suppl 9), 96.
4. Vimpat (Lacosamide). UCB, Inc. US Prescribing information, February 2012.
5. Vimpat (Lacosamide). UCB Pharma Ltd. UK Summary of product characteristics, July 2012.
6. Horstmann R, Bonn R, Cawello W, Doty P, Rudd D. SPM 927 does not interact with valproic acid and carbamazepine. *Epilepsia* (2003) 44 (Suppl 9), 97.

Lamotrigine + Antimycobacterials

Rifampicin markedly increased the clearance of lamotrigine in a pharmacokinetic study. A case report described a similar finding, and also included some limited evidence suggesting that isoniazid may inhibit lamotrigine metabolism.

Clinical evidence

In a pharmacokinetic study in 10 healthy subjects, **rifampicin (rifampin)** 600 mg daily for 5 days increased the clearance of a single 25-mg dose of lamotrigine by 97% and decreased its AUC by 44%. The amount of lamotrigine glucuronide recovered in the urine was increased by 36%.[1] Similarly, a case report describes a 56-year-old woman taking lamotrigine 150 mg daily who had unexpectedly low serum lamotrigine levels of 1.3 mg/L after starting **rifampicin**, **isoniazid** and pyrazinamide. The lamotrigine dose was therefore increased to 250 mg daily. After rifampicin and pyrazinamide were stopped, isoniazid continued and ethambutol started, the lamotrigine serum levels rose to 12.4 mg/L but no toxicity was seen.[2] It is unclear whether there is any relationship between lamotrigine plasma levels and toxicity.[3]

Mechanism

Rifampicin (rifampin) increases the loss of lamotrigine from the body, probably by inducing glucuronidation via glucuronyltransferases.[1] It was suggested that isoniazid may have inhibited lamotrigine metabolism.[2]

Importance and management

Information appears to be limited to these reports, but the interaction between lamotrigine and rifampicin (rifampin) would appear to be established. Be aware that rifampicin could reduce the efficacy of lamotrigine, and that increased lamotrigine doses are likely to be required.

The case report also raises the possibility of an interaction between lamotrigine and isoniazid. If isoniazid is added to or withdrawn from lamotrigine treatment, be alert for the need to adjust the lamotrigine dosage.

1. Ebert U, Thong NQ, Oertel R, Kirch W. Effects of rifampicin and cimetidine on pharmacokinetics and pharmacodynamics of lamotrigine in healthy subjects. *Eur J Clin Pharmacol* (2000) 56, 299–304.
2. Armijo JA, Sánchez B, Peralta FG, Cuadrado A, Leno C. Lamotrigine interaction with rifampicin and isoniazid. A case report. *Methods Find Exp Clin Pharmacol* (1996) 18 (Suppl C), 59.
3. Chong E, Dupuis LL. Therapeutic drug monitoring of lamotrigine. *Ann Pharmacother* (2002) 36, 917–20.

Lamotrigine + Cimetidine

In a study in 10 healthy subjects, cimetidine 400 mg twice daily for 5 days had no effect on the pharmacokinetics of a single 25-mg dose of lamotrigine. No lamotrigine dose adjustment therefore appears to be needed on the concurrent use of cimetidine.[1]

1. Ebert U, Thong NQ, Oertel R, Kirch W. Effects of rifampicin and cimetidine on pharmacokinetics and pharmacodynamics of lamotrigine in healthy subjects. *Eur J Clin Pharmacol* (2000) 56, 299–304.

Lamotrigine + Felbamate

Felbamate does not have a clinically relevant effect on the pharmacokinetics of lamotrigine.

Clinical evidence, mechanism, importance and management

In a study in 21 healthy subjects, felbamate 1.2 g twice daily had minimal effects on the pharmacokinetics of lamotrigine 100 mg twice daily, when both drugs were given together for 10 days. The AUC of lamotrigine was increased by 14%, which was not considered to be clinically relevant.[1] Similarly, there was no difference in the pharmacokinetics of lamotrigine in 6 patients receiving lamotrigine with felbamate and 5 patients taking lamotrigine alone.[2] Therefore the dose of lamotrigine does not need to be adjusted if felbamate is given.

1. Colucci R, Glue P, Holt B, Banfield C, Reidenberg P, Meehan JW, Pai S, Nomeir A, Lim J, Lin C-C, Affrime MB. Effect of felbamate on the pharmacokinetics of lamotrigine. *J Clin Pharmacol* (1996) 36, 634–8.
2. Gidal BE, Kanner A, Maly M, Rutecki P, Lensmeyer GL. Lamotrigine pharmacokinetics in patients receiving felbamate. *Epilepsy Res* (1997) 27, 1–5.

Lamotrigine + Fluconazole

An isolated case report suggests that fluconazole does not affect lamotrigine concentrations.

Clinical evidence, mechanism, importance and management

A patient who had been taking carbamazepine, lamotrigine and barbexaclone for many years, was given fluconazole 150 mg with her morning dose of antiepileptics. Although she developed symptoms of carbamazepine toxicity and raised carbamazepine concentrations, her lamotrigine concentrations were almost unchanged by the concurrent use of fluconazole.[1]

1. Ulivelli M, Rubegni P, Nuti D, Bartalini S, Giannini F, Rossi S. Clinical evidence of fluconazole-induced carbamazepine toxicity. *J Neurol* (2004) 251, 622–3.

Lamotrigine + Methadone

A report describes lamotrigine-associated rash and blood dyscrasias, which might have been associated with methadone use.

Clinical evidence, mechanism, importance and management

Lamotrigine-associated rash and blood dyscrasias occurred in a 40-year-old opioid-dependent woman with hepatitis C. Lamotrigine was considered to be the causal factor as haematological values returned to normal 53 days after the lamotrigine was stopped. However, the woman was also receiving methadone maintenance and it was thought that the methadone, together with liver impairment, might possibly have caused elevated lamotrigine concentrations (but note that these were not measured).[1]

It is unclear whether the methadone or the liver impairment contributed to the lamotrigine-associated rash and blood dyscrasias, and therefore this isolated case is of unknown general importance.

1. Alleyne S, Alao A, Batki SL. Lamotrigine-associated rash and blood dyscrasias in a methadone-treatment patient with hepatitis C. *Psychosomatics* (2006) 47, 257–8.

Lamotrigine + Phenobarbital or Primidone

Phenobarbital has been associated with reduced lamotrigine concentrations. Lamotrigine does not appear to affect phenobarbital and primidone concentrations. A case report describes leucopenia and thrombocytopenia when lamotrigine was given to a patient taking phenobarbital.

Clinical evidence

In a retrospective study, the lamotrigine serum concentration-to-dose ratio was lower in patients also taking phenobarbital than in those taking lamotrigine alone (0.52 versus 0.99),[1] suggesting that phenobarbital lowers lamotrigine concentrations. Similar findings have been reported in other studies.[2-4]

No changes in the serum concentrations of phenobarbital or primidone were seen in a study in 12 patients also given lamotrigine 75 to 400 mg daily.[5]

A patient with epilepsy taking phenobarbital 100 mg daily had an increase in complex partial seizures and lamotrigine 50 mg daily was started, increased to 100 mg twice daily 2 weeks later. About one month later, a routine blood test found that the patient had leucopenia and thrombocytopenia. Phenobarbital was stopped and her full blood count normalised about 20 days later. A rechallenge with phenobarbital produced the same response, which resolved within 25 days of stopping phenobarbital.[6]

Mechanism

Lamotrigine is metabolised by glucuronidation which appears to be induced by phenobarbital. The authors of the case report suggest that this induction might have increased the production of toxic metabolites, resulting in the reported blood dyscrasias.[6] However, both drugs have been reported to cause blood dyscrasias alone, and therefore additive adverse effects might also have been responsible.

Importance and management

Evidence for a pharmacokinetic interaction between lamotrigine and phenobarbital is limited; however, an interaction appears to be established. The manufacturers of lamotrigine recommend that the starting dose and the long-term maintenance dose of lamotrigine in patients already taking phenobarbital or primidone is twice that of patients receiving lamotrigine monotherapy.[7,8] However, note that if patients are also taking valproate in addition to enzyme-inducing antiepileptics such as phenobarbital or primidone, the recommended dose of lamotrigine is lower, see 'Lamotrigine + Valproate', p.587.

The case report describing blood dyscrasias in a patient taking phenobarbital and lamotrigine appears to be isolated. However, as both lamotrigine and phenobarbital alone have been associated with blood dyscrasias it would seem prudent to consider an interaction should this adverse effect develop in a patient taking both drugs.

1. May TW, Rambeck B, Jürgens U. Serum concentrations of lamotrigine in epileptic patients: the influence of dose and comedication. *Ther Drug Monit* (1996) 18, 523–31.
2. Armijo JA, Bravo J, Cuadrado A, Herranz JL. Lamotrigine serum concentration-to-dose ratio: influence of age and concomitant antiepileptic drugs and dosage implications. *Ther Drug Monit* (1999) 21, 182–190.
3. Yamamoto Y, Inoue Y, Matsuda K, Takahashi Y, Kagawa Y. Influence of concomitant antiepileptic drugs on plasma lamotrigine concentration in adult Japanese epilepsy patients. *Biol Pharm Bull* (2012) 35, 487–93.
4. Reimers A, Skogvoll E, Sund JK, Spigset O. Drug interactions between lamotrigine and psychoactive drugs: evidence from a therapeutic drug monitoring service. *J Clin Psychopharmacol* (2005) 25, 342–8.
5. Jawad S, Richens A, Goodwin G, Yuen WC. Controlled trial of lamotrigine (Lamictal) for refractory partial seizures. *Epilepsia* (1989) 30, 356–63.
6. Siniscalchi A, Gallelli L, Calabrò G, Tolotta GA, De Sarro G. Phenobarbital/lamotrigine coadministration–induced blood dyscrasia in a patient with epilepsy. *Ann Pharmacother* (2010) 44, 2031–4.
7. Lamictal (Lamotrigine). GlaxoSmithKline UK. UK Summary of product characteristics, July 2012.
8. Lamictal (Lamotrigine). GlaxoSmithKline. US Prescribing information, November 2011.

Lamotrigine + Phenytoin

Phenytoin has been associated with reduced lamotrigine serum concentrations. Lamotrigine has no effect on phenytoin concentrations.

Clinical evidence

In a retrospective study, the lamotrigine serum concentration-to-dose ratio was much lower in patients also taking phenytoin than in those taking lamotrigine alone (0.32 versus 0.98),[1] suggesting that phenytoin lowers lamotrigine concentrations. Other studies in patients taking lamotrigine with phenytoin have reported similar findings.[2-5] In another study, the mean lamotrigine concentrations were approximately doubled when phenytoin was withdrawn.[6]

One study suggests that the serum concentration of phenytoin is unchanged in patients taking lamotrigine 75 to 400 mg daily.[7]

Mechanism

Lamotrigine is metabolised by glucuronidation which appears to be induced by phenytoin, leading to a reduction in lamotrigine concentrations.

Importance and management

Evidence for a pharmacokinetic interaction between lamotrigine and phenytoin is limited; however, a clinically relevant interaction appears to be established. The manufacturers of lamotrigine recommend that the starting dose and the long-term maintenance dose of lamotrigine in patients already taking phenytoin is twice that of patients receiving lamotrigine monotherapy.[8,9] However, note that if patients are also taking valproate in addition to enzyme-inducing antiepileptics such as phenytoin, the recommended dose of lamotrigine is lower, see 'Lamotrigine + Valproate', p.587.

Note that **fosphenytoin**, a prodrug of phenytoin, would be expected to interact with lamotrigine in the same way as phenytoin.

1. May TW, Rambeck B, Jürgens U. Serum concentrations of lamotrigine in epileptic patients: the influence of dose and comedication. *Ther Drug Monit* (1996) 18, 523–31.
2. Armijo JA, Bravo J, Cuadrado A, Herranz JL. Lamotrigine serum concentration-to-dose ratio: influence of age and concomitant antiepileptic drugs and dosage implications. *Ther Drug Monit* (1999) 21, 182–90.
3. Böttiger Y, Svensson J-O, Ståhle L. Lamotrigine drug interactions in a TDM material. *Ther Drug Monit* (1999) 21, 171–4.
4. Yamamoto Y, Inoue Y, Matsuda K, Takahashi Y, Kagawa Y. Influence of concomitant antiepileptic drugs on plasma lamotrigine concentration in adult Japanese epilepsy patients. *Biol Pharm Bull* (2012) 35, 487–93.
5. Reimers A, Skogvoll E, Sund JK, Spigset O. Drug interactions between lamotrigine and psychoactive drugs: evidence from a therapeutic drug monitoring service. *J Clin Psychopharmacol* (2005) 25, 342–8.
6. Anderson GD, Gidal BE, Messenheimer J, Gilliam FG. Time course of lamotrigine de-induction: impact of step-wise withdrawal of carbamazepine or phenytoin. *Epilepsy Res* (2002) 49, 211–17.
7. Jawad S, Richens A, Goodwin G, Yuen WC. Controlled trial of lamotrigine (Lamictal) for refractory partial seizures. *Epilepsia* (1989) 30, 356–63.
8. Lamictal (Lamotrigine). GlaxoSmithKline UK. UK Summary of product characteristics, July 2012.
9. Lamictal (Lamotrigine). GlaxoSmithKline. US Prescribing information, November 2011.

Lamotrigine + SSRIs or SNRIs

An isolated report describes two cases in which sertraline appeared to increase lamotrigine concentrations and cause toxicity. However, retrospective studies suggest that sertraline, citalopram, paroxetine, and venlafaxine are unlikely to affect lamotrigine concentrations, whereas fluoxetine might lower them.

Clinical evidence

A retrospective analysis of 1733 serum samples from 829 patients taking lamotrigine found that lamotrigine concentrations were lower in 15 patients also taking **fluoxetine**, when compared with the reference group not taking fluoxetine. In the same analysis, **citalopram**, **paroxetine**, **sertraline** and **venlafaxine** were briefly reported to have no statistically significant effect on lamotrigine concentration-to-dose ratios.[1]

In a small case-control study, 7 patients taking lamotrigine and **sertraline** appeared to have slightly higher dose-adjusted lamotrigine concentrations, when compared with 44 patients not taking sertraline; however, the difference was not statistically significant.[2]

In contrast, a case report describes two patients in whom an interaction was considered possible. The lamotrigine concentration of one of the patients was found to have doubled, and symptoms of toxicity were noted (confusion, cognitive impairment), 6 weeks after **sertraline** 25 mg daily was started. The lamotrigine dose was halved, and the sertraline dose titrated to 50 mg daily. Symptoms of toxicity resolved, but the lamotrigine concentrations were still 24% higher than before sertraline was started. In the other patient lamotrigine toxicity developed. The sertraline dose was reduced by 33%, which resulted in a halving of the lamotrigine concentration even though the lamotrigine dose was increased by 33%.[3]

A study investigating the clinical effects on depressive symptom scores of adding lamotrigine to **paroxetine** briefly reported that lamotrigine had no effect on paroxetine concentrations.[4]

Mechanism

The authors of the study involving fluoxetine[1] suggested that fluoxetine or its active metabolite, norfluoxetine, might have induced the glucuronidation of lamotrigine, leading to a reduction in lamotrigine concentrations. The authors of the case report suggested that sertraline might inhibit the glucuronidation of lamotrigine,[3] leading to increased lamotrigine toxicity, but this is not established.

Importance and management

The limited evidence suggests that, in general, the SSRIs, and possibly venlafaxine, do not affect lamotrigine concentrations to a clinically relevant extent. However, the isolated cases of increased lamotrigine concentrations with sertraline and the limited data suggesting that fluoxetine might lower lamotrigine concentrations introduce a note of caution and indicate that further controlled prospective studies might be warranted to properly exclude the possibility of an interaction. Therefore, until more is known, bear the possibility of an interaction in mind if lamotrigine adverse effects become troublesome or if lamotrigine concentrations are lower than anticipated.

1. Reimers A, Skogvoll E, Sund JK, Spigset O. Drug interactions between lamotrigine and psychoactive drugs: evidence from a therapeutic drug monitoring service. *J Clin Psychopharmacol* (2005) 25, 342–8.
2. Christensen J, Sandgaard AP, Sidenius P, Linnet K, Licht RW. Lack of interaction between sertraline and lamotrigine in psychiatric patients: a retrospective study. *Pharmacopsychiatry* (2012) 45, 119–21.
3. Kaufman KR, Gerner R. Lamotrigine toxicity secondary to sertraline. *Seizure* (1998) 7, 163–5.
4. Normann C, Hummel B, Schärer LO, Hörn M, Grunze H, Walden J. Lamotrigine as adjunct to paroxetine in acute depression: a placebo-controlled double-blind study. *J Clin Psychiatry* (2002) 63, 337–44.

Lamotrigine + Topiramate

Although one study suggested that topiramate reduces lamotrigine concentrations, in general a clinically relevant interaction would not be expected. Lamotrigine has no effect on topiramate concentrations.

Clinical evidence, mechanism, importance and management

In the preliminary report of one study, it was found that serum lamotrigine concentrations of 4 of 7 patients who were stable taking lamotrigine 350 to 800 mg daily decreased by 40 to 50% when they were given topiramate, titrated to 800 mg daily.[1] Similarly, in a review of routine lamotrigine therapeutic drug monitoring, topiramate was found to lower the lamotrigine concentration-to-dose ratio, suggesting that topiramate reduces lamotrigine concentrations.[2] In contrast, a prospective study in 24 patients reported that the addition of topiramate 75 to 800 mg daily had little effect on the steady-state serum concentrations of lamotrigine 100 to 950 mg daily. The mean lamotrigine concentration before topiramate was 10.4 mg/L and during topiramate was 9.7 mg/L. Only 2 of the patients had reductions of greater than 30% (40% and 43%).[3] A further study by the same research group similarly found that topiramate did not affect lamotrigine pharmacokinetics.[4] The authors of the second study[3] note that there is some evidence that peak-to-trough variations of as much as 30 to 40% can occur during the use of lamotrigine, and therefore timing of blood sampling might be a factor in the findings of the first study.[1]

In one study in 13 patients lamotrigine had no effect on topiramate pharmacokinetics. The oral clearance of topiramate 400 mg daily was 2.6 L/hour when given alone, and 2.7 L/hour when given with lamotrigine, and the AUC and plasma concentrations of topiramate were also similar.[4]

The balance of the evidence suggests that there is no clinically important pharmacokinetic interaction between topiramate and lamotrigine. No dose adjustments of either drug appear to be necessary on their concurrent use.

1. Wnuk W, Volanski A, Foletti G. Topiramate decreases lamotrigine concentrations. *Ther Drug Monit* (1999) 21, 449.
2. Reimers A, Skogvoll E, Sund JK, Spigset O. Drug interactions between lamotrigine and psychoactive drugs: evidence from a therapeutic drug monitoring service. *J Clin Psychopharmacol* (2005) 25, 342–8.
3. Berry DJ, Besag FMC, Pool F, Natarajan J, Doose D. Lack of an effect of topiramate on lamotrigine serum concentrations. *Epilepsia* (2002) 43, 818–23.
4. Doose DR, Brodie MJ, Wilson EA, Chadwick D, Oxbury J, Berry DJ, Schwabe S, Bialer M. Topiramate and lamotrigine pharmacokinetics during repetitive monotherapy and combination therapy in epilepsy patients. *Epilepsia* (2003) 44, 917–22.

Lamotrigine + Valproate

The serum concentrations of lamotrigine can be increased by valproate. Lamotrigine has been found to cause either small increases, decreases or no changes in valproate concentrations. The concurrent use of valproate and lamotrigine has been associated with skin rashes, tremor and other toxic reactions.

Clinical evidence

(a) Effects on lamotrigine concentrations

In a study in 6 healthy subjects, sodium valproate 200 mg every 8 hours reduced the clearance of lamotrigine by 20% and increased its AUC by 30%.[1] In another study in 18 healthy subjects taking valproate 500 mg twice daily, the clearance of lamotrigine 50, 100 or 150 mg daily was reduced and its half-life increased.[2] In a retrospective study, the lamotrigine serum concentration-to-dose ratio was higher in patients also taking valproate than in those taking lamotrigine monotherapy (3.57 versus 0.98), suggesting that valproate increases lamotrigine concentrations. In patients also taking phenytoin, the effects of valproate on lamotrigine were offset (0.99 versus 0.98). However, the effects of valproate on lamotrigine were not completely offset by either carbamazepine or phenobarbital (1.67 or 1.8, respectively, versus 0.98).[3] Other studies have reported broadly similar findings.[4-8] Three studies have found that the effect of valproate on lamotrigine was independent of the valproate dose or serum concentration (that is, it is maximal within the usual therapeutic dose range of valproate).[6,7,9,10] Another study has shown that the inhibition of lamotrigine clearance by valproate begins at very low valproate doses (less than 125 mg daily), and is maximal at doses of about 500 mg daily.[11]

A case report describes a 35-year-old man taking lamotrigine 250 mg daily and valproate 1.5 g daily who had been hospitalised due to seizures, vomiting and abnormal weight loss. He was found to have a raised lamotrigine concentration (11.4 micrograms/mL, almost three times the upper limit of the reference range). This was assumed to be as a result of an interaction with the valproate, and over the course of about 2 months he required numerous reductions in the lamotrigine dose to bring the lamotrigine concentrations within their accepted therapeutic range.[12] Three patients taking lamotrigine developed neurotoxicity (confusion, lethargy) after starting to take valproate (an intravenous bolus dose of valproic acid then oral use). Lamotrigine concentrations had risen 2.9- to 6.9-fold.[13] Confusion, disorientation, visual disturbances and behavioural changes were reported in a patient 4 days after valproate was added to her treatment with lamotrigine. Lamotrigine concentrations were found to be 22.9 micrograms/mL (reference range 1 to 13 micrograms/mL). She recovered within 2 days of the discontinuation of both drugs.[14]

A study in women found that valproate appears to reduce the induction of lamotrigine metabolism associated with pregnancy or the use of oral contraceptives thus resulting in higher lamotrigine plasma concentrations.[15] Consider also 'Combined hormonal contraceptives + Lamotrigine', p.1178.

(b) Effects on valproate concentrations

In one study, 18 healthy subjects taking valproate 500 mg twice daily were also given lamotrigine 50, 100 or 150 mg daily. Lamotrigine caused a 25% decrease in valproate serum concentrations and a 25% increase in valproate oral clearance.[2] In a study in 76 patients with epilepsy, who were between 6 and 20 years of age and taking a stable dose of sodium valproate for at least 2 weeks, the addition of lamotrigine increased the valproic acid concentration in 62% of patients and decreased it in the other 38% of the patients. Some patients had an increase in valproic acid concentrations of more than 25% (26 patients), or even 50% (13 patients) whereas fewer patients had a notable decrease in concentrations (4 patients had a decrease of more than 25%, with none showing a decrease of greater than 50%).[16] A study in 11 children taking valproate and other antiepileptics noted that no clinically important changes in valproate serum concentrations occurred when lamotrigine was added.[17] A retrospective analysis found that lamotrigine was associated with only a 7% reduction in valproate concentrations, which would not be expected to be clinically significant.[18]

(c) Toxic reactions

1. Rash. In a survey of adult patients with epilepsy who had lamotrigine added to their existing treatment, 33 were also taking valproate. Of these, 10 patients (30%) developed a rash, whereas only 6 of the 70 (8%) not taking valproate did so.[19] In another analysis of rash in patients taking lamotrigine, 11 of 12 patients with serious rash were also taking sodium valproate, and all but one had a lamotrigine starting dose that is higher than currently recommended.[20] However, in another study in which patients taking valproate were given lower initial doses of lamotrigine, there was no difference in incidence of rash when compared with those taking lamotrigine and other antiepileptics (13% versus 14.2%).[21]

2. Tremor. In 3 patients severe and disabling tremor (sometimes preventing them from feeding themselves) occurred when they were given lamotrigine and sodium valproate. The problem resolved when the doses were reduced.[22] In a study of 13 adult patients, all developed upper limb tremor when given lamotrigine with valproate, which could be minimised by reducing the dose of either or both drugs.[23] Other studies have found similar effects.[9,13,24]

3. Other. Severe multiorgan dysfunction and disseminated intravascular coagulation was seen in 2 children when they took lamotrigine with valproate.[25] A 72-year-old woman taking valproate 900 mg daily and clozapine 125 mg daily developed hyperammonaemic encephalopathy (weakness, tremor, lethargy, asterixis) 3 weeks after lamotrigine was started at a dose of 12.5 mg daily, increased every 3 days by 12.5 mg, to a dose of 75 mg daily. Valproate was stopped and her symptoms resolved. She was subsequently given valproate alone without a recurrence of the hyperammonaemia.[26]

One study reported that the formation of hepatotoxic metabolites of valproate was unaffected by lamotrigine.[2]

Mechanism

Not fully understood. It is thought that valproate reduces lamotrigine glucuronidation by competitive inhibition, which results in a decreased lamotrigine clearance.[1,2,27,28] Raised lamotrigine concentrations have been implicated in the development of rash; concurrent valproate appears to increase the risk.[21,29]

Increased valproate clearance might be due to enzyme induction. Tremor might be the result of a pharmacodynamic interaction.[9,23] It was suggested that competition for metabolism by glucuronyltransferases, causing valproate to be metabolised by an alternative route resulting in increased concentrations of 4-en valproic acid, which affected the urea cycle resulting in raised ammonia concentrations.[26]

Importance and management

The interaction between lamotrigine and valproate is established and well documented. Concurrent use can be therapeutically valuable, but the lamotrigine dose should be reduced by about half when valproate is added to avoid possible toxicity (sedation, tremor, ataxia, fatigue, rash).[2,9-11,21,22,30] In patients already taking valproate, the manufacturers of lamotrigine recommend a lamotrigine starting dose that is half that of lamotrigine monotherapy, with a more gradual dose-escalation rate.[31,32] In the UK, they recommend this irrespective of whether patients are also receiving enzyme-inducing antiepileptics.[31] The outcome should be very closely monitored and the lamotrigine dose adjusted as necessary. The CSM in the UK has suggested that the concurrent use of sodium valproate is one of the main risk factors for the development of serious skin reactions to lamotrigine, because it prolongs the half-life of lamotrigine.[29] Rashes are potentially serious and should be evaluated promptly.[21,31,32] The reports cited above[22,25] also suggest that sometimes other serious reactions (disabling tremor, multiorgan dysfunction) can occur.

1. Yuen AWC, Land G, Weatherley BC, Peck AW. Sodium valproate acutely inhibits lamotrigine metabolism. *Br J Clin Pharmacol* (1992) 33, 511–13.
2. Anderson GD, Yau MK, Gidal BE, Harris SJ, Levy RH, Lai AA, Wolf KB, Wargin WA, Dren AT. Bidirectional interaction of valproate and lamotrigine in healthy subjects. *Clin Pharmacol Ther* (1996) 60, 145–56.
3. May TW, Rambeck B, Jürgens U. Serum concentrations of lamotrigine in epileptic patients: the influence of dose and comedication. *Ther Drug Monit* (1996) 18, 523–31.
4. Armijo JA, Bravo J, Cuadrado A, Herranz JL. Lamotrigine serum concentration-to-dose ratio: influence of age and concomitant antiepileptic drugs and dosage implications. *Ther Drug Monit* (1999) 21, 182–190.
5. Böttiger Y, Svensson J-O, Ståhle L. Lamotrigine drug interactions in a TDM material. *Ther Drug Monit* (1999) 21, 171–4.
6. Gidal BE, Anderson GD, Rutecki PR, Shaw R, Lanning A. Lack of effect of valproate concentration on lamotrigine pharmacokinetics in developmentally disabled patients with epilepsy. *Epilepsy Res* (2000) 42, 23–31.
7. Yamamoto Y, Inoue Y, Matsuda K, Takahashi Y, Kagawa Y. Influence of concomitant antiepileptic drugs on plasma lamotrigine concentration in adult Japanese epilepsy patients. *Biol Pharm Bull* (2012) 35, 487–93.
8. Reimers A, Skogvoll E, Sund JK, Spigset O. Drug interactions between lamotrigine and psychoactive drugs: evidence from a therapeutic drug monitoring service. *J Clin Psychopharmacol* (2005) 25, 342–8.
9. Kanner A, Frey M. Adding valproate to lamotrigine: a study of their pharmacokinetic interaction. *Neurology* (2000) 55, 588–91.
10. Decerce J, McJilton JS, Nadkarni MA, Ramsay RE. Lamotrigine-valproate interaction: relationship to the dose of valproate. *Epilepsia* (2000) 41(Suppl. 7), 220–1.
11. Gidal BE, Sheth R, Parnell J, Maloney K, Sale M. Evaluation of VPA dose and concentration effects on lamotrigine pharmacokinetics: implications for conversion to monotherapy. *Epilepsy Res* (2003) 57, 85–93.
12. Greiner C, Wittmann M, Haen E. Lamotrigine serum concentrations under valproate comedication: "contraindication" or "safe combination"? A case report. *Pharmacopsychiatry* (2007) 40, 287–9.
13. Voudris K, Mastroyianni S, Skardoutsou A, Katsarou E, Mavrommatis P. Disabling tremor in epileptic children receiving sodium valproate after addition of lamotrigine. P2197. *Eur J Neurol* (2003) 10 (Suppl. 1), 180.
14. Mueller TH, Beeber AR. Delirium from valproic acid with lamotrigine. *Am J Psychiatry* (2004) 161, 1128–9.
15. Tomson T, Luef G, Sabers A, Pittschieler S, Öhman I. Valproate effects on kinetics of lamotrigine in pregnancy and treatment with oral contraceptives. *Neurology* (2006) 67, 1297–9.
16. Martin AC, Besag FMC, Berry DJ, Besag FP. The effect of lamotrigine on valproic acid concentrations. *Curr Drug Saf* (2011) 6, 23–9.
17. Eriksson A-S, Hoppu K, Nergårdh A, Boreus L. Pharmacokinetic interactions between lamotrigine and other antiepileptic drugs in children with intractable epilepsy. *Epilepsia* (1996) 37, 769–73.
18. Mataringa M-I, May TW, Rambeck B. Does lamotrigine influence valproate concentrations? *Ther Drug Monit* (2002) 24, 631–6.
19. Li LM, Russo M, O'Donoghue MF, Duncan JS, Sander JWAS. Allergic skin rash and concomitant valproate therapy: evidence for an increased risk. *Arq Neuropsiquiatr* (1996) 54, 47–9.
20. Wong ICK, Mawer GE, Sander JWAS. Factors influencing the incidence of lamotrigine-related skin rash. *Ann Pharmacother* (1999) 33, 1037–42.
21. Faught E, Morris G, Jacobson M, French J, Harden C, Montouris G, Rosenfeld W. Adding lamotrigine to valproate: incidence of rash and other adverse effects. Postmarketing antiepileptic drug survey (PADS) Group. *Epilepsia* (1999) 40, 1135–40.
22. Reutens DC, Duncan JS, Patsalos PN. Disabling tremor after lamotrigine with sodium valproate. *Lancet* (1993) 342, 185–6.
23. Pisani F, Oteri G, Russo MF, Di Perri R, Perucca E, Richens A. The efficacy of valproate-lamotrigine comedication in refractory complex partial seizures: evidence for a pharmacodynamic interaction. *Epilepsia* (1999) 40, 1141–6.
24. Burneo JG, Limdi N, Kuzniecky RI, Knowlton RC, Mendez M, Lawn N, Faught E, Welty TE, Prasad A. Neurotoxicity following addition of intravenous valproate to lamotrigine therapy. *Neurology* (2003) 60, 1991–2.
25. Chattergoon DS, McGuigan M, Koren G, Hwang P, Ito S. Multiorgan dysfunction and disseminated intravascular coagulation in children receiving lamotrigine and valproic acid. *Neurology* (1997) 49, 1442–4.
26. Fan CC, Huang MC, Liu HC. Lamotrigine might potentiate valproic acid-induced hyperammonemic encephalopathy. *Prog Neuropsychopharmacol Biol Psychiatry* (2008) 32, 1747–8.
27. Panayiotopoulos CP, Ferrie CD, Knott C, Robinson RO. Interaction of lamotrigine with sodium valproate. *Lancet* (1993) 341, 445.
28. Rowland A, Elliot DJ, Williams JA, Mackenzie PI, Dickinson RG, Miners JO. In vitro characterization of lamotrigine *N*2-glucuronidation and the lamotrigine-valproic acid interaction. *Drug Metab Dispos* (2006) 34, 1055–62.
29. Committee on the Safety of Medicines/Medicines Control Agency. *Current Problems* (1996) 22, 12.

30. Pisani F, Di Perri R, Perucca E, Richens A. Interaction of lamotrigine with sodium valproate. *Lancet* (1993) 341, 1224.
31. Lamictal (Lamotrigine). GlaxoSmithKline UK. UK Summary of product characteristics, July 2012.
32. Lamictal (Lamotrigine). GlaxoSmithKline. US Prescribing information, November 2011.

Levetiracetam + Food

The oral absorption of levetiracetam is not significantly affected by food.

Clinical evidence, mechanism, importance and management

In a study, 10 healthy subjects were given a 500-mg tablet of levetiracetam with 120 mL of water or crushed and mixed with either 4 oz (about 113 g) of apple sauce or 120 mL of an enteral nutrition formulation (*Sustacal*). The overall rate and extent of absorption of oral levetiracetam were not significantly affected by crushing and mixing the tablet with either apple sauce or an enteral nutrition preparation, although the peak serum level of levetiracetam may be slightly reduced if it is mixed with enteral nutrition.[1] The clinical relevance of any effect seems likely to be small.

1. Fay MA, Sheth RD, Gidal BE. Oral absorption kinetics of levetiracetam: the effect of mixing with food or enteral nutrition formulas. *Clin Ther* (2005) 27, 594–8.

Levetiracetam + Meropenem

Levetiracetam plasma concentrations are not altered by meropenem.

Clinical evidence, mechanism, importance and management

In a prospective study in 12 patients taking levetiracetam, the addition of meropenem was not associated with any changes in levetiracetam plasma concentrations after 3 days of concurrent use.[1] Evidence is limited to this study, but it would not seem necessary to advise any additional monitoring on concurrent use.

1. Mink S, Muroi C, Suele M, Bjeljac M, Keller E. Levetiracetam compared to valproic acid: plasma concentration levels, adverse effects and interactions in aneurysmal subarachnoid hemorrhage. *Clin Neurol Neurosurg* (2011) 113, 644–8.

Levetiracetam + Other antiepileptics

There is some evidence that the enzyme-inducing antiepileptics (carbamazepine, phenobarbital, phenytoin, and primidone) might reduce the serum concentration of levetiracetam. Levetiracetam does not usually alter the serum concentrations of these antiepileptics. However, some studies have found increased serum phenytoin concentrations, and cases of possible carbamazepine toxicity have also been reported. There appears to be no pharmacokinetic interaction between levetiracetam and eslicarbazepine, gabapentin, lamotrigine, oxcarbazepine, topiramate, or valproate.

Clinical evidence, mechanism, importance and management

(a) Carbamazepine

Evidence from clinical studies suggests that levetiracetam does not affect the serum concentration of carbamazepine.[1-3] A study in 187 children treated with antiepileptic drugs, either alone or in combination, found that levetiracetam did not affect the plasma concentration of carbamazepine.[4] However, one report describes 4 patients who experienced disabling symptoms compatible with carbamazepine toxicity when levetiracetam was added. The symptoms resolved after a decrease in the carbamazepine dose or withdrawal of levetiracetam. A pharmacodynamic interaction was suggested, because the blood concentrations of carbamazepine and its metabolite, carbamazepine-10,11-epoxide, were not affected.[5]

Some evidence suggests that patients taking levetiracetam with enzyme-inducing antiepileptics, such as carbamazepine, had lower levetiracetam concentrations (24% lower) when compared with those also taking antiepileptics not considered to be enzyme-inducers (gabapentin, lamotrigine, vigabatrin), but this finding was not considered clinically relevant.[6] Similarly, another retrospective analysis of patient data found that the serum levetiracetam concentration-to-dose ratio was lower in patients also receiving carbamazepine than those receiving monotherapy (0.32 versus 0.52),[7] suggesting that carbamazepine minimally lowers the concentration of levetiracetam.

In general, there is no need to modify the dose of either carbamazepine or levetiracetam when used together. However, the report of possible carbamazepine toxicity introduces a note of caution.

(b) Phenytoin

Some evidence suggests that patients taking levetiracetam with enzyme-inducing antiepileptics, such as phenytoin, had lower levetiracetam concentrations (24% lower) when compared with those taking other antiepileptics not considered to be enzyme inducers (gabapentin, lamotrigine, vigabatrin), but this finding was not considered clinically relevant.[6] A retrospective analysis of patient data found that the serum levetiracetam concentration-to-dose ratio was lower in patients also receiving phenytoin than those receiving monotherapy (0.32 versus 0.52),[7] suggesting that phenytoin modestly lowers the concentration of levetiracetam.

Evidence from clinical studies suggests that levetiracetam does not affect the serum concentration of phenytoin.[1-3] Similarly, in one study, levetiracetam 1.5 g twice daily for 12 weeks had no effect on the steady-state pharmacokinetics of phenytoin in 6 subjects with epilepsy who were taking stable doses of phenytoin.[8] However, in one clinical study the addition of levetiracetam increased the serum concentration of phenytoin by 27% to 52% in 4 patients. A further patient had a 75% increase in the serum concentration of phenytoin [estimated from figure], experienced signs of toxicity (sedation, ataxia), and required a reduction in his phenytoin dose. Another patient with an increased serum phenytoin concentration [estimated increase of 47%] had the dose of levetiracetam reduced.[9]

In general therefore, there is no need to modify the dose of either phenytoin or levetiracetam when they are used concurrently. However, the report of increased serum concentrations of phenytoin suggests that some caution is warranted.

(c) Valproate

In healthy subjects, sodium valproate 500 mg twice daily for 8 days did not affect the pharmacokinetics of a single 1.5-g dose of levetiracetam. In addition, levetiracetam did not affect the pharmacokinetics of valproate.[10] In an analysis of clinical study data, the AUC of levetiracetam in 57 patients also taking valproic acid was 11% higher than in 28 patients also taking antiepileptics not thought to affect microsomal enzymes (gabapentin, lamotrigine, vigabatrin), but this finding was not thought to be clinically relevant.[6] In another retrospective analysis of patient data, the serum levetiracetam concentration-to-dose ratio was the same in patients also receiving valproic acid than those receiving monotherapy (0.53 versus 0.52),[7] suggesting that valproate does not alter the serum concentration of levetiracetam. Furthermore, evidence from clinical studies suggests that levetiracetam does not affect the serum concentration of valproate.[1,3,4] There appears to be no need to adjust the doses of either sodium valproate or levetiracetam if these drugs are used concurrently.

(d) Other antiepileptics

The AUC of levetiracetam tended to be lower in 436 patients also taking enzyme-inducing antiepileptics (carbamazepine, phenobarbital, phenytoin, **primidone**) than in 28 patients also taking antiepileptics not thought to affect microsomal enzymes (**gabapentin, lamotrigine, vigabatrin**), but the difference was small (24%).[6] Another retrospective analysis of patient data found that the serum levetiracetam concentration-to-dose ratio did not differ between patients also taking **lamotrigine** and those taking levetiracetam alone (0.45 versus 0.52), but was lower in those taking **oxcarbazepine** (0.34 versus 0.52).[7] A study in 187 children taking antiepileptic drugs either alone or in combination found that levetiracetam did not affect the plasma concentrations of **lamotrigine** or **topiramate**.[4] Furthermore, evidence from clinical studies suggests that levetiracetam does not affect the serum concentrations of **gabapentin, lamotrigine, phenobarbital**, or **primidone**.[1-3] Exposure to **eslicarbazepine** does not appear to be altered by levetiracetam, nor is the clearance of levetiracetam affected by eslicarbazepine.[11] In general, therefore, no dose adjustments would seem to be needed if levetiracetam is used as add-on therapy with any of these antiepileptics.

1. Keppra (Levetiracetam). UCB Pharma Ltd. UK Summary of product characteristics, September 2009.
2. Patsalos PN. Pharmacokinetic profile of levetiracetam: towards ideal characteristics. *Pharmacol Ther* (2000) 85, 77–85.
3. Keppra (Levetiracetam). UCB Inc. US Prescribing information, April 2009.
4. Otoul C, De Smedt H, Stockis A. Lack of pharmacokinetic interaction of levetiracetam on carbamazepine, valproic acid, topiramate, and lamotrigine in children with epilepsy. *Epilepsia* (2007) 48, 2111–5.
5. Sisodiya SM, Sander JWAS, Patsalos PN. Carbamazepine toxicity during combination therapy with levetiracetam: a pharmacodynamic interaction. *Epilepsy Res* (2002) 48, 217–19.
6. Perucca E, Gidal BE, Baltès E. Effects of antiepileptic comedication on levetiracetam pharmacokinetics: a pooled analysis of data from randomized adjunctive therapy trials. *Epilepsy Res* (2003) 53, 47–56.
7. May TW, Rambeck B, Jürgens U. Serum concentrations of levetiracetam in epileptic patients: the influence of dose and co-medication. *Ther Drug Monit* (2003) 25, 690–9.
8. Browne TR, Szabo GK, Leppik IE, Josephs E, Paz J, Baltes E, Jensen CM. Absence of pharmacokinetic drug interaction of levetiracetam with phenytoin in patients with epilepsy determined by new technique. *J Clin Pharmacol* (2000) 40, 590–5.
9. Sharief MK, et al. Efficacy and tolerability study of ucb L059 in patients with refractory epilepsy. *J Epilepsy* (1996) 9, 106–12.
10. Coupez R, Nicolas J-M, Browne TR. Levetiracetam, a new antiepileptic agent: lack of in vitro and in vivo pharmacokinetic interaction with valproic acid. *Epilepsia* (2003) 44, 171–8.
11. Falcão A, Fuseau E, Nunes T, Almeida A, Soares-da-Silva P. Pharmacokinetics, drug interactions and exposure-response relationship of eslicarbazepine acetate in adult patients with partial-onset seizures: population pharmacokinetic and pharmacokinetic/pharmacodynamic analyses. *CNS Drugs* (2012) 26, 79–91.

Levetiracetam + Probenecid

Probenecid increases the plasma levels of an inactive metabolite of levetiracetam.

Clinical evidence, mechanism, importance and management

One report suggests that probenecid 500 mg four times daily does not affect the renal excretion of levetiracetam. However, the renal excretion of the primary and pharmacologically inactive metabolite of levetiracetam, ucb L057, was reduced by 61%, and its plasma concentrations increased 2.5-fold,[1] although the manufacturer notes that these levels are still low.[2] The clinical relevance of elevated levels of ucb L057 is not known, therefore some have suggested caution is warranted in patients given both drugs.[1] The effect of levetiracetam on probenecid has not been studied.[2,3]

1. Patsalos PN. Pharmacokinetic profile of levetiracetam: toward ideal characteristics. *Pharmacol Ther* (2000) 85, 77–85.
2. Keppra (Levetiracetam). UCB Pharma Ltd. UK Summary of product characteristics, September 2009.
3. Keppra (Levetiracetam). UCB Inc. US Prescribing information, April 2009.

Mesuximide + Other antiepileptics

Phenobarbital, phenytoin, and possibly felbamate increase the levels of the active metabolite of mesuximide, *N*-desmethylmesuximide. Mesuximide increases the levels of phenobarbital and phenytoin, and decreases the levels of lamotrigine, and to a lesser extent, valproate.

Clinical evidence

(a) Felbamate

Three adolescent patients with epilepsy taking mesuximide developed mild adverse effects within 3 days of starting to take felbamate, which became more serious after one month (decreased appetite, nausea, weight loss, insomnia, dizziness, hiccups, slurred speech). During this time the levels of the active metabolite of mesuximide, *N*-desmethylmesuximide, rose by 26% and 46% in two patients, respectively. The adverse effects disappeared and *N*-desmethylmesuximide levels fell when the mesuximide dose was reduced. Other antiepileptics being taken were carbamazepine, ethotoin and valproate.[1]

(b) Lamotrigine

In 6 patients taking mesuximide, lamotrigine levels were 53% lower (range 36 to 72%), when compared with lamotrigine levels before starting or after stopping mesuximide. In some patients deterioration in seizure control was seen while taking mesuximide, and an improvement in seizure control occurred after mesuximide was stopped.[2] In another study, lamotrigine levels were about 70% lower in 13 patients also taking mesuximide than in 64 patients taking lamotrigine alone, when corrected for dose. Note that in patients also taking valproate, the reduction in lamotrigine levels caused by mesuximide was compensated for by the increase caused by valproate, see also 'Lamotrigine + Valproate', p.587.[3]

(c) Phenobarbital or Primidone

A study in hospitalised patients with petit mal epilepsy found that when mesuximide was given to 8 patients taking phenobarbital and 13 patients taking primidone, the mean serum levels of phenobarbital rose by 38% and 40%, respectively. Dose reductions were needed in 50% and 62% of patients, respectively. It was also found that the concurrent use of phenobarbital increased the serum levels of the active metabolite of mesuximide, *N*-desmethylmesuximide.[4]

(d) Phenytoin

Mesuximide was given to 17 patients taking phenytoin, which resulted in a 78% rise in the phenytoin serum levels requiring dose reductions in about 30% of the patients. It was also found that the concurrent use of phenytoin increased the serum levels of the active metabolite of mesuximide, *N*-desmethylmesuximide.[4]

(e) Valproate

A retrospective analysis of serum valproate levels was carried out in 17 patients who started and/or stopped taking mesuximide and whose concurrent medication remained unaltered. In the 14 patients starting mesuximide, a mean decrease in valproate levels of 32% was seen. In the 8 patients who stopped mesuximide a 30% increase in valproate levels occurred.[5] Note that the related drug, ethosuximide, has also been reported to lower valproate levels, see 'Ethosuximide + Other antiepileptics', p.582.

Mechanism

It has been suggested that phenobarbital, phenytoin and felbamate compete with mesuximide for the same metabolic mechanisms (hydroxylation) in the liver. As a result each one is metabolised more slowly and therefore their levels increase. Mesuximide appears to increase the clearance of valproate and lamotrigine (which principally occurs by glucuronidation).

Importance and management

Information about these interactions is limited. Nevertheless, concurrent use should be monitored. Anticipate the need to reduce the dose of phenytoin, phenobarbital or primidone if mesuximide is given. The dose of lamotrigine may need to be increased if mesuximide is given. There is also some evidence that the dose of valproate may need to be increased.

The activity of mesuximide is thought to be due to its active metabolite, *N*-desmethylmesuximide. Therefore, it has been suggested that levels of this metabolite should also be monitored. Anticipate the need to reduce the dose of mesuximide if felbamate is added. Other antiepileptics such as phenobarbital and phenytoin may also increase levels of *N*-desmethylmesuximide.[4]

1. Patrias J, Espe-Lillo J, Ritter FJ. Felbamate-methsuximide interaction. *Epilepsia* (1992) 33 (Suppl 3) 84.
2. Besag FM, Berry DJ, Pool F. Methsuximide lowers lamotrigine blood levels: a pharmacokinetic antiepileptic drug interaction. *Epilepsia* (2000) 41, 624–7.
3. May TW, Rambeck B, Jürgens U. Influence of oxcarbazepine and methsuximide on lamotrigine concentrations in epileptic patients with and without valproic acid comedication: results of a retrospective study. *Ther Drug Monit* (1999) 21, 175–81.
4. Rambeck B. Pharmacological interactions of mesuximide with phenobarbital and phenytoin in hospitalized epileptic patients. *Epilepsia* (1979) 20, 147–56.
5. Besag FMC, Berry DJ, Vasey M. Methsuximide reduces valproic acid serum levels. *Ther Drug Monit* (2001) 23, 694–7.

Oxcarbazepine + Macrolides

Erythromycin does not appear to affect the pharmacokinetics of oxcarbazepine. A case report describes a patient taking oxcarbazepine who developed oxcarbazepine toxicity when clarithromycin was added.

Clinical evidence, mechanism, importance and management

(a) Clarithromycin

A 10-year-old boy with uncontrolled epilepsy despite taking multiple antiepileptic drugs, including oxcarbazepine 540 mg in the morning and 510 mg at night, was given clarithromycin 250 mg twice daily for a respiratory tract infection. Within one hour of the first dose he was noted to be unsteady on his feet, and about 24 hours later he was admitted to hospital with vomiting, dizziness, and drowsiness. He was noted to be ataxic and showing nystagmus, so his oxcarbazepine dose was reduced to 420 mg and the clarithromycin stopped. His symptoms resolved, and he was eventually restabilised on his original oxcarbazepine dose. It was suggested that clarithromycin, a P-glycoprotein inhibitor, had increased the CNS levels of oxcarbazepine by preventing its removal from the brain by P-glycoprotein. This resulted in the adverse effects seen.[1] The general relevance of this isolated case is unknown but it would seem prudent to suspect an interaction if oxcarbazepine adverse effects (e.g. dizziness, drowsiness, and ataxia) develop in a patient given clarithromycin.

(b) Erythromycin

In a study in 8 healthy subjects, the pharmacokinetics of a single 600-mg dose of oxcarbazepine were unaffected by erythromycin 500 mg twice daily for 7 days.[2] Erythromycin appears not to interact with oxcarbazepine, and no oxcarbazepine dose adjustments therefore seem to be necessary during concurrent use.

1. Santucci R, Fothergill H, Laugel V, Perville A, De Saint Martin A, Gerout A-C, Fischbach M. The onset of acute oxcarbazepine toxicity related to prescription of clarithromycin in a child with refractory epilepsy. *Br J Clin Pharmacol* (2009) 69, 314–16.
2. Keränen T, Jolkkonen J, Jensen PK, Menge GP, Andersson P. Absence of interaction between oxcarbazepine and erythromycin. *Acta Neurol Scand* (1992) 86, 120–3.

Paraldehyde + Disulfiram

***Animal* data suggest that disulfiram can increase paraldehyde levels and prolong its effects. There is a theoretical potential for a disulfiram reaction.**

Clinical evidence, mechanism, importance and management

It is thought that paraldehyde is depolymerised in the liver to acetaldehyde, and then oxidised by acetaldehyde dehydrogenase.[1] As disulfiram inhibits this enzyme, concurrent use would be expected to result in the accumulation of acetaldehyde and result in a modified disulfiram reaction.[2] However, studies in *animals* given disulfiram and paraldehyde found increases in the levels of paraldehyde and an increase in its hypnotic effect, with only small increases in acetaldehyde levels and no increase in toxicity.[2,3] In addition, there appear to be no reports of a disulfiram reaction involving paraldehyde in humans. However, three cases of mental confusion have been reported in patients receiving disulfiram and paraldehyde.[4] Note that, patients with liver disease are at greater risk of paraldehyde adverse effects, and the addition of disulfiram results in a further risk. Therefore it may be prudent to avoid concurrent use in this type of patient.

1. Hitchcock P, Nelson EE. The metabolism of paraldehyde: II. *J Pharmacol Exp Ther* (1943) 79, 286–94.
2. Keplinger ML, Wells JA. Effect of Antabuse on the action of paraldehyde in mice and dogs. *Fedn Proc* (1956) 15, 445–6.
3. Keplinger ML, Wells JA. The effect of disulfiram on the action and metabolism of paraldehyde. *J Pharmacol Exp Ther* (1957), 119: 19–25.
4. Christie GL. Three cases of transient confusional psychosis in patients receiving con-current antabuse and paraldehyde therapy. *Med J Aust* (1956) May 12: 789–91.

Perampanel + Miscellaneous

The metabolism of perampanel appears to be increased by a number of enzyme-inducing drugs (e.g. carbamazepine) and is predicted to be increased by others (e.g. rifampicin (rifampin)). Ketoconazole very slightly increases perampanel exposure. Perampanel slightly increases oxcarbazepine concentrations, has a negligible effect on midazolam exposure, but might decrease the exposure to progestogens. Additive CNS depression might occur if perampanel is given with alcohol.

Clinical evidence, mechanism, importance and management

(a) Alcohol

Perampanel can cause dizziness and somnolence and might therefore reduce the ability to drive or undertake other complex tasks. In a study in healthy subjects, these CNS depressant effects of perampanel were additive or synergistic with those of alcohol.[1]

(b) Antiepileptics

The UK manufacturer states that **felbamate** might reduce perampanel concentrations.[1] As perampanel should be dosed according to clinical response, it would seem prudent to monitor concurrent use, adjusting the dose of perampanel as required.

In population pharmacokinetic studies of patients with partial-onset seizures taking perampanel in doses up to 12 mg daily, no clinically relevant interaction was seen between perampanel and **clobazam**, **clonazepam**, **lamotrigine**, **levetiracetam**, **phenobarbital**, **topiramate**, **valproate** or **zonisamide**.[1] Based on this information, no dose adjustment of either drug would be expected to be necessary on concurrent use; however, this type of data gives only the broadest indication of whether or not an interaction occurs. In particular, note that many enzyme-inducing antiepileptics reduce perampanel exposure, see *Enzyme-inducing antiepileptics*, below, and therefore, until more is known about perampanel metabolism, the data given above, suggesting a lack of interaction with **phenobarbital**, should be viewed with caution.

Enzyme-inducing antiepileptics. In a study in healthy subjects, **carbamazepine** reduced perampanel concentrations by two-thirds. Similarly, in a population pharmacokinetic analysis of patients with partial-onset seizures taking perampanel in doses of up to 12 mg daily, perampanel clearance was increased by a number of enzyme-inducing antiepileptics including **carbamazepine** (3-fold increase in clearance), **phenytoin** (2-fold increase in clearance), and **oxcarbazepine** (2-fold increase in clearance).[1] It seems possible that **fosphenytoin**, a prodrug of phenytoin, might interact similarly. If any of these drugs is given with perampanel, monitor the outcome closely and consider increasing the perampanel dose according to clinical need.

Perampanel does not appear to affect the concentrations of **carbamazepine** or **phenytoin** to a clinically relevant extent. Perampanel increases the concentration of **oxcarbazepine** by 35% and decreases its clearance by 26%,[1] which would not be expected to be clinically relevant.

(c) CYP3A4 inhibitors

In a study in healthy subjects, **ketoconazole** 400 mg daily for 10 days increased the AUC of perampanel by 20%.[1] This very slight increase in exposure would not be expected to be clinically relevant. However, the UK manufacturer[1] states that larger effects cannot be excluded if perampanel is given with a CYP3A inhibitor with a longer half-life than ketoconazole or when the inhibitor is given for a longer treatment duration (note that perampanel has a long half-life). Until more is known it might be prudent to monitor the use of perampanel and potent CYP3A4 inhibitors for perampanel adverse effects (such as dizziness, blurred vision, or gait disturbances) and reduce the dose of perampanel according to clinical need. For a list of CYP3A4 inhibitors, see 'Table 1.9', p.11.

(d) CYP3A4 substrates

In a study in healthy subjects, perampanel 6 mg daily for 20 days decreased the AUC of **midazolam** by 13%,[1] which would not be expected to be clinically relevant. Note that **midazolam** can be used as a probe substrate to assess the activity of drugs on CYP3A4. This study therefore suggests that perampanel is not a clinically relevant inducer of CYP3A4. However, note that the UK manufacturer states that a larger decrease in **midazolam** exposure cannot be excluded with higher perampanel doses.[1]

(e) Enzyme inducers

The UK manufacturer predicts that potent cytochrome P450 inducers will decrease perampanel concentrations (they name **rifampicin (rifampin)** and **St John's wort**).[1] Given the effects of the enzyme-inducing antiepileptics on perampanel concentrations (see *Enzyme-inducing antiepileptics*, above) this seems a logical prediction. Until more is known it would seem prudent to monitor concurrent use for perampanel efficacy, increasing the dose according to clinical need.

(f) Hormonal contraceptives

In a study, healthy women were given perampanel 12 mg daily for 21 days with an oral combined hormonal contraceptive. Perampanel decreased the AUC of **levonorgestrel** by 40%, whereas the AUC of **ethinylestradiol** was not affected. Lower doses of perampanel 4 mg daily and 8 mg daily did not affect the pharmacokinetics of these contraceptive steroids.[1] The UK manufacturer therefore state that, in patients taking perampanel 12 mg daily, the possibility of decreased contraceptive efficacy (both combined hormonal contraceptives and progestogen-only contraceptives) should be considered, and suggest using an additional reliable method of contraception (they suggest an intra-uterine device or condom).[1] In 2013 the UK Faculty of Sexual and Reproductive Healthcare issued a statement on the use of perampanel (at any dose) with combined hormonal, or progesterone-only, contraceptives, which recommends the same advice as for women taking other liver enzyme inducers with these contraceptives.[2] Their specific recommendations on the short- and long-term use of enzyme inducers are discussed in detail under 'Combined hormonal contraceptives + Barbiturates or Phenytoin', p.1169, and these should be followed.

(g) Levodopa

In healthy subjects, perampanel 4 mg daily for 19 days had no effect on the maximum concentrations or AUC of levodopa.[1] No levodopa dose adjustments would therefore be expected to be necessary on the concurrent use of perampanel.

1. Fycompa (Perampanel). Eisai Ltd. UK Summary of product characteristics, June 2015.
2. Faculty of Sexual and Reproductive Healthcare. Update on newer antiepileptic and antiretroviral drugs and interactions with hormonal contraceptives. Clinical Effectiveness Unit Statement, March 2013 (Updated August 2013). Available at: http://www.fsrh.org/pdfs/CEUstatementUpdateNewerAntiepilepticAntiretroviralDrugs.pdf (accessed 26/08/15).

Phenobarbital or Primidone + Allopurinol

Allopurinol appears not to alter phenobarbital levels, including those derived from primidone.

Clinical evidence, mechanism, importance and management

In a study of add-on therapy, allopurinol (150 mg daily in those less than 20 kg, and 300 mg daily for other patients) for 4 months, had no effect on the phenobarbital levels in 46 patients taking antiepileptics including phenobarbital.[1] In another similar study, allopurinol 10 mg/kg increased to 15 mg/kg daily for 12 weeks had no effect on serum phenobarbital levels in 11 patients taking primidone or phenobarbital with or without other antiepileptics.[2] Therefore phenobarbital or primidone dose alterations are unlikely to be required if allopurinol is also given.

1. Zagnoni PG, Bianchi A, Zolo P, Canger R, Cornaggia C, D'Alessandro P, DeMarco P, Pisani F, Gianelli M, Verzé L, Viani F, Zaccara G. Allopurinol as add-on therapy in refractory epilepsy: a double-blind placebo-controlled randomized study. *Epilepsia* (1994) 35, 107–12.
2. Coppola G, Pascotto A. Double-blind, placebo-controlled, cross-over trial of allopurinol as add-on therapy in childhood refractory epilepsy. *Brain Dev* (1996) 18, 50–2.

Phenobarbital + Azoles

Limited evidence suggests phenobarbital causes a large decrease in itraconazole concentrations, and might decrease ketoconazole concentrations. Phenobarbital is also predicted to decrease posaconazole and voriconazole concentrations.

Clinical evidence, mechanism, importance and management

Note that primidone is metabolised to phenobarbital, and therefore **primidone** might also be expected to interact similarly with azole.

(a) Fluconazole

For a report that fluconazole does not affect the concentrations of **barbexaclone** (a compound of levopropylhexedrine with phenobarbital), see 'Carbamazepine + Azoles', p.568.

(b) Itraconazole

The serum concentrations of itraconazole 200 mg daily were very low (0.01 to 0.03 mg/L, reference range 0.25 to 2 mg/L) in a patient taking phenobarbital. Two months after stopping the phenobarbital they were higher (0.15 mg/L), but still below the therapeutic range, apparently because carbamazepine had been recently started.[1] For mention of two other patients who had very low itraconazole concentrations while taking both phenytoin and phenobarbital, see 'Phenytoin + Azoles', p.595. Based on the evidence with phenytoin, some manufacturers of itraconazole state that similar effects should be expected with phenobarbital and so do not recommended concurrent use.[2,3]

(c) Ketoconazole

Low ketoconazole concentrations in a patient with leukaemia receiving various antineoplastics was attributed to the concurrent use of phenytoin and phenobarbital.[4] It would seem prudent to monitor the efficacy of ketoconazole if phenobarbital is also given.

(d) Posaconazole

Based on the evidence with phenytoin (see 'Phenytoin + Azoles', p.595), the manufacturer of posaconazole predicts that phenobarbital will reduce posaconazole concentrations, and therefore suggests avoiding the combination unless the benefits outweigh the risks.[5] If concurrent use is necessary monitor for posaconazole efficacy.

(e) Voriconazole

Based on the evidence with phenytoin (see 'Phenytoin + Azoles', p.595), the UK and US manufacturers of voriconazole predict that phenobarbital will reduce voriconazole concentrations, and therefore contraindicate their concurrent use.[6,7] They also extend this contraindication to all long-acting barbiturates.

1. Bonay M, Jonville-Bera AP, Diot P, Lemarie E, Lavandier M, Autret E. Possible interaction between phenobarbital, carbamazepine and itraconazole. *Drug Safety* (1993) 9, 309–11.
2. Sporanox Capsules (Itraconazole). Janssen-Cilag Ltd. UK Summary of product characteristics, October 2011.
3. Sporanox Capsules (Itraconazole). Ortho-McNeill-Janssen Pharmaceuticals, Inc. US Prescribing information, June 2011.
4. Stockley RJ, Daneshmend TK, Bredow MT, Warnock DW, Richardson MD, Slade RR. Ketoconazole pharmacokinetics during chronic dosing in adults with haematological malignancy. *Eur J Clin Microbiol* (1986) 5, 513–17.
5. Noxafil (Posaconazole). Merck Sharp & Dohme Ltd. UK Summary of product characteristics, September 2014.
6. VFEND (Voriconazole). Pfizer Ltd. UK Summary of product characteristics, October 2014.
7. VFEND (Voriconazole). Pfizer Inc. US Prescribing information, February 2014.

Phenobarbital + Dextropropoxyphene (Propoxyphene)

When 4 patients with epilepsy took dextropropoxyphene 65 mg three times a day for a week there was an average 20% rise in their serum phenobarbital levels.[1] This rise is unlikely to be clinically significant in most patients.

1. Hansen BS, Dam M, Brandt J, Hvidberg EF, Angelo H, Christensen JM, Lous P. Influence of dextropropoxyphene on steady state serum levels and protein binding of three anti-epileptic drugs in man. *Acta Neurol Scand* (1980) 61, 357–67.

Phenobarbital or Primidone + Felbamate

Felbamate causes a moderate increase in phenobarbital levels (including those derived from primidone), which has resulted in phenobarbital toxicity.

Clinical evidence

When 24 healthy subjects taking phenobarbital 100 mg daily were also given felbamate 1.2 g twice daily for 10 days, the AUC and the maximum plasma levels of phenobarbital were raised by 22% and 24%, respectively. Concurrent use was said to be safe and well tolerated.[1] A 30% increase in phenobarbital plasma concentrations was seen in another 19 patients taking phenobarbital or primidone (which is metabolised to phenobarbital) when they were given felbamate (average dose 2458 mg daily).[2] A phenobarbital dose reduction of about 30% was needed in another 6 patients when they started to take felbamate.[3]

A man taking sodium valproate and phenobarbital had an almost 50% increase in phenobarbital serum levels over a 5-week period after felbamate 50 mg/kg was added, despite an initial phenobarbital dose reduction from 230 mg to 200 mg daily. He was hospitalised because of increased lethargy, anorexia and ataxia and was eventually discharged taking phenobarbital 150 mg daily.[4]

It has also been noted that felbamate levels are lower in patients taking phenobarbital than in historical control patients not taking phenobarbital.[1] The manufacturer notes that steady-state felbamate levels were 29% lower in patients also given phenobarbital, when compared with levels in newly diagnosed epileptics given felbamate 2.4 g daily.[5] However, in a modelling study, phenobarbital apparently had little or no effect on the pharmacokinetics of felbamate.[6]

Mechanism

Not established. It seems possible that the felbamate may inhibit more than one pathway in the metabolism of phenobarbital, resulting in a reduction in its loss from the body. The cytochrome P450 isoenzyme CYP2C19 may be involved.[1,7]

Importance and management

An established interaction. If felbamate is added to established treatment with phenobarbital or primidone, particularly in patients already taking substantial doses, monitor closely for any evidence of increased adverse effects (drowsiness, lethargy, anorexia, ataxia) and reduce the doses of phenobarbital or primidone if necessary.

1. Reidenberg P, Glue P, Banfield CR, Colucci RD, Meehan JW, Radwanski E, Mojavarian P, Lin C-C, Nezamis J, Guillaume M, Affime MB. Effects of felbamate on the pharmacokinetics of phenobarbital. *Clin Pharmacol Ther* (1995) 58, 279–87.
2. Kerrick JM, Wolff DL, Risinger MW, Graves NM. Increased phenobarbital plasma concentrations after felbamate initiation. *Epilepsia* (1994) 35 (Suppl 8), 96.
3. Sachdeo RC, Padela MF. The effect of felbamate on phenobarbital serum concentrations. *Epilepsia* (1994) 35 (Suppl 8), 94.
4. Gidal BE, Zupanc ML. Potential pharmacokinetic interaction between felbamate and phenobarbital. *Ann Pharmacother* (1994) 28, 455–8.
5. Felbatol (Felbamate). Meda Pharmaceuticals. US Prescribing information, June 2008.
6. Kelley MT, Walson PD, Cox S, Dusci LJ. Population pharmacokinetics of felbamate in children. *Ther Drug Monit* (1997) 19, 29–36.
7. Glue P, Banfield CR, Perhach JL, Mather GG, Racha JK, Levy RH. Pharmacokinetic interactions with felbamate. *Clin Pharmacokinet* (1997) 33, 214–24.

Phenobarbital + Influenza vaccines

Influenza vaccine can cause a moderate rise in the levels of phenobarbital.

Clinical evidence, mechanism, importance and management

The serum levels of phenobarbital rose by about 30% in 11 out of 27 children who were given 0.5 mL of a whole virus influenza vaccine USP, types A and B, (Squibb). Levels remained elevated 28 days after vaccination.[1]

It was suggested that the vaccine inhibits the liver enzymes concerned with the metabolism of phenobarbital, thereby reducing its loss from the body. Information is very limited, but note that, a similar 30% increase in phenobarbital levels with felbamate has eventually required a dose adjustment after long-term concurrent use. However, as influenza vaccines are usually given as a single dose phenobarbital accumulation seems unlikely, and the increase in levels will eventually be self-limiting. Therefore it seems unlikely that this moderate increase in phenobarbital levels will be of clinical significance.

1. Jann MW, Fidone GS. Effect of influenza vaccine on serum anticonvulsant concentrations. *Clin Pharm* (1986) 5, 817–20.

Phenobarbital + Troleandomycin

Troleandomycin caused a modest fall in the phenobarbital levels of one patient.

Clinical evidence, mechanism, importance and management

A patient taking phenobarbital and carbamazepine had a modest reduction in plasma phenobarbital levels from about 40 micrograms/mL to 31 micrograms/mL when given troleandomycin.[1] The general importance of this single report is uncertain, but this 23% fall is probably of limited clinical importance.

1. Dravet C, Mesdjian E, Cenraud B and Roger J. Interaction between carbamazepine and triacetyloleandomycin. *Lancet* (1977) i, 810–11.

Phenobarbital + Valproate

Serum phenobarbital levels can be increased by valproate, which may result in excessive sedation and lethargy. Small reductions in valproate levels have also been reported. Combined use of phenobarbital and valproate may cause an increase in serum liver enzymes.

Clinical evidence

A 6-month study in 11 patients with epilepsy taking phenobarbital 90 to 400 mg daily found that when they were also given valproic acid 11.2 to 42.7 mg/kg daily sedation developed. On average the dose of phenobarbital was reduced to 54% of the original dose with continued good seizure control. Another 2 patients who did not have their phenobarbital dose reduced had an increase in their phenobarbital levels of 12% and 48%, respectively, when valproic acid was added.[1]

Another study found that sodium valproate 1.2 g daily raised serum phenobarbital levels in 20 patients by an average of 27%. Signs of toxicity occurred in 13 patients, but the dose only needed to be reduced in 3 patients.[2] This interaction has been described in numerous other reports, and dose reductions of the phenobarbital were almost always necessary to avoid excessive drowsiness.[3-17] In one study the rise in phenobarbital levels was much greater in children (over 100%) than in adults (about 50%).[18]

A small reduction in sodium valproate levels (of about 25%) has also been reported, but the effect on seizure control was not mentioned.[19] A reduction in valproate levels caused by phenobarbital has also been reported elsewhere.[20]

The incidence of increased liver enzyme activity was found to be higher in 41 patients receiving phenobarbital with valproate than in 40 patients taking valproate alone (ALT 7.3% versus 0%). When phenytoin was also given an even greater incidence of increases (ALT 26.1% and AST 28.3% versus about 20%) occurred. However, the increases were mild and were not considered clinically important.[21]

Mechanism

The evidence indicates that valproate inhibits three steps in the metabolism of phenobarbital by the liver, leading to its accumulation in the body. The inhibited steps are the formation of *p*-hydroxyphenobarbital by the cytochrome P450 isoenzyme CYP2C9,[22] the *N*-glucosidation of phenobarbital[23] and the *O*-glucuronidation of *p*-hydroxyphenobarbital.[23]

Importance and management

An extremely well documented and well established interaction of clinical importance. The incidence seems to be high. The effects of concurrent use should be well monitored and suitable phenobarbital dose reductions made as necessary to avoid toxicity. The dose may need to be reduced by one-third to one-half.[1] The significance of the modest reduction in valproate levels is not clear, especially as valproate levels do not correlate well with efficacy of treatment. Valproate has been associated with serious hepatotoxicity, especially in children aged less than 3 years, and this has been more common in those receiving other antiepileptics. Valproate monotherapy is to be preferred in this group.

1. Wilder BJ, Willmore LJ, Bruni J, Villarreal HJ. Valproic acid: interaction with other anticonvulsant drugs. *Neurology* (1978) 28, 892–6.
2. Richens A, Ahmad S. Controlled trial of sodium valproate in severe epilepsy. *BMJ* (1975) 4, 255–6.
3. Schobben F, van der Kleijn E and Gabreëls FJM. Pharmacokinetics of di-n-propylacetate in epileptic patients. *Eur J Clin Pharmacol* (1975) 8, 97–105.
4. Gram L, Wulff K, Rasmussen KE, Flachs H, Würtz-Jørgensen A, Sommerbeck KW, Løhren V. Valproate sodium: a controlled clinical trial including monitoring of drug levels. *Epilepsia* (1977) 18, 141–8.
5. Jeavons PM, Clark JE. Sodium valproate in treatment of epilepsy. *BMJ* (1974) 2, 584–6.
6. Völzke E, Doose H. Dipropylacetate (Dépakine®, Ergenyl®) in the treatment of epilepsy. *Epilepsia* (1973) 14, 185–93.
7. Millet Y, Sainty JM, Galland MC, Sidoine R, Jouglard J. Problèmes posés par l'association thérapeutique phénobarbital-dipropylacétate de sodium. A propos d'un cas. *Eur J Toxicol Environ Hyg* (1976) 9, 381–3.
8. Jeavons PM, Clark JE, Maheshwari MC. Treatment of generalized epilepsies of childhood and adolescence with sodium valproate ('Epilim'). *Dev Med Child Neurol* (1977) 19, 9–25.
9. Vakil SD, Critchley EMR, Phillips JC, Fahim Y, Haydock C, Cocks A, Dyer T. The effect of sodium valproate (Epilim) on phenytoin and phenobarbitone blood levels. Clinical and Pharmacological Aspects of Sodium Valproate (Epilim) in the Treatment of Epilepsy. Proceedings of a Symposium held at Nottingham University, September 1975, 75–7.
10. Scott DF, Boxer CM, Herzberg JL. A study of the hypnotic effects of Epilim and its possible interaction with phenobarbitone. Clinical and Pharmacological Aspects of Sodium Valproate (Epilim) in the Treatment of Epilepsy. Proceedings of a Symposium held at Nottingham University, September 1975, 155–7.
11. Richens A, Scoular IT, Ahmad S, Jordan BJ. Pharmacokinetics and efficacy of Epilim in patients receiving long-term therapy with other antiepileptic drugs. Clinical and Pharmacological Aspects of Sodium Valproate (Epilim) in the Treatment of Epilepsy. Proceedings of a Symposium held at Nottingham University, September 1975, 78–88.
12. Loiseau P, Orgogozo JM, Brachet-Liermain A, Morselli PL. Pharmacokinetic studies on the interaction between phenobarbital and valproic acid. In Adv Epileptol Proc Cong Int League Epilepsy 13th. Edited by Meinardi H and Rowan A. (1977/8) p 261–5.
13. Fowler GW. Effect of dipropylacetate on serum levels of anticonvulsants in children. *Proc West Pharmacol Soc* (1978) 21, 37–40.
14. Patel IH, Levy RH, Cutler RE. Phenobarbital-valproic acid interaction. *Clin Pharmacol Ther* (1980) 27, 515–21.
15. Coulter DL, Wu H, Allen RJ. Valproic acid therapy in childhood epilepsy. *JAMA* (1980) 244, 785–8.
16. Kapetanovic IM, Kupferberg HJ, Porter RJ, Theodore W, Schulman E, Penry JK. Mechanism of valproate-phenobarbital interaction in epileptic patients. *Clin Pharmacol Ther* (1981) 29, 480–6.
17. Yukara E, To H, Ohdo S, Higuchi S, Aoyama T. Detection of a drug-drug interaction on population based phenobarbitone clearance using nonlinear mixed-effects modeling. *Eur J Clin Pharmacol* (1998) 54, 69–74.
18. Fernandez de Gatta MR, Alonso Gonzalez AC, Garcia Sanchez MJ, Dominguez-Gil Hurle A, Santos Borbujo J, Monzon Corral L. Effect of sodium valproate on phenobarbital serum levels in children and adults. *Ther Drug Monit* (1986) 8, 416–20.
19. May T, Rambeck B. Serum concentrations of valproic acid: influence of dose and comedication. *Ther Drug Monit* (1985) 7, 387–90.

20. Meinardi H, Bongers E. Analytical data in connection with the clinical use of di-n-propylacetate. In: Schneider H, (ed). Clinical Pharmacology of Antiepileptic Drugs. New York and Berlin: Springer-Verlag; 1975 pp. 235–41.
21. Haidukewych D, John G. Chronic valproic acid and coantiepileptic drug therapy and incidence of increases in serum liver enzymes. *Ther Drug Monit* (1986) 8, 407–410.
22. Hurst SI, Hargreaves JA, Howald WN, Racha JK, Mather GG, Labroo R, Carlson SP, Levy RH. Enzymatic mechanism for the phenobarbital-valproate interaction. *Epilepsia* (1997) 38 (Suppl 8), 111–12.
23. Bernus I, Dickinson RG, Hooper WD, Eadie MJ. Inhibition of phenobarbitone *N*-glucosidation by valproate. *Br J Clin Pharmacol* (1994) 38, 411–16.

Phenytoin + Allopurinol

A case report describes phenytoin toxicity in a boy given allopurinol. Another study found that allopurinol may raise phenytoin levels but only in some patients.

Clinical evidence, mechanism, importance and management

A 13-year-old boy with Lesch-Nyhan syndrome who was taking phenobarbital, clonazepam, valproic acid and phenytoin 200 mg daily became somnolent within 7 days of starting to take allopurinol 150 mg daily. His serum phenytoin levels were found to have increased from 7.5 micrograms/mL to 20.8 micrograms/mL.[1] In a study, 2 patients had a marked increase in phenytoin levels when they were given allopurinol (150 mg daily in those less than 20 kg, and 300 mg daily for other patients) for 4 months, which in one case led to withdrawal from the study, and in the other to a phenytoin dose reduction. However, 16 other patients had no change in phenytoin levels while taking this dose of allopurinol.[2]

The reason for this reaction is not known. An *animal* study confirmed that 50 mg/kg, but not 20 mg/kg, of allopurinol reduced phenytoin elimination, but was unable to work out the mechanism.[3]

Although information is limited, it appears that allopurinol may raise phenytoin levels in some patients. It would therefore be prudent to monitor for phenytoin toxicity (e.g. blurred vision, nystagmus, ataxia or drowsiness) when allopurinol, particularly in high doses, is added.

1. Yokochi K, Yokochi A, Chiba K, Ishizaki T. Phenytoin-allopurinol interaction: Michaelis-Menten kinetic parameters of phenytoin with and without allopurinol in a child with Lesch-Nyhan syndrome. *Ther Drug Monit* (1982) 4, 353–7.
2. Zagnoni PG, Bianchi A, Zolo P, Canger R, Cornaggia C, D'Alessandro P, DeMarco P, Pisani F, Gianelli M, Verzé L, Viani F, Zaccara G. Allopurinol as add-on therapy in refractory epilepsy: a double-blind placebo-controlled randomized study. *Epilepsia* (1994) 35, 107–12.
3. Ogiso T, Ito Y, Iwaki M, Tsunekawa K. Drug interaction between phenytoin and allopurinol. *J Pharmacobiodyn* (1990) 13, 36–43.

Phenytoin + Amiodarone

Serum phenytoin levels can be raised by amiodarone, markedly so in some individuals, and phenytoin toxicity may occur. Amiodarone serum levels are reduced by phenytoin.

Clinical evidence

(a) Phenytoin serum levels increased

Three patients had a marked rise in serum phenytoin levels 10 days to 4 weeks after being given amiodarone 400 mg to 1.2 g daily. One patient developed phenytoin toxicity (ataxia, lethargy, vertigo) within 4 weeks of starting to take amiodarone and had a serum phenytoin level of 40 micrograms/mL, representing a three to fourfold increase. Levels restabilised when the phenytoin dose was withheld and then reduced from 300 to 200 mg daily. The serum phenytoin levels of the other 2 patients were approximately doubled by amiodarone.[1] Other case reports describe 3 patients who had two- to threefold rises in serum phenytoin levels, and toxicity, 2 to 6 weeks after starting amiodarone.[2-4]

A study in healthy subjects found that amiodarone 200 mg daily for 3 weeks increased the AUC of a single 5-mg/kg intravenous dose of phenytoin by 40%.[5] Another pharmacokinetic study found that amiodarone 200 mg daily for 6 weeks raised the AUC and steady-state peak serum levels of phenytoin by 40% and 33%, respectively. In this study, phenytoin 2 to 4 mg/kg daily was given orally for 14 days before and during the last 2 weeks of amiodarone use.[6]

(b) Amiodarone serum levels reduced

A study in 5 healthy subjects given amiodarone 200 mg daily found that over a 5-week period the serum amiodarone levels gradually increased. When phenytoin 3 to 4 mg/kg daily was added for a period of 2 weeks, the serum amiodarone levels fell to concentrations that were between about 50% and 65% of those predicted.[7]

Mechanism

Uncertain. It seems possible that amiodarone inhibits the liver enzymes concerned with the metabolism of phenytoin, resulting in a rise in its serum levels.[6] It seems unlikely that drug displacement from protein binding sites had a part to play as free and bound levels of phenytoin remained constant.[6]

Phenytoin is an enzyme-inducing drug that possibly increases the metabolism of the amiodarone by the liver.

Importance and management

Information seems to be limited to the reports cited, but both interactions appear to be clinically important. Concurrent use should not be undertaken unless the effects can be well monitored.

Monitor phenytoin levels and for adverse effects (e.g. blurred vision, nystagmus, ataxia or drowsiness) and reduce the phenytoin dose as necessary. A 25 to 30% reduction has been recommended for those taking phenytoin 2 to 4 mg/kg daily, but it should be remembered that small alterations in phenytoin dose may result in a large change in phenytoin levels, as phenytoin kinetics are non-linear.[6,8,9] Note that the phenytoin levels in some individuals were doubled after only 10 days of concurrent use.[1] Amiodarone has a long half-life so that this interaction will persist for weeks after its withdrawal. Continued monitoring is important. Be aware that ataxia due to phenytoin toxicity may be confused with amiodarone-induced ataxia.[1,3]

It is not clear whether or not the amiodarone dose should be increased to accommodate this interaction because the metabolite of amiodarone (*N*-desethylamiodarone) also has important antiarrhythmic effects.[7]

1. McGovern B, Geer VR, LaRaia PJ, Garan H, Ruskin JN. Possible interaction between amiodarone and phenytoin. *Ann Intern Med* (1984) 101, 650–1.
2. Gore JM, Haffajee CI, Alpert JS. Interaction of amiodarone and diphenylhydantoin. *Am J Cardiol* (1984) 54, 1145.
3. Shackleford EJ, Watson FT. Amiodarone-phenytoin interaction. *Drug Intell Clin Pharm* (1987) 21, 921.
4. Ahmad S. Amiodarone and phenytoin: interaction. *J Am Geriatr Soc* (1995) 43, 1449–50.
5. Nolan PE, Marcus FI, Hoyer GL, Bliss M, Gear K. Pharmacokinetic interaction between intravenous phenytoin and amiodarone in healthy volunteers. *Clin Pharmacol Ther* (1989) 46, 43–50.
6. Nolan PE, Erstad BL, Hoyer GL, Bliss M, Gear K, Marcus FI. Steady-state interaction between amiodarone and phenytoin in normal subjects. *Am J Cardiol* (1990) 65, 1252–7.
7. Nolan PE, Marcus FI, Karol MD, Hoyer GL, Gear K. Effect of phenytoin on the clinical pharmacokinetics of amiodarone. *J Clin Pharmacol* (1990) 30, 1112–19.
8. Nolan PE, Erstad BL, Hoyer GL, Bliss M, Gear K, Marcus FI. Interaction between amiodarone and phenytoin. *Am J Cardiol* (1991) 67, 328–9.
9. Duffal SB, McKenzie SK. Interaction between amiodarone and phenytoin. *Am J Cardiol* (1991) 67, 328.

Phenytoin + Antacids

Some studies have found that antacids can reduce phenytoin levels and this may have been responsible for some loss of seizure control in a few patients. However other studies have not found any interaction and it seems that usually no clinically important interaction occurs.

Clinical evidence

A review briefly mentions that 3 patients taking phenytoin were found to have low serum phenytoin levels of 2 to 4 micrograms/mL when they were given phenytoin at the same time as antacids (unnamed), but when antacid administration was delayed by 2 to 3 hours the serum phenytoin levels rose two to threefold.[1]

Elsewhere, 2 patients with epilepsy are reported to have had inadequate seizure control, which coincided with the ingestion of **aluminium/magnesium hydroxide** antacids for dyspepsia.[2]

In a study in 8 healthy subjects, the AUC of a single dose of phenytoin was reduced by a modest 25% by either **aluminium/magnesium hydroxide** or **calcium carbonate**.[3] A study in 6 healthy subjects given **aluminium** or **magnesium hydroxide** did not find any change in the rate or extent of absorption of a single dose of phenytoin,[2] and a similar study found that **calcium carbonate** also had no effect on the absorption of phenytoin.[4] A controlled study in 6 patients with epilepsy found that a **magnesium trisilicate** and **aluminium hydroxide** antacid (*Gelusil*) caused a slight 12% reduction in steady-state serum phenytoin levels, which would not be expected to be clinically significant. Seizure frequency was not affected.[4] A study in 2 subjects found that the absorption of phenytoin was not altered by a mixture of **aluminium/magnesium hydroxide** and **magnesium trisilicate**, or **calcium carbonate**.[5] In another study in 6 healthy subjects, no statistically significant decrease in absorption was seen when phenytoin was given with an antacid containing **simeticone, aluminium hydroxide** and **magnesium oxide** (*Asilone*).[6]

Mechanism

Not understood. One suggestion is that diarrhoea and a general increase in peristalsis caused by some antacids may cause a reduction in phenytoin absorption. Another is that antacids may cause changes in gastric acid secretion, which could affect phenytoin solubility.

Importance and management

This possible interaction is fairly well documented, but the results are conflicting. In practice it appears not to be important in most patients, although some loss of seizure control has been seen to occur in isolated cases. Concurrent use need not be avoided but if there is any hint that phenytoin levels are reduced, separation of the doses by 2 to 3 hours may, as with other interactions caused by antacids, minimise the effects.

1. Pippinger L. Personal communication 1973, quoted by Kutt H in Interactions of antiepileptic drugs. *Epilepsia* (1975) 16, 393–402.
2. O'Brien LS, Orme ML'E, Breckenridge AM. Failure of antacids to alter the pharmacokinetics of phenytoin. *Br J Clin Pharmacol* (1978) 6, 176–7.
3. Carter BL, Garnett WR, Pellock JM, Stratton MA, Howell JR. Effect of antacids on phenytoin bioavailability. *Ther Drug Monit* (1981) 3, 333–40.
4. Kulshreshtha VK, Thomas M, Wadsworth J, Richens A. Interaction between phenytoin and antacids. *Br J Clin Pharmacol* (1978) 6, 177–9.
5. Chapron DJ, Kramer PA, Mariano SL, Hohnadel DC. Effect of calcium and antacids on phenytoin bioavailability. *Arch Neurol* (1979) 36, 436–8.
6. McElnay JC, Uprichard G, Collier PS. The effect of activated dimethicone and a proprietary antacid preparation containing this agent on the absorption of phenytoin. *Br J Clin Pharmacol* (1982) 13, 501–5.

Phenytoin + Antidiabetics

Large and toxic doses of phenytoin have been seen to cause hyperglycaemia, but normal therapeutic doses do not usually affect the control of diabetes. Two isolated cases of phenytoin toxicity have been attributed to

the use of tolazamide or tolbutamide. Miglitol does not affect the bioavailability of phenytoin.

Clinical evidence

(a) Effects on phenytoin

In a study, tolbutamide 500 mg two or three times daily was given to 17 patients taking phenytoin 100 to 400 mg daily.[1] The patients had a transient 45% rise in the amount of non-protein-bound phenytoin by day 2, which had disappeared by day 4. The introduction to this report briefly mentions a man given phenytoin and **tolazamide** who developed phenytoin toxicity, which disappeared when **tolazamide** was replaced by **insulin**.[1] A woman previously uneventfully treated with phenytoin and **tolbutamide** developed toxicity on a later occasion when she took **tolbutamide** with twice the previous dose of phenytoin.[2] One study in healthy subjects found that **miglitol** 100 mg three times daily for 5 days did not affect the bioavailability of a single 400-mg dose of phenytoin.[3]

(b) Response to antidiabetics

Phenytoin has been found in a number of reports[4-9] to raise the blood glucose levels of both diabetics and non-diabetics. However, in all but one of these cases the phenytoin dose was large (at least 8 mg/kg) or even in the toxic range (70 to 80 mg/kg). There is little evidence that a hyperglycaemic response to usual doses of phenytoin is normally large enough to interfere with the control of diabetes, either with diet alone or with conventional antidiabetic drugs. In the one case where the interaction occurred with a therapeutic dose of phenytoin (1.2 g in the 24 hours following status epilepticus), the situation was complicated by the use of many other drugs and by renal impairment.[5]

Mechanism

Studies in *animals* and man[10-13] suggest that phenytoin-induced hyperglycaemia occurs because the release of insulin from the pancreas is impaired. This implies that no interaction is possible without functional pancreatic tissue. Just why phenytoin appeared to interact with tolazamide and tolbutamide is uncertain, but it is possible that these antidiabetics competitively inhibit phenytoin hydroxylation[14,15] by the cytochrome P450 isoenzyme CYP2C9.[16]

Importance and management

The weight of evidence shows that no interaction of clinical importance normally occurs between phenytoin and the antidiabetic drugs (most of the studies involved sulfonylureas). No special precautions would generally be expected to be necessary.

1. Wesseling H, Mols-Thürkow I. Interaction of diphenylhydantoin (DPH) and tolbutamide in man. *Eur J Clin Pharmacol* (1975) 8, 75–8.
2. Beech E, Mathur SVS, Harrold BP. Phenytoin toxicity produced by tolbutamide. *BMJ* (1988) 297, 1613–14.
3. Richardt D, Rosmarin C, Havlik I, Schall R. No effect of miglitol on the oral bioavailability of single-dose phenytoin in healthy males. *Clin Drug Invest* (1997) 13, 171–4.
4. Klein JP. Diphenylhydantoin intoxication associated with hyperglycaemia. *J Pediatr* (1966) 69, 463–5.
5. Goldberg EM, Sanbar SS. Hyperglycaemic, nonketotic coma following administration of Dilantin (diphenylhydantoin). *Diabetes* (1969) 18, 101–6.
6. Peters BH, Samaan NA. Hyperglycaemia with relative hypoinsulinemia in diphenylhydantoin toxicity. *N Engl J Med* (1969) 281, 91–2.
7. Millichap JG. Hyperglycemic effect of diphenylhydantoin. *N Engl J Med* (1969) 281, 447.
8. Fariss BL, Lutcher CL. Diphenylhydantoin-induced hyperglycaemia and impaired insulin release. *Diabetes* (1971) 20, 177–81.
9. Treasure T, Toseland PA. Hyperglycaemia due to phenytoin toxicity. *Arch Dis Child* (1971) 46, 563–4.
10. Kizer JS, Vargas-Cordon M, Brendel K, Bressler R. The *in vitro* inhibition of insulin secretion by diphenylhydantoin. *J Clin Invest* (1970) 49, 1942–8.
11. Levin SR, Booker J, Smith DF, Grodsky M. Inhibition of insulin secretion by diphenylhydantoin in the isolated perfused pancreas. *J Clin Endocrinol Metab* (1970) 30, 400–1.
12. Malherbe C, Burrill KC, Levin SR, Karam JH, Forsham PH. Effect of diphenylhydantoin on insulin secretion in man. *N Engl J Med* (1972) 286, 339–42.
13. Nabe K, Fujimoto S, Shimodahira M, Kominato R, Nishi Y, Funakoshi S, Mukai E, Yamada Y, Seino Y, Inagaki N. Diphenylhydantoin suppresses glucose-induced insulin release by decreasing cytoplasmic H^+ concentration in pancreatic islets. *Endocrinology* (2006) 147, 2717–27.
14. Wesseling H, Thurkow I and Mulder GJ. Effect of sulphonylureas (tolazamide, tolbutamide and chlorpropamide) on the metabolism of diphenylhydantoin in the rat. *Biochem Pharmacol* (1973) 22, 3033–40.
15. Doecke CJ, Veronese ME, Pond SM, Miners JO, Birkett DJ, Sansom LN, McManus ME. Relationship between phenytoin and tolbutamide hydroxylations in human liver microsomes. *Br J Clin Pharmacol* (1991) 31, 125–30.
16. Tassaneeyakul W, Veronese ME, Birkett DJ, Doecke CJ, McManus ME, Sansom LN, Miners JO. Co-regulation of phenytoin and tolbutamide metabolism in humans. *Br J Clin Pharmacol* (1992) 34, 494–8.

Phenytoin + Antimycobacterials

Phenytoin levels are markedly reduced by rifampicin, but can be raised by isoniazid. Patients who are slow acetylators (slow metabolisers) of isoniazid may develop phenytoin toxicity. If rifampicin (rifampin) and isoniazid are given together, serum phenytoin levels may fall in patients who are fast acetylators of isoniazid, but may occasionally rise in those who are slow acetylators. Clofazimine may reduce serum phenytoin levels.

Clinical evidence

(a) Isoniazid

A study in 32 patients given phenytoin 300 mg daily found that within a week of starting to take isoniazid 300 mg daily and **aminosalicylic acid** 15 g daily, 6 of them had phenytoin levels almost 5 micrograms/mL higher than the rest of the group. On the following days, when the phenytoin levels of these 6 patients rose above 20 micrograms/mL, the typical signs of phenytoin toxicity were seen. All 6 patients with raised phenytoin levels had unusually high serum isoniazid levels and were identified as slow acetylators of isoniazid.[1]

Rises in serum phenytoin levels and toxicity induced by the concurrent use of isoniazid has been described in numerous other reports,[2-15] involving large numbers of patients, one of which describes a fatality.[8]

(b) Rifampicin (Rifampin)

A study in 6 patients found that the clearance of intravenous phenytoin 100 mg doubled (from 46.7 to 97.8 mL/minute), when rifampicin 450 mg daily was taken for 2 weeks.[16]

A man taking phenytoin 400 mg daily experienced a seizure 3 days after starting rifampicin 600 mg daily. His phenytoin level was low (5.1 micrograms/mL) so rifampicin was stopped and the phenytoin dose increased to 500 mg daily. His level increased slowly over the next 2 weeks, eventually ranging between 16 and 25 micrograms/mL.[17] Another man taking phenytoin needed a dose reduction from 375 to 325 mg daily to keep his serum phenytoin levels within the therapeutic range when he stopped taking rifampicin.[18] A man with AIDS taking a large number of drugs (rifampicin, clofazimine, ciprofloxacin, ethambutol, clarithromycin, diphenoxylate, bismuth, octreotide, co-trimoxazole, amphotericin, flucytosine, amikacin, zalcitabine) was also given phenytoin to control a right-sided seizure disorder. Despite taking phenytoin 1.6 g daily, and a trial of intravenous treatment, his trough phenytoin plasma levels remained almost undetectable until rifampicin was withdrawn, when they rose to 5 micrograms/mL with the oral dose. When **clofazimine** was withdrawn the levels rose even further to 10 micrograms/mL.[19]

(c) Rifampicin (Rifampin) and Isoniazid

A patient taking phenytoin 300 mg daily developed progressive drowsiness (a sign of phenytoin toxicity) during the first week of taking isoniazid, rifampicin and ethambutol. His serum phenytoin levels rose to 46.1 micrograms/mL. He slowly recovered when the phenytoin was stopped, and he was later stabilised taking phenytoin 200 mg daily. He proved to be a slow acetylator of isoniazid.[20] Another patient taking phenytoin 300 mg daily was also given isoniazid, rifampicin and ethambutol but, in anticipation of the response seen in the previous patient, his phenytoin dose was reduced to 200 mg daily. Within 3 days he developed seizures because his serum phenytoin levels had fallen to only 8 micrograms/mL. He needed to take phenytoin 400 mg daily to keep the serum levels within the therapeutic range. He was a fast acetylator of isoniazid.[20]

The clearance of phenytoin was doubled in 14 patients given rifampicin 450 mg, isoniazid 300 mg and ethambutol 900 mg to 1.2 g daily for 2 weeks. No further changes occurred in the pharmacokinetics of phenytoin after 3 months of antimycobacterial treatment. In this study, the interaction was of a similar magnitude in both the 8 slow acetylators and the 6 fast acetylators.[16]

Mechanism

Rifampicin (a known potent liver enzyme inducer) increases the metabolism and clearance of phenytoin from the body so that a larger dose is needed to maintain adequate serum levels. Isoniazid inhibits the liver microsomal enzymes that metabolise phenytoin, and as a result phenytoin accumulates and its serum levels rise.[21] Only patients who are slow acetylators (slow metabolisers) of isoniazid normally attain blood levels of isoniazid that are sufficiently high to cause extensive inhibition of phenytoin metabolism. Fast acetylators (fast metabolisers) remove the isoniazid too quickly for this to occur. Acetylator status is genetically determined. Thus some individuals will show a rapid rise in phenytoin levels, which eventually reaches toxic concentrations, whereas others will show only a relatively slow and unimportant rise to a plateau within, or only slightly above the therapeutic range.

If isoniazid and rifampicin are given together, the enzyme inhibitory effects of isoniazid may oppose the effects of rifampicin in patients who are slow acetylators of isoniazid, but in patients who are fast acetylators, the isoniazid will be cleared too quickly for it effectively to oppose the rifampicin effects. However, in one study isoniazid did not counter the effects of rifampicin in slow acetylators.[16]

The interaction involving clofazimine is not understood.

Importance and management

Direct information seems to be limited to these reports, but the interactions appear to be of clinical importance. Monitor the serum phenytoin levels and increase the dose appropriately if rifampicin alone is started. Reduce the phenytoin dose if rifampicin is stopped. If both rifampicin and isoniazid are given, the outcome may depend on the isoniazid acetylator status of the patient. Patients who are fast acetylators will probably also need an increased phenytoin dose, whereas patients who are slow acetylators may need a smaller phenytoin dose if toxicity is to be avoided. All patients should be monitored very closely as, unless acetylator status is known, the outcome is unpredictable.

The interaction with phenytoin and isoniazid alone is well documented, well established, clinically important and potentially serious. About 50% of the population are slow or relatively slow metabolisers of isoniazid,[1] but not all of them develop serum phenytoin levels in the toxic range. The reports indicate that somewhere between 10 and 33% of patients are at risk.[1-4,10] This adverse interaction may take only a few days to develop fully in some patients, but several weeks in others. Therefore concurrent use should be very closely monitored (e.g. for evidence of phenytoin adverse effects, such as blurred vision, nystagmus, ataxia or drowsiness), making suitable dose reductions as necessary. One patient was reported to have had better seizure control with fewer adverse effects while taking both drugs than with phenytoin alone.[22]

Information about clofazimine seems to be limited to one report. Monitor concurrent use, anticipating the need to increase the phenytoin dose.

1. Brennan RW, Dehejia H, Kutt H, Verebely K, McDowell F. Diphenylhydantoin intoxication attendant to slow inactivation of isoniazid. *Neurology* (1970) 20, 687–93.
2. Kutt H, Brennan R, Dehejia H, Verebely K. Diphenylhydantoin intoxication. A complication of isoniazid therapy. *Am Rev Respir Dis* (1970) 101, 377–84.

3. Murray FJ. Outbreak of unexpected reactions among epileptics taking isoniazid. *Am Rev Respir Dis* (1962) 86, 729–32.
4. Kutt H, Winters W, McDowell FH. Depression of parahydroxylation of diphenylhydantoin by antituberculosis chemotherapy. *Neurology* (1966) 16, 594–602.
5. Manigand G, Thieblot P, Deparis M. Accidents de la diphénylhydantoïne induits par les traitements antituberculeux. *Presse Med* (1971) 79, 815–16.
6. Beauvais P, Mercier D, Hanoteau J, Brissand H-E. Intoxication a la diphenylhydantoine induite par l'isoniazide. *Arch Fr Pediatr* (1973) 30, 541–6.
7. Johnson J. Epanutin and isoniazid interaction. *BMJ* (1975) 1, 152.
8. Johnson J, Freeman HL. Death due to isoniazid (INH) and phenytoin. *Br J Psychiatry* (1975) 129, 511.
9. Geering JM, Ruch W, Dettli L. Diphenylhydantoin-Intoxikation durch Diphenylhydantoin-Isoniazid-Interaktion. *Schweiz Med Wochenschr* (1974) 104, 1224–8.
10. Miller RR, Porter J, Greenblatt DJ. Clinical importance of the interaction of phenytoin and isoniazid. A report from the Boston Collaborative Drug Surveillance Program. *Chest* (1979) 75, 356–8.
11. Witmer DR, Ritschel WA. Phenytoin-isoniazid interaction: a kinetic approach to management. *Drug Intell Clin Pharm* (1984) 18, 483–6.
12. Perucca E and Richens A. Anticonvulsant drug interactions. In: Tyrer J (ed) The treatment of epilepsy. MTP Lancaster. (1980) pp 95–128.
13. Sandyk R. Phenytoin toxicity induced by antituberculosis drugs. *S Afr Med J* (1982) 61, 382.
14. Yew WW, Lau KS, Ling MHM. Phenytoin toxicity in a patient with isoniazid-induced hepatitis. *Tubercle* (1991) 72, 309–10.
15. Walubo A, Aboo A. Phenytoin toxicity due to concomitant antituberculosis therapy. *S Afr Med J* (1995) 85, 1175–6.
16. Kay L, Kampmann JP, Svendsen TL, Vergman B, Hansen JEM, Skovsted L, Kristensen M. Influence of rifampicin and isoniazid on the kinetics of phenytoin. *Br J Clin Pharmacol* (1985) 20, 323–6.
17. Wagner JC, Slama TG. Rifampin-phenytoin drug interaction. *Drug Intell Clin Pharm* (1984) 18, 497.
18. Abajo FJ. Phenytoin interaction with rifampicin. *BMJ* (1988) 297, 1048.
19. Cone LA, Woodard DR, Simmons JC, Sonnenshein MA. Drug interactions in patients with AIDS. *Clin Infect Dis* (1992) 15, 1066–8.
20. O'Reilly D, Basran GS, Hourihan B, Macfarlane JT. Interaction between phenytoin and antituberculous drugs. *Thorax* (1987) 42, 736.
21. Desta Z, Soukhova NV, Flockhart DA. Inhibition of cytochrome P450 (CYP450) isoforms by isoniazid: potent inhibition of CYP2C19 and CYP3A. *Antimicrob Agents Chemother* (2001), 45, 384–92.
22. Thulasimnay M, Kela AK. Improvement of psychomotor epilepsy due to interaction of phenytoin-isoniazid. *Tubercle* (1984) 65, 229–30.

Phenytoin + Aspirin or NSAIDs

Phenytoin concentrations can be increased by azapropazone and phenylbutazone, and phenytoin toxicity might occur. It seems likely that oxyphenbutazone will interact similarly.

Phenytoin toxicity has been seen in one patient taking ibuprofen and one taking celecoxib, although no pharmacokinetic interaction was found in controlled studies using single doses of phenytoin. High-dose aspirin can cause protein-binding displacement of phenytoin. Bromfenac, etodolac, and tolfenamic acid do not alter phenytoin pharmacokinetics.

Clinical evidence, mechanism, importance and management

(a) Aspirin

It has been suggested that if a patient has been taking large quantities of aspirin, phenytoin is 'potentiated'.[1] This comment remains unconfirmed, although a study in 10 healthy subjects did find that aspirin 975 mg every 4 hours caused protein-binding displacement of phenytoin, resulting in a 16% increase in free salivary phenytoin concentrations and a 24% decrease in its serum concentrations. However, these changes were considered unlikely to be clinically significant, and aspirin doses of 325 and 650 mg every 4 hours had no appreciable effect on phenytoin.[2] Similar effects on protein binding displacement have been seen in other studies.[3-7] However, although the ratios of free and bound phenytoin can change, there does not appear to be a clinical effect, possibly because the extra free phenytoin is metabolised by the liver.[6] A study in 10 patients with epilepsy taking phenytoin found that when they were also given aspirin 500 mg three times daily for 3 days, no statistically significant changes in serum phenytoin concentrations or antiepileptic effects occurred.[8] The extremely common use of aspirin, and the almost total silence in the literature about an adverse interaction between phenytoin and aspirin implies that no phenytoin dose adjustment is likely to be needed when both drugs are given.

(b) Azapropazone

A patient taking phenytoin developed phenytoin toxicity within 2 weeks of starting azapropazone 600 mg twice daily. Further study in 5 healthy subjects given phenytoin 125 to 250 mg daily found that azapropazone 600 mg twice daily, briefly decreased their mean serum phenytoin concentrations from 5 micrograms/mL to 3.7 micrograms/mL before they increased steadily over the next 7 days to 10.5 micrograms/mL.[9,10] An extension of this study is described elsewhere.[11] Another report describes phenytoin toxicity in a woman taking phenytoin and primidone when **fenclofenac** was replaced by azapropazone 1.2 g daily.[12]

The most likely explanation is that azapropazone inhibits the liver enzymes concerned with the metabolism of phenytoin, resulting in its accumulation. It also seems possible that azapropazone displaces phenytoin from its plasma protein binding sites so that concentrations of unbound (and active) phenytoin are increased. Information seems to be limited to the reports cited, but it appears to be a clinically important interaction. The incidence is uncertain, but an interaction occurred in all 5 of the subjects in the study cited.[9,11] The concurrent use of azapropazone and phenytoin has been contraindicated.[13]

(c) Bromfenac

Twelve healthy subjects were given bromfenac 50 mg three times daily for 4 days and then phenytoin 300 to 330 mg for up to 14 days (to achieve stable concentrations), and then both drugs for 8 days. It was found that the maximum serum concentration and AUC of phenytoin were increased by 9% and 11%, respectively, while the maximum concentration and AUC of bromfenac were reduced by 42%. The suggested reason for the reduction in bromfenac concentrations is that phenytoin increases its metabolism by the liver.[14] In practical terms, these results indicate that there is no need to adjust the dose of phenytoin if bromfenac is added, nor any need to increase the bromfenac dose unless there is any evidence that its efficacy is diminished.

(d) Celecoxib

No clinically relevant changes in the pharmacokinetics of a single oral dose of phenytoin 200 mg (given on days 7 and 14) were seen in 16 healthy subjects given either celecoxib 200 mg twice daily, or placebo, for 14 days.[15] In another study in patients with brain tumours, there was no difference in the pharmacokinetics of celecoxib between 15 patients taking phenytoin and 12 patients taking non-enzyme-inducing antiepileptics (levetiracetam, lamotrigine, or gabapentin) or no antiepileptics.[16] In this study, celecoxib 400 mg twice daily was given for a mean of about 16 weeks, and there was no mention of any change in phenytoin concentrations or dose.[16] However, an elderly woman taking phenytoin 300 mg daily who had also been taking celecoxib for the previous 6 months, developed signs of phenytoin toxicity. She was found to have a phenytoin concentration of 42 micrograms/mL, and a very slow rate of elimination.[17] Note that celecoxib is not known to be an inhibitor of drug metabolism, with the exception of weak inhibition of CYP2D6, but phenytoin is not a substrate of CYP2D6. In addition, phenytoin is not an inducer of CYP2C9, by which celecoxib is principally metabolised.

On balance, the evidence suggests that there is no pharmacokinetic interaction between celecoxib and phenytoin; therefore, no dose adjustment of either drug would be expected to be routinely needed on concurrent use. The isolated case report is unlikely to be of general clinical relevance, and its reason is unclear.

(e) Etodolac

A crossover study in 16 healthy subjects found that etodolac 200 mg every 12 hours for 3 days had no effect on the pharmacokinetics or the pharmacological effects of phenytoin (100 mg twice daily for 2 days and 100 mg on day three).[18] A phenytoin dose adjustment would seem unlikely to be necessary on the concurrent use of these drugs.

(f) Ibuprofen or Dexibuprofen

Studies in healthy subjects found that the pharmacokinetics of single 300- or 900-mg doses of phenytoin were not altered by ibuprofen 300 or 400 mg every 6 hours.[19,20] However, a report describes a woman stabilised on phenytoin 300 mg daily who developed phenytoin toxicity within a week of starting to take ibuprofen 400 mg four times daily.[21] Her serum phenytoin concentrations had increased to about 25 micrograms/mL. The phenytoin was stopped for 3 days and the ibuprofen withdrawn, and within 10 days the phenytoin concentration had dropped to about 17 micrograms/mL. Another report describes a patient stabilised taking phenytoin 300 mg daily (4.3 mg/kg daily) who developed symptoms of phenytoin toxicity 72 hours after starting dexibuprofen 800 mg daily. Phenytoin concentrations were found to be 30.6 micrograms/mL. Dexibuprofen was withdrawn and phenytoin was stopped for 3 days. Two weeks after the re-introduction of phenytoin, symptoms of toxicity had resolved and concentrations had decreased to 17.3 micrograms/mL.[22] The reasons for this apparent interaction are not understood.

Both phenytoin and ibuprofen have been available for many years. Dexibuprofen, the active enantiomer of ibuprofen, has been introduced more recently. These 2 cases, some 25 years apart, appear to be the only reports of an adverse interaction. No phenytoin dose adjustment would normally seem to be necessary.

(g) Oxyphenbutazone or Phenylbutazone

Six patients with epilepsy taking phenytoin 200 to 350 mg daily who were then also given phenylbutazone 100 mg three times daily, had a mean decrease in their phenytoin serum concentrations from 15 micrograms/mL to 13 micrograms/mL over the first 3 days, after which the concentrations increased steadily to 19 micrograms/mL over the next 11 days. One patient developed symptoms of toxicity. His concentrations of free phenytoin more than doubled.[8] Another study found that phenylbutazone increased the steady-state half-life of phenytoin from 13.7 hours to 22 hours.[23]

The predominant effect of phenylbutazone seems to be the inhibition of the enzymes concerned with the metabolism of phenytoin,[23] leading to its accumulation in the body and an increase in its serum concentrations. The initial transient decrease might possibly be related in some way to the displacement by phenylbutazone of phenytoin from its plasma protein binding sites.[24] This is an established interaction, although the documentation is very limited. Monitor the outcome of adding phenylbutazone and reduce the phenytoin dose as necessary. There is no direct evidence that oxyphenbutazone interacts like phenylbutazone, but as it is the main metabolic product of phenylbutazone in the body and has been shown to prolong the half-life of phenytoin in *animals*,[25] it would be expected to interact similarly.

(h) Tolfenamic acid

In a study in 11 patients, tolfenamic acid 300 mg daily for 3 days had no apparent effect on the serum concentrations of phenytoin.[8] No phenytoin dose adjustments seem necessary if these drugs are taken concurrently.

1. Toakley JG. Dilantin overdosage. *Med J Aust* (1968) 2, 640.
2. Leonard RF, Knott PJ, Rankin GO, Robinson DS, Melnick DE. Phenytoin-salicylate interaction. *Clin Pharmacol Ther* (1981) 29, 56–60.
3. Ehrnebo M, Odar-Cederlöf I. Distribution of pentobarbital and diphenylhydantoin between plasma and cells in blood: effect of salicylic acid, temperature and total drug concentration. *Eur J Clin Pharmacol* (1977) 11, 37–42.
4. Fraser DG, Ludden TM, Evens RP, Sutherland EW. Displacement of phenytoin from plasma binding sites by salicylate. *Clin Pharmacol Ther* (1980) 27, 165–9.
5. Paxton JW. Effects of aspirin on salivary and serum phenytoin kinetics in healthy subjects. *Clin Pharmacol Ther* (1980) 27, 170–8.
6. Olanow CW, Finn A, Prussak C. The effect of salicylate on phenytoin pharmacokinetics. *Trans Am Neurol Assoc* (1979) 104, 109–10.
7. Inoue F, Walsh RJ. Folate supplements and phenytoin-salicylate interaction. *Neurology* (1983) 33, 115–16.

8. Neuvonen PJ, Lehtovaara R, Bardy A, Elomaa E. Antipyretic analgesics in patients on antiepileptic drug therapy. *Eur J Clin Pharmacol* (1979) 15, 263–8.
9. Geaney DP, Carver JG, Aronson JK, Warlow CP. Interaction of azapropazone with phenytoin. *BMJ* (1982) 284, 1373.
10. Aronson JK, Hardman M, Reynolds DJM. ABC of monitoring drug therapy. Phenytoin. *BMJ* (1992) 305, 1215–18.
11. Geaney DP, Carver JG, Davies CL, Aronson JK. Pharmacokinetic investigation of the interaction of azapropazone with phenytoin. *Br J Clin Pharmacol* (1983) 15, 727–34.
12. Roberts CJC, Daneshmend TK, Macfarlane D, Dieppe PA. Anticonvulsant intoxication precipitated by azapropazone. *Postgrad Med J* (1981) 57, 191–2.
13. Rheumox (Azapropazone dihydrate). Goldshield Pharmaceuticals Ltd. UK Summary of product characteristics, February 2000.
14. Gumbhir-Shah K, Cevallos WH, DeCleene SA, Korth-Bradley JM. Evaluation of pharmacokinetic interaction between bromfenac and phenytoin in healthy males. *J Clin Pharmacol* (1997) 37, 160–8.
15. Pfizer Ltd. Personal communication, December 2012.
16. Grossman SA, Olson J, Batchelor T, Peereboom D, Lesser G, Desideri S, Ye X, Hammour T, Supko JG; New Approaches to Brain Tumor Therapy CNS Consortium. Effect of phenytoin on celecoxib pharmacokinetics in patients with glioblastoma. *Neuro Oncol* (2008) 10, 190–8.
17. Keeling KL, Jortani SA, Linder MW, Valdes R. Prolonged elimination half-life of phenytoin in an elderly patient also on celecoxib. *Clin Chem* (2002) 48 (Suppl.), A52–A53.
18. Zvaifler N. A review of the antiarthritic efficacy and safety of etodolac. *Clin Rheumatol* (1989) 8 (Suppl 1), 43–53.
19. Bachmann KA, Schwartz JI, Forney RB, Jauregui L, Sullivan TJ. Inability of ibuprofen to alter single dose phenytoin disposition. *Br J Clin Pharmacol* (1986) 21, 165–9.
20. Townsend RJ, Fraser DG, Scavone JM, Cox SR. The effects of ibuprofen on phenytoin pharmacokinetics. *Drug Intell Clin Pharm* (1985) 19, 447–8.
21. Sandyk R. Phenytoin toxicity induced by interaction with ibuprofen. *S Afr Med J* (1982) 62, 592.
22. Llinares-Tello F, Hernández-Prats C, Pastor-Climente I, Escrivá-Moscardó S. Toxicidad neurológica aguda por probable interacción farmacocinética entre fenitoína y dexibuprofeno. *Med Clin (Barc)* (2007) 128, 239.
23. Andreasen PB, Frøland A, Skovsted L, Andersen SA, Hague M. Diphenylhydantoin half-life in man and its inhibition by phenylbutazone: the role of genetic factors. *Acta Med Scand* (1973) 193, 561–4.
24. Lunde PKM, Rane A, Yaffe SJ, Lund L, Sjöqvist F. Plasma protein binding of diphenylhydantoin in man. Interaction with other drugs and the effect of temperature and plasma dilution. *Clin Pharmacol Ther* (1970) 11, 846–55.
25. Soda DM, Levy G. Inhibition of drug metabolism by hydroxylated metabolites: cross-inhibition and specificity. *J Pharm Sci* (1975) 64, 1928–31.

Phenytoin + Atovaquone

In 12 healthy subjects, atovaquone (1 g given twelve hours before and with a single 600-mg dose of phenytoin) did not affect the pharmacokinetics of phenytoin. It was concluded that a clinically important pharmacokinetic interaction is unlikely.[1]

1. Davis JD, Dixon R, Khan AZ, Toon S, Rolan PE, Posner J. Atovaquone has no effect on the pharmacokinetics of phenytoin in healthy male volunteers. *Br J Clin Pharmacol* (1996) 42, 246–8.

Phenytoin + Azoles

Phenytoin concentrations are increased by fluconazole and phenytoin toxicity has occurred as a result. Voriconazole and possibly miconazole interact similarly, whereas itraconazole, ketoconazole and posaconazole appear to have little effect on phenytoin concentrations.

Phenytoin decreases itraconazole and possibly ketoconazole concentrations and treatment failures have occurred as a result. Posaconazole and voriconazole are similarly affected. Fluconazole concentrations are not usually affected by phenytoin, although there is one report of reduced efficacy.

Clinical evidence

(a) Fluconazole

In a randomised, placebo-controlled study, 10 subjects taking fluconazole 200 mg daily for 14 days with phenytoin 200 mg daily for the last 3 days were compared with 10 other subjects taking phenytoin alone. Fluconazole increased the AUC of phenytoin by 75%, and increased the minimum phenytoin concentration by 128%.[1] Two other studies reported similar findings,[2,3] and there are reports describing at least 7 cases of phenytoin toxicity caused by fluconazole.[4-7] A further report describes a 59-year-old woman taking phenytoin for about 5 years with consistently low phenytoin concentrations (less than 2.5 to 5 micrograms/mL), who developed phenytoin toxicity soon after starting fluconazole 50 mg daily. Her phenytoin dose at the time was 700 mg daily and her phenytoin concentration was 34.8 micrograms/mL. Fluconazole was withdrawn and the patient quickly recovered. Eight years later she was taking phenytoin 600 mg daily, and due to lack of documentation of her previous episode of phenytoin toxicity while taking fluconazole, she was prescribed fluconazole 400 daily. After 2 to 3 days she began to develop symptoms which were later realised to be similar to those experienced previously. After taking fluconazole for 14 days, her phenytoin concentration was 60.6 micrograms/mL. Both phenytoin and fluconazole were stopped and she made a rapid recovery. The patient was tested for CYP2C9 polymorphism and was found to be an ultra-rapid metaboliser via this pathway (that is she had very high activity of CYP2C9).[8]

Some studies suggest that phenytoin does not alter fluconazole concentrations;[1,3] however, a brief report noted that 3 of 9 patients taking fluconazole and phenytoin required an increase in their fluconazole dose or the substitution of another antifungal due to a lack of efficacy. It was suggested that phenytoin might reduce fluconazole concentrations in some patients.[9]

(b) Itraconazole

In a study in 13 healthy subjects, oral phenytoin 300 mg daily for 15 days reduced the AUC of a single 200-mg dose of itraconazole by more than 90%. The half-life of itraconazole was reduced from 22.3 hours to 3.8 hours. In 15 other healthy subjects, itraconazole 200 mg for 15 days increased the AUC of a single 300-mg dose of phenytoin by 10%.[10]

Two patients taking phenytoin and two taking phenytoin with carbamazepine either did not respond to treatment with itraconazole 400 mg daily for aspergillosis, coccidioidomycosis or cryptococcosis, or suffered a relapse. All of them had undetectable or substantially reduced serum itraconazole concentrations compared with other patients taking itraconazole alone.[11] Two other patients also had very low itraconazole serum concentrations while taking phenytoin and phenobarbital.[12]

(c) Ketoconazole

A study in 9 healthy subjects found that ketoconazole 200 mg twice daily for 6 days did not alter the AUC_{0-48} of a single 250-mg dose of phenytoin.[2]

A man being treated for coccidioidal meningitis with ketoconazole 400 mg daily relapsed when he was given phenytoin 300 mg daily. A pharmacokinetic study found that his maximum serum concentration and AUC of ketoconazole were reduced, when compared with the values seen before phenytoin was started. Even though the ketoconazole dose was increased to 600 mg, and later 1.2 g, his serum concentration remained low compared with other patients taking only 400 or 600 mg of ketoconazole.[13] Coccidioidomycosis progressed in another patient taking phenytoin despite the use of ketoconazole,[11] and low serum ketoconazole concentrations were seen in one patient taking phenytoin and phenobarbital.[14]

(d) Miconazole

A man with epilepsy, well controlled with phenytoin, developed symptoms of phenytoin toxicity within one day of starting *intravenous* miconazole 500 mg every 8 hours and flucytosine. After one week of concurrent use his serum phenytoin concentration had risen by 50% (from 29 micrograms/mL to 43 micrograms/mL). He had some very mild symptoms of phenytoin toxicity before the antifungal treatment was started.[15] Another patient developed symptoms of phenytoin toxicity (nystagmus, ataxia) within 5 days of starting to take *oral* miconazole 500 mg daily. His serum phenytoin concentration increased to 40.8 micrograms/mL. After discontinuation of the miconazole the same dose of phenytoin resulted in a concentration of 14.5 micrograms/mL.[16]

(e) Posaconazole

In a randomised, parallel-group study, 36 healthy subjects were given posaconazole 200 mg daily, phenytoin 200 mg daily or both, for 10 days. The AUC and maximum plasma concentration of posaconazole were 52% and 44% lower, respectively, in those subjects who also took phenytoin. There was no statistically significant difference in phenytoin pharmacokinetics between those taking both posaconazole and phenytoin and those taking phenytoin alone (AUC 25% higher and maximum plasma concentrations 24% higher); however, there was wide inter-subject variability in the combination group, with two subjects having a 50% higher AUC of phenytoin. The authors thought that such a difference could be clinically relevant.[17]

(f) Voriconazole

Studies in healthy subjects found that phenytoin 300 mg daily decreased the maximum serum concentration and AUC of voriconazole by 49% and 69%, respectively. Also, voriconazole 400 mg twice daily increased the maximum serum concentration and AUC of phenytoin 300 mg daily by 67% and 81%, respectively.[18] A patient with systemic lupus erythematosus presented with seizures, and multiple brain lesions were found on imaging. She was given phenytoin 400 mg daily for seizure control and oral voriconazole 300 mg twice daily for a possible CNS *Aspergillus* infection. After one month, because the voriconazole minimum concentration was low (0.2 micrograms/mL) and clinical improvement had not occurred, the dose of voriconazole was increased to 400 mg twice daily. Nine days later the minimum concentration of voriconazole had increased to 0.68 micrograms/mL, but 6 weeks later the patient developed oral candidiasis. Voriconazole was increased to 400 mg three times daily. At steady-state her serum concentration was 4.08 micrograms/mL and the candidiasis improved.[19] Another report describes a 28-year-old woman with suspected invasive aspergillosis who started taking voriconazole 200 mg twice daily after a loading dose, who 4 days later required phenytoin (loading dose of 1200 mg followed by 100 mg three times daily). Her voriconazole dose was increased to 300 mg twice daily after 5 days of concurrent use, and administration was changed from oral to intravenous. Her voriconazole plasma concentration was 2.6 micrograms/mL. Phenytoin was switched to levetiracetam on day 12 after which time her voriconazole plasma concentration was 2.5 micrograms/mL. Her voriconazole dose was reduced to 240 mg twice daily on day 22 and her voriconazole concentration was subsequently 3.5 micrograms/mL.[20]

Mechanism

Fluconazole is a known inhibitor of CYP2C9, which is principally responsible for phenytoin metabolism and therefore fluconazole probably increases phenytoin concentration by inhibiting its metabolism by this isoenzyme. Voriconazole and miconazole also inhibit CYP2C9 and so probably act similarly. Ketoconazole and itraconazole do not affect CYP2C9 and therefore do not have the same effect on phenytoin concentrations. Phenytoin is an enzyme inducer, and appears to induce the metabolism of these azoles to varying degrees; in the cases of itraconazole and ketoconazole this is probably by inducing CYP3A4.

Importance and management

The increase in serum phenytoin concentrations with **fluconazole** is established and clinically important. Toxicity can develop within 2 to 7 days unless the phenytoin dose is reduced. Monitor phenytoin concentrations closely and reduce the dose appropriately. Also be alert for any evidence of reduced fluconazole effects. Evidence for increased phenytoin concentrations with **miconazole** is limited, but is consistent with its effects on CYP2C9 (see *Mechanism* above) and so it would also be prudent to monitor phenytoin concentrations. Note that, a large proportion of miconazole oral gel (both prescription and non-prescription doses) is swallowed and therefore sufficient systemic absorption could occur to produce an interaction.

The decrease in **itraconazole** concentrations with phenytoin is established, clinically important and its incidence appears to be high. Because such a large reduction in itraconazole concentrations occurs, it is difficult to predict by how much its dose should be increased, and indeed, dose increases might not be effective. The authors of one report advise using another antifungal instead,[10] and this seems prudent. The small increase in serum phenytoin concentrations caused by itraconazole is unlikely to be clinically important.

Information on the interaction between **ketoconazole** and phenytoin appears to be limited, but be alert for any signs of a reduced antifungal response. It might be necessary to increase the dose of ketoconazole, but note that this might not be wholly successful. Ketoconazole probably does not have an important effect on phenytoin concentrations.

Phenytoin appears to halve **posaconazole** concentrations, and posaconazole might increase phenytoin concentrations. The manufacturers of posaconazole suggest that concurrent use should be avoided unless the benefits outweigh the risks.[21,22] If used together it would seem sensible to consider increasing the posaconazole dose, and increase monitoring of phenytoin adverse effects (e.g. blurred vision, nystagmus, ataxia or drowsiness), monitoring phenytoin concentrations as necessary, and adjusting the phenytoin dose as appropriate.

The interaction between phenytoin and **voriconazole** is established. The UK manufacturer states that the concurrent use of voriconazole and phenytoin should be avoided unless the benefits outweigh the risks.[23] If used together, the manufacturers recommend careful monitoring of phenytoin concentrations and adverse effects, and doubling the dose of oral voriconazole (from 200 to 400 mg twice daily and from 100 mg to 200 mg twice daily in patients less than 40 kg) or increasing the dose of intravenous voriconazole (from 4 to 5 mg/kg twice daily).[23,24] However, note that there are conflicting reports of the effectiveness of this approach; this was effective in one case report described above,[20] but in another,[19] doses of voriconazole 50% greater than those recommended were required to treat breakthrough infection.

1. Blum RA, Wilton JH, Hilligoss DM, Gardner MJ, Henry EB, Harrison NJ, Schentag JJ. Effect of fluconazole on the disposition of phenytoin. *Clin Pharmacol Ther* (1991) 49, 420–5.
2. Touchette MA, Chandrasekar PH, Millad MA, Edwards DJ. Contrasting effects of fluconazole and ketoconazole on phenytoin and testosterone disposition in man. *Br J Clin Pharmacol* (1992) 34, 75–8.
3. Lazar JD, Wilner KD. Drug interactions with fluconazole. *Rev Infect Dis* (1990) 12 (Suppl 3), S327–S333.
4. Mitchell AS, Holland JT. Fluconazole and phenytoin: a predictable interaction. *BMJ* (1989) 298, 1315.
5. Howitt KM, Oziemski MA. Phenytoin toxicity induced by fluconazole. *Med J Aust* (1989) 151, 603–4.
6. Sugar AM. Quoted as Personal Communication by Grant SM, Clissold SP. Fluconazole. A review of its pharmacodynamic and pharmacokinetic properties, and therapeutic potential in superficial and system mycoses. *Drugs* (1990) 39, 877–916.
7. Cadle RM, Zenon GJ, Rodriguez-Barradas MC, Hamill RJ. Fluconazole-induced symptomatic phenytoin toxicity. *Ann Pharmacother* (1994) 28, 191–5.
8. Helldén A, Bergman U, Engström Hellgren K, Masquelier M, Nilsson Remahl I, Odar-Cederlöf I, Ramsjö M, Bertilsson L. Fluconazole-induced intoxication with phenytoin in a patient with ultra-high activity of CYP2C9. *Eur J Clin Pharmacol* (2010) 66, 791–5.
9. Tett S, Carey D, Lee H-S. Drug interactions with fluconazole. *Med J Aust* (1992) 156, 365.
10. Ducharme MP, Slaughter RL, Warbasse LH, Chandrasekar PH, Van der Velde V, Mannens G, Edwards DJ. Itraconazole and hydroxyitraconazole serum concentrations are reduced more than tenfold by phenytoin. *Clin Pharmacol Ther* (1995) 58, 617–24.
11. Tucker RM, Denning DW, Hanson LH, Rinaldi MG, Graybill JR, Sharkey PK, Pappagianis D, Stevens DA. Interaction of azoles with rifampin, phenytoin, and carbamazepine: in vitro and clinical observations. *Clin Infect Dis* (1992) 14, 165–74.
12. Hay RJ, Clayton YM, Moore MK, Midgely G. An evaluation of itraconazole in the management of onychomycosis. *Br J Dermatol* (1988) 119, 359–66.
13. Brass C, Galgiani JN, Blaschke TF, Defelice R, O'Reilly RA, Stevens DA. Disposition of ketoconazole, an oral antifungal, in humans. *Antimicrob Agents Chemother* (1982) 21, 151–8.
14. Stockley RJ, Daneshmend TK, Bredow MT, Warnock DW, Richardson MD, Slade RR. Ketoconazole pharmacokinetics during chronic dosing in adults with haematological malignancy. *Eur J Clin Microbiol* (1986) 5, 513–17.
15. Rolan PE, Somogyi AA, Drew MJR, Cobain WG, South D, Bochner F. Phenytoin intoxication during treatment with parenteral miconazole. *BMJ* (1983) 287, 1760.
16. Loupi E, Descotes J, Lery N, Evreux JC. Interactions medicamenteuses et miconazole. A propos de 10 observations. *Therapie* (1982) 37, 437–41.
17. Krishna G, Sansone-Parsons A, Kantesaria B. Drug interaction assessment following concomitant administration of posaconazole and phenytoin in healthy men. *Curr Med Res Opin* (2007) 23, 1415–22..
18. Purkins L, Wood N, Ghahramani P, Love ER, Eve MD, Fielding A. Coadministration of voriconazole and phenytoin: pharmacokinetic interaction, safety, and toleration. *Br J Clin Pharmacol* (2003) 56, 37–44.
19. Gerzenshtein L, Patel SM, Scarsi KK, Postelnick MJ, Flaherty JP. Breakthrough *Candida* infections in patients receiving voriconazole. *Ann Pharmacother* (2005) 39, 1342–5.
20. Spriet I, Meersseman P, Meersseman W, de Hoon J, Willems L. Increasing the dose of voriconazole compensates for enzyme induction by phenytoin. *Br J Clin Pharmacol* (2010) 69, 701–2.
21. Noxafil (Posaconazole). Merck Sharp & Dohme Ltd. UK Summary of product characteristics, September 2014.
22. Noxafil (Posaconazole). Merck & Co., Inc. US Prescribing information, June 2014.
23. VFEND (Voriconazole). Pfizer Ltd. UK Summary of product characteristics, October 2014.
24. VFEND (Voriconazole). Pfizer Inc. US Prescribing information, February 2014.

Phenytoin + Bile-acid binding resins

The absorption of phenytoin does not appear to be affected by colestyramine or colestipol.

Clinical evidence, mechanism, importance and management

In a study in 6 healthy subjects, colestyramine 5 g or colestipol 10 g did not have a significant effect on the absorption of a single 500-mg dose of phenytoin. Colestyramine and colestipol were given 2 minutes before and 6 and 12 hours after the phenytoin.[1] Another study in 6 healthy subjects found that colestyramine 4 g four times daily for 5 days had no significant effect on the extent of the absorption of a single 400-mg dose of phenytoin (given on day 3, two minutes after the colestyramine).[2] No special precautions would seem to be necessary if either of these drugs and phenytoin is taken concurrently.

1. Callaghan JT, Tsuru M, Holtzman JL, Hunninghake DB. Effect of cholestyramine and colestipol on the absorption of phenytoin. *Eur J Clin Pharmacol* (1983) 24, 675–8.
2. Barzaghi N, Monteleone M, Amione C, Lecchini S, Perucca E, Frigo GM. Lack of effect of cholestyramine on phenytoin bioavailability. *J Clin Pharmacol* (1988) 28, 1112–14.

Phenytoin + Calcium-channel blockers

Diltiazem can increase phenytoin serum concentrations. A single case report describes phenytoin toxicity with nifedipine and another case report describes neurological toxicity when a patient taking phenytoin (with carbamazepine) was given isradipine.

Plasma concentrations of felodipine and nisoldipine are greatly reduced by phenytoin. Case reports suggest that nimodipine and verapamil concentrations can be reduced by phenytoin. Other calcium-channel blockers might be similarly affected.

Clinical evidence

(a) Diltiazem

Increased phenytoin serum concentrations and signs of toxicity developed in 2 out of 14 patients taking phenytoin when they were also given diltiazem.[1] A patient taking phenytoin 250 mg twice daily developed signs of toxicity within 2 weeks of starting to take diltiazem 240 mg every 8 hours.[2]

(b) Felodipine

After taking felodipine 10 mg daily for 4 days, 10 patients with epilepsy (including 2 taking phenytoin alone and 3 taking phenytoin with carbamazepine) had reduced felodipine plasma concentrations (maximum concentrations of 1.6 nanomol/L compared with 8.9 nanomol/L in 12 control subjects). The bioavailability of felodipine was very markedly reduced to 6.6%.[3]

(c) Isradipine

A man taking carbamazepine and phenytoin developed neurological toxicity while also taking isradipine, which the authors attributed to a pharmacokinetic or pharmacodynamic interaction between phenytoin and isradipine.[4] However, a commentator considered that an interaction between carbamazepine and isradipine was more plausible.[5]

(d) Nifedipine

An isolated report describes phenytoin toxicity in a man taking phenytoin, 3 weeks after he started to take nifedipine 30 mg daily. His phenytoin serum concentration was 30.4 micrograms/mL. The nifedipine was stopped, and over the next 2 weeks his phenytoin serum concentrations decreased to 10.5 micrograms/mL. A further 2 weeks later all of the symptoms had resolved.[6] However, a retrospective study of 8 patients suggested that nifedipine does not usually interact with phenytoin.[1]

(e) Nimodipine

A study in 8 patients with epilepsy, one of whom was taking phenytoin with carbamazepine, found that the AUC of a single 60-mg oral dose of nimodipine was only about 15% of that obtained in a group of healthy subjects.[7]

(f) Nisoldipine

Twelve patients with epilepsy taking phenytoin long-term and 12 healthy subjects were given single 40- or 20-mg doses of nisoldipine. The AUCs of nisoldipine (normalised for a 20-mg dose) were 1.6 micrograms/L per hour for the patients, and 15.2 micrograms/L per hour for the healthy subjects.[8]

(g) Verapamil

A woman taking phenytoin who was then also given verapamil had persistently subtherapeutic verapamil plasma concentrations (less than 50 nanograms/mL) despite increases in the verapamil dose from 80 mg twice daily to 160 mg three times daily. When phenytoin was stopped, her verapamil plasma concentrations increased to the expected level.[9]

Mechanism

Diltiazem might inhibit the metabolism of phenytoin by CYP3A4, thereby increasing its serum concentration. Phenytoin also inhibits CYP3A4, and can increase the metabolism of the calcium-channel blockers by this isoenzyme, resulting in a reduction in their plasma concentrations.

Importance and management

Information about the effects of calcium-channel blockers on phenytoin is limited, but what is known indicates that if diltiazem is given with phenytoin, the dose of phenytoin might need to be reduced to avoid toxicity. However, it should be noted that there are only three case reports describing this interaction, and as not all patients appear to be affected, any effect appears to be rare. The case report of phenytoin toxicity with nifedipine is isolated, and of unknown importance.

Phenytoin greatly reduces felodipine and verapamil concentrations. Although not all calcium-channel blockers have been studied, most would be expected to interact with phenytoin similarly, as they are also metabolised by CYP3A4. A considerable increase in the dose of any calcium-channel blocker will probably be needed in the presence of phenytoin. In some cases the decreases in plasma concentrations are so large, that dose increases might not be effective, and alternatives to the calcium-channel blocker will be necessary. Note that the UK manufacturer of nimodipine[10] contraindicates the concurrent use of phenytoin because of the possibility of a large reduction in their bioavailability and efficacy.

1. Bahls FH, Ozuna J, Ritchie DE. Interactions between calcium channel blockers and the anticonvulsants carbamazepine and phenytoin. *Neurology* (1991) 41, 740–2.
2. Clarke WR, Horn JR, Kawabori I, Gurtel S. Potentially serious drug interactions secondary to high-dose diltiazem used in the treatment of pulmonary hypertension. *Pharmacotherapy* (1993) 13, 402–5.
3. Capewell S, Freestone S, Critchley JAJH, Pottage A, Prescott LF. Reduced felodipine bioavailability in patients taking anticonvulsants. *Lancet* (1988) ii, 480–2.
4. Cachat F, Tufro A. Phenytoin/isradipine interaction causing severe neurologic toxicity. *Ann Pharmacother* (2002) 36: 1399–1402.
5. Hauben M. Comment: phenytoin/isradipine interaction causing severe neurologic toxicity. *Ann Pharmacother* (2002) 36: 1974–5.
6. Ahmad S. Nifedipine-phenytoin interaction. *J Am Coll Cardiol* (1984) 3, 1582.
7. Tartara A, Galimberti CA, Manni R, Parietti L, Zucca C, Baasch H, Caresia L, Mück W, Barzaghi N, Gatti G, Perucca E. Differential effects of valproic acid and enzyme-inducing anticonvulsants on nimodipine pharmacokinetics in epileptic patients. *Br J Clin Pharmacol* (1991) 32, 335–40.
8. Michelucci R, Cipolla G, Passarelli D, Gatti G, Ochan M, Heinig R, Tassinari CA, Perucca E. Reduced plasma nisoldipine concentrations in phenytoin-treated patients with epilepsy. *Epilepsia* (1996) 37, 1107–10.
9. Woodcock BG, Kirsten R, Nelson K, Rietbrock S, Hopf R, Kaltenbach M. A reduction in verapamil concentrations with phenytoin. *N Engl J Med* (1991) 325, 1179.
10. Nimotop Tablets (Nimodipine). Bayer plc. UK Summary of product characteristics, October 2012.

Phenytoin + Carbamazepine and related drugs

Some reports describe increases in phenytoin concentrations, with toxicity, whereas others describe decreases in phenytoin concentrations, when carbamazepine is given concurrently. Decreases in the plasma concentration of carbamazepine, sometimes with increases in the carbamazepine-10,11-epoxide concentration, have also been described on the concurrent use of phenytoin.

Oxcarbazepine has been shown to have no effect on phenytoin pharmacokinetics in one study, and to increase the concentration of phenytoin at higher doses in another study. Exposure to the active metabolite of oxcarbazepine is reduced by phenytoin, but the pharmacokinetics of oxcarbazepine were unaffected by phenytoin in another study. Switching from carbamazepine to oxcarbazepine has been shown to increase the plasma concentration of phenytoin.

Exposure to phenytoin is increased by eslicarbazepine and exposure to eslicarbazepine is reduced by phenytoin.

Clinical evidence

(a) Effects on phenytoin

A study in 10 patients with epilepsy found that when **oxcarbazepine** 300 mg three times daily was added to treatment with phenytoin for 3 weeks, there were no clinically relevant changes in the pharmacokinetics of phenytoin.[1] Similarly, a population pharmacokinetic model using data from 641 patients enrolled in phase III **eslicarbazepine** studies found that eslicarbazepine did not affect the clearance of phenytoin.[2] However there are other studies showing differing effects on phenytoin pharmacokinetics with **carbamazepine**, **eslicarbazepine**, and **oxcarbazepine**.

1. Phenytoin exposure reduced. **Carbamazepine** 600 mg daily for 4 to 14 days reduced the serum concentration of phenytoin in 3 out of 7 patients, from 15 to 7 micrograms/mL, from 18 to 12 micrograms/mL, and from 16 to 10 micrograms/mL, respectively. Phenytoin serum concentrations increased again 10 days after carbamazepine was withdrawn.[3] Other reports also describe reduced serum phenytoin concentrations in patients given **carbamazepine**.[4-7]

2. Phenytoin exposure or concentrations reduced. A study in 6 patients with epilepsy taking phenytoin 350 to 600 mg daily found that, over a 12-week period, the addition of **carbamazepine** 600 to 800 mg daily increased the serum concentration of phenytoin by 35%, increased its half-life by 41%, and reduced its clearance by 37%. Neurotoxicity increased 3-fold, with additional symptoms of toxicity (sedation, ataxia, nystagmus) developing in 5 of the 6 patients. The phenytoin dose remained unchanged throughout the period of the study.[8]

Other reports have also described increases in serum phenytoin concentrations,[9-15] which were as large as 81%, and even up to 100% in some cases.[10,12] One study found that **carbamazepine** increased the free fraction of phenytoin by 39%.[16]

A case report describes a 67-year-old woman with a history of bipolar disorder and epilepsy, who was started on **oxcarbazepine** 150 mg twice daily and quetiapine in addition to her existing medication of clonazepam, phenytoin 460 mg daily, and topiramate. On day 5, her serum phenytoin concentration was 21 mg/L and on day 6 she had signs of ataxia. Her **oxcarbazepine** dose was increased in increments, reaching 900 mg daily on day 12. On day 11 she was still ataxic and had suffered several falls. It was noted that her phenytoin concentration had steadily risen with the increasing **oxcarbazepine** dose and reached 28 mg/L on day 13 when her **oxcarbazepine** dose was reduced to 750 mg daily. By day 16 she was no longer ataxic, her phenytoin dose was reduced by 30 mg, and during the following week her phenytoin concentration fell to 20 mg/L.[17]

The UK manufacturer of **eslicarbazepine** briefly notes that in a study in healthy subjects, **eslicarbazepine** 1.2 g daily caused a 31 to 35% increase in phenytoin exposure.[18]

3. Effects of replacing carbamazepine with oxcarbazepine. A double-blind, crossover comparison of oxcarbazepine and carbamazepine in patients with epilepsy found that when carbamazepine was replaced by oxcarbazepine in 7 patients also taking phenytoin, the serum concentration of phenytoin rose by 23%. In 18 patients taking carbamazepine, **valproate**, and phenytoin, replacement of carbamazepine with oxcarbazepine caused an increase in the serum phenytoin concentration of 25%. The study extended over 12 weeks to establish steady-state concentrations.[19]

(b) Effects on carbamazepine

A series of multiple regression analyses on data from a large number of patients (the precise number is not clear from the report) found that phenytoin reduced the plasma concentration of carbamazepine by, on average, 0.9 micrograms/mL for each 2 mg/kg per day of phenytoin.[9] Reduced serum carbamazepine concentrations have been described in other studies and reports.[5,13,20-23] Two studies found that phenytoin increased the plasma concentration of the active metabolite of carbamazepine, carbamazepine-10,11-epoxide.[24,25]

(c) Effects on eslicarbazepine

The manufacturer of eslicarbazepine briefly notes that, in a study in healthy subjects, exposure to eslicarbazepine 1.2 g daily was reduced by 31 to 33% by the concurrent use of phenytoin.[18] A population pharmacokinetic model using data from 641 patients enrolled in phase III eslicarbazepine studies found that the clearance of eslicarbazepine was increased by 60% by phenytoin or barbiturate use (84 patients, but no breakdown for specific drugs).[2]

(d) Effects on oxcarbazepine

A study in 10 patients with epilepsy found that when oxcarbazepine 300 mg three times daily was given with phenytoin for 3 weeks there were no clinically relevant changes in the pharmacokinetics of oxcarbazepine. Phenytoin caused a 29% reduction in the AUC of monohydroxyoxcarbazepine,[1] the active metabolite of oxcarbazepine. Another study found that the plasma concentration of monohydroxyoxcarbazepine was statistically significantly lower (exact figure not stated) in patients taking phenytoin than in patients not taking enzyme-inducing antiepileptics.[15] Another study found that the serum concentration of monohydroxyoxcarbazepine was not affected by phenytoin but its further conversion to dihydroxyoxcarbazepine was increased.[26] Correspondingly, a study found that phenytoin 100 to 375 mg daily increased the clearance of monohydroxyoxcarbazepine, by almost 40%.[27] Similarly, in a study in children, phenytoin was found to increase the apparent clearance of monohydroxyoxcarbazepine by 31 to 35%.[28]

Mechanism

Carbamazepine, oxcarbazepine, and phenytoin are enzyme inducers, and might therefore be expected to increase the metabolism of each other. However, carbamazepine and the active metabolite of oxcarbazepine, monohydroxyoxcarbazepine, are also said to *inhibit* CYP2C19, which is involved in phenytoin metabolism.[29] Carbamazepine and oxcarbazepine might therefore cause *increases* in phenytoin concentration by this mechanism. Eslicarbazepine is also a CYP2C19 inhibitor and appears to interact similarly with phenytoin. Note that CYP2C19 shows genetic polymorphism (that is, in different patients there is different activity of this isoenzyme), so an interaction by this mechanism seems unlikely to occur in all patients, and other routes of phenytoin metabolism are likely to be more important.

Importance and management

Phenytoin might decrease the plasma concentration of **carbamazepine**, but carbamazepine has a variable effect on the serum concentration of phenytoin, with both increases and decreases described. Monitor antiepileptic concentrations during concurrent use (including, where possible, the active metabolite of carbamazepine, carbamazepine-10,11-epoxide) so that steps can be taken to avoid the development of toxicity or lack of efficacy. The risk of carbamazepine-induced water intoxication is reported to be reduced in patients also taking phenytoin.[21]

From the more limited evidence with **oxcarbazepine**, it seems that phenytoin might not affect oxcarbazepine pharmacokinetics, but could decrease exposure to its active metabolite, monohydroxyoxcarbazepine, and its inactive metabolite, dihydroxyoxcarbazepine. However, while the clinical implications of reduced exposure to monohydroxyoxcarbazepine are not clear (but might be expected to be important), one group of authors suggest that there is a theoretical risk that monohydroxyoxcarbazepine concentrations might increase and become toxic if phenytoin is withdrawn.[1] As the conversion to dihydroxyoxcarbazepine is a minor step in the metabolism of monohydroxyoxcarbazepine, the overall antiepileptic action of oxcarbazepine is unlikely to be altered by this effect. Oxcarbazepine has been shown to have no effect on the pharmacokinetics of phenytoin in one study, but has also been shown to increase the plasma concentration at higher doses, and the UK and US manufacturers note that a decrease in the phenytoin dose might be required when the oxcarbazepine dose is greater than 1200 mg daily.[30,31] If oxcarbazepine is substituted for carbamazepine, be aware that the plasma concentration of phenytoin might increase.

Phenytoin exposure can be increased by **eslicarbazepine**, while eslicarbazepine exposure can be reduced by phenytoin. Plasma concentrations of both drugs should be monitored on concurrent use and the doses adjusted as necessary.

Not all patients appear to have an adverse interaction, and, at present, it does not seem possible to identify those potentially at risk.

1. McKee PJW, Blacklaw J, Forrest G, Gillham RA, Walker SM, Connelly D, Brodie MJ. A double blind, placebo-controlled interaction study between oxcarbazepine and carbamazepine, sodium valproate and phenytoin in epileptic patients. *Br J Clin Pharmacol* (1994) 37, 27–32.
2. Falcão A, Fuseau E, Nunes T, Almeida L, Soares-da-Silva P. Pharmacokinetics, drug interactions and exposure-response relationship of eslicarbazepine acetate in adult patients with partial-onset seizures:

population pharmacokinetic and pharmacokinetic/pharmacodynamic analyses. *CNS Drugs* (2012) 26, 79–91.
3. Hansen JM, Siersbæk-Nielsen K, Skovsted L. Carbamazepine-induced acceleration of diphenylhydantoin and warfarin metabolism in man. *Clin Pharmacol Ther* (1971) 12, 539–43.
4. Cereghino JJ, Van Meter JC, Brock JT, Penry JK, Smith LD, White BG. Preliminary observations of serum carbamazepine concentration in epileptic patients. *Neurology* (1973) 23, 357–66.
5. Hooper WD, Dubetz DK, Eadie MJ, Tyrer JH. Preliminary observations on the clinical pharmacology of carbamazepine ('Tegretol'). *Proc Aust Assoc Neurol* (1974) 11, 189–98.
6. Lai M-L, Lin T-S, Huang JD. Effect of single- and multiple-dose carbamazepine on the pharmacokinetics of diphenylhydantoin. *Eur J Clin Pharmacol* (1992) 43, 201–3.
7. Windorfer A, Sauer W. Drug interactions during anticonvulsant therapy in childhood: diphenylhydantoin, primidone, phenobarbitone, clonazepam, nitrazepam, carbamazepin and dipropylacetate. *Neuropadiatrie* (1977) 8, 29–41.
8. Browne TR, Szabo GK, Evans JE, Evans BA, Greenblatt DJ, Mikati MA. Carbamazepine increases phenytoin serum concentration and reduces phenytoin clearance. *Neurology* (1988) 38, 1146–50.
9. Lander CM, Eadie MJ, Tyrer JH. Interactions between anticonvulsants. *Proc Aust Assoc Neurol* (1975) 12, 111–16.
10. Gratz ES, Theodore WH, Newmark ME, Kupferberg HJ, Porter RJ, Qu Z. Effect of carbamazepine on phenytoin clearance in patients with complex partial seizures. *Neurology* (1982) 32, A223.
11. Leppik IE, Pepin SM, Jacobi J, Miller KW. Effect of carbamazepine on the Michaelis-Menten parameters of phenytoin. In Metabolism of Antiepileptic Drugs (ed Levy RH et al) Raven Press, New York. (1984) pp 217–22.
12. Zielinski JJ, Haidukewych D, Leheta BJ. Carbamazepine-phenytoin interaction: elevation of plasma phenytoin concentrations due to carbamazepine comedication. *Ther Drug Monit* (1985) 7, 51–3.
13. Hidano F, Obata N, Yahaba Y, Unno K, Fukui R. Drug interactions with phenytoin and carbamazepine. *Folia Psychiatr Neurol Jpn* (1983) 37, 342–4.
14. Zielinski JJ, Haidukewych D. Dual effects of carbamazepine-phenytoin interaction. *Ther Drug Monit* (1987) 9, 21–3.
15. Barcs G, Walker EB, Elger CE, Scaramelli A, Stefan H, Strum Y, Moore A, Flesch G, Kramer L, D'Souza JD. Oxcarbazepine placebo-controlled, dose-ranging trial in refractory partial epilepsy. *Epilepsia* (2000) 41, 1597–1607.
16. Joerger M, Huitema ADR, Boogerd W, van der Sande JJ, Schellens JHM, Beijnen JH. Interactions of serum albumin, valproic acid and carbamazepine with the pharmacokinetics of phenytoin in cancer patients. *Basic Clin Pharmacol Toxicol* (2006) 99, 133–40.
17. Soskin DP, Kane AJ, Stern TA. Phenytoin toxicity secondary to an oxcarbazepine-phenytoin 2C19 interaction. *Psychosomatics* (2010) 51, 532–5.
18. Zebinix (Eslicarbazepine acetate). Eisai Ltd. UK Summary of product characteristics, August 2012.
19. Houtkooper MA, Lammertsma A, Meyer JWA, Goedhart DM, Meinardi H, van Oorschot CAEH, Blom GF, Höppener RJEA, Hulsman JARJ. Oxcarbazepine (GP 47.680): a possible alternative to carbamazepine? *Epilepsia* (1987) 28, 693–8.
20. Cereghino JJ, Brock JT, Van Meter JC, Penry JK, Smith LD, White BG. The efficacy of carbamazepine combinations in epilepsy. *Clin Pharmacol Ther* (1975) 18, 733–41.
21. Perucca E, Richens A. Reversal by phenytoin of carbamazepine-induced water intoxication: a pharmacokinetic interaction. *J Neurol Neurosurg Psychiatry* (1980) 43, 540–5.
22. Ramsay RE, McManus DQ, Guterman A, Briggle TV, Vazquez D, Perchalski R, Yost RA, Wong P. Carbamazepine metabolism in humans: effect of concurrent anticonvulsant therapy. *Ther Drug Monit* (1990) 12, 235–41.
23. Chapron DJ, LaPierre BA, Abou-Elkair M. Unmasking the significant enzyme-inducing effects of phenytoin on serum carbamazepine concentrations during phenytoin withdrawal. *Ann Pharmacother* (1993) 27, 708–11.
24. Hagiwara M, Takahashi R, Watabe M, Amanuma I, Kan R, Takahashi Y, Kumashiro H. Influence of phenytoin on metabolism of carbamazepine. *Neurosciences* (1989) 15, 303–9.
25. Dam M, Jensen A, Christiansen J. Plasma level and effect of carbamazepine in grand mal and psychomotor epilepsy. *Acta Neurol Scand* (1975) 75 (Suppl 51), 33–8.
26. Kumps A, Wurth C. Oxcarbazepine disposition: preliminary observations in patients. *Biopharm Drug Dispos* (1990) 11, 365–70.
27. Arnoldussen W, Hulsman J, Rentmeester T. Interaction between oxcarbazepine and phenytoin. *Epilepsia* (1993) 34 (Suppl 6), 37.
28. Sallas WM, Milosavljev S, D'Souza J, Hossain M. Pharmacokinetic drug interactions in children taking oxcarbazepine. *Clin Pharmacol Ther* (2003) 74, 138–49.
29. Lakehal F, Wurden CJ, Kalhorn TF, Levy RH. Carbamazepine and oxcarbazepine decrease phenytoin metabolism through inhibition of CYP2C19. *Epilepsy Res* (2002) 52, 79–83.
30. Trileptal (Oxcarbazepine). Novartis Pharmaceuticals UK Ltd. UK Summary of product characteristics, April 2012.
31. Trileptal (Oxcarbazepine). Novartis Pharmaceuticals Corp. US Prescribing information, March 2011.

Phenytoin + Chloramphenicol

Phenytoin levels can be raised by intravenous chloramphenicol and phenytoin toxicity may occur. Other evidence indicates that phenytoin may increase or decrease chloramphenicol levels in children.

Clinical evidence

(a) Effect on chloramphenicol

A child given a 6-week course of intravenous chloramphenicol 100 mg/kg daily in four divided doses had a reduction in chloramphenicol peak and trough serum levels of 46% and 74%, respectively, within 2 days of starting phenytoin 4 mg/kg daily.[1] In contrast, 6 children (aged 1 month to 12 years) developed raised, toxic chloramphenicol levels while receiving phenytoin.[2]

(b) Effect on phenytoin

A man taking phenytoin 100 mg four times daily developed signs of phenytoin toxicity within a week of starting intravenous chloramphenicol (1 g every 6 hours for 4 doses then 2 g every 6 hours). His serum phenytoin levels had risen by about threefold, from about 7 to 24 micrograms/mL.[3]

This interaction has been described in a number of other reports.[4-12] One study found that intravenous chloramphenicol more than doubled the half-life of phenytoin.[4] The AUC of phenytoin after a single intravenous dose of **fosphenytoin** was 23% higher (not significant) in children also given intravenous chloramphenicol, when compared with those given intravenous cefotaxime. In addition, the phenytoin half-life was significantly prolonged by chloramphenicol (23.7 hours versus 15.5 hours).[13]

Mechanism

It seems probable that chloramphenicol, a known enzyme inhibitor,[14] affects the liver enzymes (possibly cytochrome P450 isoenzyme CYP2C19[15]) concerned with the metabolism of phenytoin thereby reducing its rate of clearance from the body. The changes in the pharmacokinetics of chloramphenicol in children are not understood.

Importance and management

The rise in serum phenytoin levels with intravenous chloramphenicol in adults is well documented and clinically important. A two to fourfold rise can occur within a few days. Concurrent use should be avoided unless the effects can be closely monitored and appropriate phenytoin dose reductions made as necessary. The use of a single prophylactic dose of phenytoin or fosphenytoin may be an exception to this.[13] It seems very doubtful if enough chloramphenicol is absorbed from eye drops or ointments for an interaction to occur.

The general clinical importance of the changes in serum chloramphenicol levels in children is uncertain, but the effects of concurrent use should certainly be monitored. More study is needed.

1. Powell DA, Nahata M, Durrell DC, Glazer JP and Hilty MD. Interactions among chloramphenicol, phenytoin and phenobarbitone in a pediatric patient. *J Pediatr* (1981) 98, 1001.
2. Krasinski K, Kusmiesz H, Nelson JD. Pharmacologic interactions among chloramphenicol, phenytoin and phenobarbital. *Pediatr Infect Dis* (1982) 1, 232–5.
3. Ballek RE, Reidenberg MM, Orr L. Inhibition of diphenylhydantoin metabolism by chloramphenicol. *Lancet* (1973) i, 150.
4. Christensen LK, Skovsted L. Inhibition of drug metabolism by chloramphenicol. *Lancet* (1969) ii, 1397–9.
5. Houghton GW, Richens A. Inhibition of phenytoin metabolism by other drugs used in epilepsy. *Int J Clin Pharmacol Biopharm* (1975) 12, 210–16.
6. Rose JQ, Choi HK, Schentag JJ, Kinkel WR, Jusko WJ. Intoxication caused by interaction of chloramphenicol and phenytoin. *JAMA* (1977) 237, 2630–1.
7. Koup JR, Gibaldi M, McNamara P, Hilligoss DM, Colburn WA, Bruck E. Interaction of chloramphenicol with phenytoin and phenobarbital. *Clin Pharmacol Ther* (1978) 24, 571–5.
8. Vincent FM, Mills L, Sullivan JK. Chloramphenicol-induced phenytoin intoxication. *Ann Neurol* (1978) 3, 469.
9. Harper JM, Yost RL, Stewart RB, Ciezkowski J. Phenytoin-chloramphenicol interaction. *Drug Intell Clin Pharm* (1979) 13, 425–9.
10. Greenlaw CW. Chloramphenicol-phenytoin drug interaction. *Drug Intell Clin Pharm* (1979) 13, 609–10.
11. Saltiel M, Stephens NM. Phenytoin-chloramphenicol interaction. *Drug Intell Clin Pharm* (1980) 14, 221.
12. Cosh DG, Rowett DS, Lee PC, McCarthy PJ. Case report — phenytoin therapy complicated by concurrent chloramphenicol and enteral nutrition. *Aust J Hosp Pharm* (1987) 17, 51–3.
13. Ogutu BR, Newton CRJC, Muchohi SN, Otieno GO, Kokwaro GO. Phenytoin pharmacokinetics and clinical effects in African children following fosphenytoin and chloramphenicol coadministration. *Br J Clin Pharmacol* (2002) 54, 635–42.
14. Dixon RL, Fouts JR. Inhibition of microsomal drug metabolic pathways by chloramphenicol. *Biochem Pharmacol* (1962) 11, 715–20.
15. Park J-Y, Kim K-A, Kim S-L. Chloramphenicol is a potent inhibitor of cytochrome P450 isoforms CYP2C19 and CYP3A4 in human liver microsomes. *Antimicrob Agents Chemother* (2003) 47, 3464–9.

Phenytoin + Chlorphenamine

Phenytoin toxicity was attributed to the concurrent use of chlorphenamine in two patients.

Clinical evidence, mechanism, importance and management

A woman taking phenytoin and phenobarbital developed phenytoin toxicity with serum phenytoin levels of about 65 micrograms/mL about a week after starting to take chlorphenamine 4 mg three times daily. The toxic symptoms disappeared and phenytoin levels fell when chlorphenamine was withdrawn.[1] Another woman taking antiepileptics, including phenytoin, developed slight grimacing of the face and involuntary jaw movements (but no speech slurring, ataxia or nystagmus) within 12 days of starting to take chlorphenamine 12 to 16 mg daily. Her serum phenytoin level had risen to 30 micrograms/mL but it fell when chlorphenamine was withdrawn.[2]

The reason for these reactions is not clear but it has been suggested that chlorphenamine may have inhibited the metabolism of phenytoin by the liver; however, chlorphenamine is not usually associated with enzyme inhibition. These are isolated cases, and their general relevance is uncertain, but it seems likely to be small.

1. Pugh RNH, Geddes AM, Yeoman WB. Interaction of phenytoin with chlorpheniramine. *Br J Clin Pharmacol* (1975) 2, 173–5.
2. Ahmad S, Laidlaw J, Houghton GW, Richens A. Involuntary movements caused by phenytoin intoxication in epileptic patients. *J Neurol Neurosurg Psychiatry* (1975) 38, 225–31.

Phenytoin + Coumarins and related drugs

Phenytoin levels can be increased by dicoumarol (toxicity seen) and phenprocoumon, but they are usually unchanged by warfarin and phenindione. However, a single case of phenytoin toxicity has been seen with warfarin. Phenytoin would be expected to reduce the anticoagulant effects of coumarin anticoagulants, and this has been seen with dicoumarol and warfarin. However, cases of increased effects of warfarin have been reported, and one study found that the effects of phenprocoumon were generally unaltered. A single case of severe bleeding has been described in a patient taking acenocoumarol and phenytoin.

Clinical evidence

The reports of interactions between phenytoin and various anticoagulants are summarised in 'Table 14.2', p.599, and discussed in further detail below.

Table 14.2 Summary of interactions between phenytoin and anticoagulants

Concurrent treatment with phenytoin and anticoagulant	*Effect on anticoagulant*	*Effect on serum phenytoin levels*
Acenocoumarol	Single case of increase[1]	Uncertain
Dicoumarol	Reduced[2]	Markedly increased[3-5]
Phenindione	Not documented	Usually unchanged[3,4]
Phenprocoumon	Usually unchanged[6]	Increased[4]
Warfarin	Increased[7-13] Single case of increase followed by decrease[10]	Usually unchanged[4] Increased in two cases[12,14]

1. Abad-Santos F, Carcas AJ, F-Capitán C, Frias J. Case report. Retroperitoneal haematoma in a patient treated with acenocoumarol, phenytoin and paroxetine. *Clin Lab Haematol* (1995) 17, 195-7.
2. Hansen JM, Siersbæk-Nielsen K, Kristensen M, Skovsted L, Christensen LK. Effect of diphenylhydantoin on the metabolism of dicoumarol in man. *Acta Med Scand* (1971) 189, 15-19.
3. Hansen JM, Kristensen M, Skovsted L, Christensen LK. Dicoumarol-induced diphenylhydantoin intoxication. *Lancet* (1966) ii, 265-6.
4. Skovsted L, Kristensen M, Hansen JM, Siersbæk-Nielsen K. The effect of different oral anticoagulants on diphenylhydantoin (DPH) and tolbutamide metabolism. *Acta Med Scand* (1976) 199, 513-15.
5. Franzten E, Hansen JM, Hansen OE, Kristensen M. Phenytoin (Dilantin®) intoxication. *Acta Neurol Scand* (1967) 43, 440-6.
6. Chrishe HW, Tauchert M, Hilger HH. Effect of phenytoin on the metabolism of phenprocoumon. *Eur J Clin Invest* (1974) 4, 331.
7. Nappi JM. Warfarin and phenytoin interaction. *Ann Intern Med* (1979) 90, 852.
8. Koch-Weser J. Haemorrhagic reactions and drug interactions in 500 warfarin treated patients. *Clin Pharmacol Ther* (1973) 14, 139.
9. Taylor JW, Alexander B, Lyon LW. A comparative evaluation of oral anticoagulant-phenytoin interactions. *Drug Intell Clin Pharm* (1980) 14, 669-73.
10. Levine M, Sheppard I. Biphasic interaction of phenytoin with warfarin. *Clin Pharm* (1984) 3, 200-3.
11. Panegyres PK, Rischbieth RH. Fatal phenytoin warfarin interaction. *Postgrad Med J* (1991) 67, 98.
12. Meisheri YV. Simultaneous phenytoin and warfarin toxicity on chronic concomitant therapy. *J Assoc Physicians India* (1996) 44, 661-2.
13. Hassan Y, Awaisu A, Aziz NA, Ismail O. The complexity of achieving anticoagulation control in the face of warfarin-phenytoin interaction. *Pharm World Sci* (2005) 27, 16-19.
14. Rothermich NO. Diphenylhydantoin intoxication. *Lancet* (1966) ii, 640.

(a) Acenocoumarol

A 68-year-old woman with a double mitral valve lesion, atrial fibrillation and hypertension, taking digoxin and diuretics, was stabilised taking acenocoumarol 17 mg per week in divided doses and paroxetine. Phenytoin 400 mg daily for 3 days then 300 mg daily was started because of a seizure, and 11 days later she developed ataxia, lethargy and nystagmus (free phenytoin level 12.5 micromol/L). At the same time her INR was found to have risen from a range of 2 to 4, up to 14.5 and a huge retroperitoneal haematoma was discovered. After appropriate treatment she was discharged taking acenocoumarol 13 mg per week in divided doses and half the phenytoin dose.[1]

(b) Dicoumarol

Phenytoin 300 mg daily was given to 6 subjects taking dicoumarol 40 to 160 mg daily for a week. No significant changes in the prothrombin-proconvertin concentration occurred until 3 days after stopping the phenytoin. In the following 5 days it climbed from 20 to 50%, with an accompanying drop in the serum dicoumarol levels.[2] Four other subjects taking dicoumarol 60 mg daily were also given phenytoin 300 mg daily for the first week of treatment, and then 100 mg daily for 5 more weeks. The prothrombin-proconvertin concentration had risen from 20 to 70% after 2 weeks of concurrent use, representing an antagonism of the anticoagulant effect, and only fell to previous levels 5.5 weeks after stopping phenytoin.[2]

A study in 6 subjects taking phenytoin 300 mg daily found that when they were also given dicoumarol (doses adjusted to give prothrombin values of about 30%) their serum phenytoin levels rose on average by almost 10 micrograms/mL (126%) over 7 days.[3] In another study in 3 patients the half-life of phenytoin increased by about fivefold during dicoumarol use.[4]

A patient taking dicoumarol developed phenytoin toxicity within a few days of starting to take phenytoin 300 mg daily (dose based on a weight of 62 kg). Phenytoin was withdrawn, and re-introduced at 200 mg daily, which gave satisfactory phenytoin levels.[5]

(c) Phenindione

A study in 4 patients taking phenytoin 300 mg daily found that phenindione did not affect their serum phenytoin levels.[4]

(d) Phenprocoumon

An investigation in patients taking long-term phenprocoumon found that in the majority of cases phenytoin had no significant effect on either serum phenprocoumon levels or the anticoagulant control, although a few patients had a fall and others a rise in serum anticoagulant levels, with consequent decreased or increased effects.[6]

A study in 4 patients taking phenytoin 300 mg daily found that when they were given phenprocoumon their serum phenytoin levels rose from about 10 micrograms/mL to 14 micrograms/mL over 7 days.[4] The phenytoin half-life increased from 9.9 hours to 14 hours.

(e) Warfarin

The prothrombin time of a patient taking warfarin increased from 21 to 32 seconds over a month when phenytoin 300 mg daily was also given, despite a 22% reduction in the warfarin dose. He was restabilised on the original warfarin dose when phenytoin was withdrawn. Six other reports describe this interaction.[7-12] One of them describes a patient who had an increased anticoagulant response to warfarin for the first 6 days after phenytoin was added. The anticoagulant effect then declined to less than the level seen before the addition of phenytoin.[10] Conversely, a population pharmacokinetic analysis reported that the clearance of warfarin was *increased* by 30% in 6 patients taking phenytoin or phenobarbital.[13] However, the findings were not reported separately for the two drugs, and are therefore difficult to interpret (phenobarbital is a known inducer of warfarin clearance, see 'Coumarins + Barbiturates', p.411).

A study in 2 patients taking phenytoin 300 mg daily found that their serum phenytoin levels were unaffected by warfarin given for 7 days, and the half-life of phenytoin in 4 other patients was unaffected.[4] However, a patient taking phenytoin 300 mg daily developed symptoms of toxicity shortly after starting to take warfarin.[14] Another patient developed phenytoin toxicity 6 months after starting to take phenytoin with warfarin.[12]

Mechanism

Multiple, complex and poorly understood. Dicoumarol and phenprocoumon (but not normally warfarin) appear to inhibit the metabolism of phenytoin by the liver, so that its loss from the body is reduced. Phenytoin is an inducer of the cytochrome P450 isoenzyme CYP2C9, which is involved (to varying degrees) in the metabolism of the coumarin anticoagulants. Phenytoin would therefore be expected to decrease the levels and effect of some coumarins, and this has been shown for dicoumarol. However, increased effects of warfarin have been noted, suggesting reduced metabolism of warfarin. Why this occurs is uncertain, but poor CYP2C9 metaboliser phenotype (that is, those patients genetically lacking this isoenzyme) may provide an explanation.[15] Phenytoin possibly also has a diverse depressant effect on the liver, which lowers blood clotting factor production.[16]

Importance and management

None of these interactions has been extensively studied nor are they well established, but what is known suggests that the use of dicoumarol with phenytoin should be avoided or monitored very closely. Similarly, serum phenytoin levels and anticoagulant control should be well monitored if acenocoumarol, phenprocoumon or warfarin is given with phenytoin. Dose adjustments may be needed to accommodate any interactions. Information about other anticoagulants (apart from phenindione, which had no effect on phenytoin levels) appears to be lacking, but it would clearly be prudent to monitor the effects of concurrent use.

1. Abad-Santos F, Carcas AJ, F-Capitán C, Frias J. Case report. Retroperitoneal haematoma in a patient treated with acenocoumarol, phenytoin and paroxetine. *Clin Lab Haematol* (1995) 17, 195–7.
2. Hansen JM, Siersbæk-Nielsen K, Kristensen M, Skovsted L,Christensen LK. Effect of diphenylhydantoin on the metabolism of dicoumarol in man. *Acta Med Scand* (1971) 189, 15–19.
3. Hansen JM, Kristensen M, Skovsted L, Christensen LK. Dicoumarol-induced diphenylhydantoin intoxication. *Lancet* (1966) ii, 265–6.
4. Skovsted L, Kristensen M, Hansen JM, Siersbæk-Nielsen K. The effect of different oral anticoagulants on diphenylhydantoin (DPH) and tolbutamide metabolism. *Acta Med Scand* (1976) 199, 513–15.
5. Franzten E, Hansen JM, Hansen OE, Kristensen M. Phenytoin (Dilantin®) intoxication. *Acta Neurol Scand* (1967) 43, 440–6.
6. Chrishe HW, Tauchert M, Hilger HH. Effect of phenytoin on the metabolism of phenprocoumon. *Eur J Clin Invest* (1974) 4, 331.
7. Nappi JM. Warfarin and phenytoin interaction. *Ann Intern Med* (1979) 90, 852.
8. Koch-Weser J. Haemorrhagic reactions and drug interactions in 500 warfarin treated patients. *Clin Pharmacol Ther* (1973) 14, 139.
9. Taylor JW, Alexander B, Lyon LW. A comparative evaluation of oral anticoagulant-phenytoin interactions. *Drug Intell Clin Pharm* (1980) 14, 669–73.
10. Levine M, Sheppard I. Biphasic interaction of phenytoin with warfarin. *Clin Pharm* (1984) 3, 200–3.
11. Panegyres PK, Rischbieth RH. Fatal phenytoin warfarin interaction. *Postgrad Med J* (1991) 67, 98.
12. Meisheri YV. Simultaneous phenytoin and warfarin toxicity on chronic concomitant therapy. *J Assoc Physicians India* (1996) 44, 661–2.
13. Mungall DR, Ludden TM, Marshall J, Hawkins DW, Talbert RL, Crawford MH. Population pharmacokinetics of racemic warfarin in adult patients. *J Pharmacokinet Biopharm* (1985) 13, 213–27.
14. Rothermich NO. Diphenylhydantoin intoxication. *Lancet* (1966) ii, 640.
15. Rettie AE, Haining RL, Bajpai M, Levy RH. A common genetic basis for idiosyncratic toxicity of warfarin and phenytoin. *Epilepsy Res* (1999) 35, 253–5.
16. Solomon GE, Hilgartner MW, Kutt H. Coagulation defects caused by diphenylhydantoin. *Neurology* (1972) 22, 1165–71.

Phenytoin + Dextromethorphan

Dextromethorphan appears not to affect phenytoin levels.

Clinical evidence, mechanism, importance and management

A double-blind, crossover study in 4 patients with severe complex partial seizures found that dextromethorphan 120 mg daily in liquid form (*Delsym*) over 3 months had no effect on their serum phenytoin levels. There was a non-significant alteration in the complex partial seizure and tonic-clonic seizure frequency.[1] This suggests that the dose of phenytoin does not need to be adjusted in patients also given dextromethorphan.

1. Fisher RS, Cysyk BJ, Lesser RP, Pontecorvo MJ, Ferkany JT, Schwerdt PR, Hart J, Gordon B. Dextromethorphan for treatment of complex partial seizures. *Neurology* (1990) 40, 547–9.

Phenytoin + Dextropropoxyphene (Propoxyphene)

Although no interaction generally appears to occur between phenytoin and dextropropoxyphene, a case report describes phenytoin toxicity in a patient given both drugs.

Clinical evidence, mechanism, importance and management

In a study, 6 patients taking phenytoin were given dextropropoxyphene 65 mg three times daily for 6 to 13 days. Dextropropoxyphene caused only a very small rise in phenytoin levels.[1] In contrast, a review briefly mentions one patient who developed toxic serum phenytoin levels while taking dextropropoxyphene in doses of up to 600 mg daily on an as-required basis.[2]

Concurrent use need not be avoided, but as rises in the serum levels of phenytoin can occur it would be prudent to monitor the outcome, especially if large doses of dextropropoxyphene are being taken. It is probably sufficient to monitor for increased phenytoin adverse effects (blurred vision, nystagmus, ataxia or drowsiness).

1. Hansen BS, Dam M, Brandt J, Hvidberg EF, Angelo H, Christensen JM, Lous P. Influence of dextropropoxyphene on steady state serum levels and protein binding of three anti-epileptic drugs in man. *Acta Neurol Scand* (1980) 61, 357–67.
2. Kutt H. Biochemical and genetic factors regulating Dilantin metabolism in man. *Ann N Y Acad Sci* (1971) 179, 704–22.

Phenytoin + Diazoxide

Three children and one adult had very marked reductions in their phenytoin levels when diazoxide was given, and in one case seizures developed. There is some evidence that the effects of diazoxide may be reduced by phenytoin.

Clinical evidence

A child taking phenytoin 29 mg/kg daily and an adult taking phenytoin 1 g daily were unable to achieve therapeutic phenytoin serum levels while taking diazoxide. When the diazoxide was withdrawn, satisfactory serum phenytoin levels were achieved with doses of only 6.6 mg/kg and 400 mg daily, in the child and the adult, respectively. When diazoxide was restarted experimentally in the adult, the serum phenytoin levels became undetectable after 4 days, and seizures occurred.[1] Two other reports describe this interaction.[2,3]

Limited evidence suggests that the half-life and effects of the diazoxide can be reduced by phenytoin.[2,4]

Mechanism

What is known suggests that diazoxide increases the metabolism and the clearance of phenytoin from the body.[1,2]

Importance and management

Information is limited to these reports, but the interaction would appear to be established. Given the rapid development of seizures in one case, it would seem prudent to avoid concurrent use where possible. If both drugs must be given, monitor the effects of concurrent use, being alert for the need to increase the phenytoin dose. The clinical importance of the reduced diazoxide effects is uncertain.

1. Roe TF, Podosin RL, Blaskovics ME. Drug Interaction: diazoxide and diphenylhydantoin. *J Pediatr* (1975) 87, 480–4.
2. Petro DJ, Vannucci RC, Kulin HE. Diazoxide-diphenylhydantoin interaction. *J Pediatr* (1976) 89, 331–2.
3. Turck D, Largilliere C, Dupuis B, Farriaux JP. Interaction entre le diazoxide et la phénytoïne. *Presse Med* (1986) 15, 31.
4. Pruitt AW, Dayton PG, Patterson JH. Disposition of diazoxide in children. *Clin Pharmacol Ther* (1973) 14, 73–82.

Phenytoin + Dichloralphenazone

There is some evidence that phenytoin levels may be reduced by dichloralphenazone.

Clinical evidence, mechanism, importance and management

In 5 healthy subjects, dichloralphenazone 1.3 g each night for 13 nights doubled the total body clearance of a single intravenous dose of phenytoin.[1] The phenazone component of dichloralphenazone is a known enzyme inducer and the increased clearance of phenytoin is probably due to an enhancement of its metabolism by the liver. There seem to be no additional reports of adverse effects in patients given both drugs, so that the clinical importance of this interaction is uncertain. However, it would seem prudent to be alert for a reduction in serum phenytoin levels if dichloralphenazone is also given.

1. Riddell JG, Salem SAM, McDevitt DG. Interaction between phenytoin and dichloralphenazone. *Br J Clin Pharmacol* (1980) 9, 118P.

Phenytoin + Felbamate

Felbamate causes a moderate increase in phenytoin levels. Felbamate levels are reduced by phenytoin.

Clinical evidence

A pilot study in 4 patients noted that felbamate increased plasma phenytoin levels.[1] Therefore, in a further study in 5 patients, the phenytoin dose was automatically reduced by 20% when felbamate was given. One patient needed a slight increase in phenytoin dose, whereas 2 other patients needed a further reduction in their phenytoin dose.[2] In a later full report of this study, it was noted that phenytoin dose decreases of 10 to 30% were required to maintain stable levels in the presence of felbamate.[3] Another study in patients with epilepsy found that felbamate 1.2 or 1.8 g daily increased the maximum plasma phenytoin levels by 31% and 69%, respectively. Higher felbamate doses necessitated phenytoin dose reductions of 20 to 40%.[4]

Studies in children and adults have found that phenytoin increased the clearance of felbamate by about 40%,[5,6] and decreased maximum felbamate levels by 56 to 60%, when compared with patients taking felbamate alone.[4] Another report suggested that this effect was dose-dependent.[7]

Mechanism

Uncertain but felbamate probably acts as a competitive inhibitor of phenytoin metabolism, thereby reducing its loss from the body and increasing its serum levels,[2,8] whereas phenytoin induces felbamate metabolism, thereby increasing its clearance.[7]

Importance and management

Established interactions. The phenytoin dose may need to be reduced (a 20 to 40% reduction seems to be about right[2,4,8]) if felbamate is added, and increased if felbamate is withdrawn. However, note that, as phenytoin pharmacokinetics are non-linear, any dose adjustments will need to be assessed in individual patients. The importance of the reduced felbamate levels is uncertain, but they are probably less important because felbamate has a wide therapeutic range.[4]

1. Sheridan PH, Ashworth M, Milne K, White BG, Santilli N, Lothman EW, Dreifuss FE, Jacobs MP, Martinez P, Leppik IE. Open pilot study of felbamate (ADD 03055) in partial seizures. *Epilepsia* (1986) 27, 649.
2. Fuerst RH, Graves NM, Leppik IE, Remmel RP, Rosenfeld WE, Sierzant TL. A preliminary report on alteration of carbamazepine and phenytoin metabolism by felbamate. *Drug Intell Clin Pharm* (1986) 20, 465–6.
3. Leppik IE, Dreifuss FE, Pledger GW, Graves NM, Santilli N, Drury I, Tsay JY, Jacobs MP, Bertram E, Cereghino JJ, Cooper G, Sahlroot JT, Sheridan P, Ashworth M, Lee SI, Sierzant TL. Felbamate for partial seizures: results of a controlled clinical trial. *Neurology* (1991) 41, 1785–9.
4. Sachdeo R, Wagner M, Sachdeo S, Schumaker RC, Lyness WH, Rosenberg A, Ward D, Perhach JL. Coadministration of phenytoin and felbamate: evidence of additional phenytoin dose-reduction requirements based on pharmacokinetics and tolerability with increasing doses of felbamate. *Epilepsia* (1999) 40, 1122–8.
5. Kelley MT, Walson PD, Cox S, Dusci LJ. Population pharmacokinetics of felbamate in children. *Ther Drug Monit* (1997) 19, 29–36.
6. Banfield CR, Zhu G-RR, Jen JF, Jensen PK, Schumaker RC, Perhach JL Affrime MB, Glue P. The effect of age on the apparent clearance of felbamate: a retrospective analysis using nonlinear mixed-effects modeling. *Ther Drug Monit* (1996) 18, 19–29.
7. Wagner ML, Graves NM, Marienau K, Holmes GB, Remmel RP, Leppik IE. Discontinuation of phenytoin and carbamazepine in patients receiving felbamate. *Epilepsia* (1991) 32, 398–406.
8. Fuerst RH, Graves NM, Leppik IE, Brundage RC, Holmes GB, Remmel RP. Felbamate increases phenytoin but decreases carbamazepine concentrations. *Epilepsia* (1988) 29, 488–91.

Phenytoin + Fluorouracil and related prodrugs

Phenytoin toxicity has been reported on the concurrent use of fluorouracil and fluorouracil prodrugs, such as capecitabine, doxifluridine, and tegafur.

Clinical evidence

(a) Fluorouracil

A patient with epilepsy taking phenytoin developed phenytoin toxicity when given **fluorouracil** to treat colon cancer.[1] Cases of phenytoin toxicity have been reported in 3 patients receiving **fluorouracil** with folinic acid.[2,3]

(b) Fluorouracil prodrugs

Three patients with malignant brain tumours developed acute phenytoin toxicity associated with raised phenytoin serum concentrations when they were given *UFT* (**tegafur** with uracil).[4] In one of the patients, no interaction occurred when the *UFT* was replaced with **fluorouracil**, but see *Fluorouracil,* above. Another case of phenytoin toxicity has been also reported with *UFT*.[5] Two cases of phenytoin toxicity have also been reported with another **tegafur**-containing preparation (with gimeracil and oteracil).[6,7] In the first case, a 70-year-old man taking phenytoin 100 mg three times daily, with a phenytoin serum concentration between 9.4 and 11.2 micrograms/mL, experienced light headedness, repeated falls, and unstable walking one month after starting **tegafur** with gimeracil and oteracil. The **tegafur** preparation was discontinued, and 9 days later his phenytoin serum concentration was 32.8 micrograms/mL. His phenytoin dose was reduced to 50 mg three times daily, and 2 weeks later his phenytoin serum concentration was 7.4 micrograms/mL, at which point his phenytoin dose was increased back to 100 mg three times daily. Fifteen days later, his phenytoin serum concentration was 6.9 micrograms/mL.[6] The second case developed 2 months after **tegafur** with gimeracil and oteracil (in combination with cisplatin) was given to a patient taking phenytoin and valproate.[7]

Phenytoin toxicity was also seen in a woman treated with combination therapy that included **doxifluridine**.[8] Similarly, phenytoin toxicity has occurred in a patient given **capecitabine**.[2]

Mechanism

The raised phenytoin serum concentrations possibly occur because the hepatic metabolism of phenytoin is reduced by these antineoplastics possibly as a result of the inhibition of CYP2C19 which is involved in the metabolism of phenytoin. Further study is required to establish this mechanism. Changes in plasma protein binding might also be involved.

Importance and management

Information regarding an interaction between phenytoin and fluorouracil or its prodrugs is limited to case reports, but they are consistent and show that raised serum phenytoin concentrations, possibly leading to toxicity, can occur if these drugs are given concurrently. Where possible, it would be prudent to avoid the concurrent use of phenytoin and fluorouracil, capecitabine, doxifluridine, or tegafur. If this is not possible, phenytoin serum concentrations should be closely monitored, making dose adjustments as necessary. Note that phenytoin serum concentrations might be lowered by other antineoplastics, see 'Antiepileptics + Antineoplastics; Cytotoxic', p.562, for further details.

1. Rosemergy I, Findlay M. Phenytoin toxicity as a result of 5-fluorouracil administration. *N Z Med J* (2002) 115, U124.
2. Brickell K, Parter D, Thompson P. Phenytoin toxicity due to fluoropyrimidines (5FU/capecitabine): three case reports. *Br J Cancer* (2003) 89, 615–16.
3. Gilbar PJ, Brodribb TR. Phenytoin and fluorouracil interaction. *Ann Pharmacother* (2001) 35, 1367–70.
4. Wakisaka S, Shimauchi M, Kaji Y, Nonaka A, Kinoshita K. Acute phenytoin intoxication associated with the antineoplastic agent UFT. *Fukuoka Igaku Zasshi* (1990) 81, 192–6.
5. Errea-Abad JM, González-Igual J, Eito-Cativiela JL, Gastón-Añaños J. Intoxicación aguda por fenitoína debida a interacción col el derivado fluoropirimidínico. *Rev Neurol* (1998) 27, 1066–7.
6. Tsuda A, Fujiyama J, Miki A, Hori S, Ohtani H, Sawada Y. The first case of phenytoin intoxication associated with the concomitant use of phenytoin and TS-1, a combination preparation of tegafur, gimeracil, and oteracil potassium. *Cancer Chemother Pharmacol* (2008) 62, 427–32.
7. Mimatsu K, Oida T, Kawasaki A, Kida K, Fukino N, Kuboi Y, Kano H, Amano S. Phenytoin toxicity in a patient receiving concomitant use of phenytoin and S-1 plus cisplatin chemotherapy for advanced gastric cancer. *Gan To Kagaku Ryoho* (2011) 38, 1003–6.
8. Konishi H, Morita K, Minouchi T, Nakajima M, Matsuda M, Yamaji A. Probable metabolic interaction of doxifluridine with phenytoin. *Ann Pharmacother* (2002) 36, 831–4.

Phenytoin + Food

The absorption of phenytoin can be affected by some foods. A very marked reduction in phenytoin absorption has been described when it was given with enteral feeds (e.g. *Isocal, Osmolite*), by nasogastric or jejunostomy tubes.

Clinical evidence

(a) Food by mouth

A study found that serum drug levels were lower than expected when phenytoin was disguised in **vanilla pudding** and given to children. However, when the phenytoin was mixed with **apple sauce**, 3 out of 10 patients developed serum phenytoin levels within the toxic range, and the mean levels were twice those seen when the tablets were mixed with the **vanilla pudding**.[1] The absorption of phenytoin as the acid in a micronised form (*Fenantoin*, ACO, Sweden) was faster and the peak serum levels were on average 40% higher when it was given after a **standardised breakfast**.[2] In a further study to investigate the effects of component parts of the **standardised breakfast**, the same authors found that **fat** had no measurable effect, but **carbohydrate** may enhance, and **protein** reduce, the absorption of phenytoin.[3]

Another study in 5 subjects found that the bioavailability of a single dose of phenytoin was enhanced when it was given immediately after a **'balanced' meal**. Administration after a **high-lipid meal** resulted in large inter-patient variability in phenytoin bioavailability.[4] One single-dose study found that, when taken with a **high-protein meal**, the total absorption of phenytoin was not affected, although it was slightly delayed.[5]

A patient with epilepsy had a marked fall in his serum phenytoin levels accompanied by an increased seizure frequency when phenytoin was given at bedtime with 8 oz of a food supplement (***Ensure***).[6] Another patient had reduced phenytoin serum levels when phenytoin was given as an oral suspension with oral ***Fresubin liquid food concentrate***.[7]

However, in contrast, a study in 10 healthy subjects found that when ***Ensure*** or ***Vivonex TEN*** was given every 4 hours for 24 hours, the absorption of a single 400-mg dose of phenytoin was unaffected.[8] Similarly, a single-dose study in healthy subjects found that the bioavailability of phenytoin sodium 400 mg in a capsule formulation (*Dilantin Kapseals*) was not affected by ***Ensure***.[9]

A study in healthy subjects found that phenytoin levels were reduced by enteral feeds, but that it was easier to attain therapeutic levels of phenytoin in those also receiving a **meat-based** formulation (***Compleat Modified***) rather than a **protein hydrolysate** formulation (***Osmolite***).[10]

(b) Food by nasogastric tube

A patient taking phenytoin 300 mg daily who was being fed with ***Fortison*** through a nasogastric tube, following a brain injury sustained in a road traffic accident, had a phenytoin serum level of only 1 mg/L. When phenytoin 420 mg was given diluted in water and separated from the food by 2 hours, a serum level of 6 mg/L was achieved.[11] This report describes a similar reaction in another patient with a cerebral tumour.[11]

A study in 20 patients and 5 healthy subjects found that phenytoin absorption was reduced by about 70% when it was given by nasogastric tube with an **enteral feed** product (***Isocal***) at a rate of 100 to 125 mL/hour.[12] Other reports describe the same interaction in patients given ***Ensure***,[13] ***Isocal***,[14,15] or ***Osmolite***.[13,16-18] However, another study in healthy subjects found that the absolute bioavailability of phenytoin suspension or phenytoin sodium solution given by nasogastric tube was not affected by an enteral feed product (***Isocal***).[19]

(c) Food by jejunostomy tube

A woman with a history of seizures had acceptable serum phenytoin levels when phenytoin was given intravenously, but they fell from 19.1 micrograms/mL to less than 2.5 micrograms/mL when a comparable dose of phenytoin suspension was given in the presence of an **enteral feed** product (***Jevity***), given by jejunostomy tube.[20]

Mechanism

Not fully resolved. Phenytoin can bind to some food substances, which reduces its absorption.[21,22] One study in healthy subjects failed to find any difference in phenytoin bioavailability after fasting or with *Ensure* (given hourly or every 4 hours), suggesting that factors other than direct contact of phenytoin and feed contribute to decreased phenytoin bioavailability.[23] Phenytoin can also become bound to the nasogastric tubing[24] and may also be poorly absorbed if the tubing empties into the duodenum rather than the stomach.[24] Delivery into the jejunum appears to have an even greater detrimental effect on phenytoin absorption, because there is even less time for adequate absorption.[20] Other factors that could contribute to the interaction are gastrointestinal transit time, the nitrogen source in the feed, the calcium content and pH of the feed, the dose form of phenytoin or its dilution before administration.[25]

Importance and management

Phenytoin is often taken orally with food to reduce gastric irritation. This normally appears not to have a marked effect on absorption, but the studies cited above show that some formulations and some foods can interact. If there are problems with the control of seizures or evidence of toxicity, review how and when the patient is taking the phenytoin.

Some studies in healthy subjects failed to find an interaction between phenytoin and enteral feeding.[8,9,19,23] However, many studies in patients have found a clinically important interaction between phenytoin and enteral feeds given orally or by nasogastric tube. The markedly reduced bioavailability associated with the nasogastric route has been successfully managed by giving the phenytoin diluted in water 2 hours after stopping the feed, flushing with 60 mL of water, and waiting another 2 hours before restarting the feed.[11,12] However, one limited study failed to confirm that this method is successful,[13] and some sources suggest waiting 1 hour[26] or 6 hours[14] after the phenytoin dose before restarting the feed. Some increase in the phenytoin dose may also be needed. Monitor concurrent use closely. The same problem can clearly also occur when enteral feeds are given by jejunostomy tube. Approaches on how to minimise any potential interaction have been reported,[25,27] including the development and use of an algorithm.[25] In patients requiring phenytoin and enteral nutrition, the initial use of intravenous phenytoin to establish therapeutic levels has been suggested. It may also be considered if therapeutic levels cannot be maintained without compromising nutritional intake. Stopping continuous feed 1 hour rather than 2 hours before and after phenytoin administration and the use of twice daily phenytoin rather than three times daily administration have also been suggested as methods of maintaining adequate caloric intake as well as phenytoin levels in some patients.[27]

1. Jann MW, Bean J, Fidone G. Interaction of dietary pudding with phenytoin. *Pediatrics* (1986) 78, 952–3.
2. Melander A, Brante G, Johansson Ö, Lindberg T, Wåhlin-Boll E. Influence of food on the absorption of phenytoin in man. *Eur J Clin Pharmacol* (1979) 15, 269–74.
3. Johansson Ö, Wahlin-Boll E, Lindberg T, Melander A. Opposite effects of carbohydrate and protein on phenytoin absorption in man. *Drug Nutr Interact* (1983) 2, 139–44.
4. Sekikawa H, Nakano M, Takada M, Arita T. Influence of dietary components on the bioavailability of phenytoin. *Chem Pharm Bull (Tokyo)* (1980) 28, 2443–9.
5. Kennedy MC, Wade DN. The effect of food on the absorption of phenytoin. *Aust N Z J Med* (1982) 12, 258–61.
6. Longe RL, Smith OB. Phenytoin interaction with an oral feeding results in loss of seizure control. *J Am Geriatr Soc* (1988) 36, 542–4.
7. Taylor DM, Massey CA, Willson WG, Dhillon S. Lowered serum phenytoin concentrations during therapy with liquid food concentrates. *Ann Pharmacother* (1993) 27, 369.
8. Marvel ME, Bertino JS. Comparative effects of an elemental and a complex enteral feeding formulation on the absorption of phenytoin suspension. *J Parenter Enteral Nutr* (1991) 15, 316–8.
9. Nishimura LY, Armstrong EP, Plezia PM, Iacono RP. Influence of enteral feedings on phenytoin sodium absorption from capsules. *Drug Intell Clin Pharm* (1988) 22, 130–3.
10. Guidry JR, Eastwood TF, Curry SC. Phenytoin absorption in volunteers receiving selected enteral feedings. *West J Med* (1989) 150, 659–61.
11. Summers VM, Grant R. Nasogastric feeding and phenytoin interaction. *Pharm J* (1989) 243, 181.
12. Bauer LA. Interference of oral phenytoin absorption by continuous nasogastric feedings. *Neurology* (1982) 32, 570–2.
13. Ozuna J, Friel P. Effect of enteral tube feeding on serum phenytoin levels. *J Neurosurg Nurs* (1984) 16, 289–91.
14. Pearce GA. Apparent inhibition of phenytoin absorption by an enteral nutrient formula. *Aust J Hosp Pharm* (1988) 18, 289–92.
15. Worden JP, Wood CA, Workman CH. Phenytoin and nasogastric feedings. *Neurology* (1984) 34, 132.
16. Hatton RC. Dietary interaction with phenytoin. *Clin Pharm* (1984) 3, 110–11.

17. Weinryb J, Cogen R. Interaction of nasogastric phenytoin and enteral feeding solution. *J Am Geriatr Soc* (1989) 37, 195–6.
18. Maynard GA, Jones KM, Guidry JR. Phenytoin absorption from tube feedings. *Arch Intern Med* (1987) 147, 1821.
19. Doak KK, Haas CE, Dunnigan KJ, Reiss RA, Reiser JR, Huntress J, Altavela JL. Bioavailability of phenytoin acid and phenytoin sodium with enteral feedings. *Pharmacotherapy* (1998) 18, 637–45.
20. Rodman DP, Stevenson TL, Ray TR. Phenytoin malabsorption after jejunostomy tube delivery. *Pharmacotherapy* (1995) 15, 801–5.
21. Miller SW, Strom JG. Stability of phenytoin in three enteral nutrient formulas. *Am J Hosp Pharm* (1988) 45, 2529–32.
22. Hooks MA, Longe RL, Taylor AT, Francisco GE. Recovery of phenytoin from an enteral nutrient formula. *Am J Hosp Pharm* (1986) 43, 685–8.
23. Krueger KA, Garnett WR, Comstock TJ, Fitzsimmons WE, Karnes HT, Pellock JM. Effect of two administration schedules of an enteral nutrient formula on phenytoin bioavailability. *Epilepsia* (1987) 28, 706–12.
24. Fleisher D, Sheth N, Kou JH. Phenytoin interaction with enteral feedings administered through nasogastric tubes. *J Parenter Enteral Nutr* (1990) 14, 513–16.
25. Gilbert S. How to minimize interaction between phenytoin and enteral feedings: two approaches. A Strategic approach. *Nutr Clin Pract* (1996) 11, 28–30.
26. Faraji B, Yu P-P. Serum phenytoin levels of patients on gastrostomy tube feeding. *J Neurosci Nurs* (1998) 30, 55–9.
27. Hatton J, Magnuson B. How to minimize interaction between phenytoin and enteral feedings: two approaches. B Therapeutic options. *Nutr Clin Pract* (1996) 11, 30–1.

Phenytoin + H_2-receptor antagonists

Phenytoin levels are raised by the use of cimetidine and toxicity has occurred. Limited evidence suggests that low doses of cimetidine may not interact. Very rarely bone marrow depression develops on concurrent use. Famotidine, nizatidine and ranitidine do not normally interact with phenytoin, although, rarely, cases of elevated phenytoin levels have been reported.

Clinical evidence

(a) Cimetidine

The serum phenytoin levels of 9 patients rose by 60% (from 5.7 micrograms/mL to 9.1 micrograms/mL) when they were given cimetidine 200 mg three times daily and 400 mg at night for 3 weeks. The serum phenytoin level returned to its former levels within 2 weeks of stopping the cimetidine.[1]

This interaction has been described in many reports and studies involving patients[2-7] and healthy subjects.[8-11] Phenytoin toxicity has developed in some individuals. The extent of the rise in serum levels is very variable being quoted as 13 to 33% over about 6 days in one report[2] and 22 to 280% over 3 weeks in others.[4,12] There is some evidence that the effect may be dependent on the dose of cimetidine. One study found that the effect of cimetidine 2.4 g daily was greater than that of 1.2 g daily or 400 mg daily; the effect of the lower two doses did not differ from each other.[9] In another study, cimetidine 200 mg twice daily for 2 weeks had no effect on serum phenytoin levels in 9 patients taking stable doses of phenytoin.[13]

Severe and life-threatening agranulocytosis in 2 patients[14,15] and thrombocytopenia in 6 other patients[16-18] has been attributed to the concurrent use of phenytoin and cimetidine. Severe skin reactions have also been reported in 3 patients taking phenytoin, cimetidine, and dexamethasone after resection of brain tumours, which resolved on discontinuing phenytoin.[19]

(b) Famotidine

A study in 10 subjects found that famotidine 40 mg daily for 7 days did not alter the pharmacokinetics of a single dose of phenytoin.[20] However, a single case report describes phenytoin toxicity and an almost doubled serum level (increase from 18 to 33 micrograms/mL) in a patient given famotidine. This was managed by a reduction in the phenytoin dose.[21]

(c) Nizatidine

In a study in 18 healthy subjects, nizatidine 150 mg twice daily for 9 doses had no effects on the pharmacokinetics of a single dose of phenytoin.[22]

(d) Ranitidine

A study in 4 patients found that ranitidine 150 mg twice daily for 2 weeks did not alter phenytoin levels.[4,12] Similarly, a double-blind, crossover study in healthy subjects found that ranitidine 150 mg twice daily for 6 days had no significant effect on steady-state phenytoin levels.[23] However, one patient had a 40% increase in serum phenytoin levels over a month when ranitidine 150 mg twice daily was given,[24] and two others also developed elevated serum phenytoin levels and signs of toxicity, which were attributed to the use of ranitidine.[25,26] Another patient developed a severe skin reaction when treated with phenytoin, ranitidine and dexamethasone after resection of a brain tumour, which resolved on discontinuing phenytoin.[19]

Mechanism

Cimetidine inhibits the activity of the liver enzymes concerned with the metabolism of phenytoin, thus allowing it to accumulate in the body and, in some instances, to reach toxic concentrations. Famotidine, nizatidine and ranitidine normally do not affect these enzymes. Agranulocytosis and thrombocytopenia are relatively rare manifestations of bone marrow depression caused by both phenytoin and the H_2-receptor antagonists.

Importance and management

The interaction between phenytoin and cimetidine is well documented and clinically important. It is not possible to identify individuals who will show the greatest response, but those with serum levels at the top end of the therapeutic range are most at risk. Do not give cimetidine to patients already taking phenytoin unless the serum levels can be monitored and suitable phenytoin dose reductions made as necessary. The results from one small study suggest that low doses of cimetidine (such as those available without a prescription in the UK) may not interact.[13] As there are only rare cases of an interaction with phenytoin reported for famotidine, nizatidine, and ranitidine, extra monitoring beyond that usually carried out in patients receiving phenytoin does not appear to be warranted but be alert for signs of phenytoin toxicity (e.g. blurred vision, nystagmus, ataxia or drowsiness) when these H_2-receptor antagonists are first added to established treatment with phenytoin.

1. Neuvonen PJ, Tokola R, Kaste M. Cimetidine-phenytoin interaction: effect on serum phenytoin concentration and antipyrine test. *Eur J Clin Pharmacol* (1981) 21, 215–20.
2. Hetzel DJ, Bochner F, Hallpike JF, Shearman DJC, Hann CS. Cimetidine interaction with phenytoin. *BMJ* (1981) 282, 1512.
3. Algozzine GJ, Stewart RB, Springer PK. Decreased clearance of phenytoin with cimetidine. *Ann Intern Med* (1981) 95, 244–5.
4. Watts RW, Hetzel DJ, Bochner F, Hallpike JF, Hann CS, Shearman DJC. Lack of interaction between ranitidine and phenytoin. *Br J Clin Pharmacol* (1983) 15, 499–500.
5. Phillips P, Hansky J. Phenytoin toxicity secondary to cimetidine administration. *Med J Aust* (1984) 141, 602.
6. Griffin JW, May JR, DiPiro JT. Drug interactions: theory versus practice. *Am J Med* (1984) 77 (Suppl 5B), 85–9.
7. Salem RB, Breland BD, Mishra SK, Jordan JE. Effect of cimetidine on phenytoin serum levels. *Epilepsia* (1983) 24, 284–8.
8. Iteogu MO, Murphy JE, Shleifer N, Davis R. Effect of cimetidine on single-dose phenytoin kinetics. *Clin Pharm* (1983) 2, 302–4.
9. Bartle WR, Walker SE, Shapero T. Dose-dependent effect of cimetidine on phenytoin kinetics. *Clin Pharmacol Ther* (1983) 33, 649–55.
10. Frigo GM, Lecchini S, Caravaggi M, Gatti G, Tonini M, D'Angelo L, Perucca E, Crema A. Reduction of phenytoin clearance caused by cimetidine. *Eur J Clin Pharmacol* (1983) 25, 135–7.
11. Hsieh Y-Y, Huang J-D, Lai M-L, Lin M-S, Liu R-T, Wan EC-J. The complexity of cimetidine-phenytoin interaction. *Taiwan Yi Xue Hui Za Zhi* (1986) 85, 395–402.
12. Hetzel DJ, Watts RW, Bochner F, Shearman DJC. Ranitidine, unlike cimetidine, does not interact with phenytoin. *Aust N Z J Med* (1983) 13, 324.
13. Rafi JA, Frazier LM, Driscoll-Bannister SM, O'Hara KA, Garnett WR, Pugh CB. Effect of over-the-counter cimetidine on phenytoin concentrations in patients with seizures. *Ann Pharmacother* (1999) 33, 769–74.
14. Sazie E, Jaffe JP. Severe granulocytopenia with cimetidine and phenytoin. *Ann Intern Med* (1980) 93, 151–2.
15. Al-Kawas FH, Lenes BA, Sacher RA. Cimetidine and agranulocytosis. *Ann Intern Med* (1979) 90, 992–3.
16. Wong YY, Lichtor T, Brown FD. Severe thrombocytopenia associated with phenytoin and cimetidine therapy. *Surg Neurol* (1985) 23, 169–72.
17. Yue CP, Mann KS, Chan KH. Severe thrombocytopenia due to combined cimetidine and phenytoin therapy. *Neurosurgery* (1987) 20, 963–5.
18. Arbiser JL, Goldstein AM, Gordon D. Thrombocytopenia following administration of phenytoin, dexamethasone and cimetidine: a case report and a potential mechanism. *J Intern Med* (1993) 234, 91–4.
19. Cohen AD, Reichental E, Halevy S. Phenytoin-induced severe cutaneous drug reactions: suspected interactions with corticosteroids and H2-blockers. *Isr Med Assoc J* (1999) 1, 95–7.
20. Sambol NC, Upton RA, Chremos AN, Lin ET, Williams RL. A comparison of the influence of famotidine and cimetidine on phenytoin elimination and hepatic blood flow. *Br J Clin Pharmacol* (1989) 27, 83–7.
21. Shinn AF. Unrecognized drug interactions with famotidine and nizatidine. *Arch Intern Med* (1991) 151, 810, 814.
22. Bachmann KA, Sullivan TJ, Jauregui L, Reese JH, Miller K, Levine L. Absence of an inhibitory effect of omeprazole and nizatidine on phenytoin disposition, a marker of CYP2C activity. *Br J Clin Pharmacol* (1993) 36, 380–2.
23. Mukherjee S, Wicks JFC, Dixon JS, Richens A. Absence of a pharmacokinetic interaction between ranitidine and phenytoin. *Gastroenterology* (1996) 110 (Suppl), A202.
24. Bramhall D, Levine M. Possible interaction of ranitidine with phenytoin. *Drug Intell Clin Pharm* (1988) 22, 979–80.
25. Tse CST, Akinwande KI, Biallowons K. Phenytoin concentration elevation subsequent to ranitidine administration. *Ann Pharmacother* (1993) 27, 1448–51.
26. Tse CST, Iagmin P. Phenytoin and ranitidine interaction. *Ann Intern Med* (1994) 120, 892–3.

Phenytoin + Immunoglobulins

An isolated report describes a patient taking phenytoin who died, probably from hypersensitivity myocarditis, two days after receiving immunoglobulins for Guillain-Barré syndrome.

Clinical evidence, mechanism, importance and management

A man who had been taking phenytoin for 8 years was diagnosed as having Guillain-Barré syndrome for which intravenous immunoglobulin was started at 400 mg/kg daily. On day 2 the patient complained of abdominal pain, aching shoulders and backache. He subsequently developed hypotension and died, despite resuscitation attempts. A post-mortem suggested that he had died from hypersensitivity myocarditis, which the authors of the report suggest might have resulted from the long-term use of phenytoin.[1] This hypersensitivity with phenytoin has been reported before.[2] Because this complication is so serious, the authors of this report suggest that leukocyte counts, in particular eosinophils, should be monitored if immunoglobulins and phenytoin are given concurrently.[1] The general importance of this alleged interaction is not known. However, note that, subsequent to this report, intravenous immunoglobulin has successfully been used to treat a few cases of a hypersensitivity syndrome to phenytoin,[3-5] one including eosinophilia.[3] Furthermore, intravenous immunoglobulin alone has also been associated with causing myocarditis.[6] An interaction is therefore by no means established.

1. Koehler PJ, Koudstaal J. Lethal hypersensitivity myocarditis associated with the use of intravenous gammaglobulin for Guillain-Barré syndrome, in combination with phenytoin. *J Neurol* (1996) 243, 366–7.
2. Fenoglio JJ, McAllister HA, Mullick FG. Drug related myocarditis.I. Hypersensitivity myocarditis. *Hum Pathol* (1981) 12, 900–7.
3. Scheuerman O, Nofech-Moses Y, Rachmel A, Ashkenazi S. Successful treatment of antiepileptic drug hypersensitivity syndrome with intravenous immune globulin. *Pediatrics* (2001) 107, E14.
4. Salzman MB, Smith EM. Phenytoin-induced thrombocytopenia treated with intravenous immune globulin. *J Pediatr Hematol Oncol* (1998) 20, 152–3.
5. Mostella J, Pieroni R, Jones R, Finch CK. Anticonvulsant hypersensitivity syndrome: treatment with corticosteroids and intravenous immunoglobulin. *South Med J* (2004) 97, 319–21.
6. Akhtar I, Bastani B. Acute renal failure and myocarditis associated with intravenous immunoglobulin therapy. *Ann Intern Med* (2003) 139, W65.

Phenytoin + Influenza vaccines

Influenza vaccination is reported to increase, decrease or to have no effect on phenytoin serum levels. The efficacy of the vaccine remains unchanged.

Clinical evidence

The serum phenytoin levels of 8 children with epilepsy were increased by about 50% (from 9.5 to 15.16 micrograms/mL) 7 days after they were given 0.5 mL of an influenza virus vaccine USP, types A and B, whole virus (Squibb). The phenytoin levels returned to baseline over the following 7 days.[1] Temporary rises in the serum phenytoin levels of 3 patients, apparently caused by influenza vaccination, are briefly described in another report.[2]

In contrast, another study in 16 patients given 0.5 mL of an inactivated whole-virion trivalent influenza vaccine found that 7 and 14 days later their mean serum phenytoin levels were not significantly altered, although 4 of them showed a trend towards raised levels. Subsequently, these 4 patients had serum phenytoin increases ranging from 46 to 170%, which returned to baseline between week 4 and 17 after immunisation.[3]

In yet another study, within 4 days of receiving 0.5 mL of a subvirion, trivalent influenza vaccine, the serum phenytoin levels of 7 patients were reduced by 11 to 14%, which is unlikely to have much clinical significance.[4] A further study[5] measured both free and total phenytoin levels in 8 patients receiving phenytoin. Two days after receiving 0.5 mL of a trivalent influenza vaccine, the total phenytoin level had increased by 10%, and this then returned to baseline levels by day 7. However, the free phenytoin level gradually decreased after vaccination, reaching a maximum decrease of 25% below baseline at day 14.

The efficacy of influenza vaccine is reported to be unchanged by phenytoin.[6]

Mechanism

Where an interaction occurs it is suggested that it may be due to the inhibitory effect of the vaccine on the liver enzymes concerned with the metabolism of the phenytoin, resulting in a reduced clearance from the body.[1]

Importance and management

The outcome of immunisation with influenza vaccine on phenytoin levels is uncertain. Concurrent use need not be avoided but it would be prudent to monitor the effects closely. Be aware that any alteration in levels may take a couple of weeks to develop and usually resolves spontaneously.

1. Jann MW, Fidone GS. Effect of influenza vaccine on serum anticonvulsant concentrations. *Clin Pharm* (1986) 5, 817–20.
2. Mooradian AD, Hernandez L, Tamai IC, Marshall C. Variability of serum phenytoin concentrations in nursing home patients. *Arch Intern Med* (1989) 149, 890–2.
3. Levine M, Jones MW, Gribble M. Increased serum phenytoin concentration following influenza vaccination. *Clin Pharm* (1984) 3, 505–9.
4. Sawchuk RJ, Rector TS, Fordice JJ, Leppik IE. Case report. Effect of influenza vaccination on plasma phenytoin concentrations. *Ther Drug Monit* (1979) 1, 285–8.
5. Smith CD, Bledsoe MA, Curran R, Green L, Lewis J. Effect of influenza vaccine on serum concentrations of total and free phenytoin. *Clin Pharm* (1988) 7, 828–32.
6. Levine M, Beattie BL, McLean DM, Corman D. Phenytoin therapy and immune response to influenza vaccine. *Clin Pharm* (1985) 4, 191–4.

Phenytoin + Isotretinoin

A study in 7 healthy subjects taking phenytoin 300 mg daily found that the addition of isotretinoin 40 mg twice daily for 11 days had no effect on the steady-state pharmacokinetics of phenytoin.[1] No phenytoin dose adjustments would seem to be needed if these drugs are given concurrently.

1. Oo C, Barsanti F, Zhang R. Lack of effect of isotretinoin on the pharmacokinetics of phenytoin at steady-state. *Pharm Res* (1997) 14 (11 Suppl), S-561.

Phenytoin + Loxapine

A single case report describes decreased serum phenytoin levels in a patient given loxapine.

Clinical evidence, mechanism, importance and management

The serum phenytoin levels of a patient with epilepsy were reduced by loxapine: when loxapine was withdrawn, the phenytoin levels rose markedly.[1] The general importance of this case is uncertain, but bear this interaction in mind, particularly as loxapine can lower the convulsive threshold.

1. Ryan GM, Matthews PA. Phenytoin metabolism stimulated by loxapine. *Drug Intell Clin Pharm* (1977) 11, 428.

Phenytoin + Macrolides

Erythromycin appears not to interact with phenytoin. Limited evidence suggests that clarithromycin may possibly raise phenytoin levels. Phenytoin is predicted to reduce telithromycin levels.

Clinical evidence

(a) Clarithromycin

A retrospective study of serum phenytoin levels in a group of 21 patients with AIDS and a large control group of 557 subjects suggested that the concurrent use of clarithromycin (a total of 22 samples from at least 10 patients) was associated with higher serum phenytoin levels. The concentration-to-dose ratio of the phenytoin was 1.6 without clarithromycin and 3.9 with clarithromycin.[1]

(b) Erythromycin

A single-dose study in 8 healthy subjects found that the mean clearance of phenytoin was unchanged by erythromycin 333 mg every 8 hours for 7 days. However, there were occasional large changes in phenytoin clearance.[2] Similarly, in another study in 8 healthy subjects, erythromycin 250 mg every 6 hours for 7 days had no effect on the pharmacokinetics of a single dose of phenytoin.[3]

Mechanism

Not known, but it could be that clarithromycin inhibits the metabolism of phenytoin by the liver.

Importance and management

This seems to be the first and only evidence that clarithromycin possibly interacts like this. Given that the effect was identified retrospectively any interaction seems unlikely to cause an acute problem. Erythromycin appears not to interact with phenytoin, but nevertheless caution has been recommended,[2] because of the occasional large changes in clearance that were seen.

Other macrolides appear not to have been studied. However, based on an interaction with the known enzyme inducer rifampicin (rifampin) (see 'Macrolides + Rifamycins', p.332), the manufacturers of **telithromycin** predict that its levels will be reduced by phenytoin, possibly making them sub-therapeutic. They advise avoiding telithromycin use during and for up to 2 weeks after phenytoin has been taken.[4]

1. Burger DM, Meenhorst PL, Mulder JW, Kraaijeveld CL, Koks CHW, Bult A, Beijnen JH. Therapeutic drug monitoring of phenytoin in patients with the acquired immunodeficiency syndrome. *Ther Drug Monit* (1994) 16, 616–20.
2. Bachmann K, Schwartz JI, Forney RB, Jauregui L. Single dose phenytoin clearance during erythromycin treatment. *Res Commun Chem Pathol Pharmacol* (1984) 46, 207–17.
3. Milne RW, Coulthard K, Nation RL, Penna AC, Roberts G, Sansom LN. Lack of effect of erythromycin on the pharmacokinetics of single oral doses of phenytoin. *Br J Clin Pharmacol* (1988) 26, 330–3.
4. Ketek (Telithromycin). Sanofi. UK Summary of product characteristics, November 2012.

Phenytoin + Methylphenidate

Although two small studies found that methylphenidate did not alter phenytoin levels, case reports describe raised phenytoin levels and phenytoin toxicity in patients also given methylphenidate.

Clinical evidence

A 5-year-old hyperkinetic boy with epilepsy taking phenytoin 8.9 mg/kg and **primidone** 17.7 mg/kg daily, developed ataxia without nystagmus when he was also given methylphenidate 40 mg daily. Serum levels of both of the antiepileptics were found to be toxic and only began to fall when the methylphenidate dose was reduced.[1] A further case also describes phenytoin toxicity in a child given methylphenidate.[2]

Only one other case has been reported, but this patient was later re-challenged with the two drugs and phenytoin toxicity was not seen.[3] Furthermore, this interaction has not been seen in clinical studies and observations in 3 healthy subjects[3] and more than 11 patients[4] taking phenytoin and methylphenidate.

Mechanism

Not fully understood. The suggestion is that methylphenidate acts as an enzyme inhibitor, slowing the metabolism of the phenytoin by the liver and leading to its accumulation in those individuals whose drug metabolising system is virtually saturated by phenytoin.

Importance and management

These appear to be the only reports of a possible interaction between phenytoin and methylphenidate, and an interaction is not established. The concurrent use of both drugs need not be avoided but be alert for any evidence of toxicity, particularly if the phenytoin dose is high. It would seem prudent to consider the possibility of an interaction if phenytoin toxicity (e.g. blurred vision, nystagmus, ataxia or drowsiness) develops, and take levels if necessary. The effect on primidone (and therefore **phenobarbital**, to which it is metabolised) is unclear as it seems possible that the raised primidone levels described in the case may have been a result of the rise in phenytoin levels (see 'Primidone + Phenytoin', p.611).

The manufacturer of **dexmethylphenidate**, the d-isomer of methylphenidate, notes the potential interaction between methylphenidate and phenytoin, primidone or phenobarbital, and notes that dose reductions of the antiepileptic may be required.[5]

Although they make no direct recommendation for the use of these antiepileptics with **dexmethylphenidate**, until more is known, it may be prudent to follow the same precautions given for methylphenidate.

1. Garrettson LK, Perel JM, Dayton PG. Methylphenidate interaction with both anticonvulsants and ethyl biscoumacetate. A new action of methylphenidate. *JAMA* (1969) 207, 2053–6.
2. Ghofrani M. Possible phenytoin-methylphenidate interaction. *Dev Med Child Neurol* (1988) 30, 267–8.
3. Mirkin BL, Wright F. Drug interactions: effect of methylphenidate on the disposition of diphenylhydantoin in man. *Neurology* (1971) 21, 1123–8.
4. Kupferberg HJ, Jeffery W, Hunninghake DB. Effect of methylphenidate on plasma anticonvulsant levels. *Clin Pharmacol Ther* (1972) 13, 201–4.
5. Focalin XR (Dexmethylphenidate hydrochloride). Novartis. US Prescribing information, December 2013.

Phenytoin + Metronidazole

One study found that the half-life of intravenous phenytoin was modestly prolonged by metronidazole, whereas another found that metronidazole did not affect the pharmacokinetics of oral phenytoin. An anecdotal report describes a few patients who developed toxic phenytoin levels when given metronidazole.

Clinical evidence, mechanism, importance and management

A pharmacokinetic study in 7 healthy subjects found that metronidazole 250 mg three times daily increased the half-life of a single 300-mg intravenous dose of phenytoin by about 40% (from 16 to 23 hours) and reduced its clearance by 15%.[1] In contrast, another study in 5 healthy subjects found that the pharmacokinetics of a single 300-mg oral dose of phenytoin were unaffected by metronidazole 400 mg twice daily for 6 days.[2] An anecdotal report describes several patients (exact number not stated) who developed toxic phenytoin serum levels when given metronidazole.[3] These appear to be the only reports of this potential interaction, and the reason for their discordant findings is not clear. It seems that few patients are likely to experience a clinically significant interaction.

1. Blyden GT, Scavone JM, Greenblatt DJ. Metronidazole impairs clearance of phenytoin but not of alprazolam or lorazepam. *J Clin Pharmacol* (1988) 28, 240–5.
2. Jensen JC, Gugler R. Interaction between metronidazole and drugs eliminated by oxidative metabolism. *Clin Pharmacol Ther* (1985) 37, 407–10.
3. Picard EH. Side effects of metronidazole. *Mayo Clin Proc* (1983) 58, 401.

Phenytoin + Nefazodone

Nefazodone did not affect the pharmacokinetics of phenytoin in healthy subjects.

Clinical evidence, mechanism, importance and management

Nefazodone 200 mg twice daily for 7 days had no effect on the pharmacokinetics of a single 300-mg dose of phenytoin in healthy subjects, and no changes in vital signs, ECGs or other physical measurements were seen. There was no evidence that a clinically significant interaction was likely.[1]

1. Marino MR, Langenbacher KM, Hammett JL, Nichola P, Uderman HD. The effect of nefazodone on the single-dose pharmacokinetics of phenytoin in healthy male subjects. *J Clin Psychopharmacol* (1997) 17, 27–33.

Phenytoin + Nitrofurantoin

An isolated report describes a reduction in phenytoin levels and poor seizure control in a patient given nitrofurantoin.

Clinical evidence, mechanism, importance and management

A man with seizures due to a brain tumour was taking phenytoin 300 mg daily. He had a seizure within one day of starting nitrofurantoin 200 mg daily for a urinary-tract infection and, despite a recent increase in the phenytoin dose to 350 mg, his serum phenytoin levels were found to be modestly reduced (from about 9 to 7.6 micrograms/mL). They continued to fall, and were 6.3 micrograms/mL despite a further increase in the phenytoin dose to 400 mg daily. When the nitrofurantoin was stopped the patient was restabilised on his original dose of phenytoin. The reasons for this effect are not understood but, on the basis of a noted rise in serum gamma glutamyltransferase levels during the use of the nitrofurantoin, the authors speculate that it increased the metabolism of the phenytoin by the liver.[1] The general importance of this interaction is uncertain, but probably small.

1. Heipertz R, Pilz H. Interaction of nitrofurantoin with diphenylhydantoin. *J Neurol* (1978) 218, 297–301.

Phenytoin + Orlistat

Orlistat does not alter the pharmacokinetics of phenytoin.

Clinical evidence, mechanism, importance and management

In a placebo-controlled, randomised study, 12 healthy subjects were given orlistat 120 mg three times daily for 7 days, with a single 300-mg dose of phenytoin on day 4. The pharmacokinetics of phenytoin were unchanged by orlistat,[1] and no phenytoin dose adjustments are therefore thought to be needed if these two drugs are given concurrently.

1. Melia AT, Mulligan TE, Zhi J. The effect of orlistat on the pharmacokinetics of phenytoin in healthy volunteers. *J Clin Pharmacol* (1996) 36, 654–8.

Phenytoin + Penicillins

An isolated case describes a marked reduction in serum phenytoin levels, resulting in seizures, which was attributed to the use of oxacillin.

Clinical evidence, mechanism, importance and management

An woman with epilepsy taking phenytoin 400 mg daily, hospitalised for second degree burns sustained during a generalised seizure, experienced brief clonic seizures and was found to have an marked reduction in her serum phenytoin levels, from 16.3 micrograms/mL to 3.5 micrograms/mL, which was attributed to the concurrent use of oral **oxacillin** 500 mg every 6 hours. The phenytoin dose was increased, but seizures continued and progressed to status epilepticus, and intravenous phenytoin was given. Doses of oral phenytoin of about 600 mg daily were required to maintain minimum therapeutic levels, sometimes with supplementation of small intravenous doses. Just before the **oxacillin** was withdrawn the serum phenytoin level was 22.3 micrograms/mL, but 6 months later it had risen to 39.9 micrograms/mL, and the phenytoin dose was reduced.[1] Other studies have shown that penicillins such as **oxacillin**, **cloxacillin** and **dicloxacillin** can displace phenytoin from plasma protein binding, decreasing total serum levels but increasing the free fraction of phenytoin. If anything, this would be predicted to increase phenytoin toxicity,[2,3] rather than decrease its levels, as seen in the case. This seems to be only report of an adverse interaction between phenytoin and a penicillin. Its general importance is probably small.

1. Fincham RW, Wiley DE, Schottelius DD. Use of phenytoin levels in a case of status epilepticus. *Neurology* (1976) 26, 879–81.
2. Arimori K, Nakano M, Otagiri M, Uekama K. Effects of penicillins on binding of phenytoin to plasma proteins *in vitro* and *in vivo*. *Biopharm Drug Dispos* (1984) 5, 219–27.
3. Dasgupta A, Sperelakis A, Mason A, Dean R. Phenytoin-oxacillin interactions in normal and uremic sera. *Pharmacotherapy* (1997) 17, 375–8.

Phenytoin + Pheneturide

Phenytoin levels can be increased by about 50% by pheneturide.

Clinical evidence, mechanism, importance and management

In 9 patients, the steady-state half-life of phenytoin was prolonged from 32 hours to 47 hours by pheneturide. Mean serum levels were raised by about 50% but fell rapidly over the 2 weeks after pheneturide was withdrawn.[1] This study confirms a previous report of this interaction.[2] However, the reason for this interaction is uncertain, but as the two drugs have a similar structure it is possible that they compete for the same metabolising enzymes in the liver, thereby resulting, at least initially, in a reduction in the metabolism of the phenytoin. If concurrent use is undertaken the outcome should be well monitored. Reduce the phenytoin dose as necessary.

1. Houghton GW, Richens A. Inhibition of phenytoin metabolism by other drugs used in epilepsy. *Int J Clin Pharmacol Biopharm* (1975) 12, 210–16.
2. Hulsman JW, van Heycop Ten Ham MW and van Zijl CHW. Influence of ethylphenacemide on serum levels of other anticonvulsant drugs. *Epilepsia* (1970) 11, 207.

Phenytoin + Phenobarbital

The concurrent use of phenytoin and phenobarbital is normally advantageous and uneventful. Changes in phenytoin levels (often decreases but sometimes increases) can occur if phenobarbital is added, but seizure control is not usually affected. Phenytoin toxicity following phenobarbital withdrawal has been seen. Increased phenobarbital levels and possibly toxicity may result if phenytoin is given to patients taking phenobarbital.

Clinical evidence

A study in 10 patients with epilepsy taking phenytoin 2.8 to 6.8 mg/kg daily found that while taking phenobarbital 1.1 to 2.5 mg/kg daily their serum phenytoin levels were reduced. Five patients had a mean reduction of about 65% (from 15.7 to 5.7 micrograms/mL). In most cases phenytoin levels rose when phenobarbital was withdrawn. In one patient this was so rapid and steep that he developed ataxia and a cerebellar syndrome with phenytoin levels of up to 60 micrograms/mL, despite a reduction in the phenytoin dose.[1]

This reduction in phenytoin levels by phenobarbital has been described in other reports.[2-7] Some of these reports also described a very transient and small rise[4] or no alteration[4,5] in serum phenytoin levels in individual patients. Three other studies have found that phenobarbital does not alter phenytoin levels.[8-10]

Elevated serum phenobarbital levels occurred in children with epilepsy when they were also given phenytoin. In 5 patients the phenobarbital levels were approximately doubled. In some cases mild ataxia was seen but the relatively high barbiturate levels were well tolerated.[1] A long-term study in 6 adults with epilepsy found that when phenytoin was added to phenobarbital, the level-to-dose ratio of phenobarbital gradually rose by about 60% over one year, and then gradually fell again over the next 2 years.[11] This suggests that initially, phenytoin reduces phenobarbital metabolism.

In a patient taking phenobarbital 100 mg and phenytoin 160 mg daily, the serum levels of phenobarbital increased by about 53% within about 2 days when the dose of phenytoin was increased to 490 mg daily.[12]

Mechanism

Phenobarbital can have a dual effect on phenytoin metabolism: it may cause enzyme induction, which results in a more rapid clearance of the phenytoin from the body, or with large doses it may inhibit metabolism by competing for enzyme systems. The total effect will depend on the balance between the two drugs. The reason for the elevation of serum phenobarbital levels is not fully understood, but the extent of the effect may be dependent on the serum level of phenytoin.[12,13]

Importance and management

Concurrent use can be therapeutically valuable. Changes in dose or the addition or withdrawal of either drug needs to be monitored to ensure that toxicity does not occur, or that seizure control is not worsened. The contradictory reports cited here do not provide a clear picture of what is likely to happen. Consider also 'Primidone + Phenytoin', p.611.

1. Morselli PL, Rizzo M, Garattini S. Interaction between phenobarbital and diphenylhydantoin in animals and in epileptic patients. *Ann N Y Acad Sci* (1971) 179, 88–107.
2. Cucinell SA, Conney AH, Sansur M, Burns JJ. Drug interactions in man. I. Lowering effect of phenobarbital on plasma levels of bishydroxycoumarin (Dicumarol) and diphenylhydantoin (Dilantin). *Clin Pharmacol Ther* (1965) 6, 420–9.
3. Buchanan RA, Heffelfinger JC, Weiss CF. The effect of phenobarbital on diphenylhydantoin metabolism in children. *Pediatrics* (1969) 43, 114–16.
4. Kutt H, Haynes J, Verebely K, McDowell F. The effect of phenobarbital on plasma diphenylhydantoin level and metabolism in man and rat liver microsomes. *Neurology* (1969) 19, 611–16.
5. Garrettson LK, Dayton PG. Disappearance of phenobarbital and diphenylhydantoin from serum of children. *Clin Pharmacol Ther* (1970) 11, 674–9.
6. Abarbanel J, Herishanu Y, Rosenberg P, Eylath U. In vivo interaction of anticonvulsant drugs. *J Neurol* (1978) 218, 137–44.
7. Kristensen M, Hansen JM, Skovsted L. The influence of phenobarbital on the half-life of diphenylhydantoin in man. *Acta Med Scand* (1969) 185, 347–50.
8. Diamond WD, Buchanan RA. A clinical study of the effect of phenobarbital on diphenylhydantoin plasma levels. *J Clin Pharmacol* (1970) 10, 306–11.
9. Booker HE, Tormey A, Toussaint J. Concurrent administration of phenobarbital and diphenylhydantoin: lack of an interference effect. *Neurology* (1971) 21, 383–5.
10. Browne TR, Szabo GK, Evans J, Evans BA, Greenblatt DJ, Mikati MA. Phenobarbital does not alter phenytoin steady-state serum concentration or pharmacokinetics. *Neurology* (1988) 38, 639–42.
11. Encinas MP, Santos Buelga D, Alonso González AC, García Sánchez MJ, Domínguez-Gil Hurlé A. Influence of length of treatment on the interaction between phenobarbital and phenytoin. *J Clin Pharm Ther* (1992) 17, 49–50.
12. Kuranari M, Tatsukawa H, Seike M, Saikawa T, Ashikari Y, Kodama Y, Sakata T, Takeyama M. Effect of phenytoin on phenobarbital pharmacokinetics in a patient with epilepsy. *Ann Pharmacother* (1995) 29, 83–4.
13. Lambie DG, Johnson RH. The effects of phenytoin on phenobarbitone and primidone metabolism. *J Neurol Neurosurg Psychiatry* (1981) 44, 148–51.

Phenytoin + Phenothiazines

Phenytoin levels can be raised or lowered by the use of chlorpromazine, prochlorperazine or thioridazine. Phenytoin may reduce levels of the active metabolite of thioridazine.

Clinical evidence

(a) Chlorpromazine

The serum phenytoin levels of a patient taking phenytoin, primidone and sultiame doubled after chlorpromazine 50 mg daily was taken for a month.[1] However, another 4 patients taking chlorpromazine 50 to 100 mg daily showed no interaction.[1] In another report, one out of 3 patients taking phenytoin and phenobarbital had a fall in their serum phenytoin levels when they were also given chlorpromazine.[2] A further very brief report states that in rare instances chlorpromazine has been noted to impair phenytoin metabolism.[3]

In a large study in patients taking phenytoin with various phenothiazines (chlorpromazine, **thioridazine** or **mesoridazine**), phenytoin levels were decreased by 44% when the phenothiazines were started, and decreased by 33% when the phenothiazine dose was increased. A number of patients experienced an increased frequency of seizures. In patients who had these phenothiazines discontinued or the dose *decreased*, the phenytoin levels increased by 55% and 71%, respectively, and toxic levels occurred in some patients.[4]

(b) Prochlorperazine

A single very brief report states that in rare instances prochlorperazine has been noted to impair phenytoin metabolism.[3]

(c) Thioridazine

One out of 6 patients taking phenytoin and phenobarbital had a marked rise in serum phenytoin levels when thioridazine was added, whereas 4 others had a fall in phenytoin levels.[2] Phenytoin toxicity has also been described in 2 patients after about 2 weeks of the concurrent use of thioridazine.[5] A retrospective study in 27 patients taking phenytoin found that when they were given thioridazine their serum phenytoin levels were increased by at least 4 micrograms/mL (4 patients), decreased by at least 4 micrograms/mL (2 patients), or were unchanged (21 patients).[6] Another retrospective study comparing 28 patients taking both phenytoin and thioridazine with patients taking either drug alone found no evidence that thioridazine increased the risk of phenytoin toxicity.[7] A further study found no changes in serum phenytoin or thioridazine levels in patients given both drugs, but the serum levels of mesoridazine (the active metabolite of thioridazine) were reduced, suggesting that higher doses of thioridazine may be necessary to achieve the same effect.[8] See also the study[4] in section (a), which found a decrease in phenytoin levels and an increase in seizure frequency when patients took phenothiazines including thioridazine.

Mechanism

Uncertain. Phenothiazines such as thioridazine are said to be inhibitors of the cytochrome P450 isoenzyme CYP2D6, and as such would not be expected to affect phenytoin metabolism, at least by this mechanism.

Importance and management

A confusing situation as the results are inconsistent. The concurrent use of phenytoin and these phenothiazines need not be avoided, but it would be prudent to watch for any signs of changes in serum phenytoin levels that would affect antiepileptic control. It is also worth remembering that phenothiazines may decrease the seizure threshold. In one study a trend towards increased seizure frequency was noted after phenothiazines were added, or doses increased.[4] Also note that phenytoin may reduce levels of some phenothiazines. Whether all phenothiazines interact similarly is uncertain.

1. Houghton GW, Richens A. Inhibition of phenytoin metabolism by other drugs used in epilepsy. *Int J Clin Pharmacol Biopharm* (1975) 12, 210–16.
2. Siris JH, Pippenger CE, Werner WL, Masland RL. Anticonvulsant drug-serum levels in psychiatric patients with seizure disorders. Effects of certain psychotropic drugs. *N Y State J Med* (1974) 74, 1554–6.
3. Kutt H, McDowell F. Management of epilepsy with diphenylhydantoin sodium. Dosage regulation for problem patients. *JAMA* (1968) 203, 969–72.
4. Haidukewych D, Rodin EA. Effect of phenothiazines on serum antiepileptic drug concentrations in psychiatric patients with seizure disorder. *Ther Drug Monit* (1985) 7, 401–4.
5. Vincent FM. Phenothiazine-induced phenytoin intoxication. *Ann Intern Med* (1980) 93, 56–7.
6. Sands CD, Robinson JD, Salem RB, Stewart RB, Muniz C. Effect of thioridazine on phenytoin serum concentration: a retrospective study. *Drug Intell Clin Pharm* (1987) 21, 267–72.
7. Gotz VP, Yost RL, Lamadrid ME, Buchanan CD. Evaluation of a potential interaction: thioridazine-phenytoin — negative findings. *Hosp Pharm* (1984) 19, 555–7.
8. Linnoila M, Viukari M, Vaisanen K, Auvinen J. Effect of anticonvulsants on plasma haloperidol and thioridazine levels. *Am J Psychiatry* (1980) 137, 819–21.

Phenytoin + Proton pump inhibitors

Studies have found that omeprazole either does not affect phenytoin levels, or may raise phenytoin levels: the differences may be due to the different doses and subjects involved in these studies. A study with esomeprazole suggests it may cause a minor rise in phenytoin levels. Lansoprazole does not normally affect phenytoin levels, but an isolated case report of toxicity is tentatively attributed to an interaction. Pantoprazole and rabeprazole appear not to affect the pharmacokinetics of phenytoin.

Clinical evidence

(a) Esomeprazole

The manufacturer of esomeprazole reports that, in patients with epilepsy, esomeprazole 40 mg increases the trough plasma levels of phenytoin by 13%.[1]

(b) Lansoprazole

In a group of 12 healthy subjects lansoprazole 60 mg daily for 7 days caused only a very small and clinically irrelevant rise (less than 3%) in the AUC of a single intravenous dose of phenytoin.[2,3] In contrast the manufacturer has received an isolated report of the development of blurred vision, diarrhoea, muscle pain, dizziness, abdominal pain, salivary hypersecretion, increased sweating and incoordination in a man taking phenytoin, which occurred within a day of stopping sustained-release propranolol 80 mg and starting lansoprazole.[4] The phenytoin serum levels were not measured but the symptoms might possibly have been due to phenytoin toxicity, although it should be said that if an interaction with lansoprazole was responsible, it developed unusually quickly.

(c) Omeprazole

In 8 patients with epilepsy, omeprazole 20 mg daily for 3 weeks caused no changes in the mean steady-state serum phenytoin levels.[5] Four patients had unchanged levels, 2 had falls and 2 had rises, but none of them was adversely affected by the use of omeprazole.[5]

In 10 healthy subjects, omeprazole 40 mg daily for 7 days increased the AUC of a single 300-mg dose of phenytoin by 25%.[6] In another study the clearance of a 250-mg intravenous dose of phenytoin was reduced by 15% by omeprazole 40 mg given for 7 days.[7] A further study found that 3 doses of omeprazole 40 mg had no effect on the pharmacokinetics of a single dose of phenytoin.[8]

(d) Pantoprazole

A randomised, crossover study in 23 healthy subjects found that pantoprazole 40 mg daily for 7 days did not alter the pharmacokinetics (AUC, maximum serum levels, half-life) of a single 300-mg dose of phenytoin.[9] This study has also been published elsewhere.[10]

(e) Rabeprazole

A preliminary report, which gives no details, states that when rabeprazole was used with phenytoin, no significant changes in the pharmacokinetics of phenytoin were seen.[11]

Mechanism

Not understood. A possible explanation is that if the dose of omeprazole is high enough, it may possibly reduce the metabolism of phenytoin by CYP2C19. Esomeprazole may have similar effects. However, CYP2C19 has only a minor role in phenytoin metabolism,[12] and so the effects are usually small. With lansoprazole, the overall picture is that it does not act as an enzyme inducer or inhibitor[13] (or it is only very weak) so that it would not be expected to interact with phenytoin to a clinically relevant extent (confirmed by the study cited above[2]). The same appears to be true for pantoprazole and rabeprazole.

Importance and management

Information is very limited but it seems that omeprazole 20 mg daily does not affect serum phenytoin levels, whereas 40 mg daily may possibly cause a slight increase, although this is probably of no clinical relevance in most patients. However, multiple dose studies are ideally needed to confirm this. No special precautions would normally seem necessary if lansoprazole or omeprazole is given with phenytoin.

The manufacturers of esomeprazole suggest that the concurrent use of phenytoin should be monitored,[1] although the elevation in levels seen in the study would almost certainly not be clinically significant. No special precautions would seem to be necessary if rabeprazole or pantoprazole and phenytoin are given concurrently.

1. Nexium Tablets (Esomeprazole magnesium trihydrate). AstraZeneca UK Ltd. UK Summary of product characteristics, August 2013.
2. Karol MD, Mukherji D, Cavanaugh JH. Lack of effect of concomitant multi-dose lansoprazole on single-dose phenytoin pharmacokinetics in subjects. *Gastroenterology* (1994) 106, A103.
3. Karol MD, Locke CS, Cavanaugh JH. Lack of a pharmacokinetic interaction between lansoprazole and intravenously administered phenytoin. *J Clin Pharmacol* (1999) 39, 1283–9.
4. Wyeth, personal communication, January 1998.
5. Andersson T, Lagerström P-O, Unge P. A study of the interaction between omeprazole and phenytoin in epileptic patients. *Ther Drug Monit* (1990) 12, 329–33.
6. Prichard PJ, Walt RP, Kitchingman GK, Somerville KW, Langman MJS, Williams J, Richens A. Oral phenytoin pharmacokinetics during omeprazole therapy. *Br J Clin Pharmacol* (1987) 24, 543–5.
7. Gugler R, Jensen JC. Omeprazole inhibits oxidative drug metabolism. Studies with diazepam and phenytoin in vivo and 7-ethoxycoumarin in vitro. *Gastroenterology* (1985) 89, 1235–41.
8. Bachmann KA, Sullivan TJ, Jauregui L, Reese JH, Miller K, Levine L. Absence of an inhibitory effect of omeprazole and nizatidine on phenytoin disposition, a marker of CYP2C activity. *Br J Clin Pharmacol* (1993) 36, 380–2.
9. Middle MV, Müller FO, Schall R, Groenewoud G, Hundt HKL, Huber R, Bliesath H, Steinijans VW. No influence of pantoprazole on the pharmacokinetics of phenytoin. *Int J Clin Pharmacol Ther* (1995) 33, 304–7.
10. Middle MV, Müller FO, Schall R, Groenewoud G, Hundt HKL, Huber R, Bliesath H, Steinijans VW. No influence of pantoprazole on the pharmacokinetics of phenytoin. *Int J Clin Pharmacol Ther* (1996) 34 (Suppl 1), S72–S75.
11. Humphries TJ, Nardi RV, Lazar JD, Spanyers SA. Drug-drug interaction evaluation of rabeprazole sodium: a clean/expected slate? *Gut* (1996) 39 (Suppl 3), A47.
12. Giancarlo GM, Venkatakrishnan K, Granda BW, von Moltke LL, Greenblatt DJ. Relative contributions of CYP2C9 and 2C19 to phenytoin 4-hydroxylation in vitro: inhibition by sulfaphenazole, omeprazole, and ticlopidine. *Eur J Clin Pharmacol* (2001) 57, 31–36.
13. Cavanaugh JH, Park YK, Awni WM, Mukherjee DX, Karol MD, Granneman GR. Effect of lansoprazole on antipyrine and ICG pharmacokinetics. *Gastroenterology* (1991) 100, A40.

Phenytoin + *Shankhapushpi* (SRC)

A case report, and an *animal* study, indicate that an antiepileptic Ayurvedic herbal preparation, *Shankhapushpi* (*SRC*), can markedly reduce phenytoin levels, leading to an increased seizure frequency.

Clinical evidence

An man with epilepsy taking **phenobarbital** 120 mg daily and **phenytoin** 500 mg daily developed an increase in seizure frequency when *Shankhapushpi* (*SRC*) three times daily was given. His plasma **phenytoin** levels were found to have fallen from 18.2 micrograms/mL to 9.3 micrograms/mL, whereas his **phenobarbital** levels were little changed. When the *SRC* was stopped the **phenytoin** plasma levels rose to 30.3 micrograms/mL, and toxicity was seen. A reduction in the dose of **phenytoin** to 400 mg daily resulted in levels of 16.2 micrograms/mL. Another possible case of this interaction has also been reported.[1,2]

Subsequent studies in *rats* found that *SRC* reduces the plasma levels of **phenytoin** by about half.[3] These pharmacokinetic effects were only seen after multiple doses, not single doses of **phenytoin**. A pharmacodynamic interaction, resulting in reduced antiepileptic activity was also noted.[1,3,4]

Mechanism

Not understood. There is evidence from *animal* studies that *SRC* may affect the pharmacokinetics of the phenytoin and possibly its pharmacodynamics as well,[1,3] thereby reducing its antiepileptic activity. It is also suggested that one of the ingredients of *SRC* may have some antiepileptic activity.[3]

Importance and management

Information about this interaction appears to be limited to these reports. *Shankhapushpi* (*SRC*) is given because it has some antiepileptic activity (demonstrated in *animal* studies[3,4]), but there is little point in combining it with phenytoin if the outcome is a fall in plasma phenytoin levels, accompanied by an increase in seizure frequency. For this reason concurrent use should be avoided. *SRC* is a syrup prepared from *Convolvulus pluricaulis* leaves, *Nardostachys jatamansi* rhizomes, *Onosma bracteatum* leaves and flowers and the whole plant of *Centella asiatica*, *Nepeta hindostana* and *Nepeta elliptica*.[3] The first two of these plants appear to contain compounds with antiepileptic activity.[5]

It has been suggested that adulteration of traditional medicines with various antiepileptics[6,7] may be an unexpected factor in these interactions.

1. Kshirsagar NA, Personal communication 1991.
2. Kshirsagar NA, Dalvi SS, Joshi MV, Sharma SS, Sant HM, Shah PU, Chandra RS. Phenytoin and ayurvedic preparation – clinically important interaction in epileptic patients. *J Assoc Physicians India* (1992) 40, 354–5.
3. Dandekar UP, Chandra RS, Dalvi SS, Joshi MV, Gokhale PC, Sharma AV, Shah PU, Kshirsagar NA. Analysis of a clinically important interaction between phenytoin and Shankhapushpi, an Ayurvedic preparation. *J Ethnopharmacol* (1992) 35, 285–8.
4. Kshirsagar NA, Chandra RS, Dandekar UP, Dalvi SS, Sharma AV, Joshi MV, Gokhale PC, Shah PU. Investigation of a novel clinically important interaction between phenytoin and ayurvedic preparation. *Eur J Pharmacol* (1990) 183, 519.
5. Sharma VN, Barar FSK, Khanna NK, Mahawar MM. Some pharmacological actions of *Convolvulus pluricaulis* chois: an Indian indigenous herb. *Indian J Med Res* (1965) 53, 871–6.
6. Bharucha NE. Co-prescription of conventional and 'alternative' medicines. *J R Coll Physicians Lond* (1999) 33, 285.
7. Gogtay NJ, Dalvi SS, Rane CT, Pawar HS, Narayana RV, Shah PU, Kshirsagar NA. A story of "ayurvedic" tablets and misled epileptic patients. *J Assoc Physicians India* (1999) 47, 1116.

Phenytoin + SSRIs

Phenytoin levels can be increased in some patients by fluoxetine and toxicity may occur. There are also isolated reports of phenytoin toxicity in patients taking fluvoxamine. Phenytoin and sertraline do not normally interact, but rarely patients have developed increased phenytoin levels.

Sertraline and possibly paroxetine levels may be reduced by phenytoin.

Clinical evidence

(a) Fluoxetine

A woman taking phenytoin 370 mg, diazepam 4 mg, and clonazepam 6 mg daily was given fluoxetine 20 mg for depression. Five days later her serum phenytoin levels had risen from 18 micrograms/mL to 26.5 micrograms/mL, and a further 9 days later to 30 micrograms/mL, accompanied by signs of toxicity (tremor, headache, abnormal thinking, increased partial seizure activity). Seven days after stopping the phenytoin the serum levels had fallen to 22 micrograms/mL.[1]

Two other patients, taking phenytoin 300 and 400 mg daily, respectively, had marked rises in serum phenytoin levels (from 15 to 35 micrograms/mL and from 11.5 to 47 micrograms/mL), accompanied by signs of phenytoin toxicity, within 5 to 10 days of starting fluoxetine 20 or 40 mg daily. The problem resolved when the fluoxetine was stopped or the phenytoin dose reduced.[2] Another patient only developed this interaction after taking fluoxetine for about 9 months.[3] Another case describes raised phenytoin levels with improved efficacy when fluoxetine was started, and reduced levels and possible loss of efficacy when fluoxetine was stopped.[4]

A review initiated by the FDA in the US and the manufacturers of fluoxetine briefly describes another 23 anecdotal observations of suspected interactions between phenytoin and fluoxetine (most of them incompletely documented). These suggest that a 50% increase in serum phenytoin levels, with accompanying toxicity, can occur within 1 to 42 days (mean onset time of 2 weeks) after starting fluoxetine.[5] Conversely, a retrospective review of 7 patients taking phenytoin and fluoxetine found no cases of an interaction.[6]

(b) Fluvoxamine

About one month after starting to take fluvoxamine 50 mg daily, a woman taking phenytoin 300 mg daily experienced ataxia and was found to have a threefold increase in her phenytoin levels (from 16.6 to 49.1 micrograms/mL). Fluvoxamine was subsequently discontinued, and the phenytoin dose reduced, with gradual recovery.[7] Another report describes phenytoin toxicity (serum levels of 48 micrograms/mL) in an 86-year-old woman after she took fluvoxamine 100 to 200 mg daily for 10 days.[8] However the fluvoxamine was started only 2 days after phenytoin 200 mg twice daily had been started, and the serum phenytoin levels were not checked until the toxicity had actually developed. Both drugs were then stopped and the phenytoin later successfully reinstated without the fluvoxamine. A worldwide analysis of data up to 1995 by the manufacturers of fluvoxamine identified only 2 reported cases of interactions (clinical symptoms only) between phenytoin and fluvoxamine.[9]

(c) Paroxetine

In a group of patients with epilepsy, paroxetine 30 mg daily for 16 days caused no changes in the plasma levels or therapeutic effects of phenytoin. Steady-state paroxetine plasma levels were lower in those also taking phenytoin (16 nanograms/mL) than in those taking valproate (73 nanograms/mL).[10]

The US manufacturer of paroxetine notes that phenytoin 300 mg daily for 14 days decreased the AUC and half-life of a single 30-mg dose of paroxetine by 50% and 35%, respectively. In another study, paroxetine 30 mg daily for 14 days had minimal effects on a single 300-mg dose of phenytoin (AUC reduced by 12%).[11]

(d) Sertraline

A randomised, placebo-controlled study in 30 healthy subjects taking phenytoin 100 mg three times daily, found that sertraline 50 to 200 mg daily did not affect the steady-state trough serum levels of phenytoin, nor was there any evidence that concurrent use impaired cognitive function.[12] However, another report describes 2 elderly patients whose serum phenytoin levels rose when they were given sertraline, but there was no evidence of toxicity. One of them had an almost fourfold rise in serum phenytoin levels whereas the other had a rise of only about one-third.[13]

In an analysis of plasma sertraline levels the concentration to daily dose ratio of sertraline was significantly lower in patients who had taken sertraline with phenytoin compared with those who had taken sertraline without phenytoin,[14] which suggested that phenytoin increases sertraline metabolism

Mechanism

An *in vitro* investigation found that fluoxetine and fluvoxamine inhibited the metabolism of phenytoin by the cytochrome P450 isoenzyme CYP2C9 in human liver tissue.[15] This would presumably lead to a rise in serum phenytoin levels. In this study, sertraline was a weaker inhibitor of CYP2C9, and was considered less likely to interact with phenytoin.[15] A similar study also suggested that the risk of interaction was greatest for fluoxetine, and less likely with sertraline and paroxetine.[16] Sertraline plasma levels may be reduced because of enzyme induction by phenytoin which would increase its metabolism and clearance from the body.[14]

Importance and management

The interaction between phenytoin and fluoxetine appears to be established but its incidence is not known. Because of the unpredictable nature of this interaction, if fluoxetine is added to treatment with phenytoin in any patient, be alert for the need to reduce the phenytoin dose. Ideally the phenytoin serum levels should be monitored. Similarly, to be on the safe side phenytoin levels should be monitored when fluvoxamine is first added to treatment with phenytoin so that any patient affected can be quickly identified. Although an interaction with sertraline appears less likely, be alert for any evidence of an increase in phenytoin adverse effects (e.g. blurred vision, nystagmus, ataxia or drowsiness) if sertraline is given. The clinical relevance of the reduction in paroxetine levels caused by phenytoin is unknown, but it would seem prudent to be alert for a reduction in the effects of paroxetine, and increase its dose as necessary. More study of these interactions is needed.

Note that SSRIs should be avoided in patients with unstable epilepsy, and the use of SSRIs in those with controlled epilepsy should be carefully monitored, because of the potential increased seizure risk.

1. Woods DJ, Coulter DM, Pillans P. Interaction of phenytoin and fluoxetine. *N Z Med J* (1994) 107, 19.
2. Jalil P. Toxic reaction following the combined administration of fluoxetine and phenytoin: two case reports. *J Neurol Neurosurg Psychiatry* (1992) 55, 412–13.
3. Darley J. Interaction between phenytoin and fluoxetine. *Seizure* (1994) 3, 151–2.
4. Shad MU, Preskorn SH. Drug-drug interaction in reverse: possible loss of phenytoin efficacy as a result of fluoxetine discontinuation. *J Clin Psychopharmacol* (1999) 19, 471–2.
5. Shader RI, Greenblatt DJ, von Moltke LL. Fluoxetine inhibition of phenytoin metabolism. *J Clin Psychopharmacol* (1994) 14, 375–6.
6. Bécares J, Puente M, De Juana P, García B, Bermego T. Fluoxetina y fenitoína: interacción o interpretación errónea de los niveles séricos? *Farm Clin* (1997) 14, 474–8.
7. Mamiya K, Kojima K, Yukawa E, Higuchi S, Ieiri I, Ninomiya H, Tashiro N. Case report. Phenytoin intoxication induced by fluvoxamine. *Ther Drug Monit* (2001) 23, 75–7.
8. Feldman D, Claudel B, Feldman F, Allilaire JF, Thuillier A. Cas clinique d'interaction médicamenteuse entre phénytoïne et fluvoxamine. *J Pharm Clin* (1995) 14, 296–7.
9. Wagner W, Vause EW. Fluvoxamine. A review of global drug-drug interaction data. *Clin Pharmacokinet* (1995) 29 (Suppl 1), 26–32.
10. Andersen BB, Mikkelsen M, Versterager A, Dam M, Kristensen HB, Pedersen B, Lund J, Mengel H. No influence of the antidepressant paroxetine on carbamazepine, valproate and phenytoin. *Epilepsy Res* (1991) 10, 201–4.
11. Paxil Tablets and Suspension (Paroxetine hydrochloride). GlaxoSmithKline. US Prescribing information, December 2012.
12. Rapeport WG, Muirhead DC, Williams SA, Cross M, Wesnes K. Absence of effect of sertraline on the pharmacokinetics and pharmacodynamics of phenytoin. *J Clin Psychiatry* (1996) 57 (Suppl 1), 24–8.
13. Haselberger MB, Freedman LS, Tolbert S. Elevated serum phenytoin concentrations associated with coadministration of sertraline. *J Clin Psychopharmacol* (1997) 17, 107–9.
14. Pihlsgård M, Eliasson E. Significant reduction of sertraline plasma levels by carbamazepine and phenytoin. *Eur J Clin Pharmacol* (2002) 57, 915–6.
15. Schmider J, Greenblatt DJ, von Moltke LL, Karsov D, Shader RI. Inhibition of CYP2C9 by selective serotonin reuptake inhibitors *in vitro*: studies of phenytoin *p*-hydroxylation. *Br J Clin Pharmacol* (1997) 44, 495–8.
16. Nelson MH, Birnbaum AK, Remmel RP. Inhibition of phenytoin hydroxylation in human liver microsomes by several selective serotonin re-uptake inhibitors. *Epilepsy Res* (2001) 44, 71–82.

Phenytoin + Sucralfate

The absorption of single-dose phenytoin can be modestly reduced by sucralfate, but this effect was not seen in a multiple-dose study.

Clinical evidence

In 8 healthy subjects, sucralfate 1 g was found to reduce the absorption (measured over a 24-hour period) of a single 300-mg dose of phenytoin by 20%.[1] Peak serum phenytoin levels were also reduced, but this was not statistically significant. Another single-dose study found a mean reduction in phenytoin absorption of up to 9.5%.[2] In a study in 6 healthy subjects, sucralfate 1 g four times daily for 7 days had no effect on the steady-state levels of phenytoin 5 to 7 mg/kg daily. The fourth daily dose of sucralfate was taken simultaneously with the daily phenytoin dose at bedtime. After 7 days, all phenytoin levels were within 15% of the baseline values (range, 6% decrease to 15% increase).[3]

Mechanism

Uncertain. Reduced bioavailability has been demonstrated in a single-dose study in *dogs* when the drugs were given simultaneously, and this did not occur if the phenytoin was given 2 hours after the sucralfate.[4]

Importance and management

Information about an interaction between sucralfate and phenytoin is limited. The reduction in phenytoin absorption found in single-dose studies was quite small, and was not seen in a multiple-dose study, suggesting it is unlikely to be clinically relevant.

1. Smart HL, Somerville KW, Williams J, Richens A, Langman MJS. The effects of sucralfate upon phenytoin absorption in man. *Br J Clin Pharmacol* (1985) 20, 238–40.
2. Hall TG, Cuddy PG, Glass CJ, Melethil S. Effect of sucralfate on phenytoin bioavailability. *Drug Intell Clin Pharm* (1986) 20, 607–11.
3. Malli R, Jones WN, Rindone JP, Labadie EL. The effect of sucralfate on the steady-state serum concentrations of phenytoin. *Drug Metabol Drug Interact* (1989) 7, 287–93.
4. Lacz JP, Groschang AG, Giesing DH, Browne RK. The effect of sucralfate on drug absorption in dogs. *Gastroenterology* (1982) 82, 1108.

Phenytoin + Sulfinpyrazone

Phenytoin levels may be markedly increased by sulfinpyrazone.

Clinical evidence

A review of the drug interactions of sulfinpyrazone identified two studies that found interactions with phenytoin.[1] In the first, the serum phenytoin levels of 2 out of 5 patients taking phenytoin 250 to 350 mg daily were doubled (from about 10 micrograms/mL to 20 micrograms/mL) within 11 days of starting to take sulfinpyrazone 800 mg daily. One of the remaining patients had a small increase in phenytoin levels, but the other two had no changes at all. When the sulfinpyrazone was withdrawn, the serum phenytoin concentrations fell to their former levels. The second study was a clinical study in patients with epilepsy, which found that sulfinpyrazone 800 mg daily for a week increased the phenytoin half-life from 10 hours to 16.5 hours and reduced the metabolic clearance by 46% (from 59 mL/minute to 32 mL/minute).

Mechanism

Uncertain. It seems probable that sulfinpyrazone inhibits the metabolism of phenytoin by the liver, thereby allowing it to accumulate in the body and leading to a rise in its serum levels. Displacement of phenytoin from its plasma protein binding sites may also have a small part to play.

Importance and management

Information seems to be limited to these studies. A similar interaction with phenytoin has been reported with phenylbutazone, which has a very close chemical relationship with sulfinpyrazone. Thus, what is known suggests that concurrent use should be monitored and suitable phenytoin dose reductions made if necessary.

1. Pedersen AK, Jacobsen P, Kampmann JP, Hansen JM. Clinical pharmacokinetics and potentially important drug interactions of sulphinpyrazone. *Clin Pharmacokinet* (1982) 7, 42–56.

Phenytoin + Sulfonamides and/or Trimethoprim

Phenytoin concentrations can be increased by co-trimoxazole, sulfamethizole, sulfadiazine, and trimethoprim. Phenytoin toxicity might develop in some cases. A single case of liver failure has been described in a patient taking phenytoin with co-trimoxazole. Sulfamethoxypyridazine and sulfadimethoxine are reported not to interact with phenytoin.

Clinical evidence

(a) Co-trimoxazole or Trimethoprim

A pharmacokinetic study found that co-trimoxazole 1.92 g (trimethoprim 320 mg with sulfamethoxazole 1.6 g) and trimethoprim 320 mg daily for one week increased the half-life of a single intravenous dose of phenytoin by 39% and 51%, respectively, and decreased the metabolic clearance of phenytoin by 27% and 30%, respectively.[1] Sulfamethoxazole alone had only a small effect on the half-life of phenytoin, and did not affect its clearance.[1] In 3 patients taking phenytoin 300 mg daily, the addition of co-trimoxazole for a week increased the mean steady-state serum phenytoin concentration from 9.7 to 14 micrograms/mL.[1]

Two case reports have described phenytoin toxicity with co-trimoxazole. In one, a patient taking phenytoin 400 mg daily developed signs of toxicity (ataxia, nystagmus, loss of balance) within 2 weeks of starting to take co-trimoxazole 960 mg twice daily. His serum concentrations were found to have increased to about 38 micrograms/mL (reference range 10 to 20 micrograms/mL).[2] In a second case, a child who was stable taking phenytoin and sultiame developed phenytoin toxicity within 48 hours of starting co-trimoxazole. Toxicity resolved when the antibacterial was changed to amoxicillin.[3]

In a nested case-control study in patients older than 66 years taking phenytoin continuously, the risk of hospitalisation for phenytoin toxicity was approximately doubled in those who had received a prescription for co-trimoxazole in the 30 days before hospitalisation (odds ratio 2.11). The risk was not increased by amoxicillin.[4]

An additional case report describes fatal acute hepatic failure in a 60-year-old woman 10 days after she started taking co-trimoxazole and 14 days after she started taking phenytoin.[5] This patient was also given cimetidine, which might increase phenytoin concentrations, see 'Phenytoin + H_2-receptor antagonists', p.602.

(b) Sulfadiazine

In a study in 8 patients, sulfadiazine 4 g daily for a week increased the half-life of a single intravenous dose of phenytoin by 80%. The mean metabolic clearance of phenytoin decreased by 45%.[1] In one patient taking phenytoin 300 mg daily, the addition of sulfadiazine for a week increased the mean steady-state serum phenytoin concentration from 15 to 22 micrograms/mL.[1]

(c) Sulfamethizole

The development of phenytoin toxicity in a patient taking sulfamethizole prompted a study of this interaction in 8 patients. After the concurrent use of phenytoin and sulfamethizole 1 g four times daily for 7 days, the phenytoin half-life increased from 11.8 hours to 19.6 hours. Of the 4 patients receiving long-term treatment with phenytoin, 3 had increases in their serum phenytoin concentrations from 22 micrograms/mL to 33 micrograms/mL, from 19 micrograms/mL to 23 micrograms/mL and from 4 micrograms/mL to 7 micrograms/mL, respectively. The phenytoin concentrations of the fourth patient were not affected.[6,7] In another analysis in 4 patients taking phenytoin 300 mg daily, the addition of sulfamethizole for a week increased the mean steady-state serum phenytoin concentration from 15 micrograms/mL to 19.5 micrograms/mL.[1]

In a study in 8 subjects, the half-life of a single intravenous dose of phenytoin was increased, and its mean metabolic clearance reduced by 36%, by sulfamethizole 4 g daily for a week.[1]

(d) Other sulfonamides

Pretreatment for one week with **sulfamethoxypyridazine** or **sulfadimethoxine** did not alter the pharmacokinetics of a single intravenous dose of phenytoin.[1] Similarly, in patients taking phenytoin 300 mg daily, the addition of sulfamethoxypyridazine (1 patient) or sulfadimethoxine (3 patients) for a week did not alter mean steady-state serum phenytoin concentrations.[1]

Mechanism

The sulfonamides that interact appear to do so by inhibiting the metabolism of phenytoin by the liver (probably by CYP2C9)[8]. The mechanism for the interaction with trimethoprim is unknown. Depletion of glucuronic acid by phenytoin might have increased the hepatotoxicity of co-trimoxazole.[5]

Importance and management

The documentation seems to be limited to the reports cited, but the interaction is established. Co-trimoxazole, sulfamethizole, sulfadiazine, and trimethoprim can increase serum phenytoin concentrations. The interaction probably occurs in most patients, but the small number of adverse reaction reports suggests that the risk of toxicity is small. It is clearly most likely in those with serum phenytoin concentrations at the top end of the range. If concurrent use is thought appropriate, serum phenytoin concentrations should be closely monitored and the phenytoin dose reduced if necessary. Alternatively, if appropriate, use a non-interacting antibacterial (in some circumstances penicillins (see 'Phenytoin + Penicillins', p.604) or macrolides (see 'Phenytoin + Macrolides', p.603) might be appropriate). There seems to be little information about other sulfonamides. Limited data suggests that sulfamethoxypyridazine or sulfadimethoxine might not interact, but until more is known it would seem prudent to be alert for this interaction with any of them.

1. Hansen JM, Kampmann JP, Siersbæk-Nielsen K, Lumholtz B, Arrøe M, Abildgaard U, Skovsted L. The effect of different sulfonamides on phenytoin metabolism in man. *Acta Med Scand* (1979) (Suppl 624), 106–10.
2. Wilcox JB. Phenytoin intoxication and co-trimoxazole. *N Z Med J* (1981) 94, 235–6.
3. Gillman MA, Sandyk R. Phenytoin toxicity and co-trimoxazole. *Ann Intern Med* (1985) 102, 559.
4. Antoniou T, Gomes T, Mamdani MM, Juurlink DN. Trimethoprim/sulfamethoxazole-induced phenytoin toxicity in the elderly: a population-based study. *Br J Clin Pharmacol* (2011) 71, 544–9.
5. Ilario MJ-M, Ruiz JE, Axiotis CA. Acute fulminant hepatic failure in a woman treated with phenytoin and trimethoprim-sulfamethoxazole. *Arch Pathol Lab Med* (2000) 124, 1800–3.
6. Lumholtz B, Siersbaek-Nielsen K, Skovsted L, Kampmann J, Hansen JM. Sulfamethizole-induced inhibition of diphenylhydantoin, tolbutamide and warfarin metabolism. *Clin Pharmacol Ther* (1975) 17, 731–4.
7. Siersbaek-Nielsen K, Hansen JM, Skovsted L, Lumholtz B, Kampmann J. Sulphamethizole-induced inhibition of diphenylhydantoin and tolbutamide metabolism in man. *Clin Pharmacol Ther* (1973) 14, 148.
8. Giancarlo GM, Venkatakrishnan K, Granda BW, von Moltke LL, Greenblatt DJ. Relative contributions of CYP2C9 and 2C19 to phenytoin 4-hydroxylation in vitro: inhibition by sulfaphenazole, omeprazole, and ticlopidine. *Eur J Clin Pharmacol* (2001) 57, 31–36.

Phenytoin + Sultiame

Serum phenytoin levels can be approximately doubled by sultiame and phenytoin toxicity may occur.

Clinical evidence

The serum phenytoin levels in 6 out of 7 patients with epilepsy approximately doubled within about 5 to 25 days of starting to take sultiame 400 mg daily. All experienced an increase in adverse effects and definite phenytoin toxicity occurred in 2 patients. In most of the patients, phenytoin serum levels fell back to baseline over the 2 months following the withdrawal of sultiame.[1] All of the patients were also taking **phenobarbital** and although greater variations in serum **phenobarbital** levels were seen, they were not considered to be clinically significant.[1]

A number of other reports confirm this interaction,[2-8] some of which describe the development of phenytoin toxicity.

Mechanism

The evidence suggests that sultiame interferes with the metabolism of the phenytoin by the liver, leading to its accumulation in the body.

Importance and management

A reasonably well-documented, established and clinically important interaction. The incidence seems to be high. If sultiame is added to established treatment with phenytoin, increases in serum phenytoin levels of up to 75% or more may be expected.[3,7] Phenytoin serum levels should be closely monitored and appropriate dose reductions made to prevent the development of toxicity. The changes in phenobarbital levels appear to be unimportant.

1. Olesen OV, Jensen ON, Drug-interaction between sulthiame (Ospolot (R)) and phenytoin in the treatment of epilepsy. *Dan Med Bull* (1969) 16, 154–8.
2. Houghton GW, Richens A. Inhibition of phenytoin metabolism by sulthiame. *Br J Pharmacol* (1973) 49, 157P–158P.
3. Houghton GW, Richens A. Inhibition of phenytoin metabolism by sulthiame in epileptic patients. *Br J Clin Pharmacol* (1974) 1, 59–66.
4. Richens A, Houghton GW. Phenytoin intoxication caused by sulthiame. *Lancet* (1973) ii, 1442–3.
5. Houghton GW, Richens A. Inhibition of phenytoin metabolism by other drugs used in epilepsy. *Int J Clin Pharmacol Biopharm* (1975) 12, 210–16.
6. Frantzen E, Hansen JM, Hansen OE, Kristensen M. Phenytoin (Dilantin®) intoxication. *Acta Neurol Scand* (1967) 43, 440–6.
7. Houghton GW, Richens A. Phenytoin intoxication induced by sulthiame in epileptic patients. *J Neurol Neurosurg Psychiatry* (1974) 37, 275–81.
8. Hansen JM, Kristensen M, Skovsted L. Sulthiame (Ospolot®) as inhibitor of diphenylhydantoin metabolism. *Epilepsia* (1968) 9, 17–22.

Phenytoin + Tamoxifen

Some preliminary evidence suggests that high-dose tamoxifen can increase phenytoin levels, causing toxicity. Phenytoin may lower tamoxifen levels.

Clinical evidence, mechanism, importance and management

A man who had undergone an operation 10 years previously for a brain tumour and had since remained seizure-free while taking phenytoin 200 mg twice daily began to have breakthrough seizures. It was established that his brain tumour had recurred and so tamoxifen was started as experimental treatment. The dose of tamoxifen was slowly titrated to 200 mg daily over a 6-week period. He continued to receive phenytoin and was also given **carbamazepine** as his seizures were not controlled, but when the maximum dose of tamoxifen (200 mg daily) was reached he began to develop symptoms of phenytoin toxicity with a serum level of 28 micrograms/mL. The toxicity disappeared and the phenytoin levels decreased when the phenytoin dose was reduced. The **carbamazepine** serum levels remained unchanged throughout.[1] The authors of this report say that other patients similarly treated with tamoxifen also developed phenytoin toxicity, which disappeared when the phenytoin dose was reduced by 15 to 20%.

Another study of the pharmacokinetics of high-dose tamoxifen in patients with brain tumours found that the mean tamoxifen levels in 15 patients taking phenytoin were about 60% lower than in patients not taking phenytoin, although this did not reach statistical significance due to high inter-patient variability.[2]

The reasons for these possible interactions are not known. The evidence for this interaction is very slim indeed and it may possibly only occur with high-dose tamoxifen. Consider monitoring phenytoin levels if high-dose tamoxifen is added and monitor the efficacy of the tamoxifen. More study is needed to establish an interaction.

1. Rabinowicz AL, Hinton DR, Dyck P, Couldwell WT. High-dose tamoxifen in treatment of brain tumors: interaction with antiepileptic drugs. *Epilepsia* (1995) 36, 513–15.
2. Ducharme J, Fried K, Shenouda G, Leyland-Jones B, Wainer IW. Tamoxifen metabolic patterns within a glioma patient population treated with high-dose tamoxifen. *Br J Clin Pharmacol* (1997) 43: 189–93.

Phenytoin + Ticlopidine

Ticlopidine reduces the metabolism of phenytoin. A number of case reports describe patients who developed phenytoin toxicity when ticlopidine was also taken.

Clinical evidence

A 65-year-old man taking phenytoin 200 mg daily and clobazam developed signs of phenytoin toxicity (vertigo, ataxia, somnolence) within a week of starting ticlopidine 250 mg daily. His serum phenytoin levels had risen from 18 mg/L to 34 mg/L. When the phenytoin dose was reduced to 200 mg daily the toxic symptoms disappeared within a few days and his serum phenytoin levels fell to 18 mg/L. To test whether an interaction had occurred, ticlopidine was stopped, whereupon the serum phenytoin levels fell, within about 3 weeks, to 8 mg/L, during which time the patient experienced his first seizure in 2 years. When ticlopidine was restarted, his serum phenytoin levels rose again, and within a month had reached 19 mg/L.[1] A number of other case reports describe phenytoin toxicity, which occurred within 2 to 6 weeks of starting ticlopidine 250 mg once or twice daily.[2-7] These were usually managed by reducing the phenytoin dose. One patient then experienced breakthrough seizures after the ticlopidine was stopped without re-adjusting the phenytoin dose.[6] One case in a patient also taking **phenobarbital** reported that no change in **phenobarbital** levels occurred.[4]

A study in 6 patients taking phenytoin found that ticlopidine 250 mg twice daily approximately halved the steady-state phenytoin clearance.[8]

Mechanism

The metabolism of phenytoin to 5-(4-hydroxyphenyl)-5-phenylhydantoin (HPPH) by the cytochrome P450 isoenzyme CYP2C19, and to a lesser extent by CYP2C9, in the liver is inhibited by ticlopidine.[1,3,4,9] Further metabolism of HPPH to dihydroxylated products is mediated mainly by CYP2C19 and this may also be inhibited by ticlopidine.[9]

Importance and management

The interaction is established and clinically important, but its incidence is unknown. It would seem prudent to monitor for phenytoin adverse effects (blurred vision, nystagmus, ataxia or drowsiness) and consider monitoring phenytoin levels in any patient if ticlopidine is added to established treatment, being alert for the need to reduce the phenytoin dose. If ticlopidine is discontinued, the phenytoin dose may need to be increased.

1. Riva R, Cerullo A, Albani F, Baruzzi A. Ticlopidine impairs phenytoin clearance: a case report. *Neurology* (1996) 46, 1172–3.
2. Rindone JP, Bryan G. Phenytoin toxicity associated with ticlopidine administration. *Arch Intern Med* (1996) 156, 1113.
3. Privitera M, Welty TE. Acute phenytoin toxicity followed by seizure breakthrough from a ticlopidine-phenytoin interaction. *Arch Neurol* (1996) 53, 1191–2.
4. Donahue SR, Flockhart DA, Abernethy DR, Ko J-W. Ticlopidine inhibition of phenytoin metabolism mediated by potent inhibition of CYP2C19. *Clin Pharmacol Ther* (1997) 62, 572–7.
5. López-Ariztegui N, Ochoa M, Sánchez-Migallón, Nevado C, Martín M, Intoxicación aguda por fenitoina secundaria a interacción con ticlopidina. *Rev Neurol* (1998) 26, 1017–18.
6. Klaassen SL. Ticlopidine-induced phenytoin toxicity. *Ann Pharmacother* (1998) 32, 1295–8.
7. Dahm AEA, Brørs O. Fenytoinforgiftning forårsaket av interaksjon med tiklopidin. *Tidsskr Nor Laegeforen* (2002) 122, 278–80.
8. Donahue S, Flockhart DA, Abernethy DR. Ticlopidine inhibits phenytoin clearance. *Clin Pharmacol Ther* (1999) 66, 563–8.
9. Giancarlo GM, Venkatakrishnan K, Granda BW, von Moltke LL, Greenblatt DJ. Relative contributions of CYP2C9 and 2C19 to phenytoin 4-hydroxylation in vitro: inhibition by sulfaphenazole, omeprazole, and ticlopidine. *Eur J Clin Pharmacol* (2001) 57, 31–36.

Phenytoin + Tizanidine

An isolated report describes a modest increase in serum phenytoin levels in a patient also taking tizanidine.

Clinical evidence, mechanism, importance and management

An isolated report describes a 59-year-old man whose phenytoin levels rose by one-third, from about 19 micrograms/mL to 25.5 micrograms/mL, and who experienced drowsiness within a week of starting to take tizanidine 6 mg daily. The phenytoin was stopped for 3 days and restarted at a reduced dose, but the drowsiness recurred in 3 weeks (phenytoin level 20.5 micrograms/mL). Therefore, the tizanidine was withdrawn.[1] The general importance of this interaction is unclear, but it would seem prudent to remain aware of this interaction in case of otherwise unexplained phenytoin adverse effects.

1. Ueno K, Miyai K, Mitsuzane K. Phenytoin-tizanidine interaction. *DICP Ann Pharmacother* (1991) 25, 1273.

Phenytoin + Trazodone

An isolated case report describes phenytoin toxicity in a patient given trazodone.

Clinical evidence, mechanism, importance and management

A patient taking phenytoin 300 mg daily developed progressive signs of phenytoin toxicity after taking trazodone 500 mg daily for 4 months. His serum phenytoin levels had risen from 17.8 micrograms/mL to 46 micrograms/mL.[1] Therapeutic phenytoin serum levels were restored by reducing the phenytoin dose to 200 mg daily and the trazodone dose to 400 mg daily. The reasons for this apparent interaction are not understood, and this appears to be the only reported case of an interaction. No general conclusions can be drawn.

1. Dorn JM. A case of phenytoin toxicity possibly precipitated by trazodone. *J Clin Psychiatry* (1986) 47, 89–90.

Phenytoin + Tricyclic antidepressants

Evidence from two patients suggests that imipramine can raise serum phenytoin levels, but nortriptyline and amitriptyline appear not to do so. Phenytoin possibly reduces serum desipramine levels.

Clinical evidence

(a) Phenytoin levels

The serum phenytoin levels of 2 patients rose over a 3-month period when they were given **imipramine** 75 mg daily. One patient had an increase in phenytoin levels from about 7.6 micrograms/mL to 15 micrograms/mL and developed mild toxicity (drowsiness and uncoordination). These signs disappeared and the phenytoin serum levels of both patients fell when **imipramine** was withdrawn. One of them was also taking nitrazepam and clonazepam, and the other was also taking sodium valproate and carbamazepine, but both patients were stable on these combinations before the addition of **imipramine**.[1]

Other studies have found that **nortriptyline** 75 mg daily had an insignificant effect on the serum phenytoin levels of 5 patients,[2] and that **amitriptyline** had no effect on the elimination of phenytoin in 3 subjects.[3]

(b) Tricyclic antidepressant levels

A report describes 2 patients who had low serum **desipramine** levels, despite taking standard doses, while they were also taking phenytoin.[4]

Mechanism

One suggestion is that imipramine inhibits the metabolism of phenytoin by the liver, which results in its accumulation in the body. An *in vitro* study[5] has shown that the tricyclics can inhibit the cytochrome P450 isoenzyme CYP2C19, but this isoenzyme usually has only a minor role in phenytoin metabolism (see 'Antiepileptics', p.561). The reduced desipramine levels may be a result of enzyme induction by phenytoin.

Importance and management

The documentation is very limited indeed and none of these interactions is adequately established. The results of the *in vitro* study suggest that the interaction may only assume importance in those subjects that are deficient in CYP2C9, the enzyme usually responsible for phenytoin metabolism.[5] The tricyclic antidepressants as a group lower the seizure threshold, which suggests that extra care should be taken if deciding to use them in patients with epilepsy. If concurrent use is undertaken the effects should be very well monitored.

1. Perucca E, Richens A. Interaction between phenytoin and imipramine. *Br J Clin Pharmacol* (1977) 4, 485–6.
2. Houghton GW, Richens A. Inhibition of phenytoin metabolism by other drugs used in epilepsy. *Int J Clin Pharmacol Biopharm* (1975) 12, 210–16.
3. Pond SM, Graham GG, Birkett DJ, Wade DN. Effects of tricyclic antidepressants on drug metabolism. *Clin Pharmacol Ther* (1975) 18, 191–9.
4. Fogel BS, Haltzman S. Desipramine and phenytoin: a potential drug interaction of therapeutic relevance. *J Clin Psychiatry* (1987) 48, 387–8.
5. Shin J-G, Park J-Y, Kim M-J, Shon J-H, Yoon Y-R, Cha I-J, Lee S-S, Oh S-W, Kim S-W, Flockhart DA. Inhibitory effects of tricyclic antidepressants (TCAs) on human cytochrome P450 enzymes in vitro: mechanism of drug interaction between TCAs and phenytoin. *Drug Metab Dispos* (2002) 30, 1102–7.

Phenytoin + Valproate

The concurrent use of phenytoin and valproate is common and usually uneventful. Initially total phenytoin levels may fall but this is offset by a rise in the levels of free (and active) phenytoin, which may very occasionally cause some toxicity. After continued use the total phenytoin levels rise, and there might be sustained increases in free phenytoin levels. There is also some very limited evidence to suggest that concurrent use possibly increases the incidence of valproate hepatotoxicity.

Clinical evidence

(a) Phenytoin levels

A number of reports clearly show that the total serum levels of phenytoin fall during the early concurrent use of valproate, while the concentrations of free phenytoin rise.[1-5] In one report it was noted that within 4 to 7 days the total serum phenytoin levels had fallen from 19.4 micrograms/mL to 14.6 micrograms/mL.[1] A study extending over a year in 8 patients taking phenytoin and valproate found that by the end of 8 weeks the total serum phenytoin levels of 6 of them had fallen by almost as much as 50%, but had returned to their original levels in all but one patient by the end of the year.[6] Similar results were found in another study.[7] However, in a further study, some patients had a sustained increase in the free fraction of phenytoin.[4] Another regression analysis showed that valproate increased the free fraction of phenytoin.[8] The occasional patient may have symptoms of phenytoin toxicity.[9] Delirium and an increased seizure frequency were seen in one patient taking valproic acid with phenytoin.[10]

(b) Valproate levels

Studies have found that valproate levels are reduced by the presence of phenytoin.[11,12] Another study reported that valproate levels were increased by 30 to 200% when phenytoin was discontinued in 12 patients taking both drugs, which allowed dose reductions in 6 patients. In these patients, there was no change in seizure control when phenytoin was stopped.[13]

(c) Hepatotoxicity

Epidemiological studies suggest that the risk of fatal hepatotoxicity is higher when valproate is given as polytherapy with enzyme inducers such as phenytoin than when it is given as monotherapy, especially in infants.[14,15] For mention of raised liver enzymes with concurrent use of valproate, phenobarbital and phenytoin, see 'Phenobarbital + Valproate', p.591.

Mechanism

The initial fall in total serum phenytoin levels appears to result from the displacement of phenytoin from its protein binding sites by valproate,[1-5,10] the extent being subject to the diurnal variation in valproate levels.[16] This allows more of the unbound drug to be exposed to metabolism by the liver and the total phenytoin levels fall. After several weeks the metabolism of phenytoin is inhibited by valproate and phenytoin levels rise.[2,4] This may result in sustained elevation of free (active) phenytoin levels.[17] Phenytoin reduces valproate levels, probably because it increases its metabolism by the liver. Because phenytoin is an enzyme inducer it may also possibly increase the formation of a minor but hepatotoxic metabolite of valproate (2-propyl-4-pentenoic acid or 4-ene-VPA).[18]

Importance and management

An extremely well-documented interaction (only a selection of the references being listed here). Concurrent use is common and usually advantageous, the adverse effects of the interactions between the drugs usually being of only minor practical importance. However, the outcome should still be monitored. A few patients may experience mild toxicity if valproate is started, but most patients taking phenytoin do not need a dose change. During the first few weeks total serum phenytoin levels may fall by 20 to 50%, but usually no increase in the dose is needed, because it is balanced by an increase in the levels of free (active) phenytoin levels. In the following period, the total phenytoin levels may rise again. This may result in a sustained rise in free phenytoin levels.

When monitoring concurrent use it is important to understand fully the implications of changes in 'total' and 'free' or 'unbound' serum phenytoin concentrations. Where monitoring of free phenytoin levels is not available, various nomograms have been designed for predicting unbound phenytoin concentrations during the use of valproate.[17,19] Bear in mind the evidence that the incidence of valproate-induced liver toxicity may be increased when it is given with phenytoin, especially in infants.

1. Mattson RH, Cramer JA, Williamson PD, Novelly RA. Valproic acid in epilepsy: clinical and pharmacological effects. *Ann Neurol* (1978) 3, 20–5.
2. Perucca E, Hebdige S, Frigo GM, Gatti G, Lecchini S, Crema A. Interaction between phenytoin and valproic acid: plasma protein binding and metabolic effects. *Clin Pharmacol Ther* (1980) 28, 779–89.
3. Tsanaclis LM, Allen J, Perucca E, Routledge PA, Richens A. Effect of valproate on free plasma phenytoin concentrations. *Br J Clin Pharmacol* (1984) 18, 17–20.
4. Bruni J, Gallo JM, Lee CS, Pershalski RJ, Wilder BJ. Interactions of valproic acid with phenytoin. *Neurology* (1980) 30, 1233–6.
5. Friel PN, Leal KW, Wilensky AJ. Valproic acid-phenytoin interaction. *Ther Drug Monit* (1979) 1, 243–8.
6. Bruni J, Wilder BJ, Willmore LJ, Barbour B. Valproic acid and plasma levels of phenytoin. *Neurology* (1979) 29, 904–5.
7. Vakil SD, Critchley EMR, Philips JC, Fahim Y, Haydock D, Cocks A, Dyer T. The effect of sodium valproate (Epilim) on phenytoin and phenobarbitone blood levels. In: Legge NJ (ed.) 'Clinical and Pharmacological Aspects of Sodium Valproate (Epilim) in the Treatment of Epilepsy'. Proceedings of a symposium held at Nottingham University, September 1975, MCS Consultants, England, p 75–7.
8. Mamiya K, Yukawa E, Matsumoto T, Aita C, Goto S. Synergistic effect of valproate coadministration and hypoalbuminemia on the serum-free phenytoin concentration in patients with severe motor and intellectual disabilities. *Clin Neuropharmacol* (2002) 25, 230–3.
9. Haigh D, Forsythe WI. The treatment of childhood epilepsy with sodium valproate. *Dev Med Child Neurol* (1975) 17, 743–8.
10. Tollefson GD. Delirium induced by the competitive interaction between phenytoin and dipropylacetate. *J Clin Psychopharmacol* (1981) 1, 154–8.
11. May T, Rambeck B. Serum concentrations of valproic acid: influence of dose and co-medication. *Ther Drug Monit* (1985) 7, 387–90.
12. Sackellares JC, Sato S, Dreifuss FE, Penry JK. Reduction of steady-state valproate levels by other antiepileptic drugs. *Epilepsia* (1981) 22, 437–41.
13. McNew CD, Michel NC, McCabe PH. Pharmacokinetic interaction between valproic acid and phenytoin: is combination of these drugs "rational" polypharmacy. *Epilepsia* (1998) 39 (Suppl 6), abstract 4.100.
14. Dreifuss FE, Santilli N, Langer DH, Sweeney KP, Moline KA, Menander KB. Valproic acid fatalities: a retrospective review. *Neurology* (1987) 37, 379–85.
15. Dreifuss FE, Langer DH, Moline KA, Maxwell JE. Valproic acid hepatic fatalities. II. US experience since 1984. *Neurology* (1989) 39, 201–7.
16. Riva R, Albani F, Contin M, Perucca E, Ambrosetto G, Gobbi G, Santucci M, Procaccianti G, Baruzzi A. Time-dependent interaction between phenytoin and valproic acid. *Neurology* (1985) 35, 510–15.
17. Kerrick JM, Wolff DL, Graves NM. Predicting unbound phenytoin concentrations in patients receiving valproic acid: a comparison of two predicting methods. *Ann Pharmacother* (1995) 29, 470–4.
18. Levy RH, Rettenmeier AW, Anderson GD, Wilensky AJ, Friel PN, Baillie TA, Acheampong A, Tor J, Guyot M, Loiseau P. Effects of polytherapy with phenytoin, carbamazepine, and stiripentol on formation of 4-ene-valproate, a hepatotoxic metabolite of valproic acid. *Clin Pharmacol Ther* (1990) 48, 225–35.
19. May TW, Rambeck B, Nothbaum N. Nomogram for the prediction of unbound phenytoin concentrations in patients on a combined treatment of phenytoin and valproic acid. *Eur Neurol* (1991) 31, 57–60.

Phenytoin + Vigabatrin

Vigabatrin causes a small to moderate reduction in phenytoin levels.

Clinical evidence

In one early clinical study in 19 patients, the mean plasma phenytoin levels were about 30% lower when they were given vigabatrin 2 to 3 g daily: in 2 patients phenytoin levels fell below the therapeutic range. However, the change in phenytoin levels was not correlated with the change in seizure frequency.[1] Another clinical study found that vigabatrin reduced the mean serum phenytoin levels by 20% in 53 patients; 41 patients had a decrease in phenytoin levels and 12 had an increase. In this study, some of the patients (number not stated) with decreased phenytoin levels had an increase in seizure frequency and required a phenytoin dose increase.[2,3] In another analysis, the decrease in phenytoin levels did not occur until the fifth week of vigabatrin use.[4] Three other studies have shown roughly similar decreases in phenytoin levels when vigabatrin was added.[5-7]

Mechanism

Not understood. Studies in patients found that decreases in phenytoin levels do not appear to be due to reduced metabolism or altered plasma protein binding.[4] Similarly, it is not due to altered bioavailability, as the interaction occurred with intravenous phenytoin.[5]

Importance and management

The interaction between phenytoin and vigabatrin would appear to be established. Vigabatrin causes a modest decrease in phenytoin levels in some patients, which takes a number of weeks to become apparent. A small increase in the dose of phenytoin may possibly be needed in some patients.

1. Tassinari CA, Michelucci R, Ambrosetto G, Salvi F. Double-blind study of vigabatrin in the treatment of drug-resistant epilepsy. *Arch Neurol* (1987) 44, 907–10.
2. Browne TR, Mattson RH, Penry JK, Smith DB, Treiman DM, Wilder BJ, Ben-Menachem E, Miketta RM, Sherry KM, Szabo GK. A multicentre study of vigabatrin for drug-resistant epilepsy. *Br J Clin Pharmacol* (1989) 95S–100S.
3. Browne TR, Mattson RH, Penry JK, Smith DB, Treiman DM, Wilder BJ, Ben-Menachem E, Napoliello MJ, Sherry KM, Szabo GK. Vigabatrin for refractory complex partial seizures: multicenter single-blind study with long-term follow up. *Neurology* (1987) 37, 184–9.
4. Rimmer EM, Richens A. Double-blind study of γ-vinyl GABA in patients with refractory epilepsy. *Lancet* (1984) i, 189–90.
5. Gatti G, Bartoli A, Marchiselli R, Michelucci R, Tassinari CA, Pisani F, Zaccara G, Timmings P, Richens A, Perucca E. Vigabatrin-induced decrease in serum phenytoin concentration does not involve a change in phenytoin bioavailability. *Br J Clin Pharmacol* (1993) 36, 603–6.
6. Rimmer EM, Richens A. Interaction between vigabatrin and phenytoin. *Br J Clin Pharmacol* (1989) 27, 27S–33S.
7. Bernardina BD, Fontana E, Vigevano F, Fusco L, Torelli D, Galeone D, Buti D, Cianchetti C, Gnanasakthy A, Iudice A. Efficacy and tolerability of vigabatrin in children with refractory partial seizures: a single-blind dose-increasing study. *Epilepsia* (1995) 36, 687–91.

Phenytoin + Zidovudine

Although one study found that zidovudine did not alter the pharmacokinetics of phenytoin, there is other evidence suggesting that some changes possibly occur, although these might actually be due to HIV infection.

Clinical evidence, mechanism, importance and management

Although there are said to have been 13 cases of a possible interaction between zidovudine and phenytoin, the details are not described in the report.[1] No significant changes in the pharmacokinetics of phenytoin 300 mg daily were seen in 12 asymptomatic HIV-positive patients who were taking zidovudine 200 mg every 4 hours.[1] Another study found that the mean phenytoin dose was higher in HIV-positive patients, when compared with subjects with epilepsy without the virus, while the mean phenytoin levels in the HIV-positive group were lower (i.e. a higher phenytoin dose resulted in lower serum levels in HIV-positive subjects). Zidovudine did not appear to affect the levels.[2,3] The current evidence would suggest that it is HIV infection, rather than zidovudine, that affects phenytoin levels, but more study is needed to confirm this.

1. Sarver P, Lampkin TA, Dukes GE, Messenheimer JA, Kirby MG, Dalton MJ, Hak LJ. Effect of zidovudine on the pharmacokinetic disposition of phenytoin in HIV positive asymptomatic patients. *Pharmacotherapy* (1991) 11, 108–9.
2. Burger DM, Meenhorst PL, Koks CHW, Beijnen JH. Phenytoin (PH) monitoring in HIV (+) individuals: is there an interaction with zidovudine (ZDV)? 9th International Conference on AIDS & 5th World Congress on Sexually Transmitted Diseases, Berlin. June 6–11, 1993. Abstract PO-B31–2214.
3. Burger DM, Meenhorst PL, Mulder JW, Kraaijeveld CL, Koks CHW, Bult A, Beijnen JH. Therapeutic drug monitoring of phenytoin in patients with the acquired immunodeficiency syndrome. *Ther Drug Monit* (1994) 16, 616–20.

Phenytoin + Zileuton

The pharmacokinetics of phenytoin are not affected by zileuton.

Clinical evidence, mechanism, importance and management

A controlled study in 20 healthy subjects found that the pharmacokinetics of a single 300-mg dose of phenytoin were unaltered by zileuton 600 mg every 6 hours for 5 days.[1] An *in vitro* study found that zileuton had little effect on the isoenzymes responsible for the metabolism of phenytoin.[2] These studies suggest that zileuton is unlikely to affect phenytoin levels in clinical use.

1. Samara E, Cavanaugh JH, Mukherjee D, Granneman GR. Lack of pharmacokinetic interaction between zileuton and phenytoin in humans. *Clin Pharmacokinet* (1995) 29 (Suppl 2), 84–91.
2. Lu P, Schrag ML, Slaughter DE, Raab CE, Shou M, Rodrigues AD. Mechanism-based inhibition of human liver microsomal cytochrome P450 1A2 by zileuton, a 5-lipoxygenase inhibitor. *Drug Metab Dispos* (2003) 31, 1352–60.

Piracetam + Other antiepileptics

Piracetam does not appear to alter the levels of sodium valproate or primidone. No interaction has been found between piracetam and carbamazepine, clonazepam, phenobarbital, or phenytoin.

Clinical evidence, mechanism, importance and management

The addition of piracetam (2 to 4 g three times daily, increased to a maximum of 18 to 24 g daily) did not affect plasma levels of **sodium valproate** or **primidone** in patients with myoclonus. The exact number of patients taking these drugs is unclear, as the report just states that 28 patients were taking **clonazepam**, **sodium valproate**, or **primidone**, alone or in combination.[1] Another similar report, briefly noted the same findings.[2] The manufacturer of piracetam notes that no interaction has been found between piracetam and **clonazepam**, **carbamazepine**, **phenytoin**, **phenobarbital** and **sodium valproate**, although this is based on a small number of patients.[3] No dose adjustments appear to be required if piracetam is used with these antiepileptics.

1. Obeso JA, Artieda J, Quinn N, Rothwell JC, Luquin MR, Vaamonde J, Marsden CD. Piracetam in the treatment of different types of myoclonus. *Clin Neuropharmacol* (1988) 11, 529–36.
2. Raychev I. Piracetam (pyramem) in the treatment of cortical myoclonus. 5th European Congress of Epileptology, Madrid 2002. P382.
3. Nootropil (Piracetam). UCB Pharma Ltd. UK Summary of product characteristics, December 2006.

Pregabalin + Miscellaneous

Carbamazepine, oxcarbazepine, and phenytoin may decrease serum levels of pregabalin. Levetiracetam does not affect the pharmacokinetics of pregabalin, and there appears to be no pharmacokinetic interaction between pregabalin and gabapentin, lamotrigine, phenobarbital, topir-

amate, valproate, alcohol, lorazepam, or oxycodone. However, the impairment of cognitive and gross motor function caused by oxycodone was additive with pregabalin, and pregabalin may potentiate the effects of alcohol and lorazepam.

Clinical evidence, mechanism, importance and management

(a) Alcohol or Lorazepam

The manufacturer notes that there was no clinically relevant pharmacokinetic interaction between pregabalin and lorazepam or alcohol, and that concurrent use caused no clinically important effect on respiration. However, they note that pregabalin may potentiate the effects of lorazepam and alcohol.[1]

(b) Other antiepileptics

Pregabalin 200 mg three times daily for 7 days was added to monotherapy with various antiepileptics in patients with partial epilepsy. Pregabalin did not alter the steady-state levels of **phenytoin**, **carbamazepine** (or its active metabolite, carbamazepine-10,11-epoxide), **valproate** or **lamotrigine**. In addition, the steady-state pharmacokinetics of pregabalin were not different to those seen previously in healthy subjects taking pregabalin alone, suggesting that these antiepileptics do not alter pregabalin pharmacokinetics.[2] Similarly, population pharmacokinetic analyses of clinical studies found no important changes in the pharmacokinetics of **lamotrigine**, **phenobarbital**, **phenytoin**, **topiramate** or **valproate** when they were given with pregabalin, and the pharmacokinetics of pregabalin were unaffected by these drugs.[3] However, this sort of analysis gives only the broadest impression of whether or not a drug interacts, and another study in patients with epilepsy found that pregabalin levels were 30%, 22%, and 23% lower when it was given with the enzyme-inducing drugs **carbamazepine**, **oxcarbazepine**, and **phenytoin**, respectively. In this study **levetiracetam** had no effect on the serum concentrations of pregabalin.[4] The manufacturer also notes that there is no pharmacokinetic interaction between pregabalin and **gabapentin**.[1]

(c) Oxycodone

The manufacturer notes that there was no clinically relevant pharmacokinetic interaction between pregabalin and oxycodone, and that there was no clinically important effect on respiration. However, pregabalin appeared to cause an additive impairment in cognitive and gross motor function when given with oxycodone.[1] This suggests caution is warranted during combined use.

1. Lyrica (Pregabalin). Pfizer Ltd. UK Summary of product characteristics, April 2013.
2. Brodie MJ, Wilson EA, Wesche DL, Alvey CW, Randinitis EJ, Posvar EL, Hounslow NJ, Bron NJ, Gibson GL, Bockbrader HN. Pregabalin drug interaction studies: lack of effect on the pharmacokinetics of carbamazepine, phenytoin, lamotrigine, and valproate in patients with partial epilepsy. *Epilepsia* (2005) 46, 1407–13.
3. Bockbrader HN, Burger PJ, Corrigan BW, Kugler AR, Knapp LE, Garofalo EA, Lalonde RL. Population pharmacokinetic analyses of commonly prescribed antiepileptic drugs coadministered with pregabalin in adult patients with refractory partial seizures. *Epilepsia* (2001) 42 (Suppl 7), 84.
4. May TW, Rambeck B, Neb R, Jürgens U. Serum concentrations of pregabalin in patients with epilepsy: the influence of dose, age, and comedication. *Ther Drug Monit* (2007) 29, 789–94.

Primidone + Isoniazid

A single case report describes elevated primidone levels and reduced levels of its phenobarbital metabolite when primidone was given with isoniazid.

Clinical evidence, mechanism, importance and management

A patient taking primidone had raised serum primidone levels and reduced serum phenobarbital levels. This was attributed to the concurrent use of isoniazid, which inhibited the metabolism of primidone by the liver. The half-life of primidone rose from 8.7 hours to 14 hours and the steady-state primidone levels rose by 83% in the presence of isoniazid.[1] The importance of this interaction is uncertain, but prescribers should bear this interaction in mind in case of an unexpected response to primidone.

1. Sutton G, Kupferberg HJ. Isoniazid as an inhibitor of primidone metabolism. *Neurology* (1975) 25, 1179–81.

Primidone + Miscellaneous

Primidone is substantially converted to phenobarbital within the body and it is therefore expected to interact with other drugs in the same way as phenobarbital. Some drugs may increase the conversion of primidone to phenobarbital.

Clinical evidence, mechanism, importance and management

Primidone is substantially converted to phenobarbital within the body. For example, a group of patients taking long-term primidone developed serum primidone levels of 9 micrograms/mL and serum phenobarbital levels of 31 micrograms/mL.[1] Primidone would therefore be expected to interact with other drugs in the same way as phenobarbital. Some enzyme-inducing drugs might increase the conversion of primidone to phenobarbital, and this has been demonstrated for phenytoin (see 'Primidone + Phenytoin', below), and carbamazepine (see 'Carbamazepine + Primidone', p.577). Some patients have been treated with a combination of phenobarbital and primidone. In this situation higher phenobarbital levels might be expected.

1. Booker HE, Hosokowa K, Burdette RD, Darcey B. A clinical study of serum primidone levels. *Epilepsia* (1970) 11, 395–402.

Primidone + Phenytoin

Primidone-derived serum phenobarbital levels are increased by phenytoin. This is normally an advantageous interaction, but phenobarbital toxicity occasionally occurs.

Clinical evidence

A study in 44 patients with epilepsy taking primidone and phenytoin found that their serum phenobarbital to primidone ratio was high (4.35) when compared with that in 15 other patients who were only taking primidone (1.05).[1] This suggests that in the presence of phenytoin, primidone-derived phenobarbital levels are higher than when primidone is given alone. Similar results are described in other studies.[2-7] A few patients may develop barbiturate toxicity.[8]

An initial marked decrease in phenytoin levels, then an increase to half the initial phenytoin level, was seen in the first few weeks after withdrawing primidone in an infant. Primidone-derived phenobarbital levels before discontinuing the primidone were very high, and were associated with marked sedation.[9]

Mechanism

Phenytoin increases the metabolic conversion of primidone to phenobarbital, while possibly reducing the subsequent metabolism (hydroxylation) of the phenobarbital. The net effect is a rise in phenobarbital levels.[10] Phenobarbital may increase or decrease phenytoin levels, see 'Phenytoin + Phenobarbital', p.604.

Importance and management

Well documented. This is normally an advantageous interaction because phenobarbital is itself an active antiepileptic. However, it should be noted that phenobarbital serum levels could sometimes reach toxic concentrations,[8] even if only a small dose of phenytoin is added. Changes in phenytoin levels may also occur (see 'Phenytoin + Phenobarbital', p.604).

1. Fincham RW, Schottelius DD, Sahs AL. The influence of diphenylhydantoin on primidone metabolism. *Arch Neurol* (1974) 30, 259–62.
2. Fincham RW, Schottelius DD, Sahs AL. The influence of diphenylhydantoin on primidone metabolism. *Trans Am Neurol Assoc* (1973) 98, 197–9.
3. Schmidt D. The effect of phenytoin and ethosuximide on primidone metabolism in patients with epilepsy. *J Neurol* (1975) 209, 115–23.
4. Reynolds EH, Fenton G, Fenwick P, Johnson AL, Laundy M. Interaction of phenytoin and primidone. *BMJ* (1975) 2, 594–5.
5. Callaghan N, Feeley M, Duggan F, O'Callaghan M, Seldrup J. The effect of anticonvulsant drugs which induce liver microsomal enzymes on derived and ingested phenobarbitone levels. *Acta Neurol Scand* (1977) 56, 1–6.
6. Battino D, Avanzini G, Bossi L, Croci D, Cusi C, Gomeni C, Moise A. Plasma levels of primidone and its metabolite phenobarbital: effect of age and associated therapy. *Ther Drug Monit* (1983) 5, 73–9.
7. Garrettson LK, Gomez M. Phenytoin-primidone interaction. *Br J Clin Pharmacol* (1977) 4, 693–5.
8. Galdames D, Ortiz M, Saavedra I, Aguilera L. Interaccion fenitoina-primidona: intoxicacion por fenobarbital, en un adulto tratado con ambas drogas. *Rev Med Chil* (1980) 108, 716–20.
9. Wilson JT, Wilkinson GR. Chronic and severe phenobarbital intoxication in a child treated with primidone and diphenylhydantoin. *J Pediatr* (1973) 83, 484–9.
10. Porro MG, Kupferberg HJ, Porter RJ, Theodore WH, Newmark ME. Phenytoin: an inhibitor and inducer of primidone metabolism in an epileptic patient. *Br J Clin Pharmacol* (1982) 14, 294–7.

Primidone + Valproate

Valproate has been reported to cause increases, decreases, and no change in primidone levels. Primidone-derived phenobarbital levels appear to be increased by valproate.

Clinical evidence

In a number of cases, patients taking primidone required a decrease in the primidone dose after valproate was added.[1-4] In 6 cases this was due to an increase in the primidone-derived phenobarbital level,[1] and in the other cases phenobarbital levels were not measured, but the dose reduction was needed to overcome the sedation that occurred when valproate was added.[2-4] Primidone levels were not measured in any of these cases.[1-4] In two other studies, primidone levels either decreased,[5] or did not change when valproate was added.[6] However, phenobarbital levels, where measured, had increased.[6]

In 7 children the serum levels of primidone 10 to 18 mg/kg daily rose two- to threefold when valproate (dose not stated) was also given. After 1 to 3 months of concurrent use the serum primidone levels fell in 3 of the patients but persisted in one. Follow-up primidone levels were not taken in the other 3 patients, and none of the patients had phenobarbital levels measured.[7]

In contrast, in a further study, neither phenobarbital levels nor primidone levels were significantly altered when valproate was given.[8]

Mechanism

It has been suggested that valproate decreases the conversion of primidone to phenobarbital, and decreases the metabolism of phenobarbital (see also 'Phenobarbital + Valproate', p.591). This would result in increased primidone and phenobarbital levels. However, increased renal clearance of primidone may also occur, resulting in no overall change to primidone levels. Depending on the balance between these various effects a variety of levels may result.[8] The results of one study suggest that the proposed inhibition of primidone metabolism caused by valproate may diminish over the first few months of concurrent use.[7]

Importance and management

There seems to be little consistency about the effect of valproate on primidone levels. However, in the majority of cases phenobarbital levels seem to be raised (see also 'Phenobarbital + Valproate', p.591). It would therefore seem prudent not to act on primidone levels without considering the corresponding phenobarbital levels. Monitor the patient for increased signs of sedation, which may be resolved by a reduction in the primidone dose.

1. Wilder BJ, Willmore LJ, Bruni J, Villarreal HJ. Valproic acid: interaction with other anticonvulsant drugs. *Neurology* (1978) 28, 892–6.
2. Haigh D, Forsythe WI. The treatment of childhood epilepsy with sodium valproate. *Dev Med Child Neurol* (1975) 17, 743–8.
3. Richens A, Ahmad S. Controlled trial of sodium valproate in severe epilepsy. *BMJ* (1975) 4, 255–6.
4. Völzke E, Doose H. Dipropylacetate (Dépakine®, Ergenyl®) in the treatment of epilepsy. *Epilepsia* (1973) 14, 185–93.
5. Varma R, Michos GA, Varma RS, Hoshino AY. Clinical trials of Depakene (valproic acid) coadministered with other anticonvulsants in epileptic patients. *Res Commun Psychol Psychiatr Behav* (1980) 5, 265–73.
6. Yukawa E, Higuchi S, Aoyama T. The effect of concurrent administration of sodium valproate on serum levels of primidone and its metabolite phenobarbital. *J Clin Pharm Ther* (1989) 14, 387–92.
7. Windorfer A, Sauer W, Gädeke R. Elevation of diphenylhydantoin and primidone serum concentration by addition of dipropylacetate, a new anticonvulsant drug. *Acta Paediatr Scand* (1975) 64, 771–2.
8. Bruni J. Valproic acid and plasma levels of primidone and derived phenobarbital. *Can J Neurol Sci* (1981) 8, 91–2.

Progabide + Other antiepileptics

Progabide may raise phenytoin levels and alter the levels of carbamazepine. Clonazepam, phenobarbital and valproate levels are minimally affected by progabide.

Clinical evidence

(a) Phenytoin

Marked increases in serum phenytoin levels have been seen in a few patients also given progabide,[1-4] while smaller changes have been described in some studies,[5,6] and negligible changes in others.[7]

In one study, 17 out of 26 patients with epilepsy needed a reduction in their phenytoin dose to keep the levels within 25% of the serum levels achieved in the absence of progabide. Over half the patients needed a dose reduction within 4 weeks of starting concurrent use. Most of those needing a dose reduction had a maximum increase in the serum level of 40% or more, which was sometimes accompanied by toxicity.[2,8] In a later report of this study, of a total of 32 patients with epilepsy taking carbamazepine with phenytoin and then given progabide, 22 needed a reduction in their phenytoin dose to maintain serum levels within 25% of those achieved in the absence of progabide. In addition, it appeared this effect on phenytoin serum levels continued for a while after progabide was withdrawn.[4]

(b) Other antiepileptics

Information about antiepileptics other than phenytoin is limited, but progabide is reported to minimally reduce,[1,9,10] minimally increase[1] or not to change[2,3,5-7] **carbamazepine** serum levels. An increase of up to 24% in the levels of carbamazepine-10-11-epoxide (the active metabolite of **carbamazepine**) has also been reported.[6,10] **Valproate**[3,5-7] and **clonazepam**[11] serum levels do not seem to be significantly affected by progabide. Progabide appears to cause a small increase in serum **phenobarbital** levels, which is of little clinical importance.[1,5-7]

Mechanism

Uncertain.

Importance and management

Some small to moderate changes in the serum levels of carbamazepine, clonazepam, phenobarbital, and valproate can apparently occur in the presence of progabide, but only the interaction with phenytoin appears to be clinically relevant. Be alert for evidence of phenytoin adverse effects (e.g. blurred vision, nystagmus, ataxia or drowsiness) and consider reducing the dose of phenytoin if progabide is used concurrently.

1. Schmidt D, Utech K. Progabide for refractory partial epilepsy: a controlled add-on trial. *Neurology* (1986) 36, 217–221.
2. Cloyd JC, Brundage RC, Leppik IE, Graves NM, Welty TE. Effect of progabide on serum phenytoin and carbamazepine concentrations: a preliminary report. In: LERS Monograph series, volume 3. Edited by Bartholini G et al. Epilepsy and GABA receptor agonists: basic and therapeutic research. Meeting, Paris, March 1984. Raven Press, New York. (1985) pp 271–8. ISBN: 0881671061
3. Crawford P, Chadwick D. A comparative study of progabide, valproate and placebo as add-on therapy in patients with refractory epilepsy. *J Neurol Neurosurg Psychiatry* (1986) 49, 1251–7.
4. Brundage RC, Cloyd JC, Leppik IE, Graves NM and Welty TE. Effect of progabide on serum phenytoin and carbamazepine concentrations. *Clin Neuropharmacol* (1987) 10, 545–54.
5. Bianchetti G, Thiercelin JF, Thenot JP, Feuerstein J, Lambert D, Rulliere R, Thebault JJ, Morselli PL. Effect of progabide on the pharmacokinetics of various antiepileptic drugs. *Neurology* (1984) 34 (Suppl 1), 213.
6. Bianchetti G, Padovani P, Thénot JP, Thiercelin JF, Morselli PL. Pharmacokinetic interactions of progabide with other antiepileptic drugs. *Epilepsia* (1987) 28, 68–73.
7. Thénot JP, Bianchetti G, Abriol C, Feuerstein J, Lambert D, Thébault JJ, Warrington SJ, Rowland M. Interactions between progabide and antiepileptic drugs. In: LERS Monograph series, volume 3. Edited by Bartholini G et al. Epilepsy and GABA receptor agonists: basic and therapeutic research. Meeting, Paris, March 1984. Raven Press, New York. (1985) pp 259–69. ISBN: 0881671061
8. Brundage RC, Leppik IE, Cloyd JC, Graves NM. Effect of progabide on phenytoin pharmacokinetics. *Epilepsia* (1984) 25, 656–7.
9. Dam M, Gram L, Philbert A, Hansen BS, Blatt Lyon B, Christensen JM, Angelo HR. Progabide: a controlled trial in partial epilepsy. *Epilepsia* (1983) 24, 127–34.
10. Graves NM, Fuerst RH, Cloyd JC, Brundage RC, Welty TE, Leppik IE. Progabide-induced changes in carbamazepine metabolism. *Epilepsia* (1988) 29, 775–80.
11. Warrington SJ, O'Brien C, Thiercelin JF, Orofiamma B and Morselli PL. Evaluation of pharmacodynamic interaction between progabide and clonazepam in healthy men. In: LERS Monograph series, volume 3. Edited by Bartholini G et al. Epilepsy and GABA receptor agonists: basic and therapeutic research. Meeting, Paris, March 1984. Raven Press, New York. (1985) pp 279–86. ISBN: 0881671061

Remacemide + Other antiepileptics

Remacemide causes modest increases in carbamazepine and phenytoin serum levels. Carbamazepine, phenobarbital and phenytoin moderately reduce remacemide serum levels. Valproate and lamotrigine do not appear to interact with remacemide.

Clinical evidence

(a) Carbamazepine

When a group of 10 patients taking carbamazepine were also given up to 300 mg of remacemide twice daily for 2 weeks the minimum serum levels and the AUC of carbamazepine were increased by 20% and 22%, respectively. None of the patients had symptoms of carbamazepine toxicity.[1] Another study in 11 patients taking carbamazepine found that remacemide caused a similar 20 to 30% increase in the AUC of carbamazepine, again without signs of toxicity. No consistent changes in the AUC of carbamazepine-10,11-epoxide, the main metabolite of carbamazepine, were seen.[2] Another study has reported a slight inhibitory effect of remacemide on carbamazepine metabolism, which is in line with these other findings.[3] One of these studies also reported that the AUC of remacemide was decreased by 40 to 50% and the AUC of its main metabolite by about 70% in the presence of carbamazepine, when compared with healthy subjects (presumably not taking carbamazepine).[2]

However, a further study of the efficacy of remacemide and carbamazepine in combination found that about two-thirds of the 120 patients treated needed 14 to 50% reductions in their carbamazepine dose, to ensure levels remained in the therapeutic range.[4]

(b) Lamotrigine

In a study in healthy subjects there was no clinically relevant pharmacokinetic interaction between remacemide (200 mg daily increased to 200 mg three times daily) and lamotrigine (200 mg twice daily decreased to 100 mg daily).[5]

(c) Phenobarbital

In a study in healthy subjects, phenobarbital 30 mg daily increased to 90 mg daily increased the clearance of remacemide 200 mg twice daily by 67%, and slightly increased the plasma levels of phenobarbital (by 9%).[6]

(d) Phenytoin

A group of 10 patients taking phenytoin were also given up to 300 mg remacemide twice daily for 2 weeks. On average remacemide did not affect phenytoin pharmacokinetics but 5 patients had an increase in minimum serum levels of 30% or more. None of the patients had symptoms of phenytoin toxicity.[1] In another study 10 patients with epilepsy, who had been taking phenytoin for at least 3 months, were given remacemide 300 mg twice daily for 12 days. Phenytoin maximum plasma levels were increased by 14% and the AUC was raised by 12%. Average concentrations of remacemide and its main metabolite were around only 40% and 30%, respectively, of those achieved in healthy subjects taking remacemide alone, at the same dose.[7] Another study reported a slight inhibitory effect of remacemide on phenytoin metabolism, which is in line with these other findings.[3]

(e) Valproate

A group of 10 patients taking valproate were also given remacemide up to 300 mg twice daily for 14 days. The pharmacokinetics of valproate remained unchanged.[1] Another study in 17 patients confirmed these findings,[8] and an earlier study by the same authors also noted no effect of remacemide on valproate metabolism.[3]

Mechanism

Not fully understood, but *in vitro* studies indicate that remacemide inhibits the cytochrome P450 isoenzyme CYP3A4, which in practice would be expected to result in a reduction in the metabolism of the carbamazepine resulting in an increase in its serum levels. Remacemide appears to inhibit CYP2C9 to a lesser extent, which is reflected in a smaller interaction with phenytoin. Valproate is metabolised by glucuronidation and is therefore unaffected.[1]

Carbamazepine and phenytoin, known enzyme inducers, also seem to increase the metabolism of the remacemide.[7]

Importance and management

Information is limited, but the interactions of remacemide with carbamazepine, phenobarbital and phenytoin appear to be established, but so far only the carbamazepine interaction seems to have been shown to be of clinical importance. Even so, it may be prudent to monitor the effects of concurrent use with phenytoin or phenobarbital. No interaction occurs between remacemide and valproate or lamotrigine.

1. Riley RJ, Slee D, Martin CA, Webborn PJH, Wattam DG, Jones T, Logan CJ. *In vitro* evaluation of pharmacokinetic interactions between remacemide hydrochloride and established anticonvulsants. *Br J Clin Pharmacol* (1996) 41, 461P.

2. Leach JP, Blacklaw J, Stewart M, Jamieson V, Jones T, Oxley R, Richens A, Brodie MJ. Mutual pharmacokinetic interactions between remacemide hydrochloride and carbamazepine. *Epilepsia* (1995) 36 (Suppl 3), S163.
3. Leach JP, Blacklaw J, Stewart M, Jamieson V, Oxley R, Richens A, Brodie MJ. Interactions between remacemide and the established antiepileptic drugs. *Epilepsia* (1994) 35 (Suppl 7), 75.
4. Mawer GE, Jamieson V, Lucas SB, Wild JM. Adjustment of carbamazepine dose to offset the effects of the interaction with remacemide hydrochloride in a double-blind, multicentre, add-on drug trial (CR2237) in refractory epilepsy. *Epilepsia* (1999) 40, 190–6.
5. Blakey GE, Lockton JA, Rolan IP. The effect of lamotrigine on the disposition of remacemide hydrochloride. *Epilepsia* (1999) 40 (Suppl 2), 251.
6. Hooper WD, Eadie MJ, Blakey GE, Lockton JA, Manun'Ebo M. Evaluation of a pharmacokinetic interaction between remacemide hydrochloride and phenobarbitone in healthy males. *Br J Clin Pharmacol* (2001) 51, 249–55.
7. Leach JP, Girvan J, Jamieson V, Jones T, Richens A, Brodie MJ. Mutual interaction between remacemide hydrochloride and phenytoin. *Epilepsy Res* (1997) 26, 381–8.
8. Leach JP, Girvan J, Jamieson V, Jones T, Richens A, Brodie MJ. Lack of pharmacokinetic interaction between remacemide hydrochloride and sodium valproate in epileptic patients. *Seizure* (1997) 6, 179–84.

Retigabine (Ezogabine) + Other antiepileptics

The clearance of retigabine is increased by carbamazepine and phenytoin, but not affected by phenobarbital, topiramate, or valproate. Retigabine does not alter the pharmacokinetics of any of these antiepileptics. There is a modest pharmacokinetic interaction between retigabine and lamotrigine.

Clinical evidence, mechanism, importance and management

(a) Enzyme-inducing antiepileptics

The preliminary report of a study in patients with epilepsy notes that the clearance of retigabine was increased (amount not stated) by **carbamazepine** and **phenytoin**, whereas retigabine did not alter **carbamazepine** or **phenytoin** pharmacokinetics.[1] This is consistent with the known enzyme-inducing properties of **carbamazepine** and **phenytoin**, and the fact that retigabine has not been shown to induce hepatic enzymes. In contrast, in a study in healthy subjects, **phenobarbital** 90 mg daily did not affect the pharmacokinetics of retigabine 200 mg every 8 hours, and the pharmacokinetics of **phenobarbital** were not altered by retigabine.[2] The clinical relevance of the effect of **carbamazepine** and **phenytoin** on retigabine remains to be assessed. No dose adjustments seem to be necessary with **phenobarbital**.

(b) Lamotrigine

In a study in 14 healthy subjects, lamotrigine 25 mg daily for 5 days increased the AUC of a single 200-mg dose of retigabine by 15% and decreased its clearance by 13%.[3] In another 15 subjects, retigabine (200 mg twice daily increased to 300 mg twice daily over 15 days) decreased the AUC of a single 200-mg dose of lamotrigine by 18% and increased its clearance by 22%. It was suggested that lamotrigine competes for renal elimination with retigabine, but the mechanism behind the decreased lamotrigine levels is unknown.[3] These modest changes are unlikely to be clinically important for most patients, but the authors suggest that the effects need to be assessed at the upper recommended dose ranges, and therefore advise caution.

(c) Topiramate

The preliminary report of a study notes that the pharmacokinetics of retigabine and topiramate were not altered by concurrent use in patients with epilepsy.[1] No special dosing precautions are necessary.

(d) Valproate

The preliminary report of a study notes that the pharmacokinetics of retigabine and valproic acid were not altered by concurrent use in patients with epilepsy.[1] No special dosing precautions are necessary.

1. Sachdeo RC, Ferron GM, Partiot AM, Biton V, Rosenfeld WB, Porter RJ, Fritz T, Althouse S, Troy SM. An early determination of drug-drug interaction between valproic acid, phenytoin, carbamazepine or topiramate, and retigabine in epileptic patients. *Neurology* (2001) 56 (Suppl 3). A331–A332.
2. Ferron GM, Patat A, Parks V, Rolan P, Troy SM. Lack of pharmacokinetic interaction between retigabine and phenobarbitone at steady state in healthy subjects. *Br J Clin Pharmacol* (2003) 56, 39–45.
3. Hermann R, Knebel NG, Niebch G, Richards L, Borlak J, Locher M. Pharmacokinetic interaction between retigabine and lamotrigine in healthy subjects. *Eur J Clin Pharmacol* (2003) 58, 795–802.

Rufinamide + Food

Food increases the rate and extent of absorption of rufinamide.

Clinical evidence, mechanism, importance and management

In a study to investigate the effect of food on the pharmacokinetics of rufinamide, 12 healthy subjects were given a single 600-mg dose of rufinamide after an overnight fast, or with a fat- and protein-rich breakfast. The AUC of rufinamide was increased by 44% by food, when compared with the fasted state, and the maximum plasma level was increased twofold. The time to reach the maximum plasma level was shortened from 8 hours to 6 hours in the group that took rufinamide with food. Headache was reported more frequently in the fed group, but the use of analgesics was not different between the two groups.[1] The manufacturer recommends that rufinamide is taken with food,[2] to maximise absorption.

1. Cardot J-M, Lecaillon J-B, Czendlik C, Godbillon J. The influence of food on the disposition of the antiepileptic rufinamide in healthy volunteers. *Biopharm Drug Dispos* (1998) 19, 259–62.
2. Inovelon (Rufinamide). Eisai Ltd. UK Summary of product characteristics, October 2009.

Rufinamide + Miscellaneous

Rufinamide may increase the clearance of drugs that are substrates of CYP3A4, such as triazolam. Other cytochrome P450 isoenzymes are unlikely to be affected.

Clinical evidence and mechanism

(a) CYP1A2

Rufinamide 400 mg twice daily did not affect the pharmacokinetics of **olanzapine**, a substrate of CYP1A2.[1]

(b) CYP3A4

Rufinamide has been shown to induce the cytochrome P450 isoenzyme CYP3A4 to a moderate degree. A study found that rufinamide 400 mg twice daily for 11 days increased the clearance of **triazolam**, a substrate of CYP3A4, by 55% and reduced its exposure by 36%.[1]

Importance and management

Evidence about CYP3A4 substrates is limited, but is in line with the *in vitro* effects of rufinamide, and the way in which triazolam is known to be metabolised. The manufacturers recommend that any patient taking a drug that is a substrate of CYP3A4 should be monitored for 2 weeks after starting, stopping, or changing the dose of rufinamide, and dose adjustments made as appropriate. Note that the effects of CYP3A4 substrates are likely to be diminished. For a list of known substrates of this isoenzyme, see 'Table 1.10', p.12.

The manufacturer[1] also advises that similar precautions should be taken when rufinamide is given with drugs with a narrow therapeutic margin, and specifically mentions **warfarin** and **digoxin**. However, warfarin is only metabolised to a limited extent by this isoenzyme, and moderate CYP3A4 inhibitors do not generally interact with warfarin (see diltiazem under 'Coumarins and related drugs + Calcium-channel blockers', p.415, and erythromycin under 'Coumarins + Antibacterials; Macrolides', p.387), although cases of bleeding may occur. The prediction with digoxin, a P-glycoprotein substrate, appears to be based on the fact that an effect of rufinamide on P-glycoprotein has not been excluded. Further study is needed.

No pharmacokinetic interaction would be expected with substrates of CYP1A2. For a list of known substrates of this isoenzyme, see 'Table 1.2', p.5.

1. Inovelon (Rufinamide). Eisai Ltd. UK Summary of product characteristics, October 2009.

Rufinamide + Other antiepileptics

The clearance of rufinamide is increased by phenytoin, phenobarbital and primidone. Valproate may raise rufinamide levels in some patients, particularly children. No pharmacokinetic interaction appears to occur between rufinamide and carbamazepine, clobazam, lamotrigine, oxcarbazepine or topiramate. Vigabatrin does not appear to alter the pharmacokinetics of rufinamide, and rufinamide does not alter the trough levels of clonazepam.

Clinical evidence

(a) Carbamazepine or Oxcarbazepine

Preliminary evidence suggests that the pharmacokinetics of rufinamide are not affected by the concurrent use of carbamazepine or oxcarbazepine.[1] Furthermore, rufinamide does not cause a clinically relevant alteration in the trough concentrations of carbamazepine[1,2] or oxcarbazepine.[1]

(b) Clobazam or Clonazepam

Preliminary evidence suggests that the pharmacokinetics of rufinamide are not affected by the concurrent use of clobazam, and rufinamide does not alter the trough concentrations of clobazam or clonazepam.[1]

(c) Lamotrigine

The pharmacokinetics of rufinamide and lamotrigine do not appear to be affected by concurrent use.[2,3]

(d) Phenobarbital, Phenytoin, and Primidone

It has been reported that any combination of phenobarbital, phenytoin, and primidone increased the clearance of rufinamide by about 25%, but that rufinamide had no effect on the trough concentrations of these drugs.[1] However, the manufacturer suggests that the plasma levels of phenytoin may be increased by rufinamide, and that the dose of phenytoin may need to be reduced.[3]

(e) Topiramate

The pharmacokinetics of topiramate and rufinamide do not appear to be affected by concurrent use.[2,3]

(f) Valproate

Valproate has been found to reduce the clearance of rufinamide: one paper reports a modest reduction of 22%.[1] Based on predicted plasma levels, valproate was found to increase rufinamide levels by 55 to 70% in children, 23 to 26% in adolescents, and less than 16% in adults,[4] which suggests that the magnitude of the effects depends upon the age of the patient. Rufinamide has not been found to have any effect on the trough concentrations of valproate.[1]

(g) Vigabatrin

Vigabatrin is reported not to affect the pharmacokinetics of rufinamide.[1]

Mechanism, importance and management

Evidence is limited; however, the interaction between valproate and rufinamide appears to be established. In patients taking valproate, and weighing less than 30 kg, the manufacturer advises starting rufinamide at 200 mg daily, and increasing the dose by no more than 200 mg every 2 days (according to clinical response and efficacy) until a maximum dose of 600 mg daily is achieved.[3] No dose adjustment is recommended for patients weighing more than 30 kg.

It would seem prudent to monitor the plasma levels and clinical effects of rufinamide when it is started or stopped in patients taking phenobarbital, phenytoin, and primidone. Furthermore, monitor for phenytoin adverse effects (e.g. blurred vision, nystagmus, ataxia or drowsiness) and consider taking phenytoin levels if these occur. Note that fosphenytoin is a prodrug of phenytoin, and in the absence of direct evidence it would seem prudent to follow the same precautions described for phenytoin.

1. Bialer M, Johannessen SI, Kupferberg HJ, Levy RH, Loiseau P, Perucca E. Progress report on new antiepileptic drugs: a summary of the fourth Eilat conference (EILAT IV). *Epilepsy Res* (1999) 34, 1–41.
2. Perucca E, Cloyd J, Critchley D, Fuseau E. Rufinamide: Clinical pharmacokinetics and concentration-response relationships in patients with epilepsy. *Epilepsia* (2008) 49, 1123–41.
3. Inovelon (Rufinamide). Eisai Ltd. UK Summary of product characteristics, October 2009.
4. Eisai Ltd. Personal communication, July 2008.

Stiripentol + Miscellaneous

Stiripentol inhibits the metabolism of caffeine and is therefore expected to inhibit the metabolism of other similarly metabolised drugs (e.g. theophylline).

Stiripentol might inhibit the metabolism of drugs by CYP2C19 (e.g. omeprazole) and CYP3A4 (e.g. ciclosporin, simvastatin, ergot derivatives). Stiripentol has no clinically relevant effect on the pharmacokinetics of dextromethorphan and an interaction with other CYP2D6 substrates is not expected. Food might protect stiripentol from degradation by gastric acid.

Clinical evidence, mechanism, importance and management

(a) CYP1A2 substrates

In a study, 12 healthy subjects were given **caffeine** before and after stiripentol (500 mg twice daily on day one, 1 g twice daily on day 2, and 1.5 g twice daily from day 3 to day 13) found that the AUC of a metabolite of caffeine expired in the breath was almost 8-fold lower after treatment with stiripentol.[1] Caffeine can be used as a probe drug to assess the activity of CYP1A2 and this study therefore suggests that stiripentol might inhibit this isoenzyme. The manufacturer of stiripentol therefore does not recommend that **theophylline** (and therefore probably **aminophylline**) or **caffeine** are taken with stiripentol. They extend this warning to foodstuffs containing **caffeine** or **chocolate**, and specifically name **cola** drinks.[2] Clinical evidence regarding an interaction appears to be lacking. If a patient taking stiripentol develops adverse effects such as headache, jitteriness, restlessness, insomnia, consider the inadvertent intake of caffeine as a possible cause. Note that, other drugs that are potent CYP1A2 inhibitors can usually be given with caffeine, if adverse effects are appropriately monitored, see 'Caffeine + SSRIs', p.1428.

(b) CYP2C19 substrates

An *in vitro* study has shown that stiripentol is an inhibitor of CYP2C19.[1] The manufacturer of stiripentol predicts that there might be an increased risk of adverse effects when drugs metabolised by this enzyme are also taken, and that dose adjustment might be required. They specifically name **citalopram** and **omeprazole**, and suggest caution if these drugs are required.[2] For a full list of substrates of this enzyme see 'Table 1.6', p.8. Note that the clinical relevance of any interaction does not appear to have been established.

(c) CYP2D6 substrates

In vitro studies have found that stiripentol is an inhibitor of CYP2D6,[1,2] and the manufacturer of stiripentol predicts that there might be an increased risk of adverse effects when drugs metabolised by this isoenzyme are also taken, and that dose adjustment might be required. They specifically name **propranolol**, **carvedilol**, **timolol**, **fluoxetine**, **paroxetine**, **sertraline**, **imipramine**, **clomipramine**, **haloperidol**, **codeine**, **dextromethorphan**, and **tramadol**.[2] However, in a study in 12 healthy subjects, stiripentol (500 mg twice daily on day one, 1 g twice daily on day 2, and 1.5 g twice daily from day 3 to 13) did not affect the metabolism of dextromethorphan.[1] Dextromethorphan is used as a probe drug to assess the activity of CYP2D6, and this study therefore suggests that stiripentol does not have a clinically relevant effect on drugs metabolised by this isoenzyme.

(d) CYP3A4 substrates

In a study, 12 healthy subjects were given **dextromethorphan** before and after stiripentol (500 mg twice daily on day one, 1 g twice daily on day 2, and 1.5 g twice daily on days 3 to 13). Although dextromethorphan is usually used as a probe drug for CYP2D6, its metabolism by *N*-demethylation can be used as a measure of CYP3A4 activity. This study found that stiripentol does inhibit dextromethorphan *N*-demethylation, and therefore suggests that stiripentol might inhibit CYP3A4.[1] The manufacturer of stiripentol therefore predicts that there might be an increased risk of adverse effects when drugs metabolised by this isoenzyme are also taken, and that dose adjustment might be required. They specifically name the **HIV-protease inhibitors**, **chlorphenamine**, **calcium-channel blockers**, **atorvastatin**, **simvastatin**, and **oral [hormonal] contraceptives**, and suggest caution if these drugs are required. However, for the lack of effect of stiripentol on saquinavir pharmacokinetics, see 'HIV-protease inhibitors + Stiripentol', p.943.

The manufacturer of stiripentol also advises caution if drugs that have a narrow therapeutic index and are metabolised by CYP3A4 are given with stiripentol. They name **tacrolimus**, **ciclosporin** and **sirolimus**.

The manufacturer of stiripentol also suggests that ergotism could occur if **ergot derivatives** are taken with stiripentol, with the possibility of necrosis of the extremities, and recommend that ergot preparations are not taken with stiripentol unless strictly necessary.

It is suggested that there might be an increase in the plasma concentrations of benzodiazepines that are substrates of this enzyme (they name **alprazolam**, **midazolam** and **triazolam**), resulting in excessive sedation. Caution is recommended when these drugs are used with stiripentol.[2]

For a list of CYP3A4 substrates, see 'Table 1.10', p.12.

(e) Food

Stiripentol is known to degrade in an acidic environment, and the manufacturer therefore advises that stiripentol is taken with food to avoid exposure to gastric acid. Additionally they advise avoiding milk or dairy products, carbonated drinks, and fruit juice at the same time as stiripentol,[2] but state that they have no evidence of any interaction with milk or dairy products, but have predicted this interaction based on the known ability of dairy products to complex with other drugs.[3]

1. Tran A, Rey E, Pons G, Rousseau M, d'Athis P, Olive G, Mather GG, Bishop FE, Wurden CJ, Labroo R, Trager WF, Kunze KL, Thummel KE, Vincent JC, Gillardin J-M, Lepage F, Levy RH. Influence of stiripentol in cytochrome P450-mediated metabolic pathways in humans: in vitro and in vivo comparison and calculation of in vivo inhibition constants. *Clin Pharmacol Ther* (1997) 62, 490–504.
2. Diacomit (Stiripentol). Biocodex. UK Summary of product characteristics, January 2007.
3. Alan Pharmaceuticals. Personal communication, June 2008.

Stiripentol + Other antiepileptics

Stiripentol causes marked rises in the levels of carbamazepine, clobazam, phenobarbital and phenytoin. Stiripentol causes only a small rise in the levels of valproate. Levetiracetam and topiramate do not appear to interact with stiripentol.

Clinical evidence

(a) Carbamazepine

The clearance of carbamazepine in one subject fell by 39% when stiripentol 1.2 g daily was taken and by 71% when stiripentol 2.4 g daily was taken.[1] Three other studies in adults and children confirmed that stiripentol reduces the clearance of carbamazepine by about 50 to 65%,[2-4] and significantly increases carbamazepine levels.[5] Another study found that the formation of carbamazepine-10,11-epoxide, the active metabolite of carbamazepine, was markedly reduced in children taking carbamazepine with stiripentol.[6]

In 11 patients no adverse effects on motor, perceptual or attention tests were seen when stiripentol was given with other antiepileptic drugs (carbamazepine, **clobazam**, **phenobarbital**, **phenytoin**, and **valproate**) but the doses of carbamazepine, **phenobarbital**, **phenytoin** were reduced before the combination was taken.[7]

(b) Clobazam

In a study, 41 children with myoclonic epilepsy were given valproate and clobazam for one month with stiripentol 50 mg/kg daily or placebo added for a further 2 months. The dose of clobazam was reduced from 0.5 to 0.38 mg/kg daily in those also given stiripentol because of adverse effects. Plasma levels of clobazam and norclobazam were significantly increased, and levels of hydroxynorclobazam significantly decreased, by stiripentol.[8,9]

For a small study suggesting a lack of adverse effects, see under *Carbamazepine*, above.

(c) Phenobarbital

Phenobarbital clearance in 2 subjects fell by about 30 to 40% when they took stiripentol 2.4 g daily.[1] For a further study, see under *Carbamazepine*, above.

(d) Phenytoin

Patients with epilepsy taking two or three antiepileptics (phenytoin, phenobarbital, carbamazepine, clobazam, primidone, nitrazepam) were also given stiripentol, increasing from 600 mg to 2.4 g daily. The 5 patients taking phenytoin had an average 37% reduction in the phenytoin clearance when they took stiripentol 1.2 g daily, and a 78% reduction when they took stiripentol 2.4 g daily. These changes in clearance were reflected in marked rises in the steady-state serum levels of phenytoin: for example the serum phenytoin levels of one patient rose from 14.4 mg/L to 27.4 mg/L over 30 days while he was taking stiripentol, despite a 50% reduction in his phenytoin dose. Phenytoin toxicity was seen in another two subjects.[1] For a further study, see under *Carbamazepine*, above.

(e) Valproate

In a study, 41 children with myoclonic epilepsy were given valproate and clobazam for one month with stiripentol 50 mg/kg daily or placebo for a further 2 months. The dose of valproate did not change from a baseline maximum of 30 mg/kg daily when given with stiripentol.[8,9]

Valproate 1 g daily was given to 8 subjects with or without stiripentol 1.2 g daily. The stiripentol caused a 14% increase in the peak serum levels of valproate.[10] For a small study suggesting a lack of adverse effects, see under *Carbamazepine*, above.

(f) Other antiepileptics

There is no evidence to suggest that a pharmacokinetic interaction will occur between **levetiracetam** or **topiramate** and stiripentol.[11]

Mechanism

Stiripentol inhibits the activity of various cytochrome P450 isoenzymes in the liver, including CYP1A2, CYP2C9, CYP2C19, CYP2D6 and CYP3A4, some of which are concerned with the metabolism of other antiepileptics. As a result the loss of the antiepileptic from the body is reduced and the serum levels rise accordingly.[3,9,12] In the case of valproate, cytochrome P450 is only involved in minor valproate metabolic pathways and therefore only a small rise in serum levels occurs.[10] However, there is evidence that stiripentol may reduce the formation of a minor but hepatotoxic metabolite of valproate (2-propyl-4-pentenoic acid or 4-ene-VPA).[13]

Importance and management

Established and clinically important interactions. The carbamazepine, clobazam, phenobarbital and phenytoin doses should be reduced to avoid the development of elevated serum levels and possible toxicity during the concurrent use of stiripentol. One study[3] suggests that the carbamazepine dose should be decreased incrementally over 7 to 10 days, beginning as soon as the stiripentol is started and, regardless of age, the maintenance dose of carbamazepine should aim to give serum levels of 5 to 10 micrograms/mL.

Stiripentol causes only small changes in the serum levels of valproate and dose adjustments are unlikely to be needed with this combination.

No dose adjustment is needed when stiripentol is given with levetiracetam or topiramate.

1. Levy RH, Loiseau P, Guyot M, Blehaut HM, Tor J, Morland TA. Stiripentol kinetics in epilepsy: nonlinearity and interactions. *Clin Pharmacol Ther* (1984) 36, 661–9.
2. Levy RH, Kerr BM, Farwell J, Anderson GD, Martinez-Lage JM, Tor J. Carbamazepine/stiripentol interaction in adult and pediatric patients. *Epilepsia* (1989) 30, 701.
3. Kerr BM, Martinez-Lage JM, Viteri C, Tor J, Eddy AC, Levy RH. Carbamazepine dose requirements during stiripentol therapy: influence of cytochrome P-450 inhibition by stiripentol. *Epilepsia* (1991) 32, 267–74.
4. Levy RH, Martinez-Lage JM, Tor J, Blehaut H, Gonzalez I, Bainbridge B. Stiripentol level-dose relationship and interaction with carbamazepine in epileptic patients. *Epilepsia* (1985) 26, 544–5.
5. Tran A, Vauzelle-Kervroedan F, Rey E, Pons G. d'Athis P, Chiron C, Dulac O, Renard F, Olive G. Effect of stiripentol on carbamazepine plasma concentration and metabolism in epileptic children. *Eur J Clin Pharmacol* (1996) 50, 497–500.
6. Cazali N, Tran A, Treluyer JM, Rey E, d'Athis P, Vincent J, Pons G. Inhibitory effect of stiripentol on carbamazepine and saquinavir metabolism in human. *Br J Clin Pharmacol* (2003) 56, 526–36.
7. Loiseau P, Strube E, Tor J, Levy RH, Dodrill C. Evaluation neuropsychologique et thérapeutique du stiripentol dans l'épilepsie. *Rev Neurol (Paris)* (1988) 144, 165–72.
8. Chiron C, Marchand MC, Tran A, Rey E, d'Athis P, Vincent J, Dulac O, Pons G, and the STICLO study group. Stiripentol in severe myoclonic epilepsy in infancy: a randomised placebo-controlled syndrome-dedicated trial. *Lancet* (2000) 356, 1638–42.
9. In vitro and in vivo inhibitory effect of stiripentol on clobazam metabolism. Giraud C, Treluyer J-M, Rey E, Chiron C, Vincent J, Pons G, Tran A. *Drug Metab Dispos* (2006) 34, 608–611.
10. Levy RH, Loiseau P, Guyot M, Acheampong A, Tor J, Rettenmeier AW. Effects of stiripentol on valproate plasma level and metabolism. *Epilepsia* (1987) 28, 605.
11. Diacomit (Stiripentol). Biocodex. UK Summary of product characteristics, January 2007.
12. Mather GG, Bishop FE, Trager WF, Kunze KK, Thummel KE, Shen DD, Roskos LK, Lepage F, Gillardin JM, Levy RH. Mechanisms of stiripentol interactions with carbamazepine and phenytoin. *Epilepsia* (1995) 36 (Suppl 3), S162.
13. Levy RH, Rettenmeier AW, Anderson GD, Wilensky AJ, Friel PN, Baillie TA, Acheampong A, Tor J, Guyot M, Loiseau P. Effects of polytherapy with phenytoin, carbamazepine, and stiripentol on formation of 4-ene-valproate, a hepatotoxic metabolite of valproic acid. *Clin Pharmacol Ther* (1990) 48, 225–35.

Tiagabine + Cocaine

Tiagabine does not affect the cardiovascular effects of cocaine, but may attenuate some of its subjective effects.

Clinical evidence, mechanism, importance and management

In a placebo-controlled study, 7 cocaine-users were given two oral doses of tiagabine 4 mg, ten hours apart. Two hours after the second dose they were given an injection of sodium chloride 0.9%, then two doses of cocaine (0.15 mg/kg, and then, 30 minutes later, 0.3 mg/kg). Tiagabine did not affect the cocaine-induced changes in blood pressure and heart rate, but was reported to attenuate some of the subjective effects (stimulation and craving) of cocaine.[1]

The clinical relevance of this findings is unclear, but is does suggest that concurrent use is unlikely to result in adverse cardiac effects.

1. Sofuoglu M, Poling J, Mitchell E, Kosten TR. Tiagabine affects the subjective responses to cocaine in humans. *Pharmacol Biochem Behav* (2005) 82, 569–73.

Tiagabine + Gemfibrozil

An isolated case report describes increased tiagabine concentrations after a single-dose of gemfibrozil.

Clinical evidence, mechanism, importance and management

A case report describes a 39-year-old man stable taking tiagabine 16 mg three times daily with carbamazepine, who developed grade IV hypertriglyceridaemia and started to take gemfibrozil 600 mg twice a day. Within an hour of taking the first dose of gemfibrozil, he experienced generalised weakness and confusion before 'blacking out'. He was poorly responsive to family members for several hours afterwards and presented to hospital the following day. He did not take any further doses of gemfibrozil. On presentation at hospital, all symptoms had resolved, but after other possible reasons for the symptoms were excluded, a drug interaction was suspected and he was admitted for a controlled rechallenge test. The patient was monitored for 3 days, with a single 300-mg dose of gemfibrozil given on day 2. Tiagabine and carbamazepine concentrations were monitored throughout. After gemfibrozil was given, the patient reported lightheadedness, which resolved within a few hours, but about 7 hours later he experienced two brief seizures. His tiagabine concentrations 2 hours and 5 hours after gemfibrozil was taken were 59% and 75% higher, respectively, than the previous day when no gemfibrozil was given. The tiagabine concentrations the day after gemfibrozil were similar to those measured the day before. Unbound tiagabine concentrations were undetectable on days one and 3, but were 29 nanograms/mL and 43 nanograms/mL (corresponding to a free fraction of 11.4% and 13.6%) at 2 hours and 5 hours, respectively, after gemfibrozil was taken. Carbamazepine concentrations did not vary throughout the 3 day period. The authors concluded that the temporal relationship between the lightheadedness and the concurrent use of tiagabine and gemfibrozil, and the pharmacokinetic data, suggest that an interaction occurred, although the mechanism for this is not known. They suggested that protein-binding displacement and displacement from tissue binding site might explain the effect seen.[1] This is an isolated case and as such its general relevance is not clear, but bear the possibility of an interaction in mind if tiagabine and gemfibrozil are used concurrently.

1. Burstein AH, Boudreau EA, Theodore WH. Increase in tiagabine serum concentration with coadministration of gemfibrozil. *Ann Pharmacother* (2009) 43, 379–82.

Tiagabine + Miscellaneous

The pharmacokinetics of tiagabine were not altered by cimetidine or erythromycin. No clinically relevant pharmacokinetic interactions occur between tiagabine and theophylline or warfarin.

Clinical evidence, mechanism, importance and management

In a study in 12 healthy subjects, **cimetidine** 400 mg twice daily for 5 days increased the steady-state AUC of tiagabine 4 mg twice daily by just 5%.[1,2]

In a study in 14 healthy subjects, **erythromycin** 500 mg twice daily had no clinically relevant effect on the steady-state pharmacokinetics of tiagabine 4 mg twice daily.[3]

Multiple dose studies in healthy subjects have also excluded any clinically relevant pharmacokinetic interactions between tiagabine and **theophylline** or **warfarin** but no further study details were given.[1]

1. Mengel H, Jansen JA, Sommerville K, Jonkman JHG, Wesnes K, Cohen A, Carlson GF, Marshall R, Snel S, Dirach J, Kastberg H. Tiagabine: evaluation of the risk of interaction with theophylline, warfarin, digoxin, cimetidine, oral contraceptives, triazolam, or ethanol. *Epilepsia* (1995) 36 (Suppl 3), S160.
2. Snel S, Jonkman JHG, van Heiningen PNM, Jansen JA, Mengel HB. Tiagabine: evaluation of risk of interaction with cimetidine in healthy male volunteers. *Epilepsia* (1994) 35 (Suppl 7), 74.
3. Thomsen MS, Groes L, Agersø H, Kruse T. Lack of pharmacokinetic interaction between tiagabine and erythromycin. *J Clin Pharmacol* (1998) 38, 1051–6.

Tiagabine + Other antiepileptics

Tiagabine plasma levels are reduced by enzyme-inducing antiepileptics (carbamazepine, phenytoin, phenobarbital and primidone). Tiagabine may cause a slight reduction in valproate levels, but has no effect on carbamazepine, phenytoin or vigabatrin levels.

Clinical evidence, mechanism, importance and management

In an early clinical study, tiagabine was reported to have no significant effect on the plasma levels of **carbamazepine**, **phenytoin**, **valproate**, and **vigabatrin**.[1] Similarly, in 12 patients with epilepsy, tiagabine (titrated from 8 mg up to a maximum of 48 mg daily over 18 days) did not alter the steady-state pharmacokinetics of **phenytoin** or **carbamazepine**.[2] However, in another similar study, tiagabine reduced the AUC of **valproate** by 10%, but this reduction is not expected to be clinically significant.[3]

A study in patients taking 1 to 3 other enzyme-inducing antiepileptics (**phenobarbital, phenytoin, carbamazepine, primidone**) found that tiagabine half-lives were shorter (3.8 to 4.9 hours) when compared with historical values in healthy subjects taking tiagabine alone (7.1 hours).[4] The manufacturers say that the plasma concentrations of tiagabine may be reduced 1.5- to 3-fold by these enzyme-inducing antiepileptics.[5] Based on this, they recommend that the initial maintenance dose of tiagabine in patients *not* taking enzyme-inducing drugs should be lower (15 to 30 mg daily) than in those taking these drugs (30 to 45 mg daily).[5]

1. Richens A, Chadwick DW, Duncan JS, Dam M, Gram L, Mikkelsen M, Morrow J, Mengel H, Shu V, McKelvy JF, Pierce MW. Adjunctive treatment of partial seizures with tiagabine: a placebo-controlled trial. *Epilepsy Res* (1995) 21, 37–42.
2. Gustavson LE, Cato A, Boellner SW, Cao GX, Qian JX, Guenther HJ, Sommerville KW. Lack of pharmacokinetic drug interactions between tiagabine and carbamazepine or phenytoin. *Am J Ther* (1998) 5, 9–16.
3. Gustavson LE, Sommerville KW, Boellner SW, Witt GF, Guenther HJ, Granneman GR. Lack of a clinically significant pharmacokinetic drug interaction between tiagabine and valproate. *Am J Ther* (1998) 5, 73–79.
4. So EL, Wolff D, Graves NM, Leppik IE, Cascino GD, Pixton GC, Gustavson LE. Pharmacokinetics of tiagabine as add-on therapy in patients taking enzyme-inducing drugs. *Epilepsy Res* (1995) 22, 221–6.
5. Gabitril (Tiagabine). Cephalon (UK) Ltd. UK Summary of product characteristics, June 2009.

Topiramate + Azoles

An isolated case report describes topiramate toxicity after posaconazole was added.

Clinical evidence

A case report describes a 48-year-old man taking topiramate 100 mg twice daily and valproate 700 mg twice daily, who was admitted to hospital with a 10-day history of worsening stupor, daytime somnolence, anorexia, decreased oral intake and weight loss. About 4 days before the onset of symptoms, he had started posaconazole 200 mg four times daily but this was discontinued 2 days before admission. On admission his topiramate concentrations were 27.34 micromols/L (about 5 times that expected from a 100 mg dose) and he was started on intravenous amphotericin B instead of the posaconazole. During the 10 days after admission his symptoms slowly resolved, and 11 days after the posaconazole had been stopped, his topiramate concentration had fallen to 11.5 micromols/L. Valproate concentrations were found to be within the therapeutic range at all times during his admission. The patient completed a course of **voriconazole** (details not provided) without any complications. The authors attributed the symptoms to topiramate toxicity as a result of an interaction with posaconazole. They ruled out the possibility of hyperammonemic encephalopathy due to the concurrent use of topiramate and valproate (see 'Topiramate + Valproate', p.617, for description of some cases), because the patient had been taking this combination for many years without evidence of encephalopathy.[1]

Mechanism

The authors suggest that the raised topiramate concentrations were due to inhibition of CYP3A4 by posaconazole.[1] However, the uneventful use of **voriconazole**, a more potent inhibitor of CYP3A4 than posaconazole, might suggest that other mechanisms are involved. Further study is needed.

Importance and management

Evidence for an interaction between posaconazole and topiramate is limited to an isolated case and therefore the general clinical importance of this interaction is unknown. It might be worth bearing in mind in cases of suspected topiramate toxicity in patients also taking posaconazole. There does not appear to be any evidence regarding the use of other azoles with topiramate.

1. Marriott D, Levy D, Doyle T, Ray J. Posaconazole-induced topiramate toxicity. *Ann Intern Med* (2009) 151, 143.

Topiramate + Carbamazepine and related drugs

Topiramate concentrations might be reduced by carbamazepine and oxcarbazepine. Eslicarbazepine causes a small decrease in topiramate exposure. Carbamazepine pharmacokinetics are not affected by topiramate. However, one report suggests that the toxicity seen when topiramate is added to maximum tolerated doses of carbamazepine might respond to a reduction in the carbamazepine dose. The pharmacokinetics of eslicarbazepine are not affected by topiramate.

Clinical evidence

(a) Carbamazepine

In a study in 12 patients with epilepsy, topiramate titrated up to a maximum of 400 mg twice daily had no effect on the steady-state plasma concentrations of carbamazepine 300 to 800 mg every 8 hours or its main metabolite, carbamazepine-10,11-epoxide.[1] An earlier study in patients with epilepsy also reported that topiramate does not affect the pharmacokinetics of carbamazepine.[2] In contrast, another report describes 2 patients taking a maximum tolerated dose of carbamazepine who started treatment with topiramate and subsequently developed symptoms suggestive of carbamazepine toxicity. In both these cases, the symptoms resolved when the carbamazepine dose was reduced, and this enabled continued titration of the topiramate dose in one patient. A review of the clinical use of these two drugs found another 23 cases that fitted this pattern. Carbamazepine concentrations were not reported.[3]

In a study in 12 patients with epilepsy, the topiramate plasma concentration and AUC were found to be about 40% lower in the presence of carbamazepine.[1] Similarly, a population pharmacokinetic study in patients taking topiramate, reported that the 120 patients taking concurrent carbamazepine had a 41% lower topiramate serum concentration than patients taking topiramate alone (28 patients).[4] In a study in healthy subjects, carbamazepine 600 mg daily was found to cause a 2-fold increase in the clearance of a single 200-mg dose of topiramate. The mean half-life of topiramate decreased from 29 hours to 19 hours. There was also a 2- to 3-fold increase in the formation of the two major metabolites of topiramate (2,3-diol-topiramate and 10-hydroxy-topiramate), although 41% of topiramate was excreted unchanged in the urine in the presence of carbamazepine.[5] The same group have reported similar results in a study in patients.[6] In contrast, an earlier study reported that carbamazepine did not have a major effect on the pharmacokinetics of topiramate.[2]

(b) Eslicarbazepine

In a pharmacokinetic study in 16 healthy subjects, the pharmacokinetics of eslicarbazepine (given as 600 mg daily on days one and 2, and 1.2 g daily from day 3 to 27) were not affected by topiramate (given as 100 mg daily on days 9 and 10, and 200 mg daily from day 11 to day 27).[7] In the same study, the AUC of topiramate was decreased by 18% by eslicarbazepine, which was borderline in terms of bioequivalence.[7] A population pharmacokinetic model using data from 641 patients enrolled in phase III eslicarbazepine studies, predicted that topiramate clearance was increased by up to 16% by eslicarbazepine but eslicarbazepine pharmacokinetics were not affected by topiramate.[8]

(c) Oxcarbazepine

In a population pharmacokinetic study in patients taking topiramate, the 52 patients also taking oxcarbazepine had 30% lower topiramate serum concentrations than those taking topiramate alone (28 patients).[4]

Mechanism

Carbamazepine, and possibly oxcarbazepine, appear to induce the metabolism of topiramate. Although topiramate can weakly induce CYP3A4 this does not usually appear to have a clinically relevant effect on carbamazepine metabolism, unless carbamazepine is already at the maximum tolerated dose. The increase in topiramate clearance by carbamazepine might be partly due to the stimulation of oxidative pathways resulting in the formation of 2,3-diol-topiramate and 10-hydroxy-topiramate.[6] The decreased exposure to topiramate seen with eslicarbazepine has been suggested to be due to an effect on topiramate absorption, as the half-life of topiramate was unaffected.[7]

Importance and management

The modest reduction in the topiramate plasma concentration seen on the concurrent use of carbamazepine is probably of limited clinical importance and topiramate dose adjustments would not be expected to be necessary. There is some evidence that the toxicity seen when topiramate is added to maximum tolerated doses of carbamazepine might respond to a reduction in the carbamazepine dose. Similarly, limited evidence with oxcarbazepine suggests that topiramate concentrations are reduced on concurrent use, but probably not to a clinically relevant extent and it would seem unlikely that a topiramate dose adjustment would be necessary. Eslicarbazepine does not affect topiramate pharmacokinetics to a clinically relevant extent and eslicarbazepine pharmacokinetics are not affected by topiramate, so no dose adjustments are considered necessary on concurrent use.

1. Sachdeo RC, Sachdeo SK, Walker SA, Kramer LD, Nayak RK, Doose DR. Steady-state pharmacokinetics of topiramate and carbamazepine in patients with epilepsy during monotherapy and concomitant therapy. *Epilepsia* (1996) 37, 774–80.
2. Wilensky AJ, Ojemann LM, Chemelir T, Margul BL, Doose DR. Topiramate pharmacokinetics in epileptic patients receiving carbamazepine. *Epilepsia* (1989) 30, 645–6.
3. Mack CJ, Kuc S, Mulcrone SA, Pilley A, Grünewald RA. Interaction of topiramate with carbamazepine: two case reports and a review of clinical experience. *Seizure* (2002) 11, 464–7.
4. May TW, Rambeck B, Jürgens U. Serum concentrations of topiramate in patients with epilepsy: influence of dose, age and comedication. *Ther Drug Monit* (2002) 24, 366–74.
5. Britzi M, Perucca E, Soback S, Levy RH, Fattore C, Crema F, Gatti G, Doose DR, Maryanoff BE, Bialer M. Pharmacokinetic and metabolic investigation of topiramate disposition in healthy subjects in the absence and in the presence of enzyme induction by carbamazepine. *Epilepsia* (2005) 46, 378–84.
6. Mimrod D, Specchio LM, Britzi M, Perucca E, Specchio N, La Neve A, Soback S, Levy RH, Gatti G, Doose DR, Maryanoff BE, Bialer M. A comparative study of the effect of carbamazepine and valproic acid on the pharmacokinetics and metabolic profile of topiramate at steady state in patients with epilepsy. *Epilepsia* (2005) 46, 1046–54.
7. Nunes T, Sicard E, Almeida L, Falcão A, Rocha JF, Brunet JS, Lefebvre M, Soares-da-Silva P. Pharmacokinetic interaction study between eslicarbazepine acetate and topiramate in healthy subjects. *Curr Med Res Opin* (2010) 26, 1355–62.
8. Falcão A, Fuseau E, Nunes T, Almeida A, Soares-da-Silva P. Pharmacokinetics, drug interactions and exposure-response relationship of eslicarbazepine acetate in adult patients with partial-onset seizures: population pharmacokinetic and pharmacokinetic/pharmacodynamic analyses. *CNS Drugs* (2012) 26, 79–91.

Topiramate + Phenobarbital or Primidone

Topiramate appears not to alter the pharmacokinetics of phenobarbital or primidone. Phenobarbital modestly reduces topiramate levels.

Clinical evidence, mechanism, importance and management

A review of data from double-blind, placebo-controlled studies found that over periods of 8 to 12 weeks the plasma levels of phenobarbital or primidone in patients (number not stated) with partial seizures remained unchanged when they were also given topiramate.[1]

A population pharmacokinetic study reported that patients taking phenobarbital had 31% lower morning topiramate levels than patients not taking enzyme-inducing antiepileptics.[2] Another study that grouped carbamazepine, phenobarbital and phenytoin reported that patients taking one or more of these drugs had a 50% greater topiramate clearance than patients taking lamotrigine or valproate.[3]

Phenobarbital probably induces the metabolism of topiramate thereby reducing its levels. When topiramate is added to existing treatment with phenytoin or phenobarbital its dose should be titrated to effect and therefore any interaction is automatically accounted for. If phenobarbital or primidone are withdrawn or added to established treatment with topiramate, be aware that the dose of topiramate may need adjustment.

1. Doose DR, Walker SA, Pledger G, Lim P, Reife RA. Evaluation of phenobarbital and primidone/phenobarbital (primidone's active metabolite) plasma concentrations during administration of add-on topiramate therapy in five multicenter, double-blind, placebo-controlled trials in outpatients with partial seizures. *Epilepsia* (1995) 36 (Suppl 3), S158.
2. May TW, Jürges U. Serum concentrations of topiramate in epileptic patients: the influence of dose and comedication. *Epilepsia* (1999) 40 (Suppl 2), 249.
3. Contin M, Riva R, Albani F, Avoni P, Baruzzi A. Topiramate therapeutic monitoring in patients with epilepsy: effect of concomitant antiepileptic drugs. *Ther Drug Monit* (2002) 24, 332–7.

Topiramate + Phenytoin

In some patients the plasma levels of phenytoin are slightly raised by topiramate, and topiramate plasma levels may be reduced by phenytoin.

Clinical evidence

Topiramate, titrated to a maximum of 400 mg twice daily, was given to 12 patients with epilepsy taking phenytoin 260 to 600 mg daily. When the maximum tolerated dose of topiramate was reached, the phenytoin dose was then reduced, and in some cases phenytoin was subsequently discontinued. Topiramate clearance was assessed in 2 patients and was found to be increased two- to threefold by phenytoin.[1] Similarly, a population pharmacokinetic study reported that patients taking phenytoin and topiramate had 50% lower morning topiramate levels than patients not taking enzyme-inducing antiepileptics.[2]

In the first study above, 3 of the 12 patients had a decrease in phenytoin clearance and an increase of 25 to 55% in the AUC of phenytoin when taking topiramate: the other 9 had no changes.[1] This slight increase is said not to be clinically significant based on analyses from six add-on studies.[3]

Mechanism

An *in vitro* study using human liver microsomes found that topiramate does not inhibit most hepatic cytochrome P450 isoenzymes, except for CYP2C19 at high concentrations.[1] This isoenzyme plays a minor role in phenytoin metabolism, but it has been suggested this may become important at high doses of topiramate in patients who are CYP2C9 poor metabolisers,[1] (that is, those lacking this isoenzyme). Phenytoin appears to induce the metabolism of topiramate.

Importance and management

The interaction between topiramate and phenytoin appears to be established, and topiramate dose adjustments may be required if phenytoin is added or discontinued. No reduction in the phenytoin dose seems necessary in the majority of patients, but be aware that a few patients may have increased phenytoin levels, particularly at high topiramate doses. Monitor for phenytoin adverse effects (e.g. blurred vision, nystagmus, ataxia or drowsiness), take phenytoin levels if these occur, and adjust the dose of phenytoin accordingly.

1. Sachdeo RC, Sachdeo SK, Levy RH, Streeter AJ, Bishop FE, Kunze KL, Mather GG, Roskos LK, Shen DD, Thummel KE, Trager WF, Curtin CR, Doose DR, Gisclon LG, Bialer M. Topiramate and phenytoin pharmacokinetics during repetitive monotherapy and combination therapy to epileptic patients. *Epilepsia* (2002) 43: 691–6.
2. May TW, Jürges U. Serum concentrations of topiramate in epileptic patients: the influence of dose and comedication. *Epilepsia* (1999) 40 (Suppl, 2), 249.
3. Johannessen SI. Pharmacokinetics and interaction profile of topiramate: review and comparison with other newer antiepileptic drugs. *Epilepsia* (1997) 38 (Suppl 1), S18–S23.

Topiramate + Valproate

Encephalopathy has been reported in patients given topiramate with valproate. Two studies found no clinically relevant pharmacokinetic interaction between topiramate and valproate.

Clinical evidence, mechanism, importance and management

Five patients with severe epilepsy developed stuporous encephalopathy with marked cognitive impairment when taking topiramate with valproate. A further patient experienced this effect when taking topiramate alone. Four of the patients had hyperammonaemia which resolved when topiramate or valproate was withdrawn. The toxicity was possibly due to a synergistic effect of valproate and topiramate on liver ornithine metabolism resulting in hyperammonaemia. It was also possible that the encephalopathy was due to topiramate toxicity in at-risk patients, such as those with pre-existing chronic encephalopathy.[1]

In a study in 12 patients with epilepsy, the pharmacokinetics of both topiramate, titrated to 400 mg twice daily, and valproate 1 to 4.5 g daily were slightly changed by concurrent use. The topiramate AUC was raised by about 18%, and the valproate AUC was reduced by about 11%, but these changes were not considered to be clinically relevant.[2] However, the proportion of various metabolites of valproate was altered by topiramate: metabolism to 4-ene-valproate (a putative hepatotoxin) and metabolism by oxidation increased, whereas conjugation decreased.[2] Similar changes have been seen with other enzyme-inducing antiepileptics (see *Mechanism* in 'Phenytoin + Valproate', p.609). Another study in patients with epilepsy found that valproate did not have any clinically significant effects on topiramate pharmacokinetics and metabolism.[3]

The pharmacokinetic studies suggest that dose adjustments are not required during concurrent use.[2] However, the report of encephalopathy with topiramate and valproate indicates that, particularly for at-risk patients such as those with pre-existing encephalopathy, careful monitoring is advisable.[1]

1. Latour P, Biraben A, Polard E, Bentué-Ferrer D, Beauplet A, Tribut O, Allain H. Drug induced encephalopathy in six epileptic patients: topiramate? valproate? or both? *Hum Psychopharmacol Clin Exp* (2004) 19, 193–203.
2. Rosenfeld WE, Liao S, Kramer LD, Anderson G, Palmer M, Levy RH, Nayak RK. Comparison of the steady-state pharmacokinetics of topiramate and valproate in patients with epilepsy during monotherapy and concomitant therapy. *Epilepsia* (1997) 38, 324–33.
3. Mimrod D, Specchio LM, Britzi M, Perucca E, Specchio N, La Neve A, Soback S, Levy RH, Gatti G, Doose DR, Maryanoff BE, Bialer M. A comparative study of the effect of carbamazepine and valproic acid on the pharmacokinetics and metabolic profile of topiramate at steady state in patients with epilepsy. *Epilepsia* (2005) 46, 1046–54.

Valproate + Acarbose

An isolated case report describes reduced valproate levels in a patient taking acarbose.

Clinical evidence, mechanism, importance and management

A patient with epilepsy taking sodium valproate for 10 years had a 40% reduction in his normally stable valproate levels, from 67 micrograms/mL to 40.5 micrograms/mL, when acarbose was added. No other drugs were being taken. When the acarbose was stopped and then restarted, the valproate levels rose and then fell once again. The reason for this effect is not understood but the authors of the report suggest that acarbose possibly reduces the absorption of valproate.[1] This is an isolated report and its general importance is unknown, but it would seem prudent to be alert for any evidence of reduced effects if acarbose is given to a patient taking valproate.

1. Serrano JS, Jiménez CM, Serrano MI, Garrido H, Balboa B. May acarbose impair valproate bioavailability? *Methods Find Exp Clin Pharmacol* (1996) 18 (Suppl C), 98.

Valproate + Allopurinol

Allopurinol appears not to alter the levels of valproate.

Clinical evidence, mechanism, importance and management

A study investigating allopurinol in refractory epilepsy found that allopurinol (150 mg daily in those less than 20 kg, and 300 mg daily for other patients), given for 4 months, had no effect on valproate levels in 28 patients taking antiepileptics including valproate.[1] In another similar study, allopurinol 10 mg/kg increased to 15 mg/kg daily for 12 weeks had no effect on serum valproate levels in 6 patients taking antiepileptics including valproate.[2] Therefore valproate dose alterations are unlikely to be required if allopurinol is used.

1. Zagnoni PG, Bianchi A, Zolo P, Canger R, Cornaggia C, D'Alessandro P, DeMarco P, Pisani F, Gianelli M, Verzé L, Viani F, Zaccara G. Allopurinol as add-on therapy in refractory epilepsy: a double-blind placebo-controlled randomized study. *Epilepsia* (1994) 35, 107–12.
2. Coppola G, Pascotto A. Double-blind, placebo-controlled, cross-over trial of allopurinol as add-on therapy in childhood refractory epilepsy. *Brain Dev* (1996) 18, 50–2.

Valproate + Antacids

The absorption of valproate was slightly, but not significantly, increased by an aluminium/magnesium hydroxide suspension, but was not affected by magnesium trisilicate or a calcium carbonate suspension.

Clinical evidence, mechanism, importance and management

In 7 healthy subjects the AUC of a single 500-mg dose of valproic acid, given one hour after breakfast, was increased by 12% (range 3 to 28%) by 62 mL of an **aluminium/magnesium hydroxide** suspension (*Maalox*) given with and 2 hours after valproate. Neither **magnesium trisilicate** suspension (*Trisogel*) nor **calcium carbonate** suspension (*Titralac*) had a significant effect on valproate absorption.[1] No special precautions would seem necessary during concurrent use.

1. May CA, Garnett WR, Small RE, Pellock JM. Effects of three antacids on the bioavailability of valproic acid. *Clin Pharm* (1982) 1, 244–7.

Valproate + Aspirin or NSAIDs

Valproate toxicity developed in several young patients given large and repeated doses of aspirin and in an elderly patient taking low-dose aspirin. Increased levels of free valproate were found in a number of children within hours of them taking aspirin. Conversely, a slightly reduced valproate level was reported in one patient who took ibuprofen. Modestly altered protein binding has been shown when sodium valproate was given with diflunisal or naproxen.

Clinical evidence, mechanism, importance and management

(a) Aspirin

A 17-year-old girl taking valproate 21 mg/kg daily was prescribed aspirin 18 mg/kg daily for lupus arthritis. Within a few days she developed a disabling tremor which disappeared when the aspirin was stopped. Total serum valproate levels were not significantly changed, but the free fraction fell from 24% to 14% when the aspirin was withdrawn. Similar toxic reactions (tremor, nystagmus, drowsiness, ataxia) were seen in 2 children, aged 6 and 4 years, given 12 and 20 mg/kg aspirin every 4 hours while taking valproate.[1] In 5 children with epilepsy taking valproate, free valproate levels increased by 31 to 66% (average 49%) 17 hours after starting aspirin 11.5 to 16.9 mg/kg four times daily.[2]

A 76-year-old man given valproate semisodium 750 mg daily had a total valproate blood level of 13.5 nanograms/mL, which rose to 19.3 nanograms/mL after aspirin 325 mg daily was added. The valproate semisodium dose was increased over a period of 2 months in an attempt to increase levels to the reference range. Two weeks after the dose of valproate semisodium was increased to 2.5 g daily he experienced dizziness and incoordination with difficulty standing and transferring from a bed to a wheelchair and he experienced a fall. It was found that his trough total valproate level was 64 nanograms/mL (reference range 50 to 70 nanograms/mL), but his trough free valproate level was 24.7 nanograms/mL (reference range 4.8 to 17.3 nanograms/mL). Aspirin was discontinued and 5 days later total and free trough valproate levels were 36 nanograms/mL and 3.9 nanograms/mL, respectively. Dizziness and incoordination resolved when the dose of valproate semisodium was reduced to 1.25 g daily.[3]

One case report of fatal hyperammonaemia was speculated to have been induced by valproate, and the authors also considered that concurrent use of aspirin and cimetidine may have contributed.[4]

Aspirin displaces valproate from its protein binding sites[2,3,5] and also alters its metabolism by the liver[6] so that the levels of free (and pharmacologically active) valproate rise. This could temporarily increase both the therapeutic and toxic effects of the valproate. However, there is evidence that increased hepatic elimination of valproate counterbalances this effect.

Direct information seems to be limited to the studies and case reports cited. Clinically relevant interactions appear rare, probably because in most cases the effects of aspirin on free valproate levels cancel each other out. The combination need not necessarily be avoided, but it would seem prudent to be aware of this interaction if valproate and high-dose aspirin are used.

(b) Diflunisal

In 7 healthy subjects, diflunisal 250 mg twice daily for 7 days given with sodium valproate 200 mg twice daily caused a 20% increase in the unbound fraction of valproate. There was a 35% increase in the AUC of one of the oxidation metabolites of valproate, and a small decrease in the AUC of some of the diflunisal glucuronide metabolites. This was due to changes in the renal clearance of these metabolites.[7] Whether any of these modest changes have any clinical relevance remains to be seen, but it appears unlikely.

(c) Ibuprofen

A 15-year-old boy was found to have a subtherapeutic valproate level (43 micrograms/mL) 3 days after starting to take ibuprofen 600 mg every 6 hours for post-fracture analgesia. The ibuprofen was stopped, and after one week the valproate levels were within the therapeutic range (60 micrograms/mL).[8] The general importance of this isolated case is unknown. More study is needed.

(d) Naproxen

A study in 6 healthy subjects found that naproxen 500 mg twice daily moderately decreased the AUC of a single 800-mg dose of sodium valproate by 11%.[9] Similarly, in another study, when naproxen 500 mg twice daily was given with sodium valproate 500 mg twice daily, the AUC of valproate was decreased by 20% and the AUC of naproxen was increased by 7%.[10] It is suggested that naproxen and sodium valproate displace each other from their protein binding sites.[9,10] The clinical relevance of these modest changes is uncertain, but is likely to be small.[9]

1. Goulden KJ, Dooley JM, Camfield PR, Fraser AD. Clinical valproate toxicity induced by acetylsalicylic acid. *Neurology* (1987) 37, 1392–4.
2. Farrell K, Orr JM, Abbott FS, Ferguson S, Sheppard I, Godolphin W, Bruni J. The effect of acetylsalicylic acid on serum free valproate concentrations and valproate clearance in children. *J Pediatr* (1982) 101, 142–4.
3. Sandson NB, Marcucci C, Bourke DL, Smith-Lamacchia R. An interaction between aspirin and valproate: the relevance of plasma protein displacement drug-drug interactions. *Am J Psychiatry* (2006) 163, 1891–6.
4. Ichikawa H, Amano T, Kawabata K, Kushiro M, Wada J, Nagake Y, Makino H. Fatal hyperammonemia in a patient with systemic lupus erythematosus. *Intern Med* (1998) 37, 700–3.
5. Orr JM, Abbott FS, Farrell K, Ferguson S, Sheppard I, Godolphin W. Interaction between valproic acid and aspirin in epileptic children: serum protein binding and metabolic effects. *Clin Pharmacol Ther* (1982) 31, 642–9.
6. Abbott FS, Kassam J, Orr JM, Farrell K. The effect of aspirin on valproic acid metabolism. *Clin Pharmacol Ther* (1986) 40, 94–100.
7. Addison RS, Parker-Scott SL, Eadie MJ, Hooper WD, Dickinson RG. Steady-state dispositions of valproate and diflunisal alone and coadministration to healthy volunteers. *Eur J Clin Pharmacol* (2000) 56, 715–21.
8. Mankin KP, Scanlon M. Side effect of ibuprofen and valproic acid. *Orthopedics* (1998) 21, 264, 270.
9. Grimaldi R, Lecchini S, Crema F, Perucca E. *In vivo* plasma protein binding interaction between valproic acid and naproxen. *Eur J Drug Metab Pharmacokinet* (1984) 9, 359–63.
10. Addison RS, Parker-Scott SL, Hooper WD, Eadie MJ, Dickinson RG. Effect of naproxen co-administration on valproate disposition. *Biopharm Drug Dispos* (2000) 21, 235–42.

Valproate + Bile-acid binding resins

Colestyramine causes a small reduction in the absorption of valproate. No interaction occurs if administration of the drugs is separated by 3 hours. Colesevelam does not interact with valproate.

Clinical evidence

(a) Colesevelam

In a study in 26 healthy subjects, colesevelam 4.5 g had no effect on the pharmacokinetics of a single 250-mg dose of valproic acid.[1]

(b) Colestyramine

In a study, 6 healthy subjects were given a single 250-mg dose of valproic acid either alone, at the same time as colestyramine 4 g twice daily, or 3 hours before colestyramine. The bioavailability of valproate taken alone and when separated from the colestyramine by 3 hours remained the same. When the valproate was taken at the same time as the colestyramine, the valproate AUC fell by 15% and its maximum serum levels fell by 21%.[2]

Mechanism

Colestyramine is an ion-exchange resin intended to bind with bile acids in the gut, but it can also bind with drugs, leading to a reduction in their absorption. This apparently occurs to a limited extent with valproate.

Importance and management

Direct information about an interaction between colestyramine and valproate appears to be limited to this single study. The fall in the bioavailability is small and probably of very limited clinical importance, but the interaction can apparently be totally avoided by separating administration by 3 hours so that admixture in the gut is minimised. Colesevelam does not appear to interact with valproate.

1. Donovan JM, Stypinski D, Stiles MR, Olson TA, Burke SK. Drug interactions with colesevelam hydrochloride, a novel, potent lipid-lowering agent. *Cardiovasc Drugs Ther* (2000) 14, 681–90.
2. Malloy MJ, Ravis WR, Pennell AT, Diskin CJ. Effect of cholestyramine resin on single dose valproate pharmacokinetics. *Int J Clin Pharmacol Ther* (1996) 34, 208–11.

Valproate + Carbapenems

Doripenem, ertapenem, imipenem, meropenem, and panipenem with betamipron can dramatically decrease the serum concentration of valproate. Seizures have occurred in some patients taking valproate with a carbapenem.

Clinical evidence

A large number of case reports, and a few studies, describe decreases in valproate concentrations on concurrent use with **doripenem**, **ertapenem**, **imipenem**, **meropenem**, and **panipenem** with betamipron, which are often very large and might result in concentrations so low as to be undetectable. Seizures might also occur. The cases and studies are summarised in 'Table 14.3', p.619.

In addition, in a retrospective study of 39 patients who were given valproate and **meropenem**, 10 of these were started on valproate while already receiving meropenem. Therapeutic valproate concentrations could not be achieved despite adequate loading and maintenance doses (mean 21 mg/kg and 31.5 mg/kg, respectively).[1] Clinical assessment of the interaction in 20 of the patients found worsening seizures, epileptic activity on an EEG, or both in 11 patients (55%). Similarly, a prospective study found that in 5 patients started simultaneously on valproate and **meropenem**, it was not possible to achieve therapeutic valproate concentrations during concurrent use.[2] This was also seen in a 47-year-old patient receiving **ertapenem** and started on oral valproate 400 mg three times daily. Her valproate concentration was less than 1 mg/L after 11 days of concurrent use, but increased to 33.6 mg/L 3 days after ertapenem was stopped.[3]

One report suggests that the magnitude of the interaction with **meropenem** (average 89% reduction in valproate concentrations) might be greater than that with **imipenem** or **panipenem** (average 52% reduction in valproate concentrations).[4] However, other cases have described larger decreases in valproate concentrations with both imipenem and panipenem, see 'Table 14.3', p.619.

In stark contrast to all of the above reports, a 49-year-old patient with liver cirrhosis achieved therapeutic valproate concentrations while receiving **meropenem**, and when the meropenem was stopped, valproate concentrations remained therapeutic. The authors note that the patient's liver disease might have contributed to this finding.[5] Another unusual case describes the resolution of a greatly decreased valproate concentration in a 68-year-old man while receiving **meropenem**, who had previously received **ertapenem**. During the first day of ertapenem treatment, his valproate concentration decreased by 90% but gradually increased, and eventually returned to within the therapeutic range, within a few days of switching from ertapenem to meropenem.[6]

Mechanism

Unknown and the subject of much debate. A number of mechanisms have been proposed, including accelerated renal excretion,[7] altered protein binding,[8] increased distribution of valproate into erythrocytes,[9] decreased intestinal absorption,[10] and enhanced glucuronidation of valproate.[1] However, decreased hydrolysis of the metabolite of valproate (valproate glucuronide), as a result of inhibition of the hydrolytic enzyme by carbapenems,[1,11] appears to be the most plausible explanation. One study found that the enzyme responsible for the hydrolysis of the valproate glucuronide metabolite was acylpeptide hydrolase, and that its activity was inhibited by panipenem *in vitro*.[12] Meropenem has also been shown to inhibit this enzyme *in vitro*.[13]

Importance and management

Evidence for an interaction between valproate and the carbapenems is extensive, such that an interaction is established and of clinical importance. The outcome of concurrent use can be severe, with an increase in seizure frequency reported fairly commonly. The magnitude of the reduction in plasma valproate concentrations can be considerable, resulting in concentrations of less than 1 microgram/mL in several cases. Furthermore the interaction often occurs within a just few days of concurrent use, and is not always successfully managed by an increase in the valproate dose. Therefore it would seem prudent to avoid the concurrent use of a carbapenem in a patient taking valproate.

1. Spriet I, Goyens J, Meersseman W, Wilmer A, Willems L, Van Paesschen W. Interaction between valproate and meropenem: a retrospective study. *Ann Pharmacother* (2007) 41, 1130–6.
2. Mink S, Muroi C, Seule M, Bjeljac M, Keller E. Levetiracetam compared to valproic acid: plasma concentration levels, adverse effects and interactions in aneurismal subarachnoid hemorrhage. *Clin Neurol Neurosurg* (2011) 113, 644–8.

Table 14.3 Summary of the evidence for an interaction between valproate and carbapenems

Year (study or case report)	*Patient(s)*	*Valproate dose and route (where known)*	*Carbapenem dose (duration before event†)*	*Change in valproate concentration‡*	*Breakthrough seizures?*	*Management and notes*	*Refs*
Doripenem							
2011 (case report)	54-year-old	750 mg daily orally	500 mg three times daily (2 days)	62% decrease	No	Valproate concentration remained low, despite additional intravenous bolus doses, for the duration of doripenem. Two days after stopping doripenem, and receiving further intravenous bolus doses of valproate, the valproate concentration was therapeutic	1
	54-year-old	1250 mg three times daily intravenously	500 mg three times daily (36 hours)	69% decrease	No	Valproate concentration remained low throughout doripenem administration, but valproate dose was not increased due to no seizure activity. Patient later died	
Ertapenem							
2009 (study)	49-year-old	7.5 mg/kg daily intravenously	1 g daily (2 days)	81% decrease	Yes		2
2012 (study)	2 patients	Variable orally and intravenously	1 g daily	Average 74% decrease	Yes in 1 patient		3
2007 (case report)	41-year-old	2 g daily orally	1 g daily (7 days)	46% decrease	Yes	Despite a valproate intravenous bolus dose and an oral dose increase, his valproate concentration decreased further (92%) on day 11. His valproate concentration increased to greater than baseline levels during the 5 days after ertapenem was stopped	4
2006 (case report)	80-year-old	1100 mg daily enterally	1 g daily (4 days)	49% decrease	No	During the 11 days following ertapenem discontinuation and a change to intravenous valproate, her concentration returned to therapeutic levels	5
2010 (case report)	72-year-old	400 mg three times daily either intravenously or orally, depending on the patient's condition	500 mg daily (6 days)	<1 mg/L	Yes	About 10 days after ertapenem was stopped, and the dose of valproate increased to 1600 mg daily, valproate plasma concentrations increased to acceptable therapeutic concentrations	6
Imipenem							
2009 (study)	28-year-old	25 mg/kg daily intravenously	500 mg four times daily (1 day)	39% decrease	Yes		2
2012 (study)	1 patient	720 mg daily orally	4 g daily (25 days)	73% decrease	No		3
2005 (case report)	36-year-old	800 mg daily orally	500 mg twice daily (5 days)	43% decrease	No		7
	58-year-old	200 mg three times daily orally	500 mg twice daily (7 days)	51% decrease	No		
2006 (case report)	46-year-old	2 g daily intravenously	Not stated	45% decrease	Yes		8
2007 (case report)	51-year-old	1 g daily	Not stated	71% decrease	No		9
	28-year-old	1.2 g daily	Not stated	34% decrease	No		

† Stated as duration before the event (change in valproate concentration) first occurred.
‡ Stated as either the overall change or the maximum change seen during the course of the carbapenem.
* Based on the valproate concentrations of 3 out of the 4 patients. In the fourth patient there was no difference in valproate concentrations, but, an additional bolus dose of valproate resulted in no change in concentrations, and there was an increase in valproate concentrations after meropenem was discontinued, indicating an effect.

Continued

Table 14.3 Summary of the evidence for an interaction between valproate and carbapenems (continued)

Year (study or case report)	*Patient(s)*	*Valproate dose and route (where known)*	*Carbapenem dose (duration before event†)*	*Change in valproate concentration‡*	*Breakthrough seizures?*	*Management and notes*	*Refs*
Meropenem							
2007 (study)	29 patients	Mean 1.6 g daily	Mean 2.7 g daily (1 day)	Average 66% decrease (range 34 to 92%)	Unknown	In all patients the meropenem was started while the patient was already receiving valproate. For discussion of starting valproate in patients already receiving meropenem, and the clinical effect of combined use on seizure activity, see Valproate + Carbapenems, p.618	10
2009 (study)	36 patients	Mean 2 g daily	Mean 4.9 g daily	81% decrease	Unknown	In the 8 to 14 days following discontinuation of the meropenem, valproate concentrations increased to levels that were comparable with those measured prior to meropenem initiation. No association was found between meropenem dose and size of decrease in valproate concentrations	11
2009 (study)	4 patients (47 to 67-years-old)	Average 16 mg/kg daily intravenously	Average 1625 mg daily (4 to 48 hours)	Average 55% decrease*	Yes		2
2011 (study)	6 patients	Target dose of 3 g/24 hours intravenously, then enterally	Not stated (3 days)	71% decrease	Unknown		12
2012 (study)	3 patients	900 mg to 1.8 g daily orally	2 to 6 g daily (4 to 6 days)	Average 88.7% decrease	No		3
2012 (study)	13 patients	Not stated	Not stated	73.6 to 96.3% decrease	Unknown	Retrospective study of therapeutic drug monitoring records	13
	13 patients	Not stated	Not stated	49.1 to 88.4% decrease	Unknown	Prospective study	
2003 (case report)	71-year-old	500 mg three times daily enterally	1 g three times daily (9 days)	75% decrease	Yes		14
	24-year-old	800 mg twice daily, then 500 mg twice daily, enterally	1 g three times daily (4 days)	Undetectable	No	Valproate concentration was 69 micrograms/mL about 6 weeks prior to meropenem, and returned to a similar level after it was stopped	
2007 (case report)	56-year-old	900 mg daily	Not stated	91% decrease	No		9
	79-year-old	1.2 g daily	Not stated	88% decrease	No		
	80-year-old	1 g daily	Not stated	88% decrease	No		
	28-year-old	1.2 g daily	Not stated	89% decrease	No	Note that this patient had received imipenem prior to meropenem	
1998 (case report)	65-year-old	1200 mg daily intravenously	1 g three times daily (1 day)	About 50% decrease	No		15
	57-year-old	Not stated	Not stated (1 day)	89% decrease	No	Valproate concentration decreased despite additional dosing	
2004 (case report)	15-year-old	800 mg then 400 mg four times a day intravenously	Not stated (2 days)	80% decrease	Yes		16

† Stated as duration before the event (change in valproate concentration) first occurred.
‡ Stated as either the overall change or the maximum change seen during the course of the carbapenem.
* Based on the valproate concentrations of 3 out of the 4 patients. In the fourth patient there was no difference in valproate concentrations, but, an additional bolus dose of valproate resulted in no change in concentrations, and there was an increase in valproate concentrations after meropenem was discontinued, indicating an effect.

Continued

Table 14.3 Summary of the evidence for an interaction between valproate and carbapenems (continued)

Year (study or case report)	*Patient(s)*	*Valproate dose and route (where known)*	*Carbapenem dose (duration before event†)*	*Change in valproate concentration‡*	*Breakthrough seizures?*	*Management and notes*	*Refs*
2004 (case report)	14-year-old	50 mg/kg daily	Not stated (2 days)	79% decrease	No	Valproate concentration decreased despite increasing the dose up to 200 mg/kg daily	17
	7-month-old	75 mg/kg daily	Not stated (4 days)	80% decrease	No	Valproate concentration decreased despite increasing the dose up to 130 mg/kg daily	
	14-month-old	75 mg/kg daily	Not stated (3 days)	88% decrease	No	Valproate concentration decreased despite increasing the dose up to 150 mg/kg daily	
2005 (case report)	30-year-old	150 mg/hour intravenously	8 g daily (36 hours)	72% decrease	No	Valproate concentrations were undetectable after 5 days of meropenem	18
	77-year-old	1 mg/kg per hour intravenously	6 g daily (1 day)	About 50% decrease	No	Valproate dose increases did not increase the concentration, but after meropenem was stopped the valproate concentration returned to pretreatment levels within 2 to 3 days	
2006 (case report)	12-year-old	Various	60 mg/kg daily (6 days)	74% decrease	Unknown		19
	4-year-old	Various	120 mg/kg daily (8 days)	80% decrease	Yes		
2005 (case report)	21-year-old	1 g daily intravenously	1 g three times daily (2 days)	About 87% decrease	Yes	Valproate concentration decreased despite increasing dose, but within 7 days of stopping the meropenem the valproate concentration had returned to pretreatment levels	20
2005 (case report)	9-year-old	200 mg three times daily orally	600 mg three times daily (5 days)	Undetectable	Yes	The valproate concentration decreased from 46.5 to 63.3 mg/L to undetectable levels (not stated), but returned to within the therapeutic range between 3 and 14 days after stopping the meropenem. This same pattern was repeated a month later when meropenem was given again	21
2006 (case report)	50-year-old	1 g daily orally	500 mg twice daily (5 days)	85% decrease	Yes	Valproate concentration decreased despite increasing dose	22
2007 (case report)	60-year-old	Not stated	32 mg/kg daily (1 day)	85%	No	Valproate concentration decreased despite increasing dose, and increased after stopping meropenem but did not return to therapeutic levels	10, 23
	54-year-old	Not stated	28 mg/kg daily (1 day)	72%	No	Valproate concentration decreased despite increasing dose, and increased after stopping meropenem but did not return to therapeutic levels	
2009 (case report)	85-year-old	800 mg daily orally	500 mg three times daily (1 day)	81% decrease	No	First occasion	24
		800 mg daily orally	1 g twice daily (4 days)	74% decrease	Yes	Second occasion. Valproate concentration decreased despite increasing dose and a decreased meropenem dose	
2010 (case report)	46-year-old	3.5 g daily orally	1 g three times daily (about 16 days)	Undetectable	No	Valproate concentration decreased despite increasing dose, and increased after stopping meropenem but did not return to therapeutic levels	25

† Stated as duration before the event (change in valproate concentration) first occurred.
‡ Stated as either the overall change or the maximum change seen during the course of the carbapenem.
* Based on the valproate concentrations of 3 out of the 4 patients. In the fourth patient there was no difference in valproate concentrations, but, an additional bolus dose of valproate resulted in no change in concentrations, and there was an increase in valproate concentrations after meropenem was discontinued, indicating an effect.

Continued

Table 14.3 Summary of the evidence for an interaction between valproate and carbapenems (continued)

Year (study or case report)	*Patient(s)*	*Valproate dose and route (where known)*	*Carbapenem dose (duration before event†)*	*Change in valproate concentration‡*	*Breakthrough seizures?*	*Management and notes*	*Refs*
2009 (case report)	2-month-old	50 g/kg daily orally	Not stated	98.5% decrease	Yes	Valproate was switched to phenobarbital	26
2008 (case report)	25-year-old	1 g daily orally	1 g three times daily (36 hours)	Undetectable	Yes		27
2013 (case report)	14-year-old	750 mg daily orally	Not stated (2 days)	89% decrease	Yes	Meropneem was discontinued but 2 days later she still had seizures and subtherapeutic valproate concentration despite an increased dose and an intravenous loading dose. Valproate concentration returned to that before meropenem 16 days after stopping it	28
2011 (case report)	50-year-old	500 mg twice daily orally	2 g three times daily (72 hours)	Subtherapeutic	Yes	Valproate concentration decreased despite increased dose, but returned to within the therapeutic range 29 days after the meropnem was stopped	29
Panipenem							
2007 (case report)	57-year-old	900 mg daily	Not stated	74% decrease	Yes, day 9		9
1997 (case report)	10-year-old	8.3 mg/kg three times a day orally	20 mg/kg four times a day (16 days)	93% decrease	Yes	The valproate concentration remained low despite a dose increase, but were close to therapeutic levels about 8 days after panipenem was stopped	30
	8-year-old	500 mg daily orally	20 mg/kg three times a day (1 day)	About 97% decrease	Not stated		
	10-year-old	5 mg/kg twice daily orally	20 mg/kg four times a day (2 days)	Not stated	Yes	The valproate concentration was 26.5 mg/L after panipenem was started	
1998 (case report)	3-year-old	35 mg/kg daily enterally	60 mg/kg daily (3 days)	83% decrease	Yes	Valproate concentration decreased despite increasing dose, and started to increase within 24 hours of stopping panipenem	31
	22-year-old	32 mg/kg daily enterally	30 mg/kg daily (2 days)	Undetectable	Yes	Valproate concentration decreased despite increasing dose, and gradually increased after stopping panipenem	
	4-year-old	25 mg/kg daily enterally	60 mg/kg daily (6 days)	58% decrease	No	Valproate concentration returned to therapeutic levels after panipenem was stopped	

† Stated as duration before the event (change in valproate concentration) first occurred.
‡ Stated as either the overall change or the maximum change seen during the course of the carbapenem.
* Based on the valproate concentrations of 3 out of the 4 patients. In the fourth patient there was no difference in valproate concentrations, but, an additional bolus dose of valproate resulted in no change in concentrations, and there was an increase in valproate concentrations after meropenem was discontinued, indicating an effect.

1. Hellwig TR, Onisk ML, Chapman BA. Potential interaction between valproic acid and doripenem. *Curr Drug Saf* (2011) 6, 54–8.
2. Tobin JK, Golightly LK, Kick SD, Jones MA. Valproic acid-cabapenem interaction: report of six cases and a review of the literature. *Drug Metabol Drug Interact* (2009) 24, 153–82.
3. Park MK, Lim KS, Kim TE, Han HK, Yi SJ, Shin KH, Cho JY, Shin SG, Jang IJ, Yu KS et al. Reduced valproic acid serum concentrations due to drug interactions with carbapenem antibiotics: overview of 6 cases. *Ther Drug Monit* (2012) 34, 599–603.
4. Lunde JL, Nelson RE, Storandt HF. Acute seizures in a patient receiving divalproex sodium after starting ertapenem therapy. *Pharmacotherapy* (2007) 27, 1202–5.
5. Cabanes Mariscal MA, Sánchez López P, Álvarez Herranz P, Chamorro Merino G. Pharmacokinetic interaction between valproic acid and ertapenem. *Farm Hosp* (2006) 30, 313–15.
6. Liao F-F, Huang Y-B, Chen C-Y. Decrease in serum valproic acid levels during treatment with ertapenem. *Am J Health-Syst Pharm* (2010) 67, 1260–4.
7. Omoda K, Murakami T, Yumoto R, Nagai J, Maeda Y, Kiribayashi Y, Takano M. Increased erythrocyte distribution of valproic acid in pharmacokinetic interaction with carbapenem antibiotics in rat and human. *J Pharm Sci* (2005) 94, 1685–93.
8. Perea Falomir M, Roura Poch P, Higueruelo Demasón S, García Gil VJ. Descripción de un caso de interacción farmacocinética entre ácido valproico e imipenem. *Farm Hosp* (2006) 30, 316–17.
9. Lee SG, Kim JH, Joo JY, Kwon OH, Seven cases of decreased serum valproic acid concentration during concomitant use of carbapenem antibiotics. *Korean J Lab Med* (2007) 27, 338–43.
10. Spriet I, Goyens J, Meersseman W, Wilmer A, Willems L, Van Paesschen W. Interaction between valproate and meropenem: a retrospective study. *Ann Pharmacother* (2007) 41, 1130–6.
11. Haroutiunian S, Ratz Y, Rabinovich B, Adam M, Hoffman A. Valproic acid plasma concentration decreases in a dose-independent manner following administration of meropenem: a retrospective study. *J Clin Pharmacol* (2009) 49, 1363–69.
12. Mink S, Muroi C, Seule M, Bjeljac M, Keller E. Levetiracetam compared to valproic acid: plasma concentration levels, adverse effects and interactions in aneurismal subarachnoid hemorrhage. *Clin Neurol Neurosurg* (2011) 113, 644–8.
13. Vélez-Díaz-Pallarés M, Delgado Silveira E, Álvarez Díaz AM, Pérez Menéndez-Conde C, Vicente Oliveros N, Bermejo Vicedo T. Analysis of the valproic acid-meropenem interaction in hospitalised patients. *Neurologia* (2012) 27, 34–8.
14. Llinares Tello F, Bosacoma Ros N, Hernández Prats C, Climent Grana E, Selva Otaolaurruchi J, Ordovás Baines JP. Interacción farmacocinética entre ácido valproico y antibióticos carbapenémicos: descripción de tres casos. *Farm Hosp* (2003) 27, 258–63.

Continued

Table 14.3 Summary of the evidence for an interaction between valproate and carbapenems (continued)

15. De Turck BJG, Diltoer MW, Cornelis PJWW, Maes V, Spapen HDM, Camu F, Huyghens LP. Lowering of plasma valproic acid concentrations during concomitant therapy with meropenem and amikacin. *J Antimicrob Chemother* (1998) 42, 563–4.
16. Plasencia AP, Soy D, Nicolas JM. Interacción farmacocinética entre el ácido valproico y el meropenem. *Med Clin (Barc)* (2004) 123, 38–9.
17. Nacarkucuk E, Saglam H, Okan M. Meropenem decreases serum level of valproic acid. *Pediatr Neurol* (2004) 31, 232–4.
18. Clause D, Decleire P-Y, Vanbinst R, Soyer A, Hantson P. Pharmacokinetic interaction between valproic acid and meropenem. *Intensive Care Med* (2005) 31, 1293–4.
19. Sala Piñol F, Padullés Zamora N, Hidalgo Albert E, Clemente Bautista S, Cabañas Poy MJ, Oliveras Arenas M, Balcells Ramírez J. Interacción farmacocinética entre ácido valproico y meropenem. *An Pediatr (Barc)* (2006) 64, 93–5.
20. Coves-Orts FJ, Borrás-Blasco J, Navarro-Ruiz A, Murcia-López A, Palacios-Ortega F. Acute seizures due to a probable interaction between valproic acid and meropenem. *Ann Pharmacother* (2005) 39, 533–7.
21. Santucci M, Parmeggiani A, Riva R. Seizure worsening caused by decreased serum valproate during meropenem therapy. *J Child Neurol* (2005) 20, 456–7.
22. Fudio S, Carcas A, Piñana E, Ortega R. Epileptic seizures caused by low valproic acid levels from an interaction with meropenem. *J Clin Pharm Ther* (2006) 31, 393–6.
23. Spriet I, Meersseman W, De Troy E, Wilmer A, Casteels M, Willems L. Meropenem–valproic acid interaction in patients with cefepime-associated status epilepticus. *Am J Health-Syst Pharm* (2007) 64, 54–8.
24. Gu J, Huang Y. Effect of concomitant administration of meropenem and valproic acid in an elderly Chinese patient. *Am J Geriatr Pharmacother* (2009) 7, 26–33.
25. Muzyk AJ, Candeloro CL, Christopher EJ. Drug interaction between carbapenems and extended-release divalproex sodium in a patient with schizoaffective disorder. *Gen Hosp Psychiatry* (2010) 560, e1–3.
26. San Antonio Arce V, Joyanes Abancens B. Meropenem and valproic acid. An interaction to remember. *An Pediatr (Barc)* (2009) 70, 193–4.~19217581~
27. Eimil-Ortiz M, Aguirre-Mollehuanca D, Sierra-Limpo A, Fontán-Tirado C, Villar-Villar ME. Meropenem and valproic acid: a dangerous combination. *Rev Neurol* (2008) 46, 124–5.
28. Taha FA, Hammond DN, Sheth RD. Seizures from valproate-carbapenem interaction. *Pediatr Neurol* (2013) 49, 279–81.~23932807~
29. Fernández García MI, Fernández de la Puebla Giménez RÁ, García Olid B, Torres Degayón V. Meropenem decreases valproate plasmatic concentrations. *Med Clin (Barc)* (2011) 137, 43–4.
30. Nagai K, Shimizu T, Togo A, Takeya M, Yokomizo Y, Sakata Y, Matsuishi T, Kato H. Decrease in serum levels of valproic acid during treatment with a new carbapenem, panipenem/betamipron. *J Antimicrob Chemother* (1997) 39, 295–6.
31. Yamagata T, Momoi MY, Murai K, Ikematsu K, Suwa K, Sakamoto K, Fujimura A. Panipenem—Betamipron and decreases in serum valproic acid concentration. *Ther Drug Monit* (1998) 20, 396–400.

3. Liao F-F, Huang Y-B, Chen C-Y. Decrease in serum valproic acid levels during treatment with ertapenem. *Am J Health-Syst Pharm* (2010) 67, 1260–4.
4. Lee SG, Kim JH, Joo JY, Kwon OH, Seven cases of decreased serum valproic acid concentration during concomitant use of carbapenem antibiotics. *Korean J Lab Med* (2007) 27, 338–43.
5. Spriet I, Willems L. No interaction between valproate and meropenem in cirrhotic patient. *Ann Pharmacother* (2011) 45, 1167–8.
6. Yoon H, Kim DH. Unusual drug reaction between valproate sodium and meropenem. *Int J Clin Pharmacol* (2013) 35, 316–8.
7. De Turck BJG, Diltoer MW, Cornelis PJWW, Maes V, Spapen HDM, Camu F, Huyghens LP. Lowering of plasma valproic acid concentrations during concomitant therapy with meropenem and amikacin. *J Antimicrob Chemother* (1998) 42, 563–4.
8. Hobara N, Hokama N, Ohshiro S, Kameya H, Sakanashi M. Possible mechanisms of low levels of plasma valproate concentration following simultaneous administration of sodium valproate and meropenem. *Biog Amines* (2003) 17, 409–20.
9. Omoda K, Murakami T, Yumoto R, Nagai J, Maeda Y, Kiribayashi Y, Takano M. Increased erythrocyte distribution of valproic acid in pharmacokinetic interaction with carbapenem antibiotics in rat and human. *J Pharm Sci* (2005) 94, 1685–93.
10. Tobin JK, Golightly LK, Kick SD, Jones MA. Valproic acid-cabapenem interaction: report of six cases and a review of the literature. *Drug Metabol Drug Interact* (2009) 24, 153–82.
11. Nakajima Y, Mizobuchi M, Nakamura M, Takagi H, Inagaki H, Kominami G, Koike M, Yamaguchi T. Mechanism of the drug interaction between valproic acid and carbapenem antibiotics in monkeys and rats. *Drug Metab Dispos* (2004) 32, 1383–91.
12. Suzuki E, Yamamura N, Ogura Y, Nakai D, Kubota K, Kobayashi N, Miura S, Okazaki O. Identification of valproic acid glucuronide hydrolase as a key enzyme for the interaction of valproic acid with carbapenem antibiotics. *Drug Metab Dispos* (2010) 38, 1536–44.
13. Suzuki E, Nakai D, Yamamura N, Kobayashi N, Okazaki O, Izumi T. Inhibition mechanism of carbapenem antibiotics on acylpeptide hydrolase, a key enzyme in the interaction with valproic acid. *Xenobiotica* (2011) 41, 958–63.

Valproate + Chlorpromazine

Valproate levels are slightly raised in patients given chlorpromazine, but this appears to be of minimal clinical importance. An isolated report describes severe hepatotoxicity in a patient taking chlorpromazine and valproate.

Clinical evidence, mechanism, importance and management

When 6 patients taking valproate 400 mg daily were given chlorpromazine 100 to 300 mg daily, their steady-state trough valproate serum levels rose by 22%. The half-life increased by 14% and the clearance fell by 14% (possibly due to some reduction in its liver metabolism).[1] However, these changes are modest, and this interaction would normally seem to be of minimal importance. Severe hepatotoxicity occurred in another patient given both drugs,[2] which could have been due to the combined hepatotoxic effects of both drugs.

1. Ishizaki T, Chiba K, Saito M, Kobayashi K, Iizuka R. The effects of neuroleptics (haloperidol and chlorpromazine) on the pharmacokinetics of valproic acid in schizophrenic patients. *J Clin Psychopharmacol* (1984) 4, 254–61.
2. Bach N, Thung SN, Schaffner F, Tobias H. Exaggerated cholestasis and hepatic fibrosis following simultaneous administration of chlorpromazine and sodium valproate. *Dig Dis Sci* (1989) 34, 1303–7.

Valproate + Erythromycin

Two isolated reports describe valproate toxicity in a woman and a child given erythromycin. Another report describes vitamin K deficiency in a child given valproate and erythromycin.

Clinical evidence, mechanism, importance and management

A child taking valproic acid developed a deficiency of prothrombin complex after taking erythromycin 300 mg three times daily. This resolved when the patient was given oral vitamin K. It was suggested that the effect was because the numbers of vitamin-K producing intestinal bacteria were reduced.[1] A woman taking lithium and valproate 3.5 g daily developed fatigue and walking difficulties a day after starting to take erythromycin 250 mg four times daily. Within a week she had also developed slurred speech, confusion, difficulty in concentrating and a worsening gait. Her serum valproate levels had risen from 88 mg/L (measured 2 months before) to 260 mg/L. She recovered within 24 hours of the valproate and erythromycin being withdrawn. Her serum lithium levels remained unchanged.[2] In another case, a child taking sodium valproate had a threefold increase in serum valproate levels after taking erythromycin 150 mg every 8 hours and aspirin 250 mg every 6 hours for 3 days.[3]

These case reports contrast with another study in a 10-year-old boy taking valproic acid 375 mg twice daily who had only very small and clinically unimportant changes in the pharmacokinetics of valproate, consistent with inhibition of cytochrome P450 metabolism, when given erythromycin 250 mg four times daily.[4]

The general relevance of these isolated reports is unclear, but probably small.

1. Cordes I, Buchmann S, Scheffner D. Vitamin K-mangel unter Erythromycin. Beobachtung bei einem mit Valproat behandelten Jungen. *Monatsschr Kinderheilkd* (1990) 138, 85–7.
2. Redington K, Wells C, Petito F. Erythromycin and valproate interaction. *Ann Intern Med* (1992) 116, 877–8.
3. Sanchez-Romero A, Pamirez IO. Interacción ácido valproico-eritromicina. *An Esp Pediatr* (1990) 32, 78–9.
4. Gopaul SV, Farrell K, Rakshi K, Abbott FS. A case study of erythromycin interaction with valproic acid. *Pharm Res* (1996) 13 (9 Suppl), S434.

Valproate + Felbamate

Felbamate can raise valproate serum levels causing toxicity. Valproate may slightly decrease the clearance of felbamate.

Clinical evidence

(a) Effect on sodium valproate

The average steady-state valproate serum levels in 7 patients with epilepsy were raised by 28% (from 66.9 micrograms/mL to 85.4 micrograms/mL) by felbamate 1.2 g daily, and by 54% (from 66.9 micrograms/mL to 103 micrograms/mL) by felbamate 2.4 g daily. In addition, the AUC of valproate was raised by 28% and 54% by felbamate 1.2 g and 2.4 g, respectively. Valproate clearance was correspondingly reduced by felbamate.[1] Similar effects were seen in another study,[2,3] and one of these studies suggested that in children the interaction may be more marked.[3] Many of the patients experienced nausea. Other toxic effects included lethargy, drowsiness, headaches, cognitive disturbances and low platelet counts.[1,2]

(b) Effect on felbamate

The clearance of felbamate was decreased by 21% by valproate in one study,[4] and another study reported a significantly lower felbamate clearance in the presence of valproate.[5] However, a further study noted only a minimal effect of valproate on felbamate clearance.[6]

Mechanism

Uncertain. Altered plasma protein binding of valproate is unlikely to be important.[7] Felbamate may cause inhibition of the oxidative pathway of valproate metabolism.[8]

Importance and management

An established interaction. It may be necessary to reduce the valproate dose to avoid toxicity if felbamate is given. The authors of one report suggest a 30 to 50% reduction. It may also be necessary to reduce the felbamate dose, although the effects appear modest. If both drugs are given monitor the outcome closely, being alert for valproate adverse effects (e.g. nausea, vomiting and dizziness) particularly during the initial stages of treatment.

1. Wagner ML, Graves NM, Leppik IE, Remmel RP, Shumaker RC, Ward DL, Perhach JL. The effect of felbamate on valproic acid disposition. *Clin Pharmacol Ther* (1994) 56, 494–502.

2. Liu H, Delgado MR. Significant drug interaction between valproate and felbamate in epileptic children. *Epilepsia* (1995) 36 (Suppl 3), S160.
3. Delgado MR. Changes in valproic acid concentrations and dose/level ratios by felbamate coadministration in children. *Ann Neurol* (1994) 36, 538.
4. Kelley MT, Walson PD, Cox S, Dusci LJ. Population pharmacokinetics of felbamate in children. *Ther Drug Monit* (1997) 19, 29–36.
5. Wagner ML, Leppik IE, Graves NM, Remme RP, Campbell JI. Felbamate serum concentrations: effect of valproate, carbamazepine, phenytoin and phenobarbital. *Epilepsia* (1990) 31, 642.
6. Banfield CR, Zhu G-RR, Jen JF, Jensen PK, Schumaker RC, Perhach JL Affrime MB, Glue P. The effect of age on the apparent clearance of felbamate: a retrospective analysis using nonlinear mixed-effects modeling. *Ther Drug Monit* (1996) 18, 19–29.
7. Bernus I, Dickinson RG, Hooper WD, Franklin ME, Eadie MJ. Effect of felbamate on the plasma protein binding of valproate. *Clin Drug Invest* (1995) 10, 288–95.
8. Hooper WD, Franklin ME, Glue P, Banfield CR, Radwanski E, McLaughlin DB, McIntyre ME, Dickinson RG, Eadie MJ. Effect of felbamate on valproic acid disposition in healthy volunteers: inhibition of β-oxidation. *Epilepsia* (1996) 37, 91–7.

Valproate + Fluoxetine

Isolated reports describe marked increases or modest decreases in valproate levels in a small number of patients given fluoxetine. Valproate toxicity occurred in one patient.

Clinical evidence

A woman with an atypical bipolar disorder and 'severe mental retardation' taking semisodium valproate (divalproex sodium) 3 g daily had a rise in her serum valproic acid levels from 93.5 mg/L to 152 mg/L within 2 weeks of starting to take fluoxetine 20 mg daily. The valproate dose was reduced to 2.25 g daily and 2 weeks later the serum valproic acid levels had fallen to 113 mg/L. No adverse effects were seen.[1] Another woman taking valproic acid developed elevated serum valproate levels (a rise from 78 mg/L to 126 mg/L) without any accompanying clinical symptoms within one month of starting to take fluoxetine 20 mg daily. Valproate levels fell again when the fluoxetine was stopped.[2] Similarly, a 17-year-old taking valproic acid and felbamate developed drowsiness and difficulty in being roused 2 weeks after starting fluoxetine 20 mg daily. His valproate level had increased to 141 micrograms/mL from a previous range of 100 to 110 micrograms/mL. His valproate dose was reduced by about 15%, and his consciousness improved.[3]

In contrast 2 cases of *reduced* valproate levels have also been reported in patients taking fluoxetine. In the first case, a 67-year-old woman taking valproic acid 2 g daily and fluoxetine 20 mg daily had a serum valproate level of 51.9 mg/L. This increased to 64.9 mg/L 9 days after fluoxetine was discontinued and fell to 32.6 mg/L 6 days after fluoxetine was re-started. In the second case, an 81-year-old woman was taking valproic acid 1 g with fluoxetine 20 mg daily and had serum valproate levels of 41.9 mg/L. The fluoxetine was stopped, and 6 days later valproate serum levels had risen to 56.2 mg/L. After re-introduction of fluoxetine her valproate levels fell to 45.6 mg/L.[4]

Mechanism

Not understood.

Importance and management

These reports are somewhat confusing and inconsistent. The overall picture is that concurrent use need not be avoided, but that the outcome should probably be monitored. Indicators of valproate toxicity include nausea, vomiting, and dizziness. More study is needed to establish an interaction.

1. Sovner R, Davis JM. A potential drug interaction between fluoxetine and valproic acid. *J Clin Psychopharmacol* (1991) 11, 389.
2. Lucena MI, Blanco E, Corrales MA, Berthier ML. Interaction of fluoxetine and valproic acid. *Am J Psychiatry* (1998) 155, 575.
3. Cruz-Flores S, Hayat GR, Mirza W. Valproic toxicity with fluoxetine therapy. Missouri Med 1995 Jun 92 (6) 296–7.
4. Droulers A, Bodak N, Oudjhani M, Lefevre des Noettes V, Bodak A. Decrease of valproic acid concentration in the blood when coprescribed with fluoxetine. *J Clin Psychopharmacol* (1997) 17, 139–40.

Valproate + Food

Food appears not to affect the bioavailability of valproate, although in one study, the rate of absorption was increased.

Clinical evidence, mechanism, importance and management

In a study in 12 healthy subjects, the absorption of a single dose of a sustained-release formulation containing sodium valproate 333 mg and valproic acid 145 mg (*Depakine Chrono*) was increased when it was given with a standard breakfast rather than in the fasting state. However, the extent of absorption, the AUC, the mean residence time and the elimination half-life were not changed.[1] Similarly, in another study in healthy subjects, the bioavailability of a single 300-mg dose of sustained-release sodium valproate (*Orfiril long*) was not affected when it was given with a high-energy, high-fat breakfast.[2] A further study in 12 healthy subjects found that dietary fibre (citrus pectin 14 g) did not affect the rate or extent of absorption of a single 500-mg dose of valproate.[3]

1. Royer-Morrot M-J, Zhiri A, Jacob F, Necciari J, Lascombes F, Royer RJ. Influence of food intake on the pharmacokinetics of a sustained release formulation of sodium valproate. *Biopharm Drug Dispos* (1993) 14, 511–18.
2. Retzow A, Vens-Cappell B, Wangemann M. Influence of food on the pharmacokinetics of a new multiple unit sustained release sodium valproate formulation. *Arzneimittelforschung* (1997) 47, 1347–50.
3. Issy AM, Lanchote VL, de Carvalho D, Silva HC. Lack of kinetic interaction between valproic acid and citrus pectin. *Ther Drug Monit* (1997) 19, 516–20.

Valproate + H_2-receptor antagonists

Aside from one tentative case report, cimetidine and ranitidine do not appear to have a clinically significant interaction with valproate.

Clinical evidence, mechanism, importance and management

In 6 patients, the clearance of a single oral dose of sodium valproate was reduced by 2 to 17% after a 4-week course of **cimetidine**, but was not affected by **ranitidine**.[1] It seems doubtful if the interaction between valproate and **cimetidine** is of clinical importance. However, a case of fatal hyperammonaemia in a patient with systemic lupus erythematosus was speculated to have been induced by valproate, and the authors also considered that the concurrent use of **cimetidine** and aspirin (see 'Valproate + Aspirin or NSAIDs', p.617) may have contributed.[2] The general importance of this case is unknown.

1. Webster LK, Mihaly GW, Jones DB, Smallwood RA, Phillips JA, Vajda FJ. Effect of cimetidine and ranitidine on carbamazepine and sodium valproate pharmacokinetics. *Eur J Clin Pharmacol* (1984) 27, 341–3.
2. Ichikawa H, Amano T, Kawabata K, Kushiro M, Wada J, Nagake Y, Makino H. Fatal hyperammonemia in a patient with systemic lupus erythematosus. *Intern Med* (1998) 37, 700–3.

Valproate + Isoniazid

An isolated report describes the development of raised serum valproate levels and toxicity in a child given isoniazid while taking valproate. Another report describes raised liver enzymes and drowsiness in a patient taking both drugs.

Clinical evidence, mechanism, importance and management

A 5-year-old girl with left partial seizures, successfully treated with valproate 600 mg daily and clonazepam for 7 months, developed signs of valproate toxicity (drowsiness, asthenia) shortly after starting to take isoniazid 200 mg daily because of a positive tuberculin reaction. Her serum valproate levels were found to have risen to around 121 to 139 mg/L (reference range 50 to 100 mg/L).[1] Over the next few months various changes were made in her treatment, the most significant being a 62% reduction in the dose of valproate, which was needed to maintain satisfactory therapeutic valproate levels. Later when the isoniazid was stopped her valproate levels fell below the reference range and seizures recurred. It was then found necessary to increase the valproate to its former dose. The suggested explanation for this interaction is that isoniazid inhibited the metabolism (oxidation) of valproate by the liver so that it accumulated. The child was found to be a very slow acetylator of isoniazid.[1]

Another child who had been treated with valproate for several years was given isoniazid for the treatment of tuberculosis. At the same time, seizures recurred, and the valproate was stopped and primidone 750 mg daily started. Seven months later seizures persisted, and she was admitted to hospital. Liver enzyme values were normal. She was given valproate 300 mg daily increased to 600 mg daily, and within 2 days she was vomiting and drowsy. After 5 days she had increased liver enzymes and her prothrombin time had fallen, so the valproate was stopped. Valproate levels were 81 micrograms/mL. It was speculated that the CNS effects and hepatic impairment were due to an interaction between valproate and isoniazid.[2]

The general importance of these cases is uncertain, but bear them in mind in the event of an unexpected response to treatment.

1. Jonville AP, Gauchez AS, Autret E, Billard C, Barbier P, Nsabiyumva F, Breteau M. Interaction between isoniazid and valproate: a case of valproate overdosage. *Eur J Clin Pharmacol* (1991) 40, 197–8.
2. Dockweiler U. Isoniazid-induced valproic-acid toxicity, or vice versa. *Lancet* (1987) ii, 152.

Valproate + Methylphenidate

Two children taking valproic acid rapidly developed severe dyskinesias and bruxism (teeth grinding and jaw clenching) after the first and second dose of methylphenidate, respectively. Valproate appears to potentiate the effects of methylphenidate, possibly by a pharmacokinetic mechanism, or because of additive dopaminergic effects. The authors of the report advise clinical observation while the dose of methylphenidate is being established.[1]

1. Gara L, Roberts W. Adverse response to methylphenidate in combination with valproic acid. *J Child Adolesc Psychopharmacol* (2000) 10, 39–43.

Valproate + Propranolol

One patient had a reduction in valproate clearance when propranolol was also given, but 12 other patients had no change in valproate clearance when taking propranolol.

Clinical evidence, mechanism, importance and management

An isolated report describes a 28% reduction in valproate clearance in a patient taking valproate semisodium with propranolol 40 mg, and a 35% reduction in valproate clearance with propranolol 80 mg. However, 12 other patients taking valproate had no changes in the clearance, serum levels or half-life of valproate when they were given propranolol 60 or 120 mg daily for 3 weeks.[1] This interaction would therefore not appear to be of general importance. No special precautions would seem necessary if propranolol is given to patients taking valproate.

1. Nemire RE, Toledo CA, Ramsay RE. A pharmacokinetic study to determine the drug interaction between valproate and propranolol. *Pharmacotherapy* (1996) 16, 1059–62.

Valproate + Theophylline

A study in 6 healthy subjects found that oral aminophylline 200 mg every 6 hours for 3 doses did not affect the pharmacokinetics of a single 400-mg dose of sodium valproate.[1] No dose adjustment of sodium valproate appears to be needed with concurrent use of aminophylline, and therefore theophylline.

1. Kulkarni C, Vaz J, David J, Joseph T. Aminophylline alters pharmacokinetics of carbamazepine but not that of sodium valproate — a single dose pharmacokinetic study in human volunteers. *Indian J Physiol Pharmacol* (1995) 39, 122–6.

Vigabatrin + Clomipramine

An isolated case report describes mania in a patient with epilepsy taking vigabatrin and clomipramine.

Clinical evidence, mechanism, importance and management

An isolated report describes an man with epilepsy, taking carbamazepine and clobazam, who started taking clomipramine 35 mg daily for depression. About one month later, vigabatrin 2 g daily was added to improve seizure control. After about a week, the patient progressively developed signs of mania, which required him to be hospitalised after about 10 weeks. The clomipramine was stopped, the vigabatrin continued (because of its efficacy), and haloperidol started. Within a week the patient's mood had stabilised. The authors of the report attributed the mania to an interaction between the vigabatrin and the clomipramine.[1,2] Note that both clomipramine and vigabatrin can cause psychiatric disorders including mania, and vigabatrin should be used with caution in patients with depression. No general conclusions can be based on this single report.

1. Sastre-Garau P, Thomas P, Beaussart M, Goudemand M. Accès maniaque consécutif à une association vigabatrin-clomipramine. *Encephale* (1993) 19, 351–2.
2. Sastre-Garau P, Thomas P, Beaussart M, Goudemand M. Accès maniaque consécutif à une association vigabatrin-clomipramine. *Encephale* (1994) 20, 363.

Vigabatrin + Felbamate

No clinically relevant pharmacokinetic interactions appear to occur between vigabatrin and felbamate.

Clinical evidence, mechanism, importance and management

In a study in 16 healthy subjects, felbamate 2.4 g daily increased the AUC of vigabatrin 2 g daily by 13%, which is unlikely to be clinically significant. In a second study, in a further 18 healthy subjects, vigabatrin did not affect felbamate pharmacokinetics.[1] It therefore appears that concurrent use can be undertaken without the need to adjust the dose of either drug.

1. Reidenberg P, Glue P, Banfield C, Colucci R, Meehan J, Rey E, Radwanski E, Nomeir A, Lim J, Lin C, Guillaume M, Affrime MB. Pharmacokinetic interaction studies between felbamate and vigabatrin. *Br J Clin Pharmacol* (1995) 40, 157–60.

Vigabatrin + Phenobarbital or Primidone

Vigabatrin causes a small decrease in phenobarbital and primidone levels. There is some evidence that phenobarbital may reduce the efficacy of vigabatrin in infantile spasms.

Clinical evidence

In an early clinical study in 26 patients, vigabatrin 2 to 3 g daily did not change the serum levels of phenobarbital.[1] Similarly, another study found that phenobarbital levels were not significantly altered by vigabatrin.[2] A further study found that vigabatrin caused serum level reductions of 7% with phenobarbital and 11% with primidone.[3,4] Alterations of this size would not be expected to be clinically relevant.

There is some evidence that the efficacy of vigabatrin for infantile seizures may be reduced in those taking phenobarbital. The median time to response after starting vigabatrin was 3 days in 3 infants not taking phenobarbital and 34 days in 6 patients taking phenobarbital. Three patients did not respond to vigabatrin until after phenobarbital was withdrawn.[5]

Mechanism

Not understood.

Importance and management

There appears to be no change in phenobarbital levels with vigabatrin, but some suggestion that vigabatrin may be less effective for infantile spasms in the presence of phenobarbital. Bear this possibility in mind.

1. Tassinari CA, Michelucci R, Ambrosetto G, Salvi F. Double-blind study of vigabatrin in the treatment of drug-resistant epilepsy. *Arch Neurol* (1987) 44, 907–10.
2. Bernardina BD, Fontana E, Vigevano F, Fusco L, Torelli D, Galeone D, Buti D, Cianchetti C, Gnanasakthy A, Iudice A. Efficacy and tolerability of vigabatrin in children with refractory partial seizures: a single-blind dose-increasing study. *Epilepsia* (1995) 36, 687–91.
3. Browne TR, Mattson RH, Penry JK, Smith DB, Treiman DM, Wilder BJ, Ben-Menachem E, Miketta RM, Sherry KM, Szabo GK. A multicentre study of vigabatrin for drug-resistant epilepsy. *Br J Clin Pharmacol* (1989) 95S–100S.
4. Browne TR, Mattson RH, Penry JK, Smith DB, Treiman DM, Wilder BJ, Ben-Menachem E, Napoliello MJ, Sherry KM, Szabo GK. Vigabatrin for refractory complex partial seizures: multicenter single-blind study with long-term follow up. *Neurology* (1987) 37, 184–9.
5. Spence SJ, Nakagawa J, Sankar R, Shields WD. Phenobarbital interferes with the efficacy of vigabatrin in treating infantile spasms in patients with tuberous sclerosis. *Epilepsia* (2000) 41 (Suppl 7), 189.

Vigabatrin + Valproate

No pharmacokinetic interaction appears to occur between vigabatrin and valproate, but one retrospective study found a correlation between valproate levels and vigabatrin levels.

Clinical evidence, mechanism, importance and management

In 11 children, vigabatrin 40 to 80 mg/kg daily did not change the serum levels of sodium valproate.[1] The combined use of vigabatrin and sodium valproate in 16 children with refractory epilepsy was found not to affect the steady-state serum levels of either drug and the combination reduced the frequency of seizures.[2] However, a retrospective analysis of serum samples from 53 patients found that the vigabatrin concentration-to-dose ratio was increased as the valproate trough steady-state levels increased,[3] suggesting that valproate slightly raises vigabatrin levels. Nevertheless, no dose adjustments usually appear to be necessary on concurrent use.

1. Bernardina BD, Fontana E, Vigevano F, Fusco L, Torelli D, Galeone D, Buti D, Cianchetti C, Gnanasakthy A, Iudice A. Efficacy and tolerability of vigabatrin in children with refractory partial seizures: a single-blind dose-increasing study. *Epilepsia* (1995) 36, 687–91.
2. Armijo JA, Arteaga R, Valdizán EM, Herranz JL. Coadministration of vigabatrin and valproate in children with refractory epilepsy. *Clin Neuropharmacol* (1992) 15, 459–69.
3. Armijo JA, Cuadrado A, Bravo J, Arteaga R. Vigabatrin serum concentration to dosage ratio: influence of age and associated antiepileptic drugs. *Ther Drug Monit* (1997) 19, 491–8

Zonisamide + Miscellaneous

Cimetidine does not alter zonisamide pharmacokinetics. Food has no effect on the absorption of zonisamide. A case of reduced zonisamide levels possibly caused by risperidone has been described.

Potent inhibitors of CYP3A4 are predicted to modestly decrease zonisamide clearance.

Clinical evidence, mechanism, importance and management

(a) Cimetidine

In a study in healthy subjects, cimetidine 300 mg four times daily for 13 days did not affect the clearance, half-life, apparent volume of distribution or the amount of drug recovered from the urine after a single 300-mg oral dose of zonisamide. The drugs were well tolerated.[1,2] No special precautions would seem to be needed if both drugs are used.

(b) CYP3A4 inhibitors

In vitro studies have shown that the cytochrome P450 isoenzyme CYP3A4 is the principal isoenzyme involved in the metabolism of zonisamide.[3] Based on *in vitro* data, it is predicted that **ketoconazole**, **ciclosporin**, **miconazole** and **fluconazole** may cause a modest to minor decrease in the clearance of zonisamide. Conversely, **itraconazole** and **triazolam** were not predicted to have an effect.[3] This casts some doubt on these findings as *in vivo*, **ketoconazole** and **itraconazole** usually interact similarly. *In vitro* predictions do not always mirror what happens in clinical use, and therefore further study is needed to establish an effect.

(c) Food

In a study in healthy subjects there was no difference in the pharmacokinetics of a single 300- or 400-mg dose of zonisamide when given in the fasted state or when it was given after breakfast. Zonisamide may be taken without regard to the timing of meals.[4]

(d) Risperidone

A 57-year-old man taking zonisamide was given risperidone 2 mg daily, which was gradually increased to 10 mg daily. About 2 months after starting the risperidone, the zonisamide level had fallen from 23.7 micrograms/mL to 10.7 micrograms/mL. The risperidone was stopped, and the zonisamide level had slightly increased again to 12.4 micrograms/mL about one month later. It was suggested that a metabolic interaction occurred.[5] More study is needed to establish any interaction.

1. Schentag JJ, Gengo FM, Wilton JH, Sedman AJ, Grasela TH, Brockbrader HN. Influence of phenobarbital, cimetidine, and renal disease on zonisamide kinetics. *Pharm Res* (1987) 4 (Suppl), S-79.

2. Groves L, Wallace J, Shellenberger K. Effect of cimetidine on zonisamide pharmacokinetics in healthy volunteers. *Epilepsia* (1998) 39 (Suppl 6), 191.
3. Nakasa H, Nakamura H, Ono S, Tsutsui M, Kiuchi M, Ohmori S, Kitada M. Prediction of drug-drug interactions of zonisamide metabolism in humans from in vitro data. *Eur J Clin Pharmacol* (1998) 54, 177–83.
4. Shellenberger K, Wallace J, Groves L. Effect of food on pharmacokinetics of zonisamide in healthy volunteers. *Epilepsia* (1998) 39 (Suppl 6), 191.
5. Okumura K. Decrease in plasma zonisamide concentrations after coadministration of risperidone in a patient with schizophrenia receiving zonisamide therapy. *Int Clin Psychopharmacol* (1999) 14, 55.

Zonisamide + Other antiepileptics

Phenobarbital, phenytoin and carbamazepine can cause a small to moderate reduction in the levels of zonisamide, while lamotrigine may increase zonisamide levels. Clonazepam and valproate have little or no effect.

Zonisamide has variable effects (a modest decrease, an increase, or no effect) on carbamazepine serum levels, but has no important effect on lamotrigine, phenobarbital, primidone or valproate levels. Most studies also suggest that zonisamide has no effect on phenytoin levels, but two showed a modest increase. In theory, the combination of zonisamide and topiramate may increase the risk of renal calculi.

Clinical evidence

(a) Carbamazepine

In one study the ratio of plasma level to zonisamide dose was 39% lower in 17 patients taking carbamazepine than in 28 patients taking zonisamide alone, suggesting that carbamazepine modestly reduces zonisamide levels.[1] Similarly, in another study in 12 children with epilepsy taking zonisamide 8.6 to 13.6 mg/kg daily, carbamazepine 12.1 to 18.1 mg/kg daily reduced zonisamide plasma levels by about 35 to 37%.[2] In an early study in 2 groups of patients, one taking carbamazepine and the other phenytoin, it was noted that the zonisamide AUC following a single 400-mg dose was 40% higher in the carbamazepine group than the phenytoin group.[3] However, in the first study, the plasma concentration-to-dose ratio was the same in patients taking carbamazepine as in those taking phenytoin.[1] Therefore the comparative effects of carbamazepine and phenytoin on zonisamide levels are unclear.

In one study, the ratio of carbamazepine-10,11-epoxide (the major active metabolite of carbamazepine) to carbamazepine in the plasma was 50% lower in patients also taking zonisamide, suggesting that zonisamide reduces carbamazepine metabolism. However, the plasma concentration-to-dose ratio of carbamazepine was only 20% higher, which was not significant.[1] An early pilot study in 7 patients noted a consistent rise in carbamazepine plasma levels (range 26 to 270%) after zonisamide was started.[4] The opposite effect was seen in a study of 16 paediatric patients in whom zonisamide reduced the ratio of carbamazepine serum levels to dose by up to 22% and increased the relative amount of its major metabolite in the serum by up to 100%, suggesting that zonisamide increases the metabolism of carbamazepine. However, the free fraction of carbamazepine remained unaltered.[5]

Contrasting with these three studies are four others that found no changes in the serum levels of carbamazepine or carbamazepine-10,11-epoxide when zonisamide was used,[2,6-8] although in one of the studies, the renal clearance of carbamazepine-10,11-epoxide was reduced by zonisamide.[8] A further study similarly found no change in the plasma level of carbamazepine in 41 patients also given zonisamide (7.5 micrograms/mL versus 7.4 micrograms/mL).[9]

(b) Clonazepam

In one study the ratio of plasma level to dose ratio of zonisamide did not differ between 8 patients also taking clonazepam and 28 patients taking zonisamide alone, suggesting clonazepam has no effect on zonisamide levels.[1]

(c) Lamotrigine

In 18 patients, zonisamide 100 mg daily increased to 200 mg twice daily did not alter the steady-state pharmacokinetics of lamotrigine.[10,11] Further, the pharmacokinetics of zonisamide were unaffected by lamotrigine.[11] However, in 2 patients who were stable taking zonisamide 600 mg daily or 800 mg daily, the addition of lamotrigine (incremental doses up to 400 mg daily) caused roughly twofold increases in their zonisamide levels, with symptoms of toxicity that were maximal 40 to 60 minutes after taking a zonisamide dose.[12]

(d) Phenobarbital or Primidone

In one study the ratio of plasma level to dose ratio of zonisamide was 29% lower in 11 patients also taking phenobarbital than in 28 patients taking zonisamide alone, suggesting that phenobarbital reduces zonisamide levels.[1] Similarly, another study in healthy subjects found that pretreatment with phenobarbital roughly doubled the clearance of a single dose of zonisamide.[13] A further study found no changes in the serum levels of phenobarbital or primidone in 34 and 13 patients, respectively, who were also given zonisamide.[9]

(e) Phenytoin

In one study the ratio of plasma level to dose ratio of zonisamide was 39% lower in 14 patients also taking phenytoin than in 28 patients taking zonisamide alone, suggesting phenytoin modestly reduces zonisamide levels.[1] In an early study in two groups of patients, one taking carbamazepine and the other phenytoin, it was noted that the zonisamide AUC following a single 400-mg dose was 40% higher in the carbamazepine group than the phenytoin group.[3] However, in the first study, the reduction in zonisamide level-to-dose ratio was the same for phenytoin as for carbamazepine.[1] Therefore the comparative effect of phenytoin and carbamazepine on zonisamide levels is unclear.

Other studies in both adults and children suggest that zonisamide does not affect phenytoin levels.[6,9,14] However, in a population pharmacokinetic analysis, the clearance of phenytoin at a given dose was 14% lower and the serum level 16% higher in 39 patients also taking zonisamide.[15] Similarly, the preliminary results from 9 patients in another study showed that there was a 28% increase in the steady-state AUC of phenytoin when zonisamide 100 mg daily increased to 200 mg twice daily was given,[16] although a later study by the same authors, in 19 patients, found that zonisamide did not affect the pharmacokinetics of phenytoin to a clinically relevant extent.[17]

(f) Topiramate

Zonisamide and topiramate are both weak inhibitors of carbonic anhydrase and either may increase the risk of renal calculi. However, a study in children with epilepsy found that giving either topiramate or zonisamide with a ketogenic diet (high-fat, adequate protein, low-carbohydrate used in difficult to control epilepsy) did not increase the risk of renal calculi that occurred with a ketogenic diet alone.[18] In a retrospective study including 10 patients taking zonisamide and topiramate, there were no reports of renal calculi.[19]

(g) Valproate

In one study the ratio of plasma level to dose of zonisamide was about 20% lower in 24 patients also taking valproate than in 28 taking zonisamide alone, suggesting that valproate has little effect on zonisamide levels.[1] Similarly, another study in 16 patients found that valproate did not affect the pharmacokinetics of zonisamide.[20] Further, the steady-state pharmacokinetics of valproate did not change when zonisamide 100 mg daily increased to 200 mg twice daily was given 16 patients taking valproate.[20,21]

Another study found that zonisamide did not affect the serum levels of sodium valproate in 12 children.[14] A further study similarly found no marked changes in the plasma level of valproic acid in 7 patients also given zonisamide.[9]

Mechanism

Uncertain. It seems possible that phenobarbital, phenytoin and carbamazepine can induce the metabolism of zonisamide thereby reducing its serum levels. The plasma protein binding of zonisamide is unaffected by other antiepileptics (phenobarbital, phenytoin, carbamazepine, valproate).[22]

Importance and management

None of these studies reported any major problems during concurrent use of zonisamide and these other antiepileptic drugs. Zonisamide serum levels are lower with phenobarbital, phenytoin and carbamazepine, and there is the possibility of carbamazepine or phenytoin level changes, so it would be prudent to monitor patients taking any of these combinations.

There appears to be a theoretical risk of a pharmacodynamic interaction between zonisamide and topiramate, but the limited evidence available suggests the interaction is unlikely to be of importance.

1. Shinoda M, Akita M, Hasegawa M, Hasegawa T, Nabeshima T. The necessity of adjusting the dosage of zonisamide when coadministered with other anti-epileptic drugs. *Biol Pharm Bull* (1996) 19, 1090–2.
2. Abo J, Miura H, Takanashi S, Shirai H, Sunaoshi W, Hosoda N, Abo K, Takei K. Drug interaction between zonisamide and carbamazepine: a pharmacokinetic study in children with cryptogenic localization-related epilepsies. *Epilepsia* (1995) 36 (Suppl 3), S162.
3. Ojemann LM, Shastri RA, Wilensky AJ, Friel PN, Levy RH, McLean JR, Buchanan RA. Comparative pharmacokinetics of zonisamide (CI-912) in epileptic patients on carbamazepine or phenytoin monotherapy. *Ther Drug Monit* (1986) 8, 293–6.
4. Sackellares JC, Donofrio PD, Wagner JG, Abou-Khalil B, Berent S, Aasved-Hoyt K. Pilot study of zonisamide (1,2-Benzisoxazole-3-methanesulfonamide) in patients with refractory partial seizures. *Epilepsia* (1985) 26, 206–11.
5. Minami T, Ieiri I, Ohtsubo K, Hirakawa Y, Ueda K, Higuchi S, Aoyama T. Influence of additional therapy with zonisamide (Excegran) on protein binding and metabolism of carbamazepine. *Epilepsia* (1994) 35, 1023–5.
6. Browne TR, Szabo GK, Kres J, Pylilo RJ. Drug interactions of zonisamide (CI–912) with phenytoin and carbamazepine. *J Clin Pharmacol* (1986) 26, 555.
7. Rosenfeld WE, Bergen D, Garnett W, Shah J, Floren LC, Gross J, Tupper R, Shellenberger K. Steady-state drug interaction study of zonisamide and carbamazepine in patients with epilepsy. *Neurology* (2001) 56 (Suppl 3), A336.
8. Ragueneau-Majlessi I, Levy RH, Bergen D, Garnett W, Rosenfeld W, Mather G, Shah J, Grundy JS. Carbamazepine pharmacokinetics are not affected by zonisamide: in vitro mechanistic study and in vivo clinical study in epileptic patients. *Epilepsy Res* (2004) 62, 1–11.
9. Schmidt D, Jacob R, Loiseau P, Deisenhammer E, Klinger D, Despland A, Egli M, Bauer G, Stenzel E, Blankenhorn V. Zonisamide for add-on treatment of refractory partial epilepsy: a European double-blind trial. *Epilepsy Res* (1993) 15, 67–73.
10. Brodie M, Wilson E, Smith D, Dunkley D, Shah J, Floren L, Shellenberger K. Steady-state drug interaction study of zonisamide and lamotrigine in epileptic patients. *Neurology* (2001) 56 (Suppl 3), A337.
11. Levy RH, Ragueneau-Majlessi I, Brodie MJ, Smith DF, Shah J, Pan W-J. Lack of clinically significant pharmacokinetic interactions between zonisamide and lamotrigine at steady state in patients with epilepsy. *Ther Drug Monit* (2005) 27, 193–8.
12. McJilton J, DeToledo J, DeCerce J, Huda S, Abubakr A, Ramsay RE. Cotherapy of lamotrigine/zonisamide results in significant elevation of zonisamide levels. *Epilepsia* (1996) 37 (Suppl 5), 173.
13. Schentag JJ, Gengo FM, Wilton AJ, Sedman AJ, Grasela TH, Bockbrader HN. Influence of phenobarbital, cimetidine, and renal disease on zonisamide kinetics. *Pharm Res* (1987) 4 (Suppl), S-79.
14. Tasaki K, Minami T, Ieiri I, Ohtsubo K, Hirakawa Y, Ueda K, Higuchi S. Drug interactions of zonisamide with phenytoin and sodium valproate: serum concentrations and protein binding. *Brain Dev* (1995) 17, 182–5.
15. Odani A, Hashimoto Y, Takayanagi K, Otsuki Y, Koue T, Takano M, Yasuhara M, Hattori H, Furusho K, Inui K-I. Population pharmacokinetics of phenytoin in Japanese patients with epilepsy: analysis with a dose-dependent clearance model. *Biol Pharm Bull* (1996) 19, 444–8.

16. Garnett WR, Towne AR, Rosenfeld WE, Shah J, Floren LC, Gross J, Tupper R, Shellenberger K. Steady-state pharmacokinetic interaction study of zonisamide (Zonegran) and phenytoin in subjects with epilepsy. *Neurology* (2001) 56 (Suppl 3), A336.
17. Levy RH, Ragueneau-Majlessi I, Garnett WR, Schmerler M, Rosenfeld W, Shah J, Pan W-J. Lack of a clinically significant effect of zonisamide on phenytoin steady-state pharmacokinetics in patients with epilepsy. *J Clin Pharmacol* (2004) 44, 1230–4.
18. Kossoff EH, Pyzik PL, Furth SL, Hladky HD, Freeman JM, Vining EPG. Kidney stones, carbonic anhydrase inhibitors, and the ketogenic diet. *Epilepsia* (2002) 43, 1168–71.
19. Vazquez B, Ghacibeh G, Hopkins M, Devinsky O. Zonisamide and topiramate combination therapy: safety and tolerability. *Epilepsia* (2001) 42 (Suppl. 7) 261–2.
20. Ragueneau-Majlessi I, Levy RH, Brodie M, Smith D, Shah J, Grundy JS. Lack of pharmacokinetic interactions between steady-state zonisamide and valproic acid in patients with epilepsy. *Clin Pharmacokinet* (2005) 44, 517–23.
21. Smith D, Brodie M, Dunkley D, Shah J, Floren L, Shellenberger K. Steady-state drug interaction study of zonisamide and sodium valproate in epileptic patients. *Neurology* (2001) 56 (Suppl 3), A338.
22. Kimura M, Tanaka N, Kimura Y, Miyake K, Kitaura T, Fukuchi H, Harada Y. Factors influencing serum concentration of zonisamide in epileptic patients. *Chem Pharm Bull (Tokyo)* (1992) 40, 193–5.

Zonisamide + Ritonavir

In one case report, ritonavir did not alter the serum concentration of zonisamide.

Clinical evidence, mechanism, importance and management

A 20-year-old HIV-positive man with epilepsy, who had his seizures controlled with carbamazepine 350 mg twice daily and zonisamide 140 mg twice daily, was admitted to hospital for review of his antiretroviral regimen. He started taking **ritonavir**, and after the first 200-mg dose his zonisamide serum concentration remained unchanged.[1] However, his carbamazepine serum concentration was almost doubled. For further information on the concurrent use of HIV-protease inhibitors with carbamazepine, see 'HIV-protease inhibitors + Carbamazepine', p.927.

1. Kato Y, Fujii T, Mizoguchi N, Takata N, Ueda K, Feldman MD, Kayser SR. Potential interaction between ritonavir and carbamazepine. *Pharmacotherapy* (2000) 20, 851–4.

15

Antihistamines

Antihistamines (histamine H_1-antagonists) vary in their interaction profiles by sedative potential, route of metabolism, and cardiotoxicity (QT interval prolongation).

(a) Additive effects

The older antihistamines (e.g. chlorphenamine, diphenhydramine and hydroxyzine) are also referred to as sedating antihistamines or first-generation antihistamines. As the former name suggests they have the potential to cause additive sedative effects with other sedating drugs, for example, see 'Antihistamines + Benzodiazepines and related drugs', p.632. The sedating antihistamines also tend to have antimuscarinic (also called anticholinergic) adverse effects and so therefore may interact additively with other drugs with antimuscarinic effects. This is discussed elsewhere, see 'Antimuscarinics + Antimuscarinics', p.754.

The newer (non-sedating antihistamines or second-generation antihistamines) have a low potential to cause sedative effects. This appears to be because they are substrates for P-glycoprotein, an efflux transporter found in many organs, which would have the effect of actively ejecting any drug molecules that crossed the blood-brain barrier. Nevertheless, sedation may occur on occasion and patients should be advised to be alert to the possibility of drowsiness if they have not taken the drug before. Any drowsiness is likely to become apparent after the first few doses, and would indicate that additive sedative effects with other sedating drugs might be expected. The antihistamines are listed, by sedative potential, in 'Table 15.1', below.

(b) Metabolism

Some of the sedating antihistamines, such as diphenhydramine, are inhibitors of the cytochrome P450 isoenzyme CYP2D6. None of the non-sedating antihistamines are known to inhibit cytochrome P450 isoenzymes, but some are substrates for CYP3A4 including astemizole, desloratadine, ebastine, loratadine, mizolastine, rupatadine and terfenadine, see 'Table 15.2', p.629. This has important consequences for the potential cardiotoxicity of astemizole and terfenadine, see below. Loratadine and desloratadine are also substrates for CYP2D6, and mizolastine is also metabolised by glucuronidation. Cetirizine, levocetirizine and fexofenadine are minimally metabolised. Where pharmacokinetic interactions occur with fexofenadine, these appear to be mediated by drug transporters such as P-glycoprotein and/or organic anion transport polypeptide (OATP).

(c) QT prolongation

Important drug interactions occur with the non-sedating antihistamines, astemizole and terfenadine, resulting in lengthening of the QT interval and increased risk of torsade de pointes. As these drugs have been withdrawn from many countries due to the potential fatal consequences of such interactions, they are included for completeness in the archive (see 'Archived monographs', p.1594). Apart from possibly ebastine, loratadine and mizolastine, where information is inconclusive, none of the other non-sedating antihistamines have been clearly shown to be associated with QT prolongation (see 'Table 15.2', p.629). Therefore, even when pharmacokinetic interactions result in increased levels, these are unlikely to be clinically important in terms of cardiotoxicity.

Table 15.1 Systemic antihistamines (classified by sedative potential) and topical antihistamines

Sedative potential	*Antihistamine*
Non-sedating	Acrivastine, Cetirizine, Desloratadine, Ebastine,* Fexofenadine, Levocetirizine, Loratadine, Mizolastine,* Rupatadine
Sedating	Brompheniramine, Buclizine, Chlorphenamine, Cinnarizine, Clemastine, Cyclizine, Cyproheptadine, Dexchlorpheniramine, Flunarizine, Ketotifen, Meclozine, Mepyramine, Mequitazine, Triprolidine
Significantly sedating	Alimemazine, Dimenhydrinate, Diphenhydramine, Doxylamine, Hydroxyzine, Promethazine
Topical use (mainly)	Azelastine, Bepotastine, Emedastine, Epinastine, Levocabastine, Olopatadine

*Important QT prolongation may possibly occur (ebastine, mizolastine), see Table 15.2, p.629

Table 15.2 Metabolism and cardiac effects of non-sedating antihistamines

Drug	*Drug blocks the HERG*† *potassium channel in vitro*	*QTc interval prolongation shown in pharmacological studies with drug alone*	*QTc interval prolongation shown in pharmacological studies with CYP3A4 inhibitors*	*Case reports of torsade de pointes with drug alone*	*Case reports of torsade de pointes with CYP3A4 inhibitors*
Metabolised by CYP3A4					
Astemizole	Yes[1]	Yes[2]	Yes. See Astemizole or Terfenadine + CYP3A4 inhibitors, p.1597	Several[2-8]	Yes. See Astemizole or Terfenadine + CYP3A4 inhibitors, p.1597
Desloratadine	No	No	No	No	No
Ebastine	Yes[9]	Uncertain	Yes. See Azoles, p.630 or Macrolides, p.635	No	No
Loratadine	Yes, in one study[10]	No	Yes. See Azoles, p.630 or Nefazodone, p.1606	Possible case[11-13]	Yes. See Azoles, p.630 or Macrolides, p.635
Mizolastine	Yes[14]	Uncertain	Yes. See Azoles, p.630	No	No
Rupatadine	No	No	No	Yes[15]	No
Terfenadine	Yes[10,16]	Yes	Yes. See Astemizole or Terfenadine + CYP3A4 inhibitors, p.1597	A few[17,18]	Yes. See Astemizole or Terfenadine + CYP3A4 inhibitors, p.1597
Not metabolised by CYP3A4					
Cetirizine	No	No	No	Possible case[19]	No
Fexofenadine	No	No	No	Possible case[20,21]	No
Levocetirizine	No	No	No	No	No

†The HERG (human ether-a-go-go related gene) channel is involved in cardiac action potential repolarisation and is known to be blocked by certain drugs. Blocking HERG channels results in prolongation of the QT interval.

1. Zhou Z, Vorperian VR, Gong Q, Zhang S, January CT. Block of HERG potassium channels by the antihistamine astemizole and its metabolites desmethylastemizole and norastemizole. *J Cardiovasc Electrophysiol* (1999) 10, 836–43.
2. Craft TM. Torsade de pointes after astemizole overdose. *BMJ* (1986) 292, 660.
3. Snook J, Boothman-Burrell D, Watkins J, Colin-Jones D. Torsade de pointes ventricular tachycardia associated with astemizole overdose. *Br J Clin Pract* (1988) 42, 257–9.
4. Simons FER, Kesselman MS, Giddins NG, Pelech AN, Simons KJ. Astemizole-induced torsade de pointes. *Lancet* (1988) ii, 624.
5. Bishop RO, Gaudry PL. Prolonged Q-T interval following astemizole overdose. *Arch Emerg Med* (1989) 6, 63–5.
6. Hasan RA, Zureikat GY, Nolan BM. Torsade de pointes associated with astemizole overdose treated with magnesium sulfate. *Pediatr Emerg Care* (1993) 9, 23–5.
7. Gowardman J. QT prolongation on the standard dose of astemizole. *N Z Med J* (1996) 109, 38.
8. Vorperian VR, Zhou Z, Mohammad S, Hoon TJ, Studenik C, January CT. Torsade de pointes with an antihistamine metabolite: potassium channel blockade with desmethylastemizole. *J Am Coll Cardiol* (1996) 28, 1556–61.
9. Ko CM, Ducic I, Fan J, Shuba YM, Morad M. Suppression of mammalian K+ channel family by ebastine. *J Pharmacol Exp Ther* (1997) 281, 233–44.
10. Crumb WJ. Loratadine blockade of K+ channels in human heart: comparison with terfenadine under physiological conditions. *J Pharmacol Exp Ther* (2000) 292, 261–4.
11. Kuchar DL, Walker BD, Thorburn CW. Ventricular tachycardia following ingestion of a commonly used antihistamine, *Med J Aust* (2002) 176, 429–30.
12. Sager PT, Veltri EP. Ventricular tachycardia following ingestion of a commonly used antihistamine. *Med J Aust* (2003) 178, 245–6.
13. Kuchar DL, Walker BD, Thorburn CW. In reply. *Med J Aust* (2003) 178, 246.
14. Taglialatela M, Pannaccione A, Castaldo P, Giorgio G, Annunziato L. Inhibition of HERG1 K(+) channels by the novel second-generation antihistamine mizolastine. *Br J Pharmacol* (2000) 131, 1081–8.
15. Nombela-Franco L, Ruiz-Antoran B, Toquero-Ramos J, Silva-Melchor L. Torsades de pointes associated with rupatadine. *Rev Esp Cardiol* (2008) 61, 327–33.
16. Woosley RL, Chen Y, Freiman JP, Gillis RA. Mechanism of the cardiotoxic actions of terfenadine. *JAMA* (1993) 269, 1532–6.
17. MacConnell TJ, Stanners AJ. Torsades de pointes complicating treatment with terfenadine. *Br Med J* (1991) 302, 1469.
18. June RA, Nasr I. Torsades de pointes with terfenadine ingestion. *Am J Emerg Med* (1997) 15, 542–3.
19. Renard S, Ostorero M, Yvorra S, Zerrouk Z, Bargas E, Bertocchio P, Pracchia S, Ebagosti A. Torsades de pointes caused by cetirizine overdose. *Arch Mal Coeur Vaiss* (2005) 98; 157–61.
20. Pinto YM, van Gelder IC, Heeringa M, Crijns HJ. QT lengthening and life-threatening arrhythmias associated with fexofenadine. *Lancet* (1999) 353, 980.
21. Scherer CR, Lerche C, Decher N, Dennis AT, Maier P, Ficker E, Busch AE, Wollnik B, Steinmeyer K. The antihistamine fexofenadine does not affect Ikr currents in a case report of drug-induced cardiac arrhythmia. *Br J Pharmacol* (2002) 137, 892–900.

Antihistamines + Antiepileptics; Enzyme-inducing

In two small studies carbamazepine reduced the exposure to fexofenadine. Limited evidence suggests that phenytoin and carbamazepine can reduce serum flunarizine concentrations. Flunarizine does not appear to alter phenytoin or carbamazepine concentrations.

Clinical evidence, mechanism, importance and management

(a) Fexofenadine

In a crossover study, 12 healthy subjects were given **carbamazepine** 100 mg three times daily for 7 days, with a single 60-mg dose of fexofenadine on day 7. The plasma concentration and AUC of fexofenadine were reduced by 42% and 43%, respectively, with no effect on renal clearance or half-life.[1] In another study in 12 healthy subjects, also given **carbamazepine** 100 mg three times daily for 7 days with a single 60-mg dose of fexofenadine on day 7, the AUC of fexofenadine was reduced by 52 to 61%.[2] P-glycoprotein is involved in the uptake of fexofenadine and it was thought that the effects seen in the studies were due to the induction of intestinal P-glycoprotein by carbamazepine. The clinical importance of this interaction is unclear, but until more is known it would seem prudent to monitor the efficacy of fexofenadine if it is given with carbamazepine.

(b) Flunarizine

A study found that flunarizine concentrations were lower in patients taking multiple antiepileptics than in those taking only one antiepileptic (statistically significant only for flunarizine 10 mg). The antiepileptics taken were **carbamazepine**, **phenytoin**, and sodium valproate. Flunarizine did not affect the serum concentrations of these antiepileptics.[3] In another study, involving 12 patients, four of whom were taking **phenytoin**, four **carbamazepine** and four both **phenytoin** and **carbamazepine**, there was no difference in the pharmacokinetics of a single 30-mg dose of flunarizine, or of multiple-dose flunarizine, between the three groups. However, the apparent clearance values of flunarizine were several fold greater in these patients than in historical data from healthy subjects. There were no differences in the mean steady-state concentrations of the antiepileptics before and during flunarizine use.[4]

Although not conclusive, these data suggest that **phenytoin** and **carbamazepine** increase the metabolism of flunarizine and might reduce its steady-state serum concentration. There would seem to be no reason for avoiding concurrent use, but the outcome should be monitored as an increase in the dose of flunarizine might be required. It seems likely that **fosphenytoin**, a prodrug of phenytoin, will interact with flunarizine in the same way.

1. Yamada S, Yasui-Furukori N, Akamine Y, Kaneko S, Uno T. Effects of the P-glycoprotein inducer carbamazepine on fexofenadine pharmacokinetics. *Ther Drug Monit* (2009) 31, 764–8.
2. Akamine Y, Miura M, Yasui-Furukori N, Kojima M, Uno T. Carbamazepine differentially affects the pharmacokinetics of fexofenadine enantiomers. *Br J Clin Pharmacol* (2012) 73, 478–81.
3. Binnie CD, de Beukelaar F, Meijer JWA, Meinardi H, Overweg J, Wauquier A, van Wieringen A. Open dose-ranging trial of flunarizine as add-on therapy in epilepsy. *Epilepsia* (1985) 26, 424–8.
4. Kapetanovic IM, Torchin CD, Kupferberg HJ, Treiman DM, Di Giorgio C, Barber K, Norton L, Lau M, Whitley L, Cereghino JJ. Pharmacokinetic profile of flunarizine after single and multiple dosing in epileptic patients receiving comedication. *Epilepsia* (1988) 29, 770–4.

Antihistamines + Azoles

The azoles raise the concentrations of ebastine and mizolastine, which could result in prolongation of the QT interval, but there are no case reports of this happening. Acrivastine might be similarly affected. The situation with loratadine is unclear as one study found that the concurrent use of ketoconazole caused a small increase in the QT interval.

Ketoconazole raises the concentrations of desloratadine, emedastine, fexofenadine and rupatadine but no adverse cardiac effects were seen. No interaction occurs between ketoconazole and cetirizine, intranasal levocabastine, and none is expected with azelastine or levocetirizine.

Clinical evidence

In vitro study suggests that **ketoconazole** does not affect the pharmacokinetics of **azelastine**, and single or multiple-dose controlled studies have found that **ketoconazole** had no effect on the pharmacokinetics of **cetirizine** or intranasal **levocabastine**, see 'Table 15.3', p.631.

In contrast, single and multiple-dose controlled studies with **ketoconazole** have shown increases in the plasma concentrations and AUC of **desloratadine** (27% and 21% respectively), **ebastine** (16- and 43-fold, respectively), **emedastine** (37% and 34%, respectively), **fexofenadine** (2.4-fold and 2.6-fold, respectively), **loratadine** (2.4 to 3.5-fold and 2.8 to 4.5-fold, respectively) and **mizolastine** (up to 95% increase in AUC). Similarly, **itraconazole** increases the plasma concentrations and AUC of **ebastine** (2.5-fold and 6.2-fold, respectively) and **fexofenadine** (about 2- to 3-fold). Increases in the QT interval have been seen in multiple-dose studies with **ebastine**, **loratadine** or **mizolastine**, and **ketoconazole**. Details of these studies are summarised in 'Table 15.3', p.631.

The subsections below include additional data from case reports or other studies.

(a) Desloratadine

A patient undergoing chemotherapy developed severe pruritus and was given desloratadine and clemastine. Because of pyrexia of unknown origin she was initially given meropenem and then 48 hours later **fluconazole** was added. After about 36 hours severe hepatotoxicity was detected, and, apart from the anti-infectives, the other drugs were stopped. Liver parameters recovered over the following week. Because the patient had previously received clemastine and **fluconazole** without problems, this case was attributed to a possible interaction between **fluconazole** and desloratadine.[1] However, this conclusion has been disputed by others.[2]

(b) Ebastine

A review of the safety of ebastine cites two studies assessing the potential interaction between ebastine and **ketoconazole**. A single-dose study found that concurrent use did not affect the QTc interval, whereas a multiple-dose study found that concurrent use prolonged the QTc interval by 18.1 milliseconds.[3] The multiple-dose study also found that the plasma concentration and AUC of ebastine were increased by about 15-fold and 40-fold, respectively.[3]

(c) Fexofenadine

In a single-dose study, giving **itraconazole** 200 mg one hour before fexofenadine 180 mg increased the effect of fexofenadine on a histamine-induced wheal and flare reaction.[4] In another study, fexofenadine had no effect on the pharmacokinetics of **ketoconazole**.[5]

(d) Loratadine

In one study the cardiac effects of loratadine were found to be similar to those of ebastine (see above), which caused a small increase in the QTc interval.[6]

(e) Rupatadine

A review reports a study in which the systemic exposure to rupatadine 20 mg was increased 10-fold by **ketoconazole** 200 mg daily for 7 days. The pharmacokinetics of **ketoconazole** were unaffected by rupatadine. There were no clinically relevant changes in the QTc interval, vital signs or adverse effects.[7]

Mechanism

Ebastine, loratadine, mizolastine, probably rupatadine,[8] and possibly desloratadine are metabolised to varying extents by CYP3A4. The azoles are known inhibitors of this isoenzyme and so concurrent use of these antihistamines and the azoles leads to increased antihistamine concentrations, or is predicted to lead to such an increase. The strength of the effect varies between different combinations of azoles and antihistamines according to the strength of the inhibitory effect of the azole on CYP3A4 and the degree to which the antihistamine is metabolised by this isoenzyme.

With the exception of astemizole and terfenadine, the risk of cardiac arrhythmias with non-sedating antihistamines appears to be very low (see 'Table 15.2', p.629), so any pharmacokinetic interactions do not usually result in clinically relevant cardiac toxicity. In fact, studies have shown that desloratadine at nine times the recommended dose,[9] fexofenadine in overdose,[5,10] loratadine at four times the recommended dose for 90 days,[11] and mizolastine at four times the recommended dose[12] do not affect the QT interval. However, some questions remain about ebastine, loratadine and mizolastine. Additionally, some studies have reported that ketoconazole alone is associated with a small increase in the QT interval,[6] and at least one case of torsade de pointes has been reported for ketoconazole alone.[13] Therefore the cardiac effects of ketoconazole might be additive with those of the antihistamines, and this might be important for ebastine, loratadine and mizolastine.

Fexofenadine is not metabolised by CYP3A4, but it is a substrate for P-glycoprotein and OATP,[14] therefore the azoles might increase its concentrations by altering the function of these drug transporter proteins.

Importance and management

The interactions between the azoles and the non-sedating antihistamines are established, although not all antihistamines are affected to the same degree and not all of the interactions are clinically important.

The UK manufacturer of **mizolastine** contraindicates its concurrent use with systemic imidazole antifungals [e.g. ketoconazole, miconazole], and use with other CYP3A4 inhibitors is cautioned, which would include all other azoles.[15] However, note that itraconazole, a triazole, would be expected to interact to the same extent as ketoconazole.

The manufacturer of **ebastine** does not recommend the concurrent use of ketoconazole and itraconazole, and advises caution with CYP3A4 inhibitors such as the azoles.[16] Similarly, the manufacturer of **rupatadine**[8] advises that it should be used with caution with ketoconazole, and other inhibitors of CYP3A4, which would include all the other azoles. It would seem prudent to monitor the concurrent use of rupatadine and an azole for adverse effects including dry mouth, dizziness and fatigue.

There are no data on any possible interaction between **acrivastine** and ketoconazole, and therefore the manufacturer advises caution.[17]

Ketoconazole markedly raises **loratadine** concentrations. In one study, this was associated with a small increase in QT interval, but no obvious alteration in adverse event profile. No particular precautions appear to have been recommended for the use of loratadine with an azole.

Other antihistamines

Desloratadine and emedastine concentrations are raised by ketoconazole, and fexofenadine concentrations are raised by both itraconazole and ketoconazole; but because this does not result in adverse cardiac effects, concurrent use is considered safe.

Cetirizine (and therefore probably its isomer **levocetirizine**) and levocabastine seem to be free from clinically significant pharmacokinetic interactions, and have no cardiac adverse effects, and so might therefore provide suitable alternatives if a non-sedating antihistamine is needed in a patient taking an azole. Although a pharmacokinetic interaction between ketoconazole and oral azelastine is not estab-

Table 15.3 Summary of the effects of azoles on the pharmacokinetics of antihistamines and the associated cardiovascular effects

Antihistamine (Oral unless specified)	*Azole (Oral unless specified)*	*Duration of combined use (days)*	*Subjects*	*Cmax increase*	*AUC increase*	*Effect on QTc*	*Refs*
Azelastine 4 mg twice daily	Ketoconazole 200 mg twice daily	7	12 healthy subjects	Not determined. *In vitro* tests suggest no change likely.	Not determined. *In vitro* tests suggest no change likely.	No change	1
Cetirizine 20 mg daily	Ketoconazole 400 mg daily	10	Healthy subjects	No change	No change	No change	2
Desloratadine 7.5 mg daily	Ketoconazole 200 mg twice daily	10	24 healthy subjects	27%	21%	No change	3
Ebastine 20 mg single dose	Itraconazole 200 mg daily	Single dose	10 healthy subjects	2.5-fold	6.2-fold	Not measured	4
Ebastine 20 mg daily	Ketoconazole 400 mg daily	8	55 healthy subjects	16-fold	43-fold	Mean increase of 5.25 milliseconds when antihistamine added to ketoconazole. Mean increase of 12.21 milliseconds from baseline. QTc did not exceed 500 milliseconds in any subject.[†]	5
Emedastine 4 mg daily	Ketoconazole 200 mg twice daily	5	12 healthy subjects	37%	34%	No change	6
Fexofenadine 120 mg single dose	Itraconazole 100 mg twice daily	Single dose	8 healthy subjects	93%	173%	Not measured	7
Fexofenadine 180 mg single dose	Itraconazole 200 mg single dose	Single dose	14 healthy subjects	2.7- to 3-fold	2.3- to 3-fold	Not measured	8
Fexofenadine 60 mg single dose	Itraconazole 200 mg single dose	Single dose	12 healthy subjects	About 2-fold	About 3-fold	Not measured	9
Fexofenadine 60 mg daily	Itraconazole 200 mg daily	Intermittent over 6 days	10 healthy subjects	2-fold	2-fold	Not measured	10
Fexofenadine 60 mg single dose	Itraconazole 50 mg, 100mg and 200mg	Single dose	11 healthy subjects	80%, 105% and 103%, respectively	109%, 153% and 141%, respectively	Not measured	11
Fexofenadine 120 mg twice daily	Ketoconazole 400 mg daily	7	24 healthy subjects	135%	164%	No change	12
Levocabastine 200 micrograms twice daily intranasal	Ketoconazole 200 mg single dose	Single dose	37 subjects	No change	No change	No change	13
Loratadine 10 mg daily	Ketoconazole 200 mg twice daily	10	24 healthy subjects	172% loratadine 76% desloratadine	247% loratadine 82% desloratadine	No change	14
Loratadine 20 mg single dose	Ketoconazole 200 mg twice daily	Single dose	12 healthy subjects	144% loratadine 33% desloratadine	184% loratadine 54% desloratadine	Not measured	15
Loratadine 10 mg daily	Ketoconazole 400 mg daily	8	62 healthy subjects	248% loratadine 82% desloratadine	346% loratadine 94% desloratadine	Mean increase of 3.16 milliseconds when antihistamine added to ketoconazole. Mean increase of 10.68 milliseconds from baseline. QTc did not exceed 500 milliseconds in any subject.[†]	5
Mizolastine 10 mg single dose	Ketoconazole 100 mg, 200 mg, 400 mg, single doses	Single dose	12 healthy subjects	Not measured	45%, 61% and 95%, respectively	Not measured	16
Mizolastine 10 mg daily	Ketoconazole 200 mg twice daily	5	12 healthy subjects	Not measured	Not measured	Mean increase of 7 milliseconds over mizolastine or placebo alone. None exceeded 500 milliseconds	17

[†]QTc intervals calculated using the Fridericia cube route formula, rather than the more commonly used Bazett square root formula, which the authors suggest would lead to a 5 to 6 millisecond overestimation

1. Morganroth J, Lyness WH, Perhach JL, Mather GG, Harr JE, Trager WF, Levy RH, Rosenberg A. Lack of effect of azelastine and ketoconazole coadministration on electrocardiographic parameters in healthy volunteers. *J Clin Pharmacol* (1997) 37, 1065–72.
2. UCB Pharma. Personal communication, September 1994.
3. Banfield C, Herron JM, Keung A, Pahdi D, Affrime M. Desloratadine has no clinically relevant electrocardiographic or pharmacodynamic interactions with ketoconazole. *Clin Pharmacokinet* (2002) 41 (Suppl 1), 37–44.
4. Shon J-H, Yeo C-W, Liu K-H, Lee S-S, Cha I-J, Shin J-G. Itraconazole and rifampin alter significantly the disposition and antihistamine effect of ebastine and its metabolites in healthy participants. *J Clin Pharmacol* (2010) 50, 195–204.

Continued

Table 15.3 Summary of the effects of azoles on the pharmacokinetics of antihistamines and the associated cardiovascular effects (continued)

5. Chaikin P, Gillen MS, Malik M, Pentikis H, Rhodes GR, Roberts DJ. Co-administration of ketoconazole with H1-antagonists ebastine and loratadine in healthy subjects: pharmacokinetic and pharmacodynamic effects. *Br J Clin Pharmacol* (2005) 59, 346–54.
6. Herranz U, Rusca A, Assandri A. Emedastine-ketoconazole: pharmacokinetic and pharmacodynamic interactions in healthy volunteers. *Int J Clin Pharmacol Ther* (2001) 39, 102–9.
7. Shimizu M, Uno T, Sugawara K, Tateishi T. Effects of itraconazole and diltiazem on the pharmacokinetics of fexofenadine, a substrate of P-glycoprotein. *Br J Clin Pharmacol* (2006) 61, 538–44.
8. Shon J-H, Yoon Y-R, Hong W-S, Nguyen PM, Lee S-S, Choi Y-G, Cha I-J, Shin J-G. Effect of itraconazole on the pharmacokinetics and pharmacodynamics of fexofenadine in relation to the *MDR1* genetic polymorphism. *Clin Pharmacol Ther* (2005) 78, 191–201.
9. Tateishi T, Miura M, Suzuki T, Uno T. The different effects of itraconazole on the pharmacokinetics of fexofenadine enantiomers. *Br J Clin Pharmacol* (2008) 65, 693–700.
10. Shimizu M, Uno T, Sugawara K, Tateishi T. Effects of single and multiple doses of itraconazole on the pharmacokinetics of fexofenadine, a substrate of P-glycoprotein. *Br J Clin Pharmacol* (2006) 62, 372–6.
11. Uno T, Shimizu M, Sugawara K, Tateishi T. Lack of dose-dependent effects of itraconazole on the pharmacokinetic interaction with fexofenadine. *Drug Metab Dispos* (2006) 34, 1875–9.
12. Allegra (Fexofenadine hydrochloride). Sanofi-Aventis U.S. LLC. US Prescribing Information, July 2007.
13. Pesco-Koplowitz L, Hassell A, Lee P, Zhou H, Hall N, Wiesinger B, Mechlinski W, Grover M, Hunt T, Smith R, Travers S. Lack of effect of erythromycin and ketoconazole on the pharmacokinetics of steady-state intranasal levocobastine. *J Clin Pharmacol* (1999) 39, 76–85.
14. Kosoglou T, Salfi M, Lim JM, Batra VK, Cayen MN, Affrime MB. Evaluation of the pharmacokinetics and electrocardiographic pharmacodynamics of loratadine with concomitant administration of ketoconazole or cimetidine. *Br J Clin Pharmacol* (2000) 50, 581–9.
15. Van Peer A, Crabbé R, Woestenborghs R, Heykants J, Janssens M. Ketoconazole inhibits loratadine metabolism in man. *Allergy* (1993) 48 (Suppl 16), 34.
16. Dubruc C, Gillet G, Chaufour S, Holt B, Jensen R, Maurel P, Thenot JP. Metabolic interaction studies of mizolastine with ketoconazole and erythromycin in rat, dog and man. *Clin Pharmacol Ther* (1998) 63, 228.
17. Delauche-Cavallier MC, Chaufour S, Guérault E, Lacroux A, Murrieta M, Wajman A. QT interval monitoring during clinical studies with mizolastine, a new H1 antihistamine. *Clin Exp Allergy* (1999) 29 (Suppl 3), 206–11.

lished, concurrent use did not appear to affect the QT interval in one study, and so azelastine might also be a suitable alternative antihistamine.

1. Schöttker B, Dösch A, Kraemer DM. Severe hepatotoxicity after application of desloratadine and fluconazole. *Acta Haematol (Basel)* (2003) 110, 43–44.
2. Kim H, Bindslev-Jensen C. Reported case of severe hepatotoxicity likely due to fluconazole and not desloratadine. *Acta Haematol (Basel)* (2004) 112, 177–8.
3. Moss AJ, Morganroth J. Cardiac effects of ebastine and other antihistamines in humans. *Drug Safety* (1999) 21 (Suppl 1), 69–80.
4. Shon J-H, Yoon Y-R, Hong W-S, Nguyen PM, Lee S-S, Choi Y-G, Cha I-J, Shin J-G. Effect of itraconazole on the pharmacokinetics and pharmacodynamics of fexofenadine in relation to the *MDR1* genetic polymorphism. *Clin Pharmacol Ther* (2005) 78, 191–201.
5. Allegra (Fexofenadine hydrochloride). Sanofi-Aventis US LLC. US Prescribing Information, July 2007.
6. Chaikin P, Gillen MS, Malik M, Pentikis H, Rhodes GR, Roberts DJ. Co-administration of ketoconazole with H1-antagonists ebastine and loratadine in healthy subjects: pharmacokinetic and pharmacodynamic effects. *Br J Clin Pharmacol* (2005) 59, 346–54.
7. Izquierdo I, Merlos M, García-Rafanell J. Rupatadine. A new selective histamine H_1 receptor and platelet-activating factor (PAF) antagonist. A review of pharmacological profile and clinical management of allergic rhinitis. *Drugs Today* (2003) 39, 451–68.
8. Rupafin (Rupatadine fumarate). GlaxoSmithKline UK. UK Summary of product characteristics, December 2009.
9. Neoclarityn Tablets (Desloratadine). Schering-Plough Ltd. UK Summary of product characteristics, March 2008.
10. Telfast (Fexofenadine hydrochloride). Sanofi-Aventis. UK Summary of product characteristics, June 2008.
11. Affrime MB, Lorber R, Danzig M, Cuss F, Brannan MD. Three month evaluation of electrocardiographic effects of loratadine in humans. *J Allergy Clin Immunol* (1993) 91, 259.
12. Delauche-Cavallier MC, Chaufour S, Guérault E, Lacroux A, Murrieta M, Wajman A. QT interval monitoring during clinical studies with mizolastine, a new H1 antihistamine. *Clin Exp Allergy* (1999) 29 (Suppl 3), 206–11.
13. Mok NS, Lo YK, Tsui PT, Lam CW. Ketoconazole induced torsade de pointes without concomitant use of QT-interval-prolonging drug. *J Cardiovasc Electrophysiol* (2005) 16, 1375–7.
14. Tannergren C, Knutson T, Knutson L, Lennernäs H. The effect of ketoconazole on the *in vivo* intestinal permeability of fexofenadine using a regional perfusion technique. *Br J Clin Pharmacol* (2003) 55, 182–90.
15. Mizollen (Mizolastine). Sanofi-Aventis. UK Summary of product characteristics, December 2014.
16. Kestin (Ebastine). Almirall SAS. French Prescribing information, February 2008.
17. Benadryl Allergy Relief (Acrivastine). McNeil Products Ltd. UK Summary of product characteristics, September 2014.

Antihistamines + Benzodiazepines and related drugs

Benzodiazepines impair psychomotor performance, and an enhanced sedative effect would be expected if known sedative antihistamines are given with benzodiazepines. Diphenhydramine does not alter the pharmacokinetics of zaleplon, but it did enhance the sedative effects of diazepam in one study.

In small studies, ebastine and mizolastine (non-sedating antihistamines) have not been shown to further increase the CNS depressant effects of the benzodiazepines.

Clinical evidence

(a) Diphenhydramine

1. Diazepam. A study in 13 healthy subjects who took diphenhydramine 50 mg twice daily for 5 days, with a single 300-microgram/kg dose of diazepam on day 5 found no additive effects on sedation or the performance of a number of psychomotor tests. The plasma levels of diazepam measured 100 minutes after administration were increased by 39%, but this was not statistically significant. It was suggested that the subjects may have developed tolerance to the sedative effects of the antihistamine.[1]

Oral administration of diazepam 10 mg with diphenhydramine 100 mg impaired psychomotor performance, when compared with diazepam alone, with effects lasting up to 4 hours after the two drugs had been taken. Subjects noted a significant feeling of drunkenness after taking diazepam with diphenhydramine. This persisted for 4 hours, which was double the time of diazepam alone.[2]

2. Zaleplon. A randomised, single-dose study in healthy subjects found that diphenhydramine 50 mg had no significant effect on the pharmacokinetics of a single 10-mg dose of zaleplon, despite the fact diphenhydramine is a moderate inhibitor of the primary metabolic pathway [aldehyde oxidase] of zaleplon.[3]

(b) Ebastine

In 12 healthy subjects, ebastine 20 mg daily did not impair the performance of a number of psychomotor tests, although body sway and flicker fusion tests were altered. When ebastine was given with a single 15-mg dose of **diazepam**, it did not further impair performance, when compared with diazepam alone, and did not alter plasma **diazepam** levels.[4]

(c) Mizolastine

A single 2-mg dose of oral **lorazepam** was found to impair the performance of psychomotor tests in 16 healthy subjects, and caused some sedation and amnesia, but these effects were not changed when the subjects also took mizolastine 10 mg daily for 8 days.[5]

Mechanism, importance and management

Evidence for an interaction between the benzodiazepines and the antihistamines is limited. However, a number of the older antihistamines cause sedation, and this would reasonably be expected to be increased by some of the benzodiazepines by the simple addition of their CNS depressant effects; this effect has been seen with diazepam and diphenhydramine. Non-sedating antihistamines would not be expected to have this effect when given with a benzodiazepine, and small studies have demonstrated that no interaction occurs when ebastine is given with diazepam, and when mizolastine is given with lorazepam. However, every non-sedating antihistamine has the potential to cause drowsiness in a minority of subjects, and in these subjects a clinically important effect might still occur. See also 'Antihistamines', p.628.

1. Mattila MJ, Mattila M, Konno K. Acute and subacute actions on human performance and interactions with diazepam of temelastine (SK&F93944) and diphenhydramine. *Eur J Clin Pharmacol* (1986) 31, 291–8.
2. Moser L, Hüther KJ, Koch-Weser J, Lundt PV. Effects of terfenadine and diphenhydramine alone or in combination with diazepam or alcohol on psychomotor performance and subjective feelings. *Eur J Clin Pharmacol* (1978) 14, 417–23.
3. Darwish M. Overview of drug interaction studies with zaleplon. Poster presented at 13th Annual Meeting of Associated Professional Sleep Studies (APSS), Orlando, Florida, June 23rd, 1999.
4. Mattila MJ, Aranko K, Kuitunen T. Diazepam effects on the performance of healthy subjects are not enhanced by treatment with the antihistamine ebastine. *Br J Clin Pharmacol* (1993) 35, 272–7.
5. Patat A, Perault MC, Vandel B, Ulliac N, Zieleniuk I, Rosenzweig P. Lack of interaction between a new antihistamine, mizolastine, and lorazepam on psychomotor performance and memory in healthy volunteers. *Br J Clin Pharmacol* (1995) 39, 31–8.

Antihistamines + Drugs that prolong the QT interval

Isolated case reports describe torsade de pointes in patients taking amiodarone and loratadine. One early study found that hydroxyzine caused ECG abnormalities in high doses and it was suggested that the risk of such changes might be increased if it is given with other drugs having similar effects. Hydroxyzine has a small risk of prolonging the QT-interval. The manufacturer of mizolastine notes that it has a weak potential to prolong the QT interval: this effect might be additive with other drugs that prolong the QT interval.

Clinical evidence, mechanism, importance and management

(a) Non-sedating antihistamines

The older non-sedating antihistamines astemizole and terfenadine were associated with prolongation of the QT interval and torsade de pointes, particularly when their metabolism was inhibited and this led to their withdrawal from the market. However, clinically relevant QT prolongation has not yet been shown conclusively for any of the other antihistamines (see 'Table 15.2', p.629). Nevertheless, a review of data on the use of non-sedating antihistamines from the UK General Practice Research Database[1] showed an overall relative risk of ventricular arrhythmias of 0 with acrivastine, 7.9 with cetirizine and 3.2 with **loratadine**. Furthermore, isolated cases of torsade de pointes have been described with **loratadine**. In one case report, a 73-year-old woman taking amiodarone for atrial fibrillation was given **loratadine**, and developed syncope and multiple episodes of torsade de pointes.[2] In a review of torsade de pointes in patients taking amiodarone long-term, two elderly female patients taking amiodarone 200 mg daily developed torsade de pointes 2 days and 7 days, respectively, after **loratadine** 10 mg daily was added.[3] It was suggested that amiodarone might have inhibited the metabolism of **loratadine** by CYP3A4; however, even in high-dose **loratadine** does not appear to consistently affect the QT interval. The general clinical relevance of these cases is uncertain, but the authors consider that the QT interval should be monitored if **loratadine** is given with other drugs that may potentially prolong the QT interval.[2]

The manufacturers of **mizolastine**[4] note that it has a weak potential to cause QT prolongation in some individuals and therefore they contraindicate its use with drugs that prolong the QT interval.

Consider also 'Drugs that prolong the QT interval + Other drugs that prolong the QT interval', p.272.

(b) Sedating antihistamines

A study conducted in 1958, in 25 elderly patients with psychoses taking high-dose **hydroxyzine** 300 mg daily over a 9-week period, found that ECG changes were mild, except for an alteration in T waves, which were definite in 9 patients. In each case the T waves were lower in altitude, broadened and flattened and sometimes notched. The QT interval was usually prolonged. A repeat of the study in a few patients, at least one given **hydroxyzine** 400 mg, found similar effects, with the most pronounced change being a marked attenuation of cardiac repolarisation. On the basis of these observations the authors suggest that other drugs that cause ECG abnormalities such as **thioridazine** might aggravate and exaggerate these **hydroxyzine**-induced changes and increase the risk of sudden death.[5] After decades of use of **hydroxyzine** since this study was conducted there appear to be only a few reports of arrhythmias (tachycardia) associated with its use,[6-8] however, a European review concluded that **hydroxyzine** is associated with a small risk of causing QT-interval prolongation or torsade de pointes.[9] Therefore the European Medicines Agency contraindicates the use of **hydroxyzine** in patients with risk factors for QT-interval prolongation, including concurrent use with other drugs that prolong the QT-interval.[9] See 'Drugs that prolong the QT interval + Other drugs that prolong the QT interval', p.272 for more information.

1. De Abajo FJ, García Rodríguez AL. Risk of ventricular arrhythmias associated with nonsedating antihistamine drugs. *Br J Clin Pharmacol* (1999) 47, 307–13.
2. Atar S, Freedberg NA, Antonelli D, Rosenfeld T. Torsade de pointes and QT prolongation due to a combination of loratadine and amiodarone. *Pacing Clin Electrophysiol* (2003) 26, 785–6.
3. Antonelli D, Atar S, Freedberg NA, Rosenfeld T. Torsade de pointes in patients on chronic amiodarone treatment: contributing factors and drug interactions. *Isr Med Assoc J* (2005) 7,163–5.
4. Mizollen (Mizolastine). Sanofi-Aventis. UK Summary of product characteristics, December 2014.
5. Hollister LE. Hydroxyzine hydrochloride: possible adverse cardiac interactions. *Psychopharmacol Comm* (1975) 1, 61–5.
6. Wong AR, Rasool AH. Hydroxyzine-induced supraventricular tachycardia in a nine-year-old child. *Singapore Med J* (2004) 45, 90–2.
7. Magera BE, Betlach CJ, Sweatt AP, Derrick CW. Hydroxyzine intoxication in a 13-month-old child. *Pediatrics* (1981) 67, 280–3.
8. Vigne J, Alexandre J, Fobe F, Milliez P, Loilier M, Fedrizzi S, Coquerel A. QT prolongation induced by hydroxyzine: a pharmacovigilance case report. *Eur J Clin Pharmacol* (2015) 71, 379–81.
9. European Medicines Agency. PRAC recommends new measures to minimise known heart risks of hydroxyzine-containing medicines. February 2015. Available at http://www.ema.europa.eu/docs/en_GB/document_library/Referrals_document/Hydroxyzine_31/Recommendation_provided_by_Pharmacovigilance_Risk_Assessment_Committee/WC500182461.pdf (accessed 21/08/15).

Antihistamines + Food

The bioavailability of ebastine is moderately increased by food. The pharmacokinetics of cetirizine, desloratadine, fexofenadine, loratadine and rupatadine are not affected to a clinically relevant extent by food.

Clinical evidence, mechanism, importance and management

(a) Cetirizine

The manufacturer of cetirizine notes that the extent of absorption of cetirizine is unaffected by food, but the rate of absorption is decreased.[1] This is not expected to be clinically relevant.

(b) Desloratadine

A study in 18 healthy subjects found no difference in the pharmacokinetics of a single 7.5-mg dose of desloratadine taken after a 10-hour fast, or after a high-fat, high-calorie breakfast.[2]

(c) Ebastine

A placebo controlled study in patients given ebastine 20 mg daily with food (115 patients) and without food (133 patients) for 2 weeks, found that the plasma levels of ebastine and its active metabolite carebastine were increased by 6% (not statistically significant) and 15%, respectively, when given with food compared with administration without food. There was no difference in efficacy measures or adverse effects when compared with placebo.[3] In two further crossover studies, healthy subjects were given either a single 10-mg dose of ebastine after an overnight fast, a low-fat breakfast or a high-fat breakfast (18 subjects); or a single 20-mg dose of ebastine after an overnight fast and a high-fat breakfast (12 subjects). The AUC and plasma level of the active metabolite carebastine were 40 to 50% and 30 to 40% higher, respectively, under fed conditions compared with fasting conditions.[4] In contrast, in 6 healthy subjects, food intake did not affect the pharmacokinetics of a single 20-mg dose of ebastine, when compared with fasting conditions.[5] The manufacturer advises that ebastine should be taken without food.[6]

(d) Fexofenadine

A crossover study in 24 healthy subjects given a single dose of fexofenadine 80 mg (as two 40 mg capsules) or 120 mg (as three 40 mg tablets) after a 10-hour fast or after a high-fat breakfast, found that the AUC and maximum plasma levels were reduced by 21% and 14% (with 80 mg as capsules), and 27% and 30% (with 120 mg as tablets), respectively.[7] This is unlikely to be clinically important.

(e) Loratadine

In a study, 24 healthy subjects were given a single 10-mg dose of extended-release loratadine after a 10-hour fast, or with a high-fat, high-calorie breakfast. Food increased the maximum plasma levels and AUC of loratadine by 53% and 76%, respectively. However, this was not considered to be clinically significant, and there was no significant difference in the reporting of adverse effects between the two groups.[8] The UK manufacturer of an immediate-release preparation of loratadine notes that food can slightly delay the absorption of loratadine, but that this has no clinically relevant effect.[9]

(f) Rupatadine

In a crossover study, 24 healthy subjects were given a single 20-mg dose of rupatadine after a high-fat breakfast, or when fasting. When taken with food, the AUC and half-life of rupatadine increased by 26% and 72%, respectively. The time to reach maximum plasma levels increased by 133%, although the maximum plasma levels were not significantly affected. The pharmacokinetics of desloratadine and 3-hydroxydesloratadine, two active metabolites of rupatadine, were not significantly affected by the presence of food. There was no apparent difference in the prevalence or severity of adverse effects between the two groups.[10] The UK manufacturer states that rupatadine may be taken without regard to food.[11]

1. Benadryl Allergy Oral Syrup (Cetirizine dihydrochloride). McNeil Ltd. UK Summary of product characteristics, November 2008.
2. Gupta S, Banfield C, Affrime M, Marbury T, Padhi D, Glue P. Oral bioavailability of desloratadine is unaffected by food. *Clin Pharmacokinet* (2002) 41 (Suppl 1), 7–12.
3. Hampel F, Gillen M, Rohatagi SS, Lim J, Georges G; the Ebastine Study Group. A double-blind, placebo-controlled study of the efficacy and safety of ebastine 20 mg once daily given with and without food in the treatment of seasonal allergic rhinitis. *J Clin Pharmacol* (2002) 42, 1097–104.
4. Pentikis HS, Huang M-Y, Dorr MB, Heald DL. The effect of food on the bioavailability of ebastine. *Am J Ther* (1997) 4, 80–4.
5. Yamaguchi T, Hashizume T, Matsuda M, Sakashita M, Fujii T, Sekine Y, Nakashima M, Uematsu T. Pharmacokinetics of the H1-receptor antagonist ebastine and its active metabolite carebastine in healthy subjects. *Arzneimittelforschung* (1994) 44, 59–64.
6. Kestin (Ebastine). Almirall SAS. French Prescribing information, February 2008.
7. Stoltz M, Arumugham T, Lippert C, Yu D, Bhargava V, Eller M, Weir S. Effect of food on the bioavailability of fexofenadine hydrochloride (MDL 16455A). *Biopharm Drug Dispos* (1997) 18, 645–8.
8. Nomeir AA, Mojaverian P, Kosoglou T, Affrime MB, Nezamis J, Radwanski E, Lin C-C, Cayen MN. Influence of food on the oral bioavailability of loratadine and pseudoephedrine from extended-release tablets in healthy volunteers. *J Clin Pharmacol* (1996) 36, 923–30.
9. Loratadine. Sandoz Ltd. UK Summary of product characteristics, April 2008.
10. Solans A, Carbó ML, Peña J, Nadal T, Izquierdo I, Merlos M. Influence of food on the oral bioavailability of rupatadine tablets in healthy volunteers: a single-dose, randomized, open-label, two-way crossover study. *Clin Ther* (2007) 29, 900–8.
11. Rupafin (Rupatadine fumarate). GlaxoSmithKline UK. UK Summary of product characteristics, December 2009.

Antihistamines + Grapefruit and other fruit juices

The absorption of fexofenadine is modestly reduced by grapefruit juice, orange juice, and apple juice. The metabolism of ebastine might be affected by grapefruit juice, whereas grapefruit juice does not appear to alter the pharmacokinetics of desloratadine.

Clinical evidence

(a) Desloratadine

The bioavailability of a single 5-mg dose of desloratadine was unaffected by about 240 mL (8 oz) of double-strength grapefruit juice, which was given three times daily for 2 days before the desloratadine and then 5 minutes before and 2 hours after the dose.[1]

(b) Ebastine

A study in 61 healthy subjects given a single 20-mg dose of ebastine found that the urinary excretion of the metabolite desalkylebastine was reduced by about 25% by grapefruit juice. In this study 250 mL of grapefruit juice was given three times daily for 2 days before the ebastine and then simultaneously with the dose.[2]

(c) Fexofenadine

A study in 12 healthy subjects found that 300-mL of normal strength grapefruit juice reduced the AUC of a single 120-mg dose of fexofenadine by 42% when they were given simultaneously. This effect was greater (64% reduction in AUC) when 1.2 litres of grapefruit juice was given (as 300 mL simultaneously with the fexofenadine, followed by 150 mL every 30 minutes until 3 hours after dosing).[3] An effect was apparent for 300 mL of grapefruit juice given up to 10 hours before fexofenadine 120 mg in at least some of the subjects involved in this study.[4]

In a study in 23 healthy subjects the AUC of fexofenadine 60 mg was reduced by 30% by about 240 mL (8 oz) of double-strength grapefruit juice, which was given three times daily for 2 days before the fexofenadine and then 5 minutes before and 2 hours after the dose.[1] Similarly, another study in 10 healthy subjects using 1.2 litres of juice given as described above, found that grapefruit juice at normal strength decreased the AUC of a single 120-mg dose of fexofenadine by 67%. Dilute grapefruit juice (25%) caused a smaller reduction in the AUC of fexofenadine of 23%. Normal strength **orange juice** and **apple juice** also decreased the AUC of fexofenadine, by 72% and 77%, respectively.[5]

A study in 12 healthy subjects given 300 mL of grapefruit juice with, 2 hours before, or 4 hours before a single 120-mg dose of fexofenadine found that the decrease in AUC was greatest with simultaneous administration (52%) and there was no effect when administration was separated by 4 hours.[6] A study in 14 healthy subjects given a single 60-mg dose of fexofenadine at the same time as 400 mL of **apple juice**, found that the AUC of fexofenadine decreased by 49 to 59%.[7]

(d) Rupatadine

When it was available, the UK manufacturer of rupatadine noted that the concurrent use of grapefruit juice increased the systemic exposure of rupatadine 3.5-fold.[8]

Mechanism

Ebastine is partly metabolised by CYP3A4. Grapefruit juice is a known inhibitor of this isoenzyme and this could account for the changes in ebastine metabolism that were seen on concurrent use.

Fexofenadine is a substrate for P-glycoprotein, and organic anion transporting polypeptides (OATPs), and changes in their function might affect fexofenadine uptake. OATPs in particular can be inhibited by grapefruit juice, apple juice, and orange juice, so these juices could reduce fexofenadine concentrations by preventing its absorption.[5] One study suggests that specific flavonoid components of grapefruit juice (naringin) and orange juice (hesperidin) are responsible for this inhibition of OATP.[9]

Importance and management

Evidence for an interaction between grapefruit juice and **rupatadine** appears to be limited to one study that did not appear to assess the clinical relevance of the increased rupatadine exposure. Nevertheless, the increase would be expected to be clinically relevant and (when it was available) the UK manufacturer of rupatadine advised that grapefruit juice should not be taken simultaneously.[8]

Similarly, evidence for an interaction between grapefruit juice and **ebastine** appears to be limited to one study, which also did not assess the clinical relevance of the changes in ebastine metabolism. Until more is known it might be prudent to suspect an interaction if ebastine adverse effects become troublesome in a patient drinking grapefruit juice.

Further study is required to determine the clinical relevance, if any, of the reductions in **fexofenadine** bioavailability in the presence of grapefruit juice, orange juice, and apple juice. Consider this interaction as a possible cause if fexofenadine seems less effective than expected. However, note that the amounts of fruit juice consumed in two studies were quite large (1.2 litres).

There appears to be no data regarding any possible interaction between **acrivastine** and grapefruit juice and the UK manufacturer of acrivastine therefore advises caution on their concurrent use.[10]

Desloratadine does not appear to interact with grapefruit juice and it may therefore be a suitable alternative to the interacting antihistamines.

1. Banfield C, Gupta S, Marino M, Lim J, Affrime M. Grapefruit juice reduces the oral bioavailability of fexofenadine but not desloratadine. *Clin Pharmacokinet* (2002) 41, 311–18.
2. Gervasini G, Vizcaino S, Carrillo JA, Caballero MJ, Benitez J. The effect of CYP2J2, CYP3A4, CYP3A5 and the MDR1^{C3435T} polymorphisms and gender on the urinary excretion of the metabolites of the H_1-receptor antihistamine ebastine: a pilot study. *Br J Clin Pharmacol* (2006) 62, 177–86.
3. Dresser GK, Kim RB, Bailey DG. Effect of grapefruit juice volume on the reduction of fexofenadine bioavailability: possible role of organic anion transporting polypeptides. *Clin Pharmacol Ther* (2005) 77, 170–7.
4. Dresser GK, Kim RB, Bailey DG. Duration of grapefruit juice effect on fexofenadine interaction. *Clin Pharmacol Ther* (2003) 73, P48.
5. Dresser GK, Bailey DG, Leake BF, Schwarz UI, Dawson PA, Freeman DJ, Kim RB. Fruit juices inhibit organic anion transporting polypeptide–mediated drug uptake to decrease the oral availability of fexofenadine. *Clin Pharmacol Ther* (2002) 71, 11–20.
6. Glaeser H, Bailey DG, Dresser GK, Gregor JC, Schwarz UI, McGrath JS, Jolicoeur E, Lee W, Leake BF, Tirona RG, Kim RB. Intestinal drug transporter expression and the impact of grapefruit juice in humans. *Clin Pharmacol Ther* (2007) 81, 362–70.
7. Akamine Y, Miura M, Komori H, Saito S, Kusuhara H, Tamai I, Ieiri I, Uno T, Yasui-Furukori N. Effects of one-time apple juice ingestion on the pharmacokinetics of fexofenadine enantiomers. *Eur J Clin Pharmacol* (2014) 70, 1087–95.
8. Rupafin (Rupatadine fumarate). GlaxoSmithKline UK. UK Summary of product characteristics, December 2009.
9. Bailey DG, Dresser GK, Leake BF, Kim RB. Naringin is a major and selective clinical inhibitor of organic anion-transporting polypeptide 1A2 (OATP1A2) in grapefruit juice. *Clin Pharmacol Ther* (2007) 81, 495–502.
10. Benadryl Allergy Relief (Acrivastine). McNeil Products Ltd. UK Summary of product characteristics, September 2014.

Antihistamines + H_2-receptor antagonists

Cimetidine doubles loratadine levels, without affecting its adverse effects, and moderately increases hydroxyzine exposure. The renal clearance of fexofenadine was reduced by cimetidine in one study. Cimetidine does not appear to affect the pharmacokinetics of cetirizine, desloratadine, or ebastine, and ranitidine does not appear to affect the pharmacokinetics of chlorphenamine.

Clinical evidence

A. Non-sedating antihistamines

(a) Cetirizine

Cetirizine 10 mg was given to 8 patients with chronic urticaria before and after they took **cimetidine** 600 mg every 12 hours for 10 days. The pharmacokinetics of cetirizine were statistically unaltered and its effects remained unchanged.[1]

(b) Desloratadine

In a parallel study in 18 healthy subjects, **cimetidine** 600 mg every 12 hours had little effect on the pharmacokinetics of desloratadine 5 mg daily. The desloratadine AUC was increased by about 20% and its maximum level was increased by about 10%,[2,3] and there was no change in ECG parameters, including the QTc interval.[2]

(c) Ebastine

In a study in 12 healthy subjects, **cimetidine** had little effect on the conversion of a single 20-mg dose of ebastine to its active metabolite, carebastine, and there was no evidence of sedation or other adverse effects. In this study **cimetidine** was given as 2 g in divided doses the day before the ebastine dose and 400 mg four times daily both on the day of, and the day after, the ebastine dose.[4]

(d) Fexofenadine

In 12 healthy subjects, **cimetidine** 400 mg twice daily for 6 days did not cause any changes in the plasma pharmacokinetics of a single 120-mg dose of fexofenadine. However, the renal clearance of fexofenadine was decreased by 39%.[5]

(e) Loratadine

In a study, 24 healthy subjects were given loratadine 10 mg and **cimetidine** 300 mg every 6 hours, alone and together for 10 days. The AUCs of loratadine and its metabolite were increased by 103% and 6%, respectively, but the safety profile of loratadine (clinical laboratory tests, vital signs and adverse events) was unchanged. Cardiac repolarisation and all other ECG measurements were unaltered, and no sedation or syncope were seen.[6]

B. Sedating antihistamines

(a) Chlorphenamine

A study in healthy subjects found that the pharmacokinetics of a single 4-mg dose of chlorphenamine were unaffected by **ranitidine** 75 mg twice daily for 6 days.[7]

(b) Hydroxyzine

In one study, 8 patients with chronic urticaria were given hydroxyzine 25 mg before and after taking **cimetidine** 600 mg every 12 hours for 10 days. **Cimetidine** increased the AUC of hydroxyzine by 33% and also increased its suppression of the wheal and flare response (although this was not statistically significant).[1] A previous study in 7 patients found that **cimetidine** raised serum hydroxyzine levels.[8]

Mechanism

Cimetidine is a non-specific cytochrome P450 isoenzyme inhibitor, but it would seem that in most cases, with the exception of loratadine, this does not result in a significant effect on the metabolism of these antihistamines.

Cimetidine can also affect drug transporter proteins, in particular it may inhibit organic cation transporters. However, it probably does not affect anion transporter proteins as it does not affect the plasma pharmacokinetics of fexofenadine, which is a substrate of these transporters.[5]

Importance and management

There would seem to be no good reason for avoiding the concurrent use of either cetirizine, ebastine, desloratadine, fexofenadine, hydroxyzine, or loratadine with cimetidine, or chlorphenamine with ranitidine. Other H_2-receptor antagonists would not be expected to interact with any of these antihistamines, but this does not appear to have been studied.

The manufacturer of **mizolastine** recommends caution on the concurrent use of cimetidine,[9] with the implication that cimetidine might increase mizolastine levels and prolong the QT interval.

1. Simons FER, Sussman GL, Simons KJ. Effect of the H_2-antagonist cimetidine on the pharmacokinetics and pharmacodynamics of the H_1-antagonists hydroxyzine and cetirizine in patients with chronic urticaria. *J Allergy Clin Immunol* (1995) 95, 685–93.
2. Clarinex (Desloratadine). Schering Corporation. US Prescribing information, February 2007.
3. Krishna G, Khalilieh S, Ezzet F, Marino M, Kantesaria B, Lim J, Batra V. Effect of cimetidine on the pharmacokinetics of desloratadine. *AAPS PharmSci* (2001) 3, 3. Available at: http://www.aapsj.org/abstracts/AM_2001/824.htm (accessed 21/10/15).
4. van Rooij J, Schoemaker HC, Bruno R, Reinhoudt JF, Breimer DD, Cohen AF. Cimetidine does not influence the metabolism of the H_1-receptor antagonist ebastine to its active metabolite carebastine. *Br J Clin Pharmacol* (1993) 35, 661–3.
5. Yasui-Furukori N, Uno T, Sugawara K, Tateishi T. Different effects of three transporting inhibitors, verapamil, cimetidine, and probenecid, on fexofenadine pharmacokinetics. *Clin Pharmacol Ther* (2005) 77, 17–23.
6. Kosoglou T, Salfi M, Lim JM, Batra VK, Cayen MN, Affrime MB. Evaluation of the pharmacokinetics and electrocardiographic pharmacodynamics of loratadine with concomitant administration of ketoconazole or cimetidine. *Br J Clin Pharmacol* (2000) 50, 581–9.
7. Koch KM, O'Connor-Semmes RL, Davis IM, Yin Y. Stereoselective pharmacokinetics of chlorpheniramine and the effect of ranitidine. *J Pharm Sci* (1998) 87, 1097–1100.
8. Salo OP, Kauppinen K, Männistö PT. Cimetidine increases the plasma concentration of hydroxyzine. *Acta Derm Venereol (Stockh)* (1986), 66, 349–50.
9. Mizollen (Mizolastine). Sanofi-Aventis. UK Summary of product characteristics, December 2014.

Antihistamines + HIV-protease inhibitors

Ritonavir modestly increases cetirizine concentrations. Nelfinavir and hydroxyzine have been used together without adverse effects. HIV-protease inhibitors are predicted to increase mizolastine concentrations and ritonavir is predicted to increase loratadine concentrations.

Clinical evidence, mechanism, importance and management

(a) Cetirizine

In a study in 16 healthy subjects, the concurrent use of cetirizine 10 mg daily and **ritonavir** 600 mg twice daily for 4 days (after reaching steady-state **ritonavir** concentrations), increased the AUC of cetirizine by 42% and increased its maximum plasma concentration by 9%. **Ritonavir** pharmacokinetics were minimally affected by cetirizine. It was suggested that **ritonavir** might have decreased the renal excretion of cetirizine. The increase in cetirizine concentrations was not considered to be clinically relevant.[1]

(b) Fexofenadine

For the interactions of the HIV-protease inhibitors with fexofenadine, see 'Antihistamines; Fexofenadine + HIV-protease inhibitors', below.

(c) Hydroxyzine

A report describes the uneventful use of hydroxyzine in 10 HIV-positive children, who had developed a rash thought to be related to **nelfinavir** use.[2]

(d) Loratadine

The UK manufacturer states that **ritonavir**, including **ritonavir** given to boost other HIV-protease inhibitors, is expected to increase the plasma concentrations of loratadine by inhibiting its metabolism by CYP3A4.[3] This is in line with the way loratadine has been seen to interact with other CYP3A4 inhibitors. It would seem prudent to warn patients to be alert for loratadine adverse effects (e.g. fatigue, nausea, headache) if they are also given **ritonavir**.

(e) Mizolastine

The UK manufacturer of mizolastine states that the concurrent use of potent inhibitors of CYP3A4 should be approached with caution.[4] Although not specifically named, this would be expected to include the HIV-protease inhibitors. Note that the concurrent use of the macrolides, which are generally less potent CYP3A4 inhibitors than some of the HIV-protease inhibitors, is contraindicated because of the potential for QT prolongation with raised mizolastine concentrations, see 'Antihistamines + Macrolides', below.

1. Peytavin G, Gautran C, Otoul C, Cremieux AC, Moulaert B, Delatour F, Melac M, Strolin-Benedetti M, Farinotti R. Evaluation of pharmacokinetic interaction between cetirizine and ritonavir, an HIV-1 protease inhibitor, in healthy male volunteers. *Eur J Clin Pharmacol* (2005) 61, 267–73.
2. Fortuny C, Vicente MA, Medina MM, González-Enseñat A. Rash as a side-effect of nelfinavir in children. *AIDS* (2000) 14, 335–6.
3. Norvir Soft Capsules (Ritonavir). Abbott Laboratories Ltd. UK Summary of product characteristics, October 2010.
4. Mizollen (Mizolastine). Sanofi-Aventis. UK Summary of product characteristics, December 2014.

Antihistamines; Fexofenadine + HIV-protease inhibitors

Ritonavir, indinavir (alone or boosted by ritonavir) and lopinavir boosted with ritonavir increase fexofenadine exposure. Nelfinavir reduces fexofenadine concentrations but has no effect on its exposure.

Clinical evidence

(a) Lopinavir

A study in 16 healthy subjects who took a single 120-mg dose of fexofenadine before, and after taking lopinavir boosted with ritonavir 400/100 mg daily for 11 days found that the median AUC and maximum plasma concentration of fexofenadine were increased 3.5-fold and 3-fold, respectively. In this study the pharmacokinetics of fexofenadine were evaluated in 8 of the subjects after a single dose of lopinavir with ritonavir: the increase in median AUC and maximum plasma concentration was found to be 4-fold and 3.8-fold, respectively.[1]

(b) Indinavir

In a crossover study in 12 healthy subjects, indinavir 800 mg three times daily for 15 days increased the AUC and maximum plasma concentration of a single 60-mg dose of fexofenadine 3.3- and 3.4-fold, respectively.[2] In a similar study by the same authors, 12 healthy subjects were given a single 60-mg dose of fexofenadine on days 2 (acute administration) and 15 (steady-state administration) of a 21-day course of indinavir boosted with ritonavir 800/100 mg twice daily. The AUC of fexofenadine was increased 2.5-fold and 2.8-fold by acute and steady-state indinavir boosted with ritonavir, respectively. The maximum plasma concentration of fexofenadine was increased 4.8-fold and 4.2-fold by acute and steady-state administration, respectively.[3]

(c) Nelfinavir

In a study in 12 healthy subjects, nelfinavir 1.25 g twice daily for at least 15 days, decreased the maximum plasma concentration of a single 60-mg dose of fexofenadine by 25%, but had no effect on its AUC.[4]

(d) Ritonavir

In a study, 12 healthy subjects took ritonavir in increasing doses up to 400 mg twice daily for 2 weeks, followed by a single 60-mg dose of fexofenadine. The maximum plasma concentration of fexofenadine was increased by 60% and its AUC was increased 2.8-fold after the subjects took ritonavir 200 mg three times a day for one day, but after steady-state was attained, ritonavir increased the AUC of fexofenadine by 40%, and the increase in its plasma concentration was not statistically significant.[5]

In a study in 8 healthy subjects the median AUC and maximum plasma concentration of fexofenadine were increased 2.7-fold and 2.2-fold, respectively, by ritonavir.[1]

Mechanism

Fexofenadine is not principally metabolised by the cytochrome P450 enzyme system, but is a substrate for P-glycoprotein and OATP. The HIV-protease inhibitors studied therefore increase its exposure by altering the function of these drug transporter proteins. The exception is nelfinavir, which appears to have the opposite effect to the other HIV-protease inhibitors studied, as it decreases fexofenadine concentrations, although note that fexofenadine exposure is not affected.

Importance and management

A pharmacokinetic interaction between fexofenadine and the HIV-protease inhibitors would seem to be established, although the effect is not consistent, with lopinavir boosted with ritonavir, indinavir (boosted and un-boosted) and ritonavir all increasing fexofenadine concentrations, and nelfinavir reducing fexofenadine concentrations. Large increases in fexofenadine concentrations seen in studies with erythromycin (see 'Antihistamines + Macrolides', below) and ketoconazole (see 'Antihistamines + Azoles', p.630), did not increase the adverse effects of fexofenadine and were not associated with any prolongation of the QT interval. This suggests that a clinically relevant interaction between indinavir (alone or boosted by ritonavir), ritonavir or lopinavir boosted with ritonavir and fexofenadine is unlikely. The clinical importance of the decrease in fexofenadine concentrations seen with nelfinavir is not known, but it seems likely to be small.

1. van Heeswijk RPG, Bourbeau M, Campbell P, Seguin I, Chauhan BM, Foster BC, Cameron DW. Time-dependent interaction between lopinavir/ritonavir and fexofenadine. *J Clin Pharmacol* (2006) 46, 758–67.
2. Kharasch ED, Bedynek PS, Hoffer C, Walker A, Whittington D. Lack of indinavir effects on methadone disposition despite inhibition of hepatic and intestinal cytochrome P4503A (CYP3A). *Anesthesiology* (2012) 116, 432–47.
3. Kharasch ED, Hoffer C, Whittington D, Walker A, Bedynek PS. Methadone pharmacokinetics are independent of cytochrome P4503A (CYP3A) activity and gastrointestinal drug transport: insights from methadone interactions with ritonavir/indinavir. *Anesthesiology* (2009) 110, 660–72.
4. Kharasch ED, Walker A, Whittington D, Hoffer C, Bedynek PS. Methadone metabolism and clearance are induced by nelfinavir despite inhibition of cytochrome P4503A (CYP3A) activity. *Drug Alcohol Depend* (2009) 101, 158–68.
5. Kharasch ED, Bedynek PS, Walker A, Whittington D, Hoffer C. Mechanism of ritonavir changes in methadone pharmacokinetics and pharmacodynamics: II. Ritonavir effects on CYP3A and P-glycoprotein activities. *Clin Pharmacol Ther* (2008) 84, 506–12.

Antihistamines + Macrolides

Erythromycin markedly raised ebastine levels, with a modest prolongation of the QT interval. Erythromycin also raises fexofenadine, loratadine, mizolastine and rupatadine levels, but without a clinically relevant effect on the QT interval. Acrivastine is predicted to interact similarly.

Clarithromycin raises loratadine levels, with a minor effect on the QT interval, and azithromycin raises fexofenadine levels with no clinically relevant effect on QT interval. Azithromycin has no effect on rupatadine levels.

Azelastine, cetirizine, desloratadine, and intranasal levocabastine seem to be free of clinically relevant interactions with the macrolides.

Clinical evidence

Single or multiple-dose controlled studies have found that **azithromycin** had no clinically relevant effect on the pharmacokinetics of **cetirizine**, **desloratadine**, or **rupatadine**; and **erythromycin** had no clinically relevant effect on the pharmacokinetics of **azelastine**, **cetirizine**, or intranasal **levocabastine**, see 'Table 15.4', p.636.

In contrast, multiple-dose controlled studies with **erythromycin** have shown increases in the plasma levels and AUC of **ebastine** (119% and 164%, respectively), **fexofenadine** (82% and 109%, respectively), **loratadine** (53% and 40%, respectively) or **mizolastine** (40% and 53%, respectively). Increases in QT interval have been seen in multiple-dose studies with **ebastine** and **erythromycin** (19.6 milliseconds).

Other studies have found that **azithromycin** increases the plasma level and AUC of **fexofenadine** by about 70%, and **clarithromycin** increases the plasma level and AUC of **loratadine** by 36% and 76%, respectively, with a minor effect on the QT interval (4 milliseconds).

Details of all of these studies are summarised in 'Table 15.4', p.636. In addition, a review reports a study in which the systemic exposure to **rupatadine** 20 mg daily was increased two- to threefold by **erythromycin** 500 mg three times daily for 7 days. There were no clinically relevant changes in the QT interval, vital signs or adverse effects.[1]

Mechanism

Ebastine, loratadine, mizolastine probably rupatadine,[2] and possibly desloratadine are metabolised to varying extents by the cytochrome P450 isoenzyme CYP3A4. Erythromycin and clarithromycin are known inhibitors of this isoenzyme and so concurrent use of these antihistamines and macrolides leads to increased antihistamine levels. The strength of the effect varies between different combinations of macrolides and antihistamines according to the strength of the inhibitory effect of the macrolide on CYP3A4 and the degree to which the antihistamine is metabolised by this isoenzyme.

With the exception of astemizole and terfenadine the risk of cardiac arrhythmias with non-sedating antihistamines appears to be very low (see 'Table 15.2', p.629), so any pharmacokinetic interactions do not usually result in clinically relevant cardiac toxicity. In fact, studies have shown that fexofenadine in overdose,[3,4] loratadine at four times the recommended dose for 90 days,[5] and mizolastine at four times the recommended dose[6] do not affect the QT interval. However, some questions remain about ebastine, loratadine and mizolastine.

Erythromycin and azithromycin may increase the absorption and decrease the biliary secretion of fexofenadine by an effect on drug transporters such as P-glycoprotein: this leads to an increase in fexofenadine levels.

Table 15.4 Summary of the effect of macrolides on the pharmacokinetics of non-sedating antihistamines and the associated cardiovascular effects

Antihistamine (Oral unless specified)	*Macrolide (Oral unless specified)*	*Duration of combined use (days)*	*Subjects*	*Cmax increase*	*AUC increase*	*Effect on QTc*	*Refs*
Azelastine 4 mg twice daily	Erythromycin 500 mg three times daily	7	8 healthy subjects	No clinically relevant change	No clinically relevant change	No clinically relevant change	1
Cetirizine 20 mg daily	Azithromycin 500 mg, then 250 mg daily	5	14 healthy subjects	No clinically relevant change	No clinically relevant change	No clinically relevant change	2
Cetirizine 20 mg daily	Erythromycin 500 mg three times daily	10	Healthy subjects	No clinically relevant change	No clinically relevant change	No clinically relevant change	3, 4
Cetirizine 10 mg daily in children over 30 kg	Erythromycin 50 mg/kg per day	14	10 patients aged 5 to 12 years	Not studied	Not studied	No clinically relevant change with Bazett's correction	5
Desloratadine 5 mg daily	Azithromycin 500 mg, then 250 mg daily	5	18 healthy subjects	No clinically relevant change	No clinically relevant change	No clinically relevant change	6
Desloratadine 7.5 mg daily	Erythromycin 500 mg three times daily	10	24 healthy subjects	20% desloratadine 40% 3-hydroxy desloratadine	10% desloratadine 40% 3-hydroxy desloratadine	No clinically relevant change	7
Ebastine 20 mg daily	Erythromycin 2.4 g daily	10	30 healthy subjects	119% Similar changes found for carebastine	164% Similar changes found for carebastine	Mean increase of 19.6 milliseconds	8
Fexofenadine 60 mg twice daily	Azithromycin 500 mg, then 250 mg daily	5	18 healthy subjects	69%	67%	No clinically relevant change	6
Fexofenadine 120 mg twice daily	Erythromycin 500 mg three times daily	7	24 healthy subjects	82%	109%	No clinically relevant change	9
Levocabastine 200 micrograms twice daily intranasal	Erythromycin 333 mg single dose	Single dose of macrolide	38 healthy subjects	No clinically relevant change	No clinically relevant change	No clinically relevant change	10
Loratadine 10 mg daily	Clarithromycin 500 mg twice daily	10	24 healthy subjects	36% loratadine 69% descarbo-ethoxyloratadine	76% loratadine 49% descarbo-ethoxyloratadine	Mean increase of 4 milliseconds. Maximum QTc 439 milliseconds	11
Loratadine 10 mg daily	Erythromycin 500 mg three times daily	10	24 healthy subjects	53% loratadine 61% descarbo-ethoxyloratadine	40% loratadine 46% descarbo-ethoxyloratadine	No change	12
Loratadine 5 mg daily for children less than 30 kg; 10 mg daily for children greater than or equal to 30 kg	Erythromycin 50 mg/kg per day	14	10 patients aged 5 to 12 years	Not studied	Not studied	No clinically relevant change with Bazett's correction	5
Mizolastine 10 mg daily	Erythromycin 1 g twice daily	6	12 healthy subjects	40%	53%	No clinically relevant change	13
Rupatadine 10 mg daily	Azithromycin 500 mg, then 250 mg daily	5	24 healthy subjects	No clinically relevant change	No clinically relevant change	No clinically relevant change	14

1. Sale M, Lyness W, Perhach J, Woosley R, Rosenberg A. Lack of effect of coadministration of erythromycin (ERY) with azelastine (AZ) on pharmacokinetics (PK) or ECG parameters. *Ann Allergy Asthma Immunol* (1996) 74, 91.
2. Sale M, Woosley R, Thakker K, Phillips K, Caridi F, Chung M. A randomized, placebo-controlled, multiple-dose study to evaluate the electrocardiographic and pharmacokinetic interactions of azithromycin and cetirizine. *Ann Allergy Asthma Immunol* (1996) 74, 93.
3. UCB Pharma. Personal communication, September 1994.
4. Sale M, Woosley R, Thakker K, Phillips K, Caridi F, Chung M. Effects of cetirizine and erythromycin alone and in combination on QT interval and pharmacokinetics in healthy subjects. *Ann Allergy Asthma Immunol* (1996) 74, 93.
5. Delgado LF, Pferferman A, Solé D, Naspitz CK. Evaluation of the potential cardiotoxicity of the antihistamines terfenadine, astemizole, loratadine, and cetirizine in atopic children. *Ann Allergy Asthma Immunol* (1998) 80, 333–7.
6. Gupta S, Banfield C, Kantesaria B, Marino M, Clement R, Affrime M, Batra V. Pharmacokinetic and safety profile of desloratadine and fexofenadine when coadministered with azithromycin: a randomized, placebo-controlled, parallel-group study. *Clin Ther* (2001) 23, 451–66.
7. Banfield C, Hunt T, Reyderman L, Statkevich P, Padhi D, Affrime M. Lack of clinically relevant interaction between desloratadine and erythromycin. *Clin Pharmacokinet* (2002) 41 (Suppl 1), 29–35.
8. Gillen M, Pentikis H, Rhodes G, Chaikin P, Morganroth J. Pharmacokinetic (PK) and pharmacodynamic (PD) interaction of ebastine (EBA) and erythromycin (ERY). *Clin Invest Med* (1998) (Suppl), S20.
9. Allegra (Fexofenadine hydrochloride). Sanofi-Aventis U.S. LLC. US Prescribing information, July 2007.
10. Pesco-Koplowitz L, Hassell A, Lee P, Zhou H, Hall N, Wiesinger B, Mechlinski W, Grover M, Hunt T, Smith R, Travers S. Lack of effect of erythromycin and ketoconazole on the pharmacokinetics and pharmacodynamics of steady-state intranasal levocabastine. *J Clin Pharmacol* (1999) 39, 76–85.

Continued

Table 15.4 Summary of the effect of macrolides on the pharmacokinetics of non-sedating antihistamines and the associated cardiovascular effects (continued)

11. Carr RA, Edmonds A, Shi H, Locke CS, Gustavson LE, Craft JÇ, Harris SI, Palmer R. Steady-state pharmacokinetics and electrocardiographic pharmacodynamics of clarithromycin and loratadine after individual or concomitant administration. *Antimicrob Agents Chemother* (1998) 42, 1176–80.
12. Brannan MD, Reidenberg P, Radwanski E, Shneyer L, Lin C-C, Cayen MN, Affrime MB. Loratadine administered concomitantly with erythromycin: pharmacokinetic and electrocardiographic evaluations. *Clin Pharmacol Ther* (1995) 58, 269–78.
13. Chaufour S, Holt B, Jensen R, Dubruc C, Deschamp C, Rosenzweig R. Interaction study between mizolastine, a new H1 antihistamine, and erythromycin. *Clin Pharmacol Ther* (1998) 63, 214.
14. Solans A, Izquierdo I, Donado E, Antonijoan R, Peña J, Nadal T, Carbó ML, Merlos M, Barbanoj M. Pharmacokinetic and safety profile of rupatadine when coadministered with azithromycin at steady-state levels: a randomised, open-label, two-way, crossover, phase I study. *Clin Ther* (2008) 30, 1639–50.

Importance and management

The interaction between erythromycin and a number of the non-sedating antihistamines is established and can be clinically important, although not all antihistamines are affected to the same degree.

The manufacturer of **mizolastine** contraindicates the concurrent use of the macrolides,[7] although evidence of a clinically significant interaction appears to be lacking. Furthermore, not all macrolides affect CYP3A4 to the same extent.

Erythromycin markedly raises **ebastine** levels causing a modest increase in QT interval: the manufacturer of ebastine does not recommend the concurrent use of erythromycin, clarithromycin and josamycin, and advises caution with CYP3A4 inhibitors such as the macrolides.[8]

The manufacturer of **rupatadine**[2] advises that it should be used with caution with erythromycin, and other inhibitors of CYP3A4, which would include a number of the macrolides. It would seem prudent to monitor the concurrent use of rupatadine and a macrolide (particularly erythromycin, clarithromycin and telithromycin) for adverse effects including dry mouth, dizziness and fatigue.

There are no data on any possible interaction between **acrivastine** and erythromycin, and therefore the manufacturer advises caution.[9]

Erythromycin and clarithromycin raise **loratadine** levels, which caused a very slight increase in the QTc interval with clarithromycin. However, no special precautions appear to have been recommended for the use of loratadine with macrolides.

Other antihistamines

Fexofenadine levels are raised by both azithromycin and erythromycin but because this does not result in adverse cardiac effects concurrent use is considered safe. **Azelastine**, cetirizine (and therefore probably its isomer **levocetirizine**), desloratadine and intranasal levocabastine seem to be free from clinically important pharmacokinetic interactions, and have no cardiac adverse effects, and so may therefore provide suitable alternatives if a non-sedating antihistamine is needed in a patient taking macrolides.

1. Izquierdo I, Merlos M, García-Rafanell J. Rupatadine. A new selective histamine H_1 receptor and platelet-activating factor (PAF) antagonist. A review of pharmacological profile and clinical management of allergic rhinitis. *Drugs Today* (2003) 39, 451–68.
2. Rupafin (Rupatadine fumarate). GlaxoSmithKline UK. UK Summary of product characteristics, December 2009.
3. Allegra (Fexofenadine hydrochloride). Sanofi-Aventis US LLC. US Prescribing information, July 2007.
4. Telfast (Fexofenadine hydrochloride). Sanofi-Aventis. UK Summary of product characteristics, June 2008.
5. Affrime MB, Lorber R, Danzig M, Cuss F, Brannan MD. Three month evaluation of electrocardiographic effects of loratadine in humans. *J Allergy Clin Immunol* (1993) 91, 259.
6. Chaufour S, Caplain H, Lilienthal N, L'Héritier C, Deschamps C, Rosenzweig P. Mizolastine, a new H_1 antagonist, does not affect the cardiac repolarisation in healthy volunteers. *Clin Pharmacol Ther* (1998) 63, 214.
7. Mizollen (Mizolastine). Sanofi-Aventis. UK Summary of product characteristics, December 2014.
8. Kestin (Ebastine). Almirall SAS. French Prescribing information, February 2008.
9. Benadryl Allergy Relief (Acrivastine). McNeil Products Ltd. UK Summary of product characteristics, September 2014.

Antihistamines + Rifampicin (Rifampin)

Rifampicin greatly reduces the levels and effects of ebastine and increases the oral clearance of fexofenadine.

Clinical evidence, mechanism, importance and management

(a) Ebastine

In a pharmacokinetic study, 10 healthy subjects were given rifampicin 600 mg daily for 10 days, with a single 20-mg dose of ebastine on day 9. Rifampicin reduced the maximum plasma levels and AUC of ebastine by 81% and 76%, respectively, and diminished the effects of ebastine on a histamine-induced wheal and flare reaction.[1] This was thought to be due to the effects of rifampicin, a potent enzyme inducer on the metabolism of ebastine by CYP3A4 and possible other routes.

This study suggests that the efficacy of ebastine will be greatly decreased in the presence of rifampicin; it may be prudent to consider an alternative antihistamine in patients taking rifampicin.

(b) Fexofenadine

In a study in 24 healthy subjects, a single 60-mg dose of fexofenadine was given 2 days before and on the last day of a 6-day course of rifampicin 600 mg daily. The oral clearance of fexofenadine was increased 1.3- to 5.3-fold, with no effect on the renal clearance or half-life of fexofenadine. This was thought to be due to the effect of rifampicin on P-glycoprotein, which is involved in the uptake of fexofenadine.[2] The clinical importance of this interaction does not appear to have been studied, but until more is known it would seem prudent to monitor for reduced fexofenadine efficacy if rifampicin is also given.

1. Shon J-H, Yeo C-W, Liu K-H, Lee S-S, Cha I-J, Shin J-G. Itraconazole and rifampin alter significantly the disposition and antihistamine effect of ebastine and its metabolites in healthy participants. *J Clin Pharmacol* (2010) 50, 195–204.
2. Hamman MA, Bruce MA, Haehner-Daniels BD, Hall SD. The effect of rifampin administration on the disposition of fexofenadine. *Clin Pharmacol Ther* (2001) 69, 114–21.

Antihistamines + SSRIs

A case report describes prolonged delirium in a patient who took an overdose of promethazine and fluvoxamine. There does not appear to be a pharmacokinetic interaction between desloratadine and fluoxetine.

Clinical evidence and mechanism

(a) Desloratadine

In a placebo-controlled study in healthy subjects, the concurrent use of desloratadine 5 mg daily and **fluoxetine** 20 mg daily for 7 days (after attainment of **fluoxetine** steady-state) had no clinically relevant effects on the pharmacokinetics of either drug (changes in maximum levels and AUC were less than 15%). There was no change in ECG parameters including the QTc interval, and concurrent use did not increase the incidence of adverse effects.[1]

(b) Promethazine

A case report describes a 14-year-old girl taking **fluvoxamine** 150 mg daily who took an overdose of promethazine 1150 mg and cyproheptadine 200 mg. She developed an anticholinergic delirium, which lasted for 6 days. The authors suggest that this effect was prolonged because both promethazine and **fluvoxamine** are inhibitors and metabolites of CYP2D6, and thus the clearance of both drugs may have been impaired. However, other factors, such as her small size and the use of olanzapine to control the delirium, may have been contributing factors.[2]

Importance and management

Evidence regarding interactions between antihistamines and SSRIs is limited. On the whole, there is no evidence to suggest that an interaction between the SSRIs and the majority of antihistamines is likely if they are taken at clinically appropriate doses. The absence of a pharmacokinetic interaction with desloratadine and fluoxetine has been demonstrated.

1. Gupta S, Banfield C, Kantesaria B, Flannery B, Herron J. Pharmacokinetics/pharmacodynamics of desloratadine and fluoxetine in healthy volunteers. *J Clin Pharmacol* (2004) 44, 1252–9.
2. Scott J, Pache D, Keane G, Buckle H, O'Brien N. Prolonged anticholinergic delirium following antihistamine overdose. *Australas Psychiatry* (2007) 15, 242–4.

Antihistamines; Cinnarizine + Phenylpropanolamine

In 12 healthy subjects, phenylpropanolamine 50 mg counteracted the mild sedation caused by cinnarizine 25 or 50 mg, and improved the performance of some skills related to driving.[1] The clinical relevance of this finding is unclear, but it could potentially be beneficial.

1. Savolainen K, Mattila MJ, Mattila ME. Actions and interactions of cinnarizine and phenylpropanolamine on human psychomotor performance. *Curr Ther Res* (1992) 52, 160–8.

Antihistamines; Fexofenadine + Antacids

An aluminium/magnesium hydroxide-containing antacid modestly reduced fexofenadine levels in one study.

Clinical evidence, mechanism, importance and management

The US manufacturer of fexofenadine notes that when a single 120-mg dose of fexofenadine was given within 15 minutes of an **aluminium/magnesium hydroxide** antacid (*Maalox*), the fexofenadine AUC was decreased by 41% and its maximum level was decreased by 43%.[1] Although the effect of these reductions on possible efficacy has not been assessed, the UK manufacturer recommends that it is advisable to leave 2 hours between taking fexofenadine and antacids containing **aluminium** and **magnesium hydroxide**.[2] This seems prudent advice.

1. Allegra (Fexofenadine hydrochloride). Sanofi-Aventis US LLC. US Prescribing Information, July 2007.
2. Telfast (Fexofenadine hydrochloride). Sanofi-Aventis. UK Summary of product characteristics, June 2008.

Antihistamines; Fexofenadine + Efavirenz

Efavirenz slightly reduces the exposure to fexofenadine.

Clinical evidence, mechanism, importance and management

In a study in 12 healthy subjects, efavirenz 600 mg daily for 14 days, reduced the AUC of a single 60-mg dose of fexofenadine by about 30%, but had no effect on its maximum plasma concentration.[1] Fexofenadine is not principally metabolised by the cytochrome P450 enzyme system, but is a substrate for P-glycoprotein and OATP. Efavirenz might therefore reduce the exposure to fexofenadine by altering the function of these drug transporter proteins. The clinical importance of the reduction in exposure seen is not known, but it seems likely to be small.

1. Kharasch ED, Whittington D, Ensign D, Hoffer C, Bedynek PS, Campbell S, Stubbert K, Crafford A, London A, Kim T. Mechanism of efavirenz influence on methadone pharmacokinetics and pharmacodynamics. *Clin Pharmacol Ther* (2012) 91, 673–84.

Antihistamines; Fexofenadine + Probenecid

Probenecid reduces the renal clearance of fexofenadine and increases its AUC.

Clinical evidence

In a study, 8 healthy subjects and 8 patients with cystic fibrosis were given two doses of probenecid 1 g, 12 hours apart, with a single 180-mg dose of fexofenadine one hour after the first dose of probenecid. The AUC of fexofenadine was increased by 53% and its renal clearance was reduced by 70% by probenecid.[1] Similarly, a further study in 12 healthy subjects who took a single 120-mg dose of fexofenadine alone, or after probenecid 1 g twice daily for 6 days found the renal clearance of fexofenadine was reduced by 63% and the AUC of fexofenadine was increased by 50% by probenecid. There was a marked interindividual variation in the findings.[2]

Mechanism

An *in vitro* study has demonstrated that fexofenadine is a substrate for the human organic anion transporter-3 (OAT3), which probenecid inhibits. Therefore concurrent use results in decreased clearance and an increase in exposure to fexofenadine.[3]

Importance and management

Evidence for an interaction between fexofenadine and probenecid appears to be limited to these two studies, neither of which found that probenecid increased the adverse effects of fexofenadine. Note that much greater increases in the exposure to fexofenadine are not considered harmful (see 'Antihistamines + Azoles', p.630). Therefore this interaction is unlikely to be clinically relevant.

1. Liu S, Beringer PM, Hidayat L, Rao AP, Louie S, Burckart GJ, Shapiro B. Probenecid, but not cystic fibrosis, alters the total and renal clearance of fexofenadine. *J Clin Pharmacol* (2008) 48, 957–65.
2. Yasui-Furukori N, Uno T, Sugawara K, Tateishi T. Different effects of three transporting inhibitors, verapamil, cimetidine, and probenecid, on fexofenadine pharmacokinetics. *Clin Pharmacol Ther* (2005) 77, 17–23.
3. Tahara H, Kusuhara H, Maeda K, Koepsell H, Fuse E, Sugiyama Y. Inhibition of OAT3-mediated renal uptake as a mechanism for drug-drug interaction between fexofenadine and probenecid. *Drug Metab Dispos* (2006) 34, 743–7.

Antihistamines; Fexofenadine + St John's wort (*Hypericum perforatum*)

Pretreatment with St John's wort (*Hypericum perforatum*) had no clinically relevant effect on the plasma levels of single-dose fexofenadine in one study, but markedly reduced fexofenadine levels in two other studies.

Clinical evidence

In a study in 12 healthy subjects, a single 900-mg dose of St John's wort increased the maximum plasma level and AUC of a single 60-mg dose of fexofenadine by 45% and 31%, respectively.[1] However, in the same subjects, St John's wort 300 mg three times daily for 14 days caused a slight 5 to 10% *decrease* in the maximum level and AUC of a single 60-mg dose of fexofenadine.[1] In another study in healthy subjects, 12 days of pretreatment with St John's wort increased the oral clearance of a single dose of fexofenadine by about 60%.[2] Similarly, a study in 30 healthy subjects found that 10 days of pretreatment with St John's wort 300 mg three times daily, almost doubled the oral clearance of a single 60-mg dose of fexofenadine.[3]

Mechanism

In these studies St John's wort was thought to be interacting by affecting the transport of fexofenadine by P-glycoprotein.

Importance and management

An interaction between St John's wort and fexofenadine appears to be established. The findings from the multiple-dose studies suggest that St John's wort increases the oral clearance of fexofenadine, but only one study measured the systemic exposure of fexofenadine, and this suggested that the decrease in exposure may not be clinically significant. However, until the clinical relevance of this interaction is established it may be prudent to monitor closely for signs of reduced fexofenadine efficacy in a patient taking regular St John's wort. If fexofenadine efficacy is reduced, consider St John's wort as a possible cause and consider stopping the St John's wort, or trying an alternative antihistamine.

1. Wang Z, Hamman MA, Huang S-M, Lesko LJ, Hall SD. Effect of St John's wort on the pharmacokinetics of fexofenadine. *Clin Pharmacol Ther* (2002) 71, 414–20.
2. Dresser GK, Schwarz UI, Wilkinson GR, Kim RB. Coordinate induction of both cytochrome P4503A and MDR1 by St John's wort in healthy subjects. *Clin Pharmacol Ther* (2003) 73, 41–50.
3. Xie R, Tan LH, Polasek EC, Hong C, Teillol-Foo M, Gordi T, Sharma A, Nickens DJ, Arakawa T, Knuth DW, Antal EJ. CYP3A and P-glycoprotein activity induction with St. John's wort in healthy volunteers from 6 ethnic populations. *J Clin Pharmacol* (2005) 45, 352–6.

Antihistamines; Meclozine + Metaxalone

A case report describes a patient who experienced auditory hallucinations when he took the maximum doses of both meclozine and metaxalone together. This effect disappeared when the drugs were stopped, but recurred on re-challenge.[1] Note that this is an isolated report, and its general relevance is unclear.

1. Kuykendall JR, Rhodes RS. Auditory hallucinations elicited by combined meclizine and metaxalone use at bedtime. *Ann Pharmacother* (2004) 38, 1968–9.

Antihistamines; Mizolastine + Flecainide

There are no published cases of an interaction between flecainide and non-sedating antihistamines, but it has been suggested that the concurrent use of mizolastine may increase the risk of ventricular arrhythmias.

Clinical evidence, mechanism, importance and management

The UK manufacturer of flecainide advises avoiding the concurrent use of mizolastine due to an increased risk of ventricular arrhythmias.[1] Similarly, the manufacturer of mizolastine[2] contraindicates its use with drugs known to prolong the QT interval, and gives the examples of class I and III antiarrhythmics. Note that, of the class 1 antiarrhythmics, only the class 1a antiarrhythmics are generally considered to cause QT prolongation: flecainide is a class 1c antiarrhythmic.

Mizolastine may possibly cause QT prolongation, but usually only when its levels are raised; however flecainide is not known to affect mizolastine metabolism. There appear to be no published reports of an interaction between these drugs, and therefore an interaction is not established.

1. Tambocor 50 mg Tablets (Flecainide acetate). Meda Pharmaceuticals. UK Summary of product characteristics, July 2010.
2. Mizollen (Mizolastine). Sanofi-Aventis. UK Summary of product characteristics, December 2014.

Antihistamines; Ocular + Miscellaneous

No specific interaction studies have been performed with eye-drop formulations of the antihistamines azelastine, bepotastine, emedastine, epinastine, ketotifen, or olopatadine. However, interactions are not anticipated because very little drug is expected to reach the systemic circulation.

Clinical evidence, mechanism, importance and management

The UK manufacturer of **azelastine** eye drops notes that interaction studies with high oral doses of **azelastine** bear no relevance to the eye drops, as systemic levels are only in the picogram range after administration of eye drops.[1] Similarly, the manufacturer of **epinastine** eye drops notes that no drug interactions are anticipated as systemic **epinastine** levels are extremely low after ocular use. They note that **epinastine** is also excreted mostly unchanged.[2] The manufacturer of **olopatadine** eye drops notes that *in vitro* studies showed that it was not an inhibitor of the common cytochrome P450 isoenzymes.[3] Similarly, the US manufacturer of **bepotastine** eye drops notes that *in vitro* studies showed that it was not an inhibitor of the isoenzymes CYP3A4, CYP2C9 or CYP2C19, but the effect on the isoenzymes CYP1A2, CYP2C8, and CYP2D6 was not studied.[4] No drug interactions would be anticipated between these, or any other, antihistamine eye drops and systemically administered drugs; however the UK manufacturer of **ketotifen** eye drops[5] state that an interaction with systemically administered drugs cannot be ruled out. Nevertheless they also note that plasma levels of **ketotifen** after 14 day's use of **ketotifen** were, in most cases, below the limits of detection. An interaction therefore seems unlikely.

However, note that the manufacturer of **emedastine** eye drops states that an interval of 10 minutes should be allowed after the administration of the eye drops and other ophthalmically administered medicines,[6] which is good practice for any ocular drugs. The manufacturer of **ketotifen** states that only a 5-minute interval is necessary.[5]

1. Optilast Eye Drops (Azelastine). Meda Pharmaceuticals. UK Summary of product characteristics, August 2009.
2. Relestat (Epinastine). Allergan Ltd. UK Summary of product characteristics, October 2007.
3. Opatanol (Olopatadine). Alcon Laboratories (UK) Ltd. UK Summary of product characteristics, August 2007.
4. Bepreve (Bepotastine besilate). ISTA Pharmaceuticals, Inc. US Prescribing information, August 2009.
5. Zaditen Eye Drops (Ketotifen fumarate). Novartis Pharmaceuticals UK Ltd. UK Summary of product characteristics, June 2010.
6. Emadine (Emedastine). Alcon Laboratories (UK) Ltd. UK Summary of product characteristics, February 2009.

16

Antimigraine drugs

The drugs dealt with in this section are the ergot derivatives and the triptans (or more properly the serotonin 5-HT_1 agonists), whose main use is in the treatment of migraine. 'Table 16.1', below, lists some of the drugs commonly used in migraine. Drugs such as propranolol, antiepileptics, and botulinum toxin type A, which are more commonly used in other conditions, are discussed elsewhere in this publication.

(a) Ergot derivatives

The main problem with the use of the ergot derivatives is that of ergotism. Drug interactions can result in additive effects or cause raised concentrations of ergot derivatives, which might result in the symptoms of ergot poisoning. This can include severe circulatory problems e.g. the extremities may become numb, cold to the touch, or tingle, and muscle pain can result. In extreme cases there may be no palpable pulse. Ultimately gangrene might develop, and amputation could be required. Chest pain can also occur, and in some cases myocardial infarction has been reported. As dihydroergotamine, ergotamine, and methysergide are metabolised in the liver by the isoenzyme CYP3A4, drugs which inhibit this isoenzyme, particularly potent inhibitors, such as some of the HIV-protease inhibitors, see 'Ergot derivatives + HIV-protease inhibitors', p.641, should be avoided due to the risk of precipitating ergotism.

(b) Triptans

Although the triptans would be expected to share a number of pharmacodynamic drug interactions, due to their differing metabolic pathways they will not all necessarily share the same pharmacokinetic interactions. For example, sumatriptan, which is metabolised mainly by monoamine oxidase A, is unlikely to interact with macrolides, which are inhibitors of CYP3A4. However, eletriptan, which is mainly metabolised by CYP3A4, does interact (see 'Triptans + Macrolides', p.646). Frovatriptan and zolmitriptan are substrates for CYP1A2, and their metabolism is affected by CYP1A2 inhibitors such as fluvoxamine. However, the picture with zolmitriptan is more complicated, because it is also metabolised by monoamine oxidase A. Naratriptan appears unlikely to undergo important pharmacokinetic interactions because half the dose is excreted unchanged and the rest is metabolised by a variety of isoenzymes. A summary of the enzymes involved in the metabolic pathways of the triptans can be found in 'Table 16.2', below.

Early in the development of triptans it was theorised that they might present a high risk of excess serotonergic activity and increase the risk of serotonin syndrome especially when used with other drugs with serotonergic actions. Therefore sumatriptan was contraindicated in patients taking drugs such as the SSRIs and lithium. However, with more experience of the triptans it appears that interactions resulting in serotonin syndrome are rare, and so concurrent use with these other serotonergic drugs may now be undertaken with an appropriate awareness of the potential problems. For more information on the serotonin syndrome and its management, see 'Drugs that cause serotonin syndrome + Other drugs that cause serotonin syndrome', p.1471.

Table 16.1 Antimigraine drugs

Group	*Drugs*
Antihistamines	Flunarizine, Pizotifen
Beta blockers	Atenolol, Metoprolol, Nadolol, Propranolol, Timolol
Ergot derivatives	Codergocrine, Ergotamine, Dihydroergocryptine, Dihydroergotamine, Methysergide
Triptans (Serotonin (5-HT_1) agonists)	Almotriptan, Eletriptan, Frovatriptan, Naratriptan, Rizatriptan, Sumatriptan, Zolmitriptan
Antiepileptics	Gabapentin, Topiramate, Valproate
Others	Botulinum toxin type A, p.136

Table 16.2 Principal enzymes involved in the metabolism of the triptans†

	MAO-A	*CYP1A2*	*CYP2C9*	*CYP2C19*	*CYP2D6*	*CYP3A4*
Almotriptan	Substrate				Substrate (theoretical, minor)	Substrate (minor)
Eletriptan					Substrate (theoretical, minor)	Substrate (sensitive)
Frovatriptan		Substrate (theoretical)			Substrate (theoretical, minor)	
Naratriptan		Substrate (theoretical, minor)	Substrate (theoretical, minor)	Substrate (theoretical, minor)	Substrate (theoretical, minor)	Substrate (theoretical, minor)
Rizatriptan	Substrate	Substrate (theoretical, minor)				
Sumatriptan	Substrate					
Zolmitriptan	Substrate	Substrate				Substrate (theoretical, minor)

†Other isoenzymes have been implicated, but not at clinically relevant concentrations of the triptans.

Ergot derivatives + Antidepressants

A report describes three cases in which patients developed symptoms indicative of serotonin syndrome when they took dihydroergotamine with amitriptyline; paroxetine and imipramine; or sertraline. Some antidepressants such as fluoxetine, fluvoxamine, or nefazodone are predicted to decrease the metabolism of the ergot derivatives.

Clinical evidence

A case report describes a woman taking **imipramine**, **paroxetine**, and lithium, who had a 3-week continuous headache, and so was given 300 micrograms and then 500 micrograms of **dihydroergotamine** intravenously. Within 5 minutes of the 500-microgram dose she developed dysarthria, dilated pupils, diaphoresis, diffuse weakness, and barely responded to commands. She was diffusely hyperreflexic and showed occasional myoclonic jerks. She recovered after 90 minutes.[1]

A woman with a history of migraine headaches responded well to **amitriptyline**, metoclopramide, and **dihydroergotamine**. Six weeks after the **amitriptyline** was replaced by **sertraline**, she was again successfully treated for acute migraine with intravenous metoclopramide 10 mg and intravenous **dihydroergotamine** 1 mg. However, 2 hours later she developed nausea, emesis, agitation, weakness, diaphoresis, salivation, chills, and fever. All of the symptoms subsided after 24 hours.[1]

A woman with a history of migraines (treated prophylactically with **amitriptyline** and propranolol) was admitted to hospital in status migrainosus. She was given **dihydroergotamine** 1 mg, prochlorperazine 10 mg, and metoclopramide 10 mg (all intravenously). Within 20 minutes she became diaphoretic, tachycardic, diffusely hyperreflexic, agitated, confused, and briefly lost consciousness twice. Diazepam 8 mg, given intramuscularly, calmed her agitation, and all the symptoms resolved after 6 hours. A year later she was given subcutaneous sumatriptan 6 mg while taking **nortriptyline** daily with no ill effects.[1]

Mechanism

All of these patients appeared to have developed symptoms similar to those of serotonin syndrome (see 'Drugs that cause serotonin syndrome + Other drugs that cause serotonin syndrome', p.1471), which is thought to be due to hyperstimulation of 5-HT receptors in the brain. Dihydroergotamine is a 5-HT agonist while paroxetine and sertraline are both serotonin (5-HT) reuptake inhibitors, all of which might be expected to increase 5-HT concentrations in the CNS, and thereby increase receptor stimulation.

Importance and management

The interactions between the ergot derivatives and the SSRIs and/or tricyclics appear to be isolated cases and not of general importance; nevertheless, they illustrate the potential for the development of serotonin syndrome in patients given multiple drugs that affect 5-HT receptors. Serotonin syndrome is rare and it has been suggested[1] that it might sometimes be an idiosyncratic reaction.

Note that some antidepressants e.g. **fluoxetine**, **fluvoxamine**, and **nefazodone** can inhibit CYP3A4, which is involved in the metabolism of the ergot derivatives. This might result in reduced metabolism and therefore possibly ergot toxicity. The manufacturers of dihydroergotamine[2] and **ergotamine**[3,4] suggest giving these particular antidepressants with caution; although note that fluoxetine is only a weak inhibitor of this isoenzyme. **Methysergide** is also metabolised by CYP3A4 and therefore might be expected to interact similarly if given with these particular antidepressants.

The manufacturer of **reboxetine** states that its concurrent use with ergot derivatives might result in increased blood pressure, although no clinical data are quoted.[5] The general relevance of this statement is therefore difficult to determine.

1. Mathew NT, Tietjen GE, Lucker C. Serotonin syndrome complicating migraine pharmacotherapy. *Cephalalgia* (1996) 16, 323–7.
2. Migranal (Dihydroergotamine mesylate). Valeant Pharmaceuticals Inc. US Prescribing information, June 2007.
3. Migril (Ergotamine tartrate, cyclizine hydrochloride and caffeine). Wockhardt UK Ltd. UK Summary of product characteristics, March 2008.
4. Ergomar (Ergotamine tartrate). Rosedale Therapeutics. US Prescribing information, August 2007.
5. Edronax (Reboxetine). Pfizer Ltd. UK Summary of product characteristics, July 2013.

Ergot derivatives + Beta blockers

The concurrent use of beta blockers with ergot derivatives has, rarely, resulted in severe peripheral vasoconstriction and hypertension.

Clinical evidence

A man with recurrent migraine headaches, reasonably well-controlled over a 6-year period with **ergotamine tartrate** suppositories, developed progressively painful and purple feet shortly after starting **propranolol** 30 mg daily. When he resumed using **ergotamine tartrate** suppositories alone there was no further evidence of peripheral vasoconstriction.[1]

A similar case has been reported elsewhere, although an interaction is inconclusive in this patient, as neither the **ergotamine** nor the **propranolol** were taken alone.[2] Another case occurred in a woman who had been taking **oxprenolol** and **ergotamine tartrate** (doses unknown) for some considerable time. Arteriography showed severe spasm in a number of arteries, which responded eventually to an intra-arterial infusion of glyceryl trinitrate and heparin.[3] A man experienced severe pain in the legs and feet after he took **methysergide** 3 mg and **propranolol** 120 mg daily for 2 weeks. He did not respond to various therapies, and 6 days after admission it was necessary to amputate both his legs below the knee because of gangrene.[3] A woman taking **propranolol** for migraine prophylaxis became hypertensive (blood pressure 180/120 mmHg), with a crushing substernal pain, immediately after being given oxygen, prochlorperazine 5 mg, and intravenous **dihydroergotamine** 750 micrograms for an acute migraine headache. She recovered uneventfully and was later found to be hyperthyroid, which, it was suggested, might have contributed to the interaction.[4]

These reports contrast with another stating that the use of **propranolol** with **ergotamine** was both effective and uneventful in 50 patients.[5]

Mechanism

One suggestion is that additive vasoconstriction occurs.[1,3] Ergot derivatives cause vasoconstriction, and the beta blockers do the same by blocking the normal (beta$_2$-stimulated) sympathetic vasodilatation. Beta blockers also reduce blood flow by reducing cardiac output.

Importance and management

The concurrent use of ergotamine and propranolol is usually safe and effective, and there are only a handful of reports of adverse interactions. Similarly, only a handful of case reports describe similar interactions between other ergot derivatives and beta blockers. Furthermore, it has been suggested that the disease state might have contributed to the interaction in one case,[4] and at least one of the other cases could have been due to ergotamine alone (i.e. ergotism).[5] Nevertheless, the UK manufacturer of ergotamine advises that the concurrent use of ergotamine and beta blockers should be avoided.[6] At the very least, it would be prudent to be alert for any signs of an adverse response, particularly those suggestive of reduced peripheral circulation (such as coldness, numbness or tingling of the hands and feet) in any patient given an ergot derivative and a beta blocker.

1. Baumrucker JF. Drug interaction — propranolol and cafergot. *N Engl J Med* (1973) 288, 916–17.
2. Greenberg DJ, Hallett JW. Lower extremity ischemia due to combined drug therapy for migraine. *Postgrad Med* (1982) 72, 103–7.
3. Venter CP, Joubert PH, Buys AC. Severe peripheral ischaemia during concomitant use of beta blockers and ergot alkaloids. *BMJ* (1984) 289, 288–9.
4. Gandy W. Dihydroergotamine interaction with propranolol. *Ann Emerg Med* (1990) 19, 221.
5. Diamond S. Propranolol and ergotamine tartrate (cont.). *N Engl J Med* (1973) 289, 159.
6. Cafergot Tablets (Ergotamine tartrate and caffeine). Alliance Pharmaceuticals. UK Summary of product characteristics, March 2009.

Ergot derivatives + CYP3A4 inducers

CYP3A4 inducers such as rifampicin (rifampin) would be expected to reduce the clinical effect of ergot derivatives. Efavirenz would be expected to interact in the same way; however, some have predicted that it might increase the plasma concentrations of ergot derivatives.

Clinical evidence, mechanism, importance and management

Drugs that induce CYP3A4, such as **rifampicin** (**rifampin**), would be expected to increase the metabolism of the ergot derivatives and decrease their plasma concentrations. This type of interaction might result in reduced efficacy, but is unlikely to cause serious adverse effects. In fact because **rifampicin** is a potent inducer of CYP3A4, it has been used to increase the metabolism of **ergotamine** in a patient with ergotism.[1] Therefore, in patients taking CYP3A4 inducers, it might be prudent to consider an alternative antimigraine treatment, such as one of the triptans not metabolised by CYP3A4, see 'Table 16.2', p.639. A list of CYP3A4 inducers is given in 'Table 1.9', p.11.

Efavirenz also induces CYP3A4, and would therefore also be expected to reduce the plasma concentrations of ergot derivatives. However, the UK manufacturers[2,3] advise that, due to competition for metabolism by CYP3A4, **efavirenz** might possibly increase the plasma concentrations of ergot derivatives, leading to ergot toxicity. For this reason they contraindicate concurrent use.[2,3] However, competition for metabolism by the same isoenzyme rarely appears to lead to a clinically relevant interaction and there appear to be no published reports to confirm of the outcome of this predicted interaction. Its clinical relevance is therefore unclear.

1. Richardson JD, Sorensen S. Rifampin to treat ritonavir ergotamine drug interaction. *Clin Infect Dis* (1999) 29, 1002.
2. Cafergot Tablets (Ergotamine tartrate and caffeine). Alliance Pharmaceuticals. UK Summary of product characteristics, March 2009.
3. Sustiva Film-coated Tablets (Efavirenz). Bristol-Myers Squibb Pharmaceutical Ltd. UK Summary of product characteristics, March 2014.

Ergot derivatives + CYP3A4 inhibitors

Azoles are predicted to increase the exposure to ergot derivatives, which might lead to ergotism. Other CYP3A4 inhibitors are expected to interact in the same way, although possibly to a lesser extent.

Clinical evidence, mechanism, importance and management

The ergot alkaloids are mainly metabolised by CYP3A4. The UK and US manufacturers of **ergotamine**, **dihydroergotamine**, and **methysergide** therefore logically predict that their exposure and/or toxicity will be increased by CYP3A4 inhibitors, which might lead to ergotism: this has been seen with both macrolides and HIV-protease inhibitors, see 'Ergot derivatives + Macrolides', p.642, and 'Ergot derivatives + HIV-protease inhibitors', p.641.

Drugs such as the azoles would be expected to interact similarly, although there appear to be no studies or case reports describing an interaction. Note that, of the azoles, **voriconazole**, **ketoconazole**, and **itraconazole** appear to be the most potent CYP3A4 inhibitors, and would therefore be expected to interact to the greatest extent; their use, as well as the use of **posaconazole** and **miconazole** is generally contraindicated.[1-7] Similarly, the use of **delavirdine**, which is also a CYP3A4 inhibitor, is contraindicated with **methysergide**.[2]

The concurrent use of ergot derivatives with less potent CYP3A4 inhibitors, such as **cimetidine**,[1,2] **clotrimazole**,[3-6] **fluconazole**,[3-6] **grapefruit juice**,[3-6] **quinupristin** with **dalfopristin**,[1] and **zileuton**,[4,6] should either be avoided, if possible, or undertaken with caution.

Not all of the manufacturers of the various ergot derivatives mention all combinations of CYP3A4 inhibitors, but these are all reasonable predictions, and it would therefore seem appropriate to apply them to all ergot derivatives used in the management of migraine. Therefore if any of these less potent CYP3A4 inhibitors is given with an ergot derivative, it would be prudent to be aware that increased exposure to the ergot derivative might occur. Strongly advise patients not to take any further doses and seek medical advice if early symptoms of increased exposure, such as a decreased sensitivity to touch or pain, numbness or tingling in the fingers and toes, or nausea and vomiting (unrelated to the migraine), develop.

A list of CYP3A4 inhibitors is given in 'Table 1.9', p.11.

1. Cafergot Tablets (Ergotamine tartrate and caffeine). Alliance Pharmaceuticals. UK Summary of product characteristics, March 2009.
2. Deseril (Methysergide maleate). Alliance Pharmaceuticals. UK Summary of product characteristics, December 2006.
3. Cafergot Tablets (Ergotamine tartrate and caffeine). Novartis. US Prescribing information, March 2003.
4. Migranal (Dihydroergotamine mesylate). Valeant Pharmaceuticals Inc. US Prescribing information, June 2007.
5. Migril (Ergotamine tartrate, cyclizine hydrochloride and caffeine). Wockhardt UK Ltd. UK Summary of product characteristics, March 2008.
6. Ergomar (Ergotamine tartrate). Rosedale Therapeutics. US Prescribing information, August 2007.
7. Daktarin Oral Gel (Miconazole). Janssen-Cilag Ltd. UK Summary of product characteristics, December 2014.

Ergot derivatives + Ergot derivatives

The concurrent use of more than one ergot derivative can increase the risk of severe and persistent spasm of major arteries in some patients.

Clinical evidence

A man developed loss of temperature sensitivity over the right side of his face and arm, as well as vertigo, dysphagia, and hoarseness, 7 days after starting to take **methysergide** 2 mg three times daily and subcutaneous **ergotamine tartrate** 500 micrograms at night. Continued use resulted in impaired pain, touch, and temperature sensation over the right side of his face, shoulder, and arm. Arteriography demonstrated left vertebral artery occlusion and right vertebral arterial spasm. These symptoms, apart from the loss of temperature sensitivity, resolved when the drugs were stopped.[1] Another man treated for cluster headaches with **methysergide** 2 mg, intramuscular **ergotamine tartrate** and pizotifen developed ischaemia of the right foot, with impalpable popliteal and pedal pulses. Arteriography showed that blood flow to the arteries of the right leg was reduced.[1]

Other case reports describe prolonged myocardial ischaemia when a single 2-mg sublingual dose of **ergotamine tartrate** was added to methysergide 2 mg three times daily;[2] gangrene in the toes following the use of **ergotamine tartrate** 1.8 mg and **methysergide maleate** 6 mg daily;[3] and pain and numbness of the foot, requiring vascular surgery, after the use of **ergotamine** 2 mg suppositories twice daily and **methysergide** tablets 2 mg four times daily for 6 days.[4] In one of these cases sublingual glyceryl trinitrate was successfully used to relieve the pain.[2]

Mechanism

The combined vasoconstrictor effects of methysergide and ergotamine appears to cause arterial spasm, resulting in serious tissue ischaemia. Parenteral ergotamine increases the risk of arterial spasm. All ergot derivatives would be expected to behave in this way if they are given with another ergot derivative.

Importance and management

Direct information regarding an interaction resulting from the concurrent use of multiple ergot derivatives seems to be limited to these cases. Cardiovascular complications can occur with ergot derivatives given alone, but these cases suggest that their concurrent use might unpredictably increase the risk in some patients. Clearly concurrent use should be avoided where possible and, in addition, the US manufacturers of **dihydroergotamine**[5,6] state that it should not be used within 24 hours of ergot-type medications.

Note that drugs such as bromocriptine are also ergot derivatives, and it is similarly recommended that their use with other ergot derivatives should be avoided, see 'Bromocriptine and other dopamine agonists + Ergot derivatives', p.758.

1. Joyce DA, Gubbay SS. Arterial complications of migraine treatment with methysergide and parenteral ergotamine. *BMJ* (1982) 285, 260–1.
2. Galer BS, Lipton RB, Solomon S, Newman LC, Spierings ELH. Myocardial ischemia related to ergot alkaloids: a case report and literature review. *Headache* (1991) 31, 446–50.
3. Vaughan-Lane T. Gangrene induced by methysergide and ergotamine. *J Bone Joint Surg Br* (1979) 61–B, 213–14.
4. Johnson TD. Severe peripheral arterial constriction, acute ischemia of lower extremity with use of methysergide and ergotamine. *Arch Intern Med* (1966) 117, 237–41.
5. Migranal (Dihydroergotamine mesylate). Valeant Pharmaceuticals Inc. US Prescribing information, June 2007.
6. D.H.E. 45. (Dihydroergotamine mesylate). Novartis Pharmaceuticals Corporation. US Prescribing information, April 2001.

Ergot derivatives + HIV-protease inhibitors

A patient receiving indinavir rapidly developed ergotism after taking ergotamine. Several other patients taking ritonavir (sometimes with another protease inhibitor) and ergotamine have developed the same interaction. A patient taking nelfinavir developed peripheral arterial vasoconstriction after also taking ergotamine. Other ergot derivatives and HIV-protease inhibitors are expected to interact similarly.

Clinical evidence

(a) Indinavir

An HIV-positive man who had been taking lamivudine, stavudine, co-trimoxazole, and indinavir (2.4 g daily) for more than a year was given **ergotamine tartrate** 1 mg with caffeine 100 mg for migraine. He took two doses on two consecutive days, and 5 days later presented with numbness and cyanosis of the toes of his left foot. The next day he complained of intermittent claudication of his left leg, and 6 days later was admitted to hospital because of worsening symptoms and night cramps. Examination showed a typical picture of ergotism, with vasospasm and reduced blood flow in the popliteal, tibial, and femoral arteries. He was given heparin and buflomedil (a vasodilator), and recovered after 3 days.[1]

See *Ritonavir with other HIV-protease inhibitors*, below, for details regarding a fatality involving the use of indinavir and ritonavir with ergotamine.

(b) Nelfinavir

A 40-year-old HIV-positive woman twice took **ergotamine** 2 mg for a migraine while also taking nelfinavir, zidovudine, and lamivudine. On the first occasion she developed pain and cyanosis in her toes, and on the second occasion she developed cyanosis and oedema in her hands and feet, causing pain so severe that she was unable to walk. On both occasions peripheral arterial pulses were not palpable, but each time she recovered spontaneously over a period of about 2 weeks.[2]

See also *Ritonavir with other HIV-protease inhibitors*, below.

(c) Ritonavir

A 63-year-old man with AIDS, who had taken **ergotamine tartrate** 1 to 2 mg daily for migraine headaches over the last 5 years, had his treatment with zidovudine, zalcitabine and co-trimoxazole changed to zidovudine, didanosine, and ritonavir 600 mg every 12 hours. Within 10 days he developed paraesthesias, coldness, cyanosis, and skin paleness of both arms, and when admitted to hospital his axillary, brachial, radial, and ulnar pulses were found to be absent. An arterial doppler test showed the absence of blood flow in both his radial and ulnar arteries and he was diagnosed as having ergotism. The **ergotamine** and ritonavir were stopped, and he recovered when given prostaglandin E1 and calcium nadroparin.[3]

A case report describes irreversible coma in a 34-year-old woman who was taking ritonavir 600 mg twice daily, lamivudine, and stavudine. She presented with dizziness, loss of vision, headache, vomiting, diarrhoea, and a feeling of cold in her left foot after having taken three tablets of **ergotamine** 1 mg in the preceding 4 days. Peripheral pulses were absent in her extremities. After an initial period of recovery she again experienced a loss of consciousness, with signs of stenosis and vasospasm with cerebral hypoperfusion. Despite treatment with alprostadil, and discontinuation of ritonavir her condition deteriorated, and 2 years after the initial presentation, she remained in coma vigil (a state of altered consciousness).[4]

At least 4 other cases of ergotism have been reported in patients taking ritonavir after taking ergot derivatives:[5-8] one required surgical amputation of the toes.[6] Ergotism developed in two of the patients within a few hours to 24 hours of taking a single 1- or 2-mg dose of **ergotamine tartrate**,[5,7] and in the others within about 4 to 15 days.[6,8] One was taking a combination drug (**ergotamine tartrate** 300 micrograms, belladonna extract 200 micrograms, and phenobarbital 20 mg) twice daily for gastric discomfort,[6] and another received ergotamine 10 mg rectally over 4 days.[8]

(d) Ritonavir with other HIV-protease inhibitors

A 49-year-old man taking ritonavir 200 mg twice daily and **indinavir** 800 mg twice daily (with stavudine and lamivudine) took three tablets containing **ergotamine tartrate** 1 mg and caffeine 100 mg for a headache. However, his headache worsened, he developed progressive lower extremity weakness, severe peripheral vasoconstriction, labile hypertension, and livedo reticularis (skin discoloration due to underlying capillary changes). He lapsed into coma and on day 5 was declared brain dead.[9]

A 31-year-old man, taking ritonavir 400 mg twice daily (and also taking pizotifen, **nelfinavir**, stavudine, lamivudine, co-trimoxazole, and venlafaxine), developed severe burning and numbness in both feet, and paraesthesias in his hands, after taking four tablets containing **ergotamine** 1 mg and caffeine 100 mg over 10 days. He was diagnosed as having ergotism. The drugs were stopped and he was treated effectively with intravenous alprostadil and heparin.[10]

Another man receiving ritonavir and **saquinavir** experienced numbness in his hands and feet, cyanosis of his extremities, and nausea and vomiting after taking **ergotamine** 4 mg. Four days after taking the ergotamine he was found to have no pulses (by Doppler) in any extremity and ergot toxicity was diagnosed. He was given heparin, rifampicin (rifampin), nitrate vasodilators, calcium-channel blockers, and prostaglandins: pulses returned in his hands after 24 hours and in his feet after 48 hours. The patient recovered with gangrene of all his toes, one of which required amputation. Treatment included rifampicin to induce liver enzymes and therefore increase the metabolism of the ergotamine.[11]

At least three other cases of ergotism have been reported in patients taking ergot derivatives with ritonavir and another HIV-protease inhibitor (amprenavir,[12] unspecified,[13] lopinavir[14]). However, in one of these cases the last use of **ergotamine** was said to have been one month before the HIV-protease inhibitors were started,[14] and so in this case an interaction is not established.

Mechanism

HIV-protease inhibitors can, to varying degrees, reduce the metabolism of ergotamine (and other ergot derivatives) by inhibiting CYP3A4. Therefore the plasma concentration of ergotamine is increased, which might result in toxicity. High ergotamine concentrations cause arterial spasm, which reduces and even shuts down the flow of blood in arteries.

Importance and management

Information regarding an interaction between the ergot derivatives and the HIV-protease inhibitors appears to be limited to these reports, but what happened is consistent with the way other drugs that are CYP3A4 inhibitors can interact with ergot derivatives (see 'Ergot derivatives + Macrolides', below). This interaction would appear to be established, and is clearly clinically important. It would be prudent for any patient taking indinavir or ritonavir, and probably nelfinavir, to avoid the concurrent use of ergotamine or any other ergot derivative, such as **dihydroergotamine** or **methysergide**.

Information about possible interactions between ergot derivatives and other HIV-protease inhibitors seems to be limited, but as the HIV-protease inhibitors all inhibit CYP3A4 they would be expected to interact similarly, particularly if ritonavir is given as a pharmacokinetic enhancer. Concurrent use is therefore generally contraindicated.

1. Rosenthal E, Sala F, Chichmanian R-M, Batt M, Cassuto J-P. Ergotism related to concurrent administration of ergotamine tartrate and indinavir. *JAMA* (1999) 281, 987.
2. Mortier E, Pouchot J, Vinceneux P, Lalande M. Ergotism related to interaction between nelfinavir and ergotamine. *Am J Med* (2001) 110, 594.
3. Caballero-Granado FJ, Viciana P, Cordero E, Gómez-Vera MJ, del Nozal M, López-Cortés LF. Ergotism related to concurrent administration of ergotamine tartrate and ritonavir in an AIDS patient. *Antimicrob Agents Chemother* (1997) 41, 1207.
4. Pardo Rey C, Yebra M, Borrallo M, Vega A, Ramos A, Montero MC. Irreversible coma, ergotamine, and ritonavir. *Clin Infect Dis* (2003) 37, e72–3.
5. Montero A, Giovannoni AG, Tvrde PL. Leg ischemia in a patient receiving ritonavir and ergotamine. *Ann Intern Med* (1999) 130, 329–30.
6. Liaudet L, Buclin T, Jaccard C, Eckert P. Severe ergotism associated with interaction between ritonavir and ergotamine. *BMJ* (1999) 318, 771.
7. Blanche P, Rigolet A, Gombert B, Ginsburg C, Salmon D, Sicard D. Ergotism related to a single dose of ergotamine tartrate in an AIDS patient treated with ritonavir. *Postgrad Med J* (1999) 75, 546–7.
8. Spiegel M, Schmidauer C, Kampfl A, Sarcletti M, Poewe W. Cerebral ergotism under treatment with ergotamine and ritonavir. *Neurology* (2001) 57, 743–4.
9. Tribble MA, Gregg CR, Margolis DM, Amirkhan R, Smith JW. Fatal ergotism induced by an HIV protease inhibitor. *Headache* (2002) 42, 694–5.
10. Phan TG, Agaliotis D, White G, Britton WJ. Ischaemic peripheral neuritis secondary to ergotism associated with ritonavir therapy. *Med J Aust* (1999) 171, 502, 504.
11. Richardson JD, Sorensen S. Rifampin to treat ritonavir ergotamine drug interaction. *Clin Infect Dis* (1999) 29, 1002.
12. Vila A, Mykietiuk A, Bonvehí P, Temporiti E, Urueña A, Herrera F. Clinical ergotism induced by ritonavir. *Scand J Infect Dis* (2001) 33, 788–9.
13. Baldwin ZK, Ceraldi CC. Ergotism associated with HIV antiviral protease inhibitor therapy. *J Vasc Surg* (2003) 37, 676–8.
14. Cagatay A, Guler O, Guven K. Ergotism caused by concurrent use of ritonavir and ergot alkaloids: a case report. *Acta Chir Belg* (2009) 109, 639–40.

Ergot derivatives + Macrolides

Ergot toxicity can develop rapidly in patients taking ergotamine or dihydroergotamine if they are given erythromycin, clarithromycin, and probably telithromycin. Cases of toxicity have also been reported with josamycin and oleandomycin. No cases of toxicity appear to have been reported with azithromycin; nevertheless, the manufacturers suggest an interaction could occur.

Clinical evidence

(a) Clarithromycin

A 59-year-old woman took **ergotamine tartrate** 2 mg for a typical migraine headache. After 2 hours her tongue became swollen, painful, and bluish in colour. She was moderately hypertensive (blood pressure 200/110 mmHg), and her fingers and toes were cold and cyanotic (blue): this was diagnosed as ergotism. She had taken this dose of **ergotamine** many times previously without problems, but on this occasion she had been taking clarithromycin 500 mg twice daily for the previous 5 days. Other evidence suggests that this patient might possibly have been unusually sensitive to vascular occlusion.[1] The authors of this report briefly quote another case, originating from the manufacturers of clarithromycin, of a possible interaction with **dihydroergotamine**, although this was complicated by the concurrent use of other medications (not named) used in the management of AIDS.[1] A woman who had previously uneventfully taken **ergotamine tartrate** 1 mg with caffeine 100 mg for migraine developed ergotism (leg pain, cold and cyanosed limbs, and impalpable pulses) within 3 days of starting to take clarithromycin (dose not stated). The authors suggested that smoking and the use of oxymetazoline (both of which have vasoconstrictor effects) might also have had some part to play.[2]

(b) Erythromycin

A woman who had regularly and uneventfully taken **ergotamine tartrate** 2 mg (with cyclizine hydrochloride 50 mg and caffeine 100 mg) on a number of previous occasions, took one tablet during a course of treatment with erythromycin 250 mg every 6 hours. Within 2 days she developed severe ischaemic pain in her arms and legs during exercise, with a burning sensation in her feet and hands. When admitted to hospital 10 days later, her extremities were cool and cyanosed, and her pulse could not be detected in the lower limbs.[3]

Eight other cases of acute ergotism have been reported[4-11] in which patients were taking **ergotamine tartrate** or **dihydroergotamine** with erythromycin. The reaction has been reported to develop within a few hours,[7] but it can take several days to occur.[10] One case appeared to occur when the erythromycin was started 3 days after the last dose of **dihydroergotamine**.[5]

A study involving 9 healthy subjects found that erythromycin increased the mean maximum plasma concentration and AUC of the alpha isomer of **dihydroergocryptine** 9.5-fold and greater than 13-fold, respectively.[12]

(c) Josamycin

An isolated report describes a 33-year-old woman who developed severe ischaemia of the legs within 3 days of starting to take josamycin 2 g daily and **ergotamine tartrate** 300 micrograms. Her legs and feet were cold, white and painful, and most of her peripheral pulses were impalpable.[13]

(d) Midecamycin

After 12 healthy subjects took midecamycin diacetate 800 mg twice daily for 8 days, the maximum plasma concentration of a single 9-mg dose of **dihydroergotamine** were raised 3- to 40-fold.[14]

(e) Oleandomycin

A case of ergotism developed in a 45-year-old woman who had been taking **ergotamine** 4 mg daily for 5 years, shortly after she also started taking oleandomycin.[15]

(f) Troleandomycin

A 40-year-old woman who had been taking **dihydroergotamine** 90 drops daily, for 3 years without problems, developed cramp in her legs within a few hours of starting to take troleandomycin 250 mg four times a day. Five days later she was admitted to hospital, as an emergency, with severe ischaemia of her arms and legs. Her limbs were cold and all her peripheral pulses were impalpable.[16]

There are reports of several other patients who had taken normal doses of **ergotamine tartrate** or **dihydroergotamine** for months or years without problems, who then developed severe ergotism within hours or days of starting to take normal doses of troleandomycin.[17-24] This resulted in a myocardial infarction in one patient.[25]

Mechanism

The macrolides are, to varying extents, inhibitors of CYP3A4, the main isoenzyme involved in the metabolism of the ergot derivatives. Those macrolides that are moderate to potent inhibitors of this isoenzyme, such as erythromycin and clarithromycin therefore inhibit the metabolism of the ergot derivative, leading to an increased plasma concentration. This results in vasoconstriction and ultimately ischaemia. Josamycin, and midecamycin are weaker inhibitors of CYP3A4, but the evidence suggests that on occasion they might still inhibit the metabolism of the ergot derivatives.

Importance and management

The interactions of the ergot derivatives with **erythromycin** and **troleandomycin** are well documented, well established, and clinically important. Although information about **clarithromycin** and **oleandomycin** appears to be confined to case reports, they, and any other macrolide that inhibits CYP3A4 moderately to potently (such as **telithromycin**), would be expected to interact similarly. The concurrent use of all of these macrolides and ergot derivatives should be avoided. Some of the cases cited were effectively treated with sodium nitroprusside or naftidrofuryl oxalate.[1,5,7-9,22]

Josamycin and **midecamycin** are less likely to interact with the ergot derivatives because they are weaker inhibitors of CYP3A4. However, there has been a report of ergotism with josamycin, and the increase in the plasma concentration of dihydroergotamine seen with midecamycin would be expected to be clinically relevant. It would therefore be prudent to be alert for any signs of an adverse response, particularly those suggestive of reduced peripheral circulation (such as coldness, numbness or tingling of the hands and feet).

There appears to be no evidence about other macrolides. Nevertheless, one manufacturer of ergotamine does class **azithromycin** as a potent CYP3A4 inhibitor[26] and therefore contraindicates the concurrent use of ergot derivatives. The UK manufacturer of azithromycin[27] also contraindicates concurrent use because of the theoretical possibility of ergotism; however, azithromycin is not usually considered to be a CYP3A4 inhibitor and an interaction based on this mechanism therefore seems unlikely. Furthermore the US manufacturer of azithromycin states that concurrent use can be undertaken with careful monitoring.[28]

1. Horowitz RS, Dart RC, Gomez HF. Clinical ergotism with lingual ischemia induced by a clarithromycin-ergotamine interaction. *Arch Intern Med* (1996) 156, 456–8.
2. Ausband SC, Goodman PE. An unusual case of clarithromycin associated ergotism. *J Emerg Med* (2001) 21, 411–13.
3. Francis H, Tyndall A, Webb J. Severe vascular spasm due to erythromycin-ergotamine interaction. *Clin Rheumatol* (1984) 3, 243–6.
4. Lagier G, Castot A, Riboulet G, Boesh C. Un cas d'ergotisme mineur semblant en rapport avec une potentialisation de l'ergotamine par l'éthylsuccinate d'érythromycine. *Therapie* (1979) 34, 515–21.
5. Neveux E, Lesgourgues B, Luton J-P, Guilhaume B, Bertagna, Picard J. Ergotisme aigu par association proprionate d'érythromycine-dihydroergotamine. *Nouv Presse Med* (1981) 10, 2830.
6. Collet AM, Moncharmont D, San Marco JL, Eissinger F, Pinot JJ, Laselve L. Ergotisme iatrogène: rôle de l'association tartrate d'ergotamine-propionate d'érythromycine. *Sem Hop Paris* (1982) 58, 1624–6.
7. Boucharlat J, Franco A, Carpentier P, Charignon Y, Denis B, Hommel M. Ergotisme en milieu psychiatrique par association D.H.E. propionate d'érythromycine. A propos d'une observation. *Ann Med Psychol (Paris)* (1980) 138, 292–6.
8. Leroy F, Asseman P, Pruvost P, Adnet P, Lacroix D, Thery C. Dihydroergotamine-erythromycin-induced ergotism. *Ann Intern Med* (1988) 109, 249.

9. Ghali R, De Léan J, Douville Y, Noël H-P, Labbé R. Erythromycin-associated ergotamine intoxication: arteriographic and electrophysiologic analysis of a rare cause of severe ischemia of the lower extremities and associated ischemic neuropathy. *Ann Vasc Surg* (1993) 7, 291–6.
10. Bird PA, Sturgess AD. Clinical ergotism with severe bilateral upper limb ischaemia precipitated by an erythromycin-ergotamine interaction. *Aust N Z J Med* (2000) 30, 635–6.
11. Karam B, Farah E, Ashoush R, Jebara V, Ghayad E. Ergotism precipitated by erythromycin: a rare case of vasospasm. *Eur J Vasc Endovasc Surg* (2000) 19, 96–8.
12. de Mey C, Althaus M, Ezan E, Retzow A. Erythromycin increases plasma concentrations of α-dihydroergocryptine in humans. *Clin Pharmacol Ther* (2001) 70, 142–8.
13. Grolleau JY, Martin M, de la Guerrande B, Barrier J, Peltier P. Ergotism aigu lors d'une association josamycine/tartrate d'ergotamine. *Therapie* (1981) 36, 319–21.
14. Couet W, Mathieu HP, Fourtillan JB. Effect of ponsinomycin on the pharmacokinetics of dihydroergotamine administered orally. *Fundam Clin Pharmacol* (1991) 5, 47–52.
15. Monsarrat M, Lefebvre D, Parraguette J, Vaysse C, Bastide G. Ergotisme aigu par association ergotamine-oleandomycine. *Nouv Presse Med* (1982) 11, 603.
16. Franco A, Bourlard P, Massot C, Lecoeur J, Guidicelli H, Bessard G. Ergotisme aigu par association dihydroergotamine-triacétyloléandomycine. *Nouv Presse Med* (1978) 7, 205.
17. Lesca H, Ossard D, Reynier P. Les risques de l'association tri-acétyl-oléandomycine et tartrate d'ergotamine. *Nouv Presse Med* (1976) 5, 1832–3.
18. Hayton AC. Precipitation of acute ergotism by triacetyloleandomycin. *N Z Med J* (1969) 69, 42.
19. Dupuy JC, Lardy P, Seaulau P, Kervoelen P, Paulet J. Spasmes artériels systémiques. Tartrate d'ergotamine. *Arch Mal Coeur* (1979) 72, 86–91.
20. Bigorie B, Aimez P, Soria RJ, Samama F di Maria G, Guy-Grand B, Bour H. L'association triacétyl oléandomycin-tartrate d'ergotamine est-elle dangereuse? *Nouv Presse Med* (1975) 4, 2723–5.
21. Vayssairat M, Fiessinger J-N, Becquemin M-H, Housset E. Association dihydroergotamine et triacétyloléandomycine. Rôle dans une nécrose digitale iatrogène. *Nouv Presse Med* (1978) 7, 2077.
22. Matthews NT, Havill JH. Ergotism with therapeutic doses of ergotamine tartrate. *N Z Med J* (1979) 89, 476–7.
23. Chignier E, Riou R, Descotes J, Meunier P, Courpron P, Vignon G. Ergotisme iatrogène aigu par association médicamenteuse diagnostiqué par exploration non invasive (vélocimétrie à effet Doppler). *Nouv Presse Med* (1978) 7, 2478.
24. Bacourt F, Couffinhal J-C. Ischémie des membres par association dihydroergotamine-triacétyloléandomycine. Nouvelle observation. *Nouv Presse Med* (1978) 7, 1561.
25. Baudouy PY, Mellat M, Velleteau de Moulliac M. Infarctus du myocarde provoqué par l'association tartrate d'ergotamine-troléandomycine. *Rev Med Interne* (1988) 9, 420–2.
26. Migril (Ergotamine tartrate, cyclizine hydrochloride and caffeine). Wockhardt UK Ltd. UK Summary of product characteristics, March 2008.
27. Zithromax (Azithromycin). Pfizer Ltd. UK Summary of product characteristics, January 2015.
28. Zithromax (Azithromycin). Pfizer Inc. US Prescribing information, June 2012.

Ergot derivatives + Nitrates

The ergot derivatives, such as dihydroergotamine, would be expected to oppose the anti-anginal effects of glyceryl trinitrate but there seem to be no clinical reports of this effect. Oral glyceryl trinitrate increases the exposure to dihydroergotamine; isosorbide mononitrate and isosorbide dinitrate are predicted to interact similarly.

Clinical evidence, mechanism, importance and management

There seem to be no clinical reports of adverse interactions between the ergot derivatives and glyceryl trinitrate, but as **ergot** causes vasoconstriction and can provoke angina, ergot derivatives would be expected to oppose the effects of glyceryl trinitrate when used as a vasodilator for the treatment of angina.[1] However, oral glyceryl trinitrate has been shown to increase the plasma concentration and AUC (by up to 370% in one case) of **dihydroergotamine** in 4 subjects with orthostatic hypotension, which would increase its vasoconstrictor effects.[1]

The clinical outcome of concurrent use is therefore uncertain, especially as glyceryl trinitrate has been successfully used to relieve pain and arterial spasm related to the use of ergot derivatives (see 'Ergot derivatives + Ergot derivatives', p.641, and 'Ergot derivatives + Beta blockers', p.640). Furthermore, there appear to be no clinical reports of interactions between ergot derivatives and other nitrates. Nevertheless, the UK manufacturers of **isosorbide mononitrate**[2] and **isosorbide dinitrate**[3] state that nitrates might increase the plasma concentration of dihydroergotamine and therefore enhance its hypertensive effect. Whatever the outcome of concurrent use, note that ergot derivatives are generally contraindicated in those with ischaemic heart disease, for which nitrates are commonly given.

1. Bobik A, Jennings G, Skews H, Esler M, McLean A. Low oral bioavailability of dihydroergotamine and first-pass extraction in patients with orthostatic hypotension. *Clin Pharmacol Ther* (1981) 30, 673–9.
2. Chemydur 60XL (Isosorbide mononitrate) UCB Pharma Ltd. UK Summary of product characteristics, August 2010.
3. Isoket Retard (Isosorbide dinitrate). UCB Pharma Ltd. UK Summary of product characteristics, June 2008.

Ergot derivatives + Tetracyclines

Five patients taking ergotamine or dihydroergotamine developed ergotism with concurrent use of doxycycline or tetracycline.

Clinical evidence

A woman who had previously taken **ergotamine tartrate** successfully and uneventfully for 16 years was given **doxycycline** and **dihydroergotamine** 30 drops three times daily. Five days later her hands and feet became cold and reddened, and she was diagnosed as having a mild form of ergotism.[1]

Other cases of ergotism, some of them more severe, have been described in two patients taking **ergotamine tartrate** and **doxycycline**,[2,3] and in 3 patients taking **ergotamine tartrate** and **tetracycline**-containing preparations.[4,5]

Mechanism

Unknown.

Importance and management

Information regarding an interaction between the ergot derivatives and tetracyclines is very limited. In some patients the tetracycline and ergotamine were not given separately or the ergot derivative was given long-term, and in others concurrent illnesses, including liver impairment, might have contributed to the development of ergotism. An interaction is therefore not established. Nevertheless, one UK manufacturer of ergotamine[6] recommends that the concurrent use of tetracycline should be avoided.

1. Amblard P, Reymond JL, Franco A, Beani JC, Carpentier P, Lemonnier D, Bessard G. Ergotisme. Forme mineure par association dihydroergotamine-chlorhydrate de doxycycline, étude capillaroscopique. *Nouv Presse Med* (1978) 7, 4148–9.
2. Dupuy JC, Lardy P, Seaulau P, Kervoelen P, Paulet J. Spasmes artériels systémiques. Tartrate d'ergotamine. *Arch Mal Coeur* (1979) 72, 86–91.
3. Van Gestel R, Noirhomme P. Ergotism aigu par association de tartrate d'ergotamine et de doxycycline. *Louvain Med* (1984) 103, 207–8.
4. L'Yvonnet M, Boillot A, Jacquet AM, Barale F, Grandmottet P, Zurlinden B, Gillet JY. A propos d'un cas exceptionnel d'intoxication aigue par un dérivé de l'ergot de seigle. *Gynecologie* (1974) 25, 541–3.
5. Sibertin-Blanc M. Les dangers de l'ergotisme a propos de deux observations. *Arch Med Ouest* (1977) 9, 265–6.
6. Cafergot Tablets (Ergotamine tartrate and caffeine). Alliance Pharmaceuticals. UK Summary of product characteristics, March 2009.

Ergot derivatives; Dihydroergotamine + Heparin

The use of dihydroergotamine with heparin has resulted in ergotism. In some cases, amputation of the affected limb was necessary. The rate of absorption and maximum plasma concentration of subcutaneous dihydroergotamine are reduced by heparin.

Clinical evidence, mechanism, importance and management

There have been several reports of ergotism following the combined use of **dihydroergotamine** and heparin for thromboembolic prophylaxis. In a retrospective review of 61 092 Austrian patients attending trauma units, who received **dihydroergotamine** and heparin prophylaxis, complications attributable to ergotism were seen in 142 patients. In 7 patients amputation was necessary and in a further 7 cases immediate opening of the vessel and catheter dilatation was successful.[1] Other published reports support this interaction,[2-4] including a report of two patients who experienced fatal myocardial infarctions attributed to coronary artery spasm as a complication of prophylaxis with **dihydroergotamine** and heparin.[5]

It has been found that the use of heparin results in a 25% increase in the AUC of subcutaneous **dihydroergotamine**. Giving the two drugs at the same injection site reduced the rate of dihydroergotamine absorption by 63%, delayed the time to maximum plasma concentration by 110%, and reduced the maximum plasma concentration by 15%. **Dihydroergotamine** had no effect on the pharmacokinetics of heparin.[6]

Because of the risk of peripheral ischaemia, the combination of **dihydroergotamine** and heparin is no longer widely used for thromboembolic prophylaxis. If the combination is used, the patient must be closely observed for any sign of vascular spasm.

1. Gatterer R. Ergotism as complication of thromboembolic prophylaxis with heparin and dihydroergotamine. *Lancet* (1986) II, 638–639.
2. Warmuth-Metz M. Ergotismus der unteren Extremität als Folge einer DHE-Heparin-Thromboseprophylaxe. *Radiologe* (1988) 28, 491–3.
3. Jahn R. Ergotismus – ein Risiko bei der Thromboseprophylaxe? *Zentralbl Chir* (1985) 110, 482–5.
4. Coppeneur-Krieger C, Plock EB, Neugebauer R. Verlust des replantierten Daumens durch medikamentös verursachten Ergotismus.*Handchir Mikrochir Plast Chir* (1995) 27, 137–40.
5. Rem JA, Gratzl O, Follath F, Pult I. Ergotism as complication of thromboembolic prophylaxis with heparin-dihydroergotamine. *Lancet* (1987) I, 219.
6. Schran HF, Bitz DW, DiSerio FJ, Hirsh J. The pharmacokinetics and bioavailability of subcutaneously administered dihydroergotamine, heparin and the dihydroergotamine-heparin combination. Thromb Res. (1983) 31, 51–67.

Ergot derivatives; Ergotamine + Bacampicillin

A case report describes symptoms of peripheral vasoconstriction when a woman taking ergotamine also took bacampicillin.

Clinical evidence, mechanism, importance and management

An isolated case report describes a 54-year-old woman who regularly took 3 to 4 tablets of a combination of **ergotamine** 2 mg, caffeine 91.5 mg, and cyclizine 50 mg for chronic migraines. She took two tablets of **bacampicillin** 400 mg and experienced palpitations, coldness, and pallor in her right arm which disappeared spontaneously. Several days later she took another two tablets of bacampicillin 400 mg and experienced the same symptoms. The bacampicillin was discontinued but the symptoms continued until heparin and vasodilators were given.[1]

This is an isolated case and the mechanism for the effect is not established. As such its general relevance is unclear.

1. Fukui S, Coggia M, Goëau-Brissonnière O. Acute upper extremity ischemia during concomitant use of ergotamine tartrate and ampicillin. *Ann Vasc Surg* (1997) 11, 420–4.

Triptans + Azoles

Ketoconazole markedly, and fluconazole moderately, increases the exposure to eletriptan. Ketoconazole slightly increases the exposure to

almotriptan. Itraconazole, and probably voriconazole, are expected to interact with eletriptan and almotriptan in the same way as ketoconazole.

Clinical evidence

(a) Almotriptan

In a randomised, crossover study, 16 healthy subjects were given **ketoconazole** 400 mg daily on days 1 to 3, with a single 12.5-mg dose of almotriptan on day 2. Ketoconazole increased the AUC and maximum plasma concentration of almotriptan by 57% and 61%, respectively. The renal clearance of almotriptan was also reduced, by approximately 16%.[1]

(b) Eletriptan

A pharmacokinetic study by the manufacturers of eletriptan found that **ketoconazole** 400 mg increased the maximum serum concentration and AUC of eletriptan 2.7-fold, and 5.9-fold, respectively, and prolonged its half-life from 4.8 hours to 8.3 hours. **Fluconazole** caused a 40% increase in the maximum serum concentration of eletriptan, and doubled its AUC.[2,3]

Mechanism

Ketoconazole is a potent inhibitor of CYP3A4, by which eletriptan is metabolised. Ketoconazole therefore inhibits the metabolism of eletriptan, which results in an increase in its exposure. **Fluconazole** is a moderate inhibitor of CYP3A4, and therefore has a more modest effect than ketoconazole. Almotriptan is also metabolised by CYP3A4, but this is not its only route of metabolism, and therefore inhibition of CYP3A4 by ketoconazole has a less dramatic effect on its exposure. **Itraconazole** and **voriconazole** are potent inhibitors of CYP3A4, and they are therefore expected to interact in a similar way to ketoconazole.

Importance and management

Although studies are limited, these interactions are established. In the study with **almotriptan** and ketoconazole, adverse events were not notably altered, and therefore the authors considered that no almotriptan dose adjustment is likely to be necessary in patients also given ketoconazole.[1] Nevertheless, the US manufacturers recommend using a starting dose of almotriptan 6.25 mg in patients taking potent CYP3A4 inhibitors,[4] and this would be expected to include ketoconazole, as well as itraconazole and voriconazole.

Ketoconazole markedly increases the exposure to **eletriptan**, and therefore the manufacturers advise that concurrent use should be avoided.[2,3] In addition, the US manufacturer recommends that eletriptan should not be given within 72 hours of ketoconazole.[2] Itraconazole and voriconazole are expected to interact in the same way as ketoconazole, and therefore the same precautions should be taken. Fluconazole is a moderate inhibitor of CYP3A4 and therefore could be used with caution.

Other triptans would be expected to have little or no interaction with the azoles as they are not predominantly metabolised by CYP3A4 (see 'Table 16.2', p.639).

1. Fleishaker JC, Herman BD, Carel BJ, Azie NE. Interaction between ketoconazole and almotriptan in healthy volunteers. *J Clin Pharmacol* (2003) 43, 423–7.
2. Relpax (Eletriptan hydrobromide). Pfizer Inc. US Prescribing information, May 2008.
3. Relpax (Eletriptan hydrobromide). Pfizer Ltd. UK Summary of product characteristics, February 2008.
4. Axert (Almotriptan malate). Ortho-McNeil Pharmaceutical Inc. US Prescribing information, April 2009.

Triptans + Beta blockers

Propranolol increases the exposure to rizatriptan, but it does not affect the efficacy or pharmacokinetics of almotriptan. No clinically important interactions appear to occur between other triptans and beta blockers.

Clinical evidence, mechanism, importance and management

(a) Almotriptan

In an open-label study, the efficacy of almotriptan 12.5 mg in treating acute migraine attacks was compared in 89 patients taking **propranolol** 40 mg and 100 mg daily with 92 control patients not receiving migraine prophylaxis. The concurrent use of **propranolol** appeared to increase the efficacy of almotriptan, as assessed by a greater decrease in self-assessed headache severity at 2 hours and an increase in the percentage of pain-free patients at 2 hours.[1] In 12 healthy subjects given **propranolol** 80 mg twice daily for 7 days followed by a single 12.5-mg dose of almotriptan, some negligible changes were noted in the pharmacokinetics of almotriptan (e.g. AUC increased by 7%) which were not considered to be clinically significant.[2]

These studies suggest that no particular precautions or dose adjustments are necessary on the concurrent use of almotriptan and propranolol.

(b) Eletriptan

In an interaction study, 12 healthy subjects were given a single 80-mg dose of eletriptan after taking **propranolol** 80 mg twice daily for 7 days. It was found that the AUC of eletriptan was increased by 30%, and the half-life increased from 4.9 hours to 5.2 hours. However, these changes were not considered to be clinically significant, and no notable blood pressure changes or any adverse events were seen, when compared with taking eletriptan alone.[3,4]

The UK manufacturer reports that no evidence of an interaction was seen in clinical studies when eletriptan was taken with beta blockers.[4]

(c) Frovatriptan

A single 2.5-mg oral dose of frovatriptan was given to 12 healthy subjects after they had taken **propranolol** 80 mg twice daily for 7 days. The AUC and maximum plasma concentration of frovatriptan were increased by 25% and 23%, respectively. However, these changes are small, and no changes occurred in the ECGs and vital signs of the subjects. Therefore the pharmacokinetic interaction was not thought to be of clinical significance.[5]

(d) Naratriptan

The US manufacturer of naratriptan reports that, from population pharmacokinetic analyses, beta blockers did not affect the clearance of naratriptan and the efficacy of naratriptan was unaffected by the concurrent use of beta blockers.[6]

(e) Rizatriptan

A series of double-blind, placebo-controlled studies were conducted in a total of 51 healthy subjects who were given a single 10-mg dose of rizatriptan after they had taken **propranolol** 60 or 120 mg twice daily, **nadolol** 80 mg daily, or **metoprolol** 100 mg daily, for 7 days.[7] **Nadolol** and **metoprolol** had no effect on the pharmacokinetics of rizatriptan. However, **propranolol** raised the AUC and the maximum plasma concentration of rizatriptan by 67% and 75%, respectively; in one subject there was a 4-fold increase in the AUC. Adjusting the dose of **propranolol** and separating administration by 2 hours had little effect on this interaction.[7] The AUC of the active *N*-monodesmethyl metabolite of rizatriptan was not affected by **propranolol**.[7]

In vitro studies have similarly shown that **propranolol** inhibits the metabolism of rizatriptan, whereas **atenolol**, **nadolol**, and **timolol** do not affect the metabolism of rizatriptan.[7]

The manufacturers recommend that a lower dose of rizatriptan (5 mg rather than the more usual 10 mg) should be used in the presence of **propranolol**, with a maximum of two[8] or three doses in 24 hours.[9] In the UK, they also state that administration should be separated by at least 2 hours,[8] although the rationale for this is less clear given that the above study found that such a dose separation did not appear to modify the interaction. No reduction in the rizatriptan dose would seem to be needed in the presence of **atenolol**, **metoprolol**, **nadolol**, or **timolol**.

(f) Sumatriptan

In a study in 10 healthy subjects, **propranolol** 80 mg twice daily for 7 days did not alter the pharmacokinetics of a single 300-mg dose of sumatriptan given on day 7. There was no significant effect on pulse rate or blood pressure.[10] A large prospective study found no evidence of an interaction between subcutaneous sumatriptan and propranolol (1 437 patients) or other unnamed beta blockers (951 patients).[11]

(g) Zolmitriptan

In a randomised, crossover study, 12 healthy subjects were given **propranolol** 160 mg or a placebo daily for 7 days, with a single 10-mg oral dose of zolmitriptan on day 7. **Propranolol** increased the maximum serum concentration and the AUC of zolmitriptan by 56% and 37%, respectively, and reduced the extent of its conversion to its active metabolite, probably due to inhibition of, or competition for, metabolism by cytochrome P450 isoenzymes. However, the higher zolmitriptan concentration was not associated with a greater rise in blood pressure and it was concluded that no clinically important changes in the therapeutic effects of zolmitriptan are likely, nor are any adjustments in its dose needed.[12]

The UK manufacturer states there is no evidence that the concurrent use of beta blockers has any effect on the efficacy or adverse effects of zolmitriptan.[13]

1. Bermejo PE, Dorado, R, Gomez-Arguelles JM. Variation in almotriptan effectiveness according to different prophylactic treatments. *Headache* (2009) 49, 1277–82.
2. Fleishaker JC, Sisson TA, Carel BJ, Azie NE. Lack of pharmacokinetic interaction between the anti-migraine compound, almotriptan, and propranolol in healthy volunteers. *Cephalalgia* (2001) 21, 61–65.
3. Milton KA, Tan L, Love R. The pharmacokinetic and pharmacodynamic interactions of oral eletriptan and propranolol in healthy volunteers. *Cephalalgia* (1998) 18, 412.
4. Relpax (Eletriptan hydrobromide). Pfizer Ltd. UK Summary of product characteristics, February 2008.
5. Buchan P, Ward C, Stewart AJ. The effect of propranolol on the pharmacokinetic and safety profiles of frovatriptan. *Headache* (1999) 39, 345.
6. Amerge (Naratriptan hydrochloride). GlaxoSmithKline. US Prescribing information, February 2010.
7. Goldberg MR, Sciberras D, De Smet M, Lowry R, Tomasko L, Lee Y, Olah TV, Zhao J, Vyas KP, Halpin R, Kari PH, James I. Influence of β-adrenoceptor antagonists on the pharmacokinetics of rizatriptan, a 5-$HT_{1B/1D}$ agonist: differential effects of propranolol, nadolol and metoprolol. *Br J Clin Pharmacol* (2001) 52, 69–76.
8. Maxalt (Rizatriptan benzoate). Merck Sharp & Dohme Ltd. UK Summary of product characteristics, June 2010.
9. Maxalt (Rizatriptan benzoate). Merck & Co., Inc. US Prescribing information, August 2010.
10. Scott AK, Walley T, Breckenridge AM, Lacey LF, Fowler PA. Lack of an interaction between propranolol and sumatriptan. *Br J Clin Pharmacol* (1991) 32, 581–4.
11. Putnam GP, O'Quinn S, Bolden-Watson CP, Davis RL, Gutterman DL, Fox AW. Migraine polypharmacy and the tolerability of sumatriptan: a large-scale, prospective study. *Cephalalgia* (1999) 19, 668–75.
12. Peck RW, Seaber EJ, Dixon R, Gillotin CG, Weatherley BC, Layton G, Posner J. The interaction between propranolol and the novel antimigraine agent zolmitriptan (311C90). *Br J Clin Pharmacol* (1997) 44, 595–9.
13. Zomig Tablets (Zolmitriptan). AstraZeneca UK Ltd. UK Summary of product characteristics, February 2010.

Triptans + Ergot derivatives

Theoretically, additive vasoconstriction could occur when ergot derivatives and triptans are given together, although only one study with sumatriptan has found this effect. However, one isolated case report describes myocardial infarction in a woman taking sumatriptan and methysergide.

No important additive effect has been seen in pharmacodynamic studies with ergot derivatives and almotriptan, eletriptan, frovatriptan, naratriptan, rizatriptan, or zolmitriptan, although minor increases in blood pressure were reported with eletriptan.

Clinical evidence

(a) Almotriptan

The manufacturer of almotriptan states that no additive vasospastic effects were seen in a clinical study in 12 healthy subjects given almotriptan and **ergotamine**.[1] However, they do note that such effects are theoretically possible.

(b) Eletriptan

The manufacturer reports that when oral **ergotamine** with caffeine was given one hour and 2 hours after eletriptan, minor additive increases in blood pressure were seen.[2]

(c) Frovatriptan

In a randomised, crossover study, 12 healthy subjects were given a single 5-mg dose of oral frovatriptan, a single 2-mg sublingual dose of **ergotamine**, or both drugs together. **Ergotamine** reduced the maximum plasma concentration and AUC of frovatriptan by about 25%, whereas frovatriptan had no effect on **ergotamine** pharmacokinetics. No clinically significant changes in the haemodynamics or the ECGs of the subjects were noted.[3]

(d) Naratriptan

A study in 12 healthy subjects found that intramuscular **dihydroergotamine** 1 mg reduced the AUC and the maximum serum concentration of a single 2.5-mg dose of naratriptan by 15% and 20%, respectively, but this was not considered to be clinically relevant. Concurrent use was well tolerated and no clinically significant blood pressure, heart rate or ECG effects were seen.[4]

(e) Rizatriptan

In a pharmacodynamic study in 16 healthy subjects no additive vasospastic effects were seen when oral rizatriptan 10 mg was given with intravenous **ergotamine** 250 micrograms.[5]

(f) Sumatriptan

A study in 38 migraine sufferers found that intravenous **dihydroergotamine** 1 mg caused a maximum increase in blood pressure of 13/9 mmHg, while subcutaneous sumatriptan 2 mg or 4 mg caused a smaller rise in blood pressure of 7/6 mmHg. When both drugs were given together the blood pressure rises were no greater than with **dihydroergotamine** alone.[6] A clinical study found that the adverse event profile of subcutaneous sumatriptan was not affected by the concurrent use of oral **dihydroergotamine**.[7] However, another pharmacodynamic study found that subcutaneous sumatriptan and intravenous **ergotamine** had additive vasoconstrictive effects (as assessed by decreases in toe-arm systolic blood pressure gradients).[8]

Myocardial infarction has been reported in a 43-year-old woman after she took two 2-mg doses of **methysergide** 12 hours apart, followed by sumatriptan 6 mg subcutaneously. Severe chest pain and tightness with breathlessness began 15 minutes later, and results of various tests were consistent with 'coronary spasm on an area of atherosclerosis'.[9]

(g) Zolmitriptan

In a randomised, placebo-controlled study, 12 healthy subjects were given oral **dihydroergotamine** 5 mg twice daily for 10 days, with oral zolmitriptan 10 mg (four times the usual dose) on day 10. No significant changes in blood pressure, ECGs, or zolmitriptan pharmacokinetics were seen, and concurrent use was well tolerated.[10] Another randomised, placebo-controlled study in 12 healthy subjects looked at the effects of oral zolmitriptan 20 mg (eight times the usual dose) given with oral **ergotamine** 2 mg (contained in *Cafergot* tablets; **ergotamine** 1 mg with caffeine 100 mg). Using a very detailed and thorough range of techniques, no clinically relevant cardiovascular changes were found, even at this large dose of zolmitriptan, and concurrent use was generally well tolerated. No important changes in zolmitriptan pharmacokinetics were seen.[11]

Mechanism

Vasoconstriction is a well known adverse effect of ergot derivatives, and coronary vasoconstriction can also occur rarely with the triptans. Note that in 1992, soon after the marketing of sumatriptan, the CSM in the UK had received 34 reports of chest pain or tightness caused by sumatriptan, possibly due to coronary vasoconstriction.[12] It is therefore theoretically possible that the drugs might have additive vasoconstrictive effects, although there is little evidence of this in practice.

Importance and management

Due to the theoretical risk of additive vasoconstriction, and possible significant coronary vasoconstriction, ergot derivatives (such as ergotamine, dihydroergotamine, and methysergide) are generally contraindicated with the triptans.

The UK manufacturer of sumatriptan states that ergotamine should not be given less than 6 hours after taking the triptan, and recommends that the triptan should not be taken less than 24 hours after taking ergotamine.[13] The same recommendations are made by the UK manufacturers of almotriptan,[1] rizatriptan,[14] and zolmitriptan.[15] The UK manufacturers of eletriptan,[2] frovatriptan,[16] and naratriptan[17] recommend that ergot derivatives are not given for a minimum of 24 hours after these triptans, and in general, in the US, it is recommended that triptans and ergotamine or ergot-type medication should not be taken within 24 hours of each other. In the absence of specific guidance for individual triptans and ergot derivatives, it would seem prudent to follow this advice, regardless of the route of administration.

1. Almogran (Almotriptan hydrogen malate). Almirall Ltd. UK Summary of product characteristics, June 2010.
2. Relpax (Eletriptan hydrobromide). Pfizer Ltd. UK Summary of product characteristics, February 2008.
3. Buchan P, Ward C, Oliver SD. Lack of clinically significant interactions between frovatriptan and ergotamine. *Cephalalgia* (1999) 19, 364.
4. Kempsford RD, Nicholls B, Lam R, Wintermute S. A study to investigate the potential interaction of naratriptan and dihydroergotamine. 8th International Headache Congress, Amsterdam, June 1997.
5. Tfelt-Hansen P, Seidelin K, Stepanavage M, Lines C. The effect of rizatriptan, ergotamine, and their combination on human peripheral arteries: a double-blind, placebo-controlled, crossover study in normal subjects. Br J Clin Pharmacol. (2002) 54, 38–44.
6. Fowler PA, Lacey LF, Thomas M, Keene ON, Tanner RJN, Baber NS. The clinical pharmacology, pharmacokinetics and metabolism of sumatriptan. *Eur Neurol* (1991) 31, 291–4.
7. Henry P, d'Allens H, and the French Migraine Network Bordeaux-Lyon-Grenoble. Subcutaneous sumatriptan in the acute treatment of migraine in patients using dihydroergotamine as prophylaxis. *Headache* (1993) 33, 432–5.
8. Tfelt-Hansen P, Sperling B, Winter PDO'B. Transient additional effect of sumatriptan on ergotamine-induced constriction of peripheral arteries in man. *Clin Pharmacol Ther* (1992) 51, 149.
9. Liston H, Bennett L, Usher B, Nappi J. The association of the combination of sumatriptan and methysergide in myocardial infarction in a premenopausal woman. *Arch Intern Med* (1999) 159, 511–13.
10. Veronese L, Gillotin C, Marion-Gallois R, Weatherley BC, Thebault JJ, Guillaume M, Peck RW. Lack of interaction between oral dihydroergotamine and the novel antimigraine compound zolmitriptan in healthy volunteers. *Clin Drug Invest* (1997) 14, 217–20.
11. Dixon RM, Meire HB, Evans DH, Watt H, On N, Posner J, Rolan PE. Peripheral vascular effects and pharmacokinetics of the antimigraine compound, zolmitriptan, in combination with oral ergotamine in healthy volunteers. *Cephalalgia* (1997) 17, 639–46.
12. Committee on Safety of Medicines. Sumatriptan (Imigran) and chest pain. *Current Problems* (1992) 34, 2.
13. Imigran Radis Tablets (Sumatriptan succinate). GlaxoSmithKline UK. UK Summary of product characteristics, September 2010.
14. Maxalt (Rizatriptan benzoate). Merck Sharp & Dohme Ltd. UK Summary of product characteristics, June 2010.
15. Zomig Tablets (Zolmitriptan). AstraZeneca UK Ltd. UK Summary of product characteristics, February 2010.
16. Migard (Frovatriptan succinate monohydrate). A. Menarini Pharma UK SRL. UK Summary of product characteristics, July 2008.
17. Naramig (Naratriptan hydrochloride). GlaxoSmithKline UK. UK Summary of product characteristics, April 2010.

Triptans + Flunarizine

Flunarizine does not appear to interact with eletriptan or sumatriptan, or alter the efficacy of almotriptan.

Clinical evidence, mechanism, importance and management

(a) Almotriptan

In an open-label study, the efficacy of almotriptan 12.5 mg in treating acute migraine attacks was compared in 81 patients taking an average dose of flunarizine of 6.4 mg and 92 patients not receiving migraine prophylaxis. Flunarizine was found not to alter the efficacy of almotriptan, as assessed by a decrease in self-assessed headache severity at 2 hours and the percentage of pain free patients at 2 hours.[1]

(b) Eletriptan

The UK manufacturer notes that although no formal interaction studies have been undertaken, there was no evidence of an interaction between eletriptan and flunarizine in clinical studies.[2]

(c) Sumatriptan

A double-blind study in healthy subjects found that flunarizine 10 mg daily for 8 days had no effect on the pharmacokinetics of a single dose of sumatriptan, and concurrent use caused no notable changes in blood pressure, ECG, or heart rate.[3]

1. Bermejo PE, Dorado R, Gomez-Arguelles JM. Variation in almotriptan effectiveness according to different prophylactic treatments. *Headache* (2009) 94, 1277–82.
2. Relpax (Eletriptan hydrobromide). Pfizer Ltd. UK Summary of product characteristics, February 2008.
3. Van Hecken AM, Depré M, De Schepper PJ, Fowler PA, Lacey LF, Durham JM. Lack of effect of flunarizine on the pharmacokinetics and pharmacodynamics of sumatriptan in healthy volunteers. *Br J Clin Pharmacol* (1992) 34, 82–4.

Triptans + Food

The absorption of most oral triptans does not appear to be affected by food to a clinically relevant extent.

Clinical evidence, mechanism, importance and management

(a) Almotriptan

In a randomised, crossover study, 16 healthy subjects were given a single 25-mg dose of almotriptan after an overnight fast and after a standard meal. When compared with fasting, the meal had no significant effect on the rate or extent of almotriptan absorption.[1]

(b) Eletriptan

The AUC and maximum plasma concentration of eletriptan were increased by about 20 to 30% following oral administration with a high-fat meal.[2,3]

(c) Frovatriptan

Food delayed the maximum plasma concentration of frovatriptan by about one hour, but had no significant effect on its bioavailability.[4,5]

(d) Naratriptan

The absorption of naratriptan[6,7] does not appear to be affected by food.

(e) Rizatriptan

The maximum plasma concentration of rizatriptan tablets is delayed by about one hour when the tablets are given with food.[8,9] although the extent of absorption was not affected.[9] The UK manufacturer of rizatriptan, therefore, suggests that the onset of effect of the triptan might be delayed if it is given with meals.[8] However, the US manufacturer notes that rizatriptan was given without regard to meals in clinical studies.[9] It therefore seems unlikely that food will affect the clinical efficacy of rizatriptan.

(f) Sumatriptan

In healthy subjects, a high-fat meal increased the AUC and maximum plasma concentration of sumatriptan by 12% and 15%, respectively, compared with the fasting state.[10]

(g) Zolmitriptan

In a randomised study, 12 healthy subjects were given zolmitriptan 5 mg after an overnight fast and after a standard breakfast. When compared with the fasting state, food decreased the maximum plasma concentration and AUC of zolmitriptan by 12% and 16%, respectively, but neither of these changes was statistically significant.[11] Food is therefore unlikely to affect the clinical efficacy of zolmitriptan.

1. Jansat JM, Martinez-Tobed A, Garcia E, Cabarrocas X, Costa J. Effect of food intake on the bioavailability of almotriptan, an antimigraine compound, in healthy volunteers: an open, randomized, crossover, single-dose clinical trial. *Int J Clin Pharmacol Ther* (2006) 44, 185–90.
2. Relpax (Eletriptan hydrobromide). Pfizer Ltd. UK Summary of product characteristics, February 2008.
3. Relpax (Eletriptan hydrobromide). Pfizer Inc. US Prescribing information, May 2008.
4. Migard (Frovatriptan succinate monohydrate). A. Menarini Pharma UK SRL. UK Summary of product characteristics, July 2008.
5. Frova (Frovatriptan succinate). Endo Pharmaceuticals Inc. US Prescribing information, April 2007.
6. Naramig (Naratriptan hydrochloride). GlaxoSmithKline UK. UK Summary of product characteristics, April 2010.
7. Amerge (Naratriptan hydrochloride). GlaxoSmithKline. US Prescribing information, February 2010.
8. Maxalt (Rizatriptan benzoate). Merck Sharp & Dohme Ltd. UK Summary of product characteristics, June 2010.
9. Maxalt (Rizatriptan benzoate). Merck & Co., Inc. US Prescribing information, August 2010.
10. Imitrex Tablets (Sumatriptan succinate). GlaxoSmithKline. US Prescribing information, February 2010.
11. Seaber EJ, Peck RW, Smith DA, Allanson J, Hefting NR, van Lier JJ, Sollie FAE, Werner J, Jonkman JHG. The absolute bioavailability and effect of food on the pharmacokinetics of zolmitriptan in healthy volunteers. *Br J Clin Pharmacol* (1998) 46, 433–9.

Triptans + HIV-protease inhibitors

HIV-protease inhibitors such as ritonavir, indinavir, or nelfinavir would be expected to increase the plasma concentration of eletriptan. HIV-protease inhibitors are also expected to increase the plasma concentration of almotriptan.

Clinical evidence, mechanism, importance and management

The UK and US manufacturers of **eletriptan** state that the concurrent use of ritonavir, indinavir, or nelfinavir should be avoided, because these HIV-protease inhibitors are CYP3A4 inhibitors [usually considered potent inhibitors]. CYP3A4 is involved in the metabolism of **eletriptan** and concurrent use would therefore be expected to [markedly] increase the exposure to **eletriptan**.[1,2] In addition, the US manufacturer recommends that **eletriptan** should not be given within 72 hours of ritonavir and nelfinavir.[2] This predicted interaction is based on the known interaction with the potent CYP3A4 inhibitor, ketoconazole (see 'Triptans + Azoles', p.643). Similar predictions are made by the US manufacturer of **almotriptan**; they advise that increased exposure to **almotriptan** might be expected with the use of potent CYP3A4 inhibitors (none named),[3] and this would be expected to include some HIV-protease inhibitors. They recommend that a starting dose of **almotriptan** 6.25 mg in the presence of these drugs.

1. Relpax (Eletriptan hydrobromide). Pfizer Ltd. UK Summary of product characteristics, February 2008.
2. Relpax (Eletriptan hydrobromide). Pfizer Inc. US Prescribing information, May 2008.
3. Axert (Almotriptan malate). Ortho-McNeil Pharmaceutical Inc. US Prescribing information, April 2009.

Triptans + Macrolides

Erythromycin moderately increases the exposure to eletriptan; clarithromycin and josamycin are predicted to interact in a similar way. Almotriptan might be similarly affected by these macrolides. Clarithromycin does not affect the pharmacokinetics of sumatriptan.

Clinical evidence

(a) Eletriptan

A clinical pharmacokinetic study by the manufacturer of eletriptan[1] found that **erythromycin** 1 g increased the maximum plasma concentration and AUC of eletriptan 2-fold and 3.6-fold, respectively, and prolonged its half-life from 4.6 hours to 7.1 hours.

(b) Sumatriptan

A study in which 24 healthy subjects were given sumatriptan 50 mg on the morning of the fourth day of a course of **clarithromycin** 500 mg twice daily, found that **clarithromycin** did not affect the pharmacokinetics of sumatriptan to a clinically relevant extent.[2]

Mechanism

The macrolides are, to varying degrees, inhibitors of CYP3A4, by which eletriptan is metabolised. Therefore erythromycin reduces eletriptan metabolism and increases its exposure. Sumatriptan is not metabolised by CYP3A4 and therefore does not interact with clarithromycin.

Importance and management

Eletriptan

Information is limited but an interaction between eletriptan and **erythromycin** appears to be established. Because of the increase in plasma concentration seen, the UK manufacturer advises against their concurrent use.[1] Similarly, other drugs that are moderate to potent inhibitors of CYP3A4, including **clarithromycin**[1,3] are predicted to increase the plasma concentration of eletriptan, and so should also not be used with eletriptan. The US manufacturer recommends that eletriptan should not be given within 72 hours of potent CYP3A4 inhibitors, and they specifically name **clarithromycin**.[3] **Telithromycin** would be expected to interact similarly, and some suggest that and **josamycin**[1] could also interact in this way, but direct evidence appears to be lacking.

Almotriptan

Almotriptan is metabolised by CYP3A4, and although evidence of an interaction with the macrolides is lacking, potent CYP3A4 inhibitors are known to increase the plasma concentration of almotriptan (see 'Triptans + Azoles', p.643). The US manufacturer of almotriptan recommends an almotriptan starting dose of 6.25 mg in the presence of potent CYP3A4 inhibitors,[4] and this would be expected to include **clarithromycin** and **telithromycin**.

Other triptans

Other triptans would be expected to have little or no interaction with the macrolides as they are not predominantly metabolised by CYP3A4 (see 'Table 16.2', p.639), and this has been shown for sumatriptan.

1. Relpax (Eletriptan hydrobromide). Pfizer Ltd. UK Summary of product characteristics, February 2008.
2. Moore KHP, Leese PT, McNeal S, Gray P, O'Quinn S, Bye C, Sale M. The pharmacokinetics of sumatriptan when administered with clarithromycin in healthy volunteers. *Clin Ther* (2002) 24, 583–94.
3. Relpax (Eletriptan hydrobromide). Pfizer Inc. US Prescribing information, May 2008.
4. Axert (Almotriptan malate). Ortho-McNeil Pharmaceutical Inc. US Prescribing information, April 2009.

Triptans + MAOIs

Moclobemide (a RIMA) inhibits the metabolism of rizatriptan and (to a lesser extent) zolmitriptan, and approximately doubles the bioavailability of sumatriptan. Moclobemide has no clinically significant pharmacokinetic effect on almotriptan, and is not expected to affect the pharmacokinetics of eletriptan, frovatriptan, or naratriptan. Non-selective MAOIs (e.g. phenelzine) would be expected to behave similarly.

Selegiline (an MAO-B inhibitor) does not alter the pharmacokinetics of sumatriptan or zolmitriptan, and would not be expected to alter the pharmacokinetics of the other triptans.

Some have suggested that there might be a pharmacodynamic interaction between MAOIs (both selective and non-selective) and triptans, which could result in serotonin syndrome.

Clinical evidence

(a) Almotriptan

In a study, 12 healthy subjects were given **moclobemide** 150 mg twice daily for 8 days with a single 12.5-mg dose of almotriptan on day 8. The AUC of almotriptan was increased by 37%, its clearance was decreased by 27% and its half-life was increased by 24%, but this was not considered to be clinically significant.[1]

(b) Frovatriptan

A study in 9 healthy subjects given a single 2.5-mg oral dose of frovatriptan after taking **moclobemide** 150 mg twice daily for 7 days did not find any pharmacokinetic changes, or any alterations in the vital signs and ECGs of the subjects.[2]

(c) Rizatriptan

In a randomised, placebo-controlled study, 12 healthy subjects were given **moclobemide** 150 mg three times daily for 4 days, with a single 10-mg dose of rizatriptan on day 4. **Moclobemide** increased the AUCs of rizatriptan and its active (but minor) metabolite 2.2- and 5.3-fold, respectively, and increased their maximum serum concentrations by 40% and 2.6-fold, respectively. Despite these rises, the concurrent use of these drugs was well tolerated and any adverse effects were mild and similar to those seen when rizatriptan was given with placebo.[3]

(d) Sumatriptan

Three groups of 14 subjects were given placebo, **moclobemide** 150 mg three times daily, or **selegiline** 5 mg twice daily for 8 days, with subcutaneous sumatriptan 6 mg on day 8. No statistically significant differences in pulse rates or blood pressures were seen between any of the groups. However, the AUC of sumatriptan in the **moclobemide**-treated group was approximately doubled (129% increase), its clearance was reduced by 56%, and its half-life increased by 52%. The pharmacokinetic changes seen in the **selegiline** group were not consistent. There were no differences in the adverse events experienced by any of the three groups.[4]

A comprehensive search of the literature, and reports from proprietary manufacturers, identified published reports of 31 patients taking sumatriptan and MAOIs concurrently, but no adverse events were reported.[5] Furthermore, a patient taking **moclobemide** 300 mg three times daily had no adverse effects when given oral sumatriptan 100 mg on six occasions.[6] However, a patient who had taken an *overdose* of **moclobemide**, together with sumatriptan, sertraline, and citalopram developed serotonin syndrome.[7]

(e) Zolmitriptan

In a series of randomised studies, 12 healthy subjects were given **selegiline** 10 mg daily or **moclobemide** 150 mg twice daily for 7 days, with a single 10-mg oral dose of zolmitriptan on day 7.[8] **Moclobemide** increased the AUCs of zolmitriptan and its active metabolite, by 26% and 3-fold, respectively.[9]

In another study, **selegiline** had no effect on the pharmacokinetics of zolmitriptan or its metabolites, apart from a small (7%) reduction in its renal clearance.[8]

Mechanism

Almotriptan, rizatriptan, sumatriptan, and zolmitriptan are substrates of MAO-A. Therefore moclobemide, an inhibitor of MAO-A, can reduce their metabolism, resulting in increased plasma concentrations. The effect differs between the triptans, as less than 30% of a dose of almotriptan is metabolised by MAO-A,[10] whereas MAO-A is the principal enzyme concerned with the metabolism of rizatriptan[3] and sumatriptan.[11] Frovatriptan is not metabolised by MAO-A, and therefore its pharmacokinetics are not affected by moclobemide.

Importance and management

Moclobemide and MAOIs

The interactions of moclobemide with **rizatriptan** or **sumatriptan** are established, and clinically relevant. The US manufacturers contraindicate concurrent use because of the risks of coronary vasospasm.[12,13] There seems to be no direct evidence regarding an interaction of these triptans with a non-selective MAOI, nevertheless, they would be expected to behave similarly. The UK and US manufacturers of rizatriptan[12,14] and sumatriptan[13,15] contraindicate their use both during, and for 2 weeks after, the use of a non-selective MAOI (e.g. phenelzine).

The interaction with **zolmitriptan** is slight, although exposure to its active metabolite is moderately increased. The US manufacturer contraindicates its use both during, and for 2 weeks after, the use of moclobemide,[16] whereas the UK manufacturer restricts the dose of zolmitriptan to 5 mg in 24 hours.[9] In the absence of any direct information it would seem prudent to apply these warnings to the use of non-selective MAOIs.

The interaction between moclobemide with **almotriptan** is slight, and no dose adjustments would be expected to be necessary with any selective or non-selective MAOI. However, note that is has been suggested that serotonin syndrome is possible on the concurrent use of and MAOI and a triptan, and the manufacturers of almotriptan[17] specifically warn of this possibility.

Moclobemide did not affect the pharmacokinetics of **frovatriptan**, and would not be expected to affect the pharmacokinetics of **eletriptan** or **naratriptan**, as they, like frovatriptan, are not metabolised by MAO-A, see 'Table 16.2', p.639. Similarly, non-selective MAOIs would not be expected to interact. However, note that is has been suggested that serotonin syndrome is possible on the concurrent use of an MAOI and a triptan, and the manufacturers of frovatriptan[18] specifically warn of this possibility.

For more information about serotonin syndrome and its management, see 'Drugs that cause serotonin syndrome + Other drugs that cause serotonin syndrome', p.1471.

Selegiline or Rasagiline

Selegiline, a selective inhibitor of MAO-B, does not affect the pharmacokinetics of sumatriptan or zolmitriptan, and would not be expected to alter the metabolism of any other triptan. Other MAO-B inhibitors, such as rasagiline, would also therefore not be expected to interact by a pharmacokinetic mechanism. However, note that the MAO-B selectivity of selegiline is lost at doses above 10 mg daily.

In the UK, manufacturers of selegiline contraindicate its use with triptans and recommend a time interval of 24 hours between discontinuation of selegiline and initiation of serotonin agonists.[19,20] This is probably because of a theoretical possibility of serotonin syndrome developing on concurrent use. For more information about serotonin syndrome and its management, see 'Drugs that cause serotonin syndrome + Other drugs that cause serotonin syndrome', p.1471.

1. Fleishaker JC, Ryan KK, Jansat JM, Carel BJ, Bell DJA, Burke MT, Azie NE. Effect of MAO-A inhibition on the pharmacokinetics of almotriptan, an antimigraine agent in humans. *Br J Clin Pharmacol* (2001) 51, 437–41.
2. Buchan P, Ward C, Freestone S. Lack of interaction between frovatriptan and monoamine oxidase inhibitor. *Cephalalgia* (1999) 19, 364.
3. van Haarst AD, van Gerven JMA, Cohen AF, De Smet M, Sterrett A, Birk KL, Fisher AL, De Puy ME, Goldberg MR, Musson DG. The effects of moclobemide on the pharmacokinetics of the 5-$HT_{1B/1D}$ agonist rizatriptan in healthy volunteers. *Br J Clin Pharmacol* (1999) 48, 190–96.
4. Glaxo Pharmaceuticals UK Limited. Data on file. A study to determine whether the pharmacokinetics, safety or tolerability of subcutaneously administered sumatriptan (6 mg) are altered by interaction with concurrent oral monoamine oxidase inhibitors (Protocol C92–050). 1993.
5. Gardner DM, Lynd LD. Sumatriptan contraindications and the serotonin syndrome. *Ann Pharmacother* (1998) 32, 33–38.
6. Blier P, Bergeron R. The safety of concomitant use of sumatriptan and antidepressant treatments. *J Clin Psychopharmacol* (1995) 15, 106–9.
7. Höjer J, Personne M, Skagius A-S, Hansson O. Serotoninergt syndrom: flera allvarliga fall med denna ofta förbisedda diagnos. *Lakartidningen* (2002) 99, 2054–5, 2058–60.
8. Rolan P. Potential drug interactions with the novel antimigraine compound zolmitriptan (Zomig™, 311C90). *Cephalalgia* (1997) 17 (Suppl 18), 21–7.
9. Zomig Tablets (Zolmitriptan). AstraZeneca UK Ltd. UK Summary of product characteristics, February 2010.
10. Axert (Almotriptan malate). Ortho-McNeil Pharmaceutical Inc. US Prescribing information, April 2009.
11. Dixon CM, Park GR, Tarbit MH. Characterization of the enzyme responsible for the metabolism of sumatriptan in human liver. *Biochem Pharmacol* (1994) 47, 1253–7.
12. Maxalt (Rizatriptan benzoate). Merck & Co., Inc. US Prescribing information, August 2010.
13. Imitrex Tablets (Sumatriptan succinate). GlaxoSmithKline. US Prescribing information, February 2010.
14. Maxalt (Rizatriptan benzoate). Merck Sharp & Dohme Ltd. UK Summary of product characteristics, June 2010.
15. Imigran Radis Tablets (Sumatriptan succinate). GlaxoSmithKline UK. UK Summary of product characteristics, September 2010.
16. Zomig (Zolmitriptan). AstraZeneca Pharmaceuticals LP. US Prescribing information, October 2008.
17. Almogran (Almotriptan hydrogen malate). Almirall Ltd. UK Summary of product characteristics, June 2010.
18. Migard (Frovatriptan succinate monohydrate). A. Menarini Pharma UK SRL. UK Summary of product characteristics, July 2008.
19. Zelapar (Selegiline hydrochloride). Cephalon Ltd. UK Summary of product characteristics, March 2012.
20. Eldepryl (Selegiline hydrochloride). Orion Pharma (UK) Ltd. UK Summary of product characteristics, February 2012.

Triptans + Paracetamol (Acetaminophen)

Paracetamol causes a negligible increase in the exposure to zolmitriptan and zolmitriptan causes a small reduction in the rate and extent of paracetamol absorption. Sumatriptan delays paracetamol absorption but does not affect the total amount of paracetamol absorbed.

Clinical evidence, mechanism, importance and management

In a randomised, crossover study, 15 healthy subjects were given a single 10-mg dose of **zolmitriptan**, alone or with paracetamol 1 g. Paracetamol increased the maximum plasma concentration and AUC of **zolmitriptan** by 11%, while reducing its renal clearance by 9%. The paracetamol maximum plasma concentration and AUC were reduced by 31% and 11%, respectively, and absorption was delayed (time to achieve maximum plasma concentration increased from 45 minutes to 3 hours). The presence of oral metoclopramide 10 mg did not affect the interaction between **zolmitriptan** and paracetamol.[1] The small changes in pharmacokinetics seen are not clinically relevant.

Similarly, in a study in 9 migraine patients, pretreatment with oral **sumatriptan** 100 mg delayed paracetamol absorption and reduced its maximum plasma concentration by 50%, but the total absorption of paracetamol over 8 hours was not altered.[2]

It has been suggested that **sumatriptan** and **zolmitriptan** might have some inhibitory effect on gastric emptying thereby slowing the absorption of paracetamol,[1,2] and although this appears to occur, it does not appear to be clinically relevant.

1. Seaber EJ, Ridout G, Layton G, Posner J, Peck RW. The novel anti-migraine compound zolmitriptan (Zomig 311C90) has no clinically significant interactions with paracetamol or metoclopramide. *Eur J Clin Pharmacol* (1997) 53, 229–34.
2. Rani PU, Naidu MUR, Rao TRK, Das SM, Shobha JC, Sekhar KR, Sekhar EC, Kumar TV. Sumatriptan delays paracetamol absorption in migraine patients. *Clin Drug Invest* (1996) 11, 300–4.

Triptans + Pizotifen

Pizotifen does not alter the pharmacokinetics or pharmacodynamics of sumatriptan or zolmitriptan, and it does not alter the efficacy of acute sumatriptan for migraine. It seems unlikely that any of the other triptans will interact adversely with pizotifen.

Clinical evidence

(a) Sumatriptan

Pizotifen 500 micrograms three times daily for 8 days was found to have no effect on the pharmacokinetics of sumatriptan in 14 healthy subjects. In addition, no notable changes in blood pressure or heart rate occurred.[1] In a clinical study, pizotifen prophylaxis did not alter the efficacy of acute sumatriptan for migraine relief. In this study, the combination was associated with more weight gain than sumatriptan alone, an effect that was attributed solely to the pizotifen.[2]

(b) Zolmitriptan

In a placebo-controlled, randomised study, 12 healthy subjects were given pizotifen 1.5 mg daily for 8 days, with oral zolmitriptan 10 mg on day 8. Pizotifen did not alter the pharmacokinetics of zolmitriptan, and no clinically relevant changes in heart rates, ECGs, or blood pressures were seen as a result of concurrent use.[3]

Mechanism

None.

Importance and management

Although the information is limited, it shows that no sumatriptan or zolmitriptan dose adjustments are expected to be needed if either drug is used with pizotifen, and concurrent use appears to be safe. On the basis of the information about sumatriptan and zolmitriptan it seems unlikely that any of the other triptans will interact adversely with pizotifen.

1. Fowler PA, Lacey LF, Thomas M, Keene ON, Tanner RJN, Baber NS. The clinical pharmacology, pharmacokinetics and metabolism of sumatriptan. *Eur Neurol* (1991) 31, 291–4.
2. Cleland PG, Barnes D, Elrington GM, Loizou LA, Rawes GD. Studies to assess if pizotifen prophylaxis improves migraine beyond the benefit offered by acute sumatriptan therapy alone. *Eur Neurol* (1997) 38, 31–8.
3. Seaber EJ, Gillotin C, Mohanlal R, Layton G, Posner J, Peck R. Lack of interaction between pizotifen and the novel antimigraine compound zolmitriptan in healthy volunteers. *Clin Drug Invest* (1997) 14, 221–5.

Triptans + SSRIs or SNRIs

The SSRIs generally do not interact with the triptans, but there are a few rare cases of dyskinesias when sumatriptan was given with an SSRI, and there is some evidence to suggest that serotonin syndrome might occasionally develop. The SNRIs venlafaxine, duloxetine, and milnacipran are predicted to interact similarly. Fluvoxamine inhibits the metabolism of frovatriptan and might inhibit the metabolism of zolmitriptan.

Clinical evidence

The FDA in the US has reviewed 27 reports of serotonin syndrome associated with the concurrent use of an SSRI or SNRI (e.g. **duloxetine** or **venlafaxine**) and a triptan. Two reports described life-threatening events and 13 reports stated that the patients required hospitalisation. Some of the cases occurred in patients who had previously taken an SSRI or SNRI with a triptan without experiencing serotonin syndrome. In 8 cases, recent dose increases or the addition of another serotonergic drug had occurred around the time of symptom onset: the median time to onset was one day, with a range of 10 minutes to 6 days.[1] Reports describing interactions with specific triptans are outlined in the subsections below.

(a) Almotriptan

Fluoxetine 60 mg daily was given to 14 healthy subjects for 8 days, with a single 12.5-mg dose of almotriptan on day 8. **Fluoxetine** raised the maximum plasma concentration of almotriptan by about 18%. Concurrent use was well tolerated and caused no ECG changes, so no dose alterations were considered necessary.[2]

(b) Eletriptan

A retrospective review of seven double-blind studies identified 253 patients who had received eletriptan with an SSRI and 3 908 patients who received eletriptan alone. There were no clinically significant differences, with respect to the incidence of adverse effects, between the two groups.[3]

(c) Frovatriptan

Fluvoxamine has been shown to increase the plasma concentration of frovatriptan by 27 to 49%.[4]

(d) Rizatriptan

In a placebo-controlled study, 12 healthy subjects were given a single 10-mg dose of rizatriptan after they took **paroxetine** 20 mg daily for 14 days. The plasma concentration of rizatriptan and its active metabolite were not altered by **paroxetine**, and no adverse effects were seen. Safety evaluations included blood pressure, heart rate, temperature, and a visual analogue assessment of mood. There was no evidence of serotonin syndrome.[5]

(e) Sumatriptan

A study in 11 healthy subjects found that **paroxetine** 20 mg daily for 16 days had no effect on the response to a 6-mg dose of subcutaneous sumatriptan, as measured by the plasma concentration of prolactin. The plasma concentration of sumatriptan remained unaltered, its cardiovascular effects were unchanged, and no clinically significant adverse effects occurred.[6]

Other studies report that the concurrent use of sumatriptan and SSRIs (**fluoxetine** 20 to 60 mg daily, **fluvoxamine** 200 mg daily, **paroxetine** 20 to 50 mg daily, **sertraline** 50 to 100 mg daily) was successful and uneventful.[7,8] No adverse effects have been noted in 148 other patients.[9]

A prospective study of 12 339 individuals receiving sumatriptan by injection identified 14.5% of these (1 784) who were also taking SSRIs (**fluoxetine** 8.3%, **sertraline** 5.5%, **paroxetine** 3.9%, other 0.4%) or **venlafaxine** 1.7%. Patients taking SSRIs were found to have a higher absolute frequency of adverse neurological effects, when compared with those not taking antidepressants (0.8% and 0.25%, respectively). Nevertheless, the authors concluded that there was no evidence of an interaction as the adverse events occurred more than 24 hours after sumatriptan was given.[10] However, a case report describes a 65-year-old woman who had been taking **paroxetine** 20 mg [daily] for a number of years, who developed confusion, strange behaviour, sinus tachycardia, hypertension, and hyperthermia shortly after starting sumatriptan. Serotonin syndrome was diagnosed, and she recovered completely when both drugs were withdrawn.[11] Another case report describes facial flushing in a woman taking sumatriptan and an SSRI (not stated). The symptoms subsided when either the sumatriptan or the SSRI were stopped, but reappeared when both drugs were restarted.[12]

Additionally, in Canada, post-marketing surveillance of the voluntary reports received by the manufacturers of **fluoxetine** identified 2 cases that showed good evidence, and another 4 cases that showed some, but not strong, evidence, of reactions consistent with serotonin syndrome in patients also taking sumatriptan.[13] Other cases describe a decrease in the efficacy of sumatriptan with **fluoxetine**,[14] dyskinesias and dystonias with sumatriptan and **paroxetine**,[15] and twenty possible cases of serotonin syndrome with sumatriptan and SSRIs.[9,16]

The UK manufacturers of sumatriptan also state that they have rare post-marketing reports of weakness, hyperreflexia, and incoordination following the use of sumatriptan and SSRIs.[17]

(f) Zolmitriptan

A placebo-controlled, crossover study in 20 subjects, given **fluoxetine** 20 mg daily for 28 days with zolmitriptan 10 mg on day 28, found that the pharmacokinetics of zolmitriptan were unaffected by **fluoxetine**. Only very small changes were seen in the pharmacokinetics of its active metabolite.[18] **Sertraline**, **paroxetine**, and **citalopram** are also not expected to alter the pharmacokinetics of zolmitriptan. However, **fluvoxamine**, a potent CYP1A2 inhibitor, is predicted to increase the plasma concentration of zolmitriptan,[19] based on the known interaction with cimetidine (see 'Triptans; Zolmitriptan + Cimetidine', p.650).

Mechanism

SSRIs increase the amount of 5-HT (serotonin) at post-synaptic receptors. In theory the triptans (5-HT_1 agonists) might possibly add to the effects of these increased amounts of serotonin, but in practice it is questionable whether this is normally clinically relevant. Fluvoxamine probably inhibits the metabolism of frovatriptan[20] by CYP1A2, and is predicted to interact with zolmitriptan[19] by the same mechanism.

Importance and management

The weight of evidence suggests that the concurrent use of the triptans and SSRIs is normally uneventful, but adverse reactions do occur occasionally. SSRIs have frequently been prescribed with triptans and a drug interaction causing serotonin syndrome appears to be extremely rare.[21,22] The authors of some of the reports concluded that their findings do not imply that concurrent use should be avoided, but that caution and close monitoring should be used[9,13] and this is mirrored by the advice given by the American Headache Society.[23]

Serotonin syndrome is a rare adverse effect, but because of its severity, some caution is warranted if both drugs are given. For more information on serotonin syndrome and its management, see 'Drugs that cause serotonin syndrome + Other drugs that cause serotonin syndrome', p.1471. The FDA in the US recommends that patients given a triptan with an SSRI or SNRI should be informed of the possibility of serotonin syndrome and be carefully observed.[1] Similar advice is given by most US and UK manufacturers of triptans, SSRIs, and SNRIs (including the US manufacturer of **milnacipran**[24]). In contrast, the French manufacturer of milnacipran states that it should not be used with triptans, and that one week should elapse after stopping milnacipran before starting a triptan.[25]

Fluvoxamine is predicted to have a pharmacokinetic interaction with **zolmitriptan** and therefore the manufacturer recommends a maximum dose of 5 mg in 24 hours in the presence of fluvoxamine.[19] A similar pharmacokinetic interaction might also occur between fluvoxamine and **frovatriptan**, and the manufacturer advises caution and strict adherence to the recommended dose.[20]

1. FDA Information for Healthcare Professionals. Selective serotonin reuptake inhibitors (SSRIs) selective serotonin-norepinephrine reuptake inhibitors (SNRIs) 5-hydroxytryptamine receptor agonists (triptans). July 19, 2006. Available at: http://www.fda.gov/Drugs/DrugSafety/PostmarketDrugSafetyInformationforPatientsandProviders/DrugSafetyInformationforHeathcareProfessionals/ucm085845.htm (accessed 22/10/15).
2. Fleishaker JC, Ryan KK, Carel BJ, Azie NE. Evaluation of the potential pharmacokinetic interaction between almotriptan and fluoxetine in healthy volunteers. *J Clin Pharmacol* (2001) 41, 217–23.
3. Hettiarachchi J, Turrall K. Concomitant eletriptan and selective serotonin reuptake inhibitor therapy for migraine patients: a review of seven clinical studies. *Cephalalgia* (2001) 21, 431.
4. Wade A, Buchan P, Mant T, Ward C. Frovatriptan has no clinically significant interaction with fluvoxamine. *Cephalalgia* (2001) 21, 427.
5. Goldberg MR, Lowry RC, Musson DG, Birk KL, Fisher A, DePuy ME, Shadle CR. Lack of pharmacokinetic and pharmacodynamic interaction between rizatriptan and paroxetine. *J Clin Pharmacol* (1999) 39, 192–9.
6. Wing Y-K, Clifford EM, Sheehan BD, Campling GM, Hockney RA, Cowen PJ. Paroxetine treatment and the prolactin response to sumatriptan. *Psychopharmacology (Berl)* (1996) 124, 377–9.
7. Blier P, Bergeron R. The safety of concomitant use of sumatriptan and antidepressant treatments. *J Clin Psychopharmacol* (1995) 15, 106–9.
8. Leung M, Ong M. Lack of an interaction between sumatriptan and selective serotonin reuptake inhibitors. *Headache* (1995) 35, 488–9.
9. Gardner DM, Lynd LD. Sumatriptan contraindications and the serotonin syndrome. *Ann Pharmacother* (1998) 32, 33–8.
10. Putnam GP, O'Quinn S, Bolden-Watson CP, Davis RL, Gutterman DL, Fox AW. Migraine polypharmacy and the tolerability of sumatriptan: a large-scale, prospective study. *Cephalalgia* (1999) 19, 668–75.
11. Hendrix Y, van Zagten MSG. Het serotoninesyndroom bij gelijktijdig gebruik van paroxetine en sumatriptan. *Ned Tijdschr Geneeskd* (2005) 149, 888–90.
12. Deng M, Nedorost S. Facial flushing: an uncommon presentation of serotonin toxicity. *Dermatitis* (2009) 20, 296–7.
13. Joffe RT, Sokolov STH. Co-administration of fluoxetine and sumatriptan: the Canadian experience. *Acta Psychiatr Scand* (1997) 95, 551–2.
14. Szabo CP. Fluoxetine and sumatriptan: possibly a counterproductive combination. *J Clin Psychiatry* (1995) 56, 37–8.
15. Abraham JT, Brown R, Meltzer HY. Clozapine treatment of persistent paroxysmal dyskinesia associated with concomitant paroxetine and sumatriptan use. *Biol Psychiatry* (1997) 42, 144–6.
16. Mathew NT, Tietjen GE, Lucker C. Serotonin syndrome complicating migraine pharmacotherapy. *Cephalalgia* (1996) 16, 323–7.
17. GlaxoWellcome. Personal communication, August 1997.
18. Smith DA, Cleary EW, Watkins S, Huffman CS, Polvino WJ. Zolmitriptan (311C90) does not interact with fluoxetine in healthy volunteers. *Int J Clin Pharmacol Ther* (1998) 36, 301–5.
19. Zomig Tablets (Zolmitriptan). AstraZeneca UK Ltd. UK Summary of product characteristics, February 2010.
20. Migard (Frovatriptan succinate monohydrate). A. Menarini Pharma UK SRL. UK Summary of product characteristics, July 2008.
21. Tepper S, Allen C, Sanders D, Greene A, Boccuzzi S. Coprescription of triptans with potentially interacting medications: a cohort study involving 240 268 patients. *Headache* (2003) 43, 44–8.
22. Shapiro RE, Tepper SJ. The serotonin syndrome, triptans, and the potential for drug–drug interactions. *Headache* (2007) 47, 266–9.
23. Evans RW,Tepper SJ, Shapiro RE, Sun-Edelstein C, Tietjen GE. The FDA alert on serotonin syndrome with use of triptans combined with selective serotonin reuptake inhibitors or selective serotonin-norepinephrine reuptake inhibitors: American Headache Society position paper. *Headache* (2010) 50, 1089–99.
24. Savella (Milnacipran hydrochloride). Forest Pharmaceuticals, Inc. US Prescribing information, November 2013.
25. Ixel (Milnacipran hydrochloride). Pierre Fabre Médicament. French Summary of product characteristics, February 2003.

Triptans + St John's wort (*Hypericum perforatum*)

Serotonin syndrome has been reported in a patient taking eletriptan and St John's wort.

Clinical evidence

A 28-year-old woman, who had been taking fluoxetine 60 mg daily for one year for an eating disorder and St John's wort (dose and frequency not stated) for one month, suffered a loss of consciousness, convulsions, and mental confusion after **eletriptan** 40 mg daily was started 3 days earlier for a recurrent migraine. Previous use of **eletriptan** and fluoxetine had not resulted in any reported adverse effects. After admission to hospital, the patient developed acute rhabdomyolysis and transient mild acute renal failure. Serotonin syndrome was diagnosed, all medications were stopped, and the symptoms gradually resolved over 10 days.[1]

Mechanism

Both the triptans and St John's wort have been implicated in cases of serotonin syndrome when they were given with other serotonergic drugs. Additive serotonergic effects are therefore the likely explanation for the case report with eletriptan and St John's wort.

Importance and management

Published evidence for an interaction between St John's wort and the triptans appears to be limited to the case report cited. Most UK manufacturers of triptans warn about the potential increase in undesirable effects. The possible concern is that concurrent use might result in the development of serotonin syndrome. For more information on serotonin syndrome and its management, see 'Drugs that cause serotonin syndrome + Other drugs that cause serotonin syndrome', p.1471.

1. Bonetto N, Santelli L, Battistin L, Cagnin A. Serotonin syndrome and rhabdomyolysis induced by concomitant use of triptans, fluoxetine and hypericum. *Cephalalgia* (2007) 27, 1421–3.

Triptans + Tobacco

The clearance of naratriptan, and possibly frovatriptan, is increased by smoking. One large study found no evidence of an interaction between smoking and sumatriptan.

Clinical evidence

(a) Frovatriptan

In a retrospective analysis of pharmacokinetic data from phase I studies, there was a trend for a lower frovatriptan AUC and maximum plasma concentration in smokers, when compared with non-smokers. The clearance tended to be higher but the half-life did not differ.[1]

(b) Naratriptan

The manufacturer notes that smoking increases the clearance of naratriptan by 30%.[2]

(c) Sumatriptan

A prospective study of 12 339 individuals receiving sumatriptan by injection identified 2 262 patients (18.3%) who were current smokers. There was no evidence of an interaction between sumatriptan and tobacco smoking.[3]

Mechanism

Tobacco smoke is known to induce CYP1A2, by which both naratriptan and, to some extent, frovatriptan are metabolised. **Zolmitriptan** is also a substrate of CYP1A2, but the effect of smoking on its metabolism does not appear to have been studied.

Importance and management

Although data are limited, the possible slight changes in the pharmacokinetics of frovatriptan and naratriptan with smoking are unlikely to be clinically relevant.

1. Buchan P. Effects of alcohol, smoking and oral contraceptives on the pharmacokinetics of frovatriptan. *Eur J Neurol* (2000) 7 (Suppl 3), 86–7.
2. Amerge (Naratriptan hydrochloride). GlaxoSmithKline. US Prescribing information, February 2010.
3. Putnam GP, O'Quinn S, Bolden-Watson CP, Davis RL, Gutterman DL, Fox AW. Migraine polypharmacy and the tolerability of sumatriptan: a large-scale, prospective study. *Cephalalgia* (1999) 19, 668–75.

Triptans + Topiramate

Topiramate does not affect the pharmacokinetics of oral or subcutaneous sumatriptan to a clinically relevant extent, nor does it reduce the efficacy of almotriptan.

Clinical evidence, mechanism, importance and management

(a) Almotriptan

In an open-label study, the efficacy of almotriptan 12.5 mg in treating acute migraine attacks was compared in 83 patients taking topiramate and 92 patients not receiving migraine prophylaxis. Topiramate was found not to alter the efficacy of almotriptan, as assessed by a decrease in self-assessed headache severity at 2 hours and the percentage of pain free patients at 2 hours.[1]

(b) Sumatriptan

In a study, 24 healthy subjects were given topiramate (50 mg every 12 hours increased to 100 mg every 12 hours) for a total of 7 days, with a single 100-mg oral dose of sumatriptan on day 7. It was found that topiramate reduced the AUC of sumatriptan by 10%, but this was not considered to be clinically relevant. Topiramate had no effect on the AUC of a single 6-mg subcutaneous dose of sumatriptan. The clearance of topiramate appeared to be reduced, when data from this study was compared with that from historical controls, but the magnitude of the effect was not stated.[2] The clinical significance of this effect is unclear, but it seems likely to be small.

1. Bermejo PE, Dorado R, Gomez-Arguelles JM. Variation in almotriptan effectiveness according to different prophylactic treatments. *Headache* (2009) 49, 1277–82.
2. Bialer M, Doose DR, Murthy B, Curtin C, Wang S-S, Twyman RE, Schwabe S. Pharmacokinetic interactions of topiramate. Clin Pharmacokinet. (2004) 43, 763–80.

Triptans + Verapamil

Verapamil moderately increases the exposure to eletriptan, but only causes a negligible increase in the exposure to almotriptan.

Clinical evidence, mechanism, importance and management

(a) Almotriptan

In a crossover study, 12 healthy subjects were given a single 12.5-mg dose of almotriptan, either alone or after they had taken sustained-release verapamil 120 mg twice daily for 7 days. Verapamil increased the AUC and maximum plasma concentration of almotriptan by about 20% and 24%, respectively. However, the only effect this caused was a small increase in systolic BP (8 mmHg), which occurred 2 hours after the dose. It was suggested that verapamil might inhibit the metabolism of almotriptan by CYP3A4.[1] The pharmacokinetic changes are negligible, and no dose adjustments or particular precautions would appear to be necessary on concurrent use.

(b) Eletriptan

In a clinical study, verapamil 480 mg raised the maximum plasma concentration and AUC of eletriptan 2.2-fold and 2.7-fold, respectively.[2] The UK manufacturer states that these increases are not considered to be clinically significant as there were no associated increases in blood pressure or adverse events, when compared with eletriptan alone.[2]

1. Fleishaker JC, Sisson TA, Carel BJ, Azie NE. Pharmacokinetic interaction between verapamil and almotriptan in healthy volunteers. *Clin Pharmacol Ther* (2000) 67, 498–503.
2. Relpax (Eletriptan hydrobromide). Pfizer Ltd. UK Summary of product characteristics, February 2008.

Triptans; Sumatriptan + Butorphanol

Sumatriptan given by injection appears not to interact with butorphanol nasal spray, but if both drugs are given sequentially by nasal spray a slight reduction in butorphanol exposure might occur.

Clinical evidence, mechanism, importance and management

No pharmacokinetic interactions or change in adverse effects were found to occur when 24 healthy subjects were given a single 1-mg dose of butorphanol tartrate nasal spray and a single 6-mg subcutaneous dose of sumatriptan succinate. It was concluded that concurrent use during acute migraine attacks need not be avoided.[1]

In another study, 19 healthy subjects were given a 1-mg dose of butorphanol nasal spray either one minute or 30 minutes after a 20-mg dose of sumatriptan nasal spray. When butorphanol was given one minute after sumatriptan the AUC and maximum plasma concentration of butorphanol were reduced by about 29% and 38%, respectively. When butorphanol was given 30 minutes after sumatriptan no pharmacokinetic interaction was noted. It was suggested that sumatriptan might cause a transient vasoconstriction of nasal blood vessels, leading to reduced butorphanol absorption. It would therefore seem wise to separate administration to ensure that the full effects of butorphanol are achieved.[2]

1. Srinivas NR, Shyu WC, Upmalis D, Lee JS, Barbhaiya RH. Lack of pharmacokinetic interaction between butorphanol tartrate nasal spray and sumatriptan succinate. *J Clin Pharmacol* (1995) 35, 432–7.
2. Vachharajani NN, Shyu W-C, Nichola PS, Boulton DW. A pharmacokinetic interaction study between butorphanol and sumatriptan nasal sprays in healthy subjects: importance of the timing of butorphanol administration. *Cephalalgia* (2002) 22, 282–7.

Triptans; Sumatriptan + Loxapine

An isolated report describes a woman taking loxapine who developed a severe dystonic reaction when she was given sumatriptan.

Clinical evidence, mechanism, importance and management

A case report describes a woman who was taking loxapine 10 mg twice daily for psychotic target symptoms, benzatropine for the prophylaxis of extrapyramidal effects, carbamazepine for mood stabilisation, and a combination of paracetamol (acetaminophen), caffeine, and butalbital for migraine headaches. Two days after the loxapine dose was raised to 35 mg daily she was given a single 6-mg subcutaneous dose of sumatriptan for a migraine headache. Within 15 minutes she developed torticollis, which was treated with intramuscular benzatropine and intravenous diphenhydramine. The authors of the report suggest that this reaction was possibly caused by the additive dystonic effects of the loxapine and sumatriptan, despite the presence of the benzatropine. Dystonia is not an uncommon extrapyramidal reaction associated with antipsychotics, and neck stiffness and dystonia are recognised adverse effects of sumatriptan, but of low incidence.[1] This seems to be the first and only report of this apparent interaction, and therefore its general significance is unclear.

1. Garcia G, Kaufman MB, Colucci RD. Dystonic reaction associated with sumatriptan. *Ann Pharmacother* (1994) 28, 1199.

Triptans; Sumatriptan + Naproxen

Naproxen does not affect the pharmacokinetics of sumatriptan.

Clinical evidence, mechanism, importance and management

A study in 12 healthy subjects found that a single 500-mg dose of naproxen had no effect on the pharmacokinetics of a single 100-mg oral dose of sumatriptan.[1] A 12-month tolerability study found that a tablet containing both sumatriptan and naproxen was well tolerated for the treatment of acute migraine attacks, and the adverse events did not differ from those expected for the individual components alone.[2] Note that a combination product containing sumatriptan and naproxen is available in the US.

1. Srinivasu P, Rambhau D, Rao BR, Rao YM. Lack of pharmacokinetic interaction between sumatriptan and naproxen. *J Clin Pharmacol* (2000) 40, 99–104.
2. Winner P, Cady RK, Ruoff GE, Frishberg BM, Alexander WJ, Zhang Y, Kori SH, Lener SE. Twelve-month tolerability and safety of sumatriptan-naproxen sodium for the treatment of acute migraine. *Mayo Clin Proc* (2007) 82, 61–8.

Triptans; Zolmitriptan + Cimetidine

Cimetidine slightly increases the exposure to zolmitriptan.

Clinical evidence

In a crossover study, 16 healthy subjects were given cimetidine 400 mg three times a day for 2 days, followed by a single 5-mg dose of zolmitriptan on day 2. When compared with zolmitriptan alone, cimetidine increased the AUC of zolmitriptan by 48%, and increased the maximum plasma concentration and AUC of the active metabolite of zolmitriptan by 50% and 100%, respectively.[1]

Mechanism

Cimetidine is a known weak, non-specific inhibitor of several cytochrome P450 isoenzymes, including CYP1A2, and zolmitriptan is metabolised, in part, by CYP1A2. The increased exposure to zolmitriptan therefore probably occurs as a result of CYP1A2 inhibition by cimetidine.

Importance and management

Evidence for an interaction between cimetidine and zolmitriptan comes from one pharmacokinetic study, which found a slight rise in exposure to zolmitriptan. However, the clinical relevance of this increase is unclear. Increased exposure to zolmitriptan and its active metabolite might increase adverse effects (dizziness, dry mouth, palpitations), with such effects more likely to be more apparent after repeated dosing (when accumulation might occur) rather than one-off use. It might therefore be prudent to be alert for zolmitriptan adverse effects in patients taking cimetidine, decreasing the dose of zolmitriptan if these become troublesome. However, note that the UK manufacturer recommends a maximum dose of zolmitriptan of 5 mg in 24 hours in patients taking cimetidine.[2] In contrast, the US manufacturer makes no recommendation regarding dose in the presence of cimetidine.[3]

1. Dixon R, French S, Kemp J, Sellers M, Yates R. The metabolism of zolmitriptan: effects of an inducer and an inhibitor of cytochrome P450 on its pharmacokinetics in healthy volunteers. *Clin Drug Invest* (1998) 15, 515–22.
2. Zomig Tablets (Zolmitriptan). AstraZeneca UK Ltd. UK Summary of product characteristics, February 2010.
3. Zomig (Zolmitriptan). AstraZeneca Pharmaceuticals LP. US Prescribing information, October 2008.

Triptans; Zolmitriptan + Metoclopramide

Metoclopramide does not affect the pharmacokinetics of zolmitriptan.

Clinical evidence, mechanism, importance and management

In a randomised, crossover study, 15 healthy subjects were given a single 10-mg dose of zolmitriptan, alone or with metoclopramide 10 mg. Metoclopramide had no effect on the pharmacokinetics of zolmitriptan,[1] and therefore no dose adjustments are necessary on concurrent use.

1. Seaber EJ, Ridout G, Layton G, Posner J, Peck RW. The novel anti-migraine compound zolmitriptan (Zomig 311C90) has no clinically significant interactions with paracetamol or metoclopramide. *Eur J Clin Pharmacol* (1997) 53, 229–34.

Triptans; Zolmitriptan + Quinolones

The quinolones are predicted to increase the plasma concentration of zolmitriptan by inhibiting CYP1A2, an enzyme involved in its metabolism.[1] This is based on the known interaction of zolmitriptan with cimetidine (see 'Triptans; Zolmitriptan + Cimetidine', above). The UK manufacturer recommends a maximum dose of zolmitriptan of 5 mg in 24 hours in patients taking a quinolone, such as ciprofloxacin. Note that the quinolones differ in their ability to inhibit CYP1A2; their effects on caffeine might give a useful guide to their potency in this respect, see 'Caffeine + Quinolones', p.1426.

1. Zomig Tablets (Zolmitriptan). AstraZeneca UK Ltd. UK Summary of product characteristics, February 2010.

Triptans; Zolmitriptan + Rifampicin (Rifampin)

Rifampicin increases the metabolism of zolmitriptan.

Clinical evidence

In a crossover study, 14 healthy subjects were given rifampicin 600 mg daily for 8 days, followed by a single 5-mg dose of zolmitriptan on day 8. When compared with the use of zolmitriptan alone, rifampicin reduced the maximum plasma concentration and AUC of zolmitriptan by 15% and 18%, respectively, and reduced the maximum plasma concentration of the active metabolite of zolmitriptan by 11%. The AUC of the active metabolite of zolmitriptan was reduced by 10%, but this was not statistically significant.[1]

Mechanism

Rifampicin is a known inducer of several cytochrome P450 isoenzymes, including CYP3A4, and zolmitriptan is metabolised by CYP3A4. The decrease in the plasma concentration of zolmitriptan therefore probably occur as a result of CYP3A4 induction by rifampicin, but the small changes seen suggest that CYP3A4 is not a major route of zolmitriptan metabolism.

Importance and management

Evidence for an interaction between zolmitriptan and rifampicin comes from one pharmacokinetic study, which suggests that rifampicin causes a small, but probably clinically unimportant, reduction in the plasma concentration of zolmitriptan. Therefore no zolmitriptan dose adjustment is likely to be necessary in patients also taking rifampicin.

1. Dixon R, French S, Kemp J, Sellers M, Yates R. The metabolism of zolmitriptan: effects of an inducer and an inhibitor of cytochrome P450 on its pharmacokinetics in healthy volunteers. *Clin Drug Invest* (1998) 15, 515–22.

Triptans; Zolmitriptan + Xylometazoline

In a clinical study in 18 healthy subjects, the rate and extent of absorption of intranasal zolmitriptan 5 mg was not affected when it was given 30 minutes after xylometazoline nasal spray.[1] This suggests that nasal vasoconstriction does not affect absorption of intranasal zolmitriptan.

1. Nairn K, Kemp JV, Dane AL, Roberts DW, Dixon R. Evaluation of the effect of xylometazoline on the absorption of zolmitriptan nasal spray. *Clin Drug Invest* (2002) 22, 703–7.

17

Antineoplastics

The antineoplastic drugs (some of which are also called cytotoxics or sometimes cytostatics) are used in the treatment of malignant disease, alone or in conjunction with radiotherapy, surgery, or immunosuppressants. They are also used in the treatment of a number of autoimmune disorders such as rheumatoid arthritis and psoriasis, and a few are used with other immunosuppressant drugs (ciclosporin, corticosteroids) to prevent transplant rejection. These other drugs are dealt with under the section on 'Immunosuppressants', p.1203.

Of all the drugs discussed in this publication, many of the antineoplastic drugs are amongst the most toxic, being commonly used at maximum tolerated doses and thereby having a narrow therapeutic index. This means that quite small increases in their concentrations can lead to the development of serious and life-threatening toxicity. A list of the antineoplastics and other drugs that are used in the treatment of malignancy that are featured in this section appear in 'Table 17.1', p.652, grouped by their primary mechanism of action. This table also includes a number of hormone antagonists that are used in the treatment of cancer.

Unlike most of the other interaction monographs in this publication, some of the information on the antineoplastic drugs is derived from *animal* experiments and *in vitro* studies, so confirmation of their clinical relevance is still needed. The reason for including these data is that the antineoplastic drugs as a group do not lend themselves readily to the kind of clinical studies that can be undertaken with many other drugs, and there would seem to be justification for including indirect evidence of this kind. The aim is not to make definite predictions, but to warn users of the interaction possibilities.

Antineoplastic interactions

(a) Protein kinase inhibitors

Most of the available protein kinase inhibitors are **tyrosine kinase inhibitors**. Nevertheless, they differ in the specific tyrosine kinases they inactivate and are therefore indicated for different neoplasms (for example, those inhibiting BCR-ABL, such as dasatinib, are used for chronic myeloid leukaemia; and lapatinib, which inhibits EGFR and HERs, is used for breast cancer). Ruxolitinib and tofacitinib (both inhibitors of Janus tyrosine kinase) are not indicated for neoplasms: ruxolitinib is indicated for myelofibrosis, and tofacitinib, like methotrexate, is used as a disease-modifying antirheumatic drug in the treatment of rheumatoid arthritis. Despite these differences, the tyrosine kinase inhibitors share many drug interactions. For example, all of them are substrates of CYP3A4 and interact with inhibitors and inducers of this isoenzyme. Some also inhibit CYP3A4 and other isoenzymes, such as CYP2D6 and CYP2C8. In addition, the absorption of many tyrosine kinase inhibitors is affected by antacids and other drugs that affect gastric pH, such as H_2-receptor antagonists and proton pump inhibitors.

(b) Topoisomerase inhibitors

Irinotecan is metabolised by carboxylesterases to its active metabolite, SN-38. SN-38 then inactivated by glucuronidation (via UGT1A1). Irinotecan is also partly metabolised by CYP3A4 and possibly by CYP3A5. Therefore, pharmacokinetic interactions occur with irinotecan when it is given with drugs that inhibit or induce CYP3A or UGT1A1.

Table 17.1 Antineoplastics and other drugs used in the treatment of cancer

Action	*Drugs*
Alkylating agents, and drugs that appear to have an alkylating action	
Nitrosoureas	Carmustine, Lomustine, Streptozocin
Platinum compounds	Carboplatin, Cisplatin, Oxaliplatin
Others	Altretamine, Bendamustine, Busulfan, Chlorambucil, Chlormethine (Mechlorethamine), Cyclophosphamide, Dacarbazine, Estramustine, Ifosfamide, Melphalan, Temozolomide, Thiotepa
Antimetabolites	
Folate antagonists	Methotrexate, Pemetrexed, Raltitrexed
Podophylotoxin derivatives	Etoposide, Teniposide
Purine analogues	Azathioprine, Cladribine, Clofarabine, Fludarabine, Mercaptopurine, Nelarabine, Tioguanine
Pyrimidine analogues	Capecitabine, Carmofur, Cytarabine, Fluorouracil, Gemcitabine, Tegafur
Mitotic inhibitors	
Taxanes	Cabazitaxel, Docetaxel, Paclitaxel
Topoisomerase I inhibitors	Irinotecan, Topotecan
Vinca alkaloids	Vinblastine, Vincristine, Vindesine, Vinflunine, Vinorelbine
Cytotoxic antibiotics	
Anthracyclines	Aclarubicin, Amrubicin, Daunorubicin, Doxorubicin, Epirubicin, Idarubicin, Mitoxantrone, Pixantrone
Others	Bleomycin, Dactinomycin, Mitomycin
Anti-androgens	Bicalutamide, Enzalutamide, Flutamide, Nilutamide
Anti-oestrogens	
Aromatase inhibitors	Aminoglutethimide, Anastrozole, Exemestane, Formestane, Letrozole
Oestrogen-receptor antagonists	Fulvestrant, Tamoxifen, Toremifene
Tyrosine kinase inhibitors	Axitinib, Bosutinib, Cabozantinib, Crizotinib, Dasatinib, Erlotinib, Gefitinib, Imatinib, Lapatinib, Nilotinib, Pazopanib, Ponatinib, Regorafenib, Ruxolitinib, Sorafenib†, Sunitinib, Tofacitinib, Vandetanib
Monoclonal antibodies	Alemtuzumab, Bevacizumab, Brentuximab Vedotin, Cetuximab, Panitumumab, Rituximab, Trastuzumab
Photosensitisers	5-Aminolevulinic acid, Porfimer sodium, Temoporfin
Miscellaneous	Amsacrine, Asparaginase (Colaspase, Crisantaspase, Pegaspargase), Bexarotene, Bortezomib, Enzastaurin, Hydroxycarbamide, Lenalidomide, Mifamurtide, Mitotane, Pentostatin, Pomalidomide, Procarbazine, Thalidomide, Tipifarnib, Trabectedin, Tretinoin, Vorinostat

† Inhibits other protein kinases in addition to tyrosine kinases.

Alemtuzumab + Miscellaneous

Six infection-related deaths occurred in a study of consolidation therapy with alemtuzumab after induction therapy with fludarabine and rituximab. After alemtuzumab, at least 12 months should elapse before live vaccines are given.

Clinical evidence, mechanism, importance and management

(a) Fludarabine with Rituximab

In a clinical study in patients with chronic lymphocytic leukaemia, there were six infection-related deaths out of 51 patients given consolidation alemtuzumab therapy after an induction regimen of **fludarabine** and **rituximab**.[1,2] In this study, patients received up to 6 cycles of intravenous fludarabine 25 mg/m^2 with intravenous rituximab (escalated to 375 mg/m^2) daily for 5 days every 4 weeks. Four months after their last dose of fludarabine, patients with a complete response or stable disease started subcutaneous alemtuzumab (escalated to 30 mg) three times weekly for 6 weeks. Of the six patients who died, five had achieved a complete remission after induction therapy. The infections occurred both during the use of alemtuzumab and for up to 16 months afterwards. The study was subsequently amended to restrict the use of alemtuzumab to those with a partial response to **fludarabine** and **rituximab**, with close monitoring for infection.

It is thought that the immunosuppressive properties of these drugs were additive, and that there was insufficient time allowed before alemtuzumab was given for recovery from immunosuppression from the induction therapy.[1] Note that this use of alemtuzumab is outside the current licensed indications, and this combination should not be given to patients outside the context of a clinical study.[1,2]

(b) Vaccines, live

The manufacturer advises that vaccination with live viral vaccines should not be undertaken within at least 12 months of the use of alemtuzumab, although there are no specific data on this.[3]

1. Bayer HealthCare. Important safety information. Six infection-related deaths reported after treatment with MabCampath® (alemtuzumab) following fludarabine+rituximab induction in patients with B-Cell chronic lymphocytic leukaemia (CLL). Letter to Healthcare Professionals, February 2008.
2. Lin TS, Donohue KA, Lucas MS, Byrd JC, Bengtson EM, Peterson BL, Larson RA (Cancer and Leukemia Group B USA). Consolidation therapy with subcutaneous (SC) alemtuzumab results in severe infectious toxicity in previously untreated CLL patients who achieve a complete response (CR) after fludarabine and rituximab (FR) induction therapy: interim safety analysis of the CALGB study 10101. *Blood* (2007) 110, abstract 755.
3. MabCampath (Alemtuzumab). Genzyme Therapeutics. UK Summary of product characteristics, December 2008.

Altretamine (Hexamethylmelamine) + Antidepressants

Severe orthostatic hypotension has been described in patients given altretamine with either phenelzine, amitriptyline or imipramine.

Clinical evidence, mechanism, importance and management

Four patients experienced very severe orthostatic hypotension (described by the authors as potentially life-threatening) when they were given altretamine 150 to 250 mg/m^2 with either **phenelzine** 60 mg daily, **amitriptyline** 50 mg daily or **imipramine** 50 to 150 mg daily.[1] They experienced incapacitating dizziness, severe lightheadedness, and/or fainting within a few days of taking both drugs. Standing blood pressures as low as 50/30 mmHg and 60/40 mmHg were recorded. The reasons for this hypotensive effect are not known. One of the patients had no problems when **imipramine** was replaced by **nortriptyline** 50 mg daily. One other patient who had also taken altretamine with antidepressants reported dizziness, while another noted non-specific discomfort. The incidence of this interaction is unknown, but it is clear that the concurrent use of altretamine and **tricyclics** or **MAOIs** should be closely monitored.

1. Bruckner HW, Schleifer SJ. Orthostatic hypotension as a complication of hexamethylmelamine antidepressant interaction. *Cancer Treat Rep* (1983) 67, 516.

Altretamine (Hexamethylmelamine) + Pyridoxine (Vitamin B_6)

Pyridoxine reduced the neurotoxicity associated with altretamine, but also reduced its effectiveness.

Clinical evidence, mechanism, importance and management

In a large randomised study in women with advanced ovarian cancer the neurotoxicity associated with altretamine and cisplatin chemotherapy was reduced by pyridoxine, but the response duration was also reduced.[1] In this study, cisplatin was given on day 1 (37.5 or 75 mg/m^2) and altretamine 200 mg/m^2 daily was given on days 8 to 21, and half the patients also received pyridoxine 100 mg three times daily on days 1 to 21. It is unclear how pyridoxine reduced the activity of this regimen, but the use of pyridoxine should probably be avoided in patients receiving altretamine.

1. Wiernik PH, Yeap B, Vogel SE, Kaplan BH, Comis RL, Falkson G, Davis TE, Fazzini E, Cheuvart B, Horton J. Hexamethylmelamine and low or moderate dose cisplatin with or without pyridoxine for treatment of advanced ovarian carcinoma: a study of the Eastern Cooperative Oncology Group. *Cancer Invest* (1992) 10, 1–9.

5-Aminolevulinic acid + St John's wort (*Hypericum perforatum*)

An isolated case report describes a severe phototoxic reaction attributed to a synergistic effect of oral 5-aminolevulinic acid and St John's wort.

Clinical evidence

A 47-year-old woman who was taking St John's wort (*Hyperiforce*, dose not stated) experienced a phototoxic reaction on skin areas exposed to light 6 hours after receiving oral 5-aminolevulinic acid 40 mg/kg. She developed a burning erythematous rash and severe swelling of the face, neck and hands. Treatment with oral corticosteroids resulted in complete resolution after skin desquamation.[1]

Mechanism

It was suggested that there was a synergistic photosensitivity reaction between the two drugs.

Importance and management

This appears to be the only report of such an effect, but bear it in mind in the event of an unexpected adverse reaction to oral 5-aminolevulinic acid. Note that this photosensitiser and its derivative methyl aminolevulinate are more usually applied topically, and in this situation, any interaction is unlikely to be important.

1. Ladner DP, Klein SD, Steiner RA, Walt H. Synergistic toxicity of <delta>-aminolaevulinic acid-induced protoporphyrin IX used for photodiagnosis and hypericum extract, a herbal antidepressant. *Br J Dermatol* (2001) 144, 901–22.

Anthracyclines + Ciclosporin

High-dose ciclosporin increases the serum levels and the myelotoxicity of doxorubicin. An isolated report describes severe neurotoxicity and coma in a patient who had taken ciclosporin and was subsequently given doxorubicin. Ciclosporin can also increase the levels of daunorubicin, epirubicin, idarubicin and mitoxantrone.

Clinical evidence

(a) Daunorubicin

In a randomised study in patients receiving daunorubicin, ciclosporin significantly reduced the frequency of resistance to induction therapy (31% versus 47%) and increased relapse-free and overall survival. Ciclosporin recipients had higher steady-state serum levels of daunorubicin and its active metabolite, daunorubicinol.[1]

(b) Doxorubicin

Eight patients with small cell lung cancer were given an initial course of doxorubicin (25 to 70 mg/m^2 over one hour) and a subsequent ciclosporin-modulated doxorubicin course (ciclosporin 6 mg/kg bolus, then 16 mg/kg daily for 2 days) for multidrug-resistant tumour modulation. All of the patients were also given cyclophosphamide and vincristine. Ciclosporin increased the AUC of doxorubicin by 48%, and increased the AUC of its active metabolite, doxorubicinol, by 443%. The myelotoxicity was increased by concurrent use: the leucocyte count fell by 84% after doxorubicin and by 91% after doxorubicin with ciclosporin, and the platelet counts fell by 36% and 73%, respectively. The patients had significant weight loss and severe myalgias.[2]

Three preliminary phase I studies[3-5] are consistent with this report. In these studies, ciclosporin was found to increase the doxorubicin AUC by 40 to 73%, and the doxorubicinol AUC by 250 to 285%. However, no evidence of increased cardiotoxicity was found in a study of 23 patients given ciclosporin and doxorubicin.[6]

A heart transplant patient was given ciclosporin 2 mg/kg daily for 22 months. The ciclosporin was stopped and he was given doxorubicin 60 mg, vincristine 2 mg, cyclophosphamide 600 mg and prednisone 80 mg to treat Burkitt's lymphoma stage IVB. Eight hours later he developed disturbances of consciousness, which lead to stage I coma, from which he spontaneously recovered 12 hours later. A week later a similar course of chemotherapy was started, and 10 to 15 minutes later he lost consciousness and generalised tonic clonic seizures progressively developed. He died 8 days later without recovering consciousness.[7]

(c) Epirubicin

Preliminary evidence suggests that ciclosporin can markedly increase the AUC of epirubicin (up to about fourfold) and increase bone marrow suppression in response to epirubicin.[5] In one study in 20 patients ciclosporin did not increase the cardiotoxicity of epirubicin .[6]

(d) Idarubicin

In 9 patients the concurrent use of ciclosporin and idarubicin increased the AUC of idarubicin and its active metabolite, idarubicinol, by 77% and 181%, respectively, when compared with 11 patients receiving idarubicin alone.[8] Unacceptable toxicity occurred when idarubicin 9 or 12 mg/m^2 daily was given with ciclosporin 16 mg/kg daily, when compared with idarubicin 12 mg/m^2 alone: 3 of 7 patients given the combination died. Increases in the AUC of idarubicin and idarubicinol produced by ciclosporin have also been reported elsewhere.[9]

(e) Mitoxantrone

The pharmacokinetics of mitoxantrone 10 mg/m^2 daily were compared with mitoxantrone 6 mg/m^2 (a 40% reduction in dose) with high-dose ciclosporin in children.

The ciclosporin recipients had a 42% reduction in mitoxantrone clearance, a 12% increase in mitoxantrone AUC, and similar toxicity.[10]

Mechanism

Uncertain. One reason may be that ciclosporin affects P-glycoprotein in the biliary tract so that the clearance of these anthracyclines in the bile is reduced. An additional reason may be that ciclosporin inhibits the metabolism of anthracycline metabolites, such as doxorubicinol, so that they accumulate.[2] The increased levels of both would explain the increases in toxicity. It is not clear why such severe neurotoxicity was seen in one patient.

Importance and management

An established and clinically important interaction. Ciclosporin alters the pharmacokinetics of the anthracyclines resulting in increased levels. This pharmacokinetic interaction has complicated study into the value of using ciclosporin to modulate multidrug resistance in tumours and thereby improve the response to chemotherapy. In the case of anthracyclines any benefit could simply be attributed to dose intensification. Consequently, some have suggested reducing the dose of the anthracycline.[10] The use of high-dose ciclosporin for multidrug-resistant tumour modulation remains experimental and should only be used in clinical studies. Concurrent use should be very well monitored. More study is needed to find out the possible effects of low-dose ciclosporin.

1. List AF, Kopecky KL, Willman CL, Head DR, Persons DL, Slovak ML, Dorr R, Karanes C, Hynes HE, Doroshow JH, Shurafa M, Appelbaum FR. Benefit of cyclosporine modulation of drug resistance in patients with poor-risk acute myeloid leukemia: a Southwest Oncology Group study. *Blood* (2001) 98, 3212–20.
2. Rushing DA, Raber SR, Rodvold KA, Piscitelli SC, Plank GS, Tewksbury DA. The effects of cyclosporine on the pharmacokinetics of doxorubicin in patients with small cell lung cancer. *Cancer* (1994) 74, 834–41.
3. Scheulen ME, Budach W, Skorzec M, Wiefelspütz JK, Seeber S. Influence of cyclosporin A on the pharmacokinetics and pharmacodynamics of doxorubicin. *Proc Am Assoc Cancer Res* (1993) 34, 213.
4. Bartlett NL, Lum BL, Fisher GA, Brophy NA, Ehsan MN, Halsey J, Sikic BI. Phase I trial of doxorubicin with cyclosporine as a modulator of multidrug resistance. *J Clin Oncol* (1994) 12, 835–42.
5. Eggert J, Scheulen ME, Schütte J, Budach W, Annweiler HM, Mengelkolch B, Skorzec M, Wiefelspütz J, Sack H, Seeber S. Influence of cyclosporin A on the pharmacokinetics and pharmacodynamics of doxorubicin and epirubicin. *Ann Hematol* (1994) 68, A26.
6. Eising EG, Gries P, Eggert J, Scheulen ME. Does the multi-drug resistance modulator cyclosporin A increase the cardiotoxicity of high-dose anthracycline chemotherapy. *Acta Oncol* (1997) 36, 735–40.
7. Barbui T, Rambaldi A, Parenzan L, Zucchelli M, Perico N, Remuzzi G. Neurological symptoms and coma associated with doxorubicin administration during chronic cyclosporin therapy. *Lancet* (1992) 339, 1421.
8. Pea F, Damiani D, Michieli M, Ermacora A, Baraldo M, Russo D, Fanin R, Baccarani M, Furlanut M. Multidrug resistance modulation in vivo: the effect of cyclosporin A alone or with dexverapamil on idarubicin pharmacokinetics in acute leukemia. *Eur J Clin Pharmacol* (1999) 55, 361–8.
9. Smeets M, Raymakers R, Muus P, Vierwinden G, Linssen P, Masereeuw R, de Witte T. Cyclosporin increases cellular idarubicin and idarubicinol concentrations in relapsed or refractory AML mainly due to reduced systemic clearance. *Leukemia* (2001) 15, 80–8.
10. Lacayo NJ, Lum BL, Becton DL, Weinstein H, Ravindranath Y, Chang MN, Bomgaars L, Lauer SJ, Sikic BI. Pharmacokinetic interactions of cyclosporine with etoposide and mitoxantrone in children with acute myeloid leukemia. *Leukemia* (2002) 16, 920–7.

Anthracyclines + Taxanes

Toxicity associated with combinations of paclitaxel with doxorubicin or epirubicin depends on the order of administration. Some modest pharmacokinetic changes may occur when paclitaxel and epirubicin are given together. The combination of doxorubicin and paclitaxel is more cardiotoxic than doxorubicin alone: paclitaxel increases doxorubicin levels but doxorubicin does not alter paclitaxel levels. Docetaxel may modestly affect the pharmacokinetics of epirubicin and doxorubicin.

Clinical evidence

(a) Doxorubicin

1. Docetaxel. The pharmacokinetics of doxorubicin 50 mg/m^2, given as a 30-minute infusion, were unaffected when it was given immediately before or one hour before a one-hour infusion of docetaxel 75 mg/m^2 when compared with administration alone. However, the AUC of docetaxel was increased, both when given immediately before and one hour after doxorubicin, by 50% and 75%, respectively.[1] A retrospective review of patients who were given doxorubicin followed one hour later by docetaxel found that the clearance of docetaxel was about 20% lower than in patients who had received docetaxel alone, whereas the clearance of doxorubicin did not differ when given with docetaxel.[2]

In a study, 627 patients with breast cancer were given doxorubicin 50 mg/m^2 with docetaxel 75 mg/m^2, or doxorubicin 60 mg/m^2 with cyclophosphamide 600 mg/m^2, postoperatively for 4 courses to assess disease-free survival at 5 years. The study was terminated prematurely because of the high risk of life-threatening complications in the patients given doxorubicin with docetaxel (2 deaths associated with drug toxicity and one case of perforated peritonitis in a patient with febrile neutropenia). The incidence of febrile neutropenia was 41% and 7% in the doxorubicin with docetaxel, and doxorubicin with cyclophosphamide groups, respectively.[3]

A woman with recurrence of breast cancer developed pseudomembranous colitis (non-*Clostridium difficile*) and cholestatic jaundice 6 days after completing her first cycle of treatment with doxorubicin and docetaxel and again 4 days after the second cycle, about one month later.[4]

2. Paclitaxel. Early studies in patients with breast cancer found a higher frequency of toxicity (particularly mucositis) when paclitaxel was given immediately before doxorubicin (given as 24-hour and 48-hour infusions, respectively) rather than the other way around.[5] A subsequent study with similar effects revealed that doxorubicin clearance was reduced by one-third if paclitaxel was given first.[6] In another study the peak plasma levels of doxorubicin were increased when it was given by bolus injection 15 minutes after a 3-hour infusion of paclitaxel rather than the other way around. The effect was non-linear and dependent on the dose of paclitaxel.[7] The same authors had already found that this regimen produced a higher than expected incidence of cardiac toxicity, which was not affected by sequence with the short interval between administration.[8] Subsequent studies[9,10] have found that this schedule results in unacceptable cardiotoxicity when the total cumulative doxorubicin dose exceeds 340 to 380 mg/m^2. When a bolus dose of doxorubicin was given 15 or 30 minutes before a 3-hour infusion of paclitaxel, the levels of doxorubicin were higher than when the interval was 24 hours.[7,11] Moreover, when paclitaxel and doxorubicin were given together as a 3-hour infusion the levels of doxorubicin were lower than when a bolus dose of doxorubicin was given 15 minutes before a 3-hour paclitaxel infusion.[7] Similarly, in another study, the pharmacokinetics of each drug were found to be unchanged when they were given simultaneously as a 72-hour infusion.[12]

(b) Doxorubicin, liposomal

In 10 patients the AUC of intravenous pegylated liposomal doxorubicin (*Caelyx*) 30 to 35 mg/m^2 was increased by a mean of 80% when it was given immediately before intravenous **paclitaxel** 70 or 175 mg/m^2 compared with when it was given alone. Peak plasma levels of doxorubicin were also increased and clearance was reduced by 71%. In 9 other patients given *Caelyx* then **docetaxel** 30 or 60 mg/m^2, the AUC of doxorubicin was increased by 12% and clearance reduced by only 16%.[13]

(c) Epirubicin

The pharmacokinetics of epirubicin were compared in 4 patients with breast cancer given intravenous epirubicin 90 mg/m^2 alone and in 16 patients given the same dose of epirubicin followed immediately by either **paclitaxel** 175 mg/m^2 as a 3-hour infusion or **docetaxel** 70 mg/m^2 as a one-hour infusion. No effect on epirubicin levels was detected, but the concentrations of epirubicin metabolites (epirubicinol and deoxydoxorubicinone) were increased by both **paclitaxel** and **docetaxel**.[14] In a subsequent study, 21 patients were given the same regimen of epirubicin followed immediately by **paclitaxel** and 18 patients were given the drugs in the reverse order. Non-haematological toxicity was unaffected by the order of administration, but when **paclitaxel** was given first the neutrophil and platelet nadir was lower and neutrophil recovery was slower. The AUC for epirubicin was also higher when **paclitaxel** was given first, but the pharmacokinetics of **paclitaxel** were unaffected.[15]

In one study, 21 women with breast cancer were given intravenous epirubicin 90 mg/m^2 followed 15 minutes later by a 3-hour intravenous infusion of **paclitaxel** 175 mg/m^2 (6 patients), 200 mg/m^2 (9 patients), or 225 mg/m^2 (6 patients). Six women were given **paclitaxel** 200 mg/m^2 30 hours after epirubicin. A significant increase in the AUC of epirubicin occurred with **paclitaxel** 200 mg/m^2 (23%) and 225 mg/m^2 (34%) and increases in the AUC of the metabolite of epirubicin (epirubicinol) occurred at all dose levels of **paclitaxel**, compared with those found when epirubicin was given 30 hours before **paclitaxel**.[16] In another study, exposure to epirubicin metabolites, but not epirubicin itself, was increased when it was given 15 minutes before a 3-hour infusion of **paclitaxel**, when compared with a regimen using a 24-hour interval between the two drugs. In addition, the neutrophil nadir was lower, and the clearance of **paclitaxel** was 30% slower with the former regimen, but cardiac toxicity was uncommon.[17]

Conversely, a study of the concurrent use of **docetaxel** and epirubicin did not find that the sequence of drug administration affected the pharmacokinetics of epirubicin, nor was there any difference in toxicity.[18] In another study, 16 patients with breast cancer had a transient but significant increase in epirubicin plasma levels during the subsequent infusion (after an interval of one hour) of **docetaxel** 75 mg/m^2, which was not seen if the **docetaxel** was given within 10 minutes of epirubicin.[19] A study in 43 patients who received **docetaxel**, cyclophosphamide and epirubicin found an increase in the plasma levels of epirubicinol, but this was only seen during the **docetaxel** infusion, after which levels returned to normal. The pharmacokinetics of **docetaxel** were not significantly different from historical data on its use alone.[20]

Mechanism

Studies in *mice* have found that the taxanes docetaxel and paclitaxel, and the vehicle used for paclitaxel, *Cremophor*, may all modify the distribution and metabolism of doxorubicin increasing its levels in the heart, liver and kidneys. This may contribute to the cardiac toxicity seen during use with paclitaxel.[21] Similarly, *in vitro* studies in human myocardial tissue found that paclitaxel and docetaxel increased the conversion of doxorubicin to doxorubicinol, the metabolite that is thought to be responsible for cardiotoxicity.[22] An *in vitro* study on the effect of paclitaxel and *Cremophor* on epirubicin metabolism in human blood found that paclitaxel slightly decreased the production of epirubicinol. A marked inhibition of epirubicinol production occurred in the presence of *Cremophor*, but because of the low volume of distribution of *Cremophor* this is not likely to be of clinical significance.[16] In addition, *in vitro* studies have shown that the taxanes may reduce the biliary excretion of doxorubicin and epirubicin by inhibiting P-glycoprotein,[7] and inhibition of epirubicinol excretion via competition for P-glycoprotein by paclitaxel and *Cremophor* may be significant.[16]

The case of pseudomembranous colitis and cholestatic jaundice in one patient was attributed to the combination of docetaxel and doxorubicin, but the patient was also receiving long-term treatment with erythromycin and omeprazole which may have contributed to the interaction by inhibiting docetaxel metabolism by the cytochrome P450 isoenzyme CYP3A.[4]

Importance and management

The effect of paclitaxel on doxorubicin appears to be established, and various strategies have been suggested to reduce the cardiotoxicity of this combination. These include giving doxorubicin at least 24 hours before paclitaxel; reducing the cumulative dose of doxorubicin; or adding the cytoprotective drug dexrazoxane.[23] Epirubicin is considered less cardiotoxic than doxorubicin, and may be an alternative in some situations. However, it still appears preferable to give the anthracycline before the taxane. Docetaxel appears to have little clinically relevant effect on doxorubicin or epirubicin pharmacokinetics, but doxorubicin might increase docetaxel levels. Further study is needed on the optimum scheduling of anthracyclines and taxanes to maximise efficacy and minimise toxicity.

1. D'Incalci M, Schüller J, Colombo T, Zucchetti M, Riva A. Taxoids in combination with anthracyclines and other agents: pharmacokinetic considerations. *Semin Oncol* (1998) 25 (Suppl 13), 16–20.
2. Rudek MA, Sparreboom A, Garrett-Mayer ES, Armstrong DK, Wolff AC, Verweij J, Baker SD. Factors affecting pharmacokinetic variability following doxorubicin and docetaxel-based therapy. *Eur J Cancer* (2004) 40, 1170–8.
3. Brain EGC, Bachelot T, Serin D, Kirscher S, Graic Y, Eymard J-C, Extra J-M, Combe M, Fourme E, Nogues C, Rouëssé J, RAPP-01 Trial Investigators. Life-threatening sepsis associated with adjuvant doxorubicin plus docetaxel for intermediate-risk breast cancer. *JAMA* (2005) 293, 2367–71.
4. Sundar S, Chan SY. Cholestatic jaundice and pseudomembranous colitis following combination therapy with doxorubicin and docetaxel. *Anticancer Drugs* (2003) 14, 327–9.
5. Sledge GW, Robert N, Sparano JA, Cogleigh M, Goldstein LJ, Neuberg D, Rowinsky E, Baughman C, McCaskill-Stevens W. Eastern Cooperative Oncology Group studies of paclitaxel and doxorubicin in advanced breast cancer. *Semin Oncol* (1995) 22, 105–8.
6. Holmes FA, Madden T, Newman RA, Valero V, Theriault RL, Fraschini G, Walters RS, Booser DJ, Buzdar AU, Willey J, Hortobagyi GN. Sequence-dependent alteration of doxorubicin pharmacokinetics by paclitaxel in a phase I study of paclitaxel and doxorubicin in patients with metastatic breast cancer. *J Clin Oncol* (1996) 14, 2713–21.
7. Gianni L, Viganò L, Locatelli A, Capri G, Giani A, Tarenzi E, Bonadonna G. Human pharmacokinetic characterization and in vitro study of the interaction between doxorubicin and paclitaxel in patients with breast cancer. *J Clin Oncol* (1997) 15, 1906–15.
8. Gianni L, Munzone E, Capri G, Fulfaro F, Tarenzi E, Villani F, Spreafico C, Laffranchi A, Caraceni A, Martini C, Stefanelli M, Valagussa P, Bonadonna G. Paclitaxel by 3-hour infusion in combination with bolus doxorubicin in women with untreated metastatic breast cancer: high antitumor efficacy and cardiac effects in a dose-finding and sequence-finding study. *J Clin Oncol* (1995) 13, 2688–99.
9. Gianni L, Dombernowsky P, Sledge G, Martin M, Amadori D, Arbuck SG, Ravdin P, Brown M, Messina M, Tuck D, Weil C, Winograd B. Cardiac function following combination therapy with paclitaxel and doxorubicin: an analysis of 657 women with advanced breast cancer. *Ann Oncol* (2001) 12, 1067–73.
10. Giordano SH, Booser DJ, Murray JL, Ibrahim NK, Rahman ZU, Valero V, Theriault RL, Rosales MF, Rivera E, Frye D, Ewer M, Ordonez NG, Buzdar AU, Hortobagyi GN. A detailed evaluation of cardiac toxicity: a phase II study of doxorubicin and one- or three-hour-infusion paclitaxel in patients with metastatic breast cancer. *Clin Cancer Res* (2002) 8, 3360–8.
11. Moreira A, Lobato R, Morais J, Silva S, Ribeiro J, Figueira A, Vale D, Sousa C, Araújo F, Fernandes A, Oliveira J, Passos-Coelho JL. Influence of the interval between the administration of doxorubicin and paclitaxel on the pharmacokinetics of these drugs in patients with locally advanced breast cancer. *Cancer Chemother Pharmacol* (2001) 48, 333–7.
12. Berg SL, Cowan KH, Balis FM, Fisherman JS, Denicoff AM, Hillig M, Poplack DG, O'Shaughnessy JA. Pharmacokinetics of Taxol and doxorubicin administered alone and in combination by continuous 72-hour infusion. *J Natl Cancer Inst* (1994) 86, 143–5.
13. Briasoulis E, Karavasilis V, Tzamakou E, Rammou D, Soulti K, Piperidou C, Pavlidis N. Interaction pharmacokinetics of pegylated liposomal doxorubicin (Caelyx) on coadministration with paclitaxel or docetaxel. *Cancer Chemother Pharmacol* (2004) 53, 452–7.
14. Esposito M, Venturini M, Vannozzi MO, Tolino G, Lunardi G, Garrone O, Angiolini C, Viale M, Bergaglio M, Del Mastro L, Rosso R. Comparative effects of paclitaxel and docetaxel on the metabolism and pharmacokinetics of epirubicin in breast cancer patients. *J Clin Oncol* (1999) 17, 1132–40.
15. Venturini M, Lunardi G, Del Mastro L, Vannozzi MO, Tolino G, Numico G, Viale M, Pastrone I, Angiolini C, Bertelli G, Straneo M, Rosso R, Esposito M. Sequence effect of epirubicin and paclitaxel treatment on pharmacokinetics and toxicity. *J Clin Oncol* (2000) 18, 2116–25.
16. Danesi R, Innocenti F, Fogli S, Gennari A, Baldini E, Di Paolo A, Salvadori B, Bocci G, Conte PF, Del Tacca M. Pharmacokinetics and pharmacodynamics of combination chemotherapy with paclitaxel and epirubicin in breast cancer patients. *Br J Clin Pharmacol* (2002) 53, 508–18.
17. Grasselli G, Viganò L, Capri G, Locatelli A, Tarenzi E, Spreafico C, Bertuzzi A, Giani A, Materazzo C, Cresta S, Perotti A, Valagussa P, Gianni L. Clinical and pharmacologic study of the epirubicin and paclitaxel combination in women with metastatic breast cancer. *J Clin Oncol* (2001) 19, 2222–31.
18. Lunardi G, Venturini M, Vannozzi MO, Tolino G, Del Mastro L, Bighin C, Schettini G, Esposito M. Influence of alternate sequences of epirubicin and docetaxel on the pharmacokinetic behaviour of both drugs in advanced breast cancer. *Ann Oncol* (2002) 13, 280–5.
19. Ceruti M, Tagini V, Recalenda V, Arpicco S, Cattel L, Airoldi M, Bumma C. Docetaxel in combination with epirubicin in metastatic breast cancer: pharmacokinetic interactions. *Farmaco* (1999) 54, 733–9.
20. Rischin D, Ackland SP, Smith J, Garg MB, Clarke S, Millward MJ, Toner GC, Zalcberg J. Phase I and pharmacokinetic study of docetaxel in combination with epirubicin and cyclophosphamide in advanced cancer: dose escalation possible with granulocyte colony-stimulating factor, but not with prophylactic antibiotics. *Ann Oncol* (2002) 13, 1810–18.
21. Colombo T, Parisi I, Zucchetti M, Sessa C, Goldhirsch A, D'Incalci M. Pharmacokinetic interactions of paclitaxel, docetaxel and their vehicles with doxorubicin. *Ann Oncol* (1999) 10, 391–5.
22. Minotti G, Saponiero A, Licata S, Menna P, Calafiore AM, Teodori G, Gianni L. Paclitaxel and docetaxel enhance the metabolism of doxorubicin to toxic species in human myocardium. *Clin Cancer Res* (2001) 7, 1511–15.
23. Sparano JA. Use of dexrazoxane and other strategies to prevent cardiomyopathy associated with doxorubicin-taxane combinations. *Semin Oncol* (1998) 25 (Suppl 10), 66–71.

Anthracyclines; Aclarubicin + Other antineoplastics

Myelosuppression is among the adverse effects of aclarubicin. The concurrent use of other drugs with similar myelosuppressant actions may be expected to have additive effects. Previous treatment with nitrosoureas (not specifically named) or mitomycin has been shown to increase the severity of the myelosuppression.[1,2]

1. Van Echo DA, Whitacre MY, Aisner J, Applefeld MM, Wiernik PH. Phase I trial of aclacinomycin A. *Cancer Treat Rep* (1982) 66, 1127–32.
2. Bedikian AY, Karlin D, Stroehlein J, Valdivieso M, Korinek J, Bodey G. Phase II evaluation of aclacinomycin A (ACM-A, NSC208734) in patients with metastatic colorectal cancer. *Am J Clin Oncol* (1983) 6, 187–90.

Anthracyclines; Daunorubicin + HIV-protease inhibitors

The pharmacokinetics of liposomal daunorubicin did not appear to be affected by ritonavir- or indinavir-based antiretroviral regimens.

Clinical evidence, mechanism, importance and management

In a study of the effects of the HIV-protease inhibitors **ritonavir** or **indinavir** on the pharmacokinetics of liposomal daunorubicin 40 mg/m^2 twice weekly in patients with Kaposi's sarcoma, the AUC of daunorubicin and its active metabolite, daunorubicinol, did not differ between 6 patients taking a **ritonavir**-based regimen or 9 patients taking an **indinavir**-based regimen, when compared with 6 other patients not taking a HIV-protease inhibitor. In patients for whom data were available before starting the HIV-protease inhibitor, the daunorubicin AUC was unchanged by **indinavir** in 3 patients, but was reduced by 30% after starting the **ritonavir** in 2 patients. The antiretroviral regimens used were **indinavir** 800 mg three times daily plus dual NRTIs or **ritonavir** 400 mg or 600 mg twice daily plus NRTIs. The HIV-protease inhibitors had been taken for at least a month before the pharmacokinetics of daunorubicin were assessed. The potential impact of daunorubicin on the pharmacokinetics of the antiretrovirals was not assessed. Two patients in this study were taking **saquinavir boosted with ritonavir** 400/400 mg three times daily with the same schedule of liposomal daunorubicin, however the number of patients was considered too small to draw any conclusions about a possible interaction.[1]

These data suggest that indinavir and ritonavir do not alter the pharmacokinetics of liposomal daunorubicin to a clinically relevant extent, and therefore no daunorubicin dose adjustment is needed on concurrent use.

For mention that HIV-protease inhibitor regimens have been associated with an increased risk of infection when used with various antineoplastic regimens containing cyclophosphamide, see 'Antineoplastics; Cyclophosphamide + HIV-protease inhibitors', p.659.

1. Fumagalli L, Zucchetti M, Parisi I, Grazia Viganò M, Zecca B, Careddu A, D'Incalci M, Lazzarin A. The pharmacokinetics of liposomal encapsulated daunorubicin are not modified by HAART in patients with HIV-associated Kaposi's sarcoma. *Cancer Chemother Pharmacol* (2000) 45, 495–501.

Anthracyclines; Doxorubicin + Barbiturates

The effects of doxorubicin may be reduced by the barbiturates.

Clinical evidence, mechanism, importance and management

A comparative study in patients given doxorubicin found that those also taking barbiturates had a doxorubicin plasma clearance that was 50% higher than those who were not taking barbiturates (318 mL/minute compared with 202 mL/minute).[1] This clinical study is in agreement with previous studies in *mice*.[2] A possible explanation is that the barbiturate increases the metabolism of the doxorubicin. It seems possible that the dose of doxorubicin will need to be increased in barbiturate-treated patients to achieve maximal therapeutic effects.

1. Riggs CE, Engel S, Wesley M, Wiernik PH, Bachur NR. Doxorubicin pharmacokinetics, prochlorperazine and barbiturate effects. *Clin Pharmacol Ther* (1982) 31, 263.
2. Reich SD, Bachur NR. Alterations in adriamycin efficacy by phenobarbital. *Cancer* (1976) 36, 3803–6.

Anthracyclines; Doxorubicin + Tamoxifen

Tamoxifen appears to have no significant effect on the pharmacokinetics of doxorubicin.

Clinical evidence, mechanism, importance and management

A pharmacokinetic study in patients with non-Hodgkin's lymphoma receiving CHOP (cyclophosphamide, vincristine, prednisone and doxorubicin 37.5 to 50 mg/m^2) found that the addition of tamoxifen 480 mg daily for 5 days had no significant effect on the AUC or total clearance of doxorubicin.[1]

See 'Tamoxifen + Miscellaneous', p.711, for the suggestion that prior chemotherapy with doxorubicin does not affect tamoxifen levels; and for the possible additive thromboembolic effect of doxorubicin and tamoxifen, see 'Antineoplastics + Tamoxifen', p.659.

1. El-Yazigi A, Berry J, Ezzat A, Wahab FA. Effect of tamoxifen on the pharmacokinetics of doxorubicin in patients with non-Hodgkin's lymphoma. *Ther Drug Monit* (1997) 19, 632–6.

Anthracyclines; Doxorubicin + Toremifene

In a study, 6 patients were given high-dose oral toremifene 600 mg daily for 5 days, with doxorubicin 60 mg/m^2 intravenously on day 5. The pharmacokinetics of doxorubicin were not affected by toremifene when compared with a single intravenous dose of doxorubicin 60 mg/m^2 given alone.[1] Usual doses of toremifene would not be expected to interact with doxorubicin.

1. Wurz GT, Soc L, Emshoff VD, Cadman TB, DeGregorio MW. Pharmacokinetics analysis of high-dose toremifene in combination with doxorubicin. *Cancer Chemother Pharmacol* (1998) 42, 363–6.

Anthracyclines; Epirubicin + Cimetidine

Cimetidine increases the exposure to epirubicin.

Clinical evidence, mechanism, importance and management

In a study in 8 patients, cimetidine 400 mg twice daily increased the AUC of epirubicin by 50%. At the same time the AUCs of two metabolites of epirubicin, epirubicinol and 7-deoxydoxorubicinol aglycone, increased by 41% and 4.6-fold, respectively. Liver blood flow also increased by 17%.[1] The mechanism for this effect is unknown and more study of this interaction is needed. As the increase in epirubicin exposure might increase its toxicity, the manufacturers advise avoiding concurrent use.[2,3] However, if it is essential, it would seem prudent to monitor the patient closely for signs of epirubicin adverse effects (such as myelosuppression and cardiotoxicity) and adjust treatment as necessary. Note that cimetidine is available without a prescription in some countries so that patients could unwittingly increase the toxicity of epirubicin; it would seem advisable to warn them.

1. Murray LS, Jodrell DI, Morrison JG, Cook A, Kerr DJ, Whiting B, Kaye SB, Cassidy J. The effect of cimetidine on the pharmacokinetics of epirubicin in patients with advanced breast cancer: preliminary evidence of a potentially common drug interaction. *Clin Oncol* (1998) 10, 35–8.
2. Pharmorubicin (Epirubicin hydrochloride). Pharmacia Ltd. UK Summary of product characteristics, July 2009.
3. Ellence (Epirubicin hydrochloride). Pharmacia & Upjohn Co. US Prescribing information, November 2011.

Anthracyclines; Pixantrone + Miscellaneous

Pixantrone might increase the concentrations of drugs that are substrates of CYP1A2 and CYP2C8. The concentration of pixantrone might be increased or decreased by drugs that inhibit or induce, respectively, P-glycoprotein.

Clinical evidence, mechanism, importance and management

(a) CYP1A2 substrates

The UK manufacturer briefly reports that, *in vitro* pixantrone inhibits CYP1A2, and theoretically might increase the concentrations of drugs that are substrates of this isoenzyme. In particular they warn that the concentrations of **theophylline** might be increased such that toxicity results, and advise that theophylline concentrations should be closely monitored after pixantrone has been started. They also note that **warfarin** is partially metabolised by CYP1A2, and advise that coagulation parameters, especially INR, are monitored after pixantrone is started.[1] However, note that it is only the less active *R*-warfarin that is partially metabolised by this isoenzyme, and so the clinical effect of any inhibition of this isoenzyme alone is likely to be small. The manufacturer extends its warnings about the possibility of increased concentrations to **amitriptyline, clozapine, haloperidol, ondansetron**, and **propranolol**.[1] However, note that only amitriptyline and clozapine are considered clinically relevant substrates of CYP1A2, and propranolol is only partially metabolised by this isoenzyme.

(b) CYP2C8 substrates

The UK manufacturer briefly reports that, *in vitro* pixantrone inhibits CYP2C8, and advise caution on concurrent use with drugs that are substrates of this isoenzyme. In particular, they name **repaglinide, rosiglitazone**, and **paclitaxel**, and advise monitoring for adverse effects.[1] However, note that paclitaxel is often considered a CYP2C8 substrate, but this is based on *in vitro* data, and clinical data to support this are lacking.

(c) Drug transporter proteins

The UK manufacturer briefly reports that, *in vitro* pixantrone is a substrate of the drug transporter proteins P-glycoprotein, and breast cancer resistance protein (BCRP). They predict that drugs that inhibit these transporters might increase concentrations of pixantrone and advise close monitoring on concurrent use. They name **ciclosporin, nelfinavir, ritonavir, saquinavir**, and **tacrolimus**.[1] However, note that tacrolimus is not usually considered to be an inhibitor of P-glycoprotein; see 'Table 1.12', p.14 for a list of known, clinically important P-glycoprotein inhibitors. It would therefore seem prudent to monitor for adverse effects (such as nausea, vomiting, alopecia, blood dyscrasias) on concurrent use with any of these drugs, and adjust the dose of pixantrone if necessary. Similarly, they predict that drugs that induce these transporters might decrease pixantrone concentrations and they name **carbamazepine, corticosteroids**, and **rifampicin (rifampin)**.[1] However, note that corticosteroids are not usually considered to be inducers of P-glycoprotein; see 'Table 1.12', p.14 for a list of known, clinically important P-glycoprotein inducers. It would therefore seem prudent to monitor for pixantrone efficacy on concurrent use with any of these drugs and adjust the dose if necessary.

(d) Live vaccines

Due to the immunosuppression caused by pixantrone, immunisation with **live vaccines** is contraindicated.[1] This is because immunisation in general might be ineffective when given with immunosuppressants (such as pixantrone), and in particular the use of live vaccines in patients receiving immunosuppressants might result in infection.

1. Pixuvri (Pixantrone dimaleate). CTI Life Sciences Ltd. UK Summary of product characteristics, April 2014.

Antineoplastics + Amphotericin B

Amphotericin B may delay the clearance of methotrexate, and there may be an increased risk of renal impairment. Similarly, the use of conventional amphotericin B with nephrotoxic antineoplastics such as cisplatin and ifosfamide may increase the risk of renal impairment.

Clinical evidence

Two children had delayed clearance of pulse **methotrexate** (1 g/m^2 over 24 hours) while they were receiving amphotericin B. **Methotrexate** levels were about 300 to 500% higher 48 hours after **methotrexate** when they were receiving amphotericin B, compared with **methotrexate** alone.[1] In a study, **methotrexate** clearance in 18 children given high-dose **methotrexate** (1 g/m^2 intravenously) was significantly correlated with the glomerular filtration rate (GFR). Concurrent amphotericin B in 6 of the children significantly decreased the GFR.[2] A history of heavy amphotericin B treatment (greater than 30 mg/kg) correlated with decreased **methotrexate** clearance in 24 children with relapsed leukaemia.[3]

A multivariate analysis in patients receiving high-dose **cisplatin** with saline hydration and mannitol diuresis found that the concurrent use of amphotericin B was a predictor of renal failure.[4]

Mechanism

Amphotericin B may cause renal impairment, which can result in delayed methotrexate clearance. Both cisplatin and amphotericin B are nephrotoxic, and their effects might be expected to be additive.

Importance and management

Evidence regarding an interaction between amphotericin B and methotrexate appears to be limited. Nevertheless, the adverse effects of methotrexate should be carefully monitored (e.g. patient reported symptoms, LFTs, renal function, blood counts) in patients taking amphotericin B or those previously extensively treated with the drug. In patients taking large doses of methotrexate (i.e. not the weekly doses given for conditions such as rheumatoid arthritis), the monitoring of methotrexate levels is recommended.

Similarly, evidence for an interaction between cisplatin and amphotericin B is limited, but what happens is in line with the known nephrotoxic effects of both drugs. The manufacturer of conventional amphotericin B states that nephrotoxic antineoplastics should not be given concurrently except with great caution.[5] Of the antineoplastics, cisplatin, **ifosfamide** and methotrexate are well known for their nephrotoxicity. Liposomal amphotericin B is licensed for use in the empirical treatment of presumed fungal infections in febrile neutropenic patients. It is therefore likely to be used in patients who have received antineoplastics and who may have antineoplastic-induced renal impairment. The manufacturer notes that it has been used successfully in a large number of patients with pre-existing renal impairment. Nevertheless, renal function should still be closely monitored in these patients.[6]

1. Parker RI, Mahan RM, Giugliano DA. Delayed methotrexate clearance during treatment with amphotericin B. *Pediatr Res* (2002) 51 (4 part 2), 258A.
2. Murry DJ, Synold TW, Pui C-H, Rodman JH. Renal function and methotrexate clearance in children with newly diagnosed leukemia. *Pharmacotherapy* (1995) 15, 144–9.
3. Wall AM, Gajjar A, Link A, Mahmoud H, Pui C-H, Relling MV. Individualized methotrexate dosing in children with relapsed acute lymphoblastic leukemia. *Leukemia* (2000) 14, 221–5.
4. Cooper BW, Creger RJ, Soegiarso W, Mackay WL, Lazarus HM. Renal dysfunction during high-dose cisplatin therapy and autologous hematopoietic stem cell transplantation: effect of aminoglycoside therapy. *Am J Med* (1993) 94, 497–504.
5. Fungizone Intravenous (Amphotericin B). E. R. Squibb & Sons Ltd. UK Summary of product characteristics, February 2010.
6. AmBisome (Liposomal Amphotericin B). Gilead Sciences Ltd. UK Summary of product characteristics, January 2009.

Antineoplastics + Aprepitant

Aprepitant had no effect on the pharmacokinetics of single intravenous doses of docetaxel or vinorelbine. The activation of cyclophosphamide and thiotepa was slightly lower in patients receiving aprepitant. Etoposide and paclitaxel have been commonly used with aprepitant without any dose adjustment. Fosaprepitant is rapidly converted to aprepitant after intravenous administration, and is therefore expected to share the same interactions.

Clinical evidence

(a) Cyclophosphamide

The rate of auto-induction of cyclophosphamide was 23% lower and exposure to the active metabolite, 4-hydroxycyclophosphamide, was 5% lower in 6 patients receiving aprepitant with a 4-day course of high-dose CTC (cyclophosphamide, thiotepa, carboplatin) when compared with 49 patients receiving high-dose CTC without aprepitant.[1]

(b) Docetaxel

Aprepitant 125 mg given one hour before docetaxel on day one, then 80 mg daily on days 2 and 3 had no effect on the pharmacokinetics of a single 60- to 100-mg/m^2 infusion of docetaxel in 10 patients with cancer, and did not alter the toxicity profile. Each subject acted as their own control.[2]

(c) Thiotepa

The formation clearance of thiotepa was 33% lower and exposure to the active metabolite, TEPA (triethylenephosphamide), was 20% lower in 6 patients receiving aprepitant with a 4-day course of high-dose CTC (cyclophosphamide, thiotepa, carboplatin) when compared with 49 patients receiving high-dose CTC without aprepitant.[1]

(d) Vinorelbine

In a pharmacokinetic study, in 12 patients with cancer, aprepitant 125 mg on day one and 80 mg daily on days 2 and 3 had no effect on the pharmacokinetics of intravenous vinorelbine 25 mg/m^2 given on day one or day 8.[3]

Mechanism

In the short-term, aprepitant is an inhibitor of CYP3A4, and might therefore reduce the activation of antineoplastics activated by this isoenzyme (cyclophosphamide, thiotepa), or increase the toxicity of antineoplastics metabolised by this isoenzyme (docetaxel, irinotecan). There is some evidence (with midazolam) that aprepitant has a greater effect on CYP3A4 substrates when they are given orally rather than intravenously (see under 'Benzodiazepines + Aprepitant', p.813), so this might explain the findings with the intravenous antineoplastics studied.[2]

Importance and management

The studies cited above suggest that clinically relevant pharmacokinetic interactions between aprepitant and intravenous cyclophosphamide, docetaxel, thiotepa, and vinorelbine are unlikely: in each case the effects found were modest. However, a degree of caution might be warranted if any of these antineoplastics are given orally, as greater effects can result (see *Mechanism*). These findings suggest that, despite aprepitant being an inhibitor of CYP3A4, it is unlikely to have any clinically relevant effect on the pharmacokinetics of intravenous antineoplastics that are substrates of this isoenzyme. Nevertheless, the UK and US manufacturers of aprepitant and fosaprepitant recommend caution when these drugs are used with antineoplastics that are metabolised by CYP3A4.[4-7] In the UK they limit this to antineoplastics given orally (**etoposide** and vinorelbine are named);[4,6] however, in addition, they particularly caution use with **irinotecan** (given intravenously), because of the possibility of increased toxicity with this drug.[4,6] In the US, the manufacturer mentions that **etoposide**, **paclitaxel**, and vinorelbine were commonly given with aprepitant without dose adjustment for potential interactions. They recommend particular caution with **vinblastine**, **vincristine**, and **ifosfamide**, as only a few patients have received these drugs with aprepitant, and with other antineoplastics principally metabolised by CYP3A4 that have not yet been studied (**irinotecan** is named, as is imatinib; see 'Aprepitant + Tyrosine kinase inhibitors', p.1139).[5,7]

1. de Jonge ME, Huitaema AD, Holtkamp MJ, van Dam SM, Beijnen JH, Rodenhuis S. Aprepitant inhibits cyclophosphamide bioactivation and thiotepa metabolism. *Cancer Chemother Pharmacol* (2005) 56, 370–8.
2. Nygren P, Hande K, Petty KJ, Fedgchin M, van Dyck K, Majumdar A, Panebianco D, de Smet M, Ahmed T, Murphy MG, Gottesdiener KM, Cocquyt V, van Belle S. Lack of effect of aprepitant on the pharmacokinetics of docetaxel in cancer patients. *Cancer Chemother Pharmacol* (2005) 55, 609–16.
3. Loos WJ, de Wit R, Freedman SJ, Van Dyck K, Gambale JJ, Li S, Murphy GM, van Noort C, de Bruijn P, Verweij J. Aprepitant when added to a standard antiemetic regimen consisting of ondansetron and dexamethasone does not affect vinorelbine pharmacokinetics in cancer patients. *Cancer Chemother Pharmacol* (2007) 59, 407–12.
4. EMEND (Aprepitant). Merck Sharp & Dohme Ltd. UK Summary of product characteristics, December 2013.
5. EMEND Capsules (Aprepitant). Merck & Co., Inc. US Prescribing information, August 2014.
6. IVEMEND (Fosaprepitant dimeglumine). Merck Sharp & Dohme Ltd. UK Summary of product characteristics, December 2011.
7. EMEND for Injection (Fosaprepitant dimeglumine). Merck & Co., Inc. US Prescribing information, July 2012.

Antineoplastics + Calcium-channel blockers

Verapamil can increase the efficacy of doxorubicin in tissue culture systems and increase doxorubicin levels in patients. D-verapamil can alter the pharmacokinetics of epirubicin and possibly increase its bone marrow depressant effects.

The absorption of verapamil can be modestly reduced by antineoplastic regimens containing cyclophosphamide, vincristine and procarbazine, or vindesine, doxorubicin and cisplatin.

Clinical evidence, mechanism, importance and management

(a) Antineoplastic regimens

A study in 9 patients with a variety of malignant diseases found that treatment with antineoplastics reduced the absorption of a single 160-mg oral dose of **verapamil**. The **verapamil** AUC in 8 patients was reduced by 40% (range 7 to 58%), but one patient conversely had a 26% increase. Five patients received a modified COPP regimen (**cyclophosphamide**, **vincristine**, **procarbazine**, prednisone) and 4 patients received VAC (**vindesine**, **doxorubicin**, **cisplatin**).[1]

It is believed that these antineoplastics damage the lining of the upper part of the small intestine, which impairs the absorption of **verapamil**. The clinical relevance of this reduction does not appear to have been studied but it seems likely that at least some patients will be affected. Therefore it would seem prudent to monitor concurrent use for verapamil efficacy.

(b) Doxorubicin

The efficacy of doxorubicin was increased by **verapamil** and **nicardipine** in doxorubicin-resistant tissue culture systems, while **nifedipine** had only minimal activity.[2] A study in 5 patients with small cell lung cancer given doxorubicin, vincristine, etoposide and cyclophosphamide found that when they were given **verapamil** 240 to 480 mg daily the AUC of doxorubicin was doubled, its peak serum levels were raised and its clearance was reduced. No increased toxicity was seen in this study.[3] However, although another study found no increase in doxorubicin acute toxicities, intravenous **verapamil** caused an unacceptable degree of cardiac adverse effects (heart block, hypotension, and/or heart failure) when given in doses to attain plasma levels four times the normal upper limit.[4]

(c) Epirubicin

When used to reduce multidrug resistance in patients with advanced colorectal cancer receiving epirubicin, the D-isomer of **verapamil** appears to increase the bone marrow depressant toxicity of epirubicin.[5] Another study found that **D-verapamil** halved the AUC and half-life of epirubicin, and increased its clearance,[6] while yet another study did not find these changes but found that the production of the metabolites of epirubicin was increased.[7] These changes should be taken into account if both drugs are used. More study is needed to evaluate the possible advantages and disadvantages of giving these drugs together.

1. Kuhlmann J, Woodcock B, Wilke J, Rietbrock N. Verapamil plasma concentrations during treatment with cytostatic drugs. *J Cardiovasc Pharmacol* (1985) 7, 1003–6.
2. Ramu A, Spanier R, Rahamimoff H, Fuks Z. Restoration of doxorubicin responsiveness in doxorubicin-resistant P388 murine leukaemia cells. *Br J Cancer* (1984) 50, 501–7.
3. Kerr DJ, Graham J, Cummings J, Morrison JG, Thompson GG, Brodie MJ, Kaye SB. The effect of verapamil on the pharmacokinetics of adriamycin. *Cancer Chemother Pharmacol* (1986) 18, 239–42.
4. Ozols RF, Cunnion RE, Klecker RW, Hamilton TC, Ostchega Y, Parrillo JE, Young RC. Verapamil and adriamycin in the treatment of drug-resistant ovarian cancer patients. *J Clin Oncol* (1987) 5, 641–7.
5. Scheithauer W, Kornek G, Kastner J, Raderer M, Locker G, Depisch D, Pidlich J, Tetzner C. Phase II study of d-verapamil and doxorubicin in patients with metastatic colorectal cancer. *Eur J Cancer* (1993) 29A, 2337–8.
6. Scheithauer W, Schenk T, Czejka M. Pharmacokinetic interaction between epirubicin and the multidrug resistance reverting agent D-verapamil. *Br J Cancer* (1993) 68, 8–9.
7. Mross K, Hamm K, Hossfeld DK. Effects of verapamil on the pharmacokinetics and metabolism of epirubicin. *Cancer Chemother Pharmacol* (1993) 31, 369–75.

Antineoplastics + Colony-stimulating factors

Because of the increased risk of myelosuppression, colony-stimulating factors such as filgrastim, pegfilgrastim and lenograstim should not be given at the same time as myelosuppressive cytotoxic antineoplastics.

Clinical evidence, mechanism, importance and management

Colony-stimulating factors such as filgrastim and lenograstim promote the growth of myeloid cell lines. Because rapidly dividing myeloid cells have increased sensitivity to cytotoxic chemotherapy, the manufacturers have advised that these drugs should not be used from 24 hours before until 24 hours after cytotoxic chemotherapy,[1-3] or should be avoided from 14 days before[4] to 24 hours after chemotherapy.[4,5] In support of this, the manufacturer of filgrastim notes that preliminary evidence confirmed that the severity of neutropenia could be exacerbated when patients were given **fluorouracil** and filgrastim concurrently.[2]

Note also that there is some evidence that colony-stimulating factors may potentiate the pulmonary toxicity of bleomycin (see 'Bleomycin + Colony-stimulating factors', p.664) and cyclophosphamide (see 'Cyclophosphamide + Colony-stimulating factors', p.672).

1. Granocyte (Lenograstim). Chugai Pharma UK Ltd. UK Summary of product characteristics, May 2009.
2. Neupogen (Filgrastim). Amgen Ltd. UK Summary of product characteristics, March 2011.
3. Neupogen (Filgrastim). Amgen Inc. US Prescribing information, May 2012.
4. Neulasta (Pegfilgrastim). Amgen Inc. US Prescribing information, February 2010.
5. Neulasta (Pegfilgrastim). Amgen Ltd. UK Summary of product characteristics, October 2009.

Antineoplastics + 5-HT_3-receptor antagonists

Ondansetron does not appear to affect the pharmacokinetics of cyclophosphamide and cisplatin to a clinically relevant extent. Ondansetron does not appear to affect the pharmacokinetics of carmustine or the *in vitro* activity of epirubicin, bleomycin, cisplatin or estramustine. Cisplatin and fluorouracil do not affect the pharmacokinetics of ondansetron. Granisetron potentiated the cytotoxic effects of epirubicin *in vitro*, had an additive effect on bleomycin and estramustine activity and appeared not to affect the metabolism of docetaxel and paclitaxel.

Clinical evidence, mechanism, importance and management

(a) Granisetron

1. Cytotoxicity. In an *in vitro* study, granisetron significantly potentiated the cytotoxic effects of **epirubicin** on fibroblasts, and the effect of granisetron on the cytotoxic effects of **bleomycin** and **estramustine** in lung cancer cells appeared to be additive. The clinical relevance of the effects of granisetron on **epirubicin** is not known.[1]

2. Electrocardiac effects. A review of the ECGs of 30 patients who had received granisetron and **doxorubicin** or **epirubicin** found that the antineoplastics did not cause any further change in the PR interval above that which was caused by granisetron alone. There were no clinically significant cardiac effects reported.[2]

3. Pharmacokinetics. An *in vitro* study found that granisetron did not affect the metabolism of **docetaxel** or **paclitaxel**,[3] nor did a study in 6 patients demonstrate any change in the pharmacokinetics or bone-marrow suppressant effect of **docetaxel** when given with granisetron.[4]

(b) Ondansetron

1. Cytotoxicity. An *in vitro* study found that ondansetron did not affect the cytotoxic effects of **bleomycin**, **epirubicin**, **estramustine** or **cisplatin** in fibroblasts and lung cancer cells.[1]

2. Nephrotoxicity. In a small retrospective review of patients who had received cisplatin, there was a decreased incidence of nephrotoxicity (an increase in serum creatinine of about 44 micromol/L or more) in those patients who had also received ondansetron.[5] The mechanism for this association is unclear. The data from these sorts of analyses require confirmation in a controlled study, because it is possible that the findings are due to chance alone. The general relevance of this report is therefore uncertain.

3. Pharmacokinetics. The pharmacokinetics of high-dose **cyclophosphamide**, **cisplatin** and **carmustine** in 23 patients given ondansetron, lorazepam and diphenhydramine as antiemetics were compared with those in 129 patients who received prochlorperazine instead of ondansetron. It was found that the AUCs of **cyclophosphamide** and **cisplatin**, but not that of **carmustine**, were lower (by 15% and 19%, respectively) in the ondansetron group.[6] Similarly, in another study, the pharmacokinetics of antineoplastics were analysed in 54 patients with breast cancer who were receiving high-dose **cyclophosphamide**, **cisplatin** and **carmustine** with lorazepam and ondansetron, with or without prochlorperazine, and compared with 75 matched control patients whose had been given prochlorperazine and lorazepam. In those given ondansetron the median AUC of **cyclophosphamide** was 17% lower, the **cisplatin** AUC was about 10% higher and the **carmustine** AUC was unchanged.[7]

In a crossover study in 10 patients, who received intravenous **cyclophosphamide** 600 mg/m^2 and **epirubicin** 90 mg/m^2 and either oral ondansetron 16 mg or placebo, found that the pharmacokinetic parameters of **cyclophosphamide** or its metabolite were not significantly altered by ondansetron although there was considerable variation between subjects. It was concluded that ondansetron can be safely given with **cyclophosphamide**.[8]

No significant changes in the pharmacokinetics of ondansetron occurred in 20 patients with cancer taking **cisplatin** 20 to 40 mg/m^2 and/or **fluorouracil** 1 g/m^2 for 5 days but the clearance was lower than in healthy subjects.[9]

Information seems to be limited to these studies, but any pharmacokinetic effects appear to be small, and unlikely to be clinically relevant.

1. Behnam Motlagh P, Henriksson R, Grankvist K. Interaction of the antiemetics ondansetron and granisetron with the cytotoxicity induced by irradiation, epirubicin, bleomycin, estramustine, and cisplatin in vitro. *Acta Oncol* (1995) 34, 871–5.
2. Jantunen IT, Kataja VV, Muhonen TT, Parviainen T. Effects of granisetron with doxorubicin or epirubicin on ECG intervals. *Cancer Chemother Pharmacol* (1996) 37, 502–4.
3. Watanabe Y, Nakajima K, Nozaki K, Hoshiai H, Noda K. The effect of granisetron on in vitro metabolism of paclitaxel and docetaxel. *Cancer J* (2003) 9, 67–70.
4. Miyata M, Yasuda K, Burioka N, Takane H, Suyama H, Shigeoka Y, Endo M, Kurai J, Morita M, Igishi T, Shimizu E. The influence of granisetron on the pharmacokinetics and pharmacodynamics of docetaxel in Asian lung cancer patients. *Cancer J* (2006) 12, 69–72.
5. Shord SS, Thompson DM, Krempl GA, Hanigan MH. Effect of concurrent medications on cisplatin-induced nephrotoxicity in patients with head and neck cancer. *Anticancer Drugs* (2006) 17, 207–15.
6. Cagnoni PJ, Matthes S, Day TC, Bearman SI, Shpall EJ, Jones RB. Modification of the pharmacokinetics of high-dose cyclophosphamide and cisplatin by antiemetics. *Bone Marrow Transplant* (1999) 24, 1–4.
7. Gilbert CJ, Petros WP, Vredenburgh J, Hussein A, Ross M, Rubin P, Fehdrau R, Cavanaugh C, Berry D, McKinstry C, Peters WP. Pharmacokinetic interaction between ondansetron and cyclophosphamide during high-dose chemotherapy for breast cancer. *Cancer Chemother Pharmacol* (1998) 42, 497–503.
8. Lorenz C, Eickhoff C, Baumann F, Sehouli J, Preiss R, Schunack W, Jaehde U. Does ondansetron affect the metabolism of cyclophosphamide? *Int J Clin Pharmacol Ther* (2000) 38, 143–4.
9. Hsyu P-H, Bozigian HP, Pritchard JF, Kernodle A, Panella J, Hansen LA, Griffin RH. Effect of chemotherapy on the pharmacokinetics of oral ondansetron. *Pharm Res* (1991) 8 (Suppl 10), S-257.

Antineoplastics + Megestrol

In one clinical study megestrol reduced the response rates to etoposide with cisplatin but in another had no effect on response rates to alternating cycles of cyclophosphamide, doxorubicin and vincristine, and etoposide with cisplatin.

Clinical evidence

A study in 243 patients with advanced small-cell lung cancer (SCLC) given **etoposide** and **cisplatin** found that patients who also received megestrol acetate 800 mg daily had increased non-fluid body-weight and significantly less nausea and vomiting. Although the one-year survival rate was similar in both groups patients who received megestrol had a significantly worse response rate to **cisplatin** (68% compared with 80%) and a higher incidence of thromboembolic events. However the megestrol recipients did have poorer quality of life (a prognostic factor) at the beginning of the study and this may have influenced the findings.[1] In a similar study, megestrol acetate had no effect on response rates, symptom profile or overall survival in patients with SCLC receiving chemotherapy (alternating cycles of **cyclophosphamide**, **doxorubicin** and **vincristine**, and **etoposide** with **cisplatin** for a maximum of 6 cycles). In this study, megestrol acetate was given at a dose of 160 mg three times daily for 8 days starting 3 days before each cycle of chemotherapy.[2]

Mechanism

An *in vitro* study found that megestrol may antagonise the antineoplastic activity of cisplatin by up-regulating cellular detoxification mechanisms.[3]

Importance and management

The authors of the first study suggest that megestrol acetate should not be used routinely at the time of chemotherapy.[1] Be aware that the use of megestrol may antagonise the antitumour activity of cisplatin. More study is needed.

1. Rowland KM, Loprinzi CL, Shaw EG, Maksymiuk AW, Kuross SA, Jung S-H, Kugler JW, Tschetter LK, Ghosh C, Schaefer PL, Owen D, Washburn JH, Webb TA, Mailliard JA, Jett JR. Randomized double-blind placebo-controlled trial of cisplatin and etoposide plus megestrol acetate/placebo in extensive-stage small-cell lung cancer: a North Central Cancer Treatment Group Study. *J Clin Oncol* (1996) 14, 135–41.
2. Wood L, Palmer M, Hewitt J, Urtasun R, Bruera E, Rapp E, Thaell JF. Results of a phase III, double-blind, placebo-controlled trial of megestrol acetate modulation of P-glycoprotein-mediated drug resistance in the first-line management of small-cell lung carcinoma. *Br J Cancer* (1998) 77, 627–31.
3. Pu Y-S, Cheng A-L, Chen J, Guan J-Y, Lu S-H, Lai M-K, Hsieh C-Y. Megestrol acetate antagonizes cisplatin cytotoxicity. *Anticancer Drugs* (1998) 9, 733–8.

Antineoplastics + Propofol

There are two isolated reports of severe pain occurring when patients who had previously received intravenous chemotherapy were given intravenous propofol via hand veins, and one report of excessive bradycardia after a bolus dose of propofol in a child receiving cytarabine.

Clinical evidence

Although pain on injection of propofol is well known, one group of workers noted that, on a number of occasions, patients previously given intravenous chemotherapy had marked pain, both at the site of injection and up the arm, when given propofol via hand veins.[1] This would seem to link with a report of a 15-year-old girl with acute lymphoblastic leukaemia who had been given several injections of **cyclophosphamide**, **methotrexate** and **vincristine** during the previous 6 months, and who was cannulated in her hand and given an infusion of *Plasmalyte B*. An injection of 60 micrograms of fentanyl via this cannula was painful and 20 mg of lidocaine helped, but 20 mg of propofol caused extreme pain. A further 20 mg of lidocaine was given and the propofol administration was stopped, but the pain continued. The whole hand became blue and congested, and blood began to move backwards up the drip tubing. The venous congestion gradually subsided over the next 15 minutes.[2] The authors recommended that propofol should be avoided in patients who have recently had intravenous chemotherapy.[2]

A report describes a child being given **cytarabine** and **daunorubicin** who developed significant bradycardia after receiving a bolus dose of propofol.[3]

Mechanism

Both cytarabine and propofol may cause bradycardia by blocking the sinoatrial node, and an additive or synergistic effect may have caused the bradycardia in the child described above.[3]

Importance and management

The general applicability of these reports remains to be determined. The use of propofol alone may cause pain and it should be noted that the manufacturer of propofol recommends that local pain associated with propofol during the induction phase can be minimised by the use of the larger veins on the forearm and antecubital fossa.[4]

1. Whitlock JE, Nicol ME, Pattison J. Painful injection of propofol. *Anaesthesia* (1989) 44, 618.
2. Butt AD, James MFM. Venospasm due to propofol after chemotherapy. *S Afr Med J* (1990) 77, 168.
3. Wilson SE, Boyack DA, Ezeife-Ugorji OC, Costarino AT. Propofol-induced bradycardia in a pediatric patient undergoing chemotherapy with the known cardiotoxic agent cytarabin. *Pediatr Anesth* (2006) 16, 697–706.
4. Diprivan (Propofol). AstraZeneca UK Ltd. UK Summary of product characteristics, July 2009.

Antineoplastics + Semaxanib

The combination of semaxanib, cisplatin and gemcitabine has caused an unexpectedly high incidence of thromboembolic events.

Clinical evidence, mechanism, importance and management

The pharmacokinetics of semaxanib (SU5416), **cisplatin** and **gemcitabine** were unaltered when they were given together in a phase I study but investigation of the combination was terminated after 8 of the 19 patients had thromboembolic events (transient ischaemic attacks, cerebrovascular accidents, deep vein thromboses). **Gemcitabine** 1250 mg/m^2 was given on day one, immediately followed by **cisplatin** 80 mg/m^2, then semaxanib 85 mg/m^2 (escalated to 145 mg/m^2 in some patients). **Gemcitabine** then semaxanib were given on day 8, and semaxanib alone on days 4, 11, 15, and 18. The cycle was repeated every 3 weeks.[1] The incidence of thromboembolic events in this study (42%) was much higher than that seen with **cisplatin** and **gemcitabine** (0%) or semaxanib alone (2.2%), and was thought to be a result of the drug combination.[1] **Cisplatin** in particular, due to its effects on platelets and its vasoconstrictive effects, may be the drug interacting with the semaxanib.[2] Preliminary results of other studies of semaxanib with: **irinotecan**; **fluorouracil** and folinic acid; **irinotecan**, **fluorouracil** and folinic acid; or **paclitaxel** and **carboplatin** did not report this complication.[3-6] The authors of the first study[1] caution against further clinical studies of antineoplastics with angiogenesis inhibitors such as semaxanib until the exact cause of the thromboembolic events has been elucidated.

1. Kuenen BC, Rosen L, Smit EF, Parson MRN, Levi M, Ruijter R, Huisman H, Kedde MA, Noordhuis P, van der Vijgh WJF, Peters GJ, Cropp GF, Scigalla P, Hoekman K, Pinedo HM, Giaccone G. Dose-finding and pharmacokinetic study of cisplatin, gemcitabine, and SU5416 in patients with solid tumors. *J Clin Oncol* (2002) 20, 1657–67.
2. Marx GM, Steer CB, Harper P, Pavlakis N, Rixe O, Khayat D. Unexpected serious toxicity with chemotherapy and antiangiogenic combinations: time to take stock. *J Clin Oncol* (2002) 20, 1446–8.
3. Rosen PJ, Amado R, Hecht JR, Chang D, Mulay M, Parson M Laxa B, Brown J, Cropp G, Hannah A, Rosen L. A phase I/II study of SU5416 in combination with 5-FU/leucovorin in patients with metastatic colorectal cancer. *Proc Am Soc Clin Oncol* (2000) 19, 3A.
4. Rothenberg ML, Berlin JD, Cropp GF, Fleischer AC, Schumaker RD, Hande KR, Culley A, Dorminy C, Donnelly E, Chen J, Schaaf L, Hannah AL. A phase I/II study of SU5416 in combination with irinotecan/5-FU/LV (IFL) in patients with metastatic colorectal cancer. *Proc Am Soc Clin Oncol* (2001) 20, 75A.
5. Rosen P, Kabbinavar F, Figlin RA, Parson M, Laxa B, Hernandez L, Mayers A, Cropp GF, Hannah AL, Rosen LS. A phase I/II trial and pharmacokinetic (PK) study of SU5416 in combination with paclitaxel/carboplatin. *Proc Am Soc Clin Oncol* (2001) 20, 98A.
6. Hoff PM, Wolff RA, Bogaard K, Waldrum S, Abbruzzese JL. A phase I study of escalating doses of the tyrosine kinase inhibitor semaxanib (SU5416) in combination with irinotecan in patients with advanced colorectal cancer. *Jpn J Clin Oncol* (2006) 36, 100–3.

Antineoplastics + Tamoxifen

Antineoplastics and tamoxifen are associated with an increased risk of thrombosis and there is the possibility that their combined use may further increase this risk.

Clinical evidence

A retrospective analysis of data from various Eastern Cooperative Oncology Group studies suggested that venous thromboembolic complications were more common in women given tamoxifen with adjuvant chemotherapy (CMF; **cyclophosphamide, methotrexate, fluorouracil**) than women given CMF alone (3.8% versus 0% in one study).[1] In another study of patients given tamoxifen 30 mg daily for 2 years the incidence of thromboembolic events was 2.6% compared with 13.6% in those also given 8 cycles of CMF. The authors of this study considered the rate of thromboembolic events with the combination to be higher than that usually seen with CMF, and suggested that this occurred as a result of an interaction between tamoxifen and CMF.[2] In contrast, in another study, in the first 12 weeks of therapy, thrombosis occurred in 5 of 103 patients given tamoxifen with chemotherapy (**cyclophosphamide, methotrexate, fluorouracil, vincristine**, prednisone, **doxorubicin**) compared with 4 of 102 given the same chemotherapy alone, suggesting that tamoxifen made no significant contribution to the rate of thromboembolic events.[3]

Mechanism

Tamoxifen alone is known to carry a small risk of thromboembolic events when used for primary prevention of breast cancer,[4] which may be a result of tamoxifen causing an increased calcium uptake by platelets, leading to platelet activation.[5] Antineoplastic chemotherapy also increases the risk of thrombosis,[3] and cancer *per se* increases the risk, as does surgery for cancer.[6]

Importance and management

To what extent, if any, tamoxifen further increases the risk of thrombosis with cytotoxic antineoplastics is unclear from the above studies. However, some authors recommend that serious consideration be given to the use of prophylactic anticoagulants if adjuvant CMF is given with tamoxifen in women with breast cancer,[2] and the UK manufacturer endorses this for any adjuvant chemotherapy.[7] This may be prudent with antineoplastic chemotherapy in any case. See 'Tamoxifen + Miscellaneous', p.711, for the suggestion that prior chemotherapy with cyclophosphamide, does not affect tamoxifen levels.

1. Saphner T, Tormey DC, Gray R. Venous and arterial thrombosis in patients who received adjuvant therapy for breast cancer. *J Clin Oncol* (1991) 9, 286–94.
2. Pritchard KI, Paterson AHG, Paul NA, Zee B, Fine S, Pater J. Increased thromboembolic complications with concurrent tamoxifen and chemotherapy in a randomized trial of adjuvant therapy for women with breast cancer. National Cancer Institute of Canada Clinical Trials Group Breast Cancer Site Group. *J Clin Oncol* (1996) 14, 2731–7.
3. Levine MN, Gent M, Hirsh J, Arnold A, Goodyear MD, Hryniuk W, De Pauw S. The thrombogenic effect of anticancer drug therapy in women with stage II breast cancer. *N Engl J Med* (1988) 318; 404–7.
4. Fischer B, Constantino JP, Wickerham DL, Redmond CK, Kavanah M, Cronin WM, Vogel V, Robidoux A, Dimitrov N, Atkins J, Daly M, Wieand S, Tan-Chiu E, Ford L, Wolmark N. Tamoxifen for prevention of breast cancer: report of the National Surgical Adjuvant Breast and Bowel Project P-1 Study. *J Natl Cancer Inst* (1998) 90, 1371–88.
5. Dobrydneva Y, Weatherman RV, Trebley JP, Morrell MM, Fitzgerald MC, Fichandler CE, Chatterjie N, Blackmore PF. Tamoxifen stimulates calcium entry into human platelets. *J Cardiovasc Pharmacol* (2007) 50, 380–90.
6. Rickles FR, Levine MN. Venous thromboembolism in malignancy and malignancy in venous thromboembolism. *Haemostasis* (1998) 28 (Suppl 3), 43–9.
7. Nolvadex D (Tamoxifen). AstraZeneca UK Ltd. UK Summary of product characteristics, June 2008.

Antineoplastics + Vaccines

The immune response of the body is suppressed by cytotoxic antineoplastics. The effectiveness of vaccines may be poor, and generalised infection may occur in patients immunised with live vaccines.

Clinical evidence, mechanism, importance and management

As cytotoxic antineoplastics are immunosuppressant, they reduce the response of the body to immunisation. A study[1] in 53 patients with Hodgkin's disease found that chemotherapy reduced the antibody response to a **pneumococcal vaccine** by 60% when measured 3 weeks after immunisation. The patients were taking **chlormethine** (mechlorethamine), **vincristine**, prednisone and **procarbazine**. A few of them had also been given **bleomycin, vinblastine** or **cyclophosphamide**. Subtotal radiotherapy reduced the response by a further 15%.

The response to **influenza immunisation** in children with various malignancies was also markedly suppressed by chemotherapy. The regimen included prednisone and the cytotoxic drugs **mercaptopurine, methotrexate**, and **vincristine**. Some of them were also given **dactinomycin** and **cyclophosphamide**.[2] In another study only 9 out of 17 children with leukaemia or other malignant diseases and taking **methotrexate, cyclophosphamide, mercaptopurine** and prednisone developed a significant response to immunisation with **inactivated measles vaccine**.[3]

Furthermore, immunisation with **live vaccines** may result in a potentially life-threatening infection. For example, a woman taking **methotrexate** 15 mg once a month for psoriasis developed a generalised vaccinial infection after vaccination against **smallpox**.[4] Studies in *animals* given **smallpox vaccine** confirmed that they were more susceptible to infection if they had been given **methotrexate, mercaptopurine** or **cyclophosphamide**.[5]

Live vaccines should not be given to patients who are receiving cytotoxics or other immunosuppressant antineoplastics. The UK Department of Health states that live vaccines should not be given during or within at least 6 months of treatment with immunosuppressive chemotherapy or radiotherapy for malignant disease.[6] Attenuated vaccines are also unlikely to be used during cytotoxic chemotherapy, but, bear in mind that they might have reduced efficacy if they have to be given.

1. Siber GR, Weitzman SA, Aisenberg AC, Weinstein HJ, Schiffman G. Impaired antibody response to pneumococcal vaccine after treatment for Hodgkins disease. *N Engl J Med* (1978) 299, 442–8.
2. Gross PA, Lee H, Wolff JA, Hall CB, Minnefore AB, Lazicki ME. Influenza immunization in immunosuppressed children. *J Pediatr* (1978) 92, 30–5.
3. Stiehm ER, Ablin A, Kushner JH, Zoger S. Measles vaccination in patients on immunosuppressive drugs. *Am J Dis Child* (1966) 111, 191–4.
4. Allison J. Methotrexate and smallpox vaccination. *Lancet* (1968) ii, 1250.
5. Rosenbaum EH, Cohen RA, Glatstein HR. Vaccination of a patient receiving immunosuppressive therapy for lymphosarcoma. *JAMA* (1966) 198, 737–40.
6. Department of Health. Immunisation Against Infectious Disease (updated 11th September 2013): "The Green Book". Available at: https://www.gov.uk/government/publications/green-book-the-complete-current-edition (accessed 25/09/13).

Antineoplastics; Cyclophosphamide + HIV-protease inhibitors

There is limited evidence that the incidence of chemotherapy-induced toxicities with antineoplastic regimens containing cyclophosphamide, doxorubicin, and either vincristine or etoposide, might be increased by the HIV-protease inhibitors; however, there is also limited evidence for a lack of increased toxicity. When given as part of CHOP, cyclophosphamide clearance might be slightly reduced by HIV-protease inhibitor-based therapy, whereas doxorubicin pharmacokinetics do not seem to be affected. Indinavir exposure appeared to be slightly increased by CHOP chemotherapy (cyclophosphamide, doxorubicin, and vincristine) in one study, but not in another.

Clinical evidence

(a) CDE

When compared with historical controls, the mucositis experienced by 12 patients who were given **saquinavir** and CDE (**cyclophosphamide, doxorubicin**, and **etoposide**) was more severe than **saquinavir** (grade 3 or 4, 67% versus 12%). However, the use of **saquinavir** was not associated with an effect on haematological toxicity (myelosuppression, neutropenia). All patients also received stavudine and 10 also received didanosine.[1]

In a retrospective study in 46 patients with HIV-associated non-Hodgkin's lymphoma who had been receiving CDE, the incidence of neutropenia and infection in 11 patients taking HIV-protease inhibitor-based antiretroviral treatment (not specifically named) was compared to 35 patients taking non-HIV-protease inhibitor-based regimens (mostly NNRTI-based). There was a higher incidence of infections requiring hospitalisation in the group taking a HIV-protease inhibitor than in the NNRTI-based treatment group (48% compared with 25%). There was a similar difference in the incidence of grade 4 neutropenia (54% compared with 38%), and day-10 and day-14 neutrophil counts were lower in patients receiving HIV-protease inhibitors, resulting in delays in giving chemotherapy in 16% of cycles (compared with 9% with NNRTIs). Overall, however, there was no difference in response rate, disease-free survival or overall survival between the two groups.[2]

Conversely, in an earlier study in 98 patients who had received CDE for HIV-associated non-Hodgkin's lymphoma, those patients receiving a HIV-protease inhibitor and two nucleoside analogues experienced less toxicity (including grade 4 neutropenia and infections) than the 43 patients who received didanosine alone (these were patients treated early on in the study, before combined antiretroviral regimens became accepted practice).[3]

(b) CHOP

When compared with historical controls, the clearance of cyclophosphamide, as part of CHOP (**cyclophosphamide, doxorubicin**, and **vincristine**) was about 35 to 40% lower in a study in patients taking stavudine, lamivudine, and **indinavir**. There was no appreciable difference in the clearance of doxorubicin. Excessive haematological toxicity was not noted when compared with historical controls.[4]

Conversely, in a retrospective study, there was a higher incidence of anaemia, a need for colony-stimulating factor support, and neurotoxicity in patients who were taking antiretrovirals (most including HIV-protease inhibitors) with CHOP, when compared with those receiving CHOP alone.[5] Nevertheless, in a subsequent crossover study by the same research group, no appreciable changes were noted in the pharmacokinetics of doxorubicin (given as part of CHOP) during a cycle when given with antiretrovirals, when compared with a cycle when no antiretrovirals were given. In addition, when analysed by the HIV-protease inhibitors given (**indinavir, nelfinavir**, or **saquinavir**) the pharmacokinetics of doxorubicin did not differ.[6]

When compared with historical controls, indinavir concentrations did not differ in patients taking CHOP in one study.[4] However, in a prospective study in 7 patients receiving **indinavir**-based antiretroviral therapy, the AUC of **indinavir** was 38% higher when they were receiving CHOP than when they were not (either before CHOP or 2 weeks after the last CHOP cycle). However, **indinavir** plasma concentrations with CHOP were the same as those expected from historical controls given indinavir alone, whereas the concentrations of **indinavir** given without CHOP were lower than expected. There was a trend towards higher **nelfinavir** plasma concentrations in 3 patients who also received CHOP when compared with **nelfinavir** alone.[7]

(c) Hyper-CVAD

In a study in patients with AIDS-associated Burkitt lymphoma or acute lymphoblastic leukaemia, the incidence of toxicity with the use of hyper-CVAD (**cyclophosphamide,**

dexamethasone, **doxorubicin**, and **vincristine**, alternating with **methotrexate** and **cytarabine**) given with antiretrovirals (including **amprenavir**, **indinavir**, **nelfinavir**, or **ritonavir**) was similar to that usually seen with this regimen when used in HIV-negative patients.[8]

Mechanism

Unknown. It has been speculated that HIV-protease inhibitors might reduce the metabolism or transport of antineoplastics by inhibiting cytochrome P450 isoenzymes or P-glycoprotein, and thereby increase the toxicity of chemotherapy.[2]

Importance and management

No interaction is established between antineoplastics and the HIV-protease inhibitors. None of these studies on the possible effect of HIV-protease inhibitors on the toxicity of CDE, CHOP, or hyper-CVAD were randomised prospective studies, therefore the findings are difficult to interpret, especially as they differ in whether they found toxicity to be increased or not, and which toxicities in particular were assessed. However, for a case of paralytic ileus attributed to vincristine (which is part of CHOP and hyper-CVAD) with HIV-protease inhibitors, see 'Vinca alkaloids + HIV-protease inhibitors', p.746. There is limited evidence that cyclophosphamide clearance might be slightly reduced by HIV-protease inhibitors, although the relevance of this is uncertain since no increase in toxicity was noted. In one prospective study, the pharmacokinetics of doxorubicin were not altered by HIV-protease inhibitors. In another, indinavir exposure appeared to be slightly increased by CHOP, but the increase seen was not clinically relevant.

1. Sparano JA, Wiernik PH, Hu X, Sarta C, Henry DH, Ratech H. Saquinavir enhances the mucosal toxicity of infusional cyclophosphamide, doxorubicin, and etoposide in patients with HIV-associated non-Hodgkin's lymphoma. *Med Oncol* (1998) 15, 50–7.
2. Bower M, McCall-Peat N, Ryan N, Davies L, Young AM, Gupta S, Nelson M, Gazzard B, Stebbing J. Protease inhibitors potentiate chemotherapy-induced neutropenia. *Blood* (2004) 104, 2943–46.
3. Sparano JA, Lee S, Chen MG, Nazeer T, Einzig A, Ambinder RF, Henry DH, Manalo J, Li T, Von Roenn JH. Phase II trial of infusional cyclophosphamide, doxorubicin, and etoposide in patients with HIV-associated Non-Hodgkin's lymphoma: an Eastern Cooperative Oncology Group trial (E1494). *J Clin Oncol* (2004) 22, 1491–1500.
4. Ratner L, Lee J, Tang S, Redden D, Hamzeh F, Herndier B, Scadden D, Kaplan L, Ambinder R, Levine A, Harrington W, Grochow L, Flexner C, Tan B, Straus D, for the AIDS malignancy consortium. Chemotherapy for human immunodeficiency virus–associated Non-Hodgkin's lymphoma in combination with highly active antiretroviral therapy. *J Clin Oncol* (2001) 19, 2171–8.
5. Vaccher E, Spina M, di Gennaro G, Talamini R, Nasti G, Schioppa O, Vultaggio G, Tirelli U. Concomitant cyclophosphamide, doxorubicin, vincristine, and prednisone chemotherapy plus highly active antiretroviral therapy in patients with human immunodeficiency virus-related, non-Hodgkin lymphoma. *Cancer* (2001) 91, 155–63.
6. Toffoli G, Corona G, Cattarossi G, Boiocchi M, Di Gennaro G, Tirelli U, Vaccher E. Effect of highly active antiretroviral therapy (HAART) on pharmacokinetics and pharmacodynamics of doxorubicin in patients with HIV-associated non-Hodgkin's lymphoma. *Ann Oncol* (2004) 15, 1805–9.
7. Cruciani M, Gatti G, Vaccher E, Di Gennaro G, Cinelli R, Bassetti M, Tirelli U, Bassetti D. Pharmacokinetic interaction between chemotherapy for non-Hodgkin's lymphoma and protease inhibitors in HIV-1-infected patients. *J Antimicrob Chemother* (2005) 55, 546–9.
8. Cortes J, Thomas D, Rios A, Koller C, O'Brien S, Jeha S, Faderi S, Kantarjian H. Hyperfractionated cyclophosphamide, vincristine, doxorubicin, and dexamethasone and highly active antiretroviral therapy for patients with acquired immunodeficiency syndrome-related Burkitt lymphoma/leukaemia. *Cancer* (2002) 94, 1492–9.

Aromatase inhibitors + Cimetidine

Cimetidine does not affect the pharmacokinetics of anastrozole or letrozole.

Clinical evidence, mechanism, importance and management

In a clinical study, cimetidine did not affect the pharmacokinetics of **anastrozole**.[1] This provides some evidence that **anastrozole** might not be affected by other drugs that inhibit cytochrome P450 isoenzymes,[2] although cimetidine is only a weak non-specific inhibitor of this enzyme system.

Similarly, in 17 healthy subjects the pharmacokinetics of a single 2.5-mg dose of **letrozole** were unchanged by cimetidine 400 mg every 12 hours.[3]

No pharmacokinetic interaction is anticipated if these aromatase inhibitors are used with cimetidine.

1. Zeneca. Data on file. Effect of cimetidine on anastrozole pharmacokinetics, 1995.
2. Arimidex Film-coated Tablets (Anastrozole). AstraZeneca UK Ltd. UK Summary of product characteristics, December 2010.
3. Morgan JM, Palmisano M, Spencer S, Hirschhorn W, Piraino AJ, Rackley RJ, Choi L. Pharmacokinetic effect of cimetidine on a single 2.5-mg dose of letrozole in healthy subjects. *J Clin Pharmacol* (1996) 36, 852.

Aromatase inhibitors + Food

Food increases the bioavailability of exemestane. Food does not affect the bioavailability of anastrozole or letrozole.

Clinical evidence, mechanism, importance and management

In a single-dose study in 12 healthy postmenopausal women, a high-fat meal increased the AUC of **exemestane** 25 mg by 40%. The maximum levels were increased by about 60%, but this change was not statistically significant. In addition, the pharmacodynamics of **exemestane** (estrone sulfate suppressant effect) were not affected.[1] In contrast, food had no effect on the AUC of **letrozole** in a study in healthy men, although food slightly decreased the rate of **letrozole** absorption.[2] Similarly, food had no effect on the extent of absorption (AUC) of **anastrozole**, although it delayed the time to the **anastrozole** maximum level from 2 hours to 5 hours.[3]

The effect of food on the absorption of exemestane is small. Nevertheless, the manufacturers recommend that exemestane is taken after a meal,[4,5] presumably to maximise its absorption. Anastrozole and letrozole absorption is not affected by food and therefore they may be taken with or without food.

1. Valle M, Di Salle E, Jannuzzo MG, Poggesi I, Rochetti M, Spinelli R, Verotta D. A predictive model for exemestane pharmacokinetics/pharmacodynamics incorporating the effect of food and formulation. *Br J Clin Pharmacol* (2005) 59, 355–64.
2. Sioufi A, Sandrenan N, Godbillon J, Trunet P, Czendlik C, Howald H, Pfister C, Ezzet F. Comparative bioavailability of letrozole under fed and fasting conditions in 12 healthy subjects after a 2.5 mg single oral administration. *Biopharm Drug Dispos* (1997) 18, 489–97.
3. Arimidex (Anastrozole). AstraZeneca Pharmaceuticals. US Prescribing information, April 2009.
4. Aromasin (Exemestane). Pharmacia Ltd. UK Summary of product characteristics, May 2009.
5. Aromasin (Exemestane). Pfizer. US Prescribing information, October 2008.

Aromatase inhibitors; Anastrozole + Miscellaneous

Quinapril does not affect anastrozole levels. Anastrozole does not appear to interact with risedronate. Anastrozole appears to have no effect on cytochrome P450 isoenzymes, so it is unlikely to interact with drugs that are substrates of this enzyme system.

Clinical evidence, mechanism, importance and management

(a) Phenazone (Antipyrine)

In a clinical interaction study anastrozole did not affect the pharmacokinetics of phenazone,[1] a non-specific marker of cytochrome P450 induction or inhibition. Along with *in vitro* data,[2] this suggests that anastrozole is unlikely to affect the metabolism of drugs that are substrates of this enzyme system.

(b) Quinapril

In a pharmacokinetic study, 10 elderly women with breast cancer were given anastrozole 1 mg daily for 10 weeks. Five of these subjects had hypertension and were also given quinapril for 28 days, starting after week 4. Quinapril did not affect plasma anastrozole levels and therefore anastrozole dose adjustment is not required during concurrent use.[3]

(c) Risedronate

The UK manufacturer of anastrozole notes that in clinical studies there was no evidence of any interaction between anastrozole and risedronate.[4]

1. Zeneca. Data on file. Effect of anastrozole treatment on antipyrine pharmacokinetics in postmenopausal female volunteers, 1995.
2. Grimm SW, Dyroff MC. Inhibition of human drug metabolizing cytochromes P450 by anastrozole, a potent and selective inhibitor of aromatase. *Drug Metab Dispos* (1997) 25, 598–602.
3. Repetto L, Vannozzi O, Hazini A, Sestini A, Pietropaolo M, Rosso R. Anastrozole and quinapril can be safely coadministered to elderly women with breast cancer and hypertension: a pharmacokinetic study. *Ann Oncol* (2003) 14, 1587–90.
4. Arimidex Film-coated Tablets (Anastrozole). AstraZeneca UK Ltd. UK Summary of product characteristics, December 2010.

Aromatase inhibitors; Exemestane + Celecoxib

Celecoxib does not alter the oestrogen-suppressant effect of exemestane, and possibly does not alter its pharmacokinetics.

Clinical evidence, mechanism, importance and management

A pharmacodynamic and limited pharmacokinetic analysis was carried out as part of a clinical study in which women with advanced breast cancer were randomised to receive exemestane 25 mg daily or exemestane 25 mg daily with celecoxib 400 mg twice daily. There appeared to be no difference in the pharmacokinetics of exemestane or its metabolite between the groups, although, because of a limited number of blood samples, this finding was not conclusive. There was no difference in inhibition of oestrogen synthesis between the two groups, suggesting that celecoxib does not alter the oestrogen-suppressant effect of exemestane.[1]

Celecoxib appears to have no adverse effect on the pharmacokinetics or pharmacodynamics of exemestane.

1. Dirix LY, Ignacio J, Nag S, Bapsy P, Gomez H, Raghunadharao D, Paridaens R, Jones S, Falcon S, Carpentieri M, Abbattista A, Lobelle JP. Treatment of advanced hormone-sensitive breast cancer in postmenopausal women with exemestane alone or in combination with celecoxib. *J Clin Oncol* (2008) 26, 1253–9.

Aromatase inhibitors; Exemestane + CYP3A4 inducers or inhibitors

Ketoconazole does not alter the pharmacokinetics of exemestane. Rifampicin, a potent enzyme inducer, reduces exemestane levels: other potent enzyme inducers are predicted to interact similarly.

Clinical evidence, mechanism, importance and management

(a) Ketoconazole

The manufacturers state that *in vitro* evidence shows that exemestane is metabolised by both CYP3A4 and aldoketoreductases,[1,2] followed by conjugation.[1] However, a clinical study found that ketoconazole (a specific inhibitor of CYP3A4) 200 mg daily for 6 days had no effect on the pharmacokinetics of a single 10-mg dose of exemestane.[3] This indicates that the metabolism of exemestane is unlikely to be altered by any CYP3A4 inhibitor.[1,2]

(b) Rifampicin (Rifampin)

In an interaction study, the potent enzyme inducer rifampicin, given at a dose of 600 mg daily for 14 days, reduced the AUC and maximum plasma levels of a single 25-mg dose of exemestane by 54% and 41%, respectively.[1,2] Rifampicin induces a number of enzymes, and the fact that ketoconazole (see above) did not interact with exemestane seems to suggest that rifampicin does not induce exemestane metabolism by CYP3A4.

The UK manufacturer states that the clinical relevance of the interaction between exemestane and rifampicin is unknown, but that exemestane efficacy may be reduced. However, the US manufacturer recommends that the dose of exemestane should be doubled to 50 mg daily in patients taking rifampicin, and they apply this recommendation to other *potent* CYP3A4 inducers, specifically naming **phenytoin**.[2] In addition the manufacturers advise caution on the concurrent use of exemestane and other CYP3A4 inducers, such as **carbamazepine**,[1,2] **phenobarbital**[2] and **St John's wort**.[1,2] For a list of CYP3A4 inducers, see 'Table 1.9', p.11. If the concurrent use of exemestane and a CYP3A4 inhibitor is necessary, it would seem prudent to monitor the patient more closely than normal, for signs or markers indicative of poor response or relapsing disease, and for toxicity if the exemestane dose is increased.

1. Aromasin (Exemestane). Pharmacia Ltd. UK Summary of product characteristics, May 2009.
2. Aromasin (Exemestane). Pfizer. US Prescribing information, October 2008.
3. Jannuzzo MG, Spinelli R, Poggesi I, Cicioni P, Böttiger Y, Bertilsson L. Inhibition of CYP3A4 does not influence Aromasin ® (exemestane, EXE) pharmacokinetics (PK) in healthy postmenopausal volunteers (HPV) (abstr 1184). *Eur J Cancer* (1999) 35 (Suppl 4), S294.

Bevacizumab + Miscellaneous

Bevacizumab did not alter the pharmacokinetics of capecitabine, cisplatin, interferon alfa-2a, irinotecan and its active metabolite, SN-38, or oxaliplatin. There might be an increased risk of congestive heart failure in patients receiving bevacizumab who have previously received cardiotoxic antineoplastics, such as the anthracyclines.

Clinical evidence, mechanism, importance and management

(a) Anthracyclines

A case report describes a patient who, after being given bevacizumab and capecitabine, developed severe cardiac failure. She had previously received two different courses of **epirubicin**-based chemotherapy, and also radiotherapy.[1]

Bevacizumab use alone can cause congestive heart failure, principally in patients with metastatic breast cancer, as in this case. The UK manufacturer of bevacizumab notes that the previous use of an anthracycline and/or chest radiation might be a risk factor.[2] Bear this possibility in mind when using bevacizumab. The relation of capecitabine to this case is unknown.

(b) Capecitabine

The UK manufacturer of bevacizumab states that in a study in patients with metastatic colorectal cancer given capecitabine with oxaliplatin, the pharmacokinetics of capecitabine were not significantly altered when bevacizumab was given.[2] For a case of heart failure in a patient receiving capecitabine and bevacizumab, see *Anthracyclines*, above.

(c) Interferon

Bevacizumab had no effect on the pharmacokinetics of interferon alfa-2a in patients with renal cancer.[2]

(d) Irinotecan and IFL

The UK and US manufacturers note that, in a specific drug interaction study, bevacizumab did not appear to significantly alter the pharmacokinetics of irinotecan and its active metabolite, SN-38.[2,3] However, the UK manufacturer of irinotecan states that bevacizumab appeared to increase the plasma concentration of SN-38, the active metabolite of irinotecan, by about 33% in patients who received bevacizumab with **irinotecan**, **fluorouracil**, and **folinic acid** (IFL), compared with IFL alone, but because there was a wide variability between patients, it is uncertain if this was due to bevacizumab. Nevertheless, more irinotecan dose reductions were needed in the bevacizumab recipients.[4] In addition, there was no difference in the clearance of bevacizumab when it was given with bolus IFL, when compared with its use alone.[2]

(e) Platinum compounds

The UK manufacturer of bevacizumab states that in a study in patients with metastatic colorectal cancer also given capecitabine the pharmacokinetics of **oxaliplatin** were not significantly altered when it was given with bevacizumab. In addition, the pharmacokinetics of **cisplatin** were not affected by bevacizumab in patients with lung cancer.[2]

1. Fraile Gil S, Hidalgo Correas FJ, Lara Álvarez MA, Garrote Martínez FJ. Insuficiencia cardiaca grave por bevacizumab en paciente tratado con antraciclinas. *Farm Hosp* (2007) 31, 256–7.
2. Avastin (Bevacizumab). Roche Products Ltd. UK Summary of product characteristics, February 2014.
3. Avastin (Bevacizumab). Genentech, Inc. US Prescribing information, July 2009.
4. Campto (Irinotecan hydrochloride trihydrate). Pfizer Ltd. UK Summary of product characteristics, May 2009.

Bevacizumab + Tyrosine kinase inhibitors

The pharmacokinetics of bevacizumab are not altered by the addition of axitinib. There does not appear to be any pharmacokinetic interaction between bevacizumab and erlotinib. The maximum tolerated doses of sorafenib and bevacizumab were lower when given together than when given alone, and unexpected toxicities occurred. A possible association between the use of bevacizumab with sunitinib and microangiopathic haemolytic anaemia has been suggested.

Clinical evidence, mechanism, importance and management

(a) Axitinib

In a phase I study, patients with metastatic colorectal cancer and other solid tumours were given axitinib (starting at a dose of 5 mg twice daily on day 3) and FOLFOX (fluorouracil, folinic acid, oxaliplatin), with or without bevacizumab (1, 2, or 5 mg/kg) every 2 weeks. The pharmacokinetics of bevacizumab were not altered by the addition of axitinib.[1] No dose limiting toxicities were noted when bevacizumab 2 mg/kg was given concurrently with axitinib, but hypertension, resulting in an inability to resume bevacizumab within 14 days of treatment interruption, was seen in 2 of the 4 patients receiving the 5 mg/kg dose.

(b) Erlotinib

In a pharmacokinetic study, patients with recurrent non-small cell lung cancer were given erlotinib (100 or 150 mg once daily) with bevacizumab (7.5 or 15 mg/kg on day 1 of each 21-day cycle). The pharmacokinetics of both drugs when given concurrently were similar to historical data for both drugs when given alone.[2] Although less conclusive than a direct comparative study, this suggests that no pharmacokinetic interaction occurs between erlotinib and bevacizumab.

(c) Sorafenib

In a dose-finding study, the maximum tolerated doses of sorafenib and bevacizumab were lower when they were given together compared with either drug alone. Unexpectedly severe toxicity was seen, in particular hypertension, proteinuria, and thrombocytopenia. Three-quarters of patients required a further reduction in their sorafenib dose, to 200 mg daily.[3]

(d) Sunitinib

In a phase I study of bevacizumab 10 mg/kg with escalating doses of sunitinib in patients with metastatic renal cell carcinoma, 5 out of 12 patients receiving sunitinib 50 mg daily developed microangiopathic haemolytic anaemia.[4] The UK manufacturer of bevacizumab also reports that in two studies in patients with metastatic renal carcinoma [one of which might be that described earlier], 7 of 19 patients given bevacizumab 10 mg/kg every 2 weeks and sunitinib 50 mg daily developed microangiopathic haemolytic anaemia, which was reversible upon discontinuation of bevacizumab and sunitinib.[5] It is unclear whether this was related to an interaction between the two drugs, or an adverse effect of either drug alone. Note that a subsequent phase I study in patients with advanced solid tumours given sunitinib and bevacizumab at similar doses, did not observe any clinical or laboratory signs of microangiopathic haemolytic anaemia.[6] Nevertheless, bear the possibility of this effect in mind if these two drugs are used together.

1. Sharma S, Abhyankar V, Burgess RE, Infante J, Trowbridge RC, Tarazi J, Kim S, Tortorici M, Chen Y, Robles RL. A phase I study of axitinib (AG-013736) in combination with bevacizumab plus chemotherapy or chemotherapy alone in patients with metastatic colorectal cancer and other solid tumors. *Ann Oncol* (2010) 21, 297–304.
2. Herbst RS, Johnson DH, Mininberg E, Carbone DP, Henderson T, Kim ES, Blumenschein G, Lee JJ, Liu DD, Truong MT, Hong WK, Tran H, Tsao A, Xie D, Ramies DA, Mass R, Seshagiri S, Eberhard DA, Kelley SK, Sandler A. Phase I/II trial evaluating the anti-vascular endothelial growth factor monoclonal antibody bevacizumab in combination with the HER-1/epidermal growth factor receptor tyrosine kinase inhibitor erlotinib for patients with recurrent non-small-cell lung cancer. *J Clin Oncol* (2005) 23, 2544–55.
3. Azad NS, Posadas EM, Kwitkowski VE, Steinberg SM, Jain L, Annunziata CM, Minasian L, Sarosy G, Kotz HL, Premkumar A, Cao L, McNally D, Chow C, Chen HX, Wright JJ, Figg WD, Kohn EC. Combination targeted therapy with sorafenib and bevacizumab results in enhanced toxicity and antitumor activity. *J Clin Oncol* (2008) 26, 3709–14.
4. Feldman DR, Baum MS, Ginsberg MS, Hassoun H, Flombaum CD, Velasco S, Fischer P, Ronnen E, Ishill N, Patil S, Motzer RJ. Phase I trial of bevacizumab plus escalated doses of sunitinib in patients with metastatic renal cell carcinoma. *J Clin Oncol* (2009) 27, 1432–9.
5. Avastin (Bevacizumab). Roche Products Ltd. UK Summary of product characteristics, February 2014.
6. Rini BI, Garcia JA, Cooney MM, Elson P, Tyler A, Beatty K, Bokar J, Mekhail T, Bukowski RM, Budd GT, Triozzi P, Borden E, Ivy P, Chen HX, Dowlati A, Dreicer R. A phase I study of sunitinib plus bevacizumab in advanced solid tumors. *Clin Cancer Res* (2009) 15, 6277–83.

Bexarotene + Antineoplastics

Carboplatin with paclitaxel appears to increase bexarotene exposure, whereas cisplatin with vinorelbine has no effect. Bexarotene might cause a negligible decrease in paclitaxel exposure, and has no appreciable effect on carboplatin, cisplatin, or vinorelbine exposure.

Clinical evidence, mechanism, importance and management

(a) Carboplatin with Paclitaxel

In a phase I pharmacokinetic study in 16 patients with non-small cell lung cancer, continuous use of oral bexarotene 400 mg/m^2 daily, with paclitaxel 200 mg/m^2 and carboplatin (dosed to achieve an AUC of 6 mg/min/mL) once every three weeks, increased the AUC of bexarotene almost 2-fold, when compared with bexarotene given alone. The AUC of paclitaxel was decreased by just 19%, which was not statistically significant, and there was no change in the AUC of free or total carboplatin.[1]

The decrease in paclitaxel exposure by bexarotene was negligible. Nevertheless, the US manufacturer of bexarotene considers that this interaction suggests that bexarotene is an inducer of CYP3A4.[2] For further limited evidence which also appears to suggest that bexarotene might induce CYP3A4 and increases the metabolism of efavirenz and atorvastatin, see 'Bexarotene + Efavirenz and other enzyme inducers', below, and 'Statins + Bexarotene', p.1324, respectively.

The mechanism for the increase in bexarotene exposure with carboplatin and paclitaxel is unknown. Despite the increase in bexarotene exposure, there was no evidence for increased drug-related toxicity on concurrent use.[1] Nevertheless, some caution would seem prudent until more experience is gained.

(b) Cisplatin with Vinorelbine

In a phase I pharmacokinetic study in patients with lung cancer, continuous use of bexarotene 400 mg/m² daily with vinorelbine 25 mg/m² weekly and cisplatin 100 mg/m² every 4 weeks had no appreciable effect on the AUC of vinorelbine or cisplatin. In addition, there was no evidence of altered bexarotene concentrations, and no evidence of increased toxicity.[3] No dose adjustment of these drugs is therefore necessary on concurrent use.

1. Rodon J, Jacobs CD, Chu Q, Rowinsky EK, Lopez-Anaya A, Takimoto CH, Wakelee HA. A phase I pharmacokinetic study of bexarotene with paclitaxel and carboplatin in patients with advanced non-small cell lung cancer (NSCLC). *Cancer Chemother Pharmacol* (2012) 69, 825–34.
2. Targretin Capsules (Bexarotene). Eisai Inc. US Prescribing information, November 2011.
3. Wakelee HA, Middleton G, Dunlop D, Ramlau R, Leighl N, Hao D, Lopez-Anaya A, Zatloukal P, Jacobs CD. A phase I pharmacokinetic study of bexarotene with vinorelbine and cisplatin in patients with advanced non-small-cell lung cancer (NSCLC). *Cancer Chemother Pharmacol* (2012) 69, 815–24.

Bexarotene + Efavirenz and other enzyme inducers

A single case of low bexarotene exposure with partial efficacy, and also subtherapeutic efavirenz concentrations and virological failure, occurred when oral bexarotene was started in a patient taking efavirenz. Other enzyme inducers (such as phenytoin, phenobarbital, and rifampicin (rifampin)) might possibly reduce bexarotene exposure.

Clinical evidence

A patient with HIV-infection stable taking efavirenz 400 mg daily with abacavir and lamivudine, was given oral bexarotene 300 mg daily for an acute exacerbation of mycosis fungoides. Two months later his plasma HIV RNA count had increased from below 50 copies/mL (at the time of starting bexarotene) to 120 copies/mL, indicating virological failure. Efavirenz concentrations were checked, and had become subtherapeutic. The efavirenz dose was increased to 600 mg daily then to 800 mg daily to achieve therapeutic concentrations. At the same time, bexarotene concentrations were only about half that expected from historical data, and bexarotene was only partially effective.[1]

Mechanism

In vitro data indicate that bexarotene is metabolised by CYP3A4 and might be a CYP3A4 inducer.[2] Efavirenz is partially metabolised by CYP3A4 and is a known enzyme inducer. It is possible that efavirenz induced the metabolism of bexarotene and that bexarotene induced the metabolism of efavirenz, leading to reduced efficacy of both drugs. However, due to a lack of an effect of the CYP3A4 *inhibitor* ketoconazole on bexarotene (see 'Bexarotene + Ketoconazole and other CYP3A4 inhibitors', p.662), it is possible that efavirenz induces bexarotene metabolism by another mechanism.

Importance and management

Evidence for a pharmacokinetic interaction between bexarotene and efavirenz is limited to this one case. However, the effect is as might be predicted. It would be prudent to closely monitor the efficacy and plasma concentrations of both efavirenz and bexarotene if oral bexarotene is given to any patient taking efavirenz.

The UK manufacturer states that there is a theoretical risk that other CYP3A4 inducers might increase the metabolism of bexarotene and reduce its concentrations, and they name **dexamethasone**, **phenytoin** [and therefore probably **fosphenytoin**], **phenobarbital** [and therefore probably **primidone**], and **rifampicin** (**rifampin**).[3] However, the US manufacturer of bexarotene notes that the lack of an interaction with the potent CYP3A4 *inhibitor* ketoconazole suggests that bexarotene is not substantially metabolised by CYP3A4, and they state that the effects of other CYP3A4 inducers on bexarotene have not been studied.[2] Therefore further study on the effects of other CYP3A4 inducers is needed. In addition, note, that **dexamethasone** does not usually cause a clinically relevant interaction by this mechanism.

The US manufacturer states that although no formal drug interaction studies have been carried out with topical bexarotene, drugs that affect CYP3A4 might alter its disposition. However, they state that the overall systemic exposure to bexarotene from low to moderate intensity regimens is low,[4],and so a clinically relevant interaction seems unlikely.

1. Desnoyer A, Kaied FA, Descamps D, Yeni P, Descamps V, Le Beller C, Peytavin G. Deleterious pharmacokinetic interaction between bexarotene and efavirenz. *AIDS* (2010) 24, 22968.
2. Targretin Capsules (Bexarotene). Eisai Inc. US Prescribing information, November 2011.
3. Targretin Capsules (Bexarotene). Eisai Ltd. UK Summary of product characteristics, April 2009.
4. Targretin Gel (Bexarotene). Eisai Inc. US Prescribing information, April 2010.

Bexarotene + Fibrates; Gemfibrozil

Gemfibrozil appears to increase the plasma concentration of bexarotene.

Clinical evidence, mechanism, importance and management

A population analysis of patients with cutaneous T-cell lymphoma found that the concurrent use of **gemfibrozil** in 3 patients substantially increased the plasma concentrations of oral bexarotene, and caused dose-limiting hypertriglyceridaemia. The reasons for this effect are unknown, although it was suggested that inhibition of CYP3A4 by **gemfibrozil** might be partially responsible,[1] but note that gemfibrozil is not generally recognised as an inhibitor of this isoenzyme (it is an inhibitor of CYP2C8 and of some transporter proteins including OATP). The UK and US manufacturers of bexarotene state that the concurrent use of **gemfibrozil** with oral bexarotene is not recommended.[2,3]

The US manufacturer of topical bexarotene states that, due to its low systemic exposure, any increases in concentration that occur with gemfibrozil are unlikely to be sufficient to result in adverse effects with a low to moderate intensity topical bexarotene regimen.[4]

1. Talpur R, Ward S, Apisarnthanarax N, Breuer-McHam J, Duvic M. Optimizing bexarotene therapy for cutaneous T-cell lymphoma. *J Am Acad Dermatol* (2002) 47, 672–84.
2. Targretin Capsules (Bexarotene). Eisai Ltd. UK Summary of product characteristics, April 2009.
3. Targretin Capsules (Bexarotene). Eisai Inc. US Prescribing information, November 2011.
4. Targretin Gel (Bexarotene). Eisai Inc. US Prescribing information, April 2010.

Bexarotene + Ketoconazole and other CYP3A4 inhibitors

Ketoconazole does not appear to alter the plasma concentration of oral bexarotene.

Clinical evidence, mechanism, importance and management

In vitro, bexarotene is metabolised by CYP3A4, therefore the manufacturers state that there is a theoretical risk that drugs that inhibit CYP3A4 might increase the plasma concentration of oral bexarotene. They name **clarithromycin**, **erythromycin**, **itraconazole**, **ketoconazole**, the **HIV-protease inhibitors**, and **grapefruit juice**.[1,2] However, the US manufacturer briefly notes that concurrent administration of oral bexarotene with multiple-dose **ketoconazole** did not alter bexarotene plasma concentrations. This suggests that, clinically, bexarotene elimination after oral administration is not substantially dependent on CYP3A4 metabolism.[2] No bexarotene dose adjustment would therefore be expected to be needed when taken with CYP3A4 inhibitors such as ketoconazole.

The US manufacturer of topical bexarotene states that, due to its low systemic exposure, any increases in concentration that occur with CYP3A4 inhibitors are unlikely to be sufficient to result in adverse effects with a low- to moderate-intensity topical bexarotene regimen.[3]

1. Targretin Capsules (Bexarotene). Eisai Ltd. UK Summary of product characteristics, April 2009.
2. Targretin Capsules (Bexarotene). Eisai Inc. US Prescribing information, November 2011.
3. Targretin Gel (Bexarotene). Eisai Inc. US Prescribing information, April 2010.

Bexarotene + Miscellaneous

Bexarotene might reduce the concentrations of hormonal contraceptives. Increased blood glucose-lowering effects might occur with insulin or oral antidiabetic drugs. Food increases the oral absorption of bexarotene. No interaction seems to occur between bexarotene and levothyroxine.

Systemic drug interactions are unlikely to occur with topical bexarotene; however, it might increase the toxicity of topical diethyltoluamide (DEET).

Clinical evidence, mechanism, importance and management

(a) Antidiabetic drugs

The UK and US manufacturers state that, although no cases of hypoglycaemia have been seen with bexarotene monotherapy, because of the known mode of action of bexarotene, it should be used with caution if given with **insulin** or drugs that enhance insulin secretion (e.g. **sulfonylureas**) or insulin sensitisers (e.g. **thiazolidinediones**) as it might potentiate the action of these drugs leading to hypoglycaemia.[1,2] For a list of these drugs see 'Table 13.1', p.497.

(b) Diethyltoluamide (DEET)

The US manufacturer advises that patients using topical bexarotene should avoid the concurrent use of insect repellents containing diethyltoluamide because *animal* studies have shown increased diethyltoluamide toxicity.[3]

(c) Food

Oral administration of bexarotene 75 to 300 mg with a fat-containing meal resulted in an increase in the AUC and maximum plasma concentration of bexarotene of 35% and 48%, respectively, when compared with administration with a glucose solution.[1] It is therefore recommended that bexarotene capsules are taken with food.[1,2]

(d) Hormonal contraceptives

The US manufacturer states that bexarotene might induce CYP3A4,[2] and that it might theoretically increase the metabolism of other substances metabolised by CYP3A4, such as oral or other systemic hormonal contraceptives, thereby reducing both their serum concentrations and their efficacy.[1,2] For this reason and because bexarotene is teratogenic, the UK and US manufacturers advise the use of additional non-hormonal contraception (e.g. a barrier method) during, and for at least one month after stopping, bexarotene to avoid the risk of contraceptive failure.[1,2]

For limited evidence which also appears to suggest that bexarotene might induce CYP3A4, see 'Bexarotene + Efavirenz and other enzyme inducers', p.662, and 'Statins + Bexarotene', p.1324, respectively.

(e) Levothyroxine

The UK manufacturer briefly notes that population analysis suggests that bexarotene concentrations are not affected by levothyroxine. Note that changes in thyroid function, in particular hypothyroidism, caused by bexarotene are common, and have been successfully treated with **thyroid hormones**.[1,2]

(f) Tamoxifen

The US manufacturer notes that, based on interim data, oral bexarotene reduced the plasma concentration of tamoxifen by about 35%.[2] They state that this suggests that bexarotene might possibly induce CYP3A4. For this reason, the manufacturers advise caution on the concurrent use of bexarotene and tamoxifen.[1,2]

For limited evidence which also appears to suggest that bexarotene might induce CYP3A4, see 'Bexarotene + Efavirenz and other enzyme inducers', p.662, and 'Statins + Bexarotene', p.1324, respectively.

(g) Vitamin A (Retinol)

The UK and US manufacturers recommend that because bexarotene is related to vitamin A, any vitamin A supplements should be limited to 15 000 units or less daily to avoid potentially additive toxic effects.[1-3]

1. Targretin Capsules (Bexarotene). Eisai Ltd. UK Summary of product characteristics, April 2009.
2. Targretin Capsules (Bexarotene). Eisai Inc. US Prescribing information, November 2011.
3. Targretin Gel (Bexarotene). Eisai Inc. US Prescribing information, April 2010.

Bicalutamide + CYP3A4 inhibitors or substrates

Bicalutamide causes a slight increase in the AUC of midazolam suggesting that it is a weak inhibitor of CYP3A4. Nevertheless, it is predicted to affect the levels of a number of CYP3A4 substrates (e.g. ciclosporin). Theoretically, CYP3A4 inhibitors might increase bicalutamide levels, but there is no evidence of this.

Clinical evidence, mechanism, importance and management

(a) CYP3A4 inhibitors

Bicalutamide is extensively metabolised by the cytochrome P450 enzyme system, possibly by CYP3A4.[1] Although there are no specific data, the manufacturer advises caution when bicalutamide is given with other drugs that may inhibit drug oxidation as bicalutamide plasma levels may be increased, which could increase the risk of adverse effects. They specifically name **cimetidine** and **ketoconazole**.[2] However, steady-state levels of bicalutamide are known to vary up to about 15-fold[1], and so enzyme inhibition resulting in an increase in bicalutamide levels seems unlikely to result in adverse effects in most patients. In particular, any effect of a weak CYP3A4 inhibitor, such as **cimetidine**, is therefore very unlikely to be clinically relevant. There does not appear to be any published evidence of any interactions of bicalutamide with drugs that are known CYP3A4 inhibitors.

(b) CYP3A4 substrates

In vitro, the active isomer of bicalutamide is an inhibitor of various cytochrome P450 isoenzymes, particularly CYP3A4. In an early 12-week study with **phenazone** (antipyrine), there were only minor changes in **phenazone** pharmacokinetics (half-life reduced by 16% with bicalutamide 50 mg, AUC reduced by 19% with bicalutamide 150 mg). **Phenazone** was used as an investigational marker of enzyme induction or inhibition and this study therefore suggests that, clinically, bicalutamide has little effect on the cytochrome P450 system.[3]

In a further study, a single oral dose of **midazolam** was given to men who had been randomised to receive bicalutamide 150 mg twice daily or placebo at least 3 months previously.[1] The mean AUC of **midazolam** was 27% higher, with a maximum increase of 92% in the bicalutamide recipients, although this difference was not statistically significant. In addition, the sedative effects of **midazolam** were not increased.[1] The manufacturer briefly notes that the mean **midazolam** AUC may be increased by 90%[4] or up to 80%[2] when bicalutamide is given for 28 days. **Midazolam** is used as a probe substrate to assess the effects of a drug on CYP3A4, and this information therefore suggests that, clinically, bicalutamide is only a weak CYP3A4 inhibitor, and is unlikely to cause clinically relevant interactions with substrates of this isoenzyme. Nevertheless, the UK manufacturer suggests that an interaction might occur with drugs that have a narrow therapeutic range, and advise caution when bicalutamide is given with **ciclosporin**, suggesting that plasma concentrations of **ciclosporin** should be monitored closely both during and after concurrent use. They also advise caution with the **calcium-channel blockers**.[2] The US manufacturer[4] simply advises caution with drugs that are CYP3A4 substrates. There does not appear to be any published evidence of any adverse interactions of bicalutamide with any drugs that are CYP3A4 substrates.

1. Cockshott ID. Bicalutamide: clinical pharmacokinetics and metabolism. *Clin Pharmacokinet* (2004) 43, 855–78.
2. Casodex 50 mg Film-coated Tablets (Bicalutamide). AstraZeneca UK Ltd. UK Summary of product characteristics, January 2011.
3. Kaisary A, Klarskov P, McKillop D. Absence of hepatic enzyme induction in prostate cancer patients receiving 'Casodex' (bicalutamide). *Anticancer Drugs* (1996) 7, 54–9.
4. Casodex (Bicalutamide). AstraZeneca. US Prescribing information, November 2009.

Bicalutamide + Food

In a study in 15 healthy subjects, there was no clinically relevant difference in bicalutamide pharmacokinetics when a single 50-mg dose of bicalutamide was taken after an overnight fast or after a high-fat cooked breakfast.[1] Bicalutamide can therefore be taken with or without meals.

1. Cockshott ID, Oliver SD, Young JJ, Cooper KJ, Jones DC. The effect of food on the pharmacokinetics of the bicalutamide ('Casodex') enantiomers. *Biopharm Drug Dispos* (1997) 18, 499–507.

Bicalutamide + Tamoxifen and related drugs

Tamoxifen and anastrozole do not appear to alter bicalutamide levels.

Clinical evidence, mechanism, importance and management

The mean trough levels of *R*- and *S*-bicalutamide did not differ between 7 men taking bicalutamide 150 mg daily alone and men also taking tamoxifen 20 mg daily (7 subjects) or anastrozole 1 mg daily (7 subjects). The plasma levels of tamoxifen and anastrozole were similar to those usually seen. The findings of this small study suggest that tamoxifen and anastrozole do not have a marked effect on bicalutamide pharmacokinetics, although a more minor effect cannot be ruled out.[1]

1. Boccardo F, Rubagotti A, Conti G, Potenzoni D, Manganelli A, Del Monaco D. Exploratory study of drug plasma levels during bicalutamide 150 mg therapy co-administered with tamoxifen or anastrozole for prophylaxis of gynecomastia and breast pain in men with prostate cancer. *Cancer Chemother Pharmacol* (2005) 56, 415–20.

Bleomycin + Brentuximab vedotin

Concurrent use of bleomycin with brentuximab vedotin might increase the risk of pulmonary toxicity.

Clinical evidence, mechanism, importance and management

In a clinical study in patients with Hodgkin's lymphoma, given brentuximab vedotin with bleomycin (as part of a combination regimen), cough and dyspnoea were reported as a result of interstitial infiltration and inflammation. The UK and US manufacturers therefore state that concurrent use of bleomycin with brentuximab vedotin is contraindicated.[1,2]

1. Adcetris (Brentuximab vedotin). Takeda UK Ltd. UK Summary of product characteristics, March 2015.
2. Adcetris (Brentuximab vedotin). Seattle Genetics Inc. US Prescribing information, February 2015.

Bleomycin + Cisplatin

Cisplatin can increase the pulmonary toxicity of bleomycin by reducing its renal excretion. Digital ischaemia and arterial thrombosis have also been described in patients receiving both drugs.

Clinical evidence

Thirty patients with carcinoma of the cervix and 15 patients with germ cell tumours were given combination chemotherapy including bleomycin and cisplatin. Cisplatin was given by infusion on day one, followed by bleomycin given intramuscularly every 12 hours for 4 days or by continuous infusion over 72 hours. Nine of the patients with normal renal function and no previous pulmonary disease developed serious pulmonary toxicity and 6 died from respiratory failure.[1]

In a study of 18 patients given cisplatin and bleomycin for the treatment of disseminated testicular non-seminoma, 2 patients developed pneumonitis, and it was found that the cisplatin-induced reduction in renal function was paralleled by an increase in bleomycin-induced pulmonary toxicity.[2] Similar results were found by the same group in a much larger study of 54 patients.[3] A study in 2 children found that the total plasma clearance of bleomycin was halved (from 39 to 18 mL/minute/m^2) when they were also given cisplatin in cumulative doses exceeding 300 mg/m^2. The renal clearance in one of the children fell by 73% (from 30 to 8.2 mL/minute/m^2) although there was no evidence of severe bleomycin toxicity in either child.[4] Two cases of fatal bleomycin toxicity have been described in patients with cisplatin-induced renal impairment.[5,6]

A case report describes arterial thrombosis associated with pathological vascular changes in the arteries of a man receiving cisplatin, bleomycin and etoposide.[7] Another man developed fatal thrombotic microangiopathy (characterised by microangiopathic haemolytic anaemia, thrombocytopenia, renal impairment), which was attributed to the use of bleomycin and cisplatin.[8]

In an earlier study, digital ischaemia occurred in 41% of patients given cisplatin, bleomycin and vinblastine, compared with 21% of patients given only cisplatin and vinblastine.[9]

Mechanism

Renal excretion accounts for almost half of the total body clearance of bleomycin. Cisplatin is nephrotoxic and reduces the glomerular filtration rate so that the clearance of bleomycin is reduced. The accumulating bleomycin apparently causes the pulmonary toxicity.

Importance and management

Pulmonary toxicity with bleomycin and cisplatin is an established reaction with a potentially serious, sometimes fatal, outcome. Concurrent use should be very closely monitored and renal function checked. One of the problems is that levels of creatinine may not accurately indicate the extent of renal damage both during and after cisplatin treatment. The renal toxicity of cisplatin may also develop rapidly. Other toxic effects on the vascular system can also occur.

1. Rabinowits M, Souhami L, Gil RA, Andrade CAV, Paiva HC. Increased pulmonary toxicity with bleomycin and cisplatin chemotherapy combinations. *Am J Clin Oncol* (1990) 13, 132–8.
2. van Barneveld PWC, Sleijfer D Th, van der Mark Th W, Mulder NH, Donker AJM, Meijer S, Schraffordt Koops H, Sluiter HJ, Peset R. Influence of platinum-induced renal toxicity on bleomycin-induced pulmonary toxicity in patients with disseminated testicular carcinoma. *Oncology* (1984) 41, 4–7.
3. Sleijfer S, van der Mark TW, Schraffordt Koops H, Mulder NH. Enhanced effects of bleomycin on pulmonary function disturbances in patients with decreased renal function due to cisplatin. *Eur J Cancer* (1996) 32A, 550–2.
4. Yee GC, Crom WR, Champion JE, Brodeur GM, Evans WE. Cisplatin-induced changes in bleomycin elimination. *Cancer Treat Rep* (1983) 67, 587–9.
5. Bennett WM, Pastore L, Houghton DC. Fatal pulmonary bleomycin toxicity in cisplatin-induced acute renal failure. *Cancer Treat Rep* (1980) 64, 921–4.
6. Perry DJ, Weiss RB, Taylor HG. Enhanced bleomycin toxicity during acute renal failure. *Cancer Treat Rep* (1982) 66, 592–3.
7. Garstin IWH, Cooper GG, Hood JM. Arterial thrombosis after treatment with bleomycin and cisplatin. *BMJ* (1990) 300, 1018.
8. Fields SM, Lindley CM. Thrombotic microangiopathy associated with chemotherapy: case report and review of the literature. *DICP Ann Pharmacother* (1989) 23, 582–8.
9. Vogelzang NJ, Bosl GJ, Johnson K, Kennedy BJ. Raynaud's phenomenon : a common toxicity after combination chemotherapy for testicular cancer. *Ann Intern Med* (1981) 95, 288–92.

Bleomycin + Colony-stimulating factors

The concurrent use of granulocyte colony-stimulating factor or granulocyte-macrophage colony-stimulating factor has been linked with an increased occurrence of bleomycin-induced pulmonary toxicity.

Clinical evidence, mechanism, importance and management

Pulmonary toxicity that developed at low cumulative bleomycin doses (70 to 130 units/m^2) in at least 3 of 5 patients given standard ABVD treatment (doxorubicin, bleomycin, vinblastine, and dacarbazine) was attributed by the author of the report to the synergistic action of the concurrent use of **G-CSF** (granulocyte colony-stimulating factor).[1] In another report 8 out of 40 patients with malignant non-Hodgkin's lymphoma given **G-CSF** developed drug-induced pneumonia. Three of these patients were given chemotherapy regimens including bleomycin (MACOB-B, COP-BLAM III), and all 3 died of respiratory failure. None of 35 other patients, similarly treated but without **G-CSF**, developed pneumonia.[2] Non-infectious interstitial pneumonitis developed in a patient given doxorubicin, cyclophosphamide, bleomycin, vinblastine, methotrexate and prednisone with **GM-CSF** (granulocyte-macrophage colony-stimulating factor).[3] Five further reports have identified a total of 23 other patients who developed bleomycin-pulmonary toxicity probably potentiated by **G-CSF** or **GM-CSF**, including at least 7 fatalities.[4-8]

In contrast, analysis of two placebo-controlled studies of the use of adjuvant **G-CSF (filgrastim** or **lenograstim)** with combination chemotherapy including bleomycin found no evidence of an increase in pulmonary complications. Overall 7 of 139 patients given placebo and 9 of 139 given **G-CSF** had pulmonary complications possibly related to bleomycin.[9,10] Similarly, another retrospective analysis found that 34% of patients given bleomycin and **G-CSF** developed pulmonary toxicity, compared with 33% of those given bleomycin alone.[11]

These interactions are not firmly established, but good pulmonary function monitoring appears to be advisable when colony-stimulating factors are used with antineoplastics causing pulmonary toxicity, such as bleomycin. If interstitial pneumonia occurs, the drugs should be discontinued and high-dose corticosteroids started immediately.[7]

1. Matthews JH. Pulmonary toxicity of ABVD chemotherapy and G-CSF in Hodgkin's disease: possible synergy. *Lancet* (1993) 342, 988.
2. Iki S, Yoshinaga K, Ohbayashi Y, Urabe A. Cytotoxic drug-induced pneumonia and possible augmentation by G-CSF — clinical attention. *Ann Hematol* (1993) 66, 217–18.
3. Philippe B, Couderc LJ, Balloul-Delclaux E, Janvier M, Caubarrere I. Pulmonary toxicity of chemotherapy and GM-CSF. *Respir Med* (1994) 88, 715.
4. Dirix LY, Schrijvers D, Druwè P, Van Den Brande J, Verhoeven D, Van Oosterom AT. Pulmonary toxicity and bleomycin. *Lancet* (1994) 344, 56.
5. Lei KIK, Leung WT, Johnson PJ. Serious pulmonary complications in patients receiving recombinant granulocyte colony-stimulating factor during BACOP chemotherapy for aggressive non-Hodgkin's lymphoma. *Br J Cancer* (1994) 70, 1009–13.
6. Katoh M, Shikoshi K, Takada M, Umeda M, Tsukahara T, Kitagawa S, Shirai T. Development of interstitial pneumonitis during treatment with granulocyte colony-stimulating factor. *Ann Hematol* (1993) 67, 201–2.
7. Niitsu N, Iki S, Muroi K, Motomura S, Murakami M, Takeyama H, Ohsaka A, Urabe A. Interstitial pneumonia in patients receiving granulocyte colony-stimulating factor during chemotherapy: survey in Japan 1991–96. *Br J Cancer* (1997) 76, 1661–6.
8. Couderc L-J, Stelianides S, Franchon I, Stern M, Epardeau B, Baumelou E, Caubarrere I, Hermine O. Pulmonary toxicity of chemotherapy and G/GM-CSF: a report of five cases. *Respir Med* (1999) 93, 65–8.
9. Bastion Y, Reyes F, Bosly A, Gisselbrecht C, Yver A, Gilles E, Maral J, Coiffier B. Possible toxicity with the association of G-CSF and bleomycin. *Lancet* (1994) 343, 1221–2.
10. Bastion Y, Coiffier B. Pulmonary toxicity of bleomycin: is G-CSF a risk factor? *Lancet* (1994) 344, 474.
11. Saxman SB, Nichols CR, Einhorn LH. Pulmonary toxicity in patients with advanced-stage germ cell tumors receiving bleomycin with and without granulocyte colony stimulating factor. *Chest* (1997) 111, 657–60.

Bleomycin + Oxygen

Serious and potentially fatal pulmonary toxicity can develop in patients given bleomycin who are exposed to conventional oxygen concentrations during anaesthesia.

Clinical evidence

Five patients given bleomycin, exposed to oxygen concentrations of 35 to 42% during and immediately following anaesthesia, developed a severe respiratory distress syndrome and died. Bleomycin-induced pneumonitis and lung fibrosis were diagnosed at post-mortem. Another group of 12 matched patients who underwent the same procedures but with lower oxygen concentrations (22 to 25%) had an uneventful postoperative course.[1]

Another comparative study[2] similarly demonstrated that adult respiratory distress syndrome (ARDS) in patients receiving bleomycin was reduced by a technique allowing the use of lower oxygen concentrations of 22 to 30%. Bleomycin-induced pulmonary toxicity, apparently related to oxygen concentrations, has also been described in other case reports.[3-7] Studies in *animals* have also confirmed that the severity of bleomycin-induced pulmonary toxicity is increased by oxygen.[8-10] However, in two other series of patients given bleomycin and undergoing surgery there was no obvious increase in pulmonary complications despite the use of usual concentrations of oxygen.[11,12]

Mechanism

Not understood. One suggestion is that bleomycin-injured lung tissue is less able to scavenge free oxygen radicals, which may be present, and damage occurs as a result.[3]

Importance and management

An established, well-documented, serious and potentially fatal interaction. It is advised that any patient receiving bleomycin and undergoing general anaesthesia should have their inspired oxygen concentrations limited to less than 30%, and the fluid replacement should be carefully monitored to minimise the crystalloid load. This is clearly very effective because one author has treated 700 patients following these guidelines without a single case of pulmonary failure.[13] It has also been suggested that reduced oxygen levels should be continued during the recovery period and at any time during hospitalisation.[3] If an oxygen concentration equal to or greater than 30% has to be used, the short-term use of prophylactic corticosteroids should be considered. Intravenous corticosteroids should be given at once if bleomycin toxicity is suspected.[3]

1. Goldiner PL, Carlon GC, Cvitkovic E, Schweizer O, Howland WS. Factors influencing postoperative morbidity and mortality in patients treated with bleomycin. *BMJ* (1978) 1, 1664–7.
2. El-Baz N, Ivankovich AD, Faber LP, Logas WG. The incidence of bleomycin lung toxicity after anesthesia for pulmonary resection: a comparison between HFV and IPPV. *Anesthesiology* (1984) 61, A107.
3. Gilson AJ, Sahn SA. Reactivation of bleomycin lung toxicity following oxygen administration. A second response to corticosteroids. *Chest* (1985) 88, 304–6.
4. Cersosimo RJ, Matthews SJ, Hong WK. Bleomycin pneumonitis potentiated by oxygen administration. *Drug Intell Clin Pharm* (1985) 19, 921–3.
5. Hulbert JC, Grossman JE, Cummings KB. Risk factors of anesthesia and surgery in bleomycin-treated patients. *J Urol (Baltimore)* (1983) 130, 163–4.
6. Donohue JP, Rowland RG. Complications of retroperitoneal lymph node dissection. *J Urol (Baltimore)* (1981) 125, 338–40.
7. Ingrassia TS, Ryu JH, Trastek VF, Rosenow EC. Oxygen-exacerbated bleomycin pulmonary toxicity. *Mayo Clin Proc* (1991) 66, 173–8.
8. Toledo CH, Ross WE, Hood I, Block ER. Potentiation of bleomycin toxicity by oxygen. *Cancer Treat Rep* (1982) 66, 359–62.
9. Berend N. The effect of bleomycin and oxygen on rat lung. *Pathology* (1984) 16, 136–9.
10. Rinaldo J, Goldstein RH, Snider GL. Modification of oxygen toxicity after lung injury by bleomycin in hamsters. *Am Rev Respir Dis* (1982) 126, 1030–3.
11. Douglas MJ, Coppin CML. Bleomycin and subsequent anesthesia: a retrospective study at Vancouver General Hospital. *Can Anaesth Soc J* (1980) 27, 449–52.
12. Mandelbaum I, Williams SD, Einhorn LH. Aggressive surgical management of testicular carcinoma metastatic to lungs and mediastinum. *Ann Thorac Surg* (1980) 30, 224–9.
13. Goldiner PL. Editorial comment. *J Urol (Baltimore)* (1983) 130, 164.

Bortezomib + Ciclosporin

Preliminary evidence suggests that patients who have received long-term ciclosporin might be at increased risk of severe neuropathy when given bortezomib.

Clinical evidence

In a review of 24 patients with multiple myeloma who had received bortezomib after relapse following allografting, the incidence of severe peripheral neuropathy was far higher than usually seen in non-transplant patients. Fourteen patients developed neurotoxicity; in 7 patients it was severe and 6 patients required treatment discontinuation as the neurotoxicity did not resolve following a bortezomib dose reduction. In an analysis of possible risk factors, prolonged ciclosporin use (median of 15 months) was found to be a risk factor for the development of severe neurotoxicity.[1]

Mechanism

Ciclosporin can cause neurotoxicity. Bortezomib is also very commonly associated with peripheral neuropathy, which can be dose-limiting. It was suggested that long-term ciclosporin might have caused subclinical neurotoxicity that became apparent after bortezomib was given.[1]

Importance and management

An interaction between bortezomib and ciclosporin is not established, but until more is known, be aware of the possibility of this effect if bortezomib is used in patients taking ciclosporin. The authors also suggest considering using a lower bortezomib dose in these patients.[1] Note that, any patients receiving bortezomib should be carefully monitored for symptoms of neuropathy such as a burning sensation, hyperaesthesia, hypoaesthesia, paraesthesia, discomfort, neuropathic pain or weakness. Patients experiencing new or worsening peripheral neuropathy should undergo neurological evaluation and may require the dose and schedule of bortezomib to be modified.

1. Giaccone L, Sorasio R, Patriarca F, Mattei D, Montefusco V, Peccatori J, Carnevale-Schianca F, Petrucci MT, Milone G, Guidi S, Rotta M, Fanin R, Corradini P, Boccadoro M, Bruno B. Bortezomib after allografting in multiple myeloma: association between neurotoxicity and cyclosporine treatment. *Biol Blood Marrow Transplant* (2007) 13, 497–9.

Bortezomib + Miscellaneous

Exposure to bortezomib was slightly increased by ketoconazole, a CYP3A4 inhibitor, and is predicted to be similarly affected by other CYP3A4 inhibitors. Case reports suggest that peripheral neuropathy might be increased or worsened by itraconazole, but not lansoprazole. Dexamethasone and omeprazole do not alter bortezomib pharmacokinetics, and melphalan with prednisone has no clinically relevant effect on bortezomib pharmacokinetics. Cases of hyper- and hypoglycaemia have been reported in clinical studies in patients taking antidiabetics and bortezomib. Hypotension is common in patients taking bortezomib, and the effects can be additive if used with antihypertensives or other drugs that can cause hypotension.

Clinical evidence, mechanism, importance and management

(a) Antidiabetics

The UK and US manufacturers note that during clinical studies with bortezomib, some patients who were taking oral antidiabetics (none specifically named) experienced hyper- or hypoglycaemia.[1,2] Bortezomib commonly causes hyperglycaemia (sometimes requiring treatment discontinuation[2]) and uncommonly causes hypoglycaemia,[1] and it is therefore likely that this is a drug-disease interaction rather than a drug-drug interaction. The manufacturers advise that patients taking oral antidiabetics might require close monitoring of their blood glucose and adjustment of the dose of antidiabetic drugs accordingly.[1,2]

(b) CYP2C19 inhibitors and substrates

In a study, 17 patients were given bortezomib 1.3 mg/m^2 on days 1, 4, 8, and 11 of two 21-day cycles with **omeprazole** 40 mg on the morning of days 6 to 10 and the evening of day 8 of either cycle. Omeprazole had no effect on the pharmacokinetics or pharmacodynamics of bortezomib.[3] Data from *in vitro* studies[1,2] had suggested that bortezomib is metabolised by cytochrome P450 isoenzymes, including CYP2C19. However, the clinical data above with the CYP2C19 inhibitor omeprazole suggest that inhibition of this isoenzyme does not result in a clinically relevant effect on bortezomib pharmacokinetics, and so no bortezomib dose adjustment appears to be necessary on the concurrent use of omeprazole.

On the basis of *in vitro* data showing that bortezomib weakly inhibits CYP2C19, the US manufacturer of bortezomib predicts that exposure to CYP2C19 substrates might be increased.[2] For this reason, the UK manufacturer advises caution on the concurrent use of bortezomib and CYP2C19 substrates.[1] However, there appears to be no published clinical data regarding this interaction and so it requires confirmation. For a list of CYP2C19 substrates, see 'Table 1.6', p.8

(c) CYP3A4 inhibitors

In a crossover study when 12 patients with solid tumours were given bortezomib 1 mg/m^2 on days 1, 4, 8, and 11 of two 21-day cycles with **ketoconazole** 400 mg on days 6 to 9 of either cycle, the AUC of bortezomib was increased by 35%. No increase in adverse effects was noted on concurrent use, when compared with those given bortezomib alone; however, the number of patients was small and the duration of concurrent use was short, and so no definitive conclusion can be drawn.[4]

A report describes 3 patients given bortezomib with **itraconazole** 200 mg daily, either alone (2 patients) or with lansoprazole 15 mg daily (one patient), who experienced new or worsening peripheral neuropathy, grade 4 thrombocytopenia, and grade 3, or higher, neutropenia (2 of the 3 patients). Another patient given lansoprazole alone and two given neither lansoprazole or itraconazole, did not experience the same adverse effects.[5]

Bortezomib is partly metabolised by CYP3A4, of which **ketoconazole** and **itraconazole** are known potent inhibitors, leading to an increase in bortezomib exposure, and possibly in its adverse effects, The UK and US manufacturers therefore advise close monitoring when bortezomib is given with **ketoconazole** or other drugs that inhibit CYP3A4, and they name **ritonavir**.[1,2] For a list of CYP3A4 inhibitors, see 'Table 1.9', p.11.

(d) Dexamethasone

In a clinical pharmacokinetic study 7 patients with multiple myeloma or non-Hodgkin's lymphoma were given oral dexamethasone 40 mg daily on days 1 to 4 and days 9 to 12 of the third cycle of bortezomib 1.3 mg/m^2, given on days 1, 4, 8, and 11 of a 21-day cycle for three cycles (with an optional extension fourth cycle). Dexamethasone had no effect on the AUC of bortezomib and had no clinically relevant effect on its maximum concentration.[6] No bortezomib dose adjustments therefore appear to be necessary on the concurrent use of dexamethasone.

(e) Drugs causing hypotension

Bortezomib commonly causes orthostatic hypotension, which can occur throughout treatment. The UK and US manufacturers of bortezomib advise caution when treating patients receiving drugs known to be associated with hypotension. They state that the management of orthostatic hypotension might include adjustment of **antihypertensives**. Patients should be instructed to seek medical advice if they experience symptoms of dizziness, light-headedness, or fainting spells.[1,2]

(f) Melphalan with Prednisone

The UK and US manufacturers of bortezomib note that data from 21 patients show that the concurrent use of bortezomib with melphalan and prednisone resulted in an increase in the AUC of bortezomib of 17%, which is not considered to be clinically relevant.[1,2] Bortezomib is often used with melphalan and prednisone in patients with multiple myeloma.

1. Velcade (Bortezomib mannitol boronic ester). Janssen-Cilag Ltd. UK Summary of product characteristics, September 2012.
2. Velcade (Bortezomib). Millennium Pharmaceuticals, Inc. US Prescribing information, October 2012.
3. Quinn DI, Nemunaitis J, Fuloria J, Britten CD, Bagrail N, Yee L, Acharya M, Chan K, Cohen N, Dudov A. Effect of the cytochrome P450 2C19 inhibitor omeprazole on the pharmacokinetics and safety profile of bortezomib in patients with advanced solid tumours, non-Hodgkin's lymphoma or multiple myeloma. *Clin Pharmacokinet* (2009) 48, 199–209.
4. Venkatakrishnan K, Rader M, Ramanathan RK, Ramalingam S, Chen E, Riordan W, Trepicchio W, Cooper M, Karol M, von Moltke L, Neuwirth R, Egorin M, Chatta G. Effect of the CYP3A inhibitor ketoconazole on the pharmacokinetics and pharmacodynamics of bortezomib in patients with advanced solid tumors: a prospective, multicenter, open-label, randomized, two-way crossover drug-drug interaction study. *Clin Ther* (2009) 31, 2444–58.
5. Iwamoto T, Ishibashi M, Fujieda A, Masuya M, Katayama N, Okuda M. Drug interactions between itraconazole and bortezomib: exacerbation of peripheral neuropathy and thrombocytopenia induced by bortezomib. *Pharmacotherapy* (2010) 30, 661–5.
6. Hellmann A, Rule S, Walewski J, Shpilberg O, Feng H, van de Velde H, Patel H, Skee DM, Girgis S, Louw VJ. Effect of cytochrome P450 3A4 inducers on the pharmacokinetic, pharmacodynamic and safety profiles of bortezomib in patients with multiple myeloma or non-Hodgkin's lymphoma. *Clin Pharmacokinet* (2011) 50, 781–91.

Bortezomib + Rifampicin (Rifampin) and other CYP3A4 inducers

Rifampicin slightly reduced the exposure to bortezomib in one study. A phase I clinical study found that patients taking enzyme-inducing antiepileptics tolerated higher maximum doses, and required higher doses for proteasomal inhibition by bortezomib, when compared with patients not taking these drugs. Other CYP3A4 inducers would be expected to interact similarly.

Clinical evidence

(a) Antiepileptics; Enzyme-inducing

A phase I clinical study[1] investigated the maximal tolerated dose of bortezomib in patients with malignant glioma taking enzyme-inducing antiepileptics (carbamazepine, phenytoin, phenobarbital, primidone, or oxcarbazepine), when compared with patients not taking these drugs. The maximum tolerated dose of bortezomib in the patients not taking enzyme-inducing antiepileptics was 1.7 mg/m^2 compared with the group taking enzyme-inducing antiepileptics, where the maximum tolerated dose was not reached as the dose escalation was stopped at 2.5 mg/m^2.

(b) Rifampicin (Rifampin)

In a clinical pharmacokinetic study, 6 patients with multiple myeloma or non-Hodgkin's lymphoma were given oral rifampicin 600 mg daily on days 4 to 10 of the third cycle of bortezomib (given as bortezomib 1.3 mg/m^2 on days 1, 4, 8, and 11 of a 21-day cycle for three cycles, with an optional extension fourth cycle). Rifampicin decreased the AUC_{0-72} and maximum concentration of bortezomib by 45% and 22%, respectively. No increase in adverse effects or clinically relevant reduction in proteasomal inhibition was found on concurrent use.[2]

Mechanism

Rifampicin is a non-specific enzyme inducer, which has potent effects on CYP3A4 and also induces CYP2C19, the isoenzymes by which bortezomib is metabolised. Concurrent use therefore results in a decrease in bortezomib exposure.[2]

Importance and management

Information about a pharmacokinetic interaction between bortezomib and rifampicin is limited to the study cited. However, the second study with enzyme-inducing antiepileptics also suggests that enzyme inducers will decrease bortezomib exposure. The reduction in bortezomib exposure, although apparently slight, could lead to loss in its efficacy. For this reason, the manufacturers of bortezomib advise against the concurrent use of rifampicin and other potent CYP3A4 inducers: they specifically name **carbamazepine**,[3] **phenytoin**[3] [and therefore probably **fosphenytoin**], **phenobarbital**[3] [and therefore probably **primidone**], and **St John's wort**.[3,4]

1. Phuphanich S, Supko JG, Carson KA, Grossman SA, Nabors LB, Mikkelsen T, Lesser G, Rosenfeld S, Desideri S, Olson JJ. Phase I clinical trial of bortezomib in adults with recurrent malignant glioma. *J Neurooncol* (2010) 100, 95–103.

2. Hellmann A, Rule S, Walewski J, Shpilberg O, Feng H, van de Velde H, Patel H, Skee DM, Girgis S, Louw VJ. Effect of cytochrome P450 3A4 inducers on the pharmacokinetic, pharmacodynamic and safety profiles of bortezomib in patients with multiple myeloma or non-Hodgkin's lymphoma. *Clin Pharmacokinet* (2011) 50, 781–91.
3. Velcade (Bortezomib mannitol boronic ester). Janssen-Cilag Ltd. UK Summary of product characteristics, September 2012.
4. Velcade (Bortezomib). Millennium Pharmaceuticals, Inc. US Prescribing information, October 2012.

Brentuximab vedotin + Ketoconazole and other CYP3A4 inhibitors and/or P-glycoprotein inhibitors

The exposure to monomethyl auristatin E, the active component of brentuximab vedotin, was moderately increased by ketoconazole. Other drugs that are both potent CYP3A4 inhibitors and P-glycoprotein inhibitors might interact similarly.

Clinical evidence

In a study, 14 patients with CD30-positive lymphomas received brentuximab vedotin 1.2 mg/kg intravenously on day 1 of two 21-day cycles, in combination with oral ketoconazole 400 mg from day 19 of the first cycle until day 21 of the second cycle. The AUC of brentuximab vedotin was unaffected; however, the AUC of its active component, monomethyl auristatin E (MMAE) was increased by about 34% on concurrent use with ketoconazole.[1] Similarly, the UK manufacturer of brentuximab vedotin briefly reports that concurrent use with ketoconazole did not alter the plasma concentration of brentuximab vedotin but it increased the exposure to MMAE by about 73%.[2]

Mechanism

Ketoconazole is a potent CYP3A4 inhibitor and an inhibitor of P-glycoprotein. MMAE is a substrate of CYP3A4 and has been shown to be a substrate of P-glycoprotein *in vitro*. Concurrent use therefore increases the exposure to MMAE.

Importance and management

Evidence for an interaction between brentuximab vedotin and drugs that inhibit both CYP3A4 and P-glycoprotein is limited to one study which suggests that ketoconazole moderately increases the exposure to MMAE, the active component of brentuximab vedotin. Neutropenia is a very common adverse effect of brentuximab vedotin when given alone, and an increase in MMAE exposure on the concurrent use of ketoconazole, or any other drug that is both a potent CYP3A4 inhibitor and P-glycoprotein inhibitor, might increase the risk of haematotoxicity. For a list of drugs that are both potent CYP3A4 inhibitors and P-glycoprotein inhibitors, see 'Table 1.9', p.11 'Table 1.12', p.14, respectively. Patients who are taking a drug that is both a potent CYP3A4 inhibitor and a P-glycoprotein inhibitor should be closely monitored for brentuximab vedotin adverse effects. Dose adjustment of brentuximab vedotin, a delay in brentuximab vedotin treatment, or prophylaxis with a granulocyte colony-stimulating factor during subsequent cycles of brentuximab vedotin might be required if neutropenia develops.[2]

1. Han TH, Gopal AK, Ramchandren R, Goy A, Chen R, Matous JV, Cooper M, Grove LE, Alley SC, Lynch CM, O'Connor OA. CYP3A-mediated drug-drug interaction potential and excretion of brentuximab vedotin, an antibody-drug conjugate, in patients with CD30-positive hematologic malignancies. *J Clin Pharmacol* (2013) 53, 866–77.
2. Adcetris (Brentuximab vedotin). Takeda UK Ltd. UK Summary of product characteristics, March 2015.

Brentuximab vedotin + Rifampicin (rifampin) and other CYP3A4 inducers and/or P-glycoprotein inducers

Exposure to monomethyl auristatin E, the active component of brentuximab vedotin, was slightly reduced by rifampicin. Other drugs that are both potent CYP3A4 inducers and P-glycoprotein inducers might interact similarly.

Clinical evidence

In a study, 14 patients with CD30-positive lymphomas received brentuximab vedotin 1.8 mg/kg intravenously on day 1 of two 21-day cycles, in combination with oral rifampicin 600 mg from day 14 of the first cycle to day 21 of the second cycle. The AUC of brentuximab vedotin was unaffected; however, the exposure to its active component, monomethyl auristatin E (MMAE), exposure was reduced by approximately 46% on concurrent use with rifampicin.[1] Similarly, the UK manufacturer of brentuximab vedotin briefly reports that concurrent use with rifampicin, did not alter the plasma concentrations of brentuximab vedotin but it reduced the exposure to MMAE by about 31%.[2]

Mechanism

Rifampicin is a potent CYP3A4 inducer and an inducer of P-glycoprotein. MMAE is a substrate of CYP3A4 and has been shown to be a substrate of P-glycoprotein *in vitro*. Concurrent use therefore decreases the exposure to MMAE.

Importance and management

Evidence for an interaction between rifampicin and drugs that induce both CYP3A4 and P-glycoprotein is limited, but suggests that the exposure to the active component of brentuximab vedotin, MMAE, is slightly reduced by rifampicin. Other drugs that are potent CY3A4 inducers and P-glycoprotein inducers might interact similarly. For a list of drugs that are both potent CYP3A4 inducers and P-glycoprotein inducers, see 'Table 1.9', p.11 and 'Table 1.12', p.14, respectively. The reduction in MMAE exposure, although slight, could reduce the efficacy of brentuximab vedotin, and it might be prudent to monitor the patient closely, for signs or markers indicative of poor response to treatment or relapsing disease.

1. Han TH, Gopal AK, Ramchandren R, Goy A, Chen R, Matous JV, Cooper M, Grove LE, Alley SC, Lynch CM, O'Connor OA. CYP3A-mediated drug-drug interaction potential and excretion of brentuximab vedotin, an antibody-drug conjugate, in patients with CD-30-positive hematologic malignancies. *J Clin Pharmacol* (2013) 53, 866–77.
2. Adcetris (Brentuximab vedotin). Takeda UK Ltd. UK Summary of product characteristics, March 2015.

Busulfan + Azoles

Itraconazole, but not fluconazole, modestly reduces the clearance of busulfan. There is some limited evidence to suggest that the use of busulfan with ketoconazole may increase the risk of hepatic veno-occlusive disease.

Clinical evidence, mechanism, importance and management

The pharmacokinetics of busulfan were compared in 26 bone marrow transplant patients, who had received busulfan without concurrent antifungal therapy, in 13 similar patients given busulfan with **itraconazole**, and in another 13 patients given busulfan with **fluconazole**. The busulfan clearance was decreased by 20% by **itraconazole** (probably because **itraconazole** inhibits the metabolism of busulfan by the liver) but busulfan clearance was not affected by the **fluconazole**.[1] The expected rise in serum busulfan levels is only likely to be moderate, but until more information is available it would be prudent to monitor for any signs of increased busulfan toxicity if **itraconazole** is used, but no special precautions seem to be needed with **fluconazole**. Concurrent **ketoconazole** has been identified as a possible risk factor for hepatic veno-occlusive disease after the use of high-dose busulfan.[2] Further study is needed to confirm or refute this.

1. Buggia I, Zecca N, Alessandrino EP, Locatelli F, Rosti G, Bosi A, Pession A, Rotoli B, Majolino I, Dallorso A, Regazzi MB. Itraconazole can increase systemic exposure to busulfan in patients given bone marrow transplantation. *Anticancer Res* (1996) 16, 2083–8.
2. Méresse V, Hartmann O, Vassal G, Benhamou E, Valteau-Couanet D, Brugieres L, Lemerie J. Risk factors for hepatic veno-occlusive disease after high-dose busulfan-containing regimens followed by autologous bone marrow transplantation: a study in 136 children. *Bone Marrow Transplant* (1992) 10, 135–41.

Busulfan + Benzodiazepines

Diazepam and lorazepam do not appear to alter the pharmacokinetics of busulfan.

Clinical evidence, mechanism, importance and management

In a study in patients receiving high-dose busulfan, no pharmacokinetic changes were seen in 8 patients given **diazepam**, apart from a steady decline in steady-state serum levels in just one.[1] Similarly, in another study, **lorazepam** did not alter the absorption and clearance of high-dose busulfan in children undergoing stem-cell transplantation.[2] Benzodiazepines may therefore be a suitable alternative to phenytoin for seizure prophylaxis during high-dose busulfan treatment.[2]

1. Hassan M, Öberg G, Björkholm M, Wallin I, Lindgren M. Influence of prophylactic anticonvulsant therapy on high-dose busulphan kinetics. *Cancer Chemother Pharmacol* (1993) 33, 181–6.
2. Chan KW, Mullen CA, Worth LL, Choroszy M, Koontz S, Tran H, Slopis J. Lorazepam for seizure prophylaxis during high-dose busulfan administration. *Bone Marrow Transplant* (2002) 29, 963–5.

Busulfan + Ketobemidone

Ketobemidone may increase busulfan levels.

Clinical evidence, mechanism, importance and management

A patient with acute myeloid leukaemia was given busulfan 1 mg/kg four times daily for 4 days followed by cyclophosphamide for 2 days before bone marrow transplantation. At the time he was also receiving ketobemidone 1 g daily for a rectal fissure. Busulfan plasma levels after the first dose were elevated (AUC increased by about one-third). Later, when the dose of ketobemidone was reduced and morphine substituted, busulfan levels decreased.[1] The authors suggest that ketobemidone should not be used with high-dose busulfan unless monitoring is possible: dose adjustments may be required to prevent busulfan toxicity. An alternative analgesic should be considered.

1. Hassan M, Svensson J-O, Nilsson C, Hentschke P, AL-Shurbaji A, Aschan J, Ljungman P, Ringdén O. Ketobemidone may alter busulfan pharmacokinetics during high-dose therapy. *Ther Drug Monit* (2000) 22, 383–5.

Busulfan + Metronidazole

Metronidazole increases the minimum concentration of high-dose busulfan, and increases its toxicity.

Clinical evidence

In a study, patients were given oral high-dose busulfan 1 mg/kg every six hours for 4 days (adjusted to achieve a target minimum concentration) as part of a stem cell transplant procedure. It was found that the dose-adjusted minimum concentrations of busulfan were 87% higher in 5 patients who also received metronidazole 400 mg three times daily than in 10 patients who did not take metronidazole. Furthermore, all 5 patients who had received metronidazole with busulfan developed elevated liver function tests and mucositis, and 3 developed veno-occlusive disease (moderate to severe in 2 patients, with one death). In the 10 patients who did not receive metronidazole, only 3 had elevated liver function tests, one had mucositis, and none had veno-occlusive disease.[1]

In a further group of 9 patients who received busulfan alone for 2 days and then in combination with metronidazole for 2 days, the minimum concentration of busulfan increased by 78% when given metronidazole.[1]

A 7-year old child with acute myeloid leukaemia was given a test dose of intravenous busulfan 0.5 mg/kg, which was to be followed by three therapeutic doses of 106 mg, as part of a pre-conditioning regimen prior to stem cell transplant. The day after the busulfan test dose, oral metronidazole 250 mg three times daily was started for suspected *Clostridium difficile* infection. Busulfan 106 mg was then given on each of the following two days, and therapeutic drug monitoring was conducted after the first of these therapeutic doses. The busulfan clearance was 46% lower than after the test dose and so the third busulfan therapeutic dose was not given. The AUC of busulfan was 86% higher than the daily predicted AUC and the total course busulfan AUC was 24% higher than the target total course AUC, after the first two doses.[2]

Mechanism

The reason why metronidazole might increase busulfan concentrations is unknown, but it has been suggested that it might be due to glutathione depletion.[1]

Importance and management

Although information on the interaction between busulfan and metronidazole is limited, it would appear to be established and clinically important. The authors of the study, state that metronidazole should not be given at the same time as high-dose busulfan.[1] This would appear to be prudent, and is advised by the UK manufacturers of busulfan.[3] If metronidazole is given to a patient taking conventional dose busulfan, the UK manufacturer recommends weekly blood counts to detect any increase in toxicity.[3]

1. Nilsson C, Aschan J, Hentschke P, Ringdén O, Ljungman P, Hassan M. The effect of metronidazole on busulfan pharmacokinetics in patients undergoing hematopoietic stem cell transplantation. *Bone Marrow Transplant* (2003) 31, 429–35.
2. Gulbis AM, Culotta KS, Jones RB, Andersson BS. Busulfan and metronidazole: an often forgotten but significant drug interaction. *Ann Pharmacother* (2011) 45, e39.
3. Myleran (Busulfan). Aspen. UK Summary of product characteristics, May 2012.

Busulfan + Paracetamol (Acetaminophen)

Paracetamol is predicted to decrease the clearance of busulfan.

Clinical evidence, mechanism, importance and management

Busulfan is conjugated with glutathione as part of its metabolism, and, as paracetamol is known to reduce the blood levels of glutathione it is predicted to reduce the clearance of busulfan. The manufacturers of busulfan therefore advise caution when paracetamol is given during the 72-hour period before busulfan is given, and during the use of busulfan.[1,2] Note that the clinical relevance of this proposed interaction is unclear, and only the manufacturers of intravenous busulfan appear to mention it.

1. Busilvex (Busulfan). Pierre Fabre Ltd. UK Summary of product characteristics, July 2008.
2. IVBusulfex (Busulfan). Otsuka America Pharmaceutical, Inc. US Prescribing information, August 2009.

Busulfan + Phenytoin

Phenytoin modestly increases the clearance of busulfan and lowers its levels. Subtherapeutic levels of phenytoin may occur in the presence of busulfan.

Clinical evidence

Seven patients receiving high-dose busulfan (1 mg/kg four times daily for 4 days) before bone marrow transplantation had a 19% increase in busulfan clearance, a 16% lower AUC and a shorter half-life (reduced from 3.94 to 3.03 hours) when they were given phenytoin 2.5 to 5 mg/kg daily. A continuous decline in the steady-state plasma levels of busulfan was also seen in 4 of the patients.[1]

In a study in 51 patients given busulfan and prophylactic phenytoin 300 mg daily for 5 days, 3 patients developed convulsions, and plasma phenytoin levels analysed in 2 of them were found to be subtherapeutic.[2]

Mechanism

It seems likely that phenytoin (a well recognised enzyme inducer) increases the metabolism of busulfan by the liver (possibly by induction of glutathione-S-transferase), thereby decreasing its levels. In an *animal* study, phenytoin was found to reduce the myelosuppressive effects of busulfan.[3]

Importance and management

Evidence for an interaction between phenytoin and busulfan appears to be limited to these two reports. However, the effects of phenytoin on busulfan are in line with the way phenytoin is known to interact with a number of other drugs, so an interaction would appear to be established. The authors of one study suggest that antiepileptics with fewer enzyme-inducing properties than phenytoin should be used as prophylaxis if busulfan is given for bone marrow transplant pretreatment.[1] One UK manufacturer recommends prophylaxis with a benzodiazepine rather than phenytoin if high-dose busulfan is given.[4] Clobazam has been suggested as a possible alternative to phenytoin.[5] Lorazepam and diazepam appear not to interact with busulfan (see 'Busulfan + Benzodiazepines', p.666) and they may therefore be suitable alternatives. The UK manufacturer of parenteral busulfan found no evidence that phenytoin increased its clearance, and notes that all adult patients given busulfan also received phenytoin.[6] However, the US manufacturer of parenteral busulfan gives a dose assuming that phenytoin will also be given, and notes that if other antiepileptics are used instead, the busulfan plasma levels may be increased and monitoring is recommended.[7]

To overcome the problem of reduced phenytoin levels, the authors recommended a loading dose of phenytoin 18 mg/kg on the day before the first dose of busulfan, then 300 mg daily until 48 hours after the last busulfan dose. A further loading dose was given if the phenytoin level was subtherapeutic 48 hours after the initial dose (required in 35% of patients).[2]

1. Hassan M, Öberg G, Björkholm M, Wallin I, Lindgren M. Influence of prophylactic anticonvulsant therapy on high-dose busulphan kinetics. *Cancer Chemother Pharmacol* (1993) 33, 181–6.
2. Grigg AP, Shepherd JD, Phillips GL. Busulphan and phenytoin. Ann Intern Med (1989) 111, 1049–50. Correction. *Ann Intern Med* (1989) 112, 313.
3. Fitzsimmons WE, Ghalie R, Kaizer H. The effect of hepatic enzyme inducers on busulfan neurotoxicity and myelotoxicity. *Cancer Chemother Pharmacol* (1990) 27, 226–8.
4. Myleran (Busulfan). Aspen. UK Summary of product characteristics, May 2012.
5. Schwarer AP, Opat SS, Watson AL, Cole-Sinclair MF. Clobazam for seizure prophylaxis during busulfan chemotherapy. *Lancet* (1995) 346, 1238.
6. Busilvex (Busulfan). Pierre Fabre Ltd. UK Summary of product characteristics, July 2008.
7. IVBusulfex (Busulfan). Otsuka America Pharmaceutical, Inc. US Prescribing information, August 2009.

Busulfan + Tioguanine

The long-term use of busulfan with tioguanine appears to increase the risk of nodular regenerative hyperplasia of the liver, portal hypertension and oesophageal varices.

Clinical evidence, mechanism, importance and management

Five patients receiving continuous busulfan 2 mg and tioguanine 80 mg five days weekly for chronic myeloid leukaemia (CML) developed oesophageal varices and abnormal liver function tests. Three of them had gastrointestinal haemorrhages and one died. Liver biopsy of 4 of the patients showed nodular regenerative hyperplasia, which was the cause of portal hypertension and varices.[1] A later analysis of the Medical Research Council study comparing busulfan with busulfan and tioguanine in 675 patients with CML, revealed a total of 18 cases of portal hypertension and oesophageal varices (including 4 described in the first report[1]), all 18 of which occurred in patients receiving both drugs. In addition, there was no survival advantage with the combination.[2] The risk of portal hypertension may be related to the long-term use of tioguanine, or to its combination with busulfan. It has been suggested that this drug combination should not be routinely used for the long-term maintenance of CML.[2]

1. Key NS, Kelly PMA, Emerson PM, Chapman RWG, Allan NC, McGee JO'D. Oesophageal varices associated with busulphan-thioguanine combination therapy for chronic myeloid leukaemia. *Lancet* (1987) 2, 1050–2.
2. Shepherd, PCA, Fooks J, Gray R, Allan NC. Thioguanine used in maintenance therapy of chronic myeloid leukaemia causes non-cirrhotic portal hypertension. *Br J Haematol* (1991) 79, 185–92.

Cetuximab + Irinotecan

No pharmacokinetic interaction occurs between cetuximab and irinotecan.

Clinical evidence, mechanism, importance and management

Cetuximab is used with irinotecan in the treatment of metastatic colorectal cancer. In a study, 14 patients with advanced epidermal growth factor responsive (EGFR) positive adenocarcinoma were given either irinotecan 350 mg/m^2 every 3 weeks and cetuximab 400 mg/m^2 at week 2 then 250 mg/m^2 each week, or cetuximab each week starting at week one and irinotecan starting at week 4. There was at least a one-hour period between the end of the cetuximab infusion and the start of the irinotecan infusion. No evidence was found of a pharmacokinetic interaction between cetuximab and irinotecan, nor was there any significant increase in serious toxicities for the combination, when compared with treatment with either drug alone.[1] Similar results were found in a crossover study in 8 patients who received irinotecan 350 mg/m^2 every 3 weeks and cetuximab 400 mg/m^2 on day 2, then 250 mg/m^2 each week.[2]

1. Delbaldo C, Pierga J-Y, Dieras V, Faivre S, Laurence V, Vedovato J-C, Bonnaay M, Mueser M, Nolting A, Kovar A, Raymond E. Pharmacokinetic profile of cetuximab (Erbitux) alone and in combination with irinotecan in patients with advanced EGFR-positive adenocarcinoma. *Eur J Cancer* (2005) 41, 1739–45.
2. Ettlinger DE, Mitterhauser M, Wadsak W, Ostermann E, Farkouh A, Schueller J, Czejka M. *In vivo* disposition of irinotecan (CPT-11) and its metabolites in combination with the monoclonal antibody cetuximab. *Anticancer Res* (2006) 26, 1337–42.

Chlorambucil + Prednisone

An isolated report describes seizures in a patient, which were possibly caused by the use of chlorambucil with prednisone.

Clinical evidence, mechanism, importance and management

A patient with non-Hodgkin's lymphoma experienced a syncopal episode with generalised tonic-clonic seizures 8 days after completing an initial 5-day course of chlorambucil 12 mg daily and prednisone 50 mg daily. The seizures were controlled with intravenous clonazepam. Four weeks later, on the third day of a second course, she again had generalised tonic-clonic seizures, which resolved spontaneously.

Chlorambucil-induced seizures have occurred in children with nephrotic syndrome. Cases in adults usually involve high-dose chlorambucil or are in patients with a history of seizures. The seizures in this patient may have been due to the additive effects of both drugs in reducing the seizure threshold.[1]

Note that chlorambucil and prednisone or prednisolone have been widely used together, but this case report highlights the need to assess the risk of seizures when giving drugs that lower the seizure threshold.

1. Jourdan E, Topart D, Pinzani V, Jourdan J. Chlorambucil/prednisone-induced seizures in a patient with non-Hodgkin's lymphoma. *Am J Hematol* (2001) 67, 147.

Cisplatin and other platinum compounds + Aminoglycosides

The renal toxicity of cisplatin is potentiated by aminoglycosides such as gentamicin and tobramycin. In one retrospective analysis in patients taking cisplatin, hearing loss was not associated with the concurrent use of ototoxic drugs, including tobramycin.

Clinical evidence

(a) Hypomagnesaemia

Both cisplatin and the aminoglycosides can cause excessive loss of magnesium, and it has been suggested that combined use increases this loss.[1]

(b) Nephrotoxicity

Early after the introduction of cisplatin it became apparent that aminoglycosides could increase the nephrotoxicity of this drug. In one report, 4 patients given cisplatin, in doses ranging from low to very high (eight doses of 0.5 mg/kg, one or two doses of 3 mg/kg or a single-dose of 5 mg/kg), and who were subsequently given **gentamicin** and cefalotin developed acute and fatal renal failure. Autopsy revealed extensive renal tubular necrosis.[2] Two similar cases of severe renal toxicity, attributed to the use of **gentamicin** and cefalotin in patients who had previously been given cisplatin, are described elsewhere.[3,4] Another patient given cisplatin and **gentamicin** developed acute renal failure.[5] A further 3 patients given cisplatin then **gentamicin** or **tobramycin** had greater decreases in creatinine levels than 12 others receiving cisplatin alone.[5] A retrospective comparative study confirmed that the incidence of abnormal renal function was higher in patients who had received cisplatin and an aminoglycoside than in patients who had received cisplatin alone (12 of 17 versus 19 of 50 patients, respectively), but the renal impairment was described as usually mild and not clinically significant.[6] Similarly, a brief report stated that aminoglycoside use was associated with a greater decline in renal function in children receiving high-dose cisplatin.[7] There is also evidence from a study in children to show that previous treatment with cisplatin is a risk factor for the delayed elimination of aminoglycosides (**gentamicin, amikacin, tobramycin**).[8]

Conversely, in another study, aminoglycosides were not found to be a significant factor in the development of renal impairment after the use of high-dose cisplatin-based therapy, and use of appropriate supportive care (hydration and mannitol diuresis) probably played a part in this.[9]

(c) Ototoxicity

In one small retrospective analysis of patients with cancer, the risk of developing hearing loss after low-dose, slow-infusion cisplatin did not correlate significantly with the concurrent use of other ototoxic drugs, such as furosemide or **tobramycin**.[10] Enhanced renal toxicity and ototoxicity have been reported in *guinea pigs* given cisplatin and **kanamycin** for 2 weeks.[11] In another *animal* study **gentamicin** was given for 14 days. A single dose of cisplatin given early in the course enhanced the ototoxic effects of **gentamicin** but no increase in ototoxicity occurred when cisplatin was given at the end of the **gentamicin** course.[12]

Mechanism

Cisplatin (and other platinum compounds such as **carboplatin**) are nephrotoxic and it would appear that its damaging effects on the kidney are additive with the nephrotoxic effects of the aminoglycoside. Both gentamicin and cisplatin may cause ototoxicity.[13] Previous exposure to cisplatin may delay the elimination of the aminoglycosides.

Importance and management

An established and potentially serious interaction. However, aminoglycosides remain an important group of antibacterials for the empirical treatment of febrile neutropenia in patients receiving chemotherapy,[14,15] including cisplatin-based regimens. However, in selecting an initial antibacterial regimen, it has been suggested that concurrent use of some drugs, including cisplatin and aminoglycosides, should be avoided if possible because of additive renal toxicity.[16] Good supportive care is required (e.g. pre and post-treatment hydration with mannitol diuresis), and renal function should be well monitored. Audiometric tests should be carried out when cisplatin is used, particularly when other ototoxic drugs are also given. Similar precautions would seem advisable with **carboplatin**.

1. Flombaum CD. Hypomagnesemia associated with cisplatin combination chemotherapy. *Arch Intern Med* (1984) 144, 2336–7.
2. Gonzalez-Vitale JC, Hayes DM, Cvitkovic E, Sternberg SS. Acute renal failure after *cis*-Dichlorodiammineplatinum (II) and gentamicin-cephalothin therapies. *Cancer Treat Rep* (1978) 62, 693–8.
3. Salem PA, Jabboury KW, Khalil MF. Severe nephrotoxicity: a probable complication of cis-dichlorodiammineplatinum (II) and cephalothin-gentamicin therapy. *Oncology* (1982) 39, 31–2.
4. Leite JBF, De Campelo Gentil F, Burchenal J, Marques A, Teixeira MIC, Abrão FA. Insuficiênza renal aguda após o uso de cis-diaminodicloroplatina, gentamicina e cefalosporina. *Rev Paul Med* (1981) 97, 75–7.
5. Dentino M, Luft FC, Yum MN, Williams SD, Einhorn LH. Long term effect of cis-diamminedichloride platinum (CDDP) on renal function and structure in man. *Cancer* (1978) 41, 1274–81.
6. Haas A, Anderson L, Lad T. The influence of aminoglycosides on the nephrotoxicity of *cis*-diamminedichloroplatinum in cancer patients. *J Infect Dis* (1983) 147, 363.
7. Pearson ADJ, Kohli M, Scott GW, Craft AW. Toxicity of high dose cisplatinum in children — the additive role of aminoglycosides. *Proc Am Assoc Cancer Res* (1987) 28, 221.
8. Christensen ML, Stewart CF, Crom WR. Evaluation of aminoglycoside disposition in patients previously treated with cisplatin. *Ther Drug Monit* (1989) 11, 631–6.
9. Cooper BW, Creger RJ, Soegiarso W, Mackay WL, Lazarus HM. Renal dysfunction during high-dose cisplatin therapy and autologous hematopoietic stem cell transplantation: effect of aminoglycoside therapy. *Am J Med* (1993) 94, 497–504.
10. Hallmark RJ, Snyder JM, Jusenius K, Tamimi HK. Factors influencing ototoxicity in ovarian cancer patients treated with Cis-platinum based chemotherapy. *Eur J Gynaecol Oncol* (1992) 13, 35–44.
11. Schweitzer VG, Hawkins JE, Lilly DJ, Litterst CJ, Abrams G, Davis JA, Christy M. Ototoxic and nephrotoxic effects of combined treatment with *cis*-diamminedichloroplatinum and kanamycin in the guinea pig. *Otolaryngol Head Neck Surg* (1984) 92, 38–49.
12. Riggs LC, Brummett RE, Guitjens SK, Matz GJ. Ototoxicity resulting from combined administration of cisplatin and gentamicin. *Laryngoscope* (1996) 106, 401–6.
13. Lautermann J, Dehne N, Schacht J, Jahnke K. Aminoglykosid- und cisplatin-Ototoxizität: von der Grundlagenforschung zur Klinik. *Laryngorhinootologie* (2004) 83, 317–23.
14. Ziglam HM, Gelly K, Olver W. A survey of the management of neutropenic fever in oncology units in the UK. *Int J Antimicrob Agents* (2007) 29, 430–3.
15. Tamura K. Initial empirical antimicrobial therapy: duration and subsequent modifications. *Clin Infect Dis* (2004) 39 (Suppl 1) S59–S64.
16. Hughes WT, Armstrong D, Bodey GP, Bow EJ, Brown AE, Calandra T, Feld R, Pizzo PA, Rolston KVI, Shenep JL, Young LS, for the Infectious Diseases Society of America. 2002 Guidelines for the use of antimicrobial agents in neutropenic patients with cancer. *Clin Infect Dis* (2002) 34, 730–51.

Cisplatin + Cannabis

A case report describes a fatal stroke when a young man receiving cisplatin smoked cannabis.

Clinical evidence, mechanism, importance and management

A 27-year-old man who smoked cannabis and tobacco daily developed tinnitus and paraesthesias after receiving the first course of chemotherapy consisting of cisplatin, etoposide and bleomycin for testicular cancer. Following the second course of chemotherapy, the patient reported distal paresis of the right arm and, 2 days later, about 30 minutes after cannabis inhalation, he developed headache, paresis of his right leg and aphasia. A large thrombus was found in the carotid artery. The patient died the next day. He had no cardiovascular risk factors apart from the smoking (about 4 cigarettes per day).[1]

Cisplatin is known to carry a small risk of stroke, and cases have also been reported for cannabis smoking alone. In this case it was suggested that the use of cannabis may have also contributed to the adverse outcome in this patient.[1] It might be prudent for patients receiving cisplatin to avoid smoking cannabis.

1. Russmann S, Winkler A, Lövblad KO, Stanga Z, Bassetti C. Lethal ischemic stroke after cisplatin-based chemotherapy for testicular carcinoma and cannabis inhalation. *Eur Neurol* (2002) 48, 178–80.

Cisplatin + Diuretics

A single report describes the development of renal failure in a patient given furosemide and other antihypertensives during the use of cisplatin. However, note that furosemide can be used to promote diuresis in patients given cisplatin to reduce the risk of nephrotoxicity. A small retrospective review found that cisplatin-induced nephrotoxicity was associated with hydrochlorothiazide use. Although *animal* studies show that the damaging effects of cisplatin on the ear can be markedly increased by the concurrent use of etacrynic acid or furosemide a retrospective analysis in patients did not find this effect.

Clinical evidence, mechanism, importance and management

(a) Nephrotoxicity

1. Loop diuretics. Three hours after receiving intravenous cisplatin 70 mg/m^2 a patient experienced severe nausea and vomiting and his blood pressure rose from 150/90 mmHg to 248/140 mmHg. This was managed with **furosemide** 40 mg intravenously, hydralazine 10 mg intramuscularly, diazoxide 300 mg intravenously and propranolol 20 mg orally twice daily for 2 days. Nine days later the patient had evidence of renal impairment (creatinine raised from about 88 micromol/L to 283 micromol/L), which resolved within 3 weeks. The patient was subsequently similarly treated on two occasions with cisplatin and again developed hypertension, but no treatment was given and there was no evidence of renal impairment.[1]

The reasons for the renal impairment are not known, but a study in *rats*[2] indicates that kidney damage may possibly be related to the concentrations of cisplatin, and that **furosemide** can increase cisplatin levels in the kidney. However, another study in patients found that there was no difference in the toxicity or pharmacokinetics of cisplatin when **furosemide** was used to induce diuresis, compared with mannitol.[3] Two other studies have also found that **furosemide** does not alter cisplatin pharmacokinetics.[4,5] Another study found that sodium chloride solution with or without **furosemide** was associated with less cisplatin nephrotoxicity than sodium chloride solution with mannitol.[6]

For **furosemide**, information seems to be limited to the case cited and its general clinical importance is uncertain. Although mannitol is by far the more usual drug used to induce diuresis during the use of cisplatin in order to reduce the risk of nephrotoxicity, **furosemide** may also be used for this indication.[7]

2. Thiazides. A retrospective review of 62 patients who had received cisplatin found that there was an association between those patients who had also received **hydrochlorothiazide**, and those who developed nephrotoxicity (an increase in serum creatinine of about 44 micromol/L or more). All 5 patients who had taken **hydrochlorothiazide** developed nephrotoxicity after one cycle of cisplatin.[8] It was suggested that hydrochlorothiazide and cisplatin might have additive effects on renal magnesium wasting. The mechanism for any of these associations is unclear.

The data from these sorts of analyses require confirmation in a controlled study, because it is possible that the findings are due to chance alone. The general relevance of this report is therefore uncertain.

(b) Ototoxicity

Both cisplatin and loop diuretics (particularly **etacrynic acid**) given alone can be ototoxic in man. A study[9] in *guinea pigs* found that when cisplatin 7 mg/kg or **etacrynic acid** 50 mg/kg were given alone their ototoxic effects were reversible, but when given together the damaging effects on the ear were profound, prolonged and possibly permanent. Similarly, while cisplatin-induced ototoxicity was potentiated by **furosemide** in *guinea pigs* in one study[10] in another this was only seen when a very high dose of **furosemide** was used.[11] In one small retrospective analysis of patients with cancer, the risk of developing hearing loss after low-dose slow-infusion cisplatin did not correlate significantly with concurrent use of other ototoxic drugs, such as **furosemide**.[12] Audiometric tests should be carried out when cisplatin is used, and this is of particular importance when other ototoxic drugs are also given.

1. Markman M, Trump DL. Nephrotoxicity with cisplatin and antihypertensive medications. *Ann Intern Med* (1982) 96, 257.
2. Pera MF, Zook BC, Harder HC. Effects of mannitol or furosemide diuresis on the nephrotoxicity and physiological disposition of *cis*-dichlorodiammineplatinum-(II) in rats. *Cancer Res* (1979) 39, 1269–79.
3. Ostrow S, Egorin MJ, Hahn D, Markus S, Aisner J, Chang P, LeRoy A, Bachur NR, Wiernik PH. High-dose cisplatin therapy using mannitol versus furosemide diuresis: comparative pharmacokinetics and toxicity. *Cancer Treat Rep* (1981) 65, 73–8.
4. Dumas M, d'Athis P, de Gislain C, Lautissier JL, Autissier N, Escousse A, Guerrin J. Influence of frusemide on cis-dichlorodiammineplatinum (II) pharmaco-kinetics. *Eur J Drug Metab Pharmacokinet* (1987) 12, 203–6.
5. Dumas M, de Gislain C, d'Athis P, Chadoint-Noudeau V, Escousse A, Guerrin J, Autissier N. Evaluation of the effect of furosemide on ultrafilterable platinum kinetics in patients treated with *cis*-diamminedichloroplatinum. *Cancer Chemother Pharmacol* (1989) 23, 37–40.
6. Santoso JT, Lucci JA, Coleman RL, Schafer I, Hannigan EV. Saline, mannitol, and furosemide hydration in acute cisplatin nephrotoxicity: a randomised trial. *Cancer Chemother Pharmacol* (2003) 52, 13–18.
7. Numico G, Benasso M, Vannozzi MO, Merlano M, Rosso R, Viale M, Esposito M. Hydration regimen and hematological toxicity of a cisplatin-based chemotherapy regimen. Clinical observations and pharmacokinetic analysis. *Anticancer Res* (1998) 18, 1313–18.
8. Shord SS, Thompson DM, Krempl GA, Hanigan MH. Effect of concurrent medications on cisplatin-induced nephrotoxicity in patients with head and neck cancer. *Anticancer Drugs* (2006) 17, 207–15.
9. Komune S, Snow JB. Potentiating effects of cisplatin and ethacrynic acid in ototoxicity. *Arch Otolaryngol* (1981) 107, 594–7.
10. McAlpine D, Johnstone BM. The ototoxic mechanism of cisplatin. *Hear Res* (1990) 47, 191–203.
11. Laurell G, Engström B. The combined effect of cisplatin and furosemide on hearing function in guinea pigs. *Hear Res* (1989) 38, 19–26.
12. Hallmark RJ, Snyder JM, Jusenius K, Tamimi HK. Factors influencing ototoxicity in ovarian cancer patients treated with Cis-platinum based chemotherapy. *Eur J Gynaecol Oncol* (1992) 13, 35–44.

Cisplatin + H_2-receptor antagonists

Cimetidine and ranitidine probably do not have a clinically relevant effect on the renal clearance of cisplatin.

Clinical evidence, mechanism, importance and management

Some *animal* studies have shown that organic cations such as **cimetidine** and **ranitidine** may compete with the renal tubular transport of cisplatin and thus could be useful in reducing cisplatin nephrotoxicity.[1,2] However, in a study of 10 children receiving cisplatin, **ranitidine** had no effect on the total body disposition or renal clearance of cisplatin. This finding and further studies in *dogs* showed that cisplatin may not share transport systems with organic cations to a clinically relevant extent.[3] Although information is limited, it appears that there is no pharmacokinetic interaction between cisplatin and **cimetidine** or **ranitidine**.

1. Klein J, Bentur Y, Cheung D, Moselhy G, Koren G. Renal handling of cisplatin: interactions with organic anions and cations in the dog. *Clin Invest Med* (1991) 14, 388–94.
2. Haragsim L, Zima T, Němeček K. Nephrotoxic effects of platinum cytostatics–preventive effects of nifedipine and cimetidine. *Sb Lek* (1994) 95, 173–83.
3. Ito S, Weitzman S, Klein J, Greenberg M, Lau R, Atanakovic G, Koren G. Lack of cisplatin-ranitidine kinetic interactions: *in vivo* study in children, and *in vitro* study using dog renal brush border membrane vesicles. *Life Sci* (1998) 62, PL387–PL392.

Cisplatin + Probenecid

The available clinical data suggest that the nephrotoxicity of cisplatin is reduced by probenecid, but uncertainty remains.

Clinical evidence, mechanism, importance and management

In a randomised study in patients with cancer, probenecid 2 to 4 g daily reduced the fractional clearance of free platinum after a single 60- to 100-mg/m^2 dose of cisplatin given as a 24-hour infusion, and no cases of renal impairment were seen.[1] Similarly, in a further phase I dose-escalation study, no renal impairment was seen in patients given cisplatin at doses from 100 to 160 mg/m^2 when they were also given probenecid 1 g every 6 hours for 12 doses (beginning 24 hours before the cisplatin infusion, and continuing for 24 hours after).[2] It was concluded that probenecid may protect against cisplatin-induced renal toxicity. An earlier study in *rats* had also suggested that giving probenecid before cisplatin reduced nephrotoxicity, as assessed by blood urea levels and serum creatinine.[3] Subsequently, a study in *dogs* has found that probenecid decreases the renal clearance of free cisplatin,[4] and another study in *mice* found that probenecid reduces the renal tubular damage seen with cisplatin alone.[5]

Conversely, some researchers have suggested that the combination of probenecid and cisplatin is potentially more toxic than cisplatin alone. They found that probenecid increased the fractional clearance of free platinum from cisplatin in *rats*, and that pretreatment with probenecid increased nephrotoxicity, as assessed by blood urea levels.[6] Other authors similarly reported that probenecid increased cisplatin clearance in *rats*.[7]

It is unclear why some *animal* studies show that probenecid increases cisplatin-induced nephrotoxicity whereas others show a decrease. Although the available clinical data suggest that there is a decrease, some uncertainty remains. The combination should be used with caution.

1. Jacobs C, Coleman CN, Rich L, Hirst K, Weiner MW. Inhibition of *cis*-diamminedichloroplatinum secretion by the human kidney with probenecid. *Cancer Res* (1984) 44, 3632–5.
2. Jacobs C, Kaubisch S, Halsey J, Lum BL, Gosland M, Coleman CN, Sikic BI. The use of probenecid as a chemoprotector against cisplatin nephrotoxicity. *Cancer* (1991) 67, 1518–24.
3. Ross DA, Gale GR. Reduction of the renal toxicity of *cis*-dichlorodiammineplatinum (II) by probenecid. *Cancer Treat Rep* (1979) 63, 781–7.
4. Klein J, Bentur Y, Cheung D, Moselhy G, Koren G. Renal handling of cisplatin: interactions with organic anions and cations in the dog. *Clin Invest Med* (1991) 14, 388–94.
5. Ban M, Hettich D, Huguet N. Nephrotoxicity mechanism of *cis*-platinum (II) diamine dichloride in mice. *Toxicol Lett* (1994) 71, 161–8.
6. Daley-Yates PT, McBrien DCH. Enhancement of cisplatin nephrotoxicity by probenecid. *Cancer Treat Rep* (1984) 68, 445–6.
7. Osman NM, Litterst CL. Effect of probenecid and *N'*-methylnicotinamide on renal handling of *cis*-dichlorodiammineplatinum-II in rats. *Cancer Lett* (1983) 19, 107–11.

Cyclophosphamide + Allopurinol

There is some evidence to suggest that the incidence of serious bone marrow depression caused by cyclophosphamide can be increased by allopurinol, but this was not confirmed in a controlled study.

Clinical evidence

A retrospective epidemiological survey of patients in four hospitals who, over a 4-year period, had been taking cyclophosphamide, found that the incidence of serious bone marrow depression was 58% in 26 patients who had also taken allopurinol, and 19% in 32 patients who had not taken allopurinol.[1] A pharmacokinetic study in 9 patients with malignant disease and 2 healthy subjects found that while taking allopurinol 600 mg daily the concentration of the cytotoxic metabolites of cyclophosphamide increased by an average of about 38% (range 2 to 110%).[2] Another pharmacokinetic study reported that the half-life of cyclophosphamide was more than twofold longer in 3 children also receiving allopurinol 300 mg/m^2, when compared with that in children not given allopurinol.[3] However, another study found that although allopurinol pre-treatment increased the half-life of cyclophosphamide, the plasma alkylating activity and urinary metabolite and cyclophosphamide excretion were unchanged.[4] Moreover, a randomised controlled study,[5] designed as a follow-up to the survey cited above,[1] failed to confirm that allopurinol increased the toxicity of cyclophosphamide in 81 patients with Hodgkin's or non-Hodgkin's lymphoma. In this study, there was no difference in nadirs for white blood cells and platelets during 3 cycles of cyclophosphamide-containing chemotherapy in 44 patients receiving allopurinol and in 37 patients not receiving allopurinol.

Mechanism

Not understood. Cyclophosphamide itself is inactive, but it is converted by the liver into cytotoxic metabolites.[4] Allopurinol or its metabolite oxypurinol may inhibit their renal excretion, or may alter hepatic metabolism.[2,3]

Importance and management

This interaction is not established with any certainty. The authors of the randomised study consider that, if necessary, allopurinol can be safely used to prevent hyperuricaemia with the chemotherapy regimens used for lymphomas,[5] and allopurinol is standardly given for the prevention of tumour lysis syndrome.[6]

1. Boston Collaborative Drug Surveillance Programme. Allopurinol and cytotoxic drugs. Interaction in relation to bone marrow depression. *JAMA* (1974) 227, 1036–40.
2. Witten J, Frederiksen PL, Mouridsen HT. The pharmacokinetics of cyclophosphamide in man after treatment with allopurinol. *Acta Pharmacol Toxicol (Copenh)* (1980) 46, 392–4.
3. Yule SM, Boddy AV, Cole M, Price L, Wyllie R, Tasso MJ, Pearson ADJ, Idle JR. Cyclophosphamide pharmacokinetics in children. *Br J Clin Pharmacol* (1996) 41, 13–19.
4. Bagley CM, Bostick FW, DeVita VT. Clinical pharmacology of cyclophosphamide. *Cancer Res* (1973) 33, 226–33.
5. Stolbach L, Begg C, Bennett JM, Silverstein M, Falkson G, Harris DT, Glick J. Evaluation of bone marrow toxic reaction in patients treated with allopurinol. *JAMA* (1982) 247, 334–6.
6. Coiffier B, Altman A, Pui C-H, Younes A, Cairo MS. Guidelines for the management of pediatric and adult tumor lysis syndrome: an evidence-based review. *J Clin Oncol* (2008) 26, 2767–78.

Cyclophosphamide + Amiodarone

Early-onset pulmonary toxicity occurred in one patient taking amiodarone after high-dose cyclophosphamide was given. Fatal pulmonary

toxicity occurred in another patient taking amiodarone after a single dose of cyclophosphamide.

Clinical evidence

A patient with dendritic cell carcinoma who had been taking amiodarone for 18 months, and who had received 6 cycles of chemotherapy including cyclophosphamide over the previous 12 months, was admitted to hospital with progressive shortness of breath 18 days after being given a single 4-g/m^2 dose of cyclophosphamide. He was found to have interstitial pneumonitis and a lung biopsy indicated drug-induced pulmonary toxicity. The patient's condition improved rapidly over the following 10 days with discontinuation of amiodarone and treatment with prednisolone 60 mg daily. Over the previous year he had also received vincristine, etoposide and prednisone, cisplatin, cytarabine and dexamethasone as part of his chemotherapy.[1] Similarly, another patient with non-Hodgkin's lymphoma, who had been taking amiodarone 300 mg twice daily for 4 years, developed acute respiratory distress 2 days after being given a single dose of cyclophosphamide. This was eventually fatal. Autopsy revealed lung damage consistent with the effects of amiodarone and cyclophosphamide, with the cyclophosphamide the major cause. Other drugs used as part of the chemotherapy regimen were rituximab, doxorubicin, vincristine and prednisone.[2]

Mechanism

Pulmonary toxicity may occur in about 10% of patients given amiodarone.[3,4] Pulmonary toxicity due to cyclophosphamide may occur between one to 6 months after exposure or occur as a more insidious form after about 6 months. The early onset of symptoms in the patients described above suggests accelerated mechanisms of pulmonary toxicity. Both cyclophosphamide and amiodarone pulmonary toxicity appear to be enhanced by oxygen and the combination of cyclophosphamide with amiodarone may enhance oxidative stress and therefore pulmonary toxicity.

Importance and management

Although information seems to be limited to the two case reports cited, the potential for both cyclophosphamide and amiodarone to cause pulmonary toxicity is established. Be alert to the possibility of enhanced pulmonary toxicity if these drugs are given together.

1. Bhagat R, Sporn TA, Long GD, Folz RJ. Amiodarone and cyclophosphamide: potential for enhanced lung toxicity. *Bone Marrow Transplant* (2001) 27, 1109–1111.
2. Gupta S, Mahipal A. Fatal pulmonary toxicity after a single dose of cyclophosphamide. *Pharmacotherapy* (2007) 27, 616–18.
3. Martin WJ, Rosenow EC. Amiodarone pulmonary toxicity. Recognition and pathogenesis (Part 1). *Chest* (1988) 93, 1067–75.
4. Martin WJ, Rosenow EC. Amiodarone pulmonary toxicity. Recognition and pathogenesis (Part 2). *Chest* (1988) 93, 1242–8.

Cyclophosphamide + Azathioprine

A report describes liver damage in four patients given cyclophosphamide and who had previously taken azathioprine. However, other studies have found that liver function improved when cyclophosphamide was substituted for azathioprine.

Clinical evidence, mechanism, importance and management

Four patients (two with systemic lupus erythematosus, one with Sjögren's syndrome, and one with Wegener's granulomatosis) developed liver injury when given cyclophosphamide and 3 of them had liver cell necrosis. All had previously been taking azathioprine and 2 of them had received cyclophosphamide previously without apparent liver damage. It was suggested that azathioprine and cyclophosphamide may have interacted.[1] However, in a retrospective study of heart transplant recipients, substitution of cyclophosphamide for azathioprine was associated with improvement in liver function tests in 29 patients with suspected azathioprine-induced liver impairment.[2] In a similar report 10 patients with kidney transplants who developed hepatic impairment while taking azathioprine, had an improvement in liver function when the treatment was changed to cyclophosphamide.[3]

1. Shaunak S, Munro JM, Weinbren K, Walport MJ, Cox TM. Cyclophosphamide-induced liver necrosis: a possible interaction with azathioprine. *Q J Med* (1988) New Series 67, 309–17.
2. Wagoner LE, Olsen SL, Bristow MR, O'Connell JB, Taylor DO, Lappe DL, Renlund DG. Cyclophosphamide as an alternative to azathioprine in cardiac transplant recipients with suspected azathioprine-induced hepatotoxicity. *Transplantation* (1993) 56, 1415–18.
3. Berne TV, Chatterjee SN, Craig JR, Payne JE. Hepatic dysfunction in recipients of renal allografts. *Surg Gynecol Obstet* (1975), 141, 171–5.

Cyclophosphamide or Ifosfamide + Azoles

Fluconazole and itraconazole both inhibit the metabolism of cyclophosphamide, but itraconazole might cause greater increases in cyclophosphamide toxicity. Ketoconazole inhibits the metabolism of ifosfamide: efficacy could be reduced.

Clinical evidence

(a) Cyclophosphamide

Twenty-two children with established cyclophosphamide metabolism profiles, who were not receiving other treatment known to affect drug metabolism, were included in a retrospective case series investigation. The clearance of cyclophosphamide was reduced by 43% in 9 children who were given oral or intravenous **fluconazole** 5 mg/kg daily compared with the remaining 13 children who did not receive **fluconazole**.[1] A study in patients given either intravenous or oral **fluconazole** 400 mg daily or **itraconazole** (either 200 mg daily intravenously or 2.5 mg/kg three times daily orally) for prophylaxis after allogeneic stem cell transplantation found that those given **itraconazole** developed higher bilirubin and creatinine levels in the first 20 days after transplantation than those given **fluconazole**. Highest values were in patients who received **itraconazole** with cyclophosphamide. In this study, analysis of cyclophosphamide pharmacokinetics in 9 **itraconazole** recipients and 140 **fluconazole** recipients revealed that **itraconazole** recipients had a 20% greater clearance of cyclophosphamide than fluconazole recipients, leading to greater exposure to the active metabolite of cyclophosphamide, 4-hydroxycyclophosphamide, and its metabolites.[2]

(b) Ifosfamide

Eight patients undergoing chemotherapy were also given (for the first or second cycle of treatment) **ketoconazole** 200 mg twice daily for 4 days starting one day before ifosfamide. The concurrent use of **ketoconazole** modestly decreased the clearance of ifosfamide by 11%, increased its AUC by 14%, and increased urinary elimination by 26%. The fraction of ifosfamide metabolised to the inactive, neurotoxic, dechloroethylated metabolite was not affected, whereas the fraction metabolised to the active, hydroxylated metabolite was modestly decreased.[3]

Mechanism

Cyclophosphamide is oxidised to the active metabolite 4-hydroxycyclophosphamide by the cytochrome P450 isoenzymes CYP2B6, CYP3A4, CYP2C9, and CYP2A6, and then 4-hydroxycyclophosphamide undergoes further metabolism to produce several toxic metabolites. It is also metabolised by CYP3A4 to an inactive metabolite, deschloroethylcyclophosphamide (DCCP). Itraconazole is a more potent inhibitor of CYP3A4 than fluconazole, but unlike itraconazole, fluconazole can also inhibit CYP2C9. It has been suggested that inhibition of CYP2C9 by fluconazole may decrease the formation of 4-hydroxycyclophosphamide and result in increased levels of DCCP and fewer toxic metabolites.[2] Further study is required to determine whether the inhibition of active metabolite formation by fluconazole reduces the therapeutic effect of cyclophosphamide.[1]

Ketoconazole is an inhibitor of the cytochrome P450 isoenzyme CYP3A4, an enzyme that is involved in the production of active and inactive-toxic metabolites of ifosfamide. See *Mechanism,* under 'Cyclophosphamide or Ifosfamide + Barbiturates', p.671, for more on the balance of production of these metabolites.

Importance and management

Until more is known it may be prudent to encourage caution when azoles are used in patients receiving cyclophosphamide, other than therapies established in randomised clinical studies, being alert for unexpected toxicity or reduced efficacy.

In the clinical study cited, ketoconazole modestly decreased the proportion of ifosfamide undergoing activation. It was suggested that concurrent use should be avoided, as it might result in decreased ifosfamide efficacy,[3] although this is not established.

1. Yule SM, Walker D, Cole M, Mcsorley L, Cholerton S, Daly AK, Pearson ADJ, Boddy AV. The effect of fluconazole on cyclophosphamide metabolism in children. *Drug Metab Dispos* (1999) 27, 417–21.
2. Marr KA, Leisenring W, Crippa F, Slattery JT, Corey L, Boeckh M, McDonald GB. Cyclophosphamide metabolism is affected by azole antifungals. *Blood* (2004) 103, 1557–9.
3. Kerbusch T, Jansen RLH, Mathôt RAA, Huitema ADR, Jansen M, van Rijswijk REN, Beijnen JH. Modulation of the cytochrome P450–mediated metabolism of ifosfamide by ketoconazole and rifampin. *Clin Pharmacol Ther* (2001) 70, 132–41.

Cyclophosphamide or Ifosfamide + Barbiturates

Evidence suggests that neither the toxicity nor the therapeutic effects of cyclophosphamide and ifosfamide are significantly altered by the concurrent use of barbiturates. However, an isolated report describes a girl taking phenobarbital who developed encephalopathy when given ifosfamide.

Clinical evidence

(a) Cyclophosphamide

In 4 patients **phenobarbital** 180 mg daily in divided doses for 10 days increased the mean plasma levels of cyclophosphamide total metabolites by 50% and increased their rate of urinary excretion.[1] Similarly, another study in 11 patients given cyclophosphamide reported that the peak level of normustard-like substances was increased by 50% after pretreatment with **phenobarbital**.[2] Similar changes in cyclophosphamide pharmacokinetics have been described in *animal* studies, and these have generally also shown that **phenobarbital** has no effect on the antitumour activity of cyclophosphamide (one study is cited as an example[3]) although some have shown a reduction in its effects (one study is cited as an example[4]). Another study found that the auto-induction of cyclophosphamide clearance in a patient taking **phenobarbital** with subsequent chemotherapy courses was similar to that in patients not taking **phenobarbital**.[5]

Cyclophosphamide was reported to inhibit the clearance and increase the effects of **pentobarbital** in a study in *rats*.[6]

(b) Ifosfamide

A 15-year-old girl who had been taking **phenobarbital** for epilepsy since infancy developed confusion and gradually became unconscious 6 hours after being given a first dose of ifosfamide for metastatic rhabdomyosarcoma. Her chemotherapy regimen was ifosfamide 3 g/m^2, mesna 3.6 g/m^2, vincristine 2 mg and dactinomycin. An EEG revealed signs of severe diffuse encephalopathy. She remained unconscious for 24 hours but was asymptomatic after 48 hours.[7] In a pharmacokinetic study, **phenobarbital** 60 mg daily for 3 days had no effect on the pharmacokinetics of high-dose ifosfamide (4 g/m^2 over one hour each day for 3 days). The AUC for ifosfamide decreased from day one to day 3 irrespective of **phenobarbital** use.[8]

Mechanism

Cyclophosphamide and ifosfamide are prodrugs that undergo hepatic metabolism, and it seems that they are able to induce their own metabolism. Cyclophosphamide appears to be hydroxylated by the cytochrome P450 subfamilies CYP2B and CYP2C, in particular, to form active metabolites, whereas ifosfamide appears to be principally hydroxylated by CYP3A. Both drugs also undergo dechloroethylation to produce inactive but neurotoxic metabolites, which can cause encephalopathy. For cyclophosphamide, this seems to be primarily catalysed by CYP3A, whereas for ifosfamide both CYP3A and CYP2B appear to be involved. Ifosfamide has a higher incidence of encephalopathy than cyclophosphamide.[9] Phenobarbital and other barbiturates are inducers of both CYP2B and CYP3A. Therefore it is unlikely that barbiturates will generally alter the balance between dechloroethylation and hydroxylation for cyclophosphamide,[3] although there is some evidence from *animal* studies they may do so for ifosfamide.[10]

Importance and management

The relationship between the case of encephalopathy and the use of ifosfamide with phenobarbital is not established, but it serves to emphasise the need for particular caution and good monitoring if concurrent use is undertaken. Although barbiturates can cause an increase in the rate of metabolism of cyclophosphamide, this does not appear to alter the AUC and the efficacy of this drug.

1. Jao JY, Jusko WJ, Cohen JL. Phenobarbital effects on cyclophosphamide pharmacokinetics in man. *Cancer Res* (1972) 32, 2761–4.
2. Maezawa S, Ohira S, Sakauma M, Matsuoka S, Wakui A, Saito T. Effects of inducer of liver drug-metabolizing enzyme on blood level of active metabolites of cyclophosphamide in rats and in cancer patients. *Tohoku J Exp Med* (1981) 134, 45–53.
3. Yu LJ, Drewes P, Gustafsson K, Brain EGC, Hecht JED, Waxman DJ. In Vivo modulation of alternative pathways of P-450-catalyzed cyclophosphamide metabolism: impact on pharmacokinetics and antitumor activity. *J Pharmacol Exp Ther* (1999) 288, 928–37.
4. Alberts DS, van Daalen Wetters T. The effect of phenobarbital on cyclophosphamide antitumour activity. *Cancer Res* (1976) 36, 2785–9.
5. Chen T-L, Passos-Coelho JL, Noe DA, Kennedy MJ, Black KC, Colvin M, Grochow LB. Nonlinear pharmacokinetics of cyclophosphamide in patients with metastatic breast cancer receiving high-dose chemotherapy followed by autologous bone marrow transplantation. *Cancer Res* (1995) 55, 810–16. Correction. ibid. 1600.
6. Donelli MG, Colombo T, Garattini S. Effect of cyclophosphamide on the activity and distribution of pentobarbital in rats. *Biochem Pharmacol* (1973) 22, 2609–14.
7. Ghosn M, Carde P, Leclerq B, Flamant F, Friedman S, Droz JP, Hayat M. Ifosfamide/mesna related encephalopathy: a case report with a possible role of phenobarbital in enhancing neurotoxicity. *Bull Cancer* (1988) 75, 391–2.
8. Lokiec F, Santoni J, Weill S, Tubiana-Hulin M. Phenobarbital administration does not affect high-dose ifosfamide pharmacokinetics in humans. *Anticancer Drugs* (1996) 7, 893–6.
9. Goren MP, Wright RK, Pratt CB, Pell FE. Dechloroethylation of ifosfamide and neurotoxicity. *Lancet* (1986) ii, 1219–20.
10. Brain EGC, Yu LJ, Gustafsson K, Drewes P, Waxman DJ. Modulation of P450-dependent ifosfamide pharmacokinetics: a better understanding of drug activation in vivo. *Br J Cancer* (1998) 77, 1768–76.

Cyclophosphamide or Ifosfamide + Benzodiazepines

***Animal* studies suggest that the benzodiazepines may possibly increase the metabolic activation and the toxicity of high doses of cyclophosphamide and ifosfamide. However, diazepam did not alter the pharmacokinetics of high-dose cyclophosphamide in a clinical study. Note also that lorazepam is widely used for chemotherapy-induced nausea and vomiting.**

Clinical evidence, mechanism, importance and management

Studies in *mice* found that pretreatment with benzodiazepines (**chlordiazepoxide, diazepam, oxazepam**) increased the levels of the active metabolites and the lethality of high-dose cyclophosphamide[1] and similarly increased the levels of active metabolites and enhanced the toxicity of high-dose ifosfamide.[2] However, a clinical study found that the prophylactic use of **diazepam** 5 mg daily as an antiepileptic had no effect on the pharmacokinetics of very high-dose cyclophosphamide (60 mg/kg intravenously over 2 hours for 2 days) or its neurotoxic (dechloroethylated) metabolites in 3 patients receiving cyclophosphamide and busulfan before bone marrow transplantation.[3]

In the *animal* studies, it was suggested that benzodiazepines may induce the liver enzymes concerned with the metabolism of cyclophosphamide and ifosfamide to its active cytotoxic products.

There are very limited data on this potential interaction. The widespread use of the benzodiazepine **lorazepam** in antiemetic regimens for chemotherapy-induced nausea and vomiting suggest that a significant increase in toxicity or alteration in efficacy of cyclophosphamide and ifosfamide does not occur clinically, but there do not appear to be any studies directly addressing this question.

1. Sasaki K-I, Furusawa S, Takayanagi G. Effects of chlordiazepoxide, diazepam and oxazepam on the antitumour activity, the lethality and the blood level of active metabolites of cyclophosphamide and cyclophosphamide oxidase activity in mice. *J Pharmacobiodyn* (1983) 6, 767–72.
2. Furusawa S, Fujimura T, Sasaki K, Takayanagi Y. Potentiation of ifosfamide toxicity by chlordiazepoxide, diazepam, and oxazepam. *Chem Pharm Bull (Tokyo)* (1989) 73, 3420–2.
3. Williams ML, Wainer IW, Embree L, Barnett M, Granvil CL, Ducharme MP. Enantioselective induction of cyclophosphamide metabolism by phenytoin. *Chirality* (1999) 11, 569–74.

Cyclophosphamide + Busulfan

The levels of cyclophosphamide may be increased, and those of its active metabolite decreased, if it is given within 24 hours of busulfan.

Clinical evidence, mechanism, importance and management

In one study, the ratio of the AUC of cyclophosphamide and that of its active metabolite 4-hydroxycyclophosphamide (HCY) was higher in patients also receiving phenytoin and busulfan than in those receiving irradiation (suggesting reduced cyclophosphamide activation), but variability between patients was high.[1] In a similar study, 23 bone marrow transplant patients were pretreated with busulfan 4 mg/kg daily for 4 days, followed by cyclophosphamide 60 mg/kg daily for 2 days. The interval between the last dose of busulfan and starting cyclophosphamide was 24 to 50 hours in 12 patients [group A] and 7 to 15 hours in the remaining 11 [group B]. Nine others pretreated with cyclophosphamide and total body irradiation acted as the controls. In group A the AUCs of cyclophosphamide and HCY were similar to those in the controls but in group B the AUC of cyclophosphamide was more than doubled and the AUC of HCY significantly lower (representing a reduced ratio of HCY to cyclophosphamide). In addition group B had greater toxicity.[2]

Busulfan may directly inhibit the hepatic activation of cyclophosphamide or may act indirectly by depleting glutathione. Phenytoin (given in the first study) induces the metabolism of cyclophosphamide (see 'Cyclophosphamide or Ifosfamide + Phenytoin', p.673).

It seems therefore that if the cyclophosphamide is given at least 24 hours after the last busulfan dose, its serum levels will not be greatly affected, whereas if the interval is short, activation may be decreased and toxicity increased. Further study is required to determine the optimum timing to achieve maximum efficacy and minimum drug toxicity while taking into account other concurrent medication such as phenytoin.

1. Slattery JT, Kalhorn TF, McDonald GB, Lambert K, Buckner CD, Bensinger WI, Anasetti C, Appelbaum FR. Conditioning regimen-dependent disposition of cyclophosphamide and hydroxycyclophosphamide in human marrow transplantation patients. *J Clin Oncol* (1996) 14, 1484–94.
2. Hassan M, Ljungman P, Ringdén O, Hassan Z, Öberg G, Nilsson C, Békassy A, Bielenstein M, Abdel-Rehim M, Georén S, Astner L. The effect of busulphan on the pharmacokinetics of cyclophosphamide and its 4-hydroxy metabolite: time interval influence on the therapeutic efficacy and therapy-related toxicity. *Bone Marrow Transplant* (2000) 25, 915–24.

Cyclophosphamide + Chloramphenicol

Some limited evidence suggests that chloramphenicol may reduce the production of the active metabolites of cyclophosphamide.

Clinical evidence, mechanism, importance and management

Cyclophosphamide itself is inactive, but after administration it is metabolised to active alkylating metabolites. A study in *animals*[1] found that pretreatment with chloramphenicol reduced the effects of cyclophosphamide and reduced the production of its active metabolites. Although another *animal* study also found a reduction in the lethality of cyclophosphamide with chloramphenicol, the immunosuppressive effect of cyclophosphamide was unchanged.[2] A study in 4 patients found that chloramphenicol 1 g twice daily for 12 days prolonged the mean serum half-life of a single intravenous dose of cyclophosphamide from 7.5 hours to 11.5 hours, but did not significantly affect the AUC of the metabolites.[3]

Chloramphenicol is an inhibitor of the cytochrome P450 isoenzyme subfamily CYP2B, which is partially responsible for the activation of cyclophosphamide. It therefore seems possible that a reduction in the activity of cyclophosphamide may occur, but the extent to which this affects treatment with cyclophosphamide is uncertain. Concurrent use need not be avoided, but be alert for evidence of a reduced response.

1. Dixon RL. Effect of chloramphenicol on the metabolism and lethality of cyclophosphamide in rats. *Proc Soc Exp Biol Med* (1968) 127, 1151–5.
2. Berenbaum MC, Cope WA, Double JA. The effect of microsomal enzyme inhibition on the immunosuppressive and toxic effects of cyclophosphamide. *Clin Exp Immunol* (1973) 14, 257–70.
3. Faber OK, Mouridsen HT, Skovsted L. The effect of chloramphenicol and sulphaphenazole on the biotransformation of cyclophosphamide in man. *Br J Clin Pharmacol* (1975) 2, 281–5.

Cyclophosphamide or Ifosfamide + Cisplatin

The renal toxicity of ifosfamide may be greater when used with cisplatin or in those who have previously been given cisplatin. Ifosfamide may increase the hearing loss due to cisplatin.

Clinical evidence

(a) Nephrotoxicity

A comparative study in 36 children with malignant solid tumours taking a range of drugs including some known to be potentially nephrotoxic (high dose methotrexate, aminoglycosides, cyclophosphamide), indicated that the previous use of cisplatin increased their susceptibility to ifosfamide toxicity (neurotoxicity, severe leucopenia or acute renal tubular damage).[1] Similarly, in another study the cumulative cisplatin dose given before high-dose ICE (ifosfamide, carboplatin, and etoposide) was found to be a strong risk factor for the development of nephrotoxicity.[2] The nephrotoxicity may not be reversible; 3 cases requiring long-term haemodialysis have been described.[3]

Other studies also suggested that the concurrent use of ifosfamide with cisplatin appeared to increase nephrotoxicity; one found an increase in depletion of phosphate reabsorption,[4] whereas the other found increased microglobulin excretion.[5]

(b) Ototoxicity

A retrospective comparative study found that when ifosfamide was given with cisplatin, the hearing loss caused by cisplatin was exacerbated.[6]

Mechanism

Both cisplatin and ifosfamide are commonly associated with nephrotoxicity. It is thought that concurrent or possibly previous use of cisplatin damages the renal tubules so that the clearance of the ifosfamide metabolites is reduced and their toxic effects are thereby increased. Damaged renal tubules may also be less capable of converting mesna to its active kidney-protecting form. The increase in the hearing loss is not understood.

Importance and management

These interactions appear to be established. The authors of the paper cited[1] point out that the majority of patients who develop toxicity have persistently high urinary NAG concentrations (*N*-acetyl-*β*-D-glucosaminidase, an enzyme released by renal tubular cells), even though serum creatinine levels remain within the acceptable range for ifosfamide treatment. They suggest that evidence of subclinical renal tubular damage should be sought for by monitoring the excretion of urinary NAG. Note that cisplatin and ifosfamide are widely used in combination, and the related drug **cyclophosphamide** is also routinely used with cisplatin. Amifostine may be useful in reducing the nephrotoxicity of this combination.[7] The authors who reported on hearing loss advised that serial audiograms should be done in patients given both drugs.[6]

1. Goren MP, Wright RK, Pratt CB, Horowitz ME, Dodge RK, Viar MJ, Kovnar EH. Potentiation of ifosfamide neurotoxicity, hematotoxicity, and tubular nephrotoxicity by prior *cis*-diamminedichloroplatinum(II) therapy. *Cancer Res* (1987) 47, 1457–60.
2. Caglar K, Kinalp C, Arpaci F, Turan M, Saglam K, Ozturk B, Komurcu Ş, Yavuz I, Yenicesu M, Ozet A, Vural A. Cumulative prior dose of cisplatin as a cause of the nephrotoxicity of high-dose chemotherapy followed by autologous stem-cell transplantation. *Nephrol Dial Transplant* (2002) 17, 1931–5.
3. Martinez F, Deray G, Cacoub P, Beaufils H, Jacobs C. Ifosfamide nephrotoxicity: deleterious effect of previous cisplatin administration. *Lancet* (1996) 348, 1100–1.
4. Rossi R, Danzebrink S, Hillebrand D, Linnenbürger K, Ullrich K, Jürgens H. Ifosfamide-induced subclinical nephrotoxicity and its potentiation by cisplatinum. *Med Pediatr Oncol* (1994) 22, 27–32.
5. Hacke M, Schmoll H-J, Alt JM, Baumann K, Stolte H. Nephrotoxicity of *cis*-diamminedichloroplatinum with or without ifosfamide in cancer treatment. *Clin Physiol Biochem* (1983) 1, 17–26.
6. Meyer WH, Ayers D, McHaney VA, Roberson P, Pratt CB. Ifosfamide and exacerbation of cisplatin-induced hearing loss. *Lancet* (1993) 341, 754–5.
7. Hartmann JT, Fels LM, Knop S, Stolte H, Kanz L, Bokemeyer C. A randomized trial comparing the nephrotoxicity of cisplatin/ifosfamide-based combination chemotherapy with or without amifostine in patients with solid tumors. *Invest New Drugs* (2000) 18, 281–9.

Cyclophosphamide + Colony-stimulating factors

Granulocyte colony-stimulating factor (G-CSF) used with cyclophosphamide has been associated with an increased occurrence of pulmonary toxicity.

Clinical evidence, mechanism, importance and management

A one-year-old boy with a neuroblastoma Evans stage III died of respiratory failure after being given **filgrastim** (a **G-CSF**) and normal doses of cyclophosphamide and doxorubicin. The authors of the report suggest that the pulmonary toxicity of the cyclophosphamide (normally only seen with high cumulative doses) is potentiated by **filgrastim**.[1] Six of 53 patients given CHOP (cyclophosphamide, doxorubicin, vincristine and prednisolone) and **G-CSF** developed pulmonary toxicity, which was considered a much higher incidence than is usually seen with CHOP alone. The development of toxicity correlated with the mean peak leucocyte count.[2] Another 10 cases of interstitial pneumonitis have occurred with cyclophosphamide-based regimens (not including bleomycin or methotrexate) and **G-CSF**.[3,4]

These interactions are not firmly established, but good pulmonary function monitoring appears to be advisable when colony-stimulating factors are used with antineoplastics causing pulmonary toxicity, such as cyclophosphamide. If interstitial pneumonitis occurs, the drugs should be discontinued and high-dose corticosteroids started immediately.[2] Note however, because of the increased risk of myelosuppression, colony stimulating factors should not be given within 24 hours of myelosuppressive chemotherapy, see 'Antineoplastics + Colony-stimulating factors', p.657.

1. van Woensel JBM, Knoester H, Leeuw JA, van Aalderen WMC. Acute respiratory insufficiency during doxorubicin, cyclophosphamide, and G-CSF therapy. *Lancet* (1994) 344, 759–60.
2. Yokose N, Ogata K, Tamura H, An E, Nakamura K, Kamikubo K, Kudoh S, Dan K, Nomura T. Pulmonary toxicity after granulocyte colony-stimulating factor-combined chemotherapy for non-Hodgkin's lymphoma. *Br J Cancer* (1998) 77, 2286–90.
3. Niitsu N, Iki S, Muroi K, Motomura S, Murakami M, Takeyama H, Ohsaka A, Urabe A. Interstitial pneumonia in patients receiving granulocyte colony-stimulating factor during chemotherapy: survey in Japan 1991–96. *Br J Cancer* (1997) 76, 1661–6.
4. Hasegawa Y, Ninomiya J, Kamoshita M, Ohtani K, Kobayashi T, Kojima J, Nagasawa T, Abe T. Interstitial pneumonitis related to granulocyte colony-stimulating factor administration following chemotherapy for elderly patients with non-Hodgkin's lymphoma. *Intern Med* (1997) 36, 360–4.

Cyclophosphamide or Ifosfamide + Corticosteroids

There is limited and conflicting evidence on the effect of prednisone and prednisolone on the metabolic activation of cyclophosphamide. Synergistic increases in enzyme induction may occur if cyclophosphamide is given with dexamethasone. Dexamethasone does not appear to alter ifosfamide metabolism.

Clinical evidence

(a) Dexamethasone

In an *in vitro* study it was noted that the combination of cyclophosphamide with dexamethasone resulted in a greater induction of the cytochrome P450 isoenzyme CYP3A4 than with cyclophosphamide alone; the extent of induction being dependent on baseline CYP3A4 activity.[1] In *rats*,[2] dexamethasone pretreatment caused a fourfold increase in the AUC of the inactive, neurotoxic, dechloroethylated metabolite of cyclophosphamide, and caused a 60% decrease in the AUC of the active, hydroxylated metabolite. In an earlier study in patients receiving high-dose cyclophosphamide and dexamethasone for 2 days, the total clearance of both cyclophosphamide and dexamethasone were higher on the second day than the first day, with higher concentrations of cyclophosphamide metabolites.[3]

In *rats*, dexamethasone pretreatment had no net impact on the fraction of ifosfamide undergoing activation.[4] Similarly, in a clinical study, ifosfamide metabolism was no different when patients were given dexamethasone 4 mg every 8 hours with ifosfamide for 3 days than when they received ifosfamide alone.[5]

(b) Prednisone or Prednisolone

In an early study, single doses of prednisone were found to inhibit the metabolic activation of cyclophosphamide,[6,7] whereas another study briefly mentioned that massive single doses of prednisolone given just before cyclophosphamide did not inhibit cyclophosphamide metabolism.[8] Longer-term prednisone treatment (50 mg daily for 1 to 2 weeks) increased the rate of activation of cyclophosphamide in the first study.[6,7] Conversely, another study in 7 patients with systemic vasculitis given prednisone 1 mg/kg daily and cyclophosphamide 600 mg/m^2 intravenously every 3 weeks for 6 cycles found that, by the last cycle, the AUC of cyclophosphamide had significantly increased, while that of its active metabolites had significantly decreased.[9]

Mechanism

Cyclophosphamide and ifosfamide are prodrugs that undergo hepatic metabolism to active and inactive-neurotoxic metabolites, and it appears they induce their own metabolism (see also 'Cyclophosphamide or Ifosfamide + Barbiturates', p.670). Corticosteroids are said to be inducers of the cytochrome P450 isoenzyme CYP3A4. For cyclophosphamide, the CYP3A subfamily is thought to be principally involved in the production of inactive-neurotoxic metabolites, whereas, for ifosfamide, CYP3A catalyses both the production of active and inactive-neurotoxic metabolites. On this basis, corticosteroids are predicted decrease the efficacy and increase the neurotoxicity of cyclophosphamide (although this does not take account of auto-induction), whereas for ifosfamide they would not be expected to alter the balance between efficacy and toxicity.

Importance and management

The documentation is very limited. It appears that dexamethasone does not have any appreciable effect on the metabolism of ifosfamide. The information about cyclophosphamide is conflicting, and the clinical importance of any changes remains to be established. However, it should be noted that prednisone and prednisolone have a long established use as part of chemotherapy regimens including cyclophosphamide and are also often combined in various autoimmune diseases, and dexamethasone is widely used as an antiemetic with cancer chemotherapy.

1. Lindley C, Hamilton G, McCune JS, Faucette S, Shord SS, Hawke RL, Wang H, Gilbert D, Jolley S, Yan B, LeCluyse EL. The effect of cyclophosphamide with and without dexamethasone on cytochrome P450 3A4 and 2B6 in human hepatocytes. *Drug Metab Dispos* (2002) 30, 814–22.
2. Yu LJ, Drewes P, Gustafsson K, Brain EGC, Hecht JED, Waxman DJ. In vivo modulation of alternative pathways of P-450-catalyzed cyclophosphamide metabolism: impact on pharmacokinetics and antitumor activity. *J Pharmacol Exp Ther* (1999) 288, 928–37.
3. Moore MJ, Hardy RW, Thiessen JJ, Soldin SJ, Erlichman C. Rapid development of enhanced clearance after high-dose cyclophosphamide. *Clin Pharmacol Ther* (1988) 44, 622–8.
4. Brain EGC, Yu LJ, Gustafsson K, Drewes P, Waxman DJ. Modulation of P450-dependent ifosfamide pharmacokinetics: a better understanding of drug activation in vivo. *Br J Cancer* (1998) 77, 1768–76.
5. Singer JM, Hartley JM, Brennan C, Nicholson PW, Souhami RL. The pharmacokinetics and metabolism of ifosfamide during bolus and infusional administration: a randomized cross-over study. *Br J Cancer* (1998) 77, 978–84.
6. Faber OK, Mouridsen HT. Cyclophosphamide activation and corticosteroids. *N Engl J Med* (1974) 291, 211.
7. Faber OK, Mouridsen HT, Skovsted L. The biotransformation of cyclophosphamide in man: influence of prednisone. *Acta Pharmacol Toxicol (Copenh)* (1974) 35, 195–200.
8. Bagley CM, Bostick FW, DeVita VT. Clinical pharmacology of cyclophosphamide. *Cancer Res* (1973) 33, 226–33.
9. Belfayol-Pisanté L, Guillevin L, Tod M, Fauvelle F. Possible influence of prednisone on the pharmacokinetics of cyclophosphamide in systemic vasculitis. *Clin Drug Invest* (1999) 18, 225–31.

Cyclophosphamide + H_2-receptor antagonists

Ranitidine, and probably famotidine, appear not to increase the bone marrow toxicity of cyclophosphamide. *Animal* studies suggest that cimetidine might.

Clinical evidence, mechanism, importance and management

A study in 7 patients with cancer found that although oral **ranitidine** 300 mg daily significantly prolonged the half-life and increased the AUC of intravenous cyclophosphamide 600 mg/m^2, it did not significantly affect the AUCs of the two major alkylating metabolites of cyclophosphamide, nor did it affect its bone marrow toxicity (leucopenia, granulocytopenia). The authors of the study concluded that **ranitidine** can safely be given with cyclophosphamide.[1] The same authors previously reported that **cimetidine**, when given with cyclophosphamide, increased the AUC of total alkylating metabolites of cyclophosphamide, and resulted in greater toxicity to normal bone marrow, but increased survival in leukaemia-bearing *mice*.[2,3] Other studies in *mice* have found that **cimetidine**, but not **famotidine**, increases the toxicity of cyclophosphamide to normal bone marrow cells.[4]

Cimetidine inhibits the cytochrome P450 isoenzyme CYP2C9, which has a minor role in the activation of cyclophosphamide (see 'Cyclophosphamide or Ifosfamide + Barbiturates', p.670). These results suggest that no special precautions are likely to be needed when **ranitidine** or **famotidine** are given with cyclophosphamide. The relevance of the findings with **cimetidine** is uncertain.

1. Alberts DS, Mason-Liddil N, Plezia PM, Roe DJ, Dorr RT, Struck RF, Phillips JG. Lack of ranitidine effects on cyclophosphamide bone marrow toxicity or metabolism: a placebo-controlled clinical trial. *J Natl Cancer Inst* (1991) 83, 1739–43.
2. Dorr RT, Alberts DS. Cimetidine enhancement of cyclophosphamide antitumour activity. *Br J Cancer* (1982) 45, 35–43.
3. Dorr RT, Soble MJ, Alberts DS. Interaction of cimetidine but not ranitidine with cyclophosphamide in mice. *Cancer Res* (1986) 46, 1795–9.
4. Lerza RA, Bogliolo GV, Mecoboni MP, Saviane AG, Pannacciulli IM. Effect of H2 antagonists cimetidine and famotidine on the hemotoxicity of cyclophosphamide. *Anticancer Res* (1988) 8, 1241–5.

Cyclophosphamide + Indometacin

A single case report describes acute water intoxication when a patient taking indometacin was given low-dose intravenous cyclophosphamide.

Clinical evidence, mechanism, importance and management

A patient with multiple myeloma taking indometacin 50 mg every 8 hours, developed acute water intoxication and salt retention after being given a single bolus intravenous injection of cyclophosphamide 500 mg (less than 10 mg/kg). The reasons for this effect are not understood, but it is suggested that it was due to the additive or synergistic effects of the two drugs, because water intoxication had not been noted before with this low-dose of cyclophosphamide.[1] There do not appear to be any further reports or studies on this potential interaction but water intoxication has subsequently been reported with low-dose intravenous cyclophosphamide alone.[2] The evidence does not justify any special precautions when both drugs are used.

1. Webberley M J, Murray J A. Life-threatening acute hyponatraemia induced by low dose cyclophosphamide and indomethacin. *Postgrad Med J* (1989) 65, 950–2.
2. McCarron MO, Wright GD, Roberts SD. Water intoxication after low dose cyclophosphamide. *BMJ* (1995) 311, 292.

Cyclophosphamide + Metronidazole

A case report describes encephalopathy in a girl given cyclophosphamide and metronidazole.

Clinical evidence, mechanism, importance and management

After the fourth dose of pulse intravenous cyclophosphamide, a 9-year-old girl developed pancytopenia and gastrointestinal bleeding. She was then given metronidazole for presumptive *Clostridium difficile* colitis. Within 6 hours she developed encephalopathy with seizures and visual hallucinations, requiring antipsychotics. Metronidazole is thought to cause disulfiram-like reactions by inhibiting aldehyde dehydrogenase (see 'Alcohol + Metronidazole and related drugs', p.75), and it was suggested that inhibition of this enzyme may cause toxic metabolites of cyclophosphamide to accumulate (see also 'Cyclophosphamide or Ifosfamide + Barbiturates', p.670).[1] This appears to be the only report of this potential interaction, and its general relevance is unclear.

1. Pinsk MN, Renton K, Crocker JFS, Acott PD. A proposed drug interaction leading to cyclophosphamide-induced encephalopathy. *Pediatr Res* (2002) 51, 437A.

Cyclophosphamide + Pentostatin

Two patients had an acute and fatal cardiovascular collapse when pentostatin was added to high-dose cyclophosphamide. Some studies have found the combination to be effective and safe in patients with chronic lymphocytic leukaemia.

Clinical evidence, mechanism, importance and management

A clinical study that was started to find out if pentostatin would improve the immunosuppressive effects of an ablative regimen of high-dose cyclophosphamide, carmustine and etoposide in bone marrow transplant patients was stopped when acute and fatal cardiovascular collapse developed in the first 2 patients. Both patients had been given cyclophosphamide 800 mg/m^2 and etoposide 200 mg/m^2, both every 12 hours for 8 doses, and carmustine 112 mg/m^2 daily for 4 doses. On day 3 pentostatin 4 mg/m^2, given over 4 hours, was added. Within 8 to 18 hours after completion of chemotherapy both patients developed confusion, hypothermia, hypotension, respiratory distress, pulmonary oedema, and eventually fatal ventricular fibrillation within 45 to 120 minutes of the first symptoms. A later study in *rats* similarly found that pentostatin markedly increased the acute toxicity of cyclophosphamide. The reasons for this cardiotoxicity are not understood. Neither of the 2 patients had previously shown any evidence of cardiac abnormalities.[1] In view of these findings, the UK manufacturer advises against the use of pentostatin with high-dose cyclophosphamide.[2]

Note that pentostatin 4 mg/m^2 plus cyclophosphamide 600 mg/m^2, with or without subsequent rituximab 375 mg/m^2, has been used for chronic lymphocytic leukaemia[3-5] or Waldenstrom's macroglobulinaemia[6] with acceptable toxicity, and without any cases similar to that described in the first report.[1]

1. Gryn J, Gordon R, Bapat A, Goldman N, Goldberg J. Pentostatin increases the acute toxicity of high dose cyclophosphamide. *Bone Marrow Transplant* (1993) 12, 217–20.
2. Nipent (Pentostatin). Hospira UK Ltd. UK Summary of product characteristics, January 2009.
3. Weiss MA, Maslak PG, Jurcic JG, Scheinberg DA, Aliff TB, Lamanna N, Frankel SR, Kossman SE, Horgan D. Pentostatin and cyclophosphamide: an effective new regimen in previously treated patients with chronic lymphocytic leukemia. *J Clin Oncol* (2003) 21, 1278–84.
4. Lamanna N, Kalaycio M, Maslak P, Jurcic JG, Heaney M, Brentjens R, Zelenetz AD, Horgan D, Gencarelli A, Panageas KS, Scheinberg DA, Weiss MA. Pentostatin, cyclophosphamide, and rituximab is an active, well-tolerated regimen for patients with previously treated chronic lymphocytic leukaemia. *J Clin Oncol* (2006) 24, 1575–81.
5. Kay NE, Geyer SM, Call TG, Shanafelt TD, Zent CS, Jelinek DF, Tschumper R, Bone ND, Dewald GW, Lin TS, Heerema NA, Smith L, Grever MR, Byrd JC. Combination chemoimmunotherapy with pentostatin, cyclophosphamide, and rituximab shows significant clinical activity with low accompanying toxicity in previously untreated B chronic lymphocytic leukaemia. *Blood* (2007) 109, 405–11.
6. Hensel M, Villalobos M, Kornacker M, Krasniqi F, Ho AD. Pentostatin/cyclophosphamide with or without rituximab: an effective regimen for patients with Waldenström's macroglobulinaemia/lymphoplasmacytic lymphoma. *Clin Lymphoma Myeloma* (2005) 6, 131–5.

Cyclophosphamide or Ifosfamide + Phenytoin

Phenytoin increases the metabolism of cyclophosphamide and ifosfamide, but the clinical relevance of this is uncertain. Efficacy and toxicity has been suggested to be both unchanged and increased.

Clinical evidence

(a) Cyclophosphamide

In another case report, a 42-year-old man received two courses of CTC (high-dose cyclophosphamide, thiotepa and carboplatin) with phenytoin 150 mg twice daily started 5 days before the second course for seizures. When compared with the first course, phenytoin appeared to cause a 51% increase in the AUC of 4-hydroxycyclophosphamide, the active metabolite of cyclophosphamide, and a sixfold increase in its maximum plasma level. In addition, the AUC of cyclophosphamide was reduced by 67%. On the basis of these data, the dose of cyclophosphamide was almost halved for the remaining 2 days of this course of chemotherapy, and this resulted in plasma levels within the therapeutic range.[1]

In a small pharmacokinetic study, the use of prophylactic phenytoin increased the formation of *S*-dechloroethylated cyclophosphamide in 3 patients receiving cyclophosphamide and busulfan compared with 3 patients given diazepam with the same cytotoxic regimen.[2] In yet another study, the ratio of the AUC of active 4-hydroxycyclophosphamide to cyclophosphamide was 166% higher in patients receiving phenytoin and busulfan than in those receiving irradiation.[3] It is likely that phenytoin was responsible for this effect because busulfan alone decreases cyclophosphamide metabolism (see 'Cyclophosphamide + Busulfan', p.671). In an earlier study, in patients receiving enzyme-inducing drugs (2 of whom received phenytoin), the peak plasma levels of the alkylating metabolites of cyclophosphamide were raised, but declined rapidly, so that the overall exposure was not different from those not taking these drugs.[4] Another study reported that a patient taking phenytoin had a high clearance rate for cyclophosphamide during her first chemotherapy course, and that auto-induction of cyclophosphamide clearance was not apparent during her second course.[5]

(b) Ifosfamide

A child taking phenytoin and also given ifosfamide and etoposide had a neurotoxic reaction. The plasma levels of the dechloroethylated metabolites of ifosfamide were subsequently found to be markedly altered compared with those previously seen in 14 other children receiving the same chemotherapy but not taking phenytoin. The child recovered uneventfully after 3 days, and achieved clinical remission (she had not responded to first-line chemotherapy).[6]

Mechanism

The alteration in the pattern of ifosfamide metabolites suggested that phenytoin had induced the activity of the cytochrome P450 isoenzyme CYP2B6, and to a lesser extent CYP3A4.[6] The pattern of the increase in cyclophosphamide clearance is also consistent with induction of CYP2B and CYP3A.[2] See also *Mechanism*, under 'Cyclophosphamide or Ifosfamide + Barbiturates', p.670, for more detail on the metabolism of cyclophosphamide and its metabolites.

Importance and management

The alteration in the metabolism of cyclophosphamide and ifosfamide caused by phenytoin is not surprising, but the clinical importance of any changes remains to be established. The authors of the study from the 1970s concluded that phenytoin was unlikely to have much effect on the antitumour and toxic effects of cyclophosphamide.[4] Conversely, the authors of the more recent studies suggest that phenytoin may increase the therapeutic efficacy of cyclophosphamide and ifosfamide.[2,6] Moreover, the authors of the latest case report suggest that it is preferable to avoid using phenytoin with cyclophosphamide. They suggest that, when concurrent use is unavoidable, the starting dose of cyclophosphamide should be reduced, and the levels of active metabolite should be monitored to guide further doses.[1] Further study is needed.

Note that reduced phenytoin levels and seizures have been reported in a patient receiving chemotherapy including cyclophosphamide, see 'Table 14.1', p.563.

1. de Jonge ME, Huitema ADR, van Dam SM, Beijnen JH, Rodenhuis S. Significant induction of cyclophosphamide and thiotepa metabolism by phenytoin. *Cancer Chemother Pharmacol* (2005) 55, 507–510.
2. Williams ML, Wainer IW, Embree L, Barnett M, Granvil CL, Ducharme MP. Enantioselective induction of cyclophosphamide metabolism by phenytoin. *Chirality* (1999) 11, 569–74.
3. Slattery JT, Kalhorn TF, McDonald GB, Lambert K, Buckner CD, Bensinger WI, Anasetti C, Appelbaum FR. Conditioning regimen-dependent disposition of cyclophosphamide and hydroxycyclophosphamide in human marrow transplantation patients. *J Clin Oncol* (1996) 14, 1484–94.
4. Bagley CM, Bostick FW, DeVita VT. Clinical pharmacology of cyclophosphamide. *Cancer Res* (1973) 33, 226–33.
5. Chen T-L, Passos-Coelho JL, Noe DA, Kennedy MJ, Black KC, Colvin M, Grochow LB. Nonlinear pharmacokinetics of cyclophosphamide in patients with metastatic breast cancer receiving high-dose chemotherapy followed by autologous bone marrow transplantation. *Cancer Res* (1995) 55, 810–16. Correction. ibid. 1600.
6. Ducharme MP, Bernstein ML, Granvil CP, Gehrcke B, Wainer IW. Phenytoin-induced alteration in the *N*-dechloroethylation of ifosfamide stereoisomers. *Cancer Chemother Pharmacol* (1997) 40, 531–3.

Cyclophosphamide or Ifosfamide + Rifampicin (Rifampin)

Rifampicin induced the metabolism of cyclophosphamide and ifosfamide *in vitro*. For ifosfamide, this did not improve the ratio of active to inactive-toxic metabolites in a clinical study.

Clinical evidence, mechanism, importance and management

In a clinical study, rifampicin doubled the clearance of ifosfamide. In this study, patients were given rifampicin 300 mg twice daily for 3 days before ifosfamide, for 3 days concurrently for one cycle, and then for another cycle they were given the ifosfamide alone. The fraction of ifosfamide metabolised to the inactive-neurotoxic, dechloroethylated metabolite was increased, but elimination of this metabolite was also increased resulting in reduced exposure. The fraction of ifosfamide metabolised to the active, hydroxylated metabolite, and its exposure, were not altered appreciably.[1]

An *in vitro* study in human liver cells found that rifampicin was a potent inducer of the activation (hydroxylation) of cyclophosphamide and ifosfamide.[2] Rifampicin is a clinically relevant inducer of the cytochrome P450 isoenzymes CYP3A4 and CYP2B6, which are involved in the metabolism of cyclophosphamide and ifosfamide (see also 'Cyclophosphamide or Ifosfamide + Barbiturates', p.670). In the clinical study cited,[1] rifampicin did not have a positive effect on the proportion of ifosfamide undergoing activation. In addition, as rifampicin increased metabolism overall, there is the possibility of decreased efficacy,[1] although this remains to be shown.

1. Kerbusch T, Jansen RLH, Mathôt RAA, Huitema ADR, Jansen M, van Rijswijk REN, Beijnen JH. Modulation of the cytochrome P450–mediated metabolism of ifosfamide by ketoconazole and rifampin. *Clin Pharmacol Ther* (2001) 70, 132–41.
2. Chang TKH, Yu L, Maurel P, Waxman DJ. Enhanced cyclophosphamide and ifosfamide activation in primary human hepatocyte cultures: response to cytochrome P-450 inducers and autoinduction by oxazaphosphorines. *Cancer Res* (1997) 57, 1946–54.

Cyclophosphamide + Sulfonamides

Some very limited evidence suggests that sulfaphenazole may modestly inhibit the metabolism of cyclophosphamide to its active metabolite.

Clinical evidence, mechanism, importance and management

A study in 7 patients given a 50-mg dose of cyclophosphamide with **sulfaphenazole** 1 g twice daily for 9 to 14 days found that the half-life of cyclophosphamide was unchanged in 3 patients, longer in 2 patients, and shorter in 2 patients.[1] **Sulfaphenazole** and **sulfamethoxazole** are inhibitors of the cytochrome P450 isoenzyme CYP2C9, which shows genetic polymorphism (i.e. some people produce very little, while others produce larger quantities). This enzyme has a minor role in the metabolism (and therefore activation) of cyclophosphamide, and the extent of its involvement varies between patients. For example, an *in vitro* study found that **sulfaphenazole** inhibited cyclophosphamide activation by 17 to 27% in one human liver sample, but insignificant inhibition occurred in two other samples.[2] Thus, sulfonamides such as **sulfaphenazole** and **sulfamethoxazole** may moderately inhibit the activation of cyclophosphamide in some patients, but the clinical relevance of this is uncertain. Note that **co-trimoxazole** is sometimes used for prophylaxis of infection in patients receiving chemotherapy. One study found that this did not *increase* the myelotoxicity of CAE (cyclophosphamide, doxorubicin, and etoposide).[3]

1. Faber OK, Mouridsen HT, Skovsted L. The effect of chloramphenicol and sulphaphenazole on the biotransformation of cyclophosphamide in man. *Br J Clin Pharmacol* (1975) 2, 281–5.
2. Roy P, Yu LJ, Crespi CL, Waxman DJ. Development of a substrate-activity based approach to identify the major human liver P-450 catalysts of cyclophosphamide and ifosfamide activation based on cDNA-expressed activities and liver microsomal P-450 profiles. *Drug Metab Dispos* (1999) 27, 655–66.
3. de Jongh CA, Wade JC, Finley RS, Joshi JH, Aisner J, Wiernik PH, Schimpff SC. Trimethoprim/sulfamethoxazole versus placebo: a double-blind comparison of infection prophylaxis in patients with small cell carcinoma of the lung. *J Clin Oncol* (1983) 1, 302–7.

Cyclophosphamide or Ifosfamide + Taxanes

The clearance of ifosfamide is higher when it is given after docetaxel. This results in less toxicity, but the effect on efficacy is unknown. Ifosfamide did not alter the pharmacokinetics of docetaxel. Results from one study indicate that docetaxel pharmacokinetics are unaltered by cyclophosphamide. The sequence of ifosfamide followed by paclitaxel was antagonistic *in vitro*, and there is some evidence to suggest that the toxicity associated with combinations of paclitaxel and cyclophosphamide is dependent on the order of administration.

Clinical evidence, mechanism, importance and management

(a) Docetaxel

The AUCs of ifosfamide and its metabolites were lower when ifosfamide was given immediately after docetaxel than when it was given 24 hours before docetaxel, due to increased clearance. Docetaxel pharmacokinetics were unaltered by ifosfamide.[1] This supports the evidence that the maximum tolerated dose of ifosfamide is greater when it is given after docetaxel.[2] The mechanism of this effect is unknown, but it has been suggested[3] that docetaxel may competitively inhibit the activation of ifosfamide by the cytochrome P450 isoenzyme CYP3A4. These results show that the toxicity, and possibly efficacy, of the combination are schedule-dependent, but more study is needed to determine this.

In a phase I study, the pharmacokinetics of docetaxel were not altered by pretreatment with an intravenous bolus dose of cyclophosphamide.[4]

(b) Paclitaxel

In vitro studies in human liver microsomes found that additive or synergistic cytotoxicity occurred when activated ifosfamide (hydroxyifosfamide) and paclitaxel were given together or when paclitaxel was given first followed by hydroxyifosfamide. In contrast pronounced antagonism was seen when hydroxyifosfamide was given before paclitaxel.[5] The mechanism for this effect is unknown. These results suggest that the scheduling of this combination may be important for efficacy.

A study in patients given paclitaxel as a 24-hour infusion and cyclophosphamide as an infusion over one hour found that neutropenia and thrombocytopenia were more severe when paclitaxel preceded cyclophosphamide.[6] Similarly, in another study, the concurrent use of a continuous 72-hour infusion of paclitaxel and a daily bolus of cyclophosphamide had acceptable toxicity. However, when the cyclophosphamide was given as a single intravenous dose after the end of the 72-hour paclitaxel infusion, severe haematological and gastrointestinal toxicity occurred.[7] Whether the clinical efficacy of this combination is also altered by the schedule and sequence has not been determined.

1. Schrijvers D, Pronk L, Highley M, Bruno R, Locci-Tonelli D, De Bruijn E, Van Oosterom AT, Verweij J. Pharmacokinetics of ifosfamide are changed by combination with docetaxel. *Am J Clin Oncol* (2000) 23, 358–63.
2. Pronk L, Schrijvers D, Schellens JHM, De Bruijn EA, Planting ASTh, Locci-Tonelli D, Groult V, Verweij J, Van Oosterom AT. Phase I study on docetaxel and ifosfamide in patients with advanced solid tumours. *Br J Cancer* (1998) 77, 153–8.
3. Ando Y. Possible metabolic interaction between docetaxel and ifosfamide. *Br J Cancer* (2000) 82, 497.
4. Vasey PA, Roché H, Bisset D, Terret C, Vernillet L, Riva A, Ramazeilles C, Azli N, Kaye SB, Twelves CJ. Phase I study of docetaxel in combination with cyclophosphamide as first-line chemotherapy for metastatic breast cancer. *Br J Cancer* (2002) 87, 1072–8.
5. Vanhoefer U, Schleucher N, Klaassen U, Seeber S, Harstrick A. Ifosfamide-based drug combinations: preclinical evaluation of drug interactions and translation into the clinic. *Semin Oncol* (2000) 27 (Suppl 1), 8–13.
6. Kennedy MJ, Zahurak ML, Donehower RC, Noe DA, Sartorius S, Chen T-L, Bowling K, Rowinsky EK. Phase I and pharmacologic study of sequences of paclitaxel and cyclophosphamide supported by granulocyte colony-stimulating factor in women with previously treated metastatic breast cancer. *J Clin Oncol* (1996) 14, 783–91.
7. Tolcher AW, Cowan KH, Noone MH, Denicoff AM, Kohler DR, Goldspiel BR, Barnes CS, McCabe M, Gossard MR, Zujewski J, O'Shaughnessy J. Phase I study of paclitaxel in combination with cyclophosphamide and granulocyte colony-stimulating factor in metastatic breast cancer patients. *J Clin Oncol* (1996) 14, 95–102.

Cyclophosphamide + Thiotepa

Pretreatment with thiotepa may inhibit the metabolism of cyclophosphamide to its active metabolite and decrease both its efficacy and toxicity. Cyclophosphamide might slightly increase the metabolism of thiotepa to TEPA (triethylenephosphamide), but the relevance of this is uncertain.

Clinical evidence

(a) Effect on cyclophosphamide

The proportion of cyclophosphamide excreted unchanged in the urine (i.e. never metabolically activated) was found to be higher when cyclophosphamide was given as a 96-hour infusion with thiotepa and novobiocin than when it was given alone. The authors suggested that the potential of thiotepa to inhibit the metabolism of cyclophosphamide should be investigated.[1] Later, other authors observed that the concentration of the active metabolite of cyclophosphamide, 4-hydroxycyclophosphamide, decreased sharply after thiotepa was given to 20 patients.[2] In a study to investigate this effect further, 3 patients were given high-dose cyclophosphamide 1 or 1.5 g/m^2 as a one-hour infusion, followed by carboplatin and thiotepa for 4 days. The order of infusion was reversed on one treatment day in each of 4 courses. Giving thiotepa one hour before cyclophosphamide resulted in decreases in the peak plasma levels and AUC of 4-hydroxycyclophosphamide of 62% and 26%, respectively, when compared with thiotepa given one hour after cyclophosphamide.[2]

(b) Effect on thiotepa

In an *in vitro* study using human microsomes, cyclophosphamide had no effect on the metabolism of thiotepa to TEPA (triethylenephosphamide) by cytochrome P450 at therapeutic concentrations.[2,3] However, the metabolism of thiotepa to TEPA was modestly increased in the presence of cyclophosphamide in two patients who received treatment with thiotepa and carboplatin with and then without cyclophosphamide.[4] A subsequent population pharmacokinetic modelling study found that incorporation of induction of thiotepa metabolism by cyclophosphamide improved the model. According to this model, the total clearance of thiotepa is increased by 10 to 25% with cyclophosphamide.[4]

Mechanism

In human microsomes, thiotepa was found to inhibit the conversion of cyclophosphamide to its active metabolite, 4-hydroxycyclophosphamide,[2] most likely because it is an inhibitor of the cytochrome P450 isoenzyme CYP2B6.[5] See also *Mechanism*, under 'Cyclophosphamide or Ifosfamide + Barbiturates', p.670, for further detail on the metabolism of cyclophosphamide and its metabolites. Cyclophosphamide may have induced the metabolism of thiotepa by cytochrome P450 enzymes, but the exact enzymes involved are not clear.[4]

Importance and management

These results suggest that thiotepa can decrease both the efficacy and toxicity of cyclophosphamide, and that the order of administration may be of critical importance. The authors of one study question the practice of giving cyclophosphamide and thiotepa simultaneously.[2] Cyclophosphamide may also slightly increase the metabolism of thiotepa to an active metabolite, although the clinical relevance of this remains to be determined.[4]

1. Chen T-L, Passos-Coelho JL, Noe DA, Kennedy MJ, Black KC, Colvin M, Grochow LB. Nonlinear pharmacokinetics of cyclophosphamide in patients with metastatic breast cancer receiving high-dose chemotherapy followed by autologous bone marrow transplantation. *Cancer Res* (1995) 55, 810–16. Correction. ibid.1600.
2. Huitema ADR, Kerbusch T, Tibben MM, Rodenhuis S, Beijnen JH. Reduction of cyclophosphamide bioactivation by thioTEPA: critical sequence-dependency in high-dose chemotherapy regimens. *Cancer Chemother Pharmacol* (2000) 46, 119–27.
3. Van Maanen MJ, Huitema ADR, Beijnen JH. Influence of co-medicated drugs on the biotransformation of thioTEPA to TEPA and thioTEPA-mercapturate. *Anticancer Res* (2000) 20, 1711–16.
4. de Jonge ME, Huitema ADR, Rodenhuis S, Beiknen JH. Integrated population pharmacokinetic model of both cyclophosphamide and thiotepa suggesting a mutual drug-drug interaction. *J Pharmacokinet Pharmacodyn* (2004) 31, 135–56.
5. Rae JM, Soukhova NV, Flockhart DA, Desta Z. Triethylenethiophosphoramide is a specific inhibitor of cytochrome P450 2B6: implications for cyclophosphamide metabolism. *Drug Metab Dispos* (2002) 30, 525–30.

Cytarabine + Dipyridamole

A fatal case of increased cytarabine toxicity has been attributed to the concurrent use of dipyridamole.

Clinical evidence

A case report describes a 52-year-old man who experienced a relapse of acute myeloid leukaemia and was given idarubicin daily for 3 days and cytarabine daily for 7 days. Amikacin and cefepime were also given for febrile neutropenia. In addition he was given dipyridamole 75 mg three times daily for 5 days for occlusion of the peroneal and tibialis anterior arteries. His liver function deteriorated, most notably his bilirubin increased almost 10-fold by day 5, and he died 10 days after starting treatment due to multiple organ failure.[1]

Mechanism

Dipyridamole is reported to inhibit the nucleoside transporter responsible for the extracellular transport of cytarabine and its metabolites, thus increasing the intracellular retention of cytarabine within the hepatocytes.[1] One *in vitro* study in *mouse* leukaemic cells has shown that use of dipyridamole *after* cytarabine resulted in an increase in cytarabine retention and an increase in cytotoxicity.[2] However, in a similar study using human acute myeloid leukaemia blasts, dipyridamole had little effect, possibly because these cells had few nucleoside transport carriers.[3] In yet another *in vitro* study, *pretreatment* with dipyridamole inhibited the uptake of cytarabine into both normal and leukaemic *mouse* and human cells, which suggests that dipyridamole may reduce the toxicity of cytarabine when used first.[4]

Importance and management

This appears to be the only report of an interaction between dipyridamole and cytarabine, but consider an interaction as a possible cause should unexpected toxicity occur in patients receiving both drugs.

1. Babaoglu MO, Karadag O, Saikawa Y, Altundag K, Elkiran T, Yasar U, Bozkurt A. Hepatotoxicity due to a possible interaction between cytosine arabinoside and dipyridamole: a case report. *Eur J Clin Pharmacol* (2004) 60, 455–6.
2. Yang J-L, White JC, Capizzi RL. Enhanced retention of cytosine arabinoside and its metabolites and synergistic cytotoxicity by sequential treatment with dipyridamole in L5178Y leukaemia. *Cancer Chemother Pharmacol* (1990) 26, 135–8.
3. Yang J-L, White JC, Capizzi RL. Modulation of the cellular pharmacokinetics of ara-CTP in human leukemic blasts by dipyridamole. *Cancer Chemother Pharmacol* (1992) 29, 236–40.
4. King ME, Naporn A, Young B, Howell SB. Modulation of cytarabine uptake and toxicity by dipyridamole. *Cancer Treat Rep* (1984) 68, 361–6.

Enzalutamide + Miscellaneous

Enzalutamide markedly decreases midazolam exposure and is expected to decrease the exposure to other CYP3A4 substrates. Gemfibrozil moderately increases enzalutamide exposure and other CYP2C8 inhibitors are expected to interact similarly. Itraconazole slightly increases enzalutamide exposure and other CYP3A4 inhibitors are expected to interact similarly. Inducers of CYP2C8 and inducers of CYP3A4 are predicted to reduce the exposure to enzalutamide. Enzalutamide moderately decreases the exposure to S-warfarin and omeprazole; other CYP2C9 and CYP2C19 substrates might be similarly affected. Enzalutamide is predicted to increase the exposure to P-glycoprotein substrates. Enzalutamide does not have a clinically relevant effect on pioglitazone exposure. Food does not affect enzalutamide exposure. Enzalutamide does not alter the pharmacokinetics of docetaxel but concurrent use might increase the risk of neutropenia or seizures. Enzalutamide might increase the risk of seizure and this could be additive with other drugs that lower the seizure threshold.

Clinical evidence, mechanism, importance and management

(a) CYP2C8 inducers

CYP2C8 is a major enzyme involved in the metabolism of enzalutamide, but the US manufacturer notes that the effects of CYP2C8 inducers on enzalutamide has not been studied in a clinical setting. They advise that the concurrent use of potent and moderate CYP2C8 inducers should be avoided if possible.[1] The UK manufacturer advises potent CYP2C8 inducers are avoided or used with caution.[2] Until further evidence is available, be aware that the efficacy of enzalutamide might be reduced in patients taking a CYP2C8 inducer. For a list of drugs which are known to induce CYP2C8, see 'Table 1.4', p.6.

(b) CYP2C8 inhibitors

The UK and US manufacturers[1,2] of enzalutamide briefly report that in a study in healthy subjects given a single 160-mg dose[1] of enzalutamide after **gemfibrozil** 600 mg twice daily, the AUC of enzalutamide was increased 2.2-fold, and its maximum concentration was decreased by 18%.[2] CYP2C8 is a major enzyme involved in the metabolism of enzalutamide and gemfibrozil is a potent inhibitor of CYP2C8.[2] The manufacturers therefore advise that potent inhibitors of CYP2C8 should be avoided, where possible, in patients taking enzalutamide. If a potent CYP2C8 inhibitor is given, the enzalutamide dose should be reduced to 80 mg once daily during concurrent administration.[1,2] Until further evidence is available it might be prudent to monitor patients for enzalutamide adverse effects on the concurrent use of a CYP2C8 inhibitor. For a list of drugs which are known to inhibit CYP2C8, see 'Table 1.4', p.6.

(c) CYP2C8 substrates

The UK and US manufacturers of enzalutamide report that in a study in patients with prostate cancer, enzalutamide 160 mg once daily (at steady-state) increased the AUC of a single 30-mg dose[1] of **pioglitazone** by 20%, and decreased its maximum concentration by 18%. These changes were not considered to be clinically relevant.[1,2] Pioglitazone is a moderate CYP2C8 substrate and this study might suggest that enzalutamide is unlikely to induce or inhibit CYP2C8 to a clinically relevant extent. The manufacturers state that no dose adjustment is required on concurrent use of enzalutamide and CYP2C8 substrates[1,2] (see 'Table 1.4', p.6 for a list).

(d) CYP2C9 substrates

The UK and US manufacturers of enzalutamide report that a study in patients with prostate cancer were given enzalutamide 160 mg once daily (at-steady state) with a single 10-mg dose[1] of **warfarin**. The AUC of *S*-warfarin was decreased by 56%.[1,2] *S*-warfarin can be used as a probe substrate to assess the activity of drugs on CYP2C9, and this study would suggest that enzalutamide is a moderate inducer of this isoenzyme. Enzalutamide might decrease the exposure to other CYP2C9 substrates, and the US manufacturer of enzalutamide states that the concurrent use of CYP2C9 substrates with a narrow therapeutic range should be avoided.[1] For a list of known, clinically relevant CYP2C9 substrates, see 'Table 1.5', p.7. The UK manufacturer advises that the use of enzalutamide with **warfarin** and related anticoagulants should be avoided. If enzalutamide is given with warfarin,[1,2] **acenocoumarol**,[2] or another anticoagulant that is a CYP2C9 substrate[2] then the INR should be monitored more frequently.[1,2]

(e) CYP2C19 substrates

The UK and US manufacturers of enzalutamide report that in a study in patients with prostate cancer, enzalutamide 160 mg once daily (at steady-state) decreased the AUC of a single 20-mg dose[1] of **omeprazole** by 70%.[1,2] Omeprazole can be used as a probe substrate to assess the activity of drugs on CYP2C19. This study therefore suggests that enzalutamide is a moderate inducer of this isoenzyme, and it would be expected to decrease the exposure to other substrates of CYP2C19 (see 'Table 1.6', p.8 for a list). The US manufacturer notes that concurrent use of CYP2C19 substrates with a narrow therapeutic range should be avoided,[1] and the UK manufacturer advises that sensitive substrates should generally be avoided if the dose cannot be monitored and adjusted accordingly.[2] If concurrent use of enzalutamide and a sensitive CYP2C19 substrate, or a CYP2C19 substrate with a narrow therapeutic range, is necessary, it would be prudent to monitor the clinical efficacy of the substrate, and to adjust the dose accordingly.

(f) CYP3A4 inducers

The US manufacturer notes that the effects of CYP3A4 inducers on enzalutamide has not been studied in a clinical setting, and advises that concurrent use of potent and moderate CYP3A4 inducers should be avoided if possible.[1] 'Table 1.9', p.11, includes a list of known, clinically relevant CYP3A4 inducers. In addition to the drugs listed in this table, the US manufacturer also names **etravirine** and **nafcillin**. In contrast, the UK manufacturer advises that no dose adjustment is required when a CYP3A4 inducer is given concurrently with enzalutamide.[2] CYP3A4 only has a minor role in the metabolism of enzalutamide, and until further evidence is available, it would seem prudent to be aware that the efficacy of enzalutamide might be reduced on concurrent use of a CYP3A4 inducer.

(g) CYP3A4 inhibitors

The UK and US manufacturers[1,2] of enzalutamide report that in a study in healthy subjects, when a single 160-mg dose[1] of enzalutamide was given after multiple doses of **itraconazole** 200 mg once daily, there was a 41% increase in the AUC of enzalutamide, but there was no change in its maximum plasma concentration.[2] Itraconazole is a potent inhibitor of CYP3A4, but this isoenzyme only has a minor role in the metabolism of enzalutamide.[2] The slight increase in enzalutamide exposure is not expected to be clinically relevant, and the manufacturers therefore advise that no dose adjustment is required when any CYP3A4 inhibitor is given concurrently with enzalutamide.[1,2]

(h) CYP3A4 substrates

The UK and US manufacturers of enzalutamide report that in a study in patients with prostate cancer, enzalutamide 160 mg once daily at steady-state decreased the AUC of a single 2-mg dose[1] of **midazolam** by 86%.[1,2] Midazolam can be used as a probe substrate to assess the activity of drugs on CYP3A4. This study therefore suggests that enzalutamide is a potent inducer of this isoenzyme, and it would be expected to decrease the exposure to other substrates of CYP3A4 (see 'Table 1.9', p.11 for a list). The US manufacturer states that concurrent use of CYP3A4 substrates with a narrow therapeutic range should be avoided.[1] The UK manufacturer advises that sensitive substrates should generally be avoided if the dose cannot be monitored and adjusted accordingly.[2] It would seem prudent to be alert for a reduction in efficacy of any CYP3A4 substrates on concurrent use with enzalutamide.

(i) Docetaxel

The UK manufacturer of enzalutamide notes that it does not alter the pharmacokinetics of intravenous docetaxel, but it might increase the risk of docetaxel induced neutropenia. The safety of docetaxel when combined with cytotoxic chemotherapy has not been established.[2] The US manufacturer warns that a higher incidence of seizures was observed in patients taking enzalutamide who had previously been treated with docetaxel when compared with patients taking enzalutamide who had not received chemotherapy.[1]

(j) Drugs that lower the seizure threshold

The UK manufacturer of enzalutamide states that the risk of seizure with enzalutamide might be increased in patients taking other drugs that lower the seizure threshold.[2] Until further evidence is available, it would seem prudent to carefully consider the risk of using a drug that might lower the seizure threshold with enzalutamide, and ensure that patients taking enzalutamide with a drug that lowers the seizure threshold are informed of the possible increase in risk of seizure. Such drugs might include the **tricyclics**, **SSRIs**, **phenothiazines** and **butyrophenones**, **mefloquine**, **bupropion**, and **tramadol**.

(k) Food

The US manufacturer of enzalutamide reports that in a study in healthy subjects a high fat meal did not alter the AUC of a single 160-mg dose of enzalutamide when compared with the fasted state.[1] Enzalutamide can therefore be taken without regard to food.[1,2]

(l) Paracetamol

The UK manufacturer of enzalutamide briefly notes that enzyme inducers, such as enzalutamide, can increase the risk of liver injury with paracetamol.[2] An isolated report attributes a case of liver failure to an interaction between the enzyme inducer rifampicin and paracetamol, see 'Paracetamol (Acetaminophen) + Rifampicin (Rifampin)', p.210.

(m) P-glycoprotein substrates

The UK and US manufacturers of enzalutamide report that enzalutamide[1,2] and its active metabolite, N-desmethyl enzalutamide,2 inhibit P-glycoprotein *in vitro*.[1,2] The UK manufacturer cautions the concurrent use of enzalutamide and P-glycoprotein substrates with a narrow therapeutic range and advises that dose adjustment of the P-glycoprotein substrate might be needed to maintain a therapeutic plasma concentration.[2] For a list of P-glycoprotein substrates see 'Table 1.12', p.14. Note, however, that positive *in vitro* findings do not always directly translate to the clinical situation.

(n) Other drugs

The UK manufacturer of enzalutamide also notes that drugs that might be affected by concurrent use with enzalutamide through their metabolism or by active transport, include, but are not limited to, the following; **bisoprolol**, **cabazitaxel**, **clarithromycin**, **clonazepam**, **doxycycline**, **levothyroxine**, **nicardipine**, **nifedipine**, **prednisolone**, **primidone**, **propranolol**, **tramadol**, **valproate**, and **zolpidem**.

1. Xtandi (Enzalutamide). US Prescribing information, September 2014.
2. Xtandi (Enzalutamide). Astellas Pharma Ltd. UK Summary of product characteristics, January 2015.

Enzastaurin + Antineoplastics

Capecitabine, cisplatin and gemcitabine did not alter the pharmacokinetics of enzastaurin, and enzastaurin did not appear to alter the pharmacokinetics of these antineoplastics.

Clinical evidence, mechanism, importance and management

In a study in 30 patients who received enzastaurin alone, followed by enzastaurin, **gemcitabine**, and **cisplatin**, the pharmacokinetics of enzastaurin were not altered to a clinically significant extent by cisplatin and gemcitabine. The pharmacokinetics of gemcitabine or cisplatin were not affected by enzastaurin, when compared with historical data.[1] Similarly, in a study in patients who received enzastaurin alone, or enzastaurin with **capecitabine**, there were no significant changes in the pharmacokinetics of enzastaurin in the 6 patients for whom pharmacokinetic data were available. In addition, the pharmacokinetics of capecitabine were similar to those previously reported for capecitabine alone.[2]

1. Rademaker-Lakhai JM, Beerepoot LV, Mehra N, Radema SA, van Maanen R, Vermaat JS, Witteveen EO, Visseren-Grul CM, Musib L, Enas N, van Hal G, Beijnen JH, Schellens JHM, Voest EE. Phase I pharmacokinetic and pharmacodynamic study of the oral protein kinase C β-inhibitor enzastaurin in combination with gemcitabine and cisplatin in patients with advanced cancer. *Clin Cancer Res* (2007) 13, 4474–5.
2. Camidge DR, Eckhardt SG, Gore L, O'Bryant CL, Leong S, Basche M, Holden SN, Musib L, Baldwin J, Darstein C, Thornton D, Finn RS, Britten CD. A phase I safety, tolerability, and pharmacokinetic study of enzastaurin combined with capecitabine in patients with advanced solid tumors. *Anticancer Drugs* (2008) 19, 77–84.

Eribulin + Miscellaneous

Ketoconazole, a CYP3A4 and P-glycoprotein inhibitor, does not appear to alter the exposure to eribulin; however, other P-glycoprotein inhibitors and inhibitors of other transporter proteins are predicted to increase its exposure. Rifampicin (rifampin), a CYP3A4 and P-glycoprotein inducer, does not appear to alter the exposure to eribulin; however, other enzyme-inducing drugs are predicted to decrease the exposure to eribulin. Eribulin is predicted to inhibit the metabolism of CYP3A4 substrates.

Clinical evidence, mechanism, importance and management

(a) CYP3A4 substrates

The UK manufacturer states that, based on *in vitro* data, eribulin inhibits CYP3A4, and might affect the metabolism of drugs that are substrates for this isoenzyme. They therefore advise caution if eribulin is given with CYP3A4 substrates, and specifically recommend avoiding concurrent use with CYP3A4 substrates that have a narrow therapeutic index (not specified).[1] However, this advice would seem over-cautious as eribulin has been reported to have only a weak inhibitory effect *in vitro* on the metabolism of CYP3A4 probe substrates, such as midazolam.[2] Furthermore, the US manufacturer states that eribulin does not inhibit CYP3A4 at clinically significant concentrations, and so is unlikely to cause a clinically important increase the in concentrations of drugs that are substrates of CYP3A4.[3] A clinically relevant interaction between eribulin and CYP3A4 substrates therefore seems unlikely.

(b) Drug transporter proteins

Eribulin is primarily excreted unchanged in bile and although the transporter responsible for this has yet to be clarified, preclinical studies suggest that this could be P-glycoprotein. The UK manufacturer notes that, theoretically, complete inhibition of eribulin transport could lead to a 3-fold increase in its plasma concentration.[1] Therefore, they do not recommend the concurrent use of drugs that inhibit P-glycoprotein or other drug transporter proteins, such as OATP and multidrug resistance proteins: they name **clarithromycin**, **ciclosporin**, **disopyramide**, **efavirenz**, **emtricitabine**, **lopinavir**, **quinidine**, **quinine**, **ritonavir**, **saquinavir**, and **verapamil** as examples of such drugs. However, note that ketoconazole is an inhibitor of P-glycoprotein, but did not appear to affect eribulin exposure in a clinical study, see *Ketoconazole and other CYP3A4 inhibitors*, below. Furthermore, the US manufacturer states that no drug-drug interactions are expected with P-glycoprotein inhibitors, and makes no mention of a possible interaction by other transporter proteins.[3]

(c) Enzyme inducers

A non-randomised study in 11 patients found that rifampicin (rifampin) 600 mg daily for 12 days did not affect the AUC or maximum concentration of a single 1.4-mg/m^2 dose of eribulin given on day 7.[4] No eribulin dose adjustments are therefore likely to be necessary if it is given with **rifampicin** and the authors concluded that other enzyme inducers (such as St John's wort) are also unlikely to affect eribulin exposure.

The UK manufacturer does not recommend the concurrent use of eribulin with enzyme-inducing drugs, stating that they present a risk of markedly reduced eribulin concentrations and the manufacturer specifically names **rifampicin (rifampin)**, **carbamazepine**, **phenytoin**, and **St John's wort** as examples.[1] However, note that this guidance was produced before the study with rifampicin was published.

(d) Ketoconazole and other CYP3A4 inhibitors

The US manufacturer of eribulin reports that in a crossover study in 12 patients with advanced solid tumours, ketoconazole 200 mg did not alter the exposure to a single dose of eribulin.[3] Ketoconazole is an potent inhibitor of CYP3A4, and the lack of an interaction suggests that no eribulin dose adjustments are likely to be necessary if it is given with ketoconazole or other inhibitors of CYP3A4.

1. Halaven (Eribulin mesylate). Eisai Ltd. UK Summary of product characteristics, May 2012.
2. Zhang Z-Y, King BM, Pelletier RD, Wong YN. Delineation of the interactions between the chemotherapeutic agent eribulin mesylate (E7389) and human CYP3A4. *Cancer Chemother Pharmacol* (2008) 62, 707–16.
3. Halaven (Eribulin mesylate). Eisai Inc. US Prescribing information, February 2012.
4. Devriese LA, Witteveen PO, Wanders J, Law K, Edwards G, Reyderman L, Copalu W, Peng F, Marchetti S, Beijnen JH, Huitema ADR, Voest EE, Schellens JHM. Pharmacokinetics of eribulin mesylate in patients with solid tumors receiving repeated oral rifampicin. *Br J Clin Pharmacol* (2012) [Epub ahead of print].

Estramustine + ACE inhibitors

Angioedema occurred in a man taking cilazapril after starting estramustine. The concurrent use of estramustine and ACE inhibitors might increase the risk of angioedema.

Clinical evidence, mechanism, importance and management

A patient who had taken an ACE inhibitor for 20 years experienced four episodes of swelling of the tongue and epiglottis over a period of 40 days, approximately 2 months after starting to take estramustine. Three of the episodes resolved after hydrocortisone was given; one episode was unresponsive to hydrocortisone and required a tracheotomy. After stopping the estramustine and while continuing the **cilazapril**, the patient experienced no further episodes of angioedema. He had never had angioedema while taking the ACE inhibitor.[1]

Angioedema is a rare adverse effect of both estramustine and the ACE inhibitors, and it is possible that concurrent use might increase the risk. The UK manufacturer of estramustine notes that, in many of the reported cases of angioedema with estramustine, including a fatal one, patients were also taking ACE inhibitors.[2] They recommend that treatment with estramustine should be stopped immediately if angioedema occurs.[2]

1. Kamata Y, Iwamoto M, Kamimura T, Kanashiki E, Yoshio T, Okazaki H, Morita T, Minota S. Repeated massive tongue swelling due to the combined use of estramustine phosphate and angiotensin-converting enzyme inhibitor. *J Investig Allergol Clin Immunol* (2006) 16, 388–90.
2. Estracyt (Estramustine sodium phosphate). Pharmacia Ltd. UK Summary of product characteristics, November 2008.

Estramustine + Calcium compounds

The absorption of estramustine is reduced by milk, foods, and drugs containing calcium.

Clinical evidence

A randomised three-way crossover study in 6 patients with prostate cancer found that the absorption of single-doses of estramustine disodium (equivalent to 140 mg of estramustine) was reduced by 59% when taken with 200 mL of **milk**, and by 33% when taken with a standardised breakfast (2 pieces of white bread with margarine, ham, tomato, marmalade and water). Peak serum estramustine levels were reduced by 68% and 43%, respectively.[1]

Mechanism

In vitro studies suggest that estramustine combines with calcium ions in milk and food to form a poorly-soluble complex that is not as well absorbed as the parent compound.[1]

Importance and management

An established interaction although the information is limited. The manufacturers recommend that estramustine should be taken at least one hour before or 2 hours after meals, and that it should not be taken at the same time as milk, milk products, calcium-rich foods, or drugs containing calcium (such as **calcium-containing antacids**).[2,3]

1. Gunnarsson PO, Davidsson T, Andersson S-B, Backman C, Johansson S-Å. Impairment of estramustine phosphate absorption by concurrent intake of milk and food. *Eur J Clin Pharmacol* (1990) 38, 189–93.
2. Estracyt (Estramustine sodium phosphate). Pharmacia Ltd. UK Summary of product characteristics, November 2008.
3. Emcyt (Estramustine phosphate sodium). Pfizer. US Prescribing information, June 2007.

Estramustine + Clodronate

Clodronate markedly increases the levels of estramustine.

Clinical evidence, mechanism, importance and management

In 12 patients, the bioavailability of estramustine was increased by about 80% when clodronate 800 mg four times daily was given with estramustine 280 mg twice daily for 5 days. The serum levels and AUC of clodronate were not changed by estramustine.[1] Documentation appears to be limited to this study. However, the toxicity of estramustine should be more closely monitored if clodronate is also given. The effects of other bisphosphonates do not appear to have been studied.

1. Kylmälä T, Castrén-Kortekangas P, Seppänen J, Ylitalo P, Tammela TLJ. Effect of concomitant administration of clodronate and estramustine phosphate on their bioavailability in patients with metastasized prostate cancer. *Pharmacol Toxicol* (1996) 79, 157–60.

Etoposide + Antiepileptics; Enzyme-inducing

Etoposide clearance appears to be increased by phenobarbital, phenytoin, and probably carbamazepine, and this may result in reduced efficacy.

Clinical evidence, mechanism, importance and management

The clearance of etoposide was found to be highly variable in children given etoposide 320 to 500 mg/m^2 over 6 hours on alternate days for a total of 3 doses. However, it was 77% higher in 7 children taking antiepileptics (**phenobarbital**, **phenytoin** or both) than in 22 others not taking antiepileptics.[1] In a retrospective survey, long-term antiepileptic use (**phenytoin**, **phenobarbital**, **carbamazepine**, or a combination) was associated with worse event-free survival, and greater haematological and/or CNS relapse in children receiving chemotherapy for B-lineage acute lymphoblastic leukaemia. The authors considered that the increased clearance of etoposide induced by the antiepileptics was a likely factor in these findings.[2] Be alert for the possible need to give larger doses of etoposide if these antiepileptics (and probably **primidone**, which is metabolised to phenobarbital, or **fosphenytoin**, which is metabolised to phenytoin) are used. More study is needed to establish the magnitude and clinical effects of the interaction.

Note that reduced valproate levels and phenytoin levels have been reported in patients receiving chemotherapy including etoposide, see 'Antiepileptics + Antineoplastics; Cytotoxic', p.562.

1. Rodman JH, Murry DJ, Madden T, Santana VM. Altered etoposide pharmacokinetics and time to engraftment in pediatric patients undergoing autologous bone marrow transplantation. *J Clin Oncol* (1994) 12, 2390–7.
2. Relling MV, Pui C-H, Sandlund JT, Rivera GK, Hancock ML, Boyett JM, Schuetz EG, Evans WE. Adverse effect of anticonvulsants on efficacy of chemotherapy for acute lymphoblastic leukaemia. *Lancet* (2000) 356, 285–90.

Etoposide + Atovaquone

The concurrent use of atovaquone with etoposide may modestly increase exposure to the metabolite, etoposide catechol.

Clinical evidence, mechanism, importance and management

A study in 9 children with acute lymphoblastic leukaemia or non-Hodgkin's lymphoma found that the AUC of etoposide and its metabolite, etoposide catechol, were slightly increased, by 9% and 28%, respectively, following atovaquone 45 mg/kg daily, when compared with co-trimoxazole (trimethoprim with sulfamethoxazole) 150/750 mg/m^2 daily. The mechanism by which this occurs is unclear, but the authors suggested that atovaquone may affect the metabolism of etoposide by the cytochrome P450 isoenzyme CYP3A4 or its transport by P-glycoprotein.[1] The authors considered that an interaction with co-trimoxazole was unlikely, so used it as a control; however, ideally this requires confirmation. The relevance of the minor changes seen is unclear. The authors note that the risk of etoposide-related secondary acute myeloid leukaemia has been linked to minor changes in therapy, therefore, they advise caution if atovaquone is given with etoposide, particularly if it is used with other substrates of CYP3A4 or P-glycoprotein.[1] They also say it may be possible to avoid the interaction by separating the administration by one to 2 days,[1] but this requires confirmation.

1. van de Poll MEC, Relling MV, Schuetz EG, Harrison PL, Hughes W, Flynn PM. The effect of atovaquone on etoposide pharmacokinetics in children with acute lymphoblastic leukemia. *Cancer Chemother Pharmacol* (2001) 47, 467–72.

Etoposide + Ciclosporin

High-dose ciclosporin markedly raises etoposide levels and increases the suppression of white blood cell production. Severe toxicity has been reported in one patient.

Clinical evidence

In a comparative study, 16 patients with multidrug-resistant advanced cancer were given 20 paired courses of etoposide alone or with ciclosporin. Ciclosporin levels were measured at the end of a 2-hour infusion: ciclosporin levels of greater than 2000 nanograms/mL were defined as high-dose and ciclosporin levels less than 2000 nanograms/mL were defined as low-dose. High and low-dose ciclosporin, respectively, increased the etoposide AUC by 80% and 50%, decreased the total clearance by 38% and 28%, increased its half-life by 108% and 40%, reduced the leucocyte count nadir by 64% and 37%, and altered the volume of distribution at steady state by 46% and 1.4%.[1] The patients were given 150 to 200 mg/m^2 of etoposide daily as a 2-hour intravenous infusion for 3 consecutive days and ciclosporin in doses ranging from 5 to 21 mg/kg daily as a 3-day continuous infusion.[1]

In another study, 18 children with recurrent or refractory tumours who had previously received etoposide were given high-dose ciclosporin (either a continuous infusion of 15 mg/kg per 24 hours for 60 hours (13 patients) or 30 mg/kg over 3 hours on 3 consecutive days (5 patients)) with etoposide 150 mg/m^2 over one hour for 3 days, starting one hour after the beginning of the ciclosporin infusion. The AUC and half-life of etoposide were increased by 89% and 78%, respectively, and the clearance was decreased by 48%.[2] In a further study in children, the pharmacokinetics of etoposide 100 mg/m^2 daily were compared with etoposide 60 mg/m^2 (a 40% reduction in dose) with high-dose ciclosporin. Despite the dose reduction, recipients of ciclosporin had a 71% reduction in etoposide clearance and a 47% increase in the etoposide AUC, although toxicity was similar.[3]

The leukaemic cells in the bone marrow of a patient with acute T-lymphocyte leukaemia were totally cleared when ciclosporin 8.3 mg/kg orally twice daily was given with etoposide 100 to 300 mg daily for 2 to 5 days, but the adverse effects were severe (mental confusion, renal and hepatic toxicity). The patient died from respiratory failure precipitated by a chest infection.[4]

A patient with chronic myeloid leukaemia who had responded poorly to treatment with etoposide, mitoxantrone and cytarabine for blast crisis, returned to the chronic phase when given etoposide with ciclosporin.[5] An *in vitro* study by the same authors showed that etoposide was partially toxic to blast cells but that its effect on blast cells was increased sixfold when it was given with ciclosporin.[5]

Mechanism

It is suggested that the ciclosporin inhibits the metabolism of etoposide by cytochrome P450 isoenzymes,[6] and inhibits hepatic P-glycoprotein, as well as some unknown non-renal clearance mechanism.[1] The total effect is to cause the retention of etoposide in the body, thereby increasing its effects.

Importance and management

An established interaction. Ciclosporin alters the pharmacokinetics of etoposide resulting in increased levels. This pharmacokinetic interaction has complicated the study of the value of using ciclosporin to modulate multidrug resistance in tumours to improve the response to chemotherapy: any benefit could just be attributed to dose intensification. Consequently, some,[1-3] including one manufacturer,[7] have suggested reducing the dose of etoposide by 40% or 50% in the presence of ciclosporin.[1-3] In one study, a continuous infusion of ciclosporin was better tolerated than an intermittent regimen, but it was associated with similar hepatic and renal impairment as the short schedule (transient hyperbilirubinaemia, and elevated creatinine or urea).[2] The use of high-dose ciclosporin for multidrug-resistant tumour modulation remains experimental and should only be undertaken in clinical studies. Concurrent use should be very well monitored. More study is needed to find out the possible effects of low-dose ciclosporin.

1. Lum BL, Kaubisch S, Yahanda AM, Adler KM, Jew L, Ehsan MN, Brophy NA, Halsey J, Gosland MP, Sikic BI. Alteration of etoposide pharmacokinetics and pharmacodynamics by cyclosporine in a phase I trial to modulate multidrug resistance. *J Clin Oncol* (1992) 10, 1635–42.
2. Bisogno G, Cowie F, Boddy A, Thomas HD, Dick G, Pinkerton CR. High-dose cyclosporin with etoposide—toxicity and pharmacokinetic interaction in children with solid tumours. *Br J Cancer* (1998) 77, 2304–9.
3. Lacayo NJ, Lum BL, Becton DL, Weinstein H, Ravindranath Y, Chang MN, Bomgaars L, Lauer SJ, Sikic BI. Pharmacokinetic interactions of cyclosporine with etoposide and mitoxantrone in children with acute myeloid leukemia. *Leukemia* (2002) 16, 920–7.
4. Kloke O, Osieka R. Interaction of cyclosporin A with antineoplastic agents. *Klin Wochenschr* (1985) 63, 1081–2.
5. Maia RC, Noronha H, Vasconcelos FC, Rumjanek VM. Interaction of cyclosporin A and etoposide. Clinical and *in vitro* assessment in blast phase of chronic myeloid leukaemia. *Clin Lab Haematol* (1997) 19, 215–7.
6. Kawashiro T, Yamashita K, Zhao X-J, Koyama E, Tani M, Chiba K, Ishizaki T. A study on the metabolism of etoposide and possible interaction with antitumor or supporting agents by human liver microsomes. *J Pharmacol Exp Ther* (1998) 386, 1294–1300.
7. Eposin (Etoposide). Medac GmbH. UK Summary of product characteristics, January 2005.

Etoposide + Cisplatin and other platinum compounds

The clearance of etoposide may be modestly reduced by carboplatin and cisplatin.

Clinical evidence, mechanism, importance and management

(a) Carboplatin

In one study in 4 patients, the pharmacokinetics of etoposide were unchanged when carboplatin was also given.[1] However, in another study of 14 young patients receiving etoposide and carboplatin the clearance of etoposide was lower than in previous reports in adults and children. They had been given an escalating dose regimen starting with etoposide 960 mg/m^2, and increasing to 1200 mg/m^2, and 1500 mg/m^2, given in three divided doses on alternate days, with carboplatin 400 to 700 mg/m^2 given on the other days, followed by autologous marrow rescue. The authors point out that the dose and the timing of carboplatin may be important determinants for any interaction.[2] In yet another study,[3] carboplatin did not affect the pharmacokinetics of etoposide during the first cycle of chemotherapy (etoposide was given on days 1, 2 and 3, and carboplatin on day 2, and the AUC of etoposide was compared for days 1 and 2). However, during a second cycle of chemotherapy, the etoposide AUC was 8% higher on day 2 than day 1. These changes were considered unlikely to be clinically important.[3]

(b) Cisplatin

A study in 17 children with neuroblastoma found that when intravenous cisplatin 90 mg/m^2 was given immediately before etoposide, the clearance of etoposide 780 mg/m^2 fell by 20% and its serum levels rose. However, after a cumulative dose of 360 mg/m^2 cisplatin had no effect on the clearance of etoposide.[4] In another study, cisplatin did not affect the pharmacokinetics of etoposide during the first cycle of chemotherapy (etoposide was given on days 1, 2 and 3, and cisplatin on day 2, and the AUC of etoposide was compared for days 1 and 2). However, during a second cycle of chemotherapy, the etoposide AUC was 28% higher on day 3 than day 1. These changes were considered unlikely to be clinically important.[3]

1. Newell DR, Eeles RA, Gumbrell LA, Boxall FE, Horwich A, Calvert AH. Carboplatin and etoposide pharmacokinetics in patients with testicular teratoma. *Cancer Chemother Pharmacol* (1989) 23, 376–72.
2. Rodman JH, Murry DJ, Madden T, Santana VM. Altered etoposide pharmacokinetics and time to engraftment in pediatric patients undergoing autologous bone marrow transplantation. *J Clin Oncol* (1994) 12, 2390–7.
3. Thomas HD, Porter DJ, Bartelink I, Nobbs JR, Cole M, Elliott S, Newell DR, Calvert AH, Highley M, Boddy AV. Randomized cross-over clinical trial to study potential pharmacokinetics interactions between cisplatin or carboplatin and etoposide. *Br J Clin Pharmacol* (2002) 53, 83–91.
4. Relling MV, McLeod HL, Bowman LC, Santana VM. Etoposide pharmacokinetics and pharmacodynamics after acute and chronic exposure to cisplatin. *Clin Pharmacol Ther* (1994) 56, 503–11.

Etoposide + CYP3A4 inducers or inhibitors

Ketoconazole modestly increased the AUC and decreased the clearance of etoposide in one study. Etoposide clearance was markedly increased by prednisone in one study. Etoposide bioavailability was modestly (and unexpectedly) decreased by grapefruit juice.

Clinical evidence

(a) CYP3A4 inducers

In a study, 102 children with acute lymphoblastic leukaemia were given **prednisone** 40 mg/m^2 daily for 28 days with etoposide 300 mg/m^2 on day 29. Forty-eight of the children with high risk disease were given continuation therapy and received etoposide 300 mg/m^2 at week 54, two weeks or more after the last **prednisone** dose. Etoposide clearance was 62% higher on day 29 than at week 54 and the AUC for the catechol metabolite was significantly lower (27%) on day 29 compared with week 54.[1]

(b) CYP3A4 inhibitors

1. Grapefruit juice. In a single-dose study, 6 patients were given etoposide 50 mg intravenously or orally, either alone or after drinking 100 mL of **grapefruit juice**. The bioavailability of oral etoposide was unexpectedly *reduced* by about 25% by **grapefruit juice**, but there was wide inter-individual variation in the findings.[2]

2. Ketoconazole. In a study in 27 patients, ketoconazole 200 mg daily was given with oral etoposide (escalating doses of 50 mg every other day increasing to 50 mg alternating with 100 mg daily) in cycles of 3 out of 5 weeks. The median AUC of etoposide was increased by about 20%, and its clearance reduced by about 18%, and inter-individual variation was greater than seen with etoposide alone. However, the toxicity profile of etoposide did not appear to be altered by ketoconazole, when compared with historical data.[3]

Mechanism

Etoposide is a substrate for CYP3A4. *In vitro* studies using human liver microsomes showed that ketoconazole, **prednisolone**, **troleandomycin**, **verapamil** and **vincristine** can inhibit the metabolism (3′-demethylation) of etoposide by CYP3A4.[4] The clinical study found that ketoconazole modestly inhibited etoposide metabolism; however, unexpectedly, grapefruit juice (another CYP3A4 inhibitor) appeared to decrease etoposide bioavailability. The reason for this is unknown, but may be a concentration effect, or an effect via P-glycoprotein. Also, somewhat in contrast to the *in vitro* findings, prednisone (a metabolite of prednisolone) induced etoposide metabolism, but note that corticosteroids are more usually known to be clinical inducers of CYP3A4 and possibly also P-glycoprotein.

Importance and management

There seems to be little clinical confirmation that the potential interactions with CYP3A4 inhibitors or inducers, other than prednisone have clinical relevance, but good monitoring would be a prudent precaution. Ketoconazole had only a modest and variable effect on etoposide, and grapefruit juice seemed to reduce rather than increase oral etoposide bioavailability. Further study is needed.

For mention that the HIV-protease inhibitors (CYP3A4 inhibitors) have been associated with an increased risk of infection when used with various antineoplastic regimens, including those containing etoposide, see also 'Antineoplastics; Cyclophosphamide + HIV-protease inhibitors', p.659.

1. Kishi S, Yang W, Boureau B, Morand S, Das S, Chen P, Cook EH, Rosner GL, Schuetz E, Pui C-H, Relling MV. Effects of prednisone and genetic polymorphisms on etoposide disposition in children with acute lymphoblastic leukaemia. *Blood* (2004) 103, 67–72.
2. Reif S, Nicolson MC, Bisset D, Reid M, Kloft C, Jaehde U, McLeod HL. Effect of grapefruit juice intake on etoposide bioavailability. *Eur J Clin Pharmacol* (2002) 58, 491–4.
3. Yong WP, Desai AA, Innocenti F, Ramirez J, Shepard D, Kobayashi K, House L, Fleming GF, Vogelzang NJ, Schilsky RL, Ratain MJ. Pharmacokinetic modulation of oral etoposide by ketoconazole in patients with advanced cancer. *Cancer Chemother Pharmacol* (2007) 60, 811–19.
4. Kawashiro T, Yamashita K, Zhao X-J, Koyama E, Tani M, Chiba K, Ishizaki T. A study on the metabolism of etoposide and possible interactions with antitumor or supporting agents by human liver microsomes. *J Pharmacol Exp Ther* (1998) 386, 1294–1300.

Etoposide + Food

In 8 patients with extensive small cell lung carcinoma the pharmacokinetics of a 100-mg oral dose of etoposide were unaffected when it was taken with a full breakfast, when compared with the fasting state.[1] However, the UK manufacturer recommends that oral etoposide should be taken on an empty stomach.[2]

1. Harvey VJ, Slevin ML, Joel SP, Johnston A, Wrigley PFM. The effect of food and concurrent chemotherapy on the bioavailability of oral etoposide. *Br J Cancer* (1985) 52, 363–7.
2. Vepesid Capsules (Etoposide). Bristol-Myers Pharmaceuticals. UK Summary of product characteristics, March 2008.

Etoposide + Levamisole

The manufacturers of an intravenous etoposide *phosphate* product warn that the administration with drugs known to inhibit phosphatase activity (they name levamisole) should be undertaken with caution.[1,2] This is presumably because this might reduce the conversion of etoposide phosphate to etoposide in the plasma. There does not seem to be any information on whether this interaction is clinically relevant.

1. Etopophos Injection (Etoposide phosphate). Bristol-Myers Squibb Pharmaceuticals Ltd. UK Summary of product characteristics, September 2007.
2. Etopophos Injection (Etoposide phosphate). Bristol-Myers Squibb Company. US Prescribing information, March 2005.

Etoposide + Other antineoplastics

The use of doxorubicin with cyclophosphamide has no clinically relevant effects on the pharmacokinetics of oral or intravenous etoposide. Similarly, cyclophosphamide with methotrexate, doxorubicin with procarbazine and procarbazine alone do not affect the pharmacokinetics of oral etoposide.

Clinical evidence, mechanism, importance and management

(a) Cyclophosphamide with Doxorubicin

A pharmacokinetic study in 7 patients with small cell lung cancer given cyclophosphamide 800 mg/m^2, doxorubicin 40 mg/m^2 and etoposide 100 mg/m^2 (all given intravenously) found that the protein binding, metabolism and renal clearance of etoposide were unaffected by the other antineoplastics.[1] Similarly, another study found only modest changes in the pharmacokinetics of intravenous etoposide when it was given with cyclophosphamide and doxorubicin, compared with use alone, and these changes were considered unlikely to be clinically relevant. Specifically, the AUC of etoposide was 9% higher and the clearance was 10% lower on day one of the CAE cycle (cyclophosphamide, doxorubicin, and etoposide) compared with days 2 and 3 (etoposide alone).[2] This is a commonly used regimen, and these data suggest there is no pharmacokinetic interaction.

(b) Cyclophosphamide with Methotrexate

No changes in etoposide pharmacokinetics were seen when oral etoposide 100 mg was given immediately after oral cyclophosphamide 100 mg/m^2 and oral methotrexate 12.5 mg/m^2 in 8 patients with small cell lung cancer.[3]

(c) Doxorubicin with Procarbazine

No changes in etoposide pharmacokinetics were seen when oral etoposide 400 mg was given 15 minutes after intravenous doxorubicin 35 mg/m^2 with oral procarbazine 60 mg/m^2 or after oral procarbazine alone, when compared with etoposide alone.[3]

(d) Imatinib

For the possible effect of imatinib on etoposide, see 'Tyrosine kinase inhibitors; Imatinib + Antineoplastics', p.742.

(e) Platinum compounds

For the lack of effect of platinum derivatives on etoposide pharmacokinetics, see 'Etoposide + Cisplatin and other platinum compounds', p.678.

1. Van Hoogenhuijze J, Lankelma J, Stam J, Pinedo HM. Unchanged pharmacokinetics of VP-16-213 (etoposide, NSC 141540) during concomitant administration of doxorubicin and cyclophosphamide. *Eur J Cancer Clin Oncol* (1987) 23, 807–11.
2. Busse D, Würthwein G, Hinske C, Hempel G, Fromm MF, Eichelbaum M, Kroemer HK, Busch FW. Pharmacokinetics of intravenous etoposide in patients with breast cancer: influence of dose escalation and cyclophosphamide and doxorubicin coadministration. *Naunyn Schmiedebergs Arch Pharmacol* (2002) 366, 218–25.
3. Harvey VJ, Slevin ML, Joel SP, Johnston A, Wrigley PFM. The effect of food and concurrent chemotherapy on the bioavailability of oral etoposide. *Br J Cancer* (1985) 52, 363–7.

Fludarabine + Busulfan

In 16 patients with haematological malignancies the pharmacokinetics of intravenous fludarabine were unaltered by oral high-dose busulfan.[1]

1. Bonin M, Pursche S, Bergeman T, Leopold T, Illmer T, Ehninger G, Schleyer E, Bornhauser M. F-ara-A pharmacokinetics during reduced-intensity conditioning therapy with fludarabine and busulfan. *Bone Marrow Transplant* (2007) 39, 201–6.

Fludarabine + Dipyridamole

Because fludarabine phosphate is an analogue of adenine, the UK manufacturers warn that drugs that are adenosine uptake inhibitors, such as dipyridamole, may prevent the uptake of fludarabine into cells and reduce its efficacy.[1,2] Until more is known, some caution would seem to be appropriate on concurrent use.

1. Schering Health Care Ltd. Personal communication, February 1995.
2. Fludara Tablets (Fludarabine phosphate). Genzyme Therapeutics. UK Summary of product characteristics, February 2009.

Fludarabine + Food

Food does not affect the pharmacokinetics of oral fludarabine.

Clinical evidence, mechanism, importance and management

In a randomised, crossover study, 16 patients were given fludarabine 90 mg orally either on a full stomach or after fasting on the first day of their chemotherapy cycle, followed 2 days later by intravenous fludarabine 25 mg/m^2 daily for 4 days. There was no clinically significant effect of food on the pharmacokinetics of oral fludarabine.[1] The manufacturer advises that oral fludarabine may be taken with or without food.[2]

1. Oscier D, Orchard JA, Culligan D, Cunningham D, Johnson S, Parker A, Klein M, Gieschen H. The bioavailability of oral fludarabine phosphate is unaffected by food. *Hematol J* (2001) 2, 316–21.
2. Fludara Tablets (Fludarabine phosphate). Genzyme Therapeutics. UK Summary of product characteristics, February 2009.

Fludarabine + Pentostatin

When fludarabine phosphate and pentostatin were used in the treatment of chronic lymphoid leukaemia, 4 out of 6 patients developed pulmonary toxicity consistent with interstitial pneumonitis, and 3 of them died.[1] Pentostatin should therefore not be given with fludarabine.[2,3]

1. Schering Health Care Ltd. Personal communication, February 1995.
2. Fludara Tablets (Fludarabine phosphate). Genzyme Therapeutics. UK Summary of product characteristics, February 2009.
3. Fludara (Fludarabine phosphate). Bayer HealthCare Pharmaceuticals Inc. US Prescribing information, February 2009.

Fludarabine with Cytarabine + Voriconazole

A case of fatal peripheral neuropathy was tentatively attributed to the use of voriconazole with fludarabine and cytarabine.

Clinical evidence, mechanism, importance and management

A patient experienced severe peripheral neuropathy, which progressed to poor respiratory effort and death, after receiving treatment with cytarabine, fludarabine and tretinoin. During his first course he had developed probable pulmonary invasive fungal infection, and was treated with broad-spectrum antibacterials and liposomal amphotericin B. He then started taking prophylactic voriconazole, which was stopped after a total of 7 days, two days after starting his second course of chemotherapy, because he again had a fever. After 14 days, severe distal peripheral neuropathy became apparent, which progressed, and he died after 23 days.[1] The exact cause of the neurological effects was not clear. Both cytarabine and fludarabine uncommonly cause neurological toxicity, and it has been reported with the combination.[1] In the case described, it was considered that voriconazole might have altered the metabolism of the antineoplastics, and increased the risk of toxicity.[1] However, neither cytarabine nor fludarabine are metabolised by the cytochrome P450 system, which voriconazole inhibits. The clinical relevance of this single case report is uncertain and no general recommendations can be made.

1. Osborne WL, Holyoake TL, McQuaker IG, Parker AN. Fatal peripheral neuropathy following FLA chemotherapy. *Clin Lab Haematol* (2004) 26, 295–6.

Fluorouracil + Allopurinol

Allopurinol has been studied as a modulator of the effects of fluorouracil, but has not gained an established clinical use in this setting.

Clinical evidence, mechanism, importance and management

Some early studies found that allopurinol 300 mg two to four times daily allowed the usual maximum tolerated dose of fluorouracil to be increased up to 2-fold.[1-3] The hope was that allopurinol would prove useful to decrease the toxicity and/or improve the activity of fluorouracil. However, most studies have found no increase in response rates in colorectal cancer with allopurinol,[4,5] even when the fluorouracil dose was escalated,[2,4] and some have also found no reduction in toxicity.[5-7] These are by no means all the studies, and are just cited as examples. Allopurinol mouthwash has also been investigated to reduce the incidence of stomatitis with fluorouracil. Some controlled studies have found a benefit,[8] whereas others have not.[9] Allopurinol clearly modulates some of the effects of fluorouracil; however, this has not been shown to be obviously beneficial or harmful in the clinical setting.

1. Howell SB, Wung WE, Taetle R, Hussain F, Romine JS. Modulation of 5-fluorouracil toxicity by allopurinol in man. *Cancer* (1981) 48, 1281–9.
2. Fox RM, Woods RL, Tattersall MHN, Piper AA, Sampson D. Allopurinol modulation of fluorouracil toxicity. *Cancer Chemother Pharmacol* (1981) 5, 151–5.
3. Woolley PV, Ayoob MJ, Smith FP, Lokey JL, DeGreen P, Marantz A, Schein PS. A controlled trial of the effect of 4-hydroxypyrazolopyrimidine (allopurinol) on the toxicity of a single bolus dose of 5-fluorouracil. *J Clin Oncol* (1985) 3, 103–9.
4. Tsavaris N, Bacoyannis C, Milonakis N, Sarafidou M, Zamanis N, Magoulas D, Kosmidis P. Folinic acid plus high-dose 5-fluorouracil with allopurinol protection in the treatment of advanced colorectal carcinoma. *Eur J Cancer* (1990) 26, 1054–6.
5. Merimsky O, Inbar M, Chaitchik S. Treatment of advanced colorectal cancer by 5-fluorouracil–leucovorin combination with or without allopurinol: a prospective randomized study. *Anticancer Drugs* (1991) 2, 447–51.

6. Howell SB, Pfeifle CE, Wung WE. Effect of allopurinol on the toxicity of high-dose 5-fluorouracil administered by intermittent bolus injection. *Cancer* (1983) 51, 220–5.
7. Garewal H, Ahmann FR. Failure of allopurinol to provide clinically significant protection against the hematologic toxicity of a bolus 5-FU schedule. *Oncology* (1986) 43, 216–18.
8. Porta C, Moroni M, Nastasi G. Allopurinol mouthwashes in the treatment of 5-fluorouracil-induced stomatitis. *Am J Clin Oncol* (1994) 17, 246–7.
9. Loprinzi CL, Cianflone SG, Dose AM, Etzell PS, Burnham NL, Therneau TM, Hagen L, Gainey DK, Cross M, Athmann LM, Fischer T, O'Connell MJ. A controlled evaluation of an allopurinol mouthwash as prophylaxis against 5-fluorouracil–induced stomatitis. *Cancer* (1990) 65, 1879–82.

Fluorouracil + Aminoglycosides; Oral

Neomycin can delay the gastrointestinal absorption of fluorouracil, but the clinical importance of this is uncertain.

Clinical evidence, mechanism, importance and management

Some preliminary information from a study in 12 patients treated for metastatic adenocarcinoma found that the use of oral **neomycin** 500 mg four times daily for a week delayed the absorption of fluorouracil, but the effects were generally too small to reduce the therapeutic response, except possibly in one patient.[1] It seems probable that this interaction occurs because **neomycin** can induce a malabsorption syndrome. If **neomycin**, and most probably also **paromomycin** or **kanamycin**, are used in patients receiving fluorouracil, the possibility of this interaction should be borne in mind.

1. Bruckner HW, Creasey WA. The administration of 5-fluorouracil by mouth. *Cancer* (1974) 33, 14–18.

Fluorouracil + Cisplatin and other platinum compounds

Giving low-dose cisplatin with a fluorouracil infusion markedly increased toxicity in one study. Cardiotoxicity may possibly be increased if high doses of cisplatin are given with fluorouracil. Oxaliplatin appears to moderately raise fluorouracil levels, without increasing its toxicity.

Clinical evidence, mechanism, importance and management

(a) Cisplatin

In 18 patients with advanced cancers giving low-dose cisplatin 20 mg/m^2 weekly with continuous ambulatory fluorouracil infusions of 300 mg/m^2 daily considerably increased the toxicity (nausea, vomiting, anorexia, diarrhoea, stomatitis, myelosuppression). More than half of the patients developed multiple toxicities, and severe toxicity occurred in two-thirds of the patients. Leucopenia occurred in 28% given both drugs whereas it was virtually nonexistent with fluorouracil alone. Toxicity requiring treatment interruption or dose reduction was seen in 55% of patients receiving fluorouracil alone, and this rose to 94% in the presence of cisplatin.[1]

In another study, signs of cardiotoxicity (chest pain, ST-T wave changes, arrhythmias) were seen in 12 of 80 patients given fluorouracil with cisplatin for carcinoma of the head, neck, oesophagus and stomach.[2] Studies in humans and *rats* have shown that there is a prolonged elevation of filterable platinum levels associated with the concurrent use of cisplatin and fluorouracil.[3]

The combination of a platinum compound and fluorouracil is widely used, but the optimum schedule to improve activity and reduce toxicity is not firmly established. In one study of bolus cisplatin and continuous infusion fluorouracil, modifying the dose of fluorouracil based on its AUC reduced toxicity while still maintaining response rates.[4] In another study, cisplatin pharmacokinetics were said to be optimum when it was given as a continuous infusion with a continuous infusion of fluorouracil.[5] Further study is needed.

(b) Oxaliplatin

In one study, 28 patients with advanced or metastatic colorectal cancer were given fluorouracil alone, or immediately following an 85 mg/m^2 dose of oxaliplatin given over 2 hours. Oxaliplatin did not significantly affect the pharmacokinetics of fluorouracil (either 2 cycles of a 400 mg/m^2 bolus followed by a 46-hour infusion of 2400 mg/m^2 given to 10 patients, with pharmacokinetic sampling over 46 hours; or a single cycle of a 400 mg/m^2 bolus followed by 600 mg/m^2 over 22 hours given to 18 patients, with pharmacokinetic sampling over 22 hours).[6] Similarly, a study in which patients received fluorouracil 200 mg/m^2 daily as a continuous infusion, and oxaliplatin 30 mg/m^2 daily as a 12-hour infusion on days one to 4 of each 14 day cycle found that the pharmacokinetics of both oxaliplatin or fluorouracil were unaffected by concurrent use.[7] However, in another study, 29 patients with advanced colorectal cancer were given fluorouracil in a dose adjusted to give levels of 2.5 to 3 mg/L (dose range 750 to 3500 mg/m^2 per week) either alone, or immediately after a 2-hour infusion of oxaliplatin 130 mg/m^2. In this study pharmacokinetic samples were taken on days one, 8 and 15. Oxaliplatin raised the plasma levels of fluorouracil by about one-third, with the effect appearing to last for 15 days; however, fluorouracil toxicity was not increased.[8]

The combination of fluorouracil and oxaliplatin is widely used, but one of the studies cited here suggests that the schedules could still be adjusted to optimise efficacy and minimise toxicity.[8]

1. Jeske J, Hansen RM, Libnoch JA, Anderson T. 5-Fluorouracil infusion and low-dose weekly cisplatin: an analysis of increased toxicity. *Am J Clin Oncol* (1990) 13, 485–8.
2. Jeremic B, Jevremovic S, Djuric L, Mijatovic L. Cardiotoxicity during chemotherapy treatment with 5-fluorouracil and cisplatin. *J Chemother* (1990) 2, 264–7.
3. Belliveau JF, Posner MR, Crabtree GW, Weitberg AB, Wiemann MC, Cummings FJ, O'Leary GP, Ingersoll E, Calabresi P. Clinical pharmacokinetics of 3-day continuous infusion cisplatin and daily bolus 5-fluorouracil. *Eur J Clin Pharmacol* (1991) 40, 115–17.
4. Fety R, Rolland F, Barberi-Heyob M, Hardouin A, Campion L, Conroy T, Merlin J-L, Rivière A, Perrocheau G, Etienne MC, Milano G. Clinical impact of pharmacokinetically-guided dose adaptation of 5-fluorouracil: results from a multicentric randomized trial in patients with locally advanced head and neck carcinomas. *Clin Cancer Res* (1998) 4, 2039–45.
5. Ikeda K, Terashima M, Kawamura H, Takiyama I, Koeda K, Takagane A, Sato N, Ishida K, Iwaya T, Maesawa C, Yoshinari H, Saito K. Pharmacokinetics of cisplatin in combined cisplatin and 5-fluorouracil therapy: a comparative study of three different schedules of cisplatin administration. *Jpn J Clin Oncol* (1998) 28, 168–75.
6. Joel SP, Papamichael D, Richards F, Davis T, Aslanis V, Chatelut E, Locke K, Slevin ML, Seymour MT. Lack of pharmacokinetic interaction between 5-fluorouracil and oxaliplatin. *Clin Pharmacol Ther* (2004) 76, 45–54.
7. Cattel L, La Grotta G, Infante L, Passera R, Arpicco S, Brusa P, Bumma C. Pharmacokinetic study of oxaliplatin iv chronomodulated infusion combined with 5-fluorouracil iv continuous infusion in the treatment of advanced colorectal cancer. *Farmaco* (2003) 58, 1333–8.
8. Boisdron-Celle M, Craipeau MC, Brienza S, Delva R, Guérin-Meyer V, Cvitkovic E, Gamelin E. Influence of oxaliplatin on 5-fluorouracil plasma clearance and clinical consequences. *Cancer Chemother Pharmacol* (2002) 49, 235–43.

Fluorouracil + Dipyridamole

One study suggested that *intravenous* dipyridamole may reduce the steady-state plasma levels of fluorouracil, whereas others found that *oral* dipyridamole caused no important changes in fluorouracil pharmacokinetics.

Clinical evidence, mechanism, importance and management

Numerous preclinical studies found that dipyridamole enhanced the activity of fluorouracil, leading to its investigation as a biomodulator.[1] However, unexpectedly, in one phase I study of the combination, the use of dipyridamole was associated with a lower steady state plasma level of fluorouracil, suggesting an increase of about 30% in the total body clearance or volume of distribution of fluorouracil.[2] In this study, 47 patients with advanced cancer were given fluorouracil in escalating doses ranging from 185 mg/m^2 daily to 3600 mg/m^2 daily with or without dipyridamole as a continuous infusion of 7.7 mg/kg daily for 72 hours.[2] In contrast, in a later randomised study, oral dipyridamole 75 mg three times daily for 5 days did not significantly alter the pharmacokinetics of fluorouracil, except for prolonging the half-life and slightly increasing the dose-intensity: over 5 cycles the average dose of fluorouracil was 479 mg/m^2 alone, compared with 533 mg/m^2 in the presence of dipyridamole. In this study, oral dipyridamole did not improve the antineoplastic activity of fluorouracil with folinic acid.[3] Similarly, another clinical study found that oral dipyridamole did not significantly alter the pharmacokinetics of fluorouracil.[4] Thus, despite the promise of preclinical studies, the benefits of combining dipyridamole with fluorouracil have not been realised clinically.

1. Grem JL. Biochemical modulation of fluorouracil by dipyridamole: preclinical and clinical experience. *Semin Oncol* (1992) 19 (Suppl 3), 56–65.
2. Trump DL, Egorin MJ, Forrest A, Willson JKV, Remick S, Tutsch KD. Pharmacokinetic and pharmacodynamic analysis of fluorouracil during 72-hour continuous infusion with and without dipyridamole. *J Clin Oncol* (1991) 9, 2027–35.
3. Köhne C-H, Hiddemann W, Schüller J, Weiss J, Lohrmann H-P, Schmitz-Hüber U, Bodenstein H, Schöber C, Wilke H, Grem J, Schmoll H-J. Failure of orally administered dipyridamole to enhance the antineoplastic activity of fluorouracil in combination with leucovorin in patients with advanced colorectal cancer: a prospective randomized trial. *J Clin Oncol* (1995) 13, 1201–8.
4. Czejka MJ, Jäger W, Schüller J, Fogl U, Weiss C, Schernthaner G. Clinical pharmacokinetics of fluorouracil: influence of the biomodulating agents interferon, dipyridamole and folinic acid alone and in combination. *Arzneimittelforschung* (1993) 43, 387–90.

Fluorouracil + Folic acid

Two patients developed severe fluorouracil toxicity while taking multivitamin preparations containing folic acid.

Clinical evidence

A woman who underwent surgery for carcinoma of the rectum was, a month later, given intravenous fluorouracil 500 mg/m^2 daily for 5 days. At the end of this chemotherapy she was admitted to hospital with anorexia, severe mouth ulceration, bloody diarrhoea and vaginal bleeding, which was interpreted as fluorouracil toxicity. Her concurrent medication included folic acid 5 mg daily (in *Multi-B forte*) along with loperamide, sulfasalazine, vitamins B_{12} and K, and HRT. A month later, when she was given fluorouracil without the folic acid, her treatment was well tolerated and without toxicity. A man similarly treated with fluorouracil for colonic cancer was admitted to hospital 2 days later with severe mouth ulceration and bloody diarrhoea. He too was found to be taking a multivitamin preparation, containing folic acid 500 micrograms (amount taken daily not known). Subsequent courses of fluorouracil at the same dose, but without the folic acid, were well tolerated.[1]

Mechanism

It would seem that folic acid increases fluorouracil inhibition of thymidine formation which is important for DNA synthesis, and thereby increases fluorouracil toxicity.

Importance and management

Direct information seem to be limited to these two cases and a case of fatal toxicity associated with concurrent folic acid and capecitabine, a prodrug of fluorouracil (see 'Fluorouracil prodrugs; Capecitabine + Folinates', p.683) but the interaction would appear to be established. What happened is consistent with the way folinic acid, another source of folate, is used therapeutically to increase the potency of fluorouracil. Patients given fluorouracil should therefore not be given folic acid, and should be told to avoid multivitamin preparations containing folic acid to prevent the development of severe fluorouracil adverse effects.

1. Mainwaring P, Grygiel JJ. Interaction of 5-fluorouracil with folates. *Aust N Z J Med* (1995) 25, 60.

Fluorouracil + Gemcitabine

Pharmacokinetic analysis has shown that gemcitabine enhances the systemic exposure of fluorouracil in patients with pancreatic carcinoma given folinic acid, fluorouracil, and gemcitabine.[1,2] In addition, *in vitro*, gemcitabine increases both the accumulation of fluorouracil and its cytotoxicity.[1] The use of fluorouracil with gemcitabine is being investigated for its therapeutic potential, particularly in pancreatic cancer.

1. Francini G, Correale P, Cetta F, Zuckermann M, Cerretani D, Micheli V, Bruni G, Clerici M, Pozzessere D, Petrioli R, Marsili S, Messinese S, Sabatino M, Giorgio G. Effects of gemcitabine on 5-fluorouracil activity, pharmacokinetics and pharmacodynamics in vitro and in cancer patients. *Gastroenterology* (2002) 122 (Suppl 1), A308.
2. Correale P, Cerretani D, Marsili S, Pozzessere D, Petrioli R, Messinese S, Sabatino M, Roviello F, Pinto E, Francini G, Giorgi G. Gemcitabine increases systemic 5-fluorouracil exposure in advanced cancer patients. *Eur J Cancer* (2003) 39, 1547–51.

Fluorouracil + H_2-receptor antagonists

Some data indicate that four weeks, but not one week, of treatment with cimetidine can slightly increase fluorouracil exposure. Concurrent use might have increased activity in colorectal cancer.

Clinical evidence, mechanism, importance and management

A study in 6 patients with carcinoma given fluorouracil (15 mg/kg daily for 5 days, repeated every 4 weeks) found that **cimetidine** 1 g daily for 4 weeks increased the AUC and maximum plasma concentration of fluorouracil by 72% and 74%, respectively, when fluorouracil was given orally. When fluorouracil was given intravenously, **cimetidine** increased its AUC by 27% and reduced its total body clearance by 28%. In this small group, no increased toxicity was noted. The pharmacokinetics of fluorouracil were unaltered when **cimetidine** was given for only one week.[1] **Cimetidine** had similar effects in *animal* studies but **ranitidine** had no effect on fluorouracil metabolism.[2] It is suggested that **cimetidine** reduces the hepatic metabolism of fluorouracil.[1,2] At least three clinical studies have shown some treatment benefits from giving fluorouracil with long-term **cimetidine** in colorectal cancer.[3-5] However, this benefit has been attributed to immunomodulation[3] or inhibition of adhesion,[4] rather than any pharmacokinetic interaction. Whatever the mechanism, it appears that **cimetidine** can increase the activity of fluorouracil. Concurrent treatment should be undertaken with care. **Cimetidine** can be obtained without a prescription in some countries, therefore patients can unwittingly increase the toxicity of fluorouracil. **Ranitidine** does not appear to interact but this ideally needs establishing in human subjects.

1. Harvey VJ, Slevin ML, Dilloway MR, Clark PI, Johnston A, Lant AF. The influence of cimetidine on the pharmacokinetics of 5-fluorouracil. *Br J Clin Pharmacol* (1984) 18, 421–30.
2. Dilloway MR, Lant AF. Effect of H_2-receptor antagonists on the pharmacokinetics of 5-fluorouracil in the rat and monkey. *Biopharm Drug Dispos* (1991) 12, 17–28.
3. Links M, Clingan PR, Phadke K, O'Baugh J, Legge J, Adams WJ, Ross WB, Morris DL. A randomized trial of cimetidine with 5-fluorouracil and folinic acid in metastatic colorectal cancer. *Eur J Surg Oncol* (1995) 21, 523–5.
4. Matsumoto S, Imaeda Y, Umemoto S, Kobayashi K, Suzuki H, Okamoto T. Cimetidine increases survival of colorectal cancer patients with high levels of sialyl Lewis-X and sialyl Lewis-A epitope expression on tumour cells. *Br J Cancer* (2002) 86, 159–60.
5. Yoshimatsu K, Ishibashi K, Hashimoto M, Umehara A, Yokomizo H, Yoshida K, Fujimoto T, Iwasaki K, Ogawa K. Effect of cimetidine with chemotherapy on stage IV colorectal cancer. *Gan To Kagaku Ryoho* (2003) 30, 1794–7.

Fluorouracil + Interferon alfa

Interferon alfa has increased plasma fluorouracil levels in some, but not other, studies.

Clinical evidence, mechanism, importance and management

In a pharmacokinetic study, 26 patients with colorectal cancer were given a 5-day continuous infusion of fluorouracil 750 mg/m^2 daily repeated in week 4 followed by a bolus intravenous injection of 750 mg/m^2 weekly with or without subcutaneous interferon alfa-2a (*Roferon*) 9 million units three times a week. There was considerable within-patient variation but no significant differences in steady-state plasma levels were found between the two groups.[1] Similarly, others have also reported that interferon alfa does not significantly alter fluorouracil pharmacokinetics;[2,3] however, other studies[4-8] have found a significant increase in the peak levels of fluorouracil and/or its AUC when interferon alfa is given. Despite promising early pre-clinical and clinical data indicating that interferon may improve the response to fluorouracil, this has not yet been demonstrated in randomised studies.[9]

1. Pittman K, Perren T, Ward U, Primrose J, Slevin M, Patel N, Selby P. Pharmacokinetics of 5-fluorouracil in colorectal cancer patients receiving interferon. *Ann Oncol* (1993) 4, 515–6.
2. Seymour MT, Patel N, Johnston A, Joel SP, Slevin ML. Lack of effect of interferon α2a upon fluorouracil pharmacokinetics. *Br J Cancer* (1994) 70, 724–8.
3. Kim J, Zhi J, Satoh H, Koss-Twardy SG, Passe SM, Patel IH, Pazdur R. Pharmacokinetics of recombinant human interferon-α2a combined with 5-fluorouracil in patients with advanced colorectal carcinoma. *Anticancer Drugs* (1998) 9, 689–96.
4. Schüller J, Czejka MJ, Schernthaner G, Fogl U, Jäger W, Micksche M. Influence of interferon alfa-2b with or without folinic acid on pharmacokinetics of fluorouracil. *Semin Oncol* (1992) 19 (2 suppl 3) 93–7.
5. Grem JL, McAtee N, Murphy RF, Balis FM, Steinberg SM, Hamilton JM, Sorensen JM, Sartor O, Kramer BS, Goldstein LJ, Gay LM, Caubo KM, Goldspiel B, Allegra CJ. A pilot study of interferon alfa-2a in combination with fluorouracil plus high dose leucovorin in metastatic gastrointestinal carcinoma. *J Clin Oncol* (1991) 9, 1811–20.
6. Danhauser LL, Freimann JH, Gilchrist TL, Gutterman JU, Hunter CY, Yeomans AC, Markowitz AB. Phase I and plasma pharmacokinetic study of infusional fluorouracil combined with recombinant interferon alfa-2b in patients with advanced cancer. *J Clin Oncol* (1993) 11, 751–61.
7. Larsson P-A, Glimelius B, Jeppsson B, Jönsson P-E, Malmberg M, Gustavsson B, Carlsson G, Svedberg M. A pharmacokinetic study of 5-FU/leucovorin and alpha-interferon in advanced cancer. *Acta Oncol* (2000) 39, 59–63.
8. Schüller J, Czejka M. Pharmacokinetic interaction of 5-fluorouracil and interferon alpha-2b with or without folinic acid. *Med Oncol* (1995) 12, 47–53.
9. Makower D, Wadler S. Interferons as biomodulators of fluoropyrimidines in the treatment of colorectal cancer. *Semin Oncol* (1999) 26, 663–71.

Fluorouracil + Metronidazole

The toxicity, but not the efficacy of fluorouracil, is increased by metronidazole.

Clinical evidence

A sizeable increase in fluorouracil toxicity was noted in 27 patients with metastatic colorectal cancer when they were given intravenous metronidazole 750 mg/m^2 one-hour before receiving intravenous fluorouracil 600 mg/m^2 five days per week, every 4 weeks. Granulocytopenia occurred in 74% of patients, nausea and vomiting in 48%, anaemia in 41%, stomatitis and oral ulceration in 34%, and thrombocytopenia in 19%.[1] A related pharmacokinetic study in 10 patients found that metronidazole reduced the clearance of fluorouracil by 27% over the 5-day period and increased the AUC by 34%. *In vitro* studies with human colon cancer cells did not show any increased efficacy.[1]

Studies using another nitroimidazole, **misonidazole**, in patients with colorectal cancer also found an increased incidence and severity of gastrointestinal toxicity with concurrent use,[2,3] a small increase in the incidence of leucopenia[2] and a reduction in the clearance of fluorouracil.[3]

Mechanism

Metronidazole reduces the clearance of fluorouracil, thereby increasing its toxic effects.

Importance and management

Information is limited but the interaction between fluorouracil and metronidazole appears to be established. It was hoped that metronidazole, or misonidazole (no longer in clinical use), might increase the efficacy of fluorouracil. However, the studies above show that the toxicity of fluorouracil is increased without an obvious increase in its therapeutic efficacy. Care should be taken if metronidazole is required for its antimicrobial effects in a patient receiving fluorouracil. Whether other nitroimidazoles (e.g. tinidazole) behave similarly appears not to have been studied.

1. Bardakji Z, Jolivet J, Langelier Y, Besner J-G, Ayoub J. 5-Fluorouracil-metronidazole combination therapy in metastatic colorectal cancer. *Cancer Chemother Pharmacol* (1986) 18, 140–44.
2. Spooner D, Bugden RD, Peckham MJ, Wist EA. The combination of 5-fluorouracil with misonidazole in patients with advanced colorectal cancer. *Int J Radiat Oncol Biol Phys* (1982) 8, 387–9.
3. McDermott BJ, Van den Berg HW, Martin WMC, Murphy RF. Pharmacokinetic rationale for the interaction of 5-fluorouracil and misonidazole in humans. *Br J Cancer* (1983) 48, 705–10.

Fluorouracil + Miscellaneous

A retrospective analysis of studies in a total of 250 patients given fluorouracil for the treatment of gastrointestinal cancer found that chlorprothixene, cinnarizine, prochlorperazine, sodium pentobarbital, thiethylperazine, trimethobenzamide (in antiemetic doses) did not significantly increase toxicity or decrease therapeutic effects of fluorouracil, when compared with a placebo.[1]

1. Moertel CG, Reitemeier RJ, Hahn RG. Effect of concomitant drug treatment on toxic and therapeutic activity of 5-fluorouracil (5-FU; NSC-19893). *Cancer Chemother Rep* (1972) 56, 245–7.

Fluorouracil prodrugs + Brivudine or Sorivudine

Serious and rapidly fatal toxicity, attributed to fluorouracil toxicity, has been seen in patients given tegafur, or other fluorouracil prodrugs, with sorivudine. Serious and fatal toxicity has also been seen in two patients given capecitabine with brivudine.

Clinical evidence

In 1993, the Japanese Ministry of Health reported that 15 Japanese patients with cancer and a viral disease died several days after being given a fluorouracil prodrug (e.g. **tegafur**) and sorivudine. Before death most of them developed severe toxicity, including severe anorexia, marked damage to the bone marrow with decreases in white cell and platelet counts, and marked atrophy of the intestinal membrane with diarrhoea and loss of blood. Eight other patients given both drugs developed symptoms of severe toxicity.[1,2]

More recently, two case reports describe serious toxic reactions in patients receiving **capecitabine** and brivudine;[3,4] one of which resulted in death.[3] The second patient was a 66-year-old woman with metastatic breast cancer, who was receiving **capecitabine** and developed herpes zoster infection, which was treated with brivudine 125 mg daily for 7 days. She subsequently developed medullar aplasia, serious toxic effects to the intestinal mucous membrane, hand-foot syndrome, onycholysis, and dental pigmentation.[4]

Mechanism

Sorivudine appears to be converted in the gut to a metabolite (BVU or bromovinyluracil) that is an inhibitor of dihydropyrimidine dehydrogenase (DPD), an enzyme involved in the metabolism of fluorouracil (which is derived from tegafur and other fluorouracil prodrugs) to an inactive metabolite.[1,2,5] Brivudine is also converted to BVU in the liver.[3] There is some evidence that DPD activity is genetically determined, and that there are poor fluorouracil metabolisers with low DPD activity, who would be expected to be more susceptible to this interaction.[6]

Importance and management

Information is limited to these reports but the interactions between prodrugs of fluorouracil and sorivudine or brivudine would seem to be established and of clinical importance. The concurrent use of inhibitors of dihydropyrimidine dehydrogenase (such as sorivudine and brivudine) with fluorouracil[7] and oral fluorouracil prodrugs (such as capecitabine[8] and tegafur)[9,10] is contraindicated. The manufacturer of tegafur with uracil suggests that it should not be given until 4 weeks after brivudine is stopped, to allow recovery of enzyme activity.[9] A similar warning is also given by the manufacturer of tegafur with gimeracil and oteracil.[10] Note that sorivudine was withdrawn from the market following confirmation of this interaction.

1. Okuda H, Nishiyama T, Ogura K, Nagayama S, Ikeda K, Yamaguchi S, Nakamura Y, Kawaguchi Y, Watabe T. Lethal drug interactions of sorivudine, a new antiviral drug, with oral 5-fluorouracil prodrugs. *Drug Metab Dispos* (1997) 25, 270–3.
2. Diasio RB. Sorivudine and 5-fluorouracil; a clinically significant drug-drug interaction due to inhibition of dihydropyrimidine dehydrogenase. *Br J Clin Pharmacol* (1998) 46, 1–4.
3. Rätz Bravo AE, Hofer S, Krähenbühl S, Ludwig C. Fatal drug-drug interaction of brivudine and capecitabine. *Acta Oncol* (2009) 48, 631–3.
4. Baena-Cañada JM, Martínez MJ, García-Olmedo O, Jiménez-Bárcenas R, Muriel-Cueto P. Interaction between capecitabine and brivudin in a patient with breast cancer. *Nat Rev Clin Oncol* (2010) 7, 55–8.
5. Watabe T, Okuda H, Ogura K. Lethal drug interactions of the new antiviral, sorivudine, with anticancer prodrugs of 5-fluorouracil. *Yakugaku Zasshi* (1997) 117, 910–21. (In Japanese).
6. Watabe T, Ogura K, Nishiyama T. Molecular toxicological mechanism of the lethal interactions of the new antiviral drug, sorivudine, with 5-fluorouracil prodrugs and genetic deficiency of dihydropyrimidine dehydrogenase. *Yakugaku Zasshi* (2002) 122, 527–35.
7. Fluorouracil Injection. Medac GmbH. UK Summary of product characteristics, June 2009.
8. Xeloda (Capecitabine). Roche Products Ltd. UK Summary of product characteristics, June 2011.
9. Uftoral (Tegafur and uracil). Merck Serono. UK Summary of product characteristics, April 2011.
10. Teysuno (Tegafur, gimeracil and oteracil monopotassium). Nordic Pharma Ltd. UK Summary of product characteristics, March 2011.

Fluorouracil prodrugs + Food

Food slightly reduces the exposure to capecitabine, and has a negligible effect on the exposure to its active metabolite, fluorouracil. Food slightly reduces the exposure to fluorouracil derived from tegafur when given with uracil, but has a negligible effect when tegafur is given with gimeracil and oteracil.

Clinical evidence, mechanism, importance and management

(a) Capecitabine

In a crossover study in 11 patients with colorectal cancer, oral capecitabine was given either after an overnight fast, or 30 minutes after breakfast. When normalised to a dose of capecitabine of 1255 mg/m^2, the time to reach the maximum plasma concentration was prolonged from 30 minutes to 2 hours when capecitabine was taken with food, and the maximum plasma concentration and AUC were reduced by 60% and 31%, respectively. The maximum plasma concentration and AUC of fluorouracil derived from capecitabine were reduced by 33% and 16%, respectively. The clinical relevance of these findings remains to be determined.[1] Note that, it is recommended that capecitabine is taken within 30 minutes after a meal,[1-3] because this is how it was used in clinical efficacy studies.[1]

(b) Tegafur with gimeracil and oteracil

In a crossover study in 27 patients with advanced solid tumours, a single 30-mg/m^2 dose of tegafur with gimeracil and oteracil was given with, or without, food. The AUC of tegafur was not altered by the presence of food, but the AUCs of fluorouracil, gimeracil, and oteracil were reduced by 15%, 25%, and 71%, respectively.[4] In another pharmacokinetic study in 18 patients with advanced solid tumours, a single 35-mg/m^2 dose of tegafur with gimeracil and oteracil was given without food or after a standardised breakfast. Fasting decreased the time to reach maximum plasma concentrations and increased the maximum plasma concentrations of tegafur, fluorouracil, gimeracil, and oteracil, but the 90% confidence intervals for these changes fell within those set for bioequivalence. There was no difference in the AUC of tegafur between the fasted and fed states. The AUC of fluorouracil was about 17% higher in the fasted state than the fed state, but the 90% confidence interval for this change fell within those set for bioequivalence. The AUC of oteracil was 56% higher in the fasted state than the fed state.[5] The results of both of these studies suggest that tegafur with gimeracil and oteracil could be given without regard for food; however, the authors of one study,[5] suggest that the lower exposure to oteracil in the fed state, might result in a reduced gastro-protective effect of oteracil and hence a greater incidence of gastro-intestinal adverse effects, if tegafur with gimeracil and oteracil is taken with food. The UK manufacturer of tegafur with gimeracil and oteracil advises that it should be taken at least one hour before, or one hour after, food.[6]

(c) Tegafur with uracil

In a crossover study, 22 patients received a single 200-mg dose of *Uftoral* (tegafur with uracil) with a single 30-mg dose of folinic acid after an overnight fast, or 5 minutes after a high-fat breakfast. The maximum plasma concentration and AUC of fluorouracil derived from tegafur were reduced by 70% and 37%, respectively, when tegafur with uracil was given with food, and the time to reach maximum fluorouracil concentration was delayed from 30 minutes to 2 hours.[7] Similar results were found in another study in 12 patients given a single 200-mg dose of *Uftoral* (tegafur with uracil) with a single 25-mg dose of folinic acid in the fasted state or after a low-fat Japanese breakfast.[8] This slight reduction in exposure might result in reduced efficacy. It is recommended that tegafur with uracil is taken one hour before or one hour after meals,[9] as was the procedure in clinical efficacy studies.[7]

1. Reigner B, Verweij J, Dirix L, Cassidy J, Twelves C, Allman D, Weidekamm E, Roos B, Banken L, Utoh M, Osterwalder B. Effect of food on the pharmacokinetics of capecitabine and its metabolites following oral administration in cancer patients. *Clin Cancer Res* (1998) 4, 941–8.
2. Xeloda (Capecitabine). Roche Products Ltd. UK Summary of product characteristics, June 2011.
3. Xeloda (Capecitabine). Roche Laboratories Inc. US Prescribing information, February 2011.
4. Scheulen ME, Saito K, Hilger RA, Mende B, Zergebel C, Strumberg D. Effect of food and a proton pump inhibitor on the pharmacokinetics of S-1 following oral administration of S-1 in patients with advanced solid tumors. *Cancer Chemother Pharmacol* (2012) 69, 753–61.
5. Peters GJ, Noordhuis P, van Groeningen CJ, Giaccone G, Holwerda U, Voorn D, Schrijvers A, Schornagel JH, Beijnen JH, Fumoleau P, Schellens JHM. The effect of food on the pharmacokinetics of S-1 after single oral administration to patients with solid tumours. *Clin Cancer Res* (2004) 10, 4072–6.
6. Teysuno (Tegafur, gimeracil and oteracil monopotassium). Nordic Pharma Ltd. UK Summary of product characteristics, March 2011.
7. Damle B, Ravandi F, Kaul S, Sonnichsen D, Ferreira I, Brooks D, Stewart D, Alberts D, Pazdur R. Effect of food on the oral bioavailability of UFT and leucovorin in cancer patients. *Clin Cancer Res* (2001) 7, 517–23.
8. Furuhata T, Meguro M, Nishidate T, Okita K, Ishiyama G, Iwayama Y, Hosokawa Y, Tsuruma T, Kimura Y, Mizuguchi T, Sasaki K. Effects of a low-fat meal on the oral bioavailability of UFT and leucovorin in patients with colorectal cancer. *Int J Clin Oncol* (2009) 14, 529–33.
9. Uftoral (Tegafur and uracil). Merck Serono. UK Summary of product characteristics, April 2011.

Fluorouracil prodrugs + Taxanes

There are no clinically significant pharmacokinetic interactions between capecitabine and paclitaxel, and probably not between capecitabine and docetaxel. A case report describes hand-foot syndrome in a patient who received docetaxel two days after stopping tegafur with uracil.

Clinical evidence, mechanism, importance and management

(a) Capecitabine

1. Docetaxel. A study in patients with advanced solid tumours found that the use of capecitabine with docetaxel resulted in an almost twofold decrease in the maximum plasma concentration and AUC of fluorouracil. The authors suggest that more study is needed to assess the significance of this finding. Other pharmacokinetic parameters of capecitabine were not affected by docetaxel, and the pharmacokinetics of docetaxel were not significantly affected by capecitabine or its metabolites.[1]

Another study in similar patients also found that capecitabine did not alter the pharmacokinetics of docetaxel.[2] However, in a multiple regression analysis, the clearance of docetaxel appeared to be modestly increased in 32 patients who had received treatment with capecitabine and docetaxel when compared with 27 other patients who had received docetaxel alone,[3] but this was probably not clinically significant.

2. Paclitaxel. In a study in 17 patients, the concurrent use of paclitaxel and capecitabine did not significantly alter the pharmacokinetics of either drug.[4]

(b) Tegafur with uracil

A 30-year old patient received treatment with **docetaxel** 50 mg/m^2 two days after stopping tegafur with uracil, which she had been taking for the previous 14 months. Seven days later she developed hand-foot syndrome which increased to such an extent that she could not walk due to severe pain. A later subsequent dose of **docetaxel** did not result in hand-foot syndrome. Both fluoropyrimidines and taxanes have been associated with hand-foot syndrome. The authors suggested that a longer period of time is required between the two drugs to reduce the risk of this adverse effect occurring.[5] However, the combination of tegafur and docetaxel is being investigated, and other fluoropyrimidines are used with docetaxel in established regimens, suggesting that any additive interaction is rare.

1. Pronk LC, Vasey P, Sparreboom A, Reigner B, Planting AST, Gordon RJ, Osterwalder B, Verweij J. A phase I and pharmacokinetic study of the combination of capecitabine and docetaxel in patients with advanced solid tumours. *Br J Cancer* (2000) 83, 22–9.
2. Ramanathan RK, Ramalingam S, Egorin MJ, Belani P, Potter DM, Fakih M, Jung LL, Strychor S, Jacobs SA, Friedland DM, Shin DM, Chatta GS, Tutchko S, Zamboni WC. Phase I study of weekly (day 1 and 8) docetaxel in combination with capecitabine in patients with advanced solid malignancies. *Cancer Chemother Pharmacol* (2005) 55, 354–60.
3. Rudek MA, Sparreboom A, Garrett-Mayer ES, Armstrong DK, Wolff AC, Verweij J, Baker SD. Factors affecting pharmacokinetic variability following doxorubicin and docetaxel-based therapy. *Eur J Cancer* (2004) 40, 1170–8.
4. Villalona-Calero MA, Weiss GR, Burris HA, Kraynak M, Rodrigues G, Drengler RL, Eckhardt SG, Reigner B, Moczygemba J, Burger HU, Griffin T, Von Hoff DD, Rowinsky EK. Phase I and pharmacokinetic study of the oral fluoropyrimidine capecitabine in combination with paclitaxel in patients with advanced solid malignancies. *J Clin Oncol* (1999) 17, 1915–25.
5. Kanaji N, Bandoh S. Hand-foot syndrome associated with uracil/tegafur and docetaxel in a patient with lung cancer. *Nihon Kokyuki Gakkai Zasshi* (2007) 45, 474–8.

Fluorouracil prodrugs; Capecitabine + Allopurinol

The activity of capecitabine is predicted to be decreased by allopurinol.

Clinical evidence, mechanism, importance and management

Capecitabine is a prodrug, which is activated by several enzymatic steps to produce active fluorouracil within the body. Because allopurinol is reported to modulate fluorouracil, with possible decreased efficacy (although note an adverse effect is not established, see 'Fluorouracil + Allopurinol', p.679), the UK manufacturers of capecitabine say that the concurrent use of allopurinol should be avoided.[1]

1. Xeloda (Capecitabine). Roche Products Ltd. UK Summary of product characteristics, June 2011.

Fluorouracil prodrugs; Capecitabine + Antacids

The absorption of capecitabine was not affected by an aluminium/magnesium hydroxide antacid.

Clinical evidence, mechanism, importance and management

A study in 12 patients found that 20 mL of an **aluminium/magnesium hydroxide** antacid (*Maalox*) caused a small increase in the plasma levels of a single 1250-mg/m^2 oral dose of capecitabine and one metabolite (5′-DFCR) but it had no effect on the other 3 major metabolites (5′-DFUR, 5-FU and FBAL).[1] There would therefore seem to be no reason for taking special precautions if capecitabine and an antacid of this type are used concurrently.

1. Reigner B, Clive S, Cassidy J, Jodrell D, Schulz R, Goggin T, Banken L, Roos B, Utoh M, Mulligan T, Weidekamm E. Influence of the antacid Maalox on the pharmacokinetics of capecitabine in cancer patients. *Cancer Chemother Pharmacol* (1999) 43, 309–15.

Fluorouracil prodrugs; Capecitabine + Folinates

A patient died after treatment with capecitabine possibly because the concurrent use of folic acid enhanced capecitabine toxicity. The maximum tolerated dose of capecitabine is decreased by folinic acid.

Clinical evidence, mechanism, importance and management

(a) Folic acid

A 51-year-old woman with metastatic breast cancer started treatment with capecitabine 2500 mg/m^2 daily for 14 days every 21 days. Treatment was stopped after 8 days because she developed diarrhoea, vomiting, and hand-foot syndrome. She improved with parenteral hydration and symptomatic treatment, but 3 weeks later still had diarrhoea, leg oedema, and hand-foot syndrome. She was found to have been taking folic acid 15 mg daily for several weeks before starting capecitabine and had continued to take it during and after capecitabine treatment. The patient's condition improved when the folic acid was stopped, but she then developed diarrhoea and fever followed by necrotic colitis and she died from septic shock and vascular collapse. It is possible that the concurrent use of folic acid enhanced the toxicity of capecitabine.[1]

(b) Folinic acid

Studies in patients with refractory advanced cancer have found that folinic acid 30 mg twice daily does not have a major effect on the pharmacokinetics of capecitabine.[2] However, the pharmacodynamics of capecitabine were affected as determined by the more frequent occurrence of dose-limiting gastrointestinal disorders or hand-foot syndrome.[2] The UK manufacturer states that the maximum tolerated capecitabine dose when used alone in the intermittent regimen is 3 g/m^2, but this is reduced to 2 g/m^2 if folinic acid 30 mg twice daily is also given.[3]

1. Clippe C, Freyer G, Milano G, Trillet-Lenoir V. Lethal toxicity of capecitabine due to abusive folic acid prescription? *Clin Oncol* (2003) 15, 1–2.
2. Cassidy J, Dirix L, Bissett D, Reigner B, Griffin T, Allman D, Osterwalder B, Van Oosterom AT. A phase I study of capecitabine in combination with oral leucovorin in patients with intractable solid tumours. *Clin Cancer Res* (1998) 4, 2755–61.
3. Xeloda (Capecitabine). Roche Products Ltd. UK Summary of product characteristics, June 2011.

Fluorouracil prodrugs; Capecitabine + Miscellaneous

The maximum tolerated dose of capecitabine is decreased by interferon alfa. No pharmacokinetic interaction appears to occur between capecitabine and oxaliplatin.

Clinical evidence, mechanism, importance and management

(a) Interferon alfa

The UK manufacturer[1] says that the maximum tolerated capecitabine dose when used alone is 3 g/m^2, but when combined with interferon alfa-2a (3 million units/m^2 daily) the maximum tolerated dose is 2 g/m^2. Capecitabine is a prodrug of fluorouracil, the activity of which is thought to be modulated by interferon alfa. See also 'Fluorouracil + Interferon alfa', p.681.

(b) Oxaliplatin

The manufacturer notes there were no clinically significant changes in the exposure to capecitabine and its metabolites, or to the exposure to platinum (free or total) when capecitabine was given with oxaliplatin.[1]

1. Xeloda (Capecitabine). Roche Products Ltd. UK Summary of product characteristics, June 2011.

Fluorouracil prodrugs; Capecitabine + Vinca alkaloids

The concurrent use of vinflunine or vinorelbine with capecitabine does not appear to affect the pharmacokinetics of either drug.

Clinical evidence

(a) Vinflunine

In a small phase I dose-finding study, patients with breast cancer were given intravenous vinflunine (280 or 320 mg/m^2) on day 1 and oral capecitabine (1.65 or 2 g/m^2) daily from day 1 to 14, every 3 weeks. The pharmacokinetics of vinflunine did not differ from those of historical controls. However, the AUC of capecitabine and its metabolite 5-fluorouracil were 1.35- to 3-fold higher on day 14 when taken alone, compared with day 1 when vinflunine was also given, although there was high variability in the findings.[1]

(b) Vinorelbine

A study in which 44 patients received escalating doses of oral capecitabine for 14 days, every 3 or 4 weeks, and vinorelbine weekly, or on days one and 8 of a 3- or 4-week cycle, found that the pharmacokinetics of vinorelbine were unaffected by capecitabine, when compared with historical data. The pharmacokinetics of capecitabine and its metabolites were highly variable, but were generally unchanged by the use of vinorelbine, although the AUC of the 5-fluorouracil metabolite of capecitabine increased from day 1 to day 7.[2]

Mechanism

Although the AUC of fluorouracil was lower on day one (when capecitabine was given with vinorelbine or vinflunine), than on day 7 or 14 (when capecitabine was given alone), this was attributed to the repeated dosing of capecitabine, and was not considered to have been affected by the vinca alkaloid.[1,2]

Importance and management

No clinically relevant pharmacokinetic interaction appears to occur between capecitabine and vinflunine or vinorelbine.

1. Campone M, Isambert N, Bourbouloux E, Roché H, Bonneterre J, Milano G, Fumoleau P. A phase I study of vinflunine in combination with capecitabine in patients with metastatic breast cancer previously treated with anthracyclines and taxanes. *Cancer Chemother Pharmacol* (2012) 69, 871–9.
2. Nolè F, Catania C, Sanna G, Imadalou K, Munzone E, Adamoli L, Longerey B, Blanchot G, Goldhirsch A. Dose-finding and pharmacokinetic study of an all-oral combination regimen of oral vinorelbine and capecitabine for patients with metastatic breast cancer. *Ann Oncol* (2006) 19, 322–9.

Fluorouracil prodrugs; Tegafur + Miscellaneous

Tegafur is partially metabolised by CYP2A6, and the manufacturers advise caution with CYP2A6 inhibitors (such as tranylcypromine and methoxsalen). The pharmacokinetics of tegafur are not affected by gemcitabine and the pharmacokinetics of gemcitabine were not affected by tegafur. Cimetidine, folinic acid and methotrexate are predicted to increase the toxicity of a tegafur-containing preparation and allopurinol is predicted to reduce its efficacy. The haematological toxicity of tegafur-containing preparations might be additive with that of clozapine.

Clinical evidence, mechanism, importance and management

(a) Allopurinol

The UK manufacturer of tegafur with gimeracil and oteracil predicts that allopurinol might decrease the activity of this drug combination by suppressing the phosphorylation of fluorouracil [the main metabolite of tegafur], and advises that concurrent use should be avoided.[1] However, based on the effects of allopurinol on fluorouracil, the clinical importance of this would be expected to be limited, see 'Fluorouracil + Allopurinol', p.679.

(b) Cimetidine

The UK manufacturer of tegafur with gimeracil and oteracil predicts that concurrent use with cimetidine might result in decreased clearance of fluorouracil [the main metabolite of tegafur] and thus increase its plasma concentrations. Caution is advised on concurrent use due to the increased risk of toxicity.[1] For discussion of the effects of cimetidine on fluorouracil plasma concentrations, see 'Fluorouracil + H_2-receptor antagonists', p.681.

(c) Clozapine

The UK manufacturer of tegafur with gimeracil and oteracil predicts that additive myelotoxicity can occur on the concurrent use of clozapine, and advises caution due to the increased risk and severity of haematological toxicity.[1] For discussion of the additive effects of clozapine with other drugs that also suppress bone marrow, see 'Clozapine + Drugs that cause bone marrow suppression', p.850.

(d) CYP2A6 inhibitors

In vitro studies indicate that tegafur is partially metabolised by CYP2A6.[2,3] In one report, a patient who was a CYP2A6 poor metaboliser (that is, lacking or deficient in this isoenzyme) had 4-fold higher concentrations of tegafur than other patients.[4] Therefore, it is possible that tegafur might not be as effective in CYP2A6 poor metabolisers, or if it is given with drugs that are inhibitors of CYP2A6, because of reduced metabolism to active fluorouracil. In addition, the toxicity profile might be different. However, tegafur is also metabolised to fluorouracil by cytosolic thymidine phosphorylase and some other isoenzymes (CYP1A2 and CYP2C8), so it is likely that fluorouracil can still be produced in the absence of CYP2A6.[2,5] Nevertheless, one manufacturer of a tegafur-containing preparation advises that tegafur should not be used in patients with a known deficiency of hepatic CYP2A6,[2] although note that they do not advise testing for this, and a patient's CYP450 phenotype is rarely known outside of the clinical research situation. The manufacturers of tegafur-containing preparations also advise caution if they are given with other drugs that are substrates[2] or inhibitors[1,2] of CYP2A6. One manufacturer specifically includes **methoxsalen** and the azoles **clotrimazole**, **ketoconazole**, and **miconazole**.[2] The clinical relevance of any of these interactions and of CYP2A6 metaboliser status remains to be determined. However, note that **ketoconazole** did not inhibit the formation of fluorouracil from tegafur *in vitro*.[3] **Methoxsalen** is an inhibitor of CYP2A6,[6] and so might theoretically interact with tegafur, but as it has a specialist use in phototherapy it seems unlikely to be used with tegafur. The MAOI **tranylcypromine** is also considered to be a CYP2A6 inhibitor.

(e) Folinic acid

The UK manufacturer of tegafur with gimeracil and oteracil predicts that the toxicity of fluorouracil [the main metabolite of tegafur] might be increased if it is given with folinic acid and advises caution on concurrent use.[1] For discussion of decreased tolerability of **capecitabine** in the presence of folinic acid, see 'Fluorouracil prodrugs; Capecitabine + Folinates', p.683.

(f) Gemcitabine

A pharmacokinetic study in 5 patients with pancreatic cancer, given *S-1* (a combination of tegafur, gimeracil and oteracil potassium) at a dose of 30 mg/m^2 twice daily for 28 days and gemcitabine 800 mg/m on days 1, 15 and 29, found no difference in the pharmacokinetics of fluorouracil (the main metabolite of tegafur) or gemcitabine, when compared with monotherapy.[7] Further research is needed to confirm the clinical relevance of this small study.

(g) Methotrexate

The UK manufacturer of tegafur, gimeracil and oteracil predicts that the inhibition of thymidylate synthase and dihydrofolate reductase by methotrexate might increase the cytotoxicity of fluorouracil [the main metabolite of tegafur], and they advise caution on their concurrent use.[1] For discussion of the interaction between methotrexate and fluorouracil, see 'Methotrexate + Fluorouracil', p.698.

1. Teysuno (Tegafur, gimeracil and oteracil monopotassium). Nordic Pharma Ltd. UK Summary of product characteristics, March 2011.
2. Uftoral (Tegafur and uracil). Merck Serono. UK Summary of product characteristics, April 2011.
3. Komatsu T, Yamazaki H, Shimada N, Nakajima M, Yokoi T. Roles of cytochromes P450 1A2, 2A6, and 2C8 in 5-fluorouracil formation from tegafur, an anticancer prodrug, in human liver microsomes. *Drug Metab Dispos* (2000) 28, 1457–63.
4. Daigo S, Takahashi Y, Fujieda M, Ariyoshi N, Yamazaki H, Koizumi W, Tanabe S, Saigenji K, Nagayama S, Ikeda K, Nishioka Y, Kamataki T. A novel mutant allele of the CYP2A6 gene (CYP2A6*11) found in a cancer patient who showed poor metabolic phenotype towards tegafur. *Pharmacogenetics* (2002) 12, 299–306.
5. Komatsu T, Yamazaki H, Shimada N, Nagayama S, Kawaguchi Y, Nakajima M, Yokoi T. Involvement of microsomal cytochrome P450 and cytosolic thymidine phosphorylase in 5-fluorouracil formation from tegafur in human liver. *Clin Cancer Res* (2001) 7, 675–81.
6. Kharasch ED, Hankins DC, Taraday JK. Single-dose methoxsalen effects on human cytochrome P-450 2A6 activity. *Drug Metab Dispos* (2000) 28, 28–33.
7. Nakata B, Amano R, Nakao S, Tamura T, Shinto O, Hirakawa T, Okita Y, Yamada N, Hirakawa K. Plasma pharmacokinetics after combined therapy of gemcitabine and oral S-1 for unresectable pancreatic cancer. *J Exp Clin Cancer Res* (2010) 29, 15.

Fulvestrant + Miscellaneous

Rifampicin (rifampin) and ketoconazole do not alter the pharmacokinetics of fulvestrant, and fulvestrant does not alter the pharmacokinetics of midazolam.

Clinical evidence, mechanism, importance and management

The pharmacokinetics of intravenous fulvestrant were not affected by pretreatment with rifampicin (rifampin) 600 mg daily (a potent, non-specific inducer of CYP3A4), or pretreatment with ketoconazole 400 mg daily (a potent inhibitor of CYP3A4) in studies in healthy men.[1,2] This indicates that fulvestrant dose adjustment is unlikely to be needed in those taking inducers or inhibitors of CYP3A4.[1]

In addition, a low dose of intramuscular fulvestrant (36 mg), did not affect the pharmacokinetics of a single 7.5-mg dose of oral midazolam (a substrate of CYP3A4) given 24 hours later.[1,2] It is therefore unlikely that fulvestrant will alter the metabolism of drugs that are substrates of this isoenzyme.[1]

1. Robertson JFR, Harrison M. Fulvestrant: pharmacokinetics and pharmacology. *Br J Cancer* (2004) 90 (Suppl. 1), S7–S10.
2. Laight A, Yates R, Rose A, Dale A, McCormack P, Clark D, Harrison M. Fulvestrant is unlikely to be involved in clinically significant drug interactions–results of clinical trials in healthy male volunteers. *Proc Am Soc Clin Oncol* (2003) 22, abstract 133.

Gemcitabine + Anthracyclines

The concurrent use of gemcitabine and doxorubicin or epirubicin does not appear to affect the pharmacokinetics of either drug. An *in vitro* study found that the efficacy of the combination of gemcitabine and epirubicin may be schedule-dependent.

Clinical evidence, mechanism, importance and management

(a) Doxorubicin

The pharmacokinetics of gemcitabine did not differ when it was given immediately before doxorubicin, when compared with historical data of its use alone in patients with breast cancer.[1] Similarly the pharmacokinetics of gemcitabine were unchanged when it was given with paclitaxel the day after liposomal doxorubicin, when compared with historical data.[2] Another study also found that when doxorubicin was given immediately before gemcitabine on day one, the pharmacokinetics of gemcitabine were unaltered, when compared with gemcitabine alone on day 8. However, the activation of gemcitabine to its phosphorylated forms in peripheral blood mononuclear cells was reduced by doxorubicin. As the combination was poorly tolerated and no more effective than doxorubicin alone, the authors suggested that this sequence of dosing should not be further investigated in sarcomas.[3]

(b) Epirubicin

Gemcitabine pharmacokinetics were unchanged by the concurrent use of epirubicin and paclitaxel in patients with breast cancer,[4] and gemcitabine did not alter the interaction between epirubicin and paclitaxel (see 'Anthracyclines + Taxanes', p.654).

An *in vitro* study using human bladder cancer cells found that both gemcitabine and epirubicin alone exerted a cytotoxic effect but the efficacy of the combination of epirubicin and gemcitabine depended on the schedule used. When the drugs were given concurrently or if gemcitabine was given before epirubicin, there was an antagonistic interaction. There was synergistic cytotoxic activity when epirubicin was used before gemcitabine. This schedule is being investigated in clinical studies.[5]

1. Pérez-Manga G, Lluch A, Alba E, Moreno-Nogueira JA, Palomero M, García-Conde J, Khayat D, Rivelles N. Gemcitabine in combination with doxorubicin in advanced breast cancer: final results of a phase II pharmacokinetic trial. *J Clin Oncol* (2000) 18, 2545–52.
2. Bozionelou V, Vamvakas L, Pappas P, Agelaki S, Androulakis N, Kalykaki A, Nikolaidou M, Kentepozidis N, Giassas S, Marselos M, Georgoulias V, Mavroudis D. A dose escalation and pharmacokinetic study of biweekly pegylated liposomal doxorubicin, paclitaxel and gemcitabine in patients with advanced solid tumours. *Br J Cancer* (2007) 97, 43–9.
3. López-Pousa A, Losa R, Martín J, Fra J, Sierra M, Casado A, García del Muro J, Poveda A, Balañá C, Martínez-Trufero J, Esteban E, Buesa JM. Phase I/II trial if doxorubicin and fixed dose-rate infusion gemcitabine in advanced soft tissue sarcomas: a GEIS study. *Br J Cancer* (2006) 94, 1797–1802.
4. Conte PF, Gennari A, Donati S, Salvadori B, Baldini E, Bengala C, Pazzagli I, Orlandini C, Danesi R, Fogli S, Del Tacca M. Gemcitabine plus epirubicin plus taxol (GET) in advanced breast cancer: a phase II study. *Breast Cancer Res Treat* (2001) 68, 171–9.
5. Zoli W, Ricotti L, Tesei A, Ulivi P, Campani AG, Fabbri F, Gunelli R, Frassineti GL, Amadori D. Schedule-dependent cytotoxic interaction between epidoxorubicin and gemcitabine in human bladder cancer cells *in vitro*. *Clin Cancer Res* (2004) 10, 1500–1507.

Gemcitabine + Cisplatin and other platinum compounds

The toxicity and pharmacokinetics of gemcitabine combined with platinum drugs such as cisplatin is dependent upon the order in which they are given.

Clinical evidence, mechanism, importance and management

(a) Carboplatin

Gemcitabine 1 g/m^2 on days one, 8, and 15 has been given with carboplatin (maximum tolerated dose, giving an AUC of 5.2 mg/mL per minute) on day one, in a monthly cycle. No difference was detected in toxicity or tolerated dose when the gemcitabine was given before or after the carboplatin.[1] However, subsequent authors reported that this same dose schedule, with carboplatin given immediately after the gemcitabine, caused unexpected and severe thrombocytopenia, and could not be recommended.[2] Nevertheless, in clinical use,[3] it is recommended that carboplatin is given after gemcitabine 1 g/m^2.

(b) Cisplatin

When gemcitabine was given 4 hours before or after cisplatin there were no major differences in the plasma pharmacokinetics of gemcitabine, deaminated gemcitabine and platinum. Similarly, cisplatin given 24 hours before gemcitabine did not significantly change gemcitabine and deaminated gemcitabine levels, although there was a trend towards an increased AUC of gemcitabine triphosphate.[4] Gemcitabine given 24 hours before cisplatin decreased the platinum AUC twofold,[4] and caused the least leucopenia of the schedules.[5] Anaemia, thrombocytopenia, nausea and vomiting, and fatigue were not sequence dependent.[5] On the basis of these findings, the authors further evaluated the schedule of cisplatin given 24 hours before gemcitabine but found no clear evidence for the best sequence of these drugs.[6] Note that the combination of cisplatin and gemcitabine is commonly used for the treatment of various cancers, usually with cisplatin given after gemcitabine on the same day.[3]

(c) Oxaliplatin

The pharmacokinetics of gemcitabine 800 to 1500 mg/m^2 and its main metabolite did not appear to be affected by oxaliplatin 70 to 100 mg/m^2 when oxaliplatin was given immediately after gemcitabine once every 2 weeks.[7] Similarly, in a study in 10 patients with advanced solid tumours,[8] the pharmacokinetics of gemcitabine did not differ when it was given immediately before oxaliplatin on day one and when it was given alone on day 8. Furthermore, in a study in which 10 patients received either gemcitabine followed 24 hours later by oxaliplatin, or the two drugs in the reverse order, the sequence of administration had no effect on the pharmacokinetics of either gemcitabine or oxaliplatin.[9]

1. Langer CJ, Claver P, Ozols RF. Gemcitabine and carboplatin in combination: phase I and phase II studies. *Semin Oncol* (1998) 25 (Suppl 9), 51–4.
2. Ng EW, Sandler AB, Robinson L, Einhorn LH. A phase II study of carboplatin plus gemcitabine in advanced non-small-cell lung cancer (NSCLC): a Hoosier Oncology Group study. *Am J Clin Oncol* (1999) 22, 550–3.
3. Gemzar (Gemcitabine). Eli Lilly and Company. US Prescribing information, May 2007.
4. van Moorsel CJ, Kroep JR, Pinedo HM, Veerman G, Voorn DA, Postmus PE, Vermorken JB, van Groeningen CJ, van der Vijgh WJ, Peters GJ. Pharmacokinetic schedule finding study of the combination of gemcitabine and cisplatin in patients with solid tumors. *Ann Oncol* (1999) 10, 441–8.
5. Kroep JR, Peters GJ, van Moorsel CJA, Catik A, Vermorken JB, Pinedo HM, van Groeningen CJ. Gemcitabine-cisplatin: a schedule finding study. *Ann Oncol* (1999) 10, 1503–10.
6. Kroep JR, Pinedo HM, Giaccone G, Van Bochove A, Peters GJ, Van Groeningen CJ. Phase II study of cisplatin preceding gemcitabine in patients with advanced oesophageal cancer. *Ann Oncol* (2004) 15, 230–5.
7. Faivre S, Le Chevalier T, Monnerat C, Lokiec F, Novello S, Taieb J, Pautier P, Lhommé C, Ruffié P, Kayitalire L, Armand J-P, Raymond E. Phase I-II and pharmacokinetic study of gemcitabine combined with oxaliplatin in patients with advanced non-small-cell lung cancer and ovarian carcinoma. *Ann Oncol* (2002) 13, 1479–89.
8. Pappas P, Mavroudis D, Nikolaidou M, Georgoulias V, Marselos M. Coadministration of oxaliplatin does not influence the pharmacokinetics of gemcitabine. *Anticancer Drugs* (2006) 17, 1185–91.
9. Airoldi M, Cattel L, Passera R, Pedani F, Delprino L, Micari C. Gemcitabine and oxaliplatin in patients with metastatic breast cancer resistant to or pretreated with both anthracyclines and taxanes. *Am J Clin Oncol* (2006) 29, 490–4.

Gemcitabine + Taxanes

One study found that giving paclitaxel before gemcitabine increased gemcitabine levels, but other studies did not find a pharmacokinetic interaction. Gemcitabine distribution may be altered by docetaxel, but docetaxel pharmacokinetics are not affected by gemcitabine. The clinical response to the combination of gemcitabine and a taxane may depend on the sequence of administration.

Clinical evidence, mechanism, importance and management

(a) Docetaxel

In a study of gemcitabine and docetaxel, given on days one and 8 of a 21-day cycle, drug toxicity and pharmacokinetics were unaffected by the relative order of their administration.[1] However, in another study, it appeared that while docetaxel pharmacokinetics were unaffected, the distribution of gemcitabine was altered by docetaxel, although there was no clear relationship between this and toxicity.[2]

A favourable response rate of 43% was reported in a study in which 35 patients with sarcomas were given gemcitabine 675 mg/m^2 over 90 minutes on days one and 8, followed by docetaxel 100 mg/m^2, given over 60 minutes, on day 8. The possible synergistic antitumour effect may have been secondary to both the prolonged gemcitabine infusion and the sequence of drug administration.[3] More study is needed.

(b) Paclitaxel

A study in 18 patients with non small cell lung cancer found that when they were given gemcitabine 1000 mg/m^2 on days one and 8 and paclitaxel 150 to 200 mg/m^2 on day one as a 3-hour infusion immediately before the gemcitabine, the plasma levels of gemcitabine and the AUC of its deaminated metabolite were unchanged, as was the AUC of paclitaxel. However, paclitaxel increased gemcitabine triphosphate levels, potentially improving efficacy.[4] In a study in 14 patients with non small cell lung cancer, gemcitabine 800 mg/m^2 was given on days one and 8 of a 21-day cycle and paclitaxel 110 mg/m^2 was given 3 hours before the second dose of gemcitabine on day 8. When paclitaxel was given first the clearance, volume of distribution and interpatient pharmacokinetic variability of gemcitabine were decreased. Plasma levels of gemcitabine were increased by 25%, but there was no correlation between these changes and toxicity, and the clinical significance of the interaction is uncertain.[5] In another study, no pharmacokinetic interactions were detected between gemcitabine and paclitaxel given weekly, although gemcitabine showed saturation kinetics at higher doses.[6,7] Another study in patients with advanced breast cancer given gemcitabine, epirubicin and paclitaxel also found no pharmacokinetic interaction between gemcitabine and paclitaxel:[8] a similar lack of pharmacokinetic interaction was found in a further study in patients receiving liposomal doxorubicin, gemcitabine and paclitaxel.[9]

The high overall response rate of 71% in a phase II study[10] in patients with advanced breast cancer given gemcitabine and paclitaxel, prompted an *in vitro* study,[11] which found that giving paclitaxel followed by gemcitabine resulted in synergistic cytotoxic activity, whereas gemcitabine followed by paclitaxel had antagonistic activity. Phase III studies are being carried out to further evaluate the effects of order of administration of these drugs in patients with metastatic breast cancer.[12] As of 2009, paclitaxel is given before gemcitabine, with both drugs given on the same day.[13,14]

1. Bhargava P, Marshall JL, Fried K, Williams M, Lefebvre P, Dahut W, Hanfelt J, Gehan E, Figuera M, Hawkins MJ, Rizvi NA. Phase I and pharmacokinetic study of two sequences of gemcitabine and docetaxel administered weekly to patients with advanced cancer. *Cancer Chemother Pharmacol* (2001) 48, 95–103.
2. Dumez H, Louwerens M, Pawinsky A, Planting AST, de Jonge MJA, Van Oosterom AT, Highley M, Guetens G, Mantel M, De Boeck G, de Bruijn E, Verweij J. The impact of drug administration sequence and pharmacokinetic interaction in a phase I study of the combination of docetaxel and gemcitabine in patients with advanced solid tumors. *Anticancer Drugs* (2002) 13, 583–93.
3. Leu KM, Ostruszka LJ, Shewach D, Zalupski M, Sondak V, Biermann JS, Lee JS-J, Couwlier C, Palazzolo K, Baker LH. Laboratory and clinical evidence of synergistic cytotoxicity of sequential treatment with gemcitabine followed by docetaxel in the treatment of sarcoma. *J Clin Oncol* (2004) 22, 1706–12.
4. Kroep JR, Giaccone G, Voorn DA, Smit EF, Beijnen JH, Rosing H, van Moorsel CJA, van Groeningen CJ, Postmus PE, Pinedo HM, Peters GJ. Gemcitabine and paclitaxel: pharmacokinetic and pharmacodynamic interactions in patients with non-small-cell lung cancer. *J Clin Oncol* (1999) 17, 2190–7.
5. Shord SS, Faucette SR, Gillenwater HH, Pescatore SL, Hawke RL, Socinski MA, Lindley C. Gemcitabine pharmacokinetics and interaction with paclitaxel in patients with advanced non-small-cell lung cancer. *Cancer Chemother Pharmacol* (2003) 51, 328–36.
6. De Pas T, de Braud F, Danesi R, Sessa C, Catania C, Curigliano G, Fogli S, del Tacca M, Zampino G, Sbanotto A, Rocca A, Cinieri S, Marrocco E, Milani A, Goldhirsch A. Phase I and pharmacologic study of weekly gemcitabine and paclitaxel in chemo-naïve patients with advanced non-small-cell lung cancer. *Ann Oncol* (2000) 11, 821–7.
7. Fogli S, Danesi R, De Braud F, De Pas T, Curigliano G, Giovannetti G, Del Tacca M. Drug distribution and pharmacokinetic/pharmacodynamic relationship of paclitaxel and gemcitabine in patients with non-small-cell lung cancer. *Ann Oncol* (2001) 12, 1553–9.
8. Fogli S, Danesi R, Gennari A, Donati S, Conte PF, Del Tacca M. Gemcitabine, epirubicin and paclitaxel: pharmacokinetic and pharmacodynamic interactions in advanced breast cancer. *Ann Oncol* (2002) 13, 919–27.
9. Bozionelou V, Vamvakas L, Pappas P, Agelaki S, Androulakis N, Kalykaki A, Nikolaidou M, Kentepozidis N, Giassas S, Marselos M, Georgoulias V, Mavroudis D. A dose escalation and pharmacokinetic study of biweekly pegylated liposomal doxorubicin, paclitaxel and gemcitabine in patients with advanced solid tumours. *Br J Cancer* (2007) 97, 43–9.
10. Colomer R, Llombart-Cussac A, Lluch A, Barnadas A, Ojeda B, Carañana V, Fernández Y, García-Conde J, Alonso S, Montero S, Hornedo J, Guillem V. Biweekly paclitaxel plus gemcitabine in advanced breast cancer: phase II trial and predictive value of HER2 extracellular domain. *Ann Oncol* (2004) 15, 201–206.
11. Oliveras C, Vázquez-Martin A, Ferrer L, de Llorens R, Colomer R. Gemcitabine plus paclitaxel, is there a better schedule for treatment? *Breast Cancer Res Treat* (2004) 88 (Suppl 1) S205.
12. Colomer R. What is the best schedule for administration of gemcitabine-taxane? *Cancer Treat Rev* (2005) 31 (Suppl 4) S23–S28.
13. Gemzar (Gemcitabine). Eli Lilly and Company. US Prescribing information, May 2007.
14. Gemzar (Gemcitabine). Eli Lilly and Co Ltd. UK Summary of product characteristics, February 2009.

Hydroxycarbamide (Hydroxyurea) + Interferon alfa

When hydroxycarbamide is used with interferon alfa, the risk of vasculitis might be increased.

Clinical evidence, mechanism, importance and management

Hydroxycarbamide alone has been associated with cutaneous vasculitic ulceration and gangrene, and interferons alone have also been associated with vasculitis. In one review of serious vasculopathic adverse effects associated with interferon alfa in 13 patients, 5 patients were also taking hydroxycarbamide, 4 of whom had digital ulcerations and gangrene, and one of whom had pulmonary vasculitis. Most cases improved on stopping interferon alfa and adding immunosuppressants. The authors considered that the distribution of the ulcers was different from that seen with hydroxycarbamide alone. They say that whether the use of hydroxycarbamide, concurrently or use at any time, can potentiate these vascular events is a matter of debate.[1] Nevertheless, the manufacturer of hydroxycarbamide notes that the risk of cutaneous vasculitis may be increased when interferon is given with or before hydroxycarbamide,[2,3] and one UK manufacturer of interferon alfa also includes a similar warning.[4] Bear this possibility in mind. Hydroxycarbamide should be stopped if cutaneous vasculitic ulcers occur.[2,3]

1. Al-Zahrani H, Gupta V, Minden MD, Messner HA, Lipton JH. Vascular events associated with alpha interferon therapy. *Leuk Lymphoma* (2003) 44, 471–5.
2. Hydrea (Hydroxycarbamide). E. R. Squibb & Sons Ltd. UK Summary of product characteristics, December 2005.
3. Hydrea (Hydroxyurea). Bristol-Myers Squibb Company. US Prescribing information, December 2006.
4. Schering-Plough Ltd. UK Summary of product characteristics, March 2009.

Irinotecan + Antiepileptics

Enzyme-inducing antiepileptics (carbamazepine, phenobarbital, phenytoin) markedly increase the clearance of irinotecan and its active metabolite SN-38.

Limited evidence suggests that some non-enzyme inducing antiepileptics (particularly gabapentin) might be associated with modestly increased irinotecan clearance. One case report with valproate found hepatotoxicity and *decreased* active irinotecan metabolite (SN-38) levels, whereas another study found no appreciable difference in irinotecan pharmacokinetics with valproate.

Clinical evidence

(a) Enzyme-inducing antiepileptics

In a study in adult patients with malignant glioma, the clearance of irinotecan was 60% higher in 18 patients taking enzyme-inducing antiepileptics (**phenytoin**, **carbamazepine**, **phenobarbital**, or combinations) than in 22 patients who were not taking these drugs. The maximum tolerated dose of irinotecan in these patients was double that in those not receiving enzyme-inducing antiepileptics, but there was no relationship between the dose and the AUC of the active metabolite, SN-38.[1] Similarly, in 32 patients given irinotecan infusions for malignant glioma and taking antiepileptics (29 patients were taking **phenytoin**, **carbamazepine** or **phenobarbital**), the AUCs of irinotecan, SN-38, and SN-38 glucuronide were about 40%, 25% and 25% lower, respectively, than in historical controls not taking antiepileptics.[2] In another study, the clearance of irinotecan was about 57% higher in 5 patients taking **carbamazepine** or **phenobarbital** when compared with 2 patients not taking antiepileptics.[3]

In a similar study in paediatric patients, the clearance of irinotecan lactone was 49% higher and the AUC of the lactone forms of irinotecan and SN-38 were 27% and 51% lower, respectively, in 10 children taking enzyme-inducing antiepileptics than in 21 children not taking these antiepileptics.[4] The enzyme-inducing antiepileptics used were **phenytoin** alone in 6 children, **carbamazepine**, **oxcarbazepine** and **phenobarbital** in one child each, and **phenytoin** with **carbamazepine** in one child. In a subsequent study by the same authors, increasing the dose of irinotecan increased the AUC of SN-38 in 3 of 5 children taking stable doses of enzyme-inducing antiepileptics, but no increase was seen in 2 children, despite a three- to fourfold increase in the irinotecan dose.[5]

1. Carbamazepine. In a preliminary report of studies in patients with malignant glioma, the clearance of irinotecan was increased almost twofold in the presence of carbamazepine. The peak plasma levels and AUCs of irinotecan and its active metabolite SN-38 were decreased to a clinically relevant extent.[1]

2. Phenobarbital. In a preliminary report of studies in patients with malignant glioma, the clearance of irinotecan was increased by about 70% in the presence of phenobarbital. The authors state that in the presence of any enzyme inducing antiepileptic (phenytoin, phenobarbital or carbamazepine), the AUC and peak plasma levels of irinotecan and its active metabolite, SN-38, were significantly decreased.[1]

In a phase I study in patients given ciclosporin and irinotecan, giving phenobarbital 90 mg daily for 2 weeks before irinotecan allowed a dose escalation of irinotecan from 75 mg/m^2 to 144 mg/m^2. Phenobarbital increased irinotecan clearance by 27% and reduced the AUC of SN-38 by 75%, when compared with irinotecan pharmacokinetics in patients given irinotecan and ciclosporin. Further clinical studies are needed to assess the effects of phenobarbital on the antitumour response and toxicity of irinotecan.[6]

3. Phenytoin. A 14-year-old girl with glioblastoma was given irinotecan 20 to 60 mg/m^2 daily for 5 days on 2 consecutive weeks every 21 days for 2 cycles. During the first cycle she also received phenytoin 300 mg and dexamethasone 6 mg daily. Irinotecan clearance was 2.5-fold higher compared with that in other patients receiving irinotecan alone, and there was lower exposure to the active metabolite of irinotecan, SN-38. The effect on clearance decreased slowly over 8 days after she stopped taking phenytoin.[7] Another patient taking phenytoin and irinotecan was found to have much lower AUCs for irinotecan and SN-38, when compared with data from patients not taking phenytoin.[8] Similarly, a third patient had a threefold increase in irinotecan clearance and about a 60% reduction in the AUCs of irinotecan and SN-38 after starting phenytoin.[9] In a preliminary report of studies in patients with malignant glioma, the clearance of irinotecan was increased about twofold in the presence of phenytoin. The authors state that in the presence of any enzyme inducing antiepileptic (phenytoin, phenobarbital or carbamazepine), the peak plasma levels and AUCs of irinotecan and SN-38 were decreased to a clinically relevant extent.[1]

(b) Non-enzyme-inducing antiepileptics

A preliminary report of studies in patients with malignant gliomas found that in a small number of patients also taking non-enzyme-inducing antiepileptics (**gabapentin**, **lamotrigine**, **levetiracetam**, **tiagabine**, **topiramate**, **valproate**, or **zonisamide**, mostly in combination) there was a small but statistically significant increase in irinotecan clearance (about 40%) when compared with patients not taking any antiepileptics. The authors stated that this was especially so for **gabapentin**. They also noted that in the 4 patients taking **valproate** (also in combination with other non-enzyme-inducing antiepileptics), there was no difference in irinotecan clearance or the AUC of its active metabolite, SN-38,[1] but see *Valproate*, below.

1. Valproate. In a study in patients with glioblastoma receiving irinotecan, the clearance of irinotecan was about 30% higher (not statistically significant) in 20 patients taking valproate 20 to 30 mg/kg daily compared with 2 patients not taking valproate, and there was no difference in the clearance of the active metabolite, SN-38. Also, there was no difference between irinotecan pharmacokinetics and the incidence of SN-38 related toxicity (neutropenia and diarrhoea) in these 20 patients when compared with data from historical controls.[3] However, a case report describes a patient taking sodium valproate 600 mg who was given an irinotecan 600 mg infusion, and who experienced dose-limiting hepatotoxicity. During a subsequent, uneventful, course, the dose of irinotecan was reduced to 300 mg; and in further courses the valproate was discontinued and the irinotecan dose returned to 600 mg. In this patient, pharmacokinetic analysis found that during valproate treatment the AUC of SN-38, was 42% lower. There were no changes in the pharmacokinetics of the valproate.[10]

Mechanism

Irinotecan (which is inactive) is metabolised to inactive metabolites by the subfamily CYP3A and an active metabolite, SN-38, by carboxylesterases. SN-38 is inactivated by glucuronidation (via UGT1A1) to SN-38G. Enzyme-inducing antiepileptics probably induce both of these routes of metabolism, leading to decreased exposure to the active metabolite.[8,11]

Conversely, *animal* data show that valproate inhibits glucuronidation and therefore is likely to increase the AUC of the active metabolite, SN-38 (and possibly increase toxicity),[11] although no change was reported in two studies, and a decrease was seen in the one case report of this interaction. Species differences and differences in scheduling of doses of valproate might explain this.[3]

Importance and management

The pharmacokinetic interaction between enzyme-inducing antiepileptics and irinotecan is established. The enzyme-inducing antiepileptics induce the metabolism of irinotecan and reduce the exposure to its active metabolite, SN-38. Increasing the dose of irinotecan may not increase the exposure to SN-38. Further study is needed to establish the most appropriate dose of irinotecan to use in patients requiring treatment with these drugs. The manufacturers advise that their use with irinotecan should be avoided,[12,13] and that, where possible, non-enzyme-inducing drugs should be substituted at least 2 weeks before irinotecan is given.[13] This would seem prudent. Note that as **fosphenytoin** is metabolised to phenytoin, and **primidone** is metabolised to phenobarbital, similar advice should probably apply to their use with irinotecan.

With valproate, evidence from clinical studies seems to show that there is no important pharmacokinetic interaction with valproate, although there is one case study of an apparent interaction. Some caution might therefore be appropriate.

The relevance of the apparent greater clearance of irinotecan in patients taking a variety of non-enzyme inducing antiepileptics is unclear, and further study of these potential interactions is needed.

1. Kuhn JG. Influence of anticonvulsants on the metabolism and elimination of irinotecan: A North American Brain Tumor Consortium Preliminary Report. *Oncology* (2002) 16 (Suppl) 33–40.
2. Friedman HS, Petros WP, Friedman AH, Schaaf LJ, Kerby T, Lawyer J, Parry M, Houghton PJ, Lovell S, Rasheed K, Cloughsey T, Stewart ES, Colvin OM, Provenzale JM, McLendon RE, Bigner DD, Cokgor I, Haglund M, Rich J, Ashley D, Malczyn J, Elfring GL, Miller LL. Irinotecan therapy in adults with recurrent or progressive malignant glioma. *J Clin Oncol* (1999) 17, 1516–25.
3. Raymond E, Fabbro M, Boige V, Rixe O, Frenay M, Vassal G, Faivre S, Sicard E, Germa C, Rodier JM, Vernillet L, Armand JP. Multicentre phase II study and pharmacokinetic analysis of irinotecan in chemotherapy-naïve patients with glioblastoma. *Ann Oncol* (2003) 14, 603–14.
4. Crews KR, Stewart CF, Jones-Wallace D, Thompson SJ, Houghton PJ, Heideman RL, Fouladi M, Bowers DC, Chintagumpala MM, Gajjar A. Altered irinotecan pharmacokinetics in pediatric high-grade glioma patients receiving enzyme-inducing anticonvulsant therapy. *Clin Cancer Res* (2002) 8, 2202–9.
5. Gajjar A, Chintagumpala MM, Bowers DC, Jones-Wallace D, Stewart CF, Crews KR. Effect of intrapatient dosage escalation of irinotecan on its pharmacokinetics in pediatric patients who have high grade gliomas and receive enzyme-inducing anticonvulsant therapy. *Cancer* (2003) 97 (Suppl), 2374–80.
6. Innocenti F, Undevia SD, Ramírez J, Mani S, Schilsky RL, Vogelzang NJ, Prado M, Ratain MJ. A phase I trial of pharmacologic modulation of irinotecan with cyclosporine and phenobarbital. *Clin Pharmacol Ther* (2004) 76, 490–502.
7. Radomski KM, Gajjar AJ, Kirstein MN, Ma MK, Wimmer P, Thompson SJ, Houghton PJ, Stewart CF. Irinotecan clearance is increased after concomitant administration of enzyme inducers in a patient with glioblastoma multiforme. *Pharmacotherapy* (2000) 20, 353.
8. Mathijssen RHJ, Sparreboom A, Dumez J, van Oosterom AT, de Bruijn EA. Altered irinotecan metabolism in a patient receiving phenytoin. *Anticancer Drugs* (2002) 13, 139–40.
9. Murry DJ, Cherrick I, Salama V, Berg S, Bernstein M, Kuttesch N, Blaney SM. Influence of phenytoin on the disposition of irinotecan: a case report. *J Pediatr Hematol Oncol* (2002) 24, 130–3.
10. de Jong FA, van der Bol JM, Mathijssen RHJ, Loos WJ, Mathôt RAA, Kitzen JJEM, van den Bent MJ, Verweij J. Irinotecan chemotherapy during valproic acid treatment. Pharmacokinetic interaction and hepatotoxicity. *Cancer Biol Ther* (2007) 6, 1368–74.
11. Gupta E, Wang X, Ramirez J, Ratain MJ. Modulation of the glucuronidation of SN-38, the active metabolite of irinotecan, by valproic acid and phenobarbital. *Cancer Chemother Pharmacol* (1997) 39, 440–4.
12. Campto (Irinotecan hydrochloride trihydrate). Pfizer Ltd. UK Summary of product characteristics, May 2009.
13. Camptosar (Irinotecan hydrochloride). Pfizer Inc. US Prescribing information, June 2010.

Irinotecan + Azoles

Ketoconazole doubles the levels of the active metabolite of irinotecan, SN-38. Other azoles may interact similarly.

Clinical evidence

In a study in 7 patients, ketoconazole 200 mg given one hour before and 23 hours after an infusion of a low dose of irinotecan (100 mg/m^2) decreased the dose-normalised AUC of the inactive metabolite, APC, by 87% and increased the AUC of the active metabolite, SN-38, by 109%, when compared with a standard dose of irinotecan 350 mg/m^2 given alone. There was no difference in degree of myelosuppression between this low dose of irinotecan given with ketoconazole and the 3.5-fold higher dose of irinotecan given alone.[1]

Mechanism

Ketoconazole is a potent inhibitor of CYP3A4, which is involved in the metabolism of irinotecan (itself inactive) to its inactive metabolites, of which APC is one. More irinotecan would therefore be available to be metabolised by carboxylesterases to the active metabolite, SN-38. Ketoconazole had no effect on the subsequent glucuronidation of SN-38 to SN-38G.[1] Other azoles are, to varying degrees, inhibitors of CYP3A4, and would therefore be expected to interact similarly.

Importance and management

The pharmacokinetic interaction between ketoconazole and irinotecan is established, and likely to be clinically important. Excess toxicity (potentially fatal[1]) would be expected if the dose of irinotecan were not markedly reduced on concurrent use. The manufacturers of irinotecan recommend that the concurrent use of ketoconazole should be avoided,[2,3] and the US manufacturer specifies that ketoconazole should be stopped at least one week before starting irinotecan.[3] It is likely that other drugs that are potent inhibitors of CYP3A4, such as **itraconazole** and **voriconazole**, will also affect the metabolism of irinotecan, and the UK manufacturer advises avoiding concurrent use.[2]

1. Kehrer DFS, Mathijssen RHJ, Verweij J, de Bruijn P, Sparreboom A. Modulation of irinotecan metabolism by ketoconazole. *J Clin Oncol* (2002) 20, 3122–9.
2. Campto (Irinotecan hydrochloride trihydrate). Pfizer Ltd. UK Summary of product characteristics, May 2009.
3. Camptosar (Irinotecan hydrochloride). Pfizer Inc. US Prescribing information, June 2010.

Irinotecan + Cannabis

In one study, the pharmacokinetics of irinotecan were not altered by a herbal tea containing cannabis.

Clinical evidence

In a crossover study, 24 patients were given intravenous irinotecan 600 mg before and 12 days after starting a 15-day course of 200 mL daily of a herbal tea containing cannabis 1 g/L. This was prepared from medicinal-grade cannabis (*Cannabis sativa* L. Flos, Bedrocan®) containing Δ^9-tetrahydrocannabinol 18% and cannabidiol 0.8% (both cannabinoids). The clearance and the AUC of irinotecan and its metabolites, SN-38 (the active metabolite) and SN-38G (the inactive glucuronide metabolite of SN-38), were not notably altered by the presence of cannabis.[1]

Mechanism

Irinotecan is partly metabolised by CYP3A4 to inactive metabolites, but this isoenzyme does not appear to be affected by oral cannabis. The formation of the active metabolite, SN-38, via carboxylesterases; and SN-38G (the inactive glucuronide metabolite of SN-38) via UGT1A1 also seems to be unaffected by cannabis.

Importance and management

This study suggests that cannabis taken orally will not affect the pharmacokinetics of irinotecan. No dose adjustments are likely to be needed if irinotecan is given with cannabis tea.

1. Engels FK, de Jong FA, Sparreboom A, Mathot RA, Loos WJ, Kitzen JJEM, de Bruijn P, Verweij J, Mathijssen RHJ. Medicinal cannabis does not influence the clinical pharmacokinetics of irinotecan and docetaxel. *Oncologist* (2007) 12, 291–300.

Irinotecan + Celecoxib

Celecoxib appeared to increase irinotecan clearance in one study and decrease it in another, but these changes are not expected to be clinically relevant.

Clinical evidence, mechanism, importance and management

In a phase I study in patients given docetaxel followed by irinotecan on days one and 8 of a 21-day cycle, the addition of celecoxib 400 mg twice daily, started on day 2, appeared to increase the clearance of irinotecan by 18% and decrease the AUC of its active metabolite, SN-38, by 22% (day one of the first cycle compared with day one of the second cycle). Docetaxel pharmacokinetics were unaffected.[1] Conversely, in a similar study in 4 patients given FOLFIRI (irinotecan, fluorouracil and folinic acid), the addition of continuous celecoxib 400 mg twice daily, started on day 2, appeared to slightly decrease the clearance of irinotecan by 31% and decreased the clearance of SN-38 by 18%.[2] The reason for these changes is unclear. The authors considered that the changes are probably not large enough to be of clinical relevance.[1,2]

1. Argiris A, Kut V, Luong L, Avram MJ. Phase I and pharmacokinetic study of docetaxel, irinotecan, and celecoxib in patients with advanced non-small cell lung cancer. *Invest New Drugs* (2006) 24, 203–12.
2. Javle MM, Cao S, Durrani FA, Pendyala L, Lawrence DD, Smith PF, Creaven PJ, Noel DC, Iyer RV, Rustum YM. Celecoxib and mucosal protection: translation from an animal model to a phase I clinical trial of celecoxib, irinotecan, and 5-fluorouracil. *Clin Cancer Res* (2007) 13, 965–71.

Irinotecan + Ciclosporin

Ciclosporin reduces the clearance of irinotecan and increases the exposure to its active metabolite, SN-38, but also appears to reduce irinotecan-induced gastrointestinal toxicity.

Clinical evidence

In a phase I study in patients with refractory solid tumours or lymphomas, ciclosporin 5 to 10 mg/kg was given as a 6-hour infusion beginning 3 hours before irinotecan (initial dose 25 mg/m² increased to 72 mg/m² weekly). Ciclosporin increased the AUC of the active metabolite of irinotecan, SN-38, by 23 to 630% and reduced irinotecan clearance by 39 to 64%, when compared with historical controls.[1] Similar pharmacokinetic findings have been reported in further phase I and II studies using intravenous or oral ciclosporin; and these studies have generally found a reduction in the irinotecan-induced gastrointestinal toxicity (diarrhoea), when compared with historical controls.[2-4]

Mechanism

The effects of ciclosporin on irinotecan pharmacokinetics may be due to inhibition of irinotecan- and SN-38-related biliary transporters,[1,3] and this suggestion is supported by a study in *rats*.[5] It is suggested that this results in a reduction in the gastrointestinal toxicity of irinotecan.

Importance and management

Ciclosporin clearly alters the pharmacokinetics of irinotecan. In the studies described, ciclosporin was being used to try to improve the toxicity profile of irinotecan without affecting its efficacy, which would be of clinical benefit rather than an adverse drug interaction. However, bear this pharmacokinetic interaction in mind if irinotecan is used in a patient already taking ciclosporin for other reasons: in this situation, the toxicity profile and drug levels might be different from that expected.

1. Innocenti F, Undevia SD, Ramírez J, Mani S, Schilsky RL, Vogelzang NJ, Prado M, Ratain MJ. A phase I trial of pharmacologic modulation of irinotecan with cyclosporine and phenobarbital. *Clin Pharmacol Ther* (2004) 76, 490–502.
2. Desai AA, Kindler HL, Taber D, Agamah E, Mani S, Wade-Oliver K, Ratain MJ, Vokes EE. Modulation of irinotecan with cyclosporine: a phase II trial in advanced colorectal cancer. *Cancer Chemother Pharmacol* (2005) 56, 421–6.
3. Chester JD, Joel SP, Cheeseman SL, Hall GD, Braun MS, Perry J, Davis T, Button CJ, Seymour MT. Phase I and pharmacokinetic study of intravenous irinotecan plus oral ciclosporin in patients with fluorouracil-refractory metastatic colon cancer. *J Clin Oncol* (2003) 21, 1125–32.
4. Vasudev NS, Jagdev S, Anthoney DA, Seymour MT. Intravenous irinotecan plus oral ciclosporin. *Clin Oncol* (2005) 19, 646–9.
5. Gupta E, Safa AR, Wang X, Ratain MJ. Pharmacokinetic modulation of irinotecan and metabolites by cyclosporin A. *Cancer Res* (1996) 56, 1309–14.

Irinotecan + Dexamethasone

In one small study, dexamethasone did not appear to alter the pharmacokinetics of irinotecan or its active metabolite, SN-38.

Clinical evidence, mechanism, importance and management

In a study in paediatric patients with gliomas, there did not appear to be any differences in irinotecan pharmacokinetics (in the AUC of irinotecan and its active metabolite, SN-38, and in the clearance of irinotecan) between 17 patients receiving dexamethasone (1 to 16 mg daily) and 4 patients not receiving dexamethasone. None of these 21 patients were taking enzyme-inducing antiepileptics.[1] Although this study was small and non-randomised, it provides some reassurance that dexamethasone might not have an important effect on irinotecan pharmacokinetics.

1. Crews KR, Stewart CF, Jones-Wallace D, Thompson SJ, Houghton PJ, Heideman RL, Fouladi M, Bowers DC, Chintagumpala MM, Gajjar A. Altered irinotecan pharmacokinetics in pediatric high-grade glioma patients receiving enzyme-inducing anticonvulsant therapy. *Clin Cancer Res* (2002) 8, 2202–9.

Irinotecan + Fluorouracil

Some studies suggest that giving fluorouracil after irinotecan reduces the exposure to SN-38, the active metabolite of irinotecan, whereas others have found no interaction.

Clinical evidence, mechanism, importance and management

A study in 33 patients with metastatic colorectal cancer found that the toxicity and pharmacokinetics of irinotecan given with fluorouracil depended upon the order of administration of the two drugs.[1] When irinotecan was given before fluorouracil, the AUC of the active metabolite of irinotecan, SN-38, was about 40% lower, and toxicity was lower. In this study, patients were randomised to receive a 60-minute infusion of irinotecan (150 mg/m² starting dose, escalated by 50 mg/m² increments) immediately before or after a folinic acid modified 48-hour infusion of fluorouracil 3500 mg/m² in the first cycle, then given in the reverse sequence in the second cycle.

Another study, using historical controls, similarly found that the AUC of SN-38 was about 28% lower and the AUC of irinotecan about 35% higher when irinotecan was given over 90 minutes immediately before a 7-day fluorouracil infusion, compared with irinotecan alone.[2]

In contrast, one study found that fluorouracil did not substantially affect the pharmacokinetics of irinotecan and SN-38. The AUC of irinotecan and SN-38 did not differ between irinotecan alone, irinotecan immediately followed by folinic acid and fluorouracil, and irinotecan immediately after folinic acid and fluorouracil. In this study, irinotecan 100 to 150 mg/m² was given as a 90-minute infusion, and fluorouracil 210 to 500 mg/m² by rapid intravenous injection.[3] Similarly, preliminary reports from another research group found that the clearance of irinotecan did not differ when it was given one day before or one day after 5 daily bolus doses of fluorouracil.[4,5]

From this information it is unclear whether or not fluorouracil alters the pharmacokinetics of irinotecan. A key difference between the main studies is the use of bolus[3] or continuous infusion[1] fluorouracil. The combination is in established clinical usage, where the recommendation is to give irinotecan before fluorouracil and folinic acid.[6,7] This combination has been shown to be more effective than fluorouracil and folinic acid alone.[6,7] Whether this is the optimal schedule remains to be determined.

1. Falcone A, Di Paolo A, Masi G, Allegrini G, Danesi R, Lencioni M, Pfanner E, Comis S, Del Tacca M, Conte P. Sequence effect of irinotecan and fluorouracil treatment on pharmacokinetics and toxicity in chemotherapy-naive metastatic colorectal cancer patients. *J Clin Oncol* (2001) 19, 3456–62.
2. Sasaki Y, Ohtsu A, Shimada Y, Ono K, Saijo N. Simultaneous administration of CPT-11 and fluorouracil: alteration of the pharmacokinetics of CPT-11 and SN-38 in patients with advanced colorectal cancer. *J Natl Cancer Inst* (1994) 86 1096–8.
3. Salz LB, Kanowitz J, Kemeny NE, Schaaf L, Spriggs D, Staton BA, Berkery R, Steger C, Eng M, Dietz A, Locker P, Kelsen DP. Phase I clinical and pharmacokinetic study of irinotecan, fluorouracil, and leucovorin in patients with advanced solid tumors. *J Clin Oncol* (1996) 14, 2959–67.
4. Grossin F, Barbault H, Benhammouda A, Rixe O, Antoine E, Auclerc G, Weil M, Nizri D, Farabos C, Mignard D, Mahjoubi M, Khayat D, Bastian G. A phase I pharmacokinetics study of concomitant CPT-11 and 5FU combination. *Proc Am Assoc Cancer Res* (1996) 37, 168.
5. Benhammouda A, Bastian G, Rixe O, Antoine E, Gozy M, Auclerc G, Grossin F, Nizri D, Gil-Delgado M, Weil M, Bismuth H, Mignard DM, Mahjoubi M, Lenseigne S, Khayat D. A phase I pharmacokinetic study of CPT-11 and 5-FU combination. *Proc Am Soc Clin Oncol* (1997) 16, 202a.
6. Campto (Irinotecan hydrochloride trihydrate). Pfizer Ltd. UK Summary of product characteristics, May 2009.
7. Camptosar (Irinotecan hydrochloride). Pfizer Inc. US Prescribing information, June 2010.

Irinotecan + Fluorouracil prodrugs

The pharmacokinetics of irinotecan and its active metabolite, SN-38, do not appear to be affected by capecitabine. In one small study, tegafur appeared to reduce the exposure to SN-38.

Clinical evidence, mechanism, importance and management

(a) Capecitabine

In a phase I study, irinotecan was given to 12 patients on days one and 8 of a 21-day cycle, alone, and with capecitabine on days one to 14, started immediately after the irinotecan infusion on day one. Capecitabine did not alter the pharmacokinetics of irinotecan or its active metabolite, SN-38 (AUC and maximum levels unchanged). The time to reach maximum plasma levels of SN-38 was increased from 0.88 hours to 1.23 hours, suggesting a slight delay in the conversion of irinotecan to SN-38.[1] In another similar study, capecitabine was started immediately before the irinotecan infusion in one phase and immediately after irinotecan in another phase. There was no difference in irinotecan pharmacokinetics in either phase. In addition, there was no difference in 5-fluorouracil exposure in either phase, although there was a 72% increased AUC of capecitabine, when it was given immediately after irinotecan.[2] In another study, there was no pharmacokinetic interaction when irinotecan was given on day one and capecitabine was started on day two.[3] A further study in 10 patients who received a weekly infusion of irinotecan for 6 weeks, and capecitabine twice daily for 2 weeks, starting the day after the first irinotecan infusion, also indicated that capecitabine might delay the conversion of irinotecan to SN-38, but that there was no appreciable effect on other irinotecan pharmacokinetic parameters.[4]

In yet another study, there was no pharmacokinetic interaction between *oral* irinotecan and capecitabine in patients with solid tumours.[5]

Both irinotecan and capecitabine require activation by carboxylesterases, and it had been suggested that this might result in a pharmacokinetic interaction. The studies cited here suggest that no interaction of clinical relevance occurs.

(b) Tegafur

In a small study in 4 patients, an intravenous dose of irinotecan was given alone and on the last day of a tegafur-containing preparation (*S-1*: a combination of tegafur, gimestat and the potassium salt of oxonic acid in the molar ratio 10:4:10) given orally for 4 to 7 days.[6] The tegafur preparation appeared to reduce the AUC of the active metabolite of irinotecan, SN-38, by 50% without affecting that of irinotecan or SN-38G (the inactive glucuronide metabolite of SN-38). It was suggested that the tegafur might induce the enzyme responsible for the biliary excretion of SN-38. These findings need confirmation, particularly as studies are unclear as to whether or not 5-fluorouracil itself affects irinotecan pharmacokinetics, see 'Irinotecan + Fluorouracil', p.687.

1. Goel S, Desai K, Karri S, Gollamudi R, Chaudhary I, Bulgaru A, Kaubisch A, Goldberg G, Einsetin M, Camacho F, Baker S, Mani S. Pharmacokinetic and safety study of weekly irinotecan and oral capecitabine in patients with advanced solid cancers. *Invest New Drugs* (2007) 25, 237–45.
2. Rea DW, Nortier JW, Ten Bokkel Huinink WW, Falk S, Richel DJ, Maughan T, Groenewegen G, Smit JM, Steven N, Bakker JM, Semiond D, Kerr DJ, Punt CJ. A phase I/II and pharmacokinetic study of irinotecan in combination with capecitabine as first-line therapy for advanced colorectal cancer. *Ann Oncol* (2005)16, 1123–32.
3. Delord JP, Pierga JY, Dieras V, Bertheault-Cvitkovic F, Turpin FL, Lokiec F, Lochon I, Chatelut E, Canal P, Guimbaud R, Mery-Mignard D, Cornen X, Mouri Z, Bugat R. A phase I clinical and pharmacokinetic study of capecitabine (Xeloda) and irinotecan combination therapy (XELIRI) in patients with metastatic gastrointestinal tumours. *Br J Cancer* (2005) 92, 820–6.
4. Czejka M, Schueller J, Hauer K, Ostermann E. Pharmacokinetics and metabolism of irinotecan combined with capecitabine in patients with advanced colorectal cancer. *Anticancer Res* (2005) 25, 2985–90.
5. Soepenberg O, Dumez H, Verweij J, Semiond D, deJonge MJ, Eskens FA, ter Steeg J, Selleslach J, Assadourian S, Sanderink GJ, Sparreboom A, van Oosterom AT. Phase I and pharmacokinetic study of oral irinotecan given once daily for 5 days every 3 weeks in combination with capecitabine in patients with solid tumors. *J Clin Oncol* (2005) 23, 889–98.
6. Yokoo K, Hamada A, Tazoe K, Sasaki Y, Saito H. Effects of oral administration of S-1 on the pharmacokinetics of SN-38, irinotecan active metabolite, in patients with advanced colorectal cancer. *Ther Drug Monit* (2009) 31, 400–3.

Irinotecan + Food

In a study in 25 patients who received an *oral* preparation of irinotecan, formulated as a semi-solid matrix capsule, the pharmacokinetics of irinotecan and its active metabolite, SN-38, did not differ when the oral preparation was taken either with food or after an overnight fast.[1]

1. Soepenberg O, Dumez H, Verweij J, de Jong FA, de Jonge MJA, Thomas J, Eskens FALM, van Schaik RHN, Selleslach J, ter Steeg J, Lefebvre P, Assadourian S, Sanderink G-J, Sparreboom A, van Oosterom AT. Phase I pharmacokinetic, food effect, and pharmacogenetic study of oral irinotecan given as semisolid matrix capsules in patients with solid tumours. *Clin Cancer Res* (2005) 11, 1504–11.

Irinotecan + Gemcitabine

Gemcitabine does not appear to alter the pharmacokinetics of the active metabolite of irinotecan, SN-38.

Clinical evidence, mechanism, importance and management

In a phase I, dose-escalation study, a 24-hour infusion of gemcitabine, given before a 24-hour infusion of irinotecan, appeared to increase the AUC and maximum plasma levels of irinotecan (100 mg/m^2) at higher doses of gemcitabine (100 to 150 mg/m^2) about twofold and by 50%, respectively, although there was high variability in these findings. However, the pharmacokinetics of the active metabolite of irinotecan, SN-38, did not appear to be affected.[1]

1. Saif MW, Sellers S, Li M, Wang W, Cusimano L, Wang H, Zhang R. A phase I study of bi-weekly administration of 24-h gemcitabine followed by 24-h irinotecan in patients with solid tumours. *Cancer Chemother Pharmacol* (2007) 60, 871–82.

Irinotecan + HIV-protease inhibitors

Lopinavir boosted with ritonavir moderately increased the concentrations of the active metabolite of irinotecan, SN-38, in one study. Other HIV-protease inhibitors would be expected to interact similarly.

Clinical evidence

A patient taking antiretrovirals including **lopinavir boosted with ritonavir** 400/135 mg twice daily received irinotecan 150 mg/m^2 alone after a 2-day HIV-protease inhibitor washout then irinotecan at a reduced dose of 75 mg/m^2 with his antiretrovirals. The dose-normalised AUC of the active metabolite of irinotecan, SN-38, was increased by 121%, and the AUC of the inactive metabolite, APC, was reduced by 93%. In this patient, a 50% reduction in the irinotecan dose was necessary for the second cycle because of grade 2 neutropenia, and, because grade 2 neutropenia occurred again during the second cycle, no further irinotecan was given.[1]

Similar pharmacokinetic findings were later reported by the same researchers in 7 patients taking **lopinavir boosted with ritonavir** and irinotecan: this study found a 204% increase in the AUC of SN-38 and an 81% decrease in the AUC of APC. There was also a decrease in the formation of SN-38G (the inactive glucuronide metabolite of SN-38).[2]

Mechanism

It appears that the metabolism of irinotecan to the inactive metabolite APC, by CYP3A4 was inhibited by the HIV-protease inhibitors. Therefore more irinotecan is available to be metabolised by carboxylesterases to the active metabolite, SN-38.[1] In addition, it has been suggested that glucuronyltransferases (UGT1A1), which are involved in the inactivation of SN-38, and inhibited by the HIV-protease inhibitors, might also have contributed to greater SN-38 concentrations; however, note that ritonavir is usually a clinically important *inducer* of UGT1A1 (see 'Combined hormonal contraceptives + HIV-protease inhibitors', p.1177).

Importance and management

Although information is limited, what is known suggests that HIV-protease inhibitors are likely to modestly increase the AUC of the active metabolite of irinotecan, SN-38. However, SN-38 is known to be associated with irinotecan toxicity (e.g. haematological toxicity, diarrhoea), and therefore these changes suggest that an irinotecan dose reduction may be necessary to avoid such effects. Note that the US manufacturer of **atazanavir** contraindicates concurrent use with irinotecan because of this predicted interaction,[3] whereas the UK manufacturer of atazanavir[4] advises close monitoring for irinotecan adverse effects (e.g. haematological toxicity, diarrhoea).

1. Corona G, Vaccher E, Cattarossi G, Sartor I, Toffoli G. Potential hazard of pharmacokinetic interactions between lopinavir-ritonavir protease inhibitors and irinotecan. *AIDS* (2005) 19, 2043–4.
2. Corona G, Vaccher E, Sandron S, Sartor I, Tirelli U, Innocenti F, Toffoli G. Lopinavir-ritonavir dramatically affects the pharmacokinetics of irinotecan in HIV patients with Kaposi's sarcoma. *Clin Pharmacol Ther* (2008) 83, 601–6.
3. Reyataz (Atazanavir sulfate). Bristol-Myers Squibb. US Prescribing information, March 2012.
4. Reyataz (Atazanavir sulfate). Bristol-Myers Squibb Pharmaceuticals Ltd. UK Summary of product characteristics, August 2012.

Irinotecan + Ifosfamide

Ifosfamide appears to markedly reduce the level of the active metabolite of irinotecan, SN-38, when ifosfamide is given daily immediately after irinotecan.

Clinical evidence, mechanism, importance and management

The pharmacokinetics of irinotecan were investigated in 3 paediatric patients who received irinotecan 20 mg/m^2 daily for 5 days, and ifosfamide 2.65 g/m^2 daily immediately after irinotecan on days one to 3. In all 3 patients, the AUC of the active metabolite of irinotecan, SN-38, was markedly lower on day 3 when compared with day one: in 2 patients the plasma levels of SN-38 were below the limit of detection. In two of the patients, the AUC of SN-38 on day 12 was still below that measured on day one. The AUC of an inactive metabolite, APC, was also reduced on day 3, but returned to day one levels by day 12. The study was stopped in view of the low exposure to SN-38.[1]

The reason for this possible interaction is unknown, but it was suggested that ifosfamide might have induced the metabolism of irinotecan.[1]

The authors concluded that the use of daily ifosfamide with daily irinotecan in a protracted regimen such as this should be avoided, because of the marked reduction in the levels of the active metabolite of irinotecan, SN-38. They note that other administration schedules might not cause the same interaction.[1]

1. Crews KR, Stewart CF, Liu T, Rodriguez-Galindo C, Santana VM, Daw NC. Effect of fractionated ifosfamide on the pharmacokinetics of irinotecan in pediatric patients with osteosarcoma. *J Pediatr Hematol Oncol* (2004) 26, 764–7.

Irinotecan + Milk thistle

Milk thistle does not appear to affect the pharmacokinetics of irinotecan.

Clinical evidence, mechanism, importance and management

A pharmacokinetic study was undertaken in 6 patients who were receiving intravenous irinotecan 125 mg/m^2 weekly for 4 weeks, followed by a 2-week rest period. Four days before the second dose of irinotecan, a 14-day course of milk thistle seed extract 200 mg (containing silymarin 80%) three times daily was started. The pharmacokinetics of irinotecan and its metabolites did not differ between week one (no milk thistle), week two (4 days of milk thistle) or week three (12 days of milk thistle).[1] No dose alterations would therefore be expected to be needed if milk thistle (standardised with silymarin 80%) is given with irinotecan.

1. van Erp NPH, Baker SD, Zhao M, Rudek MA, Guchelaar H-J, Nortier JWR, Sparreboom A, Gelderblom H. Effect of milk thistle (*Silybum marianum*) on the pharmacokinetics of irinotecan. *Clin Cancer Res* (2005) 11, 7800–6.

Irinotecan + Miscellaneous

***In vitro* data suggest that vinorelbine and physostigmine might decrease the formation of the active metabolite of irinotecan, SN-38.**

Clinical evidence, mechanism, importance and management

In studies in human liver microsomes, **nifedipine**, **clonazepam**, **methylprednisolone**, and **vinorelbine** had substantial effects on the metabolism of irinotecan. However, only the effect of **vinorelbine** occurred at a concentration considered clinically relevant.[1] Similarly, of various potential carboxylesterase inhibitors, only **physostigmine** was considered sufficiently potent to possibly inhibit irinotecan activation.[2] Further study is needed to assess the clinical relevance of these findings.

1. Charasson V, Haaz M-C, Robert J. Determination of drug interactions occurring with the metabolic pathways of irinotecan. *Drug Metab Dispos* (2002) 30, 731–3.
2. Slatter JG, Su P, Sams JP, Schaaf LJ, Wienkers LC. Bioactivation of the anticancer agent CPT-11 to SN-38 by human hepatic microsomal carboxylesterases and the *in vitro* assessment of potential drug interactions. *Drug Metab Dispos* (1997) 25, 1157–64.

Irinotecan + Omeprazole

The pharmacokinetics of irinotecan are not affected by omeprazole.

Clinical evidence, mechanism, importance and management

In a study in 14 patients given irinotecan 600 mg for two cycles, 3-weeks apart, omeprazole 40 mg daily (started 14 days before the second irinotecan cycle and continued until 3 days after the irinotecan dose) had no effect on the pharmacokinetics of irinotecan or its active metabolite, SN-38.[1] No dose adjustment would appear necessary on concurrent use. Other proton pump inhibitors do not appear to have been studied.

1. van der Bol JM, Loos WJ, de Jong FA, van Meerten E, Konings IRHM, Lam MH, de Bruijn P, Wiemer EAC, Verweij J, Mathijssen RHJ. Effect of omeprazole on the pharmacokinetics and toxicities of irinotecan in cancer patients: a prospective cross-over drug-drug interaction study. *Eur J Cancer* (2011) 47, 831–8.

Irinotecan + Oxaliplatin

An isolated report suggests that the cholinergic toxicity associated with irinotecan may be enhanced by oxaliplatin. There does not appear to be a pharmacokinetic interaction between irinotecan and oxaliplatin.

Clinical evidence, mechanism, importance and management

One of 15 patients given a one-hour infusion of irinotecan 80 mg/m^2 following a 2-hour infusion of oxaliplatin 85 mg/m^2 experienced hypersalivation and abdominal pain, which was successfully treated with atropine. In this patient, symptoms did not recur during subsequent treatment with irinotecan alone, nor when drugs were separated by one day, but rechallenge with the original regimen again produced cholinergic toxicity.[1] Two studies have found that the combination of irinotecan with oxaliplatin does not appear to alter the pharmacokinetics of either drug.[2,3]

The cholinergic effects in the patient may have been due to a pharmacodynamic interaction.[4] It has been suggested that the cholinergic effects of irinotecan, which is a potent inhibitor of acetylcholinesterase,[5] may be enhanced by oxaliplatin, which may, like other alkylating drugs, inhibit acetylcholinesterase.[4]

The clinical relevance of this report is unknown. The combination of irinotecan and oxaliplatin has been extensively evaluated in clinical studies, and this appears to be the only report of cholinergic toxicity. However, it has been noted that the prophylactic use of atropine with irinotecan could mask any increase in cholinergic effects.[4,6]

1. Valencak J, Raderer M, Kornek GV, Henja MH, Scheithauer W. Irinotecan-related cholinergic syndrome induced by coadministration of oxaliplatin. *J Natl Cancer Inst* (1998) 90, 160.
2. Wasserman E, Cuvier C, Lokiec F, Goldwasser F, Kalla S, Méry-Mignard D, Ouldkaci M, Besmaine A, Dupont-André G, Mahjoubi M, Marty M, Misset JL, Cvitkovic E. Combination of oxaliplatin plus irinotecan in patients with gastrointestinal tumors: results of two independent phase I studies with pharmacokinetics. *J Clin Oncol* (1999) 17, 1751–9.
3. Gil-Delgado MA, Bastian G, Guijnet F, Spano JP, Taillibert S, Rocher MA, Castaing D, Adam R, Urien S, Bismuth H, Khayat D. Oxaliplatin plus irinotecan and FU-FOL combination and pharmacokinetic analysis in advanced colorectal cancer patients. *Am J Clin Oncol* (2004) 27, 294–8.
4. Dodds HM, Bishop JF, Rivory LP. More about: irinotecan-related cholinergic syndrome induced by coadministration of oxaliplatin. *J Natl Cancer Inst* (1999) 91, 91–2.
5. Dodds HM, Rivory LP. The mechanism of the inhibition of acetylcholinesterase by irinotecan (CPT-11)–a lead in explaining the cholinergic toxicity of CPT-11 and its time-course. *Proc Am Assoc Cancer Res* (1998) 39, 327.
6. Cvitkovic E, Marty M, Wasserman E, Cuvier C, Goldwasser F, Misset JL. Re: irinotecan-related cholinergic syndrome induced by coadministration of oxaliplatin. *J Natl Cancer Inst* (1998) 90, 1016–17.

Irinotecan + Pemetrexed or Raltitrexed

There do not appear to be any pharmacokinetic interactions between irinotecan and pemetrexed or raltitrexed.

Clinical evidence, mechanism, importance and management

(a) Pemetrexed

In a phase I, dose-finding study in 51 patients with advanced malignancies when irinotecan 175 mg/m^2 to 350 mg/m^2 was given after pemetrexed 300 mg/m^2 to 500 mg/m^2, the pharmacokinetics of these drugs did not differ when compared with historical data for either drug alone.[1] Although less conclusive than a direct comparative study, the information suggests that a marked pharmacokinetic interaction between the drugs is unlikely.

(b) Raltitrexed

In a phase I study in patients with advanced cancer given irinotecan as a 30-minute infusion, and then 30 minutes later, raltitrexed as a 15-minute infusion, the pharmacokinetics of both drugs did not differ when compared with historical data for either drug alone.[2] Similar results were reported in a further study.[3] Although less conclusive than a direct comparative study, the information suggests that a marked pharmacokinetic interaction between the drugs is unlikely. In the second study, the maximum tolerated dose of irinotecan was 25% lower when raltitrexed was given 24 hours after the irinotecan when compared with administration immediately after the irinotecan. This suggests that schedule-dependent synergy occurs.[3]

1. Rowinsky EK, Beeram M, Hammond LA, Schwartz G, De Bono J, Forouzesh B, Chu Q, Latz JE, Hong S, John W, Nguyen B. A phase I and pharmacokinetic study of pemetrexed plus irinotecan in patients with advanced solid malignancies. *Clin Cancer Res* (2007) 13, 532–9.
2. Ford HE, Cunningham D, Ross PJ, Rao S, Aherne GW, Benepal TS, Price T, Massey A, Vernillet L, Gruia G. Phase I study of irinotecan and raltitrexed in patients with advanced gastrointestinal tract adenocarcinoma. *Br J Cancer* (2000) 83, 146–52.
3. Lewis NL, Scher R, Gallo JM, Engstrom PF, Szarka CE, Litwin S, Adams AL, Kilpatrick D, Brady D, Weiner LM, Meropol NJ. Phase I and pharmacokinetic study of irinotecan in combination with raltitrexed. *Cancer Chemother Pharmacol* (2002) 50, 257–65.

Irinotecan + Rifampicin (Rifampin)

A single case report found that rifampicin reduced the formation of the active metabolite of irinotecan, SN-38.

Clinical evidence

A case report describes a 54-year-old man with small cell lung cancer and *Mycobacterium* infection who was uneventfully treated with rifampicin 450 mg daily, isoniazid, streptomycin and pyrazinamide. After 2 weeks of antimycobacterial treatment he was given 4 cycles of irinotecan 75 mg/m^2 on days one and 8, with cisplatin 60 mg/m^2 on day one, and during the first cycle rifampicin was stopped for a 4-day period. There was no difference in the pharmacokinetic profile of irinotecan with or without concurrent rifampicin; however, the AUC of the active metabolite of irinotecan, SN-38, and SN-38G (the inactive glucuronide metabolite of SN-38) were reduced by 20% and 58%, respectively, in the presence of rifampicin.[1]

Mechanism

Irinotecan (itself inactive) is metabolised by CYP3A4 to inactive metabolites, and rifampicin probably induces this pathway of metabolism. This would result in less irinotecan being available for conversion to the active metabolite SN-38.

Importance and management

Evidence for an interaction between irinotecan and rifampicin appears to be limited to one case report and the reduction in the levels of active metabolite of irinotecan, SN-38, in this patient was only modest. However, note that the inductive effects of rifampicin can persist for some time after it is stopped and therefore a 4-day period may not have been sufficient for any effect to have completely reversed. The UK manufacturer of irinotecan notes that the use of irinotecan with potent enzyme-inducers such as rifampicin should be avoided.[2] If concurrent use is unavoidable, it would seem wise to consider the possibility of reduced irinotecan efficacy, and to closely monitor the patient accordingly.

There does not seem to be any information regarding **rifabutin**, but, based on the way rifampicin interacts, similar precautions may be prudent if rifabutin is given to a patient taking irinotecan.

1. Yonemori K, Takeda Y, Toyota E, Kobayashi N, Kudo K. Potential interactions between irinotecan and rifampin in a patient with small-cell lung cancer. *Int J Clin Oncol* (2004) 9, 206–9.
2. Campto (Irinotecan hydrochloride trihydrate). Pfizer Ltd. UK Summary of product characteristics, May 2009.

Irinotecan + Selenium

Selenium, at a dose of 2.2 mg daily, does not appear to alter the pharmacokinetics of irinotecan, nor does it attenuate the toxicity of irinotecan.

Clinical evidence, mechanism, importance and management

In a study in 13 patients with metastatic or unresectable solid tumours **selenomethionine**, at a dose of elemental selenium of 2.2 mg daily, was given with irinotecan weekly, in escalating doses from 125 mg/m^2 to 160 mg/m^2 for 4 weeks of a 6-week cycle (to assess whether the addition of selenium would attenuate irinotecan toxicity and allow higher irinotecan dosing). Irinotecan doses above the previously recommended maximum tolerated dose (125 mg/m^2) were still considered intolerable, with 3 of 4 patients receiving a dose of 160 mg/m^2 developing dose-limiting diarrhoea. There were no notable alterations in the pharmacokinetics of irinotecan, its active metabolite, SN-38, or SN-38G (the inactive glucuronide metabolite of SN-38).[1]

1. Fakih MG, Pendyala L, Smith PF, Creaven PJ, Reid ME, Badmaev V, Azrak RG, Prey JD, Lawrence D, Rustum YM. A phase I and pharmacokinetic study of fixed-dose selenomethionine and irinotecan in solid tumors. *Clin Cancer Res* (2006) 12, 1237–44.

Irinotecan + Sodium bicarbonate

Alkalinisation of the gastrointestinal contents with oral sodium bicarbonate, and the concurrent use of domperidone and magnesium oxide, did not affect the pharmacokinetics of irinotecan or its metabolites in one study, and patients tended to have less diarrhoea.

Clinical evidence, mechanism, importance and management

In a crossover study, 10 patients with colorectal cancer who had not previously been treated with irinotecan were given irinotecan 120 mg/m^2 intravenously every 2 weeks until disease progression occurred. The patients also received sodium bicarbonate 3 g daily, **domperidone** 30 mg daily, **magnesium oxide** up to 3 g daily and at least 1.5 litres of water daily, with either the first or second course of irinotecan. Sodium bicarbonate was given to alkalinise the gastrointestinal contents, domperidone to increase gastrointestinal motility, and magnesium oxide for its laxative effects. The aim was to try to reduce the delayed toxic effect of irinotecan on the bowel that can lead to severe diarrhoea.

The AUC of irinotecan and an inactive glucuronide metabolite, SN-38G, were equivalent between the two groups, and there was no appreciable change in the AUC of the active metabolite of irinotecan, SN-38. The incidence of diarrhoea tended to be lower with alkalinisation treatment (0 of 10 patients) than without (3 of 10 patients), although this was not statistically significant, but there were no differences in the incidence of nausea and vomiting, anorexia and alopecia with or without the additional drug treatment. Concurrent alkalinisation of the gastrointestinal contents is therefore unlikely to alter the efficacy of irinotecan but it might reduce the incidence of delayed diarrhoea.[1]

Note that the current recommended treatment for delayed diarrhoea is prompt treatment with loperamide and fluid and electrolyte replacement.[2,3] The use of drugs with laxative properties [which would include **magnesium oxide**] should be avoided in case they exacerbate the diarrhoea.[3] Although alkalinisation of the gastrointestinal contents is not an accepted form of therapy with irinotecan, this study does show that sodium bicarbonate and **domperidone** do not alter the pharmacokinetics of irinotecan.

1. Tamura T, Yasutake K, Nishisaki H, Nakashima T, Horita K, Hirohata S, Ishii A, Hamano K, Aoyama N, Shirasaka D, Kamigaki T, Kasuga M. Prevention of irinotecan-induced diarrhoea by oral sodium bicarbonate and influence on pharmacokinetics. *Oncology* (2004) 67, 327–37.
2. Campto (Irinotecan hydrochloride trihydrate). Pfizer Ltd. UK Summary of product characteristics, May 2009.
3. Camptosar (Irinotecan hydrochloride). Pfizer Inc. US Prescribing information, June 2010.

Irinotecan + St John's wort (*Hypericum perforatum*)

St John's wort increases the metabolism of irinotecan, which may decrease its efficacy.

Clinical evidence

In a randomised, crossover study, St John's wort decreased the AUC of the active metabolite of irinotecan, SN-38, by 42%, but had no statistically significant effect on the AUC of the inactive metabolite, APC. Myelosuppression was also reduced; with irinotecan alone the leucocyte and neutrophil counts decreased by 56% and 63%, respectively, but in the presence of St John's wort the decreases were only 8.6% and 4.3%, respectively. In this study, irinotecan was given as a single 350-mg/m^2 intravenous dose every 3 weeks, and during one cycle a St John's wort preparation was given three times daily, beginning 14 days before and stopping 4 days after the irinotecan.[1]

Mechanism

St John's wort induces CYP3A4 and P-glycoprotein, which are both involved in the metabolism and transport of irinotecan. The evidence suggests that St John's wort increases the metabolism of irinotecan to an unknown inactive metabolite (other than APC), rather than the active metabolite, SN-38, thereby reducing its effects.[1]

Importance and management

Evidence for an interaction between irinotecan and St John's wort appears to be limited. Irinotecan has a narrow therapeutic range, and as it is a prodrug that is metabolised to its active metabolite, SN-38, the lower levels of SN-38 suggest that its efficacy will be reduced in the presence of St John's wort. It would therefore seem sensible to warn patients who are about to receive irinotecan to avoid St John's wort. Note that the manufacturers state that the use of St John's wort with irinotecan should be avoided,[2,3] and that St John's wort should be stopped at least 2 weeks before irinotecan is given.[3] It seems likely that **topotecan**, a related drug that is also a substrate for CYP3A4, will be similarly affected by St John's wort, but evidence for this is lacking.

1. Mathijssen RHJ, Verweij J, de Bruijn P, Loos WJ, Sparreboom A. Effects of St John's wort on irinotecan metabolism. *J Natl Cancer Inst* (2002) 94, 1247–9.
2. Campto (Irinotecan hydrochloride trihydrate). Pfizer Ltd. UK Summary of product characteristics, May 2009.
3. Camptosar (Irinotecan hydrochloride). Pfizer Inc. US Prescribing information, June 2010.

Irinotecan + Taxanes

In two studies paclitaxel appeared to slightly increase the exposure to irinotecan and its active metabolite, SN-38, whether it was given before the irinotecan or after, but not all studies have found this. There does not appear to be any pharmacokinetic interaction between irinotecan and docetaxel.

Clinical evidence, mechanism, importance and management

(a) Docetaxel

In phase I studies in patients with advanced malignancies given intravenous docetaxel with irinotecan, the pharmacokinetics of these drugs did not differ when compared with historical data for both drugs given alone, irrespective of whether the irinotecan was given first,[1] or the docetaxel was given first.[2] Similarly, in another study, there was no obvious pharmacokinetic interaction when irinotecan was given on days one, 8 and 15, with docetaxel on day two.[3] Although less conclusive than direct comparative studies, the information suggests that a marked pharmacokinetic interaction between the drugs is unlikely.

(b) Paclitaxel

In a pharmacokinetic study in patients, irinotecan was given as a 90-minute infusion immediately followed by paclitaxel 75 mg/m^2, once weekly for 4 weeks of a 6-week cycle, then for the subsequent cycles the sequence of drug administration was reversed. There was no difference in the pharmacokinetics of irinotecan or its active metabolite, SN-38, between the two sequences (11 patients were evaluated in cycle 1 and 6 in cycle 2), and irinotecan pharmacokinetics were similar to historical data for irinotecan alone.[4] However, in another similar study, the AUC of irinotecan tended to be higher (by about 28%) when paclitaxel 40 to 60 mg/m^2 was given before irinotecan than the reverse sequence, although just 3 patients were evaluated and the difference was not statistically significant.[5]

In another dose-finding study in patients, paclitaxel 120 to 210 mg/m^2 (given as an infusion ending 2 hours before starting irinotecan) slightly increased the AUC of irinotecan by about 10% when compared with irinotecan alone. The AUC of SN-38 was also increased at higher paclitaxel doses.[6] In yet another study in 31 patients, the AUC of irinotecan and SN-38 were 32% and 40% higher, respectively, when a 3-hour infusion of paclitaxel 135 to 200 mg/m^2 was started 90 minutes after the end of a 90-minute infusion of irinotecan when compared with irinotecan alone. The pharmacokinetics of paclitaxel were not different from historical data.[7]

It is unclear why paclitaxel might alter irinotecan levels. The pharmacokinetic findings from these studies are variable, and it is difficult to compare the studies because of differences in administration schedules and doses, and there appears to be no clear pattern in the findings. Bear in mind the possibility that paclitaxel might alter the pharmacokinetics of irinotecan whether it is given before[6] or after the irinotecan[7] when compared with irinotecan alone.

1. Adjei AA, Klein CE, Kastrissios H, Goldberg RM, Alberts SR, Pitot HC, Sloan JA, Reid JM, Hanson LJ, Atherton P, Rubin J, Erlichman C. Phase I and pharmacokinetic study of irinotecan and docetaxel in patients with advanced solid tumors: preliminary evidence of clinical activity. *J Clin Oncol* (2000) 18, 1116–23.
2. Couteau C, Risse ML, Ducreux M, Lefresne-Soulas F, Riva A, Lebecq A, Ruffié P, Rougier P, Lokiec F, Bruno R, Armand JP. Phase I and pharmacokinetic study of docetaxel and irinotecan in patients with advanced solid tumors. *J Clin Oncol* (2000) 18, 3545–52.
3. Masuda N, Negoro S, Kudoh S, Sugiura T, Nakagawa K, Saka H, Takada M, Niitani H, Fukuoka M. Phase I and pharmacologic study of docetaxel and irinotecan in advanced non-small-cell lung cancer. *J Clin Oncol* (2000) 18, 2996–3003.
4. Murren JR, Peccerillo K, DiStasio SA, Li X, Leffert JJ, Pizzorno G, Burtness BA, McKeon A, Cheng Y. Dose escalation and pharmacokinetic study of irinotecan in combination with paclitaxel in patients with advanced cancer. *Cancer Chemother Pharmacol* (2000) 46, 43–50.
5. Hotta K, Ueoka H, Kiura K, Tabata M, Kuyama S, Satoh K, Kozuki T, Hisamoto A, Hosokawa S, Fujiwara K, Tanimoto M. A phase I study and pharmacokinetics of irinotecan (CPT-11) and paclitaxel in patients with advanced non-small cell lung cancer. *Lung Cancer* (2004) 45, 77–84.
6. Kasai T, Oka M, Soda H, Tsurutani J, Fukuda M, Nakamura Y, Kawabata S, Nakatomi K, Nagashima S, Takatani H, Fukuda M, Kinoshita A, Kohno S. Phase I and pharmacokinetic study of paclitaxel and irinotecan for patients with advanced non-small cell lung cancer. *Eur J Cancer* (2002) 38, 1871–8.
7. Asai G, Yamamoto N, Kurata T, Tamura K, Uejima H, Nakagawa K, Fukuoka. Phase I and pharmacokinetic study of combination chemotherapy using irinotecan and paclitaxel in patients with lung cancer. *J Thorac Oncol* (2006) 1, 226–30.

Irinotecan + Temozolomide

Temozolomide does not appear to alter the pharmacokinetics of irinotecan or its active metabolite, SN-38. Irinotecan does not alter the pharmacokinetics of temozolomide.

Clinical evidence, mechanism, importance and management

In a study in paediatric patients, there was no change in the pharmacokinetics of irinotecan, its active metabolite SN-38, or temozolomide when oral temozolomide 100 mg/m^2 daily was given one hour before irinotecan 10 or 15 mg/m^2 daily, both for 5 days.[1] Similarly, in 6 patients also taking enzyme-inducing antiepileptic drugs, the pharmacokinetics of irinotecan and its active metabolite, SN-38, were not affected by temozolomide, when compared with historical data from patients taking irinotecan and enzyme-inducing antiepileptic drugs.[2] For details of the interaction of irinotecan with enzyme-inducing antiepileptic drugs see 'Irinotecan + Antiepileptics', p.685.

1. Wagner LM, Crews KR, Iacono LC, Houghton PJ, Fuller CE, McCarville MB, Goldsby RE, Albritton K, Stewart CF, Santana VM. Phase I trial of temozolomide and protracted irinotecan in pediatric patients with refractory solid tumors. *Clin Cancer Res* (2004) 10, 840–8.

2. Loghin ME, Prados MD, Wen P, Junck L, Lieberman F, Fine H, Fink KL, Metha M, Kuhn J, Lamborn K, Chang SM, Cloughesy T, DeAngelis LM, Robins IH, Aldape KD, Yung WK. Phase I study of temozolomide and irinotecan for recurrent malignant gliomas in patients receiving enzyme-inducing antiepileptic drugs: a North American brain tumor consortium study. *Clin Cancer Res* (2007) 13, 7133–8.

Irinotecan + Thalidomide

Thalidomide slightly increased the exposure to irinotecan and slightly decreased the exposure to its active metabolite, SN-38, in one study. In contrast, in another study, thalidomide had no effect on SN-38 exposure.

Clinical evidence, mechanism, importance and management

Patients with solid tumours given irinotecan 350 mg/m^2 on day one of a 3-week cycle were also given thalidomide 400 mg daily from days one to 14 of the first cycle. In the 16 evaluable patients, thalidomide slightly increased the AUC of irinotecan by 21% (not statistically significant), decreased the AUC of its active metabolite, SN-38, by 26%, and increased the AUC of SN-38G (the inactive glucuronide metabolite of SN-38) by 28%. There was no difference in the toxicities seen when irinotecan was given with or without thalidomide.[1] In another study, patients were given intravenous irinotecan 125 mg/m^2 on days one and 8 of a 21-day cycle with oral thalidomide 200 mg or 400 mg given daily from day 3, at least one hour before the irinotecan. There was no change in the AUC of SN-38, in 17 evaluable patients, although the maximum plasma levels of irinotecan and SN-38 were reduced by about 12%.[2] These changes are slight, and unlikely to be clinically relevant.

1. Allegrini G, Di Paolo A, Cerri E, Cupini S, Amatori F, Masi G, Danesi R, Marcucci L, Bocci G, Del Tacca M, Falcone A. Irinotecan in combination with thalidomide in patients with advanced solid tumors: a clinical study with pharmacodynamic and pharmacokinetic evaluation. *Cancer Chemother Pharmacol* (2006) 58, 585–93.
2. Villalona-Calero M, Schaaf L, Phillips G, Otterson G, Panico K, Duan W, Kleiber B, Shah M, Young D, Wu W-H, Kuhn J. Thalidomide and celecoxib as potential modulators of irinotecan's activity in cancer patients. *Cancer Chemother Pharmacol* (2007) 59, 23–33.

Irinotecan + Tobacco

Retrospective data suggests that tobacco smoking might increase the clearance of irinotecan and reduce the levels of its active metabolite, SN-38; as well as reducing its toxicity, and presumably therefore, its efficacy.

Clinical evidence

In a retrospective analysis, the pharmacokinetics of irinotecan were compared between 49 patients who were smokers and 141 patients who were non-smokers, who had all received intravenous irinotecan 175 to 350 mg/m^2 (or a fixed dose of 600 mg) once every 3 weeks. The clearance of irinotecan was 18% faster in the group of patients who smoked, and these patients had a 40% lower AUC of the active metabolite of irinotecan, SN-38, and also had more extensive conversion of SN-38, to SN-38G (the inactive glucuronide metabolite of SN-38). Smokers experienced less haematological toxicity than non-smokers (grade 3 to 4 neutropenia 6% versus 38%), possibly as a result of the increased rate of clearance.[1]

Mechanism

Uncertain. One suggestion is that smoking might induce glucuronyltransferases, which are responsible for glucuronidation of the active metabolite, SN-38.[1]

Importance and management

The findings of this retrospective analysis suggest that smoking might reduce the efficacy of irinotecan. However, the evidence is insufficient to make recommendations regarding smoking cessation or an increased irinotecan dose.[1] Further study is required.

1. van der Bol JM, Mathijssen RHJ, Loos WJ, Friberg LE, van Schaik RHN, de Jonge MJA, Planting AST, Verweij J, Sparreboom A, de Jong FA. Cigarette smoking and irinotecan treatment: pharmacokinetic interaction and effects on neutropenia. *J Clin Oncol* (2007) 25, 2719–26.

Irinotecan + Tyrosine kinase inhibitors

In phase I studies, the concurrent use of irinotecan with imatinib, erlotinib, gefitinib, lapatinib, or sunitinib resulted in dose-limiting toxicities at low doses of irinotecan. In pharmacokinetic studies, imatinib, gefitinib, lapatinib, regorafenib, and sorafenib increased the exposure to irinotecan and/or its active metabolite, SN-38: nilotinib, pazopanib, and ponatinib are predicted to interact with irinotecan similarly. In addition, irinotecan increases gefitinib and sorafenib exposure.

Clinical evidence

(a) Erlotinib

In a phase I study, the combination of erlotinib and FOLFIRI (irinotecan, folinic acid, and fluorouracil) was poorly tolerated at the lowest dose, and the study was halted. However, erlotinib did not appear to alter the pharmacokinetics of irinotecan or its active metabolite, SN-38, and irinotecan did not appear to alter erlotinib pharmacokinetics.[1]

(b) Gefitinib

In a phase I study, the addition of irinotecan to gefitinib increased gefitinib exposure by about 50%, but no change was seen in irinotecan pharmacokinetics. Dose-limiting toxicities of neutropenia and diarrhoea occurred at an unexpectedly low dose of irinotecan.[2] Similarly, in another phase I study, gefitinib did not appear to alter the pharmacokinetics of irinotecan, but the combination was associated with similar dose-limiting toxicities.[3] Another earlier study also found the combination of FOLFIRI (irinotecan, folinic acid, and fluorouracil) with gefitinib to be associated with excessive toxicity.[4] In a study in paediatric patients,[5] gefitinib appeared to increase the bioavailability of *oral* irinotecan 4-fold, and decreased clearance of both irinotecan and its active metabolite, SN-38.

(c) Imatinib

In a phase I study, imatinib 300 mg daily for 20 days increased the exposure to a single intravenous dose of irinotecan by 67% and decreased its clearance by 36% when compared with irinotecan without imatinib. There was an unexpected high frequency of neutropenia and diarrhoea, which precluded a planned imatinib dose escalation.[6]

(d) Lapatinib

The pharmacokinetics of lapatinib 1.25 g daily were unaffected when it was given with FOLFIRI (irinotecan, folinic acid, and fluorouracil). In addition, there was no change in the pharmacokinetics of irinotecan. However, there was a 41% increase in the AUC of the active metabolite of irinotecan, SN-38, and a 32% increase in its maximum concentration. In this study, toxicity necessitated dose reductions rather than the planned dose escalations, and the optimally tolerated regimen was found to be FOLFIRI at 60% of the standard doses.[7]

(e) Regorafenib

In a phase I study, regorafenib 160 mg daily for 7 days was given 4 days after FOLFIRI (irinotecan, folinic acid, and fluorouracil) in the second cycle of treatment. The AUC of irinotecan and its active metabolite, SN-38 were 28% and 44% higher, respectively, after regorafenib was added but the maximum concentrations were unaffected.[8]

(f) Sorafenib

In a phase I dose-escalation study, sorafenib 100 mg, 200 mg, or 400 mg twice daily was given continuously from day 4 of the first cycle with an intravenous infusion of irinotecan 125 mg/m^2 weekly for 4 out of 6 weeks.[9,10] The pharmacokinetics of irinotecan and its active metabolite, SN-38, were not affected by sorafenib at the two lower doses (100 mg and 200 mg twice daily). In addition, sorafenib pharmacokinetics at these dose levels were not affected by irinotecan.[9,10] However, the maximum plasma concentration of sorafenib was increased by 78% and its AUC was increased by 68% in the patients who received the highest dose of sorafenib (400 mg twice daily) with irinotecan 125 mg/m^2, but this was not seen with a lower fixed dose of irinotecan 140 mg. At both doses of irinotecan, the patients who had received the highest dose of sorafenib experienced a 26 to 42% increase in the AUC of irinotecan, and a 67 to 120% increase in the AUC of SN-38.[10]

(g) Sunitinib

In a phase I dose-finding study in patients with solid tumours, there were no apparent changes in the pharmacokinetics of sunitinib (dose corrected to maximum tolerated dose, 25 mg daily on days 1 to 14) or irinotecan (250 mg/m^2 on day 1 as part of FOLFIRI: irinotecan, folinic acid and fluorouracil).[11] In another similar study in patients with metastatic colorectal cancer, there was also no apparent pharmacokinetic interaction between sunitinib (given as 37.5 or 50 mg daily for 4 weeks of each 6 week cycle, or as 25 or 37.5 mg daily, continuously) or irinotecan (180 mg/m^2 on day 1 as part of FOLFIRI).[12] These combinations were associated with dose-limiting toxicities and planned sunitinib dose-escalation (from 37.5 mg daily to 50 mg daily) was not possible;[11,12] in one study dose reductions were necessary (from 37.5 mg daily to 25 mg daily).[11]

Mechanism

In vitro, sorafenib[9] and regorafenib[8] inhibit the glucuronidation of the active metabolite of irinotecan, SN-38, by UGT1A1, which would result in reduced SN-38 metabolism (and hence increased exposure) and increased adverse effects. *In vitro* evidence suggests that erlotinib has the same potential.[13] Gefitinib does not appear to affect UGT1A1 and lapatinib does not appreciably inhibit UGT *in vitro*,[14] which suggests that other mechanisms (such as the drug transporter, breast cancer resistance protein, BCRP[2]), might be involved in these interactions.

Importance and management

The pharmacokinetic interaction of some tyrosine kinase inhibitors (**gefitinib, imatinib, lapatinib, sorafenib**) with irinotecan would appear to be established, and a number of studies have shown increased toxicity for the combinations. Irinotecan also increases gefitinib and sorafenib concentrations. Caution is required on concurrent use of any of these tyrosine kinase inhibitors with irinotecan, with consideration given to starting at lower doses. It would also seem prudent to monitor closely for evidence of toxicity.

Although no pharmacokinetic interaction was apparent with irinotecan and **erlotinib**, or **sunitinib** in phase I studies, the poor tolerability of these combinations suggests a similar interaction is occurring, and caution would be appropriate on concurrent use.

Direct information with other tyrosine kinase inhibitors is lacking. Until more is known, caution would also be appropriate with **nilotinib**[15] and **pazopanib**,[16] which have been shown to inhibit UGT1A1 *in vitro*, and also **ponatinib** which has been shown to inhibit BCRP *in vitro*, although the US manufacturer notes that the effects of concurrent use with substrates of BCRP, such as irinotecan, have not been evaluated.[17] The UK manufacturer of **crizotinib** states that its effects on UGT1A1 are not established and advises caution with substrates such as irinotecan.[18] **Axitinib** does not inhibit UGT1A1 *in vitro*,[19,20] and so would not be expected to affect the pharmacokinetics of irinotecan by this mechanism, but this requires confirmation. **Ruxolitinib** does not inhibit BCRP *in vitro*,[21] but the UK manufacturer notes that it might inhibit BCRP in the intestine.[22] Further study is required to determine whether it has any effect on the pharmacokinetics of irinotecan.

1. Messersmith WA, Laheru DA, Senzer NN, Donehower RC, Grouleff P, Rogers T, Kelley SK, Ramies DA, Lum BL, Hidalgo M. Phase I trial of irinotecan, infusional 5-fluorouracil, and leucovorin (FOLFIRI) with erlotinib (OSI-774): early termination due to increased toxicities. *Clin Cancer Res* (2004) 10, 6522–7.
2. Chau I, Cunningham D, Hickish T, Massey A, Higgins L, Osborne R, Botwood N, Swaisland A. Gefitinib and irinotecan in patients with fluoropyrimidine-refractory, irinotecan-naive advanced colorectal cancer: a phase I-II study. *Ann Oncol* (2007) 18, 730–7.
3. Meyerhardt JA, Clark JW, Supko JG, Eder JP, Ogino S, Stewart CF, D'Amato F, Dancey J, Enzinger PC, Zhu AX, Ryan DP, Earle CC, Mayer RJ, Michelini A, Kinsella K, Fuchs CS. Phase I study of gefitinib, irinotecan, 5-fluorouracil and leucovorin in patients with metastatic colorectal cancer. *Cancer Chemother Pharmacol* (2007) 661–70.
4. Veronese ML, Sun W, Giantonio B, Berlin J, Shults J, Davis L, Haller DG, O'Dwyer PJ. A phase II trial of gefitinib with 5-fluorouracil, leucovorin, and irinotecan in patients with colorectal cancer. *Br J Cancer* (2005) 92, 1846–9.
5. Furman WL, Navid F, Daw NC, McCarville MB, McGregor LM, Spunt SL, Rodriguez-Galindo C, Panetta JC, Crews KR, Wu J, Gajjar AJ, Houghton PJ, Santana VM, Stewart CF. Tyrosine kinase inhibitor enhances the bioavailability of oral irinotecan in pediatric patients with refractory solid tumors. *J Clin Oncol* (2009) 27, 4599–604.
6. Johnson FM, Krug LM, Tran HT, Shoaf S, Prieto VG, Tamboli P, Peeples B, Patel J, Glisson BS. Phase I studies of imatinib mesylate combined with cisplatin and irinotecan in patients with small cell lung carcinoma. *Cancer* (2006) 106, 366–74.
7. Midgley RS, Kerr DJ, Flaherty KT, Stevenson JP, Pratap SE, Koch KM, Smith DA, Versola M, Fleming RA, Ward C, O'Dwyer PJ, Middleton MR. A phase I and pharmacokinetic study of lapatinib in combination with infusional 5-fluorouracil, leucovorin and irinotecan. *Ann Oncol* (2007) 18, 2025–9.
8. Schultheis B, Folprecht G, Kuhlmann, Ehrenberg R, Hacker UT, Köhne CH, Kornacker M, Boix O, Lettieri J, Krauss J, Fischer R, Hamann S, Strumberg D, Mross KB. Regorafenib in combination with FLOFOX or FOLFIRI as first- or second-line treatment of colorectal cancer: results of a multicenter, phase Ib study. *Ann Oncol* (2013) 24, 1560–7.
9. Mross K, Steinbild S, Baas F, Reil M, Buss P, Mersmann S, Voliotis D, Schwartz B, Brendel E. Drug-drug interaction pharmacokinetic study with the Raf kinase inhibitor (RKI) BAY 43-9006 administered in combination with irinotecan (CPT-11) in patients with solid tumors. *Int J Clin Pharmacol Ther* (2003) 41, 618–19.
10. Mross K, Steinbild S, Baas F, Gmehling D, Radtke M, Voliotis D, Brendel E, Christensen O, Unger C. Results from an *in vitro* and a clinical/pharmacological phase I study with the combination irinotecan and sorafenib. *Eur J Cancer* (2007) 43, 55–63.
11. Boven E, Massard C, Armand JP, Tillier C, Hartog V, Brega NM, Countouriotis AM, Ruiz-Garcia A, Soria JC. A phase I, dose-finding study of sunitinib in combination with irinotecan in patients with advanced solid tumours. *Br J Cancer* (2010) 103, 993–1000.
12. Starling N, Vázquez-Mazón F, Cunningham D, Chau I, Tabernero J, Ramos FJ, Iveson TJ, Saunders MP, Aranda E, Countouriotis AM, Ruiz-Garcia A, Wei G, Tursi JM, Guillen-Ponce C, Carrato A. A phase I study of sunitinib in combination with FOLFIRI in patients with untreated metastatic colorectal cancer. *Ann Oncol* (2012) 23, 119–27.
13. Liu Y, Ramírez J, House L, Ratain MJ. The UGT1A1 *28 polymorphism correlates with erlotinib's effect on SN-38 glucuronidation. *Eur J Cancer* (2010) Epub.
14. Tyverb (Lapatinib ditosylate monohydrate). GlaxoSmithKline UK. UK Summary of product characteristics, March 2014.
15. Fujita K, Sugiyama M, Akiyama Y, Ando Y, Sasaki Y. The small-molecule tyrosine kinase inhibitor nilotinib is a potent noncompetitive inhibitor of the SN-38 glucuronidation by human UGT1A1. *Cancer Chemother Pharmacol* (2011) 67, 237–41.
16. Votrient (Pazopanib hydrochloride). GlaxoSmithKline. US Prescribing information, November 2013.
17. Iclusig (Ponatinib). ARIAD Pharmaceuticals, Inc. US Prescribing information, January 2014.
18. Xalkori (Crizotinib). Pfizer Ltd. UK Summary of product characteristics, April 2013.
19. Inlyta (Axitinib). Pfizer Ltd. UK Summary of product characteristics, May 2015.
20. Inlyta (Axitinib). Pfizer Inc. US Prescribing information, September 2013.
21. Jakafi (Ruxolitinib phosphate). Incyte Corporation. US Prescribing information, November 2013.
22. Jakavi (Ruxolitinib phosphate). Novartis Pharmaceuticals UK Ltd. UK Summary of product characteristics, June 2013.

Lenalidomide + Miscellaneous

Lenalidomide may slightly increase digoxin levels. The concurrent use of lenalidomide and epoetins may increase the risk of thromboembolism. No interaction is anticipated when lenalidomide is taken with warfarin.

Clinical evidence, mechanism, importance and management

(a) Digoxin

The maximum level of a single 500-microgram dose of digoxin was very slightly increased by 14% by lenalidomide 10 mg daily, and the AUC of digoxin was unchanged.[1] This increase is not clinically relevant, but, as doses of lenalidomide can be higher than this (up to 25 mg daily), the possibility that higher doses might have a greater clinically relevant effect cannot be entirely excluded.[2] Note that lenalidomide is normally given with dexamethasone, consider also 'Digoxin and related drugs + Drugs that lower potassium concentrations', p.1095.

(b) Epoetins

Patients given lenalidomide and dexamethasone for multiple myeloma have an increased risk of deep vein thrombosis and pulmonary embolism. The use of epoetins may further increase this risk and therefore the UK manufacturer advises that these drugs should be used with caution.[2]

(c) Warfarin

Lenalidomide 10 mg daily did not affect the pharmacokinetics of a single dose of warfarin, nor were the pharmacokinetics of lenalidomide affected by a single 25-mg dose of warfarin.[1,2] However, the UK manufacturer mentions that an interaction cannot be excluded in clinical use, because dexamethasone is also given, and the effect of dexamethasone on warfarin is unknown.[2] Consider also 'Coumarins and related drugs + Corticosteroids or Corticotropin', p.419.

1. Revlimid (Lenalidomide). Celgene Corp. US Prescribing information, May 2012.
2. Revlimid (Lenalidomide). Celgene Ltd. UK Summary of product characteristics, March 2015.

Lenalidomide + Statins

Rhabdomyolysis has been reported in patients taking lenalidomide with pravastatin. Other statins might be associated with the same risk.

Clinical evidence, mechanism, importance and management

A case report describes a 49-year-old multiple myeloma patient taking **pravastatin** (dose not stated) for about 4 years, who developed rhabdomyolysis with lenalidomide. She was given lenalidomide as part of a course of chemotherapy, which was then continued as maintenance treatment, initially at a dose of 5 mg daily and then increased to 10 mg daily after 3 months. Eight days after the dose increase the patient complained of muscle soreness and cramping. Her creatine kinase concentration was 1051 units/L, and the pravastatin and lenalidomide were stopped. Over the following few weeks, her creatine kinase concentration slowly decreased and lenalidomide was restarted at 10 mg daily. Her creatine kinase concentration and renal function fluctuated during the next few months, and lenalidomide was stopped and restarted several times before being maintained on 5 mg daily for 6 weeks.[1] A similar case describes rhabdomyolysis in a multiple myeloma patient taking lenalidomide with dexamethasone and **pravastatin**. Symptoms developed 6 days after the lenalidomide and dexamethasone were started, when his creatine kinase concentration was 3445 units/L. The lenalidomide and pravastatin were stopped, and 2 days later the creatine kinase concentration had increased to 16126 units/L. His symptoms resolved 10 days after their initial appearance.[2]

Rhabdomyolysis and myopathy are well-known adverse effects of statin use, and rhabdomyolysis has also been rarely reported with lenalidomide, both alone and with a statin.[3] These cases therefore most likely represent an additive effect of using two drugs causing similar adverse effects, rather than a drug-drug interaction. However, because of the clinical consequences of myopathy or rhabdomyolysis, the UK manufacturer of lenalidomide advises that enhanced clinical and laboratory monitoring is undertaken if **statins** and lenalidomide are given together, particularly during the first weeks of combined use.[3] The advice to report any symptoms suggestive of myopathy and rhabdomyolysis (i.e. otherwise unexplained muscle pain, tenderness, or weakness or dark coloured urine) should be specifically reinforced to patients. Note that routine monitoring of creatine kinase in the absence of clinical signs of myopathy has been reported to be of little clinical value, see *Muscle and liver toxicity*, under 'Lipid regulating drugs', p.1309, for this and for further general guidance on monitoring, and risk factors for muscle toxicity.

1. Shahan JL, Panu LD, Hildebrandt GC. Rhabdomyolysis in a multiple myeloma patient secondary to concurrent treatment with lenalidomide and pravastatin and to lenalidomide alone. *Int J Hematol* (2012) 96, 818–9.
2. Urata C, Yoshimura M, Itamura H, Hisatomi T, Kubota Y, Fukushima N, Sueoka E, Kimura S. Lenalidomide in combination with dexamethasone induced rhabdomyolysis in a multiple myeloma patient treated with pravastatin. *Int J Hematol* (2011) 94, 216–7.
3. Revlimid (Lenalidomide). Celgene Ltd. UK Summary of product characteristics, March 2015.

Melphalan + Cimetidine

Cimetidine modestly reduces the bioavailability of melphalan.

Clinical evidence, mechanism, importance and management

A study in 8 patients with multiple myeloma or monoclonal gammopathy found that pretreatment with cimetidine 1 g daily for 6 days reduced the bioavailability of a 10-mg oral dose of melphalan by 30%. The melphalan half-life was reduced from 1.94 hours to 1.57 hours. The interindividual variation in melphalan pharmacokinetics was high.[1] Note that, because of the variability in melphalan absorption, the dose of oral melphalan is usually cautiously increased until myelosuppression is seen, to ensure therapeutic levels. Therefore, this modest interaction with cimetidine is unlikely to have many clinical consequences.

1. Sviland L, Robinson A, Proctor SJ, Bateman DN. Interaction of cimetidine with oral melphalan. *Cancer Chemother Pharmacol* (1987) 20, 173–5.

Melphalan + Food

The absorption of melphalan can be reduced by food.

Clinical evidence, mechanism, importance and management

A study in 10 patients with multiple myeloma found that the half-life of oral melphalan 5 mg/m^2 was unaffected when it was taken with a standardised breakfast, but its AUC was reduced by 39%. In one patient, no melphalan was detectable in the plasma when it was given with food. In 8 of the patients who had also been given intravenous melphalan at the same dose, the bioavailability of oral melphalan was calculated to be 85% (range 26 to 96%) when fasting and 58% (7 to 99%) when given with food.[1] A similar reduction in absorption was noted in a study in 5 patients who were given melphalan orally with food, compared with doses given while fasting, or intravenously.[2]

The authors of these studies recommend that melphalan should not be taken with food,[1] or that it should be taken first thing in the morning on an empty stomach.[2] However, the manufacturers make no specific recommendations about intake in relation to food.[3,4] They note that absorption after oral administration is highly variable, and that the dose should be adjusted based on frequent monitoring of blood counts.[4]

1. Reece PA, Kotasek D, Morris RG, Dale BM, Sage RE. The effect of food on oral melphalan absorption. *Cancer Chemother Pharmacol* (1986) 16, 194–7.
2. Bosanquet AG, Gilby ED. Comparison of the fed and fasting states on the absorption of melphalan in multiple myeloma. *Cancer Chemother Pharmacol* (1984) 12, 183–6.
3. Alkeran Tablets (Melphalan). GlaxoSmithKline UK. UK Summary of product characteristics, July 2007.
4. Alkeran (Melphalan). GlaxoSmithKline. US Prescribing information, October 2008.

Melphalan + Interferon alfa

Interferon alfa modestly decreases the AUC of melphalan, but melphalan cytotoxicity is possibly increased because of interferon-induced fever.

Clinical evidence, mechanism, importance and management

In 10 myeloma patients, the AUC of melphalan 250 microgram/kg was reduced by 13% when it was given 5 hours after the administration of human interferon alfa (7×10^6 units/m^2), possibly due to fever caused by the interferon.[1] The clinical importance of this is uncertain but the authors of the report suggest that, despite this small reduction in the AUC, the cytotoxicity of the melphalan may be increased by the fever. The use of interferon alfa with melphalan and prednisone in multiple myeloma has been associated with more adverse effects.[2-4]

1. Ehrsson H, Eksborg S, Wallin I, Österborg A, Mellstedt H. Oral melphalan pharmacokinetics: influence of interferon-induced fever. *Clin Pharmacol Ther* (1990) 47, 86–90.
2. Österborg A, Björkholm M, Björeman M, Brenning G, Carlson K, Celsing F, Gahrton G, Grimfors G, Gyllenhammar J, Hast R. Natural interferon-α in combination with melphalan/prednisone versus melphalan/prednisone in the treatment of multiple myeloma stages II and III: a randomized study from the Myeloma Group of Central Sweden. *Blood* (1993) 81, 1428–34.
3. Cooper MR, Dear K, McIntyre OR, Ozer H, Ellerton J, Canellos G, Bernhardt B, Duggan D, Faragher D, Schiffer C. A randomized clinical trial comparing melphalan/prednisone with or without interferon alfa-2b in newly diagnosed patients with multiple myeloma: a Cancer and Leukemia Group B study. *J Clin Oncol* (1993) 11, 155–60.
4. The Nordic Myeloma Study Group. Interferon-α 2b added to melphalan-prednisone for initial and maintenance therapy in multiple myeloma: a randomized, controlled trial. *Ann Intern Med* (1996) 124, 212–22.

Methotrexate + Amiodarone

An isolated case report tentatively attributes the development of methotrexate toxicity to the concurrent use of amiodarone.

Clinical evidence, mechanism, importance and management

An elderly woman, whose psoriasis was effectively controlled for 2 years with methotrexate, developed ulceration of the psoriatic plaques within 2 weeks of starting treatment with amiodarone. The reason for this effect is not understood. A modest increase in her dose of furosemide is a suggested contributory factor because it might have interfered with the excretion of the methotrexate.[1] This appears to be an isolated case, and therefore no general recommendations can be made.

1. Reynolds NJ, Jones SK, Crossley J, Harman RRM. Methotrexate induced skin necrosis: a drug interaction with amiodarone? *BMJ* (1989) 299, 980–1.

Methotrexate + Antibacterials; Aminoglycosides, oral

Limited evidence suggests that the gastrointestinal absorption of methotrexate can be reduced by paromomycin, neomycin and possibly other oral aminoglycosides, but increased by kanamycin.

Clinical evidence

A study in 10 patients with small cell bronchogenic carcinoma taking methotrexate found that when they were also given a range of oral anti-infectives (**paromomycin**, vancomycin, polymyxin B, nystatin) the urinary recovery of methotrexate was reduced by over one-third (from 69% to 44%).[1] The **paromomycin** was believed to have been responsible. In another study the concurrent use of **neomycin** 500 mg four times daily for 3 days reduced the AUC of methotrexate and its 72-hour cumulative excretion by 50%.[2] In contrast, the same report suggests that **kanamycin** can *increase* the absorption of methotrexate, but no details are given.

Mechanism

Oral aminoglycosides reduce the activity of the gut flora, which metabolise methotrexate, so that more is available for absorption. However, paromomycin[3] and neomycin, in common with other oral aminoglycosides, can cause a malabsorption syndrome, which reduces drug absorption and presumably negates any effect altering the gut flora has. Kanamycin may possibly be different because it causes less malabsorption.

Importance and management

The documentation of these interactions is sparse, but it would seem prudent to be on the alert for a reduction in the response to methotrexate if patients are given oral aminoglycosides such as paromomycin or neomycin. An increased response may possibly occur with kanamycin. No interaction would be expected if aminoglycosides are given parenterally.

1. Cohen MH, Creaven PJ, Fossieck BE, Johnston AV, Williams CL. Effect of oral prophylactic broad spectrum nonabsorbable antibiotics on the gastrointestinal absorption of nutrients and methotrexate in small cell bronchogenic carcinoma patients. *Cancer* (1976) 38, 1556–9.
2. Shen DD, Azarnoff D. Clinical pharmacokinetics of methotrexate. *Clin Pharmacokinet* (1978) 3, 1–13.
3. Keusch GT, Troncale FJ, Buchanan RD. Malabsorption due to paromomycin. *Arch Intern Med* (1970) 125, 273–6.

Methotrexate + Antibacterials; Cefotiam

Pancytopenia and pseudomembraneous colitis occurred when a patient taking low-dose methotrexate and loxoprofen was given cefotiam.

Clinical evidence, mechanism, importance and management

An elderly woman who had been taking low-dose methotrexate 5 mg weekly and loxoprofen for one month developed acute pyelonephritis. Intravenous cefotiam was started, and on day 7 she developed severe watery diarrhoea. Analysis showed pancytopenia and *Clostridium difficile* infection. Methotrexate and cefotiam were stopped, and vancomycin started, and the patient recovered.[1] It was suggested that the combination of the antineoplastic drug and the antibacterial increased the risk of *Clostridium difficile* diarrhoea. In addition, the NSAID (see 'Methotrexate + NSAIDs, Aspirin or other Salicylates', p.700) and renal impairment from the pyelonephritis could have contributed to the methotrexate toxicity.[1] This appears to be an isolated case, and any interaction between methotrexate and cefotiam is not established.

1. Nanke Y, Kotake S, Akama H, Tomii M, Kamatani N. Pancytopenia and colitis with *Clostridium difficile* in a rheumatoid arthritis patient taking methotrexate, antibiotics and non-steroidal anti-inflammatory drugs. *Clin Rheumatol* (2001) 20, 73–5.

Methotrexate + Antibacterials; Ciprofloxacin

A report describes two patients who developed methotrexate toxicity when they were given ciprofloxacin.

Clinical evidence

Two patients with osteosarcoma, receiving high-dose methotrexate 12 g/m^2 per course, were given ciprofloxacin 500 mg twice daily, either during or 2 days before the start of the methotrexate course. Methotrexate elimination was delayed, resulting in raised serum levels, severe cutaneous toxicity and renal impairment. The first patient also had hepatic injury and haematological toxicity. Increased folinic acid rescue normalised methotrexate levels after several days. In earlier courses without ciprofloxacin in the first patient and subsequent courses without ciprofloxacin in the second patient, methotrexate elimination was normal.[1] This preliminary report has subsequently been published in full.[2,3]

Mechanism

Not fully understood. Ciprofloxacin may displace methotrexate from its plasma-protein binding sites resulting in a rise in levels of unbound methotrexate. Ciprofloxacin may also cause a decrease in the renal clearance of methotrexate.

Importance and management

Information about an interaction between methotrexate and ciprofloxacin appears to be limited to one report, but it would seem prudent to monitor for raised methotrexate levels if concurrent use is necessary. More study is needed.

1. Dalle JH, Auvrignon A, Vassal G, Leverger G. Possible ciprofloxacin-methotrexate interaction: a report of 2 cases. *Intersci Conf Antimicrob Agents Chemother* (2000) 40, 477.
2. Dalle JH, Auvrignon A, Vassal G, Leverger G, Kalifa C. Interaction méthotrexate–ciprofloxacine: à propos de deux cas d'intoxication sévère. *Arch Pediatr* (2001) 8, 1078–81.
3. Dalle J-H, Auvrignon A, Vassal G, Leverger G. Interaction between methotrexate and ciprofloxacin. *J Pediatr Hematol Oncol* (2002) 24, 321–2.

Methotrexate + Antibacterials; Co-trimoxazole or Trimethoprim

Several cases of severe bone marrow depression (some of which were fatal) have been reported in patients given low-dose methotrexate and trimethoprim or co-trimoxazole (sulfamethoxazole with trimethoprim). Pancytopenia has also been reported in a few patients given co-trimoxazole shortly after stopping methotrexate.

Clinical evidence

A 61-year-old patient with rheumatoid arthritis, taking methotrexate 7.5 mg weekly, developed generalised bone marrow hypoplasia over 2 months after a 10-day course of treatment with co-trimoxazole for a urinary tract infection. She had taken a total of 775 mg of methotrexate when the hypoplasia appeared.[1] Twelve other cases of severe bone marrow depression, four of them fatal,[2-4] have been described in patients taking low-dose weekly methotrexate with co-trimoxazole[2,5-9] or trimethoprim.[3,7,10,11] Life-threatening complications (no details given) are said to have occurred in two other patients taking low-dose methotrexate with unnamed sulfonamides.[12] A 10-year (1981 to 1991) regional survey in Ottawa identified co-trimoxazole as one of four factors associated with serious pancytopenia in patients taking low-dose methotrexate. The other factors were elevated BUN or creatinine levels, increased mean corpuscular volumes and increasing age.[13]

Three cases of severe pancytopenia, one of them fatal, have been reported in patients given treatment dose co-trimoxazole for pneumocystis pneumonia shortly after stopping low-dose methotrexate.[14-16] A fatal case of severe agranulocytosis and toxic epidermal necrolysis occurred in a patient receiving co-trimoxazole for prophylaxis of pneumocystis pneumonia after high-dose methotrexate.[17]

Mechanism

Not fully understood. Both drugs can suppress the activity of dihydrofolate reductase and it seems possible that they can act additively to produce folate deficiency, which could lead to some of the bone marrow changes seen. There may also be a pharmacokinetic mechanism. An early study found that the concurrent use of co-trimoxazole had no effect on the pharmacokinetics of methotrexate in children;[18] however, another study reported that co-trimoxazole caused an increase in 'free' methotrexate from about 37% to 52% while the renal clearance was more than halved.[19] This was calculated to increase the exposure to methotrexate by 66%.[19] Another sulfonamide, **sulfafurazole** (sulfisoxazole),[20] has been found to cause a small reduction in the clearance of methotrexate by the kidneys.

Importance and management

Information seems to be limited to the reports cited but the interactions between methotrexate and co-trimoxazole or trimethoprim are established. Low-dose co-trimoxazole is commonly given without problem to patients taking methotrexate as prophylaxis of pneumocystis pneumonia. This type of patient should be having regular blood monitoring as a matter of course. However, the situation with higher doses of either drug is potentially more hazardous. Some have recommended avoiding the combination. If both drugs must be used, the haematological picture should be very closely monitored because the outcome can be life-threatening.

1. Thomas MH, Gutterman LA. Methotrexate toxicity in a patient receiving trimethoprim-sulfamethoxazole. *J Rheumatol* (1986) 13, 440–1.
2. Groenendal H, Rampen FHJ. Methotrexate and trimethoprim-sulphamethoxazole — a potentially hazardous combination. *Clin Exp Dermatol* (1990) 15, 358–60.
3. Steuer A, Gumpel JM. Methotrexate and trimethoprim: a fatal interaction. *Br J Rheumatol* (1998) 37, 105–6.
4. Bartha P, Bron R, Levy Y. Fatal pancytopenia and methotrexate-trimethoprim-sulfamethoxazole interaction. *Harefuah* (2004) 143, 398–400.
5. Thevenet JP, Ristori JM, Cure H, Mizony MH, Bussiere JL. Pancytopénie au cours due traitement d'une polyarthrite rheumatoïde par méthotrexate après administration de triméthoprime-sulfaméthoxazole. *Presse Med* (1987) 16, 1487.
6. Maricic M, Davis M, Gall EP. Megaloblastic pancytopenia in a patient receiving concurrent methotrexate and trimethoprim-sulphamethoxazole treatment. *Arthritis Rheum* (1986) 29, 133–5.
7. Jeurissen ME, Boerbooms AM, van de Putte LB. Pancytopenia and methotrexate with trimethoprim-sulfamethoxazole. *Ann Intern Med* (1989) 111, 261.
8. Liddle BJ, Marsden JR. Drug interactions with methotrexate. *Br J Dermatol* (1989) 120, 582–3.
9. Govert JA, Patton S, Fine RL. Pancytopenia from using trimethoprim and methotrexate. *Ann Intern Med* (1992) 117, 877–8.
10. Ng HWK, Macfarlane AW, Graham RM, Verbov JL. Near fatal drug interactions with methotrexate given for psoriasis. *BMJ* (1987) 295, 752–3.
11. Saravana S, Lalukotta K. Myelotoxicity due to methotrexate—an iatrogenic cause. *Eur J Haematol* (2003) 71, 315–16.
12. Zachariae H. Methotrexate and non-steroidal anti-inflammatory drugs. *Br J Dermatol* (1992) 126, 95.
13. Al-Awadhi A, Dale P, McKendry RJR. Pancytopenia associated with low dose methotrexate therapy. A regional survey. *J Rheumatol* (1993) 20, 1121–5.
14. Dan M, Shapira I. Possible role of methotrexate in trimethoprim- sulfamethoxazole-induced acute megaloblastic anemia. *Isr J Med Sci* (1984) 20, 262–3.
15. Kobrinsky NL, Ramsay NKC. Acute megaloblastic anemia induced by high-dose trimethoprim-sulfamethoxazole. *Ann Intern Med* (1981) 94, 780–1.
16. Chevrel G, Brantus JF, Sainte-Laudy, Miossec P. Allergic pancytopenia to trimethoprim-sulphamethoxazole for *Pneumocystis carinii* pneumonia following methotrexate treatment for rheumatoid arthritis. *Rheumatology (Oxford)* (1999) 38, 475–6.
17. Yang CH, Yang LJ, Jaing TH, Chan HL. Toxic epidermal necrolysis following combination of methotrexate and trimethoprim-sulfamethoxazole. *Int J Dermatol* (2000) 39, 621–3.
18. Beach BJ, Woods WG, Howell SB. Influence of co-trimoxazole on methotrexate pharmacokinetics in children with acute lymphoblastic leukemia. *Am J Pediatr Hematol Oncol* (1981) 3, 115–19.
19. Ferrazzini G, Klein J, Sulh H, Chung D, Griesbrecht E, Koren G. Interaction between trimethoprim-sulfamethoxazole and methotrexate in children with leukemia. *J Pediatr* (1990) 117, 823–6.
20. Liegler DG, Henderson ES, Hahn MA, Oliverio VT. The effect of organic acids on renal clearance of methotrexate in man. *Clin Pharmacol Ther* (1969) 10, 849–57.

Methotrexate + Antibacterials; Penicillins

Reduced methotrexate clearance and acute methotrexate toxicity has been attributed to the concurrent use of various penicillins (amoxicillin, benzylpenicillin, carbenicillin, dicloxacillin, flucloxacillin, mezlocillin, oxacillin, penicillin, phenoxymethylpenicillin, piperacillin, ticarcillin) in a small number of case reports.

Clinical evidence

Reduced methotrexate clearance and acute methotrexate toxicity has been attributed to the concurrent use of various penicillins in a number of patients. See 'Table 17.2', p.695, for details.

A survey of the Wyeth/Lederle safety database in 1996 identified two additional unpublished cases of methotrexate toxicity (aplastic anaemia, thrombocytopenia, pneumonitis) in patients who had recently started penicillins.[1]

Mechanism

It is thought that weak acids such as the penicillins can possibly successfully compete with methotrexate in the kidney tubules for excretion so that the methotrexate is retained, thereby increasing its effects and its toxicity.[2] However, this was not demonstrated in a study with flucloxacillin,[3] and the mechanism has been disputed.[4]

Importance and management

Information seems to be limited to the reports given here, which would seem to indicate that serious interactions between methotrexate and penicillins are uncommon. It is not known why only a few patients have been affected and what other factors may have contributed, but the problem does not seem to be confined to patients receiving high-dose methotrexate. There is not enough evidence to forbid concurrent use (although some have advised against it[5]), but close monitoring is obviously advisable. One published recommendation is to carry out twice-weekly platelet and white cell counts for 2 weeks initially, with the measurement of methotrexate levels if toxicity is suspected. Folinic acid (leucovorin) rescue should be available.[6]

For the general guidelines given by the CSM in the UK on the use of methotrexate alone, see under *Importance and management* in 'Methotrexate + NSAIDs, Aspirin or other Salicylates', p.700.

1. Wyeth/Lederle. Personal communication, July 1996.
2. Iven H, Brasch H. Influence of the antibiotics piperacillin, doxycycline, and tobramycin on the pharmacokinetics of methotrexate in rabbits. *Cancer Chemother Pharmacol* (1986) 17, 218–22.
3. Herrick AL, Grennan DM, Griffen K, Aarons L, Gifford LA. Lack of interaction between flucloxacillin and methotrexate in patients with rheumatoid arthritis. *Br J Clin Pharmacol* (1996) 41, 223–7.
4. Herrick AL, Grennan DM, Aarons L. Lack of interaction between methotrexate and penicillins. *Rheumatology (Oxford)* (1999) 38, 284–5.
5. Dawson JK, Abernethy VE, Lynch MP. Methotrexate and penicillin interaction. *Br J Rheumatol* (1998) 37, 807.
6. Mayall B, Poggi G, Parkin JD. Neutropenia due to low-dose methotrexate therapy for psoriasis and rheumatoid arthritis may be fatal. *Med J Aust* (1991) 155, 480–4.

Methotrexate + Antibacterials; Pristinamycin

An isolated report describes severe methotrexate toxicity in a patient also given pristinamycin.

Clinical evidence

A 13-year-old boy with acute lymphoblastic leukaemia had a relapse and began a series of regimens with high-dose methotrexate in combination with other drugs, including dexamethasone, mercaptopurine, vincristine, cytarabine and asparaginase, tioguanine and ifosfamide. During a late cycle when he was also taking pristinamycin 2 g daily for a staphylococcal infection, the clearance of methotrexate was markedly decreased (half-life prolonged from 6 hours to 203 hours). He developed severe methotrexate toxicity (oral mucositis, anusitis, balanitis, neutropenia and thrombocytopenia) and was given folinic acid rescue and haemodialysis.[1]

Mechanism

Not understood, but on the basis of experimental evidence the authors of the report excluded the possibilities of renal impairment or reduction of liver metabolism caused by the pristinamycin.[1]

Importance and management

This appears to be the first and only report of an interaction between methotrexate and pristinamycin. Its general importance is unknown but the authors strongly advise the avoidance of pristinamycin in patients taking methotrexate.[1]

1. Thyss A, Milano G, Renée N, Cassuto-Viguier E, Jambou P, Soler C. Severe interaction between methotrexate and a macrolide-like antibiotic. *J Natl Cancer Inst* (1993) 85, 582–3.

Methotrexate + Antibacterials; Tetracyclines

Two case reports describe the development of methotrexate toxicity in patients also given tetracycline or doxycycline.

Clinical evidence, mechanism, importance and management

A man stable taking methotrexate 25 mg weekly for psoriasis was also given **tetracycline** 500 mg four times daily for a mycoplasmal infection. Within 5 days he developed recurrent fever, ulcerative stomatitis and diarrhoea, his white cell count fell to 1000, and his platelet count fell to 30 000 (units not stated, previous counts not given). These are all signs of methotrexate toxicity. The problem resolved when methotrexate was withdrawn, but the psoriasis returned.[1] A 17-year-old girl with osteosarcoma of the femur was given **doxycycline** 100 mg every 12 hours for an abscess in her left eye at the same time as her eleventh cycle of high-dose methotrexate with folinic acid rescue. She had elevated plasma methotrexate levels and she developed haematological toxicity and severe vomiting; requiring antiemetics, continued folinic acid, a prolonged stay in hospital and postponement of her next dose of methotrexate. **Doxycycline** had not been taken during the first 10 cycles of methotrexate and the pharmacokinetic changes and symptoms seen in the eleventh cycle were attributed to the concurrent use of **doxycycline**.[2] It was suggested that displacement of the methotrexate from its binding sites may be part of the explanation for the raised methotrexate levels. There appears to be the only two clinical reports of this interaction on record. Concurrent use need not be avoided, but it should be well monitored.

1. Turck M. Successful psoriasis treatment then sudden 'cytotoxicity'. *Hosp Pract* (1984) 19, 175–6.
2. Tortajada-Ituren JJ, Ordovás-Baines JP, Llopis-Salvia P, Jiménez-Torres NV. High-dose methotrexate-doxycycline interaction. *Ann Pharmacother* (1999) 33, 804–8.

Table 17.2 Reports of reduced methotrexate clearance during penicillin use

Methotrexate	*Penicillin (dose)*	*Indication (number of patients)*	*Outcome*	*Refs*
High-dose intravenous regimen (with folinic acid rescue)				
Infusion of 8 g/m^2 over 6 hours	Amoxicillin (1 g every 6 hours orally)	Osteogenic sarcoma (1)	56% reduction in methotrexate clearance; prolonged and marked enhancement of methotrexate plasma levels; acute and subacute methotrexate toxicity	1
Infusion of 6 g/m^2 (10.8 g) over one hour, then 1.2 g/m^2 per hour for 23 hours	Carbenicillin (30 g daily)	Acute lymphoblastic leukaemia (1)	Elevated plasma methotrexate levels and decreased methotrexate clearance	2
Bolus of 15 to 60 mg/m^2, then 15 to 60 mg/m^2 infusion over 36 hours	Dicloxacillin (not stated) (Indometacin also given)	Oesophageal cancer (1)	93% reduction in methotrexate clearance; prolonged folinic acid rescue necessary	3
Infusion of 12 g/m^2 over 4 hours	Mezlocillin (330 mg/kg daily)	Osteogenic sarcoma (1)	Reduced methotrexate clearance; increased gastrointestinal toxicity	4
Infusion of 15 g over 6 hours	Oxacillin (1 g every 8 hours starting 6 hours after methotrexate infusion)	Osteogenic sarcoma (1)	Plasma methotrexate levels 53-fold higher than in previous cycles without oxacillin; fatal acute toxicity (renal failure and aplastic anaemia)	5
Bolus of 15 to 60 mg/m^2, then 15 to 60 mg/m^2 infusion over 36 hours	Penicillin [sic] (not stated)	Breast cancer (1)	36% reduction in methotrexate clearance; prolonged folinic acid rescue necessary	3
Bolus of 15 to 60 mg/m^2, then 15 to 60 mg/m^2 infusion over 36 hours	Piperacillin (not stated)	Chronic myeloid leukaemia (1)	67% reduction in methotrexate clearance; prolonged folinic acid rescue necessary	3
Infusion of 3 g/m^2 over 6 hours	Piperacillin (1 g every 6 hours intravenously)	Non-Hodgkin's lymphoma (1)	Reduced methotrexate clearance	6
High-dose methotrexate as part of CODOX-M regimen (Cyclophosphamide, Doxorubicin, Vincristine)	Piperacillin/tazobactam (not stated)	Burkitt's lymphoma (1)	Methotrexate clearance reduced by 97%. Plasma methotrexate levels remained at 0.2 micromols/L (reference less than 0.05 micromols/L) for 8 days until piperacillin stopped	7
Bolus of 15 to 60 mg/m^2, then 15 to 60 mg/m^2 infusion over 36 hours	Ticarcillin (not stated)	Acute myeloid leukaemia (1)	60% reduction in methotrexate clearance; prolonged folinic acid rescue necessary	3
Low-dose regimen				
7.5 mg weekly	Amoxicillin 500 mg orally three times daily for 7 days; from day 17, intravenous flucloxacillin 2 g every 4 hours, plus intravenous benzylpenicillin 2 million units every 4 hours	Rheumatoid arthritis	Neutropenia and thrombocytopenia probably as a result of reduced methotrexate clearance; folinic acid given, but patient died	8
10 mg weekly	Amoxicillin (route and dose not stated)	Not given (1)	Severe pancytopenia, sepsis, melaena, mucositis. Treatment also included aspirin and celecoxib. Treated with folinic acid and blood transfusion, but patient died	9
7.5 mg weekly	Co-amoxiclav (amoxicillin and clavulanic acid)	Psoriasis (1)	Neutropenia and thrombocytopenia, probably as a result of reduced methotrexate clearance	8
5 mg weekly	Flucloxacillin (4 g four times daily, intravenously then orally)	Rheumatoid arthritis (1)	Suspected methotrexate-induced pneumonitis	10
5 to 15 mg weekly	Flucloxacillin (500 mg four times daily orally)	Rheumatoid arthritis (10, and 10 not given flucloxacillin)	No significant effect on methotrexate pharmacokinetics	10
2.5 mg three times each week	Flucloxacillin (1 g every 6 hours intravenously) plus piperacillin (2 g every 6 hours intravenously)	Psoriasis (1)	Neutropenia and thrombocytopenia, probably as a result of reduced methotrexate clearance; folinic acid given, but patient died	8
5 mg twice weekly	Piperacillin (intravenous; dose not stated)	Psoriasis (1)	Neutropenia and thrombocytopenia, probably as a result of reduced methotrexate clearance; folinic acid given, but patient died	8

Continued

Table 17.2 Reports of reduced methotrexate clearance during penicillin use (continued)

Methotrexate	*Penicillin (dose)*	*Indication (number of patients)*	*Outcome*	*Refs*
Other regimen				
Intravenous 50 mg weekly	Phenoxymethylpenicillin 250 mg on alternate days	Dermatomyositis (also treated with prednisone; and prostatic cancer treated with diethylstilbestrol (stilboestrol); also receiving furosemide)	Methotrexate toxicity within a week of starting phenoxymethylpenicillin; treated with folinic acid and fluid replacement (and nafcillin and tobramycin)	11

1. Ronchera CL, Hernández T, Peris JE, Torres F, Granero L, Jiménez NV, Plá JM. Pharmacokinetic interaction between high-dose methotrexate and amoxycillin. *Ther Drug Monit* (1993) 15, 375–9.
2. Gibson DL, Bleyer AW, Savitch JL. Carbenicillin potentiation of methotrexate plasma concentration during high dose methotrexate therapy. American Society of Hospital Pharmacists. Mid year clinical meeting abstracts, New Orleans, Dec 1981. p. 111.
3. Bloom EJ, Ignoffo RJ, Reis CA, Cadman E. Delayed clearance (CL) of methotrexate (MTX) associated with antibiotics and anti-inflammatory agents. *Clin Res* (1986) 34, 560A.
4. Dean R, Nachman J, Lorenzana AN. Possible methotrexate-mezlocillin interaction. *Am J Pediatr Hematol Oncol* (1992) 14, 88–9.
5. Titier K, Lagrange F, Péhourcq F, Moore N, Molimard M. Pharmacokinetic interaction between high-dose methotrexate and oxacillin. *Ther Drug Monit* (2002) 24, 570–2.
6. Yamamoto K, Sawada Y, Matsushita U, Moriwaki K, Bessho F, Iga T. Delayed elimination of methotrexate associated with piperacillin administration. *Ann Pharmacother* (1997) 31, 1261–2.
7. Zarychanski R, Wlodarczyk K, Ariano R, Bow E. Pharmacokinetic interaction between methotrexate and piperacillin/tazobactam resulting in prolonged toxic concentrations of methotrexate. *J Antimicrob Chemother* (2006) 58, 228–30.
8. Mayall B, Poggi G, Parkin JD. Neutropenia due to low-dose methotrexate therapy for psoriasis and rheumatoid arthritis may be fatal. *Med J Aust* (1991) 155, 480–4.
9. Lim AYN, Gaffney K, Scott DGI. Methotrexate-induced pancytopenia: serious and under-reported? Our experience of 25 cases in 5 years. *Rheumatology* (2005) 44, 1051–5.
10. Herrick AL, Grennan DM, Griffen K, Aarons L, Gifford LA. Lack of interaction between flucloxacillin and methotrexate in patients with rheumatoid arthritis. *Br J Clin Pharmacol* (1996) 41, 223–7.
11. Nierenberg DW, Mamelok RD. Toxic reaction to methotrexate in a patient receiving penicillin and furosemide: a possible interaction. *Arch Dermatol* (1983) 119, 449–50.

Methotrexate + Antibacterials; Vancomycin

Delayed methotrexate excretion and toxicity were seen when high-dose methotrexate was given to two patients recently treated with vancomycin. No significant interaction was found in eight other patients.

Clinical evidence, mechanism, importance and management

Two patients treated with a chemotherapy regimen containing high-dose methotrexate, cisplatin, doxorubicin and ifosfamide had delayed methotrexate excretion and methotrexate toxicity during a cycle soon after they had received vancomycin. Methotrexate levels took 170 to 231 hours to fall to 200 micromol/mL, and toxicity (mucositis) occurred. Subclinical renal impairment was found, which subsequently improved. In previous and subsequent cycles, where vancomycin was not given, serum methotrexate levels in both patients fell to 200 micromol/mL within 48 to 96 hours.[1] It was suggested that vancomycin caused subclinical nephrotoxicity, which resulted in delayed excretion of methotrexate, which is primarily renally excreted.[1] However, in another report of 8 patients who had received high-dose methotrexate following the use of vancomycin (all but one within 10 days) for previous neutropenia, there was no significant interaction in the absence of overt renal impairment. It was suggested that the difference in outcome may be due to slightly lower methotrexate doses and the fact that the drug regimen in the 8 patients did not include ifosfamide which, particularly in combination with cisplatin, may cause cumulative renal tubular damage.[2]

Vancomycin is commonly used in oncology patients with febrile neutropenia, and this appears to be the first report of this interaction. The authors of this report[1] suggest that it would be prudent to measure glomerular filtration rate with an EDTA renal scan before giving high-dose methotrexate to patients recently treated with vancomycin, to allow modification of the methotrexate dose if necessary.[1] However, the authors of the second report disagree and suggest such monitoring cannot be supported by their findings.[2] Further study is needed.

1. Blum R, Seymour JF, Toner G. Significant impairment of high-dose methotrexate clearance following vancomycin administration in the absence of overt renal impairment. *Ann Oncol* (2002) 13, 327–30.
2. Shamash J, Joel S, Lundholm L, Millard L, Oliver T. High-dose methotrexate clearance following prior vancomycin administration: no significant interaction in the absence of overt renal impairment. *Ann Oncol* (2003) 14, 169–70.

Methotrexate + Antiepileptics; Enzyme-inducing

Enzyme-inducing antiepileptics appear to increase the clearance of methotrexate given as a 24-hour infusion, and their use is associated with lower efficacy of combination therapy for B-lineage leukaemia.

Clinical evidence, mechanism, importance and management

In a retrospective survey, long-term antiepileptic use (**phenytoin**, **phenobarbital**, **carbamazepine**, or a combination) was associated with worse event-free survival, and greater haematological relapse and CNS relapse in children receiving chemotherapy for B-lineage acute lymphoblastic leukaemia. Faster clearance of high-dose methotrexate given as a 24-hour infusion was found in those receiving these enzyme-inducing antiepileptics; however, the clearance of short 4 to 6-hour methotrexate infusions and weekly low-dose methotrexate did not appear to be affected.[1] Further study is needed.

Note that reduced phenytoin, carbamazepine and valproate levels, but unaltered phenobarbital levels, have been reported in various case reports of patients receiving chemotherapy including methotrexate, see 'Table 14.1', p.563.

1. Relling MV, Pui C-H, Sandlund JT, Rivera GK, Hancock ML, Boyett JM, Schuetz EG, Evans WE. Adverse effect of anticonvulsants on efficacy of chemotherapy for acute lymphoblastic leukaemia. *Lancet* (2000) 356, 285–90.

Methotrexate + Ascorbic acid (Vitamin C)

A study in a single patient found that the urinary excretion of methotrexate was not significantly changed by large amounts of vitamin C.

Clinical evidence, mechanism, importance and management

Vitamin C 1 g three times daily was found to have no effect on the urinary excretion of intravenous methotrexate 45 mg, given to a woman with breast cancer, despite the urine becoming more acidic at pH 5.9 (see also 'Methotrexate + Urinary alkalinisers', p.704). She was also receiving oral cyclophosphamide, propranolol, amitriptyline, perphenazine and prochlorperazine.[1] Although this is an isolated report, it appears that vitamin C is unlikely to affect methotrexate excretion.

1. Sketris IS, Farmer PS, Fraser A. Effect of vitamin C on the excretion of methotrexate. *Cancer Treat Rep* (1984) 68, 446–7.

Methotrexate + Bosentan

Bosentan appeared to reduce the efficacy of oral methotrexate in three patients with scleroderma. One of these patients developed hepatotoxicity when the route of methotrexate administration was changed from oral to subcutaneous.

Clinical evidence

Two cases of reduced response to methotrexate have been reported in patients with systemic scleroderma after starting bosentan. Both patients had arthritis which had been successfully managed with methotrexate 10 mg weekly and low-dose methylprednisolone 8 mg daily. They subsequently developed dyspnoea, due to pulmonary hypertension, and were started on bosentan 62.5 mg twice daily for one month, then 125 mg daily thereafter. Within one month of starting bosentan, their arthritis symptoms worsened and their inflammatory markers (such as erythrocyte sedimentation rate, ESR, and rheumatoid factor) increased. Bosentan was stopped and 4 weeks later their arthritis symptoms improved.[1]

A 45-year old woman with scleroderma who was stable taking bosentan 125 mg twice daily for at least 13 months, was started on oral methotrexate 10 mg weekly, increased to 20 mg weekly after 2 months, for arthropathy. As there was no clinical response to oral methotrexate, it was changed to a subcutaneous injection at a dose of 25 mg weekly. After the third subcutaneous dose, her liver function tests deteriorated and she developed jaundice. Bosentan and methotrexate were stopped and her liver function improved over 4-weeks. Oral methotrexate 20 mg weekly was restarted with an improvement in her arthropathy and no further liver problems.[2]

Mechanism

The authors of both reports suggest that bosentan might possibly have reduced the efficacy of methotrexate by displacing it from its protein-binding sites, resulting in a decrease in its hepatic conversion to the active polyglutamyl derivatives.[1,2] Both methotrexate and bosentan have hepatotoxic effects, and it has been suggested that, in one case, the change in the route of administration of methotrexate might have increased its exposure, increasing the risk of toxicity.[2]

Importance and management

Evidence for an interaction between methotrexate and bosentan is limited to the case reports above, and is not established. Note that doses of methotrexate used for chemotherapy are likely to be much higher than those used in the cases cited above.

Until more is known, it would seem prudent to bear the possibility of an interaction in mind should methotrexate efficacy be reduced or abolished in patients also given bosentan. The case of hepatotoxicity serves to highlight the need for caution when two potentially hepatotoxic drugs are given concurrently.

1. Cozzi F, Ostuni PA, Marotta H, Sfriso P, Favaro M, Todesco S. Bosentan may induce arthritis flare in patients with scleroderma concomitantly treated with methotrexate. *Ann Rheum Dis* (2006) 65, 292–3.
2. Dwyer N, Jones G, Kilpatrick D. Severe hepatotoxicity in a patient on bosentan upon addition of methotrexate: reversible with resumption of methotrexate without bosentan. *J Clin Rheumatol* (2009) 15, 88–9.

Methotrexate + Caffeine

Caffeine may theoretically reduce the efficacy of low-dose methotrexate given for rheumatoid arthritis.

Clinical evidence

A study in 39 patients who had recently started taking methotrexate 7.5 mg weekly found that patients with a self-reported high caffeine intake (more than 180 mg of caffeine daily, 13 patients) had less relief in their symptoms of rheumatoid arthritis, such as swollen joints and joint pain, and smaller reductions from baseline in their erythrocyte sedimentation rate (ESR), a marker for inflammation, than patients with a low caffeine intake (less than 120 mg of caffeine daily, 13 patients).[1] A survey of 91 patients taking methotrexate 5 to 15 mg weekly for rheumatoid arthritis found that patients who were regular coffee drinkers (more than 7 cups a week) had a higher rate of methotrexate discontinuation (due to treatment failure in 80% of cases).[2]

In contrast, an analysis of data in a cohort study in 264 patients taking long-term methotrexate for rheumatoid arthritis found that the consumption of caffeinated beverages did not appear to affect the efficacy of methotrexate for rheumatoid arthritis in either low, moderate or high consumers of caffeinated drinks. The average dose of methotrexate was 16 mg weekly and the average intake of caffeine from caffeinated drinks was 212 mg daily. No difference in inflammatory markers or worsening of rheumatoid arthritis was found between the low-caffeine intake group and the high-caffeine intake group.[3] Similarly, a survey in 64 patients taking methotrexate (mean dose 13 mg weekly) for psoriasis and psoriatic arthritis found no effect on the efficacy or dose requirements of methotrexate between low caffeine intake (less than 120 mg daily) and high caffeine intake (more than 180 mg daily).[4]

Mechanism

It is not known exactly how methotrexate produces its effects in rheumatoid arthritis, but one theory is that it possibly increases the levels of adenosine by blocking a step in purine biosynthesis, leading to accumulation of adenosine, which results in anti-inflammatory effects.[1] Methotrexate also inhibits the enzyme 5-aminoimidazole-4-carboxamide ribonucleotide (AICAR) transformylase, raising levels of AICAR, which in turn increases adenosine levels. It may also contribute to the phosphorylation of adenosine nucleotides creating an accumulation of adenosine in tissues.[1,3] Caffeine is an adenosine receptor antagonist and therefore could reverse the effects of methotrexate.

Importance and management

There is limited information available regarding a potential interaction between caffeine consumption and methotrexate. The cohort study results and one patient survey seem to indicate that caffeine intake is not an issue, even with a high intake, whereas one study and another survey did find reduced efficacy in those with a higher caffeine intake. However, these results, particularly the surveys, were limited by a number of factors, including subjective reporting of caffeine consumption, lack of caffeine blood levels, and uncontrolled ingestion of both drugs. One UK manufacturer of intravenous methotrexate (licenced for rheumatoid arthritis) recommends avoiding the excessive consumption of caffeine-containing drinks.[5] There do not appear to be any case reports or studies indicating treatment failure as a result of high caffeine intake in patients receiving chemotherapy with high-dose methotrexate. More study is needed, but bear in mind that a high caffeine intake may be a factor in a reduced benefit from low-dose methotrexate given for rheumatoid arthritis.

1. Nesher G, Mates M, Zevin S. Effect of caffeine consumption on efficacy of methotrexate in rheumatoid arthritis. *Arthritis Rheum* (2003) 48, 571–2.
2. Silke C, Murphy MS, Buckley T, Busteed S, Molloy MG, Phelan M. The effect of caffeine ingestion on the efficacy of methotrexate. *Rheumatology (Oxford)* (2001) 40, 34.
3. Benito-Garcia E, Heller JE, Chibnik LB, Maher NE, Matthews HM, Bilics JA, Weinblatt ME, Shadick NA. Dietary caffeine intake does not affect methotrexate efficacy in patients with rheumatoid arthritis. *J Rheumatol* (2006) 33, 1275–81.
4. Swanson DL, Barnes SA, Mengden Koon SJ, el-Azhary RA. Caffeine consumption and methotrexate dosing requirement in psoriasis and psoriatic arthritis. *Int J Dermatol* (2007) 46, 157–9.
5. Metoject (Methotrexate). Medac GmbH. UK Summary of product characteristics, November 2008.

Methotrexate + Carbonated beverages; Cola

An isolated report describes increased plasma methotrexate concentrations in a patient who consumed cola drinks.

Clinical evidence

A 56-year old patient with non-Hodgkins lymphoma was given a 30-minute infusion of methotrexate 3 g/m², with dextrose 5% and sodium bicarbonate, as per protocol, to reduce the risk of renal methotrexate precipitation. As his urinary pH was found to be reduced (pH 6.5) prior to methotrexate being given, an additional dose of sodium bicarbonate was administered. Before starting methotrexate the patient's serum creatinine concentration was normal (78 micromols/L); however, 24 hours after methotrexate was given, the patient developed acute renal failure with an increased serum creatinine concentration (167 micromols/L).His plasma methotrexate concentration was increased to 9.92 micromols/L, 48 hours after the methotrexate dose. Urinary pH was found to be intermittently reduced and this was treated with additional infusions of sodium bicarbonate, but on one occasion, it was found to have reduced from 8.5 to 6.5 soon after the patient had consumed 330 mL of a cola drink (*Coca-Cola*). It transpired that the patient had consumed a total of 3 cola drinks since the methotrexate was given, during which time his urinary pH was found to have decreased on several occasions, and his plasma methotrexate concentrations were increased. The patient was asked to stop drinking cola and, by day 12, his plasma methotrexate concentration had returned to an acceptable level (0.1 micromols/L), with renal function returning to normal by day 56. The authors state that the patient had no other risk factors other than reduced urinary pH to explain the increased plasma methotrexate concentration.[1]

Mechanism

Methotrexate can precipitate in the kidneys if the urinary pH is less than 7. Cola beverages have been reported to reduce urinary pH, and so the authors suggest that this could have reduced methotrexate elimination, leading to an increase in the plasma concentration and its adverse effect on renal function.[1]

Importance and management

This appears to be the only report of an interaction between methotrexate and cola beverages. The authors of the report suggest that patients given high-dose methotrexate should abstain from cola beverages for 24 hours before methotrexate is given and until methotrexate has been cleared.[1] However, this is an isolated report, and given the frequency of consumption of cola drinks in the general population, it seems that the risk of an interaction, if it is such, is rare. Until further evidence arises, the possibility of this interaction might be borne in mind in cases of otherwise unexplained raised methotrexate concentrations.

1. Santucci R, Levêque D, Herbrecht R. Cola beverage and delayed elimination of methotrexate. *Br J Clin Pharmacol* (2010) 70, 762.

Methotrexate + Chloroquine and related drugs

Single-dose chloroquine caused a moderate decrease in the AUC of methotrexate in one study, but another study in children found no interaction. Conversely, hydroxychloroquine caused a minor increase in the AUC of methotrexate in one study. Methotrexate does not appear to alter hydroxychloroquine pharmacokinetics.

Clinical evidence, mechanism, importance and management

Eleven patients with rheumatoid arthritis taking methotrexate 15 mg weekly were studied after they took a single dose of methotrexate alone and after they took methotrexate with a single 250-mg dose of **chloroquine**. The chloroquine *reduced* the maximum plasma levels of methotrexate by 20% and its AUC by 28%.[1] In contrast, in a study in patients with juvenile arthritis taking long-term methotrexate 150 micrograms/kg, the addition of **chloroquine** 4 mg/kg had no significant effect on the pharmacokinetics of methotrexate, when compared with similar patients taking methotrexate alone.[2]

In a randomised, crossover study in 10 healthy subjects, **hydroxychloroquine** 200 mg *increased* the AUC of methotrexate 15 mg by 52%, and slightly decreased the maximum methotrexate level by 17%.[3] In a population pharmacokinetic analysis the clearance of **hydroxychloroquine** did not appear to differ between 49 patients also taking methotrexate and 74 patients taking hydroxychloroquine alone.[4]

The reasons for the pharmacokinetic changes seen in some studies are unknown: just why the findings of these studies differ is unclear and their clinical relevance is uncertain. However, the changes seen were small, and the combination of methotrexate and chloroquine (or hydroxychloroquine) is used in the management of rheumatoid arthritis.

1. Seideman P, Albertioni F, Beck O, Eksborg S, Peterson C. Chloroquine reduces the bioavailability of methotrexate in patients with rheumatoid arthritis. A possible mechanism of reduced hepatotoxicity. *Arthritis Rheum* (1994) 37, 830–3.
2. Kimura E, Oga S, Periera RMR. Comparative study of the pharmacokinetics of MTX in juvenile idiopathic arthritis patients receiving long-term MTX monotherapy or MTX plus chloroquine. *J Clin Pharm Ther* (2007) 32, 579–84.
3. Carmichael SJ, Beal J, Day RO, Tett SE. Combination therapy with methotrexate and hydroxychloroquine for rheumatoid arthritis increases exposure to methotrexate. *J Rheumatol* (2002) 29, 2077–83.
4. Carmichael SJ, Charles B, Tett SE. Population pharmacokinetics of hydroxychloroquine in patients with rheumatoid arthritis. *Ther Drug Monit* (2003) 25, 671–81.

Methotrexate + Cisplatin

The risk of methotrexate toxicity appears to be markedly increased by the previous use of cisplatin. Methotrexate may inhibit the clearance of cisplatin.

Clinical evidence, mechanism, importance and management

Six out of 106 patients developed clinical signs of methotrexate toxicity and died 6 to 13 days after receiving standard doses of methotrexate (20 to 50 mg/m²) in the absence of signs of renal impairment, and despite having previously been given methotrexate without serious toxicity. On this occasion all had previously been given cisplatin. Four of the patients were regarded as low-risk (i.e. methotrexate toxicity was not considered likely as they did not have renal or hepatic impairment, and their general condition was good).[1] A study in children and adolescents suggested that those who had received a cumulative dose of cisplatin greater than 360 mg/m^2 had delayed methotrexate clearance and a greater risk of methotrexate toxicity.[2] Similarly, a further report by the same authors, in 14 patients receiving high-dose methotrexate,[3] indicated that previous treatment with one course of cisplatin sharply increased the serum levels of methotrexate, particularly if the cumulative cisplatin dose exceeded 400 mg/m^2.

The picture is not totally clear but it seems possible that the previous use of cisplatin causes kidney damage that may not necessarily be detectable with the usual creatinine clearance tests. The effect is to cause a marked reduction in the clearance of the methotrexate. The serum methotrexate levels of such patients should be closely monitored so that any delay in its clearance is detected early and folinic acid rescue can be given.[2] This appears to prevent serious toxicity.[1-3]

There is also a report that suggests that methotrexate inhibits the renal clearance of cisplatin. The renal clearance of platinum in 4 of 5 patients with non-small-cell lung cancer given cisplatin 50 mg/m^2 and methotrexate 40 mg/m^2 was reduced in the first 6 hours after administration (50% lower in the first 3 hours). Apart from a transient increase in serum urea nitrogen and creatinine in one patient, there was no sign of nephrotoxicity with concurrent use.[4]

1. Haim N, Kedar A, Robinson E. Methotrexate-related deaths in patients previously treated with *cis*-diamminedichloride platinum. *Cancer Chemother Pharmacol* (1984) 13, 223–5.
2. Crom WR, Pratt CB, Green AA, Champion JE, Crom DB, Stewart CF, Evans WE. The effect of prior cisplatin therapy on the pharmacokinetics of high-dose methotrexate. *J Clin Oncol* (1984) 2, 655–61.
3. Crom WR, Teresi ME, Meyer WH, Green AA, Evans WE. The intrapatient effect of cisplatin therapy on the pharmacokinetics of high-dose methotrexate. *Drug Intell Clin Pharm* (1985) 19, 467.
4. Preiss R, Brovtsyn VK, Perevodchikova NI, Bychkov MB, Hüller H, Belova LA, Michailov P. Effect of methotrexate on the pharmacokinetics and renal clearance of cisplatin. *Eur J Clin Pharmacol* (1988) 34, 139–44.

Methotrexate + Colestyramine

The serum levels of methotrexate, given by infusion, were markedly reduced by colestyramine in several patients.

Clinical evidence

An 11-year-old girl with osteosarcoma who developed colitis when given high-dose intravenous methotrexate, was subsequently given colestyramine 2 g every 6 hours from 6 to 48 hours after the methotrexate. Serum methotrexate levels at 24 hours were approximately halved. A marked fall in serum methotrexate levels was seen in another patient similarly treated.[1] Colestyramine also reduced methotrexate levels in cases of toxicity in two other patients.[2,3]

Mechanism

Methotrexate undergoes enterohepatic recirculation, that is to say it is excreted into the gut in the bile and re-absorbed further along the gut. If colestyramine is given orally, it can bind strongly to the methotrexate in the gut, thereby preventing its reabsorption and, as a result, its serum levels fall.[1,4]

Importance and management

The documentation seems to be limited. In the cases cited[1-3] the colestyramine was deliberately used to reduce serum methotrexate levels. However, in some circumstances it might represent an unwanted interaction. As methotrexate is excreted into the gut in the bile, separating the oral doses of colestyramine and methotrexate may not necessarily prevent their coming into contact and interacting together. Monitor concurrent use.

1. Erttmann R, Landbeck G. Effect of oral cholestyramine on the elimination of high-dose methotrexate. *J Cancer Res Clin Oncol* (1985) 110, 48–50.
2. Shinozaki T, Watanabe H, Tomidokoro R, Yamamoto K, Horiuchi R, Takagishi K. Successful rescue by oral cholestyramine of a patient with methotrexate nephrotoxicity: nonrenal excretion of serum methotrexate. *Med Pediatr Oncol* (2000) 34, 226–8.
3. Fernández Megía MJ, Alós Almiñana M, Terol Castera MJ. Manejo de la intoxicación por metotrexato: a propósito de un caso. *Farm Hosp* (2004) 28, 371–4.
4. McAnena OJ, Ridge JA, Daly JM. Alteration of methotrexate metabolism in rats by administration of an elemental liquid diet. II. Reduced toxicity and improved survival using cholestyramine. *Cancer* (1987) 59, 1091–7.

Methotrexate + Corticosteroids

Methotrexate clearance may be modestly reduced by the long-term use of prednisolone, but methotrexate does not alter prednisolone pharmacokinetics. Limited evidence suggests methotrexate may alter prednisone levels. Dexamethasone may increase the acute hepatotoxicity of high-dose methotrexate.

Clinical evidence, mechanism, importance and management

There is some evidence to suggest that **prednisolone** may reduce the clearance of methotrexate: patients taking long-term **prednisolone** 15 mg daily had a 20% lower clearance of intramuscular methotrexate 10 mg and a 30% higher AUC than patients given **prednisolone** 15 mg daily for just 4 days before the methotrexate, or those not given corticosteroids.[1] In another study, methotrexate had no effect on **prednisolone** pharmacokinetics in 7 patients, or **methylprednisolone** pharmacokinetics in one patient.[2] The preliminary findings of another study suggested that methotrexate may increase plasma methylprednisolone levels in response to a dose of **prednisone**: in 2 of 4 patients given methotrexate, plasma methylprednisolone levels remained stable despite a decrease in the **prednisone** dose.[3] These findings require confirmation. Their clinical relevance is uncertain.

Dexamethasone may increase the acute hepatotoxicity of high-dose methotrexate. A retrospective comparison in children with brain tumours given methotrexate alone (24 patients), or with **dexamethasone** (33 patients), found that no serious brain oedema occurred in either of the groups and there were no differences in bone marrow toxicity or mucositis, but liver enzymes were significantly higher in the **dexamethasone** group, indicating liver toxicity (AST levels 76 units/L compared with 19 units/L, ALT levels 140 units/L compared with 39 units/L). This effect was not due to differences in serum methotrexate levels.[4] The authors recommend that **dexamethasone** should not be included in high-dose methotrexate protocols for children with brain tumours when they are not glucocorticoid dependent.[4]

1. Lafforgue P, Monjanel-Mouterde S, Durand A, Catalin J, Acquaviva PC. Is there an interaction between low doses of corticosteroids and methotrexate in patients with rheumatoid arthritis? A pharmacokinetic study in 33 patients. *J Rheumatol* (1993) 20, 263–7.
2. Glynn-Barnhart AM, Erzurum SC, Leff JA, Martin RJ, Cochran JE, Cott GR, Szefler SJ. Effect of low-dose methotrexate on the disposition of glucocorticoids and theophylline. *J Allergy Clin Immunol* (1991) 88, 180–6.
3. Sockin SM, Ostro MG, Goldman MA, Bloch KJ. The effect of methotrexate on plasma prednisolone levels in steroid dependent asthmatics. *J Allergy Clin Immunol* (1992) 89, 286.
4. Wolff JEA, Hauch H, Kühl J, Egeler RM, Jürgens H. Dexamethasone increases hepatotoxicity of MTX in children with brain tumours. *Anticancer Res* (1998) 18, 2895–9.

Methotrexate + Diuretics

Some very limited evidence suggests that triamterene may possibly increase the bone marrow suppressive effects of methotrexate. It seems doubtful if thiazides interact adversely with methotrexate.

Clinical evidence, mechanism, importance and management

A 57-year-old woman who had been treated for several years with daily doses of diclofenac 150 mg, atenolol 50 mg and **triamterene** with **hydrochlorothiazide** 50/25 mg, for rheumatoid arthritis and hypertension, additionally started taking methotrexate 5 mg weekly. After 2 months she was admitted to hospital with pancytopenia, extensive mucosal ulceration and renal impairment. The authors point out that **triamterene** is structurally similar to folate and has anti-folate activity, which may therefore have been additive with the effects of methotrexate,[1] but the diclofenac may also have contributed (see 'Methotrexate + NSAIDs, Aspirin or other Salicylates', p.700). In 1998, the manufacturer of methotrexate noted there were two other reports of pancytopenia in patients taking methotrexate and **triamterene**, but again the patients were also taking an NSAID.[2] These cases are isolated, and none of them can be directly attributed to an interaction. Nevertheless, it may be prudent to consider the use of triamterene as a possible cause of otherwise unexplained methotrexate toxicity.

A study in 9 patients found that **furosemide** and **hydroflumethiazide** did not effect the urinary clearance of methotrexate.[3] However, a study in women with breast cancer, taking methotrexate, **cyclophosphamide** and **fluorouracil** found that the concurrent use of a **thiazide diuretic** appeared to increase the myelosuppressant effects of the chemotherapy, but it is not clear which of the antineoplastics might have been affected.[4] This appears to be the only evidence of an interaction between the thiazides and methotrexate. An interaction is not established.

1. Richmond R, McRorie ER, Ogden DA, Lambert CM. Methotrexate and triamterene — a potentially fatal combination. *Ann Rheum Dis* (1997) 56, 209–10.
2. Wyeth/Lederle. Data on file. September 1998.
3. Kristensen LØ, Weismann K, Hutters L. Renal function and the rate of disappearance of methotrexate from serum. *Eur J Clin Pharmacol* (1975) 8, 439–44.
4. Orr LE. Potentiation of myelosuppression from cancer chemotherapy and thiazide diuretics. *Drug Intell Clin Pharm* (1981) 15, 967–70.

Methotrexate + Fluorouracil

Two patients taking low-dose methotrexate had a toxic skin reaction when they started to use a cream containing fluorouracil. The activity of systemic treatment with methotrexate and fluorouracil are said to be dependent on the order in which the two drugs are given.

Clinical evidence, mechanism, importance and management

(a) Topical fluorouracil

Two patients with rheumatoid arthritis taking low-dose methotrexate 7.5 to 12.5 mg weekly for 6 to 14 months were given 2% fluorouracil cream for actinic keratosis. Within 2 to 3 days both patients developed erythema, blister formation and necrosis. The cream was stopped and the lesions healed over the next 2 to 3 weeks.[1] It would seem that topical fluorouracil should be avoided in patients taking methotrexate.

(b) Systemic fluorouracil

In vitro and *animal* data indicate that methotrexate and fluorouracil can be mutually antagonistic under certain conditions.[2-4] Other studies indicate that the sequence (methotrexate first)[5,6] is important for additive or synergistic activity. However, the combination of cyclophosphamide, methotrexate and fluorouracil (CMF) has been the most commonly used adjuvant therapy in breast cancer, and the sequence of administration is said not to be important.[7]

1. Blackburn WD, Alarcón GS. Toxic response to topical fluorouracil in two rheumatoid arthritis patients receiving low dose weekly methotrexate. *Arthritis Rheum* (1990) 33, 303–4.

2. Tattersall MHN, Jackson RC, Connors TA, Harrap KR. Combination chemotherapy: the interaction of methotrexate and 5-fluorouracil. *Eur J Cancer* (1973) 9, 733–9.
3. Maugh TH. Cancer chemotherapy: an unexpected drug interaction. *Science* (1976) 194, 310.
4. Waxman S, Bruckner H. Antitumour drug interactions: additional data. *Science* (1976) 194, 672.
5. Bertino JR, Sawicki WL, Lindquist CA, Gupta VS. Schedule-dependent antitumor effects of methotrexate and 5-fluorouracil. *Cancer Res* (1977) 37, 327–8.
6. Brown I, Ward HWC. Therapeutic consequences of antitumour drug interactions: methotrexate and 5-fluorouracil in the chemotherapy of C3H mice with transplanted mammary adenocarcinoma. *Cancer Lett* (1978) 5, 291–7.
7. Summerhayes M, Daniels S, eds. Practical Chemotherapy: A Multidisciplinary Guide. 1st ed. UK: Radcliffe Medical Press; 2003 P. 91.

Methotrexate + Folinates

Folic acid or folinic acid are sometimes added to low-dose methotrexate for rheumatoid arthritis or psoriasis to reduce adverse effects. Folinic acid is frequently used as an antidote to high-dose methotrexate.

Clinical evidence, mechanism, importance and management

Methotrexate acts as a folic acid antagonist by reversibly binding to the enzyme dihydrofolate reductase, so blocking the conversion of folic acid to tetrahydrofolate. Therefore folic acid and folinic acid (a derivative of tetrahydrofolate) would be expected to interfere with both the toxic and therapeutic effects of methotrexate.

Folic acid or folinic acid are commonly used to reduce the adverse effects of low-dose methotrexate used for rheumatoid arthritis and psoriasis, although the optimum doses and schedules to maximise tolerability and efficacy remain to be determined.

Similarly, folinic acid is used in conjunction with high-dose methotrexate for various cancers to minimise toxicity, when it is typically started 24 hours after methotrexate administration (folinic acid or 'leucovorin' rescue). In this setting, the antidote effect is clearly influenced by the dose of folinate in relation to the dose of methotrexate, and the timing of folinate administration in relation to methotrexate administration.

Patients taking methotrexate for any indication should avoid the inadvertent or unsupervised use of folates, which are commonly found in multivitamin preparations.

Methotrexate + Food

The absorption of low-dose oral methotrexate does not appear to be significantly affected by food.

Clinical evidence, mechanism, importance and management

In 10 children with lymphoblastic leukaemia the peak serum levels of a 15-mg/m^2 oral dose of methotrexate (measured at 1.5 hours) were reduced by about 40% when the methotrexate was taken with a milky meal (milk, cornflakes, sugar, white bread and butter). The AUC_{0-4} was reduced by about 25%. A smaller reduction in methotrexate absorption was seen when it was taken after a citrus meal (orange juice, fresh orange, white bread, butter and jam).[1] However, a 4-hour study is too short to assess the extent of the total absorption. Another study, in 16 children given methotrexate 8 to 22.7 mg/m^2, found that the peak levels and AUC were not significantly affected if methotrexate was given before a meal.[2] A further study in 12 healthy subjects found that a high fat-content breakfast delayed the absorption of methotrexate 7.5 mg orally by about 30 minutes but the extent of the absorption was unchanged.[3] It would therefore appear that methotrexate may be taken without regard to meals.

1. Pinkerton CR, Welshman SG, Glasgow JFT, Bridges JM. Can food influence the absorption of methotrexate in children with acute lymphoblastic leukaemia? *Lancet* (1980) 2, 944–6.
2. Madanat F, Awidi A, Shaheen O, Ottman S, Al-Turk W. Effects of food and gender on the pharmacokinetics of methotrexate in children. *Res Commun Chem Pathol Pharmacol* (1987) 55, 279–82.
3. Kozloski GD, De Vito JM, Kisicki JC, Johnson JB. The effect of food on the absorption of methotrexate sodium tablets in healthy volunteers. *Arthritis Rheum* (1992) 35, 761–4.

Methotrexate + Glutamine

A case report describes nephrotoxicity in a patient taking glutamine with high-dose methotrexate. No cases of renal toxicity were seen in a small study in patients taking glutamine with low-dose methotrexate.

Clinical evidence

A 14-year-old boy taking glutamine 20 g daily, to prevent chemotherapy-related mucositis, developed nephrotoxicity after administration of high-dose methotrexate. He was found to have a high plasma methotrexate concentration 24 hours after the start of the methotrexate infusion, and this remained above 0.2 micromol/L for 10 days; in addition his serum creatinine did not stabilise for 14 days. The patient had previously had two courses of glutamine and chemotherapy, uneventfully, but for these courses his urinary pH had been monitored and he had required intravenous sodium bicarbonate in addition to the standard hydration protocol. During the course of the methotrexate infusion, when the nephrotoxicity occurred, no urine had been collected or monitored.[1] The dose of methotrexate in this case was not stated, but high-dose methotrexate chemotherapy is usually considered to be a dose above 1 g/kg.

No cases of renal toxicity were noted in a study in 9 patients given low-dose methotrexate chemotherapy (neoadjuvant therapy 40 mg/m^2 to 100 mg/m^2 weekly) with oral glutamine 0.5 g/kg daily.[2]

Mechanism

Uncertain. Methotrexate is a weak acid excreted principally unchanged via the kidneys. Drugs that increase the acidity of urine decrease methotrexate elimination and, at high methotrexate doses, can cause its precipitation in the renal tubules causing acute nephrotoxicity. Glutamine metabolism produces ammonium, some of which is excreted in the urine increasing urinary acid excretion and this reduces urinary pH (from pH 6.1 to pH 5.7 in one study[3]), which might reduce methotrexate elimination. This interaction has also been seen in a study in *animals* in which glutamine reduced methotrexate clearance by 25% and decreased its renal elimination by 65%.[4]

Importance and management

Although the data are limited, it appears that glutamine can reduce methotrexate clearance and increase the risk of its renal toxicity when methotrexate is used at high-doses. However, with high-dose methotrexate chemotherapy this can probably be prevented by closely monitoring urinary pH and giving sodium bicarbonate with hydration (see also 'Methotrexate + Urinary alkalinisers', p.704). The authors of the case report suggest that the potential benefits of glutamine should be carefully evaluated against the potential risks, when used with methotrexate.[1] Note that renal toxicity of methotrexate is generally only seen with high-dose chemotherapy, so this interaction might not apply with lower doses of methotrexate.

1. Marín Pozo JF, García JA, Muriel AC, Porras IC. Hazards of concomitant administration of methotrexate and glutamine. *Am J Health-Syst Pharm* (2010) 67, 601–2.
2. Rubio IT, Cao Y, Hutchins LF, Westbrook KC, Klimberg VS. Effect of glutamine on methotrexate efficacy and toxicity. *Ann Surg* (1998) 227, 772–8.
3. Welbourne T, Claville W, Langford M. An oral glutamine load enhances renal acid secretion and function. *Am J Clin Nutr* (1998) 67, 660–3.
4. Charland SL, Bartlett DL, Torosian MH. A significant methotrexate-glutamine pharmacokinetic interaction. *Nutrition* (1995) 11, 154–8.

Methotrexate + Isoniazid

It is possible that the risk of liver function abnormalities seen with either methotrexate or isoniazid is increased when the two drugs are given together. One small review suggested this may be the case, but other larger reviews have not confirmed these findings.

Clinical evidence

In a review of clinical studies of tumour necrosis factor (TNF) antagonists given to patients already taking methotrexate or **sulfasalazine** for rheumatoid arthritis, 8 patients were identified who were also given prophylactic isoniazid 300 mg daily for inactive (latent) tuberculosis (positive PPD skin test). Of these, 4 patients (50%) developed mild to severe hepatic impairment within 7 to 16 weeks, and in three cases this resolved on discontinuation of isoniazid. In one case, excessive alcohol consumption might have been a contributory factor. Two cases (one mild, one severe) occurred in 5 patients taking methotrexate, and 2 cases (one moderate and one severe) occurred in 3 patients taking **sulfasalazine**.[1]

In contrast, when 77 patients with rheumatoid arthritis were given methotrexate with isoniazid prophylaxis for 3 years, two patients stopped treatment due to increases in AST and ALT, but the incidence of hepatotoxic effects was no different to that found in the control group.[2] In a retrospective review of the records of 44 patients taking methotrexate for rheumatoid arthritis and given prophylactic isoniazid for inactive tuberculosis (38 patients) or isoniazid, **pyrazinamide**, rifampicin and ethambutol for a history of active tuberculosis (6 patients), just 5 patients (11.3%) had elevated liver function tests. None of these were more than twice the upper limit of normal, and all abnormalities resolved without intervention. None of the patients included in this study had experienced liver function abnormalities while taking methotrexate alone.[3] For comparison, the authors of this study[3] mention that in one large study, raised liver function tests (three times the upper limit of normal), occurred in 7.5% of patients treated with methotrexate for rheumatoid arthritis.

Mechanism

Both isoniazid and methotrexate are known to be hepatotoxic, and it has been suggested that the risk might be increased by combined use. Sulfasalazine is also hepatotoxic, as is rifampicin and, particularly, pyrazinamide.

Importance and management

An increased risk of hepatotoxicity during the concurrent use of methotrexate and isoniazid is not established, and this possible risk is not a reason to avoid the combination. Monitoring of liver function is recommended during long-term methotrexate use, and is also recommended for isoniazid. This would appear to be sufficient to identify any adverse hepatic effects.

1. Vanhoof J, Landewe S, Van Wijngaerden E, Geusens P. High incidence of hepatotoxicity of isoniazid treatment for tuberculosis chemoprophylaxis in patients with rheumatoid arthritis treated with methotrexate or sulfasalazine and anti-tumour necrosis factor inhibitors. *Ann Rheum Dis* (2003) 62, 1241–2.
2. Xie QB, Wen FQ, Yin G. Isoniazid prophylaxis for pulmonary tuberculosis in Chinese patients with rheumatoid arthritis receiving long-term methotrexate therapy. *Sichuan Da Xue Xue Bao Yi Xue Ban* (2009) 40, 138–40.
3. Mor A, Bingham CO, Kishimoto M, Izmirly PM, Greenberg JD, Reddy S, Rosenthal PB. Methotrexate combined with isoniazid treatment for latent tuberculosis is well tolerated in patients with rheumatoid arthritis: experience from an urban arthritis clinic. *Ann Rheum Dis* (2008) 67, 462–5.

Methotrexate + Miscellaneous

***Animal* studies suggested that the toxicity of methotrexate might be increased by the use of chloramphenicol, aminosalicylic acid, sodium salicylate, sulfamethoxypyridazine, tetracycline or tolbutamide, but con-**

firmation of this in man has only been seen with the salicylates, sulphonamides, and possibly tetracycline.

Clinical evidence, mechanism, importance and management

Some lists, reviews and books on interactions say that **chloramphenicol**, aminosalicylic acid, sodium salicylate, sulfamethoxypyridazine, tetracycline or **tolbutamide** interact with methotrexate, apparently based largely on the preliminary findings of a study in which male *mice* were treated for 5 days with each of 4 doses of methotrexate (1.53 to 12.25 mg/kg intravenously) and immediately afterwards with non-toxic intraperitoneal doses of the drugs listed. These drugs were said to decrease the lethal dose and/or decrease the survival time of the *mice*.[1] That is to say, the toxicity of the methotrexate was increased. The reasons are not understood, but it is suggested that displacement of the methotrexate from its plasma protein binding sites could result in a rise in the levels of unbound and active methotrexate, and in the case of sodium salicylate to a decrease in renal clearance.

These *animal* studies were done in 1968. Since then the clinical importance of the interaction with salicylates has been confirmed (see 'Methotrexate + NSAIDs, Aspirin or other Salicylates', below); there are a few cases involving sulfonamides (see 'Methotrexate + Antibacterials; Co-trimoxazole or Trimethoprim', p.693); and there are two isolated case reports of an interaction with tetracyclines (see 'Methotrexate + Antibacterials; Tetracyclines', p.694), but there appears to be no direct clinical evidence of interactions between methotrexate and **chloramphenicol** or **tolbutamide**. The results of *animal* experiments cannot be applied directly and uncritically to man and it now seems probable that some of these suggested or alleged interactions are more theoretical than real.

1. Dixon RL. The interaction between various drugs and methotrexate. *Toxicol Appl Pharmacol* (1968) 12, 308.

Methotrexate + Nitrous oxide

Methotrexate-induced stomatitis and other toxic effects may be increased by the use of nitrous oxide.

Clinical evidence, mechanism, importance and management

A study in which intravenous methotrexate, cyclophosphamide and fluorouracil (CMF) were used within 36 hours of mastectomy suggested that stomatitis may be caused by a toxic interaction between methotrexate and nitrous oxide used during anaesthesia. Stomatitis was much more common in those receiving CMF within 6 hours of surgery.[1-3] A possible reason is that the effects of methotrexate on tetrahydrofolate metabolism are increased by nitrous oxide, and this has been confirmed in *animals*.[4] It was found that the incidence of stomatitis, severe leucopenia, thrombocytopenia, and of severe systemic and local infections could be reduced by giving calcium folinate (leucovorin) and intravenous hydration.[2,3] Alternatively, the use of nitrous oxide shortly before methotrexate administration should be avoided.[4]

1. Ludwig Breast Cancer Study Group. Toxic effects of early adjuvant chemotherapy for breast cancer. *Lancet* (1983) ii, 542–4.
2. Goldhirsch A, Gelber RD, Tattersall MNH, Rudenstam C-M, Cavalli F. Methotrexate/nitrous-oxide toxic interaction in perioperative chemotherapy for early breast cancer. *Lancet* (1987) ii, 151.
3. Ludwig Breast Cancer Study Group. On the safety of perioperative adjuvant chemotherapy with cyclophosphamide, methotrexate and 5-fluorouracil in breast cancer. *Eur J Cancer Clin Oncol* (1988) 24, 1305–8.
4. Ermens AAM, Schoester M, Spijkers LJM, Lindemans J, Abels J. Toxicity of methotrexate in rats preexposed to nitrous oxide. *Cancer Res* (1989) 49, 6337–41.

Methotrexate + NSAIDs, Aspirin or other Salicylates

Increased methotrexate toxicity, sometimes life-threatening, has been seen in a few patients also taking NSAIDs, whereas other patients have taken an NSAID and methotrexate uneventfully. The pharmacokinetics of methotrexate can also be changed by some NSAIDs, aspirin or other salicylates. The development of toxicity may be dose related: the risk appears to be lowest in those taking low-dose methotrexate for psoriasis or rheumatoid arthritis who have normal renal function.

Clinical evidence

(a) Aminophenazone

Megaloblastic pancytopenia occurred in a woman with rheumatoid arthritis who took methotrexate 15 mg weekly with aminophenazone 1 to 1.5 g daily.[1]

(b) Aspirin and other salicylates

A study in 15 patients with rheumatoid arthritis given a single 10-mg bolus dose of methotrexate, either with or without aspirin 975 mg four times daily, found that the methotrexate clearance was reduced by aspirin (systemic clearance about 16%, renal clearance of unbound methotrexate about 30%). Also, the unbound fraction of methotrexate was higher during aspirin use. Despite these changes no acute toxicity was seen.[2] Another study found that aspirin did not affect the pharmacokinetics of methotrexate.[3] A further study found that, although aspirin did not alter the pharmacokinetics of methotrexate, it did increase the AUC of the metabolite 7-hydroxymethotrexate.[4]

A study in 4 patients found tha the renal clearance of methotrexate was reduced by 35% by an infusion of **sodium salicylate** (2 g initially, then 33 mg/minute).[5] A further study found that **choline magnesium trisalicylate** reduced methotrexate clearance by 24 to 41%, and increased the unbound fraction by 28%, when compared with paracetamol (acetaminophen).[6]

Lethal pancytopenia in 2 patients given methotrexate and aspirin prompted a retrospective survey of the records of other patients given intra-arterial infusions of methotrexate 50 mg daily for 10 days, for epidermoid carcinoma of the oral cavity. Six out of 7 who developed rapid and serious pancytopenia were found to have taken aspirin or other salicylates.[7] There are other case reports[8,9] of methotrexate toxicity in patients taking salicylates but whether a causal relationship exists is uncertain. It has been suggested that pneumonitis in patients receiving low-dose methotrexate may have resulted from the concurrent use of aspirin 4 to 5 g daily.[10]

See also the report about the comparative use of aspirin and other NSAIDs in the section *NSAIDs in general*, below.

(c) Azapropazone

A woman who had been taking methotrexate 25 mg weekly for 4 years for psoriasis had acute toxicity (oral and genital ulceration, bone marrow failure) shortly after starting to take azapropazone (reducing from a dose of 2.4 g on the first day, 1.8 g on the second day to 1.2 g daily for a week). She was also taking aspirin 300 mg daily.[11,12]

(d) Bromfenac

In a short-term study, 10 patients taking methotrexate weekly were given bromfenac 50 mg three times daily for 6 days. No significant changes were seen in either the pharmacokinetics of bromfenac or methotrexate. However, the AUC of the major metabolite of methotrexate, 7-hydroxymethotrexate, was increased by 30% and its renal clearance was reduced by 16%. Eight of the patients had mild to moderate adverse effects and one patient had to withdraw because of moderate hypertension. No patient had any clinically important abnormal laboratory test results.[13] Note that systemic bromfenac has been withdrawn from the market because of reports of hepatic toxicity.

(e) Celecoxib

Fourteen female patients with rheumatoid arthritis taking methotrexate 5 to 20 mg weekly for at least 3 months were also given celecoxib 200 mg or a placebo twice daily for a week. It was found that the maximum serum levels of the methotrexate, its AUC, renal clearance, and other pharmacokinetic parameters were unchanged by celecoxib.[14] The authors note that, in clinical studies, celecoxib was taken in combination with low-dose methotrexate for up to 12 weeks by over 450 patients, and the incidence of adverse effects was similar to that in patients taking methotrexate with placebo.[14]

(f) Diclofenac

A study found that diclofenac 100 mg daily did not affect the pharmacokinetics of methotrexate.[3] Five patients taking low-dose methotrexate 7.5 to 12.5 mg weekly for psoriasis or rheumatoid arthritis developed serious/fatal neutropenias. These cases probably involved other drug interactions, but diclofenac may have been an additional factor in two of them.[15] Methotrexate pneumonitis occurred in a patient who had taken methotrexate 10 mg weekly for 4 weeks. He was also taking diclofenac 75 mg twice daily, although the relevance of this to the adverse reaction is uncertain.[16] Other cases involving diclofenac are mentioned in the sections on *indometacin* and *ketoprofen*, below.

(g) Dipyrone (Metamizole sodium)

A study in a patient with osteosarcoma found that dipyrone 4 g daily more than doubled the methotrexate AUC during the first cycle of high-dose methotrexate treatment.[17]

(h) Etodolac

A pharmacokinetic study in patients with rheumatoid arthritis found that etodolac 600 mg daily did not affect the AUC of methotrexate, but the duration of exposure was lengthened (mean residence time increased from 8.5 hours to 11.4 hours). No clinical toxicity was seen.[18]

(i) Etoricoxib

A study in 12 patients taking methotrexate 7.5 to 20 mg weekly for rheumatoid arthritis found that the addition of etoricoxib 60 mg daily for 7 days had no effect on the methotrexate AUC or on its renal clearance, whereas etoricoxib 120 mg daily for 7 days increased the methotrexate AUC by 28% and reduced its clearance by 13%.[19] In a related study, in 22 patients taking methotrexate 7.5 to 20 mg weekly for rheumatoid arthritis, found that the addition of etoricoxib 90 mg for 7 days and then 120 mg for 7 days had no effect on the renal clearance or AUC of methotrexate.[19]

(j) Flurbiprofen

A study in 6 patients taking methotrexate 10 to 25 mg weekly found no important changes in methotrexate levels when they were also given flurbiprofen 100 mg three times daily.[20] In another study in 10 patients with rheumatoid arthritis taking methotrexate 7.5 to 17.5 mg weekly and flurbiprofen 3 mg/kg daily, methotrexate oral and renal clearance were similarly unaffected by flurbiprofen.[21]

A case report describes an elderly woman who had been taking methotrexate 2.5 mg three times a week for 3 years for rheumatoid arthritis, who developed haematemesis, neutropenia and thrombocytopenia (diagnosed as methotrexate toxicity) within 1 to 2 weeks of starting to take flurbiprofen 100 mg daily.[22]

(k) Ibuprofen

A study in 7 patients found that the clearance of oral methotrexate 7.5 to 15 mg was halved by ibuprofen 40 mg/kg daily, when compared with paracetamol (acetaminophen).[23] In a related study the clearance of methotrexate was reduced by 40% by ibuprofen.[6] Another study in 6 patients with rheumatoid arthritis taking methotrexate 10 to 25 mg weekly found that ibuprofen 800 mg three times daily had no effect on the pharmacokinetics of methotrexate.[20] Similar findings have been reported by other workers.[3]

A patient taking methotrexate who was given ibuprofen required prolonged folinic acid rescue because the clearance of methotrexate had fallen by two-thirds.[24] Another patient receiving high-dose methotrexate (7.5 g/m^2) had severe methotrexate-induced nephrotoxicity and delayed excretion of methotrexate while taking ibuprofen 400 mg every 4 hours.[25] A report attributes pancytopenia and resulting pneumocystis pneumonia in a 16-year-old patient taking methotrexate 5 to 10 mg weekly to the concurrent use of ibuprofen 600 mg twice daily (and also prednisolone 1 mg daily).[26]

(l) Indometacin

In a child taking methotrexate 7.5 mg/m^2 weekly for 9 months, the AUC of methotrexate was increased by 140% when indometacin and aspirin were also given.[27] Another study found that indometacin did not affect the pharmacokinetics of methotrexate.[3]

Two patients given sequential intermediate-dose methotrexate and fluorouracil, who were also taking indometacin 75 to 100 mg daily, died from acute drug toxicity, which the authors of the report attributed to indometacin-associated renal failure.[28] Another case of acute renal failure has been described,[29] but there were no cases of toxicity in 4 other patients taking methotrexate with either paracetamol (acetaminophen) or indometacin.[9] An elderly woman taking indometacin 50 mg daily rectally and **diclofenac** 100 mg daily intravenously died after being given a single 10-mg intramuscular dose of methotrexate.[30]

(m) Ketoprofen

In a study in 10 patients with rheumatoid arthritis taking methotrexate 7.5 to 17.5 mg weekly and ketoprofen 3 mg/kg daily, the methotrexate oral and renal clearance and the fraction of methotrexate unbound were unaffected by ketoprofen.[21] Similarly, in another study in 18 patients with rheumatoid arthritis who were given intravenous methotrexate 15 mg weekly, ketoprofen had no significant effect on the AUC, half-life, or clearance of methotrexate and its major metabolite, 7-hydroxymethotrexate.[31] However, a retrospective study of 118 cycles of *high-dose* methotrexate (800 to 8300 mg/m^2; mean 3200 mg/m^2) in 36 patients found that 4 out of the 9 patients who developed severe methotrexate toxicity had also taken ketoprofen 150 to 200 mg daily for 2 to 15 days. Three of them died. A marked and prolonged rise in serum methotrexate levels was observed. Another patient who had methotrexate toxicity had also been given **diclofenac** 150 mg (in one day).[32] The authors of this report state that ketoprofen should not be given at the same time as high-dose methotrexate, but it may be safe to give it 12 to 24 hours after the methotrexate because 50% of the methotrexate is excreted by the kidneys within 6 to 12 hours. This was tried in two patients without adverse effects.[32]

(n) Lumiracoxib

In a double-blind, placebo-controlled study in patients with rheumatoid arthritis given methotrexate 7.5 to 15 mg weekly, lumiracoxib 400 mg daily for 7 days had no significant effects on the pharmacokinetics of methotrexate.[33]

(o) Meloxicam

Thirteen patients with rheumatoid arthritis were given intravenous methotrexate 15 mg before and after taking meloxicam 15 mg daily for a week. The pharmacokinetics of methotrexate were unaffected by meloxicam and no increase in toxicity was seen.[34]

(p) Naproxen

Naproxen had no significant effect on the AUC, half-life, or clearance of methotrexate and its major metabolite 7-hydroxymethotrexate in 18 patients with rheumatoid arthritis given intravenous methotrexate 15 mg weekly.[31] Other studies have found that naproxen did not affect the pharmacokinetics of methotrexate and/or 7-hydroxymethotrexate.[3,35,36]

In contrast, a study found that the clearance of methotrexate was decreased by 22% by naproxen.[6,23] A further study in 9 children taking methotrexate 0.22 to 1.02 mg/kg weekly found that the clearance of methotrexate was increased in 4 children by more than 30% when they were given naproxen 14.6 to 18.8 mg/kg daily. There was also a 30% or more change in the pharmacokinetics of naproxen in 6 of the patients, but as both increases and decreases in clearance occurred, the significance of these findings are uncertain.[37] In addition, two children taking methotrexate for 1 and 2 years had increases in the AUC of methotrexate of 22% and 71% when given naproxen with aspirin or indometacin, respectively.[27] A woman died of gross methotrexate toxicity apparently exacerbated by the concurrent use of naproxen,[38] and a report attributes pneumonitis in a patient taking methotrexate 7.5 to 10 mg weekly to the concurrent use of naproxen (initially 1 g then 500 mg) daily.[39] A further report describes an infant who developed severe hepatitis while taking methotrexate and naproxen for juvenile idiopathic arthritis. Following intravenous folinic acid and cessation of methotrexate and naproxen her liver function normalised. The role of naproxen is unclear, but the authors consider that the toxicity of methotrexate may have been synergistic with naproxen.[40]

(q) Parecoxib

Studies in patients with rheumatoid arthritis found that oral valdecoxib 40 mg twice daily had no clinically significant effect on the plasma levels of methotrexate given weekly by the intramuscular route [dose not stated].[41] Note that valdecoxib is the main metabolite of parecoxib.

(r) Phenylbutazone

Two patients taking methotrexate for psoriasis developed methotrexate toxicity and skin ulceration shortly after starting to take phenylbutazone 200 to 600 mg daily. One of them died from septicaemia following bone marrow depression.[42]

(s) Piroxicam

No effect on the pharmacokinetics of either free or bound methotrexate was seen in 20 patients with rheumatoid arthritis taking methotrexate 10 mg weekly when they were given piroxicam 20 mg daily for at least 15 days.[43] In another study in 10 patients with rheumatoid arthritis taking methotrexate 7.5 to 17.5 mg weekly, methotrexate oral and renal clearance were unaffected by piroxicam 20 mg daily.[21]

(t) Rofecoxib

Rofecoxib 12.5 to 50 mg daily had no effect on the AUC and renal clearance of methotrexate or 7-hydroxymethotrexate in 19 patients taking methotrexate 7.5 to 20 mg weekly.[44] However, the authors note that in previous evaluations (data on file), higher than therapeutic doses of rofecoxib (75 mg and 250 mg) were associated with a 23% and 40% increase in the AUC of methotrexate, and an 11% and 40% decrease in its renal clearance, respectively.[44]

(u) Sulindac

Sulindac (mean dose 400 mg daily) had no effect on the pharmacokinetics of a single 10-mg/m^2 intravenous dose of methotrexate, but it slightly increased the AUC of the 7-hydroxymethotrexate metabolite.[4]

(v) Tolmetin

Three children taking methotrexate for between 6 months and 1 year had increases in the AUC of methotrexate of 42% when given tolmetin, and of 18% and 25% when given tolmetin with aspirin.[27]

(w) NSAIDs in general

In a study of 34 patients with rheumatoid arthritis taking methotrexate 5 or 10 mg/m^2 (to nearest 2.5 mg) weekly, 12 patients also took **aspirin** (average 4.5 g daily) and 22 took other NSAIDs. Twenty-one of the 34 also took prednisone. Toxicity, sometimes serious (5 patients withdrawn), was common, but no clinical differences between **aspirin** or other NSAIDs with respect to this toxicity was seen during 12 months of concurrent use.[45]

A preliminary report of a study in 87 patients receiving long-term treatment with methotrexate (mean weekly dose 8.19 mg), most of whom were also taking unspecified NSAIDs, found that the majority (72%) experienced no untoward effects and in the rest adverse effects were only relatively mild.[46] The concurrent use of methotrexate and NSAIDs in more than 450 patients with psoriatic arthritis or rheumatoid arthritis was said to be without clinical interaction problems.[47]

In a review of the records of 315 patients with rheumatoid arthritis taking low-dose methotrexate, 13 patients had low platelet counts. The thrombocytopenia was believed to have resulted from an interaction with an NSAID, or in some patients, a multiple drug interaction. If multiple drug interactions were not involved, the authors found that if the NSAID was given on a separate day, or doses spaced according to the NSAID half-life, treatment could be re-introduced avoiding the problems of thrombocytopenia.[48]

Mechanism

Methotrexate is largely cleared unchanged from the body by renal excretion. The NSAIDs as a group inhibit the synthesis of the prostaglandins (PGE_2) resulting in a fall in renal perfusion, which could lead to a rise in serum methotrexate levels, accompanied by increased toxicity. In addition, salicylates competitively inhibit the tubular secretion of methotrexate, which would further reduce its clearance.[5] NSAIDs can also cause renal impairment, which would allow the methotrexate to accumulate. The pyrazolone derivatives and related drugs (e.g. azapropazone, metamizole sodium, phenylbutazone, aminophenazone), in particular, can cause bone marrow depression, which could be additive with that of methotrexate. Protein binding displacement of methotrexate or its metabolite (7-hydroxymethotrexate) have also been suggested as possible additional mechanisms.[49,50] There is also some evidence that 7-hydroxymethotrexate is cleared more slowly in the presence of NSAIDs.[4]

Importance and management

The evidence presented here clearly shows that a few patients taking methotrexate have developed very serious toxicity, apparently due to the concurrent use of NSAIDs, whereas many other patients have experienced no problems at all. There is also other evidence that the pharmacokinetics of the methotrexate are changed (in particular reduced clearance) by some NSAIDs (aspirin, choline magnesium trisalicylate, etodolac, ibuprofen, metamizole sodium, rofecoxib (at higher than therapeutic doses), sodium salicylate, tolmetin), which might be expected to increase its toxicity.

The consensus of opinion seems to be that the risks are greatest with high-dose methotrexate (150 mg or more daily to treat neoplastic diseases) and in patients with impaired renal function, but less in those given low doses (5 to 25 mg weekly) for psoriasis or rheumatoid arthritis and with normal renal function. The manufacturers of methotrexate and the CSM in the UK do not advise the avoidance of NSAIDs (except azapropazone and non-prescription aspirin and ibuprofen), even though their use is a recognised additional risk factor for toxicity. Instead their advice is that the methotrexate dose should be well monitored, which implies that the precautions for methotrexate use should be stepped up. The advice of the CSM is that any patient given methotrexate alone should have a full blood count, renal and liver function tests before starting treatment. These should be repeated weekly until therapy is stabilised, and thereafter every 2 to 3 months. Patients should be told to report any sign or symptom suggestive of infection, particularly sore throat (which might possibly indicate that white cell counts have fallen) or dyspnoea or cough (suggestive of pulmonary toxicity).[51] Aminophenazone or metamizole sodium can cause agranulocytosis on their own (and they consequently have limited use) so their use with methotrexate should be avoided.

Some of the NSAIDs cited here have not been reported to interact (celecoxib, lumiracoxib, meloxicam, piroxicam), and information about some other NSAIDs seems to be lacking, but the same general precautions indicated above should be followed with all NSAIDs just to be on the safe side.

1. Noskov SM. Megaloblastic pancytopenia in a female patient with rheumatoid arthritis given methotrexate and amidopyrine. *Ter Arkh* (1990) 62, 122–3.
2. Stewart CF, Fleming RA, Germain BF, Seleznick MJ, Evans WE. Aspirin alters methotrexate disposition in rheumatoid arthritis patients. *Arthritis Rheum* (1991) 34, 1514–20.
3. Iqbal MP, Baig JA, Ali AA, Niazi SK, Mehboobali N, Hussain MA. The effects of non-steroidal anti-inflammatory drugs on the disposition of methotrexate in patients with rheumatoid arthritis. *Biopharm Drug Dispos* (1998) 19, 163–7.
4. Furst DE, Herman RA, Koehnke R, Erickson N, Hash L, Riggs CE, Porras A, Veng-Pedersen P. Effect of aspirin and sulindac on methotrexate clearance. *J Pharm Sci* (1990) 79, 782–6.
5. Liegler DG, Henderson ES, Hahn MA, Oliverio VT. The effect of organic acids on renal clearance of methotrexate in man. *Clin Pharmacol Ther* (1969) 10, 849–57.
6. Tracy TS, Krohn K, Jones DR, Bradley JD, Hall SD, Brater DC. The effects of salicylate, ibuprofen, and naproxen on the disposition of methotrexate in patients with rheumatoid arthritis. *Eur J Clin Pharmacol* (1992) 42, 121–5.
7. Zuik M, Mandel MA. Methotrexate-salicylate interaction: a clinical and experimental study. *Surg Forum* (1975) 26, 567–9.
8. Dubin HV, Harrell ER. Liver disease associated with methotrexate treatment of psoriatic patients. *Arch Dermatol* (1970) 102, 498–503.
9. Baker H. Intermittent high dose oral methotrexate therapy in psoriasis. *Br J Dermatol* (1970) 82, 65–9.
10. Maier WP, Leon-Perez R, Miller SB. Pneumonitis during low-dose methotrexate therapy. *Arch Intern Med* (1986) 146, 602–3.
11. Daly HM, Scott GL, Boyle J, Roberts CJC. Methotrexate toxicity precipitated by azapropazone. *Br J Dermatol* (1986) 114, 733–35.
12. Burton JL. Drug interactions with methotrexate. *Br J Dermatol* (1991) 124, 300–1.
13. Gumbhir-Shah K, Cevallos WH, Decleene SA, Korth-Bradley JM. Lack of interaction between bromfenac and methotrexate in patients with rheumatoid arthritis. *J Rheumatol* (1996) 23, 984–9.
14. Karim A, Tolbert DS, Hunt TL, Hubbard RC, Harper KM, Geis GS. Celecoxib, a specific COX-2 inhibitor, has no significant effect on methotrexate pharmacokinetics in patients with rheumatoid arthritis. *J Rheumatol* (1999) 26, 2539–43.
15. Mayall B, Poggi G, Parkin JD. Neutropenia due to low-dose methotrexate therapy for psoriasis and rheumatoid arthritis may be fatal. *Med J Aust* (1991) 155, 480–4.
16. Clearkin R, Corris PA, Thomas SHL. Methotrexate pneumonitis in a patient with rheumatoid arthritis. *Postgrad Med J* (1997) 73, 603–4.
17. Hernández de la Figuera y Gómez T, Torres NVJ, Ronchera Oms CL, Ordovás Baines JP. Interacción farmacocinética entre metotrexato a altas dosis y dipirona. *Rev Farmacol Clin Exp* (1989) 6, 77–81.
18. Anaya J-M, Fabre D, Bressolle F, Bologna C, Alric R, Cocciglio M, Dropsy R, Sany J. Effect of etodolac on methotrexate pharmacokinetics in patients with rheumatoid arthritis. *J Rheumatol* (1994) 21, 203–8.
19. Schwartz JI, Agrawal NGB, Wong PH, Miller J, Bachmann K, Marbury T, Hoelscher D, Cavanaugh PF, Gottesdiener K. Examination of the effect of increasing doses of etoricoxib on oral methotrexate pharmacokinetics in patients with rheumatoid arthritis. *J Clin Pharmacol* (2009) 49, 1202–9.
20. Skeith KJ, Russell AS, Jamali F, Coates J, Friedman H. Lack of significant interaction between low dose methotrexate and ibuprofen or flurbiprofen in patients with arthritis. *J Rheumatol* (1990) 17, 1008–10.
21. Tracy TS, Worster T, Bradley JD, Greene PK, Brater DC. Methotrexate disposition following concomitant administration of ketoprofen, piroxicam and flurbiprofen in patients with rheumatoid arthritis. *Br J Clin Pharmacol* (1994) 37, 453–6.
22. Frenia ML, Long KS. Methotrexate and nonsteroidal antiinflammatory drug interactions. *Ann Pharmacother* (1992) 26, 234–7.
23. Tracy TS, Jones DR, Hall SD, Brater DC, Bradley JD, Krohn K. The effect of NSAIDs on methotrexate disposition in patients with rheumatoid arthritis. *Clin Pharmacol Ther* (1990) 47, 138.
24. Bloom EJ, Ignoffo RJ, Reis CA, Cadman E. Delayed clearance (CL) of methotrexate (MTX) associated with antibiotics and antiinflammatory agents. *Clin Res* (1986) 34, 560A.
25. Cassano WF. Serious methotrexate toxicity caused by interaction with ibuprofen. *Am J Pediatr Hematol Oncol* (1989) 11, 481–2.
26. Carmichael AJ, Ryatt KS. *Pneumocystis carinii* pneumonia following methotrexate. *Br J Dermatol* (1990) 122, 291.
27. Dupuis LL, Koren G, Shore A, Silverman ED, Laxer RM. Methotrexate-nonsteroidal antiinflammatory drug interaction in children with arthritis. *J Rheumatol* (1990) 17, 1469–73.
28. Ellison NM, Servi RJ. Acute renal failure and death following sequential intermediate-dose methotrexate and 5-FU: a possible adverse effect due to concomitant indomethacin administration. *Cancer Treat Rep* (1985) 69, 342–3.
29. Maiche AG. Acute renal failure due to concomitant action of methotrexate and indomethacin. *Lancet* (1986) i, 1390.
30. Gabrielli A, Leoni P, Danieli G. Methotrexate and non-steroidal anti-inflammatory drugs. *BMJ* (1987) 294, 776.
31. Christophidis N, Dawson TM, Angelis P, Ryan PFJ. A double-blind, randomised, placebo controlled pharmacokinetic and clinical study of the interaction of ketoprofen and naproxen with methotrexate in rheumatoid arthritis. *Arthritis Rheum* (1994) 37 (9 Suppl), S252.
32. Thyss A, Milano G, Kubar J, Namer M, Schneider M. Clinical and pharmacokinetic evidence of a life-threatening interaction between methotrexate and ketoprofen. *Lancet* (1986) i, 256–8.
33. Hartmann SN, Rordorf CM, Milosavljev S, Branson JM, Chales GH, Juvin RR, Lafforgue P, Le Parc JM, Tavernier CG, Meyer OC. Lumiracoxib does not affect methotrexate pharmacokinetics in rheumatoid arthritis patients. *Ann Pharmacother* (2004) 38, 1582–7.
34. Hübner G, Sander D, Degner FL, Türck D, Rau R. Lack of pharmacokinetic interaction of meloxicam with methotrexate in patients with rheumatoid arthritis. *J Rheumatol* (1997) 24, 845–51.
35. Vakily M, Amer F, Kukulka MJ, Andhivarothai N. Coadministration of lansoprazole and naproxen does not affect the pharmacokinetic profile of methotrexate in adult patients with rheumatoid arthritis. *J Clin Pharmacol* (2005) 45, 1179–86.
36. Stewart CF, Fleming RA, Arkin CR, Evans WE. Coadministration of naproxen and low-dose methotrexate in patients with rheumatoid arthritis. *Clin Pharmacol Ther* (1990) 47, 540–6.
37. Wallace CA, Smith AL, Sherry DD. Pilot investigation of naproxen/methotrexate interaction in patients with juvenile rheumatoid arthritis. *J Rheumatol* (1993) 20, 1764–8.
38. Singh RR, Malaviya AN, Pandey JN, Guleria JS. Fatal interaction between methotrexate and naproxen. *Lancet* (1986) i, 1390.
39. Englebrecht JA, Calhoon SL, Scherrer JJ. Methotrexate pneumonitis after low-dose therapy for rheumatoid arthritis. *Arthritis Rheum* (1983) 26, 1275–8.
40. Ting TV, Hashkes PJ. Methotrexate/naproxen-associated severe hepatitis in a child with juvenile idiopathic arthritis. *Clin Exp Rheumatol* (2007) 25, 928–9.
41. Dynastat (Parecoxib sodium). Pfizer Ltd. UK Summary of product characteristics, June 2013.
42. Adams JD, Hunter GA. Drug interaction in psoriasis. *Aust J Dermatol* (1976) 17, 39–40.
43. Combe B, Edno L, Lafforgue P, Bologna C, Bernard J-C, Acquaviva P, Sany J, Bressolle F. Total and free methotrexate pharmacokinetics, with and without piroxicam, in rheumatoid arthritis patients. *Br J Rheumatol* (1995) 34, 421–8.
44. Schwartz JI, Agrawal NGB, Wong PH, Bachmann KA, Porras AG, Miller JL, Ebel DL, Sack MR, Holmes GB, Redfern JS, Gertz BJ. Lack of pharmacokinetic interaction between rofecoxib and methotrexate in rheumatoid arthritis patients. *J Clin Pharmacol* (2001) 41, 1120–30.
45. Rooney TW, Furst DE, Koehnke R, Burmeister L. Aspirin is not associated with more toxicity than other nonsteroidal antiinflammatory drugs in patients with rheumatoid arthritis treated with methotrexate. *J Rheumatol* (1993) 20, 1297–1302.
46. Wilke WS, Calabrese LH, Segal AM. Incidence of untoward reactions in patients with rheumatoid arthritis treated with methotrexate. *Arthritis Rheum* (1983) 26 (Suppl), S56.
47. Zachariae H. Methotrexate and non-steroidal anti-inflammatory drugs. *Br J Dermatol* (1992) 126, 95.
48. Franck H, Rau R, Herborn G. Thrombocytopenia in patients with rheumatoid arthritis on long-term treatment with low dose methotrexate. *Clin Rheumatol* (1996) 15, 163–7.
49. Slørdal L, Sager G, Aarbakke J. Pharmacokinetic interactions with methotrexate: is 7-hydroxy-methotrexate the culprit? *Lancet* (1988) i, 591–2.
50. Parish RC, Johnson V. Effect of salicylate on plasma protein binding of methotrexate. *Clin Pharmacol Ther* (1996) 59, 162.
51. The Committee on Safety of Medicines/Medicines Control Agency. Blood dyscrasias and other ADRs with low-dose methotrexate. *Current Problems* (1997) 23, 12.

Methotrexate + Paracetamol (Acetaminophen)

Paracetamol appears not to interact with methotrexate.

Clinical evidence, mechanism, importance and management

A study in patients with rheumatoid arthritis found that the clearance of oral methotrexate 7.5 to 15 mg was unaffected by the concurrent use of paracetamol.[1] In a study of patients with psoriasis taking methotrexate in doses of up to 25 mg weekly, no cases of toxicity occurred in 4 patients also taking paracetamol or indometacin.[2] In one study, methotrexate clearance was reduced by NSAIDs but not by paracetamol, which was included in the study as a control.[3]

1. Tracy TS, Jones DR, Hall SD, Brater DC, Bradley JD, Krohn K. The effect of NSAIDs on methotrexate disposition in patients with rheumatoid arthritis. *Clin Pharmacol Ther* (1990) 47, 138.
2. Baker H. Intermittent high dose oral methotrexate therapy in psoriasis. *Br J Dermatol* (1970) 82, 65–9.
3. Tracy TS, Krohn K, Jones DR, Bradley JD, Hall SD, Brater DC. The effects of salicylate, ibuprofen, and naproxen on the disposition of methotrexate in patients with rheumatoid arthritis. *Eur J Clin Pharmacol* (1992) 42, 121–5.

Methotrexate + Probenecid

Probenecid markedly increases serum methotrexate levels.

Clinical evidence

The concurrent use of oral or intravenous probenecid 500 mg to 1 g and methotrexate 200 mg/m^2 as an intravenous bolus resulted in serum methotrexate levels in 4 patients that were more than four times higher than in 4 other patients who had not been given probenecid (methotrexate levels 400 micrograms/L compared with 90 micrograms/L, measured 24-hours post-dose).[1] A three to fourfold increase in serum methotrexate levels at 24 hours was also seen in 4 patients given probenecid.[2] In another 4 patients, pretreatment with probenecid (500 mg every 6 hours for 5 doses) doubled serum methotrexate levels.[3] Severe and life-threatening pancytopenia occurred when a woman taking low-dose methotrexate 7.5 mg weekly for rheumatoid arthritis was given probenecid. She also had renal impairment, hypoalbuminaemia and was taking salsalate (a salicylic acid derivative).[4]

Mechanism

Probenecid inhibits the renal excretion of methotrexate in both *monkeys* and *rats*[5,6] and this probably also happens in man. Changes in the protein binding of methotrexate may also have some part to play.[7] The increased methotrexate levels increase the risk of serious bone marrow depression.

Importance and management

An established and clinically important interaction. A marked increase in both the therapeutic and toxic effects of methotrexate can occur, apparently even with low doses if other risk factors are present.[4] Anticipate the need to reduce the dose of methotrexate and monitor the effects well if probenecid is used concurrently. If this is not possible, avoid the combination.

1. Aherne GW, Piall E, Marks V, Mould G, White WF. Prolongation and enhancement of serum methotrexate concentrations by probenecid. *BMJ* (1978) 1, 1097–99.
2. Howell SB, Olshen RA, Rice JA. Effect of probenecid on cerebrospinal fluid methotrexate kinetics. *Clin Pharmacol Ther* (1979) 26, 641–6.
3. Lilly MB, Omura GA. Clinical pharmacology of oral intermediate-dose methotrexate with or without probenecid. *Cancer Chemother Pharmacol* (1985) 15, 220–2.
4. Basin KS, Escalante A, Beardmore TD. Severe pancytopenia in a patient taking low dose methotrexate and probenecid. *J Rheumatol* (1991) 18, 609–10
5. Bourke RS, Chheda G, Bremer A, Watanabe O, Tower DB. Inhibition of renal tubular transport of methotrexate by probenecid. *Cancer Res* (1975) 35, 110–6.
6. Kates RE, Tozer TN, Sorby DL. Increased methotrexate toxicity due to concurrent probenecid administration. *Biochem Pharmacol* (1976) 25, 1485–8.
7. Paxton JW. Interaction of probenecid with the protein binding of methotrexate. *Pharmacology* (1984) 28, 86–9.

Methotrexate + Proton pump inhibitors

Methotrexate elimination has been reported to be reduced in patients given proton pump inhibitors. However, similar elevations in methotrexate concentrations in another patient were independent of ome-

prazole use. One patient had myalgia and elevated 7-hydroxymethotrexate concentrations when given methotrexate with pantoprazole.

Clinical evidence

(a) Esomeprazole

In a retrospective analysis of 6 patients given high-dose, intravenous methotrexate, who were subsequently treated for methotrexate toxicity due to delayed methotrexate elimination, 2 had also taken concurrent esomeprazole. No delay in methotrexate elimination was seen when high-dose, intravenous methotrexate was subsequently given without a proton pump inhibitor.[1]

(b) Lansoprazole

In a study in 76 patients with solid tumours treated with high-dose methotrexate infusions (300 mg/m^2 to 12 g/m^2 over one to 24 hours), the clearance of methotrexate and its metabolite, 7-hydroxymethotrexate, was decreased and its plasma concentrations increased in the 3 patients who were also given lansoprazole 30 mg daily.[2]

(c) Omeprazole

In a study in 76 patients with solid tumours, receiving high-dose methotrexate infusions (300 mg/m^2 to 12 g/m^2 over 1 to 24 hours), the clearance of methotrexate and its metabolite, 7-hydroxymethotrexate, was decreased and its plasma concentrations increased in the 10 patients who had also been given omeprazole 20 to 40 mg daily.[2] A number of case reports support this finding. In one, a man with Hodgkin's disease developed osteosarcoma and was given cyclophosphamide, bleomycin, dactinomycin, and methotrexate, followed by folinic acid rescue. He was also taking a number of other drugs, including omeprazole. During the first cycle of treatment his serum methotrexate concentration remained elevated for several days, and suspicion fell on the omeprazole, which was stopped. The patient's serum methotrexate concentration then decreased rapidly, and during the following three cycles the methotrexate pharmacokinetics were normal.[3] In another case, an 11-year-old boy with osteoblastic osteosarcoma was given high-dose methotrexate 15 g as a 4-hour infusion. He was also given omeprazole 20 mg twice daily (for about one week before the methotrexate), megestrol acetate, sucralfate, and folinic acid rescue. Methotrexate elimination was delayed and so further folinic acid was given. When later cycles of methotrexate were given, with ranitidine instead of omeprazole, the elimination of methotrexate was normal. The elimination half-life of the initial phase after the first dose given with omeprazole was 65% longer, when compared with that of the second dose without omeprazole.[4] In a third report, a 15-year-old boy experienced methotrexate toxicity, and elevated concentrations of methotrexate despite being given folinic acid, when he was also taking omeprazole. His symptoms of methotrexate toxicity resolved rapidly once omeprazole was stopped. He had experienced no toxicity in a previous cycle when he had taken ranitidine.[5] A retrospective study of 6 patients given high-dose, intravenous methotrexate, who were subsequently treated for methotrexate toxicity due to delayed methotrexate elimination, found that 3 patients had also taken concurrent omeprazole (one was also given insufficient hydration and another was also given piperacillin with tazobactam). No delay in methotrexate elimination was seen when high-dose, intravenous methotrexate was subsequently given without a proton pump inhibitor.[1]

In contrast to these findings, a case report describes a man with chondroblastic osteosarcoma, who had been taking omeprazole, and who was given high-dose methotrexate 20 g over 6 hours with hydration, urinary alkalinisation and, after 24 hours, folinic acid rescue. The folinic acid dose was adjusted in response to elevated methotrexate concentrations and omeprazole was stopped. A second dose of methotrexate 2 weeks later, this time without omeprazole, resulted in similar elevated methotrexate concentrations. Thus the elevated methotrexate concentrations in this patient could not be attributed to the concurrent use of omeprazole.[6]

(d) Pantoprazole

Severe generalised myalgia occurred in a man taking pantoprazole 20 mg daily after he received intramuscular methotrexate 15 mg weekly. The symptoms subsided and eventually disappeared when the pantoprazole was replaced with ranitidine. The symptoms reappeared in response to rechallenge with pantoprazole, and the AUC of 7-hydroxymethotrexate was found to be increased by about 70%, although the AUC of methotrexate was unchanged.[7]

(e) Various proton pump inhibitors

Two retrospective studies[8,9] in patients given high-dose, intravenous methotrexate found that the risk of delayed methotrexate elimination was increased in patients taking proton pump inhibitors, including esomeprazole, lansoprazole, omeprazole, pantoprazole, or **rabeprazole** (adjusted odds ratios of 2.65 and 6.66).

Mechanism

Proton pump inhibitors may affect renal, and possibly hepatic, clearance of methotrexate by inhibition of methotrexate transporter proteins,[2,10] in particular the breast cancer resistance protein (BCRP).[8] It has been suggested that omeprazole may inhibit the activity of a hydrogen-ion dependent mechanism in the kidney, on which methotrexate depends for its excretion, so that its renal clearance is reduced.[3] It has also been suggested that the situation with lansoprazole may be similar, but that pantoprazole may differ because at about the pH found in the renal tubules (pH 5), pantoprazole is more slowly activated than omeprazole.[4] However, a case of an interaction with pantoprazole has also been reported.[7]

Importance and management

Information about an interaction between methotrexate and the proton pump inhibitors seems to be limited to these few reports and, with the exception of one case report, they all found that proton pump inhibitors reduced the clearance of methotrexate. Any changes in methotrexate kinetics are important in terms of the potential for increased toxicity. The authors of several studies advise against concurrent use.[1,2,9] Further, the authors of one report recommend that if omeprazole is necessary for a patient about to receive methotrexate, then omeprazole should be stopped 4 to 5 days before methotrexate administration.[4] The situation with other proton pump inhibitors might be similar. Ranitidine was found to be a suitable alternative in two of the cases.[4,7] Note that the risks would appear to be most important with high-dose methotrexate, but the case report involving a 15 mg weekly dose of methotrexate introduces a note of caution in all patients given methotrexate.

1. Santucci R, Levêque D, Kemmel V, Lutz P, Gérout A-C, N'Guyen A, Lescoute A, Schneider F, Bergerat J-P, Herbrecht R. Severe intoxication with methotrexate possibly associated with concomitant use of proton pump inhibitors. *Anticancer Res* (2010) 30, 963–6.
2. Joerger M, Huitema ADR, van den Bongard HJGD, Baas P, Schornagel JH, Schellens JHM, Beijnen JH. Determinants of the elimination of methotrexate and 7-hydroxy-methotrexate following high-dose infusional therapy to cancer patients. *Br J Clin Pharmacol* (2005) 62, 71–80.
3. Reid T, Yuen A, Catolico M, Carlson RW. Impact of omeprazole on the plasma clearance of methotrexate. *Cancer Chemother Pharmacol* (1993) 33, 82–4.
4. Beorlegui B, Aldaz A, Ortega A, Aquerreta I, Sierrasesúmega L, Giráldez J. Potential interaction between methotrexate and omeprazole. *Ann Pharmacother* (2000) 34, 1024–7.
5. Bauters TGM, Verlooy J, Robays H, Laureys G. Interaction between methotrexate and omeprazole in an adolescent with leukaemia: a case report. *Pharm World Sci* (2008) 30, 316–18.
6. Whelan J, Hoare D, Leonard P. Omeprazole does not alter plasma methotrexate clearance. *Cancer Chemother Pharmacol* (1999) 44, 88–9.
7. Tröger U, Stötzel B, Martens-Lobenhoffer J, Gollnick H, Meyer FP. Severe myalgia from an interaction between treatments with pantoprazole and methotrexate. *BMJ* (2002) 324, 1497.
8. Suzuki K, Doki K, Homma M, Tamaki H, Hori S, Ohtani H, Sawada Y, Kohda Y. Co-administration of proton pump inhibitors delays elimination of plasma methotrexate in high-dose methotrexate therapy. *Br J Clin Pharmacol* (2008) 67, 44–9.
9. Santucci R, Levêque D, Kemmel V, Herbrecht R. Delayed elimination of methotrexate associated with co-administration of proton pump inhibitors. *Anticancer Res* (2010) 30, 3807–10.
10. Breedveld P, Zelcer N, Pluim D, Sönmezer Ö, Tibben MM, Beijnen JH, Schinkel AH, van Tellingen O, Borst P, Schellens JHM. Mechanism of the pharmacokinetic interaction between methotrexate and benzimidazoles: potential role for breast cancer resistance protein in clinical drug-drug interactions. *Cancer Res* (2004) 64, 5804–11.

Methotrexate + Retinoids

The levels of methotrexate may be increased by etretinate, and cases of severe liver toxicity have been reported.

Clinical evidence

(a) Acitretin

In a review of the medical records of 18 patients who had taken methotrexate and acitretin for psoriasis, two patients (both of whom had consumed alcohol during their treatment) developed mildly raised liver function tests, four patients experienced at least one elevated gamma-glutamyl transferase level, and no patient discontinued treatment due to abnormal laboratory results.[1]

(b) Etretinate

A man was given a 48-hour infusion of methotrexate 10 mg every week, for chronic discoid psoriasis but when he was also given etretinate 30 mg daily his serum methotrexate levels almost doubled. Concentrations at 12 and 24 hours during the infusion were 0.11 mmol/L, compared with 0.07 mmol/L and 0.05 mmol/L before the etretinate.[2] A later study[3] in patients with psoriasis found that those receiving etretinate had 38% higher maximum plasma levels of methotrexate, but no difference in the clearance or elimination half-life of methotrexate (i.e. no methotrexate accumulation).

Severe toxic hepatitis has been reported in a number of cases when both etretinate and methotrexate were given.[4-6] It may take several months to develop.[6] The author of two of these cases stated that these occurred in a total of just 10 patients given both drugs, whereas they not seen any cases of severe toxic hepatitis in 531 patients given methotrexate alone or in 110 patients given etretinate alone.[4]

Mechanism

Not understood. Both etretinate and methotrexate can cause hepatotoxicity. The increased incidence of toxic hepatitis seen with etretinate and methotrexate may possibly be related to the increased maximum methotrexate plasma levels.

Importance and management

Although methotrexate and etretinate have been used together with success for psoriasis,[7-9] the risk of severe drug-induced hepatitis seems to be increased. One author says that he has decided not to use this combination in future.[4] Concurrent use should clearly be undertaken with great care. Etretinate has been largely superseded by acitretin (a metabolite of etretinate, which has a shorter half-life), but some, including the manufacturers, consider that the concurrent use of methotrexate and acitretin should also be avoided.[10-12] However, some do use this combination.[1] If the combination is used, it would be prudent to increase the frequency of monitoring of liver function tests.

1. Lowenthal KE, Horn PJ, Kalb RE. Concurrent use of methotrexate and acitretin revisited. *J Dermatolog Treat* (2008) 19, 22–26.
2. Harrison PV, Peat M, James R, Orrell D. Methotrexate and retinoids in combination for psoriasis. *Lancet* (1987) ii, 512.
3. Larsen FG, Nielsen-Kudsk F, Jakobsen P, Schrøder H, Kragballe K. Interaction of etretinate with methotrexate pharmacokinetics in psoriatic patients. *J Clin Pharmacol* (1990) 30, 802–7.
4. Zachariae H. Dangers of methotrexate/etretinate combination therapy. *Lancet* (1988) i, 422.

5. Zachariae H. Methotrexate and etretinate as concurrent therapies in the treatment of psoriasis. *Arch Dermatol* (1984) 120, 155.
6. Beck H-I, Foged EK. Toxic hepatitis due to combination therapy with methotrexate and etretinate in psoriasis. *Dermatologica* (1983) 167, 94–6.
7. Vanderveen EE, Ellis CN, Campbell JP, Case PC, Voorhees JJ. Methotrexate and etretinate as concurrent therapies in severe psoriasis. *Arch Dermatol* (1982) 118, 660–2.
8. Adams JD. Concurrent methotrexate and etretinate therapy for psoriasis. *Arch Dermatol* (1983) 119, 793.
9. Rosenbaum MM, Roenigk HH. Treatment of generalized pustular psoriasis with etretinate (Ro 10-9359) and methotrexate. *J Am Acad Dermatol* (1984) 10, 357–61.
10. van de Kerkhof PCM. Therapeutic strategies: rotational therapy and combinations. *Clin Exp Dermatol* (2001) 26, 356–61.
11. Neotigason (Acitretin). Actavis UK Ltd. UK Summary of product characteristics, February 2015.
12. Soriatane (Acitretin). Stiefel Labs, Inc. US Prescribing information, May 2015.

Methotrexate + Sulfasalazine

The pharmacokinetics of methotrexate are unaffected by sulfasalazine. Clinical studies in patients with rheumatoid arthritis suggest that the combination of methotrexate and sulfasalazine may result in folate-deficiency anaemias.

Clinical evidence, mechanism, importance and management

A study in 15 patients with rheumatoid arthritis found that when sulfasalazine 2 g was given with methotrexate 7.5 mg weekly, the pharmacokinetics of methotrexate remained unchanged. Similarly, methotrexate did not alter the trough levels of sulfasalazine.[1] Although this study suggests that there is no reason to avoid the concurrent use of sulfasalazine and methotrexate, clinical studies in patients with rheumatoid arthritis have found that concurrent use does not significantly increase therapeutic efficacy and seems to increase the development of folate-deficiency anaemias.[2] The results of an *in vitro* study suggest this may be because sulfasalazine is a potent inhibitor of the reduced folate carrier-mediated cellular uptake of methotrexate and folinate.[3] An alternative explanation is that both sulfasalazine and methotrexate promote enhanced adenosine release, which may suppress inflammation, and the combination of two drugs with the same mechanism of action may not improve the therapeutic response of either.[4]

1. Haagsma CJ, Russel FGM, Vree TB, van Riel PLCM, van de Putte LBA. Combination of methotrexate and sulphasalazine in patients with rheumatoid arthritis: pharmacokinetic analysis and relationship to clinical response. *Br J Clin Pharmacol* (1996) 42, 195–200.
2. O'Dell JR, Leff R, Paulsen G, Haire C, Mallek J, Eckhoff PJ, Fernandez A, Blakely K, Wees S, Stoner J, Hadley S, Felt J, Palmer W, Waytz P, Churchill M, Klassen L, Moore G. Treatment of rheumatoid arthritis with methotrexate and hydroxychloroquine, methotrexate and sulfasalazine, or a combination of the three medications: results of a two-year, randomized, double-blind, placebo-controlled trial. *Arthritis Rheum* (2002) 46, 1164–70.
3. Jansen G, van der Heijden J, Oerlemans R, Lems WF, Ifergan I, Scheper RJ, Assaraf YG, Dijkmans BAC. Sulfasalazine is a potent inhibitor of the reduced folate carrier: implications for combination therapies with methotrexate in rheumatoid arthritis. *Arthritis Rheum* (2004) 50, 2130–9.
4. Cronstein BN. Therapeutic cocktails for rheumatoid arthritis: the mixmaster's guide. *Arthritis Rheum* (2004) 50, 2041–3.

Methotrexate + Tacrolimus

Limited evidence suggests that tacrolimus does not affect methotrexate levels.

Clinical evidence, mechanism, importance and management

In a study in 3 bone marrow transplant patients given tacrolimus 30 micrograms/kg daily from the day before transplantation and low-dose methotrexate 15 mg/m^2 on day one, and 10 mg/m^2 on days 3, 6 and 11, methotrexate levels at 24 hours post-dose remained below the range requiring folinic acid, suggesting that no interaction of clinical significance had occurred.[1] In a later, similar report from this research group, in a total of 40 patients, tacrolimus did not appear to affect methotrexate levels.[2]

1. Dix S, Devine SM, Geller RB, Wingard JR. Re: severe interaction between methotrexate and a macrolide-like antibiotic. *J Natl Cancer Inst* (1995) 87, 1641–2.
2. Wingard JR, Nash RA, Ratanatharathorn V, Fay JW, Klein JL, Przepiorka D, Maher RM, Devine SM, Boswell G, Bekersky I, Fitzsimmons W. Lack of interaction between tacrolimus (FK506) and methotrexate in bone marrow transplant recipients. *Bone Marrow Transplant* (1997) 20, 49–51.

Methotrexate + Taxanes

Docetaxel does not alter methotrexate pharmacokinetics. Methotrexate does not appear to alter paclitaxel pharmacokinetics.

Clinical evidence, mechanism, importance and management

(a) Docetaxel

In a study in 6 patients, the pharmacokinetics of methotrexate and its metabolite, 7-hydroxymethotrexate, were unaltered when methotrexate 30 mg/m^2 was given immediately before or 24 hours before an infusion of docetaxel 75 mg/m^2, compared with methotrexate 30 mg/m^2 given alone.[1]

(b) Paclitaxel

The pharmacokinetics of paclitaxel did not appear to be changed when a 24-hour infusion of paclitaxel was started 24 hours after a bolus of methotrexate, when compared with historical data of paclitaxel alone. Myelosuppression was severe in this study.[2]

1. Sparreboom A, Loos WJ, Nooter K, Stoter G, Verweij J. Liquid chromatographic analysis and preliminary pharmacokinetics of methotrexate in cancer patients co-treated with docetaxel. *J Chromatogr B Biomed Sci Appl* (1999) 735, 111–19.
2. Huber MH, Lee JS, Newman RA, Fossella FV, Wester M, Hong WK, Lippman SM. A phase I investigation of the sequential use of methotrexate and paclitaxel with and without G-CSF for the treatment of solid tumors. *Ann Oncol* (1996) 7, 59–63.

Methotrexate + Theophylline

Methotrexate causes a modest reduction in theophylline clearance. Theophylline may reduce methotrexate-induced neurotoxicity, but there is the possibility that it may also reduce methotrexate efficacy.

Clinical evidence

(a) Effects on theophylline

In 8 patients with severe, steroid-dependent asthma, the apparent clearance of theophylline (given as oral aminophylline, choline theophyllinate or theophylline) was reduced by 19% after 6 weeks of treatment with intramuscular methotrexate 15 mg weekly. Three patients complained of nausea and the theophylline dose was reduced in one of them as the theophylline level was more than 20 micrograms/mL.[1]

(b) Effects on methotrexate

Four of 6 patients aged 3 to 16 years with acute lymphoblastic leukaemia and high-dose methotrexate-induced neurotoxicity had a complete resolution of their symptoms when they were given a 2.5-mg/kg aminophylline infusion over one hour. The other 2 patients had some improvement in symptoms. One patient also had symptom relief with rapid-release theophylline.[2] Similar results were reported in another child who developed neurotoxicity after receiving high-dose methotrexate. In this case, aminophylline was reported not to alter methotrexate levels.[3] A patient with methotrexate-induced leukoencephalopathy recovered after being given a combination of intravenous folinic acid with intravenous aminophylline 145 mg daily for 7 days.[4]

Mechanism

It is not known why theophylline clearance is altered by methotrexate. Methotrexate neurotoxicity may be linked with increased levels of adenosine. Theophylline is a competitive antagonist for adenosine receptors at serum concentrations within the therapeutic range used in respiratory disease.[2]

Importance and management

The clinical importance of the small reduction in theophylline clearance is uncertain, although it may be worth bearing this in mind in patients maintained at the higher end of the therapeutic levels for theophylline, as they may be more likely to develop toxicity. One UK manufacturer of methotrexate (licensed for rheumatoid arthritis) recommends monitoring theophylline levels with concurrent use, and avoiding excessive consumption of theophylline-containing drinks; however, this recommendation appears to be based on studies and surveys that looked at the effects of caffeine intake in patients taking low-dose, weekly methotrexate for rheumatoid arthritis or psoriasis.[5,6] Consider also, 'Methotrexate + Caffeine', p.697.

Aminophylline may reduce methotrexate-induced neurotoxicity, and, although there is some evidence that theophylline does not alter the cytotoxic effects of methotrexate, this requires confirmation.[2]

1. Glynn-Barnhart AM, Erzurum SC, Leff JA, Martin RJ, Cochran JE, Cott GR, Szefler SJ. Effect of low-dose methotrexate on the disposition of glucocorticoids and theophylline. *J Allergy Clin Immunol* (1991) 88, 180–6.
2. Bernini JC, Fort DW, Griener JC, Kane BJ, Chappell WB, Kamen BA. Aminophylline for methotrexate-induced neurotoxicity. *Lancet* (1995) 345, 544–7.
3. Peyriere H, Poiree M, Cociglio M, Margueritte G, Hansel S, Hillaire-Buys D. Reversal of neurologic disturbances related to high-dose methotrexate by aminophylline. *Med Pediatr Oncol* (2001) 36, 662–4.
4. Jaksic W, Veljkovic D, Pozza C, Lewis I. Methotrexate-induced leukoencephalopathy reversed by aminophylline and high-dose folinic acid. *Acta Haematol (Basel)* (2004) 111, 230–2.
5. Metoject (Methotrexate). Medac GmbH. UK Summary of product characteristics, November 2008.
6. Medac UK. Personal Communication, March 2007.

Methotrexate + Urinary alkalinisers

Alkalinisation of the urine increases the urinary excretion of methotrexate.

Clinical evidence, mechanism, importance and management

Methotrexate is much more soluble in alkaline than in acidic fluids, therefore urinary alkalinisers such as **sodium bicarbonate** and **acetazolamide** (and ample fluids) are often given to patients receiving high-dose methotrexate to prevent the precipitation of methotrexate in the renal tubules, which would cause damage. However alkalinisation also increases the loss of methotrexate in the urine because at high pH values more of the drug exists in the ionised form, which is not readily reabsorbed by the tubules. This increased clearance was clearly shown in about 70 patients in whom alkalinisation of the urine (to pH greater than 7) with **sodium bicarbonate** and hydration reduced the serum methotrexate levels at 48 hours and 72 hours by 73% and 76%, respectively.[1] In this instance the interaction was being exploited therapeutically to avoid toxicity. This interaction has also been shown by others.[2,3] However, the possible consequences should be recognised if concurrent use is undertaken in other situations (e.g. if sodium bicarbonate is given as an antacid).

For the effects of acidic urine on methotrexate excretion see 'Methotrexate + Ascorbic acid (Vitamin C)', p.696.

1. Nirenberg A, Mosende C, Mehta BM, Gisolfi AL, Rosen G. High dose methotrexate with citrovorum factor rescue: predictive value of serum methotrexate concentrations and corrective measures to avert toxicity. *Cancer Treat Rep* (1977) 61, 779–83.
2. Sand TE, Jacobsen S. Effect of urine pH and flow on renal clearance of methotrexate. *Eur J Clin Pharmacol* (1981) 19, 453–6.
3. Shamash J, Earl H, Souhami R. Acetazolamide for alkalinisation of urine in patients receiving high-dose methotrexate. *Cancer Chemother Pharmacol* (1991) 28, 150–1.

Mifamurtide + Miscellaneous

Mifamurtide does not increase the renal toxicity of cisplatin or ifosfamide, nor the hepatic toxicity of ifosfamide or high-dose methotrexate. Ciclosporin, corticosteroids, and high-dose NSAIDs might interfere with the actions of mifamurtide.

Clinical evidence, mechanism, importance and management

(a) Ciclosporin

The concurrent use of ciclosporin or other calcineurin inhibitors [such as **tacrolimus**] is contraindicated due to a theoretical conflict in their mechanisms of action.[1]

(b) Cisplatin

The UK manufacturer of mifamurtide briefly notes that, in a study, it did not increase the renal toxicity of cisplatin, and that no mifamurtide dose adjustment is necessary on concurrent use.[1]

(c) Corticosteroids

The use of mifamurtide with corticosteroids (either long-term or routinely) should be avoided because the effects of corticosteroids on the immune system might antagonise those of mifamurtide and reduce its efficacy.[1]

(d) Doxorubicin

The UK manufacturer of mifamurtide recommends that its administration with doxorubicin or **other lipophilic drugs or products** should be separated if used as part of the same chemotherapy regime.[1]

(e) Ifosfamide

The UK manufacturer of mifamurtide briefly notes that, in a study, it did not increase the renal or hepatic toxicity of ifosfamide, and no mifamurtide dose adjustment is necessary on concurrent use.[1]

(f) Methotrexate

The manufacturer briefly notes that, in a study, mifamurtide did not increase the hepatic toxicity of high-dose methotrexate, and no mifamurtide dose adjustment is necessary on concurrent use.[1]

(g) NSAIDs

The UK manufacturer of mifamurtide briefly notes that, *in vitro*, high-dose NSAIDs can block the macrophage activating effects of mifamurtide and therefore concurrent use is contraindicated.[1]

1. Mepact (Mifamurtide). Takeda UK Ltd. UK Summary of product characteristics, December 2013.

Mitomycin + Doxorubicin

An increased incidence of cardiotoxicity has been seen in patients receiving mitomycin who were previously or simultaneously given doxorubicin.

Clinical evidence, mechanism, importance and management

Fourteen out of 91 patients (15.3%) with advanced breast cancer who had previously not responded to doxorubicin developed congestive heart failure when they were later given a combination of intravenous mitomycin 20 mg/m^2 every 4 to 6 weeks and megestrol acetate 160 mg daily. None of them had any pre-existing heart disease. This compares with only 3 out of 89 patients (3.5%) from another group who had received doxorubicin but no mitomycin. The maximum cumulative dose of doxorubicin was 450 mg/m^2 and all of the patients had also been given cyclophosphamide. Some of them also received other drugs during the doxorubicin phase. These included fluorouracil, methotrexate, tegafur and vincristine. The heart failure developed slowly (mean time of 8.5 months) compared with those in the control group (1.5 months).[1]

Other studies have also suggested that the combination of mitomycin and doxorubicin may increase cardiotoxicity.[2,3] In a randomised study, 2 of 39 patients given doxorubicin 45 mg/m^2 every 3 weeks and mitomycin 10 mg/m^2 every 6 weeks developed cardiomyopathy, compared with none of 42 patients given doxorubicin 75 mg/m^2 every 3 weeks alone.[4]

The reasons for this apparent synergistic cardiotoxicity are not understood, but it may be related to free radical generation. This interaction is not established with certainty. The authors of one report suggest that its incidence is probably less than 10%, and that it does not occur until a cumulative mitomycin dose of 30 mg/m^2 or more.[3] It may be prudent to monitor patients given mitomycin more closely if they have previously received anthracyclines.[1] Note that the combination (FAM, fluorouracil, doxorubicin and mitomycin) has been widely used for gastric cancer.

1. Buzdar AU, Legha SS, Tashima CK, Hortobagyi GN, Yap HY, Krutchik AN, Luna MA, Blumenschein GR. Adriamycin and mitomycin C: possible synergistic cardiotoxicity. *Cancer Treat Rep* (1978) 62, 1005–8.
2. Villani F, Comazzi R, Lacaita G, Guindani A, Genitoni V, Volonterio A, Brambilla MC. Possible enhancement of the cardiotoxicity of doxorubicin when combined with mitomycin C. *Med Oncol Tumor Pharmacother* (1985) 2, 93–7.
3. Verweij J, Funke-Küpper AJ, Teule GJJ, Pinedo HM. A prospective study on the dose dependency of cardiotoxicity induced by mitomycin C. *Med Oncol Tumor Pharmacother* (1988) 5, 159–63.
4. Andersson M, Daugaard S, von der Maase H, Mouridsen HT. Doxorubicin versus mitomycin versus doxorubicin plus mitomycin in advanced breast cancer: a randomized study. *Cancer Treat Rep* (1986) 70, 1181–6.

Mitomycin + Fluorouracil

Rarely, serious and potentially life-threatening intravascular haemolysis and renal failure may develop after the long-term use of mitomycin and fluorouracil.

Clinical evidence, mechanism, importance and management

Two patients developed chronic haemolysis and progressive renal impairment after the long-term use of mitomycin and fluorouracil following partial or total gastrectomy for gastric cancer. The haemolysis was exacerbated by blood transfusions. The authors of the report[1] suggested that these two cases were extreme examples of a syndrome that was becoming increasingly apparent in their pretransfusion patients, after the maintenance use of these drugs for 6 months or more. A similar syndrome occurred in 2 other patients, one with gastric carcinoma and one without, when given these two drugs.[2,3] This severe and potentially fatal syndrome has also been seen with mitomycin alone.[4,5] Its incidence is not known, but note that a regimen of fluorouracil, doxorubicin and mitomycin (FAM) has been widely used in gastric cancer and there are only a few reports of this syndrome. The authors of one report suggest that the drugs should be stopped at the first sign of intravascular haemolysis, persistent proteinuria and rising urea levels (two consecutive values above 8 mmol/L).[1] The syndrome has also occurred when tamoxifen was given to patients who had been treated with mitomycin, see 'Mitomycin + Tamoxifen', p.705.

1. Jones BG, Fielding JW, Newman CE, Howell A, Brookes VS. Intravascular haemolysis and renal impairment after blood transfusion in two patients on long-term 5-fluorouracil and mitomycin-C. *Lancet* (1980) i, 1275–7.
2. Krauss S, Sonoda T, Solomon A. Treatment of advanced gastrointestinal carcinoma with 5-fluorouracil and mitomycin C. *Cancer* (1979) 43, 1598–1603.
3. Lempert KD. Haemolysis and renal impairment syndrome in patients on 5-fluorouracil and mitomycin-C. *Lancet* (1980) ii, 369–70.
4. Rumpf KW, Reiger J, Lankisch PG, von Heyden HW, Nagel GA, Scheler F. Mitomycin-induced haemolysis and renal failure. *Lancet* (1980) ii, 1037–8.
5. Schiebe ME, Hoffmann W, Belka C, Bamberg M. Mitomycin C-related hemolytic uremic syndrome in cancer patients. *Anticancer Drugs* (1998) 9, 433–5.

Mitomycin + Furosemide

A study in 5 patients with advanced solid tumours receiving mitomycin C 10 mg/m^2 found that furosemide given as a 40 mg intravenous bolus either 120 minutes or 200 minutes after the mitomycin had no effect on its pharmacokinetics.[1]

1. Verweij J, Kerpel-Fronius S, Stuurman M, de Vries J, Pinedo HM. Absence of interaction between furosemide and mitomycin C. *Cancer Chemother Pharmacol* (1987) 19, 84–6.

Mitomycin + Tamoxifen

Haemolytic anaemia, thrombocytopenia and renal impairment, leading to potentially fatal haemolytic uraemic syndrome, has occurred in a few patients given tamoxifen with, or shortly after, mitomycin.

Clinical evidence, mechanism, importance and management

After a woman with metastatic breast cancer who had previously been given mitomycin, mitoxantrone and methotrexate, developed rapidly fatal acute renal failure 21 days after starting tamoxifen, a retrospective survey was undertaken of other patients who had also received all four of these drugs.[1] Nine out of 94 patients (9.6%) developed anaemia, thrombocytopenia and renal impairment, compared with none in another group of 45 patients not given tamoxifen. One of the 9 died from renal failure. The doses used were mitomycin 7 mg/m^2 intravenously every 42 days for four courses; mitoxantrone 7 mg/m^2 and methotrexate 35 mg/m^2 intravenously every 21 days for eight courses; and tamoxifen 20 mg orally daily.[1] A few other reports describe cases of haemolytic uraemic syndrome in patients given mitomycin and tamoxifen.[2-4]

The authors of the first study suggested that this haemolytic uraemic syndrome was due to a combination of subclinical endothelial damage induced by mitomycin, and a thrombotic effect on platelets caused by tamoxifen.[1] They advise the avoidance of tamoxifen with or shortly after mitomycin unless concurrent use can be carefully monitored. Erythropoietin may be useful in managing the syndrome.[4] This syndrome has also occurred rarely with mitomycin alone, and when mitomycin was given with fluorouracil, see 'Mitomycin + Fluorouracil', p.705.

1. Montes A, Powles TJ, O'Brien MER, Ashley SE, Luckit J, Treleaven J. A toxic interaction between mitomycin C and tamoxifen causing the haemolytic uraemic syndrome. *Eur J Cancer* (1993) 29A, 1854–7.
2. Ellis PA, Luckitt J, Treleaven J, Smith IE. Haemolytic uraemic syndrome in a patient with lung cancer: further evidence for a toxic interaction between mitomycin-C and tamoxifen. *Clin Oncol (R Coll Radiol)* (1996) 8, 402–3.
3. Arola O, Aho H, Asola M, Kauppila M, Nikkanen V, Voipio-Pulkki LM. Hemolyyttis-ureeminen oireyhtymä-mitomysiinihoidon vakava komplikaatio. *Duodecim* (1997) 113, 1923–9.
4. O'Brien MER, Casey S, Treleaven J, Powles TJ. Use of erythropoietin in the management of the haemolytic uraemic syndrome induced by mitomycin C/tamoxifen. *Eur J Cancer* (1994) 30A, 894–5.

Mitotane + Miscellaneous

The manufacturer advises that mitotane might reduce the plasma levels of drugs that are cytochrome P450 substrates. The absorption of mitotane may be increased when taken with food.

Clinical evidence, mechanism, importance and management

(a) Cytochrome P450 substrates

The manufacturer advises that mitotane may induce the activity of cytochrome P450 isoenzymes.[1,2] This appears to be based on a case report of decreased efficacy of warfarin (see 'Coumarins + Antineoplastics; Cytotoxic', p.403), and on studies in *rats*.[3] On this basis, the manufacturers give a general caution about the concurrent use of drugs influenced by hepatic enzyme induction.[1,2] However, if mitotane were an important enzyme inducer it might have been expected to have come to light by now, but there do not appear to be any case reports supporting this effect, other than the one case already mentioned with warfarin. On the basis of this proposed interaction, the UK manufacturer specifically recommends caution with **antiepileptics**, **griseofulvin**, **rifabutin**, **rifampicin**, and **St John's wort** (*Hypericum perforatum*).[1] However, most of these drugs are also enzyme inducers, with some being potent (e.g. rifampicin), and the effect of adding another modest enzyme-inducer is probably unlikely to be clinically relevant.

In summary, there is too little information available to warrant a general caution for the use of mitotane with all cytochrome P450 substrates that have a narrow therapeutic index. Further study is needed.

(b) Food

The UK manufacturer notes that the absorption of mitotane was increased when it was given with food (although they say the relative bioavailability was not calculated), and they say that mitotane should be preferably taken with meals.[1] The US information does not mention this effect, nor give any advice about administration in relation to meals.[2]

1. Lysodren (Mitotane). HRA Pharma UK Ltd. UK Summary of product characteristics, April 2009.
2. Lysodren (Mitotane). Bristol-Myers Squibb Company. US Prescribing information, February 2009.
3. EMEA Scientific discussion. 2005, 1–45.

Mitotane + Spironolactone

In an isolated report, the effects of mitotane appeared to be inhibited by spironolactone in a patient with Cushing's disease.

Clinical evidence, mechanism, importance and management

A woman with Cushing's disease taking chlorpropamide, digoxin and furosemide was given spironolactone 50 mg four times daily to control hypokalaemia. She was also given mitotane 3 g daily for 5 months to control the elevated cortisol levels, but this had no effect.[1] When an interaction was suspected (on the basis of *animal* studies[1]) it was decided to withdraw the spironolactone, whereupon severe nausea and profuse diarrhoea developed within 24 to 48 hours, suggesting mitotane toxicity. This subsided, and then redeveloped when the mitotane was stopped, and then restarted a week later. The mechanism of this apparent interaction is not understood. It would seem that mitotane can become ineffective in the management of Cushing's syndrome in the presence of spironolactone. The UK manufacturer of mitotane contraindicates its use with spironolactone,[2] while the US manufacturer does not mention this interaction.[3]

1. Wortsman J, Soler NG. Mitotane. Spironolactone antagonism in Cushing's syndrome. *JAMA* (1977) 238, 2527.
2. Lysodren (Mitotane). HRA Pharma UK Ltd. UK Summary of product characteristics, April 2009.
3. Lysodren (Mitotane). Bristol-Myers Squibb Company. US Prescribing information, February 2009.

Nitrosoureas + Cimetidine

The bone marrow depressant effects of carmustine and lomustine are possibly increased by cimetidine.

Clinical evidence

Nine patients given **carmustine** 80 mg/m^2 daily for 3 days, cimetidine 300 mg four times daily for one to 4 weeks, steroids, and cranial irradiation over 6 weeks, had marked leucopenia during the first cycle. Bone marrow aspirates confirmed the marked decrease in granulocytic elements in 2 patients. In comparison, 31 patients similarly treated, but without cimetidine, had no significant white cell depression.[1,2]

Neutropenia was found in a man taking regular cimetidine, phenytoin, phenobarbital, and dexamethasone, 53 days after he was given **lomustine** 120 mg, and 16 days after he was given **lomustine** 160 mg. The cimetidine was discontinued and the neutropenia rapidly reversed within 14 days. The neutrophil nadir from the **lomustine** 160 mg dose occurred after a further 16 to 19 days and was much less severe than the first episode.[3]

Mechanism

Studies in *animals* suggest that cimetidine impairs the clearance of carmustine.[4]

Importance and management

Information appears to be limited to the reports cited, but it seems to be an established reaction. Patients given both lomustine or carmustine and cimetidine should be closely monitored for changes in blood cell counts. Because of its immunomodulatory effects, cimetidine has been used as an adjunct to carmustine in the treatment of malignant melanoma, but this did not improve outcomes.[5]

1. Selker RG, Moore P, LoDolce D. Bone-marrow depression with cimetidine plus carmustine. *N Engl J Med* (1978) 299, 834.
2. Volkin RL, Shadduck RK, Winkelstein A, Zeigler ZR, Selker RG. Potentiation of carmustine-cranial irradiation-induced myelosuppression by cimetidine. *Arch Intern Med* (1982) 142, 243–5.
3. Hess WA, Kornblith PL. Combination of lomustine and cimetidine in the treatment of a patient with malignant glioblastoma: a case report. *Cancer Treat Rep* (1985) 69, 733.
4. Dorr RT, Soble MJ. H_2-Antagonists and carmustine. *J Cancer Res Clin Oncol* (1989) 115, 41–6.
5. Morton RF, Creagan ET, Schaid DJ, Kardinal CG, McCormack GW, McHale MS, Wiesenfeld M. Phase II trial of recombinant leukocyte A interferon (IFN-α2A) plus 1,3-bis(2-chloroethyl)-1-nitrosourea (BCNU) and the combination cimetidine with BCNU in patients with disseminated malignant melanoma. *Am J Clin Oncol* (1991) 14, 152–5.

Nitrosoureas; Lomustine + Phenobarbital

***Animal* studies have shown that the antitumour effects and the toxicity of lomustine are markedly reduced by phenobarbital. It is suggested that the metabolism of lomustine is accelerated by the enzyme-inducing effects of phenobarbital.[1] There appears to be no clinical data confirming this; nevertheless, it would be prudent to bear the possibility of an interaction in mind if both drugs are given.**

1. Siemann DW. Effect of pretreatment with phenobarbital or SKF 525A on the toxicity and antitumor activity of lomustine. *Cancer Treat Rep* (1983) 67, 259–65.

Nitrosoureas; Lomustine + Theophylline

A single case report describes thrombocytopenia and bleeding, which was attributed to the concurrent use of lomustine and theophylline.

Clinical evidence, mechanism, importance and management

An woman with asthma taking theophylline and given lomustine, prednisone and vincristine for medulloblastoma, developed severe nose bleeding and thrombocytopenia 3 weeks after the third cycle of chemotherapy.[1] This was attributed to the concurrent use of lomustine and theophylline. The suggested explanation for this effect is that theophylline inhibited the activity of phosphodiesterase within the platelets, thereby increasing cyclic AMP levels and disrupting normal platelet function (which seems to be supported by an experimental study[2]) while lomustine causes thrombocytopenia. What is known is far too limited to act as more than a warning of the possibility of increased thrombocytopenia during the concurrent use of theophylline and lomustine.

1. Zeltzer PM, Feig SA. Theophylline-induced lomustine toxicity. *Lancet* (1979) ii, 960–1.
2. DeWys WD, Bathina S. Synergistic anti-tumour effect of cyclic AMP elevation (induced by theophylline) and cytotoxic drug treatment. *Proc Am Assoc Cancer Res* (1978) 19, 104.

Panitumumab + Antineoplastics

The efficacy of panitumumab was reduced and the toxicity increased when it was given with bevacizumab-containing chemotherapy regimens. When panitumumab was given with irinotecan, bolus fluorouracil plus folinic acid (IFL) there was a high incidence of severe diarrhoea.

Clinical evidence

(a) Bevacizumab with chemotherapy

In an interim analysis of a study of 823 patients randomised to receive bevacizumab plus **oxaliplatin**-based regimens, with or without panitumumab, there was an increased incidence of adverse effects (skin toxicity, diarrhoea, infections, pulmonary embolism), a shortened progression-free survival time (10 months versus 11.4 months) and increased deaths (from pulmonary embolism) in those receiving panitumumab.[1] In a smaller cohort receiving panitumumab with bevacizumab plus **irinotecan**-based regimens similar increased toxicity without improved efficacy was seen. Patients receiving panitumumab received a lower dose-intensity of the cytotoxics (**oxaliplatin**, **irinotecan**, **fluorouracil**) because of the toxicities experienced.[2]

(b) IFL and FOLFIRI

A high incidence of severe (grade 3 to 4) diarrhoea (58%) was noted when panitumumab was given to 19 patients who also received the IFL regimen (irinotecan, bolus fluorouracil and folinic acid): the concurrent use of these drugs was considered to be poorly tolerated.[3] In another arm of this study a 25% incidence of grade 3 diarrhoea was seen when panitumumab was added to the FOLFIRI regimen (irinotecan, folinic acid and infusional fluorouracil).[3]

Mechanism

Unknown. A pharmacokinetic interaction would not be anticipated.

Importance and management

Panitumumab is currently indicated for use only as monotherapy after the failure of chemotherapy.[2,4] One study shows that the effect of combining it with another monoclonal antibody, bevacizumab, plus chemotherapy is detrimental, and this combination should not be used. A high incidence of severe diarrhoea was also seen in the study with IFL, and the UK manufacturer advises against using this combination.[4]

1. Hecht JR, Mitchell E, Chidiac T, Scroggin C, Hagenstad C, Spigel D, Marshall J, Cohn A, McCollum D, Stella P, Deeter R, Shahin S, Amado RG. A randomized phase IIIB trial of chemotherapy, bevacizumab, and panitumumab compared with chemotherapy and bevacizumab alone for metastatic colorectal cancer. *J Clin Oncol* (2009) 27, 672–80.
2. Vectibix (Panitumumab). Amgen Inc. US Prescribing information, July 2009.
3. Berlin J, Posey J, Tchekmedyian S, Hu E, Chan D, Malik I, Yang L, Amado RG, Hecht JR. Panitumumab with irinotecan/leucovorin/5-fluorouracil for first-line treatment of metastatic colorectal cancer. *Clin Colorectal Cancer* (2007) 6, 427–32.
4. Vectibix (Panitumumab). Amgen Ltd. UK Summary of product characteristics, April 2009.

Pemetrexed + Aspirin or NSAIDs

NSAIDs are predicted to decrease the renal excretion of pemetrexed. However, aspirin and ibuprofen had little effect on pemetrexed clearance in patients with normal renal function.

Clinical evidence

In a study in 27 patients with advanced cancer, aspirin 325 mg every 6 hours for 9 doses, starting 2 days before pemetrexed, and with the last dose one hour before an infusion of pemetrexed 500 mg/m^2, had no effect on the pharmacokinetics of pemetrexed.[1] In a similar study, **ibuprofen** 400 mg four times daily caused a 16% decrease in the clearance of pemetrexed, and increased its AUC by 20%.[1]

Mechanism

Pemetrexed is largely cleared unchanged from the body by renal excretion. The NSAIDs as a group inhibit the synthesis of the prostaglandins (PGE_2) resulting in a reduction in renal perfusion, which could lead to a rise in pemetrexed serum concentrations, accompanied by increased toxicity.

Importance and management

The modest increase in pemetrexed exposure seen with ibuprofen 1.6 g daily or aspirin 1.3 g daily is unlikely to be clinically relevant in patients with *normal renal function*, and they may be used in these patients. However, the effects of higher doses of aspirin or ibuprofen are not known, and they could be greater. Because of this, in patients with normal renal function, the manufacturer recommends caution when pemetrexed is used with high doses of NSAIDs (e.g. ibuprofen greater than 1.6 g daily) or high-dose aspirin (greater than 1.3 g daily).[2] Moreover, the manufacturers state that in patients with *mild to moderate renal impairment* (creatinine clearance from 45 to 79 mL/minute), NSAIDs with short half-lives, such as ibuprofen, higher dose aspirin,[2] **diclofenac** or **indometacin**[3] should be completely avoided from 2 days before to 2 days after pemetrexed use.

Because of the lack of data on pemetrexed clearance with NSAIDs with longer half-lives (the manufacturers name **meloxicam**, **nabumetone**, and **piroxicam**), they recommend that all patients taking these NSAIDs should stop them from 5 days before to 2 days after pemetrexed.[2,3] If the use of pemetrexed with an NSAID is necessary, the UK manufacturer advises close monitoring for adverse effects, especially myelosuppression and gastrointestinal toxicity.[2]

1. Sweeney CJ, Takimoto CH, Latz JE, Baker SD, Murry DJ, Krull JH, Fife K, Battiato L, Cleverly A, Chaudhary AK, Chaudhuri T, Sandler A, Mita AC, Rowinsky EK. Two drug interaction studies evaluating the pharmacokinetics and toxicity of pemetrexed when coadministered with aspirin or ibuprofen in patients with advanced cancer. *Clin Cancer Res* (2006) 12, 536–42.
2. Alimta (Pemetrexed disodium). Eli Lilly and Company Ltd. UK Summary of product characteristics, July 2012.
3. Alimta (Pemetrexed disodium). Eli Lilly and Company. US Prescribing information, October 2012.

Pemetrexed + Gemcitabine

The concurrent use of pemetrexed and gemcitabine does not affect the pharmacokinetics of either drug.

Clinical evidence, mechanism, importance and management

In one study in 4 patients, the pharmacokinetics of pemetrexed were not affected when pemetrexed was given 90 minutes after gemcitabine on day one, when compared with its use alone on day 8.[1] Similarly, another report describes a study in 14 patients in which there was no pharmacokinetic interaction between pemetrexed and gemcitabine when a single dose of pemetrexed was given immediately after gemcitabine (gemcitabine 1.25 g/m^2 was given on days 1 and 8 of a 21-day cycle, with pemetrexed 500 mg/m^2 on day 8, for 84 cycles).[2]

1. Adjei AA, Erlichman C, Sloan JA, Reid JM, Pitot HC, Goldberg RM, Peethambaram P, Atherton P, Hanson LJ, Alberts SR, Jett J. Phase I and pharmacologic study of sequences of gemcitabine and the multitargeted antifolate agent in patients with advanced solid tumors. *J Clin Oncol* (2000) 18, 1748–57.
2. Adjei AA. Clinical studies of pemetrexed and gemcitabine combinations. *Ann Oncol* (2006) 17, v29–v32.

Pemetrexed + Miscellaneous

Caution is recommended if pemetrexed is given with nephrotoxic drugs such as the aminoglycosides, cisplatin, loop diuretics, and ciclosporin, and drugs that are secreted by the renal tubules, such as probenecid and penicillin. No pharmacokinetic interaction occurs between pemetrexed and cisplatin.

Clinical evidence, mechanism, importance and management

(a) Cisplatin

The US manufacturer states that there is no pharmacokinetic interaction between pemetrexed and cisplatin,[1] but there is the possibility that cisplatin-induced nephrotoxicity could decrease pemetrexed clearance and increase its toxicity.[1,2] However, it should be noted that the use of pemetrexed with cisplatin is licensed for some indications (e.g. mesothelioma).[1,2]

(b) Folic acid and Vitamin B_{12}

Oral folic acid and intramuscular vitamin B_{12} do not alter the pharmacokinetics of pemetrexed[1] and because these vitamins were found to decrease pemetrexed toxicity, it is recommended that all patients receiving pemetrexed should receive folic acid and vitamin B_{12} supplements.[1,2]

(c) Nephrotoxic drugs

The manufacturers consider that the concurrent use of nephrotoxic drugs could potentially decrease the clearance of pemetrexed and therefore increase its toxicity.[1,2] In the UK, the manufacturer specifically mentions **aminoglycosides**, **loop diuretics**, **platinum compounds** (see also *Cisplatin*, above) and **ciclosporin**, and recommends caution on concurrent use, and, if necessary, close monitoring of creatinine clearance.[2]

(d) Probenecid and other drugs secreted by the renal tubules

It is possible that drugs that are secreted by the renal tubules (e.g. probenecid, **penicillin**) could decrease the clearance of pemetrexed, which is also secreted by this mechanism. For this reason, the manufacturer recommends caution on concurrent use, and, if necessary, close monitoring of creatinine clearance.[2]

1. Alimta (Pemetrexed disodium). Eli Lilly and Company. US Prescribing information, October 2012.
2. Alimta (Pemetrexed disodium). Eli Lilly and Company Ltd. UK Summary of product characteristics, July 2012.

Pomalidomide + Carbamazepine

Carbamazepine does not have a clinically relevant effect on the exposure to pomalidomide.

Clinical evidence

In a study, 16 healthy subjects were given carbamazepine 100 mg twice daily for 5 doses, then 200 mg twice daily for 8 days, with a single 4-mg dose of pomalidomide on the penultimate day. It was found that carbamazepine decreased the AUC of pomalidomide by about 25%, and decreased its maximum concentration by 25%, when compared with pomalidomide given alone.[1]

Mechanism

Pomalidomide is primarily metabolised by CYP1A2 and CYP3A4, and it is also a substrate for P-glycoprotein.[1] Carbamazepine is an inducer of both CYP3A4 and P-glycoprotein, and therefore decreases pomalidomide exposure.

Importance and management

The evidence for an interaction between pomalidomide and carbamazepine is limited to one study, and is not established. However, the slight decrease in pomalidomide exposure seen is unlikely to be clinically relevant and no pomalidomide dose adjustment appears to be necessary on concurrent use. The US manufacturer of pomalidomide predicts that other CYP3A4 inducers might increase its exposure,[2] but on the basis of the interaction with carbamazepine, any increase might not be expected to be clinically relevant. For a list of CYP3A4 inducers, see 'Table 1.9', p.11.

1. Kasserra C, Assaf M, Hoffmann M, Li Y, Liu L, Wang X, Kumar G, Palmisano M. Pomalidomide: evaluation of cytochrome P450 and transporter-mediated drug-drug interaction potential in vitro and in healthy subjects. *J Clin Pharmacol* (2015) 55, 168–78.
2. Pomalyst (Pomalidomide). Celgene Corporation. US Prescribing information, April 2015.

Pomalidomide + Fluvoxamine

Concurrent use of fluvoxamine appears to moderately increase pomalidomide exposure. Other potent CYP1A2 inhibitors are predicted to interact similarly.

Clinical evidence

In a study, 12 healthy subjects were given fluvoxamine 50 mg twice daily (with **ketoconazole** 200 mg twice daily) for 7 days, with a single 4-mg dose of pomalidomide on day 5. The AUC and maximum concentration of pomalidomide were increased about 2-fold and by 13%, respectively, when compared with pomalidomide and ketoconazole without fluvoxamine.[1]

Mechanism

Pomalidomide is primarily metabolised by CYP1A2 and CYP3A4.[1] Fluvoxamine is a potent inhibitor of CYP1A2, and therefore increases pomalidomide exposure.

Importance and management

An interaction between pomalidomide and fluvoxamine, a potent CYP1A2 inhibitor, is limited to a single study and is not established. However, the moderate increase in pomalidomide exposure seen on concurrent use of fluvoxamine is likely to be clinically relevant. The US manufacturer of pomalidomide recommends that the concurrent use of potent CYP1A2 inhibitors should be avoided, but if both drugs are given, monitor for pomalidomide adverse effects and reduce the pomalidomide dose if necessary.[2] The US manufacturer also states that if pomalidomide must be given with a potent CYP1A2 inhibitor *and* a drug that is both a potent CYP3A4 inhibitor and a P-glycoprotein inhibitor (such as **ketoconazole**), the dose of pomalidomide should be halved[2] (for a list of potent CYP3A4 inhibitors see 'Table 1.9', p.11, and for a list of P-glycoprotein inhibitors see 'Table 1.12', p.14). However, note that in a study, ketoconazole did not have a clinically relevant effect on the exposure to pomalidomide, see 'Pomalidomide + Ketoconazole and other CYP3A4 inhibitors or P-glycoprotein inhibitors', p.708. Until further evidence is available, it would seem prudent to closely monitor patients for pomalidomide adverse effects on the concurrent use of fluvoxamine or other potent CYP1A2 inhibitors, and to reduce the pomalidomide dose if necessary. For a list of potent CYP1A2 inhibitors, see 'Table 1.2', p.5. Note that both the UK and US manufacturers specifically name **ciprofloxacin** as a potent CYP1A2 inhibitor,[2,3] but it is generally considered to be a moderate inhibitor.

1. Kasserra C, Assaf M, Hoffmann M, Li Y, Liu L, Wang X, Kumar G, Palmisano M. Pomalidomide: evaluation of cytochrome P450 and transporter-mediated drug-drug interaction potential in vitro and in healthy subjects. *J Clin Pharmacol* (2015) 55, 168–78.
2. Pomalyst (Pomalidomide). Celgene Corporation. US Prescribing information, April 2015.
3. Imnovid (Pomalidomide). Celgene Ltd. UK Summary of product characteristics, May 2015.

Pomalidomide + Ketoconazole and other CYP3A4 inhibitors or P-glycoprotein inhibitors

Ketoconazole does not have a clinically relevant effect on the exposure to pomalidomide. Other CYP3A4 or P-glycoprotein inhibitors might act similarly.

Clinical evidence

In a study, 16 healthy subjects were given ketoconazole 200 mg twice daily for a week, with a single 4-mg dose of pomalidomide on day 5. Ketoconazole increased the AUC of pomalidomide by almost 19%, and increased the maximum concentration of pomalidomide by about 7%, when compared with pomalidomide given alone.[1]

Mechanism

Pomalidomide is primarily metabolised by CYP1A2 and CYP3A4, and is also a substrate of P-glycoprotein.[1] Ketoconazole, a potent inhibitor of CYP3A4 and a known inhibitor of P-glycoprotein, therefore increases pomalidomide exposure.

Importance and management

An interaction between pomalidomide and CYP3A4 or P-glycoprotein inhibitors is limited to one study with ketoconazole. The negligible increase in pomalidomide exposure seen is unlikely to be clinically relevant, and no dose adjustment would be considered to be necessary on concurrent use. However, note that the ketoconazole dose used in the study was a starting dose, therefore some caution might be prudent if larger doses of ketoconazole are given. Other CYP3A4 or P-glycoprotein inhibitors would not be expected to interact with pomalidomide to a clinically relevant extent via these mechanisms.

1. Kasserra C, Assaf M, Hoffmann M, Li Y, Liu L, Wang X, Kumar G, Palmisano M. Pomalidomide: evaluation of cytochrome P450 and transporter-mediated drug-drug interaction potential in vitro and in healthy subjects. *J Clin Pharmacol* (2015) 55, 168–78.

Pomalidomide + Miscellaneous

CYP1A2 inducers might reduce the exposure to pomalidomide. A high-fat, high-calorie meal did not affect pomalidomide exposure to a clinically relevant extent. Dexamethasone had no clinically relevant effect on the pharmacokinetics of pomalidomide, but thrombotic events have been reported on concurrent use; the risk might be further increased by the concurrent use of epoetins.

Clinical evidence, mechanism, importance and management

(a) CYP1A2 inducers

The US manufacturer of pomalidomide briefly notes that CYP1A2 inducers (such as **tobacco smoke**) might reduce the exposure to pomalidomide.[1] Pomalidomide is a substrate for this isoenzyme. Until evidence for an interaction becomes available, it would seem prudent to be alert for a reduction in pomalidomide efficacy on the concurrent use of CYP1A2 inducers. For a list of CYP1A2 inducers, see 'Table 1.2', p.5.

(b) Dexamethasone

The UK and US manufacturers of pomalidomide note that in patients with multiple myeloma taking pomalidomide 4 mg daily, concurrent use of **dexamethasone** 20 to 40 mg daily did not affect the pharmacokinetics of pomalidomide, when compared to pomalidomide given alone.[1,2] Therefore no pomalidomide dose adjustment appears necessary on concurrent use. Note that pomalidomide is licensed for use with dexamethasone.[1,2]

(c) Epoetins

The UK and US manufacturers of pomalidomide note that deep vein thrombosis, pulmonary embolism, and arterial thrombotic events have been reported in patients taking pomalidomide (with dexamethasone). The UK manufacturer states that the concurrent use of erythropoetic agents (which would include the epoetins) might further increase this risk, and therefore patients should be monitored for signs or symptoms of thrombotic events on the concurrent use of pomalidomide (with dexamethasone) and drugs which stimulate erythropoiesis, or with other drugs which can increase the risk of thrombosis.[2]

(d) Food

The UK manufacturer briefly reports that, in a study, giving pomalidomide with a high-fat, high-calorie meal decreased its maximum concentration and AUC by about 25% and 8%, respectively. This small reduction in exposure is unlikely to be clinically relevant, therefore they advise that pomalidomide can be taken with or without food.[2] In contrast, the US manufacturer advises that it should be taken at least 2 hours before or 2 hours after a meal.[1]

1. Pomalyst (Pomalidomide). Celgene Corporation. US Prescribing information, April 2015.
2. Imnovid (Pomalidomide). Celgene Ltd. UK Summary of product characteristics, May 2015.

Procarbazine + Antiepileptics; Enzyme-inducing

The use of phenytoin, phenobarbital or carbamazepine might increase the risk of procarbazine hypersensitivity reactions, and at high doses of procarbazine, a few cases of severe hepatotoxicity were seen with phenytoin and carbamazepine plus zolpidem. The pharmacokinetics of procarbazine did not appear to differ when given with phenytoin, phenobarbital or carbamazepine.

Clinical evidence

A retrospective study of the records of 83 patients with primary brain tumours who were given procarbazine between 1981 and 1996 found that 20 of them had experienced procarbazine hypersensitivity reactions. Of these 20, 95% had also taken antiepileptics, compared with 71% of those not developing hypersensitivity. In addition, there was a significant dose-response association between the development of hypersensitivity reactions and the serum levels of the antiepileptics used (**phenytoin, phenobarbital**, or **carbamazepine**, with or without valproate).[1]

In a prospective study, the pharmacokinetics of procarbazine did not differ between 31 patients taking enzyme-inducing antiepileptics (**carbamazepine**, **oxcarbazepine**, **phenobarbital** or **phenytoin**) and 18 patients taking non-enzyme-inducing antiepileptics or no antiepileptics. Procarbazine was given daily for 5 days every 4 weeks at a starting dose of 200 mg/m² escalated to the maximum tolerated dose. At procarbazine doses of 393 mg/m² and 429 mg/m², there were two cases of severe hepatic dysfunction in patients taking **phenytoin** (one of which was fatal), and one in a patient taking **carbamazepine** and **zolpidem** (this resolved on stopping the **zolpidem**). In addition, at a dose of procarbazine 343 mg/m², there was one case of liver dysfunction in a patient not taking enzyme-inducing antiepileptics, at which point the study was halted. In this study, the concurrent use of **dexamethasone** with or without enzyme-inducing antiepileptics also did not affect procarbazine pharmacokinetics.[2]

Mechanism

It was suggested that the enzyme-inducing antiepileptics may increase the metabolism of procarbazine to metabolites causing hypersensitivity.[1] However, no change in the pharmacokinetics of procarbazine itself was seen; suggesting this is unlikely.[2] Procarbazine clearly inhibited its own metabolism, which suggests that it might also inhibit the metabolism of the antiepileptics and this might have increased the risk of hepatotoxicity. However, hepatotoxicity may have also been a result of the high dose of procarbazine. Further study is needed.[2]

Importance and management

Enzyme-inducing antiepileptics do not appear to alter the pharmacokinetics of procarbazine, and, in clinical practice, the dose of procarbazine is not modified in patients taking these drugs.[2] There is some evidence that the incidence of procarbazine-induced hypersensitivity is higher in patients receiving enzyme-inducing antiepileptics. In one dose-finding study, an unexpectedly high incidence of hepatotoxicity was seen with high-dose procarbazine, and a possible interaction with enzyme-inducing antiepileptics could not be ruled out.

1. Lehmann DF, Hurteau TE, Newman N, Coyle TE. Anticonvulsant usage is associated with an increased risk of procarbazine hypersensitivity reactions in patients with brain tumours. *Clin Pharmacol Ther* (1997) 62, 225–9.
2. Grossman SA, Carson KA, Batchelor TT, Lesser G, Mikkelsen T, Alavi JB, Phuphanich S, Hammour T, Fisher JD, Supko JG. The effect of enzyme-inducing antiseizure drugs on the pharmacokinetics and tolerability of procarbazine hydrochloride. *Clin Cancer Res* (2006) 12, 5174–81.

Procarbazine + Chlormethine (Mechlorethamine)

A report suggests that, in two patients, the use of high doses of procarbazine with chlormethine may result in neurological toxicity.

Clinical evidence, mechanism, importance and management

Two patients with acute myelogenous leukaemia admitted to hospital for bone marrow transplantation and who were given *high doses* of procarbazine 12.5 mg/kg and 15 mg/kg with chlormethine 0.75 mg/kg and 1 mg/kg on the same day became lethargic, somnolent and disorientated for about a week. Two other patients who received the same drugs, but not on the same day, had no neurological complications. In addition, only one of 45 patients given high-dose procarbazine alone had similar persistent lethargy. Although no interaction has been proved, the authors suggest that the chlormethine may have enhanced the neurotoxic effects of the procarbazine, and advise that it would be prudent to avoid high-doses of these drugs on the same day.[1] Note that lower doses of the combination have been widely used in the MOPP regimen (mechlorethamine, vincristine, procarbazine, and prednisone) without problems.

1. Weiss GB, Weiden PL, Thomas ED. Central nervous system disturbances after combined administration of procarbazine and mechlorethamine. *Cancer Treat Rep* (1977) 61, 1713–14.

Procarbazine + Miscellaneous

The effects of drugs that can cause CNS depression or lower blood pressure may possibly be increased by the presence of procarbazine. Some caution might be appropriate with tricyclics, as procarbazine is a weak MAOI.

Clinical evidence, mechanism, importance and management

(a) Antihypertensives

In one early clinical study, 4 of 48 patients developed postural hypotension when given procarbazine. In addition, another patient with hypertension (180/110 mmHg) had a progressive fall in blood pressure (to 110/80 mmHg) while taking procarbazine.[1] Additive hypotensive effects may therefore be expected if procarbazine is given to patients taking antihypertensives.

(b) CNS depressants

Procarbazine can cause CNS depression ranging from mild drowsiness to profound stupor. In early clinical studies, the incidence was variously reported as 8%, 14%, and 31% (when combined with prochlorperazine).[1-3] Additive CNS depression may therefore be expected if other drugs possessing CNS-depressant activity are given with procarbazine. The US manufacturer names **barbiturates**, **antihistamines**, **narcotics** and **phenothiazines**.[4]

(c) Prochlorperazine

An isolated report describes an acute dystonic reaction (difficulty in speaking or moving, intermittent contractions of muscles on the left side of the neck) in a patient taking procarbazine with prochlorperazine.[5] Prochlorperazine was thought to have contributed to the sedative effects of procarbazine in one early clinical study.[3]

(d) Tricyclics

Procarbazine is a weak inhibitor of MAO (see 'Procarbazine + Sympathomimetics', p.709), and it could therefore theoretically interact with tricyclics, in a similar way to the conventional MAOIs (see 'MAOIs or RIMAs + Tricyclic and related antidepressants', p.1403). On this basis, the US manufacturer specifically advises avoiding the concurrent use of tricyclics such as amitriptyline and imipramine,[4] whereas the UK manufacturer advises caution.[6]

1. Samuels ML, Leary WV, Alexanian R, Howe CD, Frei E. Clinical trials with N-isopropyl-α-(2-methylhydrazino)-p-toluamide hydrochloride in malignant lymphoma and other disseminated neoplasia. *Cancer* (1967) 20. 1187–94.
2. Stolinsky DC, Solomon J, Pugh RP, Stevens AR, Jacobs EM, Irwin LE, Wood DA, Steinfeld JL, Bateman JR. Clinical experience with procarbazine in Hodgkin's disease, reticulum cell sarcoma, and lymphosarcoma. *Cancer* (1970) 26, 984–90.
3. Brunner KW, Young CW. A methylhydrazine derivative in Hodgkin's disease and other malignant neoplasms: therapeutic and toxic effects studied in 51 patients. *Ann Intern Med* (1965) 63, 69–86.
4. Matulane (Procarbazine hydrochloride). Sigma-tau Pharmaceuticals Inc. US Prescribing information, March 2008.
5. Poster DS. Procarbazine-prochlorperazine interaction: an underreported phenomenon. *J Med* (1978) 9, 519–24.
6. Procarbazine (Procarbazine hydrochloride). Cambridge Laboratories. UK Summary of product characteristics, August 2006.

Procarbazine + Sympathomimetics

Despite warnings, it seems doubtful that the weak MAO-inhibitory properties of procarbazine can, under normal circumstances, cause a hypertensive reaction with tyramine-rich foods or sympathomimetic drugs.

Clinical evidence, mechanism, importance and management

The manufacturers say that procarbazine is a weak inhibitor of MAO and therefore predict that interactions with certain foods and drugs may occur in rare cases.[1,2] This is apparently based on the results of *animal* studies, which show that the monoamine oxidase inhibitory properties of procarbazine are weaker than pheniprazine.[3] There seem to be no formal reports of hypertensive reactions in patients taking procarbazine who have eaten tyramine-containing foods (e.g. cheese) or after using indirectly-acting sympathomimetic amines (e.g. **phenylpropanolamine**, **amfetamines**, etc.). The only account traced is purely anecdotal and unconfirmed: one author states that he can recall one patient who had a vivid reaction to wine and chicken livers when taking MOPP (mechlorethamine, vincristine, procarbazine, and prednisone) several years earlier.[4] A practical way to deal with this interaction problem has been suggested by a practitioner in an oncology unit:[4] patients taking procarbazine should ideally be given a list of the potentially interacting foodstuffs (see 'MAOIs or RIMAs + Food; Tyramine-containing', p.1389), with a warning about the nature of the possible reaction but also with the advice that it very rarely occurs. The foods may continue to be eaten, but patients should start with small quantities to ensure that they still agree with them. Those taking MOPP should also be told that any reaction is most likely to occur during the second week of a 14-day course of treatment with procarbazine, and during the week after it has been stopped.

1. Procarbazine (Procarbazine hydrochloride). Cambridge Laboratories. UK Summary of product characteristics, August 2006.
2. Matulane (Procarbazine hydrochloride). Sigma-tau Pharmaceuticals Inc. US Prescribing information, March 2008.
3. De Vita VT, Hahn MA, Oliverio VT. Monoamine oxidase inhibition by a new carcinostatic agent. N-isopropyl-α-(2-methylhydrazino)-p-toluamide (MIH). *Proc Soc Exp Biol Med* (1965) 120, 561–5.
4. Maxwell MB. Reexamining the dietary restrictions with procarbazine (an MAOI). *Cancer Nurs* (1980) 3, 451–7.

Raltitrexed + Miscellaneous

On theoretical grounds the manufacturers say that folinic acid and folic acid may possibly interfere with the action of raltitrexed. Warfarin and NSAIDs do not appear to interact with raltitrexed.

Clinical evidence, mechanism, importance and management

(a) Folinates

The antimetabolite, raltitrexed, is a folate analogue and is a potent and specific inhibitor of the enzyme thymidylate synthase. Inhibition of this enzyme ultimately interferes with the synthesis of deoxyribonucleic acid (DNA) leading to cell death. The intracellular polyglutamation of raltitrexed leads to the formation of even more potent inhibitors of thymidylate synthase. Folate (methylene tetrahydrofolate) is a co-factor required by thymidylate synthase and therefore theoretically folinic acid or folic acid may interfere with the action of raltitrexed. Clinical interaction studies have not yet been undertaken to confirm these predicted interactions.[1]

(b) Warfarin and NSAIDs

The manufacturers say that no specific clinical interaction studies have been conducted, but a review of the clinical study database did not reveal any evidence of interactions between raltitrexed and warfarin, NSAIDs or other drugs.[1]

1. Tomudex (Raltitrexed). AstraZeneca UK Ltd. UK Summary of product characteristics, August 2008.

Romidepsin + Miscellaneous

Romidepsin might increase the effects of warfarin and related drugs. CYP3A4 inhibitors and inducers are predicted to increase and decrease the plasma concentration of romidepsin, respectively. P-glycoprotein inhibitors are also predicted to increase the plasma concentration of romidepsin.

Clinical evidence, mechanism, importance and management

(a) Coumarins and related drugs

The US manufacturer of romidepsin briefly notes that, the prothrombin time and INR were increased in a patient receiving romidepsin with **warfarin**. On this basis, they advise that prothrombin time and INR should be carefully monitored in patients receiving concurrent romidepsin and warfarin or related drugs [e.g. **acenocoumarol** and **phenprocoumon**].[1]

(b) CYP3A4 inducers

The US manufacturer notes that romidepsin is predominantly metabolised by CYP3A4 and predicts that concurrent use with potent CYP3A4 inducers (they name **carbamazepine**, **dexamethasone**, **phenobarbital** (and therefore **primidone**), **phenytoin** (and therefore **fosphenytoin**), **rifabutin**, **rifampicin**, and **rifapentine**) might decrease plasma romidepsin concentrations and should be avoided,[1] presumably because romidepsin is likely to be less effective in the presence of these drugs. However, note that dexamethasone does not usually cause clinically relevant interactions by this mechanism. In addition, the use of **St John's wort** is also not recommended.[1] For a list of CYP3A4 inducers, see 'Table 1.9', p.11.

(c) CYP3A4 inhibitors

The US manufacturer notes that romidepsin is predominantly metabolised by CYP3A4 and predicts that concurrent use with potent CYP3A4 inhibitors (they name the azoles **itraconazole**, **ketoconazole**, and **voriconazole**, the macrolides **clarithromycin** and **telithromycin**, **nefazodone**, and the HIV-protease inhibitors **atazanavir**, **indinavir**, **nelfinavir**, **ritonavir**, and **saquinavir**) might increase romidepsin plasma concentrations and should be avoided.[1] Additionally, they recommend caution with moderate CYP3A4 inhibitors.[1] For a list of CYP3A4 inhibitors, see 'Table 1.9', p.11. If romidepsin is given with any of these CYP3A4 inhibitors it would seem prudent to monitor closely for romidepsin adverse effects (such as gastrointestinal disturbances, fatigue, fever) and adjust treatment accordingly.

(d) P-glycoprotein inhibitors

The US manufacturer notes that romidepsin is a substrate for the drug transporter protein P-glycoprotein and as such, drugs that inhibit P-glycoprotein have the potential to increase the plasma concentration of romidepsin. Caution on concurrent use is advised.[1] If romidepsin is given with a P-glycoprotein inhibitors it would seem prudent to monitor closely for romidepsin adverse effects (such as gastrointestinal disturbances, fatigue, fever) and adjust treatment accordingly. For a list of P-glycoprotein inhibitors, see 'Table 1.12', p.14.

1. Istodax (Romidepsin). Celgene Corporation. US Prescribing information, March 2012.

Streptozocin + Phenytoin

A single case report indicates that phenytoin can reduce or abolish the effects of streptozocin.

Clinical evidence, mechanism, importance and management

A patient with an organic hypoglycaemic syndrome, due to a metastatic apud cell carcinoma of the pancreas, who was taking streptozocin 2 g daily with phenytoin 400 mg daily for 4 days, did not have the expected response to streptozocin until phenytoin was withdrawn.[1] It would seem that the phenytoin inhibited the effects of the streptozocin by some mechanism as yet unknown. Although this is an isolated case report its authors recommend that concurrent use should be avoided.

1. Koranyi L, Gero L. Influence of diphenylhydantoin on the effect of streptozotocin. *BMJ* (1979) 1, 127.

Tamoxifen + Acitretin

A patient taking tamoxifen developed bradycardia and a prolonged QT interval when also taking acitretin.

Clinical evidence, mechanism, importance and management

A case report describes a woman taking tamoxifen 20 mg daily who experienced symptomatic bradycardia and QT prolongation 3 weeks after starting acitretin 50 mg daily for 14 days then 30 mg daily during radiation therapy. On stopping the acitretin and later the tamoxifen, her ECG returned to normal and her symptoms resolved.[1] It was suggested that the acitretin might have inhibited the metabolism of tamoxifen, thus increasing the plasma levels of tamoxifen to a level at which QT prolongation became symptomatic. However, note that acitretin is not an established inhibitor of the cytochrome P450 enzyme system (responsible for tamoxifen metabolism), and tamoxifen has only been reported to cause QT prolongation at very high doses (greater than 160 mg/m^2 daily[2,3]), making this suggestion seem unlikely.

The clinical relevance of this isolated report is uncertain. Bear it in mind in the event of an unexpected response to treatment.

1. Slovacek L, Ansorgova V, Macingova Z, Haman L, Petera J. Tamoxifen-induced QT interval prolongation. *J Clin Pharm Ther* (2008) 33, 453–5.
2. Trump DL, Smith DC, Ellis PG, Rogers MP, Schold SC, Winer EP, Panella TJ, Jordan VC, Fine RL. High-dose oral tamoxifen, a potential multidrug-resistance-reversal agent: phase I trial in combination with vinblastine. *J Natl Cancer Inst* (1992) 84, 1811–16.
3. Pollack IF, DaRosso RC, Robertson PL, Jakacki RL, Mirro JR, Blatt J, Nicholson S, Packer RJ, Allen JC, Cisneros A, Jordan VC. A phase I study of high-dose tamoxifen for the treatment of refractory malignant gliomas of childhood. *Clin Cancer Res* (1997) 3, 1109–15.

Tamoxifen + Aromatase inhibitors

Anastrozole, exemestane and letrozole do not appear to affect tamoxifen levels. Tamoxifen modestly reduces anastrozole and letrozole levels, but it does not alter the levels of exemestane, or the effects of anastrozole, exemestane or letrozole. However, the combination of tamoxifen and anastrozole was no more effective than tamoxifen alone and was slightly less effective than anastrozole alone.

Clinical evidence

(a) Anastrozole

In a preliminary double-blind, placebo-controlled study in 34 women with breast cancer, who had been taking tamoxifen 20 mg daily for at least 10 weeks, the addition of anastrozole 1 mg daily for 28 days did not affect the pharmacokinetics of tamoxifen. In addition, the estradiol suppressant effects of anastrozole did not appear to be affected by tamoxifen.[1] These findings were confirmed in a pharmacokinetic sub-protocol in the large anastrozole and tamoxifen alone or in combination (ATAC) study. However, in this study, anastrozole levels were decreased by 27% by tamoxifen (although this was not thought to be clinically relevant).[2] Furthermore, after 3 years, the combination was no more effective than tamoxifen alone and was slightly less effective than anastrozole alone,[3] and this arm of the ATAC study was discontinued.

(b) Exemestane

In a study in 32 women who had been taking tamoxifen 20 mg daily for at least 4 months, exemestane 25 mg daily for 8 weeks had no effect on the pharmacokinetics of tamoxifen or the formation of tamoxifen metabolites.[4]

Tamoxifen did not affect the plasma levels of exemestane in a pilot study in 18 postmenopausal women given exemestane 25 mg daily for 14 days, then exemestane and tamoxifen 20 mg daily for 4 weeks. In addition, tamoxifen did not affect the pharmacodynamics (estrone, estrone sulfate and estradiol suppression) of exemestane.[5]

(c) Letrozole

In 12 women, letrozole levels were reduced by 38% (range 0 to 70%) 6 weeks after tamoxifen 20 mg daily was added to letrozole 2.5 mg daily. This reduction persisted after 4 to 8 months; however, the estradiol suppressant effects of letrozole did not appear to be affected.[6] In 18 women, the pharmacokinetics of tamoxifen 20 mg daily were not affected by letrozole 2.5 mg daily.[7]

Mechanism

It is not known how tamoxifen reduces anastrozole and letrozole levels, although it may be by enzyme induction.[6] This pharmacokinetic interaction may explain why tamoxifen with anastrozole was slightly less effective than anastrozole alone (although oestradiol suppression was unaffected by reduced anastrozole levels). An alternative explanation is that the minor oestrogenic effect of tamoxifen is not affected by the oestrogen deprivation caused by anastrozole[3] and it is this oestrogenic effect that reduces the efficacy of anastrozole.

Importance and mechanism

It was originally hypothesised that the combination of an oestrogen antagonist, such as tamoxifen, and an aromatase inhibitor should provide additional benefit in the treatment of hormone-dependent cancers; however, no clinical studies have found this to be so. Rather, the anastrozole and tamoxifen alone or in combination (ATAC) study showed that the combination of tamoxifen and anastrozole was slightly *less* effective than anastrozole alone. The pharmacokinetic interactions described above may partly explain this. Based on this evidence, these drugs should not be used concurrently.

1. Dowsett M, Tobias JS, Howell A, Blackman GM, Welch H, King N, Ponzone R, von Euler M, Baum M. The effect of anastrozole on the pharmacokinetics of tamoxifen in post-menopausal women with early breast cancer. *Br J Cancer* (1999) 79, 311–15.
2. Dowsett M, Cuzick J, Howell A, Jackson I; ATAC Trialists' Group. Pharmacokinetics of anastrozole and tamoxifen alone, and in combination, during adjuvant endocrine therapy for early breast cancer in postmenopausal women: a sub-protocol of the 'Arimidex and tamoxifen alone or in combination' (ATAC) trial. *Br J Cancer* (2001) 85, 317–24.
3. Baum M, Buzdar AU, Cuzick J, Forbes J, Houghton J, Klijn JG, Sahmoud T; ATAC Trialists' Group. Anastrozole alone or in combination with tamoxifen versus tamoxifen alone for adjuvant treatment of postmenopausal women with early breast cancer: first results of the ATAC randomised trial. *Lancet* (2002) 359, 2131–9.
4. Hutson PR, Love RR, Havighurst TC, Rogers E, Cleary JF. Effect of exemestane on tamoxifen pharmacokinetics in postmenopausal women treated for breast cancer. *Clin Cancer Res* (2005) 11, 8722–7.
5. Rivera E, Valero V, Francis D, Asnis AG, Schaaf LJ, Duncan B, Hortobagyi GN. Pilot study evaluating the pharmacokinetics, pharmacodynamics, and safety of the combination of exemestane and tamoxifen. *Clin Cancer Res* (2004) 10, 1943–8.
6. Dowsett M, Pfister C, Johnston SRD, Miles DW, Houston SJ, Verbeek JA, Gundacker H, Sioufi A, Smith IE. Impact of tamoxifen on the pharmacokinetics and endocrine effects of the aromatase inhibitor letrozole in postmenopausal women with breast cancer. *Clin Cancer Res* (1999) 5, 2238–43.
7. Ingle JN, Suman VJ, Johnson PA, Krook JE, Mailliard JA, Wheeler RH, Loprinzi CL, Perez EA, Jordan VC, Dowsett M. Evaluation of tamoxifen plus letrozole with assessment of pharmacokinetic interaction in postmenopausal women with metastatic breast cancer. *Clin Cancer Res* (1999) 5, 1642–9.

Tamoxifen + Dexamethasone

The effect of dexamethasone on tamoxifen levels is unknown.

Clinical evidence, mechanism, importance and management

The steady state levels of tamoxifen and its metabolites were measured in patients with glioma being treated with high-dose tamoxifen 120 mg/m^2 twice daily; 14 of whom were also taking oral dexamethasone 8 to 24 mg daily, and 15 of whom were also taking phenytoin. The plasma levels of tamoxifen were 2.3-fold higher in the patients also taking dexamethasone, when compared with those also taking phenytoin, although this marked difference was not statistically significant due to high variability in tamoxifen levels.[1]

The authors noted that dexamethasone is both a substrate and an inducer of the cytochrome P450 subfamily CYP3A, by which tamoxifen is, in part, metabolised, and they suggested that dexamethasone, a CYP3A substrate, might inhibit the metabolism of tamoxifen by competitive inhibition.[1] However, it is now known that this is not a clinically relevant mechanism of cytochrome P450 enzyme interactions.

It is impossible to reach a conclusion about the effect of dexamethasone on tamoxifen levels from this study because there was no group who received tamoxifen alone. It is possible that dexamethasone actually reduced tamoxifen levels, but not to the same extent as phenytoin. It is equally possible that dexamethasone had no effect on tamoxifen levels. However, it seems unlikely that dexamethasone increases tamoxifen levels, as suggested. A proper randomised study would be needed to assess the true effect.

1. Ducharme J, Fried K, Shenouda G, Leyland-Jones B, Wainer IW. Tamoxifen metabolic patterns within a glioma patient population treated with high-dose tamoxifen. *Br J Clin Pharmacol* (1997) 43: 189–93.

Tamoxifen and related drugs + HRT

In one randomised controlled study, HRT increased the risk of recurrent breast cancer in women including those taking tamoxifen, but in another similar study, no increased risk was seen.

Clinical evidence

A number of observational studies (which have been have the subject of a review[1]) found no increased risk of recurrence of breast cancer, in breast cancer survivors given HRT for the management of menopausal symptoms, although most of these studies did not specifically look at women taking tamoxifen. In one cohort study which did address this, the use of continuous combined HRT (an oestrogen with a progestogen) was not associated with an increased risk of breast cancer recurrence in women taking tamoxifen.[2]

However, these observational studies cannot control for all possible confounders and are not a substitute for a prospective randomised study. A subsequent randomised, controlled study was stopped early after a median follow up of 2 years because of a 3.3-fold increased risk in breast cancer recurrence in women allocated to HRT (mostly continuous or sequential estradiol and norethisterone acetate). About one-third of women in this study were taking tamoxifen at randomisation, and the increased risk of recurrence in this group was higher, at 4.7-fold, although this increase was not statistically significant.[3] Conversely; another similar study did not find an increased risk of breast cancer recurrence with HRT (mostly cyclic estradiol and medroxyprogesterone acetate, with the progestogen given for only 14 days at 3-month intervals in about half of the women). About half of the women were also taking tamoxifen, and there was no difference in breast cancer recurrence between these women and the group as a whole. This study was also stopped early because of the findings of the other study, and because it was not sufficiently powered to detect a small increase in risk (of 6% or less).[4] It is interesting to speculate that the difference in progestogen between these studies may account for the disparate findings, but this would need to be studied.[4]

Note that adding tamoxifen to HRT is being tried as a way of reducing the risks of HRT in *healthy* women. In one study of women randomised to tamoxifen or placebo for breast cancer prevention, the risk of breast cancer in tamoxifen recipients who took HRT was similar to that in women not taking HRT.[5] In another study in 210 *healthy* postmenopausal women taking HRT for menopausal symptoms, the addition of low-dose tamoxifen 5 mg daily appeared to have a favourable effect on markers of breast cancer risk, without appreciably increasing menopausal symptoms.[6]

Mechanism

Estrogens, such as HRT, might be expected to oppose the effects of drugs that diminish oestrogenic activity, such as tamoxifen, in the treatment and prevention of breast cancer.

Importance and management

Overall, the findings suggest that the use of menopausal HRT may greatly increase the risk of breast cancer recurrence in women who have had early breast cancer, whether or not they are currently taking tamoxifen or aromatase inhibitors. This is more of a drug-disease interaction than a drug-drug interaction. The use of HRT in these women should generally be avoided. If nothing else is effective for severe menopausal symptoms, the available data (albeit limited) suggest that HRT containing medroxyprogesterone acetate might be preferred over that containing norethisterone, but ideally this requires further confirmation. In addition, the lowest dose of HRT for the shortest period of time should be used and the patient should be fully aware of the potential risks. The use of oestrogen-containing preparations (which would include HRT) is specifically contraindicated by the manufacturers in women taking **anastrozole**,[7] and **exemestane**.[8,9] This could be reasonably extended to **letrozole**, tamoxifen and **toremifene**.

Tibolone, which is also given to treat post-menopausal oestrogen deficiency, appears to interact similarly. Consider also 'Tamoxifen and related drugs + Tibolone', p.713.

1. Col NF, Kim JA, Chlebowski RT. Menopausal hormone therapy after breast cancer: a meta-analysis and critical appraisal of the evidence. *Breast Cancer Res* (2005) 7, R535–40.
2. Dew JE, Wren BG, Eden JA. Tamoxifen, hormone receptors, and hormone replacement therapy in women previously treated for breast cancer: a cohort study. *Climacteric* (2002) 5, 151–5.
3. Holmberg L, Iversen OE, Rudenstam CM, Hammar M, Kumpulainen E, Jaskiewicz J, Jassem J, Dobaczewska D, Fjosne HE, Peralta O, Arriagada R, Holmqvist M, Maenpaa J; HABITS Study Group. Increased risk of recurrence after hormone replacement therapy in breast cancer survivors. *J Natl Cancer Inst* (2008) 100, 475–82.
4. von Schoultz E, Rutqvist LE; Stockholm Breast Cancer Study Group. Menopausal hormone therapy after breast cancer: the Stockholm randomized trial. *J Natl Cancer Inst* (2005) 97, 533–5.
5. Veronesi U, Maisonneuve P, Sacchini V, Rotmensz N, Boyle P; Italian Tamoxifen Study Group. Tamoxifen for breast cancer among hysterectomised women. *Lancet* (2002) 359, 1122–4.
6. Decensi, A, Gandini S, Serrano D, Cazzaniga M, Pizzamiglio M, Maffini F, Pelosi G, Daldoss C, Omodei U, Johansson H, Macis D, Lazzeroni M, Penotti M, Sironi L, Moroni S, Bianco V, Rondanina G, Gjerde J, Guerrieri-Gonzaga A, Bonanni B. Randomized dose-ranging trial of tamoxifen at low doses in hormone replacement therapy users. *J Clin Oncol* (2007) 25, 4201–9.
7. Arimidex Film-coated Tablets (Anastrozole). AstraZeneca UK Ltd. UK Summary of product characteristics, December 2010.
8. Aromasin (Exemestane). Pharmacia Ltd. UK Summary of product characteristics, May 2009.
9. Aromasin (Exemestane). Pfizer. US Prescribing information, October 2008.

Tamoxifen + Medroxyprogesterone

High-dose medroxyprogesterone appears to reduce the levels of the desmethyl metabolite of tamoxifen.

Clinical evidence, mechanism, importance and management

In a randomised study in 20 women with breast cancer taking tamoxifen 20 mg twice daily, the addition of medroxyprogesterone acetate 500 mg twice daily only slightly reduced the tamoxifen serum levels over a 6-month period, but considerably reduced the levels of the desmethyl metabolite of tamoxifen when compared with placebo. Differences were apparent at 6 weeks and 3 months, but not at 2 weeks and 6 months.[1] The reason for this finding is uncertain, and the clinical importance of this suggested interaction is unclear.

For discussion of the potential effects of medroxyprogesterone-containing HRT in women taking tamoxifen, see 'Tamoxifen and related drugs + HRT', above.

1. Reid AD, Horobin JM, Newman EL, Preece PE. Tamoxifen metabolism is altered by simultaneous administration of medroxyprogesterone acetate in breast cancer patients. *Breast Cancer Res Treat* (1992) 22, 153–6.

Tamoxifen + Miscellaneous

Limited evidence suggests that diuretics might modestly increase tamoxifen levels, but this requires confirmation. Other data suggests that a number of drugs do not affect tamoxifen levels, but this data alone is insufficient to exclude an interaction.

Clinical evidence, mechanism, importance and management

In a study in 98 women with breast cancer taking tamoxifen, plasma levels of tamoxifen and its 4-hydroxy and *N*-desmethyl metabolites were analysed (timing of sample in relation to dose not stated) and then a multiple linear regression model was used to look at associations between the levels and medications they were taking.[1] This sort of study is limited by its non-randomised nature, and it should be noted that the more variables that are studied the greater the likelihood that statistically significant differences can be due to chance alone. In addition, in this particular study, concurrent drugs were grouped into general categories containing disparate drugs thereby limiting its ability to detect real differences. This study also did not measure levels of endoxifen (4-hydroxy-*N*-desmethyltamoxifen) a metabolite of tamoxifen that may be important for tamoxifen efficacy, see 'Tamoxifen + SSRIs and other CYP2D6 inhibitors', p.712. Nevertheless, for completeness the results are presented below.

(a) Diuretics

One study (see details and comments, above) found that tamoxifen levels were 36% higher in 21 women taking diuretics (**furosemide, hydrochlorothiazide, spironolactone, triamterene**) than in 77 women not taking diuretics, and levels of the *N*-desmethyl metabolite of tamoxifen were 43% higher.[1] A mechanism for this possible interaction is unknown. However, even if this interaction were confirmed, modest increases of this order appear unlikely to be clinically important.

(b) Drugs for pain or arthritis

One study (see details and comments, above) found a 10% lower tamoxifen level in 15 women taking drugs for pain or arthritis (**aspirin, celecoxib, glucosamine, nabumetone, naproxen, oxaprozin, paracetamol, rofecoxib**).[1] This difference in levels is too small to be of any relevance, and the large number of drugs and limited number of women precludes any meaningful conclusion.

(c) Other drugs

In one study (see details and comments, above) groups of drugs stated as having no effect on the levels of tamoxifen or its *N*-desmethyl and 4-hydroxy metabolites included:

- **ACE inhibitors** (13 women; **benazepril, enalapril, fosinopril, lisinopril, perindopril, quinapril**).[1]
- **Beta blockers** (15 women; **atenolol, metoprolol**).[1]
- **Calcium-channel blockers** (10 women; **amlodipine, diltiazem, nifedipine, verapamil**).[1] However, note that the grouping for calcium-channel blockers contains drugs that are CYP3A4 inhibitors (diltiazem, verapamil) as well as those that are not (amlodipine, nifedipine) and the numbers of women taking each drug was not stated, meaning an interaction for the inhibitors cannot be ruled out from these data.
- **Antidepressants** (25 women; **amitriptyline, bupropion, fluoxetine, paroxetine, sertraline, trazodone, venlafaxine**).[1] However, note that paroxetine specifically has been shown to have no effect on the levels of tamoxifen or its *N*-desmethyl and 4-hydroxy metabolites, but it does reduce the levels of the active metabolite, endoxifen, and is considered to reduce the efficacy of tamoxifen; bupropion and fluoxetine may behave similarly, see 'Tamoxifen + SSRIs and other CYP2D6 inhibitors', p.712.

- Prior chemotherapy (**cyclophosphamide, doxorubicin, taxanes**).[1] However, note that some antineoplastics might increase the risk of thrombosis with tamoxifen, see 'Antineoplastics + Tamoxifen', p.659.

1. Gallicchio L, Tkaczuk K, Lord G, Danton M, Lewis LM, Lim CK, Flaws JA. Medication use, tamoxifen (TAM), and TAM metabolite concentrations in women with breast cancer. *Cancer Lett* (2004) 211, 57–67.

Tamoxifen + Rifampicin (Rifampin)

Rifampicin increases the metabolism of tamoxifen.

Clinical evidence, mechanism, importance and management

In 10 healthy men, rifampicin 600 mg daily for 5 days reduced the AUC of a single 80-mg dose of tamoxifen by 86%, reduced its peak plasma levels by 55%, and reduced its half-life by 44%. Similarly, the AUC of the metabolite, *N*-desmethyltamoxifen, was reduced by 62%.[1] It is likely that rifampicin induces the metabolism of tamoxifen thereby reducing its levels. These findings suggest that the efficacy of tamoxifen may be reduced by rifampicin; however, note that tamoxifen induces its own metabolism on long-term use.[2] Thus, further study is needed to assess the clinical impact of the long-term concurrent use of these drugs. Until more is known, it would be prudent to be cautious with the use of rifampicin in women taking tamoxifen.

1. Kivistö KT, Villikka K, Nyman L, Anttila M, Neuvonen PJ. Tamoxifen and toremifene concentrations in plasma are greatly decreased by rifampin. *Clin Pharmacol Ther* (1998) 64, 648–54.
2. Desai PB, Nallani SC, Sane RS, Moore LB, Goodwin BJ, Buckley DJ, Buckley AR. Induction of cytochrome P450 3A4 in primary human hepatocytes and activation of the human pregnane X receptor by tamoxifen and 4-hydroxytamoxifen. *Drug Metab Dispos* (2002) 30, 608–12.

Tamoxifen + SSRIs and other CYP2D6 inhibitors

Paroxetine, a CYP2D6 inhibitor, reduces the metabolism of tamoxifen to one of its active metabolites and it has been suggested that this could decrease the efficacy of tamoxifen. Several case-control studies and one retrospective cohort study investigating the effects of SSRIs on tamoxifen have not found an increase in breast cancer recurrence; although one retrospective cohort study reported an increased risk of breast cancer recurrence in patients taking paroxetine with tamoxifen. In addition, one case-control study also suggested an increased risk of breast cancer recurrence with CYP2D6 inhibitors.

Clinical evidence

(a) Endoxifen concentrations

Twelve women taking tamoxifen 20 mg daily were also given **paroxetine** 10 mg daily for 4 weeks, and the plasma concentrations of tamoxifen and its metabolites were measured.[1] Before **paroxetine**, the plasma concentrations of the active tamoxifen metabolite, endoxifen (4-hydroxy-*N*-desmethyltamoxifen) were about 12 times higher than those of the 4-hydroxytamoxifen metabolite. **Paroxetine** reduced endoxifen concentrations by 56%, but those of *N*-desmethyltamoxifen and 4-hydroxytamoxifen were unchanged. The reduction in endoxifen concentrations was greatest in those who were CYP2D6 extensive metabolisers (that is, those with normal isoenzyme activity). In a further study by the same research group, 80 women starting tamoxifen 20 mg daily had plasma concentrations of tamoxifen measured after one and 4 months.[2] These were then correlated with CYP2D6 metaboliser phenotype and the concurrent use of CYP2D6 inhibitors (taken by 24 women). In women who were CYP2D6 extensive metabolisers, the use of CYP2D6 inhibitors was associated with a 58% lower endoxifen concentration, which was substantially lower in those taking **paroxetine** (a CYP2D6 inhibitor), but venlafaxine caused only a small reduction, and **sertraline** (a weak CYP2D6 inhibitor) caused an intermediate reduction.[2] In yet another similar analysis, endoxifen concentrations were 45% lower in 46 patients taking CYP2D6 inhibitors than in 94 women not taking CYP2D6 inhibitors (about 40 mmol/L versus 72 mmol/L). When classified by potency of CYP2D6 inhibitors, endoxifen concentrations were 50% lower in 19 women taking **paroxetine** or **fluoxetine** than in 14 women taking **sertraline** or **citalopram** and 13 taking celecoxib, diphenhydramine or chlorphenamine (about 25 mmol/L versus 50 mmol/L). In this analysis, venlafaxine had no effect.[3]

(b) Breast cancer recurrence

1. Case control studies. The preliminary report of a retrospective, case-control study in 1 298 patients with breast cancer, who had been taking tamoxifen for at least 24 months, found that those who were also taking a moderate or potent CYP2D6 inhibitor (353 patients, CYP2D6 inhibitor not named) had a 13.9% increased risk of breast cancer recurrence within 2 years compared with a 7.5% increased risk in those taking tamoxifen alone.[4]

In contrast, a case-control study of 28 women taking tamoxifen with recurrences of oestrogen receptor-positive breast cancer found that there was no difference in breast cancer recurrence in the women taking CYP2D6 inhibitors (said to be **fluoxetine, paroxetine, sertraline**) between the cases and controls (women taking tamoxifen with no recurrence). Similarly, there were no differences for CYP2C9 inhibitors (said to include **paroxetine** and **sertraline**).[5] Several other case-control studies have also found that **citalopram,**[6-8] **escitalopram,**[6-8] **fluoxetine,**[7-9] **fluvoxamine,**[8] **paroxetine,**[7-9] and **sertraline**[7,8] do not affect the rate of breast cancer recurrence in women taking tamoxifen. Note that the patients in one study[6] were a subset of those used in another study.[8] A large nested case-control study using the UK General Practice Research Database also reported no increased risk of breast cancer recurrence with the use of CYP2D6 inhibitor and substrates;[10] however, it is impossible to interpret the findings of this study because it mixed substrates with inhibitors (substrates of a given isoenzyme do not interact with other substrates to a clinically relevant extent unless they are also inhibitors). The effect of this would be to dilute any effect of the drugs are that known inhibitors of CYP2D6.

2. Retrospective cohort studies. A retrospective, cohort study identified 2 430 women with breast cancer taking tamoxifen and also taking a single SSRI (**citalopram, fluoxetine, fluvoxamine, paroxetine, sertraline**) or venlafaxine. Follow up over a mean period of 2.4 years identified 374 of these women who had died from breast cancer. When the relationship between these deaths and the concurrent use of a single SSRI was examined, it was found that paroxetine was associated with an increased relative risk of death, which increased as the duration of concurrent use increased. Patients who took **paroxetine** for 25%, 50% and 75% of the time they took tamoxifen had a 24%, 54% and 91% increase in the risk of death from breast cancer, respectively. It was estimated that the use of **paroxetine** for 100% of the time the patient took tamoxifen would result in an additional death for every 6.9 patients treated. No increased risk of death from breast cancer was found with the other SSRIs or venlafaxine.[11]

In contrast, another retrospective cohort study in 439 patients with breast cancer taking tamoxifen found no important increase in the risk of recurrence of breast cancer within the first 5 years of diagnosis with the concurrent use of antidepressants including SSRIs (243 patients). Although three cases of breast cancer recurrence were reported in patients taking **paroxetine** and **fluoxetine**, the study was not sufficiently powered to assess the importance of this finding.[12] Another study also found that the use of CYP2D6 inhibitors for at least 4 years did not affect disease-free survival in patients treated with tamoxifen,[13] but this study grouped drugs that are known inhibitors of CYP2D6 with many that are not, which would have diluted any effect. In a further well-designed cohort study which adjusted for CYP2D6 metaboliser status and tamoxifen compliance, use of either **fluoxetine** or **paroxetine** in just 32 women did not alter recurrence-free survival. However, because of the small numbers, this cannot be seen as conclusive.[14]

Mechanism

Tamoxifen is metabolised to 4-hydroxytamoxifen and *N*-desmethyltamoxifen principally by the cytochrome P450 subfamily CYP3A,[1] although others have found that other isoenzymes are involved.[15] *N*-desmethyltamoxifen is further metabolised to endoxifen (4-hydroxy-*N*-desmethyltamoxifen) by CYP2D6.[1] Endoxifen in particular, and another metabolite, 4-hydroxytamoxifen, are more active anti-oestrogens than tamoxifen.[1] Inhibition of the formation of endoxifen by CYP2D6 inhibitors might therefore reduce the efficacy of tamoxifen. One large analysis of metabolite concentrations did find that those women with lower endoxifen concentrations appeared to have a higher risk of cancer relapse.[16] Of the SSRIs, paroxetine and fluoxetine are moderate to potent inhibitors of CYP2D6, whereas citalopram and sertraline only weakly inhibit CYP2D6.

CYP2D6 shows genetic polymorphism with some individuals lacking or deficient in this isoenzyme (poor metabolisers). If the interaction with CYP2D6 inhibitors does lead to reduced efficacy, then individuals who are poor metabolisers would also be expected to respond less well to tamoxifen. However, the evidence for this is also conflicting. Some analyses have found that those of poor metaboliser status had higher cancer recurrence rates than extensive metabolisers[17] whereas other analyses have not, including analysis of the ATAC study[18] and the BIG 1-98 study.[19]

Note that it has been suggested that tamoxifen resistance may be more to do with altered oestrogen receptor sensitivity than reduced concentrations of tamoxifen metabolites.[5] Further it has been suggested that the plasma concentrations of tamoxifen and metabolites found in one study[1] would be sufficient to block oestrogen binding to oestrogen receptors so that a decrease in endoxifen concentrations would not substantially affect anti-oestrogen activity.[20]

Importance and management

Although information is limited, it is established that moderate to potent inhibitors of CYP2D6, such as paroxetine, can alter the metabolism of tamoxifen to its active metabolites. However, the effect this has on the clinical efficacy of tamoxifen remains to be established. All of the clinical data comes from retrospective studies, which cannot control for all possible confounders. Most of the case-control studies suggest that paroxetine and other SSRIs do not increase the risk of breast cancer recurrence in patients taking tamoxifen; however, the number of patients included in many of these studies is small,[6-9] and it therefore seems possible that they are unable to detect a statistically significant increase in breast cancer recurrence. The exception may be with citalopram, where patient numbers were sufficient to detect statistically significant differences, and therefore support the lack of interaction for this particular SSRI.[8] However, the preliminary report of one case-control study assessing the effect of CYP2D6 inhibitors (not specified) on breast cancer recurrence, suggested an increase in breast cancer recurrence, implying that the mechanism for the interaction is valid and that CYP2D6 inhibitors, such as paroxetine, do interact with tamoxifen to a clinically relevant extent. Similarly, one retrospective cohort study suggests that paroxetine may increase the risk of breast cancer recurrence; however, this study did not control for the CYP2D6 metaboliser status of the patient as well as their breast cancer stage and prognosis, although a difference in the groups would not be expected given the number of patients involved. Ideally randomised prospective studies are needed to establish the effects of the various SSRIs on breast cancer recurrence in patients taking tamoxifen.

At present, there is insufficient evidence to provide definitive guidelines for the use of SSRIs in patients taking tamoxifen. Despite the lack of conclusive evidence, many commentators suggest that paroxetine (and therefore probably fluoxetine, which has similar CYP2D6 inhibitory potential) should be avoided. Given that a number of SSRIs only weakly inhibit CYP2D6 (e.g. citalopram, see 'Table 35.2', p.1465), and given the potential seriousness of the proposed interaction, until the risks are established, it would seem prudent to use an alternative SSRI to paroxetine and fluoxetine wherever possible. A number of non-SSRI antidepressants (including venlafaxine) also have a low potential for affecting CYP2D6, and these may provide further alternative options in some cases. It has also been suggested that, in patients known not to respond to other antidepressants, fluoxetine or paroxetine should be given and tamoxifen changed to an aromatase inhibitor, if appropriate. If the mechanism is confirmed, then other CYP2D6 inhibitors will also interact, see 'Table 1.7', p.9, for a list. Based on the available evidence, the European Medicines Agency, and the MHRA in the UK, both state that the concurrent use of drugs known to be potent CYP2D6 inhibitors should be avoided whenever possible in patients taking tamoxifen, and they specifically name paroxetine, fluoxetine, **bupropion**, **cinacalcet** and **quinidine**.[21,22] Similarly, the American Society of Clinical Oncology encourages caution on the use of CYP2D6 inhibitors such as bupropion, paroxetine or fluoxetine with tamoxifen. They suggest that women taking tamoxifen may prefer to avoid the concurrent use of known CYP2D6 inhibitors if suitable alternatives are available. They also state that patients clearly benefiting from known CYP2D6 inhibitors might prefer to avoid tamoxifen[23] [and use alternatives]. Many other bodies have given similar advice.

1. Stearns V, Johnson MD, Rae JM, Morocho A, Novielli A, Bhargava P, Hayes DF, Desta Z, Flockhart DA. Active tamoxifen metabolite plasma concentrations after coadministration of tamoxifen and the selective serotonin reuptake inhibitor paroxetine. *J Natl Cancer Inst* (2003) 95, 1758–64.
2. Jin Y, Desta Z, Stearns V, Ward B, Ho H, Lee K-H, Skaar T, Storniolo AM, Li L, Araba A, Blanchard R, Nguyen A, Ullmer L, Hayden J, Lemler S, Weinshilboum RM, Rae JM, Hayes DF, Flockhart DA. CYP2D6 genotype, antidepressant use, and tamoxifen metabolism during adjuvant breast cancer treatment. *J Natl Cancer Inst* (2005) 97, 30–9.
3. Borges S, Desta Z, Li L, Skaar TC, Ward BA, Nguyen A, Jin Y, Storniolo AM, Nikoloff DM, Wu L, Hillman G, Hayes DF, Stearns V, Flockhart DA. Quantitative effect of CYP2D6 genotype and inhibitors on tamoxifen metabolism: implication for optimization of breast cancer treatment. *Clin Pharmacol Ther* (2006) 80, 61–74.
4. Aubert RE, Stanek EJ, Yao J, Teagarden JR, Subar M, Epstein RS, Skaar TC, Desta Z, Flockhart DA. Risk of breast cancer recurrence in women initiating tamoxifen with CYP2D6 inhibitors. *J Clin Oncol* (2009) 27 (Suppl), CRA508.
5. Lehmann D, Nelsen J, Ramanath V, Newman N, Duggan D, Smith A. Lack of attenuation in the antitumor effect of tamoxifen by chronic CYP isoform inhibition. *J Clin Pharmacol* (2004) 44, 861–5.
6. Lash TL, Pedersen L, Cronin-Fenton D, Ahern TP, Rosenberg CL, Lunetta KL, Silliman RA, Hamilton-Dutoit S, Garne JP, Ewertz M, Sørensen HT. Tamoxifen's protection against breast cancer recurrence is not reduced by concurrent use of the SSRI citalopram. *Br J Cancer* (2008) 99, 616–21.
7. Ahern TP, Pederson L, Cronin-Fenton DP, Sørensen HT, Lash TL. No increase in breast cancer recurrence with concurrent use of tamoxifen and some *CYP2D6*-inhibiting medications. *Cancer Epidemiol Biomarkers Prev* (2009) 18, 2562–4.
8. Lash TL, Cronin-Fenton D, Ahern TP, Rosenberg CL, Lunetta KL, Silliman RA, Hamilton-Dutoit S, Garne JP, Ewertz M, Sørensen HT, Pedersen L. Breast cancer recurrence risk related to concurrent use of SSRI antidepressants and tamoxifen. *Acta Oncol* (2010) 49, 305–12.
9. Dezentjé VO, van Blijderveen NJC, Gelderblom H, Putter H, van Herk-Sukel MPP, Casparie MK, Egberts ACG, Nortier JWR, Guchelaar H-J. Effect of concomitant CYP2D6 inhibitor use and tamoxifen adherence on breast cancer recurrence in early-stage breast cancer. *J Clin Oncol* (2010) 28, 2423–9.
10. Azoulay L, Dell'Aniello S, Huiart L, du Fort GG, Suissa S. Concurrent use of tamoxifen with CYP2D6 inhibitors and the risk of breast cancer recurrence. *Breast Cancer Res Treat* (2011) 126, 695–703.
11. Kelly CM, Juurlink DN, Gomes T, Duong-Hua M, Pritchard KI, Austin PC, Paszat LF. Selective serotonin reuptake inhibitors and breast cancer mortality in women receiving tamoxifen: a population based cohort study. *BMJ* (2010) 340, c693.
12. Chubak J, Buist DSM, Boudreau DM, Rossing MA, Lumley T, Weiss NS. Breast cancer recurrence risk in relation to antidepressant use after diagnosis. *Breast Cancer Res Treat* (2008) 112, 123–132.
13. Siegelmann-Danieli N, Kurnik D, Lomnicky Y, Vesterman-Landes J, Katzir I, Bialik M, Loebstein R. Potent CYP2D6 inhibiting drugs do not increase relapse rate in early breast cancer patients treated with adjuvant tamoxifen. *Breast Cancer Res Treat* (2011) 125, 505–10.
14. Thompson AM, Johnson A, Quinlan P, Hillman G, Fontecha M, Bray SE, Purdie CA, Jordan LB, Ferraldeschi R, Latif A, Hadfield KD, Clarke RB, Ashcroft L, Evans DG, Howell A, Nikoloff M, Lawrence J, Newman WG. Comprehensive CYP2D6 genotype and adherence affect outcome in breast cancer patients treated with tamoxifen monotherapy. *Breast Cancer Res Treat* (2011) 125, 279–87.
15. Coller JK, Krebsfaenger N, Klein K, Endrizzi K, Wolbold R, Lang T, Nüssler A, Neuhaus P, Zanger UM, Eichelbaum M, Mürdter TE. The influence of CYP2B6, CYP2C9 and CYP2D6 genotypes on the formation of the potent antioestrogen Z-4-hydroxy-tamoxifen in human liver. *Br J Clin Pharmacol* (2002) 54, 157–67.
16. Madlensky L, Natarajan L, Tchu S, Pu M, Mortimer J, Flatt SW, Nikoloff DM, Hillman G, Fontecha MR, Lawrence HJ, Parker BA, Wu AHB, Pierce JP. Tamoxifen metabolite concentrations, CYP2D6 genotype, and breast cancer outcomes. *Clin Pharmacol Ther* (2011) 89, 718–25.
17. Schroth W, Goetz MP, Hamann U, Fasching PA, Schmidt M, Winter S, Fritz P, Simon W, Suman VJ, Ames MM, Safgren SL, Kuffel MJ, Ulmer HU, Boländer J, Strick R, Beckmann MW, Koelbl H, Weinshilboum RM, Ingle JN, Eichelbaum M, Schwab M, Brauch H. Association between CYP2D6 polymorphisms and outcomes among women with early stage breast cancer treated with tamoxifen. *JAMA* (2009) 302, 1429–36.
18. Rae JM, Drury S, Hayes DF, Stearns V, Thibert JN, Haynes BP, Salter J, Sestak I, Cuzick J, Dowsett M; ATAC trialists. CYP2D6 and UGT2B7 genotype and risk of recurrence in tamoxifen-treated breast cancer patients. *J Natl Cancer Inst* (2012) 104, 452–60.
19. Regan MM, Leyland-Jones B, Bouzyk M, Pagani O, Tang W, Kammler R, Dell'orto P, Biasi MO, Thürlimann B, Lyng MB, Ditzel HJ, Neven P, Debled M, Maibach R, Price KN, Gelber RD, Coates AS, Goldhirsch A, Rae JM, Viale G; Breast International Group (BIG) 1-98 Collaborative Group. CYP2D6 genotype and tamoxifen response in postmenopausal women with endocrine-responsive breast cancer: the breast international group 1-98 trial. *J Natl Cancer Inst* (2012) 104, 441–51.
20. Ratliff B, Dietze EC, Bean GR, Moore C, Wanko S, Seewaldt VL. RE: Active tamoxifen metabolite plasma concentrations after coadministration of tamoxifen and the selective serotonin reuptake inhibitor paroxetine. *J Natl Cancer Inst* (2004) 96, 883.
21. European Medicines Agency. Pharmacovigilance working party, September 2010 meeting. Available at: http://www.ema.europa.eu/docs/en_GB/document_library/Report/2010/10/WC500097444.pdf (accessed 21/10/15).
22. Medicines and Healthcare Products Regulatory Agency and the Commission on Human Medicines. Tamoxifen for breast cancer: drug interactions involving CYP2D6, genetic variants, and variability in clinical response. *Drug Safety Update* (2010) 4, A1. Available at: http://webarchive.nationalarchives.gov.uk/20141205150130/http://www.mhra.gov.uk/home/groups/dsu/documents/publication/con099854.pdf (accessed 21/10/15).
23. Burstein HJ, Prestrud AA, Seidenfeld J, Anderson H, Buchholz TA, Davidson NE, Gelmon KE, Giordano SH, Hudis CA, Malin J, Mamounas EP, Rowden D, Solky AJ, Sowers MR, Stearns V, Winer EP, Somerfield MR, Griggs JJ. American Society of Clinical Oncology clinical practice guideline: update on adjuvant endocrine therapy for women with hormone receptor-positive breast cancer. *J Clin Oncol* (2010) 28, 3784–96.

Tamoxifen and related drugs + Tibolone

In a large randomised study, tibolone increased the risk of recurrent breast cancer in women including those taking tamoxifen or an aromatase inhibitor.

Clinical evidence

In a large randomised placebo-controlled study, the use of tibolone 2.5 mg daily for vasomotor symptoms in women who had undergone surgery for breast cancer was associated with an increased risk of breast cancer recurrence, when compared with placebo (15.2% versus 10.7%; hazard ratio 1.40). In sub-group analyses, the use of an aromatase inhibitor (6.5% of women) was associated with a greater increased risk (hazard ratio 2.42), and the use of tamoxifen (67% of women) was associated with a slightly smaller increased risk (hazard ratio 1.25), when compared with women not using drugs that diminish oestrogenic activity (hazard ratio 1.73).[1]

Mechanism

Tibolone, a synthetic steroid, which has oestrogenic, progestogenic and weak androgenic properties might be expected to oppose the effects of drugs that diminish oestrogenic activity. It has been suggested that this might be greater for aromatase inhibitors than tamoxifen, because of the differing mechanisms of action.[1]

Importance and management

Evidence for an interaction between tibolone and an aromatase inhibitor appears to come from this one study. However, the study is large, and well designed, and its findings are in line with the way menopausal HRT interacts with the aromatase inhibitors and tamoxifen (see 'Tamoxifen and related drugs + HRT', p.711). Overall, the findings suggest that the use of tibolone may greatly increase the risk of breast cancer recurrence in women who have had early breast cancer, whether or not they are currently taking tamoxifen or aromatase inhibitors. This is more of a drug-disease interaction than a drug-drug interaction. Therefore, the use of tibolone with tamoxifen, and aromatase inhibitors or related drugs that diminish oestrogenic activity would not be recommended.

1. Kenemans P, Bundred NJ, Foidart JM, Kubista E, von Schoultz B, Sismondi P, Vassilopoulou-Sellin R, Yip CH, Egberts J, Mol-Arts M, Mulder R, van Os S, Beckmann MW; LIBERATE Study Group. Safety and efficacy of tibolone in breast-cancer patients with vasomotor symptoms: a double-blind, randomised, non-inferiority trial. *Lancet Oncol* (2009) 10, 135–46.

Taxanes + Amifostine

Amifostine had no effect on docetaxel and paclitaxel pharmacokinetics, except in one study which found that amifostine extended paclitaxel plasma circulation time. Amifostine appears not to reduce the toxicity of these taxanes.

Clinical evidence, mechanism, importance and management

In a randomised study, amifostine did not alter the response to, or the pharmacokinetics of, **paclitaxel**, neither did it protect against **paclitaxel**-related neurotoxicity or myelotoxicity.[1] Another study in 8 patients has confirmed that amifostine (750 mg/m^2 as a 15-minute infusion 30 minutes before **paclitaxel**) had no effect on the pharmacokinetics of **paclitaxel** 135 to 200 mg/m^2. Six of the patients were also taking epirubicin and cisplatin.[2] Although the preliminary findings of an earlier study had suggested that pre-treatment with amifostine reduced the AUC of **paclitaxel** by 29%,[3] the full report of this study concluded that amifostine had no clinically relevant effect on **paclitaxel** pharmacokinetics.[4] In a study in which patients were given amifostine 500 mg as an infusion over 15 minutes just before low-dose **paclitaxel** 80 mg/m^2 as a one-hour infusion, amifostine reduced maximum plasma levels by about 20%. The AUC of paclitaxel was not affected, but the paclitaxel plasma circulation time was prolonged.[5]

Amifostine had no effect on the pharmacokinetics of **docetaxel**, and it did not reduce **docetaxel**-induced myelotoxicity.[6]

The finding in two of these studies[1,6] that the toxicity of taxanes was not reduced by amifostine does not support earlier *in vitro* data where amifostine protected normal tissue from **paclitaxel** toxicity.[7]

Most studies show no beneficial or adverse consequences from giving amifostine with the taxanes. Further study is needed to evaluate the possible effects of amifostine on taxane plasma circulation time.

1. Gelmon K, Eisenhauer E, Bryce C, Tolcher A, Mayer L, Tomlinson E, Zee B, Blackstein M, Tomiak E, Yau J, Batist G, Fisher B, Iglesias J. Randomized phase II study of high-dose paclitaxel with or without amifostine in patients with metastatic breast cancer. *J Clin Oncol* (1999) 17, 3038–47.
2. Van den Brande J, Nannan Panday VR, Hoekman K, Rosing H, Huijskes RVHP, Verheijen RHM, Beijnen JH, Vermorken JB. Pharmacologic study of paclitaxel administered with or without the cytoprotective agent amifostine, and given as a single agent or in combination with epirubicin and cisplatin in patients with advanced solid tumours. *Am J Clin Oncol* (2001) 24, 401–3.
3. Schüller J, Czejka M, Pietrzak C, Springer B, Wirth M, Schernthaner G. Influence of the cytoprotective agent amifostine (AMI) on pharmacokinetics (PK) of paclitaxel (PAC) and Taxotere® (TXT). *Proc Am Soc Clin Oncol* (1997) 16, 224a.
4. Czejka M, Schueller J, Eder I, Reznicek G, Kraule C, Zeleni U, Freitag R. Clinical pharmacokinetics and metabolism of paclitaxel after polychemotherapy with the cytoprotective agent amifostine. *Anticancer Res* (2000) 20, 3871–7.
5. Juan O, Rocher A, Sánchez A, Sánchez JJ, Alberola V. Influence of the cyto-protective agent amifostine on the pharmacokinetics of low-dose paclitaxel. *Chemotherapy* (2005) 51, 200–5.
6. Freyer G, Hennebert P, Awada A, Gil T, Kerger J, Selleslags J, Brassinne C, Piccart M, de Valeriola D. Influence of amifostine on the toxicity and pharmacokinetics of docetaxel in metastatic breast cancer patients: a pilot study. *Clin Cancer Res* (2002) 8, 95–102.
7. Taylor CW, Wang LM, List AF, Fernandes D, Paine-Murrieta GD, Johnson CS, Capizzi RL. Amifostine protects normal tissues from paclitaxel toxicity while cytotoxicity against tumour cells is maintained. *Eur J Cancer* (1997) 33, 1693–8.

Taxanes + Ciclosporin

Ciclosporin increases the levels of docetaxel and paclitaxel after *oral* administration.

Clinical evidence

(a) Docetaxel

One study found that the bioavailability of docetaxel after oral administration of the intravenous formulation was increased from 8% to 90% by oral ciclosporin 15 mg/kg.[1] In this study, the AUC of ciclosporin was about 50% higher than expected from previously published data, when it was given with oral docetaxel.[2]

(b) Paclitaxel

In 5 patients the plasma levels of paclitaxel were below therapeutic concentrations when they were given an oral dose (intravenous formulation) of paclitaxel 60 mg/m^2 followed by intravenous doses of 175 mg/m^2 for subsequent courses. However, therapeutic levels above 100 micromol/mL (a ninefold increase) were achieved in 9 patients who received the same regimen with ciclosporin 15 mg/kg.[3]

Mechanism

Oral paclitaxel and docetaxel have poor oral bioavailability because of a high affinity for P-glycoprotein in the gastrointestinal tract, and possibly also pre-systemic metabolism by the cytochrome P450 isoenzyme CYP3A4. Ciclosporin is a known P-glycoprotein inhibitor, and thereby increases their oral absorption, and might also interact via CYP3A4. It was suggested that docetaxel might increase ciclosporin levels because they are both substrates for CYP3A4, but this sort of competition for metabolism does not usually result in clinically relevant interactions.

Importance and management

The use of oral docetaxel or paclitaxel is not established, therefore the pharmacokinetic interaction with ciclosporin has little general relevance. The suggestion that oral docetaxel might increase ciclosporin levels requires confirmation in a prospective study.

1. Malingré MM, Richel DJ, Beijnen JH, Rosing H, Koopman FJ, Ten Bokkel Huinink WW, Schot ME, Schellens JHM. Coadministration of cyclosporine strongly enhances the oral bioavailability of docetaxel. *J Clin Oncol* (2001) 19, 1160–6.
2. Malingré MM, Ten Bokkel Huinink WW, Mackay M, Schellens JHM, Beijnen JH. Pharmacokinetics of oral cyclosporin A when co-administered to enhance the absorption of orally administered docetaxel. *Eur J Clin Pharmacol* (2001) 57, 305–7.
3. Meerum Terwogt JM, Beijnen JH, ten Bokkel Huinink WW, Rosing H, Schellens JHM. Co-administration of cyclosporin enables oral therapy with paclitaxel. *Lancet* (1998) 352, 285.

Taxanes + Cisplatin and other platinum compounds

The toxicity of paclitaxel given with cisplatin appears to be dependent on the order of administration, with more severe myelosuppression occurring if cisplatin is given first. There does not appear to be any sequence dependent interaction for the combination of docetaxel with carboplatin or docetaxel with cisplatin. Paclitaxel may reduce the thrombocytopenia associated with carboplatin. The combination of carboplatin with paclitaxel appears to be more neurotoxic than carboplatin with docetaxel.

Clinical evidence, mechanism, importance and management

(a) Carboplatin

Several clinical studies have found that the severity of thrombocytopenia with the combination of **paclitaxel** and carboplatin was less than that expected with carboplatin alone.[1-5] This does not appear to be due to any changes in carboplatin pharmacokinetics. In one study, patients were given carboplatin as a 30-minute infusion, either alone or immediately after **paclitaxel** 175 mg/m^2 as a 3-hour infusion. It was found that the pharmacokinetics of carboplatin were not significantly affected by **paclitaxel**.[6] Similarly, a pharmacokinetic interaction was not noted when **paclitaxel** and carboplatin were given in either order in another study.[1] Other studies found the AUC of carboplatin to be similar to that predicted, despite the presence of paclitaxel.[2,5] Although one study found the AUC of carboplatin to be about 12% lower in the presence of **paclitaxel**,[4] the same researchers also found that the AUC associated with a 50% decrease in platelet count increased by 68% (i.e. more carboplatin is needed to cause the same degree of thrombocytopenia), which suggests a pharmacodynamic basis for the attenuated toxicity of the combination.[7] Other researchers also reported that the AUC of carboplatin causing a 50% reduction in platelets was about 6.3 mg/mL per minute when given with **paclitaxel** compared with historical data of 4 mg/mL per minute when given alone.[8] Although thrombocytopenia may be lower than expected, myelosuppression (in the form of neutropenia) is a dose-limiting toxicity of the combination of carboplatin and **paclitaxel**.[1-4] In one study, patients given **paclitaxel** with carboplatin experienced significantly greater neurotoxicity than those given **docetaxel** with carboplatin, but the regimens were similar in efficacy.[9] Further, there appear to be no pharmacokinetic interactions between carboplatin and **docetaxel**.[10,11]

(b) Cisplatin

Early studies of the combination of cisplatin and **paclitaxel** found that the degree of myelosuppression was sequence dependent. When cisplatin was given first, a greater degree of myelosuppression was seen.[12] Pharmacokinetic studies suggest that sequence-dependent differences in myelosuppression may be due to a 25% reduction in **paclitaxel** clearance when cisplatin is given first.[12] For this reason, the manufacturers recommend that **paclitaxel** is given before cisplatin.[13,14] There is also some evidence that *myelosuppression* is greater for the combination when **paclitaxel** is given over 24 hours as opposed to 3 hours.[13] When **paclitaxel** is given with cisplatin, *neurotoxicity* (peripheral neuropathy) is common,[13] and there is some evidence that this is more severe if the **paclitaxel** is given over 3 hours as opposed to over 24 hours.[15] In one study,[16] neurotoxicity was unexpectedly severe when **paclitaxel** alone was used in patients who had relapsed after treatment with cisplatin; however, this was not the case in another similar study.[17] There is also some retrospective evidence that the use of paclitaxel with cisplatin may increase *nephrotoxicity* when compared with cisplatin alone.[18]

In contrast to **paclitaxel**, early studies did not reveal any obvious sequence dependent toxicity for the combination of **docetaxel** and cisplatin.[19] In addition, cisplatin did not cause any significant changes in **docetaxel** pharmacokinetics.[19,20] A more recent analysis confirmed that cisplatin was not associated with any changes in docetaxel clearance.[21]

1. Huizing MT, Giaccone G, van Warmerdam LJC, Rosing H, Bakker PJM, Vermorken JB, Postmus PE, van Zandwijk N, Koolen MGJ, ten Bokkel Huinink WW, van der Vijgh WJF, Bierhorst FJ, Lai A, Dalesio O, Pinedo HM, Veenhof CHN, Beijnen JH. Pharmacokinetics of paclitaxel and carboplatin in a dose-escalating and dose-sequencing study in patients with non-small-cell lung cancer. *J Clin Oncol* (1997) 15, 317–29.
2. Bookman MA, McGuire WP, Kilpatrick D, Keenan E, Hogan WM, Johnson SW, O'Dwyer P, Rowinsky E, Gallion HH, Ozols RF. Carboplatin and paclitaxel in ovarian carcinoma: a phase I study of the Gynecologic Oncology Group. *J Clin Oncol* (1996) 14, 1895–1902.
3. Huizing MT, van Warmerdam LJC, Rosing H, Schaefers MCW, Lai A, Helmerhorst TJM, Veenhof CHN, Birkhofer MJ, Rodenhuis S, Beijnen JH, ten Bokkel Huinink WW. Phase I and pharmacologic study of the combination paclitaxel and carboplatin as first-line chemotherapy in stage III and IV ovarian cancer. *J Clin Oncol* (1997) 15, 1953–64.
4. Belani CP, Kearns CM, Zuhowski EG, Erkmen K, Hiponia D, Zacharski D, Engstrom C, Ramanathan RK, Capozzoli MJ, Aisner J, Egorin MJ. Phase I trial, including pharmacokinetics and pharmacodynamic correlations, of combination paclitaxel and carboplatin in patients with metastatic non-small-cell lung cancer. *J Clin Oncol* (1999) 17, 676–84.
5. Siddiqui N, Boddy AV, Thomas HD, Bailey NP, Robson L, Lind MJ, Calvert AH. A clinical and pharmacokinetic study of the combination of carboplatin and paclitaxel for epithelial ovarian cancer. *Br J Cancer* (1997) 75, 287–94.
6. Obasaju CK, Johnson SW, Rogatko A, Kilpatrick D, Brennan JM, Hamilton TC, Ozols RF, O'Dwyer PJ, Gallo JM. Evaluation of carboplatin pharmacokinetics in the absence and presence of paclitaxel. *Clin Cancer Res* (1996) 2, 549–52.
7. Kearns CM, Belani CP, Erkmen K, Zuhowski M, Hiponia D, Ergstrom C, Ramanathan R, Trenn M, Aisner J, Ergorin MJ. Reduced platelet toxicity with combination carboplatin & paclitaxel: pharmacodynamic modulation of carboplatin associated thrombocytopenia. *Proc Am Soc Clin Oncol* (1995) 14, 170.
8. van Warmerdam LJC, Huizing MT, Giaccone G, Postmus PE, ten Bokkel Huinink WW, van Zandwijk N, Koolen MGJ, Helmerhorst TJM, van der Vijgh WJF, Veenhof CHN, Beijnen JH. Clinical pharmacology of carboplatin administered in combination with paclitaxel. *Semin Oncol* (1997) 24 (Suppl 2), S2-97–S2-104.
9. Kaye SB, Vasey PA. Docetaxel in ovarian cancer: phase III perspectives and future development. *Semin Oncol* (2002) 29 (3 Suppl 12) 22–7.
10. Oka M, Fukuda M, Nagashima S, Fukuda M, Kinoshita A, Soda H, Doi S, Narasaki F, Suenaga M, Takatani H, Nakamura Y, Kawabata S, Tsurutani J, Kanda T, Kohno S. Phase I study of second-line chemotherapy with docetaxel and carboplatin in non-small-cell lung cancer. *Cancer Chemother Pharmacol* (2001) 48, 446–50.
11. Ando M, Saka H, Ando Y, Minami H, Kuzuya T, Yamamoto M, Watanabe A, Sakai S, Shimokata K, Hasegawa Y. Sequence effect of docetaxel and carboplatin on toxicity, tumor response and pharmacokinetics in non-small-cell lung cancer patients: a phase I study of two sequences. *Cancer Chemother Pharmacol* (2005) 55, 552–8.
12. Rowkinsky EK, Gilbert M, McGuire WP, Noe DA, Grochow LB, Forastiere AA, Ettinger DS, Lubejko BG, Clarke B, Sartorius SE, Cornblath DR, Hendricks CB, Donehower RC. Sequences of taxol and cisplatin: a phase I and pharmacologic study. *J Clin Oncol* (1991) 9, 1692–1703.
13. Paclitaxel. Medac GmbH. UK Summary of product characteristics, January 2011.
14. Taxol (Paclitaxel). Bristol-Myers Squibb Company. US Prescribing information, April 2011.
15. Connelly E, Markman M, Kennedy A, Webster K, Kulp B, Peterson G, Belinson J. Paclitaxel delivered as a 3-hr infusion with cisplatin in patients with gynecologic cancers: unexpected incidence of neurotoxicity. *Gynecol Oncol* (1996) 62, 166–8.
16. Cavaletti G, Bogliun G, Marzorati L, Zincone A, Marzola M, Colombo N, Tredici G. Peripheral neurotoxicity of taxol in patients previously treated with cisplatin. *Cancer* (1995) 75, 1141–50.
17. McGuire WP, Rowinsky EK, Rosenhein NB, Grumbine FC, Ettinger DS, Armstrong DK, Donehower RC. Taxol: a unique antineoplastic agent with significant activity in advanced ovarian epithelial neoplasms. *Ann Intern Med* (1989) 111, 273–9.
18. Merouani A, Davidson SA, Schrier RW. Increased nephrotoxicity of combination taxol and cisplatin chemotherapy in gynaecologic cancers as compared to cisplatin alone. *Am J Nephrol* (1997) 17, 53–8.
19. Pronk LC, Schellens JHM, Planting AST, van den Bent MJ, Hilkens PHE, van der Burg MEL, de Boer-Dennert M, Ma J, Blanc C, Harteveld M, Bruno R, Stoter G, Verweij J. Phase I and pharmacologic study of docetaxel and cisplatin in patients with advanced solid tumors. *J Clin Oncol* (1997) 15, 1071–9.
20. Millward MJ, Zalcberg J, Bishop JF, Webster LK, Zimet A, Rischin D, Toner GC, Laird J, Cosolo W, Urch M, Bruno R, Loret C, James R, Blanc C. Phase I trial of docetaxel and cisplatin in previously untreated patients with advanced non-small-cell lung cancer. *J Clin Oncol* (1997) 15, 750–8.
21. Rudek MA, Sparreboom A, Garrett-Mayer ES, Armstrong DK, Wolff AC, Verweij J, Baker SD. Factors affecting pharmacokinetic variability following doxorubicin and docetaxel-based therapy. *Eur J Cancer* (2004) 40, 1170–8.

Taxanes + HIV-protease inhibitors

Life-threatening haematological toxicities have been reported in a few patients taking HIV-protease inhibitors when given paclitaxel, and several cases have also been reported for docetaxel. Nelfinavir and ritonavir appear to inhibit the clearance of paclitaxel, although one case report did not find this. There is conflicting evidence on whether indinavir inhibits, or has no effect on, paclitaxel clearance.

Clinical evidence

(a) Docetaxel

An HIV-positive, 64-year-old woman taking **nelfinavir** was given trastuzumab and docetaxel 36 mg/m^2 for breast cancer. Three days later she was hospitalised with early, severe myelosuppression, which was attributed to an interaction between nelfinavir and docetaxel, and she died from sepsis.[1]

A 40-year-old HIV-positive man taking **lopinavir** boosted with **ritonavir** developed febrile neutropenia 8 days after a single 25-mg/m^2 dose of docetaxel; microbiological tests were negative.[2] Another case report describes 3 patients who developed early febrile neutropenia, grade 3 mucositis, skin rash, and hand-foot syndrome, which were attributed to an interaction with a **ritonavir**-based HAART regimen.[3] This report also mentions a further two unpublished cases of febrile neutropenia and mucositis, which developed when patients taking **ritonavir** (and **indinavir** or **saquinavir**) were given docetaxel.[3]

In a single-dose study in patients with solid tumours, ritonavir 100 mg, given 60-minutes before, or at the same time as, a 100-mg *oral* dose of docetaxel, increased docetaxel exposure 30 to 50%, when compared with the same dose of intravenous docetaxel given alone. Separating the doses did not affect the outcome.[4] Pharmacokinetic modelling showed this was due to an increase in absorption from the gut and a decrease in plasma clearance.[5]

(b) Paclitaxel

1. Pharmacokinetics. The UK manufacturer of paclitaxel briefly mentions that studies in patients with Kaposi's sarcoma, who were taking multiple other drugs, suggest that the systemic clearance of paclitaxel was significantly lower in the presence of **nelfinavir** and **ritonavir**, but not with **indinavir**.[6] Consistent with this, a published study found that the pharmacokinetics of paclitaxel did not differ in 4 patients taking **indinavir**, compared with 5 patients not taking HIV-protease inhibitors.[7] However, in another published study in HIV-positive patients with Kaposi's sarcoma, the AUC of paclitaxel 100 mg/m^2 every 2 weeks was 2-fold higher in 3 patients taking **indinavir** alone, when compared with 6 patients not taking HIV-protease inhibitors. Similarly, the AUC of paclitaxel was 2-fold higher in 6 patients taking **nelfinavir** alone and was 72% higher in 6 patients taking multiple HIV-protease inhibitors (drugs not stated), when compared with 6 patients not taking HIV-protease inhibitors. In this study, the increase in paclitaxel exposure was not associated with increased toxicity,[8] see *Toxicity,* below. In contrast, in one case, the clearance of paclitaxel was modestly *increased* and its AUC slightly reduced when it was given with HIV-protease inhibitors. Over a number of cycles of paclitaxel, this patient was given various combinations of paclitaxel alone, with **ritonavir**, **indinavir**, and two NRTIs, with **ritonavir**, **saquinavir**, and two NRTIs, or with nevirapine and two NRTIs. However, the pharmacokinetics of paclitaxel during any of these regimens did not differ from each other and were not greatly different from historical data from HIV-negative patients, and the pharmacokinetics of saquinavir, ritonavir, indinavir, or nevirapine also did not differ from historical data.[9]

2. Toxicity. In a study with paclitaxel 100 mg/m^2 given every 2 weeks for the treatment of HIV-related Kaposi's sarcoma, there was no difference in haematological toxicity (including severe or life-threatening haematological toxicity) or other toxicities between patients taking HIV-protease inhibitors (mostly **indinavir**, but also **saquinavir**, **ritonavir**, or **nelfinavir**) and those not taking an HIV-protease inhibitor in each of the first 10 cycles. Grade 4 neutropenia was reported in 35% of patients. In this study, of 107 patients, 82 received HIV-protease inhibitor-based antiretroviral regimens, and HIV-protease inhibitor use had a favourable impact on survival. Nevertheless, paclitaxel-related adverse effects contributed to the deaths of 4 patients, all of whom were receiving multiple other drugs including HIV-protease inhibitors and co-trimoxazole.[10] Similarly, in another study there was no increase in paclitaxel toxicity when it was given to patients taking HIV-protease inhibitors, despite a pharmacokinetic interaction,[8] see *Pharmacokinetics,* above.

In contrast, a number of case reports describe unexpected paclitaxel-related toxicity with HIV-protease inhibitors. A 39-year-old woman taking **lopinavir** boosted with **ritonavir** was given carboplatin and paclitaxel 175 mg/m^2 for adenocarcinoma. Five days later, she was hospitalised with early, severe myelosuppression, which was attributed to an interaction between lopinavir and paclitaxel, and she later died.[1] In another report, an HIV-positive patient taking **lopinavir** boosted with **ritonavir**, delavirdine, and didanosine was also given paclitaxel 100 mg/m^2 for Kaposi's sarcoma. Within 3 days he developed myalgia and arthralgia, and 8 days later he developed fever, tachycardia, and a productive cough. He was treated with antibacterials and granulocyte colony-stimulating factor (G-CSF), but later died. Findings at post mortem included severe oesophageal mucositis, *Streptococcus viridans* pneumonia, and a massive saddle embolism (an embolism that sits across two vessels).[11] A second patient taking **indinavir**, **ritonavir**, lamivudine, and stavudine developed severe leucopenia and thrombocytopenia within 7 days of being given paclitaxel 100 mg/m^2 for Kaposi's sarcoma, and again after a second course of paclitaxel. Further courses of paclitaxel were tolerated by giving a reduced dose of 60 mg/m^2 of paclitaxel with G-CSF.[11] Similar cases have been reported in 2 patients receiving paclitaxel 100 mg/m^2 every other week for Kaposi's sarcoma when their antiretroviral regimens were changed from **indinavir** or **nelfinavir** with NRTIs to **saquinavir**, delavirdine, and didanosine. One of these patients also received intermittent fluconazole.[12] (For more information on the interaction between fluconazole and taxanes, see 'Taxanes + Ketoconazole and other CYP3A4 inhibitors', p.715).

Mechanism

Uncertain. Paclitaxel is metabolised by CYP2C8 and CYP3A4, whereas docetaxel is principally metabolised by CYP3A4. HIV-protease inhibitors such as ritonavir and indinavir are known to inhibit CYP3A4, which might result in increased taxane concentrations and toxicity, but, docetaxel is more likely to be affected by this mechanism than paclitaxel. Nevertheless, additional use of a CYP2C8 inhibitor (such as trimethoprim as part of co-trimoxazole, as is common in HIV infection) could result in an interaction with paclitaxel. *Oral* docetaxel is poorly absorbed and concurrent use with ritonavir appears to increase its absorption, probably by inhibiting intestinal CYP3A4, and also inhibiting its elimination.

Importance and management

Although there are just a few case reports of toxicity, a pharmacokinetic interaction between the HIV-protease inhibitors and **docetaxel** would be expected, based on its metabolism and known interaction with ketoconazole (see 'Taxanes + Ketoconazole and other CYP3A4 inhibitors', p.715). The US manufacturer of docetaxel states that the concurrent use of potent CYP3A4 inhibitors should be avoided, and they specifically name **atazanavir**, indinavir, nelfinavir, ritonavir, and saquinavir.[13] If a potent CYP3A4 inhibitor needs to be given with docetaxel, the manufacturers suggest reducing the docetaxel dose by 50%,[13,14] and monitoring patients closely for docetaxel toxicity (severe myelosuppression, peripheral neuropathy, and mucositis).[13] The effect of ritonavir on *oral* docetaxel exposure is of no general clinical relevance since oral formulations of docetaxel are investigational.

There is some evidence of a pharmacokinetic interaction between the HIV-protease inhibitors and **paclitaxel**, but two studies did not find an increase in paclitaxel toxicity with the concurrent use of some HIV-protease inhibitors (principally indinavir and nelfinavir). Nevertheless, the case reports of toxicity do introduce a note of caution. Until more is known, some caution would be advisable when paclitaxel is given to patients taking HIV-protease inhibitors.

1. Parameswaran R, Sweeney C, Einhorn LH. Interaction between highly active antiretroviral therapy (HAART) and taxanes: a report of two cases. *Proc Am Soc Clin Oncol* (2002) 21, abstract 2194.
2. Loulergue P, Mir O, Allali J, Viard J-P. Possible pharmacokinetic interaction involving ritonavir and docetaxel in a patient with Kaposi's sarcoma. *AIDS* (2008) 22, 1237–9.
3. Mir O, Dessard-Diana B, Louet AL-L, Loulergue P, Viard J-P, Langlois A, Durdux C, Le Beller C. Severe toxicity related to a pharmacokinetic interaction between docetaxel and ritonavir in HIV-infected patients. *Br J Clin Pharmacol* (2010) 69, 99–101.
4. Oostendorp RL, Huitema A, Rosing H, Jansen RS, ter Heine R, Keessen M, Beijnen JH, Schellens JHM. Coadministration of ritonavir strongly enhances the apparent oral bioavailability of docetaxel in patients with solid tumors. *Clin Cancer Res* (2009) 15, 4228–33.
5. Koolen SLW, Oostendorp RL, Beijnen JH, Schellens JHM, Huitema ADR. Population pharmacokinetics of intravenously and orally administered docetaxel with or without co-administration of ritonavir in patients with advanced cancer. *Br J Clin Pharmacol* (2010) 69, 465–74.
6. Paclitaxel. Medac GmbH. UK Summary of product characteristics, January 2011.
7. Duchin K, Sun J, Tan M, Ilaw M, Cabriales S, Espina BM, East D, Tulpule A, Gill PS. Pharmacokinetics of low-dose Paxene (paclitaxel) in patients with refractory or relapsed AIDS-related Kaposi's sarcoma [abstract no. 829]. 33rd Annual Meeting of the American Society of Clinical Oncology;1997 May 17-20; Denver.
8. Cianfrocca M, Lee S, Von Roenn J, Rudek MA, Dezube BJ, Krown SE, Sparano JA. Pilot study evaluating the interaction between paclitaxel and protease inhibitors in patients with human immunodeficiency virus-associated Kaposi's sarcoma: an Eastern Cooperative Oncology Group (ECOG) and AIDS Malignancy Consortium (AMC) trial. *Cancer Chemother Pharmacol* (2011) 68, 827–33.
9. Nannan Panday VR, Hoetelmans RMW, van Heeswijk RPG, Meenhorst PL, Inghels M, Mulder JW, Beijnen JH. Paclitaxel in the treatment of human immunodeficiency virus 1-associated Kaposi's sarcoma – drug-drug interactions with protease inhibitors and a nonnucleoside reverse transcriptase inhibitor: a case report study. *Cancer Chemother Pharmacol* (1999) 43, 516–9.
10. Tulpule A, Groopman J, Saville MW, Harrington W, Friedman-Kien A, Espina BM, Garces C, Mantelle L, Mettinger K, Scadden DT, Gill PS. Multicenter trial of low-dose paclitaxel in patients with advanced AIDS-related Kaposi sarcoma. *Cancer* (2002) 95, 147–54.
11. Bundow D, Aboulafia DM. Potential drug interaction with paclitaxel and highly active antiretroviral therapy in two patients with AIDS-associated Kaposi sarcoma. *Am J Clin Oncol* (2004) 27, 81–4.
12. Schwartz JD, Howard W, Scadden DT. Potential interaction of antiretroviral therapy with paclitaxel in patients with AIDS-related Kaposi's sarcoma. *AIDS* (1999) 13, 283–4.
13. Taxotere (Docetaxel). Sanofi-Aventis US LLC. US Prescribing information, May 2010.
14. Taxotere (Docetaxel trihydrate). Sanofi. UK Summary of product characteristics, July 2012.

Taxanes + Ketoconazole and other CYP3A4 inhibitors

Ketoconazole reduces the clearance of docetaxel and increases its exposure. In one patient, fluconazole reduced the clearance of paclitaxel, whereas in two patients single-dose ketoconazole did not affect the pharmacokinetics of paclitaxel. Other CYP3A4 inhibitors are predicted to increase docetaxel and paclitaxel concentrations.

Clinical evidence

(a) Docetaxel

In a study in 7 patients, ketoconazole, 200 mg daily for 3 days, started one hour before an infusion of docetaxel 10 mg/m^2, reduced the clearance of docetaxel by 49% and increased its AUC 2.2-fold.[1] Various phase I and II clinical studies have investigated the combined use of ketoconazole with docetaxel for both the pharmacokinetic interaction and for the potential synergistic effects in prostate cancer. In one such study using increasing doses of docetaxel (from 5 mg/m^2 to 43 mg/m^2) with decreasing ketoconazole doses, ketoconazole 400 mg three times daily increased docetaxel exposure 2.6-fold, ketoconazole 200 mg in the morning and afternoon with 400 mg at night increased docetaxel exposure by 60%, and ketoconazole 200 mg three times daily increased docetaxel exposure by 30 to 50%. The dose-limiting toxicity with the two higher doses of ketoconazole was hepatic toxicity.[2] In another study in patients with breast cancer, the AUC of docetaxel was similar between patients taking ketoconazole 200 mg three times daily for 3 days with a reduced flat-dose of docetaxel of 70 mg on day 3, and those receiving conventional dose docetaxel 75 mg/m^2 alone. Patients given ketoconazole with reduced dose docetaxel had higher neutrophil counts and were less likely to develop grade 4 neutropenia and febrile neutropenia, when compared with those given standard dose docetaxel alone.[3]

(b) Paclitaxel

1. Fluconazole. The clearance of paclitaxel was assessed in one patient who had taken fluconazole (dose not stated) for 2 weeks, up until one day before his first cycle of paclitaxel, and then 3 weeks later, during his second cycle of paclitaxel. The clearance of paclitaxel was 44% lower after the use of fluconazole, and concentrations of the metabolites of paclitaxel, formed by the action of CYP3A4, were lower.[4]

2. *Ketoconazole.* Five women with ovarian cancer were given 3-hour infusions of paclitaxel 175 mg/m^2 every 21 days. In 2 patients, when single 200-mg oral doses of ketoconazole were given 3 hours before, or 3 hours after, paclitaxel, the serum concentrations of paclitaxel and its principal metabolite, 6-alpha-hydroxypaclitaxel, were unchanged.[5]

Mechanism

The metabolism of docetaxel is mainly mediated by CYP3A4, which is inhibited by ketoconazole, thereby increasing docetaxel exposure. Paclitaxel is principally metabolised by CYP2C8, and to a lesser extent by CYP3A4. The findings of the study with paclitaxel[5] suggest that CYP3A4 inhibition alone might not affect its concentrations. However, this study used a single low-dose of ketoconazole given 3 hours before, or after, paclitaxel, and it is possible that a longer course with a higher dose of ketoconazole might interact differently. The data from the single case with fluconazole, which is a dose-dependent moderate inhibitor of CYP3A4, suggest that CYP3A4 might be involved in the interaction between fluconazole and paclitaxel.

Importance and management

The pharmacokinetic interaction between ketoconazole and **docetaxel** is likely to be clinically important because a 50% decrease in docetaxel clearance has been associated with a 3- to 4-fold increase in neutropenia.[1] The US manufacturer of docetaxel states that the concurrent use of potent CYP3A4 inhibitors, such as ketoconazole, should be avoided.[6] If patients do require both drugs, the UK and US manufacturers recommend close monitoring for docetaxel toxicity (severe myelosuppression, peripheral neuropathy, and mucositis) and consideration of a reduced dose of docetaxel (50% reduction suggested).[6,7] Of the CYP3A4 inhibitors for which there is no clinical information, the UK and US manufacturers specifically name azoles, such as **itraconazole** and **voriconazole**, and **nefazodone**.[6,7]

Information on the interaction of azoles with **paclitaxel** is limited and not conclusive. Based on the study with ketoconazole, the UK manufacturer of paclitaxel states that ketoconazole can be given without any paclitaxel dose adjustments.[8] However the UK and US manufacturers of paclitaxel still continue to advise caution with other drugs that are inhibitors of CYP3A4. Of the CYP3A4 inhibitors for which there is no clinical information, they specifically name **itraconazole** and **nefazodone**.[8,9] The UK manufacturer also names **fluoxetine**,[8] but note that fluoxetine is considered, at the most, a weak inhibitor of CYP3A4 and is not known to inhibit CYP2C8. Until more is known, some caution would appear to be appropriate with the concurrent use of all moderate to potent CYP3A4 inhibitors.

Note that interactions have, on occasion, been seen when docetaxel or paclitaxel were given with the HIV-protease inhibitors, which are known potent CYP3A4 inhibitors, see 'Taxanes + HIV-protease inhibitors', p.714. For a list of other CYP3A4 inhibitors, see 'Table 1.9', p.11.

1. Engels FK, ten Tije AJ, Baker SD, Lee CKK, Loos WJ, Vulto AG, Verweij J, Sparreboom A. Effect of cytochrome P450 3A4 inhibition on the pharmacokinetics of docetaxel. *Clin Pharmacol Ther* (2004) 75, 448–54.
2. Figg WD, Woo S, Zhu W, Chen X, Ajiboye AS, Steinberg SM, Price DK, Wright JJ, Parnes HL, Arlen PM, Gulley JL, Dahut WL. A phase I clinical study of high dose ketoconazole plus weekly docetaxel for metastatic castration resistant prostate cancer. *J Urol (Baltimore)* (2010) 183, 2219–26.
3. Lim Y-W, Goh B-C, Wang L-Z, Tan S-H, Chuah BY, Lim S-E, Iau P, Buhari SA, Chan C-W, Sukri NB, Cordero MT, Soo R, Lee S-C. Pharmacokinetics and pharmacodynamics of docetaxel with or without ketoconazole modulation in chemonaive breast cancer patients. *Ann Oncol* (2010) 21, 2175–82.
4. Sonnichsen DS, Liu Q, Schuetz EG, Schuetz JD, Pappo A, Relling MV. Variability in human cytochrome P450 paclitaxel metabolism. *J Pharmacol Exp Ther* (1995) 275, 566–75.
5. Jamis-Dow CA, Pearl ML, Watkins PB, Blake DS, Klecker RW, Collins JM. Predicting drug interactions in vivo from experiments in vitro: human studies with paclitaxel and ketoconazole. *Am J Clin Oncol* (1997) 20, 592–99.
6. Taxotere (Docetaxel). Sanofi-Aventis US LLC. US Prescribing information, May 2010.
7. Taxotere (Docetaxel trihydrate). Sanofi. UK Summary of product characteristics, July 2012.
8. Paclitaxel. Medac GmbH. UK Summary of product characteristics, January 2011.
9. Taxol (Paclitaxel). Bristol-Myers Squibb Company. US Prescribing information, April 2011.

Taxanes + Macrolides

An case report describes cholestatic jaundice and pseudomembranous colitis, to which an interaction of erythromycin with docetaxel was considered a contributing factor. Macrolides that inhibit CYP3A4 are predicted to increase docetaxel exposure.

Clinical evidence

A 45-year-old woman taking long-term prophylactic erythromycin after splenectomy received doxorubicin 50 mg/m^2 and **docetaxel** 75 mg/m^2 every 3 weeks for metastatic breast cancer. Six days after the first cycle, she developed a rash, neutropenic fever, vomiting, and watery diarrhoea, with no infectious aetiology found. Four days after the second cycle, she presented with the same symptoms. Her condition worsened and she developed cholestatic jaundice and pseudomembranous colitis (not due to *Clostridium difficile*). With aggressive support she slowly recovered over 6 weeks. When she died 6 months later, post-mortem analysis showed no underlying liver or bowel pathology.[1]

Mechanism

The pseudomembranous colitis and cholestatic jaundice were attributed to the combination of docetaxel and doxorubicin. However, erythromycin, which is predicted to inhibit the metabolism of docetaxel by CYP3A4, was considered a contributing factor. Note that paclitaxel is partially metabolised by CYP3A4, and might be expected to be similarly affected by erythromycin, although to a lesser extent.

Importance and management

The case report does not prove a pharmacokinetic interaction between erythromycin and **docetaxel**, but, on the basis of data with ketoconazole (see 'Taxanes + Ketoconazole and other CYP3A4 inhibitors', p.715), an interaction with erythromycin and other macrolides that inhibit CYP3A4 is predicted. The US manufacturer of docetaxel states that the concurrent use of potent CYP3A4 inhibitors such as **clarithromycin** and **telithromycin** should be avoided.[2] If patients do require concurrent use, the UK and US manufacturers recommend close monitoring for docetaxel toxicity and consideration of a reduced dose of docetaxel (50% reduction suggested).[2,3] The UK manufacturers also advise caution with **erythromycin** and **troleandomycin**.[3]

There is little information on the interaction of CYP3A4 inhibitors with **paclitaxel**. Although the potent CYP3A4 inhibitor ketoconazole had no effect on the concentrations of paclitaxel or its hydroxy metabolites, and the UK and US manufacturers of paclitaxel advise that no dose adjustment is needed on concurrent use (see 'Taxanes + Ketoconazole and other CYP3A4 inhibitors', p.715), the manufacturers still advise caution on the concurrent use of paclitaxel and the macrolides, **clarithromycin**, **erythromycin**, and **telithromycin**.[4,5]

1. Cholestatic jaundice and pseudomembranous colitis following combination therapy with doxorubicin and docetaxel. *Anticancer Drugs* (2003) 14, 3279.
2. Taxotere (Docetaxel). Sanofi-Aventis US LLC. US Prescribing information, May 2010.
3. Taxotere (Docetaxel trihydrate). Sanofi. UK Summary of product characteristics, July 2012.
4. Paclitaxel. Medac GmbH. UK Summary of product characteristics, January 2011.
5. Taxol (Paclitaxel). Bristol-Myers Squibb Company. US Prescribing information, April 2011.

Taxanes + NNRTIs

Efavirenz and nevirapine are predicted to reduce paclitaxel concentrations, although isolated case reports suggest that no pharmacokinetic interaction occurs between paclitaxel and nevirapine. Efavirenz and nevirapine might also reduce docetaxel concentrations.

Clinical evidence

In one case report, the clearance of **paclitaxel** was modestly *increased* and its AUC slightly reduced when it was given with **nevirapine**. Over a number of cycles of paclitaxel, this patient was given various combinations of paclitaxel alone, with ritonavir, indinavir, and two NRTIs, with ritonavir, saquinavir, and two NRTIs, or with **nevirapine** and two NRTIs. However, the pharmacokinetics of **paclitaxel** during any of these regimens did not differ from each other and were not greatly different from historical data from HIV-negative patients. The pharmacokinetics of nevirapine also did not differ from historical data.[1] Similarly, a 37-year old man taking **nevirapine** 200 mg twice daily (with stavudine and lamivudine) was given **paclitaxel** 100 mg/m^2 for Kaposi's sarcoma. The concurrent use of paclitaxel had no effect on the pharmacokinetics of nevirapine, when compared with nevirapine alone. In addition, **paclitaxel** exposure, and that of its hydroxyl metabolites, was reported to be similar to the mean exposure in 8 historical controls.[2]

Mechanism

Paclitaxel is principally metabolised by CYP2C8 and also, to some extent, by CYP3A4. Nevirapine has been reported to induce CYP3A4 and might be expected to reduce paclitaxel exposure; however, the case reports above suggest that this does not always occur. **Efavirenz** also induces CYP3A4 and might be expected to reduce paclitaxel exposure.

Docetaxel is known to be principally metabolised by CYP3A4, and might also be expected to be similarly affected by these NNRTIs.

Importance and management

Evidence for an interaction between taxanes and NNRTIs is limited to isolated case reports, which suggest that **nevirapine** might not affect the pharmacokinetics of paclitaxel; however, further controlled studies are needed to confirm this. Given the data with other enzyme inducers (see 'Taxanes + Rifampicin (Rifampin) and other enzyme inducers', p.717), and the consequences of a loss of paclitaxel efficacy, until more is known, some caution would seem prudent. The UK and US manufacturers[3,4] of paclitaxel advise caution with all inducers of CYP2C8 or CYP3A4, and the UK manufacturer specifically names **efavirenz** and **nevirapine**.[3] Close monitoring to ensure paclitaxel remains effective would be appropriate, increasing the paclitaxel dose if indicated.

There appears to be no published data for an interaction between **docetaxel** and **efavirenz** or **nevirapine**. However, as the potent CYP3A4 *inhibitor* ketoconazole markedly reduced the clearance of docetaxel in patients (see 'Taxanes + Ketoconazole and other CYP3A4 inhibitors', p.715), clinically relevant increases in docetaxel clearance might occur with inducers of CYP3A4, such as efavirenz and nevirapine. If concurrent use is essential, it would seem prudent to monitor closely to ensure docetaxel remains effective and increase the docetaxel dose if necessary, carefully monitoring for toxicity.

1. Nannan Panday VR, Hoetelmans RMW, van Heeswijk RPG, Meenhorst PL, Inghels M, Mulder JW, Beijnen JH. Paclitaxel in the treatment of human immunodeficiency virus 1-associated Kaposi's sarcoma – drug-drug interactions with protease inhibitors and a nonnucleoside reverse transcriptase inhibitor: a case report study. *Cancer Chemother Pharmacol* (1999) 43, 516–9.
2. Kappelhoff BS, Huitema ADR, Mairuhu ATA, Schellens JHM, Beijnen JH. No pharmacokinetic drug-drug interaction between nevirapine and paclitaxel. *Anticancer Drugs* (2005) 627–30.
3. Paclitaxel. Medac GmbH. UK Summary of product characteristics, January 2011.
4. Taxol (Paclitaxel). Bristol-Myers Squibb Company. US Prescribing information, April 2011.

Taxanes + Rifampicin (Rifampin) and other enzyme inducers

Phenytoin, carbamazepine, and phenobarbital increase the clearance of paclitaxel and increase its maximum tolerated dose. Other enzyme inducers are predicted to interact similarly. Potent CYP3A4 inducers (such as rifampicin and the barbiturates) would also be expected to reduce docetaxel concentrations.

Clinical evidence

(a) Docetaxel

There do not appear to be any published clinical data for docetaxel taken with enzyme-inducing drugs. However, an *in vitro* study found that hyperforin, a constituent of **St John's wort**, induced docetaxel metabolism in a dose-dependent manner by 2.6- to 7-fold, when compared with controls. In the same study, rifampicin increased docetaxel metabolism by 6.8- to 32-fold, when compared with controls.[1] Similarly, microsomes prepared from the livers of 3 patients taking **pentobarbital** and/or **phenobarbital** are reported to have strikingly induced docetaxel metabolism *in vitro*.[2]

In addition, the potent CYP3A4 *inhibitor* ketoconazole markedly reduces the clearance of docetaxel in patients (see 'Taxanes + Ketoconazole and other CYP3A4 inhibitors', p.715), suggesting that clinically relevant increases in docetaxel clearance might be likely with potent inducers of CYP3A4.

(b) Paclitaxel

In a study in patients with glioblastoma multiforme, the maximum tolerated dose of paclitaxel was 43% higher in patients receiving enzyme-inducing antiepileptics (**phenytoin**, **carbamazepine**, and **phenobarbital**), than in those not receiving them.[3] Another study in patients with recurrent malignant gliomas reported the same finding: a 50% increase in the maximum tolerated dose coupled with a 2-fold increase in the plasma clearance of paclitaxel in those taking enzyme-inducing antiepileptics. In addition, this study reported that the dose-limiting toxicity differed: central neurotoxicity in those taking enzyme-inducing antiepileptics and myelosuppression and/or gastrointestinal toxicity in those not taking these antiepileptics.[4]

Mechanism

It is probable that enzyme-inducing antiepileptics increase the metabolism of paclitaxel, which is principally metabolised by CYP2C8 and also, to some extent, by CYP3A4. Docetaxel is known to be principally metabolised by CYP3A4, and would also be expected to be affected by enzyme-inducing drugs.

Importance and management

Evidence for an interaction between **paclitaxel** and enzyme-inducing antiepileptics is limited to the studies described above, but appears to be established. It is likely that patients taking enzyme-inducing antiepileptics will require an increase in their paclitaxel dose. The UK and US manufacturers of paclitaxel advise caution on concurrent use of all inducers of CYP2C8 or CYP3A4, and they specifically name rifampicin and the enzyme-inducing antiepileptics **carbamazepine**, **phenobarbital**, and **phenytoin**.[5,6] Close monitoring to ensure paclitaxel remains effective would be appropriate, increasing the paclitaxel dose if indicated. Similar caution is probably warranted with **primidone**, which is metabolised to phenobarbital, and **fosphenytoin**, which is metabolised to phenytoin. For a list of inducers of CYP3A4, see 'Table 1.9', p.11, and of CYP2C8, see 'Table 1.4', p.6.

Similarly, if the concurrent use of CYP3A4 inducers with **docetaxel** is necessary, it would seem prudent to monitor closely to ensure docetaxel remains effective and increase the dose of docetaxel if necessary, carefully monitoring for toxicity.

1. Komoroski BJ, Parise RA, Egorin MJ, Strom SC, Venkataramanan R. Effect of the St. John's wort constituent hyperforin on docetaxel metabolism by human hepatocyte cultures. *Clin Cancer Res* (2005) 11, 6972–9.
2. Royer I, Monsarrat B, Sonnier M, Wright M, Cresteil T. Metabolism of docetaxel by human cytochromes P450: Interactions with paclitaxel and other antineoplastic drugs. *Cancer Res* (1996) 56, 58–65.
3. Fetell MR, Grossman SA, Fisher JD, Erlanger B, Rowinsky E, Stockel J, Piantadosi S. Preirradiation paclitaxel in glioblastoma multiforme: efficacy, pharmacology, and drug interactions. New approaches to Brain Tumor Therapy Central Nervous System Consortium. *J Clin Oncol* (1997) 15, 3121–8.
4. Chang SM, Kuhn JG, Rizzo J, Robins HI, Schold SC, Spence AM, Berger MS, Mehta MP, Bozik ME, Pollack I, Gilbert M, Fulton C, Rankin C, Malec M, Prados MD. Phase I study of paclitaxel in patients with recurrent malignant glioma: a North American Brain Tumor Consortium report. *J Clin Oncol* (1998) 16, 2188–94.
5. Paclitaxel. Medac GmbH. UK Summary of product characteristics, January 2011.
6. Taxol (Paclitaxel). Bristol-Myers Squibb Company. US Prescribing information, April 2011.

Taxanes; Cabazitaxel + Miscellaneous

Potent CYP3A4 inducers (such as carbamazepine) are predicted to decrease the plasma concentrations of cabazitaxel and reduce its efficacy. Potent CYP3A4 inhibitors (such as ketoconazole) are predicted to increase plasma concentrations of cabazitaxel and increase its toxicity. Prednisolone and prednisone do not appear to alter cabazitaxel pharmacokinetics.

Clinical evidence, mechanism, importance and management

(a) CYP3A4 inducers and inhibitors

The manufacturers note that cabazitaxel is extensively and primarily (80 to 90%) metabolised by CYP3A4. For this reason, CYP3A4 inducers are predicted to decrease the plasma concentrations of cabazitaxel and possibly reduce its efficacy.[1,2] The manufacturers therefore advise that the use of cabazitaxel with potent CYP3A4 inducers should be avoided, and they specifically name **carbamazepine**, **phenobarbital**, **phenytoin**, **rifabutin**, **rifampicin (rifampin)**, **rifapentine** and **St John's wort**.[1,2] It would seem prudent to also apply this caution to **primidone** and **fosphenytoin**, which are metabolised to phenobarbital and phenytoin, respectively.

Similarly, CYP3A4 inhibitors are predicted to increase the plasma concentrations of cabazitaxel, which would be expected to increase its toxicity. The manufacturers of cabazitaxel therefore advise that the concurrent use of potent CYP3A4 inhibitors should be avoided: they name some azoles (**itraconazole**, **ketoconazole**, **voriconazole**), some macrolides (**clarithromycin**, **telithromycin**), some HIV-protease inhibitors (**atazanavir**, **indinavir**, **nelfinavir**, **ritonavir**, **saquinavir**) and **nefazodone**.[1,2] They also recommend caution with moderate CYP3A4 inhibitors.[1,2] Anticipate that patients taking these drugs might be more likely to need a cabazitaxel dose reduction because of adverse effects, such as neutropenia. For a list of inhibitors and inducers of CYP3A4, see 'Table 1.9', p.11.

(b) Cytochrome P450 substrates

The UK manufacturer states that cabazitaxel inhibited CYP3A4 *in vitro*, and that, at clinically relevant concentrations, inhibition of the metabolism of drugs that are CYP3A4 substrates is possible.[1] Conversely, the US manufacturer states that the potential for cabazitaxel to inhibit the metabolism of drugs that are substrates of CYP3A4/5 is low.[2]

(c) Prednisone or prednisolone

The manufacturers state that prednisone or prednisolone 10 mg daily did not alter the pharmacokinetics of cabazitaxel.[1,2] Note that the concurrent use of cabazitaxel with corticosteroids is recommended to reduce the risk of hypersensitivity reactions.[1,2]

1. Jevtana (Cabazitaxel). Sanofi-Aventis U.S. LLC. US Prescribing information, June 2010.
2. Jevtana (Cabazitaxel). Sanofi-Aventis. UK Summary of product characteristics, March 2011.

Taxanes; Docetaxel + Cannabis

The pharmacokinetics of docetaxel are not altered by a herbal tea containing cannabis.

Clinical evidence

In a study investigating the effects of cannabis on docetaxel pharmacokinetics, 12 patients were given 200 mL of a herbal tea containing cannabis 1 g/L each day for 15 days. The tea was prepared from medicinal-grade cannabis (*Cannabis sativa* L. Flos, Bedrocan®) containing the cannabinoids Δ^9-tetrahydrocannabinol 18% and cannabidiol 0.8%. The clearance and the AUC of docetaxel given on day 12 of the cannabis tea were not significantly altered, when compared with docetaxel given before the cannabis tea. The dose of docetaxel used was 180 mg, reduced to 135 mg in 3 patients who experienced dose-related docetaxel toxicity.

Mechanism

Docetaxel is metabolised by the cytochrome P450 isoenzyme CYP3A4, and this does not appear to be affected by oral cannabis.

Importance and management

This study suggests that cannabis taken orally will not affect the pharmacokinetics of docetaxel. No dose adjustments are likely to be needed if docetaxel is given with cannabis tea.[1] It is not known if this applies to other drugs metabolised by CYP3A4, or to other preparations and routes of administration of cannabis.

1. Engels FK, de Jong FA, Sparreboom A, Mathot RA, Loos WJ, Kitzen JJEM, de Bruijn P, Verweij J, Mathijssen RHJ. Medicinal cannabis does not influence the clinical pharmacokinetics of irinotecan and docetaxel. *Oncologist* (2007) 12, 291–300.

Taxanes; Docetaxel + Dronedarone

Fatal grade 4 neutropenia and severe mucositis occurred in a patient given docetaxel 24 days after starting dronedarone.

Clinical evidence, mechanism, importance and management

A 79-year-old man taking fluindione and pravastatin was given docetaxel 35 mg/m^2 on days 1 and 8 of a 21-day cycle. He tolerated the first 2 cycles well, with no neutropenia or mucositis. Shortly after the second cycle he had recurrence of atrial fibrillation for which dronedarone 400 mg twice daily was started, then 24 days later he received a third, postponed, cycle of docetaxel. Eleven days after completing this course, he was admitted with fever, diarrhoea, grade 4 neutropenia, and severe mucositis, and 14 days later was still found to have detectable docetaxel plasma concentrations, suggesting a major delay in docetaxel elimination. Despite intensive therapy, he died 18 days after admission.[1]

It was considered that dronedarone probably inhibited the metabolism of docetaxel by CYP3A4, delaying its clearance and effectively causing an overdose.[1] Dronedarone is considered a moderate inhibitor of CYP3A4.

Although this is a single case, the mechanism of the interaction between docetaxel and dronedarone is plausible. However, the severity of the interaction appears to be greater than expected. The UK and US manufacturers of docetaxel[2,3] recommend considering a docetaxel dose reduction on the concurrent use of potent CYP3A4 inhibitors, but not moderate CYP3A4 inhibitors, see 'Taxanes + Ketoconazole and other CYP3A4 inhibitors', p.715. Nevertheless, given the severity of the interaction seen in this patient, until more is known, it would seem prudent to consider reducing the dose of docetaxel in any patient also taking dronedarone, especially the elderly. Closely monitor the outcome for signs of dronedarone toxicity (such as diarrhoea, nausea, rash). The same advice should probably be applied to **amiodarone**, which is structurally related to dronedarone and is also a CYP3A4 inhibitor.

1. Vodovar D, Mongardon N, Moachon L, Arnaout M, Beuzeboc P, Lokiec F, Rezai K, Pène F. Severe docetaxel overdose induced by pharmacokinetic interaction with dronedarone. *J Clin Oncol* (2011) 29, e694–5.
2. Taxotere (Docetaxel trihydrate). Sanofi. UK Summary of product characteristics, July 2012.
3. Taxotere (Docetaxel). Sanofi-Aventis US LLC. US Prescribing information, May 2010.

Taxanes; Docetaxel + Grapefruit juice

Grapefruit juice appeared to increase docetaxel exposure in one case.

Clinical evidence, mechanism, importance and management

A 52-year-old woman who was to receive pharmacokinetically-guided docetaxel dose adjustment was found to have slow docetaxel elimination after her first course of treatment (a one-hour infusion of 40 mg/m^2). The patient was not taking any CYP3A4 inhibitors apart from one 250-mL glass of grapefruit juice daily, which she had been taking for more than 3 months. She was asked to stop drinking grapefruit juice, and 2 weeks later was given another dose of docetaxel. For this second course of docetaxel, the AUC of docetaxel was 60% lower and its clearance was 36% higher than the first course.[1]

It was concluded that grapefruit juice inhibited the metabolism of intravenous docetaxel. However, grapefruit juice is known to principally inhibit intestinal CYP3A4 rather than hepatic CYP3A4, and to have the greatest effect on drugs that have poor oral bioavailability. In addition, grapefruit juice is a weak CYP3A4 inhibitor that exerts the majority of its inhibitory effect on CYP3A4 in the intestine, so it is unexpected that it appeared to have as great an effect on intravenous docetaxel as the potent CYP3A4 inhibitor, ketoconazole[1] (see 'Taxanes + Ketoconazole and other CYP3A4 inhibitors', p.715).[1]

The evidence from this one case points to an interaction between grapefruit juice and intravenous docetaxel. However, because docetaxel was given intravenously, this interaction is unexpected. Therefore the general relevance of this case is uncertain, and further study is needed. Bear the possibility of an interaction in mind in case of an unexpected response to treatment.

1. Valenzuela B, Rebollo J, Pérez T, Brugarolas A, Pérez-Ruixo JJ. Effect of grapefruit juice on the pharmacokinetics of docetaxel in cancer patients: a case report. *Br J Clin Pharmacol* (2011) 72, 978–81.

Taxanes; Docetaxel + Prednisone

Prednisone does not alter docetaxel pharmacokinetics.

Clinical evidence, mechanism, importance and management

The UK and US manufacturers of docetaxel note that, in a study in patients with metastatic prostatic cancer, prednisone did not have a statistically significant effect on the pharmacokinetics of docetaxel.[1,2] Microsomes prepared from the liver of a single patient who had been taking prednisone for a year did not inhibit docetaxel metabolism *in vitro*.[3] It had been suggested that prednisone might induce the metabolism of docetaxel by CYP3A4, but this effect was not seen. No clinically relevant pharmacokinetic interaction therefore occurs, and no docetaxel dose adjustment would be expected to be needed on the concurrent use of prednisone.

1. Taxotere (Docetaxel trihydrate). Sanofi. UK Summary of product characteristics, July 2012.
2. Taxotere (Docetaxel). Sanofi-Aventis US LLC. US Prescribing information, May 2010.
3. Royer I, Monsarrat B, Sonnier M, Wright M, Cresteil T. Metabolism of docetaxel by human cytochromes P450: Interactions with paclitaxel and other antineoplastic drugs. *Cancer Res* (1996) 56, 58–65.

Taxanes; Docetaxel + Tipifarnib

There was no pharmacokinetic interaction between tipifarnib and docetaxel in one study.

Clinical evidence, mechanism, importance and management

In a dose-finding study, docetaxel was given intravenously on day one of a 21-day cycle and oral tipifarnib 200 or 300 mg twice daily was given for 7 or 14 days starting one hour before docetaxel. There was no change in the pharmacokinetics of docetaxel or tipifarnib when compared with docetaxel given alone on day one or tipifarnib given alone on day 3.[1]

1. Awada A, Zhang S, Gil T, de Valeriola D, Lalami Y, De Porre P, Piccart-Gebhart MJ. A phase I clinical and pharmacokinetic study of tipifarnib in combination with docetaxel in patients with advanced solid malignancies. *Curr Med Res Opin* (2007) 23, 991–1003.

Taxanes; Paclitaxel + Clindamycin

Clindamycin does not appear to alter the pharmacokinetics of paclitaxel to a clinically significant extent.

Clinical evidence, mechanism, importance and management

In a study in 16 patients given intravenous paclitaxel 175 mg/m^2 over 3 hours, intravenous clindamycin 600 mg or 1.2 g over 30 minutes started 2.5 hours after the paclitaxel slightly reduced the AUC_{0-4} and maximum plasma level of paclitaxel by about 11% when compared with placebo.[1]

Paclitaxel is highly bound to alpha-1-acid glycoprotein (AGP), and levels of this protein are increased in some cancers, which might contribute to reduced efficacy. Clindamycin was predicted to displace the AGP binding of paclitaxel, and might therefore alter paclitaxel pharmacokinetics.[1] However, the slight pharmacokinetic interaction seen in this study is not likely to be clinically relevant.

1. Fruscio R, Lissoni AA, Frapolli R, Corso S, Mangioni C, D'Incalci M, Zucchetti M. Clindamycin-paclitaxel pharmacokinetic interaction in ovarian cancer patients. *Cancer Chemother Pharmacol* (2006) 58, 319–25.

Taxanes; Paclitaxel + Miscellaneous

***In vitro* studies with human liver tissue suggest that no metabolic interactions are likely to occur between paclitaxel and cimetidine, dexamethasone or diphenhydramine. *In vitro* data also suggest that *Cremophor* may inhibit the intracellular uptake and metabolism of paclitaxel. CYP2C8 inhibitors (e.g. gemfibrozil) are predicted to raise paclitaxel levels.**

Clinical evidence, mechanism, importance and management

(a) Cimetidine, Dexamethasone, or Diphenhydramine

On the basis of an *in vitro* study using human liver slices and human liver microsomes,[1] it has been concluded that the metabolism of paclitaxel is unlikely to be altered by cimetidine, dexamethasone or diphenhydramine, all of which are frequently given to prevent the hypersensitivity reactions associated with paclitaxel or its vehicle, see *Cremophor*, below. The UK manufacturers say that paclitaxel clearance in patients is not affected by cimetidine premedication.[2] Nevertheless, some authors[3] have advised caution when using cimetidine with paclitaxel, because they have found profound neutropenia, which they attributed to a possible pharmacokinetic interaction. Cimetidine is known to inhibit the cytochrome P450 isoenzyme CYP3A4, which is responsible, in part, for the metabolism of paclitaxel. However, cimetidine is a weak inhibitor of CYP3A4 (and some other isoenzymes not involved in paclitaxel metabolism), and an interaction with CYP3A4 inhibitors is not established (see 'Taxanes + Ketoconazole and other CYP3A4 inhibitors', p.715. A pharmacokinetic interaction between cimetidine and paclitaxel is therefore seems unlikely.

(b) Cremophor

In vitro, *Cremophor* was found to inhibit the metabolism of paclitaxel in human liver microsomes,[1] which might be expected to increase its toxicity. The concentration used in the *in vitro* study may be achieved clinically in patients given paclitaxel with *Cremophor* as the vehicle.[4] This may be worth bearing in mind if other drugs formulated with *Cremophor* are given with paclitaxel.

(c) CYP2C8 inhibitors

Although there do not appear to be any clinical pharmacokinetic data on the use of paclitaxel with CYP2C8 inhibitors, the manufacturers advise caution,[2,5] presumably because of the possibility of raised paclitaxel levels. They specifically name **gemfibrozil**. Note that **trimethoprim** is also a clinically relevant CYP2C8 inhibitor.

1. Jamis-Dow CA, Klecker RW, Katki AG, Collins JM. Metabolism of taxol by humans and rat liver in vitro: a screen for drug interactions and interspecies differences. *Cancer Chemother Pharmacol* (1995) 36, 107–14.
2. Paclitaxel. Medac GmbH. UK Summary of product characteristics, January 2011.
3. Clouse T, Geisler JP, Manahan KJ, Gudenkauf TJ, Linnemeier G, Wiemann MC. Should we be using cimetidine to premedicate patients receiving docetaxel or paclitaxel? *Gynecol Oncol* (2004) 95, 270–1.
4. Rischin D, Webster LK, Millward MJ, Linahan BM, Toner GC, Woollett AM, Morton CG, Bishop JF. Cremophor pharmacokinetics in patients receiving 3-, 6-, and 24-hour infusions of paclitaxel. *J Natl Cancer Inst* (1996) 88, 1297–1301.
5. Taxol (Paclitaxel). Bristol-Myers Squibb Company. US Prescribing information, April 2011.

Taxanes; Paclitaxel + Quinine

One study found that quinine markedly reduced the plasma levels of paclitaxel.

Clinical evidence, mechanism, importance and management

In a study in 12 patients, paclitaxel levels at the end of a 20 to 24-hour infusion of paclitaxel 120 mg/m^2 given on day 2 were 40% lower when given with oral quinine 400 mg three times daily for 4 days started on day one. In one patient the paclitaxel levels were undetectable at this time point. Paclitaxel clearance was estimated to have increased twofold, but the reasons for this are unclear. Quinine was used as a chemosensitiser in this study, on the basis of *in vitro* findings, but was not very effective.[1] The pharmacokinetic interaction was unexpected, and its clinical relevance is unclear. Bear the possibility of an interaction in mind in the unlikely event that quinine is used with paclitaxel.

1. Miller TP, Chase EM, Dorr R, Dalton WS, Lam KS, Salmon SE. A phase I/II trial of paclitaxel for non-Hodgkin's lymphoma followed by paclitaxel plus quinine in drug-resistant disease. *Anticancer Drugs* (1998) 9, 135–40.

Taxanes; Paclitaxel + Verapamil

High-dose *R*-verapamil reduced the clearance of paclitaxel and increased the incidence of haematological toxicity.

Clinical evidence

In a crossover study in which 24 patients were given paclitaxel up to 200 mg/m^2 over 3 hours every 21 days alone, or with high-dose oral *R*-verapamil (up to 250 mg/m^2 every 4 hours for 12 doses starting 24 hours before the paclitaxel), haematological toxicity was greater in those cycles when *R*-verapamil had also been given. In a subset of 6 patients, the pharmacokinetics of paclitaxel were assessed: the AUC and maximum plasma level of paclitaxel were increased by 90% and 122%, respectively, when *R*-verapamil was also given.[1]

Mechanism

Paclitaxel is a substrate of P-glycoprotein. It seems likely that *R*-verapamil inhibits the efflux of paclitaxel by this transporter protein.[1]

Importance and management

The clinical significance of this finding is unclear as the use of just the *R*-isomer of verapamil in such high doses is generally limited to investigational use only. However, bear in mind the possibility that verapamil might modestly increase paclitaxel levels.

1. Tolcher AW, Cowan KH, Solomon D, Ognibene F, Goldspiel B, Chang R, Noone MH, Denicoff AM, Barnes CS, Gossard MR, Fetsch PA, Berg SL, Balis FM, Venzon DJ, O'Shaughnessy JA. Phase I crossover study of paclitaxel with r-verapamil in patients with metastatic breast cancer. *J Clin Oncol* (1996) 14, 1173–84.

Temozolomide + Miscellaneous

Valproic acid may slightly reduce the clearance of temozolomide. Carbamazepine, H_2-receptor antagonists, dexamethasone, phenobarbital, phenytoin, prochlorperazine and ondansetron did not affect the clearance of temozolomide. Food, but not ranitidine, slightly reduces the extent of absorption of temozolomide.

Clinical evidence, mechanism, importance and management

(a) Antiepileptics

The manufacturer notes that the concurrent use of **carbamazepine**, **dexamethasone**, **H_2-receptor antagonists**, **ondansetron**, **phenobarbital**, **phenytoin** or **prochlorperazine** did not affect the clearance of temozolomide, based on an analysis of population pharmacokinetics from phase II studies.[1,2] **Valproic acid** modestly reduces the oral clearance of temozolomide by 5%,[2] which seems unlikely to be clinically relevant.

(b) Food

The manufacturer notes that food slightly reduces the temozolomide AUC by 9% and maximum plasma concentration by 33%. They recommend that it should be given without food.[1,2]

(c) Ranitidine

In a study in 12 patients given temozolomide 150 mg/m^2 daily, ranitidine 150 mg twice daily had no effect on the absorption or plasma pharmacokinetics of temozolomide, or that of its active metabolite.[3]

1. Temodal (Temozolomide). Schering-Plough Ltd. UK Summary of product characteristics, June 2009.
2. Temodar (Temozolomide). Schering Corporation. US Prescribing information, March 2009.
3. Beale P, Judson I, Moore S, Statkevich P, Marco A, Cutler D, Reidenberg P, Brada M. Effect of gastric pH on the relative oral bioavailability and pharmacokinetics of temozolomide. *Cancer Chemother Pharmacol* (1999) 44, 389–94.

Teniposide + Antiepileptics; Enzyme-inducing

Carbamazepine, phenytoin and phenobarbital markedly increase the clearance of teniposide. A reduction in its effects has been noted in B-lineage leukaemia.

Clinical evidence, mechanism, importance and management

In 6 children with acute lymphocytic leukaemia the clearance of teniposide was increased two- to threefold (from 13 to 32 mL/minute per m^2) when they also took **phenytoin** or **phenobarbital**.[1] Another patient had a twofold increase in teniposide clearance when **carbamazepine** was given.[1] In a retrospective survey, long-term antiepileptic use (**phenytoin**, **phenobarbital**, **carbamazepine**, or a combination) was associated with worse event-free survival, and greater haematological relapse and CNS relapse in children receiving chemotherapy for B-lineage acute lymphoblastic leukaemia. In this study, faster clearance of teniposide was found in those receiving the antiepileptics.[2]

These effects probably occur because these antiepileptics are potent liver enzyme inducers, which may increase the metabolism of teniposide by the liver and thereby reduce its levels. The authors of these reports therefore conclude that an increased dose of teniposide will be needed in the presence of these antiepileptics to achieve systemic exposure to the drug comparable to that achievable in their absence.[1] It may be preferable to use alternative antiepileptics (that are not enzyme inducers) in patients requiring teniposide.[2] Note that **primidone** is metabolised to phenobarbital, and **fosphenytoin** is metabolised to phenytoin, and therefore these drugs may be expected to interact similarly.

1. Baker DK, Relling MV, Pui C-H, Christensen ML, Evans WE, Rodman JH. Increased teniposide clearance with concomitant anticonvulsant therapy. *J Clin Oncol* (1992) 10, 311–5.
2. Relling MV, Pui C-H, Sandlund JT, Rivera GK, Hancock ML, Boyett JM, Schuetz EG, Evans WE. Adverse effect of anticonvulsants on efficacy of chemotherapy for acute lymphoblastic leukaemia. *Lancet* (2000) 356, 285–90.

Thalidomide + Doxorubicin

The concurrent use of thalidomide and chemotherapy regimens containing doxorubicin appears to be associated with an increased risk of deep-vein thrombosis in patients with multiple myeloma.

Clinical evidence, mechanism, importance and management

In a randomised study in 100 patients with newly diagnosed multiple myeloma given induction chemotherapy (dexamethasone, vincristine, doxorubicin, cyclophosphamide, etoposide and cisplatin) with or without thalidomide, deep-vein thrombosis developed in 14 of the 50 patients (28%) given thalidomide compared with 2 of 50 patients (4%) not given thalidomide.[1] In a further study by the same authors, 232 patients with multiple myeloma were given DT-PACE (dexamethasone, thalidomide, cisplatin, doxorubicin, cyclophosphamide, etoposide) if they had preceding standard dose therapy but no previous autotransplantation, or with DCEP-T (dexamethasone, cyclophosphamide, etoposide, cisplatin, thalidomide) for relapse after transplantation. Deep-vein thrombosis developed in 31 of 192 patients (16%) given the doxorubicin-containing regimen (DT-PACE) and only 1 of 40 (2.5%) given the regimen without doxorubicin (DCEP-T).[2]

In patients with multiple myeloma, the risk of deep-vein thrombosis appears to be increased when thalidomide is given with combination chemotherapy containing doxorubicin. Various strategies are recommended to reduce this risk of thrombosis including low-molecular-weight heparin, warfarin, and low-dose aspirin.[3]

1. Zangari M, Anaissie E, Barlogie B, Badros A, Desikan R, Gopal AV, Morris C, Toor A, Siegel E, Fink L, Tricot G. Increased risk of deep-vein thrombosis in patients with multiple myeloma receiving thalidomide and chemotherapy. *Blood* (2001) 98, 1614–5.
2. Zangari M, Siegel E, Barlogie B, Anaissie E, Saghafifar F, Fassas A, Morris C, Fink L, Tricot G. Thrombogenic activity of doxorubicin in myeloma patients receiving thalidomide: implications for therapy. *Blood* (2002) 100, 1168–71.
3. Palumbo A, Rajkumar SV, Dimopoulos MA, Richardson PG, San Miguel J, Barlogie B, Harousseau J, Zonder JA, Cavo M, Zangari M, Attal M, Belch A, Knop S, Joshua D, Sezer O, Ludwig H, Vesole D, Bladé J, Kyle R, Westin J, Weber D, Bringhen S, Niesvizky R, Waage A, von Lilienfeld-Toal M, Lonial S, Morgan GJ, Orlowski RZ, Shimizu K, Anderson KC, Boccadoro M, Durie BG, Sonneveld P, Hussein MA; International Myeloma Working Group. Prevention of thalidomide- and lenalidomide-associated thrombosis in myeloma. *Leukemia* (2008) 22, 414–23.

Thalidomide + Drugs that cause bradycardia

Cases of bradycardia have been reported in patients taking thalidomide and atenolol or methadone. No pharmacokinetic interaction appears to occur between thalidomide and single-dose digoxin.

Clinical evidence

(a) Beta blockers

A 76-year old man who had been stable taking **atenolol** 50 mg daily for 2 years, developed severe bradycardia with episodes of syncope one month after starting to take thalidomide 100 mg daily. On admission his blood pressure was 90/50 mmHg and his heart rate was 30 bpm, compared with about 120/70 mmHg and 70 to 80 bpm, respectively, prior to starting thalidomide. Atenolol was stopped and the bradycardia was treated with a temporary pacemaker. He was discharged when his heart rate recovered to above 60 bpm and he continued to take thalidomide with no further problems.[1] Similarly, another report describes a 72-year old man who developed sinus bradycardia during a 10-month period of taking thalidomide 200 to 400 mg daily with **atenolol**. Prior to starting thalidomide, he had been stable taking atenolol 50 mg daily with a baseline heart rate of 63 bpm. Throughout the thalidomide course he experienced light-headedness and dizziness, with fluctuations in his heart rate, which fell as low as 45 bpm at one point. After 6 months of thalidomide he was not complaining of light-headedness or dizziness but his heart rate was 56 bpm, and the atenolol was reduced to 25 mg daily. Despite the atenolol dose reduction his heart rate remained at low levels and eventually the atenolol was stopped (about 9 months after starting thalidomide). Three weeks later his heart rate had recovered slightly (to 58 bpm) but he experienced worsening light-headedness and dizziness during the following 2 weeks and the thalidomide was also stopped. One week after stopping the thalidomide, his heart rate had risen to 61 bpm and he had no symptoms.[2] Note that despite symptomatic bradycardia and heart rate recorded as low as 45 bpm, this patient's thalidomide dose was often increased.

(b) Digoxin

In a study in 18 healthy subjects, steady-state thalidomide 200 mg daily did not affect the pharmacokinetics of a single 500-microgram dose of digoxin, nor were the pharmacokinetics of thalidomide altered by this dose of digoxin.[3,4] However, the US manufacturer of thalidomide states that the long-term safety of concurrent use has not been studied.[4]

(c) Methadone

A 47-year old man with multiple myeloma and taking thalidomide 100 mg daily was given oral methadone 15 mg twice daily with additional 10-mg doses as needed for pain relief. Three days later he developed lightheadedness with an episode of presyncope on standing and was found to be bradycardic (heart rate 40 bpm). Methadone was stopped and the bradycardia resolved within the next 4 days.[5]

Mechanism

Thalidomide can cause clinically relevant bradycardia, which might be additive with the bradycardic effects of other drugs, such as the beta blockers or methadone.

Importance and management

Evidence for an interaction between thalidomide and other drugs that cause bradycardia is limited to these case reports, but the effects seen are clinically relevant and could be serious. Thalidomide is known to cause clinically relevant bradycardia, and this might be additive with the bradycardic effects of other drugs, as was seen in the case reports with atenolol and methadone. Patients should be monitored for bradycardia, which might require a dose delay, reduction, or discontinuation of thalidomide.[3,4] The UK and US manufacturers of thalidomide advise caution on the concurrent use of other drugs that can cause bradycardia, and they name drugs that are known to induce torsade de pointes (unspecified),[3] **alpha blockers**,[4] **anticholinesterases**[3], **beta blockers**,[3,4] **calcium-channel blockers**,[4] **digoxin**,[4] **H_2-receptor antagonists**,[4] **lithium**,[4] **neuromuscular blockers** (such as **suxamethonium**),[4] and **tricyclic antidepressants**.[4]

1. Yamaguchi T. Syncope and sinus bradycardia from combined use of thalidomide and β-blocker. *Pharmacoepidemiol Drug Safety* (2008) 17, 1033–5.
2. Kaur A, Yu SS, Lee AJ, Chiao T. Thalidomide-induced sinus bradycardia. *Ann Pharmacother* (2003) 37, 1040–3.
3. Thalidomide Celgene (Thalidomide). Celgene Ltd. UK Summary of product characteristics, June 2014.
4. Thalomid (Thalidomide). Celgene Corporation. US Prescribing information, June 2014.
5. Buchanan D. Sinus bradycardia related to methadone in a patient with myeloma receiving thalidomide therapy. *Palliat Med* (2010) 24, 742–3.

Thalidomide + Epoetins

A higher than expected incidence of thromboembolic events occurred in one study in patients with myelodysplastic syndrome treated with thalidomide and darbepoetin alfa; however, this was not noted in a retrospective analysis of patients with multiple myeloma given thalidomide with epoetin, although cases of DVT have been reported with epoetin alfa and thalidomide.

Clinical evidence

A phase II study to investigate the efficacy and tolerability of the concurrent use of thalidomide 100 mg daily and subcutaneous **darbepoetin alfa** 2.25 micrograms/kg per week in patients with myelodysplastic syndrome was discontinued because of an unexpectedly high incidence of thromboembolic events. Of the first 7 patients enrolled in the study, two developed deep-vein thrombosis (DVT) and one died of pulmonary embolism.[1]

In contrast to these findings, in a retrospective analysis of patients with multiple myeloma who had been taking thalidomide, thromboses were reported in 4 of 49 patients (8.1%) also given **epoetin** and in 14 of 150 patients not given **epoetin** (9.3%). These results suggest that epoetin might not increase the risk of thrombosis in patients with multiple myeloma receiving thalidomide.[2] Nevertheless, two patients with myeloid cancers who had been taking thalidomide and dexamethasone for 5 to 6 months, developed DVTs 4 and 6 weeks, respectively, after starting treatment with **epoetin alfa** for anaemia.[3]

Mechanism

Both thalidomide and epoetins increase the risk of thromboembolism, and the risk might be increased with concurrent use. There seems to be a particular risk of thrombosis when using epoetins in patients with cancer.[4]

Importance and management

There is little information on the possible increased risk of thrombosis if epoetins are used with thalidomide in myeloid cancers. The authors of the first study recommended careful monitoring and possibly thromboprophylaxis (heparin or warfarin) in patients with myelodysplastic syndrome given both thalidomide and epoetin. This seems prudent.

1. Steurer M, Sudmeier I, Stauder R, Gastl G. Thromboembolic events in patients with myelodysplastic syndrome receiving thalidomide in combination with darbepoietin-alpha. *Br J Haematol* (2003) 121, 101–3.
2. Galli M, Elice F, Crippa C, Comotti B, Rodeghiero F, Barbui T. Recombinant human erythropoietin and the risk of thrombosis in patients receiving thalidomide for multiple myeloma. *Haematologica* (2004) 89, 1141–2.
3. Chennuru S, Baumann MA. Deep vein thrombosis occurring on treatment of patients receiving thalidomide with erythropoietin. *Intern Med J* (2007) 37, 506–7.
4. Bennett CL, Silver SM, Djulbegovic B, Samaras AT, Blau CA, Gleason KJ, Barnato SE, Elverman KM, Courtney DM, McKoy JM, Edwards BJ, Tigue CC, Raisch DW, Yarnold PR, Dorr DA, Kuzel TM, Tallman MS, Trifilio SM, West DP, Lai SY, Henke M. Venous thromboembolism and mortality associated with recombinant erythropoietin and darbepoetin administration for the treatment of cancer-associated anemia. *JAMA* (2008) 299, 914–24.

Thalidomide + Interferon alfa

Severe bone marrow depression was reported in a patient given thalidomide with peginterferon alfa.

Clinical evidence, mechanism, importance and management

A patient with multiple myeloma in remission after an autologous stem cell transplantation was given thalidomide 200 mg daily. Five weeks after also being given **peginterferon alfa-2b**, severe reversible bone marrow hypoplasia developed. **Peginterferon** was probably responsible for the bone marrow depression. However, thalidomide may also cause bone marrow depression and it was suggested that the severe suppression in this patient may have been due to the combined effects of the **peginterferon** and thalidomide.[1] This should be considered in patients given both drugs.

1. Gómez-Rangel JD, Ruiz-Delgado GJ, Ruiz-Argüelles GJ. Pegylated-interferon induced severe bone marrow hypoplasia in a patient with multiple myeloma receiving thalidomide. *Am J Hematol* (2003) 74, 290–1.

Thalidomide + Miscellaneous

Rifampicin and phenobarbital did not appear to alter thalidomide clearance in one study. Thalidomide increases the sedative effect of other CNS depressants. Peripheral neuropathy is common with thalidomide, and other drugs that have this effect might have an additive effect with thalidomide.

Clinical evidence, mechanism, importance and management

(a) CNS depressants

Animal studies have shown an increase in CNS depressant activity when thalidomide was given with **alcohol**, **barbiturates**, **chlorpromazine**, and **reserpine**.[1] In clinical use, thalidomide frequently causes drowsiness, and the UK and US manufacturers advise caution with these drugs and also with **anxiolytics**, **hypnotics**, **antipsychotics**, **antihistamines**, and **opioids**, because of the possibility of enhanced sedation.[2,3]

(b) Cytochrome P450 isoenzyme inducers

There was no clear relationship between thalidomide clearance and the concurrent use of enzyme inducers, such as **rifampicin (rifampin)** or **phenobarbital**, in a study in patients with glioma.[4] For the possible additive CNS depressant effect with barbiturates, see *CNS depressants*, above.

(c) Drugs that can cause peripheral neuropathy

Thalidomide very commonly causes peripheral neuropathy, which can be severe, and might require dose modification.[2,3] Because of this, the UK and US manufacturers recommend caution with other drugs that can cause peripheral neuropathy, and they name **vincristine** and **bortezomib**.[2,3] The US manufacturer additionally lists **alcohol** (see *CNS depressants* above also), **amiodarone**, **cisplatin**, **disulfiram**, **docetaxel**, **metronidazole**, **paclitaxel**, and **phenytoin**.[2] A review of 24 patients with multiple myeloma who had received **bortezomib** after relapse following allografting, found that the incidence of severe peripheral neuropathy was far higher than usually seen in non-transplant patients. Fourteen patients developed neurotoxicity; in 7 patients it was severe and 6 patients required treatment discontinuation as the neurotoxicity did not resolve following a **bortezomib** dose reduction. However, in an analysis of possible risk factors, previous treatment with thalidomide was not found to increase the risk of peripheral neuropathy.[5]

1. Teo SK, Colburn WA, Tracewell WG, Kook KA, Stirling DI, Jaworsky MS, Scheffler MA, Thomas SD, Laskin OL. Clinical pharmacokinetics of thalidomide. *Clin Pharmacokinet* (2004) 43, 311–27.
2. Thalomid (Thalidomide). Celgene Corporation. US Prescribing information, June 2014.
3. Thalidomide Celgene (Thalidomide). Celgene Ltd. UK Summary of product characteristics, June 2014.
4. Fine HA, Figg WD, Jaeckle K, Wen PY, Kyritsis AP, Loeffler JS, Levin VA, Black PM, Kaplan R, Pluda JM, Yung WK. Phase II trial of the antiangiogenic agent thalidomide in patients with recurrent high-grade gliomas. *J Clin Oncol* (2000) 18, 708–15.
5. Giaccone L, Sorasio R, Patriarca F, Mattei D, Montefusco V, Peccatori J, Carnevale-Schianca F, Petrucci MT, Milone G, Guidi S, Rotta M, Fanin R, Corradini P, Boccadoro M, Bruno B. Bortezomib after allografting in multiple myeloma: association between neurotoxicity and cyclosporine treatment. *Biol Blood Marrow Transplant* (2007) 13, 497–9.

Thiopurines + Allopurinol

The haematological effects of azathioprine and mercaptopurine are greatly increased by allopurinol.

Clinical evidence

(a) Azathioprine

A patient taking allopurinol 300 mg daily for gout was also given azathioprine 100 mg daily to treat autoimmune haemolytic anaemia. Within 10 weeks his platelet count fell from 236×10^9/L to 45×10^9/L, his white cell count fell from 9.4×10^9/L to 0.8×10^9/L, and his haemoglobin concentration fell from 11.5 g/dL to 5.3 g/dL.[1]

A number of other reports similarly describe reversible bone marrow toxicity associated with anaemia, pancytopenia, leucocytopenia, and thrombocytopenia in patients given azathioprine with allopurinol,[1-9] and in one case a fatality occurred as a result of neutropenia and septicaemia.[8] In a retrospective analysis of 24 patients who had received both azathioprine and allopurinol, 11 developed leucopenia, 7 developed moderate anaemia, and 5 developed thrombocytopenia. Only 14 of the patients had received a greater than two-thirds reduction in their azathioprine dose when allopurinol was started, but despite this, some of these patients still developed haematological toxicity.[10]

(b) Mercaptopurine

In early studies, allopurinol 200 to 300 mg reduced the effective dose of mercaptopurine by about 4-fold in 7 patients with chronic granulocytic leukaemia or variants.[11]

Profound pancytopenia developed in the first 3 of 13 children given mercaptopurine 2.5 mg/kg daily and allopurinol 10 mg/kg daily, but when the mercaptopurine dose was halved, toxicity was manageable in the remaining 9 children.[12] Severe leucopenia and thrombocytopenia occurred in another patient given allopurinol with standard-dose mercaptopurine.[13]

A pharmacokinetic study found that allopurinol caused a 5-fold increase in the AUC and the maximum plasma concentration of mercaptopurine when mercaptopurine was given *orally*. The bioavailability of mercaptopurine increased from 12% to 59%.[14] This did not occur when mercaptopurine was given *intravenously*.[14,15]

Mechanism

Azathioprine is firstly metabolised in the liver to mercaptopurine and then enzymatically oxidised in the liver and intestinal wall by xanthine oxidase to an inactive compound (6-thiouric acid), which is excreted. Allopurinol inhibits first-pass metabolism by xanthine oxidase so that mercaptopurine accumulates, blood concentrations increase, and its toxic effects (such as leucopenia and thrombocytopenia) develop.

Importance and management

A well documented, well established, clinically important, and potentially life-threatening interaction. The doses of azathioprine and mercaptopurine should be reduced by about two-thirds or three-quarters when given orally to reduce the development of toxicity. Despite taking these precautions toxicity might still be seen,[10] and very close haematological monitoring is advisable if concurrent use is necessary. On the basis of two studies[14,15] it would seem that this precaution might not be necessary if mercaptopurine is given intravenously, but note that parenteral mercaptopurine is not routinely available.

1. Boyd IW. Allopurinol-azathioprine interaction. *J Intern Med* (1991) 229, 386.
2. Garcia-Ortiz RE, De Los Angeles Rodriguez M. Pancytopenia associated with the interaction of allopurinol and azathioprine. *J Pharm Technol* (1991) 7, 224–6.
3. Glogner P, Heni N. Panzytopenie nach Kombinationsbehandlung mit Allopurinol und Azathioprin. *Med Welt* (1976) 27, 1545–6.
4. Brooks RJ, Dorr RT, Durie BGM. Interaction of allopurinol with 6-mercaptopurine and azathioprine. *Biomedicine* (1982) 36, 217–22.
5. Klugkist H, Lincke HO. Panzytopenie unter Behandlung mit Azathioprin durch Interaktion mit Allopurinol bei Myasthenia gravis. *Akt Neurol* (1987) 14, 165–7.
6. Zazgornik J, Kopsa H, Schmidt P, Pils P, Kuschan K, Deutsch E. Increased danger of bone marrow damage in simultaneous azathioprine-allopurinol therapy. *Int J Clin Pharmacol Ther Toxicol* (1981) 19, 96–7.
7. Venkat Raman G, Sharman VL, Lee HA. Azathioprine and allopurinol: a potentially dangerous combination. *J Intern Med* (1990) 228, 69–71.
8. Adverse Drug Reactions Advisory Committee. Allopurinol and azathioprine. Fatal interaction. *Med J Aust* (1980) 2, 130.
9. Kennedy DT, Hayney MS, Lake KD. Azathioprine and allopurinol: the price of an avoidable drug interaction. *Ann Pharmacother* (1996) 30, 951–4.
10. Cummins D, Sekar M, Halil O, Banner N. Myelosuppression associated with azathioprine-allopurinol interaction after heart and lung transplantation. *Transplantation* (1996) 61, 1661–2.
11. Rundles RW, Wyngaarden JB, Hitchings GH, Elion GB, Silberman HR. Effects of xanthine oxidase inhibitor on thiopurine metabolism, hyperuricaemia and gout. *Trans Assoc Am Physicians* (1963) 76, 126–40.
12. Levine AS, Sharp HL, Mitchell J, Krivit W, Nesbit ME. Combination therapy with 6-mercaptopurine (NSC-755) and allopurinol (NSC-1390) during induction and maintenance of remission of acute leukaemia in children. *Cancer Chemother Rep* (1969) 53, 53–7.
13. Berns A, Rubenfeld S, Rymzo WI, and Calabro JJ. Hazard of combining allopurinol and thiopurine. *N Engl J Med* (1972) 286, 730–1.
14. Zimm S, Collins JM, O'Neill D, Chabner BA, Poplak DG. Inhibition of first-pass metabolism in cancer chemotherapy: interaction of 6-mercaptopurine and allopurinol. *Clin Pharmacol Ther* (1983) 34, 810–17.
15. Coffey JJ, White CA, Lesk AB, Rogers WI, Serpick AA. Effect of allopurinol on the pharmacokinetics of 6–mercaptopurine (NSC 755) in cancer patients. *Cancer Res* (1972) 32, 1283–9.

Thiopurines + 5-Aminosalicylates

The haematological toxicity of azathioprine and mercaptopurine may be increased by mesalazine, olsalazine or sulfasalazine. Balsalazide may be less likely to interact but this requires confirmation.

Clinical evidence

(a) Balsalazide

The frequency of clinically important neutropenia did not increase in 10 patients with Crohn's disease receiving **azathioprine** or **mercaptopurine** when they were given balsalazide 6.75 g daily for 8 weeks, but increases in whole blood 6-thioguanine nucleotide concentrations were seen.[1]

(b) Mesalazine

A 13-year-old boy with severe ulcerative pancolitis and cholangitis was given prednisone 60 mg daily, ursodeoxycholic acid 15 mg/kg daily and mesalazine 25 mg/kg daily. When **azathioprine** 2 mg/kg daily was added in an attempt to reduce the prednisone dose, he developed marked and prolonged **azathioprine** toxicity (severe pancytopenia), which was attributed to an interaction resulting from abnormally high, persistent levels of an **azathioprine** metabolite.[2] In another study, there was a trend towards an increased rate of clinically important neutropenia in 10 patients with Crohn's disease receiving **azathioprine** or **mercaptopurine** when they were given mesalazine 4 g daily for 8 weeks. One patient was withdrawn from the study after 6 weeks because of leucopenia. Increases in whole blood 6-thioguanine nucleotide concentrations were also seen.[1]

(c) Olsalazine

A case report describes a patient with Crohn's disease who had two separate episodes of bone marrow suppression while receiving **mercaptopurine** 50 to 75 mg daily and olsalazine 1 to 1.75 g daily. It was found necessary to reduce the **mercaptopurine** dose on the first occasion and to withdraw both drugs on the second.[3]

(d) Sulfasalazine

A decrease in leucocyte counts was seen in 4 patients taking **azathioprine** (2.1 to 3.3 mg/kg daily) after the addition of sulfasalazine. This lasted several months in one patient, and was transitory in two. The fourth patient developed agranulocytosis after 4 days, which required treatment discontinuation. When the drugs were later resumed at a lower dose, no reduction in leucocyte counts occurred.[4] Another report describes 38 patients taking **azathioprine** (mean dose 92.8 mg) and sulfasalazine (mean dose 2.1 g) for rheumatoid or psoriatic arthritis. Some patients did well, but in general the combination was poorly tolerated, and only 45% continued treatment after 6 months. Reasons for withdrawal included rash (3 patients), gastrointestinal upset (7 patients), leucopenia (one patient) and nephrotic syndrome (one patient).[5] In another study, there was a trend towards an increased rate of clinically important neutropenia in 12 patients with Crohn's disease receiving **azathioprine** or **mercaptopurine** when they were given sulfasalazine 4 g daily for 8 weeks. One patient withdrew from the study after 6 weeks because of leucopenia. Increases in whole blood 6-thioguanine nucleotide concentrations were also found.[1]

Mechanism

The metabolism of azathioprine and mercaptopurine depends on *S*-methylation by thiopurine methyltransferase (TPMT) and oxidation by xanthine oxidase. An *in vitro* study using recombinant TPMT found that both sulfasalazine and its metabolites inhibit the activity of TPMT.[6] Therefore if these drugs are used together, the clearance of azathioprine and mercaptopurine may be reduced by the sulfasalazine, resulting in an increase in their toxicity (there is only a small margin between their therapeutic and toxic levels). About 11% of patients may be at particular risk because of genetic polymorphism whereby they have TPMT enzyme activity that is only half that of the rest of the population.[1,6] *In vitro* studies confirmed that mesalazine,[7] olsalazine and its metabolite olsalazine-*O*-sulfate[3,7] and balsalazide[7] are inhibitors of recombinant TPMT. In patients, increased levels of 6-thioguanine nucleotide are probably due to inhibition of TPMT.[1] It is suggested that the reported *in vitro* concentration (IC_{50}) of balsalazide required to halve the TPMT activity is about 1000 times higher than peak plasma levels after therapeutic doses and therefore an interaction is unlikely. Mesalazine and olsalazine peak levels may also be less than the IC_{50} concentrations, but peak plasma levels of sulfasalazine are close to IC_{50} concentrations.[8]

Importance and management

These reports underline the importance of taking particular care if azathioprine or mercaptopurine is used with balsalazide, mesalazine, olsalazine, or sulfasalazine. Balsalazide may be less likely to interact, but this requires confirmation.[1] Some have postulated that the interaction may actually benefit patients, as increased whole blood 6-thioguanine nucleotide or mild leucopenia is associated with a greater chance of remission in those taking azathioprine or mercaptopurine.[1,9] Additional monitoring of white blood cell counts is required when starting the combination.[9]

1. Lowry PW, Franklin CL, Weaver AL, Szumlanski CL, Mays DC, Loftus EV, Tremaine WJ, Lipsky JJ, Weinshilboum RM, Sandborn WJ. Leucopenia resulting from a drug interaction between azathioprine or 6-mercaptopurine and mesalamine, sulphasalazine, or balsalazide. *Gut* (2001) 49, 656–64.
2. Chouraqui JP, Serre-Debeauvais F, Armari C, Savariau N. Azathioprine toxicity in a child with ulcerative colitis: interaction with mesalazine. *Gastroenterology* (1996) 110 (4 Suppl), A883.
3. Lewis LD, Benin A, Szumlanski CL, Otterness DM, Lennard L, Weinshilboum RM, Nierenberg DW. Olsalazine and 6-mercaptopurine-related bone marrow suppression: a possible drug-drug interaction. *Clin Pharmacol Ther* (1997) 62, 464–75.
4. Bliddal H, Helin P. Leucopenia in adult Still's disease during treatment with azathioprine and sulphasalazine. *Clin Rheumatol* (1987) 6, 244–50.
5. Helliwell PS. Combination therapy with sulphasalazine and azathioprine. *Br J Rheumatol* (1996) 35, 493–4.
6. Szumlanski CL, Weinshilboum RM. Sulphasalazine inhibition of thiopurine methyltransferase: possible mechanism for interaction with 6-mercaptopurine and azathioprine. *Br J Clin Pharmacol* (1995) 39, 456–9.
7. Lowry PW, Szumlanski CL, Weinshilboum RM, Sandborn WJ. Balsalazide and azathioprine or 6-mercaptopurine: evidence for a potentially serious drug interaction. *Gastroenterology* (1999) 116, 1505–6.
8. Green JRB. Balsalazide and azathioprine or 6-mercaptopurine. *Gastroenterology* (1999) 117, 1513–14.
9. Present DH. Interaction of 6-mercaptopurine and azathioprine with 5-aminosalicylic acid agents. *Gastroenterology* (2000) 119, 276–7.

Thiopurines; Azathioprine + Co-trimoxazole or Trimethoprim

There is some evidence that the risk of haematological toxicity may be increased in renal transplant patients taking azathioprine if they are given co-trimoxazole or trimethoprim, particularly for extended periods. However, other evidence suggests that the drugs may be used together safely, and the combination is commonly used in practice.

Clinical evidence

The observation that haematological toxicity often seemed to occur in renal transplant patients given azathioprine and co-trimoxazole, prompted a retrospective survey of the records of 40 patients. It was found that there was no difference in the incidence of thrombocytopenia and neutropenia in those given azathioprine, either alone, or with co-trimoxazole, (trimethoprim 160 to 320 mg and sulfamethoxazole 800 mg to 1.6 g daily) for a short time (6 to 16 days), but a significant increase occurred in the incidence and duration of thrombocytopenia and neutropenia if both drugs were given together for 22 days or more.[1]

Another report describes a marked fall in white cell counts in renal transplant recipients during the concurrent use of azathioprine with either co-trimoxazole (described as frequent) or trimethoprim (3 cases).[2] In one case the fall occurred within 5 days and was managed by temporarily withdrawing the azathioprine and reducing the trimethoprim dose from 300 mg daily to 100 mg daily.[2]

Conversely, in an early study, there was no difference in the incidence of leucopenia when renal transplant recipients were given co-trimoxazole or other antibacterials.[3] Similarly, in 252 renal transplant patients given continuous prophylaxis with co-trimoxazole or **sulfafurazole** for 12 to 25 months, toxicity was minimal: leucopenia occurred only occasionally and was reversed by temporarily withholding azathioprine. This was needed in a similar number of patients with each antibacterial.[4] In another placebo-controlled study in heart transplant recipients taking triple therapy including azathioprine; co-trimoxazole prophylaxis for 4 months did not alter total white blood cell counts: leucopenia did not occur and no change in the dose of azathioprine was required.[5]

Mechanism

Not understood. It seems possible that the bone marrow depressant effects of azathioprine, trimethoprim and sulfamethoxazole may be additive. In addition, in some patients impaired renal function may allow co-trimoxazole levels to become elevated, and haemodialysis may deplete folate levels, which could exacerbate the anti-folate effects of the co-trimoxazole. Trimethoprim has been shown to inhibit renal tubular creatinine secretion.[6]

Importance and management

Information appears to be limited and the interaction is not established. Although there is some evidence of an increased risk of haematological toxicity in renal transplant patients taking azathioprine if they are given co-trimoxazole or trimethoprim, this has not been shown in all studies. Two of the early studies suggested that the incidence of leucopenia with co-trimoxazole was related to the time after transplantation, and it improved if the dose of azathioprine was decreased or temporarily suspended.[3,7] Prophylaxis with co-trimoxazole post-transplant is commonly used in some centres.

1. Bradley PP, Warden GD, Maxwell JG, Rothstein G. Neutropenia and thrombocytopenia in renal allograft recipients treated with trimethoprim-sulfamethoxazole. *Ann Intern Med* (1980) 93, 560–2.
2. Bailey RR. Leukopenia due to a trimethoprim-azathioprine interaction. *N Z Med J* (1984) 97, 739.
3. Hall CL. Co-trimoxazole and azathioprine: a safe combination. *BMJ* (1974) 4, 15–16.
4. Peters C, Peterson P, Marabella P, Simmons RL, Najarian JS. Continuous sulfa prophylaxis for urinary tract infection in renal transplant recipients. *Am J Surg* (1983) 146, 589–93.
5. Olsen SL, Renlund DG, O'Connell JB, Taylor DO, Lassetter JE, Eastburn TE, Hammond EH, Bristow MR. Prevention of *Pneumocystis carinii* pneumonia in cardiac transplant recipients by trimethoprim sulfamethoxazole. *Transplantation* (1993) 56, 359–62.
6. Berg KJ, Gjellestad A, Nordby G, Rootwelt K, Djoseland O, Fauchald P, Mehl A, Narverud J, Talseth T. Renal effects of trimethoprim in ciclosporin- and azathioprine-treated kidney-allografted patients. *Nephron* (1989) 53, 218–22.
7. Hulme B, Reeves DS. Leucopenia associated with trimethoprim-sulphamethoxazole after renal transplantation. *BMJ* (1971) 3, 610–12.

Thiopurines; Azathioprine + Myelosuppressive drugs

Azathioprine commonly causes myelosuppression and this effect might be enhanced by other myelosuppressive drugs.

Clinical evidence, mechanism, importance and management

Azathioprine commonly causes dose-related myelosuppression, and full blood counts should be regularly monitored when this drug is used. The manufacturers note that the concurrent use of other drugs that may have a myelosuppressive effect might lead to exaggerated leucopenia.[1,2] The UK manufacturer specifically states that, where possible such use should be avoided, and they name **penicillamine** as an example.[1] Note that the myelosuppressive effect of **penicillamine** mainly results in thrombocytopenia and less frequently neutropenia, and its use also requires monitoring of full blood counts. This advice therefore seems prudent.

The UK manufacturer also says that it has been suggested that **cimetidine** and **indometacin** may have myelosuppressive effects, which may be enhanced by azathioprine.[1] Leucopenia is a rare adverse effect of cimetidine and an infrequent adverse effect of indometacin. However, there appear to be no published clinical reports of any interactions of these drugs with azathioprine. In one *animal* study, cimetidine did *not* increase the haematopoietic toxicity of azathioprine or delay bone marrow recovery after cimetidine.[3] Whether there is a real additional risk from using drugs such as cimetidine and indometacin with azathioprine is unknown, but the likelihood seems small.

1. Imuran (Azathioprine). GlaxoSmithKline UK. UK Summary of product characteristics, May 2009.
2. Imuran (Azathioprine). Prometheus Pharmaceuticals, Inc. US Prescribing information, May 2008.
3. Gamelli RL, Foster RS, Whisnant JK. Hematopoietic toxicity by cimetidine. Reexamination using the antimetabolite azathioprine. *Transplantation* (1983) 35,12–14.

Thiopurines; Mercaptopurine + Doxorubicin

One study suggested that the hepatotoxicity of *intravenous* mercaptopurine can be increased by doxorubicin.

Clinical evidence, mechanism, importance and management

One report describes 11 patients who developed liver damage after being given *intravenous* mercaptopurine 500 mg/m² daily for 5 days, with doxorubicin 50 mg/m² on the first day. The frequency and severity of liver damage was greater than the authors had previously seen with mercaptopurine alone. They suggested that doxorubicin potentiated the hepatotoxicity of mercaptopurine.[1] Mercaptopurine is no longer commonly used *intravenously*, and the dose given in this study is much higher than that currently used *orally*. The general applicability of this study is therefore unknown.

1. Minow RA, Stern MH, Casey JH, Rodriguez V, Luna MA. Clinico-pathological correlation of liver damage in patients treated with 6-mercaptopurine and adriamycin. *Cancer* (1976) 38, 1524–8.

Thiopurines; Mercaptopurine + Food

Some studies have shown that breakfast, usually including milk, may modestly reduce and delay the absorption of mercaptopurine, whereas others have not found this effect. A case report describes increased mercaptopurine dose requirements when it was taken with milk.

Clinical evidence

A study in 17 children with acute lymphoblastic leukaemia found that the absorption of mercaptopurine 5 mg/m² was reduced if it was given 15 minutes after a standard breakfast of 250 mL of **milk** and 50 g of biscuits, when compared with fasting. The AUC was reduced by 26%, the maximum plasma levels by 36%, and the time to maximum plasma levels delayed from 1.2 hours to 2.3 hours.[1] Some individuals had more marked effects than others; 11 subjects had a decrease in absorption, whereas 6 subjects had no change or a small increase.[1] Similarly, in another study in 7 children, peak plasma mercaptopurine levels were lower and were delayed when it was given with a standard breakfast (orange juice, cereal, toast) compared with those after an overnight fast.[2] Moreover, a case report describes a 4-year-old child who required a 60% increase in his calculated dose of mercaptopurine when he took it with **milk**, but no change when he took it with water lightly flavoured with fruit squash.[3]

In contrast, in a study in 10 children, mercaptopurine levels varied widely between individuals and there was no clear effect of food. The peak plasma levels were increased only 11% (range 67% decrease to 81% increase), and the AUC was increased by a mean of 3% (range 53% decrease to 86% increase) when given in the fasting state compared with after breakfast (not standardised, but consisting mainly of milk or yogurt plus cereal, or sandwiches).[4] Similarly, a further study in 15 children taking mercaptopurine found that there was a non-significant 20 to 22% decrease in the maximum plasma levels or AUC of mercaptopurine when it was taken after a standardised breakfast (milk, bread, ham, cheese) compared with after a 12 hour fast, and there was a delay in reaching the maximum plasma levels when mercaptopurine was taken after food. Again, there was wide inter-individual variation in these parameters.[5]

Mechanism

Not understood. Delayed gastric emptying is a suggested reason.[1] Alternatively, it has been suggested that xanthine oxidases in milk might inactivate mercaptopurine.[6]

Importance and management

Mercaptopurine levels vary widely, and it is not established whether food or milk is a clear factor in this variation. Some have suggested that mercaptopurine should be taken before food or without milk to optimise its absorption,[2,3,6] and the UK Acute Lymphoblastic Leukaemia (UK ALL) study requires doses to be taken at least one hour after the evening meal without milk products,[7] whereas others do not consider the evidence sufficient to make a recommendation.[4] Note that the manufacturers of mercaptopurine do not include any specific instructions regarding food or milk intake.[8,9]

1. Riccardi R, Balis FM, Ferrara P, Lasorella A, Poplak DG, Mastrangelo R. Influence of food intake on bioavailability of oral 6-mercaptopurine in children with acute lymphoblastic leukaemia. *J Pediatr Hematol Oncol* (1986) 3, 319–24.
2. Burton NK, Barnett MJ, Aherne GW, Evans J, Douglas I, Lister TA. The effect of food on the oral administration of 6-mercaptopurine. *Cancer Chemother Pharmacol* (1986) 18, 90–1.
3. Sofianou-Katsoulis A, Khakoo G, Kaczmarski R. Reduction in bioavailability of 6-mercaptopurine on simultaneous administration with cow's milk. *Pediatr Hematol Oncol* (2006) 23, 485–7.
4. Lönnerholm G, Kreuger A, Lindström B, Myrdal U. Oral mercaptopurine in childhood leukemia: influence of food intake on bioavailability. *Pediatr Hematol Oncol* (1989) 6, 105–12.
5. Lafolie P, Björk O, Hayder S, Åhström L, Peterson C. Variability of 6-mercaptopurine pharmacokinetics during oral maintenance therapy of children with acute leukaemia. *Med Oncol Tumor Pharmacother* (1989) 6, 259–65.
6. de Lemos ML, Hamata L, Jennings S, Leduc T. Interaction between mercaptopurine and milk. *J Oncol Pharm Pract* (2007) 13, 237–40.
7. Medical Research Council. Working party on leukaemia in children. UK national randomised trial for children and young adults with acute lymphoblastic leukaemia (ALL) UKALL 2003. Version 7, 2009. Available at: http://www.ctsu.ox.ac.uk/research/mega-trials/leukaemia-trials/ukall-2003/index_html (accessed 21/10/15)
8. Purinethol (Mercaptopurine). Gate Pharmaceuticals. US Prescribing information, February 2007.
9. Puri-Nethol (Mercaptopurine). GlaxoSmithKline UK. UK Summary of product characteristics, October 2009.

Thiopurines; Mercaptopurine + Methotrexate

Methotrexate can increase the bioavailability of mercaptopurine, but the contribution this makes to their synergistic action in the maintenance of remission of leukaemia is unclear.

Clinical evidence

(a) Oral mercaptopurine

In 14 children receiving maintenance therapy for leukaemia, oral low-dose methotrexate 20 mg/m² increased the AUC and peak plasma levels of mercaptopurine 75 mg/m² by 31% and 26%, respectively.[1] In another study, 10 children with acute lymphoblastic leukaemia in remission were given mercaptopurine 25 mg/m^2 daily and intravenous infusions of high-dose methotrexate 2 or 5 g/m^2 every other week for consolidation therapy. It was found that methotrexate 2 or 5 g/m^2 increased the AUC of mercaptopurine by 69% and 93%, respectively, and raised the maximum serum levels of mercaptopurine by 108% and 121%, respectively.[2] Nevertheless, the risk of relapse of leukaemia did not appear to be related to the pharmacokinetics of methotrexate or mercaptopurine, which showed considerable inter- and intrapatient variability, in one study in children.[3]

(b) Intravenous mercaptopurine

One report suggests that, with high dose induction therapy, the combination of mercaptopurine and methotrexate may not be synergistic. In this study, children with newly diagnosed acute lymphoblastic leukaemia were given *intravenous* mercaptopurine 1 g/m^2 over 6 hours, either alone, or after low-dose oral methotrexate (6 doses of 30 mg/m^2), or high-dose intravenous methotrexate (1 g/m^2 over 24 hours). Methotrexate increased the plasma levels of mercaptopurine, but, unexpectedly, it was also found that thioguanine nucleotide levels in bone marrow leukaemic lymphoblasts were 13-fold lower during methotrexate use. It is not known whether methotrexate would reduce thiopurine metabolite levels in leukaemic lymphoblasts when mercaptopurine is given as continuation therapy where the leukaemic burden is less substantial than in newly diagnosed cases. In addition, the changes in leukocyte counts over 3 days suggested that mercaptopurine alone had little effect, and although methotrexate caused a reduction in intracellular thiopurine metabolite levels, it produced a greater decrease in leukocytes than mercaptopurine alone. It was concluded that, in this particular study, the antileukaemic effect was primarily due to methotrexate.[4]

Mechanism

The reasons for the pharmacokinetic interaction are not understood, although it is thought that methotrexate is a xanthine oxidase inhibitor, which may therefore inhibit the metabolism of mercaptopurine.[1,2,5]

Importance and management

The combination of methotrexate and mercaptopurine has an established place in the maintenance therapy of leukaemia once it is in remission after successful induction and consolidation therapy. The pharmacokinetic findings may be part of the explanation for the benefits of combined use, although biochemical mechanisms may be more important.[5]

1. Balis FM, Holcenberg JS, Zimm S, Tubergen D, Collins JM, Murphy RF, Gilchrist GS, Hammond D, Poplack DG. The effect of methotrexate on the bioavailability of oral 6-mercaptopurine. *Clin Pharmacol Ther* (1987) 41, 384–7.
2. Innocenti F, Danesi R, Di Paolo A, Loru B, Favre C, Nardi M, Bocci G, Nardini D, Macchia P, Del Tacca M. Clinical and experimental pharmacokinetic interaction between 6-mercaptopurine and methotrexate. *Cancer Chemother Pharmacol* (1996) 37, 409–14.
3. Balis FM, Holcenberg JS, Poplack DG, Ge J, Sather HN, Murphy RF, Ames MM, Waskerwitz MJ, Tubergen DG, Zimm S, Gilchrist GS, Bleyer WA. Pharmacokinetics and pharmacodynamics of oral methotrexate and mercaptopurine in children with lower risk acute lymphoblastic leukemia: a joint Children's Cancer Group and Pediatric Oncology Branch study. *Blood* (1998) 92, 3569–77.
4. Dervieux T, Hancock ML, Pui C-H, Rivera GK, Sandlund JT, Ribeiro RC, Boyett J, Evans WE, Relling MV. Antagonism by methotrexate on mercaptopurine disposition in lymphoblasts during up-front treatment of acute lymphoblastic leukemia. *Clin Pharmacol Ther* (2003) 73, 506–16.
5. Giverhaug T, Loennechen T, Aarbakke J. The interaction of 6-mercaptopurine (6-MP) and methotrexate (MTX). *Gen Pharmacol* (1999) 33, 341–6.

Thiotepa + Phenytoin

The metabolism of thiotepa to its active metabolite, TEPA (triethylenephosphamide), was increased by phenytoin in one patient.

Clinical evidence

A 42-year-old man received two courses of CTC (high-dose cyclophosphamide, thiotepa and carboplatin), with phenytoin 150 mg twice daily started 5 days before the second course, for seizures. When compared with the first course, phenytoin caused a 115% increase in the AUC of TEPA (triethylenephosphamide), the active metabolite of thiotepa, and a 29% reduction in the AUC of thiotepa. On the basis of these data, the dose of thiotepa was reduced by about one-third for the remaining 2 days of the course, and this resulted in plasma levels within the therapeutic range.[1]

Mechanism

Phenytoin probably induces the cytochrome P450 isoenzyme CYP2B6, which is involved in the metabolism of thiotepa.

Importance and management

This appears to be the only case report of such an interaction, but it would seem prudent to monitor the effects of concurrent use, and reduce the dose of thiotepa if necessary.

1. de Jonge ME, Huitema ADR, van Dam SM, Beijnen JH, Rodenhuis S. Significant induction of cyclophosphamide and thiotepa metabolism by phenytoin. *Cancer Chemother Pharmacol* (2005) 55, 507–510.

Topotecan + Amifostine

In 10 women with ovarian cancer, amifostine, given daily for 5 days before topotecan, did not alter the pharmacokinetics of topotecan.[1]

1. Zackrisson A-L, Malmström H, Peterson C. No evidence that amifostine influences the plasma pharmacokinetics of topotecan in ovarian cancer patients. *Eur J Clin Pharmacol* (2002) 58, 103–8.

Topotecan + Amrubicin

Amrubicin did not affect the pharmacokinetics of topotecan in a study in which 9 patients were given topotecan as an infusion on days one to 5 of a 4-week cycle, with amrubicin on days 3 to 5 of each cycle.[1]

1. Shibayama T, Hotta K, Takigawa N, Tada A, Ueoka H, Harita S, Kiura K, Tabata M, Segawa Y, Nogami N, Kuyama S, Shinkai T, Tanimoto M. A phase I and pharmacological study of amrubicin and topotecan in patients of small-cell lung cancer with relapsed or extensive-disease small-cell lung cancer. *Lung Cancer* (2006) 53, 189–95.

Topotecan + Ciclosporin and other P-glycoprotein inhibitors

Ciclosporin (a known P-glycoprotein inhibitor) moderately increases the AUC of oral topotecan, as does elacridar, an investigational drug. Other inhibitors of P-glycoprotein and breast cancer resistance protein (BCRP) are predicted to interact similarly.

Clinical evidence

(a) Ciclosporin

The manufacturers of topotecan report that giving oral ciclosporin 15 mg/kg within 4 hours of oral topotecan increased the AUC of the metabolite, topotecan lactone, and total topotecan 2-fold, and 2.5- or 3-fold, respectively.[1,2]

(b) Elacridar

Studies have shown that elacridar (an investigational drug) increased the oral bioavailability of topotecan from 40% to 100%, but had little effect on intravenous topotecan.[3,4] In these studies, a reduced dose of topotecan was used,[3,4] and elacridar use actually appeared to be associated with a reduced incidence of dose-limiting diarrhoea, when compared with historical data.[4]

Mechanism

Ciclosporin is an inhibitor of P-glycoprotein and CYP3A4, which affect the transport and metabolism of topotecan, thereby increasing its oral bioavailability. Elacridar is a P-glycoprotein inhibitor and also an inhibitor of the breast cancer resistance protein (BCRP), for which topotecan is a substrate.

Importance and management

The pharmacokinetic interactions of ciclosporin and elacridar with topotecan would appear to be established. Patients should be carefully monitored for topotecan adverse effects if ciclosporin or other inhibitors of P-glycoprotein, or inhibitors of breast cancer resistance protein (BCRP), are used with oral topotecan.[1,2] The US manufacturer of topotecan advises avoiding P-glycoprotein inhibitors, and, in addition to ciclosporin and elacridar, they specifically name **ketoconazole**, **ritonavir** and **saquinavir**.[2] For a list of P-glycoprotein inhibitors, see 'Table 1.12', p.14.

1. Hycamtin Hard Capsule (Topotecan hydrochloride). GlaxoSmithKline UK. UK Summary of product characteristics, January 2010.
2. Hycamtin Capsules (Topotecan). GlaxoSmithKline. US Prescribing information, June 2010.
3. Kruijtzer CM, Beijnen JH, Rosing H, ten Bokkel Huinink WW, Schot M, Jewell RC, Paul EM, Schellens JH. Increased oral bioavailability of topotecan in combination with the breast cancer resistance protein and P-glycoprotein inhibitor GF120918. *J Clin Oncol* (2002) 20, 2943–50.
4. Kuppens IE, Witteveen EO, Jewell RC, Radema SA, Paul EM, Mangum SG, Beijnen JH, Voest EE, Schellens JH. A phase I, randomized, open-label, parallel cohort, dose-finding study of elacridar (GF120918) and oral topotecan in cancer patients. *Clin Cancer Res* (2007) 13, 3276–85.

Topotecan + Food

Food does not alter the extent of absorption of oral topotecan.

Clinical evidence, mechanism, importance and management

The AUC of oral topotecan was found to be similar when it was taken either in the fasted state or after a high-fat meal, although the time to maximum plasma levels was delayed from 1.5 hours to 3 hours.[1] The manufacturers advise that oral topotecan can be taken with or without food.[2,3]

1. Herben VM, Rosing H, ten Bokkel Huinink WW, van Zomeren DM, Batchelor D, Doyle E, Beusenberg FD, Beijnen JH, Schellens JH. Oral topotecan: bioavailability and effect of food co-administration. *Br J Cancer* (1999) 80, 1380–6.
2. Hycamtin Hard Capsule (Topotecan hydrochloride). GlaxoSmithKline UK. UK Summary of product characteristics, January 2010.
3. Hycamtin Capsules (Topotecan). GlaxoSmithKline. US Prescribing information, June 2010.

Topotecan + Ifosfamide

There does not appear to be any pharmacokinetic interaction between topotecan and ifosfamide, but concurrent use has been associated with marked dose-limiting toxicity.

Clinical evidence, mechanism, importance and management

In a small phase I study in patients with advanced malignancy, the pharmacokinetics of intravenous topotecan did not appear to be different when given immediately after a 1-hour infusion of ifosfamide when compared with historical data for topotecan alone.[1] Similarly, in another study in patients given intravenous topotecan with ifosfamide, the pharmacokinetics of these drugs did not differ from those in previous studies in patients given either drug alone.[2] Although less conclusive than findings from direct comparative studies, the information suggests that a marked pharmacokinetic interaction between the drugs is unlikely. However, the combination was associated with marked haematological[1] and non-haematological[2] toxicity, limiting the doses that could be given.

1. Kerbusch T, Groenewegen G, Mathôt RA, Herben VM, ten Bokkel Huinink WW, Swart M, Ambaum B, Rosing H, Jansen S, Voest EE, Beijnen JH, Schellens JH. Phase I and pharmacokinetic study of the combination of topotecan and ifosfamide administered intravenously every 3 weeks. *Br J Cancer* (2004) 90, 2268–77.
2. Schneider CP, Merkel U, Grübner U, Kath R, Höffken K, Hoffmann A. Phase I clinical and pharmacokinetic study of combination chemotherapy with topotecan and ifosfamide in patients with progressive or relapsed solid tumors. *J Cancer Res Clin Oncol* (2002) 128, 313–18.

Topotecan + Miscellaneous

Corticosteroids, co-trimoxazole, granisetron, morphine, and ondansetron are not expected to alter the pharmacokinetics of intravenous topotecan.

Clinical evidence, mechanism, importance and management

The UK manufacturer reports that, in a population pharmacokinetic analysis, the pharmacokinetics of intravenous topotecan did not appear to be significantly affected by **granisetron**, **ondansetron**, **morphine** or **corticosteroids**.[1] Similarly, in a population pharmacokinetic analysis of intravenous topotecan in children, **dexamethasone** and **co-trimoxazole** (**sulfamethoxazole** with **trimethoprim**) did not appear to alter the clearance of topotecan.[2]

1. Hycamtin Hard Capsule (Topotecan hydrochloride). GlaxoSmithKline UK. UK Summary of product characteristics, January 2010.
2. Schaiquevich P, Panetta JC, Iacono LC, Freeman BB 3rd, Santana VM, Gajjar A, Stewart CF. Population pharmacokinetic analysis of topotecan in pediatric cancer patients. *Clin Cancer Res* (2007) 13, 6703–11.

Topotecan + Phenytoin

Phenytoin might increase topotecan clearance.

Clinical evidence, mechanism, importance and management

When a 5-year-old child with medulloblastoma received a course of topotecan with phenytoin, the total clearance of topotecan was increased by 47%, when compared with a cycle of topotecan without phenytoin.[1] Similarly, in a population pharmacokinetic analysis of studies in which intravenous topotecan was given to children, topotecan clearance was higher in those receiving phenytoin (estimated mean increase of 80%).[2]

Evidence is limited, but the case report and the pharmacokinetic data suggest that an increased topotecan dose might be needed in the presence of phenytoin. It would seem prudent to monitor topotecan efficacy more closely if phenytoin is given.

1. Zamboni WC, Gajjar AJ, Heideman RL, Beijnen JH, Rosing H, Houghton PJ, Stewart CF. Phenytoin alters the disposition of topotecan and *N*-desmethyl topotecan in a patient with medulloblastoma. *Clin Cancer Res* (1998) 4, 783–9.
2. Schaiquevich P, Panetta JC, Iacono LC, Freeman BB, Santana VM, Gajjar A, Stewart CF. Population pharmacokinetic analysis of topotecan in pediatric cancer patients. *Clin Cancer Res* (2007) 13, 6703–11.

Topotecan + Platinum compounds

The myelotoxicity of the combination of topotecan with cisplatin or carboplatin is dependent on the order of administration and does not appear to be due to any pharmacokinetic interaction.

Clinical evidence

(a) Carboplatin

In a phase I study, the toxicity and pharmacokinetics of topotecan (given as a 30-minute infusion once daily for 3 days) were compared when carboplatin was given immediately before the first dose of topotecan on day one or immediately after the last dose of topotecan on day 3.The incidence of dose-limiting thrombocytopenia was greater when the carboplatin was given on day one than on day 3. There was no difference in topotecan pharmacokinetics between the two schedules.[1] In another phase I study, the toxicity and pharmacokinetics of topotecan (given as a 30-minute infusion once daily for 5 days) were compared when it was started immediately after carboplatin or 8-days afterwards. Both schedules led to myelotoxicity requiring dose reductions and delays. The topotecan AUC was about 55% higher when it was started 8 days after the carboplatin compared with immediately after the carboplatin.[2]

(b) Cisplatin

In a phase I study,[3] the toxicity and pharmacokinetics of topotecan (given as a 30-minute infusion once daily for 5 days) was compared when cisplatin was given immediately before the first dose of topotecan on day one or immediately after the last dose of topotecan on day 5. Dose-limiting neutropenia and thrombocytopenia were greater when the cisplatin was given on day one than on day 5. In addition, limited pharmacokinetic data indicated that topotecan clearance was lower and its exposure was higher when cisplatin was given on day one. Another very similar study using *oral* topotecan confirmed the sequence-dependent toxicity when cisplatin was given on day one as opposed to day 5. However, in this study, a detailed pharmacokinetic analysis did not find any difference in topotecan pharmacokinetics between the two schedules.[4] Later authors suggested that the difference in pharmacokinetic findings might be due to the cisplatin hydration schedule used in these studies (the first used a short hydration schedule whereas the second used a hyper-hydration schedule).[5] They therefore compared the pharmacokinetics of intravenous topotecan between these two hydration schedules with cisplatin given before topotecan on day one in both cases. The clearance of topotecan was slightly reduced by the cisplatin (by about 11%), and this did not differ by hydration schedule.[5]

Mechanism

It was suggested that cisplatin-induced renal impairment reduced the clearance of topotecan leading to increased toxicity when cisplatin was given immediately before the topotecan. However, more detailed study has shown the changes in topotecan pharmacokinetics to be minor and insufficient to explain the difference in haematological toxicity between the schedules.

The reason for the increased topotecan exposure when started a week after carboplatin compared with immediately after is unknown.

Importance and management

The evidence shows that the haematological toxicity of topotecan given with cisplatin or carboplatin is dependent on the order of administration and greater when the platinum compound is given immediately before the topotecan than immediately after. Reduced platinum doses are required when these drugs are given before topotecan.

1. Boss DS, Siegel-Lakhai WS, van Egmond-Schoemaker NE, Pluim D, Rosing H, ten Bokkel Huinink WW, Beijnen JH, Schellens JHM. Phase I pharmacokinetic and pharmacodynamic study of carboplatin and topotecan administered intravenously every 28 days to patients with malignant solid tumors. *Clin Cancer Res* (2009) 15, 4475–83.
2. Simpson AB, Calvert PM, Sludden JA, Boddy AV, Griffin MJ, Schätzlein A, Wilson P, Fishwick K, Wheatley A, Ross GA, Calvert AH, Twelves CJ. Topotecan in combination with carboplatin: phase I trial evaluation of two treatment schedules. *Ann Oncol* (2002) 13, 399–402.
3. Rowinsky EK, Kaufmann SH, Baker SD, Grochow LB, Chen TL, Peereboom D, Bowling MK, Sartorius SE, Ettinger DS, Forastiere AA, Donehower RC. Sequences of topotecan and cisplatin: phase I, pharmacologic, and in vitro studies to examine sequence dependence. *J Clin Oncol* (1996) 14, 3074–84.
4. de Jonge MJA, Loos WJ, Gelderblom H, Planting AST, van der Burg MEL, Sparreboom A, Brouwer E, van Beurden V, Mantel MA, Doyle E, Hearn S, Ross G, Verweij J. Phase I pharmacologic study of oral topotecan and intravenous cisplatin: sequence-dependent hematologic side effects. *J Clin Oncol* (2000) 18, 2104–15.
5. Gelderblom H, Loos WJ, Sparreboom A, Soepenberg O, de Jonge MJA, van Boven-van Zomeren DM, Verweij J. Influence of the cisplatin hydration schedule on topotecan pharmacokinetics. *Eur J Cancer* (2003) 39, 1542–6.

Topotecan + Probenecid

In *mice*, probenecid markedly inhibited the renal tubular secretion of topotecan, which led to an increase in topotecan systemic exposure.[1] The clinical relevance of this finding is unknown, but it would seem prudent to monitor for topotecan adverse effects (e.g. diarrhoea, bone marrow suppression) in patients also given probenecid. More study is needed to confirm a clinically relevant interaction.

1. Zamboni WC, Houghton PJ, Johnson RK, Hulstein JL, Crom WR, Cheshire PJ, Hanna SK, Richmond LB, Luo X, Stewart CL. Probenecid alters topotecan systemic and renal disposition by inhibiting renal tubular secretion. *J Pharmacol Exp Ther* (1998) 284, 89–94.

Topotecan + Ranitidine

Ranitidine does not alter the pharmacokinetics of topotecan.

Clinical evidence, mechanism, importance and management

In 18 patients with solid tumours, the pharmacokinetics of topotecan (given in an initial dose of 2.3 mg/m^2 daily for 5 days, repeated every 3 weeks) and its active metabolite, topotecan lactone, were not affected by the previous use of ranitidine 150 mg twice daily for 4 days.[1] No topotecan dose adjustment would seem necessary if ranitidine or other drugs that increase gastric pH are given with oral topotecan.

1. Akhtar S, Beckman RA, Mould DR, Doyle E, Fields SZ, Wright J. Pretreatment with ranitidine does not reduce the bioavailability of orally administered topotecan. *Cancer Chemother Pharmacol* (2000) 46, 204–10.

Topotecan + Tyrosine kinase inhibitors

Lapatinib causes a negligible increase in the exposure to topotecan and decreases the tolerated dose of topotecan.

Clinical evidence, mechanism, importance and management

In a phase I study in 9 patients, **lapatinib** appeared to decrease topotecan clearance causing an 18% increase in the AUC of topotecan. The tolerated dose of topotecan was somewhat lower when given with lapatinib (3.2 mg/m^2 weekly versus 4 mg/m^2 weekly). It was suggested that this was probably because lapatinib inhibits drug transporter proteins so inhibiting renal and/or biliary topotecan excretion. In addition, the AUC of lapatinib was 36% higher on the concurrent use of topotecan, although this difference was not statistically significant.[1] Evidence is limited to this small study, but, until more is known, some caution would seem appropriate on concurrent use.

1. Molina JR, Kaufmann SH, Reid JM, Rubin SD, Gálvez-Peralta M, Friedman R, Flatten KS, Koch KM, Gilmer TM, Mullin RJ, Jewell RC, Felten SJ, Mandrekar S, Adjei AA, Erlichman C. Evaluation of lapatinib and topotecan combination therapy: tissue culture, murine xenograft, and phase I clinical trial data. *Clin Cancer Res* (2008) 14, 7900–8.

Toremifene + Antiepileptics; Enzyme-inducing

Carbamazepine, phenobarbital and possibly phenytoin can reduce the serum levels of toremifene.

Clinical evidence, mechanism, importance and management

In a pharmacokinetic study, the AUC and half-life of a single 120-mg dose of toremifene in 10 patients taking enzyme-inducing antiepileptics were approximately half that of those in 10 healthy subjects. The antiepileptics used were **carbamazepine** alone (3 patients) or with clonazepam (3 patients), or **phenobarbital** alone (3 patients) or with **phenytoin** (1 patient). This interaction is thought to occur because these antiepileptics induce the liver enzymes (almost certainly CYP3A4) by which toremifene is metabolised, resulting in increased toremifene clearance.[1]

It is possible that the efficacy of toremifene might be reduced in patients taking these enzyme-inducing antiepileptics (and therefore possibly also **fosphenytoin**, a prodrug of phenytoin, and **primidone**, which is metabolised to phenobarbital); therefore, it would be prudent to monitor patients more closely than normal during concurrent use, for signs or markers indicative of poor response. The UK manufacturer of toremifene has suggested that it might be necessary to double the toremifene dose.[2]

1. Anttila M, Laakso S, Nyländen P, Sotaniemi EA. Pharmacokinetics of the novel antiestrogenic agent toremifene in subjects with altered liver and kidney function. *Clin Pharmacol Ther* (1995) 57, 628–35.
2. Fareston (Toremifene citrate). Orion Pharma (UK) Ltd. UK Summary of product characteristics, January 2009.

Toremifene + Miscellaneous

Based on theoretical considerations, thiazides might increase the risk of hypercalcaemia if given with toremifene. Ketoconazole, a CYP3A4 inhibitor, increases toremifene concentrations. Other CYP3A4 inhibitors are expected to interact similarly.

Clinical evidence, mechanism, importance and management

(a) CYP3A inhibitors

In a study in 18 healthy subjects, ketoconazole 200 mg twice daily increased the AUC and maximum serum concentrations of an 80-mg dose of toremifene 2.9-fold and by 40%, respectively.[1] Ketoconazole is a potent inhibitor of CYP3A4 by which toremifene is, in part, metabolised. Concurrent use therefore increases toremifene exposure. The US manufacturer of toremifene therefore predicts that other potent CYP3A4 inhibitors, and grapefruit juice, will interact similarly and suggest that concurrent use should be avoided. If the use of these drugs is unavoidable, they state that toremifene should be temporarily stopped or that patients should be closely monitored for QT prolongation. For a list of known potent CYP3A4 inhibitors, see 'Table 1.9', p.11, and for more information about drugs that prolong the QT interval, see 'Drugs that prolong the QT interval + Other drugs that prolong the QT interval', p.272.

(b) Thiazides

Hypercalcaemia is a recognised adverse effect of toremifene, and it is suggested that drugs such as the **thiazides**, which decrease renal calcium excretion, may increase the risk of hypercalcaemia.[1,2] This warning is based on indirect evidence and theoretical considerations so its clinical importance awaits confirmation.

1. Fareston (Toremifene citrate). GTx, Inc. US Prescribing information, March 2011.
2. Fareston (Toremifene citrate). Orion Pharma (UK) Ltd. UK Summary of product characteristics, January 2009.

Toremifene + Rifampicin (Rifampin)

Rifampicin, which is known to induce CYP3A4, decreases toremifene exposure, and might be expected to reduce its efficacy.

Clinical evidence

A study in 9 healthy men found that rifampicin 600 mg daily for 5 days reduced the AUC, peak plasma levels, and half-life of a single 120-mg dose of toremifene by 87%, 55%, and 44%, respectively. Similarly, the AUC of the metabolite *N*-demethyltoremifene was reduced by 80%.[1]

Mechanism

Toremifene is metabolised to *N*-demethyltoremifene by CYP3A4, of which rifampicin is a known inducer.

Importance and management

Evidence for an interaction between toremifene and rifampicin appears to be limited to this study, but the findings are in line with the known effects of rifampicin and the known metabolism of toremifene: an interaction is therefore established. The magnitude of the reduction in toremifene exposure seen in the study would be expected to result in a reduction in its efficacy. Therefore, if this combination is necessary, it would seem prudent to monitor the patient more closely than normal for signs or markers indicative of a poor response. In addition, note that the UK manufacturer of toremifene states that it may be necessary to double the toremifene dose.[2]

1. Kivistö KT, Villikka K, Nyman L, Anttila M, Neuvonen PJ. Tamoxifen and toremifene concentrations in plasma are greatly decreased by rifampin. *Clin Pharmacol Ther* (1998) 64, 648–54.
2. Fareston (Toremifene citrate). Orion Pharma (UK) Ltd. UK Summary of product characteristics, January 2009.

Trabectedin + Miscellaneous

Trabectedin is mainly metabolised by CYP3A4 and therefore inhibitors of this isoenzyme are predicted to raise its levels, whereas inducers of this isoenzyme are predicted to reduce its levels. Trabectedin is also a substrate for P-glycoprotein, and therefore inhibitors of this transporter are expected to raise trabectedin levels. The concurrent use of trabectedin with statins is expected to increase the risks of rhabdomyolysis, and the concurrent use of hepatotoxic drugs is expected to increase the risks of hepatotoxicity. Trabectedin may reduce the absorption of phenytoin. The use of live vaccines should be avoided.

Clinical evidence, mechanism, importance and management

(a) Alcohol

The manufacturer warns that because of the risk of additive hepatotoxicity, the use of trabectedin with hepatotoxic drugs is not recommended. They specifically advise that alcohol consumption must be avoided during treatment with trabectedin.[1]

(b) CYP3A4 inducers and inhibitors

Trabectedin is mainly metabolised by the cytochrome P450 isoenzyme CYP3A4. The manufacturer therefore predicts that inducers of this enzyme (they name **phenobarbital**, **rifampicin (rifampin)** and **St John's wort**) may decrease trabectedin levels, and that inhibitors of this isoenzyme (they name **ketoconazole**, **fluconazole**, **ritonavir**, **aprepitant** and **clarithromycin**) may increase trabectedin levels.[1]

Patients should be monitored to ensure that the trabectedin is effective if inducers of CYP3A4 are taken concurrently (see also *Phenytoin*, below). The manufacturers advise that potent CYP3A4 inhibitors should be avoided, but suggest that, if concurrent use cannot be avoided, patients should be closely monitored for trabectedin toxicity and consideration should be given to reducing its dose.[1]

(c) P-glycoprotein inhibitors

Trabectedin is a substrate of P-glycoprotein. The manufacturer therefore advises caution when inhibitors of P-glycoprotein are given to patients taking trabectedin. They specifically name **ciclosporin** and **verapamil**.[1]

(d) Phenytoin

The manufacturer warns that trabectedin may reduce the absorption of phenytoin and therefore increase the risk of seizures. This is predicted on the basis that trabectedin is a cytotoxic and can damage the gastric mucosa and may therefore reduce phenytoin absorption.[2] They therefore do not recommend the combination.[1] There are a few cases of this having occurred with other cytotoxics, see 'Antiepileptics + Antineoplastics; Cytotoxic', p.562; however, it is by no means an established interaction mechanism, and therefore the advice seems over cautious. Note that phenytoin would also be predicted to decrease trabectedin levels, see *CYP3A4 inducers*, above. If both drugs are required, it would seem prudent to monitor phenytoin levels more closely and monitor for trabectedin efficacy.

(e) Statins

In rare cases trabectedin has been associated with rhabdomyolysis. The manufacturers therefore advise caution if other drugs that cause rhabdomyolysis are also given, and they specifically name the statins.[1]

(f) Vaccines

The manufacturer warns that patients receiving trabectedin should not also receive live attenuated vaccines, presumably because of the risks of a generalised infection developing. They specifically contraindicate **yellow fever vaccine**.[1]

1. Yondelis (Trabectedin). Pharma Mar, S.A. UK Summary of product characteristics, October 2009.
2. PharmaMar S. A. Personal communication, March 2009.

Tretinoin + Antifibrinolytics

In acute promyelocytic leukaemia the combination of oral tretinoin and intravenous antifibrinolytics such as tranexamic acid and aprotinin has been associated with fatal thrombotic complications.

Clinical evidence, mechanism, importance and management

In an analysis of 31 patients with acute promyelocytic leukaemia (APL) treated over a 7-year period, intravenous **tranexamic acid** 1 to 2 g daily for 6 days was given for prophylaxis of haemorrhage to 15 of 24 patients receiving tretinoin and chemotherapy, all 4 receiving tretinoin only and 2 of 3 receiving chemotherapy only. Seven of the patients receiving tretinoin died during the study period and 4 of them, who had received the combination of tretinoin and **tranexamic acid**, died within 42 days (early deaths). Three of the early deaths were attributed to thrombotic complications.[1] Another earlier report describes a similar fatal case of thromboembolism in a patient given oral tretinoin and intravenous **tranexamic acid**,[2] and another in a patient given tretinoin and an infusion of **aprotinin**.[3] A further report describes acute renal cortex necrosis as a result of arterial thrombosis in a patient given tretinoin and **tranexamic acid**.[4] Tretinoin alone causes a procoagulant tendency in APL, and this may be exacerbated by the use of antifibrinolytics. Although antifibrinolytics and chemotherapy may be safely used concurrently in APL, the combination of tretinoin and antifibrinolytics can cause fatal thrombotic complications and should be used with caution. The use of blood, platelets and plasma rather than **tranexamic acid** for prophylaxis of haemorrhage has been advocated for APL patients.[1]

1. Brown JE, Olujohungbe A, Chang J, Ryder WDJ, Chopra R, Scarffe JH. All-*trans* retinoic acid (ATRA) and tranexamic acid: a potentially fatal combination in acute promyelocytic leukaemia. *Br J Haematol* (2000) 110, 1010–12.
2. Hashimoto S, Koike T, Tatewaki W, Seki Y, Sato N, Azegami T, Tsukada N, Takahashi H, Kimura H, Ueno M, Arakawa M, Shibata A. fatal thromboembolism in acute promyelocytic leukemia during all-*trans* retinoic acid therapy combined with antifibrinolytic therapy for prophylaxis of hemorrhage. *Leukemia* (1994) 8, 1113–15.
3. Mahendra P, Keeling DM, Hood IM, Baglin TP, Marcus RE. Fatal thromboembolism in acute promyelocytic leukaemia treated with a combination of all-trans retinoic acid and aprotinin. *Clin Lab Haematol* (1996) 18, 51–2.
4. Levin M-D, Betjes MGH, v d Kwast TH, Wenberg BL, Leebeek FWG. Acute renal cortex necrosis caused by arterial thrombosis during treatment for acute promyelocytic leukemia. *Haematologica* (2003) 88, ECR21.

Tretinoin or Alitretinoin + Azoles

The metabolism of tretinoin can be inhibited by single-dose fluconazole and ketoconazole, although one study found that concurrent ketoconazole did not reverse tretinoin auto-induction. Case reports describe tretinoin toxicity in a child treated with fluconazole and a woman treated with voriconazole. The metabolism of alitretinoin can also be inhibited by ketoconazole, whereas the pharmacokinetics of ketoconazole are not altered by alitretinoin.

Clinical evidence

(a) Alitretinoin

In a study in 18 healthy subjects, a single 200-mg dose of ketoconazole increased the maximum plasma concentration and AUC of a single and repeated doses of oral alitretinoin 30 mg by up to 60% and 50%, respectively. In this study, single and repeated doses of alitretinoin did not affect the pharmacokinetics of ketoconazole.[1]

(b) Tretinoin

1. Fluconazole. In 2 patients taking tretinoin 22.5 mg/m^2 twice daily, fluconazole 400 mg (as a loading dose) and then 200 mg daily thereafter, increased the AUC of tretinoin about two- to fourfold, after the second fluconazole dose, when compared with the AUC 8 days after starting tretinoin, but tretinoin levels were similar to those on the first day of use.[2] A 4-year-old boy with acute promyelocytic leukaemia was given induction chemotherapy consisting of cytarabine, daunorubicin and tretinoin 45 mg/m^2 daily in two divided doses. Febrile neutropenia was treated with meropenem and amphotericin B for periods up to day 20. On day 20 he started antifungal prophylaxis with fluconazole 100 mg daily. The next day he complained of headache and a week later he had headache, vomiting and papilloedema. His CT scan was normal. Pseudotumor cerebri was diagnosed and symptoms of increased intracranial pressure resolved within a day of stopping tretinoin. Restarting tretinoin on day 30, at 75% of the previous dose, resulted in headache and vomiting, and the treatment was continued from day 35 with an even lower dose (30%), which caused headache but only one episode of vomiting. Fluconazole was stopped on day 41 and within 24 hours the patient had improved clinically with the headache and vomiting fully resolved. He was then able to tolerate the full dose of tretinoin without adverse effects.[3]

2. Ketoconazole. In 6 patients with lung cancer, a single 400-mg dose of ketoconazole given one hour before tretinoin on day 29 increased the AUC of tretinoin by 115% (compared with day 28 when tretinoin was given alone), but a 200 mg dose of ketoconazole had little effect on the AUC of tretinoin. Ketoconazole had no effect on the AUC of tretinoin when given on day 2 (compared with tretinoin alone on day one).[4] A further study investigated the effect of prolonged ketoconazole administration (400 mg then 200 mg daily for 14 days) on plasma tretinoin levels in patients given tretinoin 45 mg/m^2 twice daily for 14 days. The AUC of tretinoin showed a marked decline by 14 days, and this was not altered by ketoconazole. However, the concurrent use of ketoconazole appeared to be associated with more vomiting.[5]

3. Voriconazole. A 21-year-old woman with acute promyelocytic leukaemia taking tretinoin 40 mg twice daily and fluconazole 200 mg daily was admitted into hospital with fever and neutropenia. Due to a lack of response to treatment (including several antibacterials) she was changed from fluconazole to intravenous voriconazole 500 mg every 12 hours on day one, then 340 mg every 12 hours for a further 17 days, after which she was given oral voriconazole 200 mg twice daily. On day 15, the patient reported blurred vision, farsightedness, generalised itching and skin dryness. She was diagnosed with papilloedema, and, as no other cause was identified, this was attributed to the tretinoin, which was stopped. Three days later her symptoms had improved and she was subsequently discharged taking tretinoin without voriconazole, and no further papilloedema was reported during 4 months of follow up.[6]

Mechanism

Fluconazole and voriconazole inhibit CYP3A4 and CYP2C9, and ketoconazole inhibits CYP3A4. *In vitro* fluconazole and ketoconazole inhibited the oxidative metabolism of tretinoin, with ketoconazole being more potent.[2] Tretinoin induces its own metabolism over time, and the effect of these azoles is not as great on the first day of tretinoin administration as after a week or more of use.[2,4] However, in one study, continuous ketoconazole did not reverse tretinoin auto-induction.[5] Alitretinoin is also a substrate of CYP3A4 and therefore the concurrent use of ketoconazole inhibits its metabolism, resulting in increased exposure.

Importance and management

The pharmacokinetic findings from two single-dose studies with **tretinoin** suggested that drugs such as fluconazole and ketoconazole may be useful in overcoming clinical resistance to tretinoin,[2,4] whereas one multiple-dose study found that ketoconazole had little effect on tretinoin auto-induction and the combination was poorly tolerated.[5] It has been suggested that the concurrent use of tretinoin with drugs that affect its metabolism should be avoided if possible, or patients should be carefully monitored.[3] Given the reaction described in the case report of the child, this seems advisable. Although evidence for an interaction between tretinoin and voriconazole is limited to a case report, it would seem prudent to apply similar caution to their concurrent use.

Evidence for an interaction between **alitretinoin** and ketoconazole appears to be limited to one study. Although the clinical relevance of this interaction is unknown, it is possible that the increase in alitretinoin exposure may lead to symptoms of retinoid toxicity. The UK manufacturer suggests a dose reduction of alitretinoin may be necessary on the concurrent use of ketoconazole.[7] If both drugs are given it may be prudent to monitor for alitretinoin adverse effects (flushing, eye irritation, arthralgia), reducing the dose according to response.

There seems to be no evidence regarding an effect of ketoconazole on topical alitretinoin or tretinoin, but as systemic absorption from these formulations is low, no interaction would be expected.

1. Schmitt-Hoffmann AH, Roos B, Baumgaertner E, Thomann P, Brown T, Maares J. Alitretinoin (9-*cis* retinoic acid): pharmacokinetic interactions between alitretinoin, ketoconazole, simvastatin and ciclosporin A. European Academy of Dermatology and Venereology. 16th Annual Congress, Vienna, 2007. Poster 286.
2. Schwartz EL, Hallam S, Gallagher RE, Wiernik PH. Inhibition of all-trans retinoic acid metabolism by fluconazole in vitro and in patients with acute promyelocytic leukaemia. *Biochem Pharmacol* (1995) 50, 923–8.
3. Vanier KL, Mattiussi AJ, Johnston DL. Interaction of all-trans-retinoic acid with fluconazole in acute promyelocytic leukaemia. *J Pediatr Hematol Oncol* (2003) 25, 403–4.
4. Rigas JR, Francis PA, Muindi JRF, Kris MG, Huselton C, DeGrazia F, Orazem JP, Young CW, Warrell RP. Constitutive variability in the pharmacokinetics of the natural retinoid, all-trans-retinoic acid, and its modulation by ketoconazole. *J Natl Cancer Inst* (1993) 85, 1921–6.
5. Lee JS, Newman RA, Lippman SM, Fossella FV, Calayag M, Raber MN, Krakoff IH, Hong WK. Phase I evaluation of all-trans retinoic acid with and without ketoconazole in adults with solid tumors. *J Clin Oncol* (1995) 13, 1501–8.
6. Dixon KS, Hassoun A. Pseudotumor cerebri due to the potentiation of all-*trans* retinoic acid by voriconazole. *J Am Pharm Assoc* (2010) 50, 742–4.
7. Toctino (Alitretinoin). Basilea Pharmaceutica. UK Summary of product characteristics, July 2014.

Tyrosine kinase inhibitors + Antacids

Nilotinib and dasatinib exposure is not affected by aluminium/magnesium hydroxide when administration of the antacid is separated. Exposure to bosutinib, erlotinib, gefitinib, lapatinib, and pazopanib, is predicted to be reduced by antacids. Imatinib exposure is not affected by aluminium/magnesium hydroxide.

Clinical evidence

(a) Dasatinib

In a single-dose study, the AUC and maximum plasma concentration of dasatinib 50 mg were reduced by 55% and 58%, respectively, when it was given at the same time as 30 mL of an **aluminium/magnesium hydroxide** antacid. However, when the antacid was given 2 hours before dasatinib, there was no change in the AUC of dasatinib.[1]

(b) Imatinib

In a single-dose study in healthy subjects, there was no effect on imatinib exposure (AUC) when it was taken 15 minutes after 20 mL of an **aluminium/magnesium hydroxide** antacid (*Maalox Max*).[2]

(c) Nilotinib

In a randomised, crossover study in healthy subjects, the pharmacokinetics of a single 400-mg dose of nilotinib were not affected by the administration of 30 mL of an **aluminium/magnesium hydroxide** antacid (*Maalox*) 2 hours before, or 2 hours after, the nilotinib.[3]

Mechanism

The solubilities of dasatinib and nilotinib are pH-dependent, therefore drugs that reduce gastric acidity, such as antacids, reduce their absorption. Imatinib absorption does not appear to be affected by changes to gastric pH.

Importance and management

An interaction between **dasatinib** and antacids is established, but the extent of the reduction in dasatinib exposure appears to be influenced by the timing of concurrent administration. When the doses of **nilotinib** and an antacid were separated by 2 hours, the antacid had no effect on the exposure to nilotinib. Therefore, a similar separation between the doses of antacids and **dasatinib** might reduce the effect on dasatinib exposure; the UK and US manufacturers of both **dasatinib**[4,5] and **nilotinib**[6,7] state that antacids should be given at least 2 hours before, or 2 hours after, the tyrosine kinase inhibitor dose.

The pharmacokinetics of **imatinib** are not affected by antacids, therefore no additional precautions are necessary on concurrent use.

There does not appear to be any information on an interaction between other tyrosine kinase inhibitors and antacids, however the UK and US manufacturers of **bosutinib**,[8,9] **erlotinib**,[10,11] and **pazopanib**[12,13] make similar recommendations as for dasatinib and nilotinib regarding the separation of doses when they are given with antacids. On the basis of the effect of high-dose ranitidine on **gefitinib** (see 'Tyrosine kinase inhibitors + H_2-receptor antagonists', p.733), the concurrent use of gefitinib and antacids should probably be undertaken with caution. If both gefitinib and an antacid are given, it would be prudent to separate the doses by several hours (the US manufacturer of gefitinib recommends 6 hours before or after the antacid[14]) and to monitor for a reduction in gefitinib efficacy. The UK manufacturer of **lapatinib** advises that drugs that increase gastric pH might reduce the absorption of lapatinib and should be avoided.[15]

The UK manufacturers of **cabozantinib**[16] and **crizotinib**[17] state that no dose adjustment is required on concurrent use of antacids.

1. Eley T, Luo FR, Agrawal S, Sanil A, Manning J, Li T, Blackwood-Chirchir A, Bertz R. Phase I study of the effect of gastric acid pH modulators on the bioavailability of oral dasatinib in healthy subjects. *J Clin Pharmacol* (2009) 49, 700–9.
2. Sparano BA, Egorin MJ, Parise RA, Walters J, Komazec KA, Redner RL, Beumer JH. Effect of antacid on imatinib absorption. *Cancer Chemother Pharmacol* (2009) 63, 525–8.
3. Yin OQ, Bédoucha V, McCulloch T, Zheng C, Zhou W, Hussaini A, Novick S. Effects of famotidine or an antacid preparation on the pharmacokinetics of nilotinib in healthy volunteers. *Cancer Chemother Pharmacol* (2013) 71, 219–26.
4. Sprycel (Dasatinib monohydrate). Bristol-Myers Squibb Pharmaceutical Ltd. UK Summary of product characteristics, March 2015.
5. Sprycel (Dasatinib monohydrate). Bristol-Myers Squibb Company. US Prescribing information, August 2015.
6. Tasigna (Nilotinib hydrochloride monohydrate). Novartis Pharmaceuticals UK Ltd. UK Summary of product characteristics, June 2015.
7. Tasigna (Nilotinib hydrochloride monohydrate). Novartis Pharmaceuticals Corp. US Prescribing information, January 2015.
8. Bosulif (Bosutinib monohydrate). Pfizer Inc. US Prescribing information, November 2014.
9. Bosulif (Bosutinib monohydrate). Pfizer Ltd. UK Summary of product characteristics, July 2015
10. Tarceva (Erlotinib hydrochloride). OSI Pharmaceuticals LLC. US Prescribing information, April 2015.
11. Tarceva (Erlotinib hydrochloride). Roche Products Ltd. UK Summary of product characteristics, December 2013.
12. Votrient (Pazopanib hydrochloride). Novartis Pharmaceuticals UK Ltd. UK Summary of product characteristics, July 2015.
13. Votrient (Pazopanib hydrochloride). GlaxoSmithKline. US Prescribing information, April 2015.
14. Iressa (Gefitinib). AstraZeneca Pharmaceuticals LP. US Prescribing information, July 2015.
15. Tyverb (Lapatinib ditosylate monohydrate). GlaxoSmithKline UK. UK Summary of product characteristics, June 2015.
16. Cometriq (Cabozantinib malate). Swedish Orphan Biovitrum Ltd. UK Summary of product characteristics June 2015.
17. Xalkori (Crizotinib). Pfizer Ltd. UK Summary of product characteristics. April 2015.

Tyrosine kinase inhibitors + Anthracyclines

Dasatinib, lapatinib, and sorafenib have been reported to cause QT prolongation, and because of this, the manufacturers advise caution on their concurrent use with cumulative high-dose anthracycline chemotherapy.[1-4]

1. Sprycel (Dasatinib monohydrate). Bristol-Myers Squibb Pharmaceutical Ltd. UK Summary of product characteristics, November 2013.
2. Sprycel (Dasatinib monohydrate). Bristol-Myers Squibb Company. US Prescribing information, April 2014.
3. Tykerb (Lapatinib ditosylate monohydrate). GlaxoSmithKline. US Prescribing information, October 2013.
4. Nexavar (Sorafenib tosylate). Bayer plc. UK Summary of product characteristics, February 2013.

Tyrosine kinase inhibitors + Antiepileptics; Enzyme-inducing

Enzyme-inducing antiepileptics reduce the exposure to erlotinib, gefitinib, and imatinib and appear to reduce the exposure to lapatinib and pazopanib. Carbamazepine reduces lapatinib exposure. A single case report describes increased phenytoin concentrations in a patient given erlotinib. Enzyme-inducing antiepileptics are also predicted to reduce the exposure to other tyrosine kinase inhibitors.

Clinical evidence

(a) Effect on tyrosine kinase inhibitor pharmacokinetics

1. Erlotinib. As part of a phase I study in 33 patients with glioma, the pharmacokinetics of erlotinib 100 mg daily increasing to 500 mg daily were compared in patients taking enzyme-inducing antiepileptics and those not taking these antiepileptics. There was a 33 to 71% lower exposure to erlotinib when it was given with an enzyme-inducing antiepileptic drug, with the exposure to erlotinib at 400 to 500 mg daily with these antiepileptics being similar to erlotinib alone at 100 to 150 mg daily. The antiepileptic drugs taken were **carbamazepine**, **oxcarbazepine**, **phenytoin**, **fosphenytoin**, **phenobarbital**, and **primidone**. Patients taking these drugs tolerated a higher dose of erlotinib.[1] Similarly, in a phase II study in glioma patients, the AUC of erlotinib 200 mg daily in those not taking antiepileptics was similar to that in those patients taking erlotinib 500 mg daily with antiepileptics (**carbamazepine**, **oxcarbazepine**, **phenytoin**, **phenobarbital**, and **primidone**).[2] Likewise, another phase II study in glioblastoma patients found that on the first day of concurrent treatment, the AUC of erlotinib was comparable in 9 patients taking erlotinib 300 mg daily with enzyme-inducing antiepileptics (not stated) to that in another 45 patients taking erlotinib 150 mg daily without enzyme-inducing antiepileptics. However by day 8 the AUC of erlotinib in those patients taking antiepileptics was 55% lower than in those not taking antiepileptics.[3] In a phase I dose-escalating study in 32 patients with cerebral carcinomas who were also receiving antiepileptics (**carbamazepine**, **oxcarbazepine**, **phenytoin**, **phenobarbital**, and **primidone**), the AUC of erlotinib 150 mg daily in 6 patients was 55% lower than in another group of 76 patients not receiving antiepileptics. The conversion of erlotinib to its metabolite, OSI-420, was 2.5-fold higher than in those not taking antiepileptics. The maximum tolerated erlotinib dose in those taking antiepileptics was 650 mg daily, although note there was wide interindividual variability in the AUC of erlotinib at this dose.[4]

2. Gefitinib. In a study in healthy subjects, **phenytoin** 5 mg/kg daily for 5 days decreased the AUC of a single 250-mg dose of gefitinib by 47%. The oral clearance of gefitinib was increased 2.3-fold but there was no change in elimination half-life.[5] In a phase I study in patients with glioma taking temozolamide, the dose-normalised gefitinib AUC and maximum concentration were 55% and 33% lower, respectively, in 8 patients taking antiepileptics (**carbamazepine**, **fosphenytoin**, **oxcarbazepine**, **phenytoin**, **phenobarbital**, and **primidone**) than in 5 patients not taking antiepileptics. The maximum tolerated dose was 250 mg gefitinib daily for those not taking antiepileptics, compared with 1 g gefitinib daily in those taking antiepileptics.[6]

3. Imatinib. In a study in 224 patients with malignant gliomas, the steady-state minimum concentration of imatinib was 68% lower in 85 patients taking enzyme-inducing antiepileptics than in 111 patients not taking antiepileptics and 28 patients taking non-enzyme inducing antiepileptics (valproate, levetiracetam, or lamotrigine).[7] When analysed by individual drug, the reduction in steady-state concentrations was 73% in 15 patients taking **phenytoin**, 66% in 63 patients taking **carbamazepine**, 61% in 6 patients taking **oxcarbazepine**, and 49% in one patient taking **topiramate**. There was no reduction in imatinib concentrations in the patients taking valproate, levetiracetam, or lamotrigine. Similarly, in a phase I study in patients with glioma, the steady-state minimum concentration of imatinib was 79% lower in those taking antiepileptics (**carbamazepine**, **oxcarbazepine**, **phenytoin**, **phenobarbital**, and **primidone**) than in those not taking antiepileptics. In addition, the dose-normalised imatinib AUC and maximum concentration were 72% and 61% lower, respectively, in those taking antiepileptics. The maximum tolerated dose was 800 mg daily for those not taking antiepileptics, but in those taking antiepileptics dose-limiting toxicities were not seen until the dose reached 1.2 g daily.[8]

4. Lapatinib. In a study in 23 healthy subjects who received **carbamazepine** 100 mg twice daily for 3 days followed by 200 mg twice daily for a further 17 days, with a single 250-mg dose of lapatinib on day one and day 21, the AUC and maximum plasma concentration of lapatinib were reduced by 72% and 59%, respectively.[9] In a phase I study in patients with glioblastoma multiforme, the apparent oral clearance of lapatinib was 10-fold higher based on data from 5 patients taking enzyme-inducing antiepileptics (**carbamazepine** and **phenytoin**) than in patients not taking antiepileptics.[10] For mention of a phase I study in patients given lapatinib and pazopanib, see under *Pazopanib* below.

5. Pazopanib. A phase I study in patients with gliomas to determine the maximum tolerated doses for a combination of pazopanib and lapatinib when taking enzyme-inducing antiepileptics (**carbamazepine**, **phenobarbital**, **phenytoin**, **primidone**), found that the exposure to both pazopanib and lapatanib was lower when compared with patients not taking enzyme-inducing antiepileptics in phase II of the study.[11]

6. Sorafenib. As part of a phase II study in patients with glioblastoma, the pharmacokinetics of sorafenib 400 mg twice daily were compared in patients taking enzyme-inducing antiepileptics and those taking non-enzyme inducing antiepileptics. For the patients taking non-enzyme inducing antiepileptics, the sorafenib AUC and maximum concentrations were 2- to 3-fold higher on day 28 compared with day one, but in those taking enzyme-inducing antiepileptics, there was no difference between day 28 and day one values. Furthermore, the sorafenib AUC on day 28 in patients taking non-enzyme inducing antiepileptics was 2.7-fold higher than in those taking enzyme-inducing antiepileptics. The enzyme-inducing antiepileptic drugs taken were **carbamazepine**, **oxcarbazepine**, **phenytoin**, **phenobarbital**, and **primidone**. The non-enzyme inducing antiepileptics taken were not stated.[12]

(b) Effect on antiepileptic concentrations

A case report describes a 52-year-old woman, stabilised on **phenytoin** 100 mg twice daily, with a plasma concentration of 5 to 6 mg/dL, who experienced signs of **phenytoin** toxicity, and an elevated plasma **phenytoin** concentration (19.8 mg/dL) after starting to take **erlotinib** 150 mg daily. Despite a reduction in her **phenytoin** dose, to 100 mg daily alternating with 200 mg daily, her **phenytoin** concentration increased to 25.3 mg/dL. Three weeks after a further reduction in her **phenytoin** dose, to 100 mg daily, her phenytoin concentration was 13.5 mg/dL.[13]

Mechanism

The tyrosine kinase inhibitors are substrates of CYP3A4, and therefore their exposure is reduced by the enzyme-inducing antiepileptics, which are potent inducers of this isoenzyme. The data for gefitinib suggest that the interaction might involve inhibition of intestinal CYP3A-mediated metabolism, but further study is needed.[5]

The reason for the increase in phenytoin concentrations is uncertain as erlotinib would not be expected to alter the pharmacokinetics of phenytoin by inhibiting CYP2C9, by which phenytoin is metabolised.

Importance and management

The reduction in **erlotinib**, **gefitinib**, **lapatinib**, **imatinib**, and **sorafenib** exposure with the enzyme-inducing antiepileptics (carbamazepine, fosphenytoin, oxcarbazepine, phenobarbital, phenytoin, and primidone) is established, and likely to be clinically important. The use of these tyrosine kinase inhibitors with enzyme-inducing antiepileptics should be avoided, where possible. However, if concurrent use is necessary, some manufacturers give specific advice, see *Importance and management* in 'Tyrosine kinase inhibitors + Rifampicin (Rifampin)', p.737.

Additionally, the authors of the glioma study suggest that, for further studies in this disease, the dose of erlotinib should be at least 500 mg daily in those already taking enzyme-inducing antiepileptics and 200 mg daily in those patients not taking these drugs.[7]

Direct evidence for other tyrosine kinase inhibitors is lacking, nevertheless some manufacturers similarly recommend avoiding enzyme-inducing antiepileptics. If concurrent use is unavoidable, some give specific advice, see *Importance and management* in 'Tyrosine kinase inhibitors + Rifampicin (Rifampin)', p.737. Note that, **eslicarbazepine** is also an enzyme-inducing antiepileptic, so in the absence of specific data similar precautions would also be prudent. If making dose adjustments, remember that when the inducing drug is stopped, the dose of the tyrosine kinase inhibitor should be reduced to the indicated dose.

The case of increased **phenytoin** concentrations with erlotinib appears to be the only report of such an interaction, and its general relevance is unclear.[13]

1. Prados MD, Lamborn KR, Chang S, Burton E, Butowski N, Malec M, Kapadia A, Rabbitt J, Page MS, Fedoroff A, Xie D, Kelley SK. Phase 1 study of erlotinib HCl alone and combined with temozolomide in patients with stable or recurrent malignant glioma. *Neuro Oncol* (2006) 8, 67–78.
2. Sathornsumetee S, Desjardins A, Vredenburgh JJ, McLendon RE, Marcello J, Herndon JE, Mathe A, Hamilton M, Rich JN, Norfleet JA, Gururangan S, Friedman HS, Reardon DA. Phase II trial of bevacizumab and erlotinib in patients with recurrent malignant glioma. *Neuro Oncol* (2010) 12, 1300–10.
3. van den Bent MJ, Brandes AA, Rampling R, Kouwenhoven MCM, Kros JM, Carpentier AF, Clement PM, Frenay M, Campone M, Baurain J-F, Armand J-P, Taphoorn MJ, Tosoni A, Kletzl H, Klughammer B, Lacombe D, Gorlia T. Randomized phase II trial of erlotinib versus temozolomide or carmustine in recurrent glioblastoma: EORTC Brain tumor group study 26034. *J Clin Oncol* (2009) 27, 1268–74.
4. Raizer JJ, Abrey LE, Lassman AB, Chang SM, Lamborn KR, Kuhn JG, Yung WK, Gilbert MR, Aldape KD, Wen PY, Fine HA, Mehta M, De Angelis LM, Lieberman F, Cloughesy TF, Robins HI, Dancey J, Prados MD. A phase I trial of erlotinib in patients with nonprogressive glioblastoma multiforme postradiation therapy, and recurrent malignant gliomas and meningiomas. *Neuro Oncol* (2010) 12, 87–94.
5. Chhun S, Verstuyft C, Rizzo-Padoin N, Simoneau G, Becquemont L, Peretti I, Swaisland A, Wortelboer R, Bergmann JF, Mouly S. Gefitinib-phenytoin interaction is not correlated with the ^{14}C-erythromycin breath test in healthy male volunteers. *Br J Clin Pharmacol* (2009) 68, 226–37.
6. Prados MD, Yung WKA, Wen PY, Junck L, Cloughesy T, Fink K, Chang S, Robins HI, Dancey J, Kuhn J. Phase-1 trial of gefitinib and temozolomide in patients with malignant glioma: a North American brain tumor consortium study. *Cancer Chemother Pharmacol* (2008) 61, 1059–67.
7. Pursche S, Schleyer E, von Bonin M, Ehninger G, Said SM, Prondzinsky R, Illmer T, Wang Y, Hosius C, Nikolova Z, Bornhäuser M, Dresemann G. Influence of enzyme-inducing antiepileptic drugs on trough level of imatinib in glioblastoma patients. *Curr Clin Pharmacol* (2008) 3, 198–203.
8. Wen PY, Yung WK, Lamborn KR, Dahia PL, Wang Y, Peng B, Abrey LE, Raizer J, Cloughesy TF, Fink K, Gilbert M, Chang S, Junck L, Schiff D, Lieberman F, Fine HA, Mehta M, Robins HI, DeAngelis LM, Groves MD, Puduvalli VK, Levin V, Conrad C, Maher EA, Aldape K, Hayes M, Letvak L, Egorin MJ, Capdeville R, Kaplan R, Murgo AJ, Stiles C, Prados MD. Phase I/II study of imatinib mesylate for recurrent malignant gliomas: North American Brain Tumor Consortium Study 99-08. *Clin Cancer Res* (2006) 12, 4899–907.
9. Smith DA, Koch KM, Arya N, Bowen CJ, Herendeen JM, Beelen A. Effects of ketoconazole and carbamazepine on lapatinib pharmacokinetics in healthy subjects. *Br J Clin Pharmacol* (2009) 67, 421–6.
10. Thiessen B, Stewart C, Tsao M, Kamel-Reid S, Schaiquevich P, Mason W, Easaw J, Belanger K, Forsyth P, McIntosh L, Eisenhauer E. A phase I/II trial of GW572016 (lapatinib) in recurrent glioblastoma multiforme: clinical outcomes, pharmacokinetics and molecular correlation. *Cancer Chemother Pharmacol* (2010) 65, 353–61.
11. Reardon DA, Groves MD, Wen PY, Nabors L, Mikkelson T, Rosenfeld S, Raizer J, Barriuso J, McLendon RE, Suttle AB, Ma B, Curtis CM, Dar MM, de Bono J. A phase I/II trial of pazopanib in combination with lapatanib in adult patients with relapsed malignant glioma. *Clin Cancer Res* (2013) 19, 900–908.
12. Reardon DA, Vredenburgh JJ, Desjardins A, Peters K, Gururangan S, Sampson JH, Marcello J, Herndon JE, McLendon RE, Janney D, Friedman AH, Bigner DD, Friedman HS. Effect of CYP3A-inducing anti-epileptics on sorafenib exposure: results of a phase II study of sorafenib plus daily temozolomide in adults with recurrent glioblastoma. *J Neurooncol* (2011) 101, 57–66.
13. Grenader T, Gipps M, Shavit L, Gabizon A. Significant drug interaction: phenytoin toxicity due to erlotinib. *Lung Cancer* (2007) 57, 404–6.

Tyrosine kinase inhibitors + Azoles

Ketoconazole markedly increases the exposure to bosutinib and dasatinib; moderately increases the exposure to axitinib, crizotinib, lapatinib, and nilotinib; slightly to moderately increases exposure to tofacitinib, and slightly increases the exposure to cabozantinib, erlotinib, imatinib, pazopanib, ponatinib, regorafenib, ruxolitinib, and sunitinib. Ketoconazole has no effect on sorafenib pharmacokinetics. Itraconazole slightly increases gefitinib exposure, and has a negligible effect on vandetanib exposure.

Fluconazole slightly increases tofacitinib exposure. A case report describes an adverse skin reaction attributed to a pharmacokinetic interaction between voriconazole and imatinib. Other moderate and potent CYP3A4 inhibitors would be expected to interact similarly with these tyrosine kinase inhibitors.

Clinical evidence

(a) Fluconazole, itraconazole, and ketoconazole

Studies of the pharmacokinetic interactions of the tyrosine kinase inhibitors with fluconazole, itraconazole, and ketoconazole are summarised in 'Table 17.3', p.729. This shows that the size of the effect of **ketoconazole** varies between the tyrosine kinase inhibitors, with **bosutinib** and **dasatinib** being affected the most, followed by **axitinib**, **crizotinib**, **lapatinib**, **nilotinib** and **tofacitinib**; **cabozantinib**, **erlotinib**, **imatinib**, **pazopanib**, **ponatinib**, **regorafenib**, **ruxolitinib** and **sunitinib** are affected the least. Although no effect was seen on **sorafenib** exposure, a decrease in the inactive *N*-oxide metabolite was noted.[1]

Giving healthy subjects a single dose of **pazopanib** *eye drops* with ketoconazole increased the maximum plasma concentration and AUC of **pazopanib** 1.5-fold and 2.2-fold, respectively.[2] This is similar to the effect seen with ketoconazole and oral pazopanib, see 'Table 17.3', p.729.

The effects of **fluconazole** and **itraconazole** on **tofacitinib**, and **gefitinib** or **vandetanib**, respectively, are smaller than those of ketoconazole on other tyrosine kinase inhibitors.

(b) Voriconazole

A patient with chronic myeloid leukaemia developed a pustular eruption while taking **imatinib** 800 mg daily, 12 weeks after starting to take voriconazole for pulmonary aspergillosis. His imatinib plasma concentrations were about twice the predicted concentrations while taking both drugs. His condition improved within 3 weeks of stopping both voriconazole and imatinib, and did not recur with the use of voriconazole alone.[3]

Mechanism

Ketoconazole, voriconazole, itraconazole, and to a lesser extent, fluconazole inhibit CYP3A4 by which the tyrosine kinase inhibitors are metabolised; this results in increased exposure to the tyrosine kinase inhibitor, with the exception of sorafenib, which is unaffected by ketoconazole. The reason for the lack of effect on sorafenib has been suggested to be that other metabolic routes (possibly glucuronidation) compensate when this route is inhibited so ketoconazole has little effect.[1] Vandetanib is primarily metabolised by CYP3A4 to the *N*-desmethyl metabolite, but unexpectedly itraconazole had only a very minor effect on its metabolism. There is insufficient evidence to assess the importance of CYP3A4 to imatinib metabolism (see also 'Tyrosine kinase inhibitors + HIV-protease inhibitors', p.734), although the possible case with voriconazole (which also inhibits CYP3A4), suggests that it could be relevant.

Ketoconazole is also an inhibitor of the drug transporter P-glycoprotein, and the lack of change in elimination half-life of erlotinib with ketoconazole suggests that inhibition of this transporter protein in the gut might also be involved.[4] Other tyrosine kinase inhibitors have also been shown to be substrates of P-glycoprotein *in vitro*, and so it cannot be ruled out that this mechanism might be involved in the effect of ketoconazole on crizotinib, lapatinib, and tofacitinib.

Fluconazole is also an inhibitor of CYP2C9 and CYP2C19, by which ruxolitinib and tofacitinib, respectively, are additionally metabolised. Involvement of CYP2C19 in the effect seen with fluconazole and tofacitinib cannot be ruled out, but requires further study.

Importance and management

In general terms, a pharmacokinetic interaction between the azoles and tyrosine kinase inhibitors is established, but the size of the effect, and hence the clinical relevance, varies. However, note that tyrosine kinase inhibitors are relatively toxic and some also have a narrow therapeutic range, such that even modest effects could result in increased adverse effects. Many manufacturers recommend dose adjustments for the use of potent CYP3A4 inhibitors with tyrosine kinase inhibitors and some also suggest dose reductions for moderate CYP3A4 inhibitors. Note that, where dose adjustments are made, note that if the CYP3A4 inhibitor is stopped, a washout period of about a week should be allowed before increasing the dose of the tyrosine kinase inhibitor.

Potent CYP3A4 inhibitors

The potent CYP3A4 inhibitor, **ketoconazole**, markedly increases the exposure to **bosutinib** and **dasatinib**, and moderately increases the exposure to **axitinib**, **crizotinib**, **lapatinib**, and **nilotinib**; changes which are all likely to be clinically important. Ketoconazole slightly to moderately increases exposure to **tofacitinib**, and slightly increases the exposure to **cabozantinib**, **erlotinib**, **imatinib**, **pazopanib**, **ponatinib**, **regorafenib**, **ruxolitinib**, and **sunitinib**. The concurrent use of the tyrosine kinase inhibitors with all potent CYP3A4 inhibitors (this would include **itraconazole** and **voriconazole**; see 'Table 1.9', p.11 for a list) is generally best avoided. However, some manufacturers give specific advice if concurrent use is necessary.

- Decrease the **axitinib** dose by about half[5,6] (e.g. reduce the starting dose from 5 mg to 2 mg[5]). Subsequent doses can be increased or decreased depending on safety and tolerability.[6] Note that some adverse reactions might necessitate temporary or permanent discontinuation of axitinib.[5,6]
- Consider interrupting **bosutinib** treatment or reducing the dose.[7]
- Reduce the daily dose of **cabozantinib** by 40 mg.[8]
- The dose of **dasatinib** should be reduced to 20 mg daily in those taking 100 mg daily [a 5-fold reduction] and to 40 mg daily in those taking 140 mg daily [a 3.5-fold reduction].[9]
- Reduce the **erlotinib** dose by 50 mg decrements if severe reactions occur on concurrent use.[10]
- If the concurrent use of **gefitinib** is necessary, patients should be closely monitored for signs of increased toxicity.[11]
- Consider reducing the **lapatinib** dose to 500 mg daily.[12]
- With **nilotinib**, if concurrent use is unavoidable, the nilotinib dose should be reduced by about two-thirds, depending on the indication,[13] and close monitoring of the QT interval is advised.[13,14]
- Reduce the **pazopanib** dose to 400 mg daily, with close monitoring for adverse effects. If adverse effects suspected, reduce the dose further.[15,16]

Table 17.3 Summary of the studies assessing the effect of azoles on the pharmacokinetics of tyrosine kinase inhibitors

Tyrosine kinase inhibitor	*Study*	*Dose*	*Azole*	*Cmax increase*	*AUC increase*	*Refs*
Axitinib	Healthy subjects	5 mg single dose day 4	Ketoconazole 400 mg daily for 7 days	50%	2-fold	1
Bosutinib	Healthy subjects	100 mg single dose	Ketoconazole 400 mg daily for 5 days	5.2-fold	8.6-fold	2
Cabozantinib	Healthy subjects	Single dose	Ketoconazole 400 mg daily for 27 days		38%	3
Crizotinib		150 mg single dose	Ketoconazole 200 mg twice daily	40%	3.2-fold	4,5
Dasatinib	Patients	20 mg once daily	Ketoconazole 200 mg twice daily	4-fold	5-fold	6
Erlotinib	Healthy subjects	100 mg single dose day 2	Ketoconazole 200 mg twice daily for 5 days	52%	69%	7
Gefitinib	Healthy subjects	250 mg or 500 mg single dose day 4	Itraconazole 200 mg twice daily for 12 days	51% or 32%	78% or 61%	8
Imatinib	Healthy subjects	200 mg single dose	Ketoconazole 400 mg single dose	26%	40%	9
Lapatinib	Healthy subjects	100 mg single dose day 4	Ketoconazole 200 mg twice daily for 7 days	2.2-fold	3.6-fold	10
Nilotinib	Healthy subjects	200 mg single dose day 4	Ketoconazole 400 mg daily for 6 days	80%	3-fold	11
Pazopanib	Patients	400 mg daily for 5 days	Ketoconazole 400 mg daily for 5 days	45%	66%	12
Ponatinib	Healthy subjects	15 mg single dose	Ketoconazole 400 mg daily for 5 days	47%	78%	13
Regorafenib	Healthy subjects	160 mg single dose day 5	Ketoconazole 400 mg daily for 18 days		33%	14
Ruxolitinib	Healthy subjects	10 mg single dose day 4	Ketoconazole 200 mg twice daily for 4 days	33%	91%	15
Sorafenib	Healthy subjects	50 mg single dose day 4	Ketoconazole 400 mg daily for 7 days		No effect	16
Sunitinib	Healthy subjects	Single dose	Ketoconazole	49%	51%	17,18
Tofacitinib			Ketoconazole	About 10%	About 2-fold About 75%	19
			Fluconazole	About 25%	About 75%	
Vandetanib	Healthy subjects	300 mg single dose day 4	Itraconazole 200 mg daily for 24 days	No effect	9%	20

1. Pithavala YK, Tong W, Mount J, Rahavendran SV, Garrett M, Hee B, Selaru P, Sarapa N, Klamerus KJ. Effect of ketoconazole on the pharmacokinetics of axitinib in healthy volunteers. *Invest New Drugs* (2012) 30, 273–81.
2. Abbas R, Hug BA, Leister C, Burns J, Sonnichsen D. Effect of ketoconazole on the pharmacokinetics of oral bosutinib in healthy subjects. *J Clin Pharmacol* (2011) 51, 1721–7.
3. Cometriq (Cabozantinib malate). Exelixis, Inc. US Prescribing information, November 2012.
4. Xalkori (Crizotinib). Pfizer Inc. US Prescribing information, May 2013.
5. Xalkori (Crizotinib). Pfizer Ltd. UK Summary of product characteristics, April 2013.
6. Johnson FM, Agrawal S, Burris H, Rosen L, Dhillon N, Hong D, Blackwood-Chirchir A, Luo FR, Sy O, Kaul S, Chiappori AA. Phase 1 pharmacokinetic and drug-interaction study of dasatinib in patients with advanced solid tumors. *Cancer* (2010) 116, 1582–91.
7. Rakhit A, Pantze MP, Fettner S, Jones HM, Charoin J-E, Riek M, Lum BL, Hamilton M. The effects of CYP3A4 inhibition on erlotinib pharmacokinetics: computer-based simulation (SimCYP[TM]) predicts in vivo metabolic inhibition. *Eur J Clin Pharmacol* (2008) 64, 31–41.
8. Swaisland HC, Ranson M, Smith RP, Leadbetter J, Laight A, McKillop D, Wild MJ. Pharmacokinetic drug interactions of gefitinib with rifampicin, itraconazole and metoprolol. *Clin Pharmacokinet* (2005) 44, 1067–81.
9. Dutriex C, Peng B, Mehring G, Hayes M, Capdeville R, Porkony R, Seiberling M. Pharmacokinetic interaction between ketoconazole and imatinib mesylate (Glivec) in healthy subjects. *Cancer Chemother Pharmacol* (2004) 54, 290–4.
10. Smith DA, Koch KM, Arya N, Bowen CJ, Herendeen JM, Beelen A. Effects of ketoconazole and carbamazepine on lapatinib pharmacokinetics in healthy subjects. *Br J Clin Pharmacol* (2009) 67, 421–6.
11. Tanaka C, Yin OQ, Smith T, Sethuraman V, Grouss K, Galitz L, Harrell R, Schran H. Effects of rifampicin and ketoconazole on the pharmacokinetics of nilotinib in healthy participants. *J Clin Pharmacol* (2011)51, 75–83.
12. Tan AR, Gibbon DG, Stein MN, Lindquist D, Edenfield JW, Martin JC, Gregory C, Suttle AB, Tada H, Bothyl J, Stephenson JJ. Effects of ketoconazole and esomeprazole on the pharmacokinetics of pazopanib in patients with solid tumors. *Cancer Chemother Pharmacol* (2013) 71, 1635–43.
13. Narasimhan NI, Dorer DJ, Niland K, Haluska F, Sonnichsen D. Effects of ketoconazole on the pharmacokinetics of ponatinib in healthy subjects. *J Clin Pharmacol* (2013) 53, 974–81.
14. Stivarga (Regorafenib). Bayer HealthCare Pharmaceuticals Inc. US Prescribing information, August 2013.
15. Shi JG, Chen X, Emm T, Scherle PA, McGee RF, Lo Y, Landman RR, McKeever EG, Punwani NG, Williams WV, Yeleswaram S. The effect of CYP3A4 inhibition or induction on the pharmacokinetics and pharmacodynamics of orally administered ruxolitinib (INCB018424 phosphate) in healthy volunteers. *J Clin Pharmacol* (2012) 52, 809–18.
16. Lathia C, Lettieri J, Cihon F, Gallentine M, Radtke M, Sundaresan P. Lack of effect of ketoconazole-mediated CYP3A inhibition on sorafenib clinical pharmacokinetics. *Cancer Chemother Pharmacol* (2006) 57, 685–92.
17. Sutent (Sunitinib malate). Pfizer Ltd. UK Summary of product characteristics, August 2011.
18. Sutent (Sunitinib malate). Pfizer Inc. US Prescribing information, May 2011.
19. Xeljanz (Tofacitinib citrate). Pfizer Inc. US Prescribing information, November 2012.
20. Martin P, Oliver S, Robertson J, Kennedy SJ, Read J, Duvauchelle T. Pharmacokinetic drug interactions with vandetanib during coadministration with rifampicin or itraconazole. *Drugs R D* (2011) 11, 37–51.

- Reduce the **ponatinib** dose to 30 mg once daily.[17,18]
- The UK Manufacturer of **ruxolitinib** recommends reducing the dose by 50%, closely monitoring (e.g. twice weekly) for cytopenias, and adjusting the dose based on safety and efficacy.[19] However, the US manufacturer states that a starting dose of 5 mg twice daily should be given to patients with polycythemia vera. In patients with myelofibrosis, if the platelet count is greater or equal to 100 x 10^9/L, they recommend a starting dose of 10 mg twice daily, but if the platelet count is less than 100 x 10^9/L, they recommend a starting dose of 5 mg once daily. In patients already stable on ruxolitinib, they recommend reducing the dose by 50% in those stable on at least 10 mg twice daily or reducing the dose to 5 mg once daily in those stable on 5 mg twice daily.[20]
- Ketoconazole has no effect on the exposure to **sorafenib**, therefore no dose adjustments would seem necessary on concurrent use with potent CYP3A4 inhibitors.
- Reduce the **sunitinib** dose by one quarter to one third depending on the indication.[21,22]
- Reduce the **tofacitinib** dose to 5 mg daily.[23]
- The effect of itraconazole on **vandetanib** exposure was negligible, and is unlikely to be clinically relevant. Other CYP3A4 inhibitors would not be expected to affect the exposure to vandetanib to a clinically relevant extent via this mechanism.

Note that the small increase in **imatinib** exposure seen in the single-dose study is likely an under estimate of the effect of ketoconazole, as it is unlikely that the full inhibitory effect of ketoconazole was achieved by this study design, and a greater effect with multiple doses of ketoconazole cannot be excluded.

Moderate CYP3A4 inhibitors

Fluconazole is a moderate CYP3A4 inhibitor and a potent CYP2C19 inhibitor, and slightly increased **tofacitinib** exposure. The US manufacturer of tofacitinib recommends reducing the dose to 5 mg daily on concurrent use with fluconazole.[23] The US manufacturer of **ruxolitinib** advises avoiding concurrent use of fluconazole at doses over 200 mg daily. For fluconazole doses of 200 mg or less, the manufacturer recommends that a starting dose of 5 mg twice daily should be given to patients with polycythemia vera. In patients with myelofibrosis, if the platelet count is greater or equal to 100 x 10^9/L, they recommend a starting dose of 10 mg twice daily, but if the platelet count is between 50 x 10^9/L and 100 x 10^9/L, they recommend a starting dose of 5 mg once daily. In patients already stable on ruxolitinib, they recommend reducing the dose by 50% in those stable on at least 10 mg twice daily or reducing the dose to 5 mg once daily in those stable on 5 mg twice daily. Patients stable on ruxolitinib 5 mg once daily should avoid concurrent use of fluconazole 200 mg or less, or interrupt ruxolitinib treatment for the duration of fluconazole use.[20] The concurrent use of bosutinib with moderate CYP3A4 inhibitors, which would include **fluconazole** and **posaconazole**, should be avoided.[7]

The exposure to other tyrosine kinase inhibitors might be increased by moderate CYP3A4 inhibitors (see 'Table 1.9', p.11 for a list). Until more is known, it would seem prudent to monitor for tyrosine kinase inhibitor efficacy and adjust the dose of the tyrosine kinase inhibitor accordingly on concurrent use.

1. Lathia C, Lettieri J, Cihon F, Gallentine M, Radtke M, Sundaresan P. Lack of effect of ketoconazole-mediated CYP3A inhibition on sorafenib clinical pharmacokinetics. *Cancer Chemother Pharmacol* (2006) 57, 685–92.
2. Votrient (Pazopanib hydrochloride). GlaxoSmithKline. US Prescribing information, August 2013.
3. Gambillara E, Laffitte E, Widmer N, Decosterd LA, Duchosal MA, Kovacsovics T, Panizzon RG. Severe pustular eruption associated with imatinib and voriconazole in a patient with chronic myeloid leukaemia. *Dermatology* (2005) 211, 363–5.
4. Rakhit A, Pantze MP, Fettner S, Jones HM, Charoin J-E, Riek M, Lum BL, Hamilton M. The effects of CYP3A4 inhibition on erlotinib pharmacokinetics: computer-based simulation (SimCYP™) predicts in vivo metabolic inhibition. *Eur J Clin Pharmacol* (2008) 64, 31–41.
5. Inlyta (Axitinib). Pfizer Ltd. UK Summary of product characteristics, May 2015.
6. Inlyta (Axitinib). Pfizer Inc. US Prescribing information, August 2014.
7. Bosulif (Bosutinib monohydrate). Pfizer Ltd. UK Summary of product characteristics, July 2015.
8. Cometriq (Cabozantinib malate). Exelixis, Inc. US Prescribing information) November 2012.
9. Sprycel (Dasatinib monohydrate). Bristol-Myers Squibb Company. US Prescribing information, August 2015.
10. Tarceva (Erlotinib hydrochloride). OSI Pharmaceuticals, LLC. US Prescribing information, April 2015.
11. Iressa (Gefitinib monohydrate). AstraZeneca UK Ltd. UK Summary of product characteristics, June 2013.
12. Tykerb (Lapatinib ditosylate monohydrate). GlaxoSmithKline. US Prescribing information, March 2015..
13. Tasigna (Nilotinib hydrochloride monohydrate). Novartis Pharmaceuticals Corp. US Prescribing information, January 2015.
14. Tasigna (Nilotinib hydrochloride monohydrate). Novartis Pharmaceuticals UK Ltd. UK Summary of product characteristics, June 2015.
15. Votrient (Pazopanib hydrochloride). GlaxoSmithKline. US Prescribing information, April 2015.
16. Votrient (Pazopanib hydrochloride). Novartis Pharmaceuticals UK Ltd. UK Summary of product characteristics, July 2015.
17. Iclusig (Ponatinib). ARIAD Pharmaceuticals, Inc. US Prescribing information, September 2014.
18. Iclusig (Ponatinib). ARIAD Pharmaceuticals Ltd. UK Summary of product characteristics, April 2015.
19. Jakavi (Ruxolitinib phosphate). Novartis Pharmaceuticals UK Ltd. UK Summary of product characteristics, April 2015.
20. Jakafi (Ruxolitinib phosphate). Incyte Corporation. US Prescribing information, December 2014.
21. Sutent (Sunitinib malate). Pfizer Ltd. UK Summary of product characteristics, June 2015.
22. Sutent (Sunitinib malate). Pfizer Inc. US Prescribing information, April 2015.
23. Xeljanz (Tofacitinib citrate). Pfizer Inc. US prescribing information, June 2015.

Tyrosine kinase inhibitors + Cisplatin and other platinum compounds

No clinically relevant pharmacokinetic interaction occurs between erlotinib and carboplatin or oxaliplatin. Gefitinib does not alter the pharmacokinetics of carboplatin, but exposure to gefitinib was increased. Sorafenib did not alter the pharmacokinetics of carboplatin, but sorafenib exposure increased in one study but another found no interaction. No pharmacokinetic interaction occurs between gefitinib and cisplatin. Imatinib did not alter the pharmacokinetics of cisplatin. Cisplatin exposure was slightly increased when given with vandetanib and dose-limiting toxicities were seen. No pharmacokinetic interaction appears to occur between lapatinib or sorafenib and oxaliplatin.

Clinical evidence, mechanism, importance and management

(a) Carboplatin

1. Erlotinib. In a phase I study in patients given paclitaxel and carboplatin, the AUC of platinum was increased by about 10% when erlotinib was given, but this is not considered to be clinically relevant. The pharmacokinetics of erlotinib were not altered by carboplatin when compared with historical controls.[1] In another study, there was no obvious difference in erlotinib exposure when it was taken alone or in combination with docetaxel and carboplatin.[2] Similarly, in a pharmacokinetic study as part of a phase III study, the addition of erlotinib 150 mg daily to a standard regimen of paclitaxel and carboplatin had no effect on the AUC of carboplatin when compared with placebo, and the pharmacokinetics of erlotinib did not appear to be altered.[3]

2. Gefitinib. In 24 patients with advanced non-small cell lung cancer there was no change in the pharmacokinetics of carboplatin when gefitinib 250 or 500 mg daily was also given. There was a 56% increase in the AUC of gefitinib 250 mg and a 30% increase in the AUC of gefitinib 500 mg; the minimum plasma concentrations were increased by 85% and 33%, respectively, but no increase in toxicity was noted.[4]

3. Sorafenib. The UK manufacturer notes that the concurrent use of carboplatin and paclitaxel (225 mg/m^2, once every 3 weeks) with sorafenib 400 mg twice daily, resulted in a 47% increase in sorafenib exposure. The pharmacokinetics of carboplatin were unaffected.[5] In a phase I study, 13 patients with non-small cell lung cancer were given sorafenib 400 mg either once or twice daily on days 2 to 19 of a 21-day cycle, with paclitaxel and carboplatin given on day one. There was no change in the pharmacokinetics of sorafenib or carboplatin.[6]

(b) Cisplatin

1. Gefitinib. In an open study, 18 patients were given gemcitabine 1250 mg/m^2 on days one and 8 of a 21-day cycle, with cisplatin 80 mg/m^2 on day one and gefitinib 250 mg or 500 mg from day 2 onwards. The pharmacokinetics of gefitinib were unchanged by the combination chemotherapy, and cisplatin pharmacokinetics were not affected by gefitinib.[7]

2. Imatinib. In a phase I study in patients with small cell lung cancer given cisplatin with irinotecan and imatinib, the pharmacokinetics of cisplatin did not appear to be altered by imatinib.[8] For mention that the clearance of irinotecan might possibly be reduced by imatinib, see 'Irinotecan + Tyrosine kinase inhibitors', p.691.

3. Vandetanib. The pharmacokinetic analysis of a phase I study combining vandetanib with vinorelbine and cisplatin, or gemcitabine and cisplatin, in patients with advanced non-small cell lung cancer, found that exposure to vandetanib was not affected by concurrent use, but the AUC of cisplatin was increased by 33%. The combination was not tolerated, with thromboembolic effects being the main dose-limiting toxicity, and the authors concluded that these combinations were not a feasible first-line therapy for non-small cell lung cancer.[9]

(c) Oxaliplatin

1. Erlotinib. In a study in patients taking erlotinib, capecitabine, and oxaliplatin, there was no obvious difference in the AUC of erlotinib when capecitabine and oxaliplatin were also taken, compared with erlotinib alone. Also, there were no obvious differences in the pharmacokinetics of oxaliplatin when erlotinib was also taken.[10] In addition, erlotinib pharmacokinetics did not appear to be affected by the concurrent use of FOLFOX (fluorouracil, folinic acid, oxaliplatin) when compared with erlotinib monotherapy. Similarly, the pharmacokinetics of oxaliplatin did not appear to be affected by erlotinib.[11]

2. Lapatinib. In 19 patients with solid tumours, the pharmacokinetics of lapatinib 1.5 g daily were unaffected when it was given just before starting oxaliplatin in the FOLFOX4 regimen (oxaliplatin, folinic acid, and fluorouracil), when compared with days when lapatinib was given alone. In addition, lapatinib had no effect on the pharmacokinetics of oxaliplatin.[12] Lapatinib can be given with the full-dose FOLFOX regimen.

3. Sorafenib. In a phase I clinical study, sorafenib 200 mg or 400 mg twice daily was given continuously with intravenous oxaliplatin given on day one of a 3-week cycle. No pharmacokinetic interaction was detected between sorafenib and oxaliplatin compared with either drug alone.[13]

1. Patnaik A, Wood D, Tolcher AW, Hamilton M, Kreisberg JI, Hammond LA, Schwartz G, Beeram M, Hidalgo M, Mita MM, Wolf J, Nadler P, Rowinsky EK. Phase I, pharmacokinetic, and biological study of erlotinib in combination with paclitaxel and carboplatin in patients with advanced solid tumours. *Clin Cancer Res* (2006) 12, 7406–13.
2. Vasey PA, Gore M, Wilson R, Rustin G, Gabra H, Guastalla JP, Lauraine EP, Paul J, Carty K, Kaye S; Scottish Gynaecological Cancer Trials Group. A phase Ib trial of docetaxel, carboplatin and erlotinib in ovarian, fallopian tube and primary peritoneal cancers. *Br J Cancer* (2008) 98, 1774–80.
3. Tran HT, Zinner RG, Blumenschein GR Jr, Oh YW, Papadimitrakopoulou VA, Kim ES, Lu C, Malik M, Lum BL, Herbst RS. Pharmacokinetic study of the phase III, randomized, double-blind, multicenter trial (TRIBUTE) of paclitaxel and carboplatin combined with erlotinib or placebo in patients with advanced non-small cell lung cancer (NSCLC). *Invest New Drugs* (2010) Epub.
4. Miller VA, Johnson DH, Krug LM, Pizzo B, Tyson L, Perez W, Krozely P, Sandler A, Carbone D, Heelan RT, Kris MG, Smith R, Ochs J. Pilot trial of the epidermal growth factor receptor tyrosine kinase inhibitor gefitinib plus carboplatin and paclitaxel in patients with stage IIIB or IV non-small-cell lung cancer. *J Clin Oncol* (2003) 21, 2094–100.

5. Nexavar (Sorafenib tosylate). Bayer plc. UK Summary of product characteristics, February 2013.
6. Okamoto I, Miyazaki M, Morinaga R, Kaneda H, Ueda S, Hasegawa Y, Satoh T, Kawada A, Fukuoka M, Fukino K, Tanigawa T, Nakagawa K. Phase I clinical and pharmacokinetic study of sorafenib in combination with carboplatin and paclitaxel in patients with advanced non-small cell lung cancer. *Invest New Drugs* (2010) 28, 844–53.
7. Giaccone G, González-Larriba JL, van Oosterom AT, Alfonso R, Smit EF, Martens M, Peters GJ, van der Vijgh WJ, Smith R, Averbuch S, Fandi A. Combination therapy with gefitinib, an epidermal growth factor receptor tyrosine kinase inhibitor, gemcitabine and cisplatin in patients with advanced solid tumors. *Ann Oncol* (2004) 15, 831–8.
8. Johnson FM, Krug LM, Tran HT, Shoaf S, Prieto VG, Tamboli P, Peeples B, Patel J, Glisson BS. Phase I studies of imatinib mesylate combined with cisplatin and irinotecan in patients with small cell lung carcinoma. *Cancer* (2006) 106, 366–74.
9. Blackhall FH, O'Brien M, Schmid P, Nicolson M, Taylor P, Milenkova T, Kennedy SJ, Thatcher N. A phase I study of vandetanib in combination with vinorelbine/cisplatin or gemcitabine/cisplatin as first-line treatment for advanced non-small cell lung cancer. *J Thorac Oncol* (2010) 5, 1285–8.
10. Van Cutsem E, Verslype C, Beale P, Clarke S, Bugat R, Rakhit A, Fettner SH, Brennscheidt U, Feyereislova A, Delord JP. A phase Ib dose-escalation study of erlotinib, capecitabine and oxaliplatin in metastatic colorectal cancer patients. *Ann Oncol* (2008) 19, 332–9.
11. Hanauske AR, Cassidy J, Sastre J, Bolling C, Jones RJ, Rakhit A, Fettner S, Brennscheidt U, Feyereislova A, Díaz-Rubio E. Phase 1b dose escalation study of erlotinib in combination with infusional 5-Fluorouracil, leucovorin, and oxaliplatin in patients with advanced solid tumors. *Clin Cancer Res* (2007) 13, 523–31.
12. Siegel-Lakhai WS, Beijnen JH, Vervenne WL, Boot H, Keessen M, Versola M, Koch KM, Smith DA, Pandite L, Richel DJ, Schellens JHM. Phase I pharmacokinetic study of the safety and tolerability of lapatinib (GW572016) in combination with oxaliplatin/fluorouracil/leucovorin (FOLFOX4) in patients with solid tumours. *Clin Cancer Res* (2007) 13, 4495–4502.
13. Kupsch P, Henning BF, Passarge K, Richly H, Wiesemann K, Hilger RA, Scheulen ME, Christensen O, Brendel E, Schwartz B, Hofstra E, Voigtmann R, Seeber S, Strumberg D. Results of a phase I trial of sorafenib (BAY 43-9006) in combination with oxaliplatin in patients with refractory solid tumors, including colorectal cancer. *Clin Colorectal Cancer* (2005) 5, 188–96.

Tyrosine kinase inhibitors + Fluorouracil and related prodrugs

There appears to be no pharmacokinetic interaction between erlotinib or lapatinib and capecitabine or fluorouracil-based regimens. The pharmacokinetics of sorafenib were not affected by administration with capecitabine, but exposure to capecitabine and fluorouracil was increased.

Clinical evidence, mechanism, importance and management

(a) Capecitabine

1. Erlotinib. The UK manufacturer notes that erlotinib has no effect on the pharmacokinetics of capecitabine, but that the AUC of erlotinib was higher when given with capecitabine (amount not stated) compared with historical controls.[1] However, in a study in which patients received capecitabine, docetaxel, and erlotinib, there was no change in the AUC of erlotinib when it was given with these two drugs compared with when it was given alone.[2] Similarly, in a study in patients taking erlotinib, capecitabine, and oxaliplatin, there was no obvious difference in the AUC of erlotinib when capecitabine and oxaliplatin were also taken, compared with erlotinib alone. However, the AUC and maximum concentration of capecitabine were 12% and 27% lower, respectively, while taking erlotinib when compared with taking capecitabine and oxaliplatin alone, although this difference was not statistically significant.[3]

2. Lapatinib. In a phase I study in 19 patients with solid tumours who were given lapatinib 1.25 g daily and capecitabine 2 g/m^2, the AUC and maximum plasma concentration of lapatinib were increased by 20% and 34%, respectively, when capecitabine was also given, although these changes were not statistically significant. The maximum plasma concentration of fluorouracil was reduced by 30% when capecitabine was given with lapatinib.[4] These changes were not considered clinically relevant. Note that lapatinib is licensed for concurrent use with capecitabine.

3. Sorafenib. The UK manufacturer notes that the concurrent use of capecitabine (750 to 1 050 mg/m^2 twice daily for 14 days every 21 days) and sorafenib (200 or 400 mg twice daily continuously) did not alter sorafenib exposure, but increased capecitabine exposure by 15 to 50%, and increased fluorouracil exposure by 0 to 52%. They state that the clinical relevance of these small to modest increases in capecitabine and fluorouracil exposure is unknown.[5] Some caution would seem appropriate on their concurrent use, being aware of the possibility of increased capecitabine toxicity.

(b) Fluorouracil and fluorouracil-based regimens

1. Erlotinib. Erlotinib pharmacokinetics did not appear to be affected by the concurrent use of FOLFOX (fluorouracil, folinic acid, oxaliplatin) when compared with erlotinib monotherapy. Similarly, the pharmacokinetics of fluorouracil did not appear to be affected by erlotinib.[6]

2. Lapatinib. The pharmacokinetics of lapatinib 1.25 g daily were unaffected when it was given with the FOLFIRI regimen (irinotecan, folinic acid, fluorouracil). In addition, there was no change in the steady-state concentration of fluorouracil.[7] However, for mention of increased exposure to the active metabolite of irinotecan, and increased toxicity of this regimen, see 'Irinotecan + Tyrosine kinase inhibitors', p.691.

In 19 patients the pharmacokinetics of lapatinib 1.5 g daily were unaffected when it was given just before starting oxaliplatin in the FOLFOX4 regimen (oxaliplatin, folinic acid, fluorouracil), when compared with days when lapatinib was given alone. Lapatinib had no effect on the pharmacokinetics of fluorouracil.[8] Lapatinib can be given with the full-dose FOLFOX regimen.

1. Tarceva (Erlotinib hydrochloride). Roche Products Ltd. UK Summary of product characteristics, December 2013.
2. Twelves C, Trigo JM, Jones R, De Rosa F, Rakhit A, Fettner S, Wright T, Baselga J. Erlotinib in combination with capecitabine and docetaxel in patients with metastatic breast cancer: a dose escalation study. *Eur J Cancer* (2008) 44, 419–26.
3. Van Cutsem E, Verslype C, Beale P, Clarke S, Bugat R, Rakhit A, Fettner SH, Brennscheidt U, Feyereislova A, Delord JP. A phase Ib dose-escalation study of erlotinib, capecitabine and oxaliplatin in metastatic colorectal cancer patients. *Ann Oncol* (2008) 19, 332–9.
4. Chu QS, Schwartz G, de Bono J, Smith DA, Koch KM, Versola MJ, Pandite L, Arya N, Curtright J, Fleming RA, Ho PT, Rowinsky EK. Phase I and pharmacokinetic study of lapatinib in combination with capecitabine in patients with advanced solid malignancies. *J Clin Oncol* (2007) 25, 3753–8.
5. Nexavar (Sorafenib tosylate). Bayer plc. UK Summary of product characteristics, February 2013.
6. Hanauske AR, Cassidy J, Sastre J, Bolling C, Jones RJ, Rakhit A, Fettner S, Brennscheidt U, Feyereislova A, Díaz-Rubio E. Phase 1b dose escalation study of erlotinib in combination with infusional 5-Fluorouracil, leucovorin, and oxaliplatin in patients with advanced solid tumors. *Clin Cancer Res* (2007) 13, 523–31.
7. Midgley RS, Kerr DJ, Flaherty KT, Stevenson JP, Pratap SE, Koch KM, Smith DA, Versola M, Fleming RA, Ward C, O'Dwyer PJ, Middleton MR. A phase I and pharmacokinetic study of lapatinib in combination with infusional 5-fluorouracil, leucovorin and irinotecan. *Ann Oncol* (2007) 18, 2025–9.
8. Siegel-Lakhai WS, Beijnen JH, Vervenne WL, Boot H, Keessen M, Versola M, Koch KM, Smith DA, Pandite L, Richel DJ, Schellens JHM. Phase I pharmacokinetic study of the safety and tolerability of lapatinib (GW572016) in combination with oxaliplatin/fluorouracil/leucovorin (FOLFOX4) in patients with solid tumours. *Clin Cancer Res* (2007) 13, 4495–4502.

Tyrosine kinase inhibitors + Food

Food increases the extent of absorption of bosutinib, erlotinib, lapatinib, nilotinib, regorafenib, and pazopanib. A high-fat meal decreased the absorption of sorafenib, and increased the absorption of cabozantinib. Food has no relevant effect on the absorption of axitinib, crizotinib, dasatinib, gefitinib, imatinib, ponatinib, ruxolitinib, sunitinib, tofacitinib, or vandetanib.

Clinical evidence, mechanism, importance and management

(a) Axitinib

In a pharmacokinetic study, 30 healthy subjects received a single 5-mg dose of axitinib after an overnight fast, or with a high-fat, high-calorie, or a moderate-fat, standard-calorie, meal. Administration with a high-fat, high-calorie meal increased the AUC and maximum concentration of axitinib by 19% and 11%, respectively, compared with the fasted state. A moderate-fat, standard-calorie meal reduced the AUC and maximum concentration by 10% and 16%, respectively, compared with the fasted state. These changes were not considered clinically important.[1] Axitinib can be given without regard to food.

(b) Bosutinib

In a phase I study in healthy subjects, the AUC and maximum concentration of a single 400-mg dose of bosutinib were about 40% and 50% higher, respectively, in subjects who had received a standard high-fat meal, when compared with those who had fasted overnight.[2] The UK and US manufacturers briefly report that, in a study, the AUC and maximum concentration of bosutinib were increased by 80% and 70%, respectively, by the presence of food, when compared with the fasted state. It is recommended that bosutinib is given with food.[3,4]

(c) Cabozantinib

The US manufacturer briefly reports that, in healthy subjects, the maximum concentration and AUC of a single 140-mg dose of cabozantinib were increased by 41% and 57%, respectively, by a high-fat meal, when compared with the fasted state. Cabozantinib should not be administered with food, and further, patients should be advised to avoid food for at least 2 hours before, and 1 hour after, taking cabozantinib.[5]

(d) Crizotinib

A preliminary report of a pharmacokinetic study in cancer patients, reports that administration with a standard high-fat meal did not appear to alter the mean AUC and maximum concentration of a single 250-mg dose of crizotinib.[6] The UK and US manufacturers briefly report that, in healthy subjects the maximum concentration and AUC of a single 250-mg dose of crizotinib were reduced by about 14% when administered with a high-fat meal.[7,8] Crizotinib can be administered without regard to food.

(e) Dasatinib

The UK and US manufacturers state that in a study in healthy subjects given a single 100-mg dose of dasatinib, there was a 14% increase in the AUC of dasatinib when it was given 30 minutes after a high-fat meal.[9,10] When given 30 minutes after a low-fat meal in another study, the increase in the AUC of dasatinib was 21%.[9] The observed food effects do not represent clinically relevant changes in exposure and dasatinib can be taken with or without food.[9,10]

(f) Erlotinib

In a pharmacokinetic study, 18 healthy subjects received a single 150-mg dose of erlotinib after a 10-hour fast or with a high-fat, high-calorie breakfast. When taken with the meal, the maximum plasma concentration and AUC of erlotinib were increased by 52% and 97%, respectively. The effects of food on multiple doses of erlotinib were then investigated in 22 healthy subjects who took erlotinib 100 mg daily for 7 days after either a 10-hour fast or with a high-fat, high-calorie breakfast. On day one of the study, the AUC of erlotinib was increased by 66% when taken with food, but at day 7 of the study, there was only a 34% increase in AUC of erlotinib when it was taken with food, which was not statistically significant.[11]

The data suggest that the effect of food is less important after multiple dosing, although there is some uncertainty about this.[11] Therefore, because of the risk of dose-limiting toxicities, it is recommended that erlotinib is taken on an empty stomach, at least one hour before or 2 hours after any food.[11-13]

(g) Gefitinib

In a study in 17 healthy subjects, taking gefitinib 50 mg with a high-fat breakfast decreased the AUC by 14% when compared with the fasted state, although this difference was not statistically significant. The maximum concentration of gefitinib was decreased by 34%.[14] Gefitinib can therefore be taken without regard to food.

(h) Imatinib

In a study in patients taking imatinib, there was minimal change in the rate and extent of absorption of imatinib 400 mg when it was taken with a high-fat meal compared with fasting conditions (7% reduction in AUC, 15% decrease in maximum concentration, and prolongation of time to maximum concentration by one hour).[15] Nevertheless, the UK and US manufacturers recommend that imatinib is taken with a meal and a large glass of water to minimise gastrointestinal irritation.[16,17]

(i) Lapatinib

In a randomised, crossover study, 22 patients with cancer were given a single 1.5-g dose of lapatinib after a high-fat breakfast (50 g fat; 1000 kcal) or a low-fat breakfast (2 g fat; 500 kcal), or in the fasted state. The high-fat breakfast increased the AUC and maximum plasma concentration of lapatinib 4.3-fold and 3-fold, respectively, when compared with the fasted state. The low-fat meal increased the AUC and maximum plasma concentration of lapatinib 2.7-fold and 2.4-fold, respectively, when compared with the fasted state. In this small study, the differences appeared to have no effect on incidence of diarrhoea or QT prolongation.[18]

However, this increase in lapatinib exposure would be expected to be of clinical relevance, and therefore the UK and US manufacturers recommend taking lapatinib at least one hour before, or one hour after, food[19,20] (which was how it was taken in key clinical studies). Note that, given the findings of the food-effect study above, there is likely to be a large difference in absorption between taking lapatinib one hour before breakfast, compared with one hour after a high-fat breakfast, when a substantial effect of food is still likely, but this does not appear to have been studied. The UK manufacturer further recommends that, to minimise variability, patients should take the drug at the same time in relation to meals (that is, for example, always one hour before meals).[20] The manufacturers' recommendation has caused some controversy. Some consider that taking lapatinib with food could greatly reduce the required dose and hence the cost of treatment, and that this should be studied further.[21] However, others consider that taking lapatinib with food might result in more variable absorption because of the differences in type and quantity of food taken at meals.[22,23] However, this appears equally likely if patients switch between taking lapatinib one hour before and one hour after a high-fat breakfast, as is currently permitted by the US manufacturer's recommendation.

(j) Nilotinib

In a study in 44 healthy subjects, a high-fat meal increased the AUC of nilotinib by 82% and increased its maximum concentration by 112% when the dose was given 30 minutes after the meal, compared with the fasted state. However, when nilotinib was taken 30 minutes or 2 hours after a light meal, its AUC was increased by just 32% and 15%, respectively.[24] In a study in patients, the AUC of nilotinib 400 mg and 600 mg twice daily was increased by about 50% when taken after a high-fat meal.[24] In a crossover study, 45 healthy subjects were given 400 mg of nilotinib (as two 200 mg capsules) alone, with the contents of each capsule dispersed in one teaspoon of non-fat, plain yoghurt, and with the contents of each capsule dispersed in one teaspoon of apple sauce. The maximum concentration and AUC of nilotinib were increased by 31% and about 10%, respectively, after administration with yoghurt. Administration with apple sauce did not alter the pharmacokinetics of the nilotinib.[25]

The UK and US manufacturers[26,27] therefore state that nilotinib should be taken on an empty stomach, at least one hour before, and 2 hours after, food. Furthermore, they state that the increased exposure resulting from administration with food might prolong the QT interval. For patients who are unable to swallow nilotinib capsules, administration of each capsule with one teaspoon of apple sauce is acceptable, but it is recommended that this should be taken immediately[26,27] (or within 15 minutes).[26]

(k) Pazopanib

In a phase I study in cancer patients, a high-fat or low-fat meal increased the AUC and maximum plasma concentrations of a single 800-mg dose of pazopanib about 2-fold. Pazopanib should therefore be taken in the fasted state, at least one hour before, or 2 hours after, a meal.[28]

(l) Ponatinib

The US manufacturer briefly reports that, in 22 healthy subjects, administration of ponatinib with a high-fat or low-fat meal, did not alter its pharmacokinetics when compared with the fasted state.[29] Ponatinib can be given without regard to food.

(m) Regorafenib

The US manufacturer briefly reports that 24 healthy subjects were given a single 160-mg dose of regorafenib under fasting conditions, with a high-fat meal (54.6 g fat, 945 calories), and with a low-fat meal (8.2 g fat, 319 calories). The high-fat meal increased the AUC of regorafenib by 48% and decreased the AUC of its active metabolites M-2 and M-5 by 20% and 51%, respectively, when compared with the fasted state. The low-fat meal increased the AUC of regorafenib, M-2, and M-5 by 36%, 40%, and 23%, respectively, when compared with the fasted state. They comment that in the key clinical studies, regorafenib was taken with a low-fat meal and recommend that this is adhered to by patients. Further, they state that the meal should contain less than 30% fat (and give examples, such as 2 slices of white toast with 1 tablespoon each of low-fat margarine and jam, and about 240 mL (8 oz) of skimmed milk).[30]

(n) Ruxolitinib

The UK and US manufacturers briefly report that, in a study, administration of ruxolitinib with a high-fat meal decreased the maximum concentration and AUC by 24% and 4%, but did not alter its pharmacokinetics to a clinically relevant extent.[31,32] Ruxolitinib can be given without regard to food.

(o) Sorafenib

The US manufacturer notes that when given with a moderate-fat meal (30% fat; 700 calories), the bioavailability of sorafenib was similar to that in the fasted state. However, a high-fat meal (50% fat; 900 calories) reduced sorafenib bioavailability by 29%, when compared with the fasted state. They recommend that sorafenib should be given without food (at least one hour before, or 2 hours after, a meal).[33] However, the UK manufacturer permits taking sorafenib with a low or moderate-fat meal, and states that if a high-fat meal is to be consumed, sorafenib should be taken at least one hour before, or 2 hours after, the meal.[34]

(p) Sunitinib

In a randomised study, 16 healthy subjects were given a single 50-mg dose of sunitinib following a 10-hour fast, or within 30 minutes of a high-fat, high-calorie breakfast. The rate of formation of the active metabolite, SU12662, was slightly decreased resulting in a 23% reduction in its maximum concentration. However, the overall bioavailability of both sunitinib and the active metabolite were unaffected by food.[35] Sunitinib can therefore be taken with or without food.

(q) Tofacitinib

The US manufacturer briefly notes that, administration of tofacitinib with a high-fat meal did not alter its AUC, but its maximum concentration was reduced by 32%.[36] Tofacitinib can be given without regard to food.

(r) Vandetanib

In a crossover study, 15 healthy subjects were given a single 300-mg dose of vandetanib under fed and fasted conditions. The AUC and maximum concentration of vandetanib were not affected by food.[37] Vandetanib can be given without regard to food.

1. Pithavala YK, Chen Y, Toh M, Selaru P, LaBadie RR, Garrett M, Hee B, Mount J, Ni G, Klamerus KJ, Tortorici MA. Evaluation of the effect of food on the pharmacokinetics of axitinib in healthy volunteers. *Cancer Chemother Pharmacol* (2012) 70, 103–12.
2. Abbas R, Hug BA, Leister C, El Gaaloul M, Chalon S, Sonnichsen D. A phase I ascending single-dose study of the safety, tolerability, and pharmacokinetics of bosutinib (SKI-606) in healthy adult subjects. *Cancer Chemother Pharmacol* (2012) 69, 221–7.
3. Bosulif (Bosutinib monohydrate). Pfizer Ltd. UK Summary of product characteristics, July 2015.
4. Bosulif (Bosutinib monohydrate). Pfizer Inc. US Prescribing information, November 2014.
5. Cometriq (Cabozantinib malate). Exelixis, Inc. US Prescribing information, November 2012.
6. Tan W, Wilner KD, Bang Y, Kwak EL, Maki RG, Camidge DR, Solomon BJ, Ou SI, Salgia R, Clark JW. Pharmacokinetics (PK) of PF-02341066, a dual ALK/MET inhibitor after multiple oral doses to advanced cancer patients. *J Clin Oncol* (2010) 28 (Suppl), Abstract 2596.
7. Xalkori (Crizotinib). Pfizer Inc. US Prescribing information, May 2013.
8. Xalkori (Crizotinib). Pfizer Ltd. UK Summary of product characteristics, April 2013.
9. Sprycel (Dasatinib monohydrate). Bristol-Myers Squibb Pharmaceutical Ltd. UK Summary of product characteristics, November 2013.
10. Sprycel (Dasatinib monohydrate). Bristol-Myers Squibb Company. US Prescribing information, April 2014.
11. Ling J, Fettner S, Lum BL, Riek M, Rakhit A. Effect of food on the pharmacokinetics of erlotinib, an orally active epidermal growth factor receptor tyrosine-kinase inhibitor, in healthy individuals. *Anticancer Drugs* (2008) 19, 209–16.
12. Tarceva (Erlotinib hydrochloride). OSI Pharmaceuticals, LLC. US Prescribing information, April 2014.
13. Tarceva (Erlotinib hydrochloride). Roche Products Ltd. UK Summary of product characteristics, December 2013.
14. Swaisland H, Laight A, Stafford L, Jones H, Morris C, Dane A, Yates R. Pharmacokinetics and tolerability of the orally active selective epidermal growth factor receptor tyrosine kinase inhibitor ZD1839 in healthy volunteers. *Clin Pharmacokinet* (2001) 40, 297–306.
15. Reckmann AH, Fischer T, Peng B, Hayes M, Mehring G, Reese SF, Resta D, Ben-Am M, Gschaidmeier H, Huber C, Capdeville R. Effect of food on STI571 GLivec pharmacokinetics and bioavailability. *Proc Am Soc Clin Oncol* (2001) 20, abstract 1223.
16. Glivec (Imatinib mesilate). Novartis Pharmaceuticals UK Ltd. UK Summary of product characteristics, October 2013.
17. Gleevec (Imatinib mesylate). Novartis Pharmaceuticals Corp. US Prescribing information, October 2013.
18. Koch KM, Reddy NJ, Cohen RB, Lewis NL, Whitehead B, Mackay K, Stead A, Beelen AP, Lewis LD. Effects of food on the relative bioavailability of lapatinib in cancer patients. *J Clin Oncol* (2009) 27, 1191–6.
19. Tykerb (Lapatinib ditosylate monohydrate). GlaxoSmithKline. US Prescribing information, October 2013.
20. Tyverb (Lapatinib ditosylate monohydrate). GlaxoSmithKline UK. UK Summary of product characteristics, March 2014.
21. Ratain MJ, Cohen EE. The value meal: how to save $1,700 per month or more on lapatinib. *J Clin Oncol* (2007) 25, 3397–8.
22. Rahman A, Pazdur R, Wang Y, Huang SM, Lesko L. The value meal: effect of food on lapatinib bioavailability. J Clin Oncol. (2007) 25, 5333–4; author reply 5334–5.
23. Koch KM, Beelen AP, Ho PT, Roychowdhury DF. The value of label recommendations: how to dose lapatinib. *J Clin Oncol* (2007) 25, 5331–2; author reply 5334–5.
24. Tanaka C, Yin OQ, Sethuraman V, Smith T, Wang X, Grouss K, Kantarjian H, Giles F, Ottmann OG, Galitz L, Schran H. Clinical pharmacokinetics of the BCR-ABL tyrosine kinase inhibitor nilotinib. *Clin Pharmacol Ther* (2010) 87, 197–203.
25. Yin OQ, Rudoltz M, Galetic I, Filian J, Krishna A, Zhou W, Custodio J, Golor G, Schran H. Effects of yogurt and applesauce on the oral bioavailability of nilotinib in healthy volunteers. *J Clin Pharmacol* (2011) 51, 1580–6.
26. Tasigna (Nilotinib hydrochloride monohydrate). Novartis Pharmaceuticals Corp. US Prescribing information, January 2014..
27. Tasigna (Nilotinib hydrochloride monohydrate). Novartis Pharmaceuticals UK Ltd. UK Summary of product characteristics, December 2013.
28. Heath EI, Chiorean EG, Sweeney CJ, Hodge JP, Lager JJ, Forman K, Malburg L, Arumugham T, Dar MM, Suttle AB, Gainer SD, LoRusso P. A phase I study of the pharmacokinetic and safety profiles of oral pazopanib with a high-fat or low-fat meal in patients with advanced solid tumours. *Clin Pharmacol Ther* (2010) 88, 818–23.
29. Iclusig (Ponatinib). ARIAD Pharmaceuticals, Inc. US Prescribing information, January 2014.
30. Stivarga (Regorafenib). Bayer HealthCare Pharmaceuticals Inc. US Prescribing information, August 2013.
31. Jakavi (Ruxolitinib phosphate). Novartis Pharmaceuticals UK Ltd. UK Summary of product characteristics, June 2013.
32. Jakafi (Ruxolitinib phosphate). Incyte Corporation. US Prescribing information, November 2013.

33. Nexavar (Sorafenib tosylate). Bayer HealthCare Pharmaceuticals Inc. US Prescribing information, November 2013.
34. Nexavar (Sorafenib tosylate). Bayer plc. UK Summary of product characteristics, February 2013.
35. Bello CL, Sherman L, Zhou J, Verkh L, Smeraglia J, Mount J, Klamerus KJ. Effect of food on the pharmacokinetics of sunitinib malate (SU11248), a multi-targeted receptor tyrosine kinase inhibitor: results from a phase I study in healthy subjects. *Anticancer Drugs* (2006) 17, 353–8.
36. Xeljanz (Tofacitinib citrate). Pfizer Inc. US Prescribing information, November 2012.
37. Martin P, Oliver S, Kennedy SJ, Partridge E, Hutchison M, Clarke D, Giles P. Pharmacokinetics of vandetanib: three phase I studies in healthy subjects. *Clin Ther* (2012) 34, 221–37.

Tyrosine kinase inhibitors + Gemcitabine

Erlotinib did not alter the pharmacokinetics of gemcitabine and the pharmacokinetics of erlotinib did not appear to be different from historical controls. The pharmacokinetics of gefitinib were not altered by gemcitabine, but the exposure to gemcitabine was increased. Imatinib did not appear to alter the pharmacokinetics of gemcitabine, after modification for dose-limiting toxicities. The pharmacokinetics of sorafenib and gemcitabine were not altered when given together. The pharmacokinetics of vandetanib and gemcitabine did not appear to be altered when given concurrently, but their use was associated with dose-limiting toxicities.

Clinical evidence, mechanism, importance and management

(a) Erlotinib

In a phase I study in patients with cancer, there was no change in the pharmacokinetics of gemcitabine when erlotinib 100 mg or 150 mg daily was also given. There was also no difference in the pharmacokinetics of erlotinib when compared with historical controls.[1]

(b) Gefitinib

In an open study, 18 patients were given gemcitabine 1250 mg/m^2 on days one and 8 of a 21-day cycle, with cisplatin 80 mg/m^2 on day one and gefitinib 250 mg or 500 mg from day 2 onwards. The pharmacokinetics of gefitinib were unchanged by the combination chemotherapy. However, there was a small increase in exposure to gemcitabine on day 8 in those given the higher dose of gefitinib 500 mg daily, compared with day one (gemcitabine and cisplatin only).[2]

(c) Imatinib

In a phase I study in patients with cancer given gemcitabine and imatinib, the pharmacokinetics of gemcitabine did not appear to be altered by imatinib. However, the initial regimen was modified because of dose-limiting toxicity.[3]

(d) Sorafenib

In a phase I study,[4] the pharmacokinetics of gemcitabine and sorafenib were not altered in 27 patients who received gemcitabine weekly and sorafenib daily from day 2.

(e) Vandetanib

The pharmacokinetic analysis of a phase I study combining vandetanib with gemcitabine and cisplatin in patients with advanced non-small cell lung cancer, found that the exposure to both vandetanib and gemcitabine was not affected by concurrent use. However, the combination was not tolerated (with thromboembolic effects being the main dose-limiting toxicity) and the authors concluded that this combination was not a feasible first-line therapy for non-small cell lung cancer.[5]

1. Dragovich T, Huberman M, Von Hoff DD, Rowinsky EK, Nadler P, Wood D, Hamilton M, Hage G, Wolf J, Patnaik A. Erlotinib plus gemcitabine in patients with unresectable pancreatic cancer and other solid tumours: phase IB trial. *Cancer Chemother Pharmacol* (2007) 60, 295–303.
2. Giaccone G, González-Larriba JL, van Oosterom AT, Alfonso R, Smit EF, Martens M, Peters GJ, van der Vijgh WJ, Smith R, Averbuch S, Fandi A. Combination therapy with gefitinib, an epidermal growth factor receptor tyrosine kinase inhibitor, gemcitabine and cisplatin in patients with advanced solid tumors. *Ann Oncol* (2004) 15, 831–8.
3. Ali Y, Lin Y, Gharibo MM, Gounder MK, Stein MN, Lagattuta TF, Egorin MJ, Rubin EH, Poplin EA. Phase I and pharmacokinetic study of imatinib mesylate (Gleevec) and gemcitabine in patients with refractory solid tumors. *Clin Cancer Res* (2007) 13, 5876–82.
4. Siu LL, Awada A, Takimoto CH, Piccart M, Schwartz B, Giannaris T, Lathia C, Petrenciuc O, Moore MJ. Phase I trial of sorafenib and gemcitabine in advanced solid tumors with an expanded cohort in advanced pancreatic cancer. *Clin Cancer Res* (2006) 12, 144–51.
5. Blackhall FH, O'Brien M, Schmid P, Nicolson M, Taylor P, Milenkova T, Kennedy SJ, Thatcher N. A phase I study of vandetanib in combination with vinorelbine/cisplatin or gemcitabine/cisplatin as first-line treatment for advanced non-small cell lung cancer. *J Thorac Oncol* (2010) 5, 1285–8.

Tyrosine kinase inhibitors + Grapefruit juice

Grapefruit juice slightly increased the exposure to a single dose of nilotinib, and slightly increased steady-state sunitinib exposure. No pharmacokinetic interaction was seen with imatinib and grapefruit juice in a small study. Grapefruit juice is predicted to increase the exposure to other tyrosine kinase inhibitors.

Clinical evidence

(a) Imatinib

In a small study in 4 patients, giving imatinib with 250 mL of grapefruit juice did not alter the pharmacokinetics of imatinib.[1]

(b) Nilotinib

In a single-dose crossover study in 21 healthy subjects, taking nilotinib 400 mg at the same time as double-strength grapefruit juice 240 mL increased nilotinib exposure (AUC) by 29% and increased the maximum concentration by 60% without changes in the time to maximum concentration or the elimination half-life. There was high intersubject variability in the findings. No subjects had an increase in QTcF of greater than 60 milliseconds.[2]

(c) Sunitinib

In a study in 8 patients with cancer receiving sunitinib, the derived steady-state AUC of sunitinib was increased by just 11% when patients drank 200 mL of grapefruit juice three times daily for 3 days (the daily dose of sunitinib was taken with the first glass of grapefruit juice each day). Grapefruit juice increased oral midazolam exposure (used as a positive control) by 50% (which is consistent with other studies, see 'Benzodiazepines + Grapefruit and other fruit juices', p.822). The batch of grapefruit juice used in this study was selected as being high in furanocoumarins.[3]

Mechanism

Tyrosine kinase inhibitors are metabolised by CYP3A4. Grapefruit juice probably increased the oral absorption of nilotinib by inhibiting intestinal CYP3A4.[2] Sunitinib is less affected.[3] The lack of effect on imatinib was suggested to be due to the high oral bioavailability of imatinib (almost 100%), such that grapefruit juice could not inhibit intestinal CYP3A4 sufficiently to increase absorption.[1] However, note that this study was conducted in a very small number of patients.

Importance and management

Evidence for an interaction between grapefruit juice and the tyrosine kinase inhibitors appears to be limited to information regarding imatinib, nilotinib, and sunitinib. The increase in **nilotinib** exposure was slight, but variable. Because of this, and the known problems of possible variability of constituents between batches of grapefruit juice, the UK and US manufacturers of nilotinib advise against the concurrent use of grapefruit juice[4,5] or grapefruit products,[5] which would be prudent.

On the basis of its interaction with ketoconazole (see 'Tyrosine kinase inhibitors + Azoles', p.728), and the possibility of dose-related increases in the QT interval, the manufacturers of **sunitinib** advise avoiding grapefruit juice.[6,7] However, the study cited suggests that this advice is probably unnecessary, because the increased exposure seen was negligible and not likely to be clinically relevant.

Data regarding other tyrosine kinase inhibitors is lacking. However, **axitinib**, **bosutinib**, **crizotinib**, **dasatinib**, **lapatinib**, and **regorafenib** exposure is predicted to be similarly increased by grapefruit juice (or grapefruit products) and some of the manufacturers recommend avoiding concurrent use.[8-16] Similar advice is given for **cabozantinib**,[17] **imatinib**[18] and **pazopanib**[19,20] for which the potential for an interaction is less certain. **Erlotinib** might be affected to a small extent, and the US manufacturer simply advises caution with grapefruit and grapefruit juice.[21] On the basis of the effect of ketoconazole, the US manufacturers of **ponatinib**[22] and **ruxolitinib**[23] advise the same dose adjustments with concurrent grapefruit juice as with potent CYP3A4 inhibitors (see *Importance and management* in 'Tyrosine kinase inhibitors + Azoles', p.728). However, note that grapefruit juice is only a weak inhibitor of CYP3A4.

1. Kimura S-i, Kako S, Wada H, Sakamoto K, Ashizawa M, Sato M, Terasako K, Kikuchi M, Nakasone H, Okuda S, Yamazaki R, Oshima K, Nishida J, Watanabe T, Kanda Y. Can grapefruit juice decrease the cost of imatinib for the treatment of chronic myelogenous leukaemia? *Leuk Res* (2011) 35, e11–e12.
2. Yin OQ, Gallagher N, Li A, Zhou W, Harrell R, Schran H. Effect of grapefruit juice on the pharmacokinetics of nilotinib in healthy participants. *J Clin Pharmacol* (2010) 50, 188–94.
3. van Erp NP, Baker SD, Zandvliet AS, Ploeger BA, den Hollander M, Chen Z, den Hartigh J, König-Quartel JM, Guchelaar HJ, Gelderblom H. Marginal increase of sunitinib exposure by grapefruit juice. *Cancer Chemother Pharmacol* (2011) 67, 695–703..
4. Tasigna (Nilotinib hydrochloride monohydrate). Novartis Pharmaceuticals UK Ltd. UK Summary of product characteristics, July 2013.
5. Tasigna (Nilotinib hydrochloride monohydrate). Novartis Pharmaceuticals Corp. US Prescribing information, June 2013.
6. Sutent (Sunitinib malate). Pfizer Ltd. UK Summary of product characteristics, June 2015.
7. Sutent (Sunitinib malate). Pfizer Inc. US Prescribing information, August 2013.
8. Sprycel (Dasatinib monohydrate). Bristol-Myers Squibb Company. US Prescribing information, June 2013.
9. Tyverb (Lapatinib ditosylate monohydrate). GlaxoSmithKline UK. UK Summary of product characteristics, July 2013
10. Tykerb (Lapatinib ditosylate monohydrate). GlaxoSmithKline. US Prescribing information, June 2013.
11. Inlyta (Axitinib). Pfizer Ltd. UK Summary of product characteristics, May 2015.
12. Inlyta (Axitinib). Pfizer Inc. US Prescribing information, September 2013.
13. Bosulif (Bosutinib monohydrate). Pfizer Inc. US Prescribing information, November 2014.
14. Xalkori (Crizotinib). Pfizer Inc. US Prescribing information, May 2013.
15. Xalkori (Crizotinib). Pfizer Ltd. UK Summary of product characteristics, April 2013.
16. Stivarga (Regorafenib). Bayer HealthCare Pharmaceuticals Inc. US Prescribing information, August 2013.
17. Cometriq (Cabozantinib malate). Exelixis, Inc. US Prescribing information, November 2012
18. Gleevec (Imatinib mesylate). Novartis Pharmaceuticals Corp. US Prescribing information, February 2013.
19. Votrient (Pazopanib hydrochloride). GlaxoSmithKline UK. UK Summary of product characteristics, July 2013.
20. Votrient (Pazopanib hydrochloride). GlaxoSmithKline. US Prescribing information, August 2013.
21. Tarceva (Erlotinib hydrochloride). OSI Pharmaceuticals, LLC. US Prescribing information, May 2013.
22. Iclusig (Ponatinib). ARIAD Pharmaceuticals, Inc. US Prescribing information, December 2012.
23. Jakafi (Ruxolitinib phosphate). DSM Pharmaceuticals Inc. US Prescribing information, June 2013.

Tyrosine kinase inhibitors + H_2-receptor antagonists

H_2-receptor antagonists reduce the exposure to dasatinib, erlotinib, and gefitinib, but the extent varies. Nilotinib pharmacokinetics do not appear to be affected when administration of the H_2-receptor antagonist is

separated. The exposure to bosutinib and lapatinib is predicted to be reduced by H_2-receptor antagonists.

Clinical evidence

(a) Dasatinib

In a study in healthy subjects, a single dose of **famotidine** 40 mg was given 2 hours after dasatinib 50 mg and 10 hours before a second dose of dasatinib 50 mg. The AUC of the second dose of dasatinib was reduced by 61%, but the AUC of the first dose was not affected. In this study, it was anticipated that the timing of **famotidine** administration would have had a minimal effect on the exposure to dasatinib from both doses. The reduction in exposure to the second dose indicates that regular use of famotidine is likely to also have this effect.[1] In a retrospective pharmacokinetic analysis of 18 leukaemia patients taking lansoprazole (5 patients) or an H_2-receptor antagonist (**famotidine** 20 to 40 mg daily (4 patients) or **nizatidine** 300 mg daily (3 patients)), the dasatinib dose-adjusted AUC was 58% lower than in 6 patients not taking any acid suppressants.[2] A case report describes a 79-year-old woman with leukaemia who was receiving dasatinib 100 mg daily but whose response was sub-optimal. Dasatinib concentrations were measured to try and ascertain a possible reason for this reduced response, and were found to be considerably lower than in historical control subjects. The dasatinib dose was increased to 70 mg twice daily with no effect, and further, no dasatinib could be detected 8 hours post-dose. It was found that the patient was also receiving **famotidine** 20 mg daily for peptic ulcer prophylaxis, and after this was stopped, the dasatinib AUC increased 3.6-fold.[3]

(b) Erlotinib

Giving erlotinib with **ranitidine** 300 mg decreased the AUC and maximum concentration of erlotinib by 33% and 54%, respectively.[4,5] However, when erlotinib was given 2 hours before, or 10 hours after, **ranitidine** 150 mg twice daily, the AUC and maximum concentration of erlotinib decreased by only 15% and 17%, respectively.[4,5]

(c) Gefitinib

The UK and US manufacturers briefly note that giving gefitinib with high-dose **ranitidine** (to achieve sustained elevations in gastric pH of greater than 5), resulted in a reduction in the AUC of gefitinib of 47% in healthy subjects.[6,7]

(d) Nilotinib

In a randomised, crossover study in healthy subjects, pre-treatment with **famotidine** 20 mg twice daily for 3 days had no effect on the pharmacokinetics of a single 400-mg dose of nilotinib, given 10 hours after and 2 hours before the final famotidine dose.[8] A retrospective population pharmacokinetic analysis of data from a subgroup of 23 patients with chronic myeloid leukaemia who were given nilotinib 300 mg or 400 mg twice daily, found that the concurrent use of H_2-receptor antagonists (**cimetidine, famotidine,** or **ranitidine**) did not affect the steady-state minimum concentration of nilotinib, when compared with patients who did not take an H_2-receptor antagonist (or a proton pump inhibitor). However, this study does not state whether or not the doses of nilotinib and the H_2-receptor antagonist were separated.[9]

Mechanism

The solubility of dasatinib, erlotinib, gefitinib, and nilotinib is pH-dependent, so drugs that reduce gastric acidity, such as the H_2-receptor antagonists, reduce their absorption.

Importance and management

An interaction resulting in a reduction in the exposure to **dasatinib**, **erlotinib**, and **gefitinib** with H_2-receptor antagonists is established, but the clinical relevance varies and might be influenced by the timing of concurrent administration, such that separating the doses might reduce the size of the effect. However, the UK and US manufacturers of **dasatinib** do not recommend the concurrent use of H_2-receptor antagonists,[10,11] and suggest giving an antacid instead (but see also 'Tyrosine kinase inhibitors + Antacids', p.726). The UK and US manufacturers of **erlotinib** recommend that it is given at least 2 hours before, or 10 hours after, ranitidine.[4,5] It would be prudent to extend this advice to the concurrent use of other H_2-receptor antagonists. As high-dose ranitidine might reduce the efficacy of **gefitinib**, concurrent use should probably be avoided. If both gefitinib and a H_2-receptor antagonist are given, it would be prudent to separate the doses by several hours (the US manufacturer of gefitinib recommends 6 hours before or after the H_2-receptor antagonist[7]) and to monitor for a reduction in gefitinib efficacy.

A reduction in the exposure to **nilotinib** would also be expected on the concurrent use of H_2-receptor antagonists, but based on one study it appears to be prevented by separating the doses. The UK and US manufacturers of nilotinib therefore recommend that it should be administered about 10 hours before, or about 2 hours after, nilotinib.[12,13]

The UK manufacturer of **lapatinib** advises that drugs that increase gastric pH [such as the H_2-receptor antagonists] might reduce the solubility and absorption of lapatinib and should be avoided.[14] The US manufacturer of **bosutinib** recommends separating the doses by more than 2 hours.[15]

The UK manufacturers of **cabozantinib**[16] and **crizotinib**[17] state that no dose adjustment is required on concurrent use of H_2-receptor antagonists, and the UK manufacturer of **vandetinib** states that no dose adjustment is required when it is given with ranitidine.[18]

1. Eley T, Luo FR, Agrawal S, Sanil A, Manning J, Li T, Blackwood-Chirchir A, Bertz R. Phase I study of the effect of gastric acid pH modulators on the bioavailability of oral dasatinib in healthy subjects. *J Clin Pharmacol* (2009) 49, 700–9.
2. Takahashi N, Miura M, Niioka T, Sawada K. Influence of H2-receptor antagonists and proton pump inhibitors on dasatinib pharmacokinetics in Japanese leukemia patients. *Cancer Chemother Pharmacol* (2012) 69, 999–1004.
3. Matsuoka A, Takahashi N, Miura M, Niioka T, Kawakami K, Matsunaga T, Sawada K. H2-receptor antagonist influences dasatinib pharmacokinetics in a patient with Philadelphia-positive acute lymphoblastic leukemia. *Cancer Chemother Pharmacol* (2012) 70, 351–2.
4. Tarceva (Erlotinib hydrochloride). OSI Pharmaceuticals LLC. US Prescribing information, April 2015.
5. Tarceva (Erlotinib hydrochloride). Roche Products Ltd. UK Summary of product characteristics, December 2013.
6. Iressa (Gefitinib monohydrate). AstraZeneca UK Ltd. UK Summary of product characteristics, September 2014.
7. Iressa (Gefitinib). AstraZeneca Pharmaceuticals LP. US Prescribing information, July 2015.
8. Yin OQ, Bédoucha V, McCulloch T, Zheng C, Zhou W, Hussaini A, Novick S. Effects of famotidine or an antacid preparation on the pharmacokinetics of nilotinib in healthy volunteers. *Cancer Chemother Pharmacol* (2013) 71, 219–26.
9. Yin OQ, Giles FJ, Baccarani M, le Coutre P, Chiparus O, Gallagher N, Saglio G, Hughes TP, Hochhaus A, Kantarjian HM, Larson RA. Concurrent use of proton pump inhibitors or H2 blockers did not adversely affect nilotinib efficacy in patients with chronic myeloid leukaemia. *Cancer Chemother Pharmacol* (2012) 70, 345–50.
10. Sprycel (Dasatinib monohydrate). Bristol-Myers Squibb Pharmaceuticals Ltd. UK Summary of product characteristics, March 2015.
11. Sprycel (Dasatinib monohydrate). Bristol-Myers Squibb Company. US Prescribing information, August 2015.
12. Tasigna (Nilotinib hydrochloride monohydrate). Novartis Pharmaceuticals UK Ltd. UK Summary of product characteristics, June 2015.
13. Tasigna (Nilotinib hydrochloride monohydrate). Novartis Pharmaceuticals Corp. US Prescribing information, January 2015.
14. Tyverb (Lapatinib ditosylate monohydrate). Novartis Pharmaceuticals UK Ltd. UK Summary of product characteristics, June 2015.
15. Bosulif (Bosutinib monohydrate). Pfizer Inc. US Prescribing information, November 2014.
16. Cometriq (Cabozantinib malate). Swedish Orphan Biovitrum Ltd. UK Summary of product characteristics, June 2015.
17. Xalkori (Crizotinib). Pfizer Ltd. UK Summary of product characteristics. April 2015.
18. Caprelsa (Vandetanib). AstraZeneca UK Ltd. UK Summary of product characteristics, October 2014.

Tyrosine kinase inhibitors + HIV-protease inhibitors

Ritonavir had little effect on imatinib concentrations at steady-state but did slightly increase the exposure to the active metabolite of imatinib. However, on the basis of theoretical data, an interaction between imatinib and HIV-protease inhibitors boosted with ritonavir does appear possible. The HIV-protease inhibitors are predicted to inhibit the metabolism of other tyrosine kinase inhibitors, with the exception of sorafenib and vandetanib. However, an isolated case report describes severe adverse effects in a patient receiving atazanavir boosted with ritonavir, shortly after sorafenib was added.

Clinical evidence

(a) Imatinib

In a study, 11 patients who had been taking imatinib 400 to 800 mg daily for at least 2 months were also given **ritonavir** 600 mg daily for 3 days, with a 50% reduction in the imatinib dose. Unexpectedly, the dose-normalised pharmacokinetics of imatinib were unaltered by ritonavir. However, the AUC of the active metabolite of imatinib was increased by about 40%.[1]

(b) Sorafenib

A case report describes a 47-year-old HIV-positive man who had been receiving HAART containing **atazanavir boosted with ritonavir** for 2 years with no problems, who was started on sorafenib 400 mg twice daily after developing hepatocellular carcinoma. Twenty-four hours later he complained of asthenia, nausea, and anorexia, and 5 days later he stopped taking the sorafenib due to profuse diarrhoea and abdominal pain. He was admitted on day 6 and was found to have lost 6 kg in weight. His liver function tests were further deranged than before the sorafenib was started, but all plasma drug concentrations were within normal limits, and his symptoms resolved within 24 hours. The atazanavir and ritonavir were changed to didanosine and abacavir, and sorafenib was restarted at 200 mg daily. No noticeable adverse effects were seen.[2]

Mechanism

Ritonavir is a known inhibitor of CYP3A4, which is the main isoenzyme involved in the metabolism of imatinib; however it did not increase imatinib concentrations. This might be because imatinib is itself a CYP3A4 inhibitor, so at steady-state it is less affected by other CYP3A4 inhibitors. However, it could also be due to ritonavir inhibiting or inducing other enzymes involved in the metabolism of imatinib. Sorafenib does not appear to be metabolised by CYP3A4, of which atazanavir boosted with ritonavir is an inhibitor and therefore the reason for the increase in sorafenib adverse effects seen in the case cited is unknown.

Importance and management

Evidence for an interaction between **imatinib** and the HIV-protease inhibitors appears limited to one study with ritonavir. Ritonavir is a known, potent inhibitor of CYP3A4, but the study unexpectedly found only a minimal effect of ritonavir on imatinib at steady-state, although the exposure to the active metabolite was slightly increased. This suggests that no imatinib dose adjustment is likely to be needed if ritonavir is also given. However, because an interaction with CYP3A4 inhibitors would be expected on the basis of data with the potent CYP3A4 inhibitor, ketoconazole (see 'Tyrosine kinase inhibitors + Azoles', p.728), the manufacturers of imatinib advise caution with (potent[3]) CYP3A4 inhibitors,[4] which includes the HIV-protease inhibitors boosted with ritonavir. Until further evidence is available this seems prudent, particularly in light of the increased exposure to the active metabolite.

The general importance of the isolated case report with **sorafenib** and atazanavir boosted with ritonavir is not known. As ketoconazole has no clinically relevant effect on the pharmacokinetics of sorafenib (see 'Tyrosine kinase inhibitors + Azoles', p.728), the UK manufacturer advises that other potent CYP3A4 inhibitors would also not be expected to interact with sorafenib.[5] Similarly, as the pharmacokinetics of **vandetanib** are unaffected by itraconazole, a potent CYP3A4 inhibitor, a clinically relevant interaction with the HIV-protease inhibitors by this mechanism would not be expected.

Evidence for an interaction between the HIV-protease inhibitors and other tyrosine kinase inhibitors is lacking, but as all HIV-protease inhibitors boosted with ritonavir are potent CYP3A4 inhibitors, they are expected to increase tyrosine kinase inhibitor exposure. For discussion of the management of the interactions between potent CYP3A4 inhibitors and the tyrosine kinase inhibitors, see under *Importance and Management* in 'Tyrosine kinase inhibitors + Azoles', p.728.

1. van Erp NP, Gelderblom H, Karlsson MO, Li J, Zhao M, Ouwerkerk J, Nortier JW, Guchelaar H-J, Baker SD, Sparreboom A. Influence of CYP3A4 inhibition on the steady-state pharmacokinetics of imatinib. *Clin Cancer Res* (2007) 13, 7394–7400.
2. Ozenne V, Gervais A, Peytavin G, Castelnau C, Valla DC, Degos F. Suspected interaction between sorafenib and HAART in an HIV-1 infected patient: a case report. *Hepatogastroenterology* (2011) 58, 161–2
3. Gleevec (Imatinib mesylate). Novartis Pharmaceuticals Corp. US Prescribing information, February 2013.
4. Glivec (Imatinib mesilate). Novartis Pharmaceuticals UK Ltd. UK Summary of product characteristics, July 2013.
5. Nexavar (Sorafenib tosylate). Bayer plc. UK Summary of product characteristics, November 2014.

Tyrosine kinase inhibitors + Macrolides

Erythromycin slightly increased ruxolitinib exposure. Macrolides that are inhibitors of CYP3A4 (such as clarithromycin) are predicted to increase the exposure to other tyrosine kinase inhibitors. A case report describes a man taking sunitinib who developed severe lethargy and loss of appetite when he was also given spiramycin.

Clinical evidence

(a) Ruxolitinib

In a crossover study in 14 healthy subjects, **erythromycin** 500 mg twice daily for 4 days increased the maximum plasma concentration and AUC of a single 10-mg dose of ruxolitinib given on day 4 by 8% and 27%, respectively.[1]

(b) Sunitinib

A case report describes a 56-year-old man with metastatic liver cancer who developed severe weakness and loss of appetite 12 days after starting sunitinib 50 mg daily for 4 weeks out of every 6 weeks. The previous day he had also started taking **spiramycin** with metronidazole (*Bi-spirogyl*) for a dental abscess. The patient was hospitalised, and the antibacterial was changed, replacing spiramycin with amoxicillin while continuing metronidazole. The symptoms resolved and the patient was able to resume normal activities. Sunitinib was continued without further problems.[2]

Mechanism

Erythromycin is an inhibitor of CYP3A4, by which ruxolitinib is metabolised and concurrent use results in increased ruxolitinib exposure. It was suggested that spiramycin inhibited the metabolism of sunitinib by CYP3A4 thereby increasing sunitinib concentrations and causing the adverse effects seen.[2] However, note that spiramycin is generally considered a less potent CYP3A4 inhibitor than other macrolides and is not known to cause clinically important interactions via this mechanism.

Importance and management

Evidence for a pharmacokinetic interaction between the tyrosine kinase inhibitors and the macrolides is limited. The slight increase in ruxolitinib exposure seen with erythromycin is unlikely to be clinically relevant and no ruxolitinib dose adjustment would seem necessary on concurrent use. In contrast, the case report with sunitinib and spiramycin suggests that a clinically relevant interaction could occur; although note that the mechanism for this effect is not clear and this appears to be an isolated report.

All tyrosine kinase inhibitors are metabolised by CYP3A4, albeit to varying extents. Of the macrolides, **clarithromycin** and **telithromycin** are both potent inhibitors of CYP3A4, **erythromycin** is a moderate inhibitor, and **roxithromycin** is a weak inhibitor. On the basis that the pharmacokinetics of most (but not all) tyrosine kinase inhibitors are affected by the potent CYP3A4 inhibitor, ketoconazole, see 'Tyrosine kinase inhibitors + Azoles', p.728, a number of the manufacturers of other tyrosine kinase inhibitors predict that the macrolides will interact similarly. For discussion of the management of the interaction between the tyrosine kinase inhibitors and potent and moderate CYP3A4 inhibitors, and details of the manufacturers' recommendations, see under *Importance and Management* in 'Tyrosine kinase inhibitors + Azoles', p.728. Note that although erythromycin is generally considered a moderate CYP3A4 inhibitor, it is often stated to be a potent inhibitor.

Note that some tyrosine kinase inhibitors and macrolides are known to prolong the QT interval and concurrent use could increase the risk of serious arrhythmias, see 'Drugs that prolong the QT interval + Other drugs that prolong the QT interval', p.272, for further discussion.

1. Shi JG, Chen X, Emm T, Scherle PA, McGee RF, Lo Y, Landman RR, McKeever EG, Punwani NG, Williams WV, Yeleswaram S. The effect of CYP3A4 inhibition or induction on the pharmacokinetics and pharmacodynamics of orally administered ruxolitinib (INCB018424 phosphate) in healthy volunteers. *J Clin Pharmacol* (2012) 52, 809–18.
2. Trabelsi S, Boussen H, Gaïes E, Salouage I, El Aïdli S, Daghfous R, Loueslati MH, Lakhal M, Belkahia C. Interaction médicamenteuse entre Sutent (sunitinib) et Bi-spirogyl (spiramycine-métronidazole): risque de toxicité. *Therapie* (2008) 63, 475–6.

Tyrosine kinase inhibitors + Paracetamol (Acetaminophen)

No pharmacokinetic interaction appears to occur between imatinib and paracetamol. Fatal acute liver failure has rarely been reported with imatinib, sometimes associated with concurrent paracetamol use. A case of liver failure has also been reported when sunitinib was taken with paracetamol.

Clinical evidence

(a) Imatinib

In a pharmacokinetic study in 12 patients, the pharmacokinetics of a single 1-g dose of paracetamol (and its metabolites paracetamol glucuronide and paracetamol sulphate) were unaffected by imatinib 400 mg daily for 7 days. The pharmacokinetics of imatinib were also unaffected.[1]

In an early phase II study, one patient who had been regularly taking paracetamol 3 to 3.5 g daily for about a month, developed elevated bilirubin and transaminases, upper quadrant discomfort and jaundice 6 days after starting to take imatinib. Imatinib was stopped on day 7 and the patient died of acute liver failure 5 days later.[2] Another case report describes acute liver failure that developed 5 months after starting imatinib, and which progressively deteriorated. The patient died about 3 weeks later. The report notes that paracetamol 500 mg to 1 g daily was taken after the onset of symptoms.[3]

(b) Sunitinib

A case report describes fatal acute liver failure in a woman taking about 4.5 g of paracetamol weekly after she had received 8 cycles of sunitinib. During the 8th cycle she had also taken levothyroxine.[4]

Mechanism

A pharmacokinetic interaction has been suggested and an *in vitro* study showed that **dasatinib**, **imatinib**, and **sorafenib** inhibited paracetamol glucuronidation. **Erlotinib**, **gefitinib**, **lapatinib**, **nilotinib**, and **vandetanib** also showed inhibition, but to a lesser extent.[5] However, the study in patients suggests no pharmacokinetic interaction occurs between imatinib and paracetamol.[1] Both imatinib and paracetamol alone can cause hepatotoxicity, and there is some evidence from an *animal* study that this effect might be additive.[6]

Importance and management

Evidence is limited but no pharmacokinetic interaction appears to occur between imatinib and paracetamol. The UK and US manufacturers of imatinib note that doses of imatinib higher than 400 mg and chronic paracetamol use have not been studied.[7,8] Given the seriousness of the cases, and until more is known about the effect on chronic paracetamol use, some caution would seem prudent on the concurrent use of imatinib in patients taking paracetamol long-term. Note that liver function should be routinely monitored during the use of imatinib. The general relevance of the case of liver failure with sunitinib and paracetamol is uncertain, as sunitinib alone can, rarely, cause hepatic failure. Evidence for other tyrosine kinase inhibitors is lacking. The UK manufacturer of **crizotinib** notes that its inhibitory effect on UGTs, especially UGT1A1, is not established and advises caution on concurrent use with UGT substrates, such as paracetamol.[9] Further study is needed.

1. Kim DW, Tan EY, Jin Y, Park S, Hayes M, Demirhan E, Schran H, Wang Y. Effects of imatinib mesylate on the pharmacokinetics of paracetamol (acetaminophen) in Korean patients with chronic myelogenous leukaemia. *Br J Clin Pharmacol* (2011) 71, 199–206.
2. Talpaz M, Silver RT, Druker BJ, Goldman JM, Gambacorti-Passerini C, Guilhot F, Schiffer CA, Fischer T, Deininger MW, Lennard AL, Hochhaus A, Ottmann OG, Gratwohl A, Baccarani M, Stone R, Tura S, Mahon FX, Fernandes-Reese S, Gathmann I, Capdeville R, Kantarjian HM, Sawyers CL. Imatinib induces durable hematologic and cytogenetic responses in patients with accelerated phase chronic myeloid leukemia: results of a phase 2 study. *Blood* (2002) 99, 1928–37.
3. Ridruejo E, Cacchione R, Villamil AG, Marciano S, Gadano AC, Mandó OG. Imatinib-induced fatal acute liver failure. *World J Gastroenterol* (2007) 13, 6608–11.
4. Weise AM, Liu CY, Shields AF. Fatal liver failure in a patient on acetaminophen treated with sunitinib malate and levothyroxine. Ann Pharmacother. (2009) 43, 761–6.
5. Liu Y, Ramírez J, Ratain MJ. Inhibition of paracetamol glucuronidation by tyrosine kinase inhibitors. *Br J Clin Pharmacol* (2011) 71, 917–20.
6. Nassar I, Pasupati T, Judson JP, Segarra I. Histopathological study of the hepatic and renal toxicity associated with the co-administration of imatinib and acetaminophen in a preclinical mouse model. *Malays J Pathol* (2010) 32, 1–11.
7. Glivec (Imatinib mesilate). Novartis Pharmaceuticals UK Ltd. UK Summary of product characteristics, October 2013.
8. Gleevec (Imatinib mesylate). Novartis Pharmaceuticals Corp. US Prescribing information, October 2013.
9. Xalkori (Crizotinib). Pfizer Ltd. UK Summary of product characteristics, April 2013.

Tyrosine kinase inhibitors + Pemetrexed

There appears to be no pharmacokinetic interaction between erlotinib or sunitinib and pemetrexed. Pazopanib does not appear to affect the exposure to pemetrexed.

Clinical evidence, mechanism, importance and management

(a) Erlotinib

In a phase I dose-finding study in patients with non-small cell lung cancer, the pharmacokinetics of erlotinib and pemetrexed were not affected when pemetrexed was given within 5 minutes of erlotinib compared with either drug given alone.[1]

(b) Pazopanib

In a small phase I dose-finding study in patients with advanced solid tumours, a pharmacokinetic analysis found that pazopanib 800 mg daily caused no change in the AUC, and a negligible increase in the maximum concentration, of pemetrexed 500 mg/m^2 every 21 days.[2]

(c) Suntinib

In a pharmacokinetic analysis of a phase I dose-finding study in patients with advanced solid tumours, the pharmacokinetics of sunitinib and pemetrexed were not affected when given together as suntinib 37.5 to 50 mg daily and pemetrexed 300-500 mg/m^2 every 21-days.[3] In another similar phase I study, the pharmacokinetics of sunitinib and pemetrexed were no different to historical controls.[4]

1. Ranson M, Reck M, Anthoney A, Hanauske AR, Dean E, Melezinek I, Klingelschmitt G, Kletzl H, Blatter J, Twelves C. Erlotinib in combination with pemetrexed for patients with advanced non-small-cell lung cancer (NSCLC): a phase I dose-finding study. *Ann Oncol* (2010) 21, 2233–9.
2. Infante JR, Novello S, Ma WW, Dy GK, Bendell JC, Huff A, Wang Q, Suttle AB, Allen R, Xu CF, Ottesen LH, Burris HA, Adjei AA. Phase Ib trial of the oral angiogenesis inhibitor pazopanib administered concurrently with pemetrexed in patients with advanced solid tumors. *Invest New Drugs* (2013) 31, 927–36.
3. Chow LQ, Blais N, Jonker DJ, Laurie SA, Diab SG, Canil C, McWilliam M, Thall A, Ruiz-Garcia A, Zhang K, Tye L, Chao RC. Camidge DR. A phase I dose-escalation and pharmacokinetic study of sunitinib in combination with pemetrexed in patients with advanced solid malignancies, with an expanded cohort in non-small cell lung cancer. *Cancer Chemother Pharmacol* (2012) 69, 709–22.
4. Okamoto I, Shimizu T, Miyazaki M, Tsurutani J, Ichikawa Y, Terashima M, Takeda M, Fumita S, Ohki E, Kimura N, Hashimoto J, Nakagawa K. Feasibility of two schedules of sunitinib in combination with pemetrexed in patients with advanced solid tumors. *Invest New Drugs* (2012) 30, 639–46.

Tyrosine kinase inhibitors + Proton pump inhibitors

Proton pump inhibitors reduce the exposure to axitinib, bosutinib, dasatinib, erlotinib, lapatinib, nilotinib, pazopanib, and ponatinib, although the extent of the interaction varies. The exposure to gefitinib is also predicted to be reduced by proton pump inhibitors. The exposure to single-dose crizotinib or single-dose cabozantinib was not affected by esomeprazole, and the exposure to imatinib, sorafenib and vandetanib does not appear to be affected by omeprazole. Pazopanib, regorafenib, and sorafenib do not affect the pharmacokinetics of omeprazole.

Clinical evidence

(a) Effects on tyrosine kinase inhibitors

1. Axitinib. In a phase I study in a cohort of 6 patients with solid tumours, **rabeprazole** 20 mg daily for 5 days reduced the maximum concentration and AUC of axitinib by about 40% and 5% respectively, however there was wide interpatient variability.[1]

2. Bosutinib. A pharmacokinetic study in 23 healthy subjects found that **lansoprazole** 60 mg daily for 2 days reduced the AUC and maximum concentration of a single dose of bosutinib 400 mg taken on day 2 by 24% and 39%, respectively.[2]

3. Cabozantinib. The UK manufacturer of cabozantinib briefly notes that **esomeprazole** 40 mg twice daily for 6 days had no clinically relevant effect on the AUC of a single 100-mg dose of cabozantinib.[3]

4. Crizotinib. The UK and US manufacturers of crizotinib briefly note that **esomeprazole** 40 mg daily for 5 days reduced the AUC of a single 250-mg dose of crizotinib by 10%, but had no effect on its maximum concentration.[4,5]

5. Dasatinib. A study in 14 healthy subjects found that the AUC and maximum plasma concentration of a single 100-mg dose of dasatinib were reduced by 43% and 42%, respectively, when given 22 hours after a 4-day course of **omeprazole** 40 mg daily.[6,7] In a retrospective pharmacokinetic analysis of 18 patients with leukaemia taking **lansoprazole** 30 mg daily (5 patients) or an H_2-receptor antagonist (7 patients), the dasatinib dose-adjusted AUC was 58% lower than in 6 patients not taking any acid suppressants.[8]

6. Erlotinib. **Omeprazole** reduces the AUC and maximum plasma concentration of erlotinib by 46% and 61%, respectively.[9,10] A case report describes subtherapeutic minimum erlotinib concentrations during a 2-day course of high-dose intravenous **pantoprazole** (8 mg/hour). Erlotinib concentrations returned to within the therapeutic range after the pantoprazole was given orally, at a dose of 40 mg twice daily.[11]

7. Imatinib. In a crossover study in healthy subjects,[12] pretreatment with **omeprazole** 40 mg daily for 5 days had no effect on the AUC or maximum plasma concentration of a single 400-mg dose of imatinib given on day 5. A patient with a recurrence of a gastrointestinal stromal tumour was given imatinib 400 mg daily without adverse effect. However, after 2 months, **lansoprazole** 15 mg daily was also given for dyspepsia and the patient developed bilateral eyelid oedema with hyperaemic conjunctivae and labial oedema. Both drugs were stopped, but on reintroduction the symptoms reappeared and she developed Stevens-Johnson syndrome. Both drugs were again stopped and she recovered after treatment with methylprednisolone and desloratadine for one month. Two months later, she took a single dose of **lansoprazole** on the day before taking imatinib 300 mg daily (with prednisone and desloratadine). One day later she developed eyelid and labial oedema and a generalised rash. She recovered after imatinib was stopped.[13]

8. Lapatinib. The UK manufacturer briefly notes that pre-treatment with **esomeprazole** resulted in a 27% decrease in lapatinib exposure.[14]

9. Nilotinib. In a study in 15 healthy subjects, **esomeprazole** 40 mg daily for 6 days reduced the AUC and maximum plasma concentration of nilotinib by 34% and 27%, respectively, when a single 400-mg dose of nilotinib was given on day 6, one hour after esomeprazole. The time to reach the maximum plasma concentration was increased, from 4 hours to 6 hours, but the half-life of nilotinib was unaffected by **esomeprazole.**[15] A retrospective population pharmacokinetic analysis of data from a subgroup of 33 patients with chronic myeloid leukaemia who received nilotinib 300 mg or 400 mg twice daily, found that the use of proton pump inhibitors (**esomeprazole, lansoprazole, omeprazole, pantoprazole**, or **rabeprazole**) did not alter the steady-state minimum concentration of nilotinib, when compared with patients who did not take a proton pump inhibitor (or an H_2-receptor antagonist).[16]

10. Pazopanib. In a pharmacokinetic study in 12 patients with solid tumours given pazopanib 800 mg daily for 7 days, followed by pazopanib 800 mg daily (in the morning) with **esomeprazole** 40 mg daily (in the evening) for 5 days, the pazopanib AUC and maximum concentration were reduced by 40% and 42%, respectively.[17]

11. Ponatinib. The US manufacturer of ponatinib briefly notes that, in 18 healthy subjects, **lansoprazole** 60 mg daily reduced the AUC and maximum concentration of a single 45-mg dose of ponatinib by 6% and 25%, respectively, when compared to ponatinib alone.[18]

12. Sorafenib. The US manufacturer of sorafenib briefly notes that **omeprazole** 40 mg daily for 5 days, did not produce a clinically relevant effect on the exposure to a single dose of sorafenib.[19]

13. Vandetanib. The UK manufacturer of vandetanib briefly notes that its concurrent use with **omeprazole** had no effect on the vandetanib AUC, but reduced its maximum concentration by 15%.[20]

(b) Effects on proton pump inhibitors

1. Pazopanib. In a pharmacokinetic study in patients with cancer, pazopanib 800 mg daily for 17 days had no effect on the pharmacokinetics of a single 40-mg dose of **omeprazole.**[21]

2. Regorafenib. The US manufacturer briefly notes that in a study in 11 patients with advanced solid tumours, regorafenib 160 mg daily for 14 days did not alter the plasma concentration of a single 40-mg dose of **omeprazole.**[22]

3. Sorafenib. In a phase I/II pharmacokinetic study in 18 patients with advanced melanoma, sorafenib 400 mg twice daily for 28 days did not alter the pharmacokinetics of a single 20-mg oral dose of **omeprazole.**[23]

Mechanism

The solubility of some tyrosine kinase inhibitors, including axitinib, bosutinib, crizotinib, dasatinib, erlotinib, gefitinib, lapatinib, nilotinib, ponatinib, sorafenib, and pazopanib is pH-dependent. Drugs that reduce gastric acidity, such as the proton pump inhibitors, therefore reduce their absorption.

The authors of the case of subtherapeutic minimum concentrations of erlotinib with intravenous pantoprazole, but not oral pantoprazole, suggest that this might have been due to far greater acid suppression achieved by the high dose and intravenous route than by the lower dose and oral route, such that the solubility of erlotinib with oral pantoprazole was sufficient for adequate absorption.[16]

The case of adverse effects with imatinib and lansoprazole is unexplained. Although the adverse effects could be attributed to either drug alone, the authors suggested it was possible that they might have been the result of increased imatinib concentrations as a result of CYP3A4 inhibition by lansoprazole, which they state is a weak inhibitor of CYP3A4.[13] However, note that lansoprazole does not cause clinically important interactions with CYP3A4 substrates.

Importance and management

An interaction resulting in a reduction in the exposure to axitinib, bosutinib, crizotinib, dasatinib, erlotinib, gefitinib, and nilotinib with proton pump inhibitors is established, but the clinical relevance varies greatly. In general, the manufacturers of these tyrosine kinase inhibitors recommend caution, and suggest that the concurrent use of these drugs with proton pump inhibitors should be avoided. However the UK manufacturer of nilotinib states that it can be taken with proton pump inhibitors if necessary,[24] and the US manufacturer of gefitinib recommends that it can be given 12 hours before or after a proton pump inhibitor if concurrent use is unavoidable.[25] Some recommend the use of alternatives, such as antacids[26,27] or H_2-receptor antagonists[27] with bosutinib (but see also 'Tyrosine kinase inhibitors + Antacids', p.726 and 'Tyrosine kinase inhibitors + H_2-receptor antagonists', p.733).

The UK manufacturer of **lapatinib** advises that drugs that increase gastric pH [such as the proton pump inhibitors] might reduce the solubility and absorption of lapatinib and should be avoided.[14] However, note that the US manufacturer states that a clinically meaningful reduction in lapatinib exposure was not seen with esomeprazole and offers no cautionary advice as a result.[28]

The UK and US manufacturers of **pazopanib** state that concurrent use of proton pump inhibitors should be avoided,[29,30] and the US manufacturer[30] recommends that use of antacids should be considered as an alternative (but see also 'Tyrosine kinase inhibitors + Antacids', p.726). However the UK manufacturer recommends that if a proton pump inhibitor must be given, the dose of pazopanib should be taken once daily in the evening, without food, at the same time as the proton pump inhibitor.[29]

The decreases in exposure seen with **axitinib, crizotinib, ponatinib**, and **sorafenib** are unlikely to be clinically relevant, and no dose adjustment of the tyrosine kinase inhibitor would seem necessary on concurrent use.

No dose adjustments are expected to be necessary on the concurrent use of cabozantinib and esomeprazole, regorafenib and omeprazole, and vandetanib and omeprazole. The pharmacokinetics of **imatinib** are not affected by omeprazole. The general relevance of the case report of adverse effects on the concurrent use of imatinib and lansoprazole is uncertain.

Note that omeprazole can be used as a probe substrate to assess the activity of drugs on CYP2C19. The studies with pazopanib, regorafenib, and sorafenib therefore suggest that these drugs are not inhibitors or inducers of CYP2C19.

1. Rugo HS, Herbst RS, Liu G, Park JW, Kies MS, Steinfeldt HM, Pithavala YK, Reich SD, Freddo JL, Wilding G. Phase I trial of the oral antiangiogenesis agent AG-013736 in patients with advanced solid tumors: pharmacokinetic and clinical results. *J Clin Oncol* (2005) 23, 5474–83.
2. A clinical study to examine the potential effect of lansoprazole on the pharmacokinetics of bosutinib when administered concomitantly to healthy subjects. *Clin Drug Investig* (2013) 33, 589–95.
3. Cometriq (Cabozantinib malate). Swedish Orphan Biovitrum Ltd. UK Summary of product characteristics, June 2015.
4. Xalkori (Crizotinib). Pfizer Inc. US Prescribing information, March 2015.
5. Xalkori (Crizotinib). Pfizer Ltd. UK Summary of product characteristics, April 2015.
6. Sprycel (Dasatinib monohydrate). Bristol-Myers Squibb Pharmaceutical Ltd. UK Summary of product characteristics, March 2015.
7. Sprycel (Dasatinib monohydrate). Bristol-Myers Squibb Company. US Prescribing information, July 2015.
8. Takahashi N, Miura M, Niioka T, Sawada K. Influence of H2-receptor antagonists and proton pump inhibitors on dasatinib pharmacokinetics in Japanese leukemia patients. *Cancer Chemother Pharmacol* (2012) 69, 999–1004.
9. Tarceva (Erlotinib hydrochloride). OSI Pharmaceuticals LLC. US Prescribing information, April 2015.
10. Tarceva (Erlotinib hydrochloride). Roche Products Ltd. UK Summary of product characteristics, December 2013.
11. ter Heine R, Fanggiday JC, Lankheet NAG, Beijnen JH, van der Westerlaken MML, Staaks GHA, Malingré MM. Erlotinib and pantoprazole: a relevant pharmacokinetic interaction or not? *Br J Clin Pharmacol* (2010) 70, 908–11.
12. Egorin MJ, Shah DD, Christner SM, Yerk MA, Komazec KA, Appleman LR, Redner RL, Miller BM, Beumer JH. Effect of a proton pump inhibitor on the pharmacokinetics of imatinib. *Br J Clin Pharmacol* (2009) 68, 370–4.
13. Severino G, Chillotti C, De Lisa R, Del Zompo M, Ardau R. Adverse reactions during imatinib and lansoprazole treatment in gastrointestinal stromal tumors. *Ann Pharmacother* (2005) 39, 162–4.
14. Tyverb (Lapatinib ditosylate monohydrate). GlaxoSmithKline UK. UK Summary of product characteristics, June 2015.
15. Yin OQ, Gallagher N, Fischer D, Demirhan E, Zhou W, Golor G, Schran H. Effect of the proton pump inhibitor esomeprazole on the oral absorption and pharmacokinetics of nilotinib. *J Clin Pharmacol* (2010) 50, 960–7.
16. Yin OQ, Giles FJ, Baccarani M, le Coutre P, Chiparus O, Gallagher N, Saglio G, Hughes TP, Hochhaus A, Kantarjian HM, Larson RA. Concurrent use of proton pump inhibitors or H2 blockers did not adversely affect nilotinib efficacy in patients with chronic myeloid leukaemia. *Cancer Chemother Pharmacol* (2012) 70, 345–50.
17. Tan AR, Gibbon DG, Stein MN, Lindquist D, Edenfield JW, Martin JC, Gregory C, Suttle AB, Tada H, Bothyl J, Stephenson JJ. Effects of ketoconazole and esomeprazole on the pharmacokinetics of pazopanib in patients with solid tumors. *Cancer Chemother Pharmacol* (2013) 71, 1635–43.
18. Iclusig (Ponatinib). ARIAD Pharmaceuticals, Inc. US Prescribing information, September 2014.
19. Nexavar (Sorafenib tosylate). Bayer Healthcare Pharmaceuticals Inc. US Prescribing information, November 2013.
20. Caprelsa (Vandetanib). AstraZeneca UK Ltd. UK Summary of product characteristics, October 2014.
21. Goh BC, Reddy NJ, Dandamudi UB, Laubscher KH, Peckham T, Hodge JP, Suttle AB, Arumugham T, Xu Y, Xu C-F, Lager J, Dar MM, Lewis LD. An evaluation of the drug interaction potential of pazopanib, an oral vascular endothelial growth factor receptor tyrosine kinase inhibitor, using a modified Cooperstown 5 +1 cocktail in patients with advanced solid tumours. *Clin Pharmacol Ther* (2010) 88, 652–9.
22. Stivarga (Regorafenib). Bayer HealthCare Pharmaceuticals Inc. US Prescribing information, April 2015.
23. Flaherty KT, Lathia C, Frye RF, Schuchter L, Redlinger M, Rosen M, O'Dwyer PJ. Interaction of sorafenib and cytochrome P450 isoenzymes in patients with advanced melanoma: a phase I/II pharmacokinetic interaction study. *Cancer Chemother Pharmacol* (2011) 68, 1111–8.
24. Tasigna (Nilotinib hydrochloride monohydrate). Novartis Pharmaceuticals UK Ltd. UK Summary of product characteristics, June 2015.
25. Iressa (Gefitinib). AstraZeneca Pharmaceuticals LP. US Prescribing information, July 2015.
26. Bosulif (Bosutinib monohydrate). Pfizer Ltd. UK Summary of product characteristics, July 2015
27. Bosulif (Bosutinib monohydrate). Pfizer Inc. US Prescribing information, November 2014.
28. Tykerb (Lapatinib ditosylate monohydrate). GlaxoSmithKline. US Prescribing information, March 2015.
29. Votrient (Pazopanib hydrochloride). GlaxoSmithKline UK. UK Summary of product characteristics, July 2015.
30. Votrient (Pazopanib hydrochloride). GlaxoSmithKline. US Prescribing information, April 2015.

Tyrosine kinase inhibitors + Rifampicin (Rifampin)

Rifampicin very markedly reduces the exposure to bosutinib; markedly reduces the exposure to crizotinib, dasatinib, gefitinib, nilotinib, and tofacitinib; markedly to moderately reduces the exposure to erlotinib; moderately reduces the exposure to axitinib, cabozantinib, imatinib, regorafenib, and ruxolitinib, and slightly reduces the exposure to sorafenib, sunitinib, and vandetanib. Rifampicin is predicted to reduce the exposure to lapatinib, pazopanib, and ponatinib; and other potent CYP3A4 inducers would be expected to interact with all of these tyrosine kinase inhibitors similarly to rifampicin.

Clinical evidence

Studies of the pharmacokinetic interactions of the tyrosine kinase inhibitors with rifampicin are summarised in 'Table 17.4', p.738. These show that rifampicin very markedly reduces the exposure to **bosutinib**; markedly reduces the exposure to **crizotinib**, **dasatinib**, **gefitinib**, **nilotinib**, and **tofacitinib**; moderately to markedly reduces exposure to **erlotinib**; moderately reduces the exposure to **axitinib**, **cabozantinib**, **imatinib**, **regorafenib**, and **ruxolitinib**, and slightly reduces the exposure to **sunitinib**, **sorafenib**, and **vandetanib**.

In a study with **erlotinib**, a 3-fold dose increase (to 450 mg) still resulted in a 43% lower exposure when **erlotinib** was taken after 11 days of treatment with rifampicin when compared with **erlotinib** 150 mg taken without rifampicin.[1,2].

Exposure to the *N*-desmethyl metabolite of **vandetanib** was increased almost 4-fold and its maximum plasma concentration was increased 5-fold by rifampicin.[3]

Mechanism

Rifampicin is a known non-specific enzyme inducer, with potent effects on CYP3A4, by which all of the tyrosine kinase inhibitors are metabolised. Induction of other enzymes cannot be excluded.

Importance and management

An interaction between the potent CYP3A4 inducer, rifampicin, and the tyrosine kinase inhibitors is established. The size of the reductions in the exposure to **axitinib**, **bosutinib**, **cabozantinib**, **crizotinib**, **dasatinib**, **erlotinib**, **gefitinib**, **imatinib**, **nilotinib**, **regorafenib**, **ruxolitinib**, and **tofacitinib** with rifampicin is likely to result in therapeutic failure. Rifampicin should therefore be avoided in patients taking these drugs, where possible. However, if concurrent use of rifampicin or other potent CYP3A4 inducers (see 'Table 1.9', p.11 for a list) is necessary, some manufacturers give specific advice, which is listed below. Note that some manufacturers additionally list **dexamethasone** as a potent inducer of CYP3A4, however evidence for dexamethasone having clinically relevant interactions as a result of this mechanism is generally lacking.

Note, it is important to remember that if the CYP3A4 inducer is stopped, the dose of the tyrosine kinase inhibitor will need to be reduced back to the indicated dose.

- The **axitinib** dose should be gradually increased and the patient monitored carefully for toxicity. Note that some adverse reactions might necessitate temporary or permanent discontinuation of axitinib and/or a dose reduction.[4]
- The UK manufacturer of **bosutinib** states that increasing the bosutinib dose is unlikely to sufficiently compensate for the likely reduced exposure.[5]
- The US manufacturer of **cabozantinib** recommends increasing the dose by 40 mg, according to tolerability, up to a maximum of 180 mg daily.[6]
- The US manufacturer of **dasatinib** recommends increasing the dose and monitoring for toxicity.[7]
- The starting dose of **erlotinib** should be increased (the US manufacturer recommends 50 mg increments at 2-week intervals and the UK manufacturer suggests increasing to 300 mg) with close monitoring, and if tolerated, further increased to a maximum of 450 mg.[1,2]
- Concurrent use of rifampicin and **lapatinib**, based on the effect of carbamazepine on **lapatinib** exposure (see 'Tyrosine kinase inhibitors + Antiepileptics; Enzyme-inducing', p.727) should also be avoided, however if concurrent use of a potent CYP3A4 inducer is necessary, the US manufacturer of lapatinib recommends that its dose can be gradually titrated from 1.25 g daily up to 4.5 g daily or from 1.5 g daily up to 5.5 g daily dependent on indication and tolerability.[8]
- Increase the **imatinib** dose by at least 50% and monitor clinical response carefully. Doses up to 600 mg twice daily have been given.[9]
- The US manufacturer of **nilotinib** notes that a dose increase is unlikely to be effective in correcting the reduced exposure caused by rifampicin, due to the non-linear pharmacokinetics of nilotinib.[10]
- Evidence for an interaction between rifampicin and **ponatinib** or **pazopanib** is lacking, but based on the known metabolism of these drugs their use with rifampicin or other CYP3A4 inducers is generally not recommended. If concurrent use is unavoidable, the US manufacturer of ponatinib recommends monitoring for signs of reduced efficacy.[11]
- The UK and US manufacturers of **ruxolitinib** recommend close monitoring and titration of the dose based on safety and efficacy.[12,13]
- The UK and US manufacturer of **sunitinib** recommend increasing its dose (in 12.5 mg increments[14]) up to 62.5 mg or 87.5 mg daily depending on the indication, based on monitoring and tolerability.[14,15]
- The effect of rifampicin on **sorafenib** and **vandetanib** exposure is only slight, but it would be prudent to monitor concurrent use of any potent CYP3A4 inducer for tyrosine kinase inhibitor efficacy, and adjust the dose if necessary.

Some manufacturers suggest **rifabutin** and **rifapentine** might interact in a similar way to rifampicin, and, until more is known, similar caution to that advised with rifampicin would be prudent, even though their effects are not as potent as those of rifampicin.

1. Tarceva (Erlotinib hydrochloride). Roche Products Ltd. UK Summary of product characteristics, December 2013.
2. Tarceva (Erlotinib hydrochloride). OSI Pharmaceuticals, LLC. US Prescribing information, April 2015.
3. Martin P, Oliver S, Robertson J, Kennedy SJ, Read J, Duvauchelle T. Pharmacokinetic drug interactions with vandetanib during coadministration with rifampicin or itraconazole. *Drugs R D* (2011) 11, 37–51.
4. Inlyta (Axitinib). Pfizer Ltd. UK Summary of product characteristics, May 2015.
5. Bosulif (Bosutinib monohydrate). Pfizer Ltd. UK Summary of product characteristics, July 2015.
6. Cometriq (Cabozantinib malate). Exelixis, Inc. US Prescribing information) November 2012.
7. Sprycel (Dasatinib monohydrate). Bristol-Myers Squibb Company. US Prescribing information, August 2015.
8. Tykerb (Lapatinib ditosylate monohydrate). GlaxoSmithKline. US Prescribing information, March 2015.
9. Gleevec (Imatinib mesylate). Novartis Pharmaceuticals Corp. US Prescribing information, January 2015.
10. Tasigna (Nilotinib hydrochloride monohydrate). Novartis Pharmaceuticals Corp. US Prescribing information, January 2015.
11. Iclusig (Ponatinib). ARIAD Pharmaceuticals, Inc. US Prescribing information, September 2014.
12. Jakavi (Ruxolitinib phosphate). Novartis Pharmaceuticals UK Ltd. UK Summary of product characteristics, April 2015.
13. Jakafi (Ruxolitinib phosphate). Incyte Corporation. US Prescribing information, December 2014.
14. Sutent (Sunitinib malate). Pfizer Ltd. UK Summary of product characteristics, June 2015.
15. Sutent (Sunitinib malate). Pfizer Inc. US Prescribing information, April 2015.

Table 17.4 Summary of the studies assessing the effect of rifampicin (rifampin) on the pharmacokinetics of tyrosine kinase inhibitors

Tyrosine kinase inhibitor	*Study*	*Dose*	*Rifampicin*	*Cmax reduction*	*AUC reduction*	*Refs*
Axitinib	Healthy subjects	5 mg single dose day 8	600 mg daily for 9 days	71%	79%	1
Bosutinib	Healthy subjects	500 mg single dose	600 mg daily for 6 days	86%	94%	2,3
Cabozantinib	Healthy subjects	Single dose	600 mg daily for 31 days		77%	4
Crizotinib		250 mg single dose	600 mg daily	69%	82%	5,6
Dasatinib		Single dose	600 mg daily for 8 days	81%	82%	7
Erlotinib			600 mg daily for 7 days		66% to 80%	8,9
Gefitinib	Healthy subjects	500 mg single dose day 10	600 mg daily for 16 days	65%	83%	10
Imatinib	Healthy subjects	400 mg single dose day 8	600 mg daily for 11 days	54%	74%	11
Nilotinib	Healthy subjects	400 mg single dose day 9	600 mg daily for 12 days	64%	80%	12
Regorafenib	Healthy subjects	160 mg single dose day 7	600 mg daily for 9 days		50%	13
Ruxolitinib	Healthy subjects	50 mg single dose day 11	600 mg daily for 11 days	52%	71%	14
Sorafenib		Single dose	5 days		37%	15
Sunitinib	Healthy subjects	Single dose		23%	46%	16,17
Tofacitinib				About 75%	About 85%	18
Vandetanib	Healthy subjects	300 mg single dose day 10	600 mg daily for 31 days	No effect	40%	19

1. Pithavala YK, Tortorici M, Toh M, Garrett M, Hee B, Kuruganti U, Ni G, Klamerus KJ. Effect of rifampin on the pharmacokinetics of axitinib (AG-013736) in Japanese and Caucasian healthy volunteers. *Cancer Chemother Pharmacol* (2010) 65, 563–70.
2. Bosulif (Bosutinib monohydrate). Pfizer Inc. US Prescribing information, April 2013.
3. Bosulif (Bosutinib monohydrate). Pfizer Ltd. UK Summary of product characteristics, March 2013.
4. Cometriq (Cabozantinib malate). Exelixis, Inc. US Prescribing information, November 2012.
5. Xalkori (Crizotinib). Pfizer Inc. US Prescribing information, May 2013.
6. Xalkori (Crizotinib). Pfizer Ltd. UK Summary of product characteristics, April 2013.
7. Sprycel (Dasatinib monohydrate). Bristol-Myers Squibb Company. US Prescribing information, October 2011.
8. Tarceva (Erlotinib hydrochloride). Roche Registration Ltd. UK Summary of product characteristics, August 2011.
9. Tarceva (Erlotinib hydrochloride). OSI Pharmaceuticals, Inc., and Genentech, Inc. US Prescribing information, April 2010.
10. Swaisland HC, Ranson M, Smith RP, Leadbetter J, Laight A, McKillop D, Wild MJ. Pharmacokinetic drug interactions of gefitinib with rifampicin, itraconazole and metoprolol. *Clin Pharmacokinet* (2005) 44, 1067–81.
11. Bolton AE, Peng B, Hubert M, Krebs-Brown A, Capdeville R, Keller U, Seiberling M. Effect of rifampicin on the pharmacokinetics of imatinib mesylate (Gleevec, STI571) in healthy subjects. *Cancer Chemother Pharmacol* (2004) 53, 102–6.
12. Tanaka C, Yin OQ, Smith T, Sethuraman V, Grouss K, Galitz L, Harrell R, Schran H. Effects of rifampicin and ketoconazole on the pharmacokinetics of nilotinib in healthy participants. *J Clin Pharmacol* (2011) 51, 75–83.
13. Stivarga (Regorafenib). Bayer HealthCare Pharmaceuticals Inc. US Prescribing information, August 2013.
14. Shi JG, Chen X, Emm T, Scherle PA, McGee RF, Lo Y, Landman RR, McKeever EG, Punwani NG, Williams WV, Yeleswaram S. The effect of CYP3A4 inhibition or induction on the pharmacokinetics and pharmacodynamics of orally administered ruxolitinib (INCB018424 phosphate) in healthy volunteers. *J Clin Pharmacol* (2012) 52, 809–18.
15. Nexavar (Sorafenib tosylate). Bayer Schering Pharma AG. UK Summary of product characteristics, August 2011.
16. Sutent (Sunitinib malate). Pfizer Ltd. UK Summary of product characteristics, August 2011.
17. Sutent (Sunitinib malate). Pfizer Inc. US Prescribing information, May 2011.
18. Xeljanz (Tofacitinib citrate). Pfizer Inc. US Prescribing information, November 2012.
19. Martin P, Oliver S, Robertson J, Kennedy SJ, Read J, Duvauchelle T. Pharmacokinetic drug interactions with vandetanib during coadministration with rifampicin or itraconazole. *Drugs R D* (2011) 11, 37–51.

Tyrosine kinase inhibitors + St John's wort (*Hypericum perforatum*)

St John's wort slightly decreases the exposure to imatinib. Other tyrosine kinase inhibitors are expected to be similarly affected by St John's wort.

Clinical evidence

In a study in 12 healthy subjects, the pharmacokinetics of a single dose of **imatinib** was determined before and on day 12 of 2 weeks of treatment with St John's wort extract (Kira [LI 160], Lichtwer Pharma) 300 mg three times daily. The AUC and maximum plasma concentration of imatinib were decreased by 30% and 15%, respectively. Imatinib clearance was increased by 43% and its half-life was decreased from 12.8 hours to 9 hours.[1] Similar results were found in another study.[2,3]

Mechanism

St John's wort induces CYP3A4 in the intestine and it therefore increases the metabolism of imatinib, which is a substrate of this isoenzyme. This results in the reduction in exposure seen.

Importance and management

Evidence for an interaction between St John's wort and **imatinib** appears to be limited to one study, but the results are consistent with the moderate CYP3A4-inducing potential of St John's wort and the known metabolism of imatinib. The slight changes in imatinib exposure seen, could be sufficient to impair the efficacy of imatinib. Furthermore, it is possible that the extent of the interaction might vary between different St John's wort products. It has therefore been suggested that concurrent use should be avoided,[1] which seems prudent.

Direct evidence for an interaction between St John's wort and **other tyrosine kinase inhibitors** appears to be lacking, but given that they are also metabolised by CYP3A4, avoidance of concurrent use would also seem prudent.

1. Frye RF, Fitzgerald SM, Lagattuta TF, Hruska MW, Egorin MJ. Effect of St John's wort on imatinib mesylate pharmacokinetics. *Clin Pharmacol Ther* (2004) 76, 323–9.
2. Smith P. The influence of St John's wort on the pharmacokinetics and protein binding of imatinib mesylate. *Pharmacotherapy* (2004) 24, 1508–14.
3. Smith PF, Bullock JM, Booker BM, Haas CE, Berenson CS, Jusko WJ. Induction of imatinib metabolism by hypericum perforatum. *Blood* (2004) 104, 1229–30.

Tyrosine kinase inhibitors + Tamoxifen and related drugs

Anastrozole and tamoxifen do not alter the pharmacokinetics of gefitinib. Gefitinib does not appear to alter tamoxifen concentrations. There is no pharmacokinetic interaction between letrozole and lapatinib.

Clinical evidence, mechanism, importance and management

(a) Gefitinib

1. Anastrozole. In a study in which 53 patients received gefitinib alone or with anastrozole, the authors briefly mention that the pharmacokinetics of gefitinib were not affected by anastrozole. The addition of anastrozole did not exacerbate the adverse effects of gefitinib.[1]

A case report describes an increase in liver transaminases in a woman given gefitinib and anastrozole, which resolved when gefitinib was stopped and recurred on rechallenge. However, the authors concluded that this was likely to be an adverse effect of gefitinib, and not due to a pharmacokinetic drug interaction with anastrozole.[2] Gefitinib is principally metabolised by CYP3A4 and although anastrozole weakly inhibited CYP3A4 *in vitro*, this was not considered likely to be important at clinically attainable concentrations.[3]

2. *Tamoxifen.* In a pharmacokinetic study, 18 healthy male subjects were given tamoxifen 60 mg daily for 4 days, then 20 mg daily for at least 10 days with a single 250-mg dose of gefitinib on day 14. The pharmacokinetics of gefitinib were not altered by tamoxifen.[4] In a phase II study, women with hormone receptor-positive metastatic breast cancer were given tamoxifen 20 mg daily, with gefitinib 250 mg daily or placebo. The minimum concentration of tamoxifen did not appear to be different in those patients given gefitinib when compared with those patients given placebo.[5]

(b) Lapatinib

In a phase I study in patients with advanced breast cancer, there was no clinically relevant difference in the pharmacokinetics of lapatinib and letrozole when they were given together compared with either drug given alone. The AUCs tended to be lower with the combination (a 16% reduction for lapatinib and a 6% reduction for letrozole), but these differences were not statistically significant.[6] Note that lapatinib is licensed for concurrent use with letrozole.

1. Polychronis A, Sinnett HD, Hadjiminas D, Singhal H, Mansi JL, Shivapatham D, Shousha S, Jiang J, Peston D, Barrett N, Vigushin D, Morrison K, Beresford E, Ali S, Slade MJ, Coombes RC. Preoperative gefitinib versus gefitinib and anastrozole in postmenopausal patients with oestrogen-receptor positive and epidermal-growth-factor-receptor-positive primary breast cancer: a double-blind placebo-controlled phase II randomised trial. *Lancet Oncol* (2005) 6, 383–91.
2. Carlini P, Papaldo P, Fabi A, Felici A, Ruggeri EM, Milella M, Ciccarese M, Nuzzo C, Cognetti F, Ferretti G. Liver toxicity after treatment with gefitinib and anastrozole: drug-drug interactions through cytochrome p450? *J Clin Oncol* (2006) 24, e60–e61.
3. Grimm SW, Dyroff MC. Inhibition of human drug metabolizing cytochromes P450 by anastrozole, a potent and selective inhibitor of aromatase. *Drug Metab Dispos* (1997) 25, 598–602.
4. Cantarini MV, Macpherson MP, Marshall AL, Robinson AV, Bailey CJ. A phase I study to determine the effect of tamoxifen on the pharmacokinetics of a single 250 mg oral dose of gefitinib (IRESSA) in healthy male volunteers. *Cancer Chemother Pharmacol* (2005) 56, 557–62.
5. Osborne CK, Neven P, Dirix LY, Mackey JR, Robert J, Underhill C, Schiff R, Gutierrez C, Migliaccio I, Anagnostou VK, Rimm DL, Magill P, Sellers M. Gefitinib or placebo in combination with tamoxifen in patients with hormone receptor –positive metastatic breast cancer: a randomized phase II study. *Clin Cancer Res* (2011) 17, 1147–59.
6. Chu QS, Cianfrocca ME, Goldstein LJ, Gale M, Murray N, Loftiss J, Arya N, Koch KM, Pandite L, Fleming RA, Paul E, Rowinsky EK. A phase I and pharmacokinetic study of lapatinib in combination with letrozole in patients with advanced cancer. *Clin Cancer Res* (2008) 14, 4484–90.

Tyrosine kinase inhibitors + Taxanes

Sorafenib slightly increases docetaxel exposure. The pharmacokinetics of erlotinib were not changed by administration with docetaxel. There appears to be no pharmacokinetic interaction between lapatanib or sunitinib and docetaxel. The pharmacokinetics of erlotinib and paclitaxel were not changed by administration together. The pharmacokinetics of paclitaxel were not altered by administration with gefitinib, but the exposure to gefitinib was slightly increased. Paclitaxel exposure is slightly increased by pazopanib and negligibly increased by lapatinib. The exposure to both sorafenib and paclitaxel are slightly increased when given together.

Clinical evidence, mechanism, importance and management

(a) Docetaxel

1. *Erlotinib.* In a study in which patients received capecitabine, docetaxel, and erlotinib, there was no change in the pharmacokinetics of erlotinib when it was given with these two drugs, when compared with when it was given alone. A trend towards a modest reduction in the AUC and maximum concentration of docetaxel (with capecitabine) was seen when erlotinib was also given, compared with docetaxel and capecitabine without erlotinib. However, the authors state that this did not confirm an interaction due to variability in docetaxel pharmacokinetics. The relevance of this is therefore uncertain and further study is needed.[1] In another study, there was no obvious difference in erlotinib exposure when it was taken alone or in combination with docetaxel and carboplatin.[2] Similarly, the pharmacokinetics of erlotinib did not appear to be altered by the addition of docetaxel in a pharmacokinetic analysis performed as part of a phase I study. The study found dose-limiting toxicity, but the pharmacokinetics of docetaxel were not studied.[3]

2. *Lapatinib.* In a phase I study of lapatinib and docetaxel in patients with advanced cancer, the pharmacokinetics of lapatinib and docetaxel did not differ when given together compared with each drug given separately. The combination caused dose-limiting neutropenia, which was managed with filgrastim.[4]

3. *Sorafenib.* Sorafenib 200 mg or 400 mg twice daily on days 2 to 19 of a 21-day cycle increased the AUC and maximum concentration of docetaxel 75 or 100 mg/m^2 given on day one every 21 days, by 36 to 80%, and by 16 to 32%, respectively.[5] This scheduling allowed a 3-day break in sorafenib administration around the dose of docetaxel.[5] The reason for this interaction is unclear. Sorafenib does not inhibit CYP3A4, by which docetaxel is principally metabolised, but it might inhibit P-glycoprotein by which docetaxel is transported. The UK manufacturer recommends caution on the concurrent use of these drugs.[5]

4. *Sunitinib.* In a phase I dose-finding study in patients with advanced cancer, no pharmacokinetic interaction was observed between sunitinib (given for 4 weeks of a 6-week cycle or 2 weeks of a 3-week cycle) and docetaxel (given intravenously once every 3 weeks).[6]

(b) Paclitaxel

1. *Erlotinib.* The pharmacokinetics of paclitaxel were not altered by erlotinib in a phase I study in patients given paclitaxel and carboplatin, nor were the pharmacokinetics of erlotinib affected by paclitaxel when compared with historical controls.[7] Similarly, in a pharmacokinetic study as part of a phase III clinical study, no pharmacokinetic interaction was noted after the addition of erlotinib to a standard regimen of paclitaxel and carboplatin.[8]

2. *Gefitinib.* In 24 patients with advanced non-small cell lung cancer, there was no change in the pharmacokinetics of paclitaxel when gefitinib 250 or 500 mg daily was also given. There was a 56% and 30% increase in the AUC of gefitinib 250 mg and 500 mg, respectively, and an increase in maximum concentration of 85% and 33%, respectively, but no increase in toxicity was noted.[9]

3. *Lapatinib.* The UK and US manufacturers briefly note that lapatinib increased the exposure (AUC) of paclitaxel by 23% in cancer patients.[10,11] This is thought to be because lapatinib is an inhibitor of CYP2C8, by which paclitaxel is metabolised. Inhibition of P-glycoprotein might also be involved.[10] The US manufacturer notes that this increase could be an underestimation due to the design of the study.[11] In addition, an increase in the incidence and severity of diarrhoea and neutropenia has been observed with this combination in clinical studies.[10] Caution is advised if lapatinib is used with paclitaxel.[10]

4. *Pazopanib.* A pharmacokinetic analysis of a phase I dose-finding study in patients with advanced solid tumors, given pazopanib 800 mg daily and paclitaxel 80 mg/m^2 once weekly, found that the AUC and maximum concentration of paclitaxel were 26% and 36% higher, respectively than with paclitaxel administration alone.[12] This slight increase in exposure is probably not likely to be clinically relevant in most patients, but, because paclitaxel has a narrow therapeutic range, some might experience an increase in adverse effects, therefore caution would seem appropriate.

5. *Sorafenib.* *In vitro*, sorafenib inhibits CYP2C8, by which paclitaxel is metabolised, to its 6-hydroxy metabolite.[5] However, the UK manufacturer notes that the concurrent use of paclitaxel (225 mg/m^2, once every 3 weeks) and carboplatin with sorafenib 400 mg twice daily (without a break in sorafenib dosing) resulted in a 47% increase in sorafenib exposure, a 29% increase in paclitaxel exposure, and a 50% increase in 6-hydroxy-paclitaxel exposure.[5] The greater increase in 6-hydroxy-paclitaxel exposure in this study, relative to the increase in paclitaxel exposure, shows that sorafenib is not an inhibitor of CYP2C8 *in vivo*. In one published clinical study, there was no change in the pharmacokinetics of paclitaxel when there was a 3-day break in sorafenib administration for 2 days before, and on the day of, paclitaxel administration. In this study, sorafenib 100 mg, 200 mg, or 400 mg twice daily was given on days 2 to 19 of a 21-day cycle, and paclitaxel and carboplatin were given on day one.[13] In another similar study of this schedule, there was no change in the pharmacokinetics of sorafenib or paclitaxel.[14] The clinical relevance of the increase in paclitaxel and sorafenib exposure on concurrent use is uncertain, but it could result in an increase in adverse effects. The lack of a pharmacokinetic interaction with a 3-day break in sorafenib administration around the time of the paclitaxel dose, suggests that this should be the preferred schedule, and the UK manufacturer advises that no dose adjustment with this schedule would seem to be necessary.[5]

1. Twelves C, Trigo JM, Jones R, De Rosa F, Rakhit A, Fettner S, Wright T, Baselga J. Erlotinib in combination with capecitabine and docetaxel in patients with metastatic breast cancer: a dose escalation study. *Eur J Cancer* (2008) 44, 419–26.
2. Vasey PA, Gore M, Wilson R, Rustin G, Gabra H, Guastalla JP, Lauraine EP, Paul J, Carty K, Kaye S; Scottish Gynaecological Cancer Trials Group. A phase Ib trial of docetaxel, carboplatin and erlotinib in ovarian, fallopian tube and primary peritoneal cancers. *Br J Cancer* (2008) 98, 1774–80.
3. Kraut EH, Rhoades C, Zhang Y, Cheng H, Aimiumu J, Chen P, Lang J, Young DC, Agrawal A, Dancey J, Chan KK, Grever MR. Phase I and pharmacokinetic study of erlotinib (OSI-774) in combination with docetaxel in squamous cell carcinoma of the head and neck (SSCHN). *Cancer Chemother Pharmacol* (2011) 67, 579–86.
4. LoRusso PM, Jones SF, Koch KM, Arya N, Fleming RA, Loftiss J, Pandite L, Gadgeel S, Weber BL, Burris HA 3rd. Phase I and pharmacokinetic study of lapatinib and docetaxel in patients with advanced cancer. *J Clin Oncol* (2008) 26, 3051–6.
5. Nexavar (Sorafenib tosylate). Bayer plc. UK Summary of product characteristics, February 2013.
6. Robert F, Sandler A, Schiller JH, Liu G, Harper K, Verkh L, Huang X, Ilagan J, Tye L, Chao R, Traynor AM. Sunitinib in combination with docetaxel in patients with advanced solid tumors: a phase I dose-escalation study. *Cancer Chemother Pharmacol* (2010) 66, 669–80.
7. Patnaik A, Wood D, Tolcher AW, Hamilton M, Kreisberg JI, Hammond LA, Schwartz G, Beeram M, Hidalgo M, Mita MM, Wolf J, Nadler P, Rowinsky EK. Phase I, pharmacokinetic, and biological study of erlotinib in combination with paclitaxel and carboplatin in patients with advanced solid tumours. *Clin Cancer Res* (2006) 12, 7406–13.
8. Tran HT, Zinner RG, Blumenschein GR, Oh YW, Papadimitrakopoulou VA, Kim ES, Lu C, Malik M, Lum BL, Herbst RS. Pharmacokinetic study of the phase III, randomized, double-blind, multicenter trial (TRIBUTE) of paclitaxel and carboplatin combined with erlotinib or placebo in patients with advanced non-small cell lung cancer (NSCLC). *Invest New Drugs* (2010) Epub.
9. Miller VA, Johnson DH, Krug LM, Pizzo B, Tyson L, Perez W, Krozely P, Sandler A, Carbone D, Heelan RT, Kris MG, Smith R, Ochs J. Pilot trial of the epidermal growth factor receptor tyrosine kinase inhibitor gefitinib plus carboplatin and paclitaxel in patients with stage IIIB or IV non-small-cell lung cancer. *J Clin Oncol* (2003) 21, 2094–100.
10. Tyverb (Lapatinib ditosylate monohydrate). GlaxoSmithKline UK. UK Summary of product characteristics, March 2014.
11. Tykerb (Lapatinib ditosylate monohydrate). GlaxoSmithKline. US Prescribing information, October 2013.
12. Tan AR, Dowlati A, Jones SF, Infante JR, Nishioka J, Fang L, Hodge JP, Gainer SD, Arumugham T, Suttle AB, Dar MM, Lager JJ, Burris HA. Phase I study of pazopanib in combination with weekly paclitaxel in patients with advanced solid tumors. *Oncologist* (2010) 15, 1253–61.
13. Flaherty KT, Schiller J, Schuchter LM, Liu G, Tuveson DA, Redlinger M, Lathia C, Xia C, Petrenciuc O, Hingorani SR, Jacobetz MA, Van Belle PA, Elder D, Brose MS, Weber BL, Albertini MR, O'Dwyer PJ. A phase I trial of the oral, multikinase inhibitor sorafenib in combination with carboplatin and paclitaxel. *Clin Cancer Res* (2008) 14, 4836–42.
14. Okamoto I, Miyazaki M, Morinaga R, Kaneda H, Ueda S, Hasegawa Y, Satoh T, Kawada A, Fukuoka M, Fukino K, Tanigawa T, Nakagawa K. Phase I clinical and pharmacokinetic study of sorafenib in combination with carboplatin and paclitaxel in patients with advanced non-small cell lung cancer. *Invest New Drugs* (2010) 28, 844–53.

Tyrosine kinase inhibitors + Tyrosine kinase inhibitors

Lapatinib increases pazopanib exposure, and sorafenib decreases gefitinib and probably also erlotinib exposure. Neither erlotinib nor gefitinib appeared to alter sorafenib pharmacokinetics, and dasatinib does not alter erlotinib pharmacokinetics.

Clinical evidence, mechanism, importance and management

(a) Dasatinib

In a study in patients with non-small cell lung cancer, the addition of dasatinib 100 to 140 mg daily to **erlotinib** 100 to 150 mg daily had no effect on **erlotinib** pharmacokinetics.[1]

(b) Erlotinib

In a phase I study in patients, the effect of **sorafenib** 400 mg twice daily on the pharmacokinetics of erlotinib 150 mg daily was not assessed, but compared with historical data, the steady-state concentration of erlotinib seemed to be lower (although this was based on a small sample).[2] In this same study and also in another similar study, the pharmacokinetics of **sorafenib** did not appear to be affected by the addition of erlotinib.[2,3] Another study also found that erlotinib concentrations were below the estimated therapeutic concentration in all patients also given **sorafenib**, and that erlotinib concentrations decreased over the duration of concurrent use.[4] The effect of **sorafenib** on erlotinib pharmacokinetics needs to be studied directly.

(c) Gefitinib

In a phase I study in patients, the AUC of gefitinib 250 mg daily was reduced by 38% when given with **sorafenib** 400 mg twice daily, when compared with when it was given alone. The pharmacokinetics of **sorafenib** were not altered by gefitinib.[5] The mechanism for the decreased exposure to gefitinib is unknown and the clinical relevance of this slight reduction in exposure is uncertain, but the authors speculate that it could well result in subtherapeutic concentrations.[5] Further study is needed.

(d) Lapatinib

The UK and US manufacturers of pazopanib note that lapatinib 1.5 g daily increased the mean AUC and maximum concentration of **pazopanib** 800 mg daily by about 50 to 60% compared with the use of **pazopanib** alone.[6,7] They suggest that inhibition of the drug transporter proteins P-glycoprotein and/or the breast cancer resistance protein (BCRP) by lapatinib probably contributed to the increased exposure to pazopanib.[6] The clinical relevance of this change is uncertain, but it seems possible that pazopanib adverse effects might be increased. Note that clinical studies on the concurrent use of pazopanib with pemetrexed and lapatinib were stopped early because of concerns of increased toxicity and/or mortality.[6]

1. Haura EB, Tanvetyanon T, Chiappori A, Williams C, Simon G, Antonia S, Gray J, Litschauer S, Tetteh L, Neuger A, Song L, Rawal B, Schell MJ, Bepler G. Phase I/II study of the Src inhibitor dasatinib in combination with erlotinib in advanced non-small-cell lung cancer. *J Clin Oncol* (2010) 28, 1387–94.
2. Quintela-Fandino M, Le Tourneau C, Duran I, Chen EX, Wang L, Tsao M, Bandarchi-Chamkhaleh B, Pham NA, Do T, MacLean M, Nayyar R, Tusche MW, Metser U, Wright JJ, Mak TW, Siu LL. Phase I combination of sorafenib and erlotinib therapy in solid tumors: safety, pharmacokinetic, and pharmacodynamic evaluation from an expansion cohort. *Mol Cancer Ther* (2010) 9, 751–60.
3. Duran I, Hotté SJ, Hirte H, Chen EX, MacLean M, Turner S, Duan L, Pond GR, Lathia C, Walsh S, Wright JJ, Dancey J, Siu LL. Phase I targeted combination trial of sorafenib and erlotinib in patients with advanced solid tumors. *Clin Cancer Res* (2007) 13, 4849–57.
4. Lind JS, Dingemans AM, Groen HJ, Thunnissen FB, Bekers O, Heideman DA, Honeywell RJ, Giovannetti E, Peters GJ, Postmus PE, van Suylen RJ, Smit EF. A multicenter phase II study of erlotinib and sorafenib in chemotherapy-naïve patients with advanced non-small cell lung cancer. *Clin Cancer Res* (2010) 16, 3078–87.
5. Adjei AA, Molina JR, Mandrekar SJ, Marks R, Reid JR, Croghan G, Hanson LJ, Jett JR, Xia C, Lathia C, Simantov R. Phase I trial of sorafenib in combination with gefitinib in patients with refractory or recurrent non-small cell lung cancer. *Clin Cancer Res* (2007) 13, 2684–91.
6. Votrient (Pazopanib hydrochloride). GlaxoSmithKline UK. UK Summary of product characteristics, December 2013.
7. Votrient (Pazopanib hydrochloride). GlaxoSmithKline. US Prescribing information, November 2013.

Tyrosine kinase inhibitors; Axitinib + Miscellaneous

The manufacturer predicts that axitinib will increase theophylline concentrations. Axitinib exposure might be increased by drugs that are potent inhibitors of CYP1A2 and CYP2C19.

Clinical evidence, mechanism, importance and management

(a) CYP1A2 and CYP2C19 inhibitors

The UK manufacturer notes that although the effects of potent inhibitors of CYP1A2 and CYP2C19 have not been studied, concurrent use of axitinib and such drugs should be undertaken with caution.[1] However, as CYP1A2 and CYP2C19 are both minor routes of metabolism for axitinib,[1,2] a clinically relevant interaction would appear unlikely. For a list of drugs that are inhibitors of CYP1A2 and CYP2C19, see "Table 1.6', p.8, respectively.

(b) CYP1A2 substrates

In vitro studies[1,2] have shown that axitinib inhibits CYP1A2 but the clinical relevance of this is unclear. Nevertheless, the UK manufacturer predicts that axitinib might increase the concentrations of CYP1A2 substrates (see 'Table 1.2', p.5 for a list) and they specifically name **theophylline**.[1] Until more is known, consider the possibility of increased theophylline concentrations on their concurrent use. As aminophylline is metabolised to theophylline, it seems likely to be similarly affected.

1. Inlyta (Axitinib). Pfizer Ltd. UK Summary of product characteristics, May 2015.
2. Inlyta (Axitinib). Pfizer Inc. US Prescribing information, September 2013.

Tyrosine kinase inhibitors; Cabozantinib + Miscellaneous

Cabozantinib had no effect on the pharmacokinetics of rosiglitazone in one study, and is predicted to increase the plasma concentrations of P-glycoprotein substrates.

Clinical evidence, mechanism, importance and management

(a) P-glycoprotein substrates

Cabozantinib is an inhibitor of the drug transporter protein P-glycoprotein *in vitro*,[1] and the US manufacturer therefore predicts that cabozantinib might increase the plasma concentrations of drugs that are P-glycoprotein substrates (see 'Table 1.12', p.14 for a list). The clinical relevance of this prediction is unclear, but until more is known consider the possibility of an interaction on the concurrent use of cabozantinib and drugs that are P-glycoprotein substrates.

(b) Rosiglitazone

In a study in patients with solid tumours, cabozantinib at doses of 100 mg or more daily for at least 21 days had no effect on the pharmacokinetics of a single-dose of the CYP2C8 substrate, **rosiglitazone**.[1]

1. Cometriq (Cabozantinib malate). Exelixis, Inc. US Prescribing information, November 2012.

Tyrosine kinase inhibitors; Crizotinib + Miscellaneous

Crizotinib might increase the concentrations of drugs that are CYP2B6 substrates or P-glycoprotein substrates.

Clinical evidence, mechanism, importance and management

(a) CYP2B6 substrates

In vitro studies have shown that crizotinib is an inhibitor of CYP2B6, and the UK and US manufacturers predict that it might therefore increase the concentrations of drugs that are CYP2B6 substrates.[1,2] See 'Table 1.3', p.6 for a list; the UK manufacturer additionally names **efavirenz**.[1]

(b) P-glycoprotein substrates

Crizotinib is an inhibitor of the drug transporter protein P-glycoprotein *in vitro*.[1,2] Crizotinib might therefore increase the plasma concentrations of other drugs that are P-glycoprotein substrates (see 'Table 1.12', p.14 for a list); the UK manufacturer additionally names **pravastatin**.[1] The clinical relevance of this prediction is unclear, but until more is known consider the possibility of an interaction on the concurrent use of crizotinib and drugs that are P-glycoprotein substrates.

1. Xalkori (Crizotinib). Pfizer Ltd. UK Summary of product characteristics, April 2013.
2. Xalkori (Crizotinib). Pfizer Inc. US Prescribing information, May 2013.

Tyrosine kinase inhibitors; Dasatinib + Miscellaneous

Dasatinib might increase the concentrations of CYP3A4 substrates. Dasatinib commonly causes thrombocytopenia and bleeding, and its effects might be additive with antiplatelet drugs and NSAIDs.

Clinical evidence, mechanism, importance and management

(a) Antiplatelet drugs and NSAIDs

Dasatinib adverse effects reported in clinical studies include haemorrhages, with severe gastrointestinal haemorrhages (some of which were fatal) occurring in 4% of patients, and CNS bleeds (some of which were fatal) occurring in less than 1% of patients.[1,2] Most of these events were associated with thrombocytopenia, which is a dose-limiting toxicity of dasatinib.[2] Patients were excluded from initial clinical studies if they were taking antiplatelet drugs but in subsequent studies, if the platelet count was greater than 50 to 75 $\times$ 10^9/L the use of aspirin or NSAIDs was permitted.[1,2] The UK and US manufacturers advise caution when drugs that have antiplatelet activity are given with dasatinib.[1,2] This seems a sensible precaution. For use with anticoagulants, see 'Coumarins and related drugs + Tyrosine kinase inhibitors', p.480.

(b) CYP3A4 substrates

Dasatinib is an inhibitor of CYP3A4, based on the effect of a single-dose on the pharmacokinetics of the sensitive CYP3A4 substrate, simvastatin, (see 'Statins + Tyrosine kinase inhibitors', p.1357), and it might therefore increase the plasma concentrations of other drugs that are substrates of CYP3A4. The UK and US manufacturers recommend caution with CYP3A4 substrates that have a narrow therapeutic range.[1,2] For a list of CYP3A4 substrates see 'Table 1.10', p.12. Further study is needed to establish the magnitude of any effect on multiple dosing.

1. Sprycel (Dasatinib monohydrate). Bristol-Myers Squibb Pharmaceutical Ltd. UK Summary of product characteristics, November 2013.
2. Sprycel (Dasatinib monohydrate). Bristol-Myers Squibb Company. US Prescribing information, April 2014.

Tyrosine kinase inhibitors; Erlotinib + Miscellaneous

CYP1A2 inhibitors (such as ciprofloxacin) slightly increase erlotinib exposure. P-glycoprotein inhibitors (such as verapamil) might also increase erlotinib exposure. Erlotinib might increase the concentrations of drugs glucuronidated by UGT1A1 (such as irinotecan). Cases of gastrointestinal bleeding have occurred in patients taking erlotinib, and some of these patients were also taking NSAIDs.

Clinical evidence, mechanism, importance and management

(a) CYP1A2 inhibitors

The AUC of erlotinib was increased by 39% when it was given with **ciprofloxacin**, and its maximum plasma concentration was increased by 17%, but this was not statistically significant.[1,2] The AUC and maximum plasma concentration of the active metabolite of erlotinib were increased by 60% and 48%, respectively.[2] Erlotinib is partially metabolised by CYP1A2, of which ciprofloxacin is a moderate inhibitor. Therefore concurrent use reduces erlotinib metabolism, resulting in a slight increase in exposure.

The UK manufacturer of erlotinib notes that the clinical relevance of these pharmacokinetic changes is unclear, but advises caution when **ciprofloxacin** or potent inhibitors of CYP1A2 are given with erlotinib, and they specifically name **fluvoxamine**.[2] It might be necessary to reduce the dose of erlotinib if adverse effects (rash, diarrhoea) occur.[1,2] This seems a sensible precaution. For a list of CYP1A2 inhibitors, see 'Table 1.2', p.5.

(b) NSAIDs

Cases of gastrointestinal bleeding have been reported in patients taking erlotinib, and in some cases patients were also taking NSAIDs. Gastrointestinal perforation has also been reported for erlotinib alone.[1,2] It would seem prudent to be aware of the possibility of additive adverse effects if erlotinib is given with an NSAID.

(c) P-glycoprotein inhibitors

Erlotinib is a substrate for the drug transporter protein P-glycoprotein. The UK manufacturer suggests that drugs that are inhibitors of P-glycoprotein might alter the pharmacokinetics (absorption and/or distribution) of erlotinib, and advise caution with their concurrent use.[2] Note that many CYP3A4 inhibitors are also inhibitors of P-glycoprotein, and both mechanisms might be involved in their interactions with erlotinib. For a list of drugs that are inhibitors of P-glycoprotein, see 'Table 1.12', p.14.

(d) UDP-glucuronyltransferase substrates

Erlotinib is a strong inhibitor of glucuronidation by UGT1A1 *in vitro*.[2,3] Theoretically, erlotinib might cause clinically relevant interactions with drugs that are substrates of UGT1A1 and that have a narrow therapeutic range. Examples include irinotecan (see 'Irinotecan + Tyrosine kinase inhibitors', p.691) and **etoposide**.[3]

1. Tarceva (Erlotinib hydrochloride). OSI Pharmaceuticals, LLC US Prescribing information, April 2014.
2. Tarceva (Erlotinib hydrochloride). Roche Products Ltd. UK Summary of product characteristics, December 2013.
3. Wen Z, Tallman MN, Ali SY, Smith PC. UDP-Glucuronosyltransferase 1A1 is the principle enzyme responsible for etoposide glucuronidation in human liver and intestinal microsomes: structural characterization of phenolic and alcoholic glucuronides of etoposide and estimation of enzyme kinetics. *Drug Metab Dispos* (2007) 35, 371–80.

Tyrosine kinase inhibitors; Erlotinib + Temozolomide

The effect of temozolomide on erlotinib pharmacokinetics is unclear.

Clinical evidence, mechanism, importance and management

As part of a phase I study, 16 patients with glioma were given erlotinib (100 mg daily increasing to 250 mg daily) alone, and 14 patients were given erlotinib with temozolomide 150 mg/m^2, increasing to 200 mg/m^2 for 5 days in each 28-day cycle. There was some variability in the pharmacokinetics of erlotinib between the patients taking the combination and those taking erlotinib alone at the different doses. For example, at the lowest dose of erlotinib (100 mg daily), in the group also taking temozolomide (3 patients), the maximum plasma concentration of erlotinib was 49% lower, and the AUCs of both erlotinib and its metabolite OSI-420 were almost 50% lower. Whereas, at a dose of erlotinib 200 mg daily, the difference was reversed, with the temozolomide group (3 patients) having a 45% higher AUC of erlotinib. However, with erlotinib 150 mg and 250 mg, no differences were apparent.[1] The reason for these paradoxical findings is unclear, and could be attributed to the small group sizes and an imbalance in some factors between the groups. In another similar study in paediatric patients, there was no apparent effect of temozolomide on erlotinib pharmacokinetics.[2] Further study is needed to assess whether an interaction actually occurs and if it does, the clinical relevance of this.

1. Prados MD, Lamborn KR, Chang S, Burton E, Butowski N, Malec M, Kapadia A, Rabbitt J, Page MS, Fedoroff A, Xie D, Kelley SK. Phase 1 study of erlotinib HCl alone and combined with temozolomide in patients with stable or recurrent malignant glioma. *Neuro-oncol* (2006) 8, 67–78.
2. Jakacki RI, Hamilton M, Gilbertson RJ, Blaney SM, Tersak J, Krailo MD, Ingle AM, Voss SD, Dancey JE, Adamson PC. Pediatric phase I and pharmacokinetic study of erlotinib followed by the combination of erlotinib and temozolomide: a Children's Oncology Group Phase I Consortium Study. *J Clin Oncol* (2008) 26, 4921–7.

Tyrosine kinase inhibitors; Erlotinib + Tobacco

Smoking moderately reduces the exposure to erlotinib.

Clinical evidence

In an analysis of erlotinib concentrations from a large phase III study of erlotinib in non-small cell lung cancer, the steady-state minimum plasma concentration of erlotinib was about 50% lower in smokers than in former smokers or patients who had never smoked.[1-3]

In a single-dose pharmacokinetic study in healthy subjects, 12 smokers and 14 non-smokers were given oral erlotinib 150 mg on day one and 300 mg on day 15. The subjects who smoked had a lower exposure to erlotinib; the AUC was 65% lower after the 150 mg dose and 57% lower after the 300 mg dose. The minimum plasma concentration was also lower after both the 150 mg dose (88%) and the 300 mg dose (70%), but the maximum plasma concentration of erlotinib was less affected (35% lower after the 150 mg dose and 20% lower after the 300 mg dose).[4] Using the same group of patients as a comparison, a subsequent pharmacokinetic study in patients who continued to smoke while receiving erlotinib, found that the median steady-state erlotinib concentrations while taking erlotinib 300 mg daily were similar to those of former smokers or those who have never smoked receiving erlotinib 150 mg daily. In addition, the maximum tolerated dose of erlotinib in smokers was 300 mg, which produced comparable toxicity (incidence of rash and diarrhoea) to the standard 150 mg dose in all patients in the earlier large phase III study of erlotinib.[5]

A population pharmacokinetic analysis of phase II and phase III single agent studies, found that the clearance of erlotinib in smokers was 24% faster than in former smokers or those who had never smoked.[6]

Mechanism

Cigarette smoking induces CYP1A1 and CYP1A2, which are involved in the metabolism of erlotinib, resulting in reduced exposure.

Importance and management

The pharmacokinetic interaction between smoking and erlotinib appears to be established, and is likely to be clinically important because smokers gain less benefit from erlotinib than non-smokers in clinical studies, although they do experience less toxicity.[7,8] Therefore, consideration should be given to the smoking status of a patient when planning treatment with erlotinib. The UK and US manufacturers state that patients should be encouraged to stop smoking[2,3] as early as possible before starting erlotinib.[3] In patients who continue to smoke, the dose of erlotinib should be cautiously increased to a maximum of 300 mg. In patients who stop smoking while taking erlotinib, the erlotinib dose should be immediately reduced to the recommended starting dose.[2]

1. Hamilton M, Wolf JL, Zborowski D, Lu J, Lum BL, Ding K, Clark GM, Rakhit A, Seymour L, Ptaszynski AM, Rusk J, Shepherd F. Tarceva (erlotinib) exposure/effects (EE) analysis from a phase III study in advanced NSCLC: effect of smoking on the PK of erlotinib. *Proc Am Assoc Cancer Res* (2005) 46, 1451.
2. Tarceva (Erlotinib hydrochloride). OSI Pharmaceuticals, LLC. US Prescribing information, April 2014.
3. Tarceva (Erlotinib hydrochloride). Roche Products Ltd. UK Summary of product characteristics, December 2013.
4. Hamilton M, Wolf JL, Rusk J, Beard SE, Clark GM, Witt K, Cagnoni PJ. Effects of smoking on the pharmacokinetics of erlotinib. *Clin Cancer Res* (2006) 12, 2166–71.
5. Hughes AN, O'Brien ME, Petty WJ, Chick JB, Rankin E, Woll PJ, Dunlop D, Nicolson M, Boinpally R, Wolf J, Price A. Overcoming CYP1A1/1A2 mediated induction of metabolism by escalating erlotinib dose in current smokers. *J Clin Oncol* (2009) 27, 1220–6.
6. Lu JF, Eppler SM, Wolf J, Hamilton M, Rakhit A, Bruno R, Lum BL. Clinical pharmacokinetics of erlotinib in patients with solid tumors and exposure-safety relationship in patients with non-small cell lung cancer. *Clin Pharmacol Ther* (2006) 80, 136–45.
7. Florescu M, Hasan B, Seymour L, Ding K, Shepherd FA; National Cancer Institute of Canada Clinical Trials Group. A clinical prognostic index for patients treated with erlotinib in National Cancer Institute of Canada Clinical Trials Group study BR.21. *J Thorac Oncol* (2008) 3, 590–8.
8. Faehling M, Eckert R, Kuom S, Kamp T, Stoiber KM, Schumann C. Benefit of erlotinib in patients with non-small-cell lung cancer is related to smoking status, gender, skin rash and radiological response but not to histology and treatment line. *Oncology* (2010) 78, 249–58.

Tyrosine kinase inhibitors; Gefitinib + Antineoplastics

Gefitinib does not alter the pharmacokinetics of cisplatin, carboplatin or paclitaxel, and these antineoplastics do not alter gefitinib pharmacokinetics. High-dose gefitinib slightly increases the exposure to gemcitabine.

Clinical evidence, mechanism, importance and management

(a) Carboplatin and Paclitaxel

In 24 patients with advanced non-small cell lung cancer there was no change in the pharmacokinetics of carboplatin or paclitaxel when gefitinib 250 or 500 mg daily was also given. There was a slight increase in the exposure to gefitinib, but no increase in toxicity was noted.[1]

(b) Cisplatin and Gemcitabine

Eighteen patients were given gemcitabine 1250 mg/m^2 on days one and 8 of a 21-day cycle, with cisplatin 80 mg/m^2 on day one and gefitinib 250 mg or 500 mg daily throughout. The pharmacokinetics of gefitinib were unchanged by the combination chemotherapy, and cisplatin pharmacokinetics were not affected by gefitinib. However, there was a small increase in exposure to gemcitabine on day 8 when gefitinib 500 mg daily was also given, compared with day one (gemcitabine and cisplatin only).[1]

1. Hammond LA. Pharmacokinetic evaluation of gefitinib when administered with chemotherapy. *Clin Lung Cancer* (2003) 5 (Suppl. 1), S18–S21.

Tyrosine kinase inhibitors; Gefitinib + CYP2D6 inhibitors

Inhibitors of CYP2D6 are predicted to increase gefitinib exposure.

Clinical evidence, mechanism, importance and management

The UK manufacturer notes that *in vitro* studies have shown that gefitinib is metabolised to its major metabolite by CYP2D6, and that in a clinical study in healthy subjects, exposure to gefitinib was 2-fold higher in CYP2D6 poor metabolisers (that is, those with little or no activity of this isoenzyme) than in CYP2D6 extensive metabolisers (those with normal activity of this isoenzyme). They state that this higher than average exposure achieved by CYP2D6 poor metabolisers might be clinically relevant because adverse effects are related to dose and exposure. Consequently, they also predict that potent inhibitors of CYP2D6 could increase gefitinib concentrations about 2-fold in extensive metabolisers.[1] Note, extensive metabolisers constitute about 90 to 95% of any given population, and an individual's CYP2D6 metaboliser status is rarely known. Therefore, the manufacturer advises that all patients should be closely monitored for adverse effects (e.g. diarrhoea and skin reactions) on starting a potent CYP2D6 inhibitor.[1] Until more is known, this would seem prudent. For a list of CYP2D6 inhibitors, see 'Table 1.7', p.9. It is also important to note that a patient already taking a potent CYP2D6 inhibitor before starting gefitinib is in a similar situation to a patient of poor metaboliser status, and might not tolerate the standard dose. Similar close monitoring for adverse effects would therefore seem a sensible precaution in these patients.

1. Iressa (Gefitinib monohydrate). AstraZeneca UK Ltd. UK Summary of product characteristics, June 2013.

Tyrosine kinase inhibitors; Imatinib + Antineoplastics

Data from *animal* studies suggest that imatinib moderately increases etoposide exposure and increases the plasma concentration of ifosfamide. The use of imatinib with asparaginase might be associated with increased hepatotoxicity.

Clinical evidence, mechanism, importance and management

(a) Asparaginase

The UK manufacturer states that the concurrent use of imatinib with asparaginase could be associated with increased hepatotoxicity. They therefore recommend caution on their concurrent use.[1]

(b) Etoposide and Ifosfamide

In a study in *mice*, a 5-fold increase in the maximum plasma concentration of etoposide and a 60% increase in the maximum plasma concentration of ifosfamide occurred when these antineoplastics were given by intraperitoneal injection with imatinib, compared with when they were given alone. In a further study, there was a 3.4-fold increase in the AUC_{0-3} of etoposide when it was given with imatinib. In yet another study, the AUC of etoposide was increased by 92% and its clearance reduced by about 50% when it was given with imatinib. In a lymphoma model, an increased antitumour effect was observed with the combination, but this was not seen in a small cell lung cancer model.[2]

Imatinib is an inhibitor of CYP3A4, and etoposide and ifosfamide are both metabolised by this isoenzyme. It therefore seems likely that the concentrations of both drugs were increased as a result of this effect on CYP3A4.

Although these data are from *animals*, and therefore preliminary, they suggest that caution is necessary if imatinib is used, particularly with etoposide, and possibly with ifosfamide.

1. Glivec (Imatinib mesilate). Novartis Pharmaceuticals UK Ltd. UK Summary of product characteristics, October 2013.
2. Rezaï K, Lokiec F, Grandjean I, Weill S, de Cremoux P, Bordier V, Ekue R, Garcia M, Poupon M-F, Decaudin D. Impact of imatinib on the pharmacokinetics and *in vivo* efficacy of etoposide and/or ifosfamide. *BMC Pharmacol* (2007) 7, 13.

Tyrosine kinase inhibitors; Imatinib + Cocaine

In two patients, relapse during treatment with imatinib occurred after they began to abuse cocaine.

Clinical evidence, mechanism, importance and management

Two patients with chronic myeloid leukaemia took imatinib and achieved a complete haematological response after 3 and 7 weeks, but then relapsed after 12 and 14 weeks and also experienced more severe imatinib adverse effects. Both patients had started to abuse cocaine 2 to 4 weeks before they relapsed. It was suggested that cocaine might have interfered with imatinib metabolism; however, the mechanism for this possible interaction is unclear.[1] The general relevance of this report is uncertain.

1. Breccia M, Gentilini F, Alimena G. Cocaine abuse may influence the response to imatinib in CML patients. *Haematologica* (2007) 92, e41–e42.

Tyrosine kinase inhibitors; Lapatinib + Miscellaneous

Lapatinib is predicted to increase the concentrations of CYP2C8 substrates, but some evidence with paclitaxel (a CYP2C8 substrate) suggests that the effect of lapatinib is only minor. Lapatinib moderately increased the exposure to digoxin (a P-glycoprotein substrate) and would be expected to increase the exposure to other P-glycoprotein substrates. In addition, lapatinib concentrations are expected to be affected by inducers and inhibitors of P-glycoprotein.

Clinical evidence, mechanism, importance and management

(a) CYP2C8 substrates

In vitro, lapatinib is an inhibitor of CYP2C8 at clinically relevant concentrations, and the UK manufacturer[1] therefore advises avoiding the concurrent use of oral drugs that have a narrow therapeutic range and are substrates of this isoenzyme (they name **repaglinide**), whereas the US manufacturer advises caution.[2] For a list of CYP2C8 substrates, see 'Table 1.4', p.6. However, in a study in patients with cancer, lapatinib had only a minor effect on the exposure to paclitaxel (a CYP2C8 substrate); see 'Tyrosine kinase inhibitors + Taxanes', p.739, so the clinical relevance of the predicted interaction with CYP2C8 substrates, such as **repaglinide**, requires confirmation.

(b) P-glycoprotein inducers, inhibitors, and substrates

In vitro lapatinib is an inhibitor of P-glycoprotein at clinically relevant concentrations, and it is therefore predicted to increase the exposure to P-glycoprotein substrates.[1,2] The UK manufacturer briefly notes that lapatinib increased the exposure to the P-glycoprotein substrate, **digoxin** (AUC increased by 80%),[1] while the US manufacturer states that concurrent use increased digoxin exposure 2.8-fold.[2] The magnitude of this increase is clinically relevant, and reduced **digoxin** dose requirements would be expected to be necessary when lapatinib is given. All patients taking digoxin with lapatinib should be monitored for digoxin adverse effects (such as bradycardia), have their digoxin concentrations measured, and their digoxin dose reduced if necessary. The US manufacturers of lapatanib specifically advise that digoxin serum concentrations be checked before, and throughout, concurrent use with lapatinib, and that if the digoxin serum concentration exceeds 1.2 nanograms/mL, the digoxin dose should be reduced by half.[2]

Caution is also recommended with other P-glycoprotein substrates with a narrow therapeutic range. For a list of P-glycoprotein substrates see 'Table 1.12', p.14.

Lapatinib is also a substrate of P-glycoprotein, and the UK and US manufacturers therefore state that caution is warranted with drugs that are inhibitors or inducers of P-glycoprotein, as altered lapatinib concentrations are likely to result.[1,2] For a list of drugs that are inhibitors or inducers of P-glycoprotein see 'Table 1.12', p.14. Note that many CYP3A4 inhibitors are also inhibitors of P-glycoprotein, and both mechanisms might be involved in their interactions with lapatinib.

1. Tyverb (Lapatinib ditosylate monohydrate). GlaxoSmithKline UK. UK Summary of product characteristics, March 2014.
2. Tykerb (Lapatinib ditosylate monohydrate). GlaxoSmithKline. US Prescribing information, October 2013.

Tyrosine kinase inhibitors; Lapatinib + Trastuzumab

There appears to be no pharmacokinetic interaction between lapatinib and trastuzumab.

Clinical evidence, mechanism, importance and management

In a phase I study in women with advanced breast cancer, the pharmacokinetics of lapatinib and trastuzumab did not differ when these drugs were given together, compared with each drug given separately.[1]

1. Storniolo AM, Pegram MD, Overmoyer B, Silverman P, Peacock NW, Jones SF, Loftiss J, Arya N, Koch KM, Paul E, Pandite L, Fleming RA, Lebowitz PF, Ho PT, Burris HA. Phase I dose escalation and pharmacokinetic study of lapatinib in combination with trastuzumab in patients with advanced ErbB2-positive breast cancer. *J Clin Oncol* (2008) 26, 3317–23.

Tyrosine kinase inhibitors; Nilotinib + Miscellaneous

Theoretically, nilotinib might increase the concentrations of drugs that are substrates of P-glycoprotein, and might alter the concentrations of CYP2C9 substrates.

Clinical evidence, mechanism, importance and management

(a) CYP2C9 substrates

The UK and US manufacturers[1,2] state that, *in vitro*, nilotinib is a relatively strong inhibitor of CYP2C9, although the US manufacturer[1] notes that *in vitro* studies showed it might also induce CYP2C9. The clinical importance of its effects on CYP2C9 remain to be established, particularly as a single-dose of nilotinib had no effect on the pharmacokinetics of *S*-warfarin, a moderate CYP2C9 substrate (see 'Coumarins and related drugs + Tyrosine kinase inhibitors', p.480). Nevertheless, because an effect at steady-state cannot be ruled out, the US manufacturer of nilotinib advises caution if it is given with drugs that are substrates of CYP2C9, particularly those with a narrow therapeutic range.[1] Until more is known, this might be prudent. For a list of CYP2C9 substrates, see 'Table 1.5', p.7.

(b) P-glycoprotein inhibitors and substrates

Nilotinib is a substrate of P-glycoprotein, and the UK and US manufacturers therefore predict that inhibitors of P-glycoprotein will increase nilotinib concentrations, and they advise caution on their concurrent use.[1,2] For a list of drugs that are inhibitors of P-glycoprotein, see 'Table 1.12', p.14.

The US manufacturer also states that nilotinib is a P-glycoprotein inhibitor and therefore predicts that the concurrent use of nilotinib with drugs that are substrates of P-glycoprotein might lead to an increase in their concentrations;[1] however, the clinical relevance of this prediction needs confirming. For a list of drugs that are substrates of P-glycoprotein, see 'Table 1.12', p.14.

1. Tasigna (Nilotinib hydrochloride monohydrate). Novartis Pharmaceuticals Corp. US Prescribing information, January 2014.
2. Tasigna (Nilotinib hydrochloride monohydrate). Novartis Pharmaceuticals UK Ltd. UK Summary of product characteristics, December 2013.

Tyrosine kinase inhibitors; Pazopanib + Miscellaneous

Pazopanib has no effect on caffeine exposure but might increase the exposure to CYP2C8 substrates.

Clinical evidence, mechanism, importance and management

(a) Caffeine

In a pharmacokinetic study in patients with cancer, pazopanib 800 mg daily for 17 days had no effect on the pharmacokinetics of a single 200-mg dose of **caffeine**.[1] Caffeine can be used as a probe substrate to assess the activity of drugs on CYP1A2. This study therefore suggests that pazopanib is not a clinically relevant inducer or inhibitor of this isoenzyme.

(b) CYP2C8 substrates

Based on its effect on paclitaxel, a substrate of CYP2C8 and CYP3A4 (see 'Tyrosine kinase inhibitors + Taxanes', p.739), the US manufacturer states that the use of pazopanib with CYP2C8 substrates that have a narrow therapeutic range is not recommended.[2] Few drugs are known to be CYP2C8 substrates (see 'Table 1.4', p.6 for a list), and, with the exception of paclitaxel, none are known to have a narrow therapeutic range.

1. Goh BC, Reddy NJ, Dandamudi UB, Laubscher KH, Peckham T, Hodge JP, Suttle AB, Arumugham T, Xu Y, Xu C-F, Lager J, Dar MM, Lewis LD. An evaluation of the drug interaction potential of pazopanib, an oral vascular endothelial growth factor receptor tyrosine kinase inhibitor, using a modified Cooperstown 5 +1 cocktail in patients with advanced solid tumours. *Clin Pharmacol Ther* (2010) 88, 652–9.
2. Votrient (Pazopanib hydrochloride). GlaxoSmithKline. US Prescribing information, November 2013.

Tyrosine kinase inhibitors; Ponatinib + Miscellaneous

Ponatinib is predicted to increase the concentrations of drugs that are substrates of P-glycoprotein and breast cancer resistance protein.

Clinical evidence, mechanism, importance and management

Ponatinib has been shown *in vitro*, to be an inhibitor of the drug transporter proteins P-glycoprotein and breast cancer resistance protein (BCRP). However the clinical relevance of this in relation to the effect on drugs that are substrates of these transporter proteins has not been studied.[1] Theoretically the concentrations of such drugs could be increased. See 'Table 1.12', p.14 for a list of drugs that are P-glycoprotein substrates; the US manufacturer of ponatinib additionally names **ambrisentan**, **imatinib**, **lapatinib**, **maraviroc**, **nilotinib**, **posaconazole**, **ranolazine**, **saxagliptin**, **sitagliptin**, and **tolvaptan**. The US manufacturer names **imatinib**, **lapatinib**, **methotrexate**, **mitoxantrone**, **rosuvastatin**, **sulfasalazine**, and **topotecan** as examples of BCRP substrates.[1]

Until more is known consider the possibility of an interaction on the concurrent use of ponatinib and any of these drugs.

1. Iclusig (Ponatinib). ARIAD Pharmaceuticals, Inc. US Prescribing information, January 2014.

Tyrosine kinase inhibitors; Regorafenib + Rosiglitazone

The pharmacokinetics of rosiglitazone are not affected by regorafenib.

Clinical evidence, mechanism, importance and management

In a study in patients with advanced solid tumours, regorafenib 160 mg daily for 14 days had no effect on the pharmacokinetics of a single 4-mg dose of rosiglitazone.[1]

1. Stivarga (Regorafenib). Bayer HealthCare Pharmaceuticals Inc. US Prescribing information, August 2013.

Tyrosine kinase inhibitors; Ruxolitinib + Miscellaneous

The UK manufacturer predicts that ruxolitinib might increase the concentrations of P-glycoprotein substrates.

Clinical evidence, mechanism, importance and management

The UK manufacturer of ruxolitinib states that *in vitro* data indicate that it might inhibit intestinal P-glycoprotein and this might result in increased concentrations of drugs that are substrates of this transporter;[1] for a list of drugs that are P-glycoprotein substrates see 'Table 1.12', p.14. Further, they advise that the potential inhibition might be minimised by separating administration by as long as possible.[1] However the US manufacturer states that ruxolitinib is not an inhibitor of P-glycoprotein *in vitro*.[2]

1. Jakavi (Ruxolitinib phosphate). Novartis Pharmaceuticals UK Ltd. UK Summary of product characteristics, June 2013.
2. Jakafi (Ruxolitinib phosphate). Incyte Corporation. US Prescribing Information, November 2013.

Tyrosine kinase inhibitors; Sorafenib + Doxorubicin

Sorafenib can cause a small increase doxorubicin exposure. Doxorubicin does not appear to alter sorafenib pharmacokinetics.

Clinical evidence, mechanism, importance and management

In a phase I study in which sorafenib (in increasing doses from 100 mg to 400 mg twice daily) was given continuously with intravenous doxorubicin on day one of a 3-week cycle, sorafenib either had no effect on the exposure (AUC) to doxorubicin or caused up to a 47% increase in exposure. However, this did not appear to increase the degree of myelosuppression.[1] The UK manufacturer notes that a 21% increase in the AUC of intravenous doxorubicin occurred when it was given with sorafenib.[2] Doxorubicin did not alter the pharmacokinetics of sorafenib.[1] The clinical relevance of the increases in doxorubicin exposure seen is unknown.

1. Richly H, Henning BF, Kupsch P, Passarge K, Grubert M, Hilger RA, Christensen O, Brendel E, Schwartz B, Ludwig M, Flashar C, Voigtmann R, Scheulen ME, Seeber S, Strumberg D. Results of a Phase I trial of sorafenib (BAY 43-9006) in combination with doxorubicin in patients with refractory solid tumors. *Ann Oncol* (2006) 17, 866–73.
2. Nexavar (Sorafenib tosylate). Bayer plc. UK Summary of product characteristics, February 2013.

Tyrosine kinase inhibitors; Sorafenib + Neomycin

Neomycin reduces sorafenib exposure.

Clinical evidence, mechanism, importance and management

The UK and US manufacturers of sorafenib note that, in healthy subjects, a 5-day regimen of neomycin reduced sorafenib exposure by 54%.[1,2] This is because neomycin reduces the enterohepatic recycling of sorafenib by eradicating gastrointestinal bacteria with glucuronidase activity, which split the glucuronide conjugates of sorafenib allowing reabsorption of unconjugated sorafenib. Other antibacterials have not been studied and their effect is likely to depend on their ability to eradicate bacteria with glucuronidase activity.[1]

It is likely that neomycin will reduce the efficacy of sorafenib, and the possibility of this should be taken into account if neomycin or another antibacterial with similar effects on gut bacteria is required.[1] It would seem prudent to monitor concurrent use for sorafenib efficacy.

1. Nexavar (Sorafenib tosylate). Bayer plc. UK Summary of product characteristics, February 2013.
2. Nexavar (Sorafenib tosylate). Bayer HealthCare Pharmaceuticals Inc. US Prescribing information, November 2013.

Tyrosine kinase inhibitors; Sunitinib + Ifosfamide

The concurrent use of ifosfamide might modestly decrease sunitinib exposure, and might also increase the risk of neutropenia.

Clinical evidence, mechanism, importance and management

In a phase I dose-finding study in patients with advanced cancer, an infusion of ifosfamide (9 g/m^2 over 3 days or 6 g/m^2 over 5 days) reduced the AUC of sunitinib by about 40% and 23% with the 3-day and 5-day schedules, respectively, with a corresponding increase in exposure of the active metabolite SU12262.[1,2] Ifosfamide pharmacokinetics were not affected by sunitinib.[1,2] It was suggested that ifosfamide auto-induction of metabolism might also have increased metabolism of sunitinib to its active metabolite. In this study the maximum tolerated dose of continuous sunitinib with ifosfamide was just 12.5 mg daily, with the dose-limiting toxicity being neutropenia, which suggests that synergistic toxicity might occur.[1] Further study is needed.

1. Hamberg P, Steeghs N, Loos WJ, van de Biessen D, den Hollander M, Tascilar M, Verweij J, Gelderblom H, Sleijfer S. Decreased exposure to sunitinib due to concomitant administration of ifosfamide: results of a phase I and pharmacokinetic study on the combination of sunitinib and ifosfamide in patients with advanced solid malignancies. *Br J Cancer* (2010) 102, 1699–706.
2. Loos W, Hamberg P, Steeghs N, Kroep J, Tascilar M, Verweij J, den Hollander M, van der Biessen D, Gelderblom H, Sleijfer S. Pharmacokinetic interaction between intravenous ifosfamide and oral sunitinib. *Clin Pharmacol Ther* (2010) 87 (Suppl 1), S78.

Tyrosine kinase inhibitors; Tofacitinib + Immunosuppressants

There is a risk of additive immunosuppression if tofacitinib is given with azathioprine.

Clinical evidence, mechanism, importance and management

The US manufacturer of tofacitinib briefly notes that there is a risk of increased immunosuppression when tofacitinib is given with potent immunosuppressants, including **azathioprine**, but that this has not been studied in patients with rheumatoid arthritis.[1] Some caution is therefore required on concurrent use with azathioprine, including monitoring for signs of excessive immunosuppression, such as infection.

1. Xeljanz (Tofacitinib citrate). Pfizer Inc. US Prescribing information, November 2012.

Tyrosine kinase inhibitors; Tofacitinib + Methotrexate

The pharmacokinetics of tofacitinib and methotrexate are not altered by concurrent use.

Clinical evidence, mechanism, importance and management

In a pharmacokinetics study, 12 rheumatoid arthritis patients were given tofacitinib 30 mg twice daily for 4 days alone, with a single 30-mg dose of methotrexate the following day which was given 5 minutes after a further 30 mg dose of tofacitinib. The pharmacokinetics of tofacitinib were not altered, whereas the AUC and maximum concentration of methotrexate were reduced by 10% and 13%, respectively. However, these small changes were not considered clinically relevant.[1] No dose adjustments of either drug are therefore necessary on concurrent use.

1. Cohen S, Zwillich SH, Chow V, LaBadie RR, Wilkinson B. Co-administration of the JAK inhibitor CP-960,550 and methotrexate is well tolerated in patients with rheumatoid arthritis without need for dose adjustment. *Br J Clin Pharmacol* (2010) 69, 143–51.

Vinca alkaloids + Anthracyclines

There appears to be no pharmacokinetic interaction between vinflunine and non-liposomal doxorubicin, but the combination caused a high incidence of neutropenia. The combination of liposomal doxorubicin and vinflunine might increase vinflunine exposure and decrease doxorubicin exposure. There is evidence from *in vitro* and animal studies suggesting that anthracyclines and vinca alkaloids might be antagonistic and that this might be sequence-dependent.

Clinical evidence

(a) Vinblastine

In an *in vitro* study in primary leukaemia cells from children, **doxorubicin** inhibited vinblastine-induced apoptosis.[1]

(b) Vincristine

In vitro and animal studies suggest that **doxorubicin** can inhibit the antitumour effect of vincristine, and that this effect might be sequence-dependent.[1] *In vitro* inhibition of vincristine-induced apoptosis was also seen with **daunorubicin**, **epirubicin**, and **idarubicin**.[1]

(c) Vinflunine

In a phase I clinical study, patients with breast cancer were given either vinflunine 250 mg/m^2 and **doxorubicin** 40 mg/m^2 on day 1 of a 3-week cycle, or vinflunine 120 mg/m^2 and doxorubicin 25 mg/m^2 twice (on days 1 and 8) of a 3-week cycle. Vinflunine was infused over 20 minutes followed by doxorubicin infused over 30 minutes. The concentrations of vinflunine and doxorubicin, and their metabolites, did not differ from reference data for each drug used alone. The planned dose escalation in this study was not possible because of dose-limiting neutropenia.[2]

The UK manufacturer of vinflunine notes that, in another study using *liposomal* **doxorubicin**, there was an apparent 15% to 30% increase in vinflunine AUC and an apparent 50 to 66% decrease in doxorubicin AUC, with no change in the concentration of the metabolite, doxorubicinol.[3]

(d) Vinorelbine

In an *in vitro* study in primary leukaemia cells from children, **doxorubicin** inhibited vinorelbine-induced apoptosis.[1]

Mechanism

Doxorubicin and other anthracyclines appear to induce cell cycle arrest, whereas vinca alkaloids appear to require active cell cycling for their antitumour effect. Therefore anthracyclines might reduce the activity of vinca alkaloids if the anthracycline is given before the vinca alkaloid.[1] The UK manufacturer of vinflunine speculates that it might adsorb onto *liposomal* doxorubicin leading to the pharmacokinetic changes seen.[3]

Importance and management

No pharmacokinetic interaction appears to occur between vinflunine and non-liposomal doxorubicin, but the combination had a high incidence of neutropenia. Bear this in mind if these drugs are given concurrently. Caution is required on the concurrent use of *liposomal* doxorubicin and vinflunine because of the possible pharmacokinetic interaction, which might increase vinflunine toxicity and decrease doxorubicin efficacy.

Doxorubicin and vincristine are commonly used together on the same day in various chemotherapy protocols. However, the authors of the *in vitro* study state that these two drugs might be better given on different days,[1] and note that the sequencing of anthracyclines and vinca alkaloids was never optimised in controlled studies.

1. Ehrhardt H, Schrembs D, Moritz C, Wachter F, Haldar S, Graubner U, Nathrath M, Jeremias I. Optimized anti-tumor effects of anthracyclines plus Vinca alkaloids using a novel, mechanism-based application schedule. *Blood* (2011) 118, 6123–31.
2. Zaman K, Durando X, Baurain JF, Humblet Y, Mazzeo F, Bostnavaron M, Meheust N, Monnoyer-Favrel S, Machiels JP, Bauer J. A phase I clinical and pharmacological study evaluating vinflunine in combination with doxorubicin as first line treatment in metastatic breast cancer. *Breast Cancer Res Treat* (2011) 127, 689–96.
3. Javlor (Vinflunine ditartrate). Pierre Fabre Ltd. UK Summary of product characteristics, June 2012.

Vinca alkaloids + Antiepileptics; Enzyme-inducing

Carbamazepine and phenytoin appear to reduce vincristine exposure, and appear to reduce its efficacy. Phenobarbital is expected to interact with vincristine in the same way. Other vinca alkaloids might be similarly affected when given with enzyme-inducing antiepileptics.

Clinical evidence

(a) Effect on vincristine

The systemic clearance of vincristine 2 mg was 63% higher, and the AUC was 43% lower, in 9 patients receiving **carbamazepine** or **phenytoin**, than in 6 patients not taking antiepileptics. In this study, patients were being treated with procarbazine, lomustine, and vincristine for brain tumours.[1] In a retrospective cohort analysis of chemotherapy for B-lineage acute lymphoblastic leukaemia, 28 children receiving long-term antiepileptics (**phenytoin**, **phenobarbital**, **carbamazepine**, or a combination) had worse event-free survival (hazard ratio 2.7), and greater haematological relapse (hazard ratio 3.4) and CNS relapse (hazard ratio 2.9), than 574 children not taking these antiepileptics. The authors considered that the increased clearance of vincristine induced by the antiepileptics was a likely factor in these findings.[2] However, this increased risk or relapse was not seen in 114 children with T-cell leukaemia, 12 of whom were taking these antiepileptics.[2]

(b) Effect on phenytoin

For reports of reduced phenytoin concentrations in patients receiving chemotherapy that included vinca alkaloids, see 'Table 14.1', p.563.

Mechanism

These enzyme-inducing antiepileptics increase the metabolism of vincristine by CYP3A4. Other vinca alkaloids are also metabolised by this route and are therefore likely to be similarly affected.

Importance and management

Although evidence is limited, **carbamazepine**, **phenobarbital**, and **phenytoin** would be expected to reduce the efficacy of vincristine and other vinca alkaloids. Where possible, it would seem prudent to try to avoid the use of these enzyme-inducing antiepileptics in patients requiring vinca alkaloids. However, if concurrent use is unavoidable, monitor closely for antineoplastic efficacy, being aware that it might be necessary to increase the dose of the vinca alkaloid. Also note that **primidone** is metabolised to phenobarbital and **fosphenytoin** is metabolised to phenytoin, and these drugs are therefore also expected to reduce the efficacy of the vinca alkaloids.

Due to the risk of decreased phenytoin concentrations in patients also given a vinca alkaloid (see 'Table 14.1', p.563), if concurrent use is considered essential, it would be prudent to monitor phenytoin concentrations. Until more is known, similar precautions might also be warranted with fosphenytoin.

1. Villikka K, Kivistö KT, Mäenpää H, Joensuu H, Neuvonen PJ. Cytochrome P450-inducing antiepileptics increase the clearance of vincristine in patients with brain tumors. *Clin Pharmacol Ther* (1999) 66, 589–93.
2. Relling MV, Pui CH, Sandlund JT, Rivera GK, Hancock ML, Boyett JM, Schuetz EG, Evans WE. Adverse effect of anticonvulsants on efficacy of chemotherapy for acute lymphoblastic leukaemia. *Lancet* (2000) 356, 285–90.

Vinca alkaloids + Azoles

Itraconazole can increase the toxicity of vincristine, and there is some limited evidence that this is particularly likely with the oral liquid formulation of itraconazole and at higher doses. There are case reports of itraconazole increasing the toxicity of vinblastine, vindesine, and vinorelbine. A similar interaction has been reported in patients given vincristine and fluconazole, ketoconazole, posaconazole, or voriconazole. Ketoconazole appears to increase vinflunine exposure.

Clinical evidence

(a) Vinblastine

Acute neurotoxicity and myelotoxicity occurred in a boy with Hodgkin's lymphoma receiving vinblastine, doxorubicin, and methotrexate when he was also given **itraconazole**. The toxicity did not occur when he was given the same chemotherapy without itraconazole.[1]

(b) Vincristine

A retrospective study in 50 patients with acute lymphoblastic leukaemia given vincristine-based treatment, found that the numbers of patients discontinuing vincristine, or requiring dose modifications, was higher in 29 patients also given an azole (**fluconazole**, **posaconazole**, or **voriconazole**) than in those who were not: 48% compared with about 10% and 59% compared with 24%, respectively. Overall 66% of patients taking azoles developed symptoms of decreased peristalsis, compared with 29% of those not given an azole. Specifically, this was seen in 50% of the patients given **fluconazole** 100 to 400 mg daily, two thirds of those given **posaconazole** 400 mg twice daily, and 75% of those given oral **voriconazole** 200 to 300 mg twice daily or intravenous **voriconazole** 4 mg/kg twice daily.[2] Similarly, in a retrospective study, vincristine-induced toxicity in 20 children with ALL given vincristine and an azole (16 taking **itraconazole**, one taking **fluconazole**, two taking **voriconazole** and one taking both itraconazole and voriconazole, mainly in prophylactic doses) was compared with a period where the same children were given vincristine alone. In the presence of an azole there were 12 cases of peripheral neuropathy (at least grade 3) and 6 cases of CNS toxicity (seizures, toxic encephalopathy, syndrome of inappropriate secretion of antidiuretic hormone (SIADH)), compared with no cases when vincristine was given alone. In addition constipation was more frequently reported when the children were also given an azole.[3] Another retrospective analysis also reported a higher incidence of paralytic ileus, severe constipation and peripheral neuropathy in patients treated with vincristine and given an azole (predominantly **itraconazole**).[4]

For discussion of studies and case reports of the effects of individual azoles in vincristine-treated patients, see below.

1. Itraconazole. Four out of 14 adults with acute lymphoblastic leukaemia (ALL) given induction chemotherapy with weekly injections of vincristine (with prednisone, daunorubicin, and asparaginase) and antifungal prophylaxis with oral itraconazole capsules 400 mg daily, developed severe and early vincristine-induced neurotoxicity (paraesthesia and muscle weakness of the hands and feet, paralytic ileus, mild laryngeal nerve paralysis). The degree and early onset of these neurotoxic reactions were unusual, and were all reversible except for mild paraesthesia in one patient. The complications were more serious than in a previous series of 460 patients given vincristine without itraconazole (29% compared with 6%).[5] Similarly, five consecutive children with ALL enrolled in an open study of prophylactic oral itraconazole 2.5 mg/kg daily (presumably as a liquid formulation) developed severe vincristine toxicity (constipation, abdominal pain, hypertension, ileus, hyponatraemia, seizures) attributed to the concurrent use of itraconazole. They were also receiving nifedipine, which also appears to reduce the clearance of vincristine (see 'Vinca alkaloids + Nifedipine', p.748), and which could have made things worse.[6] Since these two reports, cases of severe vincristine neurotoxicity have been reported in five other children[7-11] and two adults[12] with ALL when they were given oral (liquid formulation where stated[11,12]) or intravenous[9] itraconazole. In a further series of 9 children given weekly vincristine and oral itraconazole 5 mg/kg (liquid formulation), all developed increased vincristine toxicity, with 4 patients experiencing seizures.[13] Similarly, in yet another study, 5 of 7 adults given vincristine as part of CHOP (cyclophosphamide, doxorubicin, vincristine, and prednisolone) for lymphoma developed vincristine neurotoxicity when receiving oral itraconazole 200 mg daily as a solution. Of note, none of the patients who received vincristine and itraconazole 200 mg daily as capsules developed neurotoxicity.[14] A study in children with haematological malignancies given vincristine reported that 3 of 22 patients also given itraconazole 25 to 200 mg daily (liquid formulation) developed non-alcoholic steatohepatitis (2 patients) or syndrome of inappropriate antidiuretic hormone secretion (SIADH, one patient).[15]

2. Ketoconazole. Vincristine-induced neurotoxicity (peripheral neuropathy, constipation, urinary retention, seizures, transient blindness) was attributed to malnutrition by the authors of one study in 10 children with cancer.[16] However, others consider that the concurrent use of ketoconazole in these patients is a more likely explanation of the toxicity seen.[17]

3. Posaconazole. A patient given posaconazole 400 mg twice daily who also received four doses of vincristine 2 mg at weekly intervals developed bilateral foot paraesthesia and was unable to walk unassisted. Treatment with posaconazole and any vinca alkaloids was stopped, but 5 months later, the patient showed little signs of improvement.[18] A 9-year-old girl with acute lymphoblastic leukaemia was given two doses of vincristine 1.5 mg/m^2 on days 1 and 6 as part of a chemotherapy regimen (which included dexamethasone, asparaginase, and methotrexate) having started posaconazole 50 mg three times daily as prophylaxis 5 days earlier. Six days after the last dose of vincristine she developed severe peripheral neuropathy, abdominal cramps, and constipation. One week later, this had progressed to severe neurotoxicity (reduced consciousness, agitation, confusion) and seizures due to syndrome of inappropriate antidiuretic hormone secretion (SIADH). Vincristine toxicity was suspected (although vincristine concentrations were not measured), and posaconazole was stopped. All symptoms resolved within 7 days of discontinuing the posaconazole. The possibility of methotrexate toxicity was ruled out as methotrexate concentrations and renal function were not increased.[19] Two similar cases of vincristine-induced neurotoxicity with SIADH in patients also given posaconazole have been reported: one in a 4-year-old boy and the other in a 19-year-old woman.[20,21]

4. Voriconazole. A 5-year-old girl with acute lymphoblastic leukaemia was given 4 doses of weekly vincristine as part of a chemotherapy induction regimen. A fungal infection was suspected and an 8-week course of voriconazole (dose not stated) with levofloxacin was started. She had two further doses of vincristine, at weeks 2 and 3 of the voriconazole course, but at week 5, she developed a severe foot drop. Vincristine-induced peripheral neuropathy was suspected and the following 10 vincristine doses were withheld. The voriconazole course was completed during this time, and the neuropathy recovered over the next few months. She was also found to have a genetic disorder (Charcot-Marie-Tooth, CMT1X) which could have predisposed her to developing vincristine-induced neuropathy; however, she was subsequently given reduced and full-dose vincristine and did not develop neuropathy.[22] In contrast, none of the eight patients who received antifungal prophylaxis with voriconazole 200 mg twice daily during the initial phase of treatment, for acute lymphoblastic leukaemia with vincristine and other chemotherapy, developed neurotoxicity.[23]

(c) Vindesine

Two cases of vindesine-associated neuropathy were reported in two adult patients. In the first case, paralytic ileus developed 9 days after the patient started to take **itraconazole** solution; vindesine was given 2 and 9 days after itraconazole was started. On stopping the itraconazole, his symptoms improved rapidly. The second case was that of a 37-year-old woman who received vindesine on days one, 8 and 15. Intravenous **itraconazole** was given from day 9, and 5 days after this she developed symptoms of neurotoxicity, which resolved rapidly on stopping itraconazole and vindesine.[24]

(d) Vinflunine

The UK manufacturer briefly reports that, in a study, **ketoconazole** 400 mg daily for 8 days increased the exposure to vinflunine (dose not stated) and its active metabolite, 4-O-deacetylvinflunine, by 30% and 50%, respectively.[25]

(e) Vinorelbine

A 72-year-old man with fungal pneumonia and lung cancer received **itraconazole** (dose not stated) and vinorelbine with cisplatin. After chemotherapy he developed constipation, oral mucositis, and leucopenia, and he progressively deteriorated and died 12 days later.[26]

Mechanism

The reasons for these interactions are not fully understood, but it has been suggested that itraconazole inhibits the metabolism of vincristine by the CYP3A subfamily.[5] Another possible explanation is that itraconazole inhibits P-glycoprotein,[5] and increased vincristine neurotoxicity might be the result of the inhibition of this pump in endothelial cells of the blood-brain barrier.[27] All of the other clinically used vinca alkaloids (vinblastine, vindesine, vinflunine, and vinorelbine) are known to be metabolised by CYP3A4. Vinblastine and, to a lesser extent, vinflunine, are also substrates for P-glycoprotein. All azoles are known inhibitors of CYP3A4, albeit to varying degrees, see 'Table 1.9', p.11, for a categorisation.

Importance and management

The interaction between vinca alkaloids and the azoles is reasonably well documented, and although largely limited to case reports and retrospective analyses, is clinically important. The interaction between itraconazole and vincristine is the best established. The authors of many of the reports[3,5,7,11-13,17] suggest that itraconazole should be avoided in patients taking vincristine (an alternative non-azole antifungal should be used[17,28]), or that treatment with itraconazole should be interrupted when vincristine is given.[9,10,28] There is some evidence that the liquid oral formulations of itraconazole might be more likely to interact (because of higher oral bioavailability for a given dose)[14] and that the interaction might be dose-related (less likely with 200 mg daily than 400 mg daily as capsules,[14] and less likely with monthly vincristine than weekly vincristine[7]). Although less well documented, itraconazole might interact similarly with vinblastine, vindesine, and vinorelbine.

Data for the other azoles and vinca alkaloids is less conclusive, but what is known suggests that all pairs might interact in the same way, but to a greater or lesser extent. If the mechanism is correct, the azoles that are potent CYP3A4 inhibitors will have the greatest effect (**itraconazole**, **ketoconazole**, **voriconazole**), particularly if they also inhibit P-glycoprotein, as with itraconazole. Given the severity of the possible outcome, it would seem prudent to avoid the concurrent use of these azoles with any vinca alkaloid, or, if this is not possible, monitor for an increase in toxicity. Some authors do not recommend reducing the dose of the vinca alkaloid because of the lack of pharmacokinetic studies and therapeutic drug monitoring to guide dose adjustment, and because of the importance of dose intensity in many chemotherapy protocols.[17]

Fluconazole and **posaconazole** are moderate CYP3A4 inhibitors, and as such, are unlikely to interact to the same extent as the potent CYP3A4 inhibitors. Nevertheless, the case reports illustrate that serious adverse effects, such as neurotoxicity, do occur, and therefore the same precautions recommended for the potent CYP3A4 inhibitors should be followed.

Although there are no data for **miconazole** oral gel, it is known that maximum doses of miconazole oral gel are sufficiently absorbed to potentially have systemic effects. It would therefore seem prudent to be alert for any evidence of vinca alkaloid toxicity in patients also using miconazole oral gel.

1. Bashir H, Motl S, Metzger ML, Howard SC, Kaste S, Krasin MP, Hudson MM. Itraconazole-enhanced chemotherapy toxicity in a patient with Hodgkin lymphoma. *J Pediatr Hematol Oncol* (2006) 28, 33–5.
2. Harnicar S, Adel N, Jurcic J. Modification of vincristine dosing during concomitant azole therapy in adult acute lymphoblastic leukemia patients. *J Oncol Pharm Pract* (2009) 15, 175–82.
3. van Schie RM, Brüggemann RJ, Hoogerbrugge PM, te Loo DM. Effect of azole antifungal therapy on vincristine toxicity in childhood acute lymphoblastic leukaemia. *J Antimicrob Chemother* (2011) 66, 1853–6.
4. Osato Y, Yokoyama T, Saito Y, Kani R, Hayabe H, Miyamatsu H, Ohyashiki K. [A retrospective analysis of neurotoxicity induced by vinca alkaloids combined with azole anti-fungal agents in hematological malignancies]. *Gan To Kagaku Ryoho* (2011) 38, 1667–72.
5. Böhme A, Ganser A, Hoelzer D. Aggravation of vincristine-induced neurotoxicity by itraconazole in the treatment of adult ALL. *Ann Hematol* (1995) 71, 311–12.
6. Murphy JA, Ross LM, Gibson BES. Vincristine toxicity in five children with acute lymphoblastic leukaemia. *Lancet* (1995) 346, 443.
7. Jeng MR, Feusner J. Itraconazole-enhanced vincristine neurotoxicity in a child with acute lymphoblastic leukemia. *Pediatr Hematol Oncol* (2001) 18, 137–42.
8. Sathiapalan RK, El-Solh H. Enhanced vincristine neurotoxicity from drug interactions: case report and review of the literature. *Pediatr Hematol Oncol* (2001) 18, 543–6.
9. Sathiapalan RK, Al-Nasser A, El-Sohl H, Al-Mohsen I, Al-Jumaah S. Vincristine-itraconazole interaction: cause for increasing concern. *J Pediatr Hematol Oncol* (2002) 24, 591.
10. Ariffin H, Omar KZ, Ang EL, Shekhar K. Severe vincristine neurotoxicity with concomitant use of itraconazole. *J Paediatr Child Health* (2003) 39, 638–9.
11. Bermúdez, Fuster JL, Llinares E, Galera A, Gonzalez C. Itraconazole-related increased vincristine neurotoxicity. Case report and review of literature. *J Pediatr Hematol Oncol* (2005) 27, 389–92.
12. Gillies J, Hung KA, Fitzsimons E, Soutar R. Severe vincristine toxicity in combination with itraconazole. *Clin Lab Haematol* (1998) 20, 123–4.
13. Kamaluddin M, McNally P, Breatnach F, O'Marcaigh A, Webb D, O'Dell E, Scanlon P, Butler K, O'Meara A. Potentiation of vincristine toxicity by itraconazole in children with lymphoid malignancies. *Acta Paediatr* (2001) 90, 1204–7.
14. Takahashi N, Kameoka Y, Yamanaka Y, Ubukawa K, Saito K, Fujishima M, Fujishima N, Saito H, Hirokawa M, Scott SA, Sawada K. Itraconazole oral solution enhanced vincristine neurotoxicity in five patients with malignant lymphoma. *Intern Med* (2008) 47, 651–3.
15. Kobayashi R, Suzuki D, Yasuda K, Kobayashi K. Itraconazole for invasive fungal infection with pediatric malignancies. *Pediatr Int* (2010) 52, 707–10.

16. Gomber S, Dewan P, Chhonker D. Vincristine induced neurotoxicity in cancer patients. *Indian J Pediatr* (2010) 77, 97–100.
17. Moriyama B, Henning SA, Leung J, Falade-Nwulia O, Jarosinski P, Penzak SR, Walsh TJ. Adverse interactions between antifungal azoles and vincristine: review and analysis of cases. *Mycoses* (2012) 55, 290–7.
18. Mantadakis E, Amoiridis G, Kondi A, Kalmanti M. Possible increase of the neurotoxicity of vincristine by the concurrent use of posaconazole in a young adult with leukemia. *J Pediatr Hematol Oncol* (2007) 29, 130.
19. Eiden C, Palenzuela G, Hillaire-buys D, Margueritte G, Cociglio M, Hansel-esteller S, Peyriere H. Posaconazole-increased vincristine neurotoxicity in a child: a case report. *J Pediatr Hematol Oncol* (2009) 31, 292–5.
20. Jain S, Kapoor G. Severe life threatening neurotoxicity in a child with acute lymphoblastic leukemia receiving posaconazole and vincristine. *Pediatr Blood Cancer* (2010) 54, 783.
21. Hamdy DA, El-Geed H, El-Salem S, Zaiden M. Posaconazole-vincristine coadministration triggers seizures in a young female adult: a case report. *Case Rep Hematol* (2012) Epub.
22. Porter CC, Carver AE, Albano EA. Vincristine induced peripheral neuropathy potentiated by voriconazole in a patient with previously undiagnosed CMT1X. *Pediatr Blood Cancer* (2009) 52, 298–300.
23. Whittle AM, Ali S. Primary prophylaxis with voriconazole in patients receiving induction chemotherapy on the MRC adult acute lymphoblastic leukaemia trial (UK-ALL XII) to avoid itraconazole-enhanced vinca neurotoxicity. *Int J Lab Hematol* (2008) 30, 173–4.
24. Chen S, Wu D, Sun A, Qiu H, Jin Z, Tang X, Miao M, Fu Z, Ma X, Han Y, Hu X. Itraconazole-enhanced vindesine neurotoxicity in adult acute lymphoblastic leukaemia. *Am J Hematol* (2007) 82, 942.
25. Javlor (Vinflunine ditartrate). Pierre Fabre Ltd. UK Summary of product characteristics, June 2012.
26. Bosque E. Possible drug interaction between itraconazole and vinorelbine tartrate leading to death after one dose of chemotherapy. *Ann Intern Med* (2001) 134, 427.
27. Muenchow N, Janka G, Ertmann R, Looft G, Bielack S, Winkler K. Increased vincristine neurotoxicity during treatment with itraconazole in 3 pediatric patients with acute myelogenous leukaemia. *Blood* (1999) 94 (Suppl 1, part 2) 234b.
28. Moriyama B, Falade-Nwulia O, Leung J, Penzak SR, JJingo C, Huang X, Henning SA, Wilson WH, Walsh TJ. Prolonged half-life of voriconazole in a CYP2C19 homozygous poor metabolizer receiving vincristine chemotherapy: avoiding a serious adverse drug interaction. *Mycoses* (2011) 54, e877–e879.

Vinca alkaloids + Ciclosporin

The toxicity of vinblastine and vincristine might be increased by ciclosporin.

Clinical evidence

(a) Vinblastine

In a phase I dose-finding study, 60 patients were given a continuous intravenous infusion of ciclosporin in doses of 1 to 15.6 mg/kg daily for 5 days, starting 12 hours before a continuous intravenous infusion of vinblastine 2 mg/m^2 daily for 4 days. Unexpectedly severe myelosuppression and neurotoxicity occurred when the dose of ciclosporin was increased to 2 mg/kg daily, requiring a reduction in the vinblastine dose to 1.6 mg/kg daily before the ciclosporin dose could be escalated further. At a ciclosporin dose of 8 mg/kg daily, neurotoxicity was seen, and the vinblastine dose was further reduced to 1.2 mg/kg daily. At this vinblastine dose, the maximum tolerated dose of ciclosporin was 12.5 mg/kg daily.[1]

For a report of vinblastine toxicity with ciclosporin and erythromycin that was attributed to erythromycin, see 'Vinca alkaloids + Macrolides', p.747.

(b) Vincristine

A study in 7 patients with multiple myeloma, who were given ciclosporin 10 mg/kg daily and chemotherapy which included vincristine, doxorubicin, and dexamethasone (VAD), found that neutropenia was more severe than anticipated. Gastrointestinal effects including severe constipation (6 patients), paralytic ileus (3 patients), and small bowel obstruction (1 patient) did not occur during previous courses of treatment when ciclosporin was not given. An increase in bilirubin and liver enzymes occurred in all 7 patients when they were given ciclosporin and VAD. All patients developed severe musculoskeletal pain.[2] In a later randomised clinical study, patients with progressive myeloma were given the VAD regimen every 4 weeks for 4 cycles, with or without intravenous ciclosporin (2 mg/kg given 2 hours before VAD, followed by a continuous infusion of 7.5 mg/kg daily for 4 days). Nausea, mucositis, and infection occurred more frequently in the ciclosporin recipients than in those patients receiving VAD alone. Note that the addition of ciclosporin did not improve outcomes or survival in this study.[3]

A case report describes a 10-year-old boy who developed severe neurotoxicity 7 days after receiving chemotherapy for acute lymphoblastic leukaemia which included vincristine and ciclosporin (doses not stated) in addition to high-dose methotrexate, cyclophosphamide, doxorubicin, and methylprednisolone.[4]

Mechanism

Uncertain. Ciclosporin was used in these studies as a P-glycoprotein inhibitor, and vinblastine and vincristine are thought to be substrates for P-glycoprotein. Therefore ciclosporin might interact with these vinca alkaloids by this mechanism, or it might directly increase their toxicity.

Importance and management

An interaction between vinca alkaloids and ciclosporin is not firmly established, but it appears that vincristine and vinblastine toxicity is increased by ciclosporin. Intravenous ciclosporin was investigated for multidrug resistant tumour modulation, but has not gained a place in clinical use. More study is needed to find out the possible effects of lower conventional doses of oral ciclosporin on vinca alkaloids. Note that the UK manufacturer of vinorelbine considers that concurrent use of ciclosporin results in excessive immunodepression with risk of lymphoproliferation.[5] Bear in mind that an increased risk of immunosuppression would apply to the concurrent use of any vinca alkaloid with any immunosuppressant.

1. Samuels BL, Mick R, Vogelzang NJ, Williams SF, Schilsky RL, Safa AR, O'Brien SM, Ratain MJ. Modulation of vinblastine resistance with cyclosporine: A phase I study. *Clin Pharmacol Ther* (1993) 54, 421–9.
2. Weber DM, Dimopoulos MA, Alexanian R. Increased neurotoxicity with VAD-cyclosporin in multiple myeloma. *Lancet* (1993) 341, 558–9.
3. Sonneveld P, Suciu S, Weijermans P, Beksac M, Neuwirtova R, Solbu G, Lokhorst H, van der Lelie J, Dohner H, Gerhartz H, Segeren CM, Willemze R, Lowenberg B. Cyclosporin A combined with vincristine, doxorubicin and dexamethasone (VAD) compared with VAD alone in patients with advanced refractory multiple myeloma: an EORTC-HOVON randomized phase III study (06914). *Br J Haematol* (2001) 115, 895–902.
4. Bertrand Y, Capdeville R, Balduck N, Philippe N. Cyclosporin A used to reverse drug resistance increases vincristine neurotoxicity. *Am J Hematol* (1992) 40, 158–9.
5. Navelbine Soft Capsules (Vinorelbine tartrate). Pierre Fabre Ltd. UK Summary of product characteristics, July 2011.

Vinca alkaloids + Gemcitabine

Gemcitabine appears not to alter vinflunine concentrations, whereas gemcitabine exposure was negligibly higher when given with vinflunine. The exposure to both gemcitabine and vinorelbine appear to be decreased on concurrent use, and their efficacy appears to be affected by the order in which they are given.

Clinical evidence

(a) Vinflunine

In a phase I dose-finding study, 19 patients were given vinflunine on day 1 and gemcitabine on days 1 and 8, every 21 days. Gemcitabine did not appear to alter vinflunine concentrations or those of its active metabolite. The AUCs of gemcitabine were 19% higher on day 1 than day 8, but as they were highly variable, a larger study would be needed to show if there is a real effect.[1]

(b) Vinorelbine

In a study in 9 patients, the AUC of gemcitabine tended to be lower by about 30% (not statistically significant) when gemcitabine 1200 mg/m^2 was given over 30 minutes followed by a bolus dose of vinorelbine 30 mg/ m^2 on days 1 and 8 every 3 weeks when compared with another group of 5 patients given gemcitabine 1200 mg/m^2 alone.[2] This research group then conducted another study where patients with cancer were given gemcitabine 1 g/m^2 followed by vinorelbine 25 mg/m^2 (9 patients), vinorelbine 25 mg/m^2 followed by gemcitabine 1 g/m^2 (17 patients), or gemcitabine 1 g/m^2 alone (5 patients). The AUC of gemcitabine was highest when gemcitabine was given alone. Of the combination treatments, the AUC of gemcitabine was higher when it was given after vinorelbine. The AUC of vinorelbine varied depending on the order of administration, but in both regimens it was 3 to 5 times lower than has been previously reported for vinorelbine alone.[3] The efficacy of the combination of gemcitabine and vinorelbine appears to be sequence related, and this is illustrated in another study, in which gemcitabine 1200 mg/m^2 followed immediately by vinorelbine 30 mg/m^2 on days 1 and 15 of a 28-day cycle was thought to be inactive.[4]

Mechanism

Unknown.

Importance and management

There appears to be no clinically relevant pharmacokinetic interaction between vinflunine and gemcitabine. In contrast, there appears to be a pharmacokinetic interaction between vinorelbine and gemcitabine, and the sequence in which the two drugs are given might be important in determining the magnitude of any effect. Further study is needed to establish this.

1. Tournoux-Facon C, Senellart H, Lemarie E, Tourani JM, Favrel S, Pouget JC, Pinel MC, Bennouna J. Phase I and pharmacokinetic study of IV vinflunine in combination with gemcitabine for treatment of advanced non-small cell lung cancer in Chemonaive patients. *J Thorac Oncol* (2011) 6, 1247–53.
2. Airoldi M, Cattel L, Cortesina G, Giordano C, Passera R, Pedani F, Novello S, Bumma C, Gabriele P. Gemcitabine and vinorelbine in recurrent head and neck cancer: pharmacokinetic and clinical results. *Anticancer Res* (2003) 23, 2845–52.
3. Cattel L, Airoldi M, Passera R, Cagliero E, Stella B, Goffredo F. Gemcitabine plus vinorelbine chemotherapy regimens: a pharmacokinetic study of alternate administration sequences. *Pharm World Sci* (2004) 26, 238–41.
4. Juergens R, Brahmer J, Ettinger D. Gemcitabine and vinorelbine in recurrent advanced non-small cell lung cancer: sequence does matter. *Cancer Chemother Pharmacol* (2007) 59, 621–9.

Vinca alkaloids + HIV-protease inhibitors

The risk of severe neutropenia with vinblastine appears to be increased in patients also taking atazanavir or lopinavir boosted with ritonavir. Paralytic ileus occurred in another patient taking lopinavir boosted with ritonavir and given a chemotherapy regimen including vincristine. In this patient, no problems occurred when vincristine was replaced with etoposide.

Clinical evidence

(a) Vinblastine

In a retrospective analysis of 16 patients with HIV-associated Hodgkin's lymphoma taking antiretrovirals and given vinblastine-containing chemotherapy regimens, the mean nadir neutrophil count was lower in 5 patients taking **atazanavir** or **lopinavir** boosted with **ritonavir** than in 7 patients taking NNRTI- or raltegravir-based antiretroviral regimens, despite routine use of granulocyte colony-stimulating factor (G-CSF). Two patients taking **lopinavir** boosted with **ritonavir** died of sepsis during the first chemotherapy cycle. In addition, there was an inverse correlation with the dose of ritonavir given to boost the HIV-protease inhibitor and the nadir neutrophil count: ritonavir 200 mg daily (given with lopinavir) caused a lower nadir neutrophil count than ritonavir 100 mg daily (given with atazanavir).[1] Similarly, in another retrospective analysis of 32 patients with HIV-associated Hodgkin's lymphoma mostly receiving ABVD (doxorubicin, bleomycin, vinblastine, and dacarbazine), the use of **lopinavir** and **ritonavir** was associated with severe neurotoxicity, and **ritonavir** was associated with haematological toxicity.[2]

Other case reports have also described this interaction. A 55-year-old HIV-positive man who was taking zidovudine, lamivudine, abacavir, nevirapine, and **lopinavir** boosted with **ritonavir** experienced unexpected severe gastrointestinal and haematological toxicities and moderate renal failure after the second and third intravenous injections of vinblastine 10 mg given to treat multicentric Castleman's disease (MCD). Subsequently, the antiretrovirals were stopped and the patient did not experience these symptoms when vinblastine was given alone. When the MCD was under control, the antiretrovirals were restarted, and the vinblastine dose reduced to 3 mg every 3 weeks without problems.[3] A second HIV-positive patient who was taking **lopinavir** boosted with **ritonavir** developed life-threatening neutropenia when given ABVD (doxorubicin, bleomycin, vinblastine, and dacarbazine) for Hodgkin's lymphoma. Further courses of vinblastine were successfully given by stopping the HIV-protease inhibitors around the time the chemotherapy was given.[4] Another report describes 3 patients taking **lopinavir** boosted with **ritonavir** who experienced severe vinblastine-associated neurotoxicity (early onset autonomic neuropathy or painful peripheral neuropathy).[5]

(b) Vincristine

A 39-year-old man taking **lopinavir** boosted with **ritonavir** 400/100 mg twice daily, abacavir, and lamivudine, developed paralytic ileus 12 days after starting the first cycle of a course of chemotherapy for Burkitt lymphoma (CODOX-M: cyclophosphamide, doxorubicin, methotrexate, cytarabine, and vincristine). This was attributed to an interaction between lopinavir boosted with ritonavir and vincristine. After he recovered, the patient was given a further course of CODOX-M, with etoposide replacing vincristine, without any problems.[6] For other reports of HIV-protease inhibitors increasing the risk of toxicity when given with various antineoplastic regimens, including those containing vincristine, see 'Antineoplastics; Cyclophosphamide + HIV-protease inhibitors', p.659.

Mechanism

Not established. Lopinavir boosted with ritonavir is a potent inhibitor of CYP3A4, and an inhibitor of P-glycoprotein, and there is some evidence that both CYP3A4 and P-glycoprotein are involved in the metabolism and transport of vinblastine and vincristine, which might increase their concentrations, resulting in increased toxicity. Vindesine and vinorelbine are also metabolised by CYP3A4, and might be similarly affected.

Importance and management

These appear to be the only reports of a possible interaction between the vinca alkaloids and the HIV-protease inhibitors. Nevertheless, given the suggested mechanism, if concurrent use is unavoidable, it would seem prudent to carefully monitor any patient taking an HIV-protease inhibitor who is also given vinblastine. Similar caution would seem prudent with all vinca alkaloids. For vinblastine, one suggestion is to temporarily stop the HIV-protease inhibitor when the chemotherapy is given, but this carries the increased risk of antiviral drug resistance.[1] Another option is a reduction of the vinblastine dose, but, at present there is no information to guide this and it is important not to under-treat patients as this could impair their prognosis. HIV-protease inhibitor regimens using a lower dose of ritonavir (100 mg) might be preferable.[1] Further study is needed to establish the best management options for this interaction.

1. Cingolani A, Torti L, Pinnetti C, de Gaetano Donati K, Murri R, Tacconelli E, Larocca LM, Teofili L. Detrimental clinical interaction between ritonavir-boosted protease inhibitors and vinblastine in HIV-infected patients with Hodgkin's lymphoma. *AIDS* (2010) 24, 2408–12.
2. Ezzat HM, Cheung MC, Hicks LK, Boro J, Montaner JSG, Lima VD, Harris M, Leitch HA. Incidence, predictors and significance of severe toxicity in patients with human immunodeficiency virus-associated Hodgkin lymphoma. *Leuk Lymphoma* (2012) 53, 2390–6.
3. Kotb R, Vincent I, Dulioust A, Peretti D, Taburet A-M, Delfraissy J-F, Goujard C. Life-threatening interaction between antiretroviral therapy and vinblastine in HIV-associated multicentric Castleman's disease. *Eur J Haematol* (2006) 76, 269–71.
4. Makinson A, Martelli N, Peyrière H, Turriere C, Le Moing V, Reynes J. Profound neutropenia resulting from interaction between antiretroviral therapy and vinblastine in a patient with HIV-associated Hodgkin's disease. *Eur J Haematol* (2007) 78, 358–60.
5. Cheung MC, Hicks LK, Leitch HA. Excessive neurotoxicity with ABVD when combined with protease inhibitor-based antiretroviral therapy in the treatment of AIDS-related Hodgkin lymphoma. *Clin Lymphoma Myeloma Leuk* (2010) 10, E22–E25.
6. Levêque D, Santucci R, Pavillet J, Herbrecht R, Bergerat JP. Paralytic ileus possibly associated with interaction between ritonavir/lopinavir and vincristine. *Pharm World Sci* (2009) 31, 619–21.

Vinca alkaloids + Macrolides

Erythromycin increased the toxicity of vinblastine in three patients. Clarithromycin was associated with an increased risk of severe neutropenia with vinorelbine. Other vinca alkaloids are predicted to be similarly affected by these macrolides.

Clinical evidence

(a) Clarithromycin

The observation of severe neutropenia in patients given **vinorelbine** and clarithromycin prompted a retrospective cohort study. In 25 patients treated with 59 courses of chemotherapy that included **vinorelbine**, there was a 4.5-fold increased risk of grade 3/4 neutropenia associated with the use of clarithromycin during the period between 7 days before the first **vinorelbine** dose and 1 day after the last **vinorelbine** dose. The incidence of grade 3/4 neutropenia for 19 **vinorelbine** courses with clarithromycin was 63.2% compared with 27.5% for 40 courses without clarithromycin. Four patients had **vinorelbine** courses with and without clarithromycin, and neutrophil counts were lower when clarithromycin was given.[1]

Other authors report that they have used clarithromycin with standard doses of vinca alkaloids (**vinblastine** and **vincristine**) in at least 6 patients without any evidence of increased toxicity, although it is probable these patients also received rifabutin, an enzyme inducer (which would attenuate or negate the enzyme-inhibiting effects of clarithromycin).[2]

(b) Erythromycin

Three patients with renal cell carcinoma given ciclosporin 10 or 13 mg/kg daily and erythromycin 1 g daily for 3 days developed severe toxicity when given **vinblastine** 7 to 10 mg/m^2 on the third day. Ciclosporin was used to reverse multidrug resistance and erythromycin was given to achieve higher ciclosporin concentrations at a lower dose. To rule out increased ciclosporin toxicity, one patient was given erythromycin without ciclosporin but he still developed **vinblastine** toxicity (severe neutropenia, constipation, myositis, severe myalgia) typical of much higher doses of **vinblastine**. Of the other 2 patients, only mild toxicity (muscle pain) developed in one when he was later given **vinblastine** alone, and the other had received ciclosporin and **vinblastine** on two previous occasions without problems.[3]

Mechanism

Uncertain, but clarithromycin and erythromycin inhibit CYP3A4, by which vinblastine, vinorelbine, and other vinca alkaloids are metabolised. This would be expected to reduce their metabolism resulting in an increase in toxicity.

Importance and management

Information about an interaction between vinca alkaloids and macrolides seems to be limited to this case report and small retrospective cohort study. On the basis of their findings, the authors of the case report suggest that erythromycin should be avoided at the time of vinblastine infusion.[3] The UK manufacturers of **vincristine** and **vindesine** state that caution is warranted in patients taking any drugs known to inhibit the CYP3A subfamily of isoenzymes because of the risk of an earlier onset and/or increased severity of adverse effects,[4,5] whereas the manufacturer of **vinorelbine** restricts this caution to *potent* CYP3A4 inhibitors,[6] and the manufacturer of **vinflunine** advises avoiding the concurrent use of potent CYP3A4 inhibitors.[7] Note that clarithromycin and **telithromycin** are potent CYP3A4 inhibitors and erythromycin is a moderate CYP3A4 inhibitor. If concurrent use of any macrolide that potently inhibits CYP3A4 with a vinca alkaloid is considered essential, the careful monitoring of adverse effects, such as myelosuppression, would seem prudent. Note that, because QT interval prolongation has been seen with vinflunine, the manufacturers advise caution with other drugs that prolong the QT interval, which includes some macrolides, see 'Table 9.2', p.273. This seems likely to be particularly important where vinflunine concentrations are also increased.

1. Yano R, Tani D, Watanabe K, Tsukamoto H, Igarashi T, Nakamura T, Masada M. Evaluation of potential interaction between vinorelbine and clarithromycin. *Ann Pharmacother* (2009) 43, 453–8.
2. Torresin A, Cassola G, Penco G, Crisalli MP, Piersantelli N. Vinca alkaloids and macrolides in human immunodeficiency virus-related malignancies: a safe association. *Cancer Chemother Pharmacol* (1996) 39, 176–7.
3. Tobe SW, Siu LL, Jamal SA, Skorecki KL, Murphy GF, Warner E. Vinblastine and erythromycin: an unrecognized serious drug interaction. *Cancer Chemother Pharmacol* (1995) 35, 188–190.
4. Eldisine (Vindesine). Genus Pharmaceuticals Ltd. UK Summary of product characteristics, July 2008.
5. Vincristine sulphate. Hospira UK Ltd. UK Summary of product characteristics, January 2008.
6. Navelbine Soft Capsules (Vinorelbine tartrate). Pierre Fabre Ltd. UK Summary of product characteristics, July 2011.
7. Javlor (Vinflunine ditartrate). Pierre Fabre Ltd. UK Summary of product characteristics, June 2012.

Vinca alkaloids + Mitomycin

A syndrome of acute pulmonary toxicity, characterised by severe shortness of breath, can occur when vinblastine, vindesine or vinorelbine is given with mitomycin. Fatalities have occurred.

Clinical evidence, mechanism, importance and management

There are numerous reports describing acute lung disease in patients given mitomycin with vinca alkaloids, which appears to be different to the chronic pulmonary fibrosis seen with mitomycin alone. Sudden onset of acute shortness of breath has been described shortly after administration of the vinca alkaloid as part of a vinca alkaloid and mitomycin-containing regimen. Chest radiographs have shown diffuse lung damage characterised by interstitial infiltrates and pulmonary oedema. The acute syndrome has usually improved over 24 hours, although some patients have chronic respiratory impairment (60% in one case series[1]). Fatalities have occurred.[2-4] The syndrome has been reported with mitomycin and **vinblastine**,[1-9] **vindesine**,[1,8,10-12] or intravenous **vinorelbine**.[12-15] The incidence is reported to be about 3 to 6%.[1,7,12]

The potential hazards of combining these drugs should be recognised, and in view of the unpredictability of the reaction, close observation of patients receiving this combination is recommended.[1,3] If the reaction occurs, supportive measures such as supplemental oxygen and mechanical ventilation might be needed. Corticosteroids are also often used in an attempt to treat the acute symptoms, and to possibly decrease the risk of chronic respiratory impairment.[1] It has been suggested that, in patients who have developed acute pulmonary toxicity, the use of both mitomycin and vinca alkaloids should subsequently be avoided.[1]

1. Rivera MP, Kris MG, Gralla RJ, White DA. Syndrome of acute dyspnea related to combined mitomycin plus vinca alkaloid chemotherapy. *Am J Clin Oncol* (1995) 18, 245–50.
2. Ozols RF, Hogan WM, Ostchega T, Young RC. MVP (mitomycin, vinblastine, progesterone): a second-line regimen in ovarian cancer with a high incidence of pulmonary toxicity. *Cancer Treat Rep* (1983) 67, 721–2.
3. Rao SX, Ramaswamy G, Levin M, McCravey JW. Fatal acute respiratory failure after vinblastine-mitomycin therapy in lung carcinoma. *Arch Intern Med* (1985) 145, 1905–7.
4. Ballen KK, Weiss ST. Fatal acute respiratory failure following vinblastine and mitomycin administration for breast cancer. *Am J Med Sci* (1988) 295, 558–60.
5. Israel RH, Olsen JP. Pulmonary edema associated with intravenous vinblastine. *JAMA* (1978) 240, 1585.
6. Konits PH, Aisner J, Sutherland JC, Wiernik PH. Possible pulmonary toxicity secondary to vinblastine. *Cancer* (1982) 50, 2771–4.
7. Hoelzer KL, Harrison BR, Luedke SW, Luedke DW. Vinblastine-associated pulmonary toxicity in patients receiving combination therapy with mitomycin and cisplatin. *Drug Intell Clin Pharm* (1986) 20, 287–9.
8. Kris MG, Pablo D, Gralla J, Burke MT, Prestifillippo J, Lewin D. Dyspnea following vinblastine or vindesine administration in patients receiving mitomycin plus vinca alkaloid combination therapy. *Cancer Treat Rep* (1984) 68, 1029–31.
9. Lagler U, Gattiker HH. Akute Dyspnoe nach intravenöser Gabe von Vinblastin/Mitomycin. *Schweiz Med Wochenschr* (1989) 119, 290–2.
10. Dyke RW. Acute bronchospasm after a vinca alkaloid in patients previously treated with mitomycin. *N Engl J Med* (1984) 310, 389.
11. Luedke D, McLaughlin TT, Daughaday C, Luedke S, Harrison B, Reed G, Martello O. Mitomycin C and vindesine associated pulmonary toxicity with variable clinical expression. *Cancer* (1985) 55, 542–5.
12. Thomas P, Pradal M, Le Caer H, Montcharmont D, Vervolet D, Kleisbauer JP. Bronchospasme aigu dû à l'association alcaloïde de la pervenche-mitomycine. *Rev Mal Respir* (1993) 10, 268–70.
13. Raderer M, Kornek G, Hejna M, Vorbeck F, Weinlaender G, Scheithauer W. Acute pulmonary toxicity associated with high-dose vinorelbine and mitomycin C. *Ann Oncol* (1996) 7, 973–5.
14. Rouzaud P, Estivals M, Pujazon MC, Carles P, Lauque D. Complications respiratoires de l'association vinorelbine-mitomycine. *Rev Mal Respir* (1999) 16, 81–4.
15. Uoshima N, Yoshioka K, Tegoshi J, Wada S, Fujiwara Y. Acute respiratory failure caused by vinorelbine tartrate in a patient with non-small cell lung cancer. *Intern Med* (2001) 40, 779–82.

Vinca alkaloids + Nifedipine

In one small study, nifedipine appeared to reduce the clearance of vincristine, but no increased toxicity was seen. Nifedipine did not increase the toxicity of vinblastine in another small study.

Clinical evidence, mechanism, importance and management

In a study in 12 patients, nifedipine reduced the clearance of a single 2-mg intravenous dose of **vincristine** by 68%, and increased its AUC 3-fold, when compared with 14 patients receiving **vincristine** alone. Nifedipine was given at a dose of 10 mg three times daily for 3 days before, and 7 days after, vincristine was given. However, no important adverse effects were noted in either group of patients, suggesting that these pharmacokinetic changes did not notably increase vincristine toxicity.[1] Similarly, in another small study, nifedipine (20 mg three times daily increased to 40 mg three times daily, starting 3 days before chemotherapy, and continued during, and for 2 days after stopping, chemotherapy) did not increase the haematological toxicity of a chemotherapy regimen including **vinblastine**.[2]

The mechanism of the pharmacokinetic interaction between vinca alkaloids and nifedipine is unknown, but the authors of the first study hypothesised that nifedipine might inhibit the outward transport of **vincristine** from intracellular sites.[1] Further study is needed to establish any the pharmacokinetic interaction and its relevance. Note that nifedipine has been considered to be a possible factor in some case reports of **vincristine** toxicity caused by itraconazole, see 'Vinca alkaloids + Azoles', p.744.

1. Fedeli L, Colozza M, Boschetti E, Sabalich I, Aristei C, Guerciolini R, Del Favero A, Rossetti R, Tonato M, Rambotti P, Davis S. Pharmacokinetics of vincristine in cancer patients treated with nifedipine. *Cancer* (1989) 64, 1805–11.
2. Holmes FA, Lopez A, Mavligit G, Fraschini G, Frye D, Hortobagyi GN. Secondary drug resistance in breast cancer: failure to reverse with oral nifedipine. *Int J Cancer* (1997) 73, 184–6.

Vinca alkaloids + Platinum compounds

There is no apparent pharmacokinetic interaction between vinflunine and either carboplatin or cisplatin. The pharmacokinetics of intravenous and oral vinorelbine do not appear to be altered by cisplatin. The incidence of granulocytopenia is reported to be higher when vinorelbine is given with cisplatin than when given alone.

Clinical evidence, mechanism, importance and management

(a) Vinflunine

In a phase I dose-finding study in 21 patients with non-small cell lung cancer, there was no apparent pharmacokinetic interaction when vinflunine 280 or 320 mg/m^2 was given with carboplatin (dosed to achieve an AUC of 5 or 6 mg/mL), both on day 1 of a 3-week cycle.[1] In a similar study in 12 patients, there was no apparent pharmacokinetic interaction between vinflunine 250 to 320 mg/m^2 and cisplatin 80 mg/m^2, when compared with historical data.[2]

(b) Vinorelbine

In a study, the pharmacokinetics of vinorelbine did not differ between 4 patients who received a single 30-mg/m^2 *infusion* of vinorelbine given over 15 minutes and 4 patients who were also given a single 80-mg/m^2 dose of cisplatin given one hour after the start of the vinorelbine infusion.[3] Similarly, another study, in 11 patients, showed no appreciable difference in vinorelbine pharmacokinetics between *oral* vinorelbine 60 mg/m^2 given 2 hours before intravenous cisplatin 100 mg/m^2 on day 1 and given alone on day 8, every 3 weeks.[4]

The incidence of granulocytopenia is reported to be higher when vinorelbine is given with cisplatin, than when given alone.[5,6] In one large clinical study, the incidence of grade 3 to 4 neutropenia was 79% in patients receiving intravenous vinorelbine 30 mg/m^2 weekly with cisplatin (120 mg/m^2 on days 1 and 29, and then every 6 weeks) compared with an incidence of 53% in patients receiving vinorelbine 30 mg/m^2 weekly alone. However, the combination regimen improved survival.[7]

The combination of vinorelbine and cisplatin is in established use. Note that close monitoring for neutropenia and appropriate dose adjustment, or a delay in treatment, is important if neutropenia develops with vinorelbine alone.

1. Tournoux-Facon C, Robinet G, Pinel MC, Ferre P, Tourani JM. Phase I and pharmacokinetic study of IV vinflunine in combination with carboplatin in chemonaive patients with advanced non-small cell lung cancer. *Am J Clin Oncol* (2012) 35, 378–85.
2. Souquet PJ, Krzakowski M, Ramlau R, Sun XS, Lopez-Vivanco G, Puozzo C, Pouget JC, Pinel MC, Rosell R. Phase I/II and pharmacokinetic study of intravenous vinflunine in combination with cisplatin for the treatment of chemonaive patients with advanced non-small-cell lung cancer. *Clin Lung Cancer* (2010) 11, 105–13.
3. Levêque D, Jehl F, Quoix E, Breillout F. Clinical pharmacokinetics of vinorelbine alone and combined with cisplatin. *J Clin Pharmacol* (1992) 32, 1096–8.
4. Delord JP, Puozzo C, Lefresne F, Bugat R. Combination chemotherapy of vinorelbine and cisplatin: a phase I pharmacokinetic study in patients with metastatic solid tumors. *Anticancer Res* (2009) 29, 553–60.
5. Navelbine Soft Capsules (Vinorelbine tartrate). Pierre Fabre Ltd. UK Summary of product characteristics, July 2011.
6. Navelbine (Vinorelbine tartrate). Pierre Fabre Pharmaceuticals Inc. US Prescribing information, October 2007.
7. Le Chevalier T, Brisgand D, Pujol JL, Douillard JY, Monnier A, Rivière A, Chomy P, Le Groumellec A, Ruffie P, Gottfried M, Gaspard MH, Chevreau C, Alberola V, Cigolari S, Besson F, Martinez A, Besenval M, Berthaud P, Tursz T. Résultats d'une étude randomisée comparant l'association Navelbine-cisplatinum à l'association vindésine-cisplatinum et à la Navelbine seule chez 612 malades porteurs d'un carcinome bronchique non à petites cellules inopérable. *Bull Cancer* (1996) 83, 385–94.

Vinca alkaloids + Rifampicin (Rifampin)

The concentrations of vinflunine and vinorelbine might be reduced by rifampicin.

Clinical evidence

In a small study in 4 *pigs*, there was no difference in the clearance of **vinorelbine** when a single 500-micrograms/kg intravenous dose was given alone, or just after, intravenous rifampicin 600 mg (given daily for 7 days). Rifampicin increased the AUC of **vinorelbine** by 69%, but this was not statistically significant,[1] possibly because of the small sample size. Pigs were chosen for this study because porcine CYP3A is reportedly similar to that of humans.[1]

Mechanism

Uncertain. Vinorelbine is known to be metabolised by CYP3A4, of which rifampicin is a known potent inducer, therefore rifampicin would be expected to increase the clearance of vinorelbine and reduce its exposure; however, this is contrary to the findings reported, suggesting that CYP3A4 is not the most important factor in this interaction. Rifampicin is also an inhibitor of some drug transporters; an effect most apparent during simultaneous administration, and this can result in increased exposure of some drugs under certain circumstances, see 'Statins + Rifampicin (Rifampin)', p.1355.

Importance and management

There appear to be no data from human studies, and the small animal study suggests that a slight increase in **vinorelbine** exposure might occur on the concurrent use of rifampicin, the general relevance of which is unknown. The UK manufacturer of vinorelbine advises caution with potent inducers of the CYP3A subfamily, including rifampicin, because of the possibility of *decreased* vinorelbine concentrations.[2] Until more is known, caution seems prudent. There are no data for other vinca alkaloids, but the UK manufacturer of **vinflunine** advises avoidance of potent CYP3A inducers such as rifampicin because of the possibility of reduced vinflunine concentrations.[3]

For a list of clinically relevant potent CYP3A4 inducers, see 'Table 1.9', p.11.

1. Leveque D, Wisniewski S, Renault C, Peter JD, Le Corre P, Monteil H, Jehl F. The effect of rifampin on the pharmacokinetics of vinorelbine in the micropig. *Anticancer Res* (2003) 23, 2741–4.
2. Navelbine Soft Capsules (Vinorelbine tartrate). Pierre Fabre Ltd. UK Summary of product characteristics, July 2011.
3. Javlor (Vinflunine ditartrate). Pierre Fabre Ltd. UK Summary of product characteristics, June 2012.

Vinca alkaloids + Taxanes

There appears to be no pharmacokinetic interaction between docetaxel and vinorelbine, although haematological toxicity might be increased. There appears to be no pharmacokinetic interaction between paclitaxel and vinorelbine. Docetaxel and paclitaxel appear to minimally reduce the metabolism of vinflunine *in vitro*.

Clinical evidence, mechanism, importance and management

In studies where an infusion of vinorelbine was given immediately before an infusion of **docetaxel**, there was no apparent pharmacokinetic interaction,[1,2] but haematological toxicity prevented dose escalation in one study.[2] However, in another analysis, the AUC of vinorelbine was found to be higher, and haematological toxicity appeared to be greater, in patients who received vinorelbine immediately before **docetaxel** than in patients who received **docetaxel** immediately before vinorelbine.[3] **Docetaxel** pharmacokinetics did not vary between the two sequences.[3] Nevertheless, the UK manufacturer notes that there was no clinically relevant pharmacokinetic interaction when vinorelbine was given with **paclitaxel** or **docetaxel**.[4] The US manufacturer states that patients who receive vinorelbine and **paclitaxel**, either concurrently or sequentially, should be monitored for development of neuropathy.[5]

Clinical data regarding other vinca alkaloids appears to be lacking. The UK manufacturer of vinflunine states that in an *in vitro* study, **docetaxel** and **paclitaxel** minimally reduced the metabolism of vinflunine.[6] Further study is needed to confirm whether a clinically relevant interaction occurs.

1. Campone M, Fumoleau P, Delecroix V, Deporte-Fety R, Perrocheau G, Vernillet L, Borg-Olivier O, Louboutin JP, Bissery MC, Riva A, Azli N. Phase I dose-finding and pharmacokinetic study of docetaxel and vinorelbine as first-line chemotherapy for metastatic breast cancer. *Ann Oncol* (2001) 12, 909–18.
2. Delord JP, Dalenc F, Pinguet F, Nguyen L, Lochon I, Poublanc M, Chatelut E, Roche H. A phase I dose-escalating and pharmacokinetic study of docetaxel and vinorelbine as first-line chemotherapy for metastatic breast cancer. *Oncology* (2007) 72, 322–5.
3. Cattel L, Recalenda V, Airoldi M, Tagini V, Arpicco S, Brusa P, Bumma C. A sequence-dependent combination of docetaxel and vinorelbine: pharmacokinetic interactions. *Farmaco* (2001) 56, 779–84.
4. Navelbine Soft Capsules (Vinorelbine tartrate). Pierre Fabre Ltd. UK Summary of product characteristics, July 2011.
5. Navelbine (Vinorelbine tartrate). Pierre Fabre Pharmaceuticals Inc. US Prescribing information, October 2007.
6. Javlor (Vinflunine ditartrate). Pierre Fabre Ltd. UK Summary of product characteristics, June 2012.

Vinca alkaloids + Tyrosine kinase inhibitors

There appears to be no pharmacokinetic interaction between gefitinib and vinorelbine, but the combination was associated with a high incidence of neutropenia. Similarly, erlotinib with vinflunine caused unacceptable toxicity despite reduced doses. Lapatinib appears to reduce vinorelbine clearance. There appears to be no pharmacokinetic interaction between vandetanib and vinorelbine but the combination was not tolerated.

Clinical evidence

(a) Erlotinib

Unexpectedly severe toxicity, predominantly bone marrow suppression, was seen in a study in which erlotinib was added to **vinflunine** therapy in patients with solid tumours. Initially **vinflunine** 280 mg/m2 was infused on day 1 every 21 days and erlotinib 75 mg daily was given on days 2 to 21. The **vinflunine** dose was then reduced to 250 mg/m^2, and the erlotinib duration was reduced to 14 days, before the study was terminated. **Vinflunine** 250 mg/m^2 is 75% of the usual dose, and erlotinib 75 mg daily is half the usual dose.[1]

(b) Gefitinib

An unacceptable rate of febrile neutropenia was seen in a study in patients with non-small cell lung cancer in which gefitinib (250 mg daily from day 2) was given as part of a 28-day cycle with **vinorelbine** (30 mg/m^2 on days 1, 8, 15, and 22), or as part of a 21-day cycle with **vinorelbine** (30 mg/m^2 on day 1 and 8) and cisplatin (80 mg/m^2 on day 1). There was no evidence of a change in the pharmacokinetics of any of the drugs. Because of the toxicity in this study, and the lack of efficacy reported in another study in non-small cell lung cancer (NSCLC), a planned phase II study of the combination did not go ahead.[2] Similar toxicity findings were reported in another study.[3]

(c) Lapatinib

In a dose-finding study combining lapatinib with **vinorelbine**, lapatinib reduced the clearance of **vinorelbine**.[4] Similarly, in another study by this research group, lapatinib 1 g or 1.25 g daily reduced the clearance of **vinorelbine** (on days 1 and 8 of a 21-day cycle) by 30 to 40% when compared with lapatinib 750 mg daily, although this was not statistically significant. The maximum tolerated doses in this study were lapatinib 1 g with **vinorelbine** 22.5 mg/m^2: the dose-limiting toxicity was neutropenia.[5] These doses are 20% and 25% lower, respectively, than those generally used.

(d) Vandetanib

The pharmacokinetic analysis of a phase I study combining vandetanib with **vinorelbine** and cisplatin in patients with advanced non-small cell lung cancer, found that exposure to vandetanib and vinorelbine was not affected by concurrent use. However, the combination was not tolerated, with thromboembolic effects being the main dose-limiting toxicity.[6] For mention of the effect of combined administration on cisplatin exposure see 'Tyrosine kinase inhibitors + Cisplatin and other platinum compounds', p.730.

Mechanism

The reason for the toxicity seen when erlotinib and vinflunine, and gefitinib and vinorelbine, were given concurrently is not clear, and there is no known mechanism for a pharmacokinetic interaction. Lapatinib probably reduces vinorelbine clearance because it inhibits CYP3A4 by which vinorelbine is metabolised.

Importance and management

In the dosage schedules used, erlotinib with vinflunine and gefitinib with vinorelbine were too toxic for use in patients.[1,2] Given these data, it might be prudent to avoid combining these two tyrosine kinase inhibitors with any vinca alkaloid. Further study of the mechanisms for the toxicity seen is required.

Lapatinib reduces the clearance of vinorelbine, and might increase the risk of bone marrow suppression. The authors recommend that reduced doses of both drugs are used when they are given concurrently.[5]

Although no pharmacokinetic interaction was seen when vinorelbine and vandetanib were given together, the combination (with cisplatin) was not tolerated, and the authors concluded that this combination was not a feasible first-line therapy for non-small cell lung cancer.[6]

1. Sanoff HK, Davies JM, Walko C, Irvin W, Buie L, Keller K, Ivanova A, Chiu WK, O'Neil BH, Stinchcombe TE, Dees EC. A phase I evaluation of the combination of vinflunine and erlotinib in patients with refractory solid tumors. *Invest New Drugs* (2011) 29, 978–83.
2. Pujol JL, Viens P, Rebattu P, Laurie SA, Feld R, Deneulin A, Fandi A. Gefitinib (IRESSA) with vinorelbine or vinorelbine/cisplatin for chemotherapy-naive non-small cell lung cancer patients. *J Thorac Oncol* (2006) 1, 417–24.
3. Yoshimura M, Nakamura S, Imamura F, Ueno K, Yamamoto S, Igarashi T. Severe myelotoxicity in a combination of gefitinib and vinorelbine. *Lung Cancer* (2004) 45, 121–3.
4. Rezai K, Urien S, Isambert N, Roche H, Dieras V, Berille J, Bonneterre J, Brain E, Lokiec F. Pharmacokinetic evaluation of the vinorelbine-lapatinib combination in the treatment of breast cancer patients. *Cancer Chemother Pharmacol* (2011) 68, 1529–36.
5. Brain E, Isambert N, Dalenc F, Diéras V, Bonneterre J, Rezai K, Jimenez M, Mefti-Lacheraf F, Cottura E, Tresca P, Vanlemmens L, Mahier-Aït Oukhatar C, Lokiec F, Fumoleau P. Phase I study of lapatinib plus vinorelbine in patients with locally advanced or metastatic breast cancer overexpressing HER2. *Br J Cancer* (2012) 106, 673–7.
6. Blackhall FH, O'Brien M, Schmid P Nicolson M, Taylor P, Milenkova T, Kennedy SJ, Thatcher N. A phase I study of vandetanib in combination with vinorelbine/cisplatin or gemcitabine/cisplatin as first-line treatment for advanced non-small cell lung cancer. *J Thorac Oncol* (2010) 5, 1285–8.

Vinca alkaloids; Vinblastine + Bleomycin

In one study, the combination of vinblastine and bleomycin, with or without cisplatin, was commonly associated with Raynaud's phenomenon. Rarely, it also appeared to cause serious life-threatening vascular events.

Clinical evidence, mechanism, importance and management

Five men (aged 23 to 58 years) treated for germ cell tumours died from unexpected acute life-threatening vascular events (myocardial infarction, rectal infarction, cerebrovascular accident) after treatment with VBP (vinblastine, bleomycin, cisplatin). A survey of the literature by the authors of this paper revealed 14 other cases of both acute and long-term vascular problems (myocardial infarction, coronary heart disease, cerebrovascular accident) in patients given VBP.[1]

Raynaud's phenomenon is common, occurring in one-third to one-half of those given vinblastine and bleomycin, or VBP, for testicular cancer,[2,3] and there is evidence that blood vessels are pathologically altered.[2] Cisplatin might contribute to the effect.[3] Analysis of late vascular toxicity after chemotherapy for testicular cancer revealed that the use of VBP carried a higher risk of Raynaud's phenomenon than BEP (bleomycin with etoposide and cisplatin).[4]

The use of the VBP (PVB) regimen for testicular cancer has largely been replaced by the BEP (PEB) regimen, because of its reduced toxicity.

1. Samuels BL, Vogelzang NJ, Kennedy BJ. Severe vascular toxicity associated with vinblastine, bleomycin and cisplatin chemotherapy. *Cancer Chemother Pharmacol* (1987) 19, 253–6.
2. Vogelzang NJ, Bosl GJ, Johnson K, Kennedy BJ. Raynaud's phenomenon: a common toxicity after combination chemotherapy for testicular cancer. *Ann Intern Med* (1981) 95, 288–92.
3. Hansen SW. Late-effects after treatment for germ-cell cancer with cisplatin, vinblastine, and bleomycin. *Dan Med Bull* (1992) 39, 391–9.
4. Berger CC, Bokemeyer C, Schneider M, Kuczyk MA, Schmoll H-J. Secondary Raynaud's phenomenon and other late vascular complications following chemotherapy for testicular cancer. *Eur J Cancer* (1995) 31A, 2229–38.

Vinca alkaloids; Vincristine + Asparaginase

A case report suggests that vincristine neurotoxicity might be increased by the subsequent use of asparaginase. Limited evidence suggests that vincristine does not increase the incidence of anaphylaxis to asparaginase.

Clinical evidence, mechanism, importance and management

A single report describes a patient who had received a total dose of vincristine of 18.6 mg over a 6 week period and who developed severe neuropathy when subsequently given asparaginase (total dose 512 000 units) several weeks later. The authors hypothesised that the neurotoxic effects of the drugs were additive.[1,2] Limited evidence from a retrospective study found that there was no statistically significant difference in the incidence of anaphylaxis to asparaginase between 11 patients given vincristine and 89 not given vincristine. None of these patients received prednisone, but in another 92 patients receiving prednisone and vincristine, there was a lower incidence of anaphylaxis to asparaginase,[3] probably due to the corticosteroid.

Note that the UK manufacturer of vincristine recommends that it should be given 12 to 24 hours before asparaginase in order to minimise toxicity.[4] Regimens including both drugs are commonly used in treating leukaemia.

1. Hildebrand J, Kenis Y. Vincristine neurotoxicity. *N Engl J Med* (1972) 287, 517.
2. Hildebrand J, Kenis Y. Additive toxicity of vincristine and other drugs for the peripheral nervous system. *Acta Neurol Belg* (1971) 71, 486–91.
3. Evans WE, Tsiatis A, Rivera G, Murphy SB, Dahl GV, Denison M, Crom WR, Barker LF, Mauer AM. Anaphylactoid reactions to *Escherichia coli* and *Erwinia* asparaginase in children with leukemia and lymphoma. *Cancer* (1982) 49, 1378–83.
4. Vincristine sulphate. Hospira UK Ltd. UK Summary of product characteristics, January 2008.

Vinca alkaloids; Vincristine + Isoniazid

Isolated reports suggest that vincristine neurotoxicity might be increased by isoniazid.

Clinical evidence, mechanism, importance and management

An 85-year-old woman with Hodgkin's disease was given COPP and ABVD (doxorubicin, bleomycin, vinblastine, and dacarbazine), alternating every 28 days. She started COPP (cyclophosphamide and 2 mg vincristine on day one, with procarbazine and prednisone on days one to 14) and was also given isoniazid 300 mg daily as prophylaxis of tuberculosis. Five days after the start of this treatment she experienced tingling in her fingers and weakness in her legs, which was interpreted by the authors of this report as being vincristine toxicity (paraesthesia of the feet and/or hands being a recognised early sign of vincristine toxicity) brought about by the concurrent use of isoniazid. Their reasoning was that such a small dose of vincristine on its own was unlikely to cause severe neurotoxicity of this kind, but it is not clear why isoniazid should apparently interact like this. The authors suggest that the age of this patient and the fact that she had diabetes (well controlled) might have contributed to this increase in vincristine neurotoxicity.[1]

This report is consistent with another much earlier report of 2 patients who also developed peripheral neurotoxicity when they were given vincristine after starting to take isoniazid and pyridoxine, the cumulative doses of vincristine being 11 mg and 11.2 mg, respectively.[2,3] Similarly, another case describes severe neurotoxicity with an overdose of isoniazid and high-dose vincristine.[4]

These reports appear to be the only ones implicating isoniazid in an increase in vincristine neurotoxicity, but they suggest that close neurological supervision would be appropriate in anyone given both drugs.

1. Carrión C, Espinosa E, Herrero A, García B. Possible vincristine-isoniazid interaction. *Ann Pharmacother* (1995) 29, 201.
2. Hildebrand J, Kenis Y. Vincristine neurotoxicity. *N Engl J Med* (1972) 287, 517.
3. Hildebrand J, Kenis Y. Additive toxicity of vincristine and other drugs for the peripheral nervous system. *Acta Neurol Belg* (1971) 71, 486–91.
4. Frappaz D, Biron P, Biron E, Amrane A, Philip T, Brunat-Mentigny M. Toxicite neurologique severe (coma, convulsions, neuropathie motrice distale) secondaire a l'association d'une intoxication accidentelle a l'isoniazide (INH) et d'un protocole comportant de fortes doses de vincristine (VCR). *Pediatrie* (1984) 39, 133–40.

Vinca alkaloids; Vincristine + Piperacillin with Tazobactam

A case of autonomic neuropathy and cholestasis with vincristine was attributed to concurrent use of piperacillin with tazobactam.

Clinical evidence, mechanism, importance and management

An 11-year-old girl with leukaemia was given a chemotherapy regimen, including vincristine on days 9, 15, 22, and 29, and daunorubicin, cyclophosphamide, asparaginase, and prednisolone (doses not stated). She complained of jaw and abdominal pain from the first vincristine injection. Piperacillin with tazobactam was started on day 17 as an empirical treatment for febrile neutropenia, and was continued until day 45. Vincristine was still given on days 22 and 29. Abdominal pain and constipation worsened, and at day 31 she developed acute intestinal obstruction. She also developed cholestasis from day 22.

The authors hypothesised that piperacillin might inhibit the drug transporter multidrug resistance protein 2 (MRP2), thereby reducing vincristine elimination and increasing its toxicity.[1] No vincristine concentrations were measured.

This is the first report of this potential interaction. Considering the length of time that both piperacillin and vincristine have been in clinical use, and the lack of any other reports, an interaction is by no means certain. However, the authors do note that it is rare to continue the vincristine while receiving treatment for neutropenic fever.[1] Bear this case in mind in the event of unexpected toxicity on the concurrent use of vincristine and piperacillin.

1. Le Guellec C, Benz-de Bretagne I, Jonville-Bera AP, Tarfaoui N, Andres CR, Gendrot C, Jourdain A. A case of severe toxicity during coadministration of vincristine and piperacillin: are drug transporters involved in vincristine hypersensitivity and drug-drug interactions? *J Pediatr Hematol Oncol* (2012) 34, e341–e343.

Vinca alkaloids; Vinflunine + Miscellaneous

St John's wort is predicted to reduce vinflunine concentrations, and grapefruit juice is predicted to increase vinflunine concentrations.

Clinical evidence, mechanism, importance and management

(a) Grapefruit juice

The UK manufacturer of vinflunine advises against the concurrent use of potent CYP3A4 inhibitors, and they name grapefruit juice as an example.[1] However, grapefruit juice is generally a weak inhibitor of CYP3A4 and has most effect on drugs that are given orally, therefore a clinically relevant interaction with vinflunine (which is given intravenously) seems unlikely.

(b) St John's wort (Hypericum perforatum)

The UK manufacturer of vinflunine advises against the concurrent use of potent CYP3A4 inducers, and they name St John's wort as an example.[1] St John's wort is generally a moderate inducer of CYP3A4, but it is possible that it might reduce vinflunine exposure and reduce its efficacy. Where possible it would seem prudent to avoid concurrent use, as it is difficult to standardise for the effects of herbal medicines, which can vary in their composition. If concurrent use is considered essential, monitor efficacy closely.

1. Javlor (Vinflunine ditartrate). Pierre Fabre Ltd. UK Summary of product characteristics, June 2012.

Vinca alkaloids; Vinorelbine + Food

Food does not notably alter the exposure to oral vinorelbine.

Clinical evidence, mechanism, importance and management

In a crossover study in 13 patients with cancer, taking vinorelbine 80 mg/m^2, as soft-gel capsules, after a continental breakfast had no effect on the AUC or maximum concentration of vinorelbine when compared with the fasted state.[1] This differs from an earlier study using a liquid-filled capsule (formulation not currently marketed), which found a 22% reduction in the AUC of vinorelbine when taken with a standard breakfast (eggs, bacon, and hash-browns).[2]

It appears that food has no effect on vinorelbine exposure after oral administration of the soft-gel capsule formulation. The UK manufacturer advises administration with a little food because this reduces the incidence of nausea.[3]

1. Bugat R, Variol P, Roché H, Fumoleau P, Robinet G, Senac I. The effects of food on the pharmacokinetic profile of oral vinorelbine. *Cancer Chemother Pharmacol* (2002) 50, 285–90.
2. Rowinsky EK, Lucas VS, Hsieh AL, Wargin WA, Hohneker JA, Lubejko B, Sartorius SE, Donehower RC. The effects of food and divided dosing on the bioavailability of oral vinorelbine. *Cancer Chemother Pharmacol* (1996) 39, 9–16.
3. Navelbine Soft Capsules (Vinorelbine tartrate). Pierre Fabre Ltd. UK Summary of product characteristics, July 2011.

Vinca alkaloids; Vinorelbine + Ondansetron with Dexamethasone

A chemotherapy regimen containing ondansetron with dexamethasone does not appear to alter the pharmacokinetics of a single intravenous dose of vinorelbine.

Clinical evidence, mechanism, importance and management

In a pharmacokinetic study in 12 patients with cancer, an antiemetic regimen, including aprepitant, **dexamethasone** (12 mg on day one and 8 mg on days 2 to 4) and **ondansetron** 32 mg on day one, had no effect on the pharmacokinetics of intravenous vinorelbine 25 mg/m^2 given on day one or day 8 when compared with vinorelbine given alone.[1]

Although the drugs were not given individually in this study, the findings suggest that neither dexamethasone nor ondansetron alter the pharmacokinetics of vinorelbine: aprepitant is known not to affect vinorelbine pharmacokinetics (see 'Antineoplastics + Aprepitant', p.656). These drugs can be used for prophylaxis against vinorelbine-induced nausea and vomiting without expectation of a pharmacokinetic interaction.

1. Loos WJ, de Wit R, Freedman SJ, Van Dyck K, Gambale JJ, Li S, Murphy GM, van Noort C, de Bruijn P, Verweij J. Aprepitant when added to a standard antiemetic regimen consisting of ondansetron and dexamethasone does not affect vinorelbine pharmacokinetics in cancer patients. *Cancer Chemother Pharmacol* (2007) 59, 407–12.

Vinca alkaloids; Vinorelbine + Vorinostat

Vorinostat appears to have no effect on vinorelbine exposure.

Clinical evidence, mechanism, importance and management

In a small study, 7 patients with advanced cancer were given vorinostat 200 mg daily for 7 days, every 21 days, and intravenous vinorelbine 25 mg/m^2 once weekly started 4 hours after the first vorinostat dose. The AUC of vinorelbine did not differ between day 1 (4 hours after the first vorinostat dose) and day 8 (one day after stopping the vorinostat), and did not differ from historical control data. This suggests that vorinostat does not alter vinorelbine pharmacokinetics. However, the vorinostat AUC on day 1 was about 30 to 50% higher than that seen in other published pharmacokinetic studies, and was associated with a higher incidence of hyperglycaemia. The authors discounted an interaction with vinorelbine as the explanation because plasma vorinostat concentrations were already higher than expected in the 4-hour time period before vinorelbine was administered. This explanation seems reasonable. No pharmacokinetic interaction would therefore be expected between vorinostat and vinorelbine. It has been suggested that unknown patient factors were responsible for the unexpectedly high vorinostat exposure;[1] this requires further investigation.

1. Gandia P, Arellano C, Chalret du Rieu Q, Lochon I, Campone M, Pierga JY, Poublanc M, Hennebelle I, Filleron T, Chatelut E, Delord JP. Unexpected high levels of vorinostat when combined with vinorelbine in patients with advanced cancer. *Curr Clin Pharmacol* (2011) 6, 274–9.

Vorinostat + Antineoplastics; Cytotoxic

The use of paclitaxel and carboplatin with vorinostat slightly increased the exposure to vorinostat in one study. Paclitaxel pharmacokinetics appeared to be unaffected by vorinostat.

Clinical evidence, mechanism, importance and management

In a study in 28 patients with solid tumours, the AUC and half-life of vorinostat were increased by 37% and 61%, respectively, when given with **carboplatin** and **paclitaxel**.

In this study, patients received intravenous **paclitaxel** 175 mg/m^2 increased to 200 mg/m^2 over 3 hours then **carboplatin** (dose adjusted to reach a target exposure) as a 30-minute infusion every 3 weeks. Oral vorinostat 200 mg daily for 14 days was given, starting 4 days before chemotherapy in the first cycle, then in increasing doses of 300 mg daily then 400 mg daily for 14 days starting on day one for subsequent cycles. The pharmacokinetics of **paclitaxel** were unaffected by vorinostat when compared with historical data, but the pharmacokinetics of **carboplatin** were not assessed. The incidence of grade 4 neutropenia was higher in this study (50%) than historical data for **carboplatin** with **paclitaxel**.[1]

The reason for the apparent alteration in vorinostat pharmacokinetics is uncertain. There was no definite relationship between vorinostat dose and the incidence of neutropenia, but it is possible that the use of vorinostat with paclitaxel contributed to this. Further study is needed to establish the effects of concurrent use.

1. Ramalingam SS, Parise RA, Ramananthan RK, Lagattuta TF, Musguire LA, Stoller RG, Potter DM, Argiris AE, Zwiebel JA, Egorin MJ, Belani CP. Phase I and pharmacokinetic study of vorinostat, a histone deacetylase inhibitor, in combination with carboplatin and paclitaxel for advanced solid malignancies. *Clin Cancer Res* (2007) 16, 3605–10.

Vorinostat + Food

The absorption of oral vorinostat is modestly increased by food.

Clinical evidence, mechanism, importance and management

The pharmacokinetics of vorinostat were investigated in 23 patients who received a single 400-mg oral dose of vorinostat in the fasted state, and again after a standardised high-fat meal. There was a 38% increase in the AUC of vorinostat when taken with food, and a delay of 2.5 hours in reaching the maximum plasma levels. This modest effect of food was not considered to be clinically relevant.[1] However, note that the manufacturer advises that the daily dose is taken with food, as this is how the clinical studies were conducted.[2]

1. Rubin EH, Agrawal NGB, Friedman EJ, Scott P, Mazina KE, Sun L, Du L, Ricker JL, Frankel SR, Gottesdiener KM, Wagner JA, Iwamoto M. A study to determine the effects of food and multiple dosing on the pharmacokinetics of vorinostat given orally to patients with advanced cancer. *Clin Cancer Res* (2006) 12, 7039–45.
2. Zolinza (Vorinostat). Merck & Co., Inc. US Prescribing information, September 2009.

Vorinostat + Miscellaneous

Severe thrombocytopenia and gastrointestinal bleeding have been reported in patients who took vorinostat and valproic acid. Increased INRs have occurred in patients taking vorinostat with coumarins.

Clinical evidence, mechanism, importance and management

(a) Valproate

The manufacturer notes that severe thrombocytopenia and gastrointestinal bleeding have been reported in patients who took vorinostat and other drugs that are histone deacetylase inhibitors. They specifically name **valproic acid**.[1] Note that thrombocytopenia is common with vorinostat alone.

(b) Warfarin and related drugs

The manufacturer notes that prolongation of the prothrombin time and raised INRs have been observed in patients receiving vorinostat with coumarin anticoagulants. They recommend close monitoring of the prothrombin time and INR in these patients.[1]

1. Zolinza (Vorinostat). Merck & Co., Inc. US Prescribing information, September 2009.

18

Antiparkinsonian and related drugs

The drugs in this section are considered together because their major therapeutic application is in the treatment of Parkinson's disease, although some of the related antimuscarinic (anticholinergic) drugs included here are also used for other conditions. Parkinson's disease is named after Dr James Parkinson who originally described the four main signs of the disease, namely rigidity, tremor, dystonias and dyskinesias (movement disorders). Similar symptoms may also be displayed as the unwanted adverse effects of certain drugs.

The basic cause of the disease lies in the basal ganglia of the brain, particularly the striatum and the substantia nigra, where the normal balance between dopaminergic nerve fibres (those that use dopamine as the chemical transmitter) and cholinergic nerve fibres (those that use acetylcholine as the transmitter) is lost, because the dopaminergic fibres degenerate. As a result the cholinergic fibres end up in relative excess. Much of the treatment of Parkinson's disease is based on an attempt to redress the balance, and there are several groups of drugs that can be used to this end. These are listed in 'Table 18.1' (below), and discussed below.

Levodopa

Levodopa can pass the blood-brain barrier (unlike dopamine), where it is converted into dopamine, and thus acts by 'topping up' the CNS dopaminergic system. Levodopa is most usually given with **carbidopa** or **benserazide** (dopa-decarboxylase inhibitors), which prevent the 'wasteful' peripheral metabolism of levodopa. This allows lower doses of levodopa to be given, which results in fewer adverse effects.

Amantadine

Amantadine may augment dopaminergic activity in the brain.

Dopamine agonists

Bromocriptine, cabergoline, pergolide, ropinirole and similar drugs act as dopamine agonists and so also have the effect of increasing dopaminergic activity in the brain.

Entacapone and Tolcapone

The catechol-*O*-methyltransferase (COMT) inhibitors work by inhibiting the peripheral metabolism of levodopa by COMT. Note that this enzyme is the major metabolising enzyme for levodopa when a decarboxylase inhibitor (e.g. benserazide) is being used.

Rasagiline and Selegiline

The selective irreversible MAO-B inhibitors enhance dopamine activity by preventing dopamine degradation. These drugs sometimes interact like non-selective MAOIs, and the reader is cross-referred to the information under MAOIs when appropriate. Selegiline undergoes rapid first-pass metabolism to produce amfetamine metabolites. A buccal tablet has been developed, which markedly reduces this first-pass metabolism, and is consequently given as a smaller dose.

Antimuscarinics

Benzhexol, orphenadrine, procyclidine and other antimuscarinic (anticholinergic) drugs work by correcting the relative cholinergic excess.

The interactions that affect the antimuscarinic effects of these drugs are discussed in this section. However, the antimuscarinics also affect the actions of other drugs (such as the centrally-acting anticholinesterases) and these are therefore discussed elsewhere in the publication.

Table 18.1 Antiparkinsonian drugs

Group	*Drugs*
Dopaminergic drugs	
Amino-acid precursor of dopamine	Levodopa
Levodopa combined with a peripheral dopa-decarboxylase inhibitor	Co-beneldopa (levodopa with benserazide) Co-careldopa (levodopa with carbidopa)
COMT-inhibitors	Entacapone, Tolcapone
Dopamine agonists	
Ergot derivatives	Bromocriptine, Cabergoline, Lisuride, Pergolide
Non-ergot dopamine agonists	Piribedil, Pramipexole, Quinagolide, Ropinirole, Rotigotine
Other dopamine agonists	Apomorphine
MAO-B inhibitors	Rasagiline, Selegiline
Other	Amantadine
Other	
Peripheral dopa-decarboxylase inhibitors	Benserazide, Carbidopa
Antimuscarinics	Benzatropine, Biperiden, Bornaprine, Dexetimide, Metixene, Orphenadrine, Procyclidine, Profenamine, Trihexyphenidyl, Tropatepine

Amantadine + Co-trimoxazole

An interaction between amantadine and co-trimoxazole is thought to have caused acute confusion in an elderly man, and amantadine toxicity in a patient with end-stage renal disease. However, in both cases other factors could have been responsible for the adverse reactions.

Clinical evidence, mechanism, importance and management

An 84-year-old man with parkinsonism, COPD and chronic atrial fibrillation, had been taking amantadine 100 mg twice daily and digoxin 125 micrograms daily for at least 2 years. Within 72 hours of starting co-trimoxazole twice daily for bronchitis he became mentally confused, incoherent and combative. He also had cogwheel rigidity and a resting tremor. Within 24 hours of stopping the amantadine and co-trimoxazole, the patient's mental status returned to normal.[1] The reasons for this reaction are not understood, but on the basis of *animal* studies, the authors suggest that the **trimethoprim** component of co-trimoxazole may have competed with amantadine for renal secretion. This resulted in an accumulation of amantadine and led to the adverse effects seen.[1] This interaction is more likely in the elderly because ageing results in a decreased clearance of these and many other drugs. However, it should be noted that both drugs can cause some mental confusion, and also that mental confusion is not an uncommon symptom of infection in the elderly. Another case of amantadine toxicity has been reported in a 27-year-old woman with end-stage renal disease who was also taking co-trimoxazole. As in the other case the authors suggest that the **trimethoprim** component of co-trimoxazole may have competed with amantadine for renal secretion. However, they also note that amantadine toxicity occurred 5 days after the amantadine dose was increased, and during an episode of acute renal failure, which could also account for the toxicity.[2]

These seem to be the only reports of a possible interaction, and therefore their general importance remains uncertain.

1. Speeg KV, Leighton JA, Maldonado AL. Case report: toxic delirium in a patient taking amantadine and trimethoprim-sulfamethoxazole. *Am J Med Sci* (1989) 298, 410–12.
2. Michalski LS, Hantsch CE, Hou SH. Amantadine toxicity in a renal transplant patient. Abstracts of the 2003 North American Congress of Clinical Toxicology Annual Meeting, 93.

Amantadine + Diuretics

A patient has been described who developed amantadine toxicity when given hydrochlorothiazide with triamterene, and another patient taking amantadine developed myoclonic jerks after starting to take spironolactone and altizide.

Clinical evidence

Amantadine toxicity (ataxia, agitation, hallucinations) developed in a patient within a week of starting to take two tablets of *Dyazide* (**hydrochlorothiazide** with **triamterene**) daily. The symptoms rapidly disappeared when all the drugs were withdrawn. In a later study the amantadine plasma levels of this patient rose by about 50% (from 156 to 243 nanograms/mL) after taking the diuretic for 7 days.[1] A further case describes myoclonic jerks in a 64-year-old man after the addition of **spironolactone** and **altizide** to established treatment for Parkinson's disease, which included levodopa with benserazide, amantadine, orphenadrine, imipramine and diazepam. The diuretics were stopped, but the myoclonic jerks only resolved after the amantadine was also stopped.[2]

Mechanism

Uncertain. Amantadine is largely excreted unchanged in the urine and it seems probable that these diuretics reduce its renal clearance.[1]

Importance and management

Published information about an adverse interaction between amantadine and diuretics appears to be limited. There seems to be little reason for avoiding concurrent use, but bear these cases in mind in the event of an unexpected response to treatment.

1. Wilson TW, Rajput AH. Amantadine–Dyazide interaction. *Can Med Assoc J* (1983) 129, 974–5.
2. Chevalier JF, Renier E, Brion S. <OE-DIPTHONG>dème et myoclonies chez un parkinsonien traité par Mantadix®. Problème des associations médicamenteuses. *Encephale* (1980) 6, 381–4.

Amantadine + MAOIs or MAO-B inhibitors

An isolated report describes a rise in blood pressure in a patient taking amantadine within 72 hours of taking phenelzine. The use of selegiline with amantadine may increase adverse effects.

Clinical evidence, mechanism, importance and management

A 49-year-old woman taking amantadine 200 mg daily, haloperidol 5 mg daily and flurazepam 30 mg at night was given **phenelzine** 15 mg twice daily for depression. Within 72 hours her blood pressure rose from 140/90 mmHg to 160/110 mmHg. The **phenelzine** was withdrawn, and 24 hours later, the amantadine and haloperidol were withdrawn. The blood pressure remained elevated for a further 72 hours.[1] In contrast, a woman is reported to have successfully and uneventfully taken amantadine 200 mg daily for Parkinson's disease and **phenelzine** 45 mg daily for depression.[2]

The first case appears to be the only reported interaction with amantadine. Its general importance is therefore uncertain, but bear it in mind in case of an unusual response to treatment.

One manufacturer of **selegiline** states that concurrent use of amantadine can lead to an increased occurrence of adverse effects,[3] but no further information is given.

1. Jack RA, Daniel DG. Possible interaction between phenelzine and amantadine. *Arch Gen Psychiatry* (1984) 41, 726.
2. Greenberg R, Meyers BS. Treatment of major depression and Parkinson's disease with combined phenelzine and amantadine. *Am J Psychiatry* (1985) 142, 273–4.
3. Zelapar (Selegiline hydrochloride). Cephalon Ltd. UK summary of product characteristics, September 2008.

Amantadine + Miscellaneous

Amantadine has antimuscarinic adverse effects and therefore may interact in the same way as the antimuscarinics.

Clinical evidence, mechanism, importance and management

The adverse effects of amantadine resemble those of antimuscarinic drugs. The manufacturers of amantadine note[1,2] that it may interact with a number of drugs, presumably somewhat based on the way these antimuscarinics are known to interact. They name alcohol (consider 'Alcohol + Antimuscarinics', p.56), antimuscarinics (consider 'Antimuscarinics + Antimuscarinics', p.754), antipsychotics (consider 'Antipsychotics + Antimuscarinics', p.805), and levodopa (consider 'Levodopa + Antimuscarinics', p.762).

1. Symmetrel (Amantadine hydrochloride). Alliance Pharmaceuticals. UK Summary of product characteristics, January 2008.
2. Symmetrel (Amantadine hydrochloride). Endo Pharmaceuticals Inc. US Prescribing information, May 2007.

Amantadine + Phenylpropanolamine

The use of amantadine in a patient also taking phenylpropanolamine resulted in psychosis, and concurrent use in another patient resulted in intense and recurrent déjà vu experiences.

Clinical evidence, mechanism, importance and management

A case report describes the development of severe psychosis in a woman within 7 to 8 days of starting amantadine 100 mg [frequency unclear but possibly twice daily] and phenylpropanolamine 80 mg daily. The reasons are not known, but both drugs alone, and in high doses sometimes cause psychosis, and concurrent use may enhance this effect.[1] Another report describes intense and recurrent déjà vu experiences in a 39-year-old man taking amantadine 100 mg twice daily and phenylpropanolamine 25 mg twice daily during a viral infection. These experiences stopped the day he discontinued the drugs. He had previously taken phenylpropanolamine without this effect. The authors considered the déjà vu experiences to be related to increased dopamine activity caused by both drugs.[2]

Concurrent use need not be avoided, but remain aware of the potential for this interaction.

1. Stroe AE, Hall J, Amin F. Psychotic episode related to phenylpropanolamine and amantadine in a healthy female. *Gen Hosp Psychiatry* (1995) 17, 457–8.
2. Taiminen T, Jääskeläinen SK. Intense and recurrent déjà vu experiences related to amantadine and phenylpropanolamine in a healthy male. *J Clin Neurosci* (2001) 8, 460–2.

Amantadine + Quinidine or Quinine

In a single-dose study, quinidine and quinine modestly reduced the loss of amantadine in the urine in men, but not women.

Clinical evidence, mechanism, importance and management

Single-dose studies into the renal excretion of amantadine in healthy subjects found that quinine sulfate 200 mg and quinidine sulfate 200 mg reduced the renal clearance of oral amantadine 3 mg/kg by about 30%, but only in male subjects.[1] Whether the long-term use of these drugs would therefore cause a clinically relevant rise in serum amantadine levels is uncertain. However, the absence of any clinical reports suggests it is unlikely. Nevertheless, be aware that amantadine toxicity (e.g. headache, nausea, or dizziness) could possibly result from the concurrent use of quinine or quinidine.

1. Gaudry SE, Sitar DS, Smyth DD, McKenzie JK, Aoki FY. Gender and age as factors in the inhibition of renal clearance of amantadine by quinine and quinidine. *Clin Pharmacol Ther* (1993) 54, 23–7.

Amantadine + Tobacco

Amantadine clearance was not altered by tobacco smoking in one study.

Clinical evidence, mechanism, importance and management

The elimination of a single 3-mg/kg dose of amantadine was compared between heavy smokers (20 or more cigarettes daily) and non-smokers.

Although a higher apparent volume of distribution was noted in the heavy smokers, renal and plasma clearances were unchanged, suggesting that no interaction of note occurs.[1]

1. Wong LTY, Sitar DS, Aoki FY. Chronic tobacco smoking and gender as variables affecting amantadine disposition in healthy subjects. *Br J Clin Pharmacol* (1995) 39, 81–4.

Antimuscarinics + Antimuscarinics

Additive antimuscarinic effects, both peripheral and central, can develop if two or more drugs with antimuscarinic effects are used together. The outcome might be harmful.

Clinical evidence, mechanism, importance and management

The antimuscarinic (sometimes called anticholinergic) effects of some drugs are exploited therapeutically. These include antimuscarinic bronchodilators, gastrointestinal antispasmodics, mydriatics, urological antimuscarinics, and drugs such as **trihexyphenidyl** and **benzatropine** (see 'Table 18.1', p.752), which are used for the control of parkinsonian symptoms. Other drugs, such as some antiemetics, sedating antihistamines, antipsychotics, and tricyclic antidepressants, (see 'Table 18.2', below), might also possess some antimuscarinic effects that are unwanted and troublesome, but usually not serious, unless they are worsened by the addition of another drug with similar properties.

The easily recognised and common peripheral antimuscarinic effects are blurred vision, dry mouth, constipation, difficulty in urination, reduced sweating, and tachycardia. Central effects include confusion, disorientation, visual hallucinations, agitation, irritability, delirium, memory problems, belligerence, and even aggressiveness. Problems are most likely to arise in patients with particular physical conditions such as glaucoma, prostatic hypertrophy or constipation, in whom antimuscarinic drugs should be used with caution, if at all. It has been pointed out that the antimuscarinic adverse effects can mimic the effects of normal ageing.

'Table 18.1', p.752 and 'Table 18.2', below list many of the drugs with antimuscarinic effects, which might be expected to be additive if used together, but apart from some reports describing life-threatening reactions (see 'Antipsychotics + Antimuscarinics', p.805) there are very few reports describing this simple additive interaction, probably because the outcome is so obvious. Many of these interactions are therefore theoretical but their probability is high.

Table 18.2 Drugs with antimuscarinic effects (main or adverse effects)

Group	*Drugs*
Antiarrhythmics	Disopyramide, Propafenone
Antiemetics	Cyclizine, Dimenhydrinate, Hyoscine (Scopolamine), Meclozine
Antihistamines	Brompheniramine, Chlorphenamine, Cyproheptadine, Diphenhydramine, Hydroxyzine, Promethazine, Tripelennamine, Triprolidine
Antiparkinsonian drugs (Antimuscarinics)	see Table 18.1, p.752
Antipsychotics	Chlorpromazine, Chlorprothixene, Clozapine, Loxapine, Mesoridazine, Perphenazine, Pimozide, Thioridazine, Trifluoperazine
Antispasmodics	Anisotropine, Atropine, Belladonna alkaloids, Dicycloverine (Dicyclomine), Flavoxate, Hyoscine (Scopolamine), Hyoscyamine, Isopropamide, Propantheline
Antiulcer drugs	Clidinium, Hexocyclium, Isopropamide, Mepenzolate, Methanthelinium, Oxyphencyclimine, Pirenzepine, Tridihexethyl
Bronchodilators	Aclidinium, Ipratropium, Tiotropium
Cycloplegic mydriatics	Atropine, Cyclopentolate, Homatropine, Hyoscine (Scopolamine), Tropicamide
Muscle relaxants	Baclofen, Cyclobenzaprine, Orphenadrine
Peripheral vasodilator	Papaverine
Tricyclic and related antidepressants	Amitriptyline, Amoxapine, Clomipramine, Desipramine, Doxepin, Imipramine, Maprotiline, Nortriptyline, Protriptyline, Trimipramine
Urinary antimuscarinics	Darifenacin, Fesoterodine, Oxybutynin, Solifenacin, Tolterodine, Trospium

After Barkin RL, Stein ZLG. *South Med J* (1989) 82, 1547, and others.
The categorization is not exclusive; some of these drugs are used for a range of effects. There are many other antimuscarinic drugs.

Some drugs with only minimal antimuscarinic properties sometimes cause difficulties if given with other antimuscarinics. A patient taking **isopropamide iodide** developed urinary retention needing catheterisation, only when **trazodone** 75 mg daily was also taken, but not when either drug was taken alone.[1] **Trazodone** is usually regarded as having minimal antimuscarinic effects. Another case describes acute psychosis in an elderly woman taking **hyoscine** and **meclozine**, both of which have antimuscarinic effects.[2]

If the central antimuscarinic effects caused by the use of antimuscarinic drugs are not clearly recognised for what they are, there is the risk that antipsychotics might be prescribed to treat them. Many antipsychotics also have antimuscarinic adverse effects so that matters are simply made worse. If the patient then demonstrates dystonias, akathisia, tremor, and rigidity, even more antimuscarinics might be added to control the extrapyramidal effects, which merely adds to the continuing downward cycle of drug-induced problems.

In addition to the obvious and very well recognised drugs with antimuscarinic effects, a study of the 25 drugs most commonly prescribed for the elderly identified detectable antimuscarinic activity (using an antimuscarinic radioreceptor assay) in 14 of them, 9 of which (**codeine**, **digoxin**, **dipyridamole**, **isosorbide dinitrate**, **nifedipine**, **prednisolone**, **ranitidine**, **theophylline**, and **warfarin**) produced levels of antimuscarinic activity that have been shown to cause significant impairment in tests of memory and attention in the elderly.[3] Thus the problem may not necessarily be confined to those drugs that have well recognised antimuscarinic properties.

1. Chan CH, Ruskiewicz RJ. Anticholinergic side effects of trazodone combined with another pharmacologic agent. *Am J Psychiatry* (1990) 147, 533.
2. Osterholm RK, Camoriano JK. Transdermal scopolamine psychosis. *JAMA* (1982) 247, 3081.
3. Tune L, Carr S, Hoag E, Cooper T. Anticholinergic effects of drugs commonly prescribed for the elderly: potential means for assessing risk of delirium. *Am J Psychiatry* (1992) 149, 1393–4.

Antimuscarinics + Areca (Betel nuts)

The control of the extrapyramidal (parkinsonian) adverse effects of fluphenazine and flupenthixol with procyclidine was lost in two patients when they began to chew areca.

Clinical evidence

An Indian patient receiving depot fluphenazine (50 mg every 3 weeks) for schizophrenia, and with mild parkinsonian tremor controlled with **procyclidine** 5 mg twice daily, developed marked rigidity, bradykinesia and jaw tremor when he began to chew areca. The symptoms were so severe he could barely speak. When he stopped chewing areca his stiffness and abnormal movements disappeared. Another patient receiving depot flupenthixol developed marked stiffness, tremor and akathisia when he began to chew areca, despite taking up to 20 mg of **procyclidine** daily. The symptoms vanished within 4 days of stopping the areca.[1]

Mechanism

Areca contains arecoline, an alkaloid with cholinergic activity, which could therefore oppose the antimuscarinic (anticholinergic) actions of procyclidine. As the procyclidine was being used to control the extrapyramidal adverse effects of the two antipsychotics, opposing its action allowed the adverse effects to re-emerge and worsen.

Importance and management

Direct information seems to be limited to this report but the interaction would seem to be established and clinically important. Patients taking antimuscarinic drugs for the control of drug-induced extrapyramidal (parkinsonian) adverse effects, or Parkinson's disease, should avoid areca (betel nuts). Betel is traditionally chewed by those from the continent of Asia, and the East Indies. The authors of this report suggest that a dental inspection for the characteristic red stains of the areca may possibly provide a simple explanation for the sudden and otherwise mysterious deterioration in the symptoms of patients. Symptoms seem to develop over a period of 2 weeks, and resolve fairly rapidly (within a week).

1. Deahl M. Betel nut-induced extrapyramidal syndrome: an unusual drug interaction. *Mov Disord* (1989) 4, 330–3.

Antimuscarinics + SSRIs

Nine patients developed delirium when given fluoxetine, paroxetine or sertraline with benzatropine, in the presence of an antipsychotic (usually perphenazine or haloperidol). Paroxetine appears to increase the exposure to procyclidine.

Clinical evidence

Five patients became confused and developed delirium when given an antipsychotic, an SSRI (4 taking **fluoxetine** and one taking **paroxetine**) and **benzatropine**. No peripheral antimuscarinic toxicity was seen. The delirium developed within 2 days in two cases, but took several weeks to appear in another. The authors also very briefly mention two other patients who became delirious when given an unnamed antipsychotic and either **sertraline** or **paroxetine** with **benzatropine**.[1] Another case describes delirium in a 17-year-old boy, 8 days after **paroxetine** was added to his medication, which included **benzatropine** and haloperidol. Serum levels of **benzatropine** were markedly increased.[2] A further case report describes delirium in a 26-year-old woman taking **sertraline** 200 mg daily, haloperidol up to 9 mg daily, and lithium 900 mg daily after **benzatropine** 5 mg daily was added to her medication, to treat an episode of parkinsonism.[3] In contrast, another report describes 12 patients taking **fluoxetine** and perphenazine who also received **benzatropine** 1 mg daily without showing signs of delirium.[4,5]

The manufacturers note that **paroxetine** 30 mg daily increased the AUC, maximum, and minimum plasma concentrations of **procyclidine** 5 mg daily by 35%, 37%, and 67%, respectively.[6]

Mechanism

The authors of the first report attributed these effects to an interaction between the SSRIs and benzatropine, speculating that the SSRIs may have inhibited the metabolism of the benzatropine thereby increasing its toxicity. Alternatively they suggest a possible additive central antimuscarinic effect. It is noteworthy that 4 of the first group of patients were given perphenazine and one haloperidol,[1] which have been involved in additive antimuscarinic interactions (see 'Antipsychotics + Antimuscarinics', p.805). Also note that adverse interactions have been reported with the use of haloperidol and SSRIs, see 'Haloperidol + SSRIs', p.863. The reason for the increase in procyclidine exposure on concurrent use of paroxetine is unknown.

Importance and management

The general clinical importance of this interaction is uncertain, but it would seem prudent to be alert for evidence of confusion and possible delirium in patients given SSRIs with benzatropine, particularly if they are also taking other psychotropics that may have antimuscarinic actions. The authors of the first report say that they have not seen delirium with combinations of SSRIs (not named) and other antimuscarinic drugs such as **biperiden** and **diphenhydramine**.[1] If antimuscarinic effects are seen in patients taking paroxetine and procyclidine, the dose of procyclidine should be reduced.[6,7]

1. Roth A, Akyol S, Nelson JC. Delirium associated with the combination of a neuroleptic, an SSRI, and benztropine. *J Clin Psychiatry* (1994) 55, 492–5.
2. Armstrong SC, Schweitzer SM. Delirium associated with paroxetine and benztropine combination. *Am J Psychiatry* (1997) 154, 581–2.
3. Byerly MJ, Christensen RC, Evans DL. Delirium associated with a combination of sertraline, haloperidol, and benztropine. *Am J Psychiatry* (1996) 153, 965–6.
4. Rothschild AJ, Samson JA, Bessette MP, Carter-Campbell JT. Efficacy of the combination of fluoxetine and perphenazine in the treatment of psychotic depression. *J Clin Psychiatry* (1993) 54, 338–42.
5. Rothschild AJ. Delirium: an SSRI-benztropine adverse effect? *J Clin Psychiatry* (1995) 56, 537.
6. Paxil Tablets and Suspension (Paroxetine hydrochloride). GlaxoSmithKline. US Prescribing information, December 2012.
7. Kemadrin (Procyclidine hydrochloride). GlaxoSmithKline UK. UK Summary of product characteristics, May 2008.

Apomorphine + Antihypertensives

The hypotensive adverse effects of apomorphine may possibly be increased by nitrates, calcium-channel blockers and alpha blockers. There is some evidence that ACE inhibitors, beta blockers and diuretics do not generally increase the risk of hypotension with apomorphine.

Clinical evidence

(a) ACE inhibitors

A single 5-mg sublingual dose of apomorphine produced no clinically relevant changes in heart rate or blood pressure in 25 patients taking ACE inhibitors [not specifically named]. One patient experienced symptomatic hypotension.[1]

(b) Alpha blockers

A single 5-mg sublingual dose of apomorphine caused a greater decrease in systolic blood pressure from supine to standing in 24 patients taking alpha blockers [not specifically named] when compared with placebo (decrease in systolic blood pressure of 23 mmHg versus 13 mmHg at 40 minutes post dose). One patient experienced symptomatic hypotension.[1]

(c) Beta blockers

A single 5-mg sublingual dose of apomorphine produced no clinically relevant changes in heart rate or blood pressure in 26 patients taking beta blockers [not specifically named]. One patient experienced syncope and one had symptomatic hypotension.[1]

(d) Calcium-channel blockers

A single 5-mg sublingual dose of apomorphine caused a greater decrease in systolic blood pressure from supine to standing in 26 patients taking calcium-channel blockers [not specifically named] when compared with placebo (decreased in systolic blood pressure of 17 mmHg versus 11 mmHg at 20 minutes post dose).[1]

(e) Diuretics

A single 5-mg sublingual dose of apomorphine produced no clinically relevant changes in heart rate or blood pressure in 21 patients taking diuretics [not specifically named]. One patient experienced symptomatic hypotension.[1]

(f) Nitrates

1. Short-acting. A single 5-mg sublingual dose of apomorphine produced no clinically relevant changes in heart rate or blood pressure in 20 patients taking short-acting nitrates. The apomorphine was given 30 minutes before the patient took their short-acting nitrate. Two patients experienced symptomatic hypotension after their sublingual glyceryl trinitrate.[1]

2. Long-acting. A single 5-mg sublingual dose of apomorphine caused a greater decrease in systolic blood pressure from supine to standing in 20 patients taking long-acting nitrates when compared with placebo (decrease in systolic blood pressure of 12 mmHg versus 6 mmHg at 50 minutes post dose). Two patients experienced symptomatic hypotension.[1]

Mechanism

Apomorphine alone may cause postural hypotension, and this is potentially additive with the effects of vasoactive antihypertensives and nitrates.

Importance and management

A potentially clinically relevant interaction resulting in orthostatic hypotension may occur when sublingual apomorphine is given to patients taking calcium-channel blockers or alpha blockers. Similarly, symptomatic hypotension on standing may be more common in patients taking nitrates. Note that the 5-mg dose used in the study was slightly higher than the recommended 2- to 3-mg sublingual dose commonly used for erectile dysfunction. All the patients who had symptomatic hypotension experienced a prodrome of symptoms such as nausea, dizziness, pallor, and/or sweating.[1] The manufacturer of apomorphine used subcutaneously for Parkinson's disease suggests caution in patients taking antihypertensives[2] and on the basis of the study mentioned above[1], particular caution should be taken with nitrates. In practice, this means telling patients what may possibly happen and what to do if adverse effects occur (i.e. do not attempt to stand up, but lie down and raise their legs until the symptoms resolve). Note that apomorphine should be given with caution to patients with cardiovascular disease.[2]

1. Fagan TC, Buttler S, Marbury T, Taylor A, Edmonds A, and the SL APO study group. Cardiovascular safety of sublingual apomorphine in patients on stable doses of oral antihypertensive agents and nitrates. *Am J Cardiol* (2001) 88, 760–6.
2. APO-go Ampoules (Apomorphine hydrochloride). Britannia Pharmaceuticals Ltd. UK Summary of product characteristics, July 2009.

Apomorphine + COMT inhibitors

Entacapone had no effect on the pharmacokinetics or efficacy of apomorphine in a single-dose study. Similarly, tolcapone had no relevant effect on the pharmacokinetics of a single dose of apomorphine.

Clinical evidence

(a) Entacapone

In a placebo-controlled, crossover study in 24 patients with Parkinson's disease a single dose of entacapone 200 mg or 400 mg given 30 minutes before a subcutaneous injection of apomorphine had no effect on the pharmacokinetics of apomorphine. In addition, entacapone had no effect on measures of apomorphine efficacy (tapping test and incidence of dyskinesias).[1]

(b) Tolcapone

In 5 patients with Parkinson's disease, tolcapone 200 mg three times daily for 5 days then 200 mg one hour before sublingual apomorphine 40 mg caused a non-significant increase in the AUC of apomorphine of about 13%.[2]

Mechanism

In vitro and *animal* data suggested that the enzyme catechol-*O*-methyl transferase (COMT) is involved in the metabolism of apomorphine[3] and that COMT inhibitors might increase apomorphine bioavailability. However, the single dose studies above suggest that this metabolic pathway for apomorphine may not be important in humans.

Importance and management

The evidence from these single-dose studies suggest that there is no pharmacokinetic interaction between entacapone or tolcapone and apomorphine, and that the drugs can be used together without alteration of the apomorphine dose. However, further data are required from longer-term concurrent use to confirm this. Until more is known, increased monitoring during concurrent use of COMT inhibitors and apomorphine may be prudent, in order to detect any apomorphine adverse effects that may develop.

1. Zijlmans JCM, Debilly B, Rascol O, Lees AJ, Durif F. Safety of entacapone and apomorphine coadministration in levodopa-treated Parkinson's disease patients: pharmacokinetic and pharmacodynamic results of a multicenter, double-blind, placebo-controlled, cross-over study. *Mov Disord* (2004) 19, 1006–11.
2. Ondo WG, Hunter C, Vuong KD, Jankovic VJ. The pharmacokinetic and clinical effects of tolcapone on a single dose of apomorphine in Parkinson's disease. *Parkinsonism Relat Disord* (2000) 6, 237–40.
3. Coudoré F, Durif F, Duroux E, Eschalier A, Fialip J. Effect of tolcapone on plasma and striatal apomorphine disposition in rats. *Neuroreport* (1997) 8, 877–80.

Apomorphine + Hormonal contraceptives

The sedative effects of apomorphine were decreased by an oral combined hormonal contraceptive in one study.

Clinical evidence, mechanism, importance and management

A study in a group of 9 women found that the sedative effects of a single 5-micrograms/kg subcutaneous dose of apomorphine were decreased when they were taking an oral combined hormonal contraceptive (**ethinylestradiol**

30 micrograms, **levonorgestrel** 150 or 250 micrograms).[1] The clinical importance of this is uncertain.

1. Chalmers JS, Fulli-Lemaire I, Cowen PJ. Effects of the contraceptive pill on sedative responses to clonidine and apomorphine in normal women. *Psychol Med* (1985) 15, 363–7.

Apomorphine + Miscellaneous

The concurrent use of apomorphine and other drugs used for erectile dysfunction or dopamine antagonists is not recommended. Domperidone and prochlorperazine are said not to interact when apomorphine is used for erectile dysfunction, and domperidone is the recommended antiemetic when apomorphine is used for Parkinson's disease. There have been reports of profound hypotension when ondansetron was used with apomorphine. There appears to be no evidence that antidepressants or antiepileptics interact adversely with apomorphine.

Clinical evidence, mechanism, importance and management

(a) Antidepressants

An analysis of phase II/III studies found no difference in the efficacy of sublingual apomorphine for erectile dysfunction in patients receiving antidepressants, nor was there any significant difference in the adverse effects reported, when compared with the general study population.[1] In a study in 7 patients with Parkinson's disease, **fluoxetine** 20 mg given twice daily for about 11 days did not alter the apomorphine-induced decrease in parkinsonian motor disability, but it did result in an improvement in the dyskinesias induced by apomorphine.[2]

(b) Antiemetics

The small doses of apomorphine used for erectile dysfunction (2 to 3 mg) do not normally cause vomiting, but nausea does occur in about 7% of patients and the manufacturer reported that interaction studies and/or clinical experience has shown that **domperidone**, **ondansetron** or **prochlorperazine** can safely be given as antiemetics in this patient group (but see below for use in Parkinson's disease).[3] Studies with other antiemetics have not been carried out, so concurrent use was not recommended.[3]

Note that **prochlorperazine** should not be given if apomorphine is used for Parkinson's disease, as its dopamine antagonist actions can worsen the disease. It is possible that the use of the dopamine antagonist, **metoclopramide**, may diminish the effects of apomorphine[4] (see also 'Levodopa + Antiemetics', p.761). Because apomorphine is highly emetogenic at the doses required for the treatment of Parkinson's disease (1 to 4 mg/hour by subcutaneous infusion), patients with Parkinson's disease requiring apomorphine should be pretreated with **domperidone** 20 mg three times daily for at least 2 days.[5] Rarely, extrapyramidal adverse effects have been reported with **ondansetron**,[6] which may be of relevance in patients with Parkinson's disease. However, the US manufacturer of apomorphine injection, indicated for the management of Parkinson's disease, contraindicates the concurrent use of 5-HT_3 receptor antagonists based on reports of profound hypotension and loss of consciousness when **ondansetron** was given with apomorphine; they name **alosetron**, **dolasetron**, **granisetron**, **ondansetron** and **palonosetron**.[4]

(c) Antiepileptics

The manufacturer of a preparation of apomorphine used for erectile dysfunction noted that no studies about interactions between apomorphine and antiepileptics have been undertaken, but clinical experience in erectile dysfunction suggests that no interaction occurs.[3]

(d) Antipsychotics

The manufacturer of a preparation of apomorphine used for erectile dysfunction, advised that apomorphine should not be given with centrally-acting dopamine antagonists[3] because potentially they may antagonise the effects of apomorphine. Such drugs would include some antipsychotics. Some manufacturers recommend that if neuroleptics are necessary in patients with Parkinson's disease receiving dopamine agonists, the dopamine agonist should be progressively reduced (and then stopped[7]), as sudden withdrawal may cause neuroleptic malignant syndrome.[5,7]

The manufacturer of *APO-go* specifically notes that there is a potential interaction between **clozapine** and apomorphine, although they say that **clozapine** may also be used to reduce the symptoms of neuropsychiatric complications of Parkinson's disease.[5]

(e) Other dopamine agonists

One manufacturer advised that apomorphine, used for erectile dysfunction, should not be given with other centrally-acting dopamine agonists.[3] See 'Table 18.1', p.752 for a list of these drugs.

(f) Other drugs used for erectile dysfunction

One manufacturer reported that although no formal studies had been done with a combination of apomorphine and other drugs used for erectile dysfunction, there seemed to be no evidence of problems, nevertheless concurrent use was not recommended.[3] Other drugs used for this condition include **alprostadil**, **moxisylyte**, **papaverine**, **phentolamine**, and the **phosphodiesterase type-5 inhibitors** such as **sildenafil**. A study using a combination of up to three of apomorphine, **papaverine** and **phentolamine**, found that the lowest incidence of treatment-related adverse effects occurred with apomorphine and **phentolamine** (9.8%), a higher incidence with **papaverine** and **phentolamine** (16.7%) and the highest incidence with all three drugs (17.5%).[8]

1. Heaton J, Sleep D, Perdok R, Rescek ME. Uprima (apomorphine SL) 2 and 3 mg is well-tolerated and effective in men with erectile dysfunction (ED) concurrently taking antidepressant medication. *Eur Urol Suppl* (2002) (Suppl 1), 153.
2. Durif F, Vidailhet M, Bonnet AM, Blin J, Agid Y. Levodopa-induced dyskinesias are improved by fluoxetine. *Neurology* (1995) 45, 1855–8.
3. Uprima (Apomorphine hydrochloride). Abbott Laboratories Ltd. UK Summary of product characteristics, September 2004.
4. Apokyn (Apomorphine hydrochloride). Tercica Inc. US Prescribing information, February 2012.
5. APO-go Ampoules (Apomorphine hydrochloride). Britannia Pharmaceuticals Ltd. UK Summary of product characteristics, July 2009
6. Zofran (Ondansetron hydrochloride dihydrate). GlaxoSmithKline UK. UK Summary of product characteristics, October 2009.
7. Britannia Pharmaceuticals Ltd. Personal Communication, March 2006.
8. Lammers PI, Rubio-Aurioles E, Castell R, Castaneda J, Ponce de Leon R, Hurley D, Lipezker M, Loehr LA, Lowrey F. Combination therapy for erectile dysfunction: a randomized, double blind, unblinded active-controlled, cross-over study of the pharmacodynamics and safety of combined oral formulations of apomorphine hydrochloride, phentolamine mesylate and papaverine hydrochloride in men with moderate to severe erectile dysfunction. *Int J Impot Res* (2002) 14, 54–9.

Bromocriptine and other dopamine agonists + ACE inhibitors

A single report describes severe hypotension when a patient taking lisinopril was given pergolide. Dopamine agonists are well known to be associated with hypotensive reactions during the first few days of treatment.

Clinical evidence

A man successfully treated for hypertension with **lisinopril** 10 mg daily experienced a severe hypotensive reaction within 4 hours of taking a single 50-microgram dose of **pergolide** for periodic leg movements during sleep. He needed hospitalisation and treatment with intravenous fluids.[1]

Mechanism

All dopamine agonists can cause hypotensive reactions during the first few days of treatment. It is not clear whether this patient was extremely sensitive to pergolide or whether what occurred was due to an interaction. However, it is not unreasonable to assume that the hypotensive effects of dopamine agonists and ACE inhibitors might be additive.

Importance and management

Evidence for an interaction between the dopamine agonists and ACE inhibitors appears to be limited to this isolated case, but what happened is in line with the known effects of both classes of drug. Postural hypotension on starting dopamine agonists is a well recognised adverse effect, but this appears to be the only report that this might be of more concern in patients taking antihypertensives. The manufacturers of pergolide recommend caution when it is given with antihypertensives because of the risk of postural and/or sustained hypotension. The authors of the case report suggest that in patients taking antihypertensives the initial dose of pergolide should be 25 micrograms.[1] It would seem prudent to exercise extra caution with the initial use of pergolide and other dopamine agonists in patients taking ACE inhibitors.

1. Kando JC, Keck PE, Wood PA. Pergolide-induced hypotension. *Ann Pharmacother* (1990) 24, 543.

Bromocriptine and other dopamine agonists + Antiemetics

Domperidone and metoclopramide would be expected to reduce the prolactin-lowering effect of bromocriptine. The hypotensive effect of bromocriptine has also been reduced by metoclopramide and domperidone. Metoclopramide, but not domperidone, would be expected to reduce the antiparkinsonian effect of any dopamine agonist.

Metoclopramide does not affect the overall bioavailability of bromocriptine. The pharmacokinetics of ropinirole or rotigotine are not affected by domperidone.

Clinical evidence, mechanism, importance and management

(a) Effect on Parkinson's disease

Dopamine agonists frequently cause nausea and vomiting on starting treatment. The manufacturers of bromocriptine,[1] **lisuride**,[2] and **pergolide**[3] state that, if necessary, this may be reduced by taking a peripheral dopamine antagonist such as **domperidone**. **Metoclopramide** is not considered a suitable antiemetic for use in Parkinson's disease because it crosses the blood brain barrier and has central dopamine antagonist effects, and may therefore reduce the efficacy of dopamine agonists in this condition, see also 'Levodopa + Antiemetics', p.761. In a single-dose study in 10 patients with Parkinson's disease, giving **metoclopramide** before bromocriptine resulted in a slight reduction in clinical response to bromocriptine in some patients.[4] The manufacturers of **cabergoline**,[5] **ropinirole**,[6] and **rotigotine**[7] advise against the use of metoclopramide for this reason.

(b) Pharmacokinetic effects

In a study, 7 healthy subjects were given a single 7.5-mg dose of bromocriptine alone or with a single 500-microgram/kg intravenous dose of **metoclopramide**, after a standardised breakfast and after an overnight fast. The bioavailability of bromocriptine was unaffected by the concurrent use of **metoclopramide**, but the time to reach the maximum plasma level of bromocriptine, after fasting, was reduced by 30% by metoclopramide.[8]

In a study in 10 patients with Parkinson's disease, giving a single 60-mg dose of **metoclopramide** before single doses of up to 100 mg of bromocriptine caused a slight increase in peak plasma bromocriptine levels in some patients, which occurred a little earlier than when bromocriptine was given alone. However, these changes did not result in any change in clinical outcomes.[4]

In a single-dose study in 9 healthy subjects, giving **domperidone** 20 mg one hour before **ropinirole** 800 micrograms did not alter the pharmacokinetics of **ropinirole**.[9]

In a crossover study, 16 healthy subjects applied a **rotigotine** patch 2 mg/24 hours daily for 4 days with or without **domperidone** 10 mg three times daily for 5 days. The pharmacokinetics of rotigotine were not affected by concurrent domperidone, and no dose adjustment is likely to be required on concurrent use.[10]

(c) Prolactin-lowering effect

Both **domperidone** and **metoclopramide** are dopamine antagonists and can raise prolactin levels, sometimes causing galactorrhoea, gynaecomastia or mastalgia.[11,12] They would therefore be expected to reduce the prolactin-lowering effect of bromocriptine.[1] However, an early study in 10 patients with Parkinson's disease given single doses of bromocriptine 12.5 to 100 mg found that pretreatment with a single 60-mg dose of **metoclopramide** had no consistent effect on plasma bromocriptine levels or on the clinical or hormonal response,[4] although this does not seem to have been studied in a multiple dose study. Further, in a single-dose study in 9 healthy subjects, a single 20-mg dose of **domperidone** increased the plasma level of prolactin whereas a single 800-microgram dose of **ropinirole** given alone reduced it. Giving **ropinirole** one hour after **domperidone** tended to blunt the response of prolactin to domperidone, but the differences were small and not likely to be clinically significant.[9] Nevertheless, it would be prudent to monitor the efficacy of bromocriptine and other dopamine agonists used for their effect on prolactin if **domperidone** or **metoclopramide** are required.

(d) Other effects

In a placebo-controlled study, 9 patients with hypertension received a single 2.5-mg dose of bromocriptine after taking **metoclopramide** 30 mg daily for one week. Bromocriptine alone reduced blood pressure from 163/93 mmHg to 143/82 mmHg, three hours after administration, but this hypotensive effect was not seen after pretreatment with **metoclopramide**. Plasma renin activity and plasma aldosterone levels were reduced after taking bromocriptine alone, but after pretreatment with **metoclopramide**, bromocriptine did not cause any significant changes in these hormonal parameters.[13] Similar results were seen in a study in which a single 2.5-mg dose of bromocriptine was given after the subjects took **domperidone** 30 mg daily for a week.[14]

In a placebo-controlled, crossover study, 9 healthy subjects took a single 20-mg dose of **domperidone** followed, one hour later, by a single 800-microgram dose of **ropinirole**. There was no significant difference in the effects on supine blood pressure when each drug was taken alone or together, but pretreatment with **domperidone** prevented orthostatic reactions to **ropinirole** in all but one subject.[9]

1. Parlodel (Bromocriptine mesilate). Meda Pharmaceuticals. UK Summary of product characteristics, November 2007.
2. Lisuride. Cambridge Laboratories. UK Summary of product characteristics, January 2001.
3. Celance (Pergolide mesilate). Eli Lilly and Company Ltd. UK Summary of product characteristics, August 2009.
4. Price P, Debono A, Parkes JD, Marsden CD, Roenthaler J. Plasma bromocriptine levels, clinical and growth hormone responses in parkinsonism. *Br J Clin Pharmacol* (1978) 6, 303–9.
5. Cabaser (Cabergoline). Pharmacia Ltd. UK Summary of product characteristics, December 2008.
6. Requip Tablets (Ropinirole hydrochloride). GlaxoSmithKline UK. UK Summary of product characteristics, April 2012.
7. Neupro (Rotigotine). UCB Pharma Ltd. UK Summary of product characteristics, August 2009.
8. Kopitar Z, Vrhovac B, Povšič L, Plavšić F, Francetić I, Urbančič J. The effect of food and metoclopramide on the pharmacokinetics and side effects of bromocriptine. *Eur J Drug Metab Pharmacokinet* (1991) 16, 177–81.
9. de Mey C, Enterling D, Meineke I, Yeulet S. Interactions between domperidone and ropinirole, a novel dopamine D_2-receptor agonist. *Br J Clin Pharmacol* (1991) 32, 483–8.
10. Braun M, Cawello W, Boekens H, Horstmann R. Influence of domperidone on pharmacokinetics, safety and tolerability of the dopamine agonist rotigotine. *Br J Clin Pharmacol* (2009) 67, 209–15.
11. Motilium Suppositories (Domperidone). Winthrop Pharmaceuticals UK Ltd. UK Summary of product characteristics, January 2009.
12. Metoclopramide injection (Metoclopramide hydrochloride). Hameln Pharmaceuticals Ltd. UK Summary of product characteristics, December 2008.
13. Luchsinger A, Grilli M, Forte P, Morales E, Velasco M. Metoclopramide blocks bromocriptine induced antihypertensive effect in hypertensive patients. *Int J Clin Pharmacol Ther* (1995) 33, 509–512.
14. Luchsinger A, Grilli M, Velasco M. Metoclopramide and domperidone block the antihypertensive effect of bromocriptine in hypertensive patients. *Am J Ther* (1998) 5, 81–8.

Bromocriptine and other dopamine agonists + Antipsychotics

Many antipsychotics are dopamine antagonists. Therefore if they are given with dopamine agonists, such as bromocriptine, the effects of both drugs may be expected to be reduced. In particular the antipsychotics are associated with extrapyramidal adverse effects, which would be expected to oppose the effects of bromocriptine and related drugs in treating Parkinsonian symptoms. Case reports describe a reduction in prolactin-lowering effects and the emergence of schizophrenic symptoms in patients given an antipsychotic with a dopamine agonist.

Clinical evidence, mechanism, importance and management

(a) Effect on antipsychotic drug activity

A woman with schizoaffective schizophrenia, taking **molindone** 100 mg and imipramine 200 mg daily, relapsed within 5 days of starting to take bromocriptine 2.5 mg three times daily for amenorrhoea and galactorrhoea.[1] Within 3 days of stopping the bromocriptine the symptoms of relapse (agitation, delusions, and auditory hallucinations) vanished. The reason suggested by the authors of the report is that the bromocriptine (a dopamine agonist) opposed the actions of the antipsychotic medication (dopamine antagonists) thereby allowing the schizophrenia to re-emerge. Limited evidence suggests that levodopa may antagonise the effects of antipsychotics (see 'Levodopa + Antipsychotics', p.762), which adds weight to this theory.

(b) Effect on prolactin levels

A case of reduced prolactin levels has been reported in a man taking **fluphenazine** and **benzatropine** who was given bromocriptine to treat a pituitary tumour. His prolactin level became undetectable, and his psychiatric status was unchanged, although no reduction in tumour size was seen with the bromocriptine.[2] The prolactin levels of a patient with a prolactin-secreting pituitary adenoma fell from almost 8000 nanograms/mL to 400 nanograms/mL when bromocriptine was started, but increased again to 1000 nanograms/mL when he started to take **thioridazine** 25 mg twice daily. As the **thioridazine** dose was increased to 200 mg daily, his prolactin level increased further, to 2000 nanograms/mL, and his visual fields deteriorated. Normal vision returned within 5 days of stopping the **thioridazine**, and his prolactin levels fell to below 500 nanograms/mL.[3]

Other dopamine agonists used for their prolactin-lowering effects would be expected to be similarly affected.

(c) Extrapyramidal effects

Many antipsychotics have dopamine antagonist properties and can cause movement disorders (extrapyramidal effects). For this reason, these drugs can reduce the efficacy of dopamine agonists used in Parkinson's disease, and exacerbate the disorder. This interaction is well established for levodopa: see 'Levodopa + Antipsychotics', p.762, which discusses the relative tendency for various classical and atypical antipsychotics to cause this effect. It would equally well be anticipated for any dopamine agonist.

If an antipsychotic is required for psychosis in Parkinson's disease, the risk-benefit ratio should be carefully assessed, and an antipsychotic chosen that has a lower risk of extrapyramidal effects such as an atypical antipsychotic.

1. Frye PE, Pariser SF, Kim MH, O'Shaughnessy RW. Bromocriptine associated with symptom exacerbation during neuroleptic treatment of schizoaffective schizophrenia. *J Clin Psychiatry* (1982) 43, 252–3.
2. Kellner C, Harris P, Blumhardt C. Concurrent use of bromocriptine and fluphenazine. *J Clin Psychiatry* (1985) 46, 455.
3. Robbins RK, Kern PA, Thompson TL. Interactions between thioridazine and bromocriptine in a patient with a prolactin-secreting pituitary adenoma. *Am J Med* (1984) 76, 921–3.

Bromocriptine and other dopamine agonists + Azoles

Two patients taking cabergoline had improvements in their Parkinson's disease symptoms while taking itraconazole. In one case a 300% increase in cabergoline levels occurred, and the other patient reduced the dose of her medications without adversely affecting disease control. All azoles may interact to a greater or lesser extent. Bromocriptine is predicted to interact in the same way as cabergoline.

Clinical evidence

A man with Parkinson's disease taking cabergoline 4 mg daily and selegiline 5 mg twice daily was prescribed pulse itraconazole (200 mg twice daily for one week out of four) for a fungal nail infection. At the end of the first week the patient reported improvements in his parkinsonism, which was confirmed by clinical investigation. The improvement gradually decreased during the weeks without itraconazole, and re-emerged while taking the itraconazole. Analysis of cabergoline blood levels found a 300% increase in levels after he had taken itraconazole for a week.[1]

Another similar patient taking cabergoline 2 mg twice daily, selegiline, entacapone, and levodopa with carbidopa, experienced symptoms of overdose (hyperkinesia of the extremities) 3 days after starting itraconazole 200 mg twice daily. She reduced the dose of her Parkinson's medication, and had marked improvement in her usual Parkinson's symptoms, which then gradually reduced after stopping the itraconazole. This was repeated following two additional periods of itraconazole use.[1]

Mechanism

Cabergoline is metabolised by the cytochrome P450 isoenzyme CYP3A4. Itraconazole is a potent inhibitor of this isoenzyme, and would therefore be expected to increase cabergoline levels.

Importance and management

Although evidence is limited, this interaction would be predicted on the basis of the known pharmacokinetics of cabergoline and enzyme-inhibitory effects of itraconazole. It would be prudent to monitor toxicity and efficacy in any patient taking cabergoline requiring itraconazole, or similar potent inhibitors of CYP3A4, which include a number of the azole antifungals. Bromocriptine is metabolised in a similar way to cabergoline, and would be expected to interact similarly. The manufacturer of bromocriptine advises caution on the concurrent use of azole antifungals.[2]

1. Christensen J, Dupont E, Østergaard K. Cabergoline plasma concentration is increased during concomitant treatment with itraconazole. *Mov Disord* (2002) 17, 1360–2.
2. Parlodel (Bromocriptine mesilate). Meda Pharmaceuticals. UK Summary of product characteristics, November 2007.

Bromocriptine and other dopamine agonists + Ergot derivatives

Because cabergoline is an ergot derivative, the manufacturers have looked at what happens if other ergot derivatives are used concurrently, but have so far found no evidence of changes in the efficacy or safety of cabergoline. Nevertheless they do not recommend their concurrent use during long-term treatment with cabergoline.[1] Similarly, the manufacturer of bromocriptine does not recommend concurrent use of other ergot derivatives during the puerperium.[2] It would seem prudent to use similar caution with other dopamine agonists that are ergot derivatives (e.g. lisuride, pergolide), although there appears to be no information available. See also 'Ergot derivatives + Ergot derivatives', p.641, for a description of a number of adverse effects that have occurred as a result of the concurrent use of two ergot derivatives.

1. Dostinex (Cabergoline). Pharmacia Ltd. UK Summary of product characteristics, April 2009.
2. Parlodel (Bromocriptine mesilate). Meda Pharmaceuticals. UK Summary of product characteristics, November 2007.

Bromocriptine and other dopamine agonists + Food

Food does not alter the pharmacokinetics of bromocriptine, cabergoline or lisuride and has little effect on the extent of absorption of ropinirole.

Clinical evidence

(a) Bromocriptine

In a study in 7 healthy subjects, taking a single 7.5-mg dose of bromocriptine after breakfast did not alter the bromocriptine AUC, when compared with the fasted state, although it slightly reduced the maximum plasma level.[1]

(b) Cabergoline

In a study in healthy subjects, the pharmacokinetics of cabergoline did not change when a single 1-mg dose of cabergoline was taken after breakfast, when compared with the fasting state.[2]

(c) Lisuride

Thirty healthy subjects were given lisuride 200 micrograms orally while fasting or with food. It was found that food did not significantly modify either the pharmacokinetics or the pharmacodynamics of lisuride.[3]

(d) Ropinirole

In a study, 12 patients who had achieved ropinirole steady-state levels took a single 2-mg dose after an overnight fast, or after a high-fat breakfast. The mean maximum ropinirole plasma levels were reduced by about 25%, and the median time to reach maximum plasma levels was delayed from 1.25 hours to 4 hours, in the presence of food. The AUC_{0-8} was reduced by 11% after a high-fat breakfast. The effect of these changes on the patients' Parkinson's disease was not monitored.[4] A study involving 20 patients with Parkinson's disease who received ropinirole 8 mg as a prolonged-release tablet, after fasting or after a high-fat breakfast, found that the AUC and maximum plasma levels of ropinirole were similar when given in the fed or fasted state. Reports of adverse effects were similar between the two groups.[5]

Mechanism

None.

Importance and management

Food had no effect on the pharmacokinetics of the dopamine agonists studied. Food decreased the rate of absorption of ropinirole, but had little effect on the extent of absorption. The manufacturers of bromocriptine, cabergoline, lisuride and ropinirole recommend that they are taken with food.[6-9] These drugs commonly cause nausea and vomiting, especially when they are newly started, and taking them with food may improve tolerability.[7-9] As **rotigotine** is given transdermally, food is not expected to affect its pharmacokinetics.[10]

1. Kopitar Z, Vrhovac B, Povšič L, Plavšić F, Francetić I, Urbančič J. The effect of food and metoclopramide on the pharmacokinetics and side effects of bromocriptine. *Eur J Drug Metab Pharmacokinet* (1991) 16, 177–81.
2. Persiani S, Rocchetti M, Pacciarini MA, Holt B, Toon S, Strolin-Benedetti M. The effect of food on cabergoline pharmacokinetics and tolerability in healthy volunteers. *Biopharm Drug Dispos* (1996) 17, 443–55.
3. Gandon JM, Le Coz F, Kühne G, Hümpel M, Allain H. PK/PD interaction studies of lisuride with erythromycin and food in healthy volunteers. *Clin Pharmacol Ther* (1995) 57, 191.
4. Brefel C, Thalamas C, Rayet S, Lopez-Gil A, Fitzpatrick K, Bullman S, Citerone DR, Taylor AC, Montastruc JL, Rascol O. Effect of food on the pharmacokinetics of ropinirole in parkinsonian patients. *Br J Clin Pharmacol* (1998) 45, 412–15.
5. Tompson DJ, Vearer D. Steady-state pharmacokinetic properties of a 24-hour prolonged-release formulation of ropinirole: results of two randomized studies in patients with Parkinson's disease. *Clin Ther* (2007) 29, 2654–66.
6. Lisuride. Cambridge Laboratories. UK Summary of product characteristics, January 2001.
7. Parlodel (Bromocriptine mesilate). Meda Pharmaceuticals. UK Summary of product characteristics, November 2007.
8. Cabaser (Cabergoline). Pharmacia Ltd. UK Summary of product characteristics, December 2008.
9. Requip Tablets (Ropinirole hydrochloride). GlaxoSmithKline UK. UK Summary of product characteristics, April 2012.
10. Neupro (Rotigotine). UCB Pharma Ltd. UK Summary of product characteristics, August 2009.

Bromocriptine and other dopamine agonists + Macrolides

Erythromycin markedly increases bromocriptine levels, and a case of toxicity has been reported. Bromocriptine toxicity also occurred in a patient given josamycin. Clarithromycin increases cabergoline levels, and erythromycin would be expected to interact similarly. Erythromycin has no effect on lisuride levels.

Clinical evidence

(a) Bromocriptine

1. Erythromycin. In 5 healthy subjects, erythromycin estolate 250 mg four times daily for 4 days increased the peak plasma levels and the AUC of a single 5-mg oral dose of bromocriptine by about 360% and 268%, respectively.[1] Another report describes 2 women taking levodopa with carbidopa and bromocriptine for parkinsonism in whom the disease was better controlled when erythromycin was added. Bromocriptine plasma levels were found to be 40 to 50% higher while they were taking erythromycin.[2] An elderly woman taking levodopa and bromocriptine 15 mg developed psychotic symptoms when she took erythromycin, which were attributed to bromocriptine toxicity.[3]

2. Josamycin. An elderly man with Parkinson's disease, which was well-controlled for 10 months with levodopa with benserazide, bromocriptine 70 mg daily and domperidone, was given josamycin 2 g daily for a respiratory infection. Shortly after the first dose he became drowsy with visual hallucinations, and began to have involuntary movements of his limbs, similar to the dystonic and dyskinetic movements seen in choreoathetosis. These adverse effects (interpreted as bromocriptine toxicity) disappeared within a few days of withdrawing the josamycin.[4]

(b) Cabergoline

In a crossover study, 10 healthy subjects received cabergoline 1 mg daily with or without **clarithromycin** 200 mg twice daily for 6 days. The AUC of cabergoline was increased by 162% and its maximum plasma level increased by 176%. The study was repeated with 7 patients with Parkinson's disease already taking cabergoline, and this found that **clarithromycin** increased the average plasma level of cabergoline by about 70%. Three of the patients experienced an improvement in their Parkinson's disease symptoms; none of the patients had adverse effects.[5]

(c) Lisuride

Twelve healthy subjects were given lisuride 200 micrograms orally or 50 micrograms as a 30 minute intravenous infusion after taking **erythromycin** (dose unknown) twice daily for 4 days. Preliminary results showed that **erythromycin** did not significantly modify either the pharmacokinetics or the pharmacodynamics of the lisuride.[6]

Mechanism

The ergot dopamine agonists, bromocriptine and cabergoline, undergo extensive metabolism, most likely by the cytochrome P450 isoenzyme CYP3A4. Erythromycin and clarithromycin (and potentially other macrolides, see 'Ergot derivatives + Macrolides', p.642) inhibit this metabolism, thus significantly elevating bromocriptine and cabergoline plasma levels.[1] *In vitro* study has suggested that bromocriptine is also a substrate of OATP-C (organic anion transporting polypeptide C), which may be inhibited by erythromycin, resulting in reduced hepatic uptake and thus metabolism of bromocriptine.[7] It is also possible that P-glycoprotein may be involved in the transport of these ergot dopamine agonists and that inhibition of P-glycoprotein-mediated excretion by macrolides such as clarithromycin may result in increased plasma levels.[5]

Importance and management

Information seems to be limited to these reports, but the pharmacokinetic interaction would appear to be established. Concurrent use should be well monitored if any of these macrolides (clarithromycin, erythromycin, josamycin) is added to bromocriptine or cabergoline treatment. Note that **azithromycin** does not normally cause enzyme inhibition and so may not interact. Moderately increased levels may be therapeutically advantageous, but grossly elevated levels can be toxic. The authors of one report[1] suggest reducing the bromocriptine dose, while in another case the dose was reduced by 50% to avoid toxicity.[3] The manufacturer of cabergoline advises avoiding the concurrent use of macrolides, and specifically names erythromycin.[8] Preliminary data suggest that dose adjustments are not needed if lisuride is given with erythromycin.

1. Nelson MV, Berchou RC, Kareti D, LeWitt PA. Pharmacokinetic evaluation of erythromycin and caffeine administered with bromocriptine. *Clin Pharmacol Ther* (1990) 47, 694–7.
2. Sibley WA, Laguna JF. Enhancement of bromocriptine clinical effect and plasma levels with erythromycin. *Excerpta Med* (1981) 548, 329–30.
3. Alegre M, Noé E, Martínez Lage JM. Psicosis por interacción de eritromicina con bromocriptina en enfermedad de Parkinson. *Neurologia* (1997) 12, 429.
4. Montastruc JL, Rascol A. Traitement de la maladie de Parkinson par doses élevées de bromocriptine. Interaction possible avec la josamycine. *Presse Med* (1984) 13, 2267–8.

5. Nakatsuka A, Nagai M, Yabe H, Nishikawa N, Nomura T, Moritoyo H, Moritoyo T, Nomoto M. Effect of clarithromycin on the pharmacokinetics of cabergoline in healthy controls and in patients with Parkinson's disease. *J Pharmacol Sci* (2006) 100, 59–64.
6. Gandon JM, Le Coz F, Kühne G, Hümpel M, Allain H. PK/PD interaction studies of lisuride with erythromycin and food in healthy volunteers. *Clin Pharmacol Ther* (1995) 57, 191.
7. Lu W-J, Huang K, Lai M-L, Huang J-D. Erythromycin alters the pharmacokinetics of bromocriptine by inhibition of organic anion transporting polypeptide C-mediated uptake. *Clin Pharmacol Ther* (2006) 80, 421–2.
8. Cabaser (Cabergoline). Pharmacia Ltd. UK Summary of product characteristics, December 2008.

Bromocriptine and other dopamine agonists + Proton pump inhibitors

A single case describes worsening mobility, which was attributed to an interaction between lansoprazole and bromocriptine. The same patient later received bromocriptine and omeprazole without problems. No pharmacokinetic interaction occurred when omeprazole was taken with rotigotine.

Clinical evidence, mechanism, importance and management

(a) Bromocriptine

A 73-year-old man taking levodopa with benserazide and bromocriptine for Parkinson's disease was given **lansoprazole** 15 mg daily to treat reflux oesophagitis. Two days later, the patient exhibited akinesia (more motor difficulties and slowness in movements) associated with frequent falls. **Lansoprazole** was discontinued, and the symptoms had resolved by the following day. About 3 months later the patient took **omeprazole** 20 mg daily, which caused no aggravation of Parkinson's disease over the following 6 months. The authors attribute this case to a possible interaction between **lansoprazole** and bromocriptine,[1] although any mechanism is unclear, especially as **omeprazole** was given without problems. This single unexplained case seems unlikely to be of general significance.

(b) Rotigotine

The pharmacokinetics of rotigotine were unaltered by **omeprazole** 40 mg daily, in healthy subjects.[2]

1. Anglès A, Bagheri H, Saivin S, Montastruc JL. Interaction between lansoprazole and bromocriptine in a patient with Parkinson's disease. *Therapie* (2002) 57, 408–10.
2. Neupro (Rotigotine). UCB Pharma Ltd. UK Summary of product characteristics, August 2009.

Bromocriptine + Griseofulvin

Evidence from a single patient, who was taking bromocriptine for acromegaly, suggests that the effects of bromocriptine can be opposed by griseofulvin.

Clinical evidence, mechanism, importance and management

In a study of the effects of bromocriptine used for the treatment of acromegaly, one patient who initially had a good response to bromocriptine developed resistance to the drug. After a number of months it was found that this patient had subsequently been given griseofulvin 500 mg daily for the treatment of a fungal nail infection. When the griseofulvin was stopped, the bromocriptine was again effective.[1] The mechanism of this interaction and its general importance are unknown.

1. Schwinn G, Dirks H, McIntosh C, Köbberling J. Metabolic and clinical studies on patients with acromegaly treated with bromocriptine over 22 months. *Eur J Clin Invest* (1977) 7, 101–7.

Bromocriptine + Nasal decongestants and related drugs

Adverse effects, including hypertension, severe headache, seizures and psychosis, have been seen in patients taking phenylpropanolamine, pseudoephedrine or isometheptene with or shortly after the use of bromocriptine.

Clinical evidence

Two healthy women who had given birth 3 to 4 days previously, developed severe headaches while taking bromocriptine 2.5 mg twice daily for milk suppression. After additionally taking three 65-mg doses of **isometheptene mucate**, the headache of one of them markedly worsened, and hypertension with life-threatening ventricular tachycardia and cardiac dysfunction developed. The other woman took two 75-mg doses of **phenylpropanolamine**, and developed grand mal seizures and cerebral vasospasm.[1]

A 32-year-old woman took two 5-mg doses of bromocriptine for milk suppression without any adverse effects following the birth of a child. Within 2 hours of taking a third dose with **phenylpropanolamine** 50 mg she awoke with a very severe headache and was found to have a blood pressure of 240/140 mmHg. She was given 5 mg of intramuscular morphine and her blood pressure became normal within 24 hours. Another 5-mg dose of bromocriptine taken 48 hours after the original dose of **phenylpropanolamine** had the same effect, but the blood pressure rise was less severe (160/120 mmHg).[2]

A case report describes a 37-year-old woman who took bromocriptine for 17 days. Nine days later, she took *Rinurel*, a preparation for colds containing **phenylpropanolamine**, and 90 minutes later she developed a severe headache: cerebral haemorrhagic lesions were detected. It was thought that the phenylpropanolamine was mainly responsible for the vascular effects, but it was also suggested that the recent use of bromocriptine may have contributed to this effect.[3]

A woman who had recently given birth and who had taken bromocriptine 2.5 mg twice daily for 9 days without problems became psychotic shortly after starting to take **pseudoephedrine** 60 mg four times daily.[4]

Mechanism

Not understood. Severe hypertension occasionally occurs with either bromocriptine or phenylpropanolamine given alone. Shortly after giving birth some individuals show increased vascular reactivity, and it could be that all of these factors conspired together to cause the adverse effects seen.[2] Psychosis occasionally occurs after giving birth or with bromocriptine alone, so that in the latter case the addition of pseudoephedrine may have been coincidental.[4]

Importance and management

Direct information seems to be limited to these cases, but the severity of the reactions suggests that it might be prudent for postpartum patients to avoid indirectly-acting sympathomimetics like these (e.g. phenylpropanolamine, ephedrine, pseudoephedrine) while taking bromocriptine. Note that bromocriptine is not recommended for the routine suppression of lactation postpartum.

1. Kulig K, Moore LL, Kirk M, Smith D, Stallworth J, Rumack B. Bromocriptine-associated headache: possible life-threatening sympathomimetic interaction. *Obstet Gynecol* (1991) 78, 941–3.
2. Chan JCN, Critchley JAJH, Cockram CS. Postpartum hypertension, bromocriptine and phenylpropanolamine. *Drug Invest* (1994) 8, 254–6.
3. Veyrac G, Huguenin H, Guillon B, Chiffoleau A, Thajte N, Bourin M, Jolliet P. Hémorragie cérébroméningée et angiopathie cérébrale aiguë associées à la prise de phénylpropanolamine: un nouveau cas. *Therapie* (2001) 56, 323–7.
4. Reeves RR, Pinkofsky HB. Postpartum psychosis induced by bromocriptine and pseudoephedrine. *J Fam Pract* (1997) 45, 164–6.

Bromocriptine + Octreotide

Octreotide modestly increases the bioavailability of bromocriptine, whereas bromocriptine does not appear to alter octreotide pharmacokinetics.

Clinical evidence, mechanism, importance and management

The concurrent use of bromocriptine 5 mg twice daily and subcutaneous octreotide 200 micrograms twice daily increased the bioavailability of bromocriptine by about 40%, without altering its clearance or half-life. The pharmacokinetics of octreotide were unchanged.[1] This effect may contribute to the increased efficacy of concurrent use in acromegaly, which has been seen in some studies. It seems unlikely that any particular precautions are necessary on concurrent use.

1. Fløgstad AK, Halse J, Grass P, Abisch E, Djøseland O, Kutz K, Bodd E, Jervell J. A comparison of octreotide, bromocriptine, or a combination of both drugs in acromegaly. *J Clin Endocrinol Metab* (1994) 79, 461–5.

Cabergoline + Grapefruit juice

Grapefruit juice increases cabergoline levels.

Clinical evidence, mechanism, importance and management

When 5 patients with Parkinson's disease were given grapefruit juice (quantity not specified) with cabergoline, the plasma levels of cabergoline were increased by about 70%. No adverse events were reported by the patients.[1]

Grapefruit juice is an inhibitor of the cytochrome P450 isoenzyme CYP3A4 in the gut, which is involved in the metabolism of cabergoline. Therefore the concurrent use of grapefruit reduces the metabolism of cabergoline in the gut, increasing its bioavailability.

Evidence for an interaction appears to be limited to this study, but the interaction is established. However, there appear to be no reports of adverse effects in patients receiving grapefruit juice and cabergoline, so its clinical relevance is not established. The authors suggest that, as cabergoline has a large therapeutic index, concurrent use need not be avoided, and may even be beneficial.[1]

1. Nagai M, Nakatsuka A, Yabe H, Moritoyo T, Nomoto M. Effect of grapefruit juice on cabergoline pharmacokinetics in patients with Parkinson's disease. *Clin Pharmacol Ther* (2005) 77, P84.

COMT inhibitors + Inotropes and Vasopressors

Entacapone potentiated the increase in heart rate and arrhythmogenic effects of isoprenaline (isoproterenol) and adrenaline (epinephrine) in a study in healthy subjects. Therefore, the manufacturers of entacapone and tolcapone issue a caution about the concurrent use of adrenaline, isoprenaline, and a number of other inotropes and vasopressors.

Clinical evidence

In a study in healthy subjects, the maximal increase in heart rate during an infusion of **adrenaline (epinephrine)** was about 80% greater (25 bpm versus 14 bpm) after pretreatment with a single 400-mg dose of **entacapone**. Similarly, the maximal increase in heart rate during **isoprenaline (isoproterenol)** infusion was about 50%

greater (40 bpm versus 27 bpm) after pretreatment with the same dose of **entacapone**. Moreover, more subjects experienced palpitations when pretreated with **entacapone**, and this study was terminated early because of two cases of ventricular arrhythmias, one requiring treatment with propranolol. There was no change in blood pressure, nor any increase in plasma levels of the **adrenaline** or **isoprenaline**.[1]

Mechanism

Tolcapone and entacapone inhibit the enzyme catechol-*O*-methyl transferase (COMT), which is concerned with the metabolism of drugs such as adrenaline (epinephrine) and isoprenaline (isoproterenol). There is therefore a possibility of increased plasma levels and related adverse effects of these drugs.

Importance and management

The evidence from this single-dose study confirms the theoretical prediction that COMT inhibitors might potentiate the effects of adrenaline (epinephrine). Because of this, the manufacturers of entacapone and tolcapone suggest caution if drugs known to be metabolised by COMT are given to patients taking COMT inhibitors.[2-5] Adrenaline (epinephrine), **dobutamine**, **dopamine**, isoprenaline (isoproterenol) and **noradrenaline (norepinephrine)**, are specifically named in one or more of the lists,[2-5] and one manufacturer of entacapone also lists **bitolterol** and **isoetarine (isoetharine)**, which are usually used in asthma, and specifically includes the inhaled route of administration.[5]

1. Illi A, Sundberg S, Ojala-Karlsson P, Korhonen P, Scheinin M, Gordin A. The effect of entacapone on the disposition and hemodynamic effects of intravenous isoproterenol and epinephrine. *Clin Pharmacol Ther* (1995) 58, 221–7.
2. Tasmar (Tolcapone). Meda Pharmaceuticals. UK Summary of product characteristics, January 2009.
3. Tasmar (Tolcapone). Valeant Pharmaceuticals North America. US Prescribing information, June 2009.
4. Comtess (Entacapone). Orion Pharma (UK) Ltd. UK Summary of product characteristics, September 2008.
5. Comtan (Entacapone). Novartis. US Prescribing information, March 2009.

COMT inhibitors + MAOIs

In a single-dose study, there was no adverse effect on heart rate or blood pressure when entacapone was given with moclobemide. The COMT inhibitors may be used with the MAO-B inhibitors (such as selegiline). However, the manufacturers of entacapone and tolcapone contraindicate concurrent use of non-selective MAOIs or a combination of both a RIMA and an MAO-B inhibitor.

Clinical evidence

In a single-dose, placebo-controlled study, **moclobemide** 150 mg did not change the heart rate or blood pressure at rest or during exercise, when given with **entacapone** 200 mg, compared with either drug alone or placebo. In addition, the plasma concentrations of endogenous noradrenaline (norepinephrine) and adrenaline (epinephrine) were not altered.[1] In 13 patients with Parkinson's disease, the addition of **selegiline** 10 mg daily to treatment with **entacapone** 200 mg three or four times daily, and levodopa with benserazide 200/50 mg three or four times daily, did not result in any clinically significant changes in haemodynamic parameters or adverse effects.[2]

Mechanism

Monoamine oxidase and COMT are the two major enzyme systems involved in the metabolism of catecholamines. Therefore it is theoretically possible that the combination of a COMT inhibitor and a non-selective MAOI would result in inhibition of the normal metabolism of catecholamines, with an increase in their effects (e.g. hypertension). Using an MAO-B inhibitor with a RIMA is similar to giving a non-selective MAOI and therefore using these two drugs with a COMT inhibitor would also be likely to inhibit the normal metabolism of catecholamines.

Importance and management

The results of the single-dose study with entacapone and moclobemide suggest that no adverse haemodynamic interaction occurs. Nevertheless, this finding needs confirmation in a clinical setting. Until further information is available, caution would be advisable on concurrent use. The manufacturers of entacapone and **tolcapone** contraindicate or advise against the use of non-selective MAOIs (e.g. **phenelzine**, **tranylcypromine**)[3-6] and combinations of both a RIMA [e.g. moclobemide] plus an MAO-B inhibitor (e.g. **selegiline**).[3,5] However, they state that **selegiline** alone is compatible with the COMT inhibitors provided not more than 10 mg daily is used.[3,5] At this dose, **selegiline** is likely to remain selective for MAO-B.

1. Illi A, Sundberg S, Ojala-Karlsson P, Scheinin M, Gordin A. Simultaneous inhibition of catechol-*O*-methyltransferase and monoamine oxidase A: effects on hemodynamics and catecholamine metabolism in healthy volunteers. *Clin Pharmacol Ther* (1996) 59, 450–7.
2. Lyytinen J, Kaakkola S, Ahtila S, Tuomainen P, Teräväinen H. Simultaneous MAO-B and COMT inhibition in L-dopa-treated patients with Parkinson's disease. *Mov Disord* (1997) 12, 497–505.
3. Tasmar (Tolcapone). Meda Pharmaceuticals. UK Summary of product characteristics, January 2009.
4. Tasmar (Tolcapone). Valeant Pharmaceuticals North America. US Prescribing information, June 2009.
5. Comtess (Entacapone). Orion Pharma (UK) Ltd. UK Summary of product characteristics, September 2008.
6. Comtan (Entacapone). Novartis. US Prescribing information, March 2009.

COMT inhibitors + Nasal decongestants

A single case report describes severe hypertension in a patient given entacapone and intravenous ephedrine. Tolcapone did not alter the effect of ephedrine in one study.

Clinical evidence

(a) Entacapone

A 76-year-old woman with Parkinson's disease taking levodopa with carbidopa and entacapone 200 mg five times daily, was given 3 mg of intravenous **ephedrine** during cataract surgery to correct a low blood pressure of 85/35 mmHg. Her blood pressure immediately rose to 225/125 mmHg. The patient needed several doses of hydralazine over the following 140 minutes before her blood pressure returned to normal.[1]

(b) Tolcapone

The manufacturer notes that tolcapone did not alter the effect of **ephedrine** (route of administration not stated) on haemodynamic parameters or plasma catecholamine levels, either at rest or during exercise.[2,3]

Mechanism

COMT inhibitors may inhibit the normal metabolism of ephedrine (and the catecholamines it releases at adrenergic nerve endings), which could result in a marked exaggeration of its normal effects.[1]

Importance and management

The single case report with entacapone and intravenous ephedrine appears to be the only evidence that COMT inhibitors could potentiate the effect of indirectly-acting sympathomimetics such as ephedrine. The manufacturer of tolcapone states that ephedrine and tolcapone can be used concurrently.[2,3] Nevertheless, some caution may be warranted with intravenous ephedrine.

1. Renfrew C, Dickson R, Schwab C. Severe hypertension following ephedrine administration in a patient receiving entacapone. *Anesthesiology* (2000) 93, 1562.
2. Tasmar (Tolcapone). Meda Pharmaceuticals. UK Summary of product characteristics, January 2009.
3. Tasmar (Tolcapone). Valeant Pharmaceuticals North America. US Prescribing information, June 2009.

COMT inhibitors + Tricyclic and related antidepressants

Entacapone and imipramine did not interact adversely in a single-dose study. Similarly, in another study, tolcapone and desipramine did not interact adversely.

Clinical evidence

(a) Entacapone

In a single-dose, crossover study, 12 healthy women were given entacapone 200 mg with **imipramine** 75 mg, either drug alone, or placebo. Although both drugs can impair the inactivation of catecholamines the study found no evidence that concurrent use had any relevant effect on haemodynamics or on free adrenaline (epinephrine) or noradrenaline (norepinephrine) plasma levels. The combination was well tolerated in all subjects.[1]

(b) Tolcapone

In one study, healthy subjects were given **desipramine** 25 mg three times daily for 3 days then 50 mg three times daily for 10 days. For the last 5 days they were also given levodopa with carbidopa 100/25 mg three times daily and either a placebo or tolcapone 200 mg three times daily. The addition of tolcapone to the use of levodopa with carbidopa and **desipramine** did not lead to any changes in haemodynamics or catecholamine levels, or to any changes in **desipramine** pharmacokinetics.[2]

Mechanism

Both COMT inhibitors and drugs with noradrenaline re-uptake inhibitory activity (e.g. the tricyclics) can impair the inactivation of catecholamines, so in theory the effects of catecholamines may be increased by concurrent use. However, this did not appear to occur in the above studies.

Importance and management

In these pharmacological studies, no important interaction between entacapone and imipramine or between tolcapone and desipramine was detected. Nevertheless, the manufacturer of entacapone says there is limited clinical experience of the use of entacapone with tricyclic antidepressants, and they therefore recommend caution.[3] Similarly, the manufacturers of tolcapone suggest that caution should be exercised with desipramine[4,5] and any drugs that are potent noradrenaline uptake inhibitors such as **maprotiline** and **venlafaxine**.[4]

1. Illi A, Sundberg S, Ojala-Karlsson P, Scheinin M, Gordin A. Simultaneous inhibition of catecholamine-*O*-methylation by entacapone and neuronal uptake by imipramine: lack of interactions. *Eur J Clin Pharmacol* (1996) 51, 273–6.
2. Jorga KM, Fotteler B, Modi M, Rabbia M. Effect of tolcapone on the haemodynamic effects and tolerability of desipramine. *Eur Neurol* (2000) 44, 94–103.
3. Comtess (Entacapone). Orion Pharma (UK) Ltd. UK Summary of product characteristics, September 2008.
4. Tasmar (Tolcapone). Meda Pharmaceuticals. UK Summary of product characteristics, January 2009.
5. Tasmar (Tolcapone). Valeant Pharmaceuticals North America. US Prescribing information, June 2009.

COMT inhibitors; Entacapone + Iron compounds

Entacapone formed chelates with iron *in vitro*.

Clinical evidence, mechanism, importance and management

An *in vitro* study[1] found that entacapone formed chelates with iron. Although the clinical relevance of this does not appear to have been assessed, the UK manufacturer recommends that entacapone and iron compounds should be taken at least 2 to 3 hours apart.[2]

1. Orama M, Tilus P, Taskinen J, Lotta T. Iron (III)-chelating properties of the novel catechol *O*-methyltransferase inhibitor entacapone in aqueous solution. *J Pharm Sci* (1997) 86, 827–31.
2. Comtess (Entacapone). Orion Pharma (UK) Ltd. UK Summary of product characteristics, September 2008.

COMT inhibitors; Tolcapone + Clozapine

A case report describes neuroleptic malignant-like syndrome and acute hepatitis in a patient who took tolcapone and clozapine.

Clinical evidence, mechanism, importance and management

A case report describes a 70-year-old woman taking levodopa with benserazide who developed a neuroleptic malignant-like syndrome, with a temperature of 40.5°C, coma, and muscular rigidity, and fulminant hepatitis about 2 weeks after starting to take tolcapone, and about 10 days after also starting to take clozapine. Twelve hours after stopping tolcapone and clozapine her temperature normalised, and within 2 days she had regained consciousness. Clozapine was restarted with no recurrence of these symptoms.[1] Tolcapone alone can cause increases in liver transaminases, hepatocellular injury, and a neuroleptic malignant-like syndrome, and therefore an interaction is not established.

1. Blum MW, Siegel AM, Meier R, Hess K. Neuroleptic malignant-like syndrome and acute hepatitis during tolcapone and clozapine medication. *Eur Neurol* (2001) 46, 158–60.

Levodopa + Antacids

Antacids do not appear to interact significantly with immediate-release levodopa, but they may reduce the bioavailability of modified-release preparations of levodopa.

Clinical evidence

(a) Immediate-release levodopa

One study found that 15 mL of an **aluminium/magnesium hydroxide** antacid, given 30 minutes before levodopa, to a patient with a prolonged gastric emptying time, caused a threefold increase in levodopa serum levels, which was associated with a marked improvement in symptoms.[1] Another patient was able to reduce his levodopa dose when taking antacids, without affecting symptom control.[1] A further study found that the maximum plasma concentration of levodopa was raised by 20% when 20 mL of an antacid was given before the levodopa.[2]

However, when 8 patients (only 3 with Parkinson's disease) were given *Mylanta* (containing **aluminium/magnesium hydroxide** and simeticone), 30 minutes before, and/or with levodopa, only occasional increases in bioavailability were seen. One of the 3 patients with Parkinson's disease who had shown improved bioavailability while taking antacids had his levodopa dose lowered and continued to take *Mylanta*, but the parkinsonian symptoms worsened and the levodopa was increased back to the original dose.[3] Another study, in 15 patients taking dopamine agonists (e.g. bromocriptine) and levodopa with carbidopa who were given six 30-mL doses of **aluminium hydroxide** daily, inferred that the antacid had no significant effect on levodopa bioavailability, because of the lack of clinical fluctuations in effect.[4]

(b) Sustained-release levodopa

In a study in healthy subjects, using *Madopar HBS*, a sustained-release preparation of levodopa with benserazide, the concurrent use of an unnamed antacid reduced the levodopa bioavailability by about one-third.[5] The manufacturer of *Madopar CR* states that antacids reduce the bioavailability of levodopa from the controlled-release preparation in comparison with conventional *Madopar*.[6]

Mechanism

The small intestine is the major site of absorption for levodopa, and delayed gastric emptying appears to result in low plasma levodopa levels, probably because levodopa can be metabolised in the stomach. In theory, antacids may reduce gastric emptying time, and increase levodopa absorption.[1] It is not known why antacids reduced absorption from the slow-release preparation.[5]

Importance and management

The overall picture is that the concurrent use of antacids need not be avoided with standard preparations of levodopa (with a dopa-decarboxylase inhibitor), although some individuals may be affected so the outcome should be monitored. With modified-release preparations it would seem advisable to avoid concurrent administration (one to 2 hours is usually enough in other similar cases of interactions with antacids). Again, the outcome should be monitored.

1. Rivera-Calimlim L, Dujovne CA, Morgan JP, Lasagna L, Bianchine JR. Absorption and metabolism of L-dopa by the human stomach. *Eur J Clin Invest* (1971) 1, 313–20.
2. Pocelinko R, Thomas GB, Solomon HM. The effect of an antacid on the absorption and metabolism of levodopa. *Clin Pharmacol Ther* (1972) 13, 149.
3. Leon AS, Spiegel HE. The effect of antacid administration on the absorption and metabolism of levodopa. *J Clin Pharmacol* (1972) 12, 263–7.
4. Lau E, Waterman K, Glover R, Schulzer M, Calne DB. Effect of antacid on levodopa therapy. *Clin Neuropharmacol* (1986) 9, 477–9.
5. Malcolm SL, Allen JG, Bird H, Quinn NP, Marion MH, Marsden CD, O'Leary CG. Single-dose pharmacokinetics of Madopar HBS in patients and effect of food and antacid on the absorption of Madopar HBS in volunteers. *Eur Neurol* (1987) 27 (Suppl 1), 28–35.
6. Madopar CR (Levodopa and Benserazide hydrochloride). Roche Products Ltd. UK Summary of product characteristics, April 2009.

Levodopa + Anticholinesterases; Centrally acting

Reports describe cases of a worsening of Parkinson's disease in a few patients given donepezil, rivastigmine or tacrine. Other centrally acting anticholinesterases may exacerbate or induce extrapyramidal symptoms, including worsening of Parkinson's disease. In contrast, one study found that donepezil did not affect the control of Parkinson's disease.

Clinical evidence

(a) Donepezil

In a placebo-controlled study in 23 patients with Parkinson's disease taking levodopa with carbidopa, donepezil 5 mg daily for 15 days caused a modest 30% increase in the AUC_{0-4} of levodopa. There was no change in carbidopa pharmacokinetics, and the pharmacokinetics of donepezil did not differ between the patients with Parkinson's disease and a control group of healthy subjects. There was no obvious difference in adverse effects between patients with Parkinson's disease and the control subjects, and no evidence that donepezil significantly altered motor activity in patients taking levodopa with carbidopa.[1] This latter finding is in contrast to a report that found a worsening of Parkinson's disease, which responded to levodopa with carbidopa, in 3 of 9 patients who had taken donepezil for 24 weeks.[2]

(b) Rivastigmine

A case report describes a 71-year-old woman taking levodopa with carbidopa and tolcapone, who experienced a worsening of her Parkinson's disease after taking a single 3-mg dose of rivastigmine. She became anxious and dysphoric, had severe bradykinesia and rigidity, and felt nauseous. Note that this dose is higher than the usual starting dose of rivastigmine, and this may have contributed to the effects seen.[3]

(c) Tacrine

The mild parkinsonism of an elderly woman with Alzheimer's disease worsened, leading to severe tremor, stiffness and gait dysfunction within 2 weeks of doubling her tacrine dose from 10 mg to 20 mg four times daily. This improved when levodopa with carbidopa was started, but the tremor returned when tacrine was increased to 30 mg four times daily. The symptoms disappeared when the tacrine dose was reduced to 20 mg four times daily.[4]

Mechanism

Parkinsonism is due to an imbalance between two neurotransmitters, dopamine and acetylcholine, in the basal ganglia of the brain. Centrally acting anticholinesterases increase the amount of acetylcholine in the brain, which could lead to an exacerbation of parkinsonian symptoms. Levodopa improves the situation by increasing the levels of dopamine. It is not known why donepezil modestly increased the levels of levodopa.

Importance and management

Direct information seems to be limited, but the reports of worsening Parkinson's disease are consistent with the known pharmacology of these drugs and the biochemical pathology of Parkinson's disease. Be aware that if centrally acting anticholinesterases are given to any patient with parkinsonism, whether taking levodopa or any other anti-parkinson drug, the disease may possibly worsen. The antiparkinson drug dose may need increasing and/or the dose of the anticholinesterase may need reducing.

1. Okereke CS, Kirby L, Kumar D, Cullen EI, Pratt RD, Hahne WA. Concurrent administration of donepezil HCl and levodopa/carbidopa in patients with Parkinson's disease: assessment of pharmacokinetic changes and safety following multiple oral doses. *Br J Clin Pharmacol* (2004) 58 (Suppl 1): 41–9.
2. Shea C, MacKnight C, Rockwood K. Donepezil for treatment of dementia with Lewy bodies: a case series of nine patients. *Int Psychogeriatr* (1998) 10, 229–38.
3. Richard IH, Justus AW, Greig NH, Marshall F, Kurlan R. Worsening of motor function and mood in a patient with Parkinson's disease after pharmacologic challenge with oral rivastigmine. *Clin Neuropharmacol* (2002) 25, 296–9.
4. Ott BR, Lannon MC. Exacerbation of parkinsonism by tacrine. *Clin Neuropharmacol* (1992) 15, 322–5.

Levodopa + Antiemetics

Although metoclopramide can increase the rate of levodopa absorption, it may also antagonise its effects by aggravating symptoms of Parkinson's disease, although some studies have found no evidence of this effect. Phenothiazine antiemetics such as prochlorperazine are also generally considered to be contraindicated in Parkinson's disease. In one small

study, promethazine did not affect the control of Parkinson's disease in patients taking levodopa. Domperidone is the antiemetic of choice to prevent and treat nausea and vomiting caused by levodopa. Other antiemetics that are generally considered useful include cyclizine and 5-HT$_3$ receptor antagonists.

Clinical evidence, mechanism, importance and management

(a) Domperidone

Domperidone is a dopamine antagonist similar to metoclopramide.[1] However, as it acts on the dopamine receptors in the stomach wall, and unlike metoclopramide, it does not readily cross the blood-brain barrier, it does not appear to oppose the effects of levodopa within the brain, although some extrapyramidal symptoms have been observed. It may even slightly increase the bioavailability and effects of levodopa (by stimulating gastric emptying).[2] Domperidone can therefore be used to control the nausea and vomiting associated with levodopa treatment of Parkinson's disease.

(b) Metoclopramide

Metoclopramide is a dopamine antagonist that can cause extrapyramidal disturbances (parkinsonian symptoms), especially in children and young adults, and possibly also in the elderly, where the effects may be misdiagnosed as Parkinson's disease.[3] On the other hand, metoclopramide stimulates gastric emptying, which can result in an increase in the bioavailability of levodopa.[4,5] The outcome of these two effects (possible antagonism resulting in aggravation of Parkinson's disease, or potentiation resulting in increased bioavailability) is uncertain, and it is generally considered that metoclopramide should be avoided in Parkinson's disease. However, in one open study, metoclopramide 30 to 60 mg daily in divided doses for a range of 4 to 16 weeks caused no change in mean total disability scores in 10 patients with Parkinson's disease taking levodopa.[6] Similarly, in a controlled study in 7 patients, the incidence and severity of levodopa-induced involuntary movements were unchanged and additional acute dyskinesias did not appear when metoclopramide was also given.[6] Furthermore, in a retrospective analysis, by the same authors, there was no worsening of parkinsonian symptoms in 40 patients with Parkinson's disease taking levodopa who were also given metoclopramide up to 80 mg daily.[7] Nevertheless, if alternative antiemetics are unsuitable for a patient with Parkinson's disease and consequently metoclopramide is given, it would seem prudent to monitor the outcome closely.

(c) Phenothiazine antiemetics

Phenothiazines block the dopamine receptors in the brain and can therefore upset the balance between cholinergic and dopaminergic components within the striatum and substantia nigra. As a consequence they may not only induce the development of extrapyramidal (parkinsonian) symptoms, but they can aggravate parkinsonism and antagonise the effects of levodopa used in its treatment. See 'Levodopa + Antipsychotics', below. Phenothiazines, used in smaller doses as antiemetics, such as **prochlorperazine**,[8,9] can also behave in this way. For this reason, drugs of this kind are generally regarded as contraindicated in patients with Parkinson's disease, and there are other more suitable alternatives, see *Non-interacting antiemetics*, below. However, one small controlled study found that **promethazine** (a phenothiazine derivative with few extrapyramidal effects) did not change the total disability score or alter the incidence or severity of levodopa-induced involuntary movements in 6 patients with Parkinson's disease taking levodopa.[6]

(d) Non-interacting antiemetics

Antiemetics that are generally considered useful in patients with Parkinson's disease include **cyclizine** and 5-HT$_3$ antagonists such as **granisetron** and **ondansetron**,[3] which do not affect dopamine, and **domperidone** as discussed above. However, note that rare cases of extrapyramidal adverse effects have been reported with **ondansetron**, which may be of relevance in patients with Parkinson's disease.[10]

1. Bradbrook ID, Gillies HC, Morrison PJ, Rogers HJ. The effects of domperidone on the absorption of levodopa in normal subjects. *Eur J Clin Pharmacol* (1986) 29, 721–3.
2. Shindler JS, Finnerty GT, Towlson K, Dolan AL, Davies CL, Parkes JD. Domperidone and levodopa in Parkinson's disease. *Br J Clin Pharmacol* (1984) 18, 959–62.
3. Avorn J, Gurwitz JH, Bohn RL, Mogun H, Monane M, Walker A. Increased incidence of levodopa therapy following metoclopramide usage. *JAMA* (1995) 274, 1780–2.
4. Berkowitz DM, McCallum RW. Interaction of levodopa and metoclopramide on gastric emptying. *Clin Pharmacol Ther* (1980) 27, 414–20.
5. Mearrick PT, Wade DN, Birkett DJ, Morris J. Metoclopramide, gastric emptying and L-dopa absorption. *Aust N Z J Med* (1974) 4, 144–8.
6. Tarsy D, Parkes JD, Marsden CD. Metoclopramide and pimozide in Parkinson's disease and levodopa-induced dyskinesias. *J Neurol Neurosurg Psychiatry* (1975) 38, 331–5.
7. Tarsy D, Parkes JD, Marsden CD. Metoclopramide in parkinsonism. *Lancet* (1975) 1, 1244–5.
8. Duvoisin RC. Diphenidol for levodopa induced nausea and vomiting. *JAMA* (1972) 221, 1408.
9. Campbell JB. Long-term treatment of Parkinson's disease with levodopa. *Neurology* (1970) 20, 18–22.
10. Zofran (Ondansetron hydrochloride dihydrate). GlaxoSmithKline UK. UK Summary of product characteristics, October 2009.

Levodopa + Antimuscarinics

Antimuscarinics and other drugs with antimuscarinic effects, such as the tricyclics, may modestly reduce the rate, and possibly the extent, of absorption of levodopa. One case describes levodopa toxicity, which occurred after the withdrawal of an antimuscarinic.

Clinical evidence

A study in 6 healthy subjects and 6 patients with Parkinson's disease found that **trihexyphenidyl** 2 mg twice daily for 3 days lowered the peak plasma levels of a 500-mg dose of levodopa by 42% in the healthy subjects and by 17% in the patients, although the interaction was present in only about half of the subjects. The AUC was reduced in both groups by less than 20%.[1] Similarly, a study in 10 healthy subjects found that the initial levodopa plasma levels were lowered when a single 250-mg dose of levodopa was taken 90 minutes after a single 5-mg dose of **trihexyphenidyl**. The absorption of levodopa was slower, but the overall bioavailability was not significantly altered. Carbidopa 100 mg was given one hour before the levodopa, and a 50-mg dose was given 5 hours after the levodopa.[2]

A study in 6 patients with Parkinson's disease taking levodopa with carbidopa or benserazide found that **orphenadrine** caused either a delay, a reduction, or an increase in levodopa absorption in 3 patients.[3] A patient who needed 7 g of levodopa daily while taking **homatropine** developed levodopa toxicity when the **homatropine** was withdrawn, and he was subsequently restabilised on only 4 g of levodopa daily.[4]

A study in 4 healthy subjects[5] found that **imipramine** 25 mg four times daily for 3 days reduced the peak plasma concentration of a single 500-mg dose of levodopa by about 50%, but did not appear to alter the extent of absorption. See also 'Levodopa + Tricyclic antidepressants', p.770, for other non-antimuscarinic interactions of the tricyclics.

Mechanism

The small intestine is the major site of absorption for levodopa. Delayed gastric emptying, which can be caused by antimuscarinics, appears to result in lower plasma levodopa levels and thus lower brain levodopa levels. This is because the gastric mucosa has more time to metabolise the levodopa to dopamine and therefore less is available for absorption.[6]

Importance and management

Antimuscarinics are commonly given with levodopa, and they are of established benefit. However, limited evidence suggests they might sometimes reduce levodopa efficacy. Levodopa preparations are now more usually given in conjunction with a dopa decarboxylase inhibitor to minimise metabolism in the gastric mucosa. This would be expected to minimise the effects of any interaction. However, note that two of the above studies included a dopa-decarboxylase inhibitor, yet still found an effect on levodopa absorption. There is certainly no need to avoid concurrent use, but it would be prudent to be alert for any evidence of a reduced levodopa response if antimuscarinics are added, or for levodopa toxicity if they are withdrawn.

1. Algeri S, Cerletti C, Curcio M, Morselli PL, Bonollo L, Buniva G, Minazzi M, Minoli G. Effect of anticholinergic drugs on gastro-intestinal absorption of L-dopa in rats and in man. *Eur J Pharmacol* (1976) 35, 293–9.
2. Roberts J, Waller DG, Renwick AG, O'Shea N, Macklin BS, Bulling M. The effects of co-administration of benzhexol on the peripheral pharmacokinetics of oral levodopa in young volunteers. *Br J Clin Pharmacol* (1996) 41, 331–7.
3. Contin M, Riva R, Martinelli P, Procaccianti G, Albani F, Baruzzi A. Combined levodopa-anticholinergic therapy in the treatment of Parkinson's disease. *Clin Neuropharmacol* (1991) 14, 148–55.
4. Fermaglich J, O'Doherty DS. Effect of gastric motility on levodopa. *Dis Nerv Syst* (1972) 33, 624–5.
5. Morgan JP, Rivera-Calimlim L, Messiha F, Sundaresan PR, Trabert N. Imipramine-mediated interference with levodopa absorption from the gastrointestinal tract in man. *Neurology* (1975) 25, 1029–34.
6. Rivera-Calimlim L, Dujovne CA, Morgan JP, Lasagna L, Bianchine JR. Absorption and metabolism of L-dopa by the human stomach. *Eur J Clin Invest* (1971) 1, 313–20.

Levodopa + Antipsychotics

Phenothiazines, butyrophenones, thioxanthenes and pimozide can oppose the effects of levodopa because of their dopamine antagonist properties, causing deterioration of motor function in Parkinson's disease. The antipsychotic effects and extrapyramidal adverse effects of these drugs can be opposed by levodopa. Of the atypical antipsychotics, risperidone and olanzapine cause deterioration in motor function in Parkinson's disease. Ziprasidone and paliperidone may act similarly, and there have been reports of mild motor deterioration with quetiapine. Clozapine does not have this effect.

Clinical evidence, mechanism, importance and management

(a) Classical antipsychotics

Phenothiazines (e.g. fluphenazine, perphenazine, prochlorperazine, and trifluoperazine), **butyrophenones** (e.g. droperidol and haloperidol), **thioxanthenes** (e.g. flupentixol and zuclopenthixol) and pimozide block the dopamine receptors in the brain and can therefore upset the balance between cholinergic and dopaminergic components within the striatum and substantia nigra. As a consequence they may not only induce the development of extrapyramidal (parkinsonian) symptoms, but they can aggravate parkinsonism and antagonise the effects of levodopa used in its treatment.[1-5] For this reason drugs of this kind are generally regarded as contraindicated in patients being treated for Parkinson's disease, or only used with great caution in carefully controlled conditions. The extrapyramidal symptoms that frequently occur with the **phenothiazines** have in the past been treated without much success with levodopa. However, the levodopa may also antagonise the antipsychotic effects of the **phenothiazines**,[6] and other dopamine-antagonist antipsychotics. Phenothiazines used as antiemetics may also act in this way. Consider also 'Levodopa + Antiemetics', p.761.

(b) Atypical antipsychotics

Of the atypical antipsychotics, both **risperidone** and **olanzapine** have caused deterioration of motor function in patients with Parkinson's disease.[7,8] **Paliperidone**, the active metabolite of risperidone, is expected to have similar effects.[9,10] There have also been reports of deterioration in motor function with **quetiapine**, but in general this effect seems to be mild[7] and, in patients with Parkinson's disease, quetiapine appears to be better tolerated than risperidone or olanzapine.[8] There is far less experience with **ziprasidone**, but it may have a propensity to cause extrapyramidal adverse effects that is similar to **olanzapine**.

Low-dose **clozapine** appears to cause little deterioration in motor function, and may improve tremor. It is therefore a preferred antipsychotic for patients with Parkinson's disease and levodopa-induced psychosis. Note that individual reports and studies of the use of these antipsychotics in patients with Parkinson's disease are numerous. Reviews on the topic have been published.[7,8]

1. Duvoisin RC. Diphenidol for levodopa induced nausea and vomiting. *JAMA* (1972) 221, 1408.
2. Klawans HL, Weiner WJ. Attempted use of haloperidol in the treatment of L-dopa induced dyskinesias. *J Neurol Neurosurg Psychiatry* (1974) 37, 427–30.
3. Hunter KR, Stern GM, Laurence DR. Use of levodopa and other drugs. *Lancet* (1970) ii, 1283–5.
4. Lipper S. Psychosis in a patient on bromocriptine and levodopa with carbidopa. *Lancet* (1976) ii, 571–2.
5. Tarsy D, Parkes JD, Marsden CD. Metoclopramide and pimozide in Parkinson's disease and levodopa-induced dyskinesias. *J Neurol Neurosurg Psychiatry* (1975) 38, 331–5.
6. Yaryura-Tobias JA, Wolpert A, Dana L, Merlis S. Action of L-dopa in drug induced extrapyramidalism. *Dis Nerv Syst* (1970) 1, 60–3.
7. Fernandez HH, Trieschmann ME, Friedman JH. Treatment of psychosis in Parkinson's disease: safety considerations. *Drug Safety* (2003) 26, 643–59.
8. Zahodne LB, Fernandez HH. Pathophysiology and treatment of psychosis in Parkinson's disease: a review. *Drugs Aging* (2008) 25, 665–82.
9. Invega (Paliperidone). Janssen-Cilag Ltd. UK Summary of product characteristics, June 2012.
10. Invega (Paliperidone). Janssen Pharmaceuticals, Inc. US Prescribing information, June 2011.

Levodopa + Ascorbic acid (Vitamin C)

Ascorbic acid does not appear to alter the pharmacokinetics of levodopa.

Clinical evidence, mechanism, importance and management

In a study, 67 elderly patients with Parkinson's disease took a single dose of levodopa 100 mg with carbidopa 10 mg alone, and with a single 200-mg dose of ascorbic acid. The AUC, maximum plasma levels, and time to reach maximum levodopa plasma levels were increased when ascorbic acid was also given, but these increases were not statistically significant. However, there was a trend towards a larger effect in those patients with lower baseline levodopa bioavailability.[1] Based on the available evidence, there would appear to be no reason for patients taking levodopa to avoid modest doses of ascorbic acid.

1. Nagayama H, Hamamoto M, Ueda M, Nito C, Yamaguchi H, Katayama Y. The effect of ascorbic acid on the pharmacokinetics of levodopa in elderly patients with Parkinson disease. *Clin Neuropharmacol* (2004) 27, 270–3.

Levodopa + Baclofen

Unpleasant adverse effects (hallucinations, confusion, headache, nausea) and worsening of the symptoms of parkinsonism have occurred in patients taking levodopa who were given baclofen.

Clinical evidence

Twelve patients with parkinsonism taking levodopa with a dopa-decarboxylase inhibitor were also given baclofen. The eventual baclofen dose was intended to be 90 mg daily, but the adverse effects were considerable (visual hallucinations, a toxic confusional state, headaches, nausea) so that only 2 patients reached this dose, and 2 patients withdrew because they could not tolerate these adverse effects. The mean dose for those who continued was 45 mg daily. Rigidity was aggravated by an average of 46% and functional capacity deteriorated by 21%.[1]

A patient with Parkinson's disease taking levodopa with carbidopa, orphenadrine and diazepam became acutely confused, agitated, incontinent and hallucinated when given a third dose of baclofen (in all 15 mg). The baclofen was stopped, but on the following night she again hallucinated and became confused. The next day she was given two 2.5-mg doses of baclofen but she became anxious and hallucinated with paranoid ideas.[2]

Mechanism

Not understood. The toxicity seen appears to be an exaggeration of the known adverse effects of baclofen.

Importance and management

Information appears to be limited to these reports, but they suggest that baclofen should be used very cautiously in patients taking levodopa.

1. Lees AJ, Shaw KM, Stern GM. Baclofen in Parkinson's disease. *J Neurol Neurosurg Psychiatry* (1978) 41, 707–8.
2. Skausig OB, Korsgaard S. Hallucinations and baclofen. *Lancet* (1977) 1, 1258.

Levodopa + Benzodiazepines and related drugs

On rare occasions it seems that the therapeutic effects of levodopa can be reduced by chlordiazepoxide, diazepam or nitrazepam.

Clinical evidence

Various benzodiazepines (dose unstated) were given to 8 patients with Parkinson's disease taking levodopa. In 5 of the patients (3 taking **chlordiazepoxide**, one taking **nitrazepam**, one taking **oxazepam**) no interactions were seen. However, the other 3 patients (one taking **diazepam**, 2 taking **nitrazepam**) experienced transient disturbances in the control of their Parkinson's disease, which lasted up to 3 weeks in the case of the patient taking **diazepam**.[1] Other cases of a reversible loss of control of Parkinson's disease have been seen in 3 patients taking **diazepam**[2] and 4 patients taking **chlordiazepoxide**.[3,4] In one further case, a patient taking **chlordiazepoxide** experienced falls associated with a worsening of parkinsonian symptoms while taking **chlordiazepoxide**. She recovered 5 days after the **chlordiazepoxide** was withdrawn.[5]

In contrast, a case-control study of patients with Parkinson's disease taking levodopa did not find a statistically significant increase in the required dose of antiparkinsonian drug treatment in the 180 days after starting a benzodiazepine.[6]

Mechanism

Not understood, although *animal* studies have shown that benzodiazepines can decrease the levels of dopamine in the striatum.[6]

Importance and management

Not established. Given the widespread use of benzodiazepines in patients taking levodopa,[7] any major or common interaction would be expected to have come to light by now. It would therefore seem that any interaction is fairly rare, and on the basis of one of the reports cited above, possibly only transient. There is no need to avoid concurrent use, but bear these reports in mind in the case of an unexpected response to treatment.

1. Hunter KR, Stern GM, Laurence DR. Use of levodopa with other drugs. *Lancet* (1970) ii, 1283–5.
2. Wodak J, Gilligan BS, Veale JL, Dowty BJ. Review of 12 months' treatment with L-dopa in Parkinson's disease, with remarks on unusual side effects. *Med J Aust* (1972) 2, 1277–82.
3. Mackie L. Drug antagonism. *BMJ* (1971) 2, 651.
4. Schwarz GA, Fahn S. Newer medical treatments in parkinsonism. *Med Clin North Am* (1970) 54, 773–85.
5. Yosselson-Superstine S, Lipman AG. Chlordiazepoxide interaction with levodopa. *Ann Intern Med* (1982) 96, 259–60.
6. van de Vijver DAMC, Roos RAC, Jansen PAF, Porsius AJ, de Boer A. Influence of benzodiazepines on antiparkinsonian drug treatment in levodopa users. *Acta Neurol Scand* (2002) 105, 8–12.
7. van de Vijver DAMC, de Boer A, Herings RMC, Roos RAC, Porsius AJ. Increased use of psychotropic drugs by patients with Parkinson's disease. *Br J Clin Pharmacol* (1999) 47, 476P.

Levodopa + Beta blockers

The concurrent use of levodopa and beta blockers normally appears to be favourable, but be aware that, as with all antihypertensives, additive hypotensive effects can occur.

Clinical evidence, mechanism, importance and management

Most of the effects of the concurrent use of levodopa and beta blockers seem to be favourable, although additive hypotension can be a problem. Dopamine derived from levodopa stimulates beta-receptors in the heart, which can cause arrhythmias.[1] These receptors are blocked by **propranolol** and other beta blockers. An enhancement of the effects of levodopa and a reduction in tremor has been described in 23 out of 25 patients taking **propranolol**,[2] but not in 9 patients taking **oxprenolol**,[3] or in another placebo-controlled study in 18 patients taking **propranolol**.[4] Early evidence found that growth hormone levels were substantially raised by **propranolol**[5,6] or **practolol**[6] [now withdrawn due to fatal reactions] in conjunction with levodopa, but no clinical relevance for this has been demonstrated.

1. Goldberg LI, Whitsett TL. Cardiovascular effects of levodopa. *Clin Pharmacol Ther* (1971) 12, 376–82.
2. Kissel P, Tridon P, André JM. Levodopa-propranolol therapy in parkinsonian tremor. *Lancet* (1974) ii, 403–4.
3. Sandler M, Fellows LE, Calne DB, Findley LJ. Oxprenolol and levodopa in parkinsonian patients. *Lancet* (1975) i, 168.
4. Marsden CD, Parkes JD, Rees JE. Propranolol in Parkinson's disease. *Lancet* (1974) ii, 410.
5. Camanni F, Massara F. Enhancement of levodopa-induced growth-hormone stimulation by propranolol. *Lancet* (1974) i, 942.
6. Lotti G, Delitala G, Masala A. Enhancement of levodopa-induced growth-hormone stimulation by practolol. *Lancet* (1974) 2, 1329.

Levodopa + Bromocriptine and other dopamine agonists

The concurrent use of levodopa and dopamine agonists can increase efficacy and adverse effects in Parkinson's disease. Bromocriptine may sometimes alter levodopa levels and levodopa may lower bromocriptine levels. There appears to be no pharmacokinetic interaction between levodopa and cabergoline, pramipexole or ropinirole. An isolated report describes the development of serotonin syndrome when levodopa with carbidopa was added to treatment with bromocriptine.

Clinical evidence

(a) Bromocriptine

A study in 20 patients with Parkinson's disease taking levodopa with carbidopa found that overall there was no difference in plasma levodopa levels after bromocriptine was also taken, although some patients had either significant elevations or significant reductions in levels. However, the only adverse clinical change found was an increase in dyskinesias in the patients with elevated levodopa levels.[1] An earlier study found no pharmacokinetic interaction between levodopa with carbidopa and bromocriptine, but it should be noted that this was a single-dose study and may not reflect long-term concurrent use.[2] A further study in 7 patients with Parkinson's disease taking long-term levodopa with benserazide found that the addition of bromocriptine, 15 mg daily in three divided doses for 6 months, had no effect on the pharmacokinetics of levodopa.[3] Steady-state bromocriptine plasma levels were found to be reduced by levodopa in a study in 10 patients with Parkinson's disease. The patients normally took levodopa, but this was withheld to give baseline bromocriptine pharmacokinetics.[4]

A patient with parkinsonism, who had been taking bromocriptine 60 mg daily for nearly 3 years, was also given levodopa with carbidopa (250/25 mg daily increasing over a week to 750/75 mg) while the bromocriptine dose was reduced to 20 mg daily. On the seventh day he started shivering, and developed myoclonus of the trunk and limbs, hyperreflexia, patellar clonus, tremor, diaphoresis, anxiety, diarrhoea, tachycardia and had a temperature of 37.9°C with a blood pressure of 180/100 mmHg. Serotonin syndrome was suspected. The patient responded to treatment with the 5-HT antagonist methysergide.[5]

A case of pathological gambling in a 54-year-old woman was attributed to the concurrent use of bromocriptine and levodopa with carbidopa.[6]

(b) Cabergoline

Levodopa with carbidopa 250/25 mg daily did not cause a clinically significant change in the pharmacokinetics of cabergoline 2 mg daily when the combination was given to patients newly diagnosed with Parkinson's disease. Similarly, cabergoline (in increasing doses up to 4 mg daily) for 8 weeks had no effect on the absorption, AUC or elimination half-life of levodopa in another group of patients with fluctuating Parkinson's disease who were taking levodopa with carbidopa.[7]

(c) Pergolide

The manufacturer notes that the use of pergolide in patients taking levodopa may cause and/or exacerbate pre-existing states of dyskinesia, confusion, and hallucinations. Also, they say that stopping pergolide abruptly in patients taking levodopa may precipitate the onset of hallucinations and confusion.[8]

(d) Pramipexole

Patients taking a stable dose of levodopa with carbidopa were given increasing doses of pramipexole or placebo for 7 weeks. Pramipexole 1.5 mg daily and 4.5 mg daily had no effect on levodopa bioavailability.[9] Several cases of pathological gambling have been reported in patients taking pramipexole, usually in association with levodopa.[10]

(e) Ropinirole

In patients taking a stable dose of levodopa with a dopa-decarboxylase inhibitor, ropinirole had no effect on the pharmacokinetics of levodopa, except for a small clinically irrelevant 16% increase in its maximum level. Levodopa also had no effect on the pharmacokinetics of ropinirole in another group of patients.[11] Similarly, in a single-dose study in healthy subjects, levodopa with benserazide had no significant effect on the pharmacokinetics of ropinirole.[12]

(f) Rotigotine

The manufacturer of rotigotine reports that levodopa and carbidopa had no effect on the pharmacokinetics of rotigotine and similarly, rotigotine had no effect on the pharmacokinetics of either levodopa or carbidopa. However, as with other dopamine agonists, rotigotine may cause and/or exacerbate dyskinesia in patients taking levodopa and may potentiate the dopaminergic adverse reactions of levodopa.[13]

Mechanism

Additive dopaminergic effects would be expected. Serotonin syndrome is thought to occur because of increased stimulation of the 5-HT receptors in the brainstem and spinal cord. A syndrome resembling neuroleptic malignant syndrome (which has similar symptoms to serotonin syndrome) can occur when a dopamine agonist like bromocriptine is withdrawn abruptly. It is therefore possible that the effects of reducing the bromocriptine dose were additive with those of levodopa, which can displace serotonin from the nerve endings.[5]

Importance and management

The concurrent use of levodopa and dopamine agonists can increase efficacy in Parkinson's disease, but adverse effects such as hallucinations and dyskinesias may also be increased, and the dose of both drugs should be gradually adjusted to optimise therapy. The manufacturer of ropinirole suggests a total reduction in the levodopa dose of about 20%.[14] If the decision is made to withdraw the dopamine agonist, this should be done slowly, over several days.

Serotonin syndrome described with levodopa and bromocriptine appears to be an isolated incident and not of general importance. A number of cases of pathological gambling have been reported in patients taking dopamine agonists with levodopa. It has been suggested that pathological gambling may be a class effect of dopamine agonists, although levodopa may have contributed in patients receiving both drugs.[10]

1. Rabey JM, Schwartz M, Graff E, Harsat A, Vered Y. The influence of bromocriptine on the pharmacokinetics of levodopa in Parkinson's disease. *Clin Neuropharmacol* (1991) 14, 514–22.
2. Bentué-Ferrer D, Allain H, Reymann JM, Sabouraud O, Van den Driessche J. Lack of pharmacokinetic influence on levodopa by bromocriptine. *Clin Neuropharmacol* (1988) 11, 83–6.
3. Contin M, Riva R, Martinelli P, Albani F, Baruzzi A. No effect of chronic bromocriptine therapy on levodopa pharmacokinetics in patients with Parkinson's disease. *Clin Neuropharmacol* (1992) 15, 505–8.
4. Rabey JM, Oberman Z, Scharf M, Isakov A, Bar M, Graff E. The influence of levodopa in the pharmacokinetics of bromocriptine in Parkinson's disease. *Clin Neuropharmacol* (1989) 12, 440–7.
5. Sandyk R. L-Dopa induced "serotonin syndrome" in a parkinsonian patient on bromocriptine. *J Clin Psychopharmacol* (1986) 6, 194–5.
6. Polard E, Trioux E, Flet L, Colin F, Allain H. Ludopathie induite par la lévodopa associée à la bromocriptine. *Presse Med* (2003) 32, 1223.
7. Del Dotto P, Colzi A, Musatti E, Benedetti MS, Persiani S, Fariello R, Bonuccelli U. Clinical and pharmacokinetic evaluation of L-dopa and cabergoline cotreatment in Parkinson's disease. *Clin Neuropharmacol* (1997) 20, 455–65.
8. Celance (Pergolide mesilate). Eli Lilly and Company Ltd. UK Summary of product characteristics, August 2009.
9. Kompoliti K, Adler CH, Raman R, Pincus JH, Leibowitz MT, Ferry JJ, Blasucci L, Caviness JN, Leurgans S, Chase WM, Yones LC, Tan E, Carvey P, Goetz CG. Gender and pramipexole effects on levodopa pharmacokinetics and pharmacodynamics. *Neurology* (2002) 58, 1418–22.
10. Anon. Dopamine agonists: pathological gambling and increased libido. Public Assessment Report. Medicines and Healthcare products Regulatory Agency. November 2006. Available at: http://www.mhra.gov.uk/home/idcplg?IdcService=GET_FILE&dDocName=CON2025150&RevisionSelectionMethod=LatestReleased (accessed 21/10/15).
11. Taylor AC, Beerahee A, Citerone DR, Cyronak MJ, Leigh TJ, Fitzpatrick KL, Lopez-Gil A, Vakil SD, Burns E, Lennox G. Lack of a pharmacokinetic interaction at steady state between ropinirole and L-dopa in patients with Parkinson's disease. *Pharmacotherapy* (1999) 19, 150–6.
12. Wen A-D, Jia Y-Y, Luo X-X, Bi L-L, Chen X-Y, Zhong D-F. The effect of Madopar on the pharmacokinetics of ropinirole in healthy Chinese volunteers. *J Pharm Biomed Anal* (2007) 43, 774–8.
13. Neupro (Rotigotine). UCB Pharma Ltd. UK Summary of product characteristics, August 2009.
14. Requip Tablets (Ropinirole hydrochloride). GlaxoSmithKline UK. UK Summary of product characteristics, April 2012.

Levodopa + Caffeine

Caffeine increased the rate of absorption of levodopa, but not its overall bioavailability.

Clinical evidence, mechanism, importance and management

In a crossover study, 12 patients with Parkinson's disease were given a single 200-mg dose of caffeine or placebo 15 minutes before receiving levodopa 250 mg with carbidopa 25 mg. The rate of absorption of levodopa was increased by caffeine, with maximum levodopa plasma levels being achieved at one hour, compared with 1.5 hours when taken with placebo. There was also a shortening of the time to detect a motor response to levodopa when caffeine was taken. However, the maximum plasma levels and the $AUC_{0\text{-}3}$ of levodopa were not significantly altered by caffeine.[1]

A study in 4 patients with Parkinson's disease investigated the therapeutic benefit of adding caffeine to levodopa with carbidopa. Doses of up to 1.4 g of caffeine daily did not potentiate the antiparkinsonian action of levodopa, but there was an increase in the duration of involuntary movements during the use of high doses of caffeine, and signs or symptoms of caffeine toxicity appeared in all 6 patients.[2]

These studies suggest that caffeine need not be avoided in patients taking levodopa, but high doses may increase movement disorders in response to levodopa. If this becomes troublesome, it may be prudent to try to decrease caffeine intake.

1. Deleu D, Jacob P, Chand P, Sarre S, Colwell A. Effects of caffeine on levodopa pharmacokinetics and pharmacodynamics in Parkinson disease. *Neurology* (2006) 67, 897–9.
2. Shoulson I, Chase TN. Caffeine and the antiparkinsonian response to levodopa or piribedil. *Neurology* (1975) 25, 722–4.

Levodopa + Clonidine

Limited evidence suggests that clonidine may oppose the effects of levodopa. Be aware that, as with the use of all antihypertensives with levodopa, additive hypotensive effects may occur.

Clinical evidence

A study in 2 patients taking levodopa with carbidopa found that the concurrent use of clonidine (up to 1.5 mg daily for 10 to 24 days) caused a worsening of parkinsonism (an exacerbation of rigidity and akinesia). The concurrent use of antimuscarinic drugs reduced the effects of this interaction.[1]

Another report on 10 hypertensive and 3 normotensive patients with Parkinson's disease, 9 of them taking levodopa and 4 of them not, suggested that the concurrent use of clonidine did not affect the control of the parkinsonism. However, 2 patients stopped taking clonidine because of an increase in tremor and gait disturbances.[2]

Mechanism

Not understood. One suggestion is that clonidine opposes the antiparkinson effects by stimulating alpha-receptors in the brain. Another idea is that clonidine directly stimulates post-synaptic dopaminergic receptors.

Importance and management

Information seems to be limited to these reports. Be alert for a reduction in the control of the Parkinson's disease during the concurrent use of levodopa and clonidine. The effects of this interaction appear to be reduced if antimuscarinic drugs are also being used.[1] Also note, that as with all antihypertensives, additive hypotensive effects may occur.

1. Shoulson I, Chase TN. Clonidine and the anti-parkinsonian response to L-dopa or piribedil. *Neuropharmacology* (1976) 15, 25–7.
2. Tarsy D, Parkes JD, Marsden CD. Clonidine in Parkinson disease. *Arch Neurol* (1975) 32, 134–6.

Levodopa + COMT inhibitors

Entacapone and tolcapone increase the AUC of levodopa given with benserazide or carbidopa. This may require a reduction in the levodopa dose to avoid symptoms of dopamine excess when first starting the

COMT inhibitor. Tolcapone increases the levels of benserazide, but neither entacapone nor tolcapone alters carbidopa pharmacokinetics.

Clinical evidence

(a) Levodopa

Entacapone[1-3] and **tolcapone**[4,5] have been shown to increase the AUC and/or prolong the elimination half-life of levodopa (given with benserazide or carbidopa) without significantly altering the maximum levodopa level. However, in some studies, the maximum levodopa plasma levels have also been increased by **entacapone** or **tolcapone**.[6,7]

COMT inhibitors can therefore improve the clinical condition of patients with Parkinson's disease, which is mainly seen as a decrease in 'off' time.[8] However, as levodopa levels are raised, there may be an accompanying increase in the adverse effects of levodopa (e.g. dyskinesias, nausea, vomiting, orthostatic hypotension, hallucinations).[9-11]

(b) Benserazide or Carbidopa

The effects of COMT inhibitors on the pharmacokinetics of dopa-decarboxylase inhibitors have also been studied. Neither **entacapone**[2] nor **tolcapone**[12] altered the pharmacokinetics of carbidopa. However, **tolcapone** increased the plasma levels of benserazide in patients with Parkinson's disease.[13] The benserazide levels remained within the usual range in patients taking levodopa with benserazide 25 mg and **tolcapone** 200 mg three times daily. However, with a 50-mg dose of benserazide the AUC of benserazide was increased 4.8-fold with standard-release preparation and 2.3-fold with a controlled-release preparation.[13]

Mechanism

When levodopa is given with a dopa-decarboxylase inhibitor such as carbidopa or benserazide, COMT becomes the major enzyme for metabolising levodopa, so inhibiting COMT delays the breakdown of levodopa.

Importance and management

When starting a COMT inhibitor, all patients should be informed of the symptoms of excess levodopa, and what to do if they occur. The manufacturers of entacapone suggest that if entacapone is started, the daily dose of levodopa should be reduced by about 10 to 30% (within the first few days or weeks) to accommodate these potential adverse effects.[10,14] This can be done by either extending the dosing intervals and/or by reducing the amount of levodopa per dose. Patients taking levodopa with benserazide may require a greater dose reduction than those taking levodopa with carbidopa because entacapone increases the bioavailability of standard levodopa with benserazide preparations by 5 to 10% more than standard levodopa with carbidopa.[10] The manufacturers of tolcapone say that the average reduction in the daily dose of levodopa required on starting tolcapone was 30%, and that greater than 70% of patients taking levodopa doses above 600 mg daily required such a reduction.[11,15] The clinical significance of the increase in benserazide levels is unknown, but the manufacturers advise good monitoring for benserazide adverse effects.[15]

1. Myllylä VV, Sotaniemi KA, Illi A, Suominen K, Keränen T. Effect of entacapone, a COMT inhibitor, on the pharmacokinetics of levodopa and on cardiovascular responses in patients with Parkinson's disease. *Eur J Clin Pharmacol* (1993) 45, 419–23.
2. Keränen T, Gordin A, Harjola V-P, Karlsson M, Korpela K, Pentikäinen PJ, Rita H, Seppälä L, Wikberg T. The effect of catechol-*O*-methyl transferase inhibition by entacapone on the pharmacokinetics and metabolism of levodopa in healthy volunteers. *Clin Neuropharmacol* (1993) 16, 145–56.
3. Contin M, Martinelli P, Scaglione C, Avoni P, Albani F, Riva R, Baruzzi A. The effect of entacapone on levodopa rate of absorption and latency to motor response in patients with Parkinson disease. *Clin Neuropharmacol* (2008) 31, 267–71.
4. Dingemanse J, Jorga K, Zürcher G, Schmitt M, Sedek G, da Prada M, van Brummelen P. Pharmacokinetic-pharmacodynamic interaction between the COMT inhibitor tolcapone and single-dose levodopa. *Br J Clin Pharmacol* (1995) 40, 253–62.
5. Sêdek G, Jorga K, Schmitt M, Burns RS, Leese P. Effect of tolcapone on plasma levodopa concentrations after coadministration with levodopa/carbidopa to healthy volunteers. *Clin Neuropharmacol* (1997) 20, 531–41.
6. Brusa L, Pierantozzi M, Bassi A, Fedele E, Lunardi G, Giacomini P, Stanzione P. Temporal administration of entacapone with slow release L-dopa: pharmacokinetic profile and clinical outcome. *Neurol Sci* (2004) 25, 53–6.
7. Baas H, Zehrden F, Selzer R, Kohnen R, Loetsch J, Harder S. Pharmacokinetic-pharmacodynamic relationship of levodopa with and without tolcapone in patients with Parkinson's disease. *Clin Pharmacokinet* (2001) 40, 383–93.
8. Heikkinen H, Nutt JG, LeWitt PA, Koller WC, Gordin A. The effects of different repeated doses of entacapone on the pharmacokinetics of L-dopa and on the clinical response to L-dopa in Parkinson's disease. *Clin Neuropharmacol* (2001) 24, 150–7.
9. Ruottinen HM, Rinne UK. Entacapone prolongs levodopa response in a one month double blind study in parkinsonian patients with levodopa related fluctuations. *J Neurol Neurosurg Psychiatry* (1996) 60, 36–40.
10. Comtess (Entacapone). Orion Pharma (UK) Ltd. UK Summary of product characteristics, September 2008.
11. Tasmar (Tolcapone). Valeant Pharmaceuticals North America. US Prescribing information, June 2009.
12. Jorga KM, Nicholl DJ. COMT inhibition with tolcapone does not affect carbidopa pharmacokinetics in parkinsonian patients on levodopa/carbidopa (Sinemet). *Br J Clin Pharmacol* (1999) 48, 449–52.
13. Jorga KM, Larsen JP, Beiske A, Schleimer M, Fotteler B, Schmitt M, Moe B. The effect of tolcapone on the pharmacokinetics of benserazide. *Eur J Neurol* (1999) 6, 211–19.
14. Comtan (Entacapone). Novartis. US Prescribing information, March 2009.
15. Tasmar (Tolcapone). Meda Pharmaceuticals. UK Summary of product characteristics, January 2009.

Levodopa + Dacarbazine

An isolated report describes a reduction in the effects of levodopa caused by dacarbazine.

Clinical evidence, mechanism, importance and management

A patient who had been treated surgically for melanoma, continued to receive dacarbazine 200 mg intravenously daily, intermittently, for sporadic positive melanuria. He later developed Parkinson's disease, and was given levodopa, which had no effect on his melanoma. However, each time he was given dacarbazine he complained that the effects of the levodopa with benserazide were reduced and his Schwab and England score (measures of activities of daily living) fell by as much as 25%. A subsequent double-blind study in this patient, using a modified Columbia Score, confirmed this.[1] The reasons are not understood, but as the serum dopamine levels remained unchanged it is suggested that competition between the two drugs at the blood-brain barrier may be the explanation.[1] Be alert for the need to modify levodopa treatment if dacarbazine is used concurrently. However, note also that the manufacturers contraindicate levodopa in those with a history of malignant melanoma because there is some suggestion that levodopa may activate this malignancy,[2] although some consider that, from the available evidence, this is unlikely.[3]

1. Merello M, Esteguy M, Perazzo F, Leiguarda R. Impaired levodopa response in Parkinson's disease during melanoma therapy. *Clin Neuropharmacol* (1992) 15, 69–74.
2. Madopar Capsules (Levodopa and Benserazide hydrochloride). Roche Products Ltd. UK Summary of product characteristics, April 2009.
3. Siple JF, Schneider DC, Wanlass WA, Rosenblatt BK. Levodopa therapy and the risk of malignant melanoma. *Ann Pharmacother* (2000) 34, 382–5.

Levodopa + Food

The fluctuations in response to levodopa experienced by some patients may be due to the timing of meals and the type of diet, particularly the protein content, both of which can reduce the effects of levodopa. The effects of levodopa can be reduced by the amino acid methionine, and the blood levels of levodopa can be reduced by the amino acid tryptophan.

Clinical evidence

(a) Effects of meals

A study in patients with Parkinson's disease taking levodopa found that if taken with a meal, the mean absorption of levodopa from the gut and its peak plasma levels were reduced by 27% and 29%, respectively, and the peak plasma level was delayed by 34 minutes.[1] Other studies have found that the absorption of levodopa is delayed and peak plasma levels are reduced if the levodopa is taken with food rather than when fasting.[2-4]

(b) Effects of protein

1. Levodopa levels. A study in healthy subjects found that a low-protein meal (protein 10.5 g) caused a small reduction in levodopa absorption when compared with the fasting state, but also found that a high-protein meal (protein 30.5 g) was no different to the fasting state.[5] In another study, the protein content of the diet appeared to have little effect on levodopa pharmacokinetics.[6]

In contrast, other studies have found that a high daily intake of protein reduces the effects of levodopa (with or without a dopa-decarboxylase inhibitor), compared with a lower intake of protein.[7-9]

2. Subjective or clinical response. A study in 20 patients with Parkinson's disease who took levodopa with carbidopa four times daily with no-, low-, or high-protein snacks, each for one day, found no difference in markers of their Parkinson's disease (such as functional activity, dyskinesias, mental status).[10]

In a study, 11 patients with Parkinson's disease followed a restricted-protein diet in which they ingested up to about 10 g of protein during the day, but their intake was unrestricted during the evening. After following this diet for 6 weeks, 7 patients reported an improvement in their daytime mobility, and 6 patients indicated that they would continue with such a diet.[11]

A case report describes a patient with Parkinson's disease, receiving levodopa with carbidopa, who was admitted to an intensive care unit and developed severe rigidity after he was given continuous **enteral nutrition** with 1.4 g/kg of protein daily, despite continuing with his antiparkinsonian medication via the gastric tube. The protein content of the feed was reduced to 900 mg/kg per day, and given as bolus doses, with the levodopa given between the boluses. His parkinsonian symptoms improved with this feeding regime.[12]

(c) Effects of specific amino acids

A study found that the clinical response to a constant intravenous infusion of levodopa in 4 patients was unchanged by **glycine** and **lysine** but was reduced by **phenylalanine**, **leucine** and **isoleucine**, although the plasma levodopa levels remained unchanged.[1]

Fourteen patients taking levodopa for Parkinson's disease were given a **low-methionine** diet (0.5 g daily) for a period of 8 days. Seven patients were given additional **methionine** (4.5 g daily), while the other 7 were given placebo. Five out of the 7 given **methionine** 4.5 g daily had a definite worsening of their symptoms (gait, tremor, rigidity, etc.). The symptoms subsided when the **methionine** was withdrawn, although this took 7 to 10 days in one patient. Three out of the 7 given placebo (while following the low-methionine diet) had some subjective improvement.[13]

The blood levels of levodopa were markedly reduced in healthy subjects when levodopa 500 mg was taken with 1 g of **tryptophan**.[14] The clinical importance of this was not assessed.

(d) Broad bean pods (Vicia faba)

In a study, patients who took levodopa with carbidopa or benserazide additionally ate a portion (approximately 250 g) of cooked broad beans at least twice a day for up to 3 months. Three patients completed diary cards, and it was found that their 'on' periods were prolonged. One patient experienced an improvement in his 'on' periods each day even when he ate the broad beans on alternate days, and another patient reduced his dose of levodopa with carbidopa, from 500/50 mg to 375/37.5 mg each day.[15]

(e) Dietary fibre

In a study, 16 patients with Parkinson's disease and severe constipation took dietary fibre, to achieve a diet high in insoluble fibre (mean 28 g daily), with their usual medications. Plasma levodopa levels were increased significantly after increasing the fibre content of the diet, and there was improvement in constipation and motor function.[16]

Mechanism

Meals that delay gastric emptying increase the potential for peripheral metabolism of levodopa in the gut, which reduces the amount available for absorption. Conversely, a diet high in insoluble fibre may possibly increase levodopa absorption due to improved gastrointestinal motility. In addition some large neutral amino acids arising from the digestion of proteins can compete with levodopa for transport into the brain so that the therapeutic response may be reduced, whereas other amino acids do not have this effect.[1,5,8,17] Broad bean pods have been shown to contain a significant amount of levodopa, which may have contributed to the beneficial effect.

Importance and management

An established interaction, but unpredictable. As the fluctuations in the response of patients to levodopa may be influenced by what is eaten and when, a change in the pattern of drug and food administration on a trial-and-error basis may be helpful. Note that the manufacturer of *Madopar* recommends taking this preparation with food or slowly increasing the dose in the early stages of treatment to control anorexia, nausea, vomiting, and diarrhoea.[18] Multiple small doses of levodopa and distributing the intake of proteins may also diminish the effects of these interactions. Diets that conform to the recommended daily allowance of protein (said to be 800 mg/kg in this report) are reported to reduce this adverse drug-food interaction.[8]

The amino acid methionine is used therapeutically, and although information about its interaction with levodopa is very limited, the available data indicate that large doses of methionine should be avoided in patients taking levodopa.

1. Anon. Timing of meals may affect clinical response to levodopa. *Am Pharm* (1985) 25, 34–5.
2. Morgan JP, Bianchine JR, Spiegel HE, Nutley NJ, Rivera-Calimlim L, Hersey RM. Metabolism of levodopa in patients with Parkinson's disease. *Arch Neurol* (1971) 25, 39–44.
3. Baruzzi A, Contin M, Riva R, Procaccianti G, Albani F, Tonello C, Zoni E, Martinelli P. Influence of meal ingestion time on pharmacokinetics of orally administered levodopa in Parkinsonian patients. *Clin Neuropharmacol* (1987) 10, 527–37.
4. Crevoisier C, Zerr P, Calvi-Gries F, Nilsen T. Effects of food on the pharmacokinetics of levodopa in a dual-release formulation. *Eur J Pharm Biopharm* (2003) 55, 71–6.
5. Robertson DRC, Higginson I, Macklin BS, Renwick AG, Waller DG, George CF. The influence of protein containing meals on the pharmacokinetics of levodopa in healthy volunteers. *Br J Clin Pharmacol* (1991) 31, 413–17.
6. Simon N, Gantcheva R, Bruguerolle B, Viallet F. The effects of a normal protein diet on LevoDOPA plasma kinetics in advanced Parkinson's disease. *Parkinsonism Relat Disord* (2004) 10, 137–42.
7. Gillespie NG, Mena I, Cotzias GC, Bell MA. Diets affecting treatment of parkinsonism with levodopa. *J Am Diet Assoc* (1973) 62, 525–8.
8. Juncos JL, Fabbrini G, Mouradian MM, Serrati C, Chase TN. Dietary influences on the antiparkinsonian response to levodopa. *Arch Neurol* (1987) 44, 1003–1005.
9. Carter JH, Nutt JG, Woodward WR, Hatcher LF, Trotman TL. Amount and distribution of dietary protein affects clinical response to levodopa in Parkinson's disease. *Neurology* (1989) 39, 552–6.
10. Bozek CB, Suchowersky O, Purves S, Calne S, Calne DB. Sinemet in Parkinson's disease: efficacy with and without food. *Clin Neuropharmacol* (1986) 9, 196–9.
11. Paré S, Barr SI, Ross SE. Effect of daytime protein restriction on nutrient intakes of free-living Parkinson's disease patients. *Am J Clin Nutr* (1992) 55, 701–7.
12. Cooper MK, Brock DG, McDaniel CM. Interaction between levodopa and enteral nutrition. *Ann Pharmacother* (2008) 42, 439–42.
13. Pearce LA, Waterbury LD. L-methionine: a possible levodopa antagonist. *Neurology* (1974) 24, 640–1.
14. Weitbrecht W-U, Weigel K. Der einfluß von L-tryptophan auf die L-dopa-resorption. *Dtsch Med Wochenschr* (1976) 101, 20–2.
15. Apaydin H, Ertan S, Özekmekçi S. Broad bean (*Vicia faba*) – a natural source of L-dopa – prolongs "on" periods in patients with Parkinson's disease who have "on-off" fluctuations. *Mov Disord* (2000) 15, 164–6.
16. Astarloa R, Mena MA, Sánchez V, de la Vega L, de Yébenes JG. Clinical and pharmacokinetic effects of a diet rich in insoluble fiber on Parkinson disease. *Clin Neuropharmacol* (1992) 15, 375–80.
17. Daniel PM, Moorhouse SR, Pratt OE. Do changes in blood levels of other aromatic aminoacids influence levodopa therapy? *Lancet* (1976) i, 95.
18. Madopar Capsules (Levodopa and Benserazide hydrochloride). Roche Products Ltd. UK Summary of product characteristics, April 2009.

Levodopa + Indinavir

An isolated report describes a man taking levodopa who developed severe dyskinesias when given indinavir.

Clinical evidence, mechanism, importance and management

A 66-year-old man with idiopathic Parkinson's disease and AIDS was free of dyskinesias when taking levodopa with a dopa-decarboxylase inhibitor, although he had unpredictable fluctuations. One month after starting indinavir 2.4 g daily, lamivudine and zidovudine, he developed severe peak-dose dyskinesias, and the 'on' periods lasted all day, with no fluctuations. The antivirals were stopped and the dyskinesias improved within 5 days. Each antiviral was then given separately for 2 weeks. Only indinavir induced dyskinesias, which started after 3 days of concurrent use.[1]

The mechanism of this interaction is uncertain, but may be related to the inhibition of cytochrome P450 by HIV-protease inhibitors such as indinavir.[1]

This appears to be the only report of this possible interaction. Bear in mind the possibility that the levodopa dose may need to be decreased if a HIV-protease inhibitor such as indinavir is required.

1. Caparros-Lefebvre D, Lannuzel A, Tiberghien F, Strobel M. Protease inhibitors enhance levodopa effects in Parkinson's disease. *Mov Disord* (1999) 14, 535.

Levodopa + Iron compounds

Ferrous sulfate can reduce the bioavailability of levodopa and carbidopa, and may possibly reduce the control of Parkinson's disease.

Clinical evidence

A study in 9 patients with Parkinson's disease found that a single 325-mg dose of **ferrous sulfate** reduced the AUC of levodopa by 30% and reduced the AUC of carbidopa by more than 75%. There was a trend towards an increase in disability, suggesting a worsening of disease, but this did not reach statistical significance. Some, but not all of the patients had some deterioration in the control of their disease.[1]

In another study, 8 healthy subjects were given a single 250-mg dose of levodopa, with and without a single 325-mg dose of **ferrous sulfate**, and the plasma levodopa levels were measured for the following 6 hours. Peak plasma levodopa levels and the levodopa AUC were reduced by 55% and 51%, respectively. Those subjects who had the highest peak levels and greatest absorption when given levodopa alone, had the greatest reductions when they were also given **ferrous sulfate**.[2]

Mechanism

Ferrous iron rapidly oxidises to ferric iron at the pH values found in the gastrointestinal tract. Ferric iron binds strongly to carbidopa and levodopa to form chelation complexes that are poorly absorbed.[2-4]

Importance and management

Information appears to be limited to these single-dose and *in vitro* studies. The importance of this interaction in patients taking both drugs long-term does not appear to have been studied, but the extent of the reductions in absorption (30 to 50%), and the hint of worsening control,[1] suggests that this interaction may be of clinical importance in some patients. Be alert for any evidence of this. Separating the administration of the iron and levodopa as much as possible is likely to prove effective, as this appears to be an absorption interaction.

1. Campbell NRC, Rankine D, Goodridge AE, Hasinoff BB, Kara M. Sinemet-ferrous sulphate interaction in patients with Parkinson's disease. *Br J Clin Pharmacol* (1990) 30, 599–605.
2. Campbell NRC, Hasinoff B. Ferrous sulfate reduces levodopa bioavailability: chelation as a possible mechanism. *Clin Pharmacol Ther* (1989) 45, 220–5.
3. Campbell RRA, Hasinoff B, Chernenko G, Barrowman J, Campbell NRC. The effect of ferrous sulfate and pH on L-dopa absorption. *Can J Physiol Pharmacol* (1990) 68, 603–7.
4. Greene RJ, Hall AD, Hider RC. The interaction of orally administered iron with levodopa and methyldopa therapy. *J Pharm Pharmacol* (1990) 42, 502–4.

Levodopa + Isoniazid

There is evidence that isoniazid can reduce the control of Parkinson's disease in patients taking levodopa. An isolated case report describes hypertension, tachycardia, flushing and tremor in a patient, which was attributed to the use of levodopa with isoniazid.

Clinical evidence

Following the observation that levodopa-induced dyskinesias were reduced by isoniazid in one patient, a further study was undertaken in 20 other patients taking levodopa with a dopa-decarboxylase inhibitor. It was found that isoniazid (average dose 290 mg daily, range 100 to 800 mg daily) reduced the dyskinesias of 18 of the 20 patients. However, the reduction in dyskinesias was accompanied by an intolerable worsening of parkinsonism, shown by decreased mobility and greater 'off' periods. The reduction in mobility was so severe that the isoniazid had to be stopped immediately in several cases and was discontinued after an average of 5.2 weeks in all the patients. Control of parkinsonism was then restored.[1] Another patient taking levodopa with carbidopa similarly had a deterioration in the control of parkinsonism within one to 2 weeks of starting isoniazid with rifampicin (*Rifinah*). When the antitubercular drugs were stopped, the patient's motor performance improved ('on' period lengthened by 75%), the levodopa AUC rose by 37%, its half-life doubled, and its maximum plasma levels fell by 33%.[2]

An isolated report describes a patient taking levodopa who developed hypertension, agitation, tachycardia, flushing and severe non-parkinsonian tremor after starting to take isoniazid. He recovered when the isoniazid was stopped.[3]

Mechanism

Not understood. Metabolic studies in one patient suggest that isoniazid inhibits dopa-decarboxylase,[2] although other mechanisms have been proposed.[1,2] The isolated case of hypertension and tachycardia is also not understood, but it has been suggested that it may have been due to a weak monoamine oxidase inhibitory effect of the isoniazid metabolites. See 'MAOIs or RIMAs + Levodopa', p.1393, for further explanation.

Importance and management

Information seems to be limited to the reports cited. If concurrent use is thought to be necessary, be alert for any evidence of a reduction in the control of the parkinsonism, and be aware that drug treatment may need to be modified. One of the reports suggests that it may take 15 to 20 days or more for the deterioration in parkinsonian symptoms to occur.[1] The isolated case seems not to be of general importance.

1. Gershanik OS, Luquin MR, Scipioni O, Obeso JA. Isoniazid therapy in Parkinson's disease. *Mov Disord* (1988) 3, 133–9.

2. Wenning GK, O'Connell MT, Patsalos PN, Quinn NP. A clinical and pharmacokinetic case study of an interaction of levodopa and antituberculous therapy in Parkinson's disease. *Mov Disord* (1995) 10, 664–7.
3. Morgan JP. Isoniazid and levodopa. *Ann Intern Med* (1980) 92, 434.

Levodopa + MAO-B inhibitors

No serious interaction usually occurs between levodopa and selegiline, although the dose of levodopa may need to be reduced when selegiline is added. Levodopa does not affect rasagiline clearance.

Clinical evidence

(a) Rasagiline

The manufacturer notes that levodopa had no effect on rasagiline clearance.[1]

(b) Selegiline

The combination of levodopa and selegiline has been very extensively used. No serious hypertensive reactions of the kind seen with non-selective MAOIs (see 'MAOIs or RIMAs + Levodopa', p.1393) seem to occur. No adverse pharmacokinetic interactions have been reported,[2,3] and serious adverse interactions are said to be lacking.[4,5] Many studies have reported the beneficial effects of this combination,[6-11] but one has suggested that it may result in increased mortality in patients with early, mild Parkinson's disease.[12] Although no clear reason for this increase in mortality could be found, it appeared that patients receiving selegiline with levodopa were more likely to have possible dementia and have had recent falls, postural dizziness, and shortness of breath.[13] Urinary retention has also been suggested as being associated with this drug combination.[14] Selegiline potentiates the effects of levodopa, so the usual adverse effects (dyskinesias, nausea, agitation, confusion, hallucinations, headache, postural hypotension, cardiac arrhythmias, and vertigo) may be increased, particularly if the levodopa dose is too high.[15]

Mechanism

MAO-B inhibitors prevent the metabolism of dopamine, therefore additive dopaminergic effects occur with levodopa.

Importance and management

No adverse interactions usually occur if levodopa and selegiline are given concurrently. However, the manufacturers say that after adding selegiline a reduction in the dose of levodopa is usually required to avoid symptoms of levodopa excess (about 10 to 30% is suggested).[15-17] Reduction of the levodopa dose should be gradual, in steps of 10% every 3 to 4 days.[16] It has been suggested that the concurrent use is probably best avoided in patients with postural hypotension, frequent falls, confusion and dementia.[13]

1. Azilect (Rasagiline mesilate). Teva Pharmaceuticals Ltd. UK Summary of product characteristics, November 2009.
2. Roberts J, Waller DG, O'Shea N, Macklin BS, Renwick AG. The effect of selegiline on the peripheral pharmacokinetics of levodopa in young volunteers. *Br J Clin Pharmacol* (1995) 40, 404–6.
3. Cedarbaum JM, Silvestri M, Clark M, Harts A, Kutt H. L-Deprenyl, levodopa pharmacokinetics, and response fluctuations in Parkinson's disease. *Clin Neuropharmacol* (1990) 13, 29–35.
4. Birkmayer W, Riederer P, Ambrozi L, Youdim MBH. Implications of combined treatment with 'Madopar' and L-deprenil in Parkinson's disease. *Lancet* (1977) i, 439–43.
5. Elsworth JD, Glover V, Reynolds GP, Sandler M, Lees AJ, Phuapradit P, Shaw KM, Stern GM, Kumar P. Deprenyl administration in man: a selective monoamine oxidase B inhibitor without the 'cheese effect'. *Psychopharmacology (Berl)* (1978) 57, 33–8.
6. Shan DE, Yeh SI. An add-on study of selegiline to Madopar in the treatment of parkinsonian patients with dose-related fluctuations: comparison between Jumexal and Parkryl. *Zhonghua Yi Xue Za Zhi (Taipei)* (1996), 58, 264–8.
7. Brannan T, Yahr MD. Comparative-study of selegiline plus L-dopa–carbidopa versus L-dopa–carbidopa alone in the treatment of Parkinson's disease. *Ann Neurol* (1995) 37, 95–8.
8. Golbe LI, Lieberman AN, Muenter MD, Ahlslog JE, Gopinathan G, Neophytides AN, Foo SH, Duvoisin RC. Deprenyl in the treatment of symptom fluctuations in advanced Parkinson's disease. *Clin Neuropharmacol* (1988) 11, 45–55.
9. Presthus J, Berstad J, Lien K. Selegiline (l-deprenyl) and low-dose levodopa treatment of Parkinson's disease. *Acta Neurol Scand* (1987) 76, 200–3.
10. Birkmayer W, Birkmayer GD. Effect of (–)deprenyl in long-term treatment of Parkinson's disease. A 10-years experience. *J Neural Transm* (1986) 22 (Suppl), 219–25.
11. Birkmayer W, Knoll J, Riederer P, Youdim MBH, Hars V, Marton J. Increased life expectancy resulting from addition of L-deprenyl to Madopar® treatment in Parkinson's disease: a longterm study. *J Neural Transm* (1985) 64, 113–127.
12. Parkinson's Disease Research Group of the United Kingdom. Comparison of therapeutic effects and mortality data of levodopa and levodopa combined with selegiline in patients with early, mild Parkinson's disease. *BMJ* (1995) 311, 1602–7.
13. Ben-Shlomo Y, Churchyard A, Head J, Hurwitz B, Overstall P, Ockelford J, Lees AJ. Investigation by Parkinson's Disease Research Group of United Kingdom into excess mortality seen with combined levodopa and selegiline treatment in patients with early, mild Parkinson's disease: further results of randomised trial and confidential inquiry. *BMJ* (1998) 316, 1191–6.
14. Waters CH. Side effects of selegiline (Eldepryl). *J Geriatr Psychiatry Neurol* (1992) 5, 31–34.
15. Eldepryl (Selegiline hydrochloride). Orion Pharma (UK) Ltd. UK Summary of product characteristics, February 2012.
16. Zelapar (Selegiline hydrochloride). Cephalon Ltd. UK Summary of product characteristics, March 2012.
17. Selegiline hydrochloride tablets USP. Apotex Inc. US Prescribing information, June 2009.

Levodopa + Methyldopa

Methyldopa can increase the effects of levodopa and permit a reduction in the dose in some patients taking levodopa alone, but the benefit may only be temporary and dyskinesias may be worsened in some patients. This interaction would not be expected to be significant in a patient taking levodopa with benserazide or carbidopa but this does not appear to have been studied. A small increase in the hypotensive actions of methyldopa may also occur.

Clinical evidence

(a) Effects on the response to levodopa

A double-blind, crossover study in 10 patients with Parkinson's disease who had been taking levodopa alone for 12 to 40 months, found that the optimum daily dose of levodopa fell by 68% with methyldopa 1.92 g daily, and by 50% with methyldopa 800 mg daily.[1]

Other reports in patients taking levodopa alone describe reductions in the levodopa dose of up to 30%[2] and 70%[3] during the concurrent use of methyldopa. Another report states that the control of Parkinson's disease improved during the concurrent use of methyldopa in some patients taking levodopa alone, but the dyskinesias were worsened in others.[4] Similar findings have been reported elsewhere: in some cases an initial improvement was followed by a loss of benefit.[5] Methyldopa on its own can cause a reversible parkinsonian-like syndrome.[6-8]

(b) Effects on the response to methyldopa

A study in 18 patients with Parkinson's disease taking levodopa alone found that the concurrent use of levodopa and methyldopa lowered the blood pressure. The doses used did not affect the systolic blood pressure when given alone, whereas daily doses of 1 to 2.5 g of levodopa with methyldopa 500 mg caused a 12/6 mmHg fall in blood pressure. No change in the control of the Parkinson's disease was seen, but the study lasted only a few days.[9] In a study of 41 patients who took methyldopa in daily doses of 125 mg to 1.25 g with levodopa 1 g to 7 g daily, two patients experienced a significant drop in blood pressure.[5]

Mechanism

Methyldopa inhibits the breakdown of levodopa outside the brain (by dopa decarboxylase) so that more is available to exert its therapeutic effects.

The increased hypotension may simply be due to the additive effects of the two drugs.

Importance and management

Well documented. Concurrent use need not be avoided but the outcome should be well monitored. In patients taking levodopa alone, the use of methyldopa may allow a reduction in the dose of the levodopa (the reports cited[1-3] give figures of 30 to 70%) and may enhance the control of Parkinson's disease, but it should also be borne in mind that in some patients dyskinesias may be worsened. However, in the presence of carbidopa or benserazide the dopa decarboxylase effects of methyldopa would be expected to be less significant and so it seems unlikely that a dose reduction of levodopa would be required. The increased hypotensive effects seem to be small, but they too should be checked.

1. Fermaglich J, Chase TN. Methyldopa or methyldopahydrazine as levodopa synergists. *Lancet* (1973) i, 1261–2.
2. Mones RJ. Evaluation of alpha methyl dopa and alpha methyl dopa hydrazine with L-dopa therapy. *N Y State J Med* (1974) 74, 47–51.
3. Fermaglich J, O'Doherty DS. Second generation of L-dopa therapy. *Neurology* (1971) 21, 408–9.
4. Sweet RD, Lee JE, McDowell FH. Methyldopa as an adjunct to levodopa treatment of Parkinson's disease. *Clin Pharmacol Ther* (1972) 13, 23–7.
5. Kofman OS. A therapeutic paradox? Combined treatment of Parkinson's disease with levodopa and methyldopa. *Arch Neurol* (1973) 29, 120–1.
6. Groden BM. Parkinsonism occurring with methyldopa treatment. *BMJ* (1963) 1, 1001.
7. Peaston MJT. Parkinsonism associated with alpha-methyldopa therapy. *BMJ* (1964) 2, 168.
8. Strang RR. Parkinsonism occurring during methyldopa therapy. *Can Med Assoc J* (1966) 95, 928–9.
9. Gibberd FB, Small E. Interaction between levodopa and methyldopa. *BMJ* (1973) 2, 90–1.

Levodopa + Methylphenidate

Methyldopa does not appear to affect the levels of levodopa or the response to levodopa.

Clinical evidence, mechanism, importance and management

A study in 12 patients with Parkinson's disease who took methylphenidate 400 micrograms/kg three times daily in addition to their normal antiparkinsonian medicines which included levodopa, found that methylphenidate had no clinically significant effect on the response to levodopa as measured by tapping speed, a walking test or the presence of dyskinesia. Methylphenidate did not significantly alter the plasma levels of levodopa.[1]

1. Nutt JG, Carter JH, Carlson NE. Effects of methylphenidate on response to oral levodopa. A double-blind clinical trial. *Arch Neurol* (2007) 64, 319–23.

Levodopa + Mirtazapine

An isolated report describes the development of serious psychosis, which was attributed to an interaction between levodopa and mirtazapine.

Clinical evidence, mechanism, importance and management

A 44-year-old woman taking levodopa with carbidopa, pergolide, selegiline and memantine for Parkinson's disease, started taking mirtazapine, in increasing doses rising from 15 to 60 mg daily over 24 days, for depression, labile mood, anxiety, social withdrawal and sleep disturbance. She initially improved, but then major depression and psychosis developed, and on day 26 she attempted self-strangulation. She recovered when the mirtazapine, memantine and selegiline were stopped and low-dose clozapine started. The authors concluded that the reaction was attributable to dopamine-induced psychosis triggered by the addition of mirtazapine to levodopa.[1] This appears to be an isolated case, and as such, no general conclusions can be drawn.

1. Normann C, Hesslinger B, Frauenknecht S, Berger M, Walden J. Psychosis during chronic levodopa therapy triggered by the new antidepressive drug mirtazapine. *Pharmacopsychiatry* (1997) 30, 263–5.

Levodopa + Papaverine

Case reports describe a deterioration in the control of parkinsonism when patients taking levodopa were given papaverine, but a controlled study did not find an interaction.

Clinical evidence

(a) Levodopa effects reduced

A woman with long-standing parkinsonism, well controlled with levodopa (and the later addition of carbidopa), began to have a steady worsening of her parkinsonism within a week of starting papaverine 100 mg daily for cerebral vascular insufficiency. The deterioration continued until the papaverine was withdrawn. The normal response to levodopa returned within a week. Four other patients had a similar response.[1] Two other similar cases have been described in another report.[2]

(b) Levodopa effects unchanged

A double-blind, crossover study in 9 patients with parkinsonism, taking levodopa (range 100 to 750 mg daily) with a dopa-decarboxylase inhibitor, did not find any changes in disease control when they also took papaverine hydrochloride 150 mg daily for 3 weeks. Two patients were also taking bromocriptine 40 mg daily and two patients were also taking trihexyphenidyl 15 mg daily.[3]

A study in 6 healthy subjects, who took a single 500-mg dose of levodopa before and after taking papaverine 150 mg twice daily for 2 weeks, found that papaverine did not affect the increase in serum growth hormone and the decrease in prolactin levels caused by levodopa.[4]

Mechanism

Not understood. One suggestion is that papaverine blocks the dopamine receptors in the striatum of the brain, thereby inhibiting the effects of the levodopa.[1,5] Another is that papaverine may have a reserpine-like action on the vesicles of adrenergic neurones[1,6] (i.e. it can deplete dopamine stores).

Importance and management

Direct information seems to be limited to the reports cited. Concurrent use can apparently be uneventful. However, in the light of the reports of adverse interactions it would be prudent to monitor the outcome closely. Carefully controlled studies can provide a good picture of the general situation, but may not necessarily identify the occasional patient who may be affected by an interaction.

1. Duvoisin RC. Antagonism of levodopa by papaverine. *JAMA* (1975) 231, 845.
2. Posner DM. Antagonism of levodopa by papaverine. *JAMA* (1975) 233, 768.
3. Montastruc JL, Rascol O, Belin J, Ane M, Rascol A. Does papaverine interact with levodopa in Parkinson's disease? *Ann Neurol* (1987) 22, 558–9.
4. Cooper DS, Jacobs LS. Failure of papaverine to alter L-dopa-influenced GH and PRL secretion. *J Clin Endocrinol Metab* (1977) 44, 585–7.
5. Gonzalez-Vegas JA. Antagonism of dopamine-mediated inhibition in the nigro-striatal pathway: a mode of action of some catatonia-inducing drugs. *Brain Res* (1974) 80, 219–28.
6. Cubeddu L, Weiner N. Relationship between a granular effect and exocytotic release of norepinephrine by nerve stimulation. *Pharmacologist* (1974) 16, 190.

Levodopa + Penicillamine

Penicillamine can raise levodopa levels in a few patients. This may improve the control of the parkinsonism but the adverse effects of levodopa may also be increased.

Clinical evidence, mechanism, importance and management

A patient with Parkinson's disease taking levodopa with a dopa-decarboxylase inhibitor [probably carbidopa] had a 60% increase in his levodopa plasma levels after taking penicillamine 600 mg daily. This resulted in improved control of symptoms but with an increase in dyskinesia. It was noted that this patient had slightly low serum copper and ceruloplasmin levels.[1] In another study 2 patients with Parkinson's disease taking levodopa also improved when they also took penicillamine, but levodopa levels were apparently not measured. Again it was noted that the patients had slightly low copper and ceruloplasmin levels. In another 4 similar patients the effects of penicillamine on levodopa seemed absent in the presence of normal copper and ceruloplasmin levels.[2] The authors of this report[2] attribute the improvement in parkinsonism to the copper chelating properties of penicillamine. However, the authors of the other report[1] suggest that the effect of penicillamine would not be this rapid, and suggested that penicillamine must be affecting levodopa pharmacokinetics.

This limited evidence suggests that the concurrent use of levodopa and penicillamine need not be avoided, and in some patients parkinsonian symptoms may be improved. However, if both drugs are given, monitor the effects as an increase in the adverse effects of levodopa is also possible.

1. Mizuta E, Kuno S. Effect of D-penicillamine on pharmacokinetics of levodopa in Parkinson's disease. *Clin Neuropharmacol* (1993) 16, 448–50.
2. Sato M, Yamane K, Oosawa Y, Tanaka H, Shirata A, Nagayama T, Maruyama S. Two cases of Parkinson's disease whose symptoms were markedly improved by D-penicillamine. A study with emphasis on cases displaying a slightly low level of serum copper and ceruloplasmin. *Neurol Ther Chiba* (1992) 9, 555–9.

Levodopa + Phenylbutazone

A single case report describes antagonism of the effects of levodopa by phenylbutazone.

Clinical evidence, mechanism, importance and management

A patient (who was very sensitive to levodopa) found that he was only able to prevent the involuntary movements of his tongue, jaw, neck and limbs caused by levodopa, by taking frequent small doses (125 mg) of levodopa. He was able to suppress the levodopa adverse effects with phenylbutazone. However, the phenylbutazone also lessened the therapeutic effect of the levodopa.[1] The reason is not understood. This interaction has not been confirmed, and its general importance is not known.

1. Wodak J, Gilligan BS, Veale JL, Dowty BJ. Review of 12 months' treatment with L-dopa in Parkinson's disease, with remarks on unusual side effects. *Med J Aust* (1972) 2, 1277–82.

Levodopa + Phenytoin

The therapeutic effects of levodopa can be reduced or abolished by phenytoin.

Clinical evidence, mechanism, importance and management

A study in 5 patients taking levodopa 630 to 4600 mg (four also taking carbidopa 150 to 225 mg daily) for Parkinson's disease, found that when they also took phenytoin in doses of up to 500 mg daily for 5 to 19 days the levodopa-induced dyskinesias were relieved, but the beneficial effects of the levodopa on parkinsonism were reduced or abolished. The patients became slow, rigidity re-emerged, and some of them became unable to get out of a chair. Within 2 weeks of stopping the phenytoin, their parkinsonism was again well controlled by the levodopa.[1] Despite many suggestions, the mechanism of this interaction is not understood. Information relating to a reduction in efficacy of levodopa seems to be limited to this study, nevertheless it would seem prudent to monitor concurrent use for any evidence of reduced levodopa efficacy.

1. Mendez JS, Cotzias GC, Mena I, Papavasiliou PS. Diphenylhydantoin blocking of levodopa effects. *Arch Neurol* (1975) 32, 44–6.

Levodopa + Pyridoxine (Vitamin B_6)

The effects of levodopa are reduced or abolished by pyridoxine, but this interaction does not occur when levodopa is given with the dopa-decarboxylase inhibitors carbidopa or benserazide, as is usual clinical practice.

Clinical evidence

A study in 25 patients taking levodopa alone found that if they were given high doses of pyridoxine (750 mg to 1 g daily), the effects of the levodopa were reduced within 24 hours, and were completely abolished within 3 to 4 days. Daily doses of pyridoxine 50 to 100 mg also reduced or abolished the effects of levodopa, and an increase in the signs and symptoms of parkinsonism occurred in 8 out of 10 patients taking only 5 to 10 mg of pyridoxine daily.[1]

The antagonism of the effects of levodopa (given without a dopa-decarboxylase inhibitor) by pyridoxine has been described in numerous other reports.[1-6]

In contrast, a study in 15 patients with Parkinson's disease taking long-term levodopa found that a single 250-mg oral dose of levodopa produced a peak dopa level of 600 nanograms/mL. When pyridoxine 50 mg was also given, the peak plasma levels of dopa fell by almost 70%. When the levodopa was given with carbidopa 50 mg the peak plasma dopa levels were 1300 nanograms/mL, and were not significantly affected by pyridoxine.[6] The results from a subset of these patients have been reported elsewhere.[7] The absence of an interaction in the presence of a dopa-decarboxylase inhibitor is confirmed in another report.[8]

Mechanism

The conversion of levodopa to dopamine within the body requires the presence of pyridoxal-5-phosphate (derived from pyridoxine) as a co-factor. When dietary amounts of pyridoxine are high, the peripheral metabolism of levodopa by dopa-decarboxylase is increased so that less is available for entry into the CNS, and its effects are reduced accordingly. Pyridoxine may also alter levodopa metabolism by Schiff-base formation. However, in the presence of dopa-decarboxylase inhibitors such as carbidopa or benserazide, this peripheral metabolism of levodopa is reduced and much larger amounts are available for entry into the CNS, even if quite small doses are given. Therefore, even in the presence of large amounts of pyridoxine, the peripheral metabolism remains unaffected and the serum levels of levodopa are virtually unaltered.

Importance and management

A clinically important, well documented and well established interaction, but principally of historical interest now as levodopa is rarely used alone. The problem of this interaction can be totally solved by giving levodopa with a dopa-decarboxylase inhibitor such as carbidopa or benserazide. In the rare cases that levodopa is used alone, pyridoxine in doses as low as 5 mg daily can reduce the effects of levodopa and should therefore be avoided. Warn patients about proprietary pyridoxine-containing preparations such as multivitamins and supplements. Some breakfast cereals are fortified with pyridoxine and other vitamins, but the amounts are usually too small to matter (e.g. a 30 g serving of *Kellogg's Corn Flakes* or *Rice Krispies* (UK products) contains only about 0.5 mg of pyridoxine). There is no good clinical evidence to suggest that a low-pyridoxine diet is desirable, and indeed it may be harmful as the normal dietary requirements are about 2 mg daily.

1. Duvoisin RC, Yahr MD, Coté LD. Pyridoxine reversal of L-dopa effects in parkinsonism. *Trans Am Neurol Assoc* (1969) 94, 81–4.
2. Celesia GG, Barr AN. Psychosis and other psychiatric manifestations of levodopa therapy. *Arch Neurol* (1970) 23, 193–200.
3. Carter AB. Pyridoxine and parkinsonism. *BMJ* (1973) 4, 236.
4. Cotzias GC, Papavasiliou PS. Blocking the negative effects of pyridoxine on patients receiving levodopa. *JAMA* (1971) 215, 1504–5.
5. Leon AS, Spiegel HE, Thomas G, Abrams WB. Pyridoxine antagonism of levodopa in parkinsonism. *JAMA* (1971) 218, 1924–7.
6. Mars H. Levodopa, carbidopa, and pyridoxine in Parkinson disease: metabolic interactions. *Arch Neurol* (1974) 30, 444–7.
7. Mars H. Metabolic interactions of pyridoxine, levodopa, and carbidopa in Parkinson's disease. *Trans Am Neurol Assoc* (1973) 98, 241–5.
8. Papavasiliou PS, Cotzias GC, Düby SE, Steck AJ, Fehling C, Bell MA. Levodopa in parkinsonism: potentiation of central effects with a peripheral inhibitor. *N Engl J Med* (1972) 285, 8–14.

Levodopa + Rauwolfia alkaloids

The effects of levodopa are opposed by rauwolfia alkaloids such as reserpine.

Clinical evidence, mechanism, importance and management

Reserpine and other rauwolfia alkaloids deplete the brain of monoamines, including dopamine, thereby reducing their effects.[1] This can lead to parkinsonian-like symptoms, and may oppose the actions of levodopa. There are not only sound pharmacological reasons for believing this to be an interaction of clinical importance, but a reduction in the antiparkinsonian activity of levodopa has been observed in patients given **reserpine**.[2] The rauwolfia alkaloids should be avoided in patients with Parkinson's disease, whether or not they are taking levodopa.

1. Bianchine JR, Sunyapridakul L. Interactions between levodopa and other drugs: significance in the treatment of Parkinson's disease. *Drugs* (1973) 6, 364–88.
2. Yahr MD. Personal communication, February 1977.

Levodopa + Sildenafil

A single case report describes a patient taking levodopa with carbidopa who developed choreoathetotic movements and a prolonged erection after he also took sildenafil.

Clinical evidence, mechanism, importance and management

A case report describes a patient with well-controlled Parkinson's disease who took a single 100-mg dose of sildenafil and developed involuntary movements (choreoathetosis) which persisted for about 12 hours, and a prolonged erection (3 hours). He was taking levodopa with carbidopa and selegiline, and had taken his last dose of a slow-release preparation of levodopa with carbidopa about 50 minutes before the sildenafil. The authors speculated that the choreoathetotic dyskinesias were due to an interaction between the levodopa and sildenafil, resulting in an increased level of levodopa-derived dopamine in the brain,[1] but a mechanism for such an effect is unclear: the high dose of sildenafil and the close timing of administration in relation to the levodopa may have been factors. Note that sildenafil has been used successfully for the treatment of erectile dysfunction in patients with Parkinson's disease, and this appears to be the only report of movement disorders. Its general relevance is therefore uncertain, but probably limited.

1. Perkovic O, Vitezic D, Rudez J, Vitezic M, Kovacevic M, Mrsic-Pelcic J, Ljubicic D, Jurjevic A. Sildenafil induced choreoathetosis in men with Parkinson's disease. *Int J Clin Pharmacol Ther* (2010) 48, 76–8.

Levodopa + Spiramycin

The plasma levels of levodopa (given with carbidopa) are reduced by spiramycin, thereby reducing its therapeutic effects.

Clinical evidence

The observation of a patient with Parkinson's disease taking levodopa with carbidopa whose condition became less well-controlled when spiramycin was taken, prompted further study. Levodopa 250 mg with carbidopa 25 mg was given to 7 healthy subjects after they had taken spiramycin 1 g twice daily for 3 days. The spiramycin reduced the AUC of levodopa by 57%, and its maximum plasma levels fell by about 20%, which was not statistically significant. The relative bioavailability of levodopa was only 43%. The plasma levels of the carbidopa were barely detectable.[1]

Mechanism

Not fully established. In some way spiramycin markedly reduces the absorption of carbidopa, possibly by forming a non-absorbable complex in the gut or by accelerating its transit through the gut. As a result, not enough carbidopa is absorbed to inhibit the peripheral metabolism of the levodopa by dopa-decarboxylase, so that the effects of the levodopa are reduced.[1]

Importance and management

Information is very limited, but the interaction appears to be established and of clinical importance. The management of this interaction is unclear, but as it appears to be due to an effect on absorption it would seem prudent to try to separate the dosing of these two drugs by as much as possible, although this may be difficult with some levodopa regimens. Monitor the outcome of concurrent use on the control of Parkinson's disease. It is not known whether other macrolide antibacterials behave in a similar way, or whether spiramycin affects levodopa with benserazide. More study is needed.

1. Brion N, Kollenbach K, Marion MH, Grégoire A, Advenier C, Pays M. Effect of a macrolide (spiramycin) on the pharmacokinetics of L-dopa and carbidopa in healthy volunteers. *Clin Neuropharmacol* (1992) 15, 229–35.

Levodopa + SSRIs and related antidepressants

The use of an SSRI is often beneficial in parkinsonian patients taking levodopa, to treat the depression associated with the disease. However, sometimes parkinsonian symptoms are worsened.

Clinical evidence

A number of reviews have been published about the extrapyramidal effects of SSRIs.[1,2] A retrospective study of patients taking levodopa, found that 15 patients taking an SSRI (**fluoxetine**, **fluvoxamine**, **paroxetine**) required faster increases in their antiparkinsonian drugs than 31 patients taking a tricyclic antidepressant, or 304 patients taking antiparkinsonian drugs only.[3] However, a retrospective study of the effect of SSRIs or serotonergic antidepressants, in patients taking levodopa, found that the change in antiparkinsonian medication in 90 patients taking SSRIs was similar to that in 99 patients taking tricyclic antidepressants. Furthermore, initiation of antidepressants with a high inhibition of serotonin reuptake was not associated with a change in antiparkinsonian drug treatment compared with antidepressants with a low inhibition of serotonin reuptake.[4] Other cases and studies outlined below have shown conflicting outcomes.

(a) Citalopram

A case report describes an 81-year-old woman who experienced an increase in the duration of her tremor and 'off' periods 2 days after starting to take citalopram 20 mg daily. She was also taking levodopa with benserazide 1 g daily and alprazolam 1.5 mg daily. One month after stopping citalopram, her parkinsonian symptoms had improved.[5]

A study in 44 patients with Parkinson's disease taking levodopa with carbidopa, 30 of whom received citalopram 10 mg daily increasing to 20 mg daily, found an improvement in bradykinesia in those patients taking citalopram.[6]

(b) Fluoxetine

Four patients taking levodopa 375 to 990 mg daily, a dopa-decarboxylase inhibitor (drug and dose not stated) and amantadine (dose not stated), had a deterioration in the control of their parkinsonism when they were also given fluoxetine 20 mg daily for 8 to 11 weeks. The fluoxetine was withdrawn and their motor performance was restored. The antidepressant efficacy of fluoxetine was not found to be substantial in any of the 4 patients.[7] A case report describes a 34-year-old woman whose dystonia was well controlled by levodopa with carbidopa 100/25 mg three times daily. Five days after starting to take fluoxetine 20 mg daily her dystonia and torticollis returned. Two days after stopping the fluoxetine her symptoms started to improve, and had resolved in about a week.[8] Another patient taking levodopa developed frequent hallucinations after the addition of fluoxetine. They resolved when the fluoxetine was withdrawn.[9]

In a retrospective study of 23 parkinsonian patients who were given fluoxetine up to 40 mg daily, 20 patients had no change in the control of their parkinsonism but 3 others experienced a worsening in their Parkinson's disease signs.[10]

However, in a study, 14 patients with Parkinson's disease whose treatment included levodopa, started to take fluoxetine 20 mg daily for one month. One patient dropped out because of intolerable asthenia. Of the remaining 13 patients there was no change in rigidity or bradykinesia, but tremor was significantly reduced.[11]

(c) Nefazodone

A case report describes a 70-year-old man whose Parkinson's disease was well controlled by levodopa with benserazide and bromocriptine, but when he started to take nefazodone, he developed severe bradykinesia, rigidity, gait instability and akathisia. He stopped taking nefazodone, and the dose of levodopa with benserazide was increased to 500 mg daily with improvement in his condition.[12] However, in a small study, nefazodone was found to be of benefit in treating depression in 9 patients taking levodopa for Parkinson's disease, and motor symptoms also improved.[13]

(d) Paroxetine

In a placebo-controlled study in 14 patients with Parkinson's disease, paroxetine 10 mg daily for 5 days and then 20 mg daily for 9 days did not significantly alter the response to an infusion of levodopa 1 mg/kg per hour given for 2 hours. Several patients reported a reduction in their sense of balance, and one patient fell, resulting in a pelvic fracture.[14]

A case report describes visual hallucinations in a 79-year-old woman taking levodopa with carbidopa when she started to take paroxetine 20 mg daily. The hallucinations stopped when paroxetine was withdrawn.[15] It has been suggested that the hallucinations may have been related to the Parkinson's disease and use of levodopa, rather than an interaction with paroxetine.[16]

(e) Sertraline

A review of 101 patients receiving treatment for Parkinson's disease and who also took an antidepressant, identified 5 patients who experienced a worsening of their Parkinson's disease, possibly attributed to the use of an SSRI. Three of these patients were taking sertraline, one **fluoxetine**, and one took **fluoxetine** followed by sertraline. Four of the 5 patients who experienced a worsening of their symptoms were also taking selegiline.[17] See also 'MAO-B inhibitors + SSRIs or SNRIs', p.772 for details of possible interactions between selegiline and the SSRIs.

(f) Venlafaxine

A case report describes a 32-year-old woman who took levodopa with carbidopa 50/1.25 mg twice daily to treat tremor, dystonia and rigidity. She started to take venlafaxine, and within 4 days her dystonia and trembling returned. Two days after stopping the venlafaxine her symptoms started to improve, and had resolved in about a week.[8]

Mechanism

Not understood. The mechanism is likely to involve a complex interaction between various neurotransmitters.[2] Extrapyramidal effects are rare but recognised adverse effects of SSRIs.[1,2]

Importance and management

Although the information is conflicting, it seems that in some cases parkinsonism can be worsened by SSRIs, venlafaxine or nefazodone. Concurrent use is valuable and need not be avoided, but monitor the outcome and withdraw the antidepressant if necessary.

1. Anonymous. Extrapyramidal effects of SSRI antidepressants. *Prescrire Int* (2001) 10, 118–19.
2. Gerber PE, Lynd LD. Selective serotonin-reuptake inhibitor-induced movement disorders. *Ann Pharmacother* (1998) 32, 692–8.
3. van de Vijver DAMC, Roos RAC, Jansen PAF, Porsius AJ, de Boer A. Start of a selective serotonin reuptake inhibitor (SSRI) and increase of antiparkinsonian drug treatment in patients on levodopa. *Br J Clin Pharmacol* (2002) 54, 168–70.
4. Arbouw MEL, Movig KLL, Neef C, Guchelaar H-J, Egberts TCG. Influence of initial use of serotonergic antidepressants on antiparkinsonian drug use in levodopa-using patients. *Eur J Clin Pharmacol* (2007) 63, 181–7.
5. Linazasoro G. Worsening of Parkinson's disease by citalopram. *Parkinsonism Relat Disord* (2000) 6, 111–13.
6. Rampello L, Chiechio S, Raffaele R, Vecchio I, Nicoletti F. The SSRI, citalopram, improves bradykinesia in patients with Parkinson's disease treated with L-dopa. *Clin Neuropharmacol* (2002) 25, 21–4.
7. Jansen Steur ENH. Increase of Parkinson disability after fluoxetine medication. *Neurology* (1993) 43, 211–13.
8. Mathen D, Marsden CD, Bhatia KP. SSRI-induced reversal of levodopa benefit in two patients with dopa-responsive dystonia. *Mov Disord* (1999) 14, 874–6.
9. Lauterbach EC. Dopaminergic hallucinosis with fluoxetine in Parkinson's disease. *Am J Psychiatry* (1993) 150, 1750.
10. Caley CF, Friedman JH. Does fluoxetine exacerbate Parkinson's disease? *J Clin Psychiatry* (1992) 53, 278–282.
11. Montastruc J-L, Fabre N, Blin O, Senard J-M, Rascol O, Rascol A. Does fluoxetine aggravate Parkinson's disease? A pilot prospective study. *Mov Disord* (1995) 10, 355–7.
12. Benazzi F. Parkinson's disease worsened by nefazodone. *Int J Geriatr Psychiatry* (1997) 12, 1195.
13. Avila A, Cardona X, Martin-Baranera M, Maho P, Sastre F, Bello J. Does nefazodone improve both depression and Parkinson disease? A pilot randomized trial. *J Clin Psychopharmacol* (2003) 23, 509–13.
14. Chung KA, Carlson NE, Nutt JG. Short-term paroxetine treatment does not alter the motor response to levodopa in PD. *Neurology* (2005) 64, 1797–8.
15. Freijzer PL, Brenninkmeijer JHE. Hallucinaties veroorzaakt door paroxetine bij gebruik van de combinatie levodopa-carbidopa. *Ned Tijdschr Geneeskd* (2002) 146, 574–5.
16. Jansen Steur ENH. Hallucinaties veroorzaakt door paroxetine bij gebruik van de combinatie levodopa-carbidopa. *Ned Tijdschr Geneeskd* (2002) 146, 1056–7.
17. Richard IH, Maughn A, Kurlan R. Do serotonin reuptake inhibitor antidepressants worsen Parkinson's disease? A retrospective case series. *Mov Disord* (1999) 14, 155–7.

Levodopa + Tetrabenazine

Tetrabenazine may interfere with the effects of levodopa.

Clinical evidence, mechanism, importance and management

Caution is advised when tetrabenazine is given with levodopa, because it can deplete dopamine and can cause parkinsonian adverse effects. Tetrabenazine may therefore be expected to diminish the effects of levodopa and interfere with its use in the management of Parkinson's disease. One manufacturer of levodopa states that concurrent use should be avoided where possible, but if both drugs are considered essential, extreme care should be exercised and patients should be monitored for any signs of potentiation, antagonism or other unusual adverse effects.[1]

1. Madopar Capsules (Levodopa and Benserazide hydrochloride). Roche Products Ltd. UK Summary of product characteristics, April 2009.

Levodopa + Tricyclic antidepressants

The concurrent use of levodopa and the tricyclics is usually uneventful although two unexplained hypertensive crises have occurred when imipramine or amitriptyline was given with levodopa and carbidopa.

Clinical evidence

A hypertensive crisis (blood pressure 210/110 mmHg) associated with agitation, tremor and generalised rigidity developed in a woman taking 6 tablets of levodopa 100 mg with carbidopa 10 mg daily the day after she started to take **imipramine** 25 mg three times daily. The **imipramine** was stopped and she recovered over the following 24 hours. The same reaction occurred again when she was later accidentally given **amitriptyline** 25 mg three times daily.[1] A similar hypertensive reaction (a rise in blood pressure from 190/110 mmHg to 270/140 mmHg) occurred over 34 hours in another woman taking **amitriptyline** 20 mg at night when she was given levodopa 50 mg with carbidopa 5 mg and metoclopramide 10 mg, both three times daily. This resolved when all the drugs were stopped.[2]

Mechanism

Not understood.

Importance and management

Information seems to be limited to these reports. Concurrent use is normally successful and uneventful.[3-5] However, be alert for the possibility of a hypertensive reaction, which resolves if the tricyclic antidepressant is withdrawn. See also 'Levodopa + Antimuscarinics', p.762 for interactions due to the antimuscarinic adverse effects of tricyclic antidepressants.

1. Edwards M. Adverse interaction of levodopa with tricyclic antidepressants. *Practitioner* (1982) 226, 1447 and 1449.
2. Rampton DS. Hypertensive crisis in a patient given Sinemet, metoclopramide, and amitriptyline. *BMJ* (1977) 3, 607–8.
3. Yahr MD. The treatment of Parkinsonism. Current concepts. *Med Clin North Am* (1972) 56, 1377–92.
4. Calne DB, Reid JL. Antiparkinsonian drugs: pharmacological and therapeutic aspects. *Drugs* (1972) 4, 49–74.
5. van Wieringen A, Wright J. Observations on patients with Parkinson's disease treated with L-dopa. I. Trial and evaluation of L-dopa therapy. *S Afr Med J* (1972) 46, 1262–6.

MAO-B inhibitors + Dextromethorphan

The concurrent use of MAO-B inhibitors and dextromethorphan might lead to the serotonin syndrome.

Clinical evidence, mechanism, importance and management

The manufacturer of rasagiline[1] suggests that its use with dextromethorphan should be avoided. Similarly, some consider that patients taking selegiline should try to avoid dextromethorphan.[2] These warnings are based on the serious adverse reactions (serotonin syndrome or similar) that have rarely occurred when dextromethorphan has been used with non-selective MAOIs, see 'MAOIs or RIMAs + Dextromethorphan and related cough suppressants', p.1387. The likelihood of any interaction with MAO-B inhibitors would appear to be very small, but because of the potential severity, some caution would appear to be prudent. For more information on serotonin syndrome and its management, see 'Drugs that cause serotonin syndrome + Other drugs that cause serotonin syndrome', p.1471.

1. Azilect (Rasagiline mesilate). Teva Pharmaceuticals Ltd. UK Summary of product characteristics, November 2009.
2. Jacob JE, Wagner ML, Sage JI. Safety of selegiline with cold medications. *Ann Pharmacother* (2003) 37, 438–41.

MAO-B inhibitors + Food; Tyramine-containing

No dietary restrictions are required with the doses of rasagiline and selegiline recommended for use in Parkinson's disease. An isolated report describes a hypertensive reaction in a patient taking selegiline 20 mg daily. Thus, at higher doses of selegiline, restriction of the amount of tyramine in the diet may be necessary.

Clinical evidence

(a) Rasagiline

In a study in which 72 patients with Parkinson's disease were given rasagiline, there was no statistically significant change in the cardiovascular response to a single 50-mg or 75-mg dose of tyramine when compared with 38 patients not taking rasagiline. Three patients taking rasagiline and one taking placebo experienced an asymptomatic increase in systolic blood pressure of 30 mmHg or more, after the tyramine challenge.[1]

The manufacturer notes that the results of four tyramine challenge studies, together with the results of home monitoring of blood pressure after meals (from 464 patients taking rasagiline 0.5 or 1 mg daily or placebo without tyramine restrictions), and the lack of reported problems in clinical studies without tyramine restriction, indicate that no dietary restrictions are necessary with rasagiline.[2]

(b) Selegiline

1. Oral selegiline. The pressor response to oral tyramine was not altered by pretreatment with selegiline 10 mg daily in healthy subjects and patients with Parkinson's disease.[3] However, another study[4] found that selegiline 5 mg daily for at least 14 days reduced the dose of oral tyramine required to achieve the cardiovascular threshold (increase in systolic blood pressure of greater than 30 mmHg, a diastolic blood pressure greater than 100 mmHg or a fall in heart rate of greater than 20%) by a factor of 2.8. Nevertheless, this reduction was less than that found with the RIMA moclobemide (4.3) and the MAOI phenelzine (10.3).[4] In other studies, higher doses of selegiline (20 or 30 mg daily) increased the sensitivity to oral tyramine by 2- to 4.5-fold.[5,6] A patient taking selegiline 20 mg daily was reported to have had a hypertensive reaction (severe headache and rise in blood pressure) after eating macaroni and cheese,[7] but this appears to be the only published report of this type of hypertensive reaction with selegiline.

2. Buccal and transdermal selegiline. The dose of tyramine required to elicit a pressor effect was not altered by pretreatment with buccal selegiline 1.25 mg in healthy subjects.[8] Similarly, the pressor response to tyramine up to 200 mg was not significantly altered by pretreatment with a single 24-hour application of transdermal selegiline 7.8 mg/24 hour in healthy subjects.[9] Another study in 12 healthy subjects who applied selegiline transdermal patches 6 mg/24 hours daily for 13 days, in order to achieve steady-state levels, similarly found no clinically significant blood pressure response to meals containing up to 400 mg of tyramine.[10] A study by the same authors, in which the use of selegiline was extended to 33 days also found no clinically meaningful change in the pressor sensitivity to tyramine.[11]

Mechanism

Rasagiline and selegiline specifically inhibit MAO-B, which leaves MAO-A still available to metabolise any tyramine in foodstuffs. However, at higher doses the selectivity of selegiline diminishes, and inhibition of the metabolism of tyramine is more likely. Nevertheless, the 2- to 4.5-fold increase in effect of tyramine seen with selegiline 5 to 30 mg daily is still less than that seen with the non-selective MAOIs, see 'MAOIs or RIMAs + Food; Tyramine-containing', p.1389.

Importance and management

The absence of an interaction between rasagiline or selegiline and tyramine is well established, and the manufacturer of rasagiline states that no dietary tyramine restrictions are necessary.[2] Similarly, at the recommended doses of conventional or buccal selegiline used in Parkinson's disease the manufacturers say that no dietary restrictions are necessary,[12-14] and this is supported by the scarcity of any published reports of reactions. If higher doses of selegiline are used, MAO-B selectivity may be lost, and patients should be advised to avoid large amounts of tyramine-rich foods. This is reflected by the advice given by one manufacturer of a transdermal selegiline patch who suggests that restrictions on tyramine ingestion are only necessary with a daily dose of 9 mg/24 hours or more.[15] For a list of the possible tyramine-content of some foods, see 'Table 32.3', p.1390.

1. deMarcaida JA, Schwid SR, White WB, Blindauer K, Fahn S, Kieburtz K, Stern M, Shoulson I, and the Parkinson Study Group TEMPO and PRESTO Tyramine Substudy Investigators and Coordinators. Effects of tyramine administration in Parkinson's disease patients treated with selective MAO-B inhibitor rasagiline. *Mov Disord* (2006) 21, 1716–1721.
2. Azilect (Rasagiline mesilate). Teva Pharmaceuticals Ltd. UK Summary of product characteristics, November 2009.
3. Elsworth JD, Glover V, Reynolds GP, Sandler M, Lees AJ, Phuapradit P, Shaw KM, Stern GM, Kumar P. Deprenyl administration in man: a selective monoamine oxidase B inhibitor without the 'cheese effect'. *Psychopharmacology (Berl)* (1978) 57, 33–8.
4. Warrington SJ, Turner P, Mant TGK, Morrison P, Haywood G, Glover V, Goodwin BL, Sandler M, St John-Smith P, McClelland GR. Clinical pharmacology of moclobemide, a new reversible monoamine oxidase inhibitor. *J Psychopharmacol* (1991) 5, 82–91.
5. Prasad A, Glover V, Goodwin BL, Sandler M, Signy M, Smith SE. Enhanced pressor sensitivity to oral tyramine challenge following high dose selegiline treatment. *Psychopharmacology (Berl)* (1988) 95, 540–3.
6. Bieck PR, Antonin KH. Tyramine potentiation during treatment with MAO inhibitors: brofaromine and moclobemide vs irreversible inhibitors. *J Neural Transm* (1989) (Suppl 28), 21–31.
7. McGrath PJ, Stewart JW, Quitkin FM. A possible l-deprenyl induced hypertensive reaction. *J Clin Psychopharmacol* (1989) 9, 310–11.
8. Clarke A, Johnson ES, Mallard N, Corn TH, Johnston A, Boyce M, Warrington S, MacMahon DG. A new low-dose formulation of selegiline: clinical efficacy, patient preference and selectivity for MAO-B inhibition. *J Neural Transm* (2003) 110, 1273–8.
9. Barrett JS, Hochadel TJ, Morales RJ, Rohatagi S, DeWitt KE, Watson SK, Darnow J, Azzaro AJ, DiSanto AR. Pressor response to tyramine after single 24-hour application of a selegiline transdermal system in healthy males. *J Clin Pharmacol* (1997) 37, 238–47.
10. Blob LF, Sharoky M, Campbell BJ, Kemper EM, Gilmor M, VanDenBerg CM, Azzaro AJ. Effects of a tyramine-enriched meal on blood pressure response in healthy male volunteers treated with selegiline transdermal system 6 mg/24 hour. *CNS Spectr* (2007) 12, 25–34.
11. Azzaro AJ, VanDenBerg CM, Blob LF, Kemper EM, Sharoky M, Oren DA, Campbell BJ. Tyramine pressor sensitivity during treatment with the selegiline transdermal system 6 mg/24 h in healthy subjects. *J Clin Pharmacol* (2006) 46, 933–44.
12. Eldepryl (Selegiline hydrochloride). Orion Pharma (UK) Ltd. UK Summary of product characteristics, February 2012.
13. Zelapar (Selegiline hydrochloride). Cephalon Ltd. UK Summary of product characteristics, March 2012.
14. Selegiline hydrochloride tablets USP. Apotex Inc. US Prescribing information, June 2009.
15. Emsam (Selegiline). Somerset Pharmaceuticals Inc. US Prescribing information, May 2009.

MAO-B inhibitors + MAOIs or RIMAs

Marked orthostatic hypotension has been seen in two patients taking iproniazid or tranylcypromine with trifluoperazine when they were given selegiline. When moclobemide is given with selegiline, restriction of dietary tyramine is necessary, and there may be an increased risk of hypotensive reactions. Some manufacturers of MAO-B inhibitors contraindicate the concurrent use of MAOIs or RIMAs.

Clinical evidence, mechanism, importance and management

(a) MAOIs

In a pilot study, one patient taking **iproniazid** 150 mg daily developed severe orthostatic hypotension on two occasions within an hour of taking **selegiline** 5 mg. Two other patients (one taking **tranylcypromine** with trifluoperazine and one taking **tranylcypromine** with trifluoperazine and **isocarboxazid**) did not have this reaction to **selegiline** 5 mg twice daily. The authors mention another patient who similarly developed postural hypotension on two occasions within 2 hours of taking **selegiline** 5 mg. He had stopped taking **tranylcypromine** with trifluoperazine, 4 weeks previously.[1] This evidence suggests that **selegiline** should be given with caution to patients taking, or who have recently stopped, non-selective MAOIs. One UK manufacturer of **selegiline**[2] and the manufacturer of **rasagiline**[3] contraindicate the concurrent use of non-selective MAOIs. The manufacturer of rasagiline includes **St John's wort** (*Hypericum perforatum*) in this contraindication, because they state that it has MAO inhibitory properties.[3] At least 14 days should elapse between stopping **rasagiline** or **selegiline** and starting an MAOI.[2,3]

Note that the MAO-B inhibitors, MAOIs, and **St John's wort** have serotonergic effects. Concurrent use of MAO-B inhibitors and either an MAOI or St John's wort might lead to the serotonin syndrome. Serotonin syndrome is a rare adverse effect, but because of its severity, some caution is warranted if both drugs are given. For more information on serotonin syndrome and its management, see 'Drugs that cause serotonin syndrome + Other drugs that cause serotonin syndrome', p.1471.

(b) RIMAs

A study in 24 healthy subjects, designed to assess the safety and tolerability of giving **moclobemide** 100 to 400 mg and **selegiline** 5 mg twice daily, sequentially or concurrently, found that the adverse effects were no greater under steady-state conditions than with either drug alone, but the sensitivity to tyramine was considerably increased. The mean tyramine sensitivity factor for **moclobemide** alone was 2 to 3, for **selegiline** alone was 1.4, and for **moclobemide** with **selegiline** was 8 to 9 (and even 18 in one subject).[4,5] The reason for this effect is, that when taken together, the **moclobemide** inhibits MAO-A while **selegiline** inhibits MAO-B, so that little or no MAO activity remains available to metabolise the tyramine. However, unexpectedly, the combined effect was more than additive.[5] **Selegiline** had no effect on the pharmacokinetics of **moclobemide**.[6] In a clinical study using tyramine restriction, one of 5 subjects taking **selegiline** and one of 5 subjects taking **selegiline** with **moclobemide** reported symptomatic hypotension, and there was no increase in blood pressure in any patient.[7]

In practical terms this means that patients taking **moclobemide** with **selegiline** should be given the same dietary restrictions for tyramine-rich foods and drinks (see 'MAOIs or RIMAs + Food; Tyramine-containing', p.1389), that relate to the non-selective MAOIs such as phenelzine and tranylcypromine.[5] However, because of the potential risks the manufacturer of **moclobemide**[8] contraindicates the concurrent use of **selegiline**. It has been suggested that if **selegiline** is replaced by **moclobemide**, the dietary restrictions can be relaxed after a wash-out period of about 2 weeks. If switching from **moclobemide** to **selegiline**, a wash-out period of one to 2 days is sufficient.[4]

For a case report describing serotonin syndrome in a patient taking selegiline, who was changed from paroxetine to moclobemide, see 'MAOIs or RIMAs + SSRIs', p.1401.

1. Pare CMB, Al Mousawi M, Sandler M, Glover V. Attempts to attenuate the 'cheese effect'. Combined drug therapy in depressive illness. *J Affect Disord* (1985) 9, 137–41.
2. Zelapar (Selegiline hydrochloride). Cephalon Ltd. UK Summary of product characteristics, March 2012.
3. Azilect (Rasagiline mesilate). Teva Pharmaceuticals Ltd. UK Summary of product characteristics, November 2009.
4. Dingemanse J. An update of recent moclobemide interaction data. *Int Clin Psychopharmacol* (1993) 7, 167–80.
5. Korn A, Wagner B, Moritz E, Dingemanse J. Tyramine pressor sensitivity in healthy subjects during combined treatment with moclobemide and selegiline. *Eur J Clin Pharmacol* (1996) 49, 273–8.
6. Dingemanse J, Kneer J, Wallnöfer A, Kettler R, Zürcher G, Koulu M, Korn A. Pharmacokinetic-pharmacodynamic interactions between two selective monoamine oxidase inhibitors: moclobemide and selegiline. *Clin Neuropharmacol* (1996) 19, 399–414.
7. Jansen Steur ENH, Ballering LAP. Moclobemide and selegiline in the treatment of depression in Parkinson's disease. *J Neurol Neurosurg Psychiatry* (1997) 63, 547.
8. Manerix (Moclobemide). Meda Pharmaceuticals. UK Summary of product characteristics, September 2009.

MAO-B inhibitors + Nasal decongestants

An isolated report describes a hypertensive crisis, which was attributed to an interaction between selegiline, ephedrine, and maprotiline. Selegiline does not appear to affect the pharmacokinetics of pseudoephedrine or phenylpropanolamine.

Clinical evidence

An isolated case report describes a man taking **selegiline** 10 mg daily, levodopa with carbidopa, lisuride, maprotiline 75 mg daily, and theophylline with **ephedrine** 180/32 mg daily who developed hypertensive crises (blood pressure up to 300/150 mmHg), intense vasoconstriction, confusion, abdominal pain, sweating, and tachycardia (110 bpm) within 2 days of raising the dose of theophylline with **ephedrine** to 270/48 mg daily. All of the drugs were stopped, and the patient was treated with intravenous nicardipine. He recovered uneventfully.[1]

In a study, 10 healthy subjects received **selegiline** via a transdermal patch delivering 6 mg/24 hours, applied daily, and **pseudoephedrine** 60 mg up to three times daily, for 3 days. **Selegiline** did not cause any significant changes in the cardiovascular pharmacodynamics or the pharmacokinetics of **pseudoephedrine**. In a separate part of this study, 11 healthy subjects received **selegiline** via a transdermal patch delivering 6 mg/24 hours and **phenylpropanolamine** 25 mg up to six times daily. Selegiline did not cause any clinically significant changes in the pharmacodynamics or pharmacokinetics of **phenylpropanolamine**.[2]

Mechanism

It is thought that this reaction described in the case report occurred as a result of excess sympathomimetic amines: ephedrine is an indirectly-acting sympathomimetic that causes increased release of noradrenaline; selegiline has some MAO-A inhibitory activity and may therefore inhibit noradrenaline metabolism; and maprotiline inhibits reuptake of noradrenaline.[1] Compare also 'MAOIs or RIMAs + Nasal decongestants and related drugs', p.1396 and 'MAOIs or RIMAs + Tricyclic and related antidepressants', p.1403.

Importance and management

This appears to be the only report of a hypertensive reaction in a patient taking selegiline and ephedrine, and the concurrent maprotiline was also implicated in this reaction. In general, if selegiline is used at recommended doses it is selective for MAO-B and no restrictions are required in the use of nasal decongestants with indirect sympathomimetic actions, such as ephedrine and pseudoephedrine. Nevertheless, this report suggests that, rarely, interactions are still possible, and some consider that patients taking selegiline should try to avoid pseudoephedrine or other related drugs.[2,3] The manufacturers of both **rasagiline**[4] and selegiline[5] contraindicate, or suggest avoiding, the concurrent use of sympathomimetics such as those present in decongestants or cold medications containing ephedrine or pseudoephedrine.[4]

1. Lefebvre H, Noblet C, Moore N, Wolf LM. Pseudo-phaeochromocytoma after multiple drug interactions involving the selective monoamine oxidase inhibitor selegiline. *Clin Endocrinol (Oxf)* (1995) 42, 95–9.
2. Azzaro AJ, VanDenBerg CM, Ziemniak J, Kemper EM, Blob LF, Campbell BJ. Evaluation of the potential for pharmacodynamic and pharmacokinetic drug interactions between selegiline transdermal system and two sympathomimetic agents (pseudoephedrine and phenylpropanolamine) in healthy volunteers. *J Clin Pharmacol* (2007) 47, 978–90.
3. Jacob JE, Wagner ML, Sage JI. Safety of selegiline with cold medications. *Ann Pharmacother* (2003) 37, 438–41.
4. Azilect (Rasagiline mesilate). Teva Pharmaceuticals Ltd. UK Summary of product characteristics, November 2009.
5. Zelapar (Selegiline hydrochloride). Cephalon Ltd. UK Summary of product characteristics, March 2012.

MAO-B inhibitors + Opioids

A case of fluctuating stupor and agitation, with muscle rigidity, sweating and a raised temperature has been reported when pethidine was used with selegiline. Rasagiline is expected to interact similarly. The concurrent use of rasagiline or selegiline with opioids that have serotonergic effects might result in the serotonin syndrome.

Clinical evidence, mechanism, importance and management

A patient taking **selegiline** 5 mg twice daily, pergolide, levodopa with carbidopa, imipramine and desipramine was given **pethidine (meperidine)** beginning on post-operative day one for 4 days in doses of 75 to 150 mg daily. On the second day he became increasingly restless and irritable, progressing to delirium on the fourth day, with fluctuations between stupor and severe agitation associated with muscular rigidity, sweating and a raised temperature. The patient remained normotensive. Both pethidine and then **selegiline** were stopped, with full recovery.[1] This case is similar to various cases described with non-selective MAOIs and pethidine, see 'MAOIs or RIMAs + Opioids; Pethidine (Meperidine)', p.1399. The US manufacturer of selegiline states that other serious reactions including death have occurred when **selegiline** was given with pethidine.[2]

Both the MAO-B inhibitors and some opioids (see 'Table 35.3', p.1472) have serotonergic effects, and concurrent use might lead to the serotonin syndrome. Serotonin syndrome is a rare adverse effect, but because of its severity, some caution is warranted if both drugs are given. For more information on serotonin syndrome and its management, see 'Drugs that cause serotonin syndrome + Other drugs that cause serotonin syndrome', p.1471. On the basis of the above evidence, the manufacturers of **selegiline**[2-4] and **rasagiline**[5] contraindicate the concurrent use of **pethidine (meperidine)**, which is a prudent precaution. Some UK manufacturers of **rasagiline** and **selegiline** additionally state that pethidine should not be given until 14 days after stopping these drugs,[3-5] which makes sense because they are irreversible inhibitors of MAO-B.

Some UK manufacturers of **selegiline** also contraindicate concurrent use with all opioids,[3,4] which is probably not always necessary, based on the evidence that generally suggests an interaction does not occur between non-selective MAOIs and some opioids, see 'MAOIs or RIMAs + Opioids; Miscellaneous', p.1398.

1. Zornberg GL, Bodkin JA, Cohen BM. Severe adverse interaction between pethidine and selegiline. *Lancet* (1991) 337, 246.
2. Selegiline hydrochloride tablets USP. Apotex Inc. US Prescribing information, June 2009.
3. Zelapar (Selegiline hydrochloride). Cephalon Ltd. UK Summary of product characteristics, March 2012.
4. Eldepryl (Selegiline hydrochloride). Orion Pharma (UK) Ltd. UK Summary of product characteristics, February 2012.
5. Azilect (Rasagiline mesilate). Teva Pharmaceuticals Ltd. UK Summary of product characteristics, November 2009.

MAO-B inhibitors + SSRIs or SNRIs

A few cases of serotonin syndrome and other serious CNS disturbances have been seen when selegiline was given with fluoxetine or venlafaxine. Other SSRIs and SNRIs are expected to interact with selegiline similarly. Rasagiline is expected to interact in the same way as selegiline.

Clinical evidence

(a) Citalopram

In a double-blind, randomised study, 18 healthy subjects were given citalopram 20 mg or placebo daily for 10 days, with **selegiline** 10 mg daily added for a further 4 days. There was no evidence of changes in vital signs or in the frequency of adverse events, but the bioavailability of **selegiline** was slightly reduced by about 30% by citalopram. The authors of this report concluded that no clinically relevant interaction occurred between **selegiline** and citalopram.[1]

(b) Fluoxetine

A woman with Parkinson's disease taking **selegiline**, bromocriptine and levodopa with carbidopa was also given fluoxetine 20 mg. Several days later she developed episodes of shivering and sweating in the mid-afternoon, which lasted several hours. Her hands became blue, cold and mottled and her blood pressure was elevated (200/120 mmHg). These episodes disappeared when both fluoxetine and **selegiline** were stopped, and did not reappear when the fluoxetine alone was restarted.[2] A case of mild serotonin syndrome has been described in a woman taking levodopa and **selegiline**, which developed a few days after she started fluoxetine,[3] and a possible case of serotonin syndrome has been described in another patient taking selegiline and fluoxetine.[4] A further case of serotonin syndrome, which was fatal, developed in a patient taking levodopa with carbidopa and fluoxetine when **selegiline** was added and the dose of levodopa increased.[5] Other patients have become hyperactive and apparently manic,[2,6] have developed ataxia,[7] or developed a tonic-clonic seizure and headache, flushes, palpitations, and a blood pressure of 250/130 mmHg (a pseudophaeochromocytoma syndrome),[8] all after the concurrent use of fluoxetine and **selegiline**.

These reports contrast with a retrospective study of 23 patients with parkinsonism, who received both **selegiline** and fluoxetine without any serious adverse effects occurring, although worsening confusion was noted in 5 patients.[9]

(c) Fluvoxamine

The manufacturer of **selegiline** notes that serious reactions similar to those seen with fluoxetine have occurred in patients receiving **selegiline** and fluvoxamine.[10] Fluvoxamine may be expected to inhibit the metabolism of **rasagiline**, see 'MAO-B inhibitors; Rasagiline + Miscellaneous', p.773.

(d) Paroxetine

A retrospective study of patients with Parkinson's disease taking **selegiline** 5 to 10 mg daily (and other antiparkinsonian drugs such as levodopa with carbidopa, bromocriptine, amantadine, pergolide, and antimuscarinics) noted that the addition of paroxetine 10 to 40 mg daily caused no adverse effects and the patients appeared to obtain overall benefit, including some improvement in parkinsonian symptoms.[11] However, the manufacturers of **selegiline** note that serious reactions similar to those seen with fluoxetine have occurred in patients receiving **selegiline** and paroxetine.[10,12]

For a case report describing serotonin syndrome in a patient taking selegiline, who was changed from paroxetine to moclobemide, see 'MAOIs or RIMAs + SSRIs', p.1401.

(e) Sertraline

A retrospective study of patients with Parkinson's disease taking **selegiline** 5 to 10 mg daily (and other antiparkinsonian drugs such as levodopa with carbidopa, bromocriptine, amantadine, pergolide, and antimuscarinics) noted that the addition of sertraline 25 to 100 mg daily caused no adverse effects and the patients appeared to obtain overall benefit, including some improvement in parkinsonian symptoms.[11] However, the manufacturers of **selegiline** note that serious reactions similar to those seen with concurrent fluoxetine have occurred in patients receiving **selegiline** and sertraline.[10,12]

(f) Venlafaxine

A man developed serotonin syndrome 15 days after stopping **selegiline** 50 mg [daily] and within 30 minutes of starting venlafaxine 37.5 mg.[13]

Mechanism

Not fully understood. In some cases the symptoms seen appear to be consistent with serotonin syndrome, which is typified by CNS irritability, increased muscle tone, shivering, altered consciousness and myoclonus, and appears to be associated with the use of more than one serotonergic drug. This syndrome has also occurred when non-selective MAOIs were given with SSRIs or venlafaxine (see 'MAOIs or RIMAs + SSRIs', p.1401, and 'MAOIs or RIMAs + SNRIs', p.1401). Note that selegiline might have some non-selective MAOI activity, especially at higher doses.

Importance and management

The possibility of serotonin syndrome or similar occurring with selegiline and SSRIs or venlafaxine would appear to be established, although the incidence is very rare. Nevertheless, the manufacturers of selegiline recommend that these drug combinations should be avoided, or specifically contraindicate concurrent use.[10,12,14] In addition, selegiline should not be started for 5 weeks after stopping fluoxetine, 2 weeks after stopping sertraline, and one week after stopping other SSRIs, and SSRIs should not be started for 2 weeks after stopping selegiline.[10,14]

Similarly, the manufacturers of **rasagiline** recommend avoiding the concurrent use of fluoxetine and fluvoxamine. Rasagiline should not be started for 5 weeks after stopping fluoxetine, and fluoxetine or fluvoxamine should not be started for 2 weeks after stopping rasagiline.[15]

For more information on serotonin syndrome and its management, see 'Drugs that cause serotonin syndrome + Other drugs that cause serotonin syndrome', p.1471.

1. Laine K, Anttila M, Heinonen E, Helminen A, Huupponen R, Mäki-Ikola O, Reinikainen K, Scheinin M. Lack of adverse interactions between concomitantly administered selegiline and citalopram. *Clin Neuropharmacol* (1997) 20, 419–33.
2. Suchowersky O, deVries JD. Interaction of fluoxetine and selegiline. *Can J Psychiatry* (1990) 35, 571–2.
3. Garcia-Monco JC, Padierna A, Gomez Beldarrain M. Selegiline, fluoxetine, and depression in Parkinson's disease. *Mov Disord* (1995) 10, 352–8.
4. Ritter JL, Alexander B. Retrospective study of selegiline-antidepressant drug interactions and a review of the literature. *Ann Clin Psychiatry* (1997) 9, 7–13.
5. Bilbao Garay J, Mesa Plaza N, Castilla Castellano V, Dhimes Tejada P. Síndrome serotoninérgico: presentación de un caso de evolución letal y revisión de la literatura. *Rev Clin Esp* (2002) 202, 209–11.
6. Kurlan R, Dimitsopulos T. Selegiline and manic behavior in Parkinson's disease. *Arch Neurol* (1992) 49, 1231.

7. Jermain DM, Hughes PL, Follender AB. Potential fluoxetine-selegiline interaction. *Ann Pharmacother* (1992) 26, 1300.
8. Montastruc JL, Chamontin B, Senard JM, Tran MA, Rascol O, Llau ME, Rascol A. Pseudophaeochromocytoma in parkinsonian patient treated with fluoxetine plus selegiline. *Lancet* (1993) 341, 555.
9. Waters CH. Fluoxetine and selegiline — lack of significant interaction. *Can J Neurol Sci* (1994) 21, 259–61.
10. Eldepryl (Selegiline hydrochloride). Orion Pharma (UK) Ltd. UK Summary of product characteristics, February 2012.
11. Toyama SC, Iacono RP. Is it safe to combine a selective serotonin reuptake inhibitor with selegiline? *Ann Pharmacother* (1994) 28, 405–6.
12. Selegiline hydrochloride tablets, USP. Apotex Inc. US prescribing information, June 2009.
13. Gitlin MJ. Venlafaxine, monoamine oxidase inhibitors, and the serotonin syndrome. *J Clin Psychopharmacol* (1997) 17, 66–67.
14. Zelapar (Selegiline hydrochloride). Cephalon Ltd. UK Summary of product characteristics, March 2012.
15. Azilect (Rasagiline mesilate). Teva Pharmaceuticals Ltd. UK Summary of product characteristics, November 2009.

MAO-B inhibitors + Tricyclic and related antidepressants

The concurrent use of selegiline and tricyclics might lead to adverse effects such as serotonin syndrome. Trazodone might interact similarly, although evidence for this is lacking. Rasagiline is expected to interact in the same way as selegiline.

Clinical evidence

(a) Trazodone

A retrospective study of patients with Parkinson's disease taking **selegiline** 5 to 10 mg daily (and other antiparkinson drugs such as levodopa with carbidopa, bromocriptine, amantadine, pergolide, and antimuscarinics) noted that the addition of trazodone 25 to 150 mg daily caused no adverse effects and the patients appeared to obtain overall benefit, including some improvement in parkinsonian symptoms.[1]

(b) Tricyclic antidepressants

Between 1989 and 1994 the FDA in the US received 16 reports of adverse interactions between **selegiline** and tricyclic antidepressants, which were attributed to serotonin syndrome.[2] The manufacturers of **selegiline** very briefly describe severe CNS toxicity in one patient given **selegiline** and **amitriptyline** (hyperpyrexia and death), and in another given **selegiline** and **protriptyline** (tremor, agitation, restlessness, followed by unresponsiveness and death).[3-5] They state that related adverse events including hypertension, syncope, asystole, diaphoresis, seizures, changes in behavioural and mental status, and muscular rigidity have also been reported in some patients receiving **selegiline** and various tricyclics.[3,4] A further report describes serotonin syndrome in a woman given **nortriptyline** with **selegiline**.[6] Another report describes hypomania occurring in a woman taking **selegiline** and **nortriptyline**;[7] the contribution of a drug interaction is unclear in this case. However, these warnings need to be balanced by other reports indicating that these reactions are uncommon. One study based on the findings of 47 investigators treating 4 568 patients with **selegiline** and antidepressants [not specifically named but possibly including the tricyclics and related antidepressants] found that only 11 patients (0.24%) experienced symptoms considered to represent serotonin syndrome, and only 2 patients (0.04%) experienced symptoms considered to be serious.[8] Another small retrospective study designed to evaluate the tolerability and efficacy of combining **selegiline** and tricyclic antidepressants (not specifically named) identified 28 patients who had taken both drugs.[2] In total, 17 patients definitely benefited and 6 patients possibly benefited from taking the combination. Another retrospective study of 25 occasions of the use of a tricyclic with **selegiline** found no cases of serotonin syndrome.[9]

Mechanism

Not fully understood. In some cases the symptoms seen appear to be consistent with serotonin syndrome, which is typified by CNS irritability, increased muscle tone, shivering, altered consciousness and myoclonus, and appears to be associated with the use of more than one serotonergic drug, see 'Drugs that cause serotonin syndrome + Other drugs that cause serotonin syndrome', p.1471. This syndrome has also occurred with non-selective MAOIs and tricyclics or trazodone (see 'MAOIs or RIMAs + Tricyclic and related antidepressants', p.1403, and 'MAOIs or RIMAs + Trazodone', p.1403). Note that selegiline may have some non-selective MAOI activity, especially at high doses.

Importance and management

Evidence for an interaction between the tricyclic and related antidepressants and **selegiline** is sparse, and needs to be balanced by the reports of safe and uneventful concurrent use. Serotonin syndrome is a rare adverse effect, but because of its severity, some caution is warranted if both selegiline and a tricyclic or a related antidepressant (such as **trazodone**) are given. For more information on serotonin syndrome and its management, see 'Drugs that cause serotonin syndrome + Other drugs that cause serotonin syndrome', p.1471. If the decision is made to use selegiline with any of the tricyclic antidepressants, the outcome should be well monitored, but the likelihood of problems seems to be small. Nevertheless, some manufacturers of selegiline advise avoiding all tricyclic antidepressants,[4,5] or specifically contraindicate concurrent use.[3]

Rasagiline might also have serotonergic effects which could be additive with those of the tricyclic and related antidepressants (including **trazodone**). The manufacturers of **rasagiline** advise caution if it is given with antidepressants.[10] See 'Drugs that cause serotonin syndrome + Other drugs that cause serotonin syndrome', p.1471 for information on the management of serotonin syndrome.

1. Toyama SC, Iacono RP. Is it safe to combine a selective serotonin reuptake inhibitor with selegiline? *Ann Pharmacother* (1994) 28, 405–6.
2. Yu LJ, Zweig RM. Successful combination of selegiline and antidepressants in Parkinson's disease. *Neurology* (1996) 46 (2 Suppl), A374.
3. Eldepryl (Selegiline hydrochloride). Orion Pharma (UK) Ltd. UK Summary of product characteristics, February 2012.
4. Selegiline hydrochloride tablets, USP. Apotex Inc. US prescribing information, June 2009.
5. Zelapar (Selegiline hydrochloride). Cephalon Ltd. UK Summary of product characteristics, March 2012.
6. Hinds NP, Hillier CEM, Wiles CM. Possible serotonin syndrome arising from an interaction between nortriptyline and selegiline in a lady with parkinsonism. *J Neurol* (2000) 247, 811.
7. Kurlan R, Dimitsopulos T. Selegiline and manic behavior in Parkinson's disease. *Arch Neurol* (1992) 49, 1231.
8. Richard IH, Kurlan R, Tanner C, Factor S, Hubble J, Suchowersky O, Waters C, and the Parkinson Study Group. Serotonin syndrome and the combined use of deprenyl and an antidepressant in Parkinson's disease. *Neurology* (1997) 48, 1070–7.
9. Ritter JL, Alexander B. Retrospective study of selegiline-antidepressant drug interactions and a review of the literature. *Ann Clin Psychiatry* (1997) 9, 7–13.
10. Azilect (Rasagiline mesilate). Teva Pharmaceuticals Ltd. UK Summary of product characteristics, November 2009.

MAO-B inhibitors; Rasagiline + Miscellaneous

Ciprofloxacin increases the AUC of rasagiline by inhibiting CYP1A2. Other inhibitors of CYP1A2 are predicted to interact similarly. There is a theoretical possibility that tobacco smoke, may reduce the plasma levels of rasagiline. Rasagiline does not affect the pharmacokinetics of theophylline.

Clinical evidence, mechanism, importance and management

(a) CYP1A2 inhibitors

The manufacturer notes that concurrent use of rasagiline and **ciprofloxacin** increased the AUC of rasagiline by 83%.[1] **Ciprofloxacin** inhibits the cytochrome P450 isoenzyme CYP1A2, which is the major enzyme responsible for the metabolism of rasagiline. The clinical relevance of this increase has not been assessed, but until more is known caution is warranted. Be alert for rasagiline adverse effects (e.g. headache, dyspepsia). This caution should be extended to other potent inhibitors of CYP1A2, such as **enoxacin**. Note that fluvoxamine is also a CYP1A2 inhibitor, but concurrent use with, and for 2 weeks after, rasagiline should be avoided, see 'MAO-B inhibitors + SSRIs or SNRIs', p.772.

(b) Theophylline

The US manufacturer of rasagiline reports that, in 24 healthy subjects, the concurrent use of rasagiline 1 mg daily and theophylline up to 500 mg twice daily did not affect the pharmacokinetics of either drug.[1] No dose adjustment of either drug is therefore needed on the concurrent use. There appears to be no direct evidence regarding aminophylline, but as it is metabolised to theophylline, no adverse interaction would be expected with rasagiline. Note that theophylline is a CYP1A2 substrate and therefore rasagiline would not be expected to affect the metabolism of other drugs by this route.

(c) Tobacco

Rasagiline is a substrate of the cytochrome P450 isoenzyme CYP1A2, and the manufacturer advises that the plasma levels of rasagiline may be lowered in patients who smoke, due to the inducing effect of tobacco smoke on CYP1A2.[1] Bear this theoretical interaction in mind if rasagiline seems less effective than anticipated.

1. Azilect (Rasagiline mesilate). Teva Pharmaceuticals Ltd. UK Summary of product characteristics, November 2009.

MAO-B inhibitors; Selegiline + Alprazolam

In a study in 12 healthy subjects, the concurrent use of transdermal selegiline patches 6 mg/24 hours and alprazolam 500 micrograms three times daily did not affect the steady-state pharmacokinetics of either drug.[1]

1. Azzaro AJ, Ziemniak J, Kemper E, Campbell BJ, VanDenBerg C. Selegiline transdermal system: an examination of the potential for CYP450-dependent pharmacokinetic interactions with 3 psychotropic medications. *J Clin Pharmacol* (2007) 47, 146–58.

MAO-B inhibitors; Selegiline + Antipsychotics

When healthy subjects were given selegiline transdermal patches 6 mg/24 hours either alone, or with olanzapine 5 mg daily or risperidone 1 mg twice daily, the steady-state pharmacokinetics of olanzapine, risperidone and selegiline were not affected.[1]

1. Azzaro AJ, Ziemniak J, Kemper E, Campbell BJ, VanDenBerg C. Selegiline transdermal system: an examination of the potential for CYP450-dependent pharmacokinetic interactions with 3 psychotropic medications. *J Clin Pharmacol* (2007) 47, 146–58.

MAO-B inhibitors; Selegiline + Cocaine

Cocaine and selegiline appear not to interact adversely.

Clinical evidence, mechanism, importance and management

In a study to establish the safety of using selegiline to prevent relapse in cocaine addiction, 5 otherwise healthy intravenous cocaine users were given 0, 20 and 40 mg intravenous doses of cocaine one hour apart after receiving selegiline 10 mg or placebo orally. The cocaine increased the heart rate, blood pressure, pupil diameter and subjective indices of euphoria as expected. However, the presence of selegiline reduced pupillary diameter, but did not alter the pupil dilation or other effects normally caused by cocaine.[1] In another study, transdermal selegiline did not alter the pharmacokinetics of intravenous cocaine in cocaine-dependent subjects. Some physiological effects (blood pressure and heart rate) and subjective effects of cocaine were attenuated by selegiline.[2]

The authors of the first study[1] concluded that concurrent use is safe and unlikely to increase the reinforcing effects of cocaine.

1. Haberny KA, Walsh SL, Ginn DH, Wilkins JN, Garner JE, Setoda D, Bigelow GE. Absence of acute cocaine interactions with the MAO-B inhibitor selegiline. *Drug Alcohol Depend* (1995) 39, 55–62.
2. Houtsmuller EJ, Notes LD, Newton T, van Sluis N, Chiang N, Elkashef A, Bigelow GE. Transdermal selegiline and intravenous cocaine: safety and interactions. *Psychopharmacology (Berl)* (2004) 172, 31–40.

MAO-B inhibitors; Selegiline + Dopamine agonists

No pharmacokinetic interaction occurs between selegiline and cabergoline, pramipexole or ropinirole.

Clinical evidence, mechanism, importance and management

(a) Cabergoline

In a study in 6 subjects with Parkinson's disease, no pharmacokinetic interaction was found to occur between cabergoline 1 mg daily and selegiline 10 mg daily after 22 days of concurrent use.[1]

(b) Pramipexole

The manufacturer of pramipexole says that no pharmacokinetic interaction occurs with selegiline.[2]

(c) Ropinirole

The manufacturer of ropinirole notes that a population pharmacokinetic analysis showed a lack of relevant effects of selegiline on ropinirole.[3]

1. Dostert P, Benedetti MS, Persiani S, La Croix R, Bosc M, Fiorentini F, Deffond D, Vernay D, Dordain G. Lack of pharmacokinetic interaction between the selective dopamine agonist cabergoline and the MAO-B inhibitor selegiline. *J Neural Transm* (1995) 45 (Suppl), 247–57.
2. Mirapexin (Pramipexole dihydrochloride monohydrate). Boehringer Ingelheim Ltd. UK Summary of product characteristics, October 2009.
3. SmithKline Beecham. Personal Communication, September 1996.

MAO-B inhibitors; Selegiline + Hormonal contraceptives or HRT

In a small study, the bioavailability of selegiline was markedly higher (mean of about 20-fold) in women taking oral combined hormonal contraceptives than in those not taking contraceptives. A controlled study found that the effect of HRT was more modest.

Clinical evidence

(a) Combined oral contraceptives

The AUCs of single doses of selegiline 5 to 40 mg were 16- to 45-fold higher in 4 women taking oral combined hormonal contraceptives than in 4 women who were not taking contraceptives. Three subjects were taking **ethinylestradiol** 30 micrograms with **gestodene** 75 micrograms, and one was taking a triphasic preparation of **ethinylestradiol** with **levonorgestrel**.[1]

(b) HRT

In a crossover study in 12 young healthy women, the AUC of a single 10-mg dose of selegiline was increased by 60% (which was not statistically significant) following 10 days of HRT (containing **estradiol valerate** 2 mg with **levonorgestrel** 250 micrograms). There was marked variability in selegiline levels with two women having a threefold increase in AUC, and 3 having a decrease. Other changes in pharmacokinetics of selegiline or its metabolites were small.[2]

Mechanism

It was suggested that the combined hormonal contraceptive inhibited the first pass metabolism of selegiline and so markedly increased its bioavailability.[1] However, this was not found for HRT containing a different estrogenic hormone.

Importance and management

Although data are limited, it appears that combined hormonal contraceptives may markedly increase the bioavailability of selegiline. Some UK manufacturers suggest that the concurrent use of oral contraceptives should be avoided.[3,4] Although the short-term use of HRT also increased the AUC of selegiline, the changes were modest and were not considered clinically relevant. Nevertheless, the results perhaps need confirming with longer term concurrent use, and some UK manufacturers of selegiline advises avoiding concurrent HRT.[3,4]

1. Laine K, Anttila M, Helminen A, Karnani H, Huupponen R. Dose linearity study of selegiline pharmacokinetics after oral administration: evidence for strong drug interaction with female sex steroids. *Br J Clin Pharmacol* (1999) 47, 249–54.
2. Palovaara S, Anttila M, Nyman L, Laine K. Effect of concomitant hormone replacement therapy containing estradiol and levonorgestrel on the pharmacokinetics of selegiline. *Eur J Clin Pharmacol* (2002) 58: 259–63.
3. Zelapar (Selegiline hydrochloride). Cephalon Ltd. UK Summary of product characteristics, March 2012.
4. Eldepryl (Selegiline hydrochloride). Orion Pharma (UK) Ltd. UK Summary of product characteristics, February 2012.

MAO-B inhibitors; Selegiline + Itraconazole

The concurrent use of selegiline and itraconazole does not appear to alter the pharmacokinetics of either drug.

Clinical evidence, mechanism, importance and management

In a randomised, placebo-controlled, crossover study, 12 healthy subjects were given selegiline 10 mg after taking itraconazole 200 mg daily for 4 days. Itraconazole did not have any significant effects on the pharmacokinetics of selegiline, although the AUC of desmethylselegiline, a primary metabolite, was increased by 11%. The pharmacokinetics of itraconazole were also unaffected. There would appear to be no reason for avoiding concurrent use.[1]

1. Kivistö KT, Wang J-S, Backman JT, Nyman L, Taavitsainen P, Anttila M, Neuvonen PJ. Selegiline pharmacokinetics are unaffected by the CYP3A4 inhibitor itraconazole. *Eur J Clin Pharmacol* (2001) 57, 37–42.

MAO-B inhibitors; Selegiline + Metamfetamine

Selegiline does not alter the pharmacokinetics of metamfetamine.

Clinical evidence, mechanism, importance and management

In a study, 5 subjects who used metamfetamine at least twice a week, took selegiline 5 mg twice daily for 12 days, and 4 subjects took placebo. During this time they received intravenous metamfetamine 15 mg and 30 mg given 2 days apart. When compared with placebo, selegiline did not affect either the pharmacokinetics of metamfetamine and its metabolite, d-amfetamine or the cardiovascular effects of metamfetamine. Subjects reported greater metamfetamine-associated "bad effects" while taking selegiline than while taking placebo, but other subjective effects were not altered.[1]

Note that both selegiline and the amfetamines have serotonergic effects, and concurrent use might lead to the serotonin syndrome. Serotonin syndrome is a rare adverse effect, but because of its severity, some caution is warranted if both drugs are given. For more information on serotonin syndrome and its management, see 'Drugs that cause serotonin syndrome + Other drugs that cause serotonin syndrome', p.1471.

1. Newton TF, De La Garza R, Fong T, Chiang N, Holmes TH, Bloch DA, Anderson A, Elkashef A. A comprehensive assessment of the safety of intravenous methamphetamine administration during treatment with selegiline. *Pharmacol Biochem Behav* (2005) 82, 704–11.

Piribedil + Clonidine

Clonidine is reported to oppose the effects of piribedil.

Clinical evidence, mechanism, importance and management

A study in 5 patients taking piribedil found that the concurrent use of clonidine (up to 1.5 mg daily for 10 to 24 days) caused a worsening of parkinsonism (an exacerbation of rigidity and akinesia). The concurrent use of antimuscarinic drugs reduced the effects of this interaction.[1] The reason is uncertain, and the general relevance of this small study is unclear.

1. Shoulson I, Chase TN. Clonidine and the anti-parkinsonian response to L-dopa or piribedil. *Neuropharmacology* (1976) 15, 25–7.

Pramipexole + Drugs that affect renal clearance

Cimetidine, and possibly amantadine modestly reduce the clearance of pramipexole. Probenecid had a minor effect on pramipexole clearance in one study.

Clinical evidence, mechanism, importance and management

A study in 12 healthy subjects found that multiple doses of **cimetidine** reduced the total oral clearance of a single 250-microgram dose of pramipexole by about 35% and increased its half-life by 40%. A similar reduction in the renal clearance of pramipexole was noted. The authors suggest that **cimetidine** reduces the renal excretion of pramipexole by inhibiting the active renal organic cation transport system.[1] The manufacturers say that **cimetidine** and other drugs that are eliminated by this route such as **amantadine** may interact with pramipexole to reduce excretion of either or both drugs.[2] The clinical significance of these interactions is uncertain, and as yet there appear to be no reports of any adverse interactions. Nevertheless, the manufacturers suggest a reduction of the pramipexole dose should be considered when **amantadine** or **cimetidine** are given with pramipexole.[2]

In a study in 12 healthy subjects, multiple doses of **probenecid** reduced the clearance of a single 250-microgram dose of pramipexole by 10%.[1] This change is not clinically relevant.

1. Wright CE, Lasher Sisson T, Ichhpurani AK, Peters GR. Influence of probenecid (PR) and cimetidine (C) on pramipexole (PX) pharmacokinetics. *Clin Pharmacol Ther* (1996) 59, 183.
2. Mirapexin (Pramipexole dihydrochloride monohydrate). Boehringer Ingelheim Ltd. UK Summary of product characteristics, October 2009.

Ropinirole + CYP1A2 inhibitors

Ciprofloxacin increased the AUC of ropinirole by 84%, by inhibiting CYP1A2: other CYP1A2 inhibitors are predicted to interact similarly.

Clinical evidence

In a study in 12 patients **ciprofloxacin** 500 mg twice daily increased the AUC of ropinirole 2 mg three times daily by 84% and increased the maximum plasma level by 60%.[1]

Mechanism

Ropinirole is principally metabolised by the cytochrome P450 isoenzyme CYP1A2, of which ciprofloxacin is a known inhibitor.

Importance and management

Although the clinical relevance of this pharmacokinetic interaction has not been assessed, it would seem possible that the effects of ropinirole may be increased. The manufacturers suggest that if a known potent inhibitor of CYP1A2 is stopped or started in a patient taking ropinirole, adjustment of the ropinirole dose may be required.[1,2] The UK manufacturer specifically mentions **cimetidine** (which is not usually considered a potent CYP1A2 inhibitor) and **fluvoxamine** in addition to ciprofloxacin.[2] Note that enoxacin is usually also considered to be a potent CYP1A2 inhibitor.

1. Requip (Ropinirole hydrochloride). GlaxoSmithKline. US Prescribing information, May 2009.
2. Requip Tablets (Ropinirole hydrochloride). GlaxoSmithKline UK. UK Summary of product characteristics, April 2012.

Ropinirole + Miscellaneous

Estrogens (HRT) may reduce the clearance and tobacco smoking may increase the clearance of ropinirole.

Clinical evidence, mechanism, importance and management

(a) Oestrogens

Population pharmacokinetic analysis of clinical study data showed that estrogens (mainly ethinylestradiol[1]) used in HRT reduced ropinirole clearance by one-third.[1-4] In another analysis it was found that women taking HRT received a slightly lower daily dose of ropinirole than those not taking HRT, with no difference in adverse effects.[4] Therefore, in women already receiving HRT, ropinirole treatment may be started using the usual dose titration.[1,3] However, it is suggested that an adjustment [reduction] in the ropinirole dose may be needed if HRT is started.[1,3]

(b) Tobacco

The manufacturer notes that, in a study in patients with restless leg syndrome, 7 tobacco smokers were found to have a 38% lower ropinirole AUC and a 30% lower maximum level than 11 non-smokers.[1] Tobacco induces the cytochrome P450 isoenzyme CYP1A2, by which ropinirole is extensively metabolised. Because the dose of ropinirole is titrated to effect, this interaction is unlikely to be clinically relevant, except perhaps if patients stop or start smoking while taking ropinirole, when further dose titration may be necessary.

(c) Other drugs

The manufacturer notes that population analysis revealed that **amantadine, antimuscarinics, antihistamines, benzodiazepines, ibuprofen, thiazides, tricyclic antidepressants**, and **trihexyphenidyl** did not have any relevant effects on the pharmacokinetics and/or clearance of ropinirole.[1,2,5]

1. Requip (Ropinirole hydrochloride). GlaxoSmithKline. US Prescribing information, May 2009.
2. SmithKline Beecham. Personal Communication, September 1996.
3. Requip Tablets (Ropinirole hydrochloride). GlaxoSmithKline UK. UK Summary of product characteristics, April 2012.
4. SmithKline Beecham. Personal Communication, May 1999.
5. Kaye CM, Nicholls B. Clinical pharmacokinetics of ropinirole. *Clin Pharmacokinet* (2000) 39, 243–54.

19

Antiplatelet drugs and Thrombolytics

This section is primarily concerned with those interactions where the activities of antiplatelet drugs or thrombolytics are changed by the presence of another drug. Note that the interactions of high-dose aspirin are covered under analgesics.

Mode of action of antiplatelet drugs and thrombolytics

Platelets usually circulate in the plasma in an inactive form, but following injury to blood vessels they become activated and adhere to the site of injury. Platelet aggregation then occurs, which contributes to the haemostatic plug. Platelet aggregation involves the binding of fibrinogen with a glycoprotein IIb/IIIa receptor on the platelet surface. The activated platelets secrete substances such as adenosine diphosphate (ADP) and thromboxane A_2 and this results in additional platelet aggregation and also causes vasoconstriction. Finally a number of platelet-derived factors stimulate the production of thrombin, and hence fibrin, through the coagulation cascade (see *The blood clotting process* under 'Anticoagulants', p.371). Opposing this process is the fibrinolysis pathway, which is initiated during clot formation by a number of mediators such as tissue plasminogen activator (tPA) and urokinase. These proteins convert plasminogen to plasmin, which in turn degrades fibrin, the main component of the clot.

Antiplatelet drugs (see 'Table 19.1', below) reduce platelet aggregation and are used to prevent thromboembolic events. They act through a wide range of mechanisms including:

- prevention of thromboxane A_2 synthesis or inhibition of thromboxane receptors e.g. aspirin, which inhibits platelet cyclo-oxygenase, preventing the synthesis of thromboxane A_2
- interference with ADP-mediated platelet activation e.g. thienopyridines such as clopidogrel and prasugrel
- inhibition of adenosine reuptake e.g. dipyridamole
- interference with adenosine metabolism by inhibiting cyclic adenosine monophosphate (cAMP) phosphodiesterase e.g. cilostazol
- interference in the final step in platelet aggregation by stopping fibrinogen binding with the glycoprotein IIb/IIIa receptor on the platelet surface e.g. abciximab

Therefore some antiplatelet drugs can have beneficial additive effects with other antiplatelet drugs that act via different mechanisms. Furthermore, other drugs, such as dextrans, heparin, some prostaglandins and sulfinpyrazone, also have some antiplatelet activity. It should be noted that the additive bleeding effects of using two drugs with antiplatelet and/or thrombolytic properties should always be considered, and patients monitored appropriately. Consideration should also be given when using these types of drugs with other drugs that may cause bleeding such as the NSAIDs (see 'NSAIDs + Aspirin', p.145, or the SSRIs (see 'Antiplatelet drugs + SSRIs or SNRIs', p.780). Note that some of the antiplatelet drugs act irreversibly (e.g. aspirin, clopidogrel, prasugrel): normalisation of platelet aggregation then depends on the rate of turnover of platelets and may take 7 to 10 days.

Thrombolytics (see 'Table 19.1', below) are used in the treatment of thromboembolic disorders. Thrombolytics activate plasminogen to form plasmin, which is a proteolytic enzyme that degrades fibrin and therefore produces clot dissolution.

The metabolism of oral antiplatelet drugs

(a) Phosphodiesterase type-3 inhibitors

Cilostazol is primarily metabolised by CYP3A4 and to a lesser extent CYP2C19. Its main active metabolite, 3,4-dehydro-cilostazol metabolite (primarily formed by CYP3A4), is four- to sevenfold more potent than cilostazol, whereas the 4-trans-hydroxymetabolite (primarily formed by CYP2C19) is only one-fifth as potent as cilostazol.[1,2]

(b) Thienopyridines

The thienopyridines clopidogrel, prasugrel and ticlopidine are prodrugs and need to be metabolised to their active thiol metabolites to have an antiplatelet effect.

Clopidogrel is metabolised through two different metabolic pathways. Its main metabolic pathway is via hepatic carboxylesterase and actually produces an inactive metabolite with no antiplatelet action (this carboxylic acid metabolite was measured in pharmacokinetic studies before an assay became available for the active metabolite). Clopidogrel is also metabolised to a minor extent through a second pathway by cytochrome P450 isoenzymes. *In vitro* this has shown to be firstly to an intermediate metabolite, 2-oxo-clopidogrel by CYP2C19, CYP2B6, and CYP1A2, and then to the active thiol metabolite by CYP3A4, CYP2C19, CYP2C9 and CYP2B6.[3]

Prasugrel is initially metabolised, principally in the intestine, by a carboxylesterase to an inactive thiolactone metabolite (R-95913). This is further metabolised to its active metabolite, R-138727, primarily by CYP3A4 and CYP2B6, and to a lesser extent by CYP2C9 and CYP2C19.[3]

Ticlopidine is thought to be metabolised by CYP2C19 and CYP2B6 to its 2-oxo-ticlopidine intermediate metabolite; however, the mechanism of metabolism to its active metabolite is as yet unknown.[3] Ticlopidine is also known to be an inhibitor of CYP2B6, CYP2C19 and also CYP1A2.

Pharmacogenetics and thienopyridine metabolism. CYP2C19 is subject to genetic variation (see *Genetic factors in drug metabolism*, under 'Drug metabolism interactions', p.4). This means that some patients (about 2% of Caucasians, 4% of Blacks and 14% of Chinese) will have non-functional forms of this isoenzyme (termed CYP2C19 poor metabolisers). This reduces the patients' ability to metabolise clopidogrel to its active metabolite and therefore reduces the antiplatelet effects of clopidogrel: some recent studies have linked poor metaboliser status to a reduced clinical benefit from clopidogrel (a higher than expected rate of cardiovascular events).[4,5] In patients with normal levels of this isoenzyme (termed CYP2C19 extensive metabolisers) complete inhibition of CYP2C19, by giving a potent inhibitor of CYP2C19, would effectively turn them into poor metabolisers, potentially

Table 19.1 Antiplatelet drugs and thrombolytics

Group	Drugs
Antiplatelet drugs	
Adenosine reuptake inhibitors/ Phosphodiesterase inhibitors	Cilostazol, Dipyridamole
Cyclo-oxygenase inhibitors	Aspirin, Indobufen, Triflusal
Glycoprotein IIb/IIIa-receptor antagonists	Abciximab, Eptifibatide, Tirofiban
Thienopyridines (inhibitors of adenosine diphosphate mediated platelet aggregation)	Clopidogrel, Prasugrel, Ticagrelor, Ticlopidine
Thromboxane receptor antagonists	Picotamide
Miscellaneous	Ditazole, Trapidil
Thrombolytics (Fibrinolytics)	
Thrombolytics	Alteplase, Anistreplase, Defibrotide, Reteplase, Streptokinase, Tenecteplase, Urokinase

reducing the benefit of clopidogrel, and this is the main proposed mechanism for the reported effects of omeprazole on clopidogrel metabolism, see 'Clopidogrel + Proton pump inhibitors and other CYP2C19 inhibitors', p.788. In contrast, genetic differences in the isoenzymes that metabolise prasugrel do not appear to affect the pharmacokinetics of its active metabolite or its effects on platelet aggregation.[6,7] These differences are thought to be due to the fact that higher concentrations of the active metabolite of prasugrel are produced relative to clopidogrel, and that prasugrel is only reliant on cytochrome P450 isoenzymes at one point in its metabolic pathway, whereas clopidogrel requires metabolism by cytochrome P450, particularly CYP2C19, from parent drug to intermediate metabolite and then again to the active metabolite.[3]

1. Pletal (Cilostazol). Otsuka Pharmaceuticals (UK) Ltd. UK Summary of product characteristics, October 2013.
2. Pletal (Cilostazol). Otsuka America Pharmaceutical, Inc. US Prescribing information, May 2007.
3. Farid NA, Kurihara A, Wrighton SA. Metabolism and disposition of the thienopyridine antiplatelet drugs ticlopidine, clopidogrel, and prasugrel in humans. *J Clin Pharmacol* (2010) 50, 126–42.
4. Plavix (Clopidogrel hydrogen sulphate). Sanofi-Aventis. UK Summary of product characteristics, January 2014.
5. Plavix (Clopidogrel bisulfate). Bristol-Myers Squibb/Sanofi Pharmaceuticals Partnership. US Prescribing information, December 2011.
6. Efient (Prasugrel hydrochloride). Eli Lilly and Company Ltd. UK Summary of product characteristics, December 2013.
7. Effient (Prasugrel). Eli Lilly and Company. US Prescribing information, November 2013.

Anagrelide + Miscellaneous

The concurrent use of anagrelide with other phosphodiesterase III inhibitors (e.g. milrinone) is predicted to lead to additive inotropic effects. Inhibitors of CYP1A2 (e.g. fluvoxamine) are predicted to increase anagrelide levels. Anagrelide is predicted to weakly inhibit the metabolism of substrates of CYP1A2 (e.g. theophylline). The concurrent use of aspirin with anagrelide does not appear to increase bleeding times; however, additive antiplatelet effects and clinically relevant bleeding might occur. Isolated reports suggest that sucralfate and hydroxycarbamide might interact with anagrelide. No clinically relevant interaction occurs between anagrelide and digoxin, food or warfarin.

Clinical evidence, mechanism, importance and management

(a) Aspirin

The manufacturers report that, in a clinical interaction study, the concurrent use of anagrelide 1 mg daily and aspirin 75 mg daily resulted in greater platelet aggregation compared with aspirin alone.[1,2] Similarly, the concurrent use of single doses of anagrelide 1 mg and aspirin 900 mg resulted in greater platelet aggregation, although no changes in the bleeding time, aPTT or PT were seen.[1] Nevertheless, in a randomised study in patients with essential thrombocythaemia, the concurrent use of anagrelide with aspirin 75 mg or 100 mg daily was associated with a 2.6-fold increased risk of serious haemorrhage (particularly gastrointestinal haemorrhage) when compared with hydroxycarbamide (hydroxyurea) and aspirin, and it was speculated that this was due to synergistic interference with platelet function between anagrelide and aspirin.[3] The manufacturers recommend that the risk/benefit ratio should be assessed before aspirin is used with anagrelide in patients at high risk of haemorrhage.[1,2]

(b) CYP1A2 inhibitors

Anagrelide is principally metabolised by CYP1A2. Drugs that are inhibitors of this isoenzyme are therefore predicted to reduce the clearance of anagrelide, and the manufacturers specifically name **fluvoxamine**.[1,2] Be aware that increased anagrelide effects, both beneficial and adverse, might occur. The UK manufacturer[2] also names **omeprazole**; however, **omeprazole** is only a weak CYP1A2 inhibitor, and would not be expected to have much effect on anagrelide metabolism. For a list of CYP1A2 inhibitors, see 'Table 1.2', p.5.

(c) CYP1A2 substrates

Anagrelide is a weak inhibitor of CYP1A2, and therefore the manufacturers suggest that it might theoretically interact with CYP1A2 substrates, such as **theophylline**.[1,2] The clinical relevance of this is unknown, but it seems likely to be small. Note that **aminophylline**, which is metabolised to theophylline, is also unlikely to be affected.

(d) Food

In a study in healthy subjects, food slightly decreased the maximum level of anagrelide 1 mg by 14%; however, the AUC of anagrelide was *increased* by 20%.[1,2] Food also reduced the maximum level of the active metabolite of anagrelide, but had no notable effect on its AUC.[2] These slight changes in the pharmacokinetics of anagrelide are not expected to be clinically relevant.[1,2]

(e) Hydroxycarbamide (Hydroxyurea)

In a preclinical study in *dogs*, there was no pharmacokinetic interaction between hydroxycarbamide and anagrelide, therefore no clinical pharmacokinetic interaction is expected.[2] A patient taking hydroxycarbamide for 7 years developed severe hypersensitivity pneumonitis soon after anagrelide was started.[4] The clinical relevance of this isolated case is unknown, although there has been another case report of hypersensitivity pneumonitis with anagrelide alone.[5]

(f) Phosphodiesterase inhibitors

Anagrelide is a cyclic AMP phosphodiesterase III inhibitor, and consequently has positive inotropic effects. The manufacturer recommends against its concurrent use with other phosphodiesterase III inhibitors, because of the potential increased inotropic effects, and they specifically mention **amrinone**, **enoximone**, **milrinone**, **olprinone** and **cilostazol**.[1,2]

(g) Sucralfate

The US manufacturer briefly mentions that an isolated case report suggested that sucralfate may interfere with the absorption of anagrelide;[1] however, the clinical relevance of this is unclear. In general, if an interaction is suspected with sucralfate, it is usual practice to separate administration by 2 hours.

(h) Other medications

The manufacturers briefly mention that anagrelide did not alter the pharmacokinetics of **digoxin** or **warfarin**, nor did **digoxin** or **warfarin** alter the pharmacokinetics of anagrelide.[1,2]

1. Agrylin (Anagrelide hydrochloride). Shire US Inc. US Prescribing information, August 2010.
2. Xagrid (Anagrelide hydrochloride). Shire Pharmaceuticals, Ltd. UK Summary of product characteristics, November 2010.
3. Harrison CN, Campbell PJ, Buck G, Wheatley K, East CL, Bareford D, Wilkins BS, van der Walt JD, Reilly JT, Grigg AP, Revell P, Woodcock BE, Green AR; United Kingdom Medical Research Council Primary Thrombocythemia 1 Study. Hydroxyurea compared with anagrelide in high-risk essential thrombocythemia. *N Engl J Med* (2005) 353, 33–45.
4. Raghavan M, Mazer MA, Brink DJ. Severe hypersensitivity pneumonitis associated with anagrelide. *Ann Pharmacother* (2003) 37, 1228–31.
5. Spencer EM, Lawrence DS. 'Double hit' from streptococcal pneumonia and hypersensitivity pneumonitis associated with anagrelide. *Clin Lab Haematol* (2006) 28, 63–5.

Antiplatelet drugs + Fish oils

The concurrent use of aspirin and fish oils caused at least additive effects on bleeding time in healthy subjects, but clinical studies in patients taking aspirin alone and with clopidogrel have found no evidence of an increase in incidence of bleeding episodes.

Clinical evidence

In a study in 8 healthy subjects, **aspirin** (325 mg on day one followed by 80 mg daily on days 2 and 3) prolonged the bleeding time by a mean of 2.2 minutes, whereas fish oils 4.5 g daily for 14 days prolonged the bleeding time by a mean of just 0.6 minutes, which was not statistically significant. The combination of aspirin and fish oils prolonged the bleeding time by a mean of 5 minutes, although this was stated to not be different from a purely additive effect.[1] In this, and a later study by the same researchers, fish oil did not increase the antiplatelet effect of aspirin.[1,2]

In a large placebo-controlled, randomised study of the effect of fish oils taken with either **aspirin** or warfarin over 9 months, there was no difference in the frequency of bleeding episodes between 119 patients taking **aspirin** 300 mg daily and fish oils 4 g daily, and 106 patients taking **aspirin** alone (10 episodes versus 8 episodes, respectively).[3]

Similarly, in another randomised study in 226 patients taking **aspirin** 325 mg daily with fish oils 8 g daily for 6 months, there was no difference in the incidence of bleeding when compared with 221 patients taking aspirin with placebo (corn oil).[4] In a retrospective, case-control study of patients prescribed omega-3 fatty acids with **aspirin** and **clopidogrel**, there was no statistically significant difference in the incidence of major bleeding (defined as bleeding that resulted in a decrease in haemoglobin of >2g, an intracerebral haemorrhage, or that which required hospitalisation) or minor bleeding (defined as epistaxis, abnormal bruising, or gastrointestinal bleeding that did not require hospitalisation or result in a decrease in haemoglobin of >2 g), when compared with control patients taking aspirin and clopidogrel only.[5] In another study, 28 healthy subjects were given escalating doses of *Lovaza* from 1 to 8 g daily (1 g approximately equivalent to **eicosapentaenoic acid** 465 mg and **docosahexaenoic acid** 375 mg) over 24 weeks, alone, with up to 325 mg **aspirin** daily, or with up to 325 mg **aspirin** daily and **clopidogrel** 75 mg daily. There was a general trend towards increased bleeding times compared with baseline across all three groups. However, only the increases seen in the group taking *Lovaza* alone were statistically significant (median bleeding time 150 seconds at baseline compared with up to 255 seconds in those taking *Lovaza* 4 g daily). The greatest proportional increase in bleeding time was seen in the patients taking *Lovaza* and **aspirin** (median bleeding time at baseline 240 seconds compared with 390 seconds in those taking *Lovaza* 2 g daily), and the smallest proportional increase was seen in the patients taking *Lovaza* with **aspirin** and **clopidogrel** (median bleeding time at baseline 570 seconds compared with 720 seconds in those taking *Lovaza* 1 g daily).[6] Bleeding times were also not increased by a single 325-mg dose of **aspirin** in healthy subjects taking *Promega* (omega-3 fatty acids) 8 g daily, when compared to a control group who were given a placebo (olive oil).[7] Note that an effect with multiple doses cannot be excluded by this result, although based on the studies cited above, this would seem unlikely. Furthermore, a review and associated commentary (which include some of the studies cited here), conclude that the risk of bleeding is not increased by omega-3 fatty acids in patients taking antiplatelets.[8,9]

For a case of life-threatening bleed after a minor fall in a patient who had been taking omega-3 fatty acids 6 g daily, together with aspirin and warfarin for a year, see 'Coumarins + Fish oils', p.427.

Mechanism

Uncertain. Fish oils contain omega-3 fatty acids, particularly **eicosapentaenoic acid** and **docosahexaenoic acid**. These are considered to have some antiplatelet activity, and might prolong the bleeding time. The exact mechanism by which they exert this effect is the subject of much research and debate. For example, one study suggests that the effect is brought about by an increase in the negative platelet surface charge,[6] and another suggests that changes to the platelet cell membrane structure might reduce platelet activation and thrombus formation.[10] Further study is needed. Theoretically, this antiplatelet activity could be additive with that of other antiplatelet drugs such as aspirin or clopidogrel.

Importance and management

It appears that the concurrent use of aspirin and fish oils might increase bleeding times, particularly at high doses of fish oils, but several clinical studies found no evidence of an increased incidence of bleeding episodes in patients taking aspirin with or without clopidogrel. The manufacturer of one prescription product, *Omacor* (omega-3-acid ethyl esters), notes that at high doses of 4 g daily it might increase the bleeding time, and advises caution in patients at a high risk of bleeding, but the only example they give is with anticoagulants.[11] Some caution on the concurrent use of fish oils with antiplatelets might be appropriate.

Note that *Omacor* is also licensed to be used with other standard therapies, including antiplatelets, as adjuvant treatment after myocardial infarction, but at a lower dose of just 1 g daily.[11]

1. Harris WS, Silveira S, Dujovne CA. The combined effects of N-3 fatty acids and aspirin on hemostatic parameters in man. *Thromb Res* (1990) 57, 517–26.
2. Larson MK, Ashmore JH, Harris KA, Vogelaar JL, Pottala JV, Sprehe M, Harris WS. Effects of omega-3 acid ethyl esters and aspirin, alone and in combination, on platelet function in healthy subjects. *Thromb Haemost* (2008) 100, 634–41.
3. Eritsland J, Arnesen H, Seljeflot I, Kierulf P. Long-term effects of *n*-3 polyunsaturated fatty acids on haemostatic variables and bleeding episodes in patients with coronary artery disease. *Blood Coag Fibrinol* (1995) 6, 17–22.

4. Leaf A, Jorgensen MB, Jacobs AK, Cote G, Schoenfeld DA, Scheer J, Weiner BH, Slack JD, Kellett MA, Raizner AE, Weber PC, Mahrer PR, Rossouw JE. Do fish oils prevent restenosis after coronary angioplasty? *Circulation* (1994) 90, 2248–57.
5. Watson PD, Joy PS, Nkonde C, Hessen SE, Karalis DG. Comparison of bleeding complications with omega-3 fatty acids + aspirin + clopidogrel–versus–aspirin + clopidogrel in patients with cardiovascular disease. *Am J Cardiol* (2009) 104, 1052–4.
6. Cohen MG, Rossi JS, Garbarino J, Bowling R, Motsinger-Reif AA, Schuler C, Dupont AG, Gabriel D. Insights into the inhibition of platelet activation by omega-3 polyunsaturated fatty acids: beyond aspirin and clopidogrel. *Thromb Res* (2011) 128, 335–40.
7. Mueller BA, Talbert RL, Tegeler CH, Prihoda TJ. The bleeding time effects of a single dose of aspirin in subjects receiving omega-3 fatty acid dietary supplementation. *J Clin Pharmacol* (1991) 31, 185–90.
8. Bays HE. Safety considerations with omega-3 fatty acid therapy. *Am J Cardiol* (2007) 99 (Suppl), 35C–43C.
9. Harris WS. Expert opinion: omega-3 fatty acids and bleeding-cause for concern? *Am J Cardiol* (2007) Mar 99 (Suppl), 44C–46C.
10. Larson MK, Tormoen GW, Weaver LJ, Luepke KJ, Patel IA, Hjelmen CE, Ensz NM, McComas LS, McCarty OJT. Exogenous modification of platelet membranes with the omega-3 fatty acids EPA and DHA reduces platelet procoagulant activity and thrombus formation. *Am J Physiol Cell Physiol* (2013) 304, C273–9.
11. Omacor (Omega-3-acid ethyl esters 90). Abbott Healthcare Products Ltd. UK Summary of product characteristics, April 2013.

Antiplatelet drugs + Ginkgo (*Ginkgo biloba*)

Ginkgo has been associated with platelet, bleeding, and clotting disorders, and there are isolated reports of serious adverse reactions after its concurrent use with antiplatelet drugs such as aspirin, clopidogrel, and ticlopidine.

Clinical evidence

A study in 10 healthy subjects found no significant increase in the antiplatelet effects of single doses of **clopidogrel** 75 mg or **cilostazol** 100 mg when a single dose of ginkgo 120 mg was added. However, the bleeding time was significantly increased when **cilostazol** was combined with ginkgo, although none of the subjects developed any significant adverse effects.[1] Another study[2] in 8 healthy subjects found that ginkgo 40 mg three times daily had no significant effect on the pharmacokinetics of a single dose of **ticlopidine** 250-mg taken on day 4.

A randomised, double-blind study in 55 patients with established peripheral artery disease (PAD) or with risk factors for developing PAD, found that the addition of ginkgo extract 300 mg (EGb 761) in divided doses to **aspirin** 325 mg daily did not have a significant effect on platelet aggregation. Five of the patients taking combined therapy reported nosebleeds or minor bleeding; however, 4 patients from the **aspirin**-only group also reported minor bleeding.[3] Similarly, a study in 41 healthy subjects found that 120-mg ginkgo coated-tablets (EGb 761) twice daily had no effect on the antiplatelet activity of **aspirin** 500 mg daily given for seven days. Minor bleeding was seen in a few subjects but this was attributed to the use of **aspirin**.[4] In an analysis of supplement use, 23% of 123 patients were currently taking supplements, and 4 patients were found to be taking ginkgo and **aspirin**. However, no problems from this use were found on review of the patients' notes.[5]

Nevertheless, a number of cases of clinically significant bleeding have been reported. A 70-year-old man developed spontaneous bleeding from the iris into the anterior chamber of his eye within one week of starting to take a ginkgo supplement (*Ginkoba*) tablet twice daily. He experienced recurrent episodes of blurred vision in one eye lasting about 15 minutes, during which he could see a red discoloration through his cornea. Each tablet contained 40 mg of concentrated (50:1) extract of ginkgo. He was also taking **aspirin** 325 mg daily, which he had taken uneventfully for 3 years since having coronary bypass surgery. He stopped taking the ginkgo but continued with the **aspirin**, and 3 months later had experienced no recurrence of the bleeding.[6] Another case reports persistent postoperative bleeding from a hip arthroplasty wound, which continued despite stopping **aspirin**. On closer questioning, the patient had continued to take ginkgo extract 120 mg daily postoperatively. The oozing from the wound gradually reduced when the ginkgo was stopped.

A search of Health Canada's database of spontaneous adverse reactions for the period January 1999 to June 2003 found 21 reports of suspected adverse reactions associated with ginkgo. Most of these involved platelet, bleeding, and clotting disorders. One report of a fatal gastrointestinal haemorrhage was associated with **ticlopidine** and ginkgo, both taken over 2 years along with other medications. Another report was of a stroke in a patient taking multiple drugs, including **clopidogrel**, **aspirin**, and a herbal product containing ginkgo.[7]

Mechanism

The reason for the bleeding is not known, but ginkgo extract contains ginkgolide B, which is a potent inhibitor of platelet-activating factor *in vitro*, which is needed for arachidonate-independent platelet aggregation. However, in one controlled study in healthy subjects, taking a ginkgo preparation alone for two weeks had no effect on platelet function.[8] Nevertheless, there are case reports of ginkgo supplements, on their own, being associated with prolonged bleeding times,[9-11] left and bilateral subdural haematomas,[9,12] a right parietal haematoma,[13] a retrobulbar haemorrhage,[14] post-laparoscopic cholecystectomy bleeding,[15] and subarachnoid haemorrhage.[10] Therefore it seems that the effects of ginkgo and conventional antiplatelet drugs can be additive, leading to bleeding complications on rare occasions.

Importance and management

The evidence from these case reports is too slim to advise patients taking aspirin, clopidogrel, or ticlopidine to avoid ginkgo, but some do recommend caution,[7] which seems prudent, especially as this is generally advised with most combinations of conventional antiplatelet drugs. There may also be a theoretical risk of increased bleeding if ginkgo is taken with other antiplatelet drugs; interactions have been reported with NSAIDs, some of which have antiplatelet effects (see 'NSAIDs + Ginkgo (*Ginkgo biloba*)', p.151).

1. Aruna D, Naidu MUR. Pharmacodynamic interaction studies of *Ginkgo biloba* with cilostazol and clopidogrel in healthy human subjects. *Br J Clin Pharmacol* (2007) 63, 333–8.
2. Lu W-J, Huang J-D, Lai M-L. The effects of ergoloid mesylates and Ginkgo biloba on the pharmacokinetics of ticlopidine. *J Clin Pharmacol* (2006) 46, 628–34.
3. Gardner CD, Zehnder JL, Rigby AJ, Nicholus JR, Farquhar JW. Effect of Ginkgo biloba (EGb 761) and aspirin on platelet aggregation and platelet function analysis among older adults at risk of cardiovascular disease: a randomized clinical trial. *Blood Coag Fibrinol* (2007) 18, 787–93.
4. Wolf HRD. Does *Ginkgo biloba* special extract EGb 761® provide additional effects on coagulation and bleeding when added to acetylsalicylic acid 500 mg daily? *Drugs R D* (2006) 7, 163–72.
5. Ly J, Percy L, Dhanani S. Use of dietary supplements and their interactions with prescription drugs in the elderly. *Am J Health-Syst Pharm* (2002) 59, 1759–62.
6. Rosenblatt M, Mindel J. Spontaneous hyphema associated with ingestion of *Ginkgo biloba* extract. *N Engl J Med* (1997) 336, 1108.
7. Griffiths J, Jordan S, Pilon S. Natural health products and adverse reactions. *Can Adverse React News* (2004) 14, 2–3.
8. Beckert BW, Concannon MJ, Henry SL, Smith DS, Puckett CL. The effect of herbal medicines on platelet function: an in vivo experiment and review of the literature. *Plast Reconstr Surg* (2007) 120, 2044–50.
9. Rowin J, Lewis SL. Spontaneous bilateral subdural hematomas associated with chronic *Ginkgo biloba* ingestion. *Neurology* (1996) 46, 1775–6.
10. Vale S. Subarachnoid haemorrhage associated with *Ginkgo biloba*. *Lancet* (1998) 352, 36.
11. Bebbington A, Kulkarni R, Roberts P. Ginkgo biloba: persistent bleeding after total hip arthroplasty caused by herbal self-medication. *J Arthroplasty* (2005) 20, 125–6.
12. Gilbert GJ. *Ginkgo biloba*. *Neurology* (1997) 48, 1137.
13. Benjamin J, Muir T, Briggs K, Pentland B. A case of cerebral haemorrhage – can *Ginkgo biloba* be implicated? *Postgrad Med J* (2001) 77, 112–13.
14. Fong KCS, Kinnear PE. Retrobulbar haemorrhage associated with chronic *Gingko* [sic] *biloba* ingestion. *Postgrad Med J* (2003) 79, 531–2.
15. Fessenden JM, Wittenborn W, Clarke L. Gingko biloba: a case report of herbal medicine and bleeding postoperatively from a laparoscopic cholecystectomy. *Am Surg* (2001) 67, 33–5.

Antiplatelet drugs + Laropiprant

Laropiprant appears to cause a transitory increase in the prolongation of bleeding time and inhibition of platelet aggregation caused by clopidogrel. Laropiprant had no clinically relevant effect on the prolongation of bleeding time and inhibition of platelet aggregation caused by aspirin, but laropiprant might increase the bleeding time if it is given with both aspirin and clopidogrel.

Clinical evidence

(a) Aspirin

In a randomised, placebo-controlled, crossover study in 14 healthy subjects, laropiprant 40 mg daily was given with aspirin 81 mg daily for 7 days. Laropiprant had no effect on aspirin-induced prolongation of bleeding time and inhibition of collagen-induced platelet aggregation.[1]

(b) Clopidogrel

In a randomised, placebo-controlled, crossover study in 20 healthy subjects, laropiprant 40 mg daily was given with clopidogrel 75 mg daily for 7 days. Although there was a slight increase in clopidogrel-induced bleeding time and ADP-induced platelet aggregation at 4 hours post-dose, when compared with clopidogrel alone, laropiprant did not have a statistically significant effect on bleeding times or platelet aggregation at 24 hours post-dose.[1]

(c) Clopidogrel with Aspirin

The UK manufacturer briefly notes that in a clinical study in patients taking aspirin 81 mg daily with clopidogrel 75 mg daily, a transient increase in platelet aggregation was seen at 4 hours post-dose; however, this was effect was not seen across the dosing interval.[2]

Mechanism

Laropiprant is an antagonist of prostaglandin D_2 receptor 1, and therefore it was suggested it might have some effect on platelet function (enhancement or inhibition). The findings with clopidogrel suggest it has some inhibitory activity of the thromboxane A_2 receptor.[1]

Importance and management

Evidence for an interaction between laropiprant and antiplatelet drugs is limited, but the studies cited were well designed. The evidence suggests that laropiprant might cause a transient increase in the pharmacological effects of **clopidogrel**; however, bearing in mind that the increase in bleeding time was not sustained it seems unlikely that dose adjustments of these antiplatelet drugs would be necessary. Furthermore, the manufacturer considers this interaction unlikely to be clinically important.[2] Clopidogrel is often used in combination with antiplatelet doses of aspirin, and it appears that there might be a risk of prolongation of bleeding time when laropiprant is used with both **clopidogrel and aspirin**. Therefore, until more is known, it would seem prudent to be alert for signs of bleeding whenever clopidogrel is used with laropiprant.

The pharmacological evidence suggests that it is unlikely that antiplatelet doses of **aspirin** would be affected by concurrent use with laropiprant.

Laropiprant is only available as a combination product with nicotinic acid, to reduce the incidence of nicotinic acid-induced flushing.

1. Dallob A, Luo W-L, Luk JM, Ratcliffe L, Johnson-Levonas AO, Schwartz JI, Dishy V, Kraft WK, De Hoon JN, Van Hecken A, Lepeleire ID, Radziszewski W, Wagner JA, Lai E. The effects of laropiprant, a selective prostaglandin D2 receptor 1 antagonist, on the antiplatelet activity of clopidogrel or aspirin. *Platelets* (2011) 22, 495–503.
2. Tredaptive (Nicotinic acid with Laropiprant). Merck Sharp & Dohme Ltd. UK Summary of product characteristics, April 2012.

Antiplatelet drugs + Policosanol

Policosanol has antiplatelet effects, which may be additive with those of other antiplatelet drugs.

Clinical evidence

In a randomised study, four groups, each containing 10 or 11 subjects, were given placebo, policosanol 20 mg daily, **aspirin** 100 mg daily, or both drugs together, for 7 days. Adrenaline-induced platelet aggregation was reduced in the group given **aspirin** and policosanol by about 35% more than in the group given **aspirin** alone: the effects of **aspirin** and policosanol were approximately additive. Furthermore, collagen-induced platelet aggregation was reduced in the group given **aspirin** and policosanol by about 10% more than in the group given **aspirin** alone. One patient taking both drugs suffered from bleeding gums. There was no significant effect on coagulation time.[1] A 3-year study, primarily designed to assess the safety and efficacy of policosanol in patients taking beta blockers, included 32 patients taking antiplatelet drugs (mainly **aspirin**). No adverse effects related to bleeding were reported.[2]

Mechanism

Additive antiplatelet effects.

Importance and management

The concurrent use of two conventional antiplatelet drugs is not uncommon, and so concurrent use of policosanol and aspirin need not be avoided. However, because platelet aggregation was reduced significantly, and a bleeding event was experienced, caution is perhaps warranted when taking policosanol supplements with aspirin or any other antiplatelet drug.

1. Arruzazabala ML, Valdés S, Más R, Carbajal D, Fernández L. Comparative study of policosanol, aspirin and the combination therapy policosanol-aspirin on platelet aggregation in healthy volunteers. *Pharmacol Res* (1997) 36, 293–7.
2. Castaño G, Mas R, Gámez R, Fernández J, Illnait J, Fernández L, Mendoza S, Mesa M, Gutiérrez JA, López E. Concomitant use of policosanol and *β*-blockers in older patients. *Int J Clin Pharmacol Res* (2004) 24, 65–77.

Antiplatelet drugs + SSRIs or SNRIs

The bleeding risk associated with antiplatelet drugs such as aspirin, clopidogrel and ticlopidine might be further increased by the concurrent use of an SSRI, although the data appears to be conflicting. The SNRIs are predicted to interact similarly.

Clinical evidence

A retrospective study[1] of the UK general practice research database identified 1 651 cases of upper gastrointestinal bleeding diagnosed between 1993 and 1997. The concurrent use of an SSRI increased the risk of bleeding 3-fold, when compared with 10 000 control patients. In addition, the concurrent use of an SSRI with **aspirin** was associated with a relative excess risk of upper gastrointestinal bleeding of 3.5. Another retrospective study found that the observed-expected ratio of an upper gastrointestinal bleed was 3.6 in patients taking an SSRI (17 320 patients), 2.5 in patients taking low-dose **aspirin** (26 762 patients), but increased to 5.2 in patients taking both an SSRI and low-dose **aspirin** (2 640 patients).[2] A retrospective case-control study in 579 patients diagnosed with gastrointestinal bleeding (upper and lower) found that the concurrent use of SSRIs with low-dose **aspirin** increased the risk of gastrointestinal bleeding above the risk found with each drug separately (odds ratio 2.1 for the combination, compared with 1.8 and 1.5 for **aspirin** and an SSRI, respectively).[3] In addition, a case report describes gastrointestinal haemorrhage in a 73-year-old patient taking **clopidogrel** 75 mg daily, which occurred 2 weeks after starting **paroxetine** 20 mg daily.[4]

In contrast, a case-control study of hospital admissions for gastrointestinal bleeding reported no substantial increase in the risk of a gastrointestinal bleed in patients taking an SSRI. Furthermore, an interaction with low-dose **aspirin** was not seen.[5] Another retrospective study using the UK general practice research database, found no evidence of an interaction between the SSRIs and **clopidogrel**.[6] Some workers have agreed with these results and found no evidence to suggest that SSRIs are more likely to cause gastrointestinal bleeding than other drugs.[7] In the SADHART study, which looked at the efficacy and cardiac safety of **sertraline** in the treatment of depression in patients with acute coronary syndromes, bleeding was not reported as an adverse effect of concurrent use, even though 170 of the 186 patients randomised to treatment with sertraline were also taking **aspirin**. Thirty-five (19%) of the **sertraline** group were taking other antiplatelet drugs such as **clopidogrel** and **ticlopidine**.[8] A sub-study of SADHART, which included 25 patients taking **sertraline**, found that the use of **sertraline** was associated with a decrease in platelet/endothelial activation, suggesting that **sertraline** did not have an additional antiplatelet effect.[9] Similarly, a randomised, placebo-controlled study in patients with coronary artery disease found no increased risk in reported bleeding in those taking **citalopram** 20 to 40 mg daily, when compared with placebo. Of the patients taking **citalopram**, 80% were also taking **aspirin** and 25% were taking other antiplatelet drugs (not specified).[10] A study in 20 healthy male smokers found that **paroxetine** 20 mg daily for 21 days did not increase the platelet inhibition produced by **aspirin** 100 mg daily from days 18 to 21.[11]

An Australian study of 4 136 coronary artery bypass graft (CABG) patients found that in the 105 patients who were taking an SSRI (**citalopram, escitalopram, fluoxetine, fluvoxamine, paroxetine**, or **sertraline**) or an SNRI (**duloxetine** or **venlafaxine**) at the time of surgery, the risk of bleeding events was not increased. Similarly, taking an SSRI or SNRI with concurrent antiplatelet medications did not increase this risk.[12] Another study in CABG patients similarly found that the use of an SSRI (**citalopram, escitalopram, fluoxetine, paroxetine**, or **sertraline**), **duloxetine**, and **venlafaxine** was not associated with an increased risk of in-hospital mortality or any bleeding event during a 3-year period, when compared with use of a non-SSRI antidepressant.[13] A further study on CABG patients found that current use (within 90 days of surgery) or former use (more than 90 days prior to surgery) of an SSRI (**citalopram, fluoxetine, fluvoxamine, paroxetine**, or **sertraline**) or **venlafaxine** did not increase the risk of requiring red blood cell transfusion post-surgery, when compared with those who had never taken an SSRI.[14]

Mechanism

Serotonin is not synthesised by platelets but is taken up into platelets from the bloodstream. At therapeutic doses, SSRIs can block this uptake leading to serotonin depletion within the platelet. Serotonin released from platelets has an important role in regulating the haemostatic response to injury as it potentiates platelet aggregation. Therefore SSRIs might impair the haemostatic function of the platelets, which might increase the risk of bleeding,[15] particularly in the presence of other antiplatelet drugs.

Importance and management

There appears to be an association between the use of antidepressant drugs that interfere with serotonin reuptake and the occurrence of bleeding, including gastrointestinal bleeding: **citalopram, fluoxetine, fluvoxamine, paroxetine**, and **sertraline** have all been reported to cause bleeding.[15] It therefore seems reasonable to anticipate that the risks of bleeding with an antiplatelet drug might be increased by an SSRI. However, the overall evidence for an increased risk of bleeding when giving an SSRI with low-dose aspirin or clopidogrel is conflicting, with some studies demonstrating an increased risk and others suggesting no additional antiplatelet effect occurs. There appears to be no published data assessing the risk of the concurrent use of SSRIs with other antiplatelet drugs, such as **prasugrel, ticagrelor**, or the **glycoprotein IIb/IIIa-receptor antagonists**; however, given the suggested mechanism, an interaction would seem possible.

In general, the UK manufacturers of SSRIs advise caution on the concurrent use of drugs that affect platelet function (they name aspirin[16-21], **dipyridamole**,[17,18] and **ticlopidine**[17,18]). Similarly, the manufacturers of the SNRIs, **desvenlafaxine, duloxetine, milnacipran, levomilnacipran** and **venlafaxine**, advise caution on their use in patients taking aspirin,[22-24] antiplatelet drugs,[25,26] or other drugs that affect coagulation.[22-26] This would seem prudent, particularly in patients taking more than one antiplatelet drug, such as aspirin and clopidogrel for acute coronary syndromes or coronary stents, where the risk of bleeding from this combination alone appears to be important (see 'Aspirin and/or Clopidogrel + Cilostazol', p.781). Note that in 2012 the FDA advised that the maximum dose of **citalopram** in patients taking a CYP2C19 inhibitor [which would include **ticagrelor**] should be 20 mg daily because concurrent use can lead to increased citalopram concentrations and increase the risk of QT interval prolongation and Torsade de pointes.[27]

Consideration should be given to prescribing gastroprotective drugs in those at high risk of gastrointestinal bleeding, such as elderly patients or those with a history of gastrointestinal bleeding. Note that this advice would also apply to those patients taking analgesic-dose aspirin with an SSRI or SNRI.

For a discussion on the theoretical pharmacokinetic interaction of fluoxetine and fluvoxamine with clopidogrel, see 'Clopidogrel + Proton pump inhibitors and other CYP2C19 inhibitors', p.788.

1. De Abajo FJ, Rodríguez LAG, Montero D. Association between selective serotonin reuptake inhibitors and upper gastrointestinal bleeding: population based case-control study. *BMJ* (1999) 319, 1106–9.
2. Dalton SO, Johansen C, Mellemkjær L, Nørgård B, Sørensen HT, Olsen JH. Use of selective serotonin reuptake inhibitors and risk of upper gastrointestinal tract bleeding. A population-based cohort study. *Arch Intern Med* (2003) 163, 59–64.
3. Wessinger S, Kaplan M, Choi L, Williams M, Lau C, Sharp L, Crowell MD, Keshavarzian A, Jones MP. Increased use of selective serotonin reuptake inhibitors in patients admitted with gastrointestinal haemorrhage: a multicentre retrospective analysis. *Aliment Pharmacol Ther* (2006) 23, 937–44.
4. Fernández-Fernández FJ, Ameneiros-Lago E, Martínez-Calvo L, Sesma P. Hemorragia digestiva alta asociada a tratamiento con clopidogrel y paroxetina. *Med Clin (Barc)* (2008) 131, 357–8.
5. Vidal X, Ibáñez L, Vendrell L, Conforti A, Laporte J-R, on behalf of the Spanish-Italian collaborative group for the epidemiology of gastrointestinal bleeding. *Drug Safety* (2008), 31, 159–68.
6. Opatrny L, Delaney JA, Suissa S. Gastro-intestinal haemorrhage risks of selective serotonin receptor antagonist therapy: a new look. *Br J Clin Pharmacol* (2008) 66, 76–81.
7. Dunn NR, Pearce GL, Shakir SAW. Association between SSRIs and upper gastrointestinal bleeding. SSRIs are no more likely than other drugs to cause such bleeding. *BMJ* (2000) 320, 1405–6.
8. Glassman AH, O'Connor CM, Califf RM, Swedberg K, Schwartz P, Bigger JT, Krishnan KRR, van Zyl LT, Swenson JR, Finkel MS, Landau C, Shapiro PA, Pepine CJ, Mardekian J, Harrison WM, for the Sertraline Antidepressant Heart Attack Randomized Trial (SADHART) group. Sertraline treatment of major depression in patients with acute MI or unstable angina. *JAMA* (2002) 288, 701–9.
9. Serebruany VL, Glassman AH, Malinin AI, Nemeroff CB, Musselman DL, van Zyl LT, Finkel MS, Krishnan KRR, Gaffney M, Harrison W, Califf RM, O'Connor CM; for the SADHART study group. Platelet/ endothelial biomarkers in depressed patients treated with the selective serotonin reuptake inhibitor sertraline after acute coronary events: the Sertraline AntiDepressant Heart Attack Randomized Trial (SADHART) platelet substudy. *Circulation* (2003) 108, 939–44.
10. Lespérance F, Frasure-Smith N, Koszycki D, Laliberté M-A, van Zyl LT, Baker B, Swenson JR, Ghatavi K, Abramson BL, Dorian P, Guertin M-C for the CREATE investigators. Effects of citalopram and interpersonal psychotherapy on depression in patients with coronary artery disease: the Canadian Cardiac Randomized Evaluation of Antidepressant and Psychotherapy Efficacy (CREATE) trial. *JAMA* (2007) 297, 367–79.
11. Kotzailias N, Andonovski T, Dukic A, Serebruany VL, Jilma B. Antiplatelet activity during coadministration of the selective serotonin reuptake inhibitor paroxetine and aspirin in male smokers: a randomized, placebo-controlled, double-blind trial. *J Clin Pharmacol* (2006) 46, 468–75.
12. Tully PJ, Cardinal T, Bennetts JS, Baker RA. Selective serotonin reuptake inhibitors, venlafaxine and duloxetine are associated with in hospital morbidity but not bleeding or late mortality after coronary artery bypass graft surgery. *Heart Lung Circ* (2012) 21, 206–14.
13. Kim DH, Daskalakis C, Whellan DJ, Whitman IR, Hohmann S, Medvedev S, Kraft WK. Safety of selective serotonin reuptake inhibitor in adults undergoing coronary artery bypass grafting. *Am J Cardiol* (2009) 103, 1391–5.

14. Andreasen JJ, Riis Am Hjortdal VE, Jørgensen J, Sørensen HT, Johnsen SP. Effect of selective serotonin reuptake inhibitors on requirement for allogeneic red blood cell transfusion following coronary artery bypass surgery. *Am J Cardiovasc Drugs* (2006) 6, 243–50.
15. De Abajo FJ, Montero D, Rodríguez LA, Madurga M. Antidepressants and risk of upper gastrointestinal bleeding. *Basic Clin Pharmacol Toxicol* (2006) 98, 304–10.
16. Prozac (Fluoxetine hydrochloride). Eli Lilly and Company Ltd. UK Summary of product characteristics, October 2014.
17. Cipramil Tablets (Citalopram hydrobromide). Lundbeck Ltd. UK Summary of product characteristics, July 2015.
18. Cipralex Tablets (Escitalopram oxalate). Lundbeck Ltd. UK Summary of product characteristics, September 2013.
19. Paroxetine Film-Coated Tablets (Paroxetine hydrochloride anhydrous). Actavis UK Ltd. UK Summary of product characteristics, June 2015.
20. Faverin (Fluvoxamine maleate). BGP Products Ltd. UK Summary of product characteristics, August 2015.
21. Lustral (Sertraline hydrochloride). Pfizer Ltd. UK Summary of product characteristics, March 2015.
22. Pristiq (Desvenlafaxine succinate). Wyeth Pharmaceuticals Inc. US Prescribing information, July 2014.
23. Savella (Milnacipran hydrochloride). Forest Pharmaceuticals, Inc. US Prescribing information, November 2013.
24. Fetzima (Levomilnacipran hydrochloride). Forest Pharmaceuticals, Inc. US Prescribing information, July 2014.
25. Cymbalta. (Duloxetine hydrochloride). Eli Lilly and Company Ltd. UK Summary of product characteristics, March 2014.
26. Efexor XL (Venlafaxine hydrochloride). Pfizer Ltd. UK Summary of product characteristics, December 2013.
27. FDA. Drug safety communication: Revised recommendations for Celexa (citalopram hydrochloride) related to a potential risk of abnormal heart rhythms with high doses. March 28, 2012. Available at: http://www.fda.gov/Drugs/DrugSafety/ucm297391.htm (accessed 06/10/15).

Aspirin and/or Clopidogrel + Cilostazol

The concurrent use of more than one antiplatelet drug might increase the risk of bleeding. However, the incidence of bleeding does not appear to be further increased if cilostazol is added to low-dose aspirin or to clopidogrel. In contrast, in patients taking clopidogrel and aspirin, the addition of cilostazol might increase the risk of bleeding.

Clinical evidence

A. Dual antiplatelet therapy

(a) Aspirin with Cilostazol

In a randomised, placebo-controlled study in 11 healthy subjects, giving aspirin 325 mg daily for 5 days with cilostazol 100 mg twice daily increased the inhibition of ADP-induced platelet aggregation by 23 to 35%, when compared with the use of cilostazol alone. Aspirin also appeared to cause a 22% increase in the AUC of cilostazol. However, there were no statistically significant additive effects on arachidonic acid-induced platelet aggregation, and no clinically relevant effects on prothrombin time, aPTT, or bleeding times.[1] Similarly, as part of a study designed to investigate the bleeding effects of the concurrent use of multiple antiplatelet drugs, 26 patients with peripheral arterial disease were given single and dual combinations of aspirin 325 mg daily, cilostazol 100 mg twice daily, consecutively, with a 14-day washout period between each phase. There was no difference in bleeding time on the concurrent use of cilostazol and aspirin, compared with aspirin alone. Note that, cilostazol alone had little effect on bleeding time, whereas aspirin alone prolonged bleeding time.[2]

In addition, the US manufacturer reports that in 8 randomised, placebo-controlled clinical studies of cilostazol, a total of 201 patients also received aspirin, and the incidence of bleeding in these patients was no greater than that seen with equivalent doses of aspirin and placebo. The most frequent doses and mean duration of aspirin use were 75 to 81 mg daily for 137 days (107 patients) and 325 mg daily for 54 days (85 patients).[3] Furthermore, the large post-marketing randomised, placebo-controlled CASTLE study found that, in the subset of patients also taking aspirin, the concurrent use of cilostazol 100 mg twice daily did not increase the risk of serious bleeding, when compared with placebo (2.1 % versus 2.1%).[4]

(b) Clopidogrel with Cilostazol

The UK manufacturer of cilostazol notes that, in healthy subjects, the concurrent use of cilostazol and clopidogrel did not have an effect on platelet count, prothrombin time, or aPTT. Clopidogrel alone prolonged bleeding time, and the addition of cilostazol did not increase this further.[5] The US manufacturer of cilostazol notes that multiple-dose clopidogrel does not have an important effect on the steady-state plasma concentration of cilostazol.[3]

As part of a study designed to investigate the bleeding effects of the concurrent use of multiple antiplatelet drugs, 26 patients with peripheral arterial disease were given either clopidogrel 75 mg daily or cilostazol 100 mg twice daily then both drugs together. There was no difference in bleeding time with the concurrent use of cilostazol and clopidogrel, when compared with clopidogrel alone. Note that, cilostazol alone had little effect on bleeding time, whereas clopidogrel alone more than doubled bleeding time.[2]

B. Triple antiplatelet therapy

Various studies have looked at whether adding cilostazol to aspirin and clopidogrel further increases bleeding risk over what you would expect with the concurrent use of aspirin and clopidogrel alone, see 'Aspirin + Clopidogrel and related drugs', p.782.

As part of one pharmacological study designed to investigate the bleeding effects of the concurrent use of multiple antiplatelet drugs, 26 patients with peripheral arterial disease were given the dual combination of aspirin 325 mg daily and clopidogrel 75 mg daily, and then the triple combination including the addition of cilostazol 100 mg twice daily. Adding cilostazol to aspirin and clopidogrel did not further increase bleeding times compared with aspirin and clopidogrel (17.9 minutes versus 17.4 minutes).[2] Another study found that the addition of cilostazol to aspirin and clopidogrel increased the inhibition of ADP-induced platelet aggregation in patients undergoing primary percutaneous coronary intervention, although cilostazol had no additive effect on aspirin-induced antiplatelet activity. There was no major bleeding and no discontinuation of cilostazol because of adverse drug reactions.[6] Similar findings were reported in another study.[7]

A variety of clinical studies have investigated the beneficial effects of adding cilostazol to the concurrent use of aspirin with clopidogrel. Although these studies were primarily designed to assess the benefits of concurrent use they did also report on bleeding events. The key findings of some of them were:

- The randomised DECLARE-Long study evaluated the efficacy of cilostazol 100 mg twice daily with clopidogrel 75 mg and aspirin 200 mg daily (triple therapy) in 250 patients with drug-eluting stents by comparing treatment with 250 similar patients taking just aspirin and clopidogrel (dual therapy). No major bleeding requiring transfusion occurred in either the triple or dual therapy group. Only 2 patients in the triple therapy group developed minor bleeding (ecchymoses) compared with 4 in the dual therapy group. However, the incidence of rash and gastrointestinal adverse effects (known adverse effects of cilostazol) was more common in the group that also took cilostazol (24 compared with 5 patients). There was also a higher discontinuation rate in the triple therapy patients.[8] A similar study by the same authors in patients with diabetes (DECLARE-DIABETES) also found similar results.[9]
- The randomised CREST study found no difference in bleeding rates (major or minor) between 354 patients taking aspirin, clopidogrel and cilostazol after percutaneous coronary intervention compared with those taking aspirin and clopidogrel (351 patients). Compliance with the triple therapy was similar to dual therapy and the only increased adverse effect reported in the triple therapy group was headache.[10]
- A randomised study found no increase in bleeding when cilostazol was added to dual therapy with aspirin and clopidogrel.[11]
- An observational cohort study in patients undergoing coronary intervention and given aspirin 200 mg daily, clopidogrel 75 mg daily for at least 6 months and cilostazol 100 mg twice daily for at least 4 weeks found no increase in the risk of major or minor bleeding compared with aspirin and clopidogrel only.[12]
- In the large post-marketing randomised, placebo-controlled CASTLE study in patients with peripheral arterial disease, the concurrent use of cilostazol 100 mg twice daily with aspirin and clopidogrel did not increase the risk of serious bleeding, when compared with patients taking placebo.[4]

Mechanism

Antiplatelet drugs prolong the bleeding time, and the risks might be additive with the combinations, which might increase the risk of clinically relevant bleeding. However, note that the extent of prolongation in bleeding time varies between the individual drugs. For example, in one small study, clopidogrel 75 mg daily prolonged the bleeding time 2.37-fold, aspirin 325 mg daily prolonged the bleeding time 1.55-fold and cilostazol 100 mg twice daily prolonged the bleeding time 1.26-fold (not statistically significant).[2]

Importance and management

The concurrent use of multiple antiplatelet drugs would generally be expected to increase the risk of bleeding; however, the likelihood and severity of bleeding appears to depend on the antiplatelet combinations given. Based on clinical trial data, the addition of cilostazol to aspirin or clopidogrel does not appear to further increase the risk of bleeding, relative to aspirin or clopidogrel alone. Triple therapy regimens containing cilostazol, aspirin, and clopidogrel also do not appear to further increase bleeding risks, when compared with the concurrent use of aspirin and clopidogrel. However, in 2013 the European Medicines Agency conducted a review of all available evidence (including reports of serious suspected adverse effects such as serious bleeding) on the risks and benefits of cilostazol. It concluded that there might be an increased risk of bleeding when cilostazol is taken with aspirin and clopidogrel, but that cilostazol with aspirin or clopidogrel alone is not likely to increase the risk. As a result, in the EU the use of cilostazol with two or more other antiplatelet drugs or anticoagulants is contraindicated.[13] In the US, caution is advised if cilostazol is given with any other antiplatelet drug.[3]

1. Mallikaarjun S, Forbes WP, Bramer SL. Interaction potential and tolerability of the coadministration of cilostazol and aspirin. *Clin Pharmacokinet* (1999) 37 (Suppl 2), 87–93.
2. Wilhite DB, Comerota AJ, Schmeider FA, Throm RC, Gaughan JP, Rao AK. Managing PAD with multiple antiplatelet inhibitors: the effect of combination therapy on bleeding time. *J Vasc Surg* (2008) 38, 710–3.
3. Pletal (Cilostazol). Otsuka America Pharmaceutical, Inc. US Prescribing information, May 2007.
4. Hiatt WR, Money SR, Brass EP. Long-term safety of cilostazol in patients with peripheral artery disease: the CASTLE study (Cilostazol: A Study in Long-Term Effects). *J Vasc Surg* (2008) 47, 330–6.
5. Pletal (Cilostazol). Otsuka Pharmaceuticals (UK) Ltd. UK Summary of product characteristics, October 2013.
6. Kim J-Y, Lee K, Shin M, Ahn M, Choe H, Yoo B-S, Yoon J, Choe K-H, Lee S-H. Cilostazol could ameliorate platelet responsiveness to clopidogrel in patients undergoing primary percutaneous coronary intervention. *Circ J* (2007) 71, 1867–72.
7. Lee B-K, Lee S-W, Park S-W, Lee S-W, Park D-W, Kim Y-H, Lee CW, Hong M-K, Kim J-J, Jang S, Chi H-S, Park S-J. Effects of triple antiplatelet therapy (aspirin, clopidogrel, and cilostazol) on platelet aggregation and P-selectin expression in patients undergoing coronary artery stent implantation. *Am J Cardiol* (2007) 100, 610–14.
8. Lee S-W, Park S-W, Kim Y-H, Yun S-C, Park D-W, Lee CW, Hong M-K, Kim H-S, Ko J-K, Park J-H, Lee J-H, Choi SW, Seong I-W, Cho YH, Lee N-H, Kim JH, Chun K-J, Park S-J for the DECLARE-Long study investigators. Comparison of triple versus dual antiplatelet therapy after drug-eluting stent implantation (from the DECLARE-Long trial). *Am J Cardiol* (2007) 100, 1103–8.
9. Lee S-W, Park S-W, Kim Y-H, Yun S-C, Park D-W, Lee CW, Hong M-K, Kim H-S, Ko J-K, Park J-H, Lee J-H, Choi SW, Seong I-W, Cho YH, Lee N-H, Kim JH, Chun K-J, Park S-J. Drug-eluting stenting

followed by cilostazol treatment reduces late restenosis in patients with diabetes mellitus. The DECLARE-DIABETES trial (a randomized comparison of triple antiplatelet therapy with dual antiplatelet therapy after drug-eluting stent implantation in diabetic patients). *J Am Coll Cardiol* (2008) 51, 1181–7.
10. Douglas JS, Holmes DR, Kereiakes DJ, Grines CL, Block E, Ghazzal ZMB, Morris DC, Liberman H, Parker K, Jurkovitz C, Murrah N, Foster J, Hyde P, Mancini GBJ, Weintraub WS for the Cilostazol for Restenosis Trial (CREST) Investigators. Coronary stent restenosis in patients treated with cilostazol. *Circulation* (2005) 112, 2826–32.
11. Han Y, Li Y, Wang S, Jing Q, Wang Z, Wang D, Shu Q, Tang X. Cilostazol in addition to aspirin and clopidogrel improves long-term outcomes after percutaneous coronary intervention in patients with acute coronary syndromes: a randomized, controlled study. *Am Heart J* (2009) 157, 733–9.
12. Lee S-W, Park S-W, Yun S-C, Kim Y-H, Park D-W, Kim W-J, Lee J-Y, Lee CW, Hong M-K, Kim J-J, Park S-J. Triple antiplatelet therapy reduces ischemic events after drug-eluting stent implantation: Drug-eluting stenting followed by Cilostazol treatment Reduces Adverse Serious cardiac Events (DECREASE registry). *Am Heart J* (2010) 159, 284–91.
13. European Medicines Agency. European Medicines Agency recommends restricting use of cilostazol-containing medicines. June 2013. Available at: http://www.ema.europa.eu/docs/en_GB/document_library/Referrals_document/Cilostazol_31/WC500148975.pdf (accessed 22/10/15).

Aspirin + Clopidogrel and related drugs

The concurrent use of more than one antiplatelet drug might increase the risk of bleeding. There is a further increased risk of bleeding if clopidogrel, prasugrel, or ticlopidine are given with low-dose aspirin, and the risk with prasugrel appears to be greater than that with clopidogrel.

Clinical evidence

A. Dual antiplatelet therapy

(a) Aspirin with Clopidogrel

As part of a study to assess short-term prolongation of bleeding, 26 patients with peripheral arterial disease were given either aspirin 325 mg daily or clopidogrel 75 mg daily or both drugs together for 14 days. Concurrent use increased bleeding time compared with either drug alone (17.4 minutes versus 6.6 minutes for aspirin alone and 10.2 minutes for clopidogrel alone).[1] Similarly, in a study in 7 healthy subjects, clopidogrel 75 mg and aspirin 150 mg daily for 2 days caused a 3.4-fold increase in bleeding time relative to baseline, and when the clopidogrel dose was increased to 300 mg there was a 5-fold increase in bleeding time.[2]

A variety of clinical studies have investigated the beneficial effects of using the combination of aspirin with clopidogrel. Although these studies were primarily designed to assess the benefits of concurrent use they did also report on bleeding events. The key findings of some of them were:

- In patients with recent acute coronary syndrome (CURE) there was a higher incidence of major bleeding events on the concurrent use of clopidogrel 75 mg daily and aspirin 75 to 325 mg daily compared with aspirin alone (3.7% versus 2.7%, respectively).[3]
- In patients with recent stroke or transient ischaemic attack (MATCH) there was a higher incidence of life-threatening bleeding events following the use of clopidogrel 75 mg daily with aspirin 75 mg daily, when compared with clopidogrel alone (2.6% versus 1.3%, respectively).[4]
- In patients with clinically evident cardiovascular disease or multiple atherosclerotic risk factors (CHARISMA) there was a higher incidence in the risk of moderate and severe bleeding following the use of clopidogrel 75 mg daily with aspirin 75 to 162 mg daily, when compared with aspirin alone (moderate 2.1% and 1.3%, respectively, severe 1.7% and 1.3%, respectively).[5] A post-hoc analysis of this trial found that the hazard ratio for severe or life-threatening bleeding was greater for aspirin doses above 100 mg, than for doses of 100 mg (1.05 versus 0.85, respectively), but neither was statistically significant.[6]
- In patients with atrial fibrillation (ACTIVE A) there was a higher incidence of bleeding in patients taking clopidogrel 75 mg daily with aspirin 75 to 100 mg daily, compared with aspirin alone. The relative risk of major and minor bleeding with concurrent use compared with aspirin alone was 1.57 and 2.42, respectively.[7]
- In patients undergoing percutaneous coronary intervention (CREDO) the risk of major bleeding at 1 year was higher in those patients given clopidogrel 75 mg daily with aspirin 81 to 325 mg daily, when compared with placebo (8.8% versus 6.7%), but this was not statistically significant.[8]
- In the large COMMIT study in patients with acute myocardial infarction, the addition of clopidogrel 75 mg daily to aspirin 162 mg daily did not increase the incidence of fatal or non-fatal cerebral, and major non-cerebral, bleeding, when compared with placebo (0.58% versus 0.55%, respectively).[9]

In addition, a retrospective, population based, case-control study identified 1 443 cases of serious upper gastrointestinal bleeding, and in 380 of these cases, patients were taking antiplatelet drugs and/or anticoagulants. The study found that the adjusted odds ratio for serious upper gastrointestinal bleeding with clopidogrel alone was 1.1 and, for low-dose aspirin alone was 1.8, but that this rose to 7.4 in patients taking clopidogrel with aspirin.[10]

Furthermore, a number of case reports describe adverse effects when using the combination:

- Spontaneous haemarthrosis of the knee has been associated with the concurrent use of aspirin and clopidogrel in one patient.[11]
- A report describes two surgical cases, which were complicated by bleeding associated with the combination of aspirin and clopidogrel. In both cases the bleeding was delayed, in that it was not obvious until the end of surgery, causing unanticipated surgical re-exploration.[12]
- Further reports describe increased peri-operative bleeding in patients taking both aspirin and clopidogrel.[13,14]

(b) Aspirin with Prasugrel

The US manufacturer of prasugrel reports that the concurrent use of aspirin 150 mg daily did not alter the antiplatelet effects of prasugrel, but increased the bleeding time compared with either drug alone.[15]

In the TRITON-TIMI 38 study, 13 608 patients with acute coronary syndromes taking aspirin 75 to 162 mg daily and undergoing percutaneous coronary intervention were randomised to receive a 60-mg loading dose of prasugrel followed by 10 mg daily or a 300-mg loading dose of clopidogrel, followed by 75 mg daily. The overall incidence of major bleeding was 2.4% in patients given prasugrel compared with 1.8% in those given clopidogrel, with a hazard ratio of 1.32. Life-threatening bleeding was also higher in the prasugrel group (hazard ratio 1.52), as was fatal bleeding (hazard ratio 4.19).In a post-hoc analysis, patients over 75 years of age, weighing less than 60 kg, or with a history of transient ischaemic attacks or stroke appeared to be at particular risk of bleeding events with prasugrel when compared with clopidogrel.[16]

(c) Aspirin with Ticagrelor

The UK and US manufacturers of ticagrelor state that patients with acute coronary syndromes given ticagrelor and aspirin had an increased risk of major bleeding and bleeds requiring medical attention. Furthermore, the efficacy of ticagrelor is decreased by higher doses of aspirin.[17,18]

(d) Aspirin with Ticlopidine

Aspirin given with ticlopidine appears to inhibit platelet aggregation more than either drug alone.[19,20] The rate of haemorrhagic complications at 30 days in the STARS study for ticlopidine 250 mg twice daily with low-dose aspirin was 5.5% compared with 1.8% for aspirin alone.[21]

Mechanism

Antiplatelet drugs prolong the bleeding time, and the risks might be additive with the combinations, which might increase the risk of clinically relevant bleeding. However, note that the extent of prolongation in bleeding time varies between the individual drugs.

Importance and management

The concurrent use of multiple antiplatelet drugs would generally be expected to increase the risk of bleeding; however, the likelihood and severity of bleeding appears to depend on the antiplatelet combinations given. The clinical benefit of giving **clopidogrel** with aspirin is established for some indications; however, it is known to increase the risk of bleeding relative to either drug alone. For this reason, the UK manufacturer of clopidogrel recommends that the dose of aspirin should not exceed 100 mg daily, as higher doses are associated with higher bleeding risks.[22] Similarly, although **prasugrel** and aspirin might have a beneficial effect on cardiovascular outcomes, the risk of haemorrhage is higher than that seen with clopidogrel and aspirin. The US manufacturer of **ticlopidine** warns that the safety of the concurrent use of aspirin beyond 30 days has not been established.[21] Patients taking low-dose aspirin with clopidogrel or related drugs should be warned regarding a possible increased risk of bleeding, and advised to report any unusual or excessive bleeding; however, it is also important to make sure the patient is aware of the clinical benefits of concurrent use as well as the risk of bleeding, to reduce the risk of inappropriate non-compliance.

Ticagrelor is specifically licensed for use with aspirin. The UK manufacturer states that an aspirin dose of 75 to 150 mg daily should be used, and, because of the potential for a decrease in the efficacy of ticagrelor, aspirin doses above 300 mg daily are not recommended.[17] However, in the US, doses of aspirin above 100 mg daily are not recommended, and the US manufacturer states that a maintenance dose of aspirin of 75 to 100 mg daily should be used with ticagrelor.[18]

Note that the UK manufacturer of **prasugrel** advises that its use with clopidogrel might increase the risk of bleeding;[23] however, as both drugs have the same mechanism of action, concurrent use is not clinically indicated.

1. Wilhite DB, Comerota AJ, Schmeider FA, Throm RC, Gaughan JP, Rao AK. Managing PAD with multiple antiplatelet inhibitors: the effect of combination therapy on bleeding time. *J Vasc Surg* (2008) 38, 710–3.
2. Payne DA, Hayes PD, Jones CI, Belham P, Naylor AR, Goodall AH. Combined therapy with clopidogrel and aspirin significantly increases the bleeding time through a synergistic antiplatelet action. *J Vasc Surg* (2002) 35, 1204–9.
3. Yusuf S, Zhao F, Mehta SR, Chrolavicius S, Tognoni G, Fox KK; The Clopidogrel in Unstable Angina to Prevent Recurrent Events (CURE) Trial Investigators. Effects of clopidogrel in addition to aspirin in patients with acute coronary syndromes without ST-segment elevation. *N Engl J Med* (2001) 345, 494–502.
4. Diener H-C, Bogousslavsky J, Brass LM, Cimminiello C, Csiba L, Kaste M, Leys D, Matias-Guiu J, Rupprecht H-J, on behalf of the MATCH investigators. Aspirin and clopidogrel compared with clopidogrel alone after recent ischaemic stroke or transient ischaemic attack in high-risk patients (MATCH): randomised, double-blind, placebo-controlled trial. *Lancet* (2004) 364, 331–7.
5. Bhatt DL, Fox KAA, Hacke W, Berger PB, Black HR, Boden WE, Cacoub P, Cohen EA, Creager MA, Easton JD, Flather MD, Haffner SM, Hamm CW, Hankey GJ, Johnston SC, Mak K-H, Mas J-L, Montalescot G, Pearson TA, Steg PG, Steinhubl SR, Weber MA, Brennan DM, Fabry-Ribaudo L, Booth J, Topol EJ for the CHARISMA Investigators. Clopidogrel and aspirin versus aspirin alone for the prevention of atherothrombotic events. *N Engl J Med* (2006) 354, 1706–17.
6. Steinhubl SR, Bhatt DL, Brennan DM, Montalescot G, Hankey GJ, Eikelboom JW, Berger PB, Topol EJ. Aspirin to prevent cardiovascular disease: the association of aspirin dose and clopidogrel with thrombosis and bleeding. *Ann Intern Med* (2009) 150, 379–86.
7. Connolly SJ, Pogue J, Hart RG, Hohnloser SH, Pfeffer M, Chrolavicius S, Yusuf S, for the Atrial Fibrillation Clopidogrel Trial with Irbesartan for Prevention of Vascular Events (ACTIVE A) investigators. Effect of clopidogrel added to aspirin in patients with atrial fibrillation. *N Engl J Med* (2009) 360, 2066–78.
8. Steinbuhl SR, Berger PB, Mann JT, Fry ET, DeLago A, Wilmer C, Topol EJ for the CREDO investigators. Early and sustained dual oral antiplatelet therapy following percutaneous coronary intervention: a randomised controlled trial. *JAMA* (2002) 288, 2411–20.
9. Chen ZM, Jiang LX, Chen YP, Xie JX, Pan HC, Peto R, Collins R, Liu LS for the COMMIT collaborative group. Addition of clopidogrel to aspirin in 45,852 patients with acute myocardial infarction: randomised placebo-controlled trial. *Lancet* (2005) 5, 1607–21.

10. Hallas J, Dall M, Andries A, Andersen BS, Aalykke C, Hansen JM, Andersen M, Lassen AT. Use of single and combined antithrombotic therapy and risk of serious upper gastrointestinal bleeding: population based case-control study. *BMJ* (2006) 333, 726.
11. Gille J, Bernotat J, Böhm S, Behrens P, Löhr JF. Spontaneous hemarthrosis of the knee associated with clopidogrel and aspirin treatment. *Z Rheumatol* (2003) 62, 80–1.
12. Moore M, Power M. Perioperative hemorrhage and combined clopidogrel and aspirin therapy. *Anesthesiology* (2004) 101, 792–4.
13. Yende S, Wunderink RG. Effect of clopidogrel on bleeding after coronary artery bypass surgery. *Crit Care Med* (2001) 29, 2271–5.
14. Chapman TWL, Bowley DMG, Lambert AW, Walker AJ, Ashley SA, Wilkins DC. Haemorrhage associated with combined clopidogrel and aspirin therapy. *Eur J Vasc Endovasc Surg* (2001) 22, 478–9.
15. Effient (Prasugrel). Eli Lilly and Company. US Prescribing information, November 2013.
16. Wiviott SD, Braunwald E, McCabe CH, Montalescot G, Ruzyllo W, Gottlieb S, Neumann F-J, Ardissino D, De Servi S, Murphy SA, Riesmeyer J, Weerakkody G, Gibson CM, Antman EM, for the TRITON-TIMI 38 investigators. Prasugrel versus clopidogrel in patients with acute coronary syndromes. *N Engl J Med* (2007) 357, 2001–15.
17. Brilique (Ticagrelor). AstraZeneca UK Ltd. UK Summary of product characteristics, July 2015.
18. Brilinta (Ticagrelor). AstraZeneca. US Prescribing information, September 2015.
19. Splawinska B, Kuzniar J, Malinga K, Mazurek AP, Splawinski J. The efficacy and potency of antiplatelet activity of ticlopidine is increased by aspirin. *Int J Clin Pharmacol Ther* (1996) 34, 352–6.
20. Gryglewski RJ, Uracz W, Świês J. Unusual effects of aspirin on ticlopidine induced thrombolysis. *Thorax* (2000) 55 (Suppl 2) S17–S19.
21. Ticlopidine hydrochloride. Apotex Corp. US Prescribing information, September 2010.
22. Plavix (Clopidogrel hydrogen sulphate). Sanofi. UK Summary of product characteristics, January 2014.
23. Efient (Prasugrel hydrochloride). Eli Lilly and Company Ltd. UK Summary of product characteristics, December 2013.

Aspirin + Dipyridamole

The concurrent use of more than one antiplatelet drug might increase the risk of bleeding. However, the addition of dipyridamole to low-dose aspirin does not appear to further increase the incidence of bleeding.

Clinical evidence

One early study in 10 healthy subjects found that dipyridamole 50 mg three times daily given with a single 180-mg dose of aspirin, or dipyridamole 75 mg three times daily given with aspirin 120 mg, maximally inhibited platelet functions, but did not prolong the bleeding time.[1] Two major studies in stroke patients (ESPRIT and ESPS-2) reported no difference in risk of bleeding on the concurrent use of aspirin and dipyridamole, when compared with aspirin alone;[2,3] however, the incidence of bleeding was higher with aspirin alone or aspirin with dipyridamole than with dipyridamole alone (8.2%, 8.8% versus 4.7%, respectively).[3] In a retrospective, population based, case-control study of cases of serious upper gastrointestinal bleeding, the adjusted odds ratio for serious upper gastrointestinal bleeding for dipyridamole plus aspirin (2.3) was slightly higher than for aspirin alone (1.8) or for dipyridamole alone (1.9), but this difference was not statistically significant.[4]

Mechanism

Antiplatelet drugs prolong the bleeding time, and the risks might be additive with combinations, which might increase the risk of clinically relevant bleeding. However, note that the extent of prolongation in bleeding time varies between the individual drugs.

Importance and management

The concurrent use of multiple antiplatelet drugs would generally be expected to increase the risk of bleeding; however, the likelihood and severity of bleeding appears to depend on the antiplatelet combinations given.

No further increased bleeding occurs when dipyridamole is given with aspirin. Nevertheless, the manufacturers of many antiplatelet drugs generally advise caution with the use of other drugs that affect platelet aggregation as this might increase the risk of bleeding: concurrent use should be closely monitored. This would seem prudent, particularly with combinations of antiplatelet drugs that are associated with an increased risk of bleeding, and also in patients at a high risk of bleeding. Note that both drugs can successfully be used together; NICE guidelines in the UK recommend the combination as an option for the prevention of occlusive vascular events.[5]

1. Rajah SM, Penny AF, Crow MJ, Pepper MD, Watson DA. The interaction of varying doses of dipyridamole and acetyl salicylic acid on the inhibition of platelet functions and their effect on bleeding time. *Br J Clin Pharmacol* (1979) 8, 483–9.
2. Halkes PHA, van Gijn J, Kappelle LJ, Koudstaal PJ, Algra A for the ESPRIT Study Group. Aspirin plus dipyridamole versus aspirin alone after cerebral ischaemia of arterial origin (ESPRIT): randomised controlled trial. *Lancet* (2006) 367, 1665–73.
3. Diener HC, Cunha L, Forbes C, Sivenius J, Smets P, Lowenthal A. European Stroke Prevention Study 2. Dipyridamole and acetylsalicylic acid in the secondary prevention of stroke. *J Neurol Sci* (1996) 143, 1–13.
4. Hallas J, Dall M, Andries A, Andersen BS, Aalykke C, Hansen JM, Andersen M, Lassen AT. Use of single and combined antithrombotic therapy and risk of serious upper gastrointestinal bleeding: population based case-control study. *BMJ* (2006) 333, 726.
5. National Institute for Clinical Excellence. Clopidogrel and modified-release dipyridamole for the prevention of occlusive vascular events (issued December 2010). Available at: http://www.nice.org.uk/guidance/TA210/ (accessed 21/10/15).

Aspirin + Phosphodiesterase type-5 inhibitors

Sildenafil, tadalafil, and vardenafil do not potentiate the increased bleeding time seen with aspirin. Avanafil would be predicted to also have no effect.

Clinical evidence

(a) Sildenafil

In a pharmacological study, sildenafil 50 mg did not potentiate the increase in bleeding time seen with aspirin 150 mg.[1]

(b) Tadalafil

A randomised, parallel-group study in a total of 28 subjects found that a single 10-mg dose of tadalafil did not increase the bleeding time after aspirin 300 mg daily was taken for 5 days.[2] Similarly, the US manufacturer reports that tadalafil 10 or 20 mg daily did not augment the increase in bleeding time seen with aspirin.[3]

(c) Vardenafil

The UK manufacturer briefly reports that population pharmacokinetic analysis suggests that aspirin had no effect on vardenafil pharmacokinetics.[4] In addition, the UK and US manufacturers note that in a study, vardenafil 10 mg and 20 mg did not potentiate the bleeding time caused by aspirin 162 mg.[4,5]

Mechanism

Phosphodiesterase type-5 is found in platelets. *In vitro*, sildenafil and vardenafil potentiated the antiplatelet effect of nitroprusside, however, an antiplatelet effect has not been seen clinically.[1,4]

Importance and management

No interaction appears to occur between aspirin and the phosphodiesterase type-5 inhibitors sildenafil, tadalafil, or vardenafil, and no additional precautions would seem necessary if they are given with antiplatelet doses of aspirin. This could also reasonably be applied to **avanafil**.

1. Viagra (Sildenafil citrate). Pfizer Inc. US Prescribing information, March 2015.
2. Eli Lilly and Company. Personal communication, March 2003.
3. Adcirca (Tadalafil). Eli Lilly and Company. US Prescribing information, April 2015.
4. Levitra (Vardenafil hydrochloride). Bayer plc. UK Summary of product characteristics, April 2014.
5. Levitra (Vardenafil hydrochloride). Bayer Healthcare Pharmaceuticals Inc. US Prescribing information, April 2014.

Cilostazol + Food

Food increases the maximum level of cilostazol, which might increase the incidence of adverse effects.

Clinical evidence, mechanism, importance and management

A randomised, crossover study in 15 healthy subjects found that giving a single 100-mg dose of cilostazol within 10 minutes of a high-fat meal caused an increase in the rate and extent of cilostazol absorption. The maximum plasma level of cilostazol was increased by about 95%, the AUC was slightly increased by 25%, and the half-life decreased from 15.1 hours to 5.4 hours, when compared with the fasted state. A trend towards an increase in the incidence of headache was seen when cilostazol was taken with food.[1] The manufacturers state that, as this increase in maximum plasma levels of cilostazol might increase the incidence of adverse effects[2] [such as headache and diarrhoea], cilostazol should be taken 30 minutes before or 2 hours after food.[2,3]

1. Bramer SL, Forbes WP. Relative bioavailability and effects of a high fat meal on single dose cilostazol pharmacokinetics. *Clin Pharmacokinet* (1999) 37 (Suppl 2), 13–23.
2. Pletal (Cilostazol). Otsuka Pharmaceuticals (UK) Ltd. UK Summary of product characteristics, October 2013.
3. Pletal (Cilostazol). Otsuka America Pharmaceutical, Inc. US Prescribing information, May 2007.

Cilostazol + Ketoconazole and other CYP3A4 inhibitors

Ketoconazole, erythromycin and diltiazem, all inhibitors of CYP3A4, increase the plasma concentrations of cilostazol and alter the concentrations of its active metabolites. Other inhibitors of CYP3A4 are predicted to interact similarly. Grapefruit juice, an intestinal CYP3A4 inhibitor, does not appear to affect the pharmacokinetics of cilostazol to a clinically relevant extent, although an isolated case of purpura has been reported on concurrent use.

Clinical evidence

(a) Diltiazem

The manufacturer states that, in a study, diltiazem 180 mg daily increased the maximum plasma concentration and AUC of cilostazol 100 mg twice daily by about 30% and 40%, respectively.[1,2] Diltiazem also increased the AUC of the less active 4'-trans-hydroxymetabolite by 40%, but had no effect on the exposure of the more active dehydro metabolite.[1] The manufacturer additionally reports that, in population pharmacokinetic analysis of clinical study data, the concurrent use of diltiazem increased cilostazol concentrations (AUC increased by 53%).[1,2]

(b) Erythromycin

A study in 16 healthy subjects found that erythromycin 500 mg three times daily for 13 days increased the maximum plasma concentration and AUC of a single 100-mg oral dose of cilostazol given on day 8, by 47% and 73%, respectively. The maximum plasma concentration and AUC of its less active 4'-trans-hydroxymetabolite were increased by 29% and 141%, respectively, whereas the maximum concentration of the more active dehydro metabolite was slightly reduced by 24%, but its AUC was not affected.[3]

(c) Grapefruit juice

The US manufacturer reports that grapefruit juice increased the maximum concentrations of cilostazol by about 50%, but had no effect on its AUC.[2] The UK manufacturer states that 240 mL of grapefruit juice did not have a notable effect on the pharmacokinetics of a single 100-mg dose of cilostazol.[1] There has been a single, published case report of a possible interaction between grapefruit juice and cilostazol. A patient taking aspirin 100 mg daily and cilostazol 100 mg twice daily developed unexplained purpura, which resolved when the patient stopped drinking grapefruit juice. Neither aspirin nor cilostazol were stopped, and no dose adjustments of either drug were made.[4]

(d) Ketoconazole

The manufacturer briefly notes that ketoconazole 400 mg (one dose the day before and one dose with a single 100-mg dose of cilostazol[2]) increased the AUC of cilostazol and its less active 4'-trans-hydroxymetabolite by 117% (about twofold) and 87%, respectively, and reduced the AUC of the more active dehydro metabolite by 87%.[1,2] The UK manufacturer notes that this resulted in an overall increase in the pharmacological effects of cilostazol of 32%, when compared with cilostazol alone.[1]

Mechanism

Cilostazol is primarily metabolised by CYP3A4 to its active dehydro metabolite, which is four- to sevenfold more potent than cilostazol. Therefore drugs that inhibit CYP3A4, such as ketoconazole, erythromycin, and diltiazem, might affect the concentrations of both cilostazol and its potent metabolite, and alter its antiplatelet effects.[1,3] Grapefruit juice also moderately inhibits CYP3A4, principally in the intestine, and therefore the lack of an important change in cilostazol pharmacokinetics with grapefruit juice suggests that intestinal CYP3A4 has limited involvement in its metabolism.

Note that cilostazol is also metabolised to another less active 4'-trans-hydroxymetabolite by CYP2C19 (this metabolite is only one-fifth as potent as cilostazol),[1,2] and inhibition of CYP3A4 appears to result in an increased exposure to this metabolite.

Importance and management

A pharmacokinetic interaction between cilostazol and inhibitors of CYP3A4, such as ketoconazole, erythromycin and diltiazem, appears to be established. However, the pharmacological effects of cilostazol were only modestly increased by ketoconazole, and the clinical relevance of this is unknown, although it cannot be ruled out that the longer-term use of ketoconazole with cilostazol might have a different effect. Nevertheless, in view of these effects, the MHRA in the UK advises that the dose of cilostazol should be reduced to 50 mg twice daily when given concurrently with ketoconazole, itraconazole, clarithromycin, erythromycin, or other potent CYP3A4 inhibitors.[5] Note that erythromycin is generally considered to be a moderate inhibitor of CYP3A4. The UK and US manufacturers of cilostazol state that the same dose reduction should be considered on concomitant use with all CYP3A4 inhibitors, depending on individual efficacy and tolerability. They specifically name some **macrolides** (e.g. **clarithromycin**), some **azoles** (**itraconazole**, **fluconazole**, **miconazole**), **nefazodone** and the **HIV-protease inhibitors**.[1,2] For a list of clinically relevant CYP3A4 inhibitors, see 'Table 1.9', p.11. Note that, of the macrolides, **azithromycin** is not expected to interact with cilostazol by inhibiting CYP3A4.[2]

The US manufacturer also suggests that **fluoxetine**, **fluvoxamine**, and **sertraline** might also interact by this mechanism.[2] However, note that the SSRIs are, at most, weak inhibitors of CYP3A4 (see 'Table 35.2', p.1465), and therefore a clinically relevant interaction seems unlikely.

The general significance of the case report of a possible interaction between cilostazol and **grapefruit juice** is unclear, particularly as no pharmacokinetic data were reported confirming a corresponding increase in cilostazol concentrations in this patient, and pharmacokinetic studies have so far shown no increase in the overall exposure to cilostazol with grapefruit juice. At present there appears to be no good evidence for avoiding the concurrent intake of grapefruit juice with cilostazol, and given the modest increase in pharmacological activity seen with more potent CYP3A4 inhibitors, such as ketoconazole, it seems that a clinically relevant interaction between cilostazol and grapefruit juice is unlikely.

1. Pletal (Cilostazol). Otsuka Pharmaceuticals (UK) Ltd. UK Summary of product characteristics, November 2008.
2. Pletal (Cilostazol). Otsuka America Pharmaceutical, Inc. US Prescribing information, May 2007.
3. Suri A, Forbes WP, Bramer SL. Effects of CYP3A inhibition on the metabolism of cilostazol. *Clin Pharmacokinet* (1999) 37 (Suppl 2), 61–8.
4. Taniguchi K, Ohtani H, Ikemoto T, Miki A, Hori S, Sawada Y. Possible case of potentiation of the antiplatelet effect of cilostazol by grapefruit juice. *J Clin Pharm Ther* (2007) 32, 457–9.
5. Medicines and Healthcare Products Regulatory Agency and the Commission on Human Medicines. Cilostazol (Pletal): risks of cardiovascular and bleeding events—indication restricted to second-line treatment and contraindicated with some cardiovascular conditions and medicine. *Drug Safety Update* (2013) 6, 9. Available at: http://webarchive.nationalarchives.gov.uk/20150122075153/http://www.mhra.gov.uk/home/groups/dsu/documents/publication/con267913.pdf (accessed 21/10/15)

Cilostazol + Miscellaneous

Inducers of CYP3A4, such as rifampicin (rifampin), are predicted to affect the metabolism of cilostazol. An increased incidence of palpitations and tachycardia has been reported when dihydropyridine calcium-channel blockers were given with cilostazol. Tobacco smoke very slightly reduces the exposure to cilostazol. The exposure to narrow therapeutic index drugs metabolised by CYP3A4 (e.g. the ergot derivatives) might be increased by cilostazol.

Clinical evidence, mechanism, importance and management

(a) Calcium-channel blockers; dihydropyridine

The UK manufacturer of cilostazol briefly states that the concurrent use of other vasodilators that also cause reflex tachycardia, such as the dihydropyridine calcium-channel blockers, increased the incidence of palpitations and peripheral oedema.[1] They do not state how much the increase was, but note that palpitations and tachycardia are common adverse effects of cilostazol, and might lead to discontinuation of cilostazol.[1,2] On this basis, the UK manufacturer of cilostazol advises caution on the use of cilostazol with other drugs that reduce blood pressure, because of the possibility of additive hypotension with reflex tachycardia.[1] Bear the possibility of this additive interaction in mind if these drugs are used together.

(b) CYP3A4 substrates

The UK manufacturer of cilostazol advises caution on the concurrent use of cilostazol with other drugs that are substrates of CYP3A4 and that also have a narrow therapeutic index: they specifically name **halofantrine**, **pimozide** and the **ergot alkaloids** [**ergot derivatives**].[1] The data from lovastatin (see 'Statins + Cilostazol', p.1329), which is also a CYP3A4 substrate, supports the suggestion that the exposure to these drugs might be increased; nevertheless, further study is needed to establish these predicted interactions. Until more is known it would be prudent to be alert for any signs of an adverse response to these drugs. As raised levels of halofantrine and pimozide can result in QT prolongation it may be prudent to avoid concurrent use where possible. With the ergot derivatives, monitor concurrent use for adverse effects, particularly those suggestive of reduced peripheral circulation (coldness, numbness or tingling of the hands and feet).

(c) Enzyme inducers

The UK manufacturer of cilostazol[1] states that the effect of inducers of CYP3A4 (they name **carbamazepine**, **phenytoin** [and therefore **fosphenytoin**], **rifampicin** (**rifampin**) and **St John's wort**) and inducers of CYP2C19 on the pharmacokinetics and antiplatelet effects of cilostazol has not been evaluated, but could potentially be altered.[1] CYP3A4 and CYP2C19 are known to be involved in the metabolism of cilostazol to its active metabolites; for example, ketoconazole, an *inhibitor* of CYP3A4, increases the levels of cilostazol and affects the metabolism of its active metabolites (see 'Cilostazol + Ketoconazole and other CYP3A4 inhibitors', p.783). Therefore it seems likely that a clinically relevant interaction may occur with CYP3A4 inducers. The UK manufacturer therefore advises monitoring concurrent use for an alteration in the antiplatelet effects of cilostazol.[1] For a list of CYP3A4 inducers, see 'Table 1.9', p.11.

The effect of CYP2C19 inducers on cilostazol is less clear, as there are no specific CYP2C19 inducers known, and the clinical relevance of the interaction of cilostazol with CYP2C19 inhibitors (see 'Cilostazol + Proton pump inhibitors', below) is unclear.

(d) Tobacco smoking

CYP1A2, which is induced by tobacco smoke, has a minor role in the metabolism of cilostazol.[1] The manufacturer reports that population pharmacokinetic analysis suggests that tobacco smoking reduces the exposure to cilostazol by about 20%,[1,2] but this is unlikely to have much, if any, clinical relevance.

1. Pletal (Cilostazol). Otsuka Pharmaceuticals (UK) Ltd. UK Summary of product characteristics, October 2013.
2. Pletal (Cilostazol). Otsuka America Pharmaceutical, Inc. US Prescribing information, May 2007.

Cilostazol + Probucol

No pharmacokinetic interaction occurs between cilostazol and probucol.

Clinical evidence, mechanism, importance and management

In a single-dose study, 12 healthy subjects were given cilostazol 100 mg alone and then with probucol 500 mg. Probucol did not alter the pharmacokinetics of cilostazol or its two active metabolites.[1] In another single-dose study, 19 healthy subjects were given either probucol 250 mg alone or with cilostazol. Cilostazol had no effect on the pharmacokinetics of probucol.[1] Therefore, no dose adjustments of cilostazol or probucol appear to be necessary on concurrent use.

1. Kim K-P, Kim B-H, Lim KS, Kim T-E, Shin S-G, Jang I-J, Yu K-S. Potential interactions between cilostazol and probucol: a two-part, single-dose, open-label study in healthy Korean male volunteers. *Clin Ther* (2009) 10, 2098–2106.

Cilostazol + Proton pump inhibitors

Omeprazole, a CYP2C19 inhibitor, increases the bioavailability of cilostazol and its main active metabolite and increases its pharmacological activity. Other CYP2C19 inhibitors (such as esomeprazole) are predicted to interact similarly.

Clinical evidence

In a crossover study in 20 healthy subjects, **omeprazole** 40 mg daily for one week increased the AUC of a single 100-mg dose of cilostazol by 26%.[1] More importantly, the AUC of 3,4-dehydro-cilostazol (the main metabolite, which is four to seven times more potent than cilostazol) was increased by 69%.[1-3] The AUC of the other, less active cilostazol metabolite, 4'-trans-hydroxymetabolite, was reduced by 31%.[1-3] The UK manufacturer notes that this results in an overall increase in pharmacological activity of 47%, when compared with cilostazol alone.[3]

Mechanism

Cilostazol is partially metabolised by CYP2C19 to the less active 4'-trans-hydroxymetabolite, and therefore omeprazole, an inhibitor of this isoenzyme, would be expected to inhibit the metabolism of cilostazol to this metabolite. The reason for the greater increase in exposure to the more active dehydro metabolite is unknown.

Importance and management

The clinical relevance of the pharmacokinetic interaction between cilostazol and omeprazole is uncertain, but some caution would seem prudent on the basis of the increase that was seen in the pharmacological activity of cilostazol. The UK manufacturer of cilostazol suggests that the interaction could have the potential to increase cilostazol adverse effects.[3] The MHRA in the UK advises that the dose of cilostazol should be reduced to 50 mg twice daily in patients also taking omeprazole or other potent CYP2C19 inhibitors,[4] although omeprazole is generally considered to be a moderate inhibitor of CYP2C19. The UK and US manufacturers of cilostazol state that the same dose reduction should be considered on concomitant use with all CYP2C19 inhibitors (this would include **esomeprazole**), depending on individual efficacy and tolerability.[2,3] For a list of clinically relevant CYP2C19 inhibitors, see 'Table 1.6', p.8.

Note that, based on the lack of a pharmacokinetic interaction with the known CYP2C19 substrate, diazepam (consider 'Benzodiazepines + Proton pump inhibitors', p.834), **rabeprazole**, and possibly also **pantoprazole** or **lansoprazole**, would not be anticipated to interact with cilostazol by CYP2C19 inhibition.

1. Suri A, Bramer SL. Effect of omeprazole on the metabolism of cilostazol. *Clin Pharmacokinet* (1999) 37, (Suppl 2), 53–9.
2. Pletal (Cilostazol). Otsuka America Pharmaceutical, Inc. US Prescribing information, May 2007.
3. Pletal (Cilostazol). Otsuka Pharmaceuticals (UK) Ltd. UK Summary of product characteristics, October 2013.
4. Medicines and Healthcare Products Regulatory Agency and the Commission on Human Medicines. Cilostazol (Pletal): risks of cardiovascular and bleeding events—indication restricted to second-line treatment and contraindicated with some cardiovascular conditions and medicine. *Drug Safety Update* (2013) 6, 9. Available at: http://webarchive.nationalarchives.gov.uk/20150122075153/http://www.mhra.gov.uk/home/groups/dsu/documents/publication/con267913.pdf (accessed 21/10/15)

Cilostazol + Quinidine

Quinidine does not appear to affect the pharmacokinetics of cilostazol.

Clinical evidence, mechanism, importance and management

In a crossover study in 22 healthy subjects, the pharmacokinetics of a single 100-mg dose of cilostazol and its metabolites were unaffected by pretreatment with two 200-mg doses of quinidine sulfate, taken 25 hours and one hour before cilostazol.[1] Quinidine inhibits CYP2D6, and this study confirms that neither cilostazol nor its metabolites are metabolised by this isoenzyme. Therefore it appears that no cilostazol dose adjustments are necessary on the concurrent use of quinidine.

1. Bramer SL, Suri A. Inhibition of CYP2D6 by quinidine and its effects on the metabolism of cilostazol. *Clin Pharmacokinet* (1999) 37 (Suppl 2), 41–51.

Clopidogrel and related drugs + Antacids

An aluminium/magnesium-containing antacid slightly decreases the absorption of ticlopidine, but does not appear to affect the absorption of clopidogrel.

Clinical evidence, mechanism, importance and management

(a) Clopidogrel

In a randomised study, 9 healthy subjects were given two 400-mg tablets of *Maalox* (**aluminium/magnesium hydroxide**) followed, one hour later, by a single 75-mg dose of clopidogrel. The maximum levels and AUC of the inactive carboxylic acid metabolite of clopidogrel (a metabolite used as a marker of absorption) were not notably affected, suggesting that clopidogrel absorption was not altered by the antacid.[1] Therefore, no particular precautions seem necessary on the concurrent use of clopidogrel and an antacid.

(b) Ticlopidine

In a single-dose study in 12 healthy subjects, 30 mL of *Maalox* [**aluminium/magnesium hydroxide**] decreased the extent of absorption of ticlopidine 250 mg by about 20%.[2] This slight change is unlikely to be of clinical importance.

1. McEwen J, Strauch G, Perles P, Pritchard G, Moreland TE, Necciari J, Dickinson JP. Clopidogrel bioavailability: absence of influence of food or antacids. *Semin Thromb Hemost* (1999) 25 (Suppl 2), 47–50.
2. Shah J, Fratis A, Ellis D, Murakami S, Teitelbaum P. Effect of food and antacid on absorption of orally administered ticlopidine hydrochloride. *J Clin Pharmacol* (1990) 30, 733–6.

Clopidogrel + Azoles

Ketoconazole appears to modestly reduce the formation of the active metabolite of clopidogrel, and reduce its antiplatelet effect. Fluconazole and voriconazole are predicted to interact similarly. In one study, itraconazole reduced the antiplatelet effect of clopidogrel, but only in subjects of one genotype.

Clinical evidence

(a) Itraconazole

In a study to determine the effect of itraconazole on clopidogrel inhibition of platelet aggregation, 32 healthy subjects took itraconazole 200 mg daily, starting 4 days before clopidogrel was given (300 mg as a loading dose followed by 75 mg daily for 6 days). The antiplatelet effect of clopidogrel was also determined when subjects took clopidogrel alone. Inhibition of platelet aggregation was modestly to markedly reduced by itraconazole, but only in the 16 subjects who were CYP3A5 non-expresser genotypes (that is, those lacking this isoenzyme), and not in the 16 subjects who were CYP3A5 expressers. For example, at 24 hours post-dose, platelet aggregation was reduced by just 2.5% in the CYP3A5 non-expressers compared with 27.7% in CYP3A4 expressers when itraconazole was given, and at day 6 the reduction was 17.8% versus 33.5%.[1]

(b) Ketoconazole

In a controlled study, 18 healthy subjects received clopidogrel alone (300 mg on day one followed by 75 mg daily for 5 days) and then with ketoconazole 400 mg daily, which was started 3 days before the clopidogrel. Ketoconazole reduced the AUC of the active metabolite of clopidogrel by 22% and 29%, after the loading and maintenance doses of clopidogrel, respectively. Inhibition of platelet aggregation (IPA) was also significantly reduced with ketoconazole, from 43% to 15% at 4 hours after the loading dose, and from 50% to 17% at 24 hours after the last maintenance dose. Of the 19 subjects, 14 had an IPA of less than 20% following the loading dose, a level seen in non-responders to clopidogrel.[2]

Mechanism

Formation of the active thiol metabolite of clopidogrel is dependent on metabolism by CYP2C19 and CYP3A4, and is therefore likely to be reduced by azoles that inhibit these isoenzymes. Ketoconazole is an inhibitor of CYP3A4 and CYP3A5,[2] and itraconazole is principally a CYP3A4 inhibitor.[1] The interaction with itraconazole appeared to occur only in those without CYP3A5 activity, which suggests that CYP3A5 may be involved in the metabolism of clopidogrel to its active metabolite in the presence of CYP3A4 inhibition.[1] This appeared to be confirmed by a further study in patients given clopidogrel after stent implantation, which found a greater risk of atherothrombotic events in those without CYP3A5 activity.[1] Azoles that are also inhibitors of CYP2C19 (such as **fluconazole** and **voriconazole**) are also predicted to interact with clopidogrel, see 'Clopidogrel + Proton pump inhibitors and other CYP2C19 inhibitors', p.788.

Importance and management

Evidence for an interaction between clopidogrel and the azoles appears to be limited to these studies. The clinical relevance of the pharmacokinetic interaction with ketoconazole is unclear and platelet reactivity studies may not be directly relevant to clinical outcomes, but the level of inhibition of platelet aggregation in about three-quarters of healthy subjects taking ketoconazole with clopidogrel was below the level at which patients are classed as non-responders to clopidogrel, suggesting it may be important. The data with itraconazole suggest that the interaction with drugs that specifically inhibit only CYP3A4 might be of more importance in those lacking CYP3A5. Until more is known, some caution may be appropriate with azoles that are potent inhibitors of CYP3A4 (see *Azoles*, under 'Anthelmintics, Antifungals, and Antiprotozoals', p.225, for the enzyme-inhibitory effects of the azoles).

Of the azoles, **fluconazole** and **voriconazole** also have CYP2C19 inhibitory activity, and the interaction of clopidogrel with CYP2C19 inhibitors is more extensively investigated than that with CYP3A4 inhibitors (see 'Clopidogrel + Proton pump inhibitors and other CYP2C19 inhibitors', p.788). The UK manufacturer of clopidogrel discourages concurrent use of potent or moderate CYP2C19 inhibitors, specifically naming fluconazole and voriconazole.[3]

1. Suh J-W, Koo B-K, Zhang S-Y, Park K-W, Cho J-Y, Jang I-J, Lee D-S, Sohn D-W, Lee M-M, Kim H-S. Increased risk of atherothrombotic events associated with cytochrome P450 3A5 polymorphism in patients taking clopidogrel. *CMAJ* (2006) 174, 1715–22.
2. Farid NA, Payne CD, Small DS, Winters KJ, Ernest CS, Brandt JT, Darstein C, Jakubowski JA, Salazar DE. Cytochrome P450 3A inhibition by ketoconazole affects prasugrel and clopidogrel pharmacokinetics and pharmacodynamics differently. *Clin Pharmacol Ther* (2007) 81, 735–41.
3. Plavix (Clopidogrel hydrogen sulphate). Sanofi-Aventis. UK Summary of product characteristics, January 2014.

Clopidogrel + Calcium-channel blockers

Some observational studies have suggested that calcium-channel blockers, particularly amlodipine, might reduce the inhibitory effect of clopidogrel on platelet aggregation, whereas other studies have found no such effect. Single-dose verapamil and possibly nifedipine had no effect on the antiplatelet effects of clopidogrel in small controlled studies.

Clinical evidence

In three non-randomised, observational studies, the antiplatelet effect of clopidogrel appeared to be lower in those patients also taking calcium-channel blockers, particularly **amlodipine**. In the first of these studies, in patients undergoing coronary artery stenting, there was a higher platelet reactivity index (PRI) in the 45 patients also taking calcium-channel blockers compared with the 155 patients not taking a calcium-channel blocker (mean PRI 61% compared with 48%), indicating a reduced antiplatelet response to clopidogrel. Patients with a PRI greater than 69% were considered to be non-responders to clopidogrel: 40% of patients taking a calcium-channel blocker were classified as non-responders compared with 20% of patients not taking a calcium-channel blocker. A total of 93% of patients were taking dihydropyridine calcium channel blockers (**amlodipine** was the most common calcium-channel blocker (35 patients), with patients also taking **nitrendipine** (3), **nifedipine** (3) or **nisoldipine** (2)) and just 7% (3 patients) were taking **diltiazem**. Although the patients taking calcium-channel blockers had a higher incidence of cardiac risk factors (such as hypertension, diabetes, and renal impairment) and less of these patients were taking beta blockers, the higher rate of reduced antiplatelet response to clopidogrel in this group remained statistically significant when the data were adjusted to account for these risk factors. A trend towards a higher rate of revascularisation procedures was also reported in these patients.[1] A second observational study in patients admitted for coronary, carotid or peripheral artery stenting, also found similar results. In this study, patients taking calcium-channel blockers with clopidogrel (53 patients) were found to have higher ADP-induced platelet reactivity (as measured by two different methods) when compared with patients not taking clopidogrel (109 patients). Of the patients taking a calcium-channel blocker, about 41% were classified as non-responders compared with about 18% of patients not taking a calcium-channel blocker. When the data were controlled for other factors, the use of a calcium-channel blocker was found to be an independent risk factor for a reduced antiplatelet response to clopidogrel. Calcium-channel blockers taken in this study were **amlodipine** (84.6% of patients), **nifedipine** (5.8%), **nisoldipine**, **lercanidipine** (both 3.85%), **nitrendipine** and **verapamil** (both 1.9%).[2]

A further third observational study in 222 patients taking clopidogrel with calcium-channel blockers also found similar results in patients admitted for coronary artery stenting. In this study, platelet aggregation (as measured by two different methods) was higher in the 124 patients taking **amlodipine** with clopidogrel compared with 410 patients not taking a calcium-channel blocker. Similarly, in the 98 patients taking **barnidipine**, **diltiazem**, **nifedipine** or **verapamil** there was a lower antiplatelet effect of clopidogrel with one assay; however, there was no statistically significant difference in platelet reactivity with the other assay. The number of patients classified as clopidogrel poor responders was higher in those taking **amlodipine** compared with those not taking calcium-channel blockers (25.6% compared with 12.9%). However, this increased rate of poor clopidogrel responders was not found in the patients taking the other four calcium-channel blockers.[3]

In contrast, other different studies have reported no interaction between clopidogrel and the calcium-channel blockers. In a placebo-controlled study in patients undergoing coronary stenting, intra-arterial **verapamil** 5 mg given before the start of the procedure, followed by a single 600-mg dose of clopidogrel 10 minutes later, had no effect on platelet inhibition in response to clopidogrel at 2, 4 and 7 hours post-dose.[4] However, it cannot be reliably concluded from this study that multiple-dose **verapamil** would also have no effect. In another placebo-controlled study in patients with peripheral vascular or coronary artery disease, the concurrent use of clopidogrel with **nifedipine** (6 patients), atenolol (8 patients), or with both atenolol and **nifedipine** (8 patients) did not alter the control of hypertension or angina by nifedipine compared with placebo. In addition, the antiplatelet effect of clopidogrel did not appear to be altered by nifedipine as it did not differ between the groups.[5] Limited data from the CAPRIE study showed that **calcium-channel blockers** have been safely given with clopidogrel.[6]

Mechanism

Clopidogrel is a prodrug and is metabolised to its active thiol metabolite by CYP3A4 and CYP2C19, as well as CYP1A2 and CYP2B6. Diltiazem and verapamil are known inhibitors of CYP3A4 and so are predicted to inhibit the CYP3A4-mediated conversion of clopidogrel to its active metabolite.[1-3] Some of the studies suggest that as the dihydropyridine calcium-channel blockers are substrates of CYP3A4, they may interact by competing with clopidogrel for CYP3A4 metabolism.[1,3] However, note that this is not an established mechanism for pharmacokinetic drug interactions, and substrates of CYP3A4 do not cause clinically relevant interactions with other substrates of CYP3A4 unless they are also CYP3A4 inhibitors, consider also 'Clopidogrel + Statins', p.792.

The intestinal efflux of clopidogrel is also possibly mediated by P-glycoprotein. One study noted that barnidipine, diltiazem, nifedipine and verapamil are also reported to inhibit P-glycoprotein, which might be predicted to lead to raised clopidogrel levels. It has been suggested that this might counteract any CYP3A4 inhibition caused by diltiazem and verapamil.[3]

Importance and management

The evidence for an interaction between clopidogrel and the calcium-channel blockers is limited to the observational studies cited, which suggest that calcium-channel blockers, in particular amlodipine, might reduce the inhibitory effects of clopidogrel on platelet aggregation. Note that non-randomised comparisons like this cannot account for all differences between patients (e.g. genetic differences resulting in non-response to clopidogrel); however, it is worth noting that three studies have come up with similar findings. Nevertheless, observational studies should only be used to generate hypotheses, and the possibility that amlodipine reduces the effects of clopidogrel on platelet aggregation and alters clopidogrel pharmacokinetics should now be confirmed in a randomised controlled study. Furthermore, it is possible that platelet reactivity studies may not be directly relevant to clinical outcomes. Overall therefore, the relevance of any possible interaction of calcium-channel blockers to the beneficial cardiovascular effects of clopidogrel is as yet unclear. In addition, the beneficial effects of calcium-channel blockers in patients with hypertension are proven, and their use is currently recommended in clinical guidelines for both hypertension and angina. There is insufficient evidence available to suggest a change in the prescribing of calcium-channel blockers in patients also taking clopidogrel. Nevertheless, further study is needed.

1. Siller-Matula JM, Lang I, Christ G, Jilma B. Calcium-channel blockers reduce the antiplatelet effect of clopidogrel. *J Am Coll Cardiol* (2008) 52, 1557–63.
2. Gremmel T, Steiner S, Seidinger D, Koppensteiner R, Panzer S, Kopp CW. Calcium-channel blockers decrease clopidogrel-mediated platelet inhibition. *Heart* (2010) 96, 186–9.
3. Harmsze AM, Robijns K, van Werkum JW, Breet NJ, Hackeng CM, ten Berg JM, Ruven HJT, Klungel OH, de Boer A, Deneer VHM. The use of amlodipine, but not of P-glycoprotein-inhibiting calcium channel blockers is associated with clopidogrel poor-response. *Thromb Haemost* (2010) 103, 920–25.
4. Gladding P, Webster M, Zeng I, Farrell H, Stewart J, Ruygrok P, Ormiston J, El-Jack S, Armstrong G, Kay P, Scott D, Gunes A, Dalh M-L. The antiplatelet effect of higher loading and maintenance dose regimens of clopidogrel. The PRINC (Plavix Response in Coronary Intervention) trial. *JACC Cardiovasc Interv* (2008) 1, 612–19.
5. Forbes CD, Lowe GDO, Maclaren M, Shaw BG, Dickinson JP, Kieffer G. Clopidogrel compatibility with concomitant cardiac co-medications: a study of its interactions with a beta-blocker and a calcium uptake antagonist. *Semin Thromb Hemost* (1999) 25 (Suppl 2), 55–9.
6. Morais J, on behalf of the CAPRIE investigators. Use of concomitant medications in the CAPRIE trial: clopidogrel is unlikely to be associated with clinically significant drug interactions. *Eur Heart J* (1998) 19 (Abstract Suppl), 5.

Clopidogrel and related drugs + Food

Food slightly increases the absorption of ticlopidine. Food has no effect on exposure to the active metabolite of clopidogrel, and does not alter its antiplatelet effect. Food does not alter the bioavailability of prasugrel, but may slightly delay the onset of action.

Clinical evidence, mechanism, importance and management

(a) Clopidogrel

In two studies in 12 healthy subjects (one group with an average age of 67 years and the other with an average age of 23 years) given a single 75-mg dose of clopidogrel, the bioavailability of the inactive *carboxylic acid metabolite* of clopidogrel (used as a marker of absorption) did not differ when clopidogrel was taken in the fasting state or with food.[1] Another later study in 12 healthy subjects measured plasma levels of the *parent drug clopidogrel*: in this study, food delayed the absorption of a single 75-mg dose of clopidogrel, and markedly increased the clopidogrel maximum concentration and AUC about sixfold and ninefold, respectively.[2] The US manufacturer reports yet another study in which the plasma levels of the *active thiol metabolite* were measured. In this study in healthy subjects given clopidogrel 75 mg daily with a standard breakfast, the maximum level of the active thiol metabolite of clopidogrel was *reduced* by 57%, but its AUC was unchanged. More importantly, this decrease did not result in an appreciable decrease in the antiplatelet effect of clopidogrel (platelet aggregation was reduced by less than 9%). They also note that the pharmacokinetics of a 300-mg loading dose of clopidogrel were similarly affected by a high-fat breakfast.[3]

Clopidogrel is an inactive ester prodrug that is rapidly hydrolysed, principally to the inactive carboxylic acid metabolite, and plasma levels of the parent compound and of the active thiol metabolite are very low. Taken together, the data suggest that food markedly increases the absorption of clopidogrel, but that it has no effect on overall exposure to the inactive carboxylic acid metabolite or the active thiol metabolite. The lack of an effect of food on exposure to the active metabolite of clopidogrel and its antiplatelet effect suggests that there is no clinically relevant pharmacokinetic interaction of food with clopidogrel. Note that, the marked increase in parent clopidogrel levels is unlikely to be clinically important because even higher levels are seen in liver cirrhosis[2] for which no dose adjustment is needed.[2-4] The manufacturers advise that clopidogrel can be taken with or without food.[3,4]

(b) Prasugrel

The manufacturers of prasugrel report that, in a study in healthy subjects given a single 15-mg dose of prasugrel, a high-fat, high-calorie meal decreased the maximum level of the active metabolite of prasugrel by 49% and increased its time to maximum concentration by one hour (from 0.5 hours to 1.5 hours), but had no effect on its AUC.[5,6] They also note that, in the TRITON study, prasugrel was given without regard to food. They therefore advise that prasugrel may be taken with or without food.[5,6] Note that, the UK manufacturer suggests that a quicker onset of action may occur if the loading dose of prasugrel is taken on an empty stomach.[5]

(c) Ticlopidine

In a study in 12 healthy subjects, the extent of absorption of a single 250-mg dose of ticlopidine was slightly increased by 20% and occurred more rapidly when ticlopidine was taken after food, when compared with the fasting state.[7] These modest changes are unlikely to be of clinical importance, and, although it is suggested that ticlopidine is taken with food, this is to minimise gastric intolerance.[7,8]

1. McEwen J, Strauch G, Perles P, Pritchard G, Moreland TE, Necciari J, Dickinson JP. Clopidogrel bioavailability: absence of influence of food or antacids. *Semin Thromb Hemost* (1999) 25 (Suppl 2), 47–50.
2. Nirogi RVS, Kandikere VN, Mudigonda K. Effect of food on bioavailability of a single oral dose of clopidogrel in healthy male subjects. *Arzneimittelforschung* (2006) 56, 735–9.
3. Plavix (Clopidogrel bisulfate). Bristol-Myers Squibb/Sanofi Pharmaceuticals Partnership. US Prescribing information, December 2011.
4. Plavix (Clopidogrel hydrogen sulphate). Sanofi-Aventis. UK Summary of product characteristics, January 2014.
5. Efient (Prasugrel hydrochloride). Eli Lilly and Company Ltd. UK Summary of product characteristics, December 2013.
6. Effient (Prasugrel). Eli Lilly and Company. US Prescribing information, November 2013.
7. Shah J, Fratis A, Ellis D, Murakami S, Teitelbaum P. Effect of food and antacid on absorption of orally administered ticlopidine hydrochloride. *J Clin Pharmacol* (1990) 30, 733–6.
8. Ticlopidine hydrochloride. Apotex Corp. US Prescribing information, February 2006.

Clopidogrel + H_2-receptor antagonists

Ranitidine does not alter the pharmacokinetics, antiplatelet activity or efficacy of clopidogrel. Famotidine, and possibly also nizatidine, do not appear to alter the efficacy of clopidogrel. Cimetidine may theoretically inhibit the metabolism of clopidogrel to its active metabolite, and limited retrospective evidence suggests that cimetidine might possibly reduce the cardiovascular benefit of clopidogrel (increase the risk of cardiovascular

adverse events), although one retrospective study found no increased cardiovascular risk on concurrent use.

Clinical evidence

(a) Cimetidine

In a preliminary report of a retrospective study of patients taking clopidogrel after an acute myocardial infarction,[1] patients who took cimetidine had an increased risk of reinfarction within 90 days compared with those who did not take cimetidine (8.8% versus 4.7%; odds ratio 1.9). Another retrospective cohort study also found an increase in cardiovascular risk when cimetidine was given with clopidogrel. In this study, the incidence of rehospitalisation for acute coronary syndrome or death in 252 patients taking clopidogrel and an H_2-receptor antagonist (including 160 patients taking cimetidine) was increased more than twofold, when compared to patients not taking an H_2-receptor antagonist (26.8% compared with 11.6%, respectively).[2] However, in a retrospective, cohort study of patients taking clopidogrel, no increased risk of hospitalisation for a major adverse cardiovascular event was found in 472 patients taking an H_2-receptor antagonist (including 41 patients taking cimetidine), when compared with a control group taking clopidogrel alone (9 390 patients).[3]

(b) Famotidine

In a retrospective, case-control study in 734 patients taking clopidogrel post-myocardial infarction and readmitted within 90 days with a further myocardial infarction, the concurrent use of H_2-receptor antagonists (including famotidine) was not associated with an increased risk of re-infarction.[4] Similarly, in a retrospective, cohort study of patients taking clopidogrel, no increased risk of hospitalisation for a major adverse cardiovascular event was found in 472 patients taking an H_2-receptor antagonist (including 161 patients taking famotidine), when compared with a control group taking clopidogrel alone (9 390 patients).[3]

In contrast, a retrospective cohort study in patients with acute coronary syndromes, the incidence of rehospitalisation for acute coronary syndrome or death was increased more than twofold in 252 patients taking an H_2-receptor antagonist (including 47 patients taking famotidine), when compared with patients not taking an H_2-receptor antagonist (26.8% compared with 11.6%, respectively). However, note that a large proportion of patients in this study were taking cimetidine (63%) which might affect clopidogrel metabolism, see under *Mechanism*, below.[2]

(c) Nizatidine

In a retrospective case-control study in 734 patients taking clopidogrel post-myocardial infarction and readmitted within 90 days with a further myocardial infarction, the concurrent use of H_2-receptor antagonists (including nizatidine) was not associated with an increased risk of re-infarction.[4] In a retrospective cohort study in patients with acute coronary syndromes, the incidence of rehospitalisation for acute coronary syndrome or death was increased more than twofold in 252 patients taking an H_2-receptor antagonist with clopidogrel, compared with patients not taking an H_2-receptor antagonist (26.8% compared with 11.6%, respectively). However, note that only 2 patients in this study were taking nizatidine and a large proportion of patients were taking cimetidine (63%), which might affect clopidogrel metabolism, see under *Mechanism*, below.[2]

(d) Ranitidine

In a randomised study, 23 healthy subjects were given a single 600-mg loading dose of clopidogrel followed by 75 mg daily for 7 days alone and then with ranitidine 150 mg twice daily for 8 days. Ranitidine did not alter the AUC or time to maximum concentration of the active metabolite of clopidogrel, nor did it alter its antiplatelet effects.[5] In a retrospective case-control study in 734 patients taking clopidogrel post-myocardial infarction and readmitted within 90 days with a further myocardial infarction, the concurrent use of H_2-receptor antagonists (including ranitidine) was not associated with an increased risk of re-infarction.[4] Similarly, in a retrospective, cohort study of patients taking clopidogrel, there was no increased risk of hospitalisation for a major adverse cardiovascular event in 472 patients taking an H_2-receptor antagonist (including 229 patients taking ranitidine), when compared with a control group taking clopidogrel alone (9 390 patients).[3]

In a retrospective, cohort study in patients with acute coronary syndromes, 252 patients taking an H_2-receptor antagonist (including 43 patients taking ranitidine) were found to have a higher incidence of rehospitalisation for acute coronary syndrome or death, when compared with patients not taking an H_2-receptor antagonist (more than twofold, 26.8% compared with 11.6%, respectively). However, note that a large proportion of patients in this study were taking cimetidine (63%), which might affect clopidogrel metabolism, see under *Mechanism*, below.[2]

Mechanism

Clopidogrel is an inactive prodrug that is metabolised to its active metabolite by the cytochrome P450 system, with CYP2C19 known to be important, and possibly also CYP3A4. Cimetidine is a non-specific weak inhibitor of various cytochrome P450 isoenzymes, and is known to inhibit the metabolism of diazepam, a substrate of CYP2C19 (see 'Benzodiazepines and related drugs + H_2-receptor antagonists', p.822). It may therefore theoretically reduce the metabolism of clopidogrel to its active metabolite, leading to a reduction in its antiplatelet effects. None of the other H_2-receptor antagonists would be expected to have this effect as they are not enzyme inhibitors.

Importance and management

The theoretical pharmacokinetic interaction between clopidogrel and cimetidine has not been studied and the general relevance of any interaction is unclear. Cimetidine may inhibit CYP2C19 and, on the basis of the interaction with omeprazole (see 'Clopidogrel + Proton pump inhibitors and other CYP2C19 inhibitors', p.788), the UK manufacturer of clopidogrel discourages the concurrent use of potent or moderate inhibitors of CYP2C19, and specifically names cimetidine.[6] Given the conflicting and limited data, with the suggestion of a possible increased risk of reinfarction on concurrent use, and also the availability of non-interacting alternatives, this would seem a prudent precaution. However, further controlled, randomised studies are needed to confirm an interaction with cimetidine.

One study[2] reported an increased incidence of adverse cardiovascular outcomes in patients taking other H_2-receptor antagonists with clopidogrel; however, this particular study did not evaluate the effects of each individual H_2-receptor antagonist separately, and also had a large proportion of patients taking cimetidine, which might have influenced the adverse outcome. In general, it would seem that no clinically relevant interaction occurs between clopidogrel and the H_2-receptor antagonists ranitidine or famotidine, and probably also nizatidine, and they would seem to be a suitable alternative to cimetidine.

1. Wang SSW, Tsai S-S, Hsu P-C, Yang C-Y, Wu D-C. Concomitant use of clopidogrel and proton pump inhibitors or cimetidine after acute myocardial infarction would increase the risk of re-infarction. *Am J Gastroenterol* (2009) 104, 3116–7.
2. Wu C-Y, Chan FK, Wu M-S, Kuo KN, Wang C-B, Tsao C-R, Lin J-T. Histamine$_2$-receptor antagonists are an alternative to proton pump inhibitor in patients receiving clopidogrel. *Gastroenterology* (2010) 139, 1165–71.
3. Kreutz RP, Stanek EJ, Aubert R, Yao J, Breall JA, Desta Z, Skaar TC, Teagarden JR, Frueh FW, Epstein RS, Flockhart DA. Impact of proton pump inhibitors on the effectiveness of clopidogrel after coronary stent placement: the clopidogrel Medco outcomes study. *Pharmacotherapy* (2010) 30, 787–796.
4. Juurlink DN, Gomes T, Ko DT, Szmitko PE, Austin PC, Tu JV, Henry DA, Kopp A, Mamdani MM. A population-based study of the drug interaction between proton pump inhibitors and clopidogrel. *CMAJ* (2009) 180, 713–18.
5. Small DS, Farid NA, Li YG, Ernest CS, Payne CD, Salazar DE, Winters KJ. Effect of ranitidine on the pharmacokinetics and pharmacodynamics of prasugrel and clopidogrel. *Curr Med Res Opin* (2008) 24, 2251–7.
6. Plavix (Clopidogrel hydrogen sulphate). Sanofi-Aventis. UK Summary of product characteristics, January 2014.

Clopidogrel + Macrolides

Troleandomycin, and to a lesser extent erythromycin, appear to reduce the antiplatelet effect of clopidogrel.

Clinical evidence

(a) Erythromycin

In a study, 9 healthy subjects were given clopidogrel 75 mg daily alone for 6 days, then erythromycin 250 mg four times daily alone for 4 days, and then both drugs together for 6 days. Erythromycin slightly decreased inhibition of platelet aggregation by clopidogrel: platelet aggregation was increased from 42% with clopidogrel alone to 55% with the concurrent use of erythromycin and clopidogrel.[1]

(b) Troleandomycin

In a single-dose study in 8 healthy subjects, troleandomycin 500 mg given one hour before clopidogrel 450 mg reduced the antiplatelet effect of clopidogrel, increasing platelet aggregation from 45% to 78%.[1]

Mechanism

Clopidogrel is a prodrug and is metabolised to its active thiol metabolite by CYP3A4 and CYP2C19, as well as CYP1A2 and CYP2B6. Erythromycin and troleandomycin are CYP3A4 inhibitors and might therefore reduce the metabolism of clopidogrel by CYP3A4 leading to a decrease in the levels of the active metabolite, and decreased inhibition of platelet aggregation.[1]

Importance and management

The evidence for an interaction between clopidogrel and the macrolides is limited to the studies above, and is not established. It appears that some macrolides might reduce the antiplatelet effect of clopidogrel, although the clinical relevance of the reductions seen is uncertain, particularly for erythromycin. In addition, platelet reactivity might not be directly relevant to clinical outcomes, and it is as yet unclear if this correlates with a reduction in the beneficial cardiovascular effects of clopidogrel. However, until further data are available regarding an interaction, it would seem prudent to consider the possibility of a reduced antiplatelet effect in response to clopidogrel in patients taking macrolides that are potent inhibitors of CYP3A4 (such as troleandomycin).

For an isolated case report of in-stent thrombosis in a patient taking **clarithromycin**, rifampicin and ethambutol, see 'Clopidogrel + Azoles', p.785.

1. Lau WC, Waskell LA, Watkins PB, Neer CJ, Horowitz K, Hopp AS, Tait AR, Carville DGM, Guyer KE, Bates ER. Atorvastatin reduces the ability of clopidogrel to inhibit platelet aggregation. A new drug-drug interaction. *Circulation* (2003) 107, 32–7.

Clopidogrel + Miscellaneous

The antiplatelet effects of clopidogrel do not appear to be affected by acetylcysteine, atenolol or oestrogens. Clopidogrel has been given safely with insulin, ACE inhibitors, antiepileptics, beta blockers, coronary or peripheral vasodilators, and diuretics.

Clinical evidence, mechanism, importance and management

(a) Acetylcysteine

A study in 11 patients with coronary artery disease found that the inhibition of platelet aggregation by clopidogrel 75 mg daily was not reduced by a single 6 g dose of oral acetylcysteine.[1]

(b) Atenolol

In a placebo-controlled study in patients with peripheral vascular or coronary artery disease, the concurrent use of clopidogrel and either atenolol (8 patients) or nifedipine (6) or both atenolol with nifedipine (8) did not affect the control of angina or hypertension by atenolol, when compared with placebo. In addition, the antiplatelet effect of clopidogrel did not appear to be altered by atenolol because it did not differ between the groups.[2] These data suggest that no interaction is likely.

(c) Miscellaneous

The UK manufacturer briefly reports that the pharmacodynamic activity of clopidogrel was not altered by the concurrent use of **oestrogen**.[3] Data from CAPRIE and other clinical studies showed that **ACE inhibitors**, **antidiabetics (insulin** named), **antiepileptics**, **beta blockers**, **coronary** or **peripheral vasodilators**, and **diuretics** have been safely given with clopidogrel.[3,4] This suggests that no additional precautions would be necessary when clopidogrel is given with any of these drugs.

1. Campbell CL, Berger PB, Nuttall GA, Orford JL, Santrach PJ, Oliver WC, Ereth MH, Thompson CM, Murphy MK, McGlassen DL, Schrader LM, Steinhubl SR. Can *N*-acetylcysteine reverse the antiplatelet effects of clopidogrel? An in vivo and vitro study. *Am Heart J* (2005) 150, 796–9.
2. Forbes CD, Lowe GDO, Maclaren M, Shaw BG, Dickinson JP, Kieffer G. Clopidogrel compatibility with concomitant cardiac co-medications: a study of its interactions with a beta-blocker and a calcium uptake antagonist. *Semin Thromb Hemost* (1999) 25 (Suppl 2), 55–9.
3. Plavix (Clopidogrel hydrogen sulphate). Sanofi-Aventis. UK Summary of product characteristics, January 2014.
4. Morais J, on behalf of the CAPRIE investigators. Use of concomitant medications in the CAPRIE trial: clopidogrel is unlikely to be associated with clinically significant drug interactions. *Eur Heart J* (1998) 19 (Abstract Suppl), 5.

Clopidogrel and related drugs + NSAIDs

Clopidogrel increases the risk of bleeding (including gastrointestinal bleeding), and there is evidence that this may be further increased with NSAIDs. Prasugrel and ticlopidine would be expected to interact with the NSAIDs similarly. One case report attributed in-stent thrombosis in a patient taking aspirin and clopidogrel to a possible antagonistic interaction with diclofenac and meloxicam. An isolated case describes agranulocytosis in a patient taking clopidogrel and dipyrone.

Clinical evidence and mechanism

(a) Clopidogrel

1. Bleeding risk. Both clopidogrel and NSAIDs alone increase the risk of gastrointestinal bleeding, and concurrent use would be expected to further increase this risk. In one double-blind, placebo-controlled study in 30 healthy subjects given **naproxen** 250 mg twice daily, the addition of clopidogrel 75 mg daily increased faecal blood loss, when compared with **naproxen** alone. Six subjects receiving both drugs had their bleeding time prolonged by a factor of more than 5, which was greater than expected (clopidogrel alone prolongs bleeding by a factor of about 2) and one subject had subcutaneous haemorrhages of moderate intensity after taking clopidogrel with **naproxen**.[1] Similarly, a retrospective study of patient records in the UK found that the adjusted rate ratio for the risk of gastrointestinal bleeding in patients taking clopidogrel with an NSAID increased from 1.67 for clopidogrel alone, to 2.9 when clopidogrel was taken with an NSAID, and to 2.6 when clopidogrel was taken with a coxib.[2]

An isolated case report describes intracerebral haemorrhage in an 86-year-old woman who had been taking **celecoxib** 200 mg daily with clopidogrel 75 mg daily for 3 weeks. The authors comment that there may also possibly have been a pharmacokinetic interaction between clopidogrel and **celecoxib**: they suggest that a metabolite of clopidogrel may inhibit CYP2C9, by which **celecoxib** is metabolised,[3] but note that a pharmacokinetic interaction has not been found between clopidogrel and other CYP2C9 substrates. Alternatively, other factors, such as age or the individual drugs, may have also caused the haemorrhage.[3]

2. Efficacy. A case of myocardial infarction due to late stent-thrombosis has been reported in a patient taking aspirin 75 mg daily and clopidogrel 75 mg daily 6 days after starting to take **diclofenac** 75 mg twice daily and **meloxicam** 15 mg twice daily. Platelet aggregation studies indicated only a partial antiplatelet effect when the patient was taking diclofenac and meloxicam, compared with measurements taken 7 days after stopping the NSAIDs, and the authors suggest that a drug interaction might possibly have contributed to the adverse outcome.[4] Note that, NSAIDs, which are reversible inhibitors of platelet aggregation, are postulated to inhibit the antiplatelet effect of irreversible inhibitors such as aspirin, and this would also include clopidogrel. NSAIDs might therefore reduce the antithrombotic efficacy of clopidogrel and aspirin, see also 'NSAIDs + Aspirin', p.145.

3. Blood dyscrasias. A case of agranulocytosis, lasting for 10 days and requiring treatment with filgrastim, has been reported in a 75-year-old patient who started to take **clopidogrel** and was given **dipyrone (metamizole)** 500 mg three times daily for severe osteoarthritis.[5] Both clopidogrel and dipyrone rarely cause blood dyscrasias, and it is possible that the risk might be greater on concurrent use.

(b) Ticlopidine

The manufacturer briefly states that ticlopidine potentiates the effect of NSAIDs on platelet aggregation.[6]

Importance and management

The published evidence for an interaction between clopidogrel and related drugs and the non-selective NSAIDs or coxibs appears to be limited to the studies and case reports above. However, as NSAIDs alone increase the risk of bleeding, concurrent use of an antiplatelet drug (such as clopidogrel, **prasugrel**, and ticlopidine) would be expected to further increase this risk.

In addition, due to an increased thrombotic risk, the use of a coxib is contraindicated in those with ischaemic heart disease, cerebrovascular disease, and peripheral artery disease; and some evidence suggests that diclofenac, and high doses of ibuprofen, might similarly be associated with an increased risk of thrombotic events.[7] A review by the European Medicines Agency identified a small increased risk of arterial thrombotic events with diclofenac, which is similar to that for coxibs. They therefore contraindicate the use of diclofenac in patients with ischaemic heart disease, peripheral arterial disease, cerebrovascular disease, or congestive heart failure.[8] Moreover, the European Society of Cardiology guidelines on non-ST-segment elevation acute coronary syndromes recommend that patients should not be given either coxibs or non-selective NSAIDs with either aspirin or clopidogrel.[9] Therefore, the need for any NSAID should be very carefully considered in those patients taking clopidogrel or related drugs, particularly for indications such as coronary stent implantation or acute coronary syndrome. For further discussion on the adverse cardiovascular effects of NSAIDs, see 'NSAIDs + Aspirin', p.145.

The general significance of the isolated case report of agranulocytosis is unclear; however, it would seem prudent to bear the possibility of an interaction in mind should any unexpected irregularities in the full blood count occur.

1. Van Hecken A, Depré M, Wynants K, Vanbilloen H, Verbruggen A, Arnout J, Vanhove P, Cariou R, De Schepper PJ. Effect of clopidogrel on naproxen-induced gastrointestinal blood loss in healthy volunteers. *Drug Metabol Drug Interact* (1998) 14, 193–205 .
2. Delaney JA, Opatrny L, Brophy JM, Suissa S. Drug-drug interactions between antithrombotic medications and the risk of gastrointestinal bleeding. *Can Med Assoc J* (2007) 177, 347–51.
3. Fisher AA, Le Couteur DG. Intracerebral hemorrhage following possible interaction between celecoxib and clopidogrel. *Ann Pharmacother* (2001) 35, 1567–9.
4. Merkely B, Toth-Zsamboki E, Becker D, Beres BJ, Szabó G, Vargova K, Fülöp G, Kerecsen G, Preda I, Spaulding C, Kiss RG. Very late drug-eluting stent thrombosis after nonsteroidal anti-inflammatory drug treatment despite dual antiplatelet therapy. *Can J Cardiol* (2009) 25, 229–232.
5. Kummer O, Haschke M, Tuscherer D, Lampert M, Martius F, Krähenbühl S. Agranulozytose bei einem mit Metamizol und Clopidogrel behandelten Patienten. *Praxis (Bern 1994)* (2006) 95, 1743–7.
6. Ticlopidine hydrochloride. Apotex Corp. US Prescribing information, February 2006.
7. Commission on Human Medicines. Safety of selective and non-selective NSAIDs - health professional letter, October 2006. Available at: http://webarchive.nationalarchives.gov.uk/20141205150130/http://www.mhra.gov.uk/home/groups/pl-p/documents/websiteresources/con2025036.pdf (accessed 20/10/15).
8. European Medicines Agency. PRAC recommends the same cardiovascular precautions for diclofenac as for selective COX-2 inhibitors. June 2013. Available at: http://www.ema.europa.eu/docs/en_GB/document_library/Press_release/2013/06/WC500144451.pdf (accessed 20/10/15).
9. Bassand J-P, Hamm CW, Ardissino D, Boersma E, Budaj A, Fernández-Avilés F, Fox KAA, Hasdai D, Ohman EM, Wallentin L, Wijns W: The Task Force for the Diagnosis and Treatment of Non-ST-Segment Elevation Acute Coronary Syndromes of the European Society of Cardiology. Guidelines for the diagnosis and treatment of non-ST-segment elevation acute coronary syndromes. *Eur Heart J* (2007) 28, 1598–1660.

Clopidogrel + Proton pump inhibitors and other CYP2C19 inhibitors

High-dose omeprazole almost halves the exposure to the active metabolite of clopidogrel and reduces the antiplatelet effects of clopidogrel. There is some evidence to suggest that low-dose omeprazole and rabeprazole have less effect, and high-dose pantoprazole interacts minimally. Findings from the numerous retrospective studies looking at the clinical relevance of the interaction of omeprazole and other proton pump inhibitors are conflicting: some studies suggest that the concurrent use of proton pump inhibitors might reduce the efficacy of clopidogrel and increase the risk of adverse cardiovascular effects, while others have found no such interaction.

Clopidogrel slightly increases omeprazole exposure in CYP2C19 extensive metabolisers.

Clinical evidence

A. Pharmacokinetics and antiplatelet effects

(a) Controlled studies

1. Lansoprazole. In a randomised study, 24 healthy subjects were given lansoprazole 30 mg daily with a single 300-mg dose of clopidogrel on day 7. Lansoprazole had no effect on the AUC and maximum concentrations of the *inactive* carboxylic acid metabolite of clopidogrel, the major clopidogrel metabolite, formed by esterases. The authors state that this study did not look at the effect of lansoprazole on the pharmacokinetics of the *active* metabolite of clopidogrel, because an assay was not available at the time. Lansoprazole tended to slightly reduce the effects of clopidogrel on platelet aggregation, but the effect was only statistically significant at 24 hours after the single dose of clopidogrel (39% versus 49%). A post-hoc analysis suggested that this effect was more pronounced in the subjects that had the greatest antiplatelet response to clopidogrel.[1] In another crossover study, 39 healthy subjects were given clopidogrel 75 mg daily alone and then with lansoprazole 30 mg daily for 7 days. Lansoprazole had no effect on the antiplatelet action of clopidogrel in both the 15 subjects who were CYP2C19 extensive metabolisers or in the 24 subjects who were CYP2C19 'decreased' metabolisers. In those subjects classified as CYP2C19 intermediate metabolisers, lansoprazole had no effect on the number classified as low responders to clopidogrel (one becoming a non-responder and others becoming responders, with wide intersubject variability in clopidogrel responsiveness).[2] In yet another study, lansoprazole 30 mg daily for 7 days slightly reduced the platelet inhibitory response to clopidogrel 75 mg daily in 21 subjects who had previously been good responders to clopidogrel alone. Ten of the 21 had a decrease, which ranged from one to 36%, and just three 'became' poor responders.[3]

2. Omeprazole. In a crossover study in 66 healthy subjects given a 300-mg loading dose of clopidogrel then clopidogrel 75 mg daily for 5 days, high-dose omeprazole 80 mg daily for 5 days, taken at the same time as clopidogrel, reduced the exposure to the active metabolite of clopidogrel by 45% on day one and 40% on day 5. In addition, the mean inhibition of platelet aggregation in response to clopidogrel was reduced by 39% at 24 hours and reduced by 21% on day 5 by omeprazole, when compared with clopidogrel alone. Similar results were seen in a further study when the daily dose of omeprazole and clopidogrel were taken 12 hours apart. Moreover, the interaction was not prevented by doubling the clopidogrel dose to a 600-mg loading dose then 150 mg daily.[4] In another similar study, a lower dose of omeprazole 40 mg daily did not alter the antiplatelet effect 24 hours after a 600-mg loading dose of clopidogrel, but the antiplatelet effect of maintenance clopidogrel 75 mg daily was reduced, whether given at the same time as omeprazole or separated by 8 to 12 hours.[5] In yet another similar study using low-dose omeprazole 20 mg daily for 7 days, omeprazole reduced the antiplatelet effect of clopidogrel 75 mg daily in the 15 subjects classified as CYP2C19 rapid metabolisers, although this was not sufficient to make any of them low responders to clopidogrel (less than 30% platelet aggregation). Whereas, in the 24 subjects classified as CYP2C19 'decreased' metabolisers, omeprazole did not alter the antiplatelet effects of clopidogrel, and had no overall effect on the number classified as low responders to clopidogrel (5 became non-responders and others becoming responders, with wide intersubject variability in clopidogrel responsiveness). In the group as a whole, giving the omeprazole dose at night rather than at the same time as clopidogrel in the morning did not reduce the interaction.[2]

In a randomised, placebo-controlled study in 124 patients undergoing elective coronary stent insertion and taking aspirin 75 mg daily and clopidogrel (300 mg loading dose followed by 75 mg daily), 64 patients were also given omeprazole 20 mg daily for 7 days. On day 7, the group given omeprazole were found to have a higher platelet reactivity index when compared with placebo recipients (51% compared with 40%, respectively), indicating a reduced antiplatelet effect.[6] The authors note that a platelet reactivity index of greater than 50% indicates a poor response to clopidogrel. On this basis, 61% of omeprazole recipients were considered to have had a poor response to clopidogrel, compared with 27% in the placebo group.[6] Note that, in this study, CYP2C19 metaboliser status was unknown,[7] although given that it was a large randomised study in a specific population, a difference between the groups would not usually be expected. Another study found a reduction in antiplatelet effects of clopidogrel with omeprazole 20 mg which was similar in magnitude to that of rabeprazole 20 mg daily.[8]

The effect of clopidogrel on omeprazole pharmacokinetics has also been studied in healthy subjects. Clopidogrel (a 300-mg loading dose and then 75 mg daily for 3 days) slightly increased the AUC of a single 40-mg dose of omeprazole given on day 4 by 30% and decreased its clearance by 22% in CYP2C19 extensive metabolisers (that is, those with normal isoenzyme activity), but had no effect in CYP2C19 poor metabolisers (that is, those lacking or totally deficient in this isoenzyme). The degree of inhibition was slight, and omeprazole exposure in CYP2C19 extensive metabolisers given clopidogrel was still lower than in CYP2C19 poor metabolisers (with or without clopidogrel).[9]

3. Pantoprazole. In a crossover study in healthy subjects given a 300-mg loading dose of clopidogrel then clopidogrel 75 mg daily for 5 days, high-dose pantoprazole 80 mg daily for 5 days, taken at the same time as clopidogrel, slightly reduced the exposure to the active metabolite of clopidogrel by 20% on day one and by 14% on day 5. In addition, the platelet reactivity index was increased by 3.9% when compared with clopidogrel alone.[4]

4. Rabeprazole. In a study in 39 healthy subjects given clopidogrel 75 mg daily alone and then with rabeprazole 20 mg daily for 7 days, rabeprazole slightly reduced the antiplatelet effect of clopidogrel in the 15 subjects classified as CYP2C19 rapid metabolisers (53.5% versus 58.3%), and this was just sufficient to make one of them a low responder to clopidogrel (less than 30% platelet aggregation). However, in the 24 subjects classified as CYP2C19 'decreased' metabolisers, rabeprazole did not alter the antiplatelet effects of clopidogrel and had no effect on the number classified as low responders to clopidogrel (two becoming non-responders and others becoming responders, with wide intersubject variability in clopidogrel responsiveness).[2] In another randomised study in patients taking clopidogrel, the use of rabeprazole 20 mg daily for 14 days increased the platelet reactivity index from about 36% to 48%, and increased the number of clopidogrel non-responders from 29.5% to 52.3% (defined as maximal platelet aggregation of greater than 50%). In this study, the effect of rabeprazole did not differ from that of omeprazole 20 mg daily.[8]

(b) Non-randomised studies

1. Esomeprazole. A study in patients taking aspirin 100 mg daily with clopidogrel 75 mg daily for at least 5 days (average 3 months) included 74 patients taking esomeprazole. The study found no difference in the platelet reactivity index or ADP-induced platelet aggregation when these patients were compared with 74 patients not taking a proton pump inhibitor.[10] Similar findings were reported in a study including 22 patients taking esomeprazole, which used five different platelet function tests.[11] Similarly, in a study of patients with coronary artery disease taking both aspirin and clopidogrel, the proportion of patients having a poor antiplatelet response to clopidogrel was similar in 42 patients taking esomeprazole and in patients not taking a proton pump inhibitor (about 20% in both groups).[12]

In contrast to these studies, in a study in patients taking clopidogrel, maximum concentrations of the active metabolite of clopidogrel were 45% lower in 6 patients also taking esomeprazole (40 mg daily in 4 subjects or 20 mg daily in 2 subjects) than in 22 patients not taking a proton pump inhibitor. There was no change in clopidogrel concentrations or the concentration of the inactive clopidogrel metabolite, indicating altered metabolism and not reduced absorption. In addition, these 6 patients had higher platelet reactivity.[13]

2. Omeprazole. In a study in patients with coronary artery disease taking both aspirin and clopidogrel, the proportion of patients having a poor antiplatelet response to clopidogrel was about 13% higher in the 64 patients taking omeprazole, when compared with patients taking esomeprazole or pantoprazole, or not taking a proton pump inhibitor (about 33% versus 20%).[12]

3. Pantoprazole. A study in patients taking aspirin 100 mg daily with clopidogrel 75 mg daily for at least 5 days (average 3 months) included 152 patients taking pantoprazole. This study found that there was no difference in the platelet reactivity index or ADP-induced platelet aggregation in the patients taking pantoprazole when compared with 74 patients not taking a proton pump inhibitor.[10] Similar findings were reported in a study including 95 patients taking pantoprazole, which used 5 different platelet function tests.[11] Similarly, in a study of patients with coronary artery disease taking both aspirin and clopidogrel, the proportion of patients having a poor antiplatelet response to clopidogrel was similar in 162 patients taking pantoprazole and those patients not taking a proton pump inhibitor (about 20% in both groups).[12] In a study in patients taking clopidogrel, maximum concentrations of the active metabolite of clopidogrel in 22 patients also receiving pantoprazole 40 mg daily did not differ from those in patients not receiving a proton pump inhibitor.[13]

4. Unspecified proton pump inhibitors. In a study, the platelet reactivity index was measured in 105 consecutive patients taking aspirin and clopidogrel to investigate its relationship with various other concurrent drugs. A higher platelet reactivity index (indicating a poor response to aspirin and clopidogrel) was found in the 24 patients taking proton pump inhibitors, when compared with the 81 patients not taking proton pump inhibitors (about 61% versus 50%).[14] Similarly, in a post-hoc analysis of a clinical study in patients given a 600-mg loading dose of clopidogrel then clopidogrel 150 mg daily (PRINCIPLE-TIMI 44), mean inhibition of platelet aggregation was lower in those patients also taking a proton pump inhibitor. The proportion of patients with reduced platelet responsiveness to clopidogrel was 2-fold higher in patients taking a proton pump inhibitor than in patients not taking a proton pump inhibitor, when assessed at 24 hours after the 600-mg loading dose of clopidogrel.[15]

B. Clinical outcomes

There does not appear to be any evidence from placebo-controlled, randomised studies on the effect of any proton pump inhibitors on the long-term cardiovascular efficacy of clopidogrel, apart from data from the halted Cogent study, see *Randomised prospective studies*, below. All other data available are retrospective analyses, and, as it is impossible to control for all possible confounders, definitive conclusions cannot be drawn from these studies. Various meta-analyses have reviewed the many analyses of the risk of cardiovascular events and mortality with the use of proton pump inhibitors in patients taking clopidogrel.[16-18] One analysis of 13 studies in a total of 48 674 patients reported a 41% increased risk of major adverse cardiovascular events in patients taking proton pump inhibitors and an 18% increased risk of mortality, when compared with patients not taking a proton pump inhibitor.[17] Another analysis of 23 studies in a total of 93 278 patients found that, in the 12 studies where myocardial infarction or acute coronary syndrome were used as outcomes, unadjusted data from observational studies gave the highest increased risk (82%), studies with data adjusted for confounders had an increased risk of 54%, and studies based on propensity matched or study participants had the lowest increased risk (15%, which was not statistically significant).[16] A third analysis of 25 studies in 159 138 patients reported a 29% increased risk of major cardiovascular events, a 31% increased risk of myocardial infarction, but no increased risk of mortality.[18] The findings of some of the key larger studies are summarised below.

(a) Randomised prospective studies

In the COGENT-1 study , there was no apparent difference in the incidence of all cardiovascular events (including myocardial infarction or in the need for revascularisation) between 1 876 patients taking clopidogrel with omeprazole 20 mg daily and 1 885 patients taking clopidogrel with placebo (4.9% versus 5.7%), for a median follow up of 106 days (hazard ratio with omeprazole 0.99 (95% CI, 0.68 to 1.44)).[19] However, note that this large, phase III randomised clinical study was stopped before the planned enrolment and duration because of bankruptcy, and was primarily designed to investigate the gastrointestinal benefits of omeprazole formulated with clopidogrel, rather than to investigate a drug interaction between omeprazole and clopidogrel and its possible effects on cardiovascular outcomes. The authors concluded that, because the confidence interval around the hazard ratio for cardiovascular events is wide, the absence of an interaction between clopidogrel and omeprazole cannot be viewed as a definitive finding.[19] Commenting on this study, authors from the FDA in the US note that the clinical setting (fewer than half of patients had acute coronary syndrome at the time of enrolment) and the cardiovascular end point limit the interpretability of the findings.[20]

(b) Retrospective studies

1. Poorer outcomes with all proton pump inhibitors. A large, retrospective, cohort study in patients taking clopidogrel who were hospitalised with acute coronary syndrome, investigated the use of proton pump inhibitors to establish if concurrent use was associated with an increase in adverse cardiovascular outcomes. In this study, the 5 244 patients taking a proton pump inhibitor with clopidogrel were reported to have a 9% additional increase in the rate of death or rehospitalisation for acute coronary syndrome compared with the 2 961 patients not taking a proton pump inhibitor (29.8% versus 20.8%), although the patients in the proton pump inhibitor group were older and had more co-morbid conditions. After adjusting for these confounding factors, the odds ratio was 1.25. Further analysis on the secondary outcomes reported that the rate of rehospitalisation for acute coronary syndrome was 14.6% in those taking a proton pump inhibitor with clopidogrel, compared with 6.9% for those patients not taking a proton pump inhibitor with clopidogrel, with an adjusted odds ratio of 1.86. The proton pump inhibitors given included **omeprazole** (59.7%), **rabeprazole** (2.9%), **lansoprazole** (0.4%) and **pantoprazole** (0.2%), and 36.7% of patients took more than one proton pump inhibitor during follow-up (that is, they switched between different proton pump inhibitors). Individual data for **lansoprazole** and **pantoprazole** were not analysed as the patient numbers were too small, but **omeprazole** and **rabeprazole** use were reported to have an increased risk of adverse outcomes (odds ratio 1.24 and 2.83, respectively). In patients discharged after an episode of acute coronary syndrome who were not given clopidogrel, the use of proton pump inhibitors was not associated with an increased risk of death or re-admission to hospital, suggesting that any effect was the result of an interaction, rather than a factor of proton pump inhibitor use.[21] Similarly, in a cohort study of 18 565 patients who were given clopidogrel, there was a slight increased risk of hospitalisation for myocardial infarction or death (adjusted risk ratio of 1.26) in those taking a proton pump inhibitor (**omeprazole**, **esomeprazole**, **lansoprazole**, **pantoprazole**, **rabeprazole**) compared with patients not taking a proton pump inhibitor. This suggests that if an effect exists, it is unlikely to be greater than a 20% increased risk.[22] In a retrospective cohort study, there was an increased risk of hospitalisation for a major adverse cardiovascular event for all proton pump inhibitors compared with clopidogrel alone (25% versus 18%, hazard ratio 1.51). The most common proton pump inhibitors taken were **esomeprazole** (3 257 patients), **omeprazole** (2 307 patients) and **pantoprazole** (1 653 patients), with fewer patients taking **lansoprazole** (785 patients) or **rabeprazole** (298 patients). When the data was analysed by individual proton pump inhibitor, a similar increased risk of hospitalisation for a major adverse cardiovascular event was seen for **lansoprazole** (24%, hazard ratio 1.39), **esomeprazole** (25%, hazard ratio 1.57), **omeprazole** (25%, hazard ratio 1.39), and **pantoprazole** (29%, hazard ratio 1.61), when compared with patients not taking a proton pump inhibitor: the patient group taking **rabeprazole** was too small for individual statistical evaluation.[23] In a Danish cohort study, use of a proton pump inhibitor with clopidogrel was associated with a 1.29-fold increased risk of adverse cardiovascular outcomes compared with clopidogrel alone. However, in patients not taking clopidogrel, use of proton pump inhibitor was also associated with a similar risk of adverse cardiovascular outcomes, leading the authors to conclude that the increased risk with clopidogrel was not real, but was due to unknown confounding factors associated with proton pump inhibitor use.[24]

2. Poorer outcomes with some proton pump inhibitors. In a retrospective case-control study in 734 patients taking clopidogrel post myocardial infarction and readmitted within 90 days with a further myocardial infarction, the concurrent use of a proton pump inhibitor (**lansoprazole**, **omeprazole**, **pantoprazole**, or **rabeprazole**; 194 cases) was associated with a 27% increased risk of re-infarction. When the data was analysed for **pantoprazole** separately (46 cases), there was no additional risk of myocardial infarction.[25] The remaining proton pump inhibitors as a group were associated with a 40% increased risk and the data for them were not analysed separately. However, the difference between the risk for pantoprazole and the other drugs was not statistically significant. The proton pump inhibitors were grouped like this on the basis of *in vitro* CYP2C19 inhibition data; however, see under *Mechanism*, below, for further discussion of the potential relevance of this. In contrast, in a large cohort study of 10 703 patients taking clopidogrel, the increased risk of myocardial infarction associated with proton pump inhibitors was highest for **pantoprazole** (91%) intermediate with **lansoprazole** (62%) and lowest for **omeprazole** (26%), with an overall increased risk of 50% for all proton pump inhibitors.[26]

3. No effect of proton pump inhibitors. In a retrospective analysis of a large clinical study in patients taking clopidogrel or prasugrel (TRITON-TIMI 38), no association was found between proton pump inhibitor use and an increased incidence of cardiovascular death, myocardial infarction, stroke or coronary stent thrombosis in those given clopidogrel. The most common proton pump inhibitors taken in the study as a whole were **pantoprazole** (1 844 patients) and **omeprazole** (1 675 patients), with fewer patients taking **esomeprazole** (613 patients), **lansoprazole** (441 patients) and **rabeprazole** (66 patients).[15]

Similarly, in a cohort study in 20 596 patients with coronary heart disease who were given clopidogrel, the concurrent use of proton pump inhibitors (7 593 patients) did not increase the risk of serious adverse cardiovascular effects (such as myocardial infarction and stroke; hazard ratio 0.99). Further analysis also found no increased risk with high or low-dose proton pump inhibitor, or with the individual drugs (**pantoprazole** (62% of patients), **lansoprazole** (about 15%), **esomeprazole** (about 10%), **omeprazole** (9%), or **rabeprazole** (about 4%). The authors also found that concurrent use of a proton pump inhibitor in patients taking clopidogrel reduced the risk of gastrointestinal bleeding by up to 50%. The extent of the risk reduction depended on the patients risk factors for gastrointestinal bleeding: the reduction was most significant in patients with three or more risk factors, whereas patients with no risk factors had no reduction in the rate of hospitalisation for gastrointestinal bleeding.[27]

Mechanism

The most plausible mechanism for the pharmacokinetic interaction is that omeprazole inhibits the conversion of clopidogrel to its active metabolite by CYP2C19. *In vitro* data indicate that lansoprazole, esomeprazole and a metabolite of rabeprazole can all inhibit CYP2C19, but that pantoprazole does not significantly affect this isoenzyme.[28] However, *in vitro* inhibitory activity does not always translate to a clinically relevant effect *in vivo*: inhibition of CYP2C19 appears to occur between the known CYP2C19 substrate diazepam and omeprazole or esomeprazole, but a clinically important interaction does not occur with rabeprazole, lansoprazole, or pantoprazole (see 'Benzodiazepines + Proton pump inhibitors', p.834). Furthermore, CYP2C19 inhibition by the proton pump inhibitors is not entirely consistent with the available data for their suggested interaction with clopidogrel. For example, there are data suggesting that esomeprazole does not alter the antiplatelet effects of clopidogrel, and some evidence from retrospective studies that all proton pump inhibitors are associated with a similar risk of poorer outcomes in patients taking clopidogrel. However, if the proton pump inhibitors completely inhibited the activity of CYP2C19, this would effectively make CYP2C19 extensive metabolisers into poor metabolisers, who have a known reduced antiplatelet response to clopidogrel and a higher than expected rate of cardiovascular events.[29,30] Others have suggested that P-glycoprotein might also be involved;[7] *in vitro* data suggest that clopidogrel absorption might be reduced by P-glycoprotein inhibition,[31] and based on their interaction with digoxin, a key P-glycoprotein substrate (see 'Digoxin and related drugs + Proton pump inhibitors', p.1108), most proton pump inhibitors appear to affect this drug transporter protein, although the effect is mild. Another explanation for a general interaction with proton pump inhibitors in observational studies is that proton pump inhibitors are a marker for increased cardiovascular risk independent of clopidogrel use.[24]

Clopidogrel is a weak inhibitor of CYP2C19, by which omeprazole and many other proton pump inhibitors are partly metabolised. In this study, the metabolism of omeprazole to 5-hydroxyomeprazole by CYP2C19 was decreased, whereas its metabolism to omeprazole sulfone by CYP3A4 was unchanged.[9]

Importance and management

A pharmacokinetic interaction between high-dose **omeprazole** (80 mg daily) and clopidogrel appears to be established, roughly halving the exposure of the active metabolite of clopidogrel and reducing its antiplatelet effects by 30%. Separating the dose of clopidogrel and omeprazole by 12 hours did not reduce or abolish the pharmacokinetic interaction in one study. However, what is not clearly established is to what degree this might reduce the clinical efficacy of clopidogrel, and to what extent it applies to more commonly used doses of omeprazole (20 mg daily). There is some evidence to suggest that the platelet inhibitory effect of clopidogrel was less affected by omeprazole 20 mg daily, and limited evidence from one unfinished, prospective, randomised, controlled study suggests that omeprazole 20 mg daily has no effect on clopidogrel efficacy.[19] Data from retrospective analyses have varied from no effect to an increased risk of adverse cardiac outcomes, with the greatest effect being a 1.86-fold increased risk in the rate of rehospitalisation for acute coronary syndrome. This, coupled with the data showing a reduced clinical response to clopidogrel alone in patients who are CYP2C19 poor metabolisers, suggests that it is not unreasonable to suppose that omeprazole causes some reduction in the efficacy of clopidogrel.

Evidence for a class interaction between clopidogrel and the **proton pump inhibitors** is mostly based on retrospective data, some of which is contradictory, and does not appear to fit with the known CYP2C19 inhibitory activity of these proton pump inhibitors. On reviewing the available evidence, in November 2009 the FDA in the US recommended that omeprazole should be avoided in patients taking clopidogrel. A similar recommendation is made for **esomeprazole** on the basis that it is the *S*-isomer of omeprazole, and also inhibits CYP2C19.[32] At that time, the FDA stated that there was insufficient evidence to make specific recommendations about the concurrent use of clopidogrel with other proton pump inhibitors.[32] In October 2010 the FDA repeated their advice to avoid omeprazole, and suggested that **pantoprazole** might be an alternative.[33] Conversely, a 2010 consensus document of the American College of Cardiology Foundation, the American College of Gastroenterology and the American Heart Association does not preclude the use of omeprazole with clopidogrel.[34] Based on data from various studies (including COGENT and TRITON-TIMI 38), in April 2010 the MHRA in the UK revised their previous advice to avoid all proton pump inhibitors (unspecified),[35] and stated that omeprazole and esomeprazole should be discouraged in patients taking clopidogrel unless concurrent use is essential. They advised that if a proton pump inhibitor is necessary in a patient taking clopidogrel, a proton pump inhibitor other than omeprazole or esomeprazole should be considered. Alternative gastroprotective drugs to the proton pump inhibitors should also be considered, such as antacids or H_2-receptor antagonists (except cimetidine, see 'Clopidogrel + H_2-receptor antagonists', p.786). The EMEA has given similar advice.[36] If a proton pump inhibitor is considered necessary, **pantoprazole** would appear to be a suitable choice because at a high dose of 80 mg daily it caused minimal effects on the pharmacokinetics and pharmacodynamics of clopidogrel, and limited evidence suggests no effect for 40 mg daily. In addition, based on the lack of a pharmacokinetic interaction with the known CYP2C19 substrate diazepam (consider 'Benzodiazepines + Proton pump inhibitors', p.834), **rabeprazole**, and possibly also **lansoprazole**, would also seem to be appropriate options. However, the effects or lack of effect of lansoprazole or rabeprazole on clopidogrel pharmacokinetics and its antiplatelet effects is not established, and more prospective studies are needed to investigate this. In general, the individual patient's risk factors for gastrointestinal bleeding should be considered against the possible risk of an interaction with clopidogrel, as in some patients the benefit of proton pump inhibitor treatment might outweigh the possible risk of reduced clopidogrel efficacy.[34]

On the basis of the interaction with omeprazole, the FDA[32] and the manufacturers[37,38] of clopidogrel state that other drugs that inhibit CYP2C19 would also be expected to interact similarly, and they advise avoiding concurrent use of potent or moderate CYP2C19 inhibitors. The MHRA[39] also predicts that other inhibitors of CYP2C19 might affect clopidogrel efficacy and they discourage concurrent use. The MHRA[39] and the UK manufacturer[38] list a number of drugs that could inhibit CYP2C19, including **carbamazepine**, **chloramphenicol**, **ciprofloxacin**, **fluoxetine**, **fluvoxamine**, **moclobemide**, **oxcarbazepine** and **ticlopidine**. However, not all of these drugs are proven, clinically relevant CYP2C19 inhibitors. Note that, **ticlopidine**, like clopidogrel, is a thienopyridine antiplatelet drug, and concurrent use is not clinically indicated with clopidogrel as it has the same mechanism of action.

1. Small DS, Farid NA, Payne CD, Weerakkody GJ, Li YG, Brandt JT, Salazar DE, Winters KJ. Effects of the proton pump inhibitor lansoprazole on the pharmacokinetics and pharmacodynamics of prasugrel and clopidogrel. *J Clin Pharmacol* (2008) 48, 475–84.
2. Furuta T, Iwaki T, Umemura K. Influences of different proton pump inhibitors on the anti-platelet function of clopidogrel in relation to CYP2C19 genotypes. *Br J Clin Pharmacol* (2010) 70, 383–92.

3. Hulot JS, Wuerzner G, Bachelot-Loza C, Azizi M, Blanchard A, Peyrard S, Funck-Brentano C, Gaussem P. Effect of an increased clopidogrel maintenance dose or lansoprazole co-administration on the antiplatelet response to clopidogrel in CYP2C19-genotyped healthy subjects. *J Thromb Haemost* (2010) 8, 610–13.
4. Angiolillo DJ, Gibson CM, Cheng S, Ollier C, Nicolas O, Bergougnan L, Perrin L, Lacreta FP, Hurbin F, Dubar M. Differential effects of omeprazole and pantoprazole on the pharmacodynamics and pharmacokinetics of clopidogrel in healthy subjects: randomized, placebo-controlled, crossover comparison studies. *Clin Pharmacol Ther* (2011) 89, 65–74
5. Ferreiro JL, Ueno M, Capodanno D, Desai B, Dharmashankar K, Darlington A, Charlton RK, Bass TA, Angiolillo DJ. Pharmacodynamic effects of concomitant versus staggered clopidogrel and omeprazole intake: results of a prospective randomized crossover study. *Circ Cardiovasc Interv* (2010) 3, 436–41.
6. Gilard M, Arnaud B, Cornily J-C, Le Gal G, Lacut K, Le Calvez G, Mansourati J, Mottier D, Abgrall J-F, Boschat J. Influence of omeprazole on the antiplatelet action of clopidogrel associated with aspirin. The randomized, double-blind OCLA (Omeprazole CLopidogrel Aspirin) study. *J Am Coll Cardiol* (2008) 51, 256–60.
7. Gurbel PA, Lau WC, Tantry US. Omeprazole: a possible new candidate influencing the antiplatelet effect of clopidogrel. *J Am Coll Cardiol* (2008) 51, 261–3.
8. Siriswangvat S, Sansanayudh N, Nathisuwan S, Panomvana D. Comparison between the effect of omeprazole and rabeprazole on the antiplatelet action of clopidogrel. *Circ J* (2010) 74, 2187–92.
9. Chen BL, Chen Y, Tu JH, Li YL, Zhang W, Li Q, Fan L, Tan ZR, Hu DL, Wang D, Wang LS, OuYang DS, Zhou HH. Clopidogrel inhibits CYP2C19-dependent hydroxylation of omeprazole related to CYP2C19 genetic polymorphisms. *J Clin Pharmacol* (2009) 49, 574–81.
10. Siller-Matula JM, Spiel AO, Lang IM, Kreiner G, Christ G, Jilma B. Effects of pantoprazole and esomeprazole on platelet inhibition by clopidogrel. *Am Heart J* (2009) 157, 148.e1–148.e5.
11. Gremmel T, Steiner S, Seidinger D, Koppensteiner R, Panzer S, Kopp CW. The influence of proton pump inhibitors on the antiplatelet potency of clopidogrel evaluated by 5 different platelet function tests. *J Cardiovasc Pharmacol* (2010) 56, 532–9.
12. Sibbing D, Morath T, Stegherr J, Braun S, Vogt W, Hadamitzky M, Schömig A, Kastrati A, von Beckerath N. Impact of proton pump inhibitors on the antiplatelet effects of clopidogrel. *Thromb Haemost* (2009) 101, 714–19.
13. Harmsze AM, van Werkum JW, Taubert D, Hackeng CM, Deneer VHM. Esomeprazole but not pantoprazole is associated with lower plasma concentrations of clopidogrel's active metabolite. *Ann Pharmacother* (2011) 45, 542–3.
14. Gilard M, Arnaud B, Le Gal G, Abgrall JF, Boschat J. Influence of omeprazol on the antiplatelet action of clopidogrel associated to aspirin. *J Thromb Haemost* (2006) 4, 2508–9.
15. O'Donoghue ML, Braunwald E, Antman EM, Murphy SA, Bates ER, Rozenman Y, Michelson AD, Hautvast RW, Ver Lee PN, Close SL, Shen L, Mega JL, Sabatine MS, Wiviott SD. Pharmacodynamic effect and clinical efficacy of clopidogrel and prasugrel with or without a proton-pump inhibitor: an analysis of two randomised trials. *Lancet* (2009) 374, 989–97.
16. Kwok CS, Loke YK. Meta-analysis: the effects of proton pump inhibitors on cardiovascular events and mortality in patients receiving clopidogrel. *Aliment Pharmacol Ther* (2010) 31, 810–23.
17. Hulot J-S, Collet J-P, Silvain J, Pena A, Bellemain-Appaix A, Barthélémy O, Cayla G, Beygui F, Montalescot G. Cardiovascular risk in clopidogrel-treated patients according to cytochrome P450 2C19*2 loss-of-function allele or proton pump inhibitor coadministration: a systematic meta-analysis. *J Am Coll Cardiol* (2010) 56, 134–43.
18. Siller-Matula JM, Jilma B, Schrör K, Christ G, Huber K. Effect of proton pump inhibitors on clinical outcome in patients treated with clopidogrel: a systematic review and meta-analysis. *J Thromb Haemost* (2010) 8, 2624–41.
19. Bhatt DL, Cryer BL, Contant CF, Cohen M, Lanas A, Schnitzer TJ, Shook TL, Lapuerta P, Goldsmith MA, Laine L, Scirica BM, Murphy SA, Cannon CP; COGENT Investigators. Clopidogrel with or without omeprazole in coronary artery disease. *N Engl J Med* (2010) 363, 1909–17
20. Southworth MR, Temple R. Interaction of clopidogrel and omeprazole. *N Engl J Med* (2010) 363, 1977.
21. Ho PM, Maddox TM, Wang L, Fihn SD, Jesse RL, Peterson ED, Rumsfeld JS. Risk of adverse outcomes associated with concomitant use of clopidogrel and proton pump inhibitors following acute coronary syndrome. *JAMA* (2009) 301, 937–44.
22. Rassen JA, Choudhry NK, Avorn J, Schneeweiss S. Cardiovascular outcomes and mortality in patients using clopidogrel with proton pump inhibitors after percutaneous coronary intervention or acute coronary syndrome. *Circulation* (2009) 120, 2322–9.
23. Kreutz RP, Stanek EJ, Aubert R, Yao J, Breall JA, Desta Z, Skaar TC, Teagarden JR, Frueh FW, Epstein RS, Flockhart DA. Impact of proton pump inhibitors on the effectiveness of clopidogrel after coronary stent placement: the clopidogrel Medco outcomes study. *Pharmacotherapy* (2010) 30, 787–796.
24. Charlot M, Ahlehoff O, Norgaard ML, Jørgensen CH, Sørensen R, Abildstrøm SZ, Hansen PR, Madsen JK, Køber L, Torp-Pedersen C, Gislason G. Proton-pump inhibitors are associated with increased cardiovascular risk independent of clopidogrel use: a nationwide cohort study. *Ann Intern Med* (2010) 153, 378–86. Erratum ibid. (2011) 154, 76.
25. Juurlink DN, Gomes T, Ko DT, Szmitko PE, Austin PC, Tu JV, Henry DA, Kopp A, Mamdani MM. A population-based study of the drug interaction between proton pump inhibitors and clopidogrel. *CMAJ* (2009) 180, 713–18.
26. Hall NL, Mathews KD, May HT, Bair TL, Horne BD, Carlquist JF, Lappé DL, Muhlestein JB, Anderson JL. Abstract 997: cardiovascular risk associated with concurrent proton pump inhibitor and clopidogrel therapy: how much? how specific? *Circulation* (2009) 120: S422.
27. Ray WA, Murray KT, Griffin MR, Chung CP, Smalley WE, Hall K, Daugherty JR, Kaltenbach LA, Stein CM. Outcomes with concurrent use of clopidogrel and proton-pump inhibitors: a cohort study. *Ann Intern Med* (2010) 152, 337–45.
28. Comparison of inhibitory effects of the proton pump-inhibiting drugs omeprazole, esomeprazole, lansoprazole, pantoprazole, and rabeprazole on human cytochrome P450 activities. *Drug Metab Dispos* (2004) 32, 821–7.
29. Society for Cardiovascular Angiography and Interventions; Society of Thoracic Surgeons; Writing Committee Members, Holmes DR Jr, Dehmer GJ, Kaul S, Leifer D, O'Gara PT, Stein CM. ACCF/AHA Clopidogrel clinical alert: approaches to the FDA "boxed warning": a report of the American College of Cardiology Foundation Task Force on Clinical Expert Consensus Documents and the American Heart Association. *Circulation* (2010) 122, 537–57.
30. FDA drug safety communication: reduced effectiveness of Plavix (clopidogrel) in patients who are poor metabolizers of the drug. Available at: http://www.fda.gov/Drugs/DrugSafety/PostmarketDrugSafetyInformationforPatientsandProviders/ucm203888.htm (accessed 21/10/15).
31. Taubert D, von Beckerath N, Grimberg G, Lazar A, Jung N, Goeser T, Kastrati A, Schömig A, Schömig E. Impact of P-glycoprotein on clopidogrel absorption. *Clin Pharmacol Ther* (2006) 80, 486–501.
32. FDA Information for healthcare professionals: Update to the labeling of clopidogrel bisulfate (marketed as Plavix) to alert healthcare professionals about a drug interaction with omeprazole (marketed as Prilosec and Prilosec OTC) [11/17/2009]. Available at: http://www.fda.gov/Drugs/DrugSafety/PostmarketDrugSafetyInformationforPatientsandProviders/DrugSafetyInformationforHeathcareProfessionals/ucm190787.htm (accessed 21/10/15).
33. FDA reminder to avoid concomitant use of Plavix (clopidogrel) and omeprazole. Available at: http://www.fda.gov/Drugs/DrugSafety/ucm231161.htm (accessed 21/10/15).
34. Abraham NS, Hlatky MA, Antman EM, Bhatt DL, Bjorkman DJ, Clark CB, Furberg CD, Johnson DA, Kahi CJ, Laine L, Mahaffey KW, Quigley EM, Scheiman J, Sperling LS, Tomaselli GF; ACCF/ACG/AHA. ACCF/ACG/AHA 2010 expert consensus document on the concomitant use of proton pump inhibitors and thienopyridines: a focused update of the ACCF/ACG/AHA 2008 expert consensus document on reducing the gastrointestinal risks of antiplatelet therapy and NSAID use. *Am J Gastroenterol* (2010) 105, 2533–49.
35. Medicines Healthcare Products Regulatory Agency and the Commission on Human Medicines. Clopidogrel and proton pump inhibitors: interaction—clarification. *Drug Safety Update* (2009) 3, 8.
36. EMEA. Interaction between clopidogrel and proton-pump inhibitors. CHMP updates warning for clopidogrel-containing medicines. London, 17 March 2010. Available at: http://www.ema.europa.eu/docs/en_GB/document_library/Public_statement/2010/03/WC500076346.pdf (accessed 21/10/15).
37. Plavix (Clopidogrel bisulfate). Bristol-Myers Squibb/Sanofi Pharmaceuticals Partnership. US Prescribing information, December 2011.
38. Plavix (Clopidogrel hydrogen sulphate). Sanofi-Aventis. UK Summary of product characteristics, January 2014.
39. Medicines Healthcare Products Regulatory Agency and the Commission on Human Medicines. Clopidogrel and proton pump inhibitors: interaction—updated advice. *Drug Safety Update* (2010) 3, 4–5.

Clopidogrel + Rifampicin (Rifampin) and other enzyme inducers

Rifampicin moderately induces the metabolism of clopidogrel to its active metabolite, and slightly increases its antiplatelet effects. In contrast, phenobarbital is reported not to alter the antiplatelet effects of clopidogrel.

Clinical evidence

(a) Phenobarbital

The UK manufacturer of clopidogrel briefly reports that the pharmacodynamic activity of clopidogrel was not notably altered by phenobarbital.[1]

(b) Rifampicin

In a study, 10 healthy subjects were given clopidogrel 75 mg daily alone for 6 days, then rifampicin 300 mg twice daily alone for 4 days, and then both drugs together for 6 days. Rifampicin slightly increased the antiplatelet effect of clopidogrel by 23%, compared with clopidogrel alone (mean platelet aggregation 33% versus 56%). In 3 of the 4 subjects who had been previously classified as non-responders to clopidogrel (platelet inhibition of less 10%) and one of the 3 subjects who had been classified as low responders (platelet inhibition of 10 to 29%), rifampicin increased the platelet inhibition response to clopidogrel to more than 30% (i.e. they were reclassified as responders to clopidogrel).[2]

In another study, 12 healthy subjects were given a 600-mg loading dose of clopidogrel followed by 75 mg daily alone for 7 days, then rifampicin 300 mg twice daily for 14 days with the same regimen of clopidogrel restarted on day 7. After the loading dose of clopidogrel, rifampicin increased the AUC of the active metabolite of clopidogrel 3.8-fold. This lead to an increase in the amount of $P2Y_{12}$ receptors blocked, and a subsequent increase in the antiplatelet response to clopidogrel (from 69% to 92% after the loading dose, and to 83% after the last dose of clopidogrel).[3]

In contrast, there is one case report of a patient with a history of *Mycobacterium avium intracellulare* infection and taking **clarithromycin**, rifampicin and **ethambutol**, which suggested a reduced response to clopidogrel. After having a myocardial infarction, this patient underwent coronary stenting and was given clopidogrel 75 mg daily with aspirin. However, within 5 days he was readmitted with another myocardial infarction and treated for in-stent thrombosis. The maintenance dose of clopidogrel was increased to 150 mg daily, and the following 6 months were uneventful. The authors of this case report suggest that the concurrent use of these antimycobacterials led to clopidogrel treatment failure and subsequent in-stent thrombosis.[4]

Mechanism

Clopidogrel is a prodrug and is metabolised to its active thiol metabolite by CYP3A4 and CYP2C19, as well as CYP1A2 and CYP2B6. Rifampicin is a strong inducer of the cytochrome P450 enzyme system, and it appears to induce the metabolism of clopidogrel leading to an increase in the levels of the active metabolite, and increased inhibition of platelet aggregation.[2,3] The reason for the apparent clopidogrel treatment failure in the patient taking antimycobacterials is unclear. The authors suggest that clarithromycin and ethambutol might inhibit the metabolism of clopidogrel, thereby reducing its activity[4] (see also 'Clopidogrel + Macrolides', p.787). However, this seems unlikely because rifampicin is such a strong enzyme inducer that all regimens including it are expected to induce isoenzymes, and would therefore be anticipated to induce clopidogrel metabolism.

Limited evidence suggests phenobarbital (which might also be expected to induce clopidogrel metabolism) does not alter the antiplatelet activity of clopidogrel, which might mean that any induction is insufficient to cause an increase in activity.

Importance and management

Evidence for an interaction between clopidogrel and rifampicin is limited to these studies. The marked increase in the levels of the active metabolite of clopidogrel seen with rifampicin appears to increase its antiplatelet effect; however, platelet reactivity studies may not be directly relevant to clinical outcomes, and whether this results in an increase in beneficial cardiovascular effects and/or an increase in the bleeding risk with clopidogrel is as yet unclear. Until further data are available on the clinical outcomes of this interaction, caution is advised on the concurrent use of clopidogrel and rifampicin. Bear this interaction in mind should any otherwise unexplained bleeding occur in a patient taking both drugs.

The single case of clopidogrel treatment failure in a patient taking rifampicin with clarithromycin and ethambutol seems unlikely to be of general clinical relevance.

Limited evidence suggests that no clinically relevant interaction with phenobarbital (and therefore possibly **primidone**) would be anticipated.

1. Plavix (Clopidogrel hydrogen sulphate). Sanofi-Aventis. UK Summary of product characteristics, January 2014.
2. Lau WC, Gurbel PA, Watkins PB, Neer CJ, Hopp AS, Carville DGM, Guyer KE, Tait AR, Bates ER. Contribution of hepatic cytochrome P450 3A4 metabolic activity to the phenomenon of clopidogrel resistance. *Circulation* (2004) 109, 166–71.
3. Judge HM, Patil SB, Buckland RJ, Jakubowski JA, Storey RF. Potentiation of clopidogrel active metabolite formation by rifampicin leads to greater P2Y12 receptor blockade and inhibition of platelet aggregation following clopidogrel. *J Thromb Haemost* (2010) 8, 1820–7.
4. Srinivasan M, Smith D. Drug interaction with anti-mycobacterial treatment as a cause of clopidogrel resistance. *Postgrad Med J* (2008) 84, 217–19.

Clopidogrel + St John's wort (*Hypericum perforatum*)

St John's wort caused a small increase in the antiplatelet effect of clopidogrel in one study in hyporesponsive patients, and a small decrease in platelet reactivity in another.

Clinical evidence

In an open-label study, 10 healthy subjects who had been classified as hyporesponsive to clopidogrel after administration of a single 300-mg dose, were given St John's wort 300 mg (containing 1.7% hyperforin) three times daily for 14 days (after a 7-day washout period) followed by another single 300-mg dose of clopidogrel. Platelet aggregation was decreased by about 30% by St John's wort.[1] Similarly, in a randomised, double-blind study, 20 post-coronary stent patients taking clopidogrel 75 mg daily and aspirin 81 mg to 325 mg daily, and classified as hyporesponsive to clopidogrel, were given St John's wort, 300 mg three times daily for 14 days, or placebo. Platelet reactivity was decreased by 18%, and platelet inhibition was increased by 78% by St John's wort.[1]

Mechanism

Clopidogrel is a prodrug and is metabolised to its active thiol metabolite by CYP3A4 and CYP2C19, as well as by CYP1A2 and CYP2B6. St John's wort is a known inducer of CYP3A4 and CYP2C19, and might also have some effects on CYP1A2 and CYP2B6. Metabolism of clopidogrel to its active metabolite might therefore be expected to be increased by St John's wort.

Importance and management

Evidence for an interaction between clopidogrel and St John's wort is limited to these studies. The clinical importance of the increased antiplatelet effect and decreased platelet reactivity seen is unclear, particularly because platelet reactivity studies might not be directly relevant to clinical outcomes, and whether this results in an increase in beneficial cardiovascular effects and/or an increase in the bleeding risk with clopidogrel requires further study. The authors of the studies[1] suggest that St John's wort might offer a therapeutic option for increasing the antiplatelet effects of clopidogrel in hyporesponders, but this also requires further study. Until further data are available on the clinical outcomes of this interaction, caution is advised on the concurrent use of clopidogrel and St John's wort. Bear this interaction in mind should any otherwise unexplained bleeding occur in a patient taking both drugs.

1. Lau WC, Welch TD, Shields T, Rubenfire M, Tantry US, Gurbel PA. The effect of St John's wort on the pharmacodynamic response of clopidogrel in hyporesponsive volunteers and patients: increased platelet inhibition by enhancement of CYP3A4 activity. *J Cardiovasc Pharmacol* (2011) 57, 86–93.

Clopidogrel + Statins

In controlled studies atorvastatin had no clinically relevant effect on the pharmacokinetics or antiplatelet effect of clopidogrel. Similarly, pravastatin, rosuvastatin, and possibly lovastatin, do not alter the antiplatelet effect of clopidogrel. Simvastatin and fluvastatin also appear not to interact with clopidogrel, although one study showed some reduction in its antiplatelet effect. Nevertheless, clinical outcome data from numerous retrospective analyses of large studies, and from two randomised studies, does not support an interaction with any of these other statins.

Isolated cases of rhabdomyolysis have been reported in patients taking statins (atorvastatin, lovastatin, simvastatin) and given clopidogrel.

Clinical evidence

A. Clopidogrel effects

(a) Atorvastatin

1. Antiplatelet activity. In 2003, a small non-randomised study reported that 19 patients undergoing coronary artery stenting and taking atorvastatin 10 to 40 mg daily had lower clopidogrel-induced antiplatelet activity when compared with 16 patients not taking statins or 9 patients taking **pravastatin**, and the effect appeared to be dose-related.[1] Note that non-randomised comparisons like this cannot account for all differences between patients (e.g. genetic differences resulting in non-response to clopidogrel), and the smaller they are, the more likely that differences could bias the results. Since this original publication suggesting an interaction, numerous non-randomised and retrospective analyses have been conducted. Of studies looking at antiplatelet effects, only one other non-randomised study found that the antiplatelet effects of clopidogrel were lower in those receiving atorvastatin or simvastatin (grouped together),[2] whereas other non-randomised studies including atorvastatin alone[3-8] or grouped with other statins;[3,9,10] and, more importantly, eight randomised studies (atorvastatin alone),[11-18] have not found any effect. However, of these randomised studies, two used a high dose of clopidogrel (600 mg)[7,11] and one used a low dose of atorvastatin (10 mg):[12] both factors that might minimise any interaction. One analysis found that use of a statin (atorvastatin or **simvastatin**) was actually associated with a greater mean decrease in platelet reactivity index at 28 hours compared with patients not taking statins (40% versus 27.6%), indicating a better response to clopidogrel.[19]

2. Clinical outcome studies. Platelet reactivity studies might not be directly relevant to clinical outcomes, so the efficacy of clopidogrel in relation to statin type has been retrospectively analysed from a number of studies and patient cohorts. Interpretation of this sort of study is complicated by the presence of unknown confounders. In one retrospective, observational review of prescribing data, a 1.49-fold higher rate of cardiovascular events at day 30 post-procedure was noted in patients taking atorvastatin with clopidogrel, when compared with control patients, about 55% of whom were taking other statins (mostly **pravastatin** or **simvastatin**).[20] However, note that simvastatin might also be anticipated to interact, based on the original proposed mechanism. Conversely, in all other analyses, use of atorvastatin, or any other statin studied, has not been associated with reduced efficacy in patients receiving clopidogrel.[6,10,21-27] For example, a retrospective examination of data from the CREDO study found no difference in one-year outcomes in patients given atorvastatin or **pravastatin**,[21] although there appeared to be a slightly better outcome in those given a statin that is not a CYP3A4 substrate (**fluvastatin, pravastatin**) compared with statins that are (**atorvastatin**, cerivastatin, **lovastatin, simvastatin**).[28,29] Furthermore, a prospective, cohort study in 1651 patients with acute coronary syndromes found that the use of clopidogrel with a statin was associated with *lower* 6-month mortality and morbidity compared with the use of clopidogrel in the absence of a statin. There was no significant difference in clinical benefit between a statin predominantly metabolised by CYP3A4 or a statin not predominantly metabolised by CYP3A4.[23] Similarly, retrospective analysis of data from the CHARISMA study, which involved 15 603 patients and had a median duration of 28 months, also found no difference in terms of clinical outcomes between patients who received statins primarily metabolised by CYP3A4 and those who took statins not predominantly affected by CYP3A4. Also, those who took a statin had a lower risk of myocardial infarction, stroke or cardiovascular death, when compared with those who did not take a statin.[24] Also, in a retrospective analysis of the PROVE IT–TIMI 22 study, no difference in clinical outcomes was found between those patients randomised to receive **atorvastatin** 80 mg daily or **pravastatin** 40 mg daily and also receiving clopidogrel.[25] In addition, one-year outcomes did not differ between statins (**atorvastatin, simvastatin, fluvastatin** and **pravastatin**) in the EXCELSIOR study.[26]

There are very few randomised clinical outcome studies. In one prospective, placebo-controlled study, 1 015 patients who underwent coronary stenting and were given clopidogrel, were randomised to also take **pravastatin, fluvastatin, atorvastatin** or placebo. There was no difference in incidence of acute stent thrombosis between any of these groups.[14] In another study, 1275 patients who underwent coronary stenting and received clopidogrel were randomised to receive atorvastatin 20 mg daily or **pravastatin** 20 mg daily. At 12 months, there was no difference between the statin groups in incidence of cardiac and cerebral ischaemic events, or in-stent thrombosis or haemorrhagic events.[30]

3. Pharmacokinetics. In 2008, a key randomised, crossover study was published, which conclusively demonstrates, that, if anything, high-dose atorvastatin actually modestly *increases* the levels of the active metabolite of clopidogrel and slightly *increases* its antiplatelet effect. In this study, 31 healthy subjects received clopidogrel alone (300 mg loading dose then 75 mg daily for 10 days) with atorvastatin 80 mg daily started 6 days before the clopidogrel. Atorvastatin did not change the exposure (AUC) to the active metabolite of clopidogrel after the 300 mg dose, but, on day 10, there was a modest 28% increase in AUC of the active metabolite. The antiplatelet effect of clopidogrel was unchanged after the 300 mg dose, but tended to be increased on the final day. There was an increase of about 6 to 16%; differences that were statistically significant at some, but not all, time points.[31]

(b) Fluvastatin

In one crossover study in 20 healthy subjects given clopidogrel 75 mg daily, fluvastatin 80 mg daily for 7 days reduced the antiplatelet response by about 29%, with just two subjects then classified as clopidogrel non-responders.[13] However, in a randomised study in patients, fluvastatin (20 mg given 24 hours before the clopidogrel) did not alter the antiplatelet effects of clopidogrel after a 600 mg dose, when compared with placebo.[11] Similarly, two retrospective analyses found that fluvastatin did not affect the platelet activity of clopidogrel.[3,6] Clopidogrel had no effect on the pharmacokinetics of fluvastatin 80 mg daily in a controlled study in healthy subjects, and the antiplatelet effect of clopidogrel was similar to that expected for clopidogrel alone.[32] Moreover, retrospective clinical outcome studies and one placebo-controlled study have shown no detrimental effect of fluvastatin, see Clinical outcome studies under *Atorvastatin*, above.

(c) Lovastatin

In a randomised study in patients, lovastatin (given 24 hours before the clopidogrel) did not alter the antiplatelet effects of clopidogrel after a 600 mg dose, when compared with placebo.[11] Moreover, retrospective clinical outcome studies have shown no detrimental effect of lovastatin, see Clinical outcome studies under *Atorvastatin*, above. There are no studies on the effect of lovastatin on clopidogrel pharmacokinetics.

(d) Pravastatin

There do not appear to be any studies suggesting that an interaction between clopidogrel and pravastatin occurs, and a number of studies showing that no interaction occurs. In one crossover study in 20 healthy subjects given clopidogrel 75 mg daily, pravastatin 40 mg daily for 7 days did not alter the antiplatelet response of clopidogrel.[13] Similarly, in two randomised studies in patients, pravastatin (20 mg or 40 mg started 24 hours before the clopidogrel) did not alter the antiplatelet effects of clopidogrel after a 600 mg or 375 mg dose,[11,12] and other randomised studies reported the same findings.[14-16] Similarly, in non-randomised studies, pravastatin did not affect the antiplatelet activity of clopidogrel.[1,5,16] Retrospective clinical outcome studies and two randomised studies have shown no detrimental effect of pravastatin, see Clinical outcome studies under *Atorvastatin*, above. There are no studies on the effect of pravastatin on clopidogrel pharmacokinetics.

(e) Rosuvastatin

In one crossover study in 20 healthy subjects given clopidogrel 75 mg daily, rosuvastatin 10 mg daily for 7 days did not alter the antiplatelet response of clopidogrel.[13] Similarly, there was no difference in the antiplatelet effect of clopidogrel between patients receiving rosuvastatin and those not, and no difference between rosuvastatin and atorvastatin.[8] Moreover, in a randomised study in patients, rosuvastatin 10 mg daily (titrated to 40 mg daily as necessary) did not alter the antiplatelet response to clopidogrel maintenance treatment when compared with atorvastatin or simvastatin.[17]

(f) Simvastatin

In one crossover study in 20 healthy subjects given clopidogrel 75 mg daily, simvastatin 20 mg daily for 7 days reduced the antiplatelet response by about 31%, with just one subject then classified as a clopidogrel non-responder.[13] However, in a randomised study in patients, simvastatin (20 mg given 24 hours before the clopidogrel) did not alter the antiplatelet effects of clopidogrel after a 600 mg dose, when compared with placebo,[11] and another randomised study also found no effect with simvastatin 40 mg daily.[17] Of the non-randomised studies looking at antiplatelet effects, one found a lower antiplatelet response to clopidogrel after coronary artery stenting in those receiving simvastatin or atorvastatin (grouped together),[2] whereas, in other similar studies, no effect was found with simvastatin alone,[5-7] grouped with atorvastatin,[9] or grouped with other CYP3A4 metabolised statins.[10] Moreover, retrospective clinical outcome studies have shown no detrimental effect of simvastatin, see Clinical outcome studies under *Atorvastatin*, above. There are no studies on the effect of simvastatin on clopidogrel pharmacokinetics.

B. Rhabdomyolysis

Isolated cases of rhabdomyolysis precipitated by clopidogrel have been reported. Two heart transplant patients taking **simvastatin** or **lovastatin**, together with ciclosporin for several years with no reported problems, developed rhabdomyolysis within 2 weeks of starting clopidogrel.[33] Another similar report describes a patient who was stable taking ciclosporin and **atorvastatin** who developed rhabdomyolysis when a 4-week course of clopidogrel was started.[34]

Mechanism

Clopidogrel is an inactive prodrug that is metabolised to its active metabolite by the cytochrome P450 isoenzyme system, with CYP2C19 known to be important, and possibly also CYP3A4 (see 'Clopidogrel + Azoles', p.785). Several statins (lovastatin, simvastatin, atorvastatin), are principally metabolised by CYP3A4 and it has been suggested that these statins may competitively inhibit the activation of clopidogrel,[1] and this was shown *in vitro* for atorvastatin lactone.[35] However, note that this is not an established mechanism for pharmacokinetic drug interactions, and substrates of CYP3A4 do not cause clinically relevant interactions unless they are also CYP3A4 inhibitors, which none of the statins are known to be. The well-designed pharmacokinetic study with atorvastatin conclusively shows that it does not inhibit the formation of the active metabolite of clopidogrel. In fact, it actually resulted in a modest increase in active metabolite levels, the mechanism for which is unknown.

One controlled study showed a reduction in the antiplatelet effects of clopidogrel with simvastatin and fluvastatin. The mechanism for this is unknown.

Clopidogrel (a possible CYP2C9 inhibitor) does not alter the metabolism of fluvastatin (a CYP2C9 substrate).[32]

Importance and management

The possible interaction between clopidogrel and the statins has been the subject of much study and debate. The few studies showing a reduced antiplatelet effect of clopidogrel with atorvastatin are all limited by their non-randomised design and small number of patients, and the findings could therefore easily be due to confounding by unknown factors. These sorts of studies are useful in generating hypotheses, but should not be used to guide clinical decisions.[36] A subsequent well-designed study has shown that atorvastatin 80 mg daily has no inhibitory effect on the metabolism and antiplatelet effects of clopidogrel, and, in fact, slightly increased the levels and activity of clopidogrel, although probably not to a clinically relevant extent. Therefore, no interaction would be expected in clinical use. This is supported by all of the retrospective analyses of clinical outcome data except one, and by the two randomised studies.

Apart from pravastatin, which also appears to have no effect on the antiplatelet action of clopidogrel, data for other statins are limited. Of some concern, in one controlled, crossover study, the antiplatelet effect of clopidogrel was reduced with both simvastatin and fluvastatin (but not with atorvastatin, pravastatin or rosuvastatin). However, this has not been shown in other studies, and all the available retrospective outcome data show no adverse effect of either simvastatin or fluvastatin. Note that the 2007 European Society of Cardiology guidelines for non-ST-segment elevation acute coronary syndromes state that clopidogrel can be given with all statins.[37]

The general significance of the case reports describing rhabdomyolysis, when clopidogrel was given to transplant patients who were stable taking a statin with ciclosporin, is unclear.

1. Lau WC, Waskell LA, Watkins PB, Neer CJ, Horowitz K, Hopp AS, Tait AR, Carville DGM, Guyer KE, Bates ER. Atorvastatin reduces the ability of clopidogrel to inhibit platelet aggregation. A new drug–drug interaction. *Circulation* (2003) 107, 32–7.
2. Neubauer H, Günesdogan B, Hanefeld C, Spiecker M, Mügge A. Lipophilic statins interfere with the inhibitory effects of clopidogrel on platelet function – a flow cytometry study. *Eur Heart J* (2003) 24, 1744–9.
3. Serebruany VL, Malinin AI, Callahan KP, Gurbel PA, Steinhubl SR. Statins do not affect platelet inhibition with clopidogrel during coronary stenting. *Atherosclerosis* (2001) 159, 239–41.
4. Serebruany VL, Midei MG, Malinin AI, Oshrine BR, Lowry DR, Sane DC, Tanguay J-F, Steinhubl SR, Berger PB, O'Connor CM, Hennekens CH. Absence of interaction between atorvastatin or other statins and clopidogrel: results from the interaction study. *Arch Intern Med* (2004) 164, 2051–7.
5. Smith SMG, Judge HM, Peters G, Storey RF. Multiple antiplatelet effects of clopidogrel are not modulated by statin type in patients undergoing percutaneous coronary intervention. *Platelets* (2004) 15, 465–74.
6. Zürn CS, Geisler T, Paterok M, Gawaz M. Einfluss von Statinen auf die antithrombozytäre Wirkung von Clopidogrel nach Stentimplantation. *Dtsch Med Wochenschr* (2008) 133, 817–22.
7. Polena S, Gupta MP, Shaikh H, Zazzali K, Coplan N, Gintautas J, Singh Labana S, Soffer D. Platelet aggregation inhibition in patients receiving statins either fully or partially metabolized by CYP3A4. *Proc West Pharmacol Soc* (2008) 51, 60–2.
8. Riondino S, Petrini N, Donato L, Torromeo C, Tanzilli G, Pulcinelli FM, Barillà F. Effects of rosuvastatin on platelet inhibition by clopidogrel in cardiovascular patients. *J Thromb Thrombolysis* (2009) 28, 151–5.
9. Gorchakova O, von Beckerath N, Gawaz M, Mocz A, Joost A, Schömig A, Kastrati A. Antiplatelet effects of a 600 mg loading dose of clopidogrel are not attenuated in patients receiving atorvastatin or simvastatin for at least 4 weeks prior to coronary artery stenting. *Eur Heart J* (2004) 25, 1898–1902.
10. Geisler T, Zürn C, Paterok M, Göhring-Frischholz K, Bigalke B, Stellos K, Seizer P, Kraemer BF, Dippon J, May AE, Herdeg C, Gawaz M. Statins do not adversely affect post-interventional residual platelet aggregation and outcomes in patients undergoing coronary stenting treated by dual antiplatelet therapy. *Eur Heart J* (2008) 29, 1635–43.
11. Müller I, Besta F, Schulz C, Li Z, Massberg S, Gawaz M. Effects of statins on platelet inhibition by a high loading dose of clopidogrel. *Circulation* (2003) 108, 2195–7.
12. Mitsios JV, Papathanasiou AI, Rodis FI, Elisaf M, Goudevenos JA, Tselepis AD. Atorvastatin does not affect the antiplatelet potency of clopidogrel when it is administered concomitantly for 5 weeks in patients with acute coronary syndromes. *Circulation* (2004) 109, 1335–8.
13. Mach F, Senouf D, Fontana P, Boehlen F, Reber G, Daali Y, de Moerloose P, Sigwart U. Not all statins interfere with clopidogrel during antiplatelet therapy. *Eur J Clin Invest* (2005) 35, 476–81.
14. Shen J, Zhang R-Y, Zhang Q, Yang Z-K, Hu J, Zhang J-S, Zheng A-F, Zhang X, Shen W-F. Impact of statins on clopidogrel platelet inhibition in patients with acute coronary syndrome or stable angina [in Chinese]. *Zhonghua Xin Xue Guan Bing Za Zhi* (2008) 36, 807–11.
15. Han Y-L, Li C-Y, Li Y, Kang J, Yan C-H. The antiplatelet effect of clopidogrel is not attenuated by statin treatment in patients with acute coronary syndromes undergoing coronary stenting [in Chinese]. *Zhonghua Xin Xue Guan Bing Za Zhi* (2007) 35, 788–92.
16. Wenaweser P, Windecker S, Billinger M, Cook S, Togni M, Meier B, Haeberli A, Hess OM. Effect of atorvastatin and pravastatin on platelet inhibition by aspirin and clopidogrel treatment in patients with coronary stent thrombosis. *Am J Cardiol* (2007) 99, 353–6.
17. Malmström RE, Östergren J, Jørgensen L, Hjemdahl P; for the CASTOR investigators. Influence of statin treatment on platelet inhibition by clopidogrel – a randomized comparison of rosuvastatin, atorvastatin and simvastatin co-treatment. *J Intern Med* (2009) 266, 457–66.
18. Piorkowski M, Weikert U, Schwimmbeck P-L, Martus P, Schultheiss HP, Rauch U. ADP induced platelet degranulation in healthy individuals is reduced by clopidogrel after pretreatment with atorvastatin. *Thromb Haemost* (2004) 92, 614–20.
19. Motovska Z, Widimsky P, Petr R, Bilkova D, Marinov I, Simek S, Kala P, for the PRAGUE-8 study investigators. Factors influencing clopidogrel efficacy in patients with stable coronary artery disease undergoing elective percutaneous coronary intervention: statin's advantage and the smoking "paradox". *J Cardiovasc Pharmacol* (2009) 53, 368–72.
20. Brophy JM, Babapulle MN, Costa V, Rinfret S. A pharmacoepidemiology study of the interaction between atorvastatin and clopidogrel after percutaneous coronary intervention. *Am Heart J* (2006) 152, 263–9.
21. Saw J, Steinhubl SR, Berger PB, Kereiakes DJ, Serebruany VL, Brennan D, Topol EJ; for the Clopidogrel for the Reduction of Events During Observation (CREDO) Investigators. Lack of adverse clopidogrel–atorvastatin clinical interaction from secondary analysis of a randomized, placebo-controlled clopidogrel trial. *Circulation* (2003) 108, 921–4.
22. Wienbergen H, Gitt AK, Schiele R, Juenger C, Heer T, Meisenzahl C, Limbourg P, Bossaller C, Senges J, for the MITRA PLUS Study Group. Comparison of clinical benefits of clopidogrel therapy in patients with acute coronary syndromes taking atorvastatin versus other statin therapies. *Am J Cardiol* (2003) 92, 285–8.
23. Mukherjee D, Kline-Rogers E, Fang J, Munir K, Eagle KA. Lack of clopidogrel-CYP3A4 statin interaction in patients with acute coronary syndrome. Heart 2005, 91, 23–6.
24. Saw J, Brennan DM, Steinhubl SR, Bhatt DL, Mak K-H, Fox K, Topol EJ, on behalf of the CHARISMA investigators. Lack of evidence of a clopidogrel-statin interaction in the CHARISMA trial. *J Am Coll Cardiol* (2007), 50, 291–5.
25. Lotfi A, Schweiger MJ, Giugliano GR, Murphy SA, Cannon CP; TIMI 22 Investigators. High-dose atorvastatin does not negatively influence clinical outcomes among clopidogrel treated acute coronary syndrome patients—a Pravastatin or Atorvastatin Evaluation and Infection Therapy-Thrombolysis in Myocardial Infarction 22 (PROVE IT-TIMI 22) analysis. *Am Heart J* (2008) 155, 954–8.
26. Trenk D, Hochholzer W, Frundi D, Stratz C, Valina CM, Bestehorn H-P, Büttner HJ, Neumann F-J. Impact of cytochrome P450 3A4-metabolized statins on the antiplatelet effect of a 600-mg loading dose clopidogrel and on clinical outcome in patients undergoing elective coronary stent placement. *Thromb Haemost* (2008) 99, 174–81.
27. Blagojevic A, Delaney JAC, Lévesque LE, Dendukuri N, Boivin J-F, Brophy JM. Investigation of an interaction between statins and clopidogrel after percutaneous coronary intervention: a cohort study. *Pharmacoepidemiol Drug Safety* (2009) 18, 362–9.
28. Ford I, Williams D. Does the use of statins compromise the effectiveness of platelet inhibition by clopidogrel? *Platelets* (2004) 15, 201–5.
29. Bates ER, Mukherjee D, Lau WC. Drug–drug interactions involving antiplatelet agents. *Eur Heart J* (2003) 24, 1707–9.
30. Han Y-L, Zhang Z-L, Li Y, Wang S-L, Jing Q-M, Wang Z-L, Wang D-M. Comparison on long-term effects of atorvastatin or pravastatin combined with clopidogrel for patients undergoing coronary stenting: a randomized controlled trial [in Chinese]. *Zhonghua Yi Xue Za Zhi (Taipei)* (2009) 89, 2240–4.
31. Farid NA, Small DS, Payne CD, Jakubowski JA, Brandt JT, Li YG, Ernest CS, Salazar DE, Konkoy CS, Winters KJ. Effect of atorvastatin on the pharmacokinetics and pharmacodynamics of prasugrel and clopidogrel in healthy subjects. *Pharmacotherapy* (2008) 28, 1483–94.
32. Ayalasomayajula SP, Vaidyanathan S, Kemp C, Prasad P, Balch A, Dole WP. Effect of clopidogrel on the steady-state pharmacokinetics of fluvastatin. *J Clin Pharmacol* (2007) 47, 613–19.
33. Uber PA, Mehra MR, Park MH, Scott RL. Clopidogrel and rhabdomyolysis after heart transplantation. *J Heart Lung Transplant* (2003) 22, 107–8.
34. Burton JR, Burton I, Pearson GJ. Clopidogrel-precipitated rhabdomyolysis in a stable heart transplant patient. *Ann Pharmacother* (2007) 41, 133–7.
35. Clarke TA, Waskell LA. The metabolism of clopidogrel is catalyzed by human cytochrome P450 3A and is inhibited by atorvastatin. *Drug Metab Dispos* (2003) 31, 53–9.
36. Serebruany VL, Steinhubl SR, Hennekens CH. Are antiplatelet effects of clopidogrel inhibited by atorvastatin? A research question formulated but not yet adequately tested. *Circulation* (2003) 107, 1568–9.
37. Bassand J-P, Hamm CW, Ardissino D, Boersma E, Budaj A, Fernández-Avilés F, Fox KAA, Hasdai D, Ohman EM, Wallentin L, Wijns W: The Task Force for the Diagnosis and Treatment of Non-ST-Segment Elevation Acute Coronary Syndromes of the European Society of Cardiology. Guidelines for the diagnosis and treatment of non-ST-segment elevation acute coronary syndromes. *Eur Heart J* (2007) 28, 1598–1660.

Clopidogrel + Tobacco

Some studies appear to suggest that the antiplatelet effects of clopidogrel might be greater in tobacco smokers, but this might also increase the risk of bleeding.

Clinical evidence

(a) Antiplatelet studies

In a study, 20 healthy subjects (7 who smoked 10 or more cigarettes daily, 6 who smoked less than 10 cigarettes daily and 7 who were non-smokers), were given a

600-mg loading dose of clopidogrel and the platelet aggregatory response was measured. At 2 and 6 hours post-dose, those who smoked 10 or more cigarettes daily had a higher inhibitory platelet aggregatory response to 5 micromol/L ADP-induced platelet inhibition compared with non-smokers, but with 20 micromol/L ADP-induced platelet inhibition the differences were not statistically significant. The inhibitory platelet aggregatory response in those who smoked less than 10 cigarettes daily did not differ from that in non-smokers.[1]

Similarly, many, but not all, studies in patients have also shown that the antiplatelet effect of clopidogrel is greater in smokers than non-smokers. For example, in one study in 259 patients admitted for elective coronary intervention, 36 patients who were taking clopidogrel before admission and who smoked more than half a pack of cigarettes daily (for at least 2 weeks before the study) had lower platelet aggregation than 72 non-smokers (32% versus 44%). Similarly, those patients who smoked and were not taking long-term clopidogrel had greater clopidogrel-induced inhibition of platelet aggregation at least 18 to 24 hours after a 600-mg loading dose, when compared with non-smokers (46% versus 34%). This was seen in those patients who smoked at least half a pack of cigarettes daily [10 or more], whereas those who smoked less than half a pack daily [9 or less] had similar clopidogrel-induced antiplatelet responses to that of the non-smokers. Further regression analysis found that current smoking was associated with lower platelet aggregation in response to clopidogrel (odds ratio of 2.63).[2] One other study found a 24% lower ADP-induced platelet aggregation, measured 24 hours after an acute dose of clopidogrel, in smokers (greater than 10 cigarettes daily) when compared with 33 non-smokers, but no difference was seen in former smokers. In addition, of those 26 patients with high residual platelet aggregation, there was a lower proportion of current smokers, when compared with the group as a whole (19% versus 39.2%).[3] However, in another study although smokers had a quicker onset of clopidogrel antiplatelet effect (with 80% of smokers having effective platelet inhibition at 12-hours post-dose), by 28 hours there was no difference between smokers and non-smokers in the number of responders.[4] Moreover, in the largest study to date (1 092 patients), smoking status was not predictive of residual platelet activity about 24 hours after a loading dose of clopidogrel. There was no difference in the proportion of smokers in those with high residual platelet activity compared with those with the median residual platelet activity (38.5% versus 40.4%).[5]

Two studies have measured platelet aggregation 3 to 5 days after starting clopidogrel. In one of these studies in patients undergoing coronary stenting, the rate of low platelet reactivity was higher in 56 patients who had smoked greater than 10 cigarettes daily within one week of coronary stenting compared with 66 who had not smoked within one year of coronary stenting (33.9% versus 10.6%). Those who smoked more than 10 cigarettes daily were found to have lower ADP-induced platelet aggregation compared with non-smokers.[1] In the second similar study, there was a trend towards a higher rate of low platelet reactivity in 97 patients who had smoked within 2 weeks of admission compared with 37 who had not smoked within one year of admission (about 31% versus 13.5%) although this difference was not statistically significant. In addition there were no differences in ADP-induced platelet aggregation in response to clopidogrel between the smokers and non-smokers.[6]

(b) Clinical outcome studies

The relationship between smoking status and efficacy of clopidogrel has been retrospectively analysed from data from various prospective, randomised studies. In CHARISMA, current smokers (at least one cigarette daily for at least one month) had an increased risk of all-cause mortality as well as cardiovascular and cancer-related mortality, compared with non-smokers (patients who had never smoked). However, the inverse was found in those patients also given clopidogrel 75 mg daily for up to 28 months. The concurrent use of clopidogrel was found to *reduce* all-cause mortality (hazard ratio 0.68) in current smokers, whereas no reduction was seen in former smokers (those who had smoked at least one cigarette daily before stopping one month before the study) or non-smokers taking clopidogrel. However, no statistically significant difference was seen in the risk of cardiovascular death between the same groups. Current smokers taking clopidogrel were also found to have a higher risk of bleeding (hazard ratio 1.62), and a trend towards an increased risk of bleeding was also seen in non-smokers, but this was not statistically significant.[7] Another retrospective sub-analysis of data from 3 429 patients from the CLARITY-TIMI 28 study reported similar findings. In those taking clopidogrel, current smokers of at least 10 cigarettes daily had a greater reduction in the primary endpoint (closed infarct-related artery or death/myocardial infarction before angiography) than in patients who had never smoked or who smoked less than 10 cigarettes daily. In addition, current smokers had a reduced rate of myocardial infarction or cardiovascular death and also reduced composite end point at 30 days (myocardial infarction, recurrent ischaemia or cardiovascular death), whereas these indices where not reduced in non-smokers. There was no difference in the incidence of major or minor bleeding between smokers and non-smokers.[8] Similarly, in a preliminary analysis of the CREDO data, smokers had greater benefit from clopidogrel at one year (reduction in incidence of death, myocardial infarction or stroke) compared with non-smokers.[9]

(c) Pharmacokinetic studies

In a study in 76 healthy subjects, 49 of whom were non-smokers and 27 were smokers (defined as 10 or more cigarettes daily for at least one year), the AUC and half-life of the *inactive* carboxylic acid metabolite of clopidogrel were found to be 30% and 35% lower, respectively, in smokers compared with non-smokers, but its maximum level was not affected.[10] However, this study did not measure the levels of the *active* thiol metabolite of clopidogrel.

Mechanism

Unknown. Clopidogrel is a prodrug and is metabolised to its active thiol metabolite by CYP3A4 and CYP2C19, as well as CYP1A2 and CYP2B6. It has been hypothesised that, as cigarette smoke is a known inducer of CYP1A2, smoking might increase levels of the active clopidogrel metabolite and thereby increase clopidogrel platelet inhibition.[1] However, this pharmacokinetic hypothesis has not been studied. The authors of one study also suggest that, as current smokers have been reported to have impaired endogenous fibrinolysis, they are more likely to have a greater benefit from antiplatelet drugs such as clopidogrel (termed 'smokers paradox').[7] In contrast, smoking is a well established risk factor for cardiovascular disease, and might increase platelet reactivity and reduce the benefit of clopidogrel. The authors of the pharmacokinetic study suggest that reduced levels of the inactive metabolite of clopidogrel indicate reduced levels of the active metabolite (which is not proven), and they theorise that clopidogrel will be less effective in smokers.[10]

Importance and management

A clinically relevant interaction between clopidogrel and smoking is not established. Studies of the effects of smoking cannot be randomised, and therefore it is not possible to exclude all possible biases, although data from healthy subjects suggests some increase in the antiplatelet effects of clopidogrel in smokers. However, studies of clopidogrel-induced platelet reactivity may not be directly relevant to clinical outcomes. Clinical outcome data is limited to retrospective analyses, and, as it is impossible to control for all possible confounders, definitive conclusions cannot be made. Further, the possible interaction of smoking itself (the 'smokers paradox'), rather than a direct effect on CYP1A2-mediated metabolism of clopidogrel, cannot be ruled out. Smoking is a well-known and established risk factor for cardiovascular disease, and the suggestion that the antiplatelet effects, and possibly the clinical benefits, of clopidogrel may be greater in patients who smoke more than 10 cigarettes daily is controversial and seems at odds with current advice on smoking in patients with cardiovascular disease. Further study is needed to confirm if any interaction modifies the long-term cardiovascular benefits of clopidogrel.

1. Jeong YH, Cho JH, Kang MK, Koh JS, Kim IS, Park Y, Kwak CH, Hwang JY. Smoking at least 10 cigarettes per day increases platelet inhibition by clopidogrel in patients with ST-segment-elevation myocardial infarction. *Thromb Res* (2010). May 5, ahead of print.
2. Bliden KP, DiChiara J, Lawal L, Singla A, Antonino MJ, Baker BA, Bailey WL, Tantry US, Gurbel PA. The association of cigarette smoking with enhanced platelet inhibition by clopidogrel. *J Am Coll Cardiol* (2008) 52, 531–3.
3. Gremmel T, Steiner S, Seidinger D, Koppensteiner R, Panzer S, Kopp CW. Smoking promotes clopidogrel-mediated platelet inhibition in patients receiving dual antiplatelet therapy. *Thromb Res* (2009) 124, 588–91.
4. Motovska Z, Widimsky P, Petr R, Bilkova D, Marinov I, Simek S, Kala P, for the PRAGUE-8 study investigators. Factors influencing clopidogrel efficacy in patients with stable coronary artery disease undergoing elective percutaneous coronary intervention: statin's advantage and the smoking "paradox". *J Cardiovasc Pharmacol* (2009) 53, 368–72.
5. Geisler T, Graβ D, Bigalke B, Stellos K, Drosch T, Dietz K, Herdeg C, Gawaz M. The Residual Platelet Aggregation after Deployment of Intracoronary Stent (PREDICT) score. *J Thromb Haemost* (2008) 6, 54–61.
6. Cho J-H, Jeong Y-H, Ahn Y-J, Kang M-K, Koh J-S, Kim I-S, Park Y, Hwang S-J, Kwak CH, Hwang J-Y. The impact of smoking on post-clopidogrel platelet reactivity in patients with acute myocardial infarction. *Korean Circ J* (2010) 40, 119–24.
7. Berger JS, Bhatt DL, Steinhubl SR, Shao M, Steg PG, Montalescot G, Hacke W, Fox KA, Lincoff AM, Topol EJ, Berger PB, and for the CHARISMA (Clopidogrel for High Atherothrombotic Risk and Ischemic Stabilization, Management, and Avoidance) investigators. Smoking, clopidogrel, and mortality in patients with established cardiovascular disease. *Circulation* (2009) 120, 2337–44.
8. Desai NR, Mega JL, Jiang S, Cannon CP, Sabatine MS. Interaction between cigarette smoking and clinical benefit of clopidogrel. *J Am Coll Cardiol* (2009) 14, 1273–8.
9. Saraff KY, Steinhubl SR, Hsu AP, Topol EJ, for the Credo investigators. Smoking influences the effectiveness of dual antiplatelet therapy on long-term outcomes following percutaneous coronary intervention. *J Am Coll Cardiol* (2006) 47, 36B.
10. Yousef A-M, Arafat T, Bulatova NR, Al-Zumyli R. Smoking behaviour modulates pharmacokinetics of orally administered clopidogrel. *J Clin Pharm Ther* (2008) 33, 439–49.

Dipyridamole + Antihypertensives

No adverse reactions normally occur in patients taking beta blockers who undergo dipyridamole–thallium-201 scintigraphy and echocardiography, but case reports suggest that very rarely bradycardia and asystole can occur. There is some evidence that nitrates, beta blockers, calcium-channel blockers, and irbesartan can mask ischaemia with dipyridamole–thallium-201 scintigraphy and echocardiography, thereby risking an underestimation of the extent of coronary artery disease.

Additive hypotension is predicted to occur if dipyridamole is given with other antihypertensives.

Clinical evidence

(a) Beta blockers

A 71-year-old woman taking **nadolol** 120 mg daily and bendroflumethiazide, with a 3-week history of chest pain, was given a 300-mg dose of oral dipyridamole as part of a diagnostic dipyridamole-thallium imaging test for coronary artery disease. She was given thallium-201 intravenously, 50 minutes after the dipyridamole, but 3 minutes later, while exercising, she complained of chest pain and then had a cardiac arrest. Cardiopulmonary resuscitation was performed, and a normal cardiac rhythm was obtained after she was given intravenous aminophylline.[1]

Adverse interactions have been reported in another 3 patients taking beta blockers during diagnostic dipyridamole-thallium stress testing. One patient, who was taking **atenolol**, developed bradycardia and then asystole, another patient who was taking **metoprolol** developed bradycardia,[2] and a third patient, also taking **metoprolol**, developed sinus bradycardia and then asystole.[3] All three patients recovered when treated with aminophylline.[2,3]

These reports need to be set in a broad context. In a very extensive study of high-dose dipyridamole echocardiography (10 451 tests in 9 122 patients) significant adverse effects were noted in only 96 patients and major adverse reactions occurred in just 7 patients. Three of the 7 patients developed asystole and two of these patients were taking unnamed beta blockers.[4] In addition, a further two case reports describe the development of asystole or symptomatic bradycardia during dipyridamole infusion in three patients *not* taking beta blockers.[5,6] See also *Other antihypertensives*, below

(b) Other antihypertensives

In a study, 26 patients who underwent dipyridamole–thallium-201 scintigraphy and echocardiography after discontinuing their usual antianginal medication (**calcium-channel blockers** in 21 patients, **nitrates** in 19 patients and **beta blockers** in 8 patients) had the test repeated while continuing their medications. The results of the test underestimated the extent and severity of myocardial perfusion defects when anti-anginal medications where continued compared with when they were stopped.[7] Similar findings were presented in a study in which 13 patients with coronary artery disease underwent dipyridamole stress testing before and after taking **irbesartan** 150 mg daily for 2 weeks,[8] and in another study in which patients were given a single dose of intravenous **metoprolol** (up to 20 mg) ten minutes before the test.[9]

Mechanism

A possible explanation for the adverse effects reported between beta blockers and dipyridamole is that both drugs have negative chronotropic effects on the heart. Anti-anginal drugs may mask the true extent of the problems with myocardial blood flow with the dipyridamole stress test.

Importance and management

The value and safety of dipyridamole perfusion scintigraphy and echocardiography have been very extensively studied in very large numbers of patients, and reports of bradycardia and asystole, attributed to an interaction between dipyridamole and beta blockers, are sparse. It would therefore appear to be a relatively rare interaction (if such it is).

The 2005 European guidelines on myocardial perfusion imaging recommend that nitrates should be temporarily stopped before dipyridamole stress testing (for at least 5 half-lives of the drug), because of the possibility of interference with the test.[10] Some consider that calcium-channel blockers and beta blockers should also be stopped, but the guidelines state that the evidence for an improved test on interrupting these drugs is limited or not obvious.[10] The authors of the irbesartan study suggest that similar effects may possibly occur with angiotensin II receptor antagonists, and that they should also be stopped; however, the guidelines do not mention that it is necessary to stop these drugs before testing.[10]

Note that, as dipyridamole may cause peripheral vasodilation and hypotension, the UK manufacturer advises caution on its concurrent use with other drugs that affect blood pressure [such as beta blockers and angiotensin II receptor antagonists] as additive blood pressure-lowering effects may occur.[11]

1. Blumenthal MS, McCauley CS. Cardiac arrest during dipyridamole imaging. *Chest* (1988) 93, 1103–4.
2. Roach PJ, Magee MA, Freedman SB. Asystole and bradycardia during dipyridamole stress testing in patients receiving beta blockers. *Int J Cardiol* (1993) 42, 92–4.
3. Lo Mauro R, Sabella FP, Enia F. Sinus arrest associated with dipyridamole infusion. *Chest* (1994) 105, 604–5.
4. Picano E, Marini C, Pirelli S, Maffei S, Bolognese L, Chiriatti G, Chiarella F,Orlandini A, Seveso G, Colosso MQ, Sclavo MG, Magaia O, Agati L, Previtali M, Lowenstein J, Torre F, Rosselli P, Ciuti M, Ostojic M, Gandolfo N, Margaria F, Gianuzzi P, Di Bello V, Lombardi M, Gigli G, Ferrara N, Santoro F, Lusa AM, Chiaranda G, Papagna D, Coletta C, Boccardi L, De Cristofaro M, Papi L, Landi P, on behalf of the Echo-Persantine International Cooperative Study Group. Safety of intravenous high-dose dipyridamole echocardiography. *Am J Cardiol* (1992) 70, 252–8.
5. Frossard M, Weiss K, Gössinger H, Zeiner A, Leitha T. Asystole during dipyridamole infusion in patients without coronary artery disease or beta-blocker therapy. *Clin Nucl Med* (1997) 22, 97–100.
6. Pennell DJ, Underwood SR, Ell PJ. Symptomatic bradycardia complicating the use of intravenous dipyridamole for thallium-201 myocardial perfusion imaging. *Int J Cardiol* (1990) 27, 272–4.
7. Sharir T, Rabinowitz B, Livschitz S, Moalem I, Baron J, Kaplinsky E, Chouraqui P. Underestimation of extent and severity of coronary artery disease by dipyridamole stress thallium-201 single-photon emission computed tomographic myocardial perfusion imaging in patients taking antianginal drugs. *J Am Coll Cardiol* (1998) 31, 1540–6.
8. Altun GD, Altun A, Yildiz M, Firat MF, Hacimahmutoglu S, Berkarda S. Irbesartan has a masking effect on dipyridamole stress induced myocardial perfusion defects. *Nucl Med Commun* (2004) 25, 195–9.
9. Taillefer R, Ahlberg AW, Masood Y, White CM, Lamargese I, Mather JF, McGill CC, Heller GV. Acute beta-blockade reduces the extent and severity of myocardial perfusion defects with dipyridamole Tc-99m sestamibi SPECT imaging. *J Am Coll Cardiol* (2003) 42, 1475–83.
10. Hesse B, Tägil K, Cuocolo A, Anagnostopoulos C, Bardiés M, Bax J, Bengel F, Busemann Sokole E, Davies G, Dondi M, Edenbrandt L, Franken P, Kjaer A, Knuuti J, Lassmann M, Ljungberg M, Marcassa C, Marie PY, McKiddie F, O'Connor M, Prvulovich E, Underwood R, van Eck-Smit B. EANM/ESC procedural guidelines for myocardial perfusion imaging in nuclear cardiology. *Eur J Nucl Med Mol Imaging* (2005) 32, 855–97.
11. Persantin Retard (Dipyridamole). Boehringer Ingelheim Ltd. UK Summary of product characteristics, July 2010.

Dipyridamole + Drugs that affect gastric pH

Famotidine and lansoprazole appear to reduce the bioavailability of dipyridamole from immediate-release formulations. Other drugs that raise gastric pH (such as antacids) would be expected to interact similarly. Modified-release preparations of dipyridamole that are buffered do not appear to be affected.

Clinical evidence

In a study in 11 healthy elderly subjects (6 control subjects with a low fasting gastric pH and 5 achlorhydric subjects with fasting gastric pH greater than 5), those with an elevated gastric pH had a lower absorption of a single 50-mg oral dose of dipyridamole. In addition, increasing the gastric pH to above 5 for at least 3 hours by pretreating with **famotidine** 40 mg, resulted in reduced dipyridamole absorption: the AUC of dipyridamole was reduced by 37% (not statistically significant) and the maximum serum levels were significantly delayed and reduced.[1] In another study, 20 healthy subjects were given **lansoprazole** 30 mg daily for 5 days and then either a single dose of an extended-release preparation of dipyridamole 200 mg with aspirin 25 mg (formulated with tartaric acid to improve bioavailability of dipyridamole if the gastric pH is elevated) or a conventional preparation of dipyridamole 100 mg with aspirin 81 mg, followed 6 hours later by another dose of dipyridamole. **Lansoprazole** halved the relative bioavailability of conventional dipyridamole tablets compared with the buffered extended-release tablets.[2]

Mechanism

The solubility of dipyridamole depends very much on pH. It is very soluble at low pH values and almost insoluble at neutral pH.[3] As dipyridamole needs a low pH in the stomach for adequate absorption to occur, drugs that raise the gastric pH (such as the proton pump inhibitors, H_2-receptor antagonists and antacids) would be expected to reduce the bioavailability of dipyridamole from immediate-release formulations.

Importance and management

Although the evidence is limited, it seems likely that any drug that raises the stomach pH (such as **proton pump inhibitors**, **H_2-receptor antagonists** and **antacids**) would be expected to reduce the dissolution and absorption of dipyridamole from immediate-release formulations such as the *tablets* and *suspension*. This is likely to result in an overall reduction in dipyridamole bioavailability. The manufacturers of dipyridamole tablets[4] and suspension[5] state that **antacids** may reduce the efficacy of dipyridamole; however, they have no direct evidence of reduced efficacy due to this interaction.[6] The usual advice to avoid antacid interactions is to separate the doses by 2 to 3 hours. Separating administration is not usually effective in reducing the interaction with proton pump inhibitors because they are such long-acting acid suppressants. Modified-release dipyridamole capsules (*Persantin Retard*, and the formulation containing aspirin, *Asasantin Retard*) do not appear to be affected[7] and might therefore be a suitable alternative to immediate-release dipyridamole in some patients.

1. Russell TL, Berardi RR, Barnett JL, O'Sullivan TL, Wagner JG, Dressman JB. pH-related changes in the absorption of dipyridamole in the elderly. *Pharm Res* (1994) 11 136–43.
2. Derendorf H, VanderMaelen CP, Brickl R-S, MacGregor TR, Eisert W. Dipyridamole bioavailability in subjects with reduced gastric acidity. *J Clin Pharmacol* (2005) 45, 845–50.
3. Boehringer Ingelheim. Data on file. Study 1482B.
4. Persantin Tablets (Dipyridamole). Boehringer Ingelheim Ltd. UK Summary of product characteristics, May 2007.
5. Dipyridamole Oral Suspension (Dipyridamole). Rosemont Pharmaceuticals Ltd. UK Summary of product characteristics, September 2007.
6. Boehringer Ingelheim. Personal communication, June 2010.
7. Boehringer Ingelheim. Personal communication, February 2008.

Dipyridamole + Xanthines

Caffeine, theophylline and aminophylline can reduce the accuracy of dipyridamole–thallium-201 scintigraphy tests.

Clinical evidence, mechanism, importance and management

In one patient, **caffeine** 4 mg/kg intravenously (roughly equivalent to 2 to 3 cups of coffee), given before dipyridamole–thallium-201 myocardial scintigraphy, caused a false-negative test result.[1] A study in 8 healthy subjects confirmed that **caffeine** inhibits the haemodynamic response to intravenous dipyridamole,[2] and another two studies in healthy subjects similarly found that **caffeine** reduced myocardial blood flow in response to intravenous dipyridamole.[3,4]

Other xanthines appear to interact like caffeine. In one study, oral **theophylline** markedly reduced the diagnostic accuracy of myocardial imaging using dipyridamole.[5] Similarly, intravenous **aminophylline** has been found to accelerate the myocardial washout rate of thallium-201 after a dipyridamole infusion.[6]

It appears that xanthines, such as **caffeine** and **theophylline**, might antagonise some of the haemodynamic effects of intravenous dipyridamole because they act as competitive antagonists of adenosine (an endogenous vasodilator involved in the action of dipyridamole).[1,2] Due to these opposing effects, intravenous **aminophylline** may be used to treat severe adverse events associated with intravenous dipyridamole (such as chest pain and bronchospasm),[7,8] and for this reason, it is recommended that intravenous **aminophylline** should be readily available before beginning dipyridamole myocardial imaging.[8,9]

Patients should therefore abstain from **caffeine** (tea, coffee, chocolate, cocoa, cola, caffeine-containing analgesics, etc.)[1,2,9] and other xanthines, such as **theophylline**,[5] for at least 12 to 24 hours[2,8,10] before dipyridamole testing. If the haemodynamic response to intravenous dipyridamole during cardiac imaging is low (e.g. no increase in heart rate), the presence of **caffeine** should be suspected.[2]

1. Smits P, Aengevaeren WRM, Corstens FHM, Thien T. Caffeine reduces dipyridamole-induced myocardial ischemia. *J Nucl Med* (1989) 30, 1723–6.
2. Smits P, Straatman C, Pijpers E, Thien T. Dose-dependent inhibition of the hemodynamic response to dipyridamole by caffeine. *Clin Pharmacol Ther* (1991) 50, 529–37.
3. Kubo S, Tadamura E, Toyoda H, Mamede M, Yamamuro M, Magata Y, Mukai T, Kitano H, Tamaki N, Konishi J. Effect of caffeine intake on myocardial hyperemic flow induced by adenosine triphosphate and dipyridamole. *J Nucl Med* (2004) 45, 730–8.
4. Böttcher M, Czernin J, Sun KT, Phelps ME, Schelbert HR. Effect of caffeine on myocardial blood flow at rest and during pharmacological vasodilation. *J Nucl Med* (1995) 36, 2016–21.
5. Daley PJ, Mahn TH, Zielonka JS, Krubsack AJ, Akhtar R, Bamrah VS. Effect of maintenance oral theophylline on dipyridamole–thallium-201 myocardial imaging using SPECT and dipyridamole-induced hemodynamic changes. *Am Heart J* (1988) 115, 1185–92.
6. Takeishi Y, Tono-oka I, Kubota I, Ikeda K, Masakane I, Chiba J, Abe S, Tsuiki K, Tomoike H. Intravenous aminophylline affects myocardial washout of thallium-201 after dipyridamole infusion. *Am J Noninvasive Cardiol* (1992) 6, 116–21.

7. Ranhosky A, Kempthorne-Rawson J, and the Intravenous Dipyridamole Thallium Imaging Study Group. The safety of intravenous dipyridamole thallium myocardial perfusion imaging. *Circulation* (1990) 81, 1205–9.
8. Persantin Ampoules (Dipyridamole). Boehringer Ingelheim Ltd. UK Summary of product characteristics, May 2007.
9. Picano E, Marini C, Pirelli S, Maffei S, Bolognese L, Chiriatti G, Chiarella F, Orlandini A, Seveso G, Colosso MQ, Sclavo MG, Magaia O, Agati L, Previtali M, Lowenstein J, Torre F, Rosselli P, Ciuti M, Ostojic M, Gandolfo N, Margaria F, Gianuzzi P, Di Bello V, Lombardi M, Gigli G, Ferrara N, Santoro F, Lusa AM, Chiaranda G, Papagna D, Coletta C, Boccardi L, De Cristofaro M, Papi L, Landi P, on behalf of the Echo-Persantine International Cooperative Study Group. Safety of intravenous high-dose dipyridamole echocardiography. *Am J Cardiol* (1992) 70, 252–8.
10. Hesse B, Tägil K, Cuocolo A, Anagnostopoulos C, Bardiés M, Bax J, Bengel F, Busemann Sokole E, Davies G, Dondi M, Edenbrandt L, Franken P, Kjaer A, Knuuti J, Lassmann M, Ljungberg M, Marcassa C, Marie PY, McKiddie F, O'Connor M, Prvulovich E, Underwood R, van Eck-Smit B. EANM/ESC procedural guidelines for myocardial perfusion imaging in nuclear cardiology. *Eur J Nucl Med Mol Imaging* (2005) 32, 855–97.

Glycoprotein IIb/IIIa-receptor antagonists + Antiplatelet drugs

Dipyridamole has been reported not to increase bleeding with eptifibatide, and ticlopidine does not appear to add to the prolongation of bleeding time seen with tirofiban. A clinically significant adverse interaction does not appear to occur between prasugrel, ticagrelor or clopidogrel and the glycoprotein IIb/IIIa-receptor antagonists. Nevertheless, an increased risk of bleeding is generally anticipated if glycoprotein IIb/IIIa-receptor antagonists (abciximab, eptifibatide or tirofiban) are given with other drugs that have antiplatelet effects.

Clinical evidence

(a) Clopidogrel and related drugs

The UK manufacturers of clopidogrel and **prasugrel** briefly note that, in clinical studies, no clinically significant adverse interactions were reported when glycoprotein IIb/IIIa-receptor antagonists (unspecified) were also given.[1,2] Similarly, the US manufacturer of **eptifibatide** states that in one study (ESPIRIT) in patients undergoing percutaneous coronary intervention and given eptifibatide, clopidogrel or **ticlopidine** were routinely started on the same day.[3] The UK manufacturer of **tirofiban** also notes that the concurrent use of **ticlopidine** did not increase the prolongation of bleeding time seen with tirofiban alone.[4]

(b) Dipyridamole

The UK manufacturer of **eptifibatide** briefly reports that concurrent use with dipyridamole did not appear to increase the risk of major and minor bleeding.[5]

(c) Ticagrelor

The UK manufacturer of ticagrelor states that in the PLATO study, ticagrelor was given with intravenous glycoprotein IIb/IIIa inhibitors without evidence of a clinically significant adverse interaction.[6]

Mechanism

Glycoprotein IIb/IIIa-receptor antagonists have antiplatelet effects, which can be additive with other drugs that affect platelets resulting in an increased risk of bleeding.

Importance and management

Glycoprotein IIb/IIIa-receptor antagonists are generally used together with low-dose aspirin and heparin, see also 'Glycoprotein IIb/IIIa-receptor antagonists + Heparin or LMWHs', below. The manufacturers of abciximab, eptifibatide and tirofiban generally advise caution on their concurrent use with other drugs that affect haemostasis because of the likely further increased risk of bleeding.[3-5,7-9] They specifically name **adenosine,**[4,5] other **antiplatelet drugs**[7] (such as **clopidogrel,**[4,5] **dipyridamole,**[3,5,7,8] and **ticlopidine**[4,5,7,8]), **epoprostenol** (prostacyclin),[4,5] **NSAIDs,**[3,5,8] and sulfinpyrazone.[4,5] When concurrent use is undertaken it would be prudent to be alert for evidence of increased bleeding.

1. Efient (Prasugrel hydrochloride). Eli Lilly and Company Ltd. UK Summary of product characteristics, December 2013.
2. Plavix (Clopidogrel hydrogen sulphate). Sanofi-Aventis. UK Summary of product characteristics, May 2011.
3. Integrilin (Eptifibatide). Schering-Plough. US Prescribing information, March 2011.
4. Aggrastat (Tirofiban hydrochloride monohydrate). Iroko Cardio GmbH. UK Summary of product characteristics, September 2010.
5. Integrilin (Eptifibatide). GlaxoSmithKline UK. UK Summary of product characteristics, April 2011.
6. Brilique (Ticagrelor). AstraZeneca UK Ltd. UK Summary of product characteristics, July 2015.
7. ReoPro (Abciximab). Eli Lilly and Company Ltd. UK Summary of product characteristics, March 2011.
8. ReoPro (Abciximab). Centocor. US Prescribing information, November 2005.
9. Aggrastat (Tirofiban hydrochloride). Medicure Pharma, Inc. US Prescribing information, July 2008.

Glycoprotein IIb/IIIa-receptor antagonists + Dextrans

In one study, there appeared to be a high incidence of bleeding when low-molecular-weight dextran was given with abciximab. Other glycoprotein IIb/IIIa-receptor antagonists would be expected to interact similarly.

Clinical evidence, mechanism, importance and management

The US manufacturer of **abciximab** reports that, in the EPIC study, of the 11 patients given low-molecular-weight dextran with abciximab, 5 had major bleeding and 4 had minor bleeding events, whereas no bleeding occurred in the 5 patients who were given dextran and placebo.[1] They therefore contraindicate the concurrent use of intravenous dextrans with **abciximab**[1] before or during coronary revascularisation procedures, whereas the UK manufacturer of **abciximab** advises caution on the concurrent use of dextrans.[2] For other glycoprotein IIb/IIIa receptor antagonists, the UK manufacturer of **tirofiban** states that the concurrent use of dextrans is not recommended,[3] and the UK manufacturer of **eptifibatide** advises caution on concurrent use.[4] If concurrent use is considered essential, monitor closely for signs of bleeding.

1. ReoPro (Abciximab). Centocor. US Prescribing information, November 2005.
2. ReoPro (Abciximab). Eli Lilly and Company Ltd. UK Summary of product characteristics, March 2011.
3. Aggrastat (Tirofiban hydrochloride monohydrate). Iroko Cardio GmbH. UK Summary of product characteristics, September 2010.
4. Integrilin (Eptifibatide). GlaxoSmithKline UK. UK Summary of product characteristics, April 2011.

Glycoprotein IIb/IIIa-receptor antagonists + Heparin or LMWHs

The risk of bleeding with glycoprotein IIb/IIIa-receptor antagonists might be increased by the concurrent use of heparin. Whether the use of a low-molecular-weight heparin increases or decreases the bleeding risk relative to the use of heparin is unclear.

Clinical evidence

A. Pharmacokinetics

A study in patients given a single intravenous dose of **enoxaparin** 750 micrograms/kg with **abciximab** (250 micrograms/kg bolus followed by 125 nanograms/kg per minute as an infusion over 12 hours) found that abciximab had no significant effect on plasma antifactor Xa pharmacokinetics and antithrombin activity, suggesting that the pharmacokinetics of enoxaparin were not affected.[1]

In a study in 12 healthy subjects, there was no difference in the pharmacokinetics or platelet inhibitory effect of **eptifibatide** when it was given with **enoxaparin** compared with heparin.[2] The UK manufacturer of **eptifibatide** states that, in a population pharmacokinetic study, there was no evidence of a pharmacokinetic interaction between eptifibatide and heparin.[3]

The manufacturers of **tirofiban** state that, in a subset of patients in a clinical study (PRISM), there was no difference in the plasma clearance of tirofiban between patients receiving heparin and those not receiving heparin.[4]

B. Bleeding risk

(a) Heparin

1. Abciximab. In a placebo-controlled study (EPIC) in 2099 patients undergoing coronary angioplasty or atherectomy, patients were given heparin and aspirin and randomised to receive a single 250 microgram/kg bolus dose of abciximab followed by either an infusion at a rate of 10 micrograms per minute, or no further treatment. The incidence of major bleeding was approximately doubled in those patients receiving abciximab compared with the placebo recipients (14% for the bolus plus infusion, 11% for the bolus only, and 7% for placebo, with the difference between the bolus plus infusion and the placebo being statistically significantly) and the need for red cell transfusions was also approximately doubled. Note that the heparin dose used in this study was much larger than is now recommended (the dose used was an initial bolus 10 000 to 20 000 units followed by incremental boluses of up to 3 000 units to a maximum of 20 000 units during the procedure, followed by infusion with the APTT maintained between 1.5 and 2.5 times the control value, for at least 12 hours).[5] In contrast, in another placebo-controlled randomised study (EPILOG), no increase in major bleeding was found when patients were given abciximab with aspirin and standard-dose heparin, although the incidence of minor bleeding was increased (7.4% versus 3.7%). The standard-dose, weight-adjusted heparin regimen was a bolus of 100 units per kilogram to a maximum of 10 000 units, with additional bolus doses during the procedure to maintain an activated clotting time of at least 200 seconds. Moreover, when a low-dose heparin regimen was used (70 units per kilogram to a maximum of 7 000 units), there was no increase in major or minor bleeding with abciximab.[6]

2. Eptifibatide. In a randomised, placebo-controlled study (PURSUIT), in patients with acute coronary syndromes, the incidence of bleeding was higher on the concurrent use of **eptifibatide** with standard treatment (heparin plus aspirin), when compared with standard treatment alone (for example, episodes of major and minor bleeding were 23.5% versus 16.5%).[7] Similar findings were also reported in another study in patients undergoing coronary stenting.[8]

3. Tirofiban. In a placebo-controlled study (PRISM-PLUS), the incidence of bleeding was slightly higher in patients taking aspirin and randomised to receive **tirofiban** with heparin compared with tirofiban or heparin alone (56% versus 43%) although the incidence of major bleeding did not differ (4% versus 3%). Further analysis of these results noted that patients who were older, female, hypertensive, or who had a low body-weight or impaired renal function were more likely to have a bleeding episode when given both tirofiban and heparin.[9] Similarly, in a further randomised study (RESTORE), the concurrent use of **tirofiban** with heparin and aspirin did not result in a statistically significant increase in major bleeding, when compared with heparin and aspirin alone, although there was a trend towards an increase (5.3% versus 3.7%).[10]

(b) Low-molecular-weight heparins

In a randomised study in patients with high-risk non-ST elevation acute coronary syndrome undergoing percutaneous coronary intervention given **eptifibatide** and aspirin (INTERACT), there was a higher rate of major bleeding at 96 hours in the patients given heparin compared with those given enoxaparin (4.6% versus 1.8%).

Conversely, the rate of minor bleeding was higher in the enoxaparin group (30.3% versus 20.8%).[11]

In a study (ACUTE II) in patients with non-ST elevation acute coronary syndromes given **tirofiban** and aspirin with either heparin or **enoxaparin**, the overall incidence of bleeding tended to be higher in the heparin group compared with the enoxaparin group (4.8% versus 3.5%, respectively); however, the rate of cutaneous and oral bleeding was higher with enoxaparin than heparin.[12] Similar findings for rate of any grade bleeding were later reported in the larger A to Z study (3% for enoxaparin and 2.2% for heparin); however, in this study, the rate of major bleeding was slightly higher for enoxaparin (0.9% versus 0.4%), although this difference was not statistically significant.[13]

In a retrospective analysis of one study in patients with acute coronary syndrome without early revascularisation, the concurrent use of **low-molecular-weight heparin (dalteparin)** was found to be the most important risk factor for increased risk of bleeding events with **abciximab**.[14]

In an observational study of patients treated for acute coronary events, in the subset of patients who underwent percutaneous coronary intervention and also received a glycoprotein IIb/IIIa-receptor antagonist (specific drugs not stated), the incidence of major bleeding tended to be lower in those who received a low-molecular weight heparin (not specified) than in those who received heparin (2.5% versus 4.1%), although this difference was not statistically significant. In contrast, in the subset of patients given a glycoprotein IIb/IIIa-receptor antagonist who did not undergo percutaneous coronary intervention, the incidence of major bleeding was higher in those treated with a low-molecular weight heparin than those receiving heparin.[15]

Mechanism

Glycoprotein IIb/IIIa-receptor antagonists inhibit platelet aggregation and prolong bleeding times, and therefore increase the risk of bleeding. This is likely to be additive with the effects of heparin or low-molecular-weight heparins.

Importance and management

The concurrent use of heparin with a glycoprotein IIb/IIIa-receptor antagonist is recommended; however, increased bleeding may also occur. For this reason, the manufacturers of abciximab, eptifibatide and tirofiban recommend caution and close monitoring for bleeding.[3,4,16-19]

The use of low-molecular weight heparins with glycoprotein IIb/IIIa-receptor antagonists is not yet established and whether they are associated with a higher or lower risk of bleeding than heparin is currently unclear.

1. Argenti D, Hoppensteadt D, Heald D, Jensen B, Fareed J. Pharmacokinetics of enoxaparin in patients undergoing percutaneous coronary intervention with and without glycoprotein IIb/IIIa therapy. *Am J Ther* (2003) 10, 241–6.
2. Gretler DD. Pharmacokinetic and pharmacodynamic properties of eptifibatide in healthy subjects receiving unfractionated heparin or the low-molecular-weight heparin enoxaparin. *Clin Ther* (2003) 25, 2564–74.
3. Integrilin (Eptifibatide). GlaxoSmithKline UK. UK Summary of product characteristics, April 2011.
4. Aggrastat (Tirofiban hydrochloride). Medicure Pharma, Inc. US Prescribing information, July 2008.
5. The EPIC investigators. Use of a monoclonal antibody directed against the platelet glycoprotein IIb/IIIa receptor in high-risk coronary angioplasty. *N Engl J Med* (1994) 330, 956–61.
6. The EPILOG investigators. Platelet glycoprotein IIb/IIIa receptor blockade and low-dose heparin during percutaneous coronary revascularization. *N Engl J Med* (1997) 336, 1689–96.
7. The PURSUIT trial investigators. Inhibition of platelet glycoprotein IIb/IIIa with eptifibatide in patients with acute coronary syndromes. *N Engl J Med* (1998) 339, 436–43.
8. The ESPRIT investigators. Novel dosing regimen of eptifibatide in planned coronary stent implantation (ESPRIT): a randomised, placebo-controlled trail. *Lancet* (2000) 356, 2037–44.
9. Huynh T, Piazza N, DiBattiste PM, Snapinn SM, Wan Y, Pharand C, Theroux P. Analysis of bleeding complications associated with glycoprotein IIb/IIIa receptors blockade in patients with high-risk acute coronary syndromes: insights from the PRISM-PLUS study. *Int J Cardiol* (2005) 100, 73–8.
10. The RESTORE investigators. Effects of platelet glycoprotein IIb/IIIa blockade with tirofiban on adverse cardiac events in patients with unstable angina or acute myocardial infarction undergoing coronary angioplasty. *Circulation* (1997) 96, 1445–53.
11. Goodman SG, Fitchett D, Armstrong PW, Tan M, Langer A; for the Integrilin and Enoxaparin Randomized Assessment of an Acute Coronary Syndrome Treatment (INTERACT) trial investigators. Randomized evaluation of the safety and efficacy of enoxaparin versus unfractionated heparin in high-risk patients with non–ST-segment elevation acute coronary syndromes receiving the glycoprotein IIb/IIIa inhibitor eptifibatide. *Circulation* (2003) 107, 238–44.
12. Cohen M, Théroux P, Borzak S, Frey MJ, White HD, Van Mieghem W, Senatore F, Lis J, Mukherjee R, Harris K, Bigonzi F; for the ACUTE II investigators. Randomized double-blind safety study of enoxaparin versus unfractionated heparin in patients with non-ST-segment elevation acute coronary syndromes treated with tirofiban and aspirin: the ACUTE II study. The Antithrombotic Combination Using Tirofiban and Enoxaparin. *Am Heart J* (2002) 144, 470–7.
13. Blazing MA, de Lemos JA, White HD, Fox KAA, Verheugt FWA, Ardissino D, DiBattiste PM, Palmisano J, Bilheimer DW, Snapinn SM, Ramsey KE, Gardner LH, Hasselblad V, Pfeffer MA, Lewis EF, Braunwald E, Califf RM for the A to Z investigators. Safety and efficacy of enoxaparin vs unfractionated heparin in patients with non-ST-segment elevation acute coronary syndromes who receive tirofiban and aspirin: a randomized controlled trial. *JAMA* (2004) 292, 55–64.
14. Lenderink T, Boersma E, Ruzyllo W, Widimsky P, Ohman EM, Armstrong PW, Wallentin L, Simoons ML; GUSTO IV-ACS Investigators. Bleeding events with abciximab in acute coronary syndromes without early revascularization: an analysis of GUSTO IV-ACS. *Am Heart J* (2004) 147, 865–73.
15. Brieger D, Van de Werf F, Avezum A, Montalescot G, Kennelly B, Granger CB, Goodman SG, Dabbous OH, Agnelli G, for the GRACE investigators. Interactions between heparins, glycoprotein IIb/IIIa antagonists, and coronary intervention. The Global Registry of Acute Coronary Events (GRACE). *Am Heart J* (2007) 153, 960–9.
16. ReoPro (Abciximab). Eli Lilly and Company Ltd. UK Summary of product characteristics, March 2011.
17. ReoPro (Abciximab). Centocor. US Prescribing information, November 2005.
18. Integrilin (Eptifibatide). Schering-Plough. US Prescribing information, March 2011.
19. Aggrastat (Tirofiban hydrochloride monohydrate). Iroko Cardio GmbH. UK Summary of product characteristics, September 2010.

Glycoprotein IIb/IIIa-receptor antagonists + Miscellaneous

In pharmacokinetic analyses of clinical studies, levothyroxine and omeprazole appeared to increase the clearance of tirofiban, whereas various drugs, including ACE inhibitors, beta blockers, calcium-channel blockers and nitrates appeared not to interact with tirofiban, eptifibatide or abciximab.

Clinical evidence, mechanism, importance and management

(a) Abciximab

The UK manufacturer of abciximab notes that, in clinical studies, no adverse drug reactions occurred in patients also taking commonly used cardiovascular medications such as **ACE inhibitors, beta blockers, calcium-channel blockers** and **nitrates** (oral and intravenous).[1] Therefore, no additional precautions would appear to be necessary on the concurrent use of abciximab and these drugs.

(b) Eptifibatide

The UK manufacturer of eptifibatide states that, in a population pharmacokinetic study, there was no evidence of a pharmacokinetic interaction between eptifibatide and some ACE inhibitors (**captopril, enalapril, lisinopril**), beta blockers (**atenolol, metoprolol**), calcium-channel blockers (**amlodipine, diltiazem, nifedipine**), **atropine, cefazolin, diazepam, digoxin, diphenhydramine, fentanyl, furosemide, lidocaine, midazolam, morphine** and **nitrates**.[2] Therefore, no dose adjustment of eptifibatide would appear to be necessary on the concurrent use of these drugs.

(c) Tirofiban

The US manufacturer reports that, in a subset of patients in the PRISM study, the plasma clearance of tirofiban was compared between patients taking specific drugs and those not taking the drug. In this analysis, the clearance of tirofiban appeared to be increased in patients taking **levothyroxine** or **omeprazole** (amount not stated), and they state that the clinical relevance of this is unknown.[3] Conversely, in this analysis, the following drugs were reported to have no clinically relevant effects on the plasma clearance of tirofiban: **ACE inhibitors (captopril, enalapril), aspirin, beta blockers** (including **acebutolol, atenolol, metoprolol, propranolol**), **benzodiazepines** (including **alprazolam, bromazepam, diazepam, lorazepam, oxazepam, temazepam**), **calcium-channel blockers (amlodipine, diltiazem, nifedipine), digoxin, docusate sodium, furosemide, glibenclamide (glyburide), insulin, metoclopramide, morphine, nitrate** preparations, **paracetamol (acetaminophen), potassium chloride, ranitidine, statins (lovastatin, simvastatin)**, and **sucralfate**.[3,4] Therefore, no additional precautions would appear to be necessary on the concurrent use of tirofiban and these drugs.

1. ReoPro (Abciximab). Eli Lilly and Company Ltd. UK Summary of product characteristics, March 2011.
2. Integrilin (Eptifibatide). GlaxoSmithKline UK. UK Summary of product characteristics, April 2011.
3. Aggrastat (Tirofiban hydrochloride). Medicure Pharma, Inc. US Prescribing information, July 2008.
4. Aggrastat (Tirofiban hydrochloride monohydrate). Iroko Cardio GmbH. UK Summary of product characteristics, September 2010.

Glycoprotein IIb/IIIa-receptor antagonists + Thrombolytics

The risk of bleeding with glycoprotein IIb/IIIa-receptor antagonists might be increased by thrombolytics, even when used in reduced doses.

Clinical evidence and mechanism

(a) Abciximab

Limited experience of abciximab in patients who have received thrombolytics suggests an increase in the risk of bleeding.[1,2] For example, a retrospective analysis of 103 patients who presented with acute myocardial infarction and underwent angioplasty with adjunctive abciximab, found that there was a significant increase in major bleeding complications when abciximab was used with full-dose **alteplase**. A major bleed occurred in 5 of 22 (23%) patients who underwent angioplasty within 15 hours of receiving a thrombolytic, compared with 0 of 36 patients who underwent elective angioplasty more than 15 hours after fibrinolysis, and 1 of 45 (2%) without prior fibrinolysis.[3]

Early evidence from available study data suggested that the concurrent use of abciximab with reduced-dose **reteplase** or other thrombolytics was associated with less bleeding complications, when compared with full-dose thrombolytics or abciximab.[4,5] However, a large, randomised study did find an increased risk of bleeding. In the GUSTO V study, 16 588 patients with acute myocardial infarction were given standard dose **reteplase** alone or half-dose **reteplase** with abciximab. The concurrent use of abciximab with half-dose reteplase increased the risk of severe or moderate non-intracranial bleeding 2-fold compared with standard-dose reteplase alone.[6] Similarly, in the FINESSE study in patients undergoing percutaneous coronary intervention, the risk of minor or major bleeding was higher in those treated with half-dose **reteplase** and abciximab compared with abciximab alone (14.5% versus 10.1%).[7]

Similar increased bleeding rates were also seen in the ASSENT-3 study, when patients were given abciximab with half-dose **tenecteplase** (a single bolus of 15 to 25 mg) and reduced dose heparin, when compared with standard-dose **tenecteplase** (a single bolus of 30 to 50 mg) alone with heparin. Major bleeding rates were higher in the patients given abciximab with half-dose tenecteplase compared with full-dose tenecteplase (4.4% compared with 2.2%, respectively) and the rate of minor bleeding was also higher (35.3% compared with 18.7%, respectively).[8]

A case of fatal pulmonary haemorrhage has been reported in a patient admitted to hospital with acute myocardial infarction and given aspirin, standard dose **streptokinase**, low-dose heparin, and then **abciximab** (9 hours after the streptokinase). The combination of streptokinase with abciximab was considered to have contributed to this rare adverse event, as was the presence of mild pulmonary congestion before treatment.[9]

(b) Eptifibatide

In a placebo-controlled study involving 181 patients who had an acute myocardial infarction and were given **streptokinase** 1.5 million units over 60 minutes, the addition of eptifibatide increased the risk of bleeding: major and minor bleeding occurred in 14% and 27%, respectively, of the patients given eptifibatide compared with none and 5%, respectively, in the placebo-treated group. The increase in risk was dose-related, with the highest incidence of bleeding occurring at the highest eptifibatide infusion rates (1.3 and 2 micrograms/kg per minute).[10] Similarly, in another study in patients undergoing percutaneous coronary intervention (ADVANCE MI), the addition of **tenecteplase** to eptifibatide was associated with a twofold higher incidence of bleeding complications than eptifibatide alone.[11] Two small dose-finding studies in patients with acute myocardial infarction found no statistically significant increase in the risk of bleeding with the concurrent use of eptifibatide and **alteplase** when compared with alteplase alone.[12,13]

(c) Tirofiban

In a study in 313 patients undergoing percutaneous coronary intervention, there was no difference in the incidence of bleeding in patients given tirofiban with **alteplase** compared with tirofiban alone.[14] Similarly, in another dose-ranging study, there was no statistically significant difference in the incidence of bleeding with the concurrent use of half-dose **tenecteplase** and tirofiban, when compared with full-dose **tenecteplase** alone.[15]

Importance and management

Data on the concurrent use of different glycoprotein IIb/IIIa-receptor antagonists with thrombolytics is limited. However, in general, the concurrent use of a glycoprotein IIb/IIIa-receptor antagonist with a thrombolytic would be expected to increase the risk of bleeding. The manufacturers of abciximab and eptifibatide therefore advise caution on their concurrent use with thrombolytics,[1,2,16,17] whereas the UK manufacturer of tirofiban advises against concurrent use.[18]

Glycoprotein IIb/IIIa-receptor antagonists should not generally be used for indications requiring thrombolytics,[16,18] and, if thrombolytics become necessary in a patient receiving a glycoprotein IIb/IIIa-receptor antagonists, these should usually be stopped.[17,18] In patients who have already received thrombolytics, the risk of bleeding is greater the sooner abciximab is given,[1] and the manufacturer of tirofiban recommends a 48 hour interval between stopping a thrombolytic and starting tirofiban.[18]

1. ReoPro (Abciximab). Eli Lilly and Company Ltd. UK Summary of product characteristics, March 2011.
2. ReoPro (Abciximab). Centocor. US Prescribing information, November 2005.
3. Sundlof DW, Rerkpattanapitat P, Wongpraparut N, Pathi P, Kotler MN, Jacobs LE, Ledley GS, Yazdanfar S. Incidence of bleeding complications associated with *abciximab* use in conjunction with thrombolytic therapy in patients requiring percutaneous transluminal coronary angioplasty. *Am J Cardiol* (1999) 83, 1569–71.
4. Califf RM. Glycoprotein IIb/IIIa blockade and thrombolytics: early lessons from the SPEED and GUSTO IV trials. *Am Heart J* (1999) 138, S12–S15.
5. Gibson CM. Primary angioplasty compared with thrombolysis: new issues in the era of glycoprotein IIb/IIIa inhibition and intracoronary stenting. *Ann Intern Med* (1999) 130, 841–7.
6. The Gusto V Investigators. Reperfusion therapy for acute myocardial infarction with fibrinolytic therapy or combination reduced fibrinolytic therapy and platelet glycoprotein IIb/IIIa inhibition: the GUSTO V randomised trial. *Lancet* (2001) 357, 1905–14.
7. Ellis SG, Tendera M, de Belder MA, van Boven AJ, Widimsky P, Janssens L, Andersen HR, Betriu A, Savonitto S, Adamus J, Peruga JZ, Kosmider M, Katz O, Neunteufl T, Jorgova J, Dorobantu M, Grinfeld L, Armstrong P, Brodie BR, Herrmann HC, Montalescot G, Neumann F-J, Effron MB, Barnathan ES, Topol EJ; FINESSE Investigators. Facilitated PCI in patients with ST-elevation myocardial infarction. *N Engl J Med* (2008) 358, 2205–17.
8. The Assessment of the Safety and Efficacy of a New Thrombolytic Regimen (ASSENT)-3 Investigators. Efficacy and safety of tenecteplase in combination with enoxaparin, abciximab, or unfractionated heparin: the ASSENT-3 randomised trial in acute myocardial infarction. *Lancet* (2001) 358, 605–13.
9. Tan HC, Low A, Ng KS, Budiono B, Sutandar A, Chia BL, Lim YT. Fatal pulmonary haemorrhage with the combined use of abciximab and fibrinolytic agent. *Singapore Med J* (2002) 43, 587–9.
10. Ronner E, van Kesteren HAM, Zijnen P, Altmann E, Molhoek PG, van der Wieken LR, Cuffie-Jackson CA, Neuhaus KL, Simoons ML. Safety and efficacy of eptifibatide vs placebo in patients receiving thrombolytic therapy with streptokinase for acute myocardial infarction. *Eur Heart J* (2000) 21, 1530–6.
11. ADVANCE MI Investigators. Facilitated percutaneous coronary intervention for acute ST-segment elevation myocardial infarction: results from the prematurely terminated ADdressing the Value of facilitated ANgioplasty after Combination therapy or Eptifibatide monotherapy in acute Myocardial Infarction (ADVANCE MI) trial. *Am Heart J* (2005) 150, 116–22.
12. Brener SJ, Zeymer U, Adgey AAJ, Vrobel TR, Ellis SG, Neuhaus K-L, Juran N, Ivanc TB, Ohman EM, Strony J, Kitt M, Topol EJ, for the INTRO AMI investigators. Eptifibatide and low-dose tissue plasminogen activator in acute myocardial infarction: the integrilin and low-dose thrombolysis in acute myocardial infarction (INTRO AMI) trial. *J Am Coll Cardiol* (2002) 39, 377–86.
13. Ohman EM, Kleiman NS, Gacioch G, Worley SJ, Navetta FI, Talley JD, Anderson HV, Ellis SG, Cohen MD, Spriggs D, Miller M, Kereiakes D, Yakubov S, Kitt MM, Sigmon KN, Califf RM, Krucoff MW, Topol EJ, for the IMPACT-AMI investigators. Combined accelerated tissue-plasminogen activator and platelet glycoprotein IIb/IIIa integrin receptor blockade with integrilin in acute myocardial infarction. *Circulation* (1997) 95, 846–54.
14. Peters S, Truemmel M, Koehler B. Facilitated PCI by combination fibrinolysis or upstream tirofiban in acute ST-segment elevation myocardial infarction: results of the alteplase and tirofiban in acute myocardial infarction (ATAMI) trial. *Int J Cardiol* (2008) 130, 235–40.
15. Ohman EM, Van de Werf F, Antman EM, Califf RM, de Lemos JA, Gibson CM, Oliverio RL, Harrelson L, McCabe C, DiBattiste P, Braunwald E, for the FASTER (TIMI 24) investigators. Tenecteplase and tirofiban in ST-segment elevation myocardial infarction: results of a randomized trial. *Am Heart J* (2005) 150, 79–88.
16. Integrilin (Eptifibatide). GlaxoSmithKline UK. UK Summary of product characteristics, April 2011.
17. Integrilin (Eptifibatide). Schering-Plough. US Prescribing information, March 2011.
18. Aggrastat (Tirofiban hydrochloride monohydrate). Iroko Cardio GmbH. UK Summary of product characteristics, September 2010.

Prasugrel + Drugs that affect gastric pH

Lansoprazole and ranitidine have no clinically relevant effect on the pharmacokinetics or antiplatelet effects of the active metabolite of prasugrel. One retrospective analysis of two studies suggested a slight reduction in the antiplatelet effects of prasugrel, but no difference in clinical outcomes, in those patients taking a proton pump inhibitor.

Clinical evidence

(a) Proton pump inhibitors

In a randomised study, 24 healthy subjects were given **lansoprazole** 30 mg daily for 7 days with a single 60-mg dose of prasugrel on day 7. **Lansoprazole** slightly reduced the AUC of the active metabolite of prasugrel by 12% and reduced its maximum concentration by 29%; however, the antiplatelet effect of prasugrel was unaffected.[1] Similarly, in a post-hoc analysis of a clinical study in 102 patients given a 60-mg loading dose of prasugrel then 10 mg daily (PRINCIPLE-TIMI 44), the mean inhibition of platelet aggregation was a lower at 30 minutes after the loading dose in those patients also taking a proton pump inhibitor, but not at any other time point. However, after 15 days, the mean platelet aggregation was lower for patients taking a proton pump inhibitor (48% versus 66%) and there was a higher proportion of patients classified as non-responders (10% versus 0%).[2] Nevertheless, in a retrospective analysis of a large clinical study in patients taking prasugrel or clopidogrel (TRITON-TIMI 38), no association was found between proton pump inhibitor or **H_2-receptor antagonist** use and an increased incidence of cardiovascular death, myocardial infarction, stroke or coronary stent thrombosis in those taking prasugrel. The most common proton pump inhibitors taken in this study were **pantoprazole** (1 844 patients) and **omeprazole** (1 675 patients), with fewer patients taking **esomeprazole** (613 patients), **lansoprazole** (441 patients) and **rabeprazole** (66 patients).[2]

(b) Ranitidine

In a study in 23 healthy subjects, prasugrel (a single 60-mg loading dose followed by 10 mg daily for 7 days) was given alone then started on day 2 of ranitidine 150 mg twice daily for 8 days. Ranitidine slightly reduced the AUC of the active metabolite of prasugrel after the loading dose by just 10%, but had no effect after the maintenance dose. Ranitidine did not alter the time to or magnitude of the platelet inhibition response to prasugrel after the loading dose or maintenance dose.[3]

Mechanism

The active metabolite of prasugrel is principally formed by CYP3A4 and CYP2B6 and, to a lesser extent, by CYP2C9 and CYP2C19. Proton pump inhibitors that are potent inhibitors of CYP2C19 would not therefore be expected to alter the pharmacokinetics of the active metabolite of prasugrel (confirmed *in vitro* for omeprazole[4]). The lack of effect of ranitidine suggests that alterations in gastric pH have no effect on prasugrel pharmacokinetics.

Importance and management

The minor pharmacokinetic changes seen with the concurrent use of lansoprazole or ranitidine and prasugrel are not clinically relevant, and no alteration in the antiplatelet effect of prasugrel appears to occur when these drugs are given concurrently. The manufacturers of prasugrel advise that it may be taken with a **proton pump inhibitor** or **H_2-receptor antagonist**;[5,6] however, the UK manufacturer suggests that a quicker onset of action might occur if the loading dose of prasugrel is taken without the use of a proton pump inhibitor.[5]

1. Small DS, Farid NA, Payne CD, Weerakkody GJ, Li YG, Brandt JT, Salazar DE, Winters KJ. Effects of the proton pump inhibitor lansoprazole on the pharmacokinetics and pharmacodynamics of prasugrel and clopidogrel. *J Clin Pharmacol* (2008) 48, 478–84.
2. O'Donoghue ML, Braunwald E, Antman EM, Murphy SA, Bates ER, Rozenman Y, Michelson AD, Hautvast RW, Ver Lee PN, Close SL, Shen L, Mega JL, Sabatine MS, Wiviott SD. Pharmacodynamic effect and clinical efficacy of clopidogrel and prasugrel with or without a proton-pump inhibitor: an analysis of two randomised trials. *Lancet* (2009) 374, 989–97.
3. Small DS, Farid NA, Li YG, Ernest CS, Payne CD, Salazar DE, Winters KJ. Effect of ranitidine on the pharmacokinetics and pharmacodynamics of prasugrel and clopidogrel. *Curr Med Res Opin* (2008) 24, 2251–7.
4. Rehmel JL, Eckstein JA, Farid NA, Heim JB, Kasper SC, Kurihara A, Wrighton SA, Ring BJ. Interactions of two major metabolites of prasugrel, a thienopyridine antiplatelet agent, with the cytochromes P450. *Drug Metab Dispos* (2006) 34, 600–7.
5. Efient (Prasugrel hydrochloride). Eli Lilly and Company Ltd. UK Summary of product characteristics, December 2013.
6. Effient (Prasugrel). Eli Lilly and Company. US Prescribing information, November 2013.

Prasugrel + Ketoconazole and other CYP3A4 inhibitors

Ketoconazole, a CYP3A4 inhibitor, does not alter exposure to the active metabolite of prasugrel and does not appear to reduce its antiplatelet effects. Other inhibitors of CYP3A4 are also not expected to interact with prasugrel.

Clinical evidence

In a randomised study, 18 healthy subjects were given prasugrel alone (a single 60-mg loading dose followed by 15 mg daily for 6 days) and then with ketoconazole (400 mg daily for 10 days started 3 days before the prasugrel). Ketoconazole modestly reduced the maximum concentration of the active metabolite of prasugrel, by 46% after the loading dose and by 34% during maintenance doses, but had no effect on its AUC. Ketoconazole did not alter the antiplatelet effect of prasugrel after the loading dose or the maintenance doses.[1]

Mechanism

Prasugrel is metabolised to its active metabolite primarily by CYP3A4 and CYP2B6 and, to a lesser extent, by CYP2C9 and CYP2C19.[2,3] Ketoconazole is a potent inhibitor of CYP3A4, and it was therefore predicted that it may reduce the metabolism of prasugrel to its active metabolite, and reduce its efficacy.

Importance and management

Although ketoconazole causes a reduction in the maximum concentrations of the active metabolite of prasugrel this is not expected to be clinically relevant as there was no reduction in overall exposure, and also no change in the antiplatelet effects of prasugrel. The manufacturers of prasugrel therefore advise that other CYP3A4 inhibitors are also unlikely to have a clinically relevant effect on the pharmacokinetics of the active metabolite of prasugrel.[2,3] No prasugrel dose adjustments are therefore likely to be necessary on the concurrent use of prasugrel and ketoconazole or other inhibitors of CYP3A4. See 'Table 1.9', p.11, for a list of CYP3A4 inhibitors. Note that the manufacturer's additionally name **ciprofloxacin**, but it is not usually considered to be an inhibitor of CYP3A4.

1. Farid NA, Payne CD, Small DS, Winters KJ, Ernest II CS, Brandt JT, Darstein C, Jakubowski JA, Salazar DE. Cytochrome P450 3A inhibition by ketoconazole affects prasugrel and clopidogrel pharmacokinetics and pharmacodynamics differently. *Clin Pharmacol Ther* (2007) 81, 735–41.
2. Efient (Prasugrel hydrochloride). Eli Lilly and Company Ltd. UK Summary of product characteristics, December 2013.
3. Effient (Prasugrel). Eli Lilly and Company. US Prescribing information, November 2013.

Prasugrel + Miscellaneous

Prasugrel is expected to have a minimal effect on the metabolism of drugs that are principally metabolised by CYP2B6, although one manufacturer suggests that those that have a narrow therapeutic margin, such as cyclophosphamide and efavirenz might be affected.

Clinical evidence, mechanism, importance and management

The US manufacturer of prasugrel[1] notes that a clinically relevant interaction would not be expected with drugs that are primarily metabolised by CYP2B6 (they name **cyclophosphamide**, **halothane**, **propofol** and **nevirapine**). This is based on the lack of interaction seen with the CYP2B6 substrate, bupropion, see 'Bupropion + Clopidogrel and related drugs', p.1468. In contrast, the UK manufacturer suggests that caution might be needed in patients taking drugs with a narrow therapeutic margin and that are solely metabolised by CYP2B6, and they give **cyclophosphamide** and **efavirenz** as examples.[2] However, given the slight pharmacokinetic changes seen with bupropion, a clinically relevant interaction seems unlikely, even with narrow therapeutic index drugs.

1. Effient (Prasugrel). Eli Lilly and Company. US Prescribing information, November 2013.
2. Efient (Prasugrel hydrochloride). Eli Lilly and Company Ltd. UK Summary of product characteristics, December 2013.

Prasugrel + Rifampicin (Rifampin) and other enzyme inducers

Rifampicin, an inducer of cytochrome P450, does not appear to affect the pharmacokinetics of the active metabolite of prasugrel, although it markedly reduced the levels of the precursor to the active metabolite. A slight, but clinically irrelevant, reduction in the antiplatelet effect of prasugrel appears to occur on concurrent use. Other inducers of cytochrome P450 (e.g. carbamazepine) are therefore not expected to interact with prasugrel to a clinically relevant extent.

Clinical evidence

In a study to investigate the potential for an interaction between prasugrel and rifampicin, 30 healthy subjects were given prasugrel alone (a single 60-mg loading dose followed by 10 mg daily), rifampicin alone (600 mg daily), and then both drugs together for 6 days. Rifampicin did not alter the pharmacokinetics of the active metabolite of prasugrel after the loading dose or the maintenance dose of prasugrel. However, rifampicin markedly reduced the AUC of the inactive thiolactone metabolite of prasugrel (the precursor of the active metabolite) by 73% after the loading dose and by 84% after the maintenance dose of prasugrel, and increased the AUC of one inactive metabolite produced from the active metabolite by 21%. Despite the lack of pharmacokinetic effect on the active metabolite of prasugrel, rifampicin slightly reduced the inhibition of platelet aggregation produced by prasugrel.[1]

Mechanism

Prasugrel is a prodrug, which is initially metabolised to an inactive thiolactone metabolite by esterases, and is then metabolised to its active metabolite primarily by CYP3A4 and CYP2B6, and to a lesser extent by CYP2C9 and CYP2C19.[1-3] Rifampicin is a non-specific potent cytochrome P450 inducer, and so it was predicted that it might induce the metabolic conversion of prasugrel to its active metabolite, and therefore increase its antiplatelet effect. The marked reduction in the thiolactone metabolite levels without a consequent increase in the active metabolite levels suggests that rifampicin is inducing the metabolism of the thiolactone to unknown inactive metabolites by an unknown route, and that the production of the active metabolite of prasugrel is not affected by enzyme induction.[1] Rifampicin itself might also have a direct effect on the platelet receptor and so this might be the reason for the slight inhibition of the activity of prasugrel.[1]

Importance and management

Rifampicin does alter the pharmacokinetics of the active metabolite of prasugrel and does not appear to have a clinically relevant effect on its antiplatelet activity. The manufacturers therefore state that no important interaction would be expected with other CYP3A4 inducers and other inducers of cytochrome P450 isoenzymes.[2,3] For a list of other known inducers of CYP2B6 and CYP3A4, see 'Table 1.3', p.6, and 'Table 1.9', p.11, respectively. No prasugrel dose adjustments are likely to be needed if prasugrel is given with rifampicin or any other cytochrome P450 inducers.

1. Farid NA, Jakubowski JA, Payne CD, Li YG, Jin Y, Ernest II CS, Winters KJ, Brandt JT, Salazar DE, Small DS. Effect of rifampicin on the pharmacokinetics and pharmacodynamics of prasugrel in healthy male subjects. *Curr Med Res Opin* (2009) 25, 1821–9.
2. Efient (Prasugrel hydrochloride). Eli Lilly and Company Ltd. UK Summary of product characteristics, December 2013.
3. Effient (Prasugrel). Eli Lilly and Company. US Prescribing information, November 2013.

Prasugrel + Statins

High-dose atorvastatin has no clinically relevant effect on the pharmacokinetics or antiplatelet effects of the active metabolite of prasugrel. Other statins metabolised by CYP3A4 (such as simvastatin and lovastatin) are also not expected to interact.

Clinical evidence

In a randomised study, 31 healthy subjects were given **atorvastatin** 80 mg daily for 16 days with a single 60-mg loading dose of prasugrel on day 7 followed by 10 mg daily for 10 days. **Atorvastatin** had no effect on the AUC of the loading dose of prasugrel, and only slightly increased the AUC of the active metabolite of prasugrel (by 17%) on day 16. The effects of prasugrel on platelet inhibition were also unchanged by atorvastatin.[1]

Mechanism

Prasugrel is a prodrug and is initially metabolised to an inactive thiolactone metabolite by esterases, and is then metabolised to its active metabolite by cytochrome P450 isoenzymes, including CYP3A4.[1-3] Atorvastatin, a substrate but not an inhibitor of CYP3A4, would not be expected to alter the pharmacokinetics of prasugrel,[1] and this study confirms this.

Importance and management

No clinically relevant pharmacokinetic interaction occurs between atorvastatin and prasugrel, and the manufacturers[2,3] state that an interaction would also not be expected with other statins metabolised by CYP3A4, such as **simvastatin** and **lovastatin**. The US manufacturer of prasugrel also states that it may be given with statins.[3] No additional precautions therefore appear to be needed on the concurrent use of prasugrel and a statin.

1. Farid NA, Small DS, Payne CD, Jakubowski JA, Brandt JT, Li YG, Ernest CS, Salazar DE, Konkoy CS, Winters KJ. Effect of atorvastatin on the pharmacokinetics and pharmacodynamics of prasugrel and clopidogrel in healthy subjects. *Pharmacotherapy* (2008) 28, 1483–94.
2. Efient (Prasugrel hydrochloride). Eli Lilly and Company Ltd. UK Summary of product characteristics, December 2013.
3. Effient (Prasugrel). Eli Lilly and Company. US Prescribing information, November 2013.

Thrombolytics + Antiplatelet drugs

The use of antiplatelet doses of aspirin, clopidogrel or other antiplatelet drugs with thrombolytics appears to increase the risk of bleeding. The risk may be increased with higher aspirin doses and with the use of more than one antiplatelet drug.

Clinical evidence and mechanism

A. Ischaemic stroke

(a) Alteplase

1. Aspirin. There is some evidence that patients already receiving low-dose aspirin daily at the time they have a stroke have an increased risk of bleeding when they are given alteplase. For example, in a retrospective analysis of data from a randomised study in 793 patients with acute ischaemic stroke and given alteplase or placebo, the use of aspirin before the stroke was found to increase the risk of intracranial parenchymal bleeding by 15.6% in patients given alteplase, compared with those patients who had not been taking aspirin (odds ratio 4.99). An increase in the risk of symptomatic intracranial haemorrhage of 12.7% was also seen (but could not be fully analysed due to lack of events in the placebo group). However, the authors note that both of these results were only marginally statistically significant.[1] Similarly, in an analysis of a post-licensing observational study of alteplase use in stroke, aspirin therapy at stroke onset was related to a 1.58-fold increased risk of symptomatic intracranial haemorrhage, although the overall rate of this adverse effect was low.[2] An analysis of another large cohort study found a similar 1.69-fold increase in the risk of symptomatic intracranial haemorrhage with the concurrent use of aspirin.[3]

In contrast, other studies have not found an increased risk of bleeding. For example, in a prospective study in 300 consecutive patients with acute ischaemic stroke given alteplase, the risk of haemorrhagic complications in the first 48 hours was not related to the previous use of aspirin (92 patients had previously received aspirin and 202 were aspirin non-users).[4]

For further studies, in which aspirin was analysed as part of a group of antiplatelet drugs, see under *Antiplatelets, general*, below.

2. Antiplatelets, general. In a retrospective study of 11 865 patients with acute ischaemic stroke who had received alteplase, 3 782 patients were identified who had been receiving any antiplatelet drug at baseline. Of these, 3 016 were taking **aspirin**, 243 were taking **clopidogrel**, 175 were taking aspirin plus **dipyridamole**, and 151 were taking aspirin plus clopidogrel. The incidence of symptomatic intracranial bleeding was 1.1% (4.1%) for those not previously taking antiplatelet drugs and 2.5% (6.2%) for the concurrent use of any antiplatelet drug (adjusted odds ratio 1.28 (1.09)). When divided by drug the incidence of intracranial bleeding was 2.5% (5.9%) for aspirin, 1.7% (4.2%) for clopidogrel, 2.3% (5.9%) for aspirin with dipyridamole and 4.1% (13.4%) for aspirin with clopidogrel. Of these, the only increase that reached statistical significance for one measure was the concurrent use of aspirin with clopidogrel (odds ratio 2.11).[5]

In an analysis of a cohort study of patients given alteplase for acute stroke, there was a high risk of symptomatic intracranial haemorrhage in patients taking antiplatelet drugs other than aspirin (mainly **ticlopidine**) before the stroke (odds ratio 3.66), although relatively few patients were taking these antiplatelet drugs, so some caution in interpretation is necessary.[3] Conversely, in an analysis of a post-licensing observational study of alteplase use in stroke, although the use of antiplatelet drugs other than aspirin (**clopidogrel**, **dipyridamole**, unspecified) at stroke onset was related to a 1.43-fold increased risk of mortality at 3 months, this was not related to an increase in symptomatic intracranial haemorrhage.[2]

(b) Streptokinase

The only study looking at the simultaneous use of aspirin and a thrombolytic for acute stroke is the MAST-I study of streptokinase with aspirin, which showed an increase in mortality. In a post-hoc analysis of this study in 313 patients with acute ischaemic stroke given intravenous streptokinase 1.5 million units, the addition of **aspirin** 300 mg daily, started at the same time as streptokinase, increased the risk of early death. The combined regimen significantly increased early fatalities (from day 3 to 10) with 53 deaths occurring out of 156 patients (34%), compared with 30 of 157 (19%) who received streptokinase alone. This was mainly due to cerebral causes (42 versus 24) and associated with intracranial haemorrhage (25 versus 11).[6] Note that, in other studies, streptokinase alone was associated with an increased risk of intracranial haemorrhage and mortality in acute ischaemic stroke.[7,8]

B. Myocardial infarction

(a) Aspirin

A retrospective analysis of data from 48 422 patients who were enrolled in two large studies of fibrinolytic therapy in ST-elevation myocardial infarction (GUSTO I and III) looked at whether the initial dose of aspirin (given to patients immediately after diagnosis of ST-elevation myocardial infarction) was related to bleeding risk. About 76% of patients received aspirin 162 mg and 24% received aspirin 325 mg. In the unadjusted analysis there were fewer moderate/severe bleeding episodes with the 325-mg dose of aspirin, but when adjusted there was a slight increase in the risk of moderate or severe bleeding with the 325 mg dose of aspirin, when compared with the 162 mg dose of aspirin (odds ratio 1.14). The lower dose of aspirin had the same efficacy as the higher dose of aspirin.[9]

(b) Aspirin with Clopidogrel

In a study, 3491 patients with acute myocardial infarction given a thrombolytic and aspirin (150 to 325 mg as a loading dose, followed by 75 to 162 mg daily), were randomised to also receive clopidogrel (300-mg loading dose, followed by 75 mg daily) or placebo. The thrombolytics used were **tenecteplase** (about 47% of patients in each group), **streptokinase** (about 31% in each group), **reteplase** (about 12% of patients in each group), and **alteplase** (about 9% in each group). No appreciable increase in major or minor bleeding occurred when clopidogrel was given with aspirin and a thrombolytic (major or minor bleeding occurred in 2.3% of clopidogrel recipients and 1.6% of placebo recipients). Most of the patients (80%) also received heparin or low-molecular-weight heparin, or both.[10]

Importance and management

The benefits and risks associated with the use of a thrombolytic with **aspirin** is dependent on the indication for use. The same seems likely to be true for other antiplatelet drugs, although most are less well studied.

Ischaemic stroke

In acute ischaemic stroke, alteplase alone has been shown to improve clinical outcomes and its use is recommended for selected patients, as is the early use of aspirin alone for patients not eligible for alteplase.[7,8] Although some retrospective analyses appear to suggest that the previous use of aspirin may increase the risk of intracranial bleeding in patients given alteplase, overall, the data support the use of alteplase in these patients.[5] However, some caution might be appropriate in patients taking dual antiplatelets including **clopidogrel**, who might be at a higher risk of bleeding because of other factors.[5] There is currently no evidence on the simultaneous use of aspirin and alteplase for acute stroke. Because the efficacy and safety of this use is not yet established, at present, aspirin or other antiplatelet drugs should not be initiated within the first 24 hours after treatment with alteplase in patients with an acute ischaemic stroke.[8,11] Further study is needed. Note that streptokinase alone is associated with an increase risk of death in ischaemic stroke and has not been recommended for use in this indication.[8]

Myocardial infarction

In acute myocardial infarction, the concurrent use of a thrombolytic with aspirin is clinically beneficial: alteplase, reteplase, streptokinase, and tenecteplase are all recommended for concurrent use with aspirin in ST-elevation myocardial infarction. Retrospective evidence from one analysis suggests that the risk of bleeding might be related to dose, and that an initial aspirin dose of 162 mg may be preferable to 325 mg. In one study, the addition of **clopidogrel** to a thrombolytic and aspirin in patients with an acute ST-elevation myocardial infarction did not appear to increase the risk of major bleeding, and clopidogrel is also licensed for this use.[12] Note, however, that, in general, giving clopidogrel in addition to aspirin has been found to increase the risk of bleeding, when compared with aspirin only, see 'Aspirin and/or Clopidogrel + Cilostazol', p.781, for further discussion.

There appears to be no specific clinical data to confirm whether or not the risk of bleeding is increased if **prasugrel** or **ticlopidine** are given with a thrombolytic. The manufacturers therefore advise caution on their concurrent use because of the potential bleeding risk.[13-16] The manufacturer of **ticlopidine** also advises that the thrombolytic should be stopped before ticlopidine is started, as the long-term efficacy and safety of concurrent use is not yet confirmed.[14]

For a discussion on the risk of bleeding with the concurrent use a thrombolytic and the glycoprotein IIb/IIIa-receptor antagonist class of antiplatelet drugs, see 'Glycoprotein IIb/IIIa-receptor antagonists + Thrombolytics', p.797.

1. Larrue V, von Kummer R, Müller A, Bluhmki E. Risk factors for severe hemorrhagic transformation in ischemic stroke patients treated with recombinant tissue plasminogen activator: a secondary analysis of the European-Australasian Acute Stroke Study (ECASS II). *Stroke* (2001) 32, 438–41.
2. Wahlgren N, Ahmed N, Eriksson N, Aichner F, Bluhmki E, Dávalos A, Erilä T, Ford GA, Grond M, Hacke W, Hennerici MG, Kaste M, Köhrmann M, Larrue V, Lees KR, Machnig T, Roine RO, Toni D, Vanhooren G; Safe Implementation of Thrombolysis in Stroke-MOnitoring STudy Investigators. Multivariable analysis of outcome predictors and adjustment of main outcome results to baseline data profile in randomized controlled trials: Safe Implementation of Thrombolysis in Stroke-MOnitoring STudy (SITS-MOST). *Stroke* (2008) 39, 3316–22.
3. Tanne D, Kasner SE, Demchuk AM, Koren-Morag N, Hanson S, Grond M, Levine SR and the Multicenter rt-PA stroke Survey Group. Markers of increased risk of intracerebral hemorrhage after intravenous recombinant tissue plasminogen activator therapy for acute ischemic stroke in clinical practice: The Multicenter rt-PA Acute Stroke Survey. *Circulation* (2002) 105, 1679–85.
4. Schmülling S, Rudolf J, Strotmann-Tack T, Grond M, Schneweis S, Sobesky J, Thiel A, Heiss WD. Acetylsalicylic acid pre-treatment, concomitant heparin therapy and the risk of early intracranial hemorrhage following systemic thrombolysis for acute ischemic stroke. *Cerebrovasc Dis* (2003) 16, 183–90.
5. Diedler J, Ahmed N, Sykora M, Uyttenboogaart M, Overgaard K, Luijckx GJ, Soinne L, Ford GA, Lees KR, Wahlgren N, Ringleb P. Safety of intravenous thrombolysis for acute ischaemic stroke in patients receiving antiplatelet therapy at stroke onset. *Stroke* (2010) 41, 288–94.
6. Ciccone A, Motto C, Aritzu E, Piana A, Candelise L, on behalf of the MAST-I Collaborative Group. Negative interaction of aspirin and streptokinase in acute ischemic stroke: further analysis of the Multicenter Acute Stroke Trial-Italy. *Cerebrovasc Dis* (2000) 10, 61–4.
7. Wardlaw JM, del Zoppo G, Yamaguchi T, Berge E. Thrombolysis for acute ischaemic stroke (review). Available in The Cochrane Database of Systematic Reviews; Issue 3. Chichester: John Wiley; 2003 (accessed 14/04/08).
8. Albers GW, Amarenco P, Easton JD, Sacco RL, Teal P. Antithrombotic and thrombolytic therapy for ischemic stroke: American College of Chest Physicians evidence-based clinical practice guidelines (8th edition). *Chest* (2008) 133, 630S–669S.
9. Berger JS, Stebbins A, Granger CB, Ohman EM, Armstrong PW, Van de Werf F, White HD, Simes RJ, Harrington RA, Califf RM, Peterson ED. Initial aspirin dose and outcome among ST-elevation myocardial infarction patients treated with fibrinolytic therapy. *Circulation* (2008) 117, 192–9.
10. Sabatine MC, Cannon CP, Gibson CM, López-Sendón JL, Montalescot G, Theroux P, Claeys MJ, Cools F, Hill KA, Skene AM, McCabe CH, Braunwald E, for the CLARITY-TIMI 28 investigators. Addition of clopidogrel to aspirin and fibrinolytic therapy for myocardial infarction with ST-segment elevation. *N Engl J Med* (2005) 352, 1179–89.
11. Actilyse (Alteplase). Boehringer Ingelheim Ltd. UK Summary of product characteristics, November 2009.
12. Plavix (Clopidogrel hydrogen sulphate). Sanofi-Aventis. UK Summary of product characteristics, January 2014.
13. Efient (Prasugrel hydrochloride). Eli Lilly and Company Ltd. UK Summary of product characteristics, December 2013.
14. Ticlopidine hydrochloride. Apotex Corp. US Prescribing information, February 2006.
15. Metalyse (Tenecteplase). Boehringer Ingelheim Ltd. UK Summary of product characteristics, June 2010.
16. Rapilysin (Reteplase). Actavis UK Ltd. UK Summary of product characteristics, August 2008.

Thrombolytics; Alteplase + Glyceryl trinitrate (Nitroglycerin)

Glyceryl trinitrate reduced the thrombolytic efficacy of alteplase in two studies, but major studies into their use in patients with myocardial infarction suggest that any interaction is of no clinical relevance.

Clinical evidence, mechanism, importance and management

In a randomised study, 60 patients with acute anterior myocardial infarction were given intravenous alteplase 100 mg over 3 hours, as well as heparin and aspirin. In addition, 27 of the patients were also given intravenous glyceryl trinitrate 100 micrograms/minute for 8 hours. Patients given both alteplase and glyceryl trinitrate had signs of reperfusion less often (56%) than the patients who received alteplase alone (76%). In the combined treatment group time-to-reperfusion was also longer (37.8 minutes versus 19.6 minutes) and the incidence of coronary artery re-occlusion was higher (53% versus 24%). The plasma levels of tissue plasminogen activator (tPA) antigen were about two-thirds lower in those given glyceryl trinitrate with alteplase compared with alteplase alone.[1] Impaired thrombolysis has been found in another study.[2]

It was postulated that glyceryl trinitrate increased hepatic blood flow and therefore increased the metabolism of alteplase, which resulted in reduced plasma tPA levels.[1] However, an *in vitro* study found that glyceryl trinitrate enhanced the degradation of alteplase, and therefore a mechanism other than increased hepatic blood flow seems likely to be involved.[3] Given the results of subsequent major studies on thrombolytics in patients with myocardial infarction, where most patients also received intravenous or sublingual nitrates, it seems unlikely that this proposed interaction is of any clinical relevance.

1. Romeo F, Rosano GMC, Martuscelli E, De Luca F, Bianco C, Colistra C, Comito M, Cardona N, Miceli F, Rosano V, Mehta JL. Concurrent nitroglycerin administration reduces the efficacy of recombinant tissue-type plasminogen activator in patients with acute anterior wall myocardial infarction. *Am Heart J* (1995) 130, 692–7.
2. Nicolini FA, Ferrini D, Ottani F, Galvani M, Ronchi A, Behrens PH, Rusticali F, Mehta JL. Concurrent nitroglycerin therapy impairs tissue-type plasminogen activator-induced thrombolysis in patients with acute myocardial infarction. *Am J Cardiol* (1994) 74, 662–6.
3. White CM, Fan C, Chen BP, Kluger J, Chow MSS. Assessment of the drug interaction between alteplase and nitroglycerin: an in vitro study. *Pharmacotherapy* (2000) 20, 380–2.

Thrombolytics; Streptokinase + Other thrombolytics

The thrombolytic effects of streptokinase and anistreplase are likely to be reduced or abolished if either drug is given some time after a dose of streptokinase, because of persistently high levels of streptokinase antibodies. There is also an increased risk of hypersensitivity reactions. This may also be true for urokinase.

Clinical evidence

A study in 25 patients who had been given streptokinase for acute myocardial infarction, found that 12 weeks later, 24 patients had enough anti-streptokinase antibodies in circulation to neutralise an entire 1.5 million unit dose of streptokinase. After 4 to 8 months, 18 out of 20 patients still had enough antibodies to neutralise half of a 1.5 million unit dose of streptokinase.[1] Further study has suggested that, after streptokinase use, anti-streptokinase antibodies fall within 24 hours, but then increase gradually and are significantly raised by 4 days after treatment. The antibody titres reach a peak (approximately 200 times that of pretreatment levels) after 2 weeks and then subsequently decline, but remain above baseline values for at least one year.[2] Studies in patients given streptokinase[3-7] or **anistreplase**[7] have variously found that:

- antibody levels return to their pretreatment range in 92% of patients approximately 12 months after treatment,[7]
- neutralising antibody titres return to control levels by 2 years,[6]
- antibody titres may remain high enough to neutralise the effects of streptokinase for several years after a dose,[3,4]
- high titres may persist for up to 7.5 years.[5]

Increased titres of streptokinase antibodies have also been seen in patients receiving topical streptokinase for wound care,[8] intrapleural streptokinase for pleural effusions,[9] and following streptococcal infections.[10] Apart from the reduced thrombolytic effect, repeated dosing[11] or high pretreatment anti-streptokinase antibody titres[12] may increase the risk of allergic reactions.

Anistreplase, like its parent drug streptokinase, has been shown to be neutralised by anti-streptokinase antibodies.[13,14]

Of 6 patients given **urokinase** 1.5 million units infused over 30 minutes for recurrent myocardial infarction, rigors occurred in 4 patients and 2 of these also had bronchospasm; they had all previously received streptokinase.[15]

Mechanism

Streptokinase use causes the production of anti-streptokinase antibodies. These persist in the circulation so that the clot-dissolving effects of another dose of streptokinase given many months later may be ineffective, or less effective, because it becomes bound and neutralised by the antibodies. Many people already have a very low titre of antibodies resulting from previous streptococcal infections, yet this does not usually appear to influence thrombolysis.[16]

Importance and management

The interaction that results in neutralisation of these thrombolytics is established and clinically important as it could result in treatment failure. The manufacturer of streptokinase therefore advises that it should not be repeated within 5 days to one year of the initial dose.[10] Given that it has been suggested that the neutralising effects may be very persistent, it would seem prudent, if subsequent treatment is needed, to use a thrombolytic with less antigenic effects, such as alteplase. The BNF in the UK states that streptokinase should not be used again beyond 4 days of the first use of either streptokinase or anistreplase,[17] whereas the American College of Cardiology/American Heart Association guidelines recommend avoiding the readministration of streptokinase more than 5 days after giving a non-fibrin specific fibrinolytic [anistreplase, streptokinase, urokinase],[18] and the European Society of Cardiology specifically contraindicates the use of streptokinase or anistreplase in patients who have previously been treated with either drug.[19]

Little is known about the increased risk of hypersensitivity reactions.

1. Jalihal S, Morris GK. Antistreptokinase titres after intravenous streptokinase. *Lancet* (1990) 335, 184–5.
2. Lynch M, Littler WA, Pentecost BL, Stockley RA. Immunoglobulin response to intravenous streptokinase in acute myocardial infarction. *Br Heart J* (1991) 66, 139–42.
3. Elliott JM, Cross DB, Cederholm-Williams SA, White HD. Neutralizing antibodies to streptokinase four years after intravenous thrombolytic therapy. *Am J Cardiol* (1993) 71, 640–5.
4. Lee HS, Cross S, Davidson R, Reid T, Jennings K. Raised levels of antistreptokinase antibody and neutralization titres from 4 days to 54 months after administration of streptokinase or anistreplase. *Eur Heart J* (1993) 14, 84–9.
5. Squire IB, Lawley W, Fletcher S, Holme E, Hillis WS, Hewitt C, Woods KL. Humoral and cellular immune responses up to 7.5 years after administration of streptokinase for acute myocardial infarction. *Eur Heart J* (1999) 20, 1245–52.
6. McGrath K, Hogan C, Hunt D, O'Malley C, Green N, Dauer R, Dalli A. Neutralising antibodies after streptokinase treatment for myocardial infarction: a persisting puzzle. *Br Heart J* (1995) 74, 122–3.
7. Fears R, Ferres H, Glasgow E, Standring R, Hogg KJ, Gemmill JD, Burns JMA, Rae AP, Dunn FG, Hillis WS. Monitoring of streptokinase resistance titre in acute myocardial infarction patients up to 30 months after giving streptokinase or anistreplase and related studies to measure specific antistreptokinase IgG. *Br Heart J* (1992) 68, 167–70.
8. Green C. Antistreptokinase titres after topical streptokinase. *Lancet* (1993) 341, 1602–3.
9. Laisaar T, Pullerits T. Effect of intrapleural streptokinase administration on antistreptokinase antibody level in patients with loculated pleural effusions. *Chest* (2003) 123, 432–5.
10. Streptase (Streptokinase). CSL Behring UK Ltd. UK Summary of product characteristics, September 2010.
11. White HD, Cross DB, Williams BF, Norris RM. Safety and efficacy of repeat thrombolytic treatment after acute myocardial infarction. *Br Heart J* (1990) 64, 177–81.
12. Lee HS, Yule S, McKenzie A, Cross S, Reid T, Davidson R, Jennings K. Hypersensitivity reactions to streptokinase in patients with high pre-treatment antistreptokinase antibody and neutralisation titres. *Eur Heart J* (1993) 14, 1640–3.
13. Binette MJ, Agnone FA. Failure of APSAC thrombolysis. *Ann Intern Med* (1993) 119, 637.
14. Brügemann J, van der Meer J, Bom VJJ, van der Schaaf W, de Graeff PA, Lie KI. Anti-streptokinase antibodies inhibit fibrinolytic effects of anistreplase in acute myocardial infarction. *Am J Cardiol* (1993) 72, 462–4.
15. Matsis P, Mann S. Rigors and bronchospasm with urokinase after streptokinase. *Lancet* (1992) 340, 1552.
16. Fears R, Hearn J, Standring R, Anderson JL, Marder VJ. Lack of influence of pretreatment antistreptokinase antibody on efficacy in a multicenter patency comparison of intravenous streptokinase and anistreplase in acute myocardial infarction. *Am Heart J* (1992) 124, 305–14.
17. Joint Formulary Committee. *British National Formulary*. 70 ed. London: BMJ Group and Pharmaceutical Press; 2015. p.195.
18. Antman EM, Anbe DT, Armstrong PW, Bates ER, Green LA, Hand M, Hochman JS, Krumholz HM, Kushner FG, Lamas GA, Mullany CJ, Ornato JP, Pearle DL, Sloan MA, Smith SC, Alpert JS, Anderson JL, Faxon DP, Fuster V, Gibbons RJ, Gregoratos G, Halperin JL, Hiratzka LF, Hunt SA, Jacobs AK. ACC/AHA guidelines for the management of patients with ST-elevation myocardial infarction (2004). *J Am Coll Cardiol* (2004) 44, E1–E111.
19. Van de Werf F, Bax J, Betriu A, Blomstrom-Lundqvist C, Crea F, Falk V, Filippatos G, Fox K, Huber K, Kastrati A, Rosengren A, Steg PG, Tubaro M, Verheugt F, Weidinger F, Weis M; The Task Force on the Management of ST-segment elevation acute myocardial infarction of the European Society of Cardiology. Management of acute myocardial infarction in patients presenting with persistent ST-segment elevation. *Eur Heart J* (2008) 29, 2909–45.

Ticagrelor + Ketoconazole and other CYP3A4 inhibitors

Ketoconazole markedly increases the exposure to ticagrelor. Diltiazem moderately increases the exposure to ticagrelor, whereas ticagrelor does not affect the plasma concentrations of diltiazem. Other CYP3A4 inhibitors are predicted to interact with ticagrelor similarly.

Clinical evidence

(a) Diltiazem

The manufacturers of ticagrelor report that diltiazem 240 mg daily increased the maximum plasma concentration and AUC of ticagrelor by 69% and 2.7-fold, respectively. The maximum plasma concentration of the active metabolite of ticagrelor was reduced by 38%, but its AUC was unchanged. Ticagrelor did not affect diltiazem plasma concentrations.[1]

(b) Ketoconazole

The manufacturers of ticagrelor report that ketoconazole 200 mg twice daily increased the maximum plasma concentration and AUC of ticagrelor 2.4-fold and 7.3-fold, respectively. The maximum plasma concentration and AUC of the active metabolite of ticagrelor were reduced by 89% and 56%, respectively.[1]

Mechanism

Ketoconazole is a potent inhibitor of CYP3A4, whereas diltiazem is a moderate inhibitor of this isoenzyme. As ticagrelor is predominantly metabolised by CYP3A4 the concurrent use of these drugs increases ticagrelor exposure.

Importance and management

A pharmacokinetic interaction between ticagrelor and **ketoconazole** is established. The large increase in ticagrelor exposure that occurs can increase the risk of bleeding, and both the UK and the US manufacturers of ticagrelor contraindicate concurrent use with ketoconazole and other potent CYP3A4 inhibitors (see 'Table 1.9', p.11 for a list).

The clinical relevance of the more modest increase in ticagrelor exposure seen with **diltiazem** appears to be minimal, particularly as the exposure to the active metabolite was unchanged, therefore no dose adjustment seems necessary on concurrent use with diltiazem and other moderate CYP3A4 inhibitors. For a list of moderate CYP3A4 inhibitors, see 'Table 1.9', p.11.

Note that, based on findings of asymptomatic ventricular pauses and bradycardia in some patients given ticagrelor, the UK manufacturer recommends caution when ticagrelor is given with other drugs which can cause bradycardia, such as diltiazem.[1] For further information, see 'Ticagrelor + Miscellaneous', below.

1. Brilique (Ticagrelor). AstraZeneca UK Ltd. UK Summary of product characteristics, July 2015.

Ticagrelor + Miscellaneous

Ticagrelor increases the exposure to simvastatin and atorvastatin, and is predicted to have a similar effect on lovastatin. Ciclosporin moderately increases ticagrelor exposure and other P-glycoprotein inhibitors are expected to interact similarly. The manufacturer predicts that ticagrelor might increase the concentrations of the ergot alkaloids. Ticagrelor might have additive effects with drugs that are likely to cause bradycardia. There appears to be no pharmacokinetic interaction between

ticagrelor and tolbutamide and therefore a pharmacokinetic interaction is not expected with warfarin, although the risk of bleeding might be increased.

Clinical evidence, mechanism, importance and management

(a) CYP2C9 substrates

The manufacturers report that the concurrent use of ticagrelor 180 mg twice daily with **tolbutamide** 500 mg daily did not have a clinically relevant effect on the pharmacokinetics of either drug. This suggests that ticagrelor does not affect CYP2C9, the isoenzyme by which tolbutamide is metabolised. Therefore, the UK manufacturer of ticagrelor states that no interaction is expected with other CYP2C9 substrates and specifically name **warfarin**.[1] However, due to the increased risk of bleeding on concurrent use, the UK manufacturer advises caution if oral anticoagulants are given within 24 hours of taking ticagrelor.[1]

(b) CYP3A4 substrates

The UK manufacturer notes that ticagrelor is an inhibitor of CYP3A4, and they therefore recommend caution on the concurrent use of CYP3A4 substrates with a narrow therapeutic range, such as the **ergot derivatives**.[1] If concurrent use is undertaken advise patients not to take any further doses of the ergot derivative and seek medical advice if early symptoms of increased exposure, such as numbness or tingling in the fingers and toes, or nausea and vomiting (unrelated to the migraine), develop. For a list of other CYP3A4 substrates, see 'Table 1.10', p.12.

(c) Drugs that affect heart rate

Based on findings of bradycardia in some patients given ticagrelor, the UK manufacturer recommends caution when ticagrelor is given with other drugs which can cause bradycardia. However, they note that no clinically relevant adverse effects were reported in one clinical study on concurrent use of ticagrelor and **beta blockers**, **diltiazem**, **verapamil**, and **digoxin**.[1] See also 'Digoxin + Ticagrelor', p.1114, 'Ticagrelor + Ketoconazole and other CYP3A4 inhibitors', p.801, and P-glycoprotein inhibitors, below, for further discussion on the effects of concurrent use of ticagrelor with **digoxin**, **diltiazem**, and **verapamil** (a P-glycoprotein inhibitor), respectively.

(d) P-glycoprotein inhibitors

The UK manufacturer of ticagrelor notes that, in a study, the maximum plasma concentration and AUC of ticagrelor were increased 2.3-fold and 2.8-fold, respectively, when given with ciclosporin 600 mg. The AUC of the active metabolite of ticagrelor increased by 32%, and its maximum plasma concentration decreased by 15%. Ciclosporin is a P-glycoprotein inhibitor, of which ticagrelor is a substrate, and therefore it increases ticagrelor concentrations resulting in the potential for increased adverse effects. Although there do not appear to be any studies on the interaction between ticagrelor and other P-glycoprotein inhibitors, the UK manufacturer recommends that the concurrent use of ticagrelor and potent P-glycoprotein inhibitors is avoided (see 'Table 1.12', p.14 for a list). Where concurrent use is unavoidable they advise caution.[1]

(e) Statins

The manufacturers state that ticagrelor 90 mg twice daily increased the maximum plasma concentration and AUC of **atorvastatin** 80 mg daily by about 25% and 30%, respectively, with similar increases in all the active metabolites.[1] The manufacturers also state that ticagrelor 180 mg twice daily increased the maximum plasma concentration and AUC of **simvastatin** 80 mg daily by 81% and 56%, respectively. The maximum plasma concentration and AUC of the active metabolite, simvastatin acid, were increased by 64% and 52%, respectively, although some individuals had a 2- to 3-fold increase.[1] **Lovastatin** is predicted to interact similarly.[1,2]

The small increase in **atorvastatin** concentrations when given with ticagrelor is unlikely to be clinically relevant, and no dose adjustments would appear to be necessary on concurrent use. The manufacturers recommend a maximum dose of **lovastatin** 40 mg daily or **simvastatin** 40 mg daily in patients taking ticagrelor.[1,2]

(f) Other drugs

The manufacturers note that, in one clinical study, no clinically relevant adverse effects were reported on the concurrent use of ticagrelor and unspecified **proton pump inhibitors, ACE inhibitors** and **angiotensin II receptor antagonists**.[1] Note that no pharmacokinetic studies appear to have been undertaken.

1. Brilique (Ticagrelor). AstraZeneca UK Ltd. UK Summary of product characteristics, July 2015.
2. Brilinta (Ticagrelor). AstraZeneca. US Prescribing information, September 2015.

Ticagrelor + Rifampicin (Rifampin) and other CYP3A4 inducers

Rifampicin reduces ticagrelor exposure. Other CYP3A4 inducers might interact similarly.

Clinical evidence

The UK and US manufacturers of ticagrelor report that rifampicin 600 mg daily decreased the maximum plasma concentration and AUC of ticagrelor by 73% and 86%, respectively, and also decreased the AUC of its active metabolite, by 46%.[1,2]

Mechanism

Rifampicin is a potent inducer of CYP3A4, by which ticagrelor is metabolised. Concurrent use therefore leads to a decrease in ticagrelor exposure.

Importance and management

Information on an interaction between ticagrelor and rifampicin is limited to this study, but is in line with the known disposition of these drugs. Concurrent use can reduce ticagrelor exposure, and as the effect is marked, this would be expected to result in decreased ticagrelor efficacy. The UK and US manufacturers of ticagrelor state that the concurrent use of rifampicin and other potent CYP3A4 inducers should be avoided. For a list of potent CYP3A4 inducers see 'Table 1.9', p.11. The manufacturers specifically name **dexamethasone** as a potent CYP3A4 inducer, however evidence of dexamethasone having clinically relevant interactions as a result of this mechanism is generally lacking. Moderate inducers of CYP3A4 would also be expected to reduce the exposure to ticagrelor, but to a lesser extent than potent inducers. It would seem prudent to monitor patients for a decrease in ticagrelor efficacy on concurrent use. For a list of moderate CYP3A4 inducers, see 'Table 1.9', p.11.

1. Brilique (Ticagrelor). AstraZeneca UK Ltd. UK Summary of product characteristics, July 2015.
2. Brilinta (Ticagrelor). AstraZeneca. US Prescribing information, September 2015.

Ticlopidine + Codergocrine mesilate (Ergoloid mesylates)

Codergocrine mesilate slightly reduces the exposure to a single dose of ticlopidine.

Clinical evidence, mechanism, importance and management

A study in 8 healthy subjects found that codergocrine mesilate 1.5 mg three times daily for 4 days decreased both the AUC and maximum level of a single 250-mg dose of ticlopidine by about 30%. It was suggested that codergocrine mesilate inhibits the human organic anion transporting polypeptide B (OATP-B)-mediated absorption of ticlopidine from the intestine.[1]

The general relevance of this study is unclear; however, bear the potential for an interaction in mind, particularly in patients where reductions in the levels of ticlopidine may be critical, such as those with drug-eluting stents.

1. Lu W-J, Huang J-D, Lai M-L. The effects of ergoloid mesylates and Ginkgo biloba on the pharmacokinetics of ticlopidine. *J Clin Pharmacol* (2006) 46, 628–34.

Ticlopidine + Miscellaneous

Methylprednisolone and prednisolone appear to inhibit the prolongation of bleeding times in response to ticlopidine but the antiplatelet effects of ticlopidine are not affected. Ticlopidine decreases the clearance of phenazone (antipyrine). Phenobarbital does not alter the antiplatelet effects of ticlopidine. Beta blockers, calcium-channel blockers and diuretics are reported not to interact with ticlopidine.

Clinical evidence, mechanism, importance and management

(a) Corticosteroids

A study involving 14 healthy subjects found that a single 20-mg intravenous injection of **methylprednisolone**, or oral **prednisolone** 15 mg twice daily for 7 days, inhibited the prolongation of bleeding times caused by ticlopidine 250 to 500 mg twice daily for 7 days. However, the antiplatelet effects of ticlopidine were not affected.[1] The clinical importance of this interaction is therefore uncertain.

(b) Phenazone (Antipyrine)

A study in 10 healthy subjects found that ticlopidine 250 mg twice daily for 3 weeks decreased the clearance of phenazone (used as a marker of enzyme inhibition or induction) and slightly increased its AUC and half-life by 14% and 27%, respectively, suggesting that ticlopidine has some mild enzyme-inhibiting effects.[2] This is consistent with the way ticlopidine appears to inhibit the metabolism of theophylline, see 'Theophylline + Clopidogrel and related drugs', p.1441. Nevertheless, this slight change in the pharmacokinetics of phenazone would not be expected to be of clinical relevance.

Note that the concurrent use of NSAIDs and ticlopidine may increase the risk of gastrointestinal bleeding, see 'Clopidogrel and related drugs + NSAIDs', p.788.

(c) Phenobarbital

The US manufacturer of ticlopidine briefly reports that, in a study in 6 healthy subjects, multiple-dose phenobarbital did not alter the antiplatelet effects of ticlopidine.[3] As **primidone** is metabolised to phenobarbital, it would be expected to behave similarly, although this requires confirmation. For a case report that suggests that ticlopidine does not affect phenobarbital levels, see under 'Phenytoin + Ticlopidine', p.608.

(d) Other drugs

The US manufacturer of ticlopidine reports that, in clinical studies in which ticlopidine was given with **beta blockers**, **calcium-channel blockers** and **diuretics** (none of the individual drugs named), no clinically significant adverse interactions were reported.[3]

1. Thébault J, Blatrix C, Blanchard J, Panak E. A possible method to control prolongations of bleeding time under antiplatelet therapy with ticlopidine. *Thromb Haemost* (1982) 48, 6–8.
2. Knudsen JB, Bastain W, Sefton CM, Allen JG, Dickinson JP. Pharmacokinetics of ticlopidine during chronic oral administration to healthy volunteers and its effects on antipyrine pharmacokinetics. *Xenobiotica* (1992) 22, 579–89.
3. Ticlopidine hydrochloride. Apotex Corp. US Prescribing information, February 2006.

20

Antipsychotics, Anxiolytics and Hypnotics

The interactions where the effects of antipsychotic, anxiolytic, and hypnotic drugs are affected are covered in this section, but there are other monographs elsewhere in this publication where the effects of other drugs are altered by benzodiazepines or related drugs, or antipsychotics.

Antipsychotics

The antipsychotics are represented by chlorpromazine (and other phenothiazines), haloperidol (and other butyrophenones), thioxanthenes, and the atypical, or newer, antipsychotic drugs, such as clozapine, olanzapine, risperidone and its active metabolite, paliperidone (9-hydroxyrisperidone), and ziprasidone. Their major use is in the treatment of psychoses such as schizophrenia and mania; a list of these drugs is given in 'Table 20.1', below. Some of the antipsychotics are also used as antiemetics, and for motor tics and hiccups.

Many of the interactions of the older antipsychotics are pharmacodynamic, relating to their effect on dopamine, while several of the newer atypical antipsychotics are metabolised to a significant extent by cytochrome P450 isoenzymes. Therefore, the concurrent use of other drugs that are inhibitors or inducers of these isoenzymes might result in large changes in plasma concentrations. Furthermore, lifestyle factors, such as tobacco smoking, can affect the pharmacokinetics of some of these drugs, leading to adverse effects or lack of therapeutic effect. Two of the atypical antipsychotics with the most important cytochrome P450 isoenzyme interactions are clozapine and risperidone.

(a) Clozapine

The principal isoenzyme involved in the metabolism of clozapine is CYP1A2, as demonstrated by its interactions with fluvoxamine (see 'Clozapine + SSRIs', p.855) and tobacco (see 'Clozapine + Tobacco', p.856).The potent CYP3A4 inhibitor ketoconazole has not been associated with interactions, indicating that CYP3A4 has a limited role in clozapine metabolism (see 'Clozapine + Azoles', p.848). Reports of raised clozapine concentrations in some, but not all, studies in patients also taking fluoxetine or paroxetine (see 'Clozapine + SSRIs', p.855) suggests that CYP2D6 might have some role in clozapine metabolism.

(b) Risperidone

Risperidone is mainly metabolised by CYP2D6 to its main active metabolite, 9-hydroxyrisperidone (paliperidone), and known inhibitors of CYP2D6 such as fluoxetine and paroxetine (see 'Risperidone + SSRIs', p.887) have been shown to increase risperidone concentrations. CYP2D6 shows genetic polymorphism, meaning that this isoenzyme has varying activity in different people, so this interaction will vary depending on genotype. There also seems to be some involvement of CYP3A4 as demonstrated by known inhibitors (such as itraconazole, see 'Risperidone + Azoles', p.883), which have raised risperidone concentrations.

(c) Other antipsychotics

Haloperidol is metabolised to its active metabolite, reduced haloperidol (a metabolite with 20 to 50% of the activity of haloperidol), which is formed by the reduction of the ketone group to a secondary alcohol by carbonyl reductase. Reduced haloperidol can also be back-oxidised to the parent compound. Neither of these routes of metabolism are affected by drug interactions. The major metabolic pathway of haloperidol is glucuronidation by UDP-glucuronyltransferases, but there is no established evidence of drug interactions attributed to inhibition or induction of this enzyme. Haloperidol is partially metabolised by cytochrome P450 isoenzymes, with CYP3A4 being the major isoenzyme responsible (see 'Haloperidol and related drugs + Azoles', p.859). Haloperidol has generally been considered to be a substrate of CYP2D6, but the evidence for this is inconsistent and inconclusive,[1] and there are no drug interactions clearly attributed to alteration of CYP2D6 activity.

Table 20.1 Antipsychotics, anxiolytics, and hypnotics

Group	*Drugs*
Antipsychotics	
Atypical antipsychotics	Amisulpride, Aripiprazole, Clozapine, Olanzapine, Paliperidone, Quetiapine, Risperidone, Sertindole, Ziprasidone, Zotepine
Phenothiazines	Butaperazine, Chlorpromazine, Cyamemazine, Fluphenazine, Levomepromazine, Mesoridazine, Metopimazine, Pericyazine, Perphenazine, Prochlorperazine, Promazine, Thioridazine, Trifluoperazine
Butyrophenones	Benperidol, Bromperidol, Droperidol, Haloperidol, Melperone, Pipamperone
Thioxanthenes	Chlorprothixene, Flupentixol, Tiotixene, Zuclopenthixol
Miscellaneous	Loxapine, Molindone, Pimozide, Ritanserin, Sulpiride
Anxiolytics and hypnotics	
Benzodiazepines	Alprazolam, Bromazepam, Brotizolam, Chlordiazepoxide, Clobazam, Clonazepam, Clorazepate, Clotiazepam, Diazepam, Estazolam, Etizolam, Flunitrazepam, Flurazepam, Ketazolam, Loprazolam, Lorazepam, Lormetazepam, Medazepam, Midazolam, Nitrazepam, Oxazepam, Oxazolam, Quazepam, Temazepam, Triazolam
Melatonin receptor agonists	Ramelteon, Tasimelteon
Non-benzodiazepine hypnotics	Eszopiclone, Zaleplon, Zolpidem, Zopiclone
Miscellaneous	Buspirone, Clomethiazole, Cloral betaine, Cloral hydrate, Glutethimide, Hydroxyzine, Meprobamate, Promethazine, Suvorexant, Tandospirone, Triclofos

Anxiolytics and Hypnotics

Anxiolytics include the benzodiazepines (e.g. diazepam, alprazolam, lorazepam), buspirone and other drugs used to treat psychoneuroses such as anxiety and tension, and are intended to induce calm without causing drowsiness and sleep. Hypnotics include benzodiazepines such as nitrazepam or temazepam and non-benzodiazepines such as zaleplon, zolpidem or zopiclone; however, the difference in action between anxiolytics and hypnotics is mainly one of degree and, in general, the same drug or group of drugs can have both effects.

Anxiolytics and hypnotics can impair judgement and increase reaction time and they can interact with other drugs that affect the CNS, see 'CNS depressants + CNS depressants', p.1560. Some of the benzodiazepines and related drugs are also used as antiepileptics. 'Table 20.1', p.803, contains a list of the benzodiazepines and other anxiolytics and hypnotics.

(a) Benzodiazepines

Many benzodiazepines undergo phase I metabolism by *N*-dealkylation and hydroxylation and many of the metabolites are active. They may then undergo phase II conjugation, mainly to form glucuronides before being excreted. For example, diazepam is metabolised to nordazepam (desmethyldiazepam), temazepam and oxazepam. The metabolism of diazepam is mediated by cytochrome P450 isoenzymes, particularly CYP2C19, and to a lesser extent CYP3A4, and diazepam is excreted mainly as free or conjugated metabolites.

The triazolo- and related benzodiazepines, such as midazolam and triazolam, are mainly metabolised by hydroxylation, mediated by CYP3A4, to active compounds, which then rapidly undergo glucuronide conjugation. Alprazolam is also extensively metabolised, but to a lesser extent by CYP3A4, and other isoenzymes might also be involved. Midazolam and triazolam undergo pre-systemic metabolism by CYP3A4 in the gut so that their oral bioavailabilities are low (about 40%), whereas alprazolam has high oral bioavailability. Midazolam is used as a probe substrate to assess the effects of other drugs on CYP3A4 activity, oral midazolam being a marker for both intestinal and hepatic CYP3A4 activity, and intravenous midazolam being a marker for hepatic CYP3A4 activity.

Therefore, drugs that affect CYP2C19 can interact with benzodiazepines such as diazepam and those that affect CYP3A4 can interact with midazolam or triazolam. Because of their low oral bioavailability, midazolam and triazolam are affected to a greater extent when given orally compared with intravenously.

Benzodiazepines such as lorazepam, oxazepam and temazepam, which are mainly conjugated without prior phase I metabolism, are less likely to be involved in interactions with inhibitors or inducers of cytochrome P450. However, they are affected by drugs that can induce or inhibit glucuronidation.

Benzodiazepines themselves do not appear to affect cytochrome P450 isoenzymes, so interactions involving altered metabolism of other drugs are unlikely

(b) Non-benzodiazepine hypnotics

Zaleplon, zolpidem, and zopiclone are non-benzodiazepine hypnotics, but they act at the benzodiazepine receptor. They are metabolised by several cytochrome P450 isoenzymes and it has been suggested that because of this, other drugs that affect a particular isoenzyme such as CYP3A4, might have less effect on their metabolism. However, their pharmacokinetics are affected by potent CYP3A4 inducers such as rifampicin (rifampin) and by potent CYP3A4 inhibitors such as the azoles.

(c) Melatonin receptor agonists

Ramelteon and tasimelteon are melatonin receptor agonists that are primarily metabolised by CYP1A2. Their pharmacokinetics are greatly affected by potent CYP1A2 inhibitors, such as fluvoxamine. Both drugs are also metabolised by CYP3A4, and CYP2C9 also has some involvement in the metabolism of ramelteon. Ketoconazole and fluconazole therefore appear to affect their exposure, to varying extents.

(d) Miscellaneous anxiolytics and hypnotics

Buspirone is an azapirone anxiolytic that does not act on benzodiazepine receptor sites and lacks sedative, antiepileptic and muscle relaxant properties. It enhances the activity of specific dopaminergic and noradrenergic pathways, and also affects serotonin and acetylcholine systems of the brain. Buspirone is metabolised by hepatic CYP3A4.

Clomethiazole is a hypnotic and sedative with anticonvulsant effects. It is extensively metabolised in the liver.

Suvorexant is an orexin receptor antagonist used as a hypnotic in the management of insomnia. It is primarily metabolised by CYP3A4 and partly by CYP2C19.

1. Kudo S, Ishizaki T. Pharmacokinetics of haloperidol: an update. *Clin Pharmacokinet* (1999) 37, 435–56.

Amisulpride + Aripiprazole

An isolated case report describes worsening of psychotic symptoms after aripiprazole was added to amisulpride.

Clinical evidence, mechanism, importance and management

A case report describes a patient who had been taking amisulpride 800 mg daily, whose psychotic symptoms worsened after aripiprazole was added in order to switch treatment. Aripiprazole was started at 10 mg daily and increased after 2 weeks to 20 mg daily, with a corresponding decrease in amisulpride dose to 400 mg daily. After 3 days the patient experienced auditory hallucinations and the dose of aripiprazole was reduced to 10 mg daily and amisulpride was increased to 800 mg daily. His symptoms slowly improved but he then described feeling as though he was in telepathic communication with others, but this resolved several weeks later when the patient did not take aripiprazole for 5 days. He was rechallenged with aripiprazole 10 mg daily and 5 days later complained of auditory hallucinations again. Aripiprazole was discontinued and a week later the patient reported no more telepathic phenomena. The authors suggested that the dopaminergic activity of aripiprazole might have induced this effect as a result of amisulpride causing a hypodopaminergic state or hypersensitivity to dopamine agonists.[1]

This is an isolated case and as such, no general recommendations can be made for concurrent use. However, note that worsening of psychotic symptoms has also been seen when aripiprazole was given with haloperidol (see 'Aripiprazole + Haloperidol', p.808) and a case of neuroleptic malignant syndrome occurred when aripiprazole was added to olanzapine (see 'Olanzapine + Aripiprazole', p.867). In both cases the dopaminergic activity of aripiprazole was thought to be a major contributory factor.

1. Adan-Manes J, Garcia-Parajua P. Aripiprazole in combination with other antipsychotic drugs may worsen psychosis. *J Clin Pharm Ther* (2009) 34, 245–6.

Antipsychotics + Antimuscarinics

Antipsychotics and antimuscarinics are very often given together advantageously and uneventfully, but occasionally serious and even life-threatening interactions occur. These include heat stroke in hot and humid conditions, severe constipation and paralytic ileus, and atropine-like psychoses. Antimuscarinics used to counteract the extrapyramidal adverse effects of antipsychotics might also reduce or abolish their therapeutic effects.

Clinical evidence

The use of antipsychotics with antimuscarinics can result in a generalised, low grade, but not usually serious, additive increase in the antimuscarinic effects of these drugs (blurred vision, dry mouth, constipation, difficulty in urination, see 'Antimuscarinics + Antimuscarinics', p.754). However, sometimes serious intensification takes place. For the sake of clarity these effects have been divided here into the sections below:

(a) Heat stroke

Three patients were admitted to hospital in Philadelphia for drug-induced hyperpyrexia during a hot and humid period. In each case their skin and mucous membranes were dry and they were tachycardic (120 bpm). There was no evidence of infection.[1]

Drug combinations implicated in reports of heat stroke, some of them fatal, include:[1-6]

- **chlorpromazine** and **benzatropine**
- **chlorpromazine** and **trifluoperazine**
- **chlorpromazine, amitriptyline** and **benzatropine**
- **chlorpromazine, chlorprothixene** and **benzatropine**
- **chlorpromazine, fluphenazine, trihexyphenidyl** and **benzatropine**
- **chlorpromazine, trifluoperazine** and **benzatropine**
- **haloperidol** and **benzatropine**
- **promazine** and **benzatropine**
- **zuclopenthixol, quetiapine** and **benzatropine**.

The danger of heat stroke in patients taking **atropine** or **atropine-like compounds** was recognised in the 1920s, and the warning has been repeated many times.[7,8]

(b) Constipation and paralytic ileus

Paralytic ileus (adynamic ileus or complete gut stasis) with faecal impaction (fatal in 6 cases) has been reported in a number of patients taking:

- **chlorpromazine** and **amitriptyline**,[9] **imipramine**,[10] **nortriptyline**,[11] or **trihexyphenidyl**[10]
- **haloperidol** and **benzatropine**[12]
- **levomepromazine** and **imipramine** with **benzatropine**[10]
- **levomepromazine** and **trihexyphenidyl**[10]
- **mesoridazine** and **benzatropine**[13]
- **thioridazine** and **imipramine** with **trihexyphenidyl**[10]
- **trifluoperazine** and **benzatropine**[14] or **trihexyphenidyl**[10]
- **trifluoperazine** and **benzatropine** with **methylphenidate**.[15]

Severe constipation also occurred in a woman given **thioridazine, biperiden** and **doxepin**.[16]

(c) Atropine-like psychoses

In a double-blind study, 3 patients given a **phenothiazine** and **benzatropine** for parkinsonian adverse effects developed an intermittent toxic confusional state (marked disturbance of short-term memory, impaired attention, disorientation, anxiety, visual and auditory hallucinations) with peripheral antimuscarinic signs.[17] Similar reactions occurred in 3 elderly patients given **imipramine** or **desipramine**, with **trihexyphenidyl**,[18] and in another man given **chlorpromazine, benzatropine** and **doxepin**.[16]

(d) Antagonism of antipsychotic effects

A study in psychiatric patients given **chlorpromazine** 300 to 800 mg daily found that when **trihexyphenidyl** 6 to 10 mg daily was added, the plasma concentrations of **chlorpromazine** were reduced from a range of 100 to 300 nanograms/mL to less than 30 nanograms/mL. When the **trihexyphenidyl** was withdrawn the plasma concentrations of **chlorpromazine** rose again and clinical improvement was seen.[19,20]

Other studies confirm that **trihexyphenidyl**[21,22] and **orphenadrine**[23] reduce the plasma concentrations and effects of **chlorpromazine**. In another study, patients with schizophrenia taking **chlorpromazine, levomepromazine, thioridazine**, or **haloperidol** and in some cases also taking small doses of **trifluoperazine, fluphenazine, thioproperazine, perphenazine** or **tiotixene** were all taking **benzatropine, trihexyphenidyl** or **procyclidine** for extrapyramidal symptoms. These antimuscarinic antiparkinsonian drugs were gradually withdrawn in the fifth study week. Plasma concentrations of the antipsychotics increased during the next 12 weeks after which a plateau was reached, suggesting that the antimuscarinic drugs reduced the plasma concentrations of the antipsychotics.[24] In contrast to these reports, one study found that **trihexyphenidyl** increased **chlorpromazine** concentrations by 41% in 20 young patients with schizophrenia, but no clinical change was seen. The concentrations dropped again over the first 4 weeks of treatment.[25] Some of the beneficial actions of **haloperidol** on social avoidance behaviour are lost during the concurrent use of **benzatropine**, but cognitive integrative function is unaffected.[26] Other studies found that the effects of **chlorpromazine** on social, affective and cognitive dysfunctions in patients with schizophrenia were reversed by **benzatropine**[27] and that **benzatropine**[28] and **trihexyphenidyl**[29] diminished the effects of **chlorpromazine** to a greater extent than those of **haloperidol**.

A study to investigate any possible interaction between **procyclidine** 5 to 15 mg daily and **chlorpromazine, fluphenazine** or **haloperidol** found that the addition of **procyclidine** caused a transient fall in the serum concentrations of **chlorpromazine**, whilst the fall in the concentrations of **fluphenazine** and **haloperidol** was maintained for the 4-week treatment period with **procyclidine**. Two patients in the **haloperidol** group experienced a worsening of symptoms whilst taking **procyclidine**.[30]

(e) Miscellaneous effects

A study in psychotic patients found that the addition of **biperiden** 2 mg three times daily or **orphenadrine** 50 mg three times daily for 3 weeks had no effect on the steady-state concentrations of **perphenazine** 24 to 48 mg daily.[31] A study in patients with schizophrenia found that **biperiden** 6 mg daily or **trihexyphenidyl** 8 mg daily had no effect on steady-state plasma concentrations of **bromperidol** or its reduced metabolite.[32]

An isolated report describes the development of a hypoglycaemic coma in a non-diabetic patient given **chlorpromazine** and **orphenadrine**.[33]

Mechanism

Antimuscarinic (anticholinergic) drugs inhibit the parasympathetic nervous system, which innervates the sweat glands, so that when the ambient temperature rises the major heat-losing mechanism of the body can be partially or wholly lost.[34] Phenothiazines, thioxanthenes and butyrophenones might also have some antimuscarinic effects, but additionally they impair (to a varying extent) the hypothalamic thermoregulatory mechanisms that control the body's ability to keep a constant temperature when exposed to heat or cold. Thus, when the ambient temperature rises, the body temperature also rises. The tricyclics can similarly disrupt temperature control. Therefore in very hot and humid conditions, when the need to reduce the temperature is great, the additive effects of these drugs can make patients unable to control their temperature,[4] which can be fatal.

Antimuscarinic drugs also reduce peristalsis, which in the extreme can result in paralytic ileus. Additive effects can occur if two or more antimuscarinic drugs are taken.

The toxic psychoses described resemble the CNS effects of atropine or belladonna poisoning and appear to result from the additive effects of the drugs used.

The mechanism for antipsychotic antagonism is not understood. *Animal* studies suggest that the site of interaction is in the gut.[20]

Importance and management

The interactions between antipsychotics and antimuscarinics are established and well-documented. While antipsychotics and antimuscarinics (including **tricyclics**, which have antimuscarinic adverse effects) have been widely used together with apparent clinical benefit and without problems, prescribers should be aware that low-grade antimuscarinic toxicity can easily go undetected, particularly in the elderly because the symptoms can be so similar to the general complaints of this group. Also be aware of the serious problems that can sometimes develop, particularly if high doses are used. The following advice is recommended:

- Warn patients to minimise outdoor exposure and/or exercise in hot and humid climates, particularly if they are taking high doses of antipsychotic and antimuscarinic drugs.
- Be alert for severe constipation and for the development of paralytic ileus, which can be fatal.
- Be aware that the symptoms of central antimuscarinic psychosis can be confused with the basic psychotic symptoms of the patient. Withdrawal of one or more of the drugs, or a dose reduction and/or appropriate symptomatic treatment can be used to control these interactions.
- Ensure that the concurrent use of antimuscarinics to control the extrapyramidal adverse effects of neuroleptics is necessary[35,36] and be aware that the therapeutic effects might possibly be reduced as a result.

1. Westlake RJ, Rastegar A. Hyperpyrexia from drug combinations. *JAMA* (1973) 225, 1250.
2. Zelman S, Guillan R. Heat stroke in phenothiazine-treated patients: a report of three fatalities. *Am J Psychiatry* (1970) 126, 1787–90.
3. Sarnquist F, Larson CP. Drug-induced heat stroke. *Anesthesiology* (1973) 39, 348–50.
4. Reimer DR, Mohan J, Nagaswami S. Heat dyscontrol syndrome in patients receiving antipsychotic, antidepressant and antiparkinson drug therapy. *J Fla Med Assoc* (1974) 61, 573–4.
5. Mirtallo JM. Drug-induced heat stroke. *DICP Ann Pharmacother* (1978) 12, 652–7.
6. Kao RL, Kelly LM. Fatal exertional heat stroke in a patient receiving zuclopenthixol, quetiapine and benztropine. *Can J Clin Pharmacol* (2007) 14, e322–e325.
7. Willcox WH. The nature, prevention, and treatment of heat hyperpyrexia: the clinical aspect. *BMJ* (1920) 1, 392–7.
8. Litman RE. Heat sensitivity due to autonomic drugs. *JAMA* (1952) 149, 635–6.
9. Burkitt EA, Sutcliffe CK. Paralytic ileus after amitriptyline ("Tryptizol"). *BMJ* (1961) 2, 1648–9.
10. Warnes H, Lehmann HE, Ban TA. Adynamic ileus during psychoactive medication: a report of three fatal and five severe cases. *Can Med Assoc J* (1967) 96, 1112–13.
11. Milner G, Hills NF. Adynamic ileus and nortriptyline. *BMJ* (1966) 1, 841–2.
12. Sheikh RA, Prindiville T, Yasmeen S. Haloperidol and benztropine interaction presenting as acute intestinal pseudo-obstruction. *Am J Gastroenterol* (2001) 96, 934–5.
13. Wade LC, Ellenor GL. Combination mesoridazine- and benztropine mesylate- induced paralytic ileus. Two case reports. *DICP Ann Pharmacother* (1980) 14, 17–22.
14. Giordano J, Huang A, Canter JW. Fatal paralytic ileus complicating phenothiazine therapy. *South Med J* (1975) 68, 351–3.
15. Spiro RK, Kysilewskyj RM. Iatrogenic ileus secondary to medication. *J Med Soc New Jers* (1973) 70, 565–7.
16. Ayd FJ. Doxepin with other drugs. *South Med J* (1973) 66, 465–71.
17. Davis JM. Psychopharmacology in the aged. Use of psychotropic drugs in geriatric patients. *J Geriatr Psychiatry* (1974) 7, 145.
18. Rogers SC. Imipramine and benzhexol. *BMJ* (1967) 1, 500.
19. Rivera-Calimlim L, Castañeda L, Lasagna L. Effect of mode of management on plasma chlorpromazine in psychiatric patients. *Clin Pharmacol Ther* (1973) 14, 978–86.
20. Rivera-Calimlim L, Castañeda L, Lasagna L. Chlorpromazine and trihexyphenidyl interaction in psychiatric patients. *Pharmacologist* (1973) 15, 212.
21. Chan TL, Sakalis G, Gershon S. Some aspects of chlorpromazine metabolism in humans. *Clin Pharmacol Ther* (1973) 14, 133.
22. Rivera-Calimlim L, Nasrallah H, Strauss J, Lasagna L. Clinical response and plasma levels: effect of dose, dosage schedules, and drug interactions on plasma chlorpromazine levels. *Am J Psychiatry* (1976) 133, 646–52.
23. Loga S, Curry S, Lader M. Interactions of orphenadrine and phenobarbitone with chlorpromazine: plasma concentrations and effects in man. *Br J Clin Pharmacol* (1975) 2, 197–208.
24. Gautier J, Jus A, Villeneuve A, Jus K, Pires P, Villeneuve R. Influence of the antiparkinsonian drugs on the plasma level of neuroleptics. *Biol Psychiatry* (1977) 12, 389–99.
25. Rockland L, Cooper T, Schwartz F, Weber D, Sullivan T. Effects of trihexyphenidyl on plasma chlorpromazine in young schizophrenics. *Can J Psychiatry* (1990) 35, 604–7.
26. Singh MM, Smith JM. Reversal of some therapeutic effects of an antipsychotic agent by an antiparkinsonism drug. *J Nerv Ment Dis* (1973) 157, 50–8.
27. Singh MM, Kay SR. Therapeutic reversal with benztropine in schizophrenics: practical and theoretical significance. *J Nerv Ment Dis* (1975) 160, 258–66.
28. Singh MM, Kay SR. A comparative study of haloperidol and chlorpromazine in terms of clinical effects and therapeutic reversal with benztropine in schizophrenia. Theoretical implications for potency differences among neuroleptics. *Psychopharmacologia* (1975) 43, 103–13.
29. Singh MM, Kay SR. A longitudinal therapeutic comparison between two prototypic neuroleptics (haloperidol and chlorpromazine) in matched groups of schizophrenics. Non therapeutic interactions with trihexyphenidyl. Theoretical implications for potency differences. *Psychopharmacologia* (1975) 43, 115–23.
30. Bamrah JS, Kumar V, Krska J Soni SD. Interactions between procyclidine and neuroleptic drugs. Some pharmacological and clinical aspects. *Br J Psychiatry* (1986) 149, 726–733.
31. Hansen LB, Elley J, Christensen TR, Larsen N-E, Naestoft J, Hvidberg EF. Plasma levels of perphenazine and its major metabolites during simultaneous treatment with anticholinergic drugs. *Br J Clin Pharmacol* (1979) 7, 75–80.
32. Otani K, Ishida M, Yasui N, Kondo T, Mihara K, Suzuki A, Kaneko S, Inoue Y, Shibata M, Ikeda K. No effect of the anticholinergic drugs trihexyphenidyl and biperiden on the plasma concentrations of bromperidol and its reduced metabolite. *Ther Drug Monit* (1997) 19, 165–8.
33. Buckle RM, Guillebaud J. Hypoglycaemic coma occurring during treatment with chlorpromazine and orphenadrine. *BMJ* (1967) 4, 599–600.
34. Kollias J, Bullard RW. The influence of chlorpromazine on physical and chemical mechanisms of temperature regulation in the rat. *J Pharmacol Exp Ther* (1964) 145, 373–81.
35. Prien RF. Unpublished surveys from the NIMH Collaborative Project on Drug Therapy in Chronic Schizophrenia and the VA Collaborative Project on Interim Drug Therapy in Chronic Schizophrenia. *Int Drug Ther Newslett* (1974) 9, 29–32.
36. Klett CJ, Caffey EM. Evaluating the long-term need for antiparkinson drugs by chronic schizophrenics. *Arch Gen Psychiatry* (1972) 26, 374–9.

Antipsychotics + Coffee or Tea

Tea and coffee do not appear to affect the plasma concentrations of chlorpromazine, haloperidol, fluphenazine or trifluoperazine.

Clinical evidence

A clinical study in 16 patients found that the plasma concentrations of **chlorpromazine, fluphenazine, trifluoperazine**, and **haloperidol** were unaffected by stopping tea or coffee consumption for a week. The patients behaviour also remained unchanged.[1] Similarly, a pharmacokinetic study in 12 healthy subjects concluded that there was no change in the AUC and plasma concentration of a single 5-mg dose of **fluphenazine** given with either tea, coffee, or water.[2]

Mechanism

In vitro studies[3-7] found that a number of drugs (chlorpromazine, **promethazine**, fluphenazine, orphenadrine, **promazine**, **prochlorperazine**, trifluoperazine, **thioridazine, loxapine**, haloperidol, **droperidol**) form a precipitate with tea and coffee due to the formation of a drug-tannin complex, which was thought might possibly lower the absorption of these drugs in the gut. Studies with *rats* also found that tea abolished the cataleptic effects of **chlorpromazine**, which did not appear to be related to the presence of caffeine.[8] However, the drug-tannin complex gives up the drug into solution if it becomes acidified, as in the stomach.[7]

Importance and management

The limited clinical information suggests that both tea and coffee do not alter the plasma concentrations of chlorpromazine, haloperidol, fluphenazine or trifluoperazine. Therefore there appears to be no direct evidence that the *in vitro* physicochemical interaction is normally of any clinical importance.

For mention that coffee can increase clozapine concentrations, see 'Clozapine + Caffeine', p.849.

1. Bowen S, Taylor KM, Gibb IAM. Effect of coffee and tea on blood levels and efficacy of antipsychotic drugs. *Lancet* (1981) i, 1217–18.
2. Wallace SM, Suveges LG, Blackburn JL, Korchinski ED, Midha KK. Oral fluphenazine and tea and coffee drinking. *Lancet* (1981) ii, 691.
3. Kulhanek F, Linde OK, Meisenberg G. Precipitation of antipsychotic drugs in interaction with coffee or tea. *Lancet* (1979) ii, 1130.
4. Hirsch SR. Precipitation of antipsychotic drugs in interaction with tea or coffee. *Lancet* (1979) ii, 1130–1.
5. Lasswell WL, Wilkins JM, Weber SS. In vitro interaction of selected drugs with coffee, tea, and gallotannic acid. *Drug Nutr Interact* (1984) 2, 235–41.
6. Lasswell WL, Weber SS, Wilkins JM. *In vitro* interaction of neuroleptics and tricyclic antidepressants with coffee, tea, and gallotannic acid. *J Pharm Sci* (1984) 73, 1056–8.
7. Curry ML, Curry SH, Marroum PJ. Interaction of phenothiazine and related drugs and caffeinated beverages. *DICP Ann Pharmacother* (1991) 25, 437–8.
8. Cheeseman HJ, Neal MJ. Interaction of chlorpromazine with tea and coffee. *Br J Clin Pharmacol* (1981) 12, 165–9.

Antipsychotics; Miscellaneous + Lithium

The development of severe extrapyramidal adverse effects or severe neurotoxicity has been seen in one or more patients given lithium with various antipsychotics.

Clinical evidence

A large-scale retrospective study of the literature over the period 1966 to 1996 using the Medline database identified 41 cases of neurotoxic adverse effects in 41 patients with low therapeutic concentrations of lithium. Of these patients, 51.2% were also taking at least one antipsychotic drug.[1] Another retrospective study using both Medline and the spontaneous reporting system of the FDA in the US, over the period 1969 to 1994, identified 237 cases of severe neurotoxicity involving lithium, with 188 involving lithium with antipsychotics.[2,3] The sudden emergence of extrapyramidal or other adverse effects has also been described in other studies. The antipsychotics implicated in this interaction with lithium are **chlorprothixene**,[2,3] **clopenthixol**,[1] **flupentixol**,[4-6] **loxapine**,[2,3,7,8] **molindone**,[2,3] **tiotixene**,[1-3,5,9] and **zuclopenthixol**.[1]

A retrospective review of 39 patients with a diagnosis of neurotoxicity caused by the concurrent use of lithium and an antipsychotic, found that the onset of symptoms varied from 24 hours to 3 months after taking the two drugs together, with an average delay of 12.7 days.[5]

A study in 8 patients found a 4-fold increase in the half-life of **molindone** when lithium was also given.[10]

Mechanism

Not understood. It is the subject of considerable discussion and debate.[1-3,11,12]

Importance and management

The development of severe neurotoxic or severe extrapyramidal adverse effects with combinations of antipsychotics and lithium appears to be uncommon and unexplained, but be alert for any evidence of toxicity if lithium is given with any of these drugs. One recommendation is that the onset of neurological manifestations, such as excessive drowsiness or movement disorders, warrants electroencephalography without delay and withdrawal of the drugs, especially as irreversible effects have been seen. A review[13] suggests that the concurrent use of haloperidol seems to be safe if lithium concentrations are below 1 mmol/L, but it is not known whether this also applies to other antipsychotics.

At the moment there seems to be no way of identifying the apparently small number of patients who are particularly at risk, but possible likely factors include a previous history of extrapyramidal reactions with antipsychotics and the use of large doses of the antipsychotic.

1. Emilien G, Maloteaux JM. Lithium neurotoxicity at low therapeutic doses: hypotheses for causes and mechanism of action following a retrospective analysis of published case reports. *Acta Neurol Belg* (1996) 96, 281–93.
2. Goldman SA. Lithium and neuroleptics in combination: is there enhancement of neurotoxicity leading to permanent sequelae? *J Clin Pharmacol* (1996) 36, 951–62.
3. Goldman SA. FDA MedWatch Report: lithium and neuroleptics in combination: the spectrum of neurotoxicity. *Psychopharmacol Bull* (1996) 32, 299–309.
4. Kamlana SH, Kerry RJ, Khan IA. Lithium: some drug interactions. *Practitioner* (1980) 224, 1291–2.

5. Prakash R, Kelwala S, Ban TA. Neurotoxicity with combined administration of lithium and a neuroleptic. *Compr Psychiatry* (1982) 23, 567–71.
6. West A. Adverse effects of lithium treatment. *BMJ* (1977) 2, 642.
7. de la Gandara J, Dominguez RA. Lithium and loxapine: a potential interaction. *J Clin Psychiatry* (1988) 49, 126.
8. Fuller MA, Sajatovic M. Neurotoxicity resulting from a combination of lithium and loxapine. *J Clin Psychiatry* (1989) 50, 187.
9. Fetzer J, Kader G, Danahy S. Lithium encephalopathy: a clinical, psychiatric, and EEG evaluation. *Am J Psychiatry* (1981) 138, 1622–3.
10. Wolf ME, Mosnaim AD. Lithium and molindone interactions: pharmacokinetic studies. *Res Commun Psychol Psychiatr Behav* (1986) 11, 23–28.
11. Geisler A, Klysner R. Combined effect of lithium and flupenthixol on striatal adenylate cyclase. *Lancet* (1977) i, 430–1.
12. von Knorring L. Possible mechanisms for the presumed interaction between lithium and neuroleptics. *Hum Psychopharmacol* (1990) 5, 287–92.
13. Batchelor DH, Lowe MR. Reported neurotoxicity with the lithium/haloperidol combination and other neuroleptics—a literature review. *Hum Psychopharmacol* (1990) 5, 275–80.

Antipsychotics + Melatonin

The concurrent use of thioridazine and melatonin led to increased CNS effects in a pharmacodynamic study.

Clinical evidence, mechanism, importance and management

In a single-dose controlled study, there was no pharmacokinetic interaction between **thioridazine** 50 mg and melatonin 2 mg. However, there was a possible pharmacodynamic interaction, with increased feelings of 'muzzy-headedness' when compared with **thioridazine** alone.[1,2] However, in a placebo-controlled, clinical efficacy study in 22 patients with antipsychotic-induced tardive dyskinesia taking various antipsychotics (13 taking **haloperidol**, 4 taking **chlorpromazine**, 3 taking **perphenazine**, and 2 taking **zuclopenthixol**), the addition of controlled-release melatonin 10 mg in the evening for 6 weeks did not cause any apparent adverse effects.[3] It is possible that the sedative effects of melatonin and antipsychotics might be additive. Bear this possibility in mind.

1. Circadin (Melatonin). Flynn Pharma Ltd. UK Summary of product characteristics, August 2011.
2. EMEA Assessment report for Circadin. Procedure No. EMEA/H/C/695. 2007. Available at: http://www.ema.europa.eu/ema/index.jsp?curl=pages/medicines/human/medicines/000695/human_med_000701.jsp&mid=WC0b01ac058001d124 (accessed 20/10/15).
3. Shamir E, Barak Y, Shalman I, Laudon M, Zisapel N, Tarrasch R, Elizur A, Weizman R. Melatonin treatment for tardive dyskinesia: a double-blind, placebo-controlled, crossover study. *Arch Gen Psychiatry* (2001) 58, 1049–52.

Antipsychotics + Metoclopramide

The risk of extrapyramidal adverse effects is predicted to be increased if metoclopramide is given with antipsychotics that have dopamine antagonist activity. A single case report describes dystonia-related tongue swelling and respiratory obstruction in a young woman given intramuscular prochlorperazine and then intramuscular metoclopramide.

Clinical evidence, mechanism, importance and management

A 19-year-old woman experienced progressive swelling of the tongue, partial upper-airways obstruction and a sensation of choking over a period of 12 hours after she was given intramuscular doses of metoclopramide to a total of 30 mg. She had received a 12.5-mg intramuscular dose of **prochlorperazine** for nausea 24 hours earlier. On examination her tongue was strikingly blue, but within 15 minutes of receiving benzatropine 2 mg it returned to its normal size and colour. The respiratory distress also disappeared.[1] The authors of the report suggested that the dystonic adverse effects of both drugs were additive, leading to the effects seen.[1] However, it should be noted that oedema of the tongue has also been described with metoclopramide alone.[2] Young patients, especially women, are particularly susceptible to the adverse effects of metoclopramide, and this patient received the standard total daily dose over just 12 hours, so an interaction in this case is by no means established. Nevertheless, metoclopramide is a dopamine antagonist that can cause extrapyramidal adverse effects, particularly of the dystonic type, especially if used at high dose or long term. Various antipsychotics also have dopamine antagonist activity and can cause extrapyramidal adverse effects. The risk of extrapyramidal adverse effects might be increased if metoclopramide is combined with antipsychotics that can cause extrapyramidal reactions. The UK manufacturer of metoclopramide states that extrapyramidal adverse effects can occur with both metoclopramide and with antipsychotics (such as the **phenothiazines**), and they recommend particular care on their concurrent use. They also note that the risk of tardive dyskinesia, which might be persistent, is increased in the elderly when long-term metoclopramide is given with antipsychotics.[3]

1. Alroe C, Bowen P. Metoclopramide and prochlorperazine: "the blue-tongue sign". *Med J Aust* (1989) 150, 724–5.
2. Robinson OPW. Metoclopramide—side effects and safety. *Postgrad Med J* (1973) 49 (Suppl July), 77–80.
3. Maxolon High Dose (Metoclopramide hydrochloride). Amdipharm plc. UK Summary of product characteristics, January 2011.

Antipsychotics + Orlistat

No changes in the plasma concentrations of haloperidol or clozapine were seen when orlistat was also given.

Clinical evidence, mechanism, importance and management

In a study, 8 patients who had experienced weight gain as a result of treatment with **haloperidol** (2), **clozapine** (2), clomipramine (3), desipramine (1), or carbamazepine (2), were given orlistat 120 mg three times daily for 8 weeks. There were no changes in the plasma concentrations of the antipsychotic drugs, and steatorrhoea, which occurred in three patients, had no effect on their bioavailability.[1] Although an interaction appears to be unlikely, due to the small numbers involved in the study, this needs confirmation.

1. Hilger E, Quiner S, Ginzel I, Walter H, Saria L, Barnas C. The effect of orlistat on plasma levels of psychotropic drugs in patients with long-term psychopharmacotherapy. *J Clin Psychopharmacol* (2002) 22, 68–70.

Aripiprazole or Risperidone + Cocaine

A case report describes two episodes of dystonia in a cocaine-user which developed after the patient took risperidone and then subsequently after a single dose of aripiprazole.

Clinical evidence, mechanism, importance and management

A case report describes a 58-year-old cocaine user who developed acute dystonia (muscle tightness in limbs and jaw), within 2 hours of taking his first 10 mg dose of aripiprazole.[1] He had difficulty speaking and raised blood pressure (220/120 mmHg). He was given benzatropine 2 mg, which resolved his symptoms within 5 minutes. The patient had experienced a less severe dystonia one day previously, after taking 4 doses of risperidone 2 mg at night, but on this occasion no treatment was required.[1] The authors suggest that the cocaine use might have contributed to the dystonia, although they also state that it is possible that the dystonia might have occurred without cocaine use.[1] The general importance of this isolated report remains to be established.

1. Henderson JB, Labbate L, Worley M. A case of acute dystonia after single dose of aripiprazole in a man with cocaine dependence. *Am J Addict* (2007) 16, 244.

Aripiprazole + CYP3A4 inducers

Aripiprazole exposure is reduced by carbamazepine, and probably phenobarbital and phenytoin. Other CYP3A4 inducers are expected to interact similarly.

Clinical evidence

In a study, 6 patients were given aripiprazole 30 mg daily alone for 14 days, and then with **carbamazepine** in doses to produce minimum serum concentrations of 8 to 12 mg/L. After 4 to 6 weeks of concurrent use, the maximum plasma concentration and AUC of aripiprazole were reduced by 66% and 71%, respectively. The apparent oral clearance of aripiprazole was increased about 4-fold. Similar reductions in the plasma concentrations of the active metabolite, dehydroaripiprazole, were also seen.[1] Another study in 18 patients taking aripiprazole 12 to 24 mg daily found that plasma concentrations of aripiprazole and dehydroaripiprazole were reduced by 64% and 68%, respectively, after **carbamazepine** 400 mg daily was added for one week. Despite these reductions, there was a small, but statistically significant improvement in the total positive and negative syndrome scale (PANSS) score. Note however, that the clinical relevance of this finding is limited by the small number of patients and short treatment period.[2] Analysis of results from a routine therapeutic drug monitoring service found that the dose-adjusted serum concentration of aripiprazole was 88% lower in one patient taking **carbamazepine** than in the monotherapy group.[3] A similar analysis of results from another routine therapeutic drug monitoring service,[4] found that the dose-adjusted serum concentrations of aripiprazole and dehydroaripiprazole were 54% and 61% lower, respectively, in 3 patients also given **carbamazepine** (2) or **phenobarbital** and **phenytoin** (1).

A retrospective chart review of patients prescribed **carbamazepine** with an atypical antipsychotic (including aripiprazole), but who discontinued carbamazepine and continued the antipsychotic, suggests that there is an increased risk of adverse effects if the dose of antipsychotic is not reduced after carbamazepine is stopped. Two of the nine patients identified were taking aripiprazole: one of whom experienced akathisia 3 weeks after the carbamazepine was stopped, but which resolved on reduction of the aripiprazole dose from 45 mg daily to 30 mg daily.[5]

Mechanism

Aripiprazole is metabolised by CYP3A4 and CYP2D6. Carbamazepine is a known inducer of these isoenzymes, and therefore concurrent use results in reduced aripiprazole exposure.

Importance and management

The moderate pharmacokinetic interaction between aripiprazole and **carbamazepine** appears to be established and can be clinically important. The UK and US manufacturers recommended that the dose of aripiprazole should be doubled when it is taken with carbamazepine.[6,7] The authors of one study suggest that the risk of adverse effects might be increased in those taking a high dose of antipsychotic before carbamazepine discontinuation. Furthermore, they suggest that the patient should be monitored for the occurrence of adverse effects for 2 to 4 weeks after carbamazepine is stopped.[5]

Other potent inducers of CYP3A4 are expected to have similar effects and similar adjustment of aripiprazole doses might also be necessary when these drugs are started and stopped: the UK manufacturer of aripiprazole names **efavirenz**, **nevirapine**, **phenytoin** [and therefore consider also **fosphenytoin**], **phenobarbital**, **primidone**, **rifabutin**, **rifampicin** and **St John's wort**.[6] For a list of other CYP3A4 inducers, see 'Table 1.9', p.11.

1. Citrome L, Macher J-P, Salazar DE, Mallikaarjun S, Boulton DW. Pharmacokinetics of aripiprazole and concomitant carbamazepine. *J Clin Psychopharmacol* (2007), 27, 279–83.

2. Nakamura A, Mihara K, Nagai G, Suzuki T, Kondo T. Pharmacokinetic and pharmacodynamic interactions between carbamazepine and aripiprazole in patients with schizophrenia. *Ther Drug Monit* (2009) 31, 575–8.
3. Castberg I, Spigset O. Effects of comedication on the serum levels of aripiprazole: evidence from a routine therapeutic drug monitoring service. *Pharmacopsychiatry* (2007) 40, 107–10.
4. Waade RB, Christensen H, Rudberg I, Refsum H, Hermann M. Influence of comedication on serum concentrations of aripiprazole and dehydroaripiprazole. *Ther Drug Monit* (2009) 31, 233–8.
5. Strack DK, Leckband SG, Meyer JM. Antipsychotic prescribing practices following withdrawal of concomitant carbamazepine. *J Psychiatr Pract* (2009) 15, 442–8.
6. Abilify (Aripiprazole). Otsuka and Bristol-Myers Squibb. UK Summary of product characteristics, September 2011.
7. Abilify (Aripiprazole). Otsuka and Bristol-Myers Squibb Company. US Prescribing information, February 2012.

Aripiprazole + CYP3A4 inhibitors

Aripiprazole exposure is slightly raised by itraconazole and ketoconazole. Other potent CYP3A4 inhibitors are expected to interact similarly. Moderate CYP3A4 inhibitors (e.g. diltiazem) might also interact, but to a lesser degree.

Clinical evidence

(a) Darunavir

A 43-year-old HIV-positive man taking aripiprazole 50 mg daily, ritonavir-boosted darunavir 800/100 mg daily and **duloxetine** 60 mg daily was found to have an aripiprazole concentration of 1 100 nanograms/mL (usual range is 100 to 200 nanograms/mL). The patient had no signs or symptoms of aripiprazole toxicity. The CYP2D6 metaboliser status of this patient was not reported.[1]

(b) Itraconazole

In a study in 24 healthy subjects, itraconazole 100 mg daily for 7 days increased the AUC of a single 3-mg dose of aripiprazole by 48%, and increased the maximum concentration and half-life by 19%. When analysed by CYP2D6 phenotype (that is, the activity of CYP2D6, which varies between subjects), the increase in AUC was somewhat greater in 3 subjects who were intermediate metabolisers (72%) compared with 14 subjects classified as extensive metabolisers (36%). There were no subjects who were poor metabolisers. The CYP2D6 intermediate metabolisers had higher exposure to aripiprazole than the extensive metabolisers before itraconazole use.[2]

(c) Ketoconazole

The manufacturers of aripiprazole report that ketoconazole 200 mg daily for 14 days increased the AUC and maximum plasma concentration of a single 15-mg dose of aripiprazole by 63% and 37%, respectively.[3,4] The AUC and maximum plasma concentration of its active metabolite, dehydroaripiprazole, were also increased, by 77% and 43%, respectively.[3] The effect of a higher 400 mg daily dose of ketoconazole has not been studied.[4]

Mechanism

Aripiprazole is metabolised by CYP3A4 and CYP2D6. Both itraconazole and ketoconazole, and ritonavir-boosted darunavir are known inhibitors of CYP3A4, and therefore concurrent use results in reduced aripiprazole metabolism and raised exposure. Furthermore, in the case with ritonavir-boosted darunavir, duloxetine, which has CYP2D6 inhibitory effects, was also given, and this might have contributed to the increase in concentrations seen. A greater increase in aripiprazole exposure might also occur in those subjects with reduced CYP2D6 activity, for whom CYP3A4 might play a greater role in aripiprazole metabolism.

Importance and management

A pharmacokinetic interaction between **itraconazole** or **ketoconazole** and aripiprazole is established; however, the increase in aripiprazole exposure is slight and probably unlikely to be generally clinically important.[2] Nevertheless, the UK manufacturer considers that the increase seen is likely to be higher in patients who are CYP2D6 poor metabolisers,[3] but note that this is unlikely to be known in clinical practice. For this reason, the manufacturers recommend that the dose of aripiprazole should be halved when given with ketoconazole or other potent CYP3A4 inhibitors: they name the **HIV-protease inhibitors**[3] and **clarithromycin**.[4] The dose of aripiprazole should also be increased again if the drug is stopped.

For a patient known to be a CYP2D6 poor metaboliser who is also given a potent CYP3A4 inhibitor, the US manufacturer recommends a 75% reduction in the aripiprazole dose.[4] They also give similar dose recommendations when both a CYP2D6 inhibitor (see *Quinidine and other CYP2D6 inhibitors*, under 'Aripiprazole + Miscellaneous', below) and a CYP3A4 inhibitor are given together.[4]

The effect of moderate CYP3A4 inhibitors (such as **diltiazem**[3] or **erythromycin**[4]) or weak CYP3A4 inhibitors (the manufacturers name **grapefruit juice**[4]) on aripiprazole exposure has not been studied; however, given the slight effect of the potent CYP3A4 inhibitors, a clinically relevant interaction would not be expected. For a list of CYP3A4 inhibitors, see 'Table 1.9', p.11.

1. Aung GL, O'Brien JG, Tien PG, Kawamoto LS. Increased aripiprazole concentrations in an HIV-positive male concurrently taking duloxetine, darunavir, and ritonavir. *Ann Pharmacother* (2010) 44, 1850–4.
2. Kubo M, Koue T, Inaba A, Takeda H, Maune H, Fukuda T, Azuma J. Influence of itraconazole co-administration and CYP2D6 genotype on the pharmacokinetics of the new antipsychotic aripiprazole. *Drug Metab Pharmacokinet* (2005) 20, 55–64.
3. Abilify (Aripiprazole). Otsuka and Bristol-Myers Squibb. UK Summary of product characteristics, September 2011.
4. Abilify (Aripiprazole). Otsuka and Bristol-Myers Squibb Company. US Prescribing information, February 2012.

Aripiprazole + Haloperidol

One case report describes a prolonged QT interval when haloperidol was given to a patient taking aripiprazole, and another describes worsening of psychotic symptoms on concurrent use.

Clinical evidence, mechanism, importance and management

A case report describes a 30-year-old man with schizophrenia who developed worsening psychotic symptoms while taking aripiprazole 10 mg daily and haloperidol 5 mg twice daily. The symptoms worsened when the aripiprazole dose was increased to 30 mg daily, and a doubling of the haloperidol dose only achieved a marginal improvement. His psychotic symptoms and agitation improved within 4 days of stopping aripiprazole. He was later discharged taking haloperidol, and had some extrapyramidal adverse effects and an increased prolactin concentration, which had been absent when taking the aripiprazole. It was suggested that aripiprazole, a partial dopamine D_2-receptor agonist, had interfered with the effects of haloperidol, a D_2 antagonist.[1]

Another case report describes a 43-year-old woman with schizophrenia whose QTc interval increased from about 415 milliseconds while taking aripiprazole 30 mg daily alone, to 492 milliseconds 7 days after haloperidol 5 mg daily was added.[2] This resolved after withdrawal of the haloperidol, although not to baseline. The authors suggest a pharmacokinetic interaction was responsible, possibly involving CYP2D6 and CYP3A4, but this is not established.

Evidence for an interaction between aripiprazole and haloperidol appears to be limited to these two case reports. An interaction is not therefore established, particularly in the case of QT prolongation, as the haloperidol alone could have been responsible for this effect. However, the UK manufacturer of aripiprazole[3] states that it should be used with caution with other drugs that prolong the QT interval, which would include haloperidol. See 'Drugs that prolong the QT interval + Other drugs that prolong the QT interval', p.272, for further information on the concurrent use of two or more drugs that prolong the QT interval.

1. Burke MJ, Lincoln J. Aripiprazole and haloperidol: a clinically relevant interaction with a dopamine antagonist and partial agonist. *Ann Clin Psychiatry* (2006) 18, 129–30.
2. Leo R, Razzini C, Di Lorenzo G, Bianchi F, Tesauro M, Zanasi M, Siracusano A, Romeo F. Asymptomatic QTc prolongation during coadministration of aripiprazole and haloperidol. *J Clin Psychiatry* (2008) 69, 327–8.
3. Abilify (Aripiprazole). Otsuka and Bristol-Myers Squibb. UK Summary of product characteristics, September 2011.

Aripiprazole + Lamotrigine

Aripiprazole does not alter the pharmacokinetics of lamotrigine, and lamotrigine does not appear to alter the pharmacokinetics of aripiprazole.

Clinical evidence, mechanism, importance and management

In an open-label study in 16 patients with bipolar disorder, aripiprazole 10 mg daily for 3 days, 20 mg daily for 3 days, then 30 mg daily for 8 days had no effect on the steady-state pharmacokinetics of lamotrigine 100 to 400 mg daily.[1]

An analysis of results from a routine therapeutic drug monitoring service, found that the dose-adjusted serum concentrations of aripiprazole and its active metabolite, dehydroaripiprazole, were not changed to a statistically significant extent in 31 patients also given lamotrigine.[2] In contrast, a similar analysis of another routine therapeutic drug monitoring service found that the dose-adjusted serum concentrations of aripiprazole in 4 patients also taking lamotrigine was 51% higher than in the monotherapy group.[3] However, interpretation of the importance of this finding is limited by the very small number of patients.

Evidence for an interaction between lamotrigine and aripiprazole is limited. Nevertheless on the basis of the available data, which shows no effect on lamotrigine pharmacokinetics and only a small increase in aripiprazole concentrations, no dose adjustments would be expected to be necessary on the concurrent use of these drugs.

1. Schieber FC, Boulton DW, Balch AH, Croop R, Mallikaarjun S, Benson J, Carlson BX. A non-randomized study to investigate the effects of the atypical antipsychotic aripiprazole on the steady-state pharmacokinetics of lamotrigine in patients with bipolar I disorder. *Hum Psychopharmacol* (2009) 24, 145–52.
2. Waade RB, Christensen H, Rudberg I, Refsum H, Hermann M. Influence of comedication on serum concentrations of aripiprazole and dehydroaripiprazole. *Ther Drug Monit* (2009) 31, 233–8.
3. Castberg I, Spigset O. Effects of comedication on the serum levels of aripiprazole: evidence from a routine therapeutic drug monitoring service. *Pharmacopsychiatry* (2007) 40, 107–10.

Aripiprazole + Miscellaneous

Quinidine, a CYP2D6 inhibitor, increases aripiprazole exposure: other CYP2D6 inhibitors might interact similarly. Limited evidence suggests that alimemazine might increase aripiprazole concentrations. Increased sedation and orthostatic hypotension were seen with lorazepam and aripiprazole, when both were given intravenously, although there was no pharmacokinetic interaction. Food, famotidine, lorazepam injection and risperidone tablets do not affect the pharmacokinetics of aripiprazole, and aripiprazole does not affect the pharmacokinetics of dextromethorphan, omeprazole, and warfarin.

Clinical evidence, mechanism, importance and management

(a) Alimemazine

An analysis of results from a routine therapeutic drug monitoring service found that the dose-adjusted serum concentrations of aripiprazole were increased by 56% in 12 patients also given alimemazine.[1] This needs confirming in a controlled study. Until more is known, it might be prudent to be aware of the possibility of increased adverse effects if the combination is used.

(b) Famotidine

In a single-dose study, famotidine 40 mg reduced the rate of absorption of aripiprazole 15 mg, and reduced the maximum concentration and AUC of aripiprazole by 37% and 13% respectively,[2] but these effects are not clinically relevant.[2,3]

(c) Food

A study in 39 healthy subjects who took aripiprazole 15 mg either after fasting, or 5 minutes after a high-fat breakfast, found no changes in the pharmacokinetics of aripiprazole.[4] Aripiprazole can be taken without regard to the timing of meals.[2,3]

(d) Lorazepam

A study in healthy subjects given lorazepam 2 mg and aripiprazole 15 mg, both by injection, found there were no clinically important changes in the pharmacokinetics of either drug. No dose adjustment is required on combined use. However, the intensity of sedation with the combination was greater than that observed with aripiprazole alone, and orthostatic hypotension was greater with the combination than with lorazepam alone.[2] On this basis, the US manufacturer recommends that if an intravenous benzodiazepine is required in addition to parenteral aripiprazole, the patient should be monitored for excessive sedation and orthostatic hypotension.[2]

(e) Quinidine and other CYP2D6 inhibitors

The US manufacturer of aripiprazole reports that quinidine 166 mg daily for 13 days moderately increased the AUC of a single 10-mg dose of aripiprazole 2.1-fold, although the maximum aripiprazole concentration was unchanged. The AUC of its active metabolite, dehydroaripiprazole, was reduced by 35%.[2]

Quinidine is a potent inhibitor of CYP2D6, by which aripiprazole is partially metabolised. CYP2D6 shows genetic polymorphism, with some people lacking or deficient in CYP2D6 (poor metabolisers). Use of quinidine in patients who are CYP2D6 extensive metabolisers will, at most, increase aripiprazole exposure to concentrations seen in poor metabolisers, but this might be clinically relevant, especially as in the US, they recommend that the dose of aripiprazole is halved in patients who are CYP2D6 poor metabolisers.[2]. The manufacturers recommend that the dose of aripiprazole is halved if quinidine or other potent CYP2D6 inhibitors are used concurrently.[2,3] The US manufacturers further recommend a 75% reduction in the aripiprazole dose when both a CYP2D6 inhibitor and a CYP3A4 inhibitor (see 'Aripiprazole + CYP3A4 inhibitors', p.808) are given together.[2] For a list of CYP2D6 inhibitors, see 'Table 1.7', p.9. Note that, of potentially more importance, the UK manufacturer of aripiprazole[3] states that it should be used with caution with other drugs that prolong the QT interval, which would include quinidine. See 'Drugs that prolong the QT interval + Other drugs that prolong the QT interval', p.272, for further information on the concurrent use of two or more drugs that prolong the QT interval.

(f) Risperidone

Dose-adjusted serum concentrations of aripiprazole and its active metabolite dehydroaripiprazole, were unchanged in 10 patients also given risperidone tablets. However, the dose-adjusted serum concentration of the active metabolite, dehydroaripiprazole, was slightly (28%) reduced in 10 patients given risperidone injection.[1] These findings require confirmation in a controlled study. Nevertheless, a clinically relevant pharmacokinetic interaction appears to be unlikely.

(g) Other drugs

The manufacturers note that aripiprazole 10 to 30 mg daily had no effect on the metabolism of **dextromethorphan** (CYP2D6 substrate), or the pharmacokinetics of **warfarin** (CYP2C9 substrate) and **omeprazole** (CYP2C19 substrate).[2,3] In addition, aripiprazole did not alter the INR response to **warfarin**.[2] No dose adjustment of these drugs is likely to be needed while taking aripiprazole, and aripiprazole is unlikely to have clinically important interactions with other drugs that are also substrates of these isoenzymes.[2,3]

1. Waade RB, Christensen H, Rudberg I, Refsum H, Hermann M. Influence of comedication on serum concentrations of aripiprazole and dehydroaripiprazole. *Ther Drug Monit* (2009) 31, 233–8.
2. Abilify (Aripiprazole). Otsuka and Bristol-Myers Squibb Company. US Prescribing information, February 2012.
3. Abilify (Aripiprazole). Otsuka and Bristol-Myers Squibb. UK Summary of product characteristics, September 2011.
4. Mallikaarjun S, Riesgo Y, Salazar F, Bramer S, Xie J, Weston I. Time of dosing and food effect on aripiprazole pharmacokinetics. *Eur Neuropsychopharmacol* (2003) S332.

Aripiprazole + Oxcarbazepine

An isolated case describes priapism in a patient taking oxcarbazepine, aripiprazole, and lithium.

Clinical evidence, mechanism, importance and management

A case report describes a 16-year-old patient who developed painless priapism after oxcarbazepine (total daily dose of 600 mg increased to 900 mg) was added to his established treatment with lithium and aripiprazole. On discontinuing the oxcarbazepine, the patient experienced no further episodes of priapism. Priapism is a known adverse effect of aripiprazole, and it is not known if priapism occurred as an adverse reaction to this drug, or whether an interaction with oxcarbazepine or lithium was responsible.[1] This is an isolated case, and as such no general recommendations can be made. However, note that oxcarbazepine is a derivative of carbamazepine, and appears to have some similar interactions. It might therefore be expected to reduce aripiprazole exposure, see 'Aripiprazole + CYP3A4 inducers', p.807.

1. Negin B, Murphy TK. Priapism associated with oxcarbazepine, aripiprazole, and lithium. *J Am Acad Child Adolesc Psychiatry* (2005) 44, 1223–4.

Aripiprazole + SNRIs

Duloxetine, desvenlafaxine, and venlafaxine do not appear to have any effect on aripiprazole concentrations. Aripiprazole does not appear to affect the pharmacokinetics of venlafaxine. The concurrent use of aripiprazole with duloxetine and venlafaxine has led to adverse effects, such as extrapyramidal symptoms and possibly hypertension.

Clinical evidence

(a) Pharmacokinetics

1. Desvenlafaxine. The US manufacturer of **desvenlafaxine** briefly notes that the pharmacokinetics of aripiprazole (dose not specified) were not affected by desvenlafaxine 100 mg daily.[1]

2. Duloxetine. In a study analysing routine therapeutic drug monitoring samples from 7 patients taking aripiprazole, duloxetine did not increase the concentration of aripiprazole, when compared with a control group of patients not taking duloxetine who were extensive metabolisers of CYP2D6 (that is, they had normal activity of this isoenzyme).[2] However, for a case report where duloxetine might have contributed to an increase in aripiprazole concentrations in a patient also taking ritonavir-boosted darunavir, see 'Aripiprazole + CYP3A4 inhibitors', p.808.

3. Venlafaxine. An analysis of samples at a therapeutic drug monitoring service found that sertraline and venlafaxine had no effect on aripiprazole concentrations in 29 patients.[3] The US manufacturer of aripiprazole briefly notes that aripiprazole 10 to 20 mg daily for 14 days had no effect on the steady-state pharmacokinetics of venlafaxine 75 mg daily (given as a modified-release preparation), or on its *O*-desmethyl metabolite.[4]

(b) Adverse effects

A case report describes a patient taking **venlafaxine**, trazodone, and clonazepam who developed parkinsonian symptoms a few days after starting to take aripiprazole 15 mg daily. Her symptoms resolved on stopping the aripiprazole. The authors attributed this effect to an interaction, due to the low incidence of extrapyramidal adverse effects with aripiprazole alone.[5]

A case of aripiprazole-induced hypertension has been attributed to the concurrent use of aripiprazole 5 mg daily and **duloxetine** 90 mg daily. The authors suggested that aripiprazole concentrations might have been increased by **duloxetine**; however, aripiprazole concentrations were not measured to confirm this hypothesis.[6]

Mechanism

Duloxetine and venlafaxine are inhibitors of CYP2D6 (perhaps to varying extents) by which aripiprazole is partially metabolised, and so might be expected to decrease aripiprazole metabolism and increase its concentrations. However the limited data cited do not show this and hence further study is required.

Importance and management

Evidence for an interaction between aripiprazole and the SNRIs is limited, and a pharmacokinetic interaction is not established. The UK manufacturer of aripiprazole suggests that weak inhibitors of CYP2D6 would be expected to cause modest increases in aripiprazole concentrations, and therefore no aripiprazole dose adjustment would be expected to be required.[7] Duloxetine is considered a moderate CYP2D6 inhibitor, but given the moderate effect of quinidine (a potent CYP2D6 inhibitor) on aripiprazole exposure, see 'Aripiprazole + Miscellaneous', p.808, it would not seem necessary to adjust the dose of aripiprazole when duloxetine is given concurrently. **Venlafaxine** is a CYP2D6 inhibitor but (although clinical data to determine its potency is lacking) it appears to be only weak. It is therefore unlikely to interact to a clinically relevant extent with aripiprazole by this mechanism. Case reports of adverse effects with **duloxetine** and **venlafaxine**, and aripiprazole suggest that it would seem prudent to bear the possibility of an interaction in mind, especially in the case of unexpected or increased adverse effects.

Desvenlafaxine at a dose of 100 mg daily had no effect on the pharmacokinetics of aripiprazole and no interaction would therefore be expected with the usual therapeutic dose of 50 mg daily.

1. Pristiq (Desvenlafaxine succinate). Wyeth Pharmaceuticals Inc. US Prescribing information, July 2014.
2. Hendset M, Molden E, Enoksen TB, Refsum H, Hermann M. The effect of coadministration of duloxetine on steady-state serum concentration of risperidone and aripiprazole: a study based on therapeutic drug monitoring data. *Ther Drug Monit* (2010) 32, 787–90.
3. Waade RB, Christensen H, Rudberg I, Refsum H, Hermann M. Influence of comedication on serum concentrations of aripiprazole and dehydroaripiprazole. *Ther Drug Monit* (2009) 31, 233–8.
4. Abilify (Aripiprazole). Otsuka Pharmaceutical Co, Inc. US Prescribing information, June 2014.
5. Cohen ST, Rulf D, Pies R. Extrapyramidal side effects associated with aripiprazole coprescription in 2 patients. *J Clin Psychiatry* (2005) 66, 135–6.

6. Hsiao Y-L, Chen S-J, Shen T-W, Chang C-H, Chen S-T. Aripiprazole augmentation induced hypertension in major depressive disorder: a case report. *Prog Neuropsychopharmacol Biol Psychiatry* (2011) 35, 305–6.
7. Abilify (Aripiprazole). Otsuka Pharmaceuticals (UK) Ltd. UK Summary of product characteristics, March 2014.

Aripiprazole + SSRIs

Fluoxetine, paroxetine, citalopram and escitalopram can increase aripiprazole concentrations, although the extent varies, but sertraline appears to have no effect. Aripiprazole does not appear to affect the pharmacokinetics of escitalopram, fluoxetine, paroxetine or sertraline.

The concurrent use of aripiprazole with SSRIs has led to adverse effects such as neuroleptic malignant syndrome, extrapyramidal symptoms, and potentially fatal hypothyroidism.

Clinical evidence

(a) Pharmacokinetic studies

A study analysing routine samples sent for aripiprazole monitoring noted that the dose-adjusted serum concentrations of aripiprazole were 44% higher in patients taking either **fluoxetine** (2 patients) or levomepromazine (3 patients). Further, in 6 patients taking **escitalopram** or **citalopram** the plasma concentrations of aripiprazole were found to be 39% higher, when compared with patients taking aripiprazole alone.[1] A similar analysis of another routine therapeutic drug monitoring service found that the dose-adjusted serum concentrations of aripiprazole were 44% higher in patients also given **fluoxetine** (9 patients) or **paroxetine** (3 patients), and 23% higher in 26 patients also given **escitalopram**. In contrast, **sertraline** had no effect on aripiprazole concentrations in 29 patients.[2]

The US manufacturer briefly reports that oral aripiprazole 10 mg daily for 14 days had no effect on the steady-state pharmacokinetics of **escitalopram** 10 mg daily. In addition, in a population pharmacokinetic analysis in patients with major depressive disorder given aripiprazole 2 to 20 mg daily, the steady-state plasma concentrations of **fluoxetine** 20 or 40 mg daily were increased by 18%, those of **paroxetine** 37.5 or 50 mg daily were decreased by about 27%, but those of **sertraline** 100 or 150 mg daily were unchanged.[3]

(b) Adverse effects

A patient taking **sertraline** 200 mg daily developed akathisia after starting to take aripiprazole 10 mg daily. This did not respond to a reduction in the aripiprazole dose, but gradually resolved when aripiprazole was withdrawn. The authors attributed this effect to an interaction, due to the low incidence of extrapyramidal adverse effects with aripiprazole alone.[4]

Neuroleptic malignant syndrome developed in a patient within 2 weeks of starting aripiprazole 30 mg daily and **fluoxetine** 20 mg daily. The patient had stopped taking aripiprazole 2 days before admission, **fluoxetine** was stopped on admission, and he recovered within one week with symptomatic treatment. The authors suggested that **fluoxetine** might have increased the risk of this syndrome developing by increasing aripiprazole concentrations.[5]

Myxoedema coma (a rare but potentially fatal form of hypothyroidism) developed in a 41-year-old man taking aripiprazole 20 mg daily and **sertraline** 200 mg daily for an unknown duration. The patient was admitted to intensive care, and after 4 days of treatment with levothyroxine and dexamethasone was clinically stable and discharged. Treatment with aripiprazole and **sertraline** was maintained, with the addition of levothyroxine for the hypothyroidism and the patient remained clinically stable 3 months later. Known precipitating causes of myxoedema coma were ruled out by the authors, who concluded that the reaction was due to the concurrent use of aripiprazole and **sertraline** and noted that hypothyroidism is not associated with aripiprazole monotherapy.[6]

Mechanism

Fluoxetine and paroxetine are inhibitors of CYP2D6, by which aripiprazole is partially metabolised, and so decrease aripiprazole metabolism and increase its concentrations. CYP2D6 shows genetic polymorphism, with some people lacking CYP2D6 activity (poor metabolisers). Use of potent CYP2D6 inhibitors in patients who are CYP2D6 extensive metabolisers will, at most, increase aripiprazole exposure to that seen in CYP2D6 poor metabolisers, see also *Quinidine and other CYP2D6 inhibitors*, in 'Aripiprazole + Miscellaneous', p.808. CYP2D6 poor metabolisers would not be affected by these CYP2D6 inhibitors. Citalopram, escitalopram, and sertraline are weaker inhibitors of CYP2D6, and cause smaller increases in aripiprazole concentrations, or have no effect. Note that, in one study,[1] results from patients taking levomepromazine were combined with those from patients taking fluoxetine, but as levomepromazine is not known to be a potent CYP2D6 inhibitor, the true increase seen with fluoxetine might therefore have been underestimated.

Importance and management

Information is limited, but a pharmacokinetic interaction between **fluoxetine** or **paroxetine** and aripiprazole would appear to be established, although the extent requires confirmation in a controlled study. The concurrent use of aripiprazole and an SSRI can be useful, but as increased aripiprazole concentrations can occur with fluoxetine and paroxetine, it would seem prudent to be alert for adverse effects (such as constipation, anxiety, insomnia). The manufacturers recommend that the dose of aripiprazole should be halved if potent CYP2D6 inhibitors, such as fluoxetine and paroxetine, are given.[3,7] In addition, the US manufacturer also recommends a 75% reduction in the aripiprazole dose when both a CYP2D6 inhibitor and a CYP3A4 inhibitor (see 'Aripiprazole + CYP3A4 inhibitors', p.808) are given together.[3]

The UK manufacturer[7] suggests that weaker inhibitors of CYP2D6 would be expected to cause more modest increases in aripiprazole concentrations, and therefore no aripiprazole dose adjustment would be expected to be required. This advice could be reasonably extended to **citalopram**, **escitalopram**, and **sertraline**, which are considered weak CYP2D6 inhibitors, and are therefore unlikely to interact to a clinically relevant extent with aripiprazole by this mechanism.

Fluvoxamine does not inhibit CYP2D6, and is only a weak inhibitor of CYP3A4 (an isoenzyme by which aripiprazole is also partially metabolised), and so would not be expected to affect aripiprazole concentrations to a clinically relevant extent.

An interaction between aripiprazole and SSRIs resulting in extrapyramidal symptoms or hypothyroidism is not established.

1. Castberg I, Spigset O. Effects of comedication on the serum levels of aripiprazole: evidence from a routine therapeutic drug monitoring service. *Pharmacopsychiatry* (2007) 40, 107–10.
2. Waade RB, Christensen H, Rudberg I, Refsum H, Hermann M. Influence of comedication on serum concentrations of aripiprazole and dehydroaripiprazole. *Ther Drug Monit* (2009) 31, 233–8.
3. Abilify (Aripiprazole). Otsuka Pharmaceutical Co, Inc. US Prescribing information, June 2014.
4. Cohen ST, Rulf D, Pies R. Extrapyramidal side effects associated with aripiprazole coprescription in 2 patients. *J Clin Psychiatry* (2005) 66, 135–6.
5. Duggal HS, Kithas J. Possible neuroleptic malignant syndrome with aripiprazole and fluoxetine. *Am J Psychiatry* (2005) 162, 397–8.
6. Church CO, Callen EC. Myxedema coma associated with combined aripiprazole and sertraline therapy. *Ann Pharmacother* (2009) 43, 2113–16.
7. Abilify (Aripiprazole). Otsuka Pharmaceuticals (UK) Ltd. UK Summary of product characteristics, March 2014.

Aripiprazole + Valproate

Valproate slightly reduces aripiprazole exposure, whereas aripiprazole has no effect on valproate exposure.

Clinical evidence

In a controlled study in patients, aripiprazole 30 mg daily for 5 weeks, with **valproate semisodium (divalproex sodium)** daily in doses to achieve serum valproate concentrations of 50 to 125 mg/L, given for weeks 3 to 5 of the study, decreased the maximum plasma concentration of aripiprazole by 26% and decreased its AUC by 24%.[1] Similarly, analysis of results from a routine therapeutic drug monitoring service found that the dose-adjusted serum concentration of aripiprazole in 9 patients also taking valproate, was 24% lower (although this was not statistically significant) than in those taking aripiprazole alone.[2] In contrast, an analysis of results from another routine therapeutic drug monitoring service, found that dose-adjusted serum concentrations of aripiprazole and its active metabolite, dehydroaripiprazole, were unaffected in 26 patients also given valproate.[3]

The US manufacturer notes that aripiprazole 30 mg daily had no effect on the steady-state AUC or maximum concentrations of valproate 1 g daily.[4]

Mechanism

Uncertain. Aripiprazole and valproate share the same protein binding sites, and it was therefore considered likely that the valproate displaced bound aripiprazole leading to increased oral clearance.[1]

Importance and management

Evidence for an interaction between aripiprazole and valproate is limited. However, the slight change in aripiprazole exposure that occurs is not considered to be clinically important, and aripiprazole dose adjustments are not expected to be necessary on the concurrent use of valproate. Similarly, no valproate dose adjustments would be expected to be necessary in the presence of aripiprazole.

1. Citrome L, Josiassen R, Bark N, Salazar DE, Mallikaarjun S. Pharmacokinetics of aripiprazole and concomitant lithium and valproate. *J Clin Pharmacol* (2005) 45, 89–93.
2. Castberg I, Spigset O. Effects of comedication on the serum levels of aripiprazole: evidence from a routine therapeutic drug monitoring service. *Pharmacopsychiatry* (2007) 40, 107–10.
3. Waade RB, Christensen H, Rudberg I, Refsum H, Hermann M. Influence of comedication on serum concentrations of aripiprazole and dehydroaripiprazole. *Ther Drug Monit* (2009) 31, 233–8.
4. Abilify (Aripiprazole). Otsuka and Bristol-Myers Squibb Company. US Prescribing information, February 2012.

Asenapine + Miscellaneous

Fluvoxamine slightly increases asenapine exposure and asenapine increases paroxetine exposure. Carbamazepine, cimetidine, imipramine, lithium, paroxetine, and valproate do not affect the pharmacokinetics of asenapine.. Food and water slightly decrease sublingual asenapine exposure.

Clinical evidence, mechanism, importance and management

(a) Carbamazepine

In a study in healthy subjects, carbamazepine 400 mg twice daily for 15 days reduced the maximum plasma concentration and AUC of a single 5-mg dose of asenapine by 16%. Carbamazepine is a known enzyme inducer, but its effect on asenapine pharmacokinetics is negligible and of no clinical relevance. No asenapine dose adjustment is required on concurrent use.[1]

(b) Cimetidine

In a study in healthy subjects, cimetidine 800 mg twice daily for 8 days reduced the maximum plasma concentration of a single 5-mg dose of asenapine by 13% but had no effect on its AUC. Cimetidine is an inhibitor of several cytochrome P450 isoenzymes including CYP1A2, by which asenapine is partially metabolised; however, this study shows that cimetidine has no clinically relevant effect on asenapine pharmacokinetics. No asenapine dose adjustment is required on concurrent use.[1]

(c) Food

In a crossover study in 26 healthy subjects, eating food immediately before or 4 hours after a single 5-mg sublingual dose of asenapine decreased the exposure to asenapine by 20% and about 10%, respectively. The reductions were thought to be due to increased hepatic blood flow.[1] In a study in 15 healthy subjects, drinking **water** 2 minutes or 5 minutes after a single 10-mg sublingual dose of asenapine reduced the exposure to asenapine by 19% and 10%, respectively.[1,2] Although these changes are slight, the manufacturers advise that patients should not eat or drink for 10 minutes after taking sublingual asenapine.[1,2]

(d) Imipramine

In a study in healthy subjects, a single 75-mg dose of imipramine increased the maximum plasma concentration and AUC of a single 5-mg dose of asenapine by 17% and 10% respectively, and did not affect plasma concentrations of the active metabolite of imipramine, desipramine.[1,2] However, note that single-dose studies are not usually sufficient to maximise enzyme inhibition. The US manufacturer states that no asenapine dose adjustment is expected to be needed on concurrent use.[1]

(e) Lithium

The US manufacturer briefly notes that, in a population pharmacokinetic analysis, lithium had no effect on the pharmacokinetics of asenapine.[1] No asenapine dose adjustment would therefore seem necessary on concurrent use.

(f) SSRIs

1. Fluvoxamine. In a study in healthy subjects, fluvoxamine 25 mg twice daily for 8 days increased the maximum plasma concentration and AUC of a single 5-mg dose of asenapine by 13% and 29%, respectively. Asenapine is partially metabolised by CYP1A2, which is inhibited by fluvoxamine. Although this increase is slight, the manufacturers predict that higher doses of fluvoxamine would be expected to cause greater increases in asenapine concentrations and they therefore advise caution on concurrent use.[1,2] It would seem prudent to be alert for adverse effects, such as drowsiness, dizziness, or increased appetite, if both drugs are given. Other potent CYP1A2 inhibitors might also be expected to increase asenapine concentrations. For a list of CYP1A2 inhibitors, see 'Table 1.2', p.5.

2. Paroxetine. In a study in healthy subjects, paroxetine 20 mg daily for 9 days decreased the maximum plasma concentration and AUC of a single 5-mg dose of asenapine by 13% and 9%, respectively.[1] However, in a study in 15 healthy subjects, when a single 20-mg dose of paroxetine was given with asenapine 5 mg twice daily, the exposure to paroxetine was increased 2-fold.[1,2]

Paroxetine is an inhibitor and substrate of CYP2D6. Data using dextromethorphan as a CYP2D6 probe, indicates that asenapine is a weak CYP2D6 inhibitor (more than 10-fold less potent than paroxetine).[1,2] The manufacturers suggest that the effect of asenapine on paroxetine might be due to asenapine enhancing the inhibitory effect of paroxetine on its own metabolism.[1,2]

No asenapine dose adjustment is required on the concurrent use of paroxetine, but the moderate increase in paroxetine exposure could be clinically relevant. The manufacturers[1,2] advise caution if asenapine is given with drugs that are both substrates and inhibitors of CYP2D6, which would include paroxetine. Bear in mind the possibility of an increase in adverse effects. For the probable lack of effect of asenapine on imipramine, another CYP2D6 substrate that is not a CYP2D6 inhibitor, see under *Imipramine*, above.

3. Other SSRIs. **Citalopram** and **escitalopram** are associated with a dose-related prolongation in the QT interval, as is asenapine. See 'Drugs that prolong the QT interval + Other drugs that prolong the QT interval', p.272, for further information about this effect.

(g) Valproate

In a study in healthy subjects, valproate 500 mg twice daily for 9 days had no effect on the AUC or maximum plasma concentration of a single 5-mg dose of asenapine. Asenapine is partially cleared by glucuronidation by UGT1A4 and valproate is an inhibitor of this enzyme, but this study shows that no pharmacokinetic interaction occurs. No asenapine dose adjustment is required on concurrent use.[1]

1. Saphris (Asenapine). Merck & Co, Inc. US Prescribing information, May 2012.
2. Sycrest (Asenapine maleate). Lundbeck Ltd. UK Summary of product characteristics, October 2011.

Barbiturates + Amfetamines

Dexamfetamine, lisdexamfetamine and amfetamine with dexamfetamine are predicted to delay the absorption of phenobarbital.

Clinical evidence, mechanism, importance and management

The US manufacturers of **dexamfetamine**, **lisdexamfetamine** (a pro-drug of dexamfetamine) and **amfetamine** with **dexamfetamine** (*Adderall* XR) predict that these drugs might delay the intestinal absorption of phenobarbital and that concurrent use could result in a synergistic anticonvulsant affect.[1-3] However, evidence for these effects appears to be limited to *animal* studies from the 1960s which also suggested that the overall anticonvulsant activity of phenobarbital is not affected by amfetamine.[4,5] The general clinical relevance of these effects is difficult to assess, but given the historical nature of the studies cited and the lack of published reports of problems occurring in patients, a clinically important interaction would seem to be unlikely.

1. Dexedrine (Dextroamphetamine sulfate). Amedra Pharmaceuticals LLC. US Prescribing information, October 2013.
2. Vyanase (Lisdexamfetamine dimesylate). Shire US Inc. US Prescribing information, January 2012.
3. Adderall XR (Mixed salts of amphetamine and dextroamphetamine). Shire US Inc. US Prescribing information, April 2015.
4. Frey HH. Note on the interactions of amphetamine with anticonvulsant drugs. *Acta Pharmacol Toxicol (Copenh)* (1964) 21, 290–8.
5. Frey HH, Kampmann E. Interaction of amphetamine with anticonvulsant drugs. II. Effect of amphetamine on the absorption of anticonvulsant drugs. *Acta Pharmacol Toxicol (Copenh)* (1966) 24, 310–16.

Barbiturates + Miscellaneous

Miconazole increases pentobarbital exposure. The hypnotic effects of pentobarbital are reduced or abolished by the concurrent use of caffeine. The CNS depressant effects of barbiturates and nabilone are additive.

Clinical evidence, mechanism, importance and management

(a) Caffeine

In a single-dose, placebo-controlled study in 34 patients, caffeine 250 mg and **pentobarbital** 100 mg were given together and alone. It was found that the hypnotic effects of **pentobarbital** were reduced in the presence of caffeine, and indistinguishable from those of placebo.[1] Caffeine stimulates the cerebral cortex and impairs sleep, whereas **pentobarbital** depresses the cortex and promotes sleep. These mutually opposing actions would seem to explain this interaction. This seems to be the only direct study of this interaction, but it is well supported by common experience and numerous studies of the properties of each of these compounds. Patients given barbiturate hypnotics should avoid caffeine-containing drinks (tea, coffee, cola drinks, etc.) or analgesics at or near bedtime if the hypnotic is to be effective.

(b) Miconazole

High-dose intravenous pentobarbital was given to 5 patients in intensive care to decrease intracranial pressure. When miconazole was also given, all patients had sizeable increases in the plasma concentration of **pentobarbital**, and a 50 to 90% reduction in its total plasma clearance. This effect is thought to occur because miconazole inhibits the liver enzymes concerned with the metabolism of the barbiturate, thereby reducing its clearance from the body.[2] It would be prudent to monitor the effects of concurrent use to ensure that the plasma concentrations of pentobarbital do not rise too high. Note that miconazole oral gel can be absorbed in sufficient amounts to potentially interact and therefore some caution is also warranted with this product.

(c) Nabilone

The manufacturer briefly notes, that in a study in 15 patients, the CNS depressant effects of nabilone and **secobarbital sodium** were found to be additive and advises caution if nabilone is given with any CNS depressant.[3]

1. Forrest WH, Bellville JW, Brown BW. The interaction of caffeine with pentobarbital as a nighttime hypnotic. *Anesthesiology* (1972) 36, 37–41.
2. Heinemeyer G, Roots I, Schulz H, Dennhardt R. Hemmung der Pentobarbital-Elimination durch Miconazol bei Intesivtherapie des erhöhten intracraniellen Druckes. *Intensivmed* (1985) 22, 164–7.
3. Cesamet (Nabilone). Meda Pharmaceuticals Inc. US Prescribing information, April 2011.

Benzodiazepines and related drugs + Acetazolamide

Although acetazolamide can be used to treat acute mountain sickness at very high altitudes, and a study suggests concurrent use with temazepam has a beneficial effect on sleep, a case report suggests that it might potentiate the respiratory depressant effects of benzodiazepines such as triazolam. Acetazolamide did not improve symptoms of sleep apnoea worsened by flurazepam.

Clinical evidence, mechanism, importance and management

A study in elderly subjects found that sleep apnoea worsened in 4 of 10 subjects given a single 30-mg dose of **flurazepam** at night. These 4 subjects were then pretreated with acetazolamide 500 mg twice daily for 3 days, as acetazolamide has been found to improve sleep apnoea. A further dose of **flurazepam** 30 mg was given on the fourth night.[1] Treatment with acetazolamide did not block the benzodiazepine-associated increase in sleep apnoea in these subjects, possibly because the acetazolamide treatment period was not long enough.[1]

Acetazolamide is sometimes used by climbers at very high altitudes as a prophylactic against acute mountain sickness. Benzodiazepines are also used in this situation, to treat insomnia, which is common at high altitude. However, benzodiazepines are believed to depress breathing because they reduce the normal respiratory response to hypoxia. This was demonstrated by a Japanese climber in the Himalayas who took acetazolamide 500 mg daily and **triazolam** 500 micrograms, and then needed to be reminded to hyperventilate in order to relieve his hypoxia while returning from a climb. The acetazolamide did not prevent, and may possibly have increased, the central ventilatory depression of the **triazolam**, possibly by increasing its delivery to the brain. The authors of the report advise against taking these two drugs together at high altitudes,[2] thus confirming a previous warning about the risks of taking benzodiazepines at high altitude.[3] In contrast, a study in 6 climbers in the Himalayas found an improvement in sleep at altitudes below 4000 metres in 3 climbers taking acetazolamide compared with 3 taking placebo, but at altitudes greater than 4000 metres, sleep was still markedly disturbed in all climbers. At altitudes above 4000 metres, **temazepam** 10 mg for one night, improved sleep in all subjects compared with placebo for one night. In the 3 subjects taking acetazolamide and **temazepam**, sleep-onset latency was reduced and sleep efficiency increased, close to that of sea level values.[4]

Although it has been suggested that acetazolamide, **temazepam**, **zolpidem**, and **zaleplon** appear to be safe and effective for improving sleep at high altitude, there is insufficient evidence to recommend the concurrent use of acetazolamide and a hypnotic.[5] Further studies are required to determine whether such combination therapy is safe and has any benefit over acetazolamide alone.

1. Guilleminault C, Silvestri R, Mondini S, Coburn S. Aging and sleep apnea: action of benzodiazepine, acetazolamide, alcohol, and sleep deprivation in a healthy elderly group. *J Gerontol* (1984) 39, 655–61.
2. Masuyama S, Hirata K, Saito A. 'Ondine's curse': side effect of acetazolamide? *Am J Med* (1989) 86, 637.
3. Sutton JR, Powles ACP, Gray GW, Houston CS. Insomnia, sedation, and high altitude cerebral oedema. *Lancet* (1979) i, 165.
4. Nicholson AN, Smith PA, Stone BM, Bradwell AR, Coote JH. Altitude insomnia: studies during an expedition to the Himalayas. *Sleep* (1988) 11, 354–61.
5. Luks AM. Which medications are safe and effective for improving sleep at high altitude? *High Alt Med Biol* (2008) 9, 195–8.

Benzodiazepines + Alosetron

Alosetron does not alter the pharmacokinetics of alprazolam.

Clinical evidence, mechanism, importance and management

In a study in 12 healthy subjects, alosetron 1 mg twice daily for 2 days had no effect on the pharmacokinetics of a single 1-mg dose of alprazolam. No increase in adverse effects was noted with the combination.[1] No alprazolam dose adjustment therefore seems necessary on concurrent use. Note that this study suggests that alosetron is unlikely to affect the pharmacokinetics of similarly metabolised benzodiazepines (such as **midazolam** and **triazolam**), but this needs confirmation as these other benzodiazepines are more sensitive CYP3A4 substrates than **alprazolam**.

1. D'Souza DL, Levasseur LM, Nezamis J, Robbins DK, Simms L, Koch KM. Effect of alosetron on the pharmacokinetics of alprazolam. *J Clin Pharmacol* (2001) 41, 452–4.

Benzodiazepines + Amiodarone

An isolated report describes clonazepam toxicity, which was attributed to the concurrent use of amiodarone. Amiodarone is predicted to inhibit the metabolism of midazolam, triazolam, and possibly alprazolam.

Clinical evidence

A 78-year-old man with congestive heart failure and coronary artery disease was taking furosemide, potassium, and calcium supplements, a multivitamin preparation, and amiodarone 200 mg daily for sustained ventricular tachycardia. Two months after **clonazepam** 500 micrograms at night was added to treat restless leg syndrome he developed slurred speech, confusion, difficulty in walking, dry mouth and urinary incontinence. This was interpreted as **clonazepam** toxicity. The problems cleared when the **clonazepam** was stopped.[1]

Mechanism

It has been suggested that amiodarone might have inhibited the oxidative metabolism of clonazepam, thereby allowing it to accumulate. Note that amiodarone is an inhibitor of CYP3A4, which is predicted to be involved in clonazepam metabolism. The authors of the report also point out that this patient might have been more sensitive to these effects because of a degree of hypothyroidism caused by the amiodarone. Hypothyroidism is known to decrease the metabolism of drugs that undergo oxidative metabolism by the liver.[1]

Importance and management

Evidence for an interaction between amiodarone and the benzodiazepines is limited. The report with clonazepam is an unconfirmed and isolated case, although what occurred does fit with the predicted mechanism. The UK manufacturer of amiodarone reasonably predicts that amiodarone might raise the levels of **midazolam** and **triazolam**, both of which are extensively metabolised via CYP3A4.[2] **Alprazolam** might be similarly affected. It would therefore seem prudent to be alert for evidence of increased and/or prolonged sedation if patients taking amiodarone are given these benzodiazepines. Note that, because of the very long half-life of amiodarone, it is likely that its effects will take a number of weeks to become maximal, and a similar length of time to diminish after stopping the drug.

1. Witt DM, Ellsworth AJ, Leversee JH. Amiodarone–clonazepam interaction. *Ann Pharmacother* (1993) 27, 1463–4.
2. Cordarone X (Amiodarone hydrochloride). Zentiva. UK Summary of product characteristics, April 2014.

Benzodiazepines + Amisulpride

Amisulpride does not appear to alter the effects of lorazepam.

Clinical evidence, mechanism, importance and management

A single-dose study in 18 healthy subjects found that amisulpride 50 mg or 200 mg did not potentiate or antagonise the effects of a single 2-mg dose of lorazepam on psychomotor performance or memory.[1] However, both amisulpride and the benzodiazepines are known to cause drowsiness and therefore some caution is probably warranted on their concurrent use.

1. Perault MC, Bergougnan L, Paillat A, Zieleniuk I, Rosenzweig P, Vandel B. Lack of interaction between amisulpride and lorazepam on psychomotor performance and memory in healthy volunteers. *Hum Psychopharmacol* (1998) 13, 493–500.

Benzodiazepines + Antacids

Antacids can reduce the rate of absorption of chlordiazepoxide, clorazepate, and diazepam. The speed of onset of sedation with diazepam and midazolam might be altered by antacids and the level of sedation with midazolam might be increased.

Clinical evidence

(a) Chlordiazepoxide

In a crossover study in 10 healthy subjects, the absorption of a single 25-mg dose of chlordiazepoxide was delayed by 100 mL of *Maalox* (**aluminium/magnesium hydroxide** mixture), compared with administration with 100 mL of water, but the total amount of drug absorbed was not affected to a clinically relevant extent.[1]

(b) Clorazepate

In a three-period study, 10 healthy subjects were given clorazepate 7.5 mg at night, with either water, *Maalox* (**aluminium/magnesium hydroxide** mixture) 30 mL, or *Maalox* 30 mL three times daily before meals. The mean steady-state plasma concentration of the active metabolite of clorazepate, nordazepam, was not affected by *Maalox*, although it varied widely between individuals.[2] This is in line with another report,[3] but contrasts with a single-dose study, in which the maximum plasma concentration of nordazepam was delayed and reduced by about one-third by the use of *Maalox*. The AUC_{0-48} was reduced by about 10%.[4]

(c) Diazepam

In a crossover study in 9 healthy subjects, the absorption of a single 5-mg dose of diazepam was delayed by 60 mL of **aluminium hydroxide**-containing antacids (*Maalox* and *Gelusil*), compared with 60 mL of water, but the total amount of drug absorbed was not affected to a clinically relevant extent.[5] However, another study found that 40 mL of **Aluminium Hydroxide Gel BP** marginally hastened the sedative effect of diazepam 10 mg when used as an oral premedication before minor surgery.[6] **Sodium citrate** 30 mL (0.3 mmol/L) had the same effect as aluminium hydroxide,[6] whereas **Magnesium Trisilicate Mixture BPC** 30 mL tended to delay sedation with diazepam.[6]

(d) Midazolam

In a controlled study, 40 children were given midazolam 0.5 mg/kg (intravenous preparation given orally) with either up to 20 mL of **sodium citrate** antacid (pH 4.5) or up to 20 mL of a fruit punch drink (pH 3), as premedication before general anaesthesia. The onset of sedation was shortened by about 4 minutes in the group given midazolam with the antacid.[7] Another study found that the addition of **sodium citrate** 10% improved the palatability of oral midazolam 0.75 mg/kg and increased the level of sedation in children requiring premedication for dental procedures.[8] In another study, **Magnesium Trisilicate Mixture BPC** 30 mL did not affect the bioavailability of a single 15-mg dose of midazolam.[9]

(e) Temazepam

The administration of **Magnesium Trisilicate Mixture BP** 30 mL did not affect the bioavailability of a single 20-mg dose of temazepam.[9]

(f) Triazolam

In a study, 11 dialysis patients were given a single 500-microgram dose of triazolam with 120 mL of water, either alone or with 3.6 g of **aluminium hydroxide** gel, and 11 control subjects not on dialysis, were given a single 500-microgram dose of triazolam with 120 mL water. The maximum plasma concentration of triazolam when taken with water alone was lower in the dialysis patients than the control subjects and the AUC tended to be lower, but the differences were not statistically significant. However, when the dialysis patients took the triazolam with **aluminium hydroxide**, the maximum plasma concentration and AUC of triazolam were increased to the range found in the control subjects.[10]

Mechanism

The delay in the absorption of chlordiazepoxide and diazepam is attributed to the effect of the antacid on gastric emptying. Clorazepate on the other hand is a prodrug, which needs acid conditions in the stomach for conversion by hydrolysis and decarboxylation to its active form, nordazepam. Antacids are presumed to inhibit this conversion by raising the pH of the stomach contents.[11] Midazolam injection has a pH of 3.5 (because solubility is decreased at higher pHs) and increasing the pH to 4.5 allows midazolam's imidazole ring to close making it more lipophilic, resulting in faster absorption across the gastric mucosa.[8] Similarly, the reduced availability of triazolam in the dialysis patients might have been due to the relatively high basal gastric acid secretion in these patients which resulted in the formation of the open ring form. The increase in pH due to antacid might have reduced the hydrolysis of triazolam and increased the bioavailability to the range seen in non-dialysis subjects.[10]

Importance and management

Most of the reports describe single-dose studies, but what is known suggests that no adverse interaction of any clinical importance is likely if antacids are given with chlordiazepoxide, clorazepate, diazepam, midazolam, temazepam or triazolam. Whether the delay in absorption has an undesirable effect in those who only take benzodiazepines during acute episodes of anxiety, and who need rapid relief is uncertain. The slightly increased rate of sedation seen with midazolam and sodium citrate is unlikely to be clinically relevant. Information about other benzodiazepines is lacking. However, no special precautions would be expected to be necessary if antacids are also given.

1. Greenblatt DJ, Shader RI, Harmatz JS, Franke K, Koch-Weser J. Influence of magnesium and aluminum hydroxide mixture on chlordiazepoxide absorption. *Clin Pharmacol Ther* (1976) 19, 234–9.
2. Shader RI, Ciraulo DA, Greenblatt DJ, Harmatz JS. Steady-state plasma desmethyldiazepam during long-term clorazepate use: effect of antacids. *Clin Pharmacol Ther* (1982) 31, 180–3.
3. Chun AHC, Carrigan PJ, Hoffman DJ, Kershner RP, Stuart JD. Effect of antacids on absorption of clorazepate. *Clin Pharmacol Ther* (1977) 22, 329–35.
4. Shader RI, Georgotas A, Greenblatt DJ, Harmatz JS, Allen MD. Impaired absorption of desmethyldiazepam from clorazepate by magnesium aluminum hydroxide. *Clin Pharmacol Ther* (1978) 24, 308–15.
5. Greenblatt DJ, Allen MD, MacLaughlin DS, Harmatz JS, Shader RI. Diazepam absorption: effect of antacids and food. *Clin Pharmacol Ther* (1978) 24, 600–9.
6. Nair SG, Gamble JAS, Dundee JW, Howard PJ. The influence of three antacids on the absorption and clinical action of oral diazepam. *Br J Anaesth* (1976) 48, 1175–80.
7. Lammers CR, Rosner JL, Crockett DE, Chhokra R, Brock-Utne JG. Oral midazolam with an antacid may increase the speed of onset of sedation in children prior to general anaesthesia. *Paediatr Anaesth* (2002) 12, 26–8.
8. Isik B, Baygin Ö, Bodur H. Effect of drinks that are added as flavoring in oral midazolam premedication on sedation success. *Pediatr Anesth* (2008) 18, 494–500. Erratum. *ibid.*, 1016.
9. Elliott P, Dundee JW, Elwood RJ, Collier PS. The influence of H_2 receptor antagonists on the plasma concentrations of midazolam and temazepam. *Eur J Anaesthesiol* (1984) 1, 245–51.
10. Kroboth PD, Smith RB, Silver MR, Rault R, Sorkin MI, Puschett JB, Juhl RP. Effects of end stage renal disease and aluminium hydroxide on triazolam pharmacokinetics. *Br J Clin Pharmacol* (1985) 19, 839–42.
11. Abruzzo CW, Macasieb T, Weinfeld R, Rider JA, Kaplan SA. Changes in the oral absorption characteristics in man of dipotassium clorazepate at normal and elevated gastric pH. *J Pharmacokinet Biopharm* (1977) 5, 377–90.

Benzodiazepines + Antiepileptics; Miscellaneous

Pharmacokinetic interactions have been reported between clobazam and felbamate, and clonazepam and lamotrigine, but not triazolam and tiagabine or clonazepam and felbamate.

Clinical evidence

(a) Felbamate

A retrospective study compared *N*-desmethylclobazam plasma concentration to dose ratios in patients taking **clobazam** and enzyme-inducing antiepileptics, without felbamate (group B, 28 patients) or with felbamate (group C, 16 patients). When compared with 22 patients (group A) receiving **clobazam** alone or with non-enzyme-inducing antiepileptics, the *N*-desmethylclobazam concentration to dose ratio of group B was 2-fold higher and the *N*-desmethylclobazam concentration to dose ratio of group C was 5-fold higher,[1] suggesting that felbamate further increased the effect of enzyme-inducing antiepileptics on **clobazam** metabolism.

In a study in 18 healthy subjects, the pharmacokinetics of **clonazepam** 1 mg every 12 hours were not altered by felbamate 1.2 g every 12 hours for 10 days.[2]

(b) Lamotrigine

The plasma concentrations of **clonazepam** in 4 of 8 patients fell by about 38% when they were also given lamotrigine.[3]

(c) Tiagabine

A single-dose study in healthy subjects did not find any clinically important pharmacodynamic or pharmacokinetic interactions between tiagabine and **triazolam**.[4]

Mechanism

Uncertain. It has been suggested that felbamate inhibits the clearance of *N*-desmethylclobazam.[1]

Importance and management

The clinical relevance of the possible interaction between clobazam and felbamate is uncertain. If these drugs are given be aware that additive sedative or other adverse effects could occur. There might also be a potential interaction between clonazepam and lamotrigine in some patients, but the clinical relevance of the reduction in clonazepam concentration is not known. No pharmacokinetic interaction occurs between single doses of tiagabine and triazolam, or between felbamate and clonazepam.

1. Contin M, Riva R, Albani F, Baruzzi A. Effect of felbamate on clobazam and its metabolite kinetics in patients with epilepsy. *Ther Drug Monit* (1999) 21, 604–8.
2. Colucci R, Glue P, Banfield C, Reidenberg P, Meehan J, Radwanski E, Korduba C, Lin C, Dogterom P, Ebels T, Hendriks G, Jonkman JHG, Affrime M. Effect of felbamate on the pharmacokinetics of clonazepam. *Am J Ther* (1996) 3, 294–7.
3. Eriksson A-S, Hoppu K, Nergårdh A, Boreus L. Pharmacokinetic interactions between lamotrigine and other antiepileptic drugs in children with intractable epilepsy. *Epilepsia* (1996) 37, 769–73.
4. Richens A, Marshall RW, Dirach J, Jansen JA, Snel S, Pedersen PC. Absence of interaction between tiagabine, a new antiepileptic drug, and the benzodiazepine triazolam. *Drug Metabol Drug Interact* (1998) 14, 159–77.

Benzodiazepines and related drugs + Antimuscarinics

Atropine and hyoscine do not affect the absorption or the sedative effects of diazepam, but atropine might slow the absorption of zopiclone.

Clinical evidence, mechanism, importance and management

(a) Diazepam

A study in 8 healthy subjects given a single 10-mg oral dose of diazepam found that serum concentrations of diazepam were not changed by the concurrent use of **atropine** 1 mg or **hyoscine hydrobromide** 1 mg. Furthermore, the sedative effects of diazepam were not altered.[1]

(b) Zopiclone

In 12 healthy subjects the absorption of a single 7.5-mg dose of zopiclone was reduced by intravenous **atropine** 600 micrograms. The mean plasma concentration of zopiclone at one hour was reduced from 22.7 nanograms/mL to 6.5 nanograms/mL and at 2 hours from 49.3 nanograms/mL to 31.9 nanograms/mL by **atropine**. This was presumably due to altered gut motility.[2] The clinical importance of these findings is not known.

1. Gregoretti SM, Uges DRA. Influence of oral atropine or hyoscine on the absorption of oral diazepam. *Br J Anaesth* (1982) 54, 1231–4.
2. Elliott P, Chestnutt WN, Elwood RJ, Dundee JW. Effect of atropine and metoclopramide on the plasma concentrations of orally administered zopiclone. *Br J Anaesth* (1983) 55, 1159P–1160P.

Benzodiazepines + Aprepitant

Aprepitant moderately increases oral midazolam exposure, but appears to have less effect on intravenous midazolam. A few days after aprepitant treatment is stopped a transient slight reduction in midazolam exposure might occur. Triazolam, and to a lesser extent alprazolam, are expected to be affected similarly. Fosaprepitant is a prodrug of aprepitant, and has been shown to slightly increase oral midazolam exposure.

Clinical evidence

(a) Aprepitant

In a randomised study, 16 healthy subjects took either aprepitant 125 mg on day one followed by 80 mg daily for 4 days, or 40 mg on day one followed by 25 mg daily for 4 days, with a single 2-mg oral dose of **midazolam** on days one and 5. The aprepitant 40/25 mg dosing schedule had only minor effects on the pharmacokinetics of **midazolam**. However, the aprepitant 125/80 mg dosing schedule increased the AUC of oral **midazolam** 2.3-fold and 3.3-fold on days one and 5, respectively, and increased the maximum plasma concentration of midazolam by 46% and 94% on days one and 5, respectively.[1]

In a randomised study, 24 healthy subjects were given aprepitant 125 mg on day one then 80 mg daily for a further 2 days, or placebo. A single 2-mg intravenous dose of **midazolam** was given on days 4, 8, and 15. The 3-day aprepitant regimen increased the **midazolam** AUC by 20%, and decreased the clearance by 17% on day 4 when compared with placebo, but on day 8 the AUC was *decreased* by 22%, and the clearance was *increased* by 28.5% when compared with placebo. By day 15 there was no difference between the groups.[2] Another study also found that a single 125-mg oral dose of aprepitant increased the AUC of intravenous **midazolam** by 47%.[3]

(b) Fosaprepitant

The manufacturer notes that in a study, intravenous fosaprepitant 100 mg given over 15 minutes increased the AUC of a single 2-mg oral dose of **midazolam** by 60%.[4] In another study in 10 healthy subjects,[5] a single intravenous dose of fosaprepitant 150 mg given on day one increased the AUC of a single 2-mg oral dose of **midazolam** given on day one by about 80%, but did not affect the AUC of a further dose given on day 4.

Mechanism

Aprepitant is a dose-dependent inhibitor of CYP3A4 by which midazolam is metabolised; concurrent use therefore results in increased midazolam exposure. There appears to be a greater pharmacokinetic effect on oral midazolam than on intravenous midazolam indicating that aprepitant affects intestinal as well as hepatic CYP3A4 activity. Aprepitant is also an inducer of CYP3A4;[2,6] however, the induction is transient, with a maximal effect 3 to 5 days after the end of the usual prescribed 3 days of treatment. In one study described above, the initial increase in midazolam exposure followed by a decrease in exposure, is probably due to initial inhibition of CYP3A4, followed by weak and transient induction of CYP3A4 by aprepitant.[2]

Fosaprepitant is a prodrug of aprepitant, and is predicted to interact similarly. The lesser effect of fosaprepitant is probably due to the differences in recommended dose regimens between oral aprepitant and intravenous fosaprepitant.

Importance and management

Based on the way **midazolam** interacts with other moderate inhibitors of CYP3A4, aprepitant would be expected to increase the drowsiness and length of sedation and amnesia in patients given midazolam. Consider reducing the midazolam dose in patients given aprepitant and monitor the outcome of concurrent use carefully. The manufacturers note that the potential effects of increased exposure to other benzodiazepines metabolised by CYP3A4, such as **alprazolam** and **triazolam**, should be considered if they are given with aprepitant, although note that alprazolam is likely to be less affected than midazolam.[6,7] The UK manufacturer also states that the effects of aprepitant on the plasma concentration of intravenously administered CYP3A4 substrates are expected to be less than its effects on orally administered substrates.[6] The transient weak induction of midazolam metabolism seen after aprepitant was stopped, was not considered clinically relevant, and no precautions would seem necessary once the recommended regimen has been completed.

Although the effect of the single recommended dose of fosaprepitant on midazolam exposure was not considered to be clinically relevant, the manufacturer applies the same caution to fosaprepitant as for aprepitant when it is given with benzodiazepines metabolised by CYP3A4, such as midazolam, alprazolam, or triazolam.[4]

Note that midazolam is used as a probe substrate to assess the activity of drugs on CYP3A4. These studies therefore suggest that, using the recommended therapeutic regimens, aprepitant is a moderate inhibitor of CYP3A4 and a weak inducer (albeit transiently), whereas fosaprepitant is a weak inhibitor of CYP3A4. For a list of CYP3A4 substrates, see 'Table 1.10', p.12.

1. Majumdar AK, McCrea JB, Panebianco DL, Hesney M, Dru J, Constanzer M, Goldberg MR, Murphy G, Gottesdiener KM, Lines CR, Petty KJ, Blum RA. Effects of aprepitant on cytochrome P450 3A4 activity using midazolam as a probe. *Clin Pharmacol Ther* (2003) 74, 150–6.
2. Shadle CR, Lee Y, Majumdar AK, Petty KJ, Gargano C, Bradstreet TE, Evans JK, Blum RA. Evaluation of potential inductive effects of aprepitant on cytochrome P450 3A4 and 2C9 activity. *J Clin Pharmacol* (2004) 44, 215–23.
3. Majumdar AK, Yan KX, Selverian DV, Barlas S, Constanzer M, Dru J, McCrea JB, Ahmed T, Frick GS, Kraft WK, Petty KJ, Greenberg HE. Effect of aprepitant on the pharmacokinetics of intravenous midazolam. *J Clin Pharmacol* (2007) 47, 744–50.
4. EMEND for Injection (Fosaprepitant dimeglumine). Merck & Co., Inc. US Prescribing information, July 2012.
5. Shadle R, Marbury TC, Ngo PL, Jin B, Panebianco D, Caro L, Murphy G. Pharmacokinetics of oral dexamethasone and oral midazolam when coadministered with single-dose intravenous 150 mg fosaprepitant dimeglumine in healthy young adult subjects. *Clin Pharmacol Ther* (2010) 87 (Suppl 1), S85–S86.
6. Emend (Aprepitant). Merck Sharp & Dohme Ltd. UK Summary of product characteristics, November 2011.
7. EMEND Capsules (Aprepitant). Merck & Co., Inc. US Prescribing information, August 2014.

Benzodiazepines + Aspirin

The induction of anaesthesia with intravenous midazolam is more rapid in patients who have been pretreated with intravenous aspirin.

Clinical evidence

A study in patients about to undergo surgery found that pretreatment with aspirin 1 g (given as intravenous **lysine aspirin**) one minute before induction shortened the induction time with intravenous **midazolam** 300 micrograms/kg. Only 60% were 'asleep' within 3 minutes of receiving **midazolam** alone, but about 80% were 'asleep' within 3 minutes of receiving **midazolam** given after the aspirin pretreatment.[1]

Mechanism

Not understood. It has been suggested that aspirin increases the amount of free (and active) midazolam in the plasma because both drugs compete for the binding sites on the plasma albumins.[1,2]

Importance and management

Information is limited but what is known shows that the effects of midazolam are increased by aspirin, but the extent of the effect seems relatively modest, and, if the mechanism is correct, no greater effect would be expected on long-term concurrent use.

1. Dundee JW, Halliday NJ, McMurray TJ. Aspirin and probenecid pretreatment influences the potency of thiopentone and the onset of action of midazolam. *Eur J Anaesthesiol* (1986) 3, 247–51.
2. Halliday NJ, Dundee JW, Collier PS, Howard PJ. Effects of aspirin pretreatment on the *in vitro* serum binding of midazolam. *Br J Clin Pharmacol* (1985) 19, 581P–582P.

Benzodiazepines and related drugs + Azoles; Fluconazole

Fluconazole moderately increases oral midazolam and triazolam exposure, thereby increasing and prolonging their sedative and amnesic effects. Intravenous midazolam is less affected. Fluconazole moderately increases diazepam exposure but has a negligible effect on zolpidem exposure and has no effect on bromazepam exposure.

Clinical evidence

A. Benzodiazepines

(a) Bromazepam

In a study in 12 healthy subjects, fluconazole 100 mg daily for 4 days had no effect on the pharmacokinetics or pharmacodynamics of oral or rectal bromazepam.[1]

(b) Diazepam

A study in healthy subjects found that fluconazole 400 mg on the first day and 200 mg on the second day increased the AUC of a single 5-mg oral dose of diazepam 2.5-fold and prolonged its half-life from 31 hours to 73 hours.[2]

(c) Midazolam

A study in 12 healthy subjects found that fluconazole 400 mg on the first day and then 200 mg daily for 5 days increased the AUC of a single 7.5-mg oral dose of midazolam approximately 3.5-fold both on day one (2 hours after the first dose of fluconazole) and on day 6. It was found that the subjects could hardly be wakened during the first hour after taking the midazolam.[3] A single intravenous dose of midazolam (50 micrograms/kg given on day 4) was not affected to the same extent (51% decrease in clearance, and little change in sedative effect).[3] Another study found that a single 150-mg dose of fluconazole given 2 hours before a single 10-mg dose of midazolam, increased the midazolam plasma concentrations at 30 to 90 minutes by about 40%. There was only a slight increase in the sedative effect of midazolam over the 90 minutes.[4,5] Yet another study found that the route of administration of a single 400-mg dose of fluconazole made little or no difference to the extent of increase in exposure (3.4-fold with intravenous administration and 3.7-fold with oral administration) or the increase in pharmacodynamic effects of oral midazolam.[6] Fluconazole 400 mg initially and then 200 mg daily given by infusion over 30 minutes caused a 2- to 4-fold increase in the plasma concentrations of midazolam in 3 intensive care unit patients receiving stable midazolam infusions; these three patients had some renal impairment. In 7 other similar patients without renal impairment there was either no increase or only a minor increase in midazolam concentrations.[7]

(d) Triazolam

Eight healthy subjects were given fluconazole or a placebo daily for 4 days, with a single 250-microgram dose of oral triazolam on day 4. The AUC of triazolam was increased 1.6-fold, 2.1-fold, and 4.4-fold by 50 mg, 100 mg, and 200 mg fluconazole, respectively, and the maximum plasma concentration of triazolam was more than doubled by the 200-mg dose of fluconazole. The 100- and 200-mg doses of fluconazole both produced marked changes in the psychomotor tests of triazolam, but the 50-mg dose did not.[8]

B. Non-benzodiazepine hypnotics

(a) Zolpidem

In a placebo-controlled study in healthy subjects, fluconazole 100 mg twice daily for 2 days had only a small effect on the pharmacokinetics of a single 5-mg dose of zolpidem given after the third dose of fluconazole: the zolpidem AUC was increased by 31%, but this was not statistically significant. The pharmacodynamic effects of zolpidem were not altered by fluconazole.[9]

Mechanism

Fluconazole is an inhibitor of CYP3A4. The benzodiazepines, zopiclone and zolpidem are, to varying degrees, metabolised by CYP3A4, with the extent of the interaction related to how significant CYP3A4 is in their metabolism and how potent a CYP3A4 inhibitor the azole is. So, for example midazolam, which is predominantly metabolised by CYP3A4, is affected most. Other isoenzymes are also involved in the metabolism of zolpidem so it is only affected by CYP3A4 inhibitors to a limited extent. Similarly, diazepam is extensively metabolised by CYP2C19 and also CYP3A4, and so fluconazole, which inhibits both CYP2C19 and CYP3A4, can moderately decrease the elimination of diazepam.

Importance and management

The interactions between midazolam or triazolam and fluconazole are established and clinically important, and if concurrent use is undertaken, the dose of midazolam or triazolam should probably be reduced, possibly by as much as half. There is some evidence that the exposure to bolus doses of intravenous midazolam given in the presence of fluconazole are not increased to a clinically relevant extent and normal doses can be used. However, where high doses of intravenous midazolam are used long term (e.g. during intensive care treatment) it has been suggested that the dose will need to be titrated to avoid long-lasting hypnotic effects.[3,7]

Exposure to diazepam, given in single doses, is also moderately increased by fluconazole and a dose reduction might similarly be required.

Note that midazolam is used as a probe substrate to assess the activity of other drugs on CYP3A4. The data here therefore suggest that fluconazole is a moderate inhibitor of CYP3A4. For a list of CYP3A4 substrates, see 'Table 1.10', p.12.

1. Ohtani Y, Kotegawa T, Tsutsumi K, Morimoto T, Hirose Y, Nakano S. Effect of fluconazole on the pharmacokinetics and pharmacodynamics of oral and rectal bromazepam: an application of electroencephalography as the pharmacodynamic method. *J Clin Pharmacol* (2002) 42, 183–91.
2. Saari TI, Laine K, Bertilsson L, Neuvonen PJ, Olkkola KT. Voriconazole and fluconazole increase the exposure to oral diazepam. *Eur J Clin Pharmacol* (2007) 63, 941–9.
3. Olkkola KT, Ahonen J, Neuvonen PJ. The effect of the systemic antimycotics, itraconazole and fluconazole, on the pharmacokinetics and pharmacodynamics of intravenous and oral midazolam. *Anesth Analg* (1996) 82, 511–16.
4. Mattila MJ, Vainio P, Vanakoski J. Fluconazole moderately increases midazolam effects on performance. *Br J Clin Pharmacol* (1995) 39, 567P.
5. Vanakoski J, Mattila MJ, Vainio P, Idänpään-Heikkilä JJ, Törnwall M. 150 mg fluconazole does not substantially increase the effects of 10 mg midazolam or the plasma midazolam concentrations in healthy subjects. *Int J Clin Pharmacol Ther* (1995) 33, 518–23.
6. Ahonen J, Olkkola KT, Neuvonen PJ. Effect of route of administration of fluconazole on the interaction between fluconazole and midazolam. *Eur J Clin Pharmacol* (1997) 51, 415–19.
7. Ahonen J, Olkkola KT, Takala A, Neuvonen PJ. Interaction between fluconazole and midazolam in intensive care patients. *Acta Anaesthesiol Scand* (1999) 43, 509–14.
8. Varhe A, Olkkola KT, Neuvonen PJ. Effect of fluconazole dose on the extent of fluconazole-triazolam interaction. *Br J Clin Pharmacol* (1996) 42, 465–70.
9. Greenblatt DJ, von Moltke LL, Harmatz JS, Mertzanis P, Graf JA, Durol ALB, Counihan M, Roth-Schechter B, Shader RI. Kinetic and dynamic interaction study of zolpidem with ketoconazole, itraconazole, and fluconazole. *Clin Pharmacol Ther* (1998) 64, 661–71.

Benzodiazepines and related drugs + Azoles; Itraconazole or Ketoconazole

Itraconazole and ketoconazole markedly, or very markedly, increase midazolam and triazolam exposure, thereby increasing and prolonging

the sedative and amnesic effects of these benzodiazepines. Moderate increases in benzodiazepine exposure are seen with itraconazole or ketoconazole and alprazolam and with itraconazole and brotizolam. Even less effect (a slight increase in exposure) is seen with itraconazole and etizolam. Itraconazole has only a negligible effect on diazepam exposure.

Ketoconazole or itraconazole cause slight to moderate increases in the exposure to the non-benzodiazepine hypnotics, zolpidem, eszopiclone, and zopiclone.

No important interaction appears to occur between itraconazole and estazolam, quazepam or temazepam; and probably between ketoconazole and chlordiazepoxide.

Clinical evidence

A. Itraconazole

(a) Benzodiazepines

1. Alprazolam. In a study, 10 healthy subjects were given a single 800-microgram dose of alprazolam before and after itraconazole 200 mg daily for 6 days. Itraconazole increased the AUC and the half-life of alprazolam nearly 3-fold, and psychomotor function was impaired.[1]

2. Brotizolam. In a placebo-controlled study, 10 healthy subjects were given itraconazole 200 mg daily for 4 days with a single 500-microgram dose of brotizolam on day 4. Itraconazole increased the AUC_{0-24} and maximum plasma concentration of brotizolam about 2.5-fold and by 25%, respectively. The elimination half-life of brotizolam was also increased, from 4.51 hours to 23.27 hours, and sedation was increased.[2]

3. Diazepam. In a study in 10 healthy subjects, itraconazole 200 mg daily for 4 days increased the AUC of a single 5-mg oral dose of diazepam by about 15%, but there was no clinically significant effect as determined by psychomotor performance tests.[3]

4. Estazolam. A placebo-controlled study in 10 healthy subjects[4] found that itraconazole 100 mg daily for 7 days did not affect the pharmacokinetics or pharmacodynamics of a single 4-mg dose of estazolam given on day 4.

5. Etizolam. A placebo-controlled study in healthy subjects found that itraconazole 100 mg twice daily for 7 days increased the AUC of a single 1-mg dose of etizolam given on day 6 by about 50%. The elimination half-life of etizolam was also increased, from 12 hours to 17.3 hours.[5]

6. Midazolam. When 9 healthy subjects were given oral midazolam 7.5 mg, before and after taking itraconazole 200 mg daily for 4 days, the AUC of midazolam was increased about 10-fold, the maximum plasma concentration was increased about 3-fold, and the half-life was prolonged, from 2.8 hours to 7.9 hours. The subjects could hardly be wakened during the first hour after taking the midazolam and most of them experienced amnesia lasting several hours.[6] A later study found that itraconazole 100 mg daily for 4 days increased the AUC of oral midazolam 6-fold and increased its maximum plasma concentration 2.5-fold.[7] In a further study, subjects were given itraconazole 200 mg daily for 4 days with a single 7.5-mg dose of midazolam on days 4 and 8. Itraconazole increased the AUC of midazolam 8-fold when the midazolam was taken on day 4, and 2.6-fold when the midazolam was taken on day 8.[8]

Another study confirmed the marked effect of itraconazole on oral midazolam, but found that the effects of bolus doses of intravenous midazolam were not increased to a clinically significant extent, although their results suggested that long-term, high-dose infusions of midazolam need to be titrated according to effect to avoid overdose.[9] The manufacturer of midazolam reports that itraconazole increased the plasma concentration of intravenous midazolam 2- to 3-fold and increased its terminal half-life 2.4-fold.[10]

7. Quazepam. Ten healthy subjects were given itraconazole 50 mg twice daily or placebo for 14 days, with a single 20-mg dose of quazepam on day 4. Itraconazole did not affect the pharmacokinetics of quazepam, but the maximum plasma concentration and AUC of its two active metabolites, 2-oxoquazepam and *N*-desalkyl-2-oxoquazepam were decreased. However, psychomotor tests were not affected in the presence of itraconazole.[11]

8. Temazepam. In a study, 10 healthy subjects were given itraconazole 200 mg daily for 4 days, with a single 20-mg dose of temazepam on day 4. Itraconazole caused a very small increase in the AUC of temazepam, but psychomotor tests were unchanged.[12]

9. Triazolam. In a study in 9 healthy subjects, the AUC of a single 250-microgram dose of triazolam was increased about 28-fold by itraconazole 200 mg daily for 4 days. Maximum plasma concentrations were increased 3-fold. Marked changes in psychomotor and other responses were also seen. The subjects had amnesia and were still very tired and confused as long as 17 hours after taking triazolam.[13] Another study found that the interaction persists for several days after taking itraconazole.[14]

(b) Non-benzodiazepine hypnotics

1. Zolpidem. In a placebo-controlled study, 10 healthy subjects were given itraconazole 200 mg daily for 4 days with a single 10-mg oral dose of zolpidem on day 4. The maximum plasma concentration of zolpidem was increased by 11% and the AUC was increased by 34%, but the performance of a number of psychomotor tests (digit symbol substitution, critical flicker fusion, subjective drowsiness, postural sway) remained unaltered.[15] Another study similarly found that itraconazole did not interact with zolpidem to a clinically relevant extent.[16]

2. Zopiclone. In a placebo-controlled study, 10 healthy subjects were given itraconazole 200 mg daily for 4 days with a single 7.5-mg oral dose of zopiclone on day 4. Itraconazole increased the maximum plasma concentration of zopiclone by 29%, increased its AUC by 73%, and prolonged its half-life from 5 hours to 7 hours. Despite these increases, there were no statistical or clinical differences between the performance of psychomotor tests carried out during the placebo and itraconazole phases of the study.[17]

B. Ketoconazole

(a) Benzodiazepines

1. Alprazolam. A study in healthy subjects found that ketoconazole 200 mg twice daily decreased the clearance of alprazolam 1 mg by about two-thirds, and prolonged its half-life 4-fold; the maximum plasma concentration was only slightly increased, but the AUC increased almost 4-fold.[18]

2. Chlordiazepoxide. In 12 healthy subjects, ketoconazole 400 mg daily for 5 days decreased the clearance of chlordiazepoxide 600 micrograms/kg by 38%.[19]

3. Midazolam. When 9 healthy subjects were given oral midazolam 7.5 mg before and after taking ketoconazole 400 mg daily for 4 days, the AUC of midazolam was increased almost 17-fold, its maximum plasma concentration was increased about 4-fold, and its half-life was prolonged, from 2.8 hours to 8.7 hours. The subjects could hardly be wakened during the first hour after taking the midazolam and most of them experienced amnesia lasting several hours.[6] A study in healthy subjects found that three doses of oral ketoconazole 200 mg increased the AUC of a single 6-mg dose of oral midazolam 16-fold, but only increased the AUC of a single 2-mg dose of intravenous midazolam 5-fold.[20] In another study in healthy subjects, ketoconazole 400 mg daily for one, 2, or 5 days increased the AUCs of single doses of midazolam 2 mg given on day one, 2, or 5, about 10-, 13-, and 14-fold, respectively. The maximum plasma concentration was increased about 5-fold in each case, and the terminal half-life was increased from 2.6 hours when midazolam was given alone, to 4.9, 6.1, and 6.9 hours after one, 2 or 5 days of ketoconazole, respectively.[21] Another study found that the increase in the AUC of oral and intravenous midazolam was much greater after ketoconazole 400 mg for 7 days (15-fold and 4.2-fold, respectively) than after ketoconazole 200 mg daily for 7 days (11-fold and 3.4-fold, respectively).[22] Ketoconazole has been shown to reduce the metabolism of midazolam and greatly prolong its effects in further studies.[23-25]

4. Triazolam. A study in healthy subjects found that when they were given triazolam 125 micrograms, after ketoconazole 200 mg taken 17 hours and one hour earlier, the triazolam half-life was prolonged (from 4 hours to almost 18 hours in one subject) and the clearance was reduced 9-fold. Pharmacodynamic testing found an increase in the impairment of a digit-symbol substitution test, and there were increased effects on EEG beta activity.[26] In another study, the AUC of a single 250-microgram dose of triazolam was increased about 23-fold by ketoconazole 400 mg daily for 4 days. The maximum plasma concentration was increased 3-fold. Marked changes in psychomotor and other responses were seen. The subjects had amnesia and were still very tired and confused as long as 17 hours after taking the triazolam.[13] A further study similarly found that ketoconazole inhibited the metabolism of triazolam leading to an increase in its sedative effects.[27]

(b) Non-benzodiazepine hypnotics

1. Eszopiclone. In a multiple-dose, crossover study in 18 healthy subjects, ketoconazole 400 mg increased the AUC of eszopiclone 3 mg 2.2-fold and increased its maximum plasma concentration by 40%. The AUC of ketoconazole was decreased by 12% with concurrent eszopiclone, but this was not considered to be clinically important.[28]

2. Zolpidem. A study in 12 healthy subjects found that ketoconazole 200 mg twice daily for 2 days increased the AUC of a single 5-mg oral dose of zolpidem by 70% and the subjects were more sedated, as shown by the digit symbol substitution test.[16]

Mechanism

Itraconazole and ketoconazole are inhibitors of CYP3A4. The benzodiazepines and zopiclone and zolpidem are, to varying degrees, metabolised by CYP3A4, with the extent of the interaction related to how significant CYP3A4 is in their metabolism and how potent a CYP3A4 inhibitor the azole is. So, for example midazolam, which is predominantly metabolised by CYP3A4, is greatly affected by potent inhibitors (e.g. itraconazole), whereas CYP3A4 is not a significant route in the metabolism of temazepam, so it is only slightly affected. Other isoenzymes are also involved in the metabolism of zolpidem, and to some extent zopiclone, so they are only moderately affected by CYP3A4 inhibitors. Similarly, diazepam is extensively metabolised by CYP2C19 and also CYP3A4, and so itraconazole has only a minor effect on its metabolism.

The azoles inhibit CYP3A4 in the liver (hence intravenous benzodiazepines can be affected), but studies have also suggested that ketoconazole inhibits the metabolism of midazolam[20,23] and triazolam[27] by CYP3A4 in the gut wall, which explains why these benzodiazepines, which undergo significant first-pass metabolism, are more affected when given orally than when given intravenously.

Ketoconazole appears to partially inhibit the oxidation of chlordiazepoxide by the liver.[19]

Importance and management

The interactions between **midazolam** or **triazolam** and itraconazole or ketoconazole are established and clinically important. In very broad terms the dose of midazolam would need to be reduced by about 75% or more in the presence of these azoles to avoid excessive sedation, and even then the effects would still be expected to be prolonged. Unless appropriate precautions are taken (very reduced doses with careful monitoring and management) these interactions can be dangerous: most manufacturers contraindicate the concurrent use of oral midazolam or triazolam with itraconazole or ketoconazole. Patients taking these azoles should be warned about the likelihood of increased and prolonged sedation and advised not to drive (for example) after receiving midazolam until completely recovered. One study found that patients are not likely to be capable of tasks such as driving for at least 6 hours after the dose of the benzodiazepine,[9] but it could be substantially longer especially after multiple doses of these azoles. There is some evidence that bolus doses of intravenous midazolam given in the presence of itraconazole are not increased to a clinically relevant extent, and normal doses can be used. However, where high doses of intravenous midazolam are used long term (e.g. during intensive care treatment) it has been suggested that the dose will need to be titrated to avoid long-lasting hypnotic effects.[9]

The effects of **alprazolam** and **brotizolam** are increased and prolonged by ketoconazole and itraconazole, but the extent of this is less than that seen with midazolam or triazolam. However, dose reductions might still be necessary: most manufacturers suggest caution, but a few have contraindicated the concurrent use of these azoles and benzodiazepines.

Diazepam, in single doses, is not affected by itraconazole to a clinically relevant extent. **Eszopiclone** (and therefore probably **zopiclone**) is slightly to moderately affected by itraconazole and ketoconazole and it might be necessary to reduce the dose.

The effects of itraconazole on **etizolam**, **quazepam**, **temazepam**, or **zolpidem**, and ketoconazole on **chlordiazepoxide** or zolpidem are negligible to slight and seem unlikely to be clinically relevant in most patients.

Note that midazolam is used as a probe substrate to assess the activity of other drugs on CYP3A4. The data here therefore suggest that ketoconazole and itraconazole are potent inhibitors of CYP3A4. For a list of CYP3A4 substrates, see 'Table 1.10', p.12.

1. Yasui N, Kondo T, Otani K, Furukori H, Kaneko S, Ohkubo T, Nagasaki T, Sugawara K. Effect of itraconazole on the single oral dose pharmacokinetics and pharmacodynamics of alprazolam. *Psychopharmacology (Berl)* (1998) 139, 269–73.
2. Osanai T, Ohkubo T, Yasui N, Kondo T, Kaneko S. Effect of itraconazole on the pharmacokinetics and pharmacodynamics of a single dose of brotizolam. *Br J Clin Pharmacol* (2004) 58, 476–81.
3. Ahonen J, Olkkola KT, Neuvonen PJ. The effect of the antimycotic itraconazole on the pharmacokinetics and pharmacodynamics of diazepam. *Fundam Clin Pharmacol* (1996) 10, 314–18.
4. Otsuji Y, Okuyama N, Aoshima T, Fukasawa T, Kato K, Gerstenberg G, Miura M, Ohkubo T, Sugawara K, Otani K. No effect of itraconazole on the single oral dose pharmacokinetics and pharmacodynamics of estazolam. *Ther Drug Monit* (2002) 24, 375–8.
5. Araki K, Yasui-Furukori N, Fukasawa T, Aoshima T, Suzuki A, Inoue Y, Tateishi T, Otani K. Inhibition of the metabolism of etizolam by itraconazole in humans: evidence for the involvement of CYP3A4 in etizolam metabolism. *Eur J Clin Pharmacol* (2004) 60, 427–30.
6. Olkkola KT, Backman JT, Neuvonen PJ. Midazolam should be avoided in patients receiving systemic antimycotics ketoconazole or itraconazole. *Clin Pharmacol Ther* (1994) 55, 481–5.
7. Ahonen J, Olkkola KT, Neuvonen PJ. Effect of itraconazole and terbinafine on the pharmacokinetics and pharmacodynamics of midazolam in healthy volunteers. *Br J Clin Pharmacol* (1995) 40, 270–2.
8. Backman JT, Kivistö KT, Olkkola KT, Neuvonen PJ. The area under the plasma concentration-time curve for oral midazolam is 400-fold larger during treatment with itraconazole than with rifampicin. *Eur J Clin Pharmacol* (1998) 54, 53–8.
9. Olkkola KT, Ahonen J, Neuvonen PJ. The effect of the systemic antimycotics, itraconazole and fluconazole, on the pharmacokinetics and pharmacodynamics of intravenous and oral midazolam. *Anesth Analg* (1996) 82, 511–16.
10. Hypnovel (Midazolam hydrochloride). Roche Products Ltd. UK Summary of product characteristics, March 2010.
11. Kato K, Yasui-Furukori N, Fukasawa T, Aoshima T, Suzuki A, Kanno M, Otani K. Effects of itraconazole on the plasma kinetics of quazepam and its two active metabolites after a single oral dose of the drug. *Ther Drug Monit* (2003) 25, 473–7.
12. Ahonen J, Olkkola KT, Neuvonen PJ. Lack of effect of antimycotic itraconazole on the pharmacokinetics or pharmacodynamics of temazepam. *Ther Drug Monit* (1996) 18, 124–7.
13. Varhe A, Olkkola KT, Neuvonen PJ. Oral triazolam is potentially hazardous to patients receiving systemic antimycotics ketoconazole or itraconazole. *Clin Pharmacol Ther* (1994) 56, 601–7.
14. Neuvonen PJ, Varhe A, Olkkola KT. The effect of ingestion time interval on the interaction between itraconazole and triazolam. *Clin Pharmacol Ther* (1996) 60, 326–31.
15. Luurila H, Kivistö KT, Neuvonen PJ. Effect of itraconazole on the pharmacokinetics and pharmacodynamics of zolpidem. *Eur J Clin Pharmacol* (1998) 54, 163–6.
16. Greenblatt DJ, von Moltke LL, Harmatz JS, Mertzanis P, Graf JA, Durol ALB, Counihan M, Roth-Schechter B, Shader RI. Kinetic and dynamic interaction study of zolpidem with ketoconazole, itraconazole, and fluconazole. *Clin Pharmacol Ther* (1998) 64, 661–71.
17. Jalava K-M, Olkkola KT, Neuvonen PJ. Effect of itraconazole on the pharmacokinetics and pharmacodynamics of zopiclone. *Eur J Clin Pharmacol* (1996) 51, 331–4.
18. Greenblatt DJ, Wright CE, von Moltke LL, Harmatz JS, Ehrenberg BL, Harrel LM, Corbett K, Counihan M, Tobias S, Shader RI. Ketoconazole inhibition of triazolam and alprazolam clearance: differential kinetic and dynamic consequences. *Clin Pharmacol Ther* (1998) 64, 237–47.
19. Brown MW, Maldonado AL, Meredith CG, Speeg KV. Effect of ketoconazole on hepatic oxidative drug metabolism. *Clin Pharmacol Ther* (1985) 37, 290–7.
20. Tsunoda SM, Velez RL, von Moltke LL, Greenblatt DJ. Differentiation of intestinal and hepatic cytochrome P450 3A activity with use of midazolam as an in vivo probe: effect of ketoconazole. *Clin Pharmacol Ther* (1999) 66, 461–71.
21. Stoch SA, Friedman E, Maes A, Yee K, Xu Y, Larson P, Fitzgerald M, Chodakewitz J, Wagner JA. Effect of different durations of ketoconazole dosing on the single-dose pharmacokinetics of midazolam: shortening the paradigm. *J Clin Pharmacol* (2009) 49, 398–406.
22. Lucksiri A, Vuppalanchi R, Hilligoss JK, Hamman MA, Li L, Chien JY, Huang S, Hall SD. Dose dependent inhibition of midazolam elimination by ketoconazole: effect of CYP3A5 genotype. *Clin Pharmacol Ther* (2005) 77, P35.
23. Lam YWF, Alfaro CL, Ereshefsky L, Miller M. Pharmacokinetic and pharmacodynamic interactions of oral midazolam with ketoconazole, fluoxetine, fluvoxamine, and nefazodone. *J Clin Pharmacol* (2003) 43, 1274–82.
24. Chen M, Nafziger AN, Bertino JS. Drug-metabolizing enzyme inhibition by ketoconazole does not reduce interindividual variability of CYP3A activity as measured by oral midazolam. *Drug Metab Dispos* (2006) 34, 2079–82.
25. Krishna G, Moton A, Ma L, Savant I, Martinho M, Seiberling M, McLeod J. Effects of oral posaconazole on the pharmacokinetic properties of oral and intravenous midazolam: a phase I, randomized, open-label, crossover study in healthy volunteers. *Clin Ther* (2009) 31, 286–98.
26. Greenblatt DJ, von Moltke LL, Harmatz JS, Harrel LM, Tobias S, Shader RI, Wright CE. Interaction of triazolam and ketoconazole. *Lancet* (1995) 345, 191.
27. von Moltke LL, Greenblatt DJ, Harmatz JS, Duan SX, Harrel LM, Cotreau-Bibbo MM, Pritchard GA, Wright CE, Shader RI. Triazolam biotransformation by human liver microsomes *in vitro*: effects of metabolic inhibitors and clinical confirmation of a predicted interaction with ketoconazole. *J Pharmacol Exp Ther* (1996) 276, 370–9.
28. Anderson AJ, Maier G, Skolly SM. Pharmacokinetic interaction between eszopiclone and ketoconazole in healthy volunteers at steady state. *Pharmacotherapy* (2005) 25, 474.

Benzodiazepines + Azoles; Miscellaneous

Oral clotrimazole lozenges slightly increase the exposure to oral midazolam.

Clinical evidence, mechanism, importance and management

(a) Clotrimazole

In a four-way crossover study, 10 healthy subjects were given single doses of either oral **midazolam** 2 mg or intravenous **midazolam** 0.025 mg/kg alone or following administration of *oral* clotrimazole troches [lozenges] 10 mg three times daily for 5 days. Clotrimazole decreased the oral clearance of **midazolam** by 37% and increased its AUC by about 60%. Clotrimazole did not affect the clearance of intravenous midazolam.[1]

The effect of an oral clotrimazole lozenge formulation on **midazolam** exposure is slight and seems unlikely to be clinically important in most patients.

Note that **midazolam** is used as a probe substrate to assess the activity of other drugs on CYP3A4. The data here therefore suggest that, in the formulation studied, which was designed to limit systemic exposure, oral clotrimazole is a weak CYP3A4 inhibitor.

(b) Miconazole

The manufacturer of miconazole oral gel contraindicates concurrent use with **triazolam** and *oral* **midazolam**.[2] This is probably because a large proportion of miconazole oral gel (both prescription and non-prescription doses) may be swallowed and therefore adequate systemic absorption may occur to produce an interaction. **Alprazolam, brotizolam** and *intravenous* **midazolam** should also be used with caution with oral miconazole.[2]

1. Shord SS, Chan L-N, Camp JR, Vasquez M, Jeong H-Y, Molokie RE, Baum CL, Xie H. Effects of oral clotrimazole troches on the pharmacokinetics of oral and intravenous midazolam. *Br J Clin Pharmacol* (2010) 69, 160–6.
2. Daktarin Oral Gel (Miconazole). Janssen-Cilag Ltd. UK Summary of product characteristics, December 2014.

Benzodiazepines + Azoles; Posaconazole

Posaconazole moderately to markedly increases midazolam exposure. Some other benzodiazepines might be similarly affected.

Clinical evidence

In a study in healthy subjects, posaconazole 200 mg daily for 10 days increased the AUC of intravenous midazolam 50 micrograms/kg by 83%.[1] In another study, oral posaconazole 200 mg or 400 mg twice daily for 7 days increased the AUC of intravenous midazolam 4.6-fold and 6.2-fold, respectively. Similarly, both doses of posaconazole increased the AUC of a single 2-mg oral dose of midazolam about 5-fold. In addition, posaconazole 200 mg or 400 mg prolonged the mean terminal half-life of midazolam from about 3 to 4 hours to 8 to 10 hours.[2,3]

Mechanism

Posaconazole is an inhibitor of CYP3A4. Therefore midazolam, which is predominantly metabolised by CYP3A4, is greatly affected by the concurrent use of posaconazole.

The azoles generally inhibit CYP3A4 in the gut as well as in the liver (hence intravenous midazolam is generally less affected than oral midazolam), although, for posaconazole, intravenous and oral midazolam appear to be affected to a similar extent.

Importance and management

Evidence of an interaction between midazolam and posaconazole is limited to the pharmacokinetic studies with midazolam, but given the magnitude of the increased exposure seen, it seems likely to be clinically relevant. If both drugs are given, consider reducing the dose of oral midazolam to avoid excessive sedation, and even then the effects might still be prolonged. Patients taking posaconazole should be warned about the likelihood of increased and prolonged sedation and advised not to drive (for example) after receiving midazolam until completely recovered. Unlike other azoles, it appears that the effects of posaconazole are similar on both oral and intravenous midazolam. Therefore consideration should be given to reducing the dose and/or careful titration if either single intravenous doses or regular intravenous doses of midazolam are given.

The effect of posaconazole on other benzodiazepines does not appear to have been studied. However, **triazolam**, and to a lesser extent, **alprazolam**, are similarly metabolised and therefore it would be prudent to use the same precautions to those suggested for midazolam if either of these benzodiazepines is given with posaconazole.

Note that midazolam is used as a probe substrate to assess the activity of other drugs on CYP3A4. The data here therefore suggest that posaconazole is borderline between being a moderate and a potent inhibitor of CYP3A4. For a list of CYP3A4 substrates, see 'Table 1.10', p.12.

1. Noxafil (Posaconazole). Merck Sharp & Dohme Ltd. UK Summary of product characteristics, September 2014.
2. Krishna G, Moton A, Ma L, Savant I, Martinho M, Seiberling M, McLeod J. Effects of oral posaconazole on the pharmacokinetic properties of oral and intravenous midazolam: a phase I, randomized, open-label, crossover study in healthy volunteers. *Clin Ther* (2009) 31, 286–98.
3. Noxafil (Posaconazole). Merck & Co., Inc. US Prescribing information, June 2014.

Benzodiazepines and related drugs + Azoles; Voriconazole

Voriconazole markedly to very markedly increases midazolam exposure, moderately increases diazepam exposure, and slightly increases zolpidem exposure.

Clinical evidence

(a) Diazepam

A study in healthy subjects found that voriconazole 400 mg twice daily on the first day and 200 mg twice daily on the second day increased the AUC of a single 5-mg oral dose of diazepam 2.2-fold and prolonged its half-life from 31 hours to 61 hours.[1]

(b) Midazolam

A study in 10 healthy subjects found that voriconazole 400 mg twice daily on the first day and 200 mg twice daily on the second day affected the pharmacokinetics of both intravenous and oral midazolam. Voriconazole reduced the clearance of intravenous midazolam 50 micrograms/kg by 72% and increased its half-life from 2.8 hours to 8.3 hours. Voriconazole increased the maximum plasma concentration and AUC of a single 7.5-mg oral dose of midazolam 3.8-fold and 10.3-fold, respectively. The psychomotor effects of oral midazolam were profoundly increased by voriconazole, but the effects of small intravenous doses of midazolam were only slightly increased.[2]

(c) Zolpidem

In a study in 10 healthy subjects, pretreatment with voriconazole 400 mg twice daily for one day and then 200 mg twice daily for the second day increased the AUC of a single 10-mg oral dose of zolpidem by 50% and its half-life was prolonged from 3.2 hours to 4.1 hours. Voriconazole appeared to increase drowsiness in the immediate period following administration of zolpidem, but no statistically significant differences in pharmacodynamic variables were seen.[3]

Mechanism

Voriconazole is an inhibitor of CYP3A4. Midazolam and zolpidem are, to varying degrees, metabolised by CYP3A4, with the extent of the interaction related to how important CYP3A4 is in their metabolism and how potent a CYP3A4 inhibitor the azole is. So, for example, midazolam, which is predominantly metabolised by CYP3A4, is greatly affected by voriconazole. Other isoenzymes are also involved in the metabolism of zolpidem so it is only weakly affected by voriconazole. Diazepam is extensively metabolised by CYP2C19 and also CYP3A4, and so voriconazole, which has some CYP2C19 inhibitory activity as well as being a CYP3A4 inhibitor, moderately increases diazepam exposure.

Importance and management

Evidence of an interaction between midazolam and voriconazole is limited to the pharmacokinetic studies, but it is almost certainly clinically important as the magnitude of the increased exposure is similar to that seen with ketoconazole. In very broad terms the dose of midazolam would need to be reduced by about 75% or more in the presence of voriconazole to avoid excessive sedation, and even then its effects would still be expected to be prolonged. Unless appropriate precautions are taken (very reduced doses with careful monitoring and management) this interaction can be dangerous. Patients taking voriconazole should be warned about the likelihood of increased and prolonged sedation and advised not to drive (for example) after receiving midazolam until completely recovered. One study suggests that while a greater effect was seen after oral midazolam than intravenous, high intravenous doses or long-term infusions might also result in long-lasting hypnotic effects.[2] Therefore consideration should be given to reducing the dose and/or careful titration if either an infusion or regular intravenous doses of midazolam are given.

Exposure to diazepam, in single doses, is moderately increased by voriconazole and a dose reduction might also be required.

Note that midazolam is used as a probe substrate to assess the activity of other drugs on CYP3A4. The data here therefore suggest that voriconazole is a potent inhibitor of CYP3A4. For a list of CYP3A4 substrates, see 'Table 1.10', p.12.

1. Saari TI, Laine K, Bertilsson L, Neuvonen PJ, Olkkola KT. Voriconazole and fluconazole increase the exposure to oral diazepam. *Eur J Clin Pharmacol* (2007) 63, 941–9.
2. Saari TI, Laine K, Leino K, Valtonen M, Neuvonen PJ, Olkkola KT. Effect of voriconazole on the pharmacokinetics and pharmacodynamics of intravenous and oral midazolam. *Clin Pharmacol Ther* (2006) 79, 362–70.
3. Saari TI, Laine K, Leino K, Valtonen M, Neuvonen PJ, Olkkola KT. Effect of voriconazole on the pharmacokinetics and pharmacodynamics of zolpidem in healthy subjects. *Br J Clin Pharmacol* (2007) 63, 116–20.

Benzodiazepines + Beta blockers

Minor changes in benzodiazepine pharmacokinetics occur when they are given with beta blockers. There is limited evidence that some psychomotor tests might be impaired in patients taking benzodiazepines with beta blockers.

Clinical evidence, mechanism, importance and management

No clinically important *pharmacokinetic* interactions were reported to occur between:

- **alprazolam** and **propranolol**[1]
- **clorazepate** and **propranolol**[2]
- **diazepam** and **atenolol**[3] or **propranolol**[3]
- **lorazepam** and **metoprolol**[4] or **propranolol**[1]
- **oxazepam** and **labetalol**[5] or **propranolol.**[5]

Slight or negligible changes, which are unlikely to be clinically relevant, were found between:

- **diazepam** and **propranolol** (diazepam clearance reduced by 17%)[1] or **metoprolol** (diazepam clearance reduced by 18%,[6] AUC increased by 25%[3])
- **bromazepam** and **metoprolol** (bromazepam AUC increased by 35%)[4] or **propranolol** (bromazepam half-life increased by 22%).[7]

However, studies of psychomotor performance have shown that simple reaction times with **oxazepam** given with either **propranolol** or **labetalol** are increased,[5] and those taking **diazepam** and **metoprolol** have a reduced kinetic visual acuity,[3,8] which is related to driving ability.[9] Moreover, choice reaction times at 2 hours were also found to be lengthened when taking **diazepam** and **metoprolol**, **propranolol** or **atenolol**, but at 8 hours they only persisted with **diazepam** and **metoprolol.**[8]

Information about interactions between the benzodiazepines and beta blockers is very limited indeed. The current evidence does not seem to justify any additional caution, but bear the possibility of an interaction in mind in case of an unexpected response to treatment.

1. Ochs HR, Greenblatt DJ, Verburg-Ochs B. Propranolol interactions with diazepam, lorazepam, and alprazolam. *Clin Pharmacol Ther* (1984) 36, 451–5.
2. Ochs HR, Greenblatt DJ, Locniskar A, Weinbrenner J. Influence of propranolol coadministration or cigarette smoking on the kinetics of desmethyldiazepam following intravenous clorazepate. *Klin Wochenschr* (1986) 64, 1217–21.
3. Hawksworth G, Betts T, Crowe A, Knight R, Nyemitei-Addo I, Parry K, Petrie JC, Raffle A, Parsons A. Diazepam/β-adrenoceptor antagonist interactions. *Br J Clin Pharmacol* (1984) 17, 69S–76S.
4. Scott AK, Cameron GA, Hawksworth GM. Interaction of metoprolol with lorazepam and bromazepam. *Eur J Clin Pharmacol* (1991) 40, 405–9.
5. Sonne J, Døssing M, Loft S, Olesen KL, Vollmer-Larsen A, Victor MA, Hamberg O, Thyssen H. Single dose pharmacokinetics and pharmacodynamics of oral oxazepam during concomitant administration of propranolol and labetalol. *Br J Clin Pharmacol* (1990) 29, 33–7.
6. Klotz U, Reimann IW. Pharmacokinetic and pharmacodynamic interaction study of diazepam and metoprolol. *Eur J Clin Pharmacol* (1984) 26, 223–6.
7. Ochs HR, Greenblatt DJ, Friedman H, Burstein ES, Locniskar A, Harmatz JS, Shader RI. Bromazepam pharmacokinetics: influence of age, gender, oral contraceptives, cimetidine, and propranolol. *Clin Pharmacol Ther* (1987) 41, 562–70.
8. Betts TA, Crowe A, Knight R, Raffle A, Parsons A, Blake A, Hawksworth G, Petrie JC. Is there a clinically relevant interaction between diazepam and lipophilic β-blocking drugs? *Drugs* (1983) 25 (Suppl 2), 279–80.
9. Betts TA, Knight R, Crowe A, Blake A, Harvey P, Mortiboy D. Effect of β-blockers on psychomotor performance in normal volunteers. *Eur J Clin Pharmacol* (1985) 28 (Suppl), 39–49.

Benzodiazepines + Buspirone

No adverse interaction appears to occur if buspirone is given with alprazolam, flurazepam or triazolam. When buspirone is given with diazepam the adverse effects appear to be mild and short-lived.

Clinical evidence, mechanism, importance and management

In 12 healthy subjects, buspirone 10 mg every 8 hours increased the maximum plasma levels and AUC of **alprazolam** 1 mg every 8 hours by 7% and 8%, respectively. The maximum plasma concentration of buspirone were not altered, but the AUC of buspirone was increased by 29%. However, these changes were within the normal pharmacokinetic variability of these drugs, and no unexpected adverse effects were seen.[1]

In 12 healthy subjects given **diazepam** 5 mg daily for 22 days, buspirone 15 mg every 8 hours for 12 days had no effect on the plasma concentration of **diazepam**, but the concentration of the metabolite nordiazepam were raised by about 20%. Concurrent use resulted in some mild adverse effects (headache, nausea, dizziness) in all subjects, and in two cases muscle twitching was seen. These symptoms subsided after a few days.[2]

The concurrent use of buspirone with either **flurazepam** or **triazolam** did not appear to prolong or intensify the sedative effects of either benzodiazepine.[3]

There would seem to be no reason for avoiding the concurrent use of these benzodiazepines and buspirone.

1. Buch AB, Van Harken DR, Seidehamel RJ, Barbhaiya RH. A study of pharmacokinetic interaction between buspirone and alprazolam at steady state. *J Clin Pharmacol* (1993) 33, 1104–9.
2. Gammans RE, Mayol RF, Labudde JA. Metabolism and disposition of buspirone. *Am J Med* (1986) 80 (Suppl 3B), 41–51.
3. BuSpar (Buspirone hydrochloride). Bristol-Myers Squibb Company. US Prescribing information, November 2010.

Benzodiazepines and related drugs + Caffeine

Caffeine appears to antagonise the effects of the benzodiazepines (mainly sedative effects, but possibly also anxiolytic effects). The effects of zopiclone might be similarly antagonised.

Clinical evidence

(a) Benzodiazepines

In a study in healthy subjects, a single 250-mg or 500-mg dose of caffeine (added to decaffeinated coffee) counteracted the drowsiness and mental slowness induced by a single 10- to 20-mg dose of **diazepam**.[1] The same or a similar study has been reported elsewhere.[2] Conversely, in a study in 6 healthy subjects, the concurrent use of caffeine 6 mg/kg and **diazepam** 300 micrograms/kg did not antagonise the effects of either drug; however, caffeine caused a minor 22% reduction in the concentration of **diaze-**

pam.[3] In one study the sedative effects of **midazolam**[4] were moderately antagonised by caffeine 250 mg but not 125 mg, and there is also some evidence to suggest that caffeine and **clonazepam**[5] or **triazolam**[6] have mutually opposing effects.

No pharmacokinetic interaction appears to occur between caffeine and **midazolam**[7] or **alprazolam**.[8]

(b) Non-benzodiazepine hypnotics

Zopiclone 7.5 mg appears to counter the stimulant effects of caffeine 300 mg more easily than **caffeine** counters the sedative effects of **zopiclone**.[6] In one study, no pharmacokinetic interaction occurred between **zolpidem** 10 mg and caffeine 300 mg (added to decaffeinated coffee), and the hypnotic effects of **zolpidem** were unchanged.[9] However, a placebo-controlled, crossover study in 12 healthy subjects found that **caffeine** 250 mg and 500 mg reversed the pharmacodynamic effects (such as sedation, reduced tapping speed, reaction time) caused by **zolpidem** 7.5 mg. Even though the pharmacodynamic effects of **zolpidem** were reduced by caffeine, the AUC of **zolpidem** was *increased* by 41% by caffeine 500 mg, when compared with placebo.[10]

Mechanism

Uncertain. One suggestion is that caffeine can block adenosine receptors, leading to CNS stimulation, which would antagonise the CNS depressant effects of the benzodiazepines.[11] Another suggestion is that the stimulant effects of caffeine and the sedative effects of benzodiazepines are simply antagonistic.

Importance and management

The evidence suggests that caffeine, particularly at higher doses, at least partially reduces the sedative and performance-impairing effects of benzodiazepines and related hypnotics. This would appear to be a disadvantage at night, but might be useful the next morning, although caffeine should not be considered an antidote to the residual effects of these hypnotics. The extent to which caffeine reduces the anxiolytic effects of the benzodiazepines remains uncertain (it needs assessment), but be alert for reduced benzodiazepine effects if both are used.

1. Mattila MJ, Nuotto E. Caffeine and theophylline counteract diazepam effects in man. *Med Biol* (1983) 61, 337–43.
2. Mattila MJ, Palva E, Savolainen K. Caffeine antagonizes diazepam effects in man. *Med Biol* (1982) 60, 121–3.
3. Ghoneim MM, Hinrichs JV, Chiang C-K, Loke WH. Pharmacokinetic and pharmacodynamic interactions between caffeine and diazepam. *J Clin Psychopharmacol* (1986) 6, 75–80.
4. Mattila MJ, Vainio P, Nurminen M-L, Vanakoski J, Seppälä T. Midazolam 12 mg is moderately counteracted by 250 mg caffeine in man. *Int J Clin Pharmacol Ther* (2000) 38, 581–7.
5. Gaillard J-M, Sovilla J-Y, Blois R. The effects of clonazepam, caffeine and the combination of the two drugs on human sleep. In: Koella WP, Rüther E, Schulz H, eds. Sleep '84. New York: Gustav Fischer Verlag; 1985: pp. 314–15.
6. Mattila ME, Mattila MJ, Nuotto E. Caffeine moderately antagonizes the effects of triazolam and zopiclone on the psychomotor performance of healthy subjects. *Pharmacol Toxicol* (1992) 70, 286–9.
7. Blakey GE, Lockton JA, Perrett J, Norwood P, Russell M, Aherne Z, Plume J. Pharmacokinetic and pharmacodynamic assessment of a five-probe metabolic cocktail for CYPs 1A2, 3A4, 2C9, 2D6 and 2E1. *Br J Clin Pharmacol* (2004) 57, 162–9.
8. Schmider J, Brockmöller J, Arold G, Bauer S, Roots I. Simultaneous assessment of CYP3A4 and CYP1A2 activity *in vivo* with alprazolam and caffeine. *Pharmacogenetics* (1999) 9, 725–34.
9. Mattila MJ, Nurminen M-L, Vainio P, Vanakoski J. Zolpidem 10 mg given at daytime is not antagonized by 300 mg caffeine in man. *Eur J Clin Pharmacol* (1998) 54, 421–5.
10. Cysneiros RM, Farkas D, Harmatz JS, von Moltke LL, Greenblatt DJ. Pharmacokinetic and pharmacodynamic interactions between zolpidem and caffeine. *Clin Pharmacol Ther* (2007) 82, 54–62.
11. Niemand D, Martinell S, Arvidsson S, Svedmyr N, Ekström-Jodal B. Aminophylline inhibition of diazepam sedation: is adenosine blockade of GABA-receptors the mechanism? *Lancet* (1984) i, 463–4.

Benzodiazepines + Calcium-channel blockers

Diltiazem and verapamil moderately increase midazolam exposure, and diltiazem moderately increases triazolam exposure. Increased effects, such as sedation, which have been marked in some cases, have been seen in patients given these drugs. Alprazolam would be expected to interact similarly. There appear to be no clinically relevant interactions between other calcium-channel blockers and benzodiazepines.

Clinical evidence

(a) Diazepam

1. Diltiazem. In 6 healthy subjects, the concurrent use of single doses of diazepam 5 mg and diltiazem 60 mg resulted in only minor changes in the plasma concentrations of either drug.[1] In another study, poor and extensive metabolisers of CYP2C19 (that is, those lacking or deficient in this isoenzyme, and those with normal activity of this isoenzyme, respectively) were given diltiazem 200 mg daily for 3 days before and 7 days after a single 2-mg dose of diazepam. Diltiazem increased the AUC of diazepam by 25% in both poor and extensive metabolisers, when compared with placebo; however, the half-life of diazepam increased from 46 hours to 65 hours in extensive metabolisers and from 77 hours to 104 hours in poor metabolisers. The clinical effects of these pharmacokinetic changes were not assessed.[2]

2. Felodipine. In 12 healthy subjects, felodipine 10 mg daily for 12 days did not affect the pharmacokinetics of a 10-mg intravenous dose of diazepam, but the AUC and maximum plasma concentration of the diazepam metabolite, nordazepam, were raised by 14% and 16%, respectively.[3]

3. Nimodipine. In 24 healthy, elderly subjects the plasma concentration of diazepam 10 mg daily and nimodipine 30 mg three times daily were unaffected by concurrent use, and no clinically relevant changes in haemodynamics, ECG recordings, clinical chemistry or haematology occurred.[4]

(b) Midazolam

1. Diltiazem. After taking diltiazem 60 mg three times daily for 2 days, 9 healthy female subjects were given midazolam 15 mg orally. The AUC of midazolam was increased 4-fold, the maximum plasma concentration was doubled, and the half-life was increased by 49%. It was almost impossible for the subjects to stay awake for 90 minutes after taking the midazolam. They suffered several hours of amnesia and there was a considerable decrease in the performance of pharmacodynamic tests (digit symbol substitution, Maddox wing test).[5] A similar 4-fold increase in midazolam AUC was seen in 3 healthy subjects given diltiazem 120 mg twice daily for 6 days, followed by a single 4-mg dose of oral midazolam.[6] The effect was smaller with a single 0.05-mg/kg intravenous midazolam dose; the AUC was increased by 60%.[6] Diltiazem 60 mg, given to 15 patients 2 hours before induction of anaesthesia with intravenous midazolam and alfentanil, increased the AUC and half-life of midazolam by 15% and 43%, respectively. Tracheal extubation was performed on average 2.5 hours later, when compared with placebo.[7]

2. Lercanidipine. Midazolam appears to increase the absorption of lercanidipine by 40%.[8]

3. Nitrendipine. A study in 9 healthy subjects found that the pharmacokinetics and pharmacodynamics of midazolam were unaffected by a single 20-mg dose of nitrendipine.[9]

4. Verapamil. After taking verapamil 80 mg three times daily for 2 days, 9 healthy female subjects were given midazolam 15 mg orally. The AUC of the midazolam was increased 3-fold, the maximum plasma concentration was doubled, and the half-life was increased by 41%. It was almost impossible for the subjects to stay awake for 90 minutes after taking the midazolam. They suffered several hours of amnesia and there was a considerable decrease in the performance of pharmacodynamic tests (digit symbol substitution, Maddox wing test).[5] Another study found that verapamil 240 mg daily for 7 days decreased the oral clearance of midazolam 4-fold and the systemic clearance was decreased by about 60%.[10]

(c) Temazepam

In 16 healthy insomniacs, **diltiazem** 40 mg had little or no effect on the hypnotic effects of temazepam.[11]

(d) Triazolam

1. Diltiazem. A study in 7 healthy subjects found that diltiazem 60 mg three times daily for 3 days increased the AUC of a single 250-microgram dose of triazolam 2.3-fold and almost doubled its maximum plasma concentration. Pharmacodynamic tests showed an increase in the sedative effects of triazolam.[12] Another study in 10 healthy subjects found that diltiazem 60 mg three times daily for 2 days increased the AUC of a single 250-microgram dose of triazolam 3.4-fold, and approximately doubled its maximum plasma concentration and half-life. The pharmacodynamic changes were briefly described as profound and prolonged.[13] In contrast, in another study, diltiazem 40 mg was found to have little or no effect on the hypnotic effects of triazolam in 16 healthy insomniacs.[11]

2. Isradipine. In 9 healthy subjects, isradipine 5 mg daily reduced the AUC of a single 250-microgram dose of triazolam by 20%, but no difference in the pharmacodynamic effects of triazolam were seen.[14]

Mechanism

The evidence suggests that diltiazem and verapamil inhibit the metabolism of midazolam and triazolam, by CYP3A4, leading to increased exposure and increased effects. The greater increase in midazolam exposure after oral compared with intravenous administration suggests the main interaction site between oral midazolam and diltiazem is the gut wall.[6] It also appears that the intestine is the major site of the interaction between oral midazolam and verapamil.[10]

Importance and management

The interactions between midazolam and diltiazem or verapamil are established and clinically important. The authors of one report say that patients taking either diltiazem or verapamil are probably incapable of undertaking skilled tasks (e.g. driving) for up to 6 hours after taking midazolam 15 mg, and possibly even after 8 to 10 hours. They suggest that the usual dose of midazolam should be reduced by at least 50% to avoid unnecessarily deep sleep and prolonged hypnosis, and they also point out that as the half-life of the midazolam is prolonged, the effects will persist regardless of the dose.[5] The effects are smaller with intravenous midazolam, but the elimination of midazolam is still reduced and post-operative recovery might be delayed.[7] Similar precautions are likely to be needed for triazolam with diltiazem, and the interaction is also predicted to occur with triazolam and verapamil.[13] As **alprazolam** is also, at least partially, metabolised by CYP3A4, diltiazem and verapamil would also be expected to increase its exposure, but to a lesser extent than midazolam. However, there do not appear to be any clinical reports of an interaction.

No special precautions appear to be necessary when other calcium-channel blockers are given with a benzodiazepine.

Note that midazolam is used as a probe substrate to assess the activity of other drugs on CYP3A4. The data here therefore suggest that diltiazem and verapamil are moderate inhibitors of CYP3A4. For a list of CYP3A4 substrates, see 'Table 1.10', p.12.

1. Etoh A, Kohno K. Studies on the drug interaction of diltiazem. IV. Relationship between first pass metabolism of various drugs and the absorption enhancing effect of diltiazem. *Yakugaku Zasshi* (1983) 103, 581–8.
2. Kosuge K, Jun Y, Watanabe H, Kimura M, Nishimoto M, Ishizaki T, Ohashi K. Effects of CYP3A4 inhibition by diltiazem on pharmacokinetics and dynamics of diazepam in relation to CYP2C19 genotype status. *Drug Metab Dispos* (2001) 29, 1284–9.

3. Meyer BH, Müller FO, Hundt HKL, Luus HG, de la Rey N, Röthig H-J. The effects of felodipine on the pharmacokinetics of diazepam. *Int J Clin Pharmacol Ther Toxicol* (1992) 30, 117–21.
4. Heine PR, Weyer G, Breuel H-P, Mück W, Schmage N, Kuhlmann J. Lack of interaction between diazepam and nimodipine during chronic oral administration to healthy elderly subjects. *Br J Clin Pharmacol* (1994) 38, 39–43.
5. Backman JT, Olkkola KT, Aranko K, Himberg J-J, Neuvonen PJ. Dose of midazolam should be reduced during diltiazem and verapamil treatments. *Br J Clin Pharmacol* (1994) 37, 221–5.
6. Zhang X, Quinney SK, Gorski JC, Jones DR, Hall SD. Semiphysiologically based pharmacokinetic models for the inhibition of midazolam clearance by diltiazem and its major metabolite. *Drug Metab Dispos* (2009) 37, 1587–97.
7. Ahonen J, Olkkola KT, Salmenperä M, Hynynen M, Neuvonen PJ. Effect of diltiazem on midazolam and alfentanil disposition in patients undergoing coronary artery bypass grafting. *Anesthesiology* (1996) 85, 1246–52.
8. Zanidip (Lercanidipine hydrochloride). Recordati Pharmaceuticals Ltd. UK Summary of product characteristics, April 2006.
9. Handel J, Ziegler G, Gemeinhardt A, Stuber H, Fischer C, Klotz U. Lack of effect of nitrendipine on the pharmacokinetics and pharmacodynamics of midazolam during steady state. *Br J Clin Pharmacol* (1988) 25, 243–50.
10. Wang Y, Jin Y, Gorski JC, Hall SD. The intestine is the major site of interaction between midazolam and verapamil. *Clin Pharmacol Ther* (2004) 75, P86.
11. Scharf MB, Sachais BA, Mayleben DW, Jennings SW. The effects of a calcium channel blocker on the effects of temazepam and triazolam. *Curr Ther Res* (1990) 48, 516–23.
12. Kosuge K, Nishimoto M, Kimura M, Umemura K, Nakashima M, Ohashi K. Enhanced effect of triazolam with diltiazem. *Br J Clin Pharmacol* (1997) 43, 367–72.
13. Varhe A, Olkkola KT, Neuvonen PJ. Diltiazem enhances the effects of triazolam by inhibiting its metabolism. *Clin Pharmacol Ther* (1996) 59, 369–75.
14. Backman JT, Wang J-S, Wen X, Kivistö KT, Neuvonen PJ. Mibefradil but not isradipine substantially elevates the plasma concentrations of the CYP3A4 substrate triazolam. *Clin Pharmacol Ther* (1999) 66, 401–7.

Benzodiazepines and related drugs + Carbamazepine and related drugs

Carbamazepine moderately increases alprazolam clearance, and appears to markedly reduce midazolam exposure and almost abolish its effects. There is some evidence for reduced clobazam, clonazepam, diazepam, and etizolam exposure. The effect of clobazam or clonazepam on carbamazepine concentrations is uncertain. Carbamazepine moderately reduces zolpidem exposure. Single-dose studies have shown that the sedative effects of zopiclone and carbamazepine are additive; however it has been predicted that, when taken long-term, carbamazepine might reduce the effects of zopiclone. The pharmacokinetics of eslicarbazepine and clobazam do not appear to be altered by concurrent use.

Clinical evidence

A. Benzodiazepines

(a) Alprazolam

In a placebo-controlled, crossover study in 7 healthy subjects, **carbamazepine** 100 mg three times daily for 10 days moderately increased the apparent oral clearance of a single 800-microgram dose of alprazolam 2.4-fold and reduced the elimination half-life from about 17 hours to 8 hours.[1] The plasma alprazolam concentration of a patient with atypical bipolar disorder and panic attacks, taking alprazolam 7.5 mg daily, was reduced by more than 50% (from 43 to 19.3 nanograms/mL) when **carbamazepine** was given. This was accompanied by a deterioration in his clinical condition, which was managed with haloperidol.[2]

(b) Clobazam

A study in patients with epilepsy found that **carbamazepine** reduces the plasma concentration of clobazam and increases the plasma concentration of *N*-desmethylclobazam (the principal metabolite).[3] Similar results are described in other studies in healthy subjects and patients with epilepsy taking clobazam and **carbamazepine**.[4,5]

A 66-year-old man taking **carbamazepine** and topiramate experienced fatigue, ataxia, impairment of gait, and clumsiness while taking clobazam 10 mg daily. His symptoms resolved when the clobazam was stopped. When he was later given **carbamazepine**, topiramate, and clobazam 20 mg daily, his **carbamazepine** concentration increased from 36.8 micromol/L to 41.9 micromol/L. Five days after the clobazam was stopped the **carbamazepine** concentration had returned to approximately the pre-clobazam concentration (35.5 micromol/L).[6] However, another study in 15 patients with epilepsy taking **carbamazepine** alone and another 7 patients taking **carbamazepine** with clobazam, found that **carbamazepine** concentrations were similar in both groups, despite patients receiving monotherapy taking a significantly lower dose of **carbamazepine**, but concentrations of **carbamazepine** metabolites, including the active carbamazepine-10,11-epoxide, were higher in those also taking clobazam. It was suggested that clobazam increased the metabolism of **carbamazepine** by about 50%.[7]

A population pharmacokinetic model using data from 641 patients enrolled in phase III **eslicarbazepine** studies, found that concurrent use of clobazam (in 37 patients) did not alter the pharmacokinetics of **eslicarbazepine** or clobazam.[8]

(c) Clonazepam

Clonazepam, in slowly increasing doses up to a maximum of 4 to 6 mg daily given over a 6-week period, had no effect on **carbamazepine** serum concentrations. Some patients were also taking phenobarbital.[9] A study in 7 healthy subjects found that **carbamazepine** 200 mg daily given over a 3-week period reduced the plasma concentration of clonazepam 1 mg daily from a range of 4 to 7 nanograms/mL down to 2.5 to 4 nanograms/mL, and reduced the half-life of clonazepam by about one-third.[10] A retrospective analysis of this interaction in 183 patients found that clonazepam clearance was increased by 22% and **carbamazepine** clearance was decreased by 21% during concurrent use.[11]

(d) Diazepam

A study found that the plasma clearance of a single 10-mg intravenous dose of diazepam was 3-fold greater, and the half-life shorter, in a group of 9 patients with epilepsy, when compared with 6 healthy subjects. Seven of the patients with epilepsy were taking **carbamazepine.**[12]

(e) Etizolam

In healthy subjects, **carbamazepine** 200 mg daily for 6 days decreased the maximum plasma concentration and AUC of a single 1-mg dose of etizolam by about 20% and 42%, respectively. The elimination half-life was reduced from 11 hours to about 7 hours.[13]

(f) Midazolam

The pharmacokinetics and pharmacodynamics of a single 15-mg oral dose of midazolam were studied in 6 patients with epilepsy taking either **carbamazepine** (2 patients), phenytoin (1), or both drugs together (3), and in 7 control subjects not taking either antiepileptic. The AUC of midazolam in the patients with epilepsy was 94% lower, and the peak plasma concentration 93% lower, than the value in the control subjects. The pharmacodynamic effects of the midazolam (subjective drowsiness, body sway with eyes closed and open, as well as more formal tests) were also reduced. Most of the patients did not notice any effects from taking midazolam, while the control subjects were clearly sedated for 2 to 4 hours, and also experienced amnesia after taking the midazolam.[14]

B. Non-benzodiazepine hypnotics

(a) Zolpidem

In a study in 18 healthy subjects, carbamazepine 400 mg once daily for 15 days moderately reduced the AUC of a single 5-mg dose of zolpidem by 57% and reduced its half-life from 2.3 to 1.6 hours.[15]

(b) Zopiclone

A crossover study in 12 healthy subjects given single oral doses of zopiclone 7.5 mg and **carbamazepine** 600 mg found only minor changes in the plasma concentrations of both drugs. Zopiclone concentrations were higher and **carbamazepine** concentrations marginally lower.[16] However, note that a single dose of carbamazepine is insufficient to study enzyme induction. Psychomotor tests confirmed that both drugs had sedative effects, which were additive, and in a simulated driving test it was found that co-ordination was impaired and reaction times prolonged.[16]

Mechanism

Alprazolam and midazolam are both metabolised by CYP3A4, of which carbamazepine is a known inducer. Concurrent use therefore increases the metabolism of these benzodiazepines and decreases their concentrations. It seems probable that the interaction with zolpidem is also due to induction of CYP3A4.

Importance and management

The interaction between carbamazepine and midazolam appears to be of greatest clinical importance, although interpretation of the study cited is complicated because it grouped carbamazepine with phenytoin and it was a between group comparison. Nevertheless, much larger doses of midazolam are likely to be required in the presence of carbamazepine, or an alternative sedative may be needed. **Triazolam** is predicted to be affected like midazolam.[14] Alprazolam and etizolam are also affected, but to a lesser extent. The dose of these drugs may also need to be increased to ensure adequate serum concentrations.

One small study[12] suggests that enzyme-inducing antiepileptic drugs including carbamazepine may increase the clearance of diazepam; however, the clinical relevance of this does not appear to have been assessed. Nevertheless, it would seem prudent to monitor concurrent use for reduced efficacy.

As *N*-desmethylclobazam retains some of the activity of clobazam the effect of carbamazepine on clobazam metabolism probably has little clinical relevance. In addition, the case of carbamazepine toxicity appears to be isolated and is therefore probably of limited importance. Concurrent use of eslicarbazepine and clobazam does not appear to alter the pharmacokinetics of either drug.

The pharmacokinetic changes seen with clonazepam seem likely to be too small to be clinically relevant, but this needs confirmation.

Note that some benzodiazepines such as clonazepam may interfere with the metabolism of carbamazepine. However, the effects are small, and unlikely to be of clinical relevance in most patients.

The evidence for an interaction between zopiclone and carbamazepine is slim, and the effects of long-term use are unclear. Carbamazepine is a strong inducer of CYP3A4 (by which zopiclone is metabolised) and it has been predicted that the effect of long-term carbamazepine treatment might be a reduction in zopiclone plasma concentrations and hypnotic effects.[17] It would seem prudent to be alert for the need to increase the zopiclone dose in patients taking carbamazepine. More study of this potential interaction is needed. Similar considerations would also seem appropriate for zolpidem as its exposure was more than halved by carbamazepine.

1. Furukori H, Otani K, Yasui N, Kondo T, Kaneko S, Shimoyama R, Ohkubo T, Nagasaki T, Sugawara K. Effect of carbamazepine on the single oral dose pharmacokinetics of alprazolam. *Neuropsychopharmacology* (1998) 18, 364–9.
2. Arana GW, Epstein S, Molloy M, Greenblatt DJ. Carbamazepine-induced reduction of plasma alprazolam concentrations: a clinical case report. *J Clin Psychiatry* (1988) 49, 448–9.
3. Bun H, Monjanel-Mouterde S, Noel F, Durand A, Cano J-P. Effects of age and antiepileptic drugs on plasma levels and kinetics of clobazam and N-desmethylclobazam. *Pharmacol Toxicol* (1990) 67, 136–40.

4. Levy RH, Lane EA, Guyot M, Brachet-Liermain A, Cenraud B, Loiseau P. Analysis of parent drug-metabolite relationship in the presence of an inducer: application to the carbamazepine-clobazam interaction in normal man. *Drug Metab Dispos* (1983) 11, 286–92.
5. Sennoune S, Mesdjian E, Bonneton J, Genton P, Dravet C, Roger J. Interactions between clobazam and standard antiepileptic drugs in patients with epilepsy. *Ther Drug Monit* (1992) 14, 269–74.
6. Genton P, Nguyen VH, Mesdjian E. Carbamazepine intoxication with negative myoclonus after the addition of clobazam. *Epilepsia* (1998) 39, 1115–18.
7. Muñoz JJ, De Salamanca RE, Diaz-Obregón C, Timoneda FL. The effect of clobazam on steady state plasma concentrations of carbamazepine and its metabolites. *Br J Clin Pharmacol* (1990) 29, 763–5.
8. Falcão A, Fuseau E, Nunes T, Almeida L, Soares-da-Silva P. Pharmacokinetics, drug interactions and exposure-response relationship of eslicarbazepine acetate in adult patients with partial-onset seizures: population pharmacokinetic and pharmacokinetic/pharmacodynamic analyses. *CNS Drugs* (2012) 26, 79–91.
9. Johannessen SI, Strandjord RE, Munthe-Kaas AW. Lack of effect of clonazepam on serum levels of diphenylhydantoin, phenobarbital and carbamazepine. *Acta Neurol Scand* (1977) 55, 506–12.
10. Lai AA, Levy RH, Cutler RE. Time-course of interaction between carbamazepine and clonazepam in normal man. *Clin Pharmacol Ther* (1978) 24, 316–23.
11. Yukawa E, Nonaka T, Yukawa M, Ohdo S, Higuchi S, Kuroda T, Goto Y. Pharmacoepidemiologic investigation of a clonazepam-carbamazepine interaction by mixed effect modeling using routine clinical pharmacokinetic data in Japanese patients. *J Clin Psychopharmacol* (2001) 21, 588–93.
12. Dhillon S, Richens A. Pharmacokinetics of diazepam in epileptic patients and normal volunteers following intravenous administration. *Br J Clin Pharmacol* (1981) 12, 841–4.
13. Kondo S, Fukasawa T, Yasui-Furukori N, Aoshima T, Suzuki A, Inoue Y, Tateishi T, Otani K. Induction of the metabolism of etizolam by carbamazepine in humans. *Eur J Clin Pharmacol* (2005) 61, 185–88.
14. Backman JT, Olkkola KT, Ojala M, Laaksovirta H, Neuvonen PJ. Concentrations and effects of oral midazolam are greatly reduced in patients treated with carbamazepine or phenytoin. *Epilepsia* (1996) 37, 253–7.
15. Vlase L, Popa A, Neag M, Muntean D, Bâldea I, Leucuța SE. Pharmacokinetic interaction between zolpidem and carbamazepine in healthy volunteers. *J Clin Pharmacol* (2011) 51, 1233–6.
16. Kuitunen T, Mattila MJ, Seppälä T, Aranko K, Mattila ME. Actions of zopiclone and carbamazepine, alone and in combination, on human skilled performance in laboratory and clinical tests. *Br J Clin Pharmacol* (1990) 30, 453–61.
17. Villikka K, Kivistö KT, Lamberg TS, Kantola T, Neuvonen PJ. Concentrations and effects of zopiclone are greatly reduced by rifampicin. *Br J Clin Pharmacol* (1997) 43, 471–4.

Benzodiazepines + Ciclosporin

No pharmacokinetic interaction appears to occur between intravenous midazolam and ciclosporin.

Clinical evidence, mechanism, importance and management

In a study in 9 transplant patients taking ciclosporin, the pharmacokinetics of a single 75-microgram/kg dose of intravenous **midazolam** did not differ from those of historical values in healthy subjects. In addition, the duration of **midazolam** sedation did not differ from that expected. **Midazolam** did not appear to alter ciclosporin concentrations in these patients.[1] These findings suggest that there is no pharmacokinetic interaction between intravenous **midazolam** and oral ciclosporin. However, this does not rule out the possibility of an interaction with oral **midazolam** and therefore further study is required.

1. Li G, Treiber G, Meinshausen J, Wolf J, Werringloer J, Klotz U. Is cyclosporin A an inhibitor of drug metabolism? *Br J Clin Pharmacol* (1990) 30, 71–7.

Benzodiazepines and related drugs + Cobicistat

Cobicistat very markedly increases the exposure to oral midazolam and triazolam is expected to be similarly affected. Parenteral midazolam would also be expected to interact similarly, although possibly to a lesser extent. Other benzodiazepines (such as diazepam) and zolpidem are also predicted to interact.

Clinical evidence

In a study in healthy subjects, cobicistat given in multiple doses from 50 to 200 mg increased the AUC of a single 5-mg dose of oral **midazolam** 9.8- to 19-fold, and caused an 89 to 95% reduction in its apparent clearance (similar in effect to ritonavir 100 mg).[1]

Mechanism

Midazolam is a probe substrate for CYP3A4 and this data shows that cobicistat is a potent inhibitor of this isoenzyme.

Importance and management

Evidence for an interaction between midazolam and cobicistat is limited to the study above but, given the likely mechanism, it would appear to be established. The US manufacturer of elvitegravir boosted with cobicistat (in a fixed-dose combination also including emtricitabine and tenofovir disoproxil fumarate) contraindicates concurrent use with **triazolam** and *oral* **midazolam**.[2] *Parenteral* midazolam can be used, but only in a setting where the patient can be closely monitored for respiratory depression and/or prolonged sedation, and treated appropriately should these occur. Consideration should be given to reducing the dose of parenteral midazolam, especially if more than a single dose of midazolam is administered.[2] The US manufacturer also recommends clinical monitoring with other benzodiazepines and hypnotics and dose reduction as necessary: they name **clorazepate, diazepam, estazolam, flurazepam,** and **zolpidem**.[2] In addition, they predict that the plasma concentration of **clonazepam** might be increased and they recommend monitoring concurrent use.[2]

1. Mathias AA, German P, Murray BP, Wei L, Jain A, West S, Warren D, Hui J, Kearney BP. Pharmacokinetics and pharmacodynamics of GS-9350: a novel pharmacokinetic enhancer without anti-HIV activity. *Clin Pharmacol Ther* (2010) 87, 322–9.
2. Stribild (Elvitegravir, cobicistat, emtricitabine, tenofovir disoproxil fumarate). Gilead Sciences, Inc. US Prescribing information, August 2012.

Benzodiazepines + Corticosteroids

The metabolism of midazolam might be increased in patients receiving long-term treatment with corticosteroids.

Clinical evidence, mechanism, importance and management

Intravenous **midazolam** 200 micrograms/kg was given to 8 patients receiving long-term treatment with corticosteroids (6 taking **prednisolone** 2.5 mg to 15 mg daily; one taking **betamethasone** 0.5 mg daily and one taking **methylprednisolone** 48 mg daily) and to 10 other patients not taking corticosteroids. In the patients taking corticosteroids the AUC of **midazolam** was 36% lower and the clearance 28% higher, when compared with the patients not taking corticosteroids; however the differences were not statistically significant. The onset of anaesthesia between the two groups was also not notably different. It was suggested that the trend towards increased **midazolam** metabolism might be due to induction of CYP3A4 and/or UDP-glucuronyltransferase. Although the results with intravenous midazolam appeared not to be clinically relevant, the authors suggested that the metabolism of oral **midazolam** might be affected to a greater extent.[1] Other benzodiazepines metabolised in a similar way to midazolam (e.g. **triazolam**, and to a lesser extent **alprazolam**) might be similarly affected. However, further study is needed to establish if any effect is clinically relevant.

1. Nakajima M, Suzuki T, Sasaki T, Yokoi T, Hosoyamada A, Yamamoto T, Kuroiwa Y. Effects of chronic administration of glucocorticoid on midazolam pharmacokinetics in humans. *Ther Drug Monit* (1999) 21, 507–13.

Benzodiazepines + Dexamfetamine

Dexamfetamine reverses the sedative effects and some of the memory-impairing effects of triazolam. Alprazolam attenuates the behavioural effects of dexamfetamine, but oxazepam appears to have no effect on dexamfetamine pharmacodynamics.

Clinical evidence

A placebo-controlled study in 20 healthy subjects found that a single 20-mg/70 kg dose of dexamfetamine sulfate reversed the sedative effects of a single 250-microgram/70 kg dose of **triazolam**. The study also found that dexamfetamine selectively reversed some of the memory-impairing effects of **triazolam**.[1] Similar results were reported in a related study.[2]

In another study, 6 healthy subjects were trained to discriminate between placebo and dexamfetamine 15 mg. Pretreatment with single 500-microgram doses of **alprazolam** significantly attenuated the discriminative-stimulus effects of dexamfetamine, and some of the self-reported drug effects.[3] A further study in 6 healthy subjects found that **oxazepam** 20 mg was ineffective at modulating the discriminative-stimulus or subject-rated effects of dexamfetamine.[4]

Mechanism

The stimulant effects of dexamfetamine would be expected to oppose the sedative effects of benzodiazepines. It is thought that the behavioural effects of dexamfetamine are due to increased synaptic dopamine levels, which are under the inhibitory control of GABA systems, whereas benzodiazepines are $GABA_A$ receptor positive modulators. However, it appears that benzodiazepines differ in their ability to affect the behavioural effects of dexamfetamine.[3,4]

Importance and management

Although these studies were conducted principally for evaluating how benzodiazepines affect memory and sedation and how amfetamines affect behaviour, they show that if dexamfetamine and benzodiazepines are used concurrently, attenuation of some of each drugs effects would be anticipated.

1. Mintzer MZ, Griffiths RR. Triazolam-amphetamine interaction: dissociation of effects on memory versus arousal. *J Psychopharmacol* (2003) 17, 17–29.
2. Mintzer MZ, Griffiths RR. A triazolam/amphetamine dose-effect interaction study: dissociation of effects on memory versus arousal. *Psychopharmacology (Berl)* (2007) 192, 425–40.
3. Rush CR, Stoops WW, Wagner FP, Hays LR, Glaser PEA. Alprazolam attenuates the behavioral effects of d-amphetamine in humans. *J Clin Psychopharmacol* (2004) 24, 410–20.
4. Lile JA, Stoops WW, Wagner FP, Glaser PEA, Rush CR. Oxazepam does not modulate the behavioral effects of *d*-amphetamine in humans. *Pharmacol Biochem Behav* (2005) 82, 270–9.

Benzodiazepines + Disulfiram

The plasma concentrations of chlordiazepoxide and diazepam are increased by the use of disulfiram, whereas alprazolam, oxazepam, and lorazepam appear to be either not affected, or only minimally affected. There is also one case of possible temazepam toxicity in a patient taking disulfiram. The intensity of the disulfiram-alcohol reaction may possibly be decreased by diazepam.

Clinical evidence

A man taking disulfiram 200 mg daily developed confusion, drowsiness, slurred speech and an unsteady gait within a few days of starting to take **temazepam** 20 mg at night. This was interpreted as **temazepam** toxicity. The symptoms disappeared when both drugs were stopped.[1]

After taking disulfiram 500 mg daily for 14 to 16 days, the median plasma clearance of single doses of **chlordiazepoxide** and **diazepam** were reduced by 54% and 41%, respectively, and the half-lives were increased by 84% and 37%, respectively, although there was considerable interindividual variation in the findings. **Oxazepam** was also given after the use of disulfiram, but changes in **oxazepam** pharmacokinetics were minimal. There was no difference in the interaction between alcoholic subjects (without hepatic cirrhosis) and healthy subjects.[2] Other studies have found that the pharmacokinetics of **lorazepam**[3] and **alprazolam**[4] were unaffected by disulfiram.

It has been reported that the intensity of the disulfiram-alcohol reaction might be decreased by benzodiazepines.[5]

Mechanism

Disulfiram inhibits the initial metabolism (*N*-demethylation and oxidation) of chlordiazepoxide and diazepam by the liver so that an alternative but slower metabolic pathway is used. This results in the accumulation of these benzodiazepines in the body. However, alprazolam is metabolised by hepatic microsomal oxidation, but does not appear to interact with disulfiram.[4]

The metabolism (glucuronidation) of oxazepam and lorazepam is minimally affected by disulfiram so that their clearance from the body remains largely unaffected.[2,3] The possible interaction between disulfiram and temazepam is not understood, as temazepam is also mainly eliminated in the urine as the inactive glucuronide metabolite, and so its metabolism would not generally be expected to be affected by disulfiram.

Importance and management

There seems to be only one report (with temazepam) of a clinically relevant interaction between disulfiram and the benzodiazepines, and this report is unconfirmed, as the patient did not take temazepam alone. The other reports only describe potential interactions that have been identified by single-dose studies. These do not necessarily reliably predict what will happen in practice. However, it seems possible that some patients will experience increased drowsiness, maybe due to this interaction or because drowsiness is a very common adverse effect of disulfiram. Reduce the dose of the benzodiazepine if necessary. Benzodiazepines that are metabolised by similar pathways to diazepam and chlordiazepoxide might interact in the same way, but this needs confirmation. Alprazolam, oxazepam, and lorazepam might be useful alternatives as a pharmacokinetic interaction is unlikely, but they might still have additive effects with disulfiram on drowsiness.

1. Hardman M, Biniwale A, Clarke CE. Temazepam toxicity precipitated by disulfiram. *Lancet* (1994) 344, 1231–2.
2. MacLeod SM, Sellers EM, Giles HG, Billings BJ, Martin PR, Greenblatt DJ, Marshman JA. Interaction of disulfiram with benzodiazepines. *Clin Pharmacol Ther* (1978) 24, 583–9.
3. Sellers EM, Giles HG, Greenblatt DJ, Naranjo CA. Differential effects on benzodiazepine disposition by disulfiram and ethanol. *Arzneimittelforschung* (1980) 30, 882–6.
4. Diquet B, Gujadhur L, Lamiable D, Warot D, Hayoun H, Choisy H. Lack of interaction between disulfiram and alprazolam in alcoholic patients. *Eur J Clin Pharmacol* (1990) 38, 157–60.
5. Antabuse (Disulfiram). Actavis UK Ltd. UK Summary of product characteristics, December 2011.

Benzodiazepines + Ethambutol

Ethambutol appears not to affect the pharmacokinetics of diazepam.

Clinical evidence, mechanism, importance and management

A study in 6 patients, newly diagnosed with tuberculosis and receiving ethambutol 25 mg/kg daily alone for 5 days, found that although some of the pharmacokinetic parameters of intravenous **diazepam** were different to those obtained in healthy control subjects not taking ethambutol, the differences were not statistically significant.[1] There seems to be nothing in the literature to suggest that ethambutol interacts with other benzodiazepines.

1. Ochs HR, Greenblatt DJ, Roberts G-M, Dengler HJ. Diazepam interaction with antituberculosis drugs. *Clin Pharmacol Ther* (1981) 29, 671–8.

Benzodiazepines + Food

Food can considerably delay the absorption of flunitrazepam and loprazolam. Food also slows the rate of absorption of alprazolam, diazepam and nitrazepam, but does not affect their overall bioavailability. Conversely, food can markedly enhance the absorption of quazepam and increase its sedative effects.

Clinical evidence, mechanism, importance and management

(a) Alprazolam

When compared with the fasting state, food had no effect on the AUC of alprazolam 1 mg, formulated as an immediate-release orally disintegrating tablet. However, the maximum plasma concentration decreased by 23% and the time to the maximum concentration increased from 2.5 to 4 hours, suggesting a slower rate of absorption. The clinical relevance of this was thought to be minimal.[1]

(b) Diazepam

In a single-dose, crossover study, light food delayed the time to the maximum plasma concentration of diazepam by about one hour, but had no effect on its maximum plasma concentration or AUC, when compared with the fasting state. Light food did not appear to affect the CNS-depressant effects of diazepam.[2] The minor effects seen are probably unlikely to be clinically relevant.

(c) Flunitrazepam

A study in 8 healthy subjects found that when they took a single 2-mg dose of flunitrazepam 2 hours after an evening meal (spaghetti, meat, salad, an apple and wine) and one hour before going to bed, the maximum plasma concentration of flunitrazepam was reduced by 63%. The time to reach the maximum plasma concentration was delayed by 2.5 hours, and the absorption half-life was considerably prolonged.[3] It seems probable therefore that the onset of sleep with flunitrazepam might be delayed by food.

(d) Loprazolam

A study in 8 healthy subjects found that when they took a single 2-mg dose of loprazolam 2 hours after an evening meal (spaghetti, meat, salad, an apple and wine) and one hour before going to bed, the maximum plasma concentration of loprazolam was reduced by 41%. The time to reach the maximum plasma concentration was delayed by 3.6 hours, and the absorption half-life was considerably prolonged.[3] It seems probable therefore that the onset of sleep with loprazolam might be delayed by food.

(e) Nitrazepam

In a single-dose, crossover study, light food delayed the time to the maximum plasma concentration of nitrazepam by about one hour, but had no effect on its maximum plasma concentration or AUC, when compared with the fasting state. Light food did not appear to affect the CNS-depressant effects of nitrazepam.[2] The minor effects seen are probably unlikely to be clinically relevant.

(f) Quazepam

In a crossover study, 9 healthy subjects were given single 20-mg doses of quazepam immediately after a standard meal, and 3 hours after a standard meal. When compared with the fasting state, the maximum plasma concentration and $AUC_{0\text{-}8}$ for quazepam were increased 3-fold and 2.4-fold, respectively, when given 30 minutes after food, and 2.5-fold and 2.1-fold, respectively, when given 3 hours after food. The CNS-depressant effects of quazepam were enhanced to a similar extent by administration 30 minutes or 3 hours after food.[4] In another study by the same authors, it was found that both low-fat and high-fat meals increased the absorption of quazepam.[5] A further study found that a light snack increased the bioavailability of quazepam and prolonged the reaction time at 4 and 6 hours after dosing.[2] However, another study found increases in the bioavailability when quazepam was taken 2 hours after food, but did not find any significant difference in the subjective effects of quazepam, such as drowsiness, malaise, and calmness, when compared with fasting.[6] It appears that food affects the absorption of quazepam and this effect might continue for at least 3 hours after food intake.[4] In Japan, the administration of quazepam with food was contraindicated;[4-6] however, it has also been suggested that, because of the good tolerability of quazepam, it might not be necessary to adjust the dose with meal content.[5] The US manufacturer does not suggest any restrictions concerning administration with food.[7]

1. Erdman K, Stypinski D, Combs M, Witt P, Stiles M, Pollock S. Absence of food effect on the extent of alprazolam absorption from an orally disintegrating tablet. *Pharmacotherapy* (2007) 27, 1120–4.
2. Yamazaki A, Kumagai Y, Fujita T, Hasunuma T, Yokota S, Maeda M, Otani Y, Majima M. Different effects of light food on pharmacokinetics and pharmacodynamics of three benzodiazepines, quazepam, nitrazepam and diazepam. *J Clin Pharm Ther* (2007) 32, 31–9.
3. Bareggi SR, Pirola R, Truci G, Leva S, Smirne S. Effect of after-dinner administration on the pharmacokinetics of oral flunitrazepam and loprazolam. *J Clin Pharmacol* (1988) 28, 371–5.
4. Yasui-Furukori N, Takahata T, Kondo T, Mihara K, Kaneko S, Tateishi T. Time effects of food intake on the pharmacokinetics and pharmacodynamics of quazepam. *Br J Clin Pharmacol* (2003) 55, 382–8.
5. Yasui-Furukori N, Kondo T, Takahata T, Mihara K, Ono S, Kaneko S, Tateishi T. Effect of dietary fat content in meals on pharmacokinetics of quazepam. *J Clin Pharmacol* (2002) 42, 1335–40.
6. Kim Y, Morikawa M, Ohsawa H, Kou M, Ishida E, Igarashi J, Kajimoto T, Danno T, Nakata M, Yokoyama T, Tokuyama A, Nakamura Y, Kishimoto T. Effects of food on the pharmacokinetics and clinical efficacy of quazepam. *Jpn J Neuropsychopharmacol* (2003) 23, 205–10.
7. Doral (Quazepam). Questcor Pharmaceuticals, Inc. US Prescribing information, August 2011.

Benzodiazepines + Ginkgo (*Ginkgo biloba*)

Ginkgo does not affect the pharmacokinetics of alprazolam or diazepam. Studies with midazolam suggest that ginkgo might increase, decrease, or have no effect on its exposure.

Clinical evidence

(a) Alprazolam

Ginkgo leaf extract (*Ginkgold*) 120 mg twice daily for 16 days was given to 12 healthy subjects before, and with, a single 2-mg dose of alprazolam on day 14. The alprazolam AUC was decreased by 17%, but its maximum concentration was not affected.[1]

(b) Diazepam

In a study in 12 healthy subjects, ginkgo 40 mg four times daily for 28 days did not affect the metabolism of a single 10-mg dose of diazepam, or its *N*-desmethyl metabolite.[2]

(c) Midazolam

In 12 healthy subjects, ginkgo 60 mg four times daily for 28 days did not affect the metabolism of midazolam 8 mg.[3] These findings were repeated in a later study using the same criteria in 12 elderly healthy subjects,[4] and a further study in 17 healthy subjects given another ginkgo extract (EGb 761), for 8 days.[5] In contrast, in another similar study, ginkgo 120 mg twice daily decreased the AUC and maximum serum concentrations of a single 8-mg dose of midazolam by 34% and 31%, respectively.[6] Furthermore, in yet another study in 10 healthy subjects, ginkgo (*Ginkgold*) 360 mg daily for 28 days *increased* the AUC of a single 8-mg dose of oral midazolam by 25%.[7]

Mechanism

Alprazolam and midazolam are principally metabolised by CYP3A4. The studies here show that ginkgo has minimal effects on this isoenzyme, with the maximum effect on midazolam being a 33% decrease in AUC. However, it is unusual for studies to show opposite effects (one of the studies found a 25% increase in midazolam AUC), and the reasons for this are unclear, but might be to do with the methodology (use of midazolam metabolic ratios rather than midazolam exposure, and length of sampling time[6] and the fact that in one study the subjects had previously received lopinavir boosted with ritonavir for 30 days, concurrently with the ginkgo for 2 weeks, just 2 weeks before the midazolam[6]).

Importance and management

The pharmacokinetic evidence here shows that diazepam exposure is not affected by ginkgo, and alprazolam exposure is only negligibly decreased, and so no clinically relevant interaction would be expected with either of these benzodiazepines. Although the evidence with midazolam is conflicting, any effect that might occur would be slight at the most, and not clinically relevant. No dose adjustments with these or other similarly metabolised benzodiazepines and ginkgo biloba would be anticipated to be necessary on concurrent use.

Note that alprazolam and midazolam can be used as probe substrates to assess the activity of drugs on CYP3A4. These results therefore suggest that ginkgo is not an inhibitor or inducer of CYP3A4, and a clinically relevant pharmacokinetic interaction between ginkgo and other CYP3A4 substrates is unlikely.

1. Markowitz JS, Donovan JL, DeVane CL, Sipkes L, Chavin KD. Multiple-dose administration of Ginkgo biloba did not affect cytochrome P-450 2D6 or 3A4 activity in normal volunteers. *J Clin Psychopharmacol* (2003) 23, 576–81.
2. Zuo X-C, Zhang B-K, Jia S-J, Liu S-K, Zhou L-Y, Li J, Zhang J, Dai L-L, Chen B-M, Yang G-P, Yuan H. Effects of ginkgo biloba extracts on diazepam metabolism: a pharmacokinetic study in healthy Chinese male subjects. *Eur J Clin Pharmacol* (2010) 66, 503–9.
3. Gurley BJ, Gardner SF, Hubbard MA, Williams DK, Gentry WB, Cui Y, Ang CYW. Cytochrome P450 phenotypic ratios for predicting herb-drug interactions in humans. *Clin Pharmacol Ther* (2002) 72, 276–87.
4. Gurley BJ, Gardner SF, Hubbard MA, Williams DK, Gentry WB, Cui Y, Ang CYW. Clinical assessment of botanical supplementation on cytochrome P450 phenotypes in the elderly: St John's wort, garlic oil, Panax ginseng, and Ginkgo biloba. *Drugs Aging* (2005) 22, 525–39.
5. Zadoyan G, Rokitta D, Klement S, Dienel A, Hoerr R, Gramatté T, Fuhr U. Effect of Ginkgo biloba special extract EGb 761® on human cytochrome P450 activity: a cocktail interaction study in healthy volunteers. *Eur J Clin Pharmacol* (2012) 68, 553–60.
6. Robertson SM, Davey RT, Voell J, Formentini E, Alfaro RM, Penzak SR. Effect of Ginkgo biloba extract on lopinavir, midazolam and fexofenadine pharmacokinetics in healthy subjects. *Curr Med Res Opin* (2008) 24, 591–9.
7. Uchida S, Yamada H, Li DX, Maruyama S, Ohmori Y, Oki T, Watanabe H, Umegaki K, Ohashi K, Yamada S. Effects of Ginkgo biloba extract on pharmacokinetics and pharmacodynamics of tolbutamide and midazolam in healthy volunteers. *J Clin Pharmacol* (2006) 46, 1290–1298.

Benzodiazepines + Grapefruit and other fruit juices

Grapefruit juice might slightly increase midazolam, quazepam, and triazolam exposure and moderately increase diazepam exposure.

Clinical evidence

(a) Diazepam

A study in 8 healthy subjects found that simultaneous administration of 250 mL of grapefruit juice increased the AUC and maximum plasma concentration of a single 5-mg oral dose of diazepam 3.2-fold and 1.5-fold, respectively.[1]

(b) Midazolam

Grapefruit juice 200 mL was given to 8 healthy subjects followed 15 minutes later by 5 mg of intravenous midazolam or 60 minutes later by 15 mg of oral midazolam. The pharmacokinetics of intravenous midazolam remained unchanged, but the AUC of oral midazolam was increased by 52%, and its maximum plasma concentration rose by 56%. These changes were also reflected in the psychometric measurements made.[2] Grapefruit juice resulted in a similar increase in the AUC of oral midazolam in another study.[3] A further study found that the AUC of oral midazolam increased by 65% when midazolam was given 2 hours after grapefruit juice, but when the midazolam was given 26 hours, 50 hours and 74 hours after grapefruit juice, its AUC was increased by 21%, 22% and 6%, respectively. The midazolam elimination half-life was not altered by grapefruit juice.[4]

A large-scale placebo-controlled study involving a total of 120 healthy young medical students used psychomotor tests to measure the effect of benzodiazepines with and without grapefruit juice. Subjects were given midazolam 10 mg or **triazolam** 250 micrograms with 300 mL of grapefruit juice or water. Only a minor increase in the benzodiazepine effects occurred with grapefruit juice, and these effects were of little or no practical importance.[5]

(c) Quazepam

A study in 9 healthy subjects found that 250 mL of grapefruit juice three times daily for 3 days increased the AUC of a single 15-mg oral dose of quazepam and its active metabolite, 2-oxoquazepam, by 38% and 28%, respectively, although these increases were not statistically significant. The pharmacodynamic effects of quazepam, such as sedation, were not enhanced by grapefruit juice.[6]

(d) Triazolam

A single oral 250-microgram dose of triazolam was given to 10 healthy subjects with either 250 mL of grapefruit juice or water. The mean AUC of the triazolam was increased by 50% by the grapefruit juice, the peak plasma concentration was increased by 30%, and the time to reach the peak plasma concentration was prolonged from 1.5 hours to 2.5 hours. A small decrease in psychomotor performance occurred (more drowsiness and tiredness).[7]

Another study of the interaction between triazolam and grapefruit juice found that the effects of grapefruit juice were much more pronounced when multiple doses of grapefruit juice were given. The triazolam AUC and half-life were increased by about 50% and 6 to 9%, respectively, when single doses of normal or double-strength grapefruit juice were given, and by about 150% and 50%, respectively, by multiple doses (three times daily) of double-strength grapefruit juice. The effect of grapefruit juice on psychomotor tests was also greater after multiple dosing.[8] Similar increases in the AUC of triazolam were found in a study using normal-strength grapefruit juice three times daily for 3 days, and although grapefruit juice was not found to enhance the sedative effects of triazolam, it did result in deterioration of performance in the digit symbol substitution test.[6] However, in another study, 300 mL of grapefruit juice once daily for 10 days only increased the AUC of a single dose of oral triazolam by 60%, which was similar to the effects of exposure to a single dose of grapefruit juice.[9]

For another study in which grapefruit juice had little effect on the response to triazolam, see under *Midazolam*, above.

Mechanism

The evidence suggests that grapefruit juice inhibits the metabolism of these benzodiazepines by CYP3A4, so that more is left to enter the circulation.[2] Single exposure to grapefruit juice appears to mainly impair enteric, but not hepatic, metabolism and recovery of enteric CYP3A function seems to be largely complete within 3 days.[4] In one study grapefruit juice was found to have a greater effect on the bioavailability and pharmacodynamics of triazolam than on quazepam. This was considered to be because triazolam is metabolised by CYP3A4, while quazepam is metabolised by CYP2C9 as well as by CYP3A4.[6]

Importance and management

The interactions between a number of the benzodiazepines and grapefruit juice are established. These slight increases in bioavailability might be expected to increase the extent of the sedation and amnesia due to these benzodiazepines to a small extent, although multiple doses of grapefruit juice might increase the risk of adverse effects. The clinical effects of the greater interaction with diazepam appear not to have been investigated.

Note that midazolam is used as a probe substrate to assess the activity of other drugs on CYP3A4. The data here suggests that grapefruit juice is a weak inhibitor of CYP3A4.

Other fruit juices have been reported to affect CYP3A4 *in vitro*, but studies in healthy subjects have not found any clinically relevant pharmacokinetic interactions with midazolam and **cranberry juice**,[10] **pomegranate juice**[3] or **tangerine juice**.[11]

1. Özdemir M, Aktan Y, Boydağ BS, Cingi MI, Musmul A. Interaction between grapefruit juice and diazepam in humans. *Eur J Drug Metab Pharmacokinet* (1998) 23, 55–9.
2. Kupferschmidt HHT, Ha HR, Ziegler WH, Meier PJ, Krähenbühl S. Interaction between grapefruit juice and midazolam in humans. *Clin Pharmacol Ther* (1995) 58, 20–8.
3. Farkas D, Oleson LE, Zhao Y, Harmatz JS, Zinny MA, Court MH, Greenblatt DJ. Pomegranate juice does not impair clearance of oral or intravenous midazolam, a probe for cytochrome P450-3A activity: comparison with grapefruit juice. *J Clin Pharmacol* (2007) 47, 286–94.
4. Greenblatt DJ, von Moltke LL, Harmatz JS, Chen G, Weemhoff JL, Jen C, Kelley CJ, LeDuc BW, Zinny MA. Time course of recovery of cytochrome P450 3A function after single doses of grapefruit juice. *Clin Pharmacol Ther* (2003) 74, 121–9.
5. Vanakoski J, Mattila MJ, Seppälä T. Grapefruit juice does not enhance the effects of midazolam and triazolam in man. *Eur J Clin Pharmacol* (1996) 50, 501–8.
6. Sugimoto K-I, Araki N, Ohmori M, Harada K-I, Cui Y, Tsuruoka S, Kawaguchi A, Fujimura A. Interaction between grapefruit juice and hypnotic drugs: comparison of triazolam and quazepam. *Eur J Clin Pharmacol* (2006) 62, 209–15.
7. Hukkinen SK, Varhe A, Olkkola KT, Neuvonen PJ. Plasma concentrations of triazolam are increased by concomitant ingestion of grapefruit juice. *Clin Pharmacol Ther* (1995) 58, 127–31.
8. Lilja JJ, Kivistö KT, Backman JT, Neuvonen PJ. Effect of grapefruit juice dose on grapefruit juice–triazolam interaction: repeated consumption prolongs triazolam half-life. *Eur J Clin Pharmacol* (2000) 56, 411–15.
9. Culm-Merdek KE, von Moltke LL, Gan L, Horan KA, Reynolds R, Harmatz JS, Court MH, Greenblatt DJ. Effect of extended exposure to grapefruit juice on cytochrome P450 3A activity in humans: comparison with ritonavir. *Clin Pharmacol Ther* (2006) 79, 243–54.
10. Lilja JJ, Backman JT, Neuvonen PJ. Effects of daily ingestion of cranberry juice on the pharmacokinetics of warfarin, tizanidine, and midazolam–probes of CYP2C9, CYP1A2, and CYP3A4. *Clin Pharmacol Ther* (2007) 81, 833–9.
11. Backman JT, Mäenpää J, Belle DJ, Wrighton SA, Kivistö KT, Neuvonen PJ. Lack of correlation between in vitro and in vivo studies on the effects of tangeretin and tangerine juice on midazolam hydroxylation. *Clin Pharmacol Ther* (2000) 67, 382–90.

Benzodiazepines and related drugs + H_2-receptor antagonists

The plasma concentrations of many of the benzodiazepines and related drugs appear to be raised by cimetidine, and occasionally patients have experienced an increase in effects (sedation). Famotidine, nizatidine and ranitidine do not normally appear to interact with most benzodiazepines.

Clinical evidence

A. Benzodiazepines

(a) Cimetidine

In 10 patients who took cimetidine 300 mg four times daily for 2 weeks the combined plasma concentration of **diazepam** and its active metabolite, nordazepam, was found to be increased by 57%, but reaction times and other motor and intellectual tests remained unaffected.[1] Other reports describe a rise in the plasma concentrations and/or

AUC of **diazepam** (associated with increased sedation in one report[2]) due to cimetidine,[3-9] and generalised incoordination has also been described in one individual.[10]

Cimetidine also raises the plasma concentrations and/or AUC of **adinazolam**,[11] **alprazolam**,[12,13] **bromazepam**,[14] **chlordiazepoxide**,[15] **clobazam**[16,17] (this interaction was considered to be both clinically significant[16] and clinically irrelevant due to large interpatient variation in clobazam plasma concentrations[17]), **clorazepate**,[18] **flurazepam**,[19] **nitrazepam**,[20] and **triazolam**.[12,13,21,22] Liver cirrhosis increases the effects of cimetidine on the loss of **chlordiazepoxide**.[23]

Confusion has been reported in a 50-year-old man taking **clorazepate** when he was given cimetidine,[24] and increased sedation has been seen in some patients taking **adinazolam** and cimetidine.[11] Prolonged hypnosis in an elderly woman[25] and CNS toxicity (including lethargy and hallucinations) in a 49-year-old woman[26] have been attributed to an interaction between **triazolam** and cimetidine but this remains unconfirmed.

In contrast, cimetidine does not normally interact with **clotiazepam**,[27] **lormetazepam**,[28] **oxazepam**[19,29,30] or **temazepam**,[31,32] although prolonged post-operative sedation was seen in one patient given **oxazepam** and cimetidine.[33] Similarly, some studies suggest that no interaction occurs between **lorazepam** and cimetidine,[19,29] although one study found an increase in **lorazepam** concentrations, but this was only statistically significant with a 400-mg intravenous dose of cimetidine and not with a 200-mg dose.[3]

There is some controversy about whether or not **midazolam** is affected by cimetidine. An increase in sedation,[34,35] an increase in **midazolam** concentrations[36] or AUC (35% to 102%),[32,35,37] and no change in the AUC after oral or intravenous administration[38] have been reported with the combination. However, none of these studies gave cimetidine for more than one day (4 doses) before midazolam, so the maximal inhibitory effect of cimetidine might not have been achieved.

(b) Famotidine

Famotidine does not interact with **bromazepam**,[39] **clorazepate**,[39] **chlordiazepoxide**,[39] **diazepam**[9,40] or **triazolam**.[39]

(c) Nizatidine

Nizatidine does not interact with **diazepam**.[41-43]

(d) Ranitidine

Ranitidine does not interact to a clinically relevant extent with **adinazolam**,[44] **diazepam**[41,45] (although diminished absorption of diazepam may possibly occur),[46] **lorazepam**,[45] or **temazepam**,[32,47] but it can slightly increase the bioavailability (by about 10 to 30%) of oral **triazolam**,[48,49] although this is unlikely to be clinically relevant.

There is some controversy about whether or not **midazolam** is affected by ranitidine. Increases in **midazolam** concentrations[32,37] and sedation[47,50] have been reported on a few occasions, but a lack of effect has also been documented.[34,36,38]

(e) Roxatidine

Roxatidine does not interact with **diazepam** or its active metabolite, nordazepam.[51]

B. Non-benzodiazepine hypnotics

(a) Cimetidine

Cimetidine increased the plasma concentrations of a single dose of **zaleplon** by 85%.[52] There appeared to be no statistically significant pharmacokinetic interaction between cimetidine and **zolpidem** in healthy subjects, although sleep duration tended to be prolonged.[53]

(b) Ranitidine

There appeared to be no statistically significant pharmacokinetic interaction between ranitidine and **zolpidem**.[53] Ranitidine did not affect the hypnotic action of **zopiclone**.[47]

Mechanism

Cimetidine inhibits the liver enzymes concerned with the metabolism of diazepam, alprazolam, chlordiazepoxide, clorazepate, flurazepam, nitrazepam, triazolam, and zaleplon. As a result their clearance from the body is reduced and their plasma concentrations rise.

Lorazepam, oxazepam and temazepam are metabolised by a different metabolic pathway involving glucuronidation, which is not affected by cimetidine, and so they do not usually interact.

Ranitidine, famotidine and nizatidine appear not to inhibit liver microsomal enzymes. There is some evidence that ranitidine increases the absorption of triazolam, and possibly other benzodiazepines, due to changes in gastric pH,[49] although it has been suggested that this effect is unimportant.[22] Cimetidine has been said to similarly affect the absorption of diazepam and lorazepam.[3]

Importance and management

The interactions between the benzodiazepines or related drugs and cimetidine are well documented (not all the references are listed here) but normally they appear to be of little clinical importance. However, a few patients might be adversely affected (increased effects, drowsiness, etc.). If symptoms occur in any patient taking a benzodiazepine or related drug and cimetidine, reduce the benzodiazepine dose: a dose reduction of one-third or increased dosing intervals (twice daily instead of three times daily) have been suggested for alprazolam.[12] Alternatively, use a non-interacting benzodiazepine, such as lorazepam, lormetazepam, oxazepam or temazepam, or a non-interacting H_2-receptor antagonist such as ranitidine, famotidine, nizatidine or roxatidine.

Note that midazolam is used as a probe substrate to assess the activity of other drugs on CYP3A4. The data here suggest that cimetidine is possibly a weak inhibitor of CYP3A4, although the studies are not definitive. For a list of CYP3A4 substrates, see 'Table 1.10', p.12.

1. Greenblatt DJ, Abernethy DR, Morse DS, Harmatz JS, Shader RI. Clinical importance of the interaction of diazepam and cimetidine. *N Engl J Med* (1984) 310, 1639–43.
2. Klotz U, Reimann I. Delayed clearance of diazepam due to cimetidine. *N Engl J Med* (1980) 302, 1012–14.
3. McGowan WAW, Dundee JW. The effect of intravenous cimetidine on the absorption of orally administered diazepam and lorazepam. *Br J Clin Pharmacol* (1982) 14, 207–11.
4. Klotz U, Reimann I. Elevation of steady-state diazepam levels by cimetidine. *Clin Pharmacol Ther* (1981) 30, 513–17.
5. Gough PA, Curry SH, Araujo OE, Robinson JD, Dallman JJ. Influence of cimetidine on oral diazepam elimination with measurement of subsequent cognitive change. *Br J Clin Pharmacol* (1982) 14, 739–42.
6. Andersson T, Andrén K, Cederberg C, Edvardsson G, Heggelund A, Lundborg P. Effect of omeprazole and cimetidine on plasma diazepam levels. *Eur J Clin Pharmacol* (1990) 39, 51–4.
7. Bressler R, Carter D, Winters L. Enprostil, in contrast to cimetidine, does not affect diazepam pharmacokinetics. *Adv Therapy* (1988) 5, 306–12.
8. Lima DR, Santos RM, Werneck E, Andrade GN. Effect of orally administered misoprostol and cimetidine on the steady state pharmacokinetics of diazepam and nordiazepam in human volunteers. *Eur J Drug Metab Pharmacokinet* (1991) 16, 161–70.
9. Locniskar A, Greenblatt DJ, Harmatz JS, Zinny MA, Shader RI. Interaction of diazepam with famotidine and cimetidine, two H_2-receptor antagonists. *J Clin Pharmacol* (1986) 26, 299–303.
10. Anon. Court warns on interaction of drugs. *Doctor* (1979) 9, 1.
11. Hulhoven R, Desager JP, Cox S, Harvengt C. Influence of repeated administration of cimetidine on the pharmacokinetics and pharmacodynamics of adinazolam in healthy subjects. *Eur J Clin Pharmacol* (1988) 35, 59–64.
12. Pourbaix S, Desager JP, Hulhoven R, Smith RB, Harvengt C. Pharmacokinetic consequences of long term coadministration of cimetidine and triazolobenzodiazepines, alprazolam and triazolam, in healthy subjects. *Int J Clin Pharmacol Ther Toxicol* (1985) 23, 447–51.
13. Abernethy DR, Greenblatt DJ, Divoll M, Moschitto LJ, Harmatz JS, Shader RI. Interaction of cimetidine with the triazolobenzodiazepines alprazolam and triazolam. *Psychopharmacology (Berl)* (1983) 80, 275–8.
14. Ochs HR, Greenblatt DJ, Friedman H, Burstein ES, Locniskar A, Harmatz JS, Shader RI. Bromazepam pharmacokinetics: influence of age, gender, oral contraceptives, cimetidine and propranolol. *Clin Pharmacol Ther* (1987) 41, 562–70.
15. Desmond PV, Patwardhan RV, Schenker S, Speeg KV. Cimetidine impairs elimination of chlordiazepoxide (Librium) in man. *Ann Intern Med* (1980) 93, 266–8.
16. Pullar T, Edwards D, Haigh JRM, Peaker S, Feeley MP. The effect of cimetidine on the single dose pharmacokinetics of oral clobazam and *N*-desmethylclobazam. *Br J Clin Pharmacol* (1987) 23, 317–21.
17. Grigoleit H-G, Hajdú P, Hundt HKL, Koeppen D, Malerczyk V, Meyer BH, Müller FO, Witte PU. Pharmacokinetic aspects of the interaction between clobazam and cimetidine. *Eur J Clin Pharmacol* (1983) 25, 139–42.
18. Divoll M, Abernethy DR, Greenblatt DJ. Cimetidine impairs drug oxidizing capacity in the elderly. *Clin Pharmacol Ther* (1982) 31, 218.
19. Greenblatt DJ, Abernethy DR, Koepke HH, Shader RI. Interaction of cimetidine with oxazepam, lorazepam, and flurazepam. *J Clin Pharmacol* (1984) 24, 187–93.
20. Ochs HR, Greenblatt DJ, Gugler R, Müntefering G, Locniskar A, Abernethy DR. Cimetidine impairs nitrazepam clearance. *Clin Pharmacol Ther* (1983) 34, 227–30.
21. Friedman H, Greenblatt DJ, Burstein ES, Scavone JM, Harmatz JS, Shader RI. Triazolam kinetics: interaction with cimetidine, propranolol, and the combination. *J Clin Pharmacol* (1988) 28, 228–33.
22. Cox SR, Kroboth PD, Anderson PH, Smith RB. Mechanism for the interaction between triazolam and cimetidine. *Biopharm Drug Dispos* (1986) 7, 567–75.
23. Nelson DC, Schenker S, Hoyumpa AM, Speeg KV, Avant GR. The effects of cimetidine on chlordiazepoxide elimination in cirrhosis. *Clin Res* (1981) 29, 824A.
24. Bouden A, El Hechmi Z, Douki S. Cimetidine-benzodiazepine association confusiogene: a propros d'une observation. *Tunis Med* (1990) 68, 63–4.
25. Parker WA, MacLachlan RA. Prolonged hypnotic response to triazolam-cimetidine combination in an elderly patient. *Drug Intell Clin Pharm* (1984) 18, 980–1.
26. Britton ML, Waller ES. Central nervous system toxicity associated with concurrent use of triazolam and cimetidine. *Drug Intell Clin Pharm* (1985) 19, 666–8.
27. Ochs HR, Greenblatt DJ, Verburg-Ochs B, Harmatz JS, Grehl H. Disposition of clotiazepam: influence of age, sex, oral contraceptives, cimetidine, isoniazid and ethanol. *Eur J Clin Pharmacol* (1984) 26, 55–9.
28. Doenicke A, Dorow R, Täuber U. Die Pharmakokinetik von Lormetazepam nach Cimetidin. *Anaesthesist* (1991) 40, 675–9.
29. Patwardhan RV, Yarborough GW, Desmond PV, Johnson RF, Schenker S, Speeg KV. Cimetidine spares the glucuronidation of lorazepam and oxazepam. *Gastroenterology* (1980) 79, 912–16.
30. Klotz U, Reimann I. Influence of cimetidine on the pharmacokinetics of desmethyldiazepam and oxazepam. *Eur J Clin Pharmacol* (1980) 18, 517–20.
31. Greenblatt DJ, Abernethy DR, Divoll M, Locniskar A, Harmatz JS, Shader RI. Noninteraction of temazepam and cimetidine. *J Pharm Sci* (1984) 73, 399–401.
32. Elliott P, Dundee JW, Elwood RJ, Collier PS. The influence of H_2 receptor antagonists on the plasma concentrations of midazolam and temazepam. *Eur J Anaesthesiol* (1984) 1, 245–51.
33. Lam AM, Parkin JA. Cimetidine and prolonged post-operative somnolence. *Can Anaesth Soc J* (1981) 28, 450–2.
34. Sanders LD, Whitehead C, Gildersleve CD, Rosen M, Robinson JO. Interaction of H_2-receptor antagonists and benzodiazepine sedation. A double-blind placebo-controlled investigation of the effects of cimetidine and ranitidine on recovery after intravenous midazolam. *Anaesthesia* (1993) 48, 286–92.
35. Salonen M, Aantaa E, Aaltonen L, Kanto J. Importance of the interaction of midazolam and cimetidine. *Acta Pharmacol Toxicol (Copenh)* (1986) 58, 91–5.
36. Klotz U, Arvela P, Rosenkranz B. Effect of single doses of cimetidine and ranitidine on the steady-state plasma levels of midazolam. *Clin Pharmacol Ther* (1985) 38, 652–5.
37. Fee JPH, Collier PS, Howard PJ, Dundee JW. Cimetidine and ranitidine increase midazolam bioavailability. *Clin Pharmacol Ther* (1987) 41, 80–4.
38. Greenblatt DJ, Locniskar A, Scavone JM, Blyden GT, Ochs HR, Harmatz JS, Shader RI. Absence of interaction of cimetidine and ranitidine with intravenous and oral midazolam. *Anesth Analg* (1986) 65, 176–80.
39. Chichmanian RM, Mignot G, Spreux A, Jean-Girard C, Hofliger P. Tolérance de la famotidine. Étude due réseau médecins sentinelles en pharmacovigilance. *Therapie* (1992) 47, 239–43.
40. Klotz U, Arvela P, Rosenkranz B. Famotidine, a new H_2-receptor antagonist, does not affect hepatic elimination of diazepam or tubular secretion of procainamide. *Eur J Clin Pharmacol* (1985) 28, 671–5.
41. Klotz U, Gottlieb W, Keohane PP, Dammann HG. Nocturnal doses of ranitidine and nizatidine do not affect the disposition of diazepam. *J Clin Pharmacol* (1987) 27, 210–12.
42. Klotz U, Dammann HG, Gottlieb WR, Walter TA, Keohane P. Nizatidine (300 mg nocte) does not interfere with diazepam pharmacokinetics in man. *Br J Clin Pharmacol* (1987) 23, 105–6.
43. Klotz U. Lack of effect of nizatidine on drug metabolism. *Scand J Gastroenterol* (1987) 22 (Suppl 136), 18–23.
44. Suttle AB, Songer SS, Dukes GE, Hak LJ, Koruda M, Fleishaker JC, Brouwer KLR. Ranitidine does not alter adinazolam pharmacokinetics or pharmacodynamics. *J Clin Psychopharmacol* (1992) 12, 282–7.
45. Abernethy DR, Greenblatt DJ, Eshelman FN, Shader RI. Ranitidine does not impair oxidative or conjugative metabolism: noninteraction with antipyrine, diazepam, and lorazepam. *Clin Pharmacol Ther* (1984) 35, 188–92.
46. Klotz U, Reimann IW, Ohnhaus EE. Effect of ranitidine on the steady state pharmacokinetics of diazepam. *Eur J Clin Pharmacol* (1983) 24, 357–60.

47. Wilson CM, Robinson FP, Thompson EM, Dundee JW, Elliott P. Effect of pretreatment with ranitidine on the hypnotic action of single doses of midazolam, temazepam and zopiclone. A clinical study. *Br J Anaesth* (1986) 58, 483–6.
48. Vanderveen RP, Jirak JL, Peters GR, Cox SR, Bombardt PA. Effect of ranitidine on the disposition of orally and intravenously administered triazolam. *Clin Pharm* (1991) 10, 539–43.
49. O'Connor-Semmes RL, Kersey K, Williams DH, Lam R, Koch KM. Effect of ranitidine on the pharmacokinetics of triazolam and α-hydroxytriazolam in both young (19-60 years) and older (61-78 years) people. *Clin Pharmacol Ther* (2001) 70, 126–31.
50. Elwood RJ, Hildebrand PJ, Dundee JW, Collier PS. Ranitidine influences the uptake of oral midazolam. *Br J Clin Pharmacol* (1983) 15, 743–5.
51. Labs RA. Interaction of roxatidine acetate with antacids, food and other drugs. *Drugs* (1988) 35 (Suppl 3), 82–9.
52. Darwish M. Analysis of potential drug interactions with zaleplon. *J Am Geriatr Soc* (1999) 47, S62.
53. Hulhoven R, Desager JP, Harvengt C, Hermann P, Guillet P, Thiercelin JF. Lack of interaction between zolpidem and H_2 antagonists, cimetidine and ranitidine. *Int J Clin Pharmacol Res* (1988) 8, 471–6.

Benzodiazepines and related drugs + HCV-protease inhibitors

Boceprevir and telaprevir markedly increase the exposure to oral midazolam, but simeprevir only slightly increases it. Paritaprevir boosted with ritonavir (in a fixed-dose combination) is predicted to increase midazolam exposure. Telaprevir also increases the exposure to intravenous midazolam, although to a lesser extent than oral midazolam, but simeprevir has no effect. Triazolam is expected to be similarly affected by boceprevir, paritaprevir boosted with ritonavir (in a fixed-dose combination), simeprevir, and telaprevir. Alprazolam exposure is slightly increased by telaprevir and paritaprevir boosted with ritonavir (in a fixed-dose combination), and boceprevir is also expected to interact similarly. Telaprevir appears to slightly decrease the exposure to zolpidem, and zolpidem appears to slightly decrease the exposure to paritaprevir.

Clinical evidence

(a) Alprazolam

1. Paritaprevir. The UK and US manufacturers briefly report that, in a study in 12 healthy subjects, a single 500-microgram dose of alprazolam had no effect on the pharmacokinetics of paritaprevir 150 mg daily (in a fixed-dose combination with ritonavir and ombitasvir, and given with dasabuvir). The AUC of alprazolam was increased by 34%, but the maximum concentration was unaffected.[1,2]

2. Telaprevir. The UK and US manufacturers of telaprevir briefly report that, in a study in 17 healthy subjects, telaprevir 750 mg three times daily for 10 days increased the AUC of a single 500-microgram dose of alprazolam by 35%, but had no effect on its maximum plasma concentration.[3,4]

(b) Midazolam

1. Boceprevir. The UK and US manufacturers of boceprevir briefly report that in a study, boceprevir 800 mg three times daily for 6 days increased the AUC and maximum plasma concentration of a single 4-mg oral dose of midazolam about 5.3-fold and 2.8-fold, respectively.[5,6]

2. Simeprevir. The UK and US manufacturers briefly report that, in a study in 16 healthy subjects given simeprevir 150 mg daily for 10 days with *oral* midazolam 75 micrograms/kg, the AUC and maximum concentration of midazolam were increased by 45% and 31%, respectively. In contrast, when *intravenous* midazolam 25 micrograms/kg was given with the same dose of simeprevir, the AUC and maximum concentration of midazolam were unaffected.[7,8]

3. Telaprevir. In a study in 21 healthy subjects, telaprevir 750 mg three times daily for 11 days increased the AUC of a single 2-mg *oral* dose of midazolam nearly 9-fold and increased its maximum plasma concentration 2.9-fold. The AUC and maximum plasma concentration of the hydroxy metabolite were reduced by 39% and 86%, respectively. In the same study, telaprevir 750 mg three times daily for 10 days increased the AUC of a single 0.5-mg intravenous dose of midazolam 3.4-fold, but had no effect on its maximum plasma concentration. The half-life of both oral and intravenous midazolam was increased by about 13 hours.[9]

(c) Zolpidem

1. Paritaprevir. The UK manufacturer briefly reports that, in a study in healthy subjects, paritaprevir 150 mg daily (in a fixed-dose combination with ritonavir and ombitasvir, and given with dasabuvir) had no effect on the pharmacokinetics of a single 5-mg dose of zolpidem. However the AUC and maximum concentration of paritaprevir were decreased by 32% and 37%, respectively.[2]

2. Telaprevir. The UK and US manufacturers of telaprevir report that, in a study in 19 subjects, telaprevir 750 mg three times daily for 10 days reduced the AUC and maximum plasma concentration of a single 5-mg dose of zolpidem by 47% and 42%, respectively.[3,4]

Mechanism

Boceprevir, simeprevir, and telaprevir are inhibitors of CYP3A4, although it seems, to different extents. The benzodiazepines and zolpidem are, to varying degrees, metabolised by CYP3A4, with the extent of the interaction related to how important CYP3A4 is in their metabolism and how potent a CYP3A4 inhibitor the interacting drug is. So, for example midazolam, which is predominantly metabolised by CYP3A4, is greatly affected by potent inhibitors of this isoenzyme, whereas alprazolam, for which CYP3A4 is a less important route of metabolism, is only slightly affected.

The study with telaprevir,[9] suggests that it inhibits the metabolism of midazolam by CYP3A4 in the gut wall as well as the liver, because it had a greater effect on oral midazolam than intravenous midazolam. In contrast, the study with simeprevir,[7,8] suggests that it inhibits the metabolism of midazolam in the gut wall only, as it had no effect on intravenous midazolam. Paritaprevir does not appear to affect CYP3A4 itself, but it is given with ritonavir as a pharmacokinetic enhancer, and as this is a well-known potent inhibitor of CYP3A4, the effects on alprazolam seen when paritaprevir is given as part of a fixed-dose combination, would seem to be most likely due to the ritonavir.

Other isoenzymes are also involved in the metabolism of zolpidem, which is less affected by CYP3A4 inhibitors as a result, but the possible mechanism for the *reduction* in exposure by telaprevir is unknown.[6]

Importance and management

The pharmacokinetic interaction between boceprevir or telaprevir and **midazolam** appears to be established and of clinical importance. Such marked increases in midazolam exposure are likely to result in prolonged or increased sedation and respiratory depression. The UK and US manufacturers of boceprevir and telaprevir therefore contraindicate concurrent use with *oral* midazolam.[3-6] The metabolism of *intravenous* midazolam was affected by telaprevir to a lesser degree than oral, and as such the UK and US manufacturers of boceprevir and telaprevir advise close monitoring for adverse effects, such as increased or excessive sedation and for signs of respiratory depression on concurrent use, adjusting the dose of intravenous midazolam[3,5] as necessary or using a lower dose.[4,6] As simeprevir only affected midazolam exposure when given orally, and the effect was only slight, the UK and US manufacturers advise caution on concurrent use of simeprevir with oral but not intravenous midazolam.[7,8] Based on the effects of ritonavir on midazolam exposure, the UK manufacturer of paritaprevir boosted with ritonavir (in a fixed-dose combination with ombitasvir with or without dasabuvir) contraindicates concurrent use with *oral* midazolam. If *intravenous* midazolam is required, they advise close monitoring for adverse effects, such as increased or excessive sedation and for signs of respiratory depression, with consideration given to adjusting the dose of intravenous midazolam.[2]

Triazolam is also extensively metabolised by CYP3A4, like midazolam, and would therefore be expected to be similarly affected. The US manufacturers of boceprevir[6] and telaprevir[4] contraindicate the concurrent use of triazolam, whereas the UK manufacturers contraindicate the concurrent use of *oral* triazolam only.[3,5] Similarly, the UK manufacturer of paritaprevir boosted with ritonavir (in a fixed-dose combination with ombitasvir with or without dasabuvir) contraindicates concurrent use with triazolam use.[2] In the UK, it is recommended that patients given boceprevir and *intravenous* triazolam should be closely monitored for adverse effects, such as increased or excessive sedation and for signs of respiratory depression, with adjustment of the triazolam dose as necessary.[5] The UK and US manufacturers of simeprevir advise caution on concurrent use with *oral* triazolam due to the possibility of a small increase in exposure, as with midazolam.[7,8]

Similar caution is advised on the concurrent use of boceprevir, paritaprevir boosted with ritonavir (in a fixed-dose combination with ombitasvir, and given with or without dasabuvir), or telaprevir and **alprazolam**, which is also metabolised by CYP3A4,[1,2,4-6] although note that CYP3A4 is less important in the metabolism of alprazolam than midazolam and this is reflected in the slight increase in alprazolam exposure seen with telaprevir in comparison with the marked increase in midazolam exposure. The effects of simeprevir on alprazolam have not been studied, but given that simeprevir only slightly increased *oral* midazolam exposure, that CYP3A4 has a lesser role in the metabolism of alprazolam than midazolam, and the high oral bioavailability of alprazolam, a clinically relevant interaction between simeprevir and alprazolam might not be expected. Nevertheless, until more is known some caution on concurrent use might be prudent.

The clinical relevance of the *reduction* in **zolpidem** exposure by telaprevir is unknown; however, it seems possible that its efficacy might be reduced. It would therefore seem prudent to monitor concurrent use to ensure zolpidem remains effective in patients also taking telaprevir, adjusting the dose of zolpidem if necessary. The decrease in exposure to paritaprevir boosted with ritonavir (in a fixed-dose combination with ombitasvir, and given with dasabuvir) with zolpidem was only slight and unlikely to be clinically relevant, and zolpidem pharmacokinetics were unaffected. Therefore, no dose adjustments are expected to be necessary when zolpidem is given with this combination.

Note that midazolam is used as a probe substrate to assess the activity of other drugs on CYP3A4. The data here therefore suggest that boceprevir and telaprevir are potent inhibitors of CYP3A4. For a list of CYP3A4 substrates, see 'Table 1.10', p.12. Further, simeprevir would appear to be only a weak inhibitor of (intestinal) CYP3A4.

1. Viekira Pak (Ombitasvir, paritaprevir, ritonavir co-packaged with dasabuvir sodium monohydrate). AbbVie Inc. US Prescribing information, December 2014.
2. Viekirax (Ombitasvir, paritaprevir, ritonavir). AbbVie Ltd. UK Summary of product characteristics, January 2015.
3. Incivo (Telaprevir). Janssen-Cilag Ltd. UK Summary of product characteristics, July 2014.
4. Incivek (Telaprevir). Vertex Pharmaceuticals, Inc. US Prescribing information, October 2013.
5. Victrelis (Boceprevir). Merck Sharp & Dohme Ltd. UK Summary of product characteristics, August 2014.
6. Victrelis (Boceprevir). Merck & Co., Inc. US Prescribing information, July 2014.
7. Olysio (Simeprevir sodium). Janssen-Cilag Ltd. UK Summary of product characteristics, May 2014.
8. Olysio (Simeprevir sodium). Janssen Products, LP. US Prescribing information, November 2014.
9. Garg V, Chandorkar G, Farmer HF, Smith F, Alves K, van Heeswijk RPG. Effect of telaprevir on the pharmacokinetics of midazolam and digoxin. *J Clin Pharmacol* (2012) 52, 1566–73.

Benzodiazepines and related drugs + HIV-protease inhibitors

Ritonavir, nelfinavir, saquinavir and saquinavir boosted with ritonavir, lopinavir and tipranavir reduce the metabolism and/or increase the bioavailability of midazolam: other HIV-protease inhibitors boosted with ritonavir would be predicted to interact similarly. Ritonavir affects triazolam and, to a lesser extent, alprazolam and zolpidem. Increased sedative effects are predicted with several different pairs of HIV-protease inhibitors and benzodiazepines.

Clinical evidence

A. Benzodiazepines

(a) Alprazolam

A crossover study in 10 healthy subjects found that **ritonavir** 200 mg for 4 doses decreased the clearance of a single 1-mg dose of alprazolam by 59% and increased its AUC approximately 2.5-fold. The half-life of alprazolam was increased from 13.3 hours to 29.6 hours and the subjects experienced increased and prolonged sedation.[1] However, in another study when **ritonavir** 500 mg was given every 12 hours for 10 days, the AUC of a single dose of alprazolam was *decreased* by 12%.[2,3]

(b) Midazolam

1. Lopinavir. In a study, 14 healthy subjects were given intravenous midazolam 0.025 mg/kg on days one and 14 and oral midazolam 5 mg on days 2 and 15, with lopinavir boosted with ritonavir 400/100 mg twice daily for 14 days from day 4 to day 17. The clearance of intravenous and oral midazolam were reduced, by 77% and 92%, respectively.[4] Further, the manufacturer of lopinavir boosted with ritonavir notes that, in a study in 14 healthy subjects, lopinavir boosted with ritonavir raised the AUC of intravenous and oral midazolam 4-fold and 13-fold, respectively.[5]

2. Nelfinavir. In a study, 90 HIV-positive patients not taking antiretrovirals (control group) and 56 similar patients taking antiretrovirals were given a 75-microgram oral dose of midazolam. The ratio of 1-hydroxymidazolam to midazolam, assessed 30 minutes after the midazolam dose, was found to be 13-fold lower in 18 patients taking nelfinavir, when compared with the control group.[6]

3. Ritonavir. In a study, 90 HIV-positive patients not taking antiretrovirals (control group) and 56 similar patients taking antiretrovirals were given a 75-microgram oral dose of midazolam. The ratio of 1-hydroxymidazolam to midazolam, assessed 30 minutes after the midazolam dose, was found to be 50-fold lower in 4 patients taking ritonavir, but less reduced in other patients who were also taking efavirenz or nevirapine.[6] In a three-way crossover study in 13 healthy subjects, three doses of ritonavir 100 mg given over 24 hours increased the AUC of a single 3-mg oral dose of midazolam about 26-fold and reduced its oral clearance by 96%, compared with placebo.[7]

4. Saquinavir. A randomised study in 12 healthy subjects found that saquinavir (soft-gel formulation) 1.2 g three times daily increased the bioavailability of oral midazolam from 41% to 90% and increased its AUC 5.2-fold. Psychomotor tests showed impaired skills and greater sedation in the presence of saquinavir.[8] When intravenous midazolam was given with saquinavir, its sedative effects were only marginally altered.[8] However, a 32-year-old man with advanced HIV, taking zidovudine, lamivudine, co-trimoxazole and saquinavir 600 mg three times daily, did not wake spontaneously from a 5-mg intravenous dose of midazolam. He was given 300 micrograms of intravenous flumazenil to revert the prolonged sedation, but he was not free from sedation until 5 hours later. On a previous occasion, in the absence of saquinavir, he woke spontaneously 2 hours after the dose of midazolam.[9] In 18 healthy subjects, saquinavir boosted with ritonavir 1000/100 mg twice daily for 2 weeks increased the maximum plasma concentration and AUC of a single 7.5-mg oral dose of midazolam 4.3-fold and 12.4-fold, respectively.[10]

5. Tipranavir. The manufacturer of tipranavir notes that tipranavir boosted with ritonavir increased the AUCs of intravenous and oral midazolam 2.8-fold and 9.8-fold, respectively.[11]

(c) Triazolam

In a crossover study in 6 healthy subjects, **ritonavir** 200 mg for 4 doses reduced the clearance of triazolam 125 micrograms to less than 4% of control values, increased its AUC about 20-fold and increased its half-life from 3 hours to 41 hours, which resulted in increased and prolonged sedation.[12] A very brief case report also describes prolonged sedation in a patient given **ritonavir** and triazolam.[13]

B. Non-benzodiazepine hypnotics

A crossover study in 6 healthy subjects found that **ritonavir** 200 mg twice daily for four doses resulted in a 28% increase in the AUC of a single 5-mg dose of **zolpidem**. The reduction in the clearance of **zolpidem** was considered to be clinically unimportant.[12]

Mechanism

Midazolam, triazolam, and to a lesser extent, alprazolam, are metabolised by CYP3A4, which is inhibited, to varying degrees, by the HIV-protease inhibitors. Concurrent use therefore increases the exposure to these benzodiazepines and their resultant effects. However, ritonavir can also induce CYP3A and although metabolism might be inhibited following the introduction of ritonavir, it appears that for some drugs, such as alprazolam, the inhibitory effects of ritonavir on CYP3A4 decreases over time,[2,3] possibly reflecting the effect of induction from chronic exposure overcoming the inhibition due to acute exposure.[14] One study suggested that the enzyme-inducing effects of the HIV-protease inhibitors are diminished by efavirenz and nevirapine, which are known enzyme inducers.[6] Another study suggests that lopinavir boosted with ritonavir inhibits CYP3A4 in the liver and in the gut wall, resulting in a greater effect on oral midazolam than intravenous midazolam.[4]

Interactions between the HIV-protease inhibitors and the benzodiazepines that are metabolised mainly by glucuronidation, such as **lorazepam, oxazepam** or **temazepam**, are less likely, and reports are lacking. However, some HIV-protease inhibitors, such as ritonavir, also induce glucuronidation, and so in theory they could induce the metabolism of these benzodiazepines decreasing their effects.[2,15]

Importance and management

The interaction between the HIV-protease inhibitors and **midazolam** is established and of clinical importance. The UK manufacturers of the HIV-protease inhibitors contraindicate the concurrent use of *oral* midazolam, but advise that *intravenous* midazolam may be used with close monitoring within an intensive care unit or similar setting so that the appropriate management of respiratory depression is available. They also suggest that dose reductions should be considered. The authors of one study[8] suggest that continuous intravenous midazolam doses should be reduced by 50%, but do not consider dose adjustments for single intravenous doses necessary.

Triazolam would be expected to interact in the same way as midazolam, and therefore the UK manufacturers generally contraindicate its use with HIV-protease inhibitors. The US manufacturers similarly contraindicate the concurrent use of midazolam and triazolam with HIV-protease inhibitors; however, they do not always differentiate between oral or intravenous midazolam.

Alprazolam is contraindicated by the UK and US manufacturers of indinavir,[16,17] whereas the manufacturers of saquinavir advise caution.[18,19] The manufacturer of ritonavir also suggests caution during the first several days when alprazolam is given with ritonavir, before induction of alprazolam metabolism develops.[2] Careful monitoring and dose adjustment will be required. It would seem prudent to apply some caution on the concurrent use of any HIV-protease inhibitor, as alprazolam is, in part, metabolised by the same route as midazolam.

Recommendations regarding other benzodiazepines vary. **Clorazepate, diazepam, estazolam,** and **flurazepam** are contraindicated by the UK manufacturer of ritonavir[2] and indinavir,[16] whereas the US manufacturer of ritonavir states that a decrease in the dose of these benzodiazepines might be necessary on concurrent use.[3] The US manufacturer of fosamprenavir and the UK and US manufacturers of saquinavir also suggest the possibility of an interaction with clorazepate, diazepam and flurazepam, and suggest that careful monitoring is needed, with dose adjustments as required.[18-20]

The manufacturers of ritonavir state that **zolpidem** may be given concurrently with careful monitoring for excessive sedative effects[2] and consideration of reducing the dose of zolpidem.[3] Similarly, the manufacturer of **zopiclone** warns that, as zopiclone is metabolised by CYP3A4, plasma concentrations of zopiclone might be increased when it is given with CYP3A4 inhibitors such as ritonavir, and a dose reduction of zopiclone might be required.[21]

Note that midazolam is used as a probe substrate to assess the activity of other drugs on CYP3A4. The data here therefore suggests that ritonavir, and all of the HIV-protease inhibitors boosted with ritonavir so far studied (lopinavir, saquinavir, and tipranavir), are potent inhibitors of CYP3A4. Unboosted saquinavir, while having much smaller effects than ritonavir-boosted HIV-protease inhibitors, is also a potent inhibitor of CYP3A4. For a list of CYP3A4 substrates, see 'Table 1.10', p.12.

1. Greenblatt DJ, von Moltke LL, Harmatz JS, Durol ALB, Daily JP, Graf JA, Mertzanis P, Hoffman JL, Shader RI. Alprazolam-ritonavir interaction: implications for product labeling. *Clin Pharmacol Ther* (2000) 67, 335–41.
2. Norvir Soft Capsules (Ritonavir). Abbott Laboratories Ltd. UK Summary of product characteristics, October 2010.
3. Norvir Capsules (Ritonavir). Abbott Laboratories. US Prescribing information, March 2012.
4. Yeh RF, Gaver VE, Patterson KB, Rezk NL, Baxter-Meheux F, Blake MJ, Eron JJ, Klein CE, Rublein JC, Kashuba AD. Lopinavir/ritonavir induces the hepatic activity of cytochrome P450 enzymes CYP2C9, CYP2C19, and CYP1A2 but inhibits the hepatic and intestinal activity of CYP3A as measured by a phenotyping drug cocktail in healthy volunteers. *J Acquir Immune Defic Syndr* (2006) 42, 52–60.
5. Kaletra Tablets (Lopinavir with Ritonavir). AbbVie Ltd. UK Summary of product characteristics, August 2012.
6. Fellay J, Marzolini C, Decosterd L, Golay KP, Baumann P, Buclin T, Telenti A, Eap CB. Variations of CYP3A activity induced by antiretroviral treatment in HIV-1 infected patients. *Eur J Clin Pharmacol* (2005) 60, 865–73.
7. Greenblatt DJ, Peters DE, Oleson LE, Harmatz JS, MacNab MW, Berkowitz N, Zinny MA, Court MH. Inhibition of oral midazolam clearance by boosting doses of ritonavir, and by 4,4-dimethyl-benziso-(2H)-selenazine (ALT-2074), an experimental catalytic mimic of glutathione oxidase. *Br J Clin Pharmacol* (2009) 68, 920–7.
8. Palkama VJ, Ahonen J, Neuvonen PJ, Olkkola KT. Effect of saquinavir on the pharmacokinetics and pharmacodynamics of oral and intravenous midazolam. *Clin Pharmacol Ther* (1999) 66, 33–9.
9. Merry C, Mulcahy F, Barry M, Gibbons S, Back D. Saquinavir interaction with midazolam: pharmacokinetic considerations when prescribing protease inhibitors for patients with HIV disease. *AIDS* (1997) 11, 268–9.
10. Schmitt C, Hofmann C, Riek M, Patel A, Zwanziger E. Effect of saquinavir-ritonavir on cytochrome P450 3A4 activity in healthy volunteers using midazolam as a probe. *Pharmacotherapy* (2009) 29, 1175–81.
11. Aptivus Soft Capsules (Tipranavir). Boehringer Ingelheim Ltd. UK Summary of product characteristics, December 2011.
12. Greenblatt DJ, von Moltke LL, Harmatz JS, Durol AL, Daily JP, Graf JA, Mertzanis P, Hoffman JL, Shader RI. Differential impairment of triazolam and zolpidem clearance by ritonavir. *J Acquir Immune Defic Syndr* (2000) 24, 129–36.
13. Shader RI, Greenblatt DJ. Protease inhibitors and drug interaction—an alert. *J Clin Psychopharmacol* (1996) 16, 343–4.
14. Greenblatt DJ, von Moltke LL, Daily JP, Harmatz JS, Shader RI. Extensive impairment of triazolam and alprazolam clearance by short-term low-dose ritonavir: the clinical dilemma of concurrent inhibition and induction. *J Clin Psychopharmacol* (1999) 19, 293–6.
15. Antoniou T, Tseng AL. Interactions between recreational drugs and antiretroviral agents. *Ann Pharmacother* (2002) 36, 1598–1613.

16. Crixivan (Indinavir sulphate). Merck Sharp & Dohme Ltd. UK Summary of product characteristics, February 2012.
17. Crixivan (Indinavir sulfate). Merck & Co., Inc. US Prescribing information, April 2012.
18. Invirase Hard Capsules (Saquinavir mesilate). Roche Products Ltd. UK Summary of product characteristics, June 2012.
19. Invirase (Saquinavir mesylate). Genentech, Inc. US Prescribing information, February 2012.
20. Lexiva (Fosamprenavir calcium). ViiV Healthcare. US Prescribing information, April 2013.
21. Zimovane (Zopiclone). Sanofi-Aventis. UK Summary of product characteristics, August 2009.

Benzodiazepines and related drugs + Hormonal contraceptives

Combined hormonal contraceptives appear to reduce the clearance of chlordiazepoxide and diazepam, and, to a lesser extent nitrazepam. Conversely, they increase the clearance of oxazepam, lorazepam and temazepam. Alprazolam, bromazepam, clotiazepam, midazolam, triazolam, and zolpidem are only minimally affected or not affected at all by combined hormonal contraceptives. There is limited evidence that chlordiazepoxide, diazepam, nitrazepam and meprobamate can possibly increase the incidence of break-through bleeding in patients taking hormonal contraceptives.

Clinical evidence

(a) Effects on benzodiazepines and related drugs

A controlled study found that the mean half-life of intravenous **chlordiazepoxide** 600 micrograms/kg was virtually doubled (20.6 hours compared with 11.6 hours) and the total clearance was almost two-thirds lower in 6 women taking oral combined hormonal contraceptives when compared with 6 women not taking oral combined hormonal contraceptives.[1]

Similar but less notable effects were found in other studies in women taking oral combined hormonal contraceptives given **chlordiazepoxide**,[2] **diazepam**,[3,4] and to an even lesser extent with **nitrazepam**.[5] Oral combined hormonal contraceptives have also been reported to inhibit[6] or to have no significant influence[7] on the metabolism of **alprazolam**. No statistically and/or clinically significant pharmacokinetic changes were seen when **bromazepam**,[8] **clotiazepam**,[9] **midazolam** (given orally,[10,11] intramuscularly,[12] or intravenously[10,13]), **triazolam**,[6] or **zolpidem**[14] were given with combined hormonal contraceptives.

A controlled study, comparing 7 women taking an oral combined hormonal contraceptive with 8 women not taking oral combined hormonal contraceptives found that the mean half-life of intravenous **lorazepam** 2 mg was over 50% shorter in the contraceptive group (6 hours compared with 14 hours) and the total clearance was over 3-fold greater.[1] A smaller increase in the elimination rate was seen in other controlled studies in women taking oral combined hormonal contraceptives and **lorazepam**,[6,15] or **temazepam**,[6] and in two other studies small decreases in the half-life of **oxazepam** were observed.[1,15]

(b) Effects on contraceptives

A study in 72 patients taking oral combined hormonal contraceptives (*Rigevidon*, *Anteovin*) found that breakthrough bleeding occurred in 36% of patients while taking **chlordiazepoxide** 10 to 20 mg daily, **diazepam** 5 to 15 mg daily, **nitrazepam** 5 to 10 mg daily or **meprobamate** 200 to 600 mg daily, but no pregnancies occurred. Only three cases of bleeding occurred with **diazepam** or **nitrazepam**.[16] The average incidence of breakthrough bleeding with these two oral contraceptives were 9.1% for *Rigevidon* and 3.3% for *Anteovin* in the absence of other drugs. It was possible to establish a causal relationship between the bleeding and the use of the anxiolytic/hypnotic in 77% of the cases either by stopping the drug or by changing it for another.[16]

Mechanism

Combined hormonal contraceptives affect the metabolism of the benzodiazepines by the liver in different ways: oxidative metabolism (possibly by CYP1A2 and CYP2C19)[13] is reduced (chlordiazepoxide, diazepam), whereas metabolism by glucuronide conjugation is increased (lorazepam, oxazepam, temazepam). Combined hormonal contraceptives do not affect CYP3A activity, and therefore do not alter midazolam clearance,[13] and are unlikely to affect other similarly metabolised benzodiazepines. Just why these hypnotics should cause breakthrough bleeding is not understood.

Importance and management

The pharmacokinetic interactions between the combined hormonal contraceptives and the benzodiazepines and related drugs are established interactions, but of uncertain clinical importance. Long-term use of some benzodiazepines that are highly oxidised (such as chlordiazepoxide, diazepam, and possibly nitrazepam) in women taking a combined hormonal contraceptive should be monitored to ensure that the dose is not too high. Those taking benzodiazepines that are metabolised to glucuronides (such as lorazepam, oxazepam, and temazepam) might need a dose increase, but this is not proven. Alprazolam, bromazepam, clotiazepam, midazolam, triazolam and zolpidem appear to interact minimally or not at all. No firm conclusions could be drawn from the results of one study, which set out to evaluate the importance of this interaction.[17]

The possible increased incidence of breakthrough bleeding (more than one-third) due to these anxiolytics/hypnotics, is an unpleasant reaction, but no contraceptive failures have been reported.[16] Limited evidence from the study suggests that changing the anxiolytic/hypnotic or the contraceptive might avoid breakthrough bleeding. Note that the UK Family Planning Association[18] did not consider that additional contraceptive precautions were necessary with **clonazepam** or **clobazam** and it seems unlikely that they will be necessary with most benzodiazepines.

1. Patwardhan RV, Mitchell MC, Johnson RF, Schenker S. Differential effects of oral contraceptive steroids on the metabolism of benzodiazepines. *Hepatology* (1983) 3, 248–53.
2. Roberts RK, Desmond PV, Wilkinson GR, Schenker S. Disposition of chlordiazepoxide: sex differences and effects of oral contraceptives. *Clin Pharmacol Ther* (1979) 25, 826–31.
3. Giles HG, Sellers EM, Naranjo CA, Frecker RC, Greenblatt DJ. Disposition of intravenous diazepam in young men and women. *Eur J Clin Pharmacol* (1981) 20, 207–13.
4. Abernethy DR, Greenblatt DJ, Divoll M, Arendt R, Ochs HR, Shader RI. Impairment of diazepam metabolism by low-dose estrogen-containing oral-contraceptive steroids. *N Engl J Med* (1982) 306, 791–2.
5. Jochemsen R, Van der Graff M, Boeijinga JK, Breimer DD. Influence of sex, menstrual cycle and oral contraception on the disposition of nitrazepam. *Br J Clin Pharmacol* (1982) 13, 319–24.
6. Stoehr GP, Kroboth PD, Juhl RP, Wender DB, Phillips JP, Smith RB. Effect of oral contraceptives on triazolam, temazepam, alprazolam, and lorazepam kinetics. *Clin Pharmacol Ther* (1984) 36, 683–90.
7. Scavone JM, Greenblatt DJ, Locniskar A, Shader RI. Alprazolam pharmacokinetics in women on low-dose oral contraceptives. *J Clin Pharmacol* (1988) 28, 454–7.
8. Ochs HR, Greenblatt DJ, Friedman H, Burstein ES, Locniskar A, Harmatz JS, Shader RI. Bromazepam pharmacokinetics: influence of age, gender, oral contraceptives, cimetidine, and propranolol. *Clin Pharmacol Ther* (1987) 41, 562–70.
9. Ochs HR, Greenblatt DJ, Verburg-Ochs B, Harmatz JS, Grehl H. Disposition of clotiazepam: influence of age, sex, oral contraceptives, cimetidine, isoniazid and ethanol. *Eur J Clin Pharmacol* (1984) 26, 55–9.
10. Belle DJ, Callaghan JT, Gorski JC, Maya JF, Mousa O, Wrighton SA, Hall SD. The effects of an oral contraceptive containing ethinyloestradiol and norgestrel on CYP3A activity. *Br J Clin Pharmacol* (2002) 53, 67–74.
11. Palovaara S, Kivistö KT, Tapanainen P, Manninen P, Neuvonen PJ, Laine K. Effect of an oral contraceptive preparation containing ethinylestradiol and gestodene on CYP3A4 activity as measured by midazolam 1′-hydroxylation. *Br J Clin Pharmacol* (2000) 50, 333–7.
12. Holazo AA, Winkler MB, Patel IH. Effects of age, gender and oral contraceptives on intramuscular midazolam pharmacokinetics. *J Clin Pharmacol* (1988) 28, 1040–5.
13. Shelepova T, Nafziger AN, Victory J, Kashuba ADM, Rowland E, Zhang Y, Sellers E, Kearns G, Leeder JS, Gaedigk A, Bertino JS. Effect of a triphasic oral contraceptive on drug-metabolizing enzyme activity as measured by the validated Cooperstown 5+1 cocktail. *J Clin Pharmacol* (2005), 45, 1413–21.
14. Olubodun JO, Ochs HR, Trüten V, Klein A, von Moltke LL, Harmatz JS, Shader RI, Greenblatt DJ. Zolpidem pharmacokinetic properties in young females: influence of smoking and oral contraceptive use. *J Clin Pharmacol* (2002) 42, 1142–6.
15. Abernethy DR, Greenblatt DJ, Ochs HR, Weyers D, Divoll M, Harmatz JS, Shader RI. Lorazepam and oxazepam kinetics in women on low-dose oral contraceptives. *Clin Pharmacol Ther* (1983) 33, 628–32.
16. Somos P. Interaction between certain psychopharmaca and low-dose oral contraceptives. *Ther Hung* (1990) 38, 37–40.
17. Kroboth PD, Smith RB, Stoehr GP, Juhl RP. Pharmacodynamic evaluation of the benzodiazepine–oral contraceptive interaction. *Clin Pharmacol Ther* (1985) 38, 525–32.
18. Belfield T, ed. FPA Contraceptive Handbook: a guide for family planning and other health professionals. 3rd ed. London: Family Planning Association, 1999.

Benzodiazepines + 5-HT_3-receptor antagonists

Granisetron does not appear to interact with lorazepam, and ondansetron does not appear to interact with temazepam.

Clinical evidence, mechanism, importance and management

Lorazepam 2.5 mg, given to 12 healthy subjects, clearly affected the performance of a number of psychometric tests. Statistically significant increases occurred in drowsiness, feebleness, muzziness, clumsiness, lethargy, mental slowness, relaxation, dreaminess, incompetence, sadness, and withdrawal. However, there was very little evidence that **granisetron** 160 micrograms/kg alone had any effect on the performance of these tests except that clumsiness and inattentiveness were increased, nor was there evidence that granisetron added to the effects of **lorazepam** when both drugs were taken concurrently.[1]

In a placebo-controlled, crossover study in 24 healthy subjects, **ondansetron** 8 mg did not affect the pharmacokinetics of **temazepam** 20 mg. The psychomotor performances of the subjects (subjective and objective sedation, memory, and other measurements) were not influenced by the presence of the **ondansetron**.[2]

No additional precautions would seem to be necessary if either of these pairs of drugs are given.

1. Leigh TJ, Link CGG, Fell GL. Effects of granisetron and lorazepam, alone and in combination, on psychometric performance. *Br J Clin Pharmacol* (1991) 31, 333–6.
2. Preston GC, Keene ON, Palmer JL. The effect of ondansetron on the pharmacokinetics and pharmacodynamics of temazepam. *Anaesthesia* (1996) 51, 827–30.

Benzodiazepines + Influenza vaccines

The pharmacokinetics of alprazolam, chlordiazepoxide and lorazepam are not affected by influenza vaccination.

Clinical evidence, mechanism, importance and management

In a study in healthy subjects, the pharmacokinetics of single doses of oral **alprazolam** 1 mg or intravenous **lorazepam** 2 mg were not affected when the benzodiazepines were given 7 and 21 days after 0.5 mL of an intramuscular trivalent influenza vaccine.[1] Similarly, in another study, neither **lorazepam** nor **chlordiazepoxide** metabolism was altered when they were given intravenously one and 7 days after a trivalent influenza vaccine.[2] There would seem to be no reason for avoiding these benzodiazepines after influenza vaccination.

1. Scavone JM, Blyden GT, Greenblatt DJ. Lack of effect of influenza vaccine on the pharmacokinetics of antipyrine, alprazolam, paracetamol (acetaminophen) and lorazepam. *Clin Pharmacokinet* (1989) 16, 180–5.
2. Meredith CG, Christian CD, Johnson RF, Troxell R, Davis GL, Schenker S. Effects of influenza virus vaccine on hepatic drug metabolism. *Clin Pharmacol Ther* (1985) 37, 396–401.

Benzodiazepines + Isoniazid

Isoniazid reduces the clearance of diazepam and triazolam. No interaction occurs between isoniazid and oxazepam or clotiazepam.

Clinical evidence

A study in 9 healthy subjects found that isoniazid 90 mg twice daily for 3 days increased the half-life of a single 5- or 7.5-mg dose of **diazepam** from about 34 hours to 45 hours, and reduced its total clearance by 26%.[1] Similarly, in another study in 6 healthy subjects, isoniazid 90 mg twice daily for 3 days, increased the half-life of a single 500-microgram dose of **triazolam** from 2.5 hours to 3.3 hours, increased its AUC by 46%, and reduced its clearance by 42%.[2]

Conversely, in a study in 9 healthy subjects, isoniazid 90 mg twice daily for 3 days had no effect on the pharmacokinetics of a single 30-mg oral dose of **oxazepam**,[2] and in another study, the pharmacokinetics of **clotiazepam** were not altered by isoniazid.[3]

Mechanism

What is known suggests that isoniazid acts as an enzyme inhibitor, decreasing the metabolism and clearance of diazepam and triazolam, thereby increasing and prolonging their effects. Oxazepam, which is metabolised by glucuronidation, would be unlikely to interact.

Importance and management

Information is limited but the pharmacokinetic interactions between isoniazid and diazepam and triazolam appear to be established. Their clinical importance is uncertain. Nevertheless, the decreases in clearance are slight and unlikely to result in increased effects. Bear the possibility in mind if problems occur when starting isoniazid. There seems to be no direct information about other benzodiazepines, but those undergoing high first-pass extraction and/or liver microsomal metabolism (such as **alprazolam** or **midazolam**) might interact similarly. Oxazepam and clotiazepam appear not to interact.

1. Ochs HR, Greenblatt DJ, Roberts G-M, Dengler HJ. Diazepam interaction with antituberculosis drugs. *Clin Pharmacol Ther* (1981) 29, 671–8.
2. Ochs HR, Greenblatt DJ, Knüchel M. Differential effect of isoniazid on triazolam oxidation and oxazepam conjugation. *Br J Clin Pharmacol* (1983) 16, 743–6.
3. Ochs HR, Greenblatt DJ, Verburg-Ochs B, Harmatz JS, Grehl H. Disposition of clotiazepam: influence of age, sex, oral contraceptives, cimetidine, isoniazid and ethanol. *Eur J Clin Pharmacol* (1984) 26, 55–9.

Benzodiazepines + Kava

A man taking alprazolam became semicomatose a few days after starting to take kava. The pharmacokinetics of midazolam are not affected by kava.

Clinical evidence

(a) Alprazolam

A 54-year-old man taking alprazolam, cimetidine and terazosin was hospitalised in a lethargic and disorientated state 3 days after starting to take kava, which he had bought from a local health food store. He denied having overdosed with any of these drugs. The patient became alert again after several hours.[1]

(b) Midazolam

In a study in 6 subjects, who regularly took 7 to 27 g of kavalactones weekly as an aqueous kava extract, there was no change in the metabolism of a single 8-mg oral dose of midazolam before or after they *stopped* kava for 30 days.[2] Similar results were found in two further pharmacokinetic studies. In a study in 16 healthy subjects given kava root extract 1.227 g three times daily (standardised to contain 75 mg kavalactones per capsule) for 14 days before taking a single 8-mg dose of oral midazolam, the pharmacokinetics of midazolam were unaffected.[3] Likewise, in another study in 12 healthy subjects given kava root extract 1 g twice daily (with no standardisation claim) for 28 days before receiving a single 8-mg dose of oral midazolam, the pharmacokinetics of midazolam were similarly unaffected.[4]

Mechanism

The reason for what happened is not known, but the suggested explanation is that the kavalactones might have had additive sedative effects with those of the alprazolam.[1,5]

Importance and management

The alprazolam case is an isolated case and its general importance is not known, although it fits with the theoretical pharmacological interaction anticipated. Bear the possibility of increased sedation in mind if kava and benzodiazepines are used together. No pharmacokinetic interaction occurs between midazolam and kava, and would not be expected with other similarly metabolised benzodiazepines such as triazolam and possibly alprazolam

Note that midazolam is used as a probe substrate to assess the activity of other drugs on CYP3A4. The evidence here therefore suggests that kava has no effect on CYP3A4 activity.

1. Almeida JC, Grimsley EW. Coma from the health food store: interaction between kava and alprazolam. *Ann Intern Med* (1996) 125, 940–1.
2. Russmann S, Lauterburg BH, Barguil Y, Choblet E, Cabalion P, Rentsch K, Wenk M. Traditional aqueous kava extracts inhibit cytochrome P450 1A2 in humans: protective effect against environmental carcinogens? *Clin Pharmacol Ther* (2005) 77, 453–4.
3. Gurley BJ, Swain A, Hubbard MA, Hartsfield F, Thaden J, Williams DK, Gentry WB, Tong Y. Supplementation with Goldenseal (*Hydratis Canadensis*), but not Kava Kava (*Piper methysticum*), inhibits human CYP3A activity *in vivo*. *Clin Pharmacol Ther* (2008) 83, 61–9.
4. Gurley BJ, Gardner SF, Hubbard MA, Williams DK, Gentry WB, Khan IA, Shah A. In vivo effects of goldenseal, kava kava, black cohosh, and valerian on human cytochrome P450 1A2, 2D6, 2E1, and 3A4/5 phenotypes. *Clin Pharmacol Ther* (2005) 77, 415–26.
5. Jussofie A, Schmiz A, Hiemke C. Kavapyrone enriched extract from *Piper methysticum* as modulator of the GABA binding site in different regions of rat brain. *Psychopharmacology (Berl)* (1994) 116, 469–74.

Benzodiazepines + Loxapine

The concurrent use of lorazepam and loxapine has resulted in sedation and respiratory depression.

Clinical evidence, mechanism, importance and management

A woman with a manic bipolar affective disorder was admitted to hospital and given lorazepam 2 mg with loxapine 25 mg. After 2 hours she was found to be lethargic with sonorous respirations, occasional episodes of apnoea and an irregular respiration as low as 4 breaths per minute. She was given oxygen and recovered spontaneously within 12 hours. She had experienced no previous problems with lorazepam, and had none when it was later given while she was taking perphenazine.[1] Two other cases have been reported where patients given intramuscular lorazepam 1 to 2 mg and oral loxapine 50 mg developed prolonged stupor, a significantly lowered respiration rate (8 breaths per minute), and in one case hypotension. Both showed signs of recovery within 3 to 5 hours and both had taken each of these drugs alone without problems.[2]

Both the benzodiazepines and loxapine are known to cause CNS depression, which, it would appear, can be quite severe in some cases. If both drugs are given be alert for these effects.

1. Cohen S, Khan A. Respiratory distress with use of lorazepam in mania. *J Clin Psychopharmacol* (1987) 7, 199–200.
2. Battaglia J, Thornton L, Young C. Loxapine-lorazepam-induced hypotension and stupor. *J Clin Psychopharmacol* (1989) 9, 227–8.

Benzodiazepines and related drugs + Macrolides

The exposure to midazolam and triazolam, and their resulting effects are markedly increased by clarithromycin and telithromycin, and moderately increased and prolonged by erythromycin. The same interaction has been seen to a limited extent with josamycin and roxithromycin, but not with azithromycin. The exposure to other benzodiazepines, such as alprazolam and brotizolam is moderately increased by erythromycin, and so would be expected to be similarly affected by these other macrolides.

Erythromycin has only a negligible to slight effect on diazepam, flunitrazepam, nitrazepam, and the related hypnotics, zaleplon and zopiclone, and does not affect temazepam metabolism. Zolpidem metabolism is not affected by clarithromycin.

Clinical evidence

A. Benzodiazepines

(a) Alprazolam

In a randomised study, 12 healthy subjects were given **erythromycin** 400 mg three times daily for 10 days with a single 800-microgram dose of alprazolam on day 8. The AUC of alprazolam was increased 2.5-fold and its half-life was prolonged from 16 hours to 40.3 hours. However, no increase in sedation was seen.[1]

(b) Brotizolam

A randomised study in healthy subjects found that **erythromycin** 400 mg three times daily for 7 days increased the AUC of a single 500-microgram dose of brotizolam 2.5-fold. The elimination half-life was also increased, from 9.4 hours to 20.7 hours. However, **erythromycin** did not affect the changes in psychomotor function associated with brotizolam.[2]

(c) Diazepam

In a crossover study, 6 healthy subjects were given a single 5-mg oral dose of diazepam after taking **erythromycin** 500 mg three times daily for one week. The diazepam AUC_{0-42} was increased by only 15% and its pharmacodynamic effects were unchanged.[3]

(d) Flunitrazepam

In a crossover study, 5 healthy subjects were given a single 1-mg oral dose of flunitrazepam after taking **erythromycin** 500 mg three times daily for one week. The flunitrazepam AUC_{0-42} was increased by only 25%, and its pharmacodynamic effects were unchanged.[3]

(e) Midazolam

1. Azithromycin. A study in 64 healthy medical students found that azithromycin 750 mg had no effect on the metabolism of a 10- or 15-mg dose of midazolam, and did not alter the performance of a number of psychomotor tests.[4] A study in 10 healthy subjects given azithromycin 250 mg daily found that some small changes in the pharmacokinetics of midazolam 15 mg occurred (a possible small delay in its onset of action), but its pharmacodynamic effects were unaltered.[5] Other studies confirm that azithromycin does not interact with midazolam.[6,7]

2. Clarithromycin. In a study, 16 healthy subjects were given both an oral 4 mg and an intravenous 50 microgram/kg dose of midazolam, before and after they took clarithromycin 500 mg twice daily for 7 days. It was found that clarithromycin reduced the systemic clearance of midazolam by about 64%, which resulted in a doubling of the midazolam-induced sleeping time.[8] Similarly, a study in elderly subjects, aged 66 to 80 years, found that clarithromycin 500 mg twice daily for 7 days increased the AUC of intravenous midazolam about 3-fold and increased the AUC of oral midazolam 8-fold.[9] Another study reported a similar interaction.[7]

3. Erythromycin. A study in 12 healthy subjects found that erythromycin 500 mg three times daily for 6 days increased the maximum plasma concentration of a single 15-mg oral dose of midazolam 2.7-fold, more than doubled its half-life and increased its AUC 4.4-fold The subjects could hardly be wakened during the first hour after being given midazolam, and most experienced amnesia lasting several hours. The same regimen of erythromycin had less effect on a single intravenous dose of midazolam (clearance was reduced by 54%, and there was only a minor increase in sedative effects).[10] Another study found that the increase in dose-corrected AUCs for oral midazolam in subjects that had taken erythromycin 200 mg four times daily for 2, 4, or 7 days were 2.3-, 3.4- and 3.4-fold, respectively. It appeared that a plateau level of CYP3A4 inhibition could be achieved by 4 days or more of erythromycin treatment at this dose.[11] The manufacturer reports that erythromycin causes about a 2-fold increase in the plasma concentration and half-life of intravenous midazolam.[12]

The plasma concentration of a 500-microgram/kg oral dose of midazolam given to an 8-year-old boy as premedication before surgery, were approximately doubled when he was given intravenous erythromycin. He developed nausea and tachycardia, and after 40 minutes (by which point he had received 200 mg of erythromycin) he lost consciousness.[13] A patient in a coronary care unit given 300 mg of intravenous midazolam over 14 hours slept for about 6 days (apart from brief wakening when given flumazenil). The midazolam half-life was increased about 10-fold. This was attributed to an interaction due to the combined effects of erythromycin 4 g daily and amiodarone 1.7 g over 3 days.[14,15] Other studies and reports have also described this interaction.[4,6,16,17]

4. Roxithromycin. In 10 healthy subjects, roxithromycin 300 mg daily for 6 days increased the AUC of a single 15-mg dose of midazolam by about 47%, and prolonged its half-life from 1.7 hours to 2.2 hours. Only minor psychomotor changes were seen.[18] A modest increase in the effects of midazolam were seen in another study in subjects given roxithromycin 300 mg, but the effects were very much weaker than those seen with erythromycin.[17]

5. Telithromycin. When intravenous and oral midazolam were given with telithromycin, the AUC of midazolam was increased 2.2-fold and 6.1-fold, respectively. The half-life of midazolam was increased about 2.5-fold.[19]

(f) Nitrazepam

When 10 healthy subjects were given **erythromycin** 500 mg three times daily for 4 days, the AUC of a single 5-mg dose of nitrazepam was increased by 25%, its maximum plasma concentration was increased by 30% and the time to maximum concentration was reduced by over 50%. However, hardly any changes were seen in the psychomotor tests undertaken.[20]

(g) Temazepam

A randomised study in 10 healthy subjects found that **erythromycin** 500 mg three times daily for 6 days had no effect on the pharmacokinetics or psychomotor effects of a single 20-mg dose of temazepam.[21]

(h) Triazolam

1. Azithromycin. A clinical study in 12 healthy subjects found that azithromycin did not affect the pharmacokinetics of a single 125-microgram dose of triazolam.[22] These results confirmed the findings of an *in vitro* study, which suggested that azithromycin was only a weak inhibitor of triazolam metabolism.[22]

2. Clarithromycin. An *in vitro* study found clarithromycin to be a relatively potent inhibitor of triazolam metabolism. These results were confirmed in practice with 12 healthy subjects, who were given both drugs. The oral clearance of triazolam was reduced by 77% by clarithromycin and the AUC was increased about 5-fold, when compared with placebo.[22]

3. Erythromycin. A study in 16 healthy subjects found that erythromycin 333 mg three times daily for 3 days, reduced the clearance of a single 500-microgram dose of triazolam by about 50%, doubled its AUC, and increased its maximum plasma concentration by about one-third.[23] Other reports confirm a decrease in triazolam clearance and an increase in its maximum concentration in the presence of erythromycin.[22,24] A patient with acute pneumonia and chronic renal failure taking erythromycin 600 mg daily developed visual hallucinations and abnormal body sensations each time a dose of triazolam and **nitrazepam** were taken. These symptoms had not occurred before the addition of erythromycin.[25]

4. Josamycin. A patient taking josamycin experienced confusion lasting about 24 hours after taking a single dose of triazolam.[26]

5. Roxithromycin. A single-dose study found that the psychomotor effects of triazolam were only slightly affected by roxithromycin 300 mg.[17]

6. Troleandomycin. Troleandomycin 2 g daily given to 7 healthy subjects for 7 days increased the maximum concentration of triazolam 2.1-fold, increased its AUC 3.8-fold and prolonged its half-life from 1.81 hours to 6.48 hours. Apparent oral clearance was reduced by 74%. Marked psychomotor impairment and amnesia was seen.[27] Troleandomycin has been reported to interact similarly in a patient taking triazolam, causing an increase in its effects.[26] An *in vitro* study has shown troleandomycin to be a potent inhibitor of triazolam metabolism.[22]

B. Non-benzodiazepine hypnotics

(a) Zaleplon

The manufacturers of zaleplon note that a single 800-mg dose of **erythromycin** increased the maximum plasma concentration of zaleplon by 34% and increased its AUC by 20%.[28,29]

(b) Zolpidem

In a study in 10 healthy subjects 4 doses of **clarithromycin** 500 mg had no effect on the pharmacokinetics of a single 5-mg dose of zolpidem or on its sedative effects. **Clarithromycin** pharmacokinetics were unaffected by zolpidem.[30]

(c) Zopiclone

Zopiclone 7.5 mg was given to 10 healthy subjects before and after they took **erythromycin** 500 mg three times daily for 6 days. **Erythromycin** increased the plasma concentration of zopiclone 5-fold at 30 minutes and 2-fold at one hour. The maximum plasma concentration rose by about 40% and occurred at one hour instead of 2 hours. The one-hour and 2-hour AUCs were increased 3-fold and 2-fold, respectively, while the total AUC was increased by nearly 80%.[31] These pharmacokinetic changes were reflected in some small changes in a number of psychomotor tests.[31]

Mechanism

Some of the macrolides (notably clarithromycin, erythromycin and telithromycin) are moderate to potent inhibitors of CYP3A4. They therefore inhibit the metabolism of some benzodiazepines by this route, causing an increase in their exposure, and increasing and prolonging their effects. Benzodiazepines, such as midazolam, that are predominantly metabolised by CYP3A4 are affected more than those such as diazepam, where CYP3A4 plays only a minor part in the metabolism. Further, CYP3A4-mediated metabolism occurs in the liver and also in the intestines. Midazolam and triazolam undergo extensive first-pass metabolism (low bioavailability of about 40%) but alprazolam and brotizolam undergo less first-pass metabolism (bioavailabilities of about 90% and 70%, respectively). Erythromycin causes greater increases in the exposure to oral midazolam and triazolam than in those of alprazolam and brotizolam, and this might be related to the extent of first-pass metabolism,[2] but could also be associated with differing routes of metabolism for these benzodiazepines. The extent of first pass metabolism does explain why intravenous midazolam is less affected by many CYP3A4 inhibitors than oral midazolam. The non-benzodiazepine hypnotics, zaleplon and zopiclone are, to varying degrees, also metabolised by CYP3A4: they are therefore also affected by the macrolides.

Importance and management

Midazolam and Triazolam

The interactions of midazolam with clarithromycin, erythromycin and telithromycin appear to be established, and of clinical importance. Troleandomycin would be expected to interact similarly. The dose of midazolam should be reduced 50 to 75% when these antibacterials are used if excessive effects (marked drowsiness, memory loss) are to be avoided. Remember too that the hypnotic effects are also prolonged so that patients should be warned about hangover effects the following morning if they intend to drive. There is some evidence that the effects of single bolus doses of intravenous midazolam given in the presence of erythromycin are not increased to a clinically relevant degree, and normal doses can be used, although the duration of effect might be prolonged. However, where high doses of intravenous midazolam are used long term (e.g. during intensive care treatment) one Australian manufacturer of midazolam[32] suggests that the initial dose might need to be reduced by up to 50% and the dose will then need to be titrated to avoid long-lasting hypnotic effects. Triazolam appears to interact similarly, and similar precautions would seem advisable.

Other macrolides appear not to interact (azithromycin) or only interact to a slight extent (roxithromycin) with midazolam and/or triazolam. No particular precautions would therefore be expected to be necessary on their concurrent use.

Note that midazolam is used as a probe substrate to assess the activity of other drugs on CYP3A4. The data here therefore suggest that clarithromycin and telithromycin are potent inhibitors of CYP3A4, erythromycin is a moderate inhibitor of CYP3A4, and roxithromycin is a weak inhibitor of CYP3A4. For a list of CYP3A4 substrates, see 'Table 1.10', p.12.

Alprazolam, Brotizolam, and Zopiclone

Pharmacokinetic information indicates that erythromycin moderately increases alprazolam and brotizolam exposure, but only small pharmacodynamic changes were reported. Nevertheless, the extent of the pharmacokinetic effect is reasonably large, and a degree of caution is warranted as some patients may be affected. Erythromycin moderately increases zopiclone exposure, and, again, some caution might be warranted. Clarithromycin, telithromycin and troleandomycin would be expected to interact similarly. If combinations of these drugs are used, be alert for increased and prolonged sedation.

Other benzodiazepines and related drugs

The manufacturers of **zaleplon** state that patients should be advised that increased sedation is possible with erythromycin,[28] although a dose adjustment is usually not required.[28,29] The study with erythromycin and zaleplon found only a very slight increase in exposure and would not generally be expected to lead to a clinically relevant interaction, however, the study used only single doses of erythromycin, and it cannot be excluded that multiple doses of erythromycin might have a greater effect.

Other benzodiazepines and related hypnotics not significantly metabolised by CYP3A4 (**diazepam**, **flunitrazepam**, **nitrazepam**, **temazepam** and **zolpidem**) have only minor or insignificant interactions with the macrolides, suggesting that no particular precautions are necessary on their concurrent use.

1. Yasui N, Otani K, Kaneko S, Ohkubo T, Osanai T, Sugawara K, Chiba K, Ishizaki T. A kinetic and dynamic study of oral alprazolam with and without erythromycin in humans: in vivo evidence for the involvement of CYP3A4 in alprazolam metabolism. *Clin Pharmacol Ther* (1996) 59, 514–19.
2. Tokairin T, Fukasawa T, Yasui-Furukori N, Aoshima T, Suzuki A, Inoue Y, Tateishi T, Otani K. Inhibition of the metabolism of brotizolam by erythromycin in humans: *in vivo* evidence for the involvement of CYP3A4 in brotizolam metabolism. *Br J Clin Pharmacol* (2005) 60, 172–5.
3. Luurila H, Olkkola KT, Neuvonen PJ. Interaction between erythromycin and the benzodiazepines diazepam and flunitrazepam. *Pharmacol Toxicol* (1996) 78, 117–22.
4. Mattila MJ, Vanakoski J, Idänpään-Heikkilä JJ. Azithromycin does not alter the effects of oral midazolam on human performance. *Eur J Clin Pharmacol* (1994) 47, 49–52.
5. Backman JT, Olkkola KT, Neuvonen PJ. Azithromycin does not increase plasma concentrations of oral midazolam. *Int J Clin Pharmacol Ther* (1995) 33, 356–9.
6. Zimmermann T, Yeates RA, Laufen H, Scharpf F, Leitold M, Wildfeuer A. Influence of the antibiotics erythromycin and azithromycin on the pharmacokinetics and pharmacodynamics of midazolam. *Arzneimittelforschung* (1996) 46, 213–17.
7. Yeates RA, Laufen H, Zimmermann T. Interaction between midazolam and clarithromycin: comparison with azithromycin. *Int J Clin Pharmacol Ther* (1996) 34, 400–5.
8. Gorski JC, Jones DR, Haehner-Daniels BD, Hamman MA, O'Mara EM, Hall SD. The contribution of intestinal and hepatic CYP3A to the interaction between midazolam and clarithromycin. *Clin Pharmacol Ther* (1998) 64, 133–43.
9. Quinney SK, Haehner BD, Rhoades MB, Lin Z, Gorski JC, Hall SD. Interaction between midazolam and clarithromycin in the elderly. *Br J Clin Pharmacol* (2008) 65, 98–109.
10. Olkkola KT, Aranko K, Luurila H, Hiller A, Saarnivaara L, Himberg J-J, Neuvonen PJ. A potentially hazardous interaction between erythromycin and midazolam. *Clin Pharmacol Ther* (1993) 53, 298–305.
11. Okudaira T, Kotegawa T, Imai H, Tsutsumi K, Nakano S, Ohashi K. Effect of the treatment period with erythromycin on cytochrome P450 3A activity in humans. *J Clin Pharmacol* (2007) 47, 871–6.
12. Hypnovel (Midazolam hydrochloride). Roche Products Ltd. UK Summary of product characteristics, March 2010.
13. Hiller A, Olkkola KT, Isohanni P, Saarnivaara L. Unconsciousness associated with midazolam and erythromycin. *Br J Anaesth* (1990) 65, 826–8.
14. Gascon M-P, Dayer P, Waldvogel F. Les interactions médicamenteuses du midazolam. *Schweiz Med Wochenschr* (1989) 119, 1834–6.
15. Gascon M-P, Dayer P. In vitro forecasting of drugs which may interfere with the biotransformation of midazolam. *Eur J Clin Pharmacol* (1991) 41, 573–8.
16. Byatt CM, Lewis LD, Dawling S, Cochrane GM. Accumulation of midazolam after repeated dosage in patients receiving mechanical ventilation in an intensive care unit. *BMJ* (1984) 289, 799–800.
17. Mattila MJ, Idänpään-Heikkilä JJ, Törnwall M, Vanakoski J. Oral single doses of erythromycin and roxithromycin may increase the effects of midazolam on human performance. *Pharmacol Toxicol* (1993) 73, 180–5.
18. Backman JT, Aranko K, Himberg J-J, Olkkola KT. A pharmacokinetic interaction between roxithromycin and midazolam. *Eur J Clin Pharmacol* (1994) 46, 551–5.
19. Ketek (Telithromycin). Sanofi. UK Summary of product characteristics, November 2012.
20. Luurila H, Olkkola KT, Neuvonen PJ. Interaction between erythromycin and nitrazepam in healthy volunteers. *Pharmacol Toxicol* (1995) 76, 255–8.
21. Luurila H, Olkkola KT, Neuvonen PJ. Lack of interaction of erythromycin with temazepam. *Ther Drug Monit* (1994) 16, 548–51.
22. Greenblatt DJ, von Moltke LL, Harmatz JS, Counihan M, Graf JA, Durol ALB, Mertzanis P, Duan SX, Wright CE, Shader RI. Inhibition of triazolam clearance by macrolide antimicrobial agents: in vitro correlates and dynamic consequences. *Clin Pharmacol Ther* (1998) 64, 278–85.
23. Phillips JP, Antal EJ, Smith RB. A pharmacokinetic drug interaction between erythromycin and triazolam. *J Clin Psychopharmacol* (1986) 6, 297–9.
24. Hugues FC, Le Jeunne C, Munera Y. Conséquences en thérapeutique de l'inhibition microsomiale hépatique par les macrolides. *Sem Hop Paris* (1987) 63, 2280–3.
25. Tokinaga N, Kondo T, Kaneko S, Otani K, Mihara K, Morita S. Hallucinations after a therapeutic dose of benzodiazepine hypnotics with co-administration of erythromycin. *Psychiatry Clin Neurosci* (1996) 50, 337–9.
26. Carry PV, Ducluzeau R, Jourdan C, Bourrat C, Vigneau C, Descotes J. De nouvelles interactions avec les macrolides? *Lyon Med* (1982) 248, 189–90.
27. Warot D, Bergougnan L, Lamiable D, Berlin I, Bensimon G, Danjou P, Puech AJ. Troleandomycin-triazolam interaction in healthy volunteers: pharmacokinetic and psychometric evaluation. *Eur J Clin Pharmacol* (1987) 32, 389–93.
28. Sonata (Zaleplon). Meda Pharmaceuticals. UK Summary of product characteristics, February 2009.
29. Sonata (Zaleplon). King Pharmaceuticals, Inc. US Prescribing information, December 2007.
30. Farkas D, Volak LP, Harmatz JS, von Moltke LL, Court MH, Greenblatt DJ. Short-term clarithromycin administration impairs clearance and enhances pharmacodynamic effects of trazodone but not of zolpidem. *Clin Pharmacol Ther* (2005) 85, 644–50.
31. Aranko K, Luurila H, Backman JT, Neuvonen PJ, Olkkola KT. The effect of erythromycin on the pharmacokinetics and pharmacodynamics of zopiclone. *Br J Clin Pharmacol* (1994) 38, 363–7.
32. Hypnovel (Midazolam hydrochloride). Roche Products Pty Ltd. Australian product information, October 2007.

Benzodiazepines + Maraviroc

Maraviroc has no effect on the pharmacokinetics of midazolam.

Clinical evidence, mechanism, importance and management

In a placebo-controlled study in 12 healthy subjects, maraviroc 300 mg twice daily for 7 days increased the AUC and maximum plasma concentration of a single 7.5-mg dose of oral midazolam taken on day 7 by 18% and 21%, respectively. These increases are not clinically relevant,[1] and no midazolam dose adjustment is needed on concurrent use. Midazolam is not expected to affect the concentration of maraviroc.[2] Midazolam is a sensitive probe substrate for CYP3A4, and the findings suggest that maraviroc is unlikely to have a clinically important effect on other CYP3A4 substrates.

1. Abel S, Russell D, Whitlock LA, Ridgway CE, Muirhead GJ. Effect of maraviroc on the pharmacokinetics of midazolam, lamivudine/zidovudine, and ethinyloestradiol/levonorgestrel in healthy volunteers. *Br J Clin Pharmacol* (2008) 65 (Suppl 1), 19–26.
2. Celsentri (Maraviroc). ViiV Healthcare UK Ltd. UK Summary of product characteristics, April 2014.

Benzodiazepines and related drugs + Melatonin

The CNS effects of benzodiazepines and related hypnotics, such as zolpidem, might be additive with those of melatonin.

Clinical evidence

In a well-controlled, single-dose study in 16 healthy subjects aged 55 years and older, giving prolonged-release melatonin 2 mg with **zolpidem** 10 mg at bedtime enhanced the impairment of cognitive function seen with **zolpidem** alone at one hour and 4 hours post-dose, but not the next morning. Melatonin alone had no effect on cognitive function. No pharmacokinetic interaction was found.[1]

Mechanism

The activity of melatonin is thought to involve similar interactions at the GABA receptors in the brain to benzodiazepines. Melatonin might therefore enhance the activity of benzodiazepines and related drugs.

Importance and management

The evidence available suggests that melatonin might enhance the sedative properties of benzodiazepines and related hypnotics such as zolpidem. Although in the study of zolpidem, the enhanced effect was not apparent the morning after dosing, it would be wise to be aware that increased drowsiness is a possibility if melatonin is also given, especially with longer-acting hypnotics.

1. Otmani S, Demazières A, Staner C, Jacob N, Nir T, Zisapel N, Staner L. Effects of prolonged-release melatonin, zolpidem, and their combination on psychomotor functions, memory recall, and driving skills in healthy middle aged and elderly volunteers. *Hum Psychopharmacol* (2008) 23, 693–705.

Benzodiazepines + Melatonin receptor agonists

Ramelteon does not alter the pharmacokinetics of midazolam, and tasimelteon also appears to have no effect. Other benzodiazepines that are similarly metabolised are also unlikely to be affected.

Clinical evidence, mechanism, importance and management

A study in 28 healthy subjects found that **ramelteon** 32 mg daily for 9 days had no effect on the pharmacokinetics of a single 10-mg oral dose of **midazolam**.[1] Similarly, the US manufacturer of **tasimelteon** briefly notes that in a study, tasimelteon 20 mg daily for 14 days did not affect the pharmacokinetics of midazolam.[2]

No midazolam dose adjustments are therefore expected to be necessary on concurrent use of ramelteon or tasimelteon. Other benzodiazepines similarly metabolised (such as **triazolam**, and to a lesser extent **alprazolam**) are also unlikely to be affected by either of these drugs.

Note that midazolam is used as a probe substrate to assess the activity of other drugs on CYP3A4. These studies therefore suggest that ramelteon and tasimelteon are not inducers or inhibitors of this isoenzyme.

1. Karim A, Tolbert D, Cao C, Zhao Z, Sainati SM. The effect of multiple doses of ramelteon (TAK-375) on the single-dose pharmacokinetic profile of midazolam in healthy adult subjects. *Sleep* (2004) 27 (Abstract Suppl), A47.
2. Hetlioz (Tasimelteon). Vanda Pharmaceuticals Inc. US Prescribing information, December 2014.

Benzodiazepines and related drugs + Metoclopramide

Intravenous, but not oral, metoclopramide increases the rate of absorption of diazepam and raises its maximum plasma concentration. Intravenous metoclopramide increases the rate of absorption of zopiclone.

Clinical evidence

(a) Diazepam

Intravenous metoclopramide increased the maximum plasma concentration of diazepam by 38% and increased the rate of absorption (maximum concentration occurred at 30 minutes instead of 60 minutes),[1] but in another study in 6 healthy subjects oral metoclopramide 10 mg did not increase the rate of absorption of oral diazepam 0.2 mg/kg.[2]

(b) Zopiclone

In a study in 12 healthy subjects, intravenous metoclopramide 10 mg increased the rate of absorption of a single 7.5-mg dose of oral zopiclone. Metoclopramide almost doubled the plasma concentration of zopiclone (from 22.7 nanograms/mL to 44.4 nanograms/mL) at one hour, but the increase in the plasma concentration of zopiclone was only about 20% (from 49.3 nanograms/mL to 59.6 nanograms/mL) at 2 hours.[3]

Mechanism

Metoclopramide increases the gastric emptying rate and thereby alters the absorption of some drugs.

Importance and management

The possible clinical consequence of the increased rate of absorption of diazepam and zopiclone is that the onset of effect of these drugs might be quicker if intravenous metoclopramide is being used concurrently, although this would require confirmation in better designed studies. Oral metoclopramide appears not to alter the absorption of diazepam.

1. Gamble JAS, Gaston JH, Nair SG, Dundee JW. Some pharmacological factors influencing the absorption of diazepam following oral administration. *Br J Anaesth* (1976) 48, 1181–5.
2. Chapman MH, Woolner DF, Begg EJ, Atkinson HC, Sharman JR. Co-administered oral metoclopramide does not enhance the rate of absorption of oral diazepam. *Anaesth Intensive Care* (1988) 16, 202–5.
3. Elliott P, Chestnutt WN, Elwood RJ, Dundee JW. Effect of atropine and metoclopramide on the plasma concentrations of orally administered zopiclone. *Br J Anaesth* (1983) 55, 1159P–1160P.

Benzodiazepines + Metronidazole

Metronidazole does not affect the pharmacokinetics of alprazolam, diazepam, lorazepam, or midazolam.

Clinical evidence

A study in healthy subjects found that metronidazole 400 mg twice daily for 5 days had no effect on the pharmacokinetics of a single 100-microgram/kg intravenous dose of **diazepam**.[1] Another study in healthy subjects found that metronidazole 250 mg three times daily had no effect on the pharmacokinetics of single doses of oral **alprazolam** 1 mg or intravenous **lorazepam** 2 mg.[2] Similarly, metronidazole 400 mg twice daily for 3 days had no effect on the pharmacokinetics or pharmacodynamics of a single 15-mg oral dose of **midazolam** or on the formation of its 1-hydroxymetabolite.[3]

Mechanism

Midazolam is a probe substrate for CYP3A4, and the study here shows that metronidazole does not affect CYP3A4 activity. The study with diazepam suggests metronidazole does not affect CYP2C19, and that with lorazepam suggests it does not affect glucuronidation.

Importance and management

Evidence for an interaction between metronidazole and the benzodiazepines is limited to a small number of benzodiazepines but a lack of an interaction appears to be confirmed. No dose adjustment of alprazolam, diazepam, lorazepam, or midazolam is likely to be needed if metronidazole is used concurrently. Although they do not appear to have been studied, interactions with other benzodiazepines seem unlikely.

1. Jensen JC, Gugler R. Interaction between metronidazole and drugs eliminated by oxidative metabolism. *Clin Pharmacol Ther* (1985) 37, 407–10.
2. Blyden GT, Scavone JM, Greenblatt DJ. Metronidazole impairs clearance of phenytoin but not of alprazolam or lorazepam. *J Clin Pharmacol* (1988) 28, 240–5.
3. Wang J-S, Backman JT, Kivistö KT, Neuvonen PJ. Effects of metronidazole on midazolam metabolism in vitro and in vivo. *Eur J Clin Pharmacol* (2000) 56, 555–9.

Benzodiazepines + Modafinil

Modafinil moderately reduces triazolam exposure, and its *R*-isomer, armodafinil slightly reduces midazolam exposure. Conversely, it is predicted that modafinil and armodafinil might reduce diazepam elimination.

Clinical evidence

(a) Midazolam

In a study in 17 healthy subjects, the AUC of a single 5-mg oral dose of midazolam was slightly reduced by about 32% and its maximum concentration was reduced by 19%, when it was given after 3 weeks of pretreatment with armodafinil, the *R*-isomer of modafinil, given at a starting dose of 100 mg daily and increased gradually during the first week to 250 mg daily. In the same study it was found that the AUC of a single 2-mg intravenous dose of midazolam was decreased by about 17% after pretreatment with armodafinil. Exposure to the midazolam metabolite, 1′-hydroxymidazolam, was increased by about 50% and 40%, by oral and intravenous midazolam, respectively.[1]

(b) Triazolam

In a placebo-controlled study, 34 healthy women (all taking an oral combined hormonal contraceptive containing ethinylestradiol and norgestimate) were given a single 125-microgram dose of triazolam, both before and on the last day of taking modafinil 200 mg daily for 7 days then 400 mg daily for 21 days. The AUC of triazolam was reduced by almost 60%, its maximum plasma concentration was reduced by 42%, and its elimination half-life was reduced by about one hour by modafinil.[2]

Mechanism

Modafinil and armodafinil are known to induce CYP3A4, by which triazolam and midazolam are metabolised: concurrent use therefore results in reduced exposure to these benzodiazepines. The larger effect of armodafinil on the pharmacokinetics of oral midazolam compared with intravenous midazolam suggests that both gastrointestinal and hepatic CYP3A4 are induced by armodafinil.[3]

Importance and Management

Evidence for an interaction between modafinil or armodafinil and the benzodiazepines appears to be limited to these two pharmacokinetic studies, with triazolam and midazolam, respectively. It would seem prudent to monitor for a reduction in both the sedative effects and the duration of action of triazolam and midazolam in patients taking modafinil or armodafinil, and increase the dose if necessary.

There appears to be no evidence about other benzodiazepines; however, modafinil and armodafinil inhibit CYP2C19 (see *CYP2C19 substrates*, under 'Modafinil + Miscellaneous', p.222). The manufacturers therefore predict that the elimination of **diazepam** might be reduced, and they suggest that a dose reduction of **diazepam** might be necessary on concurrent use.[3-5] Be alert for diazepam adverse effects (e.g. over sedation) and adjust the dose accordingly.

Note that midazolam is used as a probe substrate to assess the activity of other drugs on CYP3A4. The evidence here therefore suggests that armodafinil is a weak inducer of CYP3A4 activity. For a list of CYP3A4 substrates, see 'Table 1.10', p.12.

1. Darwish M, Kirby M, Robertson P, Hellriegel ET. Interaction profile of armodafinil with medications metabolized by cytochrome P450 enzymes 1A2, 3A4 and 2C19 in healthy subjects. *Clin Pharmacokinet* (2008) 47, 61–74.
2. Robertson P, Hellriegel ET, Arora S, Nelson M. Effect of modafinil on the pharmacokinetics of ethinyl estradiol and triazolam in healthy volunteers. *Clin Pharmacol Ther* (2002) 71, 46–56.
3. Nuvigil (Armodafinil). Cephalon, Inc. US Prescribing information, June 2013.
4. Provigil (Modafinil). Cephalon, Inc. US Prescribing information, October 2010.
5. Provigil (Modafinil). Cephalon (UK) Ltd. UK Summary of product characteristics, August 2013.

Benzodiazepines + Nabilone

The CNS depressant effects of nabilone and diazepam are additive.

Clinical evidence, mechanism, importance and management

The manufacturer notes that in a study in 15 healthy subjects, the CNS depressant effects of nabilone and **diazepam** were found to be additive. Psychomotor function was particularly impaired and they advise caution if nabilone is given with any CNS depressant,[1] which would include any benzodiazepine.

1. Cesamet (Nabilone). Meda Pharmaceuticals Inc. US Prescribing information, April 2011.

Benzodiazepines and related drugs + Nefazodone

Nefazodone increases alprazolam, midazolam, triazolam and zopiclone exposure and effects, but does not affect lorazepam pharmacokinetics.

Clinical evidence

A. Benzodiazepines

(a) Alprazolam

A placebo-controlled study in 12 healthy subjects found that nefazodone 200 mg twice daily caused a 2-fold increase in the AUC of alprazolam 1 mg twice daily taken for 7 days.[1] Another study found that nefazodone increased the AUC of alprazolam by 47%.[2] A further study reported impairment of psychomotor performance and increased sedation when nefazodone was given with alprazolam.[3] A case report describes a woman taking alprazolam who developed benzodiazepine withdrawal symptoms after nefazodone was withdrawn following several years of concurrent use. She needed an alprazolam dose increase from 500 micrograms daily to 4 mg daily to control her symptoms.[4]

(b) Lorazepam

A placebo-controlled study in healthy subjects given nefazodone 200 mg twice daily found no changes in the pharmacokinetics of lorazepam 2 mg twice daily.[5] Another study found that psychomotor performance was not further impaired and no additional sedation occurred when nefazodone was given with lorazepam.[3]

(c) Midazolam

A study in 10 healthy subjects found that both the AUC and the maximum plasma concentration of a single 10-mg oral dose of midazolam were increased 4.6-fold and 2-fold, respectively, when they took nefazodone 200 mg twice daily.[6]

(d) Triazolam

A study in 12 healthy subjects found that the maximum plasma concentration, half-life, and AUC of a single 250-microgram dose of triazolam were increased 1.7-fold, 4.6-fold, and 4-fold, respectively, by nefazodone 200 mg twice daily.[7] Another study found that impairment of psychomotor performance and increased sedation occurred when nefazodone was given with triazolam.[3]

B. Non-benzodiazepine hypnotics

An 86-year-old woman taking diltiazem, irbesartan, lorazepam, and pravastatin started taking nefazodone 50 mg twice daily, increasing to 500 mg daily in divided doses, for the treatment of a major depressive episode. Because of associated insomnia, **zopiclone** was added, starting at 15 mg each night, but this was reduced after 5 days to 7.5 mg because of morning drowsiness. Plasma concentrations of *S*-zopiclone and *R*-zopiclone were 107 nanograms/mL and 20.6 nanograms/mL, respectively, at this time. After several months, nefazodone was replaced by venlafaxine. The *S*-zopiclone and *R*-zopiclone plasma concentrations were again measured and found to be only 16.9 nanograms/mL and 1.45 nanograms/mL, respectively.[8]

Mechanism

Nefazodone appears to inhibit the oxidative metabolism of alprazolam, midazolam, triazolam and zopiclone by CYP3A4 so that they accumulate in the body. Lorazepam is unaffected because it is primarily excreted as a glucuronide conjugate.

Importance and management

The interactions of nefazodone with alprazolam, midazolam, triazolam and zopiclone are established and clinically important; the practical consequences are that the effects of these drugs are expected to be increased to varying extents. Be alert for any evidence of any psychomotor impairment, drowsiness etc. and reduce the benzodiazepine dose if necessary. A substantial reduction (about 50%) in the initial dose of alprazolam might be required, and an even greater reduction might be needed for midazolam and triazolam; however, the manufacturer of triazolam[9] contraindicates its concurrent use with nefazodone. Nefazodone does not interact with lorazepam. There seems to be no direct information about other benzodiazepines and related drugs.

Note that midazolam is used as a probe substrate to assess the activity of other drugs on CYP3A4. The data here therefore suggest that nefazodone is a moderate inhibitor of CYP3A4, although it almost classifies as a potent inhibitor. For a list of CYP3A4 substrates, see 'Table 1.10', p.12.

1. Greene DS, Salazar DE, Dockens RC, Kroboth P, Barbhaiya RH. Coadministration of nefazodone and benzodiazepines: III. A pharmacokinetic interaction study with alprazolam. *J Clin Psychopharmacol* (1995) 15, 399–408.
2. DeVane CL, Donovan JL, Liston HL, Markowitz JS, Cheng KT, Risch SC, Willard L. Comparative CYP3A4 inhibitory effects of venlafaxine, fluoxetine, sertraline, and nefazodone in healthy volunteers. *J Clin Psychopharmacol* (2004) 24, 4–10.
3. Kroboth PD, Folan MM, Lush RM, Chaikin PC, Shukla UA, Barbhaiya R, Salazar DE. Coadministration of nefazodone and benzodiazepines: I. Pharmacodynamic assessment. *J Clin Psychopharmacol* (1995) 15, 306–19.
4. Ninan T. Pharmacokinetically induced benzodiazepine withdrawal. *Psychopharmacol Bull* (2001) 35, 94–100.
5. Greene DS, Salazar DE, Dockens RC, Kroboth P, Barbhaiya RH. Coadministration of nefazodone and benzodiazepines: IV. A pharmacokinetic interaction study with lorazepam. *J Clin Psychopharmacol* (1995) 15, 409–16.
6. Lam YWF, Alfaro CL, Ereshefsky L, Miller M. Pharmacokinetic and pharmacodynamic interactions of oral midazolam with ketoconazole, fluoxetine, fluvoxamine, and nefazodone. *J Clin Pharmacol* (2003) 43, 1274–82.
7. Barbhaiya RH, Shukla UA, Kroboth PD, Greene DS. Coadministration of nefazodone and benzodiazepines: II. A pharmacokinetic interaction study with triazolam. *J Clin Psychopharmacol* (1995) 15, 320–6.
8. Alderman CP, Gebauer MG, Gilbert AL, Condon JT. Possible interaction of zopiclone and nefazodone. *Ann Pharmacother* (2001) 35, 1378–80.
9. Halcion (Triazolam). Pfizer Inc. US Prescribing information, December 2008.

Benzodiazepines + NNRTIs

There is some limited evidence that efavirenz and nevirapine might increase the metabolism of midazolam: triazolam, and to a lesser extent alprazolam, are predicted to be similarly affected. Efavirenz has a negligible effect on lorazepam exposure.

Etravirine decreases midazolam exposure, and is predicted to increase diazepam exposure. Delavirdine is predicted to increase alprazolam, midazolam and triazolam exposure.

Clinical evidence, mechanism, importance and management

(a) Delavirdine

Delavirdine is an inhibitor of CYP3A4 and might increase the plasma concentration of drugs that are metabolised by this route. Delavirdine is contraindicated with drugs that are highly dependent on CYP3A4 for clearance including **alprazolam**, **midazolam** and **triazolam**.[1]

(b) Efavirenz or Nevirapine

In a study, 90 HIV-positive patients not taking antiretrovirals (control group) and 56 similar patients already taking antiretrovirals, were given a 75-microgram dose of oral **midazolam**. When compared with the control group, the 1-hydroxymidazolam to **midazolam** ratio was 5-fold higher in 28 patients taking efavirenz, but 17-fold lower in 3 patients taking efavirenz together with ritonavir (the ratio for ritonavir alone was 50-fold lower). Similarly, the 1-hydroxymidazolam to **midazolam** ratio was 7-fold lower in 3 patients receiving nevirapine together with ritonavir or nelfinavir or grapefruit juice. This evidence suggests that efavirenz and nevirapine *induce* the metabolism of midazolam by CYP3A4, but the inhibition of CYP3A4 by ritonavir or nelfinavir offsets the inductive effects of efavirenz or nevirapine given concurrently.[2] Other benzodiazepines metabolised via CYP3A4 may be similarly affected, such as **triazolam**, and to a lesser extent **alprazolam**. However, the manufacturers of efavirenz state that, in addition to *in vitro* data showing that efavirenz induces CYP3A, there are also *in vitro* data showing that it is an inhibitor of CYP3A4. For this reason, they contraindicate its use with **midazolam** or **triazolam** as *inhibition* of the metabolism of these benzodiazepines could potentially prolong sedation or respiratory depression.[3,4] Nevertheless, the bulk of clinical pharmacokinetic data for efavirenz suggest that when it is given with substrates of CYP3A4 it is an inducer of CYP3A4 metabolism. Reduced midazolam effects would therefore seem the most likely outcome if midazolam were given to a patient taking efavirenz.

A study in 12 subjects found that efavirenz 600 mg daily for 10 days increased the maximum plasma concentration of a single 2-mg dose of **lorazepam** by 16%[4] and increased its AUC by 7%.[3] These changes are not clinically important and no dose adjustment is considered necessary for **lorazepam**.[3]

(c) Etravirine

Etravirine is a weak inhibitor of CYP2C19, the isoenzyme by which diazepam is metabolised. The manufacturers of etravirine therefore predict that concurrent use will raise diazepam levels[5,6] (which might increase the risk of prolonged and/or excessive sedation). The UK manufacturer suggests that alternatives to diazepam should be considered,[5] whereas the US manufacturer suggests that a decrease in the dose of diazepam might be necessary.[6] Note that omeprazole, a weak to moderate inhibitor of CYP2C19, has sometimes caused increased diazepam effects (see 'Benzodiazepines + Proton pump inhibitors', p.834). Some caution would therefore seem appropriate.

In a study, 12 healthy subjects were given a single 250-micrograms/kg dose of intravenous midazolam on day one and day 14 of a 14-day course of etravirine 200 mg twice daily. Etravirine modestly reduced the ratio of the AUC of **midazolam** to its metabolite, 1-hydroxymidazolam, by 37%.[7] Etravirine is an inducer of CYP3A4, by which midazolam is metabolised. However, this modest reduction in **midazolam** exposure would not be expected to be of clinical relevance in most patients.

1. Rescriptor (Delavirdine mesylate). Pfizer Inc. US prescribing information, May 2008.
2. Fellay J, Marzolini C, Decosterd L, Golay KP, Baumann P, Buclin T, Telenti A, Eap CB. Variations of CYP3A activity induced by antiretroviral treatment in HIV-1 infected patients. *Eur J Clin Pharmacol* (2005) 60, 865–73.
3. Sustiva Film-coated Tablets (Efavirenz). Bristol-Myers Squibb Pharmaceutical Ltd. UK Summary of product characteristics, March 2014.
4. Sustiva (Efavirenz). Bristol-Myers Squibb Company. US Prescribing information, August 2012.
5. Intelence (Etravirine). Janssen-Cilag Ltd. UK Summary of product characteristics, July 2012.
6. Intelence (Etravirine). Tibotec, Inc. US Prescribing information, August 2012.
7. Schöller-Gyüre M, Kakuda TN, Stevens T, Aharchi F, De Smedt G, Peeters M, Hoetelmans RMW. Effect of etravirine on cytochrome P450 isoenzymes assessed by the Cooperstown 5+1 cocktail. 48th Annual ICAAC/ IDSA 46th General Meeting, Washington DC, 25th-28th October 2008.

Benzodiazepines and related drugs + NS5A inhibitors

No interaction appears to occur between daclatasvir and midazolam, and alprazolam does not appear to alter the pharmacokinetics of ombitasvir. No interaction is predicted to occur between daclatasvir and alprazolam or triazolam. No interaction appears to occur between zolpidem and ombitasvir.

Clinical evidence, mechanism, importance and management

(a) Daclatasvir

The UK manufacturer briefly reports that, in a study in healthy subjects given a single 5-mg dose of **midazolam** with daclatasvir 60 mg daily, the pharmacokinetics of midazolam were unaffected.[1] No dose adjustments are therefore necessary on concurrent use. Other benzodiazepines (such as **alprazolam** and **triazolam**) are predicted to be similarly unaffected and would also be expected to require no dose adjustment on concurrent use.[1]

(b) Ombitasvir

The UK and US manufacturers briefly report that, in a study in 12 healthy subjects, a single 500-microgram dose of **alprazolam** had no effect on the pharmacokinetics of ombitasvir 25 mg daily (in a fixed-dose combination with paritaprevir boosted with ritonavir, given with and without dasabuvir).[2,3] The UK manufacturer also reports that the pharmacokinetics of ombitasvir (in a fixed-dose combination with paritaprevir boosted with ritonavir, given with dasabuvir) and of **zolpidem** given as a single 5-mg dose, were unaffected when given together.[3] No ombitasvir dose adjustment is necessary on concurrent use with either alprazolam or zolpidem, and no zolpidem dose adjustment is necessary.

1. Daklinza (Daclatasvir dihydrochloride). Bristol-Myers Squibb Pharmaceutical Ltd. UK Summary of product characteristics, September 2014.
2. Viekira Pak (Ombitasvir, paritaprevir, ritonavir co-packaged with dasabuvir sodium monohydrate). AbbVie Inc. US Prescribing information, December 2014.
3. Viekirax (Ombitasvir, paritaprevir, ritonavir). AbbVie Ltd. UK Summary of product characteristics, January 2015.

Benzodiazepines and related drugs + NSAIDs

The interactions of the NSAIDs with the benzodiazepines are usually minor; however, intravenous diclofenac appears to reduce the dose of intravenous midazolam needed to produce sedation and hypnosis, and in one study, feelings of dizziness were increased when indometacin was used with diazepam.

Clinical evidence, mechanism, importance and management

(a) Diazepam

1. Diclofenac. In a study in 8 healthy subjects, diazepam increased the AUC of diclofenac by 60% and reduced its clearance by 36%.[1] The effects of diazepam on diclofenac appeared to depend on the time of administration and might reflect time-dependent effects of diazepam on gastrointestinal function. More study is needed to establish the mechanism and clinical relevance of this interaction.

2. Ibuprofen. A study in 8 healthy subjects investigating the effects of diazepam on ibuprofen pharmacokinetics found that the ibuprofen half-life was increased from 2.39 hours to 3.59 hours and its clearance was reduced by about one-third when diazepam and ibuprofen were given at 10 pm, but no effect was seen with morning dosing.[2] The clinical importance of this is uncertain.

3. Indometacin. Diazepam 10 to 15 mg impaired the performance of a number of psychomotor tests (digit symbol substitution, letter cancellation, tracking and flicker fusion) in 119 healthy medical students. It also caused subjective drowsiness, mental slowness and clumsiness. When indometacin 50 or 100 mg was given, the effects were little different from diazepam alone, except that feelings of dizziness (common to both drugs) were increased and caused subjective clumsiness.[3]

4. Naproxen. A double-blind, crossover study did not find any clinically important changes in mood or attention in healthy subjects given naproxen and diazepam.[4] A single-dose study in 10 healthy subjects found that the maximum serum concentration of naproxen 500 mg was reduced by 23%, the time to maximum concentration was increased (from 1.36 hours to 2 hours) and the absorption rate constant was decreased by 40% by diazepam 10 mg. Other pharmacokinetic parameters were not affected.[5] No special precautions appear to be necessary on concurrent use.

5. Parecoxib. Valdecoxib, the active metabolite of parecoxib is an inhibitor of CYP2C19 and might increase diazepam concentrations, see 'NSAIDs; Parecoxib + Miscellaneous', p.161.

(b) Midazolam

A clinical study found that **diclofenac** 75 mg given intravenously to 10 patients reduced the dose of intravenous midazolam needed to produce sedation and hypnosis by 35%, when compared with 10 control subjects not given **diclofenac**.[6] The clinical importance of this is uncertain.

A randomised, crossover study in 32 patients undergoing two surgical procedures for bilateral symmetrically impacted third molars, found that midazolam, in doses used for conscious sedation, had no effect on the potency or duration of action of **diflunisal** for postoperative pain relief.[7]

In a single-dose study in 12 healthy adults, there were no changes in the pharmacokinetics or pharmacodynamics of midazolam 70 micrograms/kg given an hour after a single 40-mg dose of intravenous **parecoxib**.[8] These data suggest that, when a single-dose of parecoxib is used post-operatively, no dose adjustment of intravenous midazolam is required.

(c) Oxazepam

In a study in 6 healthy subjects, **diflunisal** 500 mg twice daily decreased the maximum plasma concentration and AUC of a single 30-mg dose of oxazepam by 38% and 16%, respectively; the AUC of oxazepam glucuronide was increased by 70%. It was suggested that **diflunisal** displaced oxazepam from its plasma protein binding sites leading to a small increase in presystemic hepatic extraction and a small decrease in systemic availability. In addition, there appeared to be competition between the glucuronides of oxazepam and **diflunisal** for tubular secretion. The overall clinical relevance was thought to be small.[9]

(d) Zaleplon

A randomised, single-dose study in 17 healthy subjects found that **ibuprofen** 600 mg had no effect on the pharmacokinetics of zaleplon 10 mg.[10]

1. Mahender VN, Rambhau D, Rao BR, Rao VVS, Venkateshwarlu G. Time-dependent influence of diazepam on the pharmacokinetics of orally administered diclofenac sodium in human subjects. *Clin Drug Invest* (1995) 10, 296–301.
2. Bapuji AT, Rambhau D, Srinivasu P, Rao BR, Apte SS. Time dependent influence of diazepam on the pharmacokinetics of ibuprofen in man. *Drug Metabol Drug Interact* (1999) 15, 71–81.
3. Nuotto E, Saarialho-Kere U. Actions and interactions of indomethacin and diazepam on performance in healthy volunteers. *Pharmacol Toxicol* (1988) 62, 293–7.
4. Stitt FW, Latour R, Frane JW. A clinical study of naproxen-diazepam drug interaction on tests of mood and attention. *Curr Ther Res* (1977) 21, 149–56.
5. Rao BR, Rambhau D. Influence of diazepam on the pharmacokinetic properties of orally administered naproxen. *Drug Invest* (1992) 4, 416–21.
6. Carrero E, Castillo J, Bogdanovich A, Nalda MA. El diclofenac reduce las dosis sedante e hipnótica de midazolam. *Rev Esp Anestesiol Reanim* (1991) 38, 127.
7. Rodrigo MRC, Rosenquist JB. Does midazolam sedation in oral surgery affect the potency or duration of diflunisal analgesia? *Aust Dent J* (1990) 35, 333–7.
8. Ibrahim A, Karim A, Feldman J, Kharasch E. The influence of parecoxib, a parenteral cyclooxygenase-2 specific inhibitor, on the pharmacokinetics and clinical effects of midazolam. *Anesth Analg* (2002) 95, 667–73.
9. van Hecken AM, Tjandramaga TB, Verbesselt R, de Schepper PJ. The influence of diflunisal on the pharmacokinetics of oxazepam. *Br J Clin Pharmacol* (1985) 20, 225–34.
10. Garcia PS, Carcas A, Zapater P, Rosendo J, Paty I, Leister CA, Troy SM. Absence of an interaction between ibuprofen and zaleplon. *Am J Health-Syst Pharm* (2000) 57, 1137–41.

Benzodiazepines + Paracetamol (Acetaminophen)

Paracetamol appears to reduce the urinary excretion of diazepam with little effect on diazepam exposure. Oxazepam does not affect the pharmacokinetics of paracetamol.

Clinical evidence, mechanism, importance and management

In a pharmacokinetic study in 3 subjects, the 96-hour urinary excretion of a single 10-mg oral dose of **diazepam** and its metabolite, nordazepam, appeared to be reduced by a single 500-mg dose of paracetamol (from 44% to 12% and from 27% to 8%, respectively, in 2 female subjects, and from 11% to 4.5%, respectively, in a male subject). The reasons for these changes are not understood. The AUC of **diazepam** and its metabolite appeared to be unaffected,[1] which suggests that these changes are of limited clinical relevance.

In a study, 7 healthy subjects received a single 500-mg intravenous dose of paracetamol alone, and with a single 30-mg dose of oral **oxazepam**. The pharmacokinetics of paracetamol and its metabolites were unaffected by **oxazepam**.[2]

Although data are limited, it appears that no **diazepam** dose adjustment would be necessary on the concurrent use of paracetamol, and that no paracetamol dose adjustment would be needed on the concurrent use of **oxazepam**. There seems to be no information about other benzodiazepines.

1. Mulley BA, Potter BI, Rye RM, Takeshita K. Interactions between diazepam and paracetamol. *J Clin Pharm* (1978) 3, 25–35.
2. Sonne J, Enghusen Poulsen H, Buch Andreasen P. Single dose oxazepam has no effect on acetaminophen clearance or metabolism. *Eur J Clin Pharmacol* (1986) 30, 127–9.

Benzodiazepines and related drugs + Phenobarbital or Primidone

Phenobarbital and primidone reduce the plasma concentrations of some benzodiazepines including clobazam and clonazepam. Clobazam and clonazepam appear to reduce primidone clearance, whereas nitrazepam might increase primidone clearance. Additive adverse effects such as sedation can occur during initial use of benzodiazepines and barbiturates. More serious effects (hallucinations, violent behaviour) have been reported, but appear rare.

Clinical evidence

(a) Chlordiazepoxide

A single case report describes a man given phenobarbital, secobarbital and chlordiazepoxide who became drowsy, unsteady, and developed slurred speech, nystagmus, poor memory and hallucinations, all of which disappeared once the phenobarbital was withdrawn and the chlordiazepoxide dose reduced from 80 to 60 mg daily.[1]

(b) Clobazam

A study in patients with epilepsy receiving long-term clobazam, alone or with other antiepileptic drugs, found that phenobarbital caused a small reduction in the plasma concentrations of both clobazam and its active metabolite, *N*-desmethylclobazam.[2] Similarly, another study reported that phenobarbital reduced the plasma concentration of clobazam by 63% and reduced those of *N*-desmethylclobazam by 31%, although the effect on *N*-desmethylclobazam was not statistically significant. The plasma concentration of phenobarbital was not affected by clobazam.[3] A further study also found that clobazam plasma concentrations were decreased by phenobarbital, and that the ratio between *N*-desmethylclobazam and clobazam concentrations increased. Clobazam caused a large reduction in the apparent clearance of primidone.[4]

(c) Clonazepam

Clonazepam, in slowly increasing doses up to a maximum of 4 to 6 mg daily, given over a 6-week period to patients taking phenobarbital with or without carbamazepine, had no effect on phenobarbital concentrations.[5] A study in patients receiving various combinations of phenytoin, phenobarbital and primidone, found that their plasma concentrations were not altered by the addition of clonazepam 3 mg daily for 4 weeks, but the concentrations of clonazepam were reduced in the presence of the other antiepileptics, particularly phenobarbital and primidone. Drowsiness occurred in 44 of 66 patients in the first week after clonazepam was added to their antiepileptic treatment, but this improved in most patients; after 2 to 3 weeks only 6 patients still reported drowsiness, together with ataxia and hypotonicity. Depression was reported in one patient and personality changes with irritability and violent behaviour was reported in another.[6] A study found that phenobarbital caused some small changes in the pharmacokinetics of a single dose of clonazepam but only the small increase in clearance was statistically significant.[7] In contrast, an analysis of the serum concentrations of antiepileptics in children found that those taking clonazepam had higher primidone concentrations, and toxicity was seen.[8]

(d) Clorazepate

A report suggested that the concurrent use of primidone and clorazepate might have been responsible for the development of irritability, aggression and depression in 6 of 8 patients.[9]

(e) Diazepam

Phenobarbital 100 mg daily for 8 days had no effect on the metabolism of diazepam in a group of healthy subjects.[10]

(f) Nitrazepam

An analysis of the serum concentrations of antiepileptics in children found that those taking nitrazepam had lower primidone concentrations.[8]

Mechanism

Uncertain. Simple additive effects in some cases or changes in the drug metabolism in others seem likely. Phenobarbital probably increases the rate of metabolism of some benzodiazepines through induction of liver enzymes.

Importance and management

Phenobarbital might increase the clearance of benzodiazepines and related drugs, although none of the interactions described here appear to be of major clinical importance. However, caution might be necessary with benzodiazepines, such as **midazolam**, that are primarily metabolised by CYP3A4. Similarly, the UK manufacturer of **zopiclone** states that the concurrent use of phenobarbital might decrease the plasma concentration of **zopiclone** and a dose increase might be required.[11]

Primidone concentrations might be affected by clobazam and clonazepam and one study reported increased toxicity in children. It might be prudent to be alert for primidone adverse effects such as drowsiness, ataxia, or dysarthria, and monitor plasma concentrations should these develop.

Adverse effects such as sedation might be more evident when benzodiazepines are given with barbiturates, particularly in the initial stages of treatment, and careful dose adjustment might be required.

1. Kane FJ, McCurdy RL. An unusual reaction to combined Librium-barbiturate therapy. *Am J Psychiatry* (1964) 120, 816.
2. Bun H, Monjanel-Mouterde S, Noel F, Durand A, Cano J-P. Effects of age and antiepileptic drugs on plasma levels and kinetics of clobazam and N-desmethylclobazam. *Pharmacol Toxicol* (1990) 67, 136–40.
3. Sennoune S, Mesdjian E, Bonneton J, Genton P, Dravet C, Roger J. Interactions between clobazam and standard antiepileptic drugs in patients with epilepsy. *Ther Drug Monit* (1992) 14, 269–74.
4. Theis JGW, Koren G, Daneman R, Sherwin AL, Menzano E, Cortez M, Hwang P. Interactions of clobazam with conventional antiepileptics in children. *J Child Neurol* (1997) 12, 208–13.
5. Johannessen SI, Strandjord RE, Munthe-Kaas AW. Lack of effect of clonazepam on serum levels of diphenylhydantoin, phenobarbital and carbamazepine. *Acta Neurol Scand* (1977) 55, 506–12.

6. Nanda RN, Johnson RH, Keogh HJ, Lambie DG, Melville ID. Treatment of epilepsy with clonazepam and its effect on other anticonvulsants. *J Neurol Neurosurg Psychiatry* (1977) 40, 538–43.
7. Khoo K-C, Mendels J, Rothbart M, Garland WA, Colburn WA, Min BH, Lucek R, Carbone JJ, Boxenbaum HG, Kaplan SA. Influence of phenytoin and phenobarbital on the disposition of a single oral dose of clonazepam. *Clin Pharmacol Ther* (1980) 28, 368–75.
8. Windorfer A, Sauer W. Drug interactions during anticonvulsant therapy in childhood: diphenylhydantoin, primidone, phenobarbitone, clonazepam, nitrazepam, carbamazepin and dipropylacetate. *Neuropadiatrie* (1977) 8, 29–41.
9. Feldman RG. Chlorazepate in temporal lobe epilepsy. *JAMA* (1976) 236, 2603.
10. Brockmeyer N, Dylewicz P, Habicht H, Ohnhaus EE. The metabolism of diazepam following different enzyme inducing agents. *Br J Clin Pharmacol* (1985) 19. 544P.
11. Zimovane (Zopiclone). Sanofi-Aventis. UK Summary of product characteristics, August 2009.

Benzodiazepines and related drugs + Phenothiazines

Additive CNS depressant effects might be expected between the phenothiazines and benzodiazepines or related drugs: sedation, respiratory depression and airways obstruction has been reported. In addition, hypotension, and rare, unconfirmed cases of neuroleptic malignant syndrome have been reported. The effects vary with different drug pairs, but the parenteral use of these drugs is frequent in the more severe cases.

Clinical evidence, mechanism, importance and management

A. Benzodiazepines

(a) Diazepam and Flunitrazepam

A patient with catatonic schizophrenia was given intravenous diazepam 20 mg followed by intramuscular haloperidol 10 mg and **levomepromazine** 50 mg. Because of combative behaviour about 50 minutes later, he was given intravenous flunitrazepam 2 mg, and about 2 hours later another dose of both intravenous haloperidol 12 mg and flunitrazepam 5 mg. An hour after the last injection he became mildly cyanotic due to collapse of glossopharyngeal structures and excessive oral and nasal secretions, causing airways obstruction. Four other cases of airways obstruction associated with the combination of intramuscular **levomepromazine** in doses of 0.52 mg/kg or more and intravenous flunitrazepam or diazepam are also described. A subsequent review of all cases found that there were no cases of airways obstruction in patients who received haloperidol with either **levomepromazine** or a benzodiazepine. The interaction occurred immediately after the last intravenous injection in one patient and about 25 minutes after intramuscular **levomepromazine** but onset might be delayed by up to 2 hours or more.[1]

(b) Lorazepam

A case report describes a patient who developed neuroleptic malignant syndrome after treatment with **promethazine** and lorazepam. He had recently stopped taking haloperidol, trihexyphenidyl, and chlorpromazine due to the development of extrapyramidal symptoms. The role of **promethazine** and lorazepam is unclear, but it was suggested that they had both reduced dopaminergic activity, and the lorazepam had additionally reduced cholinergic activity.[2]

B. Non-benzodiazepine hypnotics

(a) Zaleplon

A single 50-mg dose of **thioridazine** had no effect on the pharmacokinetics of zaleplon 20 mg, and the psychomotor tests showed only short-term additive effects lasting one to 4 hours.[3] These short-term CNS additive effects are small and unlikely to be clinically relevant, and so there would seem to be no reason for avoiding concurrent use.

(b) Zolpidem

Single-dose studies found that the pharmacokinetics of 20-mg doses of zolpidem were unaffected by 50 mg of **chlorpromazine**[4,5] or 2 mg of **haloperidol**.[4] The pharmacokinetics of both of these antipsychotics were unaffected by zolpidem, except that in one study the elimination half-life of **chlorpromazine** was increased from about 5 hours to 8 hours.[5] **Chlorpromazine** increased the sedative effects of zolpidem (as indicated by impaired performances of manual dexterity and Stroop's tests).[4,5] It seems likely that additive sedation will be seen with other sedative drugs.

(c) Zopiclone

No pharmacokinetic interaction was found when 12 healthy subjects were given a single 7.5-mg oral dose of zopiclone with **chlorpromazine** 50 mg. However, the overall performance in a number of psychomotor tests (including digit symbol substitution and simulated driving) was definitely impaired more by the combination of the drugs than by **chlorpromazine** alone. Zopiclone with **chlorpromazine** impaired memory and learning, and caused a marked impairment of the performance of the tests.[6] In practical terms this means that patients given **chlorpromazine** with zopiclone should be warned that drowsiness could persist the next day and they might be less able to drive or handle potentially hazardous machinery safely.

1. Hatta K, Takahashi T, Nakamura H, Yamashiro H, Endo H, Kito K, Saeki T, Masui K, Yonezawa Y. A risk for obstruction of the airways in the parenteral use of levomepromazine with benzodiazepine. *Pharmacopsychiatry* (1998) 31, 126–30.
2. Duggal HS, Nizamie SH. Neuroleptic malignant syndrome precipitated by promethazine and lorazepam. *Aust N Z J Psychiatry* (2001) 35, 250–1.
3. Hetta J, Broman J-E, Darwish M, Troy SM. Psychomotor effects of zaleplon and thioridazine coadministration. *Eur J Clin Pharmacol* (2000) 56, 211–17.
4. Harvengt C, Hulhoven R, Desager JP, Coupez JM, Guillet P, Fuseau E, Lambert D, Warrington SJ. Drug interactions investigated with zolpidem. In: Sauvanet JP, Langer SZ, Morselli PL, eds. Imidazopyridines in Sleep Disorders. New York: Raven Press, 1988: pp. 165–73.
5. Desager JP, Hulhoven R, Harvengt C, Hermann P, Guillet P, Thiercelin JF. Possible interactions between zolpidem, a new sleep inducer and chlorpromazine, a phenothiazine neuroleptic. *Psychopharmacology (Berl)* (1988) 96, 63–6.
6. Mattila MJ, Vanakoski J, Mattila-Evenden ME, Karonen S-L. Suriclone enhances the actions of chlorpromazine on human psychomotor performance but not on memory or plasma prolactin in healthy subjects. *Eur J Clin Pharmacol* (1994) 46, 215–20.

Benzodiazepines and related drugs + Phenytoin

Reports are inconsistent: benzodiazepines can cause phenytoin concentrations to increase (toxicity has been seen), decrease, or remain unaltered. In addition phenytoin might reduce clonazepam, diazepam, midazolam, and oxazepam concentrations.

Clinical evidence

(a) Phenytoin concentrations increased

The observation that toxicity developed in patients taking phenytoin when they were given **chlordiazepoxide** or **diazepam** prompted a more detailed study. The plasma concentrations of phenytoin in 25 patients taking phenytoin 300 or 400 mg daily and **chlordiazepoxide** or **diazepam** were 80 to 90% higher than those of 99 subjects taking phenytoin without a benzodiazepine.[1]

Further reports attribute increased phenytoin plasma concentrations and phenytoin toxicity to **chlordiazepoxide**,[2] **clobazam**,[3] **clonazepam**,[4-6] and **diazepam**.[7-9]

(b) Phenytoin concentrations decreased

The plasma concentrations of phenytoin in 12 patients fell by about 30% over a 2-month period while they were taking **clonazepam** 1.5 to 12 mg daily. When data from another 12 patients were combined, the mean fall was only 18%.[10] Other studies describe similar findings with **clonazepam**[11] and **diazepam**.[12,13]

(c) Phenytoin concentrations unchanged

In one study, **alprazolam** did not affect the serum concentrations of phenytoin in healthy subjects.[14] **Clonazepam** did not alter the serum concentrations of phenytoin in one study,[15] and another study concluded that **clonazepam** produced no predictable change in phenytoin concentrations, as phenytoin concentrations were increased in 9 patients, decreased in one patient, and unchanged in 3 patients.[16] A single-dose study in healthy subjects found no pharmacokinetic interaction between intravenous **diazepam** 10 mg and intravenous **fosphenytoin** 1.125 g (or the phenytoin formed by the hydrolysis of fosphenytoin).[17]

(d) Benzodiazepine concentrations reduced

A study in 5 patients given phenytoin 250 to 400 mg daily found that plasma concentrations of **clonazepam** were reduced by more than 50%,[18] and another study found that phenytoin increased the clearance of **clonazepam** by about 50%.[19] In further studies, phenytoin reduced the plasma concentrations of **clobazam** and increased the concentrations of *N*-desmethylclobazam (the principal metabolite).[20,21] **Diazepam**[22] and **oxazepam**[23] might be similarly affected in patients with epilepsy given phenytoin.

The pharmacokinetics and pharmacodynamics of a single 15-mg oral dose of **midazolam** were studied in 6 patients with epilepsy taking carbamazepine (2 patients), phenytoin (1 patient), or both drugs together (3 patients), and in 7 control subjects not taking either of these antiepileptics. In the patients with epilepsy the AUC of **midazolam** was 94.3% lower, and the maximum plasma concentrations were 92.6% lower, than the value in the control subjects. The pharmacodynamic effects (subjective drowsiness, body sway with eyes closed and open, as well as more formal tests) were also reduced. Most of the patients did not notice any effects of the **midazolam**, while the control subjects were clearly sedated for 2 to 4 hours after taking the **midazolam** and also experienced amnesia.[24]

Mechanism

The inconsistency of these reports is not understood. Benzodiazepine-induced changes in the metabolism of phenytoin[2,7,9,13] as well as alterations in the apparent volume of distribution have been suggested as possible mechanisms. Enzyme induction by phenytoin is likely to account for the reduction in benzodiazepine plasma concentrations.

Importance and management

A confusing picture. Concurrent use certainly need not be avoided (it has proved to be valuable in many cases), but monitor the outcome of concurrent use and consider monitoring phenytoin concentrations so that undesirable changes can be detected. Only diazepam, chlordiazepoxide, clobazam, and clonazepam have been implicated, but it seems possible that other benzodiazepines could also interact. Phenytoin might induce the metabolism of some benzodiazepines including clonazepam, diazepam, midazolam, and oxazepam, causing a decrease in benzodiazepine concentrations and efficacy. The manufacturer of the non-benzodiazepine hypnotic, **zopiclone**,[25] suggests that its plasma concentration might be decreased by phenytoin. If necessary, dose adjustments should be considered. **Fosphenytoin**, a prodrug of phenytoin, seems likely to have similar effects on benzodiazepine metabolism and so similar precautions to those recommended for phenytoin would seem prudent.

1. Vajda FJE, Prineas RJ, Lovell RRH. Interaction between phenytoin and the benzodiazepines. *Br Med J* (1971) i, 346.
2. Kutt H, McDowell F. Management of epilepsy with diphenylhydantoin sodium. Dosage regulation for problem patients. *JAMA* (1968) 203, 969–72.
3. Zifkin B, Sherwin A, Andermann F. Phenytoin toxicity due to interaction with clobazam. *Neurology* (1991) 41, 313–14.

4. Eeg-Olofsson O. Experiences with Rivotril in treatment of epilepsy — particularly minor motor epilepsy — in mentally retarded children. *Acta Neurol Scand* (1973) 49 (Suppl 53), 29–31.
5. Janz D, Schneider H. Bericht über Wodadibof II (Workshop on the determination of anti-epileptic drugs in body fluids). In 'Antiepileptische Langzeitmedikation'. *Bibl Psychiatr* (1975) 151, 55–7.
6. Windorfer A, Sauer W. Drug interactions during anticonvulsant therapy in childhood: diphenylhydantoin, primidone, phenobarbitone, clonazepam, nitrazepam, carbamazepin and dipropylacetate. *Neuropadiatrie* (1977) 8, 29–41.
7. Rogers HJ, Haslam RA, Longstreth J, Lietman PS. Phenytoin intoxication during concurrent diazepam therapy. *J Neurol Neurosurg Psychiatry* (1977) 40, 890–5.
8. Kariks J, Perry SW, Wood D. Serum folic acid and phenytoin levels in permanently hospitalized epileptic patients receiving anticonvulsant drug therapy. *Med J Aust* (1971) 2, 368–71.
9. Murphy A, Wilbur K. Phenytoin–diazepam interaction. *Ann Pharmacother* (2003) 37, 659–63.
10. Edwards VE, Eadie MJ. Clonazepam — a clinical study of its effectiveness as an anticonvulsant. *Proc Aust Assoc Neurol* (1973) 10, 61–6.
11. Saavedra IN, Aguilera LI, Faure E, Galdames DG. Case report. Phenytoin/clonazepam interaction. *Ther Drug Monit* (1985) 7, 481–4.
12. Siris JH, Pippenger CE, Werner WL, Masland RL. Anticonvulsant drug-serum levels in psychiatric patients with seizure disorders. Effects of certain psychotropic drugs. *N Y State J Med* (1974) 74, 1554–6.
13. Houghton GW, Richens A. The effect of benzodiazepines and pheneturide on phenytoin metabolism in man. *Br J Clin Pharmacol* (1974) 1, P344–P345.
14. Patrias JM, DiPiro JT, Cheung RPF, Townsend RJ. Effect of alprazolam on phenytoin pharmacokinetics. *Drug Intell Clin Pharm* (1987) 21, 2A.
15. Johannessen SI, Strandjord RE, Munthe-Kaas AW. Lack of effect of clonazepam on serum levels of diphenylhydantoin, phenobarbital and carbamazepine. *Acta Neurol Scand* (1977) 55, 506–12.
16. Huang CY, McLeod JG, Sampson D, Hensley WJ. Clonazepam in the treatment of epilepsy. *Med J Aust* (1974) 2, 5–8.
17. Hussey EK, Dukes GE, Messenheimer JA, Brouwer KLR, Donn KH, Krol TF, Hak LJ. Evaluation of the pharmacokinetic interaction between diazepam and ACC-9653 (a phenytoin prodrug) in healthy male volunteers. *Pharm Res* (1990) 7, 1172–6.
18. Sjö O, Hvidberg EF, Naestoft J, Lund M. Pharmacokinetics and side-effects of clonazepam and its 7-amino-metabolite in man. *Eur J Clin Pharmacol* (1975) 8, 249–54.
19. Khoo K-C, Mendels J, Rothbart M, Garland WA, Colburn WA, Min BH, Lucek R, Carbone JJ, Boxenbaum HG, Kaplan SA. Influence of phenytoin and phenobarbital on the disposition of a single oral dose of clonazepam. *Clin Pharmacol Ther* (1980) 28, 368–75.
20. Bun H, Monjanel-Mouterde S, Noel F, Durand A, Cano J-P. Effects of age and antiepileptic drugs on plasma levels and kinetics of clobazam and N-desmethylclobazam. *Pharmacol Toxicol* (1990) 67, 136–40.
21. Sennoune S, Mesdjian E, Bonneton J, Genton P, Dravet C, Roger J. Interactions between clobazam and standard antiepileptic drugs in patients with epilepsy. *Ther Drug Monit* (1992) 14, 269–74.
22. Hepner GW, Vesell ES, Lipton A, Harvey HA, Wilkinson GR, Schenker S. Disposition of aminopyrine, antipyrine, diazepam, and indocyanine green in patients with liver disease or on anticonvulsant therapy: diazepam breath test and correlations in drug elimination. *J Lab Clin Med* (1977) 90, 440–56.
23. Scott AK, Khir ASM, Steele WH, Hawksworth GM, Petrie JC. Oxazepam pharmacokinetics in patients with epilepsy treated long-term with phenytoin alone or in combination with phenobarbitone. *Br J Clin Pharmacol* (1983) 16, 441–4.
24. Backman JT, Olkkola KT, Ojala M, Laaksovirta H, Neuvonen PJ. Concentrations and effects of oral midazolam are greatly reduced in patients treated with carbamazepine or phenytoin. *Epilepsia* (1996) 37, 253–7.
25. Zimovane (Zopiclone). Sanofi-Aventis. UK Summary of product characteristics, August 2009.

Benzodiazepines + Probenecid

Probenecid reduces the clearance of adinazolam, lorazepam, and nitrazepam. Probenecid caused a small decrease in the time to induction with midazolam. Probenecid does not appear to interact with temazepam.

Clinical evidence

(a) Adinazolam

In a single-dose study in 16 healthy subjects, probenecid 2 g increased the psychomotor effects of sustained-release adinazolam 60 mg. The tests used were symbol-digit substitution, digit span forwards and continuous performance tasks.[1] The maximum plasma concentration of adinazolam and its active metabolite, *N*-desmethyladinazolam, were increased by 37% and 49%, respectively, and the clearances were reduced by 16% and 53%, respectively, by probenecid. Both drugs have uricosuric actions, but when used together the effects appear not to be additive.[1]

(b) Lorazepam

In 9 healthy subjects, probenecid 500 mg every 6 hours approximately halved the clearance of a single 2-mg intravenous dose of lorazepam. The elimination half-life was more than doubled, from 14.3 hours to 33 hours.[2]

(c) Midazolam

In 46 patients given oral probenecid 1 g about one hour before the induction of anaesthesia with midazolam 0.3 mg/kg, induction time was shorter than in 127 control patients not given probenecid: 80% and 60%, respectively, asleep at 3 minutes.[3]

(d) Nitrazepam

In healthy subjects, probenecid 500 mg daily for 7 days reduced the clearance of nitrazepam by 25%.[4]

(e) Temazepam

In healthy subjects, probenecid 500 mg daily for 7 days did not affect the clearance of temazepam.[4]

Mechanism

Probenecid inhibits the renal tubular clearance of many drugs and their metabolites, including some of the benzodiazepines. It also inhibits the glucuronidation of nitrazepam and lorazepam by the liver.[2,4] The overall result is that these benzodiazepines accumulate and their effects are increased. The effect of probenecid on midazolam might be due to competition for plasma protein binding sites.[3] Temazepam, which also undergoes glucuronidation, was not affected by probenecid, possibly as increased sulfation compensated.[4]

Importance and management

Established interactions, but of uncertain clinical importance. Be alert for increases in the effects (sedation, antegrade amnesia) of lorazepam and possibly nitrazepam. Reduce the dose as necessary. The speed of onset of midazolam induction might be hastened by the addition of probenecid, but this is unlikely to be of clinical importance. There seems to be no direct information about other benzodiazepines, but those that are metabolised like lorazepam or nitrazepam might interact. Temazepam does not appear to interact with probenecid.

1. Golden PL, Warner PE, Fleishaker JC, Jewell RC, Millikin S, Lyon J, Brouwer KLR. Effects of probenecid on the pharmacokinetics and pharmacodynamics of adinazolam in humans. *Clin Pharmacol Ther* (1994) 56, 133–41.
2. Abernethy DR, Greenblatt DJ, Ameer B, Shader RI. Probenecid impairment of acetaminophen and lorazepam clearance: direct inhibition of ether glucuronide formation. *J Pharmacol Exp Ther* (1985) 234, 345–9.
3. Dundee JW, Halliday NJ, McMurray TJ. Aspirin and probenecid pretreatment influences the potency of thiopentone and the onset of action of midazolam. *Eur J Anaesthesiol* (1986) 3, 247–51.
4. Brockmeyer NH, Mertins L, Klimek K, Goos M, Ohnhaus EE. Comparative effects of rifampin and/or probenecid on the pharmacokinetics of temazepam and nitrazepam. *Int J Clin Pharmacol Ther Toxicol* (1990) 28, 387–93.

Benzodiazepines + Proton pump inhibitors

Diazepam exposure is slightly increased by esomeprazole and omeprazole. Gait disturbances (attributed to benzodiazepine toxicity) occurred in two patients given omeprazole with triazolam and lorazepam, or with flurazepam, and another patient taking diazepam and omeprazole became wobbly and sedated. Dexlansoprazole, lansoprazole, pantoprazole, and rabeprazole appear not to alter diazepam exposure.

Clinical evidence

(a) Dexlansoprazole

In a placebo-controlled study in 19 healthy subjects, dexlansoprazole 90 mg daily did not affect the pharmacokinetics of a single, oral 5-mg dose of **diazepam**.[1]

(b) Esomeprazole

In a placebo-controlled study, 10 healthy subjects took esomeprazole 30 mg daily for 9 days, with a single 100-microgram/kg intravenous infusion of **diazepam** on day 5. The AUC of **diazepam** was increased by 81%, its clearance was decreased by 45%, and its half-life was extended from 43 hours to 86 hours. However, increased plasma concentrations of **diazepam** were only seen 12 hours or more after dosing, at which point they were subtherapeutic. **Diazepam** did not appear to change the pharmacokinetics of esomeprazole.[2] In another similar crossover study, the AUC of a single 100 microgram/kg intravenous dose of diazepam (given on day 6) increased by 28% in healthy subjects taking oral esomeprazole 40 mg daily for 11 days, when compared with oral pantoprazole 40 mg daily for 11 days.[3] Interpretation of the findings of this study is limited by the lack of a control phase with no proton pump inhibitor.

(c) Lansoprazole

In a study in 12 healthy subjects, lansoprazole 60 mg daily for 10 days was found to have no effect on the pharmacokinetics of a single 100-microgram/kg intravenous dose of **diazepam**.[4]

(d) Omeprazole

One study in 8 healthy subjects found that omeprazole 40 mg daily for one week reduced the clearance of a single 100-microgram/kg intravenous dose of **diazepam** by 54%,[5] while another study found that a lower dose of omeprazole 20 mg daily reduced **diazepam** clearance by 27%.[6]

A further study found that omeprazole 40 mg reduced the oral clearance of **diazepam** by 38% in white American subjects, but only by 21% in Chinese subjects. All of the subjects in this study were extensive CYP2C19 metabolisers,[7] that is, they had normal activity of this isoenzyme. Metaboliser status was also found to be important in other studies of this interaction: extensive metabolisers of CYP2C19 had an increase in diazepam exposure of 26%[8] or 36%[9] whereas poor metabolisers of CYP2C19 (those deficient in or lacking CYP2C19 activity) had little change in **diazepam** exposure when given omeprazole 20 mg daily.[8,9]

Two elderly patients, both smokers, taking **triazolam** with **lorazepam**, or **flurazepam**, developed gait disturbances when they were given omeprazole 20 mg daily. They rapidly recovered when either the benzodiazepines or the omeprazole were stopped.[10] A brief report describes a patient taking omeprazole who became wobbly and sedated by small, unspecified doses of **diazepam**,[11] and another report describes a patient who developed toxic concentrations of the metabolite nordazepam and remained unconscious for 13 days after receiving a high dose of **clorazepate** (1.5 g over about 29 hours) and omeprazole 80 mg daily.[12]

(e) Pantoprazole

In a placebo-controlled study in 12 healthy subjects, intravenous pantoprazole 240 mg daily for 7 days did not change the half-life, clearance, or AUC of a 100-microgram/kg intravenous bolus dose of **diazepam**.[13]

(f) Rabeprazole

In a crossover study, rabeprazole 20 mg daily or placebo was given to 20 subjects for 35 days with a single 100-microgram/kg intravenous dose of **diazepam** on day 8. The subjects were also assessed for mephenytoin hydroxylator status [a measure of CYP2C19 activity] and 2 subjects were found to be poor metabolisers. No changes in the pharmacokinetics of **diazepam** were seen with rabeprazole, either when analyses were conducted including all the subjects or when excluding the poor metabolisers.[14] Another study similarly found that rabeprazole 20 mg daily did not affect the pharmacokinetics of **diazepam** in either 6 poor or 9 extensive metabolisers of CYP2C19.[8]

Mechanism

In vitro studies with human liver microsomes suggest that omeprazole inhibits diazepam metabolism because it inhibits CYP3A and CYP2C19.[15] Studies in humans suggest that CYP2C19 might be the most important isoenzyme in this interaction.[7] Esomeprazole, the *S*-isomer of omeprazole, also inhibits CYP2C19.[2] Further, metaboliser status can modify diazepam pharmacokinetics (see 'Genetic factors in drug metabolism', p.8). Poor metabolisers have higher concentrations and a reduced clearance of diazepam compared to extensive metabolisers. Therefore, when drugs that are CYP2C19 inhibitors are given with diazepam, extensive metabolisers will also show reduced clearance and increased concentrations (they effectively become more like poor metabolisers). Of the other proton pump inhibitors, rabeprazole, and possibly lansoprazole and pantoprazole, do not inhibit CYP2C19 to a clinically relevant extent.

Omeprazole is not expected to interact with benzodiazepines that are mainly metabolised by glucuronide conjugation such as lorazepam.[10] It has been suggested that the reaction involving lorazepam[10] might not be an interaction, but an adverse effect of giving sedating medications to markedly anaemic patients.[11]

Importance and management

The pharmacokinetic interaction between omeprazole or esomeprazole and diazepam appears to be established. However, note that the increase in diazepam exposure is slight, and is probably unlikely to be clinically relevant in most patients. Nevertheless, the case reports suggest that some patients given omeprazole with diazepam might experience increased benzodiazepine effects (such as sedation and unstable gait), and the same is likely to be true for esomeprazole. If this occurs the benzodiazepine dose should be reduced. Dexlansoprazole, lansoprazole, pantoprazole, and rabeprazole do not appear to affect the pharmacokinetics of diazepam and could be suitable alternatives in some patients if adverse effects develop with omeprazole.

Information regarding other benzodiazepines appears to be limited to case reports and no general conclusions can be drawn.

1. Vakily M, Lee RD, Wu J, Gunawardhana L, Mulford D. Drug interaction studies with dexlansoprazole modified release (TAK-390MR), a proton pump inhibitor with a dual delayed-release formulation. Results of four randomized, double-blind, crossover, placebo-controlled, single-centre studies. *Clin Drug Invest* (2009) 29, 35–50.
2. Andersson T, Hassan-Alin M, Hasselgren G, Röhss K. Drug interaction studies with esomeprazole, the (*S*)-isomer of omeprazole. *Clin Pharmacokinet* (2001) 40, 523–7.
3. Drewelow B, Schaffler K, Reitmeir P, Bethke TD. Effects of multiple-dose esomeprazole and pantoprazole on diazepam pharmacokinetic profile and pharmacodynamic effects on cognitive and psychomotor function in healthy volunteers. *Arzneimittelforschung* (2010) 60, 483–91.
4. Lefebvre RA, Flouvat B, Karolac-Tamisier S, Moerman E, Van Ganse E. Influence of lansoprazole treatment on diazepam plasma concentrations. *Clin Pharmacol Ther* (1992) 52, 458–63.
5. Gugler R, Jensen JC. Omeprazole inhibits oxidative drug metabolism. Studies with diazepam and phenytoin in vivo and 7-ethoxycoumarin in vitro. *Gastroenterology* (1985) 89, 1235–41.
6. Andersson T, Andrén K, Cederberg C, Edvardsson G, Heggelund A, Lundborg P. Effect of omeprazole and cimetidine on plasma diazepam levels. *Eur J Clin Pharmacol* (1990) 39, 51–4.
7. Caraco Y, Tateishi T, Wood AJ. Interethnic difference in omeprazole's inhibition of diazepam metabolism. *Clin Pharmacol Ther* (1995) 58, 62–72.
8. Ishizaki T, Chiba K, Manabe K, Koyama E, Hayashi M, Yasuda S, Horai Y, Tomono Y, Yamato C, Toyoki T. Comparison of the interaction potential of a new proton pump inhibitor, E3810, versus omeprazole with diazepam in extensive and poor metabolizers of *S*-mephenytoin 4′-hydroxylation. *Clin Pharmacol Ther* (1995) 58, 155–64.
9. Andersson T, Cederberg C, Edvardsson G, Heggelund A, Lundborg P. Effect of omeprazole treatment on diazepam plasma levels in slow versus normal rapid metabolizers of omeprazole. *Clin Pharmacol Ther* (1990) 47, 79–85.
10. Martí-Massó JF, López de Munain A, López de Dicastillo G. Ataxia following gastric bleeding due to omeprazole–benzodiazepine interaction. *Ann Pharmacother* (1992) 26, 429–30.
11. Shader RI. Question the experts. *J Clin Psychopharmacol* (1993) 13, 459.
12. Konrad A. Protracted episode of reduced consciousness following co-medication with omeprazole and clorazepate. *Clin Drug Invest* (2000) 19, 307–11.
13. Gugler R, Hartmann M, Rudi J, Brod I, Huber R, Steinijans VW, Bliesath H, Wurst W, Klotz U. Lack of pharmacokinetic interaction of pantoprazole with diazepam in man. *Br J Clin Pharmacol* (1996) 42, 249–52.
14. Merritt GJ, Humphries TJ, Spera AC, Hale JA, Laurent AL. Effect of rabeprazole sodium on the pharmacokinetics of diazepam in healthy male volunteers. *Pharm Res* (1997) 14 (Suppl 11), S-566.
15. Zomorodi K, Houston JB. Diazepam–omeprazole inhibition interaction: an *in vitro* investigation using human liver microsomes. *Br J Clin Pharmacol* (1996) 42, 157–62.

Benzodiazepines + Quinine

Quinine does not affect the pharmacokinetics of midazolam.

Clinical evidence, mechanism, importance and management

The manufacturer notes that, in a study in 23 healthy subjects given quinine sulfate 324 mg three times daily for 7 days and a single 2-mg oral dose of **midazolam**, the AUC and maximum plasma concentration of **midazolam** and its metabolite, 1-hydroxymidazolam were not affected by quinine.[1] Midazolam is a probe substrate for CYP3A4, and the study indicates that quinine has no clinically relevant effect on CYP3A4. Nevertheless, the manufacturer[1] still states that quinine is an inhibitor of CYP3A4.

No midazolam dose adjustment would be expected to be needed in a patient taking quinine. Other benzodiazepines that are similarly metabolised (such as **triazolam**, and to a lesser extent, **alprazolam**) would also not be expected to be affected by quinine.

1. Qualaquin (Quinine sulfate). AR Scientific Inc. US Prescribing information, April 2011.

Benzodiazepines and related drugs + Quinolones

Ciprofloxacin slightly increases the exposure to diazepam and zolpidem, but does not affect the pharmacokinetics or pharmacodynamics of temazepam. Gatifloxacin does not alter the pharmacokinetics of intravenous midazolam. Patients who are dependent on, or withdrawing from, long-term benzodiazepine use might be more susceptible to CNS adverse effects of quinolones.

Clinical evidence and mechanism

(a) Ciprofloxacin

In a study in 10 healthy subjects, ciprofloxacin 500 mg twice daily for 3 days was found to have no effect on the pharmacokinetics of a single intravenous dose of **diazepam**.[1] However, a later study in 12 healthy subjects found that ciprofloxacin 500 mg twice daily for 5 days increased the AUC of a single 5-mg intravenous dose of **diazepam** by 50%, reduced its clearance by 37%, and doubled its half-life. These changes caused no alteration in the performance of a number of psychometric tests.[2] Another study by the same group found that ciprofloxacin 500 mg twice daily for 4 days did not alter the pharmacokinetics or pharmacodynamic effects of a single 10-mg oral dose of **temazepam**.[3]

In a study in 18 healthy subjects, ciprofloxacin 500 mg once daily for 5 days slightly increased the AUC of a single 5 mg oral dose of **zolpidem** by 46%, and increased its half-life by 40%.[4]

(b) Gatifloxacin

In 14 healthy subjects, gatifloxacin 400 mg daily for 5 days had no effect on the pharmacokinetics of intravenous **midazolam**.[5]

(c) Norfloxacin

A 44-year-old woman, who had undergone withdrawal from high doses of benzodiazepines 3 months previously, experienced an acute psychotic reaction within one hour of starting norfloxacin, and she attempted suicide. Her condition quickly deteriorated and she developed repeated seizures progressing to status epilepticus. Her seizures were only controlled after norfloxacin was stopped.[6]

(d) Unnamed quinolones

Results from a survey of patients dependent on, and withdrawing from, benzodiazepines suggested an abnormally high incidence of adverse reactions to fluoroquinolones. Eleven participants reported severe or very severe adverse reactions, one participant reported a moderate adverse reaction and a further participant reported no reaction to fluoroquinolone treatment. All participants reported adverse effects similar to those of acute benzodiazepine withdrawal, which included depression, anxiety, psychosis, paranoia, severe insomnia, paraesthesia, tinnitus, hypersensitivity to light and sound, and tremors; four patients became acutely suicidal.[6] See also *Norfloxacin*, above

Mechanism

It was suggested that the clearance of diazepam was reduced because ciprofloxacin inhibited the cytochrome P450-mediated metabolism of diazepam.[2] However, although ciprofloxacin is known to be an inhibitor of CYP1A2, diazepam is not a substrate of this isoenzyme. The slight pharmacokinetic interaction of ciprofloxacin with zolpidem could be due to CYP1A2 inhibition. The study with gatifloxacin shows that gatifloxacin does not affect hepatic CYP3A4, but, to be certain it does not affect CYP3A4 (intestinal and hepatic), oral midazolam should have been used. Note that quinolones alone are known to cause psychiatric reactions and trigger seizures or lower the seizure threshold, and therefore the reports of such an interaction with the benzodiazepines are not established.

Importance and management

Evidence for an interaction between the quinolones and the benzodiazepines are restricted to a small number of drug pairs. Ciprofloxacin might slightly increase diazepam and zolpidem exposure, but it seems unlikely that any clinically relevant increases in effects such as drowsiness, etc., will occur in most patients. No pharmacokinetic interactions appear to have been reported with other benzodiazepines and quinolones. However, a few reports suggest that patients who are dependent on or withdrawing from chronic use of benzodiazepines might be more susceptible to adverse reactions to fluoroquinolones, but an interaction is not established.

1. Wijnands WJA, Trooster JFG, Teunissen PC, Cats HA, Vree TB. Ciprofloxacin does not impair the elimination of diazepam in humans. *Drug Metab Dispos* (1990) 18, 954–7.
2. Kamali F, Thomas SHL, Edwards C. The influence of steady-state ciprofloxacin on the pharmacokinetics and pharmacodynamics of a single dose of diazepam in healthy volunteers. *Eur J Clin Pharmacol* (1993) 44, 365–7.
3. Kamali F, Herd B, Edwards C, Nicholson E, Wynne H. The influence of ciprofloxacin on the pharmacokinetics and pharmacodynamics of a single dose of temazepam in the young and elderly. *J Clin Pharm Ther* (1994) 19, 105–9.
4. Vlase L, Popa A, Neag M, Muntean D, Leucuța SE. Pharmacokinetic interaction between zolpidem and ciprofloxacin in healthy volunteers. *Eur J Drug Metab Pharmacokinet* (2011) 35, 83–7.
5. Grasela DM, LaCreta FP, Kollia GD, Randall DM, Uderman HD. Open-label, nonrandomized study of the effects of gatifloxacin on the pharmacokinetics of midazolam in healthy male volunteers. *Pharmacotherapy* (2000) 20, 330–5.
6. McConnell JG. Benzodiazepine tolerance, dependency, and withdrawal syndromes and interactions with fluoroquinolone antimicrobials. *Br J Gen Pract* (2008) 58, 365–6.

Benzodiazepines + Reboxetine

There is no pharmacokinetic interaction between lorazepam and reboxetine. Reboxetine does not alter the pharmacokinetics of alprazolam.

Clinical evidence

(a) Alprazolam

In a study in 12 healthy subjects, reboxetine 4 mg twice daily had no effect on the clearance of a single 1-mg dose of alprazolam given on day 12. This study was summarised in a review paper.[1]

(b) Lorazepam

In a study in 6 healthy subjects, the AUC of lorazepam did not differ when a single 2.5-mg dose of lorazepam was given alone or with reboxetine 2 mg twice daily. There was a less than 10% change in the maximum plasma concentration and half-life of lorazepam.[2] In a further study in 6 healthy subjects, the pharmacokinetics of a single 4-mg dose of reboxetine were not altered by lorazepam 1 mg twice daily for 7 days.[3]

Mechanism

These studies suggest that reboxetine does not alter the glucuronidation of lorazepam or the metabolism of alprazolam by CYP3A4.

Importance and management

These studies show that no clinically relevant pharmacokinetic interactions occur between lorazepam or alprazolam and reboxetine. Nevertheless, the manufacturer notes that during the concurrent use of reboxetine and lorazepam, mild to moderate drowsiness and an orthostatic increase in heart rate was observed in healthy subjects,[4] but they do not state how frequently these occurred with either drug alone, and, specifically, whether the effects were actually increased on concurrent use.

1. Fleishaker JC. Clinical pharmacokinetics of reboxetine, a selective norepinephrine reuptake inhibitor for the treatment of patients with depression. *Clin Pharmacokinet* (2000) 39, 413–27.
2. Januzzo MG, Bosc M, Renoux A, Dostert P, Strolin Benedetti M. Effect of reboxetine on the pharmacokinetics of lorazepam in healthy volunteers. *Eur Neuropsychopharmacol* (1995) 5, 300–301.
3. Fiorentini F, Poggesi I, Januzzo MG, Seiberling M, Dostert P, Strolin Benedetti M. Effect of lorazepam on the pharmacokinetics of reboxetine in healthy volunteers. *Eur Neuropsychopharmacol* (1995) 5, 300.
4. Edronax (Reboxetine). Pfizer Ltd. UK Summary of product characteristics, July 2013.

Benzodiazepines and related drugs + Rifamycins

Rifampicin causes a very marked decrease in oral midazolam and triazolam exposure; a marked decrease in nitrazepam, zaleplon, and zopiclone exposure; a moderate decrease in diazepam, lorazepam, intravenous midazolam, and zolpidem exposure; but has no effect on temazepam exposure. A small study with rifapentine suggests that it very markedly decreases midazolam exposure.

Clinical evidence

A. Rifampicin (Rifampin)

(a) Benzodiazepines

1. Diazepam. In 7 patients with tuberculosis who were given daily doses of isoniazid 500 mg to 2.2 g, rifampicin 450 to 600 mg and ethambutol 25 mg/kg, the mean half-life of diazepam was longer (58 hours versus 14 hours) and the clearance 4-fold higher, when compared with healthy control subjects.[1] In 21 healthy subjects rifampicin 600 mg daily for 7 days increased the clearance of diazepam 4.3-fold and decreased its AUC by 77%. Doubling the dose of rifampicin to 1.2 g daily did not further increase its effect.[2]

In a case of overdose with diazepam and **flurazepam**, intravenous rifampicin 600 mg twice daily decreased the elimination half-life of nordazepam, the active metabolite of diazepam, from 194 hours to 63 hours.[3]

2. Lorazepam. In a study in healthy subjects, rifampicin 600 mg daily for 10 days increased the mean systemic clearance of a single intravenous dose of lorazepam about 2.4-fold. The effect of rifampicin on clearance values only minimally differed by genetic variations in uridine diphosphate glucuronyltransferase (UGT).[4]

3. Midazolam. A pharmacokinetic study in 10 healthy subjects found that rifampicin 600 mg daily for 5 days reduced the AUC of a single 15-mg oral dose of midazolam by 96%, and reduced its half-life by almost two-thirds. The psychomotor effects of the midazolam (as measured by the digit symbol substitution test, Maddox wing test, postural sway and drowsiness) were almost totally lost.[5] Similarly, in another study in 9 healthy subjects, the AUCs of single 15-mg oral doses of midazolam given before, and one and 4 days after, a 5-day course of rifampicin 600 mg daily were reduced by 98% and 87%, respectively. Four days after rifampicin, the elimination half-life was still decreased, by 60%.[6] A further study in 4 healthy subjects, found that rifampicin 450 mg daily for 4 days decreased the maximum plasma concentration and AUC of a single 7.5-mg oral dose of midazolam by 89% and 95%, respectively, and increased midazolam clearance. Similar results were obtained with a single 75-microgram dose of midazolam.[7]

The UK manufacturer notes that rifampicin 600 mg daily for 7 days decreased the [AUC] of intravenous midazolam by about 60% and decreased its half-life by about 50 to 60%.[8]

4. Nitrazepam. A study in healthy subjects found that rifampicin 600 mg daily for 7 days increased the total body clearance of a single 5-mg oral dose of nitrazepam by 83%.[9]

5. Temazepam. In a study in healthy subjects, the pharmacokinetics of temazepam, given as a single 10-mg oral dose, were unchanged by rifampicin 600 mg daily for 7 days.[9]

6. Triazolam. In a placebo-controlled study, 10 healthy subjects were given oral triazolam 500 micrograms before and after rifampicin 600 mg daily for 5 days. Rifampicin reduced the AUC of triazolam by 95% and decreased its maximum plasma concentration by 88%, when compared with placebo. The elimination half-life was reduced from 2.8 hours to 1.3 hours. Pharmacodynamic tests (drowsiness, sway, Maddox wing, etc.) showed that rifampicin abolished the effects of triazolam.[10]

(a) Non-benzodiazepine hypnotics

1. Zaleplon. A non-randomised, crossover study in healthy subjects found that rifampicin 600 mg daily for 14 days increased the clearance of a 10-mg dose of zaleplon 5.4-fold, decreasing its maximum plasma concentration and AUC by 80%.[11]

2. Zolpidem. In a randomised, placebo-controlled study, 8 healthy subjects were given rifampicin 600 mg daily for 5 days with a single 20-mg oral dose of zolpidem on day 6. It was found that rifampicin reduced the AUC of zolpidem by 73%, reduced its maximum plasma concentration by about 60% and reduced its half-life from 2.5 hours to 1.6 hours. A reduction in the effects of zolpidem was also seen, as measured by a number of psychomotor tests (digital symbol substitution, critical flicker fusion, subjective drowsiness, etc.).[12]

3. Zopiclone. In a placebo-controlled study, 8 healthy subjects were given rifampicin 600 mg for 5 days, with a single 10-mg oral dose of zopiclone on day 6. Rifampicin reduced the AUC of zopiclone by 81%, decreased its maximum plasma concentration by 71% and reduced its half-life from 3.8 hours to 2.3 hours. A reduction in the effects of zopiclone was also seen, as measured by the performance of psychomotor tests.[13]

B. Rifapentine

In a phase I dose-escalating study in 22 healthy subjects, rifapentine 5 to 20 mg/kg daily for 14 days decreased the AUC of a single 15-mg oral dose of **midazolam** given on the last day, by 93%. Rifampicin 10 mg/kg daily was used as comparator in 6 other subjects, and decreased the AUC of midazolam by 74%.[14]

Mechanism

Rifampicin is a potent non-specific liver enzyme inducer, which increases the metabolism of several benzodiazepines and the non-benzodiazepine hypnotics, zaleplon, zolpidem and zopiclone, thereby decreasing their plasma concentrations. The metabolism of midazolam by CYP3A4 in both the liver and the gut is affected.[5] The enzyme-inducing effects of rifampicin seem to predominate if isoniazid (an enzyme inhibitor) is also present. Temazepam undergoes glucuronidation and was unaffected by rifampicin. However, lorazepam glucuronidation appears to be induced by rifampicin, although lorazepam pharmacokinetics might also be influenced by drug transporter activity.[4]

Rifapentine also induces CYP3A4 and hence decreases midazolam exposure.

Importance and management

The pharmacokinetic interactions between some of the benzodiazepines and related drugs and rifampicin are established and consistent with the way rifampicin interacts with many other drugs.

The effect of rifampicin on oral **midazolam** and **triazolam** is so large that they are likely to become ineffective and an alternative should be used instead. **Alprazolam** is also predicted to interact because CYP3A is involved with its metabolism.[15]

What is known also suggests that the dose of **diazepam** and **nitrazepam** might need to be increased if rifampicin is given. Be alert for a reduction in the effects of other similarly metabolised benzodiazepines (e.g. **chlordiazepoxide**, **flurazepam**). The plasma concentration and/or the pharmacodynamic effects of the non-benzodiazepine hypnotics, **zaleplon**, **zolpidem**, and **zopiclone**, are also substantially reduced and a dose increase might also be required.

The clearance of intravenous **lorazepam** was moderately increased by rifampicin, although the clinical relevance of this is uncertain: until more is known, some caution might be warranted. The pharmacokinetics of **temazepam** were unaffected by rifampicin, and this may be a useful alternative.

The effects of rifapentine on midazolam were very marked, suggesting that the same precautions as with rifampicin above, would be prudent. However, the study reporting these effects has a number of limitations (such as a small sample size, and the use of much higher, once daily doses of rifapentine than those used therapeutically) which might explain its very marked effect on midazolam exposure. The study also found a smaller effect with rifampicin than would have been expected. Rifapentine is generally considered to have moderate effects on CYP3A4, meaning some caution on concurrent use with benzodiazepines and related drugs would be prudent, being alert for a reduction in effects and bearing in mind the need for a dose adjustment. Further study into the potency of rifapentine as a CYP3A4 inducer is required.

Evidence for **rifabutin** is lacking, but it is also known to induce CYP3A4, although perhaps only weakly. It might therefore be less likely to cause a clinically relevant reduction in exposure to benzodiazepines and related drugs metabolised by this isoenzyme, but until more is known, it might be prudent to be alert for reduced effects.

Note that midazolam is used as a probe substrate to assess the activity of other drugs on CYP3A4. The data here therefore suggest that rifampicin and rifapentine are potent inducers of CYP3A4 activity, although see comment above for rifapentine. For a list of CYP3A4 substrates, see 'Table 1.10', p.12.

1. Ochs HR, Greenblatt DJ, Roberts G-M, Dengler HJ. Diazepam interaction with antituberculosis drugs. *Clin Pharmacol Ther* (1981) 29, 671–8.
2. Ohnhaus EE, Brockmeyer N, Dylewicz P, Habicht H. The effect of antipyrine and rifampin on the metabolism of diazepam. *Clin Pharmacol Ther* (1987) 42, 148–56.
3. Panday PVN, Vischjager P, Rodgers MGG, Maurer JM, Sturkenboom MGG, Nijsten MW. Rifampicin treatment of persistently elevated benzodiazepine metabolites in a comatose patient. *Intensive Care Med* (2009) 35, 1647–8.
4. Chung J-Y, Cho J-Y, Yu K-S, Kim J-R, Jung H-R, Lim K-S, Jang I-J, Shin S-G. Effect of the *UGT2B15* genotype on the pharmacokinetics, pharmacodynamics, and drug interactions of intravenous lorazepam in healthy volunteers. *Clin Pharmacol Ther* (2005) 77, 486–94.
5. Backman JT, Olkkola KT, Neuvonen PJ. Rifampin drastically reduces plasma concentrations and effects of oral midazolam. *Clin Pharmacol Ther* (1996) 59, 7–13.
6. Backman J, Kivistö KT, Olkkola KT, Neuvonen PJ. The area under the plasma concentration-time curve for oral midazolam is 400-fold larger during treatment with itraconazole than with rifampicin. *Eur J Clin Pharmacol* (1998) 54, 53–8.
7. Eap CB, Buclin T, Cucchia G, Zullino D, Hustert E, Bleiber G, Golay KP, Aubert A-C, Baumann P, Telenti A, Kerb R. Oral administration of a low dose midazolam (75 μg) as an in vivo probe for CYP3A activity. *Eur J Clin Pharmacol* (2004) 60, 237–46.
8. Hypnovel (Midazolam hydrochloride). Roche Products Ltd. UK Summary of product characteristics, March 2010.
9. Brockmeyer NH, Mertins L, Klimek K, Goos M, Ohnhaus EE. Comparative effects of rifampin and/or probenecid on the pharmacokinetics of temazepam and nitrazepam. *Int J Clin Pharmacol Ther Toxicol* (1990) 28, 387–93.
10. Villikka K, Kivistö KT, Backman JT, Olkkola KT, Neuvonen PJ. Triazolam is ineffective in patients taking rifampin. *Clin Pharmacol Ther* (1997) 61, 8–14.
11. Darwish M. Overview of drug interaction studies with zaleplon. Poster presented at 13th Annual Meeting of Associated Professional Sleep Studies (APSS), Orlando, Florida, June 23rd, 1999.
12. Villikka K, Kivistö KT, Luurila H, Neuvonen PJ. Rifampicin reduces plasma concentrations and effects of zolpidem. *Clin Pharmacol Ther* (1997) 62, 629–34.
13. Villikka K, Kivistö KT, Lamberg TS, Kantola T, Neuvonen PJ. Concentrations and effects of zopiclone are greatly reduced by rifampicin. *Br J Clin Pharmacol* (1997) 43, 471–4.
14. Dooley KE, Bliven-Sizemore EE, Weiner M, Lu Y, Nuermberger EL, Hubbard WC, Fuchs EJ, Melia MT, Burman WJ, Dorman SE. Safety and pharmacokinetics of escalating daily doses of the antituberculosis drug rifapentine in healthy volunteers. *Clin Pharmacol Ther* (2012) 91, 881–8.
15. Greenblatt DJ, von Moltke LL, Harmatz JS, Ciraulo DA, Shader RI. Alprazolam pharmacokinetics, metabolism, and plasma levels: clinical implications. *J Clin Psychiatry* (1993) 54, 10 (Suppl), 4–11.

Benzodiazepines + Rifaximin

Rifaximin does not affect the pharmacokinetics of midazolam.

Clinical evidence, mechanism, importance and management

In a study in healthy subjects, oral rifaximin 200 mg three times daily for 8 days did not affect the pharmacokinetics of single 6-mg oral or 2-mg intravenous doses of **midazolam**.[1] Oral rifaximin has minimal gastrointestinal absorption, and therefore does not appear to affect the activity of intestinal or hepatic CYP3A4, the isoenzyme by which midazolam is metabolised. Rifaximin would therefore not be expected to affect the pharmacokinetics of other benzodiazepines metabolised similarly (such as **triazolam**, and to a lesser extent **alprazolam**). No dose adjustments of these benzodiazepines would therefore be necessary if rifaximin is also given.

Note that midazolam is used as a probe substrate to assess the activity of other drugs on CYP3A4. This study therefore suggests that oral rifaximin has no effect on CYP3A4 activity.

1. Pentikis HS, Connolly M, Trapnell CB, Forbes WP, Bettenhausen DK. The effect of multiple-dose, oral rifaximin on the pharmacokinetics of intravenous and oral midazolam in healthy volunteers. *Pharmacotherapy* (2007) 27, 1361–9.

Benzodiazepines + Roflumilast

Roflumilast does not affect the pharmacokinetics of midazolam.

Clinical evidence, mechanism, importance and management

In a study, 18 healthy subjects were given a single 2-mg oral dose of **midazolam**, and a single 1-mg intravenous dose of **midazolam** before and after taking roflumilast 500 micrograms daily for 14 days. Roflumilast did not affect the pharmacokinetics of **midazolam**.[1] These findings therefore suggest that roflumilast will not affect the metabolism of other benzodiazepines similarly metabolised (such as **triazolam**, and to a lesser extent **alprazolam**). No dose adjustments would therefore appear necessary if roflumilast is given with any of these benzodiazepines.

Note that midazolam is used as a probe substrate to assess the activity of other drugs on CYP3A4. This study therefore suggests that roflumilast has no effect on CYP3A4 activity.

1. Nassr N, Lahu G, von Richter O, Reutter F, Knoerzer D, Zech K, Erb KA, Schug B, Blume H, Hermann R. Lack of a pharmacokinetic interaction between steady-state roflumilast and single-dose midazolam in healthy subjects. *Br J Clin Pharmacol* (2007) 63, 365–70.

Benzodiazepines and related drugs + SNRIs

There is limited evidence to suggest that sedation might initially be increased by the concurrent use of duloxetine and lorazepam, although there was no pharmacokinetic interaction between the two drugs. Visual hallucinations have been seen in one patient given zolpidem and venlafaxine. Desvenlafaxine might slightly decrease the exposure to midazolam. Venlafaxine slightly decreased alprazolam exposure, negligibly decreased diazepam exposure, and had no effect on zaleplon exposure. The pharmacokinetics of duloxetine are not affected by temazepam. No pharmacokinetic interaction appears to occur between levomilnacipran and alprazolam, or between milnacipran and lorazepam.

Clinical evidence

(a) Desvenlafaxine

The US manufacturer of desvenlafaxine briefly notes that in a study, desvenlafaxine 400 mg daily decreased the AUC and maximum concentration of a single 4-mg dose of **midazolam** by about 31% and 16%, respectively.[1]

(b) Duloxetine

1. Lorazepam. In a placebo-controlled study, the pharmacokinetics of duloxetine 60 mg twice daily and lorazepam 2 mg twice daily were not affected by concurrent use. However, compared with lorazepam alone, the addition of duloxetine led to decreased vigilance on various psychomotor tests (such as digit symbol substitution test) during the first day of concurrent use, although this effect tended to lessen over the 4 days of the study.[2]

2. Temazepam. The manufacturer briefly notes that the steady-state pharmacokinetics of duloxetine 20 mg at bedtime were not affected by temazepam 30 mg at bedtime.[3]

(c) Levomilnacipran

The US manufacturer of levomilnacipran briefly notes that in a study, there was no pharmacokinetic interaction between **alprazolam** and levomilnacipran.[4]

(d) Milnacipran

The US manufacturer of milnacipran briefly notes that in a single dose study, no pharmacokinetic interaction was seen when milnacipran 50 mg was given with a 1.5 mg dose of **lorazepam**.[5]

(e) Venlafaxine

1. Alprazolam. A study in 16 healthy subjects found that venlafaxine 75 mg twice daily decreased the AUC of a single 2-mg oral dose of alprazolam by 29% and decreased its half-life by 21%. The performance of psychometric tests was only minimally changed.[6]

2. Diazepam. In a study in 18 healthy subjects, venlafaxine 50 mg every 8 hours caused a 16% decrease in the AUC of a single 10-mg dose of diazepam, but had no effect on its major active metabolite nordazepam. Diazepam affected the performance of a series of pharmacodynamic tests, but pretreatment with venlafaxine had no further effects.[7]

3. Zaleplon. The manufacturers of zaleplon describe a study in which the concurrent use of extended-release venlafaxine 150 mg daily and a single 10-mg dose of zaleplon did not result in any changes in the pharmacokinetics of either zaleplon or venlafaxine.[8,9] Additionally, there was no pharmacodynamic interaction[9] with tests for memory and psychomotor performance being unaffected.[8]

4. Zolpidem. A 27-year-old woman who had been taking venlafaxine 37.5 mg at night for a week and terfenadine for a few years, started taking zolpidem 10 mg daily. After 2 days, and within 45 minutes of the zolpidem dose, she developed visual hallucinations, which lasted for 2 to 4 hours. A similar episode occurred 2 weeks later when she had discontinued the terfenadine.[10]

Mechanism

Uncertain. Zolpidem alone is associated with hallucinations, and it has been suggested that a pharmacodynamic interaction between serotonin reuptake inhibition and zolpidem might lead to a prolongation of this effect in susceptible individuals.[10] The reason why venlafaxine caused negligible to slight decreases in alprazolam and diazepam exposure is unknown. The reason for the slight decrease in midazolam exposure seen with desvenlafaxine is unclear. In an *in vitro* study[1] desvenlafaxine did not affect CYP3A4, however it appears that it might induce CYP3A4 *in vivo*, although note that the desvenlafaxine dose used was 8-fold higher than that used clinically.

Importance and management

The studies suggest that no particular precautions are necessary during the concurrent use of venlafaxine and alprazolam or diazepam, levomilnacipran and alprazolam, milnacipran and lorazepam, or duloxetine and lorazepam or temazepam. The slight decrease in midazolam exposure seen with desvenlafaxine was not considered to be clinically relevant and no dose adjustment is required.[1] However, a pharmacodynamic interaction could occur and caution has been advised due to the potential for increased sedation.[2] Hallucinations have been seen with zolpidem alone, and they have also occurred, rarely, when zolpidem was given with some SSRIs (see 'Benzodiazepines and related drugs + SSRIs', p.838), which are related to venlafaxine. Reports of adverse effects such as these seem rare and the concurrent use of these drugs need not be avoided, but bear these possible interactions in mind if hallucinations or increased sedation occur.

1. Pristiq (Desvenlafaxine succinate). Wyeth Pharmaceuticals Inc. US Prescribing information, July 2014.
2. Chalon S, Vandenhende F, Ertle S. Combined administration of duloxetine (DU) and lorazepam (LO): a pharmacokinetic and pharmacodynamic study. *Clin Pharmacol Ther* (2005) 77, P65.
3. Cymbalta (Duloxetine hydrochloride). Eli Lilly and Company. US Prescribing information, July 2014.
4. Fetzima (Levomilnacipran hydrochloride). Forest Pharmaceuticals, Inc. US Prescribing information, July 2014.
5. Savella (Milnacipran hydrochloride). Forest Pharmaceuticals, Inc. US prescribing information, November 2013.
6. Amchin J, Zarycranski W, Taylor KP, Albano D, Klockowski PM. Effect of venlafaxine on the pharmacokinetics of alprazolam. *Psychopharmacol Bull* (1998) 34, 211–19.

7. Troy SM, Lucki I, Peirgies AA, Parker VD, Klockowski PM, Chiang ST. Pharmacokinetic and pharmacodynamic evaluation of the potential drug interaction between venlafaxine and diazepam. *J Clin Pharmacol* (1995) 35, 410–19.
8. Sonata (Zaleplon). Meda Pharmaceuticals. UK Summary of product characteristics, February 2009.
9. Sonata (Zaleplon). King Pharmaceuticals, Inc. US Prescribing information, December 2007.
10. Elko CJ, Burgess JL, Robertson WO. Zolpidem-associated hallucinations and serotonin reuptake inhibition: a possible interaction. *Clin Toxicol* (1998), 36, 195–203.

Benzodiazepines and related drugs + SSRIs

Fluvoxamine moderately increases alprazolam, bromazepam and diazepam exposure, and also increases etizolam concentrations, whereas it has a slight or no effect on lorazepam, midazolam, and quazepam exposure. There is some evidence to suggest that fluoxetine may cause a negligible to slight increase in alprazolam and diazepam exposure, and increase their psychomotor impairment. Fluoxetine has no effect on clonazepam, estazolam, midazolam, triazolam, or zolpidem metabolism.

On the whole, no pharmacokinetic interaction appears to occur between other SSRIs (citalopram, paroxetine, sertraline) and the benzodiazepines or related drugs such as zaleplon or zolpidem. However, there is limited evidence to support the suggestion that sedation could be increased by the concurrent use of any SSRI and benzodiazepines and related drugs such as cloral hydrate. Isolated cases of hallucinations have been seen with zolpidem and fluoxetine or sertraline.

Clinical evidence

(a) Citalopram

1. Alprazolam. A general study in psychiatric patients taking citalopram and benzodiazepines found a 23% increase in the serum concentration of citalopram when data on all benzodiazepines was pooled, but this is almost certainly too small to be clinically relevant. Alprazolam was the only benzodiazepine to cause an elevation of citalopram levels (by 16%) when analysed alone.[1] In another study, citalopram was found to have no effect on the maximum plasma concentration or exposure to alprazolam, although the time to the maximum concentration of alprazolam was increased by 30 minutes.[2]

2. Triazolam. A study in 17 healthy subjects found no pharmacokinetic interaction between citalopram (20 mg daily increased after one week to 40 mg daily for 3 weeks) and a single 250-microgram dose of triazolam.[3]

(b) Fluoxetine

1. Alprazolam. Fluoxetine 60 mg daily for 4 days has been found to reduce the clearance of alprazolam 1 mg four times daily by about 21% and to increase its plasma concentration by about 30%. These changes were accompanied by increased psychomotor impairment.[4] Another study using fluoxetine 20 mg daily for at least 21 days also reported a slight 32% increase in the AUC of alprazolam, although no important changes in alprazolam pharmacodynamics were found.[2] In a third study, fluoxetine 20 mg twice daily for 8 days slightly increased the AUC of alprazolam by 26%.[5]

2. Diazepam. Fluoxetine 30 mg, given either as a single dose, or daily for 8 days, had no effect on the pharmacokinetics of diazepam 10 mg.[6] In a later study by the same group, fluoxetine 60 mg daily for 8 days appeared to increase the half-life and AUC of diazepam.[7] Another study found that fluoxetine 60 mg alone did not affect psychomotor performance but fluoxetine 60 mg with diazepam 5 mg impaired the divided attention tracking test and vigilance test more than with diazepam 5 mg alone.[8]

3. Other benzodiazepines and related drugs. Other studies found that fluoxetine did not alter the pharmacokinetics and/or pharmacodynamics of **clonazepam**,[5] **estazolam**,[9] **midazolam**,[10] **triazolam**[11] and **zolpidem**.[12,13]

An isolated case of visual hallucinations lasting up to 7 hours has been reported in a patient taking **zolpidem** who was also taking fluoxetine.[14] Marked drowsiness occurred for a whole day in a patient taking fluoxetine 20 mg daily after being given **cloral hydrate** 500 mg the night before. She later tolerated **cloral hydrate** 1 g in the absence of fluoxetine without adverse effects.[15]

(c) Fluvoxamine

1. Alprazolam. In 60 healthy subjects, fluvoxamine 50 mg daily for 3 days then 100 mg daily for 7 days, increased the AUC of alprazolam 1.96-fold when alprazolam 1 mg four times daily was given on days 7 to 10. The alprazolam clearance was halved. Psychomotor performance and memory were found to be worsened, even after only one day.[16] A study in 23 Japanese patients found that fluvoxamine increased the plasma concentration of alprazolam by 58%. There was wide interpatient variability, possibly associated with differences in CYP2C19 genotype in these patients, although it is unclear exactly what impact this isoenzyme has on the interaction.[17] One study investigating interpatient variability found that the interaction between fluvoxamine and alprazolam was greater in non-smokers than in smokers.[18]

2. Bromazepam. In 12 healthy subjects, fluvoxamine 50 mg twice daily increased the plasma concentration of a single 12-mg dose of bromazepam by 36% and increased its AUC almost 2.5-fold. Some increased impairment in cognitive function was seen.[19]

3. Diazepam. In 8 healthy subjects, fluvoxamine (50 mg on day one, 100 mg on day 2, then 150 mg daily thereafter) for 16 days decreased the clearance of a single 10-mg dose of diazepam given on day 4 by about 65%. The half-life was increased from 51 hours to 118 hours, and the AUC was increased 3-fold.[20]

4. Etizolam. In a study in 17 patients taking etizolam 0.75 to 3 mg daily, fluvoxamine 25 or 50 mg daily increased the plasma concentration of etizolam (corrected to the dose) by 43% (range 0.0 to 235%). The 12 patients who had taken etizolam with fluvoxamine 25 mg daily showed an increase in the concentration of etizolam of 39% and in the 5 patients who had taken fluvoxamine 50 mg daily the concentration of etizolam increased by 55%. Three of the patients taking fluvoxamine 25 mg daily had their dose increased to 150 mg or 200 mg and increases in the plasma concentration of etizolam changed from 43%, 0%, and 81% to 86%, 146%, and 190%, respectively. The extent of the interaction depends on the dose of fluvoxamine, but there is wide interpatient variability. Increased sleepiness occurred in another patient given fluvoxamine 200 mg who had an increase in the plasma concentration of etizolam of almost 400%.[21]

5. Lorazepam. In 12 healthy subjects, fluvoxamine 50 mg twice daily caused a very small, non-significant, increase in the plasma concentration and AUC of a single 4-mg dose of lorazepam.[19]

6. Midazolam. A study in 10 healthy subjects[10] found that fluvoxamine 50 mg twice daily for 8 days then 100 mg twice daily for 6 days increased the AUC of midazolam by 39% and decreased its clearance by 38% when a single 10-mg oral dose of midazolam was given on day 12.

7. Quazepam. A placebo-controlled study in 12 healthy subjects found that fluvoxamine 25 mg twice daily for 14 days had no effect on the pharmacokinetics of a single 20-mg dose of quazepam. However, formation of the metabolite, 2-oxoquazepam, was decreased, and there was a minor decrease in the sedative effects of quazepam at 4 hours.[22]

(d) Paroxetine

1. Alprazolam. A randomised, placebo-controlled study in 22 healthy subjects reported no evidence for a pharmacokinetic or pharmacological interaction between steady-state paroxetine and alprazolam.[23]

2. Clonazepam. An isolated report describes worsening anxiety, agitation, mild abdominal cramps and diaphoresis in a woman taking paroxetine, shortly after starting clonazepam (dose stated as one tablet). This toxic response was suggested as being serotonin syndrome, although in fact many of the usual signs were absent and moreover, clonazepam has actually been used to treat the myoclonus that occurs in serotonin syndrome. The patient was effectively treated with **lorazepam**.[24]

3. Diazepam. No important changes in the pharmacokinetics of paroxetine were seen when 12 healthy subjects given paroxetine 30 mg daily were also given diazepam 5 mg three times a day. Adverse events were not increased by the combination.[25]

4. Etizolam. A report describes a patient who was admitted to hospital with symptoms of serotonin syndrome within 6 days of starting paroxetine 20 mg daily, etizolam 1 mg daily, and **brotizolam** 250 micrograms daily. Paroxetine was discontinued on day 6. Serotonin syndrome usually resolves within 24 hours of discontinuing the causative medication but symptoms in this patient continued for a total of 10 days.[26]

5. Oxazepam. One study found that paroxetine did not increase the impairment of a number of psychomotor tests caused by oxazepam.[27]

6. Zaleplon. In a double-blind study in healthy subjects it was found that paroxetine 20 mg for 9 days had no effect on the pharmacokinetics of zaleplon 20 mg, and psychomotor performance was unaffected by concurrent use.[28]

7. Zolpidem. An isolated report describes a 16-year-old girl with depression who took paroxetine 20 mg daily for 3 days, and then on the evening of the third night a single 10-mg dose of zolpidem. Within one hour she began to hallucinate, then became disorientated and was unable to recognise members of her family. She recovered spontaneously within 4 hours.[29]

(e) Sertraline

1. Alprazolam. A pharmacokinetic study in 10 healthy subjects found that sertraline 50 to 150 mg daily had no effect on the pharmacokinetics of alprazolam 1 mg and did not potentiate the psychomotor impairment produced by alprazolam alone, although there was a decrease in peak performance in the manual tracking test.[30] Similarly, in 12 healthy subjects, sertraline 50 mg daily had no effect on the pharmacokinetics of alprazolam 1 mg daily after 2 weeks of concurrent use.[31]

2. Clonazepam. A study in 13 subjects given clonazepam 1 mg daily with sertraline 100 mg daily for 10 days found that sertraline did not affect the pharmacokinetics of clonazepam. There was also no evidence that the addition of sertraline to clonazepam made the subjects more sedated or less able to carry out simple psychometric tests.[32]

3. Diazepam. In a placebo-controlled study, the systemic clearance of a single intravenous dose of diazepam was reduced by 13% after 21 days of sertraline treatment.[33,34]

4. Zolpidem. Sertraline appears to have negligible effects on the pharmacokinetics of zolpidem.[35] An isolated case of visual hallucinations lasting up to 7 hours has been reported in a patient taking zolpidem and sertraline.[14]

Mechanism

Fluvoxamine is a known potent inhibitor of CYP2C19, by which diazepam is metabolised, and therefore concurrent use results in moderately increased diazepam exposure.

The reason why fluvoxamine increases alprazolam exposure to a greater extent than midazolam exposure is uncertain, because fluvoxamine is, at most, a weak inhibitor of CYP3A4, and midazolam is a more sensitive substrate of CYP3A4 than alprazolam. Fluvoxamine is known to inhibit CYP2C19 and/or CYP1A2, which might explain the interaction with alprazolam, particularly as this appeared to vary by CYP2C19 metaboliser status and by smoking status (smoking induces CYP1A2). Fluvoxamine does not appear to interact with benzodiazepines that are principally metabolised by glucuronidation (e.g. lorazepam).

None of the other SSRIs have the same effect on CYP2C19 or CYP1A2 as fluvoxamine, and all have weak to no inhibitory activity on CYP3A4, so appear to have minimal effects on the pharmacokinetics of the benzodiazepines metabolised by these isoenzymes.

Importance and management

A well studied interaction, although the evidence regarding individual pairs of benzodiazepines and SSRIs is generally limited. Regardless of any pharmacokinetic effect it should be noted that some of the studies found pharmacodynamic effects (that is, increased sedation or clumsiness) in the absence of a pharmacokinetic interaction. Somnolence is a common side effect of all SSRIs. It might be prudent to advise patients to be aware of the possibility of these effects when first starting concurrent SSRI and a benzodiazepine or related drug.

The hallucinations seen with the SSRIs and zolpidem appear rare, and reactions of this kind have been seen with zolpidem alone. The concurrent use of these drugs need not be avoided, but bear this possible interaction in mind if hallucinations occur.

Specific issues regarding the pharmacokinetic interactions of pairs of SSRIs and benzodiazepines are discussed in the sections below.

Fluvoxamine

The available data suggests that the doses of **alprazolam**, **bromazepam**, **diazepam**, and **etizolam** should be reduced, probably by half, in the presence of fluvoxamine to avoid adverse effects (drowsiness, reduced psychomotor performance and memory). Furthermore, some US manufacturers recommend avoiding the use of fluvoxamine with diazepam as substantial diazepam accumulation could occur. They also note that fluvoxamine has non-linear kinetics, and therefore the effects of higher doses of fluvoxamine could be even more pronounced, particularly with long-term diazepam or alprazolam use.[36] Some manufacturers warn that the clearance of other oxidatively metabolised benzodiazepines (e.g. **midazolam** and **triazolam**) is likely to be decreased by fluvoxamine[36,37] and the dose of these benzodiazepines might need to be reduced;[37] however, one study with midazolam and fluvoxamine found only a minimal interaction, and there are important differences in the isoenzymes involved in the metabolism of midazolam compared with diazepam (see *Mechanism*, above). This suggests that no clinically relevant interaction is likely with fluvoxamine and midazolam or triazolam. Fluvoxamine is also unlikely to affect **lorazepam** and other benzodiazepines metabolised by glucuronidation (e.g. **oxazepam**, **temazepam**).[36]

Note that midazolam is used as a probe substrate to assess the activity of other drugs on CYP3A4. The evidence here therefore suggests that fluvoxamine is a weak inhibitor of CYP3A4 activity.

Fluoxetine

Fluoxetine has a negligible to slight effect on the pharmacokinetics and pharmacodynamics of alprazolam and diazepam, which appears unlikely to be clinically relevant. Fluoxetine also does not affect the metabolism of clonazepam, estazolam, midazolam, triazolam, and zolpidem.

Note that midazolam is used as a probe substrate to assess the activity of other drugs on CYP3A4. The evidence here therefore suggests that fluoxetine has no effect on CYP3A4 activity.

Other SSRIs

Citalopram, paroxetine, and sertraline have little to no effect on the pharmacokinetics of various benzodiazepines and they might therefore be a useful alternative to fluvoxamine in some patients.

1. Leinonen E, Lepola U, Koponen H, Kinnunen I. The effect of age and concomitant treatment with other psychoactive drugs on serum concentrations of citalopram measured with a nonenantioselective method. *Ther Drug Monit* (1996) 18, 111–17.
2. Hall J, Naranjo CA, Sproule BA, Herrmann N. Pharmacokinetic and pharmacodynamic evaluation of the inhibition of alprazolam by citalopram and fluoxetine. *J Clin Psychopharmacol* (2003) 23, 349–57.
3. Nolting A, Abramowitz W. Lack of interaction between citalopram and the CYP3A4 substrate triazolam. *Pharmacotherapy* (2000) 20, 750–5.
4. Lasher TA, Fleishaker JC, Steenwyk RC, Antal EJ. Pharmacokinetic pharmacodynamic evaluation of the combined administration of alprazolam and fluoxetine. *Psychopharmacology (Berl)* (1991) 104, 323–7.
5. Greenblatt DJ, Preskorn SH, Cotreau MM, Horst WD, Harmatz JS. Fluoxetine impairs clearance of alprazolam but not of clonazepam. *Clin Pharmacol Ther* (1992) 52, 479–86.
6. Lemberger L, Bergstrom RF, Wolen RL, Farid NA, Enas GG, Aronoff GR. Fluoxetine: clinical pharmacology and physiologic disposition. *J Clin Psychiatry* (1985) 46, 3 (Sec 2), 14–19.
7. Lemberger L, Rowe H, Bosomworth JC, Tenbarge JB, Bergstrom RF. The effect of fluoxetine on the pharmacokinetics and psychomotor responses of diazepam. *Clin Pharmacol Ther* (1988) 43, 412–19.
8. Moskowitz H, Burns M. The effects on performance of two antidepressants, alone and in combination with diazepam. *Prog Neuropsychopharmacol Biol Psychiatry* (1988) 12, 783–92.
9. Cavanaugh J, Schneck D, Eason C, Hansen M, Gustavson L. Lack of effect of fluoxetine on the pharmacokinetics (PK) and pharmacodynamics (PD) of estazolam. *Clin Pharmacol Ther* (1994) 55, 141.
10. Lam YWF, Alfaro CL, Ereshefsky L, Miller M. Pharmacokinetics and pharmacodynamic interactions of oral midazolam with ketoconazole, fluoxetine, fluvoxamine, and nefazodone. *J Clin Pharmacol* (2003) 43, 1274–82.
11. Wright CE, Lasher-Sisson TA, Steenwyk RC, Swanson CN. A pharmacokinetic evaluation of the combined administration of triazolam and fluoxetine. *Pharmacotherapy* (1992) 12, 103–6.
12. Piergies AA, Sweet J, Johnson M, Roth-Schechter BF, Allard S. The effect of co-administration of zolpidem with fluoxetine: pharmacokinetics and pharmacodynamics. *Int J Clin Pharmacol Ther* (1996) 34, 178–83.
13. Allard S, Sainati S, Roth-Schechter B, Macintyre J. Minimal interaction between fluoxetine and multiple-dose zolpidem in healthy women. *Drug Metab Dispos* (1998) 26, 617–22.
14. Elko CJ, Burgess JL, Robertson WO. Zolpidem-associated hallucinations and serotonin reuptake inhibition: a possible interaction. *J Toxicol Clin Toxicol* (1998) 36, 195–203.
15. Devarajan S. Interaction of fluoxetine and chloral hydrate. *Can J Psychiatry* (1992) 37, 590–1.
16. Fleishaker JC, Hulst LK. A pharmacokinetic and pharmacodynamic evaluation of the combined administration of alprazolam and fluvoxamine. *Eur J Clin Pharmacol* (1994) 46, 35–9.
17. Suzuki Y, Shioiri T, Muratake T, Kawashima Y, Sato S, Hagiwara M, Inoue Y, Shimoda K, Someya T. Effects of concomitant fluvoxamine on the metabolism of alprazolam in Japanese psychiatric patients: interaction with CYP2C19 mutated alleles. *Eur J Clin Pharmacol* (2003) 58, 829–33.
18. Sugahara H, Maebara C, Ohtani H, Handa M, Ando K, Mine K, Kubo C, Ieiri I, Sawada Y. Effect of smoking and CYP2D6 polymorphisms on the extent of fluvoxamine–alprazolam interactions in patients with psychosomatic disease. *Eur J Clin Pharmacol* (2009) 65, 699–704.
19. Van Harten J, Holland RL, Wesnes K. Influence of multiple-dose administration of fluvoxamine on the pharmacokinetics of the benzodiazepines bromazepam and lorazepam: a randomised, cross-over study. *Eur Neuropsychopharmacol* (1992) 2, 381.
20. Perucca E, Gatti G, Cipolla G, Spina E, Barel S, Soback S, Gips M, Bialer M. Inhibition of diazepam metabolism by fluvoxamine: a pharmacokinetic study in normal volunteers. *Clin Pharmacol Ther* (1994) 56, 471–6.
21. Suzuki Y, Kawashima Y, Shioiri T, Someya T. Effects of concomitant fluvoxamine on the plasma concentration of etizolam in Japanese psychiatric patients. Wide interindividual variation in the drug interaction. *Ther Drug Monit* (2004) 26, 638–42.
22. Kanda H, Yasui-Furukori N, Fukasawa T, Aoshima T, Suzuki A, Otani K. Interaction study between fluvoxamine and quazepam. *J Clin Pharmacol* (2003) 43, 1392–7.
23. Calvo G, García-Gea C, Luque A, Morte A, Dal-Ré R, Barbanoj M. Lack of pharmacologic interaction between paroxetine and alprazolam at steady state in healthy volunteers. *J Clin Psychopharmacol* (2004) 24, 268–76.
24. Rella JG, Hoffman RS. Possible serotonin syndrome from paroxetine and clonazepam. *Clin Toxicol* (1998) 36, 257–8.
25. Bannister SJ, Houser VP, Hulse JD, Kisicki JC, Rasmussen JGC. Evaluation of the potential for interactions of paroxetine with diazepam, cimetidine, warfarin, and digoxin. *Acta Psychiatr Scand* (1989) 80 (Suppl 350), 102–6.
26. Ochiai Y, Katsu H, Okino S, Wakutsu N, Nakayama K. A prolongation case of the serotonin syndrome by paroxetine – about the recovery process. *Seishin Shinkeigaku Zasshi* (2003) 105, 1532–8.
27. Cooper SM, Jackson D, Loudon JM, McClelland GR, Raptopoulos P. The psychomotor effects of paroxetine alone and in combination with haloperidol, amylobarbitone, oxazepam, or alcohol. *Acta Psychiatr Scand* (1989) 80 (Suppl 350), 53–55.
28. Darwish M. Overview of drug interaction studies with zaleplon. Poster presented at 13th Annual Meeting of Associated Professional Sleep Studies (APSS), Orlando, Florida, June 23rd, 1999.
29. Katz SE. Possible paroxetine-zolpidem interaction. *Am J Psychiatry* (1995) 152, 1689.
30. Hassan PC, Sproule BA, Naranjo CA, Herrmann N. Dose-response evaluation of the interaction between sertraline and alprazolam *in vivo*. *J Clin Psychopharmacol* (2000) 20, 150–8.
31. Preskorn SH, Greenblatt DJ, Harvey AT. Lack of effect of sertraline on the pharmacokinetics of alprazolam. *J Clin Psychopharmacol* (2000) 20, 585–6.
32. Bonate PL, Kroboth PD, Smith RB, Suarez E, Oo C. Clonazepam and sertraline: absence of drug interaction in a multiple-dose study. *J Clin Psychopharmacol* (2000), 20, 19–27.
33. Warrington SJ. Clinical implications of the pharmacology of sertraline. *Int Clin Psychopharmacol* (1991) 6 (Suppl 2), 11–21.
34. Gardner MJ, Baris BA, Wilner KD, Preskorn SH. Effect of sertraline on the pharmacokinetics and protein binding of diazepam in healthy volunteers. *Clin Pharmacokinet* (1997) 32 (Suppl 1), 43–9.
35. Allard S, Sainati SM, Roth-Schechter BF. Coadministration of short-term zolpidem with sertraline in healthy women. *J Clin Pharmacol* (1999) 39, 184–91.
36. Luvox CR (Fluvoxamine maleate). Jazz Pharmaceuticals, Inc. US Prescribing information, May 2011.
37. Faverin (Fluvoxamine maleate). BGP Products Ltd. UK Summary of product characteristics, August 2015.

Benzodiazepines and related drugs + St John's wort (*Hypericum perforatum*)

Long-term use of St John's wort decreases alprazolam, midazolam and quazepam exposure. The effect varies depending on the St John's wort product used, with those containing lower amounts of hyperforin having less of an effect. Long-term use of St John's wort also decreases zolpidem exposure. Zopiclone is predicted to be similarly affected.

Clinical evidence

(a) Alprazolam

In a crossover study, 12 healthy subjects were given St John's wort (*LI 160, Lichtwer Pharma*, 0.12 to 0.3% hypericin) 300 mg three times daily for 16 days with a single 2-mg dose of alprazolam on day 14. The AUC of alprazolam was reduced by 54% by St John's wort and its clearance was increased 2.3-fold.[1]

In another study, alprazolam 1 or 2 mg was given to 7 healthy subjects on the third day of a 3-day treatment period with St John's wort (*Solaray*; hypericin content standardised at 0.3%) 300 mg three times daily. The pharmacokinetics of alprazolam were unchanged by St John's wort, but the authors note that 3 days may have been an insufficient time for St John's wort to fully induce cytochrome P450 isoenzymes.[2] In another study, 16 healthy subjects were given St John's wort extract 120 mg (*Esbericum* capsules; corresponding to 0.5 mg total hypericins and 1.76 mg hyperforin) twice daily for 10 days. A single 1-mg dose of alprazolam was given on the day before treatment with St John's wort and on the last day of treatment. St John's wort extract at this low dose and low hyperforin content had no clinically relevant effects on the pharmacokinetics of alprazolam, when compared with 12 subjects given placebo.[3]

(b) Midazolam

In a study in 12 healthy subjects, St John's wort 300 mg three times daily for 14 or 15 days decreased the AUC and maximum plasma concentration of a single *oral* dose of midazolam by 52% and 42%, respectively. Intravenous midazolam was little affected, with no statistically significant changes. The St John's wort product used was stated to contain 900 micrograms of hypericin per 300 mg capsule.[4] Similar results were found in two other studies: a 2.9-fold increase in oral midazolam clearance with an unspecified product[5] and a 2.6-fold increase with *LI 160* (*Lichtwer Pharma*, 0.3% hypericins).[6] In one study, 3 of 12 subjects reported that the sedative effects of midazolam were less noticeable when St John's wort was taken at the same time.[7] However, in another study, the effect of St John's wort (*TruNature*; hypericin content standardised at about 800 micrograms) 300 mg three times daily for 14 days was much less, with just a 33% increase in oral midazolam clearance.[8] In another study, the effect of St John's wort on midazolam pharmacokinetics varied among 6 different products tested, and was correlated with hyperforin content and not the St John's wort dose. The greatest effect was an 80% reduction in the AUC of midazolam with *LI 160* and the least was a 21% reduction in the AUC of midazolam with a low-hyperforin product.[9] The same research group later reported a similar negligible decrease in the AUC of midazolam with a St John's wort preparation with low hyperforin content.[10] Note that, in one study, a single dose of St John's wort had no effect on the pharmacokinetics of midazolam.[4]

(c) Quazepam

In a placebo-controlled study, 13 healthy subjects were given St John's wort (*Tru-Nature*; hypericin content standardised at 0.3%) 300 mg three times daily for 14 days with a single 15-mg dose of quazepam on day 14. St John's wort slightly decreased the AUC and maximum plasma levels of quazepam by 26% and 29%, respectively, but the pharmacodynamic effects of quazepam were not affected.[11]

(d) Zolpidem

In study, 14 healthy subjects were given St John's wort (*LI 160, Lichtwer Pharma*) 300 mg three times daily from day 2 to day 16, with a single 10-mg dose of zolpidem on day 15. St John's wort decreased the AUC and maximum plasma concentration of zolpidem by 30% and 34%, respectively, but there was marked interindividual variability in the results.[12]

Mechanism

Midazolam and, to a lesser extent, alprazolam, are substrates of CYP3A4. St John's wort appears to induce CYP3A4 thus increasing the metabolism of *oral* midazolam and alprazolam, and reducing the bioavailability of these benzodiazepines. Zolpidem is also metabolised by CYP3A4 and therefore its exposure is reduced by St John's wort. Quazepam was also thought to be affected via CYP3A4 induction;[11] however, potent inhibitors of CYP3A4 do not interact with quazepam, so this seems unlikely.

Hyperforin appears to be the main constituent that induces CYP3A4, because high-hyperforin extracts have more of an inducing effect than low-hyperforin extracts.[3,9]

Importance and management

A pharmacokinetic interaction between St John's wort and some benzodiazepines appears to be established. St John's wort can reduce **alprazolam** and **midazolam** exposure, and the moderate effect seen in a number of studies is likely to be clinically relevant. The variable findings reported in the studies (some found no interaction) could be due to the preparation of St John's wort used and the duration of treatment.[2,9] It appears that products with a low hyperforin content are unlikely to cause a clinically relevant interaction, but St John's wort products are not always standardised for this constituent. Therefore, it would seem prudent to monitor patients taking St John's wort and requiring alprazolam or oral midazolam for any signs of reduced efficacy. Single doses of *intravenous* midazolam do not appear to be affected to a clinically relevant extent. **Triazolam** is also a substrate of CYP3A4 and is likely to be affected in the same way as alprazolam and midazolam.

The reduction in exposure to the non-benzodiazepine hypnotic, **zolpidem**, is slight and would not be expected to lead to a reduction in its efficacy. Evidence for the non-benzodiazepine hypnotic, **zopiclone**, is lacking, but as it is metabolised by CYP3A4 the manufacturer suggests that the dose might need to be increased if St John's wort is also given.[13]

The slight reduction in quazepam exposure did not reduce its efficacy; and this interaction therefore does not appear to be clinically relevant. However, in light of the variability in the interaction with midazolam, which appears to be related to different St John's wort products, it might be prudent to bear the potential for an interaction in mind should a patient taking St John's wort have a reduced response to quazepam.

Note that midazolam is used as a probe substrate to assess the activity of other drugs on CYP3A4. The evidence here therefore suggests that St John's wort is a moderate inducer of CYP3A4 activity. For a list of CYP3A4 substrates, see 'Table 1.10', p.12.

1. Markowitz JS, Donovan JL, DeVane CL, Taylor RM, Ruan Y, Wang J-S, Chavin KD. Effect of St John's wort on drug metabolism by induction of cytochrome P450 3A4 enzyme. *JAMA* (2003) 290, 1500–4.
2. Markowitz JS, DeVane CL, Boulton DW, Carson SW, Nahas Z, Risch SC. Effect of St John's wort (*Hypericum perforatum*) on cytochrome P-450 2D6 and 3A4 activity in healthy volunteers. *Life Sci* (2000) 66, 133–9.
3. Arold G, Donath F, Maurer A, Diefenbach K, Bauer S, Henneicke-von Zepelin H-H, Friede M, Roots I. No relevant interaction with alprazolam, caffeine, tolbutamide, and digoxin by treatment with a low-hyperforin St John's wort extract. *Planta Med* (2005) 71, 331–7.
4. Wang Z, Gorski JC, Hamman MA, Huang S-M, Lesko LJ, Hall SD. The effects of St John's wort (*Hypericum perforatum*) on human cytochrome P450 activity. *Clin Pharmacol Ther* (2001) 70, 317–26.
5. Xie R, Tan LH, Polasek EC, Hong C, Teillol-Foo M, Gordi T, Sharma A, Nickens DJ, Arakawa T, Knuth DW, Antal EJ. CYP3A and P-glycoprotein activity induction with St. John's wort in healthy volunteers from 6 ethnic populations. *J Clin Pharmacol* (2005) 45, 352–6.
6. Dresser GK, Schwarz UI, Wilkinson GR, Kim RB. Coordinate induction of both cytochrome P4503A and MDR1 by St John's wort in healthy subjects. *Clin Pharmacol Ther* (2003) 73, 41–50.
7. Gurley BJ, Gardner SF, Hubbard MA, Williams DK, Gentry WB, Cui Y, Ang CYW. Cytochrome P450 phenotypic ratios for predicting herb-drug interactions in humans. *Clin Pharmacol Ther* (2002) 72, 276–87.
8. Imai H, Kotegawa T, Tsutsumi K, Morimoto T, Eshima N, Nakano S, Ohashi K. The recovery time-course of CYP3A after induction by St John's wort administration. *Br J Clin Pharmacol* (2008) 65, 701–7.
9. Mueller SC, Majcher-Peszynska J, Uehleke B, Klammt S, Mundkowski RG, Miekisch W, Sievers H, Bauer S, Frank B, Kundt G, Drewelow B. The extent of induction of CYP3A by St. John's wort varies among products and is linked to hyperforin dose. *Eur J Clin Pharmacol* (2006) 62, 29–36.
10. Mueller SC, Majcher-Peszynska J, Mundkowski RG, Uehleke B, Klammt S, Sievers H, Lehnfeld R, Frank B, Thurow K, Kundt G, Drewelow B. No clinically relevant CYP3A4 induction after St John's wort with low hyperforin content in healthy volunteers. *Eur J Clin Pharmacol* (2009) 65, 81–7.
11. Kawaguchi A, Ohmori M, Tsuruoka S, Nishiki K, Harada K, Miyamori I, Yano R, Nakamura T, Masada M, Fujimura A. Drug interaction between St John's wort and quazepam. *Br J Clin Pharmacol* (2004) 58, 403–10.
12. Hojo Y, Echizenya M, Ohkubo T, Shimizu T. Drug interaction between St John's wort and zolpidem in healthy subjects. *J Clin Pharm Ther* (2011) 36, 711–15.
13. Zimovane (Zopiclone). Sanofi-Aventis. UK Summary of product characteristics, August 2009.

Benzodiazepines + Statins

Atorvastatin, pitavastatin and simvastatin appear not to affect the pharmacokinetics of oral midazolam.

Clinical evidence

In a crossover study in 11 healthy subjects, the AUC of a single 15-micrograms/kg *oral* dose of **midazolam** taken on day 14 was increased by 15%, 4%, and 24% by **atorvastatin** 10 mg, **pitavastatin** 2 mg and **simvastatin** 10 mg daily for 14 days, respectively. **Midazolam** clearance was slightly reduced. However, none of these pharmacokinetic changes were statistically significant.[1]

In a study in 14 patients given *intravenous* **midazolam** 0.15 mg/kg during elective surgery, the plasma clearance of **midazolam** was found to be one-third lower and the AUC about 40% higher in 7 of the patients who were also taking long-term **atorvastatin** 10 to 40 mg daily.[2]

Mechanism

Midazolam is metabolised by CYP3A4, and is used as a probe drug for assessing the effect of other drugs on CYP3A4 activity. The limited evidence here shows that atorvastatin, pitavastatin and simvastatin have negligible effects on CYP3A4 activity.

The reason for the possible difference in intravenous midazolam pharmacokinetics seen in patients taking long-term atorvastatin is unclear. In a small between group comparison such as this, the effects seen might equally be explained by other confounding factors, and this is particularly likely as atorvastatin did not alter oral midazolam pharmacokinetics in the controlled study.

Importance and management

The findings from the controlled study show that the statins studied are unlikely to cause any clinically relevant changes in the pharmacokinetics of oral midazolam. No midazolam dose adjustment would therefore be expected to be needed in patients taking these statins. These statins would also not be expected to affect the pharmacokinetics of other benzodiazepines metabolised similarly, such as **triazolam** and possibly **alprazolam**. The effects of statins on other benzodiazepines do not appear to have been studied.

1. Kokudai M, Inui N, Takeuchi K, Sakaeda T, Kagawa Y, Watanabe H. Effects of statins on the pharmacokinetics of midazolam in healthy volunteers. *J Clin Pharmacol* (2009), 49, 568–73.
2. Mc Donnell CG, Harte S, O'Driscoll J, O'Loughlin C, Van Pelt FNAM, Shorten GD. The effects of concurrent atorvastatin therapy on the pharmacokinetics of intravenous midazolam. *Anaesthesia* (2003) 58, 899–904.

Benzodiazepines + Sucrose polyesters

Sucrose polyesters (e.g. *Olestra*) do not appear alter the pharmacokinetics of diazepam.

Clinical evidence, mechanism, importance and management

In a study in 8 healthy subjects, a single 5-mg dose of **diazepam** was given with 18 g of sucrose polyester (*Olestra*). Sucrose polyester had no effect on the pharmacokinetics of **diazepam**.[1] Sucrose polyesters are non-absorbable, non-calorific fat replacements. It has been concluded that sucrose polyesters are unlikely to reduce the absorption of oral drugs in general.[2] No diazepam dose adjustment would be required on the concurrent use of *Olestra*.

1. Roberts RJ, Leff RD. Influence of absorbable and nonabsorbable lipids and lipidlike substances on drug bioavailability. *Clin Pharmacol Ther* (1989) 45, 299–304.
2. Goldman P. Olestra: assessing its potential to interact with drugs in the gastrointestinal tract. *Clin Pharmacol Ther* (1997) 61, 613–18.

Benzodiazepines + Tadalafil

Tadalafil does not alter the pharmacokinetics of midazolam.

Clinical evidence, mechanism, importance and management

An open label study in 12 healthy subjects found that while taking tadalafil 10 mg daily for 14 consecutive days, the pharmacokinetics of a single 15-mg oral dose of **midazolam** were unchanged.[1] **Midazolam** is metabolised by CYP3A4, and it was therefore concluded that the absence of any interaction shows that tadalafil does not inhibit or induce the activity of this isoenzyme.[1] No **midazolam** dose adjustment is likely to be needed if it is given with tadalafil. This would also apply to other benzodiazepines metabolised similarly, such as **triazolam** and possibly **alprazolam**.

1. Ring BJ, Patterson BE, Mitchell MI, Vandenbranden M, Gillespie J, Bedding AW, Jewell H, Payne CD, Forgue ST, Eckstein J, Wrighton SA, Phillips DL. Effect of tadalafil on cytochrome P450 3A4-mediated clearance: studies in vitro and in vivo. *Clin Pharmacol Ther* (2005) 77, 63–75.

Benzodiazepines + Terbinafine

Terbinafine does not interact with midazolam or triazolam.

Clinical evidence, mechanism, importance and management

In studies in healthy subjects, terbinafine 250 mg daily for 4 days had no effect on the pharmacokinetics of a single 7.5-mg oral dose of **midazolam**[1] or a single 250-microgram oral dose of **triazolam**.[2] The performance of a number of psychomotor tests was unaffected by concurrent use. No midazolam or triazolam dose adjustment would seem to be necessary on the concurrent use of terbinafine. Other similarly metabolised benzodiazepines, such as **alprazolam**, are therefore also unlikely to be affected by terbinafine.

Note that midazolam is used as a probe substrate to assess the activity of other drugs on CYP3A4. This study therefore suggests that terbinafine has no effect on CYP3A4 activity.

1. Ahonen J, Olkkola KT, Neuvonen PJ. Effect of itraconazole and terbinafine on the pharmacokinetics and pharmacodynamics of midazolam in healthy volunteers. *Br J Clin Pharmacol* (1995) 40, 270–2.
2. Varhe A, Olkkola KT, Neuvonen PJ. Fluconazole, but not terbinafine, enhances the effects of triazolam by inhibiting its metabolism. *Br J Clin Pharmacol* (1996) 41, 319–23.

Benzodiazepines and related drugs + Theophylline

Aminophylline and theophylline appear to antagonise the effects of the benzodiazepines (mainly sedative effects, but possibly also anxiolytic effects). There is some evidence to suggest that theophylline might reduce the serum concentration of alprazolam.

Clinical evidence

In a comparative study, two groups of patients were given **alprazolam** 500 micrograms twice daily for 7 days. In one group there were 6 patients with COPD who were taking theophylline; and in the other group there were 7 patients with chronic heart failure or atherosclerotic disease (one patient also with COPD) who were not taking theophylline. On day 7, those taking the theophylline were found to have a minimum serum concentration of **alprazolam** of 13.25 nanograms/mL, whereas in the group not taking theophylline,the minimum serum concentration of **alprazolam** was 43.92 nanograms/mL.[1] Note that the groups were not randomised, or equivalent in terms of disease state, and other medications taken, so other factors might have had a part to play in this finding.

A patient who was unrousable and unresponsive having been given **diazepam** 60 mg over 10 minutes and nitrous oxide/oxygen anaesthesia, rapidly returned to consciousness when given aminophylline 56 mg intravenously.[2] Other reports confirm this antagonism of **diazepam**-induced sedation by low doses of aminophylline (60 mg to 4.5 mg/kg intravenously).[3-5] Further studies report that aminophylline and theophylline counteract the drowsiness and mental slowness induced by a single 10- to 20-mg dose of **diazepam**.[6-8] **Flunitrazepam**,[9] **lorazepam**,[10] and **midazolam**[11,12] also appear to be affected; however, there is some controversy about whether or not aminophylline antagonises the effects of **midazolam**.[13]

Mechanism

Uncertain. One suggestion is that the xanthines can block adenosine receptors,[3] which regulate the release of neurotransmitters, and might therefore lead to stimulant effects, which oppose the sedative effects of the benzodiazepines. Why theophylline might reduce alprazolam concentrations is unknown.

Importance and management

An interaction whereby theophylline and aminophylline antagonise the sedative effects of benzodiazepines appears to be established. However, the extent to which these xanthines actually reduce the anxiolytic effects of the benzodiazepines remains uncertain (it needs assessment), but be alert for reduced benzodiazepine effects if either xanthine is used. Such an effect has been seen with caffeine, see 'Benzodiazepines and related drugs + Caffeine', p.817.

It is unclear whether theophylline reduces alprazolam concentrations, and a controlled study is needed to assess this.

1. Tuncok Y, Akpinar O, Guven H, Akkoclu A. The effects of theophylline on serum alprazolam levels. *Int J Clin Pharmacol Ther* (1994) 32, 642–5.
2. Stirt JA. Aminophylline is a diazepam antagonist. *Anesth Analg* (1981) 60, 767–8.
3. Niemand D, Martinell S, Arvidsson S, Svedmyr N, Ekström-Jodal B. Aminophylline inhibition of diazepam sedation: is adenosine blockade of GABA-receptors the mechanism? *Lancet* (1984) i, 463–4.
4. Arvidsson SB, Ekström-Jodal B, Martinell SAG, Niemand D. Aminophylline antagonises diazepam sedation. *Lancet* (1982) 2, 1467.
5. Kleindienst G, Usinger P. Diazepam sedation is not antagonised completely by aminophylline. *Lancet* (1984) 1, 113.
6. Mattila MJ, Nuotto E. Caffeine and theophylline counteract diazepam effects in man. *Med Biol* (1983) 61, 337–43.
7. Henauer SA, Hollister LE, Gillespie HK, Moore F. Theophylline antagonizes diazepam-induced psychomotor impairment. *Eur J Clin Pharmacol* (1983) 25, 743–7.
8. Meyer BH, Weis OF, Müller FO. Antagonism of diazepam by aminophylline in healthy volunteers. *Anesth Analg* (1984) 63, 900–2.
9. Gürel A, Elevli M, Hamulu A. Aminophylline reversal of flunitrazepam sedation. *Anesth Analg* (1987) 66, 333–6.
10. Wangler MA, Kilpatrick DS. Aminophylline is an antagonist of lorazepam. *Anesth Analg* (1985) 64, 834–6.
11. Kanto J, Aaltonen L, Himberg J-J, Hovi-Viander M. Midazolam as an intravenous induction agent in the elderly: a clinical and pharmacokinetic study. *Anesth Analg* (1986) 65, 15–20.
12. Gallen JS. Aminophylline reversal of midazolam sedation. *Anesth Analg* (1989) 69, 268.
13. Sleigh JW. Failure of aminophylline to antagonize midazolam sedation. *Anesth Analg* (1986) 65, 540.

Benzodiazepines + Tibolone

Tibolone inhibited the metabolism of midazolam to a minor extent.

Clinical evidence, mechanism, importance and management

In a crossover study in 18 postmenopausal women given tibolone 2.5 mg daily for 7 days with a single 15-mg dose of **midazolam** on day 7, the metabolic ratio of **midazolam** to its 1-OH-metabolite was reduced by 30%.[1] The **midazolam** metabolite ratio is a measure of CYP3A4 activity. This study therefore indicates that tibolone has some CYP3A4 inhibitory activity. However, in order to accurately classify its inhibitory potential on CYP3A4, **midazolam** AUC or clearance data are needed, not just the metabolic ratio.

The reduction in **midazolam** metabolism seen is probably generally unlikely to be clinically important. Nevertheless, the UK manufacturer of tibolone states that drug interactions with CYP3A4 substrates might be expected, with the clinical relevance dependent on the substrate involved.[2] However, there appears to be no published information of any such interactions. If tibolone were to affect CYP3A4 to a clinically relevant extent, it is possible that **triazolam** and possibly **alprazolam** metabolism could be affected, but this also awaits confirmation.

1. Organon Laboratories Ltd. Personal communication, November 2009.
2. Livial (Tibolone). Organon Laboratories Ltd. UK Summary of product characteristics, March 2009.

Benzodiazepines and related drugs + Tobacco

Smoking might reduce the effects of some benzodiazepines or zolpidem.

Clinical evidence

Some studies have suggested that smoking tobacco does not affect the pharmacokinetics of **chlordiazepoxide**,[1] **clorazepate**,[2] **diazepam**,[3,4] **estazolam**,[5] **lorazepam**,[4] **midazolam**,[4] **quazepam**,[6] or **triazolam**,[7] but others have found that the clearance of **alprazolam**,[8] **clorazepate**,[9] **diazepam**,[10] **lorazepam**,[4,11] **oxazepam**,[12,13] or **zolpidem**[14] is higher in smokers, although not all the changes were statistically significant,[4,8,10-12,14] often due to the small numbers of smokers involved in the studies. The Boston Collaborative Drug Surveillance Program reported a decreased frequency of drowsiness in smokers who took **diazepam** or **chlordiazepoxide**,[15] which confirmed the findings of a previous study.[16] It has also been noted that two heavy smokers had a very high clearance and did not experience any sedative effects following the use of **zolpidem**.[17]

Mechanism

The probable reason for the reduction in sedative effects with these benzodiazepines and related drugs is that some of the components of tobacco smoke are enzyme inducers, which increase the rate at which the liver metabolises these drugs, thereby reducing their effects.

Importance and management

Evidence for an interaction between tobacco smoking and **benzodiazepines** is limited to often quite small studies. Nevertheless, the inference to be drawn is that smokers might need larger doses of these drugs than non-smokers to achieve the same therapeutic effects. Smoking also possibly reduces the drowsiness that the benzodiazepines and non-benzodiazepine hypnotics, such as **zolpidem**, can cause. However, one study suggested that caffeine intake,[16] and others have suggested age, might affect the response to benzodiazepines, so the picture is not altogether clear. Whether any of these interactions has much clinical relevance awaits assessment.

1. Desmond PV, Roberts RK, Wilkinson GR, Schenker S. No effect of smoking on metabolism of chlordiazepoxide. *N Engl J Med* (1979) 300, 199–200.
2. Ochs HR, Greenblatt DJ, Locniskar A, Weinbrenner J. Influence of propranolol coadministration or cigarette smoking on the kinetics of desmethyldiazepam following intravenous clorazepate. *Klin Wochenschr* (1986) 64, 1217–21.
3. Klotz U, Avant GR, Hoyumpa A, Schenker S, Wilkinson GR. The effects of age and liver disease on the disposition and elimination of diazepam in adult man. *J Clin Invest* (1975) 55, 347–59.
4. Ochs HR, Greenblatt DJ, Knüchel M. Kinetics of diazepam, midazolam, and lorazepam in cigarette smokers. *Chest* (1985) 87, 223–6.
5. Aoshima T, Fukasawa T, Otsuji Y, Okuyama N, Gerstenberg G, Miura M, Ohkubo T, Sugawara K, Otani K. Effects of the CYP2C19 genotype and cigarette smoking on the single oral dose pharmacokinetics and pharmacodynamics of estazolam. *Prog Neuropsychopharmacol Biol Psychiatry* (2003) 27, 535–8.
6. Fukasawa T, Yasui-Furukori N, Aoshima T, Suzuki A, Tateishi T, Otani K. Single oral dose pharmacokinetics of quazepam is influenced by CYP2C19 activity. *Ther Drug Monit* (2004) 26, 529–33.
7. Ochs HR, Greenblatt DJ, Burstein ES. Lack of influence of cigarette smoking on triazolam pharmacokinetics. *Br J Clin Pharmacol* (1987) 23, 759–63.
8. Smith RB, Gwilt PR, Wright CE. Single- and multiple-dose pharmacokinetics of oral alprazolam in healthy smoking and nonsmoking men. *Clin Pharm* (1983) 2, 139–43.
9. Norman TR, Fulton A, Burrows GD, Maguire KP. Pharmacokinetics of N-desmethyldiazepam after a single oral dose of clorazepate: the effect of smoking. *Eur J Clin Pharmacol* (1981) 21, 229–33.
10. Greenblatt DJ, Allen MD, Harmatz JS, Shader RI. Diazepam disposition determinants. *Clin Pharmacol Ther* (1980) 27, 301–12.
11. Greenblatt DJ, Allen MD, Locniskar A, Harmatz JS, Shader RI. Lorazepam kinetics in the elderly. *Clin Pharmacol Ther* (1979) 26, 103–13.
12. Greenblatt DJ, Divoll M, Harmatz JS, Shader RI. Oxazepam kinetics: effects of age and sex. *J Pharmacol Exp Ther* (1980) 215, 86–91.
13. Ochs HR, Greenblatt DJ, Otten H. Disposition of oxazepam in relation to age, sex, and cigarette smoking. *Klin Wochenschr* (1981) 59, 899–903.
14. Olubodun JO, Ochs HR, Trüten V, Klein A, von Moltke LL, Harmatz JS, Shader RI, Greenblatt DJ. Zolpidem pharmacokinetic properties in young females: influence of smoking and oral contraceptive use. *J Clin Pharmacol* (2002) 42, 1142–6.
15. Boston Collaborative Drug Surveillance Program. Clinical depression of the central nervous system due to diazepam and chlordiazepoxide in relation to cigarette smoking and age. *N Engl J Med* (1973) 288, 277–80.
16. Downing RW, Rickels K. Coffee consumption, cigarette smoking and reporting of drowsiness in anxious patients treated with benzodiazepines or placebo. *Acta Psychiatr Scand* (1981) 64, 398–408.
17. Harvengt C, Hulhoven R, Desager JP, Coupez JM, Guillet P, Fuseau E, Lambert D, Warrington SJ. Drug interactions investigated with zolpidem. In: Sauvanet JP, Langer SZ, Morselli PL, eds. Imidazopyridines in Sleep Disorders. New York: Raven Press, 1988: pp. 165–73.

Benzodiazepines + Tofisopam

Tofisopam moderately increases midazolam exposure, but has a negligible effect on alprazolam exposure.

Clinical evidence

In a study, 16 healthy subjects were given a single 7.5-mg oral dose of **midazolam**. After a one-week washout period, they were given tofisopam 100 mg three times daily for 9 days and on day 7 a single 7.5-mg dose of **midazolam** was given one hour after the morning dose of tofisopam. Tofisopam increased the maximum plasma concentration and AUC of **midazolam** by 90% and 2.4-fold, respectively, and its clearance was reduced by 59%. There was increased impairment in the digit symbols substitution test.[1]

In a crossover study in 15 healthy subjects, tofisopam 100 mg three times daily increased the AUC of a single 500-microgram dose of **alprazolam** by 18%, and caused a similar reduction in **alprazolam** clearance.[2]

Mechanism

The effect on midazolam pharmacokinetics suggests that tofisopam is a moderate inhibitor of CYP3A4, the isoenzyme by which midazolam and, to a lesser extent, alprazolam are metabolised.

Importance and management

The pharmacokinetic interaction with oral midazolam is likely to be clinically important. Patients taking tofisopam are likely to be more sensitive to the effects of oral midazolam and might require a reduced dose. Intravenous midazolam is not likely to be affected by tofisopam. **Triazolam** is also metabolised by CYP3A4, and would be expected to be affected in the same way as midazolam.

The pharmacokinetic interaction with alprazolam is negligible and not expected to be clinically relevant.

Note that midazolam is used as a probe substrate to assess the activity of other drugs on CYP3A4. This study therefore suggests that tofisopam is a moderate CYP3A4 inhibitor. For a list of CYP3A4 substrates, see 'Table 1.10', p.12.

1. Tóth M, Drabant S, Varga B, Végso G, Cseh A, Szentpéteri I, Klebovich I. Tofisopam inhibits the pharmacokinetics of CYP3A4 substrate midazolam. *Eur J Clin Pharmacol* (2008) 64, 93–4.
2. Drabant S, Tóth M, Bereczki A, Bajnógel J, Tömlö J, Klebovich I. Effect of tofisopam on the single-oral-dose pharmacokinetics and pharmacodynamics of the cyp3a4 probe drug alprazolam. *Eur J Clin Pharmacol* (2006) 62, 587–8.

Benzodiazepines + Tyrosine kinase inhibitors

Crizotinib moderately increases midazolam exposure, and lapatinib, pazopanib, and single-dose nilotinib slightly increase midazolam exposure. In contrast, erlotinib slightly decreases midazolam exposure. Regorafenib, sorafenib, and tofacitinib have no effect on midazolam exposure. Triazolam and, to a lesser extent, alprazolam, would be expected to be similarly affected by these tyrosine kinase inhibitors.

Clinical evidence

(a) Crizotinib

The UK and US manufacturers briefly note that, in a study in patients, crizotinib 250 mg twice daily for 28 days increased the AUC of oral midazolam 3.7-fold.[1,2]

(b) Erlotinib

The UK manufacturer briefly states that erlotinib did not alter the clearance of midazolam, but that the AUC of oral midazolam was reduced by 24%.[3]

(c) Lapatinib

In a study in 23 patients with cancer, lapatinib 1.5 g daily for 8 days increased the AUC of a single oral dose of midazolam by 45%, but did not affect the pharmacokinetics of intravenous midazolam.[4]

(d) Nilotinib

The UK and US manufacturers briefly note that, in a study in healthy subjects, a single dose of nilotinib increased the exposure to oral midazolam by 30%.[5,6]

(e) Pazopanib

In a pharmacokinetic study in patients with cancer, pazopanib 800 mg daily for 17 days increased the exposure to a single 3-mg oral dose of midazolam by about 30%.[7]

(f) Regorafenib

The US manufacturer briefly notes that, in a study in 15 patients with advanced solid tumours, regorafenib 160 mg daily for 14 days did not alter the exposure to a single 2-mg oral dose of midazolam.[8]

(g) Sorafenib

In a phase I/II pharmacokinetic study in 18 patients with advanced melanoma, sorafenib 400 mg twice daily for 28 days did not alter the pharmacokinetics of a single 2-mg oral dose of midazolam.[9]

(h) Tofacitinib

In a phase I pharmacokinetic study in 24 healthy subjects, tofacitinib 30 mg twice daily for 7 days did not alter the pharmacokinetics of a single 2-mg oral dose of midazolam.[10]

Mechanism

Crizotinib, lapatinib, nilotinib, and pazopanib inhibit CYP3A4 by which midazolam is principally metabolised, and hence they increase its exposure. Regorafenib and sorafenib[11] inhibit CYP3A4 *in vitro*, but *in vivo* they had no effect on midazolam exposure. *In vitro*[3] erlotinib inhibits CYP3A4 and therefore would be expected to increase the exposure to midazolam, but a decrease in midazolam exposure was reported; the mechanism behind this change is not known. Tofacitinib does not inhibit CYP3A4 *in vitro*, and this was confirmed *in vivo*.[10]

Importance and management

A pharmacokinetic interaction between crizotinib, lapatinib, nilotinib, and pazopanib, and midazolam is established, but the clinical importance varies.

Crizotinib

The moderate increase in midazolam exposure seen with crizotinib is likely to be clinically important and could result in increased midazolam effects. If concurrent use is necessary, closer monitoring (e.g. for increased and or prolonged sedation) would seem prudent and consideration given to reducing the dose of midazolam.

Note that midazolam can be used as a probe substrate to assess the activity of drugs on CYP3A4. This study therefore suggests that crizotinib is a moderate inhibitor of CYP3A4. The same advice would apply to other drugs that are also sensitive substrates of CYP3A4, see 'Table 1.10', p.12, for a list.

Lapatinib and Pazopanib

The slight increase in midazolam exposure seen with lapatinib and pazopanib is unlikely to be clinically important and no special precautions would seem necessary on concurrent use. Nevertheless, the UK manufacturer of lapatinib[12] and the US manufacturer of pazopanib,[13] do not recommend use with drugs that are substrates of CYP3A4 and that have a narrow therapeutic range. However, the US manufacturer of lapatinib simply advises caution with such drugs.[14]

Note that midazolam can be used as a probe substrate to assess the activity of drugs on CYP3A4. These studies therefore suggest that lapatinib and pazopanib are weak inhibitors of CYP3A4.

Nilotinib

The effect of nilotinib on midazolam exposure was only slight, however because inhibition of isoenzymes will not be maximal after a single dose, it cannot be ruled out that its effects would be greater when nilotinib is at steady state. Until more is known, some caution on concurrent use with midazolam would seem prudent, being alert for increased and/or prolonged sedation.

Note that midazolam can be used as a probe substrate to assess the activity of drugs on CYP3A4. This study therefore suggests that nilotinib is at least a weak inhibitor of CYP3A4. Until more is known, it might be prudent to be alert for adverse effects if nilotinib is given with drugs that are sensitive substrates of CYP3A4, see 'Table 1.10', p.12 for a list.

Erlotinib

The decrease in midazolam exposure with erlotinib was unexpected, and it seems possible that mechanisms other than CYP3A4 inhibition might be involved. However, as the decrease in exposure was only slight, it would not be expected to be clinically relevant, and therefore no special precautions are necessary on concurrent use.

Other tyrosine kinase inhibitors

No pharmacokinetic interaction occurs between **regorafenib**, **sorafenib**, or **tofacitinib** and midazolam and no special precautions are necessary on concurrent use.

Information for other tyrosine kinase inhibitors is lacking, but **cabozantinib**[15] has been shown to inhibit CYP3A4 *in vitro*, and so has the potential to affect midazolam exposure. Clinical study is required, but until more is known, it would seem prudent to monitor its concurrent use with midazolam, and other drugs metabolised by CYP3A4 (see 'Table 1.10', p.12 for a list). **Imatinib** is an inhibitor of CYP3A4, as shown by the fact that it increases simvastatin concentrations (see 'Statins + Tyrosine kinase inhibitors', p.1357). As its effects seem likely to be moderate, clinically relevant interactions with midazolam are possible. If concurrent use is necessary, closer monitoring (e.g. for increased and or prolonged sedation) would seem prudent and consideration given to reducing the dose of midazolam.

Other benzodiazepines

Evidence for an effect of these tyrosine kinase inhibitors on other benzodiazepines seems generally lacking. However, **triazolam** and, to some extent, **alprazolam**, are known to be metabolised by CYP3A4. Similar precautions to those recommended for midazolam would therefore seem warranted.

1. Xalkori (Crizotinib). Pfizer Inc. US Prescribing information, May 2013.
2. Xalkori (Crizotinib). Pfizer Ltd. UK Summary of product characteristics, April 2013.
3. Tarceva (Erlotinib hydrochloride). Roche Products Ltd. UK Summary of product characteristics, December 2013.
4. GlaxoSmithKline Clinical Trials Register. A four-way cross-over study to examine the effects of lapatinib on the pharmacokinetics of orally and intravenously administered midazolam in cancer patients. Available at: http://download.gsk-clinicalstudyregister.com/files/20663.pdf (accessed 22/10/15).
5. Tasigna (Nilotinib hydrochloride monohydrate). Novartis Pharmaceuticals Corp. US Prescribing information, January 2014.
6. Tasigna (Nilotinib hydrochloride monohydrate). Novartis Pharmaceuticals UK Ltd. UK Summary of product characteristics, December 2013.
7. Goh BC, Reddy NJ, Dandamudi UB, Laubscher KH, Peckham T, Hodge JP, Suttle AB, Arumugham T, Xu Y, Xu C-F, Lager J, Dar MM, Lewis LD. An evaluation of the drug interaction potential of pazopanib, an oral vascular endothelial growth factor receptor tyrosine kinase inhibitor, using a modified Cooperstown 5 +1 cocktail in patients with advanced solid tumours. *Clin Pharmacol Ther* (2010) 88, 652–9.
8. Stivarga (Regorafenib). Bayer HealthCare Pharmaceuticals Inc. US Prescribing information, August 2013.
9. Flaherty KT, Lathia C, Frye RF, Schuchter L, Redlinger M, Rosen M, O'Dwyer PJ. Interaction of sorafenib and cytochrome P450 isoenzymes in patients with advanced melanoma: a phase I/II pharmacokinetic interaction study. *Cancer Chemother Pharmacol* (2011) 68, 1111–8.
10. Gupta P, Alvey C, Wang R, Dowty ME, Fahmi OA, Walsky RL, Riese RJ, Krishnaswami S. Lack of effect of tofacitinib (CP-690,550) on the pharmacokinetics of the CYP3A4 substrate midazolam in healthy volunteers: confirmation of *in vitro* data. *Br J Clin Pharmacol* (2012) 74, 109–15.

11. Nexavar (Sorafenib tosylate). Bayer HealthCare Pharmaceuticals Inc. US Prescribing information, November 2013.
12. Tyverb (Lapatinib ditosylate monohydrate). GlaxoSmithKline UK. UK Summary of product characteristics, March 2014.
13. Votrient (Pazopanib hydrochloride). GlaxoSmithKline. US Prescribing information, November 2013.
14. Tykerb (Lapatinib ditosylate monohydrate). GlaxoSmithKline. US Prescribing information, October 2013.
15. Cometriq (Cabozantinib malate). Exelixis, Inc. US Prescribing information, November 2012

Benzodiazepines + Ursodeoxycholic acid (Ursodiol)

Ursodeoxycholic acid does not interact with midazolam.

Clinical evidence, mechanism, importance and management

A placebo-controlled, crossover study in 14 healthy subjects found that ursodeoxycholic acid 100 mg three times daily for 9 days did not affect the pharmacokinetics or the pharmacodynamics of single doses of intravenous **midazolam** 5 micrograms/kg or oral **midazolam** 15 micrograms/kg.[1] Another study also reported that ursodeoxycholic acid had no effect on the pharmacokinetics of a single 7.5-mg oral dose of **midazolam**.[2]

No midazolam dose adjustment would be expected to be necessary in patients also taking ursodeoxycholic acid. Other benzodiazepines do not appear to have been studied, but as **triazolam**, and possibly also **alprazolam**, are metabolised in a similar way to **midazolam**, they would also not be expected to interact with ursodeoxycholic acid.

Note that midazolam is used as a probe substrate to assess the activity of other drugs on CYP3A4. These studies therefore suggest that ursodeoxycholic acid has no effect on CYP3A4 activity.

1. Yan D, Yang Y, Uchida S, Misaka S, Luo J, Takeuchi K, Inui N, Yamada S, Ohashi K, Watanabe H. Effects of ursodeoxycholic acid on the pharmacokinetics and pharmacodynamics of intravenous and oral midazolam in healthy volunteers. *Naunyn Schmiedebergs Arch Pharmacol* (2008) 377, 629–36.
2. Becquemont L, Glaeser H, Drescher S, Hitzl M, Simon N, Murdter TE, Heinkele G, Hofmann U, Schaefer C, Burk O, Verstuyft C, Eichelbaum M, Fromm MF. Effects of ursodeoxycholic acid on P-glycoprotein and cytochrome P450 3A4-dependent pharmacokinetics in humans. *Clin Pharmacol Ther* (2006) 79, 449–60.

Benzodiazepines and related drugs + Valproate

Valproate increases lorazepam exposure, and possibly also increases diazepam concentrations, while clobazam appears to raise valproate concentrations. Clonazepam clearance might increase and valproate clearance might decrease during concurrent use, and increased adverse effects have been seen. An isolated case describes sleepwalking in a patient taking valproate and zolpidem.

Clinical evidence

A. Benzodiazepines

(a) Clobazam

In a study in patients with epilepsy, the plasma concentration of clobazam appeared lower in the presence of antiepileptics including sodium valproate than when patients were given monotherapy, but sodium valproate did not affect the concentration of the main metabolite of clobazam, *N*-desmethylclobazam.[1] A study in children found that clobazam caused an 11% increase in the serum concentration of valproate, despite a reduction of at least 10% in the valproate dose.[2]

(b) Clonazepam

The addition of clonazepam to sodium valproate increased the unwanted effects (drowsiness, absence status) in 9 out of 12 paediatric and adolescent patients.[3] An analysis of the interaction between clonazepam and valproate in 317 patients with epilepsy found that concurrent use increased clonazepam clearance by 14% and decreased valproate clearance by 18%.[4]

(c) Diazepam

In 6 healthy subjects sodium valproate increased the serum concentration of free diazepam 2-fold.[5] Valproate might slightly increase the sedative effects of diazepam.[6]

(d) Lorazepam

In healthy subjects, lorazepam 1 mg every 12 hours for 3 days had no effect on the pharmacokinetics of valproate semisodium 500 mg every 12 hours. Valproate semisodium increased the AUC and maximum plasma concentration of lorazepam by 20% and 8%, respectively. Sedation scores were slightly increased by concurrent use, although this was not statistically significant.[7]

The clearance of a 2-mg intravenous bolus dose of lorazepam was decreased by 40% in 6 out of 8 healthy subjects while they were taking valproate 250 mg twice daily.[8] Similarly, in another study, valproate decreased the mean systemic clearance of intravenous lorazepam by 20%, but interindividual variability occurred and clearance values were also affected by variations in uridine diphosphate glucuronyltransferase (UGT) genotype.[9] A further study by the same authors found that UGT polymorphism influenced the pharmacodynamic interaction between valproate and lorazepam in terms of increased sedation (as measured by psychomotor coordination tests), but had less effect on the pharmacokinetic interaction.[10]

A woman taking valproate, phenytoin, and carbamazepine went into a coma after she received a total of 6 mg of intravenous lorazepam. She promptly recovered on stopping the valproate.[11] Valproate might slightly increase the sedative effects of lorazepam.[7]

B. Non-benzodiazepine hypnotics

A report describes a patient taking **zolpidem** 5 mg at night and citalopram 30 mg daily, who started sleepwalking when valproate 250 mg twice daily was started. The patient stopped the valproate and the sleepwalking episodes resolved. Later, the valproate was restarted causing the sleepwalking to recur. This time the symptoms resolved when the **zolpidem** was stopped.[12]

Mechanism

It seems that valproate reduces the glucuronidation of lorazepam,[7,8] thereby decreasing its clearance and increasing its effects. The extent of the interaction appears to vary by UGT genetic polymorphism.[9,11] Other benzodiazepines that are mainly metabolised by glucuronide conjugation, such as **oxazepam** and **temazepam** might be expected to be similarly affected.

The interaction with diazepam is not understood. It was thought that valproate might displace diazepam from plasma binding sites.[5] However, this mechanism alone rarely results in clinically relevant interactions.

Importance and management

Evidence of an adverse interaction between valproate and **clonazepam** is sparse. Although potentially clinically significant effects (sedation, absence seizures) have been seen only rarely, it has been suggested that the combination should be avoided.[3] However, a very brief letter points out that clonazepam and valproate can be given together in patients with absence seizures and some patients have an excellent response to the combination.[13] Nevertheless, the potential hazard should be borne in mind when concurrent use is considered.

It has been recommended that if **clobazam** is given with valproate it would be prudent to monitor for any increase in the valproate serum concentration.[2]

The pharmacokinetic interaction of valproate with **lorazepam** is established, although the increased lorazepam exposure seen with valproate is negligible. However, the case report describing coma with intravenous lorazepam introduces a note of caution. The manufacturer of lorazepam advises that the dose of lorazepam should be reduced in patients taking valproate.[14]

Enhanced sedation has been briefly described during the concurrent use of valproate and **diazepam**[6] or some other unnamed benzodiazepines.[15] Be aware of this potential adverse effect when valproate is given with **any benzodiazepine**.

1. Bun H, Monjanel-Mouterde S, Noel F, Durand A, Cano J-P. Effects of age and antiepileptic drugs on plasma levels and kinetics of clobazam and N-desmethylclobazam. *Pharmacol Toxicol* (1990) 67, 136–40.
2. Theis JGW, Koren G, Daneman R, Sherwin AL, Menzano E, Cortez M, Hwang P. Interactions of clobazam with conventional antiepileptics in children. *J Child Neurol* (1997) 12, 208–13.
3. Jeavons PM, Clark JE, Maheshwari MC. Treatment of generalized epilepsies of childhood and adolescence with sodium valproate ('Epilim'). *Dev Med Child Neurol* (1977) 19, 9–25.
4. Yukawa E, Nonaka T, Yukawa M, Higuchi S, Kuroda T, Goto Y. Pharmacoepidemiologic investigation of a clonazepam-valproic acid interaction by mixed effect modeling using routine clinical pharmacokinetic data in Japanese patients. *J Clin Pharm Ther* (2003) 28, 497–504.
5. Dhillon S, Richens A. Valproic acid and diazepam interaction *in vivo*. *Br J Clin Pharmacol* (1982) 13, 553–60.
6. Diazepam Solution for Injection. Wockhardt UK Ltd. UK Summary of product characteristics, April 2008.
7. Samara EE, Granneman RG, Witt GF, Cavanaugh JH. Effect of valproate on the pharmacokinetics and pharmacodynamics of lorazepam. *J Clin Pharmacol* (1997) 37, 442–50.
8. Anderson GD, Gidal BE, Kantor ED, Wilensky AJ. Lorazepam-valproate interaction: studies in normal subjects and isolated perfused rat liver. *Epilepsia* (1994) 35, 221–5.
9. Chung J-Y, Cho J-Y, Yu K-S, Kim J-R, Jung H-R, Lim K-S, Jang I-J, Shin S-G. Effect of the *UGT2B15* genotype on the pharmacokinetics, pharmacodynamics, and drug interactions of intravenous lorazepam in healthy volunteers. *Clin Pharmacol Ther* (2005) 77, 486–94.
10. Chung J-Y, Cho J-Y, Yu K-S, Kim J-R, Lim KS, Sohn D-R, Shin S-G, Jang I-J. Pharmacokinetic and pharmacodynamic interaction of lorazepam and valproic acid in relation to *UGT2B7* genetic polymorphism in healthy subjects. *Clin Pharmacol Ther* (2008) 83, 595–600.
11. Lee S-A, Lee JK, Heo K. Coma probably induced by lorazepam–valproate interaction. *Seizure* (2002) 11, 124–5.
12. Sattar SP, Ramaswamy S, Bhatia SC, Petty F. Somnambulism due to probable interaction of valproic acid and zolpidem. *Ann Pharmacother* (2003) 37, 1429–33.
13. Browne TR. Interaction between clonazepam and sodium valproate. *N Engl J Med* (1979) 300, 679.
14. Ativan Injection (Lorazepam). Wyeth Pharmaceuticals. UK Summary of product characteristics, July 2010.
15. Völzke E, Doose H. Dipropylacetate (Dépakine®, Ergenyl®) in the treatment of epilepsy. *Epilepsia* (1973) 14, 185–93.

Benzodiazepines + Vinpocetine

Vinpocetine does not affect the pharmacokinetics of oxazepam. Vinpocetine did not appear to affect the ability to sleep, or the short-term memory impairment, induced by flunitrazepam.

Clinical evidence, mechanism, importance and management

In a study in 16 healthy subjects, vinpocetine 10 mg three times daily for 7 days did not affect the steady-state pharmacokinetics of **oxazepam** 10 mg three times daily.[1] No **oxazepam** dose adjustment is therefore likely to be necessary if vinpocetine is used concurrently.

A crossover study in 8 healthy subjects found that although vinpocetine 40 mg three times daily for 2 days improved short-term memory processes, it did not affect **flunitrazepam**-induced impairment of memory. **Flunitrazepam** either alone or in combination with vinpocetine appeared to improve patients' ability to sleep.[2]

1. Storm G, Oosterhuis B, Sollie FAE, Visscher HW, Sommer W, Beitinger H, Jonkman JHG. Lack of pharmacokinetic interaction between vinpocetine and oxazepam. *Br J Clin Pharmacol* (1994) 38, 143–6.
2. Bhatti JZ, Hindmarch I. Vinpocetine effects on cognitive impairments produced by flunitrazepam. *Int Clin Psychopharmacol* (1987) 2, 325–31.

Benzodiazepines; Diazepam + Misoprostol

Misoprostol does not alter the pharmacokinetics of diazepam.

Clinical evidence, mechanism, importance and management

A study in 12 subjects found that misoprostol 200 micrograms four times daily for 7 days had no effect on the steady-state plasma concentrations of diazepam 10 mg daily or on the plasma concentrations of the metabolite, nordazepam.[1] Similar results were found in another study.[2] No dose adjustments of diazepam would therefore seem to be necessary if misoprostol is also given.

1. Lima DR, Santos RM, Werneck E, Andrade GN. Effect of orally administered misoprostol and cimetidine on the steady state pharmacokinetics of diazepam and nordiazepam in human volunteers. *Eur J Drug Metab Pharmacokinet* (1991) 16, 161–70.
2. Nicholson PA, Karim A, Smith M. Pharmacokinetics of misoprostol in the elderly, in patients with renal failure and when coadministered with NSAID or antipyrine, propranolol or diazepam. *J Rheumatol* (1990) 17 (Suppl 20), 33–7.

Benzodiazepines; Lorazepam + Colestyramine and Neomycin

The clearance of lorazepam is increased by colestyramine with neomycin.

Clinical evidence

A study in 7 healthy subjects found that neomycin 1 g every 6 hours, given with colestyramine 4 g every 4 hours, reduced the half-life of oral lorazepam from 15.8 hours to 11.7 hours, and increased the clearance of free lorazepam by 34%.[1]

Mechanism

Lorazepam undergoes glucuronidation in the liver to the inactive lorazepam glucuronide which might be subject to enterohepatic recirculation. Neomycin and colestyramine might interfere with the enterohepatic circulation of lorazepam. An *in vitro* study found that 24% of lorazepam and 74% of lorazepam glucuronide were bound to colestyramine and it was suggested that the elimination of lorazepam is increased by clearance of the cycling glucuronide from the intestine before it can be acted on by glucuronidases which would release free lorazepam for further enterohepatic circulation.[2] The effects of neomycin are possibly due to inhibition of glucuronidase-containing intestinal microflora.

In the same *in vitro* study, **colestipol** was found to have a much smaller effect than colestyramine, binding only 11% and 21% of lorazepam and lorazepam glucuronide, respectively.[2]

Importance and management

Evidence for an interaction between colestyramine and lorazepam appears to be limited to this one study, which found only very small effects on lorazepam pharmacokinetics. The clinical importance of this interaction has not been assessed but it seems likely to be minor. Other benzodiazepines do not appear to have been studied.

1. Herman RJ, Duc Van Pham J, Szakacs CBN. Disposition of lorazepam in human beings: enterohepatic recirculation and first-pass effect. *Clin Pharmacol Ther* (1989) 46, 18–25.
2. Herman RJ, Chaudhary A. *In vitro* binding of lorazepam and lorazepam glucuronide to cholestyramine, colestipol, and activated charcoal. *Pharm Res* (1991) 8, 538–40.

Benzodiazepines; Midazolam + Brentuximab vedotin

Brentuximab vedotin does not appear to alter the pharmacokinetics of midazolam.

Clinical evidence, mechanism, importance and management

In a study, 15 patients with CD30-positive lymphomas received brentuximab vedotin 1.8 mg/kg intravenously on day 1 of two 21-day cycles in combination with intravenous midazolam 1 mg, given 3 days before and on day 3 of the first cycle. The AUC of midazolam was unaffected.[1] Midazolam is used as a probe substrate to assess the activity of drugs on CYP3A4. This therefore suggests that neither brentuximab vedotin nor its active component, monomethyl auristatin E (MMAE), is an inducer or inhibitor of CYP3A4.

1. Han TH, Gopal AK, Ramchandren R, Goy A, Chen R, Matous JV, Cooper M, Grove LE, Alley SC, Lynch CM, O'Connor OA. CYP3A-mediated drug-drug interaction potential and excretion of brentuximab vedotin, an antibody-drug conjugate, in patients with CD30-positive hematologic malignancies. *J Clin Pharmacol* (2013) 53, 866–77.

Buspirone + Azoles

Buspirone exposure is very markedly increased by itraconazole. Ketoconazole and voriconazole are likely to interact similarly, and posaconazole and fluconazole might also interact in this way, but to a lesser extent.

Clinical evidence

In a placebo-controlled study, 8 healthy subjects were given buspirone 10 mg, before and after taking **itraconazole** 100 mg twice daily for 4 days. It was found that the maximum plasma concentration and AUC of buspirone were increased 13-fold and 19-fold, respectively, by **itraconazole**. This increased buspirone exposure caused a moderate impairment of psychomotor performance (digital symbol substitution, body sway, drowsiness, etc.) and an increase in adverse effects.[1]

Mechanism

Itraconazole is a potent inhibitor of CYP3A4, by which buspirone is metabolised. Itraconazole therefore increases buspirone exposure and effects.

Importance and management

Direct information appears to be limited to this study but the interaction would seem to be established. The dose of buspirone should be greatly reduced if itraconazole is given concurrently. The manufacturers recommend 2.5 mg once daily, adjusted according to response[2] or 2.5 mg twice daily.[3] **Ketoconazole** is predicted to interact similarly because it is also a potent CYP3A4 inhibitor.[1,2] Of the other azoles, **voriconazole** is also a potent inhibitor of CYP3A4 and therefore would also be expected to interact similarly, whereas **posaconazole** and **fluconazole** are moderate CYP3A4 inhibitors, and would be expected to interact to a lesser extent, although caution is still needed. With these azoles, consider starting with a low dose of buspirone or, for those already taking buspirone, reducing the dose, and adjust according to response

1. Kivistö KT, Lamberg TS, Kantola T, Neuvonen PJ. Plasma buspirone concentrations are greatly increased by erythromycin and itraconazole. *Clin Pharmacol Ther* (1997) 62, 348–54.
2. BuSpar (Buspirone hydrochloride). Bristol-Myers Squibb Company. US Prescribing information, November 2010.
3. Buspirone hydrochloride. Actavis UK Ltd. UK Summary of product characteristics, January 2009.

Buspirone + Calcium-channel blockers

Diltiazem and verapamil can moderately to markedly increase buspirone exposure.

Clinical evidence

In a randomised study in 9 healthy subjects, **diltiazem** 60 mg three times daily for 5 doses increased the AUC of a single 10-mg dose of buspirone 5.5-fold and increased its maximum plasma level 4.1-fold. However, an increase in the pharmacodynamic effects of buspirone was seen only in the subjective overall drug effect, although adverse effects of buspirone were more common.[1]

When **verapamil** 80 mg three times daily was similarly given with buspirone, the AUC and maximum plasma level of buspirone were both increased 3.4-fold. However, an increase in the pharmacodynamic effects of buspirone was seen only in the subjective overall drug effect.[1]

Mechanism

The increased buspirone exposure is thought to occur because both diltiazem and verapamil moderately inhibit CYP3A4, by which buspirone is metabolised.

Importance and management

Evidence for an interaction between buspirone and diltiazem or verapamil appears to be limited to this one study, but an interaction is established. The practical consequences of this interaction are that the effects of buspirone are likely to be increased by **diltiazem** and **verapamil**. It would therefore seem prudent to reduce the buspirone dose, or start buspirone at a lower dose. The US manufacturer suggests adjusting the dose according to response,[2] while the UK manufacturer gives no specific advice for moderate CYP3A4 inhibitors such as these calcium-channel blockers.[3] Information about other calcium-channel blockers appears to be lacking, but they do not usually appear to interact by inhibiting CYP3A4 (see 'Calcium-channel blockers', p.1029), so would not be expected to increase buspirone exposure.

1. Lamberg TS, Kivistö KT, Neuvonen PJ. Effects of verapamil and diltiazem on the pharmacokinetics and pharmacodynamics of buspirone. *Clin Pharmacol Ther* (1998) 63, 640–5.
2. BuSpar (Buspirone hydrochloride). Bristol-Myers Squibb Company. US Prescribing information, November 2010.
3. Buspar (Buspirone hydrochloride). Bristol-Myers Pharmaceuticals. UK Summary of product characteristics, May 2008.

Buspirone + Disulfiram

Mania occurred in one patient taking disulfiram with buspirone.

Clinical evidence, mechanism, importance and management

An isolated report describes mania in an alcoholic patient taking buspirone 20 mg daily, possibly due to an interaction with disulfiram 400 mg daily;[1] however, buspirone on its own has also apparently caused mania.[2,3] Therefore an interaction is not established and no general recommendations can be made.

1. McIvor RJ, Sinanan K. Buspirone-induced mania. *Br J Psychiatry* (1991) 158, 136–7.
2. Price WA, Bielefeld M. Buspirone-induced mania. *J Clin Psychopharmacol* (1989) 9, 150–1.
3. McDaniel JS, Ninan PT, Magnuson JV. Possible induction of mania by buspirone. *Am J Psychiatry* (1990) 147, 125–6.

Buspirone + Grapefruit juice

Large amounts of grapefruit juice markedly increase buspirone exposure.

Clinical evidence

In a randomised, crossover study, 10 healthy subjects were given either double-strength grapefruit juice 200 mL or water 200 mL three times daily for 2 days. On the third day, a single 10-mg dose of buspirone was given with the grapefruit juice or water, and additional grapefruit juice or water ingested 30 and 90 minutes later. Grapefruit juice increased the peak plasma concentration and AUC of buspirone 4.3-fold and 9.2-fold, respectively. The time to the maximum concentration of buspirone was also increased, from 45 minutes to 3 hours. However, an increase in the pharmacodynamic effects of buspirone was seen only in the subjective overall drug effect.[1]

Mechanism

Grapefruit juice probably inhibited the metabolism of buspirone by CYP3A4 in the gut leading to increased absorption and exposure.

Clinical evidence

The pharmacokinetic interaction between grapefruit juice and buspirone is established, and likely to be clinically relevant if patients taking buspirone consume large amounts of grapefruit juice. The authors of this study recommended that the concurrent use of buspirone and grapefruit juice should be avoided.[1] However, the US manufacturer suggests that patients should avoid drinking large quantities of grapefruit juice,[2] whereas the UK manufacturer makes dose recommendations only for potent CYP3A4 inhibitors,[3] which would generally not include grapefruit juice. If a patient taking buspirone drinks usual strength grapefruit juice in small quantities, the interaction would not be expected to be as marked. However, be alert for the possibility of increased effects.

1. Lilja JJ, Kivistö KT, Backman JT, Lamberg TS, Neuvonen PJ. Grapefruit juice substantially increases plasma concentrations of buspirone. *Clin Pharmacol Ther* (1998) 64, 655–60.
2. BuSpar (Buspirone hydrochloride). Bristol-Myers Squibb Company. US Prescribing information, November 2010.
3. Buspirone hydrochloride. Actavis UK Ltd. UK Summary of product characteristics, January 2009.

Buspirone + HIV-protease inhibitors

Ritonavir, and possibly indinavir, are predicted to inhibit the metabolism of buspirone. This resulted in Parkinson-like symptoms in one case.

Clinical evidence, mechanism, importance and management

A 54-year-old man who had been taking high-dose buspirone (40 mg every morning and 30 mg every evening) developed Parkinson-like symptoms about 6 weeks after starting to take **ritonavir** 400 mg and **indinavir** 400 mg, both twice daily. The dose of buspirone was reduced to 15 mg three times daily, **ritonavir** and **indinavir** were discontinued, and **amprenavir** 1.2 g twice daily was started. The Parkinson-like symptoms were reduced after about one week and completely resolved after 2 weeks.[1]

Buspirone is metabolised by CYP3A4, and it is probable that **ritonavir** and **indinavir** inhibited the metabolism of buspirone by this isoenzyme, resulting in toxic concentrations.

This appears to be an isolated case report, but it is in line with the way buspirone is known to interact with other CYP3A4 inhibitors. The manufacturer of buspirone recommends that a lower dose of buspirone (e.g. 2.5 mg twice daily in the UK) should be used with potent inhibitors of CYP3A4,[2] which would include **ritonavir**. All HIV-protease inhibitors are potent inhibitors of CYP3A4. Therefore, if buspirone is given with any HIV-protease inhibitor, reduce the buspirone dose, and make subsequent adjustments according to response.

1. Clay PG, Adams MM. Pseudo-Parkinson disease secondary to ritonavir-buspirone interaction. *Ann Pharmacother* (2003) 37, 202–5.
2. Buspar (Buspirone hydrochloride). Bristol-Myers Pharmaceuticals. UK Summary of product characteristics, May 2008.

Buspirone + Macrolides

Buspirone exposure is markedly increased by erythromycin. Some of the other macrolides might interact similarly.

Clinical evidence

In a placebo-controlled study buspirone 10 mg was given to 8 healthy subjects before and after they took **erythromycin** 500 mg three times daily for 4 days. It was found that the maximum plasma concentration and AUC of buspirone were increased 5-fold and 6-fold, respectively, by **erythromycin**. The increased buspirone exposure caused an increased impairment of psychomotor performance (digital symbol substitution, body sway, drowsiness, etc.) and an increase in adverse effects.[1]

Mechanism

Erythromycin is a moderate inhibitor of CYP3A4, by which buspirone is metabolised. Erythromycin therefore increases buspirone exposure and hence its effects.

Importance and management

Direct information about an interaction between buspirone and the macrolides appears to be limited to this study with **erythromycin**, but the interaction would seem to be established. The dose of buspirone should be reduced if erythromycin is given concurrently. The US manufacturers suggest using a low dose of buspirone e.g. 2.5 mg twice daily, adjusted according to response.[2]

Clarithromycin and **telithromycin** are potent inhibitors of CYP3A4 and might therefore increase buspirone exposure to a greater extent than erythromycin. The dose of buspirone should be reduced to 2.5 mg twice daily with potent CYP3A4 inhibitors,[3] or even to 2.5 mg once daily.[2]

1. Kivistö KT, Lamberg TS, Kantola T, Neuvonen PJ. Plasma buspirone concentrations are greatly increased by erythromycin and itraconazole. *Clin Pharmacol Ther* (1997) 62, 348–54.
2. BuSpar (Buspirone hydrochloride). Bristol-Myers Squibb Company. US Prescribing information, November 2010.
3. Buspirone hydrochloride. Actavis UK Ltd. UK Summary of product characteristics, January 2009.

Buspirone + Miscellaneous

Cimetidine does not appear to interact with buspirone, and buspirone does not appear to interact with amitriptyline. Nefazodone very markedly increases buspirone exposure.

Clinical evidence, mechanism, importance and management

(a) Amitriptyline

In a study in healthy subjects, buspirone 15 mg every 8 hours, given with amitriptyline 25 mg every 8 hours for 10 days, had no effect on the steady-state plasma concentrations of amitriptyline or its metabolite, nortriptyline. No evidence of a pharmacodynamic interaction was seen.[1] There would seem to be no reason for avoiding concurrent use.

(b) Cimetidine

In 10 healthy subjects, cimetidine 1 g daily for 7 days had no effect on the AUC or maximum concentration of buspirone 15 mg three times daily. The performance of three psychomotor function tests remained unaltered.[2] No buspirone dose adjustment would appear to be necessary on the concurrent use of cimetidine.

(c) Nefazodone

Nefazodone 250 mg twice daily caused a 20-fold increase in the maximum plasma concentration of buspirone 2.5 or 5 mg twice daily and a very marked 50-fold increase in its AUC. Buspirone 5 mg twice daily raised the AUC of nefazodone by 23%, which is unlikely to be clinically relevant. The manufacturers of buspirone have recommended that a lower dose of buspirone e.g. 2.5 mg once daily[3] or twice daily[4] should be used if nefazodone is also given.

1. Gammans RE, Mayol RF, Labudde JA. Metabolism and disposition of buspirone. *Am J Med* (1986) 80 (Suppl 3B), 41–51.
2. Gammans RE, Pfeffer M, Westrick ML, Faulkner HC, Rehm KD, Goodson PJ. Lack of interaction between cimetidine and buspirone. *Pharmacotherapy* (1987) 7, 72–9.
3. BuSpar (Buspirone hydrochloride). Bristol-Myers Squibb Company. US Prescribing information, November 2010.
4. Buspirone hydrochloride. Actavis UK Ltd. UK Summary of product characteristics, January 2009.

Buspirone + Rifampicin (Rifampin) and other CYP3A4 inducers

Rifampicin can cause a very marked reduction in buspirone exposure.

Clinical evidence

In a randomised study, a single 30-mg dose of buspirone was given to 10 healthy subjects, before and after they took rifampicin 600 mg daily for 5 days. It was found that rifampicin reduced the AUC of buspirone by 93% and reduced its peak plasma concentration by 84%. The pharmacodynamic effects of buspirone were reduced accordingly (as measured by digit symbol substitution, critical flicker fusion, body sway and visual analogue scales for subjective drowsiness).[1]

Mechanism

Rifampicin induces CYP3A4 in the gut and liver. Buspirone is metabolised by this isoenzyme and therefore its metabolism and clearance are increased.

Importance and management

Direct information appears to be limited to this study, but this interaction would appear to be clinically important. If both drugs are used, the buspirone dose might need to be increased, although note that the extent of this interaction is so great that this might not be effective, and therefore it would be prudent to consider alternatives to buspirone, where possible.

The manufacturer predicts that other drugs that induce CYP3A4 (they name **dexamethasone** and the antiepileptics, **phenytoin**, **phenobarbital** and **carbamazepine**), might increase the rate of buspirone metabolism.[2] They state that if a patient has been titrated to a stable dose of buspirone, a dose adjustment might be necessary to avoid reduced anxiolytic activity with a potent inducer of CYP3A4. This advice seems prudent. It also seems prudent to apply this advice to **fosphenytoin**, a prodrug of phenytoin, and **primidone**, which is metabolised to phenobarbital. For a list of CYP3A4 inducers, see 'Table 1.9', p.11.

1. Lamberg TS, Kivistö KT, Neuvonen PJ. Concentrations and effects of buspirone are considerably reduced by rifampicin. *Br J Clin Pharmacol* (1998) 45, 381–5.
2. BuSpar (Buspirone hydrochloride). Bristol-Myers Squibb Company. US Prescribing information, November 2010.

Buspirone + SSRIs

Isolated reports describe symptoms of serotonin syndrome when buspirone was given with an SSRI, although in some cases there may have been other contributing factors. In addition, isolated cases of atypical dystonia, a reduction in buspirone efficacy, and seizure have been attributed to the use of fluoxetine with buspirone. Fluvoxamine increases buspirone exposure.

Clinical evidence

(a) Citalopram

An isolated report describes the development of possible serotonin syndrome and hyponatraemia, thought to be caused by an interaction between citalopram and buspirone, which had been taken in higher doses than prescribed.[1] The general importance of this interaction when conventional doses are used is unknown.

(b) Fluoxetine

Two reports describe serotonin syndrome in patients taking fluoxetine and buspirone. A 48-year-old man developed serotonin syndrome after his dose of clomipramine was increased to 250 mg daily and buspirone 5 mg three times daily and fluoxetine 20 mg daily were added to his treatment. As all three drugs can affect brain serotonin concentrations, buspirone was considered to be partially responsible.[2] In another report, a 37-year-old man who had been taking fluoxetine 20 mg daily for 9 months for an anxiety disorder was then also given buspirone in an attempt to improve response. The dose of buspirone was started at 5 mg twice daily and titrated to 20 mg then 30 mg twice daily. After reaching full dose, he developed mild symptoms of possible serotonin syndrome. Symptoms were most prominent 2 to 4 hours after the morning doses of buspirone and fluoxetine. Buspirone was discontinued and his symptoms resolved within 2 days.[3]

Another patient developed an atypical dystonic reaction. This 36-year-old woman taking buspirone 20 mg daily and desipramine 40 mg twice daily started taking fluoxetine 20 mg every other day, two days after gradually discontinuing desipramine. After 6 doses of fluoxetine she developed anxiety, insomnia, restlessness, feeling 'wired' and irritable, with involuntary clenching of her left hand and muscle spasms in her left forearm. All symptoms resolved gradually over 3 weeks after stopping both drugs. It was suggested that fluoxetine had increased buspirone concentrations resulting in buspirone adverse effects, although the patient had previously taken buspirone in doses of up to 40 mg daily without any adverse effects.[4]

Two case reports describe a possible reduction of the anxiolytic efficacy of buspirone. A 35-year-old man with a long history of depression, anxiety and panic started taking buspirone 60 mg daily. His anxiety abated, but because of worsening depression he was also given trazodone 200 mg daily for 3 weeks. This had little effect, so fluoxetine 20 mg daily was added. Within 48 hours his usual symptoms of anxiety had returned and persisted even when the dose of buspirone was raised to 80 mg daily. Stopping the buspirone did not increase his anxiety.[5] Another patient with obsessive-compulsive disorder taking fluoxetine experienced a marked worsening of his symptoms when buspirone 5 mg twice daily was added.[6]

An isolated case describes a grand mal seizure in a patient taking fluoxetine 80 mg daily which occurred 3 weeks after buspirone 30 mg daily was added. The drugs were stopped and an EEG showed no signs of epilepsy, so the seizure was attributed to a drug interaction.[7]

(c) Fluvoxamine

Possible serotonin syndrome developed in a 48-year-old man taking fluvoxamine and haloperidol after buspirone and valproate semisodium were also given. The symptoms subsided within 24 to 36 hours after discontinuation of these medications.[8]

A double-blind study in 9 healthy subjects found that after taking fluvoxamine (mean dose 127 mg daily, range 100 to 150 mg daily) for 3 weeks, the AUC of a single 30-mg dose of buspirone was increased almost 3-fold. Even so, the psychological responses to the buspirone were reduced.[9] In another study in 10 healthy subjects given a single 10-mg dose of buspirone after taking fluvoxamine 100 mg daily for 5 days, although the AUC of buspirone was similarly increased 2.4-fold, there was no increased impairment of psychomotor performance.[10]

(d) Paroxetine

A 52-year-old woman experienced symptoms of serotonin syndrome within a month of taking the combination of buspirone, paroxetine and papaverine. The symptoms rapidly decreased after paroxetine was withdrawn.[11]

(e) Sertraline

Symptoms of serotonin syndrome occurred in a patient 11 days after buspirone, sertraline and loxapine were started for recurrent major depression. Buspirone was discontinued and the main symptoms resolved over the next day, although facial dyskinesias remained until the other two drugs were stopped. The patient had previously received buspirone together with **citalopram** or another serotonergic drug without any adverse effects.[12]

Mechanism

Buspirone is a partial agonist of the serotonin $5\text{-}HT_{1A}$ receptor. Serotonin syndrome seems to develop unpredictably in some patients given two or more serotonergic drugs and therefore, it might develop in patients given buspirone with SSRIs. For more information on serotonin syndrome and its management, see 'Drugs that cause serotonin syndrome + Other drugs that cause serotonin syndrome', p.1471.

Buspirone also has antagonistic effects at central dopamine (D_2) autoreceptors and therefore has the potential to cause acute and chronic changes in dopamine-mediated neurological function (e.g. dystonia, pseudo-parkinsonism, akathisia and tardive dyskinesia). The authors of one report suggest that the concurrent use of drugs with serotonergic and antidopaminergic properties might have produced two different effects: serotonin syndrome due to both drugs and extrapyramidal adverse effects due to buspirone.[12]

Fluvoxamine is a weak inhibitor of CYP3A4, by which buspirone is extensively metabolised. Therefore, there might be a pharmacokinetic component to the interaction with this particular SSRI. The possibility of similar pharmacokinetic interactions between fluoxetine[3,7] and sertraline[12] and buspirone, resulting in increased buspirone concentrations has also been suggested, although evidence for such an interaction is lacking.

Importance and management

Buspirone can be given with SSRIs for the treatment of depression and obsessive-compulsive disorder. For example, reports describe the effective concurrent use of fluoxetine and buspirone in patients with treatment-resistant depression[13] and with obsessive-compulsive disorder.[14,15] On the basis of the evidence here, there would seem to be little reason for avoiding concurrent use of buspirone and an SSRI. However, bear the case reports of serotonin syndrome and other adverse effects (such as seizures, dystonia, and reduced buspirone efficacy) in mind if both buspirone and an SSRI are used.

The clinical relevance of the moderate increase in buspirone exposure with fluvoxamine is uncertain, but bear in mind the possibility that fluvoxamine might increase the risk of adverse effects with buspirone.

1. Spigset O, Adielsson G. Combined serotonin syndrome and hyponatraemia caused by a citalopram–buspirone interaction. *Int Clin Psychopharmacol* (1997) 12, 61–3.
2. Nijhawan PK, Katz G, Winter S. Psychiatric illness and the serotonin syndrome: an emerging adverse drug effect leading to intensive care unit admission. *Crit Care Med* (1996) 24, 1086–9.
3. Manos GH. Possible serotonin syndrome associated with buspirone added to fluoxetine. *Ann Pharmacother* (2000) 34, 871–4.
4. Metz A. Interaction between fluoxetine and buspirone. *Can J Psychiatry* (1990) 35, 722–3.
5. Bodkin JA, Teicher MH. Fluoxetine may antagonize the anxiolytic action of buspirone. *J Clin Psychopharmacol* (1989) 9, 150.
6. Tanquary J, Masand P. Paradoxical reaction to buspirone augmentation of fluoxetine. *J Clin Psychopharmacol* (1990) 10, 377.
7. Grady TA, Pigott TA, L'Heureux F, Murphy DL. Seizure associated with fluoxetine and adjuvant buspirone therapy. *J Clin Psychopharmacol* (1992) 12, 70–1.
8. Baetz M, Malcolm D. Serotonin syndrome from fluvoxamine and buspirone. *Can J Psychiatry* (1995) 40, 428–9.
9. Anderson IM, Deakin JFW, Miller HEJ. The effect of chronic fluvoxamine on hormonal and psychological responses to buspirone in normal volunteers. *Psychopharmacology (Berl)* (1996) 128, 74–82.
10. Lamberg TS, Kivistö KT, Laitila J, Mårtensson K, Neuvonen PJ. The effect of fluvoxamine on the pharmacokinetics and pharmacodynamics of buspirone. *Eur J Clin Pharmacol* (1998) 54, 761–6.
11. Jägestedt M, von Bahr C. Kombination av serotonerga läkemedel gav kraftiga biverkningar. *Lakartidningen* (2004) 101, 1618–19.
12. Bonin B, Vandel P, Vandel S, Sechter D, Bizouard P. Serotonin syndrome after sertraline, buspirone and loxapine? *Therapie* (1999) 54, 269–71.
13. Bakish D. Fluoxetine potentiation by buspirone: three case histories. *Can J Psychiatry* (1991) 36, 749–50.
14. Markovitz PJ, Stagno SJ, Calabrese JR. Buspirone augmentation of fluoxetine in obsessive-compulsive disorder. *Am J Psychiatry* (1990) 147, 798–800.
15. Jenike MA, Baer L, Buttolph L. Buspirone augmentation of fluoxetine in patients with obsessive compulsive disorder. *J Clin Psychiatry* (1991) 52, 13–14.

Buspirone + St John's wort (*Hypericum perforatum*)

Two patients taking buspirone developed marked CNS effects after starting to take herbal medicines including St John's wort.

Clinical evidence

A 27-year-old woman who had been taking buspirone 30 mg daily for over one month started to take St John's wort (*Hypericum 2000 Plus*, Herb Valley, Australia) three tablets daily. After 2 months she complained of nervousness, aggression, hyperactivity, insomnia, confusion and disorientation, which was attributed to serotonin syndrome. St John's wort was stopped, the buspirone dose was increased to 50 mg daily and her symptoms resolved over a week.[1] A 42-year-old woman who was taking fluoxetine 20 mg twice daily and buspirone 15 mg twice daily started to develop symptoms of anxiety, with episodes of over-sleeping and memory deficits. It was discovered that she had been self-medicating with St John's wort, **ginkgo biloba** and **melatonin**. She was asked to stop the non-prescribed medication and her symptoms resolved.[2]

Mechanism

The exact mechanism of these interactions are not clear, but it is possible that they were due to the additive effects of the buspirone and the herbal medicines, either through their effects on elevating mood or through excess effects on serotonin. Fluoxetine might have had a part to play in one of the cases (see 'SSRIs + St John's wort (*Hypericum perforatum*)', p.1496). Note that St John's wort, a moderate CYP3A4 inducer, might theoretically reduce the efficacy of buspirone, a CYP3A4 substrate, see 'Buspirone + Rifampicin (Rifampin) and other CYP3A4 inducers', p.845.

Importance and management

The clinical relevance of these cases describing an interaction between buspirone and St John's wort is unclear, but they highlight the importance of considering adverse effects from herbal medicines when they are used with conventional medicines. Bear in mind the possibility that St John's wort preparations might reduce buspirone efficacy.

1. Dannawi M. Possible serotonin syndrome after combination of buspirone and St John's wort. *J Psychopharmacol* (2002) 16, 401.
2. Spinella M, Eaton LA. Hypomania induced by herbal and pharmaceutical psychotropic medicines following mild traumatic brain injury. *Brain Inj* (2002) 16, 359–67.

Buspirone + Trazodone

The concurrent use of buspirone and trazodone can result in serotonin syndrome, and might affect hepatic transaminases.

Clinical evidence, mechanism, importance and management

(a) Effect on liver enzymes

The manufacturer notes that there is one report suggesting that the concurrent use of buspirone and trazodone might have caused 3- to 6-fold elevations of ALT in a few patients. However, in a further study to investigate this, no interactive effect on hepatic transaminases was identified.[1] Note that trazodone is, rarely, known to cause hepatocellular damage, sometimes severe, when given alone and it seems likely that routine precautions for this effect would be adequate to identify any interaction.

(b) Serotonin syndrome

A report describes serotonin syndrome in a patient receiving several drugs including buspirone and trazodone.[2] Mild serotonin syndrome occurred in another patient receiving **tandospirone** (which is structurally related to buspirone) and trazodone.[3] In addition, isolated cases of serotonin syndrome have occurred when buspirone was used with other serotonergic drugs, see 'Buspirone + SSRIs', p.846. Bear the possibility of this in mind if trazodone and buspirone are used concurrently. For more information on serotonin syndrome and its management, see 'Drugs that cause serotonin syndrome + Other drugs that cause serotonin syndrome', p.1471.

1. BuSpar (Buspirone hydrochloride). Bristol-Myers Squibb Company. US Prescribing information, November 2010.
2. Goldberg RJ, Huk M. Serotonin syndrome from trazodone and buspirone. *Psychosomatics* (1992) 33, 235–6.
3. Kaneda Y, Ohmori T, Okabe H. Possible mild serotonin syndrome related to co-prescription of tandospirone and trazodone. *Gen Hosp Psychiatry* (2001) 23, 98–101.

Clomethiazole + CYP3A4 inducers

Carbamazepine increases the clearance of clomethiazole. Other enzyme inducers are expected to interact similarly.

Clinical evidence, mechanism, importance and management

The manufacturers of clomethiazole note that the clearance of intravenous clomethiazole was increased by 30% by **carbamazepine**, resulting in a similar decrease in its plasma concentration. Although this interaction has not been studied with oral clomethiazole, the concurrent use of **carbamazepine** would be expected to result in decreased clomethiazole bioavailability. Higher doses of clomethiazole might therefore be needed in the presence of **carbamazepine** or other potent inducers of CYP3A4.[1] For a list of inducers of this isoenzyme see 'Table 1.9', p.11.

1. Heminevrin Capsules (Clomethiazole). AstraZeneca UK Ltd. UK Summary of product characteristics, August 2009.

Clomethiazole + Diazoxide

Intravenous clomethiazole and diazoxide, given to pregnant women in labour, can cause marked respiratory depression in their infants for up to 36 hours after birth.

Clinical evidence

An infusion of 0.8% clomethiazole, in a dose of 4 to 24 g, was given during labour to 21 pregnant women of 28 to 40 weeks gestation for eclampsia or pre-eclamptic toxaemia. Diazoxide 75 to 150 mg was also given intravenously to 14 of the women for hypertension. All 21 babies were born alive but 13 suffered hypotonia, hypoventilation or apnoea for 24 to 36 hours after birth. All of the neonates affected, apart from one, came from the group of mothers who had been given diazoxide. Three of them died of respiratory distress syndrome; one was only 28 weeks' gestation.[1]

Mechanism

Clomethiazole has some respiratory depressant effects, and is contraindicated in patients with respiratory deficiency, but it is not clear why, having passed across the placenta into the foetus, its effects should apparently be so markedly increased by diazoxide.

Importance and management

Although use of this drug combination in eclampsia is historical, the interaction is included on account of its severity. The author of the report says that the respiratory depression was managed successfully with intermittent positive pressure ventilation, provided that respiratory distress syndrome was not also present.[1] Although there are no data on oral use in adults, the UK manufacturer of clomethiazole states that the concurrent use of diazoxide should be avoided.[2]

1. Johnson RA. Adverse neonatal reaction to maternal administration of intravenous chlormethiazole and diazoxide. *BMJ* (1976) 1, 943.
2. Heminevrin Capsules (Clomethiazole). AstraZeneca UK Ltd. UK Summary of product characteristics, August 2009.

Clomethiazole + Furosemide

Clomethiazole and furosemide appear not to interact.

Clinical evidence, mechanism, importance and management

Ten female patients aged 66 to 90 years were given clomethiazole edisilate syrup 500 mg each evening and 250 mg each morning as a sedative, with furosemide 20 to 80 mg. No changes in the plasma concentrations or effects of clomethiazole or furosemide were detected, and no other adverse reactions were seen.[1] No particular precautions therefore seem necessary on concurrent use.

1. Reid J, Judge TG. Chlormethiazole night sedation in elderly subjects receiving other medications. *Practitioner* (1980) 224, 751–3.

Clomethiazole + H_2-receptor antagonists

Increased sedation appears to occur when clomethiazole is given with cimetidine. Ranitidine does not appear to affect the pharmacokinetics of clomethiazole.

Clinical evidence

(a) Cimetidine

In a study in 8 healthy subjects, cimetidine 1 g daily for one week reduced the clearance of a single 768-mg dose of clomethiazole by 31% and prolonged its elimination half-life from 2.33 hours to 3.63 hours. Furthermore, clomethiazole produced a sleep duration of 30 to 60 minutes, but this was prolonged in most subjects to at least 2 hours after cimetidine.[1]

(b) Ranitidine

In two studies, each in 7 healthy subjects, ranitidine 150 mg twice daily did not affect the pharmacokinetics of a single 768-mg dose of oral clomethiazole, or a single 192-mg dose of intravenous clomethiazole, given over 5 minutes.[2]

Mechanism

It was suggested that cimetidine inhibits the metabolism of clomethiazole and increases the bioavailability of the drug resulting in increased pharmacodynamic effects.[1]

Importance and management

The interaction between cimetidine and clomethiazole would appear to be established, but the clinical relevance of these relatively modest effects is probably small. Ranitidine does not appear to interact and might therefore provide a useful alternative to cimetidine in some patients if an interaction were to occur.

1. Shaw G, Bury RW, Mashford ML, Breen KJ, Desmond PV. Cimetidine impairs the elimination of chlormethiazole. *Eur J Clin Pharmacol* (1981) 21, 83–5.
2. Mashford ML, Harman PJ, Morphett BJ, Breen KJ, Desmond PV. Ranitidine does not affect chlormethiazole or indocyanine green disposition. *Clin Pharmacol Ther* (1983) 34, 231–3.

Clomethiazole + Propranolol

An isolated report describes marked bradycardia when an elderly woman taking propranolol started to take clomethiazole.

Clinical evidence, mechanism, importance and management

An 84-year-old woman taking propranolol 40 mg twice daily for hypertension underwent skin grafting. Her pulse was stable (54 to 64 bpm) until the thirteenth day after the operation when she took two oral doses of clomethiazole 192 mg, 9 hours apart. Three hours after taking the second dose, her heart rate fell to 43 bpm with a PR interval of 240 milliseconds, and by 5 hours after the dose her pulse rate was down to 36 bpm. Her pulse had risen to 70 bpm twelve hours after stopping both drugs, and had restabilised 2 days later at about 60 bpm with a PR interval of 200 milliseconds. At this time the propranolol was restarted, with haloperidol.[1] This interaction appears to be an isolated case and therefore probably of limited clinical relevance.

1. Adverse Drug Reactions Advisory Committee. Chlormethiazole/propranolol interaction? *Med J Aust* (1979) 2, 553.

Clozapine + Antihypertensives

Isolated cases describe hypotensive reactions in patients taking clozapine and enalapril, lisinopril or propranolol. Additive hypotensive effects are possible with clozapine and any antihypertensive drug.

Clinical evidence, mechanism, importance and management

A patient taking **enalapril** 5 mg twice daily fainted within an hour of being given an initial 25-mg dose of clozapine. Later he was stabilised without problems taking **enalapril** 2.5 mg twice daily and clozapine, initially 12.5 mg daily, later rising to 800 mg daily. Another patient taking **enalapril** 5 mg daily fainted within 5 hours of being given clozapine 25 mg. He needed resuscitation, but was later given clozapine in doses up to 600 mg daily.[1] The clozapine blood concentration of a 39-year-old man rose from 490 nanograms/mL to 966 nanograms/mL after the addition of **lisinopril** 5 mg daily. When the **lisinopril** dose was increased to 10 mg daily, the clozapine concentration further rose to 1092 nanograms/mL. The dose of clozapine was reduced, and **lisinopril** replaced by diltiazem, after which his concentration began to return to normal.[2]

Coma developed in a woman taking **propranolol** 40 mg daily 1.5 to 2 hours after she was given a single 150-mg dose of clozapine. She had stopped taking fluphenazine 24 hours earlier. The patient recovered, and was subsequently slowly titrated up to a daily clozapine dose of 100 mg in addition to the **propranolol**, without any problems. Although the authors state that an interaction between **propranolol** and clozapine was the likely cause of the coma, the effects of fluphenazine cannot be wholly ruled out.[3]

Clozapine has alpha-blocking effects and therefore may cause orthostatic hypotension. The manufacturers note that this is more likely in the presence of other antipsychotics and during initial titration with rapid dose increases. Because of the potential for additive effects they recommend caution when giving clozapine to patients taking any hypotensive drug.[4,5]

1. Aronowitz JS, Chakos MH, Safferman AZ, Lieberman JA. Syncope associated with the combination of clozapine and enalapril. *J Clin Psychopharmacol* (1994) 14, 429–30.
2. Abraham G, Grunberg B, Gratz S. Possible interaction of clozapine and lisinopril. *Am J Psychiatry* (2001) 158, 969.
3. Vetter PH, Proppe DG. Clozapine-induced coma. *J Nerv Ment Dis* (1992) 180, 58–9.
4. Clozaril (Clozapine). Novartis Pharmaceuticals UK Ltd. UK Summary of product characteristics, March 2012.
5. Clozaril (Clozapine). Novartis Pharmaceuticals Corporation. US Prescribing information, October 2011.

Clozapine + Antimuscarinics

The antimuscarinic effects of clozapine are additive with those of other antimuscarinic drugs, which has led to urinary retention, delirium and severe (sometimes fatal) bowel obstruction.

Clinical evidence, mechanism, importance and management

The manufacturers of clozapine warn that the antimuscarinic effects of some drugs (such as those used to control hypersalivation[1]) might be additive with those of clozapine, which might lead to adverse effects such as dry mouth and constipation.[2,3] Nine fatalities associated with clozapine-related constipation and bowel obstruction have been reported in a literature review (although the authors suggest that clozapine-induced serotonin antagonism might also contribute to this effect).[4] Similarly, an analysis of the French pharmacovigilance database for cases of ischaemic colitis and gastrointestinal necrosis involving antipsychotics between 1997 and 2007, found 38 cases, 37% of which were fatal. Seven of the 38 patients had taken clozapine, 3 of whom died, including one who had also taken another antimuscarinic (exact drug not stated).[5]

Other cases of this proposed interaction have been reported. In one, a patient developed severe urinary retention while taking clozapine with **meclozine**.[6]

Another case report describes possible antimuscarinic delirium in a man with a schizoaffective disorder taking **nortriptyline**, **perphenazine** and propranolol who was also given clozapine 150 mg daily. Some improvement was seen after 8 days, and over the next week the propranolol was gradually discontinued while the clozapine dose was raised to 225 mg daily. The patient then began to complain of extreme fatigue and slurred speech, and by day 17 was delirious and confused. His serum **nortriptyline** concentrations were found to have doubled (from 93 nanograms/mL to 185 nanograms/mL) from the time the clozapine was started. He recovered within 5 days of stopping all of the drugs, after which the clozapine was restarted.[7] The authors of the report interpreted the symptoms as an antimuscarinic delirium arising from the additive antimuscarinic effects of clozapine, **nortriptyline** and **perphenazine**, made worse by the increased concentrations of **nortriptyline**.[7] It is unclear why the **nortriptyline** concentrations rose, but the authors suggest that **nortriptyline** and clozapine possibly compete for metabolism by the same liver enzymes, resulting in a reduction in the clearance of the **nortriptyline**.[7] However, note that interactions by substrate competition are rarely clinically relevant.

Note that **pirenzepine**, which has antimuscarinic activity, has been used to control clozapine-associated hypersalivation. In one study in 29 patients, there were no notable changes in the serum concentrations of clozapine or its metabolite desmethylclozapine (although concentrations were increased in 3 patients) when **pirenzepine** was also taken, and the risk of additional adverse effects was reportedly low.[8]

'Table 18.1', p.752, and 'Table 18.2', p.754, give lists of drugs that have antimuscarinic activity.

1. Davydov L, Botts SR. Clozapine-induced hypersalivation. *Ann Pharmacother* (2000) 34, 662–5.
2. Clozaril (Clozapine). Novartis Pharmaceuticals UK Ltd. UK Summary of product characteristics, March 2012.
3. Clozaril (Clozapine). Novartis Pharmaceuticals Corporation. US Prescribing information, October 2011.
4. Hibbard KR, Propst A, Frank DE, Wyse J. Fatalities associated with clozapine-related constipation and bowel obstruction: a literature review and two case reports. *Psychosomatics* (2009) 50, 416–19.
5. Peyrière H, Roux C, Ferard C, Deleau N, Kreft-Jais C, Hillaire-Buys D, Boulenger J-P, Blayac J-P The French Network of the Pharmacovigilance Centers. Antipsychotic-induced ischaemic colitis and gastro-intestinal necrosis: a review of the French pharmacovigilance database. *Pharmacoepidemiol Drug Safety* (2009) 18, 948–55.
6. Cohen MAA, Alfonso CA, Mosquera M. Development of urinary retention during treatment with clozapine and meclizine. *Am J Psychiatry* (1994) 151, 619–20.
7. Smith T, Riskin J. Effect of clozapine on plasma nortriptyline concentration. *Pharmacopsychiatry* (1994) 27, 41–2.
8. Schneider B, Weigmann H, Hiemke C, Weber B, Fritze J. Reduction of clozapine-induced hypersalivation by pirenzepine is safe. *Pharmacopsychiatry* (2004) 37, 43–5.

Clozapine + Aripiprazole

An isolated case report describes neuroleptic malignant syndrome in a patient taking clozapine after aripiprazole was started. Another suspected, but unconfirmed, case has also been reported.

Clinical evidence, mechanism, importance and management

A 27-year-old man taking clozapine 300 mg daily developed neuroleptic malignant syndrome 12 days after aripiprazole 30 mg daily was added. The patient was moderately hyperthermic (38.5°C), with confusion and extrapyramidal rigidity, and his creatine phosphokinase concentration was markedly raised (22 560 units/L). Clozapine concentrations were not measured. Both antipsychotics were stopped and the patient was admitted to intensive care where he showed some improvement after 72 hours (creatinine phosphokinase concentration 1155 units/L). After 6 weeks the patient was discharged taking olanzapine 20 mg daily.[1]

In a review of the case notes of 26 patients taking clozapine and aripiprazole, one patient was suspected to have developed neuroleptic malignant syndrome, but this was not clinically confirmed.[2]

A possible explanation for the occurrence of neuroleptic malignant syndrome is that it results from the dopaminergic activity of aripiprazole and the *N*-desmethyl metabolite of clozapine (norclozapine),[1] but this requires further study. The use of aripiprazole and clozapine can be useful in some cases and so concurrent use need not be avoided; however, bear the case reports of neuroleptic malignant syndrome in mind.

1. Dassa D, Drai-Moog D, Samuelian JC. Neuroleptic malignant syndrome with the addition of aripiprazole to clozapine. *Prog Neuropsychopharmacol Biol Psychiatry* (2010) 34, 427–28.
2. Karunakaran K, Tungaraza TE, Harborne GC. Is clozapine-aripiprazole combination a useful regime in the management of treatment-resistant schizophrenia? *J Psychopharmacol* (2007) 21,453–6.

Clozapine + Azoles

Itraconazole and ketoconazole do not appear to affect the pharmacokinetics of clozapine.

Clinical evidence, mechanism, importance and management

A small double-blind study in 7 patients with schizophrenia taking clozapine found that giving **itraconazole** 200 mg daily for a week did not affect the serum concentrations of clozapine or norclozapine, its *N*-desmethyl metabolite, when compared with placebo.[1]

In a small study, 5 patients with schizophrenia were given a single 50-mg dose of clozapine before and after a 7-day course of **ketoconazole** 400 mg daily. **Ketoconazole** reduced the maximum concentration of clozapine by 46%, and reduced its AUC by 29% (although the latter result was not statistically significant). Ketoconazole also reduced the AUC of the N-oxide metabolite of clozapine by about 48%, and reduced the AUC of the desmethylclozapine metabolite by 33%, although there was high interindividual variability and only the change in the N-oxide AUC was statistically significant.[2]

The limited evidence here suggests that CYP3A4 is of only minor importance in clozapine metabolism because no clinically relevant interaction takes place between clozapine and **itraconazole** or **ketoconazole**, which are potent inhibitors of CYP3A4.[1,2] This suggests that no clozapine dose adjustment would usually be expected to be needed if these azoles or other inhibitors of CYP3A4 are given with clozapine.

1. Raaska K, Neuvonen PJ. Serum concentrations of clozapine and *N*-desmethylclozapine are unaffected by the potent CYP3A4 inhibitor itraconazole. *Eur J Clin Pharmacol* (1998) 54, 167–70.
2. Lane H-Y, Chiu C-C, Kazmi Y, Desai H, Lam YWF, Jann MW, Chang W-H. Lack of CYP3A4 inhibition by grapefruit juice and ketoconazole upon clozapine administration *in vivo*. *Drug Metabol Drug Interact* (2001) 18, 263–78.

Clozapine + Benzodiazepines

A handful of reports describe severe hypotension, respiratory depression, and respiratory arrest (fatal in one case) in patients taking benzodiazepines and clozapine. Dizziness and sedation are also increased.

Clinical evidence

A patient with schizophrenia did not respond to treatment with fluphenazine, **diazepam**, **clobazam**, and **lormetazepam** having taken these drugs for several weeks. The fluphenazine was stopped and clozapine started at a dose of 25 mg at noon and 100 mg at night. Toxic delirium and severe hypersalivation developed 3 hours later.

The patient collapsed (systolic blood pressure 50 mmHg, diastolic blood pressure unrecordable) and stopped breathing. Resuscitation was started, and the patient remained unconscious for 30 minutes. After a few drug-free days clozapine 12.5 mg was successfully re-introduced, and very slowly titrated upwards; a low benzodiazepine dose was also given.[1] Another patient taking clozapine died suddenly and unexpectedly during the night, apparently due to respiratory arrest, after being given three 2-mg intravenous doses of **lorazepam** the previous day.[2]

There are at least 6 other cases of severe hypotension, respiratory depression or loss of consciousness in patients taking clozapine and **flurazepam**, **lorazepam**, or **diazepam**,[1,3-5] as well as other cases of marked sedation, hypersalivation, ataxia and delirium in patients taking **lorazepam** and clozapine.[6,7] Two of these reports[1,3] are from the same group of workers and it is not clear whether they are about the same or different patients.

A retrospective review of prescriptions at a mental health hospital between 2001 and 2006, found that none of the 152 patients given a benzodiazepine and clozapine died as a result of concurrent use.[8]

Mechanism

Not understood. Clozapine on its own very occasionally causes respiratory arrest and hypotension.

Importance and management

Evidence for an interaction between benzodiazepines and clozapine appears to be limited to case reports. The authors of the first of these reports[1] note that the relative risk of a cardiovascular/respiratory reaction is only 2.1%. Another report[2] states that the death they reported is the only life-threatening event among 162 patients given clozapine and benzodiazepines between 1986 and 1991 so that the incidence of serious problems is quite low. Although this is backed up by the review of 152 patients,[8] it would still seem prudent for concurrent use to be very well monitored for any evidence of CNS depression because of the severity of the reaction, even if it is rare.

1. Grohmann R, Rüther E, Sassim N, Schmidt LG. Adverse effects of clozapine. *Psychopharmacology (Berl)* (1989) 99, S101–S104.
2. Klimke A, Klieser E. Sudden death after intravenous application of lorazepam in a patient treated with clozapine. *Am J Psychiatry* (1994) 151, 780.
3. Sassim N, Grohmann R. Adverse drug reactions with clozapine and simultaneous application of benzodiazepines. *Pharmacopsychiatry* (1988) 21, 306–7.
4. Friedman LJ, Tabb SE, Worthington JJ, Sanchez CJ, Sved M. Clozapine – a novel antipsychotic agent. *N Engl J Med* (1991) 325, 518–9.
5. Tupala E, Niskanen L, Tiihonen J. Transient syncope and ECG changes associated with the concurrent administration of clozapine and diazepam. *J Clin Psychiatry* (1999) 60, 619–20.
6. Cobb CD, Anderson CB, Seidel DR. Possible interaction between clozapine and lorazepam. *Am J Psychiatry* (1991) 148, 1606–7.
7. Jackson CW, Markowitz JS, Brewerton TD. Delirium associated with clozapine and benzodiazepine combinations. *Ann Clin Psychiatry* (1995) 7, 139–41.
8. Bitter R, Demler TL, Opler L. Safety evaluation of the concomitant use of clozapine and benzodiazepines: a retrospective, cross-sectional chart review. *J Psychiatr Pract* (2008) 14, 265–70.

Clozapine + Caffeine

Caffeine minimally increases clozapine exposure, but greater increases in clozapine concentrations and adverse effects have been reported in individual cases.

Clinical evidence

In a controlled study in 12 healthy subjects,[1] caffeine 400 mg to 1 g daily increased the AUC and decreased the clearance of a single 12.5-mg dose of clozapine by 19% and 14%, respectively. In a crossover study, 6 coffee-drinking patients taking clozapine were given decaffeinated or caffeine-containing instant coffee for 7 days. The minimum plasma concentrations of clozapine were just 26% higher while the patients were taking caffeine-containing coffee.[2] However, a greater interaction was reported in a previous study in 7 patients, which found that clozapine concentrations *decreased* by 47% when the subjects *avoided* caffeine for 5 days, and increased again when caffeine consumption was resumed.[3]

A patient taking clozapine for schizophrenia had an exacerbation of his psychotic symptoms, which was attributed to caffeinated coffee (5 to 10 cups daily). The problem resolved when the patient stopped drinking caffeine-containing beverages. He had previously not had any problems with caffeine while taking haloperidol 30 mg and procyclidine 30 mg daily.[4]

A 31-year-old woman taking clozapine 550 mg daily developed increased daytime sleepiness, sialorrhoea and withdrawn behaviour after taking caffeine (about 1.2 g daily as drinks and tablets). Her plasma clozapine concentrations fell from 1500 nanograms/mL to 630 nanograms/mL when her caffeine intake was stopped.[5]

A 66-year-old woman taking clozapine 300 mg daily developed supraventricular tachycardia (180 bpm) when she was given 500 mg of intravenous caffeine sodium benzoate to increase seizure length during an ECT session. Verapamil was needed to revert the arrhythmia. Before taking clozapine she had received caffeine sodium benzoate in doses of up to 1 g during ECT sessions without problems.[6]

Mechanism

Unknown. Both caffeine and clozapine are sensitive substrates of CYP1A2, but neither are known to be inhibitors of this isoenzyme. In the best designed study, the effects were negligible.

Importance and management

The pharmacokinetic interaction between caffeine and clozapine would appear to be established. Based on the data from one of the studies[3] the UK manufacturer of clozapine states that clozapine dose adjustments might be necessary if patients change their intake of caffeine-containing beverages.[7] However, the data from the controlled studies[1,2] suggests that the effect of caffeine on clozapine pharmacokinetics is negligible to slight at most, and is unlikely to be of clinical relevance in most patients, particularly if clozapine serum concentrations are established and well monitored, and caffeine intake remains fairly stable and moderate. Possible exceptions are if large doses of caffeine are given during ECT treatment or if for some other reason the caffeine intake suddenly markedly increases or decreases. Patients taking clozapine should probably avoid taking large doses of caffeine-containing herbal preparations.

1. Hägg S, Spigset O, Mjörndal T, Dahlqvist R. Effect of caffeine on clozapine pharmacokinetics in healthy volunteers. *Br J Clin Pharmacol* (2000) 49, 59–63.
2. Raaska K, Raitasuo V, Laitila J, Neuvonen PJ. Effect of caffeine-containing versus decaffeinated coffee on serum clozapine concentrations in hospitalised patients. *Basic Clin Pharmacol Toxicol* (2004) 94, 13–18.
3. Carrillo JA, Herraiz AG, Ramos SI, Benitez J. Effects of caffeine withdrawal from the diet on the metabolism of clozapine in schizophrenic patients. *J Clin Psychopharmacol* (1998) 18, 311–16.
4. Vainer JL, Chouinard G. Interaction between caffeine and clozapine. *J Clin Psychopharmacol* (1994) 14, 284–5.
5. Odom-White A, de Leon J. Clozapine levels and caffeine. *J Clin Psychiatry* (1996) 57, 175–6.
6. Beale MD, Pritchett JT, Kellner CH. Supraventricular tachycardia in a patient receiving ECT, clozapine, and caffeine. *Convuls Ther* (1994) 10, 228–31.
7. Clozaril (Clozapine). Novartis Pharmaceuticals UK Ltd. UK Summary of product characteristics, March 2012.

Clozapine + Carbamazepine and related drugs

Clozapine serum concentrations appear to be reduced by carbamazepine. An isolated case of fatal pancytopenia has been seen in a patient taking clozapine and carbamazepine, and neuroleptic malignant syndrome occurred in another. Switching from carbamazepine to oxcarbazepine increases clozapine concentrations, suggesting that oxcarbazepine interacts to a lesser extent than carbamazepine.

Clinical evidence

(a) Carbamazepine

A study by a therapeutic drug monitoring service for clozapine found that the concentration-to-dose ratio of 17 patients taking carbamazepine was 50% lower than that found in 124 other patients taking clozapine alone.[1] This suggests that clozapine concentrations are decreased by carbamazepine. The plasma clozapine concentration of 2 patients who had been taking clozapine 600 or 800 mg daily and carbamazepine 600 or 800 mg daily for several months were *increased* from 1.4 micromol/L to 2.4 micromol/L and from 1.5 micromol/L to 3 micromol/L, respectively, within 2 weeks of *stopping* the carbamazepine.[2]

A man with mania taking carbamazepine 1.2 g daily and lithium developed muscle rigidity, mild hyperpyrexia, tachycardia, sweating, and somnolence (diagnosed as neuroleptic malignant syndrome) 3 days after his lithium was stopped and clozapine 25 mg daily started. The symptoms immediately improved when the clozapine was stopped.[3]

A patient taking carbamazepine, lithium, benzatropine, and clonazepam developed fatal pancytopenia about 10 weeks after starting clozapine 400 mg daily.[4] A retrospective study of the records of other patients given clozapine and carbamazepine found a significant increase in granulopenia.[5] A previous report had not found this, due to a statistical error.[6]

(b) Oxcarbazepine

In a study in 6 patients taking clozapine and carbamazepine, the serum concentrations of clozapine were 47% lower while they were taking carbamazepine than 8 weeks after switching to oxcarbazepine.[7] Similarly, a case report describes 2 patients with schizophrenia taking clozapine whose treatment was changed from carbamazepine to oxcarbazepine. After 3 weeks their plasma clozapine concentrations had risen from 1.4 micromol/L to 1.7 micromol/L and from 1.5 micromol/L to 2.5 micromol/L, respectively.[8]

Mechanism

Not established, but it seems likely that carbamazepine (a recognised potent enzyme inducer) increases the metabolism of clozapine by the liver, thereby reducing its effects. It has been suggested that this is because carbamazepine induces the activity of CYP1A2 by which clozapine is principally metabolised.[1] However, carbamazepine is not an established inducer of this isoenzyme. The case of pancytopenia might have been due to the additive bone marrow depressant effects of clozapine and carbamazepine.

Oxcarbazepine appears to have less effect on clozapine concentrations than carbamazepine and is not known to affect CYP1A2.

Importance and management

Information on the interaction between clozapine and carbamazepine is limited, but the available data suggests that carbamazepine probably decreases clozapine concentrations to a clinically important extent: one small sub-group analysis appears to suggest that treatment with clozapine is less effective if antiepileptics (including carbamazepine) are also taken.[9] The manufacturers of clozapine advise that carbamazepine should not be given with clozapine, although this is because of the risk of bone marrow suppression,[10,11] consider also 'Clozapine + Drugs that cause bone marrow suppression', p.850. If both drugs are necessary, monitor clozapine efficacy and be alert for the need to increase the clozapine dose. Furthermore, it would seem essential to increase the frequency of monitoring associated with the use of clozapine (e.g. white cell counts). Limited evidence suggests that oxcarbazepine does not interact to the same extent as carbamazepine, and might also have a lower risk of bone marrow suppression.

1. Jerling M, Lindström L, Bondesson U, Bertilsson L. Fluvoxamine inhibition and carbamazepine induction of the metabolism of clozapine: evidence from a therapeutic drug monitoring service. *Ther Drug Monit* (1994) 16, 368–74.
2. Raitasuo V, Lehtovaara R, Huttunen MO. Carbamazepine and plasma levels of clozapine. *Am J Psychiatry* (1993) 150, 169.
3. Müller T, Becker T, Fritze J. Neuroleptic malignant syndrome after clozapine plus carbamazepine. *Lancet* (1988) 2, 1500.
4. Gerson SL, Lieberman JA, Friedenberg WR, Lee D, Marx JJ, Meltzer H. Polypharmacy in fatal clozapine-associated agranulocytosis. *Lancet* (1991) 338, 262–3.
5. Langbehm DR, Alexander B. Increased risk of side-effects in psychiatric patients treated with clozapine and carbamazepine: a reanalysis. *Pharmacopsychiatry* (2000) 33, 196.
6. Junghan U, Albers M, Woggon B. Increased risk of hematological side-effects in psychiatric patients treated with clozapine and carbamazepine? *Pharmacopsychiatry* (1993) 26, 262.
7. Tiihonen J, Vartiainen H, Hakola P. Carbamazepine-induced changes in plasma levels of neuroleptics. *Pharmacopsychiatry* (1995) 28, 26–8.
8. Raitasuo V, Lehtovaara R, Huttunen MO. Effect of switching carbamazepine to oxcarbazepine on the plasma levels of neuroleptics: a case report. *Psychopharmacology (Berl)* (1994) 116, 115–16.
9. Wilson WH. Do anticonvulsants hinder clozapine treatment? *Biol Psychiatry* (1995) 37, 132–3.
10. Clozaril (Clozapine). Novartis Pharmaceuticals UK Ltd. UK Summary of product characteristics, March 2012.
11. Clozaril (Clozapine). Novartis Pharmaceuticals Corporation. US Prescribing information, October 2011.

Clozapine + Drugs that cause bone marrow suppression

The concurrent use of clozapine with other drugs that are well-known to cause bone marrow suppression can increase the risk of this adverse effect. Low white cell counts have been seen in patients taking clozapine with co-trimoxazole, methazolamide, nitrofurantoin, olanzapine, or thiamazole.

Clinical evidence and mechanism

Clozapine can cause blood dyscrasias and potentially fatal agranulocytosis. A systematic review of MEDLINE reports in English or German of non-chemotherapy, drug-induced agranulocytosis published between January 1996 and December 2006, identified 11 drugs including clozapine where there were more than 10 reports of definite or probable drug-associated agranulocytosis. The other drugs were **benzylpenicillin** (long-term, high dose), **carbimazole**, **dapsone**, **dipyrone (metamizole)**, **procainamide**, **propylthiouracil**, **rituximab**, **sulfasalazine**, **thiamazole**, and **ticlopidine**.[1] A number of researchers have debated the inclusion or exclusion of drugs from this review and the strength of evidence used and have suggested additional drugs,[2-4] although the review's authors have further justified their methodology.[5]

There are several cases that confirm the clinical importance of this interaction. A woman was taking **thiamazole** for Graves' disease, at times with various different antipsychotics including haloperidol, flupentixol, zuclopenthixol and perphenazine for schizophrenia. Because of the severe extrapyramidal reactions and failure to control the schizophrenia, clozapine, increased over 5 days to 250 mg daily, was started instead. Within 5 days her white cell count had fallen to 2.2×10^9/L, which rose to 4×10^9/L, one month after both drugs were stopped. Later, after the **thiamazole** was stopped, she was given the same dose of clozapine without this adverse effect.[6]

A patient who had been taking clozapine 500 mg daily for 8 months developed granulocytopenia within 8 days of starting to take **nitrofurantoin** 200 mg daily.[7]

An 86-year-old woman taking clozapine developed neutropenia 2 weeks after **methazolamide** was added for glaucoma. Both drugs were stopped and her white cell count recovered. She later restarted clozapine without problem and so the toxic effect was attributed to the concurrent use of these two drugs.[8]

A 47-year-old woman who had been uneventfully taking clozapine for 5 years developed neutropenia 4 days after **co-trimoxazole** was started. **Co-trimoxazole** was stopped and the white cell counts returned to normal over the next 2 weeks.[9]

Three patients had a delay in their recovery from clozapine-induced agranulocytosis when they were given **olanzapine**, and it has been suggested that **olanzapine** should therefore be avoided until the patient's haematological status has normalised.[10]

Importance and management

The interaction between clozapine and other drugs that also cause bone suppression is established, and can result in serious adverse effects. For this reason, the manufacturers[11,12] contraindicate the concurrent use of clozapine with other drugs that are well-known to cause agranulocytosis: the UK manufacturer specifically names **chloramphenicol**, **cytotoxics**, **penicillamine**, pyrazolone analgesics (e.g. **phenylbutazone**), and **sulfonamides** (e.g. **co-trimoxazole**) as drugs that should not be given with clozapine.[11] Furthermore, because they cannot be stopped if an adverse reaction occurs, they contraindicate the use of **depot antipsychotics** that have myelosuppressive potential.[11]

1. Andersohn F, Konzen C, Garbe E. Systematic review: agranulocytosis induced by non-chemotherapy drugs. *Ann Intern Med* (2007) 146, 657–65.
2. Ben Salem C, Slim R, Hmouda H, Bouraoui K. Agranulocytosis induced by nonchemotherapy drugs. *Ann Intern Med* (2008) 148, 319.
3. Ibáñez L, Vidal X, Laporte J-R. Agranulocytosis induced by nonchemotherapy drugs. *Ann Intern Med* (2008) 148, 319–20.
4. Mossad SB. Agranulocytosis induced by nonchemotherapy drugs. *Ann Intern Med* (2008) 148, 320.
5. Andersohn F, Garbe E, Konzen C. Agranulocytosis induced by nonchemotherapy drugs. In response. *Ann Intern Med* (2008) 148, 320–1.
6. Rocco PL. Acute granulocytopenia in concomitant treatment of clozapine and methimazole. *Postgrad Med J* (1994) 70, 312–3.
7. Juul Povlsen U, Noring U, Fog R, Gerlach J. Tolerability and therapeutic effect of clozapine. *Acta Psychiatr Scand* (1985) 71, 176–85.
8. Burke WJ, Ranno AE. Neutropenia with clozapine and methazolamide. *J Clin Psychopharmacol* (1994) 14, 357–8.
9. Henderson DC, Borba CP. Trimethoprim-sulfamethoxazole and clozapine. *Psychiatr Serv* (2001) 52, 111–12.
10. Flynn SW, Altman S, MacEwan GW, Black LL, Greenidge LL, Honer WG. Prolongation of clozapine-induced granulocytopenia associated with olanzapine. *J Clin Psychopharmacol* (1997) 17, 494–5.
11. Clozaril (Clozapine). Novartis Pharmaceuticals UK Ltd. UK Summary of product characteristics, March 2012.
12. Clozaril (Clozapine). Novartis Pharmaceuticals Corporation. US Prescribing information, October 2011.

Clozapine + Grapefruit juice

Grapefruit juice does not affect the pharmacokinetics of clozapine.

Clinical evidence, mechanism, importance and management

In a study in 21 patients with schizophrenia, 250 mL of regular strength grapefruit juice (*Ocean Spray*) did not affect the pharmacokinetics of a single 50-mg dose of clozapine when given simultaneously, although there was wide interpatient variability in the findings.[1] In a sub-set of 5 patients, 500 mL of grapefruit juice daily for 7 days also had no effect on the pharmacokinetics of a single 50-mg dose of clozapine taken with the grapefruit juice on day 7.[1] Another study in 15 patients with schizophrenia found that 250 mL of regular strength grapefruit juice (*Ocean Spray*) twice daily for 14 days had no effect on the steady-state pharmacokinetics of clozapine or its metabolites, norclozapine (*N*-desmethylclozapine) and clozapine *N*-oxide.[2] Similarly, a study in 9 patients taking clozapine (doses unknown) found that 500 mL of grapefruit juice (*Minute Maid*) daily for 2 days did not alter the plasma concentrations of clozapine or its metabolite, norclozapine (*N*-desmethylclozapine).[3]

The authors of two of these reports suggest that CYP3A4, which is known to be inhibited by grapefruit juice, does not play a major role in the metabolism of clozapine.[1,2] Therefore grapefruit juice need not be restricted or avoided in patients taking clozapine.

1. Lane H-Y, Chiu C-C, Kazmi Y, Desai H, Lam YWF, Jan MW, Chang W-H. Lack of CYP3A4 inhibition by grapefruit juice and ketoconazole upon clozapine administration *in vivo*. *Drug Metabol Drug Interact* (2001) 18, 263–78.
2. Lane H-Y, Jann MW, Chang Y-C, Chiu C-C, Huang M-C, Lee S-H, Chang W-H. Repeated ingestion of grapefruit juice does not alter clozapine's steady-state plasma levels, effectiveness, and tolerability. *J Clin Psychiatry* (2001) 62, 812–17.
3. Vandel S, Netillard C, Perault MC, Bel AM. Plasma levels of clozapine and desmethylclozapine are unaffected by concomitant ingestion of grapefruit juice. *Eur J Clin Pharmacol* (2000) 56, 347–8.

Clozapine + H_2-receptor antagonists

A case report describes increased serum clozapine concentrations and toxicity, which occurred on the concurrent use of cimetidine. The same effect was not seen with ranitidine. Another case report describes the use of cimetidine to increase concentrations of clozapine to achieve therapeutic efficacy.

Clinical evidence

A man with chronic paranoid schizophrenia was taking atenolol and clozapine 900 mg daily. When **cimetidine** 400 mg twice daily was added for gastritis, his serum clozapine concentrations rose by almost 60% (from a range of 992 to 1 081 nanograms/mL, up to a range of 1 559 to 1 701 nanograms/mL), but this did not result in any adverse effects. However, within 3 days of increasing the dose of **cimetidine** to 400 mg three times daily, he developed evidence of clozapine toxicity (marked diaphoresis, dizziness, vomiting, weakness, orthostatic hypotension), which resolved over 5 days when the clozapine dose was lowered to 200 mg daily, and the **cimetidine** was stopped. The serum clozapine concentrations during this period were not reported. When **cimetidine** was replaced by **ranitidine** 150 mg twice daily his clozapine serum concentrations were not affected.[1]

Another patient with schizophrenia who was given clozapine, titrated to a target dose of 400 mg daily, had clozapine and norclozapine (*N*-desmethylclozapine) concentrations of 120 nanograms/mL and 38 nanograms/mL, respectively. The patient refused to take a higher clozapine dose. **Cimetidine** 300 mg twice daily was started, both to treat gastro-oesophageal reflux and to increase clozapine concentrations. After one month of concurrent use, his clozapine and norclozapine concentrations had increased to 278 nanograms/mL and 122 nanograms/mL, respectively. Clozapine and norclozapine concentrations further increased to 502 nanograms/mL and 176 nanograms/mL when the dose of **cimetidine** was increased to 1.5 g daily. The symptoms of schizophrenia improved, but he also experienced increased salivation.[2]

Mechanism

Cimetidine is a weak non-specific enzyme inhibitor, which has effects on CYP1A2, by which clozapine is principally metabolised. It was therefore suggested that cimetidine reduces the metabolism of clozapine by the liver so that it accumulates, causing toxicity. Ranitidine does not cause enzyme inhibition and therefore would not be expected to interact.

Importance and management

Information regarding an interaction between clozapine and cimetidine appears to be limited to these case reports, but it is consistent with the predicted mechanism. If cimetidine is given to a patient taking clozapine, it would seem prudent to monitor the outcome closely being alert for clozapine adverse effects, and consider monitoring clozapine concentrations. Ranitidine, which did not interact, might be a useful alternative to cimetidine in some patients.

1. Szymanski S, Lieberman JA, Picou D, Masiar S, Cooper T. A case report of cimetidine-induced clozapine toxicity. *J Clin Psychiatry* (1991) 52, 21–2.
2. Sandson NB, Cozza KL, Armstrong SC, Eckermann G, Fischer BA, Phillips B. Clozapine case series. *Psychosomatics* (2007) 48, 170–5.

Clozapine + Haloperidol

Two cases of apparent interactions between clozapine and haloperidol have been reported: one describing neuroleptic malignant syndrome and the other describing raised haloperidol concentrations.

Clinical evidence, mechanism, importance and management

A 68-year-old man taking clozapine 600 mg daily and venlafaxine, lorazepam, aspirin, vitamin E, and multivitamins, was given haloperidol 4 mg daily to control persistent paranoid delusions and hallucinations. After 27 days he was found collapsed and was lethargic, tachycardic, feverish, and delirious. Neuroleptic malignant syndrome was suspected so the antipsychotics were withheld, and the patient recovered over the following 7 days. Clozapine was later restarted without a recurrence of symptoms.[1]

A case of elevated haloperidol concentrations has been reported in a 40-year-old man who was given haloperidol intramuscular injections 50 mg every 4 weeks. He was also given clozapine in increasing doses from 50 to 250 mg daily. Over this time his haloperidol concentration increased from 12 nanograms/mL to 166 nanograms/mL, although it is not clear whether he had attained steady-state concentrations when the first measurement was reported.[2]

The limited evidence provided by these two cases suggests there might be an interaction between clozapine and haloperidol. Further study is needed before general recommendations can be made.

Note that haloperidol is associated with a dose-related prolongation in the QT interval; and clozapine might also cause QT prolongation. See 'Drugs that prolong the QT interval + Other drugs that prolong the QT interval', p.272, for further information on the concurrent use of two or more drugs that prolong the QT interval.

1. Garcia G, Ghani S, Poveda RA, Dansky BL. Neuroleptic malignant syndrome with antidepressant/antipsychotic drug combination. *Ann Pharmacother* (2001) 35, 784–5.
2. Allen SA. Effect of chlorpromazine and clozapine on plasma concentrations of haloperidol in a patient with schizophrenia. *J Clin Pharmacol* (2000) 40, 1296–7.

Clozapine + Hormonal contraceptives

Two case reports describe raised clozapine concentrations with associated adverse effects in patients who also took oral combined hormonal contraceptives containing ethinylestradiol.

Clinical evidence

A 47-year-old smoker with paranoid schizophrenia taking clozapine 550 mg daily had a good therapeutic response at this dose, but also reported drowsiness, weakness and dizziness. The patient was also taking an oral combined hormonal contraceptive containing **ethinylestradiol** 35 micrograms and **norethisterone** 500 micrograms. Clozapine plasma concentrations ranged from 736 to 792 nanograms/mL. After 2 months she stopped taking her contraceptive and noted that the adverse effects of clozapine resolved: her clozapine concentrations were found to range from 378 to 401 nanograms/mL. The patient did not stop smoking during this time.[1]

A second report describes a 33-year-old woman who had taken clozapine 500 mg daily for several months. Within one week of starting to take an oral combined hormonal contraceptive containing **ethinylestradiol**, she experienced marked drowsiness, anergy, dizziness, and orthostasis. Her blood concentration of clozapine had increased from 448 nanograms/mL to 1281 nanograms/mL. The contraceptive was stopped and after 3 days the clozapine concentration fell to 577 nanograms/mL. Several weeks later, the dose of clozapine was reduced to 200 mg daily, and she restarted the contraceptive: her clozapine concentration was 531 nanograms/mL.[2]

Mechanism

It was suggested that the hormonal contraceptive inhibited CYP1A2, CYP2C19 and CYP3A4 resulting in raised clozapine plasma concentrations.[1,2] Clozapine is principally metabolised by CYP1A2 and it is known that ethinylestradiol can inhibit this isoenzyme, resulting in raised drug concentrations (see 'Caffeine + Hormonal contraceptives or HRT', p.1424).

Importance and management

Evidence of an interaction between clozapine and ethinylestradiol-containing oral hormonal contraceptives is limited to these two case reports, but is consistent with the way that ethinylestradiol-containing combined hormonal contraceptives interact with other CYP1A2 substrates. The authors note that slower titration and smaller doses of clozapine might be needed in patients taking combined hormonal contraceptives.[1,2] This advice seems prudent. Bear in mind the possibility that **HRT** might interact similarly.

1. Gabbay V, O'Dowd MA, Mamamtavrishvili M, Asnis GM. Clozapine and oral contraceptives: a possible drug interaction. *J Clin Psychopharmacol* (2002) 22, 621–2.
2. Sandson NB, Cozza KL, Armstrong SC, Eckermann G, Fischer BA, Phillips B. Clozapine case series. *Psychosomatics* (2007) 48, 170–5.

Clozapine + Lamotrigine

Lamotrigine did not alter clozapine concentrations in one study. However, two case reports describe raised clozapine plasma concentrations after lamotrigine was started.

Clinical evidence, mechanism, importance and management

In a study in 11 patients stable taking clozapine in doses of 200 mg to 500 mg daily, the addition of lamotrigine 25 mg daily increased to 200 mg daily over 8 weeks caused no changes in clozapine concentrations a week 6 (100 mg daily) or week 10 (200 mg daily), when compared with baseline values. In addition, there was no change in the concentration of the norclozapine (*N*-desmethylclozapine) metabolite. Lamotrigine concentrations in these patients did not differ from those in two other groups of patients taking risperidone or olanzapine[1] However, two case reports describe raised clozapine concentrations on starting lamotrigine. A 35-year-old man, who had been taking clozapine for 3 years, became dizzy and sedated about one month after starting to take lamotrigine. His plasma clozapine concentration was found to have increased to 1020 micrograms/L. When the lamotrigine was stopped his concentration fell to 450 micrograms/L.[2] A 43-year-old patient with bipolar disorder, who had taken clozapine 300 to 400 mg daily for 4 years (with stable clozapine concentrations of between 400 and 500 nanograms/mL) was hospitalised and started taking lamotrigine titrated to 50 mg daily in steps of 25 mg/week and lorazepam. Treatment with clozapine was continued at 350 mg daily. Thirteen days after starting lamotrigine he complained of dizziness and a day later his temperature was 39.2°C and he became disorientated. The next day he developed a rash of the trunk and face attributed to lamotrigine, and his clozapine concentration was noted to be 2427 nanograms/mL. Norclozapine (*N*-desmethylclozapine) concentrations were also raised. Clozapine, lamotrigine, and lorazepam were stopped and his clozapine concentration gradually fell to 48 nanograms/mL at day 22. On day 28 he was given clozapine 100 mg daily and 2 days later his clozapine concentration was 119 nanograms/mL.[3]

The study in patients suggests that lamotrigine does not usually alter clozapine concentrations, although the two case reports do introduce an element of caution. Nevertheless, there appears to be no sound pharmacokinetic mechanism for this interaction (some suggestions have been made[2,3] but they are very speculative). Bear these cases in mind if there is any evidence of clozapine toxicity in a patient also taking lamotrigine.

1. Spina W, D'Arrigo C, Migliardi G, Santoro V, Muscatello MR, Micò U, D'Amico G, Perucca E. Effect of adjunctive lamotrigine treatment on the plasma concentrations of clozapine, risperidone and olanzapine in patients with schizophrenia or bipolar disorder. *Ther Drug Monit* (2006) 28, 599–602.
2. Kossen M, Selten JP, Kahn RS. Elevated clozapine plasma level with lamotrigine. *Am J Psychiatry* (2001) 158, 1930.
3. Egger C, Muehlbacher M, Grohmann R, Stuppaeck C. Clozapine intoxication in a patient with lamotrigine-induced rash. *Pharmacopsychiatry* (2010) 43, 35–6.

Clozapine + Macrolides

Limited evidence suggests that erythromycin does not alter the pharmacokinetics of clozapine; however, three case reports describe clozapine toxicity (e.g. seizures drowsiness, neutropenia) when the patients were given erythromycin.

Clinical evidence

A randomised, crossover study in 12 healthy subjects found that **erythromycin** 500 mg three times daily for 2 days started 9 hours before a single 12.5-mg dose of clozapine did not alter the pharmacokinetics of clozapine or its metabolites.[1] Note that this length of pre-treatment with erythromycin is unlikely to be long enough to maximally inhibit cytochrome P450 isoenzymes.

There are three reports of clozapine toxicity in patients given erythromycin. A man with schizophrenia taking clozapine 800 mg daily was given **erythromycin** 250 mg four times daily for a fever and sore throat caused by pharyngitis. After a week he had a single tonic-clonic seizure and his serum clozapine concentration was found to be 1300 micrograms/mL. Both drugs were stopped, and the clozapine restarted 2 days later, initially at only 400 mg daily, but then, after several weeks, the dose had increased to 800 mg daily, giving serum clozapine concentrations of 700 micrograms/mL.[2] Another man with schizophrenia taking clozapine 600 mg daily became drowsy, with slurred speech, incontinence, difficulty in walking and incoordination within 2 to 3 days of starting to take **erythromycin** 333 mg three times daily. His serum clozapine concentration was found to be 1150 micrograms/L and he had leucocytosis. He recovered when both drugs were stopped. When he later restarted treatment with the same clozapine dose, but without the **erythromycin**, his steady-state minimum clozapine serum concentration was 385 micrograms/L.[3] Another case also describes a reduced white cell count when **erythromycin** was added to established treatment with clozapine, but no clozapine concentrations were available.[4]

Mechanism

Uncertain. One suggestion is that erythromycin might have inhibited CYP3A4, leading to reduced clozapine clearance, and increased serum clozapine concentrations and toxicity.[2,3] However, this does not explain the apparent large increases in clozapine concentrations because clozapine is mainly metabolised by CYP1A2, which is not known to be affected by the macrolides. In addition, the known potent CYP3A4 inhibitors ketoconazole and itraconazole have been found not to affect the pharmacokinetics of clozapine, see 'Clozapine + Azoles', p.848.

Some reports suggest that clozapine concentrations might be increased by bacterial infections *per se*,[5,6] and therefore it is possible that the effects seen were independent of erythromycin use.

Importance and management

Information regarding an interaction between clozapine and the macrolides appears to be limited to an inconclusive study and the three case reports all involving erythromycin, and there is no clear mechanism for an interaction. Whatever the reason, cases of raised clozapine concentrations with erythromycin appear to be rare. Bear these case reports in mind if clozapine adverse effects (e.g. agitation, dizziness, sedation, hypersalivation) develop in patients also given erythromycin.

There does not appear to be any information regarding a possible interaction between clozapine and other macrolides.

Note that **clarithromycin**, **erythromycin**, and **telithromycin** have been said to be associated with QT prolongation, as has clozapine. See 'Drugs that prolong the QT interval + Other drugs that prolong the QT interval', p.272, for further information on the concurrent use of two or more drugs that prolong the QT interval.

1. Hägg S, Spigset O, Mjörndal T, Granberg K, Persbo-Lundqvist G, Dahlqvist R. Absence of interaction between erythromycin and a single dose of clozapine. *Eur J Clin Pharmacol* (1999) 55, 221–6.
2. Funderburg LG, Vertrees JE, True JE, Miller AL. Seizure following addition of erythromycin to clozapine treatment. *Am J Psychiatry* (1994) 151, 1840–1.
3. Cohen LG, Chesley S, Eugenio L, Flood JG, Fisch J, Goff DC. Erythromycin-induced clozapine toxic reaction. *Arch Intern Med* (1996) 156, 675–7.
4. Usiskin SI, Nicolson R, Lenane M, Rapoport JL. Retreatment with clozapine after erythromycin-induced neutropenia. *Am J Psychiatry* (2000) 157, 1021.
5. Raaska K, Raitasuo V, Arstila M, Neuvonen PJ. Bacterial pneumonia can increase serum concentration of clozapine. *Eur J Clin Pharmacol* (2002) 58, 321–2.
6. Jecel J, Michel TM, Gutknecht L, Schmidt D, Pfuhlmann B, Jabs BE. Toxic clozapine serum levels during acute urinary tract infection: a case report. *Eur J Clin Pharmacol* (2005) 60, 909–10.

Clozapine + Miscellaneous

There are isolated cases of apparent interactions between clozapine and ampicillin, buspirone, loperamide, modafinil, nicotinic acid, perazine, tryptophan or vitamin C. Influenza vaccine and venlafaxine do not appear to interact with clozapine. Cocaine concentrations might be increased by clozapine.

Clinical evidence, mechanism, importance and management

(a) Ampicillin

An isolated report describes a 17-year-old taking clozapine (12.5 mg increased to 50 mg three times daily) who was given ampicillin 500 mg four times daily, starting on day 15 of clozapine treatment. On the next day the patient became easily distracted, very drowsy and salivated excessively. These adverse reactions stopped when the ampicillin was replaced by doxycycline.[1] The general relevance of this isolated report is unknown.

(b) Buspirone

A man who had been taking clozapine for a year developed acute and potentially lethal gastrointestinal bleeding and marked hyperglycaemia about 5 weeks after starting buspirone, and one week after the buspirone dose was raised to 20 mg daily. No gut pathology (e.g. ulceration) was detected and there were no problems when he was subsequently given clozapine alone, so the reaction was attributed to the drug combination.[2] The general relevance of this isolated report is unknown.

(c) Cocaine

A single-dose study in 8 cocaine addicts found that clozapine caused a dose-dependent rise in the serum concentrations of a 2-mg/kg intranasal dose of cocaine. Cocaine concentrations rose by 6%, 49% and 67% after clozapine was given in doses of 12.5 mg, 25 mg or 50 mg, respectively. Subjective questioning revealed a reduction in the positive effects of cocaine. One subject also experienced a near-syncopal attack which required medical attention.[3] The general relevance of this study is unclear.

(d) Influenza vaccine

In an open-label study in 14 patients the metabolism of clozapine was not altered following a single intramuscular dose of influenza vaccine (*Influvac* 2001 to 2002 formula, Solvay).[4]

(e) Loperamide

A patient taking clozapine 500 mg daily died after taking loperamide 6 mg daily during an episode of food poisoning. The authors of the report attribute the death to toxic megacolon brought on by the additive effects of clozapine and loperamide on gut transit.[5] Toxic megacolon can sometimes occur with loperamide alone, especially in the presence of an infection, and clozapine can cause fatal bowel obstruction or paralytic ileus by virtue of its antimuscarinic effects. It would therefore seem prudent to bear the possibility of this adverse effect in mind on concurrent use.

(f) Mirtazapine

A study in 9 patients taking clozapine in doses ranging from 100 to 650 mg daily found no change in the pharmacokinetics of clozapine after the addition of mirtazapine 30 mg daily.[6] Therefore, no clozapine dose adjustment seems likely to be necessary on the concurrent use of mirtazapine.

(g) Modafinil

A 42-year-old man taking clozapine 450 mg daily was given modafinil, titrated up to 300 mg daily, to combat sedation. After about one month of concurrent use he developed dizziness and an unsteady gait, and his clozapine serum concentration was found to be 1 400 nanograms/mL. His clozapine concentration had been 761 nanograms/mL while taking clozapine 400 mg daily, and because the 50 mg clozapine dose increase was not thought large enough to almost double his clozapine concentration, an interaction with modafinil was suspected.[7] However, this is an isolated case and an interaction is not yet established. Further study is needed to confirm if a pharmacokinetic interaction occurs.

(h) Nicotinic acid, Tryptophan and Ascorbic acid (Vitamin C)

A man with schizophrenia taking tryptophan, lorazepam, vitamin C, benzatropine, and nicotinic acid developed a severe urticarial rash covering his face, neck and trunk 3 days after starting clozapine 150 mg daily. All of the drugs except lorazepam were stopped, and the rash subsided. It did not recur when clozapine was restarted, even at a dose of 600 mg daily, nor when small doses of benzatropine and fluphenazine were briefly added. The authors draw the inference that tryptophan, vitamin C and nicotinic acid might have been responsible for this alleged interaction with clozapine.[8] However, an interaction is not established.

(i) Perazine

A case report describes raised clozapine concentrations in a patient also taking perazine. After discontinuing olanzapine, clozapine was started and the dose increased to 250 mg on day 21, when the patient's perazine dose was 500 mg and her serum clozapine concentration was 827 mg/L (compared with about 400 mg/L on day 15). On day 27 her perazine dose was 300 mg and her clozapine dose was still 250 mg, but her clozapine concentration had risen to 1 234 mg/L. Perazine was gradually withdrawn and the clozapine concentrations fell. After discontinuation of perazine and further increases in the clozapine dose, the clozapine concentration stabilised. The authors attributed this effect to inhibition of CYP1A2 and CYP3A4 by perazine, but they also note that the clozapine might not have been at steady state on day 15, when the first clozapine concentration was taken.[9] An interaction is therefore not established.

(j) Ritonavir

As ritonavir is a potent inhibitor of CYP3A4 and, at higher doses, of CYP2D6, the UK manufacturer of ritonavir predicts that it will increase the plasma concentrations of clozapine, which might result in an increase in adverse effects including serious haematologic abnormalities.[10] Note that clozapine is principally metabolised by CYP1A2, but CYP3A4 and CYP2D6 do have a limited role in clozapine metabolism. The magnitude of any effect and therefore its clinical relevance is unclear. However, note that the UK manufacturer contraindicates concurrent use.[10]

(k) Venlafaxine

In 11 patients, venlafaxine in doses of up to 150 mg daily did not affect the pharmacokinetics of established clozapine treatment in doses of up to 950 mg daily.[11] Therefore, no clozapine dose adjustments appear to be necessary on concurrent use.

1. Csík V, Molnár J. Possible adverse interaction between clozapine and ampicillin in an adolescent with schizophrenia. *J Child Adolesc Psychopharmacol* (1994) 4, 123–8.
2. Good MI. Lethal interaction of clozapine and buspirone? *Am J Psychiatry* (1997) 154, 1472–3.
3. Farren CK, Hameedi FA, Rosen MA, Woods S, Jatlow P, Kosten TR. Significant interaction between clozapine and cocaine in cocaine addicts. *Drug Alcohol Depend* (2000) 59, 153–63.
4. Raaska K, Raitasuo V, Neuvonen PJ. Effect of influenza vaccination on serum clozapine and its main metabolite concentrations in patients with schizophrenia. *Eur J Clin Pharmacol* (2001) 57, 705–8.
5. Eronen M, Putkonen H, Hallikainen T, Vartiainen H. Lethal gastroenteritis associated with clozapine and loperamide. *Am J Psychiatry* (2003) 160, 2242–3.
6. Zoccali R, Muscatello MR, La Torre D, Malara G, Canale A, Crucitti D, D'Arrigo C, Spina E. Lack of a pharmacokinetic interaction between mirtazapine and the newer antipsychotics clozapine, risperidone and olanzapine in patients with chronic schizophrenia. *Pharmacol Res* (2003) 48, 411–14.
7. Dequardo JR. Modafinil-associated clozapine toxicity. *Am J Psychiatry* (2002) 159, 1243–4.
8. Goumeniouk AD, Ancill RJ, MacEwan GW, Koczapski AB. A case of drug-drug interaction involving clozapine. *Can J Psychiatry* (1991) 36, 234–5.
9. Schaller G, Jacobi A, Rotter A, Kornhuber J, Hillemacher T. Perazine elevates clozapine serum levels by inhibiting metabolism. *Prog Neuropsychopharmacol Biol Psychiatry* (2009) 33, 908–9.
10. Norvir Oral Solution (Ritonavir). AbbVie Ltd. UK Summary of product characteristics, September 2012.
11. Repo-Tiihonen E, Eloranta A, Hallikainen T, Tiihonen J. Effects of venlafaxine treatment on clozapine plasma levels in schizophrenic patients. *Neuropsychobiology* (2005) 51, 173–6.

Clozapine + Nefazodone

Nefazodone did not alter clozapine concentrations in one study, although an isolated case report describes raised clozapine concentrations after nefazodone was added. An isolated report describes a possible case of neutropenia occurring after nefazodone was added to clozapine, without any change in clozapine concentrations.

Clinical evidence

In a small study in 6 patients stable taking clozapine, the addition of nefazodone 100 mg twice daily for a week, then 200 mg twice daily for 2 weeks, had no effect on clozapine concentrations or the concentrations of the norclozapine metabolite.[1] However, a 40-year-old man, who had been successfully treated with risperidone and clozapine 425 to 475 mg daily, started taking nefazodone 200 mg daily, increasing to 300 mg daily, for the treatment of persistent depression. After one week on the higher dose he became dizzy and hypotensive and it was noted that his clozapine plasma concentration had risen from 133 nanograms/mL to 233 nanograms/mL.[2]

A possible case of neutropenia was attributed to the addition of nefazodone to sodium valproate and clozapine. The patient had been taking sodium valproate and clozapine for many months when nefazodone was started, in increasing doses up to 200 mg twice daily. Within one week her neutrophil count had dropped to 1.8×10^9/L, and remained low until the nefazodone was discontinued. The patient's clozapine concentration was reported to have remained stable during this time and the patient had not had any previous episodes of leucopenia during treatment with clozapine and valproate.[3]

Mechanism

Unknown. Nefazodone is a potent inhibitor of CYP3A4, but clozapine is principally metabolised by CYP1A2, so there is no known mechanism for a pharmacokinetic interaction.

The reason for the neutropenia is unknown because nefazodone is not associated with this effect.[3] In addition, although clozapine and valproate are both known to cause neutropenia, the neutropenia resolved on discontinuing nefazodone while continuing clozapine and valproate.

Importance and management

The study in patients and one case suggests that nefazodone does not usually alter clozapine concentrations, which suggests that the single case of raised clozapine concentrations is unlikely to be of general relevance. The case of neutropenia is also unexpected. As such, no general precautions can be advised.

1. Taylor D, Bodani M, Hubbeling A, Murray R. The effect of nefazodone on clozapine plasma concentrations. *Int Clin Psychopharmacol* (1999) 14, 185–7.
2. Khan AY, Preskorn SH. Increase in plasma levels of clozapine and norclozapine after administration of nefazodone. *J Clin Psychiatry* (2001) 62, 375–6.
3. Macdonald J, Rawlins S. Neutropenia due to nefazodone, interaction or coincidence? *Aust N Z J Psychiatry* (2000) 34, 1031–2.

Clozapine + Phenobarbital

Clozapine plasma concentrations appear to be reduced by phenobarbital.

Clinical evidence

A patient had a seizure 10 days after his dose of clozapine was titrated up to 300 mg twice daily. Phenobarbital 60 mg daily was given to prevent further seizures and after 4 months the dose of clozapine was tapered down to 400 mg daily. When phenobarbital was gradually withdrawn the patient experienced moderate sedation and drowsiness and the clozapine concentration was found to have increased by about 75%, when compared with the concentration found during the concurrent use of phenobarbital.[1] Similarly, the clozapine plasma concentrations in 7 patients taking clozapine and phenobarbital were 35% lower than those of 15 patients taking clozapine alone.[2]

Mechanism

Not established, but it seems likely that phenobarbital, a known CYP1A2 inducer, increases the metabolism of clozapine by the liver, thereby reducing its plasma concentrations and effects. A mixed model analysis, estimated that the size of this effect is a 28% reduction in plasma clozapine concentrations.[3]

Importance and management

Evidence for an interaction between clozapine and phenobarbital is limited, but it appears to be clinically important: one sub-group analysis appears to suggest that treatment with clozapine is less effective if antiepileptics (including phenobarbital) are also taken.[4] Monitor clozapine efficacy and be alert for the need to increase the clozapine dose if phenobarbital is started. **Primidone** is metabolised in the body to phenobarbital and would therefore be expected to interact similarly.

1. Lane H-Y, Su K-P, Chang W-H, Jann MW. Elevated plasma clozapine concentrations after phenobarbital discontinuation. *J Clin Psychiatry* (1998) 59, 131–3.
2. Facciolà G, Avenoso A, Spina E, Perucca E. Inducing effect of phenobarbital on clozapine metabolism in patients with chronic schizophrenia. *Ther Drug Monit* (1998) 20, 628–30.
3. Diaz FJ, Santoro V, Spina E, Cogollo M, Rivera TE, Botts S, de Leon J. Estimating the size of the effects of co-medications on plasma clozapine concentrations using a model that controls for clozapine doses and confounding variables. *Pharmacopsychiatry* (2008) 41, 81–91.
4. Wilson WH. Do anticonvulsants hinder clozapine treatment? *Biol Psychiatry* (1995) 37, 132–3.

Clozapine + Phenytoin

Clozapine serum concentrations are possibly reduced by phenytoin. An isolated case report describes phenytoin toxicity on starting phenytoin in a patient taking clozapine.

Clinical evidence

Two patients taking clozapine had reduced clozapine concentrations (falls of 65 to 85%) and worsening psychoses when phenytoin was also given.[1] Another patient developed neutropenia, which was attributed to the concurrent use of phenytoin 400 mg daily and clozapine 900 mg daily. Both phenytoin and clozapine were stopped, and clozapine was eventually restarted. Clozapine concentrations at the high dose of 900 mg daily while taking phenytoin were 114 nanograms/mL compared with 137 nanograms/mL while taking 300 mg daily without phenytoin.[2]

A case of phenytoin toxicity has been described in a 40-year-old woman taking clozapine 275 mg daily with desipramine, trihexyphenidyl, oxazepam, and propranolol, who was given phenytoin to treat generalised tonic-clonic seizures. The patient experienced dizziness, nystagmus and gait ataxia about 24 hours after starting phenytoin (a 1 g intravenous loading dose of phenytoin, followed a day later by an oral maintenance dose of 300 mg). Her phenytoin serum minimum concentration was 23.8 micrograms/mL and the phenytoin was stopped. Clozapine was stopped for one day and then restarted at a lower dose of 50 mg daily. Two days later the phenytoin concentration was 15.9 micrograms/mL.[3]

Mechanism

Not established. It seems likely that phenytoin, a known potent enzyme inducer, increased the metabolism of clozapine, thereby reducing its plasma concentrations and effects. It has been suggested that this is due to induction of CYP1A2. In the phenytoin toxicity case, it was suggested that clozapine raised phenytoin concentrations by inhibiting CYP2C9, the principal isoenzyme involved in the metabolism of phenytoin.[3] However, note that clozapine is not considered to be an inhibitor of CYP2C9, and the case described might have had nothing to do with the use of clozapine.

Importance and management

Evidence for an interaction between clozapine and phenytoin is limited. The effect of phenytoin on clozapine concentrations appears to be clinically important: one sub-group analysis appears to suggest that treatment with clozapine is less effective if antiepileptics (including phenytoin) are also taken.[4] Monitor clozapine efficacy and be alert for the need to increase the clozapine dose if phenytoin is also given. From the case report of phenytoin toxicity, it is not possible to say whether the effect was anything to do with the use of clozapine, and its general relevance is therefore unclear, but an interaction resulting in raised phenytoin concentrations would seem unlikely.

1. Miller DD. Effect of phenytoin on plasma clozapine concentrations in two patients. *J Clin Psychiatry* (1991) 52, 23–5.
2. Shad MU. A complex interaction between clozapine and phenytoin. *J Pharm Technol* (2004) 20, 280–2.
3. Gandelman-Marton R, Theitler J, Klein C, Rabey JM. Phenytoin intoxication in a clozapine-related prolonged seizure. *J Emerg Med* (2008) 35, 407–9.
4. Wilson WH. Do anticonvulsants hinder clozapine treatment? *Biol Psychiatry* (1995) 37, 132–3.

Clozapine + Proton pump inhibitors

Omeprazole possibly reduces the serum concentrations of clozapine.

Clinical evidence

A retrospective study identified 13 patients taking clozapine and **omeprazole** in whom the proton pump inhibitor was subsequently changed to **pantoprazole**. This resulted in an increase in the serum concentration of clozapine from 445 nanograms/mL to 579 nanograms/mL in 3 non-smokers, but in the 10 smokers there was a slight *reduction* in the concentration of clozapine, from 364 nanograms/mL to 323 nanograms/mL.[1]

A case report describes two patients (both smokers) whose clozapine concentrations were reduced from 762 to 443 nanograms/mL and from 369 to 204 nanograms/mL, respectively, after **omeprazole** was started. However, no changes in clinical condition were noted.[2]

Mechanism

Smoking is known to induce CYP1A2, which is the major isoenzyme involved in the metabolism of clozapine. Omeprazole is possibly also a weak inducer of CYP1A2, although this is not usually considered clinically relevant (see 'Theophylline + Proton pump inhibitors', p.1454). The authors suggest that when omeprazole was stopped in the non-smokers there was no CYP1A2 induction, hence clozapine concentrations rose, whereas in the smokers CYP1A2 induction continued, so their concentrations were only slightly affected by stopping omeprazole.[1]

Importance and management

The information on the interaction between clozapine and omeprazole is limited to uncontrolled evidence, and any effect appears to be relatively modest, with clozapine concentrations effectively reduced by up to 45% by omeprazole, or even minimally increased. Nevertheless, until more is known, it would seem prudent to monitor clozapine efficacy if omeprazole is started. Other proton pump inhibitors do not appear to have been studied.

1. Mookhoek EJ, Loonen AJM. Retrospective evaluation of the effect of omeprazole on clozapine metabolism. *Pharm World Sci* (2004) 26, 180–2.
2. Frick A, Kopitz J, Bergemann N. Omeprazole reduces clozapine plasma concentrations. *Pharmacopsychiatry* (2003) 36, 121–3.

Clozapine + Quinolones

A number of case reports suggest that ciprofloxacin can increase clozapine concentrations and might cause clozapine toxicity: one report describes a case of rhabdomyolysis as a result of raised clozapine concentrations. A study supports the observations of raised clozapine concentrations.

Clinical evidence

An elderly man with multi-infarct dementia and behavioural disturbances, taking clozapine, glibenclamide (glyburide), trazodone and melatonin, was hospitalised for agitation on the last day of a 10-day course of **ciprofloxacin** 500 mg twice daily. When the **ciprofloxacin** course was completed, his plasma clozapine concentrations fell from 90 nanograms/mL to undetectable concentrations (lower limit of detection being 50 nanograms/mL).[1]

A 64-year-old woman with schizophrenia whose symptoms had been controlled with clozapine 125 mg twice daily for 5 years became dizzy and somnolent within a few days of starting **ciprofloxacin** 500 mg twice daily. Clozapine and norclozapine (*N*-desmethylclozapine) concentrations were found to be 1043 nanograms/mL and 432 nanograms/mL, respectively. It was thought that she was no longer able to tolerate the clozapine and it was discontinued and replaced with ziprasidone which did not control her psychotic symptoms. It was then suggested that the high clozapine concentrations and adverse effects could have been due to an interaction with **ciprofloxacin**. Ziprasidone was tapered and clozapine reintroduced and titrated back up to her original dose of 125 mg twice daily. Clozapine and norclozapine concentrations were found to be 686 nanograms/mL and 244 nanograms/mL and there were no symptoms of toxicity.[2] A woman who was taking clozapine developed a raised concentration (1498 nanograms/mL), confusion and irritability when she started to take **ciprofloxacin** for a urinary tract infection. Clozapine was stopped, and the symptoms resolved. Subsequently clozapine was reintroduced and a concentration of 787 nanograms/mL was achieved.[3] A similar increase in clozapine concentrations was seen in a 58-year-old patient taking clozapine 300 mg daily who was also given intravenous **ciprofloxacin** 200 mg twice daily for 2 days.[4] Clozapine plasma concentrations before and 3 days after the start of ciprofloxacin were 850 nanograms/mL and 1720 nanograms/mL, respectively. The same authors also report a case of rhabdomyolysis in a patient taking clozapine 900 mg daily that was diagnosed (creatine phosphokinase concentration 195 000 units/L) two days after completion of a 5-day course of intravenous **ciprofloxacin** 400 mg twice daily for urosepsis. Clozapine treatment was stopped and one day later the patient's clozapine plasma concentration was 890 nanograms/mL. No clozapine concentrations were available during the course of **ciprofloxacin**, but they were undetectable within 5 days of stopping the clozapine. Creatine phosphokinase concentrations returned to normal 28 days later.[4]

A 5-fold rise in clozapine concentrations (from 0.55 mg/L to 2.57 mg/L) was seen in a patient taking clozapine 750 mg daily after 4 days of a course of **ciprofloxacin** 500 mg twice daily. The clozapine dose was reduced to 450 mg daily as a result and the patient continued with the ciprofloxacin course for a further 10 days, at which point his clozapine concentrations were greatly reduced (0.13 mg/L). The patient did not experience any adverse effects as a result of the increased concentrations; rather a remarkable improvement in mental state was noted.[5]

In a study, 7 patients with schizophrenia taking clozapine were given **ciprofloxacin** 250 mg twice daily for 7 days. The mean serum clozapine and norclozapine concentrations were increased by 29% and 31%, respectively, but no additional adverse effects were reported. Interindividual variation in serum concentrations was high, so it seems likely that some patients might demonstrate a clinically important interaction.[6]

Mechanism

This interaction probably occurs because ciprofloxacin inhibits CYP1A2, the major isoenzyme involved in the metabolism of clozapine. Clozapine metabolism is therefore reduced, resulting in elevated clozapine concentrations.

Importance and management

An interaction between clozapine and ciprofloxacin is established and clinically relevant. Monitor for clozapine adverse effects (e.g. agitation, dizziness, sedation, hypersalivation) if ciprofloxacin is also given. One report suggests that a clozapine dose reduction should be considered.[5] There seem to be no other reports of an interaction between clozapine and other quinolones, but as some other quinolones inhibit CYP1A2 (see 'Caffeine + Quinolones', p.1426) some interaction seems possible.

1. Markowitz JS, Gill HS, Devane CL, Mintzer JE. Fluoroquinolone inhibition of clozapine metabolism. *Am J Psychiatry* (1997) 153, 881.
2. Sandson NB, Cozza KL, Armstrong SC, Eckermann G, Fischer BA, Phillips B. Clozapine case series. *Psychosomatics* (2007) 48, 170–5.
3. Brownlowe K, Sola C. Clozapine toxicity in smoking cessation and with ciprofloxacin. *Psychosomatics* (2008) 49, 176.
4. Brouwers EEM, Söhne M, Kuipers S, van Gorp ECM, Schellens JHM, Koks CHW, Beijnen JH, Huitema ADR. Ciprofloxacin strongly inhibits clozapine metabolism: two case reports. *Clin Drug Invest* (2009) 29, 59–63.
5. Sambhi RS, Puri R, Jones G. Interaction of clozapine and ciprofloxacin: a case report. *Eur J Clin Pharmacol* (2007) 63, 895–6.
6. Raaska K, Neuvonen PJ. Ciprofloxacin increases serum clozapine and *N*-desmethylclozapine: a study in patients with schizophrenia. *Eur J Clin Pharmacol* (2000) 56, 585–9.

Clozapine + Reboxetine

Reboxetine does not appear to alter steady-state clozapine concentrations.

Clinical evidence, mechanism, importance and management

A small study in 7 patients found that reboxetine 8 mg daily for 4 weeks had no apparent effect on the steady-state plasma concentrations of clozapine or its major metabolite, norclozapine (*N*-desmethylclozapine).[1] A mixed model analysis estimating the effect of concurrent drugs on the plasma concentration of clozapine found that reboxetine had no obvious effect.[2] This suggests that the dose of clozapine is unlikely to need adjusting if reboxetine is also given.

1. Spina E, Avenoso A, Scordo MG, Ancione M, Madia A, Levita A. No effect of reboxetine on plasma concentrations of clozapine, risperidone, and their active metabolites. *Ther Drug Monit* (2001) 23, 675–8.
2. Diaz FJ, Santoro V, Spina E, Cogollo M, Rivera TE, Botts S, de Leon J. Estimating the size of the effects of co-medications on plasma clozapine concentrations using a model that controls for clozapine doses and confounding variables. *Pharmacopsychiatry* (2008) 41, 81–91.

Clozapine + Rifampicin (Rifampin)

Two case reports suggest that rifampicin reduces clozapine concentrations.

Clinical evidence

A patient with schizophrenia taking clozapine developed tuberculosis and was given rifampicin, isoniazid, and pyrazinamide. Within 2 to 3 weeks his minimum serum clozapine concentration had fallen dramatically from about 250 nanograms/mL to 40 nanograms/mL, but rose again rapidly when the rifampicin was replaced by ciprofloxacin.[1] A second case report describes a patient who was stable taking clozapine 300 mg daily, but who had symptoms of hypersalivation and sedation. He was given rifampicin 600 mg daily for tuberculosis, and after 2 weeks the adverse effects of clozapine began to resolve, but his psychosis started to re-emerge. His clozapine dose was increased to 550 mg daily without much improvement in his condition. Rifampicin was stopped after 6 months, at which point his psychotic symptoms markedly improved and the clozapine adverse effects of sedation and hypersalivation reappeared.[2]

Mechanism

Clozapine is principally metabolised by CYP1A2, an isoenzyme of which rifampicin is a weak inducer. It therefore seems likely that rifampicin increases clozapine metabolism leading to a decrease in its concentrations.

Importance and management

Evidence for an interaction between rifampicin and clozapine is limited, but the effects seen in the cases above are consistent with the way rifampicin interacts with other CYP1A2 substrates. As clozapine has a narrow therapeutic margin, it would seem prudent to monitor serum clozapine concentrations closely if rifampicin is added. The cases indicate that an increase in the dose of clozapine might not be successful in managing this interaction, and therefore it would be prudent to consider the use of alternative drugs. In the first case, ciprofloxacin was successfully given, although note that it can *increase* clozapine concentrations, see 'Clozapine + Quinolones', p.853.

1. Joos AAB, Frank UG, Kaschka WP. Pharmacokinetic interaction of clozapine and rifampicin in a forensic patient with an atypical mycobacterial infection. *J Clin Psychopharmacol* (1998) 18, 83–5.
2. Peritogiannis V, Pappas D, Antoniou K, Hyphantis T, Mavreas V. Clozapine-rifampicin interaction in a patient with pulmonary tuberculosis. *Gen Hosp Psychiatry* (2007) 29, 280–2.

Clozapine + Risperidone

Studies show that risperidone does not affect the pharmacokinetics of clozapine, but two isolated reports describe a rise in serum clozapine concentrations when risperidone was added. Other isolated reports describe the development of atrial ectopics, agranulocytosis, and neuroleptic malignant syndrome when clozapine and risperidone were given together. Dystonia has been seen when clozapine was replaced by risperidone.

Clinical evidence

(a) Pharmacokinetic effects

A man with a schizoaffective disorder taking clozapine started to take risperidone, firstly 500 micrograms twice daily, and then after a week 1 mg twice daily. Clinical improvement was seen and it was found that after 2 weeks his serum clozapine concentration had risen by 74%, from 344 nanograms/mL to 598 nanograms/mL, without any adverse effects.[1] The serum clozapine concentration of another patient more than doubled when risperidone was given. No signs of clozapine toxicity were seen, but mild oculogyric crises were reported.[2]

Contrasting with these reports is a study in 12 patients with schizophrenia, which found that the addition of risperidone to clozapine did not notably change the serum clozapine concentration.[3] Furthermore, a retrospective study in 18 patients,[4] and a pharmacokinetic study in 10 patients,[5] also found that risperidone did not alter clozapine serum concentrations or clearance.

(b) Adverse effects

A patient with schizophrenia taking clozapine and trihexyphenidyl, who developed tachycardia of 120 bpm, which was controlled with propranolol, developed atrial ectopics when risperidone 1.5 mg daily was added. The ectopics stopped when risperidone was withdrawn and started again when it was reintroduced. Clozapine plasma concentrations were normal throughout the use of risperidone.[6]

Another report describes 4 patients who developed dystonia after their treatment was changed from clozapine to risperidone.[7]

A single case of agranulocytosis has been seen 6 weeks after risperidone was added to stable clozapine treatment. The patient needed 3 doses of granulocyte colony-stimulating factor (G-CSF) before the white cell count returned to normal.[8]

Another case report describes a 20-year-old man taking risperidone who developed neuroleptic malignant syndrome in within 2 days of clozapine being started. The drugs were stopped and he recovered over the following 10 days. He subsequently received clozapine alone without problem.[9]

Mechanism

Risperidone would not be expected to alter clozapine concentrations. The authors of the first two studies suggest that the reason for the raised clozapine concentrations is that both drugs compete for metabolism by CYP2D6, resulting in a reduction in the metabolism of the clozapine.[1,2] However, interactions by substrate competition are rarely clinically relevant and studies have not found an interaction.

The dystonias are attributed to cholinergic rebound and ongoing dopamine blockade caused by a rapid switch of medication.[7] Clozapine alone is well known to be associated with agranulocytosis, and the relevance of risperidone to this case is uncertain.

Importance and management

Evidence from several studies does not support a pharmacokinetic interaction between clozapine and risperidone, and their concurrent use can be clinically beneficial and well tolerated. The raised clozapine concentrations seen appear to be isolated cases and are therefore of doubtful general importance. No dose adjustment would therefore seem necessary on the concurrent use of clozapine and risperidone, but be alert for increased clozapine adverse effects (e.g. agitation, dizziness, sedation, hypersalivation). To avoid dystonic reactions like those described, the recommendation is that withdrawal of clozapine should be tapered, and possibly that an antimuscarinic drug should be given.[7]

The occurrence of agranulocytosis after risperidone was added to clozapine is an isolated case and its general relevance is uncertain.

Note that clozapine and risperidone have been said to be associated with QT prolongation. See 'Drugs that prolong the QT interval + Other drugs that prolong the QT interval', p.272, for further information on the concurrent use of two or more drugs that prolong the QT interval.

1. Tyson SC, Devane LC, Risch SC. Pharmacokinetic interaction between risperidone and clozapine. *Am J Psychiatry* (1995) 152, 1401–2.
2. Koreen AR, Lieberman JA, Kronig M, Cooper TB. Cross-tapering clozapine and risperidone. *Am J Psychiatry* (1995) 152, 1690.
3. Henderson DC, Goff DC. Risperidone as an adjunct to clozapine therapy in chronic schizophrenics. *J Clin Psychiatry* (1996) 57, 395–7.
4. Raaska K, Raitasuo V, Neuvonen PJ. Therapeutic drug monitoring data: risperidone does not increase serum clozapine concentration. *Eur J Clin Pharmacol* (2002) 58, 587–91.
5. Chetty M, d'Esposito F, Zhang WV, Glen J, Dore G, Stankovic Z, Edwards RJ, Ramzan I, Murray M. *In vitro* and *in vivo* evaluation of the inhibition potential of risperidone toward clozapine biotransformation. *Br J Clin Pharmacol* (2009) 68, 574–5.
6. Chong SA, Tan CH, Lee HS. Atrial ectopics with clozapine-risperidone combination. *J Clin Psychopharmacol* (1997) 17, 130–1.
7. Simpson GM, Meyer JM. Dystonia while changing from clozapine to risperidone. *J Clin Psychopharmacol* (1996) 16, 260–1.
8. Godleski LS, Sernyak MJ. Agranulocytosis after addition of risperidone to clozapine treatment. *Am J Psychiatry* (1996) 153, 735–6.
9. Kontaxakis VP, Havaki-Kontaxaki BJ, Stamouli SS, Christodoulou GN. Toxic interaction between risperidone and clozapine: a case report. *Prog Neuropsychopharmacol Biol Psychiatry* (2002) 26, 407–9.

Clozapine + SSRIs

Fluvoxamine greatly increases clozapine concentrations. Most, but not all, evidence indicates that small to modest increases in clozapine concentrations occur with fluoxetine, paroxetine and sertraline. Studies suggest that citalopram generally does not interact, although one case report describes raised clozapine concentrations in a patient taking citalopram.

Clinical evidence

(a) Citalopram

A preliminary study in 5 patients found that the plasma concentration of clozapine was unchanged by citalopram.[1] Another study in 8 patients found similar results.[2] However, a patient who was stable taking clozapine developed sedation, hypersalivation and confusion shortly after he started to take citalopram 40 mg daily. When total clozapine serum concentrations were measured they were found to be 1097 nanograms/mL. The citalopram dose was reduced to 20 mg daily, the symptoms resolved over the following 2 weeks, and the total clozapine concentration reduced to 792 nanograms/mL.[3]

(b) Fluoxetine

Several studies in patients have found higher clozapine concentrations of 30 to 75%, and higher concentrations of the metabolite norclozapine (*N*-desmethylclozapine) of 34 to 52% after fluoxetine was added to established clozapine treatment compared with patients not taking fluoxetine or compared with baseline values.[4-6] In two case reports the concentrations of clozapine and norclozapine were raised more than 5-fold by fluoxetine. One patient developed hypertension, but the other experienced no troublesome adverse effects and his mood and psychotic symptoms improved.[7,8] The death of a 44-year-old patient who was taking clozapine and fluoxetine was felt to be due to an increase in clozapine concentrations caused by fluoxetine.[9] A case has also been reported of a patient with schizophrenia and depression, whose cognitive symptoms improved when he took clozapine and fluoxetine, but when treatment was changed to sertraline, this improvement was not sustained. The authors tentatively suggested that the fluoxetine elevated plasma clozapine concentrations by inhibition of CYP2D6, whereas this effect was not seen with sertraline as it is a much weaker inhibitor of this enzyme.[10] However, this explanation has been questioned, because the role of other drug metabolising enzymes was not considered.[11] In contrast, there is a case report of no change in clozapine concentrations 8 weeks after starting fluoxetine titrated to 80 mg daily.[12]

A patient who had been taking clozapine 500 mg and lorazepam 3 mg daily, developed myoclonic jerks of his whole body 79 days after fluoxetine 20 mg was added. These decreased over the next 2 days when the fluoxetine and lorazepam were stopped.[13] Another case report attributes an SSRI withdrawal reaction to an interaction between fluoxetine and clozapine, although it is unclear what part the clozapine had to play in this.[14]

(c) Fluvoxamine

In a study, 9 healthy subjects were given fluvoxamine 100 mg daily for 9 days with a single 10-mg dose of clozapine on day 4. Fluvoxamine increased the AUC of clozapine by 41%.[15] However, up to 10-fold elevations in the plasma concentrations of clozapine have been seen in several studies and case reports when clozapine was given with fluvoxamine.[16-26] These elevations occurred as early as 14 days after concurrent use began,[25] but were often not associated with any important adverse effects, even after treatment had continued for a year in one patient.[19] Another study, which compared 12 patients taking clozapine with 11 patients taking clozapine and fluvoxamine, found that in the combined treatment group, clozapine doses were about half those used when clozapine was given alone. A trend towards decreased granulocyte concentrations was also seen in the clozapine with fluvoxamine group, but not when clozapine was used alone.[27]

Another patient had extremely high plasma clozapine concentrations of up to 4160 micrograms/L as a result of taking fluvoxamine.[28]

Other cases have also demonstrated worsening psychosis[29] or extrapyramidal adverse effects[30] (including, rigidity, tremors and akathisia) and sedation within days of giving fluvoxamine with clozapine.

A study in 68 patients taking either clozapine alone or clozapine with fluvoxamine found a trend towards less weight increase after 12 weeks of treatment in the group of patients also taking fluvoxamine. Those patients taking clozapine alone were found to have higher glucose and triglyceride concentrations.[31] Note that fluvoxamine treatment alone can result in weight loss.

Low-dose fluvoxamine has been used in 3 patients unresponsive to clozapine treatment. They had low clozapine plasma concentrations (less than 350 micrograms/L) and abnormal caffeine tests (indicating increased metabolic capacity) but responded to clozapine when low-dose fluvoxamine (up to 50 mg daily) was added.[32]

(d) Paroxetine

The serum concentrations of clozapine and norclozapine (*N*-desmethylclozapine) rose by 57% and 50%, respectively, in 16 patients with schizophrenia after they took an average of 31.2 mg of paroxetine daily. One patient taking clozapine 300 mg daily developed reversible cerebral intoxication when given paroxetine 40 mg daily.[5] Another patient with a delusional disorder, (and who was an CYP2D6 extensive metaboliser) developed an antimuscarinic syndrome with doubled serum clozapine concentrations within about 3 weeks of starting paroxetine.[33] A further study in 9 patients found that the serum concentrations of clozapine and norclozapine rose by 31% and 20%, respectively, when paroxetine 20 to 40 mg daily was given for 3 weeks. Two patients experienced mild and transient sedation 2 to 3 days after starting paroxetine. The rise in clozapine concentrations was not associated with an increase in efficacy.[34] In contrast, a study in 14 patients taking clozapine 2.5 to 3 mg/kg daily found that the addition of paroxetine 20 mg daily for 14 days had no effect on the serum concentrations of clozapine.[24] This, or similar work, has been published elsewhere.[35]

An increase in the plasma concentrations of clozapine, thought to be due to concurrent treatment with paroxetine, has been suggested as the causative factor in the development of a fatal venous thromboembolism in a 47-year-old woman.[36]

A fatal case of neuroleptic malignant syndrome, which started to develop 2 days after the introduction of clozapine 25 mg daily to established treatment with paroxetine 20 mg daily, has been reported. The patient had previously taken clozapine alone with no problem.[37]

(e) Sertraline

In 10 patients with schizophrenia the serum concentrations of clozapine and norclozapine (*N*-desmethylclozapine) increased by 30% and 52%, respectively, when they started to take an average of 92.5 mg of sertraline daily.[5] Another patient taking clozapine 600 mg daily had a 40% reduction in total clozapine serum concentrations within one month of stopping sertraline 300 mg daily.[38] The serum clozapine concentrations of a patient with schizophrenia doubled within a month of adding sertraline 50 mg daily and her psychosis worsened. When the sertraline was stopped she improved and her serum clozapine concentrations fell once again.[29] In contrast, a study in 8 patients who were taking clozapine 200 to 400 mg daily and were also given sertraline 50 to 100 mg per day for 3 weeks, found no changes in the concentrations of clozapine and its major metabolites.[34]

A case report describes sudden cardiac death in a 26-year-old man, which the authors attributed to an interaction between clozapine and sertraline.[39] However, this interaction has been questioned as it is said that the patient had other risk factors that were more likely to have caused the fatality.[40]

Mechanism

Fluvoxamine is a potent inhibitor of CYP1A2, by which clozapine is principally metabolised, therefore concurrent use raises clozapine exposure. None of the other SSRIs inhibit CYP1A2, but they are known to inhibit CYP2D6 to a varying extent. The evidence here for fluoxetine and paroxetine suggests that CYP2D6 might have a minor role in clozapine metabolism, but this is not conclusive because the available evidence from uncontrolled studies. A mixed model analysis estimated that fluoxetine, fluvoxamine and paroxetine increase the plasma concentrations of clozapine by 42%, 263%, and 30%, respectively. The study also found that citalopram and sertraline had no obvious effects of clozapine concentrations, but the possibility of an inhibitory effects of sertraline at high doses was not ruled out.[41] The concentrations of clozapine and norclozapine (*N*-desmethylclozapine) rise together, and so it has been suggested that the metabolic step inhibited is after the *N*-dealkylation step.[5]

Importance and management

The interaction of **fluvoxamine** with clozapine would appear to be established. Because the interaction is greatest with fluvoxamine, other SSRIs are likely to be preferred. However, if fluvoxamine is required, it would be prudent to monitor the outcome very closely because of the rises in serum clozapine and norclozapine (*N*-desmethylclozapine) concentrations that can occur, adjusting the clozapine dose as necessary. One group advocates exploiting the interaction with fluvoxamine in patients unresponsive to clozapine (low clozapine concentrations and proven metabolic over-activity using a caffeine test to assess CYP1A2 activity), by halving the clozapine dose, adding fluvoxamine 50 mg daily and monitoring. However, this strategy could carry some risks.[32] The exploitation of interactions in this way is rarely recommended as the effects are generally unpredictable and very close monitoring, both of clozapine concentrations and for the emergence of adverse effects would be essential.

The interaction of **fluoxetine**, **paroxetine**, and **sertraline** with clozapine is more modest, with not all of the evidence suggesting an interaction. Nevertheless, increased monitoring on the concurrent use of clozapine with these SSRIs would appear to be prudent. The authors of one study suggest particularly close monitoring if the clozapine dose exceeds 300 mg or 3.5 mg/kg daily.[5] **Citalopram** (and therefore possibly **escitalopram**) appears less likely to interact with clozapine, although a case has still been reported. Bear the possibility of an interaction in mind.

Note that **citalopram** and **escitalopram** are associated with QT prolongation, as is clozapine. See 'Drugs that prolong the QT interval + Other drugs that prolong the QT interval', p.272, for further information on the concurrent use of two or more drugs that prolong the QT interval.

1. Taylor D, Ellison Z, Ementon Shaw L, Wickham H, Murray R. Co-administration of citalopram and clozapine: effect on plasma clozapine levels. *Int Clin Psychopharmacol* (1998) 13, 19–21.
2. Avenoso A, Facciolà G, Scordo MG, Gitto C, Ferrante GD, Madia AG, Spina E. No effect of citalopram on plasma levels of clozapine, risperidone and their active metabolites in patients with chronic schizophrenia. *Clin Drug Invest* (1998) 16, 393–8.
3. Borba CP, Henderson DC. Citalopram and clozapine: potential drug interaction. *J Clin Psychiatry* (2000) 61, 301–2.
4. Centorrino F, Baldessarini RJ, Kando J, Frankenburg FR, Volpicelli SA, Puopolo PR, Flood JG. Serum concentrations of clozapine and its major metabolites: effects of cotreatment with fluoxetine or valproate. *Am J Psychiatry* (1994) 151, 123–5.
5. Centorrino F, Baldessarini RJ, Frankenburg FR, Kando J, Volpicelli SA, Flood JG. Serum levels of clozapine and norclozapine in patients treated with selective serotonin reuptake inhibitors. *Am J Psychiatry* (1996) 153, 820–2.
6. Spina E, Avenoso A, Facciolà G, Fabrazzo M, Monteleone P, Maj M, Perucca E, Caputi AP. Effect of fluoxetine on the plasma concentrations of clozapine and its major metabolites in patients with schizophrenia. *Int Clin Psychopharmacol* (1998) 13, 141–5.
7. Sloan D, O'Boyle J. Hypertension and increased serum clozapine associated with clozapine and fluoxetine in combination. *Ir J Psychol Med* (1977) 14, 149–51.
8. Sandson NB, Cozza, KL, Armstrong SC, Eckermann G, Fischer BA, Phillips B. Clozapine case series. *Psychosomatics* (2007) 48, 170–5.
9. Ferslew KE, Hagardorn AN, Harlan GC, McCormick WF. A fatal drug interaction between clozapine and fluoxetine. *J Forensic Sci* (1998) 43, 1082–5.
10. Purdon SE, Snaterse M. Selective serotonin reuptake inhibitor modulation of clozapine effects on cognition in schizophrenia. *Can J Psychiatry* (1998) 43, 84–5.
11. Chong S-A, Remington G. Re: Sertraline-clozapine interaction. *Can J Psychiatry* (1998) 43, 856–7.
12. Eggert AE, Crismon ML, Dorson PG. Lack of effect of fluoxetine on plasma clozapine concentrations. *J Clin Psychiatry* (1994) 55, 454–5.
13. Kingsbury SJ, Puckett KM. Effects of fluoxetine on serum clozapine levels. *Am J Psychiatry* (1995) 152, 473–4.
14. Lu M-L, Lane H-Y, Chang W-H. Selective serotonin reuptake inhibitor syndrome: precipitated by concomitant clozapine? *J Clin Psychopharmacol* (1999) 19, 386–7.
15. Wang C-Y, Zhang Z-J, Li W-B, Zhai Y-M, Cai Z-J, Weng Y-Z, Zhu R-H, Zhao J-P, Zhou H-H. The differential effects of steady-state fluvoxamine on the pharmacokinetics of olanzapine and clozapine in healthy volunteers. *J Clin Pharmacol* (2004) 44, 785–92.
16. Hiemke C, Weigmann H, Müller H, Dahmen N, Wetzel H, Fuchs E. Elevated clozapine plasma levels after addition of fluvoxamine. *Abstr Soc Neurosci* (1993) 19, 382.
17. Weigmann H, Müller H, Dahmen N, Wetzel H, Hiemke C. Interactions of fluvoxamine with the metabolism of clozapine. *Pharmacopsychiatry* (1993) 26, 209.
18. Jerling M, Lindström L, Bondesson U, Bertilsson L. Fluvoxamine inhibition and carbamazepine induction of the metabolism of clozapine: evidence from a therapeutic drug monitoring service. *Ther Drug Monit* (1994) 16, 368–74.
19. Dumortier G, Lochu A, Colen de Melo P, Ghribi O, Roche Rabreau D, Degrassat K, Desce JM. Elevated clozapine plasma concentrations after fluvoxamine initiation. *Am J Psychiatry* (1996) 153, 738–9.
20. Olesen OV, Starup G, Linnet K. Alvorlig lægmiddelinteraktion mellem clozapin – Leponex og fluvoxamin – Fevarin. *Ugeskr Laeger* (1996) 158, 6931–2.
21. Dequardo JR, Roberts M. Elevated clozapine levels after fluvoxamine initiation. *Am J Psychiatry* (1996) 153, 840–1.
22. Koponen HJ, Leinonen E, Lepola U. Fluvoxamine increases the clozapine serum levels significantly. *Eur Neuropsychopharmacol* (1996) 6, 69–71.
23. Hiemke C, Weigmann H, Härtter S, Dahmen N, Wetzel H, Müller H. Elevated levels of clozapine in serum after addition of fluvoxamine. *J Clin Psychopharmacol* (1994) 14, 279–81.
24. Wetzel H, Anghelescu I, Szegedi A, Wiesner J, Weigmann H, Hörtter S, Hiemke C. Pharmacokinetic interactions of clozapine with selective serotonin reuptake inhibitors: differential effects of fluvoxamine and paroxetine in a prospective study. *J Clin Psychopharmacol* (1998) 18, 2–9.
25. Lu M-L, Lane H-Y, Chen K-P, Jann MW, Su M-H, Chang W-H. Fluvoxamine reduces the clozapine dosage needed in refractory schizophrenic patients. *J Clin Psychiatry* (2000) 61, 594–9.
26. Szegedi A, Anghelescu I, Wiesner J, Schlegel S, Weigmann H, Härtter S, Hiemke C, Wetzel H. Addition of low-dose fluvoxamine to low-dose clozapine monotherapy in schizophrenia: drug monitoring and tolerability data from a prospective clinical trial. *Pharmacopsychiatry* (1999) 32, 148–53.
27. Hinze-Selch D, Deuschle M, Weber B, Heuser I, Pollmächer T. Effect of coadministration of clozapine and fluvoxamine versus clozapine monotherapy on blood cell counts, plasma levels of cytokines and body weight. *Psychopharmacology (Berl)* (2000) 149, 163–9.
28. Heeringa M, Beurskens R, Schouten W, Verduijn MM. Elevated plasma levels of clozapine after concomitant use of fluvoxamine. *Pharm World Sci* (1999) 21, 243–4.
29. Chong SA, Tan CH, Lee HS. Worsening of psychosis with clozapine and selective serotonin reuptake inhibitor combination: two case reports. *J Clin Psychopharmacol* (1997) 17, 68–9.
30. Kuo F-J, Lane H-Y, Chang W-H. Extrapyramidal symptoms after addition of fluvoxamine to clozapine. *J Clin Psychopharmacol* (1998) 18, 483–4.
31. Lu M-L, Lane H-S, Lin S-K, Chen K-P, Chang W-H. Adjunctive fluvoxamine inhibits clozapine-related weight gain and metabolic disturbances. *J Clin Psychiatry* (2004) 65, 766–71.
32. Papetti F, Morel-Pingault V, Buisse V, Maziere L, Banayan M, Thauby S, Besnard T, Darcourt G, Pringuey. Clozapine-resistant schizophrenia related to an increased metabolism and benefit of fluvoxamine: four case reports. *Encephale* (2007) 33, 811–8.
33. Joos AAB, König F, Frank UG, Kaschka WP, Mörike KE, Ewald R. Dose-dependent pharmacokinetic interaction of clozapine and paroxetine in an extensive metabolizer. *Pharmacopsychiatry* (1997) 30, 266–70.
34. Spina E, Avenoso A, Salemi M, Facciolá G, Scordo MG, Ancione M, Madia A. Plasma concentrations of clozapine and its major metabolites during combined treatment with paroxetine or sertraline. *Pharmacopsychiatry* (2000) 33, 213–17.
35. Anghelescu I, Szegedi A, Schlegel S, Weigmann H, Hiemke C, Wetzel H. Combination treatment with clozapine and paroxetine in schizophrenia: safety and tolerability data from a prospective open clinical trial. *Eur Neuropsychopharmacol* (1998) 8, 315–320.
36. Farah RE, Makhoul NM, Farah RE, Shai MD. Fatal venous thromboembolism associated with antipsychotic therapy. *Ann Pharmacother* (2004) 38, 1435–8.
37. Gambassi G, Capurso S, Tarsitani P, Liperito R, Bernabei R. Fatal neuroleptic malignant syndrome in a previously long-term user of clozapine following its reintroduction in combination with paroxetine. *Aging Clin Exp Res* (2006) 18, 266–70.
38. Pinniniti NR, De Leon J. Interaction of sertraline with clozapine. *J Clin Psychopharmacol* (1997) 17, 119.
39. Hoehns JD, Fouts MM, Kelly MW, Tu KB. Sudden cardiac death with clozapine and sertraline combination. *Ann Pharmacother* (2001) 35, 862–6.
40. Gillespie JA. Comment: sudden cardiac death with clozapine and sertraline combination. *Ann Pharmacother* (2001) 35, 1671.
41. Diaz FJ, Santoro V, Spina E, Cogollo M, Rivera TE, Botts S, de Leon J. Estimating the size of the effects of co-medications on plasma clozapine concentrations using a model that controls for clozapine doses and confounding variables. *Pharmacopsychiatry* (2008) 41, 81–91.

Clozapine + St John's wort (*Hypericum perforatum*)

An isolated report describes reduced clozapine concentrations in a patient stabilised on clozapine, shortly after St John's wort was started.

Clinical evidence

A case report describes a 41-year-old patient with disorganised schizophrenia who had been stable on clozapine for 6 months and had a minimum plasma clozapine concentration of 0.46 to 0.57 mg/L at a dose of 500 mg daily. Shortly after starting St John's wort 300 mg three times daily (with each tablet containing hypericin 0.36 to 0.8 mg and hyperforin 9 mg), her clozapine plasma concentration decreased to 0.19 mg/L and she showed signs of increased disorganisation. Three weeks later, her clozapine plasma concentration was found to be 0.16 mg/L. One month after stopping St John's wort her clozapine plasma concentration had increased to 0.32 mg/L and after another month it had further increased to 0.41 mg/L, and her psychiatric condition improved.[1]

Mechanism

Not established. Clozapine is principally metabolised by CYP1A2, with some involvement of other isoenzymes, such as CYP3A4. St John's wort is known to induce CYP3A4, and possibly affects CYP1A2, although evidence of clinically important interactions with St John's wort via CYP1A2 is lacking (see 'Theophylline + St John's wort (*Hypericum perforatum*)', p.1460). It is therefore possible that induction of CYP3A4 led to the decreased clozapine plasma concentrations seen.

Importance and management

The report of reduced clozapine concentrations in a patient taking St John's wort is isolated and as such its general clinical importance is not known. Nevertheless, it is consistent with the way St John's wort interacts with other drugs, and it would seem prudent to monitor clozapine concentrations in patients taking St John's wort, or consider this as a possible cause in cases of otherwise unexplained reductions in clozapine concentrations.

1. Van Strater ACP, Bogers JPAM. Interaction of St John's wort (*Hypericum perforatum*) with clozapine. *Int Clin Psychopharmacol* (2012) 27, 121–3.

Clozapine + Tobacco

Smoking tobacco appears to decrease clozapine concentrations and smokers require a higher clozapine dose. On smoking cessation, clozapine toxicity might occur due to increased concentrations, and a clozapine dose reduction might be needed.

Clinical evidence

(a) Smoking

Although one group of workers found that smoking did not affect clozapine concentrations,[1] and another found only a trend towards a reduction in clozapine concentrations in smokers,[2] the majority of the available data supports an interaction between smoking and clozapine. Several prospective studies in 34 to 148 patients have found that smokers had dose-corrected clozapine concentrations that were about 20 to 60% lower than those of non-smokers.[3-6] In one of these studies, the mean required maintenance dose of clozapine in patients who smoked at least 15 cigarettes daily was almost twice that in non-smokers (382 mg versus 197 mg).[6] In another of these studies, there was no apparent difference in the dose-corrected clozapine concentrations between those who smoked 7 to 12 cigarettes daily, those who smoked 13 to 19, and those who smoked greater than 20, suggesting that 7 to 12 cigarettes might be sufficient for maximal clozapine induction.[4] In a very large cohort study using data from 3555 patients, modelling of plasma clozapine concentrations predicted that plasma clozapine were increased by 48% in non-smokers.[7]

A number of case reports also support the existence of an interaction. One case report describes 2 patients with psychoses resistant to treatment with clozapine. Both patients were heavy smokers and one also consumed large amounts of caffeine, which might increase plasma clozapine concentrations (see also 'Clozapine + Caffeine', p.849), but it was considered that the CYP1A2 induction due to smoking increased clearance of both clozapine and caffeine.[8] In another report, 4 patients who were smokers were found to have low clozapine concentrations and to be of CYP1A2 ultra rapid metaboliser phenotype. One patient required a clozapine dose increase up to 1.4 g daily, whereas the others were given fluvoxamine (a CYP1A2 inhibitor) to achieve therapeutic clozapine concentrations.[9] Similarly, another case series describes two smokers aged 26 and 36 years who required a very high dose of clozapine of 1.1 g daily to maintain their plasma clozapine concentrations at about 1 mg/L and 0.6 mg/L, respectively.[10]

Another report describes a patient, stable taking clozapine 500 mg daily, who used a nicotine-containing inhaler (*Nicotrol*) as a substitute for smoking when he was admitted to hospital. He started smoking again after discharge from hospital and his paranoid symptoms and hallucinations returned. His clozapine concentrations had decreased from 417 nanograms/mL to 192 nanograms/mL.[11]

(b) Smoking cessation

One retrospective study of 11 patients after a hospital-imposed ban on smoking found a mean increase in clozapine concentrations of about 72% on smoking cessation.[12] In another similar retrospective study, after a ban on smoking there was an increase in toxic plasma clozapine concentrations: 42% of patients had plasma clozapine concentrations greater than 1 mg/L, despite dose reductions, compared with just 4% before the ban.[13] At least 4 case reports describe elevations in clozapine plasma concentrations when patients stopped smoking abruptly;[14-17] in one case this was associated with seizures and in another, loss of consciousness. Another three case reports suggest that smoking cessation might have resulted in clozapine adverse effects, including seizures, although no plasma concentrations were available.[18-20]

A 37-year-old man who smoked both tobacco and **cannabis** daily, and took clozapine 700 mg daily, experienced elevated clozapine plasma concentrations and signs of clozapine toxicity one month after he stopped smoking both tobacco and **cannabis**. One week after reducing the dose of clozapine to 500 mg daily, his psychotic symptoms disappeared and plasma concentrations returned to normal.[21]

Mechanism

Tobacco smoke contains aromatic hydrocarbons that are inducers of CYP1A2, which is the major isoenzyme involved in clozapine metabolism. Smoking therefore increases clozapine metabolism and lower concentrations result. Nicotine patches and other nicotine products used as replacement therapy do not induce CYP1A2.[11]

Importance and management

An interaction between tobacco smoking and clozapine is established. It has been suggested that smoking 7 to 12 cigarettes daily is probably sufficient for maximum induction of clozapine metabolism.[4] In smokers who are resistant to clozapine, using single doses of clozapine at night when the patients are not smoking, or augmentation of treatment with another drug, such as low-dose amisulpride, has been suggested.[8] It has also been suggested that if a patient taking clozapine starts to smoke, a 50% increase in the clozapine dose should be anticipated. Likewise, a patient who stops smoking might experience a 50% increase in clozapine concentrations within 2 to 4 weeks of stopping smoking. One report recommends that patients with high baseline clozapine concentrations should be monitored if they stop smoking.[12] Note that all these recommendations are based on approximations, and that, in all cases, dose adjustments should be guided by the clinical status of the patient and clozapine concentrations.[8,22]

1. Hasegawa M, Gutierrez-Esteinou R, Way L, Meltzer HY. Relationship between clinical efficacy and clozapine concentrations in plasma in schizophrenia: effect of smoking. *J Clin Psychopharmacol* (1993) 13, 383–90.
2. Palego L, Biondi L, Giannaccini G, Sarno N, Elmi S, Ciapparelli A, Cassano GB, Luchacchini A, Martini C, Dell'Osso L. Clozapine, norclozapine plasma levels, their sum and ratio in 50 psychotic patients. Influence of patient-related variables. *Prog Neuropsychopharmacol Biol Psychiatry* (2002) 26, 473–80.
3. Haring C, Meise U, Humpel C, Fleischhacker WW, Hinterhuber H. Dose-related plasma effects of clozapine: influence of smoking behaviour, sex and age. *Psychopharmacology (Berl)* (1989) 99, S38–S40.
4. Haslemo T, Eikeseth PH, Tanum L, Molden E, Refsum H. The effect of variable cigarette consumption on the interaction with clozapine and olanzapine. *Eur J Clin Pharmacol* (2006) 62, 1049–53.
5. Dettling M, Sachse C, Brockmöller J, Schley J, Müller-Oerlinghausen B, Pickersgill I, Rolfs A, Schaub RT, Schmider J. Long-term therapeutic drug monitoring of clozapine and metabolites in psychiatric in- and outpatients. *Psychopharmacology (Berl)* (2000) 152, 80–6.
6. van der Weide J, Steijns LSW, van Weelden MJM. The effect of smoking and cytochrome P450 *CYP1A2* genetic polymorphism on clozapine clearance and dose requirement. *Pharmacogenetics* (2003) 13, 169–72.
7. Rostami-Hodjegan A, Amin AM, Spencer EP, Lennard MS, Tucker GT, Flanagan RJ. Influence of dose, cigarette smoking, age, sex, and metabolic activity on plasma clozapine concentrations: a predictive model and nomograms to aid clozapine dose adjustment and to assess compliance in individual patients. *J Clin Psychopharmacol* (2004) 24, 70–8.
8. Dratcu L, Grandison A, McKay G, Bamidele A, Vasudevan V. Clozapine-resistant psychosis, smoking, and caffeine: managing the neglected effects of substances that our patients consume every day. *Am J Ther* (2007) 14, 314–18.
9. Eap CB, Bender S, Jaquenoud Sirot E, Cucchia G, Jonzier-Perey M, Baumann P, Allorge D, Broly F. Nonresponse to clozapine and ultrarapid CYP1A2 activity: clinical data and analysis of CYP1A2 gene. *J Clin Psychopharmacol* (2004) 24, 214–9.
10. MacCall C, Billcliff N, Igbrude W, Natynczuk S, Spencer EP, Flanagan RJ. Clozapine: more than 900 mg/day may be needed. *J Psychopharmacol* (2009) 23, 206–10.
11. Sandson NB, Cozza KL, Armstrong C, Eckermann G, Fischer A, Phillips B. Clozapine case series. *Psychosomatics* (2007) 48, 170–5.
12. Meyer JM. Individual changes in clozapine levels after smoking cessation: results and a predictive model. *J Clin Psychopharmacol* (2001) 21, 569–74.
13. Cormac I, Brown A, Creasey S, Ferriter M, Huckstep B. A retrospective evaluation of the impact of total smoking cessation on psychiatric inpatients taking clozapine. *Acta Psychiatr Scand* (2010) 121, 393–7.
14. Bondolfi G, Morel F, Crettol S, Rachid F, Baumann P, Eap CB. Increased clozapine plasma concentrations and side effects induced by smoking cessation in 2 *CYP1A2* genotyped patients. *Ther Drug Monit* (2005) 27, 539–43.
15. Skogh E, Bengtsson F, Nordin C. Could discontinuing smoking be hazardous for patients administered clozapine medication? A case report. *Ther Drug Monit* (1999) 21, 580–2.
16. Ruissen A, van Schaik AM, Beijnen JH. Clozapinegebruik en abrupt stoppen met roken; een potentieel levensbedreigende combinatie. *Tijdschr Psychiatr* (2009) 51, 699–703.
17. Derenne JL, Baldessarini RJ. Clozapine toxicity associated with smoking cessation: case report. *Am J Ther* (2005) 12, 469–71.
18. Oyewumi LK. Smoking cessation and clozapine side effects. *Can J Psychiatry* (1998) 43, 748.
19. Brownlowe K, Sola C. Clozapine toxicity in smoking cessation and with ciprofloxacin. *Psychosomatics* (2008) 49, 176.
20. McCarthy RH. Seizures following smoking cessation in a clozapine responder. *Pharmacopsychiatry* (1994) 27, 210–11.
21. Zullino DF, Delessert D, Eap CB, Preisig M, Baumann P. Tobacco and cannabis smoking cessation can lead to intoxication with clozapine or olanzapine. *Int Clin Psychopharmacol* (2002) 17, 141–3.
22. de Leon J. Atypical antipsychotic dosing: the effect of smoking and caffeine. *Psychiatr Serv* (2004) 55, 491–3.

Clozapine + Topiramate

Topiramate does not appear to affect the steady-state plasma concentration of clozapine.

Clinical evidence, mechanism, importance and management

In a study, 10 patients receiving long-term treatment with clozapine 250 to 500 mg daily were given topiramate in a dose that was increased gradually to 200 mg daily over 6 to 8 weeks. The steady-state plasma concentrations of clozapine and its metabolite norclozapine (*N*-desmethylclozapine) did not appear to be affected by topiramate.[1] Similarly, the steady-state clozapine concentration was not affected by topiramate 300 mg daily in 12 treatment-resistant patients with schizophrenia.[2] These studies suggests that the dose of clozapine is unlikely to need adjusting if topiramate is also given.

1. Migliardi G, D'Arrigo C, Santoro V, Bruno A, Cortese L, Campolo D, Cacciola M, Spina E. Effect of topiramate on plasma concentrations of clozapine, olanzapine, risperidone, and quetiapine in patients with psychotic disorders. *Clin Neuropharmacol* (2007) 30, 107–13.
2. Tiihonen J, Halonen P, Wahlbeck K, Repo-Tiihonen E, Hyvärinen S, Eronen M, Putkonen H, Takala P, Mehtonen O-P, Puck M, Oksanen J, Koskelainen P, Joffe G, Aer J, Hallikainen T, Ryynänen O-P, Tupala E. Topiramate add-on in treatment-resistant schizophrenia: a randomized, double-blind, placebo-controlled, crossover trial. *J Clin Psychiatry* (2005) 66, 1012–5.

Clozapine + Valproate

Valproate appears to increase or decrease serum clozapine concentrations, but any effects are minor. Isolated cases of additive adverse effects, such as sedation, have been reported on concurrent use.

Clinical evidence

A controlled study found that when valproate (at an average dose of 1.06 g daily) was given with clozapine (11 patients), the steady-state serum clozapine concentrations were increased by 39% and the concentrations of the demethylated metabolite of clozapine (norclozapine) were increased by 23%. However, correction of these concentrations for dose and weight reduced the total clozapine metabolite values to only 6% above those of the control group taking clozapine and not given valproate (17 patients). No increase in clozapine adverse effects was seen.[1] Another study in non-smokers found that the concurrent use of sodium valproate and clozapine had no statistically significant effect on the pharmacokinetics of either drug, although there was a trend towards increased clozapine and decreased norclozapine concentrations.[2]

In contrast, a study in 4 patients with schizophrenia taking clozapine 550 to 650 mg daily found that when **valproate semisodium** (**divalproex sodium**) 750 mg to 1 g daily was added, the serum clozapine concentrations began to fall, and by 3 weeks had fallen by an average of 41%. However, no deterioration in clinical condition occurred.[3] In another study in 7 patients given clozapine, the clozapine concentrations were decreased by a more modest 15% when valproic acid was given.[4]

An isolated report describes a 37-year-old man taking clozapine who developed sedation, confusion, slurred speech and impaired functioning on two occasions when **valproate semisodium** was added.[5] Clozapine concentrations were doubled in a patient (a heavy smoker, more than 20 cigarettes per day) after valproic acid treatment was stopped.[6] The authors of an analysis of reports on the use of mood stabiliser combinations obtained from a MEDLINE search noted that there might be additive adverse effects of weight gain and drowsiness with the combination of clozapine and valproate.[7]

Mechanism

Unclear. It has been suggested that valproate might increase the metabolism of clozapine, although it is unclear which pathway is affected. Alternatively it has been suggested that valproate impairs clozapine absorption.[6] Further it has been suggested that the induction of clozapine metabolism in smokers (see 'Clozapine + Tobacco', p.856) might be enhanced by valproate. Mixed model analysis estimated that valproate increases plasma clozapine concentrations in non-smokers by 16% by inhibiting clozapine metabolism, but decreases concentrations in smokers by 22% by inducing clozapine metabolism, and this might partly explain the inconsistent results found in the literature.[8]

Importance and management

Evidence for an interaction between clozapine and valproate appears to be limited to these reports, and the outcome of concurrent use is not entirely clear. A subgroup analysis of 20 patients who received clozapine and antiepileptics including valproate suggested that this group of patients showed less clinical improvement than patients who were not also taking an antiepileptic. However, the effects of valproate were not separated from those of the enzyme-inducing antiepileptics, which are known to reduce clozapine concentrations. Also, the indication for the antiepileptic drug was not always clear and concurrent use might have been undertaken in patients who were more severely ill, or less responsive to clozapine alone.[9] Further, an analysis[8] reported that the interaction between valproate and clozapine might be also affected by smoking status (see under *Mechanism*, above), but this requires further study. In general, the effects of valproate on clozapine concentrations in the case reports were relatively modest, and the studies suggesting a lack of interaction indicate that most patients are unlikely to experience a clinically relevant effect. Nevertheless, the isolated cases suggest that it might be prudent to be alert for additive adverse effects (such as weight gain and CNS depressant effects) if both drugs are given.

1. Centorrino F, Baldessarini RJ, Kando J, Frankenburg FR, Volpicelli SA, Puopolo PR, Flood JG. Serum concentrations of clozapine and its major metabolites: effects of cotreatment with fluoxetine or valproate. *Am J Psychiatry* (1994) 151, 123–5.
2. Facciolà G, Avenoso A, Scordo MG, Madia AG, Ventimiglia A, Perucca E, Spina E. Small effects of valproic acid on the plasma concentrations of clozapine and its major metabolites in patients with schizophrenic or affective disorders. *Ther Drug Monit* (1999) 21, 341–5.
3. Finley P, Warner D. Potential impact of valproic acid therapy on clozapine disposition. *Biol Psychiatry* (1994) 36, 487–8.
4. Longo LP, Salzman C. Valproic acid effects on serum concentrations of clozapine and norclozapine. *Am J Psychiatry* (1995) 152, 650.
5. Costello LE, Suppes T. A clinically significant interaction between clozapine and valproate. *J Clin Psychopharmacol* (1995) 15, 139–141.
6. Conca A, Beraus W, König P, Waschgler R. A case of pharmacokinetic interference in comedication of clozapine and valproic acid. *Pharmacopsychiatry* (2000) 33, 234–5.
7. Freeman MP, Stoll AL. Mood stabilizer combinations: a review of safety and efficacy. *Am J Psychiatry* (1998) 155, 12–21.
8. Diaz FJ, Santoro V, Spina E, Cogollo M, Rivera TE, Botts S, de Leon J. Estimating the size of the effects of co-medications on plasma clozapine concentrations using a model that controls for clozapine doses and confounding variables. *Pharmacopsychiatry* (2008) 41, 81–91.
9. Wilson WH. Do anticonvulsants hinder clozapine treatment? *Biol Psychiatry* (1995) 37, 132–3.

Flupentixol and related drugs + Carbamazepine

Carbamazepine possibly decreases the steady-state concentrations of zuclopenthixol and flupentixol.

Clinical evidence

A retrospective analysis of results from a routine therapeutic drug monitoring service found that the concentration-to-dose ratio of **zuclopenthixol** was 2-fold lower in patients also given carbamazepine, when compared with those given zuclopenthixol alone.[1] A similar effect was seen for flupentixol, but it was not statistically significant. For both drugs, the number of patients receiving each was small (6 patients and 3 patients, respectively).[1] In another similar analysis, samples taken from patients given oral or intramuscular depot **zuclopenthixol** alone or with non-interacting drugs (216 samples from 216 patients and 247 samples from 247 patients, respectively) were compared with those from patients also taking carbamazepine (105 samples from 68 patients and 50 samples from 32 patients, respectively). The concurrent use of carbamazepine resulted in lower dose-corrected oral and depot **zuclopenthixol** concentrations of 67% and 14%, respectively. The authors note that the daily dose of carbamazepine was higher in those taking oral zuclopenthixol than intramuscular depot zuclopenthixol (693 mg daily and 526 mg daily, respectively).[2]

Mechanism

In vitro study[2] has shown that zuclopenthixol is a substrate for CYP2D6 and CYP3A4. Carbamazepine is an inducer of both these isoenzymes.

Importance and management

The information regarding an interaction between carbamazepine and flupentixol or zuclopenthixol is limited to retrospective and uncontrolled data, and, although a pharmacokinetic interaction seems to occur, its true magnitude remains to be established. The clinical relevance of the interaction is also uncertain. However, if zuclopenthixol or flupentixol are given with carbamazepine, bear in mind the possibility of reduced concentrations and efficacy.

1. Gex-Fabry M, Balant-Gorgia AE. Balant LP. Therapeutic drug monitoring databases for postmarketing surveillance of drug-drug interactions: evaluation of a paired approach for psychotropic medication. *Ther Drug Monit* (1997) 19, 1–10.
2. Davies SJC, Westin AA, Castberg I, Lewis G, Lennard MS, Taylor S, Spigset O. Characterisation of zuclopenthixol metabolism by *in vitro* and therapeutic drug monitoring studies. *Acta Psychiatr Scand* (2010) 122, 444–53.

Flupentixol and related drugs + SSRIs

Fluoxetine and paroxetine appear to raise steady-state zuclopenthixol concentrations. The pharmacokinetics of zuclopenthixol do not appear to be affected by citalopram. There is an isolated reported of parkinsonian-like symptoms in a patient taking amitriptyline, flupentixol, and fluoxetine.

Clinical evidence

(a) Flupentixol

Parkinson-like symptoms developed in a patient taking amitriptyline and flupentixol when **fluoxetine** was given.[1]

(b) Zuclopenthixol

1. Citalopram. A study in patients with schizophrenia found that over a 12-week period the serum concentrations of zuclopenthixol did not appear to be altered by citalopram 40 mg daily.[2]

2. Fluoxetine, Paroxetine, and other CYP2D6 inhibitors. In a retrospective analysis of serum samples from a therapeutic drug monitoring service, dose-corrected oral zuclopenthixol concentrations were 79% higher in samples from patients taking fluoxetine, 93% higher in those taking paroxetine, and 43% higher in those taking **levomepromazine**. Findings for intramuscular depot zuclopenthixol were similar for fluoxetine and **levomepromazine**, but less for paroxetine (46%).[3] In another similar analysis, the steady-state zuclopenthixol concentration-to-dose ratio was 44% higher in 38 patients genotyped as CYP2D6 extensive metabolisers taking drugs said to inhibit CYP2D6 (tricyclic antidepressants, citalopram, fluoxetine, and neuroleptics (mainly **levomepromazine**)) than in 58 extensive metabolisers taking no interacting drugs (1.8 nanomol/L per mg versus 1.25 nanomol/L per mg). In the 38 extensive metabolisers taking potentially interacting drugs, the concentration-to-dose ratio was similar to that in 12 poor metabolisers (2 nanomol/L per mg). However, the ratio varied almost 10-fold between all the patients.[4]

Mechanism

Paroxetine and fluoxetine are known potent inhibitors of CYP2D6, and these SSRIs apparently reduce zuclopenthixol metabolism, whereas citalopram, a weak CYP2D6 inhibitor, appears to have no effect. Levomepromazine has also been reported to be a CYP2D6 inhibitor. *In vitro* study has shown that zuclopenthixol is a substrate for CYP2D6 and CYP3A4.[3] Note that CYP2D6 is subject to genetic polymorphism, with some individuals lacking activity (poor metabolisers).

The pharmacokinetic interaction might increase the risk of movement disorders, but movement disorders might also occur simply as a result of the additive adverse effects of antipsychotics and SSRIs. Fluoxetine alone has been shown to occasionally cause movement disorders.[5,6]

Importance and management

The information on the pharmacokinetic interaction of fluoxetine and paroxetine with **zuclopenthixol** is limited to retrospective and uncontrolled data, and although an interaction seems likely to occur, its true magnitude remains to be established. The clinical relevance of the interaction is not yet established; however, the case report with zuclopenthixol and high-dose fluoxetine serves to highlight the possibility of severe adverse effects, possibly exacerbated by the pharmacokinetic interaction, on concurrent use. In one analysis, the increase in concentrations seen with the potentially interacting drugs was less than the variability between patients.[4] However, not all of the drugs included are known to be potent CYP2D6 inhibitors and as such the magnitude of the effect might have been underestimated. Furthermore, there is some evidence that poor metabolisers have a tendency to an increased risk of zuclopenthixol adverse effects,[7] and as potent CYP2D6 inhibitors would make extensive metabolisers more like poor metabolisers,[3] it is possible that potent CYP2D6 inhibitors might increase the risk of zuclopenthixol adverse effects. If patients stabilised on zuclopenthixol require a potent CYP2D6 inhibitor, such as paroxetine or fluoxetine, it would seem prudent to bear this possibility in mind, and consider monitoring serum concentrations, where possible, if adverse effects occur, and reducing the zuclopenthixol dose as necessary. Similarly, in those taking a potent CYP2D6 inhibitor and requiring zuclopenthixol, bear in mind that a lower dose of zuclopenthixol dose might be sufficient. For a list of CYP2D6 inhibitors, see 'Table 1.7', p.9. Note that weak CYP2D6 inhibitors such as citalopram appear unlikely to cause a clinically relevant pharmacokinetic interaction, therefore zuclopenthixol dose adjustments are unlikely to be necessary on concurrent use.

The general relevance of the isolated case of a possible interaction of **flupentixol** and fluoxetine is uncertain; however, bear it in mind if extrapyramidal effects become troublesome.

1. Touw DJ, Gernaat HBPE, van der Woude J. Parkinsonisme na toevoeging van fluoxetine aan behandeling met neuroleptica of carbamazepine. *Ned Tijdschr Geneeskd* (1992) 136, 332–4.
2. Syvälahti EKG, Taiminen T, Saarijärvi S, Lehto H, Niemi H, Ahola V, Dahl M-L, Salokangas RKR. Citalopram causes no significant alterations in plasma neuroleptic levels in schizophrenic patients. *J Int Med Res* (1997) 25, 24–32.
3. Davies SJC, Westin AA, Castberg I, Lewis G, Lennard MS, Taylor S, Spigset O. Characterisation of zuclopenthixol metabolism by *in vitro* and therapeutic drug monitoring studies. *Acta Psychiatr Scand* (2010) 122, 444–53.
4. Linnet K, Wiborg O. Influence of Cyp2D6 genetic polymorphism on ratios of steady-state serum concentration to dose of the neuroleptic zuclopenthixol. *Ther Drug Monit* (1996) 18, 629–34.
5. Coulter DM, Pillans PI. Fluoxetine and extrapyramidal side effects. *Am J Psychiatry* (1995) 152, 122–5.
6. Bouchard RH, Pourcher E, Vincent P. Fluoxetine and extrapyramidal side effects. *Am J Psychiatry* (1989) 146, 1352–3.
7. Jaanson P, Marandi T, Kiivet R-A, Vasar V, Vään S, Svensson J-O, Dahl M-L. Maintenance therapy with zuclopenthixol decanoate: associations between plasma concentrations, neurological side effects and CYP2D6 genotype. *Psychopharmacology (Berl)* (2002) 162, 67–73.

Haloperidol + Alosetron

Alosetron does not alter the pharmacokinetics of haloperidol.

Clinical evidence, mechanism, importance and management

A placebo-controlled study in 10 patients taking haloperidol found that alosetron 1 mg daily, given during weeks 2 and 3 of the 8-week study period, did not alter the pharmacokinetics of haloperidol.[1] No haloperidol dose adjustment would be expected to be needed on starting alosetron.

1. Gupta SK, Kunka RL, Metz A, Lloyd T, Rudolph G, Perel JM. Effect of alosetron (a new 5-HT_3 receptor antagonist) on the pharmacokinetics of haloperidol in schizophrenic patients. *J Clin Pharmacol* (1995) 35, 202–7.

Haloperidol + Amfetamines

Acute dystonia occurred in two healthy subjects when they were given haloperidol with dexamfetamine. Haloperidol inhibits the central stimulant effects of amfetamines.

Clinical evidence, mechanism, importance and management

Two healthy young women were given haloperidol 5 mg and **dexamfetamine** 5 mg as part of a neuropharmacological study. After 29 hours one of them developed stiffness of her neck and limbs, parkinsonian facies, her tongue protruded, and she had oropharyngeal spasm. After 34 hours the other woman developed an oculogyric crisis and acute dystonia of the neck with her back slightly arched. Both recovered rapidly after being given 10 mg of intramuscular procyclidine.[1]

The reasons for this interaction are not fully understood, but it might be due to acute dopamine receptor blockade with a secondary increase in dopamine release on supersensitive receptors. The general importance of these isolated cases is unclear.

The manufacturers of **amfetamine**, **dexamfetamine** and **lisdexamfetamine** state that haloperidol inhibits the central stimulant effects of amfetamines by blocking dopamine and noradrenaline re-uptake.[2-4] Therefore these amfetamines might be less effective in those taking haloperidol. Be alert for this effect on concurrent use.

1. Capstick C, Checkley S, Gray J, Dawe S. Dystonia induced by amphetamine and haloperidol. *Br J Psychiatry* (1994) 165, 276.
2. Adderall XR (Mixed salts of amphetamine and dextroamphetamine). Shire US Inc. US Prescribing information, April 2015.
3. Dexedrine (Dextroamphetamine sulfate). Amedra Pharmaceuticals, LLC. US Prescribing information, October 2013.
4. Vyvanse (Lisdexamfetamine dimesylate). Shire US Inc. US Prescribing information, January 2012.

Haloperidol + Antacids

Anecdotal evidence suggests that antacids might reduce the effects of haloperidol, but there seem to be no clinical studies or reports confirming this.

Clinical evidence, mechanism, importance and management

In 1982 a questioner in a letter asked whether haloperidol interacts with antacids because he had a patient responding well to treatment with haloperidol who had begun to deteriorate when **aluminium hydroxide** (*Amphojel*) was added. In a written answer it was stated[1] that there are no reports of this interaction but several clinicians had said that based on clinical impressions oral haloperidol and antacids should not be given together.

With other antacid interactions, separating the doses by as much as possible (one to 2 hours) to avoid admixture in the gut usually minimises any effects. This might be of use if haloperidol appears to be less effective when an antacid is taken.

1. Goldstein BJ. Interaction of antacids with psychotropics. *Hosp Community Psychiatry* (1982) 33, 96.

Haloperidol and related drugs + Azoles

Itraconazole increases the plasma concentration of haloperidol and bromperidol, and their reduced metabolites.

Clinical evidence

(a) Bromperidol

A study in 8 patients found that the plasma concentration of bromperidol 12 mg or 24 mg daily were increased by **itraconazole** 200 mg daily for 7 days. The average increase was about 87%, but there was wide variation between patients, with some being unaffected and others having increases of up to 4-fold. Concentrations of the reduced metabolite (formed by reduction of the ketone group to a secondary alcohol; also called reduced bromperidol), were also increased, up to 5.2-fold.[1]

(b) Haloperidol

A study in 13 patients with schizophrenia taking haloperidol 6 mg or 12 mg twice daily found an increase in the concentration of haloperidol and its reduced metabolite, reduced haloperidol, when **itraconazole** 200 mg daily was given for 7 days. Haloperidol concentrations were increased by 30%, and the concentration of its reduced metabolite was increased by 24%. There was also an increase in neurological adverse effects during the use of **itraconazole.**[2]

In a randomised study, 15 healthy subjects were given **itraconazole** 200 mg twice daily for 10 days with a single 5-mg dose of haloperidol on day 7. **Itraconazole** increased the AUC of haloperidol by 55% in the 8 subjects with normal CYP2D6 activity and increased it nearly 2-fold in the 7 subjects with reduced CYP2D6 activity (intermediate metabolisers). Itraconazole tended to increase neurological adverse effect scores in those subjects with reduced CYP2D6 activity. No important changes in QT prolongation were seen.[3]

Mechanism

It is likely that itraconazole inhibited the metabolism of bromperidol and haloperidol by CYP3A4. It has been suggested that this interaction might be of more importance in those patients who have lower CYP2D6 activity, (which is generally considered to be involved in the metabolism of haloperidol), because CYP3A4, which is inhibited by itraconazole, will then become more important in haloperidol metabolism.[3]

Importance and management

The clinical importance of the raised butyrophenone concentrations with itraconazole is unclear, although one study found an increase in neurological adverse effects on concurrent use. It might be prudent to monitor concurrent use, decreasing the haloperidol or bromperidol dose if adverse effects (e.g. sedation, agitation, movement disorders) become troublesome. It is likely that other azoles that are potent inhibitors of CYP3A4, such as **ketoconazole**, would interact similarly, but this does not appear to have been studied. See *Azoles*, under 'Anthelmintics, Antifungals, and Antiprotozoals', p.225) for more on the enzyme-inhibitory properties of the azoles.

1. Furukori H, Kondo T, Yasui N, Otani K, Tokinaga N, Nagashima U, Kaneko S, Inoue Y. Effects of itraconazole on the steady-state plasma concentrations of bromperidol and reduced bromperidol in schizophrenic patients. *Psychopharmacology (Berl)* (1999) 145, 189–92.
2. Yasui N, Kondo T, Otani K, Furukori H, Mihara K, Suzuki A, Kaneko S, Inoue Y. Effects of itraconazole on the steady-state plasma concentrations of haloperidol and its reduced metabolite in schizophrenic patients: in vivo evidence of the involvement of CYP3A4 for haloperidol metabolism. *J Clin Psychopharmacol* (1999) 19, 149–54.
3. Park J-Y, Shon J-H, Kim K-A, Jung H-J, Shim J-C, Yoon Y-R, Cha I-J, Shin J-G. Combined effects of itraconazole and CYP2D6*10 genetic polymorphism on the pharmacokinetics and pharmacodynamics of haloperidol in healthy subjects. *J Clin Psychopharmacol* (2006) 26, 135–42.

Haloperidol + Buspirone

Two studies found that buspirone appeared to cause a minor increase in the plasma concentrations of haloperidol, whereas another study suggested that no interaction occurred.

Clinical evidence, mechanism, importance and management

In a pharmacokinetic study in 11 patients with schizophrenia taking haloperidol 10 to 30 mg daily found that buspirone 5 mg three times daily for 2 weeks, followed by 10 mg three times daily for 4 weeks, did not alter the pharmacokinetics of haloperidol or its reduced metabolite.[1] In a further study in 27 patients, the same dose of buspirone increased the steady-state plasma concentration of haloperidol by 6% from baseline values, which was not statistically significant.[1]

These findings contrast with those of a study in which there was an increase in the steady-state concentration of haloperidol of 26% six weeks after starting buspirone: 6 out of 7 patients with schizophrenia had 15 to 122% rises in their plasma concentration of haloperidol, and one patient had a 5% decrease.[2] The authors also mention a single-dose study in healthy subjects, which found a 30% rise in haloperidol concentrations when subjects were given buspirone.[2]

The interaction between haloperidol and buspirone is not established, with the findings principally from uncontrolled studies. The increases in haloperidol concentrations seen were generally minor, and no adverse reactions have been reported. Until more is known, bear the possibility of a pharmacokinetic interaction in mind when interpreting clinical changes after giving buspirone to a patient taking haloperidol.[2]

1. Huang HF, Jann MW, Wei F-C, Chang T-P, Chen J-S, Juang D-J, Lin S-K, Lam YFW, Chien C-P, Chang W-H. Lack of pharmacokinetic interaction between buspirone and haloperidol in patients with schizophrenia. *J Clin Pharmacol* (1996) 36, 963–9.
2. Goff DC, Midha KK, Brotman AW, McCormick S, Waites M, Amico ET. An open trial of buspirone added to neuroleptics in schizophrenic patients. *J Clin Psychopharmacol* (1991) 11, 193–7.

Haloperidol and related drugs + Carbamazepine and related drugs

Haloperidol and bromperidol plasma concentrations are reduced by carbamazepine. The plasma concentration of haloperidol increased after carbamazepine was switched to oxcarbazepine. One study found that haloperidol raises carbamazepine concentrations.

Neurotoxicity has been seen in patients taking haloperidol and carbamazepine.

Clinical evidence

(a) Bromperidol

When 13 patients with schizophrenia taking bromperidol 12 or 24 mg daily were given carbamazepine 200 mg twice daily for 4 weeks, the plasma concentrations of bromperidol and reduced bromperidol (a metabolite formed by the reduction of the ketone group of bromperidol to a secondary alcohol) were decreased by 37% and 23%, respectively. Despite this reduction in plasma concentration, the Clinical Global Impression scores (a measure of illness severity) fell slightly, suggesting an improvement in disease control.[1]

(b) Haloperidol

A study in 9 patients with schizophrenia taking haloperidol (average dose 30 mg daily) found a 55% reduction in plasma haloperidol concentrations (from 45.5 nanograms/mL to 21.2 nanograms/mL) when they were given carbamazepine for 5 weeks (precise dose not stated). They also took trihexyphenidyl 10 mg daily and oxazepam 30 mg at night, as necessary. Carbamazepine serum concentrations and the control of the disease remained unchanged.[2] In another study, 11 patients taking haloperidol 6 mg twice daily were given carbamazepine, with the daily dose increased at fortnightly intervals from 100 to 300 and then 600 mg. Carbamazepine caused a dose-dependent reduction in haloperidol concentrations: reductions of 25% (9 patients), 61% (10 patients), and 82% (11 patients), with 100 mg, 300 mg and 600 mg respectively.[3]

Three patients had 2- to 5-fold increases in plasma haloperidol concentrations with clinical improvement when carbamazepine 1.2 to 1.4 g daily was stopped, but extrapyramidal adverse effects developed within one to 30 days.[4] Similarly, a report describes 3 patients with difficult to treat schizophrenia taking haloperidol, whose treatment was changed from carbamazepine to oxcarbazepine. After 2 weeks their plasma haloperidol concentrations had dramatically risen (from 6 nanomol/L to 18 nanomol/L, from 6 nanomol/L to 14 nanomol/L, and from 17 nanomol/L to 27 nanomol/L, respectively). This was also accompanied by severe extrapyramidal adverse effects, which necessitated dose reductions in 2 of the patients.[5]

Other studies and reports have found 40 to 60% reductions in plasma haloperidol concentrations in patients taking carbamazepine,[6-10] with the occasional patient having undetectable concentrations.[7,11] Decreases in plasma haloperidol concentrations of unspecified amounts have also been described.[12-15] Haloperidol clearance was found to be increased by 32% in a retrospective study in 48 patients who were also taking enzyme-inducing antiepileptics, which included carbamazepine.[16]

A few patients have had clinical worsening or increased adverse effects,[7-9,11] and three cases of neurotoxicity (drowsiness, slurred speech, confusion)[12,17,18] have also been described in patients taking haloperidol and carbamazepine. One retrospective study found that the incidence of QT prolongation in patients taking haloperidol and carbamazepine was 52% compared with 7% in those taking haloperidol without carbamazepine.[19]

A study in Japanese patients with schizophrenia found that haloperidol raised serum carbamazepine concentrations by about 30%, despite a 25% dose reduction.[13]

Mechanism

Carbamazepine is a recognised enzyme inducer and therefore it seems likely that the reduced plasma bromperidol and haloperidol concentrations occur because their metabolism is increased by carbamazepine.

The reason for the raised carbamazepine concentration with haloperidol is not understood.

Importance and management

The interactions of haloperidol with **carbamazepine** are well documented and appear to be clinically important, but only a few patients have been reported to show clinical worsening. Although there are advantages in giving carbamazepine with haloperidol in some patients[20] be alert for the need to increase the haloperidol dose. A study, in which intramuscular haloperidol was used, recommended shortening the interval between injections rather than raising the dose, but it was not stated by how much.[21] Also be alert for the development of dystonic reactions and for a rise in serum carbamazepine concentrations. Similar precautions might be needed with bromperidol, but this needs confirmation.

The situation with **oxcarbazepine** is not clear. The limited evidence from the case reports above suggest that it might not interact with haloperidol to the same extent as carbamazepine; however, further controlled study is needed to confirm this.

1. Otani K, Ishida M, Yasui N, Kondo T, Mihara K, Suzuki A, Furukori H, Kaneko S, Inoue Y. Interaction between carbamazepine and bromperidol. *Eur J Clin Pharmacol* (1997) 53, 219–22.
2. Kidron R, Averbuch I, Klein E, Belmaker RH. Carbamazepine-induced reduction of blood levels of haloperidol in chronic schizophrenia. *Biol Psychiatry* (1985) 20, 219–22.
3. Yasui-Furukori N, Kondo T, Mihara K, Suziki A, Inoue Y, Kaneko S. Significant dose effect of carbamazepine on reduction of steady-state plasma concentration of haloperidol in schizophrenic patients. *J Clin Psychopharmacol* (2003) 23, 435–40.
4. Jann MW, Fidone GS, Hernandez JM, Amrung S, Davis CM. Clinical implications of increased antipsychotic plasma concentrations upon anticonvulsant cessation. *Psychiatry Res* (1989) 28, 153–9.
5. Raitasuo V, Lehtovaara R, Huttunen MO. Effect of switching carbamazepine to oxcarbazepine on the plasma levels of neuroleptics. A case report. *Psychopharmacology (Berl)* (1994) 116, 115–16.
6. Jann MW, Ereshefsky L, Saklad SR, Seidel DR, Davis CM, Burch NR, Bowden CL. Effects of carbamazepine on plasma haloperidol levels. *J Clin Psychopharmacol* (1985) 5, 106–9.
7. Arana GW, Goff DC, Friedman H, Ornsteen M, Greenblatt DJ, Black B, Shader RI. Does carbamazepine-induced reduction of plasma haloperidol levels worsen psychotic symptoms? *Am J Psychiatry* (1986) 143, 650–1.
8. Kahn EM, Schulz SC, Perel JM, Alexander JE. Change in haloperidol level due to carbamazepine—a complicating factor in combined medication for schizophrenia. *J Clin Psychopharmacol* (1990) 10, 54–7.
9. Hesslinger B, Normann C, Langosch JM, Klose P, Berger M, Walden J. Effects of carbamazepine and valproate on haloperidol plasma levels and on psychopathologic outcome in schizophrenic patients. *J Clin Psychopharmacol* (1999) 19, 310–15.
10. Nisijima K, Kusakabe Y, Ohtuka K, Ishiguro T. Addition of carbamazepine to long-term treatment with neuroleptics may induce neuroleptic malignant syndrome. *Biol Psychiatry* (1998) 44, 930–1.
11. Fast DK, Jones BD, Kusalic M, Erickson M. Effect of carbamazepine on neuroleptic plasma levels and efficacy. *Am J Psychiatry* (1986) 143, 117–18.
12. Brayley J, Yellowlees P. An interaction between haloperidol and carbamazepine in a patient with cerebral palsy. *Aust N Z J Psychiatry* (1987) 21, 605–7.
13. Iwahashi K, Miyatake R, Suwaki H, Hosokawa K, Ichikawa Y. The drug–drug interaction effects of haloperidol on plasma carbamazepine levels. *Clin Neuropharmacol* (1995) 18, 233–6.
14. Jann MW, Chang W-H, Lane H-Y. Differences in haloperidol epidemiologic pharmacokinetic studies. *J Clin Psychopharmacol* (2001) 21, 628–30.
15. Hirokane G, Someya T, Takahashi S, Morita S, Shimoda K. Interindividual variation of plasma haloperidol concentrations and the impact of concomitant medications: the analysis of therapeutic drug monitoring data. *Ther Drug Monit* (1999) 21, 82–6.
16. Yukawa E, Hokazono T, Funakoshi A, Yukawa M, Ohdo S, Higuchi S, Ichimaru R, Maki T, Matsunaga K, Anai M, Goto Y. Epidemiologic investigation of the relative clearance of haloperidol by mixed-effect modelling using routine clinical pharmacokinetic data in Japanese patients. *J Clin Psychopharmacol* (2000) 20, 685–90.
17. Kanter GL, Yerevanian BI, Ciccone JR. Case report of a possible interaction between neuroleptics and carbamazepine. *Am J Psychiatry* (1984) 141, 1101–2.
18. Yerevanian BI, Hodgman CH. A haloperidol-carbamazepine interaction in a patient with rapid-cycling bipolar disorder. *Am J Psychiatry* (1985) 142, 785–6.
19. Iwahashi K, Nakamura K, Miyatake R, Suwaki H, Hosokawa K. Cardiac effects of haloperidol and carbamazepine treatment. *Am J Psychiatry* (1996) 153, 135.
20. Klein E, Bental E, Lerer B, Belmaker RH. Carbamazepine and haloperidol *v* placebo and haloperidol in excited psychoses: a controlled study. *Arch Gen Psychiatry* (1984) 41, 165–70.
21. Pupeschi G, Agenet C, Levron J-C, Barges-Bertocchio M-H. Do enzyme inducers modify haloperidol decanoate rate of release? *Prog Neuropsychopharmacol Biol Psychiatry* (1994) 18, 1323–32.

Haloperidol + Chlorpromazine

Some patients might have a large increase in haloperidol concentrations when they are also given chlorpromazine. A single case report describes severe tardive dyskinesia in a patient taking haloperidol long-term and given chlorpromazine.

Clinical evidence

In a study, haloperidol was given to 43 patients in doses of 2 to 21 mg daily for 2 months, and then chlorpromazine 50 to 300 mg daily was added for a further 2 months. Haloperidol plasma concentrations were increased by 29% on concurrent use and the concentrations of its reduced metabolite, reduced haloperidol, were increased 2.6-fold. However, the variation in effect was large.[1]

A case report describes a 37-year-old woman with schizophrenia, taking chlorpromazine 100 mg at night long-term and depot injections of haloperidol 50 mg monthly, who developed lip smacking and orofacial movements, which were mild and intermittent at first, but progressively worsened. On admission, a diagnosis of catatonic schizophrenia was made. Both haloperidol and chlorpromazine were stopped and she was given trihexyphenidyl. Subsequently, a diagnosis of tardive dyskinesia due to the combined effects of haloperidol and chlorpromazine was made, and trihexyphenidyl (which might induce or aggravate this condition) was also stopped. She was treated with diazepam and discharged at the request of her family, despite little improvement in her condition. The outcome is unknown as the patient did not return for follow-up appointments.[2]

Mechanism

Unknown. It was suggested that chlorpromazine might raise haloperidol concentrations by inhibiting haloperidol metabolism by CYP2D6. In addition, this isoenzyme is known to be associated with genetic polymorphism (see 'Genetic factors in drug metabolism', p.8), and this might contribute to the large inter-individual variation seen.[1] However, note that chlorpromazine is not an established inhibitor of CYP2D6, and the involvement of CYP2D6 in the metabolism of haloperidol is inconclusive, see under *Haloperidol*, in 'Antipsychotics, Anxiolytics, and Hypnotics', p.803.

Importance and management

Information on the effect of chlorpromazine on the pharmacokinetics of haloperidol is limited. Nevertheless, it seems possible that some patients might be at risk of developing adverse effects related to increased haloperidol concentrations when taking chlorpromazine. Concurrent use need not be avoided, but consider this interaction if haloperidol adverse effects (e.g. sedation, agitation, movement disorders) become troublesome.

Tardive dyskinesia is a known adverse effect of antipsychotics such as haloperidol and chlorpromazine; however, whether this case represents an interaction is unknown.

Haloperidol is a well known QT-prolonger, and there are isolated reports of torsade de pointes with chlorpromazine, therefore, bear in mind the potential for additive effects on the QT interval, see 'Drugs that prolong the QT interval + Other drugs that prolong the QT interval', p.272.

1. Suzuki Y, Someya T, Shimoda K, Hirokane G, Morita S, Yokono A, Inoue Y, Takahashi S. Importance of the cytochrome P450 2D6 genotype for the drug metabolic interaction between chlorpromazine and haloperidol. *Ther Drug Monit* (2001) 23, 363–8.
2. Atwoli L, Manguro G, Owiti P, Ndambuki D. Neuroleptic induced tardive dyskinesia in a patient on treatment for schizophrenia: case report. *East Afr Med J* (2009) 86, 354–6.

Haloperidol + Granisetron

Granisetron does not appear to increase the sedating effects of haloperidol.

Clinical evidence, mechanism, importance and management

A study in 12 healthy subjects found that, while haloperidol 3 mg alone caused some impaired psychometric performance (increased drowsiness, muzziness, lethargy, mental slowness, etc.), the addition of granisetron 160 micrograms/kg did not seem to worsen performance to a clinically relevant extent.[1] If granisetron is required in a patient taking haloperidol, no additional sedative effects would be expected.

Note that haloperidol can cause QT-interval prolongation, and granisetron has, rarely, been reported to prolong the QT interval; see '5-HT_3-receptor antagonists + Drugs that prolong the QT interval', p.1146, for further information.

1. Leigh TJ, Link CGG, Fell GL. Effects of granisetron and haloperidol, alone and in combination, on psychometric performance and the EEG. *Br J Clin Pharmacol* (1992) 34, 65–70.

Haloperidol + Grapefruit juice

Grapefruit juice does not alter the steady-state concentration of haloperidol.

Clinical evidence, mechanism, importance and management

In a study in 12 patients with schizophrenia taking oral haloperidol 6 mg twice daily, the consumption of 200 mL of regular-strength grapefruit juice three times daily for 7 days (with the morning and evening drink taken at the same time as the haloperidol) did not affect the steady-state concentration of haloperidol.[1] No haloperidol dose adjustment would be expected to be needed if a patient starts drinking grapefruit juice.

1. Yasui N, Kondo T, Suzuki A, Otani K, Mihara K, Furukori H, Kaneko S, Inoue Y. Lack of significant pharmacokinetic interaction between haloperidol and grapefruit juice. *Int Clin Psychopharmacol* (1999) 14, 113–18.

Haloperidol + Imipenem

Marked but transient hypotension was seen when three patients receiving intravenous imipenem were given intravenous haloperidol.

Clinical evidence, mechanism, importance and management

Three patients in intensive care who were receiving intravenous imipenem 500 mg (with cilastatin) every 6 hours for 2, 3, and 7 days, respectively, developed a rapid and short-lived episode of hypotension when they were given a 2.5-mg dose of intravenous haloperidol. For example, the blood pressure of one of the patients fell from 117/75 mmHg to 91/49 mmHg. After 30 minutes her blood pressure had risen to 100/57 mmHg. No treatment for hypotension was given to any of the patients and the reaction was brief and self-limiting. Two of the patients were also taking famotidine and erythromycin. No acute ECG changes were seen.[1]

The reason for this fall in blood pressure is not understood, but the authors attribute what happened to the concurrent use of haloperidol and imipenem, although they point out that intravenous haloperidol alone can cause orthostatic hypotension. One suggestion is that competitive protein binding displacement might have transiently increased the concentration of free haloperidol,[1] although this has been questioned. Furthermore, it has been suggested that the clinical condition of the patients could have had a greater part to play in the development of hypotension than any drug interaction.[2]

The authors advise that if intravenous haloperidol is given to patients receiving imipenem, low doses should be used, and the outcome well monitored. They state that no pressor agent was needed in these cases, but they suggest the possible use of metaraminol, phenylephrine or noradrenaline (norepinephrine) rather than dopamine, the vasopressor effects of which might be blocked or reversed by haloperidol.[1]

1. Franco-Bronson K, Gajwani P. Hypotension associated with intravenous haloperidol and imipenem. *J Clin Psychopharmacol* (1999) 19, 480–1.
2. Hauben M. Comments on "Hypotension associated with intravenous haloperidol and imipenem". *J Clin Psychopharmacol* (2001) 21, 345–7.

Haloperidol + Indometacin

Profound drowsiness and confusion has developed in patients given haloperidol with indometacin.

Clinical evidence, mechanism, importance and management

A crossover study in 20 patients, designed to find out the possible advantages of giving haloperidol 5 mg daily with indometacin 25 mg three times daily, was eventually abandoned because 13 patients (11 taking haloperidol and 2 taking placebo) failed to complete the study. Profound drowsiness or tiredness caused 6 of the patients taking haloperidol to withdraw. The authors of this paper stated that the concurrent use of indometacin produced drowsiness and confusion greater than anything expected with haloperidol alone, which was sufficiently severe that in some cases independent functioning was affected.[1]

Evidence for an interaction between haloperidol and indometacin appears to be very limited. If concurrent use is thought appropriate, consider warning patients about this potentially severe effect. It might be wiser to avoid concurrent use because many patients requiring this type of treatment might not be hospitalised and under the day-to-day scrutiny of the prescriber.

1. Bird HA, Le Gallez P, Wright V. Drowsiness due to haloperidol/indomethacin in combination. *Lancet* (1983) i, 830–1.

Haloperidol and related drugs + Lithium

The development of severe extrapyramidal adverse effects and severe neurotoxicity has been seen in one or more patients given lithium with bromperidol or haloperidol. Successful and uneventful use of haloperidol and lithium has also been described.

Clinical evidence

A large-scale retrospective study of the literature over the period 1966 to 1996 using the Medline database identified 41 cases of neurotoxic adverse effects in 41 patients with low therapeutic concentrations of lithium. Of these patients, 10 were taking haloperidol.[1] Another retrospective study using both Medline and the spontaneous reporting system of the FDA in the US, over the period 1969 to 1994, identified 237 cases of severe neurotoxicity involving lithium, of which one also involved the concurrent use of **bromperidol** and 59 also involved the concurrent use of haloperidol.[2,3]

Other reports describe encephalopathic syndromes (lethargy, fever, tremulousness, confusion, extrapyramidal and cerebellar dysfunction),[4] neuromuscular symptoms, impaired consciousness and hyperthermia,[5] delirium, severe extrapyramidal symptoms and organic brain damage,[6-17] and neuroleptic malignant syndrome[18] in patients taking haloperidol with lithium. In one study it was found that of the 13 patients who were taking haloperidol, 5 developed neurotoxic reactions, and they were receiving higher doses of haloperidol (average dose was 59 mg) than the 8 patients who did not develop such symptoms (average dose was 34.9 mg).[19] In another study in 10 patients with extrapyramidal symptoms, 3 of whom were taking haloperidol, the addition of lithium worsened their symptoms.[20] The sudden emergence of extrapyramidal or other adverse effects with lithium and haloperidol has also been described in other studies.[1,6,21]

In contrast to the reports cited above, there are others describing successful and uneventful use.[4,22-25] A retrospective search of Danish hospital records found that 425 patients had taken both drugs and none of them had developed serious adverse reactions.[26] For mention of a patient who took haloperidol and lithium without problem, but subsequently experienced neurotoxicity with fluphenazine and lithium, see 'Phenothiazines + Lithium', p.873.

A small rise in serum lithium concentrations occurs in the presence of haloperidol, but it is almost certainly of little or no clinical importance.[27]

Mechanism

Not understood. Just why severe neurotoxicity and other adverse effects sometimes develop in patients taking lithium and antipsychotics is not understood. It is the subject of considerable discussion and debate.[1-3,28,29]

Importance and management

The development of severe neurotoxic or severe extrapyramidal adverse effects with haloperidol and lithium appears to be uncommon and unexplained; and the evidence of an interaction between bromperidol and lithium is limited to one case. However, be alert for any evidence of toxicity if lithium is given with either of these drugs. One recommendation is that the onset of neurological manifestations, such as excessive drowsiness or movement disorders, warrants electroencephalography without delay and withdrawal of the drugs, especially as irreversible effects have been seen. A review[30] suggests that the concurrent use of haloperidol seems to be safe if lithium concentrations are below 1 mmol/L.

At the moment there seems to be no way of identifying the apparently small number of patients who are particularly at risk, but possible likely factors include a previous history of extrapyramidal reactions with antipsychotics and the use of large doses of the antipsychotic.

1. Emilien G, Maloteaux JM. Lithium neurotoxicity at low therapeutic doses: hypotheses for causes and mechanism of action following a retrospective analysis of published case reports. *Acta Neurol Belg* (1996) 96, 281–93.
2. Goldman SA. Lithium and neuroleptics in combination: is there enhancement of neurotoxicity leading to permanent sequelae? *J Clin Pharmacol* (1996) 36, 951–62.
3. Goldman SA. FDA MedWatch Report: lithium and neuroleptics in combination: the spectrum of neurotoxicity. *Psychopharmacol Bull* (1996) 32, 299–309.
4. Cohen WJ, Cohen NH. Lithium carbonate, haloperidol, and irreversible brain damage. *JAMA* (1974) 230, 1283–7.
5. Thornton WE, Pray BJ. Lithium intoxication: a report of two cases. *Can Psychiatr Assoc J* (1975) 20, 281–2.
6. Kamlana SH, Kerry RJ, Khan IA. Lithium: some drug interactions. *Practitioner* (1980) 224, 1291–2.
7. Fetzer J, Kader G, Danahy S. Lithium encephalopathy: a clinical, psychiatric, and EEG evaluation. *Am J Psychiatry* (1981) 138, 1622–3.
8. Marhold J, Zimanová J, Lachman M, Král J, Vojtěchovský M. To the incompatibility of haloperidol with lithium salts. *Act Nerv Super (Praha)* (1974) 16, 199–200.
9. Wilson WH. Addition of lithium to haloperidol in non-affective antipsychotic non-responsive schizophrenia: a double blind, placebo controlled, parallel design clinical trial. *Psychopharmacology (Berl)* (1993) 111, 359–66.
10. Loudon JB, Waring H. Toxic reactions to lithium and haloperidol. *Lancet* (1976) ii, 1088.
11. Juhl RP, Tsuang MT, Perry PJ. Concomitant administration of haloperidol and lithium carbonate in acute mania. *Dis Nerv Syst* (1977) 38, 675.
12. Spring G, Frankel M. New data on lithium and haloperidol incompatibility. *Am J Psychiatry* (1981) 138, 818–21.
13. Menes C, Burra P, Hoaken PCS. Untoward effects following combined neuroleptic-lithium therapy. *Can J Psychiatry* (1980) 25, 573–6.
14. Keitner GI, Rahman S. Reversible neurotoxicity with combined lithium-haloperidol administration. *J Clin Psychopharmacol* (1984) 4, 104–5.
15. Thomas CJ. Brain damage with lithium/haloperidol. *Br J Psychiatry* (1979) 134, 552.
16. Thomas C, Tatham A, Jakubowski S. Lithium/haloperidol combinations and brain damage. *Lancet* (1982) i, 626.
17. Sandyk R, Hurwitz MD. Toxic irreversible encephalopathy induced by lithium carbonate and haloperidol. A report of 2 cases. *S Afr Med J* (1983) 64, 875–6.
18. Susman VL, Addonizio G. Reinduction of neuroleptic malignant syndrome by lithium. *J Clin Psychopharmacol* (1987) 7, 339–41.
19. Miller F, Menninger J. Correlation of neuroleptic dose and neurotoxicity in patients given lithium and a neuroleptic. *Hosp Community Psychiatry* (1987) 38, 1219–21.
20. Addonizio G, Roth SD, Stokes PE, Stoll PM. Increased extrapyramidal symptoms with addition of lithium to neuroleptics. *J Nerv Ment Dis* (1988) 176, 682–5.

21. Prakash R, Kelwala S, Ban TA. Neurotoxicity with combined administration of lithium and a neuroleptic. *Compr Psychiatry* (1982) 23, 567–71.
22. Garfinkel PE, Stancer HC, Persad E. A comparison of haloperidol, lithium carbonate and their combination in the treatment of mania. *J Affect Disord* (1980) 2, 279–88.
23. Baptista T. Lithium-neuroleptics combination and irreversible brain damage. *Acta Psychiatr Scand* (1986) 73, 111.
24. Goldney RD, Spence ND. Safety of the combination of lithium and neuroleptic drugs. *Am J Psychiatry* (1986) 143, 882–4.
25. Biederman J, Lerner Y, Belmaker H. Combination of lithium and haloperidol in schizo-affective disorder. A controlled study. *Arch Gen Psychiatry* (1979) 36, 327–33.
26. Baastrup PC, Hollnagel P, Sørensen R, Schou M. Adverse reactions in treatment with lithium carbonate and haloperidol. *JAMA* (1976) 236, 2645–6.
27. Schaffer CB, Batra K, Garvey MJ, Mungas DM, Schaffer LC. The effect of haloperidol on serum levels of lithium in adult manic patients. *Biol Psychiatry* (1984) 19, 1495–9.
28. Geisler A, Klysner R. Combined effect of lithium and flupenthixol on striatal adenylate cyclase. *Lancet* (1977) i, 430–1.
29. von Knorring L. Possible mechanisms for the presumed interaction between lithium and neuroleptics. *Hum Psychopharmacol* (1990) 5, 287–92.
30. Batchelor DH, Lowe MR. Reported neurotoxicity with the lithium/haloperidol combination and other neuroleptics—a literature review. *Hum Psychopharmacol* (1990) 5, 275–80.

Haloperidol + Nefazodone

Nefazodone slightly increases haloperidol exposure.

Clinical evidence, mechanism, importance and management

In a placebo-controlled study in 12 healthy subjects, nefazodone 200 mg twice daily for about 8 days increased the AUC of haloperidol 5 mg daily, given on days 7 and 8, by 36%, but its maximum plasma concentrations were unaltered.[1] Nefazodone is an inhibitor of CYP3A4, by which haloperidol is partially metabolised. It seems unlikely that this change in haloperidol exposure is enough to be of clinical relevance and therefore no haloperidol dose adjustment seems necessary on concurrent use.

1. Barbhaiya RH, Shukla UA, Greene DS, Breuel H-P, Midha KK. Investigation of pharmacokinetic and pharmacodynamic interactions after coadministration of nefazodone and haloperidol. *J Clin Psychopharmacol* (1996) 16, 26–34.

Haloperidol + Phenobarbital and/or Phenytoin

Haloperidol plasma concentrations are reduced by phenobarbital and phenytoin.

Clinical evidence

A study in patients with epilepsy, 2 taking phenobarbital, 3 taking phenytoin, and 4 taking both drugs, found that after taking haloperidol 10 mg three times daily for 6 weeks their serum haloperidol concentrations were about half of those in a control group who were not taking antiepileptics (19.4 nanograms/mL compared with 36.6 nanograms/mL). Antiepileptic concentrations remained unchanged.[1] Another report describes a patient who had a large rise in serum haloperidol concentrations and clinical improvement when phenytoin 300 mg daily was stopped.[2] Haloperidol clearance was increased by 32% in a study in patients who were also taking enzyme-inducing antiepileptics, which included phenobarbital or phenytoin.[3] A retrospective study found that phenobarbital reduced the haloperidol concentration-to-dose ratio, suggesting that phenobarbital might affect the metabolism of haloperidol.[4]

Mechanism

Phenobarbital and phenytoin are recognised enzyme inducers, therefore it seems highly likely that the reduced plasma haloperidol concentrations occur because its metabolism is increased by these antiepileptics.

Importance and management

The pharmacokinetic interactions of haloperidol with phenytoin and phenobarbital are moderately well documented, but the clinical outcome does not appear to have been studied. Be alert for the need to increase the haloperidol dose if either of these antiepileptics is also given. The authors of one study suggest a 2- to 3-fold increase in the haloperidol dose might be needed.[1] Another study, in which intramuscular haloperidol was used, recommended shortening the interval between injections rather than raising the dose, but it was not stated by how much.[5]

1. Linnoila M, Viukari M, Vaisanen K, Auvinen J. Effect of anticonvulsants on plasma haloperidol and thioridazine levels. *Am J Psychiatry* (1980) 137, 819–21.
2. Jann MW, Fidone GS, Hernandez JM, Amrung S, Davis CM. Clinical implications of increased antipsychotic plasma concentrations upon anticonvulsant cessation. *Psychiatry Res* (1989) 28, 153–9.
3. Yukawa E, Hokazono T, Funakoshi A, Yukawa M, Ohdo S, Higuchi S, Ichimaru R, Maki T, Matsunaga K, Anai M, Goto Y. Epidemiologic investigation of the relative clearance of haloperidol by mixed-effect modelling using routine clinical pharmacokinetic data in Japanese patients. *J Clin Psychopharmacol* (2000) 20, 685–90.
4. Hirokane G, Someya T, Takahashi S, Morita S, Shimoda K. Interindividual variation of plasma haloperidol concentrations and the impact of concomitant medications: the analysis of therapeutic drug monitoring data. *Ther Drug Monit* (1999) 21, 82–6.
5. Pupeschi G, Agenet C, Levron J-C, Barges-Bertocchio M-H. Do enzyme inducers modify haloperidol decanoate rate of release? *Prog Neuropsychopharmacol Biol Psychiatry* (1994) 18, 1323–32.

Haloperidol + Quinidine

Haloperidol exposure is increased by single-dose quinidine.

Clinical evidence

In a single-dose study in 12 healthy subjects (11 of whom were CYP2D6 extensive metabolisers), quinidine bisulfate 250 mg, taken about one hour before a single 5-mg dose of haloperidol, approximately doubled the maximum plasma concentration and the AUC of haloperidol and increased the AUC of its metabolite, reduced haloperidol, 2.8-fold, without altering its elimination half-life.[1]

Mechanism

Uncertain. Quinidine is a potent inhibitor of CYP2D6, for which haloperidol is generally considered a substrate, although this is not established, see under *Haloperidol*, in 'Antipsychotics, Anxiolytics, and Hypnotics', p.803. However, the lack of effect on elimination half-life in this single-dose study shows that the inter-conversion of haloperidol to reduced haloperidol is not mediated by CYP2D6.[1]

Importance and management

The clinical importance of the interaction between haloperidol and quinidine has not been assessed, but it seems likely that the beneficial and adverse effects of haloperidol will be increased if quinidine is added. Concurrent use need not be avoided, but consider this interaction if haloperidol adverse effects (e.g. sedation, agitation, movement disorders) become troublesome. Of more concern is the potential for additive effects on the QT interval, see 'Drugs that prolong the QT interval + Other drugs that prolong the QT interval', p.272.

1. Young D, Midha KK, Fossler MJ, Hawes EM, Hubbard JW, McKay G, Korchinski ED. Effect of quinidine on the interconversion kinetics between haloperidol and reduced haloperidol in humans: implications for the involvement of cytochrome P450IID6. *Eur J Clin Pharmacol* (1993) 44, 433–8.

Haloperidol + Rifampicin (Rifampin) and/or Isoniazid

The serum concentrations of haloperidol can be reduced by rifampicin alone and when rifampicin is given with isoniazid. High concentrations of haloperidol were seen in some (but not all) patients taking isoniazid alone in one study.

Clinical evidence

In a study in patients with schizophrenia taking haloperidol, the 7 patients taking rifampicin with isoniazid (3 were additionally taking ethambutol) had lower steady-state haloperidol concentrations than those not taking any antimycobacterials. The half-life of haloperidol in 3 patients taking rifampicin with isoniazid was 4.9 hours compared with 9.4 hours in 2 other patients not taking antimycobacterial drugs. In 15 of 18 patients taking isoniazid alone, steady-state haloperidol concentrations did not differ from those in patients not taking antimycobacterials, but the remaining 3 had abnormally high serum haloperidol concentrations.[1]

The minimum serum haloperidol concentration of 15 patients with schizophrenia fell to 37% of the expected concentration after they took rifampicin 600 mg daily for 7 days.[2] After 28 days the serum concentration had dropped further, to 30% of the expected concentration. In another group of 5 patients taking haloperidol and rifampicin, the serum haloperidol concentrations were about 3.3-fold greater than the previous concentration 7 days after rifampicin was stopped, and were 4.3-fold greater 28 days after rifampicin was stopped.[2] The clinical effects of haloperidol appeared to be reduced by rifampicin.[2]

Mechanism

The likeliest explanation for the reduced haloperidol concentrations is that rifampicin, a recognised potent enzyme inducer, increases the metabolism of haloperidol. The reason for the abnormally high haloperidol concentrations seen in just 3 of the 18 patients taking isoniazid alone is unclear. The authors suggest it might be related to acetylator status as the patients with raised haloperidol concentrations were also slow acetylators[1] and this is important in isoniazid metabolism. However, this was not a controlled study, and the finding might be coincidental.

Importance and management

The interaction between haloperidol and rifampicin would appear to be established and clinically important. Be alert for any evidence of reduced haloperidol effects if rifampicin is also given, either alone, or with isoniazid and/or ethambutol, and adjust the haloperidol dose if necessary.

Isoniazid alone did not appear to affect haloperidol concentrations in the majority of patients, but the three cases of high concentrations raises the question of whether it might have an effect in some patients. Nothing further appears to have been published on this possible interaction. Until more is known, it would seem prudent to bear this possibility in mind.

1. Takeda M, Nishinuma K, Yamashita S, Matsubayashi T, Tanino S, Nishimura T. Serum haloperidol levels of schizophrenics receiving treatment for tuberculosis. *Clin Neuropharmacol* (1986) 9, 386–97.
2. Kim Y-H, Cha I-J, Shim J-C, Shin J-G, Yoon Y-R, Kim Y-K, Kim J-I, Park G-H, Jang I-J, Woo J-I, Shin S-G. Effect of rifampin on the plasma concentration and the clinical effect of haloperidol concomitantly administered to schizophrenic patients. *J Clin Psychopharmacol* (1996) 16, 247–52.

Haloperidol + Risperidone

A case report describes neuroleptic malignant syndrome in a patient taking risperidone and haloperidol.

Clinical evidence, mechanism, importance and management

A case report describes a 57-year-old man who had been taking haloperidol 4 mg three times daily uneventfully for several years. At a review, his treatment was changed to risperidone, in increasing doses to 3 mg twice daily, and mirtazapine 15 mg at night. Despite being advised to stop haloperidol when he started risperidone, the patient continued to take haloperidol, and by the third day of concurrent use he had become pyrexial, and exhibited rigidity of his trunk and extremities. He was diagnosed as having neuroleptic malignant syndrome, and so he was given dantrolene, bromocriptine and lorazepam: he recovered over the next 2 months.

The effects seen in this patient were thought to be due to the additive dopamine antagonism caused by both haloperidol and risperidone. Mirtazapine might have also contributed, although the patient only took 2 doses before he was admitted. The authors suggest that if antipsychotic treatment is to be changed, it is advisable to slowly reduce the dose of the old antipsychotic and, simultaneously, slowly increase the dose of the new drug to avoid the risk of a psychotic relapse, and the patient should be closely monitored during this time for signs of neuroleptic malignant syndrome.[1]

1. Reeves RR, Mack JE, Torres RA. Neuroleptic malignant syndrome during a change from haloperidol to risperidone. *Ann Pharmacother* (2001) 35, 698–701.

Haloperidol + Ritonavir

Ritonavir is predicted to raise haloperidol concentrations.

Clinical evidence, mechanism, importance and management

The UK manufacturer of ritonavir predicts that antiretroviral doses of ritonavir might increase the plasma concentrations of haloperidol by inhibiting its metabolism by CYP2D6.[1] Note that ritonavir is also a potent inhibitor of CYP3A4, and there is better evidence that haloperidol is a substrate of CYP3A4 (see 'Haloperidol and related drugs + Azoles', p.859) although it is often considered a substrate of CYP2D6. The manufacturer advises monitoring for haloperidol adverse effects (e.g. sedation, agitation, movement disorders) during concurrent use.[1] Until more is known, this seems a prudent precaution.

1. Norvir Tablets (Ritonavir). AbbVie Ltd. UK Summary of product characteristics, September 2012.

Haloperidol + SSRIs

Fluoxetine and fluvoxamine appear to raise haloperidol concentrations, which might increase its adverse effects. A number of case reports describe extrapyramidal adverse effects following the use of fluoxetine and haloperidol. Sertraline caused a minor increase in haloperidol concentrations in one study, but not another. Sertraline and paroxetine do not alter the impairment of psychomotor performance by haloperidol. Citalopram appears not to alter haloperidol concentrations. Additive QT prolongation is predicted if citalopram, or possibly escitalopram, are given with haloperidol.

Clinical evidence

(a) Citalopram

A study in patients with schizophrenia found that, over a 12-week period, the serum concentrations of haloperidol did not appear to be altered by citalopram 40 mg daily.[1]

(b) Fluoxetine

A woman taking haloperidol 2 to 5 mg daily for 2 years with only occasional mild extrapyramidal symptoms began to experience severe extrapyramidal symptoms (tongue stiffness, parkinsonism, akathisia) shortly after starting to take fluoxetine 40 mg twice daily and was virtually incapacitated for 3 days. Both drugs were stopped and she recovered over a period of one week.[2] Three other patients developed movement disorders after taking both drugs:[3-5] in one case severe antimuscarinic adverse effects also occurred.[4]

A report describes 8 patients who had a 20% rise in plasma haloperidol concentrations when fluoxetine 20 mg daily was added. Although no overall increase in extrapyramidal effects was seen, one patient developed tremor, and another developed akathisia.[6] Similarly 15 patients had an increase of nearly 30% in their haloperidol plasma concentrations after fluoxetine was given, and 5 of the 17 patients had aggravated parkinsonian symptoms.[7] Another report describes a more than 2-fold rise in plasma haloperidol concentrations, accompanied by clinical improvement, in 7 patients given fluoxetine 20 to 40 mg with haloperidol.[8]

(c) Fluvoxamine

A study in 12 patients with schizophrenia found that haloperidol concentrations were increased by 20%, 39%, and 60% by fluvoxamine 25, 75, and 150 mg daily, respectively, which suggested the extent of the interaction was related to the dose of fluvoxamine.[9] A study in 3 patients with schizophrenia found that the addition of fluvoxamine caused their serum haloperidol concentrations to rise, and when fluvoxamine was stopped the concentrations fell. This was not a formal pharmacokinetic study, but while taking fluvoxamine 150 to 200 mg daily, the haloperidol serum concentrations of one patient rose from 17 nanograms/mL to 38 nanograms/mL. The fluvoxamine was then stopped and 54 days later his serum haloperidol concentrations had fallen to 9 nanograms/mL. This patient became lethargic and showed worsening of all of the clinical and cognitive functions assessed while taking these drugs.[10] It should be noted that all three patients were also taking benzatropine, which can cause additive antimuscarinic effects when given with SSRIs (see 'Antimuscarinics + SSRIs', p.754). Another limited study also observed a rise in the serum concentrations of haloperidol in patients taking fluvoxamine.[11]

(d) Paroxetine

In one study the sedative effects and impairment of psychomotor performance caused by haloperidol 3 mg were not increased by paroxetine 30 mg.[12]

(e) Sertraline

In a randomised, placebo-controlled study, 21 healthy subjects were given sertraline 50 mg daily, increased over 7 days to 200 mg daily for 17 days, with a single 2-mg dose of haloperidol on the last day. Overall, sertraline did not appear to worsen the cognitive impairment caused by haloperidol, when compared with placebo.[13]

In a study in 36 hospitalised patients stable taking haloperidol, the addition of sertraline 50 mg daily for 8 weeks had no effect on steady-state haloperidol concentrations or the concentrations of its metabolite, reduced haloperidol, when compared with placebo.[14] In contrast, in an uncontrolled study from the same research group in 16 hospitalised patients who were taking haloperidol, it was reported that the addition of sertraline 50 mg daily for 2 weeks resulted in a 28% increase in plasma haloperidol concentrations, and a 30% reduction in the plasma concentrations of its metabolite, reduced haloperidol.[15]

Mechanism

Uncertain. Movement disorders and raised haloperidol serum concentrations seem most common with fluoxetine, possibly because it inhibits the metabolism of haloperidol by CYP2D6.[16] However, if raised haloperidol concentrations were due to inhibition of CYP2D6 by fluoxetine, then they would also be expected with paroxetine, and a pharmacokinetic interaction with haloperidol does not appear to have been reported for paroxetine. Sertraline has only weak effects on CYP2D6 and an interaction has been reported in one uncontrolled study. Note that, although haloperidol has generally been considered to be a substrate for CYP2D6, the involvement of this isoenzyme in its metabolism is not established, see *Other antipsychotics* under 'Antipsychotics, Anxiolytics, and Hypnotics', p.803.

Fluvoxamine does not inhibit CYP2D6, but it is possible that it might increase haloperidol concentrations by inhibiting other cytochrome P450 isoenzymes.

Importance and management

On the whole, clinically important interactions between haloperidol and **fluoxetine** or **fluvoxamine** appear rare. The combination can be useful and so the isolated cases of extrapyramidal adverse effects should not prevent concurrent use. However, if extrapyramidal effects become troublesome, bear this interaction in mind as a possible cause. The general relevance of the rise in haloperidol concentrations caused by fluoxetine and fluvoxamine is unclear; however, be aware that haloperidol adverse effects (e.g. sedation, agitation, movement disorders) might be increased in some patients and consider reducing the haloperidol dose if problems occur.

Citalopram does not appear to alter haloperidol concentrations; however, the UK manufacturer of citalopram and **escitalopram** predicts that raised haloperidol concentrations might occur.[17,18] In addition, citalopram and escitalopram are associated with a dose-related prolongation in the QT interval and therefore it might be prudent to use an alternative SSRI which is not known to be associated with QT prolongation. For further information on the concurrent use of two or more drugs that prolong the QT interval, see 'Drugs that prolong the QT interval + Other drugs that prolong the QT interval', p.272.

1. Syvälahti EKG, Taiminen T, Saarijärvi S, Lehto H, Niemi H, Ahola V, Dahl M-L, Salokangas RKR. Citalopram causes no significant alterations in plasma neuroleptic levels in schizophrenic patients. *J Int Med Res* (1997) 25, 24–32.
2. Tate JL. Extrapyramidal symptoms in a patient taking haloperidol and fluoxetine. *Am J Psychiatry* (1989) 146, 399–400.
3. Coulter DM, Pillans PI. Fluoxetine and extrapyramidal side effects. *Am J Psychiatry* (1995) 152, 122–5.
4. Benazzi F. Urinary retention with fluoxetine–haloperidol combination in a young patient. *Can J Psychiatry* (1996) 41, 606–7.
5. D'Souza DC, Bennett A, Abi-Dargham A, Krystal JH. Precipitation of a psychoneuromotor syndrome by fluoxetine in a haloperidol-treated schizophrenic patient. *J Clin Psychopharmacol* (1994) 14, 361–3.
6. Goff DC, Midha KK, Brotman AW, Waites M, Baldessarini RJ. Elevation of plasma concentrations of haloperidol after the addition of fluoxetine. *Am J Psychiatry* (1991) 148, 790–2.
7. Shim J-C, Kelly DL, Kim Y-H, Yoon Y-R, Park J-H, Shin J-G, Conley RR. Fluoxetine augmentation of haloperidol in chronic schizophrenia. *J Clin Psychopharmacol* (2003) 23, 520–2.
8. Viala A, Aymard N, Leyris A, Caroli F. Corrélations pharmacocliniques lors de l'administration de fluoxétine chez des patients schizophrènes déprimés traités par halopéridol décanoate. *Therapie* (1996) 51, 19–25.
9. Yasui-Furukori N, Kondo T, Mihara K, Inoue Y, Kaneko S. Fluvoxamine dose-dependent interaction with haloperidol and the effects on negative symptoms in schizophrenia. *Psychopharmacology (Berl)* (2004) 171, 223–7.
10. Daniel DG, Randolph C, Jaskiw G, Handel S, Williams T, Abi-Dargham A, Shoaf S, Egan M, Elkashef A, Liboff S, Linnoila M. Coadministration of fluvoxamine increases serum concentrations of haloperidol. *J Clin Psychopharmacol* (1994) 14, 340–3.
11. Vandel S, Bertschy G, Baumann P, Bouquet S, Bonin B, Francois T, Sechter D, Bizouard P. Fluvoxamine and fluoxetine: Interaction studies with amitriptyline, clomipramine and neuroleptics in phenotyped patients. *Pharmacol Res* (1995) 31, 347–53.
12. Cooper SM, Jackson D, Loudon JM, McClelland GR, Raptopoulos P. The psychomotor effects of paroxetine alone and in combination with haloperidol, amylobarbitone, oxazepam, or alcohol. *Acta Psychiatr Scand* (1989) 80 (Suppl 350), 53–5.
13. Williams SA, Wesnes K, Oliver SD, Rapeport WG. Absence of effect of sertraline on time-based sensitization of cognitive impairment with haloperidol. *J Clin Psychiatry* (1996) 57 (Suppl 1), 7–11.
14. Lee MS, Kim YK, Lee SK, Suh KY. A double-blind study of adjunctive sertraline in haloperidol-stabilized patients with chronic schizophrenia. *J Clin Psychopharmacol* (1998) 18, 399–403.
15. Lee M-S, Han C-S, You Y-W, Kim S-H. Co-administration of sertraline and haloperidol. *Psychiatry Clin Neurosci* (1998) 52, S193–8.
16. Özdemir V, Naranjo CA, Herrmann N, Reed K, Sellers EM, Kalow W. Paroxetine potentiates the central nervous system side effects of perphenazine: contribution of cytochrome P4502D6 inhibition in vivo. *Clin Pharmacol Ther* (1997) 62, 334–47.
17. Cipralex Tablets (Escitalopram oxalate). Lundbeck Ltd. UK Summary of product characteristics, September 2013.
18. Cipramil Tablets (Citalopram hydrobromide). Lundbeck Ltd. UK Summary of product characteristics, July 2015.

Haloperidol + Tobacco

Haloperidol concentrations appear to be reduced by tobacco smoking.

Clinical evidence

In a retrospective review of 50 patients with schizophrenia, steady-state haloperidol concentrations were found to be lower in the 23 patients who were cigarette smokers than in the 27 non-smokers (16.83 nanograms/mL compared with 28.8 nanograms/mL) and the clearance was 44% higher, but there was no difference in the therapeutic effect or adverse effects of haloperidol between the groups. The plasma concentrations of the reduced metabolite, reduced haloperidol, were also lower in the smokers than in the non-smokers (16.76 nanograms/mL compared with 34.23 nanograms/mL).[1] A similar higher haloperidol clearance (61%) was also seen in smokers in another study.[2] Lower dose-normalised haloperidol concentrations of about 24% were seen in 56 smokers receiving either oral or intramuscular haloperidol when compared with concentrations in 36 non-smokers. However, no difference in the plasma concentration of the reduced metabolite, reduced haloperidol, was seen. Note that 19 smokers and 15 non-smokers were also taking concurrent drugs known to be inhibitors or inducers of haloperidol metabolism.[3] A dose-dependent effect of smoking on haloperidol concentrations has been seen in two studies: at doses of haloperidol less than 0.2 mg/kg per day[4] or less than 0.5 mg/kg per day,[5] its plasma concentrations were lower in smokers, but this effect was not seen at higher doses.

In a sub-group of 16 patients receiving intramuscular haloperidol who were also CYP2D6 extensive metabolisers, and not taking interacting drugs, dose-normalised haloperidol concentrations were 40% lower in the smokers than in the non-smokers.[3] The effect of CYP2D6 polymorphism and smoking on haloperidol pharmacokinetics has also been studied in 110 patients with schizophrenia. No difference in the haloperidol concentration-to-dose ratio was seen between smokers and non-smokers. Similarly, in patients with reduced CYP2D6 activity, there was no difference between smokers and non-smokers. However smokers who had reduced CYP2D6 activity had higher haloperidol concentration-to-dose ratios than those who were extensive metabolisers, but there was no difference between the corresponding groups in non-smokers.[6]

Mechanism

Although the reason for the lower haloperidol concentrations has not been established, it seems likely that some of the components of tobacco smoke act as enzyme inducers. Smoking induces CYP1A2, but haloperidol is not known to be metabolised by this isoenzyme. It has been suggested that smoking induces the glucuronyltransferase involved in the glucuronidation of haloperidol,[3,6] which would increase haloperidol metabolism, thereby reducing its serum concentrations. The effect of smoking on haloperidol concentrations might differ depending on CYP2D6 genotype, but this requires further study.

Importance and management

The effect of smoking on haloperidol concentrations appears to be established and might possibly reduce its clinical effects, although this was not seen in one study. Be alert for the need to increase the dose of haloperidol in patients who smoke, and reduce the dose if smoking is stopped.

1. Jann MW, Saklad SR, Ereshefsky L, Richards AL, Harrington CA, Davis CM. Effects of smoking on haloperidol and reduced haloperidol plasma concentrations and haloperidol clearance. *Psychopharmacology (Berl)* (1986) 90, 468–70.
2. Miller DD, Kelly MW, Perry PJ, Coryell WH. The influence of cigarette smoking on haloperidol pharmacokinetics. *Biol Psychiatry* (1990) 28, 529–31.
3. Pan L, Vander Stichele R, Rosseel MT, Berlo JA, De Schepper N, Belpaire FM. Effects of smoking, CYP2D6 genotype, and concomitant drug intake on the steady state plasma concentrations of haloperidol and reduced haloperidol in schizophrenic inpatients. *Ther Drug Monit* (1999) 21, 489–97.
4. Shimoda K, Someya T, Morita S, Hirokane G, Noguchi T, Yokono A, Shibasaki M, Takahashi S. Lower plasma levels of haloperidol in smoking than in non-smoking schizophrenic patients. *Ther Drug Monit* (1999) 21, 293–6.
5. Perry PJ, Miller DD, Arndt SV, Smith DA, Holman TL. Haloperidol dosing requirements: the contribution of smoking and nonlinear pharmacokinetics. *J Clin Psychopharmacol* (1993) 13, 46–51.
6. Ohara K, Tanabu S, Yoshida K, Ishibashi K, Ikemoto K, Shubuya H. Effects of smoking and cytochrome P450 2D6*10 allele on the plasma haloperidol concentration/dose ratio. *Prog Neuropsychopharmacol Biol Psychiatry* (2003) 27, 945–9.

Haloperidol + Topiramate

Topiramate slightly increases the exposure to a metabolite of haloperidol, reduced haloperidol.

Clinical evidence, mechanism, importance and management

In a study published in a review paper, healthy subjects were given topiramate 50 mg twice daily, titrated over 2 days to 100 mg twice daily, with a single 5-mg dose of haloperidol, both 4 days before starting topiramate and on day 7 of topiramate use. The AUC of haloperidol and its active reduced metabolite (which possesses 20 to 50% of the activity of haloperidol) were increased by 11% and 31%, respectively by topiramate.[1] In another study, the mean AUC of a single 2-mg dose of haloperidol was increased by 15% in the presence of topiramate 50 to 100 mg twice daily.[2]

Evidence for an interaction between haloperidol and topiramate appears to be limited to these pharmacokinetic studies. The rise in haloperidol and reduced haloperidol exposure is slight at most, and not clinically important. Nevertheless, the authors of these reports suggest that a haloperidol dose adjustment [reduction] should be considered if adverse effects occur during concurrent use.[1,2]

1. Bialer M, Doose DR, Murthy B, Curtin C, Wang S-S, Twyman RE, Schwabe S. Pharmacokinetic interactions of topiramate. *Clin Pharmacokinet* (2004) 43, 763–80.
2. Doose DR, Kohl KA, Desai-Krieger D, Natarajan J, van Kammen DP. No clinically significant effect of topiramate on haloperidol concentration. *Eur Neuropsychopharmacol* (1999) 9, S357.

Haloperidol + Valproate

No pharmacokinetic interaction appears to occur between haloperidol and valproate.

Clinical evidence, mechanism, importance and management

A study in 6 patients taking valproic acid 400 mg daily, found that haloperidol 6 to 10 mg daily did not affect the pharmacokinetics of valproic acid.[1] A controlled study in 18 patients given haloperidol alone or with valproic acid for 4 weeks, found that plasma haloperidol concentrations increased by 32% with haloperidol alone and by 64% with valproic acid, but the difference between the groups was not statistically significant.[2]

Evidence is limited, but based on these studies no clinically relevant interaction seems to occur between haloperidol and valproic acid and no dose adjustments would therefore seem necessary on concurrent use.

1. Ishizaki T, Chiba K, Saito M, Kobayashi K, Iizuka R. The effects of neuroleptics (haloperidol and chlorpromazine) on the pharmacokinetics of valproic acid in schizophrenic patients. *J Clin Psychopharmacol* (1984) 4, 254–61.
2. Hesslinger B, Normann C, Langosch JM, Klose P, Berger M, Walden J. Effects of carbamazepine and valproate on haloperidol plasma levels and on psychopathologic outcome in schizophrenic patients. *J Clin Psychopharmacol* (1999) 19, 310–15.

Haloperidol + Venlafaxine

Venlafaxine increases haloperidol exposure. An isolated report describes a man taking haloperidol who developed urinary retention when venlafaxine was added.

Clinical evidence

A study in 24 healthy subjects found that steady-state venlafaxine 75 mg every 12 hours reduced the total oral clearance of a single 2-mg dose of haloperidol by 42%. This resulted in a 70% rise in the AUC of haloperidol and an 88% rise in its maximum serum concentrations, without increasing its elimination half-life.[1-3] An isolated report describes a 75-year-old man taking haloperidol 1 mg and alprazolam 500 micrograms daily, who suddenly developed urinary retention when venlafaxine 37.5 mg daily was added. Urinary retention resolved spontaneously when all the drugs were stopped.[4]

Mechanism

The reason why venlafaxine reduces haloperidol clearance is not known. The lack of effect on elimination half-life suggests that inhibition of haloperidol metabolism is unlikely. It was suggested that raised concentrations of haloperidol could increase its antimuscarinic effects,[4] which in the case described resulted in urinary retention. However, note that urinary retention is also an adverse effect (uncommon) of venlafaxine alone.

Importance and management

The evidence for a pharmacokinetic interaction between haloperidol and venlafaxine is limited but it appears to be established. Be aware that increased haloperidol adverse effects (e.g. sedation, agitation, movement disorders) might occur if venlafaxine is also given, and that it might be necessary to reduce the haloperidol dose.

1. Efexor XL (Venlafaxine hydrochloride). Pfizer Ltd. UK Summary of product characteristics, December 2013.
2. Wyeth, Personal communication, April 2001.
3. Effexor XR (Venlafaxine hydrochloride). Wyeth Pharmaceuticals Inc. US Prescribing information, March 2014.
4. Benazzi F. Urinary retention with venlafaxine-haloperidol combination. *Pharmacopsychiatry* (1997) 30, 27.

Iloperidone + Miscellaneous

Ketoconazole (a CYP3A4 inhibitor) and fluoxetine and paroxetine (CYP2D6 inhibitors) increase the steady-state concentrations of iloperidone and increase its effect on the QT interval. Other potent inhibitors of CYP3A4 and CYP2D6 are predicted to interact similarly. Iloperidone does not appear to affect the pharmacokinetics of dextromethorphan to a clinically relevant extent. Food appears to delay iloperidone absorption, but has no effect on its overall bioavailability. Tobacco smoking is not expected to affect the pharmacokinetics of iloperidone.

Clinical evidence, mechanism, importance and management

(a) CYP3A4 inhibitors

In a study in 19 healthy subjects, **ketoconazole** 200 mg twice daily for 4 days slightly increased the AUC of a single 3-mg dose of iloperidone by 57%. The AUC of the active metabolite of iloperidone, P88, increased by 55%, and the AUC of the other major metabolite, P95, increased by 35%.[1] When both **ketoconazole** 200 mg twice daily and paroxetine 20 mg twice daily (see *CYP2D6 inhibitors*, below) were given together, the effect on the steady-state concentrations of iloperidone (a 40% increase) was similar to either drug alone, and not additive. However, giving both **ketoconazole** and paroxetine with iloperidone increased the QTc interval by a further 10 milliseconds, when compared with iloperidone alone (19 milliseconds versus 9 milliseconds).[1]

Iloperidone is metabolised by several pathways, including CYP3A4, an isoenzyme that is potently inhibited by **ketoconazole**. Although the increase in exposure with ketoconazole is slight, it results in a potentially important increase in the QT interval. The effects of giving both a CYP3A4 inhibitor and a CYP2D6 inhibitor do not appear to be additive.

Because of the increase in the QT interval, caution is necessary when giving **ketoconazole** with iloperidone. The US manufacturer recommends that the dose of iloperidone should be halved when given with potent CYP3A4 inhibitors (they specifically name ketoconazole, **itraconazole** and **clarithromycin**).[1] A similar halving of the iloperidone dose is recommended on the concurrent use of both a potent CYP3A4 inhibitor and a potent CYP2D6 inhibitor. The effect of less potent CYP3A4 inhibitors (they name **erythromycin** and **grapefruit juice**) has not been studied,[1] and as they would be expected to produce smaller increases in iloperidone concentrations, no dose adjustment is suggested, but the possibility of an interaction should be borne in mind on concurrent use. For a list of drugs that are inhibitors of CYP3A4, see 'Table 1.9', p.11.

(b) CYP2D6 inhibitors

In a study in 23 healthy subjects, **fluoxetine** 20 mg twice daily for 21 days increased the AUC of a single 3-mg dose of iloperidone and increased the AUC of its active metabolite, P88, about 2- to 3-fold. All subjects were considered to be extensive CYP2D6 metabolisers (that is, those with normal CYP2D6 activity). The AUC of the other major metabolite of iloperidone, P95, was decreased by about 50%.[1] The pharmacokinetics of **fluoxetine** 20 mg twice daily were unaffected by a single 3-mg dose of iloperidone.[1]

In another study, patients with schizophrenia were given iloperidone 8 mg or 12 mg twice daily with **paroxetine** 20 mg daily for 5 to 8 days. The steady-state maximum concentration of iloperidone and its active metabolite, P88, were increased by about 60%, whereas the maximum concentration of its metabolite P95 was decreased by 50%.[1] When **ketoconazole** and paroxetine were given together the effect on iloperidone was similar to either drug alone, and not additive; however, the effect on the QT interval was greater (see *CYP3A4 inhibitors*, above).

Iloperidone is metabolised by several pathways, including by CYP2D6,[1] which is subject to genetic polymorphism, meaning that patients have varying activity of this isoenzyme. Fluoxetine and paroxetine are inhibitors of CYP2D6, and although the increase in steady-state concentrations with paroxetine is not large, it results in a potentially important increase in the QT interval. The effects of giving both a CYP3A4 inhibitor and a CYP2D6 inhibitor do not appear to be additive.

Because of the increase in the QT interval, caution is necessary when using **paroxetine** with iloperidone. The US manufacturer recommends that the dose of iloperidone should be halved when given with **fluoxetine** or **paroxetine**.[1] Other potent inhibitors of CYP2D6 would be expected to interact similarly, and similar iloperidone dose reductions are recommended on concurrent use.[1] For a list of drugs that are CYP2D6 inhibitors, see 'Table 1.7', p.9.

When iloperidone is given with both a potent CYP3A4 inhibitor and a potent CYP2D6 inhibitor, a similar halving of the iloperidone dose is recommended.[1]

(c) Dextromethorphan

A study in healthy subjects found that a single dose of iloperidone 3 mg increased the AUC and maximum concentrations of a single 80-mg dose of dextromethorphan by 17% and 26%, respectively. This change in exposure is negligible, and suggests that iloperidone is not a CYP2D6 inhibitor. However, note that single dose studies are not generally sufficient to maximise enzyme inhibition. Nevertheless, the manufacturer considers that an interaction between iloperidone and other CYP2D6 substrates is unlikely.[1]

(d) Food

In a study in 21 healthy subjects, a single 3-mg dose of iloperidone was given after an overnight fast or 15 minutes after a standard breakfast. Food delayed the time to reach maximum plasma concentrations by 2.1 hours, but this was not statistically significant. There were no statistically significant changes in other pharmacokinetic parameters.[2] The US manufacturer advises that iloperidone can be taken without regard to meals,[1] but the study found that when iloperidone was given with food the incidence and severity of common adverse effects, including orthostatic hypotension, dizziness and somnolence, was reduced.[2]

(e) Tobacco

In vitro studies have found that iloperidone is not a substrate of CYP1A2. Tobacco smoke is known to contain inducers of this isoenzyme, and so the US manufacturer predicts that smoking will be unlikely to affect the pharmacokinetics of iloperidone.[1]

1. Fanapt (Iloperidone). Vanda Pharmaceuticals Inc. US Prescribing information, January 2012.
2. Sainati SM, Hubbard JW, Chi E, Grasing K, CityplaceBrecherStateMBSafety, tolerability, and effect of food on the pharmacokinetics of iloperidone (HP873), a potential atypical antipsychotic. *J Clin Pharmacol* (1995) 35, 713–20.

Loxapine + SSRIs

Galactorrhoea and amenorrhoea developed in a patient given loxapine and fluvoxamine.

Clinical evidence, mechanism, importance and management

A 38-year-old woman developed amenorrhoea, followed shortly by galactorrhoea, about 6 weeks after starting to take **fluvoxamine** and loxapine. The galactorrhoea resolved within 3 weeks of stopping the **fluvoxamine**, and menstruation occurred one week later. Her prolactin concentration was found to be 80 micrograms/L (reference range 4 to 30 micrograms/L).[1]

Galactorrhoea is a known adverse effect of loxapine, and the SSRIs can increase prolactin levels,[2] which might have triggered this adverse effect.

The general relevance of this isolated case is unclear. Consider an interaction as a possible cause if a patient taking loxapine and an SSRI develops galactorrhoea.

1. Jeffries J, Bezchlibnyk-Butler K, Remington G. Amenorrhea and galactorrhea associated with fluvoxamine in a loxapine-treated patient. *J Clin Psychopharmacol* (1992) 12, 296–7.
2. Rosen RC, Lane RM, Menza M. Effects of SSRIs on sexual function: a critical review. *J Clin Psychopharmacol* (1999) 19, 67–85.

Melatonin receptor agonists + Azoles

Ketoconazole appears to slightly increase the exposure to ramelteon and tasimelteon. Fluconazole appears to moderately increase ramelteon exposure. Other azoles might interact similarly.

Clinical evidence

(a) Fluconazole

The preliminary report of a study in 28 healthy subjects notes that fluconazole 400 mg on day one then 200 mg daily for 3 days increased the AUC and maximum plasma concentration of a single 16-mg dose of **ramelteon**, given on day 4, about 2.5-fold.[1]

(b) Ketoconazole

The preliminary report of a study in 28 healthy subjects found that ketoconazole 200 mg daily for 4 days increased the AUC and maximum plasma concentration of a single 16-mg dose of **ramelteon** by 84% and 36%, respectively.[1]

The US manufacturer of **tasimelteon** briefly reports that, in a study, ketoconazole 400 mg daily for 5 days, increased the AUC of tasimelteon by 50%.[2]

Mechanism

Ramelteon and tasimelteon are both extensively metabolised by CYP1A2, with some involvement of CYP3A4. CYP2C9 is also involved in the metabolism of ramelteon. Fluconazole and ketoconazole are both well-known CYP3A4 inhibitors, and fluconazole additionally inhibits CYP2C9. Concurrent use of these azoles with ramelteon therefore results in increased exposure. A similar effect is seen when ketoconazole is given with tasimelteon.

Importance and management

Evidence for an interaction between the melatonin receptor agonists and the azoles appears to be limited. The clinical relevance of the pharmacokinetic changes seen with ramelteon and fluconazole and ketoconazole has not been assessed, but the moderate increase in ramelteon exposure with **fluconazole** might be clinically relevant. The US manufacturer[3] suggests that ramelteon should be given with caution with fluconazole (which they classify as a potent CYP2C9 inhibitor, but it is usually considered to be a weak to moderate inhibitor depending on the dose given). It would therefore be prudent to be alert for an increase in sedative effects, and the duration of effects, of ramelteon, and consider a reduction in dose if the effects become excessive.

The slight increase in exposure of ramelteon and tasimelteon with **ketoconazole** is unlikely to be clinically important, and no dose adjustments would seem necessary on concurrent use. However the US manufacturer of ramelteon advises caution on the concurrent use of ketoconazole and other potent CYP3A4 inhibitors (see 'Table 1.9', p.11 for a list).[3] Until more is known it might be prudent to follow the same advice given for fluconazole and ramelteon.

Information about other azoles generally appears to be lacking, but all of them would be expected to interact with ramelteon and tasimelteon to some extent. Therefore for ramelteon, until more is known, it might be prudent to also follow the same advice given for fluconazole with **itraconazole**, **voriconazole**, and possibly **posaconazole**. No dose adjustments would be predicted to be necessary for tasimelteon. In addition, note that a large proportion of **miconazole** oral gel (both prescription and non-prescription doses) can be swallowed and therefore adequate systemic absorption might occur to produce some interaction.

1. Karim A, Tolbert D, Cao C, Zhao Z, Sainati SM. Effects of fluconazole and ketoconazole on the pharmacokinetics of ramelteon (TAK-375) in normal healthy male and female subjects. *Sleep* (2004) 27 (Abstract Suppl), A53–54.
2. Hetlioz (Tasimelteon). Vanda Pharmaceuticals Inc. US Prescribing information, December 2014.
3. Rozerem (Ramelteon). Takeda Pharmaceuticals America, Inc. US Prescribing information, November 2010.

Melatonin receptor agonists + SSRIs

Fluvoxamine appears to very markedly increase the exposure to ramelteon, and appears to markedly increase the exposure to tasimelteon.

Other potent CYP1A2 inhibitors might be expected to interact similarly. Fluoxetine appears to slightly increase ramelteon exposure. Escitalopram and sertraline do not appear to affect ramelteon exposure.

Clinical evidence

(a) Escitalopram

The US manufacturer briefly notes that there was no clinically relevant pharmacokinetic interaction between escitalopram and **ramelteon**.[1]

(b) Fluoxetine

The preliminary report of a study in 28 healthy subjects notes that fluoxetine 40 mg daily for 11 days increased the AUC and maximum plasma concentration of a single 16-mg dose of **ramelteon** by 50% and 40%, respectively.[2]

(c) Fluvoxamine

The US manufacturer of **ramelteon** reports that the AUC and maximum plasma concentration of a single-dose of ramelteon were increased about 190-fold and 70-fold, respectively, by fluvoxamine 100 mg twice daily for 3 days.[1]

The US manufacturer of **tasimelteon** briefly reports that in a study, fluvoxamine 50 mg daily for 6 days increased the AUC and maximum concentration of tasimelteon 7-fold and 2-fold, respectively.[3]

(d) Sertraline

The US manufacturer briefly notes that there was no clinically relevant pharmacokinetic interaction between sertraline and **ramelteon**.[1]

Mechanism

Fluvoxamine is an inhibitor of CYP1A2 by which ramelteon and tasimelteon are principally metabolised. Concurrent use therefore decreases their metabolism resulting in increased exposure.

Fluoxetine is an inhibitor of CYP2D6, and the results of the study[2] suggest that it might have a minor role in ramelteon metabolism.

Importance and management

Evidence for an interaction between the melatonin receptor agonists and the SSRIS is limited, but a pharmacokinetic interaction between **fluvoxamine** and both ramelteon and tasimelteon would appear to be established. Fluvoxamine is a potent inhibitor of CYP1A2, which is a major isoenzyme in the metabolism of ramelteon and tasimelteon, and hence concurrent use results in very marked and marked, increases in their exposure, respectively. The US manufacturers therefore advise that concurrent use of ramelteon and tasimelteon with potent CYP1A2 inhibitors should be avoided.[1,3] For a list of potent CYP1A2 inhibitors see 'Table 1.2', p.5.

The slight increase in ramelteon exposure with **fluoxetine** was not considered to be clinically important[1] as ramelteon has high interindividual variability and a wide therapeutic window. No dose adjustment of ramelteon is considered to be necessary if fluoxetine is also taken. **Paroxetine** generally interacts in a similar way to fluoxetine, so a clinically important interaction would not be expected. There also appears to be no clinically relevant interaction between ramelteon and **escitalopram** or **sertraline**. Data for other SSRIS with tasimelteon is lacking.

1. Rozerem (Ramelteon). Takeda Pharmaceuticals America, Inc. US Prescribing information, November 2010.
2. Sainati SM, Karim A, Tolbert D, Cao C. Effects of multiple doses of fluoxetine on the systemic exposure of a single dose of ramelteon (TAK-375) in healthy adults. *Sleep* (2004) 27 (Abstract Suppl), A48.
3. Hetlioz (Tasimelteon). Vanda Pharmaceuticals Inc. US Prescribing information, December 2014.

Melatonin receptor agonists; Ramelteon + Dextromethorphan

The concurrent use of ramelteon and dextromethorphan does not affect the pharmacokinetics of either drug.

Clinical evidence, mechanism, importance and management

A study in 36 healthy subjects found that giving ramelteon 32 mg with dextromethorphan 30 mg had no effect on the pharmacokinetics of either drug.[1] Ramelteon does not, therefore, appear to affect the metabolism of CYP2D6 substrates by this mechanism. Dextromethorphan dose adjustments would not be expected to be necessary if ramelteon is also given.

1. Tolbert D, Karim A, Cao C, Zhao Z, Johnson J, Sainati SM. Study to assess drug interaction between ramelteon (TAK-375) and dextromethorphan in healthy adults. *Sleep* (2004) 27 (Abstract Suppl), A50.

Melatonin receptor agonists; Ramelteon + Miscellaneous

Rifampicin (rifampin) and to a much lesser extent food, decrease ramelteon exposure. CYP1A2 inhibitors (such as some quinolones) are expected to increase ramelteon exposure. Donepezil moderately and doxepin slightly increases ramelteon exposure. No clinically relevant pharmacokinetic interaction occurs with gabapentin, omeprazole, venlafaxine or zolpidem, although additive CNS depressant effects would be expected if ramelteon and zolpidem are given concurrently and additive CNS depressant effects occur with alcohol. Ramelteon does not alter the pharmacokinetics of digoxin or warfarin.

Clinical evidence, mechanism, importance and management

(a) Alcohol

Alcohol had no effect on the maximum concentration or exposure to ramelteon. However, an additive effect was seen in some tests of psychomotor performance.[1] The manufacturer states that patients taking ramelteon should avoid alcohol.[1]

(b) CYP1A2 inhibitors

Ramelteon is extensively metabolised by CYP1A2. Based on the profound interaction with the potent CYP1A2 inhibitor fluvoxamine (see 'Melatonin receptor agonists + SSRIs', p.865), for which concurrent use of ramelteon is contraindicated, the manufacturer advises caution with other less potent CYP1A2 inhibitors.[1] Note that many of the quinolones can, to varying extents, inhibit CYP1A2, most notably **enoxacin** (moderate to potent) and **ciprofloxacin** (weak to moderate). Concurrent use of these drugs and ramelteon should be closely monitored for increased sedation, and the dose of ramelteon reduced as necessary. A list of clinically relevant CYP1A2 inhibitors is given in 'Table 1.2', p.5.

(c) Digoxin

The manufacturer briefly notes that ramelteon had no clinically relevant effect on the pharmacokinetics of digoxin.[1] No digoxin dose adjustments would therefore be expected to be necessary on concurrent use.

(d) Donepezil

Donepezil 10 mg daily for 26 days increased the exposure to a single 8-mg dose of ramelteon 2-fold.[1] This might result in increased ramelteon effects (e.g. sedation, dizziness, and fatigue) and the manufacturer states that patients taking both drugs should be closely monitored.[1]

(e) Doxepin

Doxepin 10 mg daily for 23 days increased the exposure to a single 8-mg dose of ramelteon by 66%.[1] The clinical relevance of this slight increase does not appear to have been studied; however, the manufacturer recommends that patients taking the combination should be closely monitored.[1] Be alert for increased ramelteon effects (e.g. sedation, dizziness, and fatigue) on the concurrent use of doxepin.

(f) Food

A high-fat meal increased the AUC of a single 16-mg dose of ramelteon by 31% and decreased the maximum plasma concentration by 22%, compared with the fasted state. The time to maximum plasma concentration was also delayed by about 45 minutes when ramelteon was given with food. This slight increase in ramelteon exposure seems unlikely to be clinically relevant. Nevertheless, the manufacturer recommends that ramelteon should not be taken with or immediately after a high-fat meal.[1]

(g) Rifampicin (Rifampin)

Rifampicin 600 mg daily for 11 days decreased the exposure to a single 32-mg dose of ramelteon and its active metabolite by about 80%. Efficacy is likely to be reduced when ramelteon is used in combination with potent enzyme inducers such as rifampicin.[1] Be alert for a reduction in ramelteon effects in patients also taking rifampicin and adjust the ramelteon dose according to clinical need.

(h) Warfarin

The manufacturer briefly notes that ramelteon had no clinically relevant effect on the pharmacokinetics of warfarin.[1] No warfarin dose adjustments would expect to be needed on concurrent use.

(i) Zolpidem

Ramelteon 8 mg daily for 11 days had no effect on the AUC of a single 10-mg dose of zolpidem. Zolpidem did not alter ramelteon exposure.[1] The manufacturer notes that ordinarily these two hypnotics would not be used together.[1] If concurrent use is undertaken be alert for increased CNS depressant effects.

(j) Other drugs

The manufacturer briefly notes that there was no clinically relevant pharmacokinetic interaction between gabapentin, omeprazole, or venlafaxine and ramelteon.[1]

1. Rozerem (Ramelteon). Takeda Pharmaceuticals America, Inc. US Prescribing information, November 2010.

Melatonin receptor agonists; Tasimelteon + Miscellaneous

Tobacco smoke might slightly decrease the exposure to tasimelteon, and other CYP1A2 inducers might also interact similarly. Rifampicin appears to markedly decrease the exposure to tasimelteon, and other potent CYP3A4 inducers are expected to interact similarly. A high-fat meal

decreased the concentration of tasimelteon. Tasimelteon does not appear to affect the exposure to rosiglitazone.

Clinical evidence, mechanism, importance and management

(a) CYP1A2 inducers

The US manufacturer briefly reports that in a study, the exposure of tasimelteon in smokers was 40% lower than in non-smokers, suggesting that the efficacy of tasimelteon might be reduced in smokers.[1] **Tobacco smoke** is a known inducer of CYP1A2, which is the principal enzyme involved in the metabolism of tasimelteon, and therefore, it would seem prudent to bear this possible interaction in mind in cases of otherwise unexplained reduced efficacy in smokers and/or patients taking CYP1A2 inducers (see 'Table 1.2', p.5 for a list). For the effects of **fluvoxamine**, a potent inhibitor of CYP1A2, see 'Melatonin receptor agonists + SSRIs', p.865.

(b) CYP2C8 substrates

The US manufacturer briefly reports that in a study, tasimelteon 20 mg daily for 16 days did not affect the pharmacokinetics of **rosiglitazone**.[1] Note that rosiglitazone can be used as a probe substrate to assess the activity of drugs on CYP2C8. This study therefore suggests that tasimelteon is not an inducer or inhibitor of this isoenzyme, and other drugs that are also metabolised by CYP2C8 are also unlikely to be affected.

(c) CYP3A4 inducers

The US manufacturer briefly reports that in a study, **rifampicin** 600 mg daily for 11 days decreased the AUC of tasimelteon by 90%.[1] Rifampicin is a potent inducer of CYP3A4, which is a major isoenzyme in the metabolism of tasimelteon, and hence concurrent use results in a marked decrease in its exposure. The manufacturer therefore advises that concurrent use of tasimelteon with potent CYP3A4 inducers should be avoided.[1] If they are taken concurrently, be alert for a possible decrease in the clinical effect of tasimelteon. For a list of potent CYP3A4 inducers see 'Table 1.9', p.11.

(d) Food

The US manufacturer briefly notes that, when administered with a high-fat meal, the maximum concentration of tasimelteon was decreased by 44%, and the time to reach maximum concentration was delayed by almost 2 hours, when compared with administration in the fasted state.[1] Therefore tasimelteon should be taken without food.

1. Hetlioz (Tasimelteon). Vanda Pharmaceuticals Inc. US Prescribing information, December 2014.

Molindone + SSRIs

An isolated report describes extrapyramidal adverse effects following the use of paroxetine with molindone.

Clinical evidence, mechanism, importance and management

An elderly woman taking molindone 10 mg twice daily developed severe and disabling extrapyramidal symptoms (severe bradykinesia, tremor, inability to feed herself, delirium) within about 2 weeks of starting **paroxetine** 10 mg daily. The symptoms resolved when molindone was stopped, and no problems occurred when **fluoxetine** alone was started.[1]

Movement disorders might be a result of the additive adverse effects of molindone and SSRIs. **Fluoxetine** alone has been shown to occasionally cause movement disorders.[2,3] However, movement disorders might just be due to the antipsychotic alone.

The combination of an antipsychotic and an SSRI can be useful and so the isolated case of extrapyramidal adverse effects should not prevent concurrent use. However, if extrapyramidal effects become troublesome bear this interaction in mind as a possible cause.

1. Malek-Ahmadi P, Allen SA. Paroxetine-molindone interaction. *J Clin Psychiatry* (1995) 56, 82–3.
2. Coulter DM, Pillans PI. Fluoxetine and extrapyramidal side effects. *Am J Psychiatry* (1995) 152, 122–5.
3. Bouchard RH, Pourcher E, Vincent P. Fluoxetine and extrapyramidal side effects. *Am J Psychiatry* (1989) 146, 1352–3.

Olanzapine + Aripiprazole

An isolated case report describes neuroleptic malignant syndrome occurring after aripiprazole was given to a patient taking olanzapine.

Clinical evidence, mechanism, importance and management

A case report describes a 33-year-old man who had been taking olanzapine 10 mg daily for 9 months, and who developed neuroleptic malignant syndrome 2 weeks after aripiprazole was added and the dose was increased from 5 mg daily to 10 mg daily. The patient was also taking benzatropine (dose unknown).[1] Most of his symptoms had resolved after 5 weeks of hospital care. The authors suggested that the addition of aripiprazole, which has high dopamine receptor affinity, was a key factor in this case. This is an isolated case and as such, no general recommendations can be made.

1. Marshall PB, Mellman TA, Nguyen SXC. Neuroleptic malignant syndrome with the addition of aripiprazole to olanzapine. *Am J Psychiatry* (2008) 165, 1488–9.

Olanzapine + Benzodiazepines

Excessive sedation and hypotension can occur if parenteral benzodiazepines are given with intramuscular olanzapine. There appears to be no pharmacokinetic interaction between olanzapine and lorazepam, and olanzapine does not appear to alter the pharmacokinetics of diazepam.

Clinical evidence

Intramuscular olanzapine has been associated with hypotension, bradycardia, respiratory depression, and rarely death, particularly in patients who have also received benzodiazepines. A review of the manufacturer's safety database for intramuscular olanzapine for the period January 2004 to September 2005, found 160 spontaneously reported cases of adverse events in patients receiving olanzapine, 39% of which involved the concurrent use of a benzodiazepine. Of the 29 fatalities reported, 52% involved olanzapine and benzodiazepines and 31% involved olanzapine, benzodiazepines, and antipsychotics.[1] One case report describes hypotension occurring following the intramuscular use of a single 2-mg dose of **lorazepam** in a patient receiving intramuscular olanzapine 10 mg, the most recent dose being given 30 minutes before the **lorazepam**. His blood pressure dropped from 124/74 mmHg to 66/30 mmHg; 12 hours later his blood pressure had returned to normal.[2]

In a controlled study, intramuscular **lorazepam** 2 mg, given one hour after intramuscular olanzapine 5 mg increased the drowsiness seen with either drug alone. The pharmacokinetics of both drugs were not affected.[3,4]

The US manufacturer of olanzapine briefly states that the concurrent use of **diazepam** (route not stated) has been reported to increase orthostatic hypotension[3] and both the UK and US manufacturers also note that olanzapine did not alter the pharmacokinetics of **diazepam**[3,5] or its active metabolite, nordazepam.[3] It was noted that mild increases in heart rate, sedation and dry mouth were seen in patients taking both drugs, but no dose adjustments were thought to be necessary.[6]

Mechanism

The sedative and hypotensive effects of benzodiazepines and olanzapine appear to be additive, particularly with parenteral use. Olanzapine does not appear to alter diazepam metabolism by CYP2C19 or lorazepam metabolism by glucuronidation.

Importance and management

Evidence for an interaction between olanzapine and the benzodiazepines is limited, but an interaction would appear to be established. The authors of one report concluded that the combination of intramuscular olanzapine and parenteral benzodiazepines should be used with caution,[1] but the manufacturers state that concurrent use is not recommended.[3,4] If both drugs are needed, parenteral benzodiazepines should not be given for at least one hour after intramuscular olanzapine. If a parenteral benzodiazepine has already been given, intramuscular olanzapine should only be given with careful consideration and monitoring of sedation and for cardiac and respiratory depression.[4]

1. Marder SR, Sorsaburu S, Dunayevich, Karagianis JL, Dawe IC, Falk DM, Dellva MA, Carlson JL, Cavazzoni PA, Baker RW. Case reports of postmarketing adverse event experiences with olanzapine intramuscular treatment in patients with agitation. *J Clin Psychiatry* (2010) 71, 433–41..
2. Zacher JL, Roche-Desilets J. Hypotension secondary to the combination of intramuscular olanzapine and intramuscular lorazepam. *J Clin Psychiatry* (2005) 66, 1614–15.
3. Zyprexa (Olanzapine). Eli Lilly and Company. US Prescribing information, June 2011.
4. Zyprexa Powder for Solution for Injection (Olanzapine). Eli Lilly and Company Ltd. UK Summary of product characteristics, November 2011.
5. Zyprexa Tablets (Olanzapine). Eli Lilly and Company Ltd. UK Summary of product characteristics, November 2011.
6. Zyprexa (Olanzapine). Eli Lilly. Clinical and Laboratory Experience A Comprehensive Monograph. August 1996.

Olanzapine + Carbamazepine and related drugs

Carbamazepine appears to lower olanzapine concentrations, whereas oxcarbazepine does not appear to affect the pharmacokinetics of olanzapine. Olanzapine does not appear to affect carbamazepine concentrations.

Clinical evidence

(a) Carbamazepine

Multiple-dose studies in healthy subjects have shown that carbamazepine increases the metabolism of olanzapine. The clearance of olanzapine was increased by 44% and its elimination half-life was reduced by 20% by carbamazepine, but these changes were not considered to necessitate dose adjustments.[1] In another study in healthy subjects, pretreatment with carbamazepine 200 mg twice daily for 2 weeks increased the clearance of a single 10-mg dose of olanzapine by 46%. The maximum plasma concentration and AUC were decreased by about 25% and 34%, respectively.[2] Another study found that 5 patients taking olanzapine and carbamazepine had a concentration-to-dose ratio 36% lower than 22 patients taking olanzapine alone.[3] A later study by the same authors found similar results, but also found that the median glucuronidated olanzapine concentration was 79% in patients also receiving carbamazepine and 43% in patients receiving olanzapine alone.[4]

A retrospective study identified 10 patients taking olanzapine and carbamazepine. The patients taking carbamazepine were taking olanzapine doses that were double those of subjects taking olanzapine alone. When corrected for dose it was found that the concentration-to-dose ratio of olanzapine was 71% lower in those also taking carbamazepine, when compared with those not taking carbamazepine.[5] A 23-year-old woman required an olanzapine dose reduction from 15 mg daily to 10 mg daily to maintain a similar serum olanzapine concentration after stopping carbamazepine 600 mg daily.[6]

A controlled study in 81 patients found that the median concentration-to-dose ratio of olanzapine 20 to 30 mg daily was about 39% lower in the patients also taking carbamazepine (400 mg daily titrated to the highest individual tolerated dose to a maximum daily dose of 1.2 g daily), when compared with historical controls taking olanzapine alone, at a lower dose of 15 mg. There was no difference in the concentration of carbamazepine or carbamazepine-10,11-epoxide between those taking olanzapine and carbamazepine and those taking olanzapine alone.[7] A study found that the dose-corrected olanzapine plasma concentration in patients also receiving carbamazepine were no different than those in patients receiving olanzapine alone.[8]

(b) Oxcarbazepine

A study in 13 patients stable taking olanzapine 5 to 20 mg daily found that the addition of oxcarbazepine for 5 weeks (at an initial dose of 300 mg daily increased to a range of 900 mg to 1.2 g after one week) had no effect on the steady-state plasma concentration of olanzapine.[9]

Mechanism

Uncertain. Olanzapine is principally metabolised by glucuronidation, and one study[4] suggests that this is induced by carbamazepine, resulting in reduced olanzapine levels. Further study is needed.

Importance and management

Evidence for an interaction between carbamazepine and olanzapine is limited and conflicting. On balance, it seems that carbamazepine might decrease olanzapine concentrations and, in some patients at least, the decrease caused might be clinically relevant. Until more is known, it would seem prudent to monitor the outcome of concurrent use for olanzapine efficacy and adjust the olanzapine dose if necessary.

The evidence with oxcarbazepine is limited to one study, but this appears to suggest that no olanzapine dose adjustment is necessary if oxcarbazepine is also given.

1. Zyprexa (Olanzapine). Eli Lilly. Clinical and Laboratory Experience A Comprehensive Monograph, August 1996.
2. Lucas RA, Gilfillan DJ, Bergstrom RF. A pharmacokinetic interaction between carbamazepine and olanzapine: observations on possible mechanism. *Eur J Clin Pharmacol* (1998) 54, 639–43.
3. Olesen OV, Linnet K. Olanzapine serum concentrations in psychiatric patients given standard doses: the influence of comedication. *Ther Drug Monit* (1999) 21, 87–90.
4. Linnet K, Olesen OV. Free and glucuronidated olanzapine serum concentrations in psychiatric patients: influence of carbamazepine comedication. *Ther Drug Monit* (2002) 24, 512–17.
5. Skogh E, Reis M, Dahl M-L, Lundmark J, Bengtsson F. Therapeutic drug monitoring data on olanzapine and its N-demethyl metabolite in the naturalistic clinical setting. *Ther Drug Monit* (2002) 24, 518–26.
6. Licht RW, Olesen OV, Friis P, Laustsen T. Olanzapine serum concentrations lowered by concomitant treatment with carbamazepine. *J Clin Psychopharmacol* (2000) 20, 110–12.
7. Tohen M, Bowden CL, Smulevich AB, Bergstrom R, Quinlan T, Osuntokun O, Wang WV, Oliff HS, Martenyi F, Kryzhanovskaya LA, Greil W. Olanzapine plus carbamazepine v. carbamazepine alone in treating manic episodes. *Br J Psychiatry* (2008) 192, 135–43.
8. Bergemann N, Frick A, Parzer P, Kopitz J. Olanzapine plasma concentration, average daily dose, and interaction with co-medication in schizophrenic patients. *Pharmacopsychiatry* (2004) 37, 63–8.
9. Muscatello MR, Pacetti M, Cacciola M, La Torre D, Zoccali R, D'Arrigo C, Migliardi G, Spina E. Plasma concentrations of risperidone and olanzapine during coadministration with oxcarbazepine. *Epilepsia* (2005) 46, 771–4.

Olanzapine + Hormonal contraceptives

Ethinylestradiol-containing contraceptives appear not to affect olanzapine plasma concentrations, but they might decrease the plasma concentration of a metabolite of olanzapine.

Clinical evidence

In a prospective study in patients taking olanzapine and attending a therapeutic drug monitoring service, the plasma concentrations of olanzapine were compared in 10 patients taking an ethinylestradiol-containing contraceptive, 10 patients taking a progestogen-based contraceptive, and 129 patients not taking a contraceptive. The plasma concentrations of olanzapine were not statistically significantly different in the three groups; however, the plasma concentrations of *N*-desmethyl olanzapine (an inactive major metabolite) were lower in the patients taking ethinylestradiol-containing contraceptives than in the other two groups.[1]

Mechanism

The authors of this study suggest that ethinylestradiol inhibits CYP1A2, by which olanzapine is partially metabolised, leading to a decrease in olanzapine metabolism and thus, lower concentrations of its metabolite, *N*-desmethyl olanzapine.[1]

Importance and management

Evidence for an interaction between olanzapine and ethinylestradiol is limited to one study and an interaction is not established. Ethinylestradiol does not appear to alter olanzapine plasma concentrations and the changes in *N*-desmethyl olanzapine concentrations are considered unlikely to be clinically relevant.[1]

1. Haslemo T, Refsum H, Molden E. The effect of ethinylestradiol-containing contraceptives on the serum concentration of olanzapine and *N*-desmethyl olanzapine. *Br J Clin Pharmacol* (2011) 71, 611–15.

Olanzapine + Lamotrigine

Olanzapine very slightly reduces lamotrigine exposure and lamotrigine possibly increases olanzapine concentrations, but any effect is small.

Clinical evidence

In a pharmacokinetic study, 28 healthy subjects were given lamotrigine for 7 weeks (25 mg daily titrated to 200 mg daily) with either olanzapine (5 mg daily titrated to 15 mg daily) or placebo for the last 2 weeks. An additional 16 subjects took placebo for 7 weeks with olanzapine (as before) for 2 weeks. The steady-state pharmacokinetics of olanzapine were not affected by the concurrent use of lamotrigine. However, the AUC and maximum plasma concentration of lamotrigine were 24% and 20% lower, respectively, in those receiving olanzapine.[1]

A study in 14 patients stable taking olanzapine in doses of 10 mg to 20 mg daily, and who were also given lamotrigine in increasing doses over 8 weeks to 200 mg daily, found no changes in the pharmacokinetics of olanzapine with a lamotrigine dose of 100 mg daily, but when the dose was increased to 200 mg daily, the olanzapine plasma concentrations increased by 16%, when compared with baseline.[2]

A further study in 14 healthy subjects given lamotrigine 25 mg daily increased to 50 mg daily, and a single 5-mg dose of olanzapine found no changes in the AUC and maximum plasma concentration of lamotrigine, although the time to the maximum plasma concentration of lamotrigine was increased from 1.8 hours to 4.2 hours. Note that the findings of this study are limited because it used only a single dose of olanzapine, and doses of both drugs were low.[3]

A mixed model analysis of published and unpublished data found that the effect of lamotrigine on olanzapine plasma concentrations was dependent upon smoking status.[4] In smokers taking lamotrigine, olanzapine concentrations were 35% higher than in smokers not taking lamotrigine. But in non-smokers taking lamotrigine, olanzapine concentrations were 10% *lower* than in non-smokers not taking lamotrigine. The results of this analysis are unusual and might be due to unknown confounding factors. For discussion of the effect of smoking on olanzapine concentrations, see 'Olanzapine + Tobacco', p.870.

Mechanism

Not understood. It was suggested that olanzapine might induce the glucuronidation of lamotrigine.[1] The effect of lamotrigine on olanzapine concentrations is unclear, but some involvement of glucuronidation by UGT is possible, as lamotrigine is known to affect this route of metabolism. The authors of one study suggest that lamotrigine competitively inhibits UGT resulting in raised olanzapine concentrations.[2] The effect of smoking on this interaction requires further study. The delay in gastrointestinal absorption of lamotrigine in one study was suggested to be due to antimuscarinic effects of olanzapine slowing gastrointestinal transit.[3]

Importance and management

The very slight reduction in lamotrigine exposure with olanzapine is unlikely to be clinically relevant in most patients, although the authors suggested that, because of inter-patient variability in the effect seen, it is possible that the change in lamotrigine concentrations in some patients might approach clinical relevance.[1]

Lamotrigine does not affect olanzapine concentrations to a clinically relevant extent and therefore olanzapine dose adjustments are unlikely to be necessary on concurrent use. The differing effect of lamotrigine on olanzapine concentrations depending on smoking status requires further study, but in either case the changes in olanzapine concentration seen was minor and is unlikely to be clinically important.

1. Sidhu J, Job S, Bullman J, Francis E, Abbott R, Ascher J, Theis JGW. Pharmacokinetics and tolerability of lamotrigine and olanzapine coadministered to healthy subjects. *Br J Clin Pharmacol* (2006) 61, 420–6.
2. Spina E, D'Arrigo C, Migliardi G, Santoro V, Muscatello MR, Micò U, D'Amico G, Perucca E. Effect of adjunctive lamotrigine treatment on the plasma concentrations of clozapine, risperidone and olanzapine in patients with schizophrenia or bipolar disorder. *Ther Drug Monit* (2006) 28, 599–602.
3. Jann MW, Hon YY, Shamsi SA, Zheng J, Awad EA, Spratlin V. Lack of pharmacokinetic interaction between lamotrigine and olanzapine in healthy volunteers. *Pharmacotherapy* (2006) 26, 627–633.
4. Botts S, Diaz FJ, Santoro V, Spina E, Muscatello MR, Cogollo M, Castro FE, de Leon J. Estimating the effects of co-medications on plasma olanzapine concentrations by using a mixed model. *Prog Neuropsychopharmacol Biol Psychiatry* (2008) 32, 1453–8.

Olanzapine + Mirtazapine

Mirtazapine does not affect the steady-state concentration of olanzapine. An isolated case describes status epilepticus in a patient taking mirtazapine and olanzapine.

Clinical evidence, mechanism, importance and management

In a study in 7 patients with schizophrenia taking stable doses of olanzapine, adding mirtazapine 30 mg at bedtime for 6 weeks had no effect on the steady-state concentration of olanzapine.[1] A case of status epilepticus is described in a patient, 4 days after mirtazapine 30 mg daily was started and 2 days after the mirtazapine dose was increased to 60 mg and quetiapine was abruptly switched to olanzapine. Seizures appeared about 48 hours after the first dose of olanzapine 10 mg was given. Olanzapine and mirtazapine were both discontinued and the patient was given intravenous phenytoin for one month after which she remained seizure free. Due to the lack of activity of quetiapine on CYP1A2, which is the principal isoenzyme involved in the metabolism of olanzapine, the authors ruled out an association with quetiapine.[2]

No dose adjustments would seem to be necessary if olanzapine is given with mirtazapine, but be aware that both drugs have the potential to lower the seizure threshold and that their effects might be additive. This additive effect might explain the isolated case of status epilepticus.

1. Zoccali R, Muscatello MR, La Torre D, Malara G, Canale A, Crucitti D, D'Arrigo C, Spina E. Lack of a pharmacokinetic interaction between mirtazapine and the newer antipsychotics clozapine, risperidone and olanzapine in patients with chronic schizophrenia. *Pharmacol Res* (2003) 48, 411–14.
2. Spyridi S, Sokolaki S, Nimatoudis J, Iacovides A, Kaprinis G. Status epilepticus in a patient treated with olanzapine and mirtazapine. *Int J Clin Pharmacol Ther* (2009) 47, 120–3.

Olanzapine + Miscellaneous

Venlafaxine appears to cause a small increase in olanzapine concentrations. Additive dopaminergic effects have been seen in one patient taking

olanzapine and haloperidol. Single-dose aluminium/magnesium hydroxide antacids or cimetidine do not alter olanzapine bioavailability.

Clinical evidence, mechanism, importance and management

(a) Antacids

The manufacturers of olanzapine state that single doses of an **aluminium/magnesium-containing antacid** had no effect on olanzapine bioavailability.[1,2] No particular precautions would seem to be necessary on concurrent use.

(b) Cimetidine

The manufacturers of olanzapine state that *single doses* of cimetidine had no effect on the bioavailability of olanzapine.[1,2] Note that single-dose cimetidine is not sufficient to assess any interaction by inhibition of the cytochrome P450 system. However, minimal interaction would be predicted because cimetidine is only a weak inhibitor of CYP1A2, which is the main isoenzyme involved in olanzapine metabolism. It is therefore unlikely that olanzapine dose adjustment would be needed on the concurrent use of cimetidine.

(c) Haloperidol

A 67-year-old man with a long history of bipolar disorder was taking haloperidol 10 mg daily, with valproate and benzatropine. Because he had previously had parkinsonian symptoms, olanzapine was started, to be increased as the haloperidol was decreased. On day 6 his parkinsonian symptoms became particularly marked. The haloperidol was stopped and 2 days later his symptoms had resolved. It is thought that either the small amount of dopaminergic activity of olanzapine combined with that of the haloperidol brought on these symptoms, or that olanzapine affected the metabolism of haloperidol, resulting in increased concentrations and therefore greater dopaminergic activity.[3] The general importance of this interaction is not clear, but bear it in mind in the event of an unexpected response to treatment.

Note that haloperidol can prolong the QT interval, and some suggest that olanzapine also has QT-prolonging effects. See 'Drugs that prolong the QT interval + Other drugs that prolong the QT interval', p.272 for further information on the concurrent use of two or more drugs that prolong the QT interval.

(d) Venlafaxine

A retrospective study of therapeutic drug monitoring data found that venlafaxine was associated with a small 27% increase in steady-state olanzapine plasma concentrations. The clinical importance of this finding is unclear,[4] but probably small.

1. Zyprexa Tablets (Olanzapine). Eli Lilly and Company Ltd. UK Summary of product characteristics, November 2011.
2. Zyprexa (Olanzapine). Eli Lilly and Company. US Prescribing information, June 2011.
3. Gomberg RF. Interaction between olanzapine and haloperidol. *J Clin Psychopharmacol* (1999) 19, 272–3.
4. Gex-Fabry M, Balant-Gorgia AE, Balant LP. Therapeutic drug monitoring of olanzapine: the combined effect of age, gender, smoking, and comedication. *Ther Drug Monit* (2003) 25, 46–53.

Olanzapine + Probenecid

Probenecid very slightly increases olanzapine exposure.

Clinical evidence, mechanism, importance and management

In a study, 12 healthy subjects were given a single 5-mg dose of olanzapine alone, or on day 2 of a 4-day course of probenecid 500 mg twice daily. The AUC and maximum plasma concentration of olanzapine were increased by about 20%, but overall clearance was not affected. Probenecid is thought to have caused these small effects by reducing the glucuronidation of olanzapine.[1] As this was a single dose study, the clinical implications of this interaction when olanzapine is taken regularly are unclear; however, they are probably small.

1. Markowitz JS, DeVane CL, Liston HL, Bouton DW, Risch SC. The effects of probenecid on the disposition of risperidone and olanzapine in healthy volunteers. *Clin Pharmacol Ther* (2002) 71, 30–8.

Olanzapine + Quinolones

The olanzapine concentrations of one patient were reduced when ciprofloxacin was stopped. A patient taking olanzapine developed QT interval prolongation when intravenous ciprofloxacin was also given.

Clinical evidence

The olanzapine concentrations of one patient were rapidly reduced, by more than 50%, when **ciprofloxacin** 250 mg twice daily was stopped. On the day of the last dose of a 7-day course of **ciprofloxacin** her olanzapine plasma concentration was 32.6 nanograms/mL, but within 3 days it had reduced to 14.6 nanograms/mL.[1]

A case report describes a 70-year-old woman taking azathioprine, olanzapine 10 mg daily and valsartan, who developed marked QTc interval prolongation after receiving intravenous **ciprofloxacin** 800 mg daily for 3 days. Her QTc interval returned to its initial value after **ciprofloxacin** was stopped.[2]

Mechanism

Olanzapine is partially metabolised by CYP1A2, which can be inhibited by ciprofloxacin (a weak to moderate inhibitor of CYP1A2). Concurrent use therefore decreases olanzapine metabolism, which leads to increased olanzapine concentrations. However, the extent of the change in olanzapine concentrations in the case described is greater than would be predicted from the interaction of fluvoxamine, a potent CYP1A2 inhibitor, with olanzapine, see 'Olanzapine + SSRIs', below.

Importance and management

Evidence for a pharmacokinetic interaction between olanzapine and ciprofloxacin is limited to this single case, but what was seen is in line with the predicted mechanism, although of a greater magnitude. The UK manufacturer of olanzapine recommends that a lower starting dose of olanzapine, or an olanzapine dose reduction, should be considered in patients taking a CYP1A2 inhibitor, and they name ciprofloxacin.[3] Note that other quinolones can inhibit CYP1A2 to varying degrees (for example, see 'Caffeine + Quinolones', p.1426) and might therefore be expected to interact similarly.

1. Markowitz JS, DeVane CL. Suspected ciprofloxacin inhibition of olanzapine resulting in increased plasma concentration. *J Clin Psychopharmacol* (1999) 19, 289–90.
2. Letsas KP, Sideris A, Kounas SP, Efremidis M, Korantzopoulos P, Kardaras F. Drug-induced QT interval prolongation after ciprofloxacin administration in a patient receiving olanzapine. *Int J Cardiol* (2006) 109, 273–4.
3. Zyprexa Tablets (Olanzapine). Eli Lilly and Company Ltd. UK Summary of product characteristics, November 2011.

Olanzapine + Ritonavir

Ritonavir almost halves olanzapine exposure.

Clinical evidence, mechanism, importance and management

In a study, 14 healthy non-smoking subjects were given a single 10-mg dose of olanzapine after they had taken ritonavir for 11 days (initially 300 mg twice daily, escalating to 500 mg twice daily). Ritonavir decreased the AUC and maximum plasma concentration of olanzapine by 53% and 40%, respectively, and reduced its half-life from 32 hours to 16 hours.[1]

The authors suggest that ritonavir increased the metabolism of olanzapine by inducing CYP1A2 and by inducing glucuronyltransferases (UGTs), which are the two main metabolic routes of olanzapine. Although ritonavir is widely known as a potent enzyme inhibitor, it can also induce certain metabolic pathways, including UGTs and CYP1A2.

Evidence is limited to this one study, but the pharmacokinetic interaction appears to be established. It seems likely that increased olanzapine doses might be needed in the presence of ritonavir. If concurrent use is necessary monitor olanzapine concentrations (where possible) and be alert for a reduction in its efficacy. Increase the dose of olanzapine if necessary.

1. Penzak SR, Hon YY, Lawhorn WD, Shirley KL, Spratlin V, Jann MW. Influence of ritonavir on olanzapine pharmacokinetics in healthy volunteers. *J Clin Psychopharmacol* (2002) 22, 366–70.

Olanzapine + SSRIs

Fluvoxamine increases olanzapine exposure, which can result in increased adverse effects. Fluoxetine, and possibly paroxetine appear to cause, at most, a minor rise in olanzapine concentrations, while citalopram and sertraline appear to have no effect. A case of retarded ejaculation has been seen in one patient taking olanzapine and paroxetine, and serotonin syndrome has been reported in patients taking citalopram or fluoxetine with olanzapine.

Clinical evidence

(a) Citalopram

A retrospective study of therapeutic drug monitoring data found that the dose normalised steady-state olanzapine concentration did not differ between 9 patients taking citalopram and a control group not taking citalopram.[1]

Serotonin syndrome has been reported in a patient taking olanzapine, citalopram and lithium, see 'Lithium + Olanzapine', p.1376.

(b) Fluoxetine

In a study in 15 healthy non-smokers, fluoxetine 60 mg daily for 8 days increased the maximum serum concentration and AUC of a single 5-mg dose of olanzapine by 15%, although only the change in maximum concentration reached statistical significance. In the same study, a single 60-mg dose of fluoxetine increased the maximum serum concentration and AUC of a single 5-mg dose of olanzapine by 18%.[2] For mention that higher olanzapine concentrations were associated with fluoxetine, paroxetine, and sertraline considered together, see under *Sertraline*, below.

A case report describes a patient who had been taking fluoxetine 80 mg daily for several weeks with no adverse effects who developed serotonin syndrome within 3 weeks of starting to take olanzapine 5 mg daily. His symptoms resolved after discontinuing fluoxetine, and he was later able to tolerate a 20 mg daily dose of fluoxetine and olanzapine with no further adverse effects.[3]

(c) Fluvoxamine

In a placebo-controlled study, 10 male smokers were given fluvoxamine 50 to 100 mg daily for 11 days, with olanzapine 2.5 to 7.5 mg daily on days 4 to 11. Fluvoxamine increased the olanzapine maximum plasma concentration and AUC by 84% and 119%, respectively, and the olanzapine clearance decreased by 50%. During the initial 4 days of concurrent use somnolence was increased by 19 to 115%, when compared with the group taking olanzapine and placebo, but the subjects adjusted to this over the next 4 days.[4] In a study in 12 healthy non-smoking subjects, a smaller 76% increase in the AUC of a single 10-mg dose of olanzapine was seen with fluvoxamine 100 mg daily, given for 9 days, when compared with 12 subjects given olanzapine alone.[5]

In a study 10 patients with schizophrenia were given fluvoxamine 50 mg daily from days one to 14 followed by fluvoxamine 100 mg daily from days 15 to 28. A single

10-mg dose of olanzapine was given on day 10 and again on day 24. The AUC of olanzapine was raised by 30% and 55% by 50 mg and 100 mg of fluvoxamine, respectively. Increased sedation was also seen, which was more frequent with fluvoxamine 100 mg daily.[6] Other studies in patients have found 1.7- to 2.3-fold higher steady-state olanzapine concentrations on the concurrent use of fluvoxamine. There was a marked variation between individuals in the extent of the interaction.[1,7,8] In one study, plasma concentrations of olanzapine were maintained when the dose of olanzapine was reduced by an average of 4.5 mg daily following the addition of fluvoxamine 25 mg daily.[9]

A number of case reports demonstrate the clinical relevance of this interaction. In one case, the olanzapine plasma concentration of a 21-year-old woman were 6 times the recommended upper limit while she was taking fluvoxamine. During this time she developed rigidity and tremor. After the olanzapine dose was reduced from 15 mg to 5 mg daily the concentration was still almost double the recommended concentration.[10] In another case, a patient taking fluvoxamine 200 mg daily developed hypersalivation (an adverse effect of olanzapine), without any extrapyramidal symptoms, when olanzapine 10 mg daily was also given.[11]

(d) Paroxetine

A patient taking fluvoxamine had an olanzapine concentration double the upper recommended limit. When paroxetine was substituted for fluvoxamine, the olanzapine concentration became almost normal.[10] Another patient taking paroxetine developed retarded ejaculation 2 months after he started to take olanzapine 15 mg daily. This adverse effect resolved when olanzapine was given in divided doses.[12] For mention that higher olanzapine concentrations were associated with fluoxetine, paroxetine and sertraline considered together, see under *Sertraline*, below.

(e) Sertraline

A retrospective study of therapeutic drug monitoring data found that the concentration-to-dose ratio of olanzapine did not differ between 21 patients taking sertraline and a control group not taking sertraline, suggesting that sertraline does not affect the pharmacokinetics of olanzapine.[7]

Another study of therapeutic drug monitoring data that grouped **fluoxetine, paroxetine** and sertraline, reported that the dose-normalised steady-state olanzapine concentration was 32% higher in patients taking any of these three SSRIs when compared with a control group. This value is difficult to interpret because the drugs were not considered individually.[1]

Mechanism

Olanzapine is partially metabolised by cytochrome P450 isoenzymes, and CYP1A2 is the major isoenzyme involved. Fluvoxamine is a potent inhibitor of CYP1A2 resulting in increased olanzapine exposure and adverse effects. CYP2D6 also has a minor role in olanzapine metabolism. Many SSRIs can affect CYP2D6, with fluoxetine and paroxetine having the most potent effect. These SSRIs therefore raise olanzapine concentrations, but only to a very minor extent.

Importance and management

There is a good body of evidence that demonstrates that **fluvoxamine** can raise olanzapine exposure to a clinically relevant extent. The extent of the rise seen and the case reports of adverse effects suggest that a lower dose of olanzapine is likely to be needed in the presence of fluvoxamine. Monitor for olanzapine adverse effects (e.g. somnolence, weight gain, dizziness) and adjust the olanzapine dose if necessary. The manufacturers of olanzapine recommend that a lower starting dose of olanzapine[13] or an olanzapine dose reduction should be considered for patients given a CYP1A2 inhibitor, such as fluvoxamine.[13,14]

Other SSRIs do not appear to interact to a clinically relevant extent, and olanzapine dose adjustments would not be expected to be necessary on concurrent use. However, the case report with **paroxetine** and **fluoxetine** suggests that additive adverse effects are a possibility, and this should be borne in mind if adverse effects become troublesome.

1. Gex-Fabry M, Balant-Gorgia AE, Balant LP. Therapeutic drug monitoring of olanzapine: the combined effect of age, gender, smoking, and comedication. *Ther Drug Monit* (2003) 25, 46–53.
2. Gossen D, de Suray J-M, Vandenhende F, Onkelinx C, Gangji D. Influence of fluoxetine on olanzapine pharmacokinetics. *AAPS PharmSci* (2002) 4, E11.
3. Chopra P, Ng C, Schweitzer I. Serotonin syndrome associated with fluoxetine and olanzapine. *World J Biol Psychiatry* (2004) 5, 114–15.
4. Mäenpää J, Wrighton S, Bergstrom R, Cerimele B, Tatum D, Hatcher B, Callaghan JT. Pharmacokinetic (PK) and pharmacodynamic (PD) interactions between fluvoxamine and olanzapine. *Clin Pharmacol Ther* (1997) 61, 225.
5. Wang C-Y, Zhang Z-J, Li W-B, Zhai Y-M, Cai Z-J, Weng Y-Z, Zhu R-H, Zhao J-P, Zhou H-H. The differential effects of steady-state fluvoxamine on the pharmacokinetics of olanzapine and clozapine in healthy volunteers. *J Clin Pharmacol* (2004) 44, 785–92.
6. Chiu C-C, Lane H-Y, Huang M-C, Liu H-C, Jann MW, Hon Y-Y, Chang W-H, Lu M-L. Dose-dependent alterations in the pharmacokinetics of olanzapine during coadministration of fluvoxamine in patients with schizophrenia. *J Clin Pharmacol* (2004) 44, 1385–90.
7. Weigmann H, Gerek S, Zeisig A, Müller M, Härtter S, Heimke C. Fluvoxamine but not sertraline inhibits the metabolism of olanzapine: evidence from a therapeutic drug monitoring service. *Ther Drug Monit* (2001) 23, 410–13.
8. Hiemke C, Peled A, Jabarin M, Hadjez J, Weigmann H, Härtter S, Ilan M, Ritsner M, Silver H. Fluvoxamine augmentation of olanzapine in chronic schizophrenia: pharmacokinetic interactions and clinical effects. *J Clin Psychopharmacol* (2002) 22, 502–6.
9. Albers LJ, Ozdemir V, Marder SR, Raggi MA, Aravagiri M. Endrenyi L. Reist C. Low-dose fluvoxamine as an adjunct to reduce olanzapine therapeutic dose requirements. A prospective dose-adjusted drug interaction strategy. *J Clin Psychopharmacol* (2005) 25, 170–4.
10. de Jong J, Hoogenboom B, van Troostwijk LD, de Haan L. Interaction of olanzapine with fluvoxamine. *Psychopharmacology (Berl)* (2001) 155, 219–20.
11. Hori T, Makabe K, Nemoto K, Asada T. Hypersalivation induced by olanzapine with fluvoxamine. *Prog Neuropsychopharmacol Biol Psychiatry* (2006) 30, 758–60.
12. Bizouard P, Vandel S, Kantelip JP. Olanzapine-induced retarded ejaculation: role of paroxetine comedication? A case report. *Therapie* (2001) 56, 443–5.
13. Zyprexa Tablets (Olanzapine). Eli Lilly and Company Ltd. UK Summary of product characteristics, November 2011.
14. Zyprexa (Olanzapine). Eli Lilly and Company. US Prescribing information, June 2011.

Olanzapine + Tobacco

Smoking tobacco increases the clearance of olanzapine.

Clinical evidence

Retrospective studies have found that cigarette smoking reduces olanzapine concentrations:[1-3] in one study by 12%[1] and by about 50% in another.[3] Smokers needed higher doses of olanzapine than non-smokers (12.5 mg compared with 10 mg) yet had lower olanzapine concentrations (60 nanomol/L compared with 92 nanomol/L).[4] Similarly, a study found that the clearance of olanzapine was about 50% greater in 274 smokers than in 249 non-smokers.[5] A further study in 17 psychiatric patients found that the olanzapine concentration-to-dose ratio was directly related to the activity of CYP1A2: CYP1A2 activity was 6-fold higher, and dose-normalised steady-state olanzapine concentrations were 5-fold lower, in smokers than non-smokers.[6] A mixed model analysis of published and unpublished data confirms the reduction in olanzapine concentrations by smoking, but found that the size of the inducing effect of smoking was reduced by the concurrent use of lamotrigine. In smokers not taking lamotrigine there was a 41% decrease in olanzapine concentrations compared with non-smokers not taking lamotrigine, but in smokers taking lamotrigine there was only an 11% decrease in olanzapine concentrations compared with non-smokers taking lamotrigine.[7] For discussion of the effects of lamotrigine on olanzapine concentrations, see 'Olanzapine + Lamotrigine', p.868.

A case report describes a patient whose schizophrenia was successfully managed with olanzapine 15 mg daily while in hospital and smoking up to 12 cigarettes a day. However, on discharge his cigarette consumption increased to 80 per day, and his schizophrenic symptoms worsened. Olanzapine plasma concentrations reduced from 52 nanograms/mL to 30 nanograms/mL as his cigarette consumption increased.[8]

A patient taking olanzapine 30 mg daily developed extrapyramidal symptoms, probably as a result of increased plasma concentrations of olanzapine, following a reduction of his tobacco consumption. These effects improved following a reduction in his olanzapine dose to 20 mg daily.[9]

Mechanism

Olanzapine is principally metabolised by glucuronidation and by CYP1A2, both of which are induced by smoking, leading to decreased olanzapine concentrations.

Importance and management

These findings suggest that the effects of olanzapine are reduced to some extent by smoking, but as the dose of olanzapine is individually titrated to effect it seems likely that routine dose adjustments will account for this interaction when olanzapine is started in a smoker. However, if a patient decides to stop smoking, or begins to smoke more tobacco, it would be prudent to monitor the patient more closely, as dose decreases or increases might become necessary.

1. Gex-Fabry M, Balant-Gorgia AE, Balant LP. Therapeutic drug monitoring of olanzapine: the combined effect of age, gender, smoking, and comedication. *Ther Drug Monit* (2003) 25, 46–53.
2. Theisen FM, Haberhausen M, Schulz E, Fleischhaker C, Clement H-W, Heinzel-Gutenbrunner M, Remschmidt H. Serum levels of olanzapine and its N-desmethyl and 2-hydroxymethyl metabolites in child and adolescent psychiatric disorders: effects of dose, diagnosis, age, sex, smoking, and comedication. *Ther Drug Monit* (2006) 28, 750–9.
3. Haslemo T, Eikeseth PH, Tanum L, Molden E, Refsum H. The effect of variable cigarette consumption on the interaction with clozapine and olanzapine. *Eur J Clin Pharmacol* (2006) 62, 1049–53.
4. Skogh E, Reis M, Dahl M-L, Lundmark J, Bengtsson F. Therapeutic drug monitoring data on olanzapine and its N-demethyl metabolite in the naturalistic clinical setting. *Ther Drug Monit* (2002) 24, 518–26.
5. Bigos KL, Pollock BG, Coley KC, Miller DD, Marder SR, Aravagiri M, Kirshner MA, Schneider LS, Bies RR. Sex, race and smoking impact olanzapine exposure. *J Clin Pharmacol* (2008) 48, 157–65.
6. Carillo JA, Herráiz AG, Ramos SI, Gervasini G, Vizcaíno S, Benítez J. Role of the smoking-induced cytochrome P450 (CYP)1A2 and polymorphic CYP2D6 in steady-state concentration of olanzapine. *J Clin Psychopharmacol* (2003) 23, 119–27.
7. Botts S, Diaz FJ, Santoro V, Spina E, Muscatello MR, Cogollo M, Castro FE, de Leon J. Estimating the effects of co-medications on plasma olanzapine concentrations by using a mixed model. *Prog Neuropsychopharmacol Biol Psychiatry* (2008) 32, 1453–8.
8. Chiu C-C, Lu M-L, Huang M-C, Chen K-P. Heavy smoking, reduced olanzapine levels, and treatment effects. A case report. *Ther Drug Monit* (2004) 26, 579–81.
9. Zullino DF, Delessert D, Eap CB, Preisig M, Baumann P. Tobacco and cannabis smoking cessation can lead to intoxication with clozapine or olanzapine. *Int Clin Psychopharmacol* (2002) 17, 141–3.

Olanzapine + Topiramate

Topiramate does not appear to affect steady-state concentration of olanzapine.

Clinical evidence, mechanism, importance and management

In a study, 12 patients receiving long-term treatment with olanzapine 10 mg to 20 mg daily were given topiramate in a dose that was increased gradually to 200 mg daily over 6 to 8 weeks. The steady-state plasma concentration of olanzapine did not appear to be affected by topiramate.[1] Similarly, olanzapine concentrations did not appear to be affected by topiramate 300 mg daily in 5 patients with treatment-resistant schizophrenia.[2] These studies suggest that it is unlikely that the dose of olanzapine would need adjusting if topiramate was also given.

1. Migliardi G, D'Arrigo C, Santoro V, Bruno A, Cortese L, Campolo D, Cacciola M, Spina E. Effect of topiramate on plasma concentrations of clozapine, olanzapine, risperidone, and quetiapine in patients with psychotic disorders. *Clin Neuropharmacol* (2007) 30, 107–13.

2. Tiihonen J, Halonen P, Wahlbeck K, Repo-Tiihonen E, Hyvärinen S, Eronen M, Putkonen H, Takala P, Mehtonen O-P, Puck M, Oksanen J, Koskelainen P, Joffe G, Aer J, Hallikainen T, Ryynänen O-P, Tupala E. Topiramate add-on in treatment-resistant schizophrenia: a randomized, double-blind, placebo-controlled, crossover trial. *J Clin Psychiatry* (2005) 66, 1012–5.

Olanzapine + Tricyclic and related antidepressants

No pharmacokinetic interaction occurs between single doses of imipramine and olanzapine. The additive effects of clomipramine and olanzapine were thought to have caused a seizure in one patient and serotonin syndrome in another.

Clinical evidence, mechanism, importance and management

A randomised, crossover study in 9 healthy men who were given single doses of olanzapine 5 mg and **imipramine** 75 mg found no clinically relevant pharmacokinetic or pharmacodynamic interactions between the two drugs.[1] However, note that a single dose is generally insufficient to assess the potential for a drug to alter metabolism.

One case report describes seizures, thought to be caused by the additive effects of olanzapine and **clomipramine**. Neither drug alone had produced this reaction in the patient.[2]

Another case report describes serotonin syndrome in a patient, 20 days after **clomipramine** 75 mg daily and olanzapine 20 mg daily were started. On admission the patient was pyrexial, shivering, agitated and confused. His symptoms progressed to coma, with myoclonus and hyperreflexia 3 days later and he was transferred to the intensive care unit for ventilation and supportive treatment. He was diagnosed with serotonin syndrome and treated with biperiden 5 mg twice daily and cyproheptadine 4 mg six times daily. The patient had improved sufficiently one week after admission to return to the ward and he was discharged after a further 6 days.[3]

No dose adjustments would seem to be necessary if olanzapine is given with a tricyclic, but be aware that both olanzapine and the tricyclics have the potential to lower the seizure threshold and that their effects might be additive. The case of serotonin syndrome with clomipramine and olanzapine was thought to be due to the additive effects of these two drugs on serotonin receptors, although this is not established.

1. Callaghan JT, Cerimele BJ, Kassahun KJ, Nyhart EH, Hoyes-Beehler PJ, Kondraske GV. Olanzapine: interaction study with imipramine. *J Clin Pharmacol* (1997) 37, 971–8.
2. Deshauer D, Albuquerque J, Alda M, Grof P. Seizures caused by possible interaction between olanzapine and clomipramine. *J Clin Psychopharmacol* (2000) 20, 283–4.
3. Verre M, Bossio F, Mammone A, Piccirillo M, Tancioni F, Tortorella V, Varano M. Serotonin syndrome caused by olanzapine and clomipramine. *Minerva Anestesiol* (2008) 74, 41–5.

Olanzapine + Valproate

Valproate appears to cause minor to modest reductions in olanzapine concentrations. Concurrent use appears to increase the risk of hepatic injury in children.

Clinical evidence

(a) Adverse effects

A retrospective study identified 52 children (under 18-years-old) who were taking olanzapine alone (17 patients), valproate semisodium (divalproex sodium) alone (23 patients) or both drugs together (12 patients). At least one liver enzyme measurement (ALT, AST or lactate dehydrogenase) was found to be above the normal range in 59% of those taking olanzapine alone, in 26% of those taking valproate alone, and in all of the patients taking both drugs. Liver enzymes were persistently elevated in 42% of the patients taking both drugs, and 2 of these patients had concentrations that were three times the upper limit of normal. Treatment was discontinued due to pancreatitis in one and steatohepatitis in the other.[1] Both valproate and olanzapine are known to be associated with adverse effects on the liver, and the effects might be additive or synergistic.

The authors of an analysis of reports on the use of mood stabiliser combinations noted that there might be additive adverse effects of weight gain and drowsiness when olanzapine is given with valproate.[2]

(b) Pharmacokinetic effects

A study in 18 patients stabilised on olanzapine 5 to 20 mg daily found that valproate, at a dose ranging from 600 to 2000 mg daily for 4 weeks, appeared to reduce steady-state olanzapine plasma concentrations by 18%. No patient showed signs of any worsening of their psychopathological condition.[3] In another study in 4 patients, a greater reduction in olanzapine plasma concentrations of between 32 and 79% was found when valproate was given.[4]

Mechanism

The authors suggested that this occurred due to the valproate inducing the enzymes involved in the metabolism of olanzapine.[4] However, valproate is not known to be an inducer of UGTs or CYP1A2, the principal routes of metabolism of olanzapine. Other mechanisms might be involved.[3]

Importance and management

The apparent minor reductions in steady-state olanzapine concentrations seen in one study[3] are unlikely to be clinically important and an olanzapine dose adjustment would not seem necessary if valproate is also given, although the greater reduction in olanzapine concentrations in the other study[4] introduces a note of caution.

The clinical relevance of the report of increased adverse effects[2] is uncertain, but note that several manufacturers of valproate warn of an increased risk of olanzapine adverse effects (e.g. neutropenia, tremor, dry mouth) if olanzapine is given with valproate. Bear the possibility in mind. The general relevance of the adverse hepatic effects in children is also unknown, but the authors of the study recommend measuring liver enzymes every 3 to 4 months for the first year of concurrent use, thereafter monitoring every 6 months if no adverse effects are detected.[1] This is standard advice when starting valproate, particularly in patients thought to be a risk for liver dysfunction, and is therefore prudent.

1. Gonzalez-Heydrich J, Raches D, Wilens TE, Leichtner A, Mezzacappa E. Retrospective study of hepatic enzyme elevations in children treated with olanzapine, divalproex, and their combination. *J Am Acad Child Adolesc Psychiatry* (2003) 12, 1227–33.
2. Freeman MP, Stoll AL. Mood stabilizer combinations: a review of safety and efficacy. *Am J Psychiatry* (1998) 155, 12–21.
3. Spina E, D'Arrigo C, Santoro V, Muscatello MR, Pandolfo G, Zoccali R, Diaz FJ, de Leon J. Effect of valproate on olanzapine plasma concentrations in patients with bipolar or schizoaffective disorder. *Ther Drug Monit* (2009) 31, 758–63.
4. Bergemann N, Kress KR, Abu-Tair F, Frick A, Kopitz J. Valproate lowers plasma concentrations of olanzapine. *Pharmacopsychiatry* (2005) 38, 44.

Paliperidone + Miscellaneous

Paliperidone exposure is increased by a high-fat, high-calorie meal and valproate, and decreased by carbamazepine. Trimethoprim, tobacco smoking, and paroxetine do not notably affect the pharmacokinetics of paliperidone. Additive pharmacological effects can be expected if paliperidone is taken with other drugs that lower the seizure threshold. Paliperidone does not alter valproate pharmacokinetics.

Clinical evidence, mechanism, importance and management

Note that paliperidone is 9-hydroxyrisperidone, the active metabolite of risperidone.

(a) Carbamazepine

The manufacturers report that, in a study, carbamazepine 200 mg twice daily decreased the steady-state AUC and maximum concentration of paliperidone by 37%. This was mainly due to a 35% increase in renal clearance of paliperidone,[1,2] probably associated with the induction of renal P-glycoprotein by carbamazepine.[1] It is possible that higher doses of carbamazepine might produce greater decreases in paliperidone concentrations.[1] The manufacturer advises that if carbamazepine is started, the dose of paliperidone should be reviewed and increased if necessary, with decreases in dose if carbamazepine is then stopped.[1,2] The UK manufacturer notes that the induction effects of carbamazepine on paliperidone concentrations become maximal after 2 to 3 weeks. They also note that **rifampicin** (**rifampin**) and **St John's wort** (*Hypericum perforatum*) are also P-glycoprotein inducers, and they might therefore be expected to interact similarly.[1]

(b) Drugs that lower seizure threshold

The manufacturer advises caution if paliperidone is used with other drugs known to lower the seizure threshold. They specifically name **butyrophenones**, **clozapine**, **mefloquine**, **phenothiazines**, **SSRIs**, **tramadol**, and **tricyclic antidepressants**.[1]

(c) Food

Giving extended-release paliperidone with a high-fat, high-calorie meal increased its maximum concentration and AUC by 50 to 60%, when compared with the fasting state.[1] The UK manufacturer states that paliperidone should be consistently taken either on an empty stomach or with breakfast,[1] whereas the US manufacturer advises that paliperidone can be taken without regard to food,[2] which was the protocol in the clinical efficacy studies of paliperidone.[1,2]

(d) Lithium compounds

The manufacturers of paliperidone briefly state that, although no interaction studies have been conducted,[1] a pharmacokinetic interaction between paliperidone and lithium is unlikely.[1,2] However, note that cases of adverse effects, including neurotoxicity, have been reported on the concurrent use of lithium and risperidone, see 'Lithium + Risperidone', p.1377.

(e) Paroxetine

In a randomised, crossover study in 50 healthy subjects (all CYP2D6 extensive or ultrarapid metabolisers), paroxetine 20 mg daily for 13 days caused a negligible 17% increase in the AUC of a single 3-mg dose of extended-release paliperidone given on day 10.[3] Paroxetine is a potent inhibitor of CYP2D6, and this study shows that paliperidone is not metabolised to a clinically relevant extent by CYP2D6. No paliperidone dose adjustment would seem necessary on the concurrent use of paroxetine or other inhibitors of CYP2D6.

(f) Tobacco

The UK manufacturer briefly reports that, in a population pharmacokinetic analysis, smokers had a slightly lower exposure to paliperidone, when compared with non-smokers. However, they state that this slight change is not expected to be clinically relevant. In addition, *in vitro* studies suggest that paliperidone is not a substrate of CYP1A2. Therefore smoking tobacco, which is a known inducer of CYP1A2, would not be expected to affect the pharmacokinetics of paliperidone,[1] and no paliperidone dose adjustment is expected to be necessary in patients who smoke tobacco.

(g) Trimethoprim

In a randomised crossover study, 30 healthy subjects who were given a single 6-mg dose of extended-release paliperidone alone, and on day 5 of an 8-day course of trimethoprim 200 mg twice daily. Trimethoprim caused a negligible 9% decrease in the AUC of paliperidone and a 13% increase in its renal clearance. Paliperidone is a cation at physiological pH and is principally excreted unchanged by the kidneys. Therefore this study was undertaken to assess the effect of an inhibitor of the organic cation transporter system, such as trimethoprim, on its excretion. None of these changes are clinically relevant, and no paliperidone dose adjustment would be expected to be needed on the concurrent use of trimethoprim.[4]

(h) Valproate

In a pharmacokinetic study in 13 patients stable taking extended-release **valproate semisodium (divalproex sodium)** 500 mg to 2 g daily, paliperidone 12 mg daily for 5 days did not affect the steady-state pharmacokinetics of valproate.[1,2] The US manufacturer also reports that in a clinical study in patients stable taking valproate, the addition of paliperidone 3 to 15 mg daily did not affect the mean plasma concentrations of valproate, when compared with valproate alone.[2] However, extended-release **valproate semisodium (divalproex sodium)** 1 g daily increased the AUC and maximum concentration of a single 12-mg dose of paliperidone by about 50%.[1,2] The manufacturer advises considering a dose reduction of paliperidone after clinical assessment if both drugs are given.[1,2]

1. Invega (Paliperidone). Janssen-Cilag Ltd. UK Summary of product characteristics, June 2012.
2. Invega (Paliperidone). Janssen Pharmaceuticals, Inc. US Prescribing information, June 2011.
3. Berwaerts J, Cleton A, Herben V, van de Vliet I, Chang I, van Hoek P, Eerdekens M. The effect of paroxetine on the pharmacokinetics of paliperidone extended-release tablets. *Pharmacopsychiatry* (2009) 42, 158–63.
4. Thyssen A, Cleton A, Talluri K, Leempoels J, Janssens L, Boom S, Eerdekens M. No pharmacokinetic interaction between paliperidone extended-release tablets and trimethoprim in healthy subjects. *Hum Psychopharmacol* (2009) 24, 532–9.

Perospirone + Miscellaneous

Perospirone exposure is markedly reduced by carbamazepine, and markedly increased by itraconazole.

Clinical evidence, mechanism, importance and management

(a) Carbamazepine

In a study in 10 healthy subjects, **carbamazepine** 200 mg daily for 5 days reduced the plasma concentration of a single 8-mg dose of perospirone given on day 6 to below the detection limit, and reduced the AUC of its active metabolite by 53%.[1] Carbamazepine is known to be an inducer of CYP3A4, and it seems possible that perospirone is metabolised by this isoenzyme. Therefore concurrent use reduces perospirone metabolism and exposure. Although the clinical relevance of this finding was not assessed it seems probable that carbamazepine will reduce the efficacy of perospirone. Monitor concurrent use carefully and adjust the perospirone dose if necessary.

(b) Itraconazole or Ketoconazole

In a study in 9 healthy subjects, giving **itraconazole** 200 mg daily for 5 days, with a single 8-mg dose of perospirone on day 6, resulted in a 6.8-fold increase in the AUC of perospirone. A similar increase in the maximum plasma concentration and the half-life of perospirone was also seen.[2] An *in vitro* study found that the metabolism of perospirone was markedly reduced by **ketoconazole** and it was estimated that *in vivo* perospirone clearance could be reduced by 64 to 90%.[3] As itraconazole and ketoconazole are potent inhibitors of CYP3A4, increases in concentrations of perospirone seem likely to be due to inhibition of its metabolism by this isoenzyme.

1. Masui T, Kusumi I, Takahashi Y, Koyama T. Effect of carbamazepine on the single oral dose pharmacokinetics of perospirone and its active metabolite. *Prog Neuropsychopharmacol Biol Psychiatry* (2006) 30, 1330–3.
2. Masui T, Kusumi I, Takahashi Y, Koyama T. Effects of itraconazole and tandospirone on the pharmacokinetics of perospirone. *Ther Drug Monit* (2006) 28, 73–5.
3. Shimakura J, Tani N, Mizuno Y, Komuro S, Kanamaru H. In vitro drug-drug interactions with perospirone and concomitantly administered drugs in human liver microsomes. *Eur J Drug Metab Pharmacokinet* (2003) 28, 67–72.

Phenothiazines + Antacids

An antacid containing aluminium hydroxide with magnesium trisilicate appeared to reduce the maximum serum concentration of chlorpromazine, whereas a calcium carbonate glycine antacid appeared to have no effect. An antacid containing aluminium and magnesium hydroxide appeared to have no effect on the maximum concentration of chlorpromazine in one study, but reduced urinary excretion of chlorpromazine was seen in another. *In vitro* studies suggest that this interaction might possibly also occur with other antacids and phenothiazines.

Clinical evidence

A study in 10 patients taking **chlorpromazine** 600 mg to 1.2 g daily in three divided doses found that 30 mL of *Aludrox* (**aluminium/magnesium hydroxide** gel) three times daily taken simultaneously with the chlorpromazine reduced the urinary excretion of **chlorpromazine** by 27% (10 to 45%). In 3 other patients in whom administration of the antacid was separated from the chlorpromazine, a lower 17% (8 to 27%) decrease in urinary chlorpromazine excretion was seen.[1]

A study was prompted by the observation of one psychiatric patient, taking **chlorpromazine** who relapsed within 3 days of starting to take an unnamed antacid. When 6 patients were given 30 mL of *Gelusil* (**aluminium hydroxide** with **magnesium trisilicate**) with **chlorpromazine** suspension, the serum **chlorpromazine** concentration measured 2 hours later were reduced by about 20% (from 168 nanograms/mL to 132 nanograms/mL).[2] In contrast, in yet another single-dose study in patients, neither 30 mL of an **aluminium/magnesium hydroxide antacid** nor 30 mL of a **calcium carbonate glycine antacid** had any effect on chlorpromazine concentrations 2 hours after the dose.[3]

Mechanism

Chlorpromazine and other phenothiazines become adsorbed onto these antacids,[2,3] which would seem to account for the reduced bioavailability. *In vitro* studies have also found that other phenothiazines (trifluoperazine, fluphenazine, perphenazine, thioridazine) are adsorbed to a considerable extent onto a number of antacids (magnesium trisilicate, bismuth subnitrate, aluminium hydroxide with magnesium carbonate).[4]

Importance and management

Information regarding an interaction between antacids and phenothiazines seems to be limited to the reports cited for chlorpromazine. Reductions of up to 45% in serum antipsychotic concentrations would be expected to be clinically important, but so far only one case describing reduced efficacy seems to have been reported.[2] Separating the doses as much as possible (one to 2 hours) to avoid admixture in the gut should minimise any effects. Other phenothiazines and antacids are known to interact *in vitro*,[4] but the clinical importance of these interactions awaits further study.

1. Forrest FM, Forrest IS, Serra MT. Modification of chlorpromazine metabolism by some other drugs frequently administered to psychiatric patients. *Biol Psychiatry* (1970) 2, 53–8.
2. Fann WE, Davis JM, Janowsky DS, Sekerke HJ, Schmidt DM. Chlorpromazine: effects of antacids on its gastrointestinal absorption. *J Clin Pharmacol* (1973) 13, 388–90.
3. Pinell OC, Fenimore DC, Davis CM, Moreira O, Fann WE. Drug-drug interaction of chlorpromazine and antacid. *Clin Pharmacol Ther* (1978) 23, 125.
4. Moustafa MA, Babhair SA, Kouta HI. Decreased bioavailability of some antipsychotic phenothiazines due to interactions with adsorbent antacid and antidiarrhoeal mixtures. *Int J Pharmaceutics* (1987) 36, 185–9.

Phenothiazines + Barbiturates

The concentrations of chlorpromazine, and possibly thioridazine, are decreased by phenobarbital. Phenothiazines also appear to reduce barbiturate concentrations. Pentobarbital, promethazine and hyoscine in combination are said to increase the incidence of peri-operative agitation.

Clinical evidence

(a) Phenobarbital

1. Phenothiazine concentrations reduced. A study in 12 patients with schizophrenia taking **chlorpromazine** 100 mg three times daily found that phenobarbital 50 mg three times daily reduced **chlorpromazine** plasma concentrations by 25 to 30%, which was accompanied by changes in certain physiological measurements, which clearly reflected a reduced response to chlorpromazine.[1]

In another study in 7 patients, the plasma concentrations of **thioridazine** were reduced by phenobarbital, but the clinical effects of this were uncertain.[2] However, another study found that phenobarbital caused no changes in serum **thioridazine** concentrations, but the concentrations of its active metabolite, mesoridazine, were reduced.[3]

2. Phenobarbital concentrations reduced. A study in patients with epilepsy found that their serum phenobarbital concentrations fell by 29% when they were given phenothiazines, which included **chlorpromazine**, **thioridazine** or **mesoridazine**, and increased when the phenothiazine was withdrawn.[4] This study confirms another, in which **thioridazine** 100 to 200 mg daily was found to reduce serum phenobarbital concentrations by about 25%.[5]

(b) Pentobarbital

Limited evidence suggests that the concurrent use of pentobarbital, **promethazine** and hyoscine increases the incidence of pre-operative, peri-operative and postoperative agitation, and it has been suggested that this triple combination should be avoided.[6]

Mechanism

Uncertain. The barbiturates are potent liver enzyme inducers, and so it is presumed that they increase the metabolism of the phenothiazines by the liver.

Importance and management

The interactions between phenobarbital and the phenothiazines appear to be established, but the documentation is limited. Their importance is uncertain, but be alert for evidence of reductions in response to both drugs if a phenothiazine and a barbiturate are given, and to increased responses if one of the drugs is withdrawn. The only combinations implicated are phenobarbital with chlorpromazine, mesoridazine, and thioridazine, but it seems possible that other phenothiazines and barbiturates could behave similarly.

1. Loga S, Curry S, Lader M. Interactions of orphenadrine and phenobarbitone with chlorpromazine: plasma concentrations and effects in man. *Br J Clin Pharmacol* (1975) 2, 197–208.
2. Ellenor GL, Musa MN, Beuthin FC. Phenobarbital-thioridazine interaction in man. *Res Commun Chem Pathol Pharmacol* (1978) 21, 185–8.

3. Linnoila M, Viukari M, Vaisanen K, Auvinen J. Effect of anticonvulsants on plasma haloperidol and thioridazine levels. *Am J Psychiatry* (1980) 137, 819–21.
4. Haidukewych D, Rodin EA. Effect of phenothiazines on serum antiepileptic drug concentrations in psychiatric patients with seizure disorder. *Ther Drug Monit* (1985) 7, 401–4.
5. Gay PE, Madsen JA. Interaction between phenobarbital and thioridazine. *Neurology* (1983) 33, 1631–2.
6. Macris SG, Levy L. Preanesthetic medication: untoward effects of certain drug combinations. *Anesthesiology* (1965) 26, 256.

Phenothiazines + Cannabis or Tobacco

Smokers of tobacco might possibly need larger doses of chlorpromazine, fluphenazine, perphenazine or thioridazine than non-smokers. A similar effect might occur with chlorpromazine in cannabis smokers.

Clinical evidence

(a) Chlorpromazine

A comparative study found that the frequency of drowsiness in 403 patients taking chlorpromazine was 16% in non-smokers, 11% in light smokers, and 3% in heavy smokers (more than 20 cigarettes daily).[1] Another report describes a patient taking chlorpromazine who experienced increased sedation and dizziness and higher plasma chlorpromazine concentrations when he gave up smoking.[2] A study in 31 patients found that the clearance of chlorpromazine was increased by 38% by tobacco smoking, by 50% by cannabis smoking, and by 107% when both tobacco and cannabis were smoked.[3]

(b) Fluphenazine

A retrospective study in 40 psychiatric inpatients found that the plasma fluphenazine concentrations of non-smokers were more than double those of smokers (1.83 nanograms/mL compared with 0.89 nanograms/mL) when they were given oral fluphenazine hydrochloride. The clearance of both oral and intramuscular fluphenazine was 1.67-fold and 2.33-fold greater, respectively, in the smokers than in the non-smokers.[4] No behavioural differences were seen.[4]

(c) Perphenazine

In a pharmacokinetic modelling study of plasma perphenazine concentrations from a clinical study in 156 patients receiving perphenazine 8 to 32 mg daily, smoking was associated with a 33% faster perphenazine clearance than the group as a whole.[5]

(d) Thioridazine

A study in 76 patients taking thioridazine found that the dose-corrected steady-state plasma concentrations of thioridazine were lower in smokers than in non-smokers (4 nanomol/L per mg compared with 7.4 nanomol/L per mg, respectively). Concentrations of the thioridazine metabolites, mesoridazine and sulforidazine, were also lower in smokers.[6]

Mechanism

Not established. The probable reason is that some of the components of tobacco smoke act as enzyme inducers, which increase the rate at which the liver metabolises these antipsychotics, thereby reducing their serum concentrations and clinical effects.

Importance and management

The pharmacokinetic interactions between tobacco smoking and chlorpromazine, fluphenazine, perphenazine, or thioridazine appear to be established but are of uncertain clinical importance. Be alert for the need to increase the doses of these antipsychotics in patients who smoke, and reduce the doses if smoking is stopped.

1. Swett C. Drowsiness due to chlorpromazine in relation to cigarette smoking: a report from the Boston Collaborative Drug Surveillance Program. *Arch Gen Psychiatry* (1974) 31, 211–13.
2. Stimmel GL, Falloon IRH. Chlorpromazine plasma levels, adverse effects, and tobacco smoking: case report. *J Clin Psychiatry* (1983) 44, 420–2.
3. Chetty M, Miller R, Moodley SV. Smoking and body weight influence the clearance of chlorpromazine. *Eur J Clin Pharmacol* (1994) 46, 523–6.
4. Ereshefsky L, Jann MW, Saklad SR, Davis CM, Richards AL, Burch NR. Effects of smoking on fluphenazine clearance in psychiatric inpatients. *Biol Psychiatry* (1985) 20, 329–32.
5. Jin Y, Pollock BG, Coley K, Miller D, Marder SR, Florian J, Schneider L, Lieberman J, Kirshner M, Bies RR. Population pharmacokinetics of perphenazine in schizophrenia patients from CATIE: impact of race and smoking. *J Clin Pharmacol* (2010) 50, 73–80.
6. Berecz R, de la Rubia A, Dorado P, Fernández-Salguero P, Dahl M-L, LLerena A. Thioridazine steady-state plasma concentrations are influenced by tobacco smoking and CYP2D6, but not by the *CYP2C9* genotype. *Eur J Clin Pharmacol* (2003) 59, 45–50.

Phenothiazines + Carbamazepine and related drugs

Fluphenazine concentrations are reduced by carbamazepine. Switching from carbamazepine to oxcarbazepine appeared to increase chlorpromazine concentrations in one small study. The concurrent use of thioridazine and carbamazepine does not appear to affect the pharmacokinetics of either drug. Case reports describe neuroleptic malignant syndrome in patients taking phenothiazines with carbamazepine.

Clinical evidence

(a) Chlorpromazine

Oxcarbazepine was substituted for carbamazepine in 4 patients with difficult to manage schizophrenia taking chlorpromazine, and in 3 cases other antipsychotic medication (lithium, zuclopenthixol or clozapine). After 3 weeks of taking oxcarbazepine all 4 patients had rises in their chlorpromazine concentrations of 28%, 63%, 76%, and 90%, respectively. In one case this rise was associated with increased extrapyramidal adverse effects.[1]

A case report describes a patient taking amoxapine and chlorpromazine 350 mg daily, who developed ataxia, nausea and agitation when carbamazepine, titrated to 900 mg daily, was started. The adverse effects were attributed to high concentrations of the carbamazepine metabolite, carbamazepine-10,11-epoxide.[2]

(b) Fluphenazine

A patient receiving intramuscular fluphenazine decanoate 37.5 mg weekly had a rise in his serum fluphenazine concentrations from 0.6 nanograms/mL to 1.17 nanograms/mL 6 weeks after stopping carbamazepine 800 mg daily. A moderate improvement in his schizophrenic condition occurred.[3]

(c) Levomepromazine

A 54-year old man living in a psychiatric hospital, who had been taking haloperidol, levomepromazine, sultopride, and metixene long-term was prescribed carbamazepine 400 mg daily for impulsive behaviour. The following day he became unstable on his feet, and after 3 days could no longer walk by himself. He had a fever of 40°C, muscle rigidity, diaphoresis, and serum creatine phosphokinase was elevated to 923 units/L. He was diagnosed as having neuroleptic malignant syndrome, and recovered after body cooling and administration of fluids, with symptoms resolving over 12 days.[4]

(d) Thioridazine

In a study in 8 patients with epilepsy, thioridazine 100 to 200 mg daily was found to have no effect on the steady-state concentrations of carbamazepine or carbamazepine-10,11-epoxide.[5] Carbamazepine had no effect on thioridazine plasma concentrations in 6 patients.[6]

Mechanism

Carbamazepine is a recognised enzyme inducer, therefore it seems highly likely that the reduced plasma chlorpromazine concentrations occur because its metabolism by the liver is markedly increased by carbamazepine.

In the case describing neuroleptic malignant syndrome it was suggested that carbamazepine might have reduced the concentrations of the antimuscarinic (anticholinergic) antipsychotics (levomepromazine and sultopride), resulting in cholinergic rebound, and neuroleptic malignant syndrome.[4]

Importance and management

Evidence for an interaction between the phenothiazines and carbamazepine appears to be limited to the reports cited, many of which suggest that no interaction normally occurs. Nevertheless, it would seem prudent to be alert for a diminished response to a phenothiazine if carbamazepine is added: it might be necessary to increase the dose of the phenothiazine. The situation with oxcarbazepine is not clear, but the very limited evidence from the case reports above suggest that it might not interact to the same extent as carbamazepine; however, further controlled studies are needed to confirm this.

The isolated case of high carbamazepine-10,11-epoxide concentrations in the patient taking chlorpromazine appears to be the only reported case of an interaction. Its general importance is therefore unknown. Similarly, the general relevance of the case of neuroleptic malignant syndrome is unknown.

1. Raitasuo V, Lehtovaara R, Huttunen MO. Effect of switching carbamazepine to oxcarbazepine on the plasma levels of neuroleptics. A case report. *Psychopharmacology (Berl)* (1994) 116, 115–16.
2. Pitterle ME, Collins DM. Carbamazepine-10,11-epoxide evaluation associated with coadministration of loxitane or amoxapine. *Epilepsia* (1988) 29, 654.
3. Jann MW, Fidone GS, Hernandez JM, Amrung S, Davis CM. Clinical implications of increased antipsychotic plasma concentrations upon anticonvulsant cessation. *Psychiatry Res* (1989) 28, 153–9.
4. Nisijima K, Kusakabe Y, Ohtuka K, Ishiguro T. Addition of carbamazepine to long-term treatment with neuroleptics may induce neuroleptic malignant syndrome. *Biol Psychiatry* (1998) 44, 930–1.
5. Spina E, Amendola D'Agostino AM, Ioculano MP, Oteri G, Fazio A, Pisani F. No effect of thioridazine on plasma concentrations of carbamazepine and its active metabolite carbamazepine-10,11-epoxide. *Ther Drug Monit* (1990) 12, 511–13.
6. Tiihonen J, Vartiainen H, Hakola P. Carbamazepine-induced changes in plasma levels of neuroleptics. *Pharmacopsychiatry* (1995) 28, 26–8.

Phenothiazines + Lithium

Chlorpromazine concentrations can be reduced to subtherapeutic concentrations by lithium. The development of severe extrapyramidal adverse effects or severe neurotoxicity has been seen in one or more patients given lithium with various phenothiazines. Sleep-walking has been described in some patients taking phenothiazines and lithium.

Clinical evidence

(a) Chlorpromazine

In a double-blind study in psychiatric patients it was found that chlorpromazine 400 to 800 mg daily, a dose that normally produced plasma concentrations of 100 to 300 nanograms/mL, only produced concentrations of 0 to 70 nanograms/mL when lithium carbonate was also given.[1] Other studies confirm that normal therapeutic concentrations of lithium carbonate reduce plasma chlorpromazine concentrations.[2,3] The maximum serum concentrations and AUC of chlorpromazine were reduced by 40% and 26%, respectively, in healthy subjects given lithium carbonate.[2]

A patient with paranoid schizophrenia taking chlorpromazine 200 to 600 mg daily for 5 years with no extrapyramidal symptoms developed stiffness of his face, arms and legs, and parkinsonian tremor of both hands within one day of starting to take lithium 900 mg daily. His lithium blood concentration after 3 days was 0.5 mmol/L. He was later given lithium 1.8 g daily (blood concentration 1.17 mmol/L), chlorpromazine 200 mg daily and benzatropine 2 mg daily, which improved his condition, but he still complained of stiffness and had a persistent hand tremor.[4]

A number of other reports describe the emergence of severe extrapyramidal adverse effects when chlorpromazine was given with lithium.[5-7] Ventricular fibrillation, thought to be caused by chlorpromazine toxicity, occurred in a patient taking lithium when both drugs were suddenly withdrawn.[8] Severe neurotoxicity has also been seen in a handful of other patients taking lithium and chlorpromazine.[9,10]

Consider also *Other phenothiazines*, below, for a report of sleep-walking episodes during the concurrent use of chlorpromazine and lithium, and for a report of neurotoxicity with lithium and fluphenazine, but not with chlorpromazine.

(b) Other phenothiazines

The sudden emergence of extrapyramidal or other adverse effects with lithium and other phenothiazines has also been described:

- **fluphenazine**[9,11-15]
- **levomepromazine**[9,11,12]
- **mesoridazine**[11,12]
- **perphenazine**[11,12,14]
- **pipotiazine**[16]
- **prochlorperazine**[11,12]
- **thioridazine**[9,11,12,14,17,18]
- **trifluoperazine**.[11,12]

Examples of some other cases are cited in a little more detail below.

A study in 10 patients with extrapyramidal symptoms, one of whom was taking **fluphenazine**, found that the addition of lithium worsened their extrapyramidal symptoms.[19] Neurotoxicity (tremor, rigidity, ataxia, tiredness, vomiting, confusion) attributed to an interaction between lithium and **fluphenazine** has been described in another patient. He previously took **haloperidol** and later took **chlorpromazine** with lithium, without problem.[20] Irreversible brain damage has been reported in a patient taking **fluphenazine decanoate** and lithium.[21] Severe neurotoxic complications (seizures, encephalopathy, delirium, abnormal EEGs) developed in 4 patients taking **thioridazine** 400 mg daily or more and lithium. Serum lithium concentrations remained below 1 mmol/L. Lithium and other phenothiazines had been taken by 3 of the patients for extended periods without problems, and the fourth subsequently took lithium and **fluphenazine** without problems.[22]

In one study the concurrent use of lithium and **chlorpromazine**, **perphenazine**, or **thioridazine** was associated with sleep-walking episodes in 9% of patients.[23]

Mechanism

Not understood. One suggestion to account for the reduced serum concentrations of chlorpromazine, which is based on *animal* studies,[24,25] is that chlorpromazine can be metabolised in the gut. Therefore, if lithium delays gastric emptying, more chlorpromazine will be metabolised before it reaches the circulation. It is unclear why severe neurotoxicity and other adverse effects sometimes develop in patients taking lithium and antipsychotics. It is the subject of considerable discussion and debate.[9,11,12,26,27]

Importance and management

Information about the reduction in chlorpromazine concentrations caused by lithium is limited, but it would seem to be an established interaction of clinical importance. Serum chlorpromazine concentrations below 30 nanograms/mL have been shown to be ineffective, whereas clinical improvement is usually associated with concentrations within the 150 to 300 nanogram/mL range.[28] Thus a fall in concentrations to below 70 nanograms/mL, as described in one study, would be expected to result in a reduced therapeutic response to chlorpromazine. Therefore the effects of concurrent use should be closely monitored and the chlorpromazine dose increased if necessary.

The development of severe neurotoxic or severe extrapyramidal adverse effects with combinations of chlorpromazine or other phenothiazines and lithium appears to be uncommon and unexplained, but be alert for any evidence of toxicity if lithium is given with any of these drugs. One recommendation is that the onset of neurological manifestations, such as excessive drowsiness or movement disorders, warrants electroencephalography without delay and withdrawal of the drugs, especially as irreversible effects have been seen. A review[29] suggests that the concurrent use of haloperidol seems to be safe if lithium concentrations are below 1 mmol/L. It is not known whether this also applies to other antipsychotics.

At the moment there seems to be no way of identifying the apparently small number of patients who are particularly at risk, but possible likely factors include a previous history of extrapyramidal reactions with antipsychotics and the use of large doses of the antipsychotic.

1. Kerzner B, Rivera-Calimlim L. Lithium and chlorpromazine (CPZ) interaction. *Clin Pharmacol Ther* (1976) 19, 109.
2. Rivera-Calimlim L, Kerzner B, Karch FE. Effect of lithium on plasma chlorpromazine levels. *Clin Pharmacol Ther* (1978) 23, 451–5.
3. Rivera-Calimlim L, Nasrallah H, Strauss J, Lasagna L. Clinical response and plasma levels: effect of dose, dosage schedules, and drug interactions on plasma chlorpromazine levels. *Am J Psychiatry* (1976) 133, 646–52.
4. Addonizio G. Rapid induction of extrapyramidal side effects with combined use of lithium and neuroleptics. *J Clin Psychopharmacol* (1985) 5, 296–8.
5. McGennis AJ. Hazards of lithium and neuroleptics in schizo-affective disorder. *Br J Psychiatry* (1983) 142, 99–100.
6. Yassa R. A case of lithium-chlorpromazine interaction. *J Clin Psychiatry* (1986) 47, 90–1.
7. Habib M, Khalil R, Le Pensec-Bertrand D, Ali-Cherif A, Bongrand MC, Crevat A. Syndrome neurologique persistant après traitement par les sels de lithium: toxicité de l'association lithium-neuroleptiques? *Rev Neurol (Paris)* (1986) 142, 1, 61–4.
8. Stevenson RN, Blanshard C, Patterson DLH. Ventricular fibrillation due to lithium withdrawal – an interaction with chlorpromazine? *Postgrad Med J* (1989) 65, 936–8.
9. Emilien G, Maloteaux JM. Lithium neurotoxicity at low therapeutic doses: hypotheses for causes and mechanism of action following a retrospective analysis of published case reports. *Acta Neurol Belg* (1996) 96, 281–93.
10. Boudouresques G, Poncet M, Ali Cherif A, Tafani B, Boudouresques. Encéphalopathie aiguë, au cours d'un traitement associant phenothiazine et lithium. Une nouvelle observation avec lithémie basse. *Nouv Presse Med* (1980) 9, 2580.
11. Goldman SA. Lithium and neuroleptics in combination: is there enhancement of neurotoxicity leading to permanent sequelae? *J Clin Pharmacol* (1996) 36, 951–62.
12. Goldman SA. FDA MedWatch Report: lithium and neuroleptics in combination: the spectrum of neurotoxicity. *Psychopharmacol Bull* (1996) 32, 299–309.
13. Kamlana SH, Kerry RJ, Khan IA. Lithium: some drug interactions. *Practitioner* (1980) 224, 1291–2.
14. Prakash R, Kelwala S, Ban TA. Neurotoxicity with combined administration of lithium and a neuroleptic. *Compr Psychiatry* (1982) 23, 567–71.
15. Sachdev PS. Lithium potentiation of neuroleptic-related extrapyramidal side effects. *Am J Psychiatry* (1986) 143, 942.
16. Abbar M, Petit P, Castelnau D, Blayac JP. Encéphalopathie toxique lors d'une association lithium-neuroleptiques. *Psychiatr Psychobiol* (1989) 4, 239–40.
17. Bailine SH, Doft M. Neurotoxicity induced by combined lithium–thioridazine treatment. *Biol Psychiatry* (1986) 21, 834–7.
18. Cantor CH. Encephalopathy with lithium and thioridazine in combination. *Med J Aust* (1986) 144, 164–5.
19. Addonizio G, Roth SD, Stokes PE, Stoll PM. Increased extrapyramidal symptoms with addition of lithium to neuroleptics. *J Nerv Ment Dis* (1988) 176, 682–5.
20. Alevizos B. Toxic reactions to lithium and neuroleptics. *Br J Psychiatry* (1979) 135, 482.
21. Singh SV. Lithium carbonate/fluphenazine decanoate producing irreversible brain damage. *Lancet* (1982) ii, 278.
22. Spring GK. Neurotoxicity with combined use of lithium and thioridazine. *J Clin Psychiatry* (1979) 40, 135–8.
23. Charney DS, Kales A, Soldatos CR, Nelson JC. Somnambulistic-like episodes secondary to combined lithium-neuroleptic treatment. *Br J Psychiatry* (1979) 135, 418–24.
24. Sundaresan PR, Rivera-Calimlim L. Distribution of chlorpromazine in the gastrointestinal tract of the rat and its effects on absorptive function. *J Pharmacol Exp Ther* (1975) 194, 593–602.
25. Curry SH, D'Mello A, Mould GP. Destruction of chlorpromazine during absorption in the rat *in vivo* and *in vitro*. *Br J Pharmacol* (1971) 42, 403–11.
26. Geisler A, Klysner R. Combined effect of lithium and flupenthixol on striatal adenylate cyclase. *Lancet* (1977) i, 430–1.
27. von Knorring L. Possible mechanisms for the presumed interaction between lithium and neuroleptics. *Hum Psychopharmacol* (1990) 5, 287–92.
28. Rivera-Calimlim L, Castañeda L, Lasagna L. Significance of plasma levels of chlorpromazine. *Clin Pharmacol Ther* (1973) 14, 144.
29. Batchelor DH, Lowe MR. Reported neurotoxicity with the lithium/haloperidol combination and other neuroleptics—a literature review. *Hum Psychopharmacol* (1990) 5, 275–80.

Phenothiazines + Midodrine

An isolated report describes acute dystonia after midodrine was given to a patient taking perphenazine. An increased severity of akathisia was seen in one study when promethazine and midodrine were given together.

Clinical evidence

(a) Perphenazine

A 53-year-old woman taking perphenazine 4 mg daily for 4 years without problems, developed acute dystonia 3 days after midodrine 2.5 mg three times daily was started. The patient's symptoms spontaneously resolved the day after midodrine was stopped.[1]

(b) Promethazine

A placebo-controlled study in 9 healthy subjects who received a single 10-mg oral dose of midodrine followed one hour later by a single 25-mg intravenous dose of promethazine, found that the akathisia which occurred in 6 subjects taking both midodrine and promethazine was more severe than the symptoms experienced in 4 subjects when they received promethazine alone.[2]

Mechanism

Unknown. An interaction resulting from CYP2D6 inhibition or increased central noradrenergic activity of the neuroleptics by midodrine[1] have been hypothesised.

Importance and management

Information regarding an interaction between phenothiazines and midodrine is limited to this study and case report, and its general relevance is unclear. However, if patients taking both midodrine and these phenothiazines develop akathisia or acute dystonia it would be prudent to suspect an interaction as a possible cause.

1. Castrioto A, Tambasco N, ossi A, Calabresi P. Acute dystonia induced by the combination of midodrine and perphenazine. *J Neurol* (2008) 255, 767–8.
2. Platts SH, Shi S-J, Meck JV. Akathisia with combined use of midodrine and promethazine. *JAMA* (2006) 295, 2000–1.

Phenothiazines + SSRIs

A number of case reports describe extrapyramidal adverse effects following the use of fluoxetine or paroxetine with phenothiazines. Perphenazine exposure is markedly increased by paroxetine, with an increase in adverse effects. Thioridazine concentrations are increased by fluvoxamine, and are predicted to be increased by fluoxetine or par-

oxetine, increasing the risk of QT interval prolongation. An isolated case report describes QT prolongation after fluoxetine was given to a patient taking chlorpromazine. Citalopram does not appear to alter steady-state concentrations of chlorpromazine, perphenazine or thioridazine, but is predicted to have additive QT prolonging effects with the phenothiazines.

Clinical evidence

(a) Chlorpromazine

A study in patients with schizophrenia found that over a 12-week period the serum concentrations of chlorpromazine did not appear to be altered by **citalopram** 40 mg daily.[1]

A case report describes symptomatic QTc interval prolongation in a patient taking chlorpromazine 100 mg twice daily a few weeks after **fluoxetine** was added and a few minutes after an extra night-time dose of chlorpromazine 50 mg. Her QTc interval increased from 402 milliseconds to 524 milliseconds. The QTc prolongation resolved after discontinuation of both drugs.[2]

(b) Cyamemazine

A study in patients taking cyamemazine found that **fluvoxamine** 150 mg daily had no effect on cyamemazine serum concentrations, but the authors of the report also state that no firm conclusions should be drawn from this finding because the number of patients was too small.[3]

(c) Fluphenazine

A severe dystonic reaction (painful jaw tightness and his throat described as closing up) occurred in a man taking **fluoxetine** 40 mg daily when he also took fluphenazine 2.5 mg on two consecutive nights.[4]

(d) Levomepromazine

A study in patients taking levomepromazine found that **fluvoxamine** 150 mg daily did not affect levomepromazine serum concentrations, but the authors of the report also state that no firm conclusions should be drawn from this finding because the number of patients was too small.[3] A further study in 15 patients found that levomepromazine 5 to 25 mg daily did not appear to alter **fluvoxamine** concentrations. Additionally, patients in this study found that the levomepromazine counteracted the insomnia caused by **fluvoxamine**.[5]

A study in three groups of 8 healthy subjects taking **citalopram** 40 mg daily for 10 days found that a single 50-mg oral dose of levomepromazine increased the initial steady-state concentrations of desmethylcitalopram, the primary metabolite of **citalopram**, by 10 to 20%, which was not considered to be clinically important.[6]

A study in patients with schizophrenia found that over a 12-week period the serum concentrations of levomepromazine did not appear to be altered by **citalopram** 40 mg daily.[1]

(e) Metopimazine

A French regional pharmacovigilance centre reported 37 cases of extrapyramidal adverse effects linked to the concurrent use of an SSRI and a neuroleptic. In 2 cases metopimazine was also given.[7]

(f) Pericyazine

A study describes a patient who developed extrapyramidal symptoms when given pericyazine and **fluoxetine**.[8]

(g) Perphenazine

1. Citalopram. A study in patients with schizophrenia found that, over a 12-week period, the serum concentrations of perphenazine did not appear to be altered by citalopram 40 mg daily.[1]

2. Fluoxetine. One woman developed marked extrapyramidal symptoms within 2 weeks of starting perphenazine 4 mg twice daily and fluoxetine 20 mg daily.[9]

3. Paroxetine. The effects of a single 100-microgram/kg oral dose of perphenazine on the performance of psychomotor tests were assessed after 4, 6, 8 and 10 hours in 8 subjects (all CYP2D6 extensive metabolisers, that is, those with normal CYP2D6 activity). The tests were then repeated after the subjects also took paroxetine 20 mg daily for 10 days. The scores for these tests were worsened by perphenazine, when compared with placebo, and further worsened by the presence of paroxetine. In addition to over-sedation and impairment of the performance of psychomotor tests and memory, 2 of the subjects developed akathisia 10 hours after taking both drugs. The AUC of the perphenazine was increased 7-fold and its maximum plasma concentrations were increased 6-fold.[10]

(h) Thioridazine

A study in patients with schizophrenia found that, over a 12-week period, the serum concentrations of thioridazine did not appear to be altered by **citalopram** 40 mg daily.[1]

A study in 10 patients with schizophrenia found that when **fluvoxamine** 50 mg daily was added to established treatment with thioridazine 30 to 200 mg daily, steady-state thioridazine plasma concentrations were increased 3.2-fold. There were no reported changes in either clinical status or adverse effects.[11]

(i) Trifluoperazine

A New Zealand study describes a patient who developed extrapyramidal symptoms when given trifluoperazine and **fluoxetine**.[8]

Mechanism

Fluoxetine and paroxetine can inhibit the metabolism of some phenothiazines by CYP2D6.[10] Raised phenothiazine concentrations might increase the risk of phenothiazine adverse effects, such as movement disorders, and increase the risk of QT interval prolongation. However, movement disorders might just be a result of the additive adverse effects of antipsychotics and SSRIs. Furthermore, fluoxetine alone has been shown to occasionally cause movement disorders.[8,12] Fluvoxamine is not an inhibitor of CYP2D6, and probably inhibits thioridazine metabolism by CYP2C19 and/or CYP1A2.[11]

Importance and management

General guidance

On the whole, clinically important interactions between the phenothiazines and SSRIs appear rare, and the combination can be useful and so the isolated cases of extrapyramidal adverse effects should not prevent concurrent use. However, if extrapyramidal effects become troublesome bear this interaction in mind as a possible cause. Also note that SSRIs can lower the seizure threshold, and therefore concurrent use with other drugs, which can also lower the seizure threshold, such as phenothiazines, should be undertaken with caution. Some individual drugs might pose more of a problem and further management for these drugs is discussed in the subsections below.

Chlorpromazine

The general relevance of the isolated report of QT prolongation with chlorpromazine and fluoxetine is uncertain, but bear it in mind in case of an unexpected response to treatment.

Perphenazine

The marked rise in perphenazine exposure caused by paroxetine seems to result in a greater number of more serious adverse effects, and so consideration should be given to reducing the dose of perphenazine if paroxetine is started. Citalopram might be a suitable alternative as it does not appear to affect perphenazine concentrations.

Thioridazine

Thioridazine in particular has been associated with dose-related QT prolongation, and it has been withdrawn in some countries because of this. Note that, the manufacturers of **fluoxetine**[13] and **paroxetine**[14,15] contraindicate the concurrent use of thioridazine as they suggest that its metabolism by CYP2D6 might be inhibited by these SSRIs leading to raised thioridazine concentrations and the risk of QT prolongation. The use of thioridazine is also contraindicated for 5 weeks after fluoxetine has been stopped.[13] The US manufacturer of **fluvoxamine**[16] also contraindicates concurrent use; the study cited above found a large increase in thioridazine concentrations so this seems prudent. Smaller increases would be expected with other SSRIs. The UK manufacturer states that the dose of thioridazine might need to be adjusted [reduced] when it is given with **citalopram**[17] and **escitalopram**;[18] however, given that these are only weak CYP2D6 inhibitors, a clinically important pharmacokinetic interaction seems unlikely. Nevertheless, as both citalopram and escitalopram cause QT prolongation, their concurrent use with other drugs that prolong the QT interval is contraindicated by the UK manufacturers, and phenothiazine derivatives are specifically named.[17,18] See 'Drugs that prolong the QT interval + Other drugs that prolong the QT interval', p.272, for further information on the concurrent use of two or more drugs that prolong the QT interval.

1. Syvälahti EKG, Taiminen T, Saarijärvi S, Lehto H, Niemi H, Ahola V, Dahl M-L, Salokangas RKR. Citalopram causes no significant alterations in plasma neuroleptic levels in schizophrenic patients. *J Int Med Res* (1997) 25, 24–32.
2. Adetunji B, Basil B, Mathews M, Osinowo T. Should the *Physician's Desk Reference* contraindicate the use of chlorpromazine-fluoxetine combination? A case report. *J Clin Psychopharmacol* (2006) 26, 438–9.
3. Vandel S, Bertschy G, Baumann P, Bouquet S, Bonin B, Francois T, Sechter D, Bizouard P. Fluvoxamine and fluoxetine: Interaction studies with amitriptyline, clomipramine and neuroleptics in phenotyped patients. *Pharmacol Res* (1995) 31, 347–53.
4. Ketai R. Interaction between fluoxetine and neuroleptics. *Am J Psychiatry* (1993) 150, 836–7.
5. Yoshimura R, Ueda N, Nakamura J. Low dosage of levomepromazine did not increase plasma concentrations of fluvoxamine. *Int Clin Psychopharmacol* (2000) 15, 233–5.
6. Gram LF, Hansen MG, Sindrup SH, Brøsen K, Poulsen JH, Aaes-Jørgensen T, Overø KF. Citalopram: interaction studies with levomepromazine, imipramine and lithium. *Ther Drug Monit* (1993) 15, 18–24.
7. Anon. Extrapyramidal reactions to SSRI antidepressant + neuroleptic combinations. *Prescrire Int* (2004) 13, 57.
8. Coulter DM, Pillans PI. Fluoxetine and extrapyramidal side effects. *Am J Psychiatry* (1995) 152, 122–5.
9. Lock JD, Gwirtsman HE, Targ EF. Possible adverse drug interactions between fluoxetine and other psychotropics. *J Clin Psychopharmacol* (1990) 10, 383–4.
10. Özdemir V, Naranjo CA, Herrmann N, Reed K, Sellers EM, Kalow W. Paroxetine potentiates the central nervous system side effects of perphenazine: contribution of cytochrome P4502D6 inhibition in vivo. *Clin Pharmacol Ther* (1997) 62, 334–47.
11. Carrillo JA, Ramos SI, Herraiz AG, Llerena A, Agundez JAG, Berecz R, Duran M, Benítez J. Pharmacokinetic interaction of fluvoxamine and thioridazine in schizophrenic patients. *J Clin Psychopharmacol* (1999) 19, 494–9.
12. Bouchard RH, Pourcher E, Vincent P. Fluoxetine and extrapyramidal side effects. *Am J Psychiatry* (1989) 146, 1352–3.
13. Prozac (Fluoxetine hydrochloride). Eli Lilly and Company. US Prescribing information, July 2014.
14. Paxil Tablets and Suspension (Paroxetine hydrochloride). GlaxoSmithKline. US Prescribing information, December 2012.
15. Paroxetine Film-Coated Tablets (Paroxetine hydrochloride anhydrous). Actavis UK Ltd. UK Summary of product characteristics, June 2015.
16. Luvox CR (Fluvoxamine maleate). Jazz Pharmaceuticals, Inc. US Prescribing information, May 2011.
17. Cipramil Tablets (Citalopram hydrobromide). Lundbeck Ltd. UK Summary of product characteristics, July 2015.
18. Cipralex Tablets (Escitalopram oxalate). Lundbeck Ltd. UK Summary of product characteristics, September 2013.

Phenothiazines + Trazodone

The use of trazodone with a phenothiazine has been implicated in a range of undesirable adverse effects including hypotension (with chlorpromazine or trifluoperazine) fatal jaundice and hepatic encephalopathy (with trifluoperazine and thioridazine) and neuroleptic malignant syndrome (with perphenazine). Thioridazine causes a minor rise in trazodone plasma concentrations.

Clinical evidence and mechanism

(a) Chlorpromazine

A depressed patient taking chlorpromazine began to complain of dizziness and unstable gait within 2 weeks of starting to take trazodone 100 mg one to three times daily. His blood pressure had fallen to between 92/58 and 126/72 mmHg. Within 2 days of stopping the trazodone his blood pressure had restabilised.[1] It is possible that the hypotensive effects of the two drugs were additive.

(b) Perphenazine

A case report of neuroleptic malignant syndrome with serotonin involvement in a patient taking perphenazine 16 mg daily with trazodone 200 mg daily, paroxetine 20 mg daily, benzatropine and lithium carbonate,[2] resulted in some discussion by others, suggesting that pharmacodynamic and pharmacokinetic interactions resulting from CYP2D6 inhibition by paroxetine led to the symptoms described.[3] For further discussion on the interaction between phenothiazines and SSRIs, see 'Phenothiazines + SSRIs', p.874, and trazodone and SSRIs, see 'Trazodone + SSRIs', p.1500.

(c) Trifluoperazine

A patient taking trifluoperazine was given trazodone 100 mg daily and within 2 days she complained of dizziness and was found to have a blood pressure of 86/52 mmHg. Within one day of stopping the trazodone her blood pressure was back to 100/65 mmHg.[1] It would seem that the hypotensive adverse effects of the two drugs can be additive, although an interaction was not confirmed as the trazodone was not taken alone. For mention of a case of fatal hepatic necrosis in which trifluoperazine might have had a role, see under *Thioridazine*, below

(d) Thioridazine

A study, undertaken to confirm the involvement of CYP2D6 in the metabolism of trazodone, found that when 11 patients with depression were given trazodone 150 to 300 mg at bedtime for 18 weeks, and then with thioridazine 20 mg twice daily for one week, the plasma concentrations of the trazodone and its active metabolite, *m*-chlorophenylpiperazine, rose by 36% and 54%, respectively.[4] No adverse reactions were described.

A case of fatal hepatic necrosis with cholestasis has been attributed to the concurrent use of trazodone and phenothiazines. A 72-year-old woman taking **trifluoperazine**, trazodone and lithium carbonate developed an elevated alanine aminotransferase concentration. **Trifluoperazine** was replaced with thioridazine, but 9 weeks later she became jaundiced and developed hepatic encephalopathy, and died 6 weeks after the onset of jaundice. The authors consider that the combination of the phenothiazines and trazodone were the cause of her hepatic necrosis: both phenothiazines and trazodone have been reported to individually cause hepatic adverse effects.[5]

Importance and management

Evidence for an interaction between trazodone and the phenothiazines appears to be limited. The reports of hypotensive effects are also isolated. It would seem prudent to warn patients of the possibility of additive hypotensive effects (e.g. dizziness, postural hypotension) and advise them to seek medical advice if this becomes troublesome.

The isolated case of hepatic adverse effects is of unknown general importance, but it serves as a reminder to consider the additive adverse effects of drugs when prescribing them in combination. The isolated report of neuroleptic malignant syndrome with trazodone and perphenazine is complicated by the concurrent use of paroxetine, limiting its general clinical importance.

1. Asayesh K. Combination of trazodone and phenothiazines: a possible additive hypotensive effect. *Can J Psychiatry* (1986) 31, 857–8.
2. Young C. A case of neuroleptic malignant syndrome and serotonin disturbance. *J Clin Psychopharmacol* (1997) 17, 65–6.
3. Shad MU, Preskorn SH. Pharmacodynamic and pharmacokinetic factors in a case of neuroleptic malignant syndrome. *J Clin Psychopharmacol* (1998) 18, 346–7.
4. Yasui N, Otani K, Kaneko S, Ohkubo T, Osanai T, Ishida M, Mihara K, Kondo T, Sugawara K, Fukushima Y. Inhibition of trazodone metabolism by thioridazine in humans. *Ther Drug Monit* (1995) 17, 333–5.
5. Hull M, Jones R, Bendall M. Fatal hepatic necrosis associated with trazodone and neuroleptic drugs. *BMJ* (1994) 309, 378.

Phenothiazines + Tricyclic antidepressants

Tricyclic concentrations are increased by many of the phenothiazines, and the concentrations of some phenothiazines are also increased by the tricyclics. It has been suggested that concurrent use might contribute to an increased incidence of tardive dyskinesia. Nevertheless, fixed-dose combined preparations have been marketed. Tricyclics have also been shown to reverse the therapeutic effects of chlorpromazine. Occasionally the concurrent use of a tricyclic and a phenothiazine can lead to antimuscarinic adverse effects, such as paralytic ileus.

Clinical evidence

(a) Effect of phenothiazines on tricyclic antidepressants

An extended study of 4 patients given intramuscular **fluphenazine decanoate** 12.5 mg weekly, with benzatropine 2 mg three times daily and **imipramine** 300 mg daily, found that the combined plasma concentration of **imipramine** and its metabolite, desipramine, were 850 nanograms/mL. This appeared high, when compared with 60 other patients who were taking **imipramine** 225 mg daily and had a concentration of 180 nanograms/mL.[1]

A comparative study of 99 patients taking **amitriptyline** or **nortriptyline** alone, and 60 other patients also taking **perphenazine** 10 mg daily, found that although the tricyclic antidepressant doses were the same, the plasma tricyclic antidepressant concentrations were up to 70% higher in those also taking **perphenazine.**[2]

Other studies have described increased tricyclic antidepressant concentrations with phenothiazines. There is currently evidence for this interaction between:

- **imipramine,**[3-5] and **chlorpromazine**
- **nortriptyline,**[6] and **levomepromazine**
- **amitriptyline,**[7] **imipramine,**[5,8,9] **desipramine**[10] or **nortriptyline,**[6,11-13] and **perphenazine**
- **desipramine,**[14] **imipramine**[15] or **nortriptyline,**[6] and **thioridazine**
- **nortriptyline**[16] and **thioridazine** (with paroxetine).

However, other studies have found no interaction between:

- **amitriptyline**[6,11,17] or **nortriptyline,**[18] and **perphenazine**
- **amitriptyline**[6] and **thioridazine**
- **amitriptyline**[6] and **levomepromazine.**

It should be noted that in the case of **amitriptyline,** although the concentrations were not affected, concentrations of nortriptyline, its metabolite, were raised.[6]

(b) Effect of tricyclic antidepressants on phenothiazines

In a controlled study in 8 patients with schizophrenia taking **butaperazine** 20 mg daily, the 6 patients taking **desipramine** 150 mg or more daily had a rise in serum **butaperazine** concentrations of between 50 and 300%. The other 2 patients, taking **desipramine** 100 mg or less, had no changes in **butaperazine** concentrations.[19] Other studies have found a rise in phenothiazine concentrations when tricyclic antidepressants are added. So far, interactions with **chlorpromazine** and **amitriptyline,**[20] **imipramine**[20] or **nortriptyline**[21] have been documented. One study in 23 patients found transitory increases in the concentrations of **chlorpromazine, mesoridazine, methotrimeprazine, perphenazine, thioproperazine, thioridazine,** and **trifluoperazine** when **amitriptyline** was also given for 12 weeks.[22]

One study in 7 patients with chronic schizophrenia also reported that giving **nortriptyline** 50 mg three times daily to patients taking **chlorpromazine** 100 mg three times daily resulted in profound worsening of the clinical state, with marked increases in agitation and tension, despite the fact that the **chlorpromazine** concentrations were actually raised. The **nortriptyline** was withdrawn.[21] A temporary reversion to a disruptive behaviour pattern has been seen in other patients taking **chlorpromazine** when **amitriptyline** was given.[23] One patient experienced a severe catatonic reaction that was attributed to the use of **thioridazine** and **amitriptyline,**[24] and the case of a woman who became anxious with widely staring eyes, a persistent jerking of her head and at times the inability to speak was thought to be due to the use of **imipramine** and **chlorpromazine.**[25] Ventricular tachycardia has also been reported in a 38-year-old woman taking **desipramine** and **thioridazine,** which responded to treatment with lidocaine.[26]

(c) Other effects

The tricyclic antidepressants have antimuscarinic adverse effects, which can, in conjunction with the use of an antipsychotic, lead to life-threatening interactions. These are discussed further in the monograph 'Antipsychotics + Antimuscarinics', p.805.

Mechanism

The rise in the serum concentrations of both drugs is thought to be due to a mutual inhibition of the liver enzymes concerned with the metabolism of both drugs, which results in their accumulation.[3,4,8,19,21]

Importance and management

The interactions between phenothiazines and tricyclic antidepressants are established, but the advantages and disadvantages of concurrent use are the subject of debate. These two groups of drugs have been widely used together in the treatment of patients with schizophrenia who show depression, and for mixed anxiety and depression. A number of fixed-dose combinations have been marketed (e.g. amitriptyline with perphenazine and nortriptyline with fluphenazine). However, the safety of using both drugs together has been questioned.

One of the problems of phenothiazine use is the development of tardive dyskinesias, and some evidence suggests that the higher the dose, the greater the incidence.[27] The symptoms can be transiently masked by increasing the dose,[28] and so it has been suggested that the presence of a tricyclic antidepressant might not only be a factor causing tardive dyskinesia to develop, but might also mask the condition.[19,29] It has been recommended that the addition of full antidepressant doses of nortriptyline to average antipsychotic doses of chlorpromazine should be avoided because the therapeutic actions of the chlorpromazine might be reversed.[21] See also *Antagonism of antipsychotic effects*, under 'Antipsychotics + Antimuscarinics', p.805.

Attention has also been drawn to excessive weight gain associated with several months use of amitriptyline with thioridazine for the treatment of chronic pain,[30] but note that excessive weight gain is a recognised adverse effect of the use of antipsychotics alone.

For reports of paralytic ileus with faecal impaction, or severe constipation or atropine-like psychoses in patients taking various phenothiazines and tricyclics see, 'Antipsychotics + Antimuscarinics', p.805.

The tricyclic antidepressants and many antipsychotics increase the QT interval, see 'Drugs that prolong the QT interval + Other drugs that prolong the QT interval', p.272, for further information.

1. Siris SG, Cooper TB, Rifkin AE, Brenner R, Lieberman JA. Plasma imipramine concentrations in patients receiving concomitant fluphenazine decanoate. *Am J Psychiatry* (1982) 139, 104–6.
2. Linnoila M, George L, Guthrie S. Interaction between antidepressants and perphenazine in psychiatric patients. *Am J Psychiatry* (1982) 139, 1329–31.
3. Gram LF, Overø KF. Drug interaction: inhibitory effect of neuroleptics on metabolism of tricyclic antidepressants in man. *BMJ* (1972) 1, 463–5.
4. Crammer JL, Rolfe B. Interaction of imipramine and chlorpromazine in man. *Psychopharmacologia* (1972) 26 (Suppl), 81.
5. Gram LF. Lægemiddelinteraktion: hæmmende virkning af neurolepltica på tricycliske antidepressivas metabolisering. *Nord Psykiatr Tidsskr* (1971) 25, 357–60.
6. Jerling M, Bertilsson L, Sjöqvist F. The use of therapeutic drug monitoring data to document kinetic drug interactions: an example with amitriptyline and nortriptyline. *Ther Drug Monit* (1994) 16, 1–12.
7. Perel JM, Stiller RL, Feldman BL, Lin FC, Narayanan S. Therapeutic drug monitoring (TDM) of the amitriptyline (AT)/perphenazine (PER) interaction in depressed patients. *Clin Chem* (1985) 31, 939–40.
8. Gram LF, Overø KF, Kirk L. Influence of neuroleptics and benzodiazepines on metabolism of tricyclic antidepressants in man. *Am J Psychiatry* (1974) 131, 863–6.
9. Gram LF. Effects of perphenazine on imipramine metabolism in man. *Psychopharmacol Comm* (1975) 1, 165–75.
10. Nelson JC, Jatlow PI. Neuroleptic effect on desipramine steady-state plasma concentrations. *Am J Psychiatry* (1980) 137, 1232–4.
11. Linnet K. Comparison of the kinetic interactions of the neuroleptics perphenazine and zuclopenthixol with tricyclic antidepressives. *Ther Drug Monit* (1995) 17, 308–11.
12. Mulsant BH, Foglia JP, Sweet RA, Rosen J, Lo KH, Pollock BG. The effects of perphenazine on the concentration of nortriptyline and its hydroxymetabolites in older patients. *J Clin Psychopharmacol* (1997) 17, 318–21.
13. Overø KF, Gram LF, Hansen V. Interaction of perphenazine with the kinetics of nortriptyline. *Acta Pharmacol Toxicol (Copenh)* (1977) 40, 97–105.
14. Hirschowitz J, Bennett JA, Zemlan FP, Garver DL. Thioridazine effect on desipramine plasma levels. *J Clin Psychopharmacol* (1983) 3, 376–9.
15. Maynard GL, Soni P. Thioridazine interferences with imipramine metabolism and measurement. *Ther Drug Monit* (1996) 18, 729–31.
16. Ghaemi SN, Kirkwood CK. Elevation of nortriptyline plasma levels after cotreatment with paroxetine and thioridazine. *J Clin Psychopharmacol* (1998) 18, 342–3.
17. Cooper SF, Dugal R, Elie R, Albert J-M. Metabolic interaction between amitriptyline and perphenazine in psychiatric patients. *Prog Neuropsychopharmacol* (1979) 3, 369–76.
18. Kragh-Sørensen P, Borgå O, Garle M, Bolvig Hansen L, Hansen CE, Hvidberg EF, Larsen N-E, Sjöqvist F. Effect of simultaneous treatment with low doses of perphenazine on plasma and urine concentrations of nortriptyline and 10-hydroxynortriptyline. *Eur J Clin Pharmacol* (1977) 11, 479–83.
19. El-Yousef MK, Manier DH. Tricyclic antidepressants and phenothiazines. *JAMA* (1974) 229, 1419.
20. Rasheed A, Javed MA, Nazir S, Khawaja O. Interaction of chlorpromazine with tricyclic anti-depressants in schizophrenic patients. *J Pakistan Med Assoc* (1994) 44, 233–4.
21. Loga S, Curry S, Lader M. Interaction of chlorpromazine and nortriptyline in patients with schizophrenia. *Clin Pharmacokinet* (1981) 6, 454–62.
22. Jus A, Gautier J, Villeneuve A, Jus K, Pires P, Gagnon-Binette M, Fortin C. Pharmacokinetic interaction between amitriptyline and neuroleptics. *Neuropsychobiology* (1978) 4, 305–13.
23. O'Connor JW. Personal communication, February 1983.
24. Witton K. Severe toxic reaction to combined amitriptyline and thioridazine. *Am J Psychiatry* (1965) 121, 812–13.
25. Kane FJ. An unusual reaction to combined imipramine-thorazine therapy. *Am J Psychiatry* (1963) 120, 186–7.
26. Wilens TE, Stern TA. Ventricular tachycardia associated with desipramine and thioridazine. *Psychosomatics* (1990) 31, 100–3.
27. Crane GE. Persistent dyskinesia. *Br J Psychiatry* (1973), 122, 395–405.
28. Crane GE. Tardive dyskinesia in patients treated with major neuroleptics: a review of the literature. *Am J Psychiatry* (1968) 124 (Suppl), 40–8.
29. Ayd FJ. Pharmacokinetic interaction between tricyclic antidepressants and phenothiazine neuroleptics. *Int Drug Ther Newslett* (1974) 9, 31–2.
30. Pfister AK. Weight gain from combined phenothiazine and tricyclic therapy. *JAMA* (1978) 239, 1959.

Phenothiazines; Chlorpromazine + Antimalarials

Chloroquine, amodiaquine and sulfadoxine with pyrimethamine appear to increase serum chlorpromazine concentrations.

Clinical evidence

A total of 15 patients with schizophrenia taking chlorpromazine 400 mg or 500 mg daily for at least 2 weeks were given single doses of either **chloroquine sulfate** 400 mg, **amodiaquine hydrochloride** 600 mg or three tablets of **pyrimethamine** 25 mg with **sulfadoxine** 500 mg (*Fansidar*) one hour before chlorpromazine. Serum chlorpromazine concentrations, taken 3 hours later, were found to be raised about 3-fold by **chloroquine** and **amodiaquine**, and almost 4-fold by **sulfadoxine** with **pyrimethamine**. The plasma concentration of 7-hydroxychlorpromazine, one of the major metabolites of chlorpromazine, was also elevated, but not those of its other metabolite, chlorpromazine sulfoxide. The serum chlorpromazine concentrations of the patients given **chloroquine** or **sulfadoxine** with **pyrimethamine** were, to some extent, still elevated 4 days later. There was subjective evidence that the patients were more heavily sedated when they were also given the antimalarials.[1]

Mechanism

Not understood. Both chloroquine and sulfadoxine with pyrimethamine have relatively long half-lives compared with amodiaquine, which might explain the persistence of their effects.

Importance and management

Direct information about an interaction between chlorpromazine and chloroquine, amodiaquine, and sulfadoxine with pyrimethamine seems to be limited to the study cited. Its clinical importance is uncertain but it seems possible that these antimalarials could cause chlorpromazine toxicity. Until more is known, it would seem prudent to monitor the effects of concurrent use closely and anticipate the need to reduce the chlorpromazine dose. More study is needed.

Note also, that chlorpromazine can rarely cause agranulocytosis, and it is possible that this risk might be increased if it is given with drugs that have myelosuppressive effects, such as sulfadoxine with pyrimethamine.

1. Makanjuola ROA, Dixon PAF, Oforah E. Effects of antimalarial agents on plasma levels of chlorpromazine and its metabolites in schizophrenic patients. *Trop Geogr Med* (1988) 40, 31–3.

Phenothiazines; Chlorpromazine + Cimetidine

One study found that steady-state chlorpromazine plasma concentrations are reduced by cimetidine, whereas a case report suggests that cimetidine might increase chlorpromazine sedation.

Clinical evidence, mechanism, importance and management

A study in 8 patients taking chlorpromazine 75 to 450 mg daily found that cimetidine 1 g daily in divided doses for one week decreased the steady-state chlorpromazine plasma concentrations by one-third, from 37 micrograms/mL to 24 micrograms/mL. A two-thirds reduction was noted in one patient.[1] The reasons for this effect are not understood, but a decrease in chlorpromazine absorption from the gut has been suggested.[1]

In contrast, another report describes 2 patients with schizophrenia taking chlorpromazine 100 mg four times daily who became excessively sedated when they were given cimetidine 400 mg twice daily. The sedation disappeared when the chlorpromazine dose was halved. When cimetidine was later withdrawn it was found necessary to give the original chlorpromazine dose.[2] Chlorpromazine concentrations were not measured.

There is no simple explanation for these discordant reports, but they emphasise the need to monitor the concurrent use of chlorpromazine and cimetidine. More study is needed. There seems to be no information about other phenothiazines.

1. Howes CA, Pullar T, Sourindhrin I, Mistra PC, Capel H, Lawson DH, Tilstone WJ. Reduced steady-state plasma concentrations of chlorpromazine and indomethacin in patients receiving cimetidine. *Eur J Clin Pharmacol* (1983) 24, 99–102.
2. Byrne A, O'Shea B. Adverse interaction between cimetidine and chlorpromazine in two cases of chronic schizophrenia. *Br J Psychiatry* (1989) 155, 413–15.

Phenothiazines; Chlorpromazine + Combined hormonal contraceptives

A case report describes a large rise in the serum concentration of chlorpromazine in a woman taking an oral combined hormonal contraceptive.

Clinical evidence, mechanism, importance and management

A case report describes a woman who had been taking chlorpromazine 100 mg three times daily for one week without problems when an oral combined hormonal contraceptive (**ethinylestradiol** with **norgestrel**) was started. Four days later she developed severe dyskinesias and tremor, and her chlorpromazine concentration was found to have increased about 6-fold.[1] This case was briefly mentioned in an earlier report by the same authors.[2]

The reasons for the raised chlorpromazine concentration is not understood. As this is a single uncontrolled case occurring shortly after starting chlorpromazine, it requires confirmation. There seem to be no other reports of adverse reactions between phenothiazines and contraceptives, and the available data are insufficient to justify any general precautions.

1. Chetty M, Miller R. Oral contraceptives increase the plasma concentrations of chlorpromazine. *Ther Drug Monit* (2001) 23, 556–8.
2. Chetty M, Miller R, Moodley SV. Smoking and body weight influence the clearance of chlorpromazine. *Eur J Clin Pharmacol* (1994) 46, 523–6.

Phenothiazines; Chlorpromazine + Tetrabenazine

An isolated report describes severe Parkinson-like symptoms when a woman with Huntington's chorea taking tetrabenazine was given chlorpromazine.

Clinical evidence, mechanism, importance and management

A woman with Huntington's chorea, successfully treated with tetrabenazine 100 mg daily for 9 years, became motionless, rigid, mute and only able to respond by blinking her eyes within one day of being given two intramuscular injections of chlorpromazine 25 mg. This was diagnosed as severe drug-induced parkinsonism, which rapidly responded to the withdrawal of both drugs and treatment with benzatropine given intramuscularly and orally. She had previously tolerated chlorpromazine well.[1] The reason for this reaction is not understood, and its general relevance is unclear, but probably small.

1. Moss JH, Stewart DE. Iatrogenic parkinsonism in Huntington's chorea. *Can J Psychiatry* (1986) 31, 865–6.

Phenothiazines; Fluphenazine + Ascorbic acid (Vitamin C)

An isolated case report describes a reduction in serum fluphenazine concentrations and signs of a reduction in its effects when a patient was also given ascorbic acid.

Clinical evidence, mechanism, importance and management

A man with a history of manic behaviour, taking fluphenazine 15 mg daily, had a 25% reduction in his plasma fluphenazine concentration, from 0.93 nanograms/mL to 0.705 nanograms/mL, over a 13-day period while taking ascorbic acid 500 mg twice daily. This was accompanied by a deterioration in his behaviour.[1] The reason for this effect is not understood. There seem to be no other reports of this possible interaction with fluphenazine or any other phenothiazine and therefore the general importance of this case is unclear.

1. Dysken MW, Cumming RJ, Channon RA, Davis JM. Drug interaction between ascorbic acid and fluphenazine. *JAMA* (1979) 241, 2008.

Phenothiazines; Fluphenazine + Spiramycin

Acute dystonia occurred when a man taking fluphenazine was also given spiramycin.

Clinical evidence, mechanism, importance and management

A man with a schizoaffective disorder taking lorazepam, orphenadrine, fluvoxamine and fluphenazine decanoate 12.5 mg every 2 weeks, developed acute and painful dystonia of the trunk, neck, right arm and leg about one week after his last fluphenazine injection and on the fourth day of taking spiramycin 6 million units daily for gingivitis. The problem resolved when he was given biperiden.[1] The reasons for this adverse reaction are not understood, nor is it entirely clear whether this was an interaction between fluphenazine and spiramycin, although the author suggested that a causal link existed. This seems to be the only report of an alleged interaction between fluphenazine and a macrolide antibacterial and it is therefore of little or no general importance.

1. Benazzi F. Spiramycin-associated acute dystonia during neuroleptic treatment. *Can J Psychiatry* (1997) 42, 665–6.

Phenothiazines; Perphenazine + Disulfiram

An isolated case report describes a man taking perphenazine whose psychotic symptoms re-emerged when he started to take disulfiram.

Clinical evidence, mechanism, importance and management

A man taking perphenazine 8 mg twice daily developed marked psychosis soon after starting to take disulfiram 100 mg daily. His serum perphenazine concentration had fallen from a range of 2 to 3 nanomol/L to less than 1 nanomol/L. Doubling the dose of perphenazine had little effect, and no substantial clinical improvement or rise in serum concentrations occurred until he was given intramuscular perphenazine enantate 50 mg weekly, at which point the concentrations rose to about 4 nanomol/L. The results of clinical biochemical tests suggested that the disulfiram was acting as an enzyme inducer, resulting in increased metabolism and clearance of the perphenazine.[1] However, disulfiram normally acts as an enzyme *inhibitor*. Too little is known to assess the general importance of this interaction, and there seems to be no information about an interaction with other phenothiazines.

1. Hansen LB, Larsen N-E. Metabolic interaction between perphenazine and disulfiram. *Lancet* (1982) ii, 1472.

Phenothiazines; Promazine + Attapulgite-pectin

An attapulgite-pectin antidiarrhoeal preparation caused a small reduction in the absorption of promazine in one subject, but in a study, the overall excretion of promazine was minimally altered.

Clinical evidence, mechanism, importance and management

A study in one healthy subject found that attapulgite-pectin reduced the absorption of a single 50-mg dose of promazine by about 25%, possibly due to adsorption of the phenothiazine onto the attapulgite.[1] Another study in 6 healthy subjects found that the presence of activated attapulgite reduced the initial rate of urinary excretion of a single 50-mg dose of promazine, but caused only a small decrease in the overall extent of excretion.[2]

The clinical importance of this interaction and whether other phenothiazines behave similarly does not appear to have been studied; however, the magnitude of the interaction appears small, and seems unlikely to be of clinical relevance. If a problem does occur, separating administration as much as possible (2 hours or more) to avoid admixture in the gut has been shown to minimise the effects of this type of interaction with other drugs.

1. Sorby DL, Liu G. Effects of adsorbents on drug absorption II. Effect of an antidiarrhea mixture on promazine absorption. *J Pharm Sci* (1966) 55, 504–10.
2. Sorby DL. Effects of adsorbents on drug absorption I. Modification of promazine absorption by activated attapulgite and activated charcoal. *J Pharm Sci* (1965) 54, 677–83.

Phenothiazines; Thioridazine + Naltrexone

Extreme lethargy occurred in two patients taking thioridazine when they were given naltrexone.

Clinical evidence, mechanism, importance and management

Two patients with schizophrenia taking thioridazine 50 to 200 mg three times daily for at least one year took part in a pilot project to assess the efficacy of naltrexone for the treatment of tardive dyskinesias. Both patients tolerated the first challenge dose of intravenous naltrexone 800 micrograms without problems, but experienced extreme lethargy and slept almost continuously after the second naltrexone dose of 50 to 100 mg orally. The severe lethargy resolved within 12 hours of stopping the naltrexone.[1] The reasons for this reaction are not understood. Information seems to be limited to this report and the general importance of this interaction is unknown. Note that a case report has described excessive sleepiness and lethargy in a 58-year-old man who took a single 100-mg dose of naltrexone alone,[2] so an interaction is by no means established.

1. Maany I, O'Brien CP, Woody G. Interaction between thioridazine and naltrexone. *Am J Psychiatry* (1987) 144, 966.
2. Malcolm R, Gabel T, Morton A. Idiosyncratic reaction to naltrexone augmented by thioridazine. *Am J Psychiatry* (1988) 145, 773–4.

Phenothiazines; Thioridazine + Phenylpropanolamine

An isolated case report describes fatal ventricular fibrillation, which was attributed to the concurrent use of thioridazine and phenylpropanolamine.

Clinical evidence, mechanism, importance and management

A 27-year-old woman with schizophrenia who was taking thioridazine 100 mg daily and procyclidine 2.5 mg twice daily was found dead in bed 2 hours after taking a single capsule of phenylpropanolamine 50 mg with **chlorphenamine** 4 mg (*Contac C*). The principal cause of death was attributed to ventricular fibrillation.[1] The reason for this effect is not understood, but it is suggested that it might have been due to the combined effects of the thioridazine (known to be cardiotoxic and to cause T-wave abnormalities) and the phenylpropanolamine (possibly able to cause ventricular arrhythmias).

The general importance of this alleged interaction is uncertain but the authors of the report suggest that ephedrine-like drugs such as phenylpropanolamine should not be given to patients taking thioridazine or **mesoridazine**. Note that thioridazine has been withdrawn in many countries because of its cardiotoxicity.

1. Chouinard G, Ghadirian AM, Jones BD. Death attributed to ventricular arrhythmia induced by thioridazine in combination with a single Contac C capsule. *Can Med Assoc J* (1978) 119, 729–31.

Phenothiazines; Thioridazine + Ritonavir

Antiretroviral doses of ritonavir (300 mg twice daily or more) are predicted to increase the plasma concentration of thioridazine by inhibition of CYP2D6. Monitoring for thioridazine adverse effects is recommended during concurrent use.[1] Note that thioridazine has been withdrawn in many countries because of its cardiotoxicity.

1. Norvir Soft Capsules (Ritonavir). Abbott Laboratories Ltd. UK Summary of product characteristics, October 2010.

Phenothiazines; Trifluoperazine + Venlafaxine

An isolated case report describes neuroleptic malignant syndrome in a patient taking trifluoperazine, which developed after he took a single dose of venlafaxine. It was also suggested that the symptoms might have been due to serotonin syndrome.

Clinical evidence, mechanism, importance and management

A patient who had taken trifluoperazine 1 mg three times daily for 10 years was also given venlafaxine 75 mg daily. Twelve hours after the first dose of venlafaxine he presented with profound anxiety, malaise, profuse sweating, tremor and rigidity. His blood pressure was found to fluctuate between 130/80 and 165/100 mmHg, with a pulse of 163 bpm, a temperature of 38.3°C, and a respiratory rate of 25 breaths/minute. Blood and urine tests were normal except for a high creatine phosphokinase concentration and neutrophilia. The drugs were stopped and the patient recovered after taking a single 70-mg dose of dantrolene and bromocriptine 15 mg twice daily for 48 hours.

It was suggested that the patient had developed neuroleptic malignant syndrome, which might have occurred as a result of dopamine inhibition by the two drugs.[1] It was subsequently suggested that the symptoms seen might have been due to serotonin syndrome resulting from serotonergic over-activity when the single dose of venlafaxine was added to established treatment with trifluoperazine.[2] For more information about serotonin syndrome and its management, see 'Drugs that cause serotonin syndrome + Other drugs that cause serotonin syndrome', p.1471.

1. Nimmagadda SR, Ryan DH, Atkin SL. Neuroleptic malignant syndrome after venlafaxine. *Lancet* (2000) 354, 289–90.
2. Cassidy EM, O'Kearne V. Neuroleptic malignant syndrome after venlafaxine. *Lancet* (2000) 355, 2164–5.

Pimozide + CYP3A4 inhibitors

Clarithromycin moderately increases pimozide exposure and increases QT prolongation. Two cases of sudden death have occurred on concurrent use. Other inhibitors of CYP3A4 are predicted to increase pimozide exposure and increase the risk of QT interval prolongation and the development of life-threatening arrhythmias.

Clinical evidence and mechanism

The sudden death of a patient taking pimozide and **clarithromycin** prompted a study of a possible interaction between the two drugs. Using human liver microsomes it was found that pimozide is partly metabolised by CYP3A, and that 2 micromol of **clarithromycin** inhibits this enzyme by at least 80%.[1] The practical consequences of this finding were seen in a later study in 12 healthy subjects, which found that **clarithromycin** 500 mg twice daily for 5 days more than doubled the AUC of a single 6-mg oral dose of pimozide and raised its maximum plasma concentration by almost 50%. The QTc interval was prolonged by about 17 milliseconds with pimozide alone and by 24 milliseconds when **clarithromycin** was added.[2] The CYP2D6 status of the subjects was considered, as CYP2D6 is the other main metabolic route of pimozide, but the results were the same in both poor and extensive CYP2D6 metabolisers,[2] that is, those deficient or lacking CYP2D6 activity and those with normal activity of this isoenzyme. The US manufacturer mentions a second case of sudden death when clarithromycin was added to pimozide.[3]

Pimozide alone has been associated with ventricular arrhythmias, prolongation of the QT interval, T-wave changes and sudden and unexpected death, even in the young with no previous evidence of cardiac disease.[4,5] Some **macrolides** are also associated with an increased risk of QT interval prolongation, see 'Drugs that prolong the QT interval + Other drugs that prolong the QT interval', p.272, for further information.

Importance and management

The evidence for **clarithromycin** indicates that it can increase the cardiotoxicity of pimozide during chronic use, irrespective of the CYP2D6 metaboliser status of the patient.[2] Due to the severity of this interaction the UK manufacturers contraindicate the use of macrolides with pimozide,[6] whereas the US manufacturers contraindicate pimozide with the named macrolides, **azithromycin**, **clarithromycin**, **dirithromycin**, **erythromycin** and **troleandomycin**.[3] However, note that **azithromycin** and **dirithromycin** do not usually interact with other drugs by inhibiting CYP3A4.

The use of other inhibitors of CYP3A4 with pimozide is also contraindicated as they are similarly expected to increase the plasma concentrations of pimozide, which is likely to result in QT prolongation and associated arrhythmias. The manufacturers specifically name the **azoles**, **nefazodone**, and the **HIV-protease inhibitors**.[3,6] They also advise avoiding **grapefruit juice** in patients taking pimozide, as this can also inhibit CYP3A4.[3,6] The US manufacturer[3] also advises that other relatively less potent CYP3A4 inhibitors should also be avoided and they name **zileuton** and fluvoxamine, see 'Pimozide + SSRIs', below, as examples. Drugs that are known to cause clinically relevant CYP3A4 inhibition are listed in 'Table 1.9', below.

1. Flockhart DA, Richard E, Woosely RL, Pearle PL, Drici M-D. A metabolic interaction between clarithromycin and pimozide may result in cardiac toxicity. *Clin Pharmacol Ther* (1996) 59, 189.
2. Desta Z, Kerbusch T, Flockhart DA. Effect of clarithromycin on the pharmacokinetics and pharmacodynamics of pimozide in healthy poor and extensive metabolizers of cytochrome P450 2D6 (CYP2D6). *Clin Pharmacol Ther* (1999) 65, 10–20.
3. Orap (Pimozide). Gate Pharmaceuticals. US Prescribing information, January 2008.
4. Committee on Safety of Medicines. Cardiotoxic effects of pimozide. *Current Problems* (1990) 29.
5. Flockhart DA, Drici M-D, Kerbusch T, Soukhova N, Richard E, Pearle PL, Mahal SK, Babb VJ. Studies on the mechanism of a fatal clarithromycin-pimozide interaction in a patient with Tourette syndrome. *J Clin Psychopharmacol* (2000) 20, 317–24.
6. Orap (Pimozide). Janssen-Cilag Ltd. UK Summary of product characteristics, May 2012.

Pimozide + SSRIs

Pimozide exposure is moderately increased by paroxetine, slightly increased by sertraline, and is predicted to be raised by fluoxetine, which could increase the risk of QT prolongation and potentially fatal torsade de pointes arrhythmias. Fluvoxamine is predicted to interact similarly. Although citalopram did not alter pimozide exposure, QT prolongation has been reported on concurrent use. Escitalopram is predicted to interact similarly. The use of SSRIs and pimozide has also led to extrapyramidal adverse effects, oculogyric crises and sedation in rare cases.

Clinical evidence

(a) Citalopram

The UK manufacturer reports that the concurrent use of pimozide and citalopram resulted in a mean QTc increase of 10 milliseconds, with no change in pimozide exposure or maximum concentrations.[1]

(b) Fluoxetine

A patient taking fluoxetine and pimozide had a worsening of extrapyramidal symptoms, and another patient taking both drugs developed marked sinus bradycardia of 35 to 44 bpm with somnolence.[2] Another patient also developed extrapyramidal symptoms,[3] while a further patient became stuporous when given both drugs.[4]

(c) Paroxetine

In a study, paroxetine 60 mg daily caused a 2.5-fold increase in the AUC of a single 2-mg dose of pimozide and a 62% increase in its maximum plasma concentrations.[1]

A boy aged about 10 years, with various disorders (motor tics, enuresis, attention deficit hyperactivity disorder, Tourettes's disorder, impulsivity, albinism) was given pimozide 2 mg twice daily, and later three times daily for a year.[5] Within 3 days of starting paroxetine 10 mg in the morning, he began to complain of his eyes hurting and his mother noted that about 4 hours after taking the paroxetine his eyes were rolled back in his head but the problem had resolved by the evening. This oculogyric crisis occurred on a further occasion, and so the paroxetine was stopped. There was no other evidence of either extrapyramidal or hyper-serotonergic reactions. This case needs to be viewed in its particular context (oculogyric crises are associated with albinism) so that it might not be of general importance.

(d) Sertraline

In a study in 15 healthy subjects, sertraline 200 mg daily increased the AUC and maximum plasma concentrations of a single 2-mg dose of pimozide by about 40%. No changes in the QTc interval were seen.[6]

A fatality has been reported with an overdose of moclobemide, sertraline, and pimozide, with blood concentrations suggesting that, individually, none of these drugs would have been fatal.[7]

Mechanism

The SSRIs (in particular paroxetine and fluoxetine) can inhibit CYP2D6 to varying degrees (see 'Table 1.7', p.9). Pimozide is partially metabolised by CYP2D6 and concurrent use would therefore be expected to lead to raised pimozide exposure. Fluvoxamine is a weak inhibitor of CYP3A4, which is also involved in pimozide metabolism, see 'Pimozide + CYP3A4 inhibitors', p.879. Citalopram does not alter pimozide exposure, but citalopram alone causes QT prolongation, and has an additive effect with the QT-prolonging effect of pimozide.

Importance and management

Evidence of an adverse interaction between the SSRIs and pimozide is limited; however, the pharmacokinetic interaction with paroxetine, and possibly sertraline, is potentially severe as raised pimozide concentrations can cause QT prolongation and torsade de pointes arrhythmias, which can be fatal. Fluoxetine would be expected to have a similar effect. In addition, although citalopram does not have a pharmacokinetic interaction with pimozide, it can cause QT prolongation alone, and this might be additive with the QT-prolonging effects of pimozide. This would also be expected with its isomer **escitalopram**. The UK manufacturer[1] of pimozide contraindicates the concurrent use of SSRIs as a class, and they specifically name sertraline, paroxetine, citalopram, and **escitalopram**, whereas the US manufacturer[8] contraindicates only sertraline, and additionally advises avoiding **fluvoxamine** (consider *Mechanism*, above). See 'Drugs that prolong the QT interval + Other drugs that prolong the QT interval', p.272, for further information on the concurrent use of two or more drugs that prolong the QT interval.

1. Orap (Pimozide). Janssen-Cilag Ltd. UK Summary of product characteristics, May 2012.
2. Ahmed I, Dagincourt PG, Miller LG, Shader RI. Possible interaction between fluoxetine and pimozide causing sinus bradycardia. *Can J Psychiatry* (1993) 38, 62–3.
3. Coulter DM, Pillans PI. Fluoxetine and extrapyramidal side effects. *Am J Psychiatry* (1995) 152, 122–5.
4. Hansen-Grant S, Silk KR, Guthrie S. Fluoxetine-pimozide interaction. *Am J Psychiatry* (1993) 150, 1751–2.
5. Horrigan JP, Barnhill LJ. Paroxetine–pimozide drug interaction. *J Am Acad Child Adolesc Psychiatry* (1994) 33, 1060–1.
6. Alderman J. Coadministration of sertraline with cisapride or pimozide: an open-label, nonrandomized examination of pharmacokinetics and corrected QT intervals in healthy adult volunteers. *Clin Ther* (2005) 27, 1050–63.
7. A fatality involving moclobemide, sertraline, and pimozide. *J Forensic Sci* (1997) 42, 951–3.
8. Orap (Pimozide). Gate Pharmaceuticals. US Prescribing information, January 2008.

Quetiapine + CYP3A4 inducers

The plasma concentration of quetiapine is reduced by carbamazepine, and the clearance of quetiapine is increased by phenytoin. Other potent CYP3A4 inducers, such as phenobarbital and rifampicin (rifampin), are predicted to interact similarly, although this seems unlikely with the corticosteroids. Case reports suggest that quetiapine might increase carbamazepine-10,11-epoxide concentrations.

Clinical evidence

(a) Carbamazepine

In a pharmacokinetic study, 14 patients took quetiapine 300 mg twice daily for 28 days, with carbamazepine 200 mg three times daily for 20 days. It was found that the AUC and maximum plasma concentration of quetiapine were reduced by 87% and 80%, respectively.[1] Analysis of results from a routine therapeutic drug monitoring service found that carbamazepine lowered the quetiapine concentration-to-dose ratio by 86%.[2] Similarly, the quetiapine concentration-to-dose ratio was about 90% lower in 2 patients also taking carbamazepine, when compared with 8 patients taking olanzapine alone.[3] A report describes three cases of undetectable quetiapine serum concentrations in the presence of carbamazepine. All patients received quetiapine 600 mg or 700 mg daily and carbamazepine 400 mg, 600 mg, or 800 mg daily, and all drugs were given for up to 2 weeks, under close hospital supervision.[4]

A retrospective review of patients prescribed carbamazepine and an atypical antipsychotic (including quetiapine), but who discontinued carbamazepine and continued the antipsychotic, suggests that there is an increased risk of adverse effects if the dose of antipsychotic is not reduced after carbamazepine is stopped, although this was not seen in the two patients taking quetiapine.[5]

A 52-year-old woman taking carbamazepine 700 mg twice daily was given quetiapine, increased to a dose of 700 mg daily over 5 weeks. At this point she was noted to have become more aggressive and agitated, and unsteady. Her carbamazepine concentration had increased from 7.7 micrograms/mL to 11.2 micrograms/mL and the concentration of the metabolite carbamazepine-10,11-epoxide had risen from 2.1 micrograms/mL to 5.2 micrograms/mL. Symptoms resolved when carbamazepine was replaced with **oxcarbazepine**. A second patient taking carbamazepine also had a raised carbamazepine-10,11-epoxide concentration after starting quetiapine, but was asymptomatic.[6]

(b) Phenytoin

When 17 patients taking quetiapine 250 mg three times daily were given phenytoin 100 mg three times daily for 10 days, the oral clearance of quetiapine was increased 5-fold.[7]

Mechanism

Quetiapine is metabolised by CYP3A4. Both carbamazepine and phenytoin are known potent inducers of this isoenzyme, and therefore concurrent use results in an increase in quetiapine clearance and a decrease in its concentration. Oxcarbazepine is also an inducer of CYP3A4 and might be expected to interact similarly, although in one case oxcarbazepine was successfully used to replace carbamazepine, so their effects might differ somewhat.

The reason for the raised carbamazepine-10,11-epoxide concentrations is less clear. It has been suggested that quetiapine inhibits the metabolism (glucuronidation) of this metabolite.[6]

Importance and management

An interaction between quetiapine and **carbamazepine** or **phenytoin** is established. Concurrent use would be expected to reduce quetiapine concentrations. It would seem prudent to monitor the outcome of concurrent use, and increase the quetiapine dose as necessary. The authors of one study suggest that the risk of adverse effects might be increased in those taking a high dose of antipsychotic before carbamazepine discontinuation. Furthermore, they suggest that the patient should be monitored for the occurrence of adverse effects for 2 to 4 weeks after carbamazepine is discontinued.[5] Another group of authors goes further and suggests that the effect of carbamazepine is so great, that concurrent use with quetiapine cannot be recommended,[2] but this seems somewhat over cautious. The US manufacturer of quetiapine reasonably predicts that other potent CYP3A4 inducers will interact similarly,[8] and therefore similar precautions are warranted. They name the **barbiturates**, **corticosteroids**, and **rifampicin (rifampin)**, although note that the corticosteroids rarely appear to cause clinically relevant interactions by this mechanism. The UK manufacturer[9] advises that enzyme inducers (they name carbamazepine and phenytoin) should only be given with quetiapine if the benefits outweigh the risks. They also suggest that consideration should be given to changing the enzyme inducer to a drug with no enzyme-inducing effects and name valproate (see 'Quetiapine + Valproate', p.883).

Evidence for an interaction between **oxcarbazepine** and quetiapine is generally lacking, but on the basis that oxcarbazepine reduces the levels of other drugs metabolised in the same way as quetiapine, until more is known, it might be prudent to apply the same advice as for carbamazepine and phenytoin.

The general relevance of the reports of increased carbamazepine-10,11-epoxide concentrations is unknown, and more study is warranted to establish an interaction. However, it would be prudent to consider increased carbamazepine-10,11-epoxide concentrations as a possible cause if adverse effects develop.

1. Grimm SW, Richtand NM, Winter HR, Stams KR, Reele SB. Effects of cytochrome P450 3A modulators ketoconazole and carbamazepine on quetiapine pharmacokinetics. *Br J Clin Pharmacol* (2006), 61, 58–69.
2. Castberg I, Skogvoll E, Spigset O. Quetiapine and drug interactions: evidence from a routine therapeutic drug monitoring service. *J Clin Psychiatry* (2007) 68, 1540–5.
3. Hasselstrøm J, Linnet K. Quetiapine serum concentrations in psychiatric patients: the influence of comedication. *Ther Drug Monit* (2004) 26, 486–91.
4. Nickl-Jockschat T, Paulzen M, Schneider F, Grözinger M. Drug interaction can lead to undetectable serum concentrations of quetiapine in the presence of carbamazepine. *Clin Neuropharmacol* (2009) 32, 55.
5. Strack DK, Leckband SG, Meyer JM. Antipsychotic prescribing practices following withdrawal of concomitant carbamazepine. *J Psychiatr Pract* (2009) 15, 442–8.
6. Fitzgerald BJ, Okos AJ. Elevation of carbamazepine-10,11-epoxide by quetiapine. *Pharmacotherapy* (2002) 22, 1500–1503.
7. Wong YWJ, Yeh C, Thyrum PT. The effects of concomitant phenytoin administration on the steady-state pharmacokinetics of quetiapine. *J Clin Psychopharmacol* (2001) 21, 89–93.
8. Seroquel (Quetiapine fumarate). AstraZeneca. US Prescribing information, December 2011
9. Seroquel (Quetiapine fumarate). AstraZeneca UK Ltd. UK Summary of product characteristics, April 2012.

Quetiapine + CYP3A4 inhibitors

Quetiapine exposure is markedly increased by ketoconazole, and possibly clarithromycin; and moderately increased by erythromycin. Other azoles, HIV-protease inhibitors, some macrolides, and grapefruit juice are predicted to interact similarly, although to varying degrees. Two case reports describe adverse effects in patients taking quetiapine and atazanavir boosted with ritonavir.

Clinical evidence

(a) Clarithromycin

A case report describes a highly increased quetiapine concentration (827 micrograms/L) after a patient taking quetiapine was given two 500 mg doses of clarithromycin with quetiapine doses of 400 mg and 300 mg. The patient developed severely impaired consciousness and respiratory depression requiring intensive care monitoring. The quetiapine concentration decreased to within normal limits (70 to 170 micrograms/L) during the week following quetiapine discontinuation.[1]

(b) Erythromycin

A study in 19 Chinese patients who took quetiapine 200 mg twice daily and erythromycin 500 mg three times daily found that erythromycin increased the maximum plasma concentration and AUC of quetiapine by 68% and 2.3-fold, respectively.[2]

(c) HIV-protease inhibitors

A report describes increased adverse effects in two patients taking quetiapine and a **atazanavir boosted with ritonavir**-based antiretroviral regimen.[3] One patient taking a **atazanavir boosted with ritonavir** regimen experienced rapid and severe weight gain (about 23 kg) when quetiapine, titrated to 400 mg daily, was started. The second patient, taking quetiapine 600 mg daily, developed increased sedation and mental confusion when **atazanavir boosted with ritonavir** was started. In both cases quetiapine concentrations were not measured, but symptoms resolved either when both drugs (first case), or just the quetiapine (second case), were stopped.

(d) Ketoconazole

In a study, 12 healthy subjects were given ketoconazole 200 mg daily, with a single 25-mg dose of quetiapine on day 4. The AUC and maximum plasma concentration of quetiapine were increased about 6.2-fold and 3.4-fold, respectively.[4]

Mechanism

Clarithromycin, ketoconazole and HIV-protease inhibitors boosted with ritonavir are potent inhibitors of CYP3A4, by which quetiapine is metabolised. Concurrent use therefore reduces quetiapine metabolism, increasing its concentrations and might lead to an increase in quetiapine adverse effects. Erythromycin is a moderate inhibitor of this isoenzyme, and therefore has a smaller effect on quetiapine concentrations.

Importance and management

A pharmacokinetic interaction between quetiapine and ketoconazole (marked) or erythromycin (moderate) is established, and concurrent use would be expected to lead to increased quetiapine exposure. On the basis of these findings, other potent inhibitors and moderate inhibitors of CYP3A4 are likely to interact similarly to ketoconazole and erythromycin, respectively: the case of raised concentrations with clarithromycin and the two case reports of increased adverse effects with atazanavir boosted with ritonavir would seem to support this. In the UK, the manufacturer contraindicates the concurrent use of CYP3A4 inhibitors,[5] whereas in the US[6] they advise caution and suggest that a reduced quetiapine dose might be necessary: they specifically name the **HIV-protease inhibitors**, some azoles (**itraconazole**, **fluconazole**, ketoconazole), clarithromycin, erythromycin, and **nefazodone**.[5] For a list of CYP3A4 inhibitors, see 'Table 1.9', p.11. The UK manufacturer[5] also states that consuming **grapefruit juice** is not recommended, as grapefruit juice inhibits CYP3A4 (particularly in the intestine). If quetiapine is given with any of these drugs it would seem prudent to monitor closely for quetiapine adverse effects (e.g. dizziness, anxiety, orthostatic hypotension) and monitor closely for cardiac adverse effects. Anticipate the need to reduce the quetiapine dose, particularly with potent CYP3A4 inhibitors.

Note that quetiapine and some of these CYP3A4 inhibitors have been associated with QT prolongation, see 'Drugs that prolong the QT interval + Other drugs that prolong the QT interval', p.272, for further information on the concurrent use of two or more drugs that prolong the QT interval.

1. Schulz-Du Bois C, Schulz-Du Bois AC, Bewig B, Gerstner I, Aldenhoff JB, Cascorbi I, Ufer M. Major increase of quetiapine steady-state plasma concentration following co-administration of clarithromycin: confirmation of the pharmacokinetic interaction potential of quetiapine. *Pharmacopsychiatry* (2008) 41, 258–9.
2. Li K-Y, Li X, Cheng Z-N, Zhang B-K, Peng W-X, Li H-D. Effect of erythromycin on metabolism of quetiapine in Chinese suffering from schizophrenia. *Eur J Clin Pharmacol* (2005) 60, 791–5.
3. Pollack TM, McCoy C, Stead W. Clinically significant adverse events from a drug interaction between quetiapine and atazanavir-ritonavir in two patients. *Pharmacotherapy* (2009) 29, 1386–91.
4. Grimm SW, Richtand NM, Winter HR, Stams KR, Reele SB. Effects of cytochrome P450 3A modulators ketoconazole and carbamazepine on quetiapine pharmacokinetics. *Br J Clin Pharmacol* (2006), 61, 58–69.
5. Seroquel (Quetiapine fumarate). AstraZeneca UK Ltd. UK Summary of product characteristics, April 2012.
6. Seroquel (Quetiapine fumarate). AstraZeneca. US Prescribing information, December 2011.

Quetiapine + Haloperidol

Haloperidol appears to have negligible effects on the pharmacokinetics of quetiapine.

Clinical evidence, mechanism, importance and management

In 12 patients with schizophrenia or bipolar disorder taking quetiapine 300 mg twice daily, haloperidol 7.5 mg twice daily appeared to increase quetiapine exposure by 11% and decreased clearance by 10%, but these changes are not clinically important.[1]

Quetiapine dose adjustments are therefore not expected to be necessary if haloperidol is also given. However, as cases of QT prolongation have been reported with quetiapine, the UK manufacturer advises caution on the concurrent use of quetiapine with other antipsychotics,[2] whereas in the US, concurrent use with other antipsychotics is contraindicated.[3] This would therefore apply to haloperidol, which is known to be associated with QT prolongation. See 'Drugs that prolong the QT interval + Other drugs that prolong the QT interval', p.272, for more information on the concurrent use of two or more QT-prolonging drugs.

1. Potkin SG, Thyrum PT, Alva G, Bera R, Yeh C, Arvanitis LA. The safety and pharmacokinetics of quetiapine when coadministered with haloperidol, risperidone, or thioridazine. *J Clin Psychopharmacol* (2002) 22, 121–30.
2. Seroquel (Quetiapine fumarate). AstraZeneca UK Ltd. UK Summary of product characteristics, April 2012.
3. Seroquel (Quetiapine fumarate). AstraZeneca. US Prescribing information, December 2011.

Quetiapine + Lamotrigine

Limited evidence suggests that lamotrigine might reduce quetiapine concentrations.

Clinical evidence

An analysis of 147 samples in a routine therapeutic drug monitoring service reported that lamotrigine decreased the quetiapine concentration-to-dose ratio by 17%.[1] Similarly, in a case-control study that identified 22 patients given both quetiapine and lamotrigine, the concurrent use of lamotrigine and quetiapine resulted in a median 58% lower quetiapine concentration-to-dose ratio, when compared with matched controls not taking lamotrigine.[2]

Mechanism

Quetiapine is primarily metabolised by CYP3A4, and the authors of one report suggest that glucuronidation might also be involved. They suggest that lamotrigine might have induced quetiapine glucuronidation resulting in the lower quetiapine concentrations seen in the study.[2]

Importance and management

Evidence for an interaction between quetiapine and lamotrigine is limited and an interaction is not established but based on what is known a clinically relevant interaction cannot be ruled out. Therefore until more is known, it would seem prudent to bear the possibility of an interaction in mind should quetiapine become ineffective in patients given lamotrigine.

1. Castberg I, Skogvoll E, Spigset O. Quetiapine and drug interactions: evidence from a routine therapeutic drug monitoring service. *J Clin Psychiatry* (2007) 68, 1540–5.
2. Andersson ML, Björkhem-Bergman L, Lindh JD. Possible drug–drug interaction between quetiapine and lamotrigine – evidence from a Swedish TDM database. *Br J Clin Pharmacol* (2011) 72, 153.

Quetiapine + Mirtazapine

An isolated case describes an increased prolactin concentration when mirtazapine was given to a patient taking quetiapine.

Clinical evidence, mechanism, importance and management

An isolated case report describes a woman who was taking quetiapine 400 mg daily who developed an increased prolactin concentration after the introduction of mirtazapine 15 mg daily. Her prolactin concentration normalised when the mirtazapine was stopped, but rechallenge again produced an increase in prolactin concentration, although this was transient and appeared to resolve within one month. The authors suggest that mirtazapine might have caused an increase in quetiapine-induced dopamine-receptor blockade, or alternatively an agonist action at opioid receptors altered dopamine receptor function.[1] As this is an isolated report, its general importance is unknown, but no particular precautions would seem necessary on concurrent use.

1. Orlandi V, Speca A, Salviati M, Biondi M. Abnormal prolactin elevation in a schizophrenic patient in treatment with quetiapine and mirtazapine. The role of the opioid system. *J Clin Psychopharmacol* (2003) 23, 677–9.

Quetiapine + Miscellaneous

Alimemazine, clozapine, and levomepromazine possibly raise quetiapine concentrations whereas cimetidine does not appear to alter quetiapine pharmacokinetics. Quetiapine does not interact with lorazepam. An isolated case of urinary retention has been reported when quetiapine was given with diphenhydramine and an isolated report describes QT prolongation on the concurrent use of quetiapine and lovastatin.

Clinical evidence, mechanism, importance and management

(a) Alimemazine

An analysis of results from a therapeutic drug monitoring service found that alimemazine raised the quetiapine concentration-to-dose ratio by 28%. This small increase would not expected to be clinically relevant, and no alimemazine dose adjustment is considered to be necessary on concurrent use.[1]

(b) Cimetidine

In a study in 7 men with psychotic disorders, quetiapine 150 mg three times daily was given with cimetidine 400 mg three times daily for 4 days. There were some small alterations in the pharmacokinetics of the quetiapine, but these were within the intraindividual changes seen and so were not considered important.[2] The dose of quetiapine does not need to be adjusted in patients given cimetidine.

(c) Clozapine

An analysis of results from a therapeutic drug monitoring service found that clozapine raised the quetiapine concentration-to-dose ratio by 82%. The authors note that a rise of this magnitude is clinically relevant, but suggest that it should be verified in a controlled setting as it cannot be explained.[1]

Note that quetiapine is associated with QT prolongation, as is clozapine. See 'Drugs that prolong the QT interval + Other drugs that prolong the QT interval', p.272, for further information on the concurrent use of two or more drugs that prolong the QT interval.

(d) Diphenhydramine

A patient taking diphenhydramine 100 mg daily developed urinary retention when she increased her dose of quetiapine from 900 mg daily to 2.4 g daily. When the dose of quetiapine was reduced back to 900 mg daily, her urinary retention resolved. A further episode occurred when the patient again increased her quetiapine dose. Although quetiapine does not normally have antimuscarinic adverse effects at usual therapeutic doses, it is suggested by the authors that the likelihood of these adverse effects is increased at doses of quetiapine greater than 900 mg daily. This effect might have occurred as a result of additive antimuscarinic activity of both diphenhydramine and high-dose quetiapine.[3]

(e) Levomepromazine

An analysis of results from a therapeutic drug monitoring service found that levomepromazine decreased the quetiapine concentration-to-dose ratio by 20%.[1] This is in contrast to another study which found that it had no effect,[4] although the sample size was much smaller in this study. Nevertheless, the small increase reported would not be expected to be clinically relevant, and no levomepromazine dose adjustment is necessary on concurrent use.[1]

Note that levomepromazine is associated with QT prolongation, as is clozapine. See 'Drugs that prolong the QT interval + Other drugs that prolong the QT interval', p.272, for further information on the concurrent use of two or more drugs that prolong the QT interval.

(f) Lorazepam

The pharmacokinetics and pharmacodynamic effects of a single 2-mg dose of lorazepam were studied in 10 men taking quetiapine 250 mg three times daily. It was found that the maximum serum concentration of lorazepam was not significantly changed by quetiapine, and the alterations in the performance of a number of psychometric tests were small and considered not to be clinically relevant.[5]

(g) Lovastatin

A patient taking quetiapine 800 mg daily and sertraline 100 mg daily developed a prolonged QTc interval of 569 milliseconds after starting to take lovastatin 10 mg daily. Following a reduction in the lovastatin dose to 5 mg daily, her QTc interval returned to her baseline of 424 milliseconds. It was suggested that lovastatin competitively inhibited the metabolism of quetiapine by CYP3A4, as both drugs are substrates for this enzyme, resulting in increased quetiapine concentrations.[6] However, this is not a clinically important mechanism for drug interactions and lovastatin is not an inhibitor of CYP3A4, therefore this seems unlikely. Moreover, the full contribution of sertraline to this case was only briefly considered, and full details relating to the cardiac effects and calculation of the QTc interval are not given.[7]

1. Castberg I, Skogvoll E, Spigset O. Quetiapine and drug interactions: evidence from a routine therapeutic drug monitoring service. *J Clin Psychiatry* (2007) 68, 1540–5.
2. Strakowski SM, Keck PE, Wong YWJ, Thyrum PT, Yeh C. The effect of multiple doses of cimetidine on the steady-state pharmacokinetics of quetiapine in men with selected psychotic disorders. *J Clin Psychopharmacol* (2002) 22, 201–5.
3. Sokolski KN, Brown BJ, Melden M. Urinary retention following repeated high-dose quetiapine. *Ann Pharmacother* (2004) 38, 899–900.
4. Hasselstrøm J, Linnet K. Quetiapine serum concentrations in psychiatric patients: the influence of comedication. *Ther Drug Monit* (2004) 26, 486–91.
5. Zeneca Pharma. Data on file. Potkin SG: the pharmacokinetics and pharmacodynamics of lorazepam given before and during treatment with ICI 204,636 (Seroquel) in men with selected psychotic disorders (5077IL/0027), Study 27.
6. Furst BA, Champion KM, Pierre JM, Wirshing DA, Wirshing WC. Possible association of QTc interval prolongation with co-administration of quetiapine and lovastatin. *Biol Psychiatry* (2002) 51, 264–5.
7. Geller W, Smith M, Winter H, Brecher M. Response: possible association of QTc interval prolongation with co-administration of quetiapine and lovastatin. *Biol Psychiatry* (2002) 52, 914.

Quetiapine + Olanzapine

A case report describes a seizure in a patient taking olanzapine and quetiapine.

Clinical evidence, mechanism, importance and management

A case report describes a seizure lasting 30 to 60 seconds in a 27-year-old woman, which occurred one day after quetiapine 100 mg daily was added to treatment with olanzapine 15 mg daily and sertraline 100 mg daily.[1] The seizure was attributed to an interaction between quetiapine and olanzapine, although it seems possible that the sertraline might have also contributed. This case highlights the importance of considering seizure potential when prescribing multiple antipsychotic medications.

Note that quetiapine and olanzapine have been said to be associated with QT prolongation, see 'Drugs that prolong the QT interval + Other drugs that prolong the QT interval', p.272, for further information on the concurrent use of two or more drugs that prolong the QT interval.

1. Hedges DW, Jeppson KG. New-onset seizure associated with quetiapine and olanzapine. *Ann Pharmacother* (2002) 36, 437–9.

Quetiapine + Quinolones

An isolated report describes an exacerbation of psychotic symptoms after gatifloxacin was given to a patient taking quetiapine.

Clinical evidence, mechanism, importance and management

A case report describes an exacerbation of psychotic symptoms in a 60-year-old man taking quetiapine 200 mg twice daily with glibenclamide (glyburide) after **gatifloxacin** 400 mg daily was started. The patient's symptoms gradually resolved over the 36 hours following **gatifloxacin** discontinuation.[1] This is an isolated report and as such, no general recommendations can be made. However, note that quetiapine has been said to be associated with QT prolongation and some quinolones are known to prolong the QT interval. See 'Drugs that prolong the QT interval + Other drugs that prolong the QT interval', p.272, for further information on the concurrent use of two or more drugs that prolong the QT interval.

1. Reeves RR. Exacerbation of psychotic symptoms associated with gatifloxacin. *Psychosomatics* (2007) 48, 87.

Quetiapine + Risperidone

Risperidone does not affect the pharmacokinetics of quetiapine. An isolated report describes QTc prolongation in a patient who took a small quetiapine overdose while also taking risperidone.

Clinical evidence, mechanism, importance and management

In a study in 12 patients with schizophrenia or bipolar disorder taking quetiapine 300 mg twice daily, risperidone 3 mg twice daily for 9 days had no effect on the pharmacokinetics of quetiapine.[1] Quetiapine dose adjustments are therefore not expected to be necessary if risperidone is also given.

A case report describes considerable QTc prolongation (to 537 milliseconds) in a patient who took a small overdose of quetiapine of 2 g with risperidone. The QTc prolongation resolved (reducing to 401 milliseconds) on discontinuation of all drugs. The authors consider this QTc prolongation to be clinically important as the overdose was small, and because no QTc prolongation had been reported in toxicity studies of quetiapine when doses as large as 9.6 g were used,[2] although there is a single case of a prolonged QTc interval associated with a quetiapine overdose of 9.6 g.[3]

Note that quetiapine and risperidone have been said to be associated with QT prolongation, see 'Drugs that prolong the QT interval + Other drugs that prolong the QT interval', p.272, for further information on the concurrent use of two or more drugs that prolong the QT interval.

1. Potkin SG, Thyrum PT, Alva G, Bera R, Yeh C, Arvanitis LA. The safety and pharmacokinetics of quetiapine when coadministered with haloperidol, risperidone, or thioridazine. *J Clin Psychopharmacol* (2002) 22, 121–30.
2. Beelen AP, Yeo K-TJ, Lewis LD. Asymptomatic QTc prolongation associated with quetiapine fumarate overdose in a patient being treated with risperidone. *Hum Exp Toxicol* (2001) 20, 215–19.
3. Gajwani P, Pozuelo L, Tesar GE. QT interval prolongation associated with quetiapine (Seroquel) overdose. *Psychosomatics* (2000) 41, 63–5.

Quetiapine + SSRIs

Fluvoxamine, and possibly escitalopram and citalopram, might raise quetiapine concentrations. Fluoxetine has negligible effect on quetiapine exposure. Isolated reports of weight gain, neuroleptic malignant syndrome and restless legs syndrome, have been reported when escitalopram, fluvoxamine and paroxetine, respectively, were given with quetiapine.

Clinical evidence

(a) Escitalopram

Analysis of results from a routine therapeutic drug monitoring service found that escitalopram or **citalopram** (grouped together) increased the quetiapine concentration-to-dose ratio by 16%.[1]

A case report describes a dramatic increase in weight (8 kg over one month) in an adolescent when escitalopram was added to quetiapine. Quetiapine was switched to amisulpride, resulting in a transient decrease in weight. However, due to the reappearance of psychotic symptoms, quetiapine was reintroduced and an additional 8 kg weight gain was observed over one month. The authors note that the patient was considered susceptible to weight gain due to a family history, but no weight gain was seen when the patient was taking quetiapine alone.[2]

(b) Fluoxetine

In a study in 13 patients, fluoxetine 60 mg daily for 5 days increased the AUC and maximum concentration of quetiapine 300 mg twice daily by 12% and 26%, respectively, and decreased its clearance by 11%, but only the difference in the maximum concentration was statistically significant.[3] Analysis of results from a routine therapeutic drug monitoring service found a lack of effect of fluoxetine on quetiapine concentration-to-dose ratios.[1]

A 23-year-old patient taking fluoxetine 20 mg daily for one year developed sore muscles during a period of 3 days after light physical activity, and after also taking quetiapine 25 mg daily for 2 weeks. A diagnosis of rhabdomyolysis associated with quetiapine use was made as the patient was found to have very high concentrations of serum creatinine kinase and above normal concentrations of aspartate aminotransferase and alanine aminotransferase, which steadily decreased to normal after stopping quetiapine.[4]

(c) Fluvoxamine

Analysis of results from a routine therapeutic drug monitoring service found that fluvoxamine increased the quetiapine concentration-to-dose ratio 2.6-fold.[1]

A case report describes neuroleptic malignant syndrome in a 57-year-old man which developed 13 days after fluvoxamine, titrated to 100 mg daily, was added to quetiapine 150 mg daily. The patient recovered after the drugs were stopped and intensive care treatment was given. The authors note that the patient had been given both quetiapine and fluvoxamine alone previously with no problems.[5]

(d) Paroxetine

A 47-year-old man, taking valproic acid 700 mg daily and paroxetine 12.5 mg daily was started on quetiapine 200 mg at night for persistently severe depressive symptoms and sleep impairment. After one and a half hours of sleep following the first dose of quetiapine, the patient experienced unpleasant sensations in his legs which were immediately relieved by movement. The patient did not take any further doses of quetiapine and did not experience this feeling again. The authors diagnosed restless leg syndrome resulting from the concurrent use of quetiapine and paroxetine.[6]

Mechanism

Quetiapine is principally metabolised by CYP3A4. The SSRIs do not generally inhibit CYP3A4, although fluvoxamine is a weak CYP3A4 inhibitor. Weight gain is very common with quetiapine, and has also been reported with the SSRIs.

Importance and management

There would appear to be no clinically relevant pharmacokinetic interaction between quetiapine and **fluoxetine**. No quetiapine dose adjustments would therefore seem necessary if fluoxetine and quetiapine are used concurrently.

The possible minor rise in quetiapine concentrations seen with **escitalopram** or **citalopram** is unlikely to be clinically important and a quetiapine dose reduction would not be expected to be necessary on concurrent use. The general relevance of the isolated report of weight gain is unknown. However, note that citalopram and escitalopram are associated with a dose-related prolongation of the QT interval, and quetiapine has also been associated with QT prolongation. See 'Drugs that prolong the QT interval + Other drugs that prolong the QT interval', p.272, for further information on the concurrent use of two or more drugs that prolong the QT interval.

The rise in quetiapine concentrations seen with **fluvoxamine** could be clinically important and, until more is known about this potential interaction, it would seem prudent to monitor adverse effects (such as dizziness, anxiety, orthostatic hypotension) on concurrent use, monitoring levels where possible and reducing the quetiapine dose if necessary. Due to the severity of neuroleptic malignant syndrome, it would seem prudent to be aware of this possibility if these drugs are used together.

The isolated case of restless leg syndrome with **paroxetine** is of unknown clinical importance, and as such no general recommendations can be made. Similar to fluoxetine, no clinically relevant pharmacokinetic interaction would be predicted between paroxetine and quetiapine.

1. Castberg I, Skogvoll, Spigset O. Quetiapine and drug interactions: evidence from a routine therapeutic drug monitoring service. *J Clin Psychiatry* (2007) 68, 1540–5.
2. Holzer L, Paiva G, Halfon O. Quetiapine-induced weight gain and escitalopram. *Am J Psychiatry* (2005) 162, 192–3.
3. Potkin SG, Thyrum PT, Alva G, Carreon D, Yeh C, Kalali A, Arvanitis LA. Effect of fluoxetine and imipramine on the pharmacokinetics and tolerability of the antipsychotic quetiapine. *J Clin Psychopharmacol* (2002) 22, 174–82.
4. Himmerich H, Ehrlinger M, Hackenberg M, Löhr B, Nickel T. Possible case of quetiapine-induced rhabdomyolysis in a patient with depression treated with fluoxetine. *J Clin Psychopharmacol* (2006) 26, 676–7.
5. Matsumoto R, Kitabayashi Y, Nakatomi Y, Tsuchida H, Fukui K. Neuroleptic malignant syndrome induced by quetiapine and fluvoxamine. *Am J Psychiatry* (2005) 162, 812.
6. Chou K-J, Chen P-Y, Huang M-C. Restless legs syndrome following the combined use of quetiapine and paroxetine. *Prog Neuropsychopharmacol Biol Psychiatry* (2010) 34, 1139–40.

Quetiapine + Thioridazine

Thioridazine slightly reduces quetiapine exposure.

Clinical evidence, mechanism, importance and management

A study in 12 patients with schizophrenia or bipolar disorder taking quetiapine 300 mg twice daily found that thioridazine 200 mg twice daily reduced the steady-state AUC and maximum plasma concentration of quetiapine by about 41% and 48%, respectively. It was suggested that the decreased quetiapine exposure was due to an increase in its metabolism, although the mechanism for this effect is unclear.[1] These reductions are only slight, but until more information is available it would seem prudent to monitor concurrent use for efficacy, being alert for the need to raise the quetiapine dose. However, note also that quetiapine has been said to be associated with QT prolongation whereas thioridazine is a known QT-prolonging drug. See 'Drugs that prolong the QT interval + Other drugs that prolong the QT interval', p.272, for further information on the concurrent use of two or more drugs that prolong the QT interval.

1. Potkin SG, Thyrum PT, Alva G, Bera R, Yeh C, Arvanitis LA. The safety and pharmacokinetics of quetiapine when coadministered with haloperidol, risperidone, or thioridazine. *J Clin Psychopharmacol* (2002) 22, 121–30.

Quetiapine + Topiramate

Topiramate does not appear to affect the steady-state plasma concentration of quetiapine.

Clinical evidence, mechanism, importance and management

In a study, 7 patients taking quetiapine 200 mg to 600 mg daily long-term were given topiramate in a dose that was increased gradually to 200 mg daily over 6 to 8 weeks. The plasma concentration of quetiapine did not appear to be affected by topiramate.[1] There would therefore appear to be no need to adjust the dose of quetiapine in patients also given topiramate.

1. Migliardi G, D'Arrigo C, Santoro V, Bruno A, Cortese L, Campolo D, Cacciola M, Spina E. Effect of topiramate on plasma concentrations of clozapine, olanzapine, risperidone, and quetiapine in patients with psychotic disorders. *Clin Neuropharmacol* (2007) 30, 107–13.

Quetiapine + Tricyclic antidepressants

Imipramine does not appear to affect the pharmacokinetics of quetiapine. An isolated case describes elevated quetiapine concentrations in a patient taking quetiapine with doxepin. The use of quetiapine might falsely elevate tricyclic concentrations by interfering with immunoassay results.

Clinical evidence

(a) Doxepin

A patient taking doxepin 150 mg daily and lorazepam 500 micrograms daily was admitted to hospital with confusion and depression. Quetiapine 750 mg daily and pantoprazole 40 mg daily were started, and the doses of his existing medication were adjusted to doxepin 100 mg daily and lorazepam 4.5 mg daily. At this point his quetiapine concentration was found to be 1 838 to 1 860 nanograms/mL, but as there was only slight improvement in the symptoms of schizophrenia, the dose of quetiapine was increased to 900 mg daily. Pantoprazole and doxepin were discontinued and the dose of lorazepam was reduced to 2 mg daily. At this point his quetiapine concentration was found to be just 109 nanograms/mL. The lorazepam dose was decreased further, to 500 micrograms daily, and the quetiapine concentration was found to be 68 nanograms/mL.[1]

(b) Imipramine

In a study in 13 patients, imipramine 75 mg twice daily for 5 days had no effect on the steady-state pharmacokinetics of quetiapine 300 mg twice daily.[2]

Mechanism

The reasons for the elevated quetiapine concentrations are not known but the authors suggest that they might have been due to the concurrent use of doxepin and pantoprazole. As lorazepam was given continuously and was present when quetiapine concentrations were low, it was considered unlikely to be involved in the interaction.[1]

Importance and management

Evidence for an interaction between the tricyclic antidepressants and quetiapine appears to be limited to this case report,[1] which is largely unexplained. The one pharmacokinetic study involving imipramine found no interaction. Therefore, in general, no particular precautions would appear to be necessary if quetiapine is given with a tricyclic antidepressant.

Note that immunoassay methods for identifying tricyclic antidepressants in blood and urine have given false positive results in the presence of quetiapine.[3-5] In one case, HPLC analysis gave normal results.[5]

Note that QT prolongation is predicted to occur with both the tricyclics and quetiapine, and this is potentially of more concern than any pharmacokinetic interaction. See 'Drugs that prolong the QT interval + Other drugs that prolong the QT interval', p.272, for further information on the concurrent use of two or more drugs that prolong the QT interval.

1. Härtter S, Connemann B, Schönfeldt-Lecuona C, Sachse J, Hiemke C. Elevated quetiapine serum concentrations in a patient treated concomitantly with doxepin, lorazepam, and pantoprazole. *J Clin Psychopharmacol* (2004) 24, 568–71.
2. Potkin SG, Thyrum PT, Alva G, Carreon D, Yeh C, Kalali A, Arvanitis LA. Effect of fluoxetine and imipramine on the pharmacokinetics and tolerability of the antipsychotic quetiapine. *J Clin Psychopharmacol* (2002) 22, 174–82.
3. Hayes KM. Law T, Burns MM. Quetiapine (Seroquel®) produces false positive tricyclic antidepressant screen. *Pediatr Res* (2003) 53, 104A.
4. Al-Mateen CS, Wolf CE. Falsely elevated imipramine levels in a patient taking quetiapine. *J Am Acad Child Adolesc Psychiatry* (2002) 41, 5–6.
5. Schussler JM, Juenke JM, Schussler I. Quetiapine and falsely elevated nortriptyline level. *Am J Psychiatry* (2003) 160, 589.

Quetiapine + Valproate

Valproate does not appear to alter the steady-state concentrations of quetiapine.

Clinical evidence, mechanism, importance and management

An analysis of the plasma concentrations of quetiapine in 9 patients who were also taking valproate found a 77% higher concentration-to-dose ratio of quetiapine, when compared with those patients not taking valproate.[1] However, a similar analysis in a much larger group found that valproic acid appeared not to affect the quetiapine concentration-to-dose ratio.[2] Moreover, a study in 33 patients given quetiapine 150 mg twice daily or valproate semisodium (divalproex sodium) 500 mg twice daily, either alone or concurrently, found that valproate increased the maximum plasma concentration of quetiapine by just 17%, and did not affect its AUC. The plasma concentration and AUC of valproate were decreased by 11% by quetiapine. However, none of these changes were statistically significant.[3]

Although one uncontrolled analysis suggested that valproate might increase quetiapine concentrations, no clinically relevant pharmacokinetic interaction was found in the controlled study. This suggests that a quetiapine dose adjustment is unlikely to be needed on the concurrent use of valproate.

1. Aichhorn W, Marksteiner J, Walch T, Zernig G, Saria A, Kemmler G. Influence of age, gender, body weight and valproate comedication on quetiapine plasma concentrations. *Int Clin Psychopharmacol* (2006) 21, 81–5.
2. Castberg I, Skogvoll, Spigset O. Quetiapine and drug interactions: evidence from a routine therapeutic drug monitoring service. *J Clin Psychiatry* (2007) 68, 1540–5.
3. Winter HR, DeVane CL, Figueroa C, Ennis DJ, Hamer-Maansson JE, Davis PC, Smith MA. Open-label steady-state pharmacokinetic drug interaction study on co-administered quetiapine fumarate and divalproex sodium in patients with schizophrenia, schizoaffective disorder, or bipolar disorder. *Hum Psychopharmacol* (2007) 22, 469–76.

Risperidone + Azoles

Itraconazole increases the steady-state plasma concentrations of risperidone and its active metabolite, 9-hydroxyrisperidone.

Clinical evidence

A study in 19 patients who were taking risperidone 2 to 8 mg daily found that the addition of itraconazole 200 mg daily for a week increased the plasma concentrations of risperidone and its active metabolite, 9-hydroxyrisperidone, by 82% and 70%, respectively. The concentrations returned to pre-treatment values one week after the itraconazole was stopped.[1]

Mechanism

Itraconazole is a known inhibitor of CYP3A4, an isoenzyme which is partly responsible for the metabolism of risperidone (see *Risperidone*, under 'Antipsychotics, Anxiolytics, and Hypnotics', p.803), resulting in the increased concentrations seen.

Importance and management

Evidence for an interaction between risperidone and the azoles appears to be limited to one study with itraconazole, which suggests that risperidone concentrations are expected to increase if itraconazole is given concurrently. Be aware of any signs of increased risperidone adverse effects (such as agitation, insomnia, headache), and consider reducing the risperidone dose as necessary. If the predicted mechanism is correct, then other azoles that are potent inhibitors of CYP3A4 would be expected to interact similarly, see 'Table 1.9', p.11, for a list.

1. Jung SM, Kim KA, Cho HK, Jung IG, Park PW, Byun WT, Park JY. Cytochrome P450 3A inhibitor itraconazole affects plasma concentrations of risperidone and 9-hydroxyrisperidone in schizophrenic patients. *Clin Pharmacol Ther* (2005) 78, 520–8.

Risperidone + Carbamazepine and related drugs

Carbamazepine reduces risperidone concentrations, and risperidone might cause a small increase in carbamazepine concentrations. One study suggests that oxcarbazepine might not affect the pharmacokinetics of risperidone.

Clinical evidence

(a) Carbamazepine

A 22-year-old man taking risperidone 4 mg daily and carbamazepine 600 mg daily for schizophrenia had lower than expected risperidone concentrations, so his risperidone dose was doubled and the carbamazepine tailed off. Ten days after carbamazepine had been discontinued it was noted that his plasma concentration of the major active metabolite of risperidone, 9-hydroxyrisperidone, was 49 micrograms/L; it had only been 19 micrograms/L when he was taking carbamazepine. Note that this patient was an extensive CYP2D6 metaboliser (that is, he had normal activity of this isoenzyme).[1] There are 4 other cases of this interaction between risperidone and carbamazepine.[2-4] In one case the patient was a CYP2D6 poor metaboliser (that is, he lacked or had low activity of this isoenzyme), and the addition of carbamazepine to established risperidone treatment resulted in a reduction in the risperidone and 9-hydroxyrisperidone concentrations of about 75% and 65%, respectively, accompanied by the return of the patients psychotic symptoms.[4] In two other cases, a 20-year-old and an 81-year-old man developed parkinsonian symptoms when carbamazepine was stopped. The symptoms resolved when the doses of risperidone were reduced by about two-thirds.[2]

These cases are supported by a study in 5 patients taking carbamazepine and risperidone for schizophrenia or bipolar disorders. The dose-normalised plasma concentration of risperidone and its active metabolite, 9-hydroxyrisperidone, were 68% and 64% lower, respectively, in the presence of carbamazepine, when compared with patients taking risperidone alone.[5] Another study in 11 patients who had been taking risperidone for 2 to 68 weeks found that carbamazepine 200 mg twice daily for a week approximately halved the plasma concentrations of risperidone and its active moiety (risperidone plus 9-hydroxyrisperidone). They also found that the magnitude of the effect was related to CYP2D6 metaboliser status, with those having reduced CYP2D6 activity showing the greatest effect.[6] In another study in patients with acute mania, the concentrations of active risperidone were 40% lower in patients given risperidone with carbamazepine, when compared with those given risperidone and either lithium or divalproex sodium. The efficacy of the combination of risperidone with a mood stabiliser (lithium, divalproex sodium, carbamazepine) was found to be considerably increased if patients taking carbamazepine were excluded from the analysis.[7] A retrospective chart review of patients prescribed carbamazepine with an atypical antipsychotic (including risperidone), but who discontinued carbamazepine and continued the antipsychotic, suggests that there is an increased risk of adverse effects if the dose of antipsychotic is not reduced after discontinuation of the carbamazepine. Five of the 9 patients identified were taking risperidone; one of whom experienced akathisia 3 weeks after stopping carbamazepine (self-discontinuation) and the remaining four did not experience any adverse effects. Of the 4 patients not experiencing problems, the dose of risperidone had been reduced by the prescriber upon discontinuation of the carbamazepine in only one case.[8]

Risperidone might also affect carbamazepine concentrations. In one study in 8 patients, risperidone 1 mg daily for 2 weeks raised carbamazepine concentrations by about 20%.[9]

(b) Oxcarbazepine

A study in 12 patients taking risperidone 2 to 6 mg daily found that the addition of oxcarbazepine for 5 weeks, at an initial dose of 300 mg daily, increased to 900 mg to 1.2 g after one week, had no effects on the pharmacokinetics of risperidone.[10] Note that CYP2D6 metaboliser status was not assessed.

Mechanism

Risperidone is mainly metabolised by CYP2D6, with CYP3A4 playing a more minor role. Carbamazepine is a well-known enzyme inducer, with potent effects on CYP3A4, and weak effects on CYP2D6. The extent of the interaction may be related to CYP2D6 genotype (see *Genetic factors in drug metabolism*, under 'Drug metabolism interactions', p.4), when the metabolism of risperidone by CYP3A4 could become more important, but this requires further study. Oxcarbazepine is not known to affect the metabolism of drugs by CYP2D6, but it does induce CYP3A4.

Importance and management

An interaction between carbamazepine and risperidone appears to be established and clinically important. The concurrent use of these two drugs can be clinically beneficial; however, it would seem prudent, where possible, to monitor the concentrations of risperidone and 9-hydroxyrisperidone in patients given carbamazepine, being alert for the need to raise the risperidone dose, possibly by as much as two-thirds. Any interaction might be more important in poor metabolisers (that is those with low CYP2D6 activity) than extensive metabolisers (that is those with normal CYP2D6 activity), but this is not established and because CYP2D6 metaboliser status is usually unknown in practice, the management advice should be applied to all patients.

The authors of one study[8] suggest that the risk of adverse effects might be increased in those taking a high dose of antipsychotic before stopping carbamazepine. Furthermore, they suggest that the patient should be monitored for the occurrence of adverse effects for 2 to 4 weeks after carbamazepine is stopped. The increase in carbamazepine concentrations seen with risperidone is almost certainly too small to be of clinical relevance.

From the small study cited, no risperidone dose adjustment appears to be necessary if oxcarbazepine is also given. However, as the metaboliser status of the patients studied was unknown, it would seem prudent to be aware of the possibility of an interaction in some patients (who are CYP2D6 poor metabolisers) should a lack of therapeutic response be seen.

1. de Leon J, Bork J. Risperidone and cytochrome P450 3A. *J Clin Psychiatry* (1997) 58, 450.
2. Takahashi H, Yoshida K, Higuchi H, Shimizu T. Development of parkinsonian symptoms after discontinuation of carbamazepine in patients concurrently treated with risperidone: two case reports. *Clin Neuropharmacol* (2001) 24, 358–60.
3. Alfaro CL, Nicolson R, Lenane M, Rapoport JL. Carbamazepine and/or fluvoxamine drug interaction with risperidone in a patient on multiple psychotropic medications. *Ann Pharmacother* (2000) 34, 122–3.
4. Spina E, Scordo MG, Avenoso A, Perucca E. Adverse drug interaction between risperidone and carbamazepine in a patient with chronic schizophrenia and deficient CYP2D6 activity. *J Clin Psychopharmacol* (2001) 21, 108–9.
5. Spina E, Avenoso A, Facciolà G, Salemi M, Scordo MG, Giacobello T, Madia AG, Perucca E. Plasma concentrations of risperidone and 9-hydroxyrisperidone: effect of comedication with carbamazepine or valproate. *Ther Drug Monit* (2000) 22, 481–5.
6. Ono S, Mihara K, Suzuki A, Kondo T, Yasui-Furukori N, Furukori H, de Vries R, Kaneko S. Significant pharmacokinetic interaction between risperidone and carbamazepine: its relationship with CYP2D6 genotypes. *Psychopharmacology (Berl)* (2002) 162, 50–54.
7. Yatham LN, Grossman F, Augustyns I, Vieta E, Ravindran A. Mood stabilisers plus risperidone or placebo in the treatment of acute mania. *Br J Psychiatry* (2003) 182, 141–7.
8. Strack DK, Leckband SG, Meyer JM. Antipsychotic prescribing practices following withdrawal of concomitant carbamazepine. *J Psychiatr Pract* (2009) 15, 442–8.
9. Mula M, Monaco F. Carbamazepine–risperidone interactions in patients with epilepsy. *Clin Neuropharmacol* (2002) 25, 97–100.
10. Muscatello MR, Pacetti M, Cacciola M, La Torre D, Zoccali R, D'Arrigo C, Migliardi G, Spina E. Plasma concentrations of risperidone and olanzapine during coadministration with oxcarbazepine. *Epilepsia* (2005) 46, 771–4.

Risperidone + Gatifloxacin

An isolated report describes an exacerbation of psychotic symptoms after gatifloxacin was added to risperidone.

Clinical evidence, mechanism, importance and management

A 62-year-old man with paranoid schizophrenia successfully treated with intramuscular risperidone 25 mg every 2 weeks experienced an exacerbation of his psychotic symptoms 2 days after gatifloxacin 400 mg daily was started. The patient's symptoms gradually resolved over the 48 hours following gatifloxacin discontinuation.[1] This is an isolated report and as such, no general recommendations can be made. However, note that risperidone has been said to be associated with QT prolongation and some quinolones are known to prolong the QT interval. See 'Drugs that prolong the QT interval + Other drugs that prolong the QT interval', p.272, for further information on the concurrent use of two or more drugs that prolong the QT interval.

1. Reeves RR. Exacerbation of psychotic symptoms associated with gatifloxacin. *Psychosomatics* (2007) 48, 87.

Risperidone + Ginkgo (*Ginkgo biloba*)

An isolated case describes priapism in a patient taking risperidone and ginkgo.

Clinical evidence

A 26-year-old patient with paranoid schizophrenia who had been taking risperidone 3 mg daily for the past 3 years developed priapism that lasted for 4 hours, 2 weeks after starting to take ginkgo 160 mg daily for occasional tinnitus. The priapism required treatment, and both ginkgo and risperidone were stopped. Risperidone was then restarted and the patient reported no further episodes of priapism at follow-up 6 months later.[1]

Mechanism

Unclear. Risperidone alone can rarely cause priapism, probably because of its alpha-adrenergic properties, and ginkgo might have vascular effects that could be additive with the effects of risperidone. Ginkgo is unlikely to affect the metabolism of risperidone by inhibiting CYP2D6 because it has no clinical effect on other CYP2D6 substrates.

Importance and management

Evidence for an interaction between ginkgo and risperidone appears to be limited to this isolated case. Its general relevance is therefore unclear. Bear it in mind in the event of an unexpected response to treatment.

1. Lin Y-Y, Chu S-J, Tsai S-H. Association between priapism and concurrent use of risperidone and Ginkgo biloba. *Mayo Clin Proc* (2007) 82, 1288–91.

Risperidone + HIV-protease inhibitors

Neuroleptic malignant syndrome, ataxia and severe lethargy leading to coma, and extrapyramidal adverse effects have been seen in patients given risperidone and indinavir with ritonavir.

Clinical evidence

A 35-year-old man with AIDS was diagnosed with a Tourette's-like disorder and given risperidone 1 mg twice daily. After 2 weeks the risperidone was increased to 2 mg twice daily and he was also given **indinavir** 800 mg twice daily with **ritonavir** 200 mg twice daily. He discontinued the antiretrovirals after 5 days due to nausea, but started them again one month later when the tic disorder had improved. After one week he became short of breath and fatigued, with worsening tremor and other extrapyramidal adverse effects. The antiretrovirals were stopped and the risperidone dose increased to 3 mg twice daily. Over the next 3 days his symptoms worsened and began to interfere with daily living. Risperidone was discontinued and clonazepam started, and his symptoms resolved.[1] Another patient developed neuroleptic malignant syndrome 3 days after starting to take risperidone with **indinavir** and **ritonavir**. This patient also recovered when risperidone was stopped.[2] A third patient taking **indinavir** with **ritonavir** was given risperidone 3 mg twice daily to treat symptoms of mania. After 2 doses he became ataxic, drowsy and disorientated, which further developed into lethargy and coma. He recovered 24 hours after stopping all medication.[3]

Mechanism

Indinavir and particularly ritonavir are potent inhibitors of CYP3A4; ritonavir, at high dose, is also a weak to moderate inhibitor of CYP2D6, which are the main isoenzymes involved in the metabolism of risperidone. Therefore concurrent use would be expected to raise risperidone concentrations. The symptoms reported in the cases above might have all been due to increased risperidone concentrations.[1,3]

Importance and management

These appear to be the only reports of an interaction between risperidone and the HIV-protease inhibitors, but they are in line with the predicted interaction.

If risperidone is given to any patient taking ritonavir (including ritonavir given with other HIV-protease inhibitors as a pharmacokinetic enhancer) it would seem prudent to be alert for risperidone adverse effects (such as agitation, insomnia, headache, extrapyramidal effects). If these become troublesome consider decreasing the risperidone dose. Note that risperidone and **saquinavir boosted with ritonavir** have been associated with QT prolongation, see 'Drugs that prolong the QT interval + Other drugs that prolong the QT interval', p.272, for further information on the concurrent use of two or more drugs that prolong the QT interval.

1. Kelly DV, Béïque LC, Bowmer MI. Extrapyramidal symptoms with ritonavir/indinavir plus risperidone. *Ann Pharmacother* (2002) 36, 827–30.
2. Lee SI, Klesmer J, Hirsch BE. Neuroleptic malignant syndrome associated with the use of risperidone, ritonavir and indinavir: a case report. *Psychosomatics* (2000) 41, 453–4.
3. Jover F, Cuadrado J-M, Andreu L, Merino J. Reversible coma caused by risperidone-ritonavir interaction. *Clin Neuropharmacol* (2002) 25, 251–3.

Risperidone + Lamotrigine

Lamotrigine does not appear to alter the steady-state concentrations of risperidone, although an isolated case report describes increased risperidone concentrations on increasing the dose of lamotrigine.

Clinical evidence

A study in 10 patients taking risperidone 3 to 6 mg daily, and who were also given lamotrigine (increasing over 8 weeks to 200 mg daily) found no changes in the steady-state concentrations of risperidone or its active metabolite.[1] Similarly, a retrospective review of 5 patients taking risperidone and lamotrigine, for whom risperidone concentrations were available both before and after the addition of lamotrigine, found a mean 7% decrease in risperidone concentrations (range, 41% decrease to 74% increase).[2] However, an isolated case report describes greatly increased risperidone concentrations in a patient given increasing doses of lamotrigine. When the lamotrigine dose was increased from 175 mg daily to 200 mg daily, the risperidone concentration increased almost 4-fold (from 69 nanograms/mL to 263 nanograms/mL). A further increase in the lamotrigine dose to 225 mg daily, while maintaining the risperidone dose of 8 mg daily, resulted in a further 56% increase in the plasma concentration of risperidone (to 412 nanograms/mL) and the patient complained of dizziness and tiredness.[3]

Mechanism

Risperidone is metabolised by CYP2D6, but as lamotrigine is not a known inhibitor of this enzyme, a pharmacokinetic interaction was not thought to explain the change in concentrations in the case report.[3]

Importance and management

The retrospective review and small study above did not find any evidence of a consistent effect of lamotrigine on risperidone pharmacokinetics, suggesting that a pharmacokinetic interaction is unlikely. However, the unexplained case report introduces a note of caution. Bear the possibility of an interaction in mind in the event of an increase in adverse effects on concurrent use.

1. Spina W, D'Arrigo C, Migliardi G, Santoro V, Muscatello MR, Micò U, D'Amico G, Perucca E. Effect of adjunctive lamotrigine treatment on the plasma concentrations of clozapine, risperidone and olanzapine in patients with schizophrenia or bipolar disorder. *Ther Drug Monit* (2006) 28, 599–602.
2. Castberg I, Spigset O. Risperidone and lamotrigine: no evidence of a drug interaction. *J Clin Psychiatry* (2006) 67, 1159.
3. Bienentreu SD, Kronmüller K-TH. Increase in risperidone plasma level with lamotrigine. *Am J Psychiatry* (2005) 162, 811–12.

Risperidone + Levomepromazine

Levomepromazine does not appear to affect the steady-state concentrations of risperidone. An isolated case report describes akathisia on concurrent use.

Clinical evidence, mechanism, importance and management

In a study, 20 patients who had been taking risperidone for at least 2 weeks were also given levomepromazine in doses of 5 to 75 mg daily. There were no changes in the steady-state concentrations of risperidone or its active metabolite, 9-hydroxyrisperidone, and there was no aggravation of extrapyramidal effects.[1]

A case report describes a woman with schizophrenia taking risperidone 8 mg daily who became agitated and restless at night, 3 months after starting to take levomepromazine up to 50 mg at night. Risperidone was stopped, but after 10 days her condition had not improved, and so levomepromazine was also stopped. Within a day she began to feel less agitated. The authors suggested that her symptoms represented delayed-onset akathisia, which was attributed to additive adverse effects of both drugs.[2] However, as the patient did not take levomepromazine alone, an interaction is not established in this case.

It would seem that levomepromazine can be given with risperidone without risperidone dose adjustment. Although not established, the case report serves as a reminder to consider adverse effects when prescribing two drugs with a similar adverse effect profile.

1. Yoshimura R, Shinkai K, Kakihara S, Goto M, Yamada Y, Kaji K, Ueda N, Nakamura J. Little effects of low dosage of levomepromazine on plasma risperidone levels. *Pharmacopsychiatry* (2005) 38, 98–100.
2. Shimizu E, Watanabe H, Iyo M. Delayed-onset nocturnal akathisia due to risperidone and levomepromazine: a case report. *Eur Psychiatry* (2002) 17, 294–5.

Risperidone + Melperone

Melperone appears to increase risperidone concentrations.

Clinical evidence

In a patient taking risperidone 6 mg daily and melperone 50 mg daily, risperidone concentrations decreased from 2.1 micrograms/L to 1 microgram/L and the concentrations of its active metabolite, 9-hydroxyrisperidone, increased from 21 micrograms/L to 40 micrograms/L, 8 days after melperone was changed to pipamperone 40 mg daily. This was taken to suggest that melperone had raised risperidone concentrations. This suggestion is supported by a second patient, whose dose-corrected risperidone plasma concentration decreased by about 69% and the 9-hydroxyrisperidone plasma concentration increased by about 68% after the dose of risperidone was increased from 5 mg daily to 6 mg daily, and melperone was stopped. In a third patient, taking risperidone, melperone, venlafaxine and metoprolol, the dose-corrected risperidone concentration fell by 20% when melperone was stopped: the 9-hydroxyrisperidone concentration was unchanged.[1]

Mechanism

Risperidone is metabolised by CYP2D6. It was suggested that melperone raises risperidone concentrations by inhibiting this metabolism.[1]

Importance and management

Evidence for an interaction between risperidone and melperone appears to be limited to these three cases, and the authors suggest that further study is needed to establish their clinical relevance. Until more is known, it seems prudent to be alert for risperidone adverse effects (such as agitation, insomnia, headache) if melperone is also given.

1. Köhnke MD, Lutz U, Wiatr G, Schwärzler F, Weller B, Schott K, Buchkremer G. Cytochrome P450 2D6 dependent metabolization of risperidone is inhibited by melperone. *Eur J Clin Pharmacol* (2006) 62, 333–4.

Risperidone + Midodrine

An isolated report describes acute dystonia after midodrine was given to a patients taking risperidone.

Clinical evidence, mechanism, importance and management

A case report describes acute dystonia in a 33-year-old woman taking risperidone 6 mg daily, 2 days after midodrine 4 mg daily was started to treat risperidone-induced orthostatic hypotension. Symptoms rapidly disappeared after intramuscular antimuscarinics (not stated) were given and the midodrine was stopped. Two weeks later the patient was rechallenged with midodrine 4 mg daily and again acute dystonia developed, which also responded to antimuscarinics and stopping midodrine. After a further 2 weeks, the risperidone dose was reduced to 3 mg daily to control the orthostatic hypotension. This dose reduction did not lead to a reduced clinical effect and no further dystonic reactions were seen at 3 months. The authors suggest that as both drugs cause increased noradrenergic activity, the dystonia was due to their additive effects.[1] Compare also 'Phenothiazines + Midodrine', p.874.

This is an isolated report and as such, its general importance is unclear. However, if patients taking both drugs develop acute dystonia it might be prudent to suspect an interaction as a possible cause.

1. Takahashi H. Acute dystonia induced by adding midodrine, a selective alpha 1 agonist, to risperidone in a patient with catatonic schizophrenia. *J Neuropsychiatr Clin Neurosci* (2000) 12, 285–6.

Risperidone + Mirtazapine

Mirtazapine does not appear to affect the steady-state concentrations of risperidone. An isolated case report describes pulmonary thromboembolism and rhabdomyolysis in a patient given both drugs.

Clinical evidence

A pilot study in 6 psychiatric patients taking risperidone 1 to 3 mg twice daily for one to 4 weeks followed by 2 to 4 weeks of concurrent mirtazapine 15 to 30 mg at night, found that mirtazapine did not affect the steady-state plasma concentrations of risperidone or its active 9-hydroxy metabolite. In one patient taking mirtazapine, adding risperidone did not appear to alter the steady-state plasma concentrations of mirtazapine.[1] Similarly, a later study in 8 patients taking risperidone, in doses ranging from 3 to 8 mg daily, found no change in the steady-state concentrations of risperidone and its metabolite, 9-hydroxyrisperidone, when they were also given mirtazapine 30 mg daily for 6 weeks.[2]

An isolated case report describes a 40-year-old man taking risperidone 8 mg daily who was then also given mirtazapine 45 mg daily for a major depressive episode. On admission to a psychiatric day clinic because of treatment failure he was taking risperidone 7 mg daily reduced to 3 mg daily when mirtazapine was subsequently increased to 60 mg daily. The patient improved, but 6 weeks later developed acute aching in his left leg and respiratory problems. On admission to hospital, pulmonary thromboembolism and rhabdomyolysis (creatine kinase concentration 4 795 units/L) were diagnosed. He was treated with heparin and warfarin, and mirtazapine was replaced with reboxetine, and risperidone replaced with aripiprazole.[3] Note that rhabdomyolysis is a rare adverse effect of risperidone alone.

Mechanism

Unknown.

Importance and management

Evidence for an interaction between risperidone and mirtazapine is limited, but the available data suggests that no risperidone dose adjustments would seem necessary on their concurrent use. The general relevance of the isolated case of pulmonary embolism and rhabdomyolysis is uncertain.

1. Loonen AJM, Doorschot CH, Oostelbos MCJM, Sitsen JMA. Lack of drug interactions between mirtazapine and risperidone in psychiatric patients: a pilot study. *Eur Neuropsychopharmacol* (1999) 10, 51–7.
2. Zoccali R, Muscatello MR, La Torre D, Malara G, Canale A, Crucitti D, D'Arrigo C, Spina E. Lack of a pharmacokinetic interaction between mirtazapine and the newer antipsychotics clozapine, risperidone and olanzapine in patients with chronic schizophrenia. *Pharm Res* (2003) 48, 411–14.
3. Zink M, Knopf U, Argiriou S, Kuwilsky A. A case of pulmonary thromboembolism and rhabdomyolysis during therapy with mirtazapine and risperidone. *J Clin Psychiatry* (2006) 67, 835.

Risperidone + Miscellaneous

There was an unexplained increase in mortality in dementia patients taking furosemide with risperidone. Verapamil increases risperidone concentrations, and cimetidine and ranitidine increase risperidone exposure, but erythromycin has no effect. Risperidone does not alter digoxin pharmacokinetics.

Clinical evidence, mechanism, importance and management

(a) Digoxin

The manufacturer briefly mentions that risperidone 0.25 mg twice daily has no clinically relevant effect on the pharmacokinetics of digoxin.[1,2]

(b) Drugs that inhibit CYP2D6

Paroxetine, a potent inhibitor of CYP2D6, increases the concentrations of risperidone, and to a much lesser extent, its active 9-hydroxy metabolite (see 'Risperidone + SSRIs', p.887). The manufacturers of risperidone therefore predict that other drugs that inhibit CYP2D6 might also increase the concentrations of risperidone, and they name **quinidine**.[1,2] For a list of drugs that are known to inhibit CYP2D6, see 'Table 1.7', p.9.

Note that quinidine is known to prolong the QT interval and this might be additive with the effects of risperidone, see 'Drugs that prolong the QT interval + Other drugs that prolong the QT interval', p.272, for further information on the concurrent use of two or more drugs that prolong the QT interval.

(c) Erythromycin

The UK manufacturer of risperidone briefly notes that erythromycin has no effect on the pharmacokinetics of risperidone or its active 9-hydroxy metabolite.[1] Note that erythromycin can prolong the QT interval and this might be additive with the effects of risperidone, see 'Drugs that prolong the QT interval + Other drugs that prolong the QT interval', p.272, for further information on the concurrent use of two or more drugs that prolong the QT interval.

(d) Furosemide

The UK manufacturer notes that, in 2 of 4 placebo-controlled studies in elderly patients with dementia, the concurrent use of furosemide with risperidone appeared to be associated with a higher incidence of mortality than risperidone or furosemide alone (7.3% compared with 3.1% and 4.1%, respectively). The concurrent use of risperidone with low-dose **thiazides** was not associated with similar findings.[1]

The mechanism for this possible effect is unknown. However, the UK manufacturer recommends caution on concurrent use, considering the risks and benefits. They state that, irrespective of treatment, dehydration was an overall risk factor for mortality and should therefore be carefully avoided in elderly patients with dementia.[1] Note that antipsychotics such as risperidone should generally be avoided in patients with dementia because they have been associated with increased mortality irrespective of concurrent furosemide use.[2] However, in the UK, risperidone has a specific indication for the short term (maximum 6 weeks) treatment of persistent aggression in patients with moderate to severe Alzheimer's disease.[1]

(e) H_2-receptor antagonists

The manufacturer notes that **cimetidine** increased the AUC of risperidone by 64%, but did not affect the combined AUC of risperidone and its active 9-hydroxymetabolite.[2] **Ranitidine** increased the AUC of risperidone by 26% and increased the combined AUC of risperidone and its active 9-hydroxy metabolite by 20%.[2] These increases are slight and unlikely to be of any clinical relevance. No risperidone dose adjustment is expected to be needed if it is given with **cimetidine** or **ranitidine**.

(f) Verapamil

The UK manufacturer briefly notes that verapamil increases the plasma concentrations of risperidone.[1] Verapamil is an inhibitor of CYP3A4 and risperidone is known to be partially metabolised by CYP3A4. It would be prudent to bear in mind the possibility of an increase in adverse effects on concurrent use.

1. Risperdal (Risperidone). Janssen-Cilag Ltd. UK Summary of product characteristics, February 2012.
2. Risperdal (Risperidone). Ortho-McNeil-Janssen Pharmaceuticals, Inc. US Prescribing information, September 2011.

Risperidone + Phenytoin

An isolated report describes extrapyramidal symptoms in a patient starting risperidone when he was also given a single dose of phenytoin. Phenytoin is predicted to decrease risperidone concentrations.

Clinical evidence

A 31-year-old man with schizophrenia was given risperidone and the dose was titrated up from 1 mg twice daily to 3 mg twice daily over 3 days without any adverse effects. Three days later a single 200-mg dose of phenytoin was accidentally given and 8 hours later he developed laboured breathing, with severe hyperextension of the neck and oculogyric crisis. Risperidone was temporarily discontinued and he recovered after treatment with benzatropine and diazepam. He was subsequently given risperidone 3 mg twice daily, with benzatropine for prophylaxis against further extrapyramidal symptoms.[1]

Mechanism

Unknown. The author of the case report suggested that phenytoin might have increased risperidone concentrations;[1] however, phenytoin is a known inducer of CYP2D6 by which risperidone is metabolised, and so would be expected to *reduce* its concentrations. The reaction could have been idiosyncratic: the patient had previously not tolerated other antipsychotics because of extrapyramidal adverse effects.

Importance and management

Evidence for an interaction between risperidone and phenytoin appears to be limited to this one case report of severe extrapyramidal symptoms, and its general relevance is unclear. Note that, in contrast to the prediction of this case report, the US manufacturer of risperidone predicts that phenytoin will *reduce* risperidone concentrations and those of its active metabolite.[2] This is in line with the way other enzyme-inducing drugs are known to interact with risperidone, see 'Risperidone + Carbamazepine and related drugs', p.883. In the absence of further information, if phenytoin is given it would seem appropriate to monitor for a lack of therapeutic effect, and adjust the dose accordingly. Bear the report of extrapyramidal symptoms in mind in the event of an unexpected response to treatment.

Note that **fosphenytoin** is a prodrug of phenytoin and would therefore be expected to interact in a similar way.

1. Sanderson DR. Drug interaction between risperidone and phenytoin resulting in extrapyramidal symptoms. *J Clin Psychiatry* (1996) 57, 177.
2. Risperdal (Risperidone). Ortho-McNeil-Janssen Pharmaceuticals, Inc. US Prescribing information, September 2011.

Risperidone + Probenecid

Probenecid does not appear to alter the pharmacokinetics of risperidone.

Clinical evidence, mechanism, importance and management

In a study in 12 healthy subjects, probenecid 500 mg twice daily for 4 days did not affect the pharmacokinetics of a single 1-mg dose of risperidone given on day 2.[1] Probenecid is an inhibitor of glucuronidation, and this study suggests that risperidone is not metabolised by this route. No risperidone dose adjustment would be expected to be needed on the concurrent use of probenecid.

1. Markowitz JS, DeVane CL, Liston HL, Bouton DW, Risch SC. The effects of probenecid on the disposition of risperidone and olanzapine in healthy volunteers. *Clin Pharmacol Ther* (2002) 71, 30–8.

Risperidone + Reboxetine

Reboxetine does not appear to alter the steady-state concentrations of risperidone.

Clinical evidence, mechanism, importance and management

In a study in 7 patients with schizophrenia stable taking risperidone 4 to 6 mg daily, giving reboxetine 4 mg daily for one week followed by 8 mg daily for 3 weeks had no apparent effects on the steady-state concentrations of either risperidone or its active metabolite, 9-hydroxyrisperidone.[1] This appears to be the only study investigating the concurrent use of risperidone and reboxetine. It suggests that if both drugs are given, no risperidone dose adjustments are likely to be necessary.

1. Spina E, Avenoso A, Scordo MG, Ancione M, Madia A, Levita A. No effect of reboxetine on plasma concentrations of clozapine, risperidone, and their active metabolites. *Ther Drug Monit* (2001) 23, 675–8.

Risperidone + Rifampicin (Rifampin)

The exposure to risperidone and its active metabolite is reduced by rifampicin.

Clinical evidence

In a study in 10 healthy subjects, rifampicin 600 mg daily for 5 days decreased the maximum plasma concentration and AUC of a single 4-mg dose of risperidone by 50% and 72%, respectively.[1] In another study, 10 healthy subjects were given rifampicin 600 mg daily for 7 days, with a single 1-mg dose of risperidone on day 6. Rifampicin reduced the maximum plasma concentration and AUC of risperidone by 38% and 51%, respectively, and reduced the maximum plasma concentration and AUC of its active metabolite, 9-hydroxyrisperidone, by 46% and 47%, respectively.[2]

Mechanism

Rifampicin is a potent inducer of CYP3A4, which is partly responsible for the metabolism of risperidone. Concurrent use would therefore be expected to increase risperidone metabolism and reduce its concentrations. It has also been suggested that P-glycoprotein might have played a part in this interaction.[2]

Importance and management

The interaction between risperidone and rifampicin would appear to be established. Reduced concentrations of risperidone and its active 9-hydroxy metabolite would be expected to lead to reduced efficacy. It would therefore be prudent to monitor the outcome of concurrent use for risperidone efficacy, increasing the risperidone dose if necessary.

1. Mahatthanatrakul W, Nontaput T, Ridtitid W, Wongnawa M, Sunbhanich M. Rifampin, a cytochrome P450 3A inducer, decreases plasma concentrations of antipsychotic risperidone in healthy volunteers. *J Clin Pharm Ther* (2007) 32, 161–7.
2. Kim K-A, Park P-W, Liu K-H, Kim K-B, Lee H-J, Shin J-G, Park J-Y. Effect of rifampin, an inducer of CYP3A and P-glycoprotein, on the pharmacokinetics of risperidone. *J Clin Pharmacol* (2008) 48, 66–72.

Risperidone + SSRIs

Fluoxetine and paroxetine raise steady-state risperidone concentrations and concurrent use has resulted in increased extrapyramidal adverse effects. Fluvoxamine and sertraline appear to only cause a minor increase in risperidone concentrations at high doses. Serotonin syndrome has been reported with fluvoxamine, paroxetine and sertraline given with risperidone. Citalopram does not alter risperidone concentrations, but there is a case report of QT prolongation with torsade de pointes on concurrent use. Isolated cases of priapism and nasal bleeding have been reported.

Clinical evidence

(a) Citalopram

A study in 7 patients found that citalopram 40 mg daily for 8 weeks had no apparent effect on the steady-state plasma concentrations of risperidone or its active metabolite, 9-hydroxyrisperidone.[1]

A case report describes a 29-year-old man with idiopathic priapism resulting in about one 4-hour erection every one to 2 months, which typically woke him up, who began to experience much longer bouts of priapism lasting 6 to 8 hours when he was given risperidone 4 mg daily. Within about 4 weeks of adding citalopram 40 mg daily to a slightly reduced risperidone dose (3 mg daily), he began to have almost daily erections lasting 12 hours. Three days after his doses were changed to risperidone 3 mg twice daily with citalopram 20 mg daily he had an episode of such persistent priapism that emergency detumescence was needed. When both drugs were stopped he improved markedly, and then only had occasional 4-hour erections, as before.[2]

Another case report describes a 77-year-old woman who developed torsade de pointes while taking risperidone 2 mg daily and citalopram 20 mg daily. ECG showed sinus bradycardia (48 bpm), an AV block and a QTc interval of 490 milliseconds; QRS morphology and serum potassium were normal. Both drugs were stopped and the patient's QTc interval and heart rate gradually returned to normal.[3]

(b) Fluoxetine

A pharmacokinetic study in 10 patients found that fluoxetine 20 mg daily raised the concentrations of risperidone 2 or 3 mg twice daily by 60% (from 12 nanograms/mL to 19 nanograms/mL) after 3 weeks of concurrent use and 4.6-fold (to 56 nanograms/mL) after 4 weeks of concurrent use, with no change in concentrations of the active metabolite. All patients experienced a rise in risperidone concentrations, but this varied from a 2-fold rise to a 10-fold rise. One patient withdrew from the study because of severe akathisia and another two patients needed to be given biperiden to control parkinsonian adverse effects.[4] Similar results were found in another study.[5]

Case reports describe a variety of adverse effects in patients taking risperidone with fluoxetine, including painful bilateral breast enlargement,[6] nasal bleeding,[7] and in one patient urinary retention, constipation, and sedation.[8] In addition, extrapyramidal adverse effects have developed in a number of patients taking fluoxetine with risperidone,[8-10] and, in one case, also amitriptyline, see 'Risperidone + Tricyclic and related antidepressants', p.888. A patient with obsessive-compulsive disorder, who was partially successfully treated with fluoxetine 60 mg daily, saw his condition return to his pre-fluoxetine state when risperidone 3 mg daily was started. His condition gradually improved over a 3-month period after the risperidone was stopped.[11]

(c) Fluvoxamine

A 24-year-old woman taking risperidone 3 mg twice daily developed fever, limb rigidity and confusion 3 days after starting fluvoxamine 50 mg daily. She required ventilation after her condition worsened, and she was eventually diagnosed as having either serotonin syndrome or neuroleptic malignant syndrome. Both drugs were stopped and her condition resolved. She subsequently, uneventfully took fluvoxamine 100 mg twice daily.[12]

In a study in 11 patients who had been taking risperidone 3 to 6 mg daily for at least 4 weeks, fluvoxamine 100 mg daily for 4 weeks had no apparent effect on the steady-state concentrations of risperidone or its active metabolite, 9-hydroxyrisperidone. Six patients continued to take fluvoxamine 100 mg daily for a further 4 weeks, and still had no apparent change in the concentrations of risperidone or its metabolite. However, in the 5 other patients, when the dose of fluvoxamine was increased to 200 mg daily for a further 4 weeks, there was an 85% increase in the plasma concentration of risperidone by the end of week 8, with no change in the concentrations of the active metabolite. This resulted in an overall 26% increase in the concentrations of risperidone plus its active metabolite.[13]

(d) Paroxetine

In a study, 10 patients taking risperidone 2 to 4 mg twice daily were given paroxetine 20 mg daily. After 4 weeks of concurrent use, the concentrations of risperidone and its active metabolite, 9-hydroxyrisperidone, had increased by 45% and one patient developed parkinsonian adverse effects.[14] In another study, 12 patients taking risperidone 2 mg twice daily were given paroxetine in doses increasing from 10 mg daily to 20 mg and 40 mg at 4 week intervals. The steady-state plasma concentrations of risperidone were increased 3.8-fold, 7.1-fold and 9.7-fold when given with paroxetine 10 mg, 20 mg and 40 mg daily, respectively. There was no change in the concentration of the active metabolite of risperidone, 9-hydroxyrisperidone. Negative symptoms of schizophrenia were improved, but there was an increased incidence of extrapyramidal adverse effects when patients took paroxetine 20 mg or 40 mg daily.[15]

A case report describes two elderly patients taking paroxetine who developed serotonin syndrome within a couple of days of a risperidone dose increase. One patient's treatment had recently been changed from venlafaxine to paroxetine, which might have contributed to the reaction.[16] Another case report describes a 53-year-old man who developed symptoms suggestive of serotonin syndrome 10 weeks after starting to take risperidone 3 mg daily and paroxetine 20 mg daily. A deterioration in his condition occurred within 2 hours of doubling the dose of both drugs, and his symptoms resolved 2 days after stopping both drugs.[17] Another case report describes a patient taking risperidone, paroxetine and valproate semisodium, who discontinued risperidone after developing reduced facial expressions, stiffness and akathisia. In this patient the half-life of risperidone was estimated to be almost 24 hours (expected half-life only 3 hours).[18]

(e) Sertraline

A 69-year-old man taking venlafaxine for depression with psychosis started taking risperidone 0.5 mg twice daily. Five days later trazodone was started, venlafaxine was gradually stopped and sertraline 25 mg daily was started. Over the next 2 weeks the dose of risperidone was increased to 3 mg daily and the dose of sertraline was increased to 150 mg daily. The patient became tremulous with myoclonus, had cogwheel rigidity of bilateral upper extremities, and a fine tremor. He was diagnosed with serotonin syndrome: risperidone, sertraline and trazodone were stopped, and the symptoms resolved within 24 hours.[19]

A study in 11 patients taking risperidone 4 to 6 mg daily found that sertraline 50 mg daily for 4 weeks had no apparent effect on the steady-state concentrations of risperidone or its active metabolite. Four of the patients were then maintained on sertraline 50 mg daily for a further 4 weeks, 7 had the dose increased to 100 mg daily, and, of these 2 patients had the dose further increased to 150 mg daily by week 8. At week 8, sertraline 50 mg daily had no apparent effect on risperidone concentrations, sertraline 100 mg daily had little effect (a non-significant 15% increase), whereas sertraline 150 mg daily increased risperidone concentrations by 36% and 52% in each patient, respectively. No patient developed any signs of risperidone toxicity.[20]

Mechanism

Fluoxetine and paroxetine inhibit CYP2D6, the isoenzyme by which risperidone is metabolised. Concurrent use therefore decreases risperidone metabolism, and its concentrations increase. This can lead to extrapyramidal adverse effects and, it has been suggested, the increased prolactin concentrations and gynaecomastia seen in one patient.[6] As CYP2D6 shows polymorphism, these interactions would be most apparent in patients with normal CYP2D6 activity (extensive metabolisers), effectively making them poor metabolisers (that is, those lacking or deficient in CYP2D6 activity). Sertraline is thought to have a dose-dependent effect on CYP2D6 inhibition,[20] but the effects are weak, even in high dose. Citalopram has little effect on CYP2D6. Fluvoxamine does not inhibit CYP2D6, but is a weak inhibitor of CYP3A4, which also plays a part in risperidone metabolism, and it therefore has a minor effect on risperidone concentrations at high doses.

Many of the other reactions (sedation, urinary retention, priapism) appear to be a result of additive adverse effects of the SSRIs and risperidone. An additive pharmacodynamic interaction might also contribute to the extrapyramidal adverse effects.[21] Serotonin syndrome can result when two drugs with serotonin effects are given together, see 'Drugs that cause serotonin syndrome + Other drugs that cause serotonin syndrome', p.1471. Citalopram is associated with QT prolongation and might have additive effects with risperidone.

Importance and management

The elevated risperidone concentrations seen with **fluoxetine** and **paroxetine** appear to be well-documented and clinically important. If either of these SSRIs are given to a patient taking risperidone, concurrent use should be well monitored and the risperidone dose reduced accordingly: a one-third reduction has been suggested with fluoxetine.[5] In the small group who are deficient in CYP2D6 activity (that is, CYP2D6 poor metabolisers), the addition of these SSRIs will likely have no effect.

The other SSRIs have less effect on CYP2D6 than fluoxetine and paroxetine and would therefore not be expected to have an effect, or only modest effects, on risperidone concentrations; this is borne out by the studies with citalopram (no effect), **fluvoxamine** (minor increase with high-dose fluvoxamine, due to CYP3A4 inhibition) and **sertraline** (minor increase with high-dose sertraline). It would therefore seem prudent to bear the possibility of an interaction in mind if risperidone adverse effects (e.g. agitation, insomnia, headache) occur in patients taking these SSRIs. However, note that, **citalopram** and **escitalopram** are associated with a dose-related prolongation in the QT interval and risperidone might share this effect. Therefore it might be prudent to use an alternative SSRI which is not known to be associated with QT prolongation. See 'Drugs that prolong the QT interval + Other drugs that prolong the QT interval', p.272, for further information on the concurrent use of two or more drugs that prolong the QT interval.

The case reports of serotonin syndrome appear to be rare, but they should be borne in mind when prescribing SSRIs and risperidone together. For more information on serotonin syndrome and its management, see 'Drugs that cause serotonin syndrome + Other drugs that cause serotonin syndrome', p.1471.

1. Avenoso A, Facciolà G, Scordo MG, Gitto C, Ferrante GD, Madia AG, Spina E. No effect of citalopram on plasma levels of clozapine, risperidone and their active metabolites in patients with chronic schizophrenia. *Clin Drug Invest* (1998) 16, 393–8.
2. Freudenreich O. Exacerbation of idiopathic priapism with risperidone-citalopram combination. *J Clin Psychiatry* (2002) 63, 249–50.
3. Blaschke D, Parwani AS, Huemer M, Rolf S, Boldt L-H, Dietz R, Haverkamp W. Torsade de pointes during combined treatment with risperidone and citalopram. *Pharmacopsychiatry* (2007) 40, 294–5.
4. Spina E, Avenoso A, Scordo MG, Ancione M, Madia A, Gatti G, Perucca E. Inhibition of risperidone metabolism by fluoxetine in patients with schizophrenia: a clinically relevant pharmacokinetic interaction. *J Clin Psychopharmacol* (2002) 22, 419–23.
5. Bondolfi G, Eap CB, Bertschy G, Zullino D, Vermeulen A, Baumann P. The effect of fluoxetine on the pharmacokinetics and safety of risperidone in psychotic patients. *Pharmacopsychiatry* (2002) 35, 50–56.
6. Benazzi F. Gynecomastia with risperidone-fluoxetine combination. *Pharmacopsychiatry* (1999) 32, 41.
7. Mowla A, Dastgheib SA, Ebrahimi AA, Pani A. Nasal bleeding associated with fluoxetine and risperidone interaction: a case report. *Pharmacopsychiatry* (2009) 42, 204–5.
8. Bozikas V, Petrikis P, Karavatos A. Urinary retention caused after fluoxetine-risperidone combination. *J Psychopharmacol* (2001) 15, 142–3.
9. Daniel DG, Egan M, Hyde T. Probable neuroleptic induced tardive dyskinesia in association with combined SSRI and risperidone treatment. *Schizophr Res* (1996) 18, 149.
10. Dubbelman YD, Thung FH, Heeringa M. Ernstige tardieve dyskinesieën tijdens behandeling met risperidon en fluoxetine. *Ned Tijdschr Geneeskd* (1998) 142, 1508–11.
11. Andrade C. Risperidone may worsen fluoxetine-treated OCD. *J Clin Psychiatry* (1998) 59, 255–6.
12. Reeves RR, Mack JE, Bedingfield JJ. Neurotoxic syndrome associated with risperidone and fluvoxamine. *Ann Pharmacother* (2002) 36, 440–3.
13. D'Arrigo C, Migliardi G, Santoro V, Morgante L, Muscatello MR, Ancione M, Spina E. Effect of fluvoxamine on plasma risperidone concentrations in patients with schizophrenia. *Pharmacol Res* (2005) 52, 497–501.
14. Spina E, Avenoso A, Facciolà G, Scordo MG, Ancione M, Madia AG. Plasma concentrations of risperidone and 9-hydroxyrisperidone during combined treatment with paroxetine. *Ther Drug Monit* (2001) 23, 223–7.
15. Saito M, Yasui-Furukori N, Nakagami T, Furukori H, Kaneko S. Dose-dependent interaction of paroxetine with risperidone in schizophrenic patients. *J Clin Psychopharmacol* (2005) 25, 527–32.
16. Karki SD, Masood G-R. Combination risperidone and SSRI-induced serotonin syndrome. *Ann Pharmacother* (2003) 37, 388–91.
17. Hamilton S, Malone K. Serotonin syndrome during treatment with paroxetine and risperidone. *J Clin Psychopharmacol* (2000) 20, 103–5.
18. Barnhill J, Susce MT, Diaz FJ, de Leon J. Risperidone half-life in a patient taking paroxetine. *Pharmacopsychiatry* (2005) 38, 223–5.
19. Kohen I, Gordon ML, Manu P. Serotonin syndrome in elderly patients treated for psychotic depression with atypical antipsychotics and antidepressants: two case reports. *CNS Spectr* (2007) 12, 596–8.
20. Spina E, D'Arrigo C, Migliardi G, Morgante L, Zoccali R, Ancione M, Madia A. Plasma risperidone concentrations during combined treatment with sertraline. *Ther Drug Monit* (2004) 26, 386–90.
21. Caley CF. Extrapyramidal reactions from concurrent SSRI and atypical antipsychotic use. *Can J Psychiatry* (1998) 43, 307–8.

Risperidone + Tetracycline

An isolated case report describes a patient taking risperidone and sertraline who experienced a worsening of his tics when tetracycline was added.

Clinical evidence, mechanism, importance and management

A 15-year-old boy taking risperidone 1.5 mg twice daily and sertraline 100 mg daily was given tetracycline 250 mg twice daily. His tics worsened, and did not respond to an increase in his sertraline dose from 100 mg daily to 150 mg daily. After stopping the tetracycline, his tics improved within a few weeks. The exact mechanism of this possible interaction is unclear, but it has been suggested that the tetracycline somehow reduced the activity of the risperidone. Induction of CYP2D6 by tetracycline was thought unlikely: inactivation of the risperidone or its active metabolite was considered a possible explanation.[1] This appears to be the only reported case of this interaction and its general importance is therefore unknown.

1. Steele M, Couturier J. A possible tetracycline-risperidone-sertraline interaction in an adolescent. *Can J Clin Pharmacol* (1999) 6, 15–17.

Risperidone + Topiramate

Topiramate does not appear to affect the steady-state plasma concentrations of risperidone.

Clinical evidence, mechanism, importance and management

In a study, 9 patients taking long-term risperidone 3 to 6 mg daily were given topiramate in a dose that was increased gradually to 200 mg daily over 6 to 8 weeks. The steady-state plasma concentrations of risperidone and its active metabolite, 9-hydroxyrisperidone, did not appear to be affected by topiramate.[1] No risperidone dose adjustment would therefore be expected to be needed on the concurrent use of topiramate.

1. Migliardi G, D'Arrigo C, Santoro V, Bruno A, Cortese L, Campolo D, Cacciola M, Spina E. Effect of topiramate on plasma concentrations of clozapine, olanzapine, risperidone, and quetiapine in patients with psychotic disorders. *Clin Neuropharmacol* (2007) 30, 107–13.

Risperidone + Tricyclic and related antidepressants

Amitriptyline does not appear to affect the steady-state concentrations of risperidone. Two case reports suggest that risperidone might increase the plasma concentrations of maprotiline. Extrapyramidal reactions have been reported in one patient taking amitriptyline with risperidone.

Clinical evidence, mechanism, importance and management

(a) Amitriptyline

A study in 12 patients with schizophrenia found that amitriptyline 50 to 100 mg daily had no effect on the serum concentrations of risperidone 3 mg twice daily.[1] However, a 26-year-old man taking amitriptyline 25 mg daily developed extrapyramidal reactions after his dose of risperidone was increased from 2 mg daily to 4 mg daily.[2] Later, this same patient developed extrapyramidal adverse effects after risperidone 2 mg daily was added to treatment with amitriptyline 25 mg and fluoxetine 20 mg daily, to which the fluoxetine probably contributed,[2] see 'Risperidone + SSRIs', p.887. A pharmacodynamic reason for this reaction with amitriptyline has been suggested.[3] An interaction with amitriptyline is unconfirmed, but bear this case in mind if extrapyramidal reactions occur. Of more importance, note that both the tricyclics and risperidone have been said to be associated with QT prolongation, see 'Drugs that prolong the QT interval + Other drugs that prolong the QT interval', p.272, for further information on the concurrent use of two or more drugs that prolong the QT interval.

(b) Maprotiline

A 39-year-old patient with a schizodepressive disorder taking pipamperone and lorazepam, and also taking maprotiline 175 mg daily for a severe depressive episode, had plasma concentrations of maprotiline of 145 nanograms/mL and 166 nanograms/mL after 4 and 6 weeks, respectively. After 8 weeks, she was given risperidone to treat acute psychotic symptoms. The dose of risperidone was titrated over 5 days up to 5 mg daily and the dose of pipamperone was increased from 40 to 80 mg at night. She had a rapid remission of the psychotic symptoms and almost complete remission of the depression, but gradually developed antimuscarinic adverse effects. Ten days after starting risperidone and with maprotiline at a slightly lower dose of 150 mg daily, the maprotiline plasma concentration had increased to 266 nanograms/mL. The doses of maprotiline and risperidone were reduced to 100 mg and 3 mg daily, respectively, and this reduced the severity of the adverse effects.[4]

Two other patients have been reported to have gradual increases in maprotiline concentrations over 6 to 7 weeks on the concurrent use of risperidone. One of the patients was also taking **nortriptyline**, but its concentrations were unaltered.[4]

This interaction is unconfirmed but be aware of the possibility of an interaction if maprotiline adverse effects are troublesome.

1. Sommers DK, Snyman JR, van Wyk M, Blom MW, Huang ML, Levron JC. Lack of effect of amitriptyline on risperidone pharmacokinetics in schizophrenic patients. *Int Clin Psychopharmacol* (1997) 12, 141–5.
2. Brown ES. Extrapyramidal side effects with low-dose risperidone. *Can J Psychiatry* (1997) 42, 325–6.
3. Caley CF. Extrapyramidal reactions from concurrent SSRI and atypical antipsychotic use. *Can J Psychiatry* (1998) 43, 307–8.
4. Normann C, Lieb K, Walden J. Increased plasma concentration of maprotiline by coadministration of risperidone. *J Clin Psychopharmacol* (2002) 22, 92–4.

Risperidone + Valproate

A couple of isolated case reports describe oedema in patients taking risperidone and valproate. Valproate does not appear to affect the steady-state concentrations of risperidone. Risperidone does not alter the pharmacokinetics of valproate, although two cases, of increased or decreased concentrations, have been reported.

Clinical evidence, mechanism, importance and management

A study comparing 10 patients taking sodium valproate and risperidone with 23 patients taking risperidone alone found no apparent difference in the concentrations of risperidone and its metabolite, 9-hydroxyrisperidone, between the two groups, suggesting that sodium valproate does not affect risperidone pharmacokinetics.[1] Similarly, in a study in 12 patients with schizophrenia given valproic acid 400 to 800 mg daily and risperidone 2 to 6 mg daily, valproic acid did not affect the steady-state plasma concentrations of risperidone or its active metabolite, 9-hydroxyrisperidone.[2]

The effect of risperidone on valproate concentrations has also been studied. In a study in patients with bipolar disorder who were given **valproate semisodium (divalproex sodium)** 1 g daily for 4 weeks, the addition of risperidone 2 mg daily for 2 days, increasing to 4 mg daily (9 patients), did not alter the steady-state pharmacokinetics of valproate, when compared with placebo (11 patients).[3] Two earlier case reports had suggested an interaction. In one, the valproate concentrations of a 10-year-old boy increased by 33%, from 143 micrograms/mL to 191 micrograms/mL, 5 days after he started to take risperidone, initially 2 mg daily, then later 3 mg daily.[4,5] Conversely, a 15-year-old girl experienced a 29% *reduction* in her valproate concentrations, from 80 micrograms/mL to 57 micrograms/mL, when risperidone 1 mg three times daily was added to established treatment with **valproic acid**.[6] It is quite possible that these isolated cases are not due to a drug interaction.

A case report describes the development of generalised acute oedema in a patient with schizophrenia when risperidone (titrated to 10 mg daily) was added to established **sodium valproate** treatment. The oedema was unresponsive to diuretics, but resolved when the risperidone dose was reduced to 2 mg. When the risperidone dose was later increased to 8 mg the oedema reappeared, so the risperidone was withdrawn.[7] A second case of oedema has been reported in a 35-year-old man who had taken **valproate semisodium** uneventfully for over 6 years. After taking risperidone for two-and-a-half weeks, significant oedema developed, which responded to treatment with hydrochlorothiazide and triamterene.[8] Note that both risperidone and valproate can cause oedema alone.

In general the data seem to suggest that no dose adjustments are necessary if valproate and risperidone are given together. The general relevance of the two cases of oedema is uncertain; bear them in mind in should oedema develop in a patient taking both drugs.

1. Spina E, Avenoso A, Facciolà G, Salemi M, Scordo MG, Giacobello T, Madia AG, Perucca E. Plasma concentrations of risperidone and 9-hydroxyrisperidone: effect of comedication with carbamazepine or valproate. *Ther Drug Monit* (2000) 22, 481–5.
2. Yoshimura R, Shinkai K, Ueda N, Nakamura J. Valproic acid improves psychotic agitation without influencing plasma risperidone levels in schizophrenic patients. *Pharmacopsychiatry* (2007) 40, 9–13.
3. Ravindran A, Silverstone P, Lacroix D, von Schaick E, Vermeulen A, Alexander J. Risperidone does not affect steady-state pharmacokinetics of divalproex sodium in patients with bipolar disorder. *Clin Pharmacokinet* (2004) 43, 733–40.
4. van Wattum PJ. Valproic acid and risperidone. *J Am Acad Child Adolesc Psychiatry* (2001) 40, 866–7.
5. Sund JK, Aamo T, Spigset O. Valproic acid and risperidone: a drug interaction? *J Am Acad Child Adolesc Psychiatry* (2003) 42, 1–2.
6. Bertoldo M. Valproic acid and risperidone. *J Am Acad Child Adolesc Psychiatry* (2002) 41, 632.
7. Sanders RD, Lehrer DS. Edema associated with addition of risperidone to valproate treatment. *J Clin Psychiatry* (1998) 59, 689–90.
8. Baldassano CF, Ghaemi SN. Generalized edema with risperidone: divalproex sodium treatment. *J Clin Psychiatry* (1996) 57, 422.

Risperidone + Venlafaxine

Venlafaxine possibly causes a slight rise in risperidone exposure.

Clinical evidence, mechanism, importance and management

In a study in 30 healthy subjects, steady-state venlafaxine 75 mg every 12 hours was found to increase the AUC of a single 1-mg oral dose of risperidone by about 32%, but the pharmacokinetic profile of the risperidone plus its active metabolite (9-hydroxyrisperidone) was not changed.[1]

The slight effect on risperidone exposure is not expected to be clinically important, and therefore the dose of risperidone does not need adjusting if venlafaxine is given.

1. Amchin J, Zarycranski W, Taylor KP, Albano D, Klockowski PM. Effect of venlafaxine on the pharmacokinetics of risperidone. *J Clin Pharmacol* (1999) 39, 297–309.

Ritanserin + Miscellaneous

Ritanserin does not interact with alcohol; cimetidine and ranitidine do not affect ritanserin pharmacokinetics.

Clinical evidence, mechanism, importance and management

(a) Alcohol

A study in 20 healthy subjects given ritanserin 10 mg with and without alcohol 0.5 g/kg found no pharmacokinetic or pharmacodynamic interactions between these drugs.[1]

(b) H_2-receptor antagonists

In a crossover study in 9 healthy subjects, **cimetidine** 800 mg daily or **ranitidine** 300 mg daily for 11 days caused a negligible 16% decrease in the maximum concentration of a single 10-mg dose of ritanserin given on day 3, and had no effect on its AUC. These changes were attributed to altered absorption,[2] but are of no clinical importance. No ritanserin dose adjustment would be expected to be needed on the concurrent use of **cimetidine** or **ranitidine**

1. Estevez F, Parrillo S, Giusti M, Monti JM. Single-dose ritanserin and alcohol in healthy volunteers: a placebo-controlled trial. *Alcohol* (1995) 12, 541–5.
2. Trenk D, Seiler K-U, Buschmann M, Szathmary S, Benn H-P, Jähnchen E. Effect of concomitantly administered cimetidine or ranitidine on the pharmacokinetics of the 5-HT_2-receptor antagonist ritanserin. *J Clin Pharmacol* (1993) 33, 330–4.

Sertindole + CYP3A4 inhibitors

Erythromycin, a moderate CYP3A4 inhibitor, causes a very small increase in sertindole concentrations, but additive QT prolongation is predicted. Similarly, diltiazem and verapamil might slightly reduce sertindole clearance. Other CYP3A4 inhibitors are predicted to raise sertindole exposure.

Clinical evidence

(a) Erythromycin

In a study, 10 healthy subjects were given a single 4-mg dose of sertindole before and on the third day of a 10-day course of erythromycin 250 mg every 6 hours. There was a negligible increase in AUC and maximum serum concentrations of sertindole of 13% and 15%, respectively, although only the change in maximum concentration was statistically significant. No ECG changes were seen.[1,2]

(b) Other CYP3A4 inhibitors

In a population pharmacokinetic analysis, the concurrent use of calcium channel blockers (**diltiazem**, nifedipine, or **verapamil**) appeared to be associated with a 20% reduction in sertindole clearance.[3] Note that, of these calcium-channel blockers, only diltiazem and verapamil are recognised moderate CYP3A4 inhibitors

Mechanism

Erythromycin, a moderate CYP3A4 inhibitor, probably increases sertindole concentrations by inhibiting its metabolism by CYP3A4. However, the effect is very small and suggests that sertindole is only slightly metabolised by CYP3A4. Although less conclusive, the data for diltiazem and verapamil support this minor effect.

Importance and management

The pharmacokinetic interaction of **erythromycin** with sertindole is not clinically relevant. Nevertheless the UK manufacturer of sertindole contraindicated erythromycin because of the possibility of additive effects on the QT interval,[4] which can lead to life-threatening arrhythmias. See 'Drugs that prolong the QT interval + Other drugs that prolong the QT interval', p.272, for further information on the concurrent use of two or more drugs that prolong the QT interval.

The possible pharmacokinetic interaction of diltiazem and verapamil with sertindole is also unlikely to be clinically relevant. However, the manufacturers of sertindole suggest that the effect might be greater in patients who are poor metabolisers of CYP2D6 in whom CYP3A4 might be a more important route of metabolism. For this reason, they contraindicate potent inhibitors of CYP3A4 with sertindole, and they name **clarithromycin, indinavir, itraconazole, ketoconazole, diltiazem, verapamil,** and **cimetidine**. However, note that diltiazem, verapamil, and cimetidine are not generally considered to be potent inhibitors of CYP3A4. Given the very small pharmacokinetic interaction with erythromycin, and the fact that CYP2D6 inhibitors are not contraindicated even though they have a much greater effect on sertindole concentrations (see 'Sertindole + Miscellaneous', below), this advice seems over-cautious. For a list of drugs that are CYP3A4 inhibitors, see 'Table 1.9', p.11.

Note that the manufacturer of **miconazole oral gel** predicts that it will increase the levels of sertindole by inhibiting CYP3A4 and therefore contraindicates concurrent use.[5] However, given the lack of a clinically relevant pharmacokinetic interaction between sertindole and the moderate CYP3A4 inhibitor erythromycin, an interaction between miconazole and sertindole appears unlikely.

1. Granneman GR, Wozniak P, Ereshefsky L, Silber C, Mack R. Effect of erythromycin on the pharmacokinetics of sertindole (M94–145). Poster presentation at the American College of Neuropsychopharmacology Annual Meeting, San Juan, Puerto Rico, December 1996.
2. Wong SL, Cao G, Mack RJ, Granneman GR. The effect of erythromycin on the CYP3A component of sertindole clearance in healthy volunteers. *J Clin Pharmacol* (1997) 37, 1056–61.
3. Granneman GR, Wozniak P, Ereshefsky L, Silber C, Mack R. Population pharmacokinetics of sertindole during long-term treatment of patients with schizophrenia. Poster presentation at the American College of Neuropsychopharmacology Annual Meeting, San Juan, Puerto Rico, December 1996.
4. Serdolect (Sertindole). Lundbeck Ltd. UK Summary of product characteristics, July 2007.
5. Daktarin Oral Gel (Miconazole). Janssen-Cilag Ltd. UK Summary of product characteristics, December 2014.

Sertindole + Miscellaneous

Fluoxetine and paroxetine greatly increase sertindole concentrations whereas carbamazepine, phenobarbital, phenytoin, and rifampicin (rifampin) greatly reduce sertindole concentrations. Sertindole does not alter the exposure to alprazolam. Antacids, food and tobacco smoking do not appreciably alter sertindole exposure.

Clinical evidence, mechanism, importance and management

(a) Alprazolam

A pharmacokinetic study in 14 healthy subjects found that the AUC and maximum concentration of sertindole 12 mg daily were not affected by a single 1-mg dose of alprazolam.[1] No sertindole dose adjustment is necessary on the concurrent use of alprazolam.

(b) Antacids or Food

In a study in 16 healthy subjects, a standardised breakfast or *Maalox* [**aluminium/magnesium hydroxide**] 45 mL had no effect on the AUC of a single 4-mg dose of sertindole, and only minor and clinically unimportant changes occurred in maximum serum concentrations.[2,3] No particular precautions are needed if sertindole is given with *Maalox*, and it can be given without regard to meals.

(c) CYP3A4 inducers

The metabolism of sertindole is greatly increased by enzyme inducers, such as **rifampicin (rifampin), phenobarbital, phenytoin** and **carbamazepine**, and plasma sertindole concentrations can be reduced 2- to 3-fold. The manufacturers therefore state that the daily dose of sertindole might need to be increased towards the upper end of the maximum dose range to accommodate this interaction.[4,5]

(d) SSRIs

Fluoxetine and **paroxetine** are known inhibitors of CYP2D6 and their concurrent use with sertindole results in a 2- to 3-fold increase in its plasma concentrations. The manufacturers therefore advise extreme caution on concurrent use, and state that a low maintenance dose of sertindole might be needed in patients given either of these SSRIs, with close ECG monitoring when the sertindole dose is adjusted.[4] An isolated case report describes a man with paranoid psychosis and unipolar depression whose condition unexpectedly seriously worsened when **paroxetine** was stopped while continuing to take sertindole.[6]

(e) Tobacco

In a population pharmacokinetic analysis, the clearance of sertindole appeared to be increased by about 20% by tobacco smoking (probably because of the induction of cytochrome P450 isoenzymes), but no sertindole dose alteration is thought necessary.[5]

1. Wong SL, Locke C, Staser J, Granneman GR. Lack of multiple dosing effect of sertindole on the pharmacokinetics of alprazolam in healthy volunteers. *Psychopharmacology (Berl)* (1998) 135, 236–41.
2. Granneman GR, Wozniak P, Ereshefsky L, Silber C, Mack R. Effect of food and antacid on the bioavailability of sertindole (M94–164). Poster presentation at the American College of Neuropsychopharmacology Annual Meeting, San Juan, Puerto Rico, December 1996.
3. Wong S, Linnen P, Mack R, Granneman GR. Effects of food, antacid, and dosage form on the pharmacokinetics and relative bioavailability of sertindole in healthy volunteers. *Biopharm Drug Dispos* (1997) 18, 533–41.
4. Serdolect (Sertindole). Lundbeck Ltd. UK Summary of product characteristics, July 2007.
5. Granneman GR, Wozniak P, Ereshefsky L, Silber C, Mack R. Population pharmacokinetics of sertindole during long-term treatment of patients with schizophrenia. Poster presentation at the American College of Neuropsychopharmacology Annual Meeting, San Juan, Puerto Rico, December 1996.
6. Walker-Kinnear M, McNaughton S. Paroxetine discontinuation syndrome in association with sertindole therapy. *Br J Psychiatry* (1997) 170, 389.

Sulpiride + Miscellaneous

Sucralfate and an aluminium/magnesium hydroxide antacid can reduce the absorption of sulpiride. Three case reports describe extrapyramidal adverse effects in patients taking sulpiride and fluoxetine or lithium.

Clinical evidence, mechanism, importance and management

(a) Antacids and Sucralfate

A study in 6 healthy subjects found that the bioavailability of a single 100-mg dose of sulpiride was reduced by 40% by sucralfate 1 g and by 32% by 30 mL of *Simeco* **(aluminium/magnesium hydroxide** and **simeticone)**. When either the sucralfate or the antacid were taken 2 hours before sulpiride the reduction in bioavailability was only about 25%, and no change in bioavailability was seen in one subject when the sucralfate was given 2 hours after the sulpiride.[1]

The mechanism by which antacids and sucralfate reduce sulpiride absorption has not been established, but it seems possible that sulpiride becomes adsorbed onto the antacid or sucralfate, reducing the amount available for absorption.

Information about an interaction between sulpiride and antacids appears to be limited to this one study, which did not establish the clinical relevance of the effect found. With other antacid interactions, separating the doses by as much as possible (one to 2 hours) to avoid admixture in the gut usually minimises any effects. It might be prudent to consider separating dosing if sulpiride seems less effective in a patient taking an antacid. Similar precautions seem advisable if sucralfate is given with sulpiride, with one study finding a 2-hour separation adequate.

(b) Fluoxetine

Parkinson-like symptoms developed in a patient taking sulpiride and maprotiline when fluoxetine was also given.[2] This isolated case of extrapyramidal adverse effects should not prevent concurrent use; however, if extrapyramidal effects become troublesome bear this interaction in mind as a possible cause.

(c) Lithium

The sudden emergence of extrapyramidal symptoms in patients taking sulpiride and lithium has been described in two case reports.[3] In the first case, a 21-year-old woman who was taking sulpiride 800 mg twice daily (decreased from 2 g daily) developed a severe parkinsonian syndrome (with choreiform movements of the upper limbs) after a single 800-mg dose of lithium. The lithium was discontinued and the syndrome resolved within 24 to 48 hours. In the second case, a 48-year-old man who was taking lithium 1.2 g at night, developed marked orofacial dyskinesia and acute akathisia within 12 hours of starting sulpiride 800 mg twice daily. The symptoms slowly subsided within 3 to 4 days of stopping sulpiride. These are isolated cases and should not prevent concurrent use, but bear them in mind if extrapyramidal effects occur or are particularly troublesome. Note that both lithium and sulpiride are associated with an increased risk of QT interval prolongation, see 'Drugs that prolong the QT interval + Other drugs that prolong the QT interval', p.272, for further information on the concurrent use of two or more drugs that prolong the QT interval.

1. Gouda MW, Hikal AH, Babhair SA, ElHofy SA, Mahrous GM. Effect of sucralfate and antacids on the bioavailability of sulpiride in humans. *Int J Pharmaceutics* (1984) 22, 257–63.
2. Touw DJ, Gernaat HBPE, van der Woude J. Parkinsonisme na toevoeging van fluoxetine aan behandeling met neuroleptica of carbamazepine. *Ned Tijdschr Geneeskd* (1992) 136, 332–4.
3. Dinan TG, O'Keane V. Acute extrapyramidal reactions following lithium and sulpiride co-administration: two case reports. *Hum Psychopharmacol* (1991) 6, 67–9.

Suvorexant + Miscellaneous

Suvorexant exposure is increased by ketoconazole, and other potent CYP3A4 inhibitors are expected to interact similarly. Rifampicin markedly reduces suvorexant exposure; other potent CYP3A4 inducers are predicted to interact similarly. Digoxin exposure is increased by suvorexant. Food can delay the onset of suvorexant effects. Suvorexant did not have a clinically relevant effect on the pharmacokinetics of midazolam, paroxetine, or warfarin, and paroxetine did not have a clinically relevant effect on the pharmacokinetics of suvorexant.

Clinical evidence, mechanism, importance and management

(a) Alcohol

The US manufacturer reports that a single 0.7-g/kg dose of alcohol did not affect the pharmacokinetics of a single 40-mg dose of suvorexant; the concentrations of alcohol were also unchanged. They also state that additive CNS depression might occur on concurrent use, although the degree of impairment will depend on the individual.[1] However, all patients should be warned of the potential effects, and counselled against driving or undertaking other skilled tasks. The manufacturer advises that suvorexant should not be taken if the patient has drunk alcohol that evening or before going to bed.[1]

(b) Combined hormonal contraceptives

The US manufacturer briefly reports that in a study in women taking an oral combined hormonal contraceptive containing **ethinylestradiol** 35 micrograms and **norelgestromin** 250 micrograms, suvorexant 40 mg increased the AUC of norelgestromin by about 12%, but had no effect on the AUC and maximum concentration of the ethinylestradiol component.[1] No combined hormonal contraceptive dose adjustment would seem necessary on concurrent use.

(c) CYP3A4 inducers

The US manufacturer briefly reports that in a study, **rifampicin** 600 mg daily reduced the AUC and maximum concentration of suvorexant 40 mg by about 100% and 70%, respectively.[1] Rifampicin is a potent inducer of CYP3A4, by which suvorexant is primarily metabolised, and hence concurrent use results in a very marked reduction in its exposure. The manufacturer advises a maximum dose of suvorexant 20 mg when used concurrently with potent CYP3A4 inducers; however it is likely that the efficacy of suvorexant will be so greatly decreased in the presence of potent CYP3A4 inducers that it might be prudent to consider an alternative hypnotic in patients taking potent CYP3A4 inducers. For a list of potent CYP3A4 inducers see 'Table 1.9', p.11.

(d) CYP3A4 inhibitors

The US manufacturer briefly reports that in a study, **ketoconazole** 400 mg daily increased the AUC and maximum concentration of suvorexant 40 mg almost 3-fold and about 20%, respectively.[1] Ketoconazole is a potent inhibitor of CYP3A4, by which suvorexant is primarily metabolised, and hence concurrent use results in a moderate increase in its exposure. The manufacturer therefore advises that concurrent use of suvorexant with potent CYP3A4 inhibitors is not recommended.[1] If both drugs are taken concurrently, be alert for a possible increase in suvorexant adverse effects. For a list of potent CYP3A4 inhibitors see 'Table 1.9', p.11. Note that the manufacturer additionally names **conivaptan**, **indinavir**, **nefazodone**, and **posaconazole** as potent inhibitors, but these are generally considered to be moderate inhibitors of CYP3A4.

The US manufacturer also reports that **diltiazem** 240 mg increased the AUC and maximum concentration of suvorexant 40 mg about 2-fold and about 20%, respectively.[1] Diltiazem is a moderate inhibitor of CYP3A4, by which suvorexant is primarily metabolised, and hence concurrent use results in a moderate increase in its exposure. The manufacturer recommends a starting dose of suvorexant 5 mg and a maximum dose of suvorexant 10 mg when used concurrently with moderate CYP3A4 inhibitors. For a list of moderate CYP3A4 inhibitors see 'Table 1.9', p.11. Note that the manufacturer additionally names **amprenavir**, **atazanavir**, and **fosamprenavir**, which are potent CYP3A4 inhibitors (when boosted with ritonavir); they also name **grapefruit juice**, which is considered to be a weak CYP3A4 inhibitor. They also name **ciprofloxacin** as a moderate CYP3A4 inhibitor, but it is not known to be an inhibitor of this isoenzyme.

(e) CYP3A4 substrates

The US manufacturer briefly reports that in a study of suvorexant 80 mg given with multiple doses of **midazolam** 2 mg, the AUC and maximum concentration of midazolam were increased almost 50% and about 25%, respectively.[1] The effect on midazolam pharmacokinetics suggests that suvorexant is a weak inhibitor of CYP3A4, and the slight increase in midazolam exposure seen is not expected to be clinically relevant. No midazolam dose adjustment would be expected to be needed on concurrent use with suvorexant.

(f) Digoxin

The US manufacturer briefly reports that in a study, suvorexant 40 mg increased the AUC and maximum concentration of digoxin 500 micrograms almost 3-fold and by about 25%, respectively.[1] Digoxin is a substrate of the efflux pump, P-glycoprotein. The small changes seen in digoxin exposure are possibly due to the inhibitory effects of suvorexant on P-glycoprotein.[1] Some caution on the concurrent use of digoxin with suvorexant, and monitoring of digoxin concentrations, would seem prudent.

(g) Food

The US manufacturer briefly reports that taking suvorexant with a high-fat meal resulted in no meaningful change in the AUC or maximum concentration of suvorexant, but there was a delay in the time taken to reach maximum concentration of approximately 1.5 hours. They suggest that suvorexant can be taken with or without food; however for faster sleep onset, suvorexant should not be taken with, or soon after, a meal.[1]

(h) Paroxetine

The US manufacturer briefly reports that in a study of healthy subjects given suvorexant 40 mg and paroxetine 20 mg, there was no clinically relevant pharmacokinetic or pharmacodynamic interaction.[1] No dose adjustments of either drug are therefore expected on concurrent use.

(i) Warfarin

The US manufacturer briefly reports that in a study, suvorexant 40 mg given with a 30-mg dose of warfarin had no effect on the AUC and maximum concentration of warfarin.[1] No warfarin dose adjustment is therefore expected on concurrent use.

1. Belsomra (Suvorexant). Merck Sharp & Dohme Corp. US Prescribing information, August 2014.

Tiotixene + Miscellaneous

Tiotixene concentrations are reduced by the enzyme-inducers carbamazepine, phenytoin, primidone, and tobacco smoke. Additive hypotension might occur if tiotixene is given with other drugs that can lower blood pressure. Some enzyme inhibitors might reduce the clearance of tiotixene, but paroxetine does not alter tiotixene concentrations.

Clinical evidence, mechanism, importance and management

(a) Antiepileptics; enzyme-inducing

A retrospective study in 42 patients found that the mean clearance of tiotixene in those taking enzyme-inducing drugs (**carbamazepine**, **phenytoin**, **primidone**) was 3-fold greater than in the control group. Of the group taking enzyme inducers, 5 patients had non-detectable serum concentrations of tiotixene, and not surprisingly showed no clinical response.[1] It would seem prudent to monitor the concurrent use of tiotixene with any of these antiepileptics, increasing the tiotixene dose if necessary.

(b) Paroxetine

A study in 10 healthy subjects found that paroxetine 20 mg daily for 3 days did not alter the pharmacokinetics of a single 20-mg dose of tiotixene. It was suggested that CYP2D6 is not the main isoenzyme involved in the metabolism and clearance of tiotixene.[2] No tiotixene dose adjustment is necessary on the concurrent use of paroxetine.

(c) Tobacco

Tobacco smoking increased the clearance of tiotixene in patients taking enzyme inhibitors or no other drugs, but not in patients taking enzyme inducers. Those who smoked were found to need on average 45% more tiotixene than the non-smokers taking no other interacting drugs.[1] It would therefore seem prudent to monitor the efficacy of tiotixene in patients who are smokers, adjusting the tiotixene dose if necessary.

(d) Other drugs

In a retrospective analysis of results from a routine therapeutic drug monitoring of plasma tiotixene concentrations, patients taking drugs that were classified as inhibitors of enzymes or clearance (**cimetidine**, **doxepin**, **isoniazid**, **nortriptyline**, or **propranolol**) had a tiotixene clearance of 9.51 L/minute, which was 71% less than that seen in patients taking tiotixene alone.[1] It was suggested that these drugs inhibited the metabolism of tiotixene, thereby reducing its clearance. However, not all these drugs are known inhibitors of drug clearance or metabolism, and, because they were grouped, it is not possible to know which specifically might have contributed to the effect seen. Therefore, no interaction is established, and further controlled studies are necessary. Note that there is a case report of adverse effects in a patient taking tiotixene and chlorpromazine with **propranolol**, see 'Beta blockers + Phenothiazines', p.1018.

1. Ereshefsky L, Saklad SR, Watanabe MD, Davis CM, Jann MW. Thiothixene pharmacokinetic interactions: a study of hepatic enzyme inducers, clearance inhibitors, and demographic variables. *J Clin Psychopharmacol* (1991) 11, 296–301.
2. Guthrie SK, Hariharan M, Kumar AA, Bader G, Tandon R. The effect of paroxetine on thiothixene pharmacokinetics. *J Clin Pharm Ther* (1997) 22, 221–6.

Ziprasidone + Carbamazepine

Carbamazepine slightly reduces ziprasidone exposure.

Clinical evidence, mechanism, importance and management

In a randomised study, healthy subjects were given ziprasidone 20 mg twice daily for 5 doses on the last few days of either placebo (10 subjects), or carbamazepine 200 mg twice daily (9 subjects), taken for about 3 weeks. Carbamazepine reduced the AUC and maximum serum concentration of ziprasidone by 36% and 27%, respectively.[1]

Carbamazepine, a known potent inducer of CYP3A4, probably increased the metabolism of ziprasidone by this isoenzyme, resulting in the reduction in ziprasidone exposure seen. However, this reduction is slight, and not expected to be clinically important, although it is possible that a higher dose of carbamazepine might have a greater effect. On the basis of the available evidence, no ziprasidone dose adjustment would be expected to be necessary if carbamazepine is also given.

1. Miceli JJ, Anziano RJ, Robarge L, Hansen RA. Laurent A. The effect of carbamazepine on the steady-state pharmacokinetics of ziprasidone in healthy volunteers. *Br J Clin Pharmacol* (2000) 49 (Suppl 1), 65S–70S.

Ziprasidone + Ketoconazole

Ketoconazole slightly increases ziprasidone exposure.

Clinical evidence, mechanism, importance and management

In a randomised, placebo-controlled study, 14 healthy subjects were given a 40-mg dose of ziprasidone before and after taking ketoconazole 400 mg daily for 6 days. Ketoconazole increased the AUC and maximum serum concentration of ziprasidone by 33% and 34%, respectively. This slight increase in exposure probably occurs because ketoconazole inhibits CYP3A4, by which ziprasidone is partially metabolised. However, it was concluded that the increase is not clinically relevant.[1] No ziprasidone dose adjustments would therefore seem to be needed on concurrent use.

1. Miceli JJ, Smith M, Robarge L, Morse T, Laurent A. The effects of ketoconazole on ziprasidone pharmacokinetics – a placebo-controlled crossover study in healthy volunteers. *Br J Clin Pharmacol* (2000) 49 (Suppl 1), 71S–76S.

Ziprasidone + Miscellaneous

Food can increase ziprasidone absorption. Ziprasidone does not appear to interact with an aluminium/magnesium hydroxide antacid, benzatropine, cimetidine, dextromethorphan, lorazepam, propranolol or tobacco smoking.

Clinical evidence, mechanism, importance and management

(a) Antacids or Cimetidine

A single 40-mg oral dose of ziprasidone was given to 10 healthy subjects either alone, with cimetidine 800 mg daily for 2 days, or with three 30-mL doses of ***Maalox*** (**aluminium** and **magnesium hydroxide**). The only change in the pharmacokinetics of ziprasidone was a 6% increase in the AUC with cimetidine. It was concluded that no particular precautions are needed if either of these drugs and ziprasidone are given concurrently.[1]

(b) Dextromethorphan

In a single-dose study in 8 healthy subjects, ziprasidone 80 mg did not affect the pharmacokinetics of dextromethorphan 30 mg, taken 2 hours later. This suggests that the dose of dextromethorphan does not need to be adjusted if ziprasidone is also given. Furthermore, dextromethorphan is used as a probe substrate for CYP2D6, and therefore this study also suggests that ziprasidone is unlikely to affect the pharmacokinetics of other CYP2D6 substrates.[2]

(c) Food

In a series of controlled studies in healthy subjects, a high-calorie (1000 kcal) and a medium-calorie (500 kcal) meal increased the AUC of ziprasidone by 69 to 81%, when compared with the fasting state, and there was less inter-subject variability in the AUC. A low-calorie meal (250 kcal) had a negligible effect on the AUC of ziprasidone. The fat content of the meals had little effect on the outcome.[3] The US manufacturer recommends that oral ziprasidone is always taken with food.[4]

(d) Quetiapine

A case report describes a 70-year-old man who took quetiapine and ziprasidone and who developed cardiac arrhythmias with extrasystoles, and a prolonged QTc interval of 482 milliseconds, an increase of 65 milliseconds from his value with quetiapine alone. On stopping quetiapine and reducing the dose of ziprasidone, his QTc interval normalised.[5] For further discussion on the risk of QT interval prolongation with ziprasidone, see 'Drugs that prolong the QT interval + Other drugs that prolong the QT interval', p.272.

(e) Tobacco

The US manufacturer of ziprasidone suggests that as ziprasidone is not metabolised by CYP1A2, smoking should not affect its pharmacokinetics. This is borne out by population pharmacokinetic analysis, which did not reveal any differences in the pharmacokinetics of ziprasidone between tobacco smokers and non-smokers.[4]

(f) Other drugs

The US manufacturer of ziprasidone states that population pharmacokinetic analysis of patients with schizophrenia who were enrolled in clinical studies showed that no clinically relevant pharmacokinetic interactions occurred with **benzatropine**, **lorazepam** or **propranolol**.[4]

1. Wilner KD, Hansen RA, Folger CJ, Geoffroy P. The pharmacokinetics of ziprasidone in healthy volunteers treated with cimetidine or antacid. *Br J Clin Pharmacol* (2000) 49 (Suppl 1), 57S–60S.
2. Wilner KD, Demattos SB, Anziano RJ, Apseloff G, Gerber N. Ziprasidone and the activity of cytochrome P450 2D6 in healthy extensive metabolizers. *Br J Clin Pharmacol* (2000) 49 (Suppl 1), 43S–47S.
3. Gandelman K, Alderman JA, Glue P, Lombardo I, LaBadie RR, Versavel M, Preskorn SH. The impact of calories and fat content of meals on oral ziprasidone absorption: a randomized, open-label, crossover trial. *J Clin Psychiatry* (2009) 70, 58–62.
4. Geodon (Ziprasidone). Pfizer Inc. US Prescribing information, December 2010.
5. Minov C. QTc-Zeitverlängerung unter ziprasidon in kombination mit quetiapin. *Psychiatr Prax* (2004) 31, S142–4.

Zopiclone + Gemfibrozil

Gemfibrozil does not increase zopiclone exposure, but exposure to one of its major metabolites might be increased.

Clinical evidence, mechanism, importance and management

A placebo-controlled, crossover study in 10 healthy subjects found that gemfibrozil 600 mg twice daily for 3 days did not affect the pharmacokinetics of a single 7.5-mg oral dose of zopiclone. However, the AUCs of its two major metabolites, zopiclone *N*-oxide and *N*-desmethylzopiclone, were raised 2-fold and by 20%, respectively. These metabolites appear to have some, weaker pharmacological activity than zopiclone.[1]

It appears that gemfibrozil, which is a potent CYP2C8 inhibitor, does not affect the metabolism of zopiclone, but it might affect the further metabolism of its major metabolites.

Although the pharmacodynamic effects of zopiclone, such as drowsiness, were not affected by gemfibrozil, it was suggested that, due to the increased exposure to the metabolites, slightly enhanced effects could not be excluded.[1] However, in general, it appears that a clinically relevant interaction would not be expected.

1. Tornio A, Neuvonen PJ, Backman JT. The CYP2C8 inhibitor gemfibrozil does not increase the plasma concentrations of zopiclone. *Eur J Clin Pharmacol* (2006) 62, 645–51.

Zotepine + Miscellaneous

Zotepine is predicted to increase the risk of seizures when used with other antipsychotics. Two cases of deep vein thrombosis have been reported in patients taking zotepine with paroxetine. Diazepam and fluoxetine might increase plasma concentrations of zotepine. Two cases of hypothermia have been reported in patients taking benzodiazepines, valproate and zotepine when the dose of zotepine was increased. The pharmacokinetics of zotepine do not appear to be affected by tobacco smoking.

Clinical evidence, mechanism, importance and management

(a) Antimuscarinics

In a study in 21 patients, biperiden 6 mg daily for 2 weeks was found not to affect the pharmacokinetics of zotepine.[1] No zotepine dose adjustment is necessary on concurrent use of biperiden.

(b) Antipsychotics

The UK manufacturer of zotepine advised that, as with some other antipsychotics, zotepine has clear pro-convulsive effects, which might be additive with other antipsychotics, particularly if high doses of either or both drugs are used. They therefore recommended that zotepine doses above 300 mg daily or the concurrent use of high doses of other antipsychotics with zotepine should be avoided.[2]

(c) Benzodiazepines

A study in 17 patients found that plasma zotepine concentrations were higher and its elimination half-life prolonged by **diazepam**.[3] The UK manufacturer reported that in a clinical interaction study, **diazepam** increased the plasma concentrations of zotepine by about 25%, and the plasma concentration of its equipotent active metabolite, norzotepine, was also increased. They advised caution if diazepam and zotepine are given concurrently.[2] However, increases of the magnitude would not generally be expected to be clinically relevant.

A patient who was taking zotepine 50 mg daily, **valproate** 1 g daily, and **lormetazepam** 2 mg daily had his dose of zotepine increased gradually to 200 mg daily because of persistent auditory hallucinations. The **valproate** and **lormetazepam** doses were not altered. Four weeks later he presented with poor appetite, dizziness, and a low body temperature (34.8°C). The dose of zotepine was reduced and his temperature increased to 36°C. The authors reported another case of hypothermia in a patient taking **clonazepam**, **valproic acid**, and zotepine. The patient's temperature became normal when the dose of zotepine was reduced from 200 mg to 150 mg, and fell when the dose was increased to 200 mg. It was suggested that zotepine might decrease body temperature by chronic suppression of serotonin (5-HT) transmission and by increasing the rate of metabolism of dopamine and noradrenaline. **Valproate** might also lower body temperature in a dose-dependent manner, and so it is possible that the concurrent use of three drugs in each of the patients contributed to the observed hypothermia.[4]

(d) Desipramine

No pharmacokinetic interaction was seen when zotepine was given with desipramine.[2]

(e) SSRIs

Two case reports have described mobile, elderly male patients who developed deep vein thrombosis when taking **paroxetine** and zotepine. In the first case the patient was taking **paroxetine** 40 mg daily, and zotepine was added to his treatment 3 weeks later, initially at a dose of 75 mg daily, and then increased to 150 mg daily. After 17 days of treatment with zotepine 150 mg daily, the patient developed swelling of the right leg, and a deep vein thrombosis was diagnosed by Doppler studies and venography. The second patient also took **paroxetine** 40 mg daily, to which zotepine 150 mg daily was added, and within 3 days of starting zotepine the patient had developed painful swelling of the right calf, dyspnoea, and tachycardia. A deep vein thrombosis was confirmed. These 2 patients were part of a review of 150 patients consecutively admitted to a psychiatric ward. They were the only 2 patients who were given this combination of drugs, and the only two who developed a thromboembolism. The mechanism of this interaction is unclear.[5]

In a clinical interaction study, **fluoxetine** increased the plasma concentration of zotepine by about 10% and approximately doubled those of its equipotent active metabolite norzotepine. The UK manufacturer advised caution if **fluoxetine** and zotepine are given concurrently.[2]

Note that **citalopram** and **escitalopram** are associated with a dose-related prolongation in the QT interval, as is zotepine. See 'Drugs that prolong the QT interval + Other drugs that prolong the QT interval', p.272, for further information on the concurrent use of two or more drugs that prolong the QT interval.

(f) Tobacco

A study in healthy subjects found that there were no differences in the pharmacokinetics of zotepine in smokers (8 subjects) and non-smokers (6 subjects).[3]

1. Otani K, Hirano T, Kondo T, Kaneko S, Fukushima Y, Noda K, Tashiro Y. Biperiden and piroheptine do not affect the serum level of zotepine, a new antipsychotic drug. *Br J Psychiatry* (1990) 157, 128–30.
2. Zoleptil (Zotepine). Orion Pharma UK Ltd. UK Summary of product characteristics, April 2006.
3. Tanaka O. Pharmacokinetics of zotepine and various factors affecting that of zotepine. *Nihon Shinkei Seishin Yakurigaku Zasshi* (1996) 16, 49–52.
4. Chen KC, Yang YK, Chen PS, Yeh TL, Yang MJ. Two cases of hypothermia induced by an increased dosage of zotepine in a combination therapy. *Psychiatry Clin Neurosci* (2003) 57, 369–71.
5. Pantel J, Schröder J, Eysenbach, K, Mundt Ch. Two cases of deep vein thrombosis associated with a combined paroxetine and zotepine therapy. *Pharmacopsychiatry* (1997) 30, 109–11.

21

Antivirals

This section is concerned with the drugs used to treat viral infections, including hepatitis, herpes, influenza, and HIV infection. These drugs can be grouped by the viral infections they are used to treat, and also by drug class (see 'Table 21.1', p.894). Where antivirals affect other drugs the interactions are generally covered elsewhere.

Antivirals active against hepatitis

Treatment of HCV infection requires combinations of different classes of direct acting antivirals, sometimes also in combination with peg-interferon alfa and ribavirin. Patients also often require treatment for other comorbid conditions, including HIV infection, and the potential for interactions is thus increased and their assessment can be complex.

(a) HCV-protease inhibitors

The HCV-protease inhibitors, boceprevir and telaprevir, are inhibitors of CYP3A4, and can cause clinically important interactions with drugs that are substrates of CYP3A4. Simeprevir does not appear to inhibit CYP3A4 to a clinically relevant extent, and paritaprevir itself does not affect CYP3A4 but it is boosted with ritonavir and so does have clinically important effects on CYP3A4 substrates. Boceprevir is primarily metabolised by aldoketoreductases, which does not appear to result in clinically relevant interactions; it is also partially metabolised by CYP3A4 and transported by P-glycoprotein. Telaprevir and paritaprevir are substrates of CYP3A4 and of P-glycoprotein, and simeprevir is a substrate of CYP3A4 and the organic anion transporter, OATP1B1. All the HCV-protease inhibitors inhibit P-glycoprotein (see 'Digoxin and other P-glycoprotein substrates + HCV-protease inhibitors', p.1098).

(b) NS5A inhibitors

The NS5A inhibitors daclatasvir, ledipasvir, and ombitasvir are all substrates for P-glycoprotein and breast cancer resistance protein, BCRP. Only daclatasvir is a cytochrome P450 substrate, being metabolised by CYP3A4. Both daclatasvir and ledipasvir are P-glycoprotein inhibitors, but the interaction potential of ombitasvir is limited.

(c) NS5B inhibitors

The NS5B inhibitors dasabuvir and sofosbuvir are substrates for P-glycoprotein and BCRP, and dasabuvir is additionally metabolised by CYP2C8 (see 'NS5B inhibitors; Dasabuvir + Gemfibrozil', p.994). Sofosbuvir appears not to affect cytochrome P450 isoenzymes or drug transporters and hence appears to have little potential to affect other drugs. Dasabuvir also appears to cause few interactions, but does appear to inhibit BCRP.

Antivirals active against herpes virus

The nucleoside analogues (e.g. aciclovir and related drugs, entecavir, telbivudine) and nucleotide analogues (e.g. adefovir, cidofovir) are principally eliminated unchanged by the kidneys by a process of active tubular secretion as well as glomerular filtration. The few interactions with these drugs mainly involve altered renal clearance (e.g. probenecid), but as they have a wide therapeutic range, even these interactions are of debatable clinical relevance. Cytochrome P450-mediated interactions are not important for this group of drugs. However, the possibility of effects on other transport systems cannot be ruled out, see 'Adefovir + Miscellaneous', p.897.

Antiretrovirals active against HIV

Treatment of HIV infection is based on a combination of 3, and sometimes 4, antiretrovirals, termed highly active antiretroviral therapy (HAART), and initial treatment is based on a backbone of two NRTIs plus either one NNRTI, or one HIV-protease inhibitor boosted with ritonavir, or one HIV-integrase inhibitor.[1,2] Treatment regimens in treatment-experienced patients or those with drug resistance are more complex and should be undertaken by an expert in the field. In addition, patients often take a large number of other drugs for comorbid conditions. This considerably increases the risk of drug interactions and complicates their assessment.

(a) CCR5 antagonists

CCR5 antagonists are a class of antiretrovirals referred to as entry inhibitors. Maraviroc is a substrate of CYP3A4 and because of this, CYP3A4 inducers (e.g. efavirenz) lower its concentrations, and CYP3A4 inhibitors (e.g. HIV-protease inhibitors) increase its concentrations. Maraviroc is not expected to have a clinically relevant effect on most cytochrome P450 isoenzymes, although it might possibly inhibit intestinal P-glycoprotein.

(b) HIV-fusion inhibitors

The fusion inhibitor, enfuvirtide, is a peptide. It does not cause cytochrome P450-mediated drug interactions, and is not affected by potent inducers or inhibitors of cytochrome P450 isoenzymes. However, modest interactions, for which the underlying mechanism is unknown, have been reported with some of the HIV-protease inhibitors, such as ritonavir and tipranavir, see 'Enfuvirtide + HIV-protease inhibitors', p.899.

(c) HIV-integrase inhibitors

Raltegravir and dolutegravir are metabolised by glucuronidation (primarily by UGT1A1). Hence, drugs that inhibit (e.g. atazanavir, see 'HIV-integrase inhibitors + HIV-protease inhibitors', p.912) or induce (e.g. rifampicin (rifampin) see 'HIV-integrase inhibitors + Rifamycins', p.917) this enzyme can affect their metabolism. Raltegravir is not a substrate for cytochrome P450 isoenzymes, and does not appear to inhibit or induce many of the major cytochrome P450 isoenzymes, nor does it inhibit P-glycoprotein. However, it appears that drugs that affect gastric pH might also affect the exposure to of raltegravir, see 'HIV-integrase inhibitors + Antacids', p.911, for further discussion. Dolutegravir is a minor substrate for CYP3A4, and hence is not greatly affected by known potent CYP3A4 inhibitors (e.g. boceprevir or telaprevir, see 'HIV-integrase inhibitors + HCV-protease inhibitors', p.912). It also does not appear to inhibit any of the major cytochrome P450 isoenzymes, nor does it inhibit P-glycoprotein. It might inhibit the organic cation transporter, OCT-2 and multidrug and toxin extrusion transporter, MATE-1, which are said to be involved in the renal transport of metformin (see 'Metformin + HIV-integrase inhibitors; Dolutegravir', p.533).

Elvitegravir is principally metabolised by CYP3A4 and is formulated with cobicistat as a pharmacokinetic enhancer. Many of the interactions of this preparation are therefore those of the cobicistat component due to its CYP3A4 inhibitory effects.

(d) HIV-protease inhibitors

The HIV-protease inhibitors are extensively metabolised by the cytochrome P450 isoenzyme system, particularly by CYP3A4, although nelfinavir is also metabolised by CYP2C19 (see 'HIV-protease inhibitors + Proton pump inhibitors', p.937). All HIV-protease inhibitors can inhibit CYP3A4, with ritonavir being the most potent, followed by indinavir, nelfinavir, amprenavir, and saquinavir. The HIV-protease inhibitors therefore have the potential to interact with other drugs metabolised by CYP3A4, and might also be affected by other CYP3A4 inhibitors and inducers. Ritonavir and tipranavir are predicted to also affect some other cytochrome P450 isoenzymes, as summarised in 'Table 21.2', p.894, and their effect, such as that on CYP2D6, has subsequently been demonstrated clinically. HIV-protease inhibitors therefore have the potential to interact with each other, with NNRTIs, and with the HIV-integrase inhibitor, elvitegravir; HIV-protease inhibitors are not likely to

Table 21.1 Classification of Antivirals

Group	Drugs
Antivirals for hepatitis viruses	
HCV-protease inhibitors	Boceprevir, Paritaprevir, Simeprevir, Telaprevir
NS5A inhibitors	Daclatasvir, Ledipasvir, Ombitasvir
NS5B inhibitors	Dasabuvir, Sofosbuvir
Nucleoside analogues	Entecavir, Lamivudine, Telbivudine
Nucleotide analogues	Adefovir, Tenofovir
Miscellaneous	Interferon alfa, Peginterferon alfa, Ribavirin
Antivirals for herpes viruses	
Guanine nucleoside analogues	Aciclovir, Famciclovir, Ganciclovir, Penciclovir, Valaciclovir, Valganciclovir
Other nucleoside analogues	Trifluridine, Vidarabine
Nucleotide analogues	Cidofovir, Fomivirsen
Miscellaneous	Foscarnet sodium, Inosine pranobex
Antivirals for HIV infection (antiretrovirals)	
CCR5 antagonists	Maraviroc
HIV-fusion inhibitors	Enfuvirtide
HIV-integrase inhibitors	Dolutegravir, Elvitegravir, Raltegravir
HIV-protease inhibitors	Amprenavir, Atazanavir, Darunavir, Fosamprenavir, Indinavir, Lopinavir, Nelfinavir, Ritonavir, Saquinavir, Tipranavir
Non-nucleoside reverse transcriptase inhibitors (NNRTIs)	Delavirdine, Efavirenz, Etravirine, Nevirapine, Rilpivirine
Nucleoside reverse transcriptase inhibitors (NRTIs)	Abacavir, Didanosine, Emtricitabine, Lamivudine, Stavudine, Zalcitabine, Zidovudine
Nucleotide reverse transcriptase inhibitors	Tenofovir
Antivirals for influenza	
Neuraminidase inhibitors	Oseltamivir, Zanamivir
Others	Amantadine, Rimantadine

Table 21.2 Summary of the effect of the HIV-protease inhibitors and NNRTIs on cytochrome P450 isoenzymes*

Antiviral	Substrate	Inhibits	Induces
HIV-protease inhibitors			
Amprenavir or Fosamprenavir	CYP3A4	CYP3A4	
Atazanavir	CYP3A4	CYP3A4	
Darunavir	CYP3A4	CYP3A4	
Indinavir	CYP3A4	CYP3A4	
Lopinavir	CYP3A4	CYP3A4	
Nelfinavir	CYP3A4, CYP2C19, CYP2C9, CYP2D6	CYP3A4	
Ritonavir	CYP3A4, CYP2D6	CYP3A4, CYP2D6	CYP3A4
Saquinavir	CYP3A4	CYP3A4	
Tipranavir	CYP3A4	CYP3A4, CYP2D6	CYP3A4
NNRTIs (Non-nucleoside reverse transcriptase inhibitors)			
Delavirdine	CYP3A4, CYP2D6	CYP3A4, CYP2C9, CYP2D6, CYP2C19	
Efavirenz	CYP3A4, CYP2B6	CYP3A4, CYP2C9, CYP2C19	CYP3A4
Etravirine	CYP3A4, CYP2C9, CYP2C19	CYP2C9, CYP2C19	CYP3A4
Nevirapine	CYP3A4		CYP3A4
Rilpivirine	CYP3A4		

* Note that some of the data comes from *in vitro* study and requires confirmation in clinical use. For clinically demonstrated metabolic effects, see under 'Drug metabolism interactions', p.4.

interact with NRTIs. In addition, HIV-protease inhibitors are substrates as well as inhibitors of P-glycoprotein.

The minimum plasma concentration of the HIV-protease inhibitors is thought to be important in maintaining efficacy and minimising the potential for development of viral resistance. Most HIV-protease inhibitors are usually given with a low dose of ritonavir, which has the effect of increasing the minimum concentration (reducing the potential for resistance) and of prolonging the half-life (allowing a reduction in the frequency of administration), see also 'HIV-protease inhibitors + HIV-protease inhibitors', p.931.

(e) Non-nucleoside reverse transcriptase inhibitors (NNRTIs)

The NNRTIs are metabolised by the cytochrome P450 isoenzyme system, particularly by CYP3A4. Many are also inducers (nevirapine, efavirenz, and to a lesser degree, etravirine) or inhibitors (delavirdine) of CYP3A4. These NNRTIs therefore have the potential to interact with other drugs metabolised by CYP3A4, and are affected by CYP3A4 inhibitors and inducers. Efavirenz is somewhat unique within this group in that it is also metabolised by CYP2B6, and it induces its own metabolism (autoinduction) by this isoenzyme. Delavirdine, efavirenz, and to some extent, etravirine, can also inhibit some other P450 isoenzymes. Rilpivirine does not appear to have a clinically relevant effect on CYP3A4 at the recommended dose, but it might be a P-glycoprotein inhibitor. For a summary of these effects, see 'Table 21.2', above. The NNRTIs do not tend to interact with the NRTIs, see below.

(f) Nucleoside reverse transcriptase inhibitors (NRTIs)

The NRTIs are prodrugs, which need to be activated by phosphorylation within cells to a triphosphate anabolite. Drugs can therefore interact with NRTIs by increasing or decreasing intracellular activation. NRTIs might also interact with each other by this mechanism. This interaction mechanism is studied *in vitro*, and clinical data are often not available, or the clinical relevance of any findings is unclear. Nevertheless, it is generally recommended that drugs inhibiting the intracellular activation of the NRTIs are not used concurrently (e.g. doxorubicin with stavudine, see 'NRTIs; Stavudine + Doxorubicin', p.984, or zidovudine with stavudine, see 'NRTIs + NRTIs', p.977). Hydroxycarbamide (see 'NRTIs + Hydroxycarbamide (Hydroxyurea)', p.976) can increase the intracellular activation of NRTIs.

The NRTIs are water soluble, and are mainly eliminated by the kidneys (didanosine, lamivudine, stavudine, and zalcitabine) or undergo hepatic glucuronidation (abacavir, zidovudine). The few important interactions with these drugs primarily involve altered renal clearance. For zidovudine (and possibly abacavir) some interactions are reported to occur via altered glucuronidation, but the clinical relevance of these are less clear (e.g. rifampicin (rifampin), see 'NRTIs + Rifamycins', p.981). Cytochrome P450-mediated interactions are not important for this class of drugs.

Some of the didanosine preparations (e.g. chewable tablets) are formulated with antacid buffers that are intended to facilitate didanosine absorption by minimising acid-induced hydrolysis in the stomach. These preparations can therefore alter the absorption of other drugs that are affected by antacids (e.g. azoles, quinolones, tetracyclines). This interaction can be minimised by separating administration by at least 2 hours. Alternatively, the enteric-coated preparation of didanosine (gastro-resistant capsules) can be used.

Note that some NRTIs are active against hepatitis B virus as well as HIV (e.g. lamivudine).

(g) Nucleotide reverse transcriptase inhibitors

Tenofovir is a nucleotide reverse transcriptase inhibitor, but therapeutically in HIV it is used like an NRTI, and it is often listed under NRTIs. It is given as the water soluble fumarate salt of the ester prodrug tenofovir disoproxil, and the dose is either expressed as tenofovir disoproxil or tenofovir disoproxil fumarate. Note that 300 mg of tenofovir disoproxil fumarate (US dose) is equivalent to 245 mg of tenofovir disoproxil (UK dose). Neither tenofovir, nor its prodrug are substrates for, or inhibit, cytochrome P450 isoenzymes, and tenofovir is principally eliminated unchanged by the kidneys. Tenofovir is active against hepatitis B virus as well as HIV.

Antivirals active against influenza

The oral neuraminidase inhibitor oseltamivir is metabolised by esterases in the liver, and the carboxylate metabolites are then renally excreted. A clinically relevant interaction with other drugs that affect renal tubular excretion does not usually appear to occur, see 'Oseltamivir + Drugs that affect renal clearance', p.995. It is not metabolised by cytochrome P450 isoenzymes. Zanamivir, the inhaled influenza antiviral, is also not metabolised by the liver and is not protein bound, therefore it is not expected to have any clinically important drug interactions.

1. Williams I, Churchill D, Anderson J, Boffito M, Bower M, Cairns G, Cwynarski K, Edwards S, Fidler S, Fisher M, Freedman A, Geretti AM, Gilleece Y, Horne R, Johnson M, Khoo S, Leen C, Marshall N, Nelson M, Orkin C, Paton N, Phillips A, Post F, Pozniak A, Sabin C, Trevelion R, Ustianowski A, Walsh J, Waters L, Wilkins E, Winston A, Youle M. British HIV Association guidelines for the treatment of HIV-1-positive adults with antiretroviral therapy 2012 (Updated 2013). *HIV Med* (2014), 15 (Suppl 1) 1–85. Also available at: http://www.bhiva.org/documents/Guidelines/Treatment/2012/hiv1029_2.pdf (accessed 25/09/15).
2. Panel on Antiretroviral Guidelines for Adults and Adolescents. Guidelines for the use of antiretroviral agents in HIV-1-infected adults and adolescents. US Department of Health and Human Services (April 2015). 1–288. Available at: https://aidsinfo.nih.gov/contentfiles/lvguidelines/adultandadolescentgl.pdf (accessed 25/09/15).

Aciclovir and related drugs + Antacids

An antacid containing aluminium and magnesium hydroxide did not alter the pharmacokinetics of famciclovir or valaciclovir.

Clinical evidence, mechanism, importance and management

The US manufacturer of famciclovir (a prodrug of penciclovir) briefly notes that no clinically relevant alterations in penciclovir pharmacokinetics were observed when a single 500-mg dose of **famciclovir** was given shortly after an antacid (containing **magnesium** and **aluminium hydroxide**).[1]

On three separate occasions, 18 healthy subjects were given a single 1-g oral dose of **valaciclovir**, either alone or 65 minutes before, or 30 minutes after, they took 30 mL of *Maalox* (containing **aluminium** and **magnesium hydroxide**). The pharmacokinetics of aciclovir (the active metabolite of valaciclovir) remained unchanged.[2]

No special precautions are needed if these antacids are required in patients taking famciclovir or valaciclovir, and the authors of the valaciclovir report also suggest that it is unlikely that other antacids will interact.[2]

1. Famvir (Famciclovir). Novartis. US Prescribing information, April 2013.
2. de Bony F, Bidault R, Peck R, Posner J. Lack of interaction between valaciclovir, the L-valyl ester of acyclovir, and Maalox antacid. *J Antimicrob Chemother* (1996) 37, 383–7.

Aciclovir and related drugs + Cephalosporins

Retrospective data suggest that ceftriaxone might have increased the renal toxicity of intravenous aciclovir in children. Valaciclovir might be expected to have a similar effect. Cefalexin does not appear to alter valaciclovir exposure.

Clinical evidence, mechanism, importance and management

(a) Cefalexin

In a single-dose, crossover study involving 16 healthy subjects, the concurrent use of cefalexin 500 mg and **valaciclovir** 500 mg caused only a minimal mean 7% reduction in the AUC of aciclovir (the metabolite of **valaciclovir**). However, this reduction was only seen if one subject, who had an increase in aciclovir AUC, was excluded from the analysis. Furthermore, there was considerable interindividual variability in the effects of cefalexin.

Both cefalexin and **valaciclovir** are substrates for human peptide transporter 1 (hPEPT1), and *in vitro* and *animal* data indicate that cefalexin might greatly reduce **valaciclovir** absorption.[1] However, the findings in this clinical study showed a minimal interaction. No valaciclovir dose adjustments would appear to be needed on concurrent use.

(b) Ceftriaxone

A retrospective analysis of 17 children who had received intravenous **aciclovir** and ceftriaxone for suspected meningo-encephalitis revealed that all 12 children for whom creatinine concentrations were available developed an increase in serum creatinine (range 109 to 865%), and three of these children developed acute renal failure. The rate of renal toxicity was considered higher than that seen with aciclovir alone, and was attributed to the concurrent use of ceftriaxone. The dose of aciclovir correlated with nephrotoxicity. The authors concluded that caution is required with concurrent use of aciclovir and ceftriaxone and that renal function should be closely monitored.[2] Note that **valaciclovir** is a prodrug of aciclovir, and might be expected to have a similar effect. It would therefore be prudent to follow the same advice as for aciclovir.

1. Phan DD, Chin-Hong P, Lin ET, Anderle P, Sadee W, Guglielmo BJ. Intra- and interindividual variabilities of valacyclovir oral bioavailability and effect of coadministration of an hPEPT1 inhibitor. *Antimicrob Agents Chemother* (2003) 47, 2351–3.
2. Vomiero G, Carpenter B, Robb I, Filler G. Combination of ceftriaxone and acyclovir - an underestimated nephrotoxic potential? *Pediatr Nephrol* (2002) 17, 633–7.

Aciclovir and related drugs + Cimetidine

Single-dose studies have found that cimetidine increases aciclovir and valaciclovir exposure. There is a minor increase in famciclovir exposure when given with cimetidine.

Clinical evidence

(a) Aciclovir or Valaciclovir

Twelve healthy subjects were given a 1-g dose of valaciclovir either alone, or with cimetidine 800 mg (taken 10 hours and one hour earlier). Cimetidine increased the AUC_{0-3} of valaciclovir by 73%, and the AUC_{0-24} of the active metabolite of valaciclovir, aciclovir, was increased by 27%. The renal clearance of aciclovir was reduced by 22%, although the total urinary recovery of aciclovir was unchanged.[1]

(b) Famciclovir

In a study, 12 healthy subjects were given cimetidine 400 mg twice daily for 8 days with a single 500-mg dose of famciclovir, a prodrug of penciclovir, on the last day. The AUC of penciclovir was increased by about 18% by cimetidine, but there was no change in renal clearance.[2,3]

Mechanism

The increase in aciclovir exposure with cimetidine is attributable to a reduction in its renal excretion, probably due to competition for secretion by the kidney tubules.[1] When probenecid (see 'Aciclovir and related drugs + Probenecid', below), a competitor for renal tubular secretion, and cimetidine were given concurrently, the effects on aciclovir were greater than with either drug alone.[1]

Importance and management

These interactions are established but, because aciclovir has such a wide therapeutic index, the authors of the study suggest that its interaction with cimetidine is probably clinically unimportant.[1] It seems likely that no changes in the usual doses of aciclovir or valaciclovir will be needed in patients also taking cimetidine. The US manufacturer of valaciclovir considers that no dose adjustment is necessary in patients *with normal renal function*.[4] However, the UK manufacturer states that caution is required with high doses of valaciclovir.[5] No special precautions would seem necessary if cimetidine is used with famciclovir.

1. De Bony F, Tod M, Bidault R, On NT, Posner J, Rolan P. Multiple interactions of cimetidine and probenecid with valaciclovir and its metabolite acyclovir. *Antimicrob Agents Chemother* (2002) 46, 458–63.
2. Pratt SK, Fowles SE, Pierce DM, Prince WT. An investigation of the potential interaction between cimetidine and famciclovir in non-patient volunteers. *Br J Clin Pharmacol* (1991) 32, 656P–657P.
3. Daniels S, Schentag JJ. Drug interaction studies and safety of famciclovir in healthy volunteers: a review. *Antiviral Chem Chemother* (1993) 4 (Suppl 1), 57–64.
4. Valtrex (Valaciclovir hydrochloride). GlaxoSmithKline. US Prescribing information, December 2013.
5. Valtrex (Valaciclovir hydrochloride). GlaxoSmithKline UK. UK Summary of product characteristics, April 2014.

Aciclovir + Cytarabine

High-dose cytarabine reduces the bioavailability of oral, but not intravenous, aciclovir.

Clinical evidence, mechanism, importance and management

In a study, 5 patients given high-dose intravenous cytarabine 1.5 g/m^2 twice daily for 6 days were given a single 800-mg dose of oral aciclovir, or a single 250-mg/m^2 dose of intravenous aciclovir, one or 2 days before the start of the course of cytarabine, and again on either day 14 or 15. Cytarabine did not affect the bioavailability of intravenous aciclovir. However, cytarabine reduced the maximum serum concentration of oral aciclovir by 43% and the absolute bioavailability of aciclovir was reduced by 38%. The clinical importance of this reduction is not known.[1] Until more is known, bear the possibility of this interaction in mind should a reduced response occur in a patient taking oral aciclovir and given a course of cytarabine.

1. Sitar DS, Aoki FY, Bow EJ. Acyclovir bioavailability in patients with acute myelogenous leukemia treated with daunorubicin and cytarabine. *J Clin Pharm* (2008) 48, 995–8.

Aciclovir and related drugs + Hydrochlorothiazide

Hydrochlorothiazide does not appear to affect the pharmacokinetics of valaciclovir.

Clinical evidence, mechanism, importance and management

In a study in 29 elderly subjects (65 to 83 years old), the pharmacokinetics of aciclovir after administration of **valaciclovir** 500 mg three times daily for 7 days did not differ between the 9 subjects also receiving hydrochlorothiazide 12.5 to 100 mg daily (with or without triamterene) and the 20 normotensive subjects.[1] There would seem to be no reason for avoiding the concurrent use of either **valaciclovir**, or aciclovir, and hydrochlorothiazide.

1. Wang LH, Schultz M, Weller S, Smiley ML, Blum MR. Pharmacokinetics and safety of multiple-dose valaciclovir in geriatric volunteers with and without concomitant diuretic therapy. *Antimicrob Agents Chemother* (1996) 40, 80–5.

Aciclovir and related drugs + Probenecid

Probenecid reduces renal excretion and increases the exposure to aciclovir, valaciclovir, and ganciclovir. Famciclovir and valganciclovir are predicted to interact similarly.

Clinical evidence

(a) Aciclovir or Valaciclovir

Twelve healthy subjects were given valaciclovir 1 g alone, or with probenecid 1 g, taken 2 hours earlier. Probenecid increased the AUC_{0-3} of valaciclovir by 22%, and slightly increased the AUC_{0-24} of its active metabolite, aciclovir, by 48%. The renal clearance of aciclovir was reduced by 33%, although the total urinary recovery of aciclovir was unchanged.[1] An earlier study had found that oral probenecid 1 g caused a similar increase in the AUC of intravenous aciclovir.[2]

(b) Ganciclovir

In a pharmacokinetic study, 11 HIV-positive patients were given probenecid 500 mg every 6 hours with oral ganciclovir 1 g every 8 hours. The AUC of ganciclovir was slightly increased by 53%, and the renal clearance was reduced by 19% (10 subjects only) in the presence of probenecid.[3]

Mechanism

The increases in aciclovir and ganciclovir exposure are attributable to a reduction in their renal excretion by probenecid, probably due to competition for secretion by the kidney tubules.[1,3] The effects on aciclovir of combining probenecid and cimetidine, which also affects the renal excretion of aciclovir, were greater than either drug alone (see 'Aciclovir and related drugs + Cimetidine', p.896).

Importance and management

Although the information is limited to the studies above, the pharmacokinetic interaction between probenecid and aciclovir, valaciclovir, and ganciclovir appears to be established. However, because aciclovir has such a wide therapeutic index, a clinically important interaction is not expected and it seems unlikely that a dose adjustment of **aciclovir** or **valaciclovir** will be needed in patients taking probenecid. However, the UK manufacturer of valaciclovir states that caution is required with high doses of valaciclovir.[4]

The clinical relevance of the slight increase in **ganciclovir** exposure has not been assessed. Nevertheless, the UK manufacturer of intravenous ganciclovir[5] and the UK and US manufacturers of **valganciclovir**,[6,7] a prodrug of ganciclovir, recommend that patients taking probenecid should be closely monitored for ganciclovir toxicity.

The UK and US manufacturers of **famciclovir** suggest that a similar interaction might also occur with probenecid, resulting in an increase in the plasma concentration of penciclovir (the active metabolite of famciclovir), and that patients should be monitored for toxicity,[8,9] with a famciclovir dose reduction if necessary.[8]

1. De Bony F, Tod M, Bidault R, On NT, Posner J, Rolan P. Multiple interactions of cimetidine and probenecid with valaciclovir and its metabolite acyclovir. *Antimicrob Agents Chemother* (2002) 46, 458–63.
2. Laskin OL, de Miranda P, King DH, Page DA, Longstreth JA, Rocco L, Lietman PS. Effects of probenecid on the pharmacokinetics and elimination of acyclovir in humans. *Antimicrob Agents Chemother* (1982) 21, 804–7.
3. Cimoch PJ, Lavelle J, Pollard R, Gaines Griffy K, Wong R, Tarnowski TL, Casserella S, Jung D. Pharmacokinetics of oral ganciclovir alone and in combination with zidovudine, didanosine, and probenecid in HIV-infected subjects. *J Acquir Immune Defic Syndr Hum Retrovirol* (1998) 17, 227–34.
4. Valtrex (Valaciclovir hydrochloride). GlaxoSmithKline UK. UK Summary of product characteristics, April 2014.
5. Cymevene (Ganciclovir sodium). Roche Products Ltd. UK Summary of product characteristics, August 2010.
6. Valcyte (Valganciclovir hydrochloride). Roche Products Ltd. UK Summary of product characteristics, December 2013.
7. Valcyte (Valganciclovir hydrochloride). Roche Pharmaceuticals. US Prescribing information, August 2010.
8. Famvir (Famciclovir). Novartis Pharmaceuticals UK Ltd. UK Summary of product characteristics, October 2013.
9. Famvir (Famciclovir). Novartis. US Prescribing information, April 2013.

Adefovir + Miscellaneous

Adefovir appears to reduce delavirdine and saquinavir concentrations. No pharmacokinetic interaction appears to occur between adefovir and co-trimoxazole, didanosine, ibuprofen, indinavir, lamivudine, or paracetamol (acetaminophen). No pharmacokinetic interaction occurs between tacrolimus and adefovir however, additive nephrotoxicity is predicted between adefovir and tacrolimus or ciclosporin. Drugs that can impair renal function are predicted to reduce adefovir excretion.

Clinical evidence, mechanism, importance and management

(a) Antiretrovirals

In a population pharmacokinetic analysis, the concurrent use of **saquinavir** with adefovir appeared to result in a 49% increase in the clearance of saquinavir.[1] In a further pharmacokinetic study in 37 HIV-positive patients by the same group, **saquinavir boosted with ritonavir** was given with **delavirdine** or adefovir or both drugs, and **saquinavir** with **nelfinavir** was given with **delavirdine** or adefovir or both. The addition of adefovir to **saquinavir boosted with ritonavir** and delavirdine resulted in a 50% lower plasma **saquinavir** concentration when compared to the regimen without adefovir. The plasma concentration of **delavirdine** was reduced by about 50% in patients who also received adefovir. No difference in plasma **delavirdine** concentrations occurred between the **ritonavir**- and **nelfinavir**-containing regimens. The plasma concentrations of **nelfinavir** and low-dose **ritonavir** were unchanged, and the AUC of adefovir was not appreciably affected between the different treatment groups. The authors suggest that the reductions in **saquinavir** and **delavirdine** concentrations might possibly be due to induction of P-glycoprotein by adefovir. As this appears to have resulted in a reduced virological effect in the parent study (ACTG 359), the authors advise against the concurrent use of **delavirdine** and adefovir, and suggest that further study is needed.[2] It would be prudent to use similar caution if **saquinavir boosted with ritonavir** is given with adefovir until further information is available.

The US manufacturer of adefovir reports that, in a study in 21 healthy subjects, there was no pharmacokinetic interaction between adefovir dipivoxil 10 mg daily and enteric-coated **didanosine** 400 mg.[3] For the lack of a pharmacokinetic interaction between adefovir and **lamivudine** or **tenofovir**, see *Lamivudine* and *Tenofovir*, below. However, the US manufacturer states that lactic acidosis or serious liver problems might be more likely if adefovir is used in patients who have been taking nucleoside analogues, such as the NRTIs (they name **abacavir, didanosine, emtricitabine, lamivudine, stavudine, zalcitabine,** and **zidovudine**), or **tenofovir** for a long time.[3]

(b) Ciclosporin or Tacrolimus

In a study in 16 stable liver transplant patients taking tacrolimus 2 to 10 mg daily, adefovir dipivoxil 10 mg daily taken for 14 days had no significant effect on the pharmacokinetics of tacrolimus. Adefovir pharmacokinetics were also unaffected by tacrolimus, when compared with historical data. No appreciable changes in renal function were found during concurrent use in this short-term study.[4]

The UK manufacturer of adefovir predicts that, as ciclosporin is metabolised by the same route as tacrolimus, a pharmacokinetic interaction between adefovir and ciclosporin is also unlikely.[5] However, the US manufacturer states that the effect of adefovir on ciclosporin concentrations is unknown.[3] Both manufacturers[3,5] advise close monitoring of renal function if either tacrolimus or ciclosporin is given with adefovir as both drugs can cause nephrotoxicity, see below, *Drugs affecting renal function*.

(c) Drugs affecting renal function

The UK and US manufacturers of adefovir advise caution and close monitoring of renal function with concurrent use of adefovir with drugs that can affect renal function or cause nephrotoxicity or those that are renally excreted, because impairment of renal function might lead to an increase in adefovir plasma concentrations. They specifically name intravenous **aminoglycosides**, **amphotericin B**, **ciclosporin**, **cidofovir**, **foscarnet**, **NSAIDs**, **pentamidine**, **vancomycin**, and **tacrolimus**.[3,5] This seems a prudent precaution. For the general lack of a pharmacokinetic interaction, and no change in renal function, with concurrent use of **tacrolimus** and adefovir, see *Ciclosporin or Tacrolimus*, above. Also, for mention that **ibuprofen** does not generally appear have a clinically relevant interaction with adefovir, see *Drugs undergoing, or affecting, tubular secretion*, below.

(d) Drugs undergoing, or affecting, tubular secretion

Adefovir is excreted by the kidneys through a combination of glomerular filtration and active secretion via the renal transporter, human Organic Anion Transporter 1 (hOAT1). The potential for pharmacokinetic interactions with **cidofovir**, **co-trimoxazole**, **ibuprofen**, **lamivudine**, **paracetamol**, and **tenofovir** (other drugs that also undergo, or might affect, tubular secretion) has been investigated.[3,5]

1. Co-trimoxazole (Trimethoprim with Sulfamethoxazole). The US manufacturer of adefovir notes that in a study in 18 healthy subjects, there was no pharmacokinetic interaction between adefovir dipivoxil 10 mg daily and co-trimoxazole 960 mg twice daily.[3]

2. Ibuprofen. The concurrent use of adefovir dipivoxil 10 mg and ibuprofen 800 mg three times daily increased the AUC and maximum concentration of adefovir by 23% and 33%, respectively. These changes were considered to be due to higher bioavailability, rather than a reduction in renal clearance, and are not considered clinically relevant. Adefovir did not alter ibuprofen pharmacokinetics.[3] Note that, ibuprofen-induced renal impairment would be expected to increase adefovir concentrations, see *Drugs affecting renal function*, above.

3. Lamivudine. The UK and US manufacturers of adefovir note that, in a study in 18 healthy subjects, there was no pharmacokinetic interaction between adefovir dipivoxil 10 mg daily and lamivudine 100 mg daily.[3,5] For mention of the possible increased risk of lactic acidosis and serious liver problems when adefovir is used with lamivudine, see *Antiretrovirals,* above.

4. Paracetamol (Acetaminophen). The US manufacturer of adefovir notes that in a study in 20 healthy subjects, there was no pharmacokinetic interaction between adefovir dipivoxil 10 mg daily and paracetamol 1 g four times daily.[3]

5. Tenofovir. In a study in 24 healthy subjects there was no pharmacokinetic interaction between a single 10-mg dose of adefovir dipivoxil given alone and on day 7 of tenofovir disoproxil fumarate 300 mg daily for 7 days. In particular, renal clearances of both drugs were not changed on concurrent use.[6] For mention of the possible increased risk of lactic acidosis and serious liver problems when adefovir is used with tenofovir, see *Antiretrovirals*, above. However, note that the UK and US manufacturers advise against the concurrent use of adefovir with tenofovir.[3,5]

(e) Interferons

The US manufacturer of adefovir reports that its pharmacokinetics were unaffected by pegylated interferon alpha-2a. However, the results of a study to investigate the effects of a single 10-mg dose of adefovir dipivoxil on the pharmacokinetics of pegylated interferon alpha-2a 180 micrograms were inconclusive due to the high pharmacokinetic variability of pegylated interferon.[3] The UK manufacturer still advises caution with concurrent use, even though they state that the possibility of an interaction is small as adefovir and pegylated interferons are excreted by different pathways.[5]

1. Fletcher CV, Jiang H, Brundage RC, Acosta EP, Haubrich R, Katzenstein D, Gulick RM. Sex-based differences in saquinavir pharmacology and virologic response in AIDS Clinical Trials Group Study 359. *J Infect Dis* (2004) 189, 1176–84.
2. Fletcher CV, Acosta EP, Cheng H, Haubrich R, Fischl M, Raasch R, Mills C, Hu XJ, Katzenstein D, Remmel RP, Gulick RM, for the ACTG 884 Protocol Team. *AIDS* (2000) 14, 2495–2501.
3. Hepsera (Adefovir dipivoxil). Gilead Sciences, Inc. US Prescribing information, February 2012.
4. Terrault NA, Tran TT, Schiff E, McGuire BM, Brown RS, Tupper R, Ramanathan S, Enejosa J, Zhong L, Zong J, for the Study 531 team. Pharmacokinetics of tacrolimus co-administered with adefovir dipivoxil to liver transplant patients. *Liver Int* (2009) 29, 1178–83.
5. Hepsera (Adefovir dipivoxil). Gilead Sciences Ltd. UK Summary of product characteristics, August 2012.
6. Kearney BP, Ramanathan S, Cheng AK, Ebrahimi R, Shah J. Systemic and renal pharmacokinetics of adefovir and tenofovir upon coadministration. *J Clin Pharmacol* (2005) 45, 935–40. Erratum. Ibid., 1206.

Antiretrovirals + Orlistat

Orlistat might reduce the absorption of antiretroviral drugs.

Clinical evidence

A case report describes a 34-year-old HIV-positive man whose viral load was stabilised at <50 copies/mL on a combination of **tenofovir** 300 mg, **emtricitabine** 200 mg, and **efavirenz** 600 mg daily for about a year, but increased to 722 copies/mL 3 months after taking orlistat for weight loss. Three weeks after orlistat was stopped, his viral load had decreased back to <50 copies/mL. No drug resistance mutations were observed.[1] Another case report in a 39-year-old HIV-positive woman taking **lopinavir** boosted with ritonavir monotherapy, attributes an increase in viral load from 20 to 364 copies/mL to the use of orlistat for 3 months. At the time of the higher viral load, the patient had been admitted to hospital with fever, asthenia, headaches, dizziness, altered visual field, and a stiff neck. She was diagnosed with lymphocytic meningitis and encephalitis, and her lopinavir concentration in cerebrospinal fluid was low, at 9 nanograms/mL.[2]

Mechanism

Uncertain. The authors of both cases suggest that orlistat might have reduced the absorption of the antiretrovirals, resulting in reduced efficacy.[1,2] The exact mechanism behind this is not yet known, but could be a result of the retention of lipophilic medicines in the gastrointestinal tract, or reduced gastrointestinal transit time.[3] Further study to determine the mechanism is required.

Importance and management

Evidence for an interaction between **antiretrovirals** and orlistat is very limited, however, given the potential consequences of reduced antiretroviral efficacy, and in particular drug resistance, some caution on the concurrent use of orlistat with any antiretroviral would seem prudent. Monitoring of antiretroviral drug concentrations if the combination is considered essential would seem sensible. Further, the MHRA in the UK advises that orlistat should only be started after careful consideration of the possible impact it might have on the efficacy of antiretroviral medicines.[3]

1. Kent SJ. Loss of control of HIV viremia associated with the fat malabsorption drug orlistat. *AIDS Res Hum Retroviruses* (2012) 28, 961–2.
2. de Truchis P, Mathez D, Abe E, Dinh A, Ledu D, Greder-Belan A, Alvarez JC. Cerebrospinal fluid HIV-1 virological escape with lymphocytic meningitis under lopinavir/ritonavir monotherapy. *AIDS* (2010) 24, 1235–6.
3. Medicines and Healthcare Products Regulatory Agency and the Commission on Human Medicines. Orlistat: theoretical interaction with antiretroviral HIV medicines. *Drug Safety Update* (2014) 7, A1. Available at: http://webarchive.nationalarchives.gov.uk/20141205150130/http://www.mhra.gov.uk/home/groups/dsu/documents/publication/con392897.pdf (accessed 21/10/15).

Cidofovir + Miscellaneous

Cidofovir with probenecid slightly decreases the exposure to trimethoprim and sulfamethoxazole (co-trimoxazole), and slightly increases didanosine exposure, but does not alter fluconazole pharmacokinetics. None of these drugs altered the pharmacokinetics of cidofovir. Cidofovir (without probenecid) did not alter zidovudine pharmacokinetics. The safety of giving cidofovir with other nephrotoxic drugs (e.g. the aminoglycosides) has not been established.

Clinical evidence

(a) Co-trimoxazole (Trimethoprim with Sulfamethoxazole)

In a study, 6 HIV-positive subjects were given co-trimoxazole 960 mg daily with a single 3-mg/kg dose of cidofovir with probenecid given on day 7. The AUCs and maximum plasma concentrations of both trimethoprim and sulfamethoxazole were decreased by about 30% and renal clearance was increased. The pharmacokinetics of cidofovir were not affected.[1]

(b) Didanosine

In a study, 6 HIV-positive subjects were given didanosine 100 or 200 mg twice daily for 7 days with a single 3-mg/kg dose of cidofovir with probenecid given on day 7. The AUC of didanosine was increased by 60%, but the pharmacokinetics of cidofovir were not affected.[1]

(c) Fluconazole

In a study, 6 HIV-positive subjects were given fluconazole 100 mg daily for 13 days with a single 3-mg/kg dose of cidofovir with probenecid given on day 13. The pharmacokinetics of both drugs were unaffected.[1]

(d) Nephrotoxic drugs

The UK and US manufacturers of cidofovir state that the major dose-limiting toxicity of cidofovir is nephrotoxicity, and that the safety of its use with other nephrotoxic drugs (they name adefovir, the **aminoglycosides**, **amphotericin B**, **foscarnet**, **NSAIDs**, intravenous **pentamidine**, **tenofovir**, and **vancomycin**)[2,3] has not been established.[2]

(e) Zidovudine

The UK manufacturer of cidofovir briefly notes that there was no evidence that cidofovir (without probenecid) altered the pharmacokinetics of zidovudine when intravenous cidofovir was given to 10 patients receiving zidovudine.[3]

Mechanism

It has been suggested that cidofovir with probenecid might alter the renal elimination of co-trimoxazole, didanosine, and fluconazole.[1]

Importance and management

The slight decreases in trimethoprim and sulfamethoxazole exposure, and slight increase in didanosine exposure caused by cidofovir with probenecid are considered unlikely to be clinically relevant because of the infrequent dosing schedule of cidofovir with probenecid. No dose adjustments are considered necessary.[1] Cidofovir does not interact with zidovudine; however, note that cidofovir is given with probenecid, and this does interact with zidovudine. For information on the recommendations for managing this interaction, see 'NRTIs + Probenecid', below.

The concurrent use of cidofovir and nephrotoxic drugs is contraindicated: nephrotoxic drugs should be stopped at least 7 days before starting cidofovir.[2,3] To reduce the risk of nephrotoxicity with cidofovir, it must be given with probenecid, see 'Cidofovir + Probenecid', below.

1. Luber A, Lalezari J, Rooney J, Jaffe H, Flaherty J. Drug-drug interaction study with intravenous cidofovir (CDV) and either trimethoprim/sulfamethoxazole (TMP/SMX), didanosine (DDI), or fluconazole (FLU) in HIV-infected individuals. *Intersci Conf Antimicrob Agents Chemother* (2002) 42, 27.
2. Vistide (Cidofovir). Gilead Sciences Ltd. UK Summary of product characteristics, January 2011.
3. Vistide (Cidofovir). Gilead Sciences, Inc. US Prescribing information, September 2010.

Cidofovir + Probenecid

Probenecid reduces the nephrotoxicity of cidofovir.

Clinical evidence

In a study, 24 HIV-positive patients with cytomegalovirus retinitis were given either a single, oral 2-g dose of probenecid, taken one hour before intravenous cidofovir 5 mg/kg, or the standard licensed regimen of oral probenecid 2 g taken 3 hours before the same dose of cidofovir, with a 1-g dose of probenecid taken 2 and 8 hours after cidofovir administration. No apparent difference in the pharmacokinetics of cidofovir or in the adverse effects of probenecid was reported between the two regimens, and no increase in renal toxicity was seen in the patients given the lower probenecid dose.[1]

The US manufacturer of cidofovir notes that in patients with normal renal function, about 80 to 100% of the cidofovir was excreted unchanged in the urine in 24 hours when it was given without probenecid compared with about 70 to 85% when it was given with probenecid.[2] Probenecid increased cidofovir 3 mg/kg exposure by 29% and cidofovir 5 mg/kg exposure by 44%.[2]

Mechanism

Probenecid inhibits the active renal tubular secretion of cidofovir, and this reduction in the renal elimination of cidofovir reduces the incidence of nephrotoxicity.[1,3]

Importance and management

Probenecid should always be used concurrently with cidofovir.[2,4] The recommended dose of oral probenecid is 2 g taken 3 hours before the cidofovir infusion and 1 g given 2 hours and 8 hours after completion of the cidofovir infusion (a total of 4 grams of probenecid).[2,4] The study[1] suggests that the reduced-dose probenecid regimen might also be beneficial and clinically important in reducing cidofovir nephrotoxicity. However, the authors recommend that further study using the single-dose regimen is needed, particularly with longer treatment courses and in patients with pre-existing renal impairment.[1]

When using probenecid with cidofovir the interactions of probenecid should be considered.

1. Wolf DL, Rodríguez CA, Mucci M, Ingrosso A, Duncan BA, Nickens DJ. Pharmacokinetics and renal effects of cidofovir with a reduced dose of probenecid in HIV-infected patients with cytomegalovirus retinitis. *J Clin Pharmacol* (2003) 43, 43–51.
2. Vistide (Cidofovir). Gilead Sciences, Inc. US Prescribing information, September 2010.
3. Cundy KC, Petty BG, Flaherty J, Fisher PE, Polis MA, Wachsman M, Lietman PS, Lalezari JP, Hitchcock MJM, Jaffe HS. Clinical pharmacokinetics of cidofovir in human immunodeficiency virus-infected patients. *Antimicrob Agents Chemother* (1995) 39, 1247–52.
4. Vistide (Cidofovir). Gilead Sciences Ltd. UK Summary of product characteristics, January 2011.

Enfuvirtide + Cytochrome P450 substrates

Enfuvirtide does not affect the metabolism of dapsone or debrisoquine, and caused a small change in the metabolism of caffeine, chlorzoxazone, and mephenytoin.

Clinical evidence, mechanism, importance and management

A single oral dose of five drugs (**caffeine** 100 mg, **chlorzoxazone** 250 mg, **dapsone** 100 mg, **debrisoquine** 10 mg, and **mephenytoin** 100 mg) was given to 12 HIV-positive subjects before, and after, they were given subcutaneous enfuvirtide 90 mg twice daily for 6 days. Enfuvirtide had no effect on the urinary **dapsone** recovery ratio (a measure of the activity of CYP3A4), plasma monoacetyldapsone-to-**dapsone** ratio (a measure of *N*-acetyltransferase (NAT) activity), or urinary **debrisoquine** recovery ratio (a measure of CYP2D6 activity). Enfuvirtide had little effect (less than 30% change) on the plasma paraxanthine-to-**caffeine** ratio (a measure of CYP1A2 activity), the plasma 6-hydroxychlorzoxazone-to-**chlorzoxazone** ratio (a measure of CYP2E1 activity), and urinary recovery of 4-hydroxy**mephenytoin** (a measure of CYP2C19 activity). Subjects in this study were taking up to three NRTIs in stable doses, and were not taking any NNRTIs or HIV-protease inhibitors.[1]

This type of study is being increasingly used to assess the potential for new drugs to cause clinically important cytochrome P450-mediated drug interactions. The results indicate that enfuvirtide is unlikely to cause clinically important changes in the pharmacokinetics of drugs metabolised by CYP3A4, NAT, and CYP2D6. They also give some reassurance that drugs metabolised by CYP1A2, CYP2E1, and CYP2C19 are unlikely to be significantly affected. No substrate for CYP2C9 was included in this study, but enfuvirtide does not affect CYP2C9 *in vitro*.[1]

1. Zhang X, Lalezari JP, Badley AD, Dorr A, Kolis SJ, Kinchelow T, Patel IH. Assessment of drug-drug interaction potential of enfuvirtide in human immunodeficiency virus type 1–infected patients. *Clin Pharmacol Ther* (2004) 75, 558–68.

Enfuvirtide + HIV-protease inhibitors

Ritonavir and saquinavir boosted with ritonavir minimally increase enfuvirtide exposure. Enfuvirtide appears to slightly increase darunavir exposure, and to cause a minor increase in the minimum plasma concentration of lopinavir boosted with ritonavir. Enfuvirtide appears to increase the minimum plasma concentrations of ritonavir and tipranavir boosted with ritonavir. Although a case of hepatotoxicity has been reported, the overall incidence of hepatotoxicity does not appear to be increased on the concurrent use of enfuvirtide and tipranavir boosted with ritonavir.

Clinical evidence, mechanism, importance and management

(a) Darunavir

In a study, 11 patients taking darunavir boosted with ritonavir stopped enfuvirtide and started raltegravir. Twenty-four weeks later, the darunavir minimum plasma concentration decreased by 18% and the exposure to darunavir decreased by 36%. The reason for this decrease is not known, but it was considered to be possibly due to an enfuvirtide-induced increase in HIV-protease inhibitor concentrations,[1] as has apparently been seen with lopinavir and tipranavir, see below. The apparent slight increase in darunavir exposure with enfuvirtide, if confirmed, is probably not clinically relevant, and no darunavir dose adjustment would be expected to be needed.

(b) Lopinavir

In a sub-analysis of the RESIST study data, the mean lopinavir minimum plasma concentrations in 60 patients taking lopinavir boosted with ritonavir together with enfuvirtide were only 19% higher, when compared with 240 patients taking lopinavir boosted with ritonavir without enfuvirtide.[2] This apparent minor increase in lopinavir plasma concentrations would not be expected to be clinically relevant. Therefore, no adjustment to the dose of lopinavir boosted with ritonavir appears to be needed when it is taken with enfuvirtide.

(c) Ritonavir and Saquinavir

In a study in 24 HIV-positive patients, subcutaneous enfuvirtide 90 mg twice daily was given for 7 days, with either ritonavir 200 mg twice daily or saquinavir boosted with ritonavir 1 g/100 mg twice daily given for the last 4 days. Ritonavir caused a 24% increase in the AUC of enfuvirtide, and saquinavir boosted with ritonavir caused a 14% increase in the AUC of enfuvirtide. These increases in enfuvirtide exposure are not clinically relevant, and so no enfuvirtide dose adjustments appear to be needed on concurrent use with either ritonavir 200 mg twice daily or saquinavir boosted with ritonavir.[3]

(d) Tipranavir

In a study in 55 HIV-positive patients, the mean minimum plasma concentration of tipranavir boosted with ritonavir was reported to be about 50% higher in 27 patients also given subcutaneous enfuvirtide 90 mg twice daily, compared with 28 patients not receiving enfuvirtide. Similarly, the mean minimum plasma concentration of ritonavir was nearly doubled in those patients given enfuvirtide. Two subjects who stopped enfuvirtide had a subsequent decrease in their tipranavir minimum plasma concentrations by about 25% and 50%, respectively, and a patient who started enfuvirtide while taking tipranavir had an increase in tipranavir minimum plasma concentration of about 72%.[4] Similarly, in a sub-study of the RESIST study, median tipranavir minimum plasma concentrations were 31% higher in those taking enfuvirtide.[2] In a study, 9 patients taking tipranavir boosted with ritonavir stopped enfuvirtide and started to take raltegravir. Twenty-four weeks later, the minimum tipranavir plasma concentration was decreased by 51% and the exposure to tipranavir was decreased by 33%.[1]

A patient who had been taking zidovudine 300 mg twice daily, lamivudine 150 mg twice daily, and subcutaneous enfuvirtide 90 mg twice daily for 12 months, developed hepatotoxicity 2 weeks after starting tipranavir boosted with ritonavir 500/200 mg twice daily. When enfuvirtide was stopped for 6 weeks, the patient's liver enzymes decreased by 50%. However, when enfuvirtide was restarted, the liver enzymes began to increase again, so tipranavir boosted with ritonavir was stopped, and the increase in the liver enzymes resolved. An increase in tipranavir plasma concentration caused by enfuvirtide was thought to have led to hepatotoxicity, although no plasma-drug concentrations were measured.[5] However, subsequent data from a sub-study of the RESIST study reported that despite the increases in tipranavir minimum plasma concentrations seen in patients given tipranavir boosted with ritonavir together with enfuvirtide (a median increase in tipranavir minimum plasma concentrations of 31%), no additional increase in the incidence of hepatotoxicity occurred.[2]

The mechanism for the apparent increase in tipranavir concentration with concurrent enfuvirtide is unknown. It is unlikely to be by an effect on cytochrome P450 isoenzymes as enfuvirtide has little effect on these. The available data suggest that enfuvirtide might increase the concentration of tipranavir, although this requires confirmation in a controlled study. The data from the RESIST study suggests that, in most patients, the increase in tipranavir minimum concentrations with concurrent enfuvirtide is unlikely to lead to serious adverse effects. However, due to reports of hepatotoxicity with tipranavir boosted with ritonavir alone, routine close monitoring of liver function is recommended for this HIV-protease inhibitor.

1. Goldwirt L, Braun J, de Castro N, Charreau I, Barrail-Tran A, Delaugerre C, Raffi F, Lascoux-Combe C, Aboulker JP, Taburet AM, Molina JM. Switch from enfuvirtide to raltegravir lowers plasma concentrations of darunavir and tipranavir: a pharmacokinetic substudy of the EASIER-ANRS 138 trial. *Antimicrob Agents Chemother* (2011) 55, 3613–5.
2. Raffi F, Battegay M, Rusconi S, Opravil M, Blick G, Steigbigel RT, Kraft M, Neubacher D, Sabo JP. Combined tipranavir and enfuvirtide use associated with higher plasma tipranavir concentrations but not with increased hepatotoxicity: sub-analysis from RESIST. *AIDS* (2007) 21, 1977–80.
3. Ruxrungtham K, Boyd M, Bellibas SE, Zhang X, Dorr A, Kolis S, Kinchelow T, Buss N, Patel IH. Lack of interaction between enfuvirtide and ritonavir or ritonavir-boosted saquinavir in HIV-1-infected patients. *J Clin Pharmacol* (2004) 44, 793–802.
4. González de Requena D, Calcagno A, Bonora S, Ladetto L, D'Avolio A, Sciandra M, Siccardi M, Bargiacchi O, Sinicco A, Di Perri G. Unexpected drug-drug interaction between tipranavir/ritonavir and enfuvirtide. *AIDS* (2006) 20, 1977–9.
5. Jülg B, Bogner JR, Goebel FD. Severe hepatotoxicity associated with the combination of enfuvirtide and tipranavir/ritonavir: case report. *AIDS* (2006) 20, 1563.

Enfuvirtide + Rifampicin (Rifampin)

Rifampicin does not affect the pharmacokinetics of enfuvirtide.

Clinical evidence, mechanism, importance and management

Subcutaneous enfuvirtide 90 mg twice daily for 3 days was given to 12 HIV-positive subjects before, and during, the last 3 days of a 10-day course of rifampicin 600 mg daily. The AUC of enfuvirtide and its metabolite were not altered by rifampicin.[1]

Enfuvirtide is a peptide and would not be expected to be affected by enzyme inducers such as rifampicin. The findings of this study support this. Therefore no dose adjustments of enfuvirtide are required when it is given with rifampicin.

1. Boyd MA, Zhang X, Dorr A, Ruxrungtham K, Kolis S, Nieforth K, Kinchelow T, Buss N, Patel IH. Lack of enzyme-inducing effect of rifampicin on the pharmacokinetics of enfuvirtide. *J Clin Pharmacol* (2003) 43, 1382–91.

Entecavir + Miscellaneous

Ciclosporin and tacrolimus-induced renal impairment might increase entecavir exposure. Food can slightly decrease entecavir exposure. No pharmacokinetic interaction appears to occur between entecavir and adefovir, lamivudine, or tenofovir. However, interactions with other renally excreted drugs cannot be excluded. No interactions mediated by cytochrome P450 isoenzymes are expected with entecavir.

Clinical evidence, mechanism, importance and management

(a) Ciclosporin and tacrolimus

The UK and US manufacturers of entecavir note that in a few patients with liver transplants receiving ciclosporin (5 patients) or tacrolimus (4 patients), entecavir exposure was 2-fold higher than in healthy subjects with normal renal function. However, they consider that reduced renal function was the main factor for this difference rather than a drug interaction.[1,2] Because ciclosporin and tacrolimus can alter renal function, the manufacturers recommend that if entecavir is required in a patient receiving these immunosuppressants, renal function is carefully monitored.[1,2]

(b) Cytochrome P450-mediated interactions

The UK and US manufacturers state that entecavir is not a substrate, an inducer, or an inhibitor of cytochrome P450 isoenzymes. Therefore drug interactions are unlikely to occur with entecavir by this mechanism.[1,2]

(c) Food

The UK and US manufacturers state that oral administration of 0.5 mg of entecavir with a standard high-fat meal or a light meal delayed entecavir absorption by about 15 to 45 minutes, decreased the maximum plasma concentration by 44 to 46%, and decreased the AUC by 18 to 20%.[1,2] The UK manufacturer states that these changes are unlikely to be clinically relevant in patients who have never been treated with nucleoside analogues, in whom entecavir can be taken without regard to timing of food. However, they state that for patients with lamivudine-resistant or decompensated disease, entecavir should be taken on an empty stomach at least 2 hours before, or 2 hours after, meals.[1] In the US, the advice is always to take entecavir on an empty stomach, at least 2 hours before, or 2 hours after, meals.[2]

(d) Renally excreted drugs

A study in 22 healthy subjects given entecavir 1 mg daily and/or **adefovir dipivoxil** 10 mg daily found no pharmacokinetic interaction.[3] The UK and US manufacturers of entecavir note that there was no pharmacokinetic interaction between entecavir and **lamivudine**, **adefovir**, or **tenofovir** at steady state.[1,2]

As entecavir is predominantly eliminated by the kidney, the concurrent use of drugs that reduce renal function or compete for active renal tubular secretion might increase the serum concentrations of either entecavir or the concurrent drug. However, the manufacturers state that, apart from the drugs listed above, the effects of the concurrent use of entecavir with drugs that are either excreted renally or affect renal function have not been evaluated, and they therefore recommend that patients should be monitored closely for adverse reactions when entecavir is given with any such drug.[1,2] See also *ciclosporin and tacrolimus*, above.

1. Baraclude (Entecavir). Bristol-Myers Squibb Pharmaceuticals Ltd. UK Summary of product characteristics, May 2011.
2. Baraclude (Entecavir). Bristol-Myers Squibb Company. US Prescribing information, December 2010.
3. Bifano M, Yan J-H, Smith RA, Zhang D, Grasela DM, LaCreta F. Absence of a pharmacokinetic interaction between entecavir and adefovir. *J Clin Pharmacol* (2007) 47, 1327–34.

Famciclovir + Allopurinol

Allopurinol does not alter the pharmacokinetics of penciclovir (the active metabolite of famciclovir).

Clinical evidence, mechanism, importance and management

When 12 healthy subjects were given a single dose of famciclovir 500 mg after taking **allopurinol** 300 mg daily for 5 days, there were no changes in the pharmacokinetics of penciclovir (the active metabolite of famciclovir) .[1] It was concluded that xanthine oxidase does not play an important role in the metabolism of famciclovir to penciclovir.[1,2] No famciclovir dose adjustment is likely to be needed if given with allopurinol.

1. Fowles SE, Pratt SK, Laroche J, Prince WT. Lack of a pharmacokinetic interaction between oral famciclovir and allopurinol in healthy volunteers. *Eur J Clin Pharmacol* (1994) 46, 355–9.
2. Daniels S, Schentag JJ. Drug interaction studies and safety of famciclovir in healthy volunteers: a review. *Antiviral Chem Chemother* (1993) 4 (Suppl 1), 57–64.

Famciclovir + Miscellaneous

Promethazine and food do not alter the pharmacokinetics of penciclovir (the active metabolite of famciclovir). Raloxifene is predicted to inhibit the metabolism of famciclovir to penciclovir.

Clinical evidence, mechanism, importance and management

(a) Food

The US manufacturer notes that when a capsule formulation of famciclovir was taken with food, the maximum plasma concentration of penciclovir (the active metabolite of famciclovir) decreased by approximately 50% and the time to maximum plasma concentration was delayed by 1.5 hours. However, there was no effect on the penciclovir exposure (AUC).[1] Therefore, the UK and US manufacturers of famciclovir state that the changes seen are not clinically relevant, and that famciclovir can be taken without regard to the timing of meals.[1,2]

(b) Promethazine

The US manufacturer of famciclovir briefly notes that no clinically relevant alterations in penciclovir pharmacokinetics were observed when a single 500-mg dose of famciclovir was given after pre-treatment with multiple doses of promethazine.[1] No famciclovir dose adjustment would expected to be needed on concurrent use.

(c) Raloxifene

Famciclovir is converted to its active drug, penciclovir, by aldehyde oxidase. An *in vitro* study[3] reported that **raloxifene** is a potent aldehyde oxidase inhibitor, and the UK and US manufacturers of famciclovir predict that raloxifene might affect the metabolic activation of famciclovir.[1,2] However, the US manufacturer also states that other *in vitro* inhibitors of aldehyde oxidase, such as cimetidine (see 'Aciclovir and related drugs + Cimetidine', p.896) and promethazine (see *Promethazine*, above) had no clinically relevant effects on the conversion of penciclovir to famciclovir,[1] and there appear to be no published reports of an interaction in clinical practice. Nevertheless, the UK manufacturer of famciclovir suggests monitoring antiviral efficacy if it is used concurrently with raloxifene.[2]

1. Famvir (Famciclovir). Novartis. US Prescribing information, April 2013.
2. Famvir (Famciclovir). Novartis Pharmaceuticals UK Ltd. UK Summary of product characteristics, October 2013.
3. Obach RS. Potent inhibition of human liver aldehyde oxidase by raloxifene. *Drug Metab Dispos* (2004) 32, 89–97.

Famciclovir + Theophylline

Theophylline caused a minor increase in penciclovir exposure from famciclovir in one study.

Clinical evidence, mechanism, importance and management

In a study in 12 healthy subjects, theophylline 300 mg twice daily for 6 days increased the AUC of penciclovir (the active metabolite of famciclovir) by 22% when a single 500-mg dose of famciclovir was given with the last dose of theophylline.[1] Therefore, no famciclovir dose adjustments would seem to be necessary if theophylline is given concurrently.

1. Fairless AJ, Pratt SK, Pue MA, Fowles SE, Wolf D, Daniels S, Prince WT. An investigation into the potential interaction between theophylline and oral famciclovir in healthy male volunteers. *Br J Clin Pharmacol* (1992) 34, 171P–172P.

Foscarnet + NRTIs

No pharmacokinetic interactions occur between foscarnet and didanosine, zalcitabine, or zidovudine.

Clinical evidence, mechanism, importance and management

(a) Didanosine

In a three-phase study, 12 HIV-positive patients were given 4 doses of intravenous foscarnet 90 mg/kg, 4 doses of oral didanosine 200 mg, and 4 doses of both drugs together. Based on the data obtained from these patients (drug clearance, volume of distribution, half-life, mean residence time), no pharmacokinetic interactions were said to occur between these two drugs. This suggests that no dose adjustments will be needed during concurrent use.[1]

(b) Zalcitabine

Intravenous foscarnet 90 mg/kg every 12 hours and oral zalcitabine 750 micrograms every 8 hours were given to 12 HIV-positive subjects for 2 days. There were no clinically relevant alterations in the pharmacokinetics of either drug.[2]

(c) Zidovudine

No apparent alteration in the pharmacokinetics of either foscarnet or zidovudine was seen in a 14-day study in 5 patients with AIDS given both drugs.[3] The UK manufacturer of foscarnet notes that there was no evidence of increased myelotoxicity when it was given with zidovudine.[4] No special precautions are required on concurrent use.

1. Aweeka FT, Mathur V, Dorsey R, Jacobson MA, Martin-Munley S, Pirrung D, Franco J, Lizak P, Johnson J, Gambertoglio J. Concomitant foscarnet and didanosine; a pharmacokinetic (PK) evaluation in patients with HIV disease. American Society of Microbiology 2nd National Conference on Human Retroviruses and Related infections, Washington DC, 1995. Abstract 492.
2. Aweeka FT, Brody SR, Jacobson M, Botwin K, Martin-Munley S. Is there a pharmacokinetic interaction between foscarnet and zalcitabine during concomitant administration? *Clin Ther* (1998) 20, 232–43.
3. Aweeka FT, Gambertoglio JG, van der Horst C, Raasch R, Jacobson MA. Pharmacokinetics of concomitantly administered foscarnet and zidovudine for treatment of human immunodeficiency virus infection (AIDS clinical trials group protocol 053). *Antimicrob Agents Chemother* (1992) 36, 1773–8.
4. Foscavir (Foscarnet trisodium hexahydrate). Clinigen Healthcare Ltd. UK Summary of product characteristics, May 2012.

Foscarnet + Pentamidine

Marked hypocalcaemia, including one fatality, has been reported in four patients given foscarnet with intravenous pentamidine. Additive renal impairment might also occur on concurrent use.

Clinical evidence, mechanism, importance and management

Four patients with suspected AIDS-related cytomegaloviral chest infections developed signs of hypocalcaemia within 10 days of starting treatment with foscarnet and intravenous pentamidine (doses not stated). All 4 had paraesthesia of the hands and feet, and 3 of them had Chvostek's and Trousseau's signs (signs of tetany). The serum calcium concentrations of 3 of the patients decreased, but normalised when one of the drugs was stopped. The fourth patient had severe hypocalcaemia of 1.42 mmol/L and died.[1]

Both drugs have been associated with hypocalcaemia in HIV-positive patients, and in these 4 patients their effects appear to have been additive. In addition to symptomatic hypocalcaemia, the UK manufacturer of foscarnet also reports that renal impairment has occurred on the concurrent use of intravenous pentamidine.[2] Note that hypocalcaemia is a common adverse effect of parenteral pentamidine and that acute renal failure is very common, whereas the frequency of these adverse effects with inhaled pentamidine is unknown.[3] Therefore close monitoring of calcium concentrations and renal function is advised if foscarnet is used with pentamidine, particularly if used parenterally.

1. Youle MS, Clarbour J, Gazzard B, Chanas A. Severe hypocalcaemia in AIDS patients treated with foscarnet and pentamidine. *Lancet* (1988) 1, 1455–6.
2. Foscavir (Foscarnet trisodium hexahydrate). Clinigen Healthcare Ltd. UK Summary of product characteristics, May 2012.
3. Pentacarinat (Pentamidine isetionate). Sanofi. UK Summary of product characteristics, March 2012.

Foscarnet + Probenecid

Probenecid does not alter the pharmacokinetics of foscarnet.

Clinical evidence, mechanism, importance and management

A study in 10 HIV-positive patients found that probenecid 1 g twice daily for 3 days had no effect on the pharmacokinetics of foscarnet 90 mg/kg given intravenously over 2 hours. The authors conclude that, because of the lack of interaction with probenecid, almost all of the renal elimination of foscarnet is by glomerular filtration, with only a minimal contribution of active tubular secretion.[1] No foscarnet dose adjustment is likely to be necessary if both drugs are given.

1. Noormohamed FH, Youle MS, Higgs CJ, Gazzard BG, Lant AF. Renal excretion and pharmacokinetics of foscarnet in HIV sero-positive patients: effect of probenecid pretreatment. *Br J Clin Pharmacol* (1997) 43, 112–15.

Foscarnet + Quinolones

Two patients developed tonic-clonic seizures when they were given foscarnet with ciprofloxacin.

Clinical evidence

An HIV-positive patient taking multiple drugs (including ciprofloxacin 750 mg twice daily, clarithromycin, cimetidine, fluconazole, morphine, rifampicin (rifampin), and vancomycin) was also given intravenous foscarnet 60 mg/kg every 8 hours for a cytomegalovirus infection. He was only given half of the first dose, but 9 hours later he developed a tonic-clonic seizure. On completing the infusion of the first dose he again experienced similar seizure activity. About 45 minutes after the start of the second foscarnet dose, he had a third grand mal seizure. No further seizures occurred when the foscarnet was stopped.[1] Another HIV-positive patient was given foscarnet 60 mg/kg every 8 hours for 10 days without problem, until he started ciprofloxacin 750 mg twice daily, clofazimine, ethambutol, pyrazinamide, and rifampicin for mycobacterial sepsis. Within 2 days, a few minutes after the start of the foscarnet infusion, he developed a seizure. This resolved when the foscarnet was stopped, and recurred when the foscarnet was restarted.[1]

Mechanism

Both foscarnet and ciprofloxacin have the potential to cause seizures and it seems that some enhancement of this activity might occur if they are used in combination. Subsequent study in *mice* has shown that the combination of ciprofloxacin and foscarnet does increase the likelihood of seizures, and that the interaction is likely to be due to altered GABA-receptor binding. An interaction was not found for enoxacin and foscarnet.[2] However, convulsions are listed as a common adverse effect of intravenous foscarnet, so the cases seen could be due to foscarnet alone. The UK manufacturer of foscarnet states that the reduction of ionised calcium and magnesium is, most probably, the explanation for the seizures seen during, and shortly after, the infusion of high doses of foscarnet.[3]

Importance and management

Direct information seems to be limited to these two cases. It is impossible to know for certain if the seizures were due to the combined effects of these two drugs or not, but the *animal* evidence seems to point in that direction. The general importance of this interaction is uncertain, but it would seem prudent to monitor the patient very closely if these drugs are used concurrently.

1. Fan-Havard P, Sanchorawala V, Oh J, Moser EM, Smith SP. Concurrent use of foscarnet and ciprofloxacin may increase the propensity for seizures. *Ann Pharmacother* (1994) 28, 869–72.
2. Matsuo H, Ryu M, Nagata A, Uchida T, Kawakami J-I, Yamamoto K, Iga T, Sawada Y. Neurotoxicodynamics of the interaction between ciprofloxacin and foscarnet in mice. *Antimicrob Agents Chemother* (1998) 42, 691–4.
3. Foscavir (Foscarnet trisodium hexahydrate). Clinigen Healthcare Ltd. UK Summary of product characteristics, May 2012.

Ganciclovir + Imipenem

The risk of seizures might be increased if ganciclovir or valganciclovir are used with imipenem.

Clinical evidence, mechanism, importance and management

Based on an early possible report,[1] the UK and US manufacturers of ganciclovir and its prodrug, valganciclovir, note that generalised seizures have been reported in patients who received ganciclovir and imipenem with cilastatin. They recommend that ganciclovir and valganciclovir should not be used with imipenem unless the benefits outweigh the risks.[2-4] No further reports of this interaction appear to have been published, or (as of March 2007) reported to the manufacturer.[1] Note that both ganciclovir and imipenem alone can cause seizures.

1. Roche Products Ltd. Personal communication, March 2007.
2. Cymevene IV (Ganciclovir sodium). Roche Products Ltd. UK Summary of product characteristics, August 2010.
3. Valcyte (Valganciclovir hydrochloride). Roche Products Ltd. UK Summary of product characteristics, December 2013.
4. Cytovene-IV (Ganciclovir sodium). Genentech USA, Inc. US Prescribing information, February 2010.

Ganciclovir + Miscellaneous

Ganciclovir and valganciclovir might have additive adverse effects with drugs that also inhibit rapidly dividing cell populations, such as bone marrow. Drug-induced impairment of renal function is likely to reduce ganciclovir clearance and increase its toxicity.

Clinical evidence, mechanism, importance and management

(a) Myelosuppressive and related drugs

The UK and US manufacturers of ganciclovir and its prodrug, valganciclovir, state that it is possible that ganciclovir toxicity might be increased when it is used with other drugs that also inhibit replication of rapidly dividing cell populations (such as bone marrow, testes, and germinal layers of the skin and gastrointestinal mucosa). They specifically name **dapsone**, **pentamidine**, **flucytosine**, **vincristine**, **vinblastine**, **doxorubicin**, **amphotericin B** (see also *Nephrotoxic drugs*, below), trimethoprim/sulfamethoxazole combinations (see 'Ganciclovir + Trimethoprim', below), nucleoside analogues (see 'NRTIs + Ganciclovir', p.973), and **hydroxycarbamide** (**hydroxyurea**). The manufacturers recommend that all of these drugs should only be used concurrently with ganciclovir or valganciclovir if the potential benefits outweigh the potential risks,[1-3] and that patients should be carefully monitored for toxicity.[1,3]

(b) Nephrotoxic drugs

The UK manufacturers predict that the toxicity of ganciclovir or its prodrug, valganciclovir, might be increased if they are used with drugs that might reduce the renal clearance of ganciclovir and hence increase its exposure. They state that the renal clearance of ganciclovir might be inhibited by two mechanisms. The first mechanism is drug-induced nephrotoxicity, and for this they specifically name **cidofovir** and **foscarnet**.[1,3] The US manufacturer of ganciclovir notes that there was a high incidence of impaired renal function in transplant recipients who received ganciclovir in controlled clinical trials, particularly in patients receiving concurrent nephrotoxic drugs, such as ciclosporin (see 'Ciclosporin + Aciclovir and related drugs', p.1205) and **amphotericin B** (see also *Myelosuppressive and related drugs*, above).[2] The second mechanism is competitive inhibition of active tubular secretion in the kidney, which the manufacturers[1,3] predict might occur with other nucleoside analogues (see, for example, 'NRTIs + Ganciclovir', p.973).They recommend that all of these drugs should be used concurrently with ganciclovir only if the potential benefits outweigh the potential risks,[1-3] and that renal function[2] and toxicity[1,3] should be carefully monitored.

1. Cymevene (Ganciclovir sodium). Roche Products Ltd. UK Summary of product characteristics, August 2010.
2. Cytovene-IV (Ganciclovir sodium). Genentech USA, Inc. US Prescribing information, February 2010.
3. Valcyte (Valganciclovir hydrochloride). Roche Products Ltd. UK Summary of product characteristics, December 2013.

Ganciclovir + Trimethoprim

No clinically relevant pharmacokinetic interaction occurs between ganciclovir and trimethoprim. However, there might be an increased risk of myelosuppression on concurrent use.

Clinical evidence, mechanism, importance and management

In a study in 12 HIV-positive subjects, trimethoprim 200 mg daily for 7 days reduced the clearance of ganciclovir 1 g every 8 hours by 13%, and increased its half-life by 18%. Ganciclovir increased the trimethoprim minimum plasma concentration by 13%. None of these changes were considered clinically relevant, so no dose alteration appears necessary on concurrent use.[1] However, both ganciclovir and trimethoprim are known to be myelosuppressive,[2] and the UK and US manufacturers of ganciclovir and its prodrug, **valganciclovir**, note that there is a possibility that the risk of myelosuppression might be increased when trimethoprim, or trimethoprim with **sulfamethoxazole**, are used together with ganciclovir or valganciclovir. Therefore, they recommend that the combination should only be used if the benefits outweigh the risks of treatment.[3-5] Full blood counts should be closely monitored if concurrent use is necessary.

1. Jung D, AbdelHameed MH, Hunter J, Teitelbaum P, Dorr A, Griffy K. The pharmacokinetics and safety profile of oral ganciclovir in combination with trimethoprim in HIV- and CMV-seropositive patients. *Br J Clin Pharmacol* (1999) 47, 255–9.
2. Meynard J-L, Guiguet M, Arsac S, Frottier J, Meyohas M-C. Frequency and risk factors of infectious complications in neutropenic patients infected with HIV. *AIDS* (1997) 11, 995–8.
3. Cymevene IV (Ganciclovir sodium). Roche Products Ltd. UK Summary of product characteristics, August 2010.
4. Valcyte (Valganciclovir hydrochloride). Roche Products Ltd. UK Summary of product characteristics, December 2013.
5. Cytovene-IV (Ganciclovir sodium). Genentech USA, Inc. US Prescribing information, February 2010.

HCV-protease inhibitors + Azoles

Telaprevir increases the exposure to ketoconazole. Itraconazole and posaconazole are predicted to be similarly affected, whereas the effect on the plasma concentration of voriconazole is unclear. Paritaprevir boosted with ritonavir appears to increase the exposure to ketoconazole. Boceprevir is predicted to increase the exposure to ketoconazole, itraconazole, posaconazole, and voriconazole.

Ketoconazole increases the exposure to boceprevir, paritaprevir, and telaprevir. Other azoles might interact similarly. The azoles are predicted to increase the exposure to simeprevir.

Clinical evidence

(a) Boceprevir

In a study in healthy subjects, **ketoconazole** 400 mg twice daily for 6 days increased the AUC and maximum plasma concentration of a single 400-mg dose of boceprevir 2.3-fold and by 41%, respectively.[1]

(b) Paritaprevir

The UK and US manufacturers briefly report that, in a study in 12 healthy subjects, **ketoconazole** 400 mg daily increased the AUC and maximum concentration of a single 150-mg dose of paritaprevir (in a fixed-dose combination with ritonavir and ombitasvir, and given with dasabuvir) almost 2-fold, and by 37%, respectively. The

AUC of ketoconazole was increased 2-fold but there was no effect on the maximum concentration.[2,3] In addition, the UK manufacturer reports that when given without dasabuvir, the paritaprevir AUC and maximum concentration were increased 2.2-fold and by 72%, respectively.[3]

(c) Telaprevir

In a single-dose study in 17 healthy subjects, **ketoconazole** 400 mg increased the AUC and maximum plasma concentration of telaprevir 750 mg by 62% and 24%, respectively.[4] In another study in 81 healthy subjects given telaprevir 1250 mg every 8 hours for 4 doses, a single 400-mg dose of ketoconazole (taken with the fourth dose of telaprevir) increased the AUC and maximum plasma concentration of telaprevir by 21% and 17%, respectively, when compared with a lower dose of telaprevir 1250 mg followed by 750 mg every 8 hours for 3 doses alone.[4]

The UK and US manufacturers report that, in a study in 28 subjects, telaprevir 1250 mg every 8 hours for 4 doses increased the AUC and maximum plasma concentration of a single 200-mg dose of **ketoconazole** 2.3-fold and 75%, respectively, and increased the AUC and maximum plasma concentration of a single 400-mg dose of ketoconazole by 46% and 23%, respectively.[5,6]

Mechanism

Ketoconazole, boceprevir, and telaprevir are all substrates and inhibitors of CYP3A4, and therefore concurrent use would be expected to increase the exposure to both the azole and the HCV-protease inhibitor, which was seen in the studies cited. However, other CYP3A4 inhibitors (such as clarithromycin and some HIV-protease inhibitors boosted with ritonavir) do not affect boceprevir exposure to the same extent as ketoconazole and therefore other mechanisms are probably also involved. With telaprevir, the short duration of the studies mean that enzyme inhibition would potentially not have reached a maximum and so further study is warranted to establish the outcome of longer-term use. Paritaprevir is also a CYP3A4 substrate and ketoconazole therefore increases its exposure. Paritaprevir does not appear to affect this isoenzyme itself, however, it is given with ritonavir as a pharmacokinetic enhancer, and as this is a well-known potent inhibitor of CYP3A4, the effects on ketoconazole seen would seem to be most likely due to the ritonavir.

Importance and management

Boceprevir

A pharmacokinetic interaction between boceprevir and **ketoconazole** appears to be established, although the clinical importance does not appear to have been assessed. The increases in boceprevir exposure with ketoconazole would be expected to result in an increase in its adverse effects. It would therefore seem prudent to monitor for boceprevir adverse effects (such as anaemia, neutropenia, fatigue, and dysgeusia) on the concurrent use of ketoconazole. **Itraconazole**, **posaconazole**, and **voriconazole** are predicted to interact similarly,[7,8] and therefore similar precautions are advisable. Note that boceprevir has been reported to cause prolongation of the QT interval (see 'Drugs that prolong the QT interval + Other drugs that prolong the QT interval', p.272), and any increase in its exposure might further increase this risk.

The effect of boceprevir on ketoconazole exposure was not studied, but it seems possible that ketoconazole exposure might be increased on concurrent use. Until more is known it would seem prudent to also monitor for an increase in the adverse effects of the azole (such as nausea, vomiting, and increased liver enzymes). The US manufacturer states that the maximum dose of ketoconazole or itraconazole given to patients taking boceprevir should be 200 mg daily.[8]

Telaprevir

The slight increases in telaprevir exposure with **ketoconazole** would not be expected to be clinically relevant. Telaprevir appears to increase the exposure to ketoconazole, and the UK and US manufacturers[5,6] predict that the plasma concentrations of **itraconazole** and **posaconazole** might be similarly increased on concurrent use. It would therefore seem prudent to also monitor for an increase in the adverse effects of the azole (such as nausea, vomiting, increased liver enzymes). In addition, the manufacturers state that the maximum dose of ketoconazole or itraconazole should be 200 mg daily.[5,6] The UK and US manufacturers of telaprevir also state that as there are multiple isoenzymes involved in the metabolism of **voriconazole**, it is difficult to predict the outcome of any interaction; however, they advise against concurrent use unless the benefits outweigh the risks.[5,6] Telaprevir has been reported to cause prolongation of the QT interval (see 'Drugs that prolong the QT interval + Other drugs that prolong the QT interval', p.272), and any increase in its exposure might further increase this risk. The UK manufacturer of telaprevir also suggests that any increase in ketoconazole, posaconazole, and voriconazole plasma concentrations by telaprevir might increase the risk of QT prolongation,[5] which could be additive with the possible QT prolonging effects of telaprevir itself.

Paritaprevir

Ketoconazole appears to moderately increase the exposure to paritaprevir (in a fixed-dose combination including ritonavir and ombitasvir, and given with or without dasabuvir), and the UK manufacturer thus contraindicates concurrent use with ketoconazole, and other potent CYP3A4 inhibitors.[3] This would include **itraconazole** and **voriconazole** (see 'Table 1.9', p.11 for a list of known, clinically important CYP3A4 inhibitors). Note that the manufacturer includes **posaconazole** as a potent CYP3A4 inhibitor, but it is generally considered to be moderate inhibitor. Paritaprevir boosted with ritonavir appears to moderately increase ketoconazole exposure and as a result, the US manufacturer recommends that if concurrent use with ketoconazole is required, the dose of ketoconazole should be limited to 200 mg daily.[2] Further, both manufacturers predict that the exposure to **voriconazole** could be decreased,[2,3] although the UK manufacturer suggests that the effect might be dependent on CYP2C19 metaboliser status such that those patients who are CYP2C19 extensive metabolisers (that is, those with normal activity of this isoenzyme) might have decreased voriconazole concentrations, and those that are poor CYP2C19 metabolisers (that is, those with lower than normal activity of this isoenzyme) might have increased voriconazole concentrations.[3] In the US concurrent use with voriconazole is not recommended unless the benefits outweigh the risks,[2] and in the UK the combination is contraindicated.[3]

Simeprevir

The manufacturers of simeprevir predict that because it is a CYP3A4 substrate, its concentrations could be increased by the azoles (although perhaps to varying extents), and they therefore do not recommend concurrent use of **fluconazole, itraconazole, ketoconazole, posaconazole** or **voriconazole** with simeprevir.[9,10]

1. Kasserra C, Hughes E, Treitel M, Gupta S, O'Mara E. Clinical pharmacology of BOC: metabolism, excretion, and drug-drug interactions. 18th Conference on Retroviruses and Opportunistic Infections, Boston MA, February–March 2011. Abstract 118.
2. Viekira Pak (Ombitasvir, paritaprevir, ritonavir co-packaged with dasabuvir sodium monohydrate). AbbVie Inc. US Prescribing information, December 2014.
3. Viekirax (Ombitasvir, paritaprevir, ritonavir). AbbVie Ltd. UK Summary of product characteristics, January 2015.
4. Garg V, Chandorkar G, Yang Y, Adda N, McNair L, Alves K, Smith F, van Heeswijk RPG. The effect of CYP3A inhibitors and inducers on the pharmacokinetics of telaprevir in healthy volunteers. *Br J Clin Pharmacol* (2013) 75, 431–9.
5. Incivo (Telaprevir). Janssen-Cilag Ltd. UK Summary of product characteristics, July 2014.
6. Incivek (Telaprevir). Vertex Pharmaceuticals, Inc. US Prescribing information, October 2013.
7. Victrelis (Boceprevir). Merck Sharp & Dohme Ltd. UK Summary of product characteristics, August 2014.
8. Victrelis (Boceprevir). Merck & Co., Inc. US Prescribing information, July 2014.
9. Olysio (Simeprevir sodium). Janssen-Cilag Ltd. UK Summary of product characteristics, May 2014.
10. Olysio (Simeprevir sodium). Janssen Products, LP. US Prescribing information, November 2014.

HCV-protease inhibitors + CYP3A4 substrates

Boceprevir, paritaprevir boosted with ritonavir, and telaprevir are predicted to increase the plasma concentrations of drugs that are substrates of CYP3A4. Any effect is likely to be most important with drugs that have a narrow therapeutic range (such as ergot derivatives) or drugs that are associated with toxicity if plasma concentrations are increased (such as pimozide). The effects of simeprevir on CYP3A4 substrates appear to be minimal

Clinical evidence, mechanism, importance and management

Boceprevir and **telaprevir** are potent CYP3A4 inhibitors, based on their effects on the probe substrate midazolam. They are therefore predicted to interact with other drugs that are CYP3A4 substrates, see below for details. In contrast **simeprevir** does not appear to affect CYP3A4 to any clinically relevant extent and therefore no interaction with CYP3A4 substrates would be expected. See 'Benzodiazepines and related drugs + HCV-protease inhibitors', p.824 for details of the effects of these HCV-protease inhibitors on midazolam. **Paritaprevir** is itself not a CYP3A4 inhibitor, but it is boosted with the potent CYP3A4 inhibitor, ritonavir, and thus might increase the exposure to drugs that are CYP3A4 substrates.

(a) Colchicine

The UK and US manufacturers[1,2] of **telaprevir**, the US manufacturer[3] of **boceprevir**, and the UK manufacturer of **paritaprevir** boosted with ritonavir (in a fixed-dose combination with ombitasvir, and given with or without dasabuvir)[4] predict that they will increase the plasma concentration of colchicine. The UK manufacturers of **telaprevir** and **paritaprevir**, recommend interrupting colchicine treatment or giving it at a reduced dose,[1,4] and only for a limited course.[1] This would also seem prudent on the concurrent use of **boceprevir**. The US manufacturers of **boceprevir**[3] and **telaprevir**[2] give specific dose adjustments for colchicine and these are the same as for other potent CYP3A4 inhibitors, see 'Colchicine + Macrolides', p.1562, for further details. Note that the concurrent use of colchicine should be avoided in patients taking HCV-protease inhibitors who have renal or hepatic impairment, due to the risk of colchicine toxicity in these patients.[1-3] The use of colchicine with **paritaprevir** in such patients is specifically contraindicated.[4]

(b) Phosphodiesterase type-5 inhibitors

The UK and US manufacturers[1,2] of **telaprevir** and the US manufacturer[3] of **boceprevir** predict that they will increase the plasma concentrations of **sildenafil, tadalafil**, and **vardenafil**, which might result in an increase in adverse effects (such as hypotension, syncope, visual disturbances, and priapism). They contraindicate the concurrent use of boceprevir or telaprevir with **sildenafil** or **tadalafil** when given for pulmonary hypertension.[1-3] For erectile dysfunction, the UK manufacturer of telaprevir also advises against the concurrent use of **sildenafil** and **vardenafil**, but states that **tadalafil** can be given with caution at a maximum dose of 10 mg every 72 hours.[1] In contrast, the US manufacturers of boceprevir and telaprevir advise close monitoring for adverse effects on concurrent use, and state that the following doses should not be exceeded: for **sildenafil**, a maximum dose of 25 mg every 48 hours;[2,3] for **tadalafil**, a maximum dose of 10 mg every 72 hours;[2,3] and for **vardenafil**, a maximum dose of 2.5 mg every 24 hours with **boceprevir**[3] or every 72 hours with **telaprevir**.[2] The UK and US manufacturers of **simeprevir** predict that small increases in the concentrations of **sildenafil, tadalafil**, or **vardenafil** might occur on concurrent use.[5,6] They do not recommend any dose adjustment of any of these drugs when used for erectile dysfunction, but when **sildenafil** or **tadalafil** are used for pulmonary hypertension, they recommend considering starting at the lowest dose of the phosphodiesterase type-5 inhibitor and increasing as necessary, with appropriate monitoring.[5,6] When used for the treatment of pulmonary hypertension, the UK and US manufacturers of **paritaprevir** boosted with ritonavir (in a fixed-dose combination with ombitasvir, and given with or without dasabuvir) contraindicate concurrent use of **sildenafil**.[4,7]

(c) Salmeterol

The UK and US manufacturers of **telaprevir**,[1,2] the US manufacturer of **boceprevir**,[3] and the UK and US manufacturers of **paritaprevir** boosted with ritonavir (in a fixed-dose combination with ombitasvir, and given with or without dasabuvir)[4,7] predict that they will increase concentrations of salmeterol and concurrent use is not recommended due to the risk of cardiovascular adverse effects[1-3,7] (including QT prolongation,[1,2,7]), or is contraindicated.[4]

(d) Trazodone

The UK and US manufacturers[1,2] of **telaprevir**, the US manufacturer[3] of **boceprevir**, and the UK manufacturer of **paritaprevir** boosted with ritonavir (in a fixed-dose combination with ombitasvir, and given with or without dasabuvir)[4] predict that they might increase the plasma concentration of trazodone, which could increase the risk of adverse effects such as hypotension, dizziness, and syncope. They therefore advise caution on concurrent use and suggest that a lower dose of trazodone is given to patients also taking these HCV-protease inhibitors.

(e) Other drugs

The UK and US manufacturers of **boceprevir**, **paritaprevir** boosted with ritonavir (in a fixed-dose combination with ombitasvir, and given with or without dasabuvir), and **telaprevir**[1-4,7,8] predict that they will increase the plasma concentrations of other drugs that are primarily metabolised by CYP3A4, and contraindicate the concurrent use of drugs where an increase in their plasma concentrations could result in serious or life-threatening adverse effects. They name **alfuzosin**,[1-4,7] the **ergot derivatives**,[1-4,7,8] and **pimozide**.[1-4,7,8] In addition, the UK manufacturers of **boceprevir**, **paritaprevir** boosted with ritonavir, and **telaprevir** contraindicate **quetiapine**,[1,4,8] due to the risk of quetiapine-related toxicity, including coma.[1,8] The UK manufacturer of **boceprevir** also contraindicates **halofantrine**, **lumefantrine**, and the **tyrosine kinase inhibitors**.[8] The UK manufacturer of **paritaprevir** boosted with ritonavir (in a fixed-dose combination with ombitasvir, and given with or without dasabuvir) includes **ticagrelor** in its contraindications, and lower doses of **imatinib**, with clinical monitoring, are recommended if given concurrently.[4]

The UK manufacturer of **telaprevir** also advises avoiding the concurrent use of **domperidone**.[1] Note that ketoconazole, a known potent inhibitor of CYP3A4, has been reported to markedly increase the exposure to domperidone, and increase the risk of QT prolongation. As both **boceprevir** and **telaprevir** are also potent inhibitors of CYP3A4, and have both been shown to increase the QT interval themselves, the advice provided by the MHRA (and detailed in 'Domperidone + CYP3A4 inhibitors', p.1140), applies to these drugs also.

1. Incivo (Telaprevir). Janssen-Cilag Ltd. UK Summary of product characteristics, July 2014.
2. Incivek (Telaprevir). Vertex Pharmaceuticals, Inc. US Prescribing information, October 2013.
3. Victrelis (Boceprevir). Merck & Co., Inc. US Prescribing information, July 2014.
4. Viekirax (Ombitasvir, paritaprevir, ritonavir). AbbVie Ltd. UK Summary of product characteristics, January 2015.
5. Olysio (Simeprevir sodium). Janssen-Cilag Ltd. UK Summary of product characteristics, May 2014.
6. Olysio (Simeprevir sodium). Janssen Products, LP. US Prescribing information, November 2014.
7. Viekira Pak (Ombitasvir, paritaprevir, ritonavir co-packaged with dasabuvir sodium monohydrate). AbbVie Inc. US Prescribing information, December 2014.
8. Victrelis (Boceprevir). Merck Sharp & Dohme Ltd. UK Summary of product characteristics, August 2014.

HCV-Protease inhibitors + Eltrombopag

No pharmacokinetic interaction occurs between eltrombopag and boceprevir or telaprevir. It has been suggested that eltrombopag might increase simeprevir concentrations.

Clinical evidence, mechanism, importance and management

A crossover study in healthy subjects given **boceprevir** 800 mg three times daily (26 subjects) or **telaprevir** 750 mg three times daily (26 subjects), for 11 days, with a single 200-mg dose of eltrombopag on day 11, found no effect on the pharmacokinetics of **telaprevir** or eltrombopag. There was a 20% increase in the maximum concentration of **boceprevir** but no effect on its AUC. The time to reach maximum boceprevir concentration also tended to be shorter (1 hour earlier than boceprevir alone).[1] No pharmacokinetic interaction occurs between eltrombopag and telaprevir, and the increase in boceprevir maximum concentration was not considered clinically relevant. No dose adjustment is required for any of these drugs on concurrent use.

For **simeprevir**, the UK manufacturer predicts that eltrombopag might increase its concentration due to inhibition of the organic anion transporter, OATP1B1, which is involved in its hepatic uptake.[2] This requires confirmation, but until such time, it might be prudent to consider an interaction in the case of increased simeprevir adverse effects.

1. Wire MB, Fang L, Hussaini A, Kleha JF, Theodore D. Lack of clinically significant pharmacokinetic interaction between the thrombopoietin receptor agonist eltrombopag and hepatitis C virus protease inhibitors boceprevir and telaprevir. *Antimicrob Agents Chemother* (2014) 58, 6704–9.
2. Olysio (Simeprevir sodium). Janssen-Cilag Ltd. UK Summary of product characteristics, May 2014.

HCV-Protease inhibitors + Endothelin receptor antagonists

A case report describes adverse effects and an increased bosentan concentrations after telaprevir was started. Boceprevir is predicted to interact similarly. The pharmacokinetics of ambrisentan do not appear to be affected by telaprevir. Simeprevir would not be expected to affect the pharmacokinetics of bosentan, but bosentan might increase simeprevir concentrations.

Clinical evidence

A case report describes a 58-year-old man with pulmonary arterial hypertension (PAH), hepatitis C, hepatitis B, and HIV who was admitted with major confusion, blurred vision, dizziness, hypotension, and balance and gait disorders, 17 days after starting **telaprevir** 750 mg three times daily (with ribavirin and pegylated interferon alpha). He was also taking **bosentan** 125 mg twice daily, raltegravir, emtricitabine, and tenofovir. On admission his ALT and AST concentrations were both increased and he had hyperbilirubinaemia. The telaprevir and bosentan (and ribavirin and interferon) were stopped, and 2 days later his neurological symptoms had resolved, and 5 days later his liver function tests were back within the normal ranges. Plasma concentrations of telaprevir and bosentan were measured after the last doses were taken. The concentration of telaprevir was within normal limits, but that of bosentan was about 4-fold higher than previously. Three months later, **ambrisentan** was started for the PAH, and telaprevir (with ribavirin and interferon) was restarted without further problems.[1]

Mechanism

Bosentan is metabolised (at least in part) by CYP3A4, which is inhibited by telaprevir. The concentration of bosentan might increase on concurrent use.

Importance and management

Evidence for an interaction between **telaprevir** and bosentan is limited to this case report, and hence its general clinical relevance is not known. However, as the increase in bosentan concentrations is broadly in-line with the known disposition and interactions of these drugs, some caution on concurrent use would seem prudent, although note that the similarly potent CYP3A4 inhibitor, ketoconazole, caused a smaller increase in bosentan concentration in a study and no special precautions are recommended on concurrent use (see 'Endothelin receptor antagonists + Ketoconazole and other CYP3A4 inhibitors', p.1059). Nevertheless, monitoring for increased bosentan adverse effects (such as flushing, headache, oedema) would seem sensible. Ambrisentan would appear not to be affected.

Bosentan is an inducer of CYP3A4, by which telaprevir is metabolised. Other CYP3A4 inducers, such as rifampicin (rifampin) have been reported to decrease the plasma concentration of telaprevir, see 'HCV-protease inhibitors + Rifampicin (Rifampin) and other CYP3A4 inducers', p.907. The UK manufacturer of telaprevir therefore predicts that bosentan will reduce the plasma concentration of telaprevir (although note this was not seen in the case report), and advises caution on concurrent use, with clinical monitoring [for telaprevir efficacy].[2]

Boceprevir is also a potent inhibitor of CYP3A4 and therefore the US manufacturer predicts that it will increase the plasma concentration of bosentan.[3] Boceprevir is also partially metabolised by CYP3A4, and therefore its exposure could theoretically be decreased by bosentan, however note this has yet to be shown with other known potent CYP3A4 inducers. Until more is known, it would seem sensible to follow the same precautions as for telaprevir.

Simeprevir does not appear to affect CYP3A4 to any clinically relevant extent and therefore no effect on the pharmacokinetics of bosentan would be expected. However, simeprevir is a substrate of CYP3A4 and its exposure could therefore be decreased by bosentan, as has been seen with rifampicin, see 'HCV-protease inhibitors + Rifampicin (Rifampin) and other CYP3A4 inducers', p.907.

1. Lê MP, Gervais A, Le Beller C, Long K, Larrouy L, Papy E, Mal H, Descamps D, Peytavin G. Serious neuropsychiatric adverse effects in a hepatitis C virus/hepatitis B virus/HIV-coinfected patient receiving bosentan and telaprevir. *J Antimicrob Chemother* (2013) 68, 1208–9.
2. Incivo (Telaprevir). Janssen-Cilag Ltd. UK Summary of product characteristics, July 2014.
3. Victrelis (Boceprevir). Merck & Co., Inc. US Prescribing information, July 2014.

HCV-protease inhibitors + Food

Food increases the exposure to boceprevir, paritaprevir, simeprevir, and telaprevir.

Clinical evidence, mechanism, importance and management

(a) Boceprevir

The UK and US manufacturers briefly report that, in a study, food increased the exposure to boceprevir 800 mg three times daily by 60%, when compared with the fasting state. The type of meal (such as high-fat or low-fat), or when boceprevir is taken in relation to the meal (before, during, or immediately after a meal), did not influence the effect of food on its bioavailability. Therefore, boceprevir should be taken with food (a meal or a light snack).[1,2]

(b) Paritaprevir

The US manufacturer briefly reports that, in a study, a moderate-fat meal (about 600 kilocalories, with 20-30% of calories from fat) increased the AUC of paritaprevir (in a fixed-dose combination with ombitasvir and ritonavir, and given with dasabuvir) 3-fold, compared with the fasting state. When given with a high-fat meal (about 900 kilocalories, with 60% calories from fat) the AUC was increased 2.8-fold, compared with the fasting state.[3] Both the US and UK manufacturers advise taking paritaprevir with food, but without regard for fat or calorie content.[3,4]

(c) Simeprevir

The UK and US manufacturers briefly note that, in a study in healthy subjects, the AUC of simeprevir was increased by 61% and 69% when given after a high-fat, high-calorie (928 kilocalories) meal, and a normal-calorie (533 kilocalories) meal, respectively, when compared with intake on a empty stomach. Absorption was delayed by 1 hour and 1.5 hours, respectively, but the type of food did not affect exposure. Simeprevir should therefore be taken with food.[5,6]

(d) Telaprevir

The UK manufacturer reports that a high-fat, high-calorie (56 g fat, 928 kilocalories) meal increased the exposure to telaprevir by 20%, when compared with a standard meal (21 g fat, 533 kilocalories). The exposure to telaprevir is reduced by 73% if it is taken on an empty stomach, by 26% when taken with a low-calorie, high protein meal (9 g fat, 260 kilocalories), and by 39% when taken with a low-calorie, low-fat meal (3.6 g fat, 249 kilocalories), when compared to the standard meal.[7] The US manufacturer also reports that a standard fat meal increased telaprevir exposure nearly 3.4-fold, when compared with the fasting state. They also state that a low-fat meal (as before) and a high-fat meal (as before) increase the exposure to telaprevir about 2.2-fold and 4.3-fold, respectively.[8] The UK and US manufacturers therefore recommend that telaprevir is taken with meals (but not low-fat food[8]) to maximise its absorption.[7,8]

1. Victrelis (Boceprevir). Merck Sharp & Dohme Ltd. UK Summary of product characteristics, August 2014.
2. Victrelis (Boceprevir). Merck & Co., Inc. US Prescribing information, July 2014.
3. Viekira Pak (Ombitasvir, paritaprevir, ritonavir co-packaged with dasabuvir sodium monohydrate). AbbVie Inc. US Prescribing information, December 2014.
4. Viekirax (Ombitasvir, paritaprevir, ritonavir). AbbVie Ltd. UK Summary of product characteristics, January 2015.
5. Olysio (Simeprevir sodium). Janssen-Cilag Ltd. UK Summary of product characteristics, May 2014.
6. Olysio (Simeprevir sodium). Janssen Products, LP. US Prescribing information, November 2014.
7. Incivo (Telaprevir). Janssen-Cilag Ltd. UK Summary of product characteristics, July 2014.
8. Incivek (Telaprevir). Vertex Pharmaceuticals, Inc. US Prescribing information, October 2013.

HCV-protease inhibitors + HIV-protease inhibitors

HIV-protease inhibitors boosted with ritonavir (atazanavir, darunavir, fosamprenavir, and lopinavir) generally cause slight changes in exposure to boceprevir and telaprevir). In contrast, simeprevir exposure is moderately to markedly increased by darunavir boosted with ritonavir, and ritonavir alone. Paritaprevir exposure appears to be slightly increased when given with unboosted atazanavir or darunavir, and moderately increased when given with atazanavir or lopinavir, both boosted with ritonavir. In contrast, darunavir boosted with ritonavir appears to slightly decrease paritaprevir exposure. Minimum plasma concentrations of some of the HIV-protease inhibitors (darunavir, fosamprenavir, and lopinavir, all boosted with ritonavir) are reduced if given concurrently with some of the HCV-protease inhibitors (boceprevir, paritaprevir boosted with ritonavir, or telaprevir), and these changes could be clinically relevant.

Clinical evidence

(a) Atazanavir

1. Boceprevir. In a randomised study, 11 healthy subjects were given boceprevir 800 mg three times daily for 6 days, followed by a washout period, and then atazanavir boosted with ritonavir 300/100 mg daily for 22 days with boceprevir 800 mg three times daily on days 16 to 22. Boceprevir reduced the AUC and minimum plasma concentration of atazanavir (boosted with ritonavir) by 35% and 49%, respectively. Atazanavir boosted with ritonavir had no effect on the AUC or maximum plasma concentration of boceprevir, although it reduced the minimum plasma concentration of boceprevir by 18%.[1]

2. Paritaprevir. The UK manufacturer briefly reports that, in a study in healthy subjects given paritaprevir 150 mg daily (in a fixed-dose combination with ombitasvir and ritonavir, and given with dasabuvir) and atazanavir 300 mg daily at the same time, the AUC and maximum concentration of paritaprevir were increased by 94% and 46%, respectively. The pharmacokinetics of atazanavir were unaffected. When the same regimen was given without dasabuvir, the AUC and maximum concentration of paritaprevir were increased 2.9-fold and 2.7-fold, respectively, and the pharmacokinetics of atazanavir were similarly unaffected.[2] In another study, when atazanavir boosted with ritonavir 300/100 mg daily was given 12 hours after paritaprevir 150 mg daily (in a fixed-dose combination with ombitasvir and ritonavir, and given with dasabuvir) the AUC and maximum concentration of paritaprevir were increased 3.2-fold and 2.2-fold, respectively. The pharmacokinetics of atazanavir were unaffected.[2,3]

3. Telaprevir. In a crossover study in 20 healthy subjects, atazanavir boosted with ritonavir 300/100 mg daily for 10 days reduced the AUC and minimum plasma concentration of telaprevir 750 mg three times daily by 20% and 15%, respectively. Telaprevir increased the minimum plasma concentration of atazanavir (boosted with ritonavir) by 85%.[4] A case report describes a 51-year-old HIV-positive man with hepatitis C who was stable taking tenofovir (for 2 years), emtricitabine, and atazanavir boosted with ritonavir, and was started on telaprevir as part of triple therapy. A few weeks later he experienced progressive deterioration in his renal function, such that 2 weeks after telaprevir was started, tenofovir and emtricitabine were switched to abacavir and lamivudine. At week 4 he was hospitalised for severe nausea, vomiting, and dehydration, and he had elevated liver enzymes and hyperbilirubinaemia. His plasma concentration of atazanavir, taken 60 hours after his last dose, was high at 2.7 micrograms/mL. After re-starting double therapy for hepatitis C [presumably without telaprevir], his HIV and hepatitis C viral loads remained undetectable at 12 weeks.[5]

(b) Darunavir

1. Boceprevir. In a randomised study, 11 healthy subjects were given boceprevir 800 mg three times daily for 6 days, followed by a washout period, and then darunavir boosted with ritonavir 600/100 mg twice daily for 22 days with boceprevir 800 mg three times daily on days 16 to 22. Boceprevir reduced the AUC and minimum plasma concentration of darunavir (boosted with ritonavir) by 44% and 59%, respectively. Darunavir boosted with ritonavir reduced the AUC and minimum plasma concentration of boceprevir by 32% and 35%, respectively.[1]

2. Paritaprevir. The UK and US manufacturers briefly report that, in a study in healthy subjects given paritaprevir 150 mg daily (in a fixed-dose combination with ombitasvir and ritonavir, and given with dasabuvir) and darunavir 800 mg daily at the same time, the AUC and maximum concentration of paritaprevir were increased by 29% and 54%, respectively. The AUC and minimum concentration of darunavir were decreased by 24%, and 48%, respectively, but the maximum concentration was unaffected.[2,3] When the same regimen was given without dasabuvir, the AUC and maximum concentration of paritaprevir were increased about 2-fold, and the AUC and maximum concentration of darunavir were unaffected. The minimum concentration of darunavir was decreased by 26%.[2] In another study, when darunavir 600 mg in the morning and darunavir boosted with ritonavir 600/100 mg in the evening was given with paritaprevir 150 mg daily (in a fixed-dose combination with ombitasvir and ritonavir, and given with dasabuvir), the AUC of paritaprevir was *decreased* by 41%. The AUC and minimum concentration of darunavir were decreased by 20% and 43%, respectively, but the maximum concentration was unaffected.[2,3] In a further study with darunavir boosted with ritonavir 800/100 mg daily and given 12 hours after paritaprevir 150 mg daily (in a fixed-dose combination with ombitasvir and ritonavir, and given with dasabuvir), the maximum concentration of paritaprevir was *decreased* by 30%, but the AUC was unaffected. The AUC of darunavir was increased by 34% and the maximum and minimum concentrations were decreased by 21% and 46%, respectively.[2,3]

3. Simeprevir. The UK and US manufacturers briefly note that, in a study in 25 healthy subjects given darunavir boosted with ritonavir 800/100 mg daily and simeprevir 50 mg daily, all for 7 days, the AUC and minimum concentration of darunavir were increased by 18% and 31%, respectively. The AUC and minimum and maximum concentrations of ritonavir were increased by 32%, 44%, and 23% respectively. When compared with simeprevir 150 mg given alone, the AUC and minimum and maximum concentrations of simeprevir were 2.6-fold, 79%, and 4.6-fold higher.[6,7]

4. Telaprevir. In a crossover study in 20 healthy subjects, darunavir boosted with ritonavir 600/100 mg twice daily for 10 days reduced the AUC and minimum plasma concentration of telaprevir 750 mg three times daily by 35% and 32%, respectively. Telaprevir reduced the AUC and minimum plasma concentration of darunavir (boosted with ritonavir) by 40% and 42%, respectively.[4]

The US manufacturer briefly reports that, in another study in 15 subjects given the same dose of darunavir boosted with ritonavir for 24 days with a higher dose of telaprevir 1125 mg twice daily for 4 days, telaprevir reduced the AUC and minimum plasma concentration of darunavir boosted with ritonavir by 51% and 58%, respectively.[8]

(c) Fosamprenavir

In a crossover study in 20 healthy subjects, fosamprenavir boosted with ritonavir 700/100 mg twice daily for 10 days reduced the AUC and minimum plasma concentration of telaprevir 750 mg three times daily by 32% and 30%, respectively. Telaprevir reduced the AUC and minimum plasma concentration of fosamprenavir (boosted with ritonavir) by 47% and 56%, respectively.[4]

The US manufacturer briefly reports that, in another study in 17 subjects given the same dose of fosamprenavir boosted with ritonavir for 24 days with a higher dose of telaprevir 1125 mg twice daily for 4 days, telaprevir reduced the AUC and minimum plasma concentration of fosamprenavir boosted with ritonavir by 49% and 58%, respectively.[8]

(d) Lopinavir

1. Boceprevir. In a randomised study, 13 healthy subjects were given boceprevir 800 mg three times daily for 6 days, followed by a washout period, and then lopinavir boosted with ritonavir 400/100 mg twice daily for 22 days with boceprevir 800 mg three times daily on days 16 to 22. Boceprevir reduced the AUC and minimum plasma concentration of lopinavir (boosted with ritonavir) by 34% and 43%, respectively. Lopinavir boosted with ritonavir reduced the AUC and minimum plasma concentration of boceprevir by 45% and 57%, respectively.[1]

2. Paritaprevir. The UK and US manufacturers briefly report that, in a study in healthy subjects given paritaprevir 150 mg daily (in a fixed-dose combination with ombitasvir and ritonavir, and given with dasabuvir) and lopinavir boosted with ritonavir 400/100 mg twice daily, the AUC and maximum concentration of paritaprevir were increased 2.2-fold and 2-fold, respectively. The pharmacokinetics of lopinavir were unaffected.[2,3] When the same regimen was given without dasabuvir, the AUC and maximum concentration of paritaprevir were increased 6-fold and 4.8-fold, respectively, and the pharmacokinetics of lopinavir were similarly unaffected.[2] Similar effects on the AUC were seen when lopinavir boosted with ritonavir 800/200 mg daily was given 12 hours after paritaprevir (in a fixed dose combination), both with[2,3] and without dasabuvir.[2]

3. *Telaprevir.* In a crossover study in 20 healthy subjects, lopinavir boosted with ritonavir 400/100 mg twice daily for 10 days reduced the AUC and minimum plasma concentration of telaprevir 750 mg three times daily by 54% and 52%, respectively. Telaprevir had no effect on the pharmacokinetics of lopinavir (boosted with ritonavir).[4]

(e) Ritonavir

1. *Boceprevir.* The UK and US manufacturers of boceprevir briefly report that in a study with low-dose ritonavir 100 mg daily for 12 days, the AUC and minimum plasma concentration of boceprevir 400 mg three times daily for 15 days were reduced by 19% and 27%, respectively.[9,10]

Note, that the dose of ritonavir used in this study was half the usual dose of ritonavir when it is given as a pharmacokinetic booster with other HIV-protease inhibitors. For the concurrent use of boceprevir and HIV-protease inhibitors boosted with ritonavir, see under the individual HIV-protease inhibitors, above.

2. *Simeprevir.* The UK and US manufacturers briefly report that, in a study in 12 healthy subjects given ritonavir 100 mg twice daily for 15 days with simeprevir 200 mg daily for 7 days, the AUC and maximum and minimum concentrations of simeprevir were increased 7-fold, 4.7-fold, and 14-fold, respectively.[6,7] Note that the simeprevir dose used in this study was higher than the recommended dose of 150 mg daily.

3. *Telaprevir.* The US manufacturer briefly reports that, in a single-dose study in 14 subjects, ritonavir 100 mg increased the AUC and maximum plasma concentration of telaprevir 750 mg 2-fold and by 30%, respectively. However, in a multiple-dose study in 5 subjects given telaprevir 750 mg twice daily with ritonavir 100 mg twice daily, both for 14 days, ritonavir *decreased* the AUC and minimum plasma concentration of telaprevir by 24% and 32%, respectively.[8]

In a multiple-dose, parallel-group study, healthy subjects were given telaprevir 750 mg every 8 hours alone (6 subjects), or telaprevir 250 mg twice daily (6 subjects) or telaprevir 750 mg twice daily (5 subjects) with ritonavir 100 mg twice daily, all for 14 days. The addition of ritonavir to these lower doses of telaprevir did not increase the exposure to telaprevir when compared with the standard dose of 750 mg every 8 hours. Furthermore, when ritonavir was added to telaprevir 250 mg twice daily, the maximum and minimum plasma concentrations were 59% and 75% lower, respectively, and when ritonavir was added to telaprevir 750 mg twice daily, the maximum and minimum plasma concentrations were 16% and 32% lower, respectively; both compared with the standard dose of telaprevir of 750 mg every 8 hours given alone.[11] In another study, 14 HCV- and HIV-infected patients stable taking telaprevir (with ribavirin and interferon) and atazanavir boosted with ritonavir 300/100 mg daily (with other antiretrovirals), were switched to atazanavir 200 mg twice daily (without ritonavir). The telaprevir AUC and minimum concentration were 19% and 18% higher, respectively, when taken with atazanavir alone compared with atazanavir boosted with ritonavir.[12]

For the concurrent use of telaprevir and HIV-protease inhibitors boosted with ritonavir, see under the individual HIV-protease inhibitors, above.

Mechanism

Boceprevir, simeprevir, and telaprevir are all, to differing extents, substrates and inhibitors of CYP3A4, and the HIV-protease inhibitors also inhibit and share this pathway of metabolism. The balance of these inhibitor effects are therefore difficult to predict, and in most cases the effect on the pharmacokinetics of these drugs appears to be slight. It is possible that mechanisms other than CYP3A4 might be involved, which could account for some of the larger changes seen in the pharmacokinetics of the HIV- and HCV-protease inhibitors, but this remains to be established. Note that CYP3A4 might only play a small part in the metabolism of boceprevir, however boceprevir is a potent inhibitor of CYP3A4, while simeprevir might be a more sensitive CYP3A4 substrate, but does not appear to affect this isoenzyme to a clinically relevant extent. Paritaprevir is a substrate for CYP3A4, and so its metabolism might be inhibited by the HIV-protease inhibitors resulting in increased exposure. However, it does not appear to affect CYP3A4, but it is given with ritonavir as a pharmacokinetic enhancer. The effect of this extra dose of ritonavir in regimens with HIV-protease inhibitors also boosted with ritonavir appears to be an increased effect on paritaprevir exposure, with the exception of the *decrease* seen with darunavir boosted with ritonavir, the reasons for which are unclear.

Importance and management

Evidence for an interaction between **boceprevir** or **telaprevir** and the HIV-protease inhibitors boosted with ritonavir is limited. Although the changes in exposure seen are generally slight, the reductions in the plasma concentrations of some HIV-protease inhibitors could increase the risk of antiviral failure. The UK and US manufacturers therefore advise against the concurrent use of **boceprevir** with darunavir or lopinavir (both boosted with ritonavir),[9,10] and **telaprevir** with darunavir, fosamprenavir, or lopinavir (all boosted with ritonavir).[8,13] The US manufacturer[10] of **boceprevir** also advises against the concurrent use of atazanavir boosted with ritonavir, whereas the UK manufacturer states that if concurrent use is necessary, it can be reviewed on a case by case basis in patients with suppressed HIV viral loads and with HIV viral strain without any known resistance to the HIV regimen. Nevertheless close monitoring for HIV viral suppression is still warranted.[9]

Telaprevir appears to increase atazanavir concentrations when given with atazanavir boosted with ritonavir. The UK manufacturer[13] therefore advises close monitoring on concurrent use, in particular for hyperbilirubinaemia.

Simeprevir appears to only minimally increase the exposure to darunavir boosted with ritonavir, but darunavir appears to at least moderately increase the exposure to simeprevir, and ritonavir alone markedly increased simeprevir exposure. The UK and US manufacturers therefore do not recommend concurrent use of simeprevir with darunavir boosted with ritonavir, or ritonavir alone.[6,7] Other HIV-protease inhibitors, boosted and unboosted, have not been studied and the UK and US manufacturers do not recommend concurrent use of simeprevir with any of these drugs.[6,7] Other potent CYP3A4 inhibitors (see 'Table 1.9', p.11 for a list) might be expected to interact similarly, and their use with simeprevir is also not recommended.[6,7]

The effect of atazanavir and darunavir, both unboosted, on the exposure to **paritaprevir** boosted with ritonavir (in a fixed-dose combination with ombitasvir, and given with dasabuvir) was a slight increase, but when atazanavir was boosted with ritonavir, the increase was greater (moderate). When darunavir was boosted with ritonavir, there was a slight *decrease* in paritaprevir exposure. As a result, the UK and US manufacturers of paritaprevir boosted with ritonavir recommend that atazanavir is given without ritonavir, as a 300 mg dose at the same time as the combination.[2,3] No paritaprevir dose adjustment is required, and the UK manufacturer also advises that use of atazanavir and the combination without dasabuvir is not recommended.[2] The UK manufacturer gives the same advice for darunavir as it does for atazanavir, in that it should be used unboosted, and given at the same time as the combination. The recommended dose of darunavir is 800 mg daily. Further, they state that darunavir should only be used in the absence of extensive protease inhibitor resistance, and not without dasabuvir.[2] The US manufacturer advises that concurrent use of darunavir boosted with ritonavir is not recommended (due to decreased darunavir minimum concentrations).[3] Concurrent use of lopinavir boosted with ritonavir is also not recommended by the US manufacturer (due to increased paritaprevir concentrations),[3] whilst the UK manufacturer contraindicates use of lopinavir boosted with ritonavir, as well as **indinavir**, **saquinavir**, and **tipranavir**.[2]

1. Hulskotte EG, Feng HP, Xuan F, van Zutven MG, Treitel MA, Hughes EA, O'Mara E, Youngberg SP, Wagner JA, Butterton JR. Pharmacokinetic interactions between the Hepatitis C virus protease inhibitor boceprevir and ritonavir-boosted HIV-1 protease inhibitors atazanavir, darunavir, and lopinavir. *Clin Infect Dis* (2013) 56, 718–26.
2. Viekirax (Ombitasvir, paritaprevir, ritonavir). AbbVie Ltd. UK Summary of product characteristics, January 2015.
3. Viekira Pak (Ombitasvir, paritaprevir, ritonavir co-packaged with dasabuvir sodium monohydrate). AbbVie Inc. US Prescribing information, December 2014.
4. van Heeswijk R, Vandevoorde A, Boogaerts G, Vangeneugden T, de Paepe E, Polo R, Van Solingen-Ristea R, de Backer K, Garg V, Beumont M. Pharmacokinetic interactions between ARV agents and the investigational HCV protease inhibitor TVR in healthy volunteers. 18th Conference on Retroviruses and Opportunistic Infections, Boston WA, March 2011. Abstract 119.
5. Van den Eynde E, Ferrer E, Podzamczer D. Acute renal failure and liver toxicity in an HIV/hepatitis C coinfected patient receiving telaprevir and boosted atazanavir. *AIDS* (2014) 28, 1538–9.
6. Olysio (Simeprevir sodium). Janssen-Cilag Ltd. UK Summary of product characteristics, May 2014.
7. Olysio (Simeprevir sodium). Janssen Products, LP. US Prescribing information, November 2014.
8. Incivek (Telaprevir). Vertex Pharmaceuticals, Inc. US Prescribing information, October 2013.
9. Victrelis (Boceprevir). Merck Sharp & Dohme Ltd. UK Summary of product characteristics, August 2014.
10. Victrelis (Boceprevir). Merck & Co., Inc. US Prescribing information, July 2014.
11. Garg V, Luo X, McNair L, van Heeswijk R, Kauffman RS. The effect of low-dose ritonavir on the pharmacokinetics of the investigational HCV protease inhibitor telaprevir in healthy volunteers. 18th Conference on Retroviruses and Opportunistic Infections, Boston WA, March 2011. Abstract 629.
12. Gutierrez-Valencia A, Ruiz-Valderas R, Torres-Cornejo A, Viciana P, Espinosa N, Castillo-Ferrando JR, Lopez-Cortes LF. Role of ritonavir in the drug interactions between telaprevir and ritonavir-boosted atazanavir. *Clin Infect Dis* (2014) 58, 268–73.
13. Incivo (Telaprevir). Janssen-Cilag Ltd. UK Summary of product characteristics, July 2014.

HCV-Protease inhibitors + Macrolides

Clarithromycin slightly increased boceprevir exposure. Erythromycin appears to markedly increase the exposure to simeprevir; clarithromycin and telithromycin are predicted to affect simeprevir similarly. Erythromycin, clarithromycin, and telithromycin are predicted to increase the concentrations of paritaprevir boosted with ritonavir and of telaprevir. Simeprevir appears to slightly increase the exposure to erythromycin. Boceprevir is predicted to increase the exposure to clarithromycin, and paritaprevir boosted with ritonavir and telaprevir are predicted to increase the exposure to erythromycin, clarithromycin, and telithromycin.

Clinical evidence

(a) Boceprevir

A study in healthy subjects briefly reports that **clarithromycin** (given with diflunisal, see under *NSAIDs* in 'HCV-protease inhibitors; Boceprevir + Miscellaneous', p.909), increased the AUC of boceprevir by 21%.[1] The US manufacturer predicts that boceprevir might increase the plasma concentration of **clarithromycin**.[2]

(b) Paritaprevir

The UK manufacturer predicts that the paritaprevir concentration might be increased by **erythromycin**, **clarithromycin**, and **telithromycin**. They also predict that the concentrations of these macrolides might also be increased.[3]

(c) Simeprevir

The UK and US manufacturers briefly note that, in a study in 24 healthy subjects given simeprevir 150 mg daily with **erythromycin** 750 mg three times daily, both for 7 days, the maximum concentration and AUC of simeprevir were increased 4.5- and 7.5-fold, respectively. The minimum concentration was increased 12.7-fold. The maximum concentration and AUC of **erythromycin** were increased by 60% and 90%, respectively. The minimum concentration was increased 3-fold. They also predict that the concentrations of simeprevir might be increased by **clarithromycin** and **telithromycin**.[4,5]

(d) Telaprevir

The UK and US manufacturers of telaprevir predict that the plasma telaprevir concentration might be increased by **clarithromycin**, **erythromycin**, and **telithro-**

mycin. They also predict that the plasma concentrations of **clarithromycin**, **erythromycin**, and **telithromycin** might be increased by telaprevir.[6,7]

Mechanism

The HCV-protease inhibitors and the macrolides are substrates and inhibitors of CYP3A4, to varying extents. Note that CYP3A4 might only play a small part in the metabolism of boceprevir, simeprevir does not appear to affect this isoenzyme to a clinically relevant extent, and paritaprevir has no effect on this isoenzyme. The US manufacturer of simeprevir also suggests possible involvement of P-glycoprotein in the interaction with erythromycin,[5] as does the UK manufacturer of paritaprevir boosted with ritonavir (in a fixed-dose combination) for the interaction with all the macrolides named.[3] Note however, that the proposed CYP3A4 and P-glycoprotein effects for paritaprevir boosted with ritonavir could be due to ritonavir alone, as this is a well-known inhibitor of both these pathways. Concurrent use would be expected to result in increased exposure to both the macrolide and the HCV-protease inhibitor, but this has not been fully studied, and warrants further research.

Importance and management

Evidence for an interaction between the HCV-protease inhibitors and macrolides is very limited. The negligible increase in **boceprevir** exposure seen in the study,[1] would not be expected to be clinically relevant. The US manufacturer of boceprevir advises that in patients with normal renal function, no **clarithromycin** dose adjustment is necessary if it is given to patients taking boceprevir.[2] Although in patients with renal impairment, it would seem prudent to consider monitoring concurrent use for clarithromycin adverse effects.

The increase in **simeprevir** exposure seen with **erythromycin** was marked, and the UK and US manufacturers therefore advise that concurrent use of these drugs is not recommended. They also extend this to the use of **clarithromycin** and **telithromycin**,[4,5] which would seem prudent given that they are generally considered to be more potent inhibitors of CYP3A4 than erythromycin and could have even greater effects. **Azithromycin** is predicted not to interact with simeprevir and no dose adjustment is necessary.[4] Erythromycin is generally considered a moderate inhibitor of CYP3A4, and therefore other moderate inhibitors might be expected to interact similarly (although the effect might not be as great as that seen here with erythromycin, given the possible involvement of P-glycoprotein also), see 'Table 1.9', p.11 for a list. Their concurrent use with simeprevir is also not recommended.[4,5]

The UK and US manufacturers of **telaprevir** state that monitoring is required on concurrent use with **erythromycin**, **clarithromycin**, and **telithromycin** due to the risk of increased concentrations of any of these drugs.[6,7]

The UK manufacturer of **paritaprevir** boosted with ritonavir (in a fixed-dose combination with ombitasvir, and given with or without dasabuvir) contraindicates use with **clarithromycin** and **telithromycin**, and cautions use with **erythromycin**.[3]

Note that boceprevir and telaprevir, have been associated with QT prolongation, as have clarithromycin and erythromycin; therefore any increases in their plasma concentrations might increase this risk. For further information about the risks of QT prolongation, see 'Drugs that prolong the QT interval + Other drugs that prolong the QT interval', p.272.

1. Kasserra C, Hughes E, Treitel M, Gupta S, O'Mara E. Clinical pharmacology of BOC: metabolism, excretion, and drug-drug interactions. 18th Conference on Retroviruses and Opportunistic Infections, Boston MA, February–March 2011. Abstract 118.
2. Victrelis (Boceprevir). Merck & Co., Inc. US Prescribing information, July 2014.
3. Viekirax (Ombitasvir, paritaprevir, ritonavir). AbbVie Ltd. UK Summary of product characteristics, January 2015.
4. Olysio (Simeprevir sodium). Janssen-Cilag Ltd. UK Summary of product characteristics, May 2014.
5. Olysio (Simeprevir sodium). Janssen Products, LP. US Prescribing information, November 2014.
6. Incivo (Telaprevir). Janssen-Cilag Ltd. UK Summary of product characteristics, July 2014.
7. Incivek (Telaprevir). Vertex Pharmaceuticals, Inc. US Prescribing information, October 2013.

HCV-protease inhibitors + NNRTIs

The concurrent use of telaprevir and efavirenz appears to slightly decrease the exposure to both drugs. Efavirenz appears to cause a small decrease in the minimum plasma concentration of boceprevir, and boceprevir appears to cause a negligible increase in the exposure to efavirenz. Simeprevir appears to have no effect on the exposure of efavirenz, but efavirenz moderately decreased exposure to simeprevir. Etravirine had no effect on the exposure to boceprevir, but boceprevir caused a slight decrease in exposure to etravirine. Telaprevir exposure was negligibly decreased by etravirine, but telaprevir had no effect on etravirine exposure. Rilpivirine appears to have no effect on the exposure of boceprevir, paritaprevir boosted with ritonavir (in a fixed-dose combination), simeprevir, or telaprevir, and simeprevir appears to have no effect on exposure to rilpivirine. Boceprevir and telaprevir appear to slightly increase the exposure to rilpivirine, but paritaprevir boosted with ritonavir (in a fixed-dose combination) appears to moderately increase it.

Clinical evidence

(a) Efavirenz

1. Boceprevir. The UK and US manufacturers of boceprevir briefly report that, in a study, efavirenz 600 mg daily for 16 days decreased the AUC and minimum plasma concentration of boceprevir 800 mg three times daily (taken for 6 days) by 19% and 44%, respectively. Boceprevir increased the AUC and maximum plasma concentration of efavirenz by 20% and 11%, respectively.[1,2]

2. Simeprevir. The UK and US manufacturers briefly note that, in a study in 23 healthy subjects given efavirenz 600 mg daily with simeprevir 150 mg daily, both for 14 days, the AUC, and minimum and maximum concentrations of simeprevir were decreased by 71%, 91%, and 51%, respectively. There was no effect on the pharmacokinetics of efavirenz.[3,4]

3. Telaprevir. In a study in 21 subjects, efavirenz 600 mg daily for 20 days decreased the AUC and minimum plasma concentration of telaprevir 750 mg three times daily (taken for 10 days from day 11 to 20) by 26% and 47%, respectively, but had no effect on its maximum plasma concentration. Telaprevir had no effect on the pharmacokinetics of efavirenz.[5] In a crossover study, 20 healthy subjects were given telaprevir 750 mg every 8 hours for 7 days, followed, after a washout period, by efavirenz 600 mg daily with tenofovir 300 mg daily for 7 days, followed by telaprevir 1125 mg every 8 hours or 1500 mg every 12 hours with the same dose of efavirenz and tenofovir. When given with efavirenz and tenofovir, the AUCs of telaprevir 1125 mg and 1500 mg were 18% and 20% lower, respectively, and the minimum plasma concentrations were 25% and 48% lower, respectively, when compared with telaprevir 750 mg alone. In addition, the AUC of efavirenz was found to be 18% lower on the concurrent use of efavirenz and tenofovir with telaprevir 1125 mg or 1500 mg, when compared with efavirenz and tenofovir alone.[6]

(b) Etravirine

1. Boceprevir. In a crossover study in 20 healthy subjects, etravirine 200 mg twice daily for 11 to 14 days had no effect on the pharmacokinetics of boceprevir 800 mg three times daily (also taken for 11 to 14 days). The AUC, and minimum and maximum concentrations of etravirine were decreased by 23%, 29% and 24%, respectively.[7]

2. Telaprevir. The UK manufacturer briefly notes that, in a study in healthy subjects given etravirine with telaprevir 750 mg three times daily, the AUC and minimum concentration of telaprevir were decreased by 16% and 25%, respectively but the pharmacokinetics of etravirine were unaffected.[8]

(c) Rilpivirine

1. Boceprevir. The UK and US manufacturers briefly note that, in a study in healthy subjects or subjects with hepatitis C given rilpivirine 25 mg daily with boceprevir 800 mg three times daily, for 11 days the pharmacokinetics of boceprevir were unaffected. The AUC, and minimum and maximum concentrations of rilpivirine were increased by 39%, 51% and 15%, respectively.[1,2]

2. Paritaprevir. The UK and US manufacturers briefly report that, in a study in 10 healthy subjects, rilpivirine 25 mg daily had no effect on the AUC and maximum concentration of paritaprevir 150 mg (in a fixed-dose combination with ritonavir and ombitasvir, and given with dasabuvir). The AUC and maximum concentration of rilpivirine (based on data from 8 subjects) were increased 3.3-fold and 2.6-fold, respectively.[9,10]

3. Simeprevir. The UK and US manufacturers briefly note that, in a study in 23 healthy subjects given rilpivirine 25 mg daily with simeprevir 150 mg daily for 11 days, the pharmacokinetics of both drugs were unaffected, with the exception of the minimum concentration of rilpivirine which was increased by 25%.[3,4]

4. Telaprevir. The UK manufacturer briefly notes that, in a study in subjects given rilpivirine with telaprevir 750 mg three times daily, the pharmacokinetics of telaprevir were unaffected. The AUC and minimum and maximum concentrations of rilpivirine were increased by 78%, 93%, and 49%, respectively.[8]

Mechanism

Efavirenz and etravirine are substrates and inducers of CYP3A4, and telaprevir, boceprevir, and simeprevir are substrates and inhibitors of CYP3A4, although all to varying degrees. Paritaprevir is also a substrate of CYP3A4. The metabolism of boceprevir, simeprevir, and telaprevir is increased by efavirenz, leading to a decrease in their exposure. However, etravirine did not affect boceprevir and minimally decreased telaprevir exposure, most likely because this is only a weak inducer. The metabolism of efavirenz and etravirine might be expected to be reduced by boceprevir and telaprevir, but in the studies this was only the case with boceprevir and efavirenz. The reason for the opposite effect on efavirenz seen with telaprevir, and the opposite and lack of effect on etravirine seen with boceprevir and telaprevir, respectively, is not known. Rilpivirine is also a substrate of CYP3A4, but does not appear to have any clinically relevant effects on CYP3A4, which was demonstrated by the lack of effect on all the HCV-protease inhibitors. Its exposure was increased by boceprevir, paritaprevir, and telaprevir, but not by simeprevir which most likely reflects the apparent lack of a clinically important effect of simeprevir on CYP3A4. Note also, that paritaprevir itself does not affect CYP3A4, but it is given with ritonavir (a well-known potent inhibitor of CYP3A4) as a pharmacokinetic enhancer, therefore the effects on rilpivirine seen when it was given with paritaprevir (in a fixed-dose combination with ritonavir and ombitasvir, and given with dasabuvir) would seem to be most likely due to the ritonavir.

Importance and management

The evidence for a pharmacokinetic interaction between the HCV-protease inhibitors and the NNRTIs is limited to a few studies, the results of which include some inconsistencies. Nevertheless, the interactions seen are broadly in line with the known disposition and interactions of these groups of drugs. The clinical implications of the effects seen are generally unclear.

The reduction in telaprevir exposure with **efavirenz** is slight, and until more is known, it would seem prudent to monitor concurrent use for a reduction in telaprevir efficacy. The UK manufacturer specifically advises that the dose of telaprevir should be increased to 1125 mg three times daily on concurrent use with efavirenz,[8] whereas the US manufacturer does not give any advice on adjusting the telaprevir dose.[11] The UK manufacturer of boceprevir comments that the clinical relevance of the reduction in the boceprevir minimum plasma concentration when given with **efavirenz** has not been assessed,[1] whereas the US manufacturer states that, as this could possibly result in a reduction in the antiviral effects of boceprevir, concurrent use of boceprevir and efavirenz should be avoided.[2] The UK and US manufacturers of simeprevir advise that the decrease in exposure seen with **efavirenz** could result in a reduced therapeutic effect and thus do not recommend concurrent use.[3,4] The UK and US manufacturers note that concurrent use of efavirenz-based regimens with paritaprevir boosted with ritonavir (in a fixed-dose combination with ombitasvir) and given with dasabuvir resulted in ALT increases which necessitated early discontinuation of the interaction study. As a result concurrent use with efavirenz is contraindicated.[9,10] Efavirenz might also be predicted to decrease paritaprevir exposure, such that therapeutic efficacy is reduced. For this reason, other moderate, and potent CYP3A4 inducers are also contraindicated by the UK manufacturer.[10] See 'Table 1.9', p.11 for a list of known, clinically important CYP3A4 inducers. Note that the UK manufacturer also names **etravirine** (which generally has only minor effects) and **mitotane** (which is not considered a clinically relevant enzyme inducer).[10]

As **etravirine** had no effect on boceprevir pharmacokinetics, and caused only a slight decrease in telaprevir exposure, no dose adjustment would seem necessary on concurrent use. Data for simeprevir are lacking, although note that the UK and US manufacturers advise against concurrent use.[3,4]

Rilpivirine had no effect on the pharmacokinetics of boceprevir, paritaprevir, simeprevir, or telaprevir, and simeprevir had no clinically relevant effect on the pharmacokinetics of rilpivirine. The slight increases in rilpivirine exposure seen with boceprevir and telaprevir would not be expected to be clinically important, and so no dose adjustments would seem necessary on concurrent use of rilpivirine with either of these HCV-protease inhibitors. In contrast, the moderate increase in rilpivirine exposure seen with paritaprevir boosted with ritonavir (in a fixed-dose combination with ombitasvir, and given with dasabuvir) is predicted to be clinically important due to the potential for QT-interval prolongation with higher concentrations of rilpivirine, and concurrent use of these two drugs is therefore not recommended by the US manufacturer.[9] The UK manufacturer advises that concurrent use of paritaprevir boosted with ritonavir and rilpivirine should only be considered in patients without known QT-interval prolongation, without other drugs known to prolong the QT interval (see 'Table 9.2', p.273 for a list), and without the concurrent use of HIV-protease inhibitors. If the combination is used, repeated ECG monitoring is required.[10]

Note that **nevirapine** is also known to induce CYP3A4, and **delavirdine** is known to inhibit CYP3A4. These NNRTIs might therefore be expected to alter the exposure to boceprevir, paritaprevir, simeprevir, and telaprevir. Until more is known, it would seem prudent to consider the possibility of an interaction on the concurrent use of these drugs. Note that the UK and US manufacturers of simeprevir specifically advise against concurrent use with nevirapine and delavirdine.[3,4]

The small changes in efavirenz and etravirine exposure do not appear to have been assessed, but would not be expected to be clinically relevant, and no dose adjustment would seem necessary on concurrent use. However, the UK manufacturer of boceprevir recommends increased monitoring of HIV suppression on concurrent use with etravirine.[1]

1. Victrelis (Boceprevir). Merck Sharp & Dohme Ltd. UK Summary of product characteristics, August 2014.
2. Victrelis (Boceprevir). Merck & Co., Inc. US Prescribing information, July 2014.
3. Olysio (Simeprevir sodium). Janssen-Cilag Ltd. UK Summary of product characteristics, May 2014.
4. Olysio (Simeprevir sodium). Janssen Products, LP. US Prescribing information, November 2014.
5. Garg V, Chandorkar G, Yang Y, Adda N, McNair L, Alves K, Smith F, van Heeswijk RPG. The effect of CYP3A inhibitors and inducers on the pharmacokinetics of telaprevir in healthy volunteers. *Br J Clin Pharmacol* (2013) 75, 431–9.
6. van Heeswijk R, Vandevoorde A, Boogaerts G, Vangeneugden T, de Paepe E, Polo R, Van Solingen-Ristea R, de Backer K, Garg V, Beumont M. Pharmacokinetic interactions between ARV agents and the investigational HCV protease inhibitor TVR in healthy volunteers. 18th Conference on Retroviruses and Opportunistic Infections, Seattle WA, March 2011. Abstract 119.
7. Hammond KP, Wolfe P, Burton JR, Predhomme JA, Ellis CM, Ray ML, Bushman LR, Kiser JJ. Pharmacokinetic interaction between boceprevir and etravirine in HIV/HCV seronegative volunteers. *J Acquir Immune Defic Syndr* (2013) 62, 67–73.
8. Incivo (Telaprevir). Janssen-Cilag Ltd. UK Summary of product characteristics, July 2014.
9. Viekira Pak (Ombitasvir, paritaprevir, ritonavir co-packaged with dasabuvir sodium monohydrate). AbbVie Inc. US Prescribing information, December 2014.
10. Viekirax (Ombitasvir, paritaprevir, ritonavir). AbbVie Ltd. UK Summary of product characteristics, January 2015.
11. Incivek (Telaprevir). Vertex Pharmaceuticals, Inc. US Prescribing information, October 2013.

HCV-Protease inhibitors + Proton pump inhibitors

No pharmacokinetic interaction appears to occur between boceprevir and omeprazole, or telaprevir and esomeprazole. The pharmacokinetics of simeprevir and omeprazole appeared to be unaffected by concurrent use in a study. The exposure to other proton pump inhibitors would not be expected to be affected by simeprevir. The pharmacokinetics of paritaprevir boosted with ritonavir (in a fixed-dose combination) are not altered by omeprazole, but exposure to omeprazole was slightly to moderately decreased.

Clinical evidence, mechanism, importance and management

(a) Boceprevir

In a crossover study in 24 healthy subjects, the AUC and maximum concentration of boceprevir 800 mg three times daily for 5 days were not affected by **omeprazole** 40 mg daily for 5 days. The concentration of boceprevir at 8 hours (C_8) was increased by 17%. Similarly, the AUC and maximum concentration of **omeprazole** were unaffected, and its concentration at 8 hours was increased by 12%.[1] No clinically relevant pharmacokinetic interaction occurs and no dose adjustments on concurrent use would seem necessary.

(b) Paritaprevir

The UK and US manufacturers briefly report that, in a study in 11 healthy subjects, **omeprazole** 40 mg daily had no effect on the pharmacokinetics of paritaprevir 150 mg daily (in a fixed-dose combination with ritonavir and ombitasvir, and given *with* dasabuvir). The AUC and maximum concentration of **omeprazole** were both decreased by 38%.[2,3] The UK manufacturer also notes that **omeprazole** 40 mg daily, given with paritaprevir 150 mg daily (in a fixed-dose combination with ritonavir and ombitasvir, and given *without* dasabuvir) decreased the AUC of paritaprevir by 54% and the maximum concentration by 52%. The reason for these decreases in omeprazole exposure is unclear, but the involvement of ritonavir (which is used to boost paritaprevir concentrations) cannot be ruled out, since some HIV-protease inhibitors boosted with ritonavir have been shown to have a similar effect (see 'HIV-protease inhibitors + Proton pump inhibitors', p.937 for details). The slight to moderate decrease in omeprazole exposure could reduce the efficacy of omeprazole, and the US manufacturer of paritaprevir boosted with ritonavir (in a fixed-dose combination with ombitasvir, and given with dasabuvir) advises that patients should be monitored for possible decreased efficacy of omeprazole if used concurrently, and consideration should be given to increasing the omeprazole dose if this occurs, but omeprazole doses above 40 mg daily should be avoided.[2] This would seem prudent, and similarly, the UK manufacturer advises that if given concurrently, higher omeprazole doses should be used if clinically indicated. They extend this advice to **esomeprazole** and **lansoprazole**.[3]

(c) Simeprevir

The UK and US manufacturers briefly note that, in a study in 16 healthy subjects the pharmacokinetics of a single 40-mg dose of **omeprazole** were unaffected by simeprevir 150 mg daily for 11 days.[4,5] Further, the US manufacturer predicts that no clinically relevant interaction would be expected between simeprevir and proton pump inhibitors.[5] All proton pump inhibitors can therefore be given with simeprevir without the need for dose adjustment.

(d) Telaprevir

The UK and US manufacturers of telaprevir report that, in a study in 24 subjects, **esomeprazole** 40 mg daily, taken for 6 days had no effect on the pharmacokinetics of a single 750-mg dose of telaprevir.[6,7] The UK manufacturer therefore advises that proton pump inhibitors can be given without dose adjustment.[6]

1. de Kanter CT, Colbers AP, Blonk MI, Verweij-van Wissen CP, Schouwenberg BJ, Drenth JP, Burger DM. Lack of a clinically significant drug-drug interaction in healthy volunteers between the HCV protease inhibitor boceprevir and the proton pump inhibitor omeprazole. *J Antimicrob Chemother* (2013) 68, 1415–22.
2. Viekira Pak (Ombitasvir, paritaprevir, ritonavir co-packaged with dasabuvir sodium monohydrate). AbbVie Inc. US Prescribing information, December 2014.
3. Viekirax (Ombitasvir, paritaprevir, ritonavir). AbbVie Ltd. UK Summary of product characteristics, January 2015.
4. Olysio (Simeprevir sodium). Janssen-Cilag Ltd. UK Summary of product characteristics, May 2014.
5. Olysio (Simeprevir sodium). Janssen Products, LP. US Prescribing information, November 2014.
6. Incivo (Telaprevir). Janssen-Cilag Ltd. UK Summary of product characteristics, July 2014.
7. Incivek (Telaprevir). Vertex Pharmaceuticals, Inc. US Prescribing information, October 2013.

HCV-protease inhibitors + Rifampicin (Rifampin) and other CYP3A4 inducers

Rifampicin very markedly decreases the exposure to telaprevir, and slightly decreases that of simeprevir. Boceprevir is predicted to be similarly affected. Carbamazepine and phenytoin slightly decreased the exposure to telaprevir. Carbamazepine moderately decreased exposure to paritaprevir boosted with ritonavir (in a fixed-dose combination). Other CYP3A4 inducers are predicted to interact similarly with the HCV-protease inhibitors. The pharmacokinetics of carbamazepine were unaffected by telaprevir, but the exposure to phenytoin was slightly increased by telaprevir. Boceprevir and telaprevir are predicted to increase the plasma concentration of rifabutin, and telaprevir is predicted to alter exposure to phenobarbital.

Clinical evidence

(a) Carbamazepine

1. Paritaprevir. The UK and US manufacturers briefly report that, in a study in 12 healthy subjects, carbamazepine 200 mg daily followed by 200 mg twice daily decreased the AUC and maximum concentration of a single 150-mg dose of paritaprevir (in a fixed-dose combination with ritonavir and ombitasvir, and given with dasabuvir) by 70% and 66%, respectively. The pharmacokinetics of carbamazepine were not affected, but the AUC and minimum concentration of its active metabolite, carbamazepine-10,11-epoxide were decreased by 25% and 43%, respectively.[1,2]

2. Telaprevir. The UK and US manufacturers briefly note that, in a study in 11 healthy subjects given carbamazepine 200 mg twice daily for 17 days with telaprevir 750 mg three times daily for 10 days, the AUC, and minimum and maximum concentrations of telaprevir were decreased by 32%, 47%, and 21%, respectively. The pharmacokinetics of carbamazepine were unaffected.[3,4]

(b) Phenytoin

The UK and US manufacturers briefly note that, in a study in 7 healthy subjects given phenytoin 200 mg twice daily for 17 days with **telaprevir** 750 mg three times daily for 10 days, the AUC, and minimum and maximum concentrations of **telaprevir** were decreased by 47%, 68%, and 32%, respectively. The AUC, and minimum and maximum concentrations of phenytoin were increased by 31%, 36%, and 27%, respectively.[3,4]

(c) Rifampicin (rifampin)

1. Simeprevir. The UK and US manufacturers briefly note that, in a study in 18 healthy subjects given rifampicin 600 mg daily with simeprevir 200 mg daily, for 7 days, the AUC and minimum concentration of simeprevir were decreased by 48% and 92%, respectively, and the maximum concentration was *increased* by 31%. The AUC and maximum concentration of rifampicin were unaffected.[5,6] Note that the dose of simeprevir used in this study is higher than the recommended dose of 150 mg daily.

2. Telaprevir. In a study in 16 healthy subjects, rifampicin 600 mg daily for 8 days decreased the AUC and maximum plasma concentration of a single 750-mg dose of telaprevir by 92% and 86%, respectively.[7]

Mechanism

Rifampicin is a non-specific enzyme inducer, with potent effects on CYP3A4, the main isoenzyme by which telaprevir and simeprevir are metabolised. Rifampicin also induces P-glycoprotein, of which telaprevir and simeprevir are also substrates. The induction of these systems results in a decrease in telaprevir and simeprevir exposure. The reason for the increase in simeprevir maximum concentration with rifampicin is not known. Carbamazepine and phenytoin also induce CYP3A4, and carbamazepine also induces P-glycoprotein. They therefore decrease exposure to telaprevir. The reason for the increase in phenytoin exposure is not clear, as telaprevir does not inhibit the isoenzymes involved in the metabolism of phenytoin (CYP2C9 and CYP2C19). Paritaprevir is also a substrate for CYP3A4 and P-glycoprotein, and concurrent use with carbamazepine therefore decreases its exposure. Carbamazepine is itself a CYP3A4 substrate and the effects seen on its metabolite might be due to the CYP3A4 inhibitory effects of ritonavir used as a pharmacokinetic enhancer with paritaprevir.

Importance and management

Evidence for a pharmacokinetic interaction between the HCV-protease inhibitors and rifampicin and other CYP3A4 inducers is limited; however, the effect of concurrent use is consistent with the way these drugs interact with other drugs metabolised by CYP3A4, and so this interaction would appear to be established and of clinical importance. The very marked decrease in telaprevir exposure seen with **rifampicin** is likely to result in a reduction in its antiviral efficacy. The effect of rifampicin on simeprevir exposure was only slight, but the minimum concentration was greatly decreased. Carbamazepine caused a moderate decrease in paritaprevir exposure (when given in a fixed-dose combination with ritonavir and ombitasvir, and given with dasabuvir). Boceprevir is only partially metabolised by CYP3A4, but is a substrate of P-glycoprotein and so its exposure would be expected to be similarly affected. For these reasons, the UK and US manufacturers of telaprevir, simeprevir, and boceprevir and the manufacturers of paritaprevir boosted with ritonavir (in a fixed-dose combination with ombitasvir, with and without dasabuvir) contraindicate, or advise against, the concurrent use of rifampicin.[1-6,8,9] Other potent CYP3A4 inducers (see 'Table 1.9', p.11 for a list), are also predicted to reduce the plasma concentrations of the HCV-protease inhibitors and are therefore similarly contraindicated or cautioned.[1-6,8,9] Note that the UK and US manufacturers of simeprevir also specifically name **oxcarbazepine**,[5,6] and the UK manufacturer of paritaprevir boosted with ritonavir (in a fixed-dose combination with ombitasvir, with and without dasabuvir) includes **enzalutamide** (which is not an established enzyme inducer).[2] Note that the decreases in telaprevir concentrations seen in the studies with **carbamazepine** and **phenytoin** were only slight. In addition, as telaprevir inhibits CYP3A4, the UK manufacturer predicts that it could alter the plasma concentrations of **phenobarbital**.[3]

Further, the UK and US manufacturers of telaprevir[3,4] and simeprevir,[5,6] and the US manufacturer[9] of boceprevir predict that **rifabutin** might decrease the exposure to the HCV-protease inhibitors (by inducing CYP3A4), which could reduce their antiviral effects. They also state that boceprevir and telaprevir could increase the exposure to **rifabutin**, by inhibiting CYP3A4, and so concurrent use is not recommended.[3,4,9] Note that increased exposure to rifabutin could increase the risk of rifabutin adverse effects such as uveitis and neutropenia. The US manufacturer of simeprevir does not recommend the concurrent use of **rifapentine** due to the risk of decreased simeprevir concentrations.[6]

For the effects of efavirenz and etravirine, which also induce CYP3A4, on the HCV-protease inhibitors, see 'HCV-protease inhibitors + NNRTIs', p.906.

1. Viekira Pak (Ombitasvir, paritaprevir, ritonavir co-packaged with dasabuvir sodium monohydrate). AbbVie Inc. US Prescribing information, December 2014.
2. Viekirax (Ombitasvir, paritaprevir, ritonavir). AbbVie Ltd. UK Summary of product characteristics, January 2015.
3. Incivo (Telaprevir). Janssen-Cilag Ltd. UK Summary of product characteristics, July 2014.
4. Incivek (Telaprevir). Vertex Pharmaceuticals, Inc. US Prescribing information, October 2013.
5. Olysio (Simeprevir sodium). Janssen-Cilag Ltd. UK Summary of product characteristics, May 2014.
6. Olysio (Simeprevir sodium). Janssen Products, LP. US Prescribing information, November 2014.
7. Garg V, Chandorkar G, Yang Y, Adda N, McNair L, Alves K, Smith F, van Heeswijk RP. The effect of CYP3A inhibitors and inducers on the pharmacokinetics of telaprevir in healthy volunteers. *Br J Clin Pharmacol* (2013) 75, 431–9.
8. Victrelis (Boceprevir). Merck Sharp & Dohme Ltd. UK Summary of product characteristics, August 2014.
9. Victrelis (Boceprevir). Merck & Co., Inc. US Prescribing information, July 2014.

HCV-Protease inhibitors + St John's wort

St John's wort does not appear to affect the pharmacokinetics of boceprevir, but is predicted to decrease the concentrations of paritaprevir, simeprevir, and telaprevir.

Clinical evidence

A crossover study in 17 healthy subjects, given St John's wort 600 mg daily (as *Ucalm*) for 14 days with **boceprevir** 800 mg three times daily for the last 5 days, found no effect on the pharmacokinetics of boceprevir.[1]

Mechanism

St John's wort induces CYP3A4, by which boceprevir is partially metabolised. The lack of effect seen in the study probably reflects this, and the fact that St John's wort is only a moderate CYP3A4 inducer.

Importance and management

Evidence for a pharmacokinetic interaction between the HCV-protease inhibitors and St John's wort is limited to a study with boceprevir which showed no effect. However, the US manufacturer of boceprevir contraindicates concurrent use with St John's wort preparations, because they state that it could lead to loss of virological response.[2] Given that CYP3A4 is not a major pathway for boceprevir metabolism, and the results of the study, this would seem a little over cautious. Nevertheless, some caution is warranted given the variability in the quality and constituents of preparations containing St John's wort and the uncertainty that this creates. This is highlighted by the fact that the product used in the study to induce CYP3A4 has been questioned by some,[3] as its hyperforin (the main constituent of St John's wort that is responsible for its CYP3A4 inducing potential) content was not known.

In contrast, CYP3A4 is the main isoenzyme involved in the metabolism of **simeprevir** and **telaprevir**, and so they would be expected to be interact with St John's wort. As a result, the UK and US manufacturers of these two HCV-protease inhibitors[4-7] predict that their concentrations could be decreased, and therefore concurrent use is either not recommended or contraindicated. Furthermore, the manufacturers of simeprevir warn that concurrent use could result in loss of therapeutic effect.[4,5] The UK and US manufacturers of **paritaprevir** (in a fixed-dose combination including ritonavir and ombitasvir, given with and without dasabuvir), predict that St John's wort might decrease its exposure leading to a potential loss of therapeutic efficacy and hence contraindicate concurrent use.[8,9]

1. Jackson A, D'Avolio A, Moyle G, Bonora S, Di Perri G, Else L, Simiele M, Singh GJ, Back D, Boffito M. Pharmacokinetics of the co-administration of boceprevir and St John's wort to male and female healthy volunteers. *J Antimicrob Chemother* (2014) 69, 1911–5.
2. Victrelis (Boceprevir). Merck & Co., Inc. US Prescribing information, July 2014.
3. Weiss J, Haefeli WE. Comment on: Pharmacokinetics of the co-administration of boceprevir and St John's wort to male and female healthy volunteers. *J Antimicrob Chemother* (2014) Epub.
4. Olysio (Simeprevir sodium). Janssen-Cilag Ltd. UK Summary of product characteristics, May 2014.
5. Olysio (Simeprevir sodium). Janssen Products, LP. US Prescribing information, November 2014.
6. Incivo (Telaprevir). Janssen-Cilag Ltd. UK Summary of product characteristics, July 2014.
7. Incivek (Telaprevir). Vertex Pharmaceuticals, Inc. US Prescribing information, October 2013.
8. Viekira Pak (Ombitasvir, paritaprevir, ritonavir co-packaged with dasabuvir sodium monohydrate). AbbVie Inc. US Prescribing information, December 2014.
9. Viekirax (Ombitasvir, paritaprevir, ritonavir). AbbVie Ltd. UK Summary of product characteristics, January 2015.

HCV-protease inhibitors + Tenofovir

Telaprevir appears to slightly increase the exposure to tenofovir, but tenofovir does not appear to alter the pharmacokinetics of telaprevir. Simeprevir appears to minimally increase the concentration of tenofovir, and tenofovir appears to minimally decrease the exposure to simeprevir. No clinically relevant pharmacokinetic interaction appears to occur between tenofovir and boceprevir or paritaprevir.

Clinical evidence

(a) Boceprevir

The UK and US manufacturers briefly report that, in a study, the concurrent use of boceprevir 800 mg three times daily with tenofovir 300 mg daily, both taken for 7 days, had no effect on the pharmacokinetics of either drug, with the exception of a 32% increase in the maximum plasma concentration of tenofovir.[1,2]

(b) Paritaprevir

The UK manufacturer briefly reports that, in a study in healthy subjects given tenofovir 300 mg daily with emtricitabine 200 mg daily and paritaprevir 150 mg daily (in a fixed-dose combination with ritonavir and ombitasvir, given with and without dasabuvir), the pharmacokinetics of tenofovir and paritaprevir were unaffected.[3]

(c) Simeprevir

The UK and US manufacturers of simeprevir briefly report that, in a study in 24 healthy subjects given tenofovir 300 mg daily with simeprevir 150 mg daily for 7 days, the AUC and maximum concentration of simeprevir were decreased by 14% and 15%, respectively. The AUC of tenofovir was unaffected, but the minimum and maximum concentrations were increased by 24% and 19%.[4,5]

(d) Telaprevir

In a study in 16 subjects, telaprevir 750 mg three times daily for 7 days increased both the AUC and maximum plasma concentration of tenofovir 300 mg daily for 7 days by 30%. Tenofovir had no effect on the pharmacokinetics of telaprevir.[6]

In a crossover study, 20 healthy subjects were given telaprevir 750 mg every 8 hours for 7 days, followed, after a washout period, by efavirenz 600 mg daily with tenofovir 300 mg daily for 7 days, followed by telaprevir 1125 mg every 8 hours or 1500 mg every 12 hours with the same dose of efavirenz and tenofovir. When given with efavirenz and tenofovir, the AUCs of telaprevir 1125 mg and 1500 mg were 18% and 20% lower, respectively, and the minimum plasma concentrations were 25% and 48% lower, respectively, when compared with telaprevir 750 mg alone. In addition, the AUC of tenofovir was marginally higher (by about 10%) on concurrent use with efavirenz and telaprevir 1125 mg or 1500 mg, when compared with tenofovir and efavirenz alone.[7]

A case report describes a 41-year-old man who developed a greatly increased tenofovir minimum concentration (about 4-fold) a few weeks after telaprevir was added to his existing, stable antiretroviral regimen. Several weeks later the tenofovir concentration had increased further, to about 7-fold higher than before telaprevir was started. Telaprevir was stopped, and the tenofovir concentration decreased but not to pre-telaprevir levels. This case is complicated by the development of, and subsequent improvement in, renal impairment along a similar time course, and the role of this in the increased tenofovir concentration cannot be quantified or ruled out.[8]

Mechanism

Not clear. Telaprevir inhibits P-glycoprotein, of which tenofovir has been found to be a substrate *in vitro*, and hence concurrent use might result in increased tenofovir exposure. Boceprevir and simeprevir are also P-glycoprotein inhibitors, but boceprevir had no effect on tenofovir pharmacokinetics in the study, and simeprevir did not affect its exposure. The small decrease in telaprevir exposure in the second study, despite the higher telaprevir dose, is likely to be due to the effects of efavirenz, see 'HCV-protease inhibitors + NNRTIs', p.906, for further information.

Importance and management

Evidence for a pharmacokinetic interaction between the HCV-protease inhibitors and tenofovir is limited and not consistent. The clinical relevance of the slight increase in tenofovir exposure seen with telaprevir in the study is unclear. However, the UK and US manufacturers of telaprevir advise that concurrent use should be monitored closely for an increase in tenofovir adverse effects (such as nausea, diarrhoea, renal impairment, and hypophosphataemia).[9,10] Until more is known, this would seem prudent. The isolated case report of a greatly increased tenofovir concentration after telaprevir was started, might serve as an example of the importance of this. The US manufacturer of telaprevir states that tenofovir should be stopped if toxicity occurs.[10] The pharmacokinetics of telaprevir do not appear to be altered by tenofovir, and no dose adjustment would seem necessary on concurrent use.

Simeprevir did not appear to alter the exposure to tenofovir, and the increases in minimum and maximum concentrations were small, and unlikely to be clinically important. Similarly, the decrease in simeprevir exposure when given with tenofovir was small and unlikely to be clinically relevant. No dose adjustments would seem necessary on concurrent use.

No clinically relevant pharmacokinetic interaction appears to occur between boceprevir and tenofovir or paritaprevir. No dose adjustments are therefore necessary on concurrent use.

1. Victrelis (Boceprevir). Merck Sharp & Dohme Ltd. UK Summary of product characteristics, August 2014.
2. Victrelis (Boceprevir). Merck & Co., Inc. US Prescribing information, July 2014.
3. Viekirax (Ombitasvir, paritaprevir, ritonavir). AbbVie Ltd. UK Summary of product characteristics, January 2015.
4. Olysio (Simeprevir sodium). Janssen-Cilag Ltd. UK Summary of product characteristics, May 2014.
5. Olysio (Simeprevir sodium). Janssen Products, LP. US Prescribing information, November 2014.
6. van Heeswijk R, Gysen V, Boogaerts G, de Paepe E, Vangeneugden T, de Backer K, Beumont-Mauviel M, Hoetelmans R. The pharmacokinetic (PK) interaction between tenofovir disoproxil fumarate (TDF) and the investigational HCV protease inhibitor telaprevir (TVR). *Intersci Conf Antimicrob Agents Chemother* (2008) 48, A-966.
7. van Heeswijk R, Vandevoorde A, Boogaerts G, Vangeneugden T, de Paepe E, Polo R, Van Solingen-Ristea R, de Backer K, Garg V, Beumont M. Pharmacokinetic interactions between ARV agents and the investigational HCV protease inhibitor TVR in healthy volunteers. 18th Conference on Retroviruses and Opportunistic Infections, Seattle WA, March 2011. Abstract 119.
8. Gervasoni C, Milazzo L, Pezzani D, Fucile S, Cattaneo D. Telaprevir therapy, renal impairment, and their effects on the pharmacokinetics of tenofovir in HIV/hepatitis C virus coinfected patients. *AIDS* (2014) 28, 285–7.
9. Incivo (Telaprevir). Janssen-Cilag Ltd. UK Summary of product characteristics, July 2014.
10. Incivek (Telaprevir). Vertex Pharmaceuticals, Inc. US Prescribing information, October 2013.

HCV-protease inhibitors; Boceprevir + Miscellaneous

Boceprevir is predicted to increase the plasma concentrations of amiodarone, desipramine, propafenone, and quinidine. Diflunisal and ibuprofen have no notable effect on the pharmacokinetics of boceprevir.

Clinical evidence, mechanism, importance and management

(a) Antiarrhythmics

The US manufacturer of boceprevir predicts that it will increase the plasma concentrations of **amiodarone**, **propafenone**, and **quinidine**, which could increase the risk of serious adverse effects such as arrhythmias.[1] Boceprevir is an inhibitor of CYP3A4, which is at least partially involved in the metabolism of most of these antiarrhythmics. The US manufacturer advises caution on concurrent use, with monitoring of antiarrhythmic drug concentrations.[1]

Note also that the UK manufacturer advises caution on the concurrent use of boceprevir with drugs that can cause QT prolongation such as amiodarone and quinidine, see 'Drugs that prolong the QT interval + Other drugs that prolong the QT interval', p.272, for further information.

(b) Desipramine

The US manufacturer predicts that boceprevir will increase the plasma concentration of desipramine, which could increase the risk of adverse effects such as hypotension, dizziness, and syncope. They therefore advise caution on concurrent use and suggest that a lower dose of desipramine is given to patients also taking boceprevir.[1] However, desipramine is primarily metabolised by CYP2D6, and boceprevir is not known to inhibit this isoenzyme. Therefore, despite the manufacturer's prediction, a clinically relevant interaction between boceprevir and desipramine seems unlikely.

(c) NSAIDs

The US manufacturer of boceprevir states that it is primarily metabolised by aldoketo reductase, and drugs that are inhibitors of this enzyme are expected to increase the plasma boceprevir concentration. However, in a pharmacokinetic study, **diflunisal** (which is said to inhibit aldoketo reductase) 250 mg twice daily for 7 days had no effect on the AUC and maximum plasma concentration of boceprevir 800 mg three times daily for 12 days, and increased its minimum plasma concentration by 31%.[1] Similarly, **ibuprofen** (which is also said to inhibit aldoketo reductase) 600 mg three times daily for 6 days had no effect on the pharmacokinetics of a single 400-mg dose of boceprevir.[1] Therefore, no boceprevir dose adjustment would appear to be necessary on the concurrent use of diflunisal or ibuprofen.[1,2]

1. Victrelis (Boceprevir). Merck & Co., Inc. US Prescribing information, July 2014.
2. Victrelis (Boceprevir). Merck Sharp & Dohme Ltd. UK Summary of product characteristics, August 2014.

HCV-protease inhibitors; Paritaprevir + Miscellaneous

Paritaprevir boosted with ritonavir is predicted to increase the concentrations of some antiarrhythmics (such as amiodarone and disopyramide), conivaptan, furosemide, fusidic acid, levothyroxine, fexofenadine, repaglinide, valsartan, and sulfasalazine. It is also predicted to decrease the concentration of mephenytoin. No clinically relevant interaction appears to occur with duloxetine, emtricitabine, gemfibrozil, or norethisterone.

Clinical evidence, mechanism, importance and management

(a) Antiarrhythmics

The UK and US manufacturers of paritaprevir boosted with ritonavir (in a fixed-dose combination with ombitasvir, and given with or without dasabuvir) predict that it will increase the plasma concentrations of **amiodarone** and **quinidine**.[1,2] Further, the US manufacturer predicts a similar effect with **disopyramide**, **flecainide**, systemic **lidocaine**, **mexiletine**, and **propafenone**.[2] Paritaprevir itself does not appear to inhibit CYP3A4, which is at least partially involved in the metabolism of most of these antiarrhythmics, but it is boosted with ritonavir, which is a known potent inhibitor of CYP3A4. Flecainide, mexiletine, and propafenone are also metabolised by CYP2D6 (at least in part), which is also inhibited by ritonavir. The UK manufacturer contraindicates concurrent use with amiodarone and quinidine,[1] whereas the US manufacturer advises caution, with monitoring of antiarrhythmic drug concentrations (if available), if any of these drugs are given concurrently.[2]

(b) Conivaptan

The UK manufacturer of paritaprevir (in a fixed-dose combination including ritonavir and ombitasvir, given with or without dasabuvir) predicts that potent CYP3A4 inhibitors will increase paritaprevir exposure. They also predict that the concentration of conivaptan will be increased on concurrent use.[1] Due to the risk of an increase in paritaprevir exposure, they contraindicate concurrent use with potent CYP3A4 inhibitors,[1] see 'Table 1.9', p.11 for a list. They additionally name conivaptan as a potent CYP3A4 inhibitor, however it is generally considered to be a moderate inhibitor of this isoenzyme.

(c) Duloxetine

The UK manufacturer briefly reports that, in a study in healthy subjects given a single 60-mg dose of duloxetine with paritaprevir 150 mg daily (in a fixed-dose combination with ombitasvir and ritonavir, and given with dasabuvir), the pharmacokinetics of paritaprevir were unaffected, but the AUC and maximum concentration of duloxetine were decreased by 21% and 25%, respectively. The effect of the combination when given without dasabuvir was similar.[1] Such a small decrease in duloxetine exposure is unlikely to be clinically important and so no dose adjustments are necessary on concurrent use.

(d) Furosemide

The UK and US manufacturers briefly report that, in a study in 12 healthy subjects given a single 20-mg dose of furosemide with paritaprevir 150 mg daily (in a fixed-dose combination with ombitasvir and ritonavir, and given with dasabuvir), the pharmacokinetics of paritaprevir were unaffected, but the maximum concentration of furosemide was increased by 42%. The AUC of furosemide was unaffected.[1,2] They therefore recommend that patients are monitored [for furosemide effects], with the UK manufacturer advising that a 50% decrease in furosemide dose might be required,[1] and the US manufacturer suggesting that the dose should be individualised, dependent on response.[2] No dose adjustment is required for the paritaprevir combination, and the

UK manufacturer predicts that similar effects would be expected if the combination is given without dasabuvir,[1] and the same advice would therefore apply. The mechanism behind this effect is unclear, but note that other components of the combination might also be involved.

(e) Fusidic acid

The UK manufacturer predicts that paritaprevir boosted with ritonavir (in a fixed-dose combination with ombitasvir, and given with or without dasabuvir) will increase the concentration of fusidic acid, due to CYP3A4 inhibition by ritonavir, and contra-indicates concurrent use.[1] However, note that clinical evidence of an interaction between fusidic acid and CYP3A4 inhibitors, and in particular ritonavir, is sparse (see 'HIV-protease inhibitors + Fusidic acid', p.929).

(f) Gemfibrozil

The UK and US manufacturers briefly report that, in a study in 11 healthy subjects given gemfibrozil 600 mg twice daily with a single 150-mg dose of paritaprevir (with ritonavir and dasabuvir), the AUC of paritaprevir was increased by 38% but the maximum concentration was unaffected.[1,2] This slight increase in exposure is unlikely to be clinically important and so no paritaprevir dose adjustment would seem necessary on concurrent use. However, note that due to an interaction between gemfibrozil and dasabuvir, concurrent use of paritaprevir and gemfibrozil is contra-indicated only when paritaprevir is given as part of a fixed-dose preparation with, or containing, dasabuvir.[1,2] For further information see, 'NS5B inhibitors; Dasabuvir + Gemfibrozil', p.994.

(g) Levothyroxine

The UK manufacturer predicts that paritaprevir boosted with ritonavir (in a fixed-dose combination with ombitasvir, and given with or without dasabuvir) will increase the concentration of levothyroxine, due to inhibition of the glucuronosyltransferase, UGT1A1, and advises clinical monitoring (for increased levothyroxine effects), with levothyroxine dose adjustment where necessary, on concurrent use.[1] Note that other components of the combination might also be involved in any interaction.

(h) Mephenytoin

The UK manufacturer predicts that paritaprevir boosted with ritonavir (in a fixed-dose combination with ombitasvir, and given with or without dasabuvir) will decrease the concentration of S-mephenytoin, due to CYP2C19 induction by ritonavir, and advises clinical monitoring (for reduced effects), with mephenytoin dose adjustment where necessary, on concurrent use.[1] Note that mephenytoin is rarely used clinically, and so the general relevance of this in practice is limited.

(i) Norethisterone

The UK manufacturer briefly reports that, in a study in healthy subjects given norethisterone 350 micrograms daily with paritaprevir 150 mg daily (in a fixed-dose combination with ombitasvir and ritonavir, and given with dasabuvir), the pharmacokinetics of paritaprevir and norethisterone were unaffected.[1] No dose adjustments are required on concurrent use.[1,2] Note also that progestogen-only contraceptives are recommended in preference to combined hormonal contraceptives in patients taking this combination preparation, see 'Combined hormonal contraceptives + HCV-protease inhibitors', p.1175 for details.

(j) NRTIs

The UK manufacturer briefly reports that, in a study in healthy subjects given **emtricitabine** 200 mg daily (with tenofovir) and paritaprevir 150 mg daily (in a fixed-dose combination with ombitasvir and ritonavir, and given with and without dasabuvir), the pharmacokinetics of emtricitabine and paritaprevir were unaffected.1 No dose adjustments are required on concurrent use.[1,2]

(k) Organic anion transporter substrates

Paritaprevir is an inhibitor of the organic anion transporting polypeptide, OATP1B1. The UK manufacturer therefore predicts that paritaprevir boosted with ritonavir (in a fixed-dose combination with ombitasvir, and given with or without dasabuvir) will increase the concentrations of **fexofenadine**, **repaglinide**, and **valsartan**, via this mechanism. They recommend caution and a dose reduction for fexofenadine and repaglinide, and monitoring (for adverse effects such as dizziness, headache and hypotension) and a dose reduction for valsartan.[1]

(l) Sulfasalazine

The UK manufacturer predicts that paritaprevir boosted with ritonavir (in a fixed-dose combination with ombitasvir, and given with or without dasabuvir) will increase the concentration of sulfasalazine, due to inhibition of BCRP, and advises caution on concurrent use.[1] Note that other components of the combination might also be involved in any interaction.

1. Viekirax (Ombitasvir, paritaprevir, ritonavir). AbbVie Ltd. UK Summary of product characteristics, January 2015.
2. Viekira Pak (Ombitasvir, paritaprevir, ritonavir co-packaged with dasabuvir sodium monohydrate). AbbVie Inc. US Prescribing information, December 2014.

HCV-protease inhibitors; Simeprevir + Miscellaneous

Simeprevir is predicted to increase the concentrations of oral amiodarone, disopyramide, flecainide, mexiletine, propafenone, and quinidine. Simeprevir appears to slightly increase the exposure to caffeine, but appears not to affect the pharmacokinetics of dextromethorphan. Gemfibrozil, cobicistat, and milk thistle are predicted to increase exposure to simeprevir. No interaction is expected between simeprevir and antacids, H_2-receptor antagonists, NRTIs, bedaquiline, or methylphenidate.

Clinical evidence, mechanism, importance and management

(a) Antiarrhythmics

The UK and US manufacturers[1,2] predict that simeprevir might increase the concentrations of **amiodarone**, **disopyramide**, **flecainide**, **mexiletine**, **propafenone**, and **quinidine** when given *orally*, via inhibition of intestinal CYP3A4. This isoenzyme is at least partially involved in the metabolism of most of these antiarrhythmics, but simeprevir is only a weak inhibitor of CYP3A4 in the intestine (and appears to have no effect on CYP3A4 in the liver). However, note that flecainide, mexiletine, and propafenone are mainly metabolised by CYP2D6, and simeprevir does not appear to inhibit this isoenzyme (see under *CYP2D6 substrates* below). A clinically important effect on these antiarrhythmics might therefore seem unlikely, but the manufacturers advise caution on concurrent use, with the US manufacturer recommending therapeutic drug monitoring of the antiarrhythmics, where available,[2] and the UK manufacturer recommending therapeutic drug monitoring and/or clinical monitoring (such as ECG).[1]

(b) CYP1A2 substrates

The UK and US manufacturers briefly report that, in a study in 16 healthy subjects, simeprevir 150 mg daily for 11 days increased the AUC and maximum concentration of a single 150-mg dose of **caffeine** by 26% and 12%, respectively.[1,2] Note that caffeine can be used as a probe substrate to assess the activity of CYP1A2. This study therefore suggests that simeprevir is a weak inhibitor of CYP1A2. No clinically relevant effect on other CYP1A2 substrates would be expected.

(c) CYP2D6 substrates

The UK and US manufacturers briefly report that, in a study in 16 healthy subjects, simeprevir 150 mg daily for 11 days had no effect on the pharmacokinetics of a single 30-mg dose of **dextromethorphan**.[1,2] Note that dextromethorphan can be used as a probe substrate to assess the activity of CYP2D6. This study therefore suggests that simeprevir is not a clinically relevant inhibitor CYP2D6, and would not be expected to affect the pharmacokinetics of CYP2D6 substrates.

(d) Drugs that affect gastric pH

The UK and US manufacturers[1,2] predict that no clinically relevant interaction is expected between simeprevir and **antacids** (such as **aluminium hydroxide**, **calcium carbonate**, and **magnesium hydroxide**[1]), or **H_2-receptor antagonists** (such as **cimetidine**, **nizatidine**, and **ranitidine**[1]).

(e) NRTIs

The UK and US manufacturers predict that no clinically relevant interaction is expected between simeprevir and **abacavir**, **didanosine**, **emtricitabine**, **lamivudine**, **stavudine**, or **zidovudine**.[1,2]

(f) OATP1B1 inhibitors

The UK manufacturer warns that because the organic anion transporting polypeptide, OATP1B1 is involved in the hepatic uptake of simeprevir, inhibitors of this transporter might increases its plasma concentration, and they specifically name **gemfibrozil**.[1]

(g) Sofosbuvir

The UK and US manufacturers briefly report that, in a pharmacokinetic sub-study of a phase II study in 22 patients with hepatitis C given simeprevir 150 mg daily for 11 days with sofosbuvir 400 mg daily, the AUC and maximum concentration of sofosbuvir were about 3-fold and 2-fold higher, respectively, than in historical controls. The pharmacokinetics of simeprevir were no different to those in historical controls. They advise that the higher sofosbuvir exposure was not clinically relevant.[1,2] No dose adjustments on concurrent use are necessary.

(h) Other drugs

Although not studied, the UK and US manufacturers predict that no clinically relevant interaction would be expected between simeprevir and **methylphenidate**.[1,2] The UK manufacturer additionally names **bedaquiline**.[1] The US and UK manufacturers also predict that **cobicistat**-containing products and **milk thistle** might increase the concentration of simeprevir by inhibition of CYP3A4, and do not recommend their concurrent use with simeprevir.[1,2] Note that **cobicistat** is a known potent inhibitor of CYP3A4 by which simeprevir is metabolised, and therefore this prediction would seem reasonable. However, although the CYP3A4-inhibitory potential of **milk thistle** is not established, it does not appear to have a clinically relevant effect on other known CYP3A4 substrates (for example see 'HIV-protease inhibitors; Indinavir + Milk thistle', p.946); nevertheless until more is known it might be prudent to be aware of the possibility of an interaction if milk thistle is being taken and otherwise unexplained effects are seen (such as increased simeprevir adverse effects).

1. Olysio (Simeprevir sodium). Janssen-Cilag Ltd. UK Summary of product characteristics, May 2014.
2. Olysio (Simeprevir sodium). Janssen Products, LP. US Prescribing information, November 2014.

HCV-protease inhibitors; Telaprevir + Miscellaneous

Telaprevir is predicted to increase the plasma concentrations of some antiarrhythmics (such as amiodarone and systemic lidocaine), the anti-

diabetics, repaglinide and metformin, and the NRTIs, abacavir and zidovudine.

Clinical evidence, mechanism, importance and management

(a) Antiarrhythmics

Telaprevir is an inhibitor of CYP3A4 and the manufacturers predict that it will increase the plasma concentrations of **amiodarone** and **quinidine** by inhibiting their metabolism by this isoenzyme.[1,2] The US manufacturer also predicts that telaprevir will increase the plasma concentrations of systemic **lidocaine**, **propafenone**, and **flecainide**. However, note that flecainide is mainly metabolised by CYP2D6, and telaprevir does not inhibit this isoenzyme *in vitro*.[2] The UK manufacturer contraindicates the use of telaprevir with amiodarone and quinidine, and advises caution and ECG monitoring with the concurrent use of propafenone and flecainide, but not systemic lidocaine.[1] In contrast, the US manufacturer advises caution on concurrent use of any of these drugs and that patients should be monitored closely, including ECG monitoring.[2]

For the potential interaction of antiarrhythmics that prolong the QT interval, such as amiodarone, with telaprevir, see 'Drugs that prolong the QT interval + Other drugs that prolong the QT interval', p.272..

(b) Antidiabetics

The UK and US manufacturers of telaprevir predict that concentrations of **repaglinide** might be increased (by inhibition of organic anion transporting polypeptides, OATPs)[1] on concurrent use, and advise caution and clinical monitoring.[1,2] Further, the UK manufacturer also predicts that concentrations of **metformin** might be increased (by inhibition of the multidrug and toxin extrusion proteins, MATE) and recommend close monitoring for metformin efficacy and safety when starting or stopping telaprevir. They also state that a metformin dose adjustment might be necessary.[1]

(c) NRTIs

The UK manufacturer of telaprevir states that concurrent use with **abacavir** or **zidovudine** has not been studied, but the possibility that telaprevir might increase the plasma concentrations of these NRTIs by affecting glucuronidation (by UGTs) cannot be ruled out.[1] The clinical relevance of this prediction is unclear and further study is needed.

1. Incivo (Telaprevir). Janssen-Cilag Ltd. UK Summary of product characteristics, July 2014.
2. Incivek (Telaprevir). Vertek Pharmaceuticals, Inc. US Prescribing information, October 2013.

HIV-integrase inhibitors + Antacids

Aluminium and magnesium-containing antacids moderately decrease dolutegravir exposure and appear to slightly decrease elvitegravir and raltegravir exposure. Calcium-containing antacids appear to moderately decrease raltegravir exposure.

Clinical evidence

(a) Dolutegravir

In a crossover study in 16 healthy subjects, a single 20-mL dose of an **aluminium** and **magnesium**-containing antacid (*Maalox Advanced Maximum Strength*) given simultaneously with a single 50-mg dose of dolutegravir decreased the AUC and maximum concentration of dolutegravir by 74% and 72%, respectively. When given 2 hours apart, the AUC and maximum concentration of dolutegravir were decreased by just 26% and 18%, respectively.[1]

For information on the use of dolutegravir with calcium carbonate see 'HIV-integrase inhibitors; Dolutegravir + Polyvalent cations', p.919.

(b) Elvitegravir

In a study in healthy subjects given elvitegravir boosted with ritonavir 50/100 mg daily for 10 days, simultaneously given a single 20-mL dose of an **aluminium** and **magnesium**-containing antacid (*Maalox Max*) decreased the AUC and maximum concentration of elvitegravir by 45% and 47%, respectively. When given 2 hours apart, the elvitegravir AUC was decreased by 15 to 20%, and when given 4 hours apart, there was no change in AUC.[2,3]

(c) Raltegravir

In a crossover study in 12 healthy subjects, a single 30-mL dose of an **aluminium** and **magnesium** containing antacid (*Maalox Plus Extra Strength*) given simultaneously with a single 400-mg dose of raltegravir had no effect on the AUC and maximum concentration of raltegravir, but did decrease the time to maximum concentration of raltegravir from 3 hours to 1 hour, and decreased the concentration 12 hours post-dose (C_{12}) by 67%. Note that there was high inter-individual variability in the results.[4] In contrast, the UK and US manufacturers briefly report that in a study in healthy subjects given a single 20-mL dose of an **aluminium** and **magnesium** containing antacid simultaneously with raltegravir 400 mg twice daily, the AUC and maximum concentration of raltegravir were decreased by 49% and 44%, respectively. However, the C_{12} was decreased by 63%. When the antacid was given 2 hours before the raltegravir dose, the AUC and maximum concentration were both decreased by 51%, and the C_{12} was decreased by 56%. In general, administration either 2 to 6 hours after, or 2 to 6 hours before, the raltegravir dose decreased the AUC and maximum concentration, but not the C_{12} (which remained 49 to 57% lower). Note that the decrease in the AUC and maximum concentration were not always statistically significant but were within a range that might be clinically important.[5,6] In another study, when a single 3-g dose of **calcium carbonate** was given at the same time as raltegravir 400 mg twice daily, the AUC and maximum concentration of raltegravir were decreased by 55% and 52%, respectively, and the C_{12} was decreased by 32%.[5,6]

Mechanism

It has been suggested that dolutegravir,[1] elvitegravir,[2] and raltegravir[5] form an insoluble complex with metal (divalent or trivalent) cations in the gut, thus decreasing their absorption and hence exposure.

Importance and management

The interaction between the HIV-integrase inhibitors and antacids is established and is clinically important. The greatest effect is with **dolutegravir** where an aluminium and magnesium-containing antacid moderately decreased its exposure when given simultaneously. The effect was greatly decreased by separating the doses by 2 hours. As such, the UK and US manufacturers advise that dolutegravir should be taken at least 2 hours before the antacid or 6 hours after.[7,8] The decrease in **elvitegravir** exposure given simultaneously with an aluminium and magnesium-containing antacid was slight, and the effect was also decreased by separating the doses. The UK manufacturer, therefore, advises that doses should be separated by at least 4 hours,[9] and the US manufacturer advises a gap of at least 2 hours.[3]

Raltegravir exposure might be slightly decreased by giving it simultaneously with aluminium and magnesium-containing antacids, although this appears to lessen the longer the gap between administration becomes, however, the concentration at C_{12} remains decreased by about 50% irrespective of the dosing interval. Therefore, the UK and US manufacturers of raltegravir do not recommend concurrent use of any aluminium and magnesium-containing antacids, regardless of administration timings.[5,6] In contrast, the exposure of raltegravir appears to be moderately decreased by calcium-containing antacids, but the UK and US manufacturers permit concurrent use with no raltegravir dose adjustment, or adjustment to timings of administration, necessary.[5,6] The reason for this different advice is unclear, but might be related to the effect on raltegravir C_{12} which is larger than the effect on exposure with aluminium and magnesium-containing antacids (and independent of timing), but smaller with calcium-containing antacids.

1. Patel P, Song I, Borland J, Patel A, Lou Y, Chen S, Wajima T, Peppercorn A, Min SS, Piscitelli SC. Pharmacokinetics of the HIV integrase inhibitor S/GSK1349572 co-administered with acid-reducing agents and multivitamins in healthy volunteers. *J Antimicrob Chemother* (2011) 66, 1567–72.
2. Ramanathan S, Mathias A, Wei X, Shen G, Koziara J, Cheng A, Kearney BP. Pharmacokinetics of once-daily boosted elvitegravir when administered in combination with acid-reducing agents. *J Acquir Immune Defic Syndr* (2013) 64, 45–50.
3. Vitekta (Elvitegravir). Gilead Sciences, Inc. US Prescribing information, September 2014.
4. Kiser JJ, Bumpass JB, Meditz AL, Anderson PL, Bushman L, Ray M, Predhomme JA, Rower J, MaWhinney S, Brundage R. Effect of antacids on the pharmacokinetics of raltegravir in human immunodeficiency virus-seronegative volunteers. *Antimicrob Agents Chemother* (2010) 54, 4999–5003.
5. Isentress (Raltegravir potassium). Merck Sharp & Dohme Ltd. UK Summary of product characteristics, November 2014.
6. Isentress (Raltegravir potassium). Merck & Co., Inc. US Prescribing information, February 2015.
7. Tivicay (Dolutegravir sodium). ViiV Healthcare UK Ltd. UK Summary of product characteristics, September 2014.
8. Tivicay (Dolutegravir sodium). ViiV Healthcare. US Prescribing information, December 2014.
9. Vitekta (Elvitegravir). Gilead Sciences Ltd. UK Summary of product characteristics, March 2014.

HIV-integrase inhibitors + Food

Food slightly increases exposure to dolutegravir and elvitegravir, but does not have a clinically relevant effect on the exposure to raltegravir.

Clinical evidence, mechanism, importance and management

(a) Dolutegravir

In a crossover study, 18 healthy subjects were given a single 50-mg dose of dolutegravir with a low-fat (300 kcal, 7% fat), moderate-fat (600 kcal, 30% fat), or high-fat (870 kcal, 53% fat) meal. The AUC of dolutegravir was increased by 33%, 41%, and 66%, respectively, and the maximum concentration was increased by 46%, 52%, and 67%, respectively, when compared with the fasted state. The time to maximum concentration was also increased, from 2 hours in the fasted state, to 3 hours, 4 hours, and 5 hours after low-, moderate-, and high-fat meals, respectively.[1] The UK and US manufacturers advise that dolutegravir can be given without regard to food,[2,3] but in the presence of HIV-integrase inhibitor resistance, the UK manufacturer states that it should be given with food to enhance the exposure.[2]

(b) Elvitegravir

In a crossover study in 11 healthy male subjects, given a single 150-mg dose of elvitegravir (as part of a fixed-dose combination with cobicistat, emtricitabine, and tenofovir disoproxil fumarate) in the fasted state, the AUC and maximum concentration of elvitegravir were decreased by 55% and 50%, respectively, when compared with when they were given with a standard meal (413 kcal, 9.6 g fat). In addition, elvitegravir given in the same fixed-dose combination but with a protein-rich drink (*Ensure*, 250 kcal, 8.8 g fat) was considered comparable to the standard meal as no change in bioavailability of elvitegravir was noted.[4] The preliminary report of a randomised study in 24 healthy subjects, notes that a single 150-mg dose of elvitegravir (given as part of a fixed-dose combination with cobicistat, emtricitabine, and tenofovir disoproxil fumarate) with a light meal (373 kcal, 20% fat) or a high-fat meal (800 kcal, 50% fat) increased the AUC of elvitegravir by 34% and 87%, respectively, and increased the maximum concentration by 22% and 56%, respectively, when compared with the fasted state.[5] Elvitegravir should therefore be taken with food,[6,7] although it would seem that meal type is not important.

(c) Raltegravir

In a crossover study 19 healthy subjects were given raltegravir 400 mg twice daily for 10 days with a low-fat (300 kcal, 7% fat), or moderate-fat (600 kcal, 31% fat), or high-fat (825 kcal, 57% fat) meal. The AUC of raltegravir was decreased by 46%, increased by 13%, and increased 2-fold, respectively, when compared with the fasted state. The maximum concentration was decreased by 52%, and increased by 5% and 96%, respectively, when compared with the fasted state. Note that there was considerable variability in the results.[8] The UK and US manufacturers note that in clinical studies of safety and efficacy, raltegravir was given without regard to food, and this together with the results from this study mean that raltegravir can be given with or without food.[9,10]

1. Song I, Borland J, Chen S, Patel P, Wajima T, Peppercorn A, Piscitelli SC. Effect of food on the pharmacokinetics of the integrase inhibitor dolutegravir. *Antimicrob Agents Chemother* (2012) 56, 1627–9.
2. Tivicay (Dolutegravir sodium). ViiV Healthcare UK Ltd. UK Summary of product characteristics, September 2014.
3. Tivicay (Dolutegravir sodium). ViiV Healthcare. US Prescribing information, December 2014.
4. Shiomi M, Matsuki S, Ikeda A, Ishikawa T, Nishino N, Kimura M, Irie S. Effects of a protein-rich drink or a standard meal on the pharmacokinetics of elvitegravir, cobicistat, emtricitabine and tenofovir in healthy Japanese male subjects: a randomized, three-way crossover study. *J Clin Pharmacol* (2014) 54, 640–8.
5. German P, Warren D, Wei L, Zhong L, Hui J, Kearney BP. Effect of food on pharmacokinetics (PK) of elvitegravir (EVG), emtricitabine (FTC), tenofovir DF (TDF) and the pharmacoenhancer GS-9350 as a fixed dose combination tablet. 49th Interscience Conference on Antimicrobial Agents and Chemotherapy, San Francisco, 2009. Abstract A1-1300. Available at: http://www.abstractsonline.com/Plan/ViewAbstract.aspx?mID=2392&sKey=f494b9aa-551c-47d1-b35e-61f5114d1096&cKey=84bcf88a-5f63-41d2-b5ce-b66b8d265377 (accessed 29/09/15).
6. Vitekta (Elvitegravir). Gilead Sciences Ltd. UK Summary of product characteristics, March 2014.
7. Vitekta (Elvitegravir). Gilead Sciences, Inc. US Prescribing information, September 2014.
8. Brainard DM, Friedman EJ, Jin B, Beidinger SA, Tillan MD, Wenning LA, Stone JA, Chodakewitz JA, Wagner JA, Iwamoto M. Effect of low-, moderate-, and high-fat meals on raltegravir pharmacokinetics. *J Clin Pharmacol* (2011) 51, 422–7.
9. Isentress (Raltegravir potassium). Merck Sharp & Dohme Ltd. UK Summary of product characteristics, November 2014.
10. Isentress (Raltegravir potassium). Merck & Co., Inc. US Prescribing information, February 2015.

HIV-integrase inhibitors + H_2-receptor antagonists or Proton pump inhibitors

Omeprazole modestly increases raltegravir exposure, but does not affect dolutegravir or elvitegravir exposure. Famotidine does not alter elvitegravir exposure.

Clinical evidence

(a) Dolutegravir

In a crossover study in 12 healthy subjects, **omeprazole** 40 mg daily for 5 days had no effect on the pharmacokinetics of a single 50-mg dose of dolutegravir given 2 hours after omeprazole.[1]

(b) Elvitegravir

In a crossover study in 16 healthy subjects, **famotidine** 40 mg daily given simultaneously with elvitegravir boosted with cobicistat 150/150 mg daily for 8 days had no effect on the pharmacokinetics of elvitegravir. No effect was also seen in another study in 10 healthy subjects, when **famotidine** 40 mg daily was given 12 hours after elvitegravir boosted with cobicistat 150/150 mg daily for 8 days.[2]

In a study in 11 subjects, **omeprazole** 20 mg daily for 8 days, given 2 hours before or 12 hours after elvitegravir boosted with cobicistat 150/150 mg daily, increased the AUC of elvitegravir by 10% or had no effect, respectively.[2] In another study in 12 subjects, **omeprazole** 40 mg daily given 2 hours before elvitegravir boosted with ritonavir 50/100 mg for 5 days did not affect the pharmacokinetics of elvitegravir.[2]

(c) Raltegravir

In a study in 14 healthy subjects, **omeprazole** 20 mg daily for 5 days increased the AUC and maximum plasma concentration of raltegravir 3.1-fold and 4.1-fold, respectively.[3]

Mechanism

As raltegravir is not a substrate for cytochrome P450 isoenzymes that are affected by omeprazole, and omeprazole is not known to affect glucuronidation, which is the major metabolic pathway of raltegravir, another mechanism must explain the increase in raltegravir exposure seen. The most likely explanation might be the effect of omeprazole on gastric pH, increasing the absorption of raltegravir.

Importance and management

A pharmacokinetic interaction between **raltegravir** and omeprazole would seem to be established, although the clinical relevance of the modest increase in raltegravir exposure is uncertain. Because HIV-positive patients often have reduced gastric acidity, the effect of omeprazole on raltegravir might be less in these patients than that seen in this study in healthy subjects.[3] In addition, the UK manufacturer notes that the use of raltegravir with **proton pump inhibitors** and **H_2-receptor antagonists** in patients in phase III studies did not result in important adverse outcomes. For this reason, they state that no raltegravir dose adjustment is necessary with these drugs.[4]

No pharmacokinetic interaction occurs between **elvitegravir** and omeprazole or famotidine, and so no dose adjustment would seem necessary when given with proton pump inhibitors or H_2-receptor antagonists.

No pharmacokinetic interaction occurs between **dolutegravir** and omeprazole, and no dose adjustment would seem necessary if given with this, or other proton pump inhibitors. Although not studied, H_2-receptor antagonists might also be expected not to affect dolutegravir exposure.

1. Patel P, Song I, Borland J, Patel A, Lou Y, Chen S, Wajima T, Peppercorn A, Min SS, Piscitelli SC. Pharmacokinetics of the HIV integrase inhibitor S/GSK1349572 co-administered with acid-reducing agents and multivitamins in healthy volunteers. *J Antimicrob Chemother* (2011) 66, 1567–72.
2. Ramanathan S, Mathias A, Wei X, Shen G, Koziara J, Cheng A, Kearney BP. Pharmacokinetics of once-daily boosted elvitegravir when administered in combination with acid-reducing agents. *J Acquir Immune Defic Syndr* (2013) 64, 45–50.
3. Iwamoto M, Wenning LA, Nguyen B-Y, Teppler H, Moreau AR, Rhodes RR, Hanley WD, Jin B, Harvey CM, Breidinger SA, Azrolan N, Farmer HF, Isaacs RD, Chodakewitz JA, Stone JA, Wagner JA. Effects of omeprazole on plasma levels of raltegravir. *Clin Infect Dis* (2009) 48, 489–92.
4. Isentress (Raltegravir potassium). Merck Sharp & Dohme Ltd. UK Summary of product characteristics, November 2014.

HIV-integrase inhibitors + HCV-protease inhibitors

Telaprevir slightly increases the exposure to dolutegravir and raltegravir, but dolutegravir and raltegravir appear to have no effect on telaprevir pharmacokinetics. No pharmacokinetic interaction appears to occur between boceprevir and dolutegravir or raltegravir, or between simeprevir and raltegravir. Paritaprevir appears to moderately increase raltegravir exposure, but raltegravir does not appear to alter paritaprevir pharmacokinetics.

Clinical evidence

(a) Dolutegravir

In randomised study, healthy subjects were given dolutegravir 50 mg daily alone for 5 days with **boceprevir** 800 mg three times daily (13 subjects) or **telaprevir** 750 mg three times daily (15 subjects), for 10 days. The pharmacokinetics of dolutegravir were unaffected by **boceprevir**, however, **telaprevir** increased the AUC and maximum concentration of dolutegravir by 22% and 16%, respectively. The pharmacokinetics of **boceprevir** and **telaprevir** were no different to those in historical controls not taking dolutegravir.[1]

(b) Raltegravir

1. Boceprevir. In a crossover study in 22 healthy subjects, boceprevir 800 mg three times daily for 10 days did not affect the pharmacokinetics of a single 400-mg dose of raltegravir. The pharmacokinetics of boceprevir were no different to those in historical controls not taking raltegravir.[2]

2. Paritaprevir. The UK manufacturer briefly reports that, in a study in healthy subjects given raltegravir 400 mg twice daily with paritaprevir 150 mg daily (in a fixed-dose combination with ombitasvir and ritonavir, and given with dasabuvir), the pharmacokinetics of paritaprevir were no different to historical controls, but the AUC and maximum concentration of raltegravir were increased 2.3-fold.[3]

3. Simeprevir. The UK and US manufacturers briefly report that, in a study in 24 healthy subjects given simeprevir 150 mg daily with raltegravir 400 mg twice daily for 7 days, the pharmacokinetics of both drugs were unaffected.[4,5]

4. Telaprevir. In a crossover study in 20 healthy subjects, raltegravir 400 mg twice daily had no effect on the pharmacokinetics of telaprevir 750 mg three times daily when given concurrently for 6 days, whereas telaprevir increased the AUC and maximum plasma concentration of raltegravir by 31% and 26%, respectively.[6]

Mechanism

Telaprevir is an inhibitor of P-glycoprotein and the authors of the study, suggest that this leads to the slight increase in raltegravir exposure.[6] Further, they suggest that telaprevir did not affect the glucuronosyltransferase UGT1A1-mediated glucuronidation of raltegravir, which is its main route of metabolism, as the ratio of exposure to raltegravir and its glucuronide metabolite was similar, with and without telaprevir.[6] Paritaprevir is said to inhibit UGT1A1 and involvement of this in the increase in raltegravir exposure seen cannot be ruled out, but requires further study for confirmation. Dolutegravir appears to be metabolised similarly to raltegravir, and hence P-glycoprotein or UGT1A1 inhibition by telaprevir cannot be ruled out, and also requires further study.

Importance and management

Evidence for a pharmacokinetic interaction between the HCV-protease inhibitors and the HIV-integrase inhibitors shows that there is no interaction between boceprevir and dolutegravir or raltegravir. There also appears to be no interaction between simeprevir and raltegravir. However, there was a slight increase in raltegravir exposure with telaprevir, and a moderate increase with paritaprevir, but such changes are unlikely to be of clinical relevance. Raltegravir does not appear to alter the pharmacokinetics of telaprevir or paritaprevir. No dose adjustments appear to be necessary on the concurrent use of any of these HCV-protease inhibitors with raltegravir, or on the concurrent use of boceprevir or telaprevir with dolutegravir.

1. Johnson M, Borland J, Chen S, Savina P, Wynne B, Piscitelli S. Effects of boceprevir and telaprevir on the pharmacokinetics of dolutegravir. *Br J Clin Pharmacol* (2014) 78, 1043–9.
2. de Kanter CT, Blonk MI, Colbers AP Schouwenberg BJ, Burger DM. Lack of a clinically significant drug-drug interaction in healthy volunteers between the Hepatitis C virus protease inhibitor boceprevir and the HIV integrase inhibitor raltegravir. *Clin Infect Dis* (2013) 56, 300–6.
3. Viekirax (Ombitasvir, paritaprevir, ritonavir). AbbVie Ltd. UK Summary of product characteristics, January 2015.
4. Olysio (Simeprevir sodium). Janssen-Cilag Ltd. UK Summary of product characteristics, May 2014.
5. Olysio (Simeprevir sodium). Janssen Products, LP. US Prescribing information, November 2014.
6. van Heeswijk R, Garg V, Boogaerts G, Vandebosch A, Vandevoorde A, Witek J, Dannemann B. The pharmacokinetic interaction between telaprevir and raltegravir in healthy volunteers. 51st ICAAC, Chicago, 17th-20th September 2011. Abstract A1-1738a.

HIV-integrase inhibitors + HIV-protease inhibitors

Low-dose ritonavir increases elvitegravir exposure. Darunavir and tipranavir, both boosted with ritonavir, do not appear to alter elvitegravir exposure, when compared to elvitegravir boosted with ritonavir.

Atazanavir alone and boosted with ritonavir might slightly increase raltegravir exposure, and does slightly increase dolutegravir exposure. Indinavir and saquinavir are predicted to increase raltegravir exposure, but to a lesser extent than atazanavir. Low-dose ritonavir minimally decreases raltegravir exposure. Lopinavir and tipranavir, both boosted with ritonavir, appear to decrease the minimum plasma concentration of raltegravir, but have no effect on, or cause a moderate decrease in, the exposure to dolutegravir, respectively. Darunavir boosted with ritonavir appears to slightly decrease raltegravir exposure, and was associated with a high incidence of rash in one study. Darunavir boosted with ritonavir slightly decreases exposure to dolutegravir. Fosamprenavir boosted with ritonavir halves raltegravir exposure, and slightly decreases that of dolutegravir. Raltegravir decreases amprenavir exposure.

Clinical evidence

(a) Atazanavir

1. Dolutegravir. In a randomised study, 24 healthy subjects were given dolutegravir 30 mg daily for 5 days alone and then with either atazanavir boosted with ritonavir 300/100 mg daily (12 subjects) or atazanavir 400 mg daily (12 subjects) all for 14 days. The AUC and maximum concentration of dolutegravir were increased by 62% and 34%, respectively compared with 91% and 50%, respectively. Atazanavir pharmacokinetics were similar to historical controls.[1]

2. Raltegravir. In a study in 19 healthy subjects, raltegravir 400 mg twice daily was taken with atazanavir 300 mg twice daily for 14 days. The concurrent use of atazanavir and raltegravir resulted in a 17% decrease in the AUC of atazanavir, and an increase in the AUC and maximum plasma concentration of raltegravir of 54% and 39%, respectively.[2] Similarly, in another study in 12 healthy subjects, atazanavir 400 mg daily for 9 days increased the AUC and maximum plasma concentration of a single 100-mg dose of raltegravir (taken on day 7) by 72% and 53%, respectively.[3] The increase in raltegravir concentrations with atazanavir has been confirmed in a study in patients where raltegravir concentrations were found to correlate with atazanavir concentrations.[4]

In another study by the same authors in 10 healthy subjects, raltegravir 400 mg twice daily was taken alone or with atazanavir boosted with ritonavir 300/100 mg daily for 10 days. Atazanavir boosted with ritonavir increased the AUC of raltegravir by 41%, and increased the maximum plasma concentration by 24%; however, this was not statistically significant. Atazanavir concentrations were not assessed in this study.[3] In a pilot study in 8 patients, raltegravir was given at a dose of 400 mg daily, with atazanavir boosted with ritonavir plus a nucleoside/nucleotide backbone, for 10 days. The pharmacokinetics of raltegravir were comparable to those at a dose of 800 mg daily with atazanavir or standard 400 mg twice daily dosing.[5] Another study in 17 patients taking raltegravir 800 mg with unboosted atazanavir 600 mg daily with lamivudine or emtricitabine found that the pharmacokinetics of raltegravir were comparable to a dose of 400 mg twice daily alone, and achieved an undetectable viral load at the end of the study.[6] In a crossover study in 19 healthy subjects, the minimum concentration of raltegravir 400 mg daily with unboosted atazanavir 400 mg daily was 78% lower than that of raltegravir 400 mg twice daily, but the maximum concentration and AUC were no different.[7]

A case series in 3 HIV-positive patients, taking unboosted atazanavir 300 mg twice daily with raltegravir 400 mg twice daily, reported no increase in adverse effects and no loss of therapeutic efficacy. Three other patients taking the same regimen but with additional antiretrovirals (one taking lamivudine, another patient taking abacavir with **saquinavir**, and another patient taking lamivudine and tenofovir) similarly had viral loads less than 50 copies/mL and no increase in adverse effects.[8]

(b) Darunavir

1. Dolutegravir. In a randomised crossover study, healthy subjects were given dolutegravir 30 mg daily for 5 days alone and then with darunavir boosted with ritonavir 600/100 mg twice daily for 14 days. The AUC of dolutegravir was *decreased* by 22%, but the maximum concentration was not affected. Darunavir pharmacokinetics were similar to historical controls.[9]

2. Elvitegravir. In a study in healthy subjects, the pharmacokinetics of elvitegravir when added to darunavir boosted with ritonavir were similar to those when elvitegravir was given boosted with ritonavir. The pharmacokinetics of darunavir were not altered by the addition of elvitegravir.[10]

3. Raltegravir. In a study in 18 healthy subjects, only 6 subjects finished the course of darunavir boosted with ritonavir 600/100 mg twice daily with raltegravir 400 mg twice daily for 12 days. Eight cases of a rash occurred; seven were mild to moderate in nature; however, one case progressed to a severe maculopapular rash. As insufficient subjects completed the study, no clear interpretations can be made from this data. However, the pharmacokinetic data from the remaining 6 subjects suggested that darunavir boosted with ritonavir decreased the AUC and maximum plasma concentration of raltegravir by 29% and 33%, respectively, when compared with raltegravir taken alone for 4 days. No difference was found in darunavir pharmacokinetics when compared with historical data in healthy subjects.[11] In an analysis of darunavir plasma concentrations in patients taking darunavir boosted with ritonavir plus a nucleoside/nucleotide backbone, those additionally taking raltegravir had lower darunavir plasma concentrations than those not taking raltegravir; however, viral suppression was greater in the group also taking raltegravir.[12] In two similar analyses, darunavir pharmacokinetics were no different when raltegravir was added to darunavir boosted with ritonavir (plus a nucleoside/nucleotide backbone, with or without etravirine), when compared with patients not taking raltegravir or etravirine,[13] or when raltegravir was added to darunavir boosted with ritonavir plus tenofovir and emtricitabine.[14] In another study in HIV-positive patients taking raltegravir 400 mg twice daily and darunavir boosted with ritonavir 600/100 mg twice daily (8 patients) or 800/100 mg daily (9 patients), the AUC of darunavir was 38% and 35% lower, respectively, than in 5 patients and 3 patients, respectively, taking the same doses of darunavir boosted with ritonavir but without raltegravir. Patients taking raltegravir had lower maximum plasma concentrations of darunavir, and increased darunavir clearance, compared with those not taking raltegravir, but minimum plasma concentrations were unaffected.[15] A pilot pharmacokinetic study in 15 patients given darunavir boosted with ritonavir 800/100 mg daily and raltegravir 400 mg twice daily for 15 days found that the pharmacokinetics of darunavir and raltegravir were comparable to historical controls.[16]

(c) Fosamprenavir

1. Dolutegravir. In a study in 12 healthy subjects given dolutegravir 50 mg daily for 5 days alone and then with fosamprenavir boosted with ritonavir 700/100 mg twice daily for 10 days, the AUC and maximum concentration of dolutegravir were *decreased* by 35% and 24%, respectively. Amprenavir pharmacokinetics were similar to historical controls.[17]

2. Raltegravir. The US manufacturer of fosamprenavir (the pro-drug of amprenavir) includes a number of pharmacokinetic studies in which fosamprenavir alone, or boosted with ritonavir, was given with raltegravir, either in the fasted state or with food. Amprenavir exposure and minimum plasma concentration were decreased by 17 to 50%, with the greatest decreases seen in the fasted state.[18] Raltegravir exposure was halved by fosamprenavir boosted with ritonavir.[19]

(d) Lopinavir

1. Dolutegravir. In a randomised crossover study in healthy subjects given dolutegravir 30 mg daily for 5 days alone and then with lopinavir boosted with ritonavir 400/100 mg twice daily for 14 days, the pharmacokinetics of dolutegravir were unaffected. Lopinavir pharmacokinetics were similar to historical controls.[9]

2. Raltegravir. In a study in 13 healthy subjects, lopinavir boosted with ritonavir 400/100 mg twice daily had no effect on the AUC of raltegravir 400 mg twice daily but decreased the minimum plasma raltegravir concentration by 30%. One subject had a plasma concentration below the recommended minimum for raltegravir. Lopinavir and ritonavir pharmacokinetics were similar when given alone or with raltegravir.[20]

A case report describes a 55-year-old HIV-positive man with dyslipidaemia (controlled by atorvastatin, ezetimibe, and fenofibrate for the previous 3 years) who developed lipaemia retinalis due to severe dyslipidaemia (total cholesterol 600 mg/dL, triglycerides greater than 5 000 mg/dL and HDL less than 5 mg/dL) 7 months after raltegravir (and emtricitabine) was added to his lopinavir boosted with ritonavir and tenofovir. Lopinavir boosted with ritonavir and atorvastatin were stopped, his fenofibrate dose was increased, and he was started on omega-3 fatty acids and etravirine; raltegravir and emtricitabine were continued. After 2 weeks his lipid profile normalised and the original lipid-lowering regime was resumed; his lipaemia retinalis had completely resolved 4 months later.[21] The authors of this report rule out involvement of emtricitabine, which was started at the same time as raltegravir, because it has not been associated with dyslipidaemia but raltegravir with lopinavir boosted with ritonavir has.[21]

(e) Ritonavir

1. Elvitegravir. In a study in healthy subjects, ritonavir 50 to 200 mg daily increased the exposure to elvitegravir 125 mg daily up to 2-fold, compared with the same dose of elvitegravir given with ritonavir 20 mg daily.[22]

2. Raltegravir. In a study in 10 healthy subjects, ritonavir 100 mg twice daily was taken for 16 days with a single 400-mg dose of raltegravir taken on day 14. The AUC of raltegravir was decreased by 16%, but this was not statistically significant.[23]

(f) Tipranavir

1. Dolutegravir. In a study in 14 healthy subjects given dolutegravir 50 mg daily for 5 days alone and then with tipranavir boosted with ritonavir 500/200 mg twice daily for 5 days, the AUC and maximum concentration of dolutegravir were decreased by 59% and 46%, respectively.[24]

2. Elvitegravir. In a study in healthy subjects, the pharmacokinetics of elvitegravir when added to tipranavir boosted with ritonavir were similar to those when elvitegravir was given boosted with ritonavir. The pharmacokinetics of tipranavir were not altered by the addition of elvitegravir.[10]

3. Raltegravir. In a study, 15 healthy subjects were given tipranavir boosted with ritonavir 500/200 mg twice daily for 11 days with raltegravir 400 mg twice daily from day 8 to 11. Tipranavir boosted with ritonavir decreased the minimum plasma concentration of raltegravir by 55%, with a non-statistically significant 24% decrease in its AUC.[25] However, the US manufacturer of raltegravir notes that in phase 3 clinical studies, the efficacy of raltegravir regimens containing tipranavir boosted with ritonavir was comparable to raltegravir regimens containing other antiretrovirals.[26]

Mechanism

Elvitegravir is principally metabolised by CYP3A, which is inhibited by ritonavir. It is also metabolised by glucuronidation (UGT1A1 and UGT1A3).[22] The main route of metabolism for dolutegravir and raltegravir is glucuronidation (primarily by the glucuronosyltransferase, UGT1A1), and as atazanavir is a known inhibitor of this pathway, their exposure increases with concurrent use. The UK and US manufacturers of raltegravir also suggest that less potent inhibitors of UGT1A1, such as indinavir and saquinavir, might interact to a lesser extent than atazanavir.[26,27] The US manufacturer of ritonavir reports that it can induce glucuronosyltransferases,[28] and this explains the small decreases in raltegravir and dolutegravir concentrations and/or exposure seen with ritonavir and HIV-protease inhibitors boosted with ritonavir (with the exception of atazanavir). Note also, that lopinavir boosted with ritonavir had no effect on dolutegravir pharmacokinetics, the reasons for which are not known.

Importance and management

A pharmacokinetic interaction between the HIV-integrase inhibitors and most HIV-protease inhibitors is established, although the direction of the effect (i.e. increase or decrease in exposure or concentrations) varies depending on the principle metabolic pathway of the HIV-integrase inhibitor and the effect of the HIV-protease inhibitor on this.

The pharmacokinetics of **elvitegravir** alone were no different to those of elvitegravir boosted with ritonavir, when given with darunavir or tipranavir, both boosted with ritonavir, and so elvitegravir can be given with these HIV-protease inhibitors without any dose adjustment.[10] However, the US manufacturer of elvitegravir boosted with cobicistat (in a fixed-dose combination also including emtricitabine and tenofovir disoproxil fumarate) states that this product should not be given with ritonavir or other anti-retroviral regimens containing ritonavir because of the similar action of cobicistat and ritonavir on CYP3A4.[29]

Only a minor pharmacokinetic interaction appears to occur between **raltegravir** and **darunavir** boosted with ritonavir, and one study suggests that viral suppression is maintained; however, the high incidence of rash reported in another study suggests a note of caution is warranted on concurrent use.

The slight increase in raltegravir exposure seen with **atazanavir** is not expected to be clinically relevant, and the case series of successful concurrent use appears to support this. The UK and US manufacturers therefore advise that no raltegravir dose adjustment is needed when it is given with atazanavir alone or with atazanavir boosted with ritonavir. They also suggest that no dose adjustment is likely to be needed for less potent inhibitors of UGT1A1, and they name **indinavir** and **saquinavir**.[26,27]

Although **ritonavir** would be expected to have some effect on the pharmacokinetics of **raltegravir**, as it is a known inducer of glucuronosyltransferases, the data above indicates that the impact of low doses of ritonavir (such as those used for pharmacokinetic boosting of other HIV-protease inhibitors), on the pharmacokinetics of raltegravir is unlikely to be clinically relevant. No raltegravir dose adjustment appears to be needed with low-dose ritonavir specifically; however, until further data is available, it would seem prudent to monitor concurrent use in patients taking higher doses of ritonavir. Further study is needed.

The moderate decrease in **raltegravir** and amprenavir exposure seen with raltegravir and **fosamprenavir** boosted with ritonavir could be clinically important, and might result in virological failure. Concurrent use is not recommended.[19]

Tipranavir boosted with ritonavir appears to decrease the minimum plasma concentration of **raltegravir**. However, the UK and US manufacturers advise that no raltegravir dose adjustment is needed on concurrent use.[26,27]

Lopinavir boosted with ritonavir also decreases the minimum plasma concentration of raltegravir, but to a lesser extent than tipranavir, suggesting that a raltegravir dose adjustment is unlikely to be needed on concurrent use. However, until more is known it might be prudent to monitor plasma drug concentrations, if possible, and virological efficacy.

The exposure of **dolutegravir** is only slightly increased by unboosted **atazanavir** and atazanavir boosted with ritonavir and so no dose adjustment is recommended on concurrent use. **Darunavir** boosted with ritonavir slightly decreased dolutegravir exposure, but **lopinavir** boosted with ritonavir had no effect. No dose adjustment is necessary on concurrent use with either of these HIV-protease inhibitors boosted with ritonavir. **Fosamprenavir** boosted with ritonavir also caused a slight decrease in dolutegravir exposure, but because the average minimum concentration was higher than the lower limit of clinical efficacy and viral suppression had been demonstrated in a phase 3 study in patients receiving this combination,[17] the UK manufacturer of dolutegravir states that no dose adjustment is necessary in patients without resistance to HIV-integrase inhibitor.[30] In contrast, the US manufacturer advises that the dolutegravir dose should be increased to 50 mg twice daily if given with fosamprenavir boosted with ritonavir, in HIV-integrase inhibitor-naive patients who are both treatment-naive and experienced. In those who are HIV-integrase inhibitor-experienced patients with HIV-integrase inhibitor-associated resistance substitutions or clinically suspected resistance, this combination should be avoided due to the risk of decreased therapeutic efficacy and development of resistance.[31] **Tipranavir** boosted with ritonavir caused a moderate decrease in dolutegravir exposure, which could be clinically important, and as such the dose of dolutegravir should be increased to 50 mg twice daily on concurrent use.[30,31] The US manufacturer states the same patient requirements as for fosamprenavir above, and the UK manufacturer advises that this dose might be suitable in patients who are not resistant to HIV-integrase inhibitors, but the combination should not be used in those who show HIV-integrase inhibitor resistance.[30] The UK manufacturer predicts that **nelfinavir** will have no effect on dolutegravir pharmacokinetics and advises that no dose adjustment is necessary on concurrent use.[30]

Note that the concurrent use of an HIV-integrase inhibitor with a HIV-protease inhibitor is not a recommended regimen when starting antiretrovirals in treatment-naive patients.[32,33] Current local and national guidelines should be consulted for other options in treatment-naive patients and for the management of treatment-experienced patients.

1. Song I, Borland J, Chen S, Lou Y, Peppercorn A, Wajima T, Min S, Piscitelli SC. Effect of atazanavir and atazanavir/ritonavir on the pharmacokinetics of the next-generation HIV integrase inhibitor, S/GSK1349572. *Br J Clin Pharmacol* (2011) 72, 103–8.
2. Zhu L, Butterton J, Persson A, Stonier M, Comisar W, Panebianco D, Breidinger S, Zhang J, Bertz R. Pharmacokinetics and safety of twice-daily atazanavir 300 mg and raltegravir 400 mg in healthy individuals. *Antivir Ther* (2010) 15, 1107–14.
3. Iwamoto M, Wenning LA, Mistry GC, Petry AS, Liou SY, Ghosh K, Breidinger S, Azrolan N, Gutierrez MJ, Bridson WE, Stone JA, Gottesdiener KM, Wagner JA. Atazanavir modestly increases plasma levels of raltegravir. *Clin Infect Dis* (2008) 47, 137–40.
4. Cattaneo D, Ripamonti D, Baldelli S, Cozzi V, Conti F, Clementi E. Exposure-related effects of atazanavir on the pharmacokinetics of raltegravir in HIV-1-infected patients. *Ther Drug Monit* (2010) 32, 782–6.
5. Calgano A, Tettoni MC, Simiele M, Trentini L, Montrucchio C, D'Avolio A, Di Perri G, Bonora S. Pharmacokinetics of 400 mg of raltegravir once daily in combination with atazanavir/ritonavir plus two nucleoside/nucleotide reverse transcriptase inhibitors. *J Antimicrob Chemother* (2013) 68, 482–4.
6. Jansen A, Colbers EP, van der Ven AJ, Richter C, Rockstroh JK, Wasmuth JC, van Luin M, Burger DM. Pharmacokinetics of the combination raltegravir/atazanavir in HIV-1-infected patients. *HIV Med* (2013) 14, 449–52.
7. Neely M, Decosterd L, Fayet A, Lee SF, Margol A, Kanani M, di Iulio J, von Schoen-Angerer T, Jellife R, Calmy A. Pharmacokinetics and pharmacogenomics of once-daily raltegravir and atazanavir in healthy volunteers. *Antimicrob Agents Chemother* (2010) 54, 4619–25.
8. Gupta S, Lataillade M, Farber S, Kozal MJ. Raltegravir with unboosted atazanavir 300 mg twice daily in antiretroviral treatment-experienced participants. *J Int Assoc Physicians AIDS Care (Chic Ill)* (2009) 8, 87–92.
9. Song I, Min SS, Borland J, Lou Y, Chen S, Patel P, Ishibashi T, Piscitelli SC. The effect of lopinavir/ritonavir and darunavir/ritonavir on the HIV integrase inhibitor S/GSK1349572 in healthy participants. *J Clin Pharmacol* (2011) 51, 237–42.
10. Mathias AA, Hinkle J, Shen G, Enejosa J, Piliero PJ, Sekar V, Mack R, Tomaka F, Kearney BP. Effect of ritonavir-boosted tipranavir or darunavir on the steady-state pharmacokinetics of elvitegravir. *J Acquir Immune Defic Syndr* (2008) 49, 156–62.
11. Anderson MS, Sekar V, Tomaka F, Mabalot J, Mack R, Lionti L, Zajic S, Wenning L, Vanden Abeele C, Zinny M, Lunde NM, Jin B, Wagner JA, Iwamoto M. Pharmacokinetic (PK) evaluation of darunavir/ritonavir (DRV/r) and raltegravir (RAL) in healthy subjects. 48th Annual ICAAC/IDSA 46th Annual Meeting, Washington DC, 2009. Poster A-962.
12. Fabbiani M, Di Giambenedetto S, Ragazzoni E, D'Ettorre G, Parruti G, Prosperi M, Bracciale L, Cauda R, Navarra P, De Luca A. Darunavir/ritonavir and raltegravir coadministered in routine clinical practice: potential role for an unexpected drug interaction. *Pharmacol Res* (2011) 63, 249–53.
13. Dailly E, Allavena C, Bouquié R, Deslandes G, Raffi F, Jolliet P. Effect of efavirenz, nevirapine, etravirine, and raltegravir administration on the pharmacokinetics of ritonavir-boosted darunavir in a population of HIV-infected patients. *AIDS Res Hum Retroviruses* (2013) 29, 42–6.
14. Garvey L, Latch N, Erlwein OW, Mackie NE, Walsh J, Scullard G, McClure MO, Dickinson L, Back D, Winston A. The effects of a nucleoside-sparing antiretroviral regimen on the pharmacokinetics of ritonavir-boosted darunavir in HIV type-1-infected patients. *Antivir Ther* (2010) 15, 213–8.
15. Cattaneo D, Gervasoni C, Cozzi V, Baldelli S, Fucile S, Meraviglia P, Landonio S, Boreggio G, Rizzardini G, Clementi E. Co-administration of raltegravir reduces daily darunavir exposure in HIV-1 infected patients. *Pharmacol Res* (2012) 65, 198–203.
16. Martínez-Rebollar M, Muñoz A, Pérez I, Hidalgo S, Brunet M, Laguno M, González A, Calvo M, Loncà M, Blanco JL, Martínez E, Gatell JM, Mallolas J. Pharmacokinetic study of dual therapy with raltegravir 400 mg twice daily and Darunavir/Ritonavir 800/100 mg once daily in HIV-1-infected patients. *Ther Drug Monit* (2013) 35, 552–6.
17. Song I, Borland J, Chen S, Peppercorn A, Wajima T, Piscitelli SC. Effect of fosamprenavir-ritonavir on the pharmacokinetics of dolutegravir in healthy subjects. *Antimicrob Agents Chemother* (2014) 58, 6696–700.
18. Lexiva (Fosamprenavir calcium). ViiV Healthcare. US Prescribing information, April 2013.
19. Telzir (Fosamprenavir calcium). ViiV Healthcare UK Ltd. UK Summary of product characteristics, October 2014.
20. Rhame F, Long M, Acosta E. RAL-KAL: pharmacokinetics of coadministered raltegravir and lopinavir-ritonavir in healthy adults. 9th International Workshop on Clinical Pharmacology of HIV Therapy. New Orleans, 2008. Abstract O19.
21. Huesgen E, Burgos R, Goldstein DA, Max B, Jarrett OD. Severe dyslipidaemia after the addition of raltegravir to a lopinavir/ritonavir-containing regimen. *Antivir Ther* (2012) 17, 1385–8.
22. Mathias AA, West S, Hui J, Kearney BP. Dose-response of ritonavir on hepatic CYP3A activity and elvitegravir oral exposure. *Clin Pharmacol Ther* (2009) 85, 64–70.
23. Iwamoto M, Wenning LA, Petry AS, Laethem M, De Smet M, Kost JT, Breidinger SA, Mangin E, Azrolan N, Greenberg HE, Haazen W, Stone JA, Gottesdiener KM. Minimal effects of ritonavir and efavirenz on the pharmacokinetics of raltegravir. *Antimicrob Agents Chemother* (2008) 52 4338–43.
24. Song I, Borland J, Chen S, Guta P, Lou Y, Wilfret D, Wajima T, Savina P, Peppercorn A, Castellino S, Wagner D, Hosking L, Mosteller M, Rubio JP, Piscitelli SC. Effects of enzyme inducers efavirenz and tipranavir/ritonavir on the pharmacokinetics of the HIV integrase inhibitor dolutegravir. *Eur J Clin Pharmacol* (2014) 70, 1173–9.
25. Hanley WD, Wenning LA, Moreau A, Kost JT, Mangin E, Shamp T, Stone JA, Gottesdiener KM, Wagner JA, Iwamoto M. Effect of tipranavir-ritonavir on pharmacokinetics of raltegravir. *Antimicrob Agents Chemother* (2009) 53, 2752–5.
26. Isentress (Raltegravir potassium). Merck Sharp & Dohme Ltd. UK Summary of product characteristics, November 2014.
27. Isentress (Raltegravir potassium). Merck & Co. US Prescribing information, February 2015.
28. Norvir Tablets (Ritonavir). AbbVie Ltd. UK Summary of product characteristics, November 2013.
29. Stribild (Elvitegravir, cobicistat, emtricitabine, tenofovir disoproxil fumarate). Gilead Sciences, Inc. US Prescribing information, December 2014.
30. Tivicay (Dolutegravir sodium). ViiV Healthcare UK Ltd. UK Summary of product characteristics, September 2014.
31. Tivicay (Dolutegravir sodium). ViiV Healthcare. US Prescribing information, December 2014.
32. Williams I, Churchill D, Anderson J, Boffito M, Bower M, Cairns G, Cwynarski K, Edwards S, Fidler S, Fisher M, Freedman A, Geretti AM, Gilleece Y, Horne R, Johnson M, Khoo S, Leen C, Marshall N, Nelson M, Orkin C, Paton N, Phillips A, Post F, Pozniak A, Sabin C, Trevelion R, Ustianowski A, Walsh J, Waters L, Wilkins E, Winston A, Youle M. British HIV Association guidelines for the treatment of HIV-1-positive adults with antiretroviral therapy 2012 (Updated 2013). *HIV Med* (2014), 15 (Suppl 1) 1–85.
33. Panel on Antiretroviral Guidelines for Adults and Adolescents. Guidelines for the use of antiretroviral agents in HIV-1-infected adults and adolescents. US Department of Health and Human Services (April 2015). 1–288. Available at: https://aidsinfo.nih.gov/contentfiles/lvguidelines/adultandadolescentgl.pdf (accessed 14/09/15).

HIV-integrase inhibitors + Maraviroc

Maraviroc does not alter elvitegravir pharmacokinetics, but elvitegravir boosted with ritonavir moderately increases maraviroc exposure. A small decrease in exposure of both raltegravir and maraviroc appears to occur on concurrent use.

Clinical evidence

(a) Elvitegravir

In a crossover study in healthy subjects, concurrent use of elvitegravir boosted with ritonavir 150/100 mg daily and maraviroc 150 mg twice daily did not alter the pharmacokinetics of elvitegravir or ritonavir. However, the AUC of maraviroc was increased 2- to 4-fold.[1]

(b) Raltegravir

In a study in 17 healthy subjects, the pharmacokinetics of raltegravir and maraviroc were analysed when taken separately (raltegravir 400 mg twice daily for 3 days and maraviroc 300 mg twice daily for 5 days) or when taken together for 3 days. Raltegravir decreased the AUC and minimum plasma concentration of maraviroc by 14% and 10%, respectively. Similarly, maraviroc decreased the AUC and minimum plasma concentration of raltegravir by 37% and 28%, respectively. The average plasma concentration of maraviroc did not fall below the predicted therapeutic concentration of greater than 100 nanograms/mL.[2]

Mechanism

The increase in maraviroc exposure on concurrent use with elvitegravir boosted with ritonavir is likely to be due to inhibition of CYP3A4 and P-glycoprotein by ritonavir, see 'Maraviroc + HIV-protease inhibitors', p.949. The reason for the interaction between raltegravir and maraviroc is unknown.

Importance and management

The moderate increase in maraviroc exposure seen with elvitegravir boosted with ritonavir is consistent with the effect of ritonavir and other HIV-protease inhibitors, and as such an interaction would seem to be established, and the same advice would therefore seem appropriate: the maraviroc dose should be reduced to 150 mg daily on concurrent use, see 'Maraviroc + HIV-protease inhibitors', p.949 for further details. This dose reduction should also be considered for elvitegravir boosted with cobicistat because the inhibitory effects of cobicistat on CYP3A4 are similar to those of ritonavir, and so it would be predicted to interact similarly.

The decreases in raltegravir and maraviroc plasma concentrations are unlikely to be clinically important, and no dose adjustment of either drug appears to be needed on concurrent use.[2]

Note that the concurrent use of an HIV-integrase inhibitor with maraviroc is not a recommended regimen when starting antiretrovirals in treatment-naive patients.[3,4] Current local and national guidelines should be consulted for other options in treatment-naive patients and for the management of treatment-experienced patients.

1. Ramanathan S, Abel S, Tweedy S, West S, Hui J, Kearney BP. Pharmacokinetic interaction of ritonavir-boosted elvitegravir and maraviroc. *J Acquir Immune Defic Syndr* (2010) 53, 209–14.
2. Andrews E, Glue P, Fang J, Crownover P, Tressler R, Damle B. Assessment of the pharmacokinetics of co-administered maraviroc and raltegravir. *Br J Clin Pharmacol* (2010) 69, 51–7.
3. Williams I, Churchill D, Anderson J, Boffito M, Bower M, Cairns G, Cwynarski K, Edwards S, Fidler S, Fisher M, Freedman A, Geretti AM, Gilleece Y, Horne R, Johnson M, Khoo S, Leen C, Marshall N, Nelson M, Orkin C, Paton N, Phillips A, Post F, Pozniak A, Sabin C, Trevelion R, Ustianowski A, Walsh J, Waters L, Wilkins E, Winston A, Youle M. British HIV Association guidelines for the treatment of HIV-1-positive adults with antiretroviral therapy 2012 (Updated 2013). *HIV Med* (2014), 15 (Suppl 1) 1–85.
4. Panel on Antiretroviral Guidelines for Adults and Adolescents. Guidelines for the use of antiretroviral agents in HIV-1-infected adults and adolescents. US Department of Health and Human Services (April 2015). 1–288. Available at: https://aidsinfo.nih.gov/contentfiles/lvguidelines/adultandadolescentgl.pdf (accessed14/09/15).

HIV-integrase inhibitors + NNRTIs

Dolutegravir exposure is moderately decreased by efavirenz and etravirine, while rilpivirine has no effect. However, the effect of etravirine on dolutegravir exposure is attenuated by atazanavir, darunavir, and lopinavir, all boosted with ritonavir. Efavirenz slightly decreases raltegravir exposure. Etravirine caused a minor decrease in the exposure to raltegravir in one study; however, decreased or subtherapeutic plasma raltegravir concentrations have been reported in patients taking antiretroviral drugs including etravirine. Conversely, there are reports of patients taking etravirine with therapeutic or increased plasma concentrations of raltegravir. No pharmacokinetic interaction appears to occur between elvitegravir boosted with ritonavir and etravirine. There appears to be no interaction between raltegravir and rilpivirine and no interaction is predicted to occur between raltegravir and nevirapine.

Clinical evidence

(a) Efavirenz

1. Dolutegravir. In a study in 12 healthy subjects given dolutegravir 50 mg daily for 5 days alone and then with efavirenz 600 mg daily for 5 days, the AUC and maximum concentration of dolutegravir were decreased by 57% and 39%, respectively. The pharmacokinetics of efavirenz were comparable to historical controls for 8 of the 12 patients, but in the remaining 4 patients the efavirenz exposure was higher, which was explained by the presence of a genetic polymorphism of CYP2B6 which rendered these patients poor metabolisers (that is they had lower than normal activity of CYP2B6).[1]

2. Raltegravir. In a study in 9 healthy subjects, efavirenz 600 mg daily for 14 days decreased the AUC of a single 400-mg dose of raltegravir (taken on day 12) by 36%. The minimum plasma concentration was decreased by 21%, but this was not statistically significant.[2]

(b) Etravirine

1. Dolutegravir. In a study in 15 healthy subjects given dolutegravir 50 mg daily for 5 days alone and then with etravirine 200 mg twice daily for 14 days, the AUC and maximum concentration of dolutegravir were decreased by 71% and 52%, respectively.[3] In another study by the same authors, 17 healthy subjects were given dolutegravir 50 mg daily for 5 days alone and then with etravirine 200 mg twice daily plus lopinavir boosted with ritonavir 400/100 mg twice daily, or darunavir boosted with ritonavir 600/100 mg twice daily, for 14 days. The pharmacokinetics of dolutegravir were not altered by the addition of lopinavir boosted with ritonavir, but when darunavir boosted with ritonavir was added, the AUC of dolutegravir was decreased by 25% and the maximum concentration was unaffected.[3]

2. Elvitegravir. In a study in 31 healthy subjects, the concurrent use of elvitegravir boosted with ritonavir 150/100 mg daily with etravirine 200 mg twice daily for 10 days had no effect on the pharmacokinetics of etravirine or elvitegravir, when compared with either drug alone. There was a 12% decrease in the AUC of ritonavir, and a 29% decrease in its minimum plasma concentration.[4]

3. Raltegravir. In a study in 19 healthy subjects, raltegravir 400 mg twice daily was taken alone for 4 days then etravirine 200 mg twice daily was taken for 12 days with the addition of raltegravir 400 mg twice daily from day 8 to day 12. Etravirine decreased the AUC and the minimum plasma concentration of raltegravir by 10% and 34%, respectively; however, these changes were not statistically significant. The AUC and minimum plasma concentration of etravirine were increased by 10% and 17% with raltegravir.[5]

There is one report of four patients who had decreased or subtherapeutic raltegravir minimum plasma concentrations while taking antiretroviral regimens including etravirine.[6] However, in an analysis of the efficacy of the addition of raltegravir 400 mg twice daily to optimised background antiretroviral therapy, the concurrent use of etravirine (22 patients) did not have any statistically significant effect on raltegravir pharmacokinetics, although they had slightly lower pharmacokinetic parameters (not specified). All patients had minimum plasma raltegravir concentrations that exceeded the minimum therapeutic concentration, and pharmacokinetic parameters were not predictive of virological success.[7] In another report in 10 patients taking raltegravir 400 mg twice daily with darunavir boosted with ritonavir, the addition of etravirine 200 mg twice daily increased the AUC, and the maximum and minimum plasma concentrations of raltegravir by 29%, 21% and 54%, respectively.[8]

(c) Rilpivirine

1. Dolutegravir. In a study in 16 healthy subjects given dolutegravir 50 mg daily for 5 days alone and then with rilpivirine 25 mg daily for 11 days, the AUC and maximum concentration of dolutegravir were unaltered. The pharmacokinetics of rilpivirine were similarly unaffected.[9]

2. Raltegravir. The preliminary report of a study in healthy subjects given rilpivirine 25 mg daily and raltegravir 400 mg twice daily for 11 days, notes that there was no change in raltegravir pharmacokinetics or those of the raltegravir glucuronide metabolite.[10]

Mechanism

Raltegravir and dolutegravir are primarily metabolised by the glucuronosyltransferase, UGT1A1. Efavirenz is thought to induce UGT1A1, thereby decreasing raltegravir[2,11] and dolutegravir[1,12] exposure. CYP3A4 plays a minor role in the metabolism of dolutegravir, but because efavirenz also induces this isoenzyme, the contribution of this cannot be ruled out. The reasons for the effect of etravirine on dolutegravir are not entirely clear, but induction of UGT1A1 and CYP3A4 requires confirmation from further study. Etravirine is only a weak (at best) inducer of CYP3A4 and its role in dolutegravir metabolism might be questionable especially as the more potent CYP3A4 inducer, efavirenz, had a similar effect. The attenuation of the etravirine effect by darunavir and lopinavir, both boosted with ritonavir, is likely the result of complex interplay between the inhibitory and inducing effects of all these drugs.

Importance and management

Evidence for a pharmacokinetic interaction between the HIV-integrase inhibitors and the NNRTIs is limited, but is largely consistent with the known disposition and inducing effects of these drugs, although the clinical relevance of any effects varies.

Raltegravir

The slight decrease in raltegravir exposure with **efavirenz** is not expected to be clinically relevant, and the UK and US manufacturers of raltegravir advise that no dose adjustment is required on the concurrent use.[11,13] However, it might be prudent to monitor virological efficacy more closely on concurrent use.

The effect of **etravirine** on raltegravir pharmacokinetics is uncertain, with data varying from decreased or subtherapeutic plasma raltegravir concentrations to therapeutic concentrations and even increased plasma concentrations. The authors of a pharmacokinetic study,[5] and the UK and US manufacturers[11,13] of raltegravir advise that no raltegravir dose adjustment is needed if it is taken with etravirine. However, until more is known, it would seem prudent to closely monitor virological efficacy on concurrent use. Raltegravir negligibly increased the exposure to etravirine and this would not be expected to be clinically relevant and so no etravirine dose adjustment is required.[11,13]

The UK manufacturer of raltegravir advises that no dose adjustment is needed on concurrent use of **nevirapine**.[11]

No pharmacokinetic interaction appears to occur between **rilpivirine** and raltegravir, and no dose adjustment would be expected to be necessary on concurrent use.

Elvitegravir

There is no clinically relevant pharmacokinetic interaction between **etravirine** and elvitegravir boosted with ritonavir, which suggests that no interaction is likely if elvitegravir is boosted with cobicistat, as both ritonavir and cobicistat are potent inhibitors of CYP3A4. Therefore, no dose adjustment would be expected to be necessary on concurrent use. However, note that the US manufacturer of the multi-ingredient preparation containing elvitegravir, cobicistat, emtricitabine, and tenofovir disoproxil fumarate states that, as it is a complete regimen, it should not be given with NNRTIs.[14]

Dolutegravir

Dolutegravir exposure is moderately decreased by **etravirine** when given alone, and as such the UK manufacturer advises that this could lead to reduced virological response and possible resistance.[12] As the addition of atazanavir, darunavir, or lopinavir, all boosted with ritonavir, attenuates this effect, etravirine alone should not be used with dolutegravir, but can be used if combined with one of these HIV-protease inhibitors.[12,15]

Efavirenz also moderately decreases dolutegravir exposure, but an increase in dolutegravir dose to 50 mg twice daily is recommended when given with efavirenz.[12,15] The US manufacturer adds that this applies to HIV-integrase inhibitor-naive patients who are both treatment-naive and experienced, but in those who are HIV-integrase inhibitor-experienced patients with HIV-integrase inhibitor-associated resistance substitutions or clinically suspected resistance, this combination should be avoided due to the risk of decreased therapeutic efficacy and development of resistance.[15] The UK manufacturer advises that this dose might be suitable in patients who are not resistant to HIV-integrase inhibitors, but the combination should not be used in those who show HIV-integrase inhibitor resistance.[12]

Although not studied, **nevirapine** is predicted to decrease dolutegravir exposure, and the UK manufacturer recommendations an increase in dolutegravir dose to 50 mg twice daily when given with nevirapine, except if integrase class resistance is present, in which case an alternative regimen that does not include nevirapine should be given.[12] In contrast, the US manufacturer advises that nevirapine should be avoided due to a lack of data to inform dosing recommendations.[15]

No pharmacokinetic interaction occurs between dolutegravir and **rilpivirine** and so no dose adjustment is necessary on concurrent use.

Note that the concurrent use of an NNRTI with a HIV-integrase inhibitor is not a recommended regimen when starting antiretrovirals in treatment-naive patients.[16,17] Current local and national guidelines should be consulted for options in treatment-naive patients and for the management of treatment-experienced patients.

1. Song I, Borland J, Chen S, Guta P, Lou Y, Wilfret D, Wajima T, Savina P, Peppercorn A, Castellino S, Wagner D, Hosking L, Mosteller M, Rubio JP, Piscitelli SC. Effects of enzyme inducers efavirenz and tipranavir/ritonavir on the pharmacokinetics of the HIV integrase inhibitor dolutegravir. *Eur J Clin Pharmacol* (2014) 70, 1173–9.
2. Iwamoto M, Wenning LA, Petry AS, Laethem M, De Smet M, Kost JT, Breidinger SA, Mangin E, Azrolan N, Greenberg HE, Haazen W, Stone JA, Gottesdiener KM. Minimal effects of ritonavir and efavirenz on the pharmacokinetics of raltegravir. *Antimicrob Agents Chemother* (2008) 52 4338–43.
3. Song I, Borland J, Min S, Lou Y, Chen S, Patel P, Wajima T, Piscitelli SC. Effects of etravirine alone and with ritonavir-boosted protease inhibitors on the pharmacokinetics of dolutegravir. *Antimicrob Agents Chemother* (2011) 55, 3517–21.
4. Ramanathan S, Kakuda TN, Mack R, West S, Kearney BP. Pharmacokinetics of elvitegravir and etravirine following coadministration of ritonavir-boosted elvitegravir and etravirine. *Antivir Ther* (2008) 13, 1011–17.
5. Anderson MS, Kakuda TN, Hanley W, Miller J, Kost JT, Stoltz R, Wenning LA, Stone JA, Hoetelmans RMW, Wagner JA, Iwamoto M. Minimal pharmacokinetic interaction between human immunodeficiency virus nonnucleoside reverse transcriptase inhibitor etravirine and the integrase inhibitor raltegravir in healthy subjects. *Antimicrob Agents Chemother* (2008) 52, 4228–32.
6. Ménard A, Solas C, Mokhtari S, Bregigeon S, Drogoul M-P, Tamalet C, Lacarelle B, Martin IP. Etravirine–raltegravir, a marked interaction in HIV-1-infected patients: about four cases. *AIDS* (2009) 27, 869–71.
7. Wittkop L, Breilh D, Da Silva D, Duffau P, Mercié P, Raymond I, Anies G, Fleury H, Saux M-C, Dabis F, Fagard C, Thiébaut R, Masquelier B, Pellegrin I; ANRS CO3 Aquitaine Cohort. Virological and immunological response in HIV-1-infected patients with multiple treatment failures receiving raltegravir and optimized background therapy, ANRS CO3 Aquitaine Cohort. *J Antimicrob Chemother* (2009) 63, 1251–5.
8. Barrail-Tran A, Yazdanpanah Y, Goldwirt L, Chêne G, Colin C, Piketty C, Bollens D, Katlama C, Descamps D, Molina JM, Fagard C, Taburet AM; ANRS 139 study group. Pharmacokinetics of etravirine, raltegravir and darunavir/ritonavir in treatment experienced patients. *AIDS* (2010) 24, 2581–3.
9. Ford SL, Gould E, Chen S, Margolis D, Spreen W, Crauwels H, Piscitelli S. Lack of pharmacokinetic interaction between rilpivirine and integrase inhibitors dolutegravir and GSK1265744. *Antimicrob Agents Chemother* (2013) 57, 5472–7.
10. Crauwels H, Stevens M, De La Rosa G, Boven K. Absence of pharmacokinetic interaction between the NNRTI rilpivirine (TMC278) and the integrase inhibitor raltegravir. 19th Conference on Retroviruses and Opportunistic Infections, Seattle, 2012, Paper 617.
11. Isentress (Raltegravir potassium). Merck Sharp & Dohme Ltd. UK Summary of product characteristics, November 2014.
12. Tivicay (Dolutegravir sodium). ViiV Healthcare UK Ltd. UK Summary of product characteristics, September 2014.
13. Isentress (Raltegravir potassium). Merck & Co. US Prescribing information, February 2015.
14. Stribild (Elvitegravir, cobicistat, emtricitabine, tenofovir disoproxil fumarate). Gilead Sciences, Inc. US Prescribing information, August 2012.
15. Tivicay (Dolutegravir sodium). ViiV Healthcare. US Prescribing information, December 2014.
16. Williams I, Churchill D, Anderson J, Boffito M, Bower M, Cairns G, Cwynarski K, Edwards S, Fidler S, Fisher M, Freedman A, Geretti AM, Gilleece Y, Horne R, Johnson M, Khoo S, Leen C, Marshall N, Nelson M, Orkin C, Paton N, Phillips A, Post F, Pozniak A, Sabin C, Trevelion R, Ustianowski A, Walsh J, Waters L, Wilkins E, Winston A, Youle M. British HIV Association guidelines for the treatment of HIV-1-positive adults with antiretroviral therapy 2012 (Updated 2013). *HIV Med* (2014), 15 (Suppl 1) 1–85.
17. Panel on Antiretroviral Guidelines for Adults and Adolescents. Guidelines for the use of antiretroviral agents in HIV-1-infected adults and adolescents. US Department of Health and Human Services (April 2015). 1–288. Available at: https://aidsinfo.nih.gov/contentfiles/lvguidelines/adultandadolescentgl.pdf (accessed 11/09/15).

HIV-integrase inhibitors + NRTIs

Tenofovir slightly increases raltegravir exposure, but raltegravir has no clinically relevant effect on tenofovir exposure. Raltegravir also has no clinically relevant effect on lamivudine exposure. Elvitegravir boosted with ritonavir has little or no effect on the pharmacokinetics of abacavir, didanosine, emtricitabine, stavudine, tenofovir, or zidovudine. Emtricitabine with tenofovir did not affect the pharmacokinetics of elvitegravir, when boosted with ritonavir. Zidovudine did not affect the pharmacokinetics of elvitegravir, when boosted with ritonavir. There is no interaction between dolutegravir and tenofovir.

Clinical evidence

(a) Dolutegravir

In a study in 15 healthy subjects given **tenofovir** disoproxil fumarate 300 mg once daily and dolutegravir 50 mg once daily for 5 days there were no changes to the pharmacokinetics of either drug, compared with when they were given alone.[1]

(b) Elvitegravir

1. Abacavir. In a study in 24 healthy subjects, elvitegravir boosted with ritonavir 200/100 mg daily decreased the AUC of a single 600-mg dose of abacavir by 16.5%.[2]

2. Didanosine. In a study in 32 healthy subjects, elvitegravir boosted with ritonavir 200/100 mg daily decreased the AUC of a single 300-mg dose of didanosine by 16%.[2]

3. Emtricitabine with Tenofovir. In a study, 24 healthy subjects were given emtricitabine with tenofovir disoproxil fumarate 200/300 mg daily and elvitegravir boosted with ritonavir 50/100 mg daily either alone or together. There were no changes in the pharmacokinetics of emtricitabine, tenofovir, or elvitegravir when given concurrently.[3]

4. Stavudine. In a study in 32 healthy subjects, elvitegravir boosted with ritonavir 200/100 mg daily had no clinically relevant effect on the pharmacokinetics of a single 40-mg dose of stavudine .[2]

5. Zidovudine. In a study in 24 healthy subjects, elvitegravir boosted with ritonavir 200/100 mg daily had no effect on the pharmacokinetics of zidovudine 300 mg twice daily. Similarly, zidovudine did not alter the pharmacokinetics of elvitegravir.[2]

(c) Raltegravir

1. Lamivudine. The US manufacturer of raltegravir reports that, in drug interaction studies, the pharmacokinetics of lamivudine were not affected to a clinically relevant extent by raltegravir.[4]

2. Tenofovir. In a study, 9 healthy subjects were given tenofovir disoproxil fumarate 300 mg daily with raltegravir 400 mg twice daily for 4 days. The AUC and maximum plasma concentration of raltegravir were increased by 49% and 64%, respectively, and a 10% decrease in the AUC of tenofovir was also reported. In a subsequent study by the same authors, 25 HIV-positive patients taking tenofovir disoproxil fumarate 300 mg daily and lamivudine 300 mg daily were given raltegravir 100 to 600 mg twice daily. The AUC and maximum plasma concentration of raltegravir were increased by 41% and 33%, respectively.[5]

Mechanism

The mechanism for the interaction of tenofovir with raltegravir is unknown.

Importance and management

Elvitegravir boosted with ritonavir did not have a clinically relevant effect on the pharmacokinetics of abacavir, didanosine, emtricitabine, stavudine, tenofovir, or zidovudine; these NRTIs can all be given with elvitegravir without dose adjustments. If cobicistat is used as a pharmacokinetic enhancer with elvitegravir, it is expected that no clinically relevant changes to elvitegravir pharmacokinetics are also likely to occur, as cobicistat has similar properties to ritonavir.

The slight increase in **raltegravir** exposure and minor decrease in tenofovir exposure reported on concurrent use are not expected to be of clinical relevance. No dose adjustment is needed when raltegravir is used with lamivudine, and is not expected to be needed when raltegravir is used concurrently with other NRTIs.

No interaction occurs between **dolutegravir** and tenofovir and so no dose adjustments are necessary on concurrent use.

The UK and US guidelines for starting antiretrovirals in treatment-naive patients are based on a backbone of two NRTIs (usually emtricitabine plus tenofovir *or* abacavir plus lamivudine), which can be combined with one HIV-integrase inhibitor.[6,7] Current local and national guidelines should be consulted for other options in treatment-naive patients and for the management of treatment-experienced patients.

1. Song I, Min SS, Borland J, Lou Y, Chen S, Ishibashi T, Wajima T, Piscitelli S. Lack of interaction between the HIV integrase inhibitor S/GSK1349572 and tenofovir in healthy subjects. *J Acquir Immune Defic Syndr* (2010) 55, 365–7.
2. Pharmacokinetics of coadministered ritonavir-boosted elvitegravir and zidovudine, didanosine, stavudine, or abacavir. *J Acquir Immune Defic Syndr* (2007) 46, 160–6.
3. Ramanathan S, Shen G, Cheng A, Kearney BP. Pharmacokinetics of emtricitabine, tenofovir, and GS-9137 following coadministration of emtricitabine/tenofovir disoproxil fumarate and ritonavir-boosted GS-9137. *J Acquir Immune Defic Syndr* (2007) 45, 274–9.
4. Isentress (Raltegravir potassium). Merck & Co. US Prescribing information, February 2015.
5. Wenning LA, Friedman EJ, Kost JT, Breidinger SA, Stek JE, Lasseter KC, Gottesdiener KM, Chen J, Teppler H, Wagner JA, Stone JA, Iwamoto M. Lack of a significant drug interaction between raltegravir and tenofovir. *Antimicrob Agents Chemother* (2008) 52, 3253–8.
6. Williams I, Churchill D, Anderson J, Boffito M, Bower M, Cairns G, Cwynarski K, Edwards S, Fidler S, Fisher M, Freedman A, Geretti AM, Gilleece Y, Horne R, Johnson M, Khoo S, Leen C, Marshall N, Nelson M, Orkin C, Paton N, Phillips A, Post F, Pozniak A, Sabin C, Trevelion R, Ustianowski A, Walsh J, Waters L, Wilkins E, Winston A, Youle M. British HIV Association guidelines for the treatment of HIV-1-positive adults with antiretroviral therapy 2012 (Updated 2013). *HIV Med* (2014), 15 (Suppl 1) 1–85.
7. Panel on Antiretroviral Guidelines for Adults and Adolescents. Guidelines for the use of antiretroviral agents in HIV-1-infected adults and adolescents. US Department of Health and Human Services (April 2015). 1–288. Available at: https://aidsinfo.nih.gov/contentfiles/lvguidelines/adultandadolescentgl.pdf (accessed 11/09/2015).

HIV-integrase inhibitors + NS5A inhibitors

Ombitasvir might moderately increase raltegravir exposure, but raltegravir does not appear to alter the pharmacokinetics of ombitasvir. No clinically relevant pharmacokinetic interaction appears to occur between ledipasvir and elvitegravir (when given with sofosbuvir) or raltegravir. No interaction is predicted to occur between ledipasvir and dolutegravir.

Clinical evidence, mechanism, importance and management

(a) Dolutegravir

The UK manufacturer predicts that no interaction would be expected between **ledipasvir** and dolutegravir, and that no dose adjustments would be likely to be necessary on concurrent use.[1]

(b) Elvitegravir

The UK and US manufacturers briefly report that, in a study in 29 healthy subjects given **ledipasvir** 90 mg daily (in a fixed-dose combination with sofosbuvir) with elvitegravir 150 mg daily (as part of a regimen also containing cobicistat, emtricitabine, and tenofovir), the pharmacokinetics of elvitegravir were unaltered. The AUC and maximum concentration of ledipasvir were increased by 78% and 63%, respectively.[1,2] No dose adjustments would be expected to be necessary on concurrent use, but note that taking ledipasvir with sofosbuvir and elvitegravir with cobicistat, emtricitabine, and tenofovir is not recommended, or cautioned, because of the potential for an interaction with tenofovir, see 'Tenofovir + NS5A inhibitors', p.997 for details.

(c) Raltegravir

1. Ledipasvir. The UK and US manufacturers briefly report that, in a study in 28 healthy subjects given ledipasvir 90 mg daily with raltegravir 400 mg twice daily, the pharmacokinetics of ledipasvir were unaltered.[1,2] The pharmacokinetics of raltegravir were also unaltered.[1] No dose adjustments are necessary on concurrent use.

2. Ombitasvir. The UK manufacturer briefly reports that, in study in healthy subjects given raltegravir 400 mg twice daily with ombitasvir 25 mg daily (in a fixed-dose combination with paritaprevir boosted with ritonavir, given with dasabuvir) the pharmacokinetics of ombitasvir were no different to historical controls, but the AUC and maximum concentration of raltegravir were both increased 2.3-fold. They suggest that this might be a result of inhibition of the glucuronosyltransferase, UGT1A1, involved in the metabolism of raltegravir, by ombitasvir, but the increase in raltegravir exposure would not appear to be likely to be clinically important, since no dose adjustment is deemed necessary on concurrent use.[3] Other components of the combination could also be involved. No ombitasvir dose adjustment is necessary on concurrent use.

1. Harvoni (Ledipasvir, sofosbuvir). Gilead Sciences Ltd. UK Summary of product characteristics, November 2014.
2. Harvoni (Ledipasvir, sofosbuvir). Gilead Sciences, Inc. US Prescribing information, March 2015.
3. Viekirax (Ombitasvir, paritaprevir, ritonavir). AbbVie Ltd. UK Summary of product characteristics, January 2015.

HIV-integrase inhibitors + NS5B inhibitors

Dasabuvir might moderately increase raltegravir exposure, but raltegravir does not appear to alter the pharmacokinetics of dasabuvir. No pharmacokinetic interaction appears to occur between sofosbuvir and elvitegravir (given with ledipasvir), or raltegravir. No interaction is predicted to occur between sofosbuvir (with ledipasvir) and dolutegravir.

Clinical evidence, mechanism, importance and management

(a) Dolutegravir

The UK manufacturer of sofosbuvir with ledipasvir predicts that no interaction would be expected between **sofosbuvir** and dolutegravir, and that no dose adjustments would be likely to be necessary on concurrent use.[1]

(b) Elvitegravir

The UK and US manufacturers of **sofosbuvir** with ledipasvir briefly report that, in a study in 29 healthy subjects given sofosbuvir 400 mg daily (in a fixed-dose combination with ledipasvir) with elvitegravir 150 mg daily (as part of a regimen also containing cobicistat, emtricitabine, and tenofovir), the pharmacokinetics of elvitegravir were unaltered. The AUC and maximum concentration of sofosbuvir were increased by 36% and 44%, respectively, and the AUC and maximum concentration of its major inactive metabolite were increased by 44% and 33%, respectively.[1,2] As the increase in sofosbuvir exposure was only slight, no sofosbuvir or elvitegravir dose adjustments are necessary on concurrent use, but note that taking ledipasvir with sofosbuvir and elvitegravir with cobicistat, emtricitabine, and tenofovir is not recommended, or cautioned, because of the potential for an interaction with tenofovir, see 'Tenofovir + NS5A inhibitors', p.997 for details.

(c) Raltegravir

1. Dasabuvir. The UK manufacturer briefly reports that, in a study in healthy subjects given raltegravir 400 mg twice daily with dasabuvir 250 or 400 mg twice daily (with a fixed-dose combination of ombitasvir and paritaprevir boosted with ritonavir) the pharmacokinetics of dasabuvir were no different to historical controls, but the AUC and maximum concentration of raltegravir were increased 2.3-fold. They suggest that this might be a result of inhibition of the glucuronosyltransferase, UGT1A1, involved in the metabolism of raltegravir, by dasabuvir, but the increase in raltegravir exposure would not appear to be likely to be clinically important, since no dose adjustment is deemed necessary on concurrent use.[3] Other components of the combination could also be involved. No dasabuvir dose adjustment is necessary on concurrent use.

2. Sofosbuvir. The UK and US manufacturers briefly report that, in a study in 19 healthy subjects given raltegravir 400 mg twice daily with a single 400-mg dose of sofosbuvir, the pharmacokinetics of sofosbuvir and its major inactive metabolite were unaffected. The AUC and maximum concentration of raltegravir were decreased by 27% and 43%, respectively. No dose adjustments are necessary on concurrent use.[4,5]

1. Harvoni (Ledipasvir, sofosbuvir). Gilead Sciences Ltd. UK Summary of product characteristics, November 2014.
2. Harvoni (Ledipasvir, sofosbuvir). Gilead Sciences, Inc. US Prescribing information, March 2015.
3. Exviera (Dasabuvir sodium monohydrate). AbbVie Ltd. UK Summary of product characteristics, January 2015.
4. Sovaldi (Sofosbuvir). Gilead Sciences Ltd. UK Summary of product characteristics, January 2015.
5. Sovaldi (Sofosbuvir). Gilead Sciences, Inc. US Prescribing information, March 2015.

HIV-integrase inhibitors + Rifamycins

Raltegravir exposure is slightly decreased by rifampicin and rifabutin. Rifapentine given weekly moderately increases raltegravir exposure, whereas rifapentine given daily decreases its minimum plasma concentration. Elvitegravir plasma concentrations are predicted to be decreased by rifampicin (rifampin) and rifapentine. Dolutegravir exposure is moderately decreased by rifampicin, but is not affected by rifabutin. Rifabutin does not affect the pharmacokinetics of elvitegravir boosted with ritonavir.

Clinical evidence

(a) Rifabutin

1. Dolutegravir. In a study in 9 healthy subjects given dolutegravir 50 mg daily alone for 7 days and then with rifabutin 300 mg daily for 14 days, the AUC and maximum concentration of dolutegravir were unaffected.[1]

2. Elvitegravir. The UK and US manufacturers briefly report that, rifabutin 150 mg every other day given with elvitegravir boosted with ritonavir 300/100 mg daily had no effect on the pharmacokinetics of elvitegravir.[2,3] Similarly, a preliminary report of another study in 18 patients, given the same daily dose of elvitegravir boosted with ritonavir and rifabutin 150 mg daily, found that the pharmacokinetics of elvitegravir were unaffected.[4] For information on the effect of elvitegravir boosted with cobicistat on the pharmacokinetics of rifabutin and its active metabolite, see 'Rifabutin + Cobicistat', p.356.

3. Raltegravir. In a crossover study in 16 healthy subjects, rifabutin 300 mg daily for 14 days decreased the minimum concentration of raltegravir 400 mg twice daily by 20%. However, the AUC and maximum plasma concentration of raltegravir tended to be increased by 19% and 39%, respectively, although there was wide variability in the change in these parameters.[5]

(b) Rifampicin (Rifampin)

1. Dolutegravir. In a study, 11 healthy subjects were given dolutegravir 50 mg daily for 7 days alone, followed by 50 mg twice daily for 21 days, with rifampicin 600 mg daily given on days 15 to 28. The AUC and maximum concentration of dolutegravir were decreased by 54% and 44%, respectively, when compared with dolutegravir 50 mg twice daily alone. However, when compared with dolutegravir 50 mg daily alone, the AUC was *increased* by 33% and the maximum concentration was unaffected.[1]

2. Raltegravir. In a study in 9 healthy subjects, rifampicin 600 mg daily for 15 days decreased the AUC and minimum plasma concentration of a single 400-mg dose of raltegravir given on day 14, by 40% and 61%, respectively. In a subsequent study, 17 healthy subjects were given an increased dose of raltegravir 800 mg twice daily (to try to overcome the effects of rifampicin) with rifampicin 600 mg daily for 14 days. The AUC of raltegravir was *increased* by 27% when compared with raltegravir 400 mg alone. However, doubling the raltegravir dose still resulted in a decrease in the minimum plasma concentration of raltegravir by 53%, when compared with raltegravir 400 mg alone. No important increase in adverse effects was reported on concurrent use, and all adverse effects reported were transient.[6] In another study, 16 healthy subjects were given raltegravir 400 mg twice daily for 5 days alone, and then with rifampicin 600 to 900 mg *three times weekly* for 28 days, followed by raltegravir 800 mg twice daily with rifampicin for a further 5 days. The AUC and maximum concentration of raltegravir were increased by 8% and 16%, respectively, (although neither of these changes were statistically significant) when raltegravir 400 mg twice daily with rifampicin was compared with use of raltegravir alone. When raltegravir 800 mg twice daily was given with rifampicin, the AUC and maximum concentration of raltegravir were increased by 84% and 76%, respectively, when compared with raltegravir 400 mg twice daily alone. The minimum concentration of raltegravir tended to be decreased with rifampicin, regardless of dose.[7] A phase II study in patients with tuberculosis and HIV infection taking rifampicin-based treatment found that virological suppression was achieved at 24 weeks in 76% of patients taking raltegravir 400 mg twice daily, 78% of patients taking raltegravir 800 mg twice daily, and 63% of patients taking efavirenz.[8] A letter reports that 8 patients with tuberculosis and HIV infection had continued virological suppression when a rifampicin-containing regimen was used with an increased dose of raltegravir 800 mg twice daily (combined with tenofovir and emtricitabine or abacavir and lamivudine).[9] Another report in 2 patients with tuberculosis and HIV infection also reports the successful use of the same increased raltegravir dose with rifampicin.[10]

(c) Rifapentine

In a study in 16 healthy subjects, rifapentine 900 mg weekly increased the AUC and maximum plasma concentration of **raltegravir** 400 mg twice daily by 71% and 89%, respectively, with a 12% *decrease* in its minimum plasma concentration. However, rifapentine 600 mg daily did not change the AUC or maximum plasma concentration of raltegravir, and decreased its minimum plasma concentration by 40%. Raltegravir plasma concentrations varied widely between, and within, subjects.[11]

Mechanism

Elvitegravir is principally metabolised by CYP3A isoenzymes, and also undergoes glucuronidation by glucuronosyltransferases (UGT1A1/3).[2] Raltegravir and dolutegravir are primarily metabolised by UGT1A1. Rifampicin is a potent inducer of CYP3A isoenzymes and also of glucuronosyltransferases. *In vitro*, rifabutin was generally a less potent inducer of UGT1A1 than rifampicin.[5]

Importance and management

A pharmacokinetic interaction between the HIV-integrase inhibitors and rifamycins does seem to occur, although the nature and magnitude vary, and the clinical importance is not established in all cases.

The slight decrease in **raltegravir** exposure with daily rifampicin is overcome by doubling the raltegravir dose to 800 mg twice daily. Therefore if concurrent use of raltegravir and rifampicin is necessary, the UK and US manufacturers suggests that this dose of raltegravir should be used.[12,13] However, despite the increased raltegravir dose overcoming the decreased exposure, its minimum plasma concentration still seems to be lower, and the clinical importance of this is the subject of some debate. A pharmacokinetic analysis of a phase III efficacy trial with raltegravir found that the minimum concentration correlated with virological response,[14] suggesting that doubling the dose might not be the entire answer. This suggestion appears to be in agreement with the findings of the study showing similar virological efficacy with raltegravir 400 mg twice daily and 800 mg twice daily in tuberculosis patients taking rifampicin-based treatment.[8] However, several commentaries highlight deficiencies in this study design,[15] and considerable interindividual variability in the pharmacokinetics of raltegravir,[16,17] making application of this finding to clinical practice difficult. Until more is known, even with a doubling of the dose of raltegravir if concurrent use with rifampicin is necessary, it would seem prudent to monitor the virological response closely, and this is the advice of the CDC in the US.[18] In the UK, the British HIV Association (BHIVA) advises caution.[19] Similar effects were seen with intermittent rifampicin treatment (three times weekly) as with daily, and the authors of the study suggest that the dose of raltegravir should be doubled if rifampicin is used in this way too.[7] Note that the CDC in the US recommends that rifampicin should be used daily in patients taking raltegravir.[18]

The pharmacokinetic interaction between **rifabutin** with raltegravir seems unlikely to be clinically important,[5] and the usual recommended dose for raltegravir can be given with rifabutin.[12,18,19] The interaction between **rifapentine** with raltegravir is unlikely to be clinically important if rifapentine is administered weekly. When rifapentine is given daily, the reduction in the raltegravir minimum plasma concentration might be of some concern, and virological response should be monitored closely.

The UK manufacturer of a combination preparation containing elvitegravir boosted with cobicistat (with emtricitabine and tenofovir) consider that the decrease in the minimum plasma **elvitegravir** concentration by rifabutin might reduce its antiviral efficacy and lead to the development of resistance,[20] and the UK and US manufacturers of this combination preparation do not recommend concurrent use with **rifabutin**.[20,21] Note that this is also the advice of the CDC in the US[18] and BHIVA.[19] However, the UK manufacturer advises that if the combination is necessary, rifabutin should be given at a dose of 150 mg three times weekly, on set days.[20] The US manufacturer also does not recommend the concurrent use of **rifapentine**.[21] Although there is no information, **rifampicin** is predicted to greatly decrease the plasma concentrations of elvitegravir, which might lead to loss of therapeutic effect and the manufacturers therefore contraindicate concurrent use,[20,21] and the CDC in the US also suggest this combination should not be used.[18] In contrast, when elvitegravir is boosted with ritonavir there is no change in the pharmacokinetics of elvitegravir, hence the UK manufacturer and BHIVA advise that rifabutin should be given at a dose of 150 mg three times weekly,[2,19] on set days when it is given with ritonavir as a pharmacokinetic enhancer.[2] However, the US manufacturer suggests either rifabutin 150 mg every other day or three times a week can be given.[3] The use of rifampicin with elvitegravir boosted with ritonavir is contraindicated by the UK manufacturer,[2] and is not recommended by BHIVA.[19] This combination is also contraindicated by the US manufacturer, which also extends this to rifapentine.[3]

The pharmacokinetics of **dolutegravir** are not affected by **rifabutin** and therefore no dose adjustment is necessary on concurrent use. The moderate decrease in dolutegravir exposure with **rifampicin**, is overcome by increasing the dolutegravir dose to 50 mg twice daily and hence the manufacturers advise that this dose should be used if rifampicin is required.[22,23] Furthermore, the US manufacturer adds that this applies to HIV-integrase inhibitor-naive patients who are both treatment-naive and experienced, but in those who are HIV-integrase inhibitor-experienced patients with HIV-integrase inhibitor-associated resistance substitutions or clinically suspected resistance, this combination should be avoided due to the risk of decreased therapeutic efficacy and development of resistance.[23] The UK manufacturer advises that this dose might be suitable in patients who are not resistant to HIV-integrase inhibitors, but the combination should not be used in those who show HIV-integrase inhibitor resistance.[22]

1. Dooley KE, Sayre P, Borland J, Purdy E, Chen S, Song I, Peppercorn A, Everts S, Piscitelli S, Flexner C. Safety, tolerability, and pharmacokinetics of the HIV integrase inhibitor dolutegravir given twice daily with rifampin or once daily with rifabutin: results of a phase 1 study among healthy subjects. *J Acquir Immune Defic Syndr* (2013) 62, 21–7.
2. Vitekta (Elvitegravir). Gilead Sciences Ltd. UK Summary of product characteristics, March 2014.
3. Vitekta (Elvitegravir). Gilead Sciences, Inc. US Prescribing information, September 2014.
4. German P, West S, Hui J, Kearney BP. Pharmacokinetic interaction between elvitegravir/ritonavir and dose-adjusted rifabutin. 9th International Workshop on Clinical Pharmacology of HIV Therapy. New Orleans, 2008, Abstract 19.
5. Brainard DM, Kassahun K, Wenning LA, Petry AS, Liu C, Lunceford J, Hariparsad N, Eisenhandler R, Norcross A, DeNoia EP, Stone JA, Wagner JA, Iwamoto M. Lack of a clinically meaningful pharmacokinetic effect of rifabutin on raltegravir: in vitro/in vivo correlation. *J Clin Pharmacol* (2011) 51, 943–50.
6. Wenning LA, Hanley WD, Brainard DM, Petry AS, Ghosh K, Jin B, Mangin E, Marbury TC, Berg JK, Chodakewitz JA, Stone JA, Gottesdiener KM, Wagner JA, Iwamoto M. Effect of rifampin, a potent inducer of drug metabolizing enzymes, on the pharmacokinetics of raltegravir. *Antimicrob Agents Chemother* (2009) 53, 2852–6.
7. Reynolds HE, Chrdle A, Egan D, Chaponda M, Else L, Chiong J, Back DJ, Khoo SH. Effect of intermittent rifampicin on the pharmacokinetics and safety of raltegravir. *J Antimicrob Chemother* (2015) 70, 550–4.
8. Grinsztejn B, De Castro N, Arnold V, Veloso VG, Morgado M, Pilotto JH, Brites C, Madruga JV, Barcellos NT, Santos BR, Vorsatz C, Fagard C, Santini-Oliveira M, Patey O, Delaugerre C, Chêne G, Molina JM. Raltegravir for the treatment of patients co-infected with HIV and tuberculosis (ANRS 12 180 Reflate TB): a multicentre, phase 2, non-comparative, open-label, randomised trial. *Lancet Infect Dis* (2014) 14, 459–67.
9. Mena Á, Vázquez P, Castro Á, López S, Bello L, Pedreira JD. Clinical experience of raltegravir-containing regimens in HIV-infected patients during rifampicin-containing treatment of tuberculosis. *J Antimicrob Chemother* (2011) 66, 951–2.
10. Burger DM, Magis-Escurra C, van den Berk GEL, Gelinck LBS. Pharmacokinetics of double-dose raltegravir in two patients with HIV infection and tuberculosis. *AIDS* (2010) 24, 328–30.
11. Weiner M, Egelund EF, Engle M, Kiser M, Prihoda TJ, Gelfond JA, MacKenzie W, Peloquin CA. Pharmacokinetic interaction of rifapentine and raltegravir in healthy subjects. *J Antimicrob Chemother* (2014) 69, 1079–85.
12. Isentress (Raltegravir potassium). Merck Sharp & Dohme Ltd. UK Summary of product characteristics, August 2013.
13. Isentress (Raltegravir potassium). Merck & Co. US Prescribing information, April 2014.
14. Rizk ML, Hang Y, Luo WL, Su J, Zhao J, Campbell H, Nguyen BY, Sklar P, Eron JJ, Wenning L. Pharmacokinetics and pharmacodynamics of once-daily versus twice-daily raltegravir in treatment-naive HIV-infected patients. *Antimicrob Agents Chemother* (2012) 56, 3101–6.
15. Meintjes G, Maartens G. Dosing of raltegravir when given with rifampicin. *Lancet Infect Dis* (2014) 14, 442–3.
16. Klis S, Daskapan A, Akkerman OW, Alffenaar JW, Stienstra Y. Raltegravir and rifampicin in patients with HIV and tuberculosis. *Lancet Infect Dis* (2014) 14, 1046–7.
17. Bierman WF, Riezebos-Brilman A. Raltegravir and rifampicin in patients with HIV and tuberculosis. *Lancet Infect Dis* (2014) 14, 1047.
18. Centers for Disease Control and Prevention. Managing drug interactions in the treatment of HIV-related tuberculosis. *US Department of Health and Human Services* (2013). Available at: http://www.cdc.gov/tb/publications/guidelines/TB_HIV_Drugs/pdf/tbhiv.pdf (accessed 30/09/15).
19. Pozniak AL, Coyne KM, Miller RF, Lipman MCI, Freedman AR, Ormerod LP, Johnson MA, Collins S, Lucas SB on behalf of the BHIVA Guidelines Subcommittee. British HIV Association guidelines for the treatment of TB/HIV co-infection 2011. *HIV Med* (2011) 12, 517–24.
20. Stribild (Cobicistat, emtricitabine, elvitegravir, tenofovir disoproxil fumarate). Gilead Sciences Ltd. UK Summary of product characteristics, July 2014.
21. Stribild (Cobicistat, emtricitabine, elvitegravir, tenofovir disoproxil fumarate). Gilead Sciences, Inc. US Prescribing information, December 2014.
22. Tivicay (Dolutegravir sodium). ViiV Healthcare UK Ltd. UK Summary of product characteristics, September 2014.
23. Tivicay (Dolutegravir sodium). ViiV Healthcare. US Prescribing information, December 2014.

HIV-integrase inhibitors; Dolutegravir + Miscellaneous

Dolutegravir might increase the exposure to dofetilide, and increase the risk of QT prolongation. Carbamazepine, fosphenytoin, oxcarbazepine, phenobarbital, phenytoin, primidone, and St John's wort might decrease dolutegravir exposure. Fluconazole, itraconazole, ketoconazole, posaconazole, and voriconazole are predicted to not alter dolutegravir exposure.

Clinical evidence, mechanism, importance and management

(a) Azoles

The UK manufacturer notes that, although not studied, no clinically important effect on the exposure to dolutegravir would be expected on concurrent use of the azoles, **fluconazole**, **itraconazole**, **ketoconazole**, **posaconazole**, or **voriconazole**.[1] This is based on the lack of clinically important effect of the potent CYP3A4 inhibitors, boceprevir and telaprevir (see 'HIV-integrase inhibitors + HCV-protease inhibitors', p.912), due to the minor role that CYP3A4 plays in the metabolism of dolutegravir. No dolutegravir dose adjustment would therefore seem necessary on concurrent use.

(b) Dofetilide

The UK and US manufacturers note that, although not studied, exposure to dofetilide could be increased by dolutegravir due to inhibition of the renal transportation of dofetilide. *In vitro* dolutegravir has been shown to inhibit the organic cation transporter OCT-2, and the multidrug and toxin extrusion transporter, MATE-1, which are thought to be involved in the transport of dofetilide.[1,2] Dofetilide exposure would therefore be expected to be increased on concurrent use. Because there is a linear relationship between plasma dofetilide concentrations and prolongation of the QTc interval, which is a risk factor for torsade de pointes, the UK and US manufacturers of dolutegravir contraindicate concurrent use.[1,2]

(c) Enzyme inducers

The UK and US manufacturers note that, although not studied, exposure to dolutegravir could be decreased by inducers of the glucuronosyltransferase, UGT1A1 (which is the principle route of dolutegravir metabolism), or CYP3A (a minor route), and advise that concurrent use should be avoided. They specifically name **carbamazepine**, **oxcarbazepine**, **phenobarbital**, **phenytoin**, and **St John's wort**.[1,2] This contraindication would also include **fosphenytoin**, the prodrug of phenytoin, and **primidone**, which is metabolised to phenobarbital. For the effects of rifampicin and rifabutin (both known enzyme inducers), see 'HIV-integrase inhibitors + Rifamycins', p.917.

(d) Sucralfate

Due to the effect on dolutegravir exposure of magnesium and aluminium ions contained in some antacids (see 'HIV-integrase inhibitors + Antacids', p.911), the US manufacturer advises that dolutegravir should be taken 2 hours before, or 6 hours after, sucralfate.[2]

1. Tivicay (Dolutegravir sodium). ViiV Healthcare UK Ltd. UK Summary of product characteristics, September 2014.
2. Tivicay (Dolutegravir sodium). ViiV Healthcare. US Prescribing information, December 2014.

HIV-integrase inhibitors; Dolutegravir + Polyvalent cations

Calcium and iron-containing supplements decrease the exposure to dolutegravir.

Clinical evidence

(a) Calcium supplements

In a crossover study, 12 healthy subjects were given a single 50-mg dose of dolutegravir with a single 1.2-g dose of **calcium carbonate** under fasted conditions. The AUC and maximum concentration of dolutegravir were decreased by 39% and 37%, respectively, compared with 11 healthy subjects given dolutegravir alone in the fasted state. When the same combination was given with a moderate-fat (30%) meal, the AUC and maximum concentration were comparable with dolutegravir alone in the fasted state. Similarly, the pharmacokinetics of dolutegravir given 2 hours before calcium carbonate in the fasted state were comparable with dolutegravir alone in the fasted state.[1]

(b) Iron supplements

In a crossover study, 11 healthy subjects were given a single 50-mg dose of dolutegravir with a single 324-g dose of **ferrous fumarate** under fasted conditions. The AUC and maximum concentration of dolutegravir were decreased by 54% and 57%, respectively, compared with 10 healthy subjects given dolutegravir alone in the fasted state. When the same combination was given with a moderate-fat (30%) meal, the AUC and maximum concentration were comparable with dolutegravir alone in the fasted state. Similarly, the pharmacokinetics of dolutegravir given 2 hours before ferrous fumarate in the fasted state were comparable with dolutegravir alone in the fasted state.[1]

(c) Multivitamins

In a crossover study in 16 healthy subjects, given a single 50-mg dose of dolutegravir with a single-dose of a multivitamin preparation (*One A Day Maximum MVI tablets*, containing elemental calcium 162 mg, magnesium 100 mg, and iron, zinc, and copper, doses unstated) under fasted conditions, decreased the AUC and maximum concentration of dolutegravir by 33% and 35%, respectively, compared with dolutegravir alone in the fasted state.[2]

Mechanism

It has been suggested that dolutegravir, forms an insoluble complex with metal (divalent or trivalent) cations in the gut,[1,2] thus decreasing its absorption and hence exposure.

Importance and management

An interaction between dolutegravir and polyvalent cations (**calcium** and **iron**) would seem to be established and consistent with the effect of cation-containing antacids (see 'HIV-integrase inhibitors + Antacids', p.911). The effect of food on this interaction seems to be to attenuate it, and therefore the US manufacturer of dolutegravir advises that if it is taken with food, supplements containing calcium or iron can be given at the same time.[3] Alternatively, they (and the UK manufacturer) advise that dolutegravir can be given 2 hours before, or 6 hours after, the supplement.[3,4]

1. Song I, Borland J, Arya N, Wynne B, Piscitelli S. Pharmacokinetics of dolutegravir when administered with mineral supplements in healthy adult subjects. *J Clin Pharmacol* (2014) 55, 490–6.
2. Patel P, Song I, Borland J, Patel A, Lou Y, Chen S, Wajima T, Peppercorn A, Min SS, Piscitelli SC. Pharmacokinetics of the HIV integrase inhibitor S/GSK1349572 co-administered with acid-reducing agents and multivitamins in healthy volunteers. *J Antimicrob Chemother* (2011) 66, 1567–72.
3. Tivicay (Dolutegravir sodium). ViiV Healthcare. US Prescribing information, December 2014.
4. Tivicay (Dolutegravir sodium). ViiV Healthcare UK Ltd. UK Summary of product characteristics, September 2014.

HIV-integrase inhibitors; Dolutegravir + Prednisone

Prednisone has no effect on the pharmacokinetics of dolutegravir.

Clinical evidence, mechanism, importance and management

In a study in 12 healthy subjects, prednisone 60 mg daily for 5 days, and then tapered down by 10 mg each day for a further 5 days, had no effect on the pharmacokinetics of dolutegravir 50 mg daily.[1] No dolutegravir dose adjustment is necessary on concurrent use.

1. Song IH, Borland J, Chen S, Savina P, Peppercorn AF, Piscitelli S. Effect of prednisone on the pharmacokinetics of the integrase inhibitor dolutegravir. *Antimicrob Agents Chemother* (2013) 57, 4394–7.

HIV-integrase inhibitors; Elvitegravir with Cobicistat + Azoles

Ketoconazole slightly increases the exposure to elvitegravir (when given with low-dose ritonavir as a pharmacokinetic booster) and is expected to have a similar effect when elvitegravir is boosted with cobicistat. Elvitegravir boosted with cobicistat is predicted to increase the plasma concentrations of ketoconazole, itraconazole, and voriconazole.

Clinical evidence

In a pharmacokinetic study, **ketoconazole** 200 mg twice daily increased the AUC and maximum plasma concentration of elvitegravir boosted with ritonavir 150/100 mg daily by 48% and 17%, respectively.[1]

Mechanism

Ketoconazole is a potent inhibitor of CYP3A4, and this study shows it has little additional effect when elvitegravir is already boosted with ritonavir. In addition, there is some evidence that this effect might be due to inhibition of glucuronyltransferases (UGT1A1) by ketoconazole rather than inhibition of CYP3A4.[1]

Importance and management

The increase in elvitegravir exposure (when boosted with ritonavir) by ketoconazole is not clinically important. Cobicistat has similar CYP3A4 inhibitory potency to ritonavir, therefore it seems likely that ketoconazole would cause a similar increase in elvitegravir exposure when it is boosted with cobicistat. Although the effects on the azoles have not been studied, the US manufacturer of elvitegravir with cobicistat (in a fixed-dose combination also including emtricitabine and tenofovir) reasonably predicts that it might increase the plasma concentrations of **ketoconazole**, **itraconazole**, and **voriconazole**, and they recommend a maximum dose of **ketoconazole** or **itraconazole** of 200 mg daily; with **voriconazole** only given if the benefits of use outweigh the risks.[2]

1. Ramanathan S, Mathias AA, German P, Kearney BP. Clinical pharmacokinetic and pharmacodynamic profile of the HIV integrase inhibitor elvitegravir. *Clin Pharmacokinet* (2011) 50, 229–44.
2. Stribild (Elvitegravir, cobicistat, emtricitabine, tenofovir disoproxil fumarate). Gilead Sciences, Inc. US Prescribing information, August 2012.

HIV-integrase inhibitors; Elvitegravir with Cobicistat + Miscellaneous

Elvitegravir is predicted to reduce the concentrations of warfarin; other coumarins might be similarly affected.

Cobicistat (given with elvitegravir) is predicted to increase the plasma concentrations of CYP3A4 substrates, such as some antiarrhythmics, bosentan, the calcium-channel blockers, some macrolides, sildenafil, and ciclosporin.

Drugs that induce CYP3A4 (such as carbamazepine) are predicted to reduce the exposure to elvitegravir with cobicistat. No clinically relevant drug interaction appears to occur between elvitegravir with cobicistat and entecavir, famciclovir, and ribavirin.

Clinical evidence, mechanism, importance and management

Elvitegravir is formulated with cobicistat as a pharmacokinetic booster, which does not have any antiretroviral activity. Cobicistat is a potent CYP3A4 inhibitor, with similar potency to ritonavir (see 'Table 1.9', p.11). Elvitegravir with cobicistat would therefore be predicted to have similar interactions to low-dose ritonavir, where the mechanism for the interaction is CYP3A4 inhibition. Cobicistat also weakly inhibits CYP2D6, and is said to be an inhibitor of various transporters, OATP1B1 and 1B3, and BCRP.[1] Elvitegravir is stated to be a modest inducer of CYP2C9.[1]

(a) Antiarrhythmics

Cobicistat is a potent inhibitor of CYP3A4 and also weakly inhibits CYP2D6. The US manufacturer of elvitegravir boosted with cobicistat (in a fixed-dose combination also including emtricitabine and tenofovir) therefore states that the plasma concentrations of various antiarrhythmics might be increased by concurrent use: they specifically name **amiodarone**, **disopyramide**, **flecainide**, systemic **lidocaine**, **mexiletine**, **propafenone**, and **quinidine**. They recommend caution and advise monitoring antiarrhythmic plasma concentrations, if possible.[1] Note that not all of these antiarrhythmics are CYP3A4 or CYP2D6 substrates; however, until more is known, some caution might be appropriate on their concurrent use with cobicistat.

(b) Antipsychotics

The US manufacturer of elvitegravir with cobicistat (in a fixed-dose combination also including emtricitabine and tenofovir) predicts that it might increase the plasma concentrations of antipsychotics and they name **perphenazine**, **risperidone**, and **thioridazine**. They state that a decrease in the dose of these antipsychotics might be needed on concurrent use. **Risperidone** and **thioridazine** are known substrates of CYP2D6, of which cobicistat is a weak inhibitor, so some pharmacokinetic interaction might be anticipated. Note that the concurrent use of elvitegravir with cobicistat and pimozide is contraindicated, see *CYP3A4 substrates*, below.

(c) Beta blockers

Cobicistat is a weak inhibitor of CYP2D6, the isoenzyme by which metoprolol, propranolol, and timolol are principally metabolised. The US manufacturer of elvitegravir with cobicistat (in a fixed-dose combination also including emtricitabine and tenofovir) therefore predicts that it might increase the plasma concentrations of beta blockers, and they name **metoprolol** and **timolol**. They recommend monitoring concurrent use, with a dose reduction of the beta blocker if necessary.[1] However, the increase in exposure of these beta blockers seen with other weak inhibitors of CYP2D6, such as cimetidine (see 'Beta blockers + H_2-receptor antagonists; Cimetidine', p.1011), is not usually considered to be clinically important.

(d) Bosentan

Cobicistat is a potent CYP3A4 inhibitor and the US manufacturer of elvitegravir with cobicistat (in a fixed-dose combination also including emtricitabine and tenofovir) predicts that it will increase bosentan concentrations in a similar manner to ritonavir. They therefore recommend using the same dose of bosentan given to patients taking

HIV-protease inhibitors, see under 'Endothelin receptor antagonists + Ketoconazole and other CYP3A4 inhibitors', p.1059.

(e) Bupropion

The US manufacturer of elvitegravir with cobicistat (in a fixed-dose combination also including emtricitabine and tenofovir) predicts that it will increase the plasma concentration of the *tricyclic antidepressants* (see 'Tricyclic antidepressants + Cobicistat', p.1506), and they name bupropion as an example of a tricyclic antidepressant, applying the same cautions to this drug (careful dose titration of the antidepressant and monitoring for antidepressant response).[1] However, bupropion is not a tricyclic and is mainly metabolised by CYP2B6, and the effect of elvitegravir with cobicistat on CYP2B6 is not stated.[1]

(f) Buspirone

Cobicistat is a potent inhibitor of CYP3A4, by which buspirone is metabolised. The US manufacturer of elvitegravir with cobicistat (in a fixed-dose combination also including emtricitabine and tenofovir) predicts that it will increase the plasma concentration of buspirone and recommends monitoring concurrent use, reducing the dose of buspirone if necessary.[1]

(g) Calcium-channel blockers

Cobicistat is a potent inhibitor of CYP3A4, by which many calcium-channel blockers are extensively metabolised. The US manufacturer of elvitegravir boosted with cobicistat (in a fixed-dose combination also including emtricitabine and tenofovir) predicts that it will increase the plasma concentrations of calcium-channel blockers: they name **amlodipine**, **diltiazem**, **felodipine**, **nicardipine**, **nifedipine**, and **verapamil**.[1] It is possible that a clinically relevant increase in calcium-channel blocker plasma concentrations might occur, and so the US manufacturer recommends caution and clinical monitoring on concurrent use.[1]

(h) Ciclosporin, Sirolimus, and Tacrolimus

The US manufacturer of elvitegravir boosted with cobicistat (in a fixed-dose combination also including emtricitabine and tenofovir) predicts that it will increase the plasma concentrations of **ciclosporin**, **sirolimus**, and **tacrolimus**. Until more is known, it would be prudent to increase therapeutic monitoring of these drugs to ensure their plasma concentrations remain within the target range.[1]

(i) Colchicine

The US manufacturer of elvitegravir boosted with cobicistat (in a fixed-dose combination also including emtricitabine and tenofovir)[1] predicts that it will increase plasma colchicine concentrations. This appears to be based on the interaction of CYP3A4 and/or P-glycoprotein inhibitors with colchicine. They recommend the same colchicine dose reductions as are recommended for HIV-protease inhibitors, see under 'Colchicine + HIV-protease inhibitors', p.1562.

(j) Coumarins

There are no data on the effect of elvitegravir with cobicistat on warfarin concentrations or efficacy. Elvitegravir is stated to be a modest inducer of CYP2C9, by which warfarin is metabolised. Reduced warfarin efficacy might therefore be predicted. The US manufacturer of elvitegravir with cobicistat (in a fixed-dose combination also including emtricitabine and tenofovir) therefore recommends close monitoring of the INR on concurrent use.[1] Until more is known, this seems prudent. Other coumarins are also metabolised by this isoenzyme and would be expected to be similarly affected.

(k) CYP3A4 inducers

The US manufacturer of elvitegravir with cobicistat (in a fixed-dose combination also including emtricitabine and tenofovir) predicts that drugs that induce CYP3A4, such as **carbamazepine**, **oxcarbazepine**, **phenobarbital** (and therefore probably **primidone**, which is metabolised to phenobarbital), **phenytoin** (and therefore probably its prodrug **fosphenytoin**), **dexamethasone**, and **St John's wort**, might decrease cobicistat and elvitegravir plasma concentrations to an extent leading to a loss of efficacy and development of resistance. They therefore suggest giving alternative drugs, and specifically contraindicate the concurrent use of **St John's wort**.[1] However, note that although dexamethasone is often classified as a CYP3A4 inducer, there is no good evidence that dexamethasone causes clinically relevant CYP3A4 induction.

In addition, the manufacturer predicts that plasma **carbamazepine** concentrations might be increased,[1] because cobicistat is a potent inhibitor of CYP3A4 by which carbamazepine is metabolised.

(l) CYP3A4 substrates

The US manufacturer of elvitegravir with cobicistat (in a fixed-dose combination also including emtricitabine and tenofovir disoproxil fumarate) contraindicates its use with drugs that are highly dependent on CYP3A4 for clearance and for which increased concentrations are associated with serious and/or life-threatening adverse effects. This is because cobicistat is a potent inhibitor of CYP3A4 (similar to low-dose ritonavir in potency). They specifically name **alfuzosin**, ergot derivatives (**dihydroergotamine**, **ergotamine**, **methylergometrine**), **pimozide**, and the statins, simvastatin and lovastatin (see 'Statins + Cobicistat with elvitegravir', p.1330). The concurrent use of triazolam and oral midazolam is also contraindicated, see 'Benzodiazepines and related drugs + Cobicistat', p.820.

(m) Entecavir

The US manufacturer of elvitegravir boosted with cobicistat (in a fixed-dose combination also including emtricitabine and tenofovir) states that no clinically relevant drug interaction occurs with entecavir.[1]

(n) Ethosuximide

The US manufacturer of elvitegravir with cobicistat (in a fixed-dose combination also including emtricitabine and tenofovir) predicts that it will increase the plasma concentration of ethosuximide. They therefore recommend close monitoring on concurrent use.[1]

(o) Famciclovir

The US manufacturer of elvitegravir boosted with cobicistat (in a fixed-dose combination also including emtricitabine and tenofovir) states that no clinically relevant drug interaction occurs with famciclovir.[1]

(p) Fluticasone

Fluticasone is a substrate of CYP3A4, of which cobicistat is a potent inhibitor. The US manufacturer of elvitegravir with cobicistat (in a fixed-dose combination also including emtricitabine and tenofovir) therefore predicts that it will increase the concentrations of inhaled or intranasal fluticasone, leading to reduced cortisol concentrations.[1] They recommend that alternative corticosteroids should be used, particularly in the longer term, and this seems prudent.[1]

(q) Macrolides

The US manufacturer of elvitegravir with cobicistat (in a fixed-dose combination also including emtricitabine and tenofovir) predicts that cobicistat will increase the plasma concentrations of **clarithromycin** and **telithromycin**, and that these macrolides might increase cobicistat concentrations. For clarithromycin, no dose adjustment is necessary in patients with normal renal function. However, in patients with a creatinine clearance of 50 to 60 mL/minute, they recommend that the clarithromycin dose should be halved when given with cobicistat. Further dose reductions are not given as cobicistat should be discontinued if creatinine clearance decreases below 50 mL/minute. No specific dose adjustment advice is given for telithromycin.[1]

(r) Phosphodiesterase type-5 inhibitors

The US manufacturer of elvitegravir with cobicistat (in a fixed-dose combination also including emtricitabine and tenofovir disoproxil fumarate) predicts that it will increase the plasma concentrations of the phosphodiesterase type-5 inhibitors, resulting in an increase in their adverse events, including hypotension, syncope, visual disturbances, and priapism.[1] The phosphodiesterase type-5 inhibitors are substrates of CYP3A4, of which cobicistat is a potent inhibitor. The US manufacturer[1] makes a number of recommendations based on the drug and the indication.

When phosphodiesterase type-5 inhibitors are being used for pulmonary arterial hypertension:

- The use of **sildenafil** is contraindicated;
- In patients already taking elvitegravir with cobicistat (for at least one week), start **tadalafil** at 20 mg daily, and increase the dose to 40 mg daily based on tolerability;
- In patients already taking **tadalafil**, stop tadalafil at least 24 hours before starting elvitegravir with cobicistat. After at least one week, restart tadalafil at 20 mg daily, increasing to 40 mg daily based on individual tolerability.

When phosphodiesterase type-5 inhibitors are being used for erectile dysfunction the recommended doses for use with elvitegravir boosted with cobicistat are:

- **Sildenafil** at a single dose not exceeding 25 mg in 48 hours;
- **Tadalafil** at a single dose not exceeding 10 mg in 72 hours;
- **Vardenafil** at a single dose not exceeding 2.5 mg in 72 hours.

Patients should be closely monitored for phosphodiesterase type-5 inhibitors-related adverse events.

(s) Ribavirin

The US manufacturer of elvitegravir boosted with cobicistat (in a fixed-dose combination also including emtricitabine and tenofovir) states that no clinically relevant drug interaction occurs with ribavirin.[1]

(t) SSRIs

The US manufacturer of elvitegravir boosted with cobicistat (in a fixed-dose combination also including emtricitabine and tenofovir) states that the plasma concentrations of SSRIs (they specifically name **paroxetine**) might be increased on concurrent use, and recommends careful dose titration of the antidepressant and monitoring for antidepressant response.[1]

(u) Trazodone

The US manufacturer of elvitegravir with cobicistat (in a fixed-dose combination also including emtricitabine and tenofovir) predicts that it will increase plasma trazodone concentrations.[1] Cobicistat is a potent inhibitor of CYP3A4, the isoenzyme by which trazodone is metabolised, and a clinically important interaction is likely based on its interaction with other potent CYP3A4 inhibitors . It would seem prudent to give a reduced dose of trazodone or avoid concurrent use, if possible. Note that the US manufacturer recommends careful dose titration of trazodone with monitoring for its antidepressant response.[1]

1. Stribild (Elvitegravir, cobicistat, emtricitabine, tenofovir disoproxil fumarate). Gilead Sciences, Inc. US Prescribing information, August 2012.

HIV-integrase inhibitors; Raltegravir + Atovaquone with Proguanil

A case report suggests that atovaquone with proguanil slightly decreases raltegravir exposure.

Clinical evidence, mechanism, importance and management

A patient with an allergy to ritonavir taking a salvage antiretroviral regimen including raltegravir 400 mg twice daily had a slight 23% decrease in the AUC of raltegravir 20 days after starting atovaquone with proguanil 250/100 mg daily for malaria prophylaxis, when compared with the AUC the day before starting prophylaxis.[1] The general relevance of this possible interaction is unknown as data from one patient is insufficient to exclude or prove an interaction, and further study is needed.

1. Tommasi C, Bellagamba R, Tempestilli M, D'Avolio A, Gallo AL, Ivanovic J, Nicastri E, Pucillo LP, Narciso P. Marked increase in etravirine and saquinavir plasma concentrations during atovaquone/proguanil prophylaxis. *Malar J* (2011) 10, 141.

HIV-integrase inhibitors; Raltegravir + Miscellaneous

Raltegravir does not affect the pharmacokinetics of lamotrigine and might not affect those of acenocoumarol.

Clinical evidence, mechanism, importance and management

(a) Acenocoumarol

A case report briefly describes a 51-year-old HIV-positive man whose acenocoumarol dose needed to be increased when his NRTI antiretroviral regimen was changed to an NRTI backbone plus efavirenz. A further increase in the acenocoumarol dose was needed when efavirenz was changed to atazanavir boosted with ritonavir. However, when his treatment was further changed to replace atazanavir boosted with ritonavir with raltegravir 400 mg twice daily, his acenocoumarol dose needed to be reduced, suggesting a lack of pharmacokinetic interaction between acenocoumarol and raltegravir.[1] The general relevance of this isolated case report is unclear; however, until more is known, it might be prudent to consider an interaction should any otherwise unexplained change in anticoagulant control occur on concurrent use.

(b) Lamotrigine

In a study in 24 healthy subjects, raltegravir 400 mg twice daily for 5 days had no effects on the pharmacokinetics of a single 100-mg dose of lamotrigine given on day 4. Therefore, raltegravir appears not to affect the glucuronidation of lamotrigine. No serious adverse effects were reported.[2] From this study, it appears that no lamotrigine dose adjustments are usually needed in patients also taking raltegravir.

(c) Other drugs

Raltegravir is primarily metabolised by the glucuronyltransferase, UGT1A1. The UK manufacturer of raltegravir advises that no dose adjustment is needed when it is used concurrently with drugs that are less potent inducers of UGT1A1 than rifampicin (see 'HIV-integrase inhibitors + Rifamycins', p.917), and they specifically name **glucocorticoids**, **pioglitazone**, and **St John's wort**.[3] However, pioglitazone is not known to be an inducer of glucuronyltransferases. The UK manufacturer states that the effect of other potent inducers of UGT1A1, such as **phenytoin** and **phenobarbital**, is unknown.[3] If these are essential in a patient taking raltegravir, it would be prudent to closely monitor antiviral efficacy.

1. Welzen MEB, van den Berk GEL, Hamers RL, Burger DM. Interaction between antiretroviral drugs and acenocoumarol. *Antivir Ther* (2011) 16, 249–52.
2. van Luin M, Colbers A, Verwey-van Wissen CPWGM, van Ewijk-Beneken-Kolmer EWJ, van der Kolk M, Hoitsma A, da Silva HG, Burger DM. The effect of raltegravir on the glucuronidation of lamotrigine. *J Clin Pharmacol* (2009) 49, 1220–7.
3. Isentress (Raltegravir potassium). Merck Sharp & Dohme Ltd. UK Summary of product characteristics, August 2013.

HIV-integrase inhibitors; Raltegravir + Pravastatin

Pravastatin decreases the minimum plasma concentration of raltegravir. Raltegravir does not alter pravastatin pharmacokinetics.

Clinical evidence, mechanism, importance and management

In a crossover study in 24 healthy subjects, pravastatin 40 mg daily decreased the minimum plasma concentration of raltegravir 400 mg twice daily by 41%, while the maximum plasma concentration and AUC were increased by 31% and 13%, respectively. Pravastatin pharmacokinetics were not affected, and neither was the short-term lipid effect.[1]

The reason for the decreased minimum plasma concentration of raltegravir is unknown, and the authors conclude that it is unlikely to be clinically important.[1] Until more is known, it would seem prudent to be aware of the potential for an interaction in cases of otherwise unexplained reduced virological response.

1. van Luin M, Colbers A, van Ewijk-Beneken Kolmer EWJ, Verweij-van Wissen CPWGM, Schouwenberg B, Hoitsma A, da Silva HG, Burger DM. Drug-drug interactions between raltegravir and pravastatin in healthy volunteers. *J Acquir Immune Defic Syndr* (2010) 55, 82–6.

HIV-protease inhibitors + Aciclovir and related drugs

A negligible pharmacokinetic interaction occurs between valaciclovir and tipranavir boosted with ritonavir. Concurrent use of aciclovir might increase the risk of indinavir-associated renal complications.

Clinical evidence

(a) Indinavir

In a retrospective study, 57 patients taking indinavir who developed indinavir-associated renal complications where compared with 724 patients who did not develop renal complications. Concurrent use of aciclovir (mostly 400 mg twice daily for herpes prophylaxis) was associated with a 2-fold increase in risk of development of indinavir-associated renal complications, and the risk appeared to be further increased, to 2.5-fold, in patients receiving aciclovir for longer than 26 weeks.[1]

(b) Tipranavir

In a study, 26 healthy subjects were given tipranavir boosted with ritonavir 500/200 mg twice daily, with a single 500-mg dose of **valaciclovir**, a prodrug of aciclovir. Steady-state tipranavir boosted with ritonavir negligibly increased the AUC of aciclovir by 7%. The single dose of **valaciclovir** had no effects on the pharmacokinetics of tipranavir, and negligibly decreased the AUC of ritonavir by 14%.[2]

Mechanism

Both indinavir and aciclovir are associated with drug-induced crystalluria, and these effects might be additive.[1] The reason for the negligible changes in exposure when valaciclovir and tipranavir boosted with ritonavir were given together is unknown.

Importance and management

The clinical relevance of the apparent increase in risk of **indinavir**-associated renal complications with the concurrent use of aciclovir is uncertain. Bear the possibility of additive drug-induced crystalluria in mind if the two drugs are used together. This would also apply to the aciclovir prodrug, valaciclovir. This adverse effect is particularly associated with indinavir, and not the other HIV-protease inhibitors.

None of the pharmacokinetic changes seen when valaciclovir was given with **tipranavir** boosted with ritonavir were clinically relevant. No dose adjustment is therefore needed when valaciclovir, and therefore probably aciclovir, is given with tipranavir boosted with ritonavir.

1. Herman JS, Ives NJ, Nelson M, Gazzard BG, Easterbrook PJ. Incidence and risk factors for the development of indinavir-associated renal complications. *J Antimicrob Chemother* (2001) 48, 355–60.
2. Sabo JP, Cong XJ, Kraft M-F, Wallace L, Castles MA, Mauss S, MacGregor TR. Lack of a pharmacokinetic interaction between steady-state tipranavir/ritonavir and single-dose valacyclovir in healthy volunteers. *Eur J Clin Pharmacol* (2011), 67, 277–81.

HIV-protease inhibitors + Antacids

An aluminium/magnesium hydroxide-containing antacid slightly decreased tipranavir exposure, and negligibly decreased fosamprenavir exposure. Atazanavir absorption is predicted to be reduced by antacids.

Clinical evidence

(a) Fosamprenavir

In a crossover study in healthy subjects, the AUC of amprenavir (derived from a single 1.4-g unboosted dose of fosamprenavir) was decreased by 18% and the maximum plasma concentration was decreased by 35%, but the minimum plasma concentration was not notably altered by the concurrent use of 30 mL of an **aluminium/magnesium hydroxide**-containing antacid *(Maalox TC)*.[1]

(b) Lopinavir

For mention of a study of lopinavir boosted with ritonavir in which gastric-acid reducing drugs, including antacids, had no effect on minimum lopinavir plasma concentrations, see 'HIV-protease inhibitors + H_2-receptor antagonists', p.930.

(c) Tipranavir

In a single-dose study in healthy subjects, 20 mL of an **aluminium/magnesium hydroxide**-containing antacid *(Maalox Plus)* decreased the AUC, minimum plasma concentration, and maximum plasma concentration of tipranavir by 25 to 29%, after tipranavir boosted with ritonavir 200/500 mg was taken at the same time as the antacid.[2-4]

Mechanism

Unknown. The gastrointestinal absorption of some HIV-protease inhibitors, such as atazanavir[5,6] and fosamprenavir,[1] decreases as gastric acidity is reduced, due to reduced solubility with increasing pH.[1,6] Indinavir might also require normal gastric pH for optimum absorption,[7] but most other HIV-protease inhibitors are not affected in this way.

Importance and management

The decrease in amprenavir concentrations seen when **fosamprenavir** is given with an antacid is not considered clinically relevant, and no fosamprenavir dose adjustment is considered to be necessary.[8]

Antacids slightly decreased **tipranavir** concentrations, and the UK manufacturer recommends that administration should be separated by at least 2 hours.[4]

Antacids are predicted to reduce **atazanavir** absorption, and the UK and US manufacturers recommend that atazanavir should be given 2 hours before, or one hour after, antacids or buffered medicinal products.[5,6] This would include didanosine buffered tablets (see 'NRTIs + HIV-protease inhibitors', p.974). Note that buffered didanosine, has also been shown to reduce **indinavir** concentrations, and antacids might interact similarly.

1. Ford SL, Wire MB, Lou Y, Baker KL, Stein DS. Effect of antacids and ranitidine on the single-dose pharmacokinetics of fosamprenavir. *Antimicrob Agents Chemother* (2005) 49, 467–9.
2. Boffito M, Maitland D, Pozniak A. Practical perspectives on the use of tipranavir in combination with other medications: lessons learned from pharmacokinetic studies. *J Clin Pharmacol* (2006) 46, 130–9.
3. Aptivus (Tipranavir). Boehringer Ingelheim Pharmaceuticals, Inc. US Prescribing information, April 2012.
4. Aptivus Soft Capsules (Tipranavir). Boehringer Ingelheim Ltd. UK Summary of product characteristics, December 2011.
5. Reyataz (Atazanavir sulfate). Bristol-Myers Squibb Pharmaceuticals Ltd. UK Summary of product characteristics, August 2012.
6. Reyataz (Atazanavir sulfate). Bristol-Myers Squibb. US Prescribing information, March 2012.
7. Crixivan (Indinavir sulphate). Merck Sharp & Dohme Ltd. UK Summary of product characteristics, February 2012.
8. Telzir (Fosamprenavir calcium). ViiV Healthcare UK Ltd. UK Summary of product characteristics, May 2011.

HIV-protease inhibitors + Atovaquone and/or Proguanil

Atovaquone causes a minor reduction in the minimum concentration of indinavir, and in one case moderately increased saquinavir exposure. Indinavir caused a negligible increase in atovaquone exposure, whereas atazanavir and lopinavir, both boosted with ritonavir, appear to decrease atovaquone and proguanil exposure. Ritonavir alone and when used to boost other HIV-protease inhibitors is predicted to interact similarly.

Clinical evidence

(a) Indinavir

Preliminary results from a study in healthy subjects suggest that the concurrent use of atovaquone 750 mg twice daily and indinavir 800 mg three times daily results in a 5% decrease in the AUC of indinavir, and a 13% increase in the AUC of atovaquone.[1] Similarly, the UK manufacturer of atovaquone notes that concurrent use decreased the AUC of indinavir by 9%, and decreased its minimum plasma concentration by 23%.[2]

(b) Saquinavir

A patient with a ritonavir allergy taking an antiretroviral regimen including unboosted saquinavir 1 g twice daily, had a 3.7-fold increase in the AUC of saquinavir 20 days after starting malaria prophylaxis with atovaquone with proguanil 250/100 mg daily, when compared with the AUC of saquinavir the day before staring prophylaxis.[3]

(c) Other HIV-protease inhibitors

The pharmacokinetics of a single dose of atovaquone with proguanil 250/100 mg taken with a standardised breakfast was compared between 18 healthy subjects and 19 patients taking **lopinavir** boosted with ritonavir or 19 patients taking **atazanavir** boosted with ritonavir. The AUC of atovaquone was 74% lower in the lopinavir group and 46% lower in the atazanavir group when compared with the healthy subjects. In addition, proguanil exposure was 38% lower in the lopinavir group and 41% lower in the atazanavir group when compared with the healthy subjects.[4]

Mechanism

The reason for the negligible changes in atovaquone and indinavir exposure and the apparent increase in saquinavir exposure on concurrent use is unknown. Ritonavir is known to be an inducer of glucuronidation, and it has been suggested that HIV-protease inhibitors boosted with ritonavir might induce the metabolism of atovaquone by this mechanism.[4] Proguanil is mainly metabolised by CYP2C19, which might be induced by some HIV-protease inhibitors boosted with ritonavir.[4]

Importance and management

The clinical relevance of the minor decrease in the **indinavir** minimum plasma concentration on the concurrent use of atovaquone has not been assessed, but the UK manufacturer of atovaquone recommends that caution should be exercised because of the potential risk of indinavir treatment failure.[2] This seems over cautious. No clinically relevant effect on indinavir is likely if indinavir is boosted with low-dose ritonavir. However, indinavir boosted with ritonavir might decrease atovaquone exposure, as has been seen with other HIV-protease inhibitors boosted with ritonavir.

The available evidence suggests that **atazanavir** boosted with ritonavir and **lopinavir** boosted with ritonavir might cause decreases in both atovaquone and proguanil exposure. The authors of this study suggest that the relevance of the decreased exposure is difficult to assess because there is no established minimum effective atovaquone concentration for malaria prophylaxis. In addition, they note that, despite the decrease in exposure observed, there are no published reports of the failure of malaria prophylaxis when atovaquone with proguanil is used in patients treated with HIV-protease inhibitors. Nevertheless, they state that because of the difference in exposure seen, prescribers should be alert to the possibility of prophylaxis failure. They recommend emphasising strict adherence to the prescribed regimen and also the consideration of a dose increase of atovaquone with proguanil when used with lopinavir boosted with ritonavir.[4] The US manufacturer of ritonavir states that an increase in atovaquone dose might be needed,[5] and the UK manufacturer states that careful monitoring of atovaquone serum concentrations and/or therapeutic effects is recommended.[6] However, the UK manufacturer of atovaquone with proguanil advises avoiding concurrent use with [ritonavir-] boosted HIV-protease inhibitors where possible.[7] Similarly, the US guidelines on the treatment of HIV infection recommend that patients taking atazanavir, or lopinavir, boosted with ritonavir use an alternative drug to atovaquone with proguanil for malaria prophylaxis if possible.[8]

Atovaquone with proguanil caused a moderate 3.7-fold rise in unboosted **saquinavir** exposure in a single patient. This requires confirmation, but until such time, some caution would seem appropriate bearing in mind the possibility of an increase in adverse effects.

1. Emmanuel A, Gillotin C, Farinotti R, Sadler BM. Atovaquone suspension and indinavir have minimal pharmacokinetic interactions. *Int Conf AIDS* (1998) 12, 90.
2. Wellvone Oral Suspension (Atovaquone). GlaxoSmithKline UK. UK Summary of product characteristics, April 2010.
3. Tommasi C, Bellagamba R, Tempestilli M, D'Avolio A, Gallo AL, Ivanovic J, Nicastri E, Pucillo LP, Narciso P. Marked increase in etravirine and saquinavir plasma concentrations during atovaquone/proguanil prophylaxis. *Malar J* (2011) 10, 141.
4. Van Luin M, Van der Ende ME, Richter C, Visser M, Faraj D, Van der Ven A, Gelinck L, Kroon F, Wit FW, Van Schaik RHN, Kuks PFM, Burger DM. Lower atovaquone/proguanil concentrations in patients taking efavirenz, lopinavir/ritonavir or atazanavir/ritonavir. *AIDS* (2010) 24, 1223–26.
5. Norvir Capsules (Ritonavir). Abbott Laboratories. US Prescribing information, March 2012.
6. Norvir Tablets (Ritonavir). AbbVie Ltd. UK Summary of product characteristics, September 2012.
7. Malarone (Atovaquone with Proguanil hydrochloride). GlaxoSmithKline UK. UK Summary of product characteristics, August 2012.
8. Panel on Antiretroviral Guidelines for Adults and Adolescents. Guidelines for the use of antiretroviral agents in HIV-1-infected adults and adolescents. US Department of Health and Human Services (April 2015). 1–288. Available at: https://aidsinfo.nih.gov/contentfiles/lvguidelines/adultandadolescentgl.pdf (accessed 20/09/15).

HIV-protease inhibitors + Azoles; Fluconazole

Fluconazole appears to increase the exposure to saquinavir and tipranavir boosted with ritonavir, increase the clearance of nelfinavir, and increase the minimum plasma concentrations of amprenavir, lopinavir, and ritonavir when all three HIV-protease inhibitors were given concurrently. Fluconazole does not appreciably affect the pharmacokinetics of atazanavir boosted with ritonavir, indinavir, or ritonavir. Fluconazole concentrations are not affected by atazanavir or tipranavir, both boosted with ritonavir.

Clinical evidence

(a) Amprenavir

In a study in 9 HIV-positive patients taking amprenavir 600 mg to 750 mg with both **lopinavir** 400 mg to 533 mg and ritonavir 100 mg to 233 mg, all twice daily, the addition of low-dose fluconazole 100 mg daily increased the minimum plasma concentrations of amprenavir, lopinavir, and ritonavir by 66%, 18%, and 35%, respectively.[1]

(b) Atazanavir

The US manufacturer of atazanavir reports that fluconazole 200 mg daily had no effect on the pharmacokinetics of atazanavir boosted with ritonavir 300/100 mg daily. Fluconazole concentrations were unaffected by atazanavir boosted with ritonavir.[2]

(c) Indinavir

In a placebo-controlled study in 11 HIV-positive patients, there was no change in the pharmacokinetics of either indinavir 1 g every 8 hours or fluconazole 400 mg daily when given together, except for a trend towards a decrease in the AUC of indinavir of 24%, which was not statistically significant.[3] Another study found no change in the AUC of indinavir when given with fluconazole 400 mg daily.[4]

(d) Nelfinavir

A population pharmacokinetic analysis estimated that fluconazole decreased nelfinavir clearance by 26 to 30%.[5] The effects of concurrent ritonavir on the interaction of fluconazole with nelfinavir has been reported. In one patient taking nelfinavir 1.25 g twice daily with **lopinavir** boosted with ritonavir 533.3/133.3 mg twice daily, the addition of fluconazole 100 mg twice daily for 4 weeks increased the AUC and maximum plasma concentration of nelfinavir 2.4-fold and 2.1-fold, respectively. The concentrations of the M8 metabolite of nelfinavir were barely detected in the presence of fluconazole. In 2 other patients taking nelfinavir 1.25 g twice daily with stavudine 40 mg twice daily and either efavirenz 800 mg daily or abacavir 300 mg twice daily, fluconazole 100 mg twice daily for 4 weeks had no apparent effect on the pharmacokinetics of nelfinavir or its metabolite.[6]

(e) Ritonavir

A study in 8 healthy subjects found that fluconazole 400 mg on day one, followed by 200 mg daily for 4 days did not alter any of the pharmacokinetic parameters of ritonavir 200 mg every 6 hours by more than 15%.[7] Similarly, fluconazole had no apparent effect on the pharmacokinetics of ritonavir 600 mg twice daily in 3 HIV-positive subjects.[8]

(f) Saquinavir

In a study in 5 HIV-positive subjects taking saquinavir 1.2 g three times daily, fluconazole 400 mg on day 2, followed by 200 mg daily for 6 days, slightly increased the median AUC of saquinavir by 50%, and increased its maximum plasma concentration by 56%.[8]

(g) Tipranavir

In a study in 20 healthy subjects, low-dose fluconazole 100 mg daily was given with tipranavir boosted with ritonavir 500/200 mg twice daily. The AUC of tipranavir was increased by 50% and the maximum and minimum plasma concentrations of tipranavir were increased by 32% and 69%, respectively. Fluconazole concentrations were not affected.[9]

Mechanism

Fluconazole is a moderate inhibitor of CYP3A4, by which the HIV-protease inhibitors are metabolised.[3,7] It therefore has some small effects on the plasma concentrations of the HIV-protease inhibitors.

The situation with nelfinavir is more complex, as it is metabolised by CYP3A4, CYP2C9 and CYP2C19. In addition to inhibiting CYP3A4, fluconazole also inhibits CYP2C9 and CYP2C19. One study[1] and a case report[6] suggests that in the presence of ritonavir (a potent inhibitor of CYP3A4), the effect of fluconazole on CYP2C9 and CYP2C19 will become more important and it is suggested that this accounts for fluconazole appearing to have a greater effect on nelfinavir pharmacokinetics in the presence of lopinavir boosted with ritonavir. However, this proposed mechanism needs to be established..

Importance and management

Fluconazole appears to have no clinically relevant effects on the pharmacokinetics of atazanavir boosted with ritonavir, indinavir, or ritonavir. The apparent slight increase in saquinavir exposure seen with fluconazole is also not clinically relevant. Similarly, the slight effect of fluconazole on nelfinavir clearance found in the population analysis is not expected to be of clinical relevance. The reason for, and the clinical relevance of, the one case of moderately increased nelfinavir exposure when fluconazole was given with nelfinavir and lopinavir boosted with ritonavir is uncertain, and requires further study, but it might be prudent to be alert for increased nelfinavir adverse effects if the combination is given.

Low-dose fluconazole 100 mg daily caused a slight increase in the exposure to tipranavir boosted with ritonavir, which is not clinically relevant, and so no dose adjustment is needed. However, the effect of higher doses of fluconazole might be greater, and the UK and US manufacturers of tipranavir state that doses of fluconazole greater than 200 mg daily are not recommended.[10,11]

1. Peytavin G, Dominguez S, Lamotte C, Simon A, Kirstetter M, Calvez V, Costagliola D, Katlama C. Minimization of the triple reciprocal lopinavir/ritonavir/amprenavir (LPV/RTV/AMP) interaction by low-dose fluconazole (FCZ) in experienced HIV-1 infected patients (PTS) in the Lopigen prospective study. 2nd IAS Conference on HIV Pathogenesis and Treatment, Paris, 2003. Abstract No. 864.
2. Reyataz (Atazanavir sulfate). Bristol-Myers Squibb. US Prescribing information, March 2012.
3. De Wit S, Debier M, De Smet M, McCrea J, Stone J, Carides A, Matthews C, Deutsch P, Clumeck N. Effect of fluconazole on indinavir pharmacokinetics in human immunodeficiency virus-infected patients. *Antimicrob Agents Chemother* (1998) 42, 223–7.
4. The indinavir (MK 639) pharmacokinetic study group. Indinavir (MK 639) drug interaction studies. 11th International Conference on AIDS, Vancouver, 1996. Abstract Mo.B.174.
5. Jackson KA, Rosenbaum SE, Kerr BM, Pithavala YK, Yuen G, Dudley MN. A population pharmacokinetic analysis of nelfinavir mesylate in human immunodeficiency virus-infected patients enrolled in a phase III clinical trial. *Antimicrob Agents Chemother* (2000) 44, 1832–7.
6. Garazzino S, Tettoni M, Calcagno A, D'Avolio A, Bonora S, Di Perri G. Ritonavir-dependent fluconazole boosting of nelfinavir: a report of three cases. *J Antimicrob Chemother* (2006) 58, 483–5.
7. Cato A, Cao G, Hsu A, Cavanaugh J, Leonard J, Granneman R. Evaluation of the effect of fluconazole on the pharmacokinetics of ritonavir. *Drug Metab Dispos* (1997) 25, 1104–1106.
8. Koks CHW, Crommentuyn KML, Hoetelmans RMW, Burger DM, Koopmans PP, Mathôt RAA, Mulder JW, Meenhorst PL, Beijnen JH. The effect of fluconazole on ritonavir and saquinavir pharmacokinetics in HIV-1-infected individuals. *Br J Clin Pharmacol* (2001) 51, 631–5.
9. la Porte CJ, Sabo JP, Elgadi M, Cameron DW. Interaction studies of tipranavir/ritonavir (TPV/r) with clarithromycin, fluconazole, and rifabutin in healthy volunteers. *Antimicrob Agents Chemother* (2009) 53, 162–73.
10. Aptivus (Tipranavir). Boehringer Ingelheim Pharmaceuticals, Inc. US Prescribing information, April 2012.
11. Aptivus Soft Capsules (Tipranavir). Boehringer Ingelheim Ltd. UK Summary of product characteristics, December 2011.

HIV-protease inhibitors + Azoles; Itraconazole

Itraconazole increases the plasma concentrations of indinavir and saquinavir, and might theoretically increase the concentrations of other HIV-protease inhibitors. Similarly, some HIV-protease inhibitors might also increase itraconazole concentrations: cases of increased itraconazole plasma concentrations and adverse effects have been reported with lopinavir and saquinavir, both boosted with ritonavir.

Clinical evidence

(a) Indinavir

The UK and US manufacturers of indinavir report that in a study in 12 subjects given indinavir 600 mg every 8 hours with itraconazole 200 mg twice daily, the AUC of indinavir was similar to that achieved when indinavir 800 mg every 8 hours was given alone, although its minimum concentration was increased by 49%.[1,2]

Two patients taking indinavir, who were also given itraconazole, developed eczematous eruptions and increased serum transaminases. These effects can be seen with HIV-protease inhibitors alone, but were attributed in this case to the increased concentrations of both drugs, arising from concurrent use.[3]

(b) Lopinavir

In one patient, the itraconazole dose was halved when lopinavir boosted with ritonavir was started and, after 5 weeks of concurrent use, the itraconazole half-life had increased about 10-fold with increased itraconazole plasma concentrations, although no signs of itraconazole toxicity were seen. In this patient, lopinavir and ritonavir plasma concentrations were comparable to those without itraconazole.[4]

(c) Saquinavir

In a study in 3 HIV-positive patients taking saquinavir 1.2 g three times daily, itraconazole increased the AUC of saquinavir 2.5- to 6.9-fold, and increased its maximum and minimum plasma concentrations 2- to 5.4-fold and 1.6- to 16.8-fold, respectively. The increase in saquinavir exposure was similar to that seen with saquinavir boosted with ritonavir 400/400 mg twice daily without itraconazole, and it was considered that itraconazole might be an alternative to ritonavir for boosting saquinavir concentrations.[5] In another study in 17 patients, there was no statistically significant differences between the AUC of saquinavir 1.4 g twice daily and the AUCs of saquinavir 800 mg or 1.2 g twice daily when given with itraconazole 100 mg daily.[6]

A patient taking saquinavir boosted with ritonavir, who was also given itraconazole, developed eczematous eruptions and increased serum transaminases. These effects can be seen with HIV-protease inhibitors alone, but were attributed in this case to the increased concentrations of both drugs, arising from concurrent use. The patient had a very prolonged itraconazole half-life.[3]

Mechanism

Itraconazole is a known substrate and potent inhibitor of CYP3A4, and the HIV-protease inhibitors also inhibit and share this pathway of metabolism. Thus enzyme inhibition results in increased serum concentrations of, or exposure to, both drugs.

Importance and management

Effect on HIV-protease inhibitors

Available data indicate that itraconazole increases indinavir and saquinavir concentrations (when used without ritonavir). The UK and US manufacturers of **indinavir** advise reducing the indinavir dose to 600 mg every 8 hours if it is given with itraconazole.[1,2] The UK manufacturer of **saquinavir** recommends monitoring for saquinavir toxicity if itraconazole is also given, but states that no data are available for saquinavir boosted with ritonavir.[7] There does not appear to be any data on the effect of itraconazole on any other HIV-protease inhibitors. As ritonavir is such a potent CYP3A4 inhibitor, it seems unlikely that the addition of itraconazole (another potent CYP3A4 inhibitor) will have any further clinically relevant effect on the concentrations of HIV-protease inhibitors boosted with ritonavir. Note that the potent CYP3A4 inhibitor, ketoconazole, had little effect on concentrations of some HIV-protease inhibitors boosted with ritonavir, see 'HIV-protease inhibitors + Azoles; Ketoconazole', below.

Effect on itraconazole

Some HIV-protease inhibitors, particularly when boosted with ritonavir, could increase itraconazole concentrations and most HIV-protease inhibitor manufacturers state that doses of itraconazole greater than 200 mg daily are not recommended. If itraconazole is required in patients taking HIV-protease inhibitors boosted with ritonavir, it would be prudent to monitor closely for itraconazole adverse effects. For unboosted **fosamprenavir**, the US manufacturer recommends increased monitoring for adverse effects and state that the dose of itraconazole might need to be reduced if it is greater than 400 mg daily.[8]

1. Crixivan (Indinavir sulphate). Merck Sharp & Dohme Ltd. UK Summary of product characteristics, February 2012.
2. Crixivan (Indinavir sulfate). Merck & Co., Inc. US Prescribing information, April 2012.
3. MacKenzie-Wood AR, Whitfeld MJ, Ray JE. Itraconazole and HIV protease inhibitors: an important interaction. *Med J Aust* (1999) 170, 46–7.
4. Crommentuyn KML, Mulder JW, Sparidans RW, Huitema ADR, Schellens JHM, Beijnen JH. Drug-drug interaction between itraconazole and the antiretroviral drug lopinavir/ritonavir in an HIV-1-infected patient with disseminated histoplasmosis. *Clin Infect Dis* (2004) 38, e73–e75.
5. Koks CHW, Van Heeswijk RPG, Veldkamp AI, Meenhorst PL, Mulder J-W, van der Meer JTM, Beijnen JH, Hoetelmans RMW. Itraconazole as an alternative for ritonavir liquid formulation when combined with saquinavir. *AIDS* (2000) 14, 89–90.
6. Cardiello PG, Samor T, Burger D, Hoetelmans R, Mahanontharit A, Ruxrungtham K, Lange JM, Cooper DA, Phanuphak P. Pharmacokinetics of lower doses of saquinavir soft-gel caps (800 and 1200 mg twice daily) boosted with itraconazole in HIV-1-positive patients. *Antivir Ther* (2003) 8, 245–9.
7. Invirase Hard Capsules (Saquinavir mesilate). Roche Products Ltd. UK Summary of product characteristics, June 2012.
8. Lexiva (Fosamprenavir calcium). ViiV Healthcare. US Prescribing information, April 2013.

HIV-protease inhibitors + Azoles; Ketoconazole

Most HIV-protease inhibitors increase the exposure to ketoconazole. Ketoconazole appears to increase the concentrations of the HIV-protease inhibitors.

Clinical evidence

(a) Amprenavir or Fosamprenavir

In a single-dose study, amprenavir 1.2 g caused a slight 44% increase in the AUC of ketoconazole 400 mg. The AUC of amprenavir was also slightly increased by 32%.[1]

In a study in 15 healthy subjects, fosamprenavir boosted with ritonavir 700/100 mg twice daily taken for 10 days increased the AUC and maximum plasma concentration of ketoconazole 200 mg daily (taken from days 6 to 10) 2.7-fold and by 25%, respectively. However, in this study, the pharmacokinetics of amprenavir were unaffected by ketoconazole, and the AUC and maximum plasma concentration of ritonavir were increased by 13% and 17%, respectively.[2]

(b) Atazanavir

The pharmacokinetics of atazanavir 400 mg daily were not affected by the concurrent use of ketoconazole 200 mg daily for 7 days.[3]

(c) Darunavir

In a study in healthy subjects, ketoconazole 200 mg twice daily for 13 doses increased the AUC_{0-12}, maximum plasma concentration, and minimum plasma concentration of darunavir 2.6-fold, by 78%, and 2.8-fold, respectively. However, when ritonavir 100 mg twice daily was added to darunavir 400 mg twice daily, the same dose of ketoconazole had a much less pronounced effect on darunavir pharmacokinetics: the AUC_{0-12}, maximum plasma concentration, and minimum plasma concentration of darunavir were increased by 42%, 21%, and 73%, respectively. Darunavir alone had no effect on the pharmacokinetics of ketoconazole; however, darunavir boosted with ritonavir increased the AUC_{0-12}, maximum plasma concentration, and minimum plasma concentration of ketoconazole 3.1-fold, 2.1-fold, and 9.7-fold, respectively. Ketoconazole had a minimal effect on the pharmacokinetics of ritonavir.[4]

(d) Indinavir

In a study in 10 healthy subjects, ketoconazole 400 mg daily for 4 doses slightly increased the AUC of a single 400-mg dose of indinavir by 62%.[5]

(e) Lopinavir

A single 200-mg dose of ketoconazole had no effect on the pharmacokinetics of lopinavir (when taken as lopinavir boosted with ritonavir 400/100 mg twice daily). However, the AUC of ketoconazole was increased 3-fold by lopinavir boosted with ritonavir.[6] In contrast, in an HIV-positive patient, ketoconazole 200 mg daily for 14 days was associated with a 68% increase in the minimum plasma concentration of lopinavir and a 33% increase in the plasma concentration of ritonavir.[7]

(f) Nelfinavir

In a study in healthy subjects, ketoconazole slightly increased the AUC of nelfinavir by 35%. The doses and duration of treatment with ketoconazole and nelfinavir were not reported.[8]

(g) Ritonavir

In a study in 12 subjects, ritonavir 500 mg twice daily for 10 days increased the AUC of ketoconazole 200 mg daily for 7 days 3.3-fold and increased its maximum plasma concentration by 51%. There was a negligible 18% increase in the AUC of ritonavir and a small 40% increase in its minimum plasma concentration, with no apparent effect on its maximum plasma concentration.[9]

(h) Saquinavir

In one early clinical study, patients who were given ketoconazole with saquinavir had a greater reduction in viral load after 3 months than those not given ketoconazole.[10] However, in one pharmacokinetic study in 7 HIV-positive patients, ketoconazole 200 mg daily for 7 days then 400 mg daily for 7 days had no consistent effect on saquinavir maximum and minimum plasma concentrations, although there was wide inter-individual variability. Saquinavir (as hard gelatin capsules[11]) was given at a low dose of 600 mg three times daily.[12] Conversely, when a higher dose of saquinavir (as soft gel capsules) 1.2 g three times daily was given to 12 healthy subjects with ketoconazole 400 mg daily for 7 days, the saquinavir AUC and maximum plasma concentration were increased 2.9-fold and 2.7-fold, respectively.[11] A similar study in 22 HIV-positive patients who had been taking saquinavir 1.2g three times daily found that ketoconazole 200 mg daily for 7 days increased the saquinavir AUC and maximum plasma concentration by 69% and 36%, respectively.[11]

In 12 HIV-positive patients, ketoconazole 200 mg or 400 mg increased the AUC of saquinavir and ritonavir in combination (both 400 mg twice daily) by 37% and 29%, respectively. The distribution of ritonavir was also affected, with disproportionate increases seen in CSF concentrations. All these changes appeared to be unrelated to the dose of ketoconazole used.[13]

The maximum plasma concentration of ketoconazole 400 mg daily was similar to that usually seen with ketoconazole 800 mg alone when saquinavir boosted with ritonavir was given.[13] Moreover, in this study, dose escalation to higher doses of ketoconazole was discontinued as the first patient given ketoconazole 600 mg daily stopped treatment early because of gastrointestinal adverse effects.[13] However, saquinavir alone did not affect ketoconazole pharmacokinetics.[11] A further study in 25 stable HIV-positive patients investigated the potential for using ketoconazole rather than ritonavir as a pharmacokinetic booster for saquinavir. Patients were given saquinavir boosted with ritonavir 2000 mg/100 mg daily for at least 4 weeks before ritonavir was changed to ketoconazole 400 mg daily for 2 weeks. The AUC, maximum plasma concentration, and minimum plasma concentration of saquinavir were 80%, 69%, and 67% lower, respectively, in the ketoconazole-boosted regimen than in the ritonavir-boosted regimen. Thirteen patients given ketoconazole, compared with 2 patients given ritonavir, had saquinavir concentrations below the minimum recommended concentration. A positive correlation between the AUCs of ketoconazole and saquinavir was noted.[14] In another study in 32 healthy subjects, ketoconazole 200 mg daily had no effect on the pharmacokinetics of saquinavir boosted with ritonavir 1000 mg/100 mg twice daily. However, the AUC_{0-12} and maximum plasma concentration of ketoconazole were increased 2.7-fold and 45%, respectively.[15]

Mechanism

Ketoconazole is a known substrate and a potent inhibitor of CYP3A4, and the HIV-protease inhibitors also inhibit and share this pathway of metabolism.[1,11,13] Thus enzyme inhibition results in increased plasma concentrations of both drugs. Ketoconazole might also inhibit the P-glycoprotein transport of saquinavir and ritonavir, causing a decrease in their clearance, and increasing plasma concentrations.[11,13] Inhibition of P-glycoprotein might reduce the transport of HIV-protease inhibitors out of the CSF, so increasing CSF concentrations.[13]

Importance and management

Effect on HIV-protease inhibitors

The magnitude of the changes in the pharmacokinetics of amprenavir, atazanavir, nelfinavir, or darunavir, fosamprenavir, lopinavir, or saquinavir, all boosted with ritonavir, seen with ketoconazole are unlikely to warrant dose changes of the HIV-protease inhibitors or cause an increase in their adverse effects. However, for **indinavir**, the UK and US manufacturers advise considering reducing the dose of indinavir to 600 mg every 8 hours in the presence of ketoconazole.[16,17] The clinical relevance of the moderate increase in darunavir exposure seen with unboosted **darunavir** is uncertain; however, darunavir is usually given with low-dose ritonavir, and the increase in darunavir boosted with ritonavir exposure with ketoconazole is slight.

Effect on ketoconazole

Ritonavir alone and darunavir, fosamprenavir, lopinavir, and saquinavir, all boosted with ritonavir, increase the exposure to ketoconazole and might increase its adverse effects. **Tipranavir** boosted with ritonavir is predicted to interact similarly. Conversely, unboosted amprenavir and unboosted darunavir appear to have no clinically relevant effect on ketoconazole exposure. Most HIV-protease inhibitor manufacturers state that ketoconazole in doses of greater than 200 mg daily is not recommended with HIV-protease inhibitors boosted with ritonavir. Similarly, the UK manufacturers of **ritonavir** state that, due to an increase in incidence of gastrointestinal and hepatic adverse effects, a dose reduction of ketoconazole should be considered when it is given with ritonavir, either at full dose or when it is used to boost the effects of other HIV-protease inhibitors.[18] For unboosted **fosamprenavir**, the US manufacturer states that if it is given with a dose of ketoconazole greater than 400 mg daily, the ketoconazole dose might need to be reduced: increased monitoring for ketoconazole adverse effects is advised.[19]

1. Polk RE, Crouch MA, Israel DS, Pastor A, Sadler BM, Chittick GE, Symonds WT, Gouldin W, Lou Y. Pharmacokinetic interaction between ketoconazole and amprenavir after single doses in healthy men. *Pharmacotherapy* (1999) 19, 1378–84.
2. Wire MB, Ballow CH, Borland J, Shelton MJ, Lou Y, Yuen G, Lin J, Lewis EW. Fosamprenavir plus ritonavir increases plasma ketoconazole and ritonavir exposure, while amprenavir exposure remains unchanged. *Antimicrob Agents Chemother* (2007) 51, 2982–4.
3. O'Mara EM, Randall D, Mummaneni V, Uderman H, Knox L, Schuster A, Geraldes M, Raymond R. Steady-state pharmacokinetic interaction study between BMS-232632 and ketoconazole in healthy subjects. *Intersci Conf Antimicrob Agents Chemother* (2000) 40, 335.
4. Sekar VJ, Lefebvre E, De Pauw M, Vangeneugden T, Hoetelmans RM. Pharmacokinetics of darunavir/ritonavir and ketoconazole following co-administration to HIV-healthy volunteers. *Br J Clin Pharmacol* (2008) 66, 215–21.
5. McCrea J, Woolf E, Sterrett A, Matthews C, Deutsch P, Yeh KC, Waldman S, Bjornsson T. Effects of ketoconazole and other P450 inhibitors on the pharmacokinetics of indinavir. *Pharm Res* (1996) 13 (Suppl 9), S465.
6. Bertz R, Hsu A, Lam W, Williams L, Renz C, Karol M, Dutta S, Carr R, Zhang Y, Wang Q, Schweitzer S, Foit C, Andre A, Bernstein B, Granneman GR, Sun E. Pharmacokinetic interactions between lopinavir/ritonavir (ABT-378r) and other non-HIV drugs (abstract P291). *AIDS* (2000) 14 (Suppl 4), S100.
7. Boffito M, Bonora S, Sales P, Dal Conte I, Sinicco A, Hoggard PG, Khoo S, Back DJ, Di Perri G. Ketoconazole and lopinavir/ritonavir coadministration: boosting beyond boosting. *AIDS Res Hum Retroviruses* (2003) 19, 941–2.
8. Kerr B, Lee C, Yuen G, Anderson R, Daniels R, Grettenberger H, Liang B-H, Quart B, Sandoval T, Shetty B, Wu E, Zhang K. Overview of *in-vitro* and *in-vivo* drug interaction studies of nelfinavir mesylate (NFV), a new HIV-1 protease inhibitor. 4th Conference on Retroviruses and Opportunistic Infections, Washington DC, 1997. Session 39, Slide 373.
9. Bertz R, Wong C, Carothers L, Lauva I, Dennis S, Valdes J. Evaluation of the pharmacokinetics of multiple dose ritonavir and ketoconazole in combination. *Clin Pharmacol Ther* (1998) 63, 230.
10. Jordan WC. The effectiveness of combined saquinavir and ketoconazole treatment in reducing HIV viral load. *J Natl Med Assoc* (1998) 90, 622–4.
11. Grub S, Bryson H, Goggin T, Lüdin E, Jorga K. The interaction of saquinavir (soft gelatin capsule) with ketoconazole, erythromycin and rifampicin: comparison of the effect in healthy volunteers and in HIV-infected patients. *Eur J Clin Pharmacol* (2001) 57, 115–21.
12. Collazos J, Martínez E, Mayo J, Blanco M-S. Effect of ketoconazole on plasma concentrations of saquinavir. *J Antimicrob Chemother* (2000) 46, 151–2.
13. Khaliq Y, Gallicano K, Venance S, Kravcik S, Cameron DW. Effect of ketoconazole on ritonavir and saquinavir concentrations in plasma and cerebrospinal fluid from patients infected with human immunodeficiency virus. *Clin Pharmacol Ther* (2000) 68, 637–46.
14. Autar RS, Wit FWNM, Sankote J, Sutthichom D, Kimenai E, Hassink E, Hill A, Cooper DA, Phanuphak P, Lange JMA, Burger DM, Ruxrungtham K. Ketoconazole is inferior to ritonavir as an alternative booster for saquinavir in a once daily regimen in Thai HIV-1 infected patients. *AIDS* (2007) 21, 1535–9.
15. Kaeser B, Zandt H, Bour F, Zwanziger E, Schmitt C, Zhang X. Drug-drug interaction study of ketoconazole and ritonavir-boosted saquinavir. *Antimicrob Agents Chemother* (2009) 53, 609–14.
16. Crixivan (Indinavir sulfate). Merck & Co., Inc. US Prescribing information, April 2012.
17. Crixivan (Indinavir sulphate). Merck Sharp & Dohme Ltd. UK Summary of product characteristics, February 2012.
18. Norvir Tablets (Ritonavir). AbbVie Ltd. UK Summary of product characteristics, September 2012.
19. Lexiva (Fosamprenavir calcium). ViiV Healthcare. US Prescribing information, April 2013.

HIV-protease inhibitors + Azoles; Miscellaneous

Systemic clotrimazole appears to slightly increase darunavir exposure. Miconazole oral gel is predicted to increase the concentrations of the HIV-protease inhibitors, such as saquinavir.

Clinical evidence, mechanism, importance and management

The extent of absorption from many topical or intravaginal azoles is low, and therefore the likelihood of an interaction with the HIV-protease inhibitors is small, see 'Azoles; Topical + Miscellaneous', p.242. More specific information on individual azoles that are most commonly used topically is given below.

(a) Clotrimazole

The UK manufacturer of **darunavir** reports that the concurrent use of *systemic* clotrimazole increased the AUC of **darunavir** (from **darunavir** boosted with ritonavir) by 33% (using a population pharmacokinetic model). They suggest that clotrimazole might inhibit **darunavir** metabolism by CYP3A4, and therefore advise close monitoring when clotrimazole is taken with **darunavir** boosted with ritonavir.[1] However, this slight increase in **darunavir** exposure is unlikely to be clinically relevant. The US manufacturer gives no specific advice regarding this interaction.[2] The effect of **darunavir** boosted with ritonavir on the concentrations of clotrimazole given systemically does not appear to have been studied.

(b) Miconazole

Miconazole is known to inhibit CYP3A4 and the UK manufacturer includes a list of substrates of CYP3A4 that they state should be used with caution with miconazole oral gel, and they specifically name **saquinavir**.[3] Note that a large proportion of miconazole oral gel (both prescription and non-prescription doses) can be swallowed and therefore adequate systemic absorption might occur to produce an interaction. However, saquinavir is usually used boosted with ritonavir, and ritonavir is such a potent CYP3A4 inhibitor it seems unlikely that miconazole would cause an additional effect on saquinavir concentrations by this mechanism. The effect of saquinavir boosted with ritonavir on the concentrations of miconazole given systemically does not appear to have been studied.

1. Prezista (Darunavir ethanolate). Janssen-Cilag Ltd. UK Summary of product characteristics, June 2012.
2. Prezista (Darunavir ethanolate). Janssen Pharmaceuticals, Inc. US Prescribing information, May 2012.
3. Daktarin Oral Gel (Miconazole). Janssen-Cilag Ltd. UK Summary of product characteristics, December 2014.

HIV-protease inhibitors + Azoles; Posaconazole

Posaconazole moderately increases the exposure to both unboosted atazanavir and atazanavir boosted with ritonavir. Posaconazole appears to slightly increase the exposure to amprenavir from unboosted fosamprenavir, but not to the same extent as ritonavir. Unboosted fosamprenavir reduces the exposure to posaconazole, whereas unboosted atazanavir and atazanavir boosted with ritonavir do not appear to alter posaconazole concentrations.

Clinical evidence

(a) Atazanavir

In a study in 12 healthy subjects, oral posaconazole 400 mg twice daily given with atazanavir 300 mg daily for 7 days, increased the maximum serum concentration and AUC of atazanavir 2.6-fold and 3.7-fold, respectively. When the study was repeated with atazanavir boosted with ritonavir 300/100 mg daily, the maximum serum concentration and AUC of atazanavir were increased by 50% and 2.5-fold, respectively, and the AUC of ritonavir was increased by 80%. Clinically important increases in total bilirubin concentrations occurred in 11 of the 12 subjects, and occurred with both unboosted atazanavir and atazanavir boosted with ritonavir. Posaconazole concentrations were similar between the atazanavir alone and the atazanavir boosted with ritonavir arms of this study, and did not differ from historical control data.[1]

(b) Fosamprenavir

In a crossover study, 20 healthy subjects were given three regimens: fosamprenavir 700 mg twice daily with posaconazole (200 mg daily on day one, 200 mg twice daily on day 2 and then 400 mg twice daily for 8 days), fosamprenavir boosted with ritonavir 700/100 mg twice daily alone, or posaconazole alone. Unboosted fosamprenavir reduced the AUC and maximum concentration of posaconazole by 23% and 21%, respectively, when compared with posaconazole alone. In addition, the AUC and maximum concentration of amprenavir (from unboosted fosamprenavir) were 65% and 36% lower, respectively, when compared with fosamprenavir boosted with ritonavir. However, the AUC of amprenavir (from unboosted fosamprenavir) with posaconazole was 56% higher than historical control data for amprenavir (from unboosted fosamprenavir) alone. This shows that posaconazole increases amprenavir exposure, but not to the same extent as ritonavir.[2]

Mechanism

It has been suggested that as posaconazole is a moderate inhibitor of CYP3A4, it decreases the metabolism of atazanavir by this isoenzyme leading to an increase in its exposure and possibly its adverse effects. However, unusually, posaconazole still increased atazanavir exposure when boosted with the potent CYP3A4 inhibitor ritonavir and therefore CYP3A4 inhibition might not be the mechanism for this interaction. The increase in fosamprenavir exposure with posaconazole does not appear to be as great as that seen with atazanavir. The authors of the study with fosamprenavir suggest that induction of P-glycoprotein or the glucuronyltransferase UGT1A4 by fosamprenavir might have led to the reduction in posaconazole exposure.[2]

Importance and management

Evidence for an interaction between posaconazole and the HIV-protease inhibitors appears to be limited to the data on atazanavir, unboosted or boosted with ritonavir, and unboosted fosamprenavir. The increase in atazanavir exposure (both unboosted and boosted with ritonavir) seen on concurrent use with posaconazole is likely to increase the risk of adverse effects, therefore it would seem prudent to monitor patients closely for atazanavir or ritonavir adverse effects on concurrent use.[1] Other HIV-protease inhibitors boosted with ritonavir are predicted to interact similarly, and the same precautions are advisable.

The study with fosamprenavir was conducted to see if posaconazole could be an alternative booster to ritonavir. However, the effect of posaconazole on amprenavir exposure from unboosted fosamprenavir was less than the effect of ritonavir, and the combination of posaconazole and unboosted fosamprenavir seems likely to result in antiviral failure. Therefore, posaconazole is not a suitable alternative booster to ritonavir. The effect of posaconazole on fosamprenavir boosted with ritonavir is unknown.

The reduction in posaconazole exposure with unboosted fosamprenavir is slight; nevertheless, the UK and US manufacturers recommend monitoring for a loss of antifungal effects in patients taking fosamprenavir and posaconazole.[3,4] Unboosted atazanavir and atazanavir boosted with ritonavir do not appear to alter posaconazole concentrations, although this requires confirmation.

1. Krishna G, Moton A, Ma L, Martinho M, Seiberling M, McLeod J. Effects of oral posaconazole on the pharmacokinetics of atazanavir alone and with ritonavir or with efavirenz in healthy adult volunteers. *J Acquir Immune Defic Syndr* (2009) 51, 437–44.
2. Brüggemann RJM, van Luin M, Colbers EPH, van den Dungen MW, Pharo C, Schouwenberg BJJ, Burger DM. Effect of posaconazole on the pharmacokinetics of fosamprenavir and vice versa in healthy volunteers. *J Antimicrob Chemother* (2010) 65, 2188–94.
3. Noxafil (Posaconazole). Merck Sharp & Dohme Ltd. UK Summary of product characteristics, September 2014.
4. Noxafil (Posaconazole). Merck & Co., Inc. US Prescribing information, June 2014.

HIV-protease inhibitors + Azoles; Voriconazole

Ritonavir appears to cause a dose-related decrease in voriconazole exposure in most patients, although some individuals might have increased voriconazole exposure. Voriconazole had no clear effect on ritonavir exposure. A patient taking lopinavir boosted with ritonavir required a voriconazole dose increase to obtain therapeutic concentrations. A case report describes apparently decreased ritonavir and darunavir concentrations in a patient taking voriconazole, whereas in contrast, another case report describes apparently increased darunavir concentrations in a patient taking voriconazole. No pharmacokinetic interaction appears to occur between indinavir and voriconazole.

Clinical evidence

(a) Darunavir

A case report describes a patient taking darunavir boosted with ritonavir 900/100 mg daily and etravirine, who took voriconazole 400 mg twice daily for 3 weeks. The minimum plasma concentration of ritonavir was undetectable, the minimum plasma concentration of darunavir was below the reference range, and voriconazole concentrations were at the upper end of the suggested therapeutic range. Three weeks after voriconazole was stopped, the minimum plasma concentration of ritonavir increased to within the reference range and that of darunavir increased 4-fold.[1]

In contrast, in another patient taking darunavir boosted with ritonavir 800/100 mg daily and etravirine, darunavir minimum plasma concentrations measured on three occasions while taking voriconazole 400 mg in the morning and 200 mg in the evening were within the 50 to 75th percentile range. They remained within the same range when voriconazole was stopped and the darunavir dose was increased to 1.2 g daily to compensate for the possible lack of inhibition of darunavir metabolism on stopping voriconazole. Ritonavir plasma concentrations in this patient were sufficient to boost darunavir.[2]

(b) Indinavir

In a study in 18 healthy subjects, the pharmacokinetics of both indinavir 800 mg three times daily and voriconazole 200 mg twice daily were unaffected by at least one week of concurrent use.[3]

(c) Lopinavir

A patient taking lopinavir boosted with ritonavir required a voriconazole dose increase from the standard dose of 4 mg/kg twice daily to 7 mg/kg twice daily to achieve recommended voriconazole therapeutic concentrations.[4]

(d) Ritonavir

In a study in 29 healthy subjects, ritonavir 400 mg twice daily for 10 days markedly decreased the steady-state AUC_{0-12} of oral voriconazole (400 mg twice daily for one day, then 200 mg twice daily for 9 days) by 83%. However, one subject had a 2.5-fold *increase* in the steady-state maximum plasma concentration and AUC_{0-12} of voriconazole, which was suggested to be due to a lack of CYP2C19 in this subject. Voriconazole had no apparent effect on ritonavir exposure, but there was large intersubject variability, with some subjects having a 50% decrease and others a 2-fold increase in exposure, although the overall changes were not statistically significant. Low-dose ritonavir (100 mg daily) slightly decreased the steady-state AUC_{0-12} of voriconazole by 39%. However, 4 subjects had increases in voriconazole exposure, which was negligible to slight in 3 of them (increases of between 10% and 42%), but in one subject a 3-fold increase occurred. Voriconazole caused a negligible 14% decrease in ritonavir exposure.[5]

In contrast, a study in 20 healthy subjects found that when a single 400-mg dose of voriconazole was given with the first dose of ritonavir 300 mg twice daily for 2 days, the voriconazole exposure was increased 4.5-fold. This effect was much greater in the 4 patients who were CYP2C19 poor metabolisers (that is those lacking or deficient in this isoenzyme), who had a 9-fold increase in AUC, than the 8 extensive metabolisers (that is, those with normal CYP2C19 activity), who had a 50% increase in AUC.[6]

Mechanism

Voriconazole is primarily metabolised by CYP2C9 and CYP2C19, with some minor involvement from CYP3A4. Ritonavir is known to induce CYP2C19 and inhibit CYP3A4: the overall effect at steady-state is a reduction in voriconazole exposure (CYP2C19 induction predominates),[5] whereas the effect of the first ritonavir dose is an increase in voriconazole exposure (CYP3A4 inhibition). However, the interaction is also likely to be affected by CYP2C19 genetic polymorphism (meaning that different subjects have different CYP2C19 activity). In CYP2C19 poor metabolisers (that is, those lacking or deficient in CYP2C19), CYP3A4 might have a more prominent role in voriconazole metabolism. In these individuals, the inhibitory effect of ritonavir on CYP3A4 might predominate at steady state, and it is possible that the individuals with 2.5-fold and 3-fold increases in voriconazole exposure were CYP2C19 poor metabolisers.[5] The finding that the first dose of ritonavir increased voriconazole exposure to a much greater extent in CYP2C19 poor metabolisers would seem to support this, because at this time point induction of CYP2C19 would not have occurred.

Voriconazole is a known potent inhibitor of CYP3A4 and also has CYP2C19 and CYP2C9 inhibitory activity. As such it might increase HIV-protease inhibitor exposure. However, it had variable effects on ritonavir exposure and no effect on indinavir pharmacokinetics. The reason for the case of reduced ritonavir and darunavir plasma concentrations is uncertain,[4] and does not appear to have been demonstrated in another case.[2]

Importance and management

Based on the evidence of markedly reduced voriconazole exposure and the possible risk of voriconazole treatment failure, the UK and US manufacturers of both drugs state that the concurrent use of **ritonavir** at doses of 400 mg and above twice daily is contraindicated.[7-10] The manufacturers also recommend that when low-dose ritonavir is used as a pharmacokinetic booster (usually 100 mg twice daily) voriconazole should be given only if the benefits outweigh the risks.[7-10] Conversely, it should be borne in mind that voriconazole exposure might be *increased* by ritonavir in a small proportion of individuals (those lacking CYP2C19), and voriconazole adverse effects might develop. Until more is known, it would be prudent to monitor both for the possibility of voriconazole toxicity and for loss of voriconazole efficacy on the concurrent use of HIV-protease inhibitors boosted with ritonavir. If the facility is available to monitor voriconazole concentrations, this would be useful, and could guide voriconazole dose adjustment. Most HIV-protease inhibitors are given with ritonavir as a pharmacokinetic booster; however, caution is also warranted if they are given alone, as all HIV-protease inhibitors can inhibit CYP3A4 to some extent and could therefore increase voriconazole exposure. However, **indinavir** alone did not alter voriconazole exposure. Until more is known, it would be prudent to monitor both for the possibility of voriconazole toxicity and for the loss of voriconazole efficacy with any other unboosted HIV-protease inhibitor.

Voriconazole might also affect HIV-protease inhibitor concentrations, but other than ritonavir and indinavir, which do not appear to be affected to a clinically relevant extent, this does not appear to have been studied. Be aware that some increase in their concentrations is theoretically possible if voriconazole is also given. The case of reduced ritonavir and darunavir concentrations is unexplained and unconfirmed, particularly as a further similar case suggested increased darunavir concentrations.

1. Toy J, Giguère P, Kravcik S, la Porte CJL. Drug interactions between voriconazole, darunavir/ritonavir and etravirine in an HIV-infected patient with *Aspergillus* pneumonia. *AIDS* (2011) 25, 541–2.
2. Aouri M, Decosterd LA, Buclin T, Hirschel B, Calmy A, Livio F. Drug interactions between voriconazole, darunavir/ritonavir and etravirine in an HIV-infected patient with *Aspergillus* pneumonia. *AIDS* (2012) 26, 776–8.
3. Purkins L, Wood N, Kleinermans D, Love ER. No clinically significant pharmacokinetic interactions between voriconazole and indinavir in healthy volunteers. *Br J Clin Pharmacol* (2003) 56 (Suppl 1), 62–8.
4. Nierenberg NE, Thompson GR, Lewis JS, Hogan BK, Patterson TF. Voriconazole use and pharmacokinetics in combination with interferon-gamma for refractory cryptococcal meningitis in a patient receiving low-dose ritonavir. *Med Mycol* (2010) 48, 532–6.
5. Liu P, Foster G, Gandelman K, LaBadie RR, Allison MJ, Gutierrez MJ, Sharma A. Steady-state pharmacokinetic and safety profiles of voriconazole and ritonavir in healthy male subjects. *Antimicrob Agents Chemother* (2007) 51, 3617–26.
6. Mikus G, Schöwel V, Drzewinska M, Rengelshausen J, Ding R, Riedel K-D, Burhenne J, Weiss J, Thomsen T, Haefeli WE. Potent cytochrome P450 2C19 genotype–related interaction between ritonavir and the cytochrome P450 3A4 inhibitor ritonavir. *Clin Pharmacol Ther* (2006) 80, 126–35.
7. VFEND (Voriconazole). Pfizer Ltd. UK Summary of product characteristics, October 2014.
8. VFEND (Voriconazole). Pfizer Inc. US Prescribing information, February 2014.
9. Norvir Tablets (Ritonavir). AbbVie Ltd. UK Summary of product characteristics, September 2012.
10. Norvir Capsules (Ritonavir). Abbott Laboratories. US Prescribing information, March 2012.

HIV-protease inhibitors + Barbiturates

Phenobarbital and other barbiturates are predicted to increase the metabolism of the HIV-protease inhibitors, thereby reducing their concentrations. However, one case suggests that this might not have occurred when primidone was given with ritonavir and saquinavir. Another case reported unchanged phenobarbital plasma concentrations when a patient was changed from indinavir to ritonavir and saquinavir.

Clinical evidence

There do not appear to be any controlled studies to demonstrate the extent of the pharmacokinetic interaction between **phenobarbital** and different HIV-protease inhibitors.

(a) Saquinavir with Ritonavir

In one report, a patient taking an antiretroviral regimen including ritonavir 600 mg twice daily and saquinavir 400 mg twice daily had his antiepileptic medication changed from carbamazepine to **primidone** 500 mg daily, due to increased carbamazepine serum concentrations and toxicity. The authors noted that during follow-up (duration not stated), viral load was still undetectable and seizures remained under control.[1] Another patient taking **phenobarbital**, phenytoin, and carbamazepine was found to have unchanged phenobarbital concentrations 2 days after switching from an antiretroviral regimen including **indinavir** to one containing ritonavir 300 mg twice daily and saquinavir 400 mg twice daily. His carbamazepine plasma concentration had doubled, and there was a 33% decrease in the plasma concentration of phenytoin.[2] For further discussion about the interaction of carbamazepine or phenytoin with the HIV-protease inhibitors, see 'HIV-protease inhibitors + Carbamazepine', p.927, and 'HIV-protease inhibitors + Phenytoin', p.936.

(b) Tipranavir

A patient with epilepsy taking **phenobarbital** 100 mg daily had an episode of seizures 4 weeks after starting a salvage antiretroviral regimen including tipranavir boosted with ritonavir 500/200 mg twice daily (previous antiretrovirals not stated). His **phenobarbital** plasma concentration had halved from 16 micrograms/mL to 8.1 micrograms/mL. His phenobarbital dose was increased by 50% to 150 mg daily, which increased the **phenobarbital** plasma concentration to the previous value, and no further seizures occurred.[3]

Mechanism

Barbiturates are known enzyme inducers and it is generally assumed that they might decrease the concentrations of the HIV-protease inhibitors, although there appears to be little direct evidence of this. In one case, continuing antiviral efficacy on switching from carbamazepine to primidone suggests that primidone does not have a greater inducing effect on saquinavir with ritonavir than carbamazepine.

Phenobarbital is metabolised by CYP2C9 and CYP2C19. Ritonavir is known to induce CYP2C19 (an enzyme that shows genetic polymorphism, meaning that different patients have different isoenzyme activity), and might therefore decrease phenobarbital concentrations in patients that are CYP2C19 extensive metabolisers. The one case of decreased phenobarbital concentrations on starting tipranavir boosted with ritonavir appears to support this. An interaction via this mechanism would not occur in CYP2C19 poor metabolisers (that is, those lacking or deficient in CYP2C19 activity).

Importance and management

Effect on HIV-protease inhibitors

There is no direct information on the effect of phenobarbital on HIV-protease inhibitor concentrations. The manufacturers of many of the HIV-protease inhibitors predict that their plasma concentrations might be reduced by **phenobarbital**, due to induction of CYP3A4 by which they are metabolised. The one exception to this is the US manufacturer of **darunavir**, who states that darunavir concentrations are not affected by **phenobarbital**.[4] The UK and US manufacturers of **lopinavir** boosted with ritonavir state that a once daily regimen should not be used with phenobarbital.[5,6] Therefore, if the combination is needed, the standard twice daily dose of lopinavir boosted with ritonavir should be used.

Until more is known, if phenobarbital is required in a patient taking HIV-protease inhibitors, it would be prudent to increase monitoring of antiviral efficacy, and monitor HIV-protease inhibitor concentrations, if possible.

Effect on phenobarbital

One case report suggests that 2 days of saquinavir with ritonavir did not alter phenobarbital serum concentrations. However, enzyme induction takes a number of days to develop and might not have had time to occur in this case. The other case report suggests that 4 weeks of tipranavir boosted with ritonavir halved phenobarbital plasma concentrations, requiring an increase in the phenobarbital dose. Based on the proposed mechanism, it seems likely that any HIV-protease inhibitor boosted with ritonavir might decrease phenobarbital concentrations, and this possibility is mentioned by the US manufacturer of darunavir.[4] The possible exception to this is patients who are CYP2C19 poor metabolisers, that is they lack or are deficient in CYP2C19 activity. Until more is known, if phenobarbital and a HIV-protease inhibitor are used concurrently, phenobarbital concentrations should be monitored and the dose adjusted as necessary.

1. Berbel Garcia A, Latorre Ibarra A, Porta Etessam J, Martinez Salio A, Perez Martinez DA, Saiz Diaz R, Toledo Heras M. Protease inhibitor-induced carbamazepine toxicity. *Clin Neuropharmacol* (2000) 23, 216–18.
2. Mateu-de Antonio J, Grau S, Gimeno-Bayón J-L, Carmona A. Ritonavir-induced carbamazepine toxicity. *Ann Pharmacother* (2001) 35, 125–6.
3. Bonora S, Calcagno A, Fontana S, D'Avolio A, Siccardi M, Gobbi F, Di Perri G. Clinically significant drug interaction between tipranavir-ritonavir and phenobarbital in an HIV-infected subject. *Clin Infect Dis* (2007) 45, 1654–5.
4. Prezista (Darunavir ethanolate). Janssen Pharmaceuticals, Inc. US Prescribing information, May 2012.
5. Kaletra Tablets (Lopinavir with Ritonavir). AbbVie Ltd. UK Summary of product characteristics, August 2012.
6. Kaletra (Lopinavir with Ritonavir). Abbott Laboratories. US Prescribing information, April 2012.

HIV-protease inhibitors + Cannabinoids

The short-term use of cannabis cigarettes or dronabinol (Δ^9-tetrahydrocannabinol) did not appear to adversely affect indinavir or nelfinavir

concentrations or viral loads in HIV-positive patients. Ritonavir is predicted to increase dronabinol concentrations.

Clinical evidence

In 9 HIV-positive patients on a stable regimen containing **indinavir** (mostly 800 mg every 8 hours), smoking a **cannabis cigarette** (3.95% tetrahydrocannabinol) three times daily before meals for 14 days resulted in a median 14% decrease in the AUC and maximum concentration of indinavir and a 34% decrease in the minimum concentration of indinavir. However, only the change in maximum concentration was statistically significant.[1] Similarly, **dronabinol** (Δ^9-tetrahydrocannabinol) 2.5 mg three times daily for 14 days had no effect on **indinavir** pharmacokinetics.[1]

In another 11 patients on a stable regimen containing **nelfinavir** 750 mg three times daily, there was a non-significant 10% decrease in the AUC of nelfinavir, a 17% decrease in its maximum concentration, and a 12% decrease in its minimum concentration after 14 days of smoking **cannabis cigarettes**.[1] Similarly, **dronabinol** 2.5 mg three times daily for 14 days had no effect on **nelfinavir** pharmacokinetics.[1]

There was no adverse effect on viral load or CD4+ count in the patients receiving cannabis cigarettes or dronabinol.[2]

Mechanism

Unknown.

Importance and management

The short-term use of cannabis cigarettes or dronabinol does not appear to have any important effect on the concentrations of indinavir or nelfinavir, nor on markers of HIV infection. No particular precautions would therefore seem necessary if these HIV-protease inhibitors are given to cannabis smokers or those taking dronabinol. However, the US manufacturer of ritonavir predicts that it might increase dronabinol concentrations and that a decrease in dronabinol dose might be needed.[3] It would seem prudent to be alert for this effect on concurrent use.

1. Kosel BW, Aweeka FT, Benowitz NL, Shade SB, Hilton JF, Lizak PS, Abrams DI. The effects of cannabinoids on the pharmacokinetics of indinavir and nelfinavir. *AIDS* (2002) 16, 543–50.
2. Abrams DI, Hilton JF, Leiser RJ, Shade SB, Elbeik TA, Aweeka FT, Benowitz NL, Bredt BM, Kosel B, Aberg JA, Deeks SG, Mitchell TF, Mulligan K, Bacchetti P, McCune JM, Schambelan M. Short-term effects of cannabinoids in patients with HIV-1 infection: a randomized, placebo-controlled clinical trial. *Ann Intern Med* (2003) 139, 258–66.
3. Norvir Capsules (Ritonavir). Abbott Laboratories. US Prescribing information, March 2012.

HIV-protease inhibitors + Carbamazepine

Case reports suggest that ritonavir increases carbamazepine serum concentrations sometimes resulting in toxicity. Cases of increased carbamazepine concentrations or exposure have also been reported with darunavir and lopinavir both boosted with ritonavir, nelfinavir, and saquinavir with ritonavir. Carbamazepine reduces indinavir concentrations. It also reduces ritonavir exposure when given with darunavir, and appears to reduce the minimum plasma concentration of tipranavir (when boosted with ritonavir), but does not alter the pharmacokinetics of darunavir (when boosted with ritonavir).

Clinical evidence

(a) Darunavir

The UK and US manufacturers state that darunavir boosted with ritonavir 600/100 mg twice daily increased the AUC and minimum plasma concentration of carbamazepine 200 mg twice daily by 45% and 54%, respectively, and decreased the AUC of carbamazepine-10,11- epoxide (an active metabolite of carbamazepine) by 54%. The AUC of ritonavir was reduced by 49%, but the pharmacokinetics of darunavir were unaffected by carbamazepine.[1,2]

(b) Indinavir

A report describes a 48-year-old man whose antiretrovirals (indinavir 800 mg every 8 hours, lamivudine 150 mg twice daily, and zidovudine 200 mg three times daily) became ineffective after a 10-week course of carbamazepine for postherpetic neuralgia. Over this time, indinavir concentrations were up to 16 times lower than those measured in the absence of carbamazepine.[3] In two further cases, patients taking carbamazepine had partial failure of indinavir-containing antiretroviral regimens, which prompted a change in their therapy to include ritonavir rather than indinavir.[4,5]

In three of the case reports described under *Ritonavir*, below, in which ritonavir increased carbamazepine concentrations,[4-6] patients had previously received indinavir (800 mg three times daily[4,6]) and carbamazepine (600 mg daily[4,5] or 400 mg three times daily[6]) without experiencing carbamazepine toxicity (therapeutic carbamazepine concentrations were reported in two of the cases[4,5]). This suggests that indinavir does not increase carbamazepine concentrations, or only increases them minimally. However, in the first case described above,[3] carbamazepine concentrations reached the therapeutic range for epilepsy even though the dose of carbamazepine was only 200 mg daily, suggesting that indinavir might increase carbamazepine concentrations in some patients.

(c) Lopinavir

An HIV-positive patient who had a carbamazepine serum concentration of 10.3 mg/L while taking carbamazepine 400 mg three times daily, reported feeling very drowsy within 9 days of starting to take tenofovir, lamivudine, and lopinavir boosted with ritonavir 400/100 mg twice daily. His carbamazepine serum concentration was found to have increased by 46%, to 15 mg/L. The carbamazepine dose was reduced to 400 mg twice daily, and 2 days later the carbamazepine serum concentration was 7.4 mg/L.[7]

(d) Nelfinavir

An HIV-positive patient who had a carbamazepine serum concentration of 9.8 mg/L while taking carbamazepine 400 mg three times daily started feeling more tired and unsteady on his feet 3 days after starting to take tenofovir, lamivudine, and nelfinavir 1.25 g twice daily. His carbamazepine serum concentration was found to have increased by 53%, to 15 mg/L. The carbamazepine dose was reduced to 400 mg twice daily, and 2 days later the carbamazepine serum concentration was 9.3 mg/L.[7]

(e) Ritonavir

An 20-year-old HIV-positive man with epilepsy, whose seizures had been controlled with carbamazepine 350 mg twice daily and zonisamide 140 mg twice daily, was admitted to hospital for review of his antiretrovirals. He started taking ritonavir 200 mg three times daily, but after the first dose of ritonavir his serum carbamazepine concentration increased from 9.5 mg/L to 17.8 mg/L. This was accompanied by intractable vomiting and vertigo, therefore the ritonavir was stopped after 2 days and the symptoms then resolved over the next few days. Subsequently ritonavir 200 mg daily was started, with the same effect, so the carbamazepine dose was reduced by two-thirds, which resulted in a carbamazepine serum concentration of 6.2 micrograms/mL. Concentrations of ritonavir were not measured.[8]

(f) Saquinavir with Ritonavir

Three cases document 2- to 3-fold increases in carbamazepine serum concentrations with associated toxicity caused by the addition of ritonavir 300 mg, 400 mg, or 600 mg twice daily and saquinavir 400 mg twice daily.[4-6] In one case, an increase in the carbamazepine serum concentration was not expected as the effects of efavirenz, an inducer of CYP3A4, which can reduce the carbamazepine serum concentration (see 'NNRTIs + Antiepileptics; Enzyme-inducing', p.952), was expected to balance the inhibitory effects of ritonavir and saquinavir. However, the patient needed a carbamazepine dose reduction from 600 mg daily to 100 mg daily to keep the serum concentration within the therapeutic range, before the antiretrovirals were discontinued.[5]

(g) Tipranavir

In a multiple dose study, 17 subjects were given carbamazepine 200 mg twice daily for 43 doses and tipranavir boosted with ritonavir 500/200 mg twice daily for 15 doses. The minimum concentration of carbamazepine was increased by 35% and the AUC was increased by 26%.[9] When combining the AUC of carbamazepine and its active epoxy metabolite, there was a 16% increase in exposure.[10] The UK manufacturer of tipranavir states that carbamazepine 200 mg twice daily reduced the minimum plasma concentration of tipranavir (boosted with ritonavir 500/200 mg twice daily) by 61% when compared with historical controls.[10] In another study in which carbamazepine was given at a dose of 100 mg twice daily, tipranavir boosted with ritonavir 500/200 mg did not affect carbamazepine exposure.[9]

Mechanism

Ritonavir is a potent inhibitor of CYP3A4 and consequently increases the concentrations of carbamazepine, which is metabolised by this isoenzyme. Other HIV-protease inhibitors would be expected to interact similarly, although to a lesser degree. Carbamazepine is an inducer of CYP3A4 and therefore can increase the metabolism of HIV-protease inhibitors causing their concentrations to become subtherapeutic. The use of HIV-protease inhibitors boosted with ritonavir could theoretically offset this effect, but it might lead to increased carbamazepine toxicity.

Importance and management

Although the evidence is limited, these interactions seem to be established. It would therefore appear that the use of carbamazepine with HIV-protease inhibitors should be used with caution. If concurrent use is unavoidable, close monitoring of antiviral efficacy and carbamazepine concentrations and/or signs of carbamazepine toxicity (such as nausea, vomiting, ataxia, and drowsiness) is warranted.

The UK manufacturer of **darunavir** suggests that the dose of carbamazepine might need to be reduced by 25 to 50% (based on monitoring of carbamazepine concentrations), if it is given with darunavir boosted with ritonavir; no dose adjustment of ritonavir-boosted darunavir is required.[1] The US manufacturer of darunavir advises that no dose adjustment of carbamazepine is needed when concurrent use with darunavir boosted with ritonavir is started, but the carbamazepine concentration should be monitored during concurrent use and the dose adjusted according to clinical response.[2] The UK and US manufacturers of **lopinavir** state that the once daily regimen of lopinavir boosted with ritonavir should not be used with carbamazepine.[11,12] Therefore, if the combination is needed, the standard twice daily dose should be used. The UK manufacturer also states that a dose increase of lopinavir boosted with ritonavir should be considered.[11]

Where possible, an alternative non-interacting drug to carbamazepine should be considered in patients taking HIV-protease inhibitors. The authors of one report suggest that amitriptyline or gabapentin would be possible alternatives for carbamazepine used for pain, or valproic acid or lamotrigine for carbamazepine used for seizures.[3] However, note that ritonavir is predicted to increase the concentrations of amitriptyline, so caution is needed on concurrent use (see 'Tricyclic and related antidepressants + HIV-protease inhibitors', p.1509). Furthermore, reduced lamotrigine and valproate concentrations have also been reported with ritonavir-boosted HIV-protease inhibitors (see 'HIV-protease inhibitors + Lamotrigine', p.934, and 'HIV-protease inhibitors + Valproate', p.945).

1. Prezista (Darunavir ethanolate). Janssen-Cilag Ltd. UK Summary of product characteristics, June 2012.
2. Prezista (Darunavir ethanolate). Janssen Pharmaceuticals, Inc. US Prescribing information, May 2012.
3. Hugen PWH, Burger DM, Brinkman K, ter Hofstede HJM, Schuurman R, Koopmans PP, Hekster YA. Carbamazepine-indinavir interaction causes antiretroviral therapy failure. *Ann Pharmacother* (2000) 34, 465–70.
4. Berbel Garcia A, Latorre Ibarra A, Porta Etessam J, Martinez Salio A, Perez Martinez DA, Saiz Diaz R, Toledo Heras M. Protease inhibitor-induced carbamazepine toxicity. *Clin Neuropharmacol* (2000) 23, 216–18.
5. Burman W, Orr L. Carbamazepine toxicity after starting combination antiretroviral therapy including ritonavir and efavirenz. *AIDS* (2000) 14, 2793–4.
6. Mateu-de Antonio J, Grau S, Gimeno-Bayón J-L, Carmona A. Ritonavir-induced carbamazepine toxicity. *Ann Pharmacother* (2001) 35, 125–6.
7. Bates DE, Herman RJ. Carbamazepine toxicity induced by lopinavir/ritonavir and nelfinavir. *Ann Pharmacother* (2006) 40, 1190–5.
8. Kato Y, Fujii T, Mizoguchi N, Takata N, Ueda K, Feldman MD, Kayser SR. Potential interaction between ritonavir and carbamazepine. *Pharmacotherapy* (2000) 20, 851–4.
9. Aptivus (Tipranavir). Boehringer Ingelheim Pharmaceuticals, Inc. US Prescribing information, April 2012.
10. Aptivus Soft Capsules (Tipranavir). Boehringer Ingelheim Ltd. UK Summary of product characteristics, December 2011.
11. Kaletra Tablets (Lopinavir with Ritonavir). AbbVie Ltd. UK Summary of product characteristics, August 2012.
12. Kaletra (Lopinavir with Ritonavir). Abbott Laboratories. US Prescribing information, April 2012.

HIV-protease inhibitors + Cat's claw (*Uncaria tomentosa*)

An isolated case report describes increases in the plasma concentrations of atazanavir, ritonavir, and saquinavir following the use of cat's claw.

Clinical evidence

An HIV-positive woman awaiting liver transplantation, taking **atazanavir** 300 mg daily, **ritonavir** 100 mg daily, and **saquinavir** 1 g daily, in combination with abacavir 600 mg daily and lamivudine 300 mg daily, was found to have an increased minimum plasma concentration of all three HIV-protease inhibitors. The **atazanavir** minimum plasma concentration was 1.22 micrograms/mL (expected range of 0.15 to 0.18 micrograms/mL), the **ritonavir** minimum plasma concentration was 6.13 micrograms/mL (expected concentration of 2.1 micrograms/mL), and the **saquinavir** minimum plasma concentration was 3.4 micrograms/mL (expected range 0.1 to 0.25 micrograms/mL). On further questioning, the patient reported no change in her compliance with the medication but reported that she been taking a herbal supplement containing cat's claw for the previous 2 months. No evidence of HIV-protease inhibitor related toxicity was found and the patient reported no adverse effects. The supplement was stopped and by day 15 the plasma concentrations of all three drugs had returned to within normal limits.[1]

Mechanism

In vitro studies suggested that cat's claw might inhibit CYP3A4, the main isoenzyme responsible for the metabolism of atazanavir, ritonavir, and saquinavir; however, the results of this study are questionable.

Importance and management

Evidence of an interaction between the HIV-protease inhibitors and cat's claw appears to be limited to one case report from which it is difficult to draw general conclusions. What it illustrates is that more research is needed into the use of cat's claw with HIV-protease inhibitors. Patients taking drugs for serious conditions such as HIV-infection should carefully consider the risks and benefits of taking herbal medicines with their existing regimen, where the outcome of concurrent use is unknown.

1. López Galera RM, Ribera Pascuet E, Esteban Mur JI, Montoro Ronsano JB, Juárez Giménez. Interaction between cat's claw and protease inhibitors atazanavir, ritonavir and saquinavir. *Eur J Clin Pharmacol* (2008) 64, 1235–6.

HIV-protease inhibitors + Co-trimoxazole

Minor pharmacokinetic changes have been seen when co-trimoxazole (sulfamethoxazole with trimethoprim) is given with an HIV-protease inhibitor.

Clinical evidence, mechanism, importance and management

A study in 12 healthy subjects given **indinavir** 400 mg every 6 hours with co-trimoxazole 960 mg every 12 hours found that there was no change in the AUC of **indinavir**, but a small 17% decrease in the **indinavir** minimum plasma concentration occurred. In addition, there was an 18% increase in the AUC of **trimethoprim**, and a 5% increase in the AUC of **sulfamethoxazole**. None of these changes were considered to be clinically important.[1] A retrospective cohort study in 781 patients taking **indinavir** reported that the concurrent use of prophylactic co-trimoxazole in 362 patients was not associated with an increased risk of developing **indinavir**-related renal toxicity.[2]

In a study in 15 healthy subjects, **ritonavir** 500 mg twice daily caused a 20% increase in the AUC of **trimethoprim** and a 20% decrease in the AUC of **sulfamethoxazole** from a single 960-mg dose of co-trimoxazole. These changes were considered too small to be of clinical relevance.[3] The pharmacokinetics of **ritonavir** were not assessed.

The combination of **saquinavir** 600 mg three times daily and co-trimoxazole 960 mg three times weekly caused no changes in the pharmacokinetics of **saquinavir**.[4]

There would seem to be no reason for avoiding the use of co-trimoxazole with any of the HIV-protease inhibitors.

1. Sturgill MG, Seibold JR, Boruchoff SE, Yeh KC, Haddix H, Deutsch P. Trimethoprim/sulfamethoxazole does not affect the steady-state disposition of indinavir. *J Clin Pharmacol* (1999) 39, 1077–84.
2. Herman JS, Ives NJ, Nelson M, Gazzard BG, Easterbrook PJ. Incidence and risk factors for the development of indinavir-associated renal complications. *J Antimicrob Chemother* (2001) 48, 355–60.
3. Bertz RJ, Cao G, Cavanaugh JH, Hsu A, Granneman GR, Leonard JM. Effect of ritonavir on the pharmacokinetics of trimethoprim/sulfamethoxazole. 11th International Conference on AIDS, Vancouver, 1996. Abstract Mo.B.1197.
4. Maserati R, Villani P, Cocchi L, Regazzi MB. Co-trimoxazole administered for *Pneumocystis carinii* pneumonia prophylaxis does not interfere with saquinavir pharmacokinetics. *AIDS* (1998) 12, 815–6.

HIV-protease inhibitors + Food

Food increases the bioavailability of atazanavir, darunavir, lopinavir boosted with ritonavir solution, nelfinavir, and saquinavir, but decreases that of indinavir, fosamprenavir solution, and ritonavir tablets. Food has little effect on the bioavailability of tipranavir boosted with ritonavir, but food improves its tolerability. Food only minimally affects the bioavailability of fosamprenavir tablets, indinavir boosted with ritonavir, lopinavir boosted with ritonavir tablets, and ritonavir capsules and solution. Mixing ritonavir oral solution with enteral feeds does not affect the pharmacokinetics of ritonavir.

Clinical evidence, mechanism, importance and management

(a) Atazanavir

The UK and US manufacturers of atazanavir report that a light meal increased the AUC and maximum plasma concentration of a single 300/100-mg dose of atazanavir boosted with ritonavir by 33% and 40%, respectively, compared with the fasting state, whereas a high-fat meal did not increase the absorption of atazanavir.[1,2] The US manufacturer also notes that a light meal increased the AUC and maximum plasma concentration of unboosted atazanavir 400 mg by 70% and 57%, respectively.[2] Administration with a light meal or a high-fat meal also decreased the wide variation in plasma concentrations. The UK and US manufacturers therefore recommend that atazanavir should be taken with food to enhance bioavailability and minimise variability.[1,2]

(b) Darunavir

In a study in 22 healthy subjects, the relative bioavailability of darunavir boosted with ritonavir was found to be 30% lower when it was taken on an empty stomach, compared with intake immediately after food. In this study, no difference in the effects of food on darunavir were seen between the different meals tested (a high-fat breakfast, a standard breakfast, a protein-rich drink, or a croissant and coffee). Taking darunavir with food did not affect interindividual variability in darunavir absorption.[3] Therefore, the UK and US manufacturers advise that darunavir boosted with ritonavir tablets should be taken with food.[4,5]

(c) Fosamprenavir

In a study in 24 healthy subjects, food had minimal effects on the bioavailability of a 1.73 g dose of fosamprenavir from a tablet formulation.[6] Fosamprenavir tablets can be taken without regard to food intake.[7,8]

A high-fat meal slightly reduced the AUC and maximum plasma concentration of a 1.73-g dose of fosamprenavir suspension by 20% and 41%, respectively.[6] The UK and US manufacturers advise that adults should take the oral suspension without food and on an empty stomach. However, they advise that in order to improve palatability and ensure compliance, children can take the suspension with food.[8,9]

(d) Indinavir

A single 600-mg dose of indinavir was given to 7 HIV-positive subjects immediately after various types of meal. The protein, carbohydrate, fat, and high-viscosity meals reduced the AUC of indinavir by 68%, 45%, 34%, and 30%, respectively. The fat meal was associated with the largest inter-subject variation in bioavailability. The effect of the protein meal was attributed to the fact that it increased gastric pH and therefore impaired the absorption of indinavir (a weak base). The impairment of indinavir absorption caused by the other meals, which did not alter gastric pH, might have been due to delayed gastric emptying.[10] A similar study comparing a full breakfast with light breakfasts (toast or cereal) on indinavir absorption found that the full breakfast reduced the absorption of indinavir by 78% and reduced its maximum serum concentration by 86%, while the light breakfasts had no effect.[11] However, in a study in which indinavir was boosted with ritonavir, there was no difference in indinavir exposure when taken with a high-fat meal or a low-fat meal,[12] and, in another study, giving indinavir boosted with ritonavir together with food had little effect compared with the fasting state (the indinavir maximum plasma concentration was decreased by 19% and its AUC was decreased by 12%).[13]

The UK and US manufacturers[14,15] advise that indinavir should be taken one hour before, or 2 hours after, meals or with low-fat light meals only, although the UK manufacturer also states that when indinavir is taken with **ritonavir** it can be taken with or without food.[14] The manufacturers give examples of a light meal, such as dry toast with jam, juice, and coffee with skimmed milk and sugar; or corn flakes, skimmed or fat-free milk and sugar.[14,15]

(e) Lopinavir

A moderate-fat meal slightly increased the AUC of lopinavir (given as lopinavir boosted with ritonavir tablets) by 27%, whereas a high-fat meal increased the AUC of lopinavir by 19%.[16] The corresponding AUC increases for lopinavir boosted with ritonavir solution were 80% for the moderate-fat meal, and 2.3-fold for the high-fat meal; taking lopinavir boosted with ritonavir oral solution with food minimised the pharmacokinetic variability.[16,17] The UK and US manufacturers of lopinavir boosted with ritonavir state that the oral solution should be taken with food,[16,17] whereas the tablets can be taken with or without food.[16,18]

(f) Nelfinavir

When nelfinavir 400 mg or 800 mg was given to 12 healthy subjects in the fasted state, the AUC was 50% to 73% lower than that observed when nelfinavir was taken with a meal.[19] The UK and US manufacturers report that in two studies in healthy subjects, food increased the exposure to a 1.25-g dose of nelfinavir 2- to 5-fold when compared with the fasting state, with the highest increase in the AUC and maximum plasma concentration of nelfinavir occurring with the high-calorie, high-fat meal (1000 kcal and 50% fat).[20,21] A small study in healthy subjects also found a similar effect.[22] Another study in 24 healthy subjects found that the AUC of nelfinavir 1.25 g taken twice daily for 17 days, was only reduced by 13% when it was taken with a light breakfast (250 kcal and 13 g fat) compared with a standard breakfast (800 kcal and 35 g fat).[23] As food increases the absorption of nelfinavir the UK and US manufacturers recommend that it should be taken with food.[20,21]

(g) Ritonavir

The US manufacturer notes that a meal increased the AUC of ritonavir capsules by 13%, when compared with the fasting state,[24] whereas the AUC of the oral solution was decreased by 7%.[25] Although these changes are negligible, the UK and US manufacturers state that ritonavir capsules and solution should preferably be taken with food.[24-26]

When ritonavir tablets were taken with a high-fat meal or a low-fat meal, the AUC slightly decreased by 23% and 21%, respectively, compared with the fasting state.[25] Despite these slight reductions, the UK and US manufacturers recommend that ritonavir tablets are taken with food.[25,27]

There is also some evidence that mixing ritonavir oral solution with **enteral feeds** does not affect ritonavir pharmacokinetics. A 600-mg dose of ritonavir oral solution was mixed with 240 mL of an **enteral feed** (either *Advera* or *Ensure*), **chocolate milk**, or water within one hour of dosing. When given up to 15 minutes after a low-fat meal, the pharmacokinetics of ritonavir in either of the **enteral feeds** or the **milk** were almost identical to those when ritonavir was given in water.[28]

(h) Saquinavir

The UK manufacturer of saquinavir hard capsules and tablets reports a crossover study in 22 HIV-positive patients taking saquinavir boosted with ritonavir 1000/100 mg twice daily and receiving three consecutive doses under fasting conditions or after a high-fat, high-calorie meal. The AUC, maximum and minimum plasma concentrations of saquinavir under fasting conditions were about 70% lower than with a high-fat meal. There were no clinically significant differences in the pharmacokinetic profile of ritonavir in fasting and fed conditions but the ritonavir minimum plasma concentration was about 30% lower in the fasting state, when compared with its administration with a meal.[29] Saquinavir boosted with ritonavir should be given with, or up to 2 hours after, a meal.[29,30]

(i) Tipranavir

The US manufacturer states that, in a study, the pharmacokinetics of tipranavir capsules or solution (boosted with ritonavir) were unaffected when it was taken with food (500 to 682 kcal, 23 to 25% of the calories from fat), compared with fasting conditions. They therefore state that tipranavir boosted with ritonavir capsules or oral solution can be taken with or without food. However, they state that tipranavir boosted with ritonavir tablets should be taken with meals.[31] The UK manufacturer states that food improves the tolerability of tipranavir boosted with ritonavir, and recommends that it should be taken with food.[32]

1. Reyataz (Atazanavir sulfate). Bristol-Myers Squibb Pharmaceuticals Ltd. UK Summary of product characteristics, August 2012.
2. Reyataz (Atazanavir sulfate). Bristol-Myers Squibb. US Prescribing information, March 2012.
3. Sekar V, Kestens D, Spinosa-Guzman S, De Pauw M, De Paepe E, Vangeneugden T, Lefebvre E, Hoetelmans RMW. The effect of different meal types on the pharmacokinetics of darunavir (TMC114)/ritonavir in HIV-negative healthy volunteers. *J Clin Pharmacol* (2007) 47, 479–84.
4. Prezista (Darunavir ethanolate). Janssen-Cilag Ltd. UK Summary of product characteristics, June 2012.
5. Prezista (Darunavir ethanolate). Janssen Pharmaceuticals, Inc. US Prescribing information, May 2012.
6. Falcoz C, Jenkins JM, Bye C, Hardman TC, Kenney KB, Studenberg S, Fuder H, Prince WT. Pharmacokinetics of GW433908, a prodrug of amprenavir, in healthy male volunteers. *J Clin Pharmacol* (2002) 42, 887–98.
7. Telzir (Fosamprenavir calcium). ViiV Healthcare UK Ltd. UK Summary of product characteristics, May 2011.
8. Lexiva (Fosamprenavir calcium). ViiV Healthcare. US Prescribing information, April 2013.
9. Telzir Oral Suspension (Fosamprenavir calcium). ViiV Healthcare UK Ltd. UK Summary of product characteristics, May 2011.
10. Carver PL, Fleisher D, Zhou SY, Kaul D, Kazanjian P, Li C. Meal composition effects on the oral bioavailability of indinavir in HIV-infected patients. *Pharm Res* (1999) 16, 718–24.
11. Stone JA, Ju WD, Steritt A, Woolf EJ, Yeh KC, Deutsch P, Waldman S, Bjornsson TD. Effect of food on the pharmacokinetics of indinavir in man. *Pharm Res* (1996) 13 (Suppl 9), S414.
12. Saah AJ, Winchell GA, Nessly ML, Seniuk MA, Rhodes RR, Deutsch PJ. Pharmacokinetic profile and tolerability of indinavir-ritonavir combinations in healthy volunteers. *Antimicrob Agents Chemother* (2001) 45, 2710–15.
13. Aarnoutse RE, Wasmuth J-C, Fätkenheuer G, Schneider K, Schmitz K, de Boo TM, Reiss P, Hekster YA, Burger DM, Rockstroh JK. Administration of indinavir and low-dose ritonavir (800/100 mg twice daily) with food reduces nephrotoxic peak plasma levels of indinavir. *Antivir Ther* (2003) 8, 309–14.
14. Crixivan (Indinavir sulphate). Merck Sharp & Dohme Ltd. UK Summary of product characteristics, February 2012.
15. Crixivan (Indinavir sulfate). Merck & Co., Inc. US Prescribing information, April 2012.
16. Kaletra (Lopinavir with Ritonavir). Abbott Laboratories. US Prescribing information, April 2012.
17. Kaletra Oral Solution (Lopinavir with Ritonavir). AbbVie Ltd. UK Summary of product characteristics, February 2012.
18. Kaletra Tablets (Lopinavir with Ritonavir). AbbVie Ltd. UK Summary of product characteristics, August 2012.
19. Quart BD, Chapman SK, Peterkin J, Webber S, Oliver S. Phase I safety, tolerance, pharmacokinetics and food effect studies of AG1343–a novel HIV protease inhibitor. The American Society for Microbiology in collaboration with NIH and CDC. 2nd National Conference Human Retroviruses and Related Infections, Washington DC, 1995. Abstract LB3.
20. Viracept (Nelfinavir mesylate). Agouron Pharmaceuticals, Inc. US Prescribing information, May 2013.
21. Viracept (Nelfinavir mesilate). Roche Products Ltd. UK Summary of product characteristics, June 2012.
22. Aarnoutse RE, Droste JAH, van Oosterhout JJG, Koopmans PP, Popescu M, Reiss P, Hekster YA, Burger DM. Pharmacokinetics, food intake requirements and tolerability of once-daily combinations of nelfinavir and low-dose ritonavir in healthy volunteers. *Br J Clin Pharmacol* (2002) 55, 115–25.
23. Kurowski M, Kaeser B, Sawyer A, Popescu M, Mroziekiewicz A, Arslan A, Staszewski S. Limited effect of food composition on the pharmacokinetics of nelfinavir administered twice daily. *Eur J Med Res* (2002) 7, 453–6.
24. Norvir Capsules (Ritonavir). Abbott Laboratories. US Prescribing information, March 2012.
25. Norvir Tablets and Solution (Ritonavir). Abbott Laboratories. US Prescribing information, October 2012.
26. Norvir Oral Solution (Ritonavir). AbbVie Ltd. UK Summary of product characteristics, September 2012.
27. Norvir Tablets (Ritonavir). AbbVie Ltd. UK Summary of product characteristics, September 2012.
28. Bertz R, Shi H, Cavanaugh J, Hsu A. Effect of three vehicles, Advera®, Ensure® and chocolate milk, on the bioavailability of an oral liquid formulation of Norvir (Ritonavir). *Intersci Conf Antimicrob Agents Chemother* (1996) 36, 5.
29. Invirase (Saquinavir mesilate). Roche Products Ltd. UK Summary of product characteristics, October 2013.
30. Invirase (Saquinavir mesylate). Genentech, Inc. US Prescribing information, February 2012.
31. Aptivus (Tipranavir). Boehringer Ingelheim Pharmaceuticals, Inc. US Prescribing information, April 2012.
32. Aptivus Soft Capsules (Tipranavir). Boehringer Ingelheim Ltd. UK Summary of product characteristics, December 2011.

HIV-protease inhibitors + Fusidic acid

In one case report, the combination of ritonavir and saquinavir with fusidic acid increased the plasma concentrations of all three drugs.

Clinical evidence, mechanism, importance and management

A 32-year-old HIV-positive man was admitted with suspected fusidic acid toxicity after taking fusidic acid 500 mg three times daily for one week, with his usual treatment of **ritonavir** 400 mg twice daily, **saquinavir** 400 mg twice daily, and stavudine 40 mg twice daily. His plasma fusidic acid concentration was found to be twice that expected, and his **ritonavir** and **saquinavir** concentrations were also elevated. He improved spontaneously, but 4 days later he returned with jaundice, nausea, and vomiting. All medications were stopped, but after 6 days his fusidic acid plasma concentration was still 30% greater than expected, his **saquinavir** plasma concentration was 16.3 micrograms/mL (reference range 1 to 4 micrograms/mL), and his **ritonavir** plasma concentration was 43.4 micrograms/mL (reference range 4 to 12 micrograms/mL). He was later able to restart his antiretrovirals without problem. It is possible that there was mutual inhibition of drug metabolism. The authors recommend avoiding this drug combination.[1] This appears to be the only published report, and further study is needed to confirm this interaction. However, bear this case in mind should a patient taking fusidic acid with antiretrovirals develop fusidic acid adverse effects.

1. Khaliq Y, Gallicano K, Leger R, Foster B, Badley A. A drug interaction between fusidic acid and a combination of ritonavir and saquinavir. *Br J Clin Pharmacol* (2000) 50, 82–3.

HIV-protease inhibitors + Garlic

A garlic supplement reduced saquinavir exposure by 50% in one study, but had little effect on saquinavir pharmacokinetics in another two studies. Another garlic supplement did not appreciably affect the pharmacokinetics of a single dose of ritonavir. There is a report of gastrointestinal toxicity with garlic and ritonavir.

Clinical evidence

(a) Ritonavir

In a study in 10 healthy subjects the use of a garlic extract (10 mg, equivalent to 1 g of fresh garlic) twice daily for 4 days decreased the AUC of a single 400-mg dose of ritonavir by 17%, but this was not statistically significant. The garlic was given in the form of capsules (*Natural Source Odourless Garlic Life Brand*).[1] Another report describes gastrointestinal toxicity in 2 patients taking garlic or garlic supplements when they started to take ritonavir-containing regimens.[2]

(b) Saquinavir

In a study in 9 healthy subjects, garlic reduced the AUC, and maximum and minimum plasma concentrations of saquinavir by about 50%. The garlic was taken in the form of a dietary supplement (*GarliPure, Maximum Allicin Formula* caplets) twice daily for 20 days. Saquinavir 1.2 g three times daily was given for 4-day periods before, during, and after the garlic supplement. Fourteen days after the garlic supplement was stopped the saquinavir pharmacokinetics had still not returned to baseline values. Of the 9 subjects, 6 had a substantial reduction in the AUC of saquinavir while taking garlic, then an increase when garlic was stopped. The remaining 3 had no change in the AUC of saquinavir while taking garlic, but had a reduction when garlic was stopped.[3] However, in another study, garlic extract (*Garlipure*) 1.2 g daily for 3 weeks had no effect on the mean AUC of a single 1.2-g dose of saquinavir (a decrease in AUC in 7 subjects and an increase in 3).[4] In yet another study in healthy subjects given a garlic extract for 21 days, the mean AUC of a single dose of saquinavir was reduced by 15%, although this was not statistically significant.[5]

Mechanism

Unknown. There is some evidence that garlic might increase the P-glycoprotein transport of saquinavir.[5]

Importance and management

Although information is limited, a reduction in saquinavir exposure of the magnitude seen in one study, when it was given with a garlic supplement, could diminish its antiviral efficacy. All garlic supplements should probably be avoided in those taking saquinavir as the sole HIV-protease inhibitor, but note that this is no longer generally recommended. The effect of garlic on saquinavir concentrations in the presence of ritonavir (as a pharmacokinetic booster) does not appear to have been studied. The apparent effect of garlic on single-dose ritonavir exposure was not clinically important, but this requires confirmation in a multiple-dose study.

1. Gallicano K, Foster B, Choudhri S. Effect of short-term administration of garlic supplements on single-dose ritonavir pharmacokinetics in healthy volunteers. *Br J Clin Pharmacol* (2003) 55, 199–202.
2. Laroche M, Choudhri S, Gallicano K, Foster B. Severe gastrointestinal toxicity with concomitant ingestion of ritonavir and garlic. *Can J Infect Dis* (1998) 9 (Suppl A), 76A.
3. Piscitelli SC, Burstein AH, Welden N, Gallicano KD, Falloon J. The effect of garlic supplements on the pharmacokinetics of saquinavir. *Clin Infect Dis* (2002) 34, 234–8.
4. Jacek H, Rentsch KM, Steinert HC, Pauli-Magnus C, Meier PJ, Fattinger K. No effect of garlic extract on saquinavir kinetics and hepatic CYP3A4 function measured by the erythromycin breath test. *Clin Pharmacol Ther* (2004) 75, P80.
5. Hajda J, Rentsch KM, Gubler C, Steinert H, Stieger B, Fattinger K. Garlic extract induces intestinal P-glycoprotein, but exhibits no effect on intestinal and hepatic CYP3A4 in humans. *Eur J Pharm Sci* (2010) 41, 729–35.

HIV-protease inhibitors + Ginkgo (*Ginkgo biloba*)

Ginkgo does not appear to affect the pharmacokinetics of ritonavir-boosted lopinavir.

Clinical evidence

In a study in 14 healthy subjects, ginkgo 120 mg twice daily for 2 weeks had no effect on the pharmacokinetics of **lopinavir** boosted with ritonavir 400/100 mg twice daily (given for 2 weeks alone before adding the ginkgo). The ginkgo extract was assayed and contained 29% flavonol glycosides and 5% terpene lactones.[1]

Mechanism

The authors suggest that without ritonavir, the concentration of lopinavir would have been reduced by ginkgo because they also found that ginkgo modestly reduced the concentrations of midazolam, probably by inducing CYP3A4. As ritonavir is an inhibitor of CYP3A4, they suggest that it attenuates the action of ginkgo on lopinavir metabolism. However, note that all HIV-protease inhibitors are inhibitors of CYP3A4, and note also that in other studies with midazolam, ginkgo had no effect on midazolam exposure, or even caused a minor increase in exposure, which suggests that ginkgo does not have a clinically relevant effect on CYP3A4 activity (see 'Benzodiazepines + Ginkgo (*Ginkgo biloba*)', p.821).

Importance and management

The study here shows that ginkgo does not alter the pharmacokinetics of lopinavir boosted with ritonavir, and no special precautions are required on concurrent use. This would be expected to apply to all other HIV-protease inhibitors boosted with ritonavir. In addition, the authors of this study recommend avoiding ginkgo with HIV-protease inhibitors that are not boosted by ritonavir,.[1] This seems an over-cautious approach, given that the sum of studies available show that ginkgo does not have a clinically relevant effect on the probe CYP3A4 substrate midazolam.

1. Robertson SM, Davey RT, Voell J, Formentini E, Alfaro RM, Penzak SR. Effect of Ginkgo biloba extract on lopinavir, midazolam and fexofenadine pharmacokinetics in healthy subjects. *Curr Med Res Opin* (2008) 24, 591–9.

HIV-protease inhibitors + Grapefruit and other fruit juices

Grapefruit juice does not alter either amprenavir or indinavir exposure, but might increase saquinavir exposure. Seville orange juice did not alter indinavir pharmacokinetics in one study.

Clinical evidence, mechanism, importance and management

(a) Amprenavir and Fosamprenavir

In a study in 12 healthy subjects, 200 mL of grapefruit juice (given on two occasions) slightly delayed the rate, but not the extent, of absorption of a single 1.2-g dose of amprenavir and reduced the maximum plasma concentration by 22%. These effects were not clinically relevant.[1] Note that fosamprenavir is metabolised to amprenavir in the gut, so these findings are also likely to apply to fosamprenavir. No particular precautions appear to be necessary with concurrent use.

(b) Indinavir

In a single-dose study in 10 healthy subjects, grapefruit juice (8 oz, about 200 mL) slightly reduced the AUC of indinavir 400 mg by 27%.[2] However, in another study in 13 healthy subjects, grapefruit juice or **Seville orange juice** (both about 200 mL) had no effect on the pharmacokinetics of indinavir. In this study indinavir 800 mg was given every 8 hours for 4 doses; with water, grapefruit juice, or **Seville orange juice** given with the last 2 doses.[3] Similarly, in 14 HIV-positive subjects, grapefruit juice (180 mL of double strength) had no effect on the steady-state pharmacokinetics of indinavir (a non-statistically significant 5% increase in AUC was seen and a slight delay occurred in the rate of absorption).[4]

(c) Saquinavir

In a study of the effects of the concurrent use of grapefruit juice 400 mL and saquinavir (*Invirase*; hard capsules) 600 mg, grapefruit juice was found to increase the AUC of saquinavir by 50%, possibly by affecting CYP3A4 in the intestine.[5] The UK manufacturer of saquinavir states that an increase of 100% was seen when double-strength grapefruit juice was used.[6] They also state that these increases are unlikely to be clinically relevant, and no saquinavir dose adjustment is necessary, although they note that saquinavir boosted with ritonavir has not been specifically studied.[6]

1. Demarles D, Gillotin C, Bonaventure-Paci S, Vincent I, Fosse S, Taburet AM. Single-dose pharmacokinetics of amprenavir coadministered with grapefruit juice. *Antimicrob Agents Chemother* (2002) 46, 1589–90.
2. McCrea J, Woolf E, Sterrett A, Matthews C, Deutsch P, Yeh KC, Waldman S, Bjornsson T. Effects of ketoconazole and other P-450 inhibitors on the pharmacokinetics of indinavir. *Pharm Res* (1996) 13 (Suppl 9), S485.
3. Penzak SR, Acosta EP, Turner M, Edwards DJ, Hon YY, Desai HD, Jann MW. Effect of Seville orange juice and grapefruit juice on indinavir pharmacokinetics. *J Clin Pharmacol* (2002) 42, 1165–70.
4. Shelton MJ, Wynn HE, Hewitt RG, DiFrancesco R. Effects of grapefruit juice on pharmacokinetic exposure to indinavir in HIV-positive subjects. *J Clin Pharmacol* (2001) 41, 435–42.
5. Kupferschmidt HHT, Fattinger KE, Ha HR, Follath F, Krähenbühl S. Grapefruit juice enhances the bioavailability of the HIV protease inhibitor saquinavir in man. *Br J Clin Pharmacol* (1998) 45, 355–9.
6. Invirase (Saquinavir mesilate). Roche Products Ltd. UK Summary of product characteristics, October 2013.

HIV-protease inhibitors + H_2-receptor antagonists

Famotidine and ranitidine decrease the exposure to atazanavir boosted with ritonavir, and ranitidine slightly decreases the exposure to unboosted fosamprenavir. Ranitidine had no effect on the exposure to darunavir or lopinavir, and would not be expected to affect the exposure to tipranavir (all boosted with ritonavir). In contrast, cimetidine and ranitidine have been shown to increase unboosted saquinavir exposure.

Clinical evidence

(a) Atazanavir

In a study in 40 healthy subjects, **famotidine** 40 mg daily, as either a single dose or in two divided doses, for 7 days decreased the AUC and maximum plasma concentration of atazanavir boosted with ritonavir 300/100 mg by 4 to 12% and decreased the minimum plasma concentration by about 20%. No apparent difference in this effect was seen when **famotidine** was taken at the same time as atazanavir or when it was taken 2 or 12 hours later. When atazanavir boosted with ritonavir was given 2 hours before the morning dose of **famotidine** 40 mg twice daily, the atazanavir AUC, maximum plasma concentration, and minimum plasma concentration were decreased by 21%, 26%, and 28% respectively.[1] The US manufacturer of atazanavir reports that, in another study in healthy subjects, the higher dose of **famotidine** 40 mg twice daily decreased the atazanavir AUC, maximum plasma concentration, and minimum plasma concentration by 18%, 14%, and 28%, respectively, when given simultaneously with atazanavir boosted with ritonavir 300/100 mg once daily.[2] When **tenofovir disoproxil fumarate** 300 mg daily was included in the regimen, the decreases were not appreciably different (21% decrease in AUC and 28% decrease in minimum plasma concentration).[2] Increasing the dose of atazanavir boosted with ritonavir to 400/100 mg daily attenuated the interaction.[2,3] When atazanavir 400 mg daily was given without ritonavir, a greater effect (41% decrease in AUC) was seen when famotidine was given simultaneously, but no effect was seen when it was taken 10 hours before or 2 hours after atazanavir.[2] In a further study in HIV-positive patients taking atazanavir boosted with ritonavir 300/100 mg daily, with or without **tenofovir disoproxil fumarate** 300 mg daily, the effect of **famotidine** 40 mg or 20 mg twice daily was similar to that seen in healthy subjects: without tenofovir and simultaneous administration of **famotidine** there was a 20% decrease in the AUC of atazanavir with the 40 mg dose, and an 11% decrease in the AUC of atazanavir with the 20 mg dose. With tenofovir, and administration of **famotidine** 2 hours before and 10 hours after atazanavir, there was a 24% decrease in the AUC of atazanavir with the 40 mg dose, and a 20% decrease in the AUC of atazanavir with the 20 mg dose. All individual minimum plasma concentrations of atazanavir remained at least 5-fold above the target concentration.[4]

In a randomised study in healthy subjects, a single 150-mg dose of **ranitidine** given one hour before breakfast decreased the atazanavir AUC, maximum plasma concentration, and minimum plasma concentration by 48%, 52%, and 43%, respectively, when atazanavir boosted with ritonavir 300/100 mg daily was taken 30 minutes after breakfast.[5]

(b) Darunavir

In a crossover study in 16 healthy subjects, **ranitidine** 150 mg twice daily had no effect on the AUC or minimum plasma concentration of darunavir after darunavir boosted with ritonavir 400/100 mg was given twice daily for 5 days.[6]

(c) Fosamprenavir

In a crossover study in healthy subjects, **ranitidine** 300 mg, given one hour before fosamprenavir 1.4 g, decreased the AUC of amprenavir by 30% and decreased its maximum plasma concentration by 51% without altering the minimum plasma concentration.[7]

(d) Indinavir

The US manufacturer of indinavir states that, in a study in 12 healthy subjects, **cimetidine** 600 mg twice daily for 6 days had no effect on the AUC of a single 400-mg dose of indinavir, and decreased its minimum plasma concentration by 18%.[8]

(e) Lopinavir

In a randomised study in healthy subjects, **ranitidine** 150 mg one hour before breakfast had no effect on the AUC of either lopinavir or ritonavir when lopinavir boosted with ritonavir 800/200 mg daily was taken 30 minutes after breakfast, or when lopinavir boosted with ritonavir 400/100 mg twice daily (30 minutes after a meal, as tablets) was given 1.5 hours after the acid-reducing drug.[5]

In a clinical study of lopinavir boosted with ritonavir given once daily (8 study patients, 86 control patients) or twice daily (7 study patients, 45 control patients) with tenofovir and emtricitabine, the minimum plasma concentration of lopinavir was assessed at 4, 8, 16, 24, and 48 weeks: patients taking acid-reducing drugs (proton pump inhibitors 67%, H_2-receptor antagonists, or antacids) were then compared with control patients not using acid-reducing drugs. There was no notable difference in the minimum plasma concentrations of lopinavir between the patients taking acid-reducing drugs and the controls, except that at 24 weeks the minimum plasma concentration of lopinavir was 50% higher, and at 48 weeks it was 73% higher, in users of acid-reducing drugs taking lopinavir boosted with ritonavir once daily. No difference was seen in the group taking lopinavir boosted with ritonavir twice daily.[9]

(f) Saquinavir

When **cimetidine** 400 mg twice daily was given with saquinavir, the AUC of saquinavir 1.2 g twice daily was 2.2-fold greater when compared with saquinavir 1.2 g three times daily alone.[10] In a study in 12 healthy subjects, the AUC of saquinavir given with food was 67% higher when it was given after two 150-mg doses of **ranitidine** given 12 hours apart, and one hour before the saquinavir.[11]

Mechanism

The UK manufacturer of indinavir states that a normal (acidic) gastric pH might be necessary for optimum absorption of indinavir.[12] Any drug that increases the gastric pH could therefore potentially decrease absorption. Altered gastric pH also accounts for the interaction with atazanavir.[2,3] Cimetidine probably boosts saquinavir exposure by inhibiting its first-pass metabolism.[10] It is not understood why ranitidine increases saquinavir exposure.

Importance and management

Atazanavir

Negligible to slight decreases in exposure to **atazanavir boosted with ritonavir** were seen with the simultaneous use of famotidine, whereas ranitidine, taken 1.5 hours before atazanavir boosted with ritonavir, and famotidine, taken with unboosted atazanavir, had a greater effect. The manufacturers state that atazanavir boosted with ritonavir 300/100 mg (with food) can be given with famotidine 20 mg twice daily, or the comparable dose of another H_2-receptor antagonist,[2,3] given either simultaneously and/or separated by 10 hours.[2] For higher doses of famotidine of up to 40 mg twice daily, recommendations differ. The US manufacturer states this dose of famotidine can be given to treatment-naive patients, with the same dose, and dose interval as the lower dose of famotidine. This dose of famotidine should not be given to treatment-experienced patients.[2] In the UK, the higher dose of atazanavir boosted with ritonavir is recommended for all patients taking higher doses of famotidine of up to 40 mg twice daily.[3]

In the presence of **tenofovir** the UK manufacturer advises that the dose of atazanavir should be increased to 400 mg daily boosted with ritonavir 100 mg daily, but this has not been fully evaluated.[3] The US manufacturer limits this advice to treatment-experienced patients, and suggests no dose alteration for treatment-naive patients.[2]

For **unboosted atazanavir**, in treatment-naive patients, the US manufacturer recommends a dose of 400 mg daily with food, which should be given 2 hours before, or 10 hours after, the H_2-receptor antagonist. The dose of famotidine (or equivalent) should not exceed 20 mg in any single dose or 40 mg in a day.[2]

Other HIV-protease inhibitors

The clinical relevance of the slight decrease in unboosted **fosamprenavir** exposure seen with ranitidine is probably minimal especially as the minimum plasma concentration was unchanged. The UK manufacturer of fosamprenavir[13] states that no fosamprenavir dose adjustment is needed on concurrent use with ranitidine or other H_2-receptor antagonists, whereas the US manufacturer[14] states that the combination should be used with caution as fosamprenavir might become less effective. The US guidelines on the treatment of HIV infection recommend that fosamprenavir should be given at least 2 hours before the H_2-receptor antagonist, and that consideration be given to boosting fosamprenavir with ritonavir.[15]

Cimetidine moderately increases unboosted **saquinavir** exposure, and further study is required to discover whether this occurs with saquinavir boosted with ritonavir. Ranitidine causes a slight increase in unboosted saquinavir exposure, but this is probably not clinically relevant.

Ranitidine does not appear to alter the pharmacokinetics of **darunavir** boosted with ritonavir or **lopinavir** boosted with ritonavir, and no interaction would be predicted with **tipranavir** boosted with ritonavir.[16] No HIV-protease inhibitor dose adjustment would be expected to be needed. Similarly, no clinically relevant interaction occurs between **indinavir** and cimetidine, and based on this result, the other H_2-receptor antagonists would not be expected to interact with indinavir.

1. Agarwala S, Persson A, Eley T, Child M, Filoramo D, Li T, Xu X, Bertz R. Effect of famotidine 20- and 40-mg dosing regimens on the bioavailability of atazanavir with ritonavir in combination with tenofovir in healthy subjects. 14th Conference on Retroviruses and Opportunistic Infections, Los Angeles, February 2007.
2. Reyataz (Atazanavir sulfate). Bristol-Myers Squibb. US Prescribing information, March 2012.
3. Reyataz (Atazanavir sulphate). Bristol-Myers Squibb Pharmaceuticals Ltd. UK Summary of product characteristics, August 2012.
4. Wang X, Boffito M, Zhang J, Chung E, Zhu L, Wu Y, Patterson K, Kashuba A, Tebas P, Child M, Mahnke L, Bertz R. Effects of the H2-receptor antagonist famotidine on the pharmacokinetics of atazanavir-ritonavir with or without tenofovir in HIV-infected patients. *AIDS Patient Care STDS* (2011) 25, 509–15.
5. Klein CE, Chiu Y-L, Cai Y, Beck K, King KR, Causemaker SJ, Doan T, Esslinger H-U, Podsadecki TJ, Hanna GJ. Effect of acid-reducing agents on the pharmacokinetics of lopinavir/ritonavir and ritonavir-boosted atazanavir. *J Clin Pharmacol* (2008) 48, 553–62.
6. Sekar VJ, Lefebvre E, De Paepe E, De Marez T, De Pauw M, Parys W, Hoetelmans RM. Pharmacokinetic interaction between darunavir boosted with ritonavir and omeprazole or ranitidine in human immunodeficiency virus-negative healthy volunteers. *Antimicrob Agents Chemother* (2007) 51, 958–61.
7. Ford SL, Wire MB, Lou Y, Baker KL, Stein DS. Effect of antacids and ranitidine on the single-dose pharmacokinetics of fosamprenavir. *Antimicrob Agents Chemother* (2005) 49, 467–9.
8. Crixivan (Indinavir sulfate). Merck & Co., Inc. US Prescribing information, April 2012.
9. Bertz RJ, Chiu Y-L, Naylor C, Luff K, Brun SC. Lack of effect of gastric acid reducing agents on lopinavir/ritonavir plasma concentrations in HIV-infected patients. 7th Int Cong Drug Therapy HIV, Glasgow, Nov 14–18 2004. P279.
10. Boffito M, Carriero P, Trentini L, Raiteri R, Bonora S, Sinicco A, Reynolds HE, Hoggard PG, Back DJ, Di Perri G. Pharmacokinetics of saquinavir co-administered with cimetidine. *J Antimicrob Chemother* (2002) 50, 1081–4.
11. Kakuda TN, Falcon RW. Effect of food and ranitidine on saquinavir pharmacokinetics and gastric pH in healthy volunteers. *Pharmacotherapy* (2006) 26, 1060–8.
12. Crixivan (Indinavir sulphate). Merck Sharp & Dohme Ltd. UK Summary of product characteristics, February 2012.
13. Telzir (Fosamprenavir calcium). ViiV Healthcare UK Ltd. UK Summary of product characteristics, May 2011.
14. Lexiva (Fosamprenavir calcium). ViiV Healthcare. US Prescribing information, April 2013.
15. Panel on Antiretroviral Guidelines for Adults and Adolescents. Guidelines for the use of antiretroviral agents in HIV-1-infected adults and adolescents. US Department of Health and Human Services (April 2015). 1–288. Available at: https://aidsinfo.nih.gov/contentfiles/lvguidelines/adultandadolescentgl.pdf (accessed 20/09/15).
16. Aptivus Soft Capsules (Tipranavir). Boehringer Ingelheim Ltd. UK Summary of product characteristics, December 2011.

HIV-protease inhibitors + HIV-protease inhibitors

Ritonavir is the most potent of the HIV-protease inhibitors at boosting concentrations of other HIV-protease inhibitors, and its use as a pharmacokinetic enhancer is established. Various other pairs of HIV-protease inhibitors have been tried to boost the concentrations of one of the HIV-protease inhibitors in the pair. Some HIV-protease inhibitor combinations can result in additive toxicity (indinavir and ritonavir or atazanavir).

Clinical evidence

A. Atazanavir

(a) Darunavir

The UK and US manufacturers of darunavir state that giving atazanavir 300 mg daily with darunavir boosted with ritonavir 400/100 mg twice daily did not alter the AUC and minimum plasma concentration of darunavir. In addition, the AUC of atazanavir was not changed, when compared with atazanavir boosted with ritonavir 300/100 mg daily alone, and the minimum plasma concentration of atazanavir was increased by 52%.[1,2]

(b) Fosamprenavir

The use of fosamprenavir boosted with ritonavir 700/100 mg twice daily with atazanavir 300 mg daily reduces the AUC and maximum plasma concentration of atazanavir by 22% and 24%, respectively, when compared with atazanavir boosted with ritonavir 300/100 mg daily.[3] Atazanavir had no effect on the pharmacokinetics of amprenavir.[3,4]

(c) Indinavir

There are no pharmacokinetic data on the use of atazanavir with indinavir, but it is predicted that there might be an additive risk of unconjugated hyperbilirubinaemia.[5,6]

(d) Ritonavir

In a study in 61 HIV-positive patients, in those given ritonavir 100 mg once daily with atazanavir 300 mg once daily, the AUC of atazanavir was about 3.5-fold higher, and the minimum plasma concentration about 8-fold higher, when compared with those receiving atazanavir 400 mg alone.[5]

(e) Saquinavir

In a study in 7 subjects, the addition of atazanavir 400 mg daily to saquinavir soft capsules 1.2 g daily increased the AUC of saquinavir about 5.5-fold, and increased its minimum plasma concentration about 7-fold.[6] In another study in 18 HIV-positive patients, atazanavir 300 mg daily increased the AUC and maximum plasma concentration of saquinavir boosted with ritonavir 1600/100 mg daily by 60% and 42%, respectively.[7,8] The AUC and maximum plasma concentration of ritonavir was also increased by 41% and 34%, respectively, with no change in atazanavir pharmacokinetics. The US manufacturer of atazanavir notes that an antiretroviral regimen including atazanavir 400 mg daily and saquinavir soft capsules 1.2 g daily, did not provide adequate efficacy and was less effective than the same regimen including either atazanavir boosted with ritonavir, or lopinavir boosted with ritonavir.[6] There does not appear to be any data on atazanavir with saquinavir boosted with ritonavir.

(f) Tipranavir

The UK and US manufacturers of tipranavir state that, in a study in healthy subjects, the concurrent use of atazanavir boosted with ritonavir 300/100 mg once daily with tipranavir boosted with ritonavir 500/100 mg twice daily increased tipranavir exposure (AUC increased by 20% and minimum plasma concentration increased by 75%) while moderately reducing atazanavir exposure (AUC reduced by 68% and minimum concentration reduced by 81%).[9,10]

B. Darunavir

(a) Indinavir

The UK and US manufacturers of darunavir note that, in a study in 9 subjects, giving indinavir 800 mg twice daily with darunavir boosted with ritonavir 400/100 mg twice daily increased the AUC and minimum plasma concentration of darunavir by 24% and 44%, respectively. In addition, the AUC and minimum plasma concentration of indinavir were increased by 23% and 125%, respectively, when compared with indinavir boosted with ritonavir 800/100 mg twice daily alone.[1,2]

(b) Lopinavir

The UK and US manufacturers of darunavir note that, in a study in 14 subjects, giving lopinavir boosted with ritonavir 400/100 mg with darunavir boosted with ritonavir 1200/100 mg, both twice daily, decreased the AUC and minimum plasma concentration of darunavir by 38% and 51%, respectively. When lopinavir boosted with ritonavir 533/133 mg was given with unboosted darunavir 1200 mg, both twice daily, the AUC and minimum plasma concentration of darunavir were decreased by 41% and 55%, respectively. The pharmacokinetics of lopinavir were unaffected in both studies.[1,2]

(c) Saquinavir

The UK and US manufacturers of darunavir state that giving saquinavir hard capsules 1 g twice daily with darunavir boosted with ritonavir 400/100 mg twice daily decreased the AUC and minimum plasma concentration of darunavir by 26% and 42%, respectively. The concentration of saquinavir was unchanged, when compared with using saquinavir boosted with ritonavir 1000/100 mg twice daily alone.[1,2]

C. Fosamprenavir

Note that fosamprenavir is a prodrug of **amprenavir**, and that amprenavir is no longer generally used.

(a) Indinavir

The UK manufacturer of indinavir reports that indinavir 1.2 g twice daily increased the AUC of amprenavir 1.2 g twice daily by 90%. The pharmacokinetics of indinavir were unaffected.[11] In another study, the steady-state AUC of amprenavir was 33% higher when amprenavir 750 or 800 mg three times daily was given with indinavir 800 mg three times daily; this was not considered to be clinically relevant. In this study, the AUC of indinavir was 38% lower than historical control data.[12] Similarly, in a model-based pharmacokinetic analysis of data from a clinical study, amprenavir intrinsic clearance was reduced by 54% by indinavir.[13] It has been suggested[12] that the effect of amprenavir on indinavir was due to the lipid-like formulation of amprenavir reducing the absorption of indinavir (analogous to food, see 'HIV-protease inhibitors + Food', p.928).

(b) Lopinavir

Preliminary data suggest that giving amprenavir 600 mg twice daily with lopinavir boosted with ritonavir 400/100 mg twice daily resulted in amprenavir minimum plasma concentrations that were lower than with amprenavir boosted with ritonavir alone at the same doses. Similarly the plasma lopinavir concentrations were lower when given with amprenavir than those without amprenavir.[14] Others have reported similar findings,[15] and increasing the dose of ritonavir did not prevent a decrease in amprenavir concentrations on the concurrent use of lopinavir boosted with ritonavir.[16] Further study showed that separation of doses reduced the effect of amprenavir on the plasma concentration of lopinavir boosted with ritonavir, but increased the effect on the amprenavir plasma concentration.[17] However, the US manufacturer of lopinavir boosted with ritonavir reports that concurrent use of lopinavir boosted with ritonavir 400/100 mg twice daily with amprenavir 750 mg twice daily for 10 days resulted in an increase in the amprenavir AUC, maximum plasma concentration, and minimum plasma concentration of 72%, 12%, and 457%, respectively, when compared with amprenavir 1200 mg twice daily alone.[18]

In a study in HIV-infected subjects given fosamprenavir 700 mg twice daily with lopinavir boosted with ritonavir 400/100 mg twice daily, the AUC of amprenavir was decreased by 64% and its minimum plasma concentration was decreased by 69%, when compared with fosamprenavir boosted with ritonavir 700/100 mg twice daily. The AUC of lopinavir was decreased by 48% when compared with lopinavir boosted ritonavir alone.[19] In a study using higher doses, giving fosamprenavir 1400 mg twice daily with lopinavir boosted with ritonavir 533/133 mg twice daily did not change the lopinavir AUC (compared with lopinavir boosted with ritonavir 400/100 mg twice daily alone) and decreased the AUC of amprenavir by 26% (when compared with fosamprenavir boosted with ritonavir, alone).[3] However, the UK manufacturer of lopinavir boosted with ritonavir notes that use of this combination in HIV-protease inhibitor-experienced patients resulted in a higher incidence of gastrointestinal adverse events and elevations in triglycerides without increases in virological efficacy, when compared with standard doses of fosamprenavir boosted with ritonavir.[20] The US manufacturer of fosamprenavir notes that giving lopinavir boosted with ritonavir 400/100 mg with fosamprenavir boosted with ritonavir 700/100 mg, both twice daily for 2 weeks, increased the AUC and minimum plasma concentration of lopinavir by 37% and 52%, respectively, whereas the AUC and minimum plasma concentration of amprenavir were decreased by 63% and 65%, respectively.[3,4] In addition, they state that the rate of adverse effects was higher with the combination.[4]

(c) Nelfinavir

The minimum plasma concentration of amprenavir 750 or 800 mg three times daily was increased by 189% by nelfinavir 750 mg three times daily, but the AUC and maximum plasma concentration of amprenavir were not notably altered. In this study, the pharmacokinetics of nelfinavir were not altered, when compared with historical control data.[12] In a model-based pharmacokinetic analysis of data from a clinical study, amprenavir intrinsic clearance was reduced by about 40% by nelfinavir.[13] The increase in the minimum plasma concentration of amprenavir could result in improved antiviral efficacy, but further study is needed.[12]

(d) Ritonavir

The AUC, minimum plasma concentration, and maximum plasma concentration of amprenavir 1.2 g twice daily were increased by 131%, 484%, and 33%, respectively, by ritonavir 200 mg twice daily.[21] When amprenavir was available, the UK and US manufacturer recommended that doses of both HIV-protease inhibitors be reduced when they are used together.[21,22] Based on modelling of pharmacokinetic data, a dose of amprenavir 600 mg with ritonavir 100 mg, both twice daily, has been suggested.[23] Ritonavir 100 mg twice daily increased the AUC of fosamprenavir 700 mg twice daily 2.4-fold and increased the minimum plasma concentration 11-fold.[24] Amprenavir concentrations with fosamprenavir boosted with ritonavir 700/100 mg twice daily were similar to those achieved with amprenavir boosted with ritonavir 600/100 mg twice daily.[25] The UK manufacturer advises that ritonavir oral solution should not be given with amprenavir oral solution to children due to the risk of toxicity from excipients in the two formulations.[26]

(e) Saquinavir

The steady-state AUC of amprenavir was reduced by 32% when amprenavir 750 or 800 mg three times daily was given with saquinavir (soft gel capsules) 800 mg three times daily, and the maximum plasma concentration was reduced by 37%. In this study, the pharmacokinetics of saquinavir were not changed when compared with historical control data.[12] In a model-based pharmacokinetic analysis of data from a clinical study, amprenavir intrinsic clearance was not altered by saquinavir.[13] It has been suggested that, as amprenavir was given with food in the first study, this might account for the reduced amprenavir exposure.[12] For further information on the effects of food, see 'HIV-protease inhibitors + Food', p.928.

When fosamprenavir 700 mg twice daily was given with saquinavir boosted with ritonavir 1000/100 mg twice daily, the saquinavir AUC was decreased by 15% and the minimum plasma concentration by 24%, although it remained above the target threshold for effective therapy.[7] The effect on amprenavir exposure was not given.

(f) Tipranavir

In a clinical study of dual-boosted HIV-protease inhibitors in multiple-treatment experienced HIV-positive adults, there was a 55% reduction in minimum plasma amprenavir concentrations when tipranavir boosted with ritonavir 500/200 mg twice daily was added to amprenavir boosted with ritonavir 600/100 mg twice daily and a 44% reduction in amprenavir AUC.[9,10]

D. Indinavir

(a) Lopinavir

In a study in 13 subjects, indinavir 600 mg twice daily for 10 days with lopinavir boosted with ritonavir 400/100 mg twice daily produced a similar indinavir AUC, a 3.5-fold higher indinavir minimum plasma concentration and 29% lower indinavir maximum plasma concentration when compared with indinavir 800 mg three times daily alone.[18,20] Based on historical comparisons, lopinavir concentrations were similar to that seen without indinavir.[20]

(b) Nelfinavir

The concurrent use of indinavir 1.2 g every 12 hours with nelfinavir 1.25 g every 12 hours produced plasma indinavir concentrations that were equivalent to the standard dose of indinavir 800 mg every 8 hours in HIV-positive subjects. This suggests that nelfinavir minimally inhibits indinavir metabolism. In this multiple-dose study, indinavir did not affect the pharmacokinetics of nelfinavir.[27] In contrast, a single 750-mg dose of nelfinavir given after indinavir 800 mg every 8 hours for 7 days to 6 subjects, resulted in an 83% increase in the AUC of nelfinavir and a 31% increase in its maximum plasma concentration. In addition, giving a single 800-mg dose of indinavir after nelfinavir 750 mg three times daily for 7 days to 6 subjects resulted in a 51% increase in the indinavir AUC, but no effect on the maximum or minimum plasma concentrations of indinavir.[28,29]

(c) Ritonavir

The effects of a range of doses of ritonavir (200, 300, or 400 mg every 12 hours) on indinavir pharmacokinetics were assessed in 39 healthy subjects. The AUC of indinavir 400 or 600 mg was increased 2- to 5-fold by ritonavir. It is suggested that the combination of indinavir 400 mg every 12 hours with ritonavir 400 mg every 12 hours will result in an AUC of indinavir roughly equivalent to that of indinavir 800 mg every 8 hours, without any effect on the pharmacokinetics of ritonavir.[30] In another similar study, when compared with historical data for indinavir 800 mg every 8 hours, the AUC of indinavir was at least 1.4-fold, 2.3-fold, and 3.3-fold higher when indinavir boosted with ritonavir was given in twice daily doses of 400/400 mg, 800/100 mg, and 800/200 mg, respectively. The regimens also produced much higher minimum plasma indinavir concentrations. The 800/100 mg regimen was the best tolerated.[31] In another study, indinavir 800 mg twice daily for 14 days increased the AUC, maximum plasma concentration, and minimum plasma concentration of ritonavir 100 mg twice daily, also taken for 14 days, by 72%, 61%, and 62%, respectively. Increasing the dose of ritonavir to 200 mg twice daily had a lesser effect on the maximum plasma concentration (increase of 19%) and had a similar effect on the AUC, increasing it by 96%. However, this produced a greater increase in the minimum plasma concentration of ritonavir, of 4.7-fold.[32]

(d) Saquinavir

In a study in 6 subjects, indinavir 800 mg three times daily for 2 days increased the AUC of single doses of saquinavir 600 mg (hard capsule), or 800 mg or 1.2 g (soft capsule), 6-fold, 7.2-fold, and 4.6-fold, respectively. Large increases in both the minimum and maximum plasma concentrations of saquinavir were also reported.[11,32] Concurrent use with saquinavir boosted with ritonavir has not been studied.[8]

E. Lopinavir

(a) Nelfinavir

The US manufacturer notes that, in a study in 13 subjects, the concurrent use of nelfinavir 1 g twice daily with lopinavir boosted with ritonavir 400/100 mg twice daily resulted in similar nelfinavir pharmacokinetics to nelfinavir 1.25 g twice daily alone, but with greatly increased concentrations of the M8 metabolite of nelfinavir. Lopinavir concentrations were modestly reduced (27% decrease in the AUC and 38% decrease in the minimum plasma concentration).[18]

(b) Ritonavir

Ritonavir is used to increase the plasma concentration of lopinavir, and the marketed lopinavir product is a co-formulation of lopinavir with ritonavir.[18,20] When an additional 100 mg of ritonavir twice daily was added to this combination, the AUC of lopinavir was increased by 46% and its minimum plasma concentration was approximately doubled.[18]

(c) Saquinavir

Saquinavir 800 mg twice daily given with lopinavir boosted with ritonavir produced a 9.6-fold increase in the AUC of saquinavir relative to saquinavir 1.2 g three times daily given alone. When compared with saquinavir boosted with ritonavir 1000/100 mg twice daily, the increase in the AUC of saquinavir was about 30%, and was similar to that reported after saquinavir boosted with ritonavir 400/400 mg twice daily alone. When saquinavir 1.2 g twice daily was given with lopinavir boosted with ritonavir, no further increase in saquinavir concentrations was noted. Lopinavir concentrations did not appear to be affected by saquinavir, based on historical comparison with lopinavir boosted with ritonavir alone.[20]

(d) Tipranavir

In a clinical study of dual-boosted HIV-protease inhibitors in multiple-treatment experienced HIV-positive adults there was a 70% reduction in the minimum plasma concentrations of lopinavir and a 55% reduction in the AUC of lopinavir when tipranavir boosted with ritonavir 500/200 mg twice daily was added to lopinavir boosted with ritonavir 400/100 mg twice daily.[9,10]

F. Nelfinavir

(a) Ritonavir

Single-dose data indicate that ritonavir increases the AUC of nelfinavir 1.8- to 2.5-fold, whereas the AUC of ritonavir is unchanged.[33] In a multiple-dose study in healthy subjects, ritonavir 100 or 200 mg twice daily increased the steady-state AUC of nelfinavir 1.25 g twice daily by 20% and 39%, after morning and evening doses, respectively. The AUC of the M8 metabolite of nelfinavir was increased by 74% and 86%, respectively. There was no difference in the effect of the two doses of ritonavir on the AUC of nelfinavir.[34]

(b) Saquinavir

A single 1.2-g dose of saquinavir (soft gel capsules), given after 3 days of nelfinavir 750 mg every 8 hours, had no effect on the pharmacokinetics of nelfinavir, but nelfinavir caused a 4-fold increase in the AUC of saquinavir.[35] Similar 2- to 12-fold increases in the AUC of saquinavir have been found in other studies in HIV-positive subjects.[36-39] A study in which 157 patients received 12 weeks of saquinavir with nelfinavir (doses unstated) found that concurrent use was well tolerated.[40] When nelfinavir 1250 mg twice daily was given with saquinavir boosted with ritonavir 1000/100 mg twice daily, there were negligible changes in the AUCs of saquinavir and nelfinavir (increased by 13% and decreased by 6%, respectively).[7]

G. Ritonavir

A study in 6 patients with advanced HIV infection found that while taking **saquinavir** 600 mg three times daily the addition of ritonavir 300 mg twice daily increased the saquinavir maximum plasma concentration 33-fold, and increased its AUC 58-fold at steady state.[41] A pilot study in HIV-positive patients given both drugs together (saquinavir 800 mg daily, ritonavir 400 to 600 mg daily) found that the ritonavir plasma concentrations were unaffected. However, the saquinavir plasma concentrations were substantially higher than those achieved with saquinavir alone in daily doses of 3.6 to 7.2 g.[42] A study in 57 healthy subjects covering a range of ritonavir and saquinavir *(Invirase)* doses (200 to 600 mg) found that saquinavir did not affect ritonavir pharmacokinetics, but ritonavir increased the AUC of saquinavir 50- to 132-fold. The authors suggested that giving both drugs in a dose of 400 mg every 12 hours might be optimal.[43] Subsequent study has revealed that the effect of ritonavir on saquinavir is not related to the ritonavir dose in the range of 100 to 400 mg twice daily,[44-46] and that the use of a combination with a higher dose of saquinavir and a lower dose of ritonavir might be preferable, as the lower doses of ritonavir are associated with fewer adverse effects.[46] The UK and US manufacturers of ritonavir note that higher doses of ritonavir have been associated with an increased incidence of adverse events, including a significant increase in total triglycerides and cholesterol.[24,47] The concurrent use of saquinavir and ritonavir has led to severe adverse events, mainly diabetic ketoacidosis and liver disorders, especially in patients with pre-existing liver disease.[24]

H. Saquinavir

In a clinical study of dual-boosted HIV-protease inhibitors in multiple-treatment experienced HIV-positive adults there was an 82% reduction in minimum plasma concentration of saquinavir and a 76% reduction in its AUC when **tipranavir** boosted with ritonavir 500/200 mg twice daily was added to saquinavir boosted with ritonavir 600/100 mg twice daily.[9,10]

Mechanism

HIV-protease inhibitors are inhibitors and substrates of CYP3A4, with ritonavir being the most potent inhibitor and saquinavir one of the least, although still potent. In general, they interact by inhibiting each other's gut (pre-absorption) and hepatic (post-absorption) metabolism, resulting in increased absorption and decreased elimination.[43,48] Inhibition of P-glycoprotein might also be involved.[48] However, some HIV-protease inhibitor combinations, in particular tipranavir boosted with ritonavir given with other HIV-protease inhibitors, can decrease the exposure to other HIV-protease inhibitors.

Importance and management

A pharmacokinetic interaction between ritonavir and amprenavir (and its prodrug fosamprenavir), atazanavir, darunavir, indinavir, lopinavir, nelfinavir, tipranavir, and particularly saquinavir is established and clinically important, such that low-dose (less than antiretroviral dose) ritonavir is used in combination with most HIV-protease inhibitors (with the exception of indinavir and nelfinavir) to boost their minimum plasma concentrations and prolong their half-lives. The increase in minimum plasma concentration reduces the chance of developing drug resistance (as a result of suboptimal concentrations) and the longer half-life allows for less frequent dosing, which improves patient compliance.[49] Note that the US manufacturer of **indinavir** states that the appropriate doses for concurrent use with ritonavir have not been established,[32] while the UK manufacturer recommends indinavir boosted with ritonavir 400/100 mg twice daily.[11] Caution is needed when indinavir is used at a dose of 800 mg twice daily with ritonavir 100 mg twice daily, because of the possibility of an increased risk of nephrolithiasis.[24,32] Furthermore, the UK manufacturer of **nelfinavir** notes that as it is metabolised predominantly by CYP2C19 and only partially by CYP3A4, its plasma concentrations are not greatly increased by the concurrent use of ritonavir, and therefore nelfinavir does not require boosting with low-dose ritonavir.[28] In contrast, the US manufacturer advises that the appropriate dose of nelfinavir with ritonavir is not established.[29]

HIV-protease inhibitors boosted with ritonavir (usually in a dose of 100 mg) are a major component of antiretroviral regimens in the US and UK guidelines for the treatment of HIV.[49,50]

Dual therapy with HIV-protease inhibitors for treatment-naive patients is not recommended in the US or UK treatment guidelines,[49,50] and as can be seen from the data in *Clinical evidence*, above, various combinations act to lower the concentrations of one of the HIV-protease inhibitors and should therefore be avoided. However, complicated scenarios of virological failure and/or treatment resistance in treatment-experienced patients mean that if all conventional avenues of alternative regimens have been exhausted, combinations of HIV-protease inhibitors might be considered, but should only be used under expert supervision. In these circumstances current local and national guidelines should be consulted for alternative treatment regimens.

1. Prezista (Darunavir ethanolate). Janssen-Cilag Ltd. UK Summary of product characteristics, June 2012.
2. Prezista (Darunavir ethanolate). Janssen Pharmaceuticals, Inc. US Prescribing information, May 2012.
3. Telzir (Fosamprenavir calcium). ViiV Healthcare UK Ltd. UK Summary of product characteristics, May 2011.
4. Lexiva (Fosamprenavir calcium). ViiV Healthcare. US Prescribing information, April 2013.
5. Reyataz (Atazanavir sulfate). Bristol-Myers Squibb Pharmaceuticals Ltd. UK Summary of product characteristics, August 2012.
6. Reyataz (Atazanavir sulfate). Bristol-Myers Squibb. US Prescribing information, March 2012.
7. Invirase Hard Capsules (Saquinavir mesilate). Roche Products Ltd. UK Summary of product characteristics, June 2012.
8. Invirase (Saquinavir mesylate). Genentech, Inc. US Prescribing information, February 2012.
9. Aptivus (Tipranavir). Boehringer Ingelheim Pharmaceuticals, Inc. US Prescribing information, April 2012.
10. Aptivus Soft Capsules (Tipranavir). Boehringer Ingelheim Ltd. UK Summary of product characteristics, December 2011.
11. Crixivan (Indinavir sulphate). Merck Sharp & Dohme Ltd. UK Summary of product characteristics, February 2012.
12. Sadler BM, Gillotin C, Lou Y, Eron JJ, Lang W, Haubrich R, Stein DS. Pharmacokinetic study of human immunodeficiency virus protease inhibitors used in combination with amprenavir. *Antimicrob Agents Chemother* (2001) 45, 3663–8.
13. Pfister M, Labbé L, Lu J-F, Hammer SM, Mellors J, Bennett KK, Rosenkranz S, Sheiner LB, and the AIDS Clinical Trial Group Protocol 398 Investigators. Effect of coadministration of nelfinavir, indinavir, and saquinavir on the pharmacokinetics of amprenavir. *Clin Pharmacol Ther* (2002) 72, 133–41.
14. Mauss S, Schmutz G, Kuschak D. Unfavourable interaction of amprenavir and lopinavir in combination with ritonavir? *AIDS* (2002) 16, 296–7.
15. Khanlou H, Graham E, Brill M, Farthing C. Drug interaction between amprenavir and lopinavir/ritonavir in salvage therapy. *AIDS* (2002) 16, 797–8.
16. Mauss S, Scholten S, Wolf E, Berger F, Schmutz G, Jaeger H, Kurowski M, Rockstroh JK; Klinische Arbeitsgruppe AIDS Deutschland, Germany. A prospective, controlled study assessing the effect of lopinavir on amprenavir concentrations boosted by ritonavir. *HIV Med* (2004) 5, 15–17.
17. Corbett AH, Patterson KB, Tien H-C, Kalvass LA, Eron JJ, Ngo LT, Lim ML, Kashuba ADM. Dose separation does not overcome the pharmacokinetic interaction between fosamprenavir and lopinavir/ritonavir. *Antimicrob Agents Chemother* (2006) 50, 2756–61.
18. Kaletra (Lopinavir with Ritonavir). Abbott Laboratories. US Prescribing information, April 2012.

19. Kashuba ADM, Tierney C, Downey GF, Acosta EP, Vergis EN, Klingman K, Mellors JW, Eshleman SH, Scott TR, Collier AC. Combining fosamprenavir with lopinavir/ritonavir substantially reduces amprenavir and lopinavir exposure: ACTG protocol A5143 results. *AIDS* (2005) 19, 145–52.
20. Kaletra Tablets (Lopinavir with Ritonavir). AbbVie Ltd. UK Summary of product characteristics, August 2012.
21. Agenerase (Amprenavir). GlaxoSmithKline UK. UK Summary of product characteristics, February 2007.
22. Agenerase (Amprenavir). GlaxoSmithKline. US Prescribing information, May 2005.
23. Sale M, Sadler BM, Stein DS. Pharmacokinetic modeling and simulations of interaction of amprenavir and ritonavir. *Antimicrob Agents Chemother* (2002) 46, 746–54.
24. Norvir Tablets (Ritonavir). AbbVie Ltd. UK Summary of product characteristics, September 2012.
25. Wire MB, Baker KL, Jones LS, Shelton MJ, Lou Y, Thomas GJ, Berrey MM. Ritonavir increases plasma amprenavir (APV) exposure to a similar extent when coadministered with either fosamprenavir or APV. *Antimicrob Agents Chemother* (2006) 50, 1578–80.
26. Norvir Oral Solution (Ritonavir). AbbVie Ltd. UK Summary of product characteristics, September 2012.
27. Riddler SA, Havlir D, Squires KE, Kerr B, Lewis RH, Yeh K, Hawe Wynne L, Zhong L, Peng Y, Deutsch P, Saah A. Coadministration of indinavir and nelfinavir in human immunodeficiency virus type 1-infected adults: safety, pharmacokinetics, and antiretroviral activity. *Antimicrob Agents Chemother* (2002) 46, 3877–82.
28. Viracept (Nelfinavir mesilate). Roche Products Ltd. UK Summary of product characteristics, June 2012.
29. Viracept (Nelfinavir mesylate). Agouron Pharmaceuticals, Inc. US Prescribing information, May 2013.
30. Hsu A, Granneman GR, Cao G, Carothers L, Japour A, El-Shourbagy T, Dennis S, Berg J, Erdman K, Leonard JM, Sun E. Pharmacokinetic interaction between ritonavir and indinavir in healthy volunteers. *Antimicrob Agents Chemother* (1998) 42, 2784–91.
31. Saah AJ, Winchell GA, Nessly ML, Seniuk MA, Rhodes RR, Deutsch PJ. Pharmacokinetic profile and tolerability of indinavir-ritonavir combinations in healthy volunteers. *Antimicrob Agents Chemother* (2001) 45, 2710–15.
32. Crixivan (Indinavir sulfate). Merck & Co., Inc. US Prescribing information, April 2012.
33. Washington CB, Flexner C, Sheiner LB, Rosenkranz SL, Segal Y, Aberg JA, Blaschke TF, AIDS Clinical Trials Group Protocol (ACTG 378) study team. Effect of simultaneous versus staggered dosing on pharmacokinetic interactions of protease inhibitors. *Clin Pharmacol Ther* (2003) 73, 406–16.
34. Kurowski M, Kaeser B, Sawyer A, Popescu M, Mrozikiewicz A. Low-dose ritonavir moderately enhances nelfinavir exposure. *Clin Pharmacol Ther* (2002) 72, 123–32.
35. Kerr B, Yuep G, Daniels R, Quart B, Kravcik S, Sahai J, Anderson R. Strategic approach to nelfinavir mesylate (NFV) drug interactions involving CYP3A metabolism. 6th European Conference on Clinical Aspects and Treatment of HIV-infection, Hamburg, Germany, 1997.
36. Merry C, Ryan M, Mulchay F, Halifax K, Barry M, Back D. The effect of nelfinavir on plasma saquinavir levels. 6th European Conference on Clinical Aspects and Treatment of HIV-infection, Hamburg, Germany, 1997. Abstract 455.
37. Merry C, Barry MG, Mulcahy FM, Back DJ. Saquinavir pharmacokinetics alone and in combination with nelfinavir in HIV infected patients. 5th Conference on Retroviruses and Opportunistic Infections, Chicago, 1998. Abstract 352.
38. Gallicano K, Sahai J, Kravcik S, Seguin I, Bristow N, Cameron DW. Nelfinavir (NFV) increases plasma exposure of saquinavir in hard gel capsule (SQV-HGC) in HIV+ patients. 5th Conference on Retroviruses and Opportunistic Infections, Chicago, 1998. Abstract 353.
39. Hoetelmans RMW, Reijers MHE, Wit FW, ten Kate RW, Weige HM, Frissen PHJ, Bruisten SM, Beijnen JH, Lange JMA. Saquinavir (SQV) pharmacokinetics in combination with nelfinavir (NFV) in the ADAM study. 6th European Conference on Clinical Aspects and Treatment of HIV-infection, Hamburg, Germany, 1997. Abstract 255.
40. Posniak A and the SPICE study team. Study of protease inhibitors in combination in Europe (SPICE). 6th European Conference on Clinical Aspects and Treatment of HIV-infection, Hamburg, Germany, 1997. Abstract 209.
41. Merry C, Barry MG, Mulcahy F, Ryan M, Heavey J, Tjia JF, Gibbons SE, Breckenridge AM, Back DJ. Saquinavir pharmacokinetics alone and in combination with ritonavir in HIV-infected patients. *AIDS* (1997) 11, F29–F33.
42. Cameron DW, Hsu A, Granneman GR, Sun E, McMahon D, Farthing C, Poretz D, Markowitz M, Cohen C, Follansbee S, Mellors J, Ho D, Xu Y, Rode R, Salgo M, Leonard J. Pharmacokinetics of ritonavir-saquinavir combination therapy. *AIDS* (1996) 10 (Suppl 2), S16.
43. Hsu A, Granneman GR, Cao G, Carothers L, El-Shourbagy T, Baroldi P, Erdman K, Brown F, Sun E, Leonard JM. Pharmacokinetic interactions between two human immunodeficiency virus protease inhibitors, ritonavir and saquinavir. *Clin Pharmacol Ther* (1998) 63, 453–64.
44. Kilby JM, Hill A, Buss N. The effect of ritonavir on saquinavir plasma concentration is independent of ritonavir dosage: combined analysis of pharmacokinetic data from 97 subjects. *HIV Med* (2002) 3, 97–104.
45. Kurowski M, Arslan A, Moecklinghoff C, Sawyer W, Hill A. Effects of ritonavir on saquinavir plasma concentration: analysis of 271 patients in routine clinical practice (P261A). *AIDS* (2000) 14 (Suppl 4), 591.
46. Buss N, Snell P, Bock J, Hsu A, Jorga K. Saquinavir and ritonavir pharmacokinetics following combined ritonavir and saquinavir (soft gelatin capsules) administration. *Br J Clin Pharmacol* (2001) 52, 255–64.
47. Norvir Capsules (Ritonavir). Abbott Laboratories. US Prescribing information, March 2012.
48. Lu J-F, Blaschke TF, Flexner C, Rosenkranz SL, Sheiner LB, and AIDS Clinical Trials Group protocol 378 investigators. Model-based analysis of the pharmacokinetic interactions between ritonavir, nelfinavir, and saquinavir after simultaneous and staggered oral administration. *Drug Metab Dispos* (2002) 30, 1455–61.
49. Panel on Antiretroviral Guidelines for Adults and Adolescents. Guidelines for the use of antiretroviral agents in HIV-1-infected adults and adolescents. US Department of Health and Human Services (April 2015). 1–288. Available at: https://aidsinfo.nih.gov/contentfiles/lvguidelines/adultandadolescentgl.pdf (accessed 22/09/15).
50. Williams I, Churchill D, Anderson J, Boffito M, Bower M, Cairns G, Cwynarski K, Edwards S, Fidler S, Fisher M, Freedman A, Geretti AM, Gilleece Y, Horne R, Johnson M, Khoo S, Leen C, Marshall N, Nelson M, Orkin C, Paton N, Phillips A, Post F, Pozniak A, Sabin C, Trevelion R, Ustianowski A, Walsh J, Waters L, Wilkins E, Winston A, Youle M. British HIV Association guidelines for the treatment of HIV-1-positive adults with antiretroviral therapy 2012 (Updated 2013). *HIV Med* (2014), 15 (Suppl 1) 1–85. Also available at: http://www.bhiva.org/documents/Guidelines/Treatment/2012/hiv1029_2.pdf (accessed 22/09/15).

HIV-protease inhibitors + Lamotrigine

Atazanavir and lopinavir, both boosted with ritonavir, appear to reduce lamotrigine plasma concentrations, whereas the HIV-protease inhibitor concentrations do not appear to be altered. Atazanavir alone does not appear to have any effect on the pharmacokinetics of lamotrigine. An increased dose of lamotrigine was required in a patient who was also taking saquinavir boosted with ritonavir.

Clinical evidence

(a) Atazanavir

In a study, 17 healthy subjects were given a single 100-mg dose of lamotrigine alone, after 6 days of atazanavir 400 mg daily, and after 10 days of atazanavir boosted with ritonavir 300/100 mg daily. Atazanavir alone had no effect on the pharmacokinetics of lamotrigine, apart from a negligible 12% decrease in its AUC. However, atazanavir boosted with ritonavir slightly reduced the AUC of lamotrigine by 32%. Formation of lamotrigine-2N-glucuronide, a metabolite of lamotrigine, was also increased by atazanavir boosted with ritonavir.[1]

(b) Lopinavir

In a study in 18 healthy subjects taking lamotrigine 100 mg twice daily, lopinavir boosted with ritonavir 400/100 mg twice daily for 10 days decreased the steady-state minimum plasma concentration of lamotrigine by 55%, decreased the AUC of lamotrigine by 46%, and increased its clearance by 85%. Doubling the dose of lamotrigine to 200 mg twice daily increased the AUC to a value similar to that seen with the lower dose without lopinavir boosted with ritonavir. Pharmacokinetic parameters for lopinavir and ritonavir were similar to those in historical controls.[2] The authors of a review describe a patient taking lamotrigine 25 mg twice daily who had a favourable decline in viral load 2 months after starting to take lopinavir boosted with ritonavir, lamivudine, and stavudine. There was no toxicity and no recurrence of seizures.[3]

(c) Saquinavir

A 30-year-old woman taking nevirapine, saquinavir 1.2 g daily, and ritonavir 600 mg daily with an undetectable viral load had her epilepsy medication changed from gabapentin and lorazepam to lamotrigine and phenytoin because of an increased frequency and severity of seizures. The lamotrigine dose was eventually increased to 1.8 g daily to achieve serum concentrations of 5 to 8 mg/L. The ritonavir dose was doubled and the saquinavir dose increased to 2 g daily to compensate for the enzyme-inducing effects of phenytoin. The patient's viral load remained undetectable, and her seizures decreased over the next 6 months, but she died suddenly of unexplained causes following a tonic-clonic seizure (autopsy not performed).[4]

Mechanism

Lamotrigine is a substrate for glucuronidation via UGT1A4. Ritonavir decreases lamotrigine concentrations by induction of glucuronidation, although an effect of lopinavir cannot be ruled out.[2] Atazanavir alone is known to inhibit glucuronidation by UGT1A1, but the data here with lamotrigine suggest that it does not inhibit UGT1A4.

Importance and management

The pharmacokinetic interaction between lamotrigine and ritonavir would appear to be established; however, as the relationship between lamotrigine concentration and efficacy is not clear, the clinical relevance of the slight decrease in concentrations is uncertain.[2] Lamotrigine efficacy should be monitored in patients taking ritonavir or any ritonavir-boosted antiretroviral regimen. Anticipate the need to increase the lamotrigine dose.

1. Burger DM, Huisman A, Van Ewijk N, Neisingh H, Van Uden P, Rongen GA, Koopmans P, Bertz RJ. The effect of atazanavir and atazanavir/ritonavir on UDP-glucuronosyltransferase using lamotrigine as a phenotypic probe. *Clin Pharmacol Ther* (2008) 84, 698–703.
2. van der Lee MJ, Dawood L, ter Hofstede HJM, de Graaff-Teulen MJA, van Ewijk-Beneken Kolmer EWJ, Caliskan-Yassen N, Koopmans PP, Burger DM. Lopinavir/ritonavir reduces lamotrigine plasma concentrations in healthy subjects. *Clin Pharmacol Ther* (2006) 80, 159–68.
3. Liedtke MD, Lockhart SM, Rathbun RC. Anticonvulsant and antiretroviral interactions. *Ann Pharmacother* (2004) 38, 482–9.
4. Leppik IE, Gapany S, Walczak T. An HIV-positive patient with epilepsy. *Epilepsy Behav* (2003) 4 (Suppl 1), S17–S19.

HIV-protease inhibitors + Macrolides

Nelfinavir approximately doubles the exposure to azithromycin. Single doses of azithromycin have no effect on the exposure to indinavir and nelfinavir.

Most HIV-protease inhibitors increase clarithromycin exposure and reduce the exposure to the active 14-hydroxyclarithromycin metabolite, with the possible exception of unboosted amprenavir. Clarithromycin has no effect on the pharmacokinetics of amprenavir, darunavir boosted with ritonavir, indinavir, or ritonavir, but it slightly increases the exposure to atazanavir and tipranavir boosted with ritonavir, and might moderately increase the exposure to saquinavir (from soft capsules). Erythromycin can also increase saquinavir exposure from soft capsules. HIV-protease inhibitors are predicted to increase telithromycin exposure. The concurrent use of some HIV-protease inhibitors and some macrolides might lead to QT prolongation.

Clinical evidence

(a) Azithromycin

1. Indinavir. A single 1.2-g dose of azithromycin had no effect on the pharmacokinetics of indinavir in healthy subjects who had taken indinavir 800 mg three times daily for 5 days. The pharmacokinetics of azithromycin were not assessed.[1]

2. Nelfinavir. A single 1.2-g dose of azithromycin was given to 12 healthy subjects who had taken nelfinavir 750 mg every 8 hours for 8 days. The pharmacokinetics of nelfinavir were minimally affected, but the AUC and maximum serum concentration of azithromycin were approximately doubled.[2]

(b) Clarithromycin

1. Amprenavir. In a study in 12 healthy adults, amprenavir 1.2 g twice daily was given with clarithromycin 500 mg twice daily, for 4 days. The AUC and maximum serum concentration of amprenavir were increased, by 18% and 15%, respectively, whereas the pharmacokinetics of clarithromycin were not altered.[3]

2. *Atazanavir.* The concurrent use of atazanavir 400 mg daily and clarithromycin 500 mg twice daily for 4 days increased the AUC of clarithromycin by 94%, and reduced the AUC of the active metabolite, 14-hydroxyclarithromycin, by 70%. In addition, there was a slight 28% increase in the AUC of atazanavir.[4]

3. *Darunavir.* In a study, 17 healthy subjects were given darunavir boosted with ritonavir 400/100 mg twice daily, clarithromycin 500 mg twice daily, or both drugs together, all for 13 doses. Clarithromycin had little effect on the pharmacokinetics of darunavir: the maximum plasma concentration and AUC of darunavir were reduced by 17% and 13%, respectively, and the minimum plasma concentration was unchanged. However, the AUC, maximum plasma concentration, and minimum plasma concentration of clarithromycin were increased by 57%, 26%, and 174%, respectively. The active metabolite, 14-hydroxyclarithromycin, was not detectable.[5]

4. *Indinavir.* In 11 healthy subjects clarithromycin 500 mg every 12 hours, given with indinavir 800 mg every 8 hours, caused no clinically important alterations in the pharmacokinetics of indinavir: the only statistically significant change was a 52% increase in the minimum plasma concentration. The AUC of clarithromycin was increased by about 50%, and the AUC of 14-hydroxyclarithromycin was reduced by about 50%.[6]

5. *Lopinavir.* A case of rhabdomyolysis has been reported in an HIV-positive patient taking clarithromycin, lopinavir boosted with ritonavir, and atorvastatin, see 'Statins + Macrolides', p.1348.

6. *Ritonavir.* When ritonavir 200 mg every 8 hours was given with clarithromycin 500 mg every 12 hours there were only negligible changes in ritonavir pharmacokinetics (13% increase in AUC and 15% increase in the maximum plasma concentration). However, the AUC of clarithromycin increased by 77% with an almost total inhibition of 14-hydroxyclarithromycin formation (99.7% decrease in AUC).[7]

7. *Saquinavir.* In a study in healthy subjects the concurrent use of saquinavir soft capsules *(Fortovase)* [no longer available] 1.2 g three times daily and clarithromycin 500 mg twice daily increased the AUC and maximum serum concentration of saquinavir by 177% and 187%, respectively. The AUC and maximum serum concentration of clarithromycin were about 40% higher than when it was given alone.[8,9] The UK and US manufacturers state that there are no data on the interaction using hard capsules or tablets (*Invirase*) of saquinavir boosted with ritonavir.[8,9]

8. *Tipranavir.* In a study in 21 healthy subjects, clarithromycin 500 mg twice daily was taken for 13 days with tipranavir boosted with ritonavir 500/200 mg twice daily from day 6 to 13. Tipranavir boosted with ritonavir increased the minimum plasma concentration of clarithromycin by 68%, although the AUC and maximum plasma concentration were minimally affected. The AUC_{0-12} and maximum plasma concentration of the 14-hydroxy metabolite of clarithromycin were also reduced by 97%, and its minimum plasma concentration was reduced by 95%. No increase in adverse effects was reported, although one subject taking tipranavir boosted with ritonavir and clarithromycin had a significant grade 3 increase in ALT. Clarithromycin increased the AUC, and maximum and minimum plasma concentrations of tipranavir by 66%, 40%, and 100%, respectively.[10]

(c) Erythromycin

The concurrent use of **saquinavir** soft capsules (*Fortovase*) [no longer available] 1.2 g three times daily and erythromycin 250 mg four times daily doubled the AUC and maximum serum concentration of saquinavir in HIV-infected subjects.[11] The UK and US manufacturers state that there are no data on the interaction using hard capsules or tablets (*Invirase*) of **saquinavir** boosted with ritonavir.[8,9]

Mechanism

Ritonavir is a potent inhibitor of CYP3A4 and consequently markedly to very markedly inhibits the 14-hydroxylation of clarithromycin by this isoenzyme. Other HIV-protease inhibitors would be expected to interact similarly, although to a lesser extent. Clarithromycin is a potent inhibitor of CYP3A4, but as its effects are less profound than those of ritonavir it generally has only a small effect on the HIV-protease inhibitors, except for saquinavir. The effect of clarithromycin on saquinavir, and nelfinavir on azithromycin might involve inhibition of P-glycoprotein.[2,3]

Importance and management

Azithromycin

The increase in azithromycin exposure with **nelfinavir** is likely to be of clinical significance,[2] and, although the outcome is presumed to be positive, this has yet to be assessed in practice. If concurrent use is necessary, monitor for azithromycin adverse effects (such as hepatic adverse effects, hearing impairment).[12] The effect of other HIV-protease inhibitors on azithromycin pharmacokinetics does not appear to have been assessed, however the UK and US manufacturers of **lopinavir** boosted with ritonavir do not expect a clinically significant interaction with azithromycin.[13,14]

Clarithromycin

The majority of HIV-protease inhibitors studied inhibit the metabolism of clarithromycin. Although the increases in clarithromycin exposure seen (40 to 94%) are of themselves generally not clinically relevant, the concern is that when the hepatic metabolism of clarithromycin is so strongly inhibited (as demonstrated by almost undetectable concentrations of the 14-hydroxy metabolite), clarithromycin becomes more dependent on renal clearance; therefore, the interaction might be clinically important in patients with renal failure.[7]

For **ritonavir**, the UK and US manufacturers of ritonavir and clarithromycin suggest that no dose reductions should be required in those with normal renal function, but they recommend a 50% reduction in the dose of clarithromycin for those with a creatinine clearance of 30 to 60 mL/minute and a 75% reduction for those with a creatinine clearance of less than 30 mL/minute.[15-18] Some advise avoiding clarithromycin in doses exceeding 1 g daily.[15,16] Similar clarithromycin dose reductions in renal impairment are recommended by some manufacturers of **darunavir** boosted with ritonavir,[19] **lopinavir** boosted with ritonavir[14] (but see also *QT prolongation*, below), **saquinavir** boosted with ritonavir[9] (but see also *QT prolongation*, below), and **tipranavir** boosted with ritonavir.[20,21] The UK manufacturer of **tipranavir** also advises that patients taking a dose of clarithromycin of more than 500 mg twice daily should be monitored for clarithromycin adverse effects. They also note that the low concentrations of 14-hydroxyclarithromycin, due to the interaction with tipranavir boosted with ritonavir, might be of clinical relevance in the treatment of *Haemophilus influenzae*.[21] Although there are no formal studies or specific dose recommendations for other HIV-protease inhibitors (**fosamprenavir** and **indinavir**) boosted with ritonavir, similar clarithromycin dose reductions would seem prudent.

Atazanavir also reduces the conversion of clarithromycin to its 14-hydroxy metabolite, and it is usually given with ritonavir although there are no data for the combination with ritonavir. The US manufacturer of atazanavir[22] suggests that if the combination is used, the clarithromycin dose should be reduced by 50% as clarithromycin might prolong the QT interval (see *QT prolongation*, below). As the concentration of 14-hydroxyclarithromycin are also greatly reduced, they advise that for most infections an alternative to clarithromycin should be considered with the exception of *Mycobacterium avium* complex infections[22] where this metabolite is less active. However, the UK manufacturer of atazanavir states that reducing the dose of clarithromycin to avoid a high concentration of the parent drug might result in a subtherapeutic concentration of the 14-hydroxy metabolite,[23] [which is active against e.g. *Haemophilus influenzae*] and therefore they state that no recommendations about dose reductions can be made.[23] The UK manufacturer of clarithromycin states that no dose reductions are required in those with normal renal function, but they recommend a 50% reduction in the dose of clarithromycin for those with a creatinine clearance of 30 to 60 mL/minute and a 75% reduction for those with a creatinine clearance of less than 30 mL/minute.[16] They also advise avoiding clarithromycin in doses exceeding 1 g daily.

Indinavir slightly increases the AUC of clarithromycin and moderately decreased the AUC of its metabolite, which was not thought to be clinically relevant.[6]

Erythromycin

Despite the increases in **saquinavir** concentration seen, the UK manufacturer[8] states that no dose adjustment is needed when unboosted saquinavir is given with erythromycin. However, they contraindicate the use of saquinavir boosted with ritonavir with erythromycin due to the predicted risk of QT prolongation (see also *QT prolongation*, below). The UK manufacturer of **ritonavir** suggests that because erythromycin concentrations might increase due to inhibition of its metabolism by ritonavir, care should be taken if both drugs are given.[15] On this basis, it would seem prudent to monitor for erythromycin adverse effects with any HIV-protease inhibitor boosted with ritonavir. Similar warnings about the concurrent use of erythromycin have been issued by the UK manufacturers of **fosamprenavir**[24] and **indinavir**.[25] However, the US manufacturer of atazanavir does not expect a clinically significant interaction with erythromycin.[22] For the possible risk of QT prolongation when using erythromycin and lopinavir boosted with ritonavir, see *QT prolongation*, below.

QT prolongation

Note that **clarithromycin** and **erythromycin** have rarely been associated with QT prolongation, and increases in their plasma concentration might increase this risk. However, it seems unlikely that the slight increases seen in clarithromycin exposure with the HIV-protease inhibitors will increase this risk. Nevertheless, some of the HIV-protease inhibitors are also associated with QT prolongation, particularly saquinavir boosted with ritonavir. The UK manufacturer[8] (but not the US manufacturer[9]) contraindicates the use of clarithromycin or erythromycin with saquinavir boosted with ritonavir because of the potential risk of arrhythmia associated with QT prolongation. The UK manufacturer lopinavir boosted with ritonavir states that both erythromycin and clarithromycin can prolong the QT interval and that cardiac adverse effects have also been reported with lopinavir boosted with ritonavir. As lopinavir boosted with ritonavir can also increase the concentration of these macrolides, they advise caution with concurrent use.[13] The UK manufacturer of **telithromycin** predicts that the HIV-protease inhibitors will increase its plasma concentration and, as telithromycin has been reported to cause QT prolongation, they advise caution on concurrent use, and contraindicate concurrent use in patients with severe renal or hepatic impairment.[26] **Azithromycin** has also been associated with an increased risk of QT interval prolongation. For further information about the risks of QT prolongation, see 'Drugs that prolong the QT interval + Other drugs that prolong the QT interval', p.272.

1. Foulds G, LaBoy-Goral L, Wei GCG, Apseloff G. The effect of azithromycin on the pharmacokinetics of indinavir. *J Clin Pharmacol* (1999) 39, 842–6.
2. Amsden GW, Nafziger AN, Foulds G, Cabelus LJ. A study of the pharmacokinetics of azithromycin and nelfinavir when coadministered in healthy volunteers. *J Clin Pharmacol* (2000) 40, 1522–7.
3. Brophy DF, Israel DS, Pastor A, Gillotin C, Chittick GE, Symonds WT, Lou Y, Sadler BM, Polk RE. Pharmacokinetic interaction between amprenavir and clarithromycin in healthy male volunteers. *Antimicrob Agents Chemother* (2000) 44, 978–84.
4. Mummaneni V, Randall D, Chabuel D, Geraldes M, O'Mara E. Steady-state pharmacokinetic interaction study of atazanavir with clarithromycin in healthy subjects. *Intersci Conf Antimicrob Agents Chemother* (2002) 42, 275.
5. Sekar VJ, Spinosa-Guzman S, De Paepe E, De Pauw M, Vangeneugden T, Lefebvre E, Hoetelmans RMW. Darunavir/ritonavir pharmacokinetics following coadministration with clarithromycin in healthy volunteers. *J Clin Pharmacol* (2008) 48, 60–5.
6. Boruchoff SE, Sturgill MG, Grasing KW, Seibold JR, McCrea J, Winchell GA, Kusma SE, Deutsch PJ. The steady-state disposition of indinavir is not altered by the concomitant administration of clarithromycin. *Clin Pharmacol Ther* (2000) 67, 351–9.
7. Ouellet D, Hsu A, Granneman GR, Carlson G, Cavanaugh J, Guenther H, Leonard JM. Pharmacokinetic interaction between ritonavir and clarithromycin. *Clin Pharmacol Ther* (1998) 64, 355–62.
8. Invirase (Saquinavir mesilate). Roche Products Ltd. UK Summary of product characteristics, October 2013.

9. Invirase (Saquinavir mesylate). Genentech, Inc. US Prescribing information, February 2012.
10. La Porte C, Sabo JP, Elgadi M, Cameron DW. Interaction studies of tipranavir/ritonavir (TPV/r) with clarithromycin, fluconazole, and rifabutin in healthy volunteers. *Antimicrob Agents Chemother* (2009) 53, 162–73.
11. Grub S, Bryson H, Goggin T, Lüdin E, Jorga K. The interaction of saquinavir (soft gelatin capsule) with ketoconazole, erythromycin and rifampicin: comparison of the effect in healthy volunteers and in HIV-infected patients. *Eur J Clin Pharmacol* (2001) 57, 115–21.
12. Viracept (Nelfinavir mesylate). Agouron Pharmaceuticals, Inc. US Prescribing information, May 2013.
13. Kaletra Tablets (Lopinavir with Ritonavir). AbbVie Ltd. UK Summary of product characteristics, August 2012.
14. Kaletra (Lopinavir with Ritonavir). Abbott Laboratories. US Prescribing information, April 2012.
15. Norvir Tablets (Ritonavir). AbbVie Ltd. UK Summary of product characteristics, September 2012.
16. Klaricid (Clarithromycin). Abbott Healthcare Products Ltd. UK Summary of product characteristics, July 2013.
17. Norvir Capsules (Ritonavir). Abbott Laboratories. US Prescribing information, March 2012.
18. Biaxin (Clarithromycin). Abbott Laboratories. US Prescribing information, July 2012.
19. Prezista (Darunavir ethanolate). Janssen Pharmaceuticals, Inc. US Prescribing information, May 2012.
20. Aptivus (Tipranavir). Boehringer Ingelheim Pharmaceuticals, Inc. US Prescribing information, April 2012.
21. Aptivus Soft Capsules (Tipranavir). Boehringer Ingelheim Ltd. UK Summary of product characteristics, December 2011.
22. Reyataz (Atazanavir sulfate). Bristol-Myers Squibb. US Prescribing information, March 2012.
23. Reyataz (Atazanavir sulfate). Bristol-Myers Squibb Pharmaceuticals Ltd. UK Summary of product characteristics, August 2012.
24. Telzir (Fosamprenavir calcium). ViiV Healthcare UK Ltd. UK Summary of product characteristics, May 2011.
25. Crixivan (Indinavir sulphate). Merck Sharp & Dohme Ltd. UK Summary of product characteristics, February 2012.
26. Ketek (Telithromycin). Sanofi. UK Summary of product characteristics, November 2012.

HIV-protease inhibitors + Mefloquine

Data from two patients show no apparent pharmacokinetic interaction between mefloquine and indinavir or nelfinavir. Ritonavir does not alter mefloquine pharmacokinetics, but mefloquine slightly decreases steady-state ritonavir exposure.

Clinical evidence

Two HIV-positive patients receiving HAART (one taking **indinavir** 800 mg three times daily, the other taking **nelfinavir** 1.25 g twice daily) were given mefloquine 250 mg weekly for malaria prophylaxis. Mefloquine therapeutic plasma concentrations were achieved, and its half-life was similar to that found in healthy subjects. In addition, no consistent changes in the plasma concentrations of the HIV-protease inhibitors were found.[1]

In 12 healthy subjects **ritonavir** 200 mg twice daily for one week had no effect on the pharmacokinetics of mefloquine.[2] Conversely, mefloquine (250 mg daily for 3 days, then 250 mg weekly) reduced the steady-state AUC, maximum plasma concentration, and minimum plasma concentration of **ritonavir** 200 mg twice daily by 31%, 36%, and 43%, respectively, but had no effect on the pharmacokinetics of single-dose **ritonavir**.[2]

Mechanism

Despite being inhibitors of CYP3A4, the HIV-protease inhibitors do not appear to alter mefloquine pharmacokinetics.[1,2] It has been suggested that the decrease in ritonavir exposure was due to decreased absorption, perhaps due to mefloquine-induced inhibition of bile acid production or induction of P-glycoprotein.[2]

Importance and management

The limited evidence suggests that HIV-protease inhibitors do not affect mefloquine pharmacokinetics. The data on the effect of mefloquine on ritonavir suggest that it might slightly decrease ritonavir exposure. Until further evidence is available, if concurrent use is necessary, it would seem prudent to closely monitor the ritonavir plasma concentration, if possible, and to monitor for ritonavir efficacy.

1. Schippers EF, Hugen PWH, den Hartigh J, Burger DM, Hoetelmans RMW, Visser LG, Kroon FP. No drug-drug interaction between nelfinavir or indinavir and mefloquine in HIV-1 infected patients. *AIDS* (2000) 14, 2794–5.
2. Khaliq Y, Gallicano K, Tisdale C, Carignan G, Cooper C, McCarthy A. Pharmacokinetic interaction between mefloquine and ritonavir in healthy volunteers. *Br J Clin Pharmacol* (2001) 51, 591–600.

HIV-protease inhibitors + Minocycline

Minocycline, given with atazanavir boosted with ritonavir, appears to reduce atazanavir exposure but does not appear to affect ritonavir exposure.

Clinical evidence, mechanism, importance and management

In a study, 12 HIV-positive subjects who had been taking **atazanavir** boosted with ritonavir 300/100 mg daily for at least 4 weeks as part of a HAART regimen were given minocycline 100 mg twice daily for 14 days. Minocycline reduced the AUC, maximum plasma concentration, and minimum plasma concentration of **atazanavir** by 33%, 25%, and 50%, respectively. The addition of valproic acid 250 mg twice daily for a further 14 days did not change the outcome of the interaction. Minocycline had no statistically significant effect on the pharmacokinetics of **ritonavir** in the subset of 9 subjects analysed (10% and 5% reduction in the AUC and maximum plasma concentration respectively, with a 23% increase in the minimum plasma concentration).[1]

The possible mechanism and clinical relevance of this interaction are unclear. Note that this was a small study and patients were allowed to continue their regular medication during the study, which might have influenced the outcome. However, the possibility of a clinically relevant interaction cannot be excluded. The authors suggest that further study is needed to establish the pharmacokinetic interaction, as well as its likely treatment outcomes. They also advise that although no interaction was seen with **ritonavir**, an interaction cannot be excluded due to the small sample size.[1]

1. DiCenzo R, Peterson DR, Cruttenden K, Mariuz P, Rezk NL, Hochreiter J, Gelbard H, Schifitto G. Effects of minocycline and valproic acid coadministration on atazanavir plasma concentrations in human immunodeficiency virus-infected adults receiving atazanavir-ritonavir. *Antimicrob Agents Chemother* (2008) 52, 3035–9.

HIV-protease inhibitors + Phenytoin

Nelfinavir, and fosamprenavir and lopinavir (both boosted with ritonavir) slightly reduce phenytoin exposure. In one case report, ritonavir appeared to increase phenytoin concentrations, and in two others phenytoin concentrations were decreased or unaltered when ritonavir and saquinavir were given concurrently compared with indinavir alone.

Phenytoin decreased the concentrations of lopinavir boosted with ritonavir, but minimally increased the concentrations of amprenavir (given as fosamprenavir boosted with ritonavir). There are two case reports of reduced antiviral effect when phenytoin was used with indinavir or saquinavir with ritonavir. Phenytoin is predicted to reduce the concentrations of atazanavir, darunavir, saquinavir, and tipranavir.

Clinical evidence

(a) Fosamprenavir

In a randomised, crossover study, healthy subjects were given fosamprenavir boosted with ritonavir 700/100 mg daily with phenytoin 300 mg daily for 10 days. The AUC and maximum plasma concentration of amprenavir were increased by 20% and 7%, respectively, and the AUC and maximum plasma concentration of phenytoin were decreased by 22% and 20%, respectively.[1]

(b) Indinavir

A 39-year-old HIV-positive man, taking phenytoin 300 mg daily, started to take indinavir 800 mg three times daily. When the phenytoin dose was reduced to 200 mg daily, the viral load dropped by almost half and his CD4+ count doubled.[2] For two case reports where phenytoin concentrations were unchanged or decreased when switching from indinavir to ritonavir with saquinavir, see *Saquinavir with Ritonavir*, below.

(c) Lopinavir

In studies in healthy subjects, the concurrent use of phenytoin 300 mg daily and lopinavir boosted with ritonavir 400/100 mg twice daily resulted in a 30% decrease in the AUC of lopinavir and a 23% decrease in the AUC of phenytoin.[3]

(d) Nelfinavir

An HIV-positive man taking phenytoin and phenobarbital for epilepsy had been taking nelfinavir 750 mg three times daily and stavudine 30 mg twice daily for nearly 3 months when he had a tonic-clonic seizure. After starting nelfinavir and stavudine, the phenytoin serum concentration was found to have decreased from around 10 mg/L to around 5 mg/L.[4] Similarly, in healthy subjects, nelfinavir 1.25 g twice daily for 7 days decreased the AUC of phenytoin by about 30% and the maximum serum concentration by 21%.[5]

(e) Ritonavir

A case report describes the intentional use of ritonavir 600 mg twice daily to boost phenytoin concentrations in a 14-year-old boy who had been having seizures for 28 days, despite the use of several antiepileptics. Phenytoin at 20 mg/kg daily had originally failed to produce satisfactory plasma concentrations, although it did reduce the rate of seizures. After starting ritonavir his seizures were controlled and the phenytoin concentration became therapeutic. Seizures started again after the ritonavir was stopped.[6]

(f) Saquinavir with Ritonavir

An HIV-positive patient taking carbamazepine and phenytoin had little change in his phenytoin concentrations, which remained at around 15 mg/L, 2 months after switching from an antiretroviral regimen including indinavir to one containing ritonavir 600 mg twice daily and saquinavir.[7] Another patient taking phenobarbital, phenytoin and carbamazepine had a 33% reduction in his phenytoin concentration 2 days after switching from an antiretroviral regimen including indinavir to one containing ritonavir 300 mg twice daily and saquinavir. The concentration of carbamazepine had doubled, and the concentration of phenobarbital was unchanged.[8]

A 30-year-old woman taking nevirapine, saquinavir 1.2 g daily, and ritonavir 600 mg daily with undetectable viral load, had her epilepsy medication changed from gabapentin and lorazepam to lamotrigine and phenytoin because of an increase in the frequency and severity of seizures. She required phenytoin 8 mg/kg daily to maintain therapeutic serum concentrations. The ritonavir dose was doubled and the saquinavir dose increased to 2 g daily to compensate for the enzyme-inducing effects of phenytoin. The patient's viral load remained undetectable, and her seizures decreased over the next 6 months but she died suddenly of unexplained causes following a tonic-clonic seizure (autopsy not performed).[9]

Mechanism

Phenytoin is an inducer of CYP3A4, and would be predicted to increase the metabolism of the HIV-protease inhibitors, but this has only been shown for lopinavir boosted with ritonavir. Nelfinavir concentrations were not altered, and amprenavir concentrations (from fosamprenavir boosted with ritonavir) were minimally increased.

Phenytoin is principally metabolised by CYP2C9 and CYP2C19, and would therefore, not be expected to be substantially affected by most HIV-protease inhibitors. However, some HIV-protease inhibitors boosted with ritonavir are known to be inducers of CYP2C19, an enzyme which shows polymorphism (meaning that different patients have different activity with regard to this isoenzyme), which would explain the slight decreases in phenytoin exposure in the controlled studies with lopinavir and fosamprenavir (both boosted with ritonavir). A slight decrease in phenytoin exposure was also seen with nelfinavir.

Importance and management

Effect on HIV-protease inhibitors

Information on the effect of phenytoin on the HIV-protease inhibitors is limited, and not all the interactions from controlled studies result in the effects that would be predicted. From the controlled study with **lopinavir** boosted with ritonavir, phenytoin did slightly decrease lopinavir exposure, as would be expected. The UK and US manufacturers of lopinavir boosted with ritonavir recommend caution on concurrent use and advise that a dose increase of lopinavir boosted with ritonavir might be needed. They state that the once daily regimen of lopinavir boosted with ritonavir should not be used with phenytoin.[10,11] In contrast, phenytoin caused a small *increase* in the concentrations of amprenavir (given as **fosamprenavir** boosted with ritonavir). No dose adjustment of fosamprenavir boosted with ritonavir is likely to be needed with phenytoin. However, the US manufacturer of fosamprenavir states that decreased amprenavir concentrations might occur if it is given unboosted with phenytoin.[12]

There appears to be no other data on the effect of phenytoin on other HIV-protease inhibitors apart from two case reports of apparent reduced antiviral effect when phenytoin was used with indinavir or saquinavir with ritonavir. Nevertheless, the manufacturers of **indinavir**,[13,14] **saquinavir**,[15,16] **ritonavir** (UK),[17] and **tipranavir**[18,19] predict that their concentrations might be reduced by phenytoin, and advise caution on concurrent use. Similarly, the UK manufacturer of **darunavir** predicts that phenytoin might decrease darunavir concentrations and advises against concurrent use;[20] however, the US manufacturer states that darunavir concentrations are not affected by phenytoin.[21] The UK and US manufacturers of **atazanavir** also predict that its concentrations might be reduced by inducers of CYP3A4 [not named],[22,23] and the UK manufacturer specifically advises against the concurrent use of **atazanavir** boosted with ritonavir with drugs that induce CYP3A4 [not named].[22] If phenytoin is required with any of these HIV-protease inhibitors, close monitoring of antiviral efficacy (and antiviral concentrations if possible) would seem prudent.

Effect on phenytoin

Nelfinavir, and fosamprenavir and lopinavir (both boosted with ritonavir) slightly decrease phenytoin exposure, and other HIV-protease inhibitors boosted with ritonavir would be predicted to interact similarly. If phenytoin is required in a patient taking any HIV-protease inhibitor, close monitoring of phenytoin concentrations is essential, with phenytoin dose adjustment as necessary.

1. GlaxoSmithKline. A phase I, randomized, open label, four arm, two period, two 2X2, crossover, drug interaction study to assess steady-state plasma amprenavir and phenytoin pharmacokinetics following administraction (sic) of fosamprenavir 700 mg BID + ritonavir 100 mg BID + phenytoin 300 mg QD, fosamprenavir 700 mg BID + ritonavir 1-mg BID, phenytoin 300 mg QD in healthy adult subjects. Study No: 107484. Available at http://gsk-clinicalstudyregister.com/ (accessed 22/10/15).
2. Campagna KD, Torbert A, Bedsole GD, Ravis WR. Possible induction of indinavir metabolism by phenytoin. *Pharmacotherapy* (1997) 17, 182.
3. Lim ML, Min SS, Eron JJ, Bertz RJ, Robinson M, Gaedigk A, Kashuba ADM. Coadministration of lopinavir/ritonavir and phenytoin results in two-way drug interaction through cytochrome P-450 induction. *J Acquir Immune Defic Syndr* (2004) 36, 1034–40.
4. Honda M, Yasuoka A, Aoki M, Oka S. A generalized seizure following initiation of nelfinavir in a patient with human immunodeficiency virus type 1 infection, suspected due to interaction between nelfinavir and phenytoin. *Intern Med* (1999) 38, 302–3.
5. Shelton MJ, Cloen D, Becker M, Hsyu PH, Wilton JH, Hewitt RG. Evaluation of the pharmacokinetic interaction between phenytoin and nelfinavir in healthy volunteers at steady state. *Intersci Conf Antimicrob Agents Chemother* (2000) 40, 426.
6. Broderick A, Webb DW, McMenamin J, Butler K. A novel use of ritonavir. *AIDS* (1998) 12 (Suppl 4), S29.
7. Berbel Garcia A, Latorre Ibarra A, Porta Etessam J, Martinez Salio A, Perez Martinez DA, Saiz Diaz R, Toledo Heras M. Protease inhibitor-induced carbamazepine toxicity. *Clin Neuropharmacol* (2000) 23, 216–18.
8. Mateu-de Antonio J, Grau S, Gimeno-Bayón J-L, Carmona A. Ritonavir-induced carbamazepine toxicity. *Ann Pharmacother* (2001) 35, 125–6.
9. Leppik IE, Gapany S, Walczak T. An HIV-positive patient with epilepsy. *Epilepsy Behav* (2003) 4 (Suppl 1), S17–S19.
10. Kaletra Tablets (Lopinavir with Ritonavir). AbbVie Ltd. UK Summary of product characteristics, August 2012.
11. Kaletra (Lopinavir with Ritonavir). Abbott Laboratories. US Prescribing information, April 2012.
12. Lexiva (Fosamprenavir calcium). ViiV Healthcare. US Prescribing information, April 2013.
13. Crixivan (Indinavir sulphate). Merck Sharp & Dohme Ltd. UK Summary of product characteristics, February 2012.
14. Crixivan (Indinavir sulfate). Merck & Co., Inc. US Prescribing information, April 2012.
15. Invirase (Saquinavir mesilate). Roche Products Ltd. UK Summary of product characteristics, October 2013.
16. Invirase (Saquinavir mesylate). Genentech, Inc. US Prescribing information, February 2012.
17. Norvir Tablets (Ritonavir). AbbVie Ltd. UK Summary of product characteristics, September 2012.
18. Aptivus Soft Capsules (Tipranavir). Boehringer Ingelheim Ltd. UK Summary of product characteristics, December 2011.
19. Aptivus (Tipranavir). Boehringer Ingelheim Pharmaceuticals, Inc. US Prescribing information, April 2012.
20. Prezista (Darunavir ethanolate). Janssen-Cilag Ltd. UK Summary of product characteristics, June 2012.
21. Prezista (Darunavir ethanolate). Janssen Pharmaceuticals, Inc. US Prescribing information, May 2012.
22. Reyataz (Atazanavir sulfate). Bristol-Myers Squibb Pharmaceuticals Ltd. UK Summary of product characteristics, August 2012.
23. Reyataz (Atazanavir sulfate). Bristol-Myers Squibb. US Prescribing information, March 2012.

HIV-protease inhibitors + Proton pump inhibitors

Proton pump inhibitors reduce atazanavir exposure given alone or boosted with ritonavir. Omeprazole decreases indinavir exposure. Omeprazole had no effect on the concentrations of darunavir, lopinavir, or tipranavir (all boosted with ritonavir), and esomeprazole had little effect on fosamprenavir in one study. In contrast, omeprazole has been shown to increase saquinavir concentrations. Darunavir, lopinavir, and tipranavir (all boosted with ritonavir) reduce omeprazole exposure, whereas fosamprenavir boosted with ritonavir has no effect on esomeprazole exposure, and fosamprenavir alone increases esomeprazole exposure.

Clinical evidence

(a) Atazanavir

In a study in 19 healthy subjects, the addition of **omeprazole** 20 mg daily for 7 days reduced the AUC and minimum plasma concentration of atazanavir boosted with ritonavir 300/100 mg daily by 27%, and reduced its maximum plasma concentration by 33%. A large degree of interindividual variability was reported and, in 4 subjects, the reduction in the AUC and minimum plasma concentration was greater than 50%.[1] In another study, atazanavir exposure was reduced by 42% and the minimum plasma concentration was reduced by 46% when **omeprazole** 20 mg daily was given with atazanavir boosted with ritonavir 300/100 mg daily; the reduction did not differ whether the **omeprazole** was given one hour before, or 12 hours after, the HIV-protease inhibitors.[2] In this study, when the atazanavir dose was increased to 400 mg daily (boosted with ritonavir 100 mg daily), and given with **omeprazole** 20 mg daily, the atazanavir exposure and minimum plasma concentration were about 30% lower than when the recommended dose of atazanavir boosted with ritonavir (300/100 mg daily) was given without **omeprazole**.[2]

A greater reduction in exposure to atazanavir boosted with ritonavir was seen in another study in healthy subjects given **omeprazole** 40 mg daily for 10 days; the AUC and minimum plasma concentration of atazanavir were reduced by 76% and 79%, respectively. In this study, giving the HIV-protease inhibitors with cola (to reduce the gastric pH and thereby improve absorption), or increasing the atazanavir dose by 100 mg daily, only modestly improved these values.[3] Similar reductions were found in another study in healthy subjects,[4] and an even greater effect (a very marked 94% reduction in AUC) was seen when atazanavir 400 mg alone was given with omeprazole 40 mg;[5] the same effect was seen with **lansoprazole** 60 mg.[6] However, in one study, ritonavir concentrations were not affected by **omeprazole**.[4]

Atazanavir minimum concentrations were 58% lower in patients taking a proton pump inhibitor than in those taking an H_2-receptor antagonist in another study.[7] A 65-year-old HIV-positive man taking atazanavir boosted with ritonavir had a reduction in the minimum plasma concentration of atazanavir and its AUC in a 12-hour study while taking **esomeprazole**.[8] However, in a retrospective analysis of concurrent use, 9 of 12 patients had a successful virological outcome while taking atazanavir with or without ritonavir together with a proton pump inhibitor (**esomeprazole**, **lansoprazole**, **omeprazole**, **pantoprazole**, **rabeprazole**).[9] Another retrospective analysis also found no difference in virological outcome in 10 patients taking atazanavir boosted with ritonavir with a proton pump inhibitor (**rabeprazole**, **omeprazole**) and 66 patients not taking a proton pump inhibitor.[10] In a retrospective review, 10 patients were found to be taking atazanavir with a proton pump inhibitor (**esomeprazole**, **lansoprazole**, **omeprazole**, or **pantoprazole**). Only 2 patients did not maintain adequate viral suppression. Omeprazole was stopped in one of these patients; however, this did not result in an improvement in viral load.[11] Another study in HIV-positive patients reported that the concurrent use of **omeprazole** 20 mg or 40 mg daily or **rabeprazole** 20 mg daily had no apparent effect on the pharmacokinetics of atazanavir boosted with ritonavir.[12] Similarly, in one patient taking atazanavir boosted with ritonavir 300/100 mg daily, tenofovir, lamivudine, and **lansoprazole** 30 mg twice daily, the AUC, maximum plasma concentration, and minimum plasma concentration of atazanavir were higher than those seen historically with atazanavir boosted with ritonavir and tenofovir.[13] Another 2 patients maintained virological suppression when **omeprazole** 20 mg to 40 mg daily was taken with atazanavir 150 mg twice daily or 300 mg daily, both boosted with ritonavir.[14,15] However, there is a case of virological rebound in a patient taking atazanavir boosted with ritonavir and **omeprazole** for 10 weeks.[16]

(b) Darunavir

In a crossover study in 16 healthy subjects, **omeprazole** 20 mg daily and had no effect on the AUC or minimum plasma concentration of darunavir after darunavir with ritonavir 400/100 mg was given twice daily for 5 days.[17]

In a pharmacokinetic probe study, darunavir boosted with ritonavir 600/100 mg twice daily for 7 days reduced the AUC of a single 40-mg dose of **omeprazole** given on day 7 by 42%. The ratio of omeprazole to 5-hydroxy-omeprazole decreased by 31%.[18]

(c) Fosamprenavir

In studies in healthy subjects, **esomeprazole** 20 mg daily had no effect on the steady-state pharmacokinetics of amprenavir after either fosamprenavir 1.4 g twice daily or fosamprenavir boosted with ritonavir 700/100 mg twice daily was given. However, unboosted fosamprenavir 1.4 g twice daily increased the AUC of **esomeprazole** by 55%, whereas fosamprenavir boosted with ritonavir had no effect on the AUC of esomeprazole. In this study, the daily dose of **esomeprazole** was given simultaneously with the first dose of the HIV-protease inhibitor.[19] Another study in healthy subjects given fosamprenavir boosted with ritonavir 1400/100 mg once daily for 7 days found that **omeprazole** 20 mg in the evening had no effect on the pharmacokinetics of amprenavir.[1] Similarly, no pharmacokinetic interaction was apparent in an 8-hour study in a 65-year-old HIV-positive patient who was given fosamprenavir boosted with ritonavir and **esomeprazole**.[8]

(d) Indinavir

In a randomised, controlled study in 14 healthy subjects, **omeprazole** 20 mg daily and **omeprazole** 40 mg daily for 7 days reduced the AUC of a single 800-mg dose of indinavir by 34% and 47%, respectively. However, the addition of ritonavir 200 mg to indinavir negated the effect of **omeprazole** 40 mg daily, increasing the AUC of indinavir by 55% when compared with indinavir alone.[20] In the preliminary results of an earlier study in 8 healthy subjects given **omeprazole** 40 mg daily for 14 days with a single 800-mg dose of indinavir on day 14, there was a negligible 9.5% decrease in the AUC of indinavir. However, half of the subjects had a 25% or greater decrease in the AUC of indinavir, one had a greater than 25% increase, and the others had no change in AUC.[21] In a review by the same authors, 4 of 9 patients taking **omeprazole** with indinavir had lower plasma concentrations of indinavir than expected. In 2 patients, increasing the indinavir dose from 800 mg to 1 g, three times daily, resulted in acceptable plasma concentrations.[22]

(e) Lopinavir

In a randomised study in healthy subjects, **omeprazole** 40 mg daily one hour before breakfast had no effect on the AUC of either lopinavir or ritonavir when lopinavir boosted with ritonavir 800/200 mg daily was taken 30 minutes after breakfast. **Omeprazole** 40 mg daily also had no effect on the AUC of either lopinavir or ritonavir when lopinavir boosted with ritonavir 400/100 mg twice daily was taken 30 minutes after a meal (as tablets) and 1.5 hours after the acid-reducing drug.[4] In another study in patients taking antiretroviral therapy that included lopinavir boosted with ritonavir, the addition of **omeprazole** 40 mg daily increased the AUCs of lopinavir and ritonavir by 23% and 27%, respectively.[23] For mention of a study in which gastric-acid reducing drugs including proton pump inhibitors had no effect on minimum lopinavir concentrations, see 'HIV-protease inhibitors + H_2-receptor antagonists', p.930.

In a pharmacokinetic study in 13 healthy subjects who were CYP2C19 extensive metabolisers, lopinavir boosted with ritonavir 400/100 mg twice daily for 14 days increased the metabolism of **omeprazole** to 5-hydroxy-omeprazole 2-fold when a single 40-mg dose of omeprazole was given on day 14. Unexpectedly, there was also an increase in metabolism of omeprazole in a further subject who was a CYP2C19 poor metaboliser.[24]

(f) Nelfinavir

In a pharmacokinetic study, 19 healthy subjects were given **omeprazole** 40 mg daily for 4 days with 1.25 g nelfinavir twice daily for 7 doses. **Omeprazole** reduced the AUC and maximum plasma concentration of nelfinavir by almost 40%, although in 3 patients the AUC of nelfinavir was actually *increased* by **omeprazole**. The pharmacokinetics of the active metabolite of nelfinavir, M8, were also affected, with a reduction in AUC and maximum plasma concentration of 92% and 89%, respectively. Four subjects had undetectable nelfinavir metabolite concentrations.[25]

In a retrospective cohort study in 1 147 patients taking unboosted nelfinavir, 141 of whom also received proton pump inhibitors (not specified), the use of a proton pump inhibitor had no effect on the time taken to achieve an undetectable HIV viral load. However, the use of a proton pump inhibitor was associated with a 1.51-fold increased risk of virological rebound, which was only apparent in the long-term exposure group (greater than 30 days of proton pump inhibitor use).[26]

(g) Saquinavir

In a study in 18 healthy subjects, **omeprazole** 40 mg daily increased the AUC of saquinavir by 82% when saquinavir boosted with ritonavir 1000/100 mg was given twice daily.[27] In another study in 12 HIV-positive patients taking saquinavir boosted with ritonavir 1000/100 mg twice daily, **omeprazole** 40 mg taken for one week at the same time as saquinavir, increased the AUC, maximum plasma concentration, and minimum plasma concentration of saquinavir by 54%, 55%, and 73%, respectively. Taking **omeprazole** 2 hours before saquinavir boosted with ritonavir resulted in slightly larger increases of 67%, 65%, and 97%, in the AUC, maximum plasma concentration, and minimum plasma concentration of saquinavir, respectively. The pharmacokinetics of ritonavir were not affected by **omeprazole**. Increases in saquinavir bioavailability did not result in an increase in adverse effects.[28]

(h) Tipranavir

In a study in 15 healthy subjects, **omeprazole** 40 mg daily for 5 days had no effect on tipranavir exposure after a single dose of tipranavir boosted with ritonavir 500/200 mg.[29]

In a study in 23 healthy subjects, tipranavir boosted with ritonavir 500/200 mg twice daily at steady state decreased the AUC and maximum plasma concentration of a single dose of **omeprazole** by 70% and 68%, respectively. In contrast, a single dose of tipranavir boosted with ritonavir slightly increased the AUC of omeprazole by 57%.[30]

Mechanism

The UK manufacturer of indinavir states that a normal (acidic) gastric pH might be necessary for optimum absorption of indinavir.[31] Any drug that increases the gastric pH could therefore potentially reduce absorption. Altered gastric pH also accounts for the interaction with atazanavir,[5,32] and possibly nelfinavir.[25] In addition, omeprazole might inhibit the metabolism of nelfinavir to its active M8 metabolite by CYP2C19.[25] Note that nelfinavir is the only HIV-protease inhibitor to be metabolised by CYP2C19, and not all proton pump inhibitors are inhibitors of CYP2C19 (see 'Table 1.6', p.8). It is not understood why omeprazole increases saquinavir exposure.

Tipranavir boosted with ritonavir moderately induces CYP2C19 at steady-state, reducing omeprazole exposure (omeprazole metabolism to 5-hydroxy-omeprazole occurs via CYP2C19). Lopinavir boosted with ritonavir appears to act similarly, and darunavir boosted with ritonavir weakly induces CYP2C19 at steady-state. A single dose of tipranavir boosted with ritonavir weakly inhibits omeprazole metabolism: this occurs before the enzyme inducing effects become apparent. Note that CYP2C19 shows genetic polymorphism, which means that different patients have different activity with respect to this isoenzyme. In CYP2C19 poor metabolisers (those lacking or deficient in CYP2C19 activity), no increase in omeprazole metabolism would be expected, although in one poor metaboliser an unexpected increase was seen.[24] Nevertheless, in these individuals, the inhibitory effect of ritonavir on CYP3A4 (usually a minor route of omeprazole metabolism) might predominate at steady-state.

Importance and management

Atazanavir

The dose-related pharmacokinetic interaction of omeprazole leading to reduced atazanavir exposure (greater without ritonavir) by reducing absorption is established; lansoprazole appears to act similarly. Increasing the dose of atazanavir by 25% to 400 mg daily, with the standard dose of ritonavir of 100 mg daily, and limiting the dose of omeprazole to 20 mg daily attenuated, but did not avoid, the pharmacokinetic interaction. Based on the available data, unboosted atazanavir should not be given, and atazanavir boosted with ritonavir should generally not be given, with omeprazole or other proton pump inhibitors,[5,32] and the US manufacturer of atazanavir states that proton pump inhibitors should be avoided in treatment-experienced patients.[5] If concurrent use is unavoidable, the UK manufacturer[32] advises that the dose of atazanavir should be increased to 400 mg daily boosted with ritonavir 100 mg daily, whereas the US manufacturer permits the standard dose of atazanavir boosted with ritonavir (300/100 mg daily).[5] Both the UK and US manufacturers of atazanavir advise that a maximum daily dose of 20 mg of omeprazole (or the equivalent of other proton pump inhibitors) should be used with atazanavir boosted with ritonavir.[5,32] The US manufacturers limit this advice to treatment-naive patients, and advise that the dose of the proton pump inhibitor should be taken 12 hours before atazanavir.[5] Note that the effect of atazanavir boosted with ritonavir on omeprazole exposure does not appear to have been studied.

Indinavir

The pharmacokinetic interaction between omeprazole and indinavir resulting in reduced indinavir concentrations would appear to be established. Omeprazole should probably not be used with indinavir unless ritonavir is used to boost the indinavir concentrations.[20] This would be likely apply to other proton pump inhibitors used with indinavir as well.

Nelfinavir

The reduction in the concentrations of nelfinavir and its active metabolite might lead to loss of virological activity, and therefore the UK manufacturer contraindicates its concurrent use with omeprazole [a CYP2C19 inhibitor] and recommends caution if other proton pump inhibitors are used with nelfinavir.[33] The UK manufacturer of esomeprazole [the *S*-isomer of omeprazole and also a CYP2C19 inhibitor] similarly contraindicates concurrent use with nelfinavir.[34] The authors of one paper suggest that short-term (less than 30 day) use of proton pump inhibitors with nelfinavir might be acceptable.[26]

Saquinavir

In contrast to atazanavir, indinavir, and nelfinavir, omeprazole increased the exposure to saquinavir boosted with ritonavir. Although the clinical relevance of this has not been assessed, saquinavir boosted with ritonavir is known to be associated with dose-related QT prolongation. The UK manufacturer states that omeprazole and other proton pump inhibitors should not be used concurrently with saquinavir.[35] Conversely, the US manufacturer of saquinavir advises caution on concurrent use and recommends monitoring for potential saquinavir toxicity, particularly gastrointestinal symptoms, increased triglycerides, deep vein thrombosis, and QT prolongation.[36] Separating the dose of omeprazole from saquinavir does not appear to minimise the interaction. The effect of saquinavir boosted with ritonavir on omeprazole exposure does not appear to have been studied.

Other HIV-protease inhibitors

Omeprazole does not alter the pharmacokinetics of **darunavir**, **lopinavir**, or **tipranavir**, all boosted with ritonavir, and no dose adjustment of these HIV-protease inhibitors is required. However, these HIV-protease inhibitors reduce omeprazole exposure. The slight decrease seen with darunavir boosted with ritonavir is unlikely to be clinically relevant. However, the moderate decrease seen with tipranavir boosted with ritonavir might be clinically important in some situations. If both drugs are given, consider increasing the dose of the proton pump inhibitor,[37,38] according to response, but note that the UK manufacturer of tipranavir states that the use of tipranavir with omeprazole or esomeprazole or other proton pump inhibitors is not recommended.[38] The clinical relevance of the effect of lopinavir boosted with ritonavir on omeprazole metabolism is unknown.

Esomeprazole had no effect on amprenavir exposure from **fosamprenavir** alone or boosted with ritonavir. Esomeprazole, or other proton pump inhibitors can be given at the same time as fosamprenavir.[39,40] Fosamprenavir alone slightly increased esomeprazole exposure, but this increase is not clinically relevant. Fosamprenavir boosted with ritonavir had no effect on esomeprazole exposure.

1. Luber AD, Brower R, Kim D, Silverman R, Peloquin CA, Frank I. Steady-state pharmacokinetics of once-daily fosamprenavir/ritonavir and atazanavir/ritonavir alone and in combination with 20 mg omeprazole in healthy volunteers. *HIV Med* (2007) 8, 457–64.
2. Zhu L, Persson A, Mahnke L, Eley T, Li T, Xu X, Agarwala S, Dragone J, Bertz R. Effect of low-dose omeprazole (20 mg daily) on the pharmacokinetics of multiple-dose atazanavir with ritonavir in healthy subjects. *J Clin Pharmacol* (2011) 51, 368–77.
3. Agarwala S, Gray K, Wang Y, Grasela D. Pharmacokinetic effect of omeprazole on atazanavir co-administered with ritonavir in healthy subjects. 12th Conference on Retroviruses and Opportunistic Infections, Boston, February 2005.

4. Klein CE, Chiu Y-L, Cai Y, Beck K, King KR, Causemaker SJ, Doan T, Esslinger H-U, Podsadecki TJ, Hanna GJ. Effect of acid-reducing agents on the pharmacokinetics of lopinavir/ritonavir and ritonavir-boosted atazanavir. *J Clin Pharmacol* (2008) 48, 553–62.
5. Reyataz (Atazanavir sulfate). Bristol-Myers Squibb. US Prescribing information, March 2012.
6. Tomilo DL, Smith PF, Ogundele AB, Difrancesco R, Berenson CS, Eberhardt E, Bednarczyk E, Morse GD. Inhibition of atazanavir oral absorption by lansoprazole gastric acid suppression in healthy volunteers. *Pharmacotherapy* (2006) 26, 341–6.
7. Khanlou H, Farthing C. Co-administration of atazanavir with proton-pump inhibitors and H_2 blockers. *J Acquir Immune Defic Syndr* (2005) 39, 503.
8. Kiser JJ, Lichtenstein KA, Anderson PL, Fletcher CV. Effects of esomeprazole on the pharmacokinetics of atazanavir and fosamprenavir in a patient with human immunodeficiency virus infection. *Pharmacotherapy* (2006) 26, 511–14.
9. Sahloff EG, Duggan JM. Clinical outcomes associated with concomitant use of atazanavir and proton pump inhibitors. *Ann Pharmacother* (2006) 40, 1731–6.
10. Furtek KJ, Crum NF, Olson PE, Wallace MR. Proton pump inhibitor therapy in atazanavir-treated patients: contraindicated? *J Acquir Immune Defic Syndr* (2006) 41, 394–6.
11. Antoniou T, Yoong D, Beique L, Chihrin S, Rachlis A, Gough K, Loutfy MR. Impact of acid-suppressive therapy on virologic response to atazanavir-based regimens in antiretroviral-experienced patients: a case series. *J Acquir Immune Defic Syndr* (2005) 39, 126–8.
12. Guiard-Schmid J-B, Poirier J-M, Bonnard P, Meynard J-L, Slama L, Lukiana T, Jaillon P, Pialoux G. Proton pump inhibitors do not reduce atazanavir concentrations in HIV-infected patients treated with ritonavir-boosted atazanavir. *AIDS* (2005) 19, 1937–8.
13. Kosel BW, Storey SS, Collier AC. Lack of interaction between atazanavir and lansoprazole. *AIDS* (2005) 19, 637–8.
14. Chan-Tack KM, Edozien A. Ritonavir-boosted atazanavir may be efficacious in HIV-infected patients concurrently receiving omeprazole. *Clin Infect Dis* (2006) 42, 1344.
15. Goicoechea M, Best B, Capparelli E, Caperna J, Ballard C, Haubrich R. Therapeutic ritonavir-boosted atazanavir plasma concentration and concurrent omeprazole use. *AIDS* (2006) 20, 2127–8.
16. Morales Conejo M, Moreno Cuerda VJ, Abellán Martínez J, Rubio R. Efectos secundarios graves derivados de las interacciones medicamentosas del tratamiento antirretroviral. *Rev Clin Esp* (2008) 208, 557–60.
17. Sekar VJ, Lefebvre E, De Paepe E, De Marez T, De Pauw M, Parys W, Hoetelmans RM. Pharmacokinetic interaction between darunavir boosted with ritonavir and omeprazole or ranitidine in human immunodeficiency virus-negative healthy volunteers. *Antimicrob Agents Chemother* (2007) 51, 958–61.
18. Sekar V, Spinosa-Guzman S, Meyvisch P, Stevens T, De Pauw M, Vangeneugden T, Hoetelmans R. Cocktail study to investigate the in-vivo drug interaction potential of darunavir coadministered with low-dose ritonavir (DRV/r; RTV) on cytochrome P450 enzymes 2D6, 2C9 and 2C19. 5th International workshop on Clinical Pharmacology of HIV, New Orleans, April 2008, P23.
19. Shelton MJ, Ford SL, Borland J, Lou Y, Wire MB, Min SS, Xue ZG, Yuen G. Coadministration of esomeprazole with fosamprenavir has no impact on steady-state plasma amprenavir pharmacokinetics. *J Acquir Immune Defic Syndr* (2006) 42, 61–7.
20. Tappouni HL, Rublein JC, Donovan BJ, Hollowell SB, Tien H-C, Min SS, Theodore D, Rezk NL, Smith PC, Tallman MN, Raasch RH, Kashuba ADM. Effect of omeprazole on the plasma concentrations of indinavir when administered alone and in combination with ritonavir. *Am J Health-Syst Pharm* (2008) 65, 422–8.
21. Hugen PWH, Burger DM, ter Hofstede HJM, Koopmans PP. Concomitant use of indinavir and omeprazole; risk of antiretroviral subtherapy. *AIDS* (1998) 12 (Suppl 4), S29.
22. Burger DM, Hugen PWH, Kroon FP, Groeneveld P, Brinkman K, Foudraine NA, Sprenger H, Koopmans PP, Hekster YA. Pharmacokinetic interaction between the proton pump inhibitor omeprazole and the HIV protease inhibitor indinavir. *AIDS* (1998) 12, 2080–2.
23. Overton ET, Tschampa JM, Klebert M, Royal M, Rodriguez M, Spitz T, Kim G, Mondy KE, Acosta EP. The effect of acid reduction with a proton pump inhibitor on the pharmacokinetics of lopinavir or ritonavir in HIV-infected patients on lopinavir/ritonavir-based therapy. *J Clin Pharmacol* (2010) 50,1050–5.
24. Yeh RF, Gaver VE, Patterson KB, Rezk NL, Baxter-Meheux F, Blake MJ, Eron JJ, Klein CE, Rublein JC, Kashuba AD. Lopinavir/ritonavir induces the hepatic activity of cytochrome P450 enzymes CYP2C9, CYP2C19, and CYP1A2 but inhibits the hepatic and intestinal activity of CYP3A as measured by a phenotyping drug cocktail in healthy volunteers. *J Acquir Immune Defic Syndr* (2006) 42, 52–60.
25. Fang AF, Damle BD, LaBadie RR, Crownover PH, Hewlett D, Glue PW. Significant decrease in nelfinavir systemic exposure after omeprazole coadministration in healthy subjects. *Pharmacotherapy* (2008) 28, 42–50.
26. Saberi P, Ranatunga DK, Quesenberry CP, Silverberg MJ. Clinical implications of the nelfinavir-proton pump inhibitor drug interaction in patients with human immunodeficiency virus. *Pharmacotherapy* (2011) 31, 253–61.
27. Winston A, Back D, Fletcher C, Robinson L, Unsworth J, Tolowinska I, Schutz M, Pozniak AL, Gazzard B, Boffito M. Effect of omeprazole on the pharmacokinetics of saquinavir-500 mg formulation with ritonavir in healthy male and female volunteers. *AIDS* (2006) 20, 1401–6.
28. Singh K, Dickinson L, Chaikan A, Back D, Fletcher C, Pozniak A, Moyle G, Nelson M, Gazzard B, Herath D, Boffito M. Pharmacokinetics and safety of saquinavir/ritonavir and omeprazole in HIV-infected subjects. *Clin Pharmacol Ther* (2008) 83, 867–72.
29. la Porte CJL, Cameron DW, Sabo JP, Murray GE, Fagan N, Bosisio M, Jones P, Di Perri G. The effect of omeprazole, food and formulation on the pharmacokinetics of tipranavir coadministered with ritonavir (TPV/r). 8th International Workshop on Clinical Pharmacology of HIV Therapy. Hungary, April 2007. Abstract 59.
30. Dumond JB, Vourvahis M, Rezk NL, Patterson KB, Tien H-C, White N, Jennings SH, Choi SO, Li J, Wagner MJ, La-Beck NM, Drulak M, Sabo JP, Castles MA, Macgregor TR, Kashuba ADM. A phenotype-genotype approach to predicting CYP450 and P-glycoprotein drug interactions with the mixed inhibitor/inducer tipranavir/ritonavir. *Clin Pharmacol Ther* (2010) 87, 735–42.
31. Crixivan (Indinavir sulphate). Merck Sharp & Dohme Ltd. UK Summary of product characteristics, February 2012.
32. Reyataz (Atazanavir sulphate). Bristol-Myers Squibb Pharmaceuticals Ltd. UK Summary of product characteristics, August 2012.
33. Viracept (Nelfinavir mesilate). Roche Products Ltd. UK Summary of product characteristics, June 2012.
34. Nexium Tablets (Esomeprazole magnesium trihydrate). AstraZeneca UK Ltd. UK Summary of product characteristics, August 2013.
35. Invirase (Saquinavir mesilate). Roche Products Ltd. UK Summary of product characteristics, October 2013.
36. Invirase (Saquinavir mesylate). Genentech, Inc. US Prescribing information, February 2012.
37. Aptivus (Tipranavir). Boehringer Ingelheim Pharmaceuticals, Inc. US Prescribing information, April 2012.
38. Aptivus Soft Capsules (Tipranavir). Boehringer Ingelheim Ltd. UK Summary of product characteristics, December 2011.
39. Telzir (Fosamprenavir calcium). ViiV Healthcare UK Ltd. UK Summary of product characteristics, May 2011.
40. Lexiva (Fosamprenavir calcium). ViiV Healthcare. US Prescribing information, April 2013.

HIV-protease inhibitors + Rifamycins; Rifabutin

Rifabutin exposure is moderately increased, and that of its partially active 25-*O*-desacetyl metabolite is greatly increased, by the HIV-protease inhibitors and this has led to toxicity; however, reduced rifabutin doses might not be as effective as expected.

Standard doses of rifabutin slightly decrease indinavir, nelfinavir, and particularly saquinavir exposure (all unboosted). Reduced doses of rifabutin negligibly decrease the exposure to saquinavir boosted with ritonavir and negligibly increase the exposure to lopinavir boosted with ritonavir. They can also slightly increase exposure to darunavir boosted with ritonavir and fosamprenavir boosted with ritonavir, but have no appreciable effect on unboosted atazanavir exposure.

Clinical evidence

(a) Amprenavir or Fosamprenavir

When amprenavir 1.2 g twice daily was given with rifabutin 300 mg daily to 11 healthy subjects for 10 days there was an almost 3-fold increase in the AUC of rifabutin, but the pharmacokinetics of amprenavir were not altered to a clinically relevant extent. The combination was poorly tolerated, with 5 of 11 subjects stopping treatment between days one and 9 due to adverse events.[1]

When rifabutin 150 mg every other day was given with fosamprenavir boosted with ritonavir 700/100 mg twice daily for 2 weeks to healthy subjects, the rifabutin AUC_{0-48} was unchanged and the maximum plasma concentration was decreased by 14%, when compared with rifabutin 300 mg daily given alone. However, the AUC_{0-48} and maximum plasma concentration of the 25-*O*-desacetyl metabolite of rifabutin were increased 11-fold and nearly 6-fold, respectively. The AUC, maximum plasma concentration, and minimum plasma concentration of amprenavir were increased by 36%, 35%, and 17%, respectively, compared with historical data.[2] No additional increase in adverse effects was reported on concurrent use.[2]

(b) Atazanavir

The US manufacturers of atazanavir report that in a study in 7 subjects, atazanavir 400 mg daily given with rifabutin 150 mg daily for 14 days did not alter the pharmacokinetics of atazanavir.[3] In a study in 3 subjects given atazanavir 600 mg daily, the AUC of rifabutin 150 mg daily was 2.1-fold higher than for a standard 300-mg dose of rifabutin daily, and the AUC of the 25-*O*-desacetyl metabolite of rifabutin was increased 22-fold.[3]

In another parallel group study in healthy subjects given atazanavir boosted with ritonavir 300/100 mg daily and rifabutin 150 mg twice weekly, the rifabutin AUC was 48% higher, and the AUC of the 25-*O*-desacetyl metabolite of rifabutin was 9.9-fold higher than in a group receiving rifabutin 150 mg daily taken alone. The study was stopped because subjects had more severe declines in neutrophil counts in the group given atazanavir boosted with ritonavir. The authors estimated that rifabutin exposure after a dose of 150 mg three times weekly given with atazanavir boosted with ritonavir would be comparable to that after rifabutin 300 mg daily alone.[4]

There is a report of a case of a patient successfully treated for tuberculosis with a rifampicin-based regimen which was switched to rifabutin 150 mg three times weekly on starting atazanavir boosted with ritonavir 300/100 mg once daily, who had a relapse of tuberculosis which was found to be rifamycin resistant.[5]

(c) Darunavir

In a crossover study in healthy subjects, darunavir boosted with ritonavir 600/100 mg twice daily alone, rifabutin 300 mg daily alone, and darunavir boosted with ritonavir 600/100 mg twice daily with rifabutin 150 mg on alternate days were each taken for 13 days. The AUC of the lower dose of rifabutin given with darunavir boosted with ritonavir was comparable to that of rifabutin 300 mg daily alone; however, the AUC of its 25-*O*-desacetyl metabolite was increased almost 10-fold. Rifabutin increased the AUC of both darunavir and ritonavir by 57% and 66%, respectively. A higher rate of adverse effects (headache, diarrhoea, back pain, dizziness, and vomiting) was reported with concurrent use than with either drug alone, and 18 of 27 subjects discontinued the study early.[6]

(d) Indinavir

When 10 healthy subjects were given rifabutin 300 mg daily with indinavir 800 mg every 8 hours for 10 days, the indinavir maximum serum concentration and AUC were decreased by about one-third, whereas the rifabutin maximum serum concentration and AUC were increased 2- to 3-fold.[7] When the same dose of indinavir (800 mg every 8 hours) was given with half the dose of rifabutin (150 mg daily), the AUC of indinavir was similarly decreased (by 32%), but the increase in the AUC of rifabutin was less (54%).[7] In a further study, the pharmacokinetics of indinavir 1 g every 8 hours and rifabutin 150 mg daily were investigated in healthy and HIV-positive subjects. The AUC of indinavir was the same with this higher dose as with indinavir 800 mg every 8 hours alone. However, despite giving half the usual rifabutin dose, the AUC was still up to 70% higher than with the 300-mg dose alone.[8] When the combination was used in practice, there were no treatment failures in 25 patients taking rifabutin and HAART (containing indinavir and/or nelfinavir). Rifabutin was given as 300 mg twice *weekly* and the indinavir dose was increased from 800 mg to 1.2 g every 8 hours to achieve satisfactory concentrations.[9]

(e) Lopinavir

When healthy subjects were given lopinavir boosted with ritonavir 400/100 mg twice daily with reduced-dose rifabutin 150 mg daily for 10 days, the AUC of rifabutin was increased 3-fold, and the AUC of its 25-*O*-desacetyl metabolite increased 47.5-fold, compared with a higher dose of rifabutin (300 mg daily alone). The AUC of lopinavir was increased by 17%.[10,11]

There are two clinical reports of the failure to achieve therapeutic rifabutin concentrations in patients taking lopinavir boosted with ritonavir 400/100 mg twice daily when given rifabutin 150 mg three times weekly. Eight of 10 and 2 of 5 patients required an increase in rifabutin dose to 300 mg three times a week to achieve therapeutic concentrations,[12,13] and one patient was reported as having experienced tuberculosis relapse with acquired rifamycin resistance.[13] In one of these reports, lopinavir concentrations were below the target in 2 of 5 patients.[12] However, in a further retrospective analysis, lopinavir concentrations were about twice as high in 15 patients taking lopinavir boosted with ritonavir and rifabutin, compared with those not taking rifabutin.[14] A case report describes a patient successfully treated for tuberculosis with a rifampicin-based regimen which was switched to rifabutin 150 mg three times weekly on starting lopinavir boosted with ritonavir 400/100 mg twice daily. The patient then had a relapse of tuberculosis which was found to be rifamycin resistant.[5]

A case of rifabutin-induced uveitis has been reported in an HIV-positive patient taking rifabutin 300 mg daily and also taking lopinavir boosted with ritonavir 400/100 mg twice daily.[15]

(f) Nelfinavir

When rifabutin 300 mg daily for 8 days was given with nelfinavir 750 mg every 8 hours for 7 to 8 days, the nelfinavir AUC and minimum plasma concentration were decreased by 32% and 53%, respectively. Nelfinavir increased the rifabutin AUC, maximum plasma concentration, and minimum plasma concentration 3.1-fold, 2.5-fold, and 4.1-fold, respectively.[16,17] When the same dose of nelfinavir was given with half the dose of rifabutin (150 mg daily) for 8 days, the AUC of nelfinavir was decreased by a similar amount (23%), although the minimum plasma concentration was only decreased by 25%. The rifabutin AUC and minimum plasma concentration were increased by nelfinavir, but to a lesser extent (83% and 2.8-fold, respectively), and the maximum plasma concentration of rifabutin was minimally affected.[17,18] A study in 7 HIV-positive patients taking rifabutin 300 mg twice weekly with nelfinavir 1.25 g twice daily reported an increase of 22% in the AUC of rifabutin and a 3.5-fold increase in the AUC of its 25-*O*-desacetyl metabolite. The pharmacokinetics of nelfinavir and its M8 metabolite were unaffected. However, the sample size in this study was too small to establish or exclude statistical significance.[19]

(g) Ritonavir

In a study, 5 healthy subjects were given ritonavir 500 mg twice daily with rifabutin 150 mg daily for 8 days. The maximum serum concentration of rifabutin was increased 3-fold and the AUC was increased 4-fold. The AUC of the 25-*O*-desacetyl metabolite of rifabutin was increased 35-fold. Seven subjects had to be withdrawn from the study due to adverse effects, primarily leucopenia.[20] Retrospective analysis of regimens containing ritonavir found that the concurrent use of rifabutin was associated with a higher incidence of rifabutin-related adverse effects including arthralgia, joint stiffness, uveitis, and leucopenia.[21]

(h) Saquinavir

In 12 HIV-positive subjects, the AUC of saquinavir 600 mg three times daily was decreased by about 40% by rifabutin 300 mg daily.[22] Similarly, in 14 HIV-positive patients, the AUC of saquinavir (soft capsules) 1.2 g three times daily was decreased by 47% by rifabutin 300 mg daily. In addition, the rifabutin AUC was increased by 44% by saquinavir.[23] However, the concurrent use of ritonavir and saquinavir (hard capsules), both 400 mg twice daily, with intermittent rifabutin dosing (300 mg weekly or 150 mg every 3 days) for 8 weeks was reported to be safe and manageable. Rifabutin did not alter the HIV-protease inhibitor concentrations, and the rifabutin pharmacokinetics were similar to those usually seen with rifabutin 300 mg daily alone.[24] In a further study of saquinavir boosted with ritonavir 1000/100 mg twice daily, rifabutin 150 mg once every 3 days (alternate days) decreased the AUC of saquinavir by 13% without affecting the AUC of ritonavir. Compared with rifabutin 150 mg daily given alone, the AUC of rifabutin was increased by 53%, the AUC of the active metabolite increased 15.4-fold. The same dose of saquinavir boosted with ritonavir was then given with a slightly lower rifabutin dose of 150 mg once every 4 days. Compared with rifabutin 150 mg daily given alone, the AUC of rifabutin was unchanged, and the AUC of the active metabolite increased 10.5-fold. Neutropenia was more common with the combination therapy and was the most common adverse event leading to withdrawal from the study.[25]

A case of anterior uveitis has been reported in an HIV-positive patient taking saquinavir boosted with ritonavir 1000/200 mg daily and rifabutin 300 mg daily. The patient was also taking abacavir, lamivudine, tenofovir, atovaquone, omeprazole, isoniazid, and pyridoxine. Rifabutin was stopped, and the patient's vision improved when treated with topical prednisolone.[26]

(i) Tipranavir

In a study in 20 healthy subjects, a single 150-mg dose of rifabutin was taken on day 8 of a 13-day course of tipranavir boosted with ritonavir 500/200 mg twice daily. Tipranavir boosted with ritonavir increased the AUC, maximum serum concentration, and minimum serum concentration of rifabutin 2.9-fold, 1.7-fold, and 2.1-fold, respectively. In addition, the AUC, maximum serum concentration, and minimum serum concentration of the 25-*O*-desacetyl metabolite of rifabutin were increased 20.7-fold, 3.2-fold, and 7.8-fold, respectively. The single dose of rifabutin had no effect on the pharmacokinetics of tipranavir,[27] but a single dose is insufficient to induce metabolism.

(j) Various HIV-protease inhibitors

Rifabutin concentrations were measured in 123 patients taking antiretrovirals in a study of a tuberculosis outbreak in a prison. Based on the antiretrovirals being taken, the rifabutin dose was adjusted to 150 mg once daily for regimens including unboosted HIV-protease inhibitors and 150 mg twice weekly for regimens including HIV-protease inhibitors boosted with ritonavir, with those receiving only NRTIs given 300 mg daily. In the analysis, rifabutin 150 mg twice weekly with HIV-protease inhibitors boosted with ritonavir was associated with subtherapeutic rifabutin serum concentrations (33% of 9 patients in this group had subtherapeutic rifabutin serum concentrations compared with 16% of 32 receiving an unboosted HIV-protease inhibitor, and just 9% of 35 receiving non-interacting drugs).[28]

Mechanism

The HIV-protease inhibitors are metabolised by CYP3A4, and as rifabutin is an inducer of this isoenzyme, it might reduce the concentrations of the HIV-protease inhibitors.

Rifabutin itself is partially metabolised by CYP3A4 whereas the 25-*O*-desacetyl metabolite of rifabutin is completely metabolised by CYP3A4. Therefore inhibition of CYP3A4 by the HIV-protease inhibitors can increase the concentrations of rifabutin and greatly increase the concentrations of its 25-*O*-desacetyl metabolite.[27]

Importance and management

The interactions between rifabutin and the HIV-protease inhibitors are established and of clinical importance. The HIV-protease inhibitors moderately increase rifabutin exposure and greatly increase the exposure to its partially active 25-*O*-desacetyl metabolite. In studies in healthy subjects, the combination has been poorly tolerated with an increase in adverse effects, such as reduced white blood cell count, even with reduced doses of rifabutin. Nevertheless, both US and UK guidelines state that rifabutin is the preferred rifamycin to use in patients receiving HIV-protease inhibitors boosted with ritonavir,[29,30] because rifampicin is contraindicated for use with the HIV-protease inhibitors (see 'HIV-protease inhibitors + Rifamycins; Rifampicin (Rifampin) or Rifapentine', p.941).

For patients taking **HIV-protease inhibitors boosted with ritonavir**, in the UK, the British HIV Association (BHIVA) guidelines for the treatment of tuberculosis and HIV coinfection recommend using a reduced dose of rifabutin of 150 mg three times weekly.[29] In contrast, the US guidelines for the treatment of HIV infection recommend reducing the dose to 150 mg once daily or 300 mg three times weekly [a reduction of 50% or more].[30] They state that lower rifabutin exposure has been reported in HIV-infected patients than in healthy subjects.[30] Note that subtherapeutic rifabutin concentrations have been seen with doses of rifabutin 150 mg twice weekly and 150 mg three times weekly in various studies, and cases of tuberculosis relapse with acquired rifamycin-resistance have been reported. For this reason, the CDC in the US recommends a dose of rifabutin of 150 mg daily with all HIV-protease inhibitors boosted with ritonavir, but warn that safety data with this dose and combination is limited.[31] All the guidelines advise monitoring antimycobacterial activity and considering therapeutic drug monitoring for rifabutin and its metabolite.[29-31] Patients should also be closely monitored to minimise the occurrence of rifabutin-related adverse effects, in particular uveitis and neutropenia. The rifabutin dose should be further adjusted as necessary based on efficacy and tolerability. Note that reduced-dose rifabutin has resulted in a negligible decrease (saquinavir) or a negligible (lopinavir) to slight increase (darunavir, fosamprenavir) in exposure to some HIV-protease inhibitors boosted with ritonavir. However, these changes are unlikely to be clinically important and no dose adjustment of the HIV-protease inhibitors boosted with ritonavir is needed on the concurrent use of rifabutin. Patients should be closely monitored for adherence to the HIV-protease inhibitor regimen, as non-compliance is likely to lead to a reduction in the extent of the pharmacokinetic interaction which might result in subtherapeutic rifabutin concentrations and tuberculosis treatment failure.[29,31] In the UK, it is advised that, where available, HIV-protease inhibitor concentrations should be measured.[29] Note that individual manufacturers of HIV-protease inhibitors give recommendations for the dose of rifabutin to be used concurrently when they are boosted with ritonavir, and that these doses are sometimes lower than that recommended by the guidelines cited.

With the exception of atazanavir, rifabutin (standard dose) has slightly decreased exposure to some **unboosted HIV-protease inhibitors** (indinavir, nelfinavir, and particularly saquinavir), and these should probably be avoided with rifabutin (the UK guidelines specifically advise avoiding saquinavir[29]). Note that unboosted HIV-protease inhibitors are rarely used, but if this is the case, the UK guidelines suggest that the dose of rifabutin is reduced to 150 mg daily to avoid toxicity (they specifically mention atazanavir).[29] Similarly, for unboosted atazanavir or fosamprenavir, the US guidelines recommend a dose of rifabutin of 150 mg daily, although they also state that 300 mg three times a week is an option.[30] The CDC recommends 150 mg daily with unboosted atazanavir.[31] Note that antiretroviral doses of ritonavir alone are generally considered to be contraindicated with rifabutin.

1. Polk RE, Brophy DF, Israel DS, Patron R, Sadler BM, Chittick GE, Symonds WT, Lou Y, Kristoff D, Stein DS. Pharmacokinetic interaction between amprenavir and rifabutin or rifampin in healthy males. *Antimicrob Agents Chemother* (2001) 45, 502–508.
2. Ford SL, Chen Y-C, Lou Y, Borland J, Min SS, Yuen GJ, Shelton MJ. Pharmacokinetic interaction between fosamprenavir-ritonavir and rifabutin in healthy subjects. *Antimicrob Agents Chemother* (2008) 52, 534–8.
3. Reyataz (Atazanavir sulfate). Bristol-Myers Squibb. US Prescribing information, March 2012.
4. Zhang J, Zhu L, Stonier M, Coumbis J, Xu X, Wu Y, Arikan D, Farajallah A, Bertz R. Determination of rifabutin dosing regimen when administered in combination with ritonavir-boosted atazanavir. *J Antimicrob Chemother* (2011) 66, 2075–82.
5. Jenny-Avitel ER, Joseph K. Rifamycin-resistant *Mycobacterium tuberculosis* in the highly active antiretroviral therapy era: a report of 3 relapses with acquired rifampin resistance following alternate-day rifabutin and boosted protease inhibitor therapy. *Clin Infect Dis* (2009) 48, 1471–4.
6. Sekar V, Lavreys L, Van de Casteele T, Berckmans C, Spinosa-Guzman S, Vangeneugden T, De Pauw M, Hoetelmans R. Pharmacokinetics of darunavir/ritonavir and rifabutin coadministered in HIV-negative healthy volunteers. *Antimicrob Agents Chemother* (2010) 54, 4440–5.
7. Kraft WK, McCrea JB, Winchell GA, Carides A, Lowry R, Woolf EJ, Kusma SE, Deutsch PJ, Greenberg HE, Waldman SA. Indinavir and rifabutin drug interactions in healthy volunteers. *J Clin Pharmacol* (2004) 44, 305–13.
8. Hamzeh FM, Benson C, Gerber J, Currier J, McCrea J, Deutsch P, Ruan P, Wu H, Lee J, Flexner C, for the AIDS Clinical Trials Group 365 Study Team. Steady-state pharmacokinetic interaction of modified-dose indinavir and rifabutin. *Clin Pharmacol Ther* (2003) 73, 159–69.
9. Narita M, Stambaugh JJ, Hollender ES, Jones D, Pitchenik AE, Ashkin D. Use of rifabutin with protease inhibitors for human immunodeficiency virus-infected patients with tuberculosis. *Clin Infect Dis* (2000) 30, 779–83. Correction. ibid. 992.
10. Bertz R, Hsu A, Lam W, Williams L, Renz C, Karol M, Dutta S, Carr R, Zhang Y, Wang Q, Schweitzer S, Foit C, Andre A, Bernstein B, Granneman GR, Sun E. Pharmacokinetic interactions between lopinavir/ritonavir (ABT-378r) and other non-HIV drugs (abstract P291). *AIDS* (2000) 14 (Suppl 4), S100.
11. Kaletra (Lopinavir with Ritonavir). Abbott Laboratories. US Prescribing information, April 2012.

12. Khachi H, O'Connell R, Ladenheim D, Orkin C. Pharmacokinetic interactions between rifabutin and lopinavir/ritonavir in HIV-infected patients with mycobacterial co-infection. *J Antimicrob Chemother* (2009) 64, 871–3.
13. Boulanger C, Hollender E, Farrell K, Stambaugh JJ, Maasen D, Ashkin D, Symes S, Espinoza LA, Rivero RO, Graham JJ, Peloquin CA. Pharmacokinetic evaluation of rifabutin in combination with lopinavir-ritonavir in patients with HIV infection and active tuberculosis. *Clin Infect Dis* (2009) 49, 1305–11.
14. Stöhr W, Back D, Dunn D, Sabin C, Winston A, Gilson R, Pillay D, Hill T, Ainsworth J, Gazzard B, Leen C, Bansi L, Fisher M, Orkin C, Anderson J, Johnson M, Easterbrook P, Gibbons S, Khoo S; UK CHIC Steering Committee. Factors influencing lopinavir and atazanavir plasma concentration. *J Antimicrob Chemother* (2010) 65, 129–37.
15. Lin H-C, Lu P-L, Chang C-H. Uveitis associated with concurrent administration of rifabutin and lopinavir/ritonavir (Kaletra). *Eye* (2007) 21, 1540–1.
16. Kerr B, Yuep G, Daniels R, Quart B, Kravcik S, Sahai J, Anderson R. Strategic approach to nelfinavir mesylate (NFV) drug interactions involving CYP3A metabolism. 6th European Conference on Clinical Aspects and Treatment of HIV-infection, Hamburg, 1997. 256.
17. Viracept (Nelfinavir mesylate). Agouron Pharmaceuticals, Inc. US Prescribing information, May 2013.
18. Viracept (Nelfinavir mesilate). Roche Products Ltd. UK Summary of product characteristics, June 2012.
19. Benator DA, Weiner MH, Burman WJ, Vernon AA, Zhao ZA, Khan AE, Jones BE, Sandman L, Engle M, Silva-Trigo C, Hsyu PH, Becker MI, Peloquin CA, for the Tuberculosis Trials Consortium. Clinical evaluation of the nelfinavir-rifabutin interaction in patients with tuberculosis and human immunodeficiency virus infection. *Pharmacotherapy* (2007) 27, 793–800.
20. Cato A, Cavanaugh J, Shi H, Hsu A, Leonard J, Granneman R. The effect of multiple doses of ritonavir on the pharmacokinetics of rifabutin. *Clin Pharmacol Ther* (1998) 63, 414–21.
21. Sun E, Heath-Chiozzi M, Cameron DW, Hsu A, Granneman RG, Maurath CJ, Leonard JM. Concurrent ritonavir and rifabutin increases risk of rifabutin-associated adverse events. 11th International Conference on AIDS, Vancouver, 1996. Mo.B.171.
22. Sahai J, Stewart F, Swick L, Gallicano K, Garber G, Seguin I, Tucker A, Bristow N, Cameron W. Rifabutin (RBT) reduces saquinavir (SAQ) plasma levels in HIV-infected patients. *Intersci Conf Antimicrob Agents Chemother* (1996) 36, 6.
23. Moyle GJ, Buss NE, Goggin T, Snell P, Higgs C, Hawkins DA. Interaction between saquinavir soft-gel and rifabutin in patients infected with HIV. *Br J Clin Pharmacol* (2002) 54, 178–82.
24. Gallicano K, Khaliq Y, Carignan G, Tseng A, Walmsley S, Cameron DW. A pharmacokinetic study of intermittent rifabutin dosing with a combination of ritonavir and saquinavir in patients infected with human immunodeficiency virus. *Clin Pharmacol Ther* (2001) 70, 149–58.
25. Zhang X, Fettner S, Zwanziger E, Rowell L, Salgo M. Pharmacokinetic interaction study of ritonavir-boosted saquinavir in combination with rifabutin in healthy subjects. *Antimicrob Agents Chemother* (2011) 55, 680–7.
26. Ebraert H, Salu P. Toxic uveitis caused by pharmacodynamic interactions of rifabutin and protease inhibitors: a case report. *Bull Soc Belge Ophtalmol* (2007) 303, 57–60.
27. la Porte C, Sabo JP, Elgadi M, Cameron DW. Interaction studies of tipranavir/ritonavir (TPV/r) with clarithromycin, fluconazole and rifabutin in healthy volunteers. *Antimicrob Agents Chemother* (2009) 53, 162–73.
28. Spradling P, Drociuk D, McLaughlin S, Lee LM, Peloquin CA, Gallicano K, Pozsik C, Onorato I, Castro KG, Ridzon R. Drug-drug interactions in inmates treated for human immunodeficiency virus and *Mycobacterium tuberculosis* infection or disease: an institutional tuberculosis outbreak. *Clin Infect Dis* (2002) 35, 1106–12.
29. Pozniak AL, Coyne KM, Miller RF, Lipman MCI, Freedman AR, Ormerod LP, Johnson MA, Collins S, Lucas SB on behalf of the BHIVA Guidelines Subcommittee. British HIV Association guidelines for the treatment of TB/ HIV coinfection 2011. *HIV Med* (2011) 12, 517–24. Also available at: http://www.bhiva.org/documents/Guidelines/TB/hiv_954_online_final.pdf (accessed 29/09/15).
30. Panel on Antiretroviral Guidelines for Adults and Adolescents. Guidelines for the use of antiretroviral agents in HIV-1-infected adults and adolescents. US Department of Health and Human Services (April 2015). 1–288. Available at: https://aidsinfo.nih.gov/contentfiles/lvguidelines/adultandadolescentgl.pdf (accessed 29/09/15).
31. Centers for Disease Control and Prevention. Managing drug interactions in the treatment of HIV-related tuberculosis. *US Department of Health and Human Services* (2013). Available at: http://www.cdc.gov/tb/publications/guidelines/TB_HIV_Drugs/pdf/tbhiv.pdf (accessed 29/09/15).

HIV-protease inhibitors + Rifamycins; Rifampicin (Rifampin) or Rifapentine

Rifampicin moderately to markedly decreases the exposure to amprenavir, atazanavir (both boosted with ritonavir and alone), indinavir, lopinavir boosted with ritonavir, nelfinavir, saquinavir (both boosted with ritonavir and alone), but only slightly decreases the exposure to ritonavir. Rifampicin is also predicted to decrease the concentrations of darunavir, fosamprenavir, and tipranavir, all boosted with ritonavir. Higher than standard doses of lopinavir boosted with ritonavir and saquinavir might attenuate the pharmacokinetic interaction, but have been associated with an increase in hepatotoxicity. Atazanavir boosted with ritonavir and indinavir increase rifampicin exposure. Rifapentine appears to moderately decrease exposure to indinavir.

Clinical evidence

A. Rifampicin (Rifampin)

(a) Amprenavir or Fosamprenavir

When 11 healthy subjects were given amprenavir 1.2 g twice daily with rifampicin 600 mg daily for 4 days the pharmacokinetics of rifampicin were not affected, but the AUC of amprenavir was decreased by 82%. The maximum plasma concentration of amprenavir was also decreased by 70%, from 9.2 to 2.78 micrograms/mL, and its minimum plasma concentration was decreased by 94%, from 0.32 to 0.02 micrograms/mL.[1]

It is expected that the concurrent use of fosamprenavir and rifampicin or fosamprenavir boosted with ritonavir and rifampicin will also result in large decreases in the plasma concentrations of the metabolite, amprenavir.[2,3]

(b) Atazanavir

In a study, 52 healthy subjects were given standard doses of atazanavir 400 mg daily for 6 days, followed by standard dose atazanavir boosted with ritonavir 300/100 mg daily for 10 days. They were then given rifampicin 600 mg daily for the next 10 days with atazanavir boosted with ritonavir, at 300/100 mg daily, at 300/200 mg daily, or at 400/200 mg daily. The addition of rifampicin to standard dose atazanavir boosted with ritonavir decreased the AUC, maximum plasma concentration, and minimum plasma concentration of atazanavir by 72%, 49%, and 97%, respectively. However, increasing the ritonavir dose by just 100 mg daily resulted in a smaller although still clinically relevant decrease in the AUC, maximum plasma concentration, and minimum plasma concentration of atazanavir (53%, 35%, and 93%, respectively). Similarly, increasing both the atazanavir and ritonavir doses by 100 mg again slightly attenuated the effects of rifampicin; however, the AUC and minimum plasma concentration of atazanavir were still decreased, by 46% and 92%, respectively. The AUC and maximum plasma concentration of rifampicin were increased by atazanavir boosted with ritonavir by 49 to 64% and 32 to 36%, respectively, with the effects slightly increasing with the increase in atazanavir and ritonavir doses, as before.[4]

In another study in 10 healthy subjects, the effects of rifampicin 600 mg daily on the pharmacokinetics of atazanavir 300 mg or 400 mg *twice* daily for between 8 and 11 days were investigated. Rifampicin decreased the mean AUC of atazanavir 300 mg by 79% and that of atazanavir 400 mg by 59%. The maximum and minimum plasma concentrations of atazanavir were decreased by 63% and 94%, and 40% and 87% for atazanavir 300 mg and 400 mg twice daily, respectively. No notable increases in rifampicin exposure were reported.[5] A small study in 3 HIV-positive patients also reported subtherapeutic plasma concentrations of atazanavir (given as standard doses of atazanavir boosted with ritonavir 300/100 mg daily) with rifampicin 600 mg daily: the study was stopped prematurely.[6] None of these studies reported an increase in adverse effects with the concurrent use of atazanavir or atazanavir boosted with ritonavir and rifampicin.[4-6] However, a subsequent pharmacokinetic study in 15 healthy subjects who received rifampicin 600 mg daily with atazanavir boosted with ritonavir 300/100 mg *twice* daily was stopped prematurely due to nausea and vomiting, and increases in hepatic transaminases.[7]

(c) Indinavir

A study in 11 patients with AIDS given indinavir 800 mg every 8 hours and rifampicin 600 mg daily for 14 days found that the AUC of rifampicin was increased by 73%.[8] In a similar study looking at the effects of rifampicin on indinavir, the indinavir AUC and maximum serum concentration were decreased by 92% and 86%, respectively.[9] In another study, in 6 HIV-positive patients taking indinavir boosted with ritonavir 800/100 mg twice daily, rifampicin 300 mg daily for 4 days decreased the median indinavir plasma concentration (measured 12 hours after the last dose) by 87% and the median ritonavir plasma concentration by 94%.[10]

(d) Lopinavir

1. Standard dose. In a study in healthy subjects, rifampicin 600 mg daily for 10 days decreased the AUC of lopinavir (given as the standard dose of lopinavir boosted with ritonavir 400/100 mg twice daily) by 75%.[11] Another study in patients reported a 68% and 62% decrease in the AUCs of lopinavir and ritonavir, respectively, after giving rifampicin with the standard dose of lopinavir boosted with ritonavir. In addition, 10 of 21 patients and 18 of 21 patients had subtherapeutic morning (C_0) and evening (C_{12}) minimum lopinavir plasma concentrations, respectively.[12] In a review of the clinical experience of 29 patients taking standard dose lopinavir boosted with ritonavir, 67% had subtherapeutic lopinavir plasma concentrations and 38% had a detectable viral load.[13]

2. Higher doses. A dose titration of lopinavir boosted with ritonavir was carried out in healthy subjects to try to overcome the interaction with rifampicin.[14] In 10 evaluable subjects, rifampicin 600 mg daily and lopinavir boosted with ritonavir 800/200 mg twice daily decreased the lopinavir minimum serum concentration by 57% without affecting the maximum serum concentration, when compared with standard doses of lopinavir boosted with ritonavir 400/100 mg twice daily without rifampicin. In another 9 evaluable subjects, rifampicin 600 mg daily with lopinavir boosted with ritonavir 400/400 mg twice daily did not alter the maximum or minimum serum concentration of lopinavir, but greatly *increased* ritonavir serum concentrations, when compared with standard doses of lopinavir boosted with ritonavir 400/100 mg twice daily without rifampicin. Of 29 subjects who received rifampicin with the higher doses of lopinavir boosted with ritonavir, 9 subjects had grade 2 to 3 elevations in liver enzymes, and this was more common in the 400/400 mg group than the 800/200 mg group.[14] In a subsequent study, healthy subjects were given rifampicin 600 mg daily for 5 days and then also given lopinavir boosted with ritonavir (600/150 mg or 800/200 mg twice daily). However, on day 8, the study was stopped prematurely due to a high incidence of adverse effects, including nausea, vomiting, and hepatotoxicity.[15] A further study investigated the effect of slowly increasing the dose of lopinavir boosted with ritonavir after starting rifampicin in 21 HIV-infected patients with tuberculosis with virological suppression at baseline. After taking rifampicin 600 mg daily for one week with standard dose lopinavir boosted with ritonavir (400/100 mg twice daily) the lopinavir and ritonavir AUCs were decreased by 68% and 62%, respectively, and the lopinavir minimum plasma concentration was below that recommended for efficacy in 10 of 21 patients in the morning (C_0) and 18 of 21 patients in the evening (C_{12}). After increasing the dose by 50%, to 600/150 mg twice daily, for a further week, the decrease in lopinavir and ritonavir AUCs was 42% and 17% (compared with baseline values), and the lopinavir minimum plasma concentration was below that recommended in 2 of 20 patients in the morning and 10 of 20 in the evening. After further increasing the dose, to 800/200 mg twice daily, for another week, the lopinavir and ritonavir AUCs were 14% lower and 31% higher than baseline values, with no patients with subtherapeutic lopinavir plasma concentrations in the morning and 4 of 18 in the evening. Two of the participants did not remain virologically suppressed. Two participants were withdrawn because of grade 3/4 elevations in transaminases, and one because of grade 2 nausea.[12] In a review of clinical experience, 2 of 5 patients taking rifampicin and given a higher than standard dose of lopinavir boosted with ritonavir stopped the drug combination because of adverse effects.[13]

A study in children investigated the difference between a control group taking lopinavir boosted with ritonavir in the standard ratio of 4:1 and a group taking rifampicin, and lopinavir boosted with ritonavir in a ratio of 1:1. The AUC, maximum plasma concentration, and minimum plasma concentration of lopinavir were 31%, 26%, and 15% lower in the rifampicin group, when compared with the control group. However the minimum plasma concentrations in 13 of the 15 children were still above the minimum recommended concentrations of lopinavir (greater than 1 mg/L).[16] Conversely, in a later similar study by the same research group using a double dose of lopinavir boosted with ritonavir (in the standard ratio of 4:1) inadequate lopinavir plasma concentrations were seen in 12 of 20 children taking rifampicin compared with 2 of 24 control children taking standard dose lopinavir boosted with ritonavir without rifampicin.[17]

(e) Nelfinavir

Rifampicin 600 mg daily for 7 days decreased the AUC of nelfinavir 750 mg every 8 hours for 6 days by 82%.[18] A 7-month-old infant with HIV and tuberculosis was given a rifampicin-based antimycobacterial regimen with nelfinavir-based HAART. Nelfinavir plasma concentrations were found to be very low, so ritonavir was added. This increased the nelfinavir plasma concentrations and also greatly increased those of the principal active metabolite of nelfinavir. The regimen was well tolerated and had a good clinical response.[19]

(f) Ritonavir

When ritonavir 500 mg every 12 hours was given with rifampicin 300 mg or 600 mg daily for 10 days, the AUC of ritonavir was 35% lower and the minimum serum concentration 49% lower than in subjects receiving ritonavir alone.[20]

(g) Saquinavir

Rifampicin 600 mg daily decreased the AUC of saquinavir (soft capsules, *Fortovase*) 1.2 g three times daily by 70%.[21] In a pharmacokinetic study in HIV-positive patients taking saquinavir boosted with ritonavir 1600/200 mg once daily, the concurrent use of rifampicin and isoniazid decreased the median AUC, maximum serum concentration, and minimum serum concentration of saquinavir by 40%, 35%, and 49%, respectively. Similarly, the median AUC, maximum serum concentration, and minimum serum concentration of ritonavir were also decreased, by 43%, 50%, and 64%, respectively. The ritonavir minimum serum concentration was undetectable in most of the patients. Saquinavir boosted with ritonavir had no effect on the pharmacokinetics of rifampicin or isoniazid.[22] It was suggested that the combination of ritonavir and saquinavir (both 400 mg twice daily) could cancel out the effects of rifampicin on saquinavir, so therapeutic concentrations of all three drugs could be achieved. This assumption has been confirmed in HIV-positive patients.[23,24] Five of 20 patients originally given the combination developed hepatotoxicity, 2 of whom had comorbidities.[24] However, in a further study in healthy subjects, severe hepatotoxicity (with transaminase elevations about 20 times the upper limit of normal) occurred in 11 of 17 subjects after they took saquinavir boosted with ritonavir 1000/100 mg twice daily and rifampicin 600 mg daily for one to 5 days.[25]

(h) Tipranavir

Based on historical data cited by the manufacturers, British HIV Association (BHIVA) guidelines briefly state that rifampicin decreased tipranavir concentrations by 80%.[26] The UK and US manufacturers of tipranavir predict that rifampicin will decrease the plasma concentration of tipranavir boosted with ritonavir.[27,28]

B. Rifapentine

The manufacturer briefly notes that, in a study rifapentine 600 mg twice weekly for 14 days decreased the AUC of **indinavir** 800 mg three times daily for 14 days by 70%, and decreased its maximum plasma concentrations by 55%. The clearance of indinavir was increased 3-fold. Indinavir had no effect on the pharmacokinetics of rifapentine.[29]

Mechanism

Rifampicin is a known enzyme inducer, with potent effects on CYP3A4, the isoenzyme by which the HIV-protease inhibitors are at least partially metabolised, and therefore concurrent use decreases HIV-protease inhibitor concentrations.

The mechanism for the increase in rifampicin concentrations seen with indinavir and atazanavir boosted with ritonavir is unknown. As rifampicin and its metabolite are not substrates for CYP3A4, which atazanavir inhibits, and atazanavir is only a weak inhibitor of P-glycoprotein, the authors of one study suggest that other mechanisms, such as competition for biliary excretion or other transport systems might be involved.[4] Note that increased rifampicin concentrations could result in increased rifampicin-induced hepatotoxicity.

Rifapentine is also an inducer of CYP3A4, and hence decreases exposure to indinavir.

Importance and management

Rifampicin moderately to markedly decreases the exposure of many of the HIV-protease inhibitors, particularly unboosted HIV-protease inhibitors. Therefore the use of rifampicin with unboosted HIV-protease inhibitors should be avoided, because of the risk of reduced antiviral efficacy and emergence of resistant viral strains.[26,30] The interaction with **ritonavir** alone is not as great (a slight decrease in exposure), and for ritonavir alone, the British HIV Association (BHIVA) guidelines for the treatment of tuberculosis and HIV coinfection state that rifampicin might be used with full-dose ritonavir (600 mg twice daily), but they note that this combination is poorly tolerated.[26]

Rifampicin has also decreased HIV-protease inhibitor exposure to an extent likely to reduce antiviral efficacy when used with standard doses of some HIV-protease inhibitors boosted with ritonavir (namely atazanavir, lopinavir, saquinavir), and is predicted to similarly affect **darunavir**,[31,32] fosamprenavir, and tipranavir. When higher than standard doses of ritonavir have been given with HIV-protease inhibitors (with or without increased doses of the boosted HIV-protease inhibitor), for some (lopinavir, saquinavir) this has completely attenuated the pharmacokinetic interaction with rifampicin, but for others (atazanavir) the attenuation has not been sufficient to maintain plasma concentrations at the desired level. However, higher doses of atazanavir, lopinavir, or saquinavir, all boosted with ritonavir, have been associated with poor tolerability in some studies, particularly higher rates of hepatotoxicity. In addition, of the HIV-protease inhibitors that have been studied, both indinavir and atazanavir boosted with ritonavir increased rifampicin exposure. The BHIVA guidelines recommend that HIV-protease inhibitors boosted with ritonavir should not be used with rifampicin. They recommend that, if possible, the antiretroviral regimen should be switched to one that does not contain an HIV-protease inhibitor. If this is not possible, they state that rifampicin should be switched to rifabutin.[26] Similarly, the US guidelines for the treatment of HIV, and the CDC in the US, state that the use of HIV-protease inhibitors boosted with ritonavir and rifampicin is not recommended, and that rifabutin is preferred in patients taking HIV-protease inhibitors.[30,33] Further, the CDC advises that increased lopinavir and ritonavir doses (800/200 mg or 400/400 mg twice daily) should be used with caution, and that such regimens are associated with an increased risk of hepatotoxicity.[33] The UK manufacturer of lopinavir boosted with ritonavir states that a higher dose of lopinavir boosted with ritonavir (400/400 mg twice daily) should be avoided because of the higher rate of hepatic and gastrointestinal adverse effects, they nevertheless advise that if use of this regimen is unavoidable, the dose should be increased only after rifampicin has been started and patients should be very closely monitored for adverse effects and efficacy.[34]

Rifapentine appears to moderately decrease exposure to unboosted indinavir, and as with rifampicin, concurrent use would not be recommended. The US guidelines predict that rifapentine will decrease concentrations of the HIV-protease inhibitors and advise that it should not be used with HIV-protease inhibitors outside of clinical studies.[30] However, they also say that in HIV infected individuals, rifapentine-based regimens are associated with a higher rate of tuberculosis relapse than other rifamycin-based regimens and therefore an alternative to rifapentine is recommended.[30]

1. Polk RE, Brophy DF, Israel DS, Patron R, Sadler BM, Chittick GE, Symonds WT, Lou Y, Kristoff D, Stein DS. Pharmacokinetic interaction between amprenavir and rifabutin or rifampin in healthy males. *Antimicrob Agents Chemother* (2001) 45, 502–508.
2. Telzir (Fosamprenavir calcium). ViiV Healthcare UK Ltd. UK Summary of product characteristics, May 2011.
3. Lexiva (Fosamprenavir calcium). ViiV Healthcare. US Prescribing information, April 2013.
4. Burger DM, Agarwala S, Child M, Been-Tiktak A, Wang Y, Bertz R. Effect of rifampin on steady-state pharmacokinetics of atazanavir with ritonavir in healthy volunteers. *Antimicrob Agents Chemother* (2006) 50, 3336–42.
5. Acosta EP, Kendall MA, Gerber JG, Alston-Smith B, Koletar SL, Zolopa AR, Agarwala S, Child M, Bertz R, Hosey L, Haas DW. Effect of concomitantly administered rifampin on the pharmacokinetics and safety of atazanavir administered twice daily. *Antimicrob Agents Chemother* (2007) 51, 3104–10.
6. Mallolas J, Sarasa M, Nomdedeu M, Soriano A, López-Púa, Blanco JL, Martinéz E, Gatell JM. Pharmacokinetic interaction between rifampicin and ritonavir-boosted atazanavir in HIV-infected patients. *HIV Med* (2007) 8, 131–4.
7. Haas DW, Koletar SL, Laughlin L, Kendall MA, Suckow C, Gerber JG, Zolopa AR, Bertz R, Child MJ, Hosey L, Alston-Smith B, Acosta EP, for the A5213 Study Team. Hepatotoxicity and gastrointestinal intolerance when healthy volunteers taking rifampin add twice-daily atazanavir and ritonavir. *J Acquir Immune Defic Syndr* (2009) 50, 290–3.
8. Jaruratanasirikul S, Sriwiriyajan S. Pharmacokinetics of rifampicin administered alone and with indinavir. *J Antimicrob Chemother* (1999) 44 (Suppl A), 58.
9. McCrea J, Wyss D, Stone J, Carides A, Kusma S, Kleinbloesem C, Al-Hamdan Y, Yeh K, Deutsch P. Pharmacokinetic interaction between indinavir and rifampin. *Clin Pharmacol Ther* (1997) 61, 152.
10. Justesen US, Åndersen AB, Klitgaard NA, Brøsen K, Gerstoft J, Pedersen C. Pharmacokinetic interaction between rifampin and the combination of indinavir and low-dose ritonavir in HIV-infected patients. *Clin Infect Dis* (2004) 38, 426–9.
11. Bertz R, Hsu A, Lam W, Williams L, Renz C, Karol M, Dutta S, Carr R, Zhang Y, Wang Q, Schweitzer S, Foit C, Andre A, Bernstein B, Granneman GR, Sun E. Pharmacokinetic interactions between lopinavir/ritonavir (ABT-378r) and other non-HIV drugs (abstract P291). *AIDS* (2000) 14 (Suppl 4), S100.
12. Decloedt EH, McIlleron H, Smith P, Merry C, Orrell C, Maartens G. Pharmacokinetics of lopinavir in HIV-infected adults receiving rifampin with adjusted doses of lopinavir-ritonavir tablets. *Antimicrob Agents Chemother* (2011) 55, 3195–200.
13. L'homme RF, Nijland HM, Gras L, Aarnoutse RE, van Crevel R, Boeree M, Brinkman K, Prins JM, Juttmann JR, Burger DM. Clinical experience with the combined use of lopinavir/ritonavir and rifampicin. *AIDS* (2009) 23, 863–5.
14. la Porte CJL, Colbers EPH, Bertz R, Voncken DS, Wikstrom K, Boeree MJ, Koopmans PP, Hekster YA, Burger DM. Pharmacokinetics of adjusted-dose lopinavir-ritonavir combined with rifampin in healthy volunteers. *Antimicrob Agents Chemother* (2004) 48, 1553–60.
15. Nijland HMJ, L'homme RFA, Rongen GA, van Uden P, van Crevel R, Boeree MJ, Aarnoutse RE, Koopmans PP, Burger DM. High incidence of adverse events in healthy volunteers receiving rifampicin and adjusted doses of lopinavir/ritonavir tablets. *AIDS* (2008) 22, 931–5.
16. Ren Y, Nuttall JJC, Egbers C, Eley BS, Meyers TM, Smith PJ, Maartens G, McIlleron HM. Effect of rifampicin on lopinavir pharmacokinetics in HIV-infected children with tuberculosis. *J Acquir Immune Defic Syndr* (2008) 47, 566–9.
17. McIlleron H, Ren Y, Nuttall J, Fairlie L, Rabie H, Cotton M, Eley B, Meyers T, Smith PJ, Merry C, Maartens G. Lopinavir exposure is insufficient in children given double doses of lopinavir/ritonavir during rifampicin-based treatment for tuberculosis. *Antivir Ther* (2011)16, 417–21.
18. Kerr B, Yuep G, Daniels R, Quart B, Kravcik S, Sahai J, Anderson R. Strategic approach to nelfinavir mesylate (NFV) drug interactions involving CYP3A metabolism. 6th European Conference on Clinical Aspects and Treatment of HIV-infection, Hamburg, 1997. 256.
19. Bergshoeff AS, Wolfs TFW, Geelen SPM, Burger DM. Ritonavir-enhanced pharmacokinetics of nelfinavir/M8 during rifampin use. *Ann Pharmacother* (2003) 37, 521–5.
20. Norvir Tablets and Solution (Ritonavir). Abbott Laboratories. US Prescribing information, October 2012.
21. Fortovase (Saquinavir). Roche Products Ltd. UK Summary of product characteristics, January 2005.
22. Ribera E, Azuaje C, Lopez RM, Domingo P, Curran A, Feijoo M, Pou L, Sánchez P, Sambeat MA, Colomer J, Lopez-Colomes JL, Crespo M, Falcó V, Ocaña I, Pahissa A. Pharmacokinetic interaction between rifampicin and the once-daily combination of saquinavir and low-dose ritonavir in HIV-infected patients with tuberculosis. *J Antimicrob Chemother* (2007) 59, 690–7.
23. Veldkamp AI, Hoetelmans RMW, Beijnen JH, Mulder JW, Meenhorst PL. Ritonavir enables combined therapy with rifampicin and saquinavir. *Clin Infect Dis* (1999) 29, 1586.
24. Rolla VC, da Silva Vieira MA, Pereira Pinto D, Lourenço MC, de Jesus C da S, Gonçalves Morgado M, Ferreira Filho M, Werneck-Barroso E. Safety, efficacy and pharmacokinetics of ritonavir 400 mg/saquinavir 400 mg twice daily plus rifampicin combined therapy in HIV patients with tuberculosis. *Clin Drug Invest* (2006) 26, 469–79.
25. Schmitt C, Riek M, Winters K, Schutz M, Grange S. Unexpected hepatotoxicity of rifampin and saquinavir/ritonavir in healthy male volunteers. *Arch Drug Inf* (2009) 2, 8–16.
26. Pozniak AL, Coyne KM, Miller RF, Lipman MCI, Freedman AR, Ormerod LP, Johnson MA, Collins S, Lucas SB on behalf of the BHIVA Guidelines Subcommittee. British HIV Association guidelines for the treatment of TB/ HIV coinfection 2011. *HIV Med* (2011) 12, 517–24.

27. Aptivus Soft Capsules (Tipranavir). Boehringer Ingelheim Ltd. UK Summary of product characteristics, December 2011.
28. Aptivus (Tipranavir). Boehringer Ingelheim Pharmaceuticals, Inc. US Prescribing information, April 2012.
29. Priftin (Rifapentine). Sanofi-Aventis U.S. LLC. US Prescribing information, December 2014.
30. Panel on Antiretroviral Guidelines for Adults and Adolescents. Guidelines for the use of antiretroviral agents in HIV-1-infected adults and adolescents. US Department of Health and Human Services (April 2015). 1–288. Available at: https://aidsinfo.nih.gov/contentfiles/lvguidelines/adultandadolescentgl.pdf (accessed 20/09/15).
31. Prezista (Darunavir ethanolate). Janssen-Cilag Ltd. UK Summary of product characteristics, June 2012.
32. Prezista (Darunavir ethanolate). Janssen Pharmaceuticals, Inc. US Prescribing information, May 2012.
33. Centers for Disease Control and Prevention. Managing drug interactions in the treatment of HIV-related tuberculosis. *US Department of Health and Human Services* (2013). Available at: http://www.cdc.gov/tb/publications/guidelines/TB_HIV_Drugs/pdf/tbhiv.pdf (accessed 20/09/15).
34. Kaletra Tablets (Lopinavir with Ritonavir). AbbVie Ltd. UK Summary of product characteristics, August 2012.

HIV-protease inhibitors + St John's wort (*Hypericum perforatum*)

St John's wort reduces indinavir exposure. Other HIV-protease inhibitors, whether used alone or boosted with ritonavir, are predicted to interact similarly.

Clinical evidence

In a pharmacokinetic study, 8 healthy subjects were given three 800-mg doses of **indinavir** on day one and then an 800-mg dose on day 2. For the next 14 days they were given St John's wort extract 300 mg three times daily. Starting on day 16, the indinavir dosing was repeated. It was found that St John's wort reduced the AUC of **indinavir** by 54% and decreased the 8-hour **indinavir** minimum serum concentration by 81%.[1]

Mechanism

Not fully understood, but it seems likely that St John's wort induces the activity of CYP3A4, thereby increasing the metabolism of indinavir and therefore reducing its serum concentration.

Importance and management

Direct information about an interaction between the HIV-protease inhibitors and St John's wort seems to be limited to this study with indinavir, but the interaction would appear to be established. Such a large reduction in the serum concentration of indinavir is likely to result in treatment failure and the development of viral resistance. Therefore concurrent use with St John's wort should be avoided. There seems to be no direct information about other HIV-protease inhibitors, but since they are also metabolised by CYP3A4 it is reasonable to expect that they will be similarly affected by St John's wort. The FDA in the US has suggested that concurrent use of St John's wort and HIV-protease inhibitors is not recommended.[2] Similarly, the CSM in the UK has advised that patients taking HIV-protease inhibitors should avoid St John's wort and that anyone already taking both should stop the St John's wort and have their HIV RNA viral load measured.[3] The concentrations of the HIV-protease inhibitors likely to increase as the induction effects of St John's wort diminish, usually over one to two weeks.[4] Therefore the dose of the HIV-protease inhibitor will probably need adjusting on stopping St John's wort. The US and UK manufacturers of all HIV-protease inhibitors (**amprenavir, atazanavir, darunavir, fosamprenavir,** indinavir, **lopinavir** boosted with ritonavir, **nelfinavir, ritonavir, saquinavir,** and **tipranavir**) either contraindicate, or advise against, the use of St John's wort.

1. Piscitelli SC, Burstein AH, Chaitt D, Alfaro RM, Falloon J. Indinavir concentrations and St John's wort. *Lancet* (2000) 355, 547–8. Erratum *ibid.* (2001) 357, 1210.
2. Lumpkin MM, Alpert S; FDA Public Health Advisory. Risk of drug interactions with St John's wort and indinavir and other drugs, February 10, 2000. Available at: http://www.fda.gov/drugs/drugsafety/postmarketdrugsafetyinformationforpatientsandproviders/ucm052238.htm (accessed 21/10/15).
3. Committee on Safety of Medicines. Message from Professor A Breckenridge (Chairman of CSM) and Fact Sheet for Health Care Professionals, 29th February 2000.
4. Crixivan (Indinavir sulphate). Merck Sharp & Dohme Ltd. UK Summary of product characteristics, February 2012.

HIV-protease inhibitors + SNRIs

Immediate-release venlafaxine *decreased* single-dose indinavir concentrations in one study. Extended-release venlafaxine and extended-release desvenlafaxine did not affect the pharmacokinetics of indinavir in another study. The HIV-protease inhibitors are predicted to *increase* venlafaxine exposure.

Clinical evidence

(a) Desvenlafaxine

In a pharmacokinetic study, 12 healthy subjects were given a single 800-mg dose of indinavir before and after 10 days of desvenlafaxine 50 mg daily as extended-release capsules. Desvenlafaxine did not affect the pharmacokinetics of indinavir.[1]

(b) Venlafaxine

In a study, 9 healthy subjects were given a single 800-mg dose of indinavir before and on day 10 of a 13–day course of venlafaxine (75 mg daily in divided doses for 4 days, followed by 150 mg daily in divided doses). Venlafaxine reduced the AUC and maximum plasma concentration of indinavir by 28% and 36%, respectively. The single-dose of indinavir did not affect the pharmacokinetics of venlafaxine, and did not alter the pharmacokinetics of its active metabolite *O*-desmethylvenlafaxine to a clinically relevant extent.[2] However, in another pharmacokinetic study 12 healthy subjects were given a single 800-mg dose of indinavir before and after 10 days of venlafaxine 37.5 mg daily for 4 days, followed by 75 mg daily as extended release capsules. Venlafaxine did not affect the pharmacokinetics of indinavir.[1]

Mechanism

Venlafaxine is partially metabolised by CYP3A4, and as other inhibitors of this isoenzyme have been seen to increase venlafaxine exposure (see 'SNRIs + Azoles', p.1477), indinavir, an inhibitor of CYP3A4, would also be expected to increase the exposure to venlafaxine. The mechanism by which venlafaxine might decrease indinavir exposure, as seen in the study above, is unclear. The authors of this study state that their results suggest the decrease in exposure to indinavir was due to a mechanism resulting in reduced absorption.[2] Further research is needed.

Importance and management

Evidence for an interaction between venlafaxine and indinavir is limited to two single-dose studies, one of which showed a slight decrease in indinavir exposure, which might reduce its efficacy. No pharmacokinetic interaction appears to occur with extended-release preparations of venlafaxine, however further study is required to establish this. A single dose of indinavir did not affect the pharmacokinetics of venlafaxine, but more study is needed to establish the effects of multiple doses, which are likely to have greater inhibitory effects on CYP3A4, leading to an increase in the exposure to venlafaxine. Other inhibitors of CYP3A4, including other **HIV-protease inhibitors** boosted with ritonavir are expected to interact similarly. Until more is known, it would seem prudent to monitor the concurrent use of venlafaxine with indinavir closely to ensure that indinavir remains efficacious, and to monitor concurrent use of venlafaxine with all **HIV-protease inhibitors** to ensure that the adverse effects of venlafaxine are not increased.

1. Jann MW, Spratlin V, Momary K, Zhang H, Turner D, Penzak SR, Wright A, VanDenBerg C. Lack of a pharmacokinetic drug-drug interaction with venlafaxine extended-release/indinavir and desvenlafaxine extended-release/indinavir. *Eur J Clin Pharmacol* (2012) 68, 715–21.
2. Levin GM, Nelson LA, DeVane CL, Preston SL, Eisele G, Carson SW. A pharmacokinetic drug-drug interaction study of venlafaxine and indinavir. *Psychopharmacol Bull* (2001) 35, 62–71.

HIV-protease inhibitors + Stiripentol

Stiripentol does not affect the pharmacokinetics of saquinavir.

Clinical evidence, mechanism, importance and management

In a crossover study in 12 healthy subjects,[1] stiripentol 1 g twice daily for 8 days had no effect on the pharmacokinetics of a single 400-mg dose of **saquinavir** given on day 8. Saquinavir is a substrate of CYP3A4, and *in vitro* stiripentol weakly inhibited its metabolism.[1] In addition, the manufacturer of stiripentol states that it might inhibit the metabolism of CYP3A4 substrates and states that caution is warranted on the concurrent use of HIV-protease inhibitors, see 'Stiripentol + Miscellaneous', p.614. However, this controlled study shows that no dose adjustment of unboosted saquinavir [now not recommended] is likely to be needed with the concurrent use of stiripentol. The effects of using saquinavir boosted with ritonavir with stiripentol have not been reported.

1. Cazali N, Tran A, Treluyer JM, Rey E, d'Athis P, Vincent J, Pons G. Inhibitory effect of stiripentol on carbamazepine and saquinavir metabolism in human. *Br J Clin Pharmacol* (2003) 56, 526–36.

HIV-protease inhibitors + Tenofovir

Atazanavir, darunavir, and lopinavir, all boosted with ritonavir, negligibly to slightly increase tenofovir exposure. Fosamprenavir, saquinavir, and tipranavir, all boosted with ritonavir, have no effect on tenofovir exposure. There is limited evidence of a possible greater risk of tenofovir-associated renal impairment when it is given with an HIV-protease inhibitor.

Tenofovir slightly decreases atazanavir exposure and has negligible to no effects on the exposure to darunavir, lopinavir, and tipranavir, all boosted with ritonavir. In contrast tenofovir slightly increased the exposure to saquinavir boosted with ritonavir in one study. No pharmacokinetic interaction occurs between tenofovir and indinavir or nelfinavir.

Clinical evidence

A. Pharmacokinetic studies

(a) Atazanavir

In a study in 33 subjects, tenofovir disoproxil fumarate 300 mg daily decreased the AUC and minimum plasma concentration of unboosted atazanavir 400 mg daily, taken for 14 days, by 25% and 40%, respectively. Atazanavir increased the AUC and minimum plasma concentration of tenofovir by 24% and 22%, respectively.[1] When atazanavir 300 mg daily was given with ritonavir 100 mg daily (as a pharmacokinetic booster) to 10 subjects for 42 days, the addition of tenofovir disoproxil fumarate 300 mg daily decreased the AUC of atazanavir by a similar amount (25%), but had less of an effect on the minimum plasma concentration (23% decrease), when compared with atazanavir boosted with ritonavir alone.[2] Similarly, in two studies in HIV-positive patients, the pharmacokinetics of atazanavir boosted with ritonavir did not differ appreciably between patients taking tenofovir and those not taking tenofovir.[3,4] In another study, taking atazanavir boosted with ritonavir 300/100 mg in the morning and tenofovir disoproxil fumarate 300 mg in the evening for 10 days decreased the AUC of atazanavir by 11% and increased the minimum plasma concentration by 20%. The AUC of tenofovir was increased by 37%, and its minimum plasma concentration was also increased, by 29%.[5] Simultaneous administration of tenofovir with atazanavir boosted with ritonavir at the higher dose of 400/100 mg daily increased the AUC of tenofovir by 55% and resulted in an atazanavir AUC that was 38% higher than with the standard dose of 300/100 mg daily.[5] In a study in pregnant women taking atazanavir boosted with ritonavir 300/100 mg daily, the AUC of atazanavir was below target during the third trimester in more women also receiving tenofovir (11 of 20) than women not receiving tenofovir (6 of 18).[6]

(b) Darunavir

In a study in 12 healthy subjects, the concurrent use of darunavir boosted with ritonavir 300/100 mg twice daily with tenofovir disoproxil fumarate 300 mg daily for 14 days increased the tenofovir AUC and minimum plasma concentration by 22% and 37%, respectively. The AUC of darunavir was increased by 21%, but this was not statistically significant. Tenofovir had no effect on the pharmacokinetics of ritonavir.[7] In a phase I pharmacokinetic study in 14 patients taking darunavir boosted with ritonavir with tenofovir and emtricitabine, starting raltegravir, and discontinuing tenofovir and emtricitabine, decreased the minimum plasma concentration of darunavir by 36%, which was attributed to the effect of tenofovir.[8]

(c) Fosamprenavir

The US manufacturer of fosamprenavir states that the minimum plasma concentration of amprenavir (derived from fosamprenavir) in 45 subjects receiving tenofovir disoproxil fumarate 300 mg daily with fosamprenavir boosted with ritonavir 700/100 mg twice daily and in 60 subjects receiving 1400/200 mg once daily for 4 to 48 weeks were similar to those in subjects not receiving tenofovir.[9] Similarly, in a pharmacokinetic study in 30 healthy subjects given fosamprenavir boosted with ritonavir 1400/100 mg daily or 1400/200 mg daily for 28 days, tenofovir disoproxil fumarate 300 mg daily (taken on days 15 to 28) had no effect on the pharmacokinetics of amprenavir.[10] In another study in healthy subjects, the AUC of amprenavir was increased by 16% and the tenofovir AUC was decreased by 7%, when tenofovir was given with fosamprenavir boosted with ritonavir 700/100 mg twice daily. Neither of these changes were statistically significant.[11]

For mention of a lack of association between use of fosamprenavir and tenofovir and renal adverse effects, see *Tenofovir-associated renal disease,* below.

(d) Indinavir

The UK and US manufacturers of tenofovir state that, in a study in 13 subjects, there was no change in the AUC of either tenofovir disoproxil fumarate 300 mg daily or indinavir 800 mg three times daily, when they were taken for 7 days.[12,13]

(e) Lopinavir

In a study in 24 healthy subjects, the concurrent use of lopinavir boosted with ritonavir 400/100 mg twice daily with tenofovir disoproxil fumarate 300 mg daily for 14 days, resulted in a 32% increase in the AUC and a 51% increase in the minimum plasma concentration of tenofovir, but no change in the clearance of tenofovir. The pharmacokinetics of lopinavir and ritonavir were unaffected by tenofovir.[14] Another study in 30 HIV-positive patients found that tenofovir renal clearance was 18% slower in patients taking lopinavir boosted with ritonavir compared with patients not taking HIV-protease inhibitors.[15] A study in 20 HIV-positive subjects found that concurrent use of tenofovir decreased the AUC and maximum plasma concentration of lopinavir by 26% and 28%, respectively. The AUC and maximum plasma concentration of ritonavir were also similarly affected by tenofovir, with decreases of 37% and 45%, respectively. However, the minimum plasma concentrations of both drugs were not notably decreased by tenofovir.[16]

For mention of a case report of Fanconi syndrome in a patient taking tenofovir and lopinavir boosted with ritonavir, and for a case review, see *Tenofovir-associated renal disease,* below.

(f) Nelfinavir

In a study in 29 healthy subjects, there was no pharmacokinetic interaction between tenofovir disoproxil fumarate 300 mg daily and unboosted nelfinavir 1.25 g twice daily, taken for 14 days.[17]

(g) Saquinavir

In a study in 35 healthy subjects, tenofovir disoproxil fumarate 300 mg daily increased the AUC and minimum plasma concentration of saquinavir by 29% and 47%, respectively, after administration of saquinavir boosted with ritonavir 1000/100 mg twice daily for 14 days. The minimum plasma concentration of ritonavir was also increased by 23%. The only change in tenofovir pharmacokinetics was a 23% increase in minimum plasma concentration.[18] In another study, in 18 HIV-positive patients taking saquinavir boosted with ritonavir 1000/100 mg twice daily and tenofovir disoproxil fumarate 300 mg daily, the AUC and maximum plasma concentration of saquinavir did not differ from those seen with saquinavir boosted with ritonavir alone.[19]

(h) Tipranavir

In a study in 22 subjects, tipranavir boosted with ritonavir 500/100 mg twice daily had no effect on the AUC and minimum plasma concentration of a single 300-mg dose of tenofovir disoproxil fumarate, but it decreased the maximum plasma concentration of tenofovir by 23%. The tipranavir AUC and minimum plasma concentration were decreased by 18% and 21%, respectively. With an increased dose of tipranavir boosted with ritonavir 750/200 mg twice daily, taken for 23 doses, the maximum plasma concentration of tenofovir was decreased by 38% with no notable change in the AUC, and the minimum plasma concentration was increased by 14%. The decreases in the AUC of tipranavir and its minimum plasma concentration (12%) were smaller than those seen with the lower dose of tipranavir boosted with ritonavir.[20]

B. Tenofovir-associated renal disease

In one analysis, 34% (26 of 77) of patients receiving tenofovir developed decreased renal function, although the magnitude of the decrease (greater than 15% from baseline) was considered small. However, in an adjusted analysis of baseline HIV-1 loads, the odds of developing an important decrease in renal function among tenofovir-treated patients was 3.7 times higher if an HIV-protease inhibitor boosted with ritonavir was also given than if an NNRTI was also given. Creatinine clearance did not correlate with tenofovir plasma concentrations.[21] Similarly, in another prospective observational cohort study, a greater median decrease in estimated glomerular filtration rate was reported in patients given tenofovir with HIV-protease inhibitors (boosted with ritonavir) than in patients given tenofovir with an NNRTI.[22] In another study, use of tenofovir with an HIV-protease inhibitor was associated with a 2.12-fold increased risk of a 25% decrease in glomerular filtration rate in patients of low body-weight (median 56.5 kg).[23] An observational cohort study[24] in 445 HIV-positive patients taking tenofovir reported that the concurrent use of **amprenavir** (with **ritonavir**) was associated with an increased risk of tenofovir-induced renal failure (odds ratio 3.6). Conversely, another cohort study of 1 428 HIV-positive patients including 105 patients taking tenofovir and **fosamprenavir** found no statistically significant decrease in renal function with concurrent use, and the use of HIV-protease inhibitors boosted with ritonavir did not increase the risk of renal adverse effects.[25]

In one review of 27 patients with tenofovir-associated acute and chronic kidney disease, the most common drugs given with tenofovir were **ritonavir** or **lopinavir** boosted with ritonavir (21 patients), didanosine (9 patients), and **atazanavir** (5 patients).[26] Note that, it is not possible to conclude that these drugs contributed to the kidney disease without a control group.[27] Conversely, other studies have reported that none of 94 patients receiving tenofovir developed tenofovir-related renal failure or kidney disease, including 36 receiving HIV-protease inhibitors boosted with ritonavir; namely,**lopinavir** (25), **atazanavir** (6), **tipranavir** (3), and **amprenavir** (2).[28]

A case report describes Fanconi syndrome with nephrogenic diabetes insipidus, which developed in a patient taking **lopinavir** boosted with ritonavir 800/200 mg daily, tenofovir disoproxil fumarate 300 mg daily, didanosine, and lamivudine. The tenofovir plasma concentration was 3.7-fold higher than expected and the didanosine plasma concentration was 8-fold higher than it had been before tenofovir was started. Plasma lopinavir concentrations were unchanged.[29]

Mechanism

Unknown. It has been suggested that ritonavir increases tenofovir exposure via its effect on drug transporter proteins, such as P-glycoprotein, in the renal tubuli.[29,30] However, an *in vitro* study found that most HIV-protease inhibitors have low or minimal effects on the renal excretion of tenofovir. The authors of this study instead suggest that an interaction might occur in the intestine, as tenofovir and most HIV-protease inhibitors are substrates for intestinal P-glycoprotein.[31] Another *in vitro* study reported that the overall increase in tenofovir exposure by some HIV-protease inhibitors was due to a combination of different mechanisms including inhibition of tenofovir hydrolysis in intestinal tissue, inhibition of P-glycoprotein-mediated tenofovir efflux, and induction of P-glycoprotein expression by the HIV-protease inhibitors.[32] The reason for the changes in HIV-protease inhibitor concentrations with tenofovir is unknown.

Importance and management

The negligible to slight increase in tenofovir exposure seen with **atazanavir**, **darunavir**, and **lopinavir**, all boosted with ritonavir, is unlikely to be of general clinical relevance. However, there is some evidence that the combination might be associated with a greater risk of tenofovir-associated renal impairment. For this reason, various manufacturers of tenofovir and these HIV-protease inhibitors state that adverse reactions and renal function should be closely monitored when any of these HIV-protease inhibitors boosted with ritonavir are given with tenofovir, and this seems a prudent precaution. The decrease in atazanavir concentrations with tenofovir is not of clinical importance if ritonavir is also used as a booster, and the standard dose of atazanavir boosted with ritonavir of 300/100 mg daily is recommended when it is given with tenofovir.[1] In addition, there is not expected to be any advantage in separating the dose of atazanavir boosted with ritonavir from tenofovir, and they can be given simultaneously.[5] However, in pregnant women given tenofovir, it might be necessary to increase the dose of atazanavir boosted with ritonavir to 400/100 mg daily,[6] which is recommended by the UK and US manufacturers of atazanavir.[1,33] The US manufacturers of atazanavir and tenofovir state that unboosted atazanavir should not be given with tenofovir because of the potential for reduced efficacy and development of resistance.[1,12] There is no clinically relevant change in the plasma concentrations of darunavir or lopinavir, both boosted with ritonavir, when given with tenofovir.

There is no clinically relevant pharmacokinetic interaction between tenofovir and **fosamprenavir** boosted with ritonavir. Similarly, the increase in the concentrations of **saquinavir** (boosted with ritonavir) and the minor decrease in the concentration of **tipranavir** (boosted with ritonavir) are not likely to be clinically relevant. No dose adjustment is needed when any of these HIV-protease inhibitors boosted with ritonavir are given with tenofovir. There is no clinically relevant interaction between **nelfinavir** or **indinavir** and tenofovir.

Note that, tenofovir (with emtricitabine) is a recommended NRTI backbone choice in the UK and US guidelines for starting antiretrovirals in treatment-naive patients, when it is given with an HIV-protease inhibitor boosted with ritonavir.[34,35] Current local and national guidelines should be consulted for restrictions for its use and details of the HIV-protease inhibitors it can be combined with.

1. Reyataz (Atazanavir sulfate). Bristol-Myers Squibb. US Prescribing information, March 2012.
2. Taburet A-M, Piketty C, Chazallon C, Vincent I, Gérard L, Calvez V, Clavel F, Aboulker J-P, Girard P-M, and the ANRS Protocol 107 Puzzle 2 Investigators. Interactions between atazanavir-ritonavir and tenofovir in heavily pretreated human immunodeficiency virus-infected patients. *Antimicrob Agents Chemother* (2004) 48, 2091–6.
3. Hentig NV, Haberl A, Lutz T, Klauke S, Kurowski M, Harder S, Staszewski S. Concomitant intake of tenofovir disoproxil fumarate (TDF) does not impair plasma exposure of ritonavir (RTV) boosted atazanavir (ATV) in HIV-1 infected adults. *Clin Pharmacol Ther* (2005) 77, P18.
4. von Hentig N, Dauer B, Haberl A, Klauke S, Lutz T, Staszewski S, Harder S. Tenofovir comedication does not impair the steady-state pharmacokinetics of ritonavir-boosted atazanavir in HIV-1 infected adults. *Eur J Clin Pharmacol* (2007) 63, 935–40.
5. Agarwala S, Eley T, Villegas C, Wang Y, Hughes E, Xie J, Grasela D. Pharmacokinetic interaction between tenofovir and atazanavir coadministered with ritonavir in healthy subjects. 6th International Workshop on Clinical Pharmacology of HIV Therapy, Quebec, April 2005, abstract 16.
6. Mirochnick M, Best BM, Stek AM, Capparelli EV, Hu C, Burchett SK, Rossi SS, Hawkins E, Basar M, Smith E, Read JS; IMPAACT 1026s Study Team. Atazanavir pharmacokinetics with and without tenofovir during pregnancy. *J Acquir Immune Defic Syndr* (2011) 56, 412–19.
7. Hoetelmans RMW, Mariën K, De Pauw M, Hill A, Peeters M, Sekar V, De Doncker P, Woodfall B, Lefebvre E. Pharmacokinetic interaction between TCM114/ritonavir and tenofovir disoproxil fumarate in healthy volunteers. *Br J Clin Pharmacol* (2007) 64, 655–61.
8. Garvey L, Latch N, Erlwein OW, Mackie NE, Walsh J, Scullard G, McClure MO, Dickinson L, Back D, Winston A. The effects of a nucleoside-sparing antiretroviral regimen on the pharmacokinetics of ritonavir-boosted darunavir in HIV type-1-infected patients. *Antivir Ther* (2010)15, 213–18.
9. Lexiva (Fosamprenavir calcium). ViiV Healthcare. US Prescribing information, April 2013.
10. Kurowski M, Walli RK, Breske A, Kruse G, Stocker H, Banik N, Richter H, Mazur D. Fosamprenavir/ritonavir plus tenofovir does not affect amprenavir pharmacokinetics: no effect of tenofovir. *AIDS* (2007) 21, 1368–70.
11. Luber AD, Condoluci DV, Slowinski PD, Andrews M, Olson K, Peloquin CA, Pappa KA, Pakes GE; COL104422 Study Team. Steady-state amprenavir and tenofovir pharmacokinetics after coadministration of unboosted or ritonavir-boosted fosamprenavir with tenofovir disoproxil fumarate in healthy volunteers. *HIV Med* (2010) 11, 193–9.
12. Viread (Tenofovir disoproxil fumarate). Gilead Sciences, Inc. US Prescribing information, August 2012.
13. Viread (Tenofovir disoproxil fumarate). Gilead Sciences Ltd. UK Summary of product characteristics, January 2012.
14. Kearney BP, Mathias A, Mittan A, Sayre J, Ebrahimi R, Cheng AK. Pharmacokinetics and safety of tenofovir disoproxil fumarate on coadministration with lopinavir/ritonavir. *J Acquir Immune Defic Syndr* (2006) 43, 278–83.
15. Kiser JJ, Carten ML, Aquilante CL, Anderson PL, Wolfe P, King TM, Delahunty T, Bushman LR, Fletcher CV. The effect of lopinavir/ritonavir on the renal clearance of tenofovir in HIV-infected patients. *Clin Pharmacol Ther* (2008) 83, 265–72.
16. Ofotokun I, Chuck SK, Binongo JN, Palau M, Lennox JL, Acosta EP. Lopinavir/ritonavir pharmacokinetic profile: impact of sex and other covariates following change from twice-daily to once-daily therapy. *J Clin Pharmacol* (2007) 47, 970–7.
17. Boffito M, Pozniak A, Kearney BP, Higgs C, Mathias A, Zhong L, Shah J. Lack of pharmacokinetic drug interaction between tenofovir disoproxil fumarate and nelfinavir mesylate. *Antimicrob Agents Chemother* (2005) 49, 4386–9.
18. Chittick GE, Zong J, Blum MR, Sorbel JJ, Begley JA, Adda N, Kearney BP. Pharmacokinetics of tenofovir disoproxil fumarate and ritonavir-boosted saquinavir mesylate administered alone or in combination at steady state. *Antimicrob Agents Chemother* (2006) 50, 1304–10.
19. Boffito M, Back D, Stainsby-Tron M, Hill A, Di Perri G, Moyle G, Nelson M, Tomkins J, Gazzard B, Pozniak A. Pharmacokinetics of saquinavir hard gel/ritonavir (1000/100 mg twice daily) when administered with tenofovir diproxil [sic] fumarate in HIV-1-infected subjects. *Br J Clin Pharmacol* (2005) 59, 38–42.
20. Aptivus (Tipranavir). Boehringer Ingelheim Pharmaceuticals, Inc. US Prescribing information, April 2012.
21. Goicoechea M, Liu S, Best B, Sun S, Jain S, Kemper C, Witt M, Diamond C, Haubrich R, Louie S; California Collaborative Treatment Group 578 Team. Greater tenofovir-associated renal function decline with protease inhibitor-based versus nonnucleoside reverse-transcriptase inhibitor-based therapy. *J Infect Dis* (2008) 197, 102–8.
22. Gallant JE, Moore RD. Renal function with use of a tenofovir-containing initial antiretroviral regimen. *AIDS* (2009) 23, 1971–5.
23. Chaisiri K, Bowonwatanuwong C, Kasettratat N, Kiertiburanakul S. Incidence and risk factors for tenofovir-associated renal function decline among Thai HIV-infected patients with low-body weight. *Curr HIV Res* (2010) 8, 504–9.
24. Crane HM, Kestenbaum B, Harrington RD, Kitahata MM. Amprenavir and didanosine are associated with declining kidney function among patients receiving tenofovir. *AIDS* (2007) 21, 1431–9.
25. Pedrol E, Deig E. Reply to Crane *et al*., 'Amprenavir and didanosine are associated with declining kidney function among patients receiving tenofovir'. *AIDS* (2007) 21, 2566.
26. Zimmermann AE, Pizzoferrato T, Bedford J, Morris A, Hoffman R, Braden G. Tenofovir-associated acute and chronic kidney disease: a case of multiple drug interactions. *Clin Infect Dis* (2006) 42, 283–90.
27. Winston JA, Shepp DH. The role of drug interactions and monitoring in the prevention of tenofovir-associated kidney disease. *Clin Infect Dis* (2006) 42, 1657–8.
28. Lanzafame M, Lattuada E, Rapagna F, Gottardi M, Vento S. Tenofovir-associated kidney diseases and interactions between tenofovir and other antiretrovirals. *Clin Infect Dis* (2006) 42, 1656–7.
29. Rollot F, Nazal E-M, Chauvelot-Moachon L, Kélaïdi C, Daniel N, Saba M, Abad S, Blanche P. Tenofovir-related Fanconi syndrome with nephrogenic diabetes insipidus in a patient with acquired immunodeficiency syndrome: the role of lopinavir-ritonavir-didanosine. *Clin Infect Dis* (2003) 37, e174–e176.
30. Prezista (Darunavir ethanolate). Janssen-Cilag Ltd. UK Summary of product characteristics, June 2012.
31. Cihlar T, Ray AS, Laflamme G, Vela JE, Tong L, Fuller MD, Roy A, Rhodes GR. Molecular assessment of the potential for renal drug interactions between tenofovir and HIV protease inhibitors. *Antivir Ther* (2007) 12, 267–72.
32. Tong L, Phan TK, Robinson KL, Babusis D, Strab R, Bhoopathy S, Hidalgo IJ, Rhodes GR, Ray AS. Effects of human immunodeficiency virus protease inhibitors on the intestinal absorption of tenofovir disoproxil fumarate in vitro. *Antimicrob Agents Chemother* (2007) 51, 3498–3504.
33. Reyataz (Atazanavir sulphate). Bristol-Myers Squibb Pharmaceuticals Ltd. UK Summary of product characteristics, August 2012.
34. Williams I, Churchill D, Anderson J, Boffito M, Bower M, Cairns G, Cwynarski K, Edwards S, Fidler S, Fisher M, Freedman A, Geretti AM, Gilleece Y, Horne R, Johnson M, Khoo S, Leen C, Marshall N, Nelson M, Orkin C, Paton N, Phillips A, Post F, Pozniak A, Sabin C, Trevelion R, Ustianowski A, Walsh J, Waters L, Wilkins E, Winston A, Youle M. British HIV Association guidelines for the treatment of HIV-1-positive adults with antiretroviral therapy 2012 (Updated 2013). *HIV Med* (2014), 15 (Suppl 1) 1–85.
35. Panel on Antiretroviral Guidelines for Adults and Adolescents. Guidelines for the use of antiretroviral agents in HIV-1-infected adults and adolescents. US Department of Health and Human Services (April 2015). 1–288. Available at: http://www.aidsinfo.nih.gov/ContentFiles/AdultandAdolescentGL.pdf (accessed 23/09/15).

HIV-protease inhibitors + Valproate

Lopinavir exposure appeared to be increased by valproic acid in one study in HIV-positive patients, whereas the plasma concentration of valproic acid did not appear to be appreciably affected by lopinavir boosted with ritonavir. However, in one case, starting an antiretroviral regimen including lopinavir boosted with ritonavir decreased the valproic acid plasma concentration, which resulted in an exacerbation of mania. Hepatotoxicity has occurred in a patient taking valproic acid with nevirapine and saquinavir boosted with ritonavir.

Clinical evidence

(a) Lopinavir

In a study in 8 HIV-positive patients taking lopinavir boosted with ritonavir 400/100 mg twice daily with various NRTIs, the median AUC of lopinavir increased by 75% without any change in the estimated half-life after they took valproic acid 250 mg twice daily for 7 days. Although the maximum and minimum lopinavir plasma concentrations were also higher, the difference was not statistically significant. Ritonavir plasma concentrations were not assessed. Valproic acid plasma concentrations achieved in the patients taking lopinavir boosted with ritonavir were not statistically significantly different from those in 11 HIV-positive control patients mainly taking NRTIs, even when the 3 patients taking a HIV-protease inhibitor or NNRTI (amprenavir, indinavir, or nelfinavir with nevirapine) were excluded, although they did tend to be lower.[1] However, one report describes a decrease in the plasma concentration of valproate in a 30-year-old man after he started taking lopinavir boosted with ritonavir.[2] This patient, who had been taking valproic acid 375 mg daily as valproate semisodium (divalproex sodium) for 7 months after an episode of mania, had a subtherapeutic valproic acid plasma concentration of 197 micromol/L. The dose was increased to 250 mg three times daily and after 25 days his minimum valproic acid plasma concentration had increased to 495 micromol/L. He was then started on an antiretroviral regimen of lamivudine, zidovudine, and lopinavir boosted with ritonavir, and paroxetine for depression. Four days later he was hypomanic and the paroxetine was replaced with sertraline, which the patient discontinued. Twenty-one days later he had become increasingly manic, and the valproic acid plasma concentration was found to be 238 micromol/L, about 50% lower than the previous concentration. An increase in the valproic acid dose to 1.5 g daily was eventually required to achieve a therapeutic plasma concentration of 392 micromol/L.

(b) Saquinavir with ritonavir

A case of valproate-associated hepatotoxicity occurred in a 51-year-old man about 3 weeks after he started taking nevirapine 200 mg twice daily, saquinavir 400 mg twice daily, ritonavir 400 mg twice daily, and stavudine. The valproic acid serum concentration remained therapeutic.[3]

Mechanism

Ritonavir, and possibly lopinavir, might decrease the plasma concentration of valproic acid by induction of glucuronidation.

Importance and management

It has been predicted that ritonavir might reduce the plasma concentration of valproate,[4,5] but the case report[2] appears to be the first clinical evidence of this occurring. Other evidence from the earlier study[1] suggested valproate plasma concentrations were not affected to a statistically significant extent by ritonavir, although there was a downward trend in valproic acid plasma concentrations. However, the authors subsequently noted that this study used a low-dose of valproate and that a more clinically significant interaction might occur with higher doses of valproate.[6] In addition, this study unexpectedly found that lopinavir plasma concentrations appeared to be higher in patients taking valproic acid, although the increase is probably not clinically relevant.[1] If possible, monitor the valproate plasma concentration when any antiretroviral regimen that includes ritonavir is used. Further study is needed. Note that there has been some concern about using valproate in HIV infection, but there seems to be no established reason to avoid or specifically promote the use of valproate in HIV-infection *per se*.

1. DiCenzo R, Peterson D, Cruttenden K, Morse G, Riggs G, Gelbard H, Schifitto G. Effects of valproic acid coadministration on plasma efavirenz and lopinavir concentrations in human immunodeficiency virus-infected adults. *Antimicrob Agents Chemother* (2004) 48, 4328–31.
2. Sheehan NL, Brouillette M-J, Delisle M-S, Allan J. Possible interaction between lopinavir/ritonavir and valproic acid exacerbates bipolar disorder. *Ann Pharmacother* (2006) 40, 147–50.
3. Cozza KL, Swanton EJ, Humphreys CW. Hepatotoxicity with combination of valproic acid, ritonavir, and nevirapine: a case report. *Psychosomatics* (2000) 41, 452–3.
4. Norvir Tablets (Ritonavir). AbbVie Ltd. UK Summary of product characteristics, September 2012.
5. Norvir Tablets and Solution (Ritonavir). Abbott Laboratories. US Prescribing information, October 2012.
6. DiCenzo R, Peterson DR, Cruttenden K, Mariuz P, Rezk NL, Hochreiter J, Gelbard H, Schifitto G. Effects of minocycline and valproic acid coadministration on atazanavir plasma concentrations in human immunodeficiency virus-infected adults receiving atazanavir-ritonavir. *Antimicrob Agents Chemother* (2008) 52, 3035–9.

HIV-protease inhibitors; Fosamprenavir + Miscellaneous

Fosamprenavir is a prodrug of amprenavir, and is rapidly and almost completely hydrolysed to amprenavir and inorganic phosphate primarily in the lining of the gut.[1,2] The interactions of fosamprenavir are therefore primarily those of amprenavir.

1. Telzir (Fosamprenavir calcium). ViiV Healthcare UK Ltd. UK Summary of product characteristics, May 2011.
2. Lexiva (Fosamprenavir calcium). ViiV Healthcare. US Prescribing information, April 2013.

HIV-protease inhibitors; Indinavir + Ascorbic acid (Vitamin C)

Ascorbic acid (vitamin C) caused a negligible decrease in indinavir exposure in healthy subjects.

Clinical evidence, mechanism, importance and management

In a study[1] in healthy subjects, high-dose vitamin C 1 g daily for 7 days caused a 14% reduction in the AUC of indinavir 800 mg taken every 8 hours (4 doses beginning on day 6) and a 20% reduction in its maximum plasma concentration. However, whether this is a real effect needs further study as a similar reduction in plasma concentrations after a similar indinavir regimen was thought to be a time-dependent effect, see 'HIV-protease inhibitors; Indinavir + Milk thistle', below. No recommendations can therefore be made based on this isolated report.

1. Slain D, Amsden JR, Khakoo RA, Fisher MA, Lalka D, Hobbs GR. Effect of high-dose vitamin C on the steady-state pharmacokinetics of the protease inhibitor indinavir in healthy volunteers. *Pharmacotherapy* (2005) 25, 165–70.

HIV-protease inhibitors; Indinavir + Goldenseal (*Hydrastis*)

Goldenseal root had no clinically relevant effect on the pharmacokinetics of a single dose of indinavir in one study.

Clinical evidence

In a study in 10 healthy subjects, the maximum plasma concentration and oral clearance of indinavir after a single 800-mg dose was not changed by goldenseal root (*Nature's Way*) 1.14 g twice daily for 2 weeks. In addition, there was no change in the indinavir half-life. Eight of the subjects had less than a 20% change in oral clearance, but one subject had a 46% increase and one a 46% decrease.[1]

Mechanism

Goldenseal (*Hydrastis canadensis*) was found to be an inhibitor of CYP3A4 *in vitro.*[2] This was confirmed in a clinical study using oral midazolam as a probe substrate for CYP3A4, which found a decrease of about 40% in the metabolism of midazolam to hydroxymidazolam.[3] Goldenseal root might therefore have been expected to inhibit the metabolism of indinavir.

Importance and management

This study suggests that goldenseal root has no effect on indinavir exposure, and that no clinically relevant pharmacokinetic interaction would therefore be expected on the concurrent use of this HIV-protease inhibitor.

1. Sandhu RS, Prescilla RP, Simonelli TM, Edwards DJ. Influence of goldenseal root on the pharmacokinetics of indinavir. *J Clin Pharmacol* (2003) 43, 1283–8.
2. Budzinski JW, Foster BC, Vandenhoek S, Arnason JT. An in vitro evaluation of human cytochrome P450 3A4 inhibition by selected commercial herbal extracts and tinctures. *Phytomedicine* (2000) 7, 273–82.
3. Gurley BJ, Gardner SF, Hubbard MA, Williams DK, Gentry WB, Khan IA, Shah A. In vivo effects of goldenseal, kava kava, black cohosh, and valerian on human cytochrome P450 1A2, 2D6, 2E1, and 3A4/5 phenotypes. *Clin Pharmacol Ther* (2005) 77, 415–26.

HIV-protease inhibitors; Indinavir + Influenza vaccines

The pharmacokinetics of indinavir are not affected by influenza vaccination.

Clinical evidence, mechanism, importance and management

In a study, influenza whole virus vaccine was given to 9 patients taking indinavir-based antiretroviral therapy. No apparent changes were found in indinavir pharmacokinetics.[1] Therefore, no special precautions appear to be necessary on concurrent use.

1. Maserati R, Villani P, Barasolo G, Mongiovetti M, Regazzi MB. Influenza immunization and indinavir pharmacokinetics. *Scand J Infect Dis* (2000) 32, 449–50.

HIV-protease inhibitors; Indinavir + Interleukin-2

Indinavir exposure is increased by interleukin-2.

Clinical evidence, mechanism, importance and management

In a pharmacokinetic study in 9 HIV-positive patients, the subjects continued taking their usual antiretrovirals and were given a 4-week course of indinavir 800 mg three times daily followed by infusions of 3 to 12 million units of interleukin-2, daily for 5 days. The AUC of indinavir increased in 8 of the 9 subjects (average increase 88%). During this time interleukin-6 was also elevated, so it was thought that the increased indinavir exposure was due to the inhibitory effects of interleukin-6 on CYP3A4. An increase in the minimum plasma concentration of indinavir was also seen in a further 8 patients not participating in the pharmacokinetic study.[1] Although this appears to be the only evidence regarding an interaction between interleukins and indinavir it might be prudent to monitor for indinavir adverse effects if both drugs are given.

1. Piscitelli SC, Vogel S, Figg WD, Raje S, Forrest A, Metcalf JA, Baseler M, Falloon J. Alteration in indinavir clearance during interleukin-2 infusions in patients infected with the human immunodeficiency virus. *Pharmacotherapy* (1998) 18, 1212–16.

HIV-protease inhibitors; Indinavir + Milk thistle

Milk thistle does not appear to have an important effect on the pharmacokinetics of indinavir.

Clinical evidence

Milk thistle (*Silybum marianum*) 175 mg three times daily (*Thisilyn; Nature's Way,* standardised for 80% silymarin content) for 3 weeks caused a 9% reduction in the AUC of indinavir and a 25% reduction its minimum plasma concentration after four doses of indinavir 800 mg every 8 hours, but only the value for the minimum plasma concentration reached statistical significance.[1] The authors suggested that the effect on the minimum plasma concentration could represent a time-dependent effect of indinavir pharmacokinetics, as the plasma concentrations without milk thistle were found to be similarly lowered after a washout phase.[1] In another similar study, in 10 healthy subjects, milk thistle standardised for silymarin 160 mg (*General Nutrition Corp.*) three times daily for 13 days and then with indinavir 800 mg every 8 hours for 4 doses did not cause any statistically significant changes in the indinavir pharmacokinetics (6% reduction in AUC and 32% reduction in minimum plasma concentration).[2] In yet another similar study, in 8 healthy subjects, milk thistle extract 456 mg, standardised for silymarins (*Kare and Hope Ltd*) three times daily for 28 days had no effect on the pharmacokinetics of indinavir 800 mg every 8 hours for four doses when compared with 6 subjects in a control group not receiving milk thistle extract. Both the control and indinavir group had a lower AUC of indinavir after the second and third time of administration compared with the first, and this decline was greater in the control group.[3] A meta-analysis of these three studies showed no effect of milk thistle on indinavir concentrations.[3]

Mechanism

Based on *animal* data, milk thistle might be expected to increase the plasma concentration of indinavir by inhibiting its metabolism,[1] or to have effects via P-glycoprotein.[2]

Importance and management

The available data suggest that milk thistle extract does not have an effect on the pharmacokinetics of indinavir, although it is not totally conclusive. The reduction in the minimum plasma concentration of indinavir appears to be a time-dependent effect rather than an effect of the milk thistle, and further study is needed with longer exposure to indinavir than just four doses. Evidence appears to be too slim to prohibit concurrent use, but until more is known it might be prudent to give milk thistle cautiously to patients taking indinavir.

1. Piscitelli SC, Formentini E, Burstein AH, Alfaro R, Jagannatha S, Falloon J. Effect of milk thistle on the pharmacokinetics of indinavir in healthy volunteers. *Pharmacotherapy* (2002) 22, 551–6.
2. DiCenzo R, Shelton M, Jordan K, Koval C, Forrest A, Reichman R, Morse G. Coadministration of milk thistle and indinavir in healthy subjects. *Pharmacotherapy* (2003) 23, 866–70.
3. Mills E, Wilson K, Clarke M, Foster B, Walker S, Rachlis B, DeGroot N, Montori VM, Gold W, Phillips E, Myers S, Gallicano K. Milk thistle and indinavir: a randomized controlled pharmacokinetics study and meta-analysis. *Eur J Clin Pharmacol* (2005) 61, 1–7.

HIV-protease inhibitors; Nelfinavir + Calcium compounds

Calcium supplements do not appear to affect the plasma concentration of nelfinavir.

Clinical evidence, mechanism, importance and management

Calcium supplements had no apparent effect on the plasma concentrations of nelfinavir or its M8 metabolite in 15 patients receiving nelfinavir 1.25 g twice daily as part of a HAART regimen. Calcium was given as calcium carbonate 1.35 g twice daily to 9 patients, and as calcium gluconate with calcium carbonate 2.95 g/300 mg twice daily to 6 patients, both for 14 days. The plasma concentration of nelfinavir was measured before a dose and 3 hours after a dose.[1] Similar results were reported in another study.[2] No nelfinavir dose adjustments appear necessary if calcium supplements are given.

1. Jensen-Fangel S, Justesen US, Black FT, Pedersen C, Obel N. The use of calcium carbonate in nelfinavir-associated diarrhoea in HIV-1-infected patients. *HIV Med* (2003) 4, 48–52.
2. Kopp Hutzler B, Perez-Rodriguez E, Norton S, Hsyu PH. Pharmacokinetics (PK) interactions between nelfinavir (NFV) and calcium supplements (P277). *AIDS* (2000) 14 (Suppl 4), S96.

HIV-protease inhibitors; Nelfinavir + Pancreatic enzymes

Pancreatic enzyme supplements appear not to alter nelfinavir pharmacokinetics.

Clinical evidence, mechanism, importance and management

In a study in 9 HIV-positive subjects, the concurrent use of pancreatic enzymes (pancrelipase 20 000 USP units, amylase 65 000 USP units, and protease 65 000 USP units) and nelfinavir 1.25 g twice daily for 14 days resulted in no changes in the pharmacokinetics of nelfinavir.[1]

1. Price J, Shalit P, Carlsen J, Becker MI, Frye J, Hsyu P. Pharmacokinetic interaction between Ultrase® MT-20 and nelfinavir in HIV-infected individuals. *Intersci Conf Antimicrob Agents Chemother* (1999) 39, 20.

Influenza vaccines + Paracetamol (Acetaminophen)

Paracetamol does not affect antibody production in response to influenza vaccination, and might possibly reduce the adverse effects of influenza vaccination. The pharmacokinetics of paracetamol do not appear to be affected by influenza vaccination.

Clinical evidence, mechanism, importance and management

In a study in healthy subjects, the pharmacokinetics of a single 650-mg dose of intravenous paracetamol were unaffected when it was given 7 and 21 days after 0.5 mL of trivalent influenza vaccine given intramuscularly.[1] Paracetamol 1 g four times daily for 2 days had no effect on the production of influenza virus antibodies in a group of 39 elderly patients given an inactivated influenza virus vaccine, and paracetamol appeared to reduce the adverse effects of the vaccine (e.g. fever), although this was not statistically significant.[2]

In a placebo-controlled study, 262 healthy subjects were given a single 0.5-mL intramuscular dose of inactivated, trivalent, whole-virus influenza vaccine with paracetamol 325 mg or 650 mg given at the same time as the influenza vaccine and then every 4 hours for a total of 4 doses. The incidence of sore arm at the vaccination site was reduced by 25% and 28% in the subjects given the lower and higher dose of paracetamol, respectively. The concurrent use of paracetamol also reduced the incidence of vaccine-related nausea by 20% and 90% in those subjects given the lower and higher dose of paracetamol, respectively. However, paracetamol had no statistically significant effect on other vaccine-related adverse effects such as fever, headache, and muscle pain. Paracetamol did not appear to affect the antibody response to the vaccine, as no difference in the haemagglutination inhibition antibody was reported between the placebo and paracetamol groups.[3]

From the limited data available, no special precautions appear to be necessary on the concurrent use of paracetamol and influenza vaccine.

1. Scavone JM, Blyden GT, Greenblatt DJ. Lack of effect of influenza vaccine on the pharmacokinetics of antipyrine, alprazolam, paracetamol (acetaminophen) and lorazepam. *Clin Pharmacokinet* (1989) 16, 180–5.
2. Gross PA, Levandowski RA, Russo C, Weksler M, Bonelli J, Dran S, Munk G, Deichmiller S, Hilsen R, Panush RF. Vaccine immune response and side effects with the use of acetaminophen with influenza vaccine. *Clin Diagn Lab Immunol* (1994) 1, 134–8.
3. Aoki FY, Yassi A, Cheang M, Math M, Murdzak C, Hammond GW, Sekla LH, Wright B. Effects of acetaminophen on adverse effects of influenza vaccination in health care workers. *Can Med Assoc J* (1993) 149, 1425–30.

Influenza vaccine; Live + Antivirals active against influenza

The UK and US manufacturers state that antivirals active against influenza such as oseltamivir, rimantadine, and zanamivir should not be given until 2 weeks after the administration of *live* influenza virus vaccines, and that these vaccines should not be given until 48 hours after stopping the antiviral.[1-5] This is because of the theoretical concern that these antiviral drugs will inhibit replication of live vaccine virus, and therefore reduce its effect. Note that most influenza vaccines are inactivated (split virion or surface antigen), and that these would not be expected to be affected by antivirals active against influenza.

1. FluMist (Influenza virus vaccine live, intranasal). MedImmune Vaccines, Inc. US Prescribing information, July 2014.
2. Tamiflu (Oseltamivir phosphate). Roche Pharmaceuticals. US Prescribing information, May 2014.
3. Flumadine (Rimantadine hydrochloride). Forest Pharmaceuticals, Inc. US Prescribing information, April 2010.
4. Relenza (Zanamivir). GlaxoSmithKline. US Prescribing information, October 2013.
5. Fluenz Tetra (Influenza virus vaccine live, intranasal). Astra Zeneca. UK Summary of product characteristics, August 2014.

Influenza vaccine; Live + Aspirin

The UK and US manufacturers state that *live* influenza vaccines should not be given to children or adolescents who are given aspirin. This possible interaction is linked to the association of Reye's syndrome with aspirin and wild-type influenza infection. Concurrent use is contraindicated.[1,2]

1. Fluenz Tetra (Influenza virus vaccine live, intranasal). Astra Zeneca. UK Summary of product characteristics, August 2014.
2. FluMist (Influenza virus vaccine live, intranasal). MedImmune Vaccines, Inc. US Prescribing information, July 2014.

Interferons + ACE inhibitors

A case series suggests that severe granulocytopenia can develop if ACE inhibitors and interferon are given concurrently.

Clinical evidence

Patients with cryoglobulinaemia were treated with 3 million units of recombinant **interferon alfa-2a** (35 patients) or natural **interferon beta** (3 patients), usually given daily for 3 months, then on alternate days for periods of 6 to 17 months. Severe toxicity developed in 3 patients, who were the only ones amongst the group to also be taking ACE inhibitors. Granulocytopenia developed in 2 patients within a few days of starting **enalapril** 10 mg daily or **captopril** 50 mg daily, and subsided 1 to 2 weeks after both drugs were stopped. Another patient, already taking **enalapril** 5 mg daily, developed severe granulocytopenia when interferon was started, and again when rechallenged with both drugs. None of the other 35 patients receiving interferon alone developed any clinically important haematological problems. The reasons for this severe reaction are not understood but the authors of the report suggest that it might be an autoimmune response.[1]

A follow-up letter commenting on this report described 2 further patients with hepatitis C infection, cryoglobulinaemia, and glomerulonephritis, who took **captopril** 75 mg or **enalapril** 20 mg daily for several weeks, and who had granulocytopenia within 9 days of being given 3 million units of recombinant **interferon alfa-2a**, daily or on alternate days. However, this resolved without any change in treatment. Another patient with multiple myeloma given **interferon alfa-2a** 3 million units three times weekly and long-term **benazepril** 10 mg daily had a normal granulocyte count after 3 months.[2]

Mechanism

Interferons alone are associated with myelosuppression, particularly granulocytopenia. ACE inhibitors have, rarely, caused neutropenia and agranulocytosis.

Importance and management

These two reports appear to be the only information suggesting an interaction. Regular full blood counts are generally recommended when interferons are used, and therefore, no extra precautions would appear to be required if ACE inhibitors are also given.

1. Casato M, Pucillo LP, Leoni M, di Lullo L, Gabrielli A, Sansonno D, Dammacco F, Danieli G, Bonomo L. Granulocytopenia after combined therapy with interferon and angiotensin-converting enzyme inhibitors: evidence for a synergistic hematologic toxicity. *Am J Med* (1995) 99, 386–91.
2. Jacquot C, Caudwell V, Belenfant X. Granulocytopenia after combined therapy with interferon and angiotensin-converting enzyme inhibitors: evidence for a synergistic hematologic toxicity. *Am J Med* (1996) 101, 235–6.

Interferons + Aspirin or Paracetamol

Aspirin and paracetamol might reduce the flu-like adverse effects of interferon. Paracetamol has a disparate effect on some measures of the antiviral activity of interferon, and isolated cases of acute hepatitis have been seen when interferon was given with paracetamol.

Clinical evidence, mechanism, importance and management

Single intramuscular doses of recombinant human **interferon alfa-2a** 18 million units were given to groups of 8 healthy subjects alone, or after 24 hours after starting either aspirin 650 mg every 4 hours or paracetamol 650 mg every 4 hours for a total of 8 days. Neither aspirin nor paracetamol reduced the interferon adverse effects of fever, chills, headache, or myalgia.[1] In a later similar study by the same research group, the effect of the same drugs and doses (started 3 days before the interferon) was evaluated with a lower dose of **interferon alfa-2a** (3 million units). When the data for aspirin or paracetamol were combined, the subjects had a 47% reduction in symptom score, when compared with control subjects not taking any of these three drugs. In this study, aspirin did not consistently alter measures of the antiviral activity of interferon, but paracetamol appeared to enhance them.[2] Taken together, the results of these two studies suggest that these drugs might reduce the flu-like adverse effects of interferon, perhaps more so at lower doses of interferon. The clinical relevance of the measures of antiviral activity of interferon is uncertain, so the disparate effects found with paracetamol are unclear.

The authors of a report describing an unusual acute form of hepatitis, occurring in 3 patients receiving **interferon alfa-2a**, vinblastine, and paracetamol, suggested that this might have been due to a drug interaction.[3] Another two similar cases have been reported with **interferon alfa-2b** and paracetamol, but no liver toxicity occurred when one of these patients was given **indometacin** with interferon instead.[4] The general relevance of these isolated reports is unclear.

Note that the UK manufacturers of interferon alfa-2a, **interferon beta-1a** and **interferon gamma-1b** advise that paracetamol,[5,6] NSAIDs[7] or an antipyretic analgesic[8,9] might be used to manage the flu-like adverse effects of interferon treatment. The manufacturer of interferon gamma-1b also states that the potential adverse effects of anti-inflammatory drugs, such as NSAIDs, on the efficacy of interferon gamma is unknown, however they give no specific guidance on concurrent use.[5]

1. Witter FR, Woods AS, Griffin MD, Smith CR, Nadler P, Lietman PS. Effects of prednisone, aspirin and acetaminophen on an *in vivo* biologic response to interferon in humans. *Clin Pharmacol Ther* (1988) 44, 239–43.
2. Hendrix CW, Petty BG, Woods A, Kuwahara SK, Witter FR, Soo W, Griffin DE, Lietman PS. Modulation of α-interferon's antiviral and clinical effects by aspirin, acetaminophen, and prednisone in healthy volunteers. *Antiviral Res* (1995) 28, 121–31.
3. Kellokumpu-Lehtinen P, Iisalo E, Nordman E. Hepatotoxicity of paracetamol in combination with interferon and vinblastine. *Lancet* (1989) 1, 1143.
4. Fabris P, Dalla Palma M, de Lalla F. Idiosyncratic acute hepatitis caused by paracetamol in two patients with melanoma treated with high-dose interferon-α. *Ann Intern Med* (2001) 134, 345.
5. Immukin (Interferon gamma-1b). Boehringer Ingelheim Ltd. UK Summary of product characteristics, August 2013.
6. Roferon-A (Interferon alfa-2a). Roche Products Ltd. UK Summary of product characteristics, May 2014.
7. Betaferon (Interferon beta-1b). Bayer plc. UK Summary of product characteristics, April 2014.
8. Avonex (Interferon beta-1a). Biogen Idec Ltd. UK Summary of product characteristics, May 2014.
9. Rebif (Interferon beta-1a). Merck Serono. UK Summary of product characteristics, April 2014.

Interferons + Corticosteroids

Prednisone has a disparate effect on some measures of the antiviral activity of interferon.

Clinical evidence, mechanism, importance and management

A single intramuscular dose of recombinant human **interferon alfa-2a** 18 million units was given to 8 healthy subjects alone, or to 8 similar healthy subjects 24 hours after starting **prednisone** 40 mg daily, for a total of 8 days. **Prednisone** did not reduce the interferon adverse effects of fever, chills, headache, or myalgia, but appeared to reduce one of the two measures of interferon activity.[1] In a later similar study by the same research group, the effect of the same dose of **prednisone**, started 3 days before the interferon, was evaluated with a lower dose of **interferon alfa-2a** (3 million units). Subjects taking **prednisone** had a 43% reduction in symptom score, and also had fewer hours of fever, when compared with control subjects taking **interferon alfa-2a** alone. In this study, **prednisone** did not consistently alter measures of the antiviral activity of interferon.[2] Taken together the results of these two studies suggest **prednisone** might reduce the flu-like adverse effects of interferon, perhaps more so at lower doses of interferon.

The UK manufacturers of **interferon beta-1a** and **interferon beta-1b** state that although it has not been specifically studied, corticosteroids can be used with interferon beta during relapses of multiple sclerosis,[3,4] and that concurrent use for up to 28 days has not resulted in any significant interaction.[4] The manufacturer of **interferon gamma-1b** states that it does not affect the therapeutic efficacy of corticosteroids when used to treat osteopetrosis or chronic granulomatous disease.[5] Therefore, it would appear that concurrent use of corticosteroids with interferons for specific conditions might be beneficial.

1. Witter FR, Woods AS, Griffin MD, Smith CR, Nadler P, Lietman PS. Effects of prednisone, aspirin and acetaminophen on an *in vivo* biologic response to interferon in humans. *Clin Pharmacol Ther* (1988) 44, 239–43.
2. Hendrix CW, Petty BG, Woods A, Kuwahara SK, Witter FR, Soo W, Griffin DE, Lietman PS. Modulation of α-interferon's antiviral and clinical effects by aspirin, acetaminophen, and prednisone in healthy volunteers. *Antiviral Res* (1995) 28, 121–31.
3. Betaferon (Interferon beta-1b). Bayer plc. UK Summary of product characteristics, April 2014.
4. Avonex (Interferon beta-1a). Biogen Idec Ltd. UK Summary of product characteristics, May 2014.
5. Immukin (Interferon gamma-1b). Boehringer Ingelheim Ltd. UK Summary of product characteristics, August 2013.

Interferons + Ribavirin

There was no evidence of any changes in pharmacokinetic parameters when ribavirin and interferon alfa-2b were given together.[1] Another study using peginterferon alfa-2b also found no pharmacokinetic interactions with ribavirin.[2] The combination of interferon alfa and ribavirin has enhanced efficacy against hepatitis C.

1. Khakoo S, Glue P, Grellier L, Wells B, Bell A, Dash C, Murray-Lyon I, Lypnyj D, Flannery B, Walters K, Dusheiko GM. Ribavirin and interferon alfa-2b in chronic hepatitis C: assessment of possible pharmacokinetic and pharmacodynamic interactions. *Br J Clin Pharmacol* (1998) 46, 563–70.
2. Glue P, Rouzier-Panis R, Raffanel C, Sabo R, Gupta SK, Salfi M, Jacobs S, Clement RP. A dose-ranging study of pegylated interferon alfa-2b and ribavirin in chronic hepatitis C. The Hepatitis C Intervention Therapy Group. *Hepatology* (2000) 32, 647–53.

Interferons + St John's wort (*Hypericum perforatum*)

An isolated report describes acute hepatotoxicity in a patient taking peginterferon alfa and St John's wort.

Clinical evidence, mechanism, importance and management

A case report describes a 61-year-old woman with chronic hepatitis C receiving peginterferon alfa-2a 180 micrograms weekly, who developed acute hepatitis while taking St John's wort. The patient had undetectable hepatitis C virus RNA after 8 weeks of peginterferon, but at week 8 her ALT and AST concentrations were grossly elevated (at 700 units/L and 1200 units/L respectively) and treatment with peginterferon alfa-2a was stopped. Three weeks later, her ALT and AST concentrations continued to increase, intense jaundice developed, and her prothrombin time became prolonged. On further questioning, the patient revealed she had been taking St John's wort, 2 capsules daily (exact dose not stated), for 6 weeks. Due to the worsening liver failure, the patient was admitted to hospital for treatment and was discharged 4 weeks later. The authors concluded that while the initial hepatotoxicity might have been caused by peginterferon alfa-2a, the continuation of St John's wort (including after the peginterferon was stopped) might have contributed to the severity of the reaction.[1] This is an isolated report and as such its general clinical importance is not known.

1. Piccolo P, Gentile S, Alegiani F, Angelico M. Severe drug induced acute hepatitis associated with use of St John's wort (*Hypericum perforatum*) during treatment with pegylated interferon α. *BMJ Case Rep* (2009) Epub.

Maraviroc + Atovaquone with Proguanil

Data from one case suggests that atovaquone with proguanil does not alter the exposure to maraviroc.

Clinical evidence, mechanism, importance and management

A patient with an allergy to ritonavir taking a salvage antiretroviral regimen including maraviroc 150 mg twice daily, had no change in the AUC of maraviroc 20 days after starting atovaquone with proguanil 250/100 mg daily for malaria prophylaxis, when compared with the AUC the day before starting prophylaxis. Atovaquone and proguanil plasma concentrations were not measured.[1] Data from one patient is insufficient to exclude or prove an interaction, and further study is needed.

1. Tommasi C, Bellagamba R, Tempestilli M, D'Avolio A, Gallo AL, Ivanovic J, Nicastri E, Pucillo LP, Narciso P. Marked increase in etravirine and saquinavir plasma concentrations during atovaquone/proguanil prophylaxis. *Malar J* (2011) 10, 141.

Maraviroc + Co-trimoxazole

Co-trimoxazole does not appear to affect the pharmacokinetics of maraviroc.

Clinical evidence

In a study in healthy subjects, co-trimoxazole (sulfamethoxazole with trimethoprim) 960 mg twice daily had no clinically relevant effect on the pharmacokinetics of maraviroc 300 mg twice daily (a 11% increase in AUC and a 19% increase in maximum plasma concentration).[1]

Mechanism

Maraviroc undergoes some degree of renal clearance (about 20% of its total clearance).[1] Co-trimoxazole affects renal tubular transport and so it was predicted that it might possibly affect the plasma concentration of maraviroc.[1]

Importance and management

The pharmacokinetic data indicate that no maraviroc dose adjustment is likely to be necessary if it is given with co-trimoxazole.

1. Abel S, Russell D, Whitlock LA, Ridgway CE, Muirhead GJ. The effects of cotrimoxazole or tenofovir co-administration on the pharmacokinetics of maraviroc in healthy volunteers. *Br J Clin Pharmacol* (2008) 65 (Suppl 1), 47–53.

Maraviroc + HCV-Protease inhibitors

Telaprevir markedly increases, and boceprevir moderately increases, the exposure to maraviroc. Maraviroc does not appear to alter the pharmacokinetics of boceprevir or telaprevir. Simeprevir is not expected to interact with maraviroc.

Clinical evidence

(a) Boceprevir

In a study, 14 healthy subjects were given maraviroc 150 mg twice daily, alone for 5 days, and then with boceprevir 800 mg three times daily for 10 days. The AUC and maximum concentration of maraviroc were increased about 3-fold, but the pharmacokinetics of boceprevir were no different to historical controls.[1] The preliminary report of a crossover study in 5 healthy subjects, notes that boceprevir 800 mg three times daily for 14 days increased the AUC of maraviroc 150 mg twice daily about 2-fold, but did not alter the maximum concentration.[2]

(b) Telaprevir

In a study, 14 healthy subjects were given maraviroc 150 mg twice daily, alone for 5 days, and then with telaprevir 750 mg three times daily for 10 days. The AUC and maximum concentration of maraviroc were increased about 9.5-fold and 8-fold, respectively, but the pharmacokinetics of telaprevir were no different to historical controls.[1]

Mechanism

Boceprevir and telaprevir are both inhibitors of CYP3A4, by which maraviroc is metabolised. Concurrent use therefore results in an increase in maraviroc exposure.

Importance and management

A pharmacokinetic interaction between maraviroc and boceprevir and telaprevir is established, and the moderate to marked increases in exposure seen with boceprevir and telaprevir, respectively, will be clinically important. The UK and US manufacturers of maraviroc therefore recommend that during concurrent use with either of these HCV-protease inhibitors, the maraviroc dose should be restricted to 150 mg twice daily.[3,4] Furthermore, the UK manufacturer advises that in patients with a creatinine clearance of less than 80 mL/minute, the maraviroc dose should be decreased to 150 mg daily, and in those with a creatinine clearance of less than 30 mL/minute they advise that maraviroc should be used with caution.[3] The US manufacturer does not recommend concurrent use with boceprevir or telaprevir in patients with a creatinine clearance of less than 30 mL/minute.[4]

Although not studied, the manufacturers of **simeprevir** predict that no clinically relevant interaction would be expected with maraviroc.[5,6] No dose adjustments on concurrent use would therefore seem necessary.

1. Vourvahis M, Plotka A, Kantaridis C, Fang A, Heera J. The effects of boceprevir and telaprevir on the pharmacokinetics of maraviroc: an open-label, fixed-sequence study in healthy volunteers. *J Acquir Immune Defic Syndr* (2014) 65, 564–70.
2. Martel D, Sheehan NL, Tremblay CL, Turgeon J, Tseng A, Phaneuf D, Noël GE, Thibeault D, Labbé L. Pharmacokinetic interaction of the direct acting antiviral agent boceprevir with maraviroc in healthy volunteers. 14th International Workshop on Clinical Pharmacology of HIV therapy, Amsterdam, 2013. Abstract P_04.

3. Celsentri (Maraviroc). ViiV Healthcare UK Ltd. UK Summary of product characteristics, April 2014.
4. Selzentry (Maraviroc). ViiV Healthcare. US Prescribing information, March 2014.
5. Olysio (Simeprevir sodium). Janssen-Cilag Ltd. UK Summary of product characteristics, May 2014.
6. Olysio (Simeprevir sodium). Janssen Products, LP. US Prescribing information, November 2014.

Maraviroc + HIV-protease inhibitors

Atazanavir and saquinavir, and atazanavir, darunavir, and lopinavir (all boosted with ritonavir) markedly increase the exposure to maraviroc. Saquinavir boosted with ritonavir has an even greater effect, whereas tipranavir boosted with ritonavir has no effect on maraviroc exposure. Limited evidence suggests twice daily fosamprenavir boosted with ritonavir reduces maraviroc exposure, and maraviroc reduces the exposure to amprenavir. Efavirenz and etravirine attenuate the effect of these HIV-protease inhibitors on maraviroc exposure to some extent.

Clinical evidence

(a) Atazanavir

In a study in 12 healthy subjects, atazanavir 400 mg daily increased the AUC and maximum plasma concentration of maraviroc 300 mg twice daily (both drugs taken for 7 days) 3.6-fold and 2-fold, respectively. Atazanavir boosted with ritonavir 300/100 mg daily increased the AUC of maraviroc almost 5-fold and increased the maximum plasma concentration of maraviroc about 2.5-fold.[1]

(b) Darunavir

In a study in 12 healthy subjects, darunavir boosted with ritonavir 600/100 mg twice daily increased the AUC and the maximum and minimum plasma concentrations of maraviroc 150 mg twice daily 4-fold, 2.3-fold, and 8-fold, respectively.[2] Etravirine minimally attenuated this interaction: the AUC and the maximum and minimum plasma concentrations of maraviroc were increased 3-fold, 1.8-fold, and 5.3-fold, respectively. Maraviroc appeared to have no effect on darunavir and ritonavir exposure.[2] In a retrospective case review in patients taking darunavir boosted with ritonavir 800/100 mg *once* daily, the minimum maraviroc plasma concentration was 63% higher in patients taking maraviroc 300 mg *once* daily when compared with those taking 150 mg *once* daily.[3]

(c) Fosamprenavir

Fosamprenavir boosted with ritonavir 700/100 mg twice daily reduced the AUC and minimum concentration of maraviroc by 66% and 54%, respectively, whereas fosamprenavir boosted with ritonavir 1400/100 mg *once* daily had no effect on maraviroc exposure and reduced the minimum concentration by 23%. Maraviroc reduced the amprenavir exposure from the twice daily and once daily regimens by 21% and 26%, respectively.[4] The UK manufacturer of maraviroc briefly notes that fosamprenavir boosted with ritonavir 700/100 mg twice daily increased the AUC and minimum concentration of maraviroc 300 mg twice daily 2.5-fold and 1.5-fold, respectively. The AUC and maximum plasma concentration of amprenavir were decreased by 35% and 34%, respectively.[5]

(d) Indinavir

The UK manufacturer[5] of maraviroc states that, from population pharmacokinetic analysis of phase 3 studies, the concurrent use of indinavir with the recommended reduced maraviroc dose [of 150 mg twice daily] gives an appropriate maraviroc exposure.

(e) Lopinavir

In a study in 5 HIV-positive patients taking lopinavir boosted with ritonavir 400/100 mg twice daily with stavudine and lamivudine, the AUC of a single 300-mg oral dose of maraviroc was increased 2.6-fold and the maraviroc maximum plasma concentration was increased by nearly 2-fold, when compared with HIV-positive subjects taking maraviroc 300 mg daily alone.[6] In a study in 12 healthy subjects, lopinavir boosted with ritonavir 400/100 mg twice daily increased the AUC and maximum plasma concentration of maraviroc 300 mg twice daily almost 4-fold and 2-fold, respectively.[7]

Adding efavirenz 600 mg daily nearly halved the effect of lopinavir boosted with ritonavir on the AUC and maximum plasma concentration of maraviroc (to a smaller increase of 2.5-fold and 20%, respectively), and also led to an increase in adverse effects, such as dizziness.[7] Another cohort study was planned to investigate the concurrent use of lopinavir and saquinavir (both boosted with ritonavir), and efavirenz with maraviroc; however, this was discontinued because of a high rate of gastrointestinal adverse effects.[7]

(f) Ritonavir

In a study in healthy subjects, low-dose ritonavir 100 mg twice daily alone increased the AUC of maraviroc 100 mg twice daily 3.6-fold.[1]

(g) Saquinavir

In a study in 12 healthy subjects, saquinavir 1.2 g three times daily increased the AUC and maximum plasma concentration of maraviroc 100 mg twice daily 4.2-fold and 3.3-fold, respectively.[1] In another study in healthy subjects by the same group, saquinavir boosted with ritonavir 400/100 mg twice daily for 7 days increased the AUC and maximum plasma concentration of maraviroc 100 mg twice daily by about 9.7-fold and 4.8-fold, respectively. Adding efavirenz 600 mg daily nearly halved this effect, although the AUC and maximum plasma concentration of maraviroc were still increased 5-fold and 2.3-fold, respectively.[7]

(h) Tipranavir

A study in 12 healthy subjects found that tipranavir boosted with ritonavir 500/200 mg twice daily had no effect on the AUC or maximum plasma concentration of maraviroc 150 mg twice daily. An initial increase in the minimum plasma concentration of maraviroc was seen on days one to 4, but this declined thereafter.[1]

Mechanism

Maraviroc is a substrate of CYP3A4 and P-glycoprotein. CYP3A4 is inhibited to various degrees by the HIV-protease inhibitors. Therefore, maraviroc exposure would be expected to be increased if it is taken with the HIV-protease inhibitors. Giving the CYP3A4 inducers efavirenz or etravirine at the same time reduces, but does not negate, the effects of the HIV-protease inhibitors.

Importance and management

The moderate to marked effect of many of the HIV-protease inhibitors on maraviroc exposure is established and likely to be clinically important. Increases in maraviroc exposure of this magnitude are likely to result in increased adverse effects. The UK and US manufacturers of maraviroc advise that its dose should be reduced to 150 mg twice daily when it is taken with *most* HIV-protease inhibitors (atazanavir, indinavir, **nelfinavir** and saquinavir, and atazanavir, darunavir, lopinavir, and saquinavir, all boosted with ritonavir). This dose reduction is also recommended when maraviroc is given with these HIV-protease inhibitors plus the NNRTIs **efavirenz** or **etravirine** (but not nevirapine, see 'Maraviroc + NNRTIs', p.950).[5,8] However, some HIV-protease inhibitors are exempt from this dosing recommendation. In the UK, the manufacturer[5] of maraviroc contraindicates its concurrent use with **fosamprenavir boosted with ritonavir** due to the risk of a large reduction in the minimum plasma concentration of amprenavir, leading to fosamprenavir treatment failure. In both the UK and the US, the manufacturers recommend that when maraviroc is used with **tipranavir boosted with ritonavir**, the usual dose of maraviroc 300 mg twice daily should be used.[5,8] However the UK manufacturer[5] recommends increasing the maraviroc dose to 600 mg twice daily if the NNRTI efavirenz is also added.

For information on the recommended dose of maraviroc with concurrent use of HIV-protease inhibitors and other CYP3A4 inducers, see 'Maraviroc + Rifampicin (Rifampin) and other CYP3A4 inducers', p.951.

1. Abel S, Russell D, Taylor-Worth RJ, Ridgway CE, Muirhead GJ. Effect of CYP3A4 inhibitors on the pharmacokinetics of maraviroc in healthy volunteers. *Br J Clin Pharmacol* (2008) 65 (Suppl 1), 27–37.
2. Kakuda TN, Abel S, Davis J, Hamlin J, Schöller-Gyüre M, Mack R, Ndongo N, Petit W, Ridgway C, Sekar V, Tweedy S, Hoetelmans RMW. Pharmacokinetic interactions of maraviroc with darunavir-ritonavir, etravirine, and etravirine-darunavir-ritonavir in healthy volunteers: results of two drug interaction trials. *Antimicrob Agents Chemother* (2011) 55, 2290–6.
3. Okoli C, Siccardi M, Thomas-William S, Dufty N, Khonyongwa K, Ainsworth J, Watson J, Cook R, Gandhi K, Hickinbottom G, Owen A, Taylor S. Once daily maraviroc 300 mg or 150 mg in combination with ritonavir-boosted darunavir 800/100 mg. *J Antimicrob Chemother* (2012) 67, 671–4.
4. Luber A, Condoluci D, Slowinski P, *et al.* Steady-state pharmacokinetics of maraviroc and amprenavir alone and in combination after maraviroc is given BID with unboosted or ritonavir-boosted fosamprenavir one or twice daily in fasted healthy volunteers. 10th International Workshop on Clinical Pharmacology of HIV Therapy, Amsterdam, April 2009, abstract P31.
5. Celsentri (Maraviroc). ViiV Healthcare UK Ltd. UK Summary of product characteristics, April 2014.
6. Pozniak AL, Boffito M, Russell D, Ridgway CE, Muirhead GJ. A novel probe drug interaction study to investigate the effect of selected antiretroviral combinations on the pharmacokinetics of a single oral dose of maraviroc in HIV- positive subjects. *Br J Clin Pharmacol* (2008), 65 (Suppl 1), 54–9.
7. Abel S, Jenkins TM, Whitlock LA, Ridgway CE, Muirhead GJ. Effects of CYP3A4 inducers with and without CYP3A4 inhibitors on the pharmacokinetics of maraviroc in healthy volunteers. *Br J Clin Pharmacol* (2008) 65 (Suppl 1), 38–46.
8. Selzentry (Maraviroc). ViiV Healthcare. US Prescribing information, August 2012.

Maraviroc + Ketoconazole and other CYP3A4 inhibitors

Ketoconazole markedly increases maraviroc exposure. Other potent CYP3A4 inhibitors would be expected to interact similarly. Limited data suggest that fluconazole does not interact with maraviroc to a clinically relevant extent

Clinical evidence

In a study in 12 healthy subjects, **ketoconazole** 400 mg daily increased the AUC and maximum plasma concentration of maraviroc 100 mg twice daily 5-fold and 3.4-fold, respectively. No serious adverse effects were reported.[1] Population pharmacokinetic analysis suggest that no dose adjustment of maraviroc is necessary with **fluconazole**.[2]

Mechanism

Maraviroc is a substrate of CYP3A4 and P-glycoprotein. Ketoconazole is a potent inhibitor of CYP3A4. Therefore, maraviroc exposure would be expected to be increased if it is taken with ketoconazole. Other potent inhibitors of CYP3A4 would be expected to interact similarly.[2] Fluconazole is a moderate inhibitor of CYP3A4 and appears to have much less effect. Ketoconazole also inhibits P-glycoprotein, which could further contribute to the interaction with maraviroc.

Importance and management

The effects of **ketoconazole** on maraviroc metabolism are established and likely to be clinically important. Increases in maraviroc exposure of this magnitude are likely to result in increased adverse effects. The UK and US manufacturers of maraviroc advise that the dose of maraviroc should be reduced to 150 mg twice daily in the presence of ketoconazole in those with normal renal function.[2,3] In those with renal impairment (creatinine clearance less than 80 mL/min) in the presence of ketoconazole, the advice in the UK is to increase the maraviroc dose interval to once daily,[2] whereas in the US maraviroc 150 mg twice daily is recommended for mild and moderate renal impairment, and maraviroc is contraindicated with ketoconazole in those with a creatinine clearance less than 30 mL/min.[3] **Itraconazole** is predicted to interact with maraviroc, and the same maraviroc dose reductions are advised on concurrent use.[2] A similar interaction might also be expected for **voriconazole**, and the US HIV guidelines state that consideration should be given to reducing the maraviroc dose to 150 mg twice daily.[4] **Fluconazole** has less of an effect on CYP3A4, so no dose alteration is needed when it is taken with maraviroc, although nevertheless maraviroc 300 mg twice daily should be used with caution is advised.[2]

The UK and US manufacturers of maraviroc also predict that the macrolide antibacterials **clarithromycin** and **telithromycin** will increase maraviroc exposure, and they recommend reducing the maraviroc dose to 150 mg twice daily.[2,3]

Consider also 'Maraviroc + HIV-protease inhibitors', p.949, and for a list of other inhibitors of CYP3A4, which might be expected to interact similarly, although to varying extents, see 'Table 1.9', p.11.

1. Abel S, Russell D, Taylor-Worth RJ, Ridgway CE, Muirhead GJ. Effect of CYP3A4 inhibitors on the pharmacokinetics of maraviroc in healthy volunteers. *Br J Clin Pharmacol* (2008) 65 (Suppl 1), 27–37.
2. Celsentri (Maraviroc). ViiV Healthcare UK Ltd. UK Summary of product characteristics, April 2014.
3. Selzentry (Maraviroc). ViiV Healthcare. US Prescribing information, August 2012.
4. Panel on Antiretroviral Guidelines for Adults and Adolescents. Guidelines for the use of antiretroviral agents in HIV-1-infected adults and adolescents. Department of Health and Human Services. (April 2015) 1–288. Available at: http://www.aidsinfo.nih.gov/ContentFiles/AdultandAdolescentGL.pdf (accessed 18/09/2015).

Maraviroc + Miscellaneous

Food slightly reduces the absorption of maraviroc. No interaction is expected between maraviroc and enfuvirtide. No dose adjustment of maraviroc is expected to be needed if it is taken with buprenorphine, methadone, peginterferon, or ribavirin.

Clinical evidence, mechanism, importance and management

(a) Debrisoquine

In a study in 72 healthy subjects, maraviroc 25 to 300 mg twice daily had no effect on the metabolism of debrisoquine; however, maraviroc 600 mg daily resulted in a 3.3-fold increase in the debrisoquine metabolic ratio.[1] Debrisoquine is a probe substrate for CYP2D6, and the study above indicates that maraviroc, taken at usual clinical doses, is unlikely to cause a clinically relevant increase in the exposure of drugs metabolised by CYP2D6. However, at higher exposures of maraviroc, a potential inhibition of CYP2D6 cannot be excluded.[2]

(b) Enfuvirtide

The US manufacturer advises that no maraviroc dose adjustment is needed if it is taken with enfuvirtide.[3]

(c) Food

The UK and US manufacturers report that in healthy subjects, a high-fat breakfast slightly reduced the AUC and maximum plasma concentration of a single 300-mg dose of maraviroc by about 33%. However, they state that there were no food restrictions during the clinical studies that demonstrated the efficacy and safety of maraviroc. Therefore maraviroc can be taken with or without food.[2,3]

(d) Other drugs

The UK manufacturer states that, although there have been no specific drug interaction studies, maraviroc 300 mg twice daily can be taken with **buprenorphine, methadone, peginterferon**, and **ribavirin** without any dose adjustments, as an interaction would not be expected.[2]

1. Abel S, van der Ryst E, Rosario MC, Ridgway CE, Medhurst CG, Taylor-Worth RJ, Muirhead GJ. Assessment of the pharmacokinetics, safety, tolerability of maraviroc, a novel CCR5 antagonist, in healthy volunteers. *Br J Clin Pharmacol* (2008) 65 (Suppl 1), 5–18.
2. Celsentri (Maraviroc). ViiV Healthcare UK Ltd. UK Summary of product characteristics, April 2014.
3. Selzentry (Maraviroc). ViiV Healthcare. US Prescribing information, August 2012.

Maraviroc + NNRTIs

Efavirenz and etravirine reduce maraviroc exposure. Nevirapine has no effect, and rilpivirine is predicted to have no effect, on the exposure to maraviroc. Delavirdine is predicted to increase maraviroc exposure. Maraviroc does not alter etravirine pharmacokinetics, and is not expected to alter the pharmacokinetics of efavirenz, nevirapine, or rilpivirine.

Clinical evidence

(a) Efavirenz

In a placebo-controlled study in 12 healthy subjects, efavirenz 600 mg daily for 14 days reduced the steady-state AUC and maximum plasma concentration of maraviroc 100 mg twice daily by about 45% and 51%, respectively. Doubling the dose of maraviroc to 200 mg twice daily overcame this reduction in the maraviroc plasma concentration, resulting in a minor 15% *increase* in AUC and a 16% *increase* in maximum plasma concentration, when compared with maraviroc 100 mg twice daily alone.[1] Similarly, in another study in HIV-positive patients, the AUC of a single 300-mg dose of maraviroc was about 52% lower in two groups of 8 patients, when compared with patients given maraviroc alone: one group was taking efavirenz, lamivudine, and zidovudine and the other was taking efavirenz, didanosine, and tenofovir.[2] Note that the NRTIs zidovudine, lamivudine, and tenofovir, do not have a clinically significant effect on maraviroc pharmacokinetics (see 'Maraviroc + Miscellaneous', above).

For the effect of efavirenz on the interaction of the HIV-protease inhibitors with maraviroc, see 'Maraviroc + HIV-protease inhibitors', p.949.

(b) Etravirine

In a pharmacokinetic study in healthy subjects, etravirine 200 mg twice daily halved the AUC of maraviroc 300 mg twice daily and reduced the minimum plasma concentration by 39%.[3] Maraviroc had no effect on the pharmacokinetics of etravirine.[3]

(c) Nevirapine

In a study in 8 HIV-positive patients taking nevirapine 200 mg twice daily with lamivudine and tenofovir, the AUC of a single 300-mg dose of maraviroc was unchanged but its maximum plasma concentration was about 54% *higher*, when compared with HIV-positive subjects taking maraviroc alone.[2] Note that the NRTIs lamivudine and tenofovir, do not have a clinically significant effect on maraviroc pharmacokinetics, see 'Maraviroc + Miscellaneous', above.

Mechanism

Maraviroc is a substrate of CYP3A4, hence its exposure is reduced by efavirenz and etravirine, both inducers of CYP3A4. Nevirapine also induces CYP3A4; however, the study above suggests that it does not affect maraviroc exposure.

In contrast, **delavirdine** inhibits CYP3A4, and would therefore be expected to increase the concentration of maraviroc.

Importance and management

The pharmacokinetic interaction between maraviroc and **efavirenz** is of clinical importance. The reduction in maraviroc exposure could result in a decrease in therapeutic efficacy and the development of viral resistance. In one study,[1] doubling the dose of maraviroc overcame this interaction. The UK and US manufacturers therefore recommend that the dose of maraviroc should be increased to 600 mg twice daily in patients taking efavirenz and *not* taking HIV-protease inhibitors or other potent inhibitors of CYP3A4.[4,5] Note that the UK manufacturer[4] does not recommend concurrent use of maraviroc in patients taking both efavirenz and the potent CYP3A4 inducer rifampicin, see 'Maraviroc + Rifampicin (Rifampin) and other CYP3A4 inducers', p.951, for further information. If efavirenz is given with a HIV-protease inhibitor, then the maraviroc dose reductions for the HIV-protease inhibitors should be followed, see 'Maraviroc + HIV-protease inhibitors', p.949. Maraviroc is not expected to alter the concentration of efavirenz.[4]

The reduction in maraviroc exposure when given with **etravirine** is also likely to be clinically important. The US manufacturer of maraviroc advises increasing the dose to 600 mg twice daily if it is given with etravirine *without* a potent CYP3A4 inhibitor.[5] However, **etravirine** is currently only approved for use with a HIV-protease inhibitor, and in this situation the maraviroc dose reductions for concurrent use with the HIV-protease inhibitors should be followed,[4,5] see 'Maraviroc + HIV-protease inhibitors', p.949. No dose adjustment of etravirine is required if it is taken with maraviroc and HIV-protease inhibitors.[6]

Nevirapine is also an inducer of CYP3A4; however, it appears to have no effect on the exposure to maraviroc and caused only a small *increase* in the concentration of maraviroc. Therefore, no dose adjustment of maraviroc appears to be needed in patients taking nevirapine.[4,5] Maraviroc is not expected to alter nevirapine concentrations.[4]

Delavirdine *inhibits* CYP3A4 and the US manufacturer of maraviroc predicts that delavirdine will significantly increase the concentration of maraviroc. They therefore recommend reducing the maraviroc dose to 150 mg twice daily if delavirdine is also given.[5]

Maraviroc is not expected to have an effect on efavirenz or nevirapine pharmacokinetics.[4]

The UK and US manufacturers of rilpivirine predict that no clinically relevant interaction will occur between **rilpivirine** and maraviroc,[7,8] and no dose adjustment is required.[7]

1. Abel S, Jenkins TM, Whitlock LA, Ridgway E, Muirhead GJ. Effects of CYP3A4 inducers with and without CYP3A4 inhibitors on the pharmacokinetics of maraviroc in healthy volunteers. *Br J Clin Pharmacol* (2008) 65, (Suppl 1), 38–46.
2. Pozniak AL, Boffito M, Russell D, Ridgway CE, Muirhead GJ. A novel probe drug interaction study to investigate the effect of selected antiretroviral combinations on the pharmacokinetics of a single oral dose of maraviroc in HIV-positive subjects. *Br J Clin Pharmacol* (2008), 65 (Suppl 1), 54–9.
3. Kakuda TN, Abel S, Davis J, Hamlin J, Schöller-Gyüre M, Mack R, Ndongo N, Petit W, Ridgway C, Sekar V, Tweedy S, Hoetelmans RMW. Pharmacokinetic interactions of maraviroc with darunavir-ritonavir, etravirine, and etravirine-darunavir-ritonavir in healthy volunteers: results of two drug interaction trials. *Antimicrob Agents Chemother* (2011) 55, 2290–6.
4. Celsentri (Maraviroc). ViiV Healthcare UK Ltd. UK Summary of product characteristics, April 2014.
5. Selzentry (Maraviroc). ViiV Healthcare. US Prescribing information, August 2012.
6. Intelence (Etravirine). Janssen-Cilag Ltd. UK Summary of product characteristics, July 2012.
7. Edurant (Rilpivirine hydrochloride). Janssen-Cilag Ltd. UK Summary of product characteristics, November 2011.
8. Edurant (Rilpivirine hydrochloride). Tibotec Pharmaceuticals. US Prescribing information, August 2012.

Maraviroc + NRTIs

Maraviroc has no effect on the pharmacokinetics of lamivudine with zidovudine.

Clinical evidence, mechanism, importance and management

In a placebo-controlled, crossover study in 11 healthy subjects, maraviroc 300 mg twice daily had no effect on the pharmacokinetics of **zidovudine** with **lamivudine** 300/150 mg twice daily, when they were taken concurrently for one week.[1] Therefore no dose adjustments of zidovudine with lamivudine are needed when it is taken with maraviroc 300 mg twice daily.[2] The UK and US manufacturers state that no dose adjustment of maraviroc is needed when it is used with NRTIs.[2,3]

1. Abel S, Russell D, Whitlock LA, Ridgway CE, Muirhead GJ. Effect of maraviroc on the pharmacokinetics of midazolam, lamivudine/zidovudine, and ethinyloestradiol/levonorgestrel in healthy volunteers. *Br J Clin Pharmacol* (2008) 65 (Suppl 1), 19–26.
2. Celsentri (Maraviroc). ViiV Healthcare UK Ltd. UK Summary of product characteristics, April 2014.
3. Selzentry (Maraviroc). ViiV Healthcare. US Prescribing information, August 2012.

Maraviroc + Rifampicin (Rifampin) and other CYP3A4 inducers

Rifampicin reduces maraviroc exposure. Other inducers of CYP3A4, such as carbamazepine, phenobarbital, phenytoin, rifabutin, rifapentine, and St John's wort are predicted to have a similar effect.

Clinical evidence

In a placebo-controlled study in 12 healthy subjects, **rifampicin** 600 mg daily for 14 days reduced the steady-state AUC, the maximum and minimum plasma concentrations of maraviroc 100 mg twice daily by about two-thirds. Doubling the dose of maraviroc to 200 mg twice daily overcame this increase in metabolism, resulting in an AUC comparable to that of maraviroc 100 mg twice daily alone.[1]

Mechanism

Maraviroc is a substrate of CYP3A4 and P-glycoprotein, hence its exposure is reduced by rifampicin, a potent inducer of CYP3A4 and an inducer of P-glycoprotein. Other inducers of CYP3A4 and/or P-glycoprotein would therefore also be expected to reduce maraviroc exposure. For a list of CYP3A4 inducers, see 'Table 1.9', p.11, and for a list of P-glycoprotein inducers, see 'Table 1.12', p.14.

Importance and management

The pharmacokinetic interaction between maraviroc and rifampicin is likely to be clinically relevant as the reduction in maraviroc exposure seen could result in a decrease in therapeutic efficacy and the development of viral resistance. For this reason the US HIV guidelines do not recommend concurrent use.[2] In the study, doubling the maraviroc dose negated the interaction. Therefore, if concurrent use is necessary, the UK and US manufacturers and the US HIV guidelines advise that the dose of maraviroc should be increased to 600 mg twice daily (double the recommended dose for use with non-interacting drugs) in patients taking rifampicin without a potent CYP3A4 inhibitor.[2-4] However, for those also taking a potent inhibitor of CYP3A4, the US manufacturer recommends that the maraviroc dose reduction for use with CYP3A4 inhibitors should be followed (generally 150 mg twice daily) irrespective of the use of CYP3A4 inducers,[4] although there does not appear to be any pharmacokinetic information on this. Conversely, the US HIV guidelines recommend a dose of maraviroc of 300 mg twice daily when both rifampicin and a potent CYP3A4 inhibitor are used (the recommended dose for use with non-interacting drugs)[2]. For further information on the effects of CYP3A4 inhibitors, such as ketoconazole or the HIV-protease inhibitors, on maraviroc, see 'Maraviroc + Ketoconazole and other CYP3A4 inhibitors', p.949, and 'Maraviroc + HIV-protease inhibitors', p.949.

Other inducers of CYP3A4 are also predicted to reduce maraviroc exposure. The US manufacturer[4] and the US HIV guidelines[2] specifically recommend the same dose adjustments of maraviroc in patients taking **carbamazepine**, **phenytoin**, or **phenobarbital** as they do for rifampicin. It would seem prudent to also consider this dose increase with **primidone** (which is metabolised to phenobarbital) and **fosphenytoin** (a prodrug of phenytoin). **St John's wort** is another known inducer of CYP3A4 and is expected to substantially reduce maraviroc exposure and potentially reduce its antiviral effects, and both the UK and US manufacturers and the US HIV guidelines advise against its concurrent use with maraviroc.[2-4] Note that the UK manufacturer of maraviroc[3] does not recommend the concurrent use of maraviroc in patients taking both rifampicin and efavirenz, because the effect of two enzyme inducers has not been studied. For further information on the effects of efavirenz on maraviroc, see 'Maraviroc + NNRTIs', p.950.

Rifabutin is a weaker inducer of CYP3A4 than rifampicin, and its use with maraviroc does not appear to have been studied. The US HIV guidelines recommend a dose of maraviroc of 300 mg twice daily for use with rifabutin,[2] which is the usual dose for use with non-interacting drugs. In those taking rifabutin with potent CYP3A4 inhibitors a net inhibitory effect is expected,[3] and the recommended maraviroc dose is therefore the same as the recommended dose with potent CYP3A4 inhibitors (usually 150 mg twice daily[2-4]), see 'Maraviroc + HIV-protease inhibitors', p.949, and 'Maraviroc + Ketoconazole and other CYP3A4 inhibitors', p.949.

There do not appear to be any published data for an interaction between maraviroc and **rifapentine**, which also induces CYP3A4 although to a lesser extent than rifampicin; however, it would be expected to reduce maraviroc exposure. For this reason, the US HIV guidelines do not recommend concurrent use.[2]

Note that the US manufacturer of maraviroc contraindicates concurrent use with CYP3A4 inducers in patients with a creatinine clearance less than 30 mL/min.[4]

1. Abel S, Jenkins TM, Whitlock LA, Ridgway E, Muirhead GJ. Effects of CYP3A4 inducers with and without CYP3A4 inhibitors on the pharmacokinetics of maraviroc in healthy volunteers. *Br J Clin Pharmacol* (2008) 65, (Suppl 1), 38–46.
2. Panel on Antiretroviral Guidelines for Adults and Adolescents. Guidelines for the use of antiretroviral agents in HIV-1-infected adults and adolescents. Department of Health and Human Services. (April 2015) 1–288. Available at: http://www.aidsinfo.nih.gov/ContentFiles/AdultandAdolescentGL.pdf (accessed 29/09/2015).
3. Celsentri (Maraviroc). ViiV Healthcare UK Ltd. UK Summary of product characteristics, April 2014.
4. Selzentry (Maraviroc). ViiV Healthcare. US Prescribing information, August 2012.

Maraviroc + Statins

Statins do not appear to alter the antiviral efficacy of maraviroc.

Clinical evidence, mechanism, importance and management

In a post-hoc analysis of data from clinical studies, statins had no apparent effect on the mean reduction in HIV RNA, or the proportion of patients with HIV RNA below 50 copies/mL, in patients taking maraviroc. It had been hypothesised that statins might reduce the number of lipid rafts in cell membranes, which contain the CCR5 receptors, thereby reducing the number of CCR5 receptors and reducing the activity of CCR5 antagonists such as maraviroc.[1] However, the post-hoc analysis of data suggests that the potential pharmacodynamic interaction does not occur clinically. The UK manufacturer briefly states that no interaction is expected between maraviroc and the statins, and so no dose adjustment is needed on concurrent use.[2]

1. Moyle G, Rajicic N, Goodrich J, Mayer H, Valdez H. Concurrent use of statins does not influence efficacy of maraviroc in Maraviroc versus Optimized Therapy in Viremic Antiretroviral Treatment-Experienced Patients 1 and 2 trials. *AIDS* (2009) 23, 1613.
2. Celsentri (Maraviroc). ViiV Healthcare UK Ltd. UK Summary of product characteristics, April 2014.

Maraviroc + Tenofovir

Tenofovir had no effect on the pharmacokinetics of maraviroc in one study.

Clinical evidence, mechanism, importance and management

In a placebo-controlled, crossover study in 16 healthy subjects, the concurrent use of maraviroc 300 mg twice daily and tenofovir disoproxil fumarate 300 mg daily had no effect on the pharmacokinetics of maraviroc.[1] Maraviroc undergoes some degree of renal clearance (about 20% of total clearance) and tenofovir is predominantly excreted renally, so it has been predicted that tenofovir might possibly affect the concentration of maraviroc.[1] However, the pharmacokinetic data suggest that no maraviroc dose adjustment is likely to be needed if it is given with tenofovir.

1. Abel S, Russell D, Whitlock LA, Ridgway CE, Muirhead GJ. The effects of cotrimoxazole or tenofovir co-administration on the pharmacokinetics of maraviroc in healthy volunteers. *Br J Clin Pharmacol* (2008) 65 (Suppl 1), 47–53.

NNRTIs + Antacids

Antacids roughly halve the AUC of delavirdine, and are predicted to reduce rilpivirine exposure. Aluminium/magnesium-containing antacids do not alter efavirenz or nevirapine exposure.

Clinical evidence

(a) Delavirdine

In a single-dose study in 12 healthy subjects, when delavirdine 300 mg was given 10 minutes after an antacid the AUC and maximum plasma concentrations of delavirdine were reduced by 48% and 57%, respectively.[1] Note that **didanosine** tablets are buffered with an **antacid**, and might reduce the concentrations of delavirdine. See 'NNRTIs + NRTIs', p.963, for further information.

(b) Efavirenz

The manufacturer notes that, in a single-dose study in 17 healthy subjects, 30 mL of an **aluminium/magnesium hydroxide**-containing antacid did not have any effect on the AUC or maximum plasma concentration of efavirenz.[2,3]

(c) Nevirapine

In a single-dose study in 24 subjects, 30 mL of *Maalox* (**aluminium/magnesium hydroxide**) reduced the maximum plasma concentration of nevirapine 200 mg by 15% and delayed the time to maximum concentration, but had no effect on the AUC of nevirapine.[4]

Mechanism

Delavirdine is poorly soluble at pH greater than 3, therefore administration with an antacid reduces delavirdine absorption.[1] Rilpivirine is expected to be similarly affected. However, the exposure to efavirenz and nevirapine do not appear to be affected by changes in gastric pH.

Importance and management

Halving **delavirdine** exposure is likely to reduce its efficacy and could increase the chances of resistance. The manufacturer recommends separating administration of delavirdine and antacids by at least one hour.[5] Similarly, on the basis of the interaction with omeprazole (see 'NNRTIs + Proton pump inhibitors', p.964), antacids would be predicted to reduce **rilpivirine** exposure. Therefore the manufacturers state that aluminium-, magnesium-, or calcium-containing antacids are taken at least 2 hours before or 4 hours after rilpivirine.[6,7]

It appears that **efavirenz** and **nevirapine** can be taken without regard to timing of antacids.

1. Cox SR, Della-Coletta AA, Turner SW, Freimuth WW. Single-dose pharmacokinetic (PK) studies with delavirdine (DLV) mesylate: dose proportionality and effects of food and antacid. *Intersci Conf Antimicrob Agents Chemother* (1994) 34, 82.
2. Sustiva Film-coated Tablets (Efavirenz). Bristol-Myers Squibb Pharmaceutical Ltd. UK Summary of product characteristics, March 2014.
3. Sustiva (Efavirenz). Bristol-Myers Squibb Company. US Prescribing information, August 2012.
4. Lamson M, Cort S, Macy H, Love J, Korpalski D, Pav J, Keirns J. Effects of food or antacid on the bioavailability of nevirapine 200 mg tablets. 11th International Conference on AIDS, Vancouver, 1996. Abstract Tu.B.2323.
5. Rescriptor (Delavirdine mesylate). ViiV Healthcare. US Prescribing information, August 2012.
6. Edurant (Rilpivirine hydrochloride). Janssen-Cilag Ltd. UK Summary of product characteristics, November 2011.
7. Edurant (Rilpivirine hydrochloride). Tibotec Pharmaceuticals. US Prescribing information, August 2012.

NNRTIs + Antiepileptics; Enzyme-inducing

Carbamazepine reduces the plasma concentrations of delavirdine, efavirenz, and nevirapine, and is predicted to reduce the plasma concentrations of etravirine and rilpivirine. Other enzyme-inducing antiepileptics (e.g. phenytoin and phenobarbital) are expected to interact similarly, and cases of low efavirenz plasma concentrations have been reported with phenytoin.

Efavirenz reduces carbamazepine concentrations, and nevirapine is predicted to interact similarly.

Clinical evidence

(a) Delavirdine

The manufacturer of delavirdine reports that in 8 subjects taking delavirdine 300 to 400 mg three times daily, **carbamazepine**, **phenytoin**, and **phenobarbital** reduced the minimum concentration of delavirdine by 90%. No information on other pharmacokinetic parameters is available.[1]

(b) Efavirenz

In a crossover study, 26 healthy subjects took either efavirenz 600 mg daily for 35 days with **carbamazepine** titrated from 200 mg daily to 400 mg daily from days 15 to 35, or carbamazepine titrated from 200 mg to 400 mg daily for 35 days with efavirenz 600 mg daily from days 22 to 35. **Carbamazepine** slightly reduced the AUC of efavirenz by 36%, and reduced the maximum plasma concentration and minimum plasma concentration by 21% and 47%, respectively. Efavirenz slightly reduced the AUC, maximum plasma concentration, and minimum plasma concentration of **carbamazepine** by 27%, 20%, and 35%, respectively. However, no increase was seen in the plasma concentrations of the 10,11-epoxide metabolite of carbamazepine.[2]

A case of undetectable efavirenz plasma concentrations has been reported in one HIV-positive patient taking **phenytoin** 400 mg daily with efavirenz 800 mg daily. The dose of efavirenz was increased to 600 mg twice daily but the efavirenz plasma concentration did not increase until the **phenytoin** was stopped and lamotrigine and levetiracetam were started.[3] Another case of a low efavirenz plasma concentration has been reported in a patient taking **phenytoin** 300 mg twice daily. When phenytoin was changed to levetiracetam, the patient's efavirenz plasma concentration increased from 0.58 micrograms/mL to 2.5 micrograms/mL within 3 weeks. This patient had a gradual increase in phenytoin concentrations to about double the original concentration after starting efavirenz,[4] but note that the phenytoin dose had been doubled just before starting efavirenz.

One report describes efavirenz treatment failure in a patient given **oxcarbazepine**. However, in this particular case, efavirenz plasma concentrations had been checked before and during **oxcarbazepine** treatment and were unchanged, and on further questioning the patient admitted poor adherence to the HAART regimen.[5]

(c) Nevirapine

In a study, healthy subjects were given a single dose of nevirapine alone or with a single dose of **carbamazepine** 400 mg, **phenobarbital** 200 mg or **phenytoin** 184 mg, or with a 3-day or 7-day course of **phenytoin** 184 mg daily. The half-life of nevirapine was reduced by the single dose of **carbamazepine** by 37% and the two courses of **phenytoin** (by 41% and 31%), but the decrease with the single doses of **phenytoin** (11%) and **phenobarbital** (20%) were not statistically significant. The time to first undetectable nevirapine plasma concentration was also reduced, but nevirapine plasma concentrations 8 hours after administration of the enzyme inducers were not appreciably affected.[6]

Mechanism

The NNRTIs are all primarily metabolised by CYP3A4, and so their metabolism would be expected to be increased by drugs that are potent inducers of this isoenzyme, such as carbamazepine, phenytoin and probably phenobarbital. Efavirenz is also an inducer of CYP3A4, and so it can increase the metabolism of carbamazepine. Nevirapine would be expected to interact similarly.

Importance and management

The manufacturer of **delavirdine** does not recommend the concurrent use of carbamazepine, phenytoin, or phenobarbital as it could result in the loss of efficacy of delavirdine and lead to the development of delavirdine resistance.[1] Note that primidone is metabolised to phenobarbital, and fosphenytoin is a prodrug of phenytoin, so these drugs should probably also be avoided.

From the study and case reports, the concurrent use of carbamazepine and **efavirenz** reduces the concentrations of both drugs, and this might also lead to treatment failure. The manufacturers therefore recommend that an alternative to carbamazepine should be considered.[7,8] For phenytoin and phenobarbital, the manufacturers state that when efavirenz is given with these drugs, there is the potential for a reduction in efavirenz concentrations and a potential for a reduction[7,8] or increase[7] in the plasma concentrations of the antiepileptic. They recommend periodic monitoring of the plasma concentrations of phenytoin or phenobarbital on concurrent use,[7,8] and it would seem prudent to also apply this to patients given fosphenytoin or primidone. Note that efavirenz can itself cause seizures, therefore the manufacturers recommend caution in patients with a history of convulsions.[7,8]

The US manufacturer of **nevirapine** recommends caution on the concurrent use of carbamazepine because of the potential decrease in carbamazepine concentrations.[9] Bear in mind the possibility that nevirapine concentrations might also be reduced.

Etravirine and **rilpivirine** are also metabolised by CYP3A4, and the manufacturers predict that their plasma concentrations will be reduced by carbamazepine, oxcarbazepine (rilpivirine only), phenytoin, or phenobarbital. They therefore advise against concurrent use of etravirine[10,11] or contraindicate rilpivirine[12,13] with these drugs.

A number of other antiepileptics have been suggested as alternatives to the enzyme-inducing antiepileptics in patients taking NNRTIs. These include **gabapentin, lamotrigine, levetiracetam** and **vigabatrin.**[2-4,7]

1. Rescriptor (Delavirdine mesylate). ViiV Healthcare. US Prescribing information, August 2012.
2. Ji P, Damle B, Xie J, Unger SE, Grasela DM, Kaul S. Pharmacokinetic interaction between efavirenz and carbamazepine after multiple-dose administration in healthy subjects. *J Clin Pharmacol* (2008) 48, 948–56.
3. Spak CW, Dhanireddy S, Kosel BW. Clinical interaction between efavirenz and phenytoin. *AIDS* (2008) 22, 164–5.
4. Robertson SM, Penzak SR, Lane J, Pau AK, Mican JM. A potentially significant interaction between efavirenz and phenytoin: a case report and review of the literature. *Clin Infect Dis* (2005) 41, e15–e18.
5. Goicoechea M, Best B, Capparelli E, Haubrich R, for the Californian Collaborative Treatment Group. Concurrent use of efavirenz and oxcarbazepine may not affect efavirenz plasma concentrations. *Clin Infect Dis* (2006) 43, 116–7.
6. L'homme RFA, Dijkema T, van der Ven AJAM, Burger DM. Enzyme inducers reduce elimination half-life after a single dose of nevirapine in healthy women. *J Acquir Immune Defic Syndr* (2006) 43, 193–6.
7. Sustiva Film-coated Tablets (Efavirenz). Bristol-Myers Squibb Pharmaceutical Ltd. UK Summary of product characteristics, March 2014.
8. Sustiva (Efavirenz). Bristol-Myers Squibb Company. US Prescribing information, August 2012.
9. Viramune (Nevirapine). Boehringer Ingelheim Pharmaceuticals, Inc. US Prescribing information, November 2011.
10. Intelence (Etravirine). Janssen-Cilag Ltd. UK Summary of product characteristics, July 2012.
11. Intelence (Etravirine). Tibotec, Inc. US Prescribing information, August 2012.
12. Edurant (Rilpivirine hydrochloride). Janssen-Cilag Ltd. UK Summary of product characteristics, November 2011.
13. Edurant (Rilpivirine hydrochloride). Tibotec Pharmaceuticals. US Prescribing information, August 2012.

NNRTIs + Azoles; Fluconazole

Fluconazole slightly to moderately increases nevirapine exposure, and slightly increases etravirine exposure. However, fluconazole has negligible effect on efavirenz exposure, and does not appear to alter delavirdine plasma concentrations. Fluconazole pharmacokinetics are not altered by these NNRTIs.

Clinical evidence

(a) Delavirdine

In a study, 8 HIV-positive subjects were given delavirdine mesilate 300 mg three times daily for 30 days, with fluconazole 400 mg daily on days 16 to 30. When compared with 5 HIV-positive subjects given delavirdine alone, fluconazole had no apparent effect on the pharmacokinetics of delavirdine. Fluconazole pharmacokinetics did not appear to be affected by the concurrent use of delavirdine, when compared with previously reported data for healthy subjects, HIV-positive patients, and patients with AIDS.[1]

(b) Efavirenz

In a study, 20 healthy subjects were given fluconazole 400 mg daily for one day and then 200 mg daily for 6 days with efavirenz 400 mg daily. The pharmacokinetics of fluconazole were not affected by efavirenz, but the AUC of efavirenz was negligibly raised, by 15%.[2]

(c) Etravirine

In a study in 15 healthy subjects, fluconazole 200 mg daily for 16 days increased the AUC of etravirine (200 mg twice daily, taken on days 9 to 16) by 86%, and increased its maximum and minimum plasma concentrations by 75% and 2.1-fold, respectively. Etravirine did not alter fluconazole pharmacokinetics.[3]

(d) Nevirapine

In a nested pharmacokinetic study in 49 HIV-positive patients as part of a controlled clinical study, prophylactic low-dose fluconazole 200 mg three times weekly slightly increased nevirapine exposure by 29%, increased the plasma concentration of nevirapine at 8 hours post dose by 28%, and decreased its clearance by 22% when compared with placebo.[4] In the larger cohort of the controlled clinical study, use of fluconazole with nevirapine-based HAART was not associated with an increased risk of elevated hepatic transaminases requiring treatment to be stopped (5.2% taking fluconazole and 6.3% taking placebo) or rash (2.1% taking fluconazole and 3.7% taking placebo).[4] From earlier retrospective data it was estimated that the concurrent use of a larger dose of fluconazole of 200 mg daily[5] doubled the exposure to nevirapine, compared with historical control data.[5,6] Similarly, in another retrospective study in HIV-positive patients taking nevirapine-based HAART, nevirapine minimum plasma concentrations were 50% and 87% higher (9.8 mg/L and 12.2 mg/L), in patients taking fluconazole 200 mg daily (14 patients) or 400 mg daily (27 patients), respectively, compared with 6.5 mg/L in the 81 patients not taking fluconazole. However, there was no difference in liver function tests in the patients taking fluconazole compared with the control group, although one case of hepatitis was reported with the concurrent use of fluconazole. The incidence of rash was actually higher in the control group compared with those patients also taking fluconazole (7.4% versus 0%).[7] In another retrospective study, by the same authors, in HIV-positive patients who had received nevirapine-based HAART, there was no increase in the incidence of hepatitis, elevated aminotransferases or rashes, when the outcomes of 225 patients not taking fluconazole were compared with patients taking nevirapine with fluconazole 400 mg weekly (392 subjects), or fluconazole 200 mg daily (69 subjects).[8]

In a study in 19 subjects, nevirapine 200 mg daily for 14 days and then 200 mg twice daily for 14 days had a negligible effect on the pharmacokinetics of fluconazole 200 mg daily.[6]

Mechanism

Fluconazole at higher doses is a moderate inhibitor of CYP3A4, by which the NNRTIs are metabolised. Fluconazole is also an inhibitor of CYP2C9, by which etravirine is additionally partially metabolised.

Importance and management

Fluconazole slightly increases **etravirine** exposure, which is unlikely to require any dose adjustment.[9,10] Nevertheless, the US manufacturer advises caution because of the limited safety data for etravirine at this increased exposure.[10] For **nevirapine**, the best evidence indicates that low-dose fluconazole slightly increases nevirapine exposure and that this is not clinically important. However, retrospective evidence indicates that increases in nevirapine exposure might be higher with larger doses of fluconazole, although this might still have little clinical relevance. Nevertheless, the manufacturers of nevirapine advise that, if fluconazole and nevirapine are used concurrently, patients should be closely monitored for nevirapine-associated adverse effects (such as rash and hepatitis).[5,6]

No clinically relevant pharmacokinetic interaction appears to occur if fluconazole is used with delavirdine or efavirenz and no dose adjustment of these NNRTIs would be expected to be necessary in the presence of fluconazole. On the basis of the slight interaction of high doses of **rilpivirine** with ketoconazole (see 'NNRTIs + Azoles; Ketoconazole', p.954), no dose adjustment should be necessary on concurrent use of recommended doses of rilpivirine and fluconazole.[11,12] However, given the reduction in ketoconazole exposure with high-dose rilpivirine, the US manufacturer advises that patients should be monitored to ensure the azole remains effective.[12]

1. Borin MT, Cox SR, Herman BD, Carel BJ, Anderson RD, Freimuth WW. Effect of fluconazole on the steady-state pharmacokinetics of delavirdine in human immunodeficiency virus-positive patients. *Antimicrob Agents Chemother* (1997) 41, 1892–7.
2. Benedek IH, Fiske WD, White SJ, Kornhauser DM. Plasma levels of fluconazole (FL) are not altered by coadministration of DMP 266 in healthy volunteers. *Intersci Conf Antimicrob Agents Chemother* (1997) 37, 1.
3. Kakuda TN, van Solingen-Ristea R, Aharchi F, de Smedt G, Witek J, Nijs S, Vyncke V, Hoetelmans RMW. Pharmacokinetics and short-term safety of etravirine in combination with fluconazole or voriconazole in HIV-negative volunteers. *J Clin Pharmacol* (2012), Epub.
4. Wakeham K, Parkes-Ratanshi R, Watson V, Ggayi AB, Khoo S, Lalloo DG. Co-administration of fluconazole increases nevirapine concentrations in HIV-infected Ugandans. *J Antimicrob Chemother* (2010) 65, 316–19.
5. Viramune (Nevirapine). Boehringer Ingelheim Ltd. UK Summary of product characteristics, January 2012.
6. Viramune (Nevirapine). Boehringer Ingelheim Pharmaceuticals, Inc. US Prescribing information, November 2011.
7. Manosuthi W, Athichathanabadi C, Uttayamakul S, Phoorisri T, Sungkanuparph S. Plasma nevirapine levels, adverse effects and efficacy of antiretroviral therapy among HIV-infected patients concurrently receiving nevirapine-based antiretroviral therapy and fluconazole. *BMC Infect Dis* (2007) 7, 14.
8. Manosuthi W, Chumpathat N, Chaovavanich A, Sungkanuparph S. Safety and tolerability of nevirapine-based antiretroviral therapy in HIV-infected patients receiving fluconazole for cryptococcal prophylaxis: a retrospective cohort study. *BMC Infect Dis* (2005) 5, 67.
9. Intelence (Etravirine). Janssen-Cilag Ltd. UK Summary of product characteristics, July 2012.
10. Intelence (Etravirine). Tibotec, Inc. US Prescribing information, August 2012.
11. Edurant (Rilpivirine hydrochloride). Janssen-Cilag Ltd. UK Summary of product characteristics, November 2011.
12. Edurant (Rilpivirine hydrochloride). Tibotec Pharmaceuticals. US Prescribing information, August 2012.

NNRTIs + Azoles; Itraconazole

Itraconazole had no effect on efavirenz plasma concentrations in one study, whereas efavirenz slightly decreased itraconazole exposure, and cases of subtherapeutic itraconazole concentrations have been reported. Nevirapine moderately decreases itraconazole exposure. Etravirine is predicted to decrease itraconazole concentrations, and itraconazole is expected to increase etravirine plasma concentrations.

Clinical evidence

(a) Efavirenz

In a study in 18 healthy subjects, efavirenz 600 mg daily slightly decreased the steady-state AUC of itraconazole 200 mg twice daily by 39%, and decreased its maximum and minimum plasma concentrations by 37% and 44%, respectively. There was a similar decrease in the plasma concentrations of the active metabolite, hydroxyitraconazole. The steady-state maximum plasma concentrations and the AUC of efavirenz were not affected by itraconazole.[1,2]

There is evidence of subtherapeutic itraconazole concentrations and/or failure of itraconazole therapy in patients taking itraconazole. For example, a retrospective study identified 10 HIV-positive patients taking antiretroviral drugs, with itraconazole 200 mg or 400 mg daily for disseminated histoplasmosis. The 4 patients taking NNRTI-based regimens (efavirenz or **nevirapine**) had undetectable itraconazole serum concentrations. Two patients taking an HIV-protease inhibitor with an NNRTI had subtherapeutic itraconazole serum concentrations. Three patients had their NNRTI stopped due to subtherapeutic itraconazole serum concentrations. One patient taking an HIV-protease inhibitor with an NNRTI had a 6-fold increase in itraconazole serum concentrations when the NNRTI was stopped.[3] Similarly, a case of subtherapeutic itraconazole plasma concentrations has been reported in an HIV-positive patient with disseminated histoplasmosis taking efavirenz, stavudine and lamivudine. The patient had been taking itraconazole 200 mg daily with some signs of clinical improvement, but itraconazole plasma concentrations more than one year after the start of treatment were undetectable. The dose of itraconazole was subsequently increased to 200 mg twice daily but the plasma concentrations remained undetectable and the urine concentrations of *Histoplasma* antigen remained raised. Stopping efavirenz and changing to an HIV-protease inhibitor-based regimen resulted in an increase in plasma itraconazole concentrations and a reduction in the urine concentrations of *Histoplasma* antigen.[4] Note that HIV-protease inhibitors can raise itraconazole concentrations, see 'HIV-protease inhibitors + Azoles; Itraconazole', p.923.

Another case of reduced itraconazole plasma concentrations, and an *increase* in the minimum plasma concentrations of its active metabolite, hydroxyitraconazole, has also been reported on starting an efavirenz-based regimen.[5]

(b) Nevirapine

In a study in 12 healthy subjects, itraconazole 200 mg daily for 7 days had minimal effects on the pharmacokinetics of nevirapine 200 mg daily, also taken for 7 days. However, nevirapine decreased the AUC and maximum plasma concentration of itraconazole by 61% and 38%, respectively.[6] For a report of subtherapeutic itraconazole serum concentrations in 4 patients taking NNRTI-based regimens (either efavirenz or nevirapine), see under *Efavirenz*, above.

Mechanism

The metabolism of itraconazole by CYP3A4 is probably induced by efavirenz and nevirapine. **Etravirine** might interact similarly as it also induces CYP3A4.

Importance and management

On the basis of the pharmacokinetic study, the manufacturers of **efavirenz** state that alternatives to itraconazole should be considered.[1,2] If there are no appropriate alternatives, it might be prudent to increase the dose of itraconazole, with increased monitoring for efficacy and toxicity of the combination. This approach was successful in one reported case.[5] No dose adjustments of efavirenz appear to be necessary if it is taken with itraconazole.

As **nevirapine** also appears to reduce itraconazole exposure, itraconazole efficacy should be monitored carefully; anticipate the need to increase the dose of itraconazole. Nevertheless, the US manufacturer of nevirapine advises against the concurrent use of itraconazole.[7] No dose adjustments of nevirapine appear to be necessary if it is taken with itraconazole.

The manufacturers of **etravirine** predict that itraconazole might increase the plasma concentrations of etravirine,[8,9] which seems possible as voriconazole has this effect, see 'NNRTIs + Azoles; Voriconazole', p.954. They also predict that etravirine might reduce itraconazole plasma concentrations.[8,9] The US manufacturer advises that dose adjustments of itraconazole might be required, depending on other concurrent drugs.[9] However, the UK manufacturer advises that no dose adjustment of either itraconazole or etravirine is needed on concurrent use.[8]

On the basis of the slight interaction of high-dose **rilpivirine** with *ketoconazole* (see 'NNRTIs + Azoles; Ketoconazole', p.954), no dose adjustment should be necessary on concurrent use of recommended doses of rilpivirine and itraconazole.[10,11] However, given the reduction in ketoconazole exposure with high-dose rilpivirine, the US manufacturer advises that patients should be monitored to ensure the azole remains effective.[11]

1. Sustiva Film-coated Tablets (Efavirenz). Bristol-Myers Squibb Pharmaceutical Ltd. UK Summary of product characteristics, March 2014.
2. Sustiva (Efavirenz). Bristol-Myers Squibb Company. US Prescribing information, August 2012.
3. Andrade RA, Evans RT, Hamill RJ, Zerai T, Giordano TP. Clinical evidence of an interaction between itraconazole and nonnucleoside reverse transcriptase inhibitors in HIV-infected patients with disseminated histoplasmosis. *Ann Pharmacother* (2009) 43, 908–13.
4. Koo HL, Hamill RJ, Andrade RA. Drug-drug interaction between itraconazole and efavirenz in a patient with AIDS and disseminated histoplasmosis. *Clin Infect Dis* (2007) 45, e77–e79.
5. Huet E, Hadji C, Hulin A, Botterel F, Bretagne S, Lévy Y. Therapeutic monitoring is necessary for the association itraconazole and efavirenz in a patient with AIDS and disseminated histoplasmosis. *AIDS* (2008) 22, 1885–6.

6. Jaruratanasirikul S, Sriwiriyajan S. Pharmacokinetic study of the interaction between itraconazole and nevirapine. *Eur J Clin Pharmacol* (2007) 63, 451–6.
7. Viramune (Nevirapine). Boehringer Ingelheim Pharmaceuticals, Inc. US Prescribing information, November 2011.
8. Intelence (Etravirine). Janssen-Cilag Ltd. UK Summary of product characteristics, July 2012.
9. Intelence (Etravirine). Tibotec, Inc. US Prescribing information, August 2012.
10. Edurant (Rilpivirine hydrochloride). Janssen-Cilag Ltd. UK Summary of product characteristics, November 2011.
11. Edurant (Rilpivirine hydrochloride). Tibotec Pharmaceuticals. US Prescribing information, August 2012.

NNRTIs + Azoles; Ketoconazole

Ketoconazole exposure is moderately reduced by efavirenz and nevirapine, slightly reduced by supratherapeutic doses of rilpivirine, whereas it is predicted to be increased by delavirdine. Delavirdine and rilpivirine concentrations are raised by ketoconazole, whereas nevirapine concentrations appear to be little affected.

Clinical evidence

(a) Delavirdine

The manufacturer notes that, in 26 patients taking ketoconazole, the minimum plasma concentration of delavirdine was 50% higher than population pharmacokinetic data.[1]

(b) Efavirenz

In a study in 12 HIV-positive patients, efavirenz 600 mg daily for 15 days reduced the AUC_{0-24} and maximum plasma concentration of a single 400-mg dose of ketoconazole by 72% and 44%, respectively.[2]

(c) Nevirapine

The manufacturers of nevirapine quote a study in 21 HIV-positive subjects, in which nevirapine 200 mg twice daily was given with ketoconazole 400 mg daily. The AUC of ketoconazole was moderately reduced by 72% and its maximum plasma concentration was reduced by 44%.[3,4] In addition, the nevirapine plasma concentrations were 15 to 28% higher than in historical controls.[3]

(d) Rilpivirine

The manufacturers report that, in a study in 15 subjects, ketoconazole 400 mg daily slightly increased the AUC of a supratherapeutic dose of rilpivirine 150 mg daily by 49% and increased its maximum and minimum concentrations by 30%, and 76%, respectively. In addition, in this study, high-dose rilpivirine slightly reduced the AUC of ketoconazole by 24% and reduced its minimum concentration by 66%, although its maximum concentration was unaffected.[5,6]

Mechanism

Ketoconazole is likely to inhibit the metabolism of the NNRTIs by CYP3A4. Efavirenz and nevirapine both induce the metabolism of ketoconazole by CYP3A4, as does rilpivirine at higher than therapeutic doses. In theory, **etravirine**, a weak CYP3A4 inducer, might interact similarly, whereas delavirdine is likely to inhibit ketoconazole metabolism by CYP3A4.

Importance and management

A clinically relevant pharmacokinetic interaction appears to occur between **nevirapine** or **efavirenz** and ketoconazole, which might lead to antifungal treatment failure. The manufacturers of nevirapine state that ketoconazole and nevirapine should not be used together, because of the likely reduced efficacy of ketoconazole.[3,4] When compared with historical data, ketoconazole appears to cause a small increase in nevirapine concentrations, which is unlikely to be clinically important. If ketoconazole is essential with either nevirapine or efavirenz, the antifungal efficacy should be well monitored, and the ketoconazole dose increased as appropriate.

On the basis of the slight pharmacokinetic interaction of supratherapeutic doses of **rilpivirine** with ketoconazole, no dose adjustment of either drug is expected to be necessary on concurrent use.[5,6] However, given the reduction in ketoconazole exposure with high-dose rilpivirine, the US manufacturer advises that patients should be monitored to ensure the azole remains effective.[6]

The manufacturers of **etravirine** state that, as ketoconazole is a potent inhibitor of CYP3A4, it would be expected to increase the plasma concentrations of etravirine, whereas etravirine is expected to reduce the plasma concentrations of ketoconazole.[7,8] The US manufacturer advises that dose adjustments of ketoconazole might be required, depending on other concurrently used drugs.[8] However, the UK manufacturer states that no dose adjustment of either ketoconazole or etravirine is required on concurrent use.[7] Until more is known, some caution would be prudent, monitoring both the efficacy of ketoconazole and the adverse effects of etravirine.

Delavirdine plasma concentrations appear to be raised by ketoconazole, which might increase adverse effects. Delavirdine is predicted to increase ketoconazole exposure. Cautious monitoring for an increase in the adverse effects of delavirdine and ketoconazole would be prudent if concurrent use is necessary.

1. Rescriptor (Delavirdine mesylate). ViiV Healthcare. US Prescribing information, August 2012.
2. Sriwiriyajan S, Mahatthanatrakul W, Ridtitid W, Jaruratanasirikul S. Effect of efavirenz on the pharmacokinetics of ketoconazole in HIV-infected patients. *Eur J Clin Pharmacol* (2007) 63, 479–483.
3. Viramune (Nevirapine). Boehringer Ingelheim Ltd. UK Summary of product characteristics, January 2012.
4. Viramune (Nevirapine). Boehringer Ingelheim Pharmaceuticals, Inc. US Prescribing information, November 2011.
5. Edurant (Rilpivirine hydrochloride). Janssen-Cilag Ltd. UK Summary of product characteristics, November 2011.
6. Edurant (Rilpivirine hydrochloride). Tibotec Pharmaceuticals. US Prescribing information, August 2012.
7. Intelence (Etravirine). Janssen-Cilag Ltd. UK Summary of product characteristics, July 2012.
8. Intelence (Etravirine). Tibotec, Inc. US Prescribing information, August 2012.

NNRTIs + Azoles; Posaconazole

The concurrent use of efavirenz and posaconazole reduces posaconazole exposure but does not appear to affect efavirenz exposure. Etravirine plasma concentrations are predicted to be increased by posaconazole.

Clinical evidence

In a study in 10 healthy subjects, **efavirenz** 400 mg daily for 10 days reduced the AUC of posaconazole by 50% and reduced its maximum plasma concentration by 45%.[1] Posaconazole 400 mg twice daily for 10 days had no effect on **efavirenz** exposure and caused a negligible 13% increase in its maximum plasma concentration.[1]

Mechanism

Posaconazole is a substrate for glucuronyltransferases, and it is suggested that **efavirenz** induces this route of metabolism to reduce the plasma concentrations of posaconazole.[1] Posaconazole is an inhibitor of CYP3A4, and would therefore be predicted to increase the plasma concentrations of some NNRTIs similarly to ketoconazole, see 'NNRTIs + Azoles; Ketoconazole', above.

Importance and management

The halving of posaconazole exposure by efavirenz might be clinically relevant, and reduce its antifungal efficacy. The manufacturers advise avoiding concurrent use of **efavirenz** with posaconazole unless the benefits outweigh the risks.[2,3]

Etravirine plasma concentrations are predicted to be increased by posaconazole; however, the UK manufacturer states that no dose adjustment is needed on concurrent use.[4] The US manufacturer predicts that posaconazole plasma concentrations will not be altered by etravirine; however, they still advise that dose adjustments of posaconazole might be needed depending on other concurrently used drugs.[5]

On the basis of the slight interaction of high doses of **rilpivirine** with *ketoconazole* (see 'NNRTIs + Azoles; Ketoconazole', above), no dose adjustment should be necessary on the concurrent use of recommended doses of rilpivirine and posaconazole.[6,7] However, also based on the interaction with ketoconazole, the US manufacturer advises that patients should be monitored to ensure the azole remains effective.[7]

1. Krishna G, Moton A, Ma L, Martinho M, Seiberling M, McLeod J. Effects of oral posaconazole on the pharmacokinetics of atazanavir alone and with ritonavir or with efavirenz in healthy adult volunteers. *J Acquir Immune Defic Syndr* (2009) 51, 437–44.
2. Sustiva Film-coated Tablets (Efavirenz). Bristol-Myers Squibb Pharmaceutical Ltd. UK Summary of product characteristics, March 2014.
3. Sustiva (Efavirenz). Bristol-Myers Squibb Company. US Prescribing information, August 2012.
4. Intelence (Etravirine). Janssen-Cilag Ltd. UK Summary of product characteristics, July 2012.
5. Intelence (Etravirine). Tibotec, Inc. US Prescribing information, August 2012.
6. Edurant (Rilpivirine hydrochloride). Janssen-Cilag Ltd. UK Summary of product characteristics, November 2011.
7. Edurant (Rilpivirine hydrochloride). Tibotec Pharmaceuticals. US Prescribing information, August 2012.

NNRTIs + Azoles; Voriconazole

Voriconazole slightly increases efavirenz and etravirine exposure, and is predicted to increase delavirdine and nevirapine exposure. Efavirenz decreases voriconazole concentrations and nevirapine is predicted to interact similarly. Etravirine had a negligible effect on voriconazole exposure. Delavirdine is predicted to increase voriconazole exposure.

Clinical evidence

(a) Efavirenz

In a study in 16 healthy subjects, efavirenz 400 mg daily decreased the steady-state maximum plasma concentration and the AUC of voriconazole 200 mg twice daily by 62% and 78%, respectively. At the same time, the steady-state maximum plasma concentration and the AUC of efavirenz were increased by 37% and 44%, respectively.[1] In a dose-adjustment study in 15 healthy subjects, the AUC and maximum plasma concentration of voriconazole 300 mg twice daily were 55% and 36% lower, respectively, when efavirenz 300 mg daily for 7 days was also taken when compared with a lower dose of voriconazole 200 mg twice daily alone. The efavirenz AUC was equivalent to that seen with the higher dose of efavirenz 600 mg daily alone. When the voriconazole dose was increased further to 400 mg twice daily in 14 of the subjects, the AUC of voriconazole was just 7% lower than that seen with voriconazole 200 mg twice daily alone. The AUC of efavirenz was increased by 17% and the maximum plasma concentration was equivalent, when compared with efavirenz 600 mg daily alone.[2]

A case report describes the successful use of voriconazole with efavirenz, with doses adjusted based on plasma concentrations, for the long-term suppression of cryptococcosis and HIV viraemia. In this case, target plasma concentrations were achieved with voriconazole 200 mg twice daily and efavirenz 300 mg daily.[3] Conversely, another case report describes a patient taking a variety of antiretrovirals and antibacterials who developed oral candidiasis while taking voriconazole 200 mg twice daily, which was attributed to an interaction with efavirenz. The dose of voriconazole was titrated upwards to 350 mg twice daily to achieve higher minimum concentrations. The candidiasis was eventually found to be resistant to voriconazole, and it was suggested that this developed because of under-dosing in the presence of efavirenz.[4]

(b) Etravirine

In a pharmacokinetic study in 14 healthy subjects, voriconazole 400 mg twice daily for the first two doses followed by 200 mg twice daily for 15 days was given with etravirine 200 mg twice daily on days 9 to 16. Voriconazole increased the AUC of etravirine by 36% and increased its maximum plasma concentration by 26%. Etravirine had no notable effect on the pharmacokinetics of voriconazole, although there was wide interindividual variability.[5]

In one case report of a patient taking etravirine and darunavir boosted with ritonavir, the minimum etravirine concentration was 2.3-fold higher while taking voriconazole 400 mg twice daily than 3 weeks after voriconazole was stopped. The greater increase in etravirine concentrations in this patient compared with the healthy subjects might be due to the higher voriconazole dose.[6] However, in contrast, in another similar case, etravirine minimum concentrations did not appear to be appreciably affected by voriconazole 400 mg in the morning and 200 mg in the evening.[7]

Mechanism

The metabolism of voriconazole by CYP3A4 is induced by efavirenz and therefore concurrent use lowers voriconazole exposure; however, the reduction in exposure suggests that other pathways might also be induced as voriconazole is only partially metabolised by CYP3A4. Etravirine is a weak inducer of CYP3A4, and a weak inhibitor of CYP2C9 and CYP2C19. As voriconazole is primarily metabolised by CYP2C19 as well as CYP2C9 and CYP3A4, the negligible increase in voriconazole exposure is not unexpected. All of the NNRTIs are substrates of CYP3A4, which is inhibited by voriconazole, and therefore voriconazole can increase the concentrations of the NNRTIs.

Importance and management

On the basis of the pharmacokinetic studies the manufacturers state that **efavirenz** should not be given with voriconazole, unless the doses of both drugs are adjusted.[8,9] The recommendation is to double the usual dose of voriconazole to 400 mg twice daily, and to halve the usual efavirenz dose to 300 mg daily. The dose of efavirenz should be increased back to 600 mg daily when the voriconazole course is finished.[8,9] However, it has been suggested that if concurrent use is less than 4 days, then dose adjustment is not warranted.[10]

The concentrations of both **etravirine** and voriconazole are likely to be increased on concurrent use, but the effects on the exposure to both drugs are negligible to slight, and the manufacturers reasonably state that no dose adjustment is required for either drug.[11,12] However, the US manufacturer advises caution as the safety data regarding increased etravirine exposure are limited.[12] It might therefore be prudent to be alert for any evidence of increased etravirine adverse effects on concurrent use.

Nevirapine (a potentially moderate inducer of CYP3A4) reduces the concentrations of other azoles metabolised by CYP3A4, such as ketoconazole, see 'NNRTIs + Azoles; Ketoconazole', p.954, and it might be expected to have a similar effect on voriconazole metabolism, whereas **delavirdine** (a CYP3A4 inhibitor) might increase voriconazole concentrations. Exposure to these NNRTIs might also be increased by voriconazole, which might increase adverse effects. The manufacturers of voriconazole suggest that patients given delavirdine or nevirapine should be carefully monitored for evidence of drug toxicity and/or loss of efficacy during concurrent use.[13,14]

On the basis of the slight interaction of high-dose **rilpivirine** with *ketoconazole* (see 'NNRTIs + Azoles; Ketoconazole', p.954), no dose adjustment should be necessary on concurrent use of recommended doses of rilpivirine and voriconazole.[15,16] However, given the reduction in ketoconazole exposure with high-dose rilpivirine, the US manufacturer advises that patients should be monitored to ensure the azole remains effective.[15]

1. Liu P, Foster G, LaBadie R, Gutierrez MJ, Sharma A. Pharmacokinetic interaction between voriconazole and efavirenz at steady state in healthy male subjects. *J Clin Pharmacol* (2008) 48, 73–84.
2. Damle B, LaBadie R, Crownover P, Glue P. Pharmacokinetic interactions of efavirenz and voriconazole in healthy volunteers. *Br J Clin Pharmacol* (2007) 65, 523–30.
3. Carbonara S, Regazzi M, Ciraci E, Villani P, Stano F, Cusato M, Heichen M, Monno L. Long-term efficacy and safety of TDM-assisted combination of voriconazole plus efavirenz in an AIDS patient with cryptococcosis and liver cirrhosis. *Ann Pharmacother* (2009) 43, 978–84.
4. Gerzenshtein L, Patel SM, Scarsi KK, Postelnick MJ, Flaherty JP. Breakthrough *Candida* infections in patients receiving voriconazole. *Ann Pharmacother* (2005) 39, 1342–5.
5. Kakuda TN, van Solingen-Ristea R, Aharchi F, de Smedt G, Witek J, Nijs S, Vyncke V, Hoetelmans RMW. Pharmacokinetics and short-term safety of etravirine in combination with fluconazole or voriconazole in HIV-negative volunteers. *J Clin Pharmacol* (2012), Epub.
6. Toy J, Giguère P, Kravcik S, la Porte CJL. Drug interactions between voriconazole, darunavir/ritonavir and etravirine in an HIV-infected patient with Aspergillus pneumonia. *AIDS* (2011) 25, 541–2.
7. Aouri M, Decosterd LA, Buclin T, Hirschel B, Calmy A, Livio F. Drug interactions between voriconazole, darunavir/ritonavir and etravirine in an HIV-infected patient with *Aspergillus* pneumonia. *AIDS* (2012) 26, 776–8.
8. Sustiva (Efavirenz). Bristol-Myers Squibb Company. US Prescribing information, August 2012.
9. Sustiva Film-coated Tablets (Efavirenz). Bristol-Myers Squibb Pharmaceutical Ltd. UK Summary of product characteristics, March 2014.
10. Yakiwchuk EM, Foisy MM, Hughes CA. Complexity of interactions between voriconazole and antiretroviral agents. *Ann Pharmacother* (2008) 42, 698–703.
11. Intelence (Etravirine). Janssen-Cilag Ltd. UK Summary of product characteristics, July 2012.
12. Intelence (Etravirine). Tibotec, Inc. US Prescribing information, August 2012
13. VFEND (Voriconazole). Pfizer Ltd. UK Summary of product characteristics, October 2014.
14. VFEND (Voriconazole). Pfizer Inc. US Prescribing information, February 2014.
15. Edurant (Rilpivirine hydrochloride). Janssen-Cilag Ltd. UK Summary of product characteristics, November 2011.
16. Edurant (Rilpivirine hydrochloride). Tibotec Pharmaceuticals. US Prescribing information, August 2012.

NNRTIs + Food

Food slightly increases efavirenz exposure, and this is predicted to increase the frequency of efavirenz CNS adverse effects. Food increases etravirine and rilpivirine exposure. Food does not appear to alter delavirdine or nevirapine exposure; however, orange juice might increase delavirdine absorption.

Clinical evidence, mechanism, importance and management

(a) Delavirdine

In a randomised, crossover study in 13 HIV-positive patients taking delavirdine 400 mg three times daily, there were no changes in the steady-state AUC or minimum plasma concentration of delavirdine taken with food, or taken at least one hour before or 2 hours after food, for 2 weeks. Food reduced the maximum plasma concentration of delavirdine was by just 21%.[1] This differed from a previous single-dose study in 12 healthy subjects, in which there was a slight 26% reduction in the AUC of delavirdine when it was taken with food.[2] There would appear to be no need to avoid taking delavirdine with food.

Orange juice increased delavirdine absorption by 50% to 70% in subjects with gastric hypoacidity, but had less effect (0 to 30%) in those with normal gastric acidity. However, despite the use of **orange juice**, the AUC of delavirdine was still about 50% lower in patients with gastric hypoacidity than those with normal gastric acidity.[3]

Delavirdine is a weak base that is poorly soluble at neutral pH. Therefore, in subjects with gastric hypoacidity, the absorption of delavirdine is reduced, and substances that lower gastric pH increase its absorption. The manufacturer of delavirdine recommends that, in patients with achlorhydria, delavirdine should be taken with an acidic beverage such as **orange** or **cranberry juice**, although this has not been specifically investigated.[4]

(b) Efavirenz

The manufacturers of efavirenz note that a high-fat meal slightly increased the AUC of a 600-mg efavirenz *tablet* by 28%, when compared with fasting conditions, and increased its maximum concentration by 79%.[5,6] After a similar meal, the AUC and maximum plasma concentration of the *capsule* formulation was increased by just 22% and 39%, respectively, and after a low-fat meal the increases were 17% and 51%, respectively.[6] A similar 13% increase in the AUC of efavirenz and 47% increase in its maximum plasma concentrations was seen when the fixed dose combination tablet of efavirenz, tenofovir, and emtricitabine was taken with a meal compared with the fasting state.[7] However, the manufacturers state that these increases might increase the frequency of nervous system adverse effects and they recommend that efavirenz is taken on an empty stomach, preferably at bedtime.[5,6] Note that nervous system effects are common after the first few days of use and usually resolve in a few weeks.[6] Because the increases in AUC and concentrations are slight it seems unlikely that they are generally clinically relevant, especially in the longer term. The authors of one of the studies suggest that stable patients can take the combination efavirenz tablet without meal restrictions, but that patients experiencing CNS toxicities should take the tablet without food.[7]

In another single-dose study in 21 healthy subjects, when the contents of an efavirenz capsule were taken mixed with two teaspoonfuls of **apple sauce**, **grape jelly**, **yoghurt**, or **infant formula** efavirenz exposure did not differ from when an intact capsule was taken under fasting conditions.[8] Therefore, splitting the capsule and taking the contents with a small amount of food like this is acceptable where necessary.[8]

(c) Etravirine

In a randomised, crossover study in 20 healthy subjects, a single 100-mg dose of etravirine was taken on an empty stomach, with a light breakfast (a croissant), with a standard breakfast, with a high-fibre breakfast, or with a high-fat breakfast. The AUC of etravirine was 51% lower when it was taken on an empty stomach, compared with a standard breakfast. The AUC of etravirine taken after a light breakfast or high-fibre breakfast was 20% and 25% lower respectively, than after a standard breakfast. A high-fat breakfast resulted in a slight 9% increase in the AUC of etravirine. As the absorption of etravirine was nearly halved when it was taken on an empty stomach, it is recommended that etravirine should be taken with food. The differences between the types of meals were not considered to be clinically relevant.[9]

(d) Nevirapine

In a single-dose study in 24 healthy subjects, a high-fat breakfast delayed the time to maximum plasma concentration of nevirapine 200 mg by about 2 hours, but the maximum concentration was only reduced by 5% and the AUC was not affected. None of the changes were considered to be clinically relevant.[10] Nevirapine can therefore be taken with or without food.

(e) Rilpivirine

In a study, taking rilpivirine in the fasted state reduced the exposure to rilpivirine by 40%, when compared with a standard meal or a high-fat meal. **Protein-rich drinks** also appear to reduce the exposure to rilpivirine by 50%, when compared with a standard meal. These reductions in exposure could result in a loss of rilpivirine antiviral efficacy. The manufacturers therefore state that rilpivirine must be taken with a meal to ensure optimum absorption, and that a protein-rich drink is not a substitute for a meal.[11,12]

1. Morse GD, Fischl MA, Shelton MJ, Cox SR, Thompson L, Della-Coletta AA, Freimuth WW. Effect of food on the steady-state pharmacokinetics of delavirdine in patients with HIV infection. *Clin Drug Invest* (2003) 23, 255–61.
2. Cox SR, Della-Coletta AA, Turner SW, Freimuth WW. Single-dose pharmacokinetic (PK) studies with delavirdine (DLV) mesylate: dose proportionality and effects of food and antacid. *Intersci Conf Antimicrob Agents Chemother* (1994) 34, 82.
3. Shelton MJ, Hewitt RG, Adams JM, Cox SR, Chambers JH, Morse GD. Delavirdine malabsorption in HIV-infected subjects with spontaneous gastric hypoacidity. *J Clin Pharmacol* (2003) 43, 171–9.
4. Rescriptor (Delavirdine mesylate). ViiV Healthcare. US Prescribing information, August 2012.
5. Sustiva Film-coated Tablets (Efavirenz). Bristol-Myers Squibb Pharmaceutical Ltd. UK Summary of product characteristics, March 2014.

6. Sustiva (Efavirenz). Bristol-Myers Squibb Company. US Prescribing information, August 2012.
7. Lamorde M, Byakika-Kibwika P, Tamale WS, Kiweewa F, Ryan M, Amara A, Tjia J, Back D, Khoo S, Boffito M, Kityo C, Merry C. Effect of food on the steady-state pharmacokinetics of tenofovir and emtricitabine plus efavirenz in Ugandan adults. *AIDS Res Treat* (2012) 2012, doi 105980.
8. Kaul S, Ji P, Lu M, Nguyen KL, Shangguan T, Grasela D. Bioavailability in healthy adults of efavirenz capsule contents mixed with a small amount of food. *Am J Health-Syst Pharm* (2010) 67, 217–22.
9. Schöller-Gyüre M, Boffito M, Pozniak AL, Leemans R, Kakuda TN, Woodfall B, Vyncke V, Peeters M, Vandermeulen K, Hoetelmans RMW. Effects of different meal compositions and fasted state on the oral bioavailability of etravirine. *Pharmacotherapy* (2008) 28, 1215–22.
10. Lamson MJ, Cort S, Sabo JP, MacGregor TR, Keirns JJ, Effects of food or antacid on the bioavailability of nevirapine 200 mg in 24 healthy volunteers. *Pharm Res* (1995) 12 (9 Suppl), S-101.
11. Edurant (Rilpivirine hydrochloride). Janssen-Cilag Ltd. UK Summary of product characteristics, November 2011.
12. Edurant (Rilpivirine hydrochloride). Tibotec Pharmaceuticals. US Prescribing information, August 2012.

NNRTIs + H_2-receptor antagonists

Famotidine, taken 2 hours before rilpivirine, moderately reduces its exposure and ranitidine negligibly reduces etravirine exposure. H_2-receptor antagonists are predicted to reduce delavirdine exposure. H_2-receptor antagonists do not alter efavirenz exposure or nevirapine concentrations.

Clinical evidence

(a) Efavirenz

The manufacturer notes that, in a single-dose study in 17 healthy subjects, **famotidine** 40 mg did not alter the AUC or maximum concentration of efavirenz.[1,2]

(b) Etravirine

In a study in 16 healthy subjects, **ranitidine** 150 mg twice daily for 11 days negligibly decreased the AUC of a single 100-mg dose of etravirine given on day 8 by 14%.[3]

(c) Nevirapine

The UK manufacturer briefly states that nevirapine has no significant effect on the pharmacokinetics of **cimetidine**, and **cimetidine** causes an increase of only 7% in the minimum concentrations of nevirapine.[4]

(d) Rilpivirine

In a study, a single 40-mg dose of **famotidine** taken 2 hours before a single 150-mg dose of rilpivirine (23 subjects) reduced the AUC and maximum concentration of rilpivirine by 76% and 85%, respectively. However, when the same dose of famotidine was taken 4 hours after rilpivirine (24 subjects), the AUC and maximum concentration of rilpivirine were *increased* by 13% and 21%, respectively. Taking famotidine 12 hours before rilpivirine (24 subjects) had a negligible effect on the pharmacokinetics of rilpivirine (AUC reduced by 9%).[5,6]

Mechanism

The absorption of **delavirdine** and rilpivirine is pH-dependent, and is reduced if gastric acidity is reduced by drugs such as the H_2-receptor antagonists. Absorption of efavirenz, etravirine, and nevirapine does not appear to be pH dependent. Cimetidine is a weak inhibitor of a number of cytochrome P450 isoenzymes, and might therefore be predicted to cause an increase in NNRTI concentrations, but the effect on nevirapine was small.

Importance and management

The reduction in **rilpivirine** exposure with famotidine would be expected to reduce its antiviral efficacy. Other H_2-receptor antagonists would be expected to interact similarly. The manufacturers therefore state that the H_2-receptor antagonists should be taken at least 12 hours before or 4 hours after rilpivirine. They also state that only H_2-receptor antagonists that can be taken once daily should be given with rilpivirine.[5,6] Because of its interaction with antacids (see 'NNRTIs + Antacids', p.951), **delavirdine** exposure is predicted to be reduced by H_2-receptor antagonists, and similar precautions should be taken, although the manufacturer states that their long-term use with delavirdine is not recommended.[7]

The negligible decrease in **etravirine** exposure with ranitidine is not clinically relevant, neither is the small increase in **nevirapine** concentrations with cimetidine. **Efavirenz** exposure is not affected by famotidine. It is unlikely that these NNRTIs will undergo clinically important pharmacokinetic interactions with any H_2-receptor antagonists.

1. Sustiva Film-coated Tablets (Efavirenz). Bristol-Myers Squibb Pharmaceutical Ltd. UK Summary of product characteristics, March 2014.
2. Sustiva (Efavirenz). Bristol-Myers Squibb Company. US Prescribing information, August 2012.
3. Schöller-Gyüre M, Kakuda TN, De Smedt G, Vanaken H, Bouche M-P, Peeters M, Woodfall B, Hoetelmans RMW. A pharmacokinetic study of etravirine (TMC125) co-administered with ranitidine and omeprazole in HIV-negative volunteers. *Br J Clin Pharmacol* (2008) 66, 508–516.
4. Viramune (Nevirapine). Boehringer Ingelheim Ltd. UK Summary of product characteristics, January 2012.
5. Edurant (Rilpivirine hydrochloride). Janssen-Cilag Ltd. UK Summary of product characteristics, November 2011.
6. Edurant (Rilpivirine hydrochloride). Tibotec Pharmaceuticals. US Prescribing information, August 2012.
7. Rescriptor (Delavirdine mesylate). ViiV Healthcare. US Prescribing information, August 2012.

NNRTIs + HIV-protease inhibitors

In general, efavirenz and nevirapine decrease the concentrations of the HIV-protease inhibitors, whereas delavirdine increases them. Rilpivirine has little effect, and etravirine causes minor decreases or increases in some HIV-protease inhibitor concentrations. Amprenavir and nelfinavir decrease the concentrations of delavirdine. Most HIV-protease inhibitors do not appear to affect the concentrations of efavirenz or nevirapine, whereas some decrease etravirine concentrations and some increase rilpivirine concentrations. There is some evidence of increased adverse effects with antiviral doses of ritonavir and efavirenz, or saquinavir and delavirdine, including raised liver enzymes.

Clinical evidence, mechanism, importance and management

Note that the concurrent use of an NNRTI with a HIV-protease inhibitor is not a recommended regimen when starting antiretrovirals in treatment-naive patients.[1,2]

(a) Delavirdine

For a summary of the studies of the pharmacokinetic interactions of delavirdine and various HIV-protease inhibitors, see 'Table 21.3', p.957. In general, these studies show that delavirdine can markedly increase HIV-protease inhibitor exposure. In addition, **amprenavir** and **nelfinavir** have been shown to approximately halve the AUC of delavirdine.

Delavirdine and the HIV-protease inhibitors are known to be both inhibitors of, and substrates for CYP3A4, see 'Table 21.2', p.894.

It has been suggested that delavirdine could be used clinically to boost the exposure to HIV-protease inhibitors, and this has been tried in at least one study.[3] However, this combination is complicated by the decrease in delavirdine concentrations caused by some HIV-protease inhibitors, and the combination might not be appropriate if the antiviral effect of delavirdine is required.[4] Moreover, if the combination is used, patients should be closely monitored for toxicity as in one study of **nelfinavir** and delavirdine, 4 out of 24 subjects had to stop both drugs before completing the study because of neutropenia, which resolved over several days.[5] The UK manufacturer of **saquinavir** states that liver function should be monitored frequently if delavirdine is also given, because the concurrent use of saquinavir boosted with ritonavir and delavirdine carries an increased risk of hepatotoxicity.[6] For a summary of the manufacturers' recommended regimens for use with delavirdine, see 'Table 21.4', p.961.

(b) Efavirenz

For a summary of the studies of the pharmacokinetic interactions of efavirenz and various HIV-protease inhibitors, see 'Table 21.3', p.957. The HIV-protease inhibitors had no effect or a negligible effect on efavirenz exposure or plasma concentrations. Efavirenz is an inducer of CYP3A4, by which the HIV-protease inhibitors are metabolised. With the exceptions of **nelfinavir** and **ritonavir**, which showed negligible increases in exposure, efavirenz decreases HIV-protease inhibitor exposure, often to concentrations likely to lead to reduced antiviral efficacy. Ways to overcome this include the addition of low-dose **ritonavir** to boost the concentrations of the HIV-protease inhibitor (**amprenavir**, **atazanavir**, **saquinavir**, **fosamprenavir**, **lopinavir**, **tipranavir**) and/or increasing the dose of the HIV-protease inhibitor (**fosamprenavir**, **lopinavir**, **tipranavir**). For a summary of the manufacturers' recommended regimens for use with efavirenz 600 mg daily, see 'Table 21.4', p.961. The manufacturers of efavirenz note that increased adverse effects, including dizziness, nausea, paraesthesia, and elevated liver enzyme concentrations, occurred with the concurrent use of efavirenz and **ritonavir** 500 or 600 mg twice daily (antiretroviral dose), and the combination was not well tolerated.[7,8] They recommend monitoring liver enzyme concentrations with this combination.[8] The UK manufacturer states that the tolerability of low-dose **ritonavir** with efavirenz has not been assessed, and they state that the possibility of an increase in the incidence of efavirenz-associated adverse events should be considered with any **ritonavir**-boosted regimen used with efavirenz, due to a possible pharmacodynamic interaction.[7]

With **lopinavir** boosted with ritonavir, although an increased dose of 533/133 mg twice daily with efavirenz or **nevirapine** produced similar plasma concentrations of lopinavir to those seen with the lower dose of 400/100 mg twice daily without an NNRTI, the proportion of patients with a suboptimal minimum concentration of lopinavir tended to be higher in those patients receiving the NNRTI.[9] This suggests that some patients might need a further increase in the dose of lopinavir boosted with ritonavir. Another study with **atazanavir** boosted with ritonavir also found that the increased dose of atazanavir for use with NNRTIs did not appear to overcome the inducer effect of NNRTIs (efavirenz or **nevirapine**) and led to a 43% lower median minimum concentration of atazanavir, and a greater proportion of patients with suboptimal minimum concentrations (25% versus 7%).[10]

(c) Etravirine

For a summary of the studies of the pharmacokinetic interactions of etravirine and various HIV-protease inhibitors, see 'Table 21.3', p.957. Etravirine is a weak inducer of CYP3A4, and it might also inhibit CYP2C19 and P-glycoprotein. With atazanavir, lopinavir, and saquinavir (each boosted with ritonavir), there were small decreases in concentrations, whereas etravirine appeared to increase concentrations of fosamprenavir and tipranavir (both boosted with ritonavir), and caused no change in the concentrations of darunavir (boosted with ritonavir). Etravirine concentrations were decreased by darunavir, lopinavir, saquinavir, and tipranavir, each boosted with ritonavir. However, despite the decrease with darunavir, the safety and efficacy of this combination has been established in a clinical study.[11,12] For a summary of the manufacturers' recommended regimens for use with etravirine, see 'Table 21.4', p.961.

Note that the concurrent use of an NNRTI with a HIV-protease inhibitor is not a recommended regimen when starting antiretrovirals in treatment-naive patients.[1,2]

Table 21.3 Summary of the pharmacokinetic interactions of NNRTIs and HIV-protease inhibitors

Drug combination	*No. of healthy subjects (unless specified)*	*Change in AUC (unless specified)* NNRTI	HIV-protease inhibitor	*Refs*
Delavirdine studies (usually 400 mg three times daily or 600 mg twice daily)				
Amprenavir	6 HIV-positive children		3-fold increase in Cmax* 5- to 10-fold increase in Cmin*	1
Amprenavir 1200 mg	12	21% increase	4-fold increase	2
Amprenavir 1200 mg twice daily alone then 600 mg twice daily in combination	11	47% decrease	32% increase versus twice the dose given alone	2
Amprenavir 600 mg twice daily	18	61% decrease	130% increase	3
Indinavir 800 mg alone then 600 mg in combination	14	No change	44% increase versus higher dose given alone	4,5
Nelfinavir 750 mg three times daily	24	42% decrease	92% increase	6
Ritonavir 300 mg twice daily		No change in steady state concentration	No change in steady state concentration	4
Ritonavir 600 mg twice daily	12 HIV-positive subjects	No change*	64% increase with an 81% increase in Cmin	7
Ritonavir 100 mg twice daily	19	No change	80% increase	8
Saquinavir 600 mg three times daily		No change in steady state concentration	5-fold increase in steady state concentration	4
Efavirenz studies (600 mg once daily)				
Amprenavir 1200 mg twice daily	7 HIV-positive subjects		About an 80% decrease in Cmin†	9
Amprenavir 1200 mg twice daily	11 HIV-positive subjects	No change*	24% decrease with a 43% decrease in Cmin	10
Atazanavir 400 mg once daily	27	No change	74% decrease with a 93% decrease in Cmin	11
Atazanavir/Ritonavir 300/100 mg daily (2 hours before efavirenz)	13		39% increase with a 48% increase in Cmin (atazanavir)	11
Atazanavir/Ritonavir 400/100 mg daily (simultaneous)	14		No change with a 42% decrease in Cmin (atazanavir)	11
Darunavir/Ritonavir 300/100 mg twice daily	12	21% increase	13% decrease with a 31% decrease in Cmin (darunavir)	12
Darunavir/Ritonavir 900/100 mg twice daily	12	No change in AUC or Cmin	14% decrease with a 57% decrease in Cmin (darunavir) 26% decrease with a 54% decrease in Cmin (ritonavir)	13
Fosamprenavir/Ritonavir 1395/200 mg daily	11		31% decrease in Cmin (amprenavir)	14
Fosamprenavir/Ritonavir 700/100 mg twice daily	14		Slight decrease in Cmin (amprenavir)	14
Fosamprenavir/Ritonavir 1395/300 mg daily	11		Amprenavir concentrations comparable to that seen with fosamprenavir/ritonavir 1395/200 mg alone	14
Indinavir 1000 mg three times daily			Decrease of about 31% versus lower dose given alone and a 40% decrease in Cmin (indinavir)	15
Indinavir/Ritonavir 800/100 mg twice daily	14	No change*	25% decrease (indinavir) 36% decrease (ritonavir)	16
Indinavir/Ritonavir 800/100 mg twice daily	20 HIV-positive subjects	31% increase in Cmin*	Cmin halved* (indinavir)	17
Lopinavir/Ritonavir 400/100 mg twice daily	24 HIV-positive subjects		44% decrease in Cmin* (lopinavir) 56% decrease with a 79% decrease in Cmin (lopinavir)	18 19

*Versus historical control data
†Therapeutic concentrations subsequently achieved by the addition of low-dose ritonavir
‡Versus data from 139 patients not taking nevirapine
Cmax = maximum serum concentration, Cmin = minimum serum concentration

Continued

Table 21.3 Summary of the pharmacokinetic interactions of NNRTIs and HIV-protease inhibitors (continued)

Drug combination	*No. of healthy subjects (unless specified)*	*Change in AUC (unless specified)*		*Refs*
		NNRTI	**HIV-protease inhibitor**	
Lopinavir/Ritonavir 533/133 mg twice daily	26 HIV-positive subjects		No change in Cmin versus lower dose given without efavirenz* (lopinavir) 40% decrease with a 66% decrease in Cmin (lopinavir) relative to lopinavir/ritonavir 400/100 mg twice daily	18 19
Lopinavir/Ritonavir 500/125 mg twice daily			No change in steady state concentration (lopinavir) relative to lopinavir/ritonavir 400/100 mg twice daily	20
Lopinavir/Ritonavir 600/150 mg twice daily			17% decrease with a 48% decrease in Cmin (lopinavir) relative to lopinavir/ritonavir 400/100 mg twice daily	19
Lopinavir/Ritonavir 300/75 mg/m^2 twice daily	15 HIV-positive children	No change*	No change*	21
Nelfinavir 750 mg three times daily		No change	20% increase (nelfinavir), 37% decrease in M8 metabolite of nelfinavir	22
Nelfinavir/Ritonavir 1875/200 mg daily	24	No change*	30% increase (nelfinavir) 20% decrease (ritonavir)	23
Ritonavir 500 mg twice daily		21% increase	17% increase	24
Saquinavir/Ritonavir 400/400 mg twice daily	12	No change*	No change in Cmin (ritonavir) 10% decrease in Cmin (saquinavir)	25
Tipranavir/Ritonavir 500/100 mg twice daily	24/21	No change	31% decrease with a 42% decrease in Cmin (tipranavir)*	26
Tipranavir/Ritonavir 250/200 mg twice daily	23	No change		27
Tipranavir/Ritonavir 750/100 mg twice daily	19	No change		27
Tipranavir/Ritonavir 1250/100 mg twice daily	15	No change		27
Etravirine studies (100 mg or 200 mg twice daily)				
Atazanavir/Ritonavir 300/100 mg daily		30% increase	14% decrease with a 38% decrease in Cmin (atazanavir)	28
Darunavir/Ritonavir 600/100 mg twice daily	23	37% decrease with a 49% decrease in Cmin	No change with etravirine 100 mg, 15% increase with etravirine 200 mg, no change in Cmin (darunavir)	29
Fosamprenavir/Ritonavir 700/100 mg twice daily		No change	69% increase with a 77% increase in Cmin (amprenavir)	28
Lopinavir/Ritonavir 400/100 mg twice daily		35% decrease with a 45% decrease in Cmin	13% decrease with a 20% decrease in Cmin (lopinavir)	28
Saquinavir/Ritonavir 1000/100 mg twice daily		33% decrease with a 29% decrease in Cmin	No change in AUC and a 20% decrease in Cmin (saquinavir)	28
Tipranavir/Ritonavir 500/200 mg twice daily		76% decrease with a 82% decrease in Cmin	18% increase with a 24% increase in Cmin (tipranavir)	28
Nevirapine studies (200 mg once daily increased to twice daily)				
Atazanavir/Ritonavir 300/100 mg twice daily	11 HIV-positive patients	46% increase in Cmin*	41% decrease in Cmin (atazanavir)	30
Darunavir/Ritonavir 400/100 mg twice daily		27% increase	24% increase No change in Cmin* (darunavir)	31
Fosamprenavir 1400 mg twice daily		29% increase	33% decrease with a 35% decrease in Cmin (amprenavir)	32
Fosamprenavir/Ritonavir 700/100 mg twice daily		14% increase	11% decrease with a 19% decrease in Cmin (amprenavir)	32

*Versus historical control data
†Therapeutic concentrations subsequently achieved by the addition of low-dose ritonavir
‡Versus data from 139 patients not taking nevirapine
Cmax = maximum serum concentration, Cmin = minimum serum concentration

Continued

Table 21.3 Summary of the pharmacokinetic interactions of NNRTIs and HIV-protease inhibitors (continued)

Drug combination	*No. of healthy subjects (unless specified)*	*Change in AUC (unless specified)*		*Refs*
		NNRTI	**HIV-protease inhibitor**	
Indinavir 800 mg three times daily	19 HIV-positive subjects	No change*	28% decrease with a 48% decrease in Cmin	33
Indinavir 800 mg three times daily alone or 1000 mg three times daily in combination	124 HIV-positive subjects	No change	27% decrease in Cmin versus therapy alone at lower dose	34
Indinavir/Ritonavir 800/100 mg twice daily	21 HIV-positive subjects		57% decrease in Cmin (indinavir)‡	35
Lopinavir/Ritonavir 300/75 mg/m^2 twice daily	27 HIV-positive children		22% decrease with a 55% decrease in Cmin (lopinavir)	36
Lopinavir/Ritonavir 400/100 mg twice daily			44% decrease with a 67% decrease in Cmin (lopinavir)	19
Lopinavir/Ritonavir 533/133 mg twice daily			38% decrease with a 59% decrease in Cmin (lopinavir) relative to lopinavir/ritonavir 400/100 mg twice daily	19
Lopinavir/Ritonavir 600/150 mg twice daily			No change in AUC or Cmin (lopinavir) relative to lopinavir/ritonavir 400/100 mg twice daily	19
Nelfinavir 750 mg three times daily	7 HIV-positive subjects	No change*	50% decrease possibly due to sampling before nelfinavir steady state was reached	37,38
	23 HIV-positive positive	No change*	No change	39
	13 HIV-positive subjects		No change	40
	23 HIV-positive subjects		No change; 32% decrease in Cmin, 62% decrease in M8 metabolite	41,42
Ritonavir 600 mg twice daily	18 HIV-positive subjects	No change	No change	41,42
Saquinavir 600 mg three times daily	21 HIV-positive subjects	No change	27% decrease	43
Saquinavir/Ritonavir	20 HIV-positive subjects	No change*	No change	42
Tipranavir/Ritonavir 250/200 mg twice daily	26 HIV-positive subjects	No change		22,27
Tipranavir/Ritonavir 250/200 mg twice daily	22 HIV-positive subjects	No change		27
Tipranavir/Ritonavir 750/100 mg twice daily	22 HIV-positive subjects	No change		27
Tipranavir/Ritonavir 1250/100 mg twice daily	17 HIV-positive subjects	23% decrease in Cmin		27
Rilpivirine studies (150 mg daily)				
Darunavir/Ritonavir 800/100 mg daily	16	2.3-fold increase with a 2.8-fold increase in Cmin, and a 79% increase in Cmax	11% decrease with a 11% decrease in Cmin (darunavir)	44
Lopinavir/Ritonavir 400/100 mg twice daily	15	52% increase with a 74% increase in Cmin, and a 29% increase in Cmax	No change with a 11% decrease in Cmin (lopinavir)	45,46

*Versus historical control data
†Therapeutic concentrations subsequently achieved by the addition of low-dose ritonavir
‡Versus data from 139 patients not taking nevirapine
Cmax = maximum serum concentration, Cmin = minimum serum concentration

1. Wintergerst U, Engelhorn C, Kurowski M, Hoffmann F, Notheis G, Belohradsky BH. Pharmacokinetic interaction of amprenavir in combination with efavirenz or delavirdine in HIV-infected children. *AIDS* (2000) 14, 1866–8.
2. Tran JQ, Petersen C, Garrett M, Hee B, Krr BM. Pharmacokinetic interaction between amprenavir and delavirdine: evidence of induced clearance by amprenavir. *Clin Pharmacol Ther* (2002) 72, 615–26.
3. Justesen US, Klitgaard NA, Brosen K, Pedersen C. Pharmacokinetic interaction between amprenavir and delavirdine after multiple-dose administration in healthy volunteers. *Br J Clin Pharmacol* (2003) 55, 100–6.
4. Cox SR, Ferry JJ, Batts DH, Carlson GF, Schneck DW, Herman BD, Della-Coletta AA, Chambers JH, Carel BJ, Stewart F, Buss N, Brown A. Delavirdine (D) and marketed protease inhibitors (PIs): pharmacokinetic (PK) interaction studies in healthy volunteers. 4th Conference on Retroviruses and Opportunistic Infections, Washington, 1997. Abstract 372.
5. Ferry JJ, Herman BD, Carel BJ, Carlson GF, Batts DH. Pharmacokinetic drug-drug interaction study of delavirdine and indinavir in healthy volunteers. *J Acquir Immune Defic Syndr Hum Retrovirol* (1998) 18, 252–9.
6. Cox SR, Schneck DW, Herman BD, Carel BJ, Gullotti BR, Kerr BM, Freimuth WW. Delavirdine (DLV) and nelfinavir (NFV): A pharmacokinetic (PK) drug-drug interaction study in healthy adult volunteers. 5th Conference on Retroviruses and Opportunistic Infections, Chicago, 1998. Abstract 345.
7. Shelton MJ, Hewitt RG, Adams J, Della-Coletta A, Cox S, Morse GD. Pharmacokinetics of ritonavir and delavirdine in human immunodeficiency virus-infected patients. *Antimicrob Agents Chemother* (2003) 47, 1694–9.
8. Tran JQ, Petersen C, Garrett M, Smith M, Hee B, Lillibridge J, Kerr B. Delavirdine significantly increases exposure of low dose ritonavir in healthy volunteers. *Intersci Conf Antimicrob Agents Chemother* (2001) 41, 15.
9. Duval X, Le Moing V, Longuet P, Leport C, Vildé J-L, Lamotte C, Peytavin G, Farinotti R. Efavirenz-induced decrease in plasma amprenavir levels in human immunodeficiency virus-infected patients and correction by ritonavir. *Antimicrob Agents Chemother* (2000) 44, 2593.
10. Falloon J, Piscitelli S, Vogel S, Sadler B, Mitsuya H, Kavlick MF, Yoshimura K, Rogers M, LaFon S, Manion DJ, Lane HC, Masur H. Combination therapy with amprenavir, abacavir, and efavirenz in human immunodeficiency virus (HIV)-infected patients failing a protease-inhibitor regimen: pharmacokinetic drug interactions and antiviral activity. *Clin Infect Dis* (2000) 30, 313–18.

Continued

Table 21.3 Summary of the pharmacokinetic interactions of NNRTIs and HIV-protease inhibitors (continued)

11. Reyataz (Atazanavir sulfate). Bristol-Myers Squibb. US Prescribing information, March 2012.
12. Sekar VJ, De Pauw M, Mariën K, Peeters M, Lefebvre E, Hoetelemans RMW. Pharmacokinetic interaction between TMC 114/r and efavirenz in healthy volunteers. *Antivir Ther* (2007) 12, 509–14.
13. Soon GH, Shen P, Yong E-L, Pham P, Flexner C, Lee L. Pharmacokinetics of darunavir at 900 milligrams and ritonavir at 100 milligrams once daily when coadministered with efavirenz at 600 milligrams once daily in healthy volunteers. *Antimicrob Agents Chemother* (2010) 54, 2775–80.
14. Wire MB, Ballow C, Preston SL, Hendrix CW, Piliero PJ, Lou Y, Stein DS. Pharmacokinetics and safety of GW433908 and ritonavir, with and without efavirenz, in healthy volunteers. *AIDS* (2004) 18, 897–907.
15. Sustiva Film-coated Tablets (Efavirenz). Bristol-Myers Squibb Pharmaceuticals Ltd. UK Summary of product characteristics, June 2012.
16. Aarnoutse RE, Grintjes KJT, Telgt DSC, Stek M, Hugen PWH, Reiss P, Koopmans PP, Hekster YA, Burger DM. The influence of efavirenz on the pharmacokinetics of a twice-daily combination of indinavir and low-dose ritonavir in healthy volunteers. *Clin Pharmacol Ther* (2002) 71, 57–67.
17. Boyd MA, Aarnoutse RE, Ruxrungtham K, Stek M, van Heeswijk RPG, Lange JMA, Cooper DA, Phanuphak P, Burger DM. Pharmacokinetics of indinavir/ritonavir (800/100 mg) in combination with efavirenz (600 mg) in HIV-1-infected subjects. *J Acquir Immune Defic Syndr* (2003) 34, 134–9.
18. Hsu A, Isaacson J, Brun S, Bernstein B, Lam W, Bertz R, Foit C, Rynkiewicz K, Richards B, King M, Rode R, Kempf DJ, Granneman GR, Sun E. Pharmacokinetic-pharmacodynamic analysis of lopinavir-ritonavir in combination with efavirenz and two nucleoside reverse transcriptase inhibitors in extensively pretreated human immunodeficiency virus-infected patients. *Antimicrob Agents Chemother* (2003) 47, 350–9.
19. Kityo C, Walker AS, Dickinson L, Lutwama F, Kayiwa J, Ssali F, Nalumenya R, Tumukunde D, Munderi P, Reid A, Gilks CF, Gibb DM, Khoo S; DART Trial Team. Pharmacokinetics of lopinavir-ritonavir with and without nonnucleoside reverse transcriptase inhibitors in Ugandan HIV-infected adults. *Antimicrob Agents Chemother* (2010) 54, 2965–73.
20. Kaletra Tablets (Lopinavir/Ritonavir). Abbott Laboratories Ltd. UK Summary of product characteristics, August 2012.
21. Bergshoeff AS, Fraaij PL, Ndagijimana J, Verweel G, Hartwig NG, Niehues T, De Groot R, Burger DM. Increased dose of lopinavir/ritonavir compensates for efavirenz-induced drug-drug interaction in HIV-1-infected children. *J Acquir Immune Defic Syndr* (2005) 39, 63–8.
22. Fiske WD, Benedek IH, White SJ, Pepperess KA, Joseph JL, Kornhauser DM. Pharmacokinetic interaction between efavirenz (EFV) and nelfinavir mesylate (NFV) in healthy volunteers. 5th Conference on Retroviruses and Opportunistic Infections, Chicago, 1998. Abstract 349.
23. la Porte CJL, de Graaff-Teulen MJA, Colbers EPH, Voncken DS, Ibanez SM, Koopmans PP, Hekster YA, Burger DM. Effect of efavirenz treatment on the pharmacokinetics of nelfinavir boosted by ritonavir in healthy volunteers. *Br J Clin Pharmacol* (2004) 58, 632–40.
24. Norvir Tablets (Ritonavir). Abbott Laboratories Ltd. UK Summary of product characteristics, September 2012.
25. Piliero PJ, Preston SL, Japour A, Stevens RC, Morvillo C, Drusano GL. Pharmacokinetics of the combination of ritonavir plus saquinavir, with and without efavirenz, in healthy volunteers. *Intersci Conf Antimicrob Agents Chemother* (2001) 41, 15.
26. Aptivus (Tipranavir). Boehringer Ingelheim Pharmaceuticals, Inc. US Prescribing information, April 2012.
27. Goebel FD, MacGregor TR, Sabo JP, Castles M, Johnson PA, Legg D, McCallister S. Pharmacokinetic characterization of three doses of tipranavir boosted with ritonavir on highly active antiretroviral therapy in treatment-experienced HIV-1 patients. *HIV Clin Trials* (2010) 11, 28–38.
28. Intelence (Etravirine). Janssen-Cilag Ltd. UK Summary of product characteristics, July 2012.
29. Schöller-Gyüre M, Kakuda TN, Sekar V, Woodfall B, De Smedt G, Lefebvre E, Peeters M, Hotelemans RM. Pharmacokinetics of darunavir/ritonavir and TMC125 alone and coadministered in HIV-negative volunteers. *Antivir Ther* (2007) 12, 789–96.
30. Moltó J, Deig E, Valle M, Maria Llibre J, Miranda C, Cedeño S, Valero S, Negredo E, Clotet B. Effect of nevirapine on the steady-state trough concentrations of atazanavir in HIV-infected patients receiving atazanavir/ritonavir. *Ther Drug Monit* (2010) 32, 93–6.
31. Sekar V, Lefebvre E, Mariën K, De Pauw M, Vangeneugden T, Pozniak A, Hoetelmans RMW. Pharmacokinetic interaction between nevirapine and darunavir with low-dose ritonavir in HIV-1-infected patients. *Br J Clin Pharmacol* (2009) 68, 116–19.
32. DeJesus E, Piliero PJ, Summers K, Wire MB, Stein DS, Masterman A, Lou Y, Min SS, Shelton MJ. Interaction between fosamprenavir, with and without ritonavir, and nevirapine in human immunodeficiency virus-infected subjects. *Antimicrob Agents Chemother* (2006) 50, 3157–9.
33. Murphy RL, Sommadossi J-P, Lamson M, Hall DB, Myers M, Dusek A. Antiviral effect and pharmacokinetic interaction between nevirapine and indinavir in persons infected with human immunodeficiency virus type 1. *J Infect Dis* (1999) 179, 1116–23.
34. Launay O, Peytavin G, Flandre P, Gerard L, Levy C, Joly V, Aboulker JP, Yeni P. Pharmacokinetic (PK) interaction between nevirapine (NVP) and indinavir (IDV) in ANRS 081 trial. *Intersci Conf Antimicrob Agents Chemother* (2000) 40, 331.
35. Burger DM, Prins JM, van der Ende ME, Aarnoutse RE. The effect of nevirapine on the pharmacokinetics of indinavir/ritonavir 800/100 mg BID. *J Acquir Immune Defic Syndr* (2004) 35, 97–8.
36. Hsu A, Bertz R, Renz C, Lam W, Rode R, Deetz C, Schweitzer SM, Berstein B, Brun S, Granneman GR, Sun E. Assessment of the pharmacokinetic interaction between lopinavir/ritonavir (ABT-378/r) and nevirapine (NVP) in HIV-infected pediatric subjects. *AIDS* (2000) 14 (Suppl. 4), S100.
37. Merry C, Barry MG, Mulcahy F, Ryan M, Tjia JF, Halifax KL, Breckenridge AM, Back DJ. The pharmacokinetics of combination therapy with nelfinavir plus nevirapine. *AIDS* (1998) 12, 1163–7.
38. Skowron G, Leoung G, Kerr B, Dusek A, Anderson R, Beebe S, Grosso R. Lack of pharmacokinetic interaction between nelfinavir and nevirapine. *AIDS* (1998) 12, 1243–4.
39. Skowron G, Leoung G, Hall DB, Robinson P, Lewis R, Grosso R, Jacobs M, Kerr B, MacGregor T, Stevens M, Fisher A, Odgen R, Yen-Lieberman B. Pharmacokinetic evaluation and short-term activity of stavudine, nevirapine, and nelfinavir therapy in HIV-1-infected adults. *J Acquir Immune Defic Syndr* (2004) 35, 351–8.
40. Vilaro J, Mascaro J, Colomer J, Cucurull J, Garcia D, Yanez A. The pharmacokinetics of combination therapy with nelfinavir (NFV) plus nevirapine (NVP) in HIV positive patients. *Intersci Conf Antimicrob Agents Chemother* (2001) 41, 16.
41. Viramune (Nevirapine). Boehringer Ingelheim Pharmaceuticals, Inc. US Prescribing information, November 2011.
42. Viramune (Nevirapine). Boehringer Ingelheim Ltd. UK Summary of product characteristics, January 2012.
43. Sahai J, Cameron W, Salgo M, Stewart F, Myers M, Lamson M, Gagnier P. Drug interaction study between saquinavir (SQV) and nevirapine (NVP). 4th Conference on Retroviruses and Opportunistic Infections, Washington, 1997. Abstract 613.
44. van Heeswijk R, Hoetelmans RMW, Kestens D, Stevens M, Peeters M, Williams P, Woodfall B, Boven K. The pharmacokinetic interaction (PK) between TMC278, a next generation non-nucleoside reverse transcriptase inhibitor (NNRTI), and once daily darunavir/ritonavir (DRV/r) in HIV-negative volunteers. *Intersci Conf Antimicrob Agents Chemother* (2007), abstract H-1042.
45. Edurant (Rilpivirine hydrochloride). Janssen-Cilag Ltd. UK Summary of product characteristics, November 2011.
46. Edurant (Rilpivirine hydrochloride). Tibotec Pharmaceuticals. US Prescribing information, August 2012.

(d) Nevirapine

For a summary of the studies of the pharmacokinetic interactions of nevirapine and various HIV-protease inhibitors, see 'Table 21.3', p.957. Most HIV-protease inhibitors do not appear to affect nevirapine exposure, although some caused a negligible to slight increase. In a multivariate analysis of therapeutic drug monitoring data, the concurrent use of HIV-protease inhibitors was associated with 28% higher nevirapine concentrations. When analysed by drug, the increase was 43% for atazanavir and 29% for saquinavir, with no increase for lopinavir.[13] Nevirapine is an inducer of CYP3A4, and so would be expected to decrease the concentrations of some of the HIV-protease inhibitors (see 'Table 21.3', p.957), sometimes to concentrations that are unlikely to be effective. Low-dose **ritonavir** has been used to boost the concentrations of some HIV-protease inhibitors when they were given with nevirapine. For a summary of the manufacturers' recommended regimens for use with nevirapine, see 'Table 21.4', p.961. If nevirapine is used with HIV-protease inhibitors, therapy should be closely monitored. For studies suggesting that increased doses of **lopinavir** and **atazanavir** (both boosted with ritonavir) might not be sufficient in all patients given NNRTIs (including nevirapine), see *Efavirenz*, above.

(e) Rilpivirine

For a summary of the studies of the pharmacokinetic interactions of rilpivirine and various HIV-protease inhibitors, see 'Table 21.3', p.957. Ritonavir-boosted protease inhibitors slightly (lopinavir) to moderately (darunavir) increased rilpivirine exposure, probably due to inhibition of CYP3A4. The increase seen is probably not clinically relevant for recommended doses of rilpivirine. Supratherapeutic doses of rilpivirine caused a negligible decrease in concentrations of these HIV-protease inhibitors, probably due to induction of CYP3A4. At the recommended dose of rilpivirine, no dose adjustment of either rilpivirine or the HIV-protease inhibitor is considered necessary (see 'Table 21.4', p.961). However, note that supratherapeutic doses of rilpivirine cause QT prolongation, which might be additive with other drugs that prolong the QT interval, such as **saquinavir** boosted with ritonavir, see 'Drugs that prolong the QT interval + Other drugs that prolong the QT interval', p.272.

Note that the concurrent use of an NNRTI with a HIV-protease inhibitor is not a recommended regimen when starting antiretrovirals in treatment-naive patients.[1,2]

1. Williams I, Churchill D, Anderson J, Boffito M, Bower M, Cairns G, Cwynarski K, Edwards S, Fidler S, Fisher M, Freedman A, Geretti AM, Gilleece Y, Horne R, Johnson M, Khoo S, Leen C, Marshall N, Nelson M, Orkin C, Paton N, Phillips A, Post F, Pozniak A, Sabin C, Trevelion R, Ustianowski A, Walsh J, Waters L, Wilkins E, Winston A, Youle M. British HIV Association guidelines for the treatment of HIV-1-positive adults with antiretroviral therapy 2012 (Updated 2013). *HIV Med* (2014), 15 (Suppl 1) 1–85. Also available at: http://www.bhiva.org/documents/Guidelines/Treatment/2012/hiv1029_2.pdf (accessed 25/03/15).
2. Panel on Antiretroviral Guidelines for Adults and Adolescents. Guidelines for the use of antiretroviral agents in HIV-1-infected adults and adolescents. US Department of Health and Human Services (April 2015). 1–288. Available at: https://aidsinfo.nih.gov/contentfiles/lvguidelines/adultandadolescentgl.pdf (accessed 20/09/15).

Table 21.4 Summary of the manufacturers' dose recommendations for combined use of HIV-protease inhibitors and NNRTIs

	Dose of HIV-protease inhibitor to be used with standard dose of the NNRTI				
	Delavirdine 400 mg three times daily	**Efavirenz 600 mg daily**	**Etravirine 200 mg twice daily**	**Nevirapine 200 mg twice daily**	**Rilpivirine 25 mg daily**
Amprenavir	Appropriate dose not established (amprenavir concentrations increased)	Appropriate dose not established (amprenavir concentrations reduced)	Avoid	Appropriate dose not established (amprenavir concentrations may be decreased)	
Amprenavir/Nelfinavir		No dose adjustments required			
Amprenavir/Ritonavir*	Appropriate dose not established. Care (unpredictable effect)	No dose adjustments required (amprenavir 600 mg with ritonavir 100 or 200 mg twice daily)	Dose reduction may be needed (UK) Avoid — appropriate dose not established (US)		
Amprenavir/Saquinavir		Avoid			
Atazanavir		Avoid	Avoid	Avoid	No dose adjustments required
Atazanavir/Ritonavir*		Not recommended but increase to 400/200 mg daily† if required (UK) 400/100 mg daily, separate administration (US)	No dose adjustments required (UK) Avoid (US)	In the absence of data, avoid	No dose adjustments required
Darunavir/Ritonavir*		No dose adjustments required, but monitor	No dose adjustments required	No dose adjustments required	No dose adjustments required
Fosamprenavir	Caution (delavirdine potentially subtherapeutic)	Appropriate dose not established	Avoid	Avoid	
Fosamprenavir/Ritonavir*		No dose adjustment required if twice daily 1400/300 mg if given once daily	Dose reduction might be required (UK) Avoid — appropriate dose not established (US)	No dose adjustments required if twice daily	No dose adjustments required
Indinavir	Consider reducing indinavir dose to 600 mg three times daily. Optimum dose not established	Optimum dose not known. Increasing the dose to 1 g three times daily does not compensate for induced metabolism	Avoid (indinavir concentrations decreased)	Consider increasing to 1 g three times daily. Optimum dose not known	
Indinavir/Ritonavir*		Appropriate dose not established. 800/100 mg twice daily has been tried			
Lopinavir/Ritonavir*	Appropriate dose not established	533/133 mg twice daily† or 500/125 mg twice daily. Avoid once daily regimens	No dose adjustments required	533/133 mg twice daily† or 500/125 mg twice daily. Avoid once daily regimens	No dose adjustments required
Nelfinavir	Appropriate dose not established	No dose adjustments required	Avoid (increase in nelfinavir concentrations predicted)	No dose adjustment likely (UK) Appropriate dose not established (US)	
Ritonavir*	Appropriate dose not established. Ritonavir dose reductions might be appropriate	No dose adjustments required, but not well tolerated. Monitor liver function	Avoid with ritonavir 600 mg twice daily	No dose adjustments required	
Saquinavir	Appropriate dose not established, although a dose reduction may be considered. Monitor liver function	Avoid	Avoid	Appropriate dose not established	
Saquinavir/Ritonavir*		No dose adjustments required. Monitor liver function	No dose adjustments required	Appropriate dose not established	No dose adjustments required‡
Tipranavir/Ritonavir*		No dose adjustments required	Avoid (etravirine concentrations decreased)	No dose adjustments required	No dose adjustments required

*The UK manufactuer of efavirenz advises caution, because the possibility of an increase in the incidence of efavirenz-associated adverse events should be considered with any ritonavir-boosted regimen used with efavirenz, due to a possible interaction. This is because the combination of efavirenz with ritonavir at antiviral doses caused increased dizziness, nausea, paraesthesia and elevated transaminase concentrations.

† This dose increase might not be sufficient in some patients, so some caution is required.

‡ Manufacturer recommends caution with QT prolongers, which would include saquinavir/ritonavir

3. Harris M, Alexander C, O'Shaughnessy M, Montaner JSG. Delavirdine increases drug exposure of ritonavir-boosted protease inhibitors. *AIDS* (2002) 16, 798–9.
4. Justesen US, Klitgaard NA, Brosen K, Pedersen C. Pharmacokinetic interaction between amprenavir and delavirdine after multiple-dose administration in healthy volunteers. *Br J Clin Pharmacol* (2003) 55, 100–6.
5. Cox SR, Schneck DW, Herman BD, Carel BJ, Gullotti BR, Kerr BM, Freimuth WW. Delavirdine (DLV) and nelfinavir (NFV): A pharmacokinetic (PK) drug-drug interaction study in healthy adult volunteers. 5th Conference on Retroviruses and Opportunistic Infections, Chicago, 1998. Abstract 345.
6. Invirase (Saquinavir mesilate). Roche Products Ltd. UK Summary of product characteristics, October 2013.
7. Sustiva Film-coated Tablets (Efavirenz). Bristol-Myers Squibb Pharmaceutical Ltd. UK Summary of product characteristics, June 2012.
8. Sustiva (Efavirenz). Bristol-Myers Squibb Company. US Prescribing information, August 2012.
9. Solas C, Poizot-Martin I, Drogoul M-P, Ravaux I, Dhiver C, Lafeuillade A, Allegre T, Mokhtari M, Moreau J, Lepeu G, Petit N, Durand A, Lacarelle B. Therapeutic drug monitoring of lopinavir/ritonavir given alone or with a non-nucleoside reverse transcriptase inhibitor. *Br J Clin Pharmacol* (2004) 57, 436–40.
10. Poirier J-M, Guiard-Schmid J-B, Meynard J-L, Bonnard P, Zouai O, Lukiana T, Jaillon P, Girard P-M, Pialoux G. Critical drug interaction between ritonavir-boosted atazanavir regimen and non-nucleoside reverse transcriptase inhibitors. *AIDS* (2006) 20, 1087–9.
11. Intelence (Etravirine). Tibotec, Inc. US Prescribing information, August 2012.
12. Intelence (Etravirine). Janssen-Cilag Ltd. UK Summary of product characteristics, July 2012.
13. Stöhr W, Back D, Dunn D, Sabin C, Winston A, Gilson R, Pillay D, Hill T, Ainsworth J, Pozniak A, Leen C, Bansi L, Fisher M, Orkin C, Anderson J, Johnson M, Easterbrook P, Gibbons S, Khoo S; Liverpool TDM Database; UK CHIC Study. Factors influencing efavirenz and nevirapine plasma concentration: effect of ethnicity, weight and co-medication. *Antivir Ther* (2008)13, 675–85.

NNRTIs + Macrolides

Delavirdine increases clarithromycin exposure. Efavirenz, etravirine, and nevirapine reduce clarithromycin exposure but increase that of its active hydroxy metabolite. Rilpivirine is predicted not to alter clarithromycin or erythromycin concentrations. Clarithromycin does not appear to affect the pharmacokinetics of delavirdine or efavirenz, but slightly increases etravirine and nevirapine exposure, and is predicted to increase rilpivirine concentrations. Efavirenz does not alter azithromycin exposure. A case of a neuropsychiatric reaction has been attributed to the use of clarithromycin in a man taking nevirapine.

Clinical evidence

(a) Delavirdine

In a study in 7 HIV-positive patients, **clarithromycin** 500 mg twice daily for 15 days did not cause any apparent change in the pharmacokinetics of delavirdine 300 mg three times daily, when compared with 4 other HIV-positive patients taking only delavirdine.[1] However, although delavirdine plasma concentrations appear to be unaffected, the manufacturer notes that the AUC of **clarithromycin** was doubled by delavirdine.[2]

(b) Efavirenz

The manufacturers note that in 11 subjects, the concurrent use of **clarithromycin** 500 mg twice daily and efavirenz 400 mg daily for 7 days reduced the AUC of **clarithromycin** by 39% and increased the AUC of its hydroxy metabolite by 34%. Moreover, 46% of subjects receiving the combination developed a rash.[3,4] Clarithromycin had no effect on the AUC or minimum concentration of efavirenz.[4]

The manufacturers also note that, in a study in 14 healthy subjects, efavirenz 400 mg daily for 7 days had no effect on the pharmacokinetics of a single 600-mg dose of **azithromycin**.[3,4] Efavirenz had no effect on the AUC of **azithromycin**, and caused a small 22% increase in its maximum concentration.[4]

(c) Etravirine

The manufacturer of etravirine notes that concurrent use of etravirine and **clarithromycin** 500 mg twice daily reduced the AUC, and the maximum and minimum concentrations of **clarithromycin** by 39%, 53%, and 34%, respectively. The AUC and maximum concentration of the hydroxy metabolite were increased by 21% and 33%, respectively. In addition, **clarithromycin** increased the AUC and maximum concentration of etravirine by 42% and 44%, respectively.[5,6]

(d) Nevirapine

In a study in 15 HIV-positive patients, nevirapine 200 mg twice daily reduced the AUC of **clarithromycin** by 30%, and reduced the maximum and minimum plasma concentration of **clarithromycin** by 21% and 46%, respectively. Nevirapine[7] increased the AUC of the hydroxy metabolite of **clarithromycin**, by about 27%. The manufacturers also report that the AUC of nevirapine was increased by 26% by **clarithromycin**, when compared with historical controls. The AUC of **clarithromycin**[8,9] was reduced by 31% and the AUC of its hydroxy metabolite was increased by 42%.

A man developed hyperactivity (poor concentration, anxiety, suicidal and homicidal ideation) when taking **clarithromycin** and antiretroviral drugs, including nevirapine. This was thought to be due to accumulation of the hydroxy metabolite of **clarithromycin**.[10]

Mechanism

The NNRTIs are substrates of CYP3A4, which is inhibited by clarithromycin. Delavirdine is also reported to inhibit CYP3A4, whereas efavirenz and nevirapine, and to a lesser extent, etravirine, induce CYP3A4. Therefore alterations in the metabolism of these drugs by CYP3A4 results in the altered concentrations seen.

Importance and management

Delavirdine increases clarithromycin exposure. The manufacturer of delavirdine states that when both drugs are given to patients with renal impairment, the dose of clarithromycin should be reduced.[2]

In contrast, **etravirine**, **efavirenz**, and **nevirapine** slightly decrease clarithromycin exposure and increase concentrations of the hydroxy metabolite of clarithromycin. The clinical relevance of this decrease is uncertain. However, the manufacturers of nevirapine and etravirine state that alternatives to clarithromycin should be considered for the treatment of *Mycobacterium avium* complex (MAC) infection,[5,6,8,9] as the hydroxy metabolite is not as active against this bacterium.[8,9] Some suggest azithromycin.[3,4,6] The UK manufacturer of nevirapine also advises close monitoring of liver function tests on the concurrent use of nevirapine and clarithromycin.[8]

The slight increase in etravirine exposure, and possibly also nevirapine exposure, caused by clarithromycin would not be expected to be of clinical relevance.

The interaction of **rilpivirine** with the macrolides has not been studied, but usual therapeutic doses of rilpivirine are not expected to alter clarithromycin or erythromycin exposure.[11] *Ketoconazole*, a potent inhibitor of CYP3A4, causes a slight increase in rilpivirine exposure, which is not clinically relevant (see 'NNRTIs + Azoles; Ketoconazole', p.954). Nevertheless, the manufacturer of rilpivirine predicts that clarithromycin and erythromycin might increase rilpivirine concentrations, and they advise that, where possible, alternatives such as azithromycin should be considered.[11,12] Note that supratherapeutic doses of rilpivirine are associated with QT prolongation, and the manufacturer states that caution is warranted on the concurrent use of other drugs that prolong the QT interval,[11,12] which might include erythromycin, especially when given intravenously, or azithromycin (see also 'Drugs that prolong the QT interval + Other drugs that prolong the QT interval', p.272).

1. Cox SR, Borin MT, Driver MR, Levy B, Freimuth WW. Effect of clarithromycin on the steady-state pharmacokinetics of delavirdine in HIV-1 patients. American Society for Microbiology, 2nd National Conference on Human Retroviruses, 1995. Abstract 487.
2. Rescriptor (Delavirdine mesylate). ViiV Healthcare. US Prescribing information, August 2012.
3. Sustiva Film-coated Tablets (Efavirenz). Bristol-Myers Squibb Pharmaceutical Ltd. UK Summary of product characteristics, March 2014.
4. Sustiva (Efavirenz). Bristol-Myers Squibb Company. US Prescribing information, August 2012.
5. Intelence (Etravirine). Janssen-Cilag Ltd. UK Summary of product characteristics, July 2012.
6. Intelence (Etravirine). Tibotec, Inc. US Prescribing information, August 2012.
7. Robinson P, Gigliotti M, Lamson M, Azzam S, MacGregor T. Effect of the reverse transcriptase inhibitor, nevirapine, on the steady-state pharmacokinetics of clarithromycin in HIV-positive patients. 6th Conference on Retroviruses and Opportunistic Infections, Chicago, 1999. Abstract 374.
8. Viramune (Nevirapine). Boehringer Ingelheim Ltd. UK Summary of product characteristics, January 2012.
9. Viramune (Nevirapine). Boehringer Ingelheim Pharmaceuticals, Inc. US Prescribing information, November 2011.
10. Prime K, French P. Neuropsychiatric reaction induced by clarithromycin in a patient on highly active antiretroviral therapy (HAART). *Sex Transm Infect* (2001) 77, 297–8.
11. Edurant (Rilpivirine hydrochloride). Tibotec Pharmaceuticals. US Prescribing information, August 2012.
12. Edurant (Rilpivirine hydrochloride). Janssen-Cilag Ltd. UK Summary of product characteristics, November 2011.

NNRTIs + NNRTIs

Nevirapine modestly reduces the concentrations of efavirenz, whereas efavirenz has no effect on nevirapine concentrations. Efavirenz and nevirapine might reduce the concentrations of etravirine and rilpivirine.

Clinical evidence, mechanism, importance and management

In HIV treatment guidelines, recommended regimens for treatment-naive patients usually include an NNRTI with a dual NRTI backbone.[1,2] The UK guidelines recommend efavirenz as the preferred NNRTI, with nevirapine and rilpivirine as alternatives.[1] The US guidelines do not include an NNRTI in their preferred treatment regimens, but recommend the use of efavirenz or rilpivirine in alternative regimens.[2] Current local and national guidelines should be consulted when choosing an appropriate antiretroviral regimen.

(a) Efavirenz

In a study in HIV-positive patients taking efavirenz 600 mg daily, the addition of **nevirapine** 400 mg daily resulted in a median decrease in the AUC of efavirenz of 22%, and a decrease in its minimum plasma concentration of 36%. The steady-state pharmacokinetics of **nevirapine** were not altered by efavirenz, when compared with historical control data.[3] However, the manufacturer of nevirapine does not recommend this combination as concurrent use could lead to a higher risk of adverse effects and does not improve efficacy over either NNRTI alone.[4,5]

(b) Etravirine

In a study in 24 healthy subjects, pre-dosing with **efavirenz** 600 mg daily (taken on days one to 14) reduced the AUC, maximum concentrations, and minimum concentrations of etravirine 400 mg once daily (taken on days 15 to 28) by 32%, 22%, and 42%, respectively. When etravirine was taken as 200 mg twice daily, the AUC, maximum concentrations, and minimum concentrations of etravirine were reduced (by 26%, 19%, and 34%, respectively). The authors note that etravirine is metabolised by the CYP3A4 and its bioavailability is reduced by 40% when given with **efavirenz**, an inducer of this isoenzyme. However, the pharmacokinetic changes were not considered to be of clinical relevance.[6] Nevertheless, the manufacturer of etravirine advise that **efavirenz** and **nevirapine** might reduce the concentrations of etravirine and this could cause treatment failure.[7,8] They state that concurrent use has not been shown to be beneficial and is not recommended.[7,8]

(c) Rilpivirine

Rilpivirine is metabolised by CYP3A4 and the manufacturers of rilpivirine state that, although concurrent use has not been studied, the NNRTIs, **efavirenz**, **etravirine**, and **nevirapine**, would be expected to reduce rilpivirine concentrations (by inducing CYP3A4). In addition, they also predict that **delavirdine** will increase rilpivirine concentrations by inhibiting CYP3A4. They therefore do not recommend concurrent use.[9,10]

1. Williams I, Churchill D, Anderson J, Boffito M, Bower M, Cairns G, Cwynarski K, Edwards S, Fidler S, Fisher M, Freedman A, Geretti AM, Gilleece Y, Horne R, Johnson M, Khoo S, Leen C, Marshall N, Nelson M, Orkin C, Paton N, Phillips A, Post F, Pozniak A, Sabin C, Trevelion R, Ustianowski A, Walsh J, Waters L, Wilkins E, Winston A, Youle M. British HIV Association guidelines for the treatment of HIV-1-positive adults with antiretroviral therapy 2012 (Updated 2013). *HIV Med* (2014), 15 (Suppl 1) 1–85.
2. Panel on Antiretroviral Guidelines for Adults and Adolescents. Guidelines for the use of antiretroviral agents in HIV-1-infected adults and adolescents. Department of Health and Human Services. (April 2015). Available at: https://aidsinfo.nih.gov/contentfiles/lvguidelines/adultandadolescentgl.pdf (accessed 24/09/15).
3. Veldkamp AI, Harris M, Montaner JSG, Moyle G, Gazzard B, Youle M, Johnson M, Kwakkelstein MO, Carlier H, van Leeuwen R, Beijnen JH, Lange JMA, Reiss P, Hoetelmans RMW. The steady-state pharmacokinetics of efavirenz and nevirapine when used in combination in human immunodeficiency virus type 1-infected persons. *J Infect Dis* (2001) 184, 37–42.
4. Viramune (Nevirapine). Boehringer Ingelheim Ltd. UK Summary of product characteristics, January 2012.
5. Viramune (Nevirapine). Boehringer Ingelheim Pharmaceuticals, Inc. US Prescribing information, November 2011.
6. Boffito M, Jackson A, Lamorde M, Back D, Watson V, Taylor J, Waters L, Asboe D, Gazzard B, Pozniak A. Evaluation of the pharmacokinetics (PK) and safety of etravirine (ETR) administered QD and BID following two weeks of treatment with efavirenz (EFV) in healthy volunteers. 48th Annual Interscience Conference on Antimicrobial Agents and Chemotherapy, Washington DC, 2008, Presentation H-4057.
7. Intelence (Etravirine). Janssen-Cilag Ltd. UK Summary of product characteristics, July 2012.
8. Intelence (Etravirine). Tibotec, Inc. US Prescribing information, August 2012.
9. Edurant (Rilpivirine hydrochloride). Janssen-Cilag Ltd. UK Summary of product characteristics, November 2011.
10. Edurant (Rilpivirine hydrochloride). Tibotec Pharmaceuticals. US Prescribing information, August 2012.

NNRTIs + NRTIs

Delavirdine absorption is reduced by the buffered preparation of didanosine, but probably not by the enteric-coated preparation of didanosine. Delavirdine does not affect the pharmacokinetics of zidovudine. There is no pharmacokinetic interaction between efavirenz and zidovudine, or lamivudine; or between nevirapine and didanosine, lamivudine, stavudine, or zalcitabine. No pharmacokinetic interaction occurs between didanosine and etravirine or rilpivirine. The concurrent use of nevirapine with zidovudine might slightly decrease zidovudine exposure and might increase the risk of granulocytopenia.

Clinical evidence, mechanism, importance and management

(a) Delavirdine

A study in 34 HIV-positive patients taking **zidovudine** 200 mg three times daily found that delavirdine mesilate 400 mg to 1.2 g daily for 9 days appeared to have no effect on the pharmacokinetics of **zidovudine**.[1]

In a steady-state study, 9 HIV-positive patients taking **didanosine** 200 mg twice daily were also given delavirdine mesilate 400 mg three times daily for 14 days. **Didanosine** caused a 37% reduction in the maximum serum concentrations of delavirdine and a trend towards a lower AUC, but when the drugs were given one hour apart no effect occurred. The pharmacokinetics of **didanosine** were not affected by delavirdine.[2] A single-dose study in 12 HIV-positive patients found similar results.[3] The buffered preparation of **didanosine** contains antacids to increase its absorption, and antacids decrease the absorption of delavirdine (see 'NNRTIs + Antacids', p.951). The authors of the multiple-dose study advise that as **didanosine** had no clinically relevant effect on the AUC of delavirdine, there is no reason to separate the doses.[2] However, the US manufacturer of delavirdine advises that concurrent use with buffered **didanosine** might reduce the concentrations of both delavirdine and didanosine, and they therefore recommend separating their administration by at least one hour.[4] The enteric-coated preparation of **didanosine**, which does not contain antacids, would not be expected to reduce the absorption of delavirdine.

(b) Efavirenz

The manufacturer notes that efavirenz had no effect on **lamivudine** or **zidovudine** exposure, but increased their minimum concentrations more than 3-fold.[5] No dose adjustments are required on concurrent use and no pharmacokinetic interactions are anticipated with other NRTIs.[5,6]

(c) Etravirine

The manufacturer of etravirine states that no pharmacokinetic interaction occurs between etravirine and **didanosine**. Therefore, no dose adjustment is needed on their concurrent use. They also state that no interaction would be expected with other NRTIs which are primarily renally excreted, such as **abacavir**, **emtricitabine**, **lamivudine**, **stavudine**, and **zidovudine**.[7]

(d) Nevirapine

The pharmacokinetics of **didanosine** and **zidovudine**, with or without nevirapine, were assessed in 175 HIV-positive subjects. The bioavailability of **didanosine** was not affected, but the bioavailability of **zidovudine** was decreased by about one-third by nevirapine.[8] In a steady-state study in 24 HIV-positive patients, nevirapine 200 mg every 12 hours was added to regimens of **didanosine**, **didanosine** with **zidovudine**, or **zidovudine** with **zalcitabine**, for a 4-week period. No apparent changes in the pharmacokinetics of **didanosine** or **zalcitabine** were seen. However, in the group taking **didanosine** with **zidovudine** the maximum plasma concentrations and AUC of **zidovudine** were reduced by 27% and 32%, respectively, by nevirapine. **Zidovudine** pharmacokinetics in the group taking **zidovudine** and **zalcitabine** were not affected by nevirapine.[9] The reasons for these changes are not clear, but the clinical consequences are thought to be small, and the safety data indicate that the concurrent use of these drugs is safe and well tolerated. In another study in 4 patients, the simultaneous administration of nevirapine with **didanosine** tablets containing antacids had no effect on nevirapine absorption.[10] In a study in 22 patients, nevirapine 200 mg once daily for 2 weeks then 200 mg twice daily had no effect on the AUC of **stavudine** 30 to 40 mg twice daily.[11] Nevirapine appears to have no effect on **lamivudine** clearance, based on a population pharmacokinetic study.[12] The UK manufacturer states that no dose adjustments are needed if **didanosine**, **lamivudine**, **stavudine**, **zalcitabine**, or **zidovudine** is taken with nevirapine.[13] However, note that **zidovudine** can cause granulocytopenia, and the manufacturer of nevirapine states that the concurrent use of **zidovudine** and nevirapine might further increase this risk.[13] Granulocytopenia was more common in children taking nevirapine and zidovudine.[14] The UK manufacturer therefore recommends careful haematological monitoring in patients taking nevirapine and **zidovudine** especially those who are considered at particular risk (e.g. children, those with advanced disease).[13]

(e) Rilpivirine

The manufacturers of rilpivirine report that in a study in 21 subjects, where delayed-release **didanosine** 400 mg once daily was taken 2 hours before high-dose rilpivirine 150 mg daily, there was no change pharmacokinetics of rilpivirine and a negligible 12% increase in **didanosine** exposure. Note that as **didanosine** should be taken on an empty stomach and rilpivirine should be taken with food, the manufacturers advise that **didanosine** should be taken at least 2 hours before or 4 hours after rilpivirine.[15,16]

The manufacturers also state that no clinically relevant pharmacokinetic interaction would be expected to occur between rilpivirine and **abacavir**, **emtricitabine**, **lamivudine**, **stavudine**, and **zidovudine**.[15,16]

1. Morse GD, Cox SR, DeRemer MF, Batts DH, Freimuth WW. Zidovudine (ZDV) pharmacokinetics (PK) during an escalating, multiple-dose study of delavirdine (DLV) mesylate. *Intersci Conf Antimicrob Agents Chemother* (1994) 34, 132.
2. Morse GD, Cohn SE, Shelton MJ, Greisberger C, Cox SR, Della-Coletta AA, Freimuth WW, Reichman RC. Multiple-dose pharmacokinetics of delavirdine mesylate and didanosine in HIV-infected patients. *Clin Drug Investig* (2003) 23, 323–8.
3. Morse GD, Fischl MA, Shelton MJ, Cox SR, Driver M, DeRemer M, Freimuth WW. Single-dose pharmacokinetics of delavirdine mesylate and didanosine in patients with human immunodeficiency virus infection. *Antimicrob Agents Chemother* (1997) 41, 169–74.
4. Rescriptor (Delavirdine mesylate). ViiV Healthcare. US Prescribing information, August 2012.
5. Sustiva (Efavirenz). Bristol-Myers Squibb Company. US Prescribing information, August 2012.
6. Sustiva Film-coated Tablets (Efavirenz). Bristol-Myers Squibb Pharmaceutical Ltd. UK Summary of product characteristics, March 2014.
7. Intelence (Etravirine). Janssen-Cilag Ltd. UK Summary of product characteristics, July 2012.
8. Zhou XJ, Sheiner LB, D'Aquila RT, Hughes MD, Hirsch MS, Fischl MA, Johnson VA, Myers M, Sommadossi JP and the NIAID ACTG241 Investigators. Population pharmacokinetics of nevirapine, zidovudine and didanosine after combination therapy in HIV-infected patients. *Clin Pharmacol Ther* (1998) 63,182.
9. MacGregor TR, Lamson MJ, Cort S, Pav JW, Saag MS, Elvin AT, Sommadossi J-P, Myers M, Keirns JJ. Steady state pharmacokinetics of nevirapine, didanosine, zalcitabine, and zidovudine combination therapy in HIV-1 positive patients. *Pharm Res* (1995) 12 (9 Suppl), S-101.
10. van Heeswijk RPG, Veldkamp AI, Mulder JW, Meenhorst PL, Wit FWNM, Reiss P, Lange JMA, Kwakkelstein MO, Beijnen JH, Hoetelmans RMW. Nevirapine plus didanosine: once or twice daily combination? *J Acquir Immune Defic Syndr* (2000) 25, 93–5.
11. Skowron G, Leoung G, Hall DB, Robinson P, Lewis R, Grosso R, Jacobs M, Kerr B, MacGregor T, Stevens M, Fisher A, Odgen R, Yen-Lieberman B. Pharmacokinetic evaluation and short-term activity of stavudine, nevirapine, and nelfinavir therapy in HIV-1-infected adults. *J Acquir Immune Defic Syndr* (2004) 35, 351–8.
12. Sabo JP, Lamson MJ, Leitz G, Yong C-L, MacGregor TR. Pharmacokinetics of nevirapine and lamivudine in patients with HIV-1 infection. AAPS PharmSci. (2000) 2, E1–E7.
13. Viramune (Nevirapine). Boehringer Ingelheim Ltd. UK Summary of product characteristics, January 2012.
14. Viramune (Nevirapine). Boehringer Ingelheim Pharmaceuticals, Inc. US Prescribing information, November 2011.
15. Edurant (Rilpivirine hydrochloride). Janssen-Cilag Ltd. UK Summary of product characteristics, November 2011.
16. Edurant (Rilpivirine hydrochloride). Tibotec Pharmaceuticals. US Prescribing information, August 2012.

NNRTIs + Phosphodiesterase type-5 inhibitors

Etravirine moderately reduces sildenafil exposure, whereas rilpivirine has no effect on sildenafil exposure. Other phosphodiesterase type-5 inhibitors are predicted to be similarly affected.

Clinical evidence

(a) Etravirine

The UK and US manufacturers report that etravirine reduces the AUC and maximum concentration of **sildenafil** by 57% and 45%, respectively. Similarly, the AUC and maximum concentrations of its active metabolite, *N*-desmethylsildenafil, are also reduced, by 41% and 25%, respectively.[1,2]

(b) Rilpivirine

In a pharmacokinetic study, giving a single 50-mg dose of **sildenafil** to 16 subjects taking high-dose rilpivirine 75 mg daily for 12 days had no clinically relevant effect on the pharmacokinetics of either drug.[3]

Mechanism

Etravirine induces CYP3A4, by which the phosphodiesterase type-5 inhibitors are metabolised. Rilpivirine has little effect on CYP3A4.

Importance and management

Evidence for an interaction between the NNRTIs and phosphodiesterase type-5 inhibitors appears to be limited to the studies cited. Given the reduction in sildenafil exposure seen with etravirine, some patients might require a sildenafil dose increase, according to clinical effect.[1,2] Other phosphodiesterase type-5 inhibitors (**avanafil, tadalafil,** and **vardenafil**) are predicted to be similarly affected.

No dose adjustment of sildenafil is necessary with rilpivirine, and is not expected to be necessary for tadalafil or vardenafil.[4] As **avanafil** is metabolised similarly to sildenafil, no dose adjustment would be expected to be necessary if it is used with rilpivirine.

There are no data on the effect of other NNRTIs on sildenafil or other phosphodiesterase type-5 inhibitors. However, based on their known effects on CYP3A4, **efavirenz** and **nevirapine** might be expected to interact similarly to etravirine and reduce sildenafil exposure whereas, conversely, **delavirdine** might be expected to increase sildenafil exposure. Based on this predicted interaction, the US manufacturer of delavirdine actually recommends a maximum dose of sildenafil of 25 mg in 48 hours.[5] Until more is known, some caution might be appropriate if efavirenz, nevirapine, or delavirdine is given with a phosphodiesterase type-5 inhibitor.

1. Intelence (Etravirine). Janssen-Cilag Ltd. UK Summary of product characteristics, July 2012.
2. Intelence (Etravirine). Tibotec, Inc. US Prescribing information, August 2012.
3. Crauwels HM, van Heeswijk RPG, Steven M. TMC278, a next generation non-nucleoside reverse transcriptase inhibitor, does not alter the pharmacokinetics of sildenafil. 10th International Workshop on Clinical Pharmacology of HIV Therapy, Amsterdam, April 2009.
4. Edurant (Rilpivirine hydrochloride). Janssen-Cilag Ltd. UK Summary of product characteristics, November 2011.
5. Rescriptor (Delavirdine mesylate). Viiv Healthcare. US Prescribing information, August 2012.

NNRTIs + Proton pump inhibitors

Omeprazole slightly increases etravirine exposure, and etravirine inhibits omeprazole metabolism. Omeprazole reduces rilpivirine exposure and is predicted to reduce delavirdine exposure. Efavirenz halves omeprazole exposure.

Clinical evidence

(a) Efavirenz

In a pharmacokinetic study in healthy subjects, efavirenz 600 mg daily for 17 days reduced the AUCs of a single 20-mg dose of omeprazole and its hydroxy metabolite, 5-hydroxyomeprazole, by 46% and 24%, respectively, but had no effect on the AUC of its sulfone metabolite, when compared with the effect of a single 600-mg dose of efavirenz taken one hour before omeprazole. In addition, the AUCs of the *R*- and *S*-isomers of omeprazole were reduced by 44% and 47%, respectively, when compared with the effect of a single 600-mg dose of efavirenz taken one hour before omeprazole.[1]

(b) Etravirine

In 17 healthy subjects, **omeprazole** 40 mg daily for 11 days slightly increased the AUC of a single 100-mg dose of etravirine given on day 8 by 41%, and increased its maximum concentration by just 17%.There was a decrease in exposure to the etravirine metabolite M8 with no change in the metabolite M12.[2]

In a study in 12 healthy subjects to investigate the effect of etravirine on CYP2C19, a single 40-mg dose of **omeprazole** was given on days one and 14 of a 14-day course of etravirine 200 mg twice daily. Etravirine increased the ratio of the AUC of **omeprazole** to 5-hydroxyomeprazole by 29% on day one, and 3.9-fold on day 14, of etravirine use.[3]

(c) Rilpivirine

The manufacturers report that, in a study in 16 subjects, **omeprazole** 20 mg daily slightly reduced the AUC of supratherapeutic rilpivirine 150 mg daily by 40%, and reduced its maximum and minimum concentrations by 40%, and 33%, respectively. Rilpivirine reduced the AUC and maximum concentration of omeprazole by 14% (15 subjects only).[4,5]

Mechanism

The mechanism of the slight increase in etravirine exposure with **omeprazole** is unclear. Subsequent pharmacokinetic analysis by the same group suggested that omeprazole might reduce formation of the M8 metabolite of etravirine by inhibiting CYP2C19.[2] The data on the metabolism of omeprazole to 5-hydroxyomeprazole demonstrate that etravirine is a moderate inhibitor of CYP2C19 and that efavirenz is an inducer of CYP2C19. Efavirenz also induces the metabolism of omeprazole by CYP3A4 to omeprazole sulfone.[1]

The absorption of rilpivirine, and also delavirdine, is pH dependent. Omeprazole increases the gastric pH which leads to a reduction in the absorption of rilpivirine.

Importance and management

The reduction in omeprazole exposure with **efavirenz** is probably not clinically relevant for most conditions; however, where a high degree of acid suppression is required, bear in mind the possibility that omeprazole might be less effective if given with efavirenz. Efavirenz absorption is not affected by acid-suppression (see 'NNRTIs + Antacids', p.951), and it seems unlikely that omeprazole will alter efavirenz metabolism; therefore omeprazole would not be predicted to alter efavirenz exposure.

The slight increase in **etravirine** exposure with omeprazole is not considered clinically relevant. Similarly, the moderate increase in omeprazole exposure would not be expected to be clinically relevant or result in adverse effects as omeprazole has a wide therapeutic margin.

Omeprazole increases gastric pH which leads to a reduction in the absorption of **rilpivirine**. Other proton pump inhibitors would be expected to have a similar effect. The manufacturers therefore contraindicate the concurrent use of rilpivirine with the proton pump inhibitors.[4,5] Based on the effect of antacids (see 'NNRTIs + Antacids', p.951), **delavirdine** exposure is predicted to be similarly reduced by proton pump inhibitors, and the manufacturer states that their long-term use with delavirdine is not recommended.[6]

1. Michaud V, Ogburn E, Thong N, Aregbe AO, Quigg TC, Flockhart DA, Desta Z. Induction of CYP2C19 and CYP3A activity following repeated administration of efavirenz in healthy volunteers. *Clin Pharmacol Ther* (2012) 91, 475–82.
2. Schöller-Gyüre M, Kakuda TN, De Smedt G, Vanaken H, Bouche M-P, Peeters M, Woodfall B, Hoetelmans RMW. A pharmacokinetic study of etravirine (TMC125) co-administered with ranitidine and omeprazole in HIV-negative volunteers. *Br J Clin Pharmacol* (2008) 66, 508–516.
3. Schöller-Gyüre M, Kakuda TN, Stevens T, Aharchi F, De Smedt G, Peeters M, Hoetelmans RMW. Effect of etravirine on cytochrome P450 isoenzymes assessed by the Cooperstown 5+1 cocktail. 48th Annual ICAAC/ IDSA 46th General Meeting, Washington DC, 25th-28th October 2008.
4. Edurant (Rilpivirine hydrochloride). Janssen-Cilag Ltd. UK Summary of product characteristics, November 2011.
5. Edurant (Rilpivirine hydrochloride). Tibotec Pharmaceuticals. US Prescribing information, August 2012.
6. Rescriptor (Delavirdine mesylate). ViiV Healthcare. US Prescribing information, August 2012.

NNRTIs + Rifabutin

Rifabutin causes a large reduction in delavirdine plasma concentrations but rifabutin exposure is raised when the delavirdine dose is increased to compensate for this. Rifabutin does not affect efavirenz concentrations, whereas efavirenz decreases rifabutin concentrations. Rifabutin slightly reduces etravirine exposure, but etravirine has little effect on rifabutin concentrations. There is usually no important pharmacokinetic interaction between rifabutin and nevirapine, although it is predicted that some patients might have a higher risk of rifabutin adverse effects. Rilpivirine has little effect on rifabutin concentrations, but rifabutin halves rilpivirine exposure.

Clinical evidence

(a) Delavirdine

In a controlled study in 7 HIV-positive patients taking delavirdine mesilate 400 mg three times daily for 30 days, the addition of rifabutin 300 mg daily from days 16 to 30 caused a 5-fold increase in delavirdine clearance, and an 84% reduction in its steady-state plasma concentrations. Rifabutin pharmacokinetics did not appear to be altered.[1]

In another study in 5 HIV-positive patients taking rifabutin 300 mg daily, the dose of delavirdine was titrated to achieve a minimum concentration of at least 5 micromol/L. The delavirdine dose had to be increased from 400 mg three times daily to at least 600 mg three times daily to achieve therapeutic concentrations, when compared with control patients not taking rifabutin. In these control patients similar delavirdine concentrations were achieved with delavirdine 400 mg three times daily. Delavirdine was reported to increase the AUC and minimum concentration of rifabutin 3.4-fold and 5.5-fold, respectively.[2]

(b) Efavirenz

In a study in healthy subjects, the concurrent use of efavirenz 600 mg daily and rifabutin 300 mg daily for 2 weeks resulted in a slight 38% decrease in the AUC of rifabutin and a 45% decrease in its minimum concentrations, but no change in efavirenz concentrations.[3] In one study, doubling the rifabutin dose from 300 mg twice weekly to 600 mg twice weekly when starting efavirenz resulted in an AUC of rifabutin that was 20% higher than baseline values.[4] In an analysis, 8 of 35 patients taking efavirenz and given rifabutin 450 mg daily were found to have subtherapeutic rifabutin concentrations, and they were switched to isoniazid.[5]

A case report describes treatment failure in a patient with tuberculous adenitis taking an efavirenz-containing HAART regimen with rifabutin. The patient had a persistently low rifabutin concentration (less than 0.1 micrograms/mL) despite large increases in the dose of rifabutin up to 1350 mg daily. When efavirenz was changed to nevirapine the rifabutin concentrations increased to 0.6 micrograms/mL and the patient developed rifabutin-induced iritis requiring a reduction in the rifabutin dose.[6]

Although rifabutin did not alter efavirenz concentrations one of the studies cited above,[3] there is a case of a patient with persistently low efavirenz concentrations while taking rifabutin, who had an improvement in virological response once rifabutin was stopped.[7]

(c) Etravirine

The manufacturer of etravirine reports that the concurrent use of etravirine with rifabutin 300 mg daily resulted in a reduction in the AUC, maximum and minimum concentration of etravirine of about 35%. The AUC, maximum and minimum concentration of rifabutin were also reduced, by 17%, 10%, and 24%, respectively.[8]

(d) Nevirapine

In one study in 19 patients, the pharmacokinetics of nevirapine were only minimally affected by rifabutin, when compared with historical data[9] (the manufacturer notes that there was a 9% increase in nevirapine clearance[10]). The manufacturer notes that the concurrent use of rifabutin with nevirapine caused a 17% increase in the AUC of rifabutin and a 28% increase in the steady-state maximum concentration of rifabutin, although there was high intersubject variability.[10,11] In one HIV-positive patient with low rifabutin concentrations, changing efavirenz to nevirapine resulted in high concentrations of rifabutin requiring dose reduction[6] (see under *Efavirenz*, above).

(e) Rilpivirine

In a study in 16 subjects, rifabutin 300 mg given with rilpivirine 150 mg daily reduced the AUC, maximum and minimum concentrations of rilpivirine by 46%, 35%, and 49%, respectively.[12,13] Rilpivirine had no effect on the pharmacokinetics of rifabutin.[12]

Mechanism

Efavirenz is a potent inducer of CYP3A4, by which rifabutin is metabolised, and therefore concurrent use reduces rifabutin concentrations. Delavirdine and nevirapine are inhibitors of CYP3A4 and might increase rifabutin concentrations in some situations. Etravirine and rilpivirine appear to have little effect on rifabutin. As rifabutin is also an inducer of CYP3A4, it might reduce the concentrations of the NNRTIs, which are substrates of this isoenzyme; however, reductions are not consistently seen.

Importance and management

The interactions between the NNRTIs and rifabutin are clinically important. The concurrent use of **delavirdine** and rifabutin results in a clinically relevant effect on the pharmacokinetics of both drugs, which could lead to treatment failure and an increase in adverse effects, respectively. The CDC in the US and the US manufacturer recommend that rifabutin should be not used with delavirdine.[14,15]

US guidelines advise that patients taking **efavirenz** should have the dose of rifabutin increased to 450 mg or 600 mg (taken daily or intermittently).[16] The 2011 British HIV Association (BHIVA) also recommend increasing the rifabutin dose to 450 mg daily in patients taking efavirenz.[17] Concurrent use should be closely monitored.

The US and UK guidelines state that no rifabutin dose adjustment is needed if etravirine is used without an HIV-protease inhibitor.[16,17] The slight reduction in etravirine exposure with rifabutin is not considered clinically relevant.[18] However, if etravirine is used with an HIV-protease inhibitor boosted with ritonavir (as it was in clinical studies), US guidelines state that rifabutin should not be used,[16] consider also 'HIV-protease inhibitors + Rifamycins; Rifabutin', p.939. Nevertheless, in the UK, the manufacturer of etravirine simply advises caution on the concurrent use of rifabutin with etravirine and HIV-protease inhibitors boosted with ritonavir, due to the risk of reduced concentrations of etravirine and increased concentrations of rifabutin.[8]

No clinically important pharmacokinetic interaction appears to occur between **nevirapine** and rifabutin, and no change in the dose of either drug would seem to be needed on concurrent use.[16,17] However, because of the high intersubject variability, some patients might experience large increases in rifabutin exposure and could be at higher risk of adverse effects, therefore if concurrent use is appropriate, it should be well monitored and undertaken with caution.[10,11,16,17]

The reduction in **rilpivirine** concentrations with rifabutin is likely to be clinically relevant. If concurrent use is essential, it should be well-monitored, bearing in mind that the dose of rilpivirine is likely to need increasing. Both the US and BHIVA guidelines recommend doubling the rilpivirine dose.[16,17]

1. Borin MT, Chambers JH, Carel BJ, Freimuth WW, Aksentijevich S, Piergies AA. Pharmacokinetic study of the interaction between rifabutin and delavirdine mesylate in HIV-1 infected patients. *Antiviral Res* (1997) 35, 53–63.
2. Cox SR, Herman BD, Batts DH, et al. Delavirdine and rifabutin: pharmacokinetic evaluation in HIV-1 patients with concentration-targeting of delavirdine [abstract no. 344]. 5th Conference on Retroviruses and Opportunistic Infections, Chicago, 1998.
3. Benedek IH, Fiske WD, White SJ, Stevenson D, Joseph JL, Kornhauser DM. Pharmacokinetic interaction between multiple doses of efavirenz and rifabutin in healthy volunteers [abstract no. 461]. *Clin Infect Dis* (1998) 27, 1008.
4. Weiner M, Benator D, Peloquin CA, Burman W, Vernon A, Engle M, Khan A, Zhao Z; the Tuberculosis Trials Consortium. Evaluation of the drug interaction between rifabutin and efavirenz in patients with HIV infection and tuberculosis. *Clin Infect Dis* (2005) 41, 1343–9.
5. Spradling P, Drociuk D, McLaughlin S, Lee LM, Peloquin CA, Gallicano K, Pozsik C, Onorato I, Castro KG, Ridzon R. Drug-drug interactions in inmates treated for human immunodeficiency virus and *Mycobacterium tuberculosis* infection or disease: an institutional tuberculosis outbreak. *Clin Infect Dis* (2002) 35, 1106–12.
6. Edelstein HE, Cuadros Y. Failure of treatment of tuberculous adenitis due to an unexpected drug interaction with rifabutin and efavirenz. *AIDS* (2004) 18, 1748–9.
7. Hsu O, Hill CJ, Kim M, Tan B, O'Brien JG. Decreased plasma efavirenz concentrations in a patient receiving rifabutin. *Am J Health-Syst Pharm* (2010) 67, 1611–14.
8. Intelence (Etravirine). Janssen-Cilag Ltd. UK Summary of product characteristics, July 2012.
9. Maldonado S, Lamson M, Gigliotti M, Pav JW, Robinson P. Pharmacokinetic interaction between nevirapine and rifabutin. *Intersci Conf Antimicrob Agents Chemother* (1999) 39, 21.
10. Viramune (Nevirapine). Boehringer Ingelheim Ltd. UK Summary of product characteristics, January 2012.
11. Viramune (Nevirapine). Boehringer Ingelheim Pharmaceuticals, Inc. US Prescribing information, November 2011.
12. Edurant (Rilpivirine hydrochloride). Janssen-Cilag Ltd. UK Summary of product characteristics, November 2011.
13. Edurant (Rilpivirine hydrochloride). Tibotec Pharmaceuticals. US Prescribing information, August 2012.
14. Centers for Disease Control and Prevention. Managing drug interactions in the treatment of HIV-related tuberculosis. *US Department of Health and Human Services* (2007). Available at: http://www.cdc.gov/tb/publications/guidelines/TB_HIV_Drugs/default.htm (accessed 20/09/15).
15. Rescriptor (Delavirdine mesylate). ViiV Healthcare. US Prescribing information, August 2012.
16. Panel on Antiretroviral Guidelines for Adults and Adolescents. Guidelines for the use of antiretroviral agents in HIV-1-infected adults and adolescents. Department of Health and Human Services. (April 2015). 1–288. Available at: https://aidsinfo.nih.gov/contentfiles/lvguidelines/adultandadolescentgl.pdf (accessed 20/09/15).
17. Pozniak AL, Coyne KM, Miller RF, Lipman MCI, Freedman AR, Ormerod LP, Johnson MA, Collins S, Lucas SB on behalf of the BHIVA Guidelines Subcommittee. British HIV Association guidelines for the treatment of TB/HIV co-infection 2011. Available at: http://www.bhiva.org/documents/Guidelines/TB/hiv_954_online_final.pdf (accessed 20/09/15).
18. Kakuda TN, Schöller-Gyüre M, Hoetelmans RM. Pharmacokinetic interactions between etravirine and non-antiretroviral drugs. *Clin Pharmacokinet* (2011) 50, 25–39.

NNRTIs + Rifampicin (Rifampin)

Rifampicin greatly reduces delavirdine and rilpivirine plasma concentrations, and is predicted to reduce etravirine concentrations. Neither efavirenz nor nevirapine affect rifampicin concentrations, but rifampicin modestly reduces the concentrations of efavirenz and nevirapine.

Clinical evidence

(a) Delavirdine

In 7 patients given rifampicin 600 mg daily for 2 weeks, the clearance of delavirdine was 27-fold higher, and the steady-state plasma concentrations became almost undetectable when compared with 5 control patients not given rifampicin.[1]

(b) Efavirenz

The pharmacokinetics of rifampicin are not substantially altered by efavirenz.[2] A few controlled pharmacokinetic studies have shown that rifampicin slightly reduces efavirenz exposure. In one study in 12 healthy subjects, the concurrent use of rifampicin 600 mg daily and efavirenz 600 mg daily for 7 days reduced the steady-state AUC of efavirenz by 26% and reduced its minimum concentration by 32%.[3,4] In another similar study,[5] rifampicin reduced the AUC of efavirenz by 18% and reduced its minimum concentration by 19%. Similarly, in patients with HIV and tuberculosis the concurrent use of HAART including efavirenz (600 mg daily) with antitubercular drugs including rifampicin (450 mg to 720 mg daily) decreased the AUC of efavirenz by 19% and 22% and decreased the minimum concentration by 20% and 25% (although large interpatient variability was observed, and the findings from one study[6] were not statistically significant).[2,6] In another analysis of therapeutic drug monitoring data, the concurrent use of rifampicin was associated with a 35% decrease in efavirenz concentrations.[7]

In one controlled study, when the efavirenz dose was increased to 800 mg daily with rifampicin, efavirenz pharmacokinetics were similar to those of efavirenz 600 mg daily without rifampicin.[2] Some other studies have confirmed that the pharmacokinetics or minimum efavirenz concentrations were similar between patients taking efavirenz 800 mg daily with rifampicin and those taking efavirenz 600 mg daily without rifampicin or after withdrawing rifampicin.[8,9] In contrast, in one controlled study in patients taking rifampicin, the *median* minimum efavirenz concentration did not differ appreciably between those taking standard dose efavirenz and those taking 800 mg daily.[10]

Numerous clinical studies in patients taking rifampicin have investigated the effects of an increased efavirenz dose or the standard dose on virus suppression, the minimum efavirenz concentration and/or adverse effects. Many studies have shown that the standard efavirenz dose is generally adequate. For example, in a prospective cohort study in South Africans, there was no difference in viral load or virological failure in the first 2 years of therapy between 1 074 HIV-positive patients taking efavirenz 600 mg daily with rifampicin and 961 HIV-positive patients taking efavirenz 600 mg daily without rifampicin.[11] Similarly, in a controlled study in Thai patients, with an average body-weight of about 50 kg, similar virological outcomes were seen between those randomised to standard dose efavirenz and those receiving the higher dose of 800 mg daily, both with rifampicin.[12] In a subsequent study by the same research group comparing efavirenz with nevirapine, in 71 patients (mean body-weight about 53 kg) taking rifampicin and given standard dose efavirenz 600 mg daily, the mean 12-hour concentrations of efavirenz at week 6 and week 12 of concurrent use were above those suggested for efficacy (4.27 mg/L and 3.54 mg/L, respectively), and just 2 patients were reported to have subtherapeutic 12-hour efavirenz concentrations (less than 1 mg/L) at week 12. About three-quarters of patients achieved viral suppression at 48 weeks.[13] In a further analysis of data from this study, 12-hour efavirenz concentrations decreased as body-weight increased, and the mean weight at which the concentration dropped below 1 mg/L was 57.5 kg.[14] Other small studies have reported the successful use of efavirenz 600 mg daily in patients taking a rifampicin-containing regimen for tuberculosis.[6,15] In these studies, there was wide variability in efavirenz concentrations and these were not associated with HIV clinical outcome.[6,15]

Of published data for the increased dose of efavirenz of 800 mg daily, in one small study the mean efavirenz minimum concentration when it was taken with rifampicin was 1.39 micrograms/mL, but this was not correlated with clinical outcome (4 patients were found to have concentrations of less than 0.1 micrograms/mL from 7 results, but none of these patients were non-responders to HAART and their viral loads remained below 50 copies/mL). Four patients with low body-weight (45 to 55 kg) had severe acute CNS adverse effects, but no data on efavirenz concentrations were available for these episodes.[8] Similarly, in another analysis, 7 of 9 patients receiving rifampicin and efavirenz 800 mg daily developed important clinical toxicity and were found to have efavirenz concentrations much higher than the therapeutic range.[16] In contrast, in another study in 16 patients (mean weight 64 kg), efavirenz maximum concentrations were not elevated with efavirenz 800 mg and no increase in adverse effects occurred, although the authors did advise caution due to large interpatient variability.[9]

Further studies have indicated that other efavirenz dose adjustments might be required in some patients if rifampicin is also given. For example, in one retrospective study, 10 of 20 patients taking efavirenz 600 mg daily (3 patients) or 800 mg daily (7 patients) had therapeutic efavirenz concentrations while taking rifampicin. One patient taking efavirenz 800 mg daily had greatly increased efavirenz concentrations of 24.5 micrograms/mL. Five patients had further plasma concentrations analysed. Two patients had subtherapeutic efavirenz concentrations, one patient had concentrations at the low end of the therapeutic range, and 2 patients were found to have raised efavirenz concentrations, one of which had a concentration of 23.5 micrograms/mL and developed toxicity. One of the patients with low efavirenz concentrations only achieved a therapeutic range with efavirenz dose increases from 800 mg to 1.2 g daily.[17] In another report, two patients required efavirenz dose increases from 600 mg to 1000 mg and from 800 mg to 1600 mg to achieve therapeutic concentrations while taking rifampicin.[18] In addition, in a study in 15 children given recommended doses of efavirenz, subtherapeutic efavirenz concentrations were common both during and after rifampicin treatment (9 and 8 children, respectively) and 2 children had virological failure, although inter-individual variation in efavirenz concentrations might have played a part in this.[19]

Some studies have investigated the association between CYP2B6 metaboliser status and efavirenz concentrations with the concurrent use of rifampicin. In a study 26 HIV-positive patients taking efavirenz 600 mg daily as part of a HAART regimen and rifampicin for tuberculosis, the AUC, maximum and minimum plasma concentrations of efavirenz did not differ appreciably between the patients of CYP2B6 extensive metaboliser status (that is, those with normal isoenzyme activity) and those with intermediate CYP2B6 activity, who might be expected to have slightly higher concentrations of efavirenz. Those patients who were poor metabolisers (those lacking or deficient in CYP2B6) had higher concentrations of efavirenz despite rifampicin treatment.[20] In a later study, poor metabolisers had high concentrations of efavirenz, and the effect of metaboliser status was greater than the effect of rifampicin.[6] Similarly, in other analyses in Thai and African patients, poor metaboliser status had a greater effect on efavirenz concentrations than rifampicin.[21,22] Moreover, in one post-hoc analysis, poor metabolisers actually had higher efavirenz concentrations while taking rifampicin.[23] In yet another analysis, more patients who were CYP2B6 extensive metabolisers had subtherapeutic efavirenz concentrations when taking rifampicin than patients of other metaboliser statuses.[24]

A case report of a patient subsequently found to be a CYP2B6 poor metaboliser describes *raised* efavirenz concentrations of up to 10 mg/L, with agitation and drowsiness, in a patient taking standard-dose efavirenz 600 mg daily with rifampicin. The efavirenz dose needed to be reduced to 200 mg daily.[25]

(c) Nevirapine

The manufacturer states that the AUC of nevirapine was reduced by 58% by rifampicin in 14 subjects, when compared with historical data. There was no change in steady-state rifampicin pharmacokinetics.[26,27] Similarly, in a study in 16 HIV-positive patients taking nevirapine 200 mg twice daily, 10 days or more after stopping rifampicin 450 mg or 600 mg daily the AUC, maximum and minimum plasma concentrations of nevirapine increased by 67%, 63%, and 37%, respectively.[28] In another study in 13 patients taking nevirapine 200 mg twice daily, the addition of rifampicin 450 mg or 600 mg daily caused a 46% reduction in the AUC of nevirapine, and a 53% reduction in its minimum concentrations, with 8 of the patients having a nevirapine minimum concentration below the therapeutic range (3 micrograms/mL). In 7 of the patients who had a reduction in the minimum concentrations to less than the therapeutic range, increasing the dose of nevirapine to 300 mg twice daily increased the concentrations to above the therapeutic range in all patients without increasing adverse effects.[29] In another patient study, rifampicin caused a 31% decrease in the median AUC of nevirapine and a non-significant 21% decrease in its median minimum concentration.[30] In a retrospective analysis of therapeutic drug monitoring data, the concurrent use of rifampicin was associated with about a 40% reduction in nevirapine plasma concentrations.[7]

Some studies suggest that standard doses of nevirapine might be adequate in many patients. For example, in a retrospective study, 6 of 11 patients had therapeutic nevirapine concentrations while taking rifampicin, and 5 of these were taking standard doses. In this small analysis, subtherapeutic concentrations (less than 3.4 mg/L) were not associated with virological failure.[17] Similarly, observational data from 32 patients supported the continued efficacy of standard dose nevirapine when it was used with rifampicin.[31] Others have also reported the successful use of standard dose nevirapine with twice weekly rifampicin with little effect on minimum nevirapine concentrations.[32]

In yet another study, although the concurrent use of rifampicin and nevirapine 200 mg twice daily increased the proportion of patients with minimum concentrations below the suggested recommended concentration of 3.4 mg/L (29.7% versus 6.8%) at 8 weeks, there was no difference in virological outcomes at 24 weeks between 70 rifampicin recipients and 70 control patients.[33] When these patients stopped rifampicin treatment, the nevirapine concentrations were reported to increase from 5.4 mg/L to 6.4 mg/L.[34]

In contrast, a couple of later large studies have shown that the concurrent use of standard dose nevirapine and rifampicin can result in subtherapeutic concentrations of nevirapine and possibly treatment failure. For example, In a prospective, randomised, controlled study in 71 HIV-positive Thai patients taking rifampicin and given nevirapine 200 mg twice daily, by week 12, subtherapeutic 12-hour concentrations (less than 3.4 mg/L) were found in 21.3% of patients taking nevirapine. Further analysis reported that low 12-hour concentrations, indicating low exposure to nevirapine, were associated with treatment failure.[13] Similarly, in a prospective cohort study of African patients, 209 HIV-positive patients taking nevirapine 200 mg twice daily with rifampicin had a higher risk of increased viral loads at 6 months and had a shorter time to virological failure than 1 726 HIV-positive patients taking nevirapine without rifampicin.[11] This contrasted with the finding for efavirenz in this study, see above. Nevirapine 400 mg daily was associated with an unacceptable incidence of treatment failure (10 of 57 patients) in Indian patients being treated with rifampicin.[35] Starting nevirapine at 400 mg daily rather than the usual dose titration starting with nevirapine 200 mg daily was associated with a lower frequency of sub-therapeutic concentrations, but was not considered an adequate dose for continued therapy.[36]

(d) Rilpivirine

The manufacturers report that, in a study in 16 subjects, rifampicin 600 mg daily markedly reduced the AUC of rilpivirine by 80% and reduced its maximum and minimum concentrations by 69% and 89%, respectively. Rilpivirine had no effect on the pharmacokinetics of rifampicin.[37,38]

Mechanism

Rifampicin is a potent inducer of CYP3A4, by which delavirdine and rilpivirine are metabolised, therefore reducing their exposure. Nevirapine is also partially metabolised by CYP3A4. Efavirenz is mainly metabolised by CYP2B6, and this isoenzyme is also induced by rifampicin. Note that efavirenz induces its own metabolism via CYP2B6 (autoinduction).

Importance and management

The very large reduction in **delavirdine** and **rilpivirine** concentrations on the concurrent use of rifampicin is likely to greatly reduce the efficacy activity of these NNRTIs. For rilpivirine, the 2011 British HIV Association (BHIVA) guidelines,[39] US guidelines[40] and the manufacturers[37,38] contraindicate the concurrent use of rifampicin. Similarly, it has been recommended that the combination of delavirdine and rifampicin should be considered as contraindicated.[1,41]

The manufacturers of **etravirine** predict that rifampicin will decrease the plasma concentration of etravirine. Due to the risk of therapeutic failure, they therefore contraindicate[42] or advise against[43] the concurrent use of etravirine and rifampicin. The BHIVA guidelines[39] and US guidelines[40] also state that they should not be used together, which, in the absence of any data, seems prudent.

The clinical relevance of the slight reduction in **efavirenz** exposure with rifampicin is uncertain, as the clinical evidence is conflicting. After reviewing the data in 2008, authors from the FDA concluded that there was insufficient evidence to support definitive recommendations on dose adjustments of efavirenz when taken with rifampicin,[44] and the 2011 BHIVA guidelines note that there is a lack of consensus regarding the appropriate efavirenz dose.[39] The 2015 US HIV guidelines recommend using the standard efavirenz dose while monitoring for virologic response, although they note that some clinicians suggest increasing the efavirenz dose to 800 mg daily in patients weighing more than 60 kg.[40] The 2011 BHIVA guidelines recommend increasing the efavirenz dose to 800 mg daily in patients weighing more than 60 kg, and measuring the efavirenz concentration at 2 weeks.[39] The manufacturer of efavirenz recommends a dose increase to 800 mg daily in those weighing more than 50 kg.[3,4] Efavirenz concentrations are known to vary widely between individuals, and increasing evidence suggests that CYP2B6 polymorphisms in particular might be key to this variability. Until more is known, concurrent use should be closely monitored for virological efficacy and efavirenz adverse effects, with therapeutic drug monitoring as necessary, and the efavirenz dose adjusted accordingly.

The exposure of **nevirapine** is reduced to a greater extent than that of efavirenz when given with rifampicin, but there is similarly conflicting clinical evidence as to the relevance of this. The UK and US manufacturers suggest that the concurrent use of rifampicin with nevirapine is not recommended, and that rifabutin can be considered instead, with close monitoring of adverse effects.[26,27] In the UK, the BHIVA guidelines state that rifampicin is not recommended for use with nevirapine; however, if there are no alternatives to using nevirapine with rifampicin, then standard doses should be used with monitoring of nevirapine concentrations.[39] The US HIV guidelines state that nevirapine and rifampicin should not be given together.[40] Note that in a couple of comparative studies, standard-dose efavirenz was considered more effective than standard-dose nevirapine when given with rifampicin,[11,13] and the WHO state that efavirenz should be the preferred NNRTI in patients starting antiretroviral therapy while receiving antituberculosis treatment.[45]

Rifabutin can be used with some NNRTIs as an alternative to rifampicin. For further information, see 'NNRTIs + Rifabutin', p.964.

US guidelines state that **rifapentine** is predicted to reduce concentrations of the NNRTIs and, in the absence of data, should not be used with NNRTIs outside of clinical studies.[40] However, they also state that in HIV-positive individuals, rifapentine-based regimens are associated with a higher rate of tuberculosis relapse than other rifamycin-based regimens and therefore an alternative to rifapentine is recommended.[40]

1. Borin MT, Chambers JH, Carel BJ, Gagnon S, Freimuth WW. Pharmacokinetic study of the interaction between rifampin and delavirdine mesylate. *Clin Pharmacol Ther* (1997) 61, 544–53.
2. López-Cortés LF, Ruiz-Valderas R, Viciana P, Alarcón-González A, Gómez-Mateos J, León-Jimenez E, Sarasa-Nacenta M, López-Pua Y, Pachón J. Pharmacokinetic interactions between efavirenz and rifampicin in HIV-infected patients with tuberculosis. *Clin Pharmacokinet* (2002) 41, 681–90.
3. Sustiva Film-coated Tablets (Efavirenz). Bristol-Myers Squibb Pharmaceutical Ltd. UK Summary of product characteristics, March 2014.
4. Sustiva (Efavirenz). Bristol-Myers Squibb Company. US Prescribing information, August 2012.
5. Kwara A, Tashima KT, Dumond JB, Poethke P, Kurpewski J, Kashuba ADM, Court MH, Greenblatt DJ. Modest but variable effect of rifampin on steady-state plasma pharmacokinetics of efavirenz in healthy African-American and Caucasian volunteers. *Antimicrob Agents Chemother* (2011) 55, 3527–33.
6. Ramachandran G, Hemanth Kumar AK, Rajasekaran S, Kumar P, Ramesh K, Anitha S, Narendran G, Menon P, Gomathi C, Swaminathan S. CYP2B6 G516T polymorphism but not rifampin coadministration influences steady-state pharmacokinetics of efavirenz in human immunodeficiency virus-infected patients in South India. *Antimicrob Agents Chemother* (2009) 53, 863–8.
7. Stöhr W, Back D, Dunn D, Sabin C, Winston A, Gilson R, Pillay D, Hill T, Ainsworth J, Pozniak A, Leen C, Bansi L, Fisher M, Orkin C, Anderson J, Johnson M, Easterbrook P, Gibbons S, Khoo S, for the Liverpool TDM database and UK CHIC study. Factors influencing efavirenz and nevirapine plasma concentration: effect of ethnicity, weight and co-medication. *Antivir Ther* (2008) 13, 675–85.
8. Lopez-Cortes LF, Ruiz-Valderas R, Ruiz-Morales J, Leon E, de Campos AV, Marin-Niebla A, Marquez-Solero M, Lozano F, Valiente R. Efavirenz trough levels are not associated with virological failure throughout therapy with 800 mg daily and a rifampicin-containing antituberculosis regimen. *J Antimicrob Chemother* (2006) 58, 1017–23.
9. Matteelli A, Regazzi M, Villani P, De Iaco G, Cusato M, Carvalho ACC, Caligaris S, Tomasoni L, Manfrin M, Capone S, Carosi G. Multiple-dose pharmacokinetics of efavirenz with and without the use of rifampicin in HIV-positive patients. *Curr HIV Res* (2007) 5, 349–53.

10. Manosuthi W, Sungkanuparph S, Thakkinstian A, Vibhagool A, Kiertiburanakul S, Rattanasiri S, Prasithsirikul W, Sankote J, Mahanontharit A, Ruxrungtham K. Efavirenz levels and 24-week efficacy in HIV-infected patients with tuberculosis receiving highly active antiretroviral therapy and rifampicin. *AIDS* (2005) 19, 1481–6.
11. Boulle A, Van Cutsem G, Cohen K, Hilderbrand K, Mathee S, Abrahams M, Goemaere E, Coetzee D, Maartens G. Outcomes of nevirapine- and efavirenz-based antiretroviral therapy when coadministered with rifampicin-based antitubercular therapy. *JAMA* (2008) 300, 530–9.
12. Manosuthi W, Kiertiburanakul S, Sungkanuparph S, Ruxrungtham K, Vibhagool A, Rattanasiri S, Thakkinstian A. Efavirenz 600 mg/day versus efavirenz 800 mg/day in HIV-infected patients with tuberculosis receiving rifampicin: 48 weeks results. *AIDS* (2006) 20, 131–2.
13. Manosuthi W, Sungkanuparph S, Tantanathip P, Lueangniyomkul A, Mankatitham W, Prasithsirskul W, Burapatarawong S, Thongyen S, Likanonsakul S, Thawornwa U, Prommool V, Ruxrungtham K; N_2R study team. A randomized trial comparing plasma drug concentrations and efficacies between 2 nonnucleoside reverse-transcriptase inhibitor-based regimens in HIV-infected patients receiving rifampicin: the N_2R study. *Clin Infect Dis* (2009) 48, 1752–9.
14. Manosuthi W, Sungkanuparph S, Tantanathip P, Mankatitham W, Lueangniyomkul A, Thongyen S, Eampokarap B, Uttayamakul S, Suwanvattana P, Kaewsaard S, Ruxrungtham K; N2R Study Team. Body weight cutoff for daily dosage of efavirenz and 60-week efficacy of efavirenz-based regimen in human immunodeficiency virus and tuberculosis coinfected patients receiving rifampin. *Antimicrob Agents Chemother* (2009) 53, 4545–8.
15. Friedland G, Khoo S, Jack C, Lalloo U. Administration of efavirenz (600 mg/day) with rifampicin results in highly variable levels but excellent clinical outcomes in patients treated for tuberculosis and HIV. *J Antimicrob Chemother* (2006) 58, 1299–1302.
16. Brennan-Benson P, Lyus R, Harrison T, Pakianathan M, Macallan D. Pharmacokinetic interactions between efavirenz and rifampicin in the treatment of HIV and tuberculosis: one size does not fit all. *AIDS* (2005) 19, 1541–3.
17. Sathia L, Obiorah I, Taylor G, Kon O, O'Donoghue M, Gibbins S, Walsh J, Winston A. Concomitant use of nonnucleoside analogue reverse transcriptase inhibitors and rifampicin in TB/HIV type 1-coinfected patients. *AIDS Res Hum Retroviruses* (2008) 24, 897–901.
18. Cabrera SE, Cordero M, Iglesias A, Valverde MP, Domínguea-Gil A, García MJ. Efavirenz-rifampicin interaction: therapeutic drug monitoring to efavirenz dosage optimization in HIV/TBC patients. *AIDS* (2008) 22, 2549–51.
19. Ren Y, Nuttall JJC, Eley BS, Meyers TM, Smith PJ, Maartens G, McIlleron HM. Effect of rifampicin on efavirenz pharmacokinetics in HIV-infected children with tuberculosis. *J Acquir Immune Defic Syndr* (2009) 50, 439–43.
20. Kwara A, Lartey M, Sagoe KW, Xexemeku F, Kenu E, Oliver-Commey J, Boima V, Sagoe A, Boamah I, Greenblatt DJ, Court MH. Pharmacokinetics of efavirenz when co-administered with rifampin in TB/HIV co-infected patients: pharmacogenetic effect of CYP2B6 variation. *J Clin Pharmacol* (2008) 48, 1032–40.
21. Uttayamakul S, Likanonsakul S, Manosuthi W, Wichukchinda N, Kalambaheti T, Nakayama EE, Shioda T, Khusmith S. Effects of CYP2B6 G516T polymorphisms on plasma efavirenz and nevirapine levels when co-administered with rifampicin in HIV/TB co-infected Thai adults. *AIDS Res Ther* (2010) 7, 8.
22. Cohen K, Grant A, Dandara C, McIlleron H, Pemba L, Fielding K, Charalombous S, Churchyard G, Smith P, Maartens G. Effect of rifampicin-based antitubercular therapy and the cytochrome P450 2B6 516G>T polymorphism on efavirenz concentrations in adults in South Africa. *Antivir Ther* (2009) 14, 687–95.
23. Kwara A, Lartey M, Sagoe KW, Court MH. Paradoxically elevated efavirenz concentrations in HIV/tuberculosis-coinfected patients with CYP2B6 516TT genotype on rifampin-containing antituberculous therapy. *AIDS* (2011) 25, 388–90.
24. Ngaimisi E, Mugusi S, Minzi O, Sasi P, Riedel KD, Suda A, Ueda N, Janabi M, Mugusi F, Haefeli WE, Bertilsson L, Burhenne J, Aklillu E. Effect of rifampicin and CYP2B6 genotype on long-term efavirenz autoinduction and plasma exposure in HIV patients with or without tuberculosis. *Clin Pharmacol Ther* (2011) 90, 406–13.
25. Van Luin M, Brouwer A-M, van der Ven A, de Lange W, van Schaik RHN, Burger DM. Efavirenz dose reduction to 200 mg once daily in a patient treated with rifampicin. *AIDS* (2009) 23, 742–4.
26. Viramune (Nevirapine). Boehringer Ingelheim Ltd. UK Summary of product characteristics, January 2012.
27. Viramune (Nevirapine). Boehringer Ingelheim Pharmaceuticals, Inc. US Prescribing information, November 2011.
28. Cohen K, van Cutsem G, Boulle A, McIlleron H, Goemaere E, Smith PJ, Maartens G. Effect of rifampicin-based antitubercular therapy on nevirapine plasma concentrations in South African adults with HIV-associated tuberculosis. *J Antimicrob Chemother* (2008) 61, 389–93.
29. Ramachandran G, Hemanthkumar AK, Rajasekaran S, Padmapriyadarsini C, Narendran G, Sukumar B, Sathishnarayan S, Raja K, Kumaraswami V, Swaminathan S. Increasing nevirapine dose can overcome reduced bioavailability due to rifampicin coadministration. *J Acquir Immune Defic Syndr* (2006) 42, 36–41.
30. Ribera E, Pou L, Lopez RM, Crespo M, Falco V, Ocaña I, Ruiz I, Pahissa A. Pharmacokinetic interaction between nevirapine and rifampicin in HIV-infected patients with tuberculosis. *J Acquir Immune Defic Syndr* (2001) 28, 450–3.
31. Oliva J, Moreno S, Sanz J, Ribera E, Pérez Molina JAÒ, Rubio R, Casas E, Mariño A. Co-administration of rifampin and nevirapine in HIV-infected patients with tuberculosis. *AIDS* (2003) 17, 637–8.
32. Dean GL, Back DJ, de Ruiter A. Effect of tuberculosis therapy on nevirapine trough plasma concentrations. *AIDS* (1999) 13, 2489–90.
33. Manosuthi W, Sungkanuparph S, Thakkinstian A, Rattanasiri S, Chaovavanich A, Prasithsirikul W, Likanonsakul S, Ruxrungtham K. Plasma nevirapine levels and 24-week efficacy in HIV-infected patients receiving nevirapine-based highly active antiretroviral therapy with or without rifampicin. *Clin Infect Dis* (2006) 43, 253–5.
34. Manosuthi W, Ruxrungtham K, Likanonsakul S, Prasithsirikul W, Inthong Y, Phoorishi T, Sungkanuparph S. Nevirapine levels after discontinuation of rifampicin therapy and 60-week efficacy of nevirapine-based antiretroviral therapy in HIV-infected patients with tuberculosis. *Clin Infect Dis* (2007) 44, 141–4.
35. Swaminathan S, Padmapriyadarsini C, Venkatesan P, Narendran G, Ramesh Kumar S, Iliayas S, Menon PA, Selvaraju S, Pooranagangadevi NP, Bhavani PK, Ponnuraja C, Dilip M, Ramachandran R. Efficacy and safety of once-daily nevirapine- or efavirenz-based antiretroviral therapy in HIV-associated tuberculosis: a randomized clinical trial. *Clin Infect Dis* (2011) 53, 716–24.
36. Lamorde M, Byakika-Kibwika P, Okaba-Kayom V, Ryan M, Coakley P, Boffito M, Namakula R, Kalemeera F, Colebunders R, Back D, Khoo S, Merry C. Nevirapine pharmacokinetics when initiated at 200 mg or 400 mg daily in HIV-1 and tuberculosis co-infected Ugandan adults on rifampicin. *J Antimicrob Chemother* (2011) 66, 180–3.
37. Edurant (Rilpivirine hydrochloride). Janssen-Cilag Ltd. UK Summary of product characteristics, November 2011.
38. Edurant (Rilpivirine hydrochloride). Tibotec Pharmaceuticals. US Prescribing information, August 2012.
39. Pozniak AL, Coyne KM, Miller RF, Lipman MCI, Freedman AR, Ormerod LP, Johnson MA, Collins S, Lucas SB on behalf of the BHIVA Guidelines Subcommittee. British HIV Association guidelines for the treatment of TB/ HIV co-infection 2011. Available at: http://www.bhiva.org/documents/Guidelines/TB/hiv_954_online_final.pdf (accessed 20/09/15).
40. Panel on Antiretroviral Guidelines for Adults and Adolescents. Guidelines for the use of antiretroviral agents in HIV-1-infected adults and adolescents. Department of Health and Human Services. (April 2015) 1–288. Available at https://aidsinfo.nih.gov/contentfiles/lvguidelines/adultandadolescentgl.pdf (accessed 20/09/15).
41. Rescriptor (Delavirdine mesylate). ViiV Healthcare. US Prescribing information, August 2012.
42. Intelence (Etravirine). Janssen-Cilag Ltd. UK Summary of product characteristics, July 2012.
43. Intelence (Etravirine). Tibotec, Inc. US Prescribing information, August 2012.
44. DiGiacinto JL, Chan-Tack KM, Robertson SM, Reynolds KS, Struble KA. Are literature references sufficient for dose recommendations? An FDA case study of efavirenz and rifampin. *J Clin Pharmacol* (2008) 48, 518–23.
45. WHO policy on collaborative TB/HIV activities. Guidelines for national programmes and other stakeholders. 2012. Available at: http://www.who.int/tb/publications/2012/tb_hiv_policy_9789241503006/en/index.html (accessed 20/109/15).

NNRTIs + St John's wort (*Hypericum perforatum*)

There is some evidence to suggest that St John's wort might decrease the concentrations of nevirapine. Delavirdine, efavirenz, etravirine, and rilpivirine would be expected to be similarly affected.

Clinical evidence

Nevirapine plasma concentrations, obtained by routine monitoring, were noted to be lower in 5 men who were also taking St John's wort. Based on a pharmacokinetic modelling analysis, it was estimated that St John's wort increased the oral clearance of **nevirapine** by about 35%.[1]

Mechanism

This finding supports predictions based on the known metabolism of the NNRTIs by CYP3A4 (see 'Table 21.2', p.894), of which St John's wort is a known inducer.

Importance and management

The interaction between St John's wort and nevirapine confirms advice issued by the CSM in the UK,[2] that St John's wort might decrease blood concentrations of the NNRTIs with possible loss of HIV suppression. US guidelines also mention the possible interaction and recommend that NNRTIs and St John's wort should not be given together.[3] Therefore the concurrent use of St John's wort with all NNRTIs (**delavirdine, efavirenz, etravirine**, nevirapine and **rilpivirine**) should be avoided.

1. de Maat MMR, Hoetelmans RMW, Mathôt RAA, van Gorp ECM, Meenhorst PL, Mulder JW, Beijnen JH. Drug interaction between St John's wort and nevirapine. *AIDS* (2001) 15, 420–1.
2. Committee on Safety of Medicines. Message from Professor A Breckenridge (Chairman of CSM) and Fact Sheet for Health Care Professionals, 29th February 2000.
3. Panel on Antiretroviral Guidelines for Adults and Adolescents. Guidelines for the use of antiretroviral agents in HIV-1-infected adults and adolescents. Department of Health and Human Services. (April 2015). 1–288. Available at http://www.aidsinfo.nih.gov/ContentFiles/AdultandAdolescentGL.pdf (accessed 18/09/15).

NNRTIs + Tenofovir

No pharmacokinetic interaction occurs between tenofovir and efavirenz, and nevirapine concentrations appear to be unaffected by tenofovir. There are some minor pharmacokinetic changes when tenofovir is given with etravirine or rilpivirine. Apparently increased efavirenz concentrations have been reported on the concurrent use of tenofovir in one analysis in CYP2B6 poor metabolisers, as have efavirenz neuropsychiatric adverse effects.

Clinical evidence

(a) Efavirenz

In a pharmacokinetic study in 29 subjects, there was no change in the AUC or minimum and maximum concentrations of either efavirenz 600 mg daily or tenofovir disoproxil fumarate 300 mg daily when given concurrently for 14 days.[1] In a retrospective analysis of routine therapeutic drug monitoring data, efavirenz plasma concentrations did not differ between 126 patients taking tenofovir and 118 patients not taking tenofovir. It appeared that efavirenz did not alter tenofovir plasma concentrations.[2] Another study also reported no overall difference in median efavirenz exposure in 18 HIV-positive patients also taking tenofovir, when compared with 151 HIV-positive patients taking efavirenz alone. However, further analysis found that 23 patients who were CYP2B6 poor metabolisers (those lacking or deficient in CYP2B6) had a 6-fold higher AUC of efavirenz than those who were CYP2B6 extensive metabolisers (that is, those with normal activity of this isoenzyme). Five of the 23 taking tenofovir with efavirenz were found to have a 2-fold higher AUC of efavirenz than the 18 who were not taking tenofovir. In one case, the addition of tenofovir increased the AUC of efavirenz by about 66%, resulting in neuropsychological adverse effects. These adverse effects resolved when the efavirenz dose was reduced to 200 mg daily.[3]

Nine cases of neuropsychiatric adverse effects, such as nightmares, insomnia, and dizziness, have been reported in HIV-positive patients taking efavirenz, in 5 cases these adverse effects developed within 48 hours of starting tenofovir and after 2 weeks to 2 years in the remaining 4 patients. These patients had previously been taking long-term efavirenz-based HAART with no reports of neurological adverse effects. In 6 of these patients, the symptoms resolved when tenofovir was stopped. Efavirenz concentrations were within the therapeutic range in the 4 patients assessed.[4]

(b) Etravirine

In a study, healthy subjects were given tenofovir disoproxil fumarate 300 mg daily for 16 days with etravirine 200 mg or 800 mg twice daily on days one to 8 or days 9 to 16. Tenofovir slightly reduced the AUC_{0-12} of etravirine by 19 to 31%. Etravirine negligibly increased the AUC of tenofovir by about 15%.[5]

(c) Nevirapine

In a retrospective analysis of routine therapeutic drug monitoring data, plasma concentrations of nevirapine 200 mg twice daily or 400 mg once daily did not differ between 133 patients taking tenofovir disoproxil fumarate 300 mg daily and 290 not taking tenofovir. It appeared that nevirapine did not alter tenofovir plasma concentrations.[2]

(d) Rilpivirine

In a study in 16 subjects, the concurrent use of rilpivirine 150 mg daily (supratherapeutic dose) and tenofovir disoproxil fumarate 300 mg daily increased the AUC of tenofovir by 23% and increased its maximum and minimum concentrations by 19% and 24%, respectively. Tenofovir had no effect on the pharmacokinetics of rilpivirine.[6,7]

Mechanism

Efavirenz is metabolised by CYP2B6. Patients lacking or with low concentrations of this isoenzyme (poor metabolisers) are known to have increased concentrations of efavirenz, which might increase the risk of adverse effects. However, as tenofovir is not known to have inhibitory effects on cytochrome P450 isoenzymes, the mechanism for the apparent raised efavirenz concentrations reported with tenofovir is unclear.

Importance and management

No pharmacokinetic interaction occurred between **efavirenz** and tenofovir in the one controlled study. However, the analysis[3] suggesting that patients who are CYP2B6 poor metabolisers might have higher concentrations of efavirenz when taking tenofovir warrants further investigation. Nevertheless, note that the use of efavirenz with the NRTI backbone of tenofovir and emtricitabine (available as a single combination tablet), is a preferred regimen for the treatment of antiretroviral naive patients in the UK[8] guidelines, and efavirenz or rilpivirine with this NRTI backbone are suggested alternative regimens in the US guidelines.[9] Current local and national guidelines should be consulted when choosing an appropriate antiretroviral regimen.

The changes in etravirine and tenofovir pharmacokinetics are not clinically relevant, so no dose adjustment is needed with concurrent use. Similarly, the changes in tenofovir pharmacokinetics with rilpivirine are not clinically relevant. Data for nevirapine are limited, but suggest that no pharmacokinetic interaction appears to occur between nevirapine and tenofovir.

1. Sustiva (Efavirenz). Bristol-Myers Squibb Company. US Prescribing information, August 2012.
2. Droste JAH, Kearney BP, Hekster YA, Burger DM. Assessment of drug-drug interactions between tenofovir disoproxil fumarate and the nonnucleoside reverse transcriptase inhibitors nevirapine and efavirenz in HIV-infected patients. *J Acquir Immune Defic Syndr* (2006) 41, 37–43.
3. Rotger M, Colombo S, Furrer H, Décosterd L, Buclin T, Telenti A. Does tenofovir influence efavirenz pharmacokinetics? *Antivir Ther* (2007) 12, 115–8.
4. Allavena C, Le Moal G, Michau C, Chiffoleau A, Raffi F. Neuropsychiatric adverse events after switching from an antiretroviral regimen containing efavirenz without tenofovir to an efavirenz regimen containing tenofovir: a report of nine cases. *Antivir Ther* (2006) 11, 263–5.
5. Kakuda TN, Schöller-Gyüre M, De Smedt G, Beets G, Aharchi F, Peeters MP, Vandermeulen K, Woodfall BJ, Hoetelmans RMW. Assessment of the steady-state pharmacokinetic interaction between etravirine administered as two different formulations and tenofovir disoproxil fumarate in healthy volunteers. *HIV Med* (2009) 10, 173–81.
6. Edurant (Rilpivirine hydrochloride). Janssen-Cilag Ltd. UK Summary of product characteristics, November 2011.
7. Edurant (Rilpivirine hydrochloride). Tibotec Pharmaceuticals. US Prescribing information, August 2012.
8. Williams I, Churchill D, Anderson J, Boffito M, Bower M, Cairns G, Cwynarski K, Edwards S, Fidler S, Fisher M, Freedman A, Geretti AM, Gilleece Y, Horne R, Johnson M, Khoo S, Leen C, Marshall N, Nelson M, Orkin C, Paton N, Phillips A, Post F, Pozniak A, Sabin C, Trevelion R, Ustianowski A, Walsh J, Waters L, Wilkins E, Winston A, Youle M. British HIV Association guidelines for the treatment of HIV-1-positive adults with antiretroviral therapy 2012 (Updated 2013). *HIV Med* (2014), 15 (Suppl 1) 1–85.
9. Panel on Antiretroviral Guidelines for Adults and Adolescents. Guidelines for the use of antiretroviral agents in HIV-1-infected adults and adolescents. Department of Health and Human Services. (April 2015). 1–288. Available at: https://aidsinfo.nih.gov/contentfiles/lvguidelines/adultandadolescentgl.pdf (accessed 24/09/15).

NNRTIs + Valproate

The pharmacokinetics of efavirenz were not altered by valproic acid in one study in HIV-positive patients, and valproic acid concentrations were not different to those in a control group not taking efavirenz. However, one patient had a large decrease in valproate concentrations after starting efavirenz. Hepatotoxicity has occurred in a patient taking valproic acid with nevirapine, ritonavir, and saquinavir.

Clinical evidence

In a study in 11 HIV-positive patients taking **efavirenz** 600 mg daily with various NRTIs, there was no change in the pharmacokinetics of **efavirenz** after they took valproic acid 250 mg twice daily for 7 days. Valproic acid concentrations achieved in these patients were not apparently different from those in 11 HIV-positive control patients mainly taking NRTIs, even when the 3 control patients taking an HIV-protease inhibitor or NNRTI (amprenavir, indinavir, or nelfinavir with nevirapine) were excluded.[1]

However, a patient with a bipolar disorder and multidrug addiction had a decrease in valproic acid plasma concentrations of more than 50% shortly after starting an antiretroviral regimen including **efavirenz**. Even though the valproate dose was increased to 4 g daily, it was found difficult to achieve a target plasma concentration of 50 mg/dL. About 3 months later, following a valproate dose reduction to 1.5 g daily due to adverse effects, the valproate plasma concentration was unaltered, at 52 mg/dL.[2]

A case of valproate-associated hepatotoxicity occurred in a 51-year-old man about 3 weeks after he started **nevirapine** 200 mg twice daily, ritonavir 400 mg twice daily, saquinavir 400 mg twice daily, and stavudine. Valproic acid serum concentrations remained therapeutic.[3]

Mechanism

Uncertain.

Importance and management

The findings of the study[1] suggest that valproate can be used with efavirenz-based regimens without any pharmacokinetic drug interaction. However, the case report of reduced valproic acid plasma concentrations introduces a note of caution. It might be appropriate to monitor valproate concentrations in patients taking efavirenz. It is unclear whether the case of hepatotoxicity was a result of a drug interaction. Note that there has been some concern about using valproate in HIV infection, but there seems to be no established reason to avoid or specifically promote the use of valproate in HIV-infection *per se*.

1. DiCenzo R, Peterson D, Cruttenden K, Morse G, Riggs G, Gelbard H, Schifitto G. Effects of valproic acid coadministration on plasma efavirenz and lopinavir concentrations in human immunodeficiency virus-infected adults. *Antimicrob Agents Chemother* (2004) 48, 4328–31.
2. Saraga M, Preisig M, Zullino DF. Reduced valproate plasma levels possible after introduction of efavirenz in a bipolar patient. *Bipolar Disord* (2006) 8, 415–17.
3. Cozza KL, Swanton EJ, Humphreys CW. Hepatotoxicity with combination of valproic acid, ritonavir, and nevirapine: a case report. *Psychosomatics* (2000) 41, 452–3.

NNRTIs; Delavirdine + Glutamic acid

Glutamic acid increases the absorption of delavirdine in patients with poor gastric acid production.

Clinical evidence, mechanism, importance and management

When **glutamic acid** 1.36 g three times daily was given with delavirdine 400 mg three times daily to 8 HIV-positive subjects with gastric hypoacidity, the AUC of delavirdine was increased by 50%.[1] Delavirdine is a weak base that is poorly soluble at neutral pH. Therefore, in subjects with gastric hypoacidity, the absorption of delavirdine is reduced, and substances that lower gastric pH increase its absorption. However, the clinical value of using **glutamic acid** with delavirdine to boost its absorption is unknown. The manufacturer recommends that, in patients with achlorhydria, delavirdine should be taken with an **acidic beverage** such as **orange** or **cranberry juice**.[2]

1. Morse GD, Adams JM, Shelton MJ, Hewitt RG, Cox SR, Chambers JH. Gastric acidification increases delavirdine mesylate (DLV) exposure in HIV+ subjects with gastric hypoacidity (GH). *Clin Pharmacol Ther* (1996) 59, 141.
2. Rescriptor (Delavirdine mesylate). ViiV Healthcare. US Prescribing information, August 2012.

NNRTIs; Etravirine + Miscellaneous

Etravirine is predicted to decrease the concentrations of some antiarrhythmics.

Enfuvirtide does not appear to affect the pharmacokinetics of etravirine. No pharmacokinetic interaction is expected to occur between etravirine and ribavirin.

Clinical evidence, mechanism, importance and management

(a) Antiarrhythmics

The manufacturers of etravirine predict that it will reduce the concentrations of **amiodarone**, **disopyramide**, **flecainide**, **lidocaine** (systemic use), **mexiletine**, **propafenone**, and **quinidine**. They do not state the predicted mechanism for the effect on this list of drugs, although they mention that etravirine is a weak inducer of CYP3A4 and would be predicted to decrease concentrations of drugs that are principally metabolised by CYP3A4. However, some of these antiarrhythmics are not known to be notably metabolised by CYP3A4 (e.g. flecainide and mexiletine) and none are known to be principally metabolised by CYP3A4. Therefore it remains to be established that etravirine will have clinically relevant effects on the concentrations of these drugs. Nevertheless, the manufacturers recommend caution on their concurrent use, with monitoring of the drug concentrations of the affected antiarrhythmic, if this is possible.[1,2]

(b) Enfuvirtide

The UK manufacturer reports that, based on population pharmacokinetic analysis, enfuvirtide 90 mg twice daily did not appear to alter the AUC or minimum concentration of etravirine when compared with historical control data. The concentrations of enfuvirtide are not expected to be affected by etravirine. No dose adjustment is therefore necessary on concurrent use.[1,2]

(c) Ribavirin

The UK manufacturer states that although the combination has not been studied, an interaction between etravirine and ribavirin is unlikely based on the renal elimination pathway of ribavirin. Therefore no dose adjustment of either drug is necessary on concurrent use.[1]

1. Intelence (Etravirine). Janssen-Cilag Ltd. UK Summary of product characteristics, July 2012.
2. Intelence (Etravirine). Tibotec, Inc. US Prescribing information, August 2012.

NNRTIs; Rilpivirine + Miscellaneous

A negligible pharmacokinetic interaction appears to occur between rilpivirine and paracetamol (acetaminophen). Rilpivirine is predicted

to reduce the renal excretion of metformin and to increase dabigatran exposure, but is not expected to interact with ribavirin.

Clinical evidence, mechanism, importance and management

(a) Metformin

The UK manufacturer states that rilpivirine inhibits the active renal excretion of creatine, and that it is possible that rilpivirine might inhibit the renal elimination of metformin by the same mechanism, which could lead to an increase in its exposure and its effects. Until more is known, they advise monitoring patients if either drug is started,[1] presumably for increased adverse effects.

(b) Paracetamol (Acetaminophen)

The manufacturers report that, in a study in 16 subjects taking supratherapeutic dose rilpivirine 150 mg daily and given a single 500-mg dose of paracetamol, there were negligible changes in pharmacokinetics of both drugs (a 16% increase in the AUC of rilpivirine and a 26% increase in its minimum concentration, and an 8% decrease in the AUC of paracetamol), which would not be expected to be clinically relevant. Therefore no dose adjustment of either drug is needed on concurrent use.[1,2]

(c) P-glycoprotein substrates

Rilpivirine has been reported to inhibit P-glycoprotein *in vitro*. The UK manufacturer therefore states that caution is warranted on the concurrent use of rilpivirine and drugs that are substrates for P-glycoprotein, and specifically names **dabigatran**.[1]

(d) Ribavirin

The manufacturers predict that no clinically relevant interaction will occur between rilpivirine and **ribavirin**.[1,2]

1. Edurant (Rilpivirine hydrochloride). Janssen-Cilag Ltd. UK Summary of product characteristics, November 2011.
2. Edurant (Rilpivirine hydrochloride). Tibotec Pharmaceuticals. US Prescribing information, August 2012.

NRTIs + Antacids

Aluminium/magnesium hydroxide slightly reduces the bioavailability of zalcitabine. Antacids would not be expected to have any additional pharmacokinetic effect on buffered didanosine preparations.

Clinical evidence, mechanism, importance and management

(a) Didanosine

Didanosine is acid labile, so to increase its absorption, some didanosine preparations (e.g. chewable or dispersible tablets[1] and paediatric oral powder for solution[2]) have been formulated with antacids. Additional concurrent antacids would not be expected to have any further clinically relevant effect on didanosine pharmacokinetics. However, the US manufacturers of the paediatric oral powder for solution[2] suggest that additional antacids containing **aluminium** or **magnesium** might increase the adverse effects of the antacid components of this preparation. Bear this possibility in mind.

(b) Zalcitabine

A study in 12 HIV-positive patients given a single 1.5-g dose of zalcitabine found that 30 mL of *Maalox* [**aluminium/magnesium hydroxide**] caused a 25% reduction in the bioavailability of zalcitabine.[3] These changes are slight and of uncertain clinical importance. The manufacturers recommended that zalcitabine should not be taken at the same time as **aluminium/magnesium**-containing antacids.[4,5]

1. Videx Tablets (Didanosine). Bristol-Myers Squibb Pharmaceuticals Ltd. UK Summary of product characteristics, June 2009.
2. Videx Pediatric Powder for Oral Solution (Didanosine). Bristol-Myers Squibb Company. US Prescribing information, November 2011.
3. Massarella JW, Holazo AA, Koss-Twardy S, Min B, Smith B, Nazareno LA. The effects of cimetidine and Maalox® on the pharmacokinetics of zalcitabine in HIV-positive patients. *Pharm Res* (1994) 11 (10 Suppl), S-415.
4. Hivid (Zalcitabine). Roche Products Ltd. UK Summary of product characteristics, November 2004.
5. Hivid (Zalcitabine). Roche Pharmaceuticals. US Prescribing information, September 2002.

NRTIs + Atovaquone

Slight increases in zidovudine exposure and slight decreases in didanosine exposure have been seen on the concurrent use of atovaquone. Didanosine and zidovudine do not affect the pharmacokinetics of atovaquone.

Clinical evidence

(a) Didanosine

The manufacturer of atovaquone notes that it decreased the AUC of didanosine by 24% in a multiple dose interaction study. There was no change in the pharmacokinetics of atovaquone.[1]

(b) Zidovudine

A study in 14 HIV-positive patients given atovaquone 750 mg every 12 hours and zidovudine 200 mg every 8 hours found that, under steady-state conditions, zidovudine had no effect on the pharmacokinetics of atovaquone.[2] This confirmed the findings of a previous analysis of pharmacokinetic data from a small number of patients enrolled in clinical studies.[3] However, the AUC of zidovudine was increased by about 30%, and its clearance was reduced by 25% by the concurrent use of atovaquone.[2]

Mechanism

Atovaquone might inhibit the metabolism (glucuronidation) of zidovudine.[2]

Importance and management

Evidence for an interaction between atovaquone and **didanosine** is limited. Nevertheless, the magnitude of the decrease in didanosine exposure is slight, and therefore unlikely to be clinically relevant. Similarly the increase in **zidovudine** exposure seen with atovaquone is slight and unlikely to be clinically relevant. The manufacturers state that the increased plasma concentrations of zidovudine that are likely to occur with a 3-week course of atovaquone for acute pneumocystis pneumonia are unlikely to increase the adverse effects of zidovudine.[1,4] Nevertheless, the manufacturer of atovaquone[1] recommends regular monitoring for zidovudine-associated adverse effects when the drugs are used together, particularly if atovaquone suspension is used, as this achieves higher atovaquone concentrations which might have a greater effect, whereas the UK manufacturer of zidovudine limits this monitoring to those given prolonged courses of atovaquone.[4] The authors of the study with zidovudine[2] suggest that increased concentrations could possibly be important in patients also taking other drugs causing bone marrow toxicity (such as ganciclovir, see 'NRTIs + Ganciclovir', p.973, and flucytosine, see 'NRTIs; Zidovudine + Myelosuppressive drugs', p.985). If bone marrow toxicity is seen, it has been suggested that the zidovudine dose might need to be reduced by one-third.[2]

1. Wellvone Oral Suspension (Atovaquone). GlaxoSmithKline UK. UK Summary of product characteristics, April 2010.
2. Lee BL, Täuber MG, Sadler B, Goldstein D, Chambers HF. Atovaquone inhibits the glucuronidation and increases the plasma concentrations of zidovudine. *Clin Pharmacol Ther* (1996) 59, 14–21.
3. Sadler BM, Blum MR. Relationship between steady-state plasma concentrations of atovaquone (C_{ss}) and the use of various concomitant medications in AIDS patients with *Pneumocystis carinii* pneumonia. *Int Conf AIDS* (1993) 9, 504.
4. Retrovir (Zidovudine). ViiV Healthcare UK Ltd. UK Summary of product characteristics, January 2012.

NRTIs + Azoles

Fluconazole has no effect on the pharmacokinetics of didanosine or stavudine, but it slightly increases zidovudine exposure. Fluconazole concentrations are unaffected by enteric-coated didanosine and zidovudine.

Itraconazole has no effect on the pharmacokinetics of zidovudine. The concentrations of itraconazole from capsules are greatly reduced when buffered didanosine is given at the same time, but itraconazole capsules and ketoconazole are not affected if buffered didanosine is given 2 hours later. Enteric-coated didanosine negligibly decreases itraconazole exposure and possibly slightly increases ketoconazole exposure. The frequency of haematological toxicity with zidovudine does not appear to be increased by ketoconazole.

Clinical evidence

(a) Didanosine

1. Buffered preparation. A 35-year-old patient with AIDS was given **itraconazole** capsules 200 mg twice daily following an episode of cryptococcal meningitis. When he relapsed it was noted that he had been taking **itraconazole** at the same time as his buffered didanosine. Subsequent study in this patient indicated a delay in **itraconazole** absorption when it was taken with didanosine. Two hours after the dose, **itraconazole** plasma concentrations of 1.6 micrograms/mL were seen without didanosine, but were undetectable with didanosine. An **itraconazole** maximum concentration of 1.4 micrograms/mL was seen when it was given 8 hours after a dose of didanosine.[1] In a subsequent study in 6 healthy subjects, when [buffered] didanosine was given with a single 200-mg oral dose of **itraconazole** capsules the maximum concentrations of **itraconazole** were undetectable, whereas in the absence of didanosine, **itraconazole** maximum concentrations were 0.9 micrograms/mL.[2] A later study in 12 HIV-positive patients found that the AUC of a single 200-mg dose of **itraconazole** did not differ when buffered didanosine 200 mg was given 4 hours before or 2 hours after **itraconazole**, when compared with **itraconazole** alone.[3]

Twelve HIV-positive patients were given buffered didanosine 375 mg twice daily either alone or 2 hours after **ketoconazole** 200 mg daily, for 4 days. Didanosine maximum plasma concentrations were reduced by just 12% and no changes in the pharmacokinetics of **ketoconazole** were seen when dosing was separated in this way.[4]

A group of 12 HIV-positive subjects taking buffered didanosine 100 to 250 mg twice daily were also given **fluconazole** for 7 days (two 200-mg doses on the first day, followed by 200 mg daily). The pharmacokinetics of didanosine remained unchanged in the presence of **fluconazole**, and concurrent use was well tolerated. **Fluconazole** pharmacokinetics were not assessed.[5]

2. Enteric-coated preparation. Enteric-coated didanosine 400 mg had no effect on the pharmacokinetics of **fluconazole** 200 mg tablets in 14 healthy subjects, and negligibly decreased the AUC of **itraconazole** 200 mg capsules by 12% in 25 healthy subjects.[6] In another study in 24 healthy subjects, enteric-coated didanosine 400 mg slightly increased the AUC of **ketoconazole** 200 mg by 30%. Three of the subjects had increased concentrations of **ketoconazole** with didanosine, but their values for **keto-**

conazole alone appeared unusually low. When their data were excluded, no effect on the AUC of **ketoconazole** was seen in the remaining 21 subjects.[7]

(b) Stavudine

A study in 10 HIV-positive subjects taking stavudine 40 mg twice daily found that the addition of **fluconazole** 200 mg daily for one week had no effect on the pharmacokinetics of stavudine.[8]

(c) Zidovudine

On two occasions, 12 HIV-positive men were given zidovudine 200 mg every 8 hours with and without **fluconazole** 400 mg daily for 7 days. While taking **fluconazole** the AUC of zidovudine increased by 74%, the maximum serum concentration increased by 84%, the terminal half-life was increased by 128%, and the clearance was reduced by 43%.[9] In contrast, another study in 10 HIV-positive patients found only a very small change in the pharmacokinetics of a single 500-mg dose of zidovudine given before and after 7 days of treatment with **fluconazole** (e.g. a negligible 7% increase in the AUC of zidovudine). In another 10 patients, zidovudine had no effect on the pharmacokinetics of a single dose of **fluconazole**.[10]

Itraconazole 200 mg daily for 2 weeks was reported to have no effect on the pharmacokinetics of zidovudine in 7 patients, but the serum concentrations in 2 patients were higher.[11]

A study of zidovudine use in 282 patients with AIDS found that haematological abnormalities (anaemia, leucopenia, neutropenia) were very common, but this was not increased in those patients also taking **ketoconazole**.[12]

Mechanism

Itraconazole and ketoconazole depend on stomach acidity for absorption. A raised gastric pH, caused by the antacids in the buffered didanosine formulation appears to reduce itraconazole absorption from the capsule formulation (see 'Azoles + Antacids', p.235). The didanosine itself appears to have no part to play in this interaction. The enteric-coated preparation of didanosine does not contain any antacids and therefore does not interact with these azoles.

In vitro data suggest that the altered zidovudine pharmacokinetics might, in part, occur because fluconazole inhibits zidovudine glucuronidation.[13]

Importance and management

A clinically important pharmacokinetic interaction occurs between the buffered preparation of **didanosine** and itraconazole *capsules*. Patients should avoid taking these preparations at the same time, but taking itraconazole capsules at least 2 hours before buffered didanosine appears to avoid any interaction. Any possible interaction with ketoconazole can similarly be avoided by giving ketoconazole at least 2 hours before a buffered didanosine preparation. Alternatively, the interaction could be avoided by using the enteric-coated preparation of didanosine or itraconazole *solution* (see 'Azoles + Antacids', p.235, which indicates that the solution is less affected by gastric pH changes).

There is no pharmacokinetic interaction between **stavudine** and fluconazole, and no interaction would be expected with other similar NRTIs such as **lamivudine** and **zalcitabine** (see 'Antivirals', p.893).

There is some evidence of a slight increase in **zidovudine** exposure with fluconazole, but this is unlikely to require zidovudine dose adjustment. Nevertheless, the UK manufacturer of zidovudine recommends that as limited data are available, patients also taking fluconazole should be closely monitored for zidovudine toxicity.[14]

1. Moreno F, Hardin TC, Rinaldi MG, Graybill JR. Itraconazole-didanosine excipient interaction. *JAMA* (1993) 269, 1508.
2. May DB, Drew RH, Yedinak KC, Bartlett JA. Effect of simultaneous didanosine administration on itraconazole absorption in healthy volunteers. *Pharmacotherapy* (1994) 14, 509–13.
3. Hardin TC, Sharkey-Mathis PK, Rinaldi MG, Graybill JR. Evaluation of the pharmacokinetic interaction between itraconazole and didanosine in HIV-infected subjects. *Intersci Conf Antimicrob Agents Chemother* (1995) 35, 6.
4. Knupp CA, Brater DC, Relue J, Barbhaiya RH. Pharmacokinetics of didanosine and ketoconazole after coadministration to patients seropositive for the human immunodeficiency virus. *J Clin Pharmacol* (1993) 33, 912–17.
5. Bruzzese VL, Gillum JG, Israel DS, Johnson GL, Kaplowitz LG, Polk RE. Effect of fluconazole on pharmacokinetics of 2′,3′-dideoxyinosine in persons seropositive for human immunodeficiency virus. *Antimicrob Agents Chemother* (1995) 39, 1050–53.
6. Damle B, Hess H, Kaul S, Knupp C. Absence of clinically relevant drug interactions following simultaneous administration of didanosine-encapsulated, enteric-coated bead formulation with either itraconazole or fluconazole. *Biopharm Drug Dispos* (2002) 23, 59–66.
7. Damle BD, Mummaneni V, Kaul S, Knupp C. Lack of effect of simultaneously administered didanosine encapsulated enteric bead formulation (Videx EC) on oral absorption of indinavir, ketoconazole, or ciprofloxacin. *Antimicrob Agents Chemother* (2002) 46, 385–91.
8. Piscitelli SC, Kelly G, Walker RE, Kovacs J, Falloon J, Davey RT, Raje S, Masur H, Polis MA. A multiple drug interaction study of stavudine with agents for opportunistic infections in human immunodeficiency virus-infected patients. *Antimicrob Agents Chemother* (1999) 43, 647–50.
9. Sahai J, Gallicano K, Pakuts A, Cameron DW. Effect of fluconazole on zidovudine pharmacokinetics in patients infected with human deficiency virus. *J Infect Dis* (1994) 169, 1103–7.
10. Brockmeyer NH, Tillmann I, Mertins L, Barthel B, Goos M. Pharmacokinetic interaction of fluconazole and zidovudine in HIV-positive patients. *Eur J Med Res* (1997) 2, 377–83.
11. Henrivaux P, Fairon Y, Fillet G. Pharmacokinetics of AZT among HIV infected patients treated by itraconazole. 5th Int Conf AIDS, Montreal. 1989, Abstract M.B.P.340.
12. Richman DD, Fischl MA, Grieco MH, Gottlieb MS, Volberding PA, Laskin OL, Leedom JM, Groopman JE, Mildvan D, Hirsch MS, Jackson GG, Durack DT, Nusinoff-Lehrman S and the AZT Collaborative Working Group. The toxicity of azidothymidine (AZT) in the treatment of patients with AIDS and AIDS-related complex. A double-blind, placebo-controlled trial. *N Engl J Med* (1987) 317, 192–7.
13. Asgari M, Back DJ. Effect of azoles on the glucuronidation of zidovudine by human liver UDP-glucuronyltransferase. *J Infect Dis* (1995) 172, 1634–5.
14. Retrovir (Zidovudine). ViiV Healthcare UK Ltd. UK Summary of product characteristics, January 2012.

NRTIs + Co-trimoxazole or Trimethoprim

Trimethoprim, both alone and as co-trimoxazole (trimethoprim with sulfamethoxazole), reduces the renal clearance of lamivudine, zalcitabine and zidovudine, and slightly increases their exposure. Stavudine is predicted to be similarly affected. Slight changes in renal clearance occur if didanosine is given with co-trimoxazole or trimethoprim.

Clinical evidence

(a) Didanosine

A single-dose study in 10 HIV-positive subjects investigated the pharmacokinetics of didanosine 200 mg, trimethoprim 200 mg and sulfamethoxazole 1 g in combination. When the three drugs were given together, didanosine renal clearance was decreased by 35%, trimethoprim renal clearance was decreased by 32%, and sulfamethoxazole renal clearance was increased by 39%, but there were negligible changes in their AUCs. When only two of the three drugs were given, trimethoprim caused a 27% decrease in the renal clearance of didanosine, and didanosine caused an 82% increase in the renal clearance of sulfamethoxazole.[1] Despite these alterations in renal clearance, the maximum serum concentration, AUC, and half-life of each of the three drugs were minimally affected.[1]

(b) Lamivudine

A study in 14 HIV-positive patients taking co-trimoxazole 960 mg daily for 5 days found that the AUC of a single 300-mg dose of lamivudine given on day 4 was increased by 43% and the renal clearance was decreased by 35%. The pharmacokinetics of trimethoprim and sulfamethoxazole were unaffected.[2] Similarly, in a population pharmacokinetic analysis, the concurrent use of lamivudine and co-trimoxazole was associated with a 31% reduction in the apparent oral clearance of lamivudine, and an estimated 43% increase in steady-state lamivudine concentrations.[3] The UK manufacturer notes that the interaction is due to trimethoprim, and that sulfamethoxazole did not interact.[4]

(c) Zalcitabine

In a steady-state study, 8 HIV-positive patients took zalcitabine 1.5 mg three times daily with and without trimethoprim 200 mg twice daily. Trimethoprim slightly increased the AUC and decreased the clearance of zalcitabine by about 35%.[5]

(d) Zidovudine

A study in 9 HIV-positive patients given zidovudine 3 mg/kg by infusion over one hour found that trimethoprim 150 mg or co-trimoxazole 960 mg did not affect the metabolic clearance of zidovudine. However, the renal clearance of zidovudine was reduced by 48% by trimethoprim and by 58% by co-trimoxazole, and the renal clearances of its glucuronide metabolite were reduced by 20% and 27%, respectively.[6] Another study also found that co-trimoxazole did not alter zidovudine pharmacokinetics.[7] A further 5 HIV-positive patients had a slight 30% increase in the AUC of zidovudine when they were given trimethoprim (doses not stated).[8] Zidovudine renal clearance was reduced by 58% in 8 HIV-positive subjects when they were also given trimethoprim 200 mg, but the AUC_{0-6} of the zidovudine glucuronide to zidovudine ratio was unchanged, suggesting that the metabolism was unaffected.[9]

Increases in the half-lives of trimethoprim, sulfamethoxazole, and *N*-acetyl sulfamethoxazole of 72%, 39%, and 115%, respectively, were seen when co-trimoxazole was given to 4 patients with AIDS taking zidovudine 250 mg every 8 hours for 8 days.[10]

A study of zidovudine use in 282 patients with AIDS found that haematological abnormalities (anaemia, leucopenia, neutropenia) were common. However, the frequency was not increased in the patients (number unknown) also taking co-trimoxazole.[11] However, a later study in a sub-Saharan population taking co-trimoxazole and zidovudine reported a higher than expected incidence of blood disorders.[12]

Mechanism

It is suggested that trimethoprim inhibits the secretion of both zidovudine and its glucuronide by the renal tubules thereby reducing their renal clearance. The other NRTIs that are affected are likely to interact by the same mechanism. It is not known why the half-life of co-trimoxazole is increased.

Importance and management

The interaction between co-trimoxazole or trimethoprim and **lamivudine** or zidovudine is established. **Stavudine** is predicted to interact similarly.[13] With the NRTIs that are actively excreted by the kidneys (e.g. lamivudine, stavudine, and **zalcitabine**), it is unlikely that dose alterations are necessary unless the patient has renal impairment. However, when both drugs are needed, patients should be closely monitored for signs of toxicity. However, the UK manufacturer of lamivudine recommends that the use of lamivudine with high-dose co-trimoxazole for the treatment of pneumocystis pneumonia and toxoplasmosis should be avoided.[4]

As renal clearance represents only 20 to 30% of the total clearance of **zidovudine**, the authors of two of the reports cited[6,9] suggest that this interaction is unlikely to be clinically important for zidovudine unless glucuronidation by the liver is impaired by liver disease or by other drugs. The possible increased risk of haematological adverse effects requires confirmation. The UK manufacturer[14] of zidovudine advises that although limited data suggest that there is no significant increased risk of adverse effects when zidovudine is taken with *prophylactic* co-trimoxazole, in general the concurrent use of zidovudine with drugs that are known to cause myelosuppression, such as co-trimoxazole, should be closely monitored.

Didanosine does not appear to interact with co-trimoxazole or trimethoprim to a clinically relevant extent.

1. Srinivas NR, Knupp CA, Batteiger B, Smith RA, Barbhaiya RH. A pharmacokinetic interaction study of didanosine coadministered with trimethoprim and/or sulphamethoxazole in HIV seropositive asymptomatic male patients. *Br J Clin Pharmacol* (1996) 41, 207–15.
2. Moore KHP, Yuen GJ, Raasch RH, Eron JJ, Martin D, Mydlow PK, Hussey EK. Pharmacokinetics of lamivudine administered alone and with trimethoprim-sulfamethoxazole. *Clin Pharmacol Ther* (1996) 59, 550–8.
3. Sabo JP, Lamson MJ, Leitz G, Yong C-L, MacGregor TR. Pharmacokinetics of nevirapine and lamivudine in patients with HIV-1 infection. AAPS PharmSci. (2000) 2, E1–E7.
4. Epivir (Lamivudine). ViiV Healthcare UK Ltd. UK Summary of product characteristics, October 2010.
5. Lee BL, Täuber MG, Chambers HF, Gambertoglio J, Delahunty T. The effect of trimethoprim (TMP) on the pharmacokinetics (PK) of zalcitabine (ddC) in HIV-infected patients. *Intersci Conf Antimicrob Agents Chemother* (1995) 35, 6.
6. Chatton JY, Munafo A, Chave JP, Steinhäuslin F, Roch-Ramel F, Glauser MP, Biollaz J. Trimethoprim, alone or in combination with sulphamethoxazole, decreases the renal excretion of zidovudine and its glucuronide. *Br J Clin Pharmacol* (1992) 34, 551–4.
7. Cañas E, Pachon J, Garcia-Pesquera F, Castillo JR, Viciana P, Cisneros JM, Jimenez-Mejias M. Absence of effect of trimethoprim-sulfamethoxazole on pharmacokinetics of zidovudine in patients infected with human immunodeficiency virus. *Antimicrob Agents Chemother* (1996) 40, 230–33.
8. Lee BL, Safrin S, Makrides V, Benowitz NL, Gambertoglio JG, Mills J. Trimethoprim decreases the renal clearance of zidovudine. *Clin Pharmacol Ther* (1992) 51,183.
9. Lee BL, Safrin S, Makrides V, Gambertoglio JG. Zidovudine, trimethoprim, and dapsone pharmacokinetic interactions in patients with human immunodeficiency virus infection. *Antimicrob Agents Chemother* (1996) 40, 1231–6.
10. Berson A, Happy K, Rousseau F, Grateau G, Farinotti R, Séréni D. Effect of zidovudine (AZT) on cotrimoxazole (TMP-SMX) kinetics: preliminary results. 9th International Conference on AIDS & 5th STD World Congress, Berlin, June 6–11 1993. Abstract PO-B30-2193.
11. Richman DD, Fischl MA, Grieco MH, Gottlieb MS, Volberding PA, Laskin OL, Leedom JM, Groopman JE, Mildvan D, Hirsch MS, Jackson GG, Durack DT, Nusinoff-Lehrman S and the AZT Collaborative Working Group. The toxicity of azidothymidine (AZT) in the treatment of patients with AIDS and AIDS-related complex. A double-blind, placebo-controlled trial. *N Engl J Med* (1987) 317, 192–7.
12. Moh R, Danel C, Sorho S, Sauvageot D, Anzian A, Minga A, Gomis OB, Kanga C, Inwoley A, Gabillard D, Bissagnene E, Salamon R, Anglaret X. Haematological changes in adults receiving a zidovudine-containing HAART regimen in combination with cotrimoxazole in Côte d'Ivoire. *Antivir Ther* (2005) 10, 615–24.
13. Zerit Hard Capsules (Stavudine). Bristol-Myers Squibb Pharmaceuticals Ltd. UK Summary of product characteristics, March 2011.
14. Retrovir (Zidovudine). ViiV Healthcare UK Ltd. UK Summary of product characteristics, January 2012.

NRTIs + Cytokines

Interferon alfa does not alter the pharmacokinetics of didanosine and negligibly reduces lamivudine exposure. Interferon alfa and interferon beta increase zidovudine exposure. Lamivudine does not alter interferon alfa pharmacokinetics. HIV-positive patients infected with hepatitis C and given interferon alfa with or without ribavirin might be at particular risk of NRTI-associated lactic acidosis.

Interleukin-2 does not alter zidovudine exposure.

Clinical evidence

(a) Didanosine

Interferon alfa one million to 15 million units daily was given to 26 HIV-positive patients taking didanosine sachets 100 to 375 mg twice daily. Interferon appeared to have no effect on the pharmacokinetics of didanosine.[1]

(b) Lamivudine

In a study in 19 healthy subjects, a single subcutaneous injection of **interferon alfa** 10 million units caused a negligible 10% reduction in the AUC of lamivudine after lamivudine 100 mg daily was given for 7 days. Lamivudine did not appear to alter the pharmacokinetics of **interferon alfa**.[2]

(c) Zidovudine

In a study, patients with AIDS who had been taking zidovudine 200 mg every 4 hours for 8 weeks were also given subcutaneous **recombinant beta interferon** 45 million units daily. After 3 days and 15 days the metabolism of zidovudine to its glucuronide metabolite was reduced by 75% and 97%, respectively. By day 15, the zidovudine half-life was increased about 2-fold. AUC data was not reported in this study.[3] Another study in 6 children aged 3 months to 17 years found that 5 weeks of the concurrent use of **interferon alfa** slightly increased the AUC of zidovudine by 36%, increased its maximum serum concentration by 69%, and reduced its clearance by 20%.[4]

A study found that a 4-week course of **interleukin-2** (0.25 million units/m^2 daily) by continuous infusion had no effect on the pharmacokinetics of a 100-mg intravenous dose of zidovudine.[5] Another study in 8 HIV-positive men given oral zidovudine 200 mg every 4 hours found similar results.[1]

Mechanism

Interferon beta appears to inhibit the glucuronidation of zidovudine by the liver.

Importance and management

Information on the interaction between the NRTIs and interferons or interleukins seems to be limited to these reports. Interferon alfa slightly increased **zidovudine** exposure, which is unlikely to be clinically relevant. Interferon beta appears to reduce the metabolism of zidovudine; however, the effect of this on zidovudine exposure was not reported, and therefore the clinical relevance of the changes seen are uncertain. The manufacturers of zidovudine state that the risk of haematological toxicity might be increased if zidovudine and other myelosuppressive drugs such as interferon are given together. In addition, in patients with both HIV and hepatitis C infection, they state that the concurrent use of interferon and zidovudine might increase the risk of NRTI-associated lactic acidosis or hepatic decompensation. Patients at risk should be carefully monitored, and zidovudine stopped as appropriate.[6,7]

No clinically relevant pharmacokinetic interaction occurs between interferon alfa and **didanosine** or **lamivudine**. Nevertheless, many manufacturers of NRTIs note that HIV-positive patients infected with hepatitis C and treated with interferon alfa with or without ribavirin might be particularly at risk of lactic acidosis or hepatic decompensation. Patients at increased risk should be monitored closely, and the NRTI stopped as appropriate. For the discussion of the effects of ribavirin, both alone and when used in combination with interferons, on NRTIs, see 'NRTIs + Ribavirin', p.980.

No pharmacokinetic interaction appears to occur between zidovudine and interleukin-2.

1. Piscitelli SC, Amantea MA, Vogel S, Bechtel C, Metcalf JA, Kovacs JA. Effects of cytokines on antiviral pharmacokinetics: an alternative approach to assessment of drug interactions using bioequivalence guidelines. *Antimicrob Agents Chemother* (1996) 40, 161–5.
2. Johnson MA, Jenkins JM, Bye C. A study of the pharmacokinetic interaction between lamivudine and alpha interferon. *Eur J Clin Pharmacol* (2000) 56, 289–92.
3. Nokta M, Loh JP, Douidar SM, Ahmed AE, Pollard RB. Metabolic interaction of recombinant interferon-β and zidovudine in AIDS patients. *J Interferon Res* (1991) 11, 159–64.
4. Diaz C, Yogev R, Rodriguez J, Rege A, George W, Lertora J. ACTG-153: Zidovudine pharmacokinetics when used in combination with interferon alpha. *Intersci Conf Antimicrob Agents Chemother* (1994) 34, 79.
5. Skinner MH, Pauloin D, Schwartz D, Merigan TC, Blaschke TF. IL-2 does not alter zidovudine kinetics. *Clin Pharmacol Ther* (1989) 45, 128.
6. Retrovir (Zidovudine). ViiV Healthcare UK Ltd. UK Summary of product characteristics, January 2012.
7. Retrovir (Zidovudine). ViiV Healthcare. US Prescribing information, May 2012.

NRTIs + Dapsone

Buffered didanosine does not alter the pharmacokinetics of dapsone. A single early report suggested that prophylactic dapsone was not effective in preventing pneumocystis pneumonia in patients taking buffered didanosine. Dapsone has no effect on the pharmacokinetics of zalcitabine, whereas zalcitabine causes a small rise in the concentrations of dapsone, and there is a theoretical increased risk of peripheral neuropathy with the combination. Dapsone does not appear to affect the pharmacokinetics of zidovudine, although concurrent use might be associated with an increased risk of blood dyscrasias.

Clinical evidence, mechanism, importance and management

(a) Didanosine

An early report of the use of buffered didanosine described the development of pneumocystis pneumonia in 11 out of 28 HIV-positive patients taking dapsone prophylaxis, compared with only one of 12 patients taking aerosolised pentamidine, and none of 17 patients taking co-trimoxazole (trimethoprim with sulfamethoxazole). Of the 11 patients where prophylaxis failed, 4 died from respiratory failure.[1] The authors suggested that the most likely explanation of the high failure rate of dapsone with didanosine was reduced dapsone absorption due to the citrate-phosphate buffer in the didanosine formulation.[1] This has led to some recommending that the drugs be taken at least 2 hours apart. However, in a controlled study in 6 HIV-positive subjects, dapsone pharmacokinetics were not altered when a dose of buffered didanosine was taken within 5 minutes.[2] Similarly, in 6 healthy subjects, dapsone pharmacokinetics were not altered by the aluminium/magnesium-containing antacids and other excipients contained in didanosine tablets.[2] Another study in healthy subjects similarly did not find that a large rise in gastric pH affects the absorption of dapsone, see 'Dapsone + Antacids', p.318. Furthermore, low dapsone concentrations have been found in patients receiving a weekly dapsone regimen who took dapsone at least 2 hours before or 6 hours after didanosine, and in patients taking zidovudine or no antiretrovirals (although this study did not look at whether dapsone concentrations were correlated with efficacy).[3] In a retrospective analysis, other authors found no evidence to confirm a correlation between failure of pneumocystis pneumonia prophylaxis with dapsone and the use of drugs that increase gastric pH (didanosine, H_2-receptor antagonists, antacids).[4]

It has therefore been adequately demonstrated that the buffered preparation of didanosine and antacids do not affect dapsone absorption. The explanation for the apparent failure of pneumocystis pneumonia prophylaxis in the original report[1] is unresolved. Despite the use of both didanosine and dapsone in the management of HIV and opportunistic infections there do not appear to be any further reports of problems with the combination.

(b) Zalcitabine

A pharmacokinetic study in 12 HIV-positive patients who were given zalcitabine 1.5 mg three times daily and dapsone 100 mg daily, alone or together, found that dapsone did not affect the pharmacokinetics of zalcitabine. However, zalcitabine slightly decreased the clearance of dapsone by 21%, increased its maximum serum concentrations by 19% and increased its half-life by 34%.[5] These pharmacokinetic changes are small and unlikely to have much clinical relevance. The UK manufacturer[6] recommended caution with the combination because of the possibility of an increased risk of peripheral neuropathy: the US manufacturer advised avoiding the combination where possible.[7]

(c) Zidovudine

In a study in 8 HIV-positive subjects, dapsone 100 mg daily had no effect on the pharmacokinetics of a single 200-mg dose of zidovudine.[8] In a further study, which considered the safety of dapsone given with zidovudine, dapsone was shown to increase the risk of zidovudine-related blood dyscrasias.[9] It would therefore seem that dapsone and zidovudine can be given concurrently, but monitoring for an increase in adverse events would appear advisable.

1. Metroka CE, McMechan MF, Andrada R, Laubenstein LJ, Jacobus DP. Failure of prophylaxis with dapsone in patients taking dideoxyinosine. *N Engl J Med* (1992) 325, 737.
2. Sahai J, Garber G, Gallicano K, Oliveras L, Cameron DW. Effects of the antacids in didanosine tablets on dapsone pharmacokinetics. *Ann Intern Med* (1995) 123, 584–7.
3. Opravil M, Joos B, Lüthy R. Levels of dapsone and pyrimethamine in serum during once-weekly dosing for prophylaxis of *Pneumocystis carinii* pneumonia and toxoplasmic encephalitis. *Antimicrob Agents Chemother* (1994) 38, 1197–9.
4. Huengsberg M, Castelino S, Sherrard J, O'Farrell N, Bingham J. Does drug interaction cause failure of PCP prophylaxis with dapsone? *Lancet* (1993) 341, 48.
5. Lee BL, Tauber MG, Chambers HF, Gambertoglio J, Delahunty T. Zalcitabine (DDC) and dapsone (DAP) pharmacokinetic (PK) interaction in HIV-infected patients. *Clin Pharmacol Ther* (1995) 57, 186.
6. Hivid (Zalcitabine). Roche Products Ltd. UK Summary of product characteristics, November 2004.
7. Hivid (Zalcitabine). Roche Pharmaceuticals. US Prescribing information, September 2002.
8. Lee BL, Safrin S, Makrides V, Gambertoglio JG. Zidovudine, trimethoprim, and dapsone pharmacokinetic interactions in patients with human immunodeficiency virus infection. *Antimicrob Agents Chemother* (1996) 40, 1231–6.
9. Pinching AJ, Helbert M, Peddle B, Robinson D, Janes K, Gor D, Jeffries DJ, Stoneham C, Mitchell D, Kocsis AE, Mann J, Forster SM, Harris JRW. Clinical experience with zidovudine for patients with acquired immune deficiency syndrome and acquired immune deficiency syndrome-related complex. *J Infect* (1989) 18 (Suppl 1), 33–40.

NRTIs + Drugs that cause pancreatitis

An isolated case describes additive pancreatic toxicity when zalcitabine and intravenous pentamidine were given, and is expected when didanosine or stavudine are given with other drugs that can cause pancreatitis. An isolated case describes pancreatitis in a patient taking lamivudine and azathioprine.

Clinical evidence

A single case report describes a 51-year-old woman with a kidney transplant who developed pancreatitis after starting **lamivudine**. **Azathioprine** had been discontinued only 3 days before and it is possible (although the evidence is weak) that the residual serum **azathioprine** had interacted with **lamivudine** to cause the pancreatitis.[1] In another case, fatal fulminant pancreatitis occurred in a patient given **zalcitabine** and intravenous **pentamidine**.[2]

Mechanism

The specific mechanism for NRTI-associated pancreatitis is not known but might be due to mitochondrial toxicity caused by inhibition of host mitochondrial DNA polymerise gamma.[3] Concurrent use of NRTIs known to cause pancreatitis (didanosine, stavudine, zalcitabine, and possibly lamivudine) with other drugs known to cause pancreatitis (such as pentamidine[3]) might increase the risk.

Importance and management

Of the NRTIs, didanosine, stavudine, and zalcitabine have been associated with fatal pancreatitis.[2,4-8] Pancreatitis has also occurred in patients taking lamivudine.[9,10] The concurrent use of these NRTIs with other drugs known to cause pancreatitis might possibly increase the risk of pancreatitis occurring.

The manufacturers of **didanosine** recommend that if another drug that has the potential to cause pancreatitis is required (they name **pentamidine** as an example), treatment with didanosine should be stopped whenever possible. However, if concurrent use is unavoidable, patients should be closely monitored.[4,5] The UK manufacturer of **stavudine** recommends that patients receiving concurrent treatment with drugs known to cause pancreatitis should be carefully monitored for symptoms of this condition,[6] and the US manufacturer specifically recommends avoidance of the concurrent use of didanosine and stavudine,[7] see 'NRTIs + NRTIs', p.977. The manufacturers of **zalcitabine** recommended that if a drug that has the potential to cause pancreatitis is required, treatment with zalcitabine should be interrupted.[2,8] They specifically applied this to the use of pentamidine to treat pneumocystis pneumonia.[2,8]

For mention that hydroxycarbamide (hydroxyurea) might increase the risk of pancreatitis with didanosine and stavudine, see 'NRTIs + Hydroxycarbamide (Hydroxyurea)', p.976. See also 'NRTIs + Ribavirin', p.980, and 'NRTIs + Tenofovir', p.982.

The manufacturers state that **lamivudine** is rarely associated with pancreatitis, but recommend that treatment with lamivudine should be stopped if there is any suspicion of pancreatitis.[9,10] No firm conclusions can be drawn from the case discussed with azathioprine.

1. Van Vlierberghe H, Elewaut A. Development of a necrotising pancreatitis after starting lamivudine in a kidney transplant patient with fibrosing cholestatic hepatitis: A possible role of the interaction lamivudine and azathioprine. *Gastroenterology* (1997) 112 (4 Suppl), A1407.
2. Hivid (Zalcitabine). Roche Products Ltd. UK Summary of product characteristics, November 2004.
3. Riedel DJ, Gebo KA, Moore RD, Lucas GM. A ten-year analysis of the incidence and risk factors for acute pancreatitis requiring hospitalization in an urban HIV clinical cohort. *AIDS Patient Care STDS* (2008) 22, 113–21.
4. Videx Tablets (Didanosine). Bristol-Myers Squibb Pharmaceuticals Ltd. UK Summary of product characteristics, June 2009.
5. Videx EC (Didanosine). Bristol-Myers Squibb Company. US Prescribing information, November 2011.
6. Zerit Hard Capsules (Stavudine). Bristol-Myers Squibb Pharmaceuticals Ltd. UK Summary of product characteristics, March 2011.
7. Zerit (Stavudine). Bristol-Myers Squibb Company. US Prescribing information, January 2012.
8. Hivid (Zalcitabine). Roche Pharmaceuticals. US Prescribing information, September 2002.
9. Epivir (Lamivudine). ViiV Healthcare UK Ltd. UK Summary of product characteristics, October 2010.
10. Epivir (Lamivudine). ViiV Healthcare. US Prescribing information, November 2011.

NRTIs + Famciclovir

Famciclovir does not alter the pharmacokinetics of zidovudine or emtricitabine.

Clinical evidence, mechanism, importance and management

In a study in 12 healthy subjects, no important pharmacokinetic interaction was found between single doses of **emtricitabine** 200 mg and famciclovir 500 mg.[1] Similarly, minimal changes were seen in the pharmacokinetics of **zidovudine** when 12 HIV-positive patients taking zidovudine 400 mg to 1 g daily were given a single 500-mg dose of famciclovir.[2] No dose adjustment of these NRTIs is therefore expected to be needed when famciclovir is used concurrently.

1. Wang LH, Blum MR, Hui J, Hulett L, Chittick GE, Rousseau F. Lack of significant pharmacokinetic interactions between emtricitabine and other nucleoside antivirals in healthy volunteers. *Intersci Conf Antimicrob Agents Chemother* (2001) 41, 18.
2. Rousseau F, Scott S, Pratt S, Fowles S, Sparrow P, Lascoux C, Lehner V, Sereni D. Safe coadministration of famciclovir and zidovudine. *Intersci Conf Antimicrob Agents Chemother* (1994) 34, 83.

NRTIs + Food

Food moderately reduces the extent of absorption of buffered didanosine and slightly reduces the extent of absorption of enteric-coated didanosine. The extent of absorption of zalcitabine and zidovudine is negligibly to slightly reduced by food. Food does not affect the extent of absorption of abacavir, emtricitabine, lamivudine, and stavudine.

Clinical evidence, mechanism, importance and management

(a) Abacavir

The manufacturer of abacavir notes that food delayed the rate, but not the extent, of abacavir absorption. Therefore, abacavir can be taken with or without food.[1,2]

(b) Didanosine

1. Buffered preparations. Didanosine (as two 150-mg chewable tablets) was given to 10 HIV-positive subjects on four occasions: 30 minutes before breakfast, one hour before breakfast, one hour after breakfast, and 2 hours after breakfast. When the dose was given before breakfast the results were very similar to those obtained for subjects in the fasting state. When given after breakfast, the AUC and maximum plasma concentration of didanosine were both decreased by about 50%.[3] Similar results were found in another study.[4] A further study[5] using sachets containing didanosine, sucrose, and citrate-phosphate buffer, similarly found that food reduced the AUC of didanosine by 41% (a reduction from 29% to 17%). The reason for this effect would appear to be that food delays gastric emptying so that didanosine is exposed to prolonged contact with gastric acid, which causes decomposition, with a resultant reduction in bioavailability. To achieve maximum bioavailability, didanosine buffered preparations should be taken on an empty stomach at least 30 minutes before food[6,7] or 2 hours after food.[7]

2. Enteric-coated preparation. In a study in 20 healthy subjects, a high-fat meal reduced the AUC and maximum concentration of a single 400-mg dose of didanosine (from an enteric-coated bead formulation) by 19% and 46%, respectively, and increased the time to maximum concentration by 3 hours. A light meal also reduced the maximum concentration and AUC of didanosine by 22% and 27%, respectively, and delayed the time to maximum concentration by about 2.5 hours. Slight reductions in the AUC and maximum concentration were also seen when the same enteric-coated bead didanosine was taken either after fasting, one hour before and 2 hours after a light meal, or sprinkled over yoghurt or apple sauce; however, these changes were not statistically significant.[8]

Based on these results, the manufacturer recommends that didanosine gastro-resistant capsules are taken intact on an empty stomach,[9,10] at least 2 hours before or 2 hours after a meal.[9] However, a study in 668 patients found that in those patients who adhered to their HAART regimen taking enteric-coated didanosine with food did not lead to an increase in therapeutic failure.[11] An open-label study in 21 HIV-positive patients also found that taking enteric-coated didanosine with food had no effect on its virological efficacy.[12]

(c) Emtricitabine

The manufacturers state that giving emtricitabine hard capsules with a high-fat meal did not affect the AUC of emtricitabine[13,14] but minimally reduced the maximum concentration by 29%.[14] Similarly, giving emtricitabine oral solution with a low-fat or high-fat meal did not affect the AUC or maximum concentration of emtricitabine. Therefore, both these formulations of emtricitabine can be taken with or without food.[13,14]

(d) Lamivudine

In a study in 24 healthy subjects, food minimally reduced the maximum concentration of lamivudine (from a combined tablet with zidovudine) by 15% when compared with fasting subjects, but did not significantly affect the extent of absorption (AUC).[15] The US manufacturer reports that, in a study in 12 HIV-positive patients, food delayed the absorption of lamivudine and decreased its maximum concentration by 40%, when compared with the fasted state. However, the AUC of lamivudine was unaffected.[16] Similarly, the UK manufacturer notes that food delayed the rate and reduced the maximum plasma concentration of lamivudine (by about 47%), but not the extent of absorption (AUC).[17] Therefore, lamivudine can be taken with or without food.[16,17]

(e) Stavudine

The UK manufacturer of stavudine notes that a standardised high-fat meal delayed the absorption and reduced the maximum plasma concentration (specific details not given), but did not alter the extent of systemic exposure of stavudine, when compared with the fasting state. Nevertheless, they recommend that, for optimal absorption, stavudine should be taken on an empty stomach at least one hour before meals. However, if this is not possible, they suggest giving stavudine with a light meal; in addition, the contents of the capsule may be mixed with food.[18] The US manufacturer states that stavudine can be taken with food or on an empty stomach.[19]

(f) Zalcitabine

The manufacturers of zalcitabine[20,21] noted that food decreased the maximum plasma concentration by 39% and prolonged the time to achieve maximum concentrations from 0.8 hours to 1.6 hours, when compared with the fasting state. The extent of absorption was negligibly decreased by 14%. The UK manufacturer stated that zalcitabine could be taken with or without food.[20]

(g) Zidovudine

Zidovudine was given to 13 patients with AIDS either with breakfast or when fasting. The maximum plasma concentration of zidovudine was 2.8-fold greater in the fasted patients, and the AUC was slightly reduced by 22% when zidovudine was given with food.[22] The rate and extent of zidovudine absorption was reduced in another study by a standard breakfast (a negligible 14% decrease in AUC with a 200-mg dose and slight 33% decrease with a 100-mg dose).[23] In a study[24] of 8 patients, a high-fat meal reduced the zidovudine maximum serum concentrations by about 50%. In all of these studies inter-individual variation in zidovudine absorption was high.[22-24] However, when a sustained-release formulation of zidovudine was used, the absorption was delayed, but the AUC was increased slightly, by 28%, by a high-fat meal.[25] In contrast, the AUC of zidovudine was not affected by 25 g of a protein supplement.[26] In a study in 24 healthy subjects, although food reduced the maximum concentration of zidovudine (from a combined tablet with lamivudine) by 45%, when compared with fasting subjects, it had no effect on the extent of absorption of zidovudine.[15]

Inter-individual variation in zidovudine absorption appears high and the practical consequences of the changes caused by food are uncertain, although negligible to slight changes in exposure are unlikely to be generally important. Authors of some of these early studies suggested that zidovudine should be taken on an empty stomach;[23,24] however, the US manufacturer states that zidovudine can be taken with or without food,[27] and the UK manufacturer gives no specific recommendations regarding its administration in relation to food.[28]

1. Ziagen (Abacavir sulfate). ViiV Healthcare UK Ltd. UK Summary of product characteristics, October 2011.
2. Ziagen (Abacavir sulfate). ViiV Healthcare. US Prescribing information, May 2012.
3. Knupp CA, Milbrath R, Barbhaiya RH. Effect of time of food administration on the bioavailability of didanosine from a chewable tablet formulation. *J Clin Pharmacol* (1993) 33, 568–73.
4. Shyu WC, Knupp CA, Pittman KA, Dunkle L, Barbhaiya RH. Food-induced reduction in bioavailability of didanosine. *Clin Pharmacol Ther* (1991) 50, 503–7.
5. Hartman NR, Yarchoan R, Pluda JM, Thomas RV, Wyvill KM, Flora KP, Broder S, Johns DG. Pharmacokinetics of 2′,3′-dideoxyinosine in patients with severe human immunodeficiency infection. II. The effects of different oral formulations and the presence of other medications. *Clin Pharmacol Ther* (1991) 50, 278–85.
6. Videx Tablets (Didanosine). Bristol-Myers Squibb Pharmaceuticals Ltd. UK Summary of product characteristics, June 2009.
7. Videx Pediatric Powder for Oral Solution (Didanosine). Bristol-Myers Squibb Company. US Prescribing information, November 2011.
8. Damle BD, Yan JH, Behr D, O'Mara E, Nichola P, Kaul S, Knupp C. Effect of food on the oral bioavailability of didanosine from encapsulated enteric-coated beads. *J Clin Pharmacol* (2002) 42, 419–27.
9. Videx EC (Didanosine). Bristol-Myers Squibb Pharmaceuticals Ltd. UK Summary of product characteristics, June 2009.
10. Videx EC (Didanosine). Bristol-Myers Squibb Company. US Prescribing information, November 2011.
11. Lopéz JC, Moreno S, Jiménez-Oñate F, Clotet B, Rubio R, Hernández-Quero J. A cohort study of the food effect on virological failure and treatment discontinuation in patients on HAART containing didanosine enteric-coated capsules (FOODDIe Study). *HIV Clin Trials* (2006) 7, 155–62.
12. Hernández-Novoa B, Antela A, Gutiérrez C, Pérez-Molina JA, Pérez-Elías MJ, Dronda F, Moreno A, Casado JL, Page C, Pumares M, Galán JC, Moreno S. Effect of food on the antiviral activity of didanosine enteric-coated capsules: a pilot comparative study. *HIV Med* (2008) 9, 187–91
13. Emtriva Hard Capsules (Emtricitabine). Gilead Sciences Ltd. UK Summary of product characteristics, July 2011.
14. Emtriva (Emtricitabine). Gilead Sciences, Inc. US Prescribing information, July 2012.
15. Moore KH, Shaw S, Laurent AL, Lloyd P, Duncan B, Morris DM, O'Mara MJ, Pakes GE. Lamivudine/zidovudine as a combined formulation tablet: bioequivalence compared with lamivudine and zidovudine administered concurrently and the effect of food on absorption. *J Clin Pharmacol* (1999) 39, 593–605.
16. Epivir (Lamivudine). ViiV Healthcare. US Prescribing information, November 2011.
17. Epivir (Lamivudine). ViiV Healthcare UK Ltd. UK Summary of product characteristics, October 2010.
18. Zerit Hard Capsules (Stavudine). Bristol-Myers Squibb Pharmaceuticals Ltd. UK Summary of product characteristics, March 2011.
19. Zerit (Stavudine). Bristol-Myers Squibb Company. US Prescribing information, January 2012.
20. Hivid (Zalcitabine). Roche Products Ltd. UK Summary of product characteristics, November 2004.
21. Hivid (Zalcitabine). Roche Pharmaceuticals. US Prescribing information, September 2002.
22. Lotterer E, Ruhnke M, Trautmann M, Beyer R, Bauer FE. Decreased and variable systemic availability of zidovudine in patients with AIDS if administered with a meal. *Eur J Clin Pharmacol* (1991) 40, 305–8.
23. Ruhnke M, Bauer FE, Seifert M, Trautmann M, Hille H, Koeppe P. Effects of standard breakfast on pharmacokinetics of oral zidovudine in patients with AIDS. *Antimicrob Agents Chemother* (1993) 37, 2153–8.
24. Unadkat JD, Collier AC, Crosby SS, Cummings D, Opheim KE, Corey L. Pharmacokinetics of oral zidovudine (azidothymidine) in patients with AIDS when administered with and without a high-fat meal. *AIDS* (1990) 4, 229–32.
25. Hollister AS, Frazer HA. The effects of a high fat meal on the serum pharmacokinetics of sustained-release zidovudine. *Clin Pharmacol Ther* (1994) 55, 193.
26. Sahai J, Gallicano K, Garber G, McGilveray I, Hawley-Foss N, Turgeon N, Cameron DW. The effect of a protein meal on zidovudine pharmacokinetics in HIV-infected patients. *Br J Clin Pharmacol* (1992) 33, 657–60.
27. Retrovir (Zidovudine). ViiV Healthcare. US Prescribing information, May 2012.
28. Retrovir (Zidovudine). ViiV Healthcare UK Ltd. UK Summary of product characteristics, January 2012.

NRTIs + Ganciclovir

The concurrent use of zidovudine and ganciclovir produces a substantial increase in haematological toxicity, without any apparent increase in efficacy over ganciclovir alone. No clinically relevant pharmacokinetic interaction occurs between zidovudine and ganciclovir. Didanosine exposure is raised by ganciclovir, but there is limited evidence suggesting that the efficacy of ganciclovir prophylaxis is reduced. No pharmacokinetic interaction occurs between ganciclovir and stavudine, and there is no appreciable pharmacokinetic interaction between ganciclovir and zalcitabine. Valganciclovir is a prodrug of ganciclovir and is expected to interact similarly to ganciclovir.

Clinical evidence

(a) Didanosine

In a study, buffered didanosine 200 mg twice daily was given to 12 HIV-positive patients with oral ganciclovir 1 g three times daily. When didanosine was given 2 hours before ganciclovir, the maximum serum concentrations and AUC of didanosine were increased by about 47% and 83%, respectively, and those of ganciclovir were decreased by about 26% and 22%, respectively. When didanosine was given simultaneously with ganciclovir, the maximum serum concentrations and AUC of didanosine were similarly raised, by about 53% and 77%, respectively, but those of ganciclovir were unchanged. The renal clearance of didanosine was not significantly changed by ganciclovir.[1] Similar increases in didanosine concentrations with intravenous ganciclovir[2] and high-dose oral ganciclovir 2 g every 8 hours have also been reported.[3] However, in contrast, an earlier study found that the pharmacokinetics of didanosine from a sachet were not altered by intravenous ganciclovir.[4]

Rates of dose-limiting intolerance to the use of didanosine with ganciclovir were reported to be similar to those seen with didanosine alone in one small study (15 of 32 patients tolerated usual doses of didanosine with ganciclovir).[5] However, analysis of the results of a large randomised study unexpectedly suggested that there was an increased risk of cytomegalovirus infection in those patients taking ganciclovir and didanosine, when compared with those not taking didanosine.[6]

There is a case report[7] of a persistently low CD4+ count, but with complete viral suppression, in a patient taking buffered didanosine 200 mg twice daily with valganciclovir 900 mg twice daily. When didanosine was replaced with abacavir, the CD4+ count increased, from about 80 cells/m^2 to 323 cells/m^2.

(b) Stavudine

In a study in 11 HIV-positive patients, oral ganciclovir 1 g three times daily had no notable effect on the pharmacokinetics of stavudine 40 mg twice daily, nor were the pharmacokinetics of ganciclovir affected by the stavudine.[8] There were no serious or severe adverse events attributed to the combination.

(c) Zalcitabine

In a study in 10 HIV-positive patients, zalcitabine 750 micrograms every 8 hours increased the AUC of oral ganciclovir 1 g three times daily by a negligible 22%. There was no change in zalcitabine pharmacokinetics. There were no serious or severe adverse events attributed to the combination.[8]

(d) Zidovudine

The efficacy of zidovudine 100 or 200 mg every 4 hours, given alone or with intravenous ganciclovir 5 mg/kg twice daily for 14 days, then daily for 5 days of each week, was assessed in 40 patients for the treatment of cytomegalovirus. Severe haematological toxicity occurred in all of the first 10 patients given zidovudine 1.2 g daily and ganciclovir. Consequently the dose of zidovudine was reduced to 600 mg daily. Overall 82% of the 40 patients enrolled experienced profound and rapid toxicity (anaemia, neutropenia, leucopenia, gastrointestinal disturbances). Zidovudine dose reductions to 300 mg daily were needed in many patients. No change in the pharmacokinetics of zidovudine or ganciclovir was noted.[9]

Another study in 6 patients with AIDS and cytomegalovirus retinitis, given zidovudine and ganciclovir, found increased bone marrow toxicity but no improved efficacy over ganciclovir alone.[10] Increased toxicity (myelotoxicity and pancytopenia) following the use of both drugs has also been reported elsewhere.[11,12]

In contrast to the first study,[9] a specific study on the pharmacokinetics of zidovudine and ganciclovir in HIV-positive subjects reported that oral ganciclovir increased the maximum concentration and AUC of zidovudine by 38% and 15%, respectively, without altering renal clearance. Zidovudine did not alter ganciclovir pharmacokinetics.[1]

Mechanism

Ganciclovir inhibits purine nucleoside phosphorylase-4, the enzyme involved in the breakdown of didanosine, and this might result in an increase in its concentrations. Valganciclovir is rapidly metabolised to ganciclovir and would be expected to interact similarly.[7]

The toxicity resulting from the concurrent use of zidovudine and ganciclovir might be simply additive,[9] but *in vitro* studies with three human cell lines found synergistic cytotoxicity when both drugs were used.[13]

There is some *in vitro* evidence to suggest that ganciclovir antagonises the anti-HIV activity of zidovudine and didanosine.[14]

Importance and management

The interaction between ganciclovir and **zidovudine** resulting in increased toxicity would appear to be established. Ganciclovir increases **didanosine** exposure, although there is also some evidence suggesting reduced ganciclovir efficacy in the presence of didanosine, and this requires further study. Close and careful monitoring is required if either zidovudine or didanosine is given with ganciclovir. As **valganciclovir** is a prodrug of ganciclovir, it would be prudent to use similar precaution if valganciclovir is taken with these NRTIs.

Ganciclovir does not appear to alter the pharmacokinetics of **stavudine** or **zalcitabine**. Zalcitabine increased ganciclovir concentrations to a minor extent, which is not clinically important.

1. Cimoch PJ, Lavelle J, Pollard R, Griffy KG, Wong R, Tarnowski TL, Casserella S, Jung D. Pharmacokinetics of oral ganciclovir alone and in combination with zidovudine, didanosine, and probenecid in HIV-infected subjects. *J Acquir Immune Defic Syndr Hum Retrovirol* (1998) 17, 227–34.
2. Frascino RJ, Anderson RD, Griffy KG, Jung D, Yu S. Two multiple dose crossover studies of IV ganciclovir (GCV) and didanosine (ddI) in HIV infected persons. *Intersci Conf Antimicrob Agents Chemother* (1995) 35, 6.
3. Jung D, Griffy K, Dorr A, Raschke R, Tarnowski TL, Hulse J, Kates RE. Effect of high-dose oral ganciclovir on didanosine disposition in human immunodeficiency virus (HIV)-positive patients. *J Clin Pharmacol* (1998) 38, 1057–62.
4. Hartman NR, Yarchoan R, Pluda JM, Thomas RV, Wyvill KM, Flora KP, Broder S, Johns DG. Pharmacokinetics of 2′,3′-dideoxyinosine in patients with severe human immunodeficiency infection. II. The effects of different oral formulations and the presence of other medications. *Clin Pharmacol Ther* (1991) 50, 278–85.
5. Jacobson MA, Owen W, Campbell J, Brosgart C, Abrams DI. Tolerability of combined ganciclovir and didanosine for the treatment of cytomegalovirus disease associated with AIDS. *Clin Infect Dis* (1993) 16 (Suppl 1), S69–S73.
6. Brosgart CL, Louis TA, Hillman DW, Craig CP, Alston B, Fisher E, Abrams DI, Luskin-Hawk RL, Sampson JH, Ward DJ, Thompson MA, Torres RA. A randomized, placebo-controlled trial of the safety and efficacy of oral ganciclovir for prophylaxis of cytomegalovirus disease in HIV-infected individuals. *AIDS* (1998) 12, 269–77.
7. Tseng AL, Salit IE. CD4+ cell count decline despite HIV suppression: a probably didanosine-valganciclovir interaction. *Ann Pharmacother* (2007) 41, 512–7.
8. Jung D, AbdelHameed MH, Teitelbaum P, Dorr A, Griffy K. The pharmacokinetics and safety profile of oral ganciclovir combined with zalcitabine or stavudine in asymptomatic HIV- and CMV-seropositive patients. *J Clin Pharmacol* (1999) 39, 505–12.
9. Hochster H, Dieterich D, Bozzette S, Reichman RC, Connor JD, Liebes L, Sonke RL, Spector SA, Valentine F, Pettinelli C, Richman DD. Toxicity of combined ganciclovir and zidovudine for cytomegalovirus disease associated with AIDS. An AIDS clinical trials group study. *Ann Intern Med* (1990) 113, 111–17.
10. Millar AB, Miller RF, Patou G, Mindel A, Marsh R, Semple SJG. Treatment of cytomegalovirus retinitis with zidovudine and ganciclovir in patients with AIDS: outcome and toxicity. *Genitourin Med* (1990) 66, 156–8.
11. Jacobson MA, de Miranda P, Gordon SM, Blum MR, Volberding P, Mills J. Prolonged pancytopenia due to combined ganciclovir and zidovudine therapy. *J Infect Dis* (1988) 158, 489–90.
12. Pinching AJ, Helbert M, Peddle B, Robinson D, Janes K, Gor D, Jeffries DJ, Stoneham C, Mitchell D, Kocsis AE, Mann J, Forster SM, Harris JRW. Clinical experience with zidovudine for patients with acquired immune deficiency syndrome and acquired immune deficiency syndrome-related complex. *J Infect* (1989) 18 (Suppl 1), 33–40.
13. Prichard MN, Prichard LE, Baguley WA, Nassiri MR, Shipman C. Three-dimensional analysis of the synergistic cytotoxicity of ganciclovir and zidovudine. *Antimicrob Agents Chemother* (1991) 35, 1060–5.
14. Medina DJ, Hsiung GD, Mellors JW. Ganciclovir antagonizes the anti-human immunodeficiency virus type 1 activity of zidovudine and didanosine in vitro. *Antimicrob Agents Chemother* (1992) 36, 1127–30.

NRTIs + H_2-receptor antagonists

The concurrent use of buffered didanosine and ranitidine results in a negligible increase in didanosine exposure, and a negligible decrease in ranitidine exposure. Cimetidine slightly raises zalcitabine exposure. Cimetidine and ranitidine do not alter zidovudine or lamivudine exposure.

Clinical evidence, mechanism, importance and management

(a) Didanosine

In a study in 12 HIV-positive patients, didanosine 375 mg (buffered sachet preparation) was given either alone, or 2 hours after, a single 150-mg dose of **ranitidine**. The AUC of didanosine was increased by 14% by **ranitidine**.[1] The reason for this effect is not known but **ranitidine** possibly enhanced the effects of the citrate-phosphate buffer with which the didanosine was formulated. The AUC of **ranitidine** was reduced by 16% for reasons that are not understood, but it is possible that antacids (such as the citrate-phosphate buffer) that are formulated with didanosine reduce the absorption of ranitidine,[1] see 'H_2-receptor antagonists + Antacids', p.1143. These bioavailability changes are negligible, and no particular precautions would seem necessary if the drugs are taken in this way.

(b) Lamivudine

Lamivudine is predominantly renally excreted using the organic cationic transport system; however, the UK manufacturer states that **cimetidine** and **ranitidine**, which are partially eliminated by this mechanism, do not interact with lamivudine.[2]

(c) Zalcitabine

A study in 12 HIV-positive patients given a single 1.5-mg dose of zalcitabine found that **cimetidine** 800 mg caused a 24% reduction in the renal clearance of zalcitabine (assumed to be due to a reduction in renal tubular secretion) and a 36% increase in the AUC of zalcitabine.[3] These changes are slight, and probably unlikely to be clinically important.

(d) Zidovudine

In a randomised, crossover study, zidovudine 600 mg daily was given to 5 HIV-positive men and one man with AIDS. Zidovudine was given either alone, with **cimetidine** 300 mg four times daily, or with **ranitidine** 150 mg twice daily, each for 7 days. **Cimetidine** reduced the renal elimination of zidovudine by 56%, but had no effect on its AUC. It was suggested that the reduction in clearance was due to inhibition of tubular secretion. **Ranitidine** had no effect on zidovudine pharmacokinetics. No clinical toxicity occurred and the immunological parameters measured (CD4+ count and CD8+ count) were not appreciably altered. The authors concluded that no change in the dose of zidovudine is needed if either of these H_2-receptor antagonists is given concurrently.[4]

1. Knupp CA, Graziano FM, Dixon RM, Barbhaiya RH. Pharmacokinetic-interaction study of didanosine and ranitidine in patients seropositive for human immunodeficiency virus. *Antimicrob Agents Chemother* (1992) 36, 2075–9.
2. Epivir (Lamivudine). ViiV Healthcare UK Ltd. UK Summary of product characteristics, October 2010.
3. Massarella JW, Holazo AA, Koss-Twardy S, Min B, Smith B, Nazareno LA. The effects of cimetidine and Maalox® on the pharmacokinetics of zalcitabine in HIV-positive patients. *Pharm Res* (1994) 11 (10 Suppl), S-415.
4. Fletcher CV, Henry WK, Noormohamed SE, Rhame FS, Balfour HH. The effect of cimetidine and ranitidine administration with zidovudine. *Pharmacotherapy* (1995) 15, 701–8.

NRTIs + HIV-protease inhibitors

Buffered didanosine decreases atazanavir and indinavir exposure. Atazanavir, lopinavir, and tipranavir (all boosted with ritonavir) appear to negligibly to slightly decrease abacavir exposure. Tipranavir boosted with ritonavir slightly decreases zidovudine exposure. Most other combinations of HIV-protease inhibitors with NRTIs interact minimally or not at all. HIV-protease inhibitors do not affect the intracellular activation of NRTIs.

Clinical evidence, mechanism, importance and management

The HIV-protease inhibitors **indinavir**, **ritonavir**, and **saquinavir** have no effect on intracellular activation of various NRTIs (**didanosine**, **lamivudine**, **stavudine**, **zalcitabine** and **zidovudine**).[1] No interaction would be expected by this mechanism. Other potential interactions are discussed below.

When starting antiretrovirals in treatment-naive patients, the UK and US guidelines recommend a backbone of two NRTIs (usually emtricitabine plus tenofovir *or* abacavir plus lamivudine), which can be combined with one HIV-protease inhibitor boosted with ritonavir.[2,3] Current local and national guidelines should be consulted for other options in treatment-naive patients and for the management of treatment-experienced patients.

(a) Abacavir

Abacavir (with lamivudine) is an alternative NRTI backbone choice in the UK and US guidelines for starting antiretrovirals in treatment-naive patients, when it is given with an HIV-protease inhibitor boosted with ritonavir.[2,3] Current local and national guidelines should be consulted for restrictions for its use and details of the HIV-protease inhibitor-based regimens it can be combined with.

1. Amprenavir or Fosamprenavir. A phase I study in HIV-positive patients given amprenavir 900 mg twice daily with abacavir 300 mg twice daily for 3 weeks found that concurrent use did not appear to affect the pharmacokinetics of either drug.[4] The UK manufacturer of fosamprenavir states that, based on data with amprenavir, no pharmacokinetic interaction is expected with abacavir, and no dose adjustment is necessary.[5]

2. Atazanavir. In a study in 24 HIV-positive patients, atazanavir boosted with ritonavir 300/100 mg daily decreased the AUC of abacavir 600 mg daily by 17% but had no effect on the maximum or minimum plasma concentrations of abacavir. The pharmacokinetics of atazanavir boosted with ritonavir were not affected by abacavir.[6] The decrease in abacavir exposure is thought to be due to induction of abacavir glucuronidation by ritonavir.[6]

The authors of this study state that the clinical relevance of this interaction remains unclear; however, they note that even though a larger decrease in abacavir concentrations was seen with lopinavir boosted with ritonavir (see *Lopinavir*, below) a regimen containing a NRTI backbone of abacavir and lamivudine plus lopinavir boosted with ritonavir has been shown to be effective in the management of HIV infection.[6]

3. Darunavir. The UK and US manufacturers of darunavir state that no pharmacokinetic interaction is expected between abacavir and darunavir boosted with ritonavir,[7,8] and that no dose adjustment is needed on concurrent use.[7]

4. Lopinavir. In a study in 24 HIV-positive patients, lopinavir boosted with ritonavir 400/100 mg twice daily decreased the AUC, maximum plasma concentration, and minimum plasma concentration of abacavir 600 mg daily by 31%, 34%, and 64%, respectively. The pharmacokinetics of lopinavir boosted with ritonavir were not affected by abacavir.[6] The decrease in abacavir concentrations is thought to be due to induction of abacavir glucuronidation by ritonavir, and possibly also lopinavir.[6]

The authors of this study state that the clinical relevance of this interaction remains unclear; however, a regimen containing a NRTI backbone of abacavir and lamivudine plus lopinavir boosted with ritonavir has been shown to be effective in the management of HIV infection.[6] The authors[6] suggest that further study is needed, and it would seem prudent to monitor concurrent use to ensure antiviral efficacy, until further data is available.

5. Tipranavir. Tipranavir boosted with ritonavir decreased the AUC of abacavir by about 40%. The mechanism for this interaction and its clinical relevance have not been established,[9,10] but it might decrease the efficacy of abacavir.[9] Therefore the UK manufacturer states that the concurrent use of tipranavir boosted with ritonavir and abacavir is not recommended unless there are no other available NRTIs suitable for patient management.[9]

(b) Didanosine

1. Amprenavir or Fosamprenavir. The AUC and the minimum concentration of amprenavir 600 mg twice daily were not altered when it was given simultaneously with, or one hour before, buffered didanosine; or simultaneously with enteric-coated didanosine. The only notable change was a 15% decrease in the maximum concentration of amprenavir when it was given with buffered didanosine, which was not considered clinically relevant.[11] Nevertheless, the manufacturers of amprenavir suggested that it should be given at least one hour apart from didanosine,[12,13] and this has also been recommended for regimens containing amprenavir and ritonavir.[11] However, the UK manufacturer of fosamprenavir, a prodrug of amprenavir, states that, although no specific study has been done, a clinically relevant interaction due to the antacid content of didanosine would not be expected, and that no dose adjustment or separation of doses is required. Enteric-coated didanosine is also not expected to interact with fosamprenavir.[5]

2. Atazanavir. The US manufacturer of atazanavir found that simultaneous administration of buffered didanosine decreased atazanavir exposure by 87%, but no decrease occurred if administration was separated by one hour. There was little change in didanosine concentrations.[14] Therefore, they state that administration should be separated.[14,15] Conversely, although enteric-coated didanosine did not alter atazanavir concentrations (alone and boosted with ritonavir), simultaneous administration with food decreased didanosine exposure by 34%.[14,15] Therefore, the UK manufacturer[15] recommends that atazanavir boosted with ritonavir should be taken with food, 2 hours before didanosine (both the buffered tablets and enteric-coated formulations), whereas the US manufacturer[14] advises taking atazanavir 2 hours before or one hour after didanosine. Note that didanosine is preferably taken on an empty stomach (see 'NRTIs + Food', p.972), whereas atazanavir should be taken with food (see 'HIV-protease inhibitors + Food', p.928).

3. Darunavir with Ritonavir. Didanosine 400 mg daily, given on an empty stomach 2 hours before darunavir boosted with ritonavir 600/100 mg twice daily, did not affect the pharmacokinetics of darunavir and caused a 9% decrease in the AUC of didanosine.[7,8] Therefore, the UK manufacturer of darunavir advises that no dose adjustments are required when these drugs are given together.[7] However, note that didanosine is preferably taken on an empty stomach (see 'NRTIs + Food', p.972), whereas darunavir should be taken with food (see 'HIV-protease inhibitors + Food', p.928). Therefore, the manufacturers advise taking didanosine one hour before or 2 hours after darunavir boosted with ritonavir, which is taken with food.[7,8]

4. Indinavir. The concurrent use of [buffered] didanosine and indinavir decreased the AUC of indinavir by 80%, but when indinavir was given one hour before didanosine its pharmacokinetics were not notably affected.[16] Similarly, another study found that the pharmacokinetics of indinavir 800 mg were unchanged when it was given one hour after buffered didanosine 400 mg.[17] In a single-dose study in 23 healthy subjects, an enteric-coated preparation of didanosine had no effect on the pharmacokinetics of indinavir.[18] Indinavir possibly requires a normal acidic gastric pH for optimal absorption, whereas some didanosine preparations are formulated with buffering agents to increase gastric pH. Any increase in pH would therefore be expected to reduce indinavir absorption.[19] The manufacturers of indinavir recommend that indinavir and buffered didanosine preparations should be given at least one hour apart.[19,20] This recommendation does not apply to the enteric-coated preparation of didanosine.[18] Note that both didanosine and indinavir are preferably taken on an empty stomach, see 'NRTIs + Food', p.972, and 'HIV-protease inhibitors + Food', p.928, respectively.

5. Lopinavir. The US manufacturer advises that lopinavir boosted with ritonavir *tablets* can be taken at the same time as didanosine, on an empty stomach. However, didanosine must be taken one hour before or 2 hours after the *oral solution* of lopinavir boosted with ritonavir, which should be taken with food.[21]

6. Nelfinavir. The pharmacokinetics of nelfinavir were not apparently altered after concurrent use with didanosine.[22] Note that nelfinavir should preferably be taken with food (see 'HIV-protease inhibitors + Food', p.928), and all didanosine preparations should be taken without food (see 'NRTIs + Food', p.972). The US manufacturer of didanosine states that no interaction occurred when nelfinavir was taken one hour after didanosine and therefore recommends that nelfinavir is therefore taken one hour after didanosine enteric-coated preparations.[23]

7. Ritonavir. In a study in 13 HIV-positive subjects, buffered didanosine 200 mg twice daily was given with ritonavir 600 mg twice daily. Administration of the two drugs was separated by 2.5 hours, and treatment was given for 4 days. Treatment was staggered in this way, because ritonavir should be given with food (see 'HIV-protease inhibitors + Food', p.928), and didanosine without food (see 'NRTIs + Food', p.972). There was little or no change in the pharmacokinetics of ritonavir, and the maximum serum concentrations and AUC of didanosine were reduced by 16% and 13%, respectively, which was not considered to be clinically relevant. It was suggested that these changes might have been due to altered absorption in the presence of ritonavir.[24] The UK manufacturer of ritonavir therefore recommends that ritonavir and didanosine should be taken 2.5 hours apart and that dose alterations should not be necessary.[25]

8. Saquinavir. In a study in 8 healthy subjects, a single 400-mg dose of didanosine decreased the AUC and maximum plasma concentration of saquinavir (taken as saquinavir boosted with ritonavir 1600/100 mg once daily) by about 30% and 25%, respectively, but did not affect the minimum plasma concentration of saquinavir.[26] The UK manufacturer considers that no dose adjustment is needed on concurrent use.[26] Note also that saquinavir should preferably be taken with food (see 'HIV-protease inhibitors + Food', p.928), and all didanosine preparations should be taken on an empty stomach (see 'NRTIs + Food', p.972).

9. Tipranavir. Ritonavir-boosted tipranavir caused a 33% decrease in the AUC of didanosine in one of three studies,[10] but the clinical relevance of this has not been established.[9,10] Consequently, the manufacturers recommend that dosing of enteric-coated didanosine and tipranavir boosted with ritonavir should be separated by at least 2 hours to avoid formulation incompatibility.[9,10]

(c) Emtricitabine

Emtricitabine (with tenofovir) is a recommended NRTI backbone choice given in the UK and US guidelines for starting antiretrovirals in treatment-naive patients, when it is given with an HIV-protease inhibitor boosted with ritonavir.[2,3] Current local and national guidelines should be consulted for restrictions for its use and details of the HIV-protease inhibitors based regimens it can be combined with.

The UK and US manufacturers of **darunavir** state that no interaction is expected between emtricitabine and darunavir boosted with ritonavir,[7,8] and that no dose adjustment is needed.[7] The UK manufacturer of emtricitabine also states that no clinically relevant interaction occurs on the concurrent use of **indinavir**.[27]

(d) Lamivudine

Lamivudine (with abacavir) is an alternative NRTI backbone choice in the UK and US guidelines for starting antiretrovirals in treatment-naive patients, when it is given with an HIV-protease inhibitor boosted with ritonavir.[2,3] Current local and national guidelines should be consulted for restrictions for its use and details of the HIV-protease inhibitors based regimens it can be combined with.

No clinically relevant pharmacokinetic interaction appears to occur between lamivudine and **amprenavir**,[12,13] **atazanavir**,[14,15] **indinavir**,[19,20] **lopinavir** boosted with ritonavir[21,28] and **nelfinavir**,[29,30] and no interaction is expected with **darunavir** boosted with ritonavir[7,8] or **fosamprenavir** boosted with ritonavir.[5] **Tipranavir** boosted with ritonavir does not appear to cause a clinically relevant change in the AUC of lamivudine.[9,10]

(e) Stavudine

The UK and US manufacturers of **atazanavir**[14,15] note that there was no pharmacokinetic interaction with stavudine.

The UK and US manufacturers of darunavir state that no interaction is expected between stavudine and **darunavir** boosted with ritonavir.[7,8]

The AUC of stavudine was increased by 25% when stavudine 40 mg twice daily was given with **indinavir** 800 mg every 8 hours for one week, which is not clinically relevant. The serum concentrations of **indinavir** were unchanged.[31] Similarly, in a study in 24 healthy subjects, **indinavir** boosted with ritonavir 800/100 mg twice daily increased the AUC of stavudine by 24%, but this change is not clinically relevant.[32] No dose adjustments are needed on concurrent use.[19]

The UK and US manufacturers of ritonavir-boosted **lopinavir** note that no clinically relevant interaction occurs with stavudine.[21,28]

The manufacturers of stavudine note that no clinically relevant interactions have been seen with **nelfinavir**.[33,34]

In a study in HIV-positive children, **ritonavir** oral clearance was about 50% slower and the AUC about 2.5-fold higher in 6 children who received stavudine than in 7 children who received zidovudine and lamivudine, although these differences did not reach statistical significance.[35]

Tipranavir boosted with ritonavir does not appear to cause a notable change in the AUC of stavudine.[9,10] Therefore, no dose adjustment is needed on concurrent use.[9]

(f) Zalcitabine

The UK and US manufacturers of zalcitabine noted that there is no pharmacokinetic interaction with **saquinavir**.[36,37] They stated that pharmacokinetic interactions with HIV-protease inhibitors would not be expected because zalcitabine is mainly excreted unchanged in the urine.[36] The UK and US manufacturers of **darunavir** similarly state that no interaction is expected between zalcitabine and **darunavir** boosted with ritonavir.[7,8]

(g) Zidovudine

1. Amprenavir or Fosamprenavir. The UK and US manufacturer of amprenavir noted that the AUC and maximum concentrations of zidovudine were increased by 31% and 40%, respectively, when given with amprenavir. However, the pharmacokinetics of amprenavir were unchanged.[12,13] The UK manufacturer of amprenavir stated that no dose adjustment of either drug was necessary when amprenavir and zidovudine were used together.[12] The UK manufacturer of fosamprenavir states that, based on data with amprenavir, no significant interaction is expected with zidovudine, and no dose adjustment is necessary.[5]

2. Atazanavir. The UK manufacturer of atazanavir notes that there was no clinically relevant pharmacokinetic interaction with zidovudine.[15]

3. Darunavir. The UK and US manufacturers of darunavir state that no interaction is expected between zidovudine and darunavir boosted with ritonavir.[7,8]

4. Indinavir. A study found that when zidovudine 200 mg every 8 hours and indinavir 1 g every 8 hours were given together for a week, the AUC of zidovudine was increased by 17% and the AUC of indinavir was increased by 13%.[31] In another study, the concurrent use of indinavir and zidovudine with lamivudine increased the AUC of zidovudine by 39% but did not change indinavir pharmacokinetics.[20] The manufacturers of indinavir also report that the concurrent use of zidovudine 200 mg three times daily with indinavir 1 g three times daily, both taken for 7 days, had no effect on the pharmacokinetics of indinavir or on the AUC of zidovudine, although the minimum concentration of zidovudine was increased by 51%.[19,20] These changes are not clinically relevant, and the UK manufacturer of indinavir states that no dose adjustment is needed on concurrent use.[19]

5. Lopinavir with Ritonavir. The manufacturers of ritonavir-boosted lopinavir note that it induces glucuronidation and therefore has the potential to reduce zidovudine concentrations.[21,28]

6. Nelfinavir. The US manufacturer briefly reports that, in a study in 11 subjects, nelfinavir 750 mg every 8 hours for 7 to 10 days decreased the AUC and maximum concentration of a single 200-mg dose of zidovudine by 35% and 31%, respectively.[30] The UK manufacturer states that, at present, there is no evidence of inadequate efficacy of zidovudine in the CNS that could be associated with this decrease in the plasma concentration of zidovudine when given with nelfinavir.[29]

7. Ritonavir. A crossover study in 18 HIV-positive subjects found that the pharmacokinetics of ritonavir 300 mg every 6 hours were unchanged by zidovudine 200 mg every 8 hours. However, the maximum plasma concentration and AUC of zidovudine were both decreased by about 25%. The lack of change in the other pharmacokinetic parameters suggested that these changes were not due to altered metabolism,[38] although the manufacturer of ritonavir suggests that ritonavir might have induced the glucuronidation of zidovudine.[25] Nevertheless, zidovudine dose alterations are not necessary on concurrent use.[25,39]

8. Saquinavir. The UK manufacturer of saquinavir notes that there was no pharmacokinetic interaction between unboosted saquinavir and zidovudine.[26]

9. Tipranavir. Tipranavir boosted with ritonavir decreased the AUC of zidovudine by about 35%, without affecting the concentrations of glucuronidated zidovudine. The clinical relevance of this decrease has not been established,[9,10] but it might reduce the efficacy of zidovudine.[9] Therefore, the UK manufacturer states that the concurrent use of tipranavir boosted with ritonavir and zidovudine is not recommended unless there are no other suitable NRTIs available.[9]

1. Hoggard PG, Manion V, Barry MG, Back DJ. Effect of protease inhibitors on nucleoside analogue phosphorylation *in vitro*. *Br J Clin Pharmacol* (1998) 45, 164–7.
2. Williams I, Churchill D, Anderson J, Boffito M, Bower M, Cairns G, Cwynarski K, Edwards S, Fidler S, Fisher M, Freedman A, Geretti AM, Gilleece Y, Horne R, Johnson M, Khoo S, Leen C, Marshall N, Nelson M, Orkin C, Paton N, Phillips A, Post F, Pozniak A, Sabin C, Trevelion R, Ustianowski A, Walsh J, Waters L, Wilkins E, Winston A, Youle M. British HIV Association guidelines for the treatment of HIV-1-positive adults with antiretroviral therapy 2012 (Updated 2013). *HIV Med* (2014), 15 (Suppl 1) 1–85. Also available at: http://www.bhiva.org/documents/Guidelines/Treatment/2012/hiv1029_2.pdf (accessed 16/09/15).
3. Panel on Antiretroviral Guidelines for Adults and Adolescents. Guidelines for the use of antiretroviral agents in HIV-1-infected adults and adolescents. US Department of Health and Human Services (April 2015). 1–288. Available at: https://aidsinfo.nih.gov/contentfiles/lvguidelines/adultandadolescentgl.pdf (accessed 16/09/15).
4. McDowell J, Sadler BM, Millard J, Nunnally P, Mustafa N. Evaluation of potential pharmacokinetic (PK) drug interaction between 141W94 and 1592U89 in HIV+ patients. *Intersci Conf Antimicrob Agents Chemother* (1997) 37, 13.
5. Telzir (Fosamprenavir calcium). ViiV Healthcare UK Ltd. UK Summary of product characteristics, May 2011.
6. Waters LJ, Moyle G, Bonora S, D'Avolio A, Else L, Mandalia S, Pozniak A, Nelson M, Gazzard B, Back D, Boffito M. Abacavir plasma pharmacokinetics in the absence and presence of atazanavir/ritonavir or lopinavir/ritonavir and vice versa in HIV-infected patients. *Antivir Ther* (2007) 12, 825–30.
7. Prezista (Darunavir ethanolate). Janssen-Cilag Ltd. UK Summary of product characteristics, June 2012.
8. Prezista (Darunavir ethanolate). Janssen Pharmaceuticals, Inc. US Prescribing information, May 2012.
9. Aptivus Soft Capsules (Tipranavir). Boehringer Ingelheim Ltd. UK Summary of product characteristics, December 2011.
10. Aptivus (Tipranavir). Boehringer Ingelheim Pharmaceuticals, Inc. US Prescribing information, April 2012.
11. Shelton MJ, Giovanniello AA, Cloen D, Berenson CS, Keil K, DiFrancesco R, Hewitt RG. Effects of didanosine formulations on the pharmacokinetics of amprenavir. *Pharmacotherapy* (2003) 23, 835–42.
12. Agenerase (Amprenavir). GlaxoSmithKline UK. UK Summary of product characteristics, February 2007.
13. Agenerase (Amprenavir). GlaxoSmithKline. US Prescribing information, May 2005.
14. Reyataz (Atazanavir sulfate). Bristol-Myers Squibb. US Prescribing information, March 2012.
15. Reyataz (Atazanavir sulfate). Bristol-Myers Squibb Pharmaceuticals Ltd. UK Summary of product characteristics, August 2012.
16. Mummaneni V, Kaul S, Knupp CA. Single oral dose pharmacokinetic interaction study of didanosine and indinavir sulfate in healthy subjects (abstract 34). *J Clin Pharmacol* (1997) 37, 865.
17. Shelton MJ, Mei H, Hewitt RG, Defrancesco R. If taken 1 hour before indinavir (IDV), didanosine does not affect IDV exposure, despite persistent buffering effects. *Antimicrob Agents Chemother* (2001) 45, 298–300.
18. Damle BD, Mummaneni V, Kaul S, Knupp C. Lack of effect of simultaneously administered didanosine encapsulated enteric bead formulation (Videx EC) on oral absorption of indinavir, ketoconazole, or ciprofloxacin. *Antimicrob Agents Chemother* (2002) 46, 385–91.
19. Crixivan (Indinavir sulphate). Merck Sharp & Dohme Ltd. UK Summary of product characteristics, February 2012.
20. Crixivan (Indinavir sulfate). Merck & Co., Inc. US Prescribing information, April 2012.
21. Kaletra (Lopinavir with Ritonavir). Abbott Laboratories. US Prescribing information, April 2012.
22. Pedneault L, Elion R, Adler M, Anderson R, Kelleher T, Knupp C, Kaul S, Kerr B, Cross A, Dunkle L. Stavudine (d4T), didanosine (ddI), and nelfinavir combination therapy in HIV-infected subjects: antiviral effect and safety in an ongoing pilot study. 4th Conference on Retroviruses and Opportunistic Infections, Washington, 1997. Abstract 241.
23. Videx EC (Didanosine). Bristol-Myers Squibb Company. US Prescribing information, November 2011.
24. Cato A, Qian J, Hsu A, Vomvouras S, Piergies AA, Leonard J, Granneman R. Pharmacokinetic interaction between ritonavir and didanosine when administered concurrently to HIV-infected patients. *J Acquir Immune Defic Syndr Hum Retrovirol* (1998) 18, 466–72.
25. Norvir Film-coated Tablets (Ritonavir). AbbVie Ltd. UK Summary of product characteristics, March 2014.
26. Invirase Hard Capsules (Saquinavir mesilate). Roche Products Ltd. UK Summary of product characteristics, June 2012.
27. Emtriva Hard Capsules (Emtricitabine). Gilead Sciences Ltd. UK Summary of product characteristics, July 2011.
28. Kaletra Tablets (Lopinavir with Ritonavir). AbbVie Ltd. UK Summary of product characteristics, August 2012.
29. Viracept (Nelfinavir mesilate). Roche Products Ltd. UK Summary of product characteristics, June 2012.
30. Viracept (Nelfinavir mesylate). Agouron Pharmaceuticals, Inc. US Prescribing information, May 2013.
31. The Indinavir (MK 639) Pharmacokinetic Study Group. Indinavir (MK 639) drug interaction studies. 11th International Conference on AIDS, Vancouver, 1996. Abstract Mo.B.174.
32. Kaul S, Agarwala S, Hess H, Nepal S, Gale J, O'Mara E, Stevens M. The effect of coadministration of indinavir (IDV) and ritonavir (RTV) on the pharmacokinetics of stavudine (d4T). *Intersci Conf Antimicrob Agents Chemother* (2002) 42, 26.
33. Zerit Hard Capsules (Stavudine). Bristol-Myers Squibb Pharmaceuticals Ltd. UK Summary of product characteristics, March 2011.
34. Zerit (Stavudine). Bristol-Myers Squibb Company. US Prescribing information, January 2012.
35. Fletcher CV, Yogev R, Nachman SA, Wiznia A, Pelton S, McIntosh K, Stanley K. Pharmacokinetic characteristics of ritonavir, zidovudine, lamivudine, and stavudine in children with human immunodeficiency virus infection. *Pharmacotherapy* (2004) 24, 453–9.
36. Hivid (Zalcitabine). Roche Products Ltd. UK Summary of product characteristics, November 2004.
37. Hivid (Zalcitabine). Roche Pharmaceuticals. US Prescribing information, September 2002.
38. Cato A, Qian J, Hsu A, Levy B, Leonard J, Granneman R. Multidose pharmacokinetics of ritonavir and zidovudine in human immunodeficiency virus-infected patients. *Antimicrob Agents Chemother* (1998) 42, 1788–93.
39. Retrovir (Zidovudine). ViiV Healthcare. US Prescribing information, May 2012.

NRTIs + Hydroxycarbamide (Hydroxyurea)

Hydroxycarbamide appears to increase the antiviral activity of the NRTIs, particularly didanosine. However, the concurrent use of hydroxycarbamide and didanosine appears to carry a higher risk of adverse effects including neuropathy, pancreatitis, and hepatotoxicity, especially if stavudine is also given.

Clinical evidence, mechanism, importance and management

Data from *in vitro* studies have shown that hydroxycarbamide increases the antiviral activity of NRTIs, particularly **didanosine**, possibly by increasing their intracellular activation (phosphorylation).[1,2] The combination has therefore been investigated clinically. Some randomised studies[3-5] have found that the addition of hydroxycarbamide to reverse transcriptase inhibitors improves virologic response, whereas others have not found this.[6] One of these studies, in patients taking **efavirenz** and **abacavir**, found no increased rate of adverse effects in patients taking hydroxycarbamide 500 mg twice daily compared with patients not taking hydroxycarbamide, but more subjects in the hydroxycarbamide group withdrew from the study because of adverse effects (23% versus 4%). There was no increase in the incidence of blood dyscrasias with the concurrent use of hydroxycarbamide.[5] However, a number of studies have found increased toxicity, particularly with **didanosine** and **stavudine**. One study reported that the relative risk of *neuropathy* when **didanosine** was given with hydroxycarbamide was 2.35, compared with **didanosine** alone, and increased to 7.8 when **stavudine** was also added.[7] Another study reported an increased incidence of *neuropathy*, and an increased incidence of fatigue and nausea and vomiting.[8] The risk of *pancreatitis* might also be increased. In one study, 3 patients randomised to receive indinavir, **didanosine**, **stavudine**, and hydroxycarbamide developed pancreatitis and died, compared with no deaths in those receiving the same antivirals without hydroxycarbamide.[9] Another case of pancreatitis (non-fatal) has been reported when hydroxycarbamide was given with **stavudine**, **didanosine**, and nevirapine.[10] Fatal *hepatotoxicity* and hepatic failure have also been reported in patients given hydroxycarbamide with **didanosine** and **stavudine**.[11,12] For a case of hepatotoxicity and pancreatitis in a patient taking didanosine and hydroxycarbamide attributed to use of paracetamol, see 'NRTIs + Paracetamol (Acetaminophen)', p.979.

In response to these data, the manufacturers of **didanosine** and **stavudine** specifically state that use of these two NRTIs with hydroxycarbamide should be avoided.[11-14] Moreover, the UK manufacturers of **stavudine** go as far as to say that hydroxycarbamide should not be used in the treatment of HIV infection.[14]

1. Palmer S, Cox S. Increased activation of the combination of 3'-azido-3'-deoxythymidine and 2'-deoxy-3'-thiacytidine in the presence of hydroxyurea. *Antimicrob Agents Chemother* (1997) 41, 460–4.
2. Rana KZ, Simmons KA, Dudley MN. Hydroxyurea reduces the 50% inhibitory concentration of didanosine in HIV-infected cells. *AIDS* (1999) 13, 2186–8.
3. Lafeuillade A, Hittinger G, Chadapaud S, Maillefet S, Rieu A, Poggi C. The HYDILE trial: efficacy and tolerance of a quadruple combination of reverse transcriptase inhibitors versus the same regimen plus hydroxyurea or hydroxyurea and interleukin-2 in HIV-infected patients failing protease inhibitor-based combinations. *HIV Clin Trials* (2002) 3, 263–71.
4. Rodriguez CG, Vila J, Capurro AF, Maidana MM, Boffo Lissin LD. Combination therapy with hydroxyurea versus without hydroxyurea as first line treatment options for antiretroviral-naive patients. *HIV Clin Trials* (2000) 1, 1–8.
5. Swindells S, Cohen CJ, Berger DS, Tashima KT, Liao Q, Pobiner BF, Snidow JW, Pakes GE, Hernandez JE, and the NZT4008 Study Team. *BMC Infect Dis* (2005) 5, 23.
6. Zala C, Salomon H, Ochoa C, Kijak G, Federico A, Perez H, Montaner JSG, Cahn P. Higher rate of toxicity with no increased efficacy when hydroxyurea is added to a regimen of stavudine plus didanosine and nevirapine in primary HIV infection. *J Acquir Immune Defic Syndr* (2002) 29, 368–73.
7. Moore RD, Wong W-ME, Keruly JC, McArthur JC. Incidence of neuropathy in HIV-infected patients on monotherapy versus those on combination therapy with didanosine, stavudine and hydroxyurea. *AIDS* (2000) 14, 273–8.
8. Rutschmann OT, Vernazza PL, Bucher HC, Opravil M, Ledergerber B, Telenti A, Malinverni R, Bernasconi E, Fagard C, Leduc D, Perrin L, Hirschel B. Long-term hydroxyurea in combination with didanosine and stavudine for the treatment of HIV-1 infection. *AIDS* (2000) 14, 2145–51.
9. Havlir DV, Gilbert PB, Bennett K, Collier AC, Hirsch MS, Tebas P, Adams EM, Wheat LJ, Goodwin D, Schnittman S, Holohan MK, Richman DD; ACTG 5025 Study Team. Effects of treatment intensification with hydroxyurea in HIV-infected patients with virologic suppression. *AIDS* (2001) 1379–88.
10. Longhurst HJ, Pinching AJ. Pancreatitis associated with hydroxyurea in combination with didanosine. *BMJ* (2001) 322, 81.
11. Videx EC (Didanosine). Bristol-Myers Squibb Company. US Prescribing information, November 2011.
12. Zerit (Stavudine). Bristol-Myers Squibb Company. US Prescribing information, January 2012.
13. Videx Tablets (Didanosine). Bristol-Myers Squibb Pharmaceuticals Ltd. UK Summary of product characteristics, June 2009.
14. Zerit Hard Capsules (Stavudine). Bristol-Myers Squibb Pharmaceuticals Ltd. UK Summary of product characteristics, March 2011.

NRTIs + Isoniazid

The risk of peripheral neuropathy appears to be increased if isoniazid is given with stavudine, and is predicted to be increased by didanosine and

zalcitabine. The clearance of isoniazid is increased by zalcitabine, but isoniazid does not alter zalcitabine pharmacokinetics.

Clinical evidence

(a) Stavudine

In a retrospective case review, 12 out of 22 patients taking stavudine with isoniazid developed peripheral neuropathy. In 9 of the 21, this resolved on changing antiretroviral treatment (8 switched to zidovudine and one to saquinavir boosted with ritonavir).[1]

(b) Zalcitabine

A study in 12 HIV-positive patients found that when zalcitabine 1.5 mg three times daily was given with isoniazid 300 mg daily the pharmacokinetics of zalcitabine remained unchanged, but the clearance of isoniazid was approximately doubled with a 52% reduction in the AUC of isoniazid (which was not statistically significant).[2]

In a retrospective case review, one patient taking isoniazid with zalcitabine developed peripheral neuropathy and this resolved on switching therapy.[1]

Mechanism

Isoniazid can cause peripheral neuropathy as can stavudine, and to a lesser extent **didanosine** and zalcitabine.[3] The effects of concurrent use might be additive or synergistic. The reason for the apparent increased isoniazid clearance with zalcitabine is unknown.

Importance and management

There appears to be an increased risk of peripheral neuropathy when isoniazid is given with stavudine, and this is also predicted for **didanosine** and zalcitabine. The 2011 British HIV Association (BHIVA) guidelines advise that stavudine should not be given with isoniazid because of the risk of peripheral neuropathy.[3] Similarly, BHIVA guidelines also state that alternatives to didanosine should be given to patients taking isoniazid.[3] The UK manufacturer of zalcitabine[4] recommended caution with the combination, whereas the US manufacturer recommended that the combination should be avoided where possible.[5] The clinical relevance of the apparent increased isoniazid clearance with zalcitabine is unknown.

1. Breen RAM, Lipman MCI, Johnson MA. Increased incidence of peripheral neuropathy with co-administration of stavudine and isoniazid in HIV infected individuals. *AIDS* (2000) 14, 615.
2. Lee BL, Täuber MG, Chambers HF, Gambertoglio J, Delahunty T. The effect of zalcitabine on the pharmacokinetics of isoniazid in HIV-infected patients. *Intersci Conf Antimicrob Agents Chemother* (1994) 34, 3.
3. Pozniak AL, Coyne KM, Lipman MCI, Freedman AR, Ormerod LP, Johnson MA, Collins S, Lucas SB on behalf of the BHIVA Guidelines Subcommittee. British HIV Association guidelines for the treatment of TB/ HIV co-infection 2011. *HIV Med* (2011) 12, 517.
4. Hivid (Zalcitabine). Roche Products Ltd. UK Summary of product characteristics, November 2004.
5. Hivid (Zalcitabine). Roche Pharmaceuticals. US Prescribing information, September 2002.

NRTIs + Macrolides

Clarithromycin appears to cause some slight reduction in zidovudine exposure, but it does not appear to alter the pharmacokinetics of didanosine, stavudine, or zalcitabine. Azithromycin does not alter the pharmacokinetics of didanosine or zidovudine.

Clinical evidence

(a) Didanosine

When **azithromycin** 1.2 g daily for 14 days was given to 12 HIV-positive subjects with didanosine 200 mg twice daily, there was no change in the pharmacokinetics of didanosine.[1]

Clarithromycin 1 g twice daily for 7 days was given to 4 HIV-positive patients and 8 patients with AIDS taking oral didanosine. For the group as a whole the pharmacokinetics of didanosine remained unchanged, but there were large differences in the AUC between subjects, which could have hidden an interaction.[2]

(b) Stavudine

A study in 10 HIV-positive subjects found that the addition of **clarithromycin** 500 mg twice daily to stavudine 30 or 40 mg twice daily had no apparent effect on the pharmacokinetics of stavudine.[3]

(c) Zalcitabine

A 7-day course of **clarithromycin** 500 mg twice daily was given to 12 HIV-positive subjects taking zalcitabine. The addition of **clarithromycin** caused no change in the pharmacokinetics of zalcitabine.[4]

(d) Zidovudine

In a study in 12 HIV-positive subjects, **azithromycin** 600 mg to 1.2 g daily for 14 days did not affect the pharmacokinetics of zidovudine 100 mg five times daily.[1] Similarly, **azithromycin** 1 g, given weekly to 9 HIV-positive subjects, caused no change in the pharmacokinetics of zidovudine 10 mg/kg daily. The pharmacokinetics of **azithromycin** also remained unchanged.[5]

Fifteen HIV-positive patients were given zidovudine 100 mg every 4 hours five times daily and oral **clarithromycin** 500 mg, 1 g or 2 g every 12 hours, both together and alone. The pharmacokinetics of **clarithromycin** were not substantially changed by zidovudine, but the AUC of zidovudine was negligibly to slightly reduced, by 12 to 36%, by **clarithromycin**. However, these effects were not seen in all patients.[6,7]

Another study similarly found that **clarithromycin** caused a slight reduction in the AUC of oral zidovudine (by up to 27%). No changes were seen when zidovudine was given 4 or more hours after **clarithromycin**.[8] In a study in 16 patients with AIDS, zidovudine and **clarithromycin** were given 2 hours apart for 4 days. The maximum plasma concentration of zidovudine increased by about 50%, but the minimum concentration and the AUC over 8 hours did not change.[9]

Mechanism

Not understood but the interaction between clarithromycin and zidovudine might possibly be due to changes in absorption.

Importance and management

The overall picture is slightly confusing, but it seems that some reductions in **zidovudine** exposure are likely if clarithromycin is taken at the same time, but no important changes seem to occur if the administration of the drugs is separated. The authors of one study recommend that clarithromycin is given at least 2 hours before or after zidovudine.[7] The UK manufacturer of zidovudine includes this recommendation,[10] but the US manufacturer states that routine dose modification is not needed with clarithromycin.[11] Azithromycin appears to be a potential non-interacting alternative.

The authors of the report on **didanosine** conclude that clarithromycin can be given with didanosine,[2] and it also seems likely that didanosine and azithromycin can be given together without any pharmacokinetic interaction. Similarly, **stavudine** and **zalcitabine** can be given with clarithromycin without any need for the dose of the NRTIs to be adjusted.

1. Amsden G, Flaherty J, Luke D. Lack of an effect of azithromycin on the disposition of zidovudine and dideoxyinosine in HIV-infected patients. *J Clin Pharmacol* (2001) 41, 210–16.
2. Gillum JG, Bruzzese VL, Israel DS, Kaplowitz LG, Polk RE. Effect of clarithromycin on the pharmacokinetics of 2′,3′-dideoxyinosine in patients who are seropositive for human immunodeficiency virus. *Clin Infect Dis* (1996) 22, 716–18.
3. Piscitelli SC, Kelly G, Walker RE, Kovacs J, Falloon J, Davey RT, Raje S, Masur H, Polis MA. A multiple drug interaction study of stavudine with agents for opportunistic infections in human immunodeficiency virus-infected patients. *Antimicrob Agents Chemother* (1999) 43, 647–50.
4. Pastore A, van Cleef G, Fisher EJ, Gillum JG, LeBel M, Polk RE. Dideoxycytidine (ddC) pharmacokinetics and interaction with clarithromycin in patients seropositive for HIV. 4th Conference on Retroviruses and Opportunistic Infections, Washington DC, January 22nd-26th 1997. Abstract 613.
5. Chave J-P, Munafo A, Chatton J-Y, Dayer P, Glauser MP, Biollaz J. Once-a-week azithromycin in AIDS patients: tolerability, kinetics, and effects on zidovudine disposition. *Antimicrob Agents Chemother* (1992) 36, 1013–18.
6. Gustavson LE, Chu S-Y, Mackenthun A, Gupta SD, Craft JC. Drug interaction between clarithromycin and oral zidovudine in HIV-1 infected patients. *Clin Pharmacol Ther* (1993) 53, 163.
7. Polis MA, Piscitelli SC, Vogel S, Witebsky FG, Conville PS, Petty B, Kovacs JA, Davey RT, Walker RE, Falloon J, Metcalf JA, Craft C, Lane HC, Masur H. Clarithromycin lowers plasma zidovudine levels in persons with human immunodeficiency virus infection. *Antimicrob Agents Chemother* (1997) 41, 1709–14.
8. Petty B, Polis M, Haneiwich S, Dellerson M, Craft JC, Chaisson R. Pharmacokinetic assessment of clarithromycin plus zidovudine in HIV patients. *Intersci Conf Antimicrob Agents Chemother* (1992) 32, 114.
9. Vance E, Watson-Bitar M, Gustavson L, Kazanjian P. Pharmacokinetics of clarithromycin and zidovudine in patients with AIDS. *Antimicrob Agents Chemother* (1995) 39, 1355–60.
10. Retrovir (Zidovudine). ViiV Healthcare UK Ltd. UK Summary of product characteristics, January 2012.
11. Retrovir (Zidovudine). ViiV Healthcare. US Prescribing information, May 2012.

NRTIs + NRTIs

Some combinations of NRTIs are potentially antagonistic (stavudine with zidovudine and lamivudine with zalcitabine) and some are associated with additive toxicity (didanosine with stavudine or zalcitabine, and possibly stavudine with zalcitabine). Some do not appear to result in additional benefits (emtricitabine with lamivudine or zalcitabine), and some are considered inferior to other combinations (stavudine with lamivudine, zidovudine with zalcitabine or didanosine).

Clinical evidence, mechanism, importance and management

Current local and national guidelines should be consulted when choosing NRTI combinations. The US and UK guidelines recommend tenofovir (a nucleotide (nucleoside monophosphate) analogue often classed as an NRTI) with emtricitabine as the preferred NRTI backbone (see also 'NRTIs + Tenofovir', p.982) for combination with an NNRTI or an HIV-protease inhibitor boosted with ritonavir, or an integrase inhibitor in treatment-naive patients. Abacavir with lamivudine is an alternative NRTI backbone.[1,2] In US guidelines, lamivudine can be substituted for emtricitabine, and *vice versa*.[2] Most data on the efficacy of antiretroviral regimens in pregnancy are based on zidovudine with lamivudine and as such they are the preferred NRTI backbone for pregnant women.[3,4] The UK guidelines state there is no routine role for other NRTI backbones, and they specifically state there is no place for the use of stavudine- or didanosine-containing regimens as initial therapy, due to the associations with significant mitochondrial and hepatic toxicities.[1] Note that antiretroviral regimens consisting solely of NRTIs are not recommended either as dual-NRTI combinations or triple-NRTIs regimens, because these have shown suboptimal virological activity compared with the preferred regimens.[2]

A. Dual NRTI backbones

(a) Abacavir with Lamivudine

In a study, 13 HIV-positive subjects were given a single 150-mg dose of lamivudine with abacavir 600 mg. The pharmacokinetics of abacavir were not affected, and the AUC of lamivudine was negligibly decreased by 15%, with a 35% decrease in maximum concentrations. These changes were considered to be consistent with a change in absorption. The extent of the change is not clinically relevant and so no dose alteration would seem necessary on concurrent use.[5] In the UK and US guidelines, the combination of abacavir and lamivudine is currently a recommended dual NRTI backbone.[1,2]

(b) Abacavir with Zidovudine

In a study in 13 HIV-positive patients, a single 300-mg dose of zidovudine had no effect on the pharmacokinetics of abacavir 600 mg. The maximum plasma concentration of zidovudine was decreased by 20%, but the AUC was unchanged.[5] These results were confirmed in a steady-state study in which 79 HIV-positive subjects received 8 weeks of treatment with abacavir 600 mg to 1.8 g daily, in divided doses, and zidovudine 600 mg daily, in divided doses.[6] This change is not clinically relevant, and so no dose alteration would seem necessary on the concurrent use of abacavir and zidovudine.[5]

(c) Didanosine with Emtricitabine

In US guidelines, the combination of didanosine and emtricitabine is not recommended as a dual NRTI option for the treatment of HIV-infection in treatment naive patients because of lack of clinical studies and inferior virological efficacy.[2] The UK guidelines state that there is no place for the use of didanosine-containing regimens as initial therapy, due to the associations with significant mitochondrial and hepatic toxicities.[1]

(d) Didanosine with Lamivudine

The manufacturer of lamivudine notes that as lamivudine is predominantly renally cleared using the organic cationic transport system and didanosine is not cleared in this way, an interaction between these two drugs by this mechanism is unlikely.[7] Didanosine does not affect the intracellular activation of lamivudine *in vitro*.[8] The UK guidelines state that there is no place for the use of didanosine-containing regimens as initial therapy, due to the associations with significant mitochondrial and hepatic toxicities.[1]

(e) Didanosine with Stavudine

In a study in 10 HIV-positive patients, stavudine 40 mg twice daily, taken for 9 doses, had no effect on the pharmacokinetics of didanosine 100 mg taken twice daily. The half-life of the stavudine increased from 1.56 hours to 1.96 hours, but the AUC was unchanged and adverse effects were minimal. The authors of the report concluded that no clinically relevant pharmacokinetic interaction is likely to occur on concurrent use.[9] Didanosine does not interfere with the intracellular activation of stavudine *in vitro*.[10]

However, both didanosine and stavudine can cause peripheral neuropathy and pancreatitis, and there is evidence that this risk might be additive. In one early study, stavudine and didanosine were given to 13 HIV-positive subjects for 8 weeks. Neuropathy occurred in 3 patients, with only 2 patients restarting treatment.[11] In another study, the relative risk of neuropathy was 1.39 for stavudine alone, relative to didanosine alone, and 3.5 for the concurrent use of both drugs.[12] In 1999, the manufacturer of didanosine issued a stronger warning about the risk of pancreatitis with didanosine, and noted this risk was higher in patients also taking stavudine.[13] In addition, other evidence indicated that the risk of lactic acidosis (hyperlactataemia) was greatest in patients taking didanosine with stavudine,[14] and this has resulted in fatalities in pregnant women.[2] It is now established that the concurrent use of stavudine and didanosine is associated with a higher incidence of toxicity, particularly peripheral neuropathy, pancreatitis, and lactic acidosis. The US guidelines state that the combination of didanosine and stavudine is not recommended.[2] Similarly, the UK guidelines state that stavudine is not recommended for use as one of the NRTIs for initial therapy of HIV because of its toxicity.[1]

See also 'NRTIs + Drugs that cause pancreatitis', p.972, and 'NRTIs + Ribavirin', p.980.

(f) Didanosine with Zalcitabine

In vitro, didanosine had no significant effect on the intracellular activation of zalcitabine.[15] A 29-year-old man with persistent mild neuropathy due to zalcitabine developed severe neuropathy when given didanosine 3 weeks after stopping zalcitabine. As the didanosine neuropathy developed so rapidly it was suggested that it was caused by additive toxicity with zalcitabine.[16] Note also that both drugs are associated with pancreatitis. The US manufacturer advised against use of the combination,[17] whereas the UK manufacturers advised caution and careful monitoring if drugs that share these serious adverse effects are used concurrently.[15] See also 'NRTIs + Drugs that cause pancreatitis', p.972.

The UK guidelines state there is no place for the use of didanosine-containing regimens as initial therapy, due to the associations with significant mitochondrial and hepatic toxicities.[1] Note that zalcitabine is now rarely used and has been withdrawn in many countries.

(g) Didanosine with Zidovudine

A study in 8 HIV-positive patients found that when they were given zidovudine 250 mg with didanosine 250 mg (as a buffered sachet), the pharmacokinetics of didanosine were unaltered but the AUC of zidovudine was slightly raised by 35%, possibly due to altered absorption.[18] Conversely, in another study zidovudine plasma concentrations were lower in 4 out of 5 HIV-positive patients when given didanosine (chewable tablets) and there was an negligible 14% reduction in the AUC of zidovudine. Zidovudine clearance was increased by 29% but didanosine pharmacokinetics were unchanged.[19] A study in over 50 subjects ranging in age from 3 months to 21 years found that, when compared with day 3 (start of concurrent use), no apparent changes in AUCs occurred after 4 or 12 weeks of them taking zidovudine 60 to 180 mg/m^2 every 6 hours with didanosine 60 to 180 mg/m^2 every 12 hours (given 2 minutes after an antacid).[20] Several other studies have not found a pharmacokinetic interaction or evidence of increased toxicity when didanosine and zidovudine were used concurrently.[21-23] The UK manufacturer of didanosine states that there is no evidence that concurrent use increases the myelosuppressive effects of zidovudine.[24]

The reports are slightly contradictory, but the weight of evidence seems to be that no clinically relevant pharmacokinetic interaction occurs. However, note that the UK guidelines state there is no place for the use of didanosine-containing regimens as initial therapy, due to the associations with significant mitochondrial and hepatic toxicities.[1]

(h) Emtricitabine with Lamivudine

The US guidelines state that the combination of emtricitabine and lamivudine should not be offered at any time because of the similar resistance profile of the two drugs, minimal additive antiviral activity, and the possibility of inhibition of activation by intracellular phosphorylation.[2]

(i) Emtricitabine with Stavudine

In a single-dose study in 6 healthy subjects, no important pharmacokinetic interaction occurred between emtricitabine 200 mg and stavudine 40 mg.[25] The 2012 UK guidelines state that stavudine is not recommended for use as one of the NRTIs for initial therapy of HIV because of its toxicity.[1]

(j) Emtricitabine with Zalcitabine

The manufacturer of emtricitabine states that there is no information on the concurrent use of cytidine analogues, such as emtricitabine and zalcitabine, and therefore, the combination should not be used.[26] Note that zalcitabine is now rarely used and has been withdrawn in many countries

(k) Emtricitabine with Zidovudine

In a single-dose study in 6 healthy subjects, the AUC and maximum concentration of zidovudine 300 mg were increased by 26% and 66%, respectively, by emtricitabine 200 mg. The pharmacokinetics of emtricitabine were not altered.[25] The authors suggest that these increases in zidovudine concentrations are unlikely to be clinically relevant based on experience of using the two drugs together for 48 weeks in a phase III clinical study.[25]

(l) Lamivudine with Stavudine

NRTIs such as lamivudine need to be activated by phosphorylation within the cells to a triphosphate anabolite. Because stavudine does not affect this phosphorylation *in vitro*[8] it is predicted that no interaction is likely to occur by this mechanism. The manufacturer briefly states that no clinically relevant pharmacokinetic interaction was noted between stavudine 40 mg and lamivudine 150 mg in a single-dose study.[27,28] However, they note that peripheral neuropathy has been seen with the combination.[27] The US guidelines state that the combination of stavudine and lamivudine is not recommended for use in initial antiretroviral regimens because of significant toxicities including lipoatrophy, peripheral neuropathy and serious, life-threatening lactic acidosis, hepatic steatosis, and pancreatitis.[2] Similarly, the UK guidelines state that stavudine is not recommended for use as one of the NRTIs for initial therapy of HIV because of its toxicity.[1]

(m) Lamivudine with Zalcitabine

The manufacturers state that lamivudine is not recommended to be used with zalcitabine, because lamivudine might inhibit the intracellular activation of zalcitabine.[15,17] Note that zalcitabine is now rarely used and has been withdrawn in many countries.

(n) Lamivudine with Zidovudine

In a study, lamivudine 300 mg twice daily was given to 12 HIV-positive patients for 5 doses, with a 200-mg dose of zidovudine with the last dose. No major changes in the pharmacokinetics of the zidovudine occurred and it was concluded that dose adjustments are not needed if these two drugs are given concurrently.[29] Another study found the same results,[5] and a study in over 200 patients has shown that concurrent use can be safe and effective.[30]

However, there are case reports of blood dyscrasias occurring with concurrent use. Zidovudine 500 to 600 mg daily was given with lamivudine 300 mg daily to 13 HIV-positive patients. Zidovudine or lamivudine alone had previously been given to 9 of these 13 without problem. However, when both drugs were given, blood dyscrasias occurred in all patients within 7 weeks. Significant anaemia occurred in all patients, with precipitous declines in haemoglobin concentrations and one patient developed leucopenia and thrombocytopenia. Both drugs were stopped, blood transfusions were given, and all patients improved or recovered. Zidovudine or lamivudine alone was later started in 8 patients and 2 patients tolerated the combination (with the zidovudine dose halved in one patient and the drugs added sequentially in the other) without further haematological problems.[31] Similar precipitous falls in haemoglobin occurred in another 2 patients when lamivudine 300 mg daily was added to their long-term zidovudine treatment. Again both recovered when the drugs were stopped and blood was given.[32] Anaemia is a common adverse effect of zidovudine, but these patients had no problems until the lamivudine was added. However, the available evidence indicates that concurrent use can be safe and effective, with the adverse interactions cited here being uncommon. It has been suggested that a complete baseline blood count should be done, both when concurrent use is started, and every month for the first 3 months of treatment.[32] Although the combination of zidovudine and lamivudine is not currently a recommended acceptable dual NRTI backbone option as it has greater toxicity than tenofovir with emtricitabine, or abacavir and lamivudine, and requires twice daily administration,[1,2] it remains the preferred option in pregnant women because it has the most data in the mother and newborn.[3,4]

(o) Stavudine with Zalcitabine

In vitro, stavudine had no significant effect on the intracellular activation of zalcitabine.[15,27] Both stavudine and zalcitabine have the potential to cause peripheral neuropathy and pancreatitis. The concurrent use of drugs causing these serious adverse effects should be closely monitored (see also 'NRTIs + Drugs that cause pancreatitis', p.972). The UK guidelines state that stavudine is not recommended for use as one of the NRTIs for initial therapy of HIV because of its toxicity.[1] Note that zalcitabine is now rarely used and has been withdrawn in many countries.

(p) Stavudine with Zidovudine

NRTIs such as stavudine need to be phosphorylated within the cells to a triphosphate anabolite before they become effective. *In vitro* studies using mononucleated blood cells found that zidovudine significantly inhibited this phosphorylation.[10] Antagonism between zidovudine and stavudine has also been seen in a clinical study.[33] Therefore, the manufacturers[27,28] and the US guidelines[2] do not recommend the combination. Similarly, the UK guidelines state that stavudine is not recommended as one of the NRTIs for initial therapy of HIV because of its toxicity.[1]

(q) Zalcitabine with Zidovudine

In vitro, zalcitabine had no significant effect on the intracellular activation of zidovudine.[15] In a study in 56 patients with advanced HIV infection, taking zidovudine 50 to 200 mg every 8 hours and zalcitabine 5 to 10 micrograms/kg every 8 hours, neither drug affected the pharmacokinetics of the other nor was toxicity increased.[34] No particular precautions would appear to be necessary. Note that zalcitabine is now rarely used and has been withdrawn in many countries.

B. Triple NRTI regimens

The triple NRTI combination of **abacavir**, **lamivudine**, and **zidovudine** is generally not recommended as it is less efficacious than other recommended regimens. The US guidelines recommend that it should only be used when preferred, alternative, or acceptable regimens (which include NNRTIs, HIV-protease inhibitors, or integrase inhibitors) cannot be used.[2] They advise that all other triple regimens should not be used.[2]

C. Quadruple NRTI regimens

The US guidelines state that the quadruple NRTI regimen of **abacavir**, **lamivudine**, **tenofovir**, and **zidovudine** cannot be recommended because it is less efficacious than other recommended regimens.[2]

1. Williams I, Churchill D, Anderson J, Boffito M, Bower M, Cairns G, Cwynarski K, Edwards S, Fidler S, Fisher M, Freedman A, Geretti AM, Gilleece Y, Horne R, Johnson M, Khoo S, Leen C, Marshall N, Nelson M, Orkin C, Paton N, Phillips A, Post F, Pozniak A, Sabin C, Trevelion R, Ustianowski A, Walsh J, Waters L, Wilkins E, Winston A, Youle M. British HIV Association guidelines for the treatment of HIV-1-positive adults with antiretroviral therapy 2012 (Updated 2013). *HIV Med* (2014), 15 (Suppl 1) 1–85.
2. Panel on Antiretroviral Guidelines for Adults and Adolescents. Guidelines for the use of antiretroviral agents in HIV-1-infected adults and adolescents. Department of Health and Human Services. (April 2015). 1–288. Available at: https://aidsinfo.nih.gov/contentfiles/lvguidelines/adultandadolescentgl.pdf http://www.aidsinfo.nih.gov/ContentFiles/AdultandAdolescentGL.pdf (accessed 22/09/15).
3. de Ruiter A, Taylor GP, Clayden P, Dhar J, Gandhi K, Gilleece Y, Harding K, Hay P, Kennedy J, Low-Beer N, Lyall H, Palfreeman A, O'Shea S, Tookey P, Tosswill J, Welch S, Wilkins E. British HIV Association guidelines for the management of HIV infection in pregnant women 2012 (2014 interim review). *HIV Med* (2014), 15 (Suppl 4) 1–77.
4. Panel on Treatment of HIV-Infected Pregnant Women and Prevention of Perinatal Transmission. Recommendations for use of antiretroviral drugs in pregnant HIV-1-infected women for maternal health and interventions to reduce perinatal HIV transmission in the United States. 1–236. Available at: https://aidsinfo.nih.gov/contentfiles/lvguidelines/perinatalgl.pdf (accessed 23/09/15).
5. Wang LH, Chittick GE, McDowell JA. Single-dose pharmacokinetics and safety of abacavir (1592U89), zidovudine, and lamivudine administered alone and in combination in adults with human immunodeficiency virus infection. *Antimicrob Agents Chemother* (1999) 43, 1708–15.
6. McDowell JA, Lou Y, Symonds WS, Stein DS. Multiple-dose pharmacokinetics and pharmacodynamics of abacavir alone and in combination with zidovudine in human immunodeficiency virus-infected adults. *Antimicrob Agents Chemother* (2000) 44, 2061–7.
7. Epivir (Lamivudine). ViiV Healthcare UK Ltd. UK Summary of product characteristics, October 2010.
8. Kewn S, Veal GJ, Hoggard PG, Barry MG, Back DJ. Lamivudine (3TC). Phosphorylation and drug interactions *in vitro*. *Biochem Pharmacol* (1997) 54, 589–95.
9. Seifert RD, Stewart MB, Sramek JJ, Conrad J, Kaul S, Cutler NR. Pharmacokinetics of co-administered didanosine and stavudine in HIV-seropositive male patients. *Br J Clin Pharmacol* (1994) 38, 405–10.
10. Hoggard PG, Kewn S, Barry MG, Khoo SH, Back DJ. Effects of drugs on 2',3'-dideoxy-2',3'-didehydrothymidine phosphorylation in vitro. *Antimicrob Agents Chemother* (1997) 41, 1231–6.
11. Kalathoor S, Sinclair J, Andron L, Sension MG, High K. Combination therapy with stavudine and didanosine. 4th Conference on Retroviruses and Opportunistic Infections, Washington DC, Jan 22-26 1997. Abstract 552.
12. Moore RD, Wong W-ME, Keruly JC, McArthur JC. Incidence of neuropathy in HIV-infected patients on monotherapy versus those on combination therapy with didanosine, stavudine, and hydroxyurea. *AIDS* (2000) 14, 273–8.
13. Anon. ddI, d4T, hydroxyurea: new pancreatitis warning. *AIDS Treat News* (1999) Nov 19 (No. 331), 1–3.
14. Imhof A, Ledergerber B, Günthard HF, Haupts S, Weber R; Swiss HIV Cohort Study. Risk factors for and outcome of hyperlactatemia in HIV-infected persons: is there a need for routine lactate monitoring? *Clin Infect Dis* (2005) 41, 721–8.
15. Hivid (Zalcitabine). Roche Products Ltd. UK Summary of product characteristics, November 2004.
16. LeLacheur SF, Simon GL. Exacerbation of dideoxycytidine-induced neuropathy with dideoxyinosine. *J Acquir Immune Defic Syndr* (1991) 4, 538–9.
17. Hivid (Zalcitabine). Roche Pharmaceuticals. US Prescribing information, September 2002.
18. Barry M, Howe JL, Ormesher S, Back DJ, Breckenridge AM, Bergin C, Mulcahy F, Beeching N, Nye F. Pharmacokinetics of zidovudine and dideoxyinosine alone and in combination in patients with acquired immunodeficiency syndrome. *Br J Clin Pharmacol* (1994) 37, 421–6.
19. Burger DM, Meenhorst PL, Kroon FP, Mulder JW, Koks CHW, Bult A, Beijnen JH. Pharmacokinetic interaction study of zidovudine and didanosine. *J Drug Dev* (1994) 6, 187–94.
20. Mueller BU, Pizzo PA, Farley M, Husson RN, Goldsmith J, Kovacs A, Woods L, Ono J, Church JA, Brouwers P, Jarosinski P, Venzon D, Balis FM. Pharmacokinetic evaluation of the combination of zidovudine and didanosine in children with human immunodeficiency virus infection. *J Pediatr* (1994) 125, 142–6.
21. Collier AC, Coombs RW, Fischl MA, Skolnik PR, Northfelt D, Boutin P, Hooper CJ, Kaplan LD, Volberding PA, Davis LG, Henrard DR, Weller S, Corey L. Combination therapy with zidovudine and didanosine compared with zidovudine alone in HIV-1 infection. *Ann Intern Med* (1993) 119, 786–93.
22. Sahai J, Gallicano K, Garber G, Pakuts A, Cameron W. Pharmacokinetics of simultaneously administered zidovudine and didanosine in HIV-seropositive male patients. *J Acquir Immune Defic Syndr Hum Retrovirol* (1995) 10, 54–60.
23. Gibb D, Barry M, Ormesher S, Nokes L, Seefried M, Giaquinto C, Back D. Pharmacokinetics of zidovudine and dideoxyinosine alone and combination in children with HIV infection. *Br J Clin Pharmacol* (1995) 39, 527–30.
24. Videx EC (Didanosine). Bristol-Myers Squibb Pharmaceuticals Ltd. UK Summary of product characteristics, June 2009.
25. Zhong J, Chittick GE, Wang LH, Hui J, Begley JA, Blum MR. Pharmacokinetic evaluation of emtricitabine in combination with other nucleoside antivirals in healthy volunteers. *J Clin Pharmacol* (2007) 47, 877–9.
26. Emtriva Hard Capsules (Emtricitabine). Gilead Sciences Ltd. UK Summary of product characteristics, July 2011.
27. Zerit Hard Capsules (Stavudine). Bristol-Myers Squibb Pharmaceuticals Ltd. UK Summary of product characteristics, March 2011.
28. Zerit (Stavudine). Bristol-Myers Squibb Company. US Prescribing information, January 2012.
29. Rana KZ, Horton CM, Yuen GJ, Pivarnik PE, Mikolich DM, Fisher AE, Mydlow PK, Dudley MN. Effect of lamivudine on zidovudine pharmacokinetics in asymptomatic HIV-infected individuals. *Intersci Conf Antimicrob Agents Chemother* (1994) 34, 83.
30. Staszewski S, Loveday C, Picazo JJ, Dellamonica P, Skinhøj P, Johnson MA, Danner SA, Harrigan PR, Hill AM, Verity L, McDade H; for the Lamivudine European HIV Working Group. Safety and efficacy of lamivudine-zidovudine combination therapy in zidovudine-experienced patients. A randomized controlled comparison with zidovudine monotherapy. *JAMA* (1996) 276, 111–17.
31. Tseng A, Conly J, Fletcher D, Keystone D, Salit I, Walmsley S. Precipitous declines in hemoglobin levels associated with combination zidovudine and lamivudine. *Clin Infect Dis* (1998) 27, 908–9.
32. Hester EK, Peacock JE. Profound and unanticipated anemia with lamivudine-zidovudine combination therapy in zidovudine-experienced patients with HIV infection. *AIDS* (1998) 12, 439–51.
33. Havlir DV, Tierney C, Friedland GH, Pollard RB, Smeaton L, Sommadossi JP, Fox L, Kessler H, Fife KH, Richman DD. In vivo antagonism with zidovudine plus stavudine combination therapy. *J Infect Dis* (2000) 182, 321–5.
34. Meng T-C, Fischl MA, Boota AM, Spector SA, Bennett D, Bassiakos Y, Lai S, Wright B, Richman DD. Combination therapy with zidovudine and dideoxycytidine in patients with advanced human immunodeficiency virus infection. *Ann Intern Med* (1992) 116, 13–20.

NRTIs + Paracetamol (Acetaminophen)

Limited and unconfirmed evidence suggests that paracetamol possibly increases the bone marrow suppressant effects of zidovudine. Single case reports describe severe liver toxicity when patients were given paracetamol with either zidovudine or didanosine.

Clinical evidence

(a) Didanosine

Increasing abdominal pain occurred in a 47-year-old HIV-positive man one month after he started to take didanosine (his other medications included nevirapine, **hydroxycarbamide**, aciclovir and lorazepam). He had been treating the pain with paracetamol, and had taken 4 g over 3 days. Severe hepatitis and pancreatitis were diagnosed, which slowly resolved over the following 3 weeks.[1]

(b) Zidovudine

An early study of zidovudine use in 282 patients with AIDS found that haematological abnormalities (anaemia, leucopenia, neutropenia) were very common and 21% needed multiple red cell transfusions. Some of the patients also received paracetamol, which increased the haematological toxicity (neutropenia) by an unstated amount.[2]

Short-term clinical studies using paracetamol 650 mg up to every 4 hours found that paracetamol had no appreciable effects on the pharmacokinetics of zidovudine,[3-6] although in one case zidovudine clearance was slightly increased.[7] An 8-month study in a single patient suggested that the long-term concurrent use of zidovudine and paracetamol did not affect the pharmacokinetics of either drug. However, in this individual, very rapid absorption and a high maximum serum concentration of zidovudine were seen, so as a precaution the zidovudine dose was reduced from 200 mg every 4 hours to 100 mg every 6 hours.[8]

A patient taking zidovudine and co-trimoxazole took 3.3 g of paracetamol over 36 hours. Within 2 days he developed severe hepatotoxicity, and as other causes were excluded, the reaction was attributed to paracetamol. The authors suggested that zidovudine might have augmented paracetamol toxicity.[9] However, in a single-dose study, reduced paracetamol glucuronidation and increased formation of hepatotoxic metabolites were seen in patients with advanced HIV infection compared with healthy HIV-positive subjects and those without HIV, and this effect was independent of zidovudine use.[10] In contrast, in another study, disease state (AIDS versus healthy HIV-positive subjects) was not found to alter paracetamol metabolism, and zidovudine was found to *increase* paracetamol glucuronidation in some patients.[11]

Mechanism

Not understood. Paracetamol does not increase the serum concentrations of zidovudine,[3-5,7] which might have provided an explanation for the apparent increased toxicity. One *in vitro* study found that paracetamol does not affect the glucuronidation of zidovudine,[12] whereas another found that paracetamol did inhibit zidovudine glucuronidation.[13] The effect of zidovudine on paracetamol metabolism is also unclear.

Didanosine can cause pancreatitis or hepatic disease, and zidovudine can also rarely cause hepatic disease. It has been suggested that the hepatotoxicity of these drugs are augmented when they are given with paracetamol.[1]

Importance and management

Paracetamol is a widely used non-prescription analgesic, and the cited report of potential combined toxicity with **didanosine** appears to be isolated; nevertheless, the authors suggest extreme caution when potentially hepatotoxic drugs such as paracetamol are used with didanosine.[1] Both drugs can cause hepatotoxicity alone, and didanosine itself can cause severe pancreatitis, and there is limited evidence that hepatotoxicity might be increased by their concurrent use. However, note that the case of hepatitis in question might be attributed to the concurrent use of didanosine and hydroxycarbamide, which has been reported to cause hepatotoxicity, see 'NRTIs + Hydroxycarbamide (Hydroxyurea)', p.976.

The short-term use of **zidovudine** and paracetamol does not appear to alter the pharmacokinetics of either drug. Whether paracetamol increases the haematological toxicity of zidovudine and whether the drugs have combined hepatotoxicity is unclear from the available data.

1. Lederman JC, Nawaz H. Toxic interaction of didanosine and acetaminophen leading to severe hepatitis and pancreatitis: a case report and review of the literature. *Am J Gastroenterol* (2001) 96, 3474–5.
2. Richman DD, Fischl MA, Grieco MH, Gottlieb MS, Volberding PA, Laskin OL, Leedom JM, Groopman JE, Mildvan D, Hirsch MS, Jackson GG, Durack DT, Nusinoff-Lehrman S and the AZT Collaborative Working Group. The toxicity of azidothymidine (AZT) in the treatment of patients with AIDS and AIDS-related complex. A double-blind, placebo-controlled trial. *N Engl J Med* (1987) 317, 192–7.
3. Steffe EM, King JH, Inciardi JF, Flynn NF, Goldstein E, Tonjes TS, Benet LZ. The effect of acetaminophen on zidovudine metabolism in HIV-infected patients. *J Acquir Immune Defic Syndr* (1990) 3, 691–4.
4. Ptachcinski J, Pazin G, Ho M. The effect of acetaminophen on the pharmacokinetics of zidovudine. *Pharmacotherapy* (1989) 9, 190.
5. Pazin GJ, Ptachcinski RJ, Sheehan M, Ho M. Interactive pharmacokinetics of zidovudine and acetaminophen. 5th International Conference on AIDS, Montreal, 1989. Abstract M.B.P.338.
6. Burger DM, Meenhorst PL, Underberg WJM, van der Heijde JF, Koks CHW, Beijnen JH. Short-term, combined use of paracetamol and zidovudine does not alter the pharmacokinetics of either drug. *Neth J Med* (1994) 44, 161–5.
7. Sattler FR, Ko R, Antoniskis D, Shields M, Cohen J, Nicoloff J, Leedom J, Koda R. Acetaminophen does not impair clearance of zidovudine. *Ann Intern Med* (1991) 114, 937–40.
8. Burger DM, Meenhorst PL, Koks CHW, Beijnen JH. Pharmacokinetics of zidovudine and acetaminophen in a patient on chronic acetaminophen therapy. *Ann Pharmacother* (1994) 28, 327–30.
9. Shriner K, Goetz MB. Severe hepatotoxicity in a patient receiving both acetaminophen and zidovudine. *Am J Med* (1992) 93, 94–6.
10. Esteban A, Pérez-Mateo M, Boix V, González M, Portilla J, Mora A. Abnormalities in the metabolism of acetaminophen in patients infected with the human immunodeficiency virus (HIV). *Methods Find Exp Clin Pharmacol* (1997) 19, 129–32.
11. O'Neil WM, Pezzullo JC, Di Girolamo A, Tsoukas CM, Wainer IW. Glucuronidation and sulphation of paracetamol in HIV-positive patients and patients with AIDS. *Br J Clin Pharmacol* (1999) 48, 811–18.
12. Kamali F, Rawlins MD. Influence of probenecid and paracetamol (acetaminophen) on zidovudine glucuronidation in human liver *in vitro*. *Biopharm Drug Dispos* (1992) 13, 403–9.
13. Schumann L, Unadkat JD. Does acetaminophen potentiate the hematotoxicity of zidovudine (ZDV or AZT) by inhibition of its metabolism to the glucuronide? *Pharm Res* (1988) 5 (Suppl), S-177.

NRTIs + Probenecid

Probenecid reduces the renal excretion of zalcitabine and zidovudine, increasing their exposure. The incidence of adverse effects appears to be greatly increased by the concurrent use of probenecid and zidovudine.

Clinical evidence

(a) Zalcitabine

In a single-dose study, 12 HIV-positive or patients with AIDS were given zalcitabine 1.5 mg alone or with probenecid 500 mg, given 8 and 2 hours before, then 4 hours after, zalcitabine. The renal clearance of the zalcitabine was decreased by 42% by probenecid, its half-life was increased by 47% and its AUC was increased by 54%.[1]

(b) Zidovudine

In 12 patients with AIDS or AIDS-related complex the concurrent use of zidovudine and probenecid 500 mg every 8 hours for 3 days increased the AUC of zidovudine by an average of 80% (range 14 to 192%).[2] Other studies in patients[3-5] and healthy subjects[6] found that probenecid roughly doubled the AUC of zidovudine when given in a variety of dosing schedules.[3,4] However, the effects on the pharmacokinetics of zidovudine were minimal if the two drugs were given 6 hours apart.[5] Another report describes a very high incidence of rashes in 6 out of 8 HIV-positive men given zidovudine with probenecid 500 mg every 6 hours. The rash and other symptoms (such as malaise, fever, and myalgia) were sufficiently severe for the probenecid to be withdrawn in 4 patients.[7] A later study found that when using only 250 mg of probenecid every 8 hours the AUC of zidovudine was increased by 70% but the adverse effects still occurred, although the incidence was possibly somewhat lower.[8] Conversely, others reported the successful use of probenecid 500 mg three times daily with a reduced dose of zidovudine (600 mg daily) in 7 patients without any occurrence of rash.[9]

Mechanism

Experimental clinical evidence indicates that probenecid reduces the metabolism (glucuronidation) of zidovudine by liver enzymes, and inhibits the renal secretion of the zidovudine glucuronide metabolite.[2-4,6,10,11] The interaction with zalcitabine is presumably due to inhibition of zalcitabine secretion in the renal tubules.[1]

Importance and management

The pharmacokinetic interaction of probenecid with **zidovudine** leading to a 2-fold increase in exposure would appear to be established. However, the US manufacturer states that routine zidovudine dose adjustment is not required on concurrent use.[12] The UK manufacturer advises that patients should be closely monitored for haematological toxicity.[13] Given the available data, some caution would seem appropriate. The apparent increase in other adverse effects during concurrent use, such as rash seen by one group of researchers,[7,8] should be borne in mind. In some situations, zidovudine might be used with cidofovir, which should always be taken with probenecid. In this situation the US manufacturer of cidofovir advises that zidovudine should be temporarily discontinued or the dose halved.[14]

Although probenecid also increases **zalcitabine** exposure, the increase was not as great (50%), and because the half-life of zalcitabine is short compared with its dosing schedule significant accumulation would not be expected.

It would seem prudent to monitor for any signs of toxicity if either drug combination is used long-term. The safety of concurrent use needs further assessment.

1. Massarella JW, Nazareno LA, Passe S, Min B. The effect of probenecid on the pharmacokinetics of zalcitabine in HIV-positive patients. *Pharm Res* (1996) 13, 449–52.
2. Kornhauser DM, Petty BG, Hendrix CW, Woods AS, Nerhood LJ, Bartlett JG, Lietman PS. Probenecid and zidovudine metabolism. *Lancet* (1989) 2, 473–5.
3. Hedaya MA, Elmquist WF, Sawchuk RJ. Probenecid inhibits the metabolic and renal clearances of zidovudine (AZT) in human volunteers. *Pharm Res* (1990) 7, 411–17.
4. de Miranda P, Good SS, Yarchoan R, Thomas RV, Blum MR, Myers CE, Broder S. Alteration of zidovudine pharmacokinetics by probenecid in patients with AIDS or AIDS-related complex. *Clin Pharmacol Ther* (1989) 46, 494–500.
5. McDermott J, Kennedy J, Ellis-Pegler RB, Thomas MG. Pharmacokinetics of zidovudine plus probenecid. *J Infect Dis* (1992) 166, 687–8.
6. Campion JJ, Bawdon RE, Baskin LB, Barton CI. Effect of probenecid on the pharmacokinetics of zidovudine and zidovudine glucuronide. *Pharmacotherapy* (1990) 10, 235.
7. Petty BG, Kornhauser DM, Lietman PS. Zidovudine with probenecid: a warning. *Lancet* (1990) 1, 1044–5.
8. Petty BG, Barditch-Crovo PA, Nerhood L, Kornhauser DM, Kuwahara S, Lietman PS. Unexpected clinical toxicity of probenecid (P) with zidovudine (Z) in patients with HIV infection. *Intersci Conf Antimicrob Agents Chemother* (1991) 31, 323.
9. Duckworth AS, Duckworth GW, Henderson G, Contreras G. Zidovudine with probenecid. *Lancet* (1990) 336, 441.
10. Sim SM, Back DJ, Breckenridge AM. The effect of various drugs on the glucuronidation of zidovudine (azidothymidine; AZT) by human liver microsomes. *Br J Clin Pharmacol* (1991) 32, 17–21.
11. Kamali F, Rawlins MD. Influence of probenecid and paracetamol (acetaminophen) on zidovudine glucuronidation in human liver *in vitro*. *Biopharm Drug Dispos* (1992) 13, 403–9.
12. Retrovir (Zidovudine). ViiV Healthcare. US Prescribing information, May 2012.
13. Retrovir (Zidovudine). ViiV Healthcare UK Ltd. UK Summary of product characteristics, January 2012.
14. Vistide (Cidofovir). Gilead Sciences, Inc. US Prescribing information, September 2010.

NRTIs + Ribavirin

The use of ribavirin with the NRTIs might result in increased toxicity (lactic acidosis, pancreatitis, and hepatotoxicity), which is possibly more frequent with didanosine and stavudine than other NRTIs. These effects might also be exacerbated by the additional use of interferon for hepatitis C. The use of zidovudine with ribavirin is associated with an increased risk of myelosuppression. There is conflicting evidence as to whether abacavir is associated with an increased risk of ribavirin treatment failure. Early *in vitro* data suggested that ribavirin might reduce the antiretroviral effects of some NRTIs, particularly stavudine and zidovudine, but this does not appear to have been demonstrated in practice.

Clinical evidence

In an analysis of data from the adverse event reporting system of the FDA in the US, 31 patients were identified who had adverse events suggestive of mitochondrial toxicity while taking ribavirin with an NRTI. Of these, nearly 90% had received **didanosine**, 71% **stavudine**, and 65% both **didanosine** and **stavudine**. Five patients died; all of whom were taking didanosine (with stavudine in three of these cases). The use of ribavirin with didanosine was associated with an increased risk of mitochondrial toxicity (odds ratio 12.4) compared with patients taking ribavirin with other NRTIs (odds ratios: **didanosine** and **stavudine** 8; **stavudine** 3.3; **abacavir** 1.1; **lamivudine** 0.2; **zidovudine** 0.06).[1]

There is also some evidence that patients with *cirrhotic* chronic hepatitis C and HIV-infection receiving HAART and interferon alfa-2a with or without ribavirin appear to be at increased risk for the development of hepatic decompensation, when compared with patients not receiving HAART.[2,3] One US manufacturer includes details of clinical study NR15961, in which 14 (11%) of 129 such patients receiving HAART developed hepatic decompensation resulting in 6 deaths. All 14 patients were taking NRTIs, including **stavudine, didanosine, abacavir, zidovudine,** and **lamivudine**. Because of the small number of patients, it is not possible to assess the risk for individual NRTIs.[3] However, the UK manufacturers of ribavirin note that use of **didanosine** is a possible risk factor for development of hepatic decompensation.[2,4] Specific data for NRTIs is covered in the subsections below.

(a) Abacavir

Some evidence has suggested that abacavir reduces ribavirin concentrations and response rate. For example, in a retrospective study in HIV-positive patients with hepatitis C, the use of abacavir was reported to increase the risk of therapeutic failure with interferon alfa and ribavirin, particularly in patients with ribavirin concentrations of less than 2.3 micrograms/mL.[5] Similarly, another study found that abacavir reduced the response to ribavirin.[6] Conversely, other evidence has found no interaction. For example, in 124 patients taking ribavirin and pegylated interferon, 22% of whom were taking also taking abacavir, there was no difference in the steady-state ribavirin concentrations, no difference in the rapid or early virological response rate, and no difference in the decline in HCV-RNA between abacavir users and abacavir non-users. The sustained virological response rate was higher in abacavir users, but this difference was not statistically significant.[7] Other studies have reported similar findings.[8,9]

For the possible risk of hepatic decompensation and possible lack of mitochondrial toxicity when abacavir was given with ribavirin in patients with both chronic hepatitis C and HIV infection, see above.

(b) Didanosine

In two studies, ribavirin did not alter the pharmacokinetics of didanosine in HIV-positive adults or children.[10,11] However, *in vitro*, ribavirin increases the *intracellular activation* of didanosine to its active metabolite dideoxyadenosine 5′-triphosphate,[12,13] which could result in increased adverse effects. In one early study, no increase in adverse effects was seen when ribavirin 600 mg daily was given to 16 HIV-positive patients who had already been taking didanosine 125 to 200 mg twice daily for 4 weeks. Ribavirin was given 6 hours after the morning dose of didanosine. Over the 8 or 20 weeks of the study the combination was well tolerated.[10] Nevertheless, cases of mitochondrial toxicity (hepatotoxicity, pancreatitis, lactic acidosis) have been reported when ribavirin was added to didanosine-containing antiretroviral regimens,[14-16] and fatalities have occurred.[1,14] Some other studies have shown an increased risk of mitochondrial toxicity when ribavirin was given with didanosine.[17-19]

For further evidence, and the possible risk of hepatic decompensation when didanosine was given with ribavirin in patients with both chronic hepatitis C and HIV infection, see above.

(c) Lamivudine

In vitro, ribavirin reduced the intracellular activation and antiretroviral activity of lamivudine.[20] However, in a study in 22 HIV-positive patients with hepatitis C, ribavirin 800 mg daily had no statistically significant effect on the pharmacokinetics of lamivudine (a 27% increase in AUC), and no effect on the intracellular activation of lamivudine, when compared with 24 similar patients who received placebo.[21]

For the possible risk of hepatic decompensation and possible lack of mitochondrial toxicity when lamivudine was given with ribavirin in patients with both chronic hepatitis C and HIV infection, see above.

(d) Stavudine

In vitro, ribavirin reduced the intracellular activation and antiretroviral activity of stavudine.[2,22] However, in a study in 5 HIV-positive patients with hepatitis C, ribavirin 800 mg daily had no statistically significant effect on the pharmacokinetics of stavudine (a 45% increase in AUC), and no effect on intracellular activation of stavudine, when compared with similar patients who received placebo.[21] Similarly, no decrease in the antiviral activity of stavudine (as assessed by plasma HIV-RNA loads) has been seen when ribavirin was given with interferon for hepatitis C infection in patients with HIV.[23,24]

In clinical study NR15961, the incidence of pancreatitis and/or lactic acidosis in patients concurrently treated with stavudine and interferon therapy with or without ribavirin was 3% (12 of 398 patients).[2]

For further evidence, and the possible risk of hepatic decompensation when stavudine was used with ribavirin in patients with both chronic hepatitis C and HIV infection, see above.

(e) Zidovudine

In vitro, ribavirin reduced the intracellular activation and antiretroviral activity of zidovudine.[2,25] However, in a study in 14 patients with hepatitis C and HIV infections, giving ribavirin with zidovudine 300 mg twice daily had no significant effect on the pharmacokinetics of zidovudine.[26] Similarly, an earlier study in a study in 7 HIV-positive patients with hepatitis C, ribavirin 800 mg daily had no statistically significant effect on the pharmacokinetics of zidovudine (a 22% decrease in AUC), and no effect on the intracellular activation of zidovudine, when compared with similar patients who received placebo.[21] Moreover, in a study in 8 patients taking zidovudine, there was no statistically significant variation in HIV viral load or CD4+ counts after 3 or 6 months of ribavirin treatment, when compared with baseline values.[24]

One US manufacturer of ribavirin includes details of a study (NR15961) in which patients treated with zidovudine, interferon alfa and ribavirin had a higher incidence of severe neutropenia (15% versus 9%) and severe anaemia (5% versus 1%) than other similar patients not receiving zidovudine.[3]

For the possible risk of hepatic decompensation and possible lack of mitochondrial toxicity when zidovudine was given with ribavirin in patients with both chronic hepatitis C and HIV infection, see above.

Mechanism

Unknown.

Importance and management

There is some evidence that patients with both chronic hepatitis C and HIV-infection treated with interferon, ribavirin and NRTIs, in particular didanosine or stavudine, are at increased risk of lactic acidosis. There is also some limited evidence of an increased risk of hepatic decompensation with all NRTIs. Because of the risk of lactic acidosis, in the UK, the manufacturers of many NRTIs state that patients co-infected with hepatitis C and treated with interferon alfa with or without ribavirin should be closely monitored. Similarly, because of the risk of hepatic decompensation, ribavirin manufacturers and many US manufacturers of NRTIs advise caution and suggest that these patients should be closely monitored for treatment-associated toxicities. Note that ribavirin has a very long half-life and the potential for interactions continues for 2 months after stopping treatment. Additional specific advice for individual NRTIs is as follows.

The British HIV Association (BHIVA) recommends avoiding the concurrent use of **abacavir** with ribavirin for hepatitis C infection, if possible, particularly if ribavirin cannot be used at a dose of 1 g daily or greater, because of the evidence suggesting a reduced response to low-dose ribavirin. If abacavir cannot be avoided, they recommend using the maximum weight-based dose of ribavirin.[27] However, other authors consider that abacavir use is acceptable.[7] If abacavir is used concurrently, it would seem prudent to monitor ribavirin efficacy closely.

As a result of the increased risk of mitochondrial toxicity, many manufacturers of **didanosine** and ribavirin state that concurrent use is not recommended, and the US manufacturers of didanosine[13] and ribavirin,[28] and BHIVA[27] specifically contraindicate concurrent use. Given the availability of less toxic alternatives, this seems prudent.

BHIVA recommends avoiding the concurrent use of **stavudine** and ribavirin, if at all possible, because of the risk of mitochondrial toxicity.[27] The UK manufacturers of ribavirin[2,4] give similar advice. If stavudine is given, on the basis of the antagonistic *in vitro* data, one UK manufacturer of ribavirin advises that plasma HIV-RNA loads are closely monitored in patients taking ribavirin with stavudine to ensure continued efficacy.[2] However, note that there is limited evidence that reduced stavudine efficacy does not occur.

BHIVA recommends avoiding the concurrent use of **zidovudine** with ribavirin, if at all possible, because of the increased myelosuppression seen.[27] In patients already taking zidovudine, consideration should be given to replacing it if treatment with ribavirin is required, particularly those with a previous history of zidovudine-induced anaemia.[2,4] If used concurrently, on the basis of antagonistic *in vitro* activity, one manufacturer of ribavirin advises that plasma HIV-RNA loads are closely monitored to ensure continued zidovudine efficacy.[2] However, there is limited evidence that ribavirin does not alter zidovudine efficacy.

1. Fleischer R, Boxwell D, Sherman KE. Nucleoside analogues and mitochondrial toxicity. *Clin Infect Dis* (2004) 38, e79–e80.
2. Copegus (Ribavirin). Roche Products Ltd. UK Summary of product characteristics, March 2014.
3. Copegus (Ribavirin). Genentech, Inc. US Prescribing information, August 2011.
4. Rebetol Hard Capsules (Ribavirin). Merck Sharp & Dohme Ltd. UK Summary of product characteristics, April 2014.
5. Vispo E, Barriero P, Pineda JA, Mira JA, Maida I, Martin-Carbonero L, Rodriguez-Nóvoa S, Santos I, López-Cortes LF, Merino D, Rivero A, Soriano V. Low response to pegylated interferon plus ribavirin in HIV-infected patients with chronic hepatitis C treated with abacavir. *Antivir Ther* (2008) 13, 429–37.
6. Bani-Sadr F, Denoeud L, Morand P, Lunel-Fabiani F, Pol S, Cacoub P, Perronne C, Carrat F; Agence Nationale pour la Recherche contre le SIDA et les hépatites virales HC02-Ribavic Study Team. Early virologic failure in HIV-coinfected hepatitis C patients treated with peginterferon-ribavirin combination: Does abacavir play a role? *J Acquir Immune Defic Syndr* (2007) 45, 123–5.
7. Solas C, Pambrun E, Winnock M, Salmon D, Poizot-Martin I, Dominguez S, Bani-Sadr F, Izopet J, Garraffo R, Peytavin G; for The ANRS CO-13 HEPAVIH Study Group. Ribavirin and abacavir drug interaction in HIV-HCV coinfected patients: fact or fiction? *AIDS* (2012) [Epub].
8. Amorosa VK, Slim J, Mounzer K, Bruno C, Hoffman-Terry M, Dorey-Stein Z, Ferrara T, Kostman JR, Lo Re V. The influence of abacavir and other antiretroviral agents on virological response to hepatitis C virus therapy among antiretroviral-treated HIV-infected patients. *Antivir Ther* (2010) 15, 91–9.
9. Laufer N, Laguno M, Perez I, Cifuentes C, Murillas J, Vidal F, Bonet L, Veloso S, Gatell JM, Mallolas J. Abacavir does not influence the rate of sustained virological response in HIV-HCV coinfected patients treated with pegylated interferon and weight adjusted ribavirin. *Antivir Ther* (2008) 13, 953–7.
10. Japour AJ, Lertora JJ, Meehan PM, Erice A, Connor JD, Griffith BP, Clax PA, Holden-Wiltse J, Hussey S, Walesky M, Cooney E, Pollard R, Timpone J, McLaren C, Johanneson N, Wood K, Booth DK, Bassiakos Y, Crumpacker CS, for the AIDS Clinical Trials Group 231 Protocol Team. A phase-1 study of the safety, pharmacokinetics, and antiviral activity of combination didanosine and ribavirin in patients with HIV-1 disease. *J Acquir Immune Defic Syndr Hum Retrovirol* (1996) 13, 235–46.
11. Lertora JJL, Harrison M, Dreisbach AW, Van Dyke R. Lack of pharmacokinetic interaction between DDI and ribavirin in HIV infected children. *J Investig Med* (1999) 47, 106A.
12. Videx EC (Didanosine). Bristol-Myers Squibb Pharmaceuticals Ltd. UK Summary of product characteristics, June 2009.
13. Videx EC (Didanosine). Bristol-Myers Squibb Company. US Prescribing information, November 2011.
14. Butt AA. Fatal lactic acidosis and pancreatitis associated with ribavirin and didanosine therapy. *AIDS Read* (2003) 13, 344–8.
15. Lafeuillade A, Hittinger G, Chadapaud S. Increased mitochondrial toxicity with ribavirin in HIV/HCV coinfection. *Lancet* (2001) 357, 280–1.
16. Salmon-Céron D, Chauvelot-Moachon L, Abad S, Silbermann B, Sogni P. Mitochondrial toxic effects and ribavirin. *Lancet* (2001) 357, 1803–4.
17. Moreno A, Quereda C, Moreno L, Perez-Elías MJ, Muriel A, Casado JL, Antela A, Dronda F, Navas E, Bárcena R, Moreno S. High rate of didanosine-related mitochondrial toxicity in HIV/HCV-coinfected patients receiving ribavirin. *Antivir Ther* (2004) 9, 133–8.
18. Laguno M, Milinkovic A, de Lazzari E, Murillas J, Martínez E, Blanco JL, Loncá M, Biglia A, Leon A, García M, Larrousse M, García F, Miró JM, Gatell JM, Mallolas J. Incidence and risk factors for mitochondrial toxicity in treated HIV/HCV-coinfected patients. *Antivir Ther* (2005) 10, 423–9.
19. Bani-Sadr F, Carrat F, Pol S, Hor R, Rosenthal E, Goujard C, Morand P, Lunel-Fabiani F, Salmon-Ceron D, Piroth L, Pialoux G, Bentata M, Cacoub P, Perronne C; The ANRS Hc02-Ribavic Study Team. Risk factors for symptomatic mitochondrial toxicity in HIV/hepatitis C virus-coinfected patients during interferon plus ribavirin-based therapy. *J Acquir Immune Defic Syndr* (2005) 40, 47–52.
20. Huh A, Nam J, Chang K, Yeom J, Song Y, Kim S, Lee J, Kim J. Antagonistic effect of ribavirin on lamivudine against HIV-1 infection (abstract I-1939). *Intersci Conf Antimicrob Agents Chemother* (2001) 41, 348.
21. Rodriguez-Torres M, Torriani FJ, Soriano V, Borucki MJ, Lissen E, Sulkowski M, Dieterich D, Wang K, Gries J-M, Hoggard PG, Back D; APRICOT Study Group. Effect of ribavirin on intracellular and plasma pharmacokinetics of nucleoside reverse transcriptase inhibitors in patients with human immunodeficiency virus-hepatitis C virus coinfection: results of a randomized clinical study. *Antimicrob Agents Chemother* (2005) 49, 3997–4008.
22. Hoggard PG, Kewn S, Barry MG, Khoo SH, Back DJ. Effects of drugs on 2',3'-dideoxy-2',3'-didehydrothymidine phosphorylation in vitro. *Antimicrob Agents Chemother* (1997) 41, 1231–6.
23. Salmon-Céron D, Lassalle R, Pruvost A, Benech H, Bouvier-Alias M, Payan C, Goujard C, Bonnet E, Zoulim F, Morlat P, Sogni P, Pérusat S, Tréluyer J-M, Chêne G, and the CORIST-ANRS HC1 Study Group. Interferon-ribavirin in association with stavudine has no impact on plasma human immunodeficiency virus (HIV) type 1 level in patients coinfected with HIV and hepatitis C virus: a CORIST-ANRS HC1 trial. *Clin Infect Dis* (2003) 36, 1295–1304.
24. Zylberberg H, Benhamou Y, Lagneaux JL, Landau A, Chaix M-L, Fontaine H, Bochet M, Poynard T, Katlama C, Pialoux G, Bréchot C, Pol S. Safety and efficacy of interferon-ribavirin combination therapy in HCV-HIV coinfected subjects: an early report. *Gut* (2000) 47, 694–7.
25. Vogt MW, Hartshorn KL, Furman PA, Chou TC, Fyfe JA, Coleman LA, Crumpacker C, Schooley RT, Hirsch MS. Ribavirin antagonizes the effect of azidothymidine on HIV replication. *Science* (1987) 235, 1376–9.
26. Aweeka FT, Kang M, Yu J-Y, Lizak P, Alston B, Chung RT, for the AIDS Clinical Trials Group 5092s Study Team. Pharmacokinetic evaluation of the effects of ribavirin on zidovudine triphosphate formulation: ACTG 5092s Study Team. *HIV Med* (2007) 8, 288–94.
27. Wilkins E, Nelson M, Agarwal K, Awoyemi D, Barnes E, Bhagani S, Brook G, Brown A, Castelino S, Cooke G, Fisher M, Geretti AM, James R, Kulasegaram R, Leen C, Mutimer D, Orkin C, Page E, Palfreeman A, Papineni P, Rodger A, Tong CY on behalf of the British HIV Association. British HIV Association guidelines for the management of hepatitis viruses in adults infected with HIV 2013. *HIV Med* (2013) 14 (suppl 4), 1–71.
28. Rebetol (Ribavirin). Merck Sharp and Dohme Corp. US Prescribing information, July 2014.

NRTIs + Rifamycins

Rifabutin appears to increase the clearance of zidovudine, but does not affect didanosine or stavudine exposure. Buffered didanosine did not alter rifabutin pharmacokinetics in one study, although an isolated case

describes undetectable rifabutin concentrations in a patient taking antiretrovirals including buffered didanosine.

Rifampicin (rifampin) appears to increase the clearance of zidovudine, and is predicted to interact similarly with abacavir. Marked anaemia was seen in one study in patients given rifampicin with isoniazid, pyrazinamide, and ethambutol.

Clinical evidence

(a) Didanosine

In a study in 12 patients with AIDS, **rifabutin** 300 to 600 mg daily for 12 days did not appreciably alter the pharmacokinetics of [buffered] didanosine 167 to 250 mg twice daily.[1] The steady-state pharmacokinetics of **rifabutin** were not affected by didanosine (buffered sachet),[2] which suggests that the buffer used in the didanosine preparation had no effect on **rifabutin** absorption.[2] However, a case report describes a patient taking lopinavir boosted with ritonavir, efavirenz, lamivudine and buffered didanosine who had impaired **rifabutin** absorption. When **rifabutin** was taken 30 minutes after didanosine, **rifabutin** concentrations were undetectable, but when **rifabutin** was taken 3 hours after didanosine, **rifabutin** concentrations were apparent.[3]

(b) Stavudine

A study in 10 HIV-positive subjects found that **rifabutin** 300 mg daily had no effect on the pharmacokinetics of stavudine 30 mg or 40 mg twice daily and the incidence of adverse effects did not increase.[4]

(c) Zidovudine

The pharmacokinetics of **rifabutin** are not affected by the concurrent use of zidovudine in patients with AIDS,[5] and **rifabutin** does not affect the pharmacokinetics of zidovudine in HIV-positive patients,[6] although one analysis found a trend towards increased zidovudine clearance.[7] No increase in adverse effects appears to occur when **rifabutin** is given with zidovudine.[5]

In a retrospective study of healthy subjects and HIV-positive individuals, the clearance of zidovudine was increased by 132% by **rifampicin (rifampin)** and by 50% by **rifabutin**, suggesting that the enzyme-inducing effects of **rifabutin** are less than those of **rifampicin**, so a smaller interaction would be expected.[8]

Another study in 4 HIV-positive patients found that **rifampicin** reduced the AUC and increased the clearance of zidovudine in all patients. When **rifampicin** was stopped in one patient, the AUC of zidovudine doubled.[9] A later study of the same interaction in 8 HIV-positive men found that **rifampicin** induced the glucuronidation of zidovudine and suggested that the effect wore off 14 days after stopping **rifampicin**.[10]

A comparative study in HIV-positive patients given zidovudine and a rifampicin-based antimycobacterial regimen (initially **isoniazid**, **rifampicin**, **pyrazinamide**, and **ethambutol**, and then **isoniazid** with **rifampicin**) for 8 months, found no evidence of an adverse interaction. However, marked anaemia occurred in those subjects given both groups of drugs, but it was not necessary to permanently stop zidovudine in any patient.[11]

Mechanism

The majority of NRTIs are excreted renally and would not therefore be expected to be affected by enzyme-inducing drugs such as rifampicin and rifabutin. Zidovudine and **abacavir** are partially metabolised by glucuronidation, which is induced by rifabutin and rifampicin.

Importance and management

Rifampicin, and to a lesser extent rifabutin, increase the clearance of zidovudine and would be predicted to affect **abacavir**[12] similarly. However, this interaction is not considered to be clinically important. The British HIV Association (BHIVA) advise that standard doses of zidovudine and abacavir can be used with rifabutin or rifampicin.[13] Similarly, no pharmacokinetic interaction occurs with didanosine and stavudine, and would not be expected for other NRTIs. The isolated case of undetectable rifabutin concentrations with buffered didanosine is not supported by the controlled study and is therefore not of general relevance. The British HIV Association (BHIVA) advise that standard doses of enteric-coated didanosine, emtricitabine, lamivudine and stavudine can be used with rifabutin or rifampicin.[13] However, note that alternatives to stavudine and didanosine should be used if isoniazid is part of tuberculosis therapy, see 'NRTIs + Isoniazid', p.976.

The clinical relevance of the marked anaemia seen in one small study of the use of zidovudine with a rifampicin-based regimen for tuberculosis is uncertain.

The UK manufacturer of **rifabutin** suggests that no significant interaction would be expected between **rifabutin** and zalcitabine.[14]

1. Sahai J, Foss N, Li R, Narang PK, Cameron DW. Rifabutin and didanosine interaction in AIDS patients. *Clin Pharmacol Ther* (1993) 53, 197.
2. Li RC, Narang PK, Sahai J, Cameron W, Bianchine JR. Rifabutin absorption in the gut unaltered by concomitant administration of didanosine in AIDS patients. *Antimicrob Agents Chemother* (1997) 41, 1566–70.
3. Marzolini C, Chave J-P, Telenti A, Brenas-Chinchon L, Biollaz J. Impaired absorption of rifabutin by concomitant administration of didanosine. *AIDS* (2001) 15, 2203–4.
4. Piscitelli SC, Kelly G, Walker RE, Kovacs J, Falloon J, Davey RT, Raje S, Masur H, Polis MA. A multiple drug interaction study of stavudine with agents for opportunistic infections in human immunodeficiency virus-infected patients. *Antimicrob Agents Chemother* (1999) 43, 647–50.
5. Li RC, Nightingale S, Lewis RC, Colburn DC, Narang PK. Lack of effect of concomitant zidovudine on rifabutin kinetics in patients with AIDS-related complex. *Antimicrob Agents Chemother* (1996) 40, 1397–1402.
6. Gallicano K, Sahai J, Swick L, Seguin I, Pakuts A, Cameron DW. Effect of rifabutin on the pharmacokinetics of zidovudine in patients infected with human immunodeficiency virus. *Clin Infect Dis* (1995) 21, 1008–11.
7. Narang PK, Sale M. Population based assessment of rifabutin (R) effect on zidovudine (ZDV) disposition in AIDS patients. *Clin Pharmacol Ther* (1993) 53, 219.
8. Narang PK, Gupta S, Li RC, Strolin-Benedetti M, Della Bruna C, Bianchine JR. Assessing dosing implications of enzyme inducing potential: rifabutin (RIF) vs. rifampin (RFM). *Intersci Conf Antimicrob Agents Chemother* (1993) 33, 228.
9. Burger DM, Meenhorst PL, Koks CHW, Beijnen JH. Pharmacokinetic interaction between rifampin and zidovudine. *Antimicrob Agents Chemother* (1993) 37, 1426–31.
10. Gallicano KD, Sahai J, Shukla VK, Seguin I, Pakuts A, Kwok D, Foster BC, Cameron DW. Induction of zidovudine glucuronidation and amination pathways by rifampicin in HIV-infected patients. *Br J Clin Pharmacol* (1999) 48, 168–79.
11. Antoniskis D, Easley AC, Espina BM, Davidson PT, Barnes PF. Combined toxicity of zidovudine and antituberculosis chemotherapy. *Am Rev Respir Dis* (1992) 145, 430–4.
12. Ziagen (Abacavir sulfate). ViiV Healthcare UK Ltd. UK Summary of product characteristics, October 2011.
13. Pozniak AL, Coyne KM, Miller RF, Lipman MCI, Freedman AR, Ormerod LP, Johnson MA, Collins S, Lucas SB on behalf of the BHIVA Guidelines Subcommittee. British HIV Association guidelines for the treatment of TB/ HIV co-infection 2011. *HIV Med* (2011) 12, 517.
14. Mycobutin (Rifabutin). Pfizer Ltd. UK Summary of product characteristics, December 2013.

NRTIs + Tenofovir

Tenofovir increases didanosine exposure: an increased risk of pancreatitis and peripheral neuropathy has been reported, as well as a high rate of treatment failure. No pharmacokinetic interaction occurs between tenofovir and abacavir, emtricitabine, lamivudine, or stavudine. Sole triple-NRTI regimens such as tenofovir and lamivudine with abacavir or didanosine have been associated with a high rate of treatment failure.

Clinical evidence, mechanism, importance and management

Note that tenofovir is a nucleotide (nucleoside monophosphate) analogue and is often classed as an NRTI. Current local and national guidelines should be consulted when choosing NRTI combinations. The US and UK guidelines recommend tenofovir with emtricitabine as the preferred NRTI backbone (see also 'NRTIs + NRTIs', p.977) for combination with an NNRTI or an HIV-protease inhibitor boosted with ritonavir or an integrase inhibitor in treatment-naive patients.[1,2] In US guidelines, lamivudine can be substituted for emtricitabine, and *vice versa*.[1] The UK guidelines state there is no routine role for other NRTI backbones, and they specifically state that there is no place for the use of stavudine- or didanosine-containing regimens as initial therapy, due to the associations with significant mitochondrial and hepatic toxicities.[2] Note that antiretroviral regimens consisting of solely NRTIs are not recommended, either as sole dual-NRTI combinations or triple-NRTIs regimens, because these have shown suboptimal virological activity to preferred regimens.[1]

A. Dual NRTI backbones

(a) Abacavir

In a study in HIV-positive patients taking HAART, no apparent pharmacokinetic interaction was found between tenofovir and abacavir.[3] Similarly, in a pharmacokinetic study in 8 healthy subjects, tenofovir caused a negligible 10% increase in abacavir exposure, and tenofovir pharmacokinetics did not differ from historical controls.[4] No dose adjustment would be expected to be needed if tenofovir and abacavir were used together.

(b) Didanosine

The AUC of buffered didanosine 250 mg or 400 mg was increased by 44% when it was given one hour before tenofovir.[5] Similarly, the AUC of enteric-coated didanosine 400 mg was increased by 48% and 60% when didanosine was given 2 hours before or at the same time as tenofovir disoproxil fumarate 300 mg, respectively.[6] The pharmacokinetics of tenofovir were unchanged.[5,6] Another study found that the AUC of enteric-coated didanosine 250 mg (simultaneously or 2 hours apart, fasted or with food) was about equivalent to that seen with didanosine 400 mg alone when tenofovir was given.[6]

The main concern with raised didanosine exposure is the increased risk of adverse effects, particularly pancreatitis and peripheral neuropathy. One retrospective analysis found that 5 of 185 patients receiving didanosine with tenofovir developed pancreatitis compared with one of 182 taking didanosine without tenofovir and none of 208 taking tenofovir without didanosine, suggesting an increased risk of pancreatitis with the combination. All 6 cases of pancreatitis were in women without renal impairment, who weighed less than 60 kg. Five had received a reduced dose of didanosine (250 mg) and one had received didanosine 400 mg. Pancreatitis developed after 12 to 24 weeks.[7] Similarly, another analysis found that the use of tenofovir with didanosine (400 mg daily or 250 mg daily if weight less than 60 kg) was associated with a higher incidence of peripheral neuropathy (12% versus 4%) and pancreatitis (4% versus 0%) than use with lower doses of didanosine (100 mg to 250 mg daily).[8] However, another analysis did not find an enhanced risk of toxicity with the combination of didanosine and tenofovir at full dose during the first 6 months of use.[9] Tenofovir is rarely associated with acute renal failure, and in one study,[10] the concurrent use of didanosine with tenofovir was found to be associated with an increased risk of developing renal impairment (odds ratio 3.1). In an analysis of 5 HIV-positive patients with acute renal failure and 22 cases reported in the literature, all of whom were taking tenofovir, 9 patients were also taking didanosine. It was suggested that tenofovir-associated renal failure might be due to an interaction with didanosine,[11] although others contend that this does not necessarily infer an association.[12] Cases of pancreatitis[13,14] or lactic acidosis and renal failure[15-17] have been reported (the use of ritonavir might have been a factor in at least one of these cases[17]).

Furthermore, other studies have shown a high rate of treatment failure with a once daily combination of tenofovir disoproxil fumarate 300 mg, enteric-coated didanosine 250 mg, and either efavirenz or nevirapine in treatment-naive patients with high baseline viral loads and low CD4+ counts.[18-20] A poor immune response (lack of increase in CD4+ counts) has also been seen with full-dose didanosine with tenofovir regimens in treatment-experienced patients.[21]

The pharmacokinetic interaction between didanosine and tenofovir is established. Didanosine exposure would be expected to be increased when it is given with tenofovir, which could increase the risk of didanosine-related toxicity. For this reason, and because high rates of treatment failure have been reported with didanosine in combination with tenofovir and an NNRTI or lamivudine, the US and UK guidelines state that didanosine should not be given with tenofovir.[1,2] The US manufacturers state that the dose of didanosine should be reduced to 250 mg daily when given with tenofovir in patients weighing more than 60 kg with a creatinine clearance of at least 60 mL/minute;[5,22] and to 200 mg daily in patients weighing less than 60 kg and with a creatinine clearance of at least 60 mL/minute. In patients with a creatinine clearance of less than 60 mL/minute, the dose of didanosine, when given with tenofovir, has not been established.[22] However, the UK manufacturer of tenofovir notes that reducing the didanosine dose to 250 mg has been associated with a high rate of virological failure.[23] If concurrent use is considered unavoidable, patients should be closely monitored for didanosine-related adverse effects (e.g. pancreatitis, peripheral neuropathy) and for antiviral efficacy.[23]

(c) Emtricitabine

In a study in 16 healthy subjects, no pharmacokinetic interaction was reported between tenofovir disoproxil fumarate 300 mg daily and emtricitabine 200 mg daily, both for 7 days.[24] The UK and US guidelines for treatment of HIV infections recommend the combination of tenofovir and emtricitabine as the preferred NRTI backbone of antiretroviral therapy.[1,2] Tenofovir and emtricitabine are available in a fixed dose combination product.

(d) Lamivudine

In a study in HIV-positive patients taking HAART, no apparent pharmacokinetic interaction was found between tenofovir and lamivudine.[3] The manufacturer also briefly notes that there was no pharmacokinetic interaction between tenofovir and lamivudine.[23] The US guidelines state that lamivudine can be substituted for emtricitabine for combination with tenofovir as part of preferred HIV antiretroviral regimens.[1]

(e) Stavudine

There is information to suggest that tenofovir disoproxil fumarate 300 mg does not alter concentrations of stavudine 100 mg.[25] The UK guidelines state that stavudine is not recommended for use as one of the NRTIs for initial therapy of HIV because of its toxicity.[2]

B. Triple NRTI regimens

The triple combination of tenofovir, **lamivudine**, and **abacavir** used alone was unexpectedly associated with a high rate of treatment failure (early virological nonresponse) in clinical studies.[26] Similarly, a once daily triple combination of tenofovir, **didanosine**, and **lamivudine** used alone was associated with a high rate of treatment failure (early virological non-response) in a clinical study in treatment-naive patients.[27] Use of such regimens is not recommended,[1,2] with the possible exception of tenofovir with **lamivudine** and **zidovudine**.[1]

C. Quadruple NRTI regimens

The 2012 US guidelines state that the quadruple NRTI regimen of **abacavir**, **lamivudine**, **tenofovir**, and **zidovudine** cannot be recommended because of the incidence of serious toxicity with this regimen was high.[1]

1. Panel on Antiretroviral Guidelines for Adults and Adolescents. Guidelines for the use of antiretroviral agents in HIV-1-infected adults and adolescents. Department of Health and Human Services. (April 2015). 1–288. Available at: https://aidsinfo.nih.gov/contentfiles/lvguidelines/adultandadolescentgl.pdf (accessed 22/09/15).
2. Williams I, Churchill D, Anderson J, Boffito M, Bower M, Cairns G, Cwynarski K, Edwards S, Fidler S, Fisher M, Freedman A, Geretti AM, Gilleece Y, Horne R, Johnson M, Khoo S, Leen C, Marshall N, Nelson M, Orkin C, Paton N, Phillips A, Post F, Pozniak A, Sabin C, Trevelion R, Ustianowski A, Walsh J, Waters L, Wilkins E, Winston A, Youle M. British HIV Association guidelines for the treatment of HIV-1-positive adults with antiretroviral therapy 2012 (Updated 2013). *HIV Med* (2014), 15 (Suppl 1) 1–85.
3. Pruvost A, Negredo E, Théodoro F, Puig J, Levi M, Ayen R, Grassi J, Clotet B. Pilot pharmacokinetic study of human immunodeficiency virus-infected patients receiving tenofovir disoproxil fumarate (TDF): Investigation of systemic and intracellular interactions between TDF and abacavir, lamivudine and lopinavir-ritonavir. *Antimicrob Agents Chemother* (2009) 53, 1937–43.
4. Kearney BP, Isaacson E, Sayre J, Ebrahimi R, Cheng AK. The pharmacokinetics of abacavir, a purine nucleoside analog, are not affected by tenofovir DF. *Intersci Conf Antimicrob Agents Chemother* (2003) 43, 36.
5. Viread (Tenofovir disoproxil fumarate). Gilead Sciences, Inc. US Prescribing information, August 2012.
6. Kearney BP, Sayre JR, Flaherty JF, Chen S-S, Kaul S, Cheng AK. Drug-drug and drug-food interactions between tenofovir disoproxil fumarate and didanosine. *J Clin Pharmacol* (2005) 45, 1360–7.
7. Martinez E, Milinkovic A, de Lazzari E, Ravasi G, Blanco JL, Larrousse M, Mallolas J, García F, Miró JM, Gatell JM. Pancreatic toxic effects associated with co-administration of didanosine and tenofovir in HIV-infected adults. *Lancet* (2004) 364, 65–7.
8. Young B, Weidle PJ, Baker RK, Armon C, Wood KC, Moorman AC, Holmberg SD; HIV Outpatient Study (HOPS) Investigators. Short-term safety and tolerability of didanosine combined with high- versus low-dose tenofovir disproxil [sic] fumarate in ambulatory HIV-1-infected persons. *AIDS Patient Care STDS* (2006) 20, 238–44.
9. Barrios A, Maida I, Perez-Saleme L, Negredo E, Clotet B, Vilaro J, Domingo P, Estrada V, Santos J, Asensi V, Labarga P, Terron J, Vergara A, Garcia-Benayas T, Martin-Carbonero L, Barreiro P, Gonzalez-Lahoz J, Soriano V. Safety and efficacy of combinations based on didanosine 400 mg od plus tenofovir 300 mg od. *Intersci Conf Antimicrob Agents Chemother* (2003) 43, 314.
10. Crane HM, Kestenbaum B, Harrington RD, Kitahata MM. Amprenavir and didanosine are associated with declining kidney function among patients receiving tenofovir. *AIDS* (2007) 21, 1431–9.
11. Zimmermann AE, Pizzoferrato T, Bedford J, Morris A, Hoffman R, Braden G. Tenofovir-associated acute and chronic kidney disease: a case of multiple drug interactions. *Clin Infect Dis* (2006) 42, 283–90.
12. Winston JA, Shepp DH. The role of drug interactions and monitoring in the prevention of tenofovir-associated kidney disease. *Clin Infect Dis* (2006) 42, 1657–8; author reply ibid.,1658.
13. Blanchard JN, Wohlfeiler M, Canas A, King K, Lonergan JT. Pancreatitis with didanosine and tenofovir disoproxil fumarate. *Clin Infect Dis* (2003) 37, e57–e62. Correction. ibid. 995.
14. Kirian MA, Higginson RT, Pecora Fulco P. Acute onset of pancreatitis with concomitant use of tenofovir and didanosine. *Ann Pharmacother* (2004) 38, 1660–3.
15. Murphy MD, O'Hearn M, Chou S. Fatal lactic acidosis and acute renal failure after addition of tenofovir to an antiretroviral regimen containing didanosine. *Clin Infect Dis* (2003) 36, 1082–5.
16. Guo Y, Fung HB. Fatal lactic acidosis associated with coadministration of didanosine and tenofovir disoproxil fumarate. *Pharmacotherapy* (2004) 24, 1089–94.
17. Rollot F, Nazal E-M, Chauvelot-Moachon L, Kélaidi C, Daniel N, Saba M, Abad S, Blanche P. Tenofovir-related Fanconi syndrome with nephrogenic diabetes insipidus in a patient with acquired immunodeficiency syndrome: the role of lopinavir-ritonavir-didanosine. *Clin Infect Dis* (2003) 37, e174–6.
18. Hodder SL. Re: Important new clinical data. Potential early virologic failure associated with the combination antiretroviral regimen of tenofovir disoproxil fumarate, didanosine, and either efavirenz or nevirapine in HIV treatment-naïve patients with high baseline viral loads. Bristol-Myers Squibb Company, November 2004. Available at: www.fda.gov/downloads/ForConsumers/ByAudience/ForPatientAdvocates/HIVandAIDSActivities/UCM151456.pdf (accessed 01/10/15).
19. Podzamczer D, Ferrer E, Gatell JM, Niubo J, Dalmau D, Leon A, Knobel H, Polo C, Iniguez D, Ruiz I. Early virological failure with a combination of tenofovir, didanosine and efavirenz. *Antivir Ther* (2005) 10, 171–7.
20. Maitland D, Moyle G, Hand J, Mandalia S, Boffito M, Nelson M, Gazzard B. Early virologic failure in HIV-1 infected subjects on didanosine/tenofovir/efavirenz: 12-week results from a randomized trial. *AIDS* (2005) 19, 1183–8.
21. Negredo E, Bonjoch A, Paredes R, Puig J, Clotet B. Compromised immunologic recovery in treatment-experienced patients with HIV infection receiving both tenofovir disoproxil fumarate and didanosine in the TORO studies. *Clin Infect Dis* (2005) 41, 901–5.
22. Videx EC (Didanosine). Bristol-Myers Squibb Company. US Prescribing information, November 2011.
23. Viread (Tenofovir disoproxil fumarate). Gilead Sciences Ltd. UK Summary of product characteristics, January 2012.
24. Blum MR, Chittick GE, Begley JA, Zong J. Steady-state pharmacokinetics of emtricitabine and tenofovir disoproxil fumarate administered alone and in combination in healthy volunteers. *J Clin Pharmacol* (2007) 47, 751–9.
25. Anon. E. Tenofovir drug interactions: ddI and d4T. *TreatmentUpdate* (2003) 15 (Part 2), 7.
26. Manion DJ. Important drug warning. Re: early virologic non-response in patients with HIV infection treated with lamivudine, abacavir and tenofovir. GlaxoSmithKline, July 2003. Available at: http://www.fda.gov/downloads/safety/medwatch/safetyinformation/safetyalertsforhumanmedicalproducts/ucm169506.pdf (accessed 01/10/15).
27. Toole J. Important drug warning. High rate of virologic failure in patients with HIV infection treated with a once-daily triple NRTI regimen containing didanosine, lamivudine, and tenofovir. October 2003. Available at: http://www.fda.gov/downloads/safety/medwatch/safetyinformation/safetyalertsforhumanmedical-products/ucm169505.pdf (accessed 01/10/15).

NRTIs + Valproate

Valproate increases zidovudine exposure, and one case of severe anaemia has been attributed to the interaction. A case of liver toxicity has also been reported on the concurrent use of these drugs.

Clinical evidence

In a study in 6 HIV-positive subjects, the AUC and plasma concentration of **zidovudine** 100 mg every 8 hours were increased by 80% when it was given with valproic acid 250 mg or 500 mg every 8 hours for 4 days. No adverse reactions, changes in hepatic or renal function, or alterations in the blood picture were reported.[1] A case report describes a patient with AIDS taking zidovudine 100 mg five times daily who had a 2- to 3-fold increase in the minimum and maximum serum zidovudine concentrations, and a 74% increase in the CSF concentration of zidovudine while taking valproic acid 500 mg three times daily.[2] In another report, a patient taking carbamazepine, clobazam, and gabapentin was given **zidovudine**, **lamivudine**, and **abacavir**. Nine months later, valproic acid 500 mg twice daily was added because of a seizure frequency of greater than one per month. At this time, his haemoglobin concentration was normal. About 2 months later, he was found to have severe anaemia, requiring a blood transfusion. **Stavudine** was substituted for zidovudine and 4 months later his haemoglobin was normal. The adverse haematological effects were attributed to an interaction between valproate and zidovudine.[3] Another HIV-positive patient, who had been taking valproate for 2 years, and zidovudine, developed severe encephalopathy, adult respiratory distress syndrome, and liver failure (steatosis). Both valproate and zidovudine were stopped, and the patient gradually recovered.[4]

For the possible effect of zidovudine on phenytoin concentrations, see 'Phenytoin + Zidovudine', p.610.

Mechanism

The evidence indicates that the metabolism (glucuronidation) of zidovudine is inhibited by valproate so that its bioavailability is increased.[1,2] It was suggested that this caused the haematological toxicity in the case reported.[3]

Importance and management

Information regarding an interaction between the NRTIs and valproate seems to be limited to the papers cited, but an interaction between zidovudine and valproate would appear to be established. It would therefore seem prudent to monitor for increases in zidovudine adverse effects and possible toxicity if valproate is added. With the exception of **abacavir**, the other NRTIs do not undergo significant glucuronidation (see 'Antivirals', p.893), and would therefore not be expected to interact with valproate.

Note that there has been some concern about using valproate in HIV infection, but there seems to be no established reason to avoid or specifically promote the use of valproate in HIV-infection *per se*.

1. Lertora JJL, Rege AB, Greenspan DL, Akula S, George WJ, Hyslop NE, Agrawal KC. Pharmacokinetic interaction between zidovudine and valproic acid in patients infected with human immunodeficiency virus. *Clin Pharmacol Ther* (1994) 56, 272–8.
2. Akula SK, Rege AB, Dreisbach AW, Dejace PMJT, Lertora JJL. Valproic acid increases cerebrospinal fluid zidovudine levels in a patient with AIDS. *Am J Med Sci* (1997) 313, 244–6.
3. Antoniou T, Gough K, Yoong D, Arbess G. Severe anemia secondary to a probable drug interaction between zidovudine and valproic acid. *Clin Infect Dis* (2004) 38, e38–40.
4. Leppik IE, Gapany S, Walczak T. An HIV-positive patient with epilepsy. *Epilepsy Behav* (2003) 4 (Suppl 1), S17–S19.

NRTIs; Abacavir + Antiepileptics; Enzyme-inducing

The UK manufacturer of abacavir predicts that potent enzyme inducers such as phenobarbital and phenytoin might slightly decrease abacavir concentrations by affecting glucuronyltransferases.[1] The US manufacturer however does not mention this potential interaction.[2] Bear in mind the possibility of an interaction should a patient taking enzyme-inducing antiepileptics have a reduced response to abacavir.

1. Ziagen (Abacavir sulfate). ViiV Healthcare UK Ltd. UK Summary of product characteristics, October 2011.
2. Ziagen (Abacavir sulfate). ViiV Healthcare. US Prescribing information, May 2012.

NRTIs; Didanosine + Allopurinol

Allopurinol increases didanosine exposure.

Clinical evidence

In a study, buffered didanosine 400 mg was given to 14 healthy subjects, with and without allopurinol 300 mg daily for 7 days. Allopurinol increased the AUC of didanosine 2.1-fold, and increased its maximum serum concentration by 69%.[1] Similar findings were seen in HIV-positive subjects.[2] Moreover, the addition of allopurinol 300 mg daily allowed the dose of didanosine to be halved from 400 mg daily to 200 mg daily in 4 patients taking buffered didanosine, hydroxycarbamide (hydroxyurea) and chloroquine. Didanosine plasma concentrations and antiviral efficacy were unchanged when compared with pre-treatment concentrations in patients taking didanosine 400 mg daily without allopurinol.[3] The US manufacturer also notes that, in subjects with renal impairment, allopurinol 300 mg increased the AUC and maximum plasma concentration of a single 200-mg dose of didanosine 3.1-fold and 2.3-fold, respectively.[4]

Mechanism

The UK manufacturer notes that allopurinol might increase the exposure to didanosine by inhibiting xanthine oxidase, an enzyme involved in didanosine metabolism.[5]

Importance and management

The pharmacokinetic interaction between didanosine and allopurinol would appear to be established, and was formerly studied for its therapeutic benefit.[3] However, if the dose of didanosine is not reduced, there is the potential for an increase in didanosine adverse effects. The manufacturers of didanosine state that the concurrent use of allopurinol with didanosine is contraindicated,[5] or is not recommended,[4] and that patients requiring allopurinol should be changed from didanosine to an alternative antiretroviral regimen.[5] They also state that other xanthine oxidase inhibitors (such as **febuxostat**) might interact similarly,[5] so some caution would be warranted.

1. Liang D, Breaux K, Nornoo A Phadungpojna S, Rodriguez-Barradas M, Bates TR. Pharmacokinetic interaction between didanosine (ddI) and allopurinol in healthy volunteers. *Intersci Conf Antimicrob Agents Chemother* (1999) 39, 25.
2. Liang D, Breaux K, Rodriguez-Barradas M, Bates TR. Allopurinol increases didanosine absorption in HIV-infected patients. *Intersci Conf Antimicrob Agents Chemother* (2001) 41, 16.
3. Boelaert JR, Dom GM, Huitema ADR, Beijnen JH, Lange JMA. The boosting of didanosine by allopurinol permits a halving of the didanosine dosage. *AIDS* (2002) 16, 2221–3.
4. Videx EC (Didanosine). Bristol-Myers Squibb Company. US Prescribing information, November 2011.
5. Videx EC (Didanosine). Bristol-Myers Squibb Pharmaceuticals Ltd. UK Summary of product characteristics, June 2009.

NRTIs; Didanosine + Loperamide or Metoclopramide

Loperamide and metoclopramide do not appear to alter the pharmacokinetics of didanosine.

Clinical evidence, mechanism, importance and management

In a study in 6 men and 6 women who were HIV-positive, the pharmacokinetics of oral buffered didanosine 300 mg were not altered by four 4-mg doses of loperamide, given 19, 13, 7 and one hour before the didanosine. The rate of didanosine absorption (time to maximum concentration) was decreased but the extent of absorption (AUC) was unchanged. Similarly, the pharmacokinetics of oral buffered didanosine 300 mg were found to be unaffected by 10 mg of intravenous metoclopramide.[1] It appears that neither delaying nor accelerating gastrointestinal transit time appreciably alters the pharmacokinetics of didanosine, which is acid labile. On the basis of this study the authors conclude that neither the dose nor the frequency of didanosine administration need to be altered if either loperamide or metoclopramide is given concurrently.[1]

1. Knupp CA, Milbrath RL, Barbhaiya RH. Effect of metoclopramide and loperamide on the pharmacokinetics of didanosine in HIV seropositive asymptomatic male and female patients. *Eur J Clin Pharmacol* (1993) 45, 409–13.

NRTIs; Stavudine + Doxorubicin

***In vitro* evidence suggests that doxorubicin might inhibit the activation of stavudine, but evidence from one clinical study shows that chemotherapy including doxorubicin did not alter the antiviral efficacy of a HAART regimen including stavudine.**

Clinical evidence, mechanism, importance and management

NRTIs such as stavudine need to be phosphorylated within cells before they become effective. *In vitro* studies using mononucleated blood cells found that doxorubicin might inhibit stavudine phosphorylation at clinically relevant concentrations.[1] In one clinical study comparing HAART (stavudine, lamivudine and nevirapine) alone with HAART and chemotherapy (bleomycin, doxorubicin and vincristine or alternatively oral etoposide in about one third of patients) in 112 therapy naive patients with HIV-associated Kaposi sarcoma, there was no difference in HIV viral load between the groups (82% had suppression to less than 50 copies/mL).[2]

The *in vitro* study suggests that the antiviral efficacy of stavudine might be compromised by the use of doxorubicin, and the manufacturers of stavudine recommend caution on concurrent use.[3,4] However, the clinical study shows that chemotherapy including doxorubicin did not alter the antiviral efficacy of a HAART regimen including stavudine. This suggests that the *in vitro* interaction is unlikely to be clinically important.

1. Hoggard PG, Kewn S, Barry MG, Khoo SH, Back DJ. Effects of drugs on 2',3'-dideoxy-2',3'-didehydrothymidine phosphorylation in vitro. *Antimicrob Agents Chemother* (1997) 41, 1231–6.
2. Mosam A, Shaik F, Uldrick TS, Esterhuizen T, Friedland GH, Scadden DT, Aboobaker J, Coovadia HM. A randomized controlled trial of highly active antiretroviral therapy versus highly active antiretroviral therapy and chemotherapy in therapy-naive patients with HIV-associated Kaposi sarcoma in South Africa. *J Acquir Immune Defic Syndr* (2012) 60, 150–7.
3. Zerit Hard Capsules (Stavudine). Bristol-Myers Squibb Pharmaceuticals Ltd. UK Summary of product characteristics, March 2011.
4. Zerit (Stavudine). Bristol-Myers Squibb Company. US Prescribing information, January 2012.

NRTIs; Zidovudine + Aciclovir

No pharmacokinetic interaction occurs between zidovudine and aciclovir, and none would be expected with valaciclovir. An isolated report describes overwhelming fatigue in one patient given zidovudine and intravenous aciclovir.

Clinical evidence, mechanism, importance and management

A study in 20 HIV-positive men found no pharmacokinetic interaction between **zidovudine** 100 mg and aciclovir 400 or 800 mg, both given every 4 hours, 5 times a day, and the combination was well tolerated over a 6-month period.[1] When 41 HIV-positive patients taking **zidovudine** were given aciclovir, there were no changes in the pharmacokinetics of zidovudine and the adverse effects were unchanged.[2] In a group of patients with AIDS taking **zidovudine**, some of whom were also given aciclovir, no obvious problems developed that could be attributed to the use of the aciclovir.[3]

In contrast, a man with herpes who had been treated with intravenous aciclovir 250 mg every 8 hours for 3 days, developed overwhelming fatigue and lethargy within about an hour of starting oral **zidovudine** 200 mg every 4 hours. This lessened slightly on changing from intravenous to oral aciclovir, which was continued for 3 days, and the symptoms resolved when aciclovir was withdrawn. The symptoms developed again when intravenous aciclovir was given as a test.[4] This isolated case of fatigue is not understood, and no other cases appear to have been reported. It is therefore unlikely to be of general relevance.

Note that as **valaciclovir** is a prodrug of aciclovir, no pharmacokinetic interaction would be expected when it is given with **zidovudine**.

1. Hollander H, Lifson AR, Maha M, Blum R, Rutherford GW, Nusinoff-Lehrman S. Phase I study of low-dose zidovudine and acyclovir in asymptomatic human immunodeficiency virus seropositive individuals. *Am J Med* (1989) 87, 628–32.
2. Tartaglione TA, Collier AC, Opheim K, Gianola FG, Benedetti J, Corey L. Pharmacokinetic evaluations of low- and high-dose zidovudine plus high-dose acyclovir in patients with symptomatic human immunodeficiency virus infection. *Antimicrob Agents Chemother* (1991) 35, 2225–31.
3. Richman DD, Fischl MA, Grieco MH, Gottlieb MS, Volberding PA, Laskin OL, Leedom JM, Groopman JE, Mildvan D, Hirsch MS, Jackson GG, Durack DT, Nusinoff-Lehrman S and the AZT Collaborative Working Group. The toxicity of azidothymidine (AZT) in the treatment of patients with AIDS and AIDS-related complex. A double-blind, placebo-controlled trial. *N Engl J Med* (1987) 317, 192–7.
4. Bach MC. Possible drug interaction during therapy with azidothymidine and acyclovir for AIDS. *N Engl J Med* (1987) 316, 547.

NRTIs; Zidovudine + Aspirin or NSAIDs

***In vitro* evidence suggests that indometacin and naproxen inhibit the glucuronidation of zidovudine. However, in subsequent clinical studies, indometacin and naproxen did not affect zidovudine pharmacokinetics. The concurrent use of ibuprofen and zidovudine appears to increase the risk of bleeding in patients with haemophilia.**

Clinical evidence, mechanism, importance and management

An *in vitro* study using human liver microsomes found that **indometacin** and **naproxen** inhibited the glucuronidation of zidovudine by 50% or more, and aspirin also had some inhibitory effect.[1] This suggested that these drugs might possibly increase the effects and the toxicity of zidovudine. However, clinical studies have found no changes in the pharmacokinetics of zidovudine given with **indometacin** 25 mg twice daily for 3 days[2] or **naproxen** 500 mg to 1 g daily for 3 or 4 days.[2,3] Many drugs that were reported to inhibit the glucuronidation of zidovudine *in vitro* appear to have slight or no effect on zidovudine pharmacokinetics in clinical studies, which are unlikely to be clinically relevant (see 'NRTIs; Zidovudine + Drugs that inhibit glucuronidation', p.985).

No clinically relevant pharmacokinetic interaction appears to occur between zidovudine and NSAIDs. However, in 2007, the MHRA in the UK issued minimum requirements to manufacturers regarding the content of licensed product characteristics for systemic NSAIDs. This included a statement that the concurrent use of NSAIDs increased the risk of haematological toxicity with zidovudine, and that there is evidence of an increased risk of haemarthroses and haematoma in HIV-positive patients with haemophilia taking zidovudine and ibuprofen.[4,5] This appears to be based on data from a study in 10 HIV-positive patients with haemophilia taking zidovudine 100 or 200 mg five times daily, which found a reduction in platelet adhesion and an increase in bleeding times in those patients given **ibuprofen** 400 mg four times daily for at least 2 weeks. Three patients had an excess bleeding tendency on concurrent use, although this did not correlate with platelet function defects. Neither the clearance of zidovudine or **ibuprofen** was affected by concurrent use.[6] A patient with AIDS and haemophilia taking **ibuprofen** had a 4-fold increase in spontaneous haemorrhages of the joints after starting zidovudine. This eventually resolved when zidovudine was stopped and restarted at a reduced dose of zidovudine 100 mg three times daily with once-daily **ibuprofen**.[7] Another case has also been reported of a prolonged bleeding time, with bleeding from a venous ulcer, in a patient taking zidovudine who self-medicated with **ibuprofen** 800 mg tablets. His bleeding time had returned to normal 4 weeks after stopping **ibuprofen**.[8] An earlier study of zidovudine use in 282 patients with AIDS found that haematological abnormalities were not increased by the concurrent use of aspirin in 47 patients.[9]

Although there is limited published evidence, the increased risk of bleeding reported in HIV-positive patients with haemophilia taking **ibuprofen** with zidovudine appears to be clinically relevant, and these patients require close monitoring if they are also prescribed NSAIDs. Whether this increased risk is restricted to those patients with haemophilia is unclear.

1. Sim SM, Back DJ, Breckenridge AM. The effect of various drugs on the glucuronidation of zidovudine (azidothymidine; AZT) by human liver microsomes. *Br J Clin Pharmacol* (1991) 32, 17–21.
2. Barry M, Howe J, Back D, Breckenridge A, Brettle R, Mitchell R, Beeching NJ, Nye FJ. The effects of indomethacin and naproxen on zidovudine pharmacokinetics. *Br J Clin Pharmacol* (1993) 36, 82–5.
3. Sahai J, Gallicano K, Garber G, Pakuts A, Hawley-Foss N, Huang L, McGilveray I, Cameron DW. Evaluation of the in vivo effect of naproxen on zidovudine pharmacokinetics in patients infected with human immunodeficiency virus. *Clin Pharmacol Ther* (1992) 52, 464–70.
4. Medicines and Healthcare products Regulatory Authority (MHRA). Minimum clinical particulars: non-selective POM NSAIDs for systemic administration (excludes aspirin/salicylic acid derivatives). Available at: http://webarchive.nationalarchives.gov.uk/20100304082711/http://www.mhra.gov.uk/home/groups/pl-a/documents/websiteresources/con2033954.pdf (accessed 20/10/15).
5. Medicines and Healthcare products Regulatory Authority (MHRA). Minimum clinical particulars: P and GSL ibuprofen for systemic administration (Guidance for MA holders).
6. Ragni MV, Miller BJ, Whalen R, Ptachcinski R. Bleeding tendency, platelet function, and pharmacokinetics of ibuprofen and zidovudine in HIV(+) hemophilic men. *Am J Hematol* (1992) 40, 176–82.
7. Ragni MV, Tama G, Lewis JH, Ho M. Increased frequency of haemarthroses in haemophilic patient treated with zidovudine. *Lancet* (1992) 40, 176–82.
8. Pieper B, Smitherman HC. Altered bleeding time associated with ibuprofen and zidovudine use. *Nurse Pract* (1998) 23, 74–5.
9. Richman DD, Fischl MA, Grieco MH, Gottlieb MS, Volberding PA, Laskin OL, Leedom JM, Groopman JE, Mildvan D, Hirsch MS, Jackson GG, Durack DT, Nusinoff-Lehrman S and the AZT Collaborative Working Group. The toxicity of azidothymidine (AZT) in the treatment of patients with AIDS and AIDS-related complex. A double-blind, placebo-controlled trial. *N Engl J Med* (1987) 317, 192–7.

NRTIs; Zidovudine + Benzodiazepines

Oxazepam does not appear to affect zidovudine exposure, but in one study concurrent use appeared to increase the incidence of headaches.

Clinical evidence, mechanism, importance and management

A pharmacokinetic study in 6 HIV-positive patients found that **oxazepam** 15 mg every 8 hours did not alter the steady-state AUC of oral zidovudine 100 mg every 4 hours or the AUC of a single intravenous dose of zidovudine. All of the patients were sleepy and fatigued while taking **oxazepam** (as expected), but 5 of the 6 complained of headaches while taking both drugs, compared with only one of 6 while taking zidovudine alone, and none while taking **oxazepam** alone. The authors of the report suggest that if headaches occur during concurrent use, the benzodiazepine should be stopped.[1] A previous *in vitro* study using human liver microsomes suggested that **oxazepam** inhibits the metabolism of zidovudine to its glucuronide, and **lorazepam** behaves in the same way.[2] However, the clinical study shows that no clinically relevant pharmacokinetic interaction occurs between oxazepam and zidovudine. The general relevance of the possible increase in headache in this small study is uncertain.

1. Mole L, Israelski D, Bubp J, O'Hanley P, Merigan T, Blaschke T. Pharmacokinetics of zidovudine alone and in combination with oxazepam in the HIV infected patient. *J Acquir Immune Defic Syndr* (1993) 6, 56–60.
2. Unadkat JD, Chien J. Lorazepam and oxazepam inhibit the metabolism of zidovudine (ZDV or azidothymidine) in an *in vitro* human liver microsomal system. *Pharm Res* (1988) 5 (Suppl), S177.

NRTIs; Zidovudine + Drugs that inhibit glucuronidation

***In vitro* evidence suggests that chloramphenicol inhibits the glucuronidation of zidovudine. Dipyridamole does not appear to alter the pharmacokinetics of zidovudine.**

Clinical evidence

(a) Chloramphenicol

An *in vitro* study using human liver microsomes found that chloramphenicol inhibited the glucuronidation of zidovudine by 50% or more, suggesting that the effects and toxicity of zidovudine might be increased.[1]

(b) Dipyridamole

It has been suggested that, theoretically, dipyridamole and zidovudine might inhibit the metabolism of each other by competing for glucuronidation, the major clearance mechanism for both drugs. However, a study in 11 asymptomatic HIV-positive patients found that dipyridamole 75 to 100 mg every 4 hours for 5 days caused no significant changes in the pharmacokinetics of zidovudine 500 mg daily, but the adverse effects of dipyridamole (headaches, nausea) when taking the higher dose were found to be intolerable.[2]

Mechanism, importance and management

Many drugs that have been reported to inhibit the glucuronidation of zidovudine *in vitro* (such as naproxen and indometacin, see 'NRTIs; Zidovudine + Aspirin or NSAIDs', p.984) appear to have only slight or no effects on zidovudine pharmacokinetics in clinical studies. In general, these minor pharmacokinetic interactions are unlikely to be of clinical importance. No pharmacokinetic interaction appears to occur between dipyridamole and zidovudine.

Based on data from studies with other drugs that affect the glucuronidation of zidovudine and the lack of a reported clinical interaction, it seems unlikely that a clinically relevant pharmacokinetic interaction will occur between systemic chloramphenicol and zidovudine. However, bear the possibility in mind should a patient develop zidovudine adverse effects, particularly as both drugs can cause haematological toxicity. Topical chloramphenicol would not be expected to interact.

1. Sim SM, Back DJ, Breckenridge AM. The effect of various drugs on the glucuronidation of zidovudine (azidothymidine; AZT) by human liver microsomes. *Br J Clin Pharmacol* (1991) 32, 17–21.
2. Hendrix CW, Flexner C, Szebeni J, Kuwahara S, Pennypacker S, Weinstein JN, Lietman PS. Effect of dipyridamole on zidovudine pharmacokinetics and short-term tolerance in asymptomatic human immunodeficiency virus-infected subjects. *Antimicrob Agents Chemother* (1994) 38, 1036–40.

NRTIs; Zidovudine + Lithium

Lithium can apparently oppose the neutropenic effects of zidovudine in some patients.

Clinical evidence, mechanism, importance and management

A study in 5 patients with AIDS found that lithium carbonate serum concentrations of 0.6 to 1.2 mmol/L increased their neutrophil counts sufficiently to allow the re-introduction of zidovudine, which had previously been withdrawn due to neutropenia. Withdrawal of the lithium resulted in a rapid fall in neutrophil counts in 2 patients.[1] Improvement in neutropenia occurred in another patient with AIDS taking zidovudine 1.2 g daily when lithium carbonate 300 mg three times daily was also given.[2] Lithium has been found to induce granulopoiesis, and these reports suggest that no adverse reaction appears to occur in patients taking zidovudine and lithium, and that there might be some advantages to their use. However, lithium has a narrow therapeutic range and its toxic symptoms might be difficult to distinguish from any neurological complications caused by the disease. The addition of lithium could also increase the risk of interactions with other drugs.[3,4] A study of 3 further patients found a lack of a beneficial effect with lithium in 2 of the patients and only a short-term improvement in the neutrophil count in the third. In addition, one patient experienced severe diarrhoea requiring lithium to be stopped.[5]

1. Roberts DE, Berman SM, Nakasato S, Wyle FA, Wishnow RM, Segal GP. Effect of lithium carbonate on zidovudine-associated neutropenia in the acquired immunodeficiency syndrome. *Am J Med* (1988) 85, 428–31.
2. Herbert V, Hirschman S, Jacobson J. Lithium for zidovudine-induced neutropenia in AIDS. *JAMA* (1988) 260, 3588.
3. Nathwani D, Green ST. Lithium for zidovudine-induced neutropenia in AIDS. *JAMA* (1989) 262, 775–6.
4. Klutman NE. Lithium carbonate therapy for zidovudine-associated neutropenia in patients with acquired immunodeficiency syndrome. *Am J Med* (1989) 87, 362–3.
5. Worthington M. Lack of effect of lithium carbonate on zidovudine-associated neutropenia in patients with AIDS. *J Infect Dis* (1990) 162, 777–8.

NRTIs; Zidovudine + Megestrol

Megestrol acetate does not affect the pharmacokinetics of zidovudine.

Clinical evidence, mechanism, importance and management

In a study in 12 asymptomatic HIV-positive patients, megestrol acetate 800 mg daily for 13 days had no effect on the steady-state pharmacokinetics of zidovudine or its glucuronide metabolite.[1] As megestrol does not appear to affect the metabolism of zidovudine, no dose adjustment of zidovudine appears to be necessary on concurrent use.

1. Van Harken DR, Pei JC, Wagner J, Pike IM. Pharmacokinetic interaction of megestrol acetate with zidovudine in human immunodeficiency virus-infected patients. *Antimicrob Agents Chemother* (1997) 41, 2480–3.

NRTIs; Zidovudine + Myelosuppressive drugs

There have been reports of serious myelotoxicity when zidovudine was given with vancomycin or cytotoxic antineoplastics, and, on theoretical grounds, the effects of any drug causing bone marrow suppression might be additive with the effects of zidovudine. Moderate pharmacokinetic changes have been seen when zidovudine was given with chemotherapy

regimens used for Kaposi's sarcoma, Hodgkin's disease, and non-Hodgkin's lymphoma.

Clinical evidence and mechanism

(a) Amphotericin

One UK manufacturer of amphotericin lipid complex notes that, in a study in *dogs*, the concurrent use of zidovudine exacerbated myelotoxicity and nephrotoxicity.[1]

(b) Antineoplastics

In one preliminary report, the addition of **vinblastine** to zidovudine resulted in severe bone marrow depression.[2] Similarly, 9 of 21 patients could not tolerate zidovudine while receiving a chemotherapy regimen (**cyclophosphamide, doxorubicin, teniposide, prednisone, vincristine**, and **bleomycin**) because of haematological toxicity.[3] However, a small retrospective case review in patients with Kaposi's sarcoma who were given **vincristine** 2 mg and **bleomycin** 30 mg or **vinblastine** 2.5 mg to 5 mg (every 3 to 4 weeks) found no significant increased risk of relapse or effect on survival in those also taking zidovudine. Of the patients taking zidovudine, 11 (24%) developed anaemia. Peripheral neuropathy was reported in 13 (28%) of all patients treated.[4] Similarly, another group have reported that the concurrent use of zidovudine 400 mg to 1 g daily with **vincristine** 2 mg and **bleomycin** 30 units (both given once every 2 weeks) in 19 HIV-positive patients with Kaposi's sarcoma was well-tolerated. Neutropenia occurred in 4 patients (21%) and neuropathy occurred in one patient (5%).[5] For a case of severe gastrointestinal and haematological toxicities in a patient taking HAART including zidovudine that was attributed to lopinavir boosted with ritonavir, see 'Vinca alkaloids + HIV-protease inhibitors', p.746.

The pharmacokinetic interaction of chemotherapy with zidovudine was assessed in HIV-positive patients being treated for Kaposi's sarcoma, non-Hodgkin's lymphoma, or Hodgkin's disease. The antineoplastics used were **bleomycin, cyclophosphamide, doxorubicin, epirubicin, etoposide, vinblastine, vincristine, vindesine**, and **vinorelbine**. Zidovudine metabolism was unchanged, but a 43% decrease was noted in the maximum plasma concentrations of zidovudine and the time to maximum concentration was prolonged by 51%, which was independent of the chemotherapy given.[6] The authors concluded that dose changes of zidovudine were not needed with the antineoplastics used, based on these pharmacokinetic changes alone, as the AUC of zidovudine remained unchanged and maximum plasma concentrations have not been shown to clearly correlate with its activity.[6] Thus it appears that any interaction is likely to be attributable to additive myelosuppressive effects.

(c) Vancomycin

A report describes marked neutropenia in 4 HIV-positive patients taking zidovudine when they were given vancomycin (which can also, rarely, have neutropenic effects).[7]

Importance and management

On theoretical grounds any drug causing bone marrow suppression might have additive effects with zidovudine. The manufacturers recommend that extra care be taken in monitoring haematological parameters if concurrent treatment with any myelosuppressive drug and zidovudine is required.[8,9] The UK manufacturer names several drugs including systemic **pentamidine**, amphotericin, **flucytosine**, vinblastine, and **doxorubicin**,[8] and the US manufacturer additionally names cytotoxic drugs.[9] However, the UK manufacturer[8] also states that limited clinical data do not indicate a significantly increased risk of adverse reactions to zidovudine if it is given with aerosolised pentamidine.

Note that the UK manufacturer[8] also states that the use of **vincristine** with zidovudine might also lead to additive myelosuppression, although vincristine is much less commonly associated with blood dyscrasias and anaemia than vinblastine.

1. Abelcet (Amphotericin B lipid complex). Cephalon Ltd. UK Summary of product characteristics, June 2010.
2. Gharakhanian S, De Sahb R, Vaseghi M, Cardon B, Rozenbaum W. Evaluation of the association of zidovudine and vinblastine in treatment of AIDS-related Kaposi's sarcoma. 5th International Conference on AIDS, Montreal, 1989. Abstract MBP368.
3. Tirelli U, Errante D, Oksenhendler E, Spina M, Vaccher E, Serraino D, Gastaldi R, Repetto L, Rizzardini G, Carbone A, et al. French-Italian Cooperative Study Group. Prospective study with combined low-dose chemotherapy and zidovudine in 37 patients with poor-prognosis AIDS-related non-Hodgkin's lymphoma. *Ann Oncol* (1992) 3, 843–7.
4. Gompels MM, Hill A, Jenkins P, Peters B, Tomlinson D, Harris JRW, Stewart S, Pinching AJ. Kaposi's sarcoma in HIV infection treated with vincristine and bleomycin. *AIDS* (1992) 6, 1175–80.
5. Lipman MCI, Swaden LS, Sabin CA, Collis C, Johnson MA. Kaposi's sarcoma in HIV infection treated with vincristine and bleomycin. *AIDS* (1993) 7, 592–3.
6. Toffoli G, Errante D, Corona G, Vaccher E, Bertola A, Robieux I, Aita P, Sorio R, Tirelli U, Boiocchi M. Interactions of antineoplastic chemotherapy with zidovudine pharmacokinetics in patients with HIV-related neoplasms. *Chemotherapy* (1999) 45, 418–28.
7. Kitchen LW, Clark RA, Hanna BJ, Pollock B, Valainis GT. Vancomycin and neutropenia in AZT-treated AIDS patients with staphylococcal infections. *J Acquir Immune Defic Syndr* (1990) 3, 925–6.
8. Retrovir (Zidovudine). ViiV Healthcare UK Ltd. UK Summary of product characteristics, January 2012.
9. Retrovir (Zidovudine). ViiV Healthcare. US Prescribing information, May 2012.

NRTIs; Zidovudine + Nimodipine

***Animal* studies suggest that intravenous nimodipine might slightly increase intravenous zidovudine exposure, but two small clinical studies reported no problems with concurrent oral use.**

Clinical evidence, mechanism, importance and management

Studies in *animals* have shown that the AUC of intravenous zidovudine is slightly increased by 36% and that of its glucuronide metabolite increased 2-fold when it is given with intravenous nimodipine.[1] The change in zidovudine exposure is slight, and, if similar changes were seen in humans, unlikely to be of clinical relevance. Nevertheless, as the adverse effects of zidovudine are dose-related, the UK manufacturer of nimodipine suggests that this interaction should be considered in patients given both drugs.[2] However, there is a small study comparing the concurrent use of zidovudine 250 mg twice daily and low-dose nimodipine 30 mg three times daily (15 patients) with zidovudine 250 mg twice daily alone (15 patients) for 6 months in the treatment of HIV-associated cognitive deficits. The authors state that both treatments were well tolerated and no adverse effects were reported.[3] Similarly, in another study in 38 patients, the addition of nimodipine 60 mg five times daily, nimodipine 30 mg three times daily or placebo to zidovudine (24 patients), didanosine (6 patients) or a combination of zidovudine and didanosine or zalcitabine (4 patients) for 16 weeks was not associated with any difference in adverse effects, when compared with placebo.[4] Although not pharmacokinetic studies, these small reports provide some reassurance that a clinically relevant pharmacokinetic interaction leading to a general increase in adverse effects seems unlikely to occur with nimodipine.

1. Gallo JM, Swagler AR, Mehta M, Qian M. Pharmacokinetic evaluation of drug interactions with anti-human immunodeficiency virus drugs. VI. Effect of the calcium channel blocker nimodipine on zidovudine kinetics in monkeys. *J Pharmacol Exp Ther* (1993) 264, 315–20.
2. Nimotop Tablets (Nimodipine). Bayer plc. UK Summary of product characteristics, October 2012.
3. Galgani S, Balestra P, Narciso P, Tozzi V, Sette P, Pau F, Visco G. Nimodipine plus zidovudine versus zidovudine alone in the treatment of HIV-1 associated cognitive deficits. *AIDS* (1997) 11, 1520–1.
4. Navia BA, Dafni U, Simpson D, Tucker T, Singer E, McArthur JC, Yiannoutsos C, Zaborski L, Lipton SA. A phase I/II trial of nimodipine for HIV-related neurologic complications. *Neurology* (1998) 51, 221–8.

NS5A inhibitors and NS5B inhibitors + Amiodarone

Serious and life-threatening symptomatic bradycardia can develop in patients taking amiodarone together with sofosbuvir, or sofosbuvir with ledipasvir, in combination with another direct-acting antiviral.

Clinical evidence, mechanism, importance and management

A review of reports to the FDA in the US indicates that serious and life-threatening symptomatic bradycardia can develop in patients taking amiodarone together with **sofosbuvir**, or **sofosbuvir with ledipasvir**, in combination with another direct-acting antiviral, such as **daclatasvir** or **simeprevir**. Nine patients taking amiodarone reported symptomatic bradycardia while taking either sofosbuvir, or sofosbuvir with ledipasvir, in combination with another direct acting antiviral. Of the 9 patients (7 of whom were also taking a beta blocker), 6 experienced symptoms within the first 24 hours, and 3 experienced symptoms within the first 2 to 12 days of concurrent use. One patient had a fatal cardiac arrest and 3 required pacemakers. The other patients recovered on stopping the antivirals or amiodarone, or both. The FDA note that symptomatic bradycardia has not been reported in patients taking sofosbuvir with ribavirin or with pegylated interferon and ribavirin.[1]

Mechanism

The mechanism for this effect is unknown.[1]

Importance and management

The FDA states that concurrent use of amiodarone and sofosbuvir, or sofosbuvir with ledipasvir, when combined with another direct-acting antiviral is not recommended. In those patients for whom there is no suitable alternative, cardiac monitoring for the first 48 hours after starting treatment in an in-patient setting, followed by daily out-patient or self-monitoring of the heart rate for 2 weeks is recommended. Patients should also be advised to seek medical attention immediately if they have signs and symptoms suggesting bradycardia, such as fainting or near fainting, dizziness, malaise, weakness, excessive tiredness, shortness of breath, chest pain, confusion, or memory problems. Amiodarone has a long half-life and patients who have recently (within the last few months[2]) discontinued amiodarone prior to starting treatment with either sofosbuvir, or sofosbuvir with ledipasvir, in combination with another direct-acting antiviral should also receive cardiac monitoring and be given advice on the symptoms of bradycardia as detailed above.[1] The European Medicines Agency makes similar recommendations.[2]

1. FDA. Drug Safety Communication: FDA warns of serious slowing of the heart rate when antiarrhythmic drug amiodarone is used with hepatitis C treatments containing sofosbuvir (Harvoni or Sovaldi) in combination with another direct acting antiviral drug, March 2015. Available at: http://www.fda.gov/Drugs/DrugSafety/ucm439484.htm (accessed 07/08/15).
2. European Medicines Agency. EMA recommends avoidance of certain hepatitis C medicines and amiodarone together, April 2015. Available at: http://www.ema.europa.eu/docs/en_GB/document_library/Press_release/2015/04/WC500186152.pdf (accessed 07/08/15).

NS5A inhibitors + Drugs that affect gastric pH

Antacids might decrease the concentration of ledipasvir (in a fixed-dose combination with sofosbuvir), but no interaction is predicted to occur with daclatasvir. Famotidine does not appear to affect the pharmacokinetics of dacaltasvir or ledipasvir, and other H_2-receptor antagonists might also be expected to not interact. Omeprazole does not appear to affect the pharmacokinetics of daclatasvir or ombitasvir, and other proton pump inhibitors might also be expected to not interact. Exposure to ledipasvir (in a fixed-dose combination with sofosbuvir) does not appear to be affected by simultaneous omeprazole, but when given 2 hours before ledipasvir alone, omeprazole appears to slightly decrease

ledipasvir exposure. Other proton pump inhibitors might interact similarly.

Clinical evidence, mechanism, importance and management

(a) Antacids

1. Daclatasvir. The UK manufacturer notes that no clinically relevant interaction is expected between daclatasvir and antacids.[1]

2. Ledipasvir. The UK and US manufacturers of ledipasvir in a fixed-dose combination with sofosbuvir, predict that ledipasvir concentrations will be decreased by antacids (such as **aluminium hydroxide**, **calcium carbonate**, or **magnesium hydroxide**) because ledipasvir solubility decreases with increasing pH. They therefore advise that administration is separated by 4 hours.[2,3]

(b) H_2-receptor antagonists

1. Daclatasvir. The UK manufacturer briefly reports that, in a single-dose study in healthy subjects, **famotidine** 40 mg decreased the AUC and maximum concentration of daclatasvir 60 mg, by 18% and 44%, respectively.[1] Such a small decrease in exposure is unlikely to be clinically relevant, and so no daclatasvir dose adjustment is necessary on concurrent use.[1] On this basis other H_2-receptor antagonists might also be expected not to interact.

2. Ledipasvir. The UK and US manufacturers briefly report that, in a study in 12 healthy subjects, a single 40-mg dose of **famotidine** given at the same time as, or 12 hours before, a single 90-mg dose of ledipasvir (with sofosbuvir) had no effect on the AUC of ledipasvir, but decreased its maximum concentration by about 20%. They therefore advise that ledipasvir (with sofosbuvir) can be administered simultaneously with, or separated (by 12 hours[3]) from, famotidine or other H_2-receptor antagonists, at a dose that does not exceed famotidine 40 mg twice daily, or equivalent.[2,3]

(c) Proton pump inhibitors

1. Daclatasvir. The UK manufacturer briefly reports that, in a study in healthy subjects, **omeprazole** 40 mg daily decreased the AUC and maximum concentration of a single 60-mg dose of daclatasvir by 16% and 36%, respectively.[1] Such a small decrease in exposure is unlikely to be clinically relevant, and so no daclatasvir dose adjustment is necessary on concurrent use.[1] Other proton pump inhibitors might also be expected not to interact.

2. Ledipasvir. The UK and US manufacturers briefly report that, in a study in 16 healthy subjects, **omeprazole** 20 mg daily given at the same time as a single 90-mg dose of ledipasvir (with sofosbuvir) had no effect on the ledipasvir AUC or maximum concentration.[2,3] The US manufacturer also reports that in a study in 17 healthy subjects, **omeprazole** 20 mg daily given 2 hours prior to a single 30-mg dose of ledipasvir (alone) decreased the AUC and maximum concentration by 42% and 48%, respectively.[3] It is therefore recommended that all proton pump inhibitors should be given simultaneously with ledipasvir (in a fixed-dose combination with sofosbuvir), and at doses that are comparable to omeprazole 20 mg[2] (or lower[3]).

3. Ombitasvir. The UK and US manufacturers briefly report that, in a study in 11 healthy subjects, **omeprazole** 40 mg daily had no effect on the pharmacokinetics of ombitasvir 25 mg daily (in a fixed-dose combination with paritaprevir boosted with ritonavir, with and without dasabuvir).[4,5] No ombitasvir dose adjustment is necessary on concurrent use. Other proton pump inhibitors might reasonably be expected to not affect ombitasvir pharmacokinetics.

1. Daklinza (Daclatasvir dihydrochloride). Bristol-Myers Squibb Pharmaceutical Ltd. UK Summary of product characteristics, September 2014.
2. Harvoni (Ledipasvir, sofosbuvir). Gilead Sciences Ltd. UK Summary of product characteristics, November 2014.
3. Harvoni (Ledipasvir, sofosbuvir). Gilead Sciences, Inc. US Prescribing information, March 2015.
4. Viekira Pak (Ombitasvir, paritaprevir, ritonavir co-packaged with dasabuvir sodium monohydrate). AbbVie Inc. US Prescribing information, December 2014.
5. Viekirax (Ombitasvir, paritaprevir, ritonavir). AbbVie Ltd. UK Summary of product characteristics, January 2015.

NS5A inhibitors + Food

Food appears to increase the exposure to ombitasvir, but does not appear to affect exposure to ledipasvir or daclatasvir.

Clinical evidence, mechanism, importance and management

(a) Daclatasvir

The UK manufacturer briefly reports that, in a study in healthy subjects, a high-fat meal decreased the AUC and maximum concentration of daclatasvir 60 mg by 23% and 28%, respectively, when compared with the fasting state. Administration after a light meal did not affect its exposure. They recommend that daclatasvir can be taken with or without food.[1]

(b) Ledipasvir

The UK and US manufacturers briefly report that, in a study, neither a high-fat (about 1000 kilocalories, 50% fat) or moderate-fat (about 600 kilocalories, 25-30% fat) meal altered the pharmacokinetics of ledipasvir (in a fixed-dose combination with sofosbuvir) relative to the fasted state, and it can therefore be given without regard to food.[2,3]

(c) Ombitasvir

The US manufacturer briefly reports that, in a study, a moderate-fat meal (about 600 kilocalories, 20-30% of calories from fat) increased the AUC of ombitasvir (in a fixed-dose combination with paritaprevir boosted with ritonavir, and given with dasabuvir) by 82%, relative to fasting. When given with a high-fat meal (about 900 kilocalories, 60% calories from fat) the AUC was increased by 76%, compared with the fasting state.[4] Both the UK and US manufacturers advise that ombitasvir should be taken with food, but without regard to fat or calorie content.[4,5]

1. Daklinza (Daclatasvir dihydrochloride). Bristol-Myers Squibb Pharmaceutical Ltd. UK Summary of product characteristics, September 2014.
2. Harvoni (Ledipasvir, sofosbuvir). Gilead Sciences Ltd. UK Summary of product characteristics, November 2014.
3. Harvoni (Ledipasvir, sofosbuvir). Gilead Sciences, Inc. US Prescribing information, March 2015.
4. Viekira Pak (Ombitasvir, paritaprevir, ritonavir co-packaged with dasabuvir sodium monohydrate). AbbVie Inc. US Prescribing information, December 2014.
5. Viekirax (Ombitasvir, paritaprevir, ritonavir). AbbVie Ltd. UK Summary of product characteristics, January 2015.

NS5A inhibitors + HCV-protease inhibitors

Daclatasvir exposure appears to be moderately increased by telaprevir and slightly increased by simeprevir. Boceprevir is predicted to interact similarly. Daclatasvir appears to moderately increase simeprevir exposure but have no effect on that of telaprevir. Exposure to ledipasvir and simeprevir both appear to be increased (slightly and moderately, respectively) when given together.

Clinical evidence

(a) Simeprevir

1. Daclatasvir. The UK manufacturer of daclatasvir briefly reports that, in a study in healthy subjects, simeprevir 150 mg once daily increased the AUC and maximum concentration of daclatasvir 60 mg daily almost 2-fold and by 50%, respectively. The AUC and maximum concentration of simeprevir were increased by 44% and 39%, respectively.[1]

2. Ledipasvir. The UK and US manufacturers briefly report that, in a study in 22 healthy subjects, simeprevir 150 mg daily increased the AUC and maximum concentration of ledipasvir 30 mg daily by 92% and 81%, respectively. The AUC and maximum concentration of simeprevir were increased 2.7-fold and 2.6-fold, respectively.[2,3]

(b) Telaprevir

The UK manufacturer of daclatasvir briefly reports that, in a study in healthy subjects, telaprevir 500 mg twice daily increased the AUC and maximum concentration of **daclatasvir** 20 mg daily 2.3-fold and by 46%, respectively. Similarly, telaprevir 750 mg three times daily increased the AUC and maximum concentration of **daclatasvir** 20 mg daily 2.2-fold and by 22%, respectively. The pharmacokinetics of telaprevir were unaffected at both doses.[1]

Mechanism

Daclatasvir is a substrate for CYP3A4 and P-glycoprotein, and ledipasvir is a substrate for P-glycoprotein. Both CYP3A4 (albeit to varying extents) and P-glycoprotein are inhibited by simeprevir and telaprevir, and their concurrent use with daclatasvir or ledipasvir therefore results in increased exposure of these NS5A inhibitors. Simeprevir and telaprevir are also themselves substrates for CYP3A4 and possibly P-glycoprotein. As neither daclatasvir nor ledipasvir appear to have important effects on CYP3A4, but do appear to inhibit P-glycoprotein, the role of this transporter in the increased exposure to simeprevir seen cannot be ruled out, and warrants further study. However, no increase in telaprevir exposure was seen with concurrent use of daclatasvir, the reason for which is unclear.

Importance and management

Evidence for an interaction between daclatasvir and the HCV-protease inhibitors is limited, but appears to be consistent with the disposition and interactions of these drugs. The increases in daclatasvir and simeprevir exposure when given together were slight and unlikely to be clinically important. No dose adjustments are therefore necessary on concurrent use.[1] In contrast, the increase in daclatasvir exposure with telaprevir was moderate, and it is recommended that the daclatasvir dose be reduced by 50% to 30 mg daily if given concurrently with telaprevir. As **boceprevir** is a potent CYP3A4 inhibitor (like telaprevir) it is predicted that it will have similar effects and the same dose reduction is recommended if given concurrently with daclatasvir.[1]

The effect of simeprevir on ledipasvir exposure was only slight, but the increase in simeprevir exposure was moderate. As a result, the UK and US manufacturers of ledipasvir with sofosbuvir (in a fixed-dose combination) do not recommend concurrent use.[2,3]

1. Daklinza (Daclatasvir dihydrochloride). Bristol-Myers Squibb Pharmaceutical Ltd. UK Summary of product characteristics, September 2014.
2. Harvoni (Ledipasvir, sofosbuvir). Gilead Sciences Ltd. UK Summary of product characteristics, November 2014.
3. Harvoni (Ledipasvir, sofosbuvir). Gilead Sciences, Inc. US Prescribing information, March 2015.

NS5A inhibitors + HIV-protease inhibitors

Daclatasvir exposure is moderately increased by atazanavir boosted with ritonavir. Other HIV-protease inhibitors might be expected to interact similarly. No clinically relevant pharmacokinetic interaction appears to occur between atazanavir or darunavir, both boosted with ritonavir, and ledipasvir (in a fixed-dose combination), but tipranavir is predicted to

decrease ledipasvir exposure. No pharmacokinetic interaction appears to occur between ombitasvir (in a fixed-dose combination) and atazanavir (unboosted and boosted with ritonavir), or lopinavir boosted with ritonavir. The pharmacokinetics of ombitasvir appeared to be unaffected when given with darunavir (unboosted and boosted with ritonavir), but the minimum concentration of darunavir appeared to be decreased.

Clinical evidence

(a) Atazanavir

1. Daclatasvir. In a crossover study in 14 healthy subjects given atazanavir boosted with ritonavir 300/100 mg daily for 10 days with daclatasvir 20 mg daily, the dose-normalised AUC and maximum concentration of daclatasvir were increased about 2-fold and by 35%, respectively.[1]

2. Ledipasvir. The UK and US manufacturers briefly report that, in a study in 30 healthy subjects given ledipasvir 90 mg daily (in a fixed-dose combination with sofosbuvir) and atazanavir boosted with ritonavir 300/100 mg daily, the AUC and maximum concentration of ledipasvir were increased about 2-fold. The AUC of atazanavir was increased by 33%.[2,3]

3. Ombitasvir. The UK manufacturer briefly reports that, in a study in healthy subjects given ombitasvir 25 mg daily (in a fixed-dose combination with paritaprevir and ritonavir, and given with dasabuvir) and atazanavir 300 mg daily at the same time, the AUC and maximum concentration of ombitasvir were decreased by 17% and 23%, respectively. The pharmacokinetics of atazanavir were unaffected. Similar effects were seen when the same regimen was given without dasabuvir.[4] In another study, when atazanavir boosted with ritonavir 300/100 mg daily was given 12 hours after ombitasvir 25 mg daily (in a fixed-dose combination with paritaprevir and ritonavir, and given with dasabuvir) the AUC of ombitasvir was unaffected, but the maximum concentration was decreased by 17%. The pharmacokinetics of atazanavir were unaffected.[4,5]

(b) Darunavir

1. Ledipasvir. The UK and US manufacturers briefly report that, in a study in 23 healthy subjects given ledipasvir 90 mg daily and darunavir boosted with ritonavir 800/100 mg daily, the AUC and maximum concentration of ledipasvir were increased by 39% and 45%, respectively. The pharmacokinetics of darunavir were unaffected.[2,3]

2. Ombitasvir. The UK and US manufacturers briefly report that, in a study in healthy subjects given ombitasvir 25 mg daily (in a fixed-dose combination with paritaprevir and ritonavir, and given with dasabuvir) and darunavir 800 mg daily at the same time, the pharmacokinetics of ombitasvir were unaffected. The AUC and minimum concentration of darunavir were decreased by 24%, and 48%, respectively, but the maximum concentration was unaffected.[4,5] No changes in the pharmacokinetics of ombitasvir were seen when the same regimen was given without dasabuvir, and the AUC and maximum concentration of darunavir were unaffected. The minimum concentration of darunavir was decreased by 26%.[4] In another study, when darunavir boosted with ritonavir 600/100 mg twice daily was given with ombitasvir 25 mg daily (in a fixed-dose combination with paritaprevir and ritonavir, and given with dasabuvir) the AUC and maximum concentration of ombitasvir were decreased by 27% and 24%, respectively. The AUC and minimum concentration of darunavir were decreased by 20% and 43%, respectively, but the maximum concentration was unaffected.[4,5] In a further study with darunavir boosted with ritonavir 800/100 mg daily and given 12 hours after ombitasvir 25 mg daily (in a fixed-dose combination with paritaprevir and ritonavir, and given with dasabuvir), the pharmacokinetics of ombitasvir were unaffected. The AUC of darunavir was increased by 34% and the maximum and minimum concentrations were decreased by 21% and 46%, respectively.[4,5]

(c) Lopinavir

The UK and US manufacturers briefly report that, in a study in healthy subjects given **ombitasvir** 25 mg daily (in a fixed-dose combination with paritaprevir and ritonavir, and given with dasabuvir) and lopinavir boosted with ritonavir 400/100 mg twice daily, the pharmacokinetics of ombitasvir and lopinavir were unaffected.[4,5] Similar effects were seen when the same regimen was given without dasabuvir,[4] and when lopinavir boosted with ritonavir 800/200 mg daily was given 12 hours later, both with[4,5] and without dasabuvir.[4]

Mechanism

Daclatasvir is a CYP3A4 substrate, which is inhibited by HIV-protease inhibitors boosted with ritonavir, and thus concurrent use of atazanavir boosted with ritonavir increases daclatasvir exposure. Ledipasvir is a P-glycoprotein substrate, and the reason for the increase in its exposure on concurrent use with atazanavir might be due to inhibition of P-glycoprotein by atazanavir.

Importance and management

Evidence for an interaction between **daclatasvir** and atazanavir boosted with ritonavir is consistent with the known disposition and interactions of these drugs and would therefore seem to be established, and clinically important. The daclatasvir dose should be decreased by 50% to 30 mg daily,[6] as with concurrent use of other potent CYP3A4 inhibitors. The UK manufacturer advises that due to a lack of data, darunavir and lopinavir, boosted with ritonavir are not recommended with daclatasvir.[6] However, given the known similarities in interactions between the HIV-protease inhibitors, the same advice as for atazanavir boosted with ritonavir and other potent CYP3A4 inhibitors would seem reasonable.

The increases in exposure seen with **ledipasvir** (in a fixed-dose combination with sofosbuvir) and atazanavir boosted with ritonavir, and with ledipasvir and darunavir boosted with ritonavir, are not considered to be clinically relevant,[3] and no dose adjustments are required on concurrent use. However, special precautions apply when ledipasvir (in a fixed-dose combination with sofosbuvir) is given with an HIV protease inhibitor boosted with ritonavir in regimens containing tenofovir, see 'Tenofovir + NS5A inhibitors', p.997 for details. Furthermore, the UK and US manufacturers predict that **tipranavir** boosted with ritonavir will *decrease* ledipasvir exposure[2,3] (possibly via induction of P-glycoprotein by tipranavir) leading to a decrease in therapeutic effect. Concurrent use is therefore not recommended.[2,3]

No clinically relevant change in the pharmacokinetics of **ombitasvir** (in a fixed-dose combination with paritaprevir and ritonavir and given with or without dasabuvir) appears to occur when it is given with, or 12 hours before, atazanavir (unboosted and boosted with ritonavir) or lopinavir boosted with ritonavir, and the pharmacokinetics of atazanavir and lopinavir seem to be similarly unaffected. No dose adjustments would seem necessary on concurrent use. When given with darunavir (unboosted and boosted with ritonavir) the pharmacokinetics of ombitasvir seemed to be unaffected, but the minimum concentration of darunavir appeared to be decreased. As a result the US manufacturer does not recommend use with darunavir.[5] In contrast, the UK manufacturer advises that the recommended dose of darunavir is 800 mg daily, without ritonavir, and given at the same time as the combination. Furthermore, they state that it should only be used in the absence of extensive protease inhibitor resistance, and not without dasabuvir.[4] No ombitasvir dose adjustment is necessary.

1. Bifano M, Hwang C, Oosterhuis B, Hartstra J, Grasela D, Tiessen R, Velinova-Donga M, Kandoussi H, Sevinsky H, Bertz R. Assessment of pharmacokinetic interactions of the HCV NS5A replication complex inhibitor daclatasvir with antiretroviral agents: ritonavir-boosted atazanavir, efavirenz and tenofovir. *Antivir Ther* (2013) 18, 931–40.
2. Harvoni (Ledipasvir, sofosbuvir). Gilead Sciences Ltd. UK Summary of product characteristics, November 2014.
3. Harvoni (Ledipasvir, sofosbuvir). Gilead Sciences, Inc. US Prescribing information, March 2015.
4. Viekirax (Ombitasvir, paritaprevir, ritonavir). AbbVie Ltd. UK Summary of product characteristics, January 2015.
5. Viekira Pak (Ombitasvir, paritaprevir, ritonavir co-packaged with dasabuvir sodium monohydrate). AbbVie Inc. US Prescribing information, December 2014.
6. Daklinza (Daclatasvir dihydrochloride). Bristol-Myers Squibb Pharmaceutical Ltd. UK Summary of product characteristics, September 2014.

NS5A inhibitors + Ketoconazole and other CYP3A4 inhibitors

Daclatasvir exposure appears to be moderately increased by ketoconazole. Other potent CYP3A4 inhibitors are predicted to interact similarly. Moderate CYP3A4 inhibitors are also predicted to increase daclatasvir exposure. Ketoconazole appears to have no effect on the pharmacokinetics of ombitasvir.

106 Clinical evidence

(a) Daclatasvir

The UK manufacturer briefly reports that, in a study in healthy subjects, ketoconazole 400 mg daily increased the AUC and maximum concentration of a single 10-mg dose of daclatasvir 3-fold and by 57%, respectively.[1]

(b) Ombitasvir

The UK and US manufacturers briefly report that, in a study in 12 healthy subjects, ketoconazole 400 mg daily had no effect on the AUC or maximum concentration of a single 25-mg dose of ombitasvir (in a fixed-dose combination with paritaprevir boosted with ritonavir, and given with dasabuvir).[2,3] The same lack of effect was seen in a similar study, but without dasabuvir.[3]

Mechanism

Daclatasvir is metabolised by CYP3A4 and transported by P-glycoprotein, both of which are inhibited by ketoconazole. Concurrent use therefore results in increased daclatasvir exposure.

Importance and management

Evidence for an interaction between **daclatasvir** and ketoconazole is limited, but would appear to be consistent with the disposition of daclatasvir and the well-known effects of ketoconazole on other similarly metabolised drugs. The study suggests that exposure to daclatasvir is moderately increased by ketoconazole, and the UK manufacturer advises that the daclatasvir dose should be halved to 30 mg daily if given concurrently with ketoconazole or other potent CYP3A4 inhibitors.[1] They also predict that more modest increases in daclatasvir exposure might be seen with moderate CYP3A4 inhibitors, but that no dose adjustment is necessary on concurrent use. For a list of potent and moderate CYP3A4 inhibitors see 'Table 1.9', p.11. Note that the manufacturer includes **posaconazole** as a potent CYP3A4 inhibitor, but it is generally considered as moderate.

Ketoconazole does not appear to alter the pharmacokinetics of **ombitasvir**, and no ombitasvir dose adjustment would seem necessary on concurrent use. However, note that other components of the fixed-dose preparation do interact with ketoconazole, see 'HCV-protease inhibitors + Azoles', p.901 and 'HIV-protease inhibitors + Azoles; Ketoconazole', p.923.

1. Daklinza (Daclatasvir dihydrochloride). Bristol-Myers Squibb Pharmaceutical Ltd. UK Summary of product characteristics, September 2014.
2. Viekira Pak (Ombitasvir, paritaprevir, ritonavir co-packaged with dasabuvir sodium monohydrate). AbbVie Inc. US Prescribing information, December 2014.
3. Viekirax (Ombitasvir, paritaprevir, ritonavir). AbbVie Ltd. UK Summary of product characteristics, January 2015.

NS5A inhibitors + NNRTIs

Daclatasvir exposure is slightly decreased by efavirenz. Other moderate CYP3A4 inducers are predicted to interact similarly. Ledipasvir exposure (in a fixed-dose combination with sofosbuvir) appears to be slightly decreased by efavirenz, but is not affected by rilpivirine. Rilpivirine does not appear to alter the pharmacokinetics of ombitasvir, but etravirine and nevirapine are predicted to decrease ombitasvir concentrations.

Clinical evidence

(a) Efavirenz

1. Daclatasvir. In a crossover study, 15 healthy subjects were given efavirenz 600 mg daily for 10 days with daclatasvir 60 mg daily and then for a further 4 days with daclatasvir 120 mg daily. The dose-normalised AUC and maximum concentration of daclatasvir were decreased by 32% and 17%, respectively.[1]

2. Ledipasvir. The UK and US manufacturers briefly report that, in a study in 14 healthy subjects given efavirenz 600 mg daily with emtricitabine 200 mg and tenofovir 300 mg both daily, the AUC and maximum concentration of ledipasvir 90 mg daily (given in a fixed-dose combination with sofosbuvir) were decreased by 34%.[2,3] The pharmacokinetics of efavirenz were not affected.[2,3]

(b) Rilpivirine

1. Ledipasvir. The UK manufacturer briefly reports that, in a study in healthy subjects given rilpivirine 25 mg daily with emtricitabine 200 mg and tenofovir 300 mg both daily, the pharmacokinetics of ledipasvir 90 mg daily (given in a fixed-dose combination with sofosbuvir) were not affected. The pharmacokinetics of rilpivirine were also not affected.[2] The US manufacturer states that no change was seen in the pharmacokinetics of rilpivirine or ledipasvir when given concurrently.[3]

2. Ombitasvir. The UK and US manufacturers briefly report that, in a study in 10 healthy subjects, rilpivirine 25 mg daily had no effect on the pharmacokinetics of ombitasvir 25 mg daily (in a fixed-dose combination with paritaprevir boosted with ritonavir, and given with dasabuvir).[4,5]

Mechanism

Daclatasvir is metabolised by CYP3A4, of which efavirenz is a moderate inducer. Concurrent use therefore results in decreased daclatasvir exposure.

Importance and management

Evidence for an interaction between **daclatasvir** and the NNRTIs is limited to that with efavirenz, but is consistent with the disposition of daclatasvir and the known effects of efavirenz on other similarly metabolised drugs. The study shows that exposure to daclatasvir is slightly decreased by **efavirenz**, and the UK manufacturer advises that the daclatasvir dose should be increased by 50% to 90 mg daily on concurrent use.[6] This advice is extended to other moderate CYP3A4 inducers (see 'Table 1.9', p.11 for a list), although note that even though **nevirapine** is a potentially moderate inducer of CYP3A4, the UK manufacturer of daclatasvir advises that due to a lack of data, concurrent use is not recommended.[6] **Etravirine** appears to induce CYP3A4, albeit to a lesser extent than efavirenz and nevirapine, but its use is also not recommended due to a lack of data.[6] **Rilpivirine** does not appear to affect CYP3A4 to a clinically relevant extent and therefore no interaction with daclatasvir would be expected. No dose adjustments are required on concurrent use.[6]

The decrease in **ledipasvir** exposure when given with **efavirenz**, emtricitabine, and tenofovir was only slight and the UK manufacturer of ledipasvir with sofosbuvir (in a fixed-dose combination) advises that no dose adjustments are necessary on concurrent use.[2] No interaction appears to occur between ledipasvir and **rilpivirine** and no dose adjustments are necessary on concurrent use. Other NNRTIs might also be expected not to interact with ledipasvir, but further study is required to confirm this.

Rilpivirine does not appear to alter the pharmacokinetics of **ombitasvir**, and so no ombitasvir dose adjustment is necessary on concurrent use. **Nevirapine** and **etravirine** are predicted by the UK manufacturer to decrease the concentration of ombitasvir, and concurrent use is contraindicated.[5] However, ombitasvir is not appreciably metabolised by cytochrome P450 isoenzymes and so an effect due to CYP3A4 induction by these two NNRTIs, or by efavirenz, would seem unlikely.

1. Bifano M, Hwang C, Oosterhuis B, Hartstra J, Grasela D, Tiessen R, Velinova-Donga M, Kandoussi H, Sevinsky H, Bertz R. Assessment of pharmacokinetic interactions of the HCV NS5A replication complex inhibitor daclatasvir with antiretroviral agents: ritonavir-boosted atazanavir, efavirenz and tenofovir. *Antivir Ther* (2013) 18, 931–40.
2. Harvoni (Ledipasvir, sofosbuvir). Gilead Sciences Ltd. UK Summary of product characteristics, November 2014.
3. Harvoni (Ledipasvir, sofosbuvir). Gilead Sciences, Inc. US Prescribing information, March 2015.
4. Viekira Pak (Ombitasvir, paritaprevir, ritonavir co-packaged with dasabuvir sodium monohydrate). AbbVie Inc. US Prescribing information, December 2014.
5. Viekirax (Ombitasvir, paritaprevir, ritonavir). AbbVie Ltd. UK Summary of product characteristics, January 2015.
6. Daklinza (Daclatasvir dihydrochloride). Bristol-Myers Squibb Pharmaceutical Ltd. UK Summary of product characteristics, September 2014.

NS5A inhibitors + NRTIs

No pharmacokinetic interaction appears to occur between ledipasvir and abacavir, emtricitabine, or lamivudine, or between ombitasvir and emtricitabine. No pharmacokinetic interactions are expected between daclatasvir and the NRTIs.

Clinical evidence, mechanism, importance and management

(a) Abacavir

1. Daclatasvir. The UK manufacturer notes that no pharmacokinetic interaction is expected between daclatasvir and abacavir, and that no dose adjustment is considered necessary on concurrent use.[1]

2. Ledipasvir. The UK manufacturer briefly reports that, in a study in healthy subjects given ledipasvir 90 mg daily (in a fixed-dose combination with sofosbuvir) with abacavir 600 mg daily (also with lamivudine), the pharmacokinetics of ledipasvir and abacavir were unaltered.[2] The US manufacturer also notes that the pharmacokinetics of ledipasvir and abacavir were not affected by concurrent use.[3] No dose adjustments are necessary on concurrent use.

(b) Emtricitabine

1. Daclatasvir. The UK manufacturer notes that no pharmacokinetic interaction is expected between daclatasvir and emtricitabine, and that no dose adjustment is considered necessary on concurrent use.[1]

2. Ledipasvir. The UK manufacturer briefly reports that, in several studies in healthy subjects given ledipasvir 90 mg daily (in a fixed-dose combination with sofosbuvir) with emtricitabine 200 mg daily (as part of regimens also including efavirenz, rilpivirine, tenofovir, and/or HIV-protease inhibitors), the pharmacokinetics of emtricitabine were unaltered.[2] The US manufacturer also notes that the pharmacokinetics of ledipasvir and emtricitabine were not affected by concurrent use.[3] No dose adjustments are necessary on concurrent use.

3. Ombitasvir. The UK manufacturer briefly reports that, in a study in healthy subjects given emtricitabine 200 mg daily (with tenofovir) and ombitasvir 25 mg daily (in a fixed-dose combination with paritaprevir boosted with ritonavir, given with and without dasabuvir), the pharmacokinetics of emtricitabine and ombitasvir were unaffected.[4] No dose adjustments are required on concurrent use.[4,5]

(c) Lamivudine

1. Daclatasvir. The UK manufacturer notes that no pharmacokinetic interaction is expected between daclatasvir and lamivudine, and that no dose adjustment is considered necessary on concurrent use.[1]

2. Ledipasvir. The UK manufacturer briefly reports that, in a study in healthy subjects given ledipasvir 90 mg daily (in a fixed-dose combination with sofosbuvir) with lamivudine 300 mg daily (also with abacavir), the pharmacokinetics of ledipasvir and lamivudine were unaltered.[2] The US manufacturer also notes that the pharmacokinetics of ledipasvir and lamivudine were not affected by concurrent use.[3] No dose adjustments are necessary on concurrent use.

(d) Other NRTIs

The UK manufacturer notes that no pharmacokinetic interaction is expected between daclatasvir and **didanosine**, **stavudine**, or **zidovudine**, and that no dose adjustment is considered necessary on concurrent use.[1]

1. Daklinza (Daclatasvir dihydrochloride). Bristol-Myers Squibb Pharmaceutical Ltd. UK Summary of product characteristics, September 2014.
2. Harvoni (Ledipasvir, sofosbuvir). Gilead Sciences Ltd. UK Summary of product characteristics, November 2014.
3. Harvoni (Ledipasvir, sofosbuvir). Gilead Sciences, Inc. US Prescribing information, March 2015.
4. Viekirax (Ombitasvir, paritaprevir, ritonavir). AbbVie Ltd. UK Summary of product characteristics, January 2015.
5. Viekira Pak (Ombitasvir, paritaprevir, ritonavir co-packaged with dasabuvir sodium monohydrate). AbbVie Inc. US Prescribing information, December 2014.

NS5A inhibitors + Rifampicin (Rifampin) and other CYP3A4/P-glycoprotein inducers

Daclatasvir and ledipasvir exposure appear to be moderately decreased by rifampicin. Ombitasvir exposure (when given in a fixed-dose combination) is slightly decreased by carbamazepine. Other potent CYP3A4 inducers and/or P-glycoprotein inducers are predicted to interact similarly.

Clinical evidence

(a) Daclatasvir

The UK manufacturer briefly reports that, in a study in healthy subjects, rifampicin 600 mg daily decreased the AUC and maximum concentration of a single 60-mg dose of daclatasvir by 79% and 56%, respectively.[1]

(b) Ledipasvir

The UK and US manufacturers briefly report that, in a study in 31 healthy subjects, rifampicin 600 mg daily decreased the AUC and maximum concentration of a single 90-mg dose of ledipasvir by 59% and 35%, respectively.[2,3]

(c) Ombitasvir

The UK and US manufacturers briefly report that, in a study in 12 healthy subjects, **carbamazepine** 200 mg daily followed by 200 mg twice daily decreased both the AUC and maximum concentration of a single 25-mg dose of ombitasvir (in a fixed-dose combination with paritaprevir boosted with ritonavir, and given with dasabuvir) by 31%.[4,5]

Mechanism

Daclatasvir is metabolised by CYP3A4 and transported by P-glycoprotein, and ledipasvir and ombitasvir are also P-glycoprotein substrates. Both CYP3A4 and P-glycoprotein are induced by rifampicin and carbamazepine. As a result, daclatasvir and ledipasvir exposure was decreased with rifampicin, and ombitasvir exposure was decreased with carbamazepine.

Importance and management

Evidence for an interaction between the NS5A inhibitors and rifampicin and other CYP3A4/P-glycoprotein inducers is limited, but would appear to be consistent with the disposition of the NS5A inhibitors and the well-known inducing effects of rifampicin and carbamazepine on other similarly metabolised drugs.

Daclatasvir

The study suggests that exposure to daclatasvir is moderately decreased by rifampicin, and the UK manufacturer contraindicates concurrent use with rifampicin and other potent CYP3A4 inducers due to the risk of reduced daclatasvir efficacy.[1] For a list of potent CYP3A4 inducers see 'Table 1.9', p.11. Note that the manufacturer names **rifabutin**, **rifapentine**, and **St John's wort** as potent CYP3A4 inducers, but they are generally considered as moderate. (For more information on the concurrent use of daclatasvir with moderate CYP3A4 inducers, see 'NS5A inhibitors + NNRTIs', p.989). They similarly contraindicate the concurrent use of **dexamethasone** due to its potent CYP3A4 inducing effects,[1] however, evidence of dexamethasone having clinically relevant interactions as a result of this mechanism is generally lacking. **Oxcarbazepine** is also named as a potent CYP3A4 inducer,[1] and although its potency is yet to be fully established, it does have clinically important effects on the concentrations of ethinylestradiol when taken with combined hormonal contraceptives, that are comparable to those of the well-known potent inducer carbamazepine (see 'Combined hormonal contraceptives + Carbamazepine and related drugs', p.1172).

Ledipasvir

The study suggests that exposure to ledipasvir is moderately decreased by rifampicin, and the UK and US manufacturers of ledipasvir with sofosbuvir (in a fixed-dose combination) do not recommend concurrent use with rifampicin due to the risk of reduced ledipasvir efficacy.[2,3] They extend this warning to other drugs that induce P-glycoprotein,[2,3] see 'Table 1.12', p.14 for a list. However, they also name other drugs whose P-glycoprotein-inducing effects are yet to be established: **oxcarbazepine**, **phenobarbital**, **phenytoin**, **rifabutin**, and **rifapentine**.[2]

Ombitasvir

The study suggests that exposure to ombitasvir (when given in a fixed-dose combination with paritaprevir boosted with ritonavir, and given with dasabuvir) is only slightly decreased by carbamazepine, but concurrent use is contraindicated.[4,5] The manufacturers extend this to other potent[4,5] or moderate enzyme inducers,[5] specifically naming the other enzyme-inducing antiepileptics **phenobarbital** and **phenytoin**,[4,5] as well as **enzalutamide**,[5] **mitotane**,[5] **rifampicin**,[4,5] and **St John's wort**.[4,5] It is important to note that ombitasvir is not appreciably metabolised by cytochrome P450 isoenzymes and so an effect by these inducers would seem unlikely via this mechanism. However, as ombitasvir is a P-glycoprotein substrate, an interaction via induction of this transporter cannot be ruled out; see 'Table 1.12', p.14 for a list of P-glycoprotein inducers.

1. Daklinza (Daclatasvir dihydrochloride). Bristol-Myers Squibb Pharmaceutical Ltd. UK Summary of product characteristics, September 2014.
2. Harvoni (Ledipasvir, sofosbuvir). Gilead Sciences Ltd. UK Summary of product characteristics, November 2014.
3. Harvoni (Ledipasvir, sofosbuvir). Gilead Sciences, Inc. US Prescribing information, March 2015.
4. Viekira Pak (Ombitasvir, paritaprevir, ritonavir co-packaged with dasabuvir sodium monohydrate). AbbVie Inc. US Prescribing information, December 2014.
5. Viekirax (Ombitasvir, paritaprevir, ritonavir). AbbVie Ltd. UK Summary of product characteristics, January 2015.

NS5A inhibitors + SSRIs

No interaction appears to occur between daclatasvir or ombitasvir and escitalopram.

Clinical evidence, mechanism, importance and management

(a) Daclatasvir

The UK manufacturer briefly reports that, in a study in healthy subjects given **escitalopram** 10 mg daily with daclatasvir 60 mg daily, the pharmacokinetics of both drugs were unaffected. No dose adjustments are therefore necessary on concurrent use.[1]

(b) Ombitasvir

The UK manufacturer briefly reports that, in a study in healthy subjects given a single 10-mg dose of **escitalopram** with ombitasvir 25 mg daily (in a fixed-dose combination with paritaprevir boosted with ritonavir, given with and without dasabuvir), the pharmacokinetics of both drugs were unaffected. No dose adjustments are therefore necessary on concurrent use.[2]

1. Daklinza (Daclatasvir dihydrochloride). Bristol-Myers Squibb Pharmaceutical Ltd. UK Summary of product characteristics, September 2014.
2. Viekirax (Ombitasvir, paritaprevir, ritonavir). AbbVie Ltd. UK Summary of product characteristics, January 2015.

NS5A inhibitors; Daclatasvir + Miscellaneous

Amlodipine, diltiazem, nifedipine, and verapamil might increase daclatasvir exposure. No pharmacokinetic interactions are expected between daclatasvir and the antiarrhythmics (amiodarone, disopyramide, flecainide, mexiletine, propafenone, or quinidine), azithromycin, ciprofloxacin, enfuvirtide, the HIV-integrase inhibitors (dolutegravir and raltegravir), maraviroc, mycophenolate, sirolimus, warfarin, ACE inhibitors, angiotensin II receptor antagonists, or phosphodiesterase type-5 inhibitors.

Clinical evidence, mechanism, importance and management

(a) Antiarrhythmics

The UK manufacturer notes that no pharmacokinetic interaction is expected between daclatasvir and the antiarrhythmics; **amiodarone**, **disopyramide**, **flecainide**, **mexiletine**, **propafenone**, or **quinidine**.[1] No dose adjustments would be expected to be necessary on concurrent use.

(b) Antibacterials

The UK manufacturer notes that no pharmacokinetic interaction is expected between daclatasvir and **azithromycin** or **ciprofloxacin** and that no dose adjustment is considered necessary on concurrent use.[1]

(c) Calcium-channel blockers

The UK manufacturer predicts that **amlodipine**, **diltiazem**, **nifedipine**, and **verapamil** might increase the concentrations of daclatasvir if given concurrently, and advises caution.[1] Daclatasvir is a CYP3A4 substrate, and both diltiazem and verapamil are moderate inhibitors of this isoenzyme and so could increase daclatasvir exposure. Verapamil is also an inhibitor of P-glycoprotein, for which daclatasvir is also a substrate, and might therefore have a greater effect than diltiazem. Note that amlodipine and nifedipine are not known to inhibit CYP3A4.

(d) Enfuvirtide

The UK manufacturer notes that no pharmacokinetic interaction is expected between daclatasvir and enfuvirtide, and that no dose adjustment is considered necessary on concurrent use.[1]

(e) HIV-integrase inhibitors

The UK manufacturer notes that no pharmacokinetic interaction is expected between daclatasvir and **raltegravir** or **dolutegravir**, and that no dose adjustment is considered necessary on concurrent use.[1]

(f) Maraviroc

The UK manufacturer notes that no pharmacokinetic interaction is expected between daclatasvir and maraviroc, and that no dose adjustment is considered necessary on concurrent use.[1]

(g) Mycophenolate mofetil

The UK manufacturer notes that no pharmacokinetic interaction is expected between daclatasvir and mycophenolate mofetil, and that no dose adjustment is considered necessary on concurrent use.[1]

(h) Sirolimus

The UK manufacturer notes that no pharmacokinetic interaction is expected between daclatasvir and sirolimus, and that no dose adjustment is considered necessary on concurrent use.[1] Sirolimus is a substrate for P-glycoprotein, of which daclatasvir is an inhibitor. An increase in sirolimus exposure might be expected on concurrent use, but this needs confirmation in a clinical setting.

(i) Warfarin

The UK manufacturer notes that no pharmacokinetic interaction is expected between daclatasvir and warfarin, and that no dose adjustment is considered necessary on concurrent use.[1] Daclatasvir does not appear to affect the isoenzymes involved in the metabolism of *R*- or *S*-warfarin (CYP3A4 and CYP2C9, respectively) and would therefore not be expected to alter the metabolism of warfarin.

(j) Other drugs

The UK manufacturer notes that no pharmacokinetic interaction is expected between daclatasvir and **ACE inhibitors** (they specifically name **enalapril**), **angiotensin II receptor antagonists** (they specifically name **candesartan**, **irbesartan**, **losartan**, **olmesartan**, and **valsartan**) or **phosphodiesterase type-5 inhibitors**.[1] No dose adjustments would be expected to be necessary on concurrent use.

1. Daklinza (Daclatasvir dihydrochloride). Bristol-Myers Squibb Pharmaceutical Ltd. UK Summary of product characteristics, September 2014.

NS5A inhibitors; Daclatasvir + NS5B inhibitors

No pharmacokinetic interaction appears to occur between daclatasvir and sofosbuvir.

Clinical evidence, mechanism, importance and management

The UK manufacturer briefly reports that, in a study in patients with chronic hepatitis C infection given **sofosbuvir** 400 mg daily, and daclatasvir 60 mg daily, the pharmacokinetics of the major inactive metabolite of sofosbuvir were unaffected, and the pharmacokinetics of daclatasvir were comparable to historical values in patients given dalatasvir (with ribavirin and peginterferon alfa). No dose adjustments are necessary on concurrent use.[1] Note that daclatasvir with sofosbuvir is indicated for the treatment of several genotypes of hepatitis C infection.

1. Daklinza (Daclatasvir dihydrochloride). Bristol-Myers Squibb Pharmaceutical Ltd. UK Summary of product characteristics, September 2014.

NS5A inhibitors; Daclatasvir + Peginterferon alfa

No pharmacokinetic interaction appears to occur between daclatasvir and peginterferon alfa.

Clinical evidence, mechanism, importance and management

The UK manufacturer briefly reports that, in a study in patients with chronic hepatitis C infection given peginterferon alfa 180 micrograms weekly (with ribavirin) and daclatasvir 60 mg daily, the pharmacokinetics of both drugs were comparable to historical values in patients given peginterferon alfa with ribavirin and placebo, and in patients given daclatasvir monotherapy, respectively. No dose adjustments are necessary on concurrent use.[1] Note that daclatasvir with peginterferon alfa (and ribavirin) is indicated for the treatment of genotype 4 hepatitis C infection.

1. Daklinza (Daclatasvir dihydrochloride). Bristol-Myers Squibb Pharmaceutical Ltd. UK Summary of product characteristics, September 2014.

NS5A inhibitors; Daclatasvir + Ribavirin

No pharmacokinetic interaction appears to occur between daclatasvir and ribavirin.

Clinical evidence, mechanism, importance and management

The UK manufacturer briefly reports that, in a study in patients with chronic hepatitis C infection given ribavirin 1 g or 1.2 g daily (with peginterferon alfa), and daclatasvir 60 mg daily, the pharmacokinetics of ribavirin were unaffected, and the pharmacokinetics of daclatasvir were comparable to historical values in patients given dalatasvir monotherapy. No dose adjustments are necessary on concurrent use.[1] Note that daclatasvir with ribavirin (and peginterferon alfa) is indicated for the treatment of genotype 4 hepatitis C infection.

1. Daklinza (Daclatasvir dihydrochloride). Bristol-Myers Squibb Pharmaceutical Ltd. UK Summary of product characteristics, September 2014.

NS5A inhibitors; Ledipasvir + Miscellaneous

Verapamil does not appear to alter the pharmacokinetics of ledipasvir. Other P-glycoprotein inhibitors, and inhibitors of BCRP might increase the concentrations of ledipasvir.

Clinical evidence, mechanism, importance and management

The UK and US manufacturers of ledipasvir with sofosbuvir briefly note that ledipasvir is a P-glycoprotein and BCRP substrate, thus inhibitors of these transport proteins might increase the concentrations of ledipasvir. However, they advise that P-glycoprotein and/or BCRP inhibitors can be given concurrently with ledipasvir (in a fixed-dose combination with sofosbuvir).[1,2] For a list of P-glycoprotein inhibitors, see 'Table 1.12', p.14. Further, the US manufacturer also notes that in drug interaction studies, no clinically relevant interaction was observed, or is expected, with **verapamil** [a P-glycoprotein inhibitor].[2]

1. Harvoni (Ledipasvir, sofosbuvir). Gilead Sciences Ltd. UK Summary of product characteristics, November 2014.
2. Harvoni (Ledipasvir, sofosbuvir). Gilead Sciences, Inc. US Prescribing information, March 2015.

NS5A inhibitors; Ombitasvir + Miscellaneous

Ombitasvir might increase the exposure to furosemide and is predicted to increase the concentration of levothyroxine. Amlodipine and furosemide do not appear to alter the pharmacokinetics of ombitasvir. There appears to be no pharmacokinetic interaction between ombitasvir and duloxetine, norethisterone, or warfarin.

Clinical evidence, mechanism, importance and management

(a) Amlodipine

The UK and US manufacturers briefly report, that in a study in 14 healthy subjects given a single 5-mg dose of **amlodipine** with ombitasvir 25 mg daily (in a fixed-dose combination with paritaprevir boosted ritonavir, and given with dasabuvir), the pharmacokinetics of ombitasvir were unaffected.[1,2] The UK manufacturer also notes that similar effects are expected when the combination is given without dasabuvir.[1] No ombitasvir dose adjustment is necessary on concurrent use.

(b) Duloxetine

The UK manufacturer briefly reports that, in a study in healthy subjects given a single 60-mg dose of duloxetine with ombitasvir 25 mg daily (in a fixed-dose combination with paritaprevir boosted with ritonavir, and given with dasabuvir), the pharmacokinetics of ombitasvir were unaffected, but the AUC and maximum concentration of duloxetine were decreased by 25% and 21%, respectively. The effect of the combination when given without dasabuvir was similar.[1] Such a small decrease in duloxetine exposure is unlikely to be clinically important and so no dose adjustments are necessary on concurrent use.

(c) Furosemide

The UK and US manufacturers briefly report that, in a study in 12 healthy subjects given a single 20-mg dose of furosemide with ombitasvir 25 mg daily (in a fixed-dose combination with paritaprevir boosted with ritonavir, and given with dasabuvir), the pharmacokinetics of ombitasvir were unaffected, but the maximum concentration of furosemide was increased by 42%. The AUC of furosemide was unaffected.[1,2] The UK manufacturer also notes that similar effects are expected when the combination is given without dasabuvir.[1] They therefore recommend that patients are monitored [for furosemide effects], with the UK manufacturer advising that a 50% decrease in furosemide dose might be required,[1] and the US manufacturer suggesting that the dose should be individualised, dependent on response.[2] No ombitasvir dose adjustment is required. The mechanism behind this effect is unclear, but note that other components of the combination might also be involved.

(d) Levothyroxine

The UK manufacturer predicts that ombitasvir (in a fixed-dose combination with paritaprevir boosted with ritonavir, and given with or without dasabuvir) will increase the concentration of levothyroxine, due to inhibition of the glucuronosyltransferase, UGT1A1, and advises clinical monitoring (for increased levothyroxine effects), with levothyroxine dose adjustment where necessary, on concurrent use.[1] Note that other components of the combination might also be involved.

(e) Norethisterone

The UK manufacturer briefly reports that, in a study in healthy subjects given norethisterone 350 micrograms daily with ombitasvir 25 mg daily (in a fixed-dose combination with paritaprevir boosted with ritonavir, and given with dasabuvir), the pharmacokinetics of ombitasvir and norethisterone were unaffected.[1] No dose adjustments are required on concurrent use.[1,2] Note also that progesterone-only contraceptives are recommended in preference to combined hormonal contraceptives in patients taking this combination preparation, see 'Combined hormonal contraceptives + NS5A inhibitors', p.1182 for details.

(f) Warfarin

The UK manufacturer briefly reports that, in a study in healthy subjects given a single 5-mg dose of warfarin with ombitasvir 25 mg daily (in a fixed-dose combination with paritaprevir boosted with ritonavir, and given with and without dasabuvir), there were no effects on the pharmacokinetics of *R*- and *S*-warfarin or of ombitasvir.[1] No dose adjustments are necessary on concurrent use,[1,2] but the UK manufacturer recommends appropriate monitoring of INR,[1] which is standard practice in all patients taking warfarin.

1. Viekirax (Ombitasvir, paritaprevir, ritonavir). AbbVie Ltd. UK Summary of product characteristics, January 2015.
2. Viekira Pak (Ombitasvir, paritaprevir, ritonavir co-packaged with dasabuvir sodium monohydrate). AbbVie Inc. US Prescribing information, December 2014.

NS5B inhibitors + Ciclosporin

Ciclosporin does not appear to alter the pharmacokinetics of dasabuvir, but appeared to moderately increase exposure to sofosbuvir. Sofosbuvir does not appear to alter the pharmacokinetics of ciclosporin.

Clinical evidence, mechanism, importance and management

(a) Dasabuvir

The UK manufacturer briefly reports that, in a study in healthy subjects given a single 30-mg dose of ciclosporin and dasabuvir 250 or 400 mg twice daily (with a fixed-dose combination of ombitasvir and paritaprevir boosted with ritonavir), the AUC and maximum concentration of dasabuvir were decreased by 30% and 34%, respectively.[1] The decrease in exposure is only slight and therefore no dasabuvir dose adjustment is necessary on concurrent use.

(b) Sofosbuvir

The UK and US manufacturers briefly report that, in a single-dose study in 19 healthy subjects given 600-mg of ciclosporin and 400-mg of sofosbuvir, the AUC and maximum concentration of ciclosporin were unaffected, but the AUC and maximum concentration of sofosbuvir were increased 4.5- and 2.5-fold, respectively. The exposure to the major inactive metabolite of sofosbuvir was unaffected, but the maximum concentration was decreased by 40%.[2,3] Despite this moderate increase in sofosbuvir exposure, no dose adjustment is considered necessary on concurrent use with ciclosporin, and no ciclosporin dose adjustment is necessary.[2,3]

1. Exviera (Dasabuvir sodium monohydrate). AbbVie Ltd. UK Summary of product characteristics, January 2015.
2. Sovaldi (Sofosbuvir). Gilead Sciences Ltd. UK Summary of product characteristics, January 2015.
3. Sovaldi (Sofosbuvir). Gilead Sciences, Inc. US Prescribing information, March 2015.

NS5B inhibitors + Drugs that affect gastric pH

Famotidine appears to have no effect on the pharmacokinetics of sofosbuvir, and other H_2-receptor antagonists would also be expected to have no effect. Omeprazole appears to have no effect on the pharmacokinetics of dasabuvir or sofosbuvir. Other proton pump inhibitors would also be expected to have no effect.

Clinical evidence, mechanism, importance and management

(a) H_2-receptor antagonists

The UK and US manufacturers of **sofosbuvir** (in a fixed-dose combination with ledipasvir) briefly report that, in a study in 12 healthy subjects, a single 40-mg dose of **famotidine** given at the same time as, or 12 hours before, a single 400-mg dose of sofosbuvir (with ledipasvir) had no effect on the pharmacokinetics of sofosbuvir or its major inactive metabolite. They therefore advise that sofosbuvir (with ledipasvir) can be given simultaneously with, or separated (by 12 hours[1]) from, famotidine or other H_2-receptor antagonists, at a dose that does not exceed famotidine 40 mg twice daily, or equivalent.[1,2]

(b) Proton pump inhibitors

1. Dasabuvir. The UK manufacturer briefly reports that, in a study in healthy subjects given **omeprazole** 40 mg once daily with dasabuvir 250 or 400 mg twice daily (with a fixed-dose combination of ombitasvir and paritaprevir boosted with ritonavir), the pharmacokinetics of dasabuvir were unaffected. No dasabuvir dose adjustment is necessary on concurrent use.[3] Other proton pump inhibitors might reasonably be expected to not affect dasabuvir pharmacokinetics.

2. Sofosbuvir. The UK and US manufacturers of sofosbuvir in a fixed-dose combination with ledipasvir briefly report that, in a study in 16 healthy subjects, **omeprazole** 20 mg daily given at the same time as a single 400-mg dose of sofosbuvir (with ledipasvir) had no effect on the pharmacokinetics of sofosbuvir or its major inactive metabolite.[1,2] It is therefore recommended that proton pump inhibitors should be given simultaneously with sofosbuvir (with ledipasvir), and at doses that are comparable to omeprazole 20 mg[2] (or lower[1]).

1. Harvoni (Ledipasvir, sofosbuvir). Gilead Sciences, Inc. US Prescribing information, March 2015.
2. Harvoni (Ledipasvir, sofosbuvir). Gilead Sciences Ltd. UK Summary of product characteristics, November 2014.
3. Exviera (Dasabuvir sodium monohydrate). AbbVie Ltd. UK Summary of product characteristics, January 2015.

NS5B inhibitors + Food

Food appears to slightly increase the exposure to dasabuvir and sofosbuvir.

Clinical evidence, mechanism, importance and management

(a) Dasabuvir

The UK manufacturer briefly reports that, in a study in healthy subjects, food increased the AUC of dasabuvir by 30%, relative to the fasting state, and was not affected by the fat (high- versus moderate-fat) or calorie (600 versus 1000 kilocalories) content of the meal. Dasabuvir should be taken with food, but without regard to fat or calorie content.[1]

(b) Sofosbuvir

The UK manufacturer briefly reports that, in a study, a standardised high-fat meal increased the AUC of a single dose of sofosbuvir about 2-fold, relative to the fasted state. They recommend that it should be given with food.[2] A similar effect was seen when sofosbuvir was given with ledipasvir, and a high- or moderate-fat meal.[3,4] In contrast, the US manufacturer of sofosbuvir states that a standardised high-fat meal did not substantially alter the AUC and maximum concentration of sofosbuvir, and it can be given without regard to food.[5]

1. Exviera (Dasabuvir sodium monohydrate). AbbVie Ltd. UK Summary of product characteristics, January 2015.
2. Sovaldi (Sofosbuvir). Gilead Sciences Ltd. UK Summary of product characteristics, January 2015.
3. Harvoni (Ledipasvir, sofosbuvir). Gilead Sciences Ltd. UK Summary of product characteristics, November 2014.
4. Harvoni (Ledipasvir, sofosbuvir). Gilead Sciences, Inc. US Prescribing information, March 2015.
5. Sovaldi (Sofosbuvir). Gilead Sciences, Inc. US Prescribing information, March 2015.

NS5B inhibitors + HIV-protease inhibitors

The pharmacokinetics of dasabuvir and sofosbuvir do not appear to be affected to a clinically relevant extent by atazanavir or darunavir. Dasabuvir and sofosbuvir do not appear to alter the pharmacokinetics of atazanavir to a clinically relevant extent. Dasabuvir might slightly decrease exposure to, and decrease the minimum concentration of darunavir, but sofosbuvir appears to have no effect. No interaction appears to occur between dasabuvir and lopinavir. Tipranavir is predicted to decrease the concentration of sofosbuvir.

Clinical evidence, mechanism, importance and management

(a) Atazanavir

1. Dasabuvir. The UK manufacturer briefly reports that, in a study in healthy subjects given dasabuvir 250 or 400 mg twice daily (with a fixed-dose combination of ombitasvir and paritaprevir boosted with ritonavir) and atazanavir 300 mg daily at the same time, the AUC and maximum concentration of dasabuvir were both decreased by about 18%. The pharmacokinetics of atazanavir were unaffected. Similar results were seen in another study, when atazanavir boosted with ritonavir 300/100 mg daily was given 12 hours after dasabuvir 250 or 400 mg twice daily (with a fixed-dose combination of ombitasvir and paritaprevir boosted with ritonavir).[1] No atazanavir or dasabuvir dose adjustments are required on concurrent use. For further information on the effect of other components of the fixed-dose combination preparation, see 'HCV-protease inhibitors + HIV-protease inhibitors', p.904.

2. Sofosbuvir. The UK manufacturers briefly report that, in a study in 30 healthy subjects given sofosbuvir 400 mg daily (in a fixed-dose combination with ledipasvir) and atazanavir boosted with ritonavir 300/100 mg daily, the AUC and maximum concentration of sofosbuvir and its major inactive metabolite were unaffected. The AUC of atazanavir was increased by 33%.[2,3] No dose adjustments are necessary on concurrent use.

(b) Darunavir

1. Dasabuvir. The UK manufacturer briefly reports that, in a study in healthy subjects given dasabuvir 250 or 400 mg twice daily (with a fixed-dose combination of ombitasvir and paritaprevir boosted with ritonavir) and darunavir 800 mg daily at the same time, the pharmacokinetics of dasabuvir were unaffected. The AUC and minimum concentration of darunavir were decreased by 24%, and 48%, respectively, but the maximum concentration was unaffected.[1] In another study, when darunavir boosted with ritonavir 600/100 mg twice daily was given with dasabuvir 250 or 400 mg twice daily (with a fixed-dose combination of ombitasvir and paritaprevir boosted with ritonavir) the AUC of dasabuvir was decreased by 27%, and the minimum concentration by 46%, but the maximum concentration was unaffected. The AUC and minimum concentration of darunavir were decreased by 20% and 43%, respectively, but the maximum concentration was unaffected.[1] In a further study when darunavir boosted with ritonavir 800/100 mg daily was given 12 hours after dasabuvir 250 or 400 mg twice daily (with a fixed-dose combination of ombitasvir and paritaprevir boosted with ritonavir), the AUC and maximum concentration of dasabuvir were decreased by about 25%. The AUC of darunavir was increased by 34% and the maximum and minimum concentrations were decreased by 21% and 46%, respectively.[1] No dasabuvir dose adjustment is necessary on concurrent use, but the UK manufacturer advises that the recommended dose of darunavir is 800 mg daily, without ritonavir, and given at the same time as the combination. Further, they say that it should only be used in the absence of extensive protease inhibitor resistance.[1]

2. Sofosbuvir. The UK and US manufacturers briefly report that, in a study in 18 healthy subjects given a single 400-mg dose of sofosbuvir with darunavir boosted with ritonavir 800/100 mg daily, the AUC and maximum concentration of sofosbuvir were increased by 34% and 45%, respectively, and the AUC of the major inactive metabolite was increased by 24%. The pharmacokinetics of darunavir were unaffected.[4,5] No dose adjustments are necessary on concurrent use.

(c) Lopinavir

The UK manufacturer briefly reports that, in a study in healthy subjects given **dasabuvir** 250 or 400 mg twice daily (with a fixed-dose combination of ombitasvir and paritaprevir boosted with ritonavir) and lopinavir boosted with ritonavir 400/100 mg twice daily, the pharmacokinetics of dasabuvir and lopinavir were unaffected.1 No lopinavir or dasabuvir dose adjustments are necessary on concurrent use. For further information on the effect of other components of the fixed-dose combination preparation, see 'HCV-protease inhibitors + HIV-protease inhibitors', p.904.

(d) Tipranavir

The UK and US manufacturers of **sofosbuvir** in a fixed-dose combination with ledipasvir predict that tipranavir boosted with ritonavir might decrease the concentration of sofosbuvir and reduce the therapeutic efficacy of the combination, and hence do not recommend concurrent use.[4,5]

1. Exviera (Dasabuvir sodium monohydrate). AbbVie Ltd. UK Summary of product characteristics, January 2015.
2. Harvoni (Ledipasvir, sofosbuvir). Gilead Sciences Ltd. UK Summary of product characteristics, November 2014.
3. Harvoni (Ledipasvir, sofosbuvir). Gilead Sciences, Inc. US Prescribing information, March 2015.
4. Sovaldi (Sofosbuvir). Gilead Sciences Ltd. UK Summary of product characteristics, January 2015.
5. Sovaldi (Sofosbuvir). Gilead Sciences, Inc. US Prescribing information, March 2015.

NS5B inhibitors + NNRTIs

No pharmacokinetic interaction appears to occur between sofosbuvir and efavirenz or rilpivirine. The pharmacokinetics of dasabuvir do not appear to be altered by rilpivirine. ALT elevations were seen when

dasabuvir was given with paritaprevir boosted with ritonavir, and efavirenz.

Clinical evidence, mechanism, importance and management

(a) Efavirenz

1. Dasabuvir. The UK manufacturer notes that concurrent use of efavirenz-based regimens and dasabuvir (given with paritaprevir boosted with ritonavir) resulted in ALT increases which necessitated early discontinuation of the interaction study. As a result concurrent use with efavirenz is contraindicated.[1]

2. Sofosbuvir. The UK and US manufacturers briefly report that, in a study in 16 healthy subjects given efavirenz 600 mg once daily (with emtricitabine and tenofovir) with a single 400-mg dose of sofosbuvir, the pharmacokinetics of efavirenz and sofosbuvir were unaffected.[2,3] Similar results were seen when efavirenz (in the same combination) was given with sofosbuvir in a fixed-dose combination with ledipasvir.[4,5] No dose adjustments are necessary on concurrent use.

(b) Rilpivirine

1. Dasabuvir. The UK manufacturer briefly reports that, in a study in healthy subjects, rilpivirine 25 mg daily had no effect on the pharmacokinetics of dasabuvir 250 or 400 mg twice daily (with a fixed-dose combination of ombitasvir and paritaprevir boosted with ritonavir).[1] No dasabuvir dose adjustment is required on concurrent use.

2. Sofosbuvir. The UK and US manufacturers briefly report that, in a study in 17 healthy subjects given rilpivirine 25 mg daily with a single 400-mg dose of sofosbuvir, the pharmacokinetics of rilpivirine and of sofosbuvir and its major inactive metabolite were unaffected.[2,3] Similar results were seen when sofosbuvir was given in a fixed-dose combination with ledipasvir.[4,5] No dose adjustments are necessary on concurrent use.

(c) Other NNRTIs

The UK manufacturer of **dasabuvir** predicts that **etravirine** and **nevirapine** will decrease the concentration of dasabuvir and contraindicates concurrent use.[1] However, dasabuvir is not a major substrate of CYP3A4, which is induced by these NNRTIs (albeit to varying extents), and so an interaction via this mechanism is unlikely.

1. Exviera (Dasabuvir sodium monohydrate). AbbVie Ltd. UK Summary of product characteristics, January 2015.
2. Sovaldi (Sofosbuvir). Gilead Sciences Ltd. UK Summary of product characteristics, January 2015.
3. Sovaldi (Sofosbuvir). Gilead Sciences, Inc. US Prescribing information, March 2015.
4. Harvoni (Ledipasvir, sofosbuvir). Gilead Sciences Ltd. UK Summary of product characteristics, November 2014.
5. Harvoni (Ledipasvir, sofosbuvir). Gilead Sciences, Inc. US Prescribing information, March 2015.

NS5B inhibitors + NRTIs

No pharmacokinetic interaction appears to occur between dasabuvir or sofosbuvir and emtricitabine.

Clinical evidence, mechanism, importance and management

1. Dasabuvir. The UK manufacturer briefly reports that, in a study in healthy subjects given emtricitabine 200 mg daily (with tenofovir) and dasabuvir 250 or 400 mg twice daily (with a fixed-dose combination of ombitasvir and paritaprevir boosted with ritonavir), the pharmacokinetics of emtricitabine and dasabuvir were unaffected.[1] No dose adjustments are necessary on concurrent use.[1]

2. Sofosbuvir. The UK and US manufacturers briefly report that, in a study in 16 healthy subjects given emtricitabine 200 mg once daily (with efavirenz and tenofovir) with a single 400-mg dose of sofosbuvir, the pharmacokinetics of emtricitabine and sofosbuvir (and its major inactive metabolite) were unaffected.[2,3] Similar results were seen when emtricitabine (in the same combination) was given with sofosbuvir in a fixed-dose combination with ledipasvir.[4,5] No dose adjustments are necessary on concurrent use.

1. Exviera (Dasabuvir sodium monohydrate). AbbVie Ltd. UK Summary of product characteristics, January 2015.
2. Sovaldi (Sofosbuvir). Gilead Sciences Ltd. UK Summary of product characteristics, January 2015.
3. Sovaldi (Sofosbuvir). Gilead Sciences, Inc. US Prescribing information, March 2015.
4. Harvoni (Ledipasvir, sofosbuvir). Gilead Sciences Ltd. UK Summary of product characteristics, November 2014.
5. Harvoni (Ledipasvir, sofosbuvir). Gilead Sciences, Inc. US Prescribing information, March 2015.

NS5B inhibitors + Rifampicin (Rifampin) and other enzyme/P-glycoprotein inducers

Carbamazepine appears to moderately decrease dasabuvir exposure. Other enzyme/P-glycoprotein inducers are predicted to have a similar effect. Rifampicin appears to moderately decrease sofosbuvir exposure. Other P-glycoprotein inducers are predicted to have a similar effect.

Clinical evidence

(a) Dasabuvir

The UK manufacturer briefly reports that, in a study in healthy subjects, **carbamazepine** 200 mg daily followed by 200 mg twice daily decreased the AUC and maximum concentration of a single-dose of dasabuvir (given with a fixed-dose combination of ombitasvir and paritaprevir boosted with ritonavir) by 70% and 55%, respectively.[1]

(b) Sofosbuvir

The UK manufacturer briefly reports that in a study in healthy subjects, **rifampicin** 600 mg once daily decreased the AUC and maximum concentration of a single 400-mg dose of sofosbuvir by 72% and 77%, respectively.[2]

Mechanism

Dasabuvir is a substrate of CYP2C8 and P-glycoprotein. Carbamazepine is a well-known enzyme inducer (although perhaps not of CYP2C8) and also induces P-glycoprotein. Concurrent use therefore results in decreased dasabuvir exposure. Sofosbuvir is a substrate of P-glycoprotein which is induced by rifampicin, resulting in a decrease in exposure to sofosbuvir.

Importance and management

Evidence for an interaction between the NS5B inhibitors and enzyme or P-glycoprotein inducers is limited to the two studies. The moderate decrease in dasabuvir exposure seen is consistent with the metabolism of dasabuvir and the known inducing effects of carbamazepine. Concurrent use is contraindicated by the manufacturer due to the risk of reduced therapeutic effect, and they extend this to other potent or moderate enzyme inducers, specifically naming the other enzyme-inducing antiepileptics **phenobarbital** and **phenytoin**, as well as **enzalutamide**, **mitotane**, **rifampicin**, and **St John's wort**.[1] However, it is important to note that, of these drugs only rifampicin is known to be a clinically relevant inducer of CYP2C8 (involved in the metabolism of dasabuvir), and only rifampicin and St John's wort are known to be clinically relevant inducers of P-glycoprotein (involved in the transport of dasabuvir). Interactions with these drugs can therefore not be ruled out. But, as mitotane is not considered a clinically relevant inducer of any enzymes, the inducing effects of enzalutamide are yet to be established, and phenobarbital and phenytoin are known CYP3A4 inducers (dasabuvir is not a CYP3A4 substrate), interactions with these drugs via these known mechanisms would seem unlikely.

The moderate decrease in exposure to **sofosbuvir** seen with rifampicin is also consistent with its metabolism and the known inducing effects of rifampicin. The UK and US manufacturers state that because of the risk of a decreased therapeutic effect, concurrent use of P-glycoprotein inducers is not recommended,[3,4] see 'Table 1.12', p.14 for a list. They also name **oxcarbazepine**, **phenytoin**, **phenobarbital**, **rifabutin**, and **rifapentine**, but the P-glycoprotein inducing effects of these drugs are yet to be established.

1. Exviera (Dasabuvir sodium monohydrate). AbbVie Ltd. UK Summary of product characteristics, January 2015.
2. Harvoni (Ledipasvir, sofosbuvir). Gilead Sciences Ltd. UK Summary of product characteristics, November 2014.
3. Sovaldi (Sofosbuvir). Gilead Sciences Ltd. UK Summary of product characteristics, January 2015.
4. Sovaldi (Sofosbuvir). Gilead Sciences, Inc. US Prescribing information, March 2015.

NS5B inhibitors + Tenofovir

No pharmacokinetic interaction appears to occur between tenofovir and dasabuvir or sofosbuvir.

Clinical evidence, mechanism, importance and management

(a) Dasabuvir

The UK manufacturer briefly reports that, in a study in healthy subjects given tenofovir 300 mg daily (with emtricitabine) and dasabuvir 250 or 400 mg twice daily (with a fixed-dose combination of ombitasvir and paritaprevir boosted with ritonavir), the pharmacokinetics of tenofovir and dasabuvir were unaffected.[1] No dose adjustment is necessary on concurrent use.

(b) Sofosbuvir

The UK and US manufacturers briefly report that, in a study in 16 healthy subjects given tenofovir 300 mg once daily (with efavirenz and emtricitabine) with a single 400-mg dose of sofosbuvir, the pharmacokinetics of tenofovir and sofosbuvir were unaffected.[2,3] No dose adjustments are necessary on concurrent use. Sofosbuvir was similarly unaffected when tenofovir (in the same combination) was given with sofosbuvir in a fixed-dose combination with ledipasvir.[4,5] For the effects of sofosbuvir with ledipasvir on tenofovir exposure, see 'Tenofovir + NS5A inhibitors', p.997.

1. Exviera (Dasabuvir sodium monohydrate). AbbVie Ltd. UK Summary of product characteristics, January 2015.
2. Sovaldi (Sofosbuvir). Gilead Sciences Ltd. UK Summary of product characteristics, January 2015.
3. Sovaldi (Sofosbuvir). Gilead Sciences, Inc. US Prescribing information, March 2015.
4. Harvoni (Ledipasvir, sofosbuvir). Gilead Sciences Ltd. UK Summary of product characteristics, November 2014.
5. Harvoni (Ledipasvir, sofosbuvir). Gilead Sciences, Inc. US Prescribing information, March 2015.

NS5B inhibitors; Dasabuvir + Azoles

Ketoconazole appears to slightly increase the exposure to dasabuvir.

Clinical evidence, mechanism, importance and management

The UK manufacturer briefly reports that, in a study in healthy subjects, ketoconazole 400 mg daily increased the AUC of a single-dose of dasabuvir (given with a fixed-dose combination of ombitasvir and paritaprevir boosted with ritonavir) by 42%, but had no effect on its maximum concentration.[1] This slight increase in exposure is unlikely to be clinically important and so no dasabuvir dose adjustment would seem necessary on concurrent use. However, note that concurrent use of ketoconazole with paritaprevir (which is part of the fixed dose combination) is contraindicated in the UK, see 'HCV-protease inhibitors + Azoles', p.901.

1. Exviera (Dasabuvir sodium monohydrate). AbbVie Ltd. UK Summary of product characteristics, January 2015.

NS5B inhibitors; Dasabuvir + Gemfibrozil

Gemfibrozil appears to very markedly increase the exposure to dasabuvir.

Clinical evidence

The UK manufacturer briefly reports that, in a study in healthy subjects, gemfibrozil 600 mg twice daily increased the AUC and maximum concentration of a single-dose of dasabuvir (given with paritaprevir boosted with ritonavir) 11-fold and 2-fold, respectively.[1]

Mechanism

Dasabuvir is a substrate of CYP2C8, which is inhibited by gemfibrozil. Concurrent use therefore results in increased dasabuvir exposure.

Importance and management

Evidence for a pharmacokinetic interaction between dasabuvir and gemfibrozil is limited to this one study, but given the known potent inhibitory effects of gemfibrozil on other drugs metabolised by CYP2C8, an interaction would seem to be established. The very marked increase in exposure seen, means that the interaction will be clinically important. The UK manufacturer therefore contraindicates the concurrent use of dasabuvir with gemfibrozil or other potent CYP2C8 inhibitors.[1]

1. Exviera (Dasabuvir sodium monohydrate). AbbVie Ltd. UK Summary of product characteristics, January 2015.

NS5B inhibitors; Dasabuvir + Miscellaneous

Alprazolam, amlodipine, and furosemide do not appear to alter the pharmacokinetics of dasabuvir. Deferasirox and teriflunomide are predicted to increase dasabuvir concentrations. Dasabuvir might increase the exposure to furosemide, and is predicted to increase the concentrations of sulfasalazine and imatinib. There appears to be no pharmacokinetic interaction between dasabuvir and duloxetine, escitalopram, norethisterone, warfarin, or zolpidem. Dasabuvir is predicted to increase the concentration of levothyroxine.

Clinical evidence, mechanism, importance and management

(a) Amlodipine

The UK manufacturer briefly reports, that in a study in healthy subjects given a single 5-mg dose of amlodipine with dasabuvir 250 or 400 mg twice daily (with a fixed-dose combination of ombitasvir and paritaprevir boosted with ritonavir), the pharmacokinetics of dasabuvir were unaffected.[1] No dasabuvir dose adjustment is necessary on concurrent use.

(b) Benzodiazepines and related drugs

The UK manufacturer briefly reports that, in studies in healthy subjects given a single 500-microgram dose of **alprazolam** or a single 5-mg dose of **zolpidem** with dasabuvir 250 or 400 mg twice daily (with a fixed-dose combination of ombitasvir and paritaprevir boosted with ritonavir), the pharmacokinetics of dasabuvir were unaffected, as were those of zolpidem. No dasabuvir dose adjustment is necessary on concurrent use with either alprazolam or zolpidem, and no zolpidem dose adjustment is necessary.[1]

(c) Duloxetine

The UK manufacturer briefly reports that, in a study in healthy subjects given a single 60-mg dose of duloxetine with dasabuvir 250 or 400 mg twice daily (with a fixed-dose combination of ombitasvir and paritaprevir boosted with ritonavir), the pharmacokinetics of dasabuvir were unaffected, but the AUC and maximum concentration of duloxetine were decreased by 21% and 25%, respectively.[1] Such a small decrease in duloxetine exposure is unlikely to be clinically important and so no dose adjustments are necessary on concurrent use.

(d) Escitalopram

The UK manufacturer briefly reports that, in a study in healthy subjects given a single 10-mg dose of escitalopram with dasabuvir 250 or 400 mg twice daily (with a fixed-dose combination of ombitasvir and paritaprevir boosted with ritonavir), the pharmacokinetics of dasabuvir and escitalopram were unaffected. No dose adjustments are necessary on concurrent use.[1]

(e) Furosemide

The UK manufacturer briefly reports that, in a study in healthy subjects given a single 20-mg dose of furosemide with dasabuvir 250 or 400 mg twice daily (with a fixed-dose combination of ombitasvir and paritaprevir boosted with ritonavir), the pharmacokinetics of dasabuvir were unaffected, but the maximum concentration of furosemide was increased by 42%. The AUC of furosemide was unaffected.[1] They therefore recommend that patients are monitored for furosemide effects, and that a 50% decrease in furosemide dose might be required.[1] No dasabuvir dose adjustment is required.[1] The mechanism behind this effect is unclear, but note that other components of the combination might also be involved.

(f) Levothyroxine

The UK manufacturer predicts that dasabuvir 250 or 400 mg twice daily (with a fixed-dose combination of ombitasvir and paritaprevir boosted with ritonavir) will increase the concentration of levothyroxine, due to inhibition of the glucuronosyltransferase, UGT1A1, and advises clinical monitoring (for increased levothyroxine effects), with levothyroxine dose adjustment where necessary, on concurrent use.[1] Note that other components of the combination might also be involved.

(g) Norethisterone

The UK manufacturer briefly reports that, in a study in healthy subjects given norethisterone 350 micrograms daily with dasabuvir 250 or 400 mg twice daily (with a fixed-dose combination of ombitasvir and paritaprevir boosted with ritonavir), the pharmacokinetics of dasabuvir and norethisterone were unaffected.[1] No dose adjustments are required on concurrent use.[1] Note also that progesterone-only contraceptives are recommended in preference to combined hormonal contraceptives in patients taking this combination, see 'Combined hormonal contraceptives + NS5B inhibitors', p.1182 for details.

(h) Warfarin

The UK manufacturer briefly reports that, in a study in healthy subjects given a single 5-mg dose of warfarin with dasabuvir 250 or 400 mg twice daily (with a fixed-dose combination of ombitasvir and paritaprevir boosted with ritonavir), there were no effects on the pharmacokinetics of *R*- and *S*-warfarin or dasabuvir.[1] No dose adjustments are necessary on concurrent use, but the manufacturer recommends appropriate monitoring of INR,[1] which is standard practice in all patients taking warfarin.

(i) Other drugs

Although not studied, the UK manufacturer predicts that **deferasirox** and **teriflunomide** might both increase dasabuvir concentrations and advises caution on concurrent use.[1] They also predict that dasabuvir might increase the concentrations of **sulfasalazine** and **imatinib**, via inhibition of BCRP, although note that other components of the fixed-dose combination preparation given with dasabuvir might also be involved. Caution is recommended if **sulfasalazine** is given concurrently, and clinical monitoring and lower **imatinib** doses are recommended.[1]

1. Exviera (Dasabuvir sodium monohydrate). AbbVie Ltd. UK Summary of product characteristics, January 2015.

NS5B inhibitors; Sofosbuvir + Miscellaneous

Sofosbuvir concentrations are predicted to be increased by telaprevir but not boceprevir, and decreased by modafinil. There appears to be no interaction between sofosbuvir and abacavir or lamivudine. Verapamil does not appear to alter the pharmacokinetics of sofosbuvir. Other P-glycoprotein inhibitors, and inhibitors of BCRP, are also not expected to interact.

Clinical evidence, mechanism, importance and management

(a) Drug transporter proteins

The UK and US manufacturers briefly note that sofosbuvir is a P-glycoprotein and BCRP substrate, thus inhibitors of these transport proteins might increase the concentrations of sofosbuvir, but are not expected to increase those of its major inactive metabolite. However, they advise that P-glycoprotein and BCRP inhibitors can be given concurrently with sofosbuvir.[1,2] For a list of P-glycoprotein inhibitors, see 'Table 1.12', p.14. Further, the US manufacturer of sofosbuvir with ledipasvir also notes that in drug interaction studies, no clinically relevant interaction was observed, or is expected, with **verapamil** [a P-glycoprotein inhibitor].[3]

(b) HCV-protease inhibitors

Although not studied, the UK manufacturer predicts that **boceprevir** will have no effect on the concentrations of sofosbuvir, but that **telaprevir** will increase its concentrations. Neither boceprevir nor telaprevir are predicted to affect the major inactive metabolite of sofosbuvir. In addition there are no clinical data to support the concurrent use of sofosbuvir with either of these HCV-protease inhibitors and so combined use is not recommended.[1]

(c) Modafinil

Although not studied, the UK manufacturer predicts that modafinil will decrease the concentrations of sofosbuvir and its major inactive metabolite, resulting in a decreased therapeutic effect. Concurrent use is therefore not recommended.[1] It is not clear what the mechanism for this interaction (should it occur) might be, because although modafinil is an enzyme inhibitor and inducer (of CYP2C19 and CYP3A4, respectively), sofosbuvir is not a substrate for any cytochrome P450 isoenzymes. Further study is required to establish the relevance of this prediction in practice.

(d) NRTIs

The UK manufacturer of sofosbuvir with ledipasvir briefly reports that in a study in healthy subjects given sofosbuvir 400 mg daily (in a fixed-dose combination with ledipasvir) with **abacavir** 600 mg daily and **lamivudine** 300 mg daily, the pharmacokinetics of sofosbuvir and its major inactive metabolite were unaltered, as were the pharmacokinetics of abacavir and lamivudine.[4] The US manufacturer also notes that the pharmacokinetics of all these drugs were not affected by concurrent use.[3] No dose adjustments are necessary on concurrent use.

1. Sovaldi (Sofosbuvir). Gilead Sciences Ltd. UK Summary of product characteristics, January 2015.
2. Sovaldi (Sofosbuvir). Gilead Sciences, Inc. US Prescribing information, March 2015.
3. Harvoni (Ledipasvir, sofosbuvir). Gilead Sciences, Inc. US Prescribing information, March 2015.
4. Harvoni (Ledipasvir, sofosbuvir). Gilead Sciences Ltd. UK Summary of product characteristics, November 2014.

Oseltamivir + Drugs that affect renal clearance

Probenecid inhibits the renal secretion of the active metabolite of oseltamivir and greatly increases its plasma concentration. No pharmacokinetic interaction occurs between amoxicillin and oseltamivir, and cimetidine does not appear to alter oseltamivir pharmacokinetics.

Clinical evidence

(a) Amoxicillin

In a study in healthy subjects, oseltamivir 75 mg twice daily for 4.5 days had no effect on the pharmacokinetics of a single 500-mg dose of amoxicillin given with the last dose of oseltamivir. Similarly, amoxicillin had no effect on the pharmacokinetics of the active metabolite of oseltamivir.[1]

(b) Cimetidine

In a crossover study[1] in 18 healthy subjects, cimetidine 400 mg every 6 hours for 4 days had no effect on the pharmacokinetics of a single 150-mg dose of oseltamivir given on day 2.

(c) Probenecid

In a crossover study in 18 healthy subjects, probenecid 500 mg every 6 hours for 4 days approximately halved the renal clearance of the active metabolite of oseltamivir, and increased its AUC about 2.5-fold when a single 150-mg dose of oseltamivir was given on day 2. Population pharmacokinetic data have been used to assess the possibility of using a lower dose of oseltamivir in combination with probenecid. Oseltamivir 45 mg twice daily, but not oseltamivir 30 mg twice daily, with probenecid 500 mg every 6 hours resulted in the same plasma concentration of the active metabolite as oseltamivir 75 mg twice daily alone.[2] Similarly, another study found that giving oseltamivir 75 mg every 48 hours with probenecid 500 mg four times daily produced similar plasma concentrations of oseltamivir and its carboxylate metabolite as giving oseltamivir 75 mg daily.[3] In this study, concurrent use was generally well tolerated, although one subject developed thrombocytopenia, with a platelet count of 15 x10^9/L after 14 days of concurrent use.[4]

Mechanism

Probenecid appears to completely inhibit the renal tubular secretion of the active metabolite of oseltamivir via the anionic renal transporter process. Oseltamivir does not alter amoxicillin pharmacokinetics, suggesting minimal potential to inhibit the renal anionic transport process.[1] Cimetidine, which inhibits the renal tubular secretion of drugs via the cationic secretion transport process, had no effect on oseltamivir.

Importance and management

Probenecid greatly increased the AUC of the active metabolite of oseltamivir, but because of the large therapeutic range of oseltamivir, this increase is not considered to be clinically relevant.[1,5,6] The case of thrombocytopenia reported by one of the studies seems unlikely to be generally relevant; however, if thrombocytopenia develops in a patient taking both drugs, it might be prudent to consider these drugs as a possible cause.[4] Although one study found that a reduced dose of oseltamivir with probenecid produced therapeutic oseltamivir metabolite concentrations it was suggested that the use of the combination might compromise tolerability, increase the potential for interactions, and the increased dosing requirements of the oseltamivir with probenecid regimen might reduce compliance.[2]

Oseltamivir did not alter **amoxicillin** pharmacokinetics, and is therefore unlikely to interact with other renally secreted organic acids. Other drugs that are involved in the active anionic tubular secretion mechanism are also unlikely to interact. **Cimetidine** does not interact with oseltamivir, and other drugs that are inhibitors of the renal cationic secretion transport process are unlikely to interact.[1]

Although the UK manufacturer states that clinically important drug interactions involving competition for renal tubular secretion are unlikely, they recommend care should be taken when giving oseltamivir to patients taking other similarly excreted drugs with a narrow therapeutic margin, and they give **chlorpropamide**, **methotrexate**, and **phenylbutazone** as examples.[5]

1. Hill G, Cihlar T, Oo C, Ho ES, Prior K, Wiltshire H, Barrett J, Liu B, Ward P. The anti-influenza drug oseltamivir exhibits low potential to induce pharmacokinetic drug interactions via renal secretion–correlation of in vivo and in vitro studies. *Drug Metab Dispos* (2002) 30, 13–19.
2. Rayner GR, Chanu P, Gieschke R, Boak LM, Jonsson EN. Population pharmacokinetics of oseltamivir when coadministered with probenecid. *J Clin Pharm* (2008) 48 (8) 935-47
3. Holodniy M, Penzak SR, Straight TM, Davey RT, Lee KK, Bidwell Goetz M, Raisch DW, Cunningham F, Lin ET, Olivio N, Deyton LR. Pharmacokinetics and tolerability of oseltamivir combined with probenecid. *Antimicrob Agents Chemother* (2008) 52, 3013–21.
4. Raisch DW, Straight TM, Holodniy M. Thrombocytopenia from combination treatment with oseltamivir and probenecid: case report, MedWatch data summary, and review of the literature. *Pharmacotherapy* (2009) 29, 988–92.
5. Tamiflu (Oseltamivir phosphate). Roche Products Ltd. UK Summary of product characteristics, April 2014.
6. Tamiflu (Oseltamivir phosphate). Roche Pharmaceuticals. US Prescribing information, May 2014.

Oseltamivir and Zanamivir + Miscellaneous

Antacids do not affect the pharmacokinetics of oseltamivir. There appears to be no pharmacokinetic interaction between amantadine (with or without ribavirin), aspirin, or paracetamol (acetaminophen) and oseltamivir. Aspirin, and a variety of other drugs used for influenza management, do not affect the antiviral activity of zanamivir *in vitro*.

Clinical evidence, mechanism, importance and management

(a) Oseltamivir

1. Amantadine. In a crossover study, 17 healthy subjects were given oseltamivir 75 mg twice daily alone or with amantadine 100 mg twice daily for 5 days. Amantadine did not significantly affect the pharmacokinetics of oseltamivir or its active metabolite, oseltamivir carboxylate, and the pharmacokinetics of amantadine were not significantly affected by oseltamivir.[1] In a crossover study, three groups of 14 healthy subjects were given single doses of oseltamivir 75 mg, amantadine 100 mg, or **ribavirin** 600 mg. Seven days later, all subjects were given a single dose of all three drugs. No changes in the pharmacokinetics of oseltamivir carboxylate, amantadine, or ribavirin were seen on concurrent use, compared with when each drug was given alone.[2] Therefore, no dose adjustment of these drugs appears to be necessary on concurrent use.

2. Antacids. In a single-dose study, the pharmacokinetics of oseltamivir 150 mg and its active carboxylate metabolite were not affected by antacids. The antacids used were an **aluminium/magnesium hydroxide** suspension (*Maalox*) and **calcium carbonate** tablet (*Titralac*).[3] No dose adjustment of oseltamivir appears to be necessary on concurrent use.

3. Aspirin. A pharmacokinetic interaction between oseltamivir and aspirin was predicted to occur, because both drugs are hydrolysed by esterases and secreted by anionic tubular secretion.[4] However, in a study in 12 healthy subjects given a single 900-mg dose of aspirin before, during and/or after oseltamivir 75 mg twice daily for 9 doses, no pharmacokinetic interaction occurred between aspirin and oseltamivir.[4] Therefore, no dose adjustment of either drug appears to be necessary on concurrent use.

4. Paracetamol (Acetaminophen). The UK and US manufacturers of oseltamivir note that no pharmacokinetic interaction occurs with paracetamol.[5,6] Therefore, no dose adjustment of either drug appears to be necessary with concurrent use.

(b) Zanamivir

The *in vitro* antiviral potency of zanamivir was not affected by **aspirin**, **paracetamol**, **ibuprofen**, **phenylephrine**, **oxymetazoline**, **promethazine**, or **co-amoxiclav** (amoxicillin with clavulanic acid).[7] Zanamivir is used as an inhalation, and has a low systemic bioavailability, so interactions would not generally be expected.

1. Morrison D, Roy S, Rayner C, Amer A, Howard D, Smith JR, Evans TG. A randomized, crossover study to evaluate the pharmacokinetics of amantadine and oseltamivir administered alone and in combination. *PLoS One* (2007) 2, e1305.
2. Seo S, Englund JA, Nguyen JT, Pukrittayakamee S, Lindegardh N, Tarning J, Tambyah PA, Renaud C, Went GT, de Jong MD, Boeckh MJ. Combination therapy with amantadine, oseltamivir and ribavirin for influenza A infection: safety and pharmacokinetics. *Antivir Ther* (2013) 18, 377–86.
3. Snell P, Oo C, Dorr A, Barrett J. Lack of pharmacokinetic interaction between the oral anti-influenza neuraminidase inhibitor prodrug oseltamivir and antacids. *Br J Clin Pharmacol* (2002) 54, 372–7.
4. Oo C, Barrett J, Dorr A, Liu B, Ward P. Lack of pharmacokinetic interaction between the oral anti-influenza prodrug oseltamivir and aspirin. *Antimicrob Agents Chemother* (2002) 46, 1993–5.
5. Tamiflu (Oseltamivir phosphate). Roche Products Ltd. UK Summary of product characteristics, April 2014.
6. Tamiflu (Oseltamivir phosphate). Roche Pharmaceuticals. US Prescribing information, May 2014.
7. Daniel MJ, Barnett JM, Pearson BA. The low potential for drug interactions with zanamivir. *Clin Pharmacokinet* (1999) 36 (Suppl 1), 41–50.

Oseltamivir + Rimantadine

No pharmacokinetic interactions or adverse effects appear to occur between oseltamivir and rimantadine.

Clinical evidence, mechanism, importance and management

In a crossover study, 21 healthy subjects were given either oseltamivir 75 mg twice daily, rimantadine 100 mg twice daily, or both drugs together, for 4.5 days.[1] There were no changes in the AUC or maximum plasma concentrations of either drug when given together, compared with each drug given alone. The AUC and maximum plasma concentration of oseltamivir carboxylate, the active metabolite of oseltamivir, were also unaffected. No adverse effects were seen on concurrent use.

1. Cirrincione-Dall G, Brennan BJ, Ballester-Sanchis RM, Navarro MT, Davies BE. Pharmacokinetics and safety of coadministered oseltamivir and rimantadine in healthy volunteers: an open-label, multiple-dose, randomized, crossover study. *J Clin Pharmacol* (2012) 52, 1255–64.

Ribavirin + Antacids

An antacid decreased ribavirin exposure.

Clinical evidence, mechanism, importance and management

The UK and US manufacturers of ribavirin note that there was a 14% decrease in the AUC of ribavirin 600 mg when it was given with an antacid containing aluminium, magnesium, and simeticone,[1-3] but this change is not clinically relevant.[1,2] No ribavirin dose adjustment is needed on concurrent use.

1. Copegus (Ribavirin). Roche Products Ltd. UK Summary of product characteristics, March 2014.
2. Rebetol Hard Capsules (Ribavirin). Merck Sharp & Dohme Ltd. UK Summary of product characteristics, April 2014.
3. Rebetol (Ribavirin). Merck Sharp and Dohme Corp. US Prescribing information, July 2014.

Rimantadine + Aspirin or Paracetamol (Acetaminophen)

Both aspirin and paracetamol cause a small reduction in the exposure to rimantadine, but this is unlikely to be clinically relevant.

Clinical evidence, mechanism, importance and management

(a) Aspirin

In a study in healthy subjects, rimantadine 100 mg twice daily was given for 13 days. On day 11, aspirin 650 mg four times daily was started and continued for 8 days. The maximum plasma concentration and AUC of rimantadine were reduced by about 10% in the presence of aspirin.[1] These reductions are unlikely to be clinically relevant.

(b) Paracetamol

In a study in healthy subjects, rimantadine 100 mg twice daily was given for 13 days. On day 11, paracetamol 650 mg four times daily was started and continued for 8 days. The peak plasma concentration and AUC of rimantadine were reduced by about 11% in the presence of paracetamol.[1] These reductions are unlikely to be clinically relevant.

1. Flumadine (Rimantadine hydrochloride). Forest Pharmaceuticals, Inc. US Prescribing information, April 2010.

Rimantadine + Cimetidine

Cimetidine causes a small, but probably clinically unimportant increase in the exposure to rimantadine.

Clinical evidence, mechanism, importance and management

In 23 healthy subjects, the AUC of a single 100-mg dose of rimantadine was increased by 20% and the apparent total clearance reduced by 18% when it was taken one hour after the first dose of cimetidine 300 mg four times daily for 6 days. The authors of the study suggest that these changes are likely to have little, if any, clinical consequences.[1] The effects of multiple-dose concurrent use are not known.

1. Holazo AA, Choma N, Brown SY, Lee LF, Wills RJ. Effect of cimetidine on the disposition of rimantadine in healthy subjects. *Antimicrob Agents Chemother* (1989) 33, 820–3.

Rimantadine + Food

In a study in 12 healthy subjects, the rate and extent of absorption of a single 100-mg dose of rimantadine was not altered by the absence or presence of food.[1] Therefore rimantadine can be taken without food.

1. Wills RJ, Rodriguez LC, Choma N, Oakes M. Influence of a meal on the bioavailability of rimantadine HCl. *J Clin Pharmacol* (1987) 27, 821–3.

Telbivudine + Miscellaneous

Drugs affecting renal function might alter the plasma concentration of telbivudine. It is unknown whether the risk of myopathy with telbivudine is increased by the concurrent use of other drugs that can cause myopathy. Peginterferon-alfa 2a does not alter telbivudine pharmacokinetics; however, the incidence of neuropathy with telbivudine might be increased. Food does not affect telbivudine pharmacokinetics. No pharmacokinetic interaction appears to occur between telbivudine and adefovir, ciclosporin, lamivudine, or tenofovir. No cytochrome P450-mediated interactions are expected to occur with telbivudine.

Clinical evidence, mechanism, importance and management

(a) Adefovir

In a study in healthy subjects, the concurrent use of telbivudine 600 mg daily and adefovir dipivoxil 10 mg daily for 7 days did not alter the pharmacokinetics of either drug, when compared with their use alone.[1] No dose adjustment of either drug appears to be needed on concurrent use.

(b) Ciclosporin

The UK and US manufacturers of telbivudine note that no pharmacokinetic interaction occurs between ciclosporin and telbivudine.[2,3] However, there is a possibility that additive myopathy might occur, see under *Drugs causing myopathy*, below. In addition, there is the possibility that ciclosporin-induced renal impairment will increase plasma telbivudine concentrations, see under *Drugs affecting renal function*, below.

(c) Cytochrome P450-mediated interactions

The UK and US manufacturers note that telbivudine is not metabolised by cytochrome P450 and is principally excreted unchanged by the kidneys. It is therefore unlikely to be affected by drugs that induce or inhibit cytochrome P450 isoenzymes.[2,3] Furthermore, *in vitro* studies suggest that telbivudine does not inhibit or induce cytochrome P450 isoenzymes, and is therefore unlikely to interact with drugs that are substrates for these isoenzymes.[2,3]

(d) Drugs affecting renal function

The UK and US manufacturers note that telbivudine is eliminated primarily by renal excretion.[2,3] Therefore, the concurrent use of drugs that affect renal function (the manufacturers name **aminoglycosides, loop diuretics, platinum compounds, vancomycin, amphotericin B,**[3] **ciclosporin,** and **tacrolimus**[2]) might affect the plasma concentration of telbivudine. Caution is advised,[3] and it would be sensible to closely monitor renal function during concurrent use. Note that signs of myopathy should also be monitored if ciclosporin is used with telbivudine, see *Drugs causing myopathy*, below. Note also that no pharmacokinetic interaction occurs with ciclosporin, see *Ciclosporin*, above.

(e) Drugs causing myopathy

The UK and US manufacturers of telbivudine note that it is unknown whether the risk of myopathy during treatment is increased by the concurrent use of other drugs associated with myopathy (such as **statins, fibrates,** and **ciclosporin**).[2,3] The US manufacturer also lists **corticosteroids, chloroquine, hydroxychloroquine, penicillamine, zidovudine, erythromycin, nicotinic acid,** and certain **azoles.**[2] Monitor concurrent use closely. Patients should be told to report any signs of myopathy and possible rhabdomyolysis (such as otherwise unexplained muscle pain, tenderness, or weakness or dark coloured urine).[2,3] If myopathy does occur, telbivudine should be stopped.[3] Note that renal function should also be monitored if ciclosporin is used with telbivudine, see *Drugs affecting renal function,* above. No pharmacokinetic interaction occurs with ciclosporin, see *Ciclosporin*, above.

(f) Food

In a study in healthy subjects, when a single 600-mg dose of telbivudine was given immediately after a high-fat/high-calorie meal, there was no effect on the pharmacokinetics of telbivudine when compared with the fasting state.[4] Telbivudine can be taken with or without food.

(g) Interferons

The UK and US manufacturers of telbivudine note that peginterferon-alfa 2a did not alter the pharmacokinetics of telbivudine, although no conclusion could be made about the effect of telbivudine on peginterferon-alfa 2a because of high interindividual variability in its plasma concentration.[2,3] However telbivudine causes neuropathy, and the incidence and severity of this was increased by peginterferon-alfa 2a in one study of telbivudine 600 mg once daily and peginterferon-alfa 2a 180 mg once weekly.[2] The MHRA and CHM in the UK therefore advise that the combination cannot be recommended. If both drugs are given, patients should be closely monitored for peripheral neuropathy. If peripheral neuropathy develops, telbivudine and peginterferon should be stopped.[5] The manufacturers also note that the benefit of combining interferons with telbivudine has not been established,[2,3] and advise that the increased risk of neuropathy cannot be excluded if telbivudine is used with other interferon alfa products.[2] In the UK they contraindicate all interferon alfa products,[3] whereas in the US they contraindicate just peginterferon-alfa 2a.[2]

(h) Lamivudine

In a study in healthy subjects, when telbivudine 200 mg daily and lamivudine 100 mg daily were given concurrently for 7 days, the pharmacokinetics of both drugs were unchanged.[1] No dose adjustment of either drug appears to be needed if they are used together. Nevertheless, the UK manufacturer of telbivudine notes that in a phase II study, the combination of telbivudine and lamivudine was less effective than telbivudine alone; therefore, telbivudine is not recommended to be used with lamivudine.[3]

(i) Tenofovir

The UK and US manufacturers of telbivudine note that there was no pharmacokinetic interaction between tenofovir and telbivudine.[2,3] Therefore, no dose adjustment of either drug appears to be needed if they are used together.

1. Zhou X-J, Fielman BA, Lloyd DM, Chao GC, Brown NA. Pharmacokinetics of telbivudine in healthy subjects and absence of drug interaction with lamivudine or adefovir dipivoxil. *Antimicrob Agents Chemother* (2006) 50, 2309–15.
2. Tyzeka (Telbivudine). Novartis Pharmaceuticals Corporation. US Prescribing information, December 2011.
3. Sebivo (Telbivudine). Novartis Pharmaceuticals UK Ltd. UK Summary of product characteristics, April 2012.
4. Zhou X-J, Lloyd DM, Chao GC, Brown NA. Absence of food effect on the pharmacokinetics of telbivudine following oral administration in healthy subjects. *J Clin Pharmacol* (2006) 46, 275–81.
5. Medicines Healthcare Products Regulatory Agency and the Commission on Human Medicines. Telbivudine: risk of peripheral neuropathy with pegylated interferon. *Drug Safety Update* (2008) 1 (Issue 8), 4. Available at: http://webarchive.nationalarchives.gov.uk/20141205150130/http://www.mhra.gov.uk/Publications/Safetyguidance/DrugSafetyUpdate/CON014099 (accessed 21/10/15).

Tenofovir + Miscellaneous

Tenofovir absorption is increased by high-fat food. Cases of nephrotoxicity have been reported with tenofovir and NSAIDs or vancomycin, and an increased risk of nephrotoxicity is predicted with other nephrotoxic drugs. Tenofovir does not alter the pharmacokinetics of ribavirin or

tacrolimus. Tacrolimus and rifampicin had minor effects on tenofovir pharmacokinetics.

Clinical evidence, mechanism, importance and management

(a) Cidofovir

Tenofovir is actively secreted by human organic anion transporter 1 (hOAT1) in the kidneys. Therefore, the manufacturers suggest that if it is given with other drugs that are also secreted by this renal transporter, such as cidofovir, increased concentrations of tenofovir or the other drug could result. The UK manufacturer of tenofovir states that concurrent use should be avoided, but if both drugs are necessary, renal function should be monitored weekly.[1] However, the UK manufacturer of cidofovir actually contraindicates the concurrent use of other nephrotoxic drugs, and states that use with tenofovir might increase the risk of Fanconi syndrome (a disorder of the renal tubules leading to polyuria, polydipsia, dehydration, hypophosphataemia and rickets). They state that nephrotoxic drugs should be stopped at least 7 days before starting cidofovir.[2]

(b) Food

Administration of tenofovir with a high-fat meal increased its AUC by about 40%, and its maximum concentration by about 14%, when compared with the fasted state, whereas administration with a light meal had no effect.[1,3] The UK manufacturer recommends that tenofovir is taken with food,[1] whereas the US manufacturer states that tenofovir tablets can be taken without regard to food.[3]

(c) NSAIDs

A case of acute tubular necrosis has been reported in an HIV-positive patient taking tenofovir disoproxil fumarate 300 mg daily, lopinavir boosted with ritonavir 133/33 mg daily and lamivudine 300 mg daily when **diclofenac** was started 5 days earlier for limb pain. The patient had been taking tenofovir for several years with no adverse effects on renal function, and the authors suggests that **diclofenac** affected the renal clearance of tenofovir leading to nephrotoxicity.[4] Another report describes three cases of renal failure with tenofovir. In all cases, the patients had multiple risk factors for developing renal failure secondary to tenofovir; however, the addition of an NSAID (**indometacin** suppositories in one case, **naproxen** in the other two) lead to the development of acute renal failure. In one of these cases the patient died and another developed end stage renal failure requiring regular dialysis.[5] Ten cases[6] of nephrotoxicity with tenofovir (including 2 of the 3 cases noted above[5] as well as details of a patient who had recently started taking valdecoxib) have been reported to Health Canada between March 2003 and December 2005. Another report describes a possible exacerbation of tenofovir-induced renal failure by NSAIDs: **diclofenac** in one case, and **ibuprofen** and **rofecoxib** in the other.[7]

Tenofovir has the potential to cause nephrotoxicity, and renal function should be routinely monitored during use.[1] NSAIDs reduce renal blood flow and can also rarely cause acute renal failure. From the cases reported above, it seems possible that NSAIDs might occasionally precipitate renal failure in patients taking tenofovir, particularly these with pre-existing risk factors or mild renal impairment. Further study is needed to assess this risk. The manufacturers do not give any specific warnings about the concurrent use of NSAIDs. For nephrotoxic drugs in general, they advise avoidance of the concurrent use of tenofovir.[1,3] If concurrent use of a nephrotoxic drug is unavoidable, they advise increasing the monitoring of renal function to weekly.[1]

(d) Other nephrotoxic drugs

Two cases of acute renal failure, which developed after intravenous **vancomycin** was given, have been reported in patients previously stable taking tenofovir for 6 to 10 months.[8] Tenofovir has the potential to cause nephrotoxicity, and the manufacturer recommends monthly monitoring of renal function. Although the concurrent use of other nephrotoxic drugs has not been studied, the manufacturer suggests that renal function should be monitored more frequently (weekly) if concurrent use is unavoidable. The UK manufacturer specifically names **aminoglycosides**, **amphotericin B**, cidofovir (see above), **foscarnet**, **ganciclovir**, **interleukin-2**, **pentamidine** and **vancomycin**.[1] The US manufacturer specifically names cidofovir (see above), **aciclovir**, **valaciclovir**, **ganciclovir**, and **valganciclovir**.[3] **NSAIDs** may also cause acute renal failure and cases of nephrotoxicity with tenofovir have been reported, see under *NSAIDs*, above.

(e) Ribavirin

Tenofovir disoproxil fumarate 300 mg daily did not alter the pharmacokinetics of a single 600-mg dose of ribavirin in 22 subjects, and the pharmacokinetics of tenofovir did not appear to be changed by ribavirin when compared with historical data.[9] Note that, there is evidence that HIV-positive patients co-infected with hepatitis C and treated with interferon alfa and ribavirin might be at increased risk of lactic acidosis and hepatic decompensation when receiving any including tenofovir, and increased monitoring is recommended.[1] For further details see, 'NRTIs + Ribavirin', p.980.

(f) Rifampicin (Rifampin)

In a study in 23 subjects, when rifampicin 600 mg daily was given with tenofovir disoproxil fumarate 300 mg daily, tenofovir exposure was negligibly decreased by 13%, and rifampicin pharmacokinetics did not appear to be changed when compared with historical data. One subject who was withdrawn from the study had raised liver enzymes, which is a well-known effect of rifampicin.[10] The interaction seen is unlikely to be clinically relevant and therefore no tenofovir dose adjustment appears to be necessary on the concurrent use of rifampicin.

(g) Tacrolimus

In a study in healthy subjects taking a combination of **emtricitabine** 200 mg daily and tenofovir disoproxil fumarate 300 mg daily alone or with tacrolimus 100 micrograms/kg daily, the only statistically significant change in the pharmacokinetics of all three drugs was a minor 13% increase in the maximum concentration of tenofovir, which is not clinically relevant.[11] No dose adjustment would be expected to be needed on concurrent use. However, bear in mind that both tacrolimus and tenofovir have the potential to cause nephrotoxicity. The UK manufacturer of tenofovir recommends that renal function should be monitored closely if it is used with tacrolimus.[1]

1. Viread (Tenofovir disoproxil fumarate). Gilead Sciences Ltd. UK Summary of product characteristics, January 2012.
2. Vistide (Cidofovir). Gilead Sciences Ltd. UK Summary of product characteristics, January 2011.
3. Viread (Tenofovir disoproxil fumarate). Gilead Sciences, Inc. US Prescribing information, August 2012.
4. Morelle J, Labriola L, Lambert M, Cosyns J-P, Jouret F, Jadoul M. Tenofovir-related acute kidney injury and proximal tubule dysfunction precipitated by diclofenac: a case of drug-drug interaction. *Clin Nephrol* (2009) 71, 567–70.
5. Marcotte S, Talbot A, Trottier B. Acute renal failure in four HIV-infected patients: potential association with tenofovir and nonsteroidal anti-inflammatory drugs. *Can J Infect Dis Med Microbiol* (2008) 19, 75–6.
6. McMorran M. Tenofovir (Viread) and NSAIDs: acute renal failure. *Can Adverse React News* (2006) 16, 1–2.
7. Parsonage MJ, Wilkins EGL, Snowden N, Issa BG, Savage MW. The development of hypophosphataemic osteomalacia with myopathy in two patients with HIV infection receiving tenofovir therapy. *HIV Med* (2005) 6, 341–6.
8. Psevdos G, Gonzalez E, Sharp V. Acute renal failure in patients with AIDS on tenofovir while receiving prolonged vancomycin course for osteomyelitis. *AIDS Read* (2009) 19, 235–8.
9. Ramanathan S, Cheng A, Mittan A, Ebrahimi R, Kearney BP. Absence of clinically relevant pharmacokinetic interaction between ribavirin and tenofovir in healthy subjects. *J Clin Pharmacol* (2006) 46, 559–66.
10. Droste JAH, Verweij-van Wissen CPWGM, Kearney BP, Buffels R, vanHorssen PJ, Hekster YA, Burger DM. Pharmacokinetic study of tenofovir disoproxil fumarate combined with rifampin in healthy volunteers. *Antimicrob Agents Chemother* (2005) 49, 680–4.
11. Chittick GE, Zong J, Begley JA, Alianti JR, Sorbel JJ, Blum MR. Pharmacokinetics of emtricitabine/tenofovir disoproxil fumarate and tacrolimus at steady state when administered alone or in combination. *Int J Clin Pharmacol Ther* (2008) 46, 627–36.

Tenofovir + NS5A inhibitors

Tenofovir exposure is slightly increased by ledipasvir (in a fixed-dose combination with sofosbuvir). No pharmacokinetic interaction occurs between daclatasvir and tenofovir, and none appears to occur between ombitasvir and tenofovir.

Clinical evidence

(a) Daclatasvir

In a crossover study in 20 healthy subjects, tenofovir 300 mg daily for 7 days had no effect on the pharmacokinetics of daclatasvir 60 mg daily. The pharmacokinetics of tenofovir were also unaffected.[1]

(b) Ledipasvir

The UK and US manufacturers briefly report that, in a study in healthy subjects given tenofovir 300 mg daily with efavirenz 600 mg and emtricitabine 200 mg both daily, ledipasvir 90 mg daily (in a fixed-dose combination with sofosbuvir) increased the AUC and maximum concentration of tenofovir 2-fold and by 79%, respectively. The minimum concentration of tenofovir was increased 2.6-fold. For discussion of the effects on ledipasvir pharmacokinetics, see 'NS5A inhibitors + NNRTIs', p.989. When the same dose of tenofovir was given with emtricitabine 200 mg and rilpivirine 25 mg, both daily, ledipasvir 90 mg (in a fixed-dose combination with sofosbuvir) increased the AUC and maximum concentration of tenofovir by 40% and 32%, respectively, and the minimum concentration was increased by 90%.[2,3] The UK manufacturer also reports that when tenofovir was given with emtricitabine, and atazanavir or darunavir boosted with ritonavir, ledipasvir 90 mg daily (in a fixed-dose combination with sofosbuvir),increased the AUC of tenofovir by 35% and 50%, and the maximum concentration increased by 47% and 64%, respectively.[2]

(c) Ombitasvir

The UK manufacturer briefly reports that, in a study in healthy subjects given tenofovir 300 mg daily with emtricitabine 200 mg daily and ombitasvir 25 mg daily (in a fixed-dose combination with paritaprevir boosted with ritonavir, with and without dasabuvir), the pharmacokinetics of tenofovir and ombitasvir were unaffected.[4]

Mechanism

The reason for the increased tenofovir exposure seen with ledipasvir (given with sofosbuvir) is unclear.

Importance and management

No pharmacokinetic interaction occurs between daclatasvir and tenofovir and therefore no dose adjustments are necessary on concurrent use.

Tenofovir exposure is slightly increased when given with efavirenz and emtricitabine, or emtricitabine and rilpivirine, together with ledipasvir (with sofosbuvir). The US manufacturer of ledipasvir in a fixed-dose combination with sofosbuvir advises that patients should be monitored for tenofovir adverse effects (such as nausea, diarrhoea, renal impairment) if used concurrently with tenofovir, emtricitabine, and efavirenz.[3] Slight increases in tenofovir exposure were also seen when it was given with emtricitabine, and atazanavir or darunavir boosted with ritonavir, together with ledipasvir with sofosbuvir. The UK and US manufacturers of ledipasvir with sofosbuvir both note that the safety of the increases in tenofovir exposure seen with these combinations is not established (they extend this to all HIV protease inhibitors boosted with ritonavir). They therefore advise alternative combinations be used where possible.[2,3] If this is not possible, caution should be exercised on concurrent use, particularly in patients at increased risk of renal dysfunction,[2] and all patients should be monitored for tenofovir adverse effects,[3] especially renal dysfunction.[2] Furthermore, the concurrent use of ledipasvir with sofosbuvir, and tenofovir with elvitegravir, cobicistat, and emtricitabine is predicted to increase tenofovir exposure and thus is not recommended by the US manufacturer,[3] and cautioned by the UK manufacturer, with frequent renal monitoring advised if an alternative is not possible.[2]

No pharmacokinetic interaction appears to occur between tenofovir and ombitasvir (in a fixed-dose combination with paritaprevir boosted with ritonavir, with and without dasbuvir), and no dose adjustments are necessary on concurrent use.

1. Bifano M, Hwang C, Oosterhuis B, Hartstra J, Grasela D, Tiessen R, Velinova-Donga M, Kandoussi H, Sevinsky H, Bertz R. Assessment of pharmacokinetic interactions of the HCV NS5A replication complex inhibitor daclatasvir with antiretroviral agents: ritonavir-boosted atazanavir, efavirenz and tenofovir. *Antivir Ther* (2013) 18, 931–40.
2. Harvoni (Ledipasvir, sofosbuvir). Gilead Sciences Ltd. UK Summary of product characteristics, November 2014.
3. Harvoni (Ledipasvir, sofosbuvir). Gilead Sciences, Inc. US Prescribing information, March 2015.
4. Viekirax (Ombitasvir, paritaprevir, ritonavir). AbbVie Ltd. UK Summary of product characteristics, January 2015.

Vidarabine + Allopurinol

There is some evidence to suggest that if allopurinol and vidarabine (adenine arabinoside) are given together the toxicity of vidarabine may be increased.

Clinical evidence

Two patients with chronic lymphocytic leukaemia taking allopurinol 300 mg daily developed severe neurotoxicity (coarse rhythmic tremors of the extremities and facial muscles, and impaired mentation) 4 days after vidarabine was added for the treatment of viral infections.[1] A retrospective search to find other patients who had taken both drugs for 4 days revealed a total of 17 patients, 5 of whom had experienced adverse reactions including tremors, nausea, pain, itching, and anaemia.[1] Another possible case report describes neurological toxicity in a patient taking both drugs.[2]

Mechanism

Uncertain. One suggestion is that the allopurinol causes hypoxanthine arabinoside, the major metabolite of vidarabine, to accumulate by inhibiting xanthine oxidase. A study with *rat* liver cytosol found that allopurinol greatly increased the half-life of this metabolite.[3]

Importance and management

Information seems to be limited to these reports and so the general clinical importance of this possible interaction is uncertain, but it would be prudent to exercise particular care if these drugs are used together.

1. Friedman HM, Grasela T. Adenine arabinoside and allopurinol – possible adverse drug interaction. *N Engl J Med* (1981) 304, 423.
2. Collignon PJ, Sorrell TC. Neurological toxicity associated with vidarabine (adenine arabinoside) therapy. *Aust N Z J Med* (1983) 13, 627–9.
3. Drach JC, Rentea RG, Cowen ME. The metabolic degradation of 9-β-D-arabinofuranosyladenine (ara-A) *in vitro*. *Fedn Proc* (1973) 32, 777.

22

Beta blockers

The adrenoceptors of the sympathetic nervous system are of two main types, namely alpha and beta. Drugs that block the beta adrenoceptors (better known as the beta blockers) are therapeutically exploited to reduce, for example, the normal sympathetic stimulation of the heart. The activity of the heart in response to stress and exercise is reduced, its consumption of oxygen is diminished, and in this way exercise-induced angina can be managed. Beta blockers given orally can also be used in the management of cardiac arrhythmias, hypertension, myocardial infarction, and heart failure. They may also be used for some symptoms of anxiety and for migraine prophylaxis. Some beta blockers are used in the form of eye drops for glaucoma and ocular hypertension.

Not all beta receptors are identical but can be further subdivided into two groups, $beta_1$ and $beta_2$. The former are found in the heart and the latter in the bronchi. Because one of the unwanted adverse effects of generalised beta blockade can be the loss of the normal noradrenaline-stimulated bronchodilation (leading to bronchospasm), cardioselective $beta_1$-blocking drugs (e.g. atenolol, metoprolol) were developed, which have less effect on $beta_2$ receptors. However, it should be emphasised that their selectivity is not absolute because bronchospasm can still occur with these drugs, particularly at high doses. 'Table 22.1', below, includes an indication of the cardioselectivity of commonly used systemic beta blockers.

Some beta blockers also have $alpha_1$-blocking activity, which causes vasodilatation, and this is also indicated in 'Table 22.1', below. Some beta blockers, such as celiprolol and nebivolol, also have vasodilator activity but produce this by mechanisms other than blocking $alpha_1$ receptors. Other beta blockers also possess intrinsic sympathomimetic activity in that they can *activate* beta receptors and are therefore partial agonists. Sotalol has additional class III antiarrhythmic activity, which causes it to prolong the QT interval, and this results in a range of interactions not shared by most other beta blockers.

Beta blockers may be lipophilic drugs (such as metoprolol) or hydrophilic (such as atenolol). The lipophilic beta blockers are more likely to be involved in pharmacokinetic interactions than the hydrophilic drugs. Many of the lipophilic beta blockers are principally metabolised by the cytochrome P450

Table 22.1 The actions and metabolism of widely used systemic beta blockers

Drug	*$Beta_1$-receptor selectivity*	*Alpha-blocking activity?*	*ISA**	*Lipophilicity*	*Bioavailability*	*First pass metabolism*	*Metabolism*
Acebutolol	Selective	No	Yes (weak)	Hydrophilic	50 to 70%	30 to 50%	Rapidly metabolised to an active metabolite after which about 50% is excreted by the liver and 50% excreted in the urine.
Atenolol	Selective	No	No	Hydrophilic	40 to 50%	Less than 10%	Largely excreted unchanged in the urine.
Bisoprolol	Selective	No	No	Intermediate	88%	Less than 10%	50% hepatic metabolism and 50% excreted unchanged in the urine.
Carvedilol	Non-selective	Yes ($alpha_1$)	No	Lipophilic	25 to 35%	60 to 80%	Primarily metabolised by CYP2D6, although other isoenzymes do contribute.
Celiprolol	Selective	Yes (weak $alpha_2$)	Yes	Hydrophilic	30 to 70%	Little	Mostly excreted unchanged (only 1-3% metabolised) with 50% excreted in the bile and 50% excreted in the urine.
Esmolol	Selective	No	No	Relatively hydrophilic	N/A	Extensive	Rapidly hydrolysed in red blood cells (half-life 9 minutes).
Labetalol	Non-selective	Yes (postsynaptic $alpha_2$)	No	Moderately lipophilic	25 to 40%	Extensive	Conjugated in the liver.
Metoprolol	Selective	No	No	Lipophilic	50%	About 40 to 60%	Metabolised by CYP2D6.
Nadolol	Non-selective	No	No	Hydrophilic	20 to 40%	Little	Largely excreted unchanged in the urine.
Nebivolol	Selective	No	No		12 to 96%	Extensive	Metabolised by CYP2D6.
Oxprenolol	Non-selective	No	Yes	Lipophilic	19 to 74%	25 to 80%	Extensively metabolised by the liver.
Pindolol	Non-selective	No	Yes	Moderately lipophilic	90 to 100%	Little	30 to 40% excreted unchanged in the urine, rest excreted by liver and kidney as inactive metabolites.
Propranolol	Non-selective	No	No	Lipophilic	30 to 70%	Up to 95%	Mainly metabolised by CYP2D6 with some contribution by CYP1A2.
Sotalol	Non-selective	No	No	Hydrophilic	75 to 90%	None	Largely excreted unchanged in the urine.
Timolol	Non-selective	No	No	Lipophilic	61%	About 50 to 70%	Mostly metabolised by the liver, with some involvement from CYP2D6. 20% excreted unchanged. Timolol and metabolites renally excreted.

*Intrinsic sympathomimetic activity (partial agonists)

isoenzyme CYP2D6 (see 'Table 22.1', p.999). This isoenzyme is subject to genetic polymorphism (see 'Genetic factors in drug metabolism', p.8, for a further explanation), and drugs that are inhibitors or inducers of this isoenzyme (see 'Table 1.7', p.9) increase or decrease beta blocker levels, particularly in those of extensive metaboliser phenotype. Propranolol is also metabolised in part by CYP1A2 (see 'Beta blockers + SSRIs', p.1022), which can cause it to interact differently to other extensively metabolised beta blockers. Talinolol is a substrate of P-glycoprotein, and possibly some other transporter proteins, and therefore its pharmacokinetics may be altered by inhibitors or inducers of transporter proteins.

Beta blockers may also be involved in pharmacodynamic interactions with other drugs that are based on enhancement or antagonism of pharmacological effects (such as additive blood pressure reduction).

This section is generally concerned with those drugs that affect the activity of the beta blockers. Where the beta blocker is the affecting drug, the interaction is dealt with elsewhere.

Beta blockers + 5-Alpha reductase inhibitors

Finasteride and dutasteride do not appear to interact with beta blockers.

Clinical evidence, mechanism, importance and management

In a study in healthy subjects, **finasteride** 5 mg daily for 10 days did not affect the pharmacokinetics or pharmacodynamics of a single 80-mg dose of **propranolol**.[1] Further, the US manufacturer states that **finasteride** was used with beta blockers in clinical studies without any evidence of an interaction.[2] Similarly, **dutasteride** was used with beta blockers in clinical studies without any evidence of an interaction.[3,4]

1. Gregoire S, Williams R, Gormely G, Lin E. Effect of finasteride (Mk-906), a new potent 5 alpha reductase inhibitor on the disposition of D and L-propranolol. *J Clin Pharmacol* (1990) 30, 847.
2. Proscar (Finasteride). Merck & Co., Inc. US Prescribing information, August 2010.
3. GlaxoSmithKline, Personal communication, August 2003.
4. Avodart (Dutasteride). GlaxoSmithKline. US Prescribing information, October 2012.

Beta blockers + Amiodarone

The concurrent use of amiodarone and a beta blocker (propranolol, metoprolol, or sotalol) has led to hypotension, bradycardia, ventricular fibrillation, and asystole in a few patients. Torsade de pointes developed in two patients taking amiodarone and atenolol, but other factors might have contributed to the development of the arrhythmia. Amiodarone might inhibit the metabolism of beta blockers metabolised by CYP2D6, such as metoprolol, which might be a factor in the interaction.

The concurrent use of amiodarone and sotalol increases the risk of torsade de pointes.

Clinical evidence

(a) Atenolol

In a review of torsade de pointes in patients taking amiodarone long-term, two elderly patients developed torsade de pointes 3 and 5 weeks after atenolol 25 mg daily was added. Bradycardia was observed in one patient and hypokalaemia probably contributed to the arrhythmia in the other patient.[1]

(b) Carvedilol

In a study in patients with heart failure taking carvedilol, it was found that the serum concentration to dose ratio for *R*-carvedilol was not affected by amiodarone given for 14 days. However, the serum concentration to dose ratio for *S*-carvedilol and the serum *S*- to *R*-carvedilol ratio was significantly lower in the group given carvedilol alone than in the group given carvedilol and amiodarone,[2] suggesting that amiodarone inhibits the metabolism of *S*-carvedilol.

In a retrospective analysis of the use of carvedilol in patients with chronic heart failure, there was no difference in the reduction in heart rate between 80 patients receiving amiodarone and 150 patients not receiving amiodarone (reduction of about 15 bpm in both groups). In addition, there was no difference in the incidence of withdrawal of carvedilol because of bradycardia between the two groups. However, the incidence of worsening heart failure was slightly higher in the amiodarone group (21% versus 13%), but this might have been due to underlying differences between the two groups.[3] In another similar analysis in patients given carvedilol, there was no difference in worsened heart failure or bradycardia in patients also receiving amiodarone and those not.[4]

(c) Metoprolol

In one study, 10 elderly patients (9 with symptomatic atrial fibrillation and one with an implanted defibrillator and frequent ventricular tachycardia) taking metoprolol (mean daily dose 119 mg) were also given amiodarone 1.2 g daily for 6 days. The AUC and plasma concentration of metoprolol were increased by 81% and 75%, respectively, by the amiodarone, the extent varying by CYP2D6 genotype.[5] None of the patients included in the study were poor metabolisers (that is, those with little or no CYP2D6 activity).

In another study in 120 patients with cardiac arrhythmias taking metoprolol, the concurrent use of amiodarone in an average dose of 170 mg daily for one month in 30 patients increased the metoprolol serum concentration to dose ratio. Furthermore, the metoprolol dose was higher in those patients receiving metoprolol alone.[6]

A 64-year-old woman with hypertrophic cardiomyopathy taking amiodarone 1.2 g daily and atenolol 50 mg daily had her atenolol replaced by metoprolol 100 mg daily. Within 3 hours she complained of dizziness, weakness and blurred vision. On examination she was found to be pale and sweating with a pulse rate of 20 bpm. Her systolic blood pressure was 60 mmHg. Atropine 2 mg did not produce chronotropic or haemodynamic improvement. She responded to isoprenaline (isoproterenol).[7]

Nevertheless, in a study of the use of oral amiodarone for the prevention of atrial fibrillation after open heart surgery, there was no difference in the incidence of symptomatic bradycardia between those patients receiving amiodarone and those receiving placebo (7.5% versus 7%). In this study, most patients (90%) received pre-operative beta blockers (88% were given metoprolol and 10% were given **atenolol**).[8]

(d) Propranolol

A report describes cardiac arrest in one patient taking amiodarone, and severe bradycardia and ventricular fibrillation (requiring defibrillation) in another, within 1.5 hours and 2 hours of starting to take propranolol.[9]

(e) Sotalol

Severe hypotension has been reported in a patient taking sotalol when intravenous amiodarone (total dose 250 mg) was given.[10] For a case report of an elderly woman who developed torsade de pointes after receiving amiodarone, sotalol and ciprofloxacin within the space of 4 days, see 'Amiodarone + Quinolones', p.265.

(f) Unspecified beta blockers

In a retrospective analysis of data from two large randomised clinical studies of the use of amiodarone for post-myocardial infarction arrhythmias, there was no difference in the withdrawal rate due to bradycardia between those receiving amiodarone and a beta blocker and those receiving amiodarone alone (1.2% versus 1%).[11]

Mechanism

Not understood. The clinical picture is that of excessive beta-blockade, and additive pharmacodynamic effects are possible. Bradycardia associated with beta blockers and amiodarone can induce early after-depolarisations and facilitate torsade de pointes.[1] In addition, amiodarone and its metabolite, desethylamiodarone, increase the concentration of metoprolol by inhibiting its metabolism by CYP2D6.[5,6] Other beta blockers that are also substrates of CYP2D6 (see 'Table 22.1', p.999) could therefore be similarly affected. However, the study with carvedilol suggests that other factors such as CYP2C9 and the drug transporter protein, P-glycoprotein, might also be involved.[2]

Importance and management

Reports describing an adverse pharmacodynamic interaction between the beta blockers and amiodarone are limited, but this is possibly because the effects described (bradycardia and arrhythmias) are in line with what might be expected when giving two drugs that slow heart rate. Nevertheless, these reports emphasise the need for caution when amiodarone is used with beta blockers.

A pharmacokinetic interaction between amiodarone and beta blockers that are substrates of CYP2D6, such as metoprolol, also appears to be established. Although this interaction with other moderate inhibitors of CYP2D6 is generally not thought to be clinically relevant (e.g. see 'Beta blockers + SSRIs', p.1022), it is possible that this pharmacokinetic interaction plays some part in the adverse reactions sometimes seen, or even in the clinical benefits.[5]

The manufacturers of amiodarone state that the concurrent use of amiodarone and a beta blocker is not recommended[12] or should be undertaken with caution[13] because potentiation of negative chronotropic properties and conduction-slowing effects might occur. However, the clinical benefits of concurrent use should not be overlooked, and some patients might benefit from the combination. In these patients it would seem prudent to monitor for bradycardia, adjusting the doses or stopping one drug if the heart rate becomes too slow.

Note that the concurrent use of sotalol presents a greater risk than that of other beta blockers, as it might prolong the QT interval. See also 'Drugs that prolong the QT interval + Other drugs that prolong the QT interval', p.272, for more information.

1. Antonelli D, Atar S, Freedberg NA, Rosenfeld T. Torsade de pointes in patients on chronic amiodarone treatment: contributing factors and drug interactions. *Isr Med Assoc J* (2005) 7,163–5.
2. Fukumoto K, Kobayashi T, Komamura K, Kamakura S, Kitakaze M, Ueno K. Stereoselective effect of amiodarone on the pharmacokinetics of racemic carvedilol. *Drug Metab Pharmacokinet* (2005) 20, 423–7.
3. Macdonald PS, Keogh AM, Aboyoun C, Lund M, Amor R, McCaffrey D. Impact of concurrent amiodarone treatment on the tolerability and efficacy of carvedilol in patients with chronic heart failure. *Heart* (1999) 82, 589–93.
4. Krum H, Shusterman N, MacMahon S, Sharpe N. Efficacy and safety of carvedilol in patients with chronic heart failure receiving concomitant amiodarone therapy. *J Card Fail* (1998) 4, 281–8.
5. Werner D, Wuttke H, Fromm MF, Schaefer S, Eschenhagen T, Brune K, Daniel WG, Werner U. Effect of amiodarone on the plasma levels of metoprolol. *Am J Cardiol* (2004) 94, 1319–21.
6. Fukumoto K, Kobayashi T, Tachibana K, Kato R, Tanaka K, Komamura K, Kamakura S, Kitakaze M, Ueno K. Effect of amiodarone on the serum concentration/dose ratio of metoprolol in patients with cardiac arrhythmia. *Drug Metab Pharmacokinet* (2006) 21, 501–5.
7. Leor J, Levartowsky D, Sharon C, Farfel Z. Amiodarone and β-adrenergic blockers: an interaction with metoprolol but not with atenolol. *Am Heart J* (1988) 116, 206–7.
8. Giri S, White CM, Dunn AB, Felton K, Freeman-Bosco L, Reddy P, Tsikouris JP, Wilcox HA, Kluger J. Oral amiodarone for prevention of atrial fibrillation after open heart surgery, the Atrial Fibrillation Suppression Trial (AFIST): a randomised placebo-controlled trial. *Lancet* (2001) 357, 830–6.
9. Derrida JP, Ollagnier J, Benaim R, Haiat R, Chiche P. Amiodarone et propranolol; une association dangereuse? *Nouv Presse Med* (1979) 8, 1429.
10. Warren R, Vohra J, Hunt D, Hamer A. Serious interactions of sotalol with amiodarone and flecainide. *Med J Aust* (1990) 152, 277.
11. Boutitie F, Boissel J-P, Connolly SJ, Camm AJ, Cairns JA, Julian DG, Gent M, Janse MJ, Dorian P, Frangin G. Amiodarone interaction with β-blockers: analysis of the merged EMIAT (European Myocardial Infarct Amiodarone Trial) and CAMIAT (Canadian Amiodarone Myocardial Infarction Trial) databases. *Circulation* (1999) 99, 2268–75.
12. Cordarone X (Amiodarone hydrochloride). Zentiva. UK Summary of product characteristics, April 2014.
13. Cordarone (Amiodarone hydrochloride). Wyeth Pharmaceuticals Inc. US Prescribing information, December 2014.

Beta blockers + Antacids or Kaolin-pectin

Some antacids and kaolin-pectin may cause a minor to modest reduction in the absorption of atenolol, propranolol, or sotalol, and possibly a slight increase in the absorption of metoprolol.

Clinical evidence

(a) Atenolol

In a study in 6 healthy subjects, **aluminium hydroxide** 5.6 g reduced the plasma levels of a single 100-mg dose of atenolol by 20%, which had no effect on the atenolol-induced reduction in exercising heart rate. Similarly, **aluminium hydroxide** had no significant effect on atenolol pharmacokinetics when both drugs were given together for 6 days.[1] Another study in 6 healthy subjects found that 30 mL of *Novalucol forte* (an **aluminium/magnesium-containing antacid**) reduced the peak plasma level and AUC of a single 100-mg dose of atenolol by 37% and 33%, respectively, which was considered to be of possible significance in some patients.[2]

In a study in 6 healthy subjects a single 500-mg dose of **calcium** (as the lactate, gluconate and carbonate) caused a 51% reduction in the peak plasma level of a single 100-mg dose of atenolol. **Calcium** also reduced the AUC of atenolol by 32%, and increased its elimination half-life from 6.2 to 11 hours. The effect of atenolol on heart rate was decreased by 12%. However, these changes were no longer statistically significant after 6 days of concurrent use, except for a 21% reduction in the peak plasma levels of atenolol, which would not be expected to be clinically relevant. In a further 6 hypertensive subjects, neither **calcium** 500 mg daily nor **aluminium hydroxide** 5.6 g daily had any influence on the blood pressure-lowering effect of atenolol 100 mg daily, given for 4 weeks.[1]

(b) Metoprolol

In 6 healthy subjects, 30 mL of *Novalucol forte* (an **aluminium/magnesium-containing antacid**) increased the peak plasma level and AUC of a single 100-mg dose of metoprolol by 25% and 11%, respectively.[2]

(c) Propranolol

In a study in 6 healthy subjects, **aluminium hydroxide gel** 30 mL did not affect either the plasma level of a single 40-mg dose of propranolol, or the reduction in exercise heart rate in response to propranolol.[3] In contrast, a study in 5 healthy subjects found that 30 mL of an **aluminium hydroxide gel** reduced the levels and AUC of a single 80-mg dose of propranolol by almost 60%.[4] *In vitro* and *animal* data suggest that **bismuth subsalicylate, kaolin-pectin** and **magnesium trisilicate** can also reduce the absorption of propranolol.[5,6]

(d) Sotalol

A study in 5 healthy subjects found that single doses of **aluminium hydroxide** suspension (*Neutragel*) or **calcium carbonate** suspension, given after an overnight fast, had negligible effects on the pharmacokinetics of a single 160-mg dose of sotalol.[7] However, a single dose of **magnesium hydroxide** slightly reduced the AUC of sotalol by 16%.[7] A further study in 6 healthy subjects found that when 20 mL of *Maalox* (**aluminium/magnesium hydroxide**) was given at the same time as 160 mg of sotalol, the maximum plasma level of the sotalol was reduced by 26% and its AUC was reduced by 21%. Changes in heart rates reflected these pharmacokinetic changes.[8] No interaction occurred when *Maalox* was given 2 hours after sotalol.[8]

Mechanism

Uncertain. The reduction in absorption could possibly be related to a delay in gastric emptying caused by the antacid, delayed dissolution due to an increase in gastric pH, or to the formation of a complex of the two drugs in the gut, which reduces absorption. However, one *in vitro* study indicated that sotalol was only subject to minor absorption or complexation interactions.[8] Another study found that 35 to 40% of sotalol was bound by magnesium hydroxide, but this may be reversible under physiological conditions and is therefore unlikely to be relevant during long-term clinical use.[7]

Importance and management

Evidence for an interaction between antacids and beta blockers is generally limited, and largely confined to single-dose studies, which may not reflect the situation with multiple dosing. Indeed, one study with atenolol and aluminium hydroxide found a modest pharmacokinetic interaction with single doses, but no interaction after 6 days of concurrent use. Some minor to modest changes in beta blocker absorption may possibly occur, but these are unlikely to be clinically relevant, and no study seems to have shown that there is a significant effect on the therapeutic effectiveness of the beta blockers with multiple dosing. However, bear in mind the possibility of an interaction if the effects of beta blockers are reduced, especially during the initial stages of concurrent use. Separating the doses by 2 hours was shown to avoid the interaction in one study with sotalol,[8] and this would seem a simple way of resolving problems, should they occur.

1. Kirch W, Schäfer-Korting M, Axthelm T, Köhler H, Mutschler E. Interaction of atenolol with furosemide and calcium and aluminium salts. *Clin Pharmacol Ther* (1981) 30, 429–35.
2. Regårdh CG, Lundborg P, Persson BA. The effect of antacid, metoclopramide and propantheline on the bioavailability of metoprolol and atenolol. *Biopharm Drug Dispos* (1981) 2, 79–87.
3. Hong CY, Hu SC, Lin SJ, Chiang BN. Lack of influence of aluminium hydroxide on the bioavailability and beta-adrenoceptor blocking activity of propranolol. *Int J Clin Pharmacol Ther Toxicol* (1985) 23, 244–6.
4. Dobbs JH, Skoutakis VA, Acchardio SR, Dobbs BR. Effects of aluminium hydroxide on the absorption of propranolol. *Curr Ther Res* (1977) 21, 887–92.
5. Moustafa MA, Gouda MW, Tariq M. Decreased bioavailability of propranolol due to interactions with adsorbent antacids and antidiarrhoeal mixtures. *Int J Pharmaceutics* (1986) 30, 225–8.
6. McElnay JC, D'Arcy PF, Leonard JK. The effect of activated dimethicone, other antacid constituents, and kaolin on the absorption of propranolol. *Experientia* (1982) 38, 605–7.
7. Kahela P, Anttila M, Sundqvist H. Antacids and sotalol absorption. *Acta Pharmacol Toxicol (Copenh)* (1981) 49, 181–3.
8. Läer S, Neumann J, Scholz H. Interaction between sotalol and an antacid preparation. *Br J Clin Pharmacol* (1997) 43, 269–72.

Beta blockers + Anticholinesterases

A small number of reports describe marked bradycardia and hypotension during the recovery period from anaesthesia and neuromuscular blockade, when patients taking beta blockers were given anticholinesterases. However, normally no adverse reaction seems to occur.

Clinical evidence

(a) Atenolol

A study in 8 hypertensive patients taking long-term atenolol or propranolol found no significant changes in heart rate and no serious adverse reactions when they were given low-dose oral **pyridostigmine** 30 mg three times daily for 2 days.[1] However, prolonged bradycardia and hypotension, requiring isoprenaline (isoproterenol) then adrenaline (epinephrine), were seen in an elderly woman taking atenolol 50 mg daily and nitrates when she was given **neostigmine** and atropine for the reversal of muscle relaxation at the end of general anaesthesia.[2]

(b) Labetalol

A study in 10 patients with severe hypertension due to renal ischaemia who were given propranolol 10 to 36 mg/kg daily (or equivalent doses of oxprenolol or labetalol) found that during surgery **neostigmine** consistently reduced heart rates to below 45 bpm despite atropinisation.[3]

(c) Nadolol

A patient taking nadolol 40 mg daily, recovering from surgery during which suxamethonium (succinylcholine) and pancuronium had been given, developed prolonged bradycardia of 32 to 36 bpm and hypotension (systolic blood pressure 60 to 70 mmHg) when **neostigmine** and atropine were given to reverse the neuromuscular blockade. Isoprenaline (isoproterenol) and phenylephrine infusions were required to maintain a systolic blood pressure of 90 mmHg, and were gradually reduced over 3 days. Propranolol was substituted for nadolol, and about 10 weeks later the patient underwent general anaesthesia again (this time without a neuromuscular blocker or **neostigmine**) and she recovered uneventfully.[4]

(d) Oxprenolol

A study in 10 patients with severe hypertension due to renal ischaemia who were given propranolol 10 to 36 mg/kg daily (or equivalent doses of oxprenolol or labetalol) found that during surgery **neostigmine** consistently reduced heart rates to below 45 bpm despite atropinisation.[3]

(e) Propranolol

A study in 10 patients with severe hypertension due to renal ischaemia who were given propranolol 10 to 36 mg/kg daily (or equivalent doses of oxprenolol or labetalol) found that during surgery **neostigmine** consistently reduced heart rates to below 45 bpm despite atropinisation.[3] Another report similarly describes bradycardia in a patient taking propranolol when intravenous **neostigmine** was used to reverse pancuronium-induced blockade. This responded to atropine.[5] A patient taking propranolol 20 mg twice daily, recovering from surgery during which alcuronium had been used, received glycopyrronium and **neostigmine** without any change in heart rate. However, one hour later he developed severe bradycardia (a fall from 65 to 40 bpm) and hypotension (systolic blood pressure 70 mmHg) when given intravenous **physostigmine** 2 mg over 5 minutes, for extreme drowsiness attributed to the premedication. His symptoms responded to glycopyrronium (glycopyrrolate).[6] A study in 8 hypertensive patients taking long-term atenolol or propranolol found no significant changes in heart rate and no serious adverse reactions when they were given low-dose oral **pyridostigmine** 30 mg three times daily for 2 days.[1]

Mechanism

It would appear that the bradycardic effects of the beta blockers and the acetylcholine-like effects of these anticholinesterase drugs can be additive, and inadequately controlled by the use of atropine in some of the instances cited. This bradycardic effect has also been seen with the centrally-acting anticholinesterases, see 'Beta blockers + Anticholinesterases; Centrally acting', p.1003.

Importance and management

The information available indicates that marked adverse reactions between beta blockers and anticholinesterases after surgery are uncommon, but be aware of the possibility of an interaction if a patient becomes bradycardic or hypotensive shortly after surgery.

Note that limited information suggests that beta blockers given orally or topically could, in some cases, oppose the efficacy of anticholinesterases in the treatment of myasthenia gravis, see 'Anticholinesterases + Miscellaneous', p.366.

1. Arad M, Roth A, Zelinger J, Zivner Z, Rabinowitz B, Atsmon J. Safety of pyridostigmine in hypertensive patients receiving beta blockers. *Am J Cardiol* (1992) 69, 518–22.
2. Eldor J, Hoffman B, Davidson JT. Prolonged bradycardia and hypotension after neostigmine administration in a patient receiving atenolol. *Anaesthesia* (1987) 42, 1294–7.
3. Prys-Roberts C. Hemodynamic effects of anesthesia and surgery in renal hypertensive patients receiving large doses of β-receptor antagonists. *Anesthesiology* (1979) 51, S122.
4. Seidl DC, Martin DE. Prolonged bradycardia after neostigmine administration in a patient taking nadolol. *Anesth Analg* (1984) 63, 365–7.
5. Sprague DH. Severe bradycardia after neostigmine in a patient taking propranolol to control paroxysmal atrial tachycardia. *Anesthesiology* (1975) 42, 208–10.
6. Baraka A, Dajani A. Severe bradycardia following physostigmine in the presence of beta-adrenergic blockade. *Middle East J Anesthesiol* (1984) 7, 291–3.

Beta blockers + Anticholinesterases; Centrally acting

The concurrent use of centrally-acting anticholinesterases and beta blockers may increase the risk of bradycardia.

Clinical evidence

An analysis of the French Pharmacovigilance Database for adverse drug reactions involving a centrally-acting anticholinesterase (**donepezil**, **galantamine** and **rivastigmine**), up to March 2006, found 83 potential drug interactions between anticholinesterases and beta blockers. Of these, 33 were thought to have caused adverse drug reactions, including syncope, bradycardia, arrhythmia or cardiac arrest. The concurrent use of a centrally-acting anticholinesterase drug and a drug with bradycardic effects resulted in 5 fatalities; however, it is unclear if any of these cases involved a beta blocker.[1] Two of the 3 cases of bradycardia that occurred in a study in which 131 patients were immediately switched from **donepezil** to transdermal **rivastigmine** without a break were in patients also taking **metoprolol**, the third patient had a pre-existing conduction disorder.[2]

In contrast, in a case-control study of 161 patients taking cholinesterase inhibitors (mainly **donepezil**) admitted to hospital with a diagnosis of bradycardia, there was no increased risk in those who were also taking other drugs that slow the heart rate including beta blockers, digoxin, diltiazem and verapamil. The odds ratio for hospitalisation for bradycardia was 2.13 for patients that had recently started a cholinesterase inhibitor and 2.34 in those also receiving other drugs that slow the heart rate.[3] Similarly, in an analysis of data from a large phase III study in patients with Alzheimer's disease who were given donepezil for 12 weeks, the risk of bradycardia was not significantly increased by the concurrent use of beta blockers.[4]

Mechanism

The effects of centrally-acting anticholinesterases on heart rate might be additive with those of the beta blockers, sometimes resulting in a dramatic slowing of the heart. This effect has also been seen with other anticholinesterases, see 'Beta blockers + Anticholinesterases', p.1002).

Importance and management

It appears that the increased risk of bradycardia from the concurrent use of centrally-acting anticholinesterases and beta blockers is probably low. However, it would be prudent to be alert for bradycardia if a beta blocker is given with donepezil, galantamine or rivastigmine. The effects of **tacrine** do not appear to have been studied, but it would be expected to interact similarly.

1. Tavassoli N, Sommet A, Lapeyre-Mestre M, Bagheri H, Montrastruc J-L. Drug interactions with cholinesterase inhibitors: an analysis of the French Pharmacovigilance Database and a comparison of two national drug formularies (Vidal, British National Formulary). *Drug Safety* (2007) 30, 1063–71.
2. Sadowsky CH, Dengiz A, Olin JT, Koumaras B, Meng X, Brannan S, on behalf of the US38 study group. Switching from donepezil tablets to rivastigmine transdermal patch in Alzheimer's disease. *Am J Alzheimers Dis Other Demen* (2009) 24, 267–75.
3. Park-Wyllie LY, Mamdani MM, Li P, Gill SS, Laupacis A, Juurlink DN. Cholinesterase inhibitors and hospitalisation for bradycardia: a population-based study. *PLoS Med* (2009) 6, e1000157.
4. Relkin NR, Reichman WE, Orazem J, McRae T. A large, community-based, open-label trial of donepezil in the treatment of Alzheimer's disease. Dement Geriatr Cogn Disord. (2003)16, 15–24.

Beta blockers + Aspirin or NSAIDs

There is evidence to suggest that most NSAIDs can increase blood pressure in patients taking antihypertensives, although some studies have not found the increase to be clinically relevant. Similarly, multiple-dose aspirin, both in high and low dose, did not reduce the efficacy of antihypertensives including beta blockers in three studies. However, various small studies have found some evidence of reduced beta blocker effects, either for hypertension or heart failure, in patients given NSAIDs including indometacin, piroxicam, ibuprofen and naproxen, or aspirin. Isolated case reports also describe hypertension in patients taking a beta blocker and an NSAID.

Celecoxib may decrease the metabolism of metoprolol, but in general the NSAIDs do not significantly affect the pharmacokinetics of the beta blockers.

Clinical evidence

Various large epidemiological studies and meta-analyses of clinical studies have been conducted to assess the effect of NSAIDs on blood pressure in patients taking antihypertensives, and the findings of these are summarised in 'Table 23.2', p.1031. In these studies, NSAIDs were not always associated with an increase in blood pressure, and the maximum increase was 6.2 mmHg. The effect has been shown for both COX-2 inhibitors and non-selective NSAIDs. In two meta-analyses,[1,2] the effects were evaluated by NSAID. The confidence intervals for all the NSAIDs overlapped, showing that there was no statistically significant difference between the NSAIDs, with the exception of the comparison between **indometacin** and **sulindac** in one analysis.[1] Nevertheless, an attempt was made at ranking the NSAIDs based on the means. In one analysis,[1] the effect was greatest for **piroxicam**, **indometacin**, and **ibuprofen**, intermediate for **naproxen**, and least for **sulindac** and **flurbiprofen**. In the other meta-analysis,[2] the effect was greatest for **indometacin** and **naproxen**, intermediate for **piroxicam**, and least for **ibuprofen** and **sulindac**. An attempt was also made to evaluate the effect by antihypertensive in one analysis.[1] The mean effect was greatest for beta blockers, intermediate for vasodilators (includes ACE inhibitors and calcium-channel blockers), and least for diuretics. However, the differences between the groups were not significant.

The findings of individual clinical and pharmacological studies that have studied the effects of aspirin or specific NSAIDs on systemic beta blockers are outlined in the subsections below.

(a) Aspirin and other salicylates

A small study in patients taking various antihypertensives (including beta blockers and diuretics) found that aspirin, in both low doses (650 mg daily) and high doses (3.9 g daily) for 3 or 4 weeks, did not cause clinically significant increases in blood pressure.[3] Similarly, a study in 11 patients taking a number of antihypertensives (which included a few patients taking **propranolol** or **pindolol**) found that aspirin 650 mg three times daily for 7 days did not affect the control of blood pressure.[4] In contrast, another study found that 5 g of aspirin given over 24 hours prevented the antihypertensive effects of a single 1-mg intravenous dose of **pindolol**, and a single 1- to 1.5-g dose of aspirin reduced the antihypertensive effect of a single 5-mg intravenous dose of **propranolol**.[5] Aspirin was reported not to affect the control of hypertension by **metipranolol**.[6] A retrospective study of patients with heart failure taking **carvedilol** found that aspirin did not significantly affect systolic blood pressure or heart rate but did observe that left ventricular ejection fraction improved less in those patients taking aspirin in addition to **carvedilol** The effect appeared to be dose-related.[7]

A single-dose study in 6 healthy subjects found that aspirin 500 mg did not affect the pharmacokinetics of **atenolol**.[8] Another study in 6 healthy subjects found that aspirin did not affect the pharmacokinetics of **metoprolol**, but the maximum plasma levels of aspirin were increased by **metoprolol**, although this was not considered to be clinically relevant.[9]

Sodium salicylate did not affect either the pharmacokinetics of **alprenolol** or its effects on heart rate and blood pressure during exercise in a single-dose study in healthy subjects.[10] **Imidazole salicylate** did not affect the blood pressure control of patients treated with **atenolol**.[11]

(b) Celecoxib

In a randomised, crossover study in 12 healthy subjects, celecoxib 200 mg twice daily for 7 days increased the AUC of a single 50-mg dose of **metoprolol** by 64%.[12]

(c) Diclofenac

A study in 16 patients taking **atenolol**, **metoprolol**, **propranolol** or **pindolol** and/or a diuretic found that diclofenac 50 mg three times daily had no effect on the control of blood pressure.[13]

(d) Flurbiprofen

A study in 10 patients with hypertension found that flurbiprofen 100 mg daily for 7 days did not affect the pharmacokinetics of single-doses of either **propranolol** 80 mg or **atenolol** 100 mg. However, the blood pressure-lowering effects of **propranolol** were reduced by the flurbiprofen, whereas those of **atenolol** were not affected.[14]

(e) Ibuprofen

In a randomised study in 6 hypertensive patients treated with thiazides and beta blockers, ibuprofen 400 mg every 8 hours caused significant increases in blood pressure (mean increases of about 5 to 7 mmHg).[15] The antihypertensive effect of **pindolol** was antagonised by ibuprofen in one patient.[16] However, in one randomised controlled study, ibuprofen 400 mg four times daily had no effect on the control of blood pressure in patients taking **propranolol**.[17]

(f) Indometacin

A study found that when indometacin 25 mg three times daily was given to hypertensive patients taking thiazides with or without beta blockers, their blood pressure increased by 8 to 10 mmHg.[3] The diastolic blood pressures of 7 hypertensive patients treated with **pindolol** 15 mg daily or **propranolol** 80 to 160 mg daily rose from 82 mmHg to 96 mmHg when they were given indometacin 100 mg daily over a 10-day period. Changes in systolic blood pressures were not statistically significant.[18]

In another study, indometacin 50 mg twice daily raised the blood pressure of patients taking **propranolol** 60 to 320 mg daily by 14/5 mmHg when lying and 16/9 mmHg when standing.[19] This interaction has also been seen in other studies in patients taking **atenolol**,[11,20,21] **labetalol**,[22] **metipranolol**,[6] **oxprenolol**,[23,24] and **propranolol**.[4,25] Two women with pre-eclampsia taking **propranolol** or **pindolol** became markedly hypertensive (rises in blood pressure from 135/85 mmHg to 240/140 mmHg, and from 130/70 mmHg to 230/130 mmHg, respectively) within 4 to 5 days of being given indometacin to inhibit premature contractions.[26]

(g) Naproxen

A study in hypertensive patients taking **timolol** and hydrochlorothiazide with amiloride found that naproxen 250 mg twice daily caused a 4 mmHg rise in diastolic blood pressure, but did not significantly increase systolic blood pressure.[27] Similarly, in another study, naproxen 500 mg twice daily caused an average 4 mmHg rise in systolic blood pressure in patients taking **atenolol**, but did not significantly increase diastolic blood pressure.[28] In contrast, another study found that naproxen caused no changes in hypertension controlled with **propranolol**,[29] and a study in patients taking antihypertensives (drugs not specified) found that naproxen did not cause clinically significant increases in blood pressure.[3] A case report describes one patient taking **propranolol** who had a marked rise in blood pressure when given naproxen.[30]

(h) Oxaprozin

A study in 32 hypertensive arthritic patients found that oxaprozin 1.2 g daily for 4 weeks did not affect the antihypertensive effects of **metoprolol** 100 mg twice daily, although at 2 weeks there was a significant increase in systolic blood pressure.[31]

(i) Parecoxib

In a randomised, crossover study, 15 healthy subjects were given a single 50-mg dose of **metoprolol** after taking valdecoxib (the main metabolite of parecoxib) 20 mg daily for 7 days. The AUC and maximum levels of **metoprolol**, and its effect on heart rate were unchanged by the NSAID.[32]

(j) Piroxicam

A double-blind study found that about one-quarter of the patients given piroxicam 20 mg daily and **propranolol** 80 to 160 mg daily developed diastolic pressure rises of 10 mmHg or more when lying or standing.[33,34] Increases in both systolic and diastolic blood pressures (8.1/5.2 mmHg lying and 8.5/8.9 mmHg standing) were seen in another study in 3 patients.[35] In contrast, patients taking **propranolol** and piroxicam 20 mg daily had blood pressure rises of 5.8/2.4 mmHg when lying and 3.5/0.5 mmHg when standing, after 2 weeks, but these increases were not statistically significant.[36] Blood pressure showed a trend towards higher levels in another study in 20 patients given **timolol** and piroxicam 20 mg daily.[27]

A study in 6 healthy subjects given **atenolol** 100 mg daily and piroxicam 20 mg daily for 7 days found no pharmacokinetic interaction. An associated study in another 6 healthy subjects given **metoprolol** 100 mg twice daily and piroxicam 20 mg daily for 7 days found that **metoprolol** levels were increased by piroxicam, but not to a statistically significant extent.[37]

(k) Sulindac

Sulindac 200 mg twice daily had little or no effect on the control of hypertension in patients taking hydrochlorothiazide with amiloride and **atenolol**, **metoprolol**, **propranolol** or **pindolol**.[13] In another study, diastolic blood pressure was slightly and significantly lower when sulindac was given with **timolol**.[27] No statistically significant rises in blood pressure occurred in other studies in patients taking **propranolol**[29,33-35] or **atenolol**[21,28] or unspecified antihypertensives[3] given sulindac 200 mg twice daily. In contrast, another study claimed that patients given **propranolol** with sulindac 200 mg twice daily had blood pressure rises of 10.3/4.8 mmHg when standing and 2.4/7.1 mmHg when lying, after 2 weeks, but only the increase in standing systolic blood pressure statistically significant.[36] Similarly, a crossover study in 26 hypertensive patients taking **labetalol** found that sulindac 200 mg twice daily for 7 days raised the mean systolic blood pressure by 6 mmHg when sitting, and by 9 to 14 mmHg when standing, which was considered potentially clinically significant. Diastolic blood pressure was not affected.[22]

(l) Tenoxicam

In one study, the control of hypertension in 16 patients taking **atenolol** was not affected by tenoxicam 40 mg daily.[38]

Mechanism

Indometacin alone can raise blood pressure (13 hypertensive patients given indometacin 150 mg daily for 3 days had a mean systolic blood pressure rise from 118 mmHg to 131 mmHg).[39] One suggested reason is that indometacin inhibits the synthesis and release of two prostaglandins (PGA and PGE), which have a potent dilating effect on peripheral arterioles throughout the body. In their absence the blood pressure rises. Thus the hypotensive actions of the beta blockers are opposed by the hypertensive actions of indometacin. This mechanism has been questioned and it is possible that other physiological and pharmacological mechanisms have a part to play.[3,40,41] One study found that although indometacin caused increases in blood pressure in treated hypertensive patients, other inhibitors of prostaglandin synthesis (aspirin, naproxen and sulindac) did not.[3] Further, all four drugs caused similar reductions in plasma renin activity and aldosterone concentration, which suggests that the effect of indometacin on blood pressure may not be dependent on such changes.[3]

Celecoxib inhibits the metabolism of metoprolol by the cytochrome P450 isoenzyme CYP2D6.[12]

Importance and management

Overall, the evidence suggests that some patients taking beta blockers can have a rise in blood pressure when given an NSAID, but this may not always be clinically relevant. Some have suggested that the use of NSAIDs should be kept to a minimum in patients taking antihypertensives.[42] The effects may be greater in the elderly and in those with blood pressures that are relatively high, as well as in those with high salt intake.[42] However, others consider that the clinical importance of an interaction between NSAIDs and antihypertensives is less than has previously been suggested.[43] While their findings do not rule out a 2/1 mmHg increase in blood pressure with NSAIDs in treated hypertensives, they suggest that if patients in primary care have inadequate control of blood pressure, other reasons (such as 'white-coat hypertension', poor adherence to treatment, or disease progression) may be more likely than any effect of concurrent NSAIDs.[43] There is insufficient data at present to clearly differentiate between NSAIDs, although there is some evidence that the effects of indometacin are greatest and those of sulindac least.

For the effects of NSAIDs on other antihypertensive drug classes see 'ACE inhibitors + NSAIDs', p.38, 'Calcium-channel blockers + Aspirin or NSAIDs', p.1030 and 'Thiazide diuretics + NSAIDs', p.1132.

A few multiple-dose studies have found that **aspirin** does not alter the antihypertensive effect of beta blockers, even in high doses, but one single-dose high-dose study reported an interaction. Another study suggested that aspirin might attenuate the benefit of carvedilol in heart failure, but this evidence alone does not warrant a change in practice.

Although **celecoxib** increased the levels of metoprolol, increases in plasma metoprolol levels of this size are unlikely to be clinically relevant in most patients. Those most at risk would be patients with heart failure, in whom the use of NSAIDs should generally be avoided.

Parecoxib (which is rapidly hydrolysed to valdecoxib) at low daily doses does not appear to interact with metoprolol. Nevertheless, the authors of the study suggest that the possibility of an interaction with higher doses cannot be excluded,[32] and the manufacturers of parecoxib suggest that caution is warranted.[44] However, the lack of interaction with low-dose parecoxib would seem to imply that higher doses would only have a moderate effect, if any, on metoprolol metabolism. Furthermore, metoprolol is generally considered to have a wide therapeutic index and therefore a very large rise in levels would be necessary for the interaction to become clinically relevant. The exception may be heart failure, where the beta blockers are considered to have a narrow therapeutic index, but it should be noted that NSAIDs should generally be avoided in those with heart failure.

1. Johnson AG, Nguyen TV, Day RO. Do nonsteroidal anti-inflammatory drugs affect blood pressure? A meta-analysis. *Ann Intern Med* (1994) 121, 289–300.
2. Pope JE, Anderson JJ, Felson DT. A meta-analysis of the effects of nonsteroidal anti-inflammatory drugs on blood pressure. *Arch Intern Med* (1993) 153, 477–84.
3. Chalmers JP, West MJ, Wing LMH, Bune AJC, Graham JR. Effects of indomethacin, sulindac, naproxen, aspirin, and paracetamol in treated hypertensive patients. *Clin Exp Hypertens A* (1984) 6, 1077–93.
4. Mills EH, Whitworth JA, Andrews J, Kincaid-Smith P. Non-steroidal anti-inflammatory drugs and blood pressure. *Aust N Z J Med* (1982) 12, 478–82.
5. Sziegoleit W, Rausch J, Polák G, György M, Dekov E, Békés M. Influence of acetylsalicylic acid on acute circulatory effects of the beta-blocking agents pindolol and propranolol in humans. *Int J Clin Pharmacol Ther Toxicol* (1982) 20, 423–30.
6. Macek K, Jurin I. Effects of indomethacine and aspirin on the antihypertensive action of metipranolol — a clinical study. *Eur J Pharmacol* (1990) 183, 839–40.
7. Lindenfeld J, Robertson AD, Lowes BD, Brisow MR. Aspirin impairs reverse myocardial remodelling in patients with heart failure treated with beta-blockers. *J Am Coll Cardiol* (2001) 38, 1950–6.
8. Schäfer-Korting M, Kirch W, Axthelm T, Köhler H, Mutschler E. Atenolol interaction with aspirin, allopurinol, and ampicillin. *Clin Pharmacol Ther* (1983) 33, 283–8.
9. Spahn H, Langguth P, Kirch W, Mutschler E, Ohnhaus EE. Pharmacokinetics of salicylates administered with metoprolol. *Arzneimittelforschung* (1986) 36, 1697–9.
10. Johnsson G, Regårdh CG, Sölvell L. Lack of biological interaction of alprenolol and salicylate in man. *Eur J Clin Pharmacol* (1973) 6, 9–14.
11. Abdel-Haq B, Magagna A, Favilla S, Salvetti A. The interference of indomethacin and of imidazole salicylate on blood pressure control of essential hypertensive patients treated with atenolol. *Int J Clin Pharmacol Ther Toxicol* (1987) 25, 598–600.
12. Werner U, Werner D, Rau T, Fromm MF, Hinz B, Brune K. Celecoxib inhibits metabolism of cytochrome P450 2D6 substrate metoprolol in humans. *Clin Pharmacol Ther* (2003) 74, 130–7.
13. Stokes GS, Brooks PM, Johnston HJ, Monaghan JC, Okoro EO, Kelly D. The effects of sulindac and diclofenac in essential hypertension controlled by treatment with a beta blocker and/or diuretic. *Clin Exp Hypertens A* (1991) 13, 1169–78.
14. Webster J, Petrie JC, McLean I, Hawksworth GM. Flurbiprofen interaction with single doses of atenolol and propranolol. *Br J Clin Pharmacol* (1984) 18, 861–6.
15. Radack KL, Deck CC, Bloomfield SS. Ibuprofen interferes with the efficacy of antihypertensive drugs. A Randomized, double-blind, placebo-controlled trial of ibuprofen compared with acetaminophen. *Ann Intern Med* (1987) 107, 628–35.
16. Reid ALA. Antihypertensive effect of thiazides. *Med J Aust* (1981) 2, 109–10.
17. Davies JG, Rawlins DC, Busson M. Effect of ibuprofen on blood pressure control by propranolol and bendrofluazide. *J Int Med Res* (1988) 16, 173–81.
18. Durão V, Prata MM, Gonçalves LMP. Modification of antihypertensive effects of β-adrenoceptor blocking agents by inhibition of endogenous prostaglandin synthesis. *Lancet* (1977) ii, 1005–7.
19. Watkins J, Abbott EC, Hensby CN, Webster J, Dollery CT. Attenuation of hypotensive effects of propranolol and thiazide diuretics by indomethacin. *BMJ* (1980) 281, 702–5.
20. Ylitalo P, Pitkäjärvi T, Pyykönen M-L, Nurmi A-K, Seppälä E, Vapaatalo H. Inhibition of prostaglandin synthesis by indomethacin interacts with the antihypertensive effect of atenolol. *Clin Pharmacol Ther* (1985) 38, 443–9.
21. Salvetti A, Pedrinelli R, Alberici A, Magagna A and Abdel-Haq B. The influence of indomethacin and sulindac on some pharmacological actions of atenolol in hypertensive patients. *Br J Clin Pharmacol* (1984) 17, 108S–111S.
22. Abate MA, Neeley JL, Layne RD, D'Alessandri R. Interaction of indomethacin and sulindac with labetalol. *Br J Clin Pharmacol* (1991) 31, 363–6.
23. Salvetti A, Arzilli F, Pedrinelli R, Beggi P, Motolese M. Interaction between oxprenolol and indomethacin on blood pressure in essential hypertensive patients. *Eur J Clin Pharmacol* (1982) 22, 197–201.
24. Sörgel F, Hemmerlein M, Lang E. Wirkung von Pirprofen und Indometacin auf die Effekte von Oxprenolol und Furosemid. *Arzneimittelforschung* (1984) 34, 1330–2.
25. Lopez-Ovejero JA, Weber MA, Drayer JIM, Sealey JE, Laragh JH. Effects of indomethacin alone and during diuretic or beta-adrenoceptor blockade therapy on blood pressure and the renin system in essential hypertension. *Clin Sci Mol Med* (1978) 55, 203S–205S.
26. Schoenfeld A, Freedman S, Hod M, Ovadia Y. Antagonism of antihypertensive drug therapy in pregnancy by indomethacin? *Am J Obstet Gynecol* (1989) 161, 1204–5.
27. Wong DG, Spence JD, Lamki L, Freeman D, McDonald JWD. Effect of non-steroidal anti-inflammatory drugs on control of hypertension by beta-blockers and diuretics. *Lancet* (1986) i, 997–1001.
28. Abate MA, Layne RD, Neeley JL, D'Alessandri R. Effect of naproxen and sulindac on blood pressure response to atenolol. *DICP Ann Pharmacother* (1990) 24, 810–3.
29. Schuna AA, Vejraska BD, Hiatt JG, Kochar M, Day R, Goodfriend TL. Lack of interaction between sulindac or naproxen and propranolol in hypertensive patients. *J Clin Pharmacol* (1989) 29, 524–8.
30. Anon. Adverse Drug Reactions Advisory Committee. Seven case studies. *Med J Aust* (1982) 2, 190–1.
31. Halabi A, Linde M, Zeidler H, König J, Kirch W. Double-blind study on the interaction of oxaprozin with metoprolol in hypertensives. *Cardiovasc Drugs Ther* (1989) 3, 441–3.
32. Werner U, Lamprecht C, Werner D, Schaefer S, Wuttke H, Hinz B, Fromm MF, Brune K. Valdecoxib does not interfere with the CYP2D6 substrate metoprolol. *Int J Clin Pharmacol Ther* (2006) 44, 397–400.
33. Ebel DL, Rhymer AR, Stahl E. Effect of sulindac, piroxicam and placebo on the hypotensive effect of propranolol in patients with mild to moderate essential hypertension. *Adv Therapy* (1985) 2, 131–42.
34. Ebel DL, Rhymer AR, Stahl E, Tipping R. Effect of Clinoril (sulindac, MSD), piroxicam and placebo on the hypotensive effect of propranolol in patients with mild to moderate essential hypertension. *Scand J Rheumatol* (1986) (Suppl), 62, 41–49.
35. Pugliese F, Simonetti BM, Cinotti GA, Ciabattoni G, Catella F, Vastano S, Ghidini Ottonelli A, Pierucci A. Differential interaction of piroxicam and sulindac with the anti-hypertensive effect of propranolol. *Eur J Clin Invest* (1984) 14, 54.
36. Baez MA, Alvarez CR, Weidler DJ. Effects of the non-steroidal anti-inflammatory drugs, piroxicam or sulindac, on the antihypertensive actions of propranolol and verapamil. *J Hypertens* (1987) 5 (Suppl): S563–S566.
37. Spahn H, Langguth P, Krauss D, Kirch W, Mutschler E. Pharmacokinetics of atenolol and metoprolol administered together with piroxicam. *Arch Pharm (Wienheim)* (1987) 320, 103–7.
38. Hartmann D, Stief G, Lingenfelder M, Güzelhan C, Horsch AK. Study on the possible interaction between tenoxicam and atenolol in hypertensive patients. *Arzneimittelforschung* (1995) 45, 494–8.
39. Barrientos A, Alcazar V, Ruilope L, Jarillo D, Rodicio JL. Indomethacin and beta-blockers in hypertension. *Lancet* (1978) i, 277.

40. Frölich JC, Whorten AR, Walker L, Smigel M, Oates JA, France R, Hollifield JW, Data JL, Gerber JG, Nies AS, Williams W, Robertson GL. Renal prostaglandins: regional differences in synthesis and role in renin release and ADH action. 7th Int Congr Nephrol, Montreal, 1978. 107–114.
41. Walker LA, Frölich JC. Renal prostaglandins and leukotrienes. *Rev Physiol Biochem Pharmacol* (1987) 107, 1–72.
42. Johnson AG. NSAIDs and blood pressure. Clinical importance for older patients. *Drugs Aging* (1998) 12, 17–27.
43. Sheridan R, Montgomery AA, Fahey T. NSAID use and BP in treated hypertensives: a retrospective controlled observational study. *J Hum Hypertens* (2005) 19, 445–50.
44. Dynastat (Parecoxib sodium). Pfizer Ltd. UK Summary of product characteristics, June 2013.

Beta blockers + Barbiturates

The plasma levels and the effects of beta blockers that are mainly metabolised by the liver (e.g. alprenolol, metoprolol, timolol) are reduced by the barbiturates. Alprenolol concentrations are halved by pentobarbital, but metoprolol is less affected. The serum levels of pindolol and phenobarbital do not appear to be affected by concurrent use.

Clinical evidence

(a) Pentobarbital

In a study in 6 hypertensive patients, pentobarbital 100 mg daily for 10 days at bedtime reduced the plasma levels of **alprenolol** 400 mg twice daily by 59%. On day 11, the mean pulse rate at rest had risen from 70 bpm to 74 bpm and blood pressure had risen from 134/89 mmHg to 145/97 mmHg. The changes were seen within 4 to 5 days of starting the barbiturate, and decreased within 8 to 9 days of stopping it.[1] These results are similar to those found in previous studies by the same research group using pentobarbital 100 mg daily in healthy subjects.[2,3] In one of these studies, pentobarbital reduced the plasma levels of a single 200-mg dose of **alprenolol** by 38%, 90 minutes after the **alprenolol** was given, and reduced its AUC by 43%. The elimination half-life of **alprenolol** was unchanged. There was also a 20% reduction in the effects of the beta blocker on heart rate during exercise.[3] In the other study, the AUC of oral **alprenolol** was reduced by about 80% by pentobarbital, but that of intravenous **alprenolol** was unaffected.[2]

Another study in 8 healthy subjects found that pentobarbital 100 mg daily for 10 days reduced the AUC of **metoprolol** 100 mg by 32% (range 2 to 46%).[4]

(b) Phenobarbital

In a study in 12 healthy subjects, phenobarbital 100 mg daily for 7 days slightly reduced the AUC of a single 10-mg oral dose of **timolol** by 24%, but this was not statistically significant.[5]

In a study, patients who were taking phenobarbital were given **pindolol** titrated (in 10 mg increments every 3 days) to 40 mg daily, then decreased back to zero in the same stepwise manner. None of the 3 patients for whom results were presented showed any significant changes in phenobarbital levels. In addition, in 17 patients, **pindolol** levels appeared not to be affected by phenobarbital alone or in combination with haloperidol and/or phenytoin.[6]

In a non-randomised study, the half-life of **propranolol** was 6.1 hours in 7 pregnant hypertensive women taking **propranolol** 75 mg daily for 3 days compared with 3.1 hours in 8 pregnant hypertensive women who took phenobarbital 90 mg daily for at least 7 days before starting to take **propranolol**.[7]

Mechanism

Barbiturates are potent liver enzyme inducers that can increase the metabolism and clearance of other drugs from the body. Beta blockers that are removed from the body principally by liver metabolism (e.g. alprenolol, metoprolol, timolol) can therefore possibly be cleared more quickly in the presence of a barbiturate.

Importance and management

The interaction between **alprenolol** and pentobarbital is well documented and likely to be of modest clinical importance when the beta blocker is being used to treat hypertension, and possibly angina. Monitor the effects of alprenolol and increase the dose as necessary or consider using a different beta blocker. Those beta blockers that are not hepatically metabolised (see 'Table 22.1', p.999) would not be expected to interact, but note that this does not appear to have been studied. Alternatively, where possible, it may be preferable to replace the barbiturate with a non-interacting alternative, such as one of the benzodiazepines (see 'Benzodiazepines + Beta blockers', p.817, which only have a minor effect on the beta blockers).

A reduced response is possible if any of the beta blockers that are extensively metabolised (see 'Table 22.1', p.999) are given with pentobarbital, but the effects on the AUC of **metoprolol** appear to be smaller than the effects on alprenolol. Detailed information about the clinical importance of this interaction is largely lacking, but seems likely to be minor. However, if a problem does occur consider the alternative measures suggested for alprenolol, above.

Evidence is largely lacking, but all barbiturates would be expected to interact similarly, although the extent of the interaction may vary. For example, the interaction between phenobarbital and **timolol** was modest and not statistically significant; therefore, a clinically relevant effect is unlikely.

1. Seideman P, Borg K-O, Haglund K, von Bahr C. Decreased plasma concentrations and clinical effects of alprenolol during combined treatment with pentobarbitone in hypertension. *Br J Clin Pharmacol* (1987) 23, 267–71.
2. Alvan G, Piafsky K, Lind M, von Bahr C. Effect of pentobarbital on the disposition of alprenolol. *Clin Pharmacol Ther* (1977) 22, 316–21.
3. Collste P, Seideman P, Borg K-O, Haglund K, von Bahr C. Influence of pentobarbital on effects and plasma levels of alprenolol and 4-hydroxy-alprenolol. *Clin Pharmacol Ther* (1979) 25, 423–7.
4. Haglund K, Seideman P, Collste P, Borg K-O, von Bahr C. Influence of pentobarbital on metoprolol plasma levels. *Clin Pharmacol Ther* (1979) 26, 326–9.
5. Mäntylä R, Männistö P, Nykänen S, Koponen A, Lamminsivu U. Pharmacokinetic interactions of timolol with vasodilating drugs, food and phenobarbitone in healthy human volunteers. *Eur J Clin Pharmacol* (1983) 24, 227–30.
6. Greendyke RM, Gulya A. Effect of pindolol administration on serum levels of thioridazine, haloperidol, phenytoin, and phenobarbital. *J Clin Psychiatry* (1988) 49, 105–7.
7. Hoffmann-Traeger A, Peiker G, Glöckner R, Wittmann I, Balogh A, Henschel L. The influence of phenobarbital on the pharmacokinetics of propranolol in pregnancy. *Biol Res Pregnancy Perinatol* (1987) 8, 57–9.

Beta blockers + Bile-acid binding resins

Although both colestyramine and colestipol can moderately reduce the absorption of propranolol, this does not seem to reduce its effects. Colesevelam does not appear to affect the absorption of metoprolol.

Clinical evidence

(a) Colesevelam

A single-dose study in 33 healthy subjects found that colesevelam 4.5 g did not cause a clinically relevant alteration in the plasma levels of sustained-release **metoprolol** 100 mg.[1]

(b) Colestipol

When 6 healthy subjects took a single 120-mg dose of **propranolol** with a 10-g dose of colestipol the peak plasma **propranolol** levels were *raised* by 30%. However, if an additional 10 g dose of colestipol was taken 12 hours before **propranolol** its peak plasma levels were decreased by 36% and its AUC was reduced by about 30%. No changes in blood pressure or pulse rates were seen.[2]

(c) Colestyramine

When 6 healthy subjects took a single 120-mg dose of **propranolol** with an 8-g dose of colestyramine the peak **propranolol** plasma levels were reduced by almost 25% and the AUC was reduced by 13%. An additional dose of colestyramine 12 hours before the **propranolol** reduced the AUC by 43%. However, no changes in blood pressure or pulse rate were seen.[2] Preliminary results of another study found that colestyramine (single unstated dose) caused no significant changes in the blood levels of **propranolol** in 5 patients with type II hyperlipidaemia taking **propranolol** 40 mg four times daily.[3]

Mechanism

Uncertain. It seems probable that both colestyramine and colestipol can, to some extent, bind to propranolol in the gut, thereby modestly reducing its absorption.

Importance and management

Information is limited. Even though both colestyramine and colestipol can modestly reduce the absorption of a single dose of propranolol, no changes in its effects were reported,[2] suggesting that the interaction is of minimal clinical importance. There is therefore no obvious reason for avoiding concurrent use. However, note that it is usually recommended that other drugs are given one hour before or 4 to 6 hours after colestyramine, and one hour before or 4 hours after colestipol. Colesevelam does not appear to interact with metoprolol, and no precautions regarding the timing of the administration of these drugs would therefore seem necessary.

1. Donovan JM, Stypinski D, Stiles MR, Olson TA, Burke SK. Drug interactions with colesevelam hydrochloride, a novel, potent lipid-lowering agent. *Cardiovasc Drugs Ther* (2000) 14, 681–90.
2. Hibbard DM, Peters JR, Hunninghake DB. Effects of cholestyramine and colestipol on the plasma concentrations of propranolol. *Br J Clin Pharmacol* (1984) 18, 337–42.
3. Schwartz DE, Schaeffer E, Brewer HB, Franciosa JA. Bioavailability of propranolol following administration of cholestyramine. *Clin Pharmacol Ther* (1982) 31, 268.

Beta blockers + Bupropion

A patient taking metoprolol developed bradycardia and hypotension when bupropion was also given.

Clinical evidence, mechanism, importance and management

A 50-year-old man taking **metoprolol** 75 mg twice daily and diltiazem 240 mg twice daily for hypertension developed fatigue 12 days after starting to take bupropion 150 mg twice daily. He was found to have a pulse rate of 43 bpm, a blood pressure of 102/65 mmHg, and signs of mild heart failure. He recovered within 24 hours of stopping all three drugs.[1] It was suggested that these effects had developed as a result of raised **metoprolol** levels, which had occurred because bupropion inhibited the metabolism of **metoprolol** by the cytochrome P450 isoenzyme CYP2D6.

The manufacturers of bupropion have predicted this interaction and recommend that if **metoprolol** is added to existing treatment with bupropion, doses at the lower end of the range should be used. If bupropion is added to existing treatment with **metoprolol**, decreased doses of **metoprolol** should be considered.[2,3] These precautions seem prudent, especially in patients with heart failure, where raised beta blocker levels seem most likely to cause an adverse effect.

Although direct evidence appears to be lacking, it seems likely that this interaction could occur with any of the beta blockers metabolised by CYP2D6 (see 'Table 22.1', p.999, for a list).

1. McCollum DL, Greene JL, McGuire DK. Severe sinus bradycardia after initiation of bupropion therapy: a probable drug-drug interaction with metoprolol. *Cardiovasc Drugs Ther* (2004) 18, 329–30.
2. Zyban (Bupropion hydrochloride). GlaxoSmithKline UK. UK Summary of product characteristics, November 2013.
3. Zyban (Bupropion hydrochloride). GlaxoSmithKline. US Prescribing information, March 2014.

Beta blockers + Calcium-channel blockers; Dihydropyridines

The use of beta blockers with felodipine, isradipine, lacidipine, nicardipine, nimodipine and nisoldipine normally appears to be useful and safe. However, severe hypotension and heart failure have occurred rarely when a beta blocker was given with nifedipine or nisoldipine. Changes in the pharmacokinetics of the beta blockers and calcium-channel blockers may also occur on concurrent use, but they do not appear to be clinically important.

Clinical evidence

(a) Felodipine

A double-blind, crossover study in 8 healthy subjects found that over a 5-day period, **metoprolol** 100 mg twice daily did not affect the pharmacokinetics of felodipine 10 mg twice daily. However, the bioavailability and peak plasma levels of **metoprolol** were modestly increased by 31% and 38%, respectively.[1] Another study in 10 healthy subjects given felodipine 10 mg with either **metoprolol** 100 mg, **pindolol** 5 mg, **propranolol** 80 mg, or **timolol** 10 mg found no changes in heart rate, PR interval or blood pressure that might be considered to be harmful to patients with hypertension or angina. However, 7 of the 10 subjects reported some increase in adverse effects.[2]

(b) Isradipine

A preliminary report of a study in 24 healthy subjects found that **propranolol** 40 mg twice daily given with isradipine 5 mg twice daily caused some modest changes in the pharmacokinetics of both drugs (peak **propranolol** plasma levels increased by 17%, peak isradipine plasma levels reduced by 18%), but the AUCs were not significantly altered.[3] An earlier preliminary report by the same research group in 17 subjects found a 28% increase in the AUC of **propranolol**, a 22% reduction in the AUC of isradipine, and a 59% increase in the peak **propranolol** levels.[4]

(c) Lacidipine

Twelve patients with mild to moderate hypertension not satisfactorily controlled by **atenolol** alone were given lacidipine 4 mg daily with or without **atenolol** 100 mg daily for 14 days. There was no evidence of a significant change in drug levels, but there was a significant additive reduction in blood pressure during concurrent use, when compared with the reductions observed with either drug alone.[5]

Single-dose studies in 24 healthy subjects found that **propranolol** 160 mg reduced the peak plasma levels and AUC of lacidipine 4 mg by 38% and 42%, respectively, while the peak plasma levels and AUC of **propranolol** were increased by 35% and 26%, respectively. There was a modest additive reduction in blood pressure of 4 to 6 mmHg, and the combination reduced the heart rate, but not to an extent greater than **propranolol** alone. No significant adverse effects were seen.[6] A further preliminary report of a study by the same authors, in which 12 hypertensive patients were given **propranolol** 160 mg twice daily and lacidipine 4 mg daily for 2 weeks, found a non-significant 30% increase in the systemic availability of lacidipine, and no change in **propranolol** pharmacokinetics. In addition, no clinically significant alterations in ECG recordings, blood pressure, or pulse rate were seen.[7]

(d) Lercanidipine

The manufacturer notes that when lercanidipine was given with **metoprolol**, the bioavailability of lercanidipine was reduced by 50% while the bioavailability of **metoprolol** was unchanged. They suggest that any beta blocker may alter lercanidipine bioavailability.[8]

(e) Nicardipine

In a single-dose study in healthy subjects, nicardipine 30 mg did not affect the pharmacokinetics or pharmacodynamics of **atenolol** 100 mg.[9]

In another study, 14 healthy subjects were given nicardipine 50 mg every 12 hours and **metoprolol** 100 mg every 12 hours, both together and alone, for 11 doses. **Metoprolol** plasma levels were raised by 28% by nicardipine in the 7 subjects who were CYP2D6 extensive metabolisers (that is, those with normal levels of this isoenzyme), but had no significant effect in the poor metabolisers (those lacking or deficient in CYP2D6). The extent of the beta-blockade was unchanged in all of them.[10]

Preliminary analysis of another study in healthy subjects found that the pharmacokinetics of both **propranolol** 80 mg twice daily and nicardipine 30 mg three times daily were unaffected when they were given together for 6 days.[11] However, two single-dose studies found that nicardipine 30 mg increased the AUC and peak plasma levels of **propranolol** 80 mg by 47% and 80%, respectively,[12] and raised the AUC and peak plasma levels of sustained-release **propranolol** 80 mg to a lesser extent (17% and 22%, respectively).[13] A related single-dose study found that in elderly healthy subjects nicardipine 30 mg increased the maximum plasma levels and AUC of **propranolol** 40 mg by about 100% and 80%, respectively. Nicardipine caused a further decrease in blood pressure, and attenuated the reduction in heart rate seen with **propranolol** alone.[14]

A study in 8 healthy subjects found that the increase in heart rate during exercise associated with a single 40-mg dose of nicardipine was reduced by one drop of **timolol** 0.5% put into each eye. Systolic blood pressure was also reduced during concurrent use, but nicardipine did not cause any further reduction in intraocular pressure than **timolol** alone.[15]

(f) Nifedipine

Nifedipine 10 mg three times daily did not alter the pharmacokinetics of **atenolol** 100 mg daily,[16,17] **betaxolol**,[18] **metoprolol** 100 mg twice daily[16,17] or **propranolol** 80 mg twice daily.[16] A single-dose study also found no pharmacokinetic interaction between nifedipine and **atenolol**.[19] However, a multiple-dose study found that nifedipine 10 mg three times daily increased the peak plasma level and AUC of **propranolol** 80 mg twice daily by 56% and 23%, respectively.[18] Another study found that the absorption of a single-dose of **propranolol** appeared to be faster, leading to higher initial concentrations, when it was given after nifedipine.[20]

Regardless of the pharmacokinetic changes, none of these studies in healthy subjects found any adverse haemodynamic effects as a result of giving nifedipine with any of these beta blockers.[16,18,19] Similarly, in studies in patients with normal left ventricular function there was no evidence of adverse haemodynamic effects when nifedipine (single-dose sublingual,[21,22] or intravenous[23] or oral daily dose[23]) was given with **atenolol**,[23] **celiprolol**[22] or **propranolol**.[21,24] However, there are a few earlier isolated case reports of hypotension and heart failure with the combination:

- Two patients with angina taking **alprenolol** or **propranolol** developed heart failure when they were given nifedipine 10 mg three times daily. The signs of heart failure disappeared when nifedipine was withdrawn.[25]
- One out of 15 patients with hypertension and exertional angina progressively developed hypotension (90/60 mmHg) when given nifedipine 10 mg twice daily with **atenolol** 50 mg daily and a diuretic for one month.[26]
- A patient with angina taking **propranolol** 160 mg four times daily developed severe and prolonged hypotension (blood pressure initially not recordable, then 60 mmHg systolic) 18 days after nifedipine 10 mg three times daily was substituted for 'isosorbide', and this may have been a factor that led to fatal myocardial infarction.[27]
- Heart failure developed in a patient with angina taking **atenolol** (and various other drugs) when nifedipine 20 mg three times daily was given.[28]

A further report describes a patient who developed hypotension and severe bradycardia on two occasions after being given her usual antihypertensive medication of **labetalol** and extended-release nifedipine crushed and given via a nasogastric tube. Crushing the nifedipine tablet altered its release characteristics so that the total dose was released quickly resulting in profound hypotension. The **labetalol** produced additional hypotensive effects and prevented a compensatory increase in heart rate.[29]

There was no change in the psychomotor performance of 12 healthy subjects who took a single 100-mg dose of **atenolol** with a single 20-mg dose of slow-release nifedipine when compared with either drug alone.[30]

(g) Nimodipine

In a preliminary report of a study in 12 healthy subjects, nimodipine 30 mg three times daily for 4 days had no significant effect on the changes in heart rate, blood pressure or cardiac output seen with either **propranolol** 40 mg or **atenolol** 25 mg three times daily. The pharmacokinetics of the beta blockers were also unaltered.[31]

(h) Nisoldipine

A single 20-mg dose of nisoldipine slightly increased both the steady-state AUC and peak plasma level of **atenolol** 100 mg daily by 19%. After concurrent use for 7 days, the AUC of **atenolol** was increased by 17% and its peak plasma level was increased by 20%. The combination enhanced blood pressure reduction to a small extent, but nisoldipine did not significantly reduce the effect of **atenolol** on heart rate.[32] In the same study, a single 20-mg dose of nisoldipine increased the steady-state AUC and peak plasma level of **propranolol** 160 mg daily by 35% and 55%, respectively. After concurrent use for 7 days, the AUC of **propranolol** was increased by 60% and the peak plasma level was increased by 55%. As with atenolol, the combination enhanced blood pressure reduction to a small extent, but nisoldipine did not significantly reduce the effect of **propranolol** on heart rate.[32] Similarly, another study found that a single 20-mg dose of nisoldipine increased the AUC and peak plasma level of a single 40-mg dose of **propranolol** by 43% and 68%, respectively, and that the AUC and peak plasma level of nisoldipine increased by 30% and 57%, respectively. In this study, nisoldipine was reported to enhance beta-blockade.[33] However, the same research group later found that the steady-state pharmacokinetics of **propranolol** 80 mg twice daily and nisoldipine 10 mg twice daily were not affected by concurrent use for 7 days, but nisoldipine attenuated the decrease in forearm blood flow seen with **propranolol**.[34] The US manufacturer of nisoldipine notes that **propranolol** attenuated the heart rate increase seen with immediate-release nisoldipine.[35]

The UK manufacturer of nisoldipine noted that severe hypotension can occur when it is given at the same time as beta blockers, and that, in isolated cases, signs of heart failure can also occur.[36]

Mechanism

Not understood. Where pharmacokinetic changes are seen, a possible reason is that the metabolism of the beta blockers is altered by changes in blood flow through the liver. The pharmacodynamic changes with nifedipine may be explained by the fact that nifedipine reduces the contractility of the heart muscle. This is counteracted by a sympathetic reflex increase in heart rate due to nifedipine-induced peripheral vasodilation, so that the ventricular output stays the same or is even improved. The presence of a beta blocker may oppose this to some extent by slowing the heart rate, which allows the negative inotropic effects of nifedipine to go unchecked.

The manufacturer of lercanidipine suggests that the reduction in lercanidipine bioavailability may be due to reduced hepatic blood flow caused by beta-adrenoceptor blockade.[8]

Importance and management

The concurrent use of beta blockers and the dihydropyridine calcium-channel blockers is common, and normally valuable. However, isolated cases of severe hypotension and heart failure have been seen in a few patients taking beta blockers and **nifedipine** or **nisoldipine**. It has been suggested that those likely to be most at risk are patients with impaired left ventricular function[37] (which is a caution for the use of nifedipine anyway) and/or those taking beta blockers in high dose. Bear this in mind. It should also be noted that the topical use of beta blockers (such as timolol eye drops) may reduce heart rate and blood pressure. It may also be worth noting that all but one of the cases of an adverse reaction with a beta blocker and nifedipine occurred with 'short-acting' formulations, which are now considered unsuitable for long-term management of angina or hypertension, because they are associated with larger variations in blood pressure and heart rate. The remaining case was associated with the incorrect use of an extended-release nifedipine preparation.

Changes in the pharmacokinetics of the beta blockers and calcium-channel blockers may also occur, but these do not appear to be clinically important.

The manufacturer of **lercanidipine** suggests that, as a reduction in lercanidipine bioavailability may occur with any beta blocker, some adjustment of the lercanidipine dose may be needed.[8]

1. Smith SR, Wilkins MR, Jack DB, Kendall MJ, Laugher S. Pharmacokinetic interactions between felodipine and metoprolol. *Eur J Clin Pharmacol* (1987) 31, 575–8.
2. Carruthers SG, Bailey DG. Tolerance and cardiovascular effects of single dose felodipine/β-blocker combinations in healthy subjects. *J Cardiovasc Pharmacol* (1987) 10 (Suppl 1), S169–S176.
3. Schran HF, Shepherd AM, Choc MM, Gonasun LM, Brodie CL. The effect of concomitant administration of isradipine and propranolol on their steady-state bioavailability. *Pharmacologist* (1989) 31, 153.
4. Shepherd AMM, Brodie CL, Carrillo DW, Kwan CM. Pharmacokinetic interaction between isradipine and propranolol. *Clin Pharmacol Ther* (1988) 43,194.
5. Lyons D, Fowler G, Webster J, Hall ST, Petrie JC. An assessment of lacidipine and atenolol in mild to moderate hypertension. *Br J Clin Pharmacol* (1994) 37, 45–51.
6. Hall ST, Harding SM, Hassani H, Keene ON, Pellegatti M. The pharmacokinetic and pharmacodynamic interaction between lacidipine and propranolol in healthy volunteers. *J Cardiovasc Pharmacol* (1991) 18, (Suppl 11), S13–S17.
7. Hall ST, Saul P, Keene ON, Hassani H. Pharmacodynamic and pharmacokinetic interaction between lacidipine and propranolol. *Pharm Res* (1992) 9 (10 Suppl), S88.
8. Zanidip (Lercanidipine hydrochloride). Recordati Pharmaceuticals Ltd. UK Summary of product characteristics, April 2006.
9. Vercruysse I, Schoors DF, Musch G, Massart DL, Dupont AG. Nicardipine does not influence the pharmacokinetics and pharmacodynamics of atenolol. *Br J Clin Pharmacol* (1990) 30, 499–500.
10. Laurent-Kenesi M-A, Funck-Brentano C, Poirier J-M, Decolin D, Jaillon P. Influence of CYP2D6-dependent metabolism on the steady-state pharmacokinetics and pharmacodynamics of metoprolol and nicardipine, alone and in combination. *Br J Clin Pharmacol* (1993) 36, 531–8.
11. Macdonald FC, Dow RJ, Wilson RAG, Yee KF, Finlayson J. A study to determine potential interactions between nicardipine and propranolol in healthy volunteers. *Br J Clin Pharmacol* (1987), 23, 626P.
12. Schoors DF, Vercruysse I, Musch G, Massart DL, Dupont AG. Influence of nicardipine on the pharmacokinetics and pharmacodynamics of propranolol in healthy volunteers. *Br J Clin Pharmacol* (1990) 29, 497–501.
13. Vercruysse I, Massart DL, Dupont AG. Increase in plasma propranolol caused by nicardipine is dependent on the delivery rate of propranolol. *Eur J Clin Pharmacol* (1995) 49, 121–5.
14. Hartmann C, Vercruysse I, Metz T, Massart DL, Dupont AG. Influence of nicardipine on the pharmacokinetics of propranolol in the elderly. *Br J Clin Pharmacol* (1995) 39, 540P.
15. Yatsuka YI, Tsutsumi K, Kotegawa T, Nakamura K, Nakano S, Nakatsuka K. Interaction between timolol eyedrops and oral nicardipine or oral diltiazem in healthy Japanese subjects. *Eur J Clin Pharmacol* (1998) 54, 149–54.
16. Gangji D, Juvent M, Niset G, Wathieu M, Degreve M, Bellens R, Poortmans J, Degre S, Fitzsimons TJ, Herchuelz A. Study of the influence of nifedipine on the pharmacokinetics and pharmacodynamics of propranolol, metoprolol and atenolol. *Br J Clin Pharmacol* (1984) 17, 29S–35S.
17. Kendall MJ, Jack DB, Laugher SJ, Lobo J, Smith RS. Lack of a pharmacokinetic interaction between nifedipine and the β-adrenoceptor blockers metoprolol and atenolol. *Br J Clin Pharmacol* (1984) 18, 331–5.
18. Vinceneux Ph, Canal M, Domart Y, Roux A, Cascio B, Orofiamma B, Larribaud J, Flouvat B, Carbon C. Pharmacokinetic and pharmacodynamic interactions between nifedipine and propranolol or betaxolol. *Int J Clin Pharmacol Ther Toxicol* (1986) 24, 153–8.
19. Rosenkranz B, Ledermann H, Frölich JC. Interaction between nifedipine and atenolol: pharmacokinetics and pharmacodynamics in normotensive volunteers. *J Cardiovasc Pharmacol* (1986) 8, 943–9.
20. Bauer LA, Murray K, Horn JR, Opheim K, Olsen J. Influence of nifedipine therapy on indocyanine green and oral propranolol pharmacokinetics. *Eur J Clin Pharmacol* (1989) 37, 257–60.
21. Elkayam U, Roth A, Weber L, Kulick D, Kawanishi D, McKay C, Rahimtoola SH. Effects of nifedipine on hemodynamics and cardiac function in patients with normal left ventricular ejection fraction already treated with propranolol. *Am J Cardiol* (1986) 58, 536–40.
22. Silke B, Verma SP, Guy S. Hemodynamic interactions of a new beta blocker, celiprolol, with nifedipine in angina pectoris. *Cardiovasc Drugs Ther* (1991) 5, 681–8.
23. Rowland E, Razis P, Sugrue D, Krikler DM. Acute and chronic haemodynamic and electrophysiological effects of nifedipine in patients receiving atenolol. *Br Heart J* (1983) 50, 383–9.
24. Vetrovec GW, Parker VE. Nifedipine, beta blocker interaction: effect on left ventricular function. *Clin Res* (1984) 32, 833A.
25. Anastassiades CJ. Nifedipine and beta-blocker drugs. *BMJ* (1980) 281, 1251–2.
26. Opie LH, White DA. Adverse interaction between nifedipine and β-blockade. *BMJ* (1980) 281, 1462.
27. Staffurth JS, Emery P. Adverse interaction between nifedipine and beta-blockade. *BMJ* (1981) 282, 225.
28. Robson RH, Vishwanath MC. Nifedipine and beta-blockade as a cause of cardiac failure. *BMJ* (1982) 284, 104.
29. Schier JG, Howland MA, Hoffman RS, Nelson LS. Fatality from administration of labetalol and crushed extended-release nifedipine. *Ann Pharmacother* (2003) 37, 1420–3.
30. Gerrard L, Wheeldon NM, McDevitt DG. Effect of combined atenolol and nifedipine administration on psychomotor performance in normal subjects. *Eur J Clin Pharmacol* (1995) 48, 229–33.
31. Horstmann R, Weber H, Wingender W, Rämsch K-D, Kuhlmann J. Does nimodipine interact with beta adrenergic blocking agents? *Eur J Clin Pharmacol* (1989) 36, A258.
32. Elliott HL, Meredith PA, McNally C, Reid JL. The interactions between nisoldipine and two β-adrenoceptor antagonists—atenolol and propranolol. *Br J Clin Pharmacol* (1991) 32, 379–85.
33. Levine MAH, Ogilvie RI, Leenen FHH. Pharmacokinetic and pharmacodynamic interactions between nisoldipine and propranolol. *Clin Pharmacol Ther* (1988) 43, 39–48.
34. Shaw-Stiffel TA, Walker SE, Ogilvie RI, Leenen FH. Pharmacokinetic and pharmacodynamic interactions during multiple-dose administration of nisoldipine and propranolol. *Clin Pharmacol Ther* (1994) 55, 661–9.
35. Sular (Nisoldipine). Sciele Pharma, Inc. US Prescribing information, February 2010.
36. Syscor MR (Nisoldipine). Forest Laboratories UK Ltd. UK Summary of product characteristics, August 1998.
37. Brooks N, Cattell M, Pigeon J, Balcon R. Unpredictable response to nifedipine in severe cardiac failure. *BMJ* (1980) 281, 1324.

Beta blockers + Calcium-channel blockers; Diltiazem

The cardiac depressant effects of diltiazem and the beta blockers are additive, and a number of patients, (usually those with pre-existing ventricular failure or conduction abnormalities) have developed serious and potentially life-threatening bradycardia. However, concurrent use can be beneficial. Diltiazem increases the serum levels of propranolol and metoprolol, but not those of atenolol.

Clinical evidence

(a) Cardiac depressant effects

Ten patients were admitted to an intensive coronary care unit during one year with severe bradycardia (heart rates of 24 to 44 bpm) after taking diltiazem 90 to 360 mg daily with **propranolol** 30 to 120 mg daily, **atenolol** 50 to 100 mg daily, or **pindolol** 90 mg daily. All were relatively elderly and presented with lethargy, dizziness, syncope, chest pain, and in one case, pulmonary oedema. The ECG abnormalities were localised in the sinus node, the primary rhythm disorders being junctional escape rhythms, sinus bradycardia and sinus pause. These resolved within 24 hours of withdrawing the drugs, although a temporary pacemaker was needed in 4 patients.[1]

In an analysis of drug use in cases listed in a post-mortem toxicology database in Finland for the period 2000 to 2006, drug combinations possessing potentially severe interactions were found in 267 cases (0.71% of cases). The use of a beta blocker with verapamil or diltiazem accounted for 22 possible pharmacodynamic interactions. In one case, a 63-year-old man who died in a car accident was found to have slightly elevated levels of **bisoprolol** (0.13 mg/L) and therapeutic levels of diltiazem. It was speculated that the combination could have led to bradyarrhythmias or other adverse cardiac effects, which might have contributed to the fatality.[2]

Symptomatic and severe bradyarrhythmias of this kind have been described in case reports in 16 other patients taking diltiazem with **atenolol**,[3] **carteolol**,[4] **metoprolol**,[3,5,6] **nadolol**,[7] **pindolol**,[8] **propranolol**,[3,5,7,9] or **sotalol**.[4,8] In a prospective study of hospital admissions due to cardiovascular adverse drug reactions, bradycardia, hypotension, syncope and worsening heart failure were noted in 21 patients taking beta blockers with diltiazem. The beta blockers involved were **propranolol** (13 patients), **atenolol** (5), **metoprolol** (2) and **oxprenolol** (1).[10] Similarly, severe sinus bradycardia occurred in 8 of 59 patients in three early clinical studies of the combination of diltiazem and **propranolol**.[11-13] One patient developed congestive heart failure.[13] In contrast, four other similar clinical studies did not report any adverse effects.[14-17]

In a single-dose study, one drop of **timolol** 0.5% eye drops did not cause an additional reduction in heart rate when it was given to healthy subjects with a 60-mg dose of diltiazem.[18]

(b) Pharmacokinetics

In healthy subjects, diltiazem increased the AUC of **propranolol** and **metoprolol** by 48% and 33%, respectively, and increased the maximum serum levels of these beta blockers by 45% and 71%, respectively. The pharmacokinetics of **atenolol** were not affected by diltiazem.[19] Another study found that diltiazem caused a 24 to 27% reduction in **propranolol** clearance.[20]

Mechanism

The bradycardic effects of the beta blockers can be additive with the delay in conduction through the atrioventricular node caused by diltiazem.[8] This advantageously increases the antianginal effects in most patients, but in a few these effects might exacerbate existing cardiac abnormalities. Diltiazem apparently also inhibits the metabolism of propranolol and metoprolol, but the exact mechanism for this is not clear.[19]

Importance and management

The concurrent use of a beta blocker and diltiazem is unquestionably valuable and uneventful in many patients, but severe adverse effects can develop. This is well established. On the basis of 6 reports, the incidence of symptomatic bradyarrhythmia was estimated to be about 10 to 15%.[1] It can occur with different beta blockers, even with very low doses, and at any time from within a few hours of starting treatment to 2 years of concurrent use.[1] The main risk factors seem to be ventricular dysfunction, or sinoatrial or AV nodal conduction abnormalities,[1] which are usually contraindications to the use of diltiazem. Patients with normal ventricular function and no evidence of conduction abnormalities are usually not at risk. Concurrent use should be well monitored for evidence of adverse effects. Changes in the pharmacokinetics of the beta blockers might also occur, but these changes are probably not clinically important.

1. Sagie A, Strasberg B, Kusnieck J, Sclarovsky S. Symptomatic bradycardia induced by the combination of oral diltiazem and beta blockers. *Clin Cardiol* (1991) 14, 314–16.
2. Launiainen T, Vuori E, Ojanperä I. Prevalence of adverse drug combinations in a large post-mortem toxicology database. *Int J Legal Med* (2009) 123, 109–15.
3. Yust I, Hoffman M, Aronson RJ. Life-threatening bradycardic reactions due to beta blocker-diltiazem interactions. *Isr J Med Sci* (1992) 28, 292–4.
4. Lamaison D, Vacher D, Berenfeld A, Schandrin C, Lavarenne V. Association de diltiazem à libération prolongée et d'un bêta-bloquant dans l'hypertension artérielle. Deux cas de choc cardiogénique avec bradycardie extrême. *Therapie* (1990) 45, 411–13.
5. Lan Cheong Wah LSH, Robinet G, Guiavarc'h M, Garo B, Boles JM. États de choc au cours de l'association diltiazem-β-bloquant. *Rev Med Interne* (1992) 13, 80.

6. Kjeldsen SE, Syvertsen J-O, Hedner T. Cardiac conduction with diltiazem and beta-blockade combined. A review and report on cases. *Blood Pressure* (1996) 5, 260–3.
7. Hossack KF. Conduction abnormalities due to diltiazem. *N Engl J Med* (1982) 307, 953–4.
8. Hassell AB, Creamer JE. Profound bradycardia after the addition of diltiazem to a beta-blocker. *BMJ* (1989) 298, 675.
9. Ishikawa T, Imamura T, Koiwaya Y, Tanaka K. Atrioventricular dissociation and sinus arrest induced by oral diltiazem. *N Engl J Med* (1983) 309, 1124–5.
10. Edoute Y, Nagachandran P, Svirski B, Ben-Ami H. Cardiovascular adverse drug reaction associated with combined β-adrenergic and calcium entry-blocking agents. *J Cardiovasc Pharmacol* (2000) 35, 556–9.
11. O'Hara MJ, Khurmi NS, Bowles MJ, Raftery EB. Diltiazem and propranolol combination for the treatment of chronic stable angina pectoris. *Clin Cardiol* (1987) 10, 115–23.
12. Hung J, Lamb IH, Connolly SJ, Jutzy KR, Goris ML, Schroeder JS. The effect of diltiazem and propranolol, alone and in combination, on exercise performance and left ventricular function in patients with stable effort angina: a double-blind, randomized, and placebo-controlled study. *Circulation* (1983) 68, 560–7.
13. Strauss WE, Parisi AF. Superiority of combined diltiazem and propranolol therapy for angina pectoris. *Circulation* (1985) 71, 951–7.
14. Tilmant PY, Lablanche JM, Thieuleux FA, Dupuis BA, Bertrand ME. Detrimental effect of propranolol in patients with coronary arterial spasm countered by combination with diltiazem. *Am J Cardiol* (1983) 52, 230–33.
15. Rocha P, Baron B, Delestrain A, Pathe M, Cazor J-L, Kahn J-C. Hemodynamic effects of intravenous diltiazem in patients treated chronically with propranolol. *Am Heart J* (1986) 111, 62–8.
16. Humen DP, O'Brien P, Purves P, Johnson D, Kostuk WJ. Effort angina with adequate beta-receptor blockade: comparison with diltiazem alone and in combination. *J Am Coll Cardiol* (1986) 7, 329–35.
17. Kenny J, Daly K, Bergman G, Kerkez S, Jewitt DE. Beneficial effects of diltiazem combined with beta blockade in angina pectoris. *Eur Heart J* (1985) 6, 418–23.
18. Yatsuka YI, Tsutsumi K, Kotegawa T, Nakamura K, Nakano S, Nakatsuka K. Interaction between timolol eyedrops and oral nicardipine or oral diltiazem in healthy Japanese subjects. *Eur J Clin Pharmacol* (1998) 54, 149–54.
19. Tateishi T, Nakashima H, Shitou T, Kumagai Y, Ohashi K, Hosoda S, Ebihara A. Effect of diltiazem on the pharmacokinetics of propranolol, metoprolol and atenolol. *Eur J Clin Pharmacol* (1989) 36, 67–70.
20. Hunt BA, Bottorff MB, Herring VL, Self TH, Lalonde RL. Effects of calcium channel blockers on the pharmacokinetics of propranolol stereoisomers. *Clin Pharmacol Ther* (1990) 47, 584–91.

Beta blockers + Calcium-channel blockers; Verapamil

The cardiac depressant effects of verapamil and the beta blockers are additive, and although concurrent use can be beneficial, serious cardiodepression (bradycardia, asystole, sinus arrest) sometimes occurs. An adverse interaction can also occur with beta blockers given as eye drops.

Clinical evidence

(a) Pharmacodynamic interactions

In an analysis of drug use in cases listed in a post-mortem toxicology database in Finland, for the period 2000 to 2006, drug combinations possessing potentially severe interactions were found in 267 cases (0.71% of cases). Combinations of beta blockers with verapamil or diltiazem accounted for 22 possible pharmacodynamic interactions.[1]

1. Intravenous use. Ventricular asystole developed in a 70-year-old man and a 6-month-old baby when intravenous verapamil was given after the unsuccessful use of intravenous **practolol** to treat supraventricular tachycardia.[2] In a later study, the combination of intravenous verapamil and intravenous **practolol** produced a marked reduction in cardiac contractility, which was more evident when **practolol** was given first.[3]

2. Oral use. In one series, 34 out of 42 patients taking verapamil 360 mg daily with beta blockers (daily dose: **atenolol** 100 mg (34 patients), **atenolol** 50 mg (2), **propranolol** 160 mg (4), **pindolol** 20 mg (1), or **metoprolol** 100 mg (1)) experienced a reduction in anginal episodes over a mean period of 6.5 months while taking both drugs. However, 12 patients needed a reduced dose or withdrawal of one or both drugs. One had non-specific symptoms (drugs withdrawn), 2 had bradyarrhythmias (drugs withdrawn) and 6 experienced dyspnoea (3 withdrawals and 3 dose reductions), which were presumed to be secondary to left ventricular failure. Other complications were tiredness (2 patients) and postural hypotension (1 patient), which were dealt with by reducing the dose.[4] In another study in 15 patients with angina who were taking **atenolol** with verapamil, 4 patients experienced profound lethargy, one had left ventricular failure and 4 had bradyarrhythmias.[5]

Other case reports and studies describe heart failure,[6,7] dyspnoea,[6,8,9] sinus arrest,[10,11] heart block,[10,12-14] hypotension,[6,7,9,11,14-17] and bradycardia[5,6,9,11,12,15-19] in patients taking verapamil with **alprenolol**,[10] **atenolol**,[7,10,11,13] **metoprolol**,[6,12,14,16] **propranolol**[8,9,15,17-19] or **pindolol**.[6] A number of reports noted that patients experiencing this interaction had reasonable left ventricular function.[6,11,13]

3. Ocular use. In two cases, bradycardia occurred in patients taking verapamil and using **timolol** eye drops.[20,21] Another case has been reported, but this was complicated by the presence of flecainide, which may also interact with the beta blockers, see 'Beta blockers + Flecainide', p.1010.

(b) Pharmacokinetic interactions

1. Atenolol. In one study in a single patient, the pharmacokinetics of atenolol were not altered by verapamil.[22] A study in 15 patients found that the plasma levels of verapamil and atenolol varied greatly during individual and concurrent use but mean concentrations were not significantly changed.[5] In another study, in 10 patients, the mean AUC of atenolol was not significantly increased by verapamil, but individual patients had atenolol AUC increases of up to 112%.[23]

2. Metoprolol. In a study in 10 patients, verapamil raised the metoprolol AUC by 33% and raised its peak plasma levels by 41%. The minimum pulse rate and systolic blood pressure (1 to 3 hours post dose) were also lower in those taking the combination than with metoprolol alone.[16] Similarly, in a single-dose study in 9 healthy subjects, the AUC and maximum plasma level of metoprolol were increased by 35% and 64%, respectively, and the AUC and half-life of verapamil were increased by 57% and 29%, respectively, when both drugs were given together.[24]

3. Propranolol. In healthy subjects, verapamil reduced the clearance of propranolol by 26 to 32% and increased its AUC by 46 to 58% after 6 days of concurrent use.[25] Similarly, in 5 patients, verapamil increased the peak plasma levels of propranolol by 94%, and increased its AUC by 66%.[19] Propranolol did not affect the pharmacokinetics of verapamil.[19] However, in another study in healthy subjects, no pharmacokinetic interaction was noted when propranolol and verapamil were taken together for 6 days.[26]

4. Talinolol. In a randomised, crossover study in 9 healthy subjects, a single 120-mg dose of *(R)*-verapamil reduced the bioavailability of a single 50-mg oral dose of talinolol by 25%.[27]

Mechanism

Both the beta blockers and verapamil have negative inotropic effects on the heart, which can be additive.[26] Given together they can cause marked bradycardia and may even depress the contraction of the ventricle completely. Verapamil can also raise the serum levels of the beta blockers that are extensively metabolised in the liver (e.g. metoprolol, propranolol), probably by inhibiting their metabolism,[28] although the exact mechanism for this is unclear. It is thought that verapamil affects talinolol bioavailability by modulating intestinal P-glycoprotein.[27,29]

Importance and management

The interactions between verapamil and the beta blockers are well documented and well established. Although concurrent use can be uneventful and successful, the reports cited here amply demonstrate that it may not always be safe. The difficulty is identifying the patients most at risk. In the UK, the BNF says that oral concurrent use should only be considered if myocardial function is well preserved, and that verapamil should not be injected in patients recently given beta blockers because of the risk of hypotension and asystole. They also note that, although 30 minutes has been suggested as a sufficient interval before giving a beta blocker when a verapamil injection has been given first, the safety of this has not been established.[30] The UK manufacturer of verapamil contraindicates its intravenous use in those receiving intravenous beta blockers.[31]

It has been advised that the initiation of treatment should be restricted to hospital practice, where the dose of each drug can be carefully titrated and the patient closely supervised, particularly during the first few days when adverse effects are most likely to develop.[4,5,19] Some have suggested that beta blockers that are extensively metabolised (e.g. metoprolol, propranolol) may possibly carry some additional risk because verapamil raises their serum levels.[22] However, others contend that, because the interaction occurs with atenolol (which is largely excreted unchanged in the urine), the pharmacodynamic effects are more important than any pharmacokinetic changes.[5,11,19] Note that the latter argument is probably valid, as changes in the AUC of beta blockers of this size, or even more have proved not to be clinically important, even in those patients likely to be sensitive to the effects of the beta blockers, such as those with heart failure.

1. Launiainen T, Vuori E, Ojanperä I. Prevalence of adverse drug combinations in a large post-mortem toxicology database. *Int J Legal Med* (2009) 123, 109–15.
2. Boothby CB, Garrard CS, Pickering D. Verapamil in cardiac arrhythmias. *BMJ* (1972) 2, 349.
3. Seabra-Gomes R, Rickards A, Sutton R. Hemodynamic effects of verapamil and practolol in man. *Eur J Cardiol* (1976) 4, 79–85.
4. McGourty JC, Silas JH, Solomon SA. Tolerability of combined treatment with verapamil and beta-blockers in angina resistant to monotherapy. *Postgrad Med J* (1985) 61, 229–32.
5. Findlay IN, MacLeod K, Gillen G, Elliott AT, Aitchison T, Dargie HJ. A double blind placebo controlled comparison of verapamil, atenolol, and their combination in patients with chronic stable angina pectoris. *Br Heart J* (1987) 57, 336–43.
6. Wayne VS, Harper RW, Laufer E, Federman J, Anderson ST, Pitt A. Adverse interaction between beta-adrenergic blocking drugs and verapamil-report of three cases. *Aust N Z J Med* (1982) 12, 285–9.
7. Sakurai H, Kei M, Matsubara K, Yokouchi K, Hattori K, Ichihashi R, Hirakawa Y, Tsukamoto H, Saburi Y. Cardiogenic shock triggered by verapamil and atenolol—a case report of therapeutic experience with intravenous calcium. *Jpn Circ J* (2000) 64, 893–6.
8. Balasubramian V, Bowles M, Davies AB, Rafferty EB. Combined treatment with verapamil and propranolol in chronic stable angina. *Br Heart J* (1981) 45, 349–50.
9. Leon MB, Rosing DR, Bonow RO, Lipson LC, Epstein SE. Clinical efficacy of verapamil alone and combined with propranolol in treating patients with chronic stable angina pectoris. *Am J Cardiol* (1981) 48, 131–9.
10. McQueen EG. New Zealand Committee on Adverse Reactions: fourteenth annual report 1979. *N Z Med J* (1980) 91, 226–9.
11. Misra M, Thakur R, Bhandari K. Sinus arrest caused by atenolol-verapamil combination. *Clin Cardiol* (1987) 10, 365–7.
12. Eisenberg JNH, Oakley GDG. Probable adverse interaction between oral metoprolol and verapamil. *Postgrad Med J* (1984) 60, 705–6.
13. Hutchison SJ, Lorimer AR, Lakhdar A, McAlpine SG. β-blockers and verapamil: a cautionary tale. *BMJ* (1984) 289, 659–60.
14. Lee DW, Cohan B. Refractory cardiogenic shock and complete heart block after verapamil SR and metoprolol treatment. *Angiology* (1995) 46, 517–19.
15. Ljungström A, Åberg H. Interaktion mellan betareceptorblockerare och verapamil. *Lakartidningen* (1973) 70, 3548.
16. Keech AC, Harper RW, Harrison PM, Pitt A, McLean AJ. Pharmacokinetic interaction between oral metoprolol and verapamil for angina pectoris. *Am J Cardiol* (1986) 58, 551–2.
17. Zatuchni J. Bradycardia and hypotension after propranolol HCl and verapamil. *Heart Lung* (1985) 14, 94–5.
18. Rumboldt Z, Baković Z, Bagatin J. Opasna kardiodepresivna interakcija izmedu verapamila i propranolola. *Lijec Vjesn* (1979) 101, 430–2.
19. McCourty JC, Silas JH, Tucker GT, Lennard MS. The effect of combined therapy on the pharmacokinetics and pharmacodynamics of verapamil and propranolol in patients with angina pectoris. *Br J Clin Pharmacol* (1988) 25, 349–57.
20. Sinclair NI, Benzie JL. Timolol eye drops and verapamil — a dangerous combination. *Med J Aust* (1983) 1, 548.
21. Pringle SD, MacEwen CJ. Severe bradycardia due to interaction of timolol eye drops and verapamil. *BMJ* (1987) 294, 155–6.
22. McLean AJ, Knight R, Harrison PM, Harper RW. Clearance-based oral drug interaction between verapamil and metoprolol and comparison with atenolol. *Am J Cardiol* (1985) 55, 1628–9.

23. Keech AC, Harper RW, Harrison PM, Pitt A, McLean AJ. Extent and pharmacokinetic mechanisms of oral atenolol-verapamil interaction in man. *Eur J Clin Pharmacol* (1988) 35, 363–6.
24. Bauer LA, Horn JR, Maxon MS, Easterling TR, Shen DD, Strandness DE. Effect of metoprolol and verapamil administered separately and concurrently after single doses on liver blood flow and drug disposition. *J Clin Pharmacol* (2000) 40, 533–43.
25. Hunt BA, Bottorff MB, Herring VL, Self TH, Lalonde RL. Effects of calcium channel blockers on the pharmacokinetics of propranolol stereoisomers. *Clin Pharmacol Ther* (1990) 47, 584–91.
26. Murdoch DL, Thomson GD, Thompson GG, Murray GD, Brodie MJ, McInnes GT. Evaluation of potential pharmacodynamic interactions between verapamil and propranolol in normal subjects. *Br J Clin Pharmacol* (1991) 31, 323–32.
27. Schwarz UI, Gramatté T, Krappweis J, Berndt A, Oertel R, von Richter O, Kirch W. Unexpected effect of verapamil on oral bioavailability of the β-blocker talinolol in humans. *Clin Pharmacol Ther* (1999) 65, 283–90.
28. Kim M, Shen DD, Eddy AC, Nelson WL. Inhibition of the enantioselective oxidative metabolism of metoprolol by verapamil in human liver microsomes. *Drug Metab Dispos* (1993) 21, 309–17.
29. Gramatté T, Oertel R. Intestinal secretion of intravenous talinolol is inhibited by luminal *R*-verapamil. *Clin Pharmacol Ther* (1999) 66, 239–45.
30. Joint Formulary Committee. *British National Formulary.* 70 ed. London: BMJ Group and Pharmaceutical Press; 2015. p.157.
31. Securon IV (Verapamil hydrochloride). Abbott Laboratories Ltd. UK Summary of product characteristics, January 2010.

Beta blockers + Chloroquine and related drugs

Hydroxychloroquine and possibly chloroquine may increase the blood levels of metoprolol and probably other similarly metabolised beta blockers.

Clinical evidence, mechanism, importance and management

In a study in 7 healthy subjects, hydroxychloroquine 400 mg daily for 8 days increased the AUC and peak plasma levels of a single 100-mg dose of **metoprolol** by 65% and 72%, respectively.[1] The subjects in this study were of the extensive CYP2D6 metaboliser phenotype, meaning that they had normal levels of this isoenzyme. Hydroxychloroquine may inhibit the metabolism of **metoprolol** by the cytochrome P450 isoenzyme CYP2D6. The clinical significance of this interaction is unknown, but normally the beta blockers are considered to have a wide therapeutic range, and so rises in levels are generally well tolerated. Patients with heart failure are usually more at risk, because drugs such as metoprolol need slow and careful dose titration in this condition, but even in this patient group the rise in levels seems unlikely to be generally important. There appears to be no information about other beta blockers, but all those metabolised by CYP2D6 would be expected to be affected to some extent. See 'Table 22.1', p.999, for a list.

In vitro study suggests that **chloroquine** may interact with **metoprolol** in the same way as hydroxychloroquine.[2] More study is needed to establish the clinical relevance of any interaction.

1. Somer M, Kallio J, Pesonen U, Pyykkö K, Huupponen R, Scheinin M. Influence of hydroxychloroquine on the bioavailability of oral metoprolol. *Br J Clin Pharmacol* (2000) 49, 549–54.
2. Lancaster DL, Adio RA, Tai KK, Simooya OO, Broadhead GD, Tucker GT, Lennard MS. Inhibition of metoprolol metabolism by chloroquine and other antimalarial drugs. *J Pharm Pharmacol* (1990) 42, 267–71.

Beta blockers + Dextropropoxyphene (Propoxyphene)

A single-dose study has shown that the bioavailability of metoprolol is notably increased by dextropropoxyphene and a case report of bradycardia and increased metoprolol concentrations is in line with these findings. The bioavailability of propranolol is also increased by dextropropoxyphene, but to a lesser extent than that of metoprolol.

Clinical evidence

A 48-year-old man taking **metoprolol** 100 mg daily developed dizziness and sweating 3 hours after taking dextropropoxyphene 200 mg and paracetamol (acetaminophen) 1.3 g. He was found to have a heart rate of 30 to 40 bpm and a blood pressure of 98/65 mmHg, which returned to normal over the following 8 hours. Assessment of blood samples showed that his normal **metoprolol** concentration was 89 nanograms/mL, but that this had risen to 160 nanograms/mL in the presence of dextropropoxyphene.[1]

Preliminary results of a study in healthy subjects suggest that after taking dextropropoxyphene (dose not stated) for a day the bioavailability of a single 100-mg oral dose of **metoprolol** was increased 3.6-fold and the total body clearance was reduced by 19%. The bioavailability of a single 40-mg oral dose of **propranolol** was increased by about 70% by dextropropoxyphene.[2]

Mechanism

Dextropropoxyphene inhibits the metabolism of metoprolol and propranolol by the CYP2D6, which results in increased concentrations and therefore increased effects. Propranolol is probably affected to a lesser extent as it is also metabolised by CYP1A2.

Importance and management

Evidence regarding an interaction between metoprolol or propranolol and dextropropoxyphene is limited, but an interaction seems to be established. It seems likely that this interaction could occur with any of the beta blockers metabolised by CYP2D6 (see 'Table 22.1', p.999). Therefore it would be prudent to be alert for evidence of an increased response to the beta blocker, but so far there seems to be very little evidence to suggest that concurrent use causes problems. Patients with heart failure are usually more at risk from an interaction, because drugs such as metoprolol need slow and careful dose titration in this condition, and therefore some monitoring (e.g. for shortness of breath, bradycardia, hypotension) might be prudent. No interaction would be expected with those beta blockers that are largely excreted unchanged in the urine (see 'Table 22.1', p.999).

1. Marraffa JM, Lang L, Ong G, Lehmann DF. Profound metoprolol-induced bradycardia precipitated by acetaminophen-propoxyphene. *Clin Pharmacol Ther* (2006) 79, 282–6.
2. Lundborg P, Regårdh CG. The effect of propoxyphene pretreatment on the disposition of metoprolol and propranolol. *Clin Pharmacol Ther* (1981) 29, 263–4.

Beta blockers + Diphenhydramine

Diphenhydramine moderately inhibits the metabolism of metoprolol.

Clinical evidence

In a placebo-controlled study, 16 healthy male subjects were given diphenhydramine 50 mg three times daily for 5 days, with a single 100-mg dose of **metoprolol** on day 3. Diphenhydramine decreased the clearance of **metoprolol** by 46% and increased its AUC by 61% in the 10 subjects who were of the extensive CYP2D6 metaboliser phenotype (meaning those that had normal levels of this isoenzyme), but had no significant effect in the 6 poor metabolisers (that is, those lacking or deficient in CYP2D6). However, the **metoprolol** AUC in the extensive metabolisers taking diphenhydramine was still only about one-third of that in the poor metabolisers taking placebo, suggesting a limited effect. The effect of **metoprolol** on heart rate and systolic blood pressure during exercise was also increased by diphenhydramine in extensive metabolisers. However, as before, the effect was not as great as that of **metoprolol** alone in poor metabolisers.[1] The same group of researchers repeated this study in 20 healthy women and found broadly similar results.[2]

Mechanism

Diphenhydramine modestly inhibits the cytochrome P450 isoenzyme CYP2D6, which is responsible, in part, for the metabolism of metoprolol and some other beta blockers. CYP2D6 shows polymorphism, with some individuals lacking significant CYP2D6 activity (poor metabolisers), in whom diphenhydramine would have little or no effect. See 'Genetic factors in drug metabolism', p.8, for more information on genetic polymorphism.

Importance and management

Information about an interaction between diphenhydramine and metoprolol appears to be limited to these studies. Increases in plasma metoprolol levels of this size are unlikely to be clinically relevant. However, patients with heart failure are usually more at risk, because drugs such as metoprolol need slow and careful dose titration in this condition, but even in this patient group the rise in levels seems unlikely to be generally important. Indeed, despite the likely widespread use of extensively metabolised beta blockers (see 'Table 22.1', p.999) and diphenhydramine, no problems seem to have been reported.

1. Hamelin BA, Bouayad A, Méthot J, Jobin J, Desgagnés P, Poirier P, Allaire J, Dumesnil J, Turgeon J. Significant interaction between the nonprescription antihistamine diphenhydramine and the CYP2D6 substrate metoprolol in healthy men with high or low CYP2D6 activity. *Clin Pharmacol Ther* (2000) 67, 466–77.
2. Sharma A, Pibarot P, Pilote S, Dumesnil JG, Arsenault M, Bélanger PM, Meibohn B, Hamelin BA. Modulation of metoprolol pharmacokinetics and hemodynamics by diphenhydramine coadministration during exercise testing in healthy premenopausal women. *J Pharmacol Exp Ther* (2005) 313, 1172–81.

Beta blockers + Dronedarone

Additive bradycardia may occur if dronedarone is taken with any beta blocker. In addition, dronedarone increases the AUC of metoprolol in most patients, which may further contribute to bradycardia, although in one study the additional increase in the negative inotropic effects seen as a consequence was modest. Dronedarone also increases the AUC of propranolol, and is also likely to interact with other beta blockers that are similarly metabolised. It is recommended that sotalol should not be used with dronedarone, because of the additive risk of QT prolongation.

Clinical evidence

In a study, 44 healthy subjects (39 extensive and 5 poor CYP2D6 metabolisers; that is, 39 subjects with normal levels of CYP2D6 and 5 subjects lacking or deficient in CYP2D6) were given **metoprolol** 200 mg daily for 13 days with dronedarone 800 mg, 1.2 g or 1.6 g daily from day 5. Dronedarone increased the AUC of **metoprolol** in a dose-dependent manner in the 39 subjects who were extensive metabolisers 1.63-fold, 2.08-fold and 2.53-fold, respectively, but had no effect in the 5 subjects who were poor metabolisers. Note that the metoprolol levels reached with dronedarone in the extensive metabolisers were still lower than those seen in poor metabolisers. Concurrent use resulted in an additive dose-dependent negative inotropic effect in all subjects. The negative inotropic effect of metoprolol was almost doubled by the addition of dronedarone 1.6 g daily, but at the therapeutic dose of 800 mg the effects were modest. The incidence of bradycardia of less than 45 bpm was 4% with metoprolol alone, and 17%, 33% and 45% with dronedarone 800 mg, 1.2 mg and 1.6 mg, respectively.[1]

The UK manufacturer briefly notes that when dronedarone 800 mg daily was given with a single dose of **propranolol** (dose not specified), the exposure to **propranolol** was increased by 30%.[2]

The manufacturer notes that, in clinical studies, bradycardia was seen more frequently when dronedarone was used with beta blockers than when it was used without beta blockers.[2,3]

Mechanism

A pharmacodynamic interaction occurs because both beta blockers and dronedarone slow the heart rate and their effects are additive. In addition, a pharmacokinetic interaction occurs, because dronedarone can inhibit the cytochrome P450 isoenzyme CYP2D6, by which metoprolol and propranolol are metabolised. The study with metoprolol shows that this inhibition of CYP2D6 makes extensive metabolisers more like poor metabolisers. For more information on metaboliser status, see 'Genetic factors in drug metabolism', p.8.

Importance and management

An additive effect resulting in a decreased heart rate would be expected when dronedarone is used with any beta blocker, and this appears to result in an increased incidence of bradycardia. A heart rate of less than 50 bpm is a contraindication to dronedarone use. In addition, a pharmacokinetic interaction between dronedarone and metoprolol is established, although the additional increase in negative inotropic effect seen as a consequence was considered modest at the recommended therapeutic dose of 800 mg. Other beta blockers that are metabolised by CYP2D6 (see 'Table 22.1', p.999) would be expected to interact similarly, and this was demonstrated with propranolol. The manufacturers advise that initially only low doses of beta blockers should be given with dronedarone, and that good tolerability, demonstrated by ECG, should be obtained before the dose of the beta blocker is increased.[2,3] In addition, they advise that, in patients already taking a beta blocker when starting dronedarone, an ECG should be performed and the dose adjusted if needed.[2]

For **sotalol**, an additive effect on QT prolongation is possible; with an increased risk of torsade de pointes, see also 'Drugs that prolong the QT interval + Other drugs that prolong the QT interval', p.272, for more information.

1. Damy T, Pousset F, Caplain H, Hulot J-S, Lechat P. Pharmacokinetic and pharmacodynamic interactions between metoprolol and dronedarone in extensive and poor CYP2D6 metabolizers healthy subjects. *Fundam Clin Pharmacol* (2004) 18, 113–23.
2. Multaq (Dronedarone hydrochloride). Sanofi. UK Summary of product characteristics, November 2013.
3. Multaq (Dronedarone). Sanofi-Aventis U.S. LLC. US Prescribing information, March 2014.

Beta blockers + Fingolimod

The concurrent use of atenolol and fingolimod results in a greater reduction in heart rate than that seen with either drug alone, without affecting the pharmacokinetics of either drug. Other beta blockers are also likely to affect heart rate when given with fingolimod.

Clinical evidence, mechanism, importance and management

In a randomised, placebo-controlled study, 13 healthy subjects were given **atenolol** 50 mg daily for 5 days, with a single 5-mg dose of fingolimod on day 5. Concurrent use did not alter the pharmacokinetics of either drug; however, the combination reduced heart rate by 15% more than fingolimod alone, and the heart rate nadir with fingolimod and **atenolol** (42 bpm) was lower than that seen with **atenolol** alone (55 bpm).[1] Note that the dose of fingolimod used in this study was much higher than the dose usually recommended in clinical practice. In a study in 2 282 multiple sclerosis patients given fingolimod 0.5 mg daily for 4 months, 120 patients were also taking unspecified beta blockers or calcium-channel blockers. Bradycardia in the first 2 days after starting fingolimod occurred in 15 patients and was more frequent in those taking beta blockers or calcium-channel blockers (4 patients) than in those not taking these drugs (11 patients); all patients recovered without pharmacological intervention. None of the 120 patients taking beta blockers or calcium-channel blockers developed atrioventricular block. During the 4-month follow up, 6 serious cardiac adverse events were recorded (including angina, atrioventricular block, and bradycardia) but none of these occurred in patients taking beta blockers or calcium-channel blockers.[2] Similarly, a retrospective study of 317 multiple sclerosis patients included 12 patients taking beta-blockers (unspecified), all of whom had uneventful first-dose observations when fingolimod was started.[3]

Fingolimod is known to be associated with bradycardia on initiation (including when it is re-started if treatment is suspended for 2 weeks or more), and it is generally recommended that patients should be monitored for 6 hours after their first dose.[4,5] This effect is increased in patients taking **atenolol**, although any reduction in heart rate seems likely to be detected by the routine monitoring advised for fingolimod alone, with any resulting bradycardia managed according to symptoms. However, because of the risk of severe bradycardia or atrioventricular block, the UK and US manufacturers of fingolimod advise against the concurrent use of beta blockers. If concurrent use is unavoidable, extended monitoring, including continuous overnight ECG monitoring, is recommended after the first dose of fingolimod.[4,5] Note that the maximum bradycardic effect of fingolimod alone is usually within 4 to 5 hours after the first dose, and has usually resolved within one month of starting treatment.[4,5]

For the potential interaction of **sotalol**, a beta blocker with class III antiarrhythmic activity, see 'Fingolimod + Drugs that prolong the QT interval', p.1571.

1. Kovarik JM, Lu M, Riviere G-J, Barbet I, Maton S, Goldwater DR, Schmouder RL. The effect on heart rate of combining single-dose fingolimod with steady-state atenolol or diltiazem in healthy subjects. *Eur J Clin Pharmacol* (2008) 64, 457–63.
2. Gold R, Comi G, Palace J, Siever A, Gottschalk R, Bijarnia M, von Rosenstiel P, Tomic D, Kappos L; FIRST Study Investigators. Assessment of cardiac safety during fingolimod treatment initiation in a real-world relapsing multiple sclerosis population: a phase 3b, open-label study. *J Neurol* (2014) 261, 267–76.
3. Ontaneda D1, Hara-Cleaver C, Rudick RA, Cohen JA, Bermel RA. Early tolerability and safety of fingolimod in clinical practice. J Neurol Sci. (2012) 323, 167-72.
4. Gilenya (Fingolimod hydrochloride). Novartis Pharmaceuticals UK Ltd. UK Summary of product characteristics, February 2015.
5. Gilenya (Fingolimod hydrochloride). Novartis. US Prescribing information, May 2015.

Beta blockers + Fish oils

The hypotensive effect of propranolol might be enhanced by fish oils.

Clinical evidence

In a study, 36 patients with mild hypertension were given either **propranolol** 80 mg daily or fish oils 9 g daily (as capsules and equivalent to **eicosapentaenoic acid** 1.8 g and **docosahexaenoic acid** 1.1 g daily) for 36 weeks, followed by placebo for 4 weeks. A further group of 16 patients were given **propranolol** 80 mg daily for 12 weeks, **propranolol** plus fish oils 9 g daily for 12 weeks, **propranolol** plus fish oils placebo for 12 weeks, and finally **propranolol** placebo for 4 weeks. Fish oils alone decreased blood pressure to a similar extent to **propranolol**, and decreases in blood pressure with the combination were greater than with either **propranolol** or fish oil alone.[1]

A further similar study in 14 patients taking a beta blocker found that when they were also given 4 capsules of *Omacor* (equivalent to **eicosapentaenoic acid** 1.9 g and **docosahexaenoic acid** 1.5 g) daily for 6 weeks their blood pressure decreased by a further 3.3/1.9 mmHg.[2]

Mechanism

Uncertain, but as fish oils seem to have a hypotensive effect of their own, the hypotensive effect of any beta blocker might be enhanced.

Importance and management

Evidence of an additive effect between fish oils and beta blockers is limited to the studies cited. Nevertheless, the effects are modest and so an adverse hypotensive response seems unlikely, but bear this in mind if blood pressure becomes too low.

1. Singer P, Melzer S, Goschel M, Augustin S. Fish oil amplifies the effect of propranolol in mild essential hypertension. *Hypertension* (1990) 16, 682–91.
2. Lungershausen YK, Abbey M, Nestel PJ, Howe PRC. Reduction of blood pressure and plasma triglycerides by omega-3 fatty acids in treated hypertensives. *J Hypertens* (1994) 12, 1041–5.

Beta blockers + Flecainide

The concurrent use of flecainide and beta blockers may have additive cardiac depressant effects. An isolated case of bradycardia and fatal AV block developed during the use of flecainide with sotalol, and bradycardia developed when a patient taking flecainide was given timolol eye drops.

Clinical evidence, mechanism, importance and management

A study on cardiac function and drug clearance in 10 healthy subjects found that when **propranolol** 80 mg three times daily was given with flecainide 200 mg twice daily for 4 days the AUCs of both drugs were increased by 20 to 30%, and they had some additive negative inotropic effects.[1] A report describes a patient taking flecainide 100 mg twice daily who developed bradycardia and fatal atrioventricular conduction block 3 hours after taking a second dose of **sotalol** 40 mg.[2] Another report describes a patient with chronic atrial fibrillation that had been stable for 5 years during treatment with flecainide and verapamil. Within 3 days of starting **timolol** 0.1% eye drops twice daily, she developed bradycardia with a heart rate of 35 to 40 bpm. The eye drops were stopped and 16 hours after the last dose, her heart rate had increased to 90 to 100 bpm.[3] Careful monitoring has therefore been recommended if beta blockers are given with flecainide. Note that serious cardiac depression has been seen following the use of flecainide with other drugs that have negative inotropic effects such as verapamil, see 'Flecainide + Verapamil', p.278.

1. Holtzman JL, Kvam DC, Berry DA, Mottonen L, Borrell G, Harrison LI, Conard GJ. The pharmacodynamic and pharmacokinetic interaction of flecainide acetate with propranolol: effects on cardiac function and drug clearance. *Eur J Clin Pharmacol* (1987) 33, 97–9.
2. Warren R, Vohra J, Hunt D, Hamer A. Serious interactions of sotalol with amiodarone and flecainide. *Med J Aust* (1990) 152, 277.
3. Minish T, Herd A. Symptomatic bradycardia secondary to interaction between timolol maleate, verapamil, and flecainide: a case report. *J Emerg Med* (2002) 22, 247–9.

Beta blockers + Food

Food can modestly increase, decrease or not affect the bioavailability of beta blockers.

Clinical evidence

Several studies suggest that food increases the AUC of **propranolol** by 50 to 80%,[1-3] and increases the AUC of both **metoprolol**[1] and **labetalol**[4] by about 40%. In contrast, in other studies, food did not affect the extent of absorption of a sustained-release formulation of **propranolol**,[2] and had very little effect on the absorption of **oxprenolol**,[5,6] **pindolol**[7] and orally administered **timolol**.[8] In another study, food reduced the AUC of **atenolol** by about 20%,[9] and the manufacturer of **celiprolol** briefly notes that food reduces its bioavailability.[10]

Mechanism

Food probably increases the bioavailability of propranolol, metoprolol and labetalol by changing the extent of their first pass metabolism through the liver.[2-4] It has been suggested that changes in propranolol disposition with a high protein meal may be partly due to a transient increase in hepatic blood flow[11-13] and rate of gastrointestinal absorption, which are subject to high intraindividual variation.[13] However, one study found that changes in hepatic blood flow, similar to those occurring with food consumption, had little effect on propranolol bioavailability.[14] A later study suggested that atenolol (and possibly other hydrophilic beta blockers, see 'Table 22.1', p.999) become tightly associated with bile acid micelles, preventing their absorption.[15]

Importance and management

The modest changes in beta blocker bioavailability seen in these studies are unlikely to be clinically important. Beta blocker serum levels vary widely between patients (a 20-fold difference in propranolol AUC has been noted),[1] and individualising the dose is therefore more of an issue than food intake. However, note that the manufacturer of celiprolol advises that it should be taken first thing in the morning, half-an-hour before food.[10]

1. Melander A, Danielson K, Scherstén B, Wåhlin E. Enhancement of the bioavailability of propranolol and metoprolol by food. *Clin Pharmacol Ther* (1977) 22, 108–12.
2. Liedholm H, Melander A. Concomitant food intake can increase the bioavailability of propranolol by transient inhibition of its presystemic primary conjugation. *Clin Pharmacol Ther* (1986) 40, 29–36.
3. McLean AJ, Isbister C, Bobik A, Dudley F. Reduction of first-pass hepatic clearance of propranolol by food. *Clin Pharmacol Ther* (1981) 30, 31–4.
4. Daneshmend TK, Roberts CJC. The influence of food on the oral and intravenous pharmacokinetics of a high clearance drug: a study with labetalol. *Br J Clin Pharmacol* (1982) 14, 73–8.
5. Dawes CP, Kendall MJ, Welling PG. Bioavailability of conventional and slow-release oxprenolol in fasted and nonfasted individuals. *Br J Clin Pharmacol* (1979) 7, 299–302.
6. John VA, Smith SE. Influence of food intake on plasma oxprenolol concentrations following oral administration of conventional and Oros preparations. *Br J Clin Pharmacol* (1985) 19, 191S–195S.
7. Kiger JL, Lavene D, Guillaume MF, Guerret M, Longchampt J. The effect of food and clopamide on the absorption of pindolol in man. *Int J Clin Pharmacol Biopharm* (1976) 13, 228–32.
8. Mäntylä R, Männistö P, Nykänen S, Koponen A, Lamminsivu U. Pharmacokinetic interactions of timolol with vasodilating drugs, food and phenobarbitone in healthy human volunteers. *Eur J Clin Pharmacol* (1983) 24, 227–30.
9. Melander A, Stenberg P, Liedholm H, Scherstén B, Wåhlin-Boll E. Food-induced reduction in bioavailability of atenolol. *Eur J Clin Pharmacol* (1979) 16, 327–30.
10. Celectol (Celiprolol hydrochloride). Winthrop Pharmaceuticals UK Ltd. UK Summary of product characteristics, March 2009.
11. Svensson CK, Edwards DJ, Mauriello PM, Barde SH, Foster AC, Lanc RA, Middleton E, Lalka D. Effect of food on hepatic blood flow: implications in the "food effect" phenomenon. *Clin Pharmacol Ther* (1983) 34, 316–23.
12. Olanoff LS, Walle T, Cowart TD, Walle UK, Oexmann MJ, Conradi EC. Food effects on propranolol systemic and oral clearance: support for a blood flow hypothesis. *Clin Pharmacol Ther* (1986) 40, 408–14.
13. Liedholm H, Wåhlin-Boll E, Melander A. Mechanisms and variations in the food effect on propranolol bioavailability. *Eur J Clin Pharmacol* (1990) 38, 469–75.
14. Modi MW, Hassett JM, Lalka D. Influence of posture on hepatic perfusion and the presystemic biotransformation of propranolol: simulation of the food effect. *Clin Pharmacol Ther* (1988) 44, 268–74.
15. Barnwell SG, Laudanski T, Dwyer M, Story MJ, Guard P, Cole S, Attwood D. Reduced bioavailability of atenolol in man: the role of bile acids. *Int J Pharmaceutics* (1993) 89, 245–50.

Beta blockers + Grapefruit and other fruit juices

The bioavailability of celiprolol is markedly reduced by both grapefruit juice and orange juice, the bioavailability of atenolol is moderately reduced by orange juice, and the bioavailability of talinolol is moderately reduced by grapefruit juice. Grapefruit juice does not affect the pharmacokinetics or pharmacodynamics of acebutolol to a clinically relevant extent.

Clinical evidence, mechanism, importance and management

(a) Acebutolol

In a randomised, crossover study, 10 healthy subjects were given 200-mL of normal-strength grapefruit juice three times a day for 4 days (total of 11 drinks), with a single 400-mg dose of acebutolol on the morning of day 3. Grapefruit juice decreased the maximum plasma levels and AUC of acebutolol by a modest 19% and 6%, respectively. No significant changes in heart rate or blood pressure were seen.[1] This suggests that no special precautions are required if a patient taking acebutolol wishes to drink grapefruit juice.

(b) Atenolol

In a randomised, crossover study, 10 healthy subjects were given 200 mL of **orange juice** (from concentrate) three times daily with a single 50-mg dose of atenolol on the third day. **Orange juice** reduced the AUC and maximum plasma levels of atenolol by 40% and 49%, respectively, and also attenuated the atenolol-induced reduction in heart rate. However, the effect of atenolol on blood pressure was unchanged.[2] This suggests that orange juice could make atenolol less effective when it is used for rate control, but the clinical significance of this effect is unclear.

(c) Celiprolol

In a randomised, crossover study, 12 healthy subjects were given grapefruit juice 200 mL three times daily for 2 days. On the third day celiprolol 100 mg was given with the second of four 200 mL volumes of grapefruit juice, and on day 4 two further 200 mL volumes of grapefruit juice were given. The AUC and peak plasma levels of celiprolol were reduced by about 87% and 95%, respectively, and its half-life was slightly prolonged. However, grapefruit juice did not affect the changes in blood pressure or heart rate caused by celiprolol.[3] In a similar study in 10 healthy subjects, 200 mL of normal-strength **orange juice** was given two to four times daily for 4 days, with a single 100-mg dose of celiprolol on day 3. **Orange juice** reduced the AUC and peak plasma levels of celiprolol by 83% and 89%, respectively. The half-life of celiprolol was prolonged from 4.6 to 10.8 hours and its renal excretion was reduced by 77%. However, the effects of celiprolol on blood pressure or heart rate were not altered by the **orange juice**.[4]

The mechanism of this effect is not known, but suggestions include an effect on intraduodenal pH and the lipid solubility of celiprolol, or the formation of a complex between celiprolol and an ingredient of grapefruit or **orange juice** that interfered with celiprolol absorption. Alternatively, inhibition of uptake transporter proteins in the intestine may have reduced absorption.[3,4] A study in *animals* has suggested that the presence of the flavonoid hesperidin in **orange juice** may contribute to this interaction.[5]

Although the clinical relevance of these effects has not been fully assessed, the studies suggest that the effects of celiprolol on blood pressure and heart rate are not affected. Nevertheless the marked reduction in celiprolol bioavailability in the presence of grapefruit or **orange juice** suggests this interaction may be of clinical significance in some patients.[3,4]

(d) Talinolol

Grapefruit juice 300 mL decreased the AUC of a single 50-mg dose of talinolol by 44%, decreased its maximum serum level by 42%, and increased its oral clearance by 62%. Similar results were seen after repeated administration of grapefruit juice over 6 days. However, the haemodynamic effects of talinolol were not altered.[6] Because P-glycoprotein levels did not appear to be affected by grapefruit juice, it was suggested that constituents in the juice might inhibit an uptake process other than P-glycoprotein. The decreases in talinolol levels are probably unlikely to be clinically relevant.

1. Lilja JJ, Raaska K, Neuvonen PJ. Effects of grapefruit juice on the pharmacokinetics of acebutolol. *Br J Clin Pharmacol* (2005) 60, 659–63.
2. Lilja JJ, Raaska K, Neuvonen PJ. Effects of orange juice on the pharmacokinetics of atenolol. *Eur J Clin Pharmacol* (2005) 61, 337–40.
3. Lilja JJ, Backman JT, Laitila J, Luurila H, Neuvonen PJ. Itraconazole increases but grapefruit juice greatly decreases plasma concentrations of celiprolol. *Clin Pharmacol Ther* (2003) 73, 192–8.
4. Lilja JJ, Juntti-Patinen L, Neuvonen PJ. Orange juice substantially reduces the bioavailability of the β-adrenergic-blocking agent celiprolol. *Clin Pharmacol Ther* (2004) 75, 184–90.
5. Uesawa Y, Mohri K. Hesperidin in orange juice reduces the absorption of celiprolol in rats. *Biopharm Drug Dispos* (2008) 29, 185–8.
6. Schwarz UI, Seemann D, Oertel R, Miehlke S, Kuhlisch E, Fromm MF, Kim RB, Bailey DG, Kirch W. Grapefruit juice ingestion significantly reduces talinolol bioavailability. *Clin Pharmacol Ther* (2005) 77, 291–301.

Beta blockers + H_2-receptor antagonists; Cimetidine

No clinically significant interaction appears to occur between the beta blockers and cimetidine, although the blood levels of some extensively metabolised beta blockers (e.g. metoprolol, propranolol) can be doubled by cimetidine. Isolated case reports describe bradycardia with atenolol, an irregular heart beat with metoprolol, and hypotension with labetalol, in patients also taking cimetidine.

Clinical evidence

(a) Atenolol

A report briefly mentions a patient taking a beta blocker for angina who developed profound sinus bradycardia (36 bpm) and hypotension when cimetidine was also given.[1] The beta blocker was not specified, but it was identified as atenolol elsewhere.[2] Three well controlled studies in healthy subjects and patients found that cimetidine did not significantly alter the blood levels of atenolol, nor did it alter the effect of atenolol on heart rate.[3-8] Atenolol did not affect cimetidine pharmacokinetics.[5]

(b) Betaxolol

The plasma levels and pharmacokinetics of betaxolol were unaffected by cimetidine in one study.[9]

(c) Bisoprolol

A study in 6 healthy subjects found that the maximum plasma level, AUC and clearance of bisoprolol were not significantly affected by cimetidine,[10,11] although an analysis of the results by other authors suggested that cimetidine may cause a significant reduction in the renal clearance of bisoprolol.[12]

(d) Carvedilol

The plasma levels and pharmacokinetics of carvedilol were unaffected by cimetidine in one study.[13]

(e) Labetalol

The AUC and bioavailability of a single 200-mg oral dose of labetalol was increased by 66% and 56%, respectively, in 6 healthy subjects who took cimetidine 400 mg four times daily for 4 days.[14] One subject developed orthostatic hypotension (70/40 mmHg), felt light-headed and almost fainted on standing.[14] Conversely, the AUC of intravenous labetalol was unaffected by cimetidine.[14]

(f) Metoprolol

A study in 6 healthy subjects given metoprolol 100 mg twice daily for a week found that cimetidine 1 g daily in divided doses increased the peak plasma levels and AUC of metoprolol by 70% and 61%, respectively, but this did not increase the effect of metoprolol on the heart rate during exercise.[3-5] Metoprolol did not affect cimetidine pharmacokinetics.[5] Three other studies confirmed that cimetidine increases metoprolol plasma levels after single or multiple doses, but none of the studies found that this interaction resulted in an increase in the effect of metoprolol on heart rate during exercise.[15-18] In contrast, two other studies found that cimetidine did not affect the plasma levels of a single 100-mg dose of metoprolol.[6,7]

An isolated case describes one patient who complained of a "very irregular heart beat" while taking both drugs, which was much less marked when he took the two drugs separated by as much time as possible.[19]

(g) Nadolol

A review cites a study in which the plasma levels and pharmacokinetics of nadolol were not affected by cimetidine, and the effects of the beta blocker on heart rate and blood pressure were unchanged.[20]

(h) Nebivolol

In one study, cimetidine 400 mg twice daily increased the AUC and peak plasma levels of a single 5-mg dose of nebivolol by 48% and 23%, respectively, but did not alter the effect of nebivolol on blood pressure or heart rate.[21]

(i) Penbutolol

The plasma levels and pharmacokinetics of penbutolol[8,22] were not affected by cimetidine, and the effects of the beta blocker on heart rate and blood pressure were unchanged.[22]

(j) Pindolol

Cimetidine 1 g daily in divided doses increased the AUC and peak plasma levels of pindolol 10 mg twice daily by 30% and 33%, respectively, although these changes were not statistically significant.[8] In another study, cimetidine 400 mg twice daily increased the AUC of pindolol by about 40% and decreased its renal clearance by about 35%.[23]

(k) Propranolol

In a study, 12 healthy subjects were given cimetidine 300 mg four times daily for a week with propranolol 80 mg every 12 hours from day 3 onwards. The mean steady-state blood levels and the AUC of propranolol were raised by 47%, and its half-life was prolonged by 17%, but cimetidine did not alter the effect of propranolol on heart rate.[24] A number of other single-dose and steady-state studies confirm that cimetidine causes rises of 35 to 136% in the plasma levels, AUC and clearance of propranolol,[3-5,9,20,25-31] but this does not appear to increase the effect of the beta blocker on blood pressure,[20,26,28] or on heart rate, either at rest or during exercise.[3,20,26-28]

In contrast, one study found a further reduction in heart rate when cimetidine was given with propranolol.[32] In another study, the increase in the steady-state AUC of propranolol tended to be higher when cimetidine was given simultaneously with propranolol than when they were given separated by 10 hours (41% versus 26%), but the difference was not significant.[33] A letter describes one patient who had a three- to fourfold increase in the serum levels and AUC of a single 80-mg dose of propranolol after taking cimetidine 1 g daily for 6 weeks.[1]

In one study propranolol did not affect cimetidine pharmacokinetics.[5]

(l) Timolol

A double-blind study in 12 healthy subjects found that cimetidine 400 mg twice daily for 3 days did not modify the effect of a single drop of timolol 0.5%, put into each eye, on heart rate or intraocular pressure, to either a statistically or clinically relevant extent.[34]

Mechanism

The plasma levels of the beta blockers that are extensively metabolised in the liver by the cytochrome P450 isoenzyme CYP2D6 (e.g. metoprolol, nebivolol and propranolol) are increased because cimetidine reduces their metabolism by inhibiting the activity of the liver enzymes. However, this does not seem to be a complete explanation as cimetidine does not affect carvedilol, which is metabolised by CYP2D6, but does affect labetalol, which is not metabolised by CYP2D6.[14] Pindolol is partly excreted by an active renal tubular secretion mechanism, and cimetidine increases pindolol levels by inhibiting this mechanism.[23] Cimetidine may reduce the renal clearance of bisoprolol by a similar mechanism.[11] Therefore a renal mechanism may play a part. However, those beta blockers that are largely excreted unchanged in the urine (e.g. atenolol, nadolol) are not affected by cimetidine.[7,20]

Importance and management

These are well studied and established interactions, but despite the considerable rises in plasma levels that can occur when some beta blockers are given with cimetidine, the effects are not normally clinically important: cases describing clinically relevant effects (hypotension, bradycardia) appear rare. Normally the beta blockers are considered to have a wide therapeutic range, and so raises in levels are generally well tolerated. Patients with heart failure are usually more at risk, because drugs such as metoprolol need slow and careful dose titration in this condition, but even in this patient group the rise in levels seems unlikely to be generally important. However, it has been suggested that any patient with impaired liver function who is given cimetidine with a beta blocker that is extensively metabolised in the liver (see 'Table 22.1', p.999) might possibly develop grossly elevated plasma levels, which could cause adverse effects. It would seem prudent to either monitor this type of patient (for effects such as hypotension, bradycardia, shortness of breath) or to use a non-interacting H_2-receptor antagonist, such as ranitidine (see 'Beta blockers + H_2-receptor antagonists; Ranitidine', p.1013).

1. Donovan MA, Heagerty AM, Patel L, Castleden M, Pohl JEF. Cimetidine and bioavailability of propranolol. *Lancet* (1981) i, 164.
2. Rowley-Jones D, Flind AC. Drug interactions with cimetidine. *Pharm J* (1981) 283, 659.
3. Kirch W, Spahn H, Köhler H, Mutschler E. Accumulation and adverse effects of metoprolol and propranolol after concurrent administration of cimetidine. *Arch Toxicol* (1983) (Suppl 6), 379–83.
4. Kirch W, Spahn H, Köhler H, Mutschler E. Interaction of metoprolol, propranolol and atenolol with cimetidine. *Clin Sci* (1982) 63 (Suppl 8), 451S–453S.
5. Kirch W, Spahn H, Köhler H, Mutschler E. Influence of β-receptor antagonists on the pharmacokinetics of cimetidine. *Drugs* (1983) 25 (Suppl 2), 127–30.
6. Houtzagers JJR, Streurman O, Regårdh CG. The effect of pretreatment with cimetidine on the bioavailability and disposition of atenolol and metoprolol. *Br J Clin Pharmacol* (1982) 14, 67–72.
7. Ellis ME, Hussain M, Webb AK, Barker NP, Fitzsimons TJ. The effect of cimetidine on the relative cardioselectivity of atenolol and metoprolol in asthmatic patients. *Br J Clin Pharmacol* (1984) 17, 59S–64S.
8. Mutschler E, Spahn H, Kirch W. The interaction between H2-receptor antagonists and β-adrenoceptor blockers. *Br J Clin Pharmacol* (1984) 17, 51S–57S.
9. Rey E, Jammet P, d'Athis P, de Lauture D, Christoforov B, Weber S, Olive G. Effect of cimetidine on the pharmacokinetics of the new beta-blocker betaxolol. *Arzneimittelforschung* (1987) 37, 953–6.
10. Kirch W, Rose I, Klingmann I, Pabst J, Ohnhaus EE. Interaction of bisoprolol with cimetidine and rifampicin. *Eur J Clin Pharmacol* (1986) 31, 59–62.
11. Kirch W, Ohnhaus EE, Pabst J. Reply. *Eur J Clin Pharmacol* (1987) 33, 110.
12. Somogyi A, Muirhead M. Interaction of cimetidine with bisoprolol. *Eur J Clin Pharmacol* (1987) 33, 109–110.
13. Ruffolo RR, Boyle DA, Venuti RP, Lukas MA. Carvedilol (Kredex®): a novel multiple action cardiovascular agent. *Drugs Today* (1991) 27, 465–92.
14. Daneshmend TK, Roberts CJC. The effects of enzyme induction and enzyme inhibition on labetalol pharmacokinetics. *Br J Clin Pharmacol* (1984) 18, 393–400.
15. Kendall MJ, Laugher SJ, Wilkins MR. Ranitidine, cimetidine and metoprolol: a pharmacokinetic interaction study. *Gastroenterology* (1986) 90, 1490.
16. Kirch W, Rämsch K, Janisch HD, Ohnhaus EE. The influence of two histamine H_2-receptor antagonists, cimetidine and ranitidine, on plasma levels and clinical effect of nifedipine and metoprolol. *Arch Toxicol* (1984) (Suppl 7), 256–9.
17. Chellingsworth MC, Laugher S, Akhlaghi S, Jack DB, Kendall MJ. The effects of ranitidine and cimetidine on the pharmacokinetics and pharmacodynamics of metoprolol. *Aliment Pharmacol Ther* (1988) 2, 521–7.
18. Toon S, Davidson EM, Garstang FM, Batra H, Bowes RJ, Rowland M. The racemic metoprolol H_2-antagonist interaction. *Clin Pharmacol Ther* (1988) 43, 283–9.
19. Anon. Adverse Drug Reactions Advisory Committee. Seven case studies. *Med J Aust* (1982) 2, 190–1.
20. Duchin KL, Stern MA, Willard DA, McKinstry DN. Comparison of kinetic interactions of nadolol and propranolol with cimetidine. *Am Heart J* (1984) 108, 1084–6.
21. Kamali F, Howes A, Thomas SHL, Ford GA, Snoeck E. A pharmacokinetic and pharmacodynamic interaction study between nebivolol and the H_2-receptor antagonists cimetidine and ranitidine. *Br J Clin Pharmacol* (1997) 43, 201–4.
22. Spahn H, Kirch W, Hajdu P, Mutschler E, Ohnhaus EE. Penbutolol pharmacokinetics: the influence of concomitant administration of cimetidine. *Eur J Clin Pharmacol* (1986) 29, 555–60.
23. Somogyi AA, Bochner F, Sallustio BC. Stereoselective inhibition of pindolol renal clearance by cimetidine in humans. *Clin Pharmacol Ther* (1992) 51, 379–87.
24. Donn KH, Powell JR, Rogers JF, Eshelman FN. The influence of H2-receptor antagonists on steady-state concentrations of propranolol and 4-hydroxypropranolol. *J Clin Pharmacol* (1984) 24, 500–8.
25. Kirch W, Köhler H, Spahn H, Mutschler E. Interaction of cimetidine with metoprolol, propranolol or atenolol. *Lancet* (1981) 2, 531–2.
26. Reimann IW, Klotz U, Frölich JC. Effects of cimetidine and ranitidine on steady-state propranolol kinetics and dynamics. *Clin Pharmacol Ther* (1982) 32, 749–57.
27. Reimann IW, Klotz U, Siems B, Frölich JC. Cimetidine increases steady-state plasma levels of propranolol. *Br J Clin Pharmacol* (1981) 12, 785–90.
28. Markiewicz A, Hartleb M, Lelek A, Boldys H, Nowak A. The effect of treatment with cimetidine and ranitidine on bioavailability of, and circulatory response to, propranolol. *Zbl Pharm* (1984) 123, 516–18.
29. Heagerty AM, Donovan MA, Castleden CM, Pohl JF, Patel L, Hedges A. Influence of cimetidine on pharmacokinetics of propranolol. *BMJ* (1981) 282, 1917–19.
30. Heagerty AM, Donovan MA, Casteleden CM, Pohl JEF, Patel L. The influence of histamine (H_2) antagonists on propranolol pharmacokinetics. *Int J Clin Pharmacol Res* (1982) 2, 203–5.
31. Reilly CS, Biollaz J, Koshakji RP, Wood AJJ. Enprostil, in contrast to cimetidine, does not inhibit propranolol metabolism. *Clin Pharmacol Ther* (1986) 40, 37–41.
32. Feely J, Wilkinson GR, Wood AJJ. Reduction in liver blood flow and propranolol metabolism by cimetidine. *N Engl J Med* (1981) 304, 692–5.
33. Asgharnejad M, Powell JR, Donn KH, Danis M. The effect of cimetidine dose timing on oral propranolol kinetics in adults. *J Clin Pharmacol* (1988) 28, 339–43.
34. Ishii Y, Nakamura K, Tsutsumi K, Kotegawa, Nakano S, Natasuka K. Drug interaction between cimetidine and timolol ophthalmic solution: effect on heart rate and intraocular pressure in healthy Japanese volunteers. *J Clin Pharmacol* (2000) 40, 193–9.

Beta blockers + H_2-receptor antagonists; Famotidine

Famotidine does not appear to alter the effects of the beta blockers on heart rate and blood pressure.

Clinical evidence, mechanism, importance and management

A survey of 15 patients taking beta blockers (**acebutolol, atenolol, betaxolol, nadolol, pindolol, propranolol** or **sotalol**) for 6 to 8 weeks found no evidence of changes in antihypertensive effects or bradycardia while they were taking famotidine 40 mg daily.[1] No interaction would be expected, and no special precautions would seem necessary if famotidine is taken with these or any other beta blocker.

1. Chichmanian RM, Mignot G, Spreux A, Jean-Girard C, Hofliger P. Tolérance de la famotidine. Étude due réseau médecins sentinelles en pharmacovigilance. *Therapie* (1992) 47, 239–43.

Beta blockers + H_2-receptor antagonists; Nizatidine

An isolated study suggests that the reduction in heart rate caused by atenolol is increased by nizatidine.

Clinical evidence, mechanism, importance and management

After taking **atenolol** 100 mg daily for 7 days the mean resting heart rate of 12 healthy subjects fell from about 64 bpm to 53 bpm three hours after dosing. A further fall of 6 bpm occurred when they were also given nizatidine 300 mg daily for 7 days. Nizatidine alone caused a fall in heart rate of about 8 bpm.[1] However, up to the end of 2007, the manufacturers have had only 4 reports of bradycardia with nizatidine, by which time it had been used in more than 100 million patients,[2] and the drug analysis print of the MHRA in the UK, which lists reported adverse effects of drugs, includes only one case of sinus bradycardia associated with nizatidine.[3] Further, the manufacturers note there are no interaction reports of nizatidine with other drugs that have a bradycardic potential.[2] Therefore, a clinically significant interaction between beta blockers and nizatidine seems unlikely.

1. Halabi A, Kirch W. Negative chronotropic effects of nizatidine. *Gut* (1991) 32, 630–4.
2. Flynn Pharma Ltd. Personal communication, February 2009.
3. Nizatidine, Drug analysis print. Available at: http://www.mhra.gov.uk/drug-analysis-prints/ (accessed 21/10/15).

Beta blockers + H_2-receptor antagonists; Ranitidine

Ranitidine does not alter either the steady-state plasma levels or the therapeutic effects of atenolol, nebivolol, propranolol or tertatolol. Some studies have shown moderate rises in metoprolol levels in patients also given ranitidine.

Clinical evidence

(a) Metoprolol

In a study in 12 healthy subjects the plasma levels of metoprolol 100 mg twice daily were unaffected by ranitidine 300 mg daily for 7 days.[1] Two other studies also suggest that ranitidine did not significantly affect the plasma levels of metoprolol,[2-5] although these studies did find increases of up to 38% in the AUC of single intravenous or oral doses of metoprolol.[2-5] Another study found that ranitidine increased the AUC and plasma levels of metoprolol 100 mg twice daily by 55% and 34%, respectively.[6-8] All of these studies found that ranitidine did not alter the effect of metoprolol on heart rate during exercise.[1,2,5,6]

(b) Propranolol

In a study in 5 healthy subjects, ranitidine 300 mg daily for 6 days did not affect either the steady-state plasma levels of propranolol 160 mg daily or its effects on heart rate and blood pressure.[9] Similarly no changes in plasma propranolol levels were seen in other multiple-dose[10] or single-dose studies.[11-14]

(c) Other beta blockers

Studies suggest that ranitidine 150 mg twice daily does not significantly alter the pharmacokinetic or pharmacodynamic effects of a single 5-mg dose of **nebivolol**,[15] a single 5-mg dose of **tertatolol**,[16] or **atenolol** 100 mg daily for 7 days.[6,8]

Mechanism

The rises in metoprolol serum levels caused by ranitidine in the two single-dose studies are not understood, nor is it clear why one of four studies found an increase after multiple doses.

Importance and management

The possible effects of ranitidine on the plasma levels and effects of **propranolol** and **metoprolol** have been well studied. Although some studies have shown moderate rises in metoprolol levels, particularly after single doses, the majority of the data from multiple-dose studies suggest that an interaction does not generally occur.

Less is known about **atenolol**, **nebivolol** and **tertatolol**, although no clinically relevant interactions have been seen. There is nothing to suggest that the concurrent use of ranitidine and any beta blocker should be avoided.

1. Toon S, Davidson EM, Garstang FM, Batra H, Bowers RJ, Rowland M. The racemic metoprolol H_2-antagonist interaction. *Clin Pharmacol Ther* (1988) 43, 283–9.
2. Kelly JG, Salem SAM, Kinney CD, Shanks RG, McDevitt DG. Effects of ranitidine on the disposition of metoprolol. *Br J Clin Pharmacol* (1985) 19, 219–24.
3. Kelly JG, Shanks RG, McDevitt DG. Influence of ranitidine on plasma metoprolol concentrations. *BMJ* (1983) 287, 1218–19.
4. Kendall MJ, Laugher SJ, Wilkins MR. Ranitidine, cimetidine and metoprolol-a pharmacokinetic interaction study. *Gastroenterology* (1986) 90, 1490.
5. Chellingsworth MC, Laugher S, Akhlaghi S, Jack DB, Kendall MJ. The effects of ranitidine and cimetidine on the pharmacokinetics and pharmacodynamics of metoprolol. *Aliment Pharmacol Ther* (1988) 2, 521–7.
6. Spahn H, Mutschler E, Kirch W, Ohnhaus EE, Janisch HD. Influence of ranitidine on plasma metoprolol and atenolol concentrations. *BMJ* (1983) 286, 1546–7.
7. Kirch W, Rämsch K, Janisch HD, Ohnhaus EE. The influence of two histamine H_2-receptor antagonists, cimetidine and ranitidine, on the plasma levels and clinical effect of nifedipine and metoprolol. *Arch Toxicol* (1984) 7 (Suppl), 256–9.
8. Mutschler E, Spahn H, Kirch W. The interaction between H_2-receptor antagonists and beta-adrenoceptor blockers. *Br J Clin Pharmacol* (1984) 17, 51S–57S.
9. Reimann IW, Klotz U, Frölich JC. Effects of cimetidine and ranitidine on steady-state propranolol kinetics and dynamics. *Clin Pharmacol Ther* (1982) 32, 749–57.
10. Donn KH, Powell JR, Rogers JF, Eshelman FN. The influence of H_2-receptor antagonists on steady-state concentrations of propranolol and 4-hydroxypropranolol. *J Clin Pharmacol* (1984) 24, 500–8.
11. Markiewicz A, Hartleb M, Lelek H, Boldys H, Nowak A. The effect of treatment with cimetidine and ranitidine on bioavailability of, and circulatory response to, propranolol. *Zbl Pharm* (1984) 123, 516–18.
12. Heagerty AM, Castleden CM, Patel L. Failure of ranitidine to interact with propranolol. *BMJ* (1982) 284, 1304.
13. Heagerty AM, Donovan MA, Castleden CM, Pohl JEF, Patel L. The influence of histamine (H_2) antagonists on propranolol pharmacokinetics. *Int J Clin Pharmacol Res* (1982) 2, 203–5.
14. Patel L, Weerasuriya K. Effect of cimetidine and ranitidine on propranolol clearance. *Br J Clin Pharmacol* (1983) 15, 152P.
15. Kamali F, Howes A, Thomas SHL, Ford GA, Snoeck E. A pharmacokinetic and pharmacodynamic interaction study between nebivolol and the H_2-receptor antagonists cimetidine and ranitidine. *Br J Clin Pharmacol* (1997) 43, 201–4.
16. Kirch W, Milferstädt S, Halabi A, Rocher I, Efthymiopoulos C, Jung L. Interaction of tertatolol with rifampicin and ranitidine pharmacokinetics and antihypertensive activity. *Cardiovasc Drugs Ther* (1990) 4, 487–92.

Beta blockers + Haloperidol

Carteolol may increase plasma haloperidol levels. An isolated case report describes severe hypotension and cardiopulmonary arrest in a woman shortly after she was given haloperidol and propranolol. Plasma levels of haloperidol in three patients were not significantly changed by propranolol. The concurrent use of sotalol and haloperidol is predicted to increase the risk of QT prolongation.

Clinical evidence, mechanism, importance and management

(a) Carteolol

In a single-dose study in 8 healthy subjects, oral carteolol 10 mg increased the peak plasma level and AUC of haloperidol by about 25% and 40%, respectively and decreased its clearance by 33%, possibly by altering hepatic blood flow. The pharmacokinetics of carteolol were unaffected by haloperidol. Two patients experienced sleepiness with concurrent use, but this was mild and resolved within 24 hours.[1] These increases in haloperidol levels are modest, and therefore no particular precautions seem necessary if carteolol is also given.

(b) Propranolol

A middle-aged woman with schizophrenia and hypertension experienced three episodes of severe hypotension within 30 to 120 minutes of being given propranolol 40 to 80 mg and haloperidol 10 mg.[2] On two of the occasions she had a cardiopulmonary arrest. She fainted each time, became cyanotic, had no palpable pulses and severe hypotension, but rapidly responded to cardiopulmonary resuscitation. She suffered no adverse consequences.[2] The reasons for the severe hypotension are not understood, although both drugs alone can cause hypotension.

A study found that the steady-state plasma levels of haloperidol 6 to 15 mg daily were not significantly changed in 3 patients by long-acting propranolol (given in incremental doses up to 480 mg daily).[3]

There seems to be only one case of an interaction between haloperidol and propranolol on record. Bearing in mind the widespread use of these drugs, this interaction would appear to be rare. There would therefore seem to be little reason for avoiding concurrent use.

(c) Sotalol

Both haloperidol and sotalol can prolong the QT interval and should therefore not generally be used together, see 'Drugs that prolong the QT interval + Other drugs that prolong the QT interval', p.272.

1. Isawa S, Murasaki M, Miura S, Yoshioka M, Uchiumi M, Kumagai Y, Aoki S, Hisazumi H, Kudo S. Pharmacokinetic and pharmacodynamic interactions among haloperidol, carteolol hydrochloride and biperiden hydrochloride. *Nihon Shinkei Seishin Yakurigaku Zasshi* (1999) 19, 111–18.
2. Alexander HE, McCarty K, Giffen MB. Hypotension and cardiopulmonary arrest associated with concurrent haloperidol and propranolol therapy. *JAMA* (1984) 252, 87–8.
3. Greendyke RM, Kanter DR. Plasma propranolol levels and their effect on plasma thioridazine and haloperidol concentrations. *J Clin Psychopharmacol* (1987) 7, 178–82.

Beta blockers + HIV-protease inhibitors

Ritonavir (including low-dose ritonavir used a pharmacokinetic enhancer) is predicted to increase plasma concentrations of metoprolol and propranolol, and other similarly metabolised beta blockers.

Clinical evidence, mechanism, importance and management

Some manufacturers specifically advise caution when **metoprolol**, **timolol** or **propranolol** are given with **ritonavir**, as concurrent use is predicted to result in raised beta blocker plasma concentrations.[1-5] This prediction would seem to include the use of low-dose **ritonavir** given as a pharmacokinetic enhancer.[3,4]

There do not appear to be any studies that have evaluated these predicted pharmacokinetic interactions. However, **ritonavir** is a known inhibitor of the cytochrome P450 isoenzyme CYP2D6 by which **metoprolol**, **propranolol** and some other beta blockers are metabolised, although at low-doses, when **ritonavir** is used as a pharmacokinetic enhancer, it has less effect (for example, see *Desipramine* under 'Tricyclic and related antidepressants + HIV-protease inhibitors', p.1509). Therefore it seems reasonable to assume that an interaction resulting in raised concentrations of these beta blockers may occur, although the extent of the rise is unclear. In addition, the situation with **propranolol** may be more complicated as ritonavir can induce glucuronidation and CYP1A2, by which **propranolol** is also partially metabolised; therefore, in theory, ritonavir could reduce **propranolol** concentrations by these mechanisms. The pharmacokinetic outcome of the concurrent use of **propranolol** and ritonavir is therefore unclear.

In general, interactions of beta blockers with CYP2D6 inhibitors that result in raised beta blocker concentrations are of limited clinical relevance, because the beta blockers have a wide therapeutic index, and large increases in concentrations are reasonably well tolerated in most patients. The exception may be in heart failure, where slow and careful dose titration is required, and therefore patients with this condition may be at more risk from any interaction. Until more is known, it may be prudent to monitor for symptoms such as shortness of breath, hypotension and bradycardia in patients given **metoprolol**, **timolol** or **propranolol** with **ritonavir** at any dose, reducing the dose of the beta blocker if necessary. However, note that one UK manufacturer of **tipranavir** actually contraindicates the concurrent use of **metoprolol** in heart failure.[6]

Other beta blockers that are metabolised by CYP2D6 may be similarly affected and similar precautions are warranted. See 'Table 22.1', p.999, for information on the metabolism of the commonly used systemic beta blockers.

1. Lopresor (Metoprolol tartrate). Novartis Pharmaceuticals UK Ltd. UK Summary of product characteristics, July 2008.
2. Inderal LA (Propranolol hydrochloride). Wyeth Pharmaceuticals Inc. US Prescribing information, November 2007.
3. Prezista (Darunavir ethanolate). Janssen-Cilag Ltd. UK Summary of product characteristics, June 2012.
4. Prezista (Darunavir ethanolate). Janssen Pharmaceuticals, Inc. US Prescribing information, May 2012.
5. Norvir Capsules (Ritonavir). Abbott Laboratories. US Prescribing information, March 2012.
6. Aptivus Soft Capsules (Tipranavir). Boehringer Ingelheim Ltd. UK Summary of product characteristics, December 2011.

Beta blockers + Hormonal contraceptives

The plasma levels of metoprolol were moderately higher in women taking combined hormonal contraceptives. Acebutolol, oxprenolol and propranolol pharmacokinetics are minimally affected by hormonal contraceptive use.

Clinical evidence

The peak plasma levels and the AUC of a single 100-mg dose of **metoprolol** were 36% and 70% higher, respectively, in 12 women taking oral, low-dose combined hormonal contraceptives, when compared with a similar group not taking contraceptives. The elimination half-life of **metoprolol** was unaffected.[1] In a further study by the same research group, the AUC of **metoprolol** was 71% higher, the AUC of **oxprenolol** was 26% higher, the AUC of **propranolol** was 42% higher, and the AUC of **acebutolol** was marginally lower in women taking combined hormonal contraceptives, when compared with those not taking contraceptives. However only the **metoprolol** difference was statistically significant.[2] In contrast, in another study in 8 women, the total clearance of a single 80-mg dose of **propranolol** was slightly increased by about 25% (although this was not statistically significant) by **ethinylestradiol** 50 micrograms daily: an even smaller increase was seen when they were taking a combined hormonal contraceptive containing **ethinylestradiol** and **norethisterone**.[3]

Mechanism

Uncertain. In the case of propranolol, its conjugation (by glucuronidation) and ring oxidation (by the cytochrome P450 isoenzyme CYP2D6) are increased by ethinylestradiol, whereas its side-chain oxidation (mainly by CYP1A2) is decreased, leading to little overall change in propranolol clearance.[3] However, if these findings are extrapolated to metoprolol, which is not metabolised by CYP1A2, then a lower AUC of metoprolol would have been anticipated in women taking combined hormonal contraceptives. Note that small, between-group comparisons undertaken in some of the studies cannot account for genetic differences in the women that might result in differences in beta blocker levels, so it is not possible to ascribe the differences to the contraceptive.

Importance and management

The differences in plasma levels of **propranolol**, **oxprenolol** and **acebutolol** are almost certainly too small to matter, but with **metoprolol** the apparent increase is somewhat larger. Even so, changes of this size caused by the interactions of other drugs with beta blockers are not usually clinically relevant. No special precautions are generally necessary if any of these beta blockers are given to women taking combined contraceptives containing ethinylestradiol, (or those taking ethinylestradiol alone for other indications).

If beta blockers are being used to treat hypertension, it is of note that combined hormonal contraceptives may cause increases in blood pressure (but consider also 'Antihypertensives + Hormonal contraceptives', p.1053). Stopping combined hormonal contraceptives has been suggested as an effective antihypertensive intervention in women with hypertension.[4] Also be aware that some of the indications for beta blockers, including hypertension and migraine, are cautions for, or preclude the use of, combined hormonal contraceptives.

1. Kendall MJ, Quarterman CP, Jack DB, Beeley L. Metoprolol pharmacokinetics and the oral contraceptive pill. *Br J Clin Pharmacol* (1982) 14, 120–2.
2. Kendall MJ, Jack DB, Quarterman CP, Smith SR, Zaman R. β-adrenoceptor blocker pharmacokinetics and the oral contraceptive pill. *Br J Clin Pharmacol* (1984) 17, 87S–89S.
3. Walle T, Fagan TC, Walle UK, Topmiller MJ. Stimulatory as well as inhibitory effects of ethinyloestradiol on the metabolic clearances of propranolol in young women. *Br J Clin Pharmacol* (1996) 41, 305–9.
4. Lubianca JN, Moreira LB, Gus M, Fuchs FD. Stopping oral contraceptives: an effective blood pressure-lowering intervention in women with hypertension. *J Hum Hypertens* (2005) 19, 451–5.

Beta blockers + Hydralazine

The plasma levels of propranolol and other extensively metabolised beta blockers (such as metoprolol and oxprenolol) are increased by hydralazine, but no increase in adverse effects appears to have been reported.

Clinical evidence

In a study in 5 healthy subjects, single 25- and 50-mg doses of hydralazine increased the AUC of a single 40-mg dose of **propranolol** by 60% and 110%, respectively, and raised the peak plasma levels by 144% and 240%, respectively,[1] Similarly, in another single-dose study, hydralazine increased the AUC of **propranolol** by 62 to 77%.[2] However, a further single-dose study using sustained-release **propranolol** found that hydralazine had no effect on **propranolol** pharmacokinetics.[3]

In another study, hydralazine increased the AUC of sustained-release **oxprenolol** by 41% at steady-state;[4] whereas **oxprenolol** was found not to have a significant effect on the pharmacokinetics of hydralazine.[4]

Further studies have found that hydralazine increases the AUC of **metoprolol** by 30% after a single dose,[5] and by 38% at steady-state.[6] Hydralazine did not affect the AUC of **acebutolol** or **nadolol** in single-dose studies.[5]

Mechanism

Uncertain. Hydralazine appears to increase the bioavailability of those beta blockers that undergo high hepatic extraction and not those that are largely excreted unchanged in the urine. Hepatic extraction is discussed in more detail under 'Changes in first-pass metabolism', p.4, and 'Table 22.1', p.999 lists the metabolic routes of the commonly used systemic beta blockers. It has been suggested that hydralazine may alter hepatic blood flow or inhibit hepatic enzymes,[1,5,6] although other mechanisms may also be involved.[3,7,8]

Importance and management

The pharmacokinetic interactions between hydralazine and the extensively metabolised beta blockers are moderately well documented and established, but the increased beta blocker plasma levels appear to cause no adverse clinical effect. Concurrent use is usually valuable in the treatment of hypertension (additive hypotensive effects would be expected), and it has been suggested that the concurrent use of beta blockers may provide additional benefit in patients taking hydralazine and isosorbide dinitrate for heart failure.[9]

1. Schneck DW, Vary JE. Mechanism by which hydralazine increases propranolol bioavailability. *Clin Pharmacol Ther* (1984) 35, 447–53.
2. McLean AJ, Skews H, Bobik A, Dudley FJ. Interaction between oral propranolol and hydralazine. *Clin Pharmacol Ther* (1980) 27, 726–32.
3. Byrne AJ, McNeil JJ, Harrison PM, Louis W, Tonkin AM, McLean AJ. Stable oral availability of sustained release propranolol when co-administered with hydralazine or food: evidence implicating substrate delivery rate as a determinant of presystematic drug interactions. *Br J Clin Pharmacol* (1984) 17, 45S–50S.
4. Hawksworth GM, Dart AM, Chiang K, Parry K, Petrie JC. Effect of oxprenolol on the pharmacokinetics and pharmacodynamics of hydralazine. *Drugs* (1983) 25 (Suppl 2), 136–40.
5. Jack DB, Kendall MJ, Dean S, Laugher SJ, Zaman R, Tenneson ME. The effect of hydralazine on the pharmacokinetics of three different beta adrenoceptor antagonists: metoprolol, nadolol, and acebutolol. *Biopharm Drug Dispos* (1982) 3, 47–54.
6. Lindeberg S, Holm B, Lundborg P, Regårdh CG, Sandström B. The effect of hydralazine on steady-state plasma concentrations of metoprolol in pregnant hypertensive women. *Eur J Clin Pharmacol* (1988) 35, 131–5.
7. Svensson CK, Cumella JC, Tronolone M, Middleton E, Lalka D. Effects of hydralazine, nitroglycerin, and food on estimated hepatic blood flow. *Clin Pharmacol Ther* (1985) 37, 464–8.
8. Svensson CK, Knowlton PW, Ware JA. Effect of hydralazine on the elimination of antipyrine in the rat. *Pharm Res* (1987) 4, 515–18.
9. Ghali JK, Tam SW, Ferdinand KC, Lindenfeld J, Sabolinski ML, Taylor AL, Worcel M, Curry CL, Cohn JN, the A-HeFT Investigators. Effects of ACE inhibitors or β-blockers in patients treated with the fixed-dose combination of isosorbide dinitrate/hydralazine in the African-American Heart Failure Trial. *Am J Cardiovasc Drugs* (2007) 7, 373–80.

Beta blockers + Inotropes and Vasopressors

Effects on blood pressure and heart rate: **the hypertensive effects of adrenaline (epinephrine) can be markedly increased in patients taking non-selective beta blockers such as propranolol. A severe and potentially life-threatening hypertensive reaction and/or marked bradycardia can develop. Cardioselective beta blockers such as atenolol and metoprolol interact minimally. Dobutamine would be expected to interact similarly, but some studies and case reports suggest that paradoxical effects may occur. The pressor effects of noradrenaline (norepinephrine) appear to be diminished by the beta blockers. An isolated report describes a fatal hypertensive reaction in a patient given propranolol and phenylephrine, but concurrent use normally seems to be uneventful.**

Anaphylaxis: **some evidence suggests that anaphylactic shock in patients taking beta blockers may be resistant to treatment with adrenaline (epinephrine).**

Clinical evidence

A. Effects on blood pressure and heart rate

(a) Adrenaline (Epinephrine) with non-selective beta blockers

1. Nadolol. In 24 healthy subjects given either **nadolol**, atenolol or placebo for one week followed by an infusion of adrenaline, mean arterial pressure and calf vascular resistance rose markedly in the **nadolol**-treated group and heart rate dropped (by 10 bpm at an adrenaline dose of 0.032 micrograms/kg per minute).[1] Similarly, in a study in 10 healthy subjects who were given intravenous adrenaline after taking **nadolol** or propranolol (increased up to 240 mg daily over 4 weeks), there was about an 18 mmHg increase in diastolic blood pressure and a 12 bpm decrease in heart rate at an adrenaline dose of 0.08 micrograms/kg per minute for 4 minutes.[2]

2. Pindolol. The haemodynamic response to intravenous adrenaline (0.1 micrograms/kg per minute for 30 minutes) in healthy subjects given intravenous pindolol 27 micrograms/kg (an 8 bpm drop in heart rate and an increase in blood pressure of 11/17 mmHg) was similar to that after propranolol.[3] However, when healthy subjects were pretreated with a single 5-mg oral dose of **pindolol**, there were only small reductions in blood pressure (4 mmHg) and heart rate (about 5 bpm) after the intra-oral injection of 3.6 mL of lidocaine 2% containing 1:80 000 adrenaline (45 micrograms of adrenaline).[4]

3. Propranolol. An early study in 10 healthy subjects found that intravenous adrenaline (epinephrine) 5 micrograms/minute increased heart rates and caused minimal changes in blood pressure. However, after pretreatment with intravenous **propranolol** 10 mg, the same dose of adrenaline caused a *fall* in heart rate of 12 bpm and an increase in arterial pressure of 20/10 mmHg.[5] One case series describes 6 patients taking **propranolol** 20 to 80 mg daily, undergoing plastic surgery, who experienced marked hypertensive reactions (blood pressures in the range of 190/110 to 260/150 mmHg) and bradycardia when their eyelids and/or faces were infiltrated with 8 to 40 mL of local anaesthetic solutions of lidocaine containing 1:100 000 or 1:200 000 (10 or 5 micrograms/mL) of adrenaline. Cardiac arrest occurred in one patient.[6]

Similar marked increases in blood pressure, associated with marked bradycardia, have been described with **propranolol** in other studies involving the use of intravenous adrenaline.[2,3,7-10] and in a few case reports involving the use of 0.3 mL of subcutaneous adrenaline 1:1 000 for allergic reactions[11-13] or during plastic surgery (dose not stated).[14] However, there is some evidence that the interaction is related to adrenaline dose. One dose-response study in 5 patients with hypertension found that the effect was not clinically meaningful when adrenaline was infused at a dose of 0.5 micrograms/minute for 8 minutes (diastolic blood pressure increased by 5 mmHg and heart rate decreased by 3 bpm).[15] No interaction was seen in a further study in 10 patients taking **propranolol** 40 to 160 mg daily who received 1.5 to 6 mL of a local anaesthetic containing equal parts of anaesthetic with adrenaline 1:100 000 or adrenaline 1:200 000 during skin surgery.[16]

Test doses of adrenaline have been used to check epidural catheter placement (the result being a transient rise in heart rate if the catheter is misplaced intravascularly), but two studies have shown that **propranolol** blocks this response,[17,18] and in one case with **timolol** eye drops, this resulted in the test being unreliable.[19]

(b) Adrenaline (Epinephrine) with selective beta blockers

A study in which intravenous adrenaline (epinephrine) 8 micrograms/minute for 6 minutes was given to patients taking **metoprolol**, found only a small rise in blood pressure compared with a marked rise when propranolol (5 mmHg versus 21 mmHg) was given.[8] This was confirmed in other studies in which patients given identical infusions of adrenaline developed a hypertensive/bradycardic reaction while taking propranolol but not while taking **metoprolol**.[10,15] In 24 healthy subjects given either nadolol, **atenolol** or placebo for one week followed by an infusion of adrenaline, mean arterial pressure and calf vascular resistance was not affected in the **atenolol** group.[1] Similarly, in another study in 7 healthy subjects given a single 210-microgram/kg dose of **atenolol**, there was a 10 bpm increase in heart rate and a modest 6 mmHg drop in diastolic blood pressure when adrenaline 0.1 micrograms/kg per minute was given for 30 minutes, which was in contrast to a marked drop in heart rate and increase in diastolic blood pressure with pindolol or propranolol.[3]

(c) Adrenaline (Epinephrine) with non-selective beta blockers with alpha-blocking activity

In 6 healthy subjects, giving intravenous adrenaline (epinephrine) 8, 16 and 32 micrograms/minute for 4 minutes at each dose level after intravenous **labetalol** 1 mg/kg, resulted in a 13 to 21 mmHg increase in mean arterial pressure and a very marked 23 to 29 bpm reduction in heart rate, when compared with adrenaline alone.[20]

(d) Dobutamine

A 54-year-old man with severe heart failure was given **carvedilol** 3.125 to 6.25 mg twice daily. His symptoms worsened and he was admitted for treatment with intravenous dobutamine; the **carvedilol** was discontinued and other medications apart from furosemide were withheld short-term. Dobutamine was started at 1 microgram/kg per minute and gradually increased to 5 micrograms/kg per minute. However, with each 1 microgram/kg increment the systolic blood pressure *dropped* to about 70 mmHg for 5 to 10 minutes and then quickly returned to the baseline level of 80 to 84 mmHg. When the dose of dobutamine reached 5 micrograms/kg per minute, his systolic blood pressure dropped to 56 mmHg and the dobutamine was discontinued. The blood pressure returned to normal over the next 30 minutes. Two months later when the patient was no longer taking **carvedilol** he was again given intravenous dobutamine and his systolic blood pressure increased, as would be expected.[21] Another case of hypotension (blood pressure 70/40 mmHg) has been reported with the use of **carvedilol** and dobutamine in a patient with acute coronary syndrome.[22]

(e) Isoprenaline (Isoproterenol)

In a study in patients with asthma, oral doses of the non-selective beta blockers **propranolol** 100 mg, **oxprenolol** 100 mg, **pindolol** 5 mg and **timolol** 10 mg blocked the bronchodilator response to inhaled isoprenaline 1.5 mg, but the selective beta blockers **metoprolol** 100 mg, **acebutolol** 300 mg and **atenolol** 100 mg did not interfere with bronchodilation.[23]

In a placebo-controlled study in healthy subjects, isoprenaline 0.03 micrograms/kg per minute was infused over 5 minutes, 30 minutes before single oral doses of either **metoprolol** 40 mg or 80 mg or **propranolol** 40 mg were given. Isoprenaline 0.09 micrograms/kg per minute [for 5 minutes] was then given at intervals of 30 minutes starting 60 minutes after administration of the beta blocker. Isoprenaline increased heart rate by a mean of 32 bpm. Although the dose of isoprenaline was increased threefold after administration of the beta blockers, the effect of isoprenaline after **propranolol** was very small and consistently more reduced by **propranolol** than by **metoprolol**.[24] Another study in patients with hypertension found that the blood pressure and cardiac responses to isoprenaline were attenuated or inhibited by both intravenous **propranolol** and **pindolol**.[25] In a study in 6 healthy subjects, intravenous **labetalol** 1.5 mg/kg antagonised the increases in heart rate and diastolic pressure due to isoprenaline.[26]

(f) Noradrenaline (Norepinephrine)

A study in patients with hypertension found that noradrenaline produced a fall in heart rate and rise in systolic pressure, which was not affected by **propranolol** but virtually abolished by **pindolol**.[25] Similarly, there was no alteration in the decrease in heart rate and rise in blood pressure in response to noradrenaline in another study in healthy subjects who received intravenous infusions of noradrenaline and **propranolol** (6 subjects) or **metoprolol** (4 subjects).[10] In contrast, in one earlier study, the hypertensive response to noradrenaline was increased in 10 healthy subjects when they also took **nadolol** or **propranolol** 240 mg daily.[2]

In two other studies in healthy subjects, the increase in blood pressure due to noradrenaline was antagonised by intravenous **labetalol**.[20,26]

(g) Phenylephrine

A woman taking **propranolol** 40 mg four times daily for hypertension was given phenylephrine hydrochloride 10% solution, one drop in each eye, during an ophthalmic examination. About 45 minutes later she complained of a sudden and sharp bi-temporal pain and shortly afterwards became unconscious. She later died of an intracerebral haemorrhage due to the rupture of a berry aneurysm. She had received a similar dose of phenylephrine on a previous occasion in the absence of **propranolol** without any problems.[27]

However, no change in blood pressure was seen in a study in both normotensive subjects and patients taking **metoprolol** who were given 0.5 to 4-mg intranasal doses of phenylephrine every hour, to a total of 7.5 to 15 mg (4 to 30 times the usual dose).[28] Similarly, in a placebo-controlled study in 12 hypertensive patients, **propranolol** and **metoprolol** did not significantly alter the dose of intravenous phenylephrine required to cause a 25 mmHg increase in systolic blood pressure.[29]

B. Anaphylaxis: resistance to treatment

A patient taking **propranolol** who suffered an anaphylactic reaction after receiving an allergy injection for desensitisation did not respond to adrenaline (epinephrine) and required intubation.[30] Anaphylactic shock, refractory to adrenaline, occurred in a penicillin-allergic patient taking **acebutolol** after she accidentally took amoxicillin.[31] Resistance to adrenaline treatment for anaphylaxis occurred in another patient using **timolol** eye drops,[32] in a child taking **nadolol**,[33] and in patients taking beta blockers and receiving X-ray contrast media (see 'Beta blockers + X-ray contrast media', p.1025). Severe hypertension, sometimes with bradycardia, has also been described following the use of adrenaline to treat allergic reactions, including presumed anaphylaxis, in patients taking **propranolol**.[11-13] These are also cited under *Effects on blood pressure and heart rate*, above.

It has also been proposed that the incidence and severity of anaphylactic reactions may be increased in those taking beta blockers,[34,35] one idea being that the adrenoceptors concerned with suppressing the release of the mediators of anaphylaxis may be blocked by either $beta_1$ or $beta_2$ antagonists.[34] However, one study did not find any evidence to support an increased incidence of systemic reactions in patients taking beta blockers receiving allergen immunotherapy.[36] See also 'Beta blockers + Penicillins', p.1017, and 'Beta blockers + X-ray contrast media', p.1025, for other anaphylactic reactions potentially exacerbated by beta blockers.

A beta-agonist bronchodilator, for example isoprenaline (isoproterenol) or salbutamol (albuterol), may be effective in patients taking beta blockers with anaphylaxis resistant to adrenaline,[33,34] and glucagon was effective in treating a severe anaphylactic reaction in one patient taking a beta blocker.[35]

Mechanism

Adrenaline (epinephrine) stimulates the alpha- and beta-receptors of the cardiovascular system, the former results in vasoconstriction (mainly $alpha_1$) and the latter in both vasodilation (mainly $beta_2$), and stimulation of the heart (mainly $beta_1$). The net result is usually a modest increase in heart rate and a small rise in blood pressure. However, if the beta-receptors are blocked by a non-selective beta blocker, such as propranolol or nadolol (see 'Table 22.1', p.999 for a list), the unopposed alpha vasoconstriction causes a marked rise in blood pressure, followed by reflex bradycardia. Cardioselective beta blockers such as atenolol and metoprolol, which are more selective for $beta_1$ receptors, do not prevent the vasodilator action of adrenaline at the $beta_2$ receptors to the same extent, and therefore the effect of any interaction is relatively small. Consequently, adrenaline has been used to assess the degree of beta blockade produced by propranolol and other beta blockers.[1,37]

Noradrenaline (norepinephrine) stimulates alpha receptors (although to a lesser extent than adrenaline) and $beta_1$ receptors but has minimal effects on $beta_2$ receptors. The precise mechanism for the effects of the beta blockers on the pressor effects of noradrenaline are unclear, but as beta blockers lower blood pressure and noradrenaline raises blood pressure a reduction in the response to noradrenaline is not unexpected.

Isoprenaline (isoproterenol) acts almost exclusively on beta-receptors and the increase in heart rate is due to stimulation of the heart ($beta_1$), an increase in sympathetic nerve activity secondary to peripheral vasodilation ($beta_2$), and a direct effect on the heart ($beta_2$). Nadolol, pindolol and propranolol exert their effects by blockade at both $beta_1$ and $beta_2$ receptors while bisoprolol and metoprolol, which are selective for $beta_1$ receptors, exert less effect on the isoprenaline-induced effects on heart rate or venodilation. Labetalol is also a non-selective beta blocker (and alpha blocker) and also antagonises the effects of isoprenaline.

Phenylephrine is largely an alpha stimulator, therefore beta blockers should have a minimal effect on its action.

Dobutamine is a $beta_1$, $beta_2$ and $alpha_1$ adrenergic agonist and carvedilol is a non-selective beta blocker, but at low doses it is primarily a selective $beta_1$ adrenergic antagonist and it is also an $alpha_1$ antagonist. It was proposed that the drop in blood pressure was caused by vasodilation due to vascular $beta_2$ receptor activation, which was not blocked by low doses of carvedilol.[21]

Importance and management

The interaction between propranolol and **adrenaline (epinephrine)** is established. It may be serious and potentially life-threatening, depending on the dose of adrenaline used. Marked and serious blood pressure rises and severe bradycardia have occurred in patients given 300 micrograms of adrenaline (0.3 mL of 1:1000) subcutaneously[11-13] or 40 to 400 micrograms by infiltration of the skin and eyelids during plastic surgery.[6] Adrenaline 15 micrograms given intravenously can cause an almost 40% fall in heart rate.[17] Patients taking non-selective beta blockers such as propranolol (see 'Table 22.1', p.999 for a list) should only be given adrenaline in very reduced doses because of the marked bradycardia and hypertension that can occur. Acute hypertensive episodes have been controlled with chlorpromazine or phentolamine (both of which are alpha blockers). Hydralazine,[6,14] nifedipine[12] and aminophylline[14] have also been used. Reflex bradycardia may be managed with atropine and the pre-emptive use of glycopyrrolate has also been suggested.[14] A less marked effect is likely with the cardioselective beta blockers,[8] such as atenolol and metoprolol (see 'Table 22.1', p.999 for a list). Local anaesthetics used in dental surgery usually contain very low concentrations of adrenaline (e.g. 5 to 20 micrograms/mL, i.e. 1:200 000 to 1:50 000) and only small volumes are usually given, so that an undesirable interaction is unlikely. Bear in mind that beta blockers will reduce the response to adrenaline if it is given to detect inadvertent intravascular placement of an epidural catheter.

Similar effects to those seen with adrenaline (hypertension and reflex bradycardia) are also theoretically possible if **dobutamine**, which also causes alpha- and beta-receptor stimulation, is given with a beta blocker (see adrenaline under *Mechanism*, above), but the case reports describing *hypotension* suggest that the effects may not always be predictable.

In general, the beta blockers appear to attenuate the rise in blood pressure caused by **noradrenaline (norepinephrine)**; beta blockers are often omitted in patients requiring inotropic support with noradrenaline for this reason. Some sources suggest that noradrenaline will interact with beta blockers in the same way as adrenaline, but there does not seem to be any evidence supporting this prediction. Furthermore, it should be noted that the beta effects of noradrenaline are not the same as those of adrenaline (see *Mechanism*, above).

No interaction between **phenylephrine** and the beta blockers would be expected, and apart from the single unexplained case cited above, the literature appears to support this. Concurrent use normally appears to be clinically unimportant, particularly bearing in mind the widespread use of beta blockers and the ready availability of phenylephrine in the form of non-prescription cough-and-cold remedies and nasal decongestants.

Similarly, an interaction resulting in hypertension and reflex bradycardia would not be expected if **isoprenaline (isoproterenol)** is given with a beta blocker, and the studies support this theory. However, the studies do suggest that the bronchodilator effects of isoprenaline may be antagonised by non-selective beta blockers. For more on this effect, see 'Anti-asthma drugs + Beta blockers', p.1420.

1. Hiatt WR, Wolfel EE, Stoll S, Nies AS, Zerbe GO, Brammell HL, Horwitz LD. Beta-2 Adrenergic blockade evaluated with epinephrine after placebo, atenolol, and nadolol. *Clin Pharmacol Ther* (1985) 37, 2–6.
2. Reeves RA, Boer WH, DeLeve L, Leenen FHH. Nonselective beta-blockade enhances pressor responsiveness to epinephrine, norepinephrine, and angiotensin II in normal man. *Clin Pharmacol Ther* (1984) 35, 461–6.
3. Rehling M, Svendsen TL, Maltbæk N, Tangø M, Trap-Jensen J. Haemodynamic effects of atenolol, pindolol and propranolol during adrenaline infusion in man. *Eur J Clin Pharmacol* (1986) 30, 659–63.
4. Sugimura M, Hirota Y, Shibutani T, Niwa H, Hori T, Kim Y, Matsuura H. An echocardiographic study of interactions between pindolol and epinephrine contained in a local anesthetic solution. *Anesth Prog* (1995) 42, 29–35.
5. Harris WS, Schoenfeld CD, Brooks RH, Weissler AM. Effect of beta adrenergic blockade on the hemodynamic responses to epinephrine in man. *Am J Cardiol* (1966) 17, 484–92.
6. Foster CA, Aston SJ. Propranolol-epinephrine interaction: a potential disaster. *Plast Reconstr Surg* (1983) 72, 74–8.
7. Kram J, Bourne HR, Melmon KL, Maibach H. Propranolol. *Ann Intern Med* (1974) 80, 282–3.
8. van Herwaarden CLA, Binkhorst RA, Fennis JFM, van'T Laar A. Effects of adrenaline during treatment with propranolol and metoprolol. *BMJ* (1977) 2, 1029.
9. Lampman RM, Santinga JT, Bassett DR, Savage PJ. Cardiac arrhythmias during epinephrine-propranolol infusions for measurement on in vivo insulin resistance. *Diabetes* (1981) 30, 618–20.
10. Hjemdahl P, Åkerstedt T, Pollare T, Gillberg M. Influence of β-adrenoceptor blockade by metoprolol and propranolol on plasma concentrations and effects of noradrenaline and adrenaline during i.v. infusion. *Acta Physiol Scand* (1983) 515 (Suppl), 45–53.
11. Hansbrough JF, Near A. Propranolol-epinephrine antagonism with hypertension and stroke. *Ann Intern Med* (1980) 92, 717.
12. Whelan TV. Propranolol, epinephrine and accelerated hypertension during hemodialysis. *Ann Intern Med* (1987) 106, 327.
13. Gandy W. Severe epinephrine-propranolol interaction. *Ann Emerg Med* (1989) 18, 98–9.
14. Centeno RF, Yu YL. The propranolol-epinephrine interaction revisited: a serious and potentially catastrophic adverse drug interaction in facial plastic surgery. *Plast Reconstr Surg* (2003) 111, 944–5.
15. Houben H, Thien T, Laor VA. Effect of low-dose epinephrine infusion on hemodynamics after selective and non-selective beta-blockade in hypertension. *Clin Pharmacol Ther* (1982) 31, 685.
16. Dzubow LM. The interaction between propranolol and epinephrine as observed in patients undergoing Mohs' surgery. *J Am Acad Dermatol* (1986) 15, 71–5.
17. Mackie K, Lam A. Epinephrine-containing test dose during beta-blockade. *J Clin Monit* (1991) 7, 213–6.
18. Guinard J-P, Mulroy MF, Carpenter RL, Knopes KD. Test doses: optimal epinephrine content with and without acute beta-adrenergic blockade. *Anesthesiology* (1990) 73, 386–92.
19. Li B-H, Bradshaw P. Intravascularly administered epinephrine, injected inadvertently as part of an epidural test dose, failed to elicit tachycardia in a patient using timolol eye drops. *Anesth Analg* (2007) 104, 1308–9.
20. Richards DA, Prichard BNC, Hernández R. Circulatory effects of noradrenaline and adrenaline before and after labetalol. *Br J Clin Pharmacol* (1979) 7, 371–8.
21. Lindenfield J, Lowes BD, Bristow MR. Hypotension with dobutamine: β-adrenergic antagonist selectivity at low doses of carvedilol. *Ann Pharmacother* (1999) 33, 1266–9.
22. Vural M. Akut koroner sendrom nedeniyle tedavi edilen bir olguda ciddi hipotansiyon gelişmesinde karvedilol dobutamin etkileşiminin rolü. *Anadolu Kardiyol Derg* (2007) 7, 229.
23. Decalmer PBS, Chatterjee SS, Cruickshank JM, Benson MK, Sterling GM. Beta-blockers and asthma. *Br Heart J* (1978) 40, 184–9.
24. Johnsson G, Nyberg G, Sölvell L. Influence of metoprolol and propranolol on hemodynamic effects induced by physical work and isoprenaline. *Acta Pharmacol Toxicol (Copenh)* (1975) 36 (Suppl 5) 69–75.
25. Chu D, Cocco G, Sceweda E, Haeusler G, Strozzi C. Influence of propranolol and pindolol on the hemodynamic effects of papaverine, isoprenaline and noradrenaline in hypertensive patients. *Eur J Clin Pharmacol* (1980) 18, 141–6.
26. Richards DA, Prichard BNC. Concurrent antagonism of isoproterenol and norepinephrine after labetalol. *Clin Pharmacol Ther* (1978) 23, 253–8.
27. Cass E, Kadar D, Stein HA. Hazards of phenylephrine topical medication in persons taking propranolol. *Can Med Assoc J* (1979) 120, 1261–2.
28. Myers MG, Iazzetta JJ. Intranasally administered phenylephrine and blood pressure. *Can Med Assoc J* (1982) 127, 365–8.
29. Myers MG. Beta adrenoceptor antagonism and pressor response to phenylephrine. *Clin Pharmacol Ther* (1984) 36, 57–63.
30. Newman BR, Schultz LK. Epinephrine-resistant anaphylaxis in a patient taking propranolol hydrochloride. *Ann Allergy* (1981) 47, 35–7.
31. Goddet N-S, Descatha A, Liberge O, Dolveck F, Boutet J, Baer M, Fletcher D. Templier F. Paradoxical reaction to epinephrine induced by beta-blockers in an anaphylactic shock induced by penicillin. *Eur J Emerg Med* (2006) 13, 358–60.
32. Moneret-Vautrin DA, Kanny G, Faller JP, Levan D, Kohler C.Choc anaphylactique grave avec arrêt cardiaque au café et à la gomme arabique, potentialisé par un collyre bêta-bloquant. *Rev Med Interne* (1993) 14, 107–11.
33. Momeni M, Brui B, Baele P, Matta A. Anaphylactic shock in a beta-blocked child: usefulness of isoproterenol. *Paediatr Anaesth* (2007) 17, 897–9.
34. Toogood JH. Beta-blocker therapy and the risk of anaphylaxis. *Can Med Assoc J* (1987) 136, 929–33.
35. Lang DM. Anaphylactoid and anaphylactic reactions. Hazards of beta-blockers. *Drug Safety* (1995) 12, 299–304.
36. Hepner MJ, Ownby DR, Anderson JA, Rowe MS, Sears-Ewald D, Brown EB. Risk of systemic reactions in patients taking beta-blocker drugs receiving allergen immunotherapy injections. *J Allergy Clin Immunol* (1990) 86, 407–11.
37. Varma DR, Sharma KK, Arora RC. Response to adrenaline and propranolol in hyperthyroidism. *Lancet* (1976), i, 260.

Beta blockers + Itraconazole

Itraconazole markedly increases the bioavailability of celiprolol and only slightly affects the pharmacokinetics of atenolol, without affecting heart rate or blood pressure.

Clinical evidence, mechanism, importance and management

(a) Atenolol

In a study in 10 healthy subjects, itraconazole 200 mg twice daily for 5 doses had only minor effects on the pharmacokinetics of a single 50-mg dose of atenolol and no effects on heart rate or blood pressure were seen.[1] No atenolol dose adjustment would be required in patients also given itraconazole.

(b) Celiprolol

In a study in 12 healthy subjects, itraconazole 200 mg twice daily for 5 doses increased the AUC of a single 100-mg dose of celiprolol by 80%, without increasing its half-life. However, itraconazole did not increase the effect of celiprolol on heart rate or blood pressure.[2] It was suggested that itraconazole probably increases the absorption of celiprolol by inhibiting P-glycoprotein in the intestinal wall.[2] Although the increase in plasma levels was marked, it was suggested that it is unlikely to be clinically relevant because celiprolol has a wide therapeutic range.[2]

1. Lilja JJ, Backman JT, Neuvonen PJ. Effect of itraconazole on the pharmacokinetics of atenolol. *Basic Clin Pharmacol Toxicol* (2005) 97, 395–8.
2. Lilja JJ, Backman JT, Laitila J, Luurila H, Neuvonen PJ. Itraconazole increases but grapefruit juice greatly decreases plasma concentrations of celiprolol. *Clin Pharmacol Ther* (2003) 73, 192–8.

Beta blockers + Macrolides

The bioavailability of talinolol is modestly increased by erythromycin, whereas the bioavailability of nadolol is not affected by erythromycin. The bioavailability of metoprolol is modestly increased by telithromycin.

A study suggests that telithromycin does not adversely affect sotalol-induced QT prolongation, whereas the combined use of sotalol and intravenous erythromycin should generally be avoided because of the possible additive effects on QT interval prolongation.

Clinical evidence, mechanism, importance and management

(a) Metoprolol

The peak plasma level and AUC of metoprolol are reported to be increased by about 38% by **telithromycin**, but its elimination half-life is not affected.[1] The manufacturer of **telithromycin** considers the increased exposure to metoprolol may be of clinical importance in patients with heart failure, and that in such patients, caution is suggested.[1] However, other interactions suggest that the levels of metoprolol may need to be almost doubled before an interaction becomes clinically relevant, even in patients with heart failure.

(b) Nadolol

A study, in which 7 healthy subjects were given a single 80-mg dose of nadolol after **erythromycin** 500 mg plus neomycin 500 mg every 6 hours for 2 days, suggested an increase in the rate of beta blocker absorption (reduced time to maximum plasma level and twofold increase in maximum level, but no effect on AUC). A decrease in the elimination half-life was also seen.[2] These changes are unlikely to be clinically relevant.

(c) Sotalol

Telithromycin does not appear to be associated with QT prolongation and a study in 24 healthy women found that a single 800-mg dose of **telithromycin** had no adverse effect on the QT-prolongation induced by a 160-mg dose of sotalol. **Telithromycin** slightly reduced the AUC and maximum serum levels of sotalol, which was attributed to a decrease in its absorption,[3] but this is expected to be of little clinical significance. Sotalol prolongs the QT interval and should generally not be given with other drugs that also have this effect, such as intravenous **erythromycin**, because of the increased risk of torsade de pointes (see also 'Drugs that prolong the QT interval + Other drugs that prolong the QT interval', p.272).

(d) Talinolol

A single-dose study in 8 healthy subjects found that the AUC and serum levels of talinolol 50 mg were modestly increased by 51% and 26%, respectively, by **erythromycin** 2 g. It was suggested that the increased bioavailability of talinolol was due to increased intestinal absorption caused by the inhibition of P-glycoprotein by **erythromycin**.[4] The clinical relevance of this effect is unclear, but it seems unlikely to be important.

1. Ketek (Telithromycin). Sanofi. UK Summary of product characteristics, November 2012.
2. du Souich P, Caillé G, Larochelle P. Enhancement of nadolol elimination by activated charcoal and antibiotics. *Clin Pharmacol Ther* (1983) 33, 585–90.
3. Démolis J-L, Strabach S, Vacheron F, Funck-Bretano C. Assessment of the effect of a single oral dose of telithromycin on sotalol-induced QT interval prolongation in healthy women. *Br J Clin Pharmacol* (2005) 60, 120–7.
4. Schwarz UI, Gramatté T, Krappweis J, Oertel R, Kirch W. P-glycoprotein inhibitor erythromycin increases oral bioavailability of talinolol in humans. *Int J Clin Pharmacol Ther* (2000) 38, 161–7.

Beta blockers + Metoclopramide

A patient with scleroderma suffered a fatal cardiac arrest after receiving intravenous labetalol and intravenous metoclopramide postoperatively. Metoclopramide increased the rate of absorption of metoprolol and a conventional formulation of propranolol, but did not affect atenolol or a sustained-release preparation of propranolol.

Clinical evidence, mechanism, importance and management

(a) Atenolol

In a study, 6 healthy subjects took a single 100-mg dose of atenolol alone or one hour after a single 25-mg dose of metoclopramide. The time to reach atenolol maximum plasma levels was reduced slightly, by 0.3 hours, but this was not statistically significant, and there was no effect on the overall bioavailability of atenolol.[1]

No dose adjustment of atenolol would be required in patients also given metoclopramide.

(b) Labetalol

A 38-year-old patient with scleroderma, hypertension (for which she was taking lisinopril) and gangrene of her left index finger underwent minor hand surgery. While in postoperative care her blood pressure rose to 153/120 mmHg and she was given intravenous labetalol 10 mg. About 15 minutes later she experienced nausea and vomiting, and so she was given intravenous metoclopramide 10 mg. About 5 minutes later her heart rate decreased to 38 bpm and she became unresponsive with no palpable pulse: an ECG showed junctional bradycardia. She was initially resuscitated but died about 13 hours later after a further episode of bradycardia, despite full supportive treatment. It was noted that the bradycardia did not respond well to atropine, and there was persistent hypotension, despite escalating vasopressor use.

Scleroderma and lisinopril may have contributed to the failure to resuscitate the patient; however, bradycardia or heart block and hypotension may occur with intravenous metoclopramide. In this patient the use of labetalol may have exacerbated the effects of metoclopramide by causing reductions in ventricular contractility due to its beta-adrenergic effects and limiting vasoconstrictive compensatory mechanisms due to alpha-adrenergic effects.[2] However, it has subsequently been suggested that this reaction may have been due to local anaesthetic toxicity rather than a drug interaction,[3] although this was disputed by the original authors.[4]

A study in 11 untreated hypertensive patients found that intravenous metoclopramide (7.5 micrograms/kg per minute for 30 minutes) caused a slight decrease in the responsiveness to labetalol 400 to 600 mg daily. However, as metoclopramide only attenuated the systolic blood pressure response to labetalol by 3 mmHg this effect seems unlikely to be clinically relevant in most patients.[5]

(c) Metoprolol

In a crossover study, 8 young healthy subjects (aged 27 to 39 years) and 7 elderly healthy subjects aged (67 to 94 years) received a single 10-mg intravenous dose of metoclopramide or placebo followed 15 minutes later by a single 100-mg oral dose of metoprolol. In the young subjects, there was an increase in the rate of absorption of metoprolol (the time to reach maximum plasma levels was decreased from 1.3 hours to 0.7 hours and the maximum plasma level increased by 31%) when it was given after metoclopramide, without any change in the extent of absorption (AUC). Similar findings were seen in the elderly subjects: the time the time to reach maximum plasma levels of metoprolol was decreased from 2.5 hours to 1.7 hours when it was given after metoclopramide, and the maximum plasma level increased by 48%, without any change in the AUC.[6] These changes are unlikely to be clinically relevant.

(d) Propranolol

In a study in 12 healthy subjects, metoclopramide syrup 20 mg, given 30 minutes before sustained-release propranolol 160 mg, had no effect on the pharmacokinetics of propranolol.[7] In contrast, an earlier brief report found that the rate of absorption of a conventional formulation of propranolol 80 mg was increased by intravenous metoclopramide 10 mg in 4 healthy subjects. In the first 2 hours after dosing, propranolol levels were increased by 1.3 to 2.5-fold.[8] This study did not report the overall extent of absorption (AUC). Nevertheless, these changes are unlikely to be clinically relevant.

1. Regårdh CG, Lundborg P, Persson BA. The effect of antacid, metoclopramide and propantheline on the bioavailability of metoprolol and atenolol. *Biopharm Drug Dispos* (1981) 2, 79–87.
2. Tung A, Sweitzer B, Cutter T. Cardiac arrest after labetalol and metoclopramide administration in a patient with scleroderma. *Anesth Analg* (2002) 95, 1667–8.
3. Schwartz D, VadeBoncour T, Weinberg G. Was case report a case of unrecognized local anesthetic toxicity? *Anesth Analg* (2003) 96, 1844–5.
4. Tung A, Sweitzer BJ, Cutter TW. Was case report a case of unrecognized local anesthetic toxicity? In response. *Anesth Analg* (2003) 96, 1845.
5. Blanco M, Gomez J, Negrín C, Blanco G, Rodriguez M, Torres M, Vásquez M, Alcalá I, Vargas R, Velasco M. Metoclopramide enhances labetalol-induced antihypertensive effect during handgrip in hypertensive patients. *Am J Ther* (1998) 5, 221–4.
6. Briant RH, Dorrington RE, Ferry DG, Paxton JW. Bioavailability of metoprolol in young adults and the elderly, with additional studies on the effects of metoclopramide and probanthine. *Eur J Clin Pharmacol* (1983) 25, 353–6.
7. Charles BG, Renshaw PJ, Kay JJ, Ravenscroft PJ. Effect of metoclopramide on the bioavailability of long-acting propranolol. *Br J Clin Pharmacol* (1981) 517–18.
8. George CF, Castleden M. Propranolol absorption. *BMJ* (1977) 1, 47.

Beta blockers + Morphine

Morphine may moderately raise the serum levels of esmolol in some patients. The fatal doses of morphine and propranolol are markedly reduced by concurrent use in *animals*, but the clinical relevance of this in humans is uncertain.

Clinical evidence, mechanism, importance and management

In a study in 10 healthy men, a 3-mg injection of morphine sulfate increased the steady-state levels of **esmolol**, which was given as a 300 microgram/kg per minute infusion over 4 hours. However, the increases were only statistically significant in 2 of the subjects (increase of 46%), and were considered to be of no clinical importance. The pharmacokinetics of morphine were unchanged.[1]

Studies in *animals* have shown that the median fatal dose of **propranolol** was reduced two- to sevenfold by morphine in *mice*[2] and the median lethal dose of morphine was reduced fifteen- to sixteenfold by **propranolol** in *rats*.[3] The same interaction has also been seen in *dogs*.[3] There do not appear to be any published reports of toxicity involving morphine and **propranolol**, and the clinical relevance of this interaction is uncertain.

1. Lowenthal DT, Porter RS, Saris SD, Bies CM, Slegowski MB, Staudacher A. Clinical pharmacology, pharmacodynamics and interactions with esmolol. *Am J Cardiol* (1985) 56, 14F–18F.
2. Murmann W, Almirante L, Saccani-Guelfi M. Effects of hexobarbitone, ether, morphine, and urethane upon the acute toxicity of propranolol and D-(-)-INPEA. *J Pharm Pharmacol* (1966) 18, 692–4.
3. Davis WM, Hatoum NS. Possible toxic interaction of propranolol and narcotic analgesics. *Drug Intell Clin Pharm* (1981) 15, 290–1.

Beta blockers + Penicillins

Plasma atenolol levels are halved by 1-g doses of ampicillin, but no important interaction occurs if atenolol is given with ampicillin 250 mg every 6 hours. There may be a slight reduction in the half-life of practolol when it is given with ampicillin. One brief report suggests that anaphylactic reactions to penicillins may be more severe in patients taking beta blockers.

Clinical evidence

(a) Pharmacokinetics

1. Atenolol. In a single-dose study in 6 healthy subjects, **ampicillin** 1 g reduced the AUC of atenolol 100 mg by 40%, and decreased its bioavailability from 60% to 36%.[1] Similarly, when atenolol 100 mg was given with **ampicillin** 1 g daily for 6 days, the mean steady-state plasma atenolol level was reduced by 52%, and the AUC was reduced by 52%. The blood pressure-lowering effect of atenolol at rest was not affected, but after exercise a small rise in systolic pressure of up to 17 mmHg occurred, whereas diastolic blood pressure was unchanged. The effects of atenolol on reducing heart rate during exercise were diminished from 24% to 11% at 12 hours.[1] A further single-dose study found that when atenolol 50 mg was given with oral **ampicillin** 1 g the AUC of atenolol was reduced by 52%, whereas when **ampicillin** 250 mg four times daily was given for 24 hours, the AUC was only reduced by 18%.[2]

2. Practolol. In a crossover study, 4 healthy subjects were given a single 400-mg dose of practolol, orally or intravenously, both alone and 24 hours after starting to take **ampicillin** 500 mg four times daily. There was a minor reduction in the elimination half-life of oral practolol, from 8.6 hours to 6.3 hours, in the presence of **ampicillin**, but intravenous practolol was unaffected. In a similar preliminary study in 8 healthy subjects who took a single 400-mg oral dose of practolol, there was a trend towards a reduction in the half-life of practolol when ampicillin was also given, but this was not statistically significant.[3]

(b) Anaphylaxis

A brief report describes 2 patients, one taking **nadolol** and one taking **propranolol**, who developed fatal anaphylactic shock after taking **phenoxymethylpenicillin**. The authors suggested that, as fatal reactions to penicillins are rare, the reaction had been exacerbated by the presence of a non-selective beta blocker.[4] For a report of anaphylaxis associated with **amoxicillin**, refractory to adrenaline (epinephrine), in a patient taking **acebutolol**, see 'Beta blockers + Inotropes and Vasopressors', p.1014.

Mechanism

Uncertain. Ampicillin, in large doses, apparently affects the absorption of atenolol.

Importance and management

Information about interactions between penicillins and beta blockers is limited, but the absorption interaction between a 1-g dose of ampicillin and atenolol appears to be established. The clinical importance awaits full evaluation but the modest effects on blood pressure and heart rate[1] suggest that it is limited. Similarly, the clinical relevance of the minor reduction in the half-life of practolol given orally is likely to be small. Information about other beta blockers and penicillins is lacking.

Information on potentiation of anaphylaxis is too limited to make comment, but note that there is also limited evidence that anaphylactic shock in patients taking beta blockers may be resistant to treatment with adrenaline (epinephrine), see 'Beta blockers + Inotropes and Vasopressors', p.1014.

1. Schäfer-Korting M, Kirch W, Axthelm T, Köhler H, Mutschler E. Atenolol interaction with aspirin, allopurinol, and ampicillin. *Clin Pharmacol Ther* (1983) 33, 283–8.
2. McLean AJ, Tonkin A, McCarthy P, Harrison P. Dose-dependence of atenolol-ampicillin interaction. *Br J Clin Pharmacol* (1984) 18, 969–71.
3. Kelly JG, Leahey WJ, McDevitt DG, Diddell JG. Does ampicillin affect practolol kinetics? *Br J Clin Pharmacol* (1977) 4, 396P.
4. Berkelman RL, Finton RJ, Elsea WR. Beta-adrenergic antagonists and fatal anaphylactic reactions to oral penicillins. *Ann Intern Med* (1986) 104, 134.

Beta blockers + Phenothiazines

Both beta blockers and phenothiazines can cause hypotension, and these effects could be additive: a handful of case reports suggest that this could occasionally be serious. In addition, the concurrent use of chlorpromazine with propranolol can result in a marked rise in the plasma levels of both drugs. A similar interaction appears to occur between thioridazine and pindolol. Propranolol markedly increases plasma thioridazine levels. The concurrent use of sotalol and phenothiazines that prolong the QT interval should generally be avoided.

Clinical evidence

(a) Chlorpromazine

In 4 healthy subjects and one hypertensive patient, the mean steady-state levels of **propranolol** 80 mg every 8 hours were raised by 70% when they were given chlorpromazine 50 mg every 8 hours.[1] The increase was considerable in some subjects but barely detectable in others. A sixth subject taking **propranolol** promptly fainted when getting out of bed after the first dose of chlorpromazine. He was found to have a pulse rate of 35 to 40 bpm and a blood pressure of 70/0 mmHg. He rapidly recovered, achieving a pulse rate of 85 bpm and a blood pressure of 120/70 mmHg when given atropine 3 mg. However, it is unclear whether the adverse effect was due to chlorpromazine alone, or to an interaction with **propranolol**.[1]

Propranolol (mean daily dose 8.1 mg/kg) increased the serum chlorpromazine levels of 7 patients with schizophrenia by about 100 to 500%, and raised the plasma levels of the active metabolites of chlorpromazine by about 50 to 100%.[2] The same or similar work by the same authors is described elsewhere.[3] One of the patients was withdrawn from the study because he suffered a cardiovascular collapse while taking both drugs.[3] It has been suggested that the value of **propranolol** in the treatment of schizophrenia probably results from the rise in serum chlorpromazine levels.[3]

A report briefly mentions a girl with diabetes who had an episode of minor hypotension with chlorpromazine that appeared to have been exacerbated by **sotalol**.[4] A patient with schizophrenia taking chlorpromazine and **tiotixene** experienced delirium, grand mal seizures and skin photosensitivity, attributed to a rise in the serum levels of the antipsychotic drugs caused by increasing doses of **propranolol** (up to a total of 1.2 g daily).[5]

(b) Thioridazine

Serum **pindolol** levels were 2.5-fold higher in 7 patients taking thioridazine than in 17 patients taking haloperidol, phenytoin, and/or phenobarbital.[6] Furthermore, **pindolol** 40 mg daily increased serum thioridazine levels by about 50% in 8 patients.[6]

Two patients, taking stable doses of thioridazine 600 or 800 mg daily, had three- and fivefold rises in plasma levels, respectively, when they were given **propranolol**, in increasing doses up to a total of 800 mg daily, over 26 to 40 days. No signs or symptoms of thioridazine toxicity were seen even though plasma levels had risen into the toxic range.[7] Similarly, in another study, thioridazine levels rose by about 55 to 370% in 5 patients taking **propranolol** 320 to 520 mg daily.[8]

Mechanism

Both beta blockers and phenothiazines can cause hypotension, and these effects could be additive. In addition, pharmacokinetic evidence[1] and *animal* studies[9] suggest that propranolol and chlorpromazine mutually inhibit the liver metabolism of the other drug so that both accumulate within the body. The mechanism of the interaction between propranolol and thioridazine is probably similar. Thioridazine is an inhibitor of the cytochrome P450 isoenzyme CYP2D6 and may inhibit the metabolism of propranolol and metoprolol, which are substrates for this isoenzyme.

Importance and management

The pharmacokinetic interaction between **propranolol** and chlorpromazine appears to be established although information is limited. Concurrent use should be well monitored and the doses reduced if necessary. The same precautions apply with propranolol and thioridazine.[7] The manufacturer of **metoprolol** advises caution with the concurrent use of thioridazine.[10] Normally the beta blockers are considered to have a wide therapeutic range, and so increases in levels are generally well tolerated. Patients with heart failure are usually more at risk, because drugs such as metoprolol need slow and careful dose titration in this condition, and therefore, until the magnitude of any interaction is known, some monitoring (e.g. for shortness of breath, bradycardia, hypotension) may be prudent.

There seems to be no information about any interaction between other beta blockers and phenothiazines, but if the mechanism of the pharmacokinetic interaction suggested above is true, it seems possible that other beta blockers that are mainly cleared from the body by liver metabolism might interact similarly with chlorpromazine, whereas those mainly cleared unchanged in the urine are less likely to have a pharmacokinetic interaction. See 'Table 22.1', p.999, for information on the metabolism of the commonly used systemic beta blockers. In all cases the concurrent use of a phenothiazine and a beta blocker could result in additive hypotension, and this should be borne in mind when giving the combination.

Note that **sotalol** and some phenothiazines, including chlorpromazine and thioridazine prolong the QT interval (see 'Table 9.2', p.273 for a more extensive list). Concurrent use should therefore generally be avoided, because of the increased risk of torsade de pointes. See also 'Drugs that prolong the QT interval + Other drugs that prolong the QT interval', p.272.

1. Vestal RE, Kornhauser DM, Hollifield JW, Shand DG. Inhibition of propranolol metabolism by chlorpromazine. *Clin Pharmacol Ther* (1979) 25, 19–24.
2. Peet M, Middlemiss DN, Yates RA. Pharmacokinetic interaction between propranolol and chlorpromazine in schizophrenic patients. *Lancet* (1980) ii, 978.
3. Peet M, Middlemiss DN, Yates RA. Propranolol in schizophrenia II. Clinical and biochemical aspects of combining propranolol with chlorpromazine. *Br J Psychiatry* (1981) 138, 112–17.
4. Baker L, Barcai A, Kaye R, Haque N. Beta adrenergic blockade and juvenile diabetes: acute studies and long-term therapeutic trial. *J Pediatr* (1969) 75, 19–29.
5. Miller FA, Rampling D. Adverse effects of combined propranolol and chlorpromazine therapy. *Am J Psychiatry* (1982) 139, 1198–9.
6. Greendyke RM, Gulya A. Effect of pindolol administration on serum levels of thioridazine, haloperidol, phenytoin, and phenobarbital. *J Clin Psychiatry* (1988) 49, 105–7.
7. Silver JM, Yudofsky SC, Kogan M, Katz BL. Elevation of thioridazine plasma levels by propranolol. *Am J Psychiatry* (1986) 143, 1290–2.
8. Greendyke RM, Kanter DR. Plasma propranolol levels and their effect on plasma thioridazine and haloperidol concentrations. *J Clin Psychopharmacol* (1987) 7, 178–82.
9. Shand DG, Oates JA. Metabolism of propranolol by rat liver microsomes and its inhibition by phenothiazine and tricyclic antidepressant drugs. *Biochem Pharmacol* (1971) 20, 1720–3.
10. Lopresor (Metoprolol tartrate). Novartis Pharmaceuticals UK Ltd. UK Summary of product characteristics, July 2008.

Beta blockers + Phenylpropanolamine

A rise in blood pressure may occur in patients taking beta blockers who take single doses of phenylpropanolamine, particularly with immediate-release preparations. However, there appears to be only one published case report (in a patient taking oxprenolol with methyldopa and phenylpropanolamine) that specifically describes an adverse effect from this interaction. Propranolol attenuates the blood pressure rise seen with phenylpropanolamine.

Clinical evidence

A study in 13 patients taking various antihypertensives, including 5 taking unnamed beta blockers, found that a single dose of *Dimetapp Extentabs* (phenylpropanolamine 75 mg with brompheniramine 12 mg) caused a blood pressure rise of 1.7/0.9 mmHg over a 4-hour period, which was not statistically or clinically significant.[1] Another study in 7 stabilised hypertensive patients taking beta blockers (**atenolol** 5 patients, **metoprolol** 1, **propranolol** 1) found that a single 25-mg dose of rapid-release phenylpropanolamine (*Super Odrinex*) increased the mean peak blood pressures by about 8/5 mmHg over a 6-hour period.[2] A later multiple dose study in the same subjects (only 5 of whom completed the study), taking the same beta blockers, found a greater increase in blood pressure: on day 1 phenylpropanolamine increased diastolic blood pressure by 9 to 16 mmHg, and on day 7 by up to 14 mmHg. The day 1 and day 7 results were not statistically different, which suggests that the increase in blood pressure is not enhanced by multiple dosing.[3]

In a placebo-controlled study in 6 healthy subjects, **propranolol** given either orally as a pretreatment or intravenously after phenylpropanolamine, was found to antagonise the rise in blood pressure induced by the phenylpropanolamine. Oral phenylpropanolamine 75 mg alone increased blood pressure from 116/63 mmHg to 148/83 mmHg; pretreatment with oral **propranolol** 80 mg every 6 hours reduced the baseline blood pressure to 107/62 mmHg and the increase with phenylpropanolamine was lower, reaching only 119/72 mmHg. Intravenous **propranolol** 0.3 mg/kg given after the phenylpropanolamine decreased blood pressure from 144/87 mmHg to 121/84 mmHg.[4]

Mechanism

Phenylpropanolamine is a sympathomimetic drug, with mainly indirect actions, which causes it to release noradrenaline (norepinephrine) from the nerve endings. Thus, it may raise blood pressure, and in rare cases it has caused hypertensive crises. The beta blockers lower blood pressure and therefore concurrent use can oppose the effect of either drug on blood pressure.

Importance and management

Evidence for an interaction between phenylpropanolamine and the beta blockers is relatively limited, but the pharmacological effects of both drugs are well known. The rises in blood pressure that occurred in patients taking beta blockers who were given single doses of extended-release phenylpropanolamine were small and relatively short-lived, and probably of little clinical importance. However, the larger rise in blood pressure seen in one study with an immediate-release preparation is of greater concern and suggests that some patients at least may experience a detrimental rise in blood pressure on concurrent use, especially if blood pressure is already poorly controlled. It would therefore seem prudent to avoid concurrent use unless the patient can be closely monitored and the benefits of phenylpropanolamine use are expected to outweigh the risks.

Note that a marked rise in blood pressure was seen in one patient taking methyldopa and oxprenolol when phenylpropanolamine was given, see 'Methyldopa + Nasal decongestants', p.1070.

1. Petrulis AS, Imperiale TF, Speroff T. The acute effect of phenylpropanolamine and brompheniramine on blood pressure in controlled hypertension. *J Gen Intern Med* (1991) 6, 503–6.
2. O'Connell MB, Gross CR. The effect of single-dose phenylpropanolamine on blood pressure in patients with hypertension controlled by β blockers. *Pharmacotherapy* (1990) 10, 85–91.
3. O'Connell MB, Gross CR. The effect of multiple doses of phenylpropanolamine on the blood pressure of patients whose hypertension was controlled with β blockers. *Pharmacotherapy* (1991) 11, 376–81.
4. Pentel PR, Asinger RW, Benowitz, NL. Propranolol antagonism of phenylpropanolamine-induced hypertension. *Clin Pharmacol Ther* (1985) 37, 488–94.

Beta blockers + Pilocarpine

The concurrent use of oral pilocarpine and beta blockers is said to be associated with a risk of conduction disorders (presumably bradycardia).

Clinical evidence, mechanism, importance and management

The manufacturer of *oral* pilocarpine notes that it should be given with caution to patients taking beta blockers because of the possibility of conduction disorders.[1] Note also that palpitations, hypertension, and flushing (due to vasodilation) are said to be common with the use of oral pilocarpine.[1] There do not appear to be any published reports of adverse interactions between oral pilocarpine and beta blockers; however, based on the known pharmacology of both drugs bradycardia would appear to be a possibility. Bear this in mind if pilocarpine is given to a patient taking a beta blocker.

Adverse effects from pilocarpine *eye drops* appear rare, but a couple of cases of cardiac decompensation (hypotension, sinus bradycardia, atrioventricular block) have been reported, although these followed the use of excessive doses of pilocarpine before surgery.[2]

1. Salagen (Pilocarpine hydrochloride). Novartis Pharmaceuticals UK Ltd. UK Summary of product characteristics, September 2007.
2. Everitt DE, Avorn J. Systemic effects of medications used to treat glaucoma. *Ann Intern Med* (1990) 112, 120–25.

Beta blockers + Potassium-depleting drugs

The use of potassium-depleting diuretics can precipitate the development of potentially life-threatening torsade de pointes in patients taking sotalol, unless potassium levels are maintained. This would also be expected with other potassium-depleting drugs such as corticosteroids, possibly some laxatives, and intravenous amphotericin.

Chlortalidone and hydrochlorothiazide may reduce the bioavailability of celiprolol, but the evidence for this is sparse.

Clinical evidence

(a) Pharmacokinetic effects

A study in 12 healthy subjects found that when **sotalol** 160 mg was given with **hydrochlorothiazide** 25 mg the pharmacokinetics of both drugs were unchanged.[1]

The manufacturer of **celiprolol** suggests that **chlortalidone** and **hydrochlorothiazide** reduce its bioavailability.[2] This appears to be based on a single-dose study that found that **chlortalidone** decreased the bioavailability of **celiprolol**, which is briefly mentioned in the report of an *in vitro* study,[3] which found that **chlortalidone** and **hydrochlorothiazide** blocked the active transport of **celiprolol** across the intestinal epithelium..

(b) QT-prolongation

A 4-year study in cardiac clinics in South Africa identified 13 patients who developed syncope and a prolonged QT interval while taking **sotalol** 80 to 480 mg daily. Twelve patients were taking a combined preparation (*Sotazide*) containing **sotalol** 160 mg and **hydrochlorothiazide** 25 mg. Eleven patients were being treated for hypertension, one for ventricular asystoles, and one for both. Polymorphous ventricular tachycardia was seen in 12 of the patients, and torsade de pointes was seen in 10 of these 12. Arrhythmias occurred within 72 hours of starting **sotalol** in 6 patients, and at varying intervals from 10 days to 3 years in the other 6 patients. Definite hypokalaemia (defined by the study as serum potassium of less than 3.5 mmol/L) was detected in 8 of the 13 patients. Four of the patients were also taking other drugs known to prolong the QT interval, namely disopyramide and tricyclic antidepressants. The problems resolved in all of the cases within 12 hours of stopping the **sotalol** and giving potassium supplements when indicated.[4] A further case of torsade de pointes has also been reported in a patient who developed hypokalaemia while taking **sotalol** and **hydrochlorothiazide**.[5]

Mechanism

Potassium-depleting drugs may cause hypokalaemia, which increases the potential for torsade de pointes with any drug that prolongs the QT interval, including sotalol.

Importance and management

The interaction between potassium-depleting diuretics such as hydrochlorothiazide and sotalol that results in QT prolongation is established, clinically important and potentially life threatening.

Torsade de pointes may occur in patients taking sotalol alone and who appear to have no predisposing factors.[6] One study found that there is an increased risk of proarrhythmia as the dose of sotalol is increased, with an abrupt change occurring at doses greater than 320 mg daily.[7] According to the manufacturer, the incidence of severe proarrhythmias, including torsade de pointes, in clinical study patients taking sotalol was less than 2% for doses up to 320 mg daily, but more than doubled at higher doses.[8] However, torsade de pointes can occur even with small doses of sotalol if potassium depletion is present or allowed to develop.[8,9] It is clearly very important therefore to ensure that potassium levels are maintained if potassium-depleting drugs are given with sotalol. A list of potassium-depleting diuretics is given in 'Table 26.1', p.1117. Other drugs that may cause potassium depletion include the **corticosteroids** and intravenous **amphotericin**. It has also been suggested that stimulant **laxatives**, may cause potassium depletion, but note that this generally tends to occur with abuse, or long-term use.

The interactions of chlortalidone and hydrochlorothiazide with celiprolol are poorly documented and their clinical significance is unclear, although it would be expected to be limited.

1. Sundquist H, Anttila M, Simon A, Reich JW. Comparative bioavailability and pharmacokinetics of sotalol administered alone and in combination with hydrochlorothiazide. *J Clin Pharmacol* (1979) 19, 557–64.
2. Celectol (Celiprolol hydrochloride). Winthrop Pharmaceuticals UK Ltd. UK Summary of product characteristics, March 2009.
3. Karlsson J, Kuo S-M, Zeiminak J, Artursson P. Transport of celiprolol across human intestinal epithelial (Caco-2) cells: mediation of secretion by multiple transporters including P-glycoprotein. *Br J Pharmacol* (1993) 110, 1009–1016.
4. McKibbin JK, Pocock WA, Barlow JB, Scott Millar RN, Obel IWP. Sotalol, hypokalaemia, syncope, and torsade de pointes. *Br Heart J* (1984) 51, 157–62.
5. Bennett JM, Gourassas J, Konstantinides S. Torsade de pointes induced by sotalol and hypokalaemia. *S Afr Med J* (1995) 68, 591–2.
6. D'Aloia A, Faggiano P, Brentana L, Boldini A, Pedrinazzi C, Procopio R, Dei Cas L. Sustained torsade de pointes occurring early during oral sotalol therapy for atrial fibrillation recurrence prophylaxis in a patient without heart disease. *Int J Cardiol* (2005) 105, 337–9.
7. MacNeil DJ, Davies RO, Deitchman D. Clinical safety profile of sotalol in the treatment of arrhythmias. *Am J Cardiol* (1993) 72, 44A–50A.
8. Sotacor Tablets (Sotalol hydrochloride). Bristol-Myers Pharmaceuticals. UK Summary of product characteristics, January 2010.
9. Tan HH, Hsu LF, Kam RML, Chua T, Teo WS. A case series of sotalol-induced torsade de pointes in patients with atrial fibrillation a tale with a twist. *Ann Acad Med Singapore* (2003) 32, 403–7.

Beta blockers + Propafenone

Plasma metoprolol and propranolol concentrations can be increased by propafenone. This has led to toxicity in some cases. Profound hypotension and cardiac arrest has also occurred after a patient receiving timolol eye drops was given propafenone. Transient syncope and ECG changes have been seen in a patient taking carvedilol after a single-dose of propafenone was taken.

Clinical evidence

(a) Carvedilol

A case report describes a 76-year-old woman taking carvedilol, who experienced transient syncope 3 hours after self-administering a single 600-mg dose of propafenone for atrial fibrillation. On hospital admission, an ECG showed a left bundle-branch block and a first degree AV block, which resolved in the following hours.[1]

(b) Metoprolol

Four patients with ventricular arrhythmias taking metoprolol 150 to 200 mg daily had a 2- to 5-fold increase in their steady-state metoprolol plasma concentrations when they were given propafenone 150 mg three times daily. One of them developed distressing nightmares, and another had acute left ventricular failure with pulmonary oedema and haemoptysis, which resolved when the metoprolol dose was reduced or stopped. In four other patients taking metoprolol 50 mg three times daily and propafenone 150 mg three times daily, it was found that stopping metoprolol did not affect propafenone plasma concentrations.[2] Single-dose studies in healthy subjects found a 51% decrease in the clearance of metoprolol and a further 20% reduction in exercise-induced tachycardia at 90 minutes when propafenone was also given.[2]

A patient developed neurotoxicity (including vivid nightmares, fatigue, headache) when given metoprolol 100 mg daily in divided doses, which worsened while it was being withdrawn and replaced by propafenone 300 mg daily. The symptoms disappeared when both drugs were stopped.[3]

(c) Propranolol

In a study in 12 healthy subjects, propafenone 225 mg every 8 hours increased the steady-state plasma concentrations of propranolol 50 mg every 8 hours 2.1-fold. However, the beta-blocking effects were only modestly increased and the propafenone pharmacokinetics remained unchanged.[4]

(d) Timolol

A case report describes a 59-year-old woman receiving timolol eye drops who was given propafenone 450 mg then 300 mg, 6 hours apart, for pharmacological cardioversion of atrial fibrillation. About 2.5 hours later she developed profound hypotension and cardiac arrest. The hypotension was initially resistant to treatment with cortisone, adrenaline (epinephrine) and colloid infusion. A week later an ECG showed sinus rhythm with ectopic supraventricular beats.[5]

Mechanism

Both propafenone and beta blockers have negative inotropic effects, which could be additive. In addition, propafenone appears to be an inhibitor of CYP2D6, by which carvedilol, metoprolol and propranolol are metabolised. It is therefore likely that this is the reason for the increased plasma concentrations of metoprolol and propranolol. Whether the effect seen with carvedilol and propafenone is due to altered metabolism is unclear.

Importance and management

Information about an interaction between propafenone and the beta blockers is limited, but the pharmacokinetic interaction would seem to be established. Concurrent use need not be avoided but anticipate the need to reduce the dose of metoprolol and propranolol. Monitor closely because some patients might experience adverse effects. If the suggested mechanism of interaction is correct it is possible (but not confirmed) that other beta blockers that undergo liver metabolism will interact similarly, but not those largely excreted unchanged in the urine. See 'Table 22.1', p.999 for the metabolism of some commonly used beta blockers.

The clinical relevance of the isolated cases involving carvedilol and timolol eye drops is unclear. Hypotension is known to occur with propafenone alone, but as propafenone and the beta blockers have negative inotropic effects, which could be additive and result in unwanted cardiodepression, it would seem prudent to consider the potential for adverse cardiac effects if propafenone is given with any beta blocker.

1. Patanè S, Marte F, Di Bella G. Transient syncope, left bundle branch block and first degree atrioventricular block after "pill-in-the-pocket" administration. *Int J Cardiol* (2008) 126, e19–e21.
2. Wagner F, Kalusche D, Trenk D, Jähnchen E, Roskamm H. Drug interaction between propafenone and metoprolol. *Br J Clin Pharmacol* (1987) 24, 213–20.
3. Ahmad S. Metoprolol-induced delirium perpetuated by propafenone. *Am Fam Physician* (1991) 44, 1142–3.
4. Kowey PR, Kirsten EB, Fu C-HJ, Mason WD. Interaction between propranolol and propafenone in healthy volunteers. *J Clin Pharmacol* (1989) 29, 512–17.
5. Patane S, Marte F, Di Bella G, Pugliatti P. Atrial fibrillation, pharmacological cardioversion and topical ophthalmic beta-blocker use. *Int J Cardiol* (2008) 126, e43–e46.

Beta blockers + Propantheline

Propantheline delays but modestly increases the extent of atenolol absorption. Propantheline delays but does not appear to affect the extent of metoprolol absorption.

Clinical evidence

(a) Atenolol

In a study, 6 healthy subjects took a single 100-mg dose of atenolol alone or 90 minutes after they had taken a single 30-mg dose of propantheline. The time to reach maximum plasma levels of atenolol was increased from 2.1 hours to 4.5 hours, and the AUC of atenolol was increased by 36%.[1]

(b) Metoprolol

In a crossover study, 7 healthy subjects received a single weight-adjusted intravenous dose of propantheline of 10 to 30 mg, or placebo, followed 15 minutes later by a single 100-mg oral dose of metoprolol. The time to reach the maximum plasma levels of metoprolol was increased from 1.3 hours to 4.6 hours, and its maximum plasma level was decreased by 24% when it was given after propantheline. There was no change in the AUC of metoprolol, although measurements were only made up to 8 hours, so this does not rule out a modest effect.[2]

Mechanism

Propantheline decreases gut motility, and delays the absorption of atenolol and metoprolol.

Importance and management

An interaction between propantheline and atenolol or metoprolol would appear to be established, and is generally in line with what would be expected from the known effects of propantheline on gut motility. However, the pharmacokinetic changes that occurred were small, and not clinically relevant. Therefore there seems to be no need to separate the administration of propantheline and these beta blockers.

1. Regårdh CG, Lundborg P, Persson BA. The effect of antacid, metoclopramide and propantheline on the bioavailability of metoprolol and atenolol. *Biopharm Drug Dispos* (1981) 2, 79–87.
2. Briant RH, Dorrington RE, Ferry DG, Paxton JW. Bioavailability of metoprolol in young adults and the elderly, with additional studies on the effects of metoclopramide and probanthine. *Eur J Clin Pharmacol* (1983) 25, 353–6.

Beta blockers + Proton pump inhibitors

Proton pump inhibitors do not appear to alter the pharmacokinetics or pharmacological effects of metoprolol and propranolol.

Clinical evidence

(a) Metoprolol

In a crossover study in 7 healthy subjects, **omeprazole** 40 mg daily for 8 days had no effect on the steady-state plasma concentration of metoprolol 100 mg daily.[1] Similarly, in a crossover study 18 healthy subjects, **pantoprazole** 40 mg daily for 5 days did not alter the steady-state pharmacokinetics of metoprolol 95 mg daily, and did not change the pharmacodynamics of metoprolol based on the effect on heart rate, when compared with placebo.[2]

(b) Propranolol

In a crossover study in 8 healthy subjects, **omeprazole** 20 mg daily for 8 days had no effect on the steady-state plasma concentration of propranolol 80 mg twice daily, and no effect on resting and exercising heart rates or blood pressure, when compared with placebo.[3] Similarly, in a crossover study in 18 healthy subjects, **lansoprazole** 60 mg daily for 7 days had no effect on the pharmacokinetics of a single 80-mg dose of propranolol.[4]

Mechanism

Metoprolol and propranolol are mainly metabolised by CYP2D6 and so would not be expected to be affected by lansoprazole and omeprazole, which are inhibitors of and substrates for CYP2C19. Pantoprazole would also not be anticipated to interact.

Importance and management

No interaction would be expected between the beta blockers and the proton pump inhibitors, and the studies cited here confirm the lack of interaction between metoprolol and omeprazole or pantoprazole; and propranolol and omeprazole or lansoprazole. No dose adjustments are therefore necessary if these proton pump inhibitors are given with propranolol or metoprolol.

1. Andersson T, Lundborg P, Regårdh CG. Lack of effect of omeprazole treatment on steady-state plasma levels of metoprolol. *Eur J Clin Pharmacol* (1991) 40, 61–5.
2. Koch HJ, Hartmann M, Bliesath H, Huber R, Steinijans VW, Mascher H, Wurst W. Pantoprazole has no influence on steady state pharmacokinetics and pharmacodynamics of metoprolol in healthy volunteers. *Int J Clin Pharmacol Ther* (1996) 34, 420–3.
3. Henry D, Brent P, Whyte I, Mihaly G, Devenish-Meares S. Propranolol steady-state pharmacokinetics are unaltered by omeprazole. *Eur J Clin Pharmacol* (1987) 33, 369–73.
4. Karol MD, Locke CS, Cavanaugh JH. Lack of interaction between lansoprazole and propranolol, a pharmacokinetic and safety assessment. *J Clin Pharmacol* (2000) 40, 301–8.

Beta blockers + Quinidine

An isolated report describes a patient taking quinidine who developed marked bradycardia when using timolol eye drops. Other case reports describe orthostatic hypotension when quinidine was given with atenolol, propranolol or unnamed beta blockers. Quinidine can raise plasma metoprolol, propranolol, and timolol levels.

Both sotalol and quinidine can prolong the QT interval, which may increase the risk of torsade de pointes if they are used together.

Clinical evidence

(a) Atenolol

A 56-year-old woman taking isosorbide dinitrate, diltiazem and quinidine sulfate 300 mg four times daily developed orthostatic hypotension 3 days after she started taking atenolol 50 mg daily. This resolved within 2 days of stopping the atenolol. Before starting the quinidine, she had previously taken atenolol and the other drugs without problems.[1]

(b) Metoprolol

A metabolic study in 5 healthy subjects who were extensive metabolisers of CYP2D6 (that is, those with normal levels of this isoenzyme) found that a single 50-mg dose of quinidine markedly inhibited the metabolism of a single 100-mg dose of metoprolol, which effectively made the subjects poor metabolisers (that is, those that are deficient or lacking CYP2D6). The plasma levels of metoprolol were raised about threefold. Quinidine had no effect on metoprolol pharmacokinetics in 5 poor metabolisers.[2] Similar results have been found when quinidine 50 mg daily was given with metoprolol 100 mg twice daily for 7 days,[3] and when a 20-mg dose of metoprolol was given intravenously following either a single 50-mg dose of quinidine, or quinidine slow-release tablets 250 mg twice daily for 3 days.[4] The effect on heart-rate reduction was small given the increase in metoprolol levels.[3]

(c) Propranolol

A single-dose pharmacokinetic study found that quinidine 200 mg doubled the AUC and the peak plasma levels of a 20-mg dose of propranolol. Maximum heart rates during exercise were suppressed by 45% more than with propranolol alone.[5] Other controlled studies have also found that quinidine increases the AUC of propranolol two- to threefold,[6,7] and this has resulted in increased beta-blockade.[7] In contrast, one earlier controlled study found no effect of quinidine on propranolol levels.[8]

In a non-controlled study, the peak plasma levels of a single 200-mg dose of quinidine were more than 50% higher and clearance was almost 40% lower in 7 patients taking propranolol 40 to 400 mg daily when compared with 8 patients not taking propranolol. However, the quinidine elimination half-life was unchanged.[9] In contrast, in two other controlled studies, propranolol did not alter the pharmacokinetics of quinidine.[8,10]

A man taking propranolol 40 mg four times daily developed orthostatic hypotension, with symptoms of dizziness and faintness on standing, when he took quinidine 200 mg four times daily. This resolved when quinidine was withdrawn.[11] The same authors subsequently briefly reported another two cases of orthostatic hypotension when quinidine was given with **unnamed beta blockers**.[12]

(d) Sotalol

Although one study reports the safe concurrent use of sotalol and quinidine,[13] both drugs can prolong the QT interval, which may increase the risk of torsade de pointes if they are used together. See 'Drugs that prolong the QT interval + Other drugs that prolong the QT interval', p.272, for a general review of QT prolongation and drug interactions.

(e) Timolol

An elderly man taking quinidine sulfate 500 mg three times daily for premature atrial beats was hospitalised with dizziness 12 weeks after starting to use timolol 0.5% eye drops for open-angle glaucoma. He was found to have a sinus bradycardia of 36 bpm. The symptoms abated when the drugs were withdrawn and normal sinus rhythm returned after 24 hours. The same symptoms developed within 30 hours of re-starting both drugs, but disappeared when the quinidine was withdrawn.[14]

In a later study in 13 healthy subjects, a single 50-mg oral dose of quinidine was given 30 minutes before 2 drops of timolol 0.5% ophthalmic solution, put into each *nostril*. In 8 extensive metabolisers of CYP2D6 (that is, those with normal levels of this isoenzyme), quinidine caused a further decrease in heart rate and increase in plasma timolol levels, when compared with timolol alone. Giving quinidine with timolol in these extensive metabolisers gave results similar to giving timolol alone in 5 poor metabolisers of CYP2D6 (that is, those that are deficient or lacking CYP2D6).[15] In another study, quinidine augmented the plasma levels and cardiac effects of intravenous timolol.[16]

Mechanism

Quinidine appears to increase metoprolol, propranolol and timolol plasma levels by inhibiting the cytochrome P450 isoenzyme CYP2D6, thereby reducing their clearance.[2,7,15] As CYP2D6 shows polymorphism, these interactions would be most apparent in patients with normal CYP2D6 activity (extensive metabolisers), effectively making them poor metabolisers. See 'Genetic factors in drug metabolism', p.8, for further information on genetic polymorphism.

Importance and management

The pharmacokinetic interaction between quinidine and metoprolol, propranolol and timolol would seem to be established, but it is of uncertain clinical importance. Normally the beta blockers are considered to have a wide therapeutic range, and so raises in levels are generally well tolerated. Patients with heart failure are usually more at risk, because drugs such as metoprolol need slow and careful dose titration in this condition, and therefore some monitoring in this patient group (e.g. for shortness of breath, bradycardia, hypotension) may be prudent. There appears to be no information about other beta blockers, but all those metabolised by CYP2D6 would be expected to be affected to some extent. See 'Table 22.1', p.999, for a list.

Only one isolated case of possible excessive beta-blockade has been reported (with quinidine and timolol eye drops). Concurrent use need not be avoided (and may be beneficial in the treatment of atrial fibrillation), but some care is warranted as both quinidine and the beta blockers have negative inotropic effects, which could be additive and result in unwanted cardiodepression. The general relevance of the isolated reports of orthostatic hypotension with atenolol or propranolol and quinidine is uncertain.

Both quinidine and sotalol prolong the QT interval. The general consensus is that the combination of two drugs that prolong the QT interval should usually be avoided, or only used with great caution. See 'Drugs that prolong the QT interval + Other drugs that prolong the QT interval', p.272, for more information about the concurrent use of QT-prolonging drugs.

1. Manolis AS, Estes NA. Orthostatic hypotension due to quinidine and atenolol. *Am J Med* (1987) 82, 1083–4.
2. Leemann T, Dayer P, Meyer UA. Single-dose quinidine treatment inhibits metoprolol oxidation in extensive metabolizers. *Eur J Clin Pharmacol* (1986) 29, 739–41.
3. Schlanz KD, Yingling KW, Verme CN, Lalonde RL, Harrison DC, Bottorff MB. Loss of stereoselective metoprolol metabolism following quinidine inhibition of P450IID6. *Pharmacotherapy* (1991) 11, 272.
4. Leeman TD, Devi KP, Dayer P. Similar effect of oxidation deficiency (debrisoquine polymorphism) and quinidine on the apparent volume of distribution of (±)-metoprolol. *Eur J Clin Pharmacol* (1993) 45, 65–71.
5. Sakurai T, Kawai C, Yasuhara M, Okumura K, Hori R. Increased plasma concentration of propranolol by a pharmacokinetic interaction with quinidine. *Jpn Circ J* (1983) 47, 872–3.
6. Yasuhara M, Yatsuzuka A, Yamada K, Okumura K, Hori R, Sakurai T, Kawai C. Alteration of propranolol pharmacokinetics and pharmacodynamics by quinidine in man. *J Pharmacobiodyn* (1990) 13, 681–7.
7. Zhou H-H, Anthony LB, Roden DM, Wood AJJ. Quinidine reduces clearance of (+)-propranolol more than (−)-propranolol through marked reduction in 4-hydroxylation. *Clin Pharmacol Ther* (1990) 47, 686–93.
8. Fenster P, Perrier D, Mayersohn M, Marcus FI. Kinetic evaluation of the propranolol-quinidine combination. *Clin Pharmacol Ther* (1980) 27, 450–3.
9. Kessler KM, Humphries WC, Black M, Spann JF. Quinidine pharmacokinetics in patients with cirrhosis or receiving propranolol. *Am Heart J* (1978) 96, 627–35.
10. Kates RE, Blanford MF. Disposition kinetics of oral quinidine when administered concurrently with propranolol. *J Clin Pharmacol* (1979) 19, 378–83.
11. Loon NR, Wilcox CS, Folger W. Orthostatic hypotension due to quinidine and propranolol. Am J Med (1986) 81, 1101–4. Correction. *ibid.* (1987) 82, 870.
12. Loon NR, Wilcox CS. Orthostatic hypotension due to quinidine and propranolol. The reply. *Am J Med* (1987) 82, 1277.
13. Dorian P, Newman D, Berman N, Hardy J, Mitchell J. Sotalol and type IA drugs in combination prevent recurrence of sustained ventricular tachycardia. *J Am Coll Cardiol* (1993) 22, 106–13.
14. Dinai Y, Sharir M, Naveh N, Halkin H. Bradycardia induced by interaction between quinidine and ophthalmic timolol. *Ann Intern Med* (1985) 103, 890–1.
15. Edeki TI, He H, Wood AJJ. Pharmacogenetic explanation for excessive β-blockade following timolol eye drops. *JAMA* (1995) 274, 1611–13.
16. Kaila T, Huupponen R, Karhuvaara S, Havula P, Scheinin M, Iisalo E, Salminen L. Beta-blocking effects of timolol at low plasma concentrations. *Clin Pharmacol Ther* (1991) 49, 53–8.

Beta blockers + Quinolones

Ciprofloxacin modestly reduces the clearance of metoprolol. Some quinolones prolong the QT interval and this effect may be additive with the known QT-prolonging effects of sotalol.

Clinical evidence, mechanism, importance and management

(a) Metoprolol

Preliminary evidence from 7 healthy subjects given a single 100-mg dose of metoprolol suggested that pretreatment with **ciprofloxacin** 500 mg, given every 12 hours for 5 doses, increased the AUC of *(+)*-metoprolol by 54% and reduced its clearance by 39%. The AUC of *(−)*-metoprolol was increased by 29% and its clearance reduced by 12%.[1] It has been suggested that this interaction may occur because **ciprofloxacin** inhibits the activity of the cytochrome P450 isoenzymes concerned with the metabolism and clearance of metoprolol. However, this is questionable as metoprolol is extensively metabolised by the cytochrome P450 isoenzyme CYP2D6 while **ciprofloxacin** inhibits CYP1A2. Changes of this size, or even more, in the AUC of beta blockers are not usually considered to be clinically relevant because the beta blockers have a wide therapeutic margin. Patients with heart failure are usually more at risk, because drugs such as metoprolol need slow and careful dose titration in this condition, but even in this patient group the rise in levels is unlikely to be generally important.

(b) Sotalol

In an analysis of the FDA Adverse Events Reporting System database for cases of torsade de pointes associated with fluoroquinolones, two cases of torsade de pointes were noted in patients taking a fluoroquinolone with sotalol (there were 37 cases identified, and 19 occurred in patients also taking other drugs known to prolong the QT interval).[2] Sotalol has class III antiarrhythmic effects and prolongs the QT interval, and this effect could be additive with the effects of quinolones that prolong the QT interval (e.g. **gatifloxacin**, **moxifloxacin**, **sparfloxacin**, see 'Table 9.2', p.273).The concurrent use of sotalol and these quinolones should generally be avoided (see 'Drugs that prolong the QT interval + Other drugs that prolong the QT interval', p.272). For a case report of an elderly woman who developed torsade de pointes after receiving amiodarone, sotalol and **ciprofloxacin** within the space of 4 days, see 'Amiodarone + Quinolones', p.265.

1. Waite NM, Rutledge DR, Warbasse LH, Edwards DJ. Disposition of the (+) and (−) isomers of metoprolol following ciprofloxacin treatment. *Pharmacotherapy* (1990) 10, 236.
2. Frothingham R. Rates of torsades de pointes associated with ciprofloxacin, ofloxacin, levofloxacin, gatifloxacin, and moxifloxacin. *Pharmacotherapy* (2001) 21, 1468–72.?tpb=-4pt>

Beta blockers + Rifampicin (Rifampin)

Rifampicin increases the clearance of bisoprolol, carvedilol, celiprolol, metoprolol, tertatolol and talinolol, and reduces their plasma levels. Similar but smaller effects have been seen when atenolol is given with rifampicin, but a case report suggests that occasionally the effects may be large enough to be of clinical relevance. The effects of rifampicin on propranolol appear more pronounced.

Clinical evidence

(a) Atenolol

A case report describes a man taking atenolol for angina whose exercise threshold before developing angina symptoms appreciably worsened when he was given rifampicin 600 mg daily as part of a standard antitubercular regimen. Rifampicin was stopped, and after a week **rifabutin** 300 mg daily was started. **Rifabutin** did not cause any change in his baseline exercise tolerance.[1] In a randomised, placebo-controlled, crossover study, 9 healthy subjects were given rifampicin 600 mg daily for 5 days, with a single 100-mg dose of atenolol on day 6. Although some pharmacokinetic changes were seen they were variable between subjects and in most cases slight (e.g. a 19% reduction in AUC). Heart rate and blood pressure were on average slightly higher in the presence of rifampicin (3.5 bpm and 4.3/3.9 mmHg, respectively), suggesting a modest reduction in the effects of atenolol, which was expected to be of only minor clinical relevance.[2]

(b) Bisoprolol

The AUC of bisoprolol 10 mg daily was reduced by 34% in healthy subjects given rifampicin 600 mg daily.[3]

(c) Carvedilol

Rifampicin 600 mg daily for 12 days caused a 60% decrease in the maximum serum levels and the AUC of carvedilol.[4]

(d) Celiprolol

In a study in healthy subjects, rifampicin 600 mg daily reduced the AUC of a single 200-mg dose of celiprolol by 55%.[5]

(e) Metoprolol

In a study in healthy subjects, rifampicin 600 mg daily reduced the AUC of a single 100-mg dose of metoprolol by 33%.[6]

(f) Propranolol

In a study in 6 healthy subjects, rifampicin 600 mg daily for 3 weeks increased the oral clearance of propranolol almost threefold. Increasing the rifampicin dose to 900 mg or

1.2 g daily did not further increase the clearance. Four weeks after withdrawing the rifampicin the blood levels of propranolol had returned to normal.[7] In a similar study the oral clearance of propranolol was increased by about fourfold by rifampicin 600 mg daily for 3 weeks in both poor and extensive metabolisers of propranolol.[8]

(g) Talinolol

In a study in 8 healthy subjects, rifampicin 600 mg daily decreased the AUC of a single-dose of talinolol 30 mg intravenously or 100 mg orally by 21% and 35%, respectively.[9]

(h) Tertatolol

Rifampicin 600 mg daily for a week increased the clearance of tertatolol almost threefold and reduced its half-life from 9 hours to 3.4 hours. A slight reduction in the effects of tertatolol on blood pressure was seen and heart rates were raised from 68 bpm to 74 bpm.[10]

Mechanism

Rifampicin is a potent liver-enzyme inducer that increases the metabolism and clearance of extensively metabolised beta blockers such as propranolol and metoprolol. Rifampicin may induce systems other than cytochrome P450, such as glucuronidation, which is relevant to the metabolism of propranolol.[8] Rifampicin also increases duodenal P-glycoprotein expression, so the increased clearance of talinolol (which is not hepatically metabolised) may be due to induction of P-glycoprotein, which increases the excretion of talinolol.[9] The effects on atenolol, which is not extensively metabolised, are also possibly due to induction of P-glycoprotein or some other transporter,[2] although this needs confirmation.

Importance and management

The interactions between rifampicin and the beta blockers are established. Their clinical importance is uncertain but probably small.[10] Nevertheless, they cannot be completely dismissed as the case report with atenolol shows. Consider increasing the dose of the beta blocker if there is any evidence that the therapeutic response is inadequate. Any beta blocker that undergoes extensive liver metabolism would be expected to be affected by the enzyme-inducing effects of rifampicin (see 'Table 22.1', p.999). An interaction may also occur with beta blockers that are substrates for P-glycoprotein, such as talinolol. Those beta blockers mainly lost unchanged in the urine would not be expected to be affected by rifampicin, and the minor pharmacokinetic changes seen in the study with atenolol support this suggestion. However, the case report describing reduced exercise tolerance in a patient taking rifampicin and atenolol suggests that concurrent use may not be entirely without problems, and therefore caution seems warranted in with any beta blocker and rifampicin.

1. Goldberg SV, Hanson D, Peloquin CA. Rifamycin treatment of tuberculosis in a patient receiving atenolol: less interaction with rifabutin than with rifampin. *Clin Infect Dis* (2003), 37, 607–8.
2. Lilja JJ, Juntti-Patinen L, Neuvonen PJ. Effect of rifampicin on the pharmacokinetics of atenolol. *Basic Clin Pharmacol Toxicol* (2006) 98, 555–8.
3. Kirch W, Rose I, Klingmann I, Pabst J, Ohnhaus EE. Interaction of bisoprolol with cimetidine and rifampicin. *Eur J Clin Pharmacol* (1986) 31, 59–62.
4. Ruffolo RR, Boyle DA, Venuti RP, Lukas MA. Carvedilol (Kredex®): a novel multiple action cardiovascular agent. *Drugs Today* (1991) 27, 465–92.
5. Lilja JJ, Niemi M, Neuvonen PJ. Rifampicin reduces plasma concentrations of celiprolol. *Eur J Clin Pharmacol* (2004) 59, 819–24.
6. Bennett PN, John VA, Whitmarsh VB. Effect of rifampicin on metoprolol and antipyrine kinetics. *Br J Clin Pharmacol* (1982) 13, 387–91.
7. Herman RJ, Nakamura K, Wilkinson GR, Wood AJJ. Induction of propranolol metabolism by rifampicin. *Br J Clin Pharmacol* (1983) 16, 565–9.
8. Shaheen O, Biollaz J, Koshakji RP, Wilkinson GR, Wood AJJ. Influence of debrisoquin phenotype on the inducibility of propranolol metabolism. *Clin Pharmacol Ther* (1989) 45, 439–43.
9. Westphal K, Weinbrenner A, Zschiesche M, Franke G, Knoke M, Oertel R, Fritz P, von Richter O, Warzok R, Hachenberg T, Kauffmann H-M, Schrenk D, Terhaag B, Kroemer HK, Siegmund W. Induction of P-glycoprotein by rifampin increases intestinal secretion of talinolol in human beings: a new type of drug/drug interaction. *Clin Pharmacol Ther* (2000) 68, 345–55.
10. Kirch W, Milferstädt S, Halabi A, Rocher I, Efthymiopoulos C, Jung L. Interaction of tertatolol with rifampicin and ranitidine pharmacokinetics and antihypertensive activity. *Cardiovasc Drugs Ther* (1990) 4, 487–92.

Beta blockers + SSRIs

Fluoxetine can increase pindolol and carvedilol levels, and possibly increases metoprolol and propranolol levels (isolated cases of lethargy and bradycardia have been reported). Paroxetine appears to increase carvedilol levels and may increase levels of metoprolol resulting in increased beta-blocking effects; this has led to AV block in one case, and other clinical manifestations of excessive beta-blockade in other patients. Citalopram and escitalopram may also increase metoprolol levels. Fluvoxamine probably markedly raises propranolol levels (there is a case of hypotension and bradycardia), but does not alter the pharmacokinetics of atenolol, although slight bradycardia and hypotension were reported. Sertraline does not alter the beta-blocking effects of atenolol.

Clinical evidence

(a) Citalopram

The manufacturers state that although the concurrent use of **metoprolol** and citalopram has no statistically or clinically significant effect on heart rate and blood pressure, the plasma concentrations of **metoprolol** are increased 2-fold,[1,2] which might decrease its cardioselectivity.[2]

(b) Escitalopram

The manufacturers state that escitalopram causes a 2-fold increase in the plasma concentration of **metoprolol**,[3] or a 50% increase in the plasma concentration of **metoprolol** and an 82% increase in its AUC.[4] They note that, although the concurrent use of **metoprolol** and escitalopram has no clinically significant effect on heart rate and blood pressure, this increase in plasma concentrations might decrease the cardioselectivity of **metoprolol**.[4]

(c) Fluoxetine

Metoprolol 100 mg daily improved the angina of a man who had undergone a coronary artery bypass 4 years earlier. A month later he was given fluoxetine 20 mg daily for depression. Within 2 days he complained of profound lethargy, and his resting heart rate was found to have fallen from 64 bpm to 36 bpm. The fluoxetine was withdrawn, and within 5 days his heart rate returned to 64 bpm. The **metoprolol** was replaced by **sotalol** 80 mg twice daily and fluoxetine reintroduced without problems.[5]

A patient taking **propranolol** 40 mg twice daily developed bradycardia of 30 bpm, heart block and syncope 2 weeks after starting fluoxetine 20 mg daily. This patient possibly also had some pre-existing conduction disease contributing to the effect.[6]

When 9 healthy subjects were given **pindolol** 5 mg every 6 hours with fluoxetine (20 mg daily for 3 days and then 60 mg daily for another 7 days), the **pindolol** AUC rose by about 75% and its clearance fell by about 45%, when compared with a single 5-mg dose of **pindolol**. Only mild to moderate alterations in pulse rate and blood pressure were seen.[7] A crossover study in 10 patients with heart failure, taking **carvedilol** 25 to 50 mg twice daily, found that the addition of fluoxetine 20 mg daily for 28 days increased the AUC of ***R*-carvedilol** by 77%, and decreased the clearance of both enantiomers by 44 to 56%. However, these pharmacokinetic changes were of little clinical importance, and there were no changes in blood pressure, heart rate, and heart rate variability.[8]

(d) Fluvoxamine

A 79-year-old man who had taken **propranolol** for prophylaxis of migraine for several years developed fatigue and lightheadedness within a few days of starting fluvoxamine. He was admitted to hospital with syncope and bradycardia of 38 bpm but recovered after both drugs were discontinued.[9] In healthy subjects, fluvoxamine 100 mg daily raised the plasma levels of **propranolol** 160 mg daily fivefold, but the bradycardic effects were only slightly increased (by 3 bpm). The diastolic pressure following exercise was only slightly reduced but the general hypotensive effects remained unaltered.[10] Fluvoxamine did not change the plasma levels of **atenolol** 100 mg daily, but the heart-slowing effects were slightly increased and the hypotensive effects were slightly decreased.[10]

(e) Paroxetine

In a study in 17 patients who had been diagnosed with an acute myocardial infarction, the pharmacokinetics and pharmacodynamics of metoprolol were assessed before and 8 days after starting paroxetine 20 mg daily. The AUC_{0-12} of **metoprolol** was increased 4.2-fold by paroxetine. Two patients required a reduction in the dose of **metoprolol**, one due to bradycardia and one due to postural hypotension. Excessive hypotension was also noted in 4 other patients, but because this was well tolerated it did not require a dose reduction and it may have been due to other medication.[11] A patient taking paroxetine 20 mg daily developed presyncope and complete AV block 15 days after starting **metoprolol** 50 mg daily. Both drugs were stopped and the AV block resolved over 5 days. **Metoprolol** was then reinstated for 5 days without any sign of bradyarrhythmia. Two weeks after replacing **metoprolol** with amlodipine and aspirin, paroxetine was reintroduced at 10 mg daily and gradually increased to 20 mg daily without any signs of bradyarrhythmia.[12] Another case report describes bradycardia in a 62-year-old patient taking paroxetine 20 mg daily and **metoprolol**, which persisted despite a reduction in the metoprolol dose from 100 mg daily to 25 mg daily, and eventually required the discontinuation of metoprolol.[13]

A study in 8 healthy subjects found that paroxetine 20 mg daily for 6 days increased the AUCs of *R*- and *S*-metoprolol eightfold and fivefold, respectively, after a single 100-mg dose of **metoprolol**. The maximum plasma concentration and elimination half-life were increased about twofold. The beta-blocking effects of **metoprolol** were more sustained and the reduction in exercise systolic pressure was more pronounced when paroxetine was also taken, when compared with **metoprolol** alone.[14]

In a crossover study, 11 healthy subjects were given a single 12.5-mg dose of **carvedilol** with paroxetine. Paroxetine increased the AUC of both *R*- and *S*-carvedilol 2.5-fold and 90%, respectively. However, these pharmacokinetics changes did not alter the effect of carvedilol on blood pressure, heart rate and PR interval, although there was wide interindividual variability in the pharmacokinetic parameters reported.[15]

(f) Sertraline

In a single-dose study in 10 healthy subjects, the beta-blocking effects of **atenolol** 50 mg were unchanged by sertraline 100 mg given 5 hours before the **atenolol**.[16,17]

(g) Unnamed SSRIs

In a small cohort study in 250 patients with end-stage heart failure, the risk of death from cardiovascular causes during an 18 month follow-up was lower in patients with depression who were taking a beta blocker and an SSRI, when compared with those who were taking an SSRI and no beta blocker; hazard ratio for death 2.2 for those taking an SSRI alone compared with those taking a beta blocker with an SSRI. The beta blockers being taken were **metoprolol**, **carvedilol** or **nebivolol**, but the SSRIs were unspecified.[18] In contrast, in a very large cohort study of patients who had been previously hospitalised for heart failure, the adjusted hazard ratio for death from a cardiovascular cause in 4 045 patients who were taking a beta blocker and an SSRI was slightly higher than in 11 627 patients taking an SSRI with no beta blocker (1.3 versus 1.13). Similar results were found when the analysis was performed for **metoprolol**, **carvedilol** and **bisoprolol** separately.[19]

Mechanism

Fluoxetine and paroxetine inhibit CYP2D6 thus inhibiting the metabolism of some beta blockers (e.g. propranolol, metoprolol, carvedilol) so that they accumulate, the result being that their effects, such as bradycardia, may be increased.[5] Citalopram and escitalopram may also inhibit CYP2D6. *In vitro* studies with human liver microsomes found that fluoxetine and paroxetine are potent inhibitors of metoprolol metabolism whereas fluvoxamine, sertraline and citalopram have less of an effect.[20] However, fluvoxamine also potently inhibits the metabolism of propranolol by CYP1A2.[9,21] Beta blockers that are not extensively metabolised, such as atenolol and sotalol, would not be expected to be affected by the SSRIs.

Importance and management

Pharmacokinetic interactions have been found between fluoxetine, fluvoxamine or paroxetine and some beta blockers, but despite marked pharmacokinetic changes, the clinical effects are probably not generally important. However, be aware that there are a few isolated reports of AV block with metoprolol and paroxetine and severe bradycardia with the use of a beta blocker and fluoxetine, or fluvoxamine. If problems arise, the interaction can apparently be avoided by giving a beta blocker (such as atenolol), which is not extensively metabolised. Alternatively, sertraline and citalopram seem to be less likely than the other SSRIs to interact with extensively metabolised beta blockers.[20] However, because metoprolol is considered to have a narrow therapeutic index in the treatment of heart failure, the UK manufacturers of escitalopram say that caution and possible dose adjustments are warranted on concurrent use.[3] Similarly the UK manufacturer of paroxetine suggests that concurrent use should be avoided if metoprolol is being used for heart failure.[22] Remember that fluoxetine and particularly its metabolite have long half-lives so that this interaction may possibly occur for some days after the fluoxetine has been stopped.

The conflicting findings from observational studies regarding mortality in heart failure with the combination of beta blockers and SSRIs are difficult to interpret due to the many variables involved and should therefore be used principally as hypothesis-generating studies for further randomised, controlled studies. Further study is required to consider the long term outcome of this combination.

There appears to be no information about other beta blockers, but all those metabolised by CYP2D6 would be expected to be affected by paroxetine and fluoxetine to some extent. See 'Table 22.1', p.999, for a list. Note that one of the manufacturers of **timolol**[23] lists the SSRIs as examples of CYP2D6 inhibitors that may interact; however, most SSRIs are less potent inhibitors of CYP2D6 than fluoxetine and paroxetine and are therefore less likely to interact to a clinically relevant extent.

1. Cipramil Tablets (Citalopram hydrobromide). Lundbeck Ltd. UK Summary of product characteristics, July 2015.
2. Celexa (Citalopram hydrobromide). Forest Pharmaceuticals, Inc. US Prescribing information, July 2014.
3. Cipralex Tablets (Escitalopram oxalate). Lundbeck Ltd. UK Summary of product characteristics, September 2013.
4. Lexapro (Escitalopram oxalate). Forest Pharmaceuticals Inc. US Prescribing information, July 2014.
5. Walley T, Pirmohamed M, Proudlove C, Maxwell D. Interaction of metoprolol and fluoxetine. *Lancet* (1993) 341, 967–8.
6. Drake WM, Gordon GD. Heart block in a patient on propranolol and fluoxetine. *Lancet* (1994) 343, 425–6.
7. Goldberg MJ, Bergstrom RF, Cerimele BJ, Thomassom HR, Hatcher BL, Simcox EA. Fluoxetine effects on pindolol pharmacokinetics. *Clin Pharmacol Ther* (1997) 61, 178.
8. Graff DW, Williamson KM, Pieper JA, Carson SW, Adams KF, Cascio WE, Patterson JH. Effect of fluoxetine on carvedilol pharmacokinetics, CYP2D6 activity, and autonomic balance in heart failure patients. *J Clin Pharmacol* (2001) 41, 97–106.
9. Morocco AP, Hendrickson RG. Propranolol-induced symptomatic bradycardia after initiation of fluvoxamine therapy. *J Toxicol Clin Toxicol* (2001) 39, 490–1.
10. Benfield P, Ward A. Fluvoxamine, a review of its pharmacodynamic and pharmacokinetic properties and therapeutic efficacy in depressive illness. *Drugs* (1986) 32, 313–34.
11. Goryachkina K, Burbello A, Boldueva S, Babak S, Bergman U, Bertilsson L. Inhibition of metoprolol metabolism and potentiation of its effects by paroxetine in routinely treated patients with acute myocardial infarction (AMI). *Eur J Clin Pharmacol* (2008) 64, 275–82.
12. Onalan O, Cumurcu BE, Bekar L. Complete atrioventricular block associated with concomitant use of metoprolol and paroxetine. *Mayo Clin Proc* (2008) 83, 595–9.
13. König F, Häfele M, Hauger B, Löble M, Wößner S, Wolfersdorf M. Bradykardie nach therapiebeginn mit Metoprolol und Paroxetin. *Psychiatr Prax* (1996) 23, 244–5.
14. Hemeryck A, Lefebvre RA, De Vriendt C, Belpaire FM. Paroxetine affects metoprolol pharmacokinetics and pharmacodynamics in healthy volunteers. *Clin Pharmacol Ther* (2000) 67, 283–9.
15. Stout SM, Nielsen J, Bleske BE, Shea M, Brook R, Kerber K, Welage LS. The impact of paroxetine coadministration on stereospecific carvedilol pharmacokinetics. *J Cardiovasc Pharmacol Ther* (2010) 15, 373–9.
16. Warrington SJ. Clinical implications of the pharmacology of sertraline. *Int Clin Psychopharmacol* (1991) 6 (Suppl 2), 11–21.
17. Ziegler MG, Wilner KD. Sertraline does not alter the β-adrenergic blocking activity of atenolol in healthy male volunteers. *J Clin Psychiatry* (1996) 57, (Suppl 1), 12–15.
18. Tousoulis D, Antoniades C, Drolias A, Stefanadi E, Marinou K, Vasiliadou C, Tsioufis C, Toutouzas K, Latsios G, Stefanadis C. Selective serotonin reuptake inhibitors modify the effect of β-blockers on long-term survival of patients with end-stage heart failure and major depression. *J Card Fail* (2008) 14, 456–64.
19. Fosbøl EL, Gislason GH, Poulsen HE, Hansen ML, Folke F, Schramm TK, Olesen JB, Bretler D-M, Abildstrøm SZ, Sørensen R, Hvelplund A, Køber L, Torp-Pedersen C. Prognosis in heart failure and the value of β-blockers are altered by the use of antidepressants and depend on the type of antidepressants used. *Circ Heart Fail* (2009) 2, 582–90.
20. Belpaire FM, Wijnant P, Temmerman A, Rasmussen BB, Brøsen K. The oxidative metabolism of metoprolol in human liver microsomes: inhibition by the selective serotonin reuptake inhibitors. *Eur J Clin Pharmacol* (1998) 54, 261–4.
21. Brøsen K, Skelbo E, Rasmussen BB, Poulsen HE, Loft S. Fluvoxamine is a potent inhibitor of cytochrome P4501A2. *Biochem Pharmacol* (1993) 45, 1211–14.
22. Paroxetine Film-Coated Tablets (Paroxetine hydrochloride anhydrous). Actavis UK Ltd. UK Summary of product characteristics, June 2015.
23. Cosopt Opthalmic Solution (Dorzolamide hydrochloride with Timolol maleate). Merck Sharp & Dohme Ltd. UK Summary of product characteristics, February 2010.

Beta blockers + Sulfinpyrazone

The antihypertensive effects of oxprenolol might be reduced or abolished by sulfinpyrazone. The pharmacokinetics of metoprolol are not affected by sulfinpyrazone.

Clinical evidence

Oxprenolol 80 mg twice daily was given to 10 hypertensive subjects for 15 days, which reduced their mean supine blood pressure from 161/101 mmHg to 149/96 mmHg, and their heart rate from 72 bpm to 66 bpm. When they were additionally given sulfinpyrazone 400 mg twice daily for 15 days, their mean blood pressure rose to about the former level. The reduction in mean heart rate remained unaffected. Sulfinpyrazone attenuated the reduction in cardiac workload seen with **oxprenolol** alone by about half.[1]

A study in 9 healthy subjects found that sulfinpyrazone 400 mg twice daily did not affect the pharmacokinetics of **metoprolol** 100 mg twice daily. Metoprolol did not alter the reduction in uric acid levels seen with sulfinpyrazone.[2]

Mechanism

Not understood. One idea is that the sulfinpyrazone inhibits the production of vasodilatory (antihypertensive) prostaglandins by the kidney. This would oppose the actions of the oxprenolol. If this was the case, an interaction with any beta blocker would also be expected, but there seems to be no evidence for this. Sulfinpyrazone does not appear to affect the cytochrome P450 isoenzyme CYP2D6, by which metoprolol is metabolised.

Importance and management

Information seems to be limited. If sulfinpyrazone is given to patients taking oxprenolol for hypertension, the effects should be monitored. It seems possible that this interaction could be accommodated by raising the dose of the oxprenolol but this needs confirmation. The effect of this interaction on cardiac workload appears to be less important, but it would still be prudent to monitor concurrent use if oxprenolol is used for angina. The pharmacokinetics of metoprolol do not appear to be affected by sulfinpyrazone. There appears to be no information regarding other beta blockers.

1. Ferrara LA, Mancini M, Marotta T, Pasanisi F, Fasano ML. Interference by sulphinpyrazone with the antihypertensive effects of oxprenolol. *Eur J Clin Pharmacol* (1986) 29, 717–19.
2. Cortellaro M, Boschetti C, Antoniazzi V, Polli EE, de Gaetano G, De Blasi A, Gerna M, Pezzi L, Garattini S. A pharmacokinetic and platelet function study of the combined administration of metoprolol and sulfinpyrazone to healthy volunteers. *Thromb Res* (1984) 34, 65–74.

Beta blockers + Tobacco or Nicotine ± Caffeine

Tobacco smoking can reduce the beneficial effects of the beta blockers on heart rate and blood pressure. Drinking coffee may have a similar but smaller effect, probably due to the caffeine content. Nicotine attenuates the effects of tobacco withdrawal, and this effect may be enhanced by some beta blockers.

Clinical evidence

(a) Caffeine

In a placebo-controlled study in 12 healthy subjects taking **propranolol** 240 mg or **metoprolol** 300 mg, two 150-mL cups of caffeine-containing coffee (made from 24 g of coffee) increased the mean blood pressure by 7%/22% with **propranolol** and 7%/19% with **metoprolol**. The increase with placebo was similar, at 4%/16% mmHg. The beta blockers and placebo were given in divided doses over 15 hours before the test.[1]

(b) Nicotine

A placebo-controlled, single-dose study in smokers given **carvedilol** 25 or 50 mg 140 minutes before a 4-mg nicotine lozenge found that **carvedilol** attenuated nicotine-induced increases in heart rate and blood pressure and also attenuated the self-reported 'bad effects' of nicotine but did not affect tobacco withdrawal symptoms.[2] Another similar study in 9 smokers found that a single 200-mg dose of **labetalol** attenuated the effects of a 15-mg/kg intravenous injection of nicotine on heart rate, whereas a single 100-mg dose of **labetalol** had no effect. Both doses of **labetalol** had no effect on the increase in blood pressure caused by nicotine. **Labetalol** 200 mg in conjunction with nicotine caused a greater attenuation in the symptoms of tobacco withdrawal than **labetalol** 100 mg.[3]

(c) Tobacco smoking

In a placebo-controlled study in 10 smokers with angina pectoris taking **propranolol** 240 mg daily or **atenolol** 100 mg daily, smoking reduced plasma **propranolol** levels by 25%, when compared with a non-smoking phase. Plasma **atenolol** levels were not significantly altered. Both of the beta blockers reduced heart rate at rest and during exercise, but the reductions were less when subjects smoked (effects attenuated by 8 to 14%).[4]

Other studies found that serum **propranolol** levels in smokers were about half those in non-smokers,[5,6] and that the AUC of a single 80-mg dose of **propranolol** was 38% lower in 6 smokers compared with 7 non-smokers.[7]

In another study, smoking caused an increase in blood pressure and heart rate in patients with angina and these effects were still evident, to a reduced extent, during **propranolol** treatment. In addition smoking abolished the beneficial effects of **propranolol** on ST-segment depression.[8]

(d) Tobacco smoking and caffeine

Eight patients with mild hypertension taking **propranolol** 80 mg twice daily, **oxprenolol** 80 mg twice daily or **atenolol** 100 mg daily over a 6-week period had their blood pressure monitored after smoking 2 tipped cigarettes and drinking coffee, containing 200 mg of caffeine. Their mean blood pressure rises over the following 2 hours were 8.5/8 mmHg in those taking **propranolol**, 12.1/9.1 mmHg in those taking **oxprenolol** and 5.2/4.4 mmHg in those taking **atenolol**.[9]

Mechanism

Smoking tobacco increases heart rate, blood pressure and the severity of myocardial ischaemia, probably as a direct effect of the nicotine and due to the reduced oxygen-carrying capacity of the blood.[4,8] These actions oppose the beneficial actions of the beta blockers. In addition, smoking induces the liver enzymes concerned with the metabolism of some beta blockers (e.g. propranolol[7]) so that their serum levels are reduced. However, the use of a beta blocker appears to enhance the beneficial effects of nicotine on tobacco withdrawal symptoms.

Caffeine causes the release of catecholamines, such as adrenaline (epinephrine), into the blood, which could account for the increases in heart rate and blood pressure that were seen in one study.[9] The blood pressure rise may be exaggerated in the presence of non-selective beta blockers, which block vasodilatation leaving the alpha (vasoconstrictor) effects of adrenaline unopposed. This will also oppose the actions of the beta blockers.

Importance and management

Evidence for an interaction between tobacco smoking and/or coffee intake and beta blockers is generally sparse. Smoking tobacco and (to a very much lesser extent) drinking coffee may oppose the effects of the beta blockers in the treatment of angina or hypertension, but the extent of any effect appears relatively modest. However, patients should be encouraged to stop smoking because, quite apart from its other toxic effects, it aggravates myocardial ischaemia, increases heart rate and can impair blood pressure control. If patients continue to smoke, it may be necessary to raise the doses of the beta blockers. The effects of the caffeine are quite small and there seems to be no strong reason to forbid the intake of beverages containing caffeine (e.g. tea, coffee, cola), but the excessive consumption of large amounts may not be a good idea, particularly in those who also smoke.

Evidence for an interaction between nicotine replacement therapy and beta blockers is also sparse; however, the concurrent use of nicotine and a beta blocker may actually be beneficial in minimising the effects of tobacco withdrawal. This requires further study.

1. Smits P, Hoffmann H, Thien T, Houben H, van't Laar A. Hemodynamic and humoral effects of coffee after β_1-selective and nonselective β-blockade. *Clin Pharmacol Ther* (1983) 34, 153–8.
2. Sofuoglu M, Mouratidis M, Yoo S, Kosten T. Adrenergic blocker carvedilol attenuates the cardiovascular and aversive effects of nicotine in abstinent smokers. *Behav Pharmacol* (2006) 17, 731–5.
3. Sofuoglu M, Babb D, Hatsukami DK. Labetalol treatment enhances the attenuation of tobacco withdrawal symptoms by nicotine in abstinent smokers. *Nicotin Tob Res* (2003) 5, 947–53.
4. Fox K, Deanfield J, Krikler S, Ribeiro P, Wright C. The interaction of cigarette smoking and β-adrenoceptor blockade. *Br J Clin Pharmacol* (1984) 17, 92S–93S.
5. Vestal RE, Wood AJJ, Branch RA, Shand DG, Wilkinson GR. Effects of age and cigarette smoking on propranolol disposition. *Clin Pharmacol Ther* (1979) 26, 8–15.
6. Gardner SK, Cady WJ, Ong YS. Effect of smoking on the elimination of propranolol hydrochloride. *Int J Clin Pharmacol Ther Toxicol* (1980) 18, 421–4.
7. Walle T, Walle UK, Cowart TD, Conradi EC, Gaffney TE. Selective induction of propranolol metabolism by smoking: additional effects on renal clearance of metabolites. *J Pharmacol Exp Ther* (1987) 241, 928–33.
8. Fox K, Jonathan A, Williams H, Selwyn A. Interaction between cigarettes and propranolol in treatment of angina pectoris. *BMJ* (1980) 281, 191–3.
9. Freestone S, Ramsey LE. Effect of β-blockade on the pressor response to coffee plus smoking in patients with mild hypertension. *Drugs* (1983) 25 (Suppl 2), 141–5.

Beta blockers + Tyrosine kinase inhibitors

The exposure to metoprolol is negligibly increased by imatinib. Other beta blockers metabolised by CYP2D6 might interact similarly. Gefitinib does not appear to affect metoprolol exposure.

Clinical evidence

(a) Gefitinib

In a study, 15 patients were given gefitinib 500 mg daily for 28 days, with a single 50-mg dose of **metoprolol** on day 15. The maximum plasma concentration of **metoprolol** was increased by about 10% by gefitinib. There was a 35% increase in the AUC of **metoprolol**, but this was not statistically significant.[1]

(b) Imatinib

In a pharmacokinetic study in 20 Chinese patients, a single 100-mg dose of **metoprolol** was given alone and then on day 7 of a 9-day course of imatinib 400 mg twice daily. The AUC and maximum plasma concentration of **metoprolol** were increased by about 20%, with a 24% increase in the AUC in 13 patients that were CYP2D6 extensive metabolisers (that is, those with normal activity of this isoenzyme) and a 17% increase in 7 patients that were said to be CYP2D6 intermediate metabolisers (those with lower activity of this isoenzyme). There were no clinically important changes in laboratory parameters, vital signs or ECG recordings.[2]

Mechanism

The UK manufacturer notes that *in vitro*, imatinib inhibits CYP2D6,[3] by which metoprolol is extensively metabolised. The study shows that clinically imatinib is only a very weak CYP2D6 inhibitor. Similarly, *in vitro* gefitinib inhibits CYP2D6,[1] but clinically, its effects are not clinically relevant.

Importance and management

The increase in metoprolol exposure seen with imatinib is negligible, and no clinically relevant interaction would be expected. Nevertheless, the UK manufacturer of imatinib recommends that clinical monitoring should be considered in patients taking metoprolol when given imatinib, because they consider metoprolol to be a drug with a narrow therapeutic range.[3] However, metoprolol is only usually classified as such in patients with heart failure, and even then, increases of this magnitude are not considered clinically relevant. Therefore this advice seems overly cautious.

The change in metoprolol exposure seen with gefitinib is not clinically relevant and no special precautions would seem necessary on concurrent use.

There appears to be no information about other beta blockers, but those also metabolised by CYP2D6 might be predicted to be affected by imatinib to some extent, depending on the level of involvement of CYP2D6 in their metabolism. See 'Table 22.1', p.999, for a list.

In addition, on the basis of these studies, dose adjustments are not likely to be necessary when imatinib or gefitinib are given with any other CYP2D6 substrates. Nevertheless, the UK manufacturers of both imatinib and gefitinib note that CYP2D6 substrates with a narrow therapeutic range should be given with caution,[3,4] and that a reduction in dose might be necessary.[4] Based on the available data with metoprolol, this seems over cautious.

Information about an interaction between other tyrosine kinase inhibitors and metoprolol is lacking.

1. Swaisland HC, Ranson M, Smith RP, Leadbetter J, Laight A, McKillop D, Wild MJ. Pharmacokinetic drug interactions of gefitinib with rifampicin, itraconazole and metoprolol. *Clin Pharmacokinet* (2005) 44, 1067–81.
2. Wang Y, Zhou L, Dutreix C, Leroy E, Yin Q, Sethuraman V, Riviere G-J, Yin OQP, Schran H, Shen Z-X. Effects of imatinib (Glivec) on the pharmacokinetics of metoprolol, a CYP2D6 substrate, in Chinese patients with chronic myelogenous leukaemia. *Br J Clin Pharmacol* (2008) 65, 885–92.
3. Glivec (Imatinib mesilate). Novartis Pharmaceuticals UK Ltd. UK Summary of product characteristics, October 2013.
4. Iressa (Gefitinib monohydrate). AstraZeneca UK Ltd. UK Summary of product characteristics, June 2013.

Beta blockers + Venlafaxine

Venlafaxine slightly increases metoprolol levels, but tends to decrease its blood pressure lowering effect. A case of raised venlafaxine levels has been attributed to the use of propranolol, amongst other drugs.

Clinical evidence

(a) Metoprolol

In a study in 18 healthy subjects given metoprolol 100 mg daily for 5 days and venlafaxine 50 mg three times daily for 5 days, the maximum plasma levels and AUC of metoprolol were increased by about 30 to 40%. The AUC of the metabolite alpha hydroxymetoprolol, which has some beta$_1$ receptor-blocking activity, was slightly increased by 16%, with no change in its maximum levels.[1-3] However, the blood pressure-lowering effect of metoprolol appeared to be reduced by venlafaxine.[2] There were no changes in the pharmacokinetics of venlafaxine or its active metabolite.[1,2]

(b) Propranolol

A case study reports higher than expected trough plasma levels of venlafaxine and lower than expected levels of *O*-desmethylvenlafaxine in a patient also taking propranolol and mianserin, amongst other drugs.[4]

Mechanism

Venlafaxine is a weak inhibitor of the cytochrome P450 isoenzyme CYP2D6, by which metoprolol is extensively metabolised, and therefore venlafaxine is likely to slightly increase metoprolol levels in patients with CYP2D6, and also other beta blockers that are similarly metabolised such as propranolol. However, venlafaxine alone commonly causes dose-related increases in blood pressure, and this could attenuate the blood pressure lowering effect of metoprolol and other beta blockers.

The authors of the case with propranolol suggested that propranolol and mianserin might have competitively inhibited the metabolism of venlafaxine by CYP2D6. However, neither of these drugs is known to inhibit CYP2D6, and, although they are both substrates for CYP2D6, combining substrates of an isoenzyme is not usually known to cause clinically relevant pharmacokinetic interactions. Moreover, the addition of the CYP2D6 inhibitor thioridazine further increased the venlafaxine levels in this case, suggesting that CYP2D6 was available for inhibition.

Importance and management

Evidence for an interaction between venlafaxine and metoprolol appears to be limited to the single study cited. The minor increase in metoprolol levels is probably unlikely to be of any clinical relevance; therefore, a clinically relevant pharmacokinetic interaction with other similarly metabolised beta blockers is also unlikely (see 'Table 22.1', p.999). Similarly, even if the increase in venlafaxine levels was proven to be as a result of an interaction with propranolol, an alteration in the ratio of venlafaxine to *O*-desmethylvenlafaxine is not considered clinically relevant.

Of potentially more importance is the possibility of a pharmacodynamic interaction, resulting in increases in blood pressure. The findings of the study with metoprolol appear to suggest that the rise in blood pressure caused by venlafaxine opposes any effect of the minor pharmacokinetic interaction. This effect may be of relevance with the use of any beta blocker, as venlafaxine alone commonly causes dose-related hypertension, which can be sustained. The manufacturers advise that venlafaxine should be avoided in patients with uncontrolled hypertension, and that blood pressure should be monitored in all patients receiving venlafaxine. If sustained increases in blood pressure occur, consider reducing the venlafaxine dose, or discontinuing it.[1,2]

1. Efexor XL (Venlafaxine hydrochloride). Pfizer Ltd. UK Summary of product characteristics, December 2013.
2. Effexor XR (Venlafaxine hydrochloride). Wyeth Pharmaceuticals Inc. US Prescribing information, March 2014.
3. Pfizer UK. Personal communication, May 2010.
4. Eap CB, Bertel-Laubscher R, Zullino D, Amey M, Baumann P. Marked increase of venlafaxine enantiomer concentrations as a consequence of metabolic interactions: a case report. *Pharmacopsychiatry* (2000) 33, 112–15.

Beta blockers + X-ray contrast media

There is some evidence to suggest that use of a beta blocker is a risk factor for anaphylactoid reactions such as bronchospasm to X-ray contrast media. Severe hypotension has been seen in two patients taking beta blockers who were given sodium meglumine amidotrizoate and in a further patient taking atenolol who was given iohexol, and fatal anaphylactic shock occurred in a patient taking metoprolol and given meglumine ioxitalamate.

Clinical evidence

A case-control study of anaphylactoid reactions to X-ray contrast media found that the risk of bronchospasm during intravenous contrast media procedures was associated with beta blocker use and also with asthma, while the risk of major and life-threatening anaphylactoid reactions were associated with cardiovascular disorders. The use of a beta blocker also increased the risk of hospitalisation in those patients who had a severe anaphylactoid reaction.[1] This study extended and re-analysed the data from an earlier analysis.[2]

Two patients, one taking **nadolol** and the other **propranolol**, developed severe hypotensive reactions when given **sodium meglumine amidotrizoate** as a contrast agent for X-ray urography. Both patients developed slowly progressive erythema on the face and arms followed by tachycardia and a weak pulse. Each was successfully treated with subcutaneous adrenaline (epinephrine) and hydrocortisone.[3] Another report describes two similar cases in patients taking **pindolol** and **propranolol**.[4]

A further patient who had developed a transient rash during cardiac catheterisation 6 years earlier, and who was subsequently given **atenolol**, developed generalised urticaria and severe hypotension immediately after an injection of **iohexol** for coronary angiography. However, in this case, the hypotension was refractory to aggressive standard treatment with adrenaline (epinephrine), atropine and dopamine, and the patient remained in shock (BP 60/34 mmHg). Noradrenaline (norepinephrine) infusion produced a modest improvement (BP 80/40 mmHg), but significant improvement in blood pressure occurred only after intravenous injections of glucagon 1 mg.[5] A further case describes a 47-year-old patient treated with **metoprolol** for hypertension who received **meglumine ioxitalamate** during general anaesthesia and died as a result of anaphylactic shock resistant to adrenaline (epinephrine), atropine and isoprenaline.[6] See also, *Anaphylaxis* under 'Beta blockers + Inotropes and Vasopressors', p.1014, for more information about anaphylaxis resistant to adrenaline in patients taking beta blockers.

Mechanism

Iodinated contrast media are associated with hypersensitivity reactions due to the release of histamine. It is suggested that beta blockers compromise the ability of the body to cope with the effects of histamine release.[3]

Importance and management

Limited documentation. Withdrawal of the beta blocker 2 to 3 days before use of contrast media has been suggested,[3] but because of the potential for beta blocker withdrawal syndromes this must be considered on an individual risk/benefit basis.[1] It has been suggested that pretreatment with an antihistamine such as diphenhydramine and a corticosteroid such as prednisone may reduce the risk of reactions.[5,7,8] Ephedrine and cimetidine have also been tried, but their use is controversial.[8] Use of low osmolality, non-ionic contrast media may reduce the risk of adverse reactions, including anaphylaxis.[1,8,9] However, even mild reactions to contrast media may sensitise the patient and a serious anaphylactoid reaction may occur on further exposure, despite pretreatment and the use of low osmolality contrast media.[5] Pre-testing with a small amount of the contrast media has been shown to be a poor predictor of a reaction.[8]

When anaphylactic reactions do occur in patients taking beta blockers, it may be preferable to use a beta-agonist bronchodilator such as isoprenaline (isoproterenol), rather than adrenaline (epinephrine).[3] Glucagon, which has inotropic and chronotropic actions that are only minimally antagonised by beta blockers, may also be effective in reversing anaphylactoid shock in patients taking beta blockers.[5]

1. Lang DM, Alpern MB, Visintainer PF, Smith ST. Elevated risk of anaphylactoid reaction from radiographic contrast media is associated with both β-blocker exposure and cardiovascular disorders. *Arch Intern Med* (1993) 153, 2033–40.
2. Lang DM, Alpern MB, Visintainer PF, Smith ST. Increased risk for anaphylactoid reaction from contrast media in patients on β-adrenergic blockers or with asthma. *Ann Intern Med* (1991) 115, 270–6.
3. Hamilton G. Severe adverse reactions to urography in patients taking beta-adrenergic blocking agents. *Can Med Assoc J* (1985) 133, 122.
4. Capellier G, Boillot A, Cordier A, Juilliot MC, Francois P, Barale F, Clerc P, Bonneville JF. Choc anaphylactique chez les malades sous bêtabloqueurs. *Presse Med* (1989) 18, 181.
5. Javeed N, Javeed H, Javeed S, Moussa G, Wong P, Rezai F. Refractory anaphylactoid shock potentiated by beta-blockers. *Cathet Cardiovasc Diagn* (1996) 39, 383–4.
6. Laxenaire MC, Torrens J, Moneret-Vautrin DA. Choc anaphylactoïde mortel chex un malade traité par bêta-bloquants. *Ann Fr Anesth Reanim* (1984) 3, 453–5.
7. Greenberger PA, Patterson R, Tapio CM. Prophylaxis against repeated radiocontrast media reactions in 857 cases. *Arch Intern Med* (1985) 145, 2197–2200.
8. Wittbrodt ET, Spinler SA. Prevention of anaphylactoid reactions in high-risk patients receiving radiographic contrast media. *Ann Pharmacother* (1994) 28, 236–41.
9. Greenberger PA, Patterson R. The prevention of immediate generalized reactions to radiocontrast media in high-risk patients. *J Allergy Clin Immunol* (1991) 87, 867–72.

Beta blockers + Zileuton

Zileuton appears to increase the exposure to propranolol, and this has led to a decrease in heart rate.

Clinical evidence

The manufacturer of zileuton reports a study in which 16 healthy subjects were given zileuton 600 mg every 6 hours for 5 days followed by a single 80-mg dose of propranolol. The AUC and maximum plasma level of propranolol were increased by 104% and 52%, respectively, which resulted in a decrease in heart rate (not quantified).[1]

Mechanism

Zileuton is an inhibitor of the cytochrome P450 isoenzyme CYP1A2 by which propranolol is, in part, metabolised. Concurrent use therefore decreases propranolol metabolism and increases its exposure.

Importance and management

Evidence for an interaction between propranolol and zileuton appears to be limited to this one study reported by the manufacturers, but what happened is in line with the known metabolism of these drugs. However, the clinical relevance of these findings are unclear, as the effect on heart rate was not quantified, and much greater increases in propranolol levels seen with fluvoxamine (see 'Beta blockers + SSRIs', p.1022) have led to clinically relevant bradycardia only in isolated cases. The manufacturer of zileuton[1] recommends monitoring concurrent use, presumably for bradycardia, and decreasing the dose of propranolol if necessary. Until more is known, this seems prudent.

Based on the findings with propranolol, the manufacturer also extends caution to the other beta blockers. However, as propranolol is the only beta blocker known to be metabolised by CYP1A2, an interaction between zileuton and the other beta blockers seems unlikely.

1. Zyflo CR (Zileuton). Cornerstone Therapeutics Inc. US Prescribing information, November 2011.

Beta blockers; Atenolol + Allopurinol

In a study in 6 healthy subjects, allopurinol 300 mg daily for 6 days did not affect the steady-state pharmacokinetics of atenolol 100 mg daily.[1] No atenolol dose adjustments would therefore appear to be necessary on concurrent use.

1. Schäfer-Korting M, Kirch W, Axthelm T, Köhler H, Mutschler E. Atenolol interaction with aspirin, allopurinol, and ampicillin. *Clin Pharmacol Ther* (1983) 33, 283–8.

Beta blockers; Metoprolol + Acetylcholine

An isolated case describes bronchospasm, which developed when a patient taking metoprolol was given intra-ocular acetylcholine.

Clinical evidence, mechanism, importance and management

An elderly patient with a history of hypertension, obstructive pulmonary disease and stable angina, taking several drugs including metoprolol, experienced severe bronchospasm and pulmonary oedema immediately following the intra-ocular injection of acetylcholine chloride during cataract surgery. Her blood pressure rapidly increased, and she became tachycardic. She had also received phenylephrine eye drops before surgery. The patient may have been more sensitive to the pulmonary effects of acetylcholine, such as bronchospasm, because of pre-existing disease and the presence of metoprolol.[1] It was suggested that phenylephrine may also have been involved, but cases of an interaction between phenylephrine and beta blockers are rare, see 'Beta blockers + Inotropes and Vasopressors', p.1014.

The general clinical relevance of this single case is therefore uncertain but it seems likely to be small.

1. Rasch D, Holt J, Wilson M, Smith RB. Bronchospasm following intraocular injection of acetylcholine in a patient taking metoprolol. *Anesthesiology* (1983) 59, 583–5.

Beta blockers; Metoprolol + Dulaglutide

Dulaglutide appears to slightly increase the exposure to metoprolol.

Clinical evidence, mechanism, importance and management

The UK and US manufacturer briefly report that, in a single-dose study (doses not stated), dulaglutide increased the AUC and maximum concentration of metoprolol by

19% and 32%, respectively. Such changes were not considered clinically relevant and no metoprolol dose adjustment is recommended on concurrent use.[1,2]

1. Trulicity (Dulaglutide). Eli Lilly and Company Ltd. UK Summary of product characteristics, November 2014.
2. Trulicity (Dulaglutide). Eli Lilly and Company. US Prescribing information, March 2015.

Beta blockers; Metoprolol + Lanthanum

Lanthanum carbonate does not alter the absorption of metoprolol.

Clinical evidence, mechanism, importance and management

In a crossover study in 12 healthy subjects, lanthanum 1 g (taken as the carbonate) three times daily for 4 doses had no effect on the AUC and half-life of a single 100-mg dose of metoprolol taken 30 minutes after the fourth dose of lanthanum. The only change was a slight 13% reduction in the maximum plasma level of metoprolol, but this is not clinically relevant. There were also no clinically relevant changes in ECG recordings, vital signs or physical findings.[1]

This study shows that lanthanum carbonate has no effect on the absorption of metoprolol. There is therefore no need to separate administration of these two drugs.

1. Fiddler G, Täubel J. Lanthanum carbonate has a good safety profile following concomitant administration with metoprolol and has no clinically significant effect on its pharmacokinetics. Poster presented at the National Kidney Foundation Clinical Meeting, Dallas, Texas, USA, 2-6 April, 2003.

Beta blockers; Metoprolol + Mirabegron

Mirabegron moderately increases the exposure to metoprolol.

Clinical evidence

In a phase I study in 12 healthy males given a single 100-mg dose of metoprolol before and on the last day of a 5-day course of mirabegron 160 mg daily, the AUC and maximum plasma concentration of metoprolol were increased 3.3-fold and by 90%, respectively.[1]

Mechanism

Mirabegron is a moderate inhibitor of CYP2D6, by which metoprolol is metabolised. Concurrent use therefore decreases its metabolism, resulting in increased exposure.

Importance and management

Evidence for an interaction between metoprolol and mirabegron is limited to this study, but a pharmacokinetic interaction is established and likely to be clinically important. Metoprolol exposure was moderately increased, meaning an increased response to the beta blocker might be seen. Some caution and monitoring for increased effects (e.g. shortness of breath, bradycardia, hypotension) might be prudent on concurrent use with mirabegron, particularly when the dose of metoprolol requires slow and careful titration in conditions such as heart failure.

1. Krauwinkel W, Dickinson J, Schaddelee M, Meijer J, Tretter R, van de Wetering J, Strabach G, van Gelderen M. The effect of mirabegron, a potent and selective β_3-adrenoceptor agonist, on the pharmacokinetics of CYP2D6 substrates desipramine and metoprolol. *Eur J Drug Metab Pharmacokinet* (2014) 39, 43–52.

Beta blockers; Metoprolol + Sevelamer

Sevelamer does not alter the absorption of metoprolol.

Clinical evidence, mechanism, importance and management

In a single-dose study in 31 healthy subjects, there was no change in the AUC or other pharmacokinetic parameters of metoprolol 100 mg when it was given at the same time as sevelamer 2.418 g.[1] Therefore, sevelamer does not alter the absorption of metoprolol and there is no need to separate administration of the two drugs.

1. Burke SK, Amin NS, Incerti C, Plone MA, Lee JW. Sevelamer hydrochloride (Renagel®), a phosphate-binding polymer, does not alter the pharmacokinetics of two commonly used antihypertensives in healthy volunteers. *J Clin Pharmacol* (2001) 41, 199–205.

Beta blockers; Nebivolol + Spironolactone

The concurrent use of spironolactone and nebivolol does not appear to affect the pharmacokinetics of either drug.

Clinical evidence, mechanism, importance and management

A randomised study in 36 healthy subjects given nebivolol 10 mg daily with spironolactone 25 mg daily found no clinically significant changes in the pharmacokinetics of spironolactone and its metabolites canrenone and 7α-thiomethyl spironolactone. Further, spironolactone is reported not to affect the pharmacokinetics of nebivolol.[1] No particular precautions therefore seem necessary on concurrent use, although note that both drugs can lower blood pressure, and this should be borne in mind if they are both given.

1. Morton TL, Tu HC, Lui S, Chervenick SW, Rackley RJ, Huang MY. Lack of pharmacokinetic interaction between nebivolol and spironolactone. *Clin Pharmacol Ther* (2005) 77, P46.

Beta blockers; Propranolol + Alpha-glucosidase inhibitors

Miglitol has been found to reduce the bioavailability of propranolol, but acarbose had no effect. Propranolol has no effect on the blood-glucose lowering effects of acarbose.

Clinical evidence, mechanism, importance and management

In a study in 6 healthy subjects, **acarbose** 300 mg daily for one week had no effect on the pharmacokinetics or pharmacodynamics of a single 80-mg dose of **propranolol**, and the blood-glucose lowering effects of acarbose were also unaffected.[1] Conversely, the US manufacturer of **miglitol** notes that it reduced the bioavailability of **propranolol** by 40%.[2] No propranolol dose adjustment would seem necessary on concurrent use with acarbose or miglitol.

1. Hillebrand I, Graefe KH, Bischoff H, Frank G, Raemsch KD, Berchtold P. Serum digoxin- and propranolol levels during acarbose treatment. *Diabetologia* (1981) 21, 282–3.
2. Glyset (Miglitol). Pfizer Inc. US Prescribing information, September 2012.

Beta blockers; Propranolol + Ascorbic acid (Vitamin C)

Ascorbic acid reduces the bioavailability of propranolol but the extent of the reduction is too small to be of clinical relevance.

Clinical evidence, mechanism, importance and management

A study in 5 healthy subjects given a single 80-mg dose of propranolol found that a single 2-g dose of ascorbic acid reduced the maximum plasma levels of propranolol by 28%, reduced its AUC by 37% and reduced the recovery of propranolol metabolites in the urine by 66%. The reduction in heart rate in response to propranolol was also very slightly diminished. This interaction appears to occur because ascorbic acid reduces both the absorption and the metabolic conjugation of propranolol.[1] However, none of the changes seen would appear to be of clinical relevance.

1. Gonzalez JP, Valdivieso A, Calvo R, Rodríguez-Sasiaín JM, Jimenez R, Aguirre C, du Souich P. Influence of vitamin C on the absorption and first pass metabolism of propranolol. *Eur J Clin Pharmacol* (1995) 48, 295–7.

Beta blockers; Propranolol + Dextromoramide

An early isolated report describes two patients who developed marked bradycardia and severe hypotension when they were given propranolol and dextromoramide following the induction of anaesthesia.

Clinical evidence, mechanism, importance and management

Two women about to undergo a partial thyroidectomy were given propranolol 30 mg and dextromoramide 1.25 or 4 mg by injection during the pre-operative period, after which anaesthesia was induced with a barbiturate. Each woman developed marked bradycardia and severe hypotension, which responded rapidly to intravenous atropine.[1] The authors of the report attributed this effect to the use of dextromoramide and propranolol; however, the reasons for this response are not established (e.g. the induction of anaesthesia may have played a part) and there do not appear to have been any subsequent reports; therefore the general significance of this interaction (if such it is) is unclear.

1. Cabanne F, Wilkening M, Caillard B, Foissac JC, Aupecle P. Interférences médicamenteuses induites par l'association propranolol-dextromoramide. *Anesth Analg Reanim* (1973) 30, 369–75.

Beta blockers; Propranolol + Miscellaneous

The US manufacturers predict that propranolol levels will be raised by inhibitors of CYP1A2 (such as ciprofloxacin). In addition, the US manufacturers predict that propranolol levels will be raised by inhibitors and substrates of CYP2C19 (such as fluconazole and tolbutamide, respectively).

Clinical evidence, mechanism, importance and management

(a) CYP1A2 inhibitors

As propranolol is partly metabolised by the cytochrome P450 isoenzyme CYP1A2, the US manufacturer[1] predicts that its levels may be raised by inhibitors of this isoenzyme (they name **ciprofloxacin**, **fluvoxamine** and **zileuton**). Inhibitors of CYP1A2 raise propranolol levels (as seen with **fluvoxamine**, see 'Beta blockers + SSRIs', p.1022, and **zileuton**, see 'Beta blockers + Zileuton', p.1025) and therefore an interaction with other CYP1A2 inhibitors seems likely. However, note that propranolol levels fluctuate greatly between individuals, and propranolol is only partially metabolised by CYP1A2, therefore any interaction seems likely to produce only moderate clinical effects, even with the most potent CYP1A2 inhibitors.

(b) CYP2C19 substrates or inhibitors

The US manufacturer[1] suggests that raised propranolol levels may occur with CYP2C19 inhibitors (e.g. **fluconazole**) or CYP2C19 substrates (e.g. **tolbutamide**). However, CYP2C19 plays only a very minor part in propranolol metabolism. Further, the manufacturer also notes that omeprazole (a potent inhibitor of CYP2C19) does not interact with propranolol (see 'Beta blockers + Proton pump inhibitors', p.1020), and so a clinically relevant interaction involving CYP2C19 seems unlikely.

1. Inderal LA (Propranolol hydrochloride). Wyeth Pharmaceuticals Inc. US Prescribing information, November 2007.

Beta blockers; Propranolol + Misoprostol

Misoprostol does not alter the pharmacokinetics of propranolol.

Clinical evidence, mechanism, importance and management

In 12 healthy subjects, misoprostol 400 micrograms twice daily raised the AUC of propranolol 80 mg twice daily by about 20 to 40%, and this remained raised 7 days after misoprostol was discontinued.[1] However, as these findings were unexpected, the authors conducted a randomised, crossover, placebo-controlled study and ensured that propranolol was at steady state before assessing the effect of misoprostol. Under these controlled conditions, no statistically significant effects on the pharmacokinetics of propranolol were found.[2] No dose adjustment of propranolol would therefore seem necessary if misoprostol is given.

1. Bennett PN, Fenn GC, Notarianni LJ. Potential drug interactions with misoprostol: effects on the pharmacokinetics of antipyrine and propranolol. *Postgrad Med J* (1988) 64 (Suppl 1), 21–4.
2. Bennett PN, Fenn GC, Notarianni LJ, Lee CE. Misoprostol does not alter the pharmacokinetics of propranolol. *Postgrad Med J* (1991) 67, 455–7.

Beta blockers; Propranolol + Nefazodone

Nefazodone does not affect the pharmacokinetics of propranolol to a clinically relevant extent, and propranolol does not alter the pharmacokinetics of nefazodone.

Clinical evidence, mechanism, importance and management

A study in 18 healthy subjects found that giving nefazodone 200 mg every 12 hours with propranolol 40 mg every 12 hours for 7 days, slightly reduced the AUC of propranolol by 14% and decreased its maximum plasma levels by 29%, when compared with propranolol alone. No clinically relevant changes in the heart-rate response to propranolol were seen with nefazodone. The pharmacokinetics of nefazodone were also unchanged when given with propranolol, when compared with nefazodone alone.[1] No special precautions would therefore seem to be necessary if both drugs are given.

1. Salazar DE, Marathe PH, Fulmor IE, Lee JS, Raymond RH, Uderman HD. Pharmacokinetic and pharmacodynamic evaluation during coadministration of nefazodone and propranolol in healthy men. *J Clin Pharmacol* (1995) 35, 1109–18.

Beta blockers; Propranolol + Sucrose polyesters

Sucrose polyesters (e.g. *Olestra*) do not appear to alter the absorption of propranolol.

Clinical evidence, mechanism, importance and management

In a single-dose study, 8 fasting healthy subjects were given sucrose polyester 18 g (*Olestra*) blended with fat-free milk and an unstated dose of propranolol. The sucrose polyester had no effect on the pharmacokinetics of propranolol, when compared with water.[1] Sucrose polyesters, are non-absorbable, non-calorific fat replacements, and it has been concluded that they are unlikely to reduce the absorption of oral drugs in general.[2] This study confirms that they do not alter the absorption of propranolol.

1. Roberts RJ, Leff RD. Influence of absorbable and nonabsorbable lipids and lipidlike substances on drug bioavailability. *Clin Pharmacol Ther* (1989) 45, 299–304.
2. Goldman P. Olestra: assessing its potential to interact with drugs in the gastrointestinal tract. *Clin Pharmacol Ther* (1997) 61, 613–18.

Beta blockers; Propranolol + Topiramate

There is no clinically relevant pharmacokinetic interaction between propranolol and topiramate.

Clinical evidence, mechanism, importance and management

In a pharmacokinetic study, 30 healthy subjects took propranolol (40 mg twice daily for 2 days, then 80 mg twice daily from day 3 to 22, then tapered down over days 23 to 28), with topiramate in increasing doses from 25 mg twice daily to 100 mg twice daily from day 9 to 23. There were no clinically relevant changes in the steady-state pharmacokinetics of propranolol (none of the changes were more than a 20% reduction or a 25% increase).

In another similar pharmacokinetic study using the same drugs and doses, 32 healthy subjects received topiramate alone for 10 days, and then with propranolol to day 24. The renal clearance of topiramate was reduced by 35% by propranolol, but there was little change in the AUC and steady-state maximum plasma level.[1]

These studies show there is no clinically relevant pharmacokinetic interaction between propranolol and topiramate. No dose adjustments are required for either drug if they are given together.

1. Bialer M, Doose DR, Murthy B, Curtin C, Wang S-S, Twyman RE, Schwabe S. Pharmacokinetic interactions of topiramate. *Clin Pharmacokinet* (2004) 43, 763–80.

Beta blockers; Sotalol + Oseltamivir

A report describes QT prolongation and torsade de pointes when two patients who were stable taking sotalol long-term started taking oseltamivir for influenza.

Clinical evidence

A 63-year-old woman with a history of atrial fibrillation taking sotalol 80 mg twice daily for the past year (QTc interval 506 milliseconds) was given oseltamivir 75 mg twice daily. Three days later she was found unresponsive with ventricular fibrillation and a QTc interval of 521 milliseconds. Sinus rhythm was restored and sotalol was discontinued, but she developed symptomatic torsade de pointes on two occasions. On follow up, her QTc interval was 598 milliseconds. Oseltamivir was discontinued and her QT interval gradually shortened.[1] Similarly, a 79-year-old woman with hypokalaemia, taking sotalol 40 mg twice daily for atrial fibrillation (QTc interval 460 milliseconds) was given oseltamivir 75 mg twice daily for 5 days. On day 4 her QTc interval had increased to 550 milliseconds and 6 days after stopping oseltamivir, she developed torsade de pointes with a QTc interval of 690 milliseconds. She was treated with potassium, magnesium and transvenous pacing, sotalol was discontinued, and her cardiac rhythm returned to normal.[1]

Mechanism

Sotalol is a well known cause of QT prolongation and torsade de pointes and hypokalaemia is also a risk factor for this arrhythmia (see 'Drugs that prolong the QT interval + Other drugs that prolong the QT interval', p.272). Oseltamivir is not known to cause QT prolongation. Nevertheless, the authors suggest that giving oseltamivir to patients taking sotalol might have increased the risk of QT prolongation, as might the occurrence of hypokalaemia in one case.[1]

Importance and management

Evidence is limited to these isolated reports and it is unclear whether the concurrent use of oseltamivir and sotalol increases the risk of QT prolongation and torsades de points beyond the risk posed by sotalol alone. Further study is needed. In the meantime, bear the possibility of an interaction in mind if unexpected ECG changes occur on, or shortly after, concurrent use. See also 'Drugs that prolong the QT interval + Other drugs that prolong the QT interval', p.272, for further information about QT prolongation.

1. Wells Q, Hardin B, Raj SR, Darbar D. Sotalol-induced torsades de pointes precipitated during treatment with oseltamivir for H1N1 influenza. *Heart Rhythm* (2010) 7, 1454–7.

Beta blockers; Sotalol + Paracetamol (Acetaminophen)

One isolated report suggests that paracetamol may enhance the effects of sotalol on heart rate.

Clinical evidence, mechanism, importance and management

A brief report describes 9 patients with hypertension who were given a single 240-mg dose of sotalol daily for 2 weeks. Sotalol alone reduced the heart rate by 10 bpm by day 10; however, in 5 of the patients who were also given paracetamol 2 g daily in three divided doses on days 8 to 10 (for headache) there was an average reduction in heart rate of 18 bpm.[1] This appears to be an old and isolated report and therefore the general relevance of any interaction seems likely to be small.

1. Tongia SK. Paracetamol augments the sotalol-induced bradycardia in man. *Indian J Physiol Pharmacol* (1982) 26, 97–8.

Beta blockers; Talinolol + Carbamazepine

Carbamazepine may slightly reduce the absorption of talinolol.

Clinical evidence, mechanism, importance and management

In a study in 7 healthy subjects, the concurrent use of carbamazepine 600 mg daily and talinolol 100 mg daily for 18 days decreased the AUC of talinolol by about 15%. These changes were thought to be due to changes in the intestinal transport of talinolol, caused by the effects of carbamazepine on the expression of the drug transporter protein multidrug resistance-protein 2 (MRP2). However, AUC changes of this magnitude are not clinically relevant, and therefore no talinolol dose alterations would be expected to be needed on concurrent use.[1]

1. Giessmann T, May K, Modess C, Wegner D, Hecker U, Zschiesche M, Dazert P, Grube M, Schroeder E, Warzok R, Cascorbi I, Kroemer HK, Siegmund W. Carbamazepine regulates intestinal P-glycoprotein and multidrug resistance protein MRP2 and influences disposition of talinolol in humans. *Clin Pharmacol Ther* (2004) 76, 192–200.

Beta blockers; Talinolol + Ginkgo (*Ginkgo biloba*)

Ginkgo causes a slight increase in talinolol bioavailability but this is not expected to be clinically relevant.

Clinical evidence

In a pharmacokinetic study, 10 healthy subjects took a single 100-mg dose of talinolol on three occasions; alone, with a single 120-mg oral dose of a standardised ginkgo extract, and after 14 days of taking the extract at a dose of 120 mg three times daily. The single dose of ginkgo had no effect on the pharmacokinetics of talinolol. However, after repeated doses of ginkgo, the AUC and maximum plasma levels of talinolol were increased by 22% and 36%, respectively, while there was no change in elimination half-life.[1]

In a similar study by the same research group in 12 healthy subjects, the AUC and maximum plasma level of a single 100-mg dose of talinolol were increased by 25% and 33%, respectively, after taking a standardised ginkgo extract 120 mg three times daily for 14 days.[2]

Mechanism

Uncertain. Talinolol is a substrate for P-glycoprotein and ginkgo may have some inhibitory effect on this transporter protein, thereby increasing talinolol levels after multiple dosing. However, note that ginkgo did not interact with digoxin, see 'Digoxin + Ginkgo (*Ginkgo biloba*)', p.1097, which is also a known substrate of P-glycoprotein and so an effect on P-glycoprotein alone seems unlikely to fully explain the pharmacokinetic changes seen. Talinolol is known to be affected by other transporter proteins and therefore these may also have some part to play.

Importance and management

Information regarding an interaction between ginkgo and talinolol is limited and the available studies did not assess the clinical consequences of any effect on talinolol as they were primarily designed to study the pharmacokinetics of the interaction. Nevertheless, they show that ginkgo causes only a small increase in the exposure to talinolol, which is unlikely to be clinically relevant.

1. Fan L, Tao G-Y, Wang G, Chen Y, Zhang W, He Y-J, Li Q, Lei H-P, Jiang F, Hu D-L, Huang Y-F, Zhou H-H. Effects of *Ginkgo biloba* extract ingestion on the pharmacokinetics of talinolol in healthy Chinese volunteers. *Ann Pharmacother* (2009) 43, 944–9.
2. Fan L, Mao X-Q, Tao G-Y, Wang G, Jiang F, Chen Y, Li Q, Zhang W, Lei H-P, Hu D-L, Huang Y-F, Wang D, Zhou H-H. Effect of *Schisandra chinensis* extract and *Ginkgo biloba* extract on the pharmacokinetics of talinolol in healthy volunteers. *Xenobiotica* (2009) 39, 249–54.

Beta blockers; Talinolol + St John's wort (*Hypericum perforatum*)

St John's wort modestly decreases the plasma levels of talinolol.

Clinical evidence

In a pharmacokinetic study, a single dose of talinolol (50 mg orally or 30 mg intravenously) was given to 9 healthy subjects alone and after St John's wort (*Jarsin*, Lichtwer Pharma) 900 mg daily for 12 days. St John's wort was found to reduce the AUC and oral bioavailability of talinolol by about 31% and 25%, respectively. The non-renal clearance of talinolol 30 mg given as a 30 minute infusion was increased by about 26%. Other pharmacokinetic parameters of both oral and intravenous talinolol were not significantly affected.[1]

Mechanism

Talinolol is a known substrate for P-glycoprotein. This study found that the levels of intestinal P-glycoprotein in the duodenal biopsy samples of 9 subjects were raised by St John's wort, leading to a reduction in the absorption of talinolol.

Importance and management

Information about an interaction between St John's wort and talinolol appears to be limited to this study but it is in line with the known effects of St John's wort on substrates of P-glycoprotein, such as digoxin (consider also 'Digoxin + St John's wort (*Hypericum perforatum*)', p.1111). The modest decrease in talinolol levels suggests that, in most patients, this interaction is unlikely to be clinically significant. Nevertheless, consider this interaction if blood pressure is difficult to control.

1. Schwarz UI, Hanso H, Oertel R, Miehlke S, Kuhlisch E, Glaeser H, Hitzl M, Dresser GK, Kim RB, Kirch W. Induction of intestinal P-glycoprotein by St John's wort reduces the oral bioavailability of talinolol. *Clin Pharmacol Ther* (2007) 81, 669–78.

Beta blockers; Talinolol + Sulfasalazine

Sulfasalazine markedly reduces the absorption of talinolol.

Clinical evidence

In a study in 8 healthy subjects the AUC of talinolol 50 mg was reduced by 91% by sulfasalazine 4 g. The talinolol maximum serum levels were also markedly reduced, from 112 nanograms/mL to 23 nanograms/mL in 3 subjects, and to undetectable levels in the other 5 subjects.[1]

Mechanism

Not known. It is suggested that talinolol is adsorbed onto the sulfasalazine, thereby preventing its absorption.[1]

Importance and management

Information regarding an interaction between talinolol and sulfasalazine is limited to this study, but it would appear to be an established and probably clinically important interaction. The efficacy of talinolol would be expected to be markedly reduced, but this does not appear to have been studied. If the mechanism suggested by the authors is true, their advice to separate administration by 2 to 3 hours should minimise this interaction.[1] Nevertheless, it would still be prudent to monitor the outcome of concurrent use (e.g. by monitoring blood pressure). More study is needed to confirm the clinical effects of the interaction, how effective separating the doses is, and whether other beta blockers behave similarly.

1. Terhaag B, Palm U, Sahre H, Richter K, Oertel R. Interaction of talinolol and sulfasalazine in the human gastrointestinal tract. *Eur J Clin Pharmacol* (1992) 42, 461–2.

Beta blockers; Talinolol + Surfactant excipients

The surfactant excipient d-α-Tocopheryl polyethylene glycol 1000 succinate (TPGS) increases the bioavailability of talinolol, whereas another surfactant, poloxamer 188, has no effect.

Clinical evidence, mechanism, importance and management

A study in 9 healthy subjects given talinolol 50 mg via a nasogastric tube, either alone, with **d-α-tocopheryl polyethylene glycol 1000 succinate (TPGS**; 0.04%), or with **poloxamer 188** (0.8%), found that **TPGS** increased the peak plasma level and AUC of talinolol by 100% and 39%, respectively, probably by inhibition of intestinal P-glycoprotein. **Poloxamer 188** did not significantly affect the pharmacokinetics of talinolol.[1] No relevant changes in heart rate or blood pressure were noted with either surfactant, and the increase in talinolol levels caused by **TPGS** was only modest. Therefore a clinically relevant interaction seems unlikely.

1. Bogman K, Zysset Y, Degen L, Hopfgartner G, Gutmann H, Alsenz J, Drewe J. P-glycoprotein and surfactants: effect on intestinal talinolol absorption. *Clin Pharmacol Ther* (2005) 77, 24–32.

23

Calcium-channel blockers

This section is primarily concerned with those interactions where the activity of the calcium-channel blockers is changed by the presence of another drug. Where the calcium-channel blocker is the affecting drug, the relevant monograph is usually categorised under the heading of the affected drug.

Calcium-channel blockers in current clinical usage affect the slow L-type channel. They are usually classified by their chemical structure, which determines their selectivity for vascular smooth muscle over myocardium, and hence their potential to slow the heart rate (negative inotropic activity) see 'Table 23.1', below. Interactions due to additive inotropic effects will therefore apply only to the benzothiazepine (diltiazem) and phenylalkylamine-type (verapamil) calcium-channel blockers, and usually not to the dihydropyridine-type (e.g. nifedipine) calcium-channel blockers. All three types of calcium-channel blocker will have additive hypotensive effects with other drugs with blood-pressure lowering activity.

Calcium-channel blockers also undergo interactions due to altered metabolism. Both verapamil and diltiazem are principally metabolised by the cytochrome P450 isoenzyme CYP3A4, and also inhibit this enzyme (see 'Table 1.10', p.12, and 'Table 1.9', p.11, respectively). They are therefore affected by drugs that induce or inhibit CYP3A4, and also themselves interact with drugs metabolised by CYP3A4.

Many of the dihydropyridine-type calcium-channel blockers are also metabolised by CYP3A4, and are affected by inducers or inhibitors of this isoenzyme to varying degrees. However, they do not generally inhibit CYP3A4, or other isoenzymes to a clinically relevant extent. The exception is perhaps nicardipine, which may cause a clinically relevant inhibition of CYP3A4.

Mibefradil is a calcium-channel blocker that acts on the fast T-type calcium channel. It was withdrawn soon after it was launched because of identification of an increasing number of serious drug interactions caused by its inhibitory effects on CYP3A4 and CYP2D6. It was thought that the practical problems of implementing all the warnings relating to these interactions were too difficult and risky.

Table 23.1 Classification of calcium-channel blockers that act on slow L-type channels

Class	*Rate limiting?*	*Effect on AV or SA node*	*Examples*
Dihydropyridine	No	Little or none	Amlodipine, Barnidipine, Benidipine, Felodipine, Isradipine, Lacidipine, Lercanidipine, Manidipine, Nicardipine, Nifedipine, Nilvadipine, Nimodipine,† Nisoldipine, Nitrendipine
Benzothiazepine	Yes	Depression (negative inotropic activity)	Diltiazem
Phenylalkylamine	Yes	Depression (negative inotropic activity)	Gallopamil, Verapamil

†Nimodipine crosses the blood-brain barrier and therefore affects cerebral blood vessels, and is used for cerebral ischaemia.

Calcium-channel blockers + Aliskiren

Verapamil raises aliskiren levels. The concurrent use of aliskiren and amlodipine does not result in any clinically significant pharmacokinetic changes. The use of aliskiren with calcium-channel blockers is expected to result in additive blood pressure-lowering effects.

Clinical evidence, mechanism, importance and management

(a) Amlodipine

In a study, 18 healthy subjects were given amlodipine 10 mg daily and aliskiren 300 mg daily, either alone, or together for 2 weeks. Amlodipine increased the AUC of aliskiren by 29%, but there was no significant change in the maximum plasma level of aliskiren, although the time to maximum plasma concentration increased from 1 to 3 hours. The pharmacokinetics of amlodipine were not affected by aliskiren.[1]

A change in the AUC of aliskiren of 29% would not be expected to be clinically relevant, and therefore the dose of aliskiren does not need to be adjusted if amlodipine is also given. However, as both drugs lower blood pressure, be aware that concurrent use could result in a reduction in blood pressure that might be greater than clinically desirable. Other calcium-channel blockers seem likely to interact in the same way, but see also *Verapamil*, below.

(b) Verapamil

In a study in 18 healthy subjects, aliskiren 300 mg was given before and after they had taken sustained-release verapamil 240 mg daily for 7 days. Verapamil increased the AUC and maximum levels of aliskiren twofold, whereas aliskiren had no clinically relevant effect on the pharmacokinetics of verapamil.[2] Aliskiren is a substrate of the transporter protein, P-glycoprotein, which is inhibited by verapamil. Concurrent use therefore leads to increased aliskiren levels. The authors of this study concluded that no dose adjustment of aliskiren is needed on concurrent use,[2] but it may be prudent to monitor to check that the blood pressure-lowering effects do not become excessive.

1. Vaidyanathan S, Valencia J, Kemp C, Zhao C, Yeh C-M, Bizot M-N, Denouel J, Dieterich HA, Dole WP. Lack of pharmacokinetic interactions of aliskiren, a novel direct renin inhibitor for the treatment of hypertension, with the antihypertensives amlodipine, valsartan, hydrochlorothiazide (HCTZ) and ramipril in healthy volunteers. *Int J Clin Pract* (2006) 60, 1343–56.
2. Rebello S, Leon S, Hariry S, Dahlke M, Jarugula V. Effect of verapamil on the pharmacokinetics of aliskiren in healthy participants. *J Clin Pharmacol* (2011) 51, 218–28.

Calcium-channel blockers + Antihistamines

Verapamil substantially increased the AUC of a single dose of fexofenadine in two studies, but another study found a much more modest effect. Verapamil prolonged the reaction times of subjects taking cetirizine in one small study. Diltiazem does not appear to affect the pharmacokinetics of fexofenadine. In one study no pharmacodynamic interaction occurred between diltiazem and mizolastine, and mizolastine did not alter diltiazem pharmacokinetics. Nifedipine is predicted to increase the concentrations of mizolastine.

Clinical evidence, mechanism, importance and management

(a) Cetirizine

In a crossover study, when 13 healthy subjects were given a single 15-mg dose of cetirizine with a single 120-mg dose of **verapamil,** they were found to have longer reaction times (measured during attention tests) than when given cetirizine alone, verapamil alone, or placebo. This was thought to be caused by verapamil blocking the efflux of cetirizine from the brain by the transporter P-glycoprotein, thereby increasing the CNS effects of cetirizine. The plasma concentrations of cetirizine were not notably increased when given with verapamil. The clinical relevance of this interaction needs further study but bear it in mind if CNS adverse effects are experienced with cetirizine whilst taking verapamil.[1]

(b) Fexofenadine

In a study in 12 healthy subjects **verapamil** 240 mg daily for 6 days increased the AUC of a single 120-mg dose of fexofenadine 2.5-fold and increased its maximum concentration 2.9-fold. There was marked interindividual variation in these effects.[2] Similarly, in a study in 13 healthy subjects, verapamil 80 mg three times daily for 6 days increased the AUC of a single 120-mg dose of fexofenadine 2.2 to 3.5-fold.[3] Whereas another study showed a smaller 30% increase in maximum concentration of fexofenadine when a single 60-mg dose was given to subjects who had taken **verapamil** 240 mg daily for 10 days. However, after 38 days of **verapamil**, the maximum concentration and clearance of fexofenadine was not notably changed.[4] Fexofenadine is not metabolised by cytochrome P450, and it was suggested that **verapamil** might have increased fexofenadine bioavailability by inhibiting P-glycoprotein or OATPs.[2,3] In another study, pretreatment with slow-release **diltiazem** did not affect the pharmacokinetics of fexofenadine.[5]

Note that fexofenadine has a relatively wide therapeutic range and sizeable increases in fexofenadine concentrations with erythromycin (see 'Antihistamines + Macrolides', p.635), and ketoconazole (see 'Antihistamines + Azoles', p.630), did not increase adverse effects and were not associated with any prolongation of the QT interval. This suggests that a clinically relevant interaction between **verapamil** and fexofenadine is not expected, but some caution may be warranted until further experience is gained.

(c) Mizolastine

A double-blind, crossover study in 12 healthy subjects taking **diltiazem** 60 mg three times daily found that the concurrent use of mizolastine 10 mg daily for 5 days did not alter ECGs or blood pressures. No notable increases in adverse effects were seen, and the pharmacokinetics of **diltiazem** remained unchanged. However, mizolastine pharmacokinetics were not assessed.[6] Some manufacturers of **nifedipine**[7] and mizolastine[8] suggest that concurrent use might increase mizolastine concentrations by inhibition of CYP3A4, and caution is therefore advised,[8] presumably because mizolastine has a weak potential to prolong the QT interval. If caution is required with **nifedipine**, then this should be extended to both **diltiazem** and **verapamil**, since these are both moderate inhibitors of CYP3A4. Further study is needed. However, note that nifedipine is not usually known to interact by inhibiting CYP3A4.

1. Conen S, Theunissen EL, Vermeeren A, van Ruitenbeek P, Stiers P, Mehta MA, Toennes SW, Ramaekers JG. The role of P-glycoprotein in CNS antihistamine effects. *Psychopharmacology (Berl)* (2013) 229, 9–19.
2. Yasui-Furukori N, Uno T, Sugawara K, Tateishi T. Different effects of three transporting inhibitors, verapamil, cimetidine, and probenecid, on fexofenadine pharmacokinetics. *Clin Pharmacol Ther* (2005) 77, 17–23.
3. Sakugawa T, Miura M, Hokama N, Suzuki T, Tateishi T, Uno T. Enantioselective disposition of fexofenadine with the P-glycoprotein inhibitor verapamil. *Br J Clin Pharmacol* (2009) 67, 535–40.
4. Lemma GL, Hamman MA, Hall SD, Wang Z. The effect of verapamil administration on the pharmacokinetics of fexofenadine. *Clin Pharmacol Ther* (2003), 73, P16.
5. Shimizu M, Uno T, Sugawara K, Tateishi T. Effects of itraconazole and diltiazem on the pharmacokinetics of fexofenadine, a substrate of P-glycoprotein. *Br J Clin Pharmacol* (2006) 61, 538–44.
6. Miget N, Herrmann WM, Bergougnan L, Dubruc C, Weber F, Rosenzweig P. Lack of interaction between mizolastine and diltiazem in healthy volunteers. *Methods Find Exp Clin Pharmacol* (1996) 18 (Suppl B), 204.
7. Coracten SR (Nifedipine). UCB Pharma Ltd. UK Summary of product characteristics, October 2014.
8. Mizollen (Mizolastine). Sanofi-Aventis. UK Summary of product characteristics, December 2014.

Calcium-channel blockers + Aprepitant

The concurrent use of aprepitant and diltiazem increases the levels of both drugs. Fosaprepitant moderately raises diltiazem levels. It seems likely that verapamil will interact with both drugs in the same way as diltiazem.

Clinical evidence

The US manufacturer notes that the use of aprepitant 230 mg daily with **diltiazem** 120 mg three times daily for 5 days increased the AUC of aprepitant 2-fold and increased the AUC of **diltiazem** by 70% in patients with hypertension. Nevertheless, aprepitant did not alter the effects of **diltiazem** on heart rate or blood pressure.[1] The UK manufacturer of fosaprepitant notes that when subjects with mild to moderate hypertension were given a 100-mg infusion of fosaprepitant with **diltiazem** 120 mg three times daily, the AUC of **diltiazem** was increased by 40%, and the AUC of **fosaprepitant** was increased by 50%. A small but clinically meaningful decrease in blood pressure occurred, but the heart rate and PR interval were not affected to a clinically relevant extent.[2]

Mechanism

Both aprepitant, its prodrug fosaprepitant, and diltiazem are substrates and inhibitors of the cytochrome P450 isoenzyme CYP3A4. Concurrent use therefore inhibits the metabolism of the other drug. The effects on fosaprepitant may be smaller because it is given intravenously.

Importance and management

Evidence appears to be limited to these two, apparently unpublished studies by the manufacturers, but the findings are in line with the known effects of the drugs. The US manufacturer of aprepitant recommends caution with the concurrent use of moderate inhibitors of CYP3A4, such as diltiazem.[1] Although the effects of diltiazem were not increased in the study with aprepitant, the smaller rise that occurred with fosaprepitant did have some clinically relevant effects on blood pressure, and it may therefore be prudent to be aware of a potential decrease in blood pressure if either of these antiemetics is given to a patient taking diltiazem.

It may be prudent to consider giving the lower dose of aprepitant, where possible, as a twofold increase in its levels is likely to be clinically significant. Be alert for adverse effects such as hiccups, fatigue, constipation, and headache. Furthermore, the CYP3A4 inhibitory effects are dose-dependent and using a smaller dose may minimise the effects on diltiazem. The rise in fosaprepitant levels is not expected to be clinically significant.

Evidence about other calcium-channel blockers is lacking, but note that **verapamil** is also a moderate CYP3A4 inhibitor, and therefore would be expected to interact similarly.

1. EMEND Capsules (Aprepitant). Merck & Co., Inc. US Prescribing information, August 2014.
2. IVEMEND (Fosaprepitant dimeglumine). Merck Sharp & Dohme Ltd. UK Summary of product characteristics, December 2011.

Calcium-channel blockers + Aspirin or NSAIDs

There is evidence that most NSAIDs can increase blood pressure in patients taking antihypertensives, although some studies have not found the increase to be clinically relevant. Some small pharmacokinetic interactions may occur, but they do not appear to be clinically relevant.

Table 23.2 Summary of epidemiological studies and meta-analyses of the effect of NSAIDs on blood pressure in patients taking antihypertensive drugs

Study type	*Patients*	*Antihypertensives*	*NSAIDs*	*Findings*	*Refs*
Case-control (2005)	184 cases 762 controls (UK primary care)	Not stated. Median of two different drugs.	Ibuprofen (78 cases) Diclofenac (60) Other (25)	BP control in treated hypertensives was not affected by use of NSAIDs. No evidence that either systolic BP or diastolic BP differed according to type of NSAID.	1
Retrospective analysis (2004)	8538 patients with rheumatic disease and hypertension	Not stated	NSAID (1164 patients) Celecoxib (654) Rofecoxib (417)	NSAID or celecoxib use was not associated with difficulty in controlling blood pressure, but rofecoxib use was (odds ratio 1.38).	2
Meta-analysis (1994)	50 randomised controlled studies in 771 patients or healthy subjects	Beta blockers (15) Vasodilators (18) Diuretics (12)	Indometacin (33 studies) Sulindac (7) Ibuprofen (5) Piroxicam (4) Flurbiprofen (4)	NSAIDs elevated mean supine BP by 5 mmHg. NSAIDs antagonised all antihypertensives, but only the effect on beta blockers was statistically significant (6.2 mmHg). Among the NSAIDs, only the effect of piroxicam was statistically significant, with piroxicam, indometacin and ibuprofen causing the greatest increase, and sulindac and flurbiprofen the least.	3
Case-control (1993)	133 cases 133 controls	Hydrochlorothiazide, furosemide, methyldopa, propranolol	Ibuprofen (30% of cases) Indometacin (22%) Naproxen (18%) Sulindac (13%)	Systolic BP was about 5 mmHg higher (not statistically significant) in those taking NSAIDs, but diastolic BP did not differ. Findings the same if indometacin users removed.	4
Cross-sectional cohort (1993)	2800 elderly patients (12% taking both an NSAID and antihypertensives)	Not stated	Not stated	NSAID use was associated with a 29% increased risk of hypertension in those taking antihypertensives, but not in those not taking antihypertensives.	5
Meta-analysis (1993)	54 studies with 108 NSAID treatment arms in 1213 hypertensive patients	Not stated	Indometacin (600 patients) Naproxen (72) Piroxicam (51) Ibuprofen (55) Sulindac (277)	Increase in mean arterial pressure with indometacin 3.6 mmHg, naproxen 3.7 mmHg, piroxicam 0.5 mmHg, decrease in mean arterial pressure with ibuprofen 0.8 mmHg, sulindac 0.16 mmHg. The difference between indometacin and sulindac was statistically significant.	6

1. Sheridan R, Montgomery AA, Fahey T. NSAID use and BP in treated hypertensives: a retrospective controlled observational study. *J Hum Hypertens* (2005) 19, 445–50.
2. Wolfe F, Zhao S, Pettitt D. Blood pressure destabilization and edema among 8538 users of celecoxib, rofecoxib, and nonselective nonsteroidal antiinflammatory drugs (NSAID) and nonusers of NSAID receiving ordinary clinical care. *J Rheumatol* (2004) 31, 1143–51.
3. Johnson AG, Nguyen TV, Day RO. Do nonsteroidal anti-inflammatory drugs affect blood pressure? A meta-analysis. *Ann Intern Med* (1994) 121, 289–300.
4. Chrischilles EA, Wallace RB. Nonsteroidal anti-inflammatory drugs and blood pressure in an elderly population. *J Gerontol* (1993) 48, M91–M96.
5. Johnson AG, Simons LA, Simons J, Friedlander Y, McCallum J. Non-steroidal anti-inflammatory drugs and hypertension in the elderly: a community-based cross-sectional study. *Br J Clin Pharmacol* (1993) 35, 455–9.
6. Pope JE, Anderson JJ, Felson DT. A meta-analysis of the effects of nonsteroidal anti-inflammatory drugs on blood pressure. *Arch Intern Med* (1993) 153, 477–84.

Some small studies suggest that low-dose aspirin does not alter the antihypertensive effect of felodipine, isradipine, nifedipine or nitrendipine, and long-term aspirin did not alter the cardiovascular benefits of nitrendipine.

Two reports describe abnormal bruising and prolonged bleeding times in two patients and one healthy subject taking verapamil with aspirin. There are conflicting reports as to whether or not gastrointestinal bleeding is increased by giving NSAIDs with calcium-channel blockers.

One report suggests that calcium-channel blockers, particularly nifedipine, may increase the risk of acute renal failure associated with NSAIDs.

Clinical evidence

A. Antagonism of antihypertensive effects

Various large epidemiological studies and meta-analyses of clinical studies have been conducted to assess the effect of NSAIDs on blood pressure in patients taking antihypertensives, and the findings of these are summarised in 'Table 23.2', above. In these studies, NSAIDs were not always associated with an increase in blood pressure, and the maximum increase was 6.2 mmHg. The effect has been shown for both COX-2 inhibitors and non-selective NSAIDs. In two meta-analyses,[1,2] the effects were evaluated by NSAID. The confidence intervals for all the NSAIDs overlapped, showing that there was no statistically significant difference between the NSAIDs, with the exception of the comparison between **indometacin** and **sulindac** in one analysis.[2] Nevertheless, an attempt was made at ranking the NSAIDs based on the means. In one analysis,[1] the effect was greatest for **piroxicam**, **indometacin**, and **ibuprofen**, intermediate for **naproxen**, and least for **sulindac** and **flurbiprofen**. In the other meta-analysis,[2] the effect was greatest for **indometacin** and **naproxen**, intermediate for **piroxicam**, and least for **ibuprofen** and **sulindac**. An attempt was also made to evaluate the effect by antihypertensive in one analysis.[1] The mean effect was greatest for beta blockers, intermediate for vasodilators (includes ACE inhibitors and calcium-channel blockers), and least for diuretics. However, the differences between the groups were not significant.

The findings of individual clinical and pharmacological studies that have studied the effects of aspirin or specific NSAIDs on specific calcium-channel blockers are outlined in the subsections below.

(a) Aspirin

1. Felodipine. In the Hypertension Optimal Treatment (HOT) study, 18 790 treated hypertensive patients, about 82% of whom were taking a calcium-channel blocker, usually felodipine alone or in combination, were also given either aspirin 75 mg daily or placebo for an average of 3.8 years. It was found that long-term, low-dose aspirin does not interfere with the blood pressure lowering effects of the antihypertensive drugs studied.[3]

2. Isradipine. A study in 20 patients with essential hypertension, who had been taking isradipine 2.5 mg daily for 8 weeks found that the addition of aspirin 100 mg daily for a further 8 weeks did not affect the antihypertensive efficacy of the calcium-channel blocker.[4]

3. Nifedipine. In a small study in 18 patients, low-dose aspirin 100 mg daily for 2 weeks did not alter the blood pressure lowering effect of nifedipine 30 to 60 mg daily, given as a modified-release preparation.[5]

4. Nitrendipine. A study in 19 patients with essential hypertension, who had taken nitrendipine 10 mg daily for 8 weeks found that the addition of aspirin 100 mg daily for a further 8 weeks did not affect the antihypertensive efficacy of the calcium-channel blocker.[4] A post-hoc analysis of the Syst-Eur study of nitrendipine-based antihypertensive treatment found no difference in cardiovascular outcome between 861 patients who were also taking long-term aspirin (700 patients) and/or other NSAIDs (161 patients) and 2882 patients who had never taken aspirin or NSAIDs. Patients in this study were randomised to receive nitrendipine, which could be combined or replaced by enalapril, hydrochlorothiazide, or both.[6]

5. Unnamed calcium-channel blockers. In a randomised study, the use of low-dose aspirin 100 mg daily for 3 months did not alter blood pressure control in patients taking calcium-channel blockers or ACE inhibitors, when compared with placebo.[7]

(b) Diclofenac

A study in elderly women with hypertension found that diclofenac 25 mg three times daily for one week had no effect on the control of their blood pressure with **nifedipine**.[8] In 18 healthy subjects, the AUC of **isradipine** 5 mg twice daily for a week was not affected by a single 50-mg dose of diclofenac, but the maximum plasma levels were raised by a modest 20%. Platelet aggregation was unaffected and the pharmacokinetics of the diclofenac were unchanged.[9] Hypertensive subjects taking slow-release **verapamil** 240 mg daily had a 26% reduction in the AUC of **verapamil** when they took diclofenac 75 mg twice daily.[10]

(c) Ibuprofen

A study in 12 patients with mild or moderate essential hypertension controlled with **amlodipine** 10 mg daily, found that ibuprofen 400 mg three times daily for 3 days increased the mean blood pressure by 7.8/3.9 mmHg.[11] However, 53 hypertensive patients had no changes in their blood pressure control with **verapamil** 240 or 480 mg daily when they also took ibuprofen 400 mg three times daily for 3 weeks.[12]

(d) Indometacin

In a study in 10 patients with mild to moderate essential hypertension indometacin 100 mg daily for a week did not significantly affect the hypotensive effects of **nifedipine** 20 mg twice daily.[13] In contrast, in another study, indometacin 100 mg in divided doses over 24 hours was found to raise the mean arterial pressure by 17 to 20 mmHg in 5 out of 8 hypertensive patients taking **nifedipine** 15 to 40 mg daily.[14]

Five other studies, two in healthy subjects[15,16] and 3 in patients with hypertension[17-19] found that indometacin did not alter the blood pressure lowering effects of **amlodipine**,[19] **felodipine**,[15,17] **nicardipine**[16] or **verapamil**.[18] Similarly, in 24 healthy elderly subjects, the haemodynamic effects of **nimodipine** 30 mg three times daily were not affected to a clinically relevant extent by indometacin 25 mg twice daily in, although the AUC of **nimodipine** and its maximum plasma levels were slightly increased.[20] However, in 15 patients taking **nitrendipine** 5 to 20 mg twice daily, indometacin 25 mg three times daily raised systolic and diastolic blood pressure by a mean of 4 mmHg.[21]

(e) Naproxen

A placebo-controlled study in 100 patients taking **nicardipine** 30 mg three times daily found that naproxen 375 mg twice daily caused no clinically relevant changes in the control of their blood pressure.[22] In another study, 55 hypertensive patients had no changes in their blood pressure control with **verapamil** 240 to 480 mg daily when they were given naproxen 250 mg twice daily for 3 weeks.[12] Similarly, naproxen 375 mg twice daily had no effect on the pharmacokinetics of **verapamil** in hypertensive subjects.[10]

(f) Piroxicam

A study in hypertensive patients given up to 440 mg of **verapamil** daily found that piroxicam 20 mg daily for 4 weeks did not significantly alter the antihypertensive effects of **verapamil**.[23]

(g) Sulindac

A study in elderly women with hypertension found that sulindac 100 mg three times daily for one week had no effect on the control of their blood pressure with **nifedipine**.[8]

A study in hypertensive patients given up to 440 mg of **verapamil** daily found that sulindac 200 mg twice daily for 4 weeks did not significantly alter the antihypertensive effects of **verapamil**.[23]

B. Antiplatelet effects and gastrointestinal bleeding

Abnormal bruising and prolonged bleeding times occurred in a woman taking **verapamil** 80 mg three times daily when she took **aspirin** 650 mg several times a week for headaches. The bruising ceased when the **verapamil** was stopped. Her normal bleeding time of 1 minute rose to 4.5 minutes while she was taking **verapamil**, and to 9 minutes while she was taking **verapamil** and **aspirin**. A healthy subject taking the same doses of **verapamil** and **aspirin** noticed the appearance of new petechiae and her bleeding time rose from 4.5 minutes to more than 15 minutes in the presence of both drugs.[24] An 85-year-old man taking enteric-coated **aspirin** 325 mg daily developed widespread and serious ecchymoses of his arms and legs and a retroperitoneal bleed about 3 weeks after starting to take **verapamil** 240 mg daily.[25]

A prospective cohort study[26] in 1636 elderly hypertensive patients, and a case-control study,[27] found that calcium-channel blockers were associated with an increased risk of gastrointestinal bleeding, when compared with beta blockers. In one of the studies, **verapamil** was associated with the highest rate of bleeding, followed by **diltiazem** and **nifedipine**.[26] However, two other studies indicated that gastrointestinal bleeding was not increased by calcium-channel blockers.[28,29] Furthermore, a post-hoc analysis of the Syst-Eur data found that there was no interaction between chronic NSAID intake (81% **aspirin**) and antihypertensive use (based on **nitrendipine**) in terms of the incidence of gastrointestinal bleeding. In fact, the results suggested that chronic NSAID use tended to be associated with a *lower* incidence of bleeding in patients taking **nitrendipine**-based therapy than those receiving placebo.[6]

C. Effects on renal function

A case-control study using the UK General Practice Research Database found that current NSAID use increased the risk of acute renal failure (relative risk 3.2 compared with non-NSAID use) and this risk was further increased by the concurrent use of a calcium-channel blocker (relative risk 7.8); **nifedipine** appeared to be most likely to interact.[30]

Mechanism

A. Antagonism of antihypertensive effects

There is some evidence that NSAIDs may increase blood pressure in patients taking antihypertensives. Possible explanations for this include inhibition of vasodilator and natriuretic prostaglandins in the kidney and/or a decrease in vascular or endothelial prostaglandin synthesis, resulting in salt retention and vasoconstriction.[31] In contrast, low-dose aspirin appears not to affect the blood pressure lowering effects of calcium-channel blocker-based antihypertensive therapy.[3]

B. Antiplatelet effects and gastrointestinal bleeding

The prolonged bleeding times noted with verapamil[24] may occur as a result of inhibition of platelet aggregation, because calcium-channel blockers interfere with the movement of calcium ions through cell membranes, which can affect platelet function. This appears to be additive with the effects of other antiplatelet drugs. It was suggested that vasodilation produced by calcium-channel blockers in conjunction with inhibition of platelet aggregation may increase the risk of bleeding, or at least prevent the normal vasoconstrictive response to bleeding,[26] although a protective effect of beta blockers rather than an adverse effect of calcium-channel blockers may also be the reason.[28]

C. Effects on renal function

It has been suggested that the increased adverse renal effects seen when NSAIDs are given with nifedipine may be due to nifedipine-induced potential afterload reduction (renal hypoperfusion) secondary to an excess decrease in blood pressure, particularly among the elderly. However, the use of cardiac medications might also be markers of underlying conditions such as cardiovascular disease, low circulating plasma volume and/or already compromised renal function.[30]

Importance and management

Although several studies exist, the evidence for an interaction between the calcium-channel blockers and NSAIDs or aspirin is still somewhat inconclusive. Some consider that the use of NSAIDs should be kept to a minimum in patients taking antihypertensives. The effects may be greater in the elderly and in those with relatively high blood pressure, as well as in those with a high salt intake.[32] However, others consider that the clinical importance of an interaction between NSAIDs and antihypertensives is less than has previously been suggested.[33] While their findings do not rule out a 2/1 mmHg increase in blood pressure with NSAIDs in treated hypertensives, they suggest that if patients in primary care have inadequate control of blood pressure, other reasons may be more likely than any effect of concurrent NSAIDs (e.g. poor compliance or 'white-coat' hypertension).[33] There is insufficient data at present to clearly differentiate between NSAIDs. However, there is some limited evidence to suggest that the interaction of NSAIDs with calcium-channel blockers is less than that with ACE inhibitors.[5,17,19] For the effects of NSAIDs on other antihypertensive drugs, see 'ACE inhibitors + NSAIDs', p.38, 'Beta blockers + Aspirin or NSAIDs', p.1003 and 'Thiazide diuretics + NSAIDs', p.1132.

The risk of renal failure with NSAIDs appears to be increased in patients taking calcium-channel blockers, particularly nifedipine, but it is not clear whether this is due to the drugs or the disease state. A low circulating plasma volume can increase the risk of adverse renal effects and so caution has been suggested in the elderly, especially in patients with hypertension and/or heart failure.[30]

Clinically significant interactions between NSAIDs and calcium-channel blockers that result in bleeding appear to be rare.

1. Johnson AG, Nguyen TV, Day RO. Do nonsteroidal anti-inflammatory drugs affect blood pressure? A meta-analysis. *Ann Intern Med* (1994) 121, 289–300.
2. Pope JE, Anderson JJ, Felson DT. A meta-analysis of the effects of nonsteroidal anti-inflammatory drugs on blood pressure. *Arch Intern Med* (1993) 153, 477–84.
3. Zanchetti A, Hansson L, Leonetti G, Rahn K-H, Ruilope L, Warnold I, Wedel H. Low-dose aspirin does not interfere with the blood pressure-lowering effects of antihypertensive therapy. *J Hypertens* (2002) 20, 1015–22.
4. Tison P, Ulicna L, Jakubovska Z, Oravcova J, Fetkovska N. Effects of dihydropyridines and their combination with aspirin on blood pressure and circadian platelet activity in patients with essential hypertension. *Am J Hypertens* (1994) 7, 46S–49S.
5. Polónia J, Boaventura I, Gama G, Camões I, Bernardo F, Andrade P, Nunes JP, Brandão F, Cerqueira-Gomes M. Influence of non-steroidal anti-inflammatory drugs on renal function and 24 h ambulatory blood pressure-reducing effects of enalapril and nifedipine gastrointestinal therapeutic system in hypertensive patients. *J Hypertens* (1995) 13, 925–31.
6. Celis H, Thijs L, Staessen JA, Birkenhäger WH, Bulpitt CJ, de Leeuw PW, Leonetti G, Nachev C, Tuomilehto J, Fagard RH for the Syst-Eur investigators. Interaction between nonsteroidal anti-inflammatory drug intake and calcium-channel blocker-based antihypertensive treatment in the Syst-Eur trial. *J Hum Hypertens* (2001) 15, 613–18.
7. Avanzini F, Palumbo G, Alli C, Roncaglioni MC, Ronchi E, Cristofari M, Capra A, Rossi S, Nosotti L, Costantini C, Pietrofeso R. Collaborative Group of the Primary Prevention Project (PPP)–Hypertension study. Effects of low-dose aspirin on clinic and ambulatory blood pressure in treated hypertensive patients. *Am J Hypertens* (2000) 13, 611–16.
8. Takeuchi K, Abe K, Yasujima M, Sato M, Tanno M, Sato K, Yoshinaga K. No adverse effect of non-steroidal anti-inflammatory drugs, sulindac and diclofenac sodium, on blood pressure control with a calcium antagonist, nifedipine, in elderly hypertensive patients. *Tohoku J Exp Med* (1991) 165, 201–8.
9. Sommers DK, Kovarik JM, Meyer EC, van Wyk M, Snyman JR, Blom M, Ott S, Grass P, Kutz K. Effects of diclofenac on isradipine pharmacokinetics and platelet aggregation in volunteers. *Eur J Clin Pharmacol* (1993) 44, 391–3.
10. Peterson C, Basch C, Cohen A. Differential effects of naproxen and diclofenac on verapamil pharmacokinetics. *Clin Pharmacol Ther* (1990) 49, 129.
11. Minuz P, Pancera P, Ribul M, Priante F, Degan M, Campedelli A, Arosio E, Lechi A. Amlodipine and haemodynamic effects of cyclo-oxygenase inhibition. *Br J Clin Pharmacol* (1995) 39, 45–50.
12. Houston MC, Weir M, Gray J, Ginsberg D, Szeto C, Kaihlenen PM, Sugimoto D, Runde M, Lefkowitz M. The effects of nonsteroidal anti-inflammatory drugs on blood pressures of patients with hypertension controlled by verapamil. *Arch Intern Med* (1995) 155, 1049–54.
13. Salvetti A, Pedrinelli R, Magagna A, Stornello M, Scapellato L. Calcium antagonists: interactions in hypertension. *Am J Nephrol* (1986) 6 (Suppl 1), 95–99.
14. Thatte UM, Shah SJ, Dalvi SS, Suraokar S, Temulkar P, Anklesaria P, Kshirsagar NA. Acute drug interaction between indomethacin and nifedipine in hypertensive patients. *J Assoc Physicians India* (1988) 36, 695–8.
15. Hardy BG, Bartle WR, Myers M, Bailey DG, Edgar B. Effect of indomethacin on the pharmacokinetics and pharmacodynamics of felodipine. *Br J Clin Pharmacol* (1988) 26, 557–62.
16. Debbas NMG, Raoof NT, Al Qassab HK, Jackson SHD, Turner P. Does indomethacin antagonise the effects of nicardipine? *Acta Pharmacol Toxicol (Copenh)* (1986) 59 (Suppl V), 181.
17. Morgan T, Anderson A. Interaction of indomethacin with felodipine and enalapril. *J Hypertens* (1993) 11 (Suppl 5), S338–S339.
18. Perreault MM, Foster RT, Lebel M, Du Souich P, Larochelle P, Cusson JR. Pharmacodynamic effects of indomethacin in essential hypertensive patients treated with verapamil. *Clin Invest Med* (1993) 16 (Suppl 4), B17.
19. Morgan TO, Anderson A, Bertram D. Effect of indomethacin on blood pressure in elderly people with essential hypertension well controlled on amlodipine or enalapril. *Am J Hypertens* (2000), 13, 1161–7.

20. Mück W, Heine PR, Schmage N, Niklaus H, Horkulak J, Breuel H-P. Steady-state pharmacokinetics of nimodipine during chronic administration of indometacin in elderly healthy volunteers. *Arzneimittelforschung* (1995) 45, 460–2.
21. Harvey PJ, Wing LM, Beilby J, Ramsay A, Tonkin AL, Goh SH, Russell AE, Bune AJ, Chalmers JP. Effect of indomethacin on blood pressure control during treatment with nitrendipine. *Blood Pressure* (1995) 4, 307–12.
22. Klassen DK, Jane LH, Young DY, Peterson CA. Assessment of blood pressure during naproxen therapy in hypertensive patients treated with nicardipine. *Am J Hypertens* (1995) 8, 146–53.
23. Baez MA, Alvarez CR, Weidler DJ. Effects of the non-steroidal anti-inflammatory drugs, piroxicam or sulindac, on the antihypertensive actions of propranolol and verapamil. *J Hypertens* (1987) 5 (Suppl 5) S563–S566.
24. Ring ME, Martin GV, Fenster PE. Clinically significant antiplatelet effects of calcium-channel blockers. *J Clin Pharmacol* (1986) 26, 719–20.
25. Verzino E, Kaplan B, Ashley JV, Burdette M. Verapamil–aspirin interaction. *Ann Pharmacother* (1994) 28, 536–7.
26. Pahor M, Guralnik JM, Furberg CD, Carbonin P, Havlik RJ. Risk of gastrointestinal haemorrhage with calcium antagonists in hypertensive persons over 67 years old. *Lancet* (1996) 347, 1061–5.
27. Kaplan RC, Heckbert SR, Koepsell TD, Rosendaal FR, Psaty BM. Use of calcium channel blockers and risk of hospitalized gastrointestinal tract bleeding. *Arch Intern Med* (2000) 160, 1849–55.
28. Suissa S, Bourgault C, Barkun A, Sheehy O, Ernst P. Antihypertensive drugs and the risk of gastrointestinal bleeding. *Am J Med* (1998) 105, 230–5.
29. Kelly JP, Laszlo A, Kaufman DW, Sundstrom A, Shapiro S. Major upper gastrointestinal bleeding and the use of calcium channel blockers. *Lancet* (1999) 353, 559.
30. Huerta C, Castellsague J, Varas-Lorenzo C, García Rodríguez LA. Nonsteroidal anti-inflammatory drugs and risk of ARF in the general population. *Am J Kidney Dis* (2005) 45, 531–9.
31. Beilin LJ. Non-steroidal anti-inflammatory drugs and antihypertensive drug therapy. *J Hypertens* (2002) 20, 849–50.
32. Johnson AG. NSAIDs and blood pressure. Clinical importance for older patients. *Drugs Aging* (1998) 12, 17–27.
33. Sheridan R, Montgomery AA, Fahey T. NSAID use and BP in treated hypertensives: a retrospective controlled observational study. *J Hum Hypertens* (2005) 19, 445–50.

Calcium-channel blockers + Azoles

Itraconazole can greatly increase the serum concentration of felodipine. A few case reports suggest that isradipine and nifedipine can interact similarly with itraconazole, and that fluconazole can also interact with nifedipine in this way. Ketoconazole greatly increases the plasma concentrations of lercanidipine and nisoldipine.

Clinical evidence

(a) Felodipine

In a placebo-controlled study in 9 healthy subjects, **itraconazole** 200 mg daily for 4 days, increased the AUC of a single 5-mg dose of felodipine 6-fold, and increased its maximum plasma concentrations 8-fold. The effects of the felodipine on blood pressure and heart rate were also increased.[1]

A 52-year-old woman, who had been taking felodipine 10 mg daily for hypertension for a year without problems, developed ankle and leg swelling within 7 days of starting **itraconazole** 100 mg daily for tinea pedis. The oedema disappeared within 2 to 4 days of stopping **itraconazole**.[2] Virtually the same reaction occurred in another woman taking both drugs. Later tests found that, in this patient, the $AUC_{0\text{-}6}$ of a single 5-mg dose of felodipine was increased at least 4-fold (possibly up to 10-fold) while taking **itraconazole**, and ankle swelling was noted.[2]

(b) Isradipine

Ankle swelling was noted in a patient taking isradipine 5 mg daily when **itraconazole** 200 mg twice daily was also taken.[2]

(c) Lercanidipine

The manufacturer of lercanidipine notes that an interaction study found that **ketoconazole** increased the AUC of *S*-lercanidipine and its maximum plasma concentration 15-fold and 8-fold, respectively.[3]

(d) Nifedipine

A report describes massive pitting oedema in the legs and ankles of a patient taking nifedipine when **itraconazole** 100 mg twice daily was also taken.[4] Another patient similarly had ankle oedema and large increases in the serum concentrations nifedipine (minimum concentration increased almost 5-fold) while taking **itraconazole**.[5] A patient with malignant phaeochromocytoma, and persistent hypertension controlled with nifedipine, had an increase in blood pressure when **fluconazole** 200 mg daily was *stopped*. His blood pressure decreased when the **fluconazole** was restarted. A later study found that his maximum nifedipine plasma concentrations and $AUC_{0\text{-}5}$ were increased about 3-fold by **fluconazole**.[6]

A case report describes the development of hypotension when intravenous **voriconazole** was started in a patient stable taking eplerenone 50 mg daily and nifedipine 40 mg daily. A complete resolution was achieved by stopping the eplerenone and halving the daily dose of nifedipine.[7] However, it is unclear to what extent nifedipine contributed to the hypotensive effects seen, as eplerenone concentrations can, in theory, also be increased by **voriconazole**, see 'Potassium-sparing diuretics; Eplerenone + CYP3A4 inhibitors', p.1129.

(e) Nisoldipine

A study in 7 healthy subjects found that **ketoconazole** 200 mg daily for 5 days increased the AUC and maximum plasma concentration of a single 5-mg dose of nisoldipine 24-fold and 11-fold, respectively. The concentrations of the nisoldipine metabolite were similarly increased.[8]

Mechanism

Ankle swelling due to precapillary vasodilatation is a relatively common adverse effect of the dihydropyridine calcium-channel blockers, and this effect appears to be dose-related. Calcium-channel blockers are metabolised in the gut wall and liver by CYP3A4, which is inhibited by itraconazole, ketoconazole and to a lesser extent by fluconazole. Therefore in the presence of these antifungals the concentrations of the calcium-channel blockers are increased and their adverse effects increased. In the case of felodipine, other mechanisms, such as inhibition of P-glycoprotein by itraconazole, might also have contributed.

Importance and management

The interaction between felodipine and itraconazole would appear to be established and clinically important. It also seems that isradipine, lercanidipine, nifedipine, and nisoldipine can interact similarly with itraconazole, ketoconazole, and possibly fluconazole. It is likely that all calcium-channel blockers will behave in a similar way, although probably to a greater or lesser extent. Note that fluconazole is more likely to interact in doses of 200 mg daily or more (see *Azoles*, under 'Anthelmintics, Antifungals, and Antiprotozoals', p.225).

Other azoles such as **posaconazole**, which is a potent inhibitor of CYP3A4, and **voriconazole** would be expected to interact similarly. Note that, at the maximum doses **miconazole** oral gel is sufficiently absorbed to potentially have systemic effects, and might therefore also interact. If any of these azoles is given to a patient on established treatment with a calcium-channel blocker, be alert for the need to lower the dose of the calcium-channel blocker. It would seem prudent to monitor for adverse effects, such as hypotension, headache, flushing, and oedema. However, note that in some cases, the effects are pronounced (such as with felodipine, nisoldipine, and lercanidipine) and it might prove difficult to manage the interaction. In this situation is might be prudent to consider the use of alternative drugs.

1. Jalava K-M, Olkkola KT, Neuvonen PJ. Itraconazole greatly increases plasma concentrations and effects of felodipine. *Clin Pharmacol Ther* (1997) 61, 410–15.
2. Neuvonen PJ, Suhonen R. Itraconazole interacts with felodipine. *J Am Acad Dermatol* (1995) 33, 134–5.
3. Zanidip (Lercanidipine hydrochloride). Recordati Pharmaceuticals Ltd. UK Summary of product characteristics, April 2006.
4. Rosen T. Debilitating edema associated with itraconazole therapy. *Arch Dermatol* (1994) 130, 260–1.
5. Tailor SAN, Gupta AK, Walker SE, Shear NH. Peripheral edema due to nifedipine-itraconazole interaction: a case report. *Arch Dermatol* (1996) 132, 350–2.
6. Kremens B, Brendel E, Bald M, Czyborra P, Michel MC. Loss of blood pressure control on withdrawal of fluconazole during nifedipine therapy. *Br J Clin Pharmacol* (1999) 47, 707–8.
7. Kato J, Mori T, Nakamura Y, Sakurai M, Aisa Y, Ikeda Y, Okamoto S. Hypotension due to the drug interaction of voriconazole with eplerenone and nifedipine. *Eur J Clin Pharmacol* (2009) 65, 323–4.
8. Heinig R, Adelmann HG, Ahr G. The effect of ketoconazole on the pharmacokinetics, pharmacodynamics and safety of nisoldipine. *Eur J Clin Pharmacol* (1999) 55, 57–60.

Calcium-channel blockers + Bile-acid binding resins

Colesevelam slightly reduces the bioavailability of verapamil, and colestipol slightly reduces the bioavailability of diltiazem.

Clinical evidence, mechanism, importance and management

(a) Colesevelam

A study in 31 healthy subjects found that a single 4.5-g dose of colesevelam reduced the peak plasma levels and AUC of a single 240-mg dose of **verapamil** by about 33% and about 15%, respectively. These changes were not considered to be clinically significant.[1]

(b) Colestipol

A study in 12 healthy subjects found that colestipol reduced the AUC and peak plasma levels of a single 120-mg dose of sustained-release **diltiazem** by 22% and 36%, respectively, and those of a single 120-mg dose of immediate-release **diltiazem** by 27% and 33%, respectively. In a further study sustained-release **diltiazem** 120 mg was given alone, 1 hour before or 4 hours after multiple doses of colestipol. The AUC of **diltiazem** was decreased by 17% when it was taken 1 hour before colestipol and by 22% when taken 4 hours after colestipol. This suggests that the effects of colestipol on **diltiazem** bioavailability are not reduced by separating their administration. However, these small reductions in the AUC of **diltiazem** are unlikely to result in a reduction in its efficacy. Nevertheless, the authors advise caution if these drugs are used concurrently.[2]

1. Donovan JM, Stypinski D, Stiles MR, Olson TA, Burke SK. Drug interactions with colesevelam hydrochloride, a novel, potent lipid-lowering agent. *Cardiovasc Drugs Ther* (2000) 14, 681–90.
2. Turner SW, Jungbluth GL, Knuth DW. Effect of concomitant colestipol hydrochloride administration on the bioavailability of diltiazem from immediate- and sustained-release formulations. *Biopharm Drug Dispos* (2002) 23, 369–77.

Calcium-channel blockers + Calcium compounds

An isolated report describes antagonism of the antiarrhythmic effects of oral verapamil due to the use of oral calcium. Note that intravenous calcium compounds are sometimes given before intravenous verapamil, where the hypotensive effects of verapamil would be detrimental, and calcium has been used to reverse the effects of calcium-channel blocker overdose.

Clinical evidence, mechanism, importance and management

An elderly woman with atrial fibrillation, successfully treated for over a year with **verapamil**, developed atrial fibrillation within a week of starting to take an oral calcium compound 1.2 g with calciferol (vitamin D) 3000 units daily for diffuse osteoporosis. Her serum calcium levels had risen from 2.45 to 2.7 mmol/L. Normal sinus rhythm was restored by giving 500 mL of sodium chloride 0.9% and repeated doses of furosemide 20 mg and **verapamil** 5 mg by intravenous injection.[1]

Verapamil acts by inhibiting the passage of calcium ions into cardiac muscle cells and it would appear that in this case the increased concentration of calcium ions outside the cells opposed the effects of the **verapamil**.

The general importance of this isolated case is uncertain, but bear it in mind in the event of an unexpected reduction in **verapamil** effects.

Note that intravenous calcium compounds are sometimes given before intravenous verapamil in the treatment of ventricular arrhythmias to prevent verapamil-induced hypotension in situations where this could be detrimental. This is said not to affect the antiarrhythmic efficacy.[2] Calcium, usually in the form of intravenous calcium gluconate, is used as an antidote in cases of overdose of calcium-channel blockers.

There therefore seems no reason to avoid the use of calcium in patients taking calcium-channel blockers, but, if the effects of the calcium-channel blocker are diminished, it may be prudent to consider monitoring serum calcium levels.

1. Bar-Or D, Yoel G. Calcium and calciferol antagonise effect of verapamil in atrial fibrillation. *BMJ* (1981) 282, 1585–6.
2. Moser LR, Smythe MA, Tisdale JE. The use of calcium salts in the prevention and management of verapamil-induced hypotension. *Ann Pharmacother* (2000) 34, 622–9.

Calcium-channel blockers + Calcium-channel blockers

Plasma levels of both nifedipine and diltiazem are increased by concurrent use and blood pressure is reduced accordingly. Verapamil is predicted to interact similarly with nifedipine. Amlodipine levels are raised by diltiazem (and therefore possibly verapamil). There are isolated reports of intestinal occlusion attributed to the concurrent use of nifedipine and diltiazem. Note that if nimodipine is used with another calcium-channel blocker, the hypotensive effect may be increased and careful monitoring is recommended.

Clinical evidence

Pretreatment of 6 healthy subjects with **diltiazem** 30 or 90 mg three times daily for 3 days was found to increase the AUC of a single 20-mg dose of **nifedipine** two- and threefold, respectively.[1] Similar and related results are reported elsewhere.[2,3] In another study it was found that **nifedipine** 10 mg three times daily for 3 days increased the maximum plasma levels of a single 60-mg dose of **diltiazem** by 54% and increased its AUC by 49%.[4]

One of the manufacturers of **amlodipine** briefly mentions that, in elderly patients, **diltiazem** increases the levels of **amlodipine** by 50%, and this is accompanied by an increase in its effects.[5]

A patient taking **nifedipine** 20 mg twice daily developed abdominal distension and vomiting, 2 days after starting to take **diltiazem** 100 mg twice daily. Both calcium-channel blockers were stopped and abdominal X-ray suggested paralytic ileus, which resolved, but then recurred when both drugs were restarted.[6] Another report describes a patient taking diltiazem, who developed complete or partial intestinal occlusion on three occasions, each time when **nifedipine** was added.[7]

Mechanism

The increase in nifedipine and diltiazem levels is thought to occur as a result of a reduction in the metabolism of both drugs in the liver.[4] It has been suggested that an increased relaxant effect on smooth muscle resulted in intestinal occlusion,[7] and this may related to increased the increased nifedipine levels.[6]

Importance and management

Established interactions but of uncertain clinical importance. Some manufacturers of nifedipine advise caution when it is used with diltiazem because of possible increases in nifedipine levels.[8,9] They say a reduction in the dose of nifedipine should be considered.[9] **Verapamil** is likely to interact similarly with nifedipine,[9] as it has similar effects to diltiazem on hepatic metabolism. Some caution may also be prudent if diltiazem or, in theory, verapamil are given with amlodipine. Consider increasing blood pressure monitoring.

Information about the use of combinations of other calcium-channel blockers appears to be lacking. However, the manufacturers of **nimodipine**[10,11] warn that the blood pressure lowering effect of other calcium-channel blockers could be enhanced by the addition of nimodipine: the UK manufacturer[10] advises careful monitoring of the patient.

Note that the clinical use of two calcium-channel blockers is rarely justified and consideration should be given to stopping one or other of the drugs, as appropriate.

1. Tateishi T, Ohashi K, Sudo T, Sakamoto K, Toyosaki N, Hosoda S, Toyo-oka T, Kumagai Y, Sugimoto K, Fujimura A, Ebihara A. Dose dependent effect of diltiazem on the pharmacokinetics of nifedipine. *J Clin Pharmacol* (1989) 29, 994–7.
2. Ohashi K, Tateishi T, Sudo T, Sakamoto K, Toyosaki N, Hosoda S, Toyo-oka T, Sugimoto K, Kumagai Y, Ebihara A. Effects of diltiazem on the pharmacokinetics of nifedipine. *J Cardiovasc Pharmacol* (1990) 15, 96–101.
3. Ohashi K, Sudo T, Sakamoto K, Tateishi T, Fujimura A, Kumagai Y, Ebihara A. The influence of pretreatment periods with diltiazem on nifedipine kinetics. *J Clin Pharmacol* (1993) 33, 222–5.
4. Tateishi T, Ohashi K, Sudo T, Sakamoto K, Fujimura A, Ebihara A. The effect of nifedipine on the pharmacokinetics and dynamics of diltiazem: the preliminary study in normal volunteers. *J Clin Pharmacol* (1993) 33, 738–40.
5. Exforge (Amlodipine besylate with Valsartan). Novartis Pharmaceuticals UK Ltd. UK Summary of product characteristics, June 2008.
6. Harada T, Ohtaki E, Sumiyoshi T, Hosoda S. Paralytic ileus induced by the combined use of nifedipine and diltiazem in the treatment of vasospastic angina. *Cardiology* (2002) 97, 113–14.
7. Lamaison D, Abrieu V, Fialip J, Dumas R, Andronikoff M, Lavarenne J. Occlusion intestinale aiguë et antagonistes calciques. *Therapie* (1989) 44, 201–2.
8. Adalat LA 60 (Nifedipine). Bayer plc. UK Summary of product characteristics, May 2008.
9. Adalat CC (Nifedipine). Bayer HealthCare. US Prescribing information, April 2011.
10. Nimotop Tablets (Nimodipine). Bayer plc. UK Summary of product characteristics, October 2012.
11. Nimotop Capsules (Nimodipine). Bayer HealthCare Pharmaceuticals. US Prescribing information, February 2008.

Calcium-channel blockers + Clonidine

Two hypertensive patients taking verapamil developed complete heart block after they also started to take clonidine. The hypotensive effects of nifedipine and clonidine were additive in hypertensive patients. Transdermal clonidine has been successfully used with nifedipine or diltiazem in small studies.

Clinical evidence

(a) Diltiazem

In a clinical study, transdermal clonidine decreased blood pressure in 58 of 60 patients with hypertension inadequately controlled by sustained-release diltiazem 90 mg twice daily. The addition of clonidine did not cause a significant decrease in heart rate.[1]

(b) Nifedipine

In a study in 12 patients, sustained-release clonidine 250 micrograms daily for 2 weeks increased the hypotensive effects of nifedipine 20 mg twice daily by about 5 mmHg (mean blood pressure reduction). Clonidine did not alter the slight heart rate increase seen with nifedipine.[2] In a clinical study, in 39 patients with hypertension inadequately controlled by nifedipine GITS (gastrointestinal therapeutic system) 30 to 60 mg daily, transdermal clonidine successfully decreased blood pressure in all 35 patients who completed a titration phase and then an 8-week maintenance phase.[3]

(c) Verapamil

A 54-year-old woman with refractory hypertension (blood pressure 240/140 mmHg) and hyperaldosteronism, was given verapamil 160 mg three times daily and spironolactone 100 mg daily for 10 days, and had a reduction in her blood pressure to 180/100 mmHg. Clonidine 150 micrograms twice daily was then added, and after the second dose she became confused and her blood pressure was found to have fallen to 90/70 mmHg, with a heart rate of 50 bpm. She had developed complete AV block, which resolved when all the drugs were stopped. A 65-year-old woman with persistent hypertension did not have a satisfactory reduction in blood pressure with extended-release verapamil 240 mg daily (blood pressure 165/100 mmHg). Clonidine 150 micrograms twice daily was then added, and the next day a routine ECG showed that she had a nodal rhythm of 80 bpm, which developed into complete AV block. Her blood pressure had fallen to 130/80 mmHg.[4]

Mechanism

Not fully understood. Verapamil very occasionally causes AV node disturbances, but both of these patients had normal sinus rhythm before the clonidine was added. Clonidine alone has been associated with AV node dysfunction in hypertensive patients. It would seem, therefore, that these effects were additive in these two patients.[4]

Importance and management

Information about the interaction between verapamil and clonidine seems to be limited to the one report.[4] Its authors say that a review of the literature from 1966 to 1992 revealed no reports of any adverse interactions between these drugs. Nonetheless, they suggest that it would now be prudent to give these two drugs together with caution and good monitoring in any patient, even in those without sinus or AV node dysfunction.

There was no adverse effect on heart rate in one study in patients taking diltiazem and using transdermal clonidine and the additive blood pressure lowering effect seen with nifedipine is what would be expected with the use of clonidine and any calcium-channel blocker. One US manufacturer of clonidine warns about the potential for additive effects such as bradycardia and AV block if calcium-channel blockers are also given;[5] however, this seems most likely to be a problem with diltiazem or verapamil, rather than the dihydropyridine-type calcium-channel blockers (see 'Table 23.1', p.1029).

1. Lueg MC, Herron J, Zellner S. Transdermal clonidine as an adjunct to sustained-release diltiazem in the treatment of mild-to-moderate hypertension. *Clin Ther* (1991) 13, 471–81.
2. Salvetti A, Pedrinelli R, Magagna A, Stornello M, Scapellato L. Calcium antagonists: interactions in hypertension. *Am J Nephrol* (1986) 6 (Suppl 1), 95–9.
3. Houston MC, Hays L. Transdermal clonidine as an adjunct to nifedipine-GITS therapy in patients with mild-to-moderate hypertension. *Am Heart J* (1993) 126, 918–23.
4. Jaffe R, Livshits T, Bursztyn M. Adverse interaction between clonidine and verapamil. *Ann Pharmacother* (1994) 28, 881–3.
5. Catapres Tablets (Clonidine hydrochloride). Boehringer Ingelheim Pharmaceuticals, Inc. US Prescribing information, January 2010.

Calcium-channel blockers + Dantrolene

An isolated report describes acute hyperkalaemia and cardiovascular collapse when intravenous dantrolene was given to a patient taking verapamil. Another case describes severe hyperkalaemia in a patient taking diltiazem when intravenous dantrolene was given. *Animal* studies have found similar effects with the combination of dantrolene and

verapamil or diltiazem. Nifedipine and amlodipine do not appear to interact.

Clinical evidence, mechanism, importance and management

(a) Diltiazem

A case report describes a 42-year-old patient who developed severe hyperkalaemia after being given an intravenous infusion of dantrolene sodium 200 mg, before the induction of anaesthesia for coronary artery bypass grafting. Preoperatively, the patient was taking metoprolol twice daily and diltiazem 30 mg every 6 hours.[1] One *animal* study also suggests that diltiazem may sometimes interact with dantrolene to produce hyperkalaemia and cardiovascular collapse.[2] Note that, in the UK the use of diltiazem with dantrolene infusion is generally contraindicated because the combination of a calcium-channel blocker and dantrolene is said to be potentially dangerous.

(b) Verapamil

A case report describes a 60-year-old man with insulin-dependent diabetes undergoing a right hemicolectomy. Due to inoperable coronary artery disease, which was causing angina pain, he was taking verapamil 80 mg three times daily. On the morning of surgery he was given verapamil 80 mg with his pre-operative sedation and then, 2 hours later at the start of surgery, he was given intravenous dantrolene 220 mg over 30 minutes, because he was known to have previously had malignant hypertension. After surgery, when he was in intensive care, it was found that his potassium had risen from 4.6 mmol/L before surgery to 6.1 mmol/L at the end of surgery (about 90 minutes after the dantrolene infusion). He was given 10 units of insulin, but an hour later his potassium was 7.1 mmol/L. He was given more insulin, but then developed metabolic acidosis and some cardiac depression, which resolved when he was given bicarbonate and hetastarch 5%. He received three further doses of dantrolene without incident.[3]

The authors of the report attributed the effects seen to an interaction between verapamil and dantrolene. They note that hyperkalaemia has been seen following dantrolene infusions, but the case they cite in support of this suggestion actually describes hyperkalaemia in response to *suxamethonium*. Furthermore, the UK and US manufacturers of dantrolene do not include hyperkalaemia as an adverse effect.[4,5] Nevertheless, the overall picture is that hyperkalaemia, of whatever cause, can apparently increase the myocardial depression caused by verapamil.[6,7] This case seems to be the only report of an interaction between verapamil, and several factors do not make this a clear-cut case of an interaction. However, hyperkalaemia and cardiovascular collapse have been seen in *pigs* and *dogs* given dantrolene and verapamil,[8-10] and so an interaction cannot be completely ruled out. The manufacturers of dantrolene recommend that the combination of intravenous dantrolene sodium and calcium-channel blockers, such as verapamil, is not used during the management of malignant hyperthermia crisis,[4,5] and one manufacturer of verapamil contraindicates intravenous dantrolene.[11]

(c) Miscellaneous

Studies suggest that **amlodipine**[6] and **nifedipine**[2] do not interact with dantrolene and they may therefore be safer alternatives to diltiazem or verapamil. In the case above with verapamil[3] the patient later underwent further surgery while taking **nifedipine**, without any significant adverse effect (although the potassium was moderately raised at 5.4 mmol/L).

1. Yoganathan T, Casthely PA, Lamprou M. Dantrolene-induced hyperkalemia in a patient treated with diltiazem and metoprolol. *J Cardiothorac Anesth* (1988) 2, 363–4.
2. Saltzman LS, Kates RA, Norfleet EA, Corke BC, Heath KS. Hemodynamic interactions of diltiazem-dantrolene and nifedipine and nifedipine-dantrolene. *Anesthesiology* (1984) 61, A11.
3. Rubin AS, Zablocki AD. Hyperkalemia, verapamil, and dantrolene. *Anesthesiology* (1987) 66, 246–9.
4. Dantrium Intravenous (Dantrolene sodium). SpePharm UK Ltd. UK Summary of product characteristics, July 2008.
5. Dantrium Intravenous (Dantrolene sodium). JHP Pharmaceuticals. US Prescribing information, November 2008.
6. Freysz M, Timour Q, Bernaud C, Bertrix L, Faucon G. Cardiac implications of amlodipine-dantrolene combinations. *Can J Anaesth* (1996) 43, 50–5.
7. Jolly SR, Keaton N, Movahed A, Rose GC, Reeves WC. Effect of hyperkalemia on experimental myocardial depression by verapamil. *Am Heart J* (1991) 121, 517–23.
8. Lynch C, Durbin CG, Fisher NA, Veselis RA, Althaus JS. Effects of dantrolene and verapamil on atrioventricular conduction and cardiovascular performance in dogs. *Anesth Analg* (1986) 65, 252–8.
9. San Juan AC, Port JD, Wong KC. Hyperkalemia after dantrolene administration in dogs. *Anesth Analg* (1986) 65, S131.
10. Saltzman LS, Kates RA, Corke BC, Norfleet EA, Heath KR. Hyperkalemia and cardiovascular collapse after verapamil and dantrolene administration in swine. *Anesth Analg* (1984) 63, 473–8.
11. Univer (Verapamil hydrochloride). Cephalon (UK) Ltd. UK Summary of product characteristics, March 2012.

Calcium-channel blockers + Diuretics

No pharmacokinetic interaction appears to occur between hydrochlorothiazide and diltiazem or isradipine. Similarly, spironolactone does not alter the pharmacokinetics of felodipine.

Combinations of diuretics and calcium-channel blockers are used clinically for their additive antihypertensive effects.

Clinical evidence, mechanism, importance and management

A study in 21 healthy subjects given **diltiazem** 60 mg four times daily (for 21 doses) and **hydrochlorothiazide** 25 mg twice daily (for 11 doses), either alone or in combination, found that at steady-state there was no clinically significant pharmacokinetic interaction between the two drugs.[1] **Diltiazem** and **verapamil** increase the levels of **eplerenone**, and dosage adjustments are recommended, see 'Potassium-sparing diuretics; Eplerenone + CYP3A4 inhibitors', p.1129.

The pharmacokinetics of **isradipine** and **hydrochlorothiazide** are not affected by concurrent use,[2,3] and **spironolactone** 50 mg was found not to affect either the pharmacokinetics or the clinical effects of **felodipine**.[4]

Amlodipine was found to be effective (13/11 mmHg fall in blood pressure) with an acceptable safety profile when added to **hydrochlorothiazide** in patients with inadequately controlled hypertension.[5] The manufacturers say that **amlodipine** has been safely given with **thiazides** and no dosage adjustment of **amlodipine** is required.[6,7]

Additive antihypertensive effects are expected when diuretics such as **hydrochlorothiazide** are used in combination with calcium-channel blockers, and such combinations are used clinically.

1. Weir SJ, Dimmitt DC, Lanman RC, Morrill MB, Geising DH. Steady-state pharmacokinetics of diltiazem and hydrochlorothiazide administered alone and in combination. *Biopharm Drug Dispos* (1998) 19, 365–71.
2. Prescal (Isradipine). Novartis Pharmaceuticals UK Ltd. UK Summary of product characteristics, June 2007.
3. Dynacirc CR (Isradipine). Reliant Pharmaceuticals, Inc. US prescribing information, August 2005.
4. Janzon K, Edgar B, Lundborg P, Regårdh CG. The influence of cimetidine and spironolactone on the pharmacokinetics and haemodynamic effects of felodipine in healthy subjects. *Acta Pharmacol Toxicol (Copenh)* (1986) 59 (Suppl 4), 98.
5. Glasser SP, Chrysant SG, Graves J, Rofman B, Koehn DK. Safety and efficacy of amlodipine added to hydrochlorothiazide therapy in essential hypertension. *Am J Hypertens* (1989) 2, 154–7.
6. Istin (Amlodipine besilate). Pfizer Ltd. UK Summary of product characteristics, July 2007.
7. Norvasc (Amlodipine besylate). Pfizer Inc. US Prescribing information, August 2006.

Calcium-channel blockers + Fingolimod

In one study, the concurrent use of fingolimod and diltiazem did not alter the pharmacokinetics of either drug or result in additive bradycardia. Bradycardia has been reported in patients taking calcium-channel blockers when starting fingolimod.

Clinical evidence, mechanism, importance and management

In a randomised, placebo-controlled study, 13 healthy subjects were given **diltiazem** 240 mg daily for 5 days with a single 5-mg dose of fingolimod on day 5. Concurrent use did not alter the pharmacokinetics of either drug, and had no additional effect on heart rate or blood pressure, when compared with either drug alone.[1] Note that the dose of fingolimod used in this study was much higher than the dose usually recommended in clinical practice. In a study in 2 282 multiple sclerosis patients given fingolimod 0.5 mg daily for 4 months, 120 patients were also taking unspecified beta blockers or calcium-channel blockers. Bradycardia in the first 2 days after starting fingolimod occurred in 15 patients and was more frequent in those taking beta blockers or calcium-channel blockers (4 patients) than in those not taking these drugs (11 patients); all patients recovered without pharmacological intervention. None of the 120 patients taking beta blockers or calcium-channel blockers developed atrioventricular block. During the 4-month follow up, 6 serious cardiac adverse events were recorded (including angina, atrioventricular block, and bradycardia) but none of these occurred in patients taking beta blockers or calcium-channel blockers.[2] Similarly, a retrospective study of 317 multiple sclerosis patients included 9 patients taking calcium-channel blockers (unspecified), all of whom had uneventful first-dose observations when fingolimod was started.[3]

Fingolimod is known to cause bradycardia, with a maximal effect around 4 to 5 hours after initiation (including when it is re-started if treatment is suspended for 2 weeks or more), and it is generally recommended that patients should be monitored for 6 hours after their first dose.[4,5] It is possible that additive bradycardia or atrioventricular block might occur on the concurrent use of fingolimod and calcium-channel blockers with bradycardic effects (such as **diltiazem** or **verapamil**), particularly as increased bradycardic effects have been reported with other drugs that can cause bradycardia, such as the beta blockers, see 'Beta blockers + Fingolimod', p.1010. Consequently, the UK and US manufacturers of fingolimod advise against its concurrent use with heart-rate lowering calcium-channel blockers (such as **diltiazem** or **verapamil**). If concurrent use is unavoidable, extended monitoring, including continuous overnight ECG monitoring, is recommended after the first dose of fingolimod.[4,5] Should bradycardia occur on concurrent use, patients should be managed according to their symptoms. Note that the bradycardic effect of fingolimod usually resolves within one month of starting treatment.[4,5]

1. Kovarik JM, Lu M, Riviere G-J, Barbet I, Maton S, Goldwater DR, Schmouder RL. The effect on heart rate of combining single-dose fingolimod with steady-state atenolol or diltiazem in healthy subjects. *Eur J Clin Pharmacol* (2008) 64, 457–63.
2. Gold R, Comi G, Palace J, Siever A, Gottschalk R, Bijarnia M, von Rosenstiel P, Tomic D, Kappos L; FIRST Study Investigators. Assessment of cardiac safety during fingolimod treatment initiation in a real-world relapsing multiple sclerosis population: a phase 3b, open-label study. *J Neurol* (2014) 261, 267–76.
3. Ontaneda DI, Hara-Cleaver C, Rudick RA, Cohen JA, Bermel RA. Early tolerability and safety of fingolimod in clinical practice. J Neurol Sci. (2012) 323, 167–72.
4. Gilenya (Fingolimod hydrochloride). Novartis Pharmaceuticals UK Ltd. UK Summary of product characteristics, February 2015.
5. Gilenya (Fingolimod hydrochloride). Novartis. US Prescribing information, May 2015.

Calcium-channel blockers + Food

Some modified-release preparations of felodipine, nifedipine, and nisoldipine show markedly increased levels when given with food, particularly high-fat food. The bioavailability of lercanidipine is markedly increased and the absorption of manidipine is improved by food. Food modestly decreases the rate and extent of absorption of nimodipine

capsules and food also modestly decreases the peak level of nicardipine. Food does not appear to have a clinically significant effect on the absorption of amlodipine, diltiazem, isradipine, or verapamil.

Clinical evidence

(a) Amlodipine

There was no difference in rate or extent of absorption of amlodipine capsules between the fed and fasted state in a study in healthy subjects.[1] Similarly, another study in healthy subjects found that a high-fat meal had no effect on the bioavailability of amlodipine.[2]

(b) Diltiazem

The rate and extent of absorption of both a slow-release and a conventional tablet of diltiazem were unaffected by food in healthy subjects.[3] Similarly, in a study in healthy subjects, the pharmacokinetic parameters of another sustained-release formulation of diltiazem (*Mono-Tildiem LP*) showed only minor changes when given with food.[4]

(c) Felodipine

The manufacturer of one prolonged-release tablet of felodipine (*Vascalpha*) notes that taking it with a high-fat meal markedly increased the maximum level (2- to 2.5-fold) without altering the extent of absorption.[5]

(d) Isradipine

Compared with the fasted state, the pharmacokinetic parameters of isradipine differed by less than 20% when modified-release and standard-release formulations of isradipine were given with a light meal.[6]

(e) Lercanidipine

The manufacturer notes that the oral bioavailability of lercanidipine is increased fourfold when it is taken up to 2 hours after a high-fat meal.[7]

(f) Manidipine

In a study in 12 healthy subjects, the bioavailability of single 20-mg dose of manidipine was increased by 42% when given after a standard breakfast rather than in the fasting state. Peak plasma levels were increased by about 25% by food (not statistically significant), and the rate of absorption was unaffected.[8]

(g) Nicardipine

Nicardipine peak plasma levels are reduced by 30% when given with a high-fat meal.[9] When a sustained-release preparation of nicardipine (*Cardene SR*) was given with a high-fat breakfast, the mean maximum plasma concentration was 45% lower, the AUC was 25% lower and trough levels were 75% higher, compared with the fasting state.[10]

(h) Nifedipine

Some single-dose studies suggested that food might delay the absorption of nifedipine[11] and reduce its peak levels,[12,13] but a multiple dose study found that food did not have an important effect on the steady-state levels of nifedipine in a 'biphasic' formulation.[14] A further single-dose study in healthy subjects found that the bioavailability of two modified-release preparations of nifedipine (*Adalat OROS* or *Nifedicron*) were not significantly different when they were given in the fasting state, although the maximum plasma levels were 31 micrograms/L and 53 micrograms/L, respectively. The bioavailability and maximum plasma level (38 micrograms/L) of *Adalat OROS* were similar when given after a high-fat or in the fasting state. However, the maximum plasma level of *Nifedicron* increased 2.4-fold to 128 micrograms/L after a high-fat breakfast. Although the bioavailability of *Nifedicron* was only modestly increased by food, the increase in plasma levels indicates a loss of modified-release characteristics and suggests that the effect of food on nifedipine may depend on the product formulation.[15] Similar results were found in another study.[16] The manufacturer of another modified-release preparation of nifedipine (*Adalat CC*) also notes that administration immediately after a high-fat meal increased the peak plasma level by 60% without altering the AUC.[17]

(i) Nimodipine

The US manufacturer notes that taking nimodipine capsules after a standard breakfast reduced the AUC by 38% and the peak level by 68%, when compared with the fasted state in healthy subjects.[18]

(j) Nisoldipine

The manufacturer of an extended-release nisoldipine preparation (*Sular*) notes that food with a high fat content markedly increases the maximum plasma concentration of nisoldipine (by up to 245%), but decreases total exposure by 25%.[19]

(k) Verapamil

The absorption of verapamil from a multiparticulate sustained-release preparation was not affected when it was given with food.[20]

Mechanism

The increase in bioavailability of manidipine in the presence of food may be because it is lipophilic and solubilised by food and bile secretions.[8] Other lipophilic dihydropyridine calcium-channel blockers include lercanidipine,[21] felodipine and nisoldipine.[8] Food may alter the release characteristics of modified-release preparations of drugs, increasing the rate of absorption of the drug, and thereby potentially increasing effects.

Importance and management

Some modified-release preparations of felodipine, nifedipine and nisoldipine have shown markedly increased peak levels when given with meals, particularly if they are high in fat content. Because of this increase, the manufacturers of *Vascalpha* (felodipine),[5] *Adalat CC* (nifedipine)[17] and *Sular* (nisoldipine)[19] recommend that they are taken on an empty stomach[5,17] or with a light meal,[5] avoiding high-fat meals.[5] Note that these precautions do not apply to all preparations of these calcium-channel blockers (e.g. *Plendil* (felodipine) can be taken irrespective of meals), so the manufacturer's literature needs to be consulted.

Food markedly increases the bioavailability of lercanidipine, and it should therefore be taken at least 15 minutes before meals.[7] However, food modestly increases the extent of absorption of manidipine, and it has been recommended that manidipine should be given with food.[8]

In contrast, food modestly decreases the absorption of nimodipine *capsules*, and the US manufacturer says they should preferably be taken not less than one hour before, or 2 hours after, meals.[18] Food also modestly decreases the peak level of nicardipine, and the manufacturers of the sustained release preparation suggest that taking *Cardene SR* with a meal reduces the fluctuation in plasma levels.[10,22]

Food had no clinically significant effect on the absorption of amlodipine, diltiazem, isradipine, or verapamil from the preparations studied (see *Clinical evidence*, above).

1. Faulkner JK, Hayden ML, Chasseaud LF, Taylor T. Absorption of amlodipine unaffected by food. Solid dose equivalent to solution dose. *Arzneimittelforschung* (1989) 39, 799–801.
2. Chung M, Calcagni A, Glue P, Bramson C. Effect of food on the bioavailability of amlodipine besylate/atorvastatin calcium combination tablet. *J Clin Pharmacol* (2006) 46, 1212–16.
3. Du Souich P, Lery N, Lery L, Varin F, Boucher S, Vezina M, Pilon D, Spenard J, Caillé G. Influence of food on the bioavailability of diltiazem and two of its metabolites following the administration of conventional tablets and slow-release capsules. *Biopharm Drug Dispos* (1990) 11, 137–47.
4. Bianchetti G, Bagheri H, Houin G, Dubruc C, Thénot JP. Pharmacokinetic and bioavailability of diltiazem sustained-release: influence of food and time of administration. *Fundam Clin Pharmacol* (1995) 9, 197–201.
5. Vascalpha (Felodipine). Actavis UK Ltd. UK Summary of product characteristics, March 2012.
6. Holmes DG, Kutz K. Bioequivalence of a slow-release and a non-retard formulation of isradipine. *Am J Hypertens* (1993) 6 (3 Pt 2), 70S–73S.
7. Zanidip (Lercanidipine hydrochloride). Recordati Pharmaceuticals Ltd. UK Summary of product characteristics, April 2006.
8. Rosillon D, Stockis A, Poli G, Acerbi D, Lins R, Jeanbaptiste B. Food effect on the oral bioavailability of manidipine: single dose, randomized, crossover study in healthy male subjects. *Eur J Drug Metab Pharmacokinet* (1998) 23, 197–202.
9. Cardene (Nicardipine hydrochloride). Astellas Pharma Ltd. UK Summary of product characteristics, November 2005.
10. Cardene SR (Nicardipine hydrochloride). PDL BioPharma, Inc. US Prescribing information, January 2007.
11. Ochs HR, Rämsch K-D, Verburg-Ochs B, Greenblatt DJ, Gerloff J. Nifedipine: kinetics and dynamics after single oral doses. *Klin Wochenschr* (1984) 62, 427–9.
12. Reitberg DP, Love SJ, Quercia GT, Zinny MA. Effect of food on nifedipine pharmacokinetics. *Clin Pharmacol Ther* (1987) 42, 72–5.
13. Challenor VF, Waller DG, Gruchy BS, Renwick AG, George CF. Food and nifedipine pharmacokinetics. *Br J Clin Pharmacol* (1987) 23, 248–9.
14. Rimoy GH, Idle JR, Bhaskar NK, Rubin PC. The influence of food on the pharmacokinetics of 'biphasic' nifedipine at steady state in normal subjects. *Br J Clin Pharmacol* (1989) 28, 612–15.
15. Schug BS, Brendel E, Wonnemann M, Wolf D, Wargenau M, Dingler A, Blume HH. Dosage form-related food interaction observed in a marketed once-daily nifedipine formulation after a high-fat American breakfast. *Eur J Clin Pharmacol* (2002) 58, 119–25.
16. Wonnemann M, Schug B, Schmücker K, Brendel E, van Zwieten PA, Blume H. Significant food interactions observed with a nifedipine modified-release formulation marketed in the European Union. *Int J Clin Pharmacol Ther* (2006) 44, 38–48.
17. Adalat CC (Nifedipine). Bayer HealthCare. US Prescribing information, April 2011.
18. Nimotop Capsules (Nimodipine). Bayer HealthCare Pharmaceuticals. US Prescribing information, February 2008.
19. Sular (Nisoldipine). Sciele Pharma, Inc. US Prescribing information, February 2010.
20. Devane JG, Kelly JG. Effect of food on the bioavailability of a multiparticulate sustained-release verapamil formulation. *Adv Therapy* (1991) 8, 48–53.
21. Meredith PA. Lercanidipine: a novel lipophilic dihydropyridine calcium antagonist with long duration of action and high vascular selectivity. *Expert Opin Invest Drugs* (1999) 8, 1043–62.
22. Cardene SR (Nicardipine hydrochloride). Astellas Pharma Ltd. UK Summary of product characteristics, June 2006.

Calcium-channel blockers + Glyceryl trinitrate (Nitroglycerin)

The effect of sublingual glyceryl trinitrate was not altered by pretreatment with nifedipine in two studies. Nifedipine and intravenous glyceryl trinitrate had additive vasodilator effects in one study, but the preliminary results of another study found that nifedipine may increase glyceryl trinitrate requirements.

Clinical evidence, mechanism, importance and management

In 9 patients with stable chronic angina, there was no significant haemodynamic interaction between sublingual glyceryl trinitrate and a single 20-mg dose of nifedipine, or nifedipine 20 mg three times daily for 5 days.[1] In another study in healthy subjects, the venodilatory effect of sublingual glyceryl trinitrate was not altered by pretreatment with nifedipine 10 mg.[2] No special precautions are required during concurrent use.

In 7 patients with severe congestive heart failure, a single 10-mg dose of oral nifedipine increased stroke volume, with a peak effect at 30 minutes. The addition of intravenous glyceryl trinitrate at 2 hours further increased stroke volume and increased the cardiac index.[3] Therefore the addition of glyceryl trinitrate enhanced the vasodilator action of nifedipine. Conversely, in the preliminary findings of a comparative study of 3 groups of patients undergoing coronary bypass graft surgery, those taking nifedipine 20 mg twice daily needed initial doses of intravenous glyceryl trinitrate (to reduce cardiac workload, maintain graft patency and control blood pressure) that were about 40% higher than those in the other two groups; one taking nifedipine 10 mg twice daily for hypertension, and the other a control group of normotensive patients. Moreover, these higher doses had little effect on the initial mean systolic blood pressure of half of the group taking nifedipine 20 mg twice daily, and they needed an additional infusion of nitroprusside.[4] It was suggested that as glyceryl trinitrate is converted to nitric oxide to elicit its vasodilator effect, it is possible that the nifedipine inhibits the enzymic production of the nitrous oxide. This appears to be the only study to suggest a negative interaction, and the clinical relevance of its findings is unclear. Note that this study was non-randomised, and there may have been other important differences between the patients in each group that would account for the effects seen.

Most manufacturers suggest that, as may be expected, enhanced hypotensive effects can occur when calcium-channel blockers are given with nitrates. Some manufacturers of amlodipine,[5,6] diltiazem,[7] nifedipine[8] and verapamil[9] suggest that the concurrent use of long-acting nitrates and/or sublingual glyceryl trinitrate may be safely undertaken. However, one manufacturer of diltiazem suggests caution in those also taking nitrates, as increased hypotensive effects and faintness, due to additive vasodilating effects, may occur. They recommend that the dosage of any concurrent nitrate should be increased gradually.[10]

1. Boje KM, Fung H-L, Yoshitomi K, Parker JO. Haemodynamic effects of combined oral nifedipine and sublingual nitroglycerin in patients with chronic stable angina. *Eur J Clin Pharmacol* (1987) 33, 349–54.
2. Gascho JA, Apollo WP. Effects of nifedipine on the venodilatory response to nitroglycerin. *Am J Cardiol* (1990) 65, 99–102.
3. Kubo SH, Fox SC, Prida XE, Cody RJ. Combined hemodynamic effects of nifedipine and nitroglycerin in congestive heart failure. *Am Heart J* (1985) 110, 1032–4.
4. Key BJ, Wilkes MP, Keen M. Reduced responsiveness to glyceryl trinitrate following antihypertensive treatment with nifedipine in man. *Br J Clin Pharmacol* (1993) 36, 499P.
5. Istin (Amlodipine besilate). Pfizer Ltd. UK Summary of product characteristics, July 2007.
6. Norvasc (Amlodipine besylate). Pfizer Inc. US Prescribing information, August 2006.
7. Cardizem LA (Diltiazem hydrochloride). Abbott Laboratories. US Prescribing information, September 2007.
8. Procardia (Nifedipine). Pfizer Inc. US Prescribing information, March 2006.
9. Calan (Verapamil hydrochloride). Pfizer Inc. US Prescribing information, May 2006.
10. Tildiem Retard (Diltiazem hydrochloride). Sanofi-Aventis. UK Summary of product characteristics, March 2007.

Calcium-channel blockers + Grapefruit juice

Grapefruit juice moderately increases the exposure to felodipine, manidipine, and nisoldipine and alters their haemodynamic effects. The bioavailability of nicardipine, nifedipine, nimodipine, nitrendipine, and verapamil are also increased, but the haemodynamic effects appear to be less affected, whereas the bioavailability of amlodipine and diltiazem are negligibly affected. Isolated reports involving grapefruit juice describe peripheral oedema and weight gain with nifedipine and verapamil toxicity. A few case reports suggest that amlodipine can occasionally interact with grapefruit juice.

Clinical evidence

(a) Grapefruit juice

There are several studies on the effects of grapefruit juice on calcium-channel blockers. These are summarised in 'Table 23.3', p.1038. Case reports also describe this interaction. One describes a 54-year-old black African man taking **nifedipine** retard 60 mg daily, lisinopril 5 mg daily and aspirin 75 mg who presented with peripheral oedema, weight gain, and apparently improved blood pressure control over a period of about 6 months. Over this time he had been drinking about 400 mL of freshly squeezed grapefruit juice every morning as part of a diet regimen. He was advised to stop drinking grapefruit juice, and 2 weeks later the oedema had disappeared, he had lost 2 kg in weight, and his blood pressure was slightly higher (140/85 mmHg) than when he presented (130/80 mmHg).[1] Another brief report describes a 42-year-old patient who was admitted to hospital with a 6-hour history of worsening headache, palpitations and altered perception. In the previous 2 weeks she had been taking a preparation containing butalbital, paracetamol, and caffeine for migraine in addition to her usual medication (topiramate, sumatriptan, amitriptyline, and sustained-release **verapamil** 120 mg daily). On the morning of her admission she accidentally took three **verapamil** tablets over a 6-hour period. She was found to have complete heart block with a ventricular escape rhythm of 34 bpm, a systolic blood pressure of 56 mmHg, hypoxic respiratory failure, metabolic acidosis, and hyperglycaemia. Her **verapamil** serum concentration was 2 772 nanograms/mL (therapeutic range 100 to 600 nanograms/mL); norverapamil concentrations were 1895 nanograms/mL (therapeutic range 100 to 400 nanograms/mL). The patient recovered with supportive measures. She reported that she had drunk 3 to 4 litres of grapefruit juice in the week before her admission. The elevated concentration of **verapamil** was attributed to its chronic use, which might increase its bioavailability, and its interaction with grapefruit juice.[2]

In 2002 the Adverse Drug Reactions Advisory Committee (ADRAC) in Australia reported that they had received three case reports describing an interaction between **amlodipine** and grapefruit juice. No details were given.[3]

(b) Whole grapefruit

Some studies have found that grapefruit pulp (equivalent to one fruit), grapefruit segments (including seed but devoid of vascular layer), or grapefruit segment-free extract (extract of peel and pith) can increase the AUCs of **nifedipine**, **nisoldipine** and **felodipine** by 30%, 30%, and 3-fold, respectively.[4,5] However, a case study found that ingestion of a grapefruit (300 g) before taking either **amlodipine** or **nifedipine** had no effect on the plasma concentration of either drug.[6]

Mechanism

Complex. It has been suggested that the increases in exposure are due to components of the fruit juice, particularly bergamottin, 6',7'-dihydroxybergamottin;[7-12] and naringin.[13-15] These components inhibit the activity of CYP3A4 in the intestine, by which many of the calcium channel blockers are metabolised, at least in part. This leads to an increase in their exposure and effects.

Grapefruit juice has little effect on hepatic CYP3A4 and this is borne out by the fact that it interacts with oral, but not intravenous, calcium-channel blockers. Therefore, the sensitivity of the interaction with grapefruit juice might be related to the oral bioavailability of the calcium-channel blocker.[16,17] Thus, amlodipine and diltiazem with high bioavailability are least affected, nifedipine is intermediate; and felodipine[16] and nisoldipine,[17] which have lower bioavailability, are most sensitive to the activity of grapefruit juice. The exception is verapamil, which has low bioavailability and appears to be only modestly affected by grapefruit juice, but this is possibly because isoenzymes other than CYP3A4 are involved in its metabolism.[16]. The plasma protein binding[17] or lipophilicity[18] of the calcium-channel blocker might also contribute to the strength of the interaction, as drugs with a higher plasma protein binding ratio such as manidipine[17] or highly lipophilic drugs such as **lercanidipine**[18] are predicted to interact with grapefruit juice to a greater extent than nifedipine.

Furanocoumarins and possibly other components of grapefruit juice might also increase the plasma concentrations of calcium-channel blockers by inhibition of intestinal P-glycoprotein,[7,8,16] and this might explain the more moderate effects seen with felodipine.

Importance and management

The interaction between felodipine and grapefruit juice is established, and several manufacturers of felodipine[19,20] suggest that it should not be taken with grapefruit juice. Similar advice is given for most other calcium-channel blockers. The UK manufacturer of lercanidipine[21] and one manufacturer of verapamil[22] contraindicate concurrent use with grapefruit juice, although another manufacturer of verapamil[23] suggests that this interaction appears to be of little clinical relevance in the majority of patients. It is noteworthy that only two probable case reports of the interaction appear to have been published.

Generally speaking, the studies suggest that the concurrent use of grapefruit juice and most calcium-channel blockers other than felodipine, and possibly manidipine, nifedipine or nisoldipine, need not be avoided. However, it would be worth checking the diet of any patient who complains of increased or excessive adverse effects with any calcium-channel blocker (e.g. hypotension, headache, flushing, oedema). Any problems can be solved either by avoiding grapefruit juice, or, where possible, by swapping the calcium-channel blocker for one less likely to interact (although note that cases have been reported with amlodipine, which is generally considered as unlikely to interact). Note that some studies suggest that the effects of grapefruit juice can persist for several days, and this should be taken into account when adjusting treatment.

It has also been suggested that **whole grapefruit** or products made from **grapefruit peel** such as marmalade should also be avoided in patients taking felodipine.[5]

1. Adigun AQ, Mudasiru Z. Clinical effects of grapefruit juice-nifedipine interaction in a 54-year-old Nigerian: a case report. *J Natl Med Assoc* (2002) 94, 276–8.
2. Pillai U, Muzaffar J, Sen S, Yancey A. Grapefruit juice and verapamil: a toxic cocktail. *South Med J* (2009) 102, 308–9.
3. Adverse Drug Reactions Advisory Committee (ADRAC). Interactions with grapefruit juice. *Aust Adverse Drug React Bull* (2002) 21, 14.
4. Ohtani M, Kawabata S, Kariya S, Uchino K, Itou K, Kotaki H, Kasuyama K, Morikawa A, Seo I, Nishida N. Effect of grapefruit pulp on the pharmacokinetics of the dihydropyridine calcium antagonists nifedipine and nisoldipine. *Yakugaku Zasshi* (2002) 122, 323–9.
5. Bailey DG, Dresser GK, Kreeft JH, Munoz C, Freeman DJ, Bend JR. Grapefruit-felodipine interaction: effect of unprocessed fruit and probable active ingredients. *Clin Pharmacol Ther* (2000) 68, 468–77.
6. Nakagawa K, Goto T. Effects of ingestion of grapefruit juice or grapefruit on the hypotensive effect and plasma concentrations of dihydropyridine calcium antagonists (amlodipine and nifedipine): a case study. *Clin Exp Hypertens* (2010) 32, 71–5.
7. Malhotra S, Bailey DG, Paine MF, Watkins PB. Seville orange juice-felodipine interaction: comparison with dilute grapefruit juice and involvement of furocoumarins. *Clin Pharmacol Ther* (2001) 69, 14–23.
8. Takanaga H, Ohnishi A, Murakami H, Matsuo H, Higuchi S, Urae A, Irie S, Furuie H, Matsukuma K, Kimura M, Kawano K, Orii Y, Tanaka T, Sawada Y. Relationship between time after intake of grapefruit juice and the effect on pharmacokinetics and pharmacodynamics of nisoldipine in healthy subjects. *Clin Pharmacol Ther* (2000) 67, 201–14.
9. Bailey DG, Dresser GK, Bend JR. Bergamottin, lime juice, and red wine as inhibitors of cytochrome P450 3A4 activity: comparison with grapefruit juice. *Clin Pharmacol Ther* (2003) 73, 529–37.
10. Goosen TC, Cillié D, Bailey DG, Yu C, He K, Hollenberg PF, Woster PM, Cohen L, Williams JA, Rheeders M, Dijkstra HP. Bergamottin contribution to the grapefruit juice—felodipine interaction and disposition in humans. *Clin Pharmacol Ther* (2004) 76, 607–17.
11. Paine MF, Widmer WW, Hart HL, Pusek SN, Beavers KL, Criss AB, Brown SS, Thomas BF, Watkins PB. A furanocoumarin-free grapefruit juice establishes furanocoumarins as the mediators of the grapefruit juice–felodipine interaction. *Am J Clin Nutr* (2006) 83, 1097–105.
12. Kakar SM, Paine MF, Stewart PW, Watkins PB. 6',7'-Dihydroxybergamottin contributes to the grapefruit juice effect. *Clin Pharmacol Ther* (2004) 75, 569–79.
13. Bailey DG, Spence JD, Munoz C, Arnold JMO. Interaction of citrus juices with felodipine and nifedipine. *Lancet* (1991) 337, 268–9.
14. Bailey DG, Arnold JMO, Munoz C, Spence JD. Grapefruit juice–felodipine interaction: mechanism, predictability, and effect of naringin. *Clin Pharmacol Ther* (1993) 53, 637–42.
15. Bailey DG, Arnold JMO, Strong HA, Munoz C, Spence JD. Effect of grapefruit juice and naringin on nisoldipine pharmacokinetics. *Clin Pharmacol Ther* (1993) 54, 589–94.
16. Christensen H, Åsberg A, Holmboe A-B, Berg KJ. Coadministration of grapefruit juice increases systemic exposure of diltiazem in healthy volunteers. *Eur J Clin Pharmacol* (2002) 58, 515–20.
17. Ohnishi A, Ohtani H, Sawada Y. Major determinant factors of the extent of interaction between grapefruit juice and calcium channel antagonists. *Br J Clin Pharmacol* (2006) 62, 196–9.
18. Uesawa Y, Mohri K. Relationship between lipophilicities of 1,4-dihydropyridine derivatives and pharmacokinetic interaction strengths with grapefruit juice. *Yakugaku Zasshi* (2008) 128, 117–22.
19. Plendil (Felodipine). AstraZeneca UK Ltd. UK Summary of product characteristics, July 2013.
20. Vascalpha (Felodipine). Actavis UK Ltd. UK Summary of product characteristics, March 2012.
21. Zanidip (Lercanidipine hydrochloride). Recordati Pharmaceuticals Ltd. UK Summary of product characteristics, April 2006.
22. Univer (Verapamil hydrochloride). Cephalon (UK) Ltd. UK Summary of product characteristics, March 2012.
23. Covera-HS (Verapamil hydrochloride). Pfizer Inc. US Prescribing information, October 2011.

Table 23.3 Summary of pharmacokinetic studies involving calcium-channel blockers and grapefruit juice*

Calcium-channel blocker	*Pharmacokinetic effects*	*Pharmacodynamic effects*	*Refs*
Amlodipine	AUC increased by 7 to 16%, which would not be expected to be clinically significant and no effect on plasma concentrations.	No clinically relevant changes in healthy subjects and one patient.	1-4
Diltiazem	AUC increased by10 to 20%, which would not be expected to be clinically significant.	No clinically relevant changes in healthy subjects.	5,6
Felodipine	AUC increased 2- to 3-fold in healthy subjects. Marked and variable increases in felodipine bioavailability. Effects of grapefruit juice may continue for at least 24 hours after intake. Extended-release tablets less affected; AUC increased by 60 to 100%. IV felodipine not affected.	Decreased blood pressure and increased heart rate seen. Adverse effects (headache; facial flushing; lightheadedness) also increased.	7-18
Manidipine	AUC increased 2.3- to 3-fold.	Adverse effects (headache; flushing; palpitations) more frequent.	19
Nicardipine	AUC increased by 40 to 80%. IV nicardipine not affected.	No clinically relevant effects in healthy subjects, apart from an increase in heart rate.	20
Nifedipine	AUC increased by 10 to 100%. Effects of GFJ may last at least 3 days after intake. IV nifedipine not affected.	Two patients experienced a drop in blood pressure.	4,7,21-26
Nimodipine	AUC increased by 50%. Effects of grapefruit juice may last at least 4 days after intake.	Heart rate increased in healthy subjects.	27
Nisoldipine	AUC increased 2- to 4-fold. Effects of GFJ may last 3 days after intake.	Some studies suggest blood pressure decreased and heart rate slightly increased in healthy subjects, whereas others suggest no clinically relevant effects occur.	28,29
Nitrendipine	AUC increased 2.3-fold.	No clinically relevant changes in healthy subjects.	30
Verapamil	No clinically relevant effects with a single drink of grapefruit juice, but AUC increased by 30 to 50% with multiple doses. Pharmacokinetic effect showed considerable intersubject variation.	Effects generally not clinically significant in healthy subjects, but the PR interval was prolonged in 2 subjects; this was considered to be of borderline significance (increases to above 350 milliseconds in 2 subjects, usual maximal PR intervals of 200 to 260 milliseconds).	31-33

*The usual volume of grapefruit juice used in the studies was 200 to 250 mL

1. Josefsson M, Zackrisson A-L, Ahlner J. Effect of grapefruit juice on the pharmacokinetics of amlodipine in healthy volunteers. *Eur J Clin Pharmacol* (1996) 51, 189–93.
2. Vincent J, Harris SI, Foulds G, Dogolo LC, Willavize S, Friedman HL. Lack of effect of grapefruit juice on the pharmacokinetics and pharmacodynamics of amlodipine. *Br J Clin Pharmacol* (2000) 50, 455–63.
3. Josefsson M, Ahlner J. Amlodipine and grapefruit juice. *Br J Clin Pharmacol* (2002) 53, 405.
4. Nakagawa K, Goto T. Effects of ingestion of grapefruit juice or grapefruit on the hypotensive effect and plasma concentrations of dihydropyridine calcium antagonists (amlodipine and nifedipine): a case study. *Clin Exp Hypertens* (2010) 32, 71–5.
5. Sigusch H, Henschel L, Kraul H, Merkel U, Hoffmann A. Lack of effect of grapefruit juice on diltiazem bioavailability in normal subjects. *Pharmazie* (1994) 49, 675–9.
6. Christensen H, Åsberg A, Holmboe A-B, Berg KJ. Coadministration of grapefruit juice increases systemic exposure of diltiazem in healthy volunteers. *Eur J Clin Pharmacol* (2002) 58, 515–20.
7. Bailey DG, Spence JD, Munoz C, Arnold JMO. Interaction of citrus juices with felodipine and nifedipine. *Lancet* (1991) 337, 268–9.
8. Edgar B, Bailey DG, Bergstrand R, Johnsson G, Lurje L. Formulation dependent interaction between felodipine and grapefruit juice. *Clin Pharmacol Ther* (1990) 47, 181.
9. Bailey DG, Spence JD, Edgar B, Bayliff CD, Arnold JMO. Ethanol enhances the hemodynamic effects of felodipine. *Clin Invest Med* (1989) 12, 357–62.
10. Edgar B, Bailey D, Bergstrand R, Johnsson G, Regårdh CG. Acute effects of drinking grapefruit juice on the pharmacokinetics and dynamics on felodipine – and its potential clinical relevance. *Eur J Clin Pharmacol* (1992) 42, 313–17.
11. Bailey DG, Arnold JMO, Munoz C, Spence JD. Grapefruit juice–felodipine interaction: mechanism, predictability, and effect of naringin. *Clin Pharmacol Ther* (1993) 53, 637–42.
12. Bailey DG, Bend JR, Arnold JMO, Tran LT, Spence JD. Erythromycin-felodipine interaction: magnitude, mechanism, and comparison with grapefruit juice. *Clin Pharmacol Ther* (1996) 60, 25–33.
13. Lundahl JUE, Regårdh CG, Edgar B, Johnsson G. The interaction effect of grapefruit juice is maximal after the first glass. *Eur J Clin Pharmacol* (1998) 54, 75–81.
14. Lundahl J, Regårdh CG, Edgar B, Johnsson G. Effects of grapefruit juice ingestion – pharmacokinetics and haemodynamics of intravenously and orally administered felodipine in healthy men. *Eur J Clin Pharmacol* (1997) 52, 139–45.
15. Malhotra S, Bailey DG, Paine MF, Watkins PB. Seville orange juice-felodipine interaction: comparison with dilute grapefruit juice and involvement of furocoumarins. *Clin Pharmacol Ther* (2001) 69, 14–23.
16. Dresser GK, Bailey DG, Carruthers SG. Grapefruit juice—felodipine interaction in the elderly. *Clin Pharmacol Ther* (2000) 68, 28–34.
17. Bailey DG, Arnold JMO, Bend JR, Tran LT, Spence JD. Grapefruit juice-felodipine interaction: reproducibility and characterization with the extended release drug formulation. *Br J Clin Pharmacol* (1995) 40, 135–40.
18. Lundahl J, Regårdh CG, Edgar B, Johnsson G. Relationship between time of intake of grapefruit juice and its effect on pharmacokinetics and pharmacodynamics of felodipine in healthy subjects. *Eur J Clin Pharmacol* (1995) 49, 61–7.
19. Uno T, Ohkubo T, Motomura S, Sugawara K. Effect of grapefruit juice on the disposition of manidipine enantiomers in healthy subjects. *Br J Clin Pharmacol* (2006) 61, 533–7.
20. Uno T, Ohkubo T, Sugawara K, Higashiyama A, Motomura S, Ishizaki T. Effects of grapefruit juice on the stereoselective disposition of nicardipine in humans: evidence for dominant presystemic elimination at the gut site. *Eur J Clin Pharmacol* (2000) 56, 643–9.
21. Rashid J, McKinstry C, Renwick AG, Dirnhuber M, Waller DG, George CF. Quercetin, an in vitro inhibitor of CYP3A, does not contribute to the interaction between nifedipine and grapefruit juice. *Br J Clin Pharmacol* (1993) 36, 460–3.
22. Sigusch H, Hippius M, Henschel L, Kaufmann K, Hoffmann A. Influence of grapefruit juice on the pharmacokinetics of a slow release nifedipine formulation. *Pharmazie* (1994) 49, 522–4.
23. Rashid TJ, Martin U, Clarke H, Waller DG, Renwick AG, George CF. Factors affecting the absolute bioavailability of nifedipine. *Br J Clin Pharmacol* (1995) 40, 51–8.
24. Pisarik P. Blood pressure-lowering effect of adding grapefruit juice to nifedipine and terazosin in a patient with severe renovascular hypertension. *Arch Fam Med* (1996) 5, 413–6.
25. Odou P, Ferrari N, Barthélémy C, Brique S, Lhermitte M, Vincent A, Libersa C, Robert H. Grapefruit juice–nifedipine interaction: possible involvement of several mechanisms. *J Clin Pharm Ther* (2005) 30, 153–8.
26. Azuma J, Yamamoto I, Watase T, Orii Y, Tanigawa T, Terashima S, Yoshikawa K, Tanaka T, Kawano K. Effects of grapefruit juice on the pharmacokinetics of the calcium channel blockers nifedipine and nisoldipine. *Curr Ther Res* (1998) 59, 619–34.
27. Fuhr U, Maier-Brüggemann A, Blume H, Mück W, Unger S, Kuhlmann J, Huschka C, Zaigler M, Rietbrock S, Staib AH. Grapefruit juice increases oral nimodipine bioavailability. *Int J Clin Pharmacol Ther* (1998) 36, 126–32.
28. Bailey DG, Arnold JMO, Strong HA, Munoz C, Spence JD. Effect of grapefruit juice and naringin on nisoldipine pharmacokinetics. *Clin Pharmacol Ther* (1993) 54, 589–94.

Continued

Table 23.3 Summary of pharmacokinetic studies involving calcium-channel blockers and grapefruit juice* (continued)

29. Takanaga H, Ohnishi A, Murakami H, Matsuo H, Higuchi S, Urae A, Irie S, Furuie H, Matsukuma K, Kimura M, Kawano K, Orii Y, Tanaka T, Sawada Y. Relationship between time after intake of grapefruit juice and the effect on pharmacokinetics and pharmacodynamics of nisoldipine in healthy subjects. *Clin Pharmacol Ther* (2000) 67, 201–14.
30. Soons PA, Vogels BAPM, Roosemalen MCM, Schoemaker HC, Uchida E, Edgar B, Lundahl J, Cohen AF, Breimer DD. Grapefruit juice and cimetidine inhibit stereoselective metabolism of nitrendipine in humans. *Clin Pharmacol Ther* (1991) 50, 394–403.
31. Zaidenstein R, Dishi V, Gips M, Soback S, Cohen N, Weissgarten J, Blatt A, Golik A. The effect of grapefruit juice on the pharmacokinetics of orally administered verapamil. *Eur J Clin Pharmacol* (1998) 54, 337–40.
32. Ho P-C, Ghose K, Saville D, Wanwimolruk S. Effect of grapefruit juice on pharmacokinetics and pharmacodynamics of verapamil enantiomers in healthy volunteers. *Eur J Clin Pharmacol* (2000) 56, 693–8.
33. Fuhr U, Müller-Peltzer H, Kern R, Lopez-Rojas P, Jünemann M, Harder S, Staib AH. Effects of grapefruit juice and smoking on verapamil concentrations in steady state. *Eur J Clin Pharmacol* (2002) 58, 45–53.

Calcium-channel blockers + H_2-receptor antagonists

The plasma levels of diltiazem, felodipine, isradipine, lacidipine, nifedipine, nimodipine, nisoldipine, and nitrendipine are increased by cimetidine. High doses of cimetidine may increase the bioavailability of lercanidipine. The manufacturers of nicardipine advise caution with cimetidine, although studies suggest no clinically important interactions occur. Cimetidine does not interact with amlodipine, and it is uncertain whether cimetidine interacts significantly with verapamil. Ranitidine appears to interact only minimally with calcium-channel blockers, if at all. There is no pharmacokinetic interaction between famotidine and nifedipine.

Clinical evidence

(a) Amlodipine

A crossover study in 12 healthy subjects found that **cimetidine** 400 mg twice daily for 14 days had no effect on the pharmacokinetics of amlodipine 10 mg.[1]

(b) Diltiazem

In a single-dose study, **cimetidine** increased the AUC of diltiazem by 25 to 50% and increased its serum levels by 40%.[2] In a study in 6 healthy subjects, **cimetidine** 300 mg before meals and at bedtime for a week increased the AUC of a single 60-mg oral dose of diltiazem by 50% and increased its peak plasma levels by 57%. In the same study, **ranitidine** 150 mg twice daily for a week had no significant effect on the AUC of diltiazem.[3] No adverse interaction was seen in 22 patients given calcium-channel blockers, including diltiazem, with oral **famotidine** for 6 to 8 weeks.[4]

(c) Felodipine

In a study in 12 subjects, **cimetidine** 1 g daily increased the AUC of felodipine 10 mg by 56%, and raised its peak serum level by 54%. There was a short lasting effect on heart rate but the clinical effects were minimal.[5]

(d) Isradipine

The manufacturer of isradipine[6] notes that **cimetidine** increases the bioavailability of isradipine by about 50%.

(e) Lacidipine

In a study in healthy subjects a single 800-mg dose of **cimetidine** increased the maximum plasma level of a single 4-mg dose of lacidipine by 59% and increased its AUC by 74%. Pulse rate and blood pressure were unaffected.[7]

(f) Lercanidipine

The manufacturers of lercanidipine state that **cimetidine** 800 mg daily causes no significant alteration in the plasma levels of lercanidipine;[8,9] the AUC and maximum plasma concentration were increased by a mean of 11%,[9] which would not be expected to be clinically relevant. However, they suggest that the bioavailability of lercanidipine and its hypotensive effects may be increased by higher doses of **cimetidine**.[8,9]

(g) Nicardipine

In a study in 12 healthy subjects, intravenous **cimetidine** 300 mg every 6 hours for 48 hours did not alter the pharmacokinetics or pharmacodynamics of a 12-hour intravenous infusion of nicardipine 24 mg.[10] In a review of patients prescribed H_2-receptor antagonists, no adverse interaction was seen in 22 patients given calcium-channel blockers, including nicardipine, with **famotidine** for 6 to 8 weeks.[4]

(h) Nifedipine

In a pharmacokinetic study, **cimetidine** 1 g daily for a week increased the AUC of nifedipine 40 mg daily by about 60% and increased the maximum plasma levels by about 90%. **Ranitidine** 150 mg twice daily for a week caused an insignificant rise of about 25% in maximum nifedipine plasma levels and AUC.[11] Seven hypertensive patients had a fall in mean blood pressure from 127 mmHg to 109 mmHg after taking nifedipine 40 mg daily for 4 weeks, and a further fall to 95 mmHg after they also took **cimetidine** 1 g daily for 3 weeks. When they took **ranitidine** 300 mg instead of **cimetidine**, blood pressure was not significantly affected.[11,12] Other studies clearly confirm that **cimetidine** causes a very significant rise in plasma nifedipine levels and an increase in its effects, whereas **ranitidine** interacts only minimally.[13-19] Overall, cimetidine appears to increase the AUC of nifedipine by about 1.5- to 2-fold and the maximum plasma concentration by about 1.6- to 2-fold.[20]

A study found no pharmacokinetic interaction between nifedipine and **famotidine**, but **famotidine** reversed the effects of nifedipine on systolic time intervals and significantly reduced the stroke volume and cardiac output.[21,22] In a review of patients prescribed H_2-receptor antagonists, no adverse interaction was seen in 22 patients given calcium-channel blockers, including nifedipine, with **famotidine** for 6 to 8 weeks.[4]

(i) Nimodipine

In a study in 8 healthy subjects, **cimetidine** 1 g daily for 7 days increased the bioavailability of nimodipine 30 mg three times daily by 75%, but the haemodynamic effects were unchanged. **Ranitidine** did not interact.[23]

(j) Nisoldipine

A study in 8 healthy subjects found that taking **cimetidine** 1 g in divided doses on the day before the study and then three 200 mg doses every 4 hours on the study day, increased the bioavailability of a single 10-mg dose of nisoldipine by about 50%, but the haemodynamic effects of the nisoldipine were unaltered.[24] The manufacturer reports that **cimetidine** 400 mg twice daily increases the AUC and maximum plasma concentration of nisoldipine by 30 to 45%, whereas **ranitidine** does not interact.[25]

(k) Nitrendipine

In a study, 9 healthy subjects were given **cimetidine** 800 mg before a single 20-mg dose of nitrendipine, and **cimetidine** 400 mg in divided doses after the nitrendipine. **Cimetidine** increased the bioavailability of nitrendipine by 154% but its haemodynamic effects were unchanged.[26] Another study found that the AUC of oral nitrendipine 20 mg daily for 1 week was increased by about 50% by ranitidine and its clearance was decreased, but there were no changes in the haemodynamic measurements (systolic time intervals, impedance cardiography).[27,28] A further study found that **ranitidine** increases the AUC of nitrendipine by 89%, but no adverse effects were noted as a result of this increase.[29]

(l) Verapamil

A study in 8 healthy subjects found that **cimetidine** 300 mg every 6 hours for 8 days did not affect the pharmacokinetics of a single 10-mg intravenous dose of verapamil, but the bioavailability of a 120-mg oral dose of verapamil was increased from 26% to 49%. There was, however, no significant change in oral clearance and the changes in the PR interval caused by the verapamil were unaltered in the presence of **cimetidine**.[30]

Another study found that **cimetidine** 300 mg four times daily for 5 days reduced the clearance of a single intravenous dose of verapamil by 21% and increased its elimination half-life by 50%.[31] A further study found that **cimetidine** 400 mg twice daily for a week increased the bioavailability of verapamil from 35% to 42% and its apparent oral clearance was reduced by almost 30%.[32] Yet another study found that **cimetidine** increased the bioavailability of both enantiomers of verapamil and increased the effect of verapamil on atrioventricular conduction.[33] In contrast, other studies have found that the pharmacokinetics[34,35] and pharmacodynamics[34] of verapamil were unaffected by **cimetidine**.

Mechanism

It is believed that cimetidine increases the bioavailability of nifedipine and other interacting calcium-channel blockers by inhibiting their oxidative metabolism by the liver. It has been proposed that ranitidine may increase the bioavailability of nifedipine by lowering gastric acidity.[15]

Importance and management

The interaction of cimetidine with nifedipine is established. Concurrent use need not be avoided but the increase in the calcium-channel blocker effects should be taken into account and blood pressure monitored. If necessary, a dosage reduction should be considered; a reduction of 40 to 50% has been suggested.[36,37] Cimetidine also increases the bioavailability of diltiazem, felodipine, isradipine, lacidipine, nimodipine and nitrendipine, although the haemodynamic changes usually appear minimal. Nevertheless, the dose of these calcium-channel blockers may possibly need to be reduced; it has been suggested that the dosage of diltiazem should be reduced by 30 to 50%,[36,37] and the dosage of isradipine should be reduced by 50%.[6]

The interaction between verapamil and cimetidine is not well established, but, until more is known, it may be prudent to monitor concurrent use for verapamil adverse effects. It has been suggested that the verapamil dose may need to be reduced by 50%.[37] Similarly, high doses of cimetidine may increase the hypotensive effects of lercanidipine and caution is advised.[8,9] One study indicated no interaction between nicardipine and cimetidine, but the manufacturers note that cimetidine increases nicardipine plasma levels and careful monitoring is recommended.[38,39] Amlodipine and cimetidine do not interact and one study suggests that cimetidine does not alter the clinical effects of nisoldipine.

Ranitidine does not interact significantly with diltiazem, nifedipine, nimodipine or nisoldipine, and famotidine does not interact with nifedipine. Ranitidine may therefore be a suitable non-interacting alternative to cimetidine with these and probably other calcium-channel blockers. Note that the nitrendipine AUC was increased by 50% and 89% by ranitidine, although this was not considered clinically relevant.

1. Quoted as unpublished data, Pfizer Central Research by Abernethy DR. Amlodipine: pharmacokinetic profile of a low-clearance calcium antagonist. *J Cardiovasc Pharmacol* (1991) 17 (Suppl 1), S4–S7.
2. Mazhar M, Popat KD, Sanders C. Effect of cimetidine on diltiazem blood levels. *Clin Res* (1984) 32, 741A.
3. Winship LC, McKenney JM, Wright JT, Wood JH, Goodman RP. The effect of ranitidine and cimetidine on single-dose diltiazem pharmacokinetics. *Pharmacotherapy* (1985) 5, 16–19.
4. Chichmanian RM, Mignot G, Spreux A, Jean-Girard C, Hofliger P. Tolérance de la famotidine. Étude du réseau médecins sentinelles en pharmacovigilance. *Therapie* (1992) 47, 239–43.
5. Janzon K, Edgar B, Lundborg P, Regårdh CG. The influence of cimetidine and spironolactone on the pharmacokinetics and haemodynamic effects of felodipine in healthy subjects. *Acta Pharmacol Toxicol (Copenh)* (1986) 59 (Suppl 4), 98.
6. Prescal (Isradipine). Novartis Pharmaceuticals UK Ltd. UK Summary of product characteristics, June 2007.
7. Dewland PM. A study to assess the effect of food and a single 800 mg oral dose of cimetidine on the pharmacokinetics of a single 4 mg oral dose of calcium-channel inhibitor, GR43659X (lacidipine). Boehringer Ingelheim report GMH/88/030.
8. Zanidip (Lercanidipine hydrochloride). Recordati Pharmaceuticals Ltd. UK Summary of product characteristics, April 2006.
9. Zanidip (Lercanidipine). Solvay Pharmaceuticals. Australian Product information, December 2005.
10. Lai C-M, McEntegart CM, Maher KE, Bell VA, Turlapaty P, Quon CY. The effects of iv cimetidine on the pharmacokinetics (PK) and pharmacodynamics (PD) of iv nicardipine in man. *Pharm Res* (1994) 11 (Suppl 10), S386.
11. Kirch W, Janisch HD, Heidemann H, Rämsch K, Ohnhaus EE. Einfluss von Cimetidin und Ranitidin auf Pharmakokinetik und antihypertensiven Effekt von Nifedipin. *Dtsch Med Wochenschr* (1983) 108, 1757–61.
12. Kirch W, Rämsch K, Janisch HD, Ohnhaus EE. The influence of two histamine H_2-receptor antagonists, cimetidine and ranitidine, on the plasma levels and clinical effect of nifedipine and metoprolol. *Arch Toxicol* (1984) (Suppl 7), 256–9.
13. Kirch W, Hoensch H, Ohnhaus EE, Janisch HD. Ranitidin-Nifedipin-Interaktion. *Dtsch Med Wochenschr* (1984) 109, 1223.
14. Smith SR, Kendall MJ, Lobo J, Beerahee A, Jack DB, Wilkins MR. Ranitidine and cimetidine: drug interactions with single dose and steady-state nifedipine administration. *Br J Clin Pharmacol* (1987) 23, 311–15.
15. Adams LJ, Antonow DR, McClain CJ, McAllister R. Effect of ranitidine on bioavailability of nifedipine. *Gastroenterology* (1986) 90, 1320.
16. Kirch W, Ohnhaus EE, Hoensch H, Janisch HD. Ranitidine increases bioavailability of nifedipine. *Clin Pharmacol Ther* (1985) 37, 204.
17. Schwartz JB, Upton RA, Lin ET, Williams RL, Benet LZ. Effect of cimetidine or ranitidine administration on nifedipine pharmacokinetics and pharmacodynamics. *Clin Pharmacol Ther* (1988) 43, 673–80.
18. Renwick AG, Le Vie J, Challenor VF, Waller DG, Gruchy B, George CF. Factors affecting the pharmacokinetics of nifedipine. *Eur J Clin Pharmacol* (1987) 32, 351–5.
19. Khan A, Langley SJ, Mullins FGP, Dixon JS, Toon S. The pharmacokinetics and pharmacodynamics of nifedipine at steady state during concomitant administration of cimetidine or high dose ranitidine. *Br J Clin Pharmacol* (1991) 32, 519–22.
20. Adalat CC (Nifedipine). Bayer HealthCare. US Prescribing information, April 2011.
21. Kirch W, Halabi A, Linde M, Ohnhaus EE. Negativ-inotrope Wirkung von Famotidin. *Schweiz Med Wochenschr* (1988) 118, 1912–14.
22. Kirch W, Halabi A, Linde M, Santos SR, Ohnhaus EE. Negative effects of famotidine on cardiac performance assessed by noninvasive hemodynamic measurements. *Gastroenterology* (1989) 96, 1388–92.
23. Mück W, Wingender W, Seiberling M, Woelke E, Rämsch K-D, Kuhlmann J. Influence of the H2-receptor antagonists cimetidine and ranitidine on the pharmacokinetics of nimodipine in healthy volunteers. *Eur J Clin Pharmacol* (1992) 42, 325–8.
24. Van Harten J, van Brummelen P, Lodewijks MTM, Danhof M, Breimer DD. Pharmacokinetics and hemodynamic effects of nisoldipine and its interaction with cimetidine. *Clin Pharmacol Ther* (1988) 43, 332–41.
25. Sular (Nisoldipine). Sciele Pharma, Inc. US Prescribing information, February 2010.
26. Soons PA, Vogels BAPM, Roosemalen MCM, Schoemaker HC, Uchida E, Edgar B, Lundahl J, Cohen AF, Breimer DD. Grapefruit juice and cimetidine inhibit stereoselective metabolism of nitrendipine in humans. *Clin Pharmacol Ther* (1991) 50, 394–403.
27. Kirch W, Nahoui R, Ohnhaus EE. Ranitidine/nitrendipine interaction. *Clin Pharmacol Ther* (1988) 43, 149.
28. Halabi A, Nahoui R, Kirch W. Influence of ranitidine on kinetics of nitrendipine and on noninvasive hemodynamic parameters. *Ther Drug Monit* (1990) 12, 303–4.
29. Santos SR, Storpirtis S, Moreira-Filho L, Donzella H, Kirch W. Ranitidine increases the bioavailability of nitrendipine in patients with arterial hypertension. *Braz J Med Biol Res* (1992) 25, 337–47.
30. Smith MS, Benyunes MC, Bjornsson TD, Shand DG, Pritchett ELC. Influence of cimetidine on verapamil kinetics and dynamics. *Clin Pharmacol Ther* (1984) 36, 551–4.
31. Loi C-M, Rollins DE, Dukes GE, Peat MA. Effect of cimetidine on verapamil disposition. *Clin Pharmacol Ther* (1985) 37, 654–7.
32. Mikus G, Stuber H. Influence of cimetidine treatment on the physiological disposition of verapamil. *Naunyn Schmiedebergs Arch Pharmacol* (1987) 335 (Suppl), R106.
33. Mikus G, Eichelbaum M, Fischer C, Gumulka S, Klotz U, Kroemer HK. Interaction of verapamil and cimetidine: stereochemical aspects of drug metabolism, drug disposition and drug action. *J Pharmacol Exp Ther* (1990) 253, 1042–8.
34. Abernethy DR, Schwartz JB, Todd EL. Lack of interaction between verapamil and cimetidine. *Clin Pharmacol Ther* (1985) 38, 342–9.
35. Wing LMH, Miners JO, Lillywhite KJ. Verapamil disposition—effects of sulphinpyrazone and cimetidine. *Br J Clin Pharmacol* (1985) 19, 385–91.
36. Piepho RW, Culbertson VL, Rhodes RS. Drug interactions with the calcium-entry blockers. *Circulation* (1987) 75 (Suppl V), V181–V194.
37. Piepho RW. Individualization of calcium entry–blocker dosage for systemic hypertension. *Am J Cardiol* (1985) 56, 105H–111H.
38. Cardene SR (Nicardipine hydrochloride). Astellas Pharma Ltd. UK Summary of product characteristics, June 2006.
39. Cardene SR (Nicardipine hydrochloride). PDL BioPharma, Inc. US Prescribing information, January 2007.

Calcium-channel blockers + HCV-protease inhibitors

Telaprevir moderately increases the exposure to amlodipine, paritaprevir boosted with ritonavir appears to have a similar effect; boceprevir and simeprevir are expected to interact similarly. Other calcium-channel blockers would be expected to be similarly affected by the HCV-protease inhibitors. The exposure to paritaprevir is predicted to be increased by diltiazem and verapamil.

Clinical evidence

(a) Paritaprevir

The UK and US manufacturers briefly report, that in a study in 14 healthy subjects given a single 5-mg dose of **amlodipine** with paritaprevir 150 mg daily (in a fixed-dose combination with ombitasvir and ritonavir, and given with dasabuvir), the AUC and maximum concentration of paritaprevir were decreased by about 22%. The AUC and maximum concentration of amlodipine were increased 2.6-fold, and by 26%, respectively.[1,2] The UK manufacturer also notes that similar effects are expected when the paritaprevir combination is given without dasabuvir.[1] The UK manufacturer also predicts that the exposure to paritaprevir might be increased by diltiazem and verapamil.[1]

(b) Telaprevir

In a study in 19 healthy subjects, telaprevir 750 mg three times daily for 6 days, increased the AUC and maximum plasma concentration of a single 5-mg dose of **amlodipine** (given with atorvastatin 20 mg) nearly 3-fold and by about 29%, respectively.[3]

Mechanism

Telaprevir is an inhibitor of CYP3A4, the main isoenzyme by which amlodipine is metabolised, and thus increases its exposure. Paritaprevir itself is not an inhibitor of CYP3A4, but it is boosted with ritonavir, which is a well-known inhibitor of this isoenzyme, and hence the increase in amlodipine exposure seen is most likely due to the effects of the ritonavir (see 'Calcium-channel blockers + HIV-protease inhibitors', below). Paritaprevir is a substrate of both CYP3A4 and P-glycoprotein, therefore inhibitors of CYP3A4 (such as diltiazem and verapamil) or P-glycoprotein (such as verapamil) would be expected to increase its exposure.

Importance and management

Evidence for a pharmacokinetic interaction between the HCV-protease inhibitors and the calcium-channel blockers is limited to these studies with amlodipine, but the effects seen are consistent with those seen with other inhibitors of CYP3A4, and an interaction would appear to be established. Boceprevir and simeprevir also inhibit CYP3A4 (albeit to varying extents), and would be expected to increase the exposure to amlodipine.[4-7] Other calcium-channel blockers would be expected to be similarly affected by the HCV-protease inhibitors and the manufacturers specifically name **diltiazem**,[1,4-9] **felodipine**,[4-9] **nicardipine**,[4-9] **nifedipine**,[1,4-9] **nisoldipine**,[4-9] and **verapamil**.[1,4-9] Given the moderate increase in exposure to amlodipine, it would seem prudent to monitor the concurrent use of any calcium-channel blocker with the HCV-protease inhibitors for calcium-channel blocker-related adverse effects (such as headache, flushing, hypotension, and ankle oedema), reducing the calcium-channel blocker dose if necessary. The UK manufacturer of paritaprevir boosted with ritonavir (in a fixed-dose combination with ombitasvir, and given with or without dasabuvir) specifically advises a 50% amlodipine dose reduction.[1] It would also be prudent to be alert for an increase in paritaprevir adverse effects on concurrent use with diltiazem and verapamil.

1. Viekirax (Ombitasvir, paritaprevir, ritonavir). AbbVie Ltd. UK Summary of product characteristics, January 2015.
2. Viekira Pak (Ombitasvir, paritaprevir, ritonavir co-packaged with dasabuvir sodium monohydrate). AbbVie Inc. US Prescribing information, December 2014.
3. Lee JE, van Heeswijk R, Alves K, Smith F, Garg V. Effect of the hepatitis C virus protease inhibitor telaprevir on the pharmacokinetics of amlodipine and atorvastatin. *Antimicrob Agents Chemother* (2011) 55, 4569–74.
4. Victrelis (Boceprevir). Merck & Co., Inc. US Prescribing information, July 2014.
5. Olysio (Simeprevir sodium). Janssen-Cilag Ltd. UK Summary of product characteristics, May 2014.
6. Olysio (Simeprevir sodium). Janssen Products, LP. US Prescribing information, November 2014.
7. Victrelis (Boceprevir). Merck Sharp & Dohme Ltd. UK Summary of product characteristics, August 2014.
8. Incivo (Telaprevir). Janssen-Cilag Ltd. UK Summary of product characteristics, July 2014.
9. Incivek (Telaprevir). Vertex Pharmaceuticals, Inc. US Prescribing information, October 2013.

Calcium-channel blockers + HIV-protease inhibitors

A patient taking nifedipine experienced hypotension, oedema, and acute renal failure when lopinavir boosted with ritonavir was also given. Symptomatic orthostasis occurred in another patient taking nifedipine with nelfinavir, and then ritonavir and indinavir. A further patient had similar symptoms when nelfinavir was given with felodipine. Atazanavir moderately increased diltiazem exposure with an increase in cardiac effects in a study in healthy subjects. Indinavir boosted with ritonavir caused a slight increase in diltiazem exposure (although some subjects had larger increases) and amlodipine exposure. Based on this evidence, HIV-protease inhibitors, especially ritonavir, are predicted to increase the exposure to all of the calcium-channel blockers.

Clinical evidence

(a) Amlodipine

In a study in 18 healthy subjects, **indinavir** 800 mg twice daily and **ritonavir** 100 mg twice daily given with amlodipine 5 mg daily for 7 days, increased the median AUC of amlodipine by 90%. Amlodipine had no effect on the steady-state AUCs of the HIV-protease inhibitors.[1] For mention of a patient who tolerated amlodipine and **lopinavir** boosted with **ritonavir** after serious adverse effects had occurred with nifedipine and these HIV-protease inhibitors, see under *Nifedipine*, below.

(b) Diltiazem

1. Atazanavir. A study in healthy subjects found that atazanavir 400 mg daily given with diltiazem 180 mg daily resulted in a 2- to 3-fold increase in the AUC of diltiazem and its metabolite desacetyldiltiazem. The pharmacokinetics of atazanavir were not affected by diltiazem. There was an increase in the maximum PR interval on concurrent use, when use compared with atazanavir alone.[2,3]

2. Indinavir. In a study in 13 healthy subjects, indinavir 800 mg twice daily and ritonavir 100 mg twice daily, given with diltiazem 120 mg daily for 7 days, increased the median AUC of diltiazem by 27%, which was not statistically significant. However, two of the subjects had a 4-fold increase in the AUC of diltiazem, and the AUC of desacetyldiltiazem was doubled. Diltiazem had no effect on the steady-state AUCs of the HIV-protease inhibitors.[1]

(c) Felodipine

A woman taking metoprolol 50 mg daily and felodipine 5 mg daily for hypertension developed bilateral leg oedema, orthostatic hypotension, and other symptoms including dizziness and fatigue, 3 days after starting HAART following a needle-stick injury. The antiretrovirals included zidovudine, lamivudine, and **nelfinavir** 2 g daily. Antihypertensive treatment was stopped and the adverse effects abated within 3 days. The patient was then successfully switched to a diuretic-based regimen without recurrence of oedema.[4]

(d) Nifedipine

A 51-year-old HIV-positive man with coronary artery disease, hypertension and osteoarthritis, taking atenolol, also started taking extended-release nifedipine 60 mg daily. When his blood pressure control improved he was given zidovudine 300 mg, lamivudine 150 mg, and **nelfinavir** 1.25 g all twice daily. Within 3 days of starting the antiretrovirals he experienced dizziness, weakness and hypotension and developed complete heart block with a junctional escape rhythm. His ECG returned to normal within 24 hours of stopping the antiretrovirals, but he developed orthostatic symptoms within 2 days of restarting **nelfinavir**. He later tolerated a regimen consisting of stavudine, didanosine and efavirenz without any episodes of dizziness, hypotension or bradycardia. However, when he was given zidovudine, abacavir, **ritonavir**, and **indinavir**, he experienced hypotension, decreased heart rate, weakness and fatigue. His symptoms were controlled by modifying his antihypertensives, including stopping atenolol and reduction of the dose of nifedipine to 30 mg daily.[5]

Another case report describes a patient taking antihypertensive drugs including nifedipine 30 mg twice daily, who developed malaise, severe hypotension, oliguria and progressive generalised oedema on the second day of taking **lopinavir** boosted with **ritonavir**. He had previously developed hypotension and progressive renal failure when taking nifedipine and HAART (including **lopinavir** boosted with **ritonavir**). All antihypertensive and antiretroviral drugs were discontinued and the patient improved, but the same symptoms recurred after the nifedipine and then **lopinavir** and **ritonavir** were reintroduced. All drugs were stopped, then HAART (including **lopinavir** boosted with **ritonavir**) was reintroduced again and **amlodipine** 15 mg daily was substituted for nifedipine. This regimen was well tolerated.[6]

Mechanism

The HIV-protease inhibitors, particularly ritonavir, are potent inhibitors of CYP3A4, by which many of the calcium-channel blockers are, at least in part, metabolised. It appears that some HIV-protease inhibitors can cause a clinically relevant increase in calcium-channel blocker exposure. Verapamil and diltiazem are known to inhibit CYP3A4, and might therefore theoretically reduce the metabolism of the HIV-protease inhibitors. However, the effect might depend on which is the more potent inhibitor, as, in the studies above, diltiazem did not affect atazanavir, indinavir, or ritonavir concentrations.

Importance and management

Although information is limited, the pharmacokinetic interactions between some HIV-protease inhibitors and calcium-channel blockers are predictable, and potentially serious. Clinically relevant increases in calcium-channel blocker exposure or effects have been shown for amlodipine, diltiazem, felodipine, and nifedipine. Caution would be required with any of these calcium-channel blockers given with an HIV-protease inhibitor boosted with ritonavir. Monitor patients for calcium-channel blocker adverse effects (e.g. hypotension, headache, flushing, and oedema), and anticipate the need to use lower doses of the calcium-channel blocker. Evidence for other calcium-channel blockers is generally lacking; however, as they are all metabolised, to a greater or lesser extent, by CYP3A4 it seems likely that they might interact similarly, and therefore, until more is known, similar precautions would seem advisable. Particular caution is warranted with **verapamil** because adverse cardiac effects (conduction disorders) are more commonly associated with this particular calcium-channel blocker.

Note that the UK manufacturer of **lercanidipine**[7] contraindicates the concurrent use of ritonavir or other strong inhibitors of CYP3A4, which would be expected to include most, if not all, HIV-protease inhibitors. The manufacturers of **atazanavir** specifically recommend that, if diltiazem is also given, its initial dose should be reduced by 50% with subsequent dose titration and ECG monitoring.[2,3]

It has been suggested that other antihypertensive drugs such as ACE inhibitors and diuretics, which are primarily eliminated renally, could be considered as alternatives to calcium-channel blockers:[8] this seems prudent advice.

1. Glesby MJ, Aberg JA, Kendall MA, Fichtenbaum CJ, Hafner R, Hall S, Grosskopf N, Zolopa AR, Gerber JG, for the Adult AIDS Clinical Trials Group A5159 Protocol Team. Pharmacokinetic interactions between indinavir plus ritonavir and calcium channel blockers. *Clin Pharmacol Ther* (2005) 78, 143–53.
2. Reyataz (Atazanavir sulphate). Bristol-Myers Squibb Pharmaceutical Ltd. UK Summary of product characteristics, August 2012.
3. Reyataz (Atazanavir sulfate). Bristol-Myers Squibb. US Prescribing information, March 2012.
4. Izzedine H, Launay-Vacher V, Deray G, Hulot J-S. Nelfinavir and felodipine: A cytochrome P450 3A4-mediated drug interaction. *Clin Pharmacol Ther* (2004) 75, 362–3.
5. Rossi DR, Rathbun RC, Slater LN. Symptomatic orthostasis with extended-release nifedipine and protease inhibitors. *Pharmacotherapy* (2002) 22, 1312–16.
6. Baeza MT, Merino E, Boix V, Climent E. Nifedipine–lopinavir/ritonavir severe interaction: a case report. *AIDS* (2007) 21, 119–20.
7. Zanidip (Lercanidipine hydrochloride). Recordati Pharmaceuticals Ltd. UK Summary of product characteristics, April 2006.
8. Vourvahis M, Kashuba AD. Mechanisms of pharmacokinetic and pharmacodynamic drug interactions associated with ritonavir-enhanced tipranavir. *Pharmacotherapy* (2007) 27, 888–909.

Calcium-channel blockers + Hormonal contraceptives

A 21-day course of combined hormonal contraceptives appeared to have little effect on the AUC of nifedipine, but the AUC of its metabolite was reduced. Diltiazem may slightly raise estradiol levels.

Clinical evidence

(a) Combined hormonal contraceptives

A study in 23 healthy women investigated the influence of oral contraceptives on the pharmacokinetics of a single 10-mg dose of **nifedipine**. The intake of oral contraceptives containing **dienogest** 2 mg with **ethinylestradiol** 30 micrograms or **levonorgestrel** 125 micrograms with **ethinylestradiol** 30 micrograms for 21 days did not influence the AUC of **nifedipine**, but the AUC_{0-24} of its main metabolite, dehydronifedipine, was reduced by about 25%.

(b) Estradiol

A study in 5 healthy postmenopausal women given **diltiazem** 30 mg twice daily for 4 days with a single 2-mg oral dose of estradiol on day 2, found that there was a slight but non-significant increase in the maximum levels of estrone.[1]

Mechanism

The reduction in dehydronifedipine levels suggests that the formation rate of the metabolite was reduced, probably because the contraceptive reduced the metabolism of nifedipine to dehydronifedipine by the cytochrome P450 isoenzyme CYP3A4.[2]

Diltiazem is a moderate inhibitor of the cytochrome P450 isoenzyme CYP3A4 and would be expected to decrease the metabolism of estradiol.

Importance and management

The effects of combined hormonal contraceptives on nifedipine appear minimal, but a multiple-dose study would be needed to confirm the expected lack of a clinically relevant interaction. The current data suggests that the efficacy of nifedipine would not be expected to be reduced by a pharmacokinetic mechanism; however, for further comments on the effect of hormonal contraceptives on blood pressure, see 'Antihypertensives + Hormonal contraceptives', p.1053.

The increase in oestrogen levels caused by diltiazem is small and unlikely to cause any clinically significant adverse effects. However, the dose of diltiazem given in the study was much lower than commonly prescribed doses, the number of patients involved in the study was small, and therefore these results may not accurately reflect the effect of concurrent use. The available data is insufficient to warrant any change in practice, but more study is needed to confirm the absence of a clinically relevant interaction.

1. Annas A, Carlström K, Alván G, AL-Shurbaji A. The effect of ketoconazole and diltiazem on oestrogen metabolism in postmenopausal women after single dose oestradiol treatment. *Br J Clin Pharmacol* (2003) 56, 334–6.
2. Balogh A, Gessinger S, Svarovsky U, Hippius M, Mellinger U, Klinger G, Hoffmann A, Oettel M. Can oral contraceptive steroids influence the elimination of nifedipine and its primary pyridine metabolite in humans? *Eur J Clin Pharmacol* (1998) 54, 729–34.

Calcium-channel blockers + Macrolides

Erythromycin moderately increases the exposure to felodipine. Cases reports and retrospective analyses suggest that the use of clarithromycin, erythromycin, or telithromycin with calcium-channel blockers including diltiazem, felodipine, nifedipine, and verapamil increases the risk of toxicity and adverse effects, such as hypotension and QT prolongation.

Clinical evidence

A case-control study found that 176 of 7 100 elderly patients taking a calcium-channel blocker (**amlodipine**, **diltiazem**, **felodipine**, **nifedipine**, or **verapamil**), and admitted to hospital because of hypotension, had taken a macrolide either in the 7-day risk period immediately before admission or in a 7-day control period one month earlier. The use of **erythromycin** or **clarithromycin** was associated with an increased short-term risk of hospitalisation for hypotension (odds ratio 5.8 and 3.7, respectively), whereas the use of **azithromycin** was not associated with this increased risk.[1] When the results were re-analysed for only the dihydropyridine calcium-channel blockers, similar risks were found with **erythromycin** (odds ratio 3.4) and **clarithromycin** (odds ratio, 4.25).[1] Analyses of the use of individual pairs of a calcium-channel blocker and a macrolide are covered in the following sections.

(a) Diltiazem

A patient who had marked hypotension and bradycardia when **erythromycin** was added to verapamil and propranolol (see *Verapamil*, below) had previously taken **erythromycin** with diltiazem and a beta blocker without any reported adverse effects.[2]

In a retrospective cohort study, there was one sudden cardiac death in 106 person-years among patients taking diltiazem with **erythromycin**. When combined with the findings for verapamil, patients taking these calcium-channel blockers and erythromycin had about a 5-fold increase in risk of sudden death when compared with those who were not taking CYP3A4 inhibitors or **erythromycin**.[3]

For details of a case control study that found some calcium-channel blockers, including diltiazem, were associated with a greater risk of hospitalisation for hypotension when given with **erythromycin** or **clarithromycin**, but not **azithromycin**, see above.

(b) Felodipine

In a pharmacokinetic study, 12 healthy subjects were given felodipine 10 mg before and after taking **erythromycin** 250 mg four times daily for a day.[4] The felodipine AUC was increased almost 3-fold by **erythromycin**, its maximum plasma concentration was more than doubled, and its half-life prolonged from 6.9 hours to 11.1 hours.[4]

A hypertensive woman taking felodipine 10 mg daily developed tachycardia, flushing, and massive ankle oedema within 2 to 3 days of starting to take **erythromycin** 250 mg twice daily. Her blood pressure had reduced from 120/90 mmHg to 110/70 mmHg. She fully recovered within a few days of stopping the **erythromycin**.[5]

For details of a case control study that found some calcium-channel blockers, including felodipine, were associated with a greater risk of hospitalisation for hypotension when given with **erythromycin** or **clarithromycin**, but not **azithromycin**, see above.

(c) Nifedipine

1. Clarithromycin. A 77-year-old man with slight renal impairment, taking sustained-release nifedipine 60 mg twice daily, captopril, and doxazosin, had persistent systolic hypertension (170 to 180 mmHg). Two days after starting to take clarithromycin 500 mg twice daily for breathing difficulty and cough, his blood pressure was 140/70 mmHg at a routine appointment, and so the doxazosin dose was halved and valsartan substituted for captopril. Later that day, he was admitted with hypotension (80/40 mmHg) and bradycardia (40 bpm). Clarithromycin was replaced with erythromycin and the antihypertensives stopped. After 3 days his blood pressure was stabilised with nifedipine 60 mg daily and furosemide, and clarithromycin was restarted. Septic shock was ruled out as a cause of the hypotension.[6]

For details of a case control study that found some calcium-channel blockers, including nifedipine, were associated with a greater risk of hospitalisation for hypotension when given with clarithromycin, see above.

2. Erythromycin. In a retrospective cohort study, there were no sudden deaths from cardiac causes in 114 person-years of the use of oral erythromycin with calcium-channel blockers that do not inhibit CYP3A4 to a clinically relevant extent (mostly nifedipine).[3] This was in contrast to the increased risk of sudden death with erythromycin and diltiazem (see above) or verapamil (see below).

For details of a case control study that found some calcium-channel blockers, including nifedipine, were associated with a greater risk of hospitalisation for hypotension when given with erythromycin, see above.

(d) Verapamil

1. Clarithromycin. A 53-year-old woman undergoing haemodialysis 3 times a week, taking a range of medicines including digoxin, was given clarithromycin 250 mg and verapamil 120 mg both twice daily because of an acute exacerbation of chronic obstructive pulmonary disease and a recurrence of atrial fibrillation. After 24 hours she experienced dizziness and episodes of fainting. A day later her supine blood pressure was 89/39 mmHg and her heart rate 50 bpm. Verapamil was stopped and she recovered within 2 days, after which verapamil was restarted at a dose of 40 mg before each dialysis session. The authors suggest that, although an interaction between digoxin and verapamil cannot be ruled out, the digoxin concentrations were very low before verapamil was started, and they therefore believe that the effects seen cannot entirely have been due to raised digoxin concentrations.[7] Another report[2] describes a 77-year-old woman with hypertension, taking propranolol and verapamil, who developed marked bradycardia (37 to 50 bpm), within 4 days of starting a course of clarithromycin 500 mg twice daily. The problem was solved by temporarily reducing the dose of verapamil from 80 mg twice daily to 40 mg twice daily and halving the dose of propranolol until the clarithromycin course had been finished. Essentially the same thing happened 2 years later when erythromycin was added.

For details of a case control study[1] that found some calcium-channel blockers, including verapamil, were associated with a greater risk of hospitalisation for hypotension when given with clarithromycin, see above.

2. Erythromycin. A 79-year-old woman taking verapamil 240 mg twice daily and ramipril was admitted to hospital with extreme fatigue and dizziness one week after starting a course of erythromycin 2 g daily for a respiratory tract infection. Her blood pressure was 80/60 mmHg and her respiratory rate was 18 breaths per minute. ECG showed complete AV block, escape rhythm of 50 bpm, pattern of left bundle-branch block and QTc interval prolongation (583 milliseconds compared with 436 milliseconds 20 days before admission). Verapamil and erythromycin were stopped and intravenous fluids, dopamine and calcium were given. Her blood pressure increased to 110/70 mmHg and after 4 days the QTc interval prolongation had resolved and her heart rate was 76 bpm.[8] Another patient taking verapamil and propranolol developed marked bradycardia and hypotension 2 days after starting to take erythromycin 333 mg three times daily.[2]

In a retrospective cohort study, there were two sudden cardiac deaths in 78 person-years among patients taking verapamil with erythromycin. When combined with the findings for verapamil, patients taking these calcium-channel blockers and erythromycin had a 5-fold increase in risk of sudden death when compared with those who used were not taking CYP3A4 inhibitors or erythromycin.[3]

For details of a case control study that found some calcium-channel blockers, including verapamil, were associated with a greater risk of hospitalisation for hypotension when given with erythromycin, see above.

3. Telithromycin. A 76-year-old woman taking verapamil 180 mg daily experienced shortness of breath and weakness 2 days after starting telithromycin 800 mg daily for a sinus infection. She was found to have marked hypotension (systolic blood pressure 50 to 60 mmHg) and bradycardia (30 bpm). She required a transvenous pacemaker for 3 days and pressor drugs.[9]

Mechanism

Erythromycin, clarithromycin, and telithromycin are inhibitors of CYP3A4, by which many of the calcium-channel blockers are, at least in part, metabolised, resulting in increased concentrations and adverse effects. Verapamil, erythromycin, and clarithromycin are also P-glycoprotein inhibitors, which might contribute to the pharmacokinetic interaction by reducing the elimination of the calcium-channel blocker,[7] or by increasing macrolide absorption.[8]

Erythromycin has been associated with prolongation of the QT interval; an effect that is likely to be increased by drugs that increase erythromycin concentrations such as diltiazem and verapamil.[3]

Importance and management

Information seems to be limited, but the interaction between the calcium-channel blockers and the macrolides would appear to be established and clinically important, although its incidence is probably low. Anticipate the need to reduce the felodipine or verapamil dose if erythromycin or clarithromycin, or possibly also telithromycin, is added. Evidence for other calcium-channel blockers is limited, but given the way many interact with other CYP3A4 inhibitors, until more is known it would seem prudent to be alert for increased effects if they are given with erythromycin, clarithromycin, or also telithromycin. Monitor for effects such as hypotension, headache, flushing, and oedema, and reduce the calcium-channel blocker dose where necessary. However, note that the manufacturer of **lercanidipine** contraindicates the concurrent use of erythromycin.[10]

The case control study[1] found that azithromycin did not increase the hypotensive risk and this is probably because **azithromycin** appears to have little or no effect on the CYP3A subfamily and so would be less likely to interact. However, note that an effect via P-glycoprotein is theoretically possible and so an interaction cannot entirely be excluded.

Other reports suggests that the cardiac toxicity of erythromycin might be increased by verapamil,[3,8] and diltiazem,[3] and the authors of one of these reports consider that erythromycin should not be used with CYP3A4 inhibitors (that is diltiazem and verapamil).[3]

1. Wright AJ, Gomes T, Mamdani MM, Horn JR, Juurlink DN. The risk of hypotension following co-prescription of macrolide antibiotics and calcium channel blockers. *CMAJ* (2011) 183, 303–7.
2. Steenbergen JA, Stauffer VL. Potential macrolide interaction with verapamil. *Ann Pharmacother* (1998) 32, 387–8.
3. Ray WA, Murray KT, Meredith S, Narasimhulu SS, Hall K, Stein CM. Oral erythromycin and the risk of sudden death from cardiac causes. *N Engl J Med* (2004) 351, 1089–96.
4. Bailey DG, Bend JR, Arnold JMO, Tran LT, Spence JD. Erythromycin-felodipine interaction: magnitude, mechanism, and comparison with grapefruit juice. *Clin Pharmacol Ther* (1996) 60, 25–33.
5. Liedholm H, Nordin G. Erythromycin–felodipine interaction. *DICP Ann Pharmacother* (1991) 25, 1007–8.
6. Gerónimo-Pardo M, Cuartero-del-Pozo AB, Jiménez-Vizuete JM, Cortiñas-Sáez M, Peyró-García R. Clarithromycin-nifedipine interaction as possible cause of vasodilatory shock. *Ann Pharmacother* (2005) 39, 538–42.
7. Kaeser YA, Brunner F, Drewe J, Haefeli WE. Severe hypotension and bradycardia associated with verapamil and clarithromycin. *Am J Health-Syst Pharm* (1998) 55, 2417–18.
8. Goldschmidt N, Azaz-Livshits T, Gotsman I, Nir-Paz R, Ben-Yehuda A, Muszkat M. Compound cardiac toxicity of oral erythromycin and verapamil. *Ann Pharmacother* (2001) 35, 1396–9.
9. Reed M, Wall GC, Shah NP, Heun JM, Hicklin GA. Verapamil toxicity resulting from a probable interaction with telithromycin. *Ann Pharmacother* (2005) 39, 357–60.
10. Zanidip (Lercanidipine hydrochloride). Recordati Pharmaceuticals Ltd. UK Summary of product characteristics, April 2006.

Calcium-channel blockers + Magnesium compounds

There are isolated reports of pregnant women who have developed bilateral hand contractures or muscular weakness and then paralysis, after receiving intravenous magnesium sulfate, either alone or with nifedipine or amlodipine. Profound hypotension occurred in two women when nifedipine was added to intravenous magnesium sulfate and methyldopa. However, a larger retrospective study of combined use of intravenous magnesium sulfate and nifedipine did not find these effects.

Clinical evidence

(a) Hypotension

Two women with pre-eclampsia, unsuccessfully treated with methyldopa and magnesium sulfate, experienced severe hypotension when a single 10-mg oral dose of **nifedipine** was added.[1] In contrast, a study in 10 women with severe pre-eclampsia receiving magnesium sulfate found that oral **nifedipine** 10 mg followed by 20 mg every 20 minutes, caused a steady decrease in mean arterial pressure and severe hypotension was not observed.[2] Moreover, in a retrospective study, the incidence of hypotension in 162 women given **nifedipine** and magnesium sulfate was lower than in 183 receiving magnesium sulfate and no antihypertensive (41.4% versus 53%).[3] For further details of this study, see (b) below.

(b) Neuromuscular blockade and hypocalcaemia

1. Amlodipine. A pre-eclamptic woman at 32 weeks gestation was unsuccessfully treated with intravenous magnesium sulfate (2 g loading dose then 10 g daily) and labetalol and underwent caesarean section on the third day. She continued to receive the magnesium, but the labetalol was discontinued 2 days later, and she was given amlodipine 2.5 mg orally. After 7 hours she experienced neuromuscular blockade (inability to move fingers and hands or lift her head) and was found to have low plasma calcium and high plasma magnesium. The magnesium was discontinued; she was given calcium gluconate and the symptoms resolved. She had no further symptoms while continuing amlodipine 2.5 mg twice daily.[4]

2. Nifedipine. A report describes symptomatic hypocalcaemia (serum calcium concentration of 1.35 mmol/L) in a woman at 33 weeks gestation after she received magnesium sulfate and nifedipine.[5] However, this report also describes this effect in a patient taking magnesium sulfate alone. Both women experienced bilateral hand contractures and were successfully treated with calcium gluconate.[5]

A pregnant woman at 32 weeks gestation was effectively treated for premature uterine contractions with nifedipine, 60 mg orally over 3 hours, and later 20 mg every 8 hours. When contractions began again 12 hours later, she was given magnesium sulfate 500 mg intravenously. She developed jerky movements of the extremities, complained of difficulty in swallowing, paradoxical respirations, and an inability to lift her head from the pillow. The magnesium was stopped and the muscle weakness disappeared over the next 25 minutes.[6]

A woman at 28 weeks gestation with mild pre-eclampsia was given an infusion of magnesium sulfate 2 g/hour. Her plasma magnesium was found to be high (2.75 mmol/L). No untoward reactions developed when she took a 20-mg dose of nifedipine, but 30 minutes after taking a second dose [by implication 3 to 4 hours later] she complained of flushing and sweating and had difficulty in lifting her head and limbs. Shortly afterwards almost complete muscular paralysis developed. The magnesium sulfate was stopped and a dramatic improvement followed within 15 minutes of a 1-g intravenous injection of calcium gluconate.[7]

In contrast, a retrospective analysis found no increased risk of serious magnesium-related maternal adverse effects in 162 women with pre-eclampsia who were also given nifedipine, compared with 32 women receiving another antihypertensive, or 183 who received no antihypertensive. The women receiving nifedipine had more severe pre-eclampsia and a longer magnesium sulfate infusion. However, the incidence of neuromuscular weakness was about 53% in these women, compared with 53% in those receiving another antihypertensive, and 45% in those receiving no antihypertensive. These differences were not statistically significant. Moreover, the incidence of maternal hypotension was lower in those receiving **nifedipine** than in those receiving no antihypertensive (see (a) above).[3]

Mechanism

The probable reason for neuromuscular effects is that both magnesium sulfate and calcium channel blockers can reduce the amount of calcium ions needed for normal muscular contraction. Calcium channel blockers inhibit the inflow of extracellular calcium across cell membranes. Magnesium probably acts in the same way, and also reduces intracellular calcium by activating adenyl cyclase and increasing cyclic adenosine monophosphate (cAMP). In addition magnesium stimulates calcium-dependent ATPase, which promotes calcium uptake by the sarcoplasmic reticulum. The result is muscular paralysis, which is reversed by giving large amounts of calcium. Magnesium sulfate alone is also known to have neuromuscular blocking activity if hypermagnesaemia occurs. Both drugs can also cause hypotension, which could be additive.

Importance and management

Direct information about the neuromuscular and hypotensive effects of the combination of nifedipine or amlodipine and intravenous magnesium sulfate seems to be limited. Although a few cases of possible additive effects have been reported, one large retrospective study did not find an increase in risk of neuromuscular effects, or of hypotension, with concurrent use of nifedipine. Nevertheless, one UK manufacturer of nifedipine advises particular caution when it is used in combination with intravenous magnesium sulfate in pregnant women, and recommends careful monitoring of blood pressure.[8] Plasma calcium and magnesium should also be carefully monitored when using intravenous magnesium sulfate in pregnancy. If this is an interaction, it would be expected to occur with all calcium-channel blockers. The interaction would not be expected with oral magnesium compounds because these have a low risk of causing hypermagnesaemia.

One UK manufacturer of magnesium sulfate injection states that concurrent use of **nimodipine** might very rarely lead to a calcium ion imbalance which could result in abnormal muscle function.[9]

1. Waisman GD, Mayorga LM, Cámera MI, Vignolo CA, Martinotti A. Magnesium plus nifedipine: potentiation of hypotensive effect in preeclampsia? *Am J Obstet Gynecol* (1988) 159, 308–9.
2. Scardo JA, Vermillion ST, Hogg BB, Newman RB. Hemodynamic effects of oral nifedipine in preeclamptic hypertensive emergencies. *Am J Obstet Gynecol* (1996) 175, 336–8.
3. Magee LA, Miremadi S, Li J, Cheng C, Ensom MHH, Carleton B, Coté A-M, von Dadelszen P. Therapy with both magnesium sulfate and nifedipine does not increase the risk of serious magnesium-related maternal side effects in women with preeclampsia. *Am J Obstet Gynecol* (2005) 193, 153–63.
4. Wu QA, Ye YQ. Neuromuscular blockade after therapy with magnesium sulfate and amlodipine. *Eur J Obstet Gynecol Reprod Biol* (2010) 149, 225.
5. Koontz SL, Friedman SA, Schwartz ML. Symptomatic hypocalcemia after tocolytic therapy with magnesium sulfate and nifedipine. *Am J Obstet Gynecol* (2004) 190, 1773–6.
6. Snyder SW, Cardwell MS. Neuromuscular blockade with magnesium sulfate and nifedipine. *Am J Obstet Gynecol* (1989) 161, 35–6.
7. Ben-Ami M, Giladi Y, Shalev E. The combination of magnesium sulphate and nifedipine: a cause of neuromuscular blockade. *Br J Obstet Gynaecol* (1994) 101, 262–3.
8. Adalat Retard (Nifedipine). Bayer plc. UK Summary of product characteristics, April 2012.
9. Magnesium Sulphate Injection. UCB Pharma Ltd. UK Summary of product characteristics, September 2010.

Calcium-channel blockers + Melatonin

Melatonin may have some modest effects on blood pressure in patients taking nifedipine.

Clinical evidence

Forty-seven subjects with mild to moderate hypertension well-controlled with **nifedipine** GITS 30 mg or 60 mg daily for the past 3 months were given melatonin immediate-release capsules 5 mg each evening for 4 weeks. At the end of the 4 weeks, there was a modest increase in mean 24-hour systolic and diastolic blood pressure of 6.5 mmHg and 4.9 mmHg, respectively, and an increase in heart rate of 3.9 bpm. However, there was no difference in single-time point 'clinic' blood pressure (136/85 mmHg versus 138/87 mmHg) and heart rate. While taking melatonin, there was a greater incidence of drowsiness, during the morning, and weakness. One subject dropped out of the study complaining of marked weakness.[1]

Mechanism

Unknown. Melatonin has been reported to possess blood pressure-lowering properties when used alone and was expected to have additive effects with nifedipine.[1]

Importance and management

The chronic use of melatonin appears to modestly impair the hypotensive effects of nifedipine and increase the blood pressure and heart rates of patients. However, this was only detected on 24-hour blood pressure monitoring, and was not apparent with single-measures of blood pressure at the clinic. Therefore, given that the overall change was small, the clinical relevance of the effect is probably minor. Nevertheless, it is not clear just why this change occurred, and until more is known, it may be prudent to consider the use of melatonin if blood pressure is hard to control in any patient taking a calcium-channel blocker.

1. Lusardi P, Piazza E, Fogari R. Cardiovascular effects of melatonin in hypertensive patients well controlled by nifedipine: a 24-hour study. *Br J Clin Pharmacol* (2000) 49, 423–7.

Calcium-channel blockers + NNRTIs

Efavirenz decreases the bioavailability of diltiazem, whereas diltiazem has no clinically relevant effect on the pharmacokinetics of efavirenz. Potentially, other calcium-channel blockers might be expected to interact similarly with efavirenz. Delavirdine is predicted to inhibit the metabolism of the calcium-channel blockers.

Clinical evidence, mechanism, importance and management

(a) Delavirdine

The manufacturer of delavirdine states that it might inhibit the metabolism of the calcium-channel blockers (they name **amlodipine**, **diltiazem**, **felodipine**, **isradipine**, **nifedipine**, **nicardipine**, **nimodipine**, **nisoldipine**, and **verapamil**), resulting in increased concentrations of the calcium-channel blocker. They state that caution and clinical monitoring of patients is warranted on concurrent use.[1] It would seem prudent to monitor blood pressure closely if delavirdine is given to a patient taking a calcium-channel blocker, decreasing the dose of the calcium-channel blocker if necessary. If a calcium-channel blocker is to be started in a patient taking delavirdine it would seem prudent to start with the lowest possible dose and titrate carefully, according to response. Note that this interaction probably occurs because delavirdine is an inhibitor of CYP3A4, by which the calcium-channel blockers are metabolised. Therefore if dose titration of the calcium-channel blocker proves difficult it would be prudent, where possible, to try an alternative class of drugs. Note that ACE inhibitors, angiotensin II receptor antagonists and beta blockers are not known to be affected by CYP3A4.

(b) Efavirenz

In a study in healthy subjects, efavirenz 600 mg daily decreased the steady-state AUC and maximum plasma concentration of **diltiazem** by 69% and 60%, respectively. Concentrations of diltiazem metabolites were also reduced. The pharmacokinetics of efavirenz were not altered to a clinically relevant extent.[2,3] The manufacturer of efavirenz suggests that the dose of **diltiazem** might need to be adjusted [increased], depending on clinical response.[2,3]

No data are available on the potential interaction of efavirenz with other calcium-channel blockers. However, efavirenz is known to induce CYP3A4, the main route of metabolism of many of the calcium-channel blockers, and therefore efavirenz would be expected to reduce their concentrations. The manufacturers suggest that any dose adjustments should be guided by clinical response (e.g. blood pressure).[2,3] Note that ACE inhibitors, angiotensin II receptor antagonists and beta blockers are not known to be affected by CYP3A4, and therefore they might provide a suitable alternative in some patients..

1. Rescriptor (Delavirdine mesylate). ViiV Healthcare. US Prescribing information, August 2012.
2. Sustiva Film-coated Tablets (Efavirenz). Bristol-Myers Squibb Pharmaceutical Ltd. UK Summary of product characteristics, March 2014.
3. Sustiva (Efavirenz). Bristol-Myers Squibb Company. US Prescribing information, August 2012.

Calcium-channel blockers + Phenobarbital

Phenobarbital greatly reduces the plasma concentration and/or increases the clearance of felodipine, nifedipine, nimodipine, and verapamil.

Primidone is expected to interact similarly. Other calcium-channel blockers are expected to be similarly affected by both phenobarbital and primidone.

Clinical evidence

(a) Felodipine

In a study in 10 patients with epilepsy given felodipine 10 mg daily for 4 days, maximum plasma concentrations of felodipine were found to be 1.6 nanomol/L which was much lower than that in 12 control subjects not taking antiepileptic drugs (maximum plasma concentration 8.9 nanomol/L). Of the 10 patients, one was taking phenobarbital.[1]

(b) Nifedipine

In a pharmacokinetic study in 15 healthy subjects, the clearance of a single 20-mg dose of nifedipine was increased almost 3-fold after they took phenobarbital 100 mg daily for 2 weeks. The AUC of nifedipine was reduced by about 60%.[2]

A 67-year-old patient taking several medications including nifedipine and ticlopidine was also given phenobarbital and had higher than expected serum concentrations of phenobarbital (21.4 mg/L; serum concentration-to-dose ratio 16.7) without any evidence of toxicity. It was suggested that ticlopidine and nifedipine might have interacted with phenobarbital.[3] However, note that ticlopidine did not change phenobarbital concentrations in another patient, see 'Phenytoin + Ticlopidine', p.608.

(c) Nimodipine

A study in 8 patients with epilepsy taking antiepileptics long-term (including 4 who were taking phenobarbital and 2 who were taking phenobarbital with carbamazepine) found that the AUC of a single 60-mg oral dose of nimodipine was reduced by about 85%, when compared with a group of healthy subjects.[4]

(d) Verapamil

A study in 7 healthy subjects found that phenobarbital 100 mg daily for 3 weeks increased the clearance of verapamil 80 mg every 6 hours 4-fold and reduced its bioavailability 5-fold.[5]

Mechanism

Phenobarbital is an enzyme inducer that can increase the metabolism of calcium-channel blockers by CYP3A4 in the liver. This results in lower plasma concentrations of the calcium-channel blocker.

Importance and management

Evidence for an interaction between phenobarbital and the calcium-channel blockers is limited, but the available data suggest that phenobarbital can reduce nifedipine, nimodipine, and verapamil plasma concentrations, and probably has a similar effect on felodipine concentrations. Information regarding other calcium-channel blockers is generally lacking, but as they are all, at least in part, metabolised by CYP3A4 it would seem prudent, until more is known, to consider the possibility that their effects will be reduced in patients also taking phenobarbital. Monitor the outcome of concurrent use for the effects on blood pressure and anticipate the need to increase the dose of the calcium-channel blockers. However, note that in some cases the interaction seems particularly marked, and a dose increase of the calcium-channel blocker might not be adequate to manage the interaction and other antihypertensives should be considered. The ACE inhibitors and angiotensin II receptor antagonists are not known to be affected by CYP3A4, and therefore might provide a suitable alternative to a calcium-channel blocker in some patients. The UK manufacturers of nimodipine contra-indicate[6] concurrent use.

As **primidone** is metabolised to phenobarbital, it seems likely that it will interact similarly.

1. Capewell S, Freestone S, Critchley JAJH, Pottage A, Prescott LF. Reduced felodipine bioavailability in patients taking anticonvulsants. *Lancet* (1988) ii, 480–2.
2. Schellens JHM, van der Wart JHF, Brugman M, Breimer DD. Influence of enzyme induction and inhibition on the oxidation of nifedipine, sparteine, mephenytoin and antipyrine in humans as assessed by a "cocktail" study design. *J Pharmacol Exp Ther* (1989) 249, 638–45.
3. Sánchez-Romero A, García-Delgado R, Durán-Quintana JA. ¿Puede el tratamiento asociado con ticlopidina y nifedipina aumentar los niveles séricos de fenobarbital? *Rev Neurol* (2003) 36, 433–4.
4. Tartara A, Galimberti CA, Manni R, Parietti L, Zucca C, Baasch H, Caresia L, Mück W, Barzaghi N, Gatti G, Perucca E. Differential effects of valproic acid and enzyme-inducing anticonvulsants on nimodipine pharmacokinetics in epileptic patients. *Br J Clin Pharmacol* (1991) 32, 335–40.
5. Rutledge DR, Pieper JA, Mirvis DM. Effects of chronic phenobarbital on verapamil disposition in humans. *J Pharmacol Exp Ther* (1988) 246, 7–13.
6. Nimotop Tablets (Nimodipine). Bayer plc. UK Summary of product characteristics, October 2012.

Calcium-channel blockers + Phenothiazines

The hypotensive adverse effects of the phenothiazines are expected to be additive with the known blood pressure lowering effects of the calcium-channel blockers.

Clinical evidence, mechanism, importance and management

An isolated report describes a patient taking chlorpromazine, who was given **nifedipine** the day before surgery, and then developed marked hypotension during surgery, which was eventually controlled with noradrenaline (norepinephrine).[1] It was suggested that the hypotension was due to an interaction between **nifedipine** and chlorpromazine. Although in general the hypotensive adverse effects of phenothiazines would be expected to be additive with the blood pressure lowering effects of the calcium-channel blockers there are many other factors that mean that the hypotensive effects seen in the case cannot be directly attributed to an interaction. For example, the dose of nifedipine given was not stated, the patient was additionally taking cimetidine, which can increase the bioavailability of nifedipine, see 'Calcium-channel blockers + H_2-receptor antagonists', p.1039, and, furthermore, the concurrent use of antihypertensives and general anaesthetics can also result in enhanced hypotension, for example, see 'Anaesthetics, general + ACE inhibitors or Angiotensin II receptor antagonists', p.99. Nevertheless, because of the known effects of both groups of drugs, some caution seems prudent on their concurrent use. Warn patients to take time in getting up to minimise orthostatic hypotension.

1. Stuart-Taylor ME, Crosse MM. A plea for noradrenaline. *Anaesthesia* (1989) 44, 916–17.

Calcium-channel blockers + Quinupristin with Dalfopristin

Quinupristin with dalfopristin modestly increased the AUC of nifedipine. Other calcium-channel blockers are predicted to be similarly affected.

Clinical evidence, mechanism, importance and management

The manufacturer notes that the AUC of repeated-dose **nifedipine** was increased by about 40% by quinupristin with dalfopristin, and the maximum level was increased by about 20%.[1] This is probably because quinupristin with dalfopristin inhibits the metabolism of **nifedipine** by the cytochrome P450 isoenzyme CYP3A4.[2] Although the clinical relevance of these increases have not been assessed, an increase in the AUC of nifedipine of 40% is fairly modest. The manufacturers of **nifedipine** advise blood pressure monitoring and, if necessary, a reduction of the **nifedipine** dosage during concurrent use.[1,3] It is predicted that other calcium-channel blockers[2] will also have their levels raised by quinupristin with dalfopristin, and this seem likely, as all calcium-channel blockers are metabolised, at least in part, by CYP3A4; however, the extent of the interaction is likely to vary between drugs. It may therefore be prudent to be alert for an increase in their effects (e.g. a drop in blood pressure, headache, flushing, peripheral oedema) and reduce the dose if problems occur.

1. Adalat CC (Nifedipine). Bayer HealthCare. US Prescribing information, April 2011.
2. Rubinstein E, Prokocimer P, Talbot GH. Safety and tolerability of quinupristin/dalfopristin: administration guidelines. *J Antimicrob Chemother* (1999) 44 (Suppl A), 37–46.
3. Adalat Retard (Nifedipine). Bayer plc. UK Summary of product characteristics, April 2012.

Calcium-channel blockers + Rifampicin (Rifampin)

Rifampicin greatly reduces the plasma concentrations of diltiazem, nifedipine, nilvadipine, and verapamil, and possibly reduces those of barnidipine, isradipine, lercanidipine, manidipine, nicardipine, nimodipine, and nisoldipine. Rifapentine and rifabutin would also be expected to reduce the plasma concentrations of these calcium-channel blockers.

Clinical evidence

(a) Barnidipine and Manidipine

A brief report states that elderly patients with hypertension well-controlled with calcium-channel blockers including barnidipine and manidipine had increases in their blood pressure when rifampicin was added. Increased doses or additional antihypertensives were needed to control the blood pressure, and reduced doses were required when the rifampicin was withdrawn.[1]

(b) Diltiazem

A study in 12 subjects found that the maximum plasma concentration following a single 120-mg oral dose of diltiazem was 186 nanograms/mL, but after taking rifampicin 600 mg daily for 8 days the maximum plasma concentration of diltiazem was less than 8 nanograms/mL.[2] One patient with angina controlled with diltiazem 120 mg daily began to feel chest pain at rest one month after starting rifampicin and isoniazid.[3]

(c) Nifedipine

A woman with hypertension well controlled with nifedipine 40 mg twice daily, had an increase in her blood pressure from under 160/90 mmHg to 200/110 mmHg within 2 weeks of starting to take antitubercular drugs, which included rifampicin 450 mg daily. When rifampicin was stopped and then restarted, the blood pressure decreased and then increased again. The maximum plasma concentration and AUC of nifedipine were both reduced by about 60% in the presence of rifampicin.[4] Another patient had anginal attacks refractory to nifedipine while taking rifampicin, which were controlled by nifedipine when the rifampicin was stopped. Restarting rifampicin reduced nifedipine levels (maximum plasma concentration and AUCs roughly halved) and increased the number of anginal attacks.[3] A further patient taking nifedipine had a loss of blood pressure control when given rifampicin.[5]

Six healthy subjects were given nifedipine 20 micrograms/kg intravenously and nifedipine 20 mg orally on separate days before and after taking rifampicin 600 mg daily for 7 days. The pharmacokinetics of *intravenous* nifedipine were not affected by rifampicin, but the *oral* clearance of nifedipine increased from 1.5 L/minute to 20.9 L/minute and its bioavailability was reduced from about 41% to 5%.[6] A pharmacokinetic study in 6 healthy subjects found that when a single 10-mg oral dose of nifedipine was taken 8 hours after a single 1.2-g dose of rifampicin, the bioavailability of nifedipine was reduced to 36%, its half-life was more than halved, and its clearance increased 3-fold.[7]

(d) Nilvadipine

A study in 5 healthy normotensive subjects found that rifampicin 450 mg daily for 6 days reduced the maximum plasma concentration and AUC of a single 4-mg dose of nilvadipine about 20-fold and 30-fold, respectively. The hypotensive effect and reflex tachycardia associated with nilvadipine in these subjects was abolished by rifampicin.[8]

(e) Nisoldipine

There is some evidence to suggest that nisoldipine is ineffective in reducing blood pressure in the presence of rifampicin.[1,4]

(f) Verapamil

The observation that a patient whose increased blood pressure was not reduced by verapamil while taking antitubercular drugs, prompted a study in 4 other patients.[9] No verapamil could be detected in the plasma of 3 patients who took a single 40-mg dose of verapamil with rifampicin 450 to 600 mg daily, isoniazid 5 mg/kg daily, and ethambutol 15 mg/kg daily. A verapamil maximum concentration of 20 nanograms/mL was found in the fourth patient. Six other subjects not taking antitubercular drugs had a verapamil maximum plasma concentration of 35 nanograms/mL.[9] Similar results have been reported by the same authors in another study.[10]

Supraventricular tachycardia was inadequately controlled in a patient taking rifampicin 600 mg daily and isoniazid 300 mg daily, despite a verapamil dose of 480 mg every 6 hours. Substitution of rifampicin by ethambutol resulted in a 4-fold increase in verapamil serum concentrations.[11] A later study in 6 healthy subjects found that after taking rifampicin 600 mg daily for 2 weeks the oral bioavailability of verapamil was reduced from 26% to 2%, and the effects of verapamil on the ECG were abolished.[12] A further study, in elderly patients, similarly found that rifampicin 600 mg daily greatly decreased the bioavailability of verapamil 120 mg twice daily. The effects of verapamil on AV conduction were almost abolished.[13]

Mechanism

Rifampicin is a known, potent inducer of CYP3A4 by which many of the calcium-channel blockers are metabolised, at least in part. Concurrent use therefore decreases their concentrations and effects on blood pressure. Rifampicin reduces the effectiveness of nifedipine and verapamil to a greater extent after oral than after intravenous use, suggesting that CYP3A4 metabolism is induced in the intestine as well as the liver. **Rifabutin** and **rifapentine** are also inducers of CYP3A4, although to a lesser extent than rifampicin, and would therefore also be expected to reduce the plasma concentrations of the calcium-channel blockers.

Importance and management

The interactions between diltiazem, nifedipine, or verapamil, and rifampicin are established and of clinical importance. There is some evidence that barnidipine, manidipine, nilvadipine, and nisoldipine also interact with rifampicin in this way, and, as most calcium-channel blockers are metabolised in a similar way it would seem prudent, in the absence of any specific information, to expect that they might interact similarly. Monitor the effects closely if rifampicin is given with any calcium-channel blocker, being alert for the need to make a large increase in their dose. Note that, with some of the reduction in plasma concentrations seen, it seems unlikely that blood pressure control will be possible with calcium-channel blockers in patients taking rifampicin. Therefore other drugs such as beta blockers or ACE inhibitors might be required, where appropriate. However, note that these classes of drugs are not entirely free of interactions with rifampicin, although the effects seem less important than with some of the calcium-channel blockers. See also 'Beta blockers + Rifampicin (Rifampin)', p.1021, and 'ACE inhibitors + Rifampicin (Rifampin)', p.42. However, note that some manufacturers of nifedipine,[14] and **nimodipine**[15] contraindicate their use with rifampicin.

Rifabutin and **rifapentine** would also be expected to reduce concentrations of calcium-channel blockers, although perhaps to a lesser extent than rifampicin. However, there does not appear to be any data to support this.

1. Yoshimoto H, Takahashi M, Saima S. Influence of rifampicin on antihypertensive effects of dihydropiridine calcium-channel blockers in four elderly patients. *Nippon Ronen Igakkai Zasshi* (1996) 33, 692–6.
2. Drda KD, Bastian TL, Self TH, Lawson J, Lanman RC, Burlew BS, Lalonde RL. Effects of debrisoquine hydroxylation phenotype and enzyme induction with rifampin on diltiazem pharmacokinetics and pharmacodynamics. *Pharmacotherapy* (1991) 11, 278.
3. Tsuchihashi K, Fukami K, Kishimoto H, Sumiyoshi T, Haze K, Saito M, Hiramori K. A case of variant angina exacerbated by administration of rifampicin. *Heart Vessels* (1987) 3, 214–17.
4. Tada Y, Tsuda Y, Otsuka T, Nagasawa K, Kimura H, Kusaba T, Sakata T. Case report: nifedipine-rifampicin interaction attenuates the effect on blood pressure in a patient with essential hypertension. *Am J Med Sci* (1992) 303, 25–7.
5. Takasugi T. A case of hypertension suggesting nifedipine and rifampicin drug interaction. *Igaku To Yakugaku* (1989) 22, 132–5.
6. Holtbecker N, Fromm MF, Kroemer HK, Ohnhaus EE, Heidemann H. The nifedipine-rifampin interaction: Evidence for induction of gut wall metabolism. *Drug Metab Dispos* (1996) 24, 1121–3.
7. Ndanusa BU, Mustapha A, Abdu-Aguye I. The effect of single dose of rifampicin on the pharmacokinetics of oral nifedipine. *J Pharm Biomed Anal* (1997) 15, 1571–5.
8. Saima S, Furuie K, Yoshimoto H, Fukuda J, Hayashi T, Echizen H. The effects of rifampicin on the pharmacokinetics and pharmacodynamics of orally administered nilvadipine to healthy subjects. *Br J Clin Pharmacol* (2002) 53, 203–6.
9. Rahn KH, Mooy J, Böhm R, vd Vet, A. Reduction of bioavailability of verapamil by rifampin. *N Engl J Med* (1985) 312, 920–1.
10. Mooy J, Böhm R, van Baak M, van Kemenade J, vd Vet A, Rahn KH. The influence of antituberculosis drugs on the plasma level of verapamil. *Eur J Clin Pharmacol* (1987) 32, 107–9.
11. Barbarash RA. Verapamil-rifampin interaction. *Drug Intell Clin Pharm* (1985) 19, 559–60.
12. Barbarash RA, Bauman JL, Fischer JH, Kondos GT, Batenhorst RL. Near-total reduction in verapamil bioavailability by rifampin: electrocardiographic correlates. *Chest* (1988) 94, 954–9.
13. Fromm MF, Dilger K, Busse D, Kroemer HK, Eichelbaum M, Klotz U. Gut wall metabolism of verapamil in older people: effects of rifampicin-mediated enzyme induction. *Br J Clin Pharmacol* (1998) 45, 247–55.
14. Adalat Retard (Nifedipine). Bayer plc. UK Summary of product characteristics, April 2012.
15. Nimotop Tablets (Nimodipine). Bayer plc. UK Summary of product characteristics, October 2012.

Calcium-channel blockers + SSRIs

Two patients taking verapamil and two taking nifedipine developed increased adverse effects (oedema, headaches, nausea, flushing, orthostatic hypotension) when they also took fluoxetine. Fluoxetine appears to increase nimodipine concentrations, whereas nimodipine might decrease fluoxetine concentrations. Fluoxetine does not appear to alter lercanidipine pharmacokinetics.

Clinical evidence

(a) Lercanidipine

The manufacturer notes that a study in elderly subjects found that **fluoxetine** had no clinically relevant effects on the pharmacokinetics of lercanidipine. No other details were given.[1]

(b) Nifedipine

A patient taking nifedipine 60 mg daily developed nausea and flushing after also starting to take **fluoxetine** 20 mg every other day. The adverse effects gradually disappeared over the next 2 to 3 weeks when the nifedipine dose was halved.[2] An 80-year-old woman taking nifedipine developed tachycardia, hypotension and profound weakness 10 days after starting to take **fluoxetine** 20 mg daily. On admission to hospital 8 days later she was unable to stand, her standing blood pressure was 90/50 mmHg and her heart rate was 120 bpm. She fully recovered within a week of stopping the fluoxetine.[3]

(c) Nimodipine

The UK manufacturer of nimodipine states that, in elderly patients given nimodipine 30 mg twice daily with **fluoxetine** 20 mg daily, the plasma concentration of nimodipine was increased by about 50%, and the plasma concentrations of fluoxetine were reduced, with no effect on the concentration of the metabolite norfluoxetine.[4]

(d) Verapamil

A woman taking verapamil 240 mg daily developed oedema of the feet and ankles, and neck vein distension within 6 weeks of starting to take **fluoxetine** 20 mg every other day. The oedema resolved within 2 to 3 weeks of reducing the verapamil dose to 120 mg daily.[2] Another patient taking verapamil 240 mg daily for the prophylaxis of migraine developed morning headaches (believed by the patient not to be migraine) about one week after his **fluoxetine** dose was increased from 20 to 40 mg daily. The headaches stopped when the verapamil dose was reduced and then stopped.[2]

Mechanism

The calcium-channel blockers are metabolised by CYP3A4, of which fluoxetine is said to be a weak inhibitor. This might result in a reduction in the metabolism and clearance of some calcium-channel blockers. The reactions reported appear to be the exaggeration of the adverse effects of these calcium-channel blockers, possibly due to an increase in their plasma concentrations.

Importance and management

Evidence for a pharmacokinetic interaction between **fluoxetine** and the calcium-channel blockers is limited and largely restricted to case reports, which suggests that any adverse interaction occurs only rarely. Bear the possibility of a pharmacokinetic interaction in mind if a patient shows an exaggerated response to a calcium-channel blocker after starting fluoxetine, being alert for the need to reduce the drug doses (note that reducing the fluoxetine dose resolved the interaction in some of the cases described above). The clinical relevance of the interaction between nimodipine and fluoxetine[4] is not established, however, until more is known it would be prudent to monitor for an increase in adverse effects with nimodipine, such as hypotension, and a reduction in the response to fluoxetine on concurrent use.

Information about other calcium-channel blockers with fluoxetine, or other SSRIs, appears to be lacking.

1. Zanidip (Lercanidipine hydrochloride). Recordati Pharmaceuticals Ltd. UK Summary of product characteristics, April 2006.
2. Sternbach H. Fluoxetine-associated potentiation of calcium-channel blockers. *J Clin Psychopharmacol* (1991) 11, 390–1.
3. Azaz-Livshits TLT, Danenberg HD. Tachycardia, orthostatic hypotension and profound weakness due to concomitant use of fluoxetine and nifedipine. *Pharmacopsychiatry* (1997) 30, 274–5.
4. Nimotop Tablets (Nimodipine). Bayer plc. UK Summary of product characteristics, October 2012.

Calcium-channel blockers + St John's wort (*Hypericum perforatum*)

St John's wort significantly reduces the bioavailability of nifedipine and verapamil. Other calcium-channel blockers would be expected to interact similarly.

Clinical evidence

(a) Nifedipine

In a study in 10 healthy subjects, St John's wort 900 mg daily for 14 days decreased the maximum levels and AUC of a single 10-mg oral dose of nifedipine by about 38% and 45%, respectively. The maximum levels and AUC of the active metabolite of nifedipine, dehydronifedipine, were raised by about 45% and 26%, respectively. The

St John's wort preparation used was standardised to contain hypericin 0.3% and hyperforin 5%.[1]

(b) Verapamil

In a study in 8 healthy subjects, verapamil 24 mg was given as a jejunal perfusion over 100 minutes both before and after they took St John's wort tablets *(Movina;* containing 3 to 6% hyperforin) 300 mg three times daily for 14 days. St John's wort did not affect jejunal permeability or the absorption of either *R*- or *S*-verapamil. The AUCs of *R*- and *S*-verapamil were decreased by 78% and 80%, respectively, and the peak plasma levels were decreased by 76% and 78%, respectively. The terminal half-life was not changed significantly. The AUC for *R*-verapamil was sixfold higher than that of *S*-verapamil, and St John's wort did not change this ratio.[2]

Mechanism

It appears that St John's wort decreased the bioavailability of both nifedipine and verapamil by inducing their metabolism by the cytochrome P450 isoenzyme CYP3A4 in the gut. An effect on P-glycoprotein-mediated transport is not likely, as intestinal permeability was not significantly altered.[2]

Importance and management

The general importance of this interaction is unclear, as neither study reported on the clinical outcome of these reductions in calcium-channel blocker levels. Patients taking St John's wort with nifedipine or verapamil should have their blood pressure and heart rate monitored to ensure they are still effective, and the dose should be adjusted if needed. There appears to be no information about other calcium-channel blockers, but as they are all metabolised by CYP3A4, to a greater or lesser extent, it would seem prudent to monitor concurrent use carefully. If an interaction occurs it may be prudent to use an alternative class of drugs (ACE inhibitors, angiotensin II receptor antagonists and beta blockers are not known to be affected by CYP3A4), or advise against the use of St John's wort.

1. Wang X-D, Li J-L, Lu Y, Chen X, Huang M, Chowbay B, Zhou S-F. Rapid and simultaneous determination of nifedipine and dehydronifedipine in human plasma by liquid chromatography-tandem mass spectrometry: Application to a clinical herb-drug interaction study. *J Chromatogr B Analyt Technol Biomed Life Sci* (2007) 852, 534.
2. Tannergren C, Engman H, Knutson L, Hedeland M, Bondesson U, Lennernäs H. St John's wort decreases the bioavailability of *R*- and *S*-verapamil through induction of the first-pass metabolism. *Clin Pharmacol Ther* (2004) 75, 298–309.

Calcium-channel blockers + Tyrosine kinase inhibitors

A man taking nifedipine developed a gallstone after starting imatinib, and a patient developed imatinib toxicity after starting amlodipine. The plasma concentration of sorafenib was increased in a patient, after felodipine was added. Imatinib is predicted to increase the exposure to some dihydropyridine calcium-channel blockers. Other tyrosine kinase inhibitors that also inhibit CYP3A4 might interact similarly.

Clinical evidence

(a) Imatinib

A patient taking **nifedipine** developed nausea, vomiting, and abdominal pain 8 weeks after starting to take imatinib 400 mg [daily]. Ultrasound showed a thickened gallbladder wall, dilatation of the principal bile ducts, and a gallstone. He had not previously had any gall bladder disease. Imatinib was stopped until the abdominal pain was resolved and then restarted at half the initial dose.[1]

A 74-year-old patient with chronic myeloid leukaemia taking imatinib 400 mg twice daily developed symptoms of imatinib toxicity (nausea, marked periorbital and ankle oedema) 2 weeks after starting to take **amlodipine** 10 mg daily. He was given diuretics and the oedema improved, but after 10 days the patient experienced numbness of the chin and bilateral pain and numbness of the soles of the feet, and light touch and vibration sense were reduced. The dose of imatinib was reduced to 400 mg daily and amlodipine was stopped. Apart from residual plantar numbness, the symptoms resolved and imatinib was increased to 600 mg daily without worsening of symptoms. The patient remained on imatinib 600 mg daily and the neuropathy resolved within 9 months.[2]

(b) Sorafenib

An 80-year-old man taking sorafenib 400 mg daily for two weeks, was started on **felodipine** 5 mg twice daily for hypertension. Two weeks later, his sorafenib plasma concentration had increased from 3.6 mg/L to 11.4 mg/L and he had lost 13 kg in weight since starting the sorafenib. His hypertension was controlled and, as he had no diarrhoea or cutaneous adverse effects, his sorafenib dose was maintained. Over the following 2 months, his sorafenib plasma concentration gradually reduced to about 7 mg/L, and he experienced some diarrhoea, hoarseness, and asthenia, but gained 4 kg in weight.[3]

Mechanism

In the case with imatinib and nifedipine, the authors suggest that imatinib might have inhibited the metabolism of nifedipine by CYP3A4 leading to an increase in its effects on lipids, and an increase in biliary secretion and gallstone development.[1] However, the development of gallstones would not usually be considered a sign of increased nifedipine concentrations. The authors of the report with imatinib and amlodipine suggest that inhibition of the BCRP transporter and CYP3A4 by amlodipine might have reduced the hepatic clearance of imatinib, leading to increased imatinib adverse effects, such as paraesthesia.[2] The reason for the increased sorafenib concentrations on concurrent use with felodipine is not known.

Importance and management

Evidence for an interaction between the tyrosine kinase inhibitors and the calcium-channel blockers is limited to the case reports cited, which are of unknown general relevance. However, imatinib is a moderate inhibitor of CYP3A4, and would be expected to increase the exposure to dihydropyridine calcium-channel blockers which are substrates of this isoenzyme (see 'Table 1.10', p.12). It would therefore seem prudent to monitor the concurrent use of these calcium-channel blockers and imatinib for an increase in calcium-channel blocker adverse effects, such as hypotension, headache, flushing, and oedema, and adjust the dose of the calcium-channel blocker accordingly. Other tyrosine kinase inhibitors that also inhibit CYP3A4 (see 'Table 1.9', p.11) might be predicted to interact similarly. Sorafenib does not inhibit CYP3A4, and so would not be expected to affect the exposure of calcium-channel blockers metabolised by this isoenzyme by this mechanism.

Note that **diltiazem** and **verapamil** are moderate inhibitors of CYP3A4, and might be expected to increase the exposure of tyrosine kinase inhibitors metabolised by this isoenzyme (see 'Table 1.10', p.12).

The clinical relevance of the increase in sorafenib exposure seen on the concurrent use of felodipine in the case report is unknown. It might be prudent to consider an interaction should an increase in sorafenib adverse effects occur on concurrent use.

1. Breccia M, D'Andrea M, Alimena G. Can nifedipine and estrogen interaction with imatinib be responsible for gallbladder stone development? *Eur J Haematol* (2005) 75, 89–90.
2. Ross DM. Peripheral neuropathy on imatinib treatment for chronic myeloid leukaemia: suspected adverse drug interaction with amlodipine. *Intern Med J* (2009) 39, 708.
3. Gomo C, Coriat R, Faivre L, Mir O, Ropert S, Billemont B, Dauphin A, Tod M, Goldwasser F, Blanchet B. Pharmacokinetic interaction involving sorafenib and the calcium-channel blocker felodipine in a patient with hepatocellular carcinoma. *Invest New Drugs* (2011) 29, 1511–14.

Calcium-channel blockers + Valproate

Nimodipine and possibly nifedipine levels are raised by valproate.

Clinical evidence, mechanism, importance and management

In a pharmacokinetic study, 8 patients with epilepsy who had been taking valproate alone for at least 4 months were given a single 60-mg dose of **nimodipine**. The AUC of **nimodipine** was about 50% higher, when compared with that found in a control group not taking valproate.[1] The **nimodipine** dosage may need to be reduced if it is given with valproate.

One manufacturer of **nifedipine** suggests that there is a theoretical possibility that levels of **nifedipine** may be increased in the presence of valproate,[2] and advises that blood pressure should be monitored and, if necessary, a reduction in the dose of **nifedipine** should be considered.[2] Note that they suggest that this may occur because valproate inhibits the cytochrome P450 isoenzyme CYP3A4, by which **nifedipine** is metabolised; however, clinically relevant examples of valproate interacting by this mechanism are largely lacking.

1. Tartara A, Galimberti CA, Manni R, Parietti L, Zucca C, Baasch H, Caresia L, Mück W, Barzaghi N, Gatti G, Perucca E. Differential effects of valproic acid and enzyme-inducing anticonvulsants on nimodipine pharmacokinetics in epileptic patients. *Br J Clin Pharmacol* (1991) 32, 335–40.
2. Adalat Retard (Nifedipine). Bayer plc. UK Summary of product characteristics, April 2012.

Calcium-channel blockers + X-ray contrast media

The hypotensive effects of an intravenous bolus of an ionic X-ray contrast medium can be increased by the presence of calcium-channel blockers. No interaction or only a small interaction appears to occur with non-ionic contrast media.

Clinical evidence, mechanism, importance and management

It is well recognised that ionic x-ray contrast media used for ventriculography reduce the systemic blood pressure due to peripheral vasodilation. They also have a direct depressant effect on the heart muscle. A comparative study of the haemodynamic response of 65 patients found that the hypotensive effect of a bolus dose of an ionic agent (0.5 mL/kg of **meglumine amidotrizoate** and **sodium amidotrizoate** with edetate sodium or disodium) was increased by the concurrent use of **nifedipine** or **diltiazem**. Haemodynamic effects occurred earlier (3.1 seconds compared with 12.9 seconds), were more profound (a fall in systolic pressure of 48.4 mmHg compared with 36.9 mmHg) and more prolonged (62 seconds compared with 36 seconds).[1] A similar interaction was seen in *dogs* given **verapamil**.[2] No interaction or only a minimal interaction was seen in the patients and *dogs* when non-ionic contrast media (**iopamidol** or **iohexol**) were used instead.[1,2] The clinical relevance of these findings is uncertain. Note that calcium-channel blockers have been tried to prevent the nephrotoxicity of contrast media.

1. Morris DL, Wisneski JA, Gertz EW, Wexman M, Axelrod R, Langberg JJ. Potentiation by nifedipine and diltiazem of the hypotensive response after contrast angiography. *J Am Coll Cardiol* (1985) 6, 785–91.
2. Higgins CB, Kuber M, Slutsky RA. Interaction between verapamil and contrast media in coronary arteriography: comparison of standard ionic and new nonionic media. *Circulation* (1983) 68, 628–35.

Calcium-channel blockers; Amlodipine + Chloroquine

A case report attributes an acute hypotensive episode to the use of amlodipine with chloroquine.

Clinical evidence, mechanism, importance and management

A case report describes a 48-year-old hypertensive man, who had been taking amlodipine 5 mg daily for 3 months with optimal blood pressure control. Because he had self-diagnosed malaria, he took chloroquine base 600 mg: two hours later he fainted and had a systolic blood pressure of 80 mmHg, and an unrecordable diastolic blood pressure. He was given supportive fluids and recovered over the following 2 hours. The severe adverse reaction was attributed to acute synergistic hypotensive, venodilator and cardiac effects of the two drugs.[1] However, any interaction remains unproven, as there was no re-challenge, and it seems reasonable that the faint may simply have been as a result of the fever from which he was suffering. Furthermore, the authors note that concurrent use of these two drugs would be expected to be quite frequent, and this appears to be the only case reported. No special precautions are therefore considered warranted based on this isolated case report.

1. Ajayi AAL, Adigun AQ. Syncope following oral chloroquine administration in a hypertensive patient controlled on amlodipine. *Br J Clin Pharmacol* (2002) 53, 404–5.

Calcium-channel blockers; Nifedipine + Co-trimoxazole

Adverse effects (leg cramps, facial flushing) have been reported in one patient taking nifedipine when co-trimoxazole was also taken. One study found that co-trimoxazole had no effect on the pharmacokinetics and hypotensive action of a single dose of nifedipine.

Clinical evidence, mechanism, importance and management

The observation of a patient taking nifedipine who developed leg cramps and facial flushing (possibly as a result of raised plasma nifedipine levels) when given co-trimoxazole, prompted further study of this possible interaction in 9 healthy subjects. After taking co-trimoxazole 960 mg twice daily for 3 days the pharmacokinetics and hypotensive effects of a single 20-mg dose of nifedipine were found to be unchanged.[1] No special precautions would therefore normally seem to be necessary on concurrent use.

1. Edwards C, Monkman S, Cholerton S, Rawlins MD, Idle JR, Ferner RE. Lack of effect of co-trimoxazole on the pharmacokinetics and pharmacodynamics of nifedipine. *Br J Clin Pharmacol* (1990) 30, 889–91.

Calcium-channel blockers; Nifedipine + Ginkgo (*Ginkgo biloba*)

Ginkgo may increase the levels and some of the effects of nifedipine.

Clinical evidence

In the preliminary report of a clinical study, 22 healthy subjects were given ginkgo 120 mg daily for 18 days before a single 10-mg oral dose of nifedipine. Ginkgo increased the levels of nifedipine by about 50%.[1]

In another study, a single 240-mg dose of ginkgo extract did not significantly affect the pharmacokinetics of a single 10-mg oral dose of nifedipine when they were given at the same time to 8 healthy subjects. However, the maximum level tended to increase (30% increase), and two subjects experienced a doubling of nifedipine maximum serum levels. In addition, the incidence and severity of headaches, hot flushes and dizziness tended to be higher with the combination when compared with nifedipine alone. Subjects also experienced increased heart rate with the combination although the decrease in blood pressure was unaffected.[2] The ginkgo extract used in this study contained 24% flavonoids and 6% terpene lactones.

Mechanism

Ginkgo may inhibit the cytochrome P450 isoenzyme CYP3A4, which would reduce the metabolism of nifedipine, a CYP3A4 substrate, and increase its levels. Note that simultaneous administration of single doses is probably insufficient to completely evaluate CYP3A4 inhibition. Note also that clinically relevant CYP3A4 inhibition has not been seen with ginkgo and the conventional CYP3A4 probe substrates such as midazolam.

Importance and management

Limited clinical data suggest that ginkgo may raise the levels of nifedipine and increase its effects. Until more is known, some caution might be warranted when they are used together. Monitor for signs of nifedipine adverse effects such as headaches, hot flushes, dizziness and palpitations. If they become apparent, advise the patient to stop taking ginkgo.

1. Smith M, Lin KM, Zheng YP. An open trial of nifedipine-herb interactions: nifedipine with St. John's wort, ginseng or Ginko [sic] biloba. *Clin Pharmacol Ther* (2001) 69, P86.
2. Yoshioka M, Ohnishi N, Koishi T, Obata Y, Nakagawa M, Matsumoto T, Tagagi K, Takara K, Ohkuni T, Yokoyama T, Kuroda K. Studies on interactions between functional foods or dietary supplements and medicines. IV. Effects of Ginkgo biloba leaf extract on the pharmacokinetics and pharmacodynamics of nifedipine in healthy volunteers. *Biol Pharm Bull* (2004) 27, 2006–9.

Calcium-channel blockers; Nifedipine + Terbinafine

A study in 12 healthy subjects found that terbinafine 250 mg did not alter the pharmacokinetics of nifedipine 30 mg (as *Procardia XL*).[1]

1. Cramer JA, Robbins B, Barbeito R, Bedman TC, Dreisbach A, Meligeni JA. Lamisil®: interaction study with a sustained release nifedipine formulation. *Pharm Res* (1996) 13 (9 Suppl), S436.

Calcium-channel blockers; Nifedipine + Vancomycin

An isolated case report suggests that the hypotensive effects of the rapid infusion of vancomycin may occur more readily in those who are already vasodilated with nifedipine, but it seems likely that the effects seen were solely due to the vancomycin.

Clinical evidence, mechanism, importance and management

A man with severe systemic sclerosis was hospitalised for Raynaud's phenomenon and dental extraction. After he started taking nifedipine 40 mg daily, he was given intravenous vancomycin 1 g in 200 mL of dextrose 5% over 30 minutes. After 20 minutes he experienced a severe headache and was found to have a marked macular erythema on the upper trunk, head, neck and arms. His blood pressure fell to 100/60 mmHg and his pulse rate was 90 bpm. He recovered spontaneously.[1] The authors of the report acknowledge the possibility of 'red-man syndrome' caused by the vancomycin, and suggest that it may occur more readily in those already vasodilated with nifedipine. However, given that this is an isolated report, and the vancomycin was given over 3 times faster than the recommended rate, it seems likely that this is purely an adverse effect of vancomycin.

1. Daly BM, Sharkey I. Nifedipine and vancomycin-associated red man syndrome. *Drug Intell Clin Pharm* (1986) 20, 986.

Calcium-channel blockers; Nitrendipine + Bile acids

Chenodeoxycholic acid and ursodeoxycholic acid reduce the AUC of nitrendipine.

Clinical evidence, mechanism, importance and management

In a single-dose study, 6 healthy subjects were given nitrendipine 10 mg with or without either **chenodeoxycholic acid** 200 mg or 600 mg, or **ursodeoxycholic acid** 50 mg. **Chenodeoxycholic acid** 200 mg decreased the peak plasma level and AUC of nitrendipine by about 20%, whereas **chenodeoxycholic acid** 600 mg had a greater effect, reducing the peak plasma level and AUC of nitrendipine by 54% and 68%, respectively. **Ursodeoxycholic acid** reduced the peak plasma level and AUC of nitrendipine by 54% and 75%, respectively. The reduction in the AUC of nitrendipine was possibly due to the effects of the bile acids on tablet disintegration or more probably on drug solubilisation.[1] The clinical importance of the interaction is not known, but the extent of the reduction in the AUC of nitrendipine suggests that its effects may be diminished. It may therefore be prudent to consider monitoring the outcome of concurrent use, increasing the dose of nitrendipine as necessary.

1. Sasaki M, Maeda A, Sakamoto K-I, Fujimura A. Effect of bile acids on absorption of nitrendipine in healthy subjects. *Br J Clin Pharmacol* (2001) 52, 699–701.

Calcium-channel blockers; Verapamil + Ceftriaxone and Clindamycin

An isolated report describes the development of complete heart block in a man taking verapamil, which was attributed to the use of intravenous ceftriaxone and clindamycin. However, the validity of this interaction has been questioned.

Clinical evidence, mechanism, importance and management

A 59-year-old man who had been taking sustained-release verapamil 240 mg twice daily for 2 years and phenytoin 300 mg daily for several years, developed complete heart block an hour after being given intravenous ceftriaxone 1 g and clindamycin 900 mg for bilateral pneumonia. He needed cardiopulmonary resuscitation and the insertion of a temporary pacemaker, but spontaneously recovered normal sinus rhythm after 16 hours, and subsequently made a full recovery. The reasons for this serious reaction are not known, but the authors of the report postulate that these two antibacterials precipitated acute verapamil toxicity, possibly by displacing it from its plasma protein binding sites. Although both antibacterials are highly protein-bound (93% or more),[1] they are acidic and do not bind to the same sites as the verapamil (a base), so that this mechanism of interaction seems very unlikely. This seems to be the first and only report of this reaction, and the suggestion by the authors that it was due to a drug interaction has been seriously questioned.[2] There seems to be no other evidence that either of these antibacterials interact with verapamil, either given orally or intravenously. The current evidence is insufficient to suggest that extra caution is warranted if these drugs are given concurrently.

1. Kishore K, Raina A, Misra V, Jonas E. Acute verapamil toxicity in a patient with chronic toxicity: possible interaction with ceftriaxone and clindamycin. *Ann Pharmacother* (1993) 27, 877–80.
2. Horn JR, Hansten PD. Comment: pitfalls in reporting drug interactions. *Ann Pharmacother* (1993) 27, 1545–6.

Calcium-channel blockers; Verapamil + Sulfinpyrazone

The clearance of verapamil is markedly increased by sulfinpyrazone.

Clinical evidence, mechanism, importance and management

A study in 8 healthy subjects found that sulfinpyrazone 800 mg daily for a week, increased the clearance of a single oral dose of verapamil by about threefold, possibly due to an increase in its liver metabolism.[1] The clinical importance of this effect is uncertain, but be alert for reduced verapamil effects. It seems probable that the dosage of verapamil may need to be increased, or an alternative drug considered.

1. Wing LMH, Miners JO, Lillywhite KJ. Verapamil disposition—effects of sulphinpyrazone and cimetidine. *Br J Clin Pharmacol* (1985) 19, 385–91.

24

Cardiovascular drugs, miscellaneous

The drugs dealt with in this section include the centrally acting drugs (e.g. clonidine, methyldopa), inotropes and vasopressors (e.g. adrenaline, phenylephrine), adrenergic neurone blockers (e.g. guanethidine), some vasodilator antihypertensives (e.g. hydralazine, diazoxide), nitrates (e.g. glyceryl trinitrate), potassium channel activators (e.g. nicorandil), peripheral vasodilators (e.g. pentoxifylline), calcium sensitisers (e.g. levosimendan), endothelin receptor antagonists (e.g. ambrisentan, bosentan, and macitentan), direct renin inhibitors (e.g. aliskiren), the guanylate cyclase stimulator, riociguat, and other drugs used in the management of angina (e.g. ivabradine and ranolazine).

(a) Miscellaneous antihypertensives

The combination of two antihypertensive drugs often results in an increased antihypertensive action. Likewise the combination of drugs that might have hypotension as an adverse effect, can lead to an unexpected increase in hypotension. For examples of these types of interactions see 'Antihypertensives + Other drugs that affect blood pressure', p.1054. Some drugs are known to antagonise the effect of antihypertensives, and these are also generally discussed in this monograph.

(b) Sympathomimetics

Many of the inotropes and vasopressors have actions on the sympathetic nervous system. Noradrenaline (norepinephrine) is the principal neurotransmitter involved in the final link between nerve endings of the sympathetic nervous system and the adrenergic receptors of the organs or tissues innervated. The effects of stimulating this system can be reproduced or mimicked by exogenous noradrenaline and by a number of other drugs that also stimulate these receptors. The drugs that behave in this way are described as 'sympathomimetics' and act either directly, like noradrenaline, on the adrenergic receptors, or indirectly by releasing stored noradrenaline from the nerve endings. Some drugs do both. This is very simply illustrated in 'Figure 24.1', below.

The adrenergic receptors of the sympathetic system are not identical but can be subdivided into two main types, namely alpha and beta receptors, which can then be further subdivided. The sympathomimetics are categorised in 'Table 24.1', p.1050, and a brief summary of the principal effects of stimulation of these receptors is listed below:

- $Alpha_1$ (vasoconstriction, increased blood pressure, and sometimes reflex bradycardia; contraction of smooth muscle; mydriasis in the eye)
- $Alpha_2$ (role in feedback inhibition of neurotransmitter release; inhibition of insulin release)
- $Beta_1$ (increased rate and force of contraction or the heart)
- $Beta_2$ (vasodilatation and bronchodilation; uterine relaxation and decreased gastrointestinal motility; release of insulin)

A third distinct group of receptors, which occur primarily within the CNS and may be affected by some sympathomimetics, are the dopamine receptors.

It is therefore possible to broadly categorise the sympathomimetics into groups according to their activity.

Given these wide ranging actions on a number of different receptors the group 'sympathomimetics' is clearly a very diverse collection of drugs with a wide range of uses. One should not, therefore, extrapolate the interactions seen with one drug to any other without fully taking into account their differences. For this reason, where possible, this term has been avoided and drugs have been grouped by therapeutic use. This section is generally concerned with the interactions of sympathomimetics that have predominately cardiovascular actions (mainly through stimulation of $alpha_1$ and/or $beta_1$ receptors). Those used as decongestants (through stimulation of alpha receptors with or without beta activity) are mainly discussed in 'Miscellaneous drugs', p.1552, but some of these drugs are also given intravenously for their pressor actions, in which case their interactions are discussed here. Interactions involving beta agonists, such as salbutamol, which selectively stimulate the $beta_2$ receptors in bronchi causing bronchodilation, are mainly covered in 'Respiratory drugs', p.1418 and for interactions involving dopaminergics, such as levodopa, see 'Antiparkinsonian and related drugs', p.752.

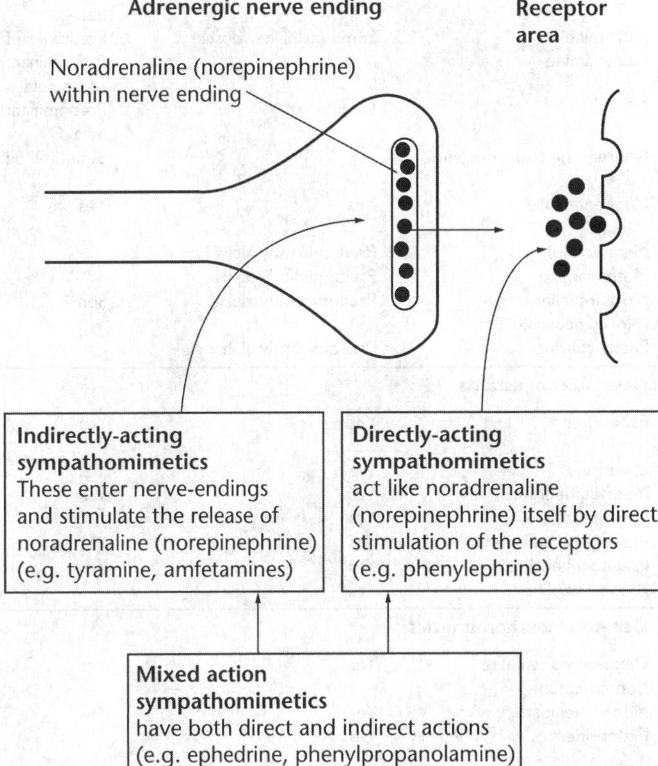

Fig. 24.1 A very simple illustration of the modes of action of indirectly-acting, directly acting and mixed action sympathomimetics at adrenergic neurones.

Table 24.1 A categorisation of some sympathomimetic drugs

Drug	*Alpha adrenoceptors affected*	*Beta adrenoceptors affected*	*Direct or indirect effect*	*Other actions of note*
Amfetamines and related drugs				
Amfetamine	Yes	Yes	Indirect (mainly)	Central stimulant
Benzfetamine	Yes	Yes	Indirect (mainly)	Central stimulant
Dexamfetamine	Yes	Yes	Indirect (mainly)	Central stimulant
Lisdexamfetamine	Yes	Yes	Indirect (mainly)	Central stimulant
Metamfetamine	Yes	Yes	Indirect (mainly)	Central stimulant
Beta agonist bronchodilators				
Arformoterol		Predominantly $beta_2$	Direct	
Bambuterol		Predominantly $beta_2$	Direct	
Clenbuterol		Predominantly $beta_2$	Direct	
Fenoterol		Predominantly $beta_2$	Direct	
Formoterol		Predominantly $beta_2$	Direct	
Hexoprenaline		Predominantly $beta_2$	Direct	
Indacaterol		Predominantly $beta_2$	Direct	
Levosalbutamol		Predominantly $beta_2$	Direct	
Orciprenaline		Predominantly $beta_2$	Direct	
Pirbuterol		Predominantly $beta_2$	Direct	
Procaterol		Predominantly $beta_2$	Direct	
Reproterol		Predominantly $beta_2$	Direct	
Salbutamol (Albuterol)		Predominantly $beta_2$	Direct	
Salmeterol		Predominantly $beta_2$	Direct	
Terbutaline		Predominantly $beta_2$	Direct	
Tretoquinol		Predominantly $beta_2$	Direct	
Tulobuterol		Predominantly $beta_2$	Direct	
Inotropes and Vasopressors				
Adrenaline (Epinephrine)	Yes (effects increase with dose)	Predominantly $beta_2$, some $beta_1$	Direct	
Dobutamine	Some	Predominantly $beta_1$, some $beta_2$	Direct (mainly)	
Dopamine	Some (at higher doses)	Predominantly $beta_1$	Direct and indirect	
Dopexamine		Predominantly $beta_2$, possibly some $beta_1$	Direct and indirect	
Etilefrine	Some	Predominantly $beta_1$, some $beta_2$	Direct	
Isoprenaline (Isoproterenol)		$Beta_1$ and $beta_2$	Direct	Also used for its **bronchodilator** actions
Mephentermine	Yes	Yes	Indirect (mainly) and some direct	Some central stimulant effects
Metaraminol	Predominantly alpha		Direct (mainly)	
Methoxamine	Predominantly alpha		Direct (mainly)	Central stimulant
Noradrenaline (Norepinephrine)	Predominantly alpha	Some	Direct (mainly)	
Phenylephrine	Predominantly alpha		Direct (mainly)	
Nasal decongestants				
Ephedrine	Yes	Yes	Direct and indirect	Also used for its **vasopressor** actions
Etafedrine	Yes	Yes	Direct and indirect	
Methylephedrine	Yes	Yes	Direct and indirect	
Oxymetazoline	Yes		Direct	Used topically
Phenylpropanolamine	Yes	Yes	Direct and indirect	
Pseudoephedrine	Yes	Yes	Direct and indirect	
Xylometazoline	Yes		Direct	Used topically
Other sympathomimetics				
Dexmethylphenidate	Yes	Yes	Indirect (mainly)	Central stimulant
Isometheptene			Indirect	Used in migraine
Methylphenidate	Yes	Yes	Indirect (mainly)	Central stimulant
Midodrine	Yes		Direct	Used for its **vasopressor** actions
Ritodrine		Predominantly $beta_2$	Direct	Used as a tocolytic
Tyramine	Yes	Yes	Indirect (mainly)	Used as a test drug; present in foods

Aliskiren + Azoles

The exposure to aliskiren is markedly increased by itraconazole and modestly increased by ketoconazole.

Clinical evidence

(a) Itraconazole

In a placebo-controlled, crossover study, 11 healthy subjects were given itraconazole 200 mg for one dose, then 100 mg twice daily for 5 days with a single 150-mg dose of aliskiren on day 3. Itraconazole increased the peak plasma concentration and AUC of aliskiren 5.8-fold and 6.5-fold respectively, although the results showed considerable inter-individual variability. Furthermore, itraconazole decreased the plasma renin activity in response to aliskiren by 68%.[1]

(b) Ketoconazole

In a study, 20 healthy subjects were given aliskiren 300 mg daily for 11 days, with the concurrent use of ketoconazole 200 mg twice daily for the last 4 days. Ketoconazole increased the AUC, peak plasma levels and minimum plasma levels of aliskiren by 76%, 81% and 64%, respectively. The clearance of aliskiren was reduced by 43%.[2] Ketoconazole is therefore predicted to effectively double the dose of aliskiren, and doses of this order (up to 600 mg of aliskiren daily) have been found to be well-tolerated.[3]

Mechanism

Aliskiren is a substrate of the efflux pump, P-glycoprotein, which is involved in the intestinal absorption and biliary excretion of aliskiren. *In vitro* studies suggest that CYP3A4 is involved in aliskiren metabolism. Ketoconazole and itraconazole inhibit P-glycoprotein and are also potent inhibitors of CYP3A4. Concurrent use therefore leads to increased aliskiren levels.

Importance and management

Evidence for an interaction between aliskiren and itraconazole or ketoconazole is limited, but in line with the way these drugs are known to interact. Moderate and potent inhibitors of P-glycoprotein cause clinically relevant increases in the plasma levels of aliskiren and it is suggested that they may have greater effects on tissue levels. The UK manufacturer advises caution if aliskiren is given with ketoconazole.[3] The effect of itraconazole is much larger, and therefore both the US and UK manufacturers of aliskiren contraindicate the concurrent use of itraconazole.[3,4]

If any of these drugs are given with aliskiren it may be prudent to be alert for aliskiren adverse effects such as diarrhoea, dyspepsia and hypotension. Adjust the aliskiren dose as necessary.

1. Tapanien T, Backman JT, Kurkinen KJ, Neuvonen PJ, Niemi M. Itraconazole, a P-glycoprotein and CYP3A4 inhibitor, markedly raises the plasma concentrations and enhances the renin-inhibiting effect of aliskiren. *J Clin Pharmacol* (2011) 51, 359–67.
2. Vaidyanathan S, Camenisch G, Schuetz H, Reynolds C, Yeh C-M, Bizot M-N, Dieterich HA, Howard D, Dole WP. Pharmacokinetics of the oral direct renin inhibitor aliskiren in combination with digoxin, atorvastatin, and ketoconazole in healthy subjects: the role of P-glycoprotein in the disposition of aliskiren. *J Clin Pharmacol* (2008) 48, 1323–38.
3. Rasilez 300 mg Tablets (Aliskiren hemifumarate). Novartis Pharmaceuticals UK Ltd. UK Summary of product characteristics, August 2012.
4. Tekturna (Aliskiren hemifumarate). Novartis. US Prescribing information, September 2012.

Aliskiren + Beta blockers

The blood pressure lowering effects of aliskiren can be enhanced by atenolol, as would be expected; other beta blockers would be expected to interact similarly. Atenolol does not appear to affect the pharmacokinetics of aliskiren.

Clinical evidence, mechanism, importance and management

In a randomised, crossover study, 15 healthy subjects were given single doses of aliskiren 150 mg, atenolol 100 mg and both drugs together. There was no statistically significant difference in plasma concentrations or AUC of aliskiren when it was given alone or with atenolol. Furthermore, aliskiren did not appear to affect the pharmacokinetics of atenolol.[1] However, the concurrent use of atenolol and aliskiren would be expected to have greater effects on systolic blood pressure than either drug alone, and therefore it may be prudent to be alert for additional hypotensive effects if both drugs are given, and adjust the doses accordingly. It seems likely that all beta blockers will have additive effects with aliskiren and it would therefore be prudent to be aware of the possibility of greater than desirable effects on blood pressure on their concurrent use.

1. Dieterle W, Corynen S, Vaidyanathan S, Mann J. Pharmacokinetic interactions of the oral renin inhibitor aliskiren with lovastatin, atenolol, celecoxib and cimetidine. *Int J Clin Pharmacol Ther* (2005) 43, 527–35.

Aliskiren + Ciclosporin

Ciclosporin markedly increases the exposure to aliskiren.

Clinical evidence

In a single-dose study, 8 healthy subjects were given aliskiren 75 mg alone, with ciclosporin 200 mg and with ciclosporin 600 mg. Ciclosporin increased the maximum plasma concentration and AUC of aliskiren about 2.5-fold and 5-fold, respectively. This was independent of the dose of ciclosporin used.[1]

Mechanism

Aliskiren is a substrate of the drug transporter, P-glycoprotein, which is involved in the intestinal absorption and biliary excretion of aliskiren. Ciclosporin inhibits P-glycoprotein, and concurrent use therefore leads to increased aliskiren concentrations. Other mechanisms might also be involved.

Importance and management

Evidence for an interaction between aliskiren and ciclosporin is limited, but consistent with the way these drugs are known to interact. Ciclosporin causes a clinically relevant increase in the exposure to aliskiren, and it is suggested that it might have greater effects on tissue concentrations. The UK and US manufacturers of aliskiren therefore contraindicate, or recommend avoiding, concurrent use.[2,3] If both drugs are considered essential, it seems likely that the dose of aliskiren will need to be very much reduced, and concurrent use should be closely monitored for aliskiren adverse effects, such as diarrhoea, dyspepsia, and hypotension.

1. Rebello S, Compain S, Feng A, Hariry S, Dieterich H-A, Jarugula V. Effect of cyclosporine on the pharmacokinetics of aliskiren in healthy subjects. *J Clin Pharmacol* (2011) 51, 1549–60.
2. Rasilez 300 mg Tablets (Aliskiren hemifumarate). Novartis Pharmaceuticals UK Ltd. UK Summary of product characteristics, August 2012.
3. Tekturna (Aliskiren hemifumarate). Novartis. US Prescribing information, September 2012.

Aliskiren + Miscellaneous

Apple juice, grapefruit juice, and orange juice appear to greatly reduce plasma aliskiren concentrations and plasma renin activity. A number of studies found that there were no clinically important pharmacokinetic interactions between aliskiren and allopurinol, cimetidine, digoxin, fenofibrate, or isosorbide mononitrate. There was no pharmacokinetic interaction between aliskiren and celecoxib, but the concurrent use of aliskiren with NSAIDs in patients with renal impairment such as the elderly, may result in further deterioration in renal function and even renal failure.

Clinical evidence, mechanism, importance and management

(a) Allopurinol

In a study in 20 healthy subjects given aliskiren 300 mg daily, allopurinol 300 mg daily for 5 days did not affect the AUC or maximum plasma concentrations of aliskiren, although there was wide variability in plasma concentrations.[1]

(b) Cimetidine

In a study in 22 healthy subjects given aliskiren 300 mg daily for 7 days, followed by aliskiren with cimetidine 800 mg daily for a further 5 days, cimetidine increased the maximum plasma concentration and AUC of aliskiren by 25% and 20%, respectively.[1] Another study in 12 healthy subjects given cimetidine 800 mg daily for 5 days, found that the AUC, maximum plasma concentration, and half-life of a single 150-mg dose of aliskiren given on day 3 were increased by 17%, 19%, and 15%, respectively.[2] These small pharmacokinetic changes would not be expected to be clinically relevant.

(c) Digoxin

In a study, 19 healthy subjects were given aliskiren 300 mg daily for 7 days, then after a washout period, digoxin 250 micrograms daily for 9 days, with aliskiren 300 mg daily added for a further 7 days. Digoxin had no effect on the pharmacokinetics of aliskiren. The AUC of digoxin was reduced by 15% by aliskiren, but the digoxin maximum concentration was unaffected.[3] This small change in digoxin exposure would not be expected to be clinically relevant.

(d) Fenofibrate

In a study in 17 healthy subjects, there was no pharmacokinetic interaction when aliskiren 300 mg daily was given with fenofibrate 200 mg daily for 5 days.[4]

(e) Food

The AUC and maximum plasma concentration of aliskiren are reduced by about 70% and 85%, respectively, when it is taken with a high-fat meal.[5,6] The UK manufacturer recommends taking aliskiren with a light meal preferably at the same time each day.[6] The US manufacturer notes that aliskiren was not taken at a fixed time in relation to meals in clinical studies, but states that patients should adopt a routine pattern for taking aliskiren with regard to meals.[5]

(f) Grapefruit and other fruit juices

In a randomised, crossover study, 11 healthy subjects were given grapefruit juice 200 mL three times daily for 5 days, with a single 150-mg dose of aliskiren on day 3. Grapefruit juice reduced the maximum plasma concentration and AUC of aliskiren by 81% and 61%, respectively.[7] In another study of the same design by the same authors, 12 healthy subjects were given 200-mL of **apple juice** or **orange juice** (both made from concentrate, normal strength) or water three times daily for 5 days, with a single 150-mg oral dose of aliskiren taken at the same time as the first drink on day 3. Apple juice reduced the AUC and maximum plasma concentration of aliskiren by 63% and 84%, respectively, while orange juice reduced the AUC and maximum plasma concentration of aliskiren by 62% and 80%, respectively.[8] The clearance and half-life of aliskiren were unaffected by either juice. However, there was wide interindividual variability in the AUC of aliskiren within each group, including those given water, although the variability with water appeared to be less than that with the fruit juices. Plasma renin activity at 24 hours post-dose was 67% and 87% higher with apple juice and orange juice, respectively, when compared with water. Blood pressure and heart rate did not differ between any of the groups; however, this is possibly because it was a single-dose study the effect of aliskiren on blood pressure can take several weeks to fully develop.[8]

The exact mechanism for this interaction is unclear, although it was considered that apple, grapefruit, and orange juices might have reduced the exposure to aliskiren by inhibiting its absorption by the drug transporter OATP2B1.[7,8] Further study is needed.

As the effect of **apple**, grapefruit, and **orange juices** on aliskiren exposure and renin activity was quite sizeable, it seems likely that concurrent use might reduce the effects of aliskiren on blood pressure. It might therefore be prudent to advise patients to avoid drinking these juices while taking aliskiren.

(g) Isosorbide mononitrate

In a study, 18 healthy subjects were given isosorbide mononitrate alone for 3 days, then after a washout period, aliskiren 300 mg daily for 7 days, followed by aliskiren with isosorbide mononitrate 40 mg daily for a further 3 days. There was no clinically important pharmacokinetic interaction, but dizziness and low blood pressure were more frequent during concurrent use than with either drug alone.[9] It might be prudent to be alert for these effects if both drugs are given, and adjust the doses accordingly.

(h) NSAIDs

In a study, aliskiren 300 mg daily was given to 22 healthy subjects for 7 days alone, and then with **celecoxib** 200 mg twice daily for a further 4.5 days. **Celecoxib** caused a very slight (14%) reduction in the AUC of aliskiren and there was wide variability in its maximum plasma concentrations. Dizziness was more frequently reported during concurrent use than with either drug alone.[1] In a single-dose study, **celecoxib** 200 mg caused a very slight increase (about 9%) in the AUC of aliskiren and increased maximum plasma concentration by 36%.[2] Although no clinically relevant pharmacokinetic interaction occurs between aliskiren and celecoxib, NSAIDs may reduce the antihypertensive effect of aliskiren through their action on the renin-angiotensin system. Furthermore, in dehydrated or elderly patients with some renal impairment, the concurrent use of aliskiren and NSAIDs could result in further deterioration of renal function, and possible renal failure. The UK manufacturer of aliskiren recommends caution if both drugs are given, especially in the elderly,[6] and the US manufacturer advises periodic monitoring of renal function on concurrent use.[5] In addition, the concurrent use of aliskiren and NSAIDs might increase the risk of hyperkalaemia, and so both the UK and US manufacturers recommend monitoring potassium concentrations on concurrent use.[5,6]

1. Ayalasomayajula S, Tchaloyan S, Yeh C-M, Bizot M-N, Dieterich HA, Howard D, Dole WP. A study of the pharmacokinetic interactions of the direct renin inhibitor aliskiren with allopurinol, celecoxib and cimetidine in healthy subjects. *Curr Med Res Opin* (2008) 24, 717–26.
2. Dieterle W, Corynen S, Vaidyanathan S, Mann J. Pharmacokinetic interactions of the oral renin inhibitor aliskiren with lovastatin, atenolol, celecoxib and cimetidine. *Int J Clin Pharmacol Ther* (2005) 43, 527–35.
3. Vaidyanathan S, Camenisch G, Schuetz H, Reynolds C, Yeh C-M, Bizot M-N, Dieterich HA, Howard D, Dole WP. Pharmacokinetics of the oral direct renin inhibitor aliskiren in combination with digoxin, atorvastatin, and ketoconazole in healthy subjects: the role of P-glycoprotein in the disposition of aliskiren. *J Clin Pharmacol* (2008) 48, 1323–8.
4. Vaidyanathan S, Maboudian M, Warren V, Yeh C-M, Dieterich HA, Howard D, Dole WP. A study of the pharmacokinetic interactions of the direct renin inhibitor aliskiren with metformin, pioglitazone and fenofibrate in healthy subjects. *Curr Med Res Opin* (2008) 24, 2313–26.
5. Tekturna (Aliskiren hemifumarate). Novartis. US Prescribing information, September 2012.
6. Rasilez 300 mg Tablets (Aliskiren hemifumarate). Novartis Pharmaceuticals UK Ltd. UK Summary of product characteristics, August 2012.
7. Tapaninen T, Neuvonen PJ, Niemi M. Grapefruit juice greatly reduces the plasma concentrations of the OATP2B1 and CYP3A4 substrate aliskiren. *Clin Pharmacol Ther* (2010) 88, 339–42.
8. Tapaninen T, Neuvonen PJ, Niemi M. Orange and apple juice greatly reduce the plasma concentrations of the OATP2B1 substrate aliskiren. *Br J Clin Pharmacol* (2011) 71, 718–26.
9. Vaidyanathan S, Bartlett M, Dieterich HA, Yeh C-M, Antunes A, Howard D, Dole WP. Pharmacokinetic interaction of the direct renin inhibitor aliskiren with furosemide and extended-release isosorbide-5-mononitrate in healthy subjects. *Cardiovasc Ther* (2008) 26, 238–46.

Aliskiren + P-glycoprotein inducers

Rifampicin (rifampin), a P-glycoprotein inducer, lowers aliskiren levels. Other P-glycoprotein inducers are predicted to interact similarly.

Clinical evidence

In a placebo-controlled, crossover study, 12 healthy subjects were given a single 150-mg dose of aliskiren before and after taking rifampicin (rifampin) 600 mg daily for 5 days. Rifampicin reduced the maximum level and AUC of aliskiren by 39% and 56%, respectively; but there was a large interindividual variability in these results. Plasma renin activity was 61% greater during rifampicin use, suggesting that rifampicin reduced the effects of aliskiren on renin activity.[1]

Mechanism

P-glycoprotein is reported to be the major efflux system involved in the intestinal absorption and biliary excretion of aliskiren. *In vitro* studies suggest that CYP3A4 is involved in aliskiren metabolism. Rifampicin (rifampin) is an inducer of both P-glycoprotein and CYP3A4 and therefore concurrent use reduces aliskiren levels.

Importance and management

Evidence for an interaction between aliskiren and rifampicin (rifampin) is limited, but in line with the way these drugs are known to interact. Although in the study the blood pressure-lowering effects of aliskiren were not affected to a statistically significant extent by rifampicin it was suggested that this was because only a single dose of aliskiren was given; the blood pressure-lowering effects of aliskiren may take several weeks to fully develop.[1] Therefore, given that rifampicin reduces aliskiren levels and reduces its effects on plasma renin, it seems likely that long-term concurrent use may reduce the blood pressure-lowering effects of aliskiren. It would therefore seem prudent to monitor concurrent use for this effect and increase the dose of aliskiren if necessary.

There appears to be no data about the concurrent use of other P-glycoprotein inducers and aliskiren, but the UK manufacturer of aliskiren[2] predicts that **St John's wort** may interact similarly. Until more is known, it may be prudent to follow similar precautions to those given for rifampicin, if St John's wort is given to a patient taking aliskiren.

1. Tapaninen T, Neuvonen PJ, Niemi M. Rifampicin reduces the plasma concentrations and the renin-inhibiting effect of aliskiren. *Eur J Clin Pharmacol* (2010) 66, 497–502.
2. Rasilez 300 mg Tablets (Aliskiren hemifumarate). Novartis Pharmaceuticals UK Ltd. UK Summary of product characteristics, August 2012.

Aliskiren + P-glycoprotein inhibitors

Inhibitors of P-glycoprotein, such as quinidine, are expected to increase aliskiren levels.

Clinical evidence, mechanism, importance and management

Aliskiren is a substrate of the efflux pump, P-glycoprotein. Some potent P-glycoprotein inhibitors have been shown to increase plasma levels of aliskiren (see 'Aliskiren + Ciclosporin', p.1051) and therefore the UK manufacturer of aliskiren contraindicates its use with other potent inhibitors of P-glycoprotein, such as **quinidine**. Similarly, some less potent inhibitors of P-glycoprotein also raise aliskiren levels (see 'Aliskiren + Azoles', p.1051) and therefore the UK manufacturer advises caution if aliskiren is given with moderate inhibitors of P-glycoprotein, and they name **amiodarone**, **clarithromycin**, **erythromycin**, and **telithromycin**.[1]

If any of these drugs are given with aliskiren it may be prudent to be alert for aliskiren adverse effects such as diarrhoea, dyspepsia and hypotension. Adjust the aliskiren dose as necessary.

1. Rasilez 300 mg Tablets (Aliskiren hemifumarate). Novartis Pharmaceuticals UK Ltd. UK Summary of product characteristics, August 2012.

Aliskiren + Statins

Atorvastatin increases the AUC and peak plasma levels of aliskiren. Lovastatin does not appear to affect the pharmacokinetics of aliskiren. Aliskiren does not affect the pharmacokinetics of either atorvastatin or lovastatin.

Clinical evidence

(a) Atorvastatin

In a study, 20 healthy subjects were given aliskiren 300 mg daily for 11 days, with atorvastatin 80 mg daily for the last 4 days. Atorvastatin increased the AUC and peak plasma levels of aliskiren by 47% and 50%, respectively, and reduced its clearance by 34%. Peak levels of atorvastatin were reduced by 23% during the concurrent use of aliskiren, but there were no clinically significant effects on the AUC of atorvastatin and its metabolites.[1]

(b) Lovastatin

In a randomised, crossover study, 15 healthy subjects were given single doses of aliskiren 150 mg, lovastatin 40 mg and both drugs together. There was no statistically significant difference in the plasma concentrations or AUC of aliskiren when it was given alone or with lovastatin. Furthermore, aliskiren did not appear to affect the pharmacokinetics of lovastatin.[2]

Mechanism

Aliskiren is a substrate of the efflux pump, P-glycoprotein, which is involved in the intestinal absorption and biliary excretion of aliskiren. Atorvastatin is a weak inhibitor of P-glycoprotein and therefore concurrent use results in an increase in aliskiren levels.

Importance and management

Evidence for an interaction between aliskiren and atorvastatin is limited, but in line with the way these drugs are known to interact. The effect of atorvastatin is modest and is not expected to be clinically relevant. However, until more is known, some caution is probably advisable if it is given with aliskiren. Be alert for aliskiren adverse effects such as diarrhoea, dyspepsia and hypotension and adjust the aliskiren dose as necessary.

Lovastatin does not affect the pharmacokinetics of aliskiren, and no dose adjustments are therefore likely to be necessary on their concurrent use.

1. Vaidyanathan S, Camenisch G, Schuetz H, Reynolds C, Yeh C-M, Bizot M-N, Dieterich HA, Howard D, Dole WP. Pharmacokinetics of the oral direct renin inhibitor aliskiren in combination with digoxin, atorvastatin, and ketoconazole in healthy subjects: the role of P-glycoprotein in the disposition of aliskiren. *J Clin Pharmacol* (2008) 48, 1323–38.
2. Dieterle W, Corynen S, Vaidyanathan S, Mann J. Pharmacokinetic interactions of the oral renin inhibitor aliskiren with lovastatin, atenolol, celecoxib and cimetidine. *Int J Clin Pharmacol Ther* (2005) 43, 527–35.

Antihypertensives + Drospirenone-containing HRT

Drospirenone-containing HRT appears to further decrease blood pressure when given with enalapril or hydrochlorothiazide.

Clinical evidence

In a study in 24 postmenopausal women with hypertension taking **enalapril** 10 mg twice daily, the use of **enalapril** with drospirenone 3 mg and estradiol 1 mg daily (12 women) produced a significant *decrease* in blood pressure of 9/5 mmHg after 14 days of treatment, when compared with the placebo group (12 patients).[1] In another study, 34 hypertensive postmenopausal women taking **hydrochlorothiazide** 25 mg daily were given either drospirenone 3 mg with estradiol 1 mg daily or placebo. Mean systolic and diastolic blood pressures were *reduced* by 7.2 mmHg and 4.5 mmHg, respectively, when compared with the placebo group, and drospirenone with estradiol also counteracted **hydrochlorothiazide**-induced potassium loss.[2,3] Drospirenone with **estradiol** did not affect the pharmacokinetics of **hydrochlorothiazide**.[2]

Mechanism

Note that drospirenone is an analogue of spironolactone, and shares its aldosterone antagonist effects, thereby lowering blood pressure and having some potassium-sparing effects. In a placebo-controlled study in women with untreated hypertension, drospirenone 2 or 3 mg combined with estradiol 1 mg daily lowered blood pressure (by 12.1 to 13.8 mmHg and 8.5 to 9.2 mmHg, compared with 8.7 mmHg and 5 mmHg for placebo, for systolic and diastolic blood pressure, respectively.[4]

Importance and management

Evidence for an interaction between drospirenone-containing HRT and antihypertensives is limited, but supported by the known effects of drospirenone alone on blood pressure. Bear in mind the possibility that drospirenone-containing HRT might further decrease blood pressure in women taking antihypertensives. It might be prudent to monitor blood pressure on starting concurrent use. Note that, conversely, hypertension has also been reported uncommonly (occurring in greater than 1 in 1 000 but less than 1 in 100 women) as an adverse effect of drospirenone-containing HRT.[5,6]

Note also that drospirenone has some potassium-sparing effects, which attenuated the effect of hydrochlorothiazide in the study cited, and might be additive with the effect of ACE inhibitors and angiotensin II receptor antagonists, see 'Drospirenone-containing contraceptives or HRT + Potassium-sparing drugs', p.1191.

1. Preston RA, Alonso A, Panzitta D, Zhang P, Karara AH. Additive effect of drospirenone/17-β-estradiol in hypertensive postmenopausal women receiving enalapril. *Am J Hypertens* (2002) 15, 816–22.
2. Karara AH, Hanes V, Alonso A, Ni P, Poola N, Silang R, Blode H, Preston RA. Pharmacokinetics and pharmacodynamics of drospirenone-estradiol combination hormone therapy product coadministered with hydrochlorothiazide in hypertensive postmenopausal women. *J Clin Pharmacol* (2007) 47, 1292–302.
3. Preston RA, Norris PM, Alonso AB, Ni P, Hanes V, Karara AH. Randomized, placebo-controlled trial of the effects of drospirenone-estradiol on blood pressure and potassium balance in hypertensive postmenopausal women receiving hydrochlorothiazide. *Menopause* (2007) 14, 408–14.
4. White WB, Hanes V, Chauhan V, Pitt B. Effects of a new hormone therapy, drospirenone and 17-β-estradiol, in postmenopausal women with hypertension. *Hypertension* (2006) 48, 246–53.
5. Angeliq (Drospirenone with Estradiol). Bayer plc. UK Summary of product characteristics, December 2011.
6. Angeliq (Drospirenone with Estradiol). Bayer HealthCare Pharmaceuticals, Inc. US Prescribing information, February 2012.

Antihypertensives + Hormonal contraceptives

Oral combined hormonal contraceptives are associated with increased blood pressure and might antagonise the efficacy of antihypertensive drugs. However, the effects are far greater with the high-dose contraceptives that were used historically, and the risks appear to be smaller with the newer low-dose contraceptives. Nevertheless, combined hormonal contraceptives are generally not considered suitable for women taking antihypertensives. The risks with progestogen-only contraceptives seem to be low.

Clinical evidence and mechanism

(a) Combined hormonal contraceptives

Early after the introduction of the oral combined hormonal contraceptives it was realised that they can cause increases in blood pressure and clinical hypertension in otherwise healthy women.[1,2] One study from the 1970s, in 83 women, found that the average rise in blood pressure was 9.2/5 mmHg, and that it was about twice as likely to occur as in those not taking a contraceptive.[3] Another study from the 1980s found that women taking an oral combined hormonal contraceptive containing **levonorgestrel** 250 micrograms and **ethinylestradiol** 50 micrograms had higher blood pressures (systolic and diastolic blood pressures were 3.6 to 5 mmHg and 1.9 to 2.7 mmHg higher, respectively) than a similar group of women using non-hormonal contraception.[4] Additionally, cases were noted where antihypertensives (at that time, commonly **guanethidine** and/or **methyldopa**) were not that effective in women with hypertension taking oral combined hormonal contraceptives.[2,5] Although modern oral combined hormonal contraceptives are lower dose, they are still associated with a small increased risk of elevated blood pressure.[6,7] A UK study found that oral combined hormonal contraceptives were associated with a 2.6/1.8 mmHg rise in blood pressure.[6] Evidence from a systematic review suggests that in women with hypertension, those using oral combined hormonal contraceptives were at higher risk for stroke and acute myocardial infarction than those not using these contraceptives.[8]

In a clinical study in 36 women with kidney transplants who had a high rate of arterial hypertension requiring treatment (80 to 88%), combined hormonal contraceptives (tablets or patch) were added for at least 18 months. Ten of 23 (42.7%) women given oral combined hormonal contraceptives and 3 of 10 (30%) given transdermal combined hormonal contraceptives required modification of the type and/or dose of antihypertensives [no specific details given] to maintain blood pressure control. Because of these adjustments, overall, there was no apparent change in mean arterial pressure over the study. Because there was no control group not given hormonal contraceptives, it is not possible to know to what extent the modification in antihypertensive therapy was due to the contraceptives or to other unrelated factors.[9]

(b) Progestogen-only contraceptives

A UK study found that, in contrast to combined hormonal contraceptives, oral progestogen-only contraceptives did not affect blood pressure.[6] A review of four studies also found no significant association between high blood pressure and the use of oral progestogen-only hormonal contraceptives during follow-up periods of 2 to 3 years.[10] A study in women who had been using depot **medroxyprogesterone** for 10 years, found that it did not raise blood pressure.[11]

Importance and management

This is only a very brief review of this subject, but the risks of hypertension with **combined hormonal contraceptives** appear to be modest. Nevertheless, it is generally advised that combined hormonal contraceptives are not used in women with hypertension with no other risk factors for cardiovascular disease, and that they should be avoided in women with hypertension and other risk factors for cardiovascular disease. The 2004 guidelines from the British Hypertension Society suggest that oral combined hormonal contraceptives are not contraindicated in women with treated hypertension if blood pressure control is good, but that progestogen-only contraceptives are usually the preferred hormonal method of contraception in women with hypertension.[12] The UK Faculty of Sexual and Reproductive Healthcare consider that the use of a combined hormonal contraceptive (tablet, transdermal patch, or vaginal ring) is not usually recommended in women with adequately controlled hypertension with no other risk factors for cardiovascular disease, unless other more appropriate methods are not available or acceptable.[13] In these women, there is no restriction on the use of oral **progestogen-only contraceptives** or progestogen-only implants, and the benefits of the use of depot medroxyprogesterone acetate or norethisterone enantate are considered to usually outweigh the theoretical risks.[13] If combined hormonal contraceptives are used in a woman taking antihypertensives, it would seem prudent to monitor blood pressure more frequently. Although **drospirenone** HRT has been shown to lower blood pressure (see 'Antihypertensives + Drospirenone-containing HRT', above), there does not appear to be any information on blood pressure in women taking the drospirenone-containing combined hormonal contraceptives.

1. Wallace MR. Oral contraceptives and severe hypertension. *Aust N Z J Med* (1971) 1, 49–52.
2. Woods JW. Oral contraceptives and hypertension. *Lancet* (1967) iii, 653–4.
3. Weir RJ, Briggs E, Mack A, Naismith L, Taylor L, Wilson E. Blood pressure in women taking oral contraceptives. *BMJ* (1974) 1, 533–5.
4. WHO Task Force on Oral Contraceptives. The WHO multicentre trial of the vasopressor effects of combined oral contraceptives: 1. comparison with IUD. *Contraception* (1989) 40, 129–45.
5. Clezy TM. Oral contraceptives and hypertension: the effect of guanethidine. *Med J Aust* (1970) 1, 638–40.
6. Dong W, Colhoun HM, Poulter NR. Blood pressure in women using oral contraceptives: results from the Health Survey for England 1994. *J Hypertens* (1997) 15, 1063–8.
7. Khaw K-T, Peart WS. Blood pressure and contraceptive use. *BMJ* (1982) 285, 403–7.
8. Curtis KM, Mohllajee AP, Martins SL, Peterson HB. Combined oral contraceptive use among women with hypertension: a systematic review. *Contraception* (2006) 73, 179–88.
9. Pietrzak B, Bobrowska K, Jabiry-Zieniewicz Z, Kaminski P, Wielgos M, Pazik J, Durlik M. Oral and transdermal hormonal contraception in women after kidney transplantation. *Transplant Proc* (2007) 39, 2759–62.
10. Hussain SF. Progestogen-only pills and high blood pressure: is there an association? A literature review. *Contraception* (2004) 69, 89–97.
11. Taneepanichskul S, Reinprayoon D, Jaisamrarn U. Effect of DMPA on weight and blood pressure in long-term acceptors. *Contraception* (1999) 59, 301–3.
12. Williams B, Poulter NR, Brown MJ, Davis M, McInnes GT, Potter JF, Sever PS, McG Thom S. British Hypertension Society Guidelines. Guidelines for management of the fourth working party of the British Hypertension Society, 2004–BHS IV. *J Hum Hypertens* (2004) 18, 139–85.
13. Faculty of Sexual and Reproductive Healthcare. UK medical eligibility criteria for contraceptive use. 2009. Available at: http://www.fsrh.org/pdfs/UKMEC2009.pdf (accessed 21/10/15)

Antihypertensives + Orlistat

In a handful of cases, patients taking enalapril and/or losartan and other antihypertensive drugs (amlodipine, atenolol, hydrochlorothiazide) had marked increases in blood pressure, hypertensive crises and, in one case, intracranial haemorrhage, within 7 to 60 days of starting orlistat.

Clinical evidence

The Argentinian System of Pharmacovigilance identified the following 3 cases of a possible interaction of orlistat with antihypertensives. An obese man whose hypertension was controlled at 120/80 mmHg with daily doses of **losartan** 100 mg, **atenolol** 100 mg, and **hydrochlorothiazide** 12.5 mg developed a hypertensive crisis (blood pressure 260/140 mmHg) 7 days after starting to take orlistat 120 mg three - times daily. The orlistat was stopped and the crisis was controlled. When later rechallenged with orlistat, his diastolic blood pressure rose to 100 to 110 mmHg after 5 days, but the systolic blood pressure increased only slightly. His blood pressure returned to baseline values 3 days after stopping the orlistat.[1] Two other patients reacted similarly. One whose blood pressure was controlled at 130/85 mmHg with **enalapril** 20 mg daily and **losartan** 50 mg daily developed an intracranial haemorrhage and hypertension (blood pressure 160/100 mmHg) with occasional systolic peaks of around 200 mmHg one week after starting orlistat 120 mg three times daily. The other patient who was taking **enalapril** 20 mg daily and **amlodipine** 5 mg daily began to develop hypertensive peaks (blood pressure 180/120 mmHg) 60 days after starting orlistat 120 mg twice daily. The hypertension responded when his medication was changed to **losartan** with **hydrochlorothiazide**, but 20 days later new hypertensive peaks developed (blood pressure 180/110 to 120 mmHg). When the orlistat was withdrawn, the hypertension was controlled within 48 hours.[1]

The Uppsala Adverse Drug Reaction database has two reports of aggravated hypertension in women taking antihypertensives and orlistat.[1] Hypertension has also been reported in previously normotensive individuals taking orlistat, which, in one case, responded to stopping orlistat.[2,3]

However, the manufacturer has found no evidence of an association between orlistat and hypertension. In clinical studies, orlistat use was associated with a small reduction in blood pressure compared with placebo, which was as a result of weight reduction. Moreover, the incidence of hypertension of new onset and hypertensive crisis did not differ between orlistat and placebo (1.2% versus 1.3%, and 0% versus 0.1%, respectively).[4] In studies in healthy subjects, orlistat had no effect on steady-state **losartan** pharmacokinetics,[5] and no clinically significant effect on the pharmacokinetics of single-dose **captopril**, **atenolol**, **furosemide**[6] or **nifedipine**.[6,7]

Mechanism

Not understood. Suggestions include a decrease in the absorption of the drugs due to accelerated gastrointestinal transit, increased defaecation, diarrhoea, or an increase in the amount of fat in the chyme.[1] An explanation for the difference between the clinical cases and pharmacokinetic studies might be that the latter tended to be single-dose studies in healthy subjects. Alternatively, these cases could just be idiosyncratic and not related to orlistat treatment.

Importance and management

The interactions between the antihypertensives and orlistat seem to be confined to the reports cited here, and their general relevance is unclear. Given that the manufacturers report that specific drug interaction studies have not found any evidence of an interaction, the incidence seems likely to be small.

1. Valsecia ME, Malgor LA, Farias EF, Figueras A, Laporte J-R. Interaction between orlistat and antihypertensive drugs. *Ann Pharmacother* (2001) 35, 1495–6.
2. Persson M, Vitols S, Yue Q-Y. Orlistat associated with hypertension. *BMJ* (2000) 321, 87.
3. Persson M, Vitols S, Yue Q-Y. Orlistat associated with hypertension. Author's reply. *BMJ* (2001) 322, 111.
4. Huber MH. Orlistat associated with hypertension. Roche concludes that there is no evidence of a causal association. *BMJ* (2001) 322, 110.
5. Zhi J, Moore R, Kanitra L, Mulligan TE. Pharmacokinetic evaluation of the possible interaction between selected concomitant medications and orlistat at steady state in healthy subjects. *J Clin Pharmacol* (2002) 42, 1011–19.
6. Weber C, Tam YK, Schmidtke-Schrezenmeier G, Jonkmann JHG, van Brummelen P. Effect of the lipase inhibitor orlistat on the pharmacokinetics of four different antihypertensive drugs in healthy volunteers. *Eur J Clin Pharmacol* (1996) 51, 87–90.
7. Melia AT, Mulligan TE, Zhi J. Lack of effect of orlistat on the bioavailability of a single dose of nifedipine extended-release tablets (Procardia X) in healthy volunteers. *J Clin Pharmacol* (1996) 36, 352–5.

Antihypertensives + Other drugs that affect blood pressure

The blood pressure-lowering effects of the antihypertensives can be enhanced by other antihypertensives, as would be expected. Although first-dose hypotension (dizziness, lightheadedness, fainting) can occur with some combinations, the additive effects are usually clinically useful. Perhaps of more concern is the use of antihypertensives with drugs that lower blood pressure as an adverse effect, where the effects may not be anticipated. Some drugs antagonise the blood pressure-lowering effects of the antihypertensives and should therefore be used with caution.

Clinical evidence, mechanism, importance and management

(a) Antihypertensive drugs

Enhanced hypotensive effects should be expected when using two antihypertensives together and it is widely acknowledged that most people require more than one antihypertensive to control blood pressure.[1,2] In the US, more than two-thirds of patients receive two or more antihypertensives in order to reach the desired target blood pressure. Not only does this improve blood pressure control, but adverse effects can also be reduced as lower doses of each drug can be used.[3]

Therefore many antihypertensive combinations produce additive hypotensive effects that are exploited clinically. Calcium-channel blockers and diuretics (see 'Calcium-channel blockers + Diuretics', p.1035) are often used together for additional blood pressure lowering in patients with hypertension. However, the side effects of the drug combinations may also be additive, and although there are only a few reports describing these additive interactions, they are highly probable, and caution is advised when using two antihypertensives together. The most common symptoms seen in hypotensive patients are dizziness, fatigue, headache, nausea, confusion, general weakness, lightheadedness, faintness and possible loss of consciousness.

Investigation of whether the effects of two antihypertensives is additive, greater than additive or less than additive is difficult to assess.[2] However, in some cases combining two or more antihypertensives has led to severe, first-dose hypotension, see 'Alpha blockers + ACE inhibitors or Angiotensin II receptor antagonists', p.90. Further, life-threatening bradycardia, asystole and sinus arrest can occur when antihypertensives that cause cardiodepression are given together (see 'Beta blockers + Calcium-channel blockers; Diltiazem', p.1007).

In contrast, a sharp and serious rise in blood pressure (rebound hypertension) can occur following the sudden withdrawal of clonidine, and this can be exacerbated in the presence of a beta blocker (see 'Clonidine and related drugs + Beta blockers', p.1056). In some cases fatalities have occurred. 'Table 24.2', p.1055 lists antihypertensive combinations that have been implicated in adverse events.

(b) Drugs with significant hypotensive adverse effects

Caution must also be used when combining two or more drugs that, although not primarily indicated for hypertension, may have blood pressure-lowering adverse effects. In fact, it is these drugs, rather than drugs commonly given for their blood pressure-lowering effects that may cause more of a problem, as the effects are less likely to be deliberately sought. These drugs are listed in 'Table 24.3', p.1055 with cross-references to the individual monographs that discuss the reports of adverse effects from these combinations.

(c) Drugs that antagonise hypotensive effects

When using antihypertensive drugs it is important to consider the implications of using drugs that antagonise their effects. The NSAIDs are the prime example of this. In the US, NSAIDs and steroids are reported to be the most common classes of drugs that raise blood pressure. Calcineurin inhibitors (ciclosporin and tacrolimus) and epoetins are reported to raise blood pressure in most patients.[4] Similarly, **danazol** is reported oppose the action of antihypertensives, possibly by increasing fluid retention.[5] Drugs that are thought to antagonise the effects of antihypertensives are listed in 'Table 24.4', p.1055, with cross-references to the individual monographs that discuss the reports of adverse effects from these combinations.

1. Williams B, Poulter NR, Brown MJ, Davis M, McInnes GT, Potter JF, Sever PS, McG Thom S. British Hypertension Society. Guidelines for management of hypertension: report of the fourth working party of the British Hypertension Society, 2004-BHS IV. *J Hum Hypertens* (2004) 18, 139–185.
2. McInnes GT. Antihypertensive drugs in combination: additive or greater than additive? *J Hum Hypertens* (2007) 21, 914–6.
3. Chobanian AV, Bakris GL, Black HR, Cushman WC, Green LA, Izzo JL, Jones DW, Materson BJ, Oparil S, Wright JT, Roccella EJ and the National High Blood Pressure Education Program Co-ordinating Committee. Seventh report of the Joint National Committee on Prevention, Detection, Evaluation, and Treatment of Blood Pressure. *Hypertension* (2003) 42, 1206–52.
4. Elliott WJ. Drug interactions and drugs that affect blood pressure. *J Clin Hypertens* (2006) 8, 731–7.
5. Danol (Danazol). Sanofi. UK Summary of product characteristics, May 2012.

Antihypertensives + Phenylpropanolamine

A single dose of a sustained-release preparation of phenylpropanolamine and brompheniramine was found to cause a minor and clinically insignificant rise in the blood pressures of patients taking various antihypertensives.

Clinical evidence, mechanism, importance and management

A randomised, double-blind, crossover study in 13 patients with hypertension controlled with unnamed **diuretics** (7), **ACE inhibitors** (6), **beta blockers** (5), **calcium-channel blockers** (1) and a **centrally acting alpha-agonist** (1) found that a single dose of *Dimetapp Extentabs* (phenylpropanolamine 75 mg with brompheniramine 12 mg) caused only a minor rise in blood pressure of 1.7/0.9 mmHg over 4 hours.[1] This sustained-release preparation in this dose has therefore no clinically important effect on blood pressure, but (as the authors point out), these results do not necessarily apply to different doses and immediate-release preparations. A marked rise in blood pressure was seen in one patient taking **methyldopa** and **oxprenolol** when given phenylpropanolamine, see 'Methyldopa + Nasal decongestants', p.1070. Consider also 'Beta blockers + Phenylpropanolamine', p.1018.

1. Petrulis AS, Imperiale TF, Speroff T. The acute effect of phenylpropanolamine and brompheniramine on blood pressure in controlled hypertension. *J Gen Intern Med* (1991) 6, 503–6.

Clonidine + Antipsychotics

The hypotensive adverse effects of the phenothiazines, and possibly haloperidol may be additive with the antihypertensive effects of clonidine. Patients may feel faint and dizzy if they stand up quickly.

Clinical evidence

One report describes a patient who experienced dizziness and hypotension (systolic blood pressure 76 mmHg) about an hour after being given **chlorpromazine** 100 mg, clonidine 100 micrograms and furosemide 40 mg. Another patient also experienced hypotension 2 hours after being given clonidine 100 micrograms and a 1-mg intramuscular dose of **haloperidol**.[1]

There is also an isolated and unexplained case of a patient with psychosis taking **fluphenazine decanoate** who began to exhibit delirium, agitation, disorientation, short-term memory loss, confusion and clouded consciousness within 10 days of starting to take clonidine 200 micrograms daily. These symptoms disappeared when the clonidine was stopped and returned when it was re-started. Previous use of **haloperidol** with clonidine had been uneventful.[2]

Mechanism

Simple addition of the hypotensive effects of both drugs seems to be the explanation for the increased hypotension and orthostasis. However, note that in contrast to the case report above, *animal* studies have shown that chlorpromazine *reduces* the antihypertensive effect of clonidine.[3]

Table 24.2 Antihypertensive + Antihypertensive drug interactions

Drugs	*Additive antihypertensive interactions*
ACE inhibitors	ACE inhibitors + Beta blockers, p.25 ACE inhibitors + Calcium-channel blockers, p.25 ACE inhibitors + Clonidine, p.26 ACE inhibitors + Diuretics; Loop, Thiazide and related, p.28 Alpha blockers + ACE inhibitors or Angiotensin II receptor antagonists, p.90
Adrenergic neurone blockers (e.g. guanethidine)	Minoxidil + Miscellaneous, p.1071
Alpha blockers	Alpha blockers + ACE inhibitors or Angiotensin II receptor antagonists, p.90 Alpha blockers + Beta blockers, p.90 Alpha blockers + Calcium-channel blockers, p.91 Alpha blockers + Diuretics, p.93
Angiotensin II receptor antagonists	Angiotensin II receptor antagonists + Beta blockers, p.44 Angiotensin II receptor antagonists + Calcium-channel blockers, p.44 Angiotensin II receptor antagonists + Diuretics; Loop, Thiazide and related, p.45
Beta blockers	ACE inhibitors + Beta blockers, p.25 Alpha blockers + Beta blockers, p.90 Angiotensin II receptor antagonists + Beta blockers, p.44 Beta blockers + Calcium-channel blockers; Dihydropyridines, p.1006 Beta blockers + Calcium-channel blockers; Diltiazem, p.1007 Beta blockers + Calcium-channel blockers; Verapamil, p.1008 Beta blockers + Hydralazine, p.1014 Clonidine and related drugs + Beta blockers, p.1056 Ketanserin + Beta blockers, p.1068
Calcium-channel blockers	ACE inhibitors, p.25 Alpha blockers + Calcium-channel blockers, p.91 Angiotensin II receptor antagonists + Calcium-channel blockers, p.44 Beta blockers + Calcium-channel blockers; Dihydropyridines, p.1006 Beta blockers + Calcium-channel blockers; Diltiazem, p.1007 Beta blockers + Calcium-channel blockers; Verapamil, p.1008 Calcium-channel blockers + Calcium-channel blockers, p.1034 Calcium-channel blockers + Diuretics, p.1035 Calcium-channel blockers + Glyceryl trinitrate (Nitroglycerin), p.1036
Centrally acting antihypertensives (e.g. clonidine, moxonidine)	ACE inhibitors + Clonidine, p.26 Clonidine + Beta blockers, p.1056 Moxonidine + Hydrochlorothiazide, p.1072
Diazoxide	Diazoxide + Hydralazine, p.1058
Diuretics	ACE inhibitors + Diuretics; Loop, Thiazide and related, p.28 Alpha blockers + Diuretics, p.93 Angiotensin II receptor antagonists + Diuretics; Loop, Thiazide and related, p.45 Calcium-channel blockers + Diuretics, p.1035
Nicorandil	Nicorandil + Miscellaneous, p.1072
Nitrates	Calcium-channel blockers + Glyceryl trinitrate (Nitroglycerin), p.1036 Sodium nitroprusside + Miscellaneous, p.1075
Rauwolfia alkaloids	—
Vasodilators (e.g. hydralazine)	Beta blockers + Hydralazine, p.1014 Diazoxide + Hydralazine, p.1058 Minoxidil + Miscellaneous, p.1071 Nicorandil + Miscellaneous, p.1072

Table 24.3 Antihypertensive drug interactions involving drugs with significant hypotensive properties or adverse effects

Drugs	*Additive antihypertensive interactions*
Alcohol	Alcohol + Antihypertensives, p.55
Anaesthetics	Anaesthetics, general + ACE inhibitors or Angiotensin II receptor antagonists, p.99 Anaesthetics, general + Beta blockers, p.103 Anaesthetics, general + MAOIs and related drugs, p.107 Anaesthetics, local + Antihypertensives, p.115
Antipsychotics Drugs specifically named as having hypotensive effects include Asenapine, Iloperidone, Paliperidone, Risperidone, Tiotixene, Ziprasidone, and Zotepine	ACE inhibitors + Antipsychotics, p.20 Beta blockers + Haloperidol, p.1013 Clonidine + Antipsychotics, p.1054 Clozapine + Antihypertensives, p.848 Guanethidine + Antipsychotics, p.1061 Methyldopa + Haloperidol, p.1070
Dopamine agonists (e.g. apomorphine, bromocriptine etc.)	Apomorphine + Miscellaneous, p.756 Bromocriptine and other dopamine agonists + ACE inhibitors, p.756
Levodopa	Guanethidine + Levodopa, p.1062 Levodopa + Methyldopa, p.767
Moxisylyte	Moxisylyte + Miscellaneous, p.1071
Phosphodiesterase type-5 inhibitors	Phosphodiesterase type-5 inhibitors + Alpha blockers, p.1538 Phosphodiesterase type-5 inhibitors + Antihypertensives, p.1539 Phosphodiesterase type-5 inhibitors + Nitrates, p.1545
Procarbazine	Procarbazine + Miscellaneous, p.709
Tizanidine	Tizanidine + Antihypertensives, p.1587
Other drugs suggested to cause hypotension but where no reports of adverse interaction found	Aldesleukin Alprostadil MAOIs

Table 24.4 Antihypertensive drugs and drugs antagonising their effect

Drugs	*Antagonising antihypertensive interactions*
Amfetamines	Guanethidine + Amfetamines and related drugs, p.1061
High-dose aspirin	ACE inhibitors + Aspirin, p.22
Carbenoxolone	Carbenoxolone + Antihypertensives, p.1602
Hormonal contraceptives	Antihypertensives + Hormonal contraceptives or HRT, p.1053
Epoetin	ACE inhibitors and Angiotensin II receptor antagonists + Epoetins, p.33
NSAIDs	ACE inhibitors + NSAIDs, p.38 Alpha blockers + Aspirin or NSAIDs, p.90 Angiotensin II receptor antagonists + Aspirin or NSAIDs, p.43 Beta blockers + Aspirin or NSAIDs, p.1003 Calcium-channel blockers + Aspirin or NSAIDs, p.1030 Guanethidine + NSAIDs, p.1062 Hydralazine + NSAIDs, p.1063 Thiazide diuretics + NSAIDs, p.1132
Phenylpropanolamine	Antihypertensives + Phenylpropanolamine, p.1054 Beta blockers + Phenylpropanolamine, p.1018
Other drugs suggested to antagonise the effects of antihypertensives	Corticosteroids

Importance and management

The increased hypotension and orthostasis that can occur if phenothiazines are used with antihypertensive drugs such as clonidine is established. Note that, of the phenothiazines, **levomepromazine** is particularly associated with postural hypotension. One report suggests that haloperidol may interact similarly. Monitor, particularly during the initial stages of concurrent use, and warn patients that if they feel faint and dizzy they should lie down, and that they should remain lying down until symptoms abate completely. Dose adjustment may be necessary.

The manufacturers of clonidine note that a reduced antihypertensive effect may occur with antipsychotics with alpha-blocking properties (e.g. chlorpromazine),.[4] but the only evidence for this appears to come from *animal* data. However, it has been suggested that the tricyclics may interact by a similar mechanism, see 'Clonidine and related drugs + Tricyclic and related antidepressants', p.1057.

1. Fruncillo RJ, Gibbons WJ, Vlasses PH, Ferguson RK. Severe hypotension associated with concurrent clonidine and antipsychotic medication. *Am J Psychiatry* (1985) 142, 274.
2. Allen RM, Flemenbaum A. Delirium associated with combined fluphenazine-clonidine therapy. *J Clin Psychiatry* (1979) 40, 236–7.
3. van Zwieten PA. The interaction between clonidine and various neuroleptic agents and some benzodiazepine tranquillizers. *J Pharm Pharmacol* (1977) 29, 229–34.
4. Catapres Tablets (Clonidine hydrochloride). Boehringer Ingelheim Ltd. UK Summary of product characteristics, July 2009.

Clonidine and related drugs + Beta blockers

The use of clonidine with beta blockers can be therapeutically valuable, but a sharp and serious rise in blood pressure (rebound hypertension) can follow the sudden withdrawal of clonidine, which may be worsened by the presence of a beta blocker. Moxonidine is predicted to interact similarly. Isolated cases of marked bradycardia and hypotension have been seen in patients given clonidine with esmolol. There are also two reports describing paradoxical hypertension when clonidine was given with a beta blocker.

Clinical evidence

(a) Antagonism of the hypotensive effects

In a study in 10 patients, the concurrent use of **sotalol** 160 mg daily and clonidine 450 micrograms daily caused a marked rise in blood pressure in 6 of the 10 patients, compared with either clonidine alone (3 patients) or **sotalol** alone (3 patients). Of the 4 patients who did not have a marked rise in blood pressure, 2 patients had blood pressures that were lower than with either drug alone, and 2 patients had no appreciable change in blood pressure.[1] Two cases of hypertension involving clonidine with **propranolol** have also been described,[2] and in some studies the concurrent use of clonidine and **nadolol**[3] or **propranolol**[4] has been no more effective than either drug alone.

(b) Bradycardia and hypotension

A man anaesthetised with thiopental and diamorphine, with oxygen, nitrous oxide, enflurane and atracurium, was given clonidine 50 micrograms to control hypertension. After 15 minutes he became tachycardic with a heart rate of up to 170 bpm. **Esmolol** 75 mg was given by slow infusion, whereupon his heart rate fell to 20 bpm. He responded to atropine 1.2 mg, adrenaline (epinephrine) 1 mg and calcium chloride 10 mL with a stable heart rate of 110 bpm.[5] In a clinical study, 32 patients were given **esmolol** during surgery: one patient developed marked hypotension and bradycardia, which responded to ephedrine 10 mg. It was noted that this patient had been receiving clonidine.[6] A subset of 5 patients involved in a study investigating the use of clonidine with **propranolol** and minoxidil had a reduction in blood pressure when clonidine (200 to 400 micrograms daily) was added. After the discontinuation of **propranolol**, blood pressure returned to that seen before clonidine was added, indicating that **propranolol** and clonidine have additive hypotensive actions.[7] Similarly, **atenolol** and clonidine have been found to have additive hypotensive effects.[3,4]

(c) Peripheral vascular disorders

The manufacturer of clonidine notes that the concurrent use of a beta blocker may possibly potentiate peripheral vascular disorders.[8] This is based on the known pharmacology of the drugs,[9] and no specific cases appear to have been reported.

(d) Rebound hypertension

A woman with a blood pressure of 180/140 mmHg was taking clonidine and **timolol**. When the clonidine was stopped in error, she developed a violent throbbing headache and became progressively confused, ataxic and semicomatose, and had a grand mal convulsion. Her blood pressure was found to have risen to over 300/185 mmHg.[10]

A number of other reports describe similar cases of hypertensive rebound (a sudden and serious rise in blood pressure) within 24 to 72 hours of stopping the clonidine, apparently worsened by the presence of **propranolol**.[11-15] The symptoms resemble those of phaeochromocytoma, and include tremor, apprehension, flushing, nausea, vomiting, severe headache, and a serious rise in blood pressure. One patient died from a cerebellar haemorrhage.[14]

Mechanism

The normal additive hypotensive effects of these drugs result from their actions at different but complementary sites in the cardiovascular system. Just why antagonism sometimes occurs is unexplained. The hypertensive rebound following clonidine withdrawal is thought to be due to an increase in the levels of circulating catecholamines. With the beta (vasodilator) effects blocked by a beta blocker, the alpha (vasoconstrictor) effects of the catecholamines are unopposed and the hypertension is further exaggerated.

Importance and management

The interaction whereby the beta blockers seriously worsen the rebound hypertension following clonidine withdrawal is well established. This adverse effect can be controlled by stopping the beta blocker several days before starting a gradual withdrawal of clonidine.[16] A successful alternative is to replace the clonidine and the beta blocker with labetalol,[17] which is both an alpha and a beta blocker: The blood catecholamine levels still rise markedly (20-fold) and the patient may experience tremor, nausea, apprehension and palpitations, but no serious blood pressure rise or headaches appear to occur.[17] The dose of labetalol will need to be titrated to effect, with regular checks on the blood pressure over 2 to 3 days. If a hypertensive episode develops, it can be managed with an alpha-blocking drug such as phentolamine.[11] Diazoxide is also said to be effective.[10,14] Re-introduction of oral or intravenous clonidine should also stabilise the situation. It is clearly important to emphasise to patients taking clonidine and beta blockers that they should not stop taking these drugs without seeking medical advice.

Clonidine and atenolol (a cardio-selective beta blocker) have additive hypotensive effects and smaller doses of clonidine can be given, which decreases its troublesome adverse effects (sedation and dry mouth). In contrast, limited evidence suggests that if clonidine is given with propranolol or nadolol (non-selective beta blockers) the blood pressure reductions were the same as with either drug alone, although this has not been confirmed in other studies. The weight of evidence suggests that paradoxical hypertension is rare.[1,2]

There appears to be no evidence regarding this interaction with **moxonidine**, which is related to clonidine. Moxonidine is reported to have less affinity for central alpha-receptors than clonidine and therefore would be expected to present less of a risk. Furthermore, no such rebound hypertension has been seen when moxonidine is withdrawn. However, to be on the safe side the manufacturers advise that any beta blocker should be stopped first, followed by the moxonidine a few days later.[18,19]

1. Saarimaa H. Combination of clonidine and sotalol in hypertension. *BMJ* (1976) i, 810.
2. Warren SE, Ebert E, Swerdlin A-H, Steinberg SM, Stone R. Clonidine and propranolol paradoxical hypertension. *Arch Intern Med* (1979) 139, 253.
3. Fogari R, Corradi L. Interaction of clonidine and beta blocking agents in the treatment of essential hypertension. In 'Low dose oral and transdermal therapy of hypertension' (Proceedings of Conference 1984), edited by Weber MA, Drayer JIM, Kolloch R. Springer-Verlag, 1985, p. 118–21.
4. Lilja M, Jounela AJ, Juustila H, Mattila MJ. Interaction of clonidine and β-blockers. *Acta Med Scand* (1980) 207, 173–6.
5. Perks D, Fisher GC. Esmolol and clonidine — a possible interaction. *Anaesthesia* (1992) 47, 533–4.
6. Kanitz DD, Ebert TJ, Kampine JP. Intraoperative use of bolus doses of esmolol to treat tachycardia. *J Clin Anesth* (1990) 2, 238–42.
7. Pettinger WA, Mitchell HC, Güllner H-G. Clonidine and the vasodilating beta blocker antihypertensive drug interaction. *Clin Pharmacol Ther* (1977) 22, 164–71.
8. Catapres Tablets (Clonidine hydrochloride). Boehringer Ingelheim Ltd. UK Summary of product characteristics, July 2009.
9. Boehringer Ingelheim. Personal communication, 29 March 2005.
10. Bailey RR, Neale TJ. Rapid clonidine withdrawal with blood pressure overshoot exaggerated by beta-blockade. *BMJ* (1976) i, 942–3.
11. Bruce DL, Croley TF, Lee JS. Preoperative clonidine withdrawal syndrome. *Anesthesiology* (1979) 51, 90–2.
12. Cairns SA, Marshall AJ. Clonidine withdrawal. *Lancet* (1976) i, 368.
13. Strauss FG, Franklin SS, Lewin AJ, Maxwell MH. Withdrawal of antihypertensive therapy. Hypertensive crisis in renovascular hypertension. *JAMA* (1977) 238, 1734–6.
14. Vernon C, Sakula A. Fatal rebound hypertension after abrupt withdrawal of clonidine and propranolol. *Br J Clin Pract* (1979) 33, 112,121.
15. Reid JL, Wing LMH, Dargie HJ, Hamilton CA, Davies DS, Dollery CT. Clonidine withdrawal in hypertension. Changes in blood pressure and plasma and urinary noradrenaline. *Lancet* (1977) i, 1171–4.
16. Harris AL. Clonidine withdrawal and blockade. *Lancet* (1976) i, 596.
17. Rosenthal T, Rabinowitz B, Boichis H, Elazar E, Brauner A, Neufeld HN. Use of labetalol in hypertensive patients during discontinuation of clonidine therapy. *Eur J Clin Pharmacol* (1981) 20, 237–40.
18. Physiotens (Moxonidine). Abbott Healthcare Products Ltd. UK Summary of product characteristics, December 2010.
19. Solvay Healthcare. Personal communication, September 1996.

Clonidine + Bupropion

In a study in 8 healthy subjects, bupropion 100 mg three times daily for 9 days did not reduce the hypotensive effect of a single 300-microgram dose of oral clonidine.[1]

1. Cubeddu LX, Cloutier G, Gross K, Grippo R, Tanner L, Lerea L, Shakarjian M, Knowlton G, Harden TK, Arendshorst W and Rogers JF. Bupropion does not antagonize cardiovascular actions of clonidine in normal subjects and spontaneously hypertensive rats. *Clin Pharmacol Ther* (1984) 35, 576–84.

Clonidine and related drugs + CNS depressants

Increased sedation may occur if alcohol or other CNS depressants are taken with clonidine, moxonidine, guanfacine or guanabenz.

Clinical evidence, mechanism, importance and management

Sedation is a common adverse effect of clonidine and other central alpha-adrenoceptor agonists such as **moxonidine**, **guanfacine** and **guanabenz**, particularly during the initial stages of treatment.[1-4] However, the effects of this in the presence of other CNS depressants does not appear to have been widely studied.

In one study with **moxonidine**, the cognitive function of 24 healthy subjects was not impaired by moxonidine 400 micrograms daily, but the presence of moxonidine was found to increase the cognitive impairment caused by **lorazepam** 1 mg daily.[5] For this reason the manufacturer warns that the sedative effects of the benzodiazepines may possibly be enhanced by moxonidine,[4] and this also seems possible with the related drugs clonidine, **guanfacine** and **guanabenz**. Patients starting treatment with these drugs should be warned that their tolerance to **alcohol** and other CNS depressant drugs may be diminished. Patients who are affected should not drive or operate machinery.

1. Catapres Tablets (Clonidine hydrochloride). Boehringer Ingelheim Ltd. UK Summary of product characteristics, July 2009.
2. Guanfacine hydrochloride. Watson Laboratories, Inc. US Prescribing information, October 2007.
3. Catapres Tablets (Clonidine hydrochloride). Boehringer Ingelheim Pharmaceuticals, Inc. US Prescribing information, January 2010.
4. Physiotens (Moxonidine). Abbott Healthcare Products Ltd. UK Summary of product characteristics, December 2010.
5. Wesnes K, Simpson PM, Jansson B, Grahnén A, Wemann H-J, Küppers H. Moxonidine and cognitive function: interactions with moclobemide and lorazepam. *Eur J Clin Pharmacol* (1997) 52, 351–8.

Clonidine + Escitalopram

An isolated case report describes severe sedation with the concurrent use of clonidine and escitalopram.

Clinical evidence, mechanism, importance and management

A case report describes a critically ill 66-year-old woman treated with clonidine for hypertension and agitation, who became increasingly drowsy to almost unconsciousness during the 3 days after escitalopram 5 mg (her regular antidepressant for the past year) was restarted, having been omitted in error. As a result, the escitalopram was stopped and the patient was alert the next morning.[1]

Evidence for an interaction between clonidine and escitalopram appears to be limited to this case report, and is unlikely to be of general clinical importance.

1. Nikolić M, Noorani A, Park G. Interaction between clonidine and escitalopram. *Br J Anaesth* (2009) 102, 567–8.

Clonidine + Hormonal contraceptives

The sedative effects of intravenous clonidine were increased in one study by an oral combined hormonal contraceptive.

Clinical evidence, mechanism, importance and management

A study[1] in a group of 10 women found that the sedative effects of a single 1.3-microgram/kg dose of intravenous clonidine were increased by an oral combined hormonal contraceptive (**ethinylestradiol** 30 micrograms with **levonorgestrel** 150 or 250 micrograms). The clinical importance of this is uncertain. Consider also 'Antihypertensives + Hormonal contraceptives', p.1053.

1. Chalmers JS, Fulli-Lemaire I, Cowen PJ. Effects of the contraceptive pill on sedative responses to clonidine and apomorphine in normal women. *Psychol Med* (1985) 15, 363–7.

Clonidine + Naloxone

Naloxone does not appear to alter the blood pressure lowering effects of clonidine, or its effects on heart rate.

Clinical evidence, mechanism, importance and management

A study in *animals* suggesting naloxone blocked the antihypertensive effects of clonidine prompted a placebo-controlled study in 6 patients with hypertension. Each patient received a single oral dose of clonidine 300 micrograms during an infusion of either naloxone 6 micrograms/kg per hour or placebo for 8 hours. Supine and standing blood pressure and heart rate were monitored. Naloxone was not found to affect the hypotensive or bradycardic effect of clonidine.[1]

1. Rogers JF, Cubeddu LX. Naloxone does not antagonize the antihypertensive effect of clonidine in essential hypertension. *Clin Pharmacol Ther* (1983) 34, 68–73.

Clonidine + Prazosin

There is some evidence to suggest that prazosin can reduce the antihypertensive effects of clonidine, whereas some other evidence suggests that this does not occur.

Clinical evidence, mechanism, importance and management

In 18 patients with essential hypertension, the hypotensive effect of a 150-microgram intravenous dose of clonidine was reduced by 47% by prazosin (mean dose 11 mg three times daily for 4 days).[1] A later crossover study by the same research group in 17 patients with essential hypertension (mean blood pressures 170/103 mmHg) found that clonidine 300 micrograms daily for 4 days reduced the mean blood pressure by 38/18 mmHg and prazosin 6 mg daily for 3 days reduced the mean blood pressure by 10/4 mmHg. However, when prazosin and clonidine were given together the mean blood pressure was only reduced to a similar extent as prazosin alone (12/6 mmHg).[2] Similarly, some earlier studies had suggested that the concurrent use of clonidine and prazosin produced only a modest,[3] or no additive antihypertensive effect.[4] Conversely, other studies using the combination have not reported a reduced antihypertensive effect.[5,6] In the presence of prazosin the rebound hypertension following clonidine withdrawal was said to be moderate (a rise from 145/85 mmHg to 169/104 mmHg).[6]

Clonidine is an alpha$_2$ agonist, whereas prazosin is an alpha$_1$ blocker. Consequently, it has been postulated that the drugs may be partially antagonistic when given together, and the authors of the first study cite a number of *animal* studies to support this.[1] Although not conclusive, it seems possible that concurrent use may not always be favourable. Therefore it would seem prudent to monitor the effects of concurrent use on blood pressure.

1. Kapocsi J, Farsang C, Vizi ES. Prazosin partly blocks clonidine-induced hypotension in patients with essential hypertension. *Eur J Clin Pharmacol* (1987) 32, 331–4.
2. Farsang C, Varga K, Kapocsi J. Prazosin-clonidine and prazosin-guanfacine interactions in hypertension. *Pharmacol Res Commun* (1988) 20 (Suppl 1), 85–6.
3. Kuokkanen K, Mattila MJ. Antihypertensive effects of prazosin in combination with methyldopa, clonidine or propranolol. *Ann Clin Res* (1979) 11, 18–24.
4. Hubbell FA, Weber MA, Drayer JIM, Rose DE. Combined central and peripheral sympathetic blockade: absence of additive antihypertensive effects. *Am J Med Sci* (1983) 285: 18–26.
5. Stokes GS, Gain JM, Mahoney JE, Raaftos J, Steward JH. Long term use of prazosin in combination or alone for treating hypertension. *Med J Aust* (1977) 2 (Suppl), 13–16.
6. Andréjak M, Fievet P, Makdassi R, Comoy E, de Fremont JF, Coevoet B, Fournier A. Lack of antagonism in the antihypertensive effects of clonidine and prazosin in man. *Clin Sci* (1981) 61, 453s–455s.

Clonidine + Rifampicin (Rifampin)

Rifampicin does not interact with clonidine.

Clinical evidence, mechanism, importance and management

In 6 subjects taking clonidine 200 micrograms twice daily the use of rifampicin 600 mg twice daily for 7 days did not affect the elimination kinetics of clonidine, or its effects on pulse rate or blood pressure.[1] No special precautions would seem necessary on concurrent use.

1. Affrime MB, Lowenthal DT, Rufo M. Failure of rifampin to induce the metabolism of clonidine in normal volunteers. *Drug Intell Clin Pharm* (1981) 15, 964–6.

Clonidine and related drugs + Tricyclic and related antidepressants

The tricyclic antidepressants reduce or abolish the antihypertensive effects of clonidine and a case report describes a hypertensive crisis as a result of this interaction. Moxonidine is expected to interact similarly. The tetracyclics, maprotiline and mianserin do not appear to alter the antihypertensive effects of clonidine, although a case report describes a hypertensive crisis in a patient taking the related drug mirtazapine with clonidine.

Clinical evidence

(a) Tetracyclic and related antidepressants

In a study in 8 healthy subjects, **maprotiline** 100 mg in four divided doses over 22 hours did not alter the effect of a single 300-microgram dose of clonidine on blood pressure or heart rate.[1] **Mianserin** 20 mg three times daily for 2 weeks had no effect on the control of blood pressure in 5 patients receiving clonidine.[2,3] Similarly, in healthy subjects, **mianserin** pretreatment did not significantly alter the hypotensive action of a single 300-microgram dose of clonidine.[2,4] In contrast, an isolated report describes hypertensive urgency in a man with end-stage renal disease taking clonidine, metoprolol and losartan when **mirtazapine** (a **mianserin** analogue) was added for depression.[5]

(b) Trazodone

A 12-year-old boy taking clonidine 100 micrograms three times daily and dexamfetamine 15 mg twice daily was given trazodone 50 mg at bedtime. After a few weeks his trazodone dose was increased to 100 mg at bedtime. Within 45 minutes of taking his first increased dose he had a hypotensive episode with bradycardia and sedation. The trazodone dose was reduced back to 50 mg, but the drug was discontinued 2 weeks later because of low blood pressure.[6]

(c) Tricyclic antidepressants

Desipramine 75 mg daily for 2 weeks caused the lying and standing blood pressures of 4 out of 5 hypertensive patients taking clonidine 600 to 1800 micrograms daily (with chlortalidone or hydrochlorothiazide) to rise by 22/15 mmHg and 12/10 mmHg respectively.[7] This interaction has been seen in other patients taking **clomipramine**, **desipramine** and **imipramine**.[8-11] In one study, the antihypertensive effects of a single intravenous dose of clonidine were reduced by about 50% in 6 patients given **desipramine** for 3 weeks.[12] Similarly, in 8 healthy subjects, the blood pressure lowering effect of a single 300-microgram dose of clonidine was reduced by 40 to 50% when it was given on day 9 of treatment with **imipramine** 25 mg three times daily.[13] An elderly woman taking clonidine 200 micrograms daily developed severe frontal headache, dizziness, chest and neck pain and tachycardia of 120 bpm with hypertension (230/124 to 130 mmHg) on the second day of taking **imipramine** 50 mg for incontinence.[14]

A case report describes a 73-year-old woman, who developed rebound hypertension and tachycardia on the withdrawal of clonidine. This may have been made worse by the presence of **amitriptyline**.[15]

A man with severe pain, well controlled with **amitriptyline**, sodium valproate and intrathecal boluses of diamorphine, experienced severe pain within 5 minutes of an intrathecal test dose of clonidine 75 micrograms. It was considered that an interaction between the tricyclic and the clonidine may have been responsible.[16]

Mechanism

Not understood. One idea is that the tricyclics desensitise or block central alpha$_2$-receptors.[17] This would explain the interaction with mirtazapine (a mianserin analogue), which also has alpha-blocking properties.[5] However, mianserin (also an alpha blocker) did not interact.[2] Another idea is that tricyclics block noradrenaline uptake. However, maprotiline, which also blocks noradrenaline uptake, did not interact.[1] Trazodone, which also has alpha-blocking properties was predicted to inhibit the effect of clonidine based on a study in *animals* where it antagonised the hypotensive effect of clonidine when given centrally (note this effect was not seen when it was given intravenously).[18] The case of hypotension described could be explained by the hypotensive effect of trazodone alone, but may have been compounded by the hypotensive effect of clonidine.

Importance and management

The interaction between clonidine and the tricyclics is established and clinically important. The incidence is uncertain but an interaction is not seen in all patients.[7] Avoid concurrent use unless the effects can be monitored. Increasing the dose of clonidine may possibly be effective. The clonidine dose was apparently successfully titrated in 10 out of 11 hypertensive patients already taking amitriptyline or imipramine.[19] Only clomipramine, desipramine and imipramine have been implicated so far, but other tricyclics would be expected to behave similarly (amitriptyline, **nortriptyline** and **protriptyline** have been shown to interact in *animals*[20]). The tetracyclic antidepressants maprotiline and mianserin do not generally appear to interact with clonidine. The isolated case of hypotension with trazodone and the isolated case of severe pain with amitriptyline and clonidine are of unknown general importance.

There appears to be no evidence regarding an interaction between **moxonidine** and the tricyclics. The manufacturer of moxonidine advises avoiding tricyclic antidepressants, as they state that moxonidine can increase the effects of the tricyclics, and the tricyclics may antagonise the effects of moxonidine.[21] Presumably, this is because moxonidine is related to clonidine. It may therefore be prudent to follow the same precautions described for clonidine.

1. Gundert-Remy U, Amann E, Hildebrandt R, Weber E. Lack of interaction between the tetracyclic antidepressant maprotiline and the centrally acting antihypertensive drug clonidine. *Eur J Clin Pharmacol* (1983) 25, 595–9.
2. Elliott HL, Whiting B, Reid JL. Assessment of the interaction between mianserin and centrally-acting antihypertensive drugs. *Br J Clin Pharmacol* (1983) 15, 323S–328S.
3. Elliott HL, McLean K, Sumner DJ, Reid JL. Absence of an effect of mianserin on the actions of clonidine or methyldopa in hypertensive patients. *Eur J Clin Pharmacol* (1983) 24, 15–19.
4. Elliott HL, McLean K, Sumner DJ, Reid JL. Pharmacodynamic studies on mianserin and its interaction with clonidine. *Eur J Clin Pharmacol* (1981) 21, 97–102.
5. Abo-Zena RA, Bobek MB, Dweik RA. Hypertensive urgency induced by an interaction of mirtazapine and clonidine. *Pharmacotherapy* (2000) 20, 476–8.
6. Bhatara VS, Kallepalli BR, Misra LK, Awadallah S. A possible clonidine-trazodone-dextroamphetamine interaction in a 12-year-old boy. *J Child Adolesc Psychopharmacol* (1996) 6, 203–9.
7. Briant RH, Reid JL, Dollery CT. Interaction between clonidine and desipramine in man. *BMJ* (1973) i, 522–3.
8. Coffler DE. Antipsychotic drug interaction. *Drug Intell Clin Pharm* (1976) 10, 114–15.
9. Andrejak M, Fournier A, Hardin J-M, Coevoet B, Lambrey G, De Fremont J-F, Quichaud J. Suppression de l'effet antihypertenseur de la clonidine par la prise simultanée d'un antidépresseur tricyclique. *Nouv Presse Med* (1977) 6, 2603.
10. Lacomblez L, Warot D, Bouche P, Derouesné C. Suppression de l'effet antihypertenseur de la clonidine par la clomipramine. *Rev Med Interne* (1988) 9, 291–3.
11. Manchon ND, Bercoff E, Lemarchand P, Chassagne P, Senant J, Bourreille J. Fréquence et gravité des interactions médicamenteuses dans une population âgée: étude prospective concernant 639 malades. *Rev Med Interne* (1989) 10, 521–5.
12. Checkley SA, Slade AP, Shur E, Dawling S. A pilot study of the mechanism of action of desipramine. *Br J Psychiatry* (1981) 138, 248–51.
13. Cubeddu LX, Cloutier G, Gross K, Grippo PA-CR, Tanner L, Lerea L, Shakarjian M, Knowlton G, Harden TK, Arendshorst W, Rogers JF. Bupropion does not antagonize cardiovascular actions of clonidine in normal subjects and spontaneously hypertensive rats. *Clin Pharmacol Ther* (1984) 35, 576–84.
14. Hui KK. Hypertensive crisis induced by interaction of clonidine with imipramine. *J Am Geriatr Soc* (1983) 31, 164–5.
15. Stiff JL, Harris DB. Clonidine withdrawal complicated by amitriptyline therapy. *Anesthesiology* (1983) 59, 73–4.
16. Hardy PAJ, Wells JCD. Pain after spinal intrathecal clonidine. An adverse interaction with tricyclic antidepressants? *Anaesthesia* (1988) 43, 1026–7.
17. van Spanning HW, van Zwieten PA. The interference of tricyclic antidepressants with the central hypotensive effect of clonidine. *Eur J Pharmacol* (1973) 24, 402–4.
18. van Zwieten PA. Inhibition of the central hypotensive effect of clonidine by trazodone, a novel antidepressant. *Pharmacology* (1977) 15, 331–6.
19. Raftos J, Bauer GE, Lewis RG, Stokes GS, Mitchell AS, Young AA, Maclachlan I. Clonidine in the treatment of severe hypertension. *Med J Aust* (1973) 1, 786–93.
20. van Zwieten PA. Interaction between centrally active hypotensive drugs and tricyclic antidepressants. *Arch Int Pharmacodyn Ther* (1975) 214, 12–30.
21. Physiotens (Moxonidine). Abbott Healthcare Products Ltd. UK Summary of product characteristics, December 2010.

Diazoxide + Hydralazine

Severe hypotension, in some cases fatal, has followed the use of high doses of intravenous diazoxide, given before or after hydralazine.

Clinical evidence

A previously normotensive 25-year-old woman had a blood pressure of 250/150 mmHg during the 34th week of pregnancy, which did not respond to intravenous magnesium sulfate 4 g. Her blood pressure fell transiently to 170/120 mmHg when she was given hydralazine 15 mg intravenously. One hour later intravenous diazoxide 5 mg/kg resulted in a blood pressure fall to 60/0 mmHg. Despite large doses of noradrenaline (norepinephrine), the hypotension persisted and the woman died.[1]

Other cases of severe hypotension in patients given high doses of intravenous diazoxide and intravenous or oral hydralazine are described in this[1] and other studies and reports.[2-4] In some instances the patients had also received other antihypertensives such as methyldopa[1] or reserpine.[1,4] At least three of the cases had a fatal outcome.[4]

Mechanism

Not fully understood. The (vasodilatory) hypotensive effects of the two drugs are additive and it would seem that in some instances the normal compensatory responses of the cardiovascular system to maintain an adequate blood pressure reach their limit. This can occur with intravenous diazoxide alone.[2]

Importance and management

The concurrent use of intravenous diazoxide and hydralazine should be undertaken extremely cautiously with thorough monitoring. Note that the doses of diazoxide used in the above reports were frequently higher than those currently recommended for hypertensive crises,[5] and there are now many more options available for the treatment of very severe hypertension. Moreover, diazoxide was frequently associated with clinically important hypotension when used in pregnancy, and is not considered a good choice in this situation.[6]

1. Henrich WL, Cronin R, Miller PD, Anderson RJ. Hypotensive sequelae of diazoxide and hydralazine therapy. *JAMA* (1977) 237, 264–5.
2. Kumar GK, Dastoor FC, Robayo JR, Razzaque MA. Side effects of diazoxide. *JAMA* (1976) 235, 275–6.
3. Tansey WA, Williams EG, Landesman RH and Schwarz MJ. Diazoxide. *JAMA* (1973) 225, 749.
4. Davey M, Moodley J, Soutter P. Adverse effects of a combination of diazoxide and hydrallazine therapy. *S Afr Med J* (1981) 59, 496–7.
5. *Martindale. The Complete Drug Reference*, [online] London: Pharmaceutical Press. https://www.medicinescomplete.com/mc/martindale/current/862-j.htm (accessed 19/10/15).
6. Duley L, Henderson-Smart DJ, Meher S. Drugs for treatment of very high blood pressure during pregnancy. Available in the Cochrane Database of Systematic Reviews; Issue 3. Chichester: John Wiley; 2006.

Diazoxide + Other drugs with hyperglycaemic activity

The risk of hyperglycaemia is increased if diazoxide is given with other drugs with hyperglycaemic activity (e.g. the thiazides, chlorpromazine, corticosteroids, combined hormonal contraceptives).

Clinical evidence, mechanism, importance and management

An isolated report[1] describes a child receiving long-term treatment for hypoglycaemia with diazoxide 8 mg/kg daily in divided doses and **bendroflumethiazide** 1.25 mg daily, who developed a diabetic pre-coma and severe hyperglycaemia after taking a single 30-mg dose of **chlorpromazine**. The reason for this reaction is not understood but one idea is that all three drugs had additive hyperglycaemic effects. Enhanced hyperglycaemia has been seen in other patients given diazoxide with **trichlormethiazide**.[2] Caution is clearly needed to ensure that the hyperglycaemic effects do not become excessive. The manufacturers of diazoxide also mention that the risk of hyperglycaemia may be increased by **corticosteroids** or oestrogen-progestogen combinations (e.g. **combined hormonal contraceptives**).[3]

1. Aynsley-Green A, Illig R. Enhancement by chlorpromazine of hyperglycaemic action of diazoxide. *Lancet* (1975) ii, 658–9.
2. Seltzer HS, Allen EW. Hyperglycemia and inhibition of insulin secretion during administration of diazoxide and trichlormethiazide in man. *Diabetes* (1969) 18, 19–28.
3. Eudemine Tablets (Diazoxide). UCB Pharma Ltd. UK Summary of product characteristics, March 2009.

Endothelin receptor antagonists + HIV-protease inhibitors

Lopinavir boosted with ritonavir markedly increases bosentan exposure. Other HIV-protease inhibitors boosted with ritonavir are predicted to interact similarly. A case of subtherapeutic indinavir concentrations has been reported in a patient after he started to take bosentan. The exposure to ambrisentan and macitentan is predicted to be increased by the concurrent use of HIV-protease inhibitors boosted ritonavir.

Clinical evidence

1. Indinavir. A 39-year old man taking an antiretroviral regimen which included indinavir 800 mg three times daily (which gave an indinavir minimum concentration of 0.24 mg/L, usual therapeutic range 0.15 to 0.8 mg/L) was found to have a reduced indinavir minimum concentration of less than 0.05 mg/L about 2.5 months after he started to take bosentan, (initially 62.5 mg increased to 125 mg twice daily). His indinavir dose was increased to 1 g three times daily, and a pharmacokinetic profile at month 8 of concurrent use found that the pharmacokinetics of indinavir were similar to those reported for a dose of 800 mg three times daily.[1]

2. Lopinavir. In a pharmacokinetic study in 8 healthy subjects, the concurrent use of bosentan 125 mg twice daily and lopinavir boosted with ritonavir 400/100 mg twice daily increased the day 10 steady-state AUC of bosentan 5.2-fold, with a similar increase in the AUC of its active metabolite. Bosentan decreased the steady-state AUCs of lopinavir and ritonavir by 14% and 17%, respectively. Minimum drug concentrations were measured daily before the morning dose, and the minimum concentration of bosentan minimum concentration was highest on day 4 (48-fold higher) coinciding with the highest minimum concentration s of lopinavir and ritonavir, reducing to about 5-fold higher at steady-state.[2]

Mechanism

Bosentan is known to be partly metabolised by CYP3A4, but the increase in exposure seen with lopinavir boosted with ritonavir is greater than would be expected from CYP3A4 inhibition alone. Bosentan is also a substrate for the transporter protein OATP1B1, and it is possible that inhibition of this transporter by ritonavir contributes to the interaction. In one study, the minimum plasma concentration of bosentan was increased to the greatest extent when the minimum plasma concentrations of lopinavir and ritonavir were highest, which occurred in the first 4 days or so of administration of these HIV-protease inhibitors.[2]

In an *in vitro* study, ritonavir inhibited hepatic uptake of ambrisentan as well as bosentan.[3] Ambrisentan is also affected by rifampicin, another OATP inhibitor, see 'Endothelin receptor antagonists + Rifampicin (Rifampin)', p.1060, but to a lesser extent than bosentan.

Importance and management

(a) Effects on endothelin receptor antagonists

The increased **bosentan** concentrations seen with lopinavir boosted with ritonavir are likely to be clinically important at steady-state, and perhaps even more so during the first few days of administration of lopinavir boosted with ritonavir. This interaction is likely to be similar for all HIV-protease inhibitors boosted with ritonavir. It would therefore be prudent to closely monitor for bosentan toxicity, including hypotension and liver function tests, on concurrent use, adjusting the bosentan dose as necessary. If an HIV-protease inhibitor boosted with ritonavir is to be started in a patient already taking bosentan, the US recommendation is that bosentan should be stopped for at least 36 hours before starting the HIV-protease inhibitors. When the HIV-protease inhibitor boosted with ritonavir has been given for at least 10 days, bosentan can be restarted at a dose of 62.5 mg daily or on alternate days, depending on tolerability.[4] Patients taking unboosted **indinavir** or **nelfinavir** need not stop bosentan, but the dose should be reduced to 62.5 mg daily or on alternate days.[5,6] In patients already taking an HIV-protease inhibitor boosted with ritonavir for at least 10 days, the US advice is to start bosentan at the reduced dose of 62.5 mg daily or on alternate days.[4]

Note that the UK and US manufacturers of bosentan advise against the concurrent use of CYP3A4 inhibitors (which would be expected to include the HIV-protease inhibitors) with CYP2C9 inhibitors, see 'Endothelin receptor antagonists + Ketoconazole and other CYP3A4 inhibitors', below.

Nothing is known about the effect of HIV-protease inhibitors boosted with ritonavir on other endothelin receptor antagonists. However, *in vitro*, **ritonavir** inhibited **ambrisentan** hepatic uptake, so because of this, and until more is known, some caution would be appropriate on concurrent use. For **maitentan**, the concurrent use of potent CYP3A4 inhibitors (which would be expected to include the HIV-protease inhibitors when boosted with ritonavir) is not recommended or should be undertaken with caution, based on the effect of ketoconazole (see 'Endothelin receptor antagonists + Ketoconazole and other CYP3A4 inhibitors', below).

(b) Effects on HIV-protease inhibitors

The negligible decrease in the exposure to lopinavir and ritonavir after 10 days of concurrent use with bosentan is not clinically relevant. However, the case report of subtherapeutic concentrations of indinavir suggests that some caution might be necessary on concurrent use until more is known. Also, the UK manufacturer of bosentan states that they cannot exclude the possibility that the effect might be greater if bosentan were continued for longer. For this reason, they recommend that antiviral efficacy be closely monitored if any HIV-protease inhibitor boosted with ritonavir is used in patients taking bosentan.[7] In the US, the manufacturer of **atazanavir** considers that bosentan will reduce its concentrations and states that the combination of unboosted atazanavir with bosentan should be avoided,[8] although they allow use of atazanavir boosted with ritonavir (however, see *Effects on endothelin receptor antagonists*, above).

1. Beau-Salinas F, Garot D, Le Guellec C, Jonville-Béra AP, Ingremeau V, Autret-Leca E. Possible reduction in indinavir serum concentrations by bosentan. *Ther Drug Monit* (2005) 27, 822–3.
2. Dingemanse J, van Giersbergen PLM, Patat A, Nilsson PN. Mutual pharmacokinetic interactions between bosentan and lopinavir/ritonavir in healthy participants. *Antivir Ther* (2010) 15, 157–63.
3. Hartman JC, Brouwer K, Mandagere A, Melvin L, Gorczynski R. Evaluation of the endothelin receptor antagonists ambrisentan, darusentan, bosentan, and sitaxsentan as substrates and inhibitors of hepatobiliary transporters in sandwich-cultured human hepatocytes. *Can J Physiol Pharmacol* (2010) 88, 682–91.
4. Tracleer (Bosentan). Actelion Pharmaceuticals US, Inc. US Prescribing information, October 2012.
5. Crixivan (Indinavir sulfate). Merck & Co., Inc. US Prescribing information, December 2013.
6. Viracept (Nelfinavir mesylate). Agouron Pharmaceuticals, Inc. US Prescribing information, May 2013.
7. Tracleer (Bosentan monohydrate). Actelion Pharmaceuticals UK Ltd. UK Summary of product characteristics, September 2013.
8. Reyataz (Atazanavir sulfate). Bristol-Myers-Squibb. US Prescribing information, June 2014.

Endothelin receptor antagonists + Ketoconazole and other CYP3A4 inhibitors

Ketoconazole moderately increases bosentan and macitentan exposure. Fluconazole is predicted to have a similar or greater effect on bosentan. Ketoconazole slightly increases the exposure to ambrisentan.

Clinical evidence

(a) Ambrisentan

A study in 16 healthy subjects found that **ketoconazole** 400 mg daily for 4 days increased the AUC and maximum concentration of a single 10-mg dose of ambrisentan by 35% and 20%, respectively.[1]

(b) Bosentan

In a crossover study, 10 healthy male subjects were given bosentan 62.5 mg twice daily for 11 doses, either alone, or with **ketoconazole** 200 mg daily. The maximum plasma concentration of bosentan was increased 2.1-fold, and the AUC was increased 2.3-fold (range 1.4- to 4-fold).[2]

(c) Macitentan

In a crossover study, 10 healthy male subjects were given a single 10-mg dose of macitentan alone, and on day 5 of ketoconazole 400 mg daily. The AUC and maximum concentration of macitentan were increased 2.3-fold and by 30%, respectively.[3]

Mechanism

Ambrisentan, bosentan, and macitentan are all metabolised to varying extents by CYP3A4, of which ketoconazole is a known, potent inhibitor. Concurrent use therefore results in increases in their exposure, albeit to varying extents.

Importance and management

A pharmacokinetic interaction between ketoconazole and ambrisentan, bosentan, and macitentan is established, however, the size and clinical importance of the increases in exposure of the endothelin receptor antagonists varies. The increase in the exposure to **bosentan** was moderate and the importance of this is unclear. Bosentan has been tolerated in single-doses of up to 2.4 g in healthy subjects, although elevations in liver transaminases have been seen during long-term, high-dose use.[2] The UK and US manufacturers suggest that no adjustment of the bosentan dose is likely to be required when it is used with **ketoconazole**,[4,5] although increased adverse effects should be considered.[5] Other potent CYP3A4 inhibitors would be expected to interact similarly.

The UK and US manufacturers note that bosentan is also metabolised by CYP2C9, and although there are no data, they predict that the concurrent use of inhibitors of CYP2C9 and inhibitors of CYP3A4 might result in a large increase in bosentan exposure; for this reason such a combination is not recommended.[4,5] For a list of CYP2C9 inhibitors, see 'Table 1.5', p.7, and for a list of CYP3A4 inhibitors, see 'Table 1.9', p.11. Note that **fluconazole** is a moderate inhibitor of CYP3A4 and a dose-dependent weak to moderate inhibitor of CYP2C9, and so concurrent use with bosentan is not recommended.[4,5] Until more is known, it would be prudent to carefully monitor liver function if the concurrent use of **fluconazole** with bosentan is necessary. Note also that **voriconazole** also inhibits both CYP3A4 and CYP2C9 (although the latter only weakly).

The slight increase in **ambrisentan** exposure when given with ketoconazole is not expected to be clinically relevant, therefore no ambrisentan dose adjustment is required if **ketoconazole** is also given.[1] It seems unlikely that other azoles will interact with ambrisentan, but this does not appear to have been studied.

Due to the moderate increase in **macitentan** exposure seen with ketoconazole, the UK manufacturer recommends caution on concurrent use,[6] whereas the US manufacturer advises avoiding the combination.[7] Both manufacturers extend their respective advice to other potent CYP3A4 inhibitors (see 'Table 1.9', p.11 for a list).[6,7] Note that the UK manufacturer includes **nefazodone** as a potent CYP3A4 inhibitor, but it is generally considered a moderate inhibitor.

1. Richards DB, Walker GA, Mandagere A, Magee MH, Henderson LS. Effect of ketoconazole on the pharmacokinetic profile of ambrisentan. *J Clin Pharmacol* (2009) 49, 719–24.
2. van Giersbergen PLM, Halabi A, Dingemanse J. Single- and multiple-dose pharmacokinetics of bosentan and its interaction with ketoconazole. *Br J Clin Pharmacol* (2002) 53, 589–95.
3. Atsmon J, Dingemanse J, Shaikevich D, Volokhov I, Sidharta PN. Investigation of the effects of ketoconazole on the pharmacokinetics of macitentan, a novel dual endothelin receptor antagonist, in healthy subjects. *Clin Pharmacokinet* (2013) 52, 685–92.
4. Tracleer (Bosentan monohydrate). Actelion Pharmaceuticals UK Ltd. UK Summary of product characteristics, September 2013.
5. Tracleer (Bosentan). Actelion Pharmaceuticals US, Inc. US Prescribing information, October 2012.
6. Opsumit (Macitentan). Actelion Pharmaceuticals UK Ltd. UK Summary of product characteristics, May 2014.
7. Opsumit (Macitentan). Actelion Pharmaceuticals US, Inc. US Prescribing information, October 2013.

Endothelin receptor antagonists + Miscellaneous

The pharmacokinetics of bosentan were not altered by losartan or nimodipine. Omeprazole does not alter the pharmacokinetics of ambrisentan. There is no pharmacokinetic interaction between ambrisentan and mycophenolate. The pharmacokinetics of tacrolimus are not altered by ambrisentan, but there might be an interaction between bosentan and tacrolimus or sirolimus. The exposure to ambrisentan and bosentan might be increased by ceftobiprole.

Clinical evidence, mechanism, importance and management

(a) Ceftobiprole

The UK manufacturer of ceftobiprole states that *in-vitro* studies indicated that ceftobiprole inhibits OATP1B1 and OATP1B3,[1] which are involved in the hepatic uptake of **ambrisentan** and **bosentan**. They therefore predict that ceftobiprole might increase the exposure to bosentan;[1] a similar effect would be expected on concurrent use with ambrisentan. However note that *in vitro* inhibitory activity does not always translate into a clinically relevant effect *in vivo*.

(b) CYP2C19 substrates

Ambrisentan is metabolised, in part, by CYP2C19, and therefore caution is advised if potent CYP2C19 inhibitors are also given, presumably because of the possibility that concentrations of ambrisentan might be increased. However, the US manufacturer notes that concurrent use with **omeprazole** (a CYP2C19 substrate and inhibitor) does not have clinically significant effects on ambrisentan pharmacokinetics,[2] and therefore a clinically relevant interaction seems unlikely.

(c) Losartan

A study in healthy subjects found that the pharmacokinetics of **bosentan** 125 mg twice daily were unaffected by the concurrent use of losartan 100 mg daily for 9 doses.[3]

(d) Mycophenolate

The US manufacturer briefly notes that **ambrisentan** minimally increased the AUC and maximum concentration of mycophenolic acid. Similarly mycophenolate had only a minimal effect on ambrisentan pharmacokinetics. No dose adjustments are necessary on concurrent use.[2]

(e) Nimodipine

In a study of 6 patients with subarachnoid haemorrhage, the pharmacokinetics of a single 500-mg intravenous dose of **bosentan** were not affected by the concurrent use of nimodipine (dose not specified).[4]

(f) Sirolimus or Tacrolimus

1. Ambrisentan. The US manufacturer briefly notes that ambrisentan had little or no effect on the AUC and maximum concentration of **tacrolimus**, and no dose adjustment is necessary on concurrent use.[2]

2. Bosentan. The concurrent use of **tacrolimus** or **sirolimus** with bosentan has not been studied. But, based on the information available for ciclosporin (see 'Ciclosporin + Endothelin receptor antagonists', p.1227), the UK manufacturer of bosentan advises against concurrent use if possible.[5] If both bosentan and tacrolimus or sirolimus are required, it would be prudent to monitor for bosentan adverse effects and closely monitor immunosuppressant concentrations.

1. Zevtera (Ceftobiprole). Basilea Pharmaceutica. UK Summary of product characteristics, November 2013.
2. Letairis (Ambrisentan). Gilead Sciences, Inc. US Prescribing information, May 2014.
3. van Giersbergen PLM, Clozel M, Bodin F. A drug interaction study between bosentan and ketoconazole and losartan. *Clin Pharmacol Ther* (2001) 69, P67
4. Dingemanse J, van Giersbergen PLM. Clinical pharmacology of bosentan, a dual endothelin receptor antagonist. *Clin Pharmacokinet* (2004) 43, 1089–1115.
5. Tracleer (Bosentan monohydrate). Actelion Pharmaceuticals UK Ltd. UK Summary of product characteristics, September 2013.

Endothelin receptor antagonists + Rifampicin (Rifampin)

In the first 2 days of starting rifampicin, large increases in the minimum concentrations of bosentan occur, but when rifampicin is at steady-state, bosentan exposure is halved. Similarly, when rifampicin is initially given simultaneously with ambrisentan, ambrisentan exposure is slightly increased, whereas at steady-state, rifampicin has no effect on ambrisentan exposure. Rifampicin moderately decreases the exposure to macitentan.

Clinical evidence

(a) Ambrisentan

In a pharmacokinetic study in 20 healthy subjects, ambrisentan 10 mg daily was given for 13 days with rifampicin 600 mg daily for the last 8 days, and taken at the same time as ambrisentan. During the first 2 days of concurrent rifampicin, the ambrisentan AUC was increased by 87%, but by day 8 of concurrent use there was no difference in the AUC of ambrisentan.[1]

(b) Bosentan

In a crossover study in 9 healthy subjects, bosentan 125 mg twice daily was given for 6 and a half days, either alone or with rifampicin 600 mg daily (which was given with the evening dose of bosentan for 6 days). Steady-state rifampicin decreased the AUC and maximum plasma concentration of bosentan by 58% and 53%, respectively. Minimum concentrations of bosentan were increased up to 15-fold on day 2 of concurrent use, but decreased with subsequent treatment, and by day 4 were lower than those with bosentan alone.[2]

(c) Macitentan

In a crossover study, 10 healthy male subjects were given macitentan 30 mg on day 1, followed by 10 mg daily, with rifampicin 600 mg daily on days 6 to 12. The AUC of macitentan was decreased by 79%, and the minimum concentration was almost reduced to zero.[3]

Mechanism

The initial increase in ambrisentan and bosentan concentrations on starting rifampicin was probably due to rifampicin inhibition of the hepatic uptake of these endothelin receptor antagonists by organic ion-transporting polypeptides (OATP1B1 and OATP1B3).[1,2,4] The decrease in bosentan exposure by rifampicin at steady-state was probably due to induction of CYP3A4 and CYP2C9 by rifampicin. The enzyme-inducing effects of rifampicin take a number of days to develop, so, when rifampicin is started, the OATP inhibitory effects predominate. When rifampicin reaches steady-state, the enzyme-inducing effects predominate. There is evidence with atorvastatin (see 'Statins + Rifampicin (Rifampin)', p.1355) that the OATP inhibitory effects of rifampicin are greatest with simultaneous administration. Therefore, if administration of rifampicin had been separated from ambrisentan and bosentan, the outcome might have been different.

Macitentan is metabolised by CYP3A4, but is not a substrate for OATP, and so its exposure is simply decreased by concurrent rifampicin.

Importance and management

The effect of rifampicin on ambrisentan and bosentan depends on the duration of rifampicin therapy. During the first couple of days of giving rifampicin with these endothelin receptor antagonists, their concentrations are increased, whereas when rifampicin is at steady-state, the exposure of bosentan is halved and that of ambrisentan remains unchanged. The clinical relevance of these findings is uncertain. For **bosentan**, the UK manufacturer notes that a decrease in efficacy cannot be excluded. However, they also warn that the risk of liver dysfunction with bosentan might be increased when it is given with inhibitors of the bile salt export pump, such as rifampicin. Concurrent use is not recommended.[5] The US manufacturer recommends increasing the monitoring of hepatic function to weekly for the first 4 weeks after starting rifampicin.[6] Note that the UK manufacturer extends its advice to other CYP3A4 inducers,[5] see 'Table 1.9', p.11 for a list; although consider that the effects would not be expected to be as great as those seen with rifampicin if they do not also inhibit OATP. For **ambrisentan**, no dose adjustment is necessary on concurrent use,[7] but the UK manufacturer recommends close monitoring when starting rifampicin.[8]

Note that, for **atorvastatin**, another substrate of OATP and CYP3A4, the effect of rifampicin at *steady-state* depended on the timing of administration (see 'Statins + Rifampicin (Rifampin)', p.1355). When administration was simultaneous (as here with ambrisentan and bosentan), atorvastatin exposure was little affected, whereas when administration was separated, atorvastatin exposure was markedly reduced. It is therefore theoretically possible that if **ambrisentan** and rifampicin administration are separated by 12 hours that ambrisentan exposure might be reduced by steady-state rifampicin. However, as **bosentan** is administered twice daily, it might be difficult to separate the doses of each drug sufficiently to have a clinically relevant effect. Nevertheless, further study is needed to confirm this.

The moderate decrease in **macitentan** exposure on concurrent use with rifampicin is likely to reduce the efficacy of macitentan, and the combination should be avoided.[9,10] This advice is also extended to other potent CYP3A4 inducers, see 'Table 1.9', p.11 for a list.

1. Harrison B, Magee MH, Mandagere A, Walker G, Dufton C, Henderson LS, Boinpally R. Effects of rifampicin (rifampin) on the pharmacokinetics and safety of ambrisentan in healthy subjects: a single-sequence, open-label study. *Clin Drug Investig* (2010) 30, 875–85.
2. van Giersbergen PLM, Treiber A, Schneiter R, Dietrich H, Dingemanse J. Inhibitory and inductive effects of rifampin on the pharmacokinetics of bosentan in healthy subjects. *Clin Pharmacol Ther* (2007) 81, 414–9.
3. Bruderer S, Aänismaa P, Homery MC, Häusler S, Landskroner K, Sidharta PN, treiber A, Dingemanse J. Effect of cyclosporine and rifampin on the pharmacokinetics of macitentan, a tissue-targeting dual endothelin receptor antagonist. *AAPS J* (2012) 14, 68–78.
4. Treiber A, Schneiter R, Häusler S, Stieger B. Bosentan is a substrate of human OATP1B1 and OATP1B3: inhibition of hepatic uptake as the common mechanism of its interactions with cyclosporin A, rifampicin, and sildenafil. *Drug Metab Dispos* (2007) 35, 1400–7.
5. Tracleer (Bosentan monohydrate). Actelion Pharmaceuticals UK Ltd. UK Summary of product characteristics, September 2013.
6. Tracleer (Bosentan). Actelion Pharmaceuticals US, Inc. US Prescribing information, October 2012.
7. Letairis (Ambrisentan). Gilead Sciences, Inc. US Prescribing information, May 2014.
8. Volibris (Ambrisentan). GlaxoSmithKline UK. UK Summary of product characteristics, September 2014.
9. Opsumit (Macitentan). Actelion Pharmaceuticals UK Ltd. UK Summary of product characteristics, May 2014.
10. Opsumit (Macitentan). Actelion Pharmaceuticals US, Inc. US Prescribing information, October 2013.

Endothelin receptor antagonists; Bosentan + Food

In a study in 16 healthy subjects the pharmacokinetics of bosentan were not significantly changed by the presence of food. Bosentan may therefore be given without regard to meal times.[1]

1. Dingemanse J, Bodin F, Weidekamm E, Kutz K, van Giersbergen P. Influence of food intake and formulation on the pharmacokinetics and metabolism of bosentan, a dual endothelin receptor antagonist. *J Clin Pharmacol* (2002) 42, 283–9.

Glyceryl trinitrate (Nitroglycerin) + Antimuscarinics

Dry mouth associated with the use of antimuscarinic drugs may reduce the dissolution and thus, the effectiveness of sublingual glyceryl trinitrate tablets.

Clinical evidence, mechanism, importance and management

There is a report of a patient taking **imipramine** who found that the effects of glyceryl trinitrate sublingual tablets for the relief of angina were delayed. The patient had a dry mouth associated with the antimuscarinic adverse effects of **imipramine** and the problem was resolved when imipramine was discontinued.[1] Another brief report notes that the dissolution of glyceryl trinitrate sublingual tablets following **atropine** may take over 5 minutes.[2] Drugs with antimuscarinic effects, such as the **tricyclic antidepressants** and **disopyramide**, depress salivation and many patients complain of having a dry mouth. In a study in patients with angina of effort, both the sublingual and oral spray formulations were equally effective if the oral mucosa was moist (7 patients), but the oral spray was found to be better than sublingual tablets in patients with dry mouth (10 patients).[3] Sublingual glyceryl trinitrate tablets will dissolve less readily under the tongue in patients with dry mouth, thereby reducing glyceryl trinitrate absorption and effects. 'Table 18.1', p.752, and 'Table 18.2', p.754 list drugs that have antimuscarinic effects. A possible alternative is to use a glyceryl trinitrate spray in patients who suffer from dry mouth.

1. Robbins LJ. Dry mouth and delayed dissolution of sublingual nitroglycerin. *N Engl J Med* (1983) 309, 985.
2. Kimchi A. Dry mouth and delayed dissolution of nitroglycerin. *N Engl J Med* (1984) 310, 1122–3.
3. Sato H, Koretsune Y, Taniguchi T, Fukui S, Shimazu T, Sugii M, Matsuyama T, Karita M, Hori M. Studies on the response of nitroglycerin oral spray compared with sublingual tablets for angina pectoris patients with dry mouth. A multicenter trial. *Arzneimittelforschung* (1997) 47, 128–31.

Glyceryl trinitrate (Nitroglycerin) + Aspirin

Some limited evidence suggests that analgesic doses of aspirin can increase the levels of glyceryl trinitrate given sublingually, possibly resulting in an increase in its adverse effects such as hypotension and headache. Paradoxically, long-term aspirin use appears to reduce the effects of intravenous glyceryl trinitrate used for vasodilatation in patients following coronary artery bypass surgery.

Clinical evidence

(a) Intravenous effects reduced

A study in patients following coronary artery bypass surgery found that those who had been taking aspirin 150 or 300 mg daily (33 patients) for at least 3 months, needed more glyceryl trinitrate to control blood pressure during the recovery period than those who had not taken aspirin (33 patients). To achieve the blood pressure criteria required, the aspirin-group needed an 8.2 micrograms/minute infusion of glyceryl trinitrate. The dose remained relatively high at 3.3 micrograms/minute even after 8 hours, whereas the non-aspirin group needed only 5.5 micrograms/minute, which was reduced to 1.9 micrograms/minute after 8 hours.[1]

(b) Sublingual effects increased

When aspirin 1 g was given to 7 healthy subjects followed one hour later by 800 micrograms of glyceryl trinitrate sublingual spray, the mean plasma glyceryl trinitrate levels 30 minutes after administration were increased by 54% (from 0.24 to 0.37 nanograms/mL). The haemodynamic effects of the glyceryl trinitrate (including heart rate and reduced diastolic blood pressure) were enhanced. Some changes were seen when aspirin 500 mg was given every 2 days (described as an anti-aggregant dose) but the effects were not statistically significant.[2,3]

(c) Sublingual effects unchanged

A study in 40 healthy subjects who were given 650 mg aspirin or placebo, followed after one to 2 hours by sublingual glyceryl trinitrate 432 micrograms found no significant alterations in the peak haemodynamic response or in the area under the time-pressure and time-pulse curves. There was a transient pressor response, which occurred one minute after glyceryl trinitrate was given: this was blunted by aspirin. Taken alone, this change was significant, but when the overall pattern of changes during the 30 minute study was considered, the differences were not significant.[4]

Mechanism

Not understood. Prostaglandin-synthetase inhibitors such as aspirin can, to some extent, suppress the vasodilator effects of glyceryl trinitrate by blocking prostaglandin release. However, it seems that a much greater pharmacodynamic interaction also occurs, in which aspirin reduces the flow of blood through the liver, so that the metabolism of the glyceryl trinitrate is reduced, thus increasing its levels, and therefore its effects.

Importance and management

A confusing and unexplained situation. It seems possible that patients taking sublingual glyceryl trinitrate may experience an exaggeration of its adverse effects such as hypotension and headaches if they are taking analgesic doses of aspirin. Also be aware that long-term aspirin use may reduce the vasodilatory effects of intravenous glyceryl trinitrate. The antiplatelet effects of aspirin and glyceryl trinitrate appear to be additive.[5]

1. Key BJ, Keen M, Wilkes MP. Reduced responsiveness to nitro-vasodilators following prolonged low dose aspirin administration in man. *Br J Clin Pharmacol* (1992) 34, 453P–454P.
2. Weber S, Rey E, Pipeau C, Lutfalla G, Richard M-O, Daoud-El-Assaf H, Olive G, Degeorges M. Influence of aspirin on the hemodynamic effects of sublingual nitroglycerin. *J Cardiovasc Pharmacol* (1983) 5, 874–7.
3. Rey E, El-Assaf HD, Richard MO, Weber S, Bourdon A, Picard G, Olive G. Pharmacological interaction between nitroglycerin and aspirin after acute and chronic aspirin treatment of healthy subjects. *Eur J Clin Pharmacol* (1983) 25, 779–82.
4. Levin RI, Feit F. The effect of aspirin on the hemodynamic response to nitroglycerin. *Am Heart J* (1988) 116, 77–84.
5. Karlberg K-E, Ahlner J, Henriksson P, Torfgård K, Sylvén C. Effects of nitroglycerin on platelet aggregation beyond the effects of acetylsalicylic acid in healthy subjects. *Am J Cardiol* (1993) 71, 361–4.

Guanethidine + Amfetamines and related drugs

The antihypertensive effects of guanethidine can be reduced or abolished by drugs including dexamfetamine, ephedrine, metamfetamine and methylphenidate. The blood pressure may even rise higher than before treatment with the antihypertensive.

Clinical evidence

When 16 hypertensive patients taking guanethidine 25 to 35 mg daily were given single-doses of **dexamfetamine** 10 mg orally, **ephedrine** 90 mg orally, **metamfetamine** 30 mg intramuscularly or **methylphenidate** 20 mg orally, the hypotensive effects of the guanethidine were completely abolished, and in some instances the blood pressures rose higher than before treatment with the guanethidine.[1] Another report describes the same interaction between guanethidine and **dexamfetamine**.[2]

Mechanism

These drugs are all indirectly-acting sympathomimetic amines, which not only prevent guanethidine-like drugs from entering the adrenergic neurones of the sympathetic nervous system, but also displace the antihypertensive drug already there.[3] As a result the blood pressure lowering effects are lost. In addition these amines release noradrenaline (norepinephrine) from the neurones, which raises the blood pressure. Thus the antihypertensive effects are not only opposed, but the pressure may even be raised higher than before treatment.[3-8]

Importance and management

Well documented, well established, and clinically important interactions. Other drugs, such as **phenylpropanolamine**, which is also an indirectly-acting sympathomimetic, are likely to interact similarly. Patients taking guanethidine should avoid indirectly-acting sympathomimetics, see 'Table 24.1', p.1050, for a list. Warn them against the temptation to use proprietary non-prescription nasal decongestants containing any of these amines to relieve the nasal stuffiness commonly associated with the use of guanethidine and related drugs. The same precautions apply to the sympathomimetics used as appetite suppressants (although note that the use of these drugs for this indication is not generally recommended). However, one brief report stated that **diethylpropion** has been used with guanethidine without any adverse events.[9] Note that the antihypertensive use of guanethidine and related adrenergic neurone blockers has largely been superseded by other antihypertensive drug classes.

Guanethidine increases the hypertensive effects of the *directly*-acting sympathomimetics used as inotropes and vasopressors, see 'Inotropes and Vasopressors + Guanethidine', p.1065.

1. Gulati OD, Dave BT, Gokhale SD, Shah KM. Antagonism of adrenergic neuron blockade in hypertensive subjects. *Clin Pharmacol Ther* (1966) 7, 510–4.
2. Ober KF, Wang RIH. Drug interactions with guanethidine. *Clin Pharmacol Ther* (1973) 14, 190–5.
3. Flegin OT, Morgan DH, Oates JA, Shand DG. The mechanism of the reversal of the effect of guanethidine by amphetamines in cat and man. *Br J Pharmacol* (1970) 39, 253P–254P.
4. Day MD, Rand MJ. Antagonism of guanethidine and bretylium by various agents. *Lancet* (1962) 2, 1282–3.
5. Day MD, Rand MJ. Evidence for a competitive antagonism of guanethidine by dexamphetamine. *Br J Pharmacol* (1963) 20, 17–28.
6. Day MD. Effect of sympathomimetic amines on the blocking action of guanethidine, bretylium and xylocholine. *Br J Pharmacol* (1962) 18, 421–39.
7. Starke K. Interactions of guanethidine and indirectly-acting sympathomimetic amines. *Arch Int Pharmacodyn Ther* (1972) 195, 309–14.
8. Boura ALA, Green AF. Comparison of bretylium and guanethidine: tolerance and effects on adrenergic nerve function and responses to sympathomimetic amines. *Br J Pharmacol* (1962) 19, 13–41.
9. Seedat YK, Reddy J. Diethylpropion hydrochloride (Tenuate Dospan) in the treatment of obese hypertensive patients. *S Afr Med J* (1974) 48, 569.

Guanethidine + Antipsychotics

Large doses of chlorpromazine may reduce or even abolish the antihypertensive effects of guanethidine, although in some patients the inherent hypotensive effects of the chlorpromazine may possibly predominate. Case reports suggest that haloperidol and tiotixene may interact similarly. Molindone is reported not to interact with guanethidine, and a single-dose of prochlorperazine did not interact with guanethidine.

Clinical evidence

Two severely hypertensive patients, with stable blood pressure while taking guanethidine 80 mg daily, were given **chlorpromazine** 200 to 300 mg daily. The diastolic blood pressure of one patient rose over 10 days from 94 mmHg to 112 mmHg and continued to rise to 116 mmHg, even when the **chlorpromazine** was withdrawn. Similarly, the diastolic pressure of the other patient rose from 105 mmHg to 127 mmHg, and then to 150 mmHg, even after the **chlorpromazine** had been withdrawn.[1] Other reports also describe marked rises in blood pressure in patients taking guanethidine with **chlorpromazine** 100 to 400 mg daily.[2-4]

Three hypertensive patients taking guanethidine 60 to 150 mg daily had an increase in their blood pressure when **haloperidol** 6 to 9 mg daily was added. The blood pressure rose from 132/95 mmHg to 149/99 mmHg in the first patient; from 125/84 mmHg to 148/100 mmHg in the second patient; and from 138/91 mmHg to 154/100 mmHg in the third patient. **Tiotixene** 60 mg daily was later given to one of the patients and the blood pressure rose from 126/87 mmHg to 156/110 mmHg.[2] These results have been reported elsewhere.[3,4]

However, a single 25-mg dose of **prochlorperazine** did not significantly antagonise the effect of guanethidine 15 to 20 mg daily in 5 patients.[5] In another study in 7 patients taking guanethidine 50 to 95 mg daily, the addition of **molindone** 30 to 120 mg daily had no effect on blood pressure.[6]

Mechanism

Chlorpromazine prevents the entry of guanethidine into the adrenergic neurones of the sympathetic nervous system resulting in a loss of its blood pressure-lowering effects. The other interacting antipsychotics probably have similar effects. This is essentially the same mechanism of interaction as that seen with the tricyclic antidepressants (consider also 'Guanethidine + Tricyclic and related antidepressants', p.1062).

Importance and management

Direct information is limited but the interaction between guanethidine and chlorpromazine is established and can be clinically important. It may take several days to develop. Not all patients may react to the same extent.[2,7] Monitor concurrent use and raise the guanethidine dose if necessary. It is uncertain how much chlorpromazine is needed before a significant effect occurs, but the smallest dose of chlorpromazine used in the studies was 100 mg with 90 mg guanethidine, which raised the blood pressure by 40/23 mmHg.[2] The inherent hypotensive effects of the chlorpromazine may possibly reduce the effects of this interaction. Other antipsychotics (particularly the phenothiazines) might be expected to interact similarly and this has been seen with tiotixene and haloperidol. The effects should be monitored. However, molindone is reported not to interact, and a single-dose of prochlorperazine did not interact. Note that the antihypertensive use of guanethidine and related adrenergic neurone blockers has largely been superseded by other antihypertensive drug classes.

1. Fann WE, Janowsky DS, Davis JM, Oates JA. Chlorpromazine reversal of the antihypertensive action of guanethidine. *Lancet* (1971) ii, 436–7.
2. Janowsky DS, El-Yousef MK, Davis JM, Fann WE, Oates JA. Guanethidine antagonism by antipsychotic drugs. *J Tenn Med Assoc* (1972) 65, 620–2.
3. Janowsky DS, El-Yousef MK, Davis JM, Fann WE. Antagonism of guanethidine by chlorpromazine. *Am J Psychiatry* (1973) 130, 808–12.
4. Davis JM. Psychopharmacology in the aged. Use of psychotropic drugs in geriatric patients. *J Geriatr Psychiatry* (1974) 7, 145–59.
5. Ober KF, Wang RIH. Drug interactions with guanethidine. *Clin Pharmacol Ther* (1973) 14, 190–5.
6. Simpson LL. Combined use of molindone and guanethidine in patients with schizophrenia and hypertension. *Am J Psychiatry* (1979) 136, 1410–14.
7. Tuck D, Hamberger B and Sjoqvist F. Drug interactions: effect of chlorpromazine on the uptake of monoamines into adrenergic neurones in man. *Lancet* (1972) ii, 492.

Guanethidine + Levodopa

Levodopa appeared to enhance the antihypertensive effects of guanethidine in two patients.

Clinical evidence, mechanism, importance and management

A brief report describes a patient taking guanethidine and a diuretic who, when given levodopa (dose not stated), required a reduction in his daily dose of guanethidine, from 60 to 20 mg. Another patient similarly treated was able to discontinue the diuretic.[1] The suggested reason is that the hypotensive adverse effects of the levodopa are additive with the effects of the guanethidine. Direct information seems to be limited to this report but it would be wise to confirm that excessive hypotension does not develop if levodopa is added to treatment with guanethidine. Note that the antihypertensive use of guanethidine and related adrenergic neurone blockers has largely been superseded by other antihypertensive drug classes, but note that any antihypertensive may interact in this way, see 'Antihypertensives + Other drugs that affect blood pressure', p.1054.

1. Hunter KR, Stern GM, Laurence DR. Use of levodopa with other drugs. *Lancet* (1970) ii, 1283–5.

Guanethidine + MAOIs

The antihypertensive effects of guanethidine can be reduced by nialamide, and probably therefore by other non-selective MAOIs.

Clinical evidence, mechanism, importance and management

Four out of 5 hypertensive patients taking guanethidine 25 to 35 mg daily had a rise in blood pressure from 140/85 mmHg to 165/100 mmHg six hours after being given a single 50-mg dose of **nialamide**.[1] The reason for this effect is not understood but one idea is that the MAOIs possibly oppose the guanethidine-induced loss of noradrenaline from sympathetic neurones. In *animal* studies, effective antagonism of guanethidine was shown by those MAOIs that also possess sympathomimetic effects (**phenelzine** and **tranylcypromine**), but not by **iproniazid** or **nialamide**,[2] and the antagonism was weaker than that seen with some other sympathomimetics.[3]

Direct clinical information seems to be limited to the single dose study,[1] but it would be prudent to monitor the effects if any non-selective MAOI is given to patients taking any guanethidine-like drug. The manufacturers of guanethidine actually contraindicate the use of MAOIs because of the possibility of the release of large quantities of catecholamines and the risk of hypertensive crisis. They recommend that at least 14 days should elapse between stopping an MAOI and starting guanethidine.[4] Note that the antihypertensive use of guanethidine and related adrenergic neurone blockers has largely been superseded by other antihypertensive drug classes.

1. Gulati OD, Dave BT, Gokhale SD, Shah KM. Antagonism of adrenergic neuron blockade in hypertensive subjects. *Clin Pharmacol Ther* (1966) 7, 510–4.
2. Day MD. Effect of sympathomimetic amines on the blocking action of guanethidine, bretylium and xylocholine. *Br J Pharmacol* (1962) 18, 421–39.
3. Day MD, Rand MJ. Antagonism of guanethidine and bretylium by various agents. *Lancet* (1962) 2, 1282–3.
4. Ismelin Ampoules (Guanethidine monosulphate). Amdipharm. UK Summary of product characteristics, April 2005.

Guanethidine + NSAIDs

Phenylbutazone and kebuzone reduce the antihypertensive effects of guanethidine.

Clinical evidence, mechanism, importance and management

When 20 patients taking guanethidine 75 mg daily were given **phenylbutazone** or **kebuzone** 750 mg daily the mean systolic blood pressure rose by 20 mmHg (from 169 mmHg to 189 mmHg).[1] This rise represents about a 35% reduction in the antihypertensive effect of guanethidine. The mechanism of this interaction is uncertain but it is probably due to salt and water retention caused by these pyrazolone compounds. Direct evidence seems to be limited to this report. Patients taking guanethidine should be monitored if **phenylbutazone** or **kebuzone** is given concurrently. There does not appear to be any information on guanethidine and other NSAIDs, but indometacin, in particular, is well known to reduce the efficacy of other classes of antihypertensives, see for example 'ACE inhibitors + NSAIDs', p.38. Some caution may therefore be warranted with other NSAIDs.

1. Polak F. Die hemmende Wirkung von Phenylbutazon auf die durch einige Antihypertonika hervorgerufene Blutdrucksenkung bei Hypertonikern. *Z Gesamte Inn Med* (1967) 22, 375–6.

Guanethidine and related drugs + Pizotifen

Pizotifen might antagonise the effects of guanethidine and related drugs.

Clinical evidence, mechanism, importance and management

The UK manufacturer of pizotifen[1] states that pizotifen antagonises the hypotensive effect of adrenergic neurone blockers (e.g. **debrisoquine, guanethidine**). Direct evidence for such an interaction is sparse, and there appears only to be one published report, which describes a loss of blood pressure control 5 weeks after a patient taking debrisoquine 30 mg three times daily started taking pizotifen 1.5 mg daily. The blood pressure was subsequently controlled on the original medication when pizotifen was stopped.[2] However, pizotifen is structurally related to the tricyclics, which are also known to antagonise the effects of adrenergic neurone blockers, see 'Guanethidine + Tricyclic and related antidepressants', below. Therefore, if guanethidine or a related drug is given for blood pressure control it may be prudent to consider the possibility of a reduction in its effects if pizotifen is also given.

1. Sanomigran Tablets (Pizotifen hydrogen maleate) Novartis Pharmaceuticals UK Ltd. UK Summary of product characteristics, August 2009.
2. Bailey, RR. Antagonism of debrisoquine sulphate by pizotifen (Sandomigran). *N Z Med J* (1976) 83, 449.

Guanethidine + Tricyclic and related antidepressants

The antihypertensive effects of guanethidine are reduced or abolished by amitriptyline, desipramine, imipramine, nortriptyline and protriptyline. Doxepin in doses of 300 mg or more daily interacts similarly, but in smaller doses appears not to do so, although one case is reported with doxepin 100 mg daily. A few case reports suggest that maprotiline and mianserin do not interact with guanethidine.

Clinical evidence

(a) Tricyclic antidepressants

Five hypertensive patients taking guanethidine sulfate 50 to 150 mg daily had a mean arterial blood pressure rise of 27 mmHg when they were also given **desipramine** 50 or 75 mg daily or **protriptyline** 20 mg daily for one to 9 days. The full antihypertensive effects of the guanethidine were not re-established until 5 days after the antidepressants were withdrawn.[1]

The same interaction has been described in other reports, with guanethidine and **desipramine**,[2,3] **imipramine**,[4] **amitriptyline**,[5-7] **protriptyline**[3] or **nortriptyline**.[8] The interaction may take several days to develop fully and can last an average of 5 days after discontinuation of the tricyclic.[2] Some studies, and clinical experience suggests that **doxepin** does not begin to interact until doses of about 200 to 250 mg daily are used, then at 300 mg or more daily it interacts to the same extent as other tricyclics.[9-13] However, in one case excessive hypertension occurred in a man taking guanethidine and **doxepin** 100 mg daily.[14]

(b) Tetracyclic antidepressants

Maprotiline 25 mg three times daily caused no appreciable change in blood pressure in 2 patients taking guanethidine.[7] Similarly, in a study in 2 patients, **mianserin** 20 mg three times daily for 2 days did not alter the antihypertensive efficacy of guanethidine.[15]

Mechanism

The guanethidine-like drugs exert their hypotensive actions by entering the adrenergic nerve endings associated with blood vessels using the noradrenaline uptake mechanism. The tricyclics successfully compete for the same mechanism so that the antihypertensives are unable to reach their site of action, and as a result, the blood pressure rises once again.[16] The differences in the rate of development, duration and extent of the interactions reflect the pharmacokinetic differences between the various tricyclics, as well as individual differences between patients.

Importance and management

A very well documented and well established interaction of clinical importance. Not every combination of guanethidine and tricyclic antidepressant has been studied but all are expected to interact similarly, to a greater or lesser extent. Concurrent use should be avoided unless the effects are very closely monitored and the interaction balanced by raising the dose of the antihypertensive. Note that the antihypertensive use of guanethidine and related adrenergic neurone blockers has largely been superseded by other antihypertensive drug classes.

1. Mitchell JR, Arias L, Oates JA. Antagonism of the antihypertensive actions of guanethidine sulfate by desipramine hydrochloride. *JAMA* (1967) 202, 973–6.

2. Oates JA, Mitchell JR, Feagin OT, Kaufmann JS, Shand DG. Distribution of guanidinium antihypertensives-mechanism of their selective action. *Ann N Y Acad Sci* (1971) 179, 302–9.
3. Mitchell JR, Cavanaugh JH, Arias L, Oates JA. Guanethidine and related agents. III. Antagonism by drugs which inhibit the norepinephrine pump in man. *J Clin Invest* (1970) 49, 1596–1604.
4. Leishman AWD, Matthews HL, Smith AJ. Antagonism of guanethidine by imipramine. *Lancet* (1963) i, 112.
5. Meyer JF, McAllister CK, Goldberg LI. Insidious and prolonged antagonism of guanethidine by amitriptyline. *JAMA* (1970) 213, 1487–8.
6. Ober KF, Wang RIH. Drug interactions with guanethidine. *Clin Pharmacol Ther* (1973) 14, 190–5.
7. Smith AJ, Bant WP. Interactions between post-ganglionic sympathetic blocking drugs and anti-depressants. *J Int Med Res* (1975) 3 (Suppl 2), 55–60.
8. McQueen EG. New Zealand Committee on Adverse Reactions: Ninth Annual Report 1974. *N Z Med J* (1974) 80, 305–11.
9. Oates JA, Fann WE, Cavanaugh JH. Effect of doxepin on the norepinephrine pump. A preliminary report. *Psychosomatics* (1969) 10 (Suppl), 12–13.
10. Fann WE, Cavanaugh JH, Kaufmann JS, Griffith JD, Davis JM, Janowsky DS, Oates JA. Doxepin: effects on transport of biogenic amines in man. *Psychopharmacologia* (1971) 22, 111–25.
11. Gerson IM, Friedman R, Unterberger H. Non-antagonism of antiadrenergic agents by dibenzoxepine (preliminary report). *Dis Nerv Syst* (1970) 31, 780–2.
12. Ayd FJ. Long-term administration of doxepin (Sinequan). *Dis Nerv Syst* (1971) 32, 617–22.
13. Ayd FJ. Doxepin with other drugs. *South Med J* (1973) 66, 465–71.
14. Poe TE, Edwards JL, Taylor RB. Hypertensive crisis possibly due to drug interaction. *Postgrad Med* (1979) 66, 235–7.
15. Burgess CD, Turner P, Wadsworth J. Cardiovascular responses to mianserin hydrochloride: a comparison with tricyclic antidepressant drugs. *Br J Clin Pharmacol* (1978) 5, 21S–28S.
16. Cairncross KD. On the peripheral pharmacology of amitriptyline. *Arch Int Pharmacodyn Ther* (1965) 154, 438–48.

Guanfacine + Phenobarbital or Phenytoin

In two patients, the concurrent use of phenobarbital or phenytoin increased the metabolism of guanfacine.

Clinical evidence, mechanism, importance and management

When a hypertensive patient with chronic renal failure who was taking guanfacine 4 mg daily, was given phenobarbital 10 mg daily the antihypertensive effects of guanfacine were noted to be reduced and its dose was progressively raised over about 18 months to 12 mg daily. Phenobarbital was eventually stopped. Single measurements of the pharmacokinetics of guanfacine, both when the patient was taking phenobarbital, and 2 months after cessation of phenobarbital, found that the half-life of guanfacine increased fourfold when the phenobarbital was stopped.[1] The manufacturer also reports a similar case with phenytoin and guanfacine.[2] Phenobarbital and phenytoin probably induce the metabolism of guanfacine. Patients taking these drugs are likely to need more frequent doses of guanfacine. Primidone is metabolised to **phenobarbital**, and **fosphenytoin** is a prodrug of phenytoin. These drugs may therefore be expected to interact similarly.

1. Kiechel JR, Lavene D, Guerret M, Comoy E, Godin M, Fillastre JP. Pharmacokinetic aspects of guanfacine withdrawal syndrome in a hypertensive patient with chronic renal failure. *Eur J Clin Pharmacol* (1983) 25, 463–6.
2. Guanfacine hydrochloride. Watson Laboratories, Inc. US Prescribing information, October 2007.

Guanfacine + Tricyclic antidepressants

A single case report describes a reduced antihypertensive response to guanfacine in a patient given amitriptyline and later imipramine. The sedative effects of guanfacine and tricyclics are predicted to be additive.

Clinical evidence

A 38-year-old woman with stable hypertension, taking guanfacine 2 mg daily, had a rise in her mean blood pressure from 138/89 mmHg to 150/100 mmHg while taking **amitriptyline** 75 mg daily for 14 days. The patient's blood pressure fell again when the **amitriptyline** was stopped. A month later her blood pressure rose to 142/98 mmHg after she had taken **imipramine** 50 mg daily for 2 days, and fell again when it was stopped.[1]

Mechanism

Uncertain. A possible reason is that, like clonidine (another alpha-2 agonist), the uptake of guanfacine into neurones within the brain is blocked by tricyclic antidepressants, thereby reducing its effects.

Importance and management

Direct information is limited to this report, but it is supported by *animal* studies[2] and consistent with the way another alpha-2 agonist interacts with tricyclic antidepressants (see 'Clonidine and related drugs + Tricyclic and related antidepressants', p.1057). Be alert for this interaction in any patient given guanfacine and any tricyclic antidepressant. **Guanabenz** is another alpha-2 agonist that might interact similarly, but as yet there is no direct clinical evidence that it does so. Note that the sedative effects of guanfacine or guanabenz and tricyclics would be predicted to be additive.

1. Buckley M, Feeley J. Antagonism of antihypertensive effect of guanfacine by tricyclic antidepressants. *Lancet* (1991) 337, 1173–4.
2. Ohkubo K, Suzuki K, Oguma T, Otorii T. Central hypotensive effects of guanfacine in anaesthetised rabbits. *Nippon Yakurigaku Zasshi* (1982) 79, 263–74.

Hydralazine + Adrenaline (Epinephrine)

The manufacturers note that patients taking hydralazine who develop hypotension while undergoing surgery should *not* be treated with adrenaline (epinephrine).[1] This is because hydralazine frequently causes tachycardia,[2] and adrenaline would enhance this.[1]

1. Apresoline (Hydralazine hydrochloride). Amdipharm. UK Summary of product characteristics, November 2007.
2. Lin M-S, McNay JL, Shepherd AMM, Musgrave GE, Keeton TK. Increased plasma norepinephrine accompanies persistent tachycardia after hydralazine. *Hypertension* (1983) 5, 257–63.

Hydralazine + Food

The effect of food on hydralazine absorption is uncertain: food increased the AUC of hydralazine in two studies, had no effect in one study, and decreased it in three others. In other studies, a bolus dose of enteral feed decreased the AUC of hydralazine, but an enteral feed infusion had no effect.

Clinical evidence, mechanism, importance and management

Food *enhanced* the bioavailability of a single 50-mg dose of hydralazine in healthy subjects by two- to threefold in one study.[1] Similar findings were reported by the same research group with conventional hydralazine tablets, but not slow-release tablets.[2] In contrast, others found that food had no effect on the AUC of hydralazine in healthy subjects.[3] Furthermore, other studies have found that food decreases the AUC of hydralazine by 46% when it is given as oral solution,[4] by 44% after conventional tablets,[5] and by 29% (not statistically significant) after a slow-release preparation.[5] A reduction in the antihypertensive effect of hydralazine was noted in the first of these studies,[4] but no significant alteration in antihypertensive effect was seen in the second.[5] Similarly, another study reported a decrease in the AUC of hydralazine of 55% when it was given with a meal, and 62% when it was given with a bolus dose of **enteral feed**, but no significant change when it was given during an **enteral feed infusion**.[6]

The widely different findings of these studies may be related to the problems in analysing hydralazine and its metabolites, all of which are unstable. All these studies were single-dose, and no studies have adequately assessed the possible clinical importance of any pharmacokinetic changes in long-term clinical use. Note that the bioavailability of hydralazine varies widely between individuals depending on their acetylator status. No recommendations can be made as to whether or not hydralazine should be taken at a set time in relation to meals.

1. Melander A, Danielson K, Hanson A, Rudell B, Schersten B, Thulin T, Wåhlin E. Enhancement of hydralazine bioavailability by food. *Clin Pharmacol Ther* (1977) 22, 104–7.
2. Liedholm H, Wåhlin-Boll E, Hanson A, Melander A. Influence of food on the bioavailability of 'real' and 'apparent' hydralazine from conventional and slow-release preparations. *Drug Nutr Interact* (1982) 1, 293–302.
3. Walden RJ, Hernadez R, Witts D, Graham BR, Prichard BN. Effect of food on the absorption of hydralazine in man. *Eur J Clin Pharmacol* (1981) 20, 53–8.
4. Shepherd AM, Irvine NA, Ludden TM. Effect of food on blood hydralazine levels and response in hypertension. *Clin Pharmacol Ther* (1984) 36, 14–18.
5. Jackson SHD, Shepherd AMM, Ludden TM, Jamieson MJ, Woodworth J, Rogers D, Ludden LK, Muir KT. Effect of food on oral bioavailability of apresoline and controlled release hydralazine in hypertensive patients. *J Cardiovasc Pharmacol* (1990) 16, 624–8.
6. Semple HA, Koo W, Tam YK, Ngo LY, Coutts RT. Interactions between hydralazine and oral nutrients in humans. *Ther Drug Monit* (1991) 13, 304–8.

Hydralazine + NSAIDs

Oral indometacin abolished the hypotensive effects of intravenous hydralazine in one study, but no effect was found in another. In patients with pulmonary hypertension, intravenous indometacin reduced the effects of intravenous hydralazine, and in patients with hypertension, intravenous diclofenac reduced the effects of intravenous dihydralazine.

Clinical evidence, mechanism, importance and management

In 9 healthy subjects, oral **indometacin** 50 mg every 6 hours for four doses abolished the hypotensive response to intravenous hydralazine 150 micrograms/kg, and the subjects only responded when given another dose of hydralazine 30 minutes later.[1] A study in 7 patients with pulmonary hypertension given **indometacin** 50 mg and hydralazine 350 micrograms/kg, both intravenously, either alone, or concurrently, also found that the effects of hydralazine (reduction in systemic arterial pressure, heart rate, cardiac index) were reduced by **indometacin**.[2] In contrast, another study in 9 healthy subjects[3] found that oral **indometacin** 25 mg four times daily for 2.5 days did not affect the hypotensive response to a single 200-microgram/kg intravenous dose of hydralazine.

Thus it is not clear if **indometacin** interacts with intravenous hydralazine, and it is uncertain if an interaction occurs when hydralazine is given orally.

On the other hand, a single-dose study in 4 hypertensive subjects found that the actions of intravenous **dihydralazine** (effects on blood pressure, urinary excretion, heart rate and sodium clearance) were reduced by intravenous **diclofenac**.[4]

NSAIDs can cause increases in blood pressure due to their effects on sodium and water retention. Various NSAIDs have been reported to reduce the efficacy of other antihypertensive drug classes, for example see 'ACE inhibitors + NSAIDs', p.38. It would therefore be prudent to monitor concurrent use of hydralazine and any NSAID.

1. Cinquegrani MP, Liang C-S. Indomethacin attenuates the hypotensive action of hydralazine. *Clin Pharmacol Ther* (1986) 39, 564–70.
2. Adnot S, Defouilloy C, Brun-Buisson C, Piquet J, De Cremoux H, Lemaire F. Effects of indomethacin on pulmonary hemodynamics and gas exchange in patients with pulmonary artery hypertension, interference with hydralazine. *Am Rev Respir Dis* (1987) 136, 1343–9.
3. Jackson SHD, Pickles H. Indomethacin does not attenuate the effects of hydralazine in normal subjects. *Eur J Clin Pharmacol* (1983) 25, 303–5.
4. Reimann IW, Ratge D, Wisser H, Fröhlich JC. Are prostaglandins involved in the antihypertensive effect of dihydralazine? *Clin Sci* (1981) 61, 319S–321S.

Inotropes and Vasopressors + Amfetamines

The manufacturers of amfetamine, dexamfetamine, and lisdexamfetamine state that amfetamines enhance the adrenergic effects of noradrenaline (norepinephrine).[1-3] This might result in increased vasoconstriction, and could enhance the pressor effects of noradrenaline (norepinephrine). Other inotropes and vasopressors with adrenergic actions might be similarly affected, but this does not appear to be specifically mentioned. Consider 'Table 24.1', p.1050, for a list of these drugs.

1. Adderall XR (Mixed salts of amphetamine and dextroamphetamine). Shire US Inc. US Prescribing information, April 2015.
2. Dexedrine (Dextroamphetamine sulfate). Amedra Pharmaceuticals, LLC. US Prescribing information, October 2013.
3. Vyvanse (Lisdexamfetamine dimesylate). Shire US Inc. US Prescribing information, January 2012.

Inotropes and Vasopressors + Antimuscarinics

The hypertensive and other serious adverse effects of intravenous phenylephrine and phenylephrine absorbed from *eye drops* can be markedly increased by intravenous or intramuscular atropine.

Clinical evidence

A brief report describes 7 cases of pseudo-phaeochromocytoma, with severe rises in blood pressure and tachycardia, which occurred in young adults and children when they underwent eye operations and were given phenylephrine 10% eye drops and atropine. Only two of them had any pre-existing cardiovascular illness (moderate hypertension). All were under general anaesthesia with propofol, phenoperidine and vecuronium, and premedicated with intramuscular **atropine**, and some were later given more intravenous **atropine** to control the bradycardia that occurred as a result of stretching the oculomotor muscles. The total atropine doses were less than 10 micrograms/kg in adults and 20 micrograms/kg in children. At least 0.4 mL of phenylephrine 10% was used. In three cases left ventricular failure and pulmonary oedema occurred, which needed monitoring in intensive care.[1] The authors say that no further cardiovascular adverse events were observed during similar procedures when steps were taken to reduce the amount of phenylephrine used and absorbed (see *Importance and Management*, below). Before this case report was made, a number of cases of cardiovascular adverse effects (severe hypertension, cardiac arrhythmias, myocardial infarction) had been reported for phenylephrine eye drops (usually 10%), or subconjunctival injection, and many of these patients had also received antimuscarinics (**atropine, cyclopentolate, homatropine, hyoscine, tropicamide**),[2-6] although the contribution, if any, of these antimuscarinics to the adverse effects is unknown.

In a study, 6 healthy subjects were given an intravenous phenylephrine infusion at incremental rates before and after being given three intravenous doses of **atropine**, 20, 10, and 10 micrograms/kg at 90, 120 and 150 minutes, respectively. It was found that phenylephrine 420 nanograms/kg per minute raised the diastolic and systolic blood pressures by 4 mmHg before using atropine, and 17 mmHg after atropine was given. For safety reasons the increases in blood pressure were limited to 30 mmHg above the baseline.[7]

Mechanism

Phenylephrine causes vasoconstriction, which can raise the blood pressure. Normally this would be limited by a baroreflex mediated by the vagus nerve, but if this cholinergic mechanism is blocked by atropine or other antimuscarinics, the rise in blood pressure is largely uncontrolled. Severe hypertension may occur, and other adverse cardiac events such as acute cardiac failure may follow.

Importance and management

A surprisingly large amount of phenylephrine can be absorbed from eye drops, and the potential cardiovascular adverse effects of this are well documented. The reports cited here suggest that these risks are clearly increased by the systemic use of atropine. The authors of one of the reports[1] found that the systemic absorption of phenylephrine can be reduced by using lower concentrations of phenylephrine, swabbing to minimise the amount that drains into the nasolachrymal duct to the nasal mucosa where rapid absorption occurs, and reducing the drop size by using a thin-walled cannula. Others have demonstrated that a cannula reduced the dose of phenylephrine given by two-thirds without loss of efficacy.[8] Other suggestions for reducing systemic absorption of phenylephrine are punctal plugging, nasolachrymal duct compression, and lid closure after instillation of the eye drop.[8] Note that phenylephrine eye drops are contra-indicated in those with cardiovascular disease.[9] Note also that topical phenylephrine is commonly used with a topical antimuscarinic to enhance mydriasis.

1. Daelman F, Andréjak M, Rajaonarivony D, Bryselbout E, Jezraoui P, Ossart M. Phenylephrine eyedrops, systemic atropine and cardiovascular adverse events. *Therapie* (1994) 49, 467.
2. Fraunfelder FT, Scafidi AF. Possible adverse effects from topical ocular 10% phenylephrine. *Am J Ophthalmol* (1978) 85, 447–53.
3. Van der Spek AFL, Hantler CB. Phenylephrine eyedrops and anesthesia. *Anesthesiology* (1986) 64, 812–14.
4. Lai Y-K. Adverse effect of intraoperative phenylephrine 10%: case report. *Br J Ophthalmol* (1989) 73, 468–9.
5. Miller SA, Mieler WF. Systemic reaction to subconjunctival phenylephrine. *Can J Ophthalmol* (1978) 13, 291–3.
6. Benatar-Haserfaty J, Tercero-López JQ. Crisis hipertensiva y coma tras la administración de colirio de escopolamina, atropine y fenilefrina durante dos casos de ciugía vitrorretiniana. *Rev Esp Anestesiol Reanim* (2002) 49, 440–1.
7. Levine MAH, Leenen FHH. Role of vagal activity in the cardiovascular responses to phenylephrine in man. *Br J Clin Pharmacol* (1992) 33, 333–6.
8. Craig EW, Griffiths PG. Effect on mydriasis of modifying the volume of phenylephrine drops. *Br J Ophthalmol* (1991) 75, 222–3.
9. Minims Phenylephrine hydrochloride 10%. Bausch & Lomb UK Ltd. UK Summary of product characteristics, November 2006.

Inotropes and Vasopressors + Calcium compounds

Calcium chloride infusions reduce the cardiotonic effects of adrenaline (epinephrine) and dobutamine, but not those of amrinone.

Clinical evidence, mechanism, importance and management

In a double-blind, randomised, crossover study in 12 patients following coronary artery bypass grafting, calcium chloride (10 mg/kg bolus followed by a 2 mg/kg per hour infusion) was found to attenuate the effects of **adrenaline (epinephrine)** 10 and 30 nanograms/kg per minute, given for 8 minutes each. **Adrenaline** alone produced a significant increase in the cardiac index, but following the calcium infusion **adrenaline** had no significant effect and the maximal **adrenaline**-induced increase in cardiac index was reduced by 70%. **Adrenaline** 30 nanograms/kg per minute alone increased mean arterial blood pressure from 87 mmHg to 95 mmHg; calcium chloride also raised blood pressure from 85 mmHg to 93 mmHg. After calcium was given, **adrenaline** had no further significant effect on blood pressure.[1]

Some of these workers also studied the mode of action of **dobutamine** in 22 patients recovering from coronary artery bypass surgery.[2] It was found that an infusion of calcium chloride (1 mg/kg per minute initially, then 0.25 mg/kg per minute) attenuated the increase in cardiac output produced by an infusion of **dobutamine** 2.5 to 5 micrograms/kg per minute by 30%. In a group of 24 similar patients the cardiotonic actions of **amrinone** (a phosphodiesterase inhibitor) were unaffected by the calcium infusion.[2]

Just how the calcium alters the effects of **adrenaline** and **dobutamine** is not known, but as they are both beta-receptor agonists a reasonable suggestion is that calcium interferes with the signal transduction through the beta-adrenergic receptor complex. The clinical importance of these findings is uncertain.

1. Zaloga GP, Strickland RA, Butterworth JF, Mark LJ, Mills SA, Lake CR. Calcium attenuates epinephrine's ß-adrenergic effects in postoperative heart surgery patients. *Circulation* (1990) 81, 196–200.
2. Butterworth JF, Zaloga GP, Prielipp RC, Tucker WY, Royster RL. Calcium inhibits the cardiac stimulating properties of dobutamine but not of amrinone. *Chest* (1992) 101, 174–80.

Inotropes and Vasopressors + Cimetidine

An exaggerated hypertensive response to dobutamine occurred during anaesthetic induction in a patient taking cimetidine. Another case report describes supraventricular tachycardia, which occurred when a patient receiving dobutamine and dopamine was given cimetidine.

Clinical evidence, mechanism, importance and management

A patient about to undergo coronary artery bypass grafting was anaesthetised with midazolam, fentanyl, vecuronium and oxygen. When a 5 micrograms/kg per minute infusion of **dobutamine** was given the patient developed unexpectedly marked hypertension of 210/100 mmHg. The infusion was stopped and over the next 15 minutes the blood pressure fell to 90/50 mmHg. A new infusion had the same hypertensive effect, and the patient's blood pressure was subsequently controlled at 120/80 mmHg with **dobutamine** 1 microgram/kg per minute.[1] The authors of the report suggest that this exaggerated response to **dobutamine** may have been due to cimetidine 1 g daily, which the patient was also taking. They postulate that the cimetidine may possibly have inhibited the metabolism and clearance of the **dobutamine** by the liver, thereby increasing its effects.[1]

A post-operative patient receiving **dopamine** and **dobutamine** infusions developed a supraventricular tachycardia 30 seconds after an intravenous injection of cimetidine. Similar episodes of tachycardia occurred on rechallenge with both drugs, but not when each drug was given separately.[2]

These are isolated cases and the general importance is not known but it seems likely to be small.

1. Baraka A, Nauphal M, Arab W. Cimetidine–dobutamine interaction? *Anaesthesia* (1992) 47, 965–6.
2. Grozel JM, Mignotte H, Descotes J. Une nouvelle interaction médicamenteuse: dopamine-cimétidine? *Nouv Presse Med* (1980) 9, 3548.

Inotropes and Vasopressors + Clonidine

Studies suggest that pretreatment with clonidine decreases the blood pressure response to small doses of dopamine; does not affect the blood pressure response to noradrenaline (norepinephrine); and can increase the blood pressure responses to dobutamine, ephedrine, isoprenaline (isoproterenol) and phenylephrine.

Clinical evidence

In a study in 70 patients undergoing elective surgery, 35 patients were given clonidine 5 micrograms/kg 90 minutes before the induction of anaesthesia and 35 patients were used as a control group. While under anaesthesia, and when haemodynamically stable for at least 10 minutes, all patients were given a 10-minute infusion of **dopamine** 3 or 5 micrograms/kg per minute or **dobutamine** 0.5, 1, or 3 micrograms/kg per minute.[1] Clonidine attenuated the response to the 5 micrograms/kg per minute dose of **dopamine** (blood pressure rise 19/10 mmHg in the control group but only 4/0 mmHg in the clonidine group). However, **dopamine** 3 micrograms/kg per minute did not significantly affect blood pressure in either the control group or the clonidine group. Conversely, clonidine enhanced the response to **dobutamine** at all 3 doses. The study had to be stopped after 2 minutes in the clonidine group receiving the highest dose of **dobutamine** as the rise in blood pressure exceed the study limits (rise 45/24 mmHg compared with 16/7 mmHg in the control group).[1] In a study of the same design, 20 clonidine-treated patients and 20 controls were given a bolus infusion of **phenylephrine** 3 micrograms/kg or **isoprenaline (isoproterenol)** 0.02 micrograms/kg. Those who received clonidine had a greater and more prolonged increase in arterial pressure and heart rate with **phenylephrine** (10 minutes compared with 2 to 3 minutes) and increase in heart rate (but not arterial pressure) with **isoprenaline (isoproterenol)**.[2]

In another similar study, 77 patients (38 premedicated with clonidine 5 micrograms/kg and famotidine 20 mg, 90 minutes before anaesthetic induction, and a control group of 39 given only famotidine) were given **noradrenaline (norepinephrine)** 0.5 micrograms/kg or **phenylephrine** 2 micrograms/kg. It was found that the overall response to **noradrenaline (norepinephrine)** was not significantly affected by clonidine, although 2 to 4 minutes after administration the mean arterial blood pressure was raised in the clonidine group. The blood pressure rise in response to **phenylephrine** was found to be augmented. There were no significant differences between the groups in terms of the incidence of hypertension, arrhythmias or bradycardia.[3] Similar results have been reported with **phenylephrine** in other studies (see below). The same group of workers repeated this study using two doses of **ephedrine** 100 micrograms/kg as the vasopressor. Clonidine prolonged the response to **ephedrine** by 2 minutes and increased the rise in blood pressure (rise in mean blood pressure in response to **ephedrine** at 3 minutes of 12.7 mmHg with clonidine, compared with 6.6 mmHg without clonidine). The rise in blood pressure was greater in both groups after a second dose of **ephedrine** was given but the effect in the clonidine group was still greater (rise in mean blood pressure in response to **ephedrine** at 4 minutes of 15 mmHg with clonidine compared with 9.4 mmHg without clonidine).[4]

Additional effects on blood pressure were found in another group of patients who were anaesthetised with enflurane and nitrous oxide/oxygen, and given intravenous **ephedrine** 100 micrograms/kg after pretreatment with clonidine (about 5 micrograms/kg).[5] A study in patients anaesthetised with propofol found premedication with clonidine enhanced the pressor and tachycardic effects of **ephedrine**, especially in elderly patients (over 60 years old) given standard dose of propofol (1 mg/kg at induction followed by 6 mg/kg per hour as maintenance).[6] In another study, 21 patients were premedicated with oral clonidine (about 5 micrograms/kg) and famotidine 20 mg, 90 minutes before spinal anaesthesia with tetracaine and a further 20 patients were given famotidine alone as premedication. All patients were given intravenous **ephedrine** 200 micrograms/kg when their systolic pressure decreased to below 100 mmHg or to less than 80% of pre-anaesthetic value. Premedication with clonidine enhanced the pressor response of **ephedrine** and its duration.[7]

Further study, using enflurane and nitrous oxide/oxygen for anaesthesia, found that the mean maximum blood pressure increased in a group of patients premedicated with clonidine and given intravenous **phenylephrine** 2 micrograms/kg by 26% and 32%, for awake and anaesthetised subjects, respectively. This was greater than the blood pressure rises seen in a group not given clonidine, which were 13% and 18%, for awake and anaesthetised subjects, respectively.[8] In a placebo-controlled study, patients with hypertension were given intravenous **phenylephrine** in increasing bolus doses or 30 to 300 micrograms on the day before surgery, before induction of anaesthesia and one and 3 hours postoperatively. Oral clonidine 6 micrograms/kg, was given 2 hours before surgery and a further dose of 3 micrograms/kg intravenously during the last hour of surgery. The pressor response calculated for a dose of **phenylephrine** 1.5 micrograms/kg was 42 mmHg in patients given clonidine before surgery compared with 27 mmHg for those given placebo. The postoperative pressor response to **phenylephrine** was 37 mmHg and 26 mmHg for the clonidine and placebo groups, respectively.[9]

Mechanism

Not understood. Clonidine is an alpha$_2$ agonist, which blocks the release of noradrenaline (norepinephrine) from the nerve endings, and most suggested mechanisms consider noradrenaline release to be involved in some way.

Importance and management

An interaction is established, although the exact outcome of the concurrent use of clonidine and these sympathomimetic vasopressors is not clear. It has been suggested that the effects may be different at different doses of dopamine.[8] The authors of the one report,[3] studying phenylephrine and noradrenaline (norepinephrine) with clonidine, suggested that the increase in pressor response was unlikely to be clinically significant.

Be aware that dobutamine, ephedrine, and phenylephrine may have a greater than expected effect if clonidine has been taken. Some of these drugs may also be used as nasal decongestants (e.g. ephedrine, and phenylephrine). The outcome of the concurrent use of clonidine in these circumstances is unclear, but a rise in blood pressure seems possible. However, note that these products are usually cautioned in patients with hypertension.

1. Ohata H, Iida H, Watanabe Y, Dohi S. Hemodynamic responses induced by dopamine and dobutamine in anesthetized patients premedicated with clonidine. *Anesth Analg* (1999) 89, 843–8.
2. Watanabe Y, Iida H, Tanabe K, Ohata H, Dohi S. Clonidine premedication modifies responses to adrenoceptor agonists and baroreflex sensitivity. *Can J Anaesth* (1998) 45, 1084–1090.
3. Tanaka M, Nishikawa T. Effects of clonidine premedication on the pressor response to α-adrenergic agonists. *Br J Anaesth* (1995) 75, 593–7.
4. Tanaka M, Nishikawa T. Enhancement of pressor response to ephedrine following clonidine medication. *Anaesthesia* (1996) 51, 123–7.
5. Nishikawa T, Kimura T, Taguchi N, Dohi S. Oral clonidine preanesthetic medication augments the pressor responses to intravenous ephedrine in awake or anesthetized patients. *Anesthesiology* (1991) 74, 705–10.
6. Ishiyama T, Kashimoto S, Oguchi T, Matsukawa T, Kumazawa T. The effects of clonidine premedication on the blood pressure and tachycardiac responses to ephedrine in elderly and young patients during propofol anesthesia. *Anesth Analg* (2003) 96, 136–41.
7. Goyagi T, Tanaka M, Nishikawa T. Oral clonidine premedication enhances the pressor response to ephedrine during spinal anesthesia. *Anesth Analg* (1998) 87, 1336–9.
8. Inomata S, Nishikawa T, Kihara S, Akiyoshi Y. Enhancement of pressor response to intravenous phenylephrine following oral clonidine medication in awake and anaesthetized patients. *Can J Anaesth* (1995) 42, 119–25.
9. Parlow JL, Sagnard P, Begou G, Viale J-P, Quintin L. The effects of clonidine on sensitivity to phenylephrine and nitroprusside in patients with essential hypertension recovering from surgery. *Anesth Analg* (1999) 88, 1239–43.

Inotropes and Vasopressors + Ergometrine (Ergonovine)

An isolated report attributes the development of gangrene and subsequently fatal septicaemia to the use of dopamine following the use of ergometrine. A similar case has been reported with ergometrine and noradrenaline (norepinephrine).

Clinical evidence, mechanism, importance and management

One patient developed gangrene of the hands and feet after being given an infusion of **dopamine** (10 micrograms/kg per minute, later doubled) started approximately 2 hours after the use of ergometrine (two 400-microgram doses).[1] This would seem to have resulted from the additive peripheral vasoconstrictor effects of both drugs, which reduced the circulation to such an extent that gangrene and then fatal septicaemia developed. Note that gangrene has been reported with the use of both drugs alone, and it is recommended that peripheral tissue perfusion should be monitored in elderly patients or patients with a history of peripheral vascular disease receiving **dopamine**.[2] This would also seem to be a prudent precaution in those who have previously received ergometrine.

A similar case report describes a pregnant woman (24-weeks gestation) with severe burns who received ergometrine to treat post-partum bleeding after spontaneous abortion and **noradrenaline (norepinephrine)** to treat hypotensive septic shock. The combination of these two vasoconstrictors is thought to have contributed to ischaemia of the fingers, resulting in loss of some digits.[3]

In the rare circumstances when it may be necessary to use both of these drugs, close attention should be paid to peripheral tissue perfusion.

1. Buchanan N, Cane RD, Miller M. Symmetrical gangrene of the extremities associated with the use of dopamine subsequent to ergometrine administration. *Intensive Care Med* (1977) 3, 55–6.
2. Dopamine Sterile Concentrate (Dopamine hydrochloride). Hospira UK Ltd. UK Summary of product characteristics, April 2003.
3. Chuang S-S. Finger ischemia secondary to the synergistic agonist effect of norepinephrine and ergonovine and in a burn patient. *Burns* (2003) 29, 92–4.

Inotropes and Vasopressors + Guanethidine

The increase in blood pressure in response to noradrenaline (norepinephrine), phenylephrine, and metaraminol can be enhanced in the presence of guanethidine. These drugs can also be used as eye drops, and in this situation their mydriatic effects are similarly enhanced and prolonged by guanethidine.

Clinical evidence

(a) Blood pressure response

A study in 6 normotensive subjects given guanethidine 200 mg on the first day of the study and 100 mg daily for the next 2 days, found that their mean arterial blood pressure in response to a range of doses of **noradrenaline (norepinephrine)**, was increased by 6 to 18% (a 6 to 20 mmHg increase). Moreover, cardiac arrhythmias appeared at lower doses of **noradrenaline** and with greater frequency than in the absence of guanethidine, and were more serious in nature.[1]

In another report, a patient taking guanethidine 20 mg daily was given intramuscular **metaraminol** 10 mg, which rapidly caused the blood pressure to rise to 220/130 mmHg accompanied by severe headache and extreme angina.[2] An increase in blood pressure from 165/90 mmHg to 170/110 mmHg was also seen in a patient taking guanethidine who, before surgery, was given **phenylephrine** eye drops.[3]

(b) Mydriatic response

The mydriasis due to **phenylephrine** given as a 10% eye drop solution was prolonged for up to 10 hours in a patient taking guanethidine for hypertension.[4] This enhanced mydriatic response has been described in another study using guanethidine eye drops with **adrenaline (epinephrine)**, **phenylephrine** or **methoxamine** eye drops.[5]

Mechanism

By preventing the release of noradrenaline from adrenergic neurones, guanethidine and other adrenergic neurone blockers cause a temporary drug-induced sympathectomy, which is also accompanied by hypersensitivity of the receptors. This results in the increased response to the stimulation of the receptors by directly-acting sympathomimetics such as noradrenaline (norepinephrine) and phenylephrine.

Importance and management

An established, well-documented and potentially serious interaction. As the increase in blood pressure can be grossly exaggerated, doses of inotropes or vasopressors with directly-acting sympathomimetic actions (alpha-agonists) should be reduced appropriately. In addition it should be remembered that the incidence and severity of cardiac arrhythmias is increased.[1] Considerable care is required. Direct evidence seems to be limited to noradrenaline (norepinephrine), phenylephrine, metaraminol, and methoxamine. **Dopamine** also possesses direct sympathomimetic activity and may be expected to interact similarly. If as a result of this interaction the blood pressure becomes grossly elevated, it can be controlled by giving an alpha-adrenergic blocker such as phentolamine.[6] Phenylephrine, which is used as a vasopressor, is also contained in a number of non-prescription cough and cold preparations, which may contain 12 mg in a dose. A single dose of this size is only likely to cause a moderate blood pressure rise. However, this requires confirmation, particularly as the non-prescription products may be taken up to four times daily for up to 7 days, and higher doses may be available in some countries.

An exaggerated pressor response is clearly much more potentially serious than enhanced and prolonged mydriasis, but the latter is also possible and undesirable. The same precautions apply with the use of smaller amounts of these drugs.

1. Mulheims GH, Entrup RW, Paiewonsky D, Mierzwiak DS. Increased sensitivity of the heart to catecholamine-induced arrhythmias following guanethidine. *Clin Pharmacol Ther* (1965) 6, 757–62.
2. Stevens FRT. A danger of sympathomimetic drugs. *Med J Aust* (1966) 2, 576.
3. Kim JM, Stevenson CE, Mathewson HS. Hypertensive reactions to phenylephrine eyedrops in patients with sympathetic denervation. *Am J Ophthalmol* (1978) 85, 862–8.
4. Cooper B. Neo-synephrine (10%) eye drops. *Med J Aust* (1968) 55, 420.
5. Sneddon JM, Turner P. The interactions of local guanethidine and sympathomimetic amines in the human eye. *Arch Ophthalmol* (1969) 81,622–7.
6. Allum W, Aminu J, Bloomfield TH, Davies C, Scales AH, Vere DW. Interaction between debrisoquine and phenylephrine in man. *Br J Clin Pharmacol* (1974) 1, 51–7.

Inotropes and Vasopressors + Lithium

The pressor effects of noradrenaline (norepinephrine) and phenylephrine are slightly reduced by lithium carbonate.

Clinical evidence, mechanism, importance and management

A study in 8 patients with manic depression found that after taking lithium carbonate for 7 to 10 days (serum level range 0.72 to 1.62 mmol/L) the dose of a **noradrenaline (norepinephrine)** infusion had to be increased by 1.8 micrograms in 7 patients to maintain a blood pressure increase of 25 mmHg. This equated to a 22% reduction in the pressor effect of **noradrenaline**.[1] Another study in 17 depressed patients with serum lithium levels in the range 0.8 to 1.2 mmol/L found that 12% more **noradrenaline** and 31% more **phenylephrine** were needed to raise the blood pressure by 30 mmHg.[2] The reasons for this interaction are not known. Results from an *animal* study suggest that lithium may increase the inactivation of **noradrenaline** and decrease the **noradrenaline** available for adrenergic receptors.[3]

These decreases in the pressor response to **noradrenaline** and to **phenylephrine** in the presence of lithium carbonate are both relatively small and it seems unlikely that they will present any problems in practice.

1. Fann WE, Davis JM, Janowsky DS, Cavanaugh JH, Kaufmann JS, Griffith JD, Oates JA. Effects of lithium on adrenergic function in man. *Clin Pharmacol Ther* (1972) 13, 71–7.
2. Ghose K. Assessment of peripheral adrenergic activity and its interactions with drugs in man. *Eur J Clin Pharmacol* (1980) 17, 233–8.
3. Sastre E, Nicolay A, Bruguerolle B, Portugal H. Effect of lithium on norepinephrine metabolic pathways. *Life Sci* (2005) 77, 758–67.

Inotropes and Vasopressors + Reserpine

The effects of adrenaline (epinephrine), noradrenaline (norepinephrine) and other related drugs are slightly increased in the presence of reserpine.

Clinical evidence

In 11 patients taking reserpine, pretreatment with **phenylephrine** 10% eye drops caused a blood pressure increase of 30/12 mmHg, whereas no significant increase in blood pressure occurred in 176 patients who were given **phenylephrine** eye drops and who were not taking reserpine.[1] After 7 healthy subjects took reserpine 0.25 to 1 mg daily for 2 weeks the increase in the blood pressure in response to **noradrenaline (norepinephrine)** was increased by 20 to 40%.[2] A man taking reserpine who became hypotensive while undergoing surgery did not respond to an intravenous injection of **ephedrine**, but did so after 30 minutes treatment with **noradrenaline**, presumably because the stores of **noradrenaline** at adrenergic neurones had become replenished.[3] The mydriatic effects of **ephedrine** have also been found to be antagonised by pretreatment with reserpine.[4] However, in contrast, one report claimed that **ephedrine** 25 mg given orally or intramuscularly, once or twice daily, proved to be an effective treatment for reserpine-induced hypotension and bradycardia in patients with schizophrenia.[5]

Studies in *dogs* have demonstrated that **adrenaline (epinephrine)**, **noradrenaline** and **phenylephrine** (all sympathomimetics with direct actions) remain effective vasopressors after treatment with reserpine, and their actions are enhanced to some extent.[6-8] **Metaraminol** has also been successfully used to raise blood pressure in reserpine-treated patients.[9]

Mechanism

The rauwolfia alkaloids (e.g. reserpine) cause adrenergic neurones to lose their stores of noradrenaline (norepinephrine), so that they can no longer stimulate adrenergic receptors and transmission ceases. Indirectly-acting sympathomimetics, which work by stimulating the release of stored noradrenaline, may therefore be expected to become ineffective. In contrast, the effects of directly-acting sympathomimetics should remain unchanged. However, their effects may be enhanced (as described above) because when the receptors are deprived of stimulation by noradrenaline for any length of time they can become supersensitive. Drugs with mixed direct and indirect actions, such as ephedrine, should fall somewhere between the two, although the reports cited seem to indicate that ephedrine has predominantly indirect activity.[3,4]

Importance and management

These are established interactions, but the paucity of clinical information suggests that in practice they do not present many problems, perhaps because the effects of these vasopressors are so closely monitored, and titrated to effect. If a pressor drug is required, a directly-acting drug such as noradrenaline (norepinephrine) or phenylephrine may be expected to be effective. The receptors may show some supersensitivity so that a dose reduction may be required. 'Table 24.1', p.1050 gives a classification of the sympathomimetics.

1. Kim JM, Stevenson CE, Mathewson HS. Hypertensive reactions to phenylephrine eyedrops in patients with sympathetic denervation. *Am J Ophthalmol* (1978) 85, 862–8.
2. Abboud FM, Eckstein JW. Effects of small oral doses of reserpine on vascular responses to tyramine and norepinephrine in man. *Circulation* (1964) 29, 219–23.
3. Ziegler CH, Lovette JB. Operative complications after therapy with reserpine and reserpine compounds. *JAMA* (1961) 176, 916–19.
4. Sneddon JM, Turner P. Ephedrine mydriasis in hypertension and the response to treatment. *Clin Pharmacol Ther* (1969) 10, 64–71.
5. Noce RH, Williams DB, Rapaport W. Reserpine (Serpasil) in the management of the mentally ill. *JAMA* (1955) 158, 11–15.
6. Stone CA, Ross CA, Wenger HC, Ludden CT, Blessing JA, Totaro JA, Porter CC. Effect of α-methyl-3,4-dihydroxyphenylalanine (methyldopa), reserpine and related agents on some vascular responses in the dog. *J Pharmacol Exp Ther* (1962) 136, 80–8.
7. Eger EI, Hamilton WK. The effect of reserpine on the action of various vasopressors. *Anesthesiology* (1959) 20, 641–5.
8. Moore JI, Moran NC. Cardiac contractile force responses to ephedrine and other sympathomimetic amines in dogs after pretreatment with reserpine. *J Pharmacol Exp Ther* (1962) 136, 89–96.
9. Smessaert AA, Hicks RG. Problems caused by rauwolfia drugs during anesthesia and surgery. *N Y State J Med* (1961) 61, 2399–2403.

Inotropes and Vasopressors; Dobutamine + Dipyridamole

The addition of dipyridamole to dobutamine for echocardiography can cause potentially hazardous hypotension.

Clinical evidence, mechanism, importance and management

Ten patients with a low probability of coronary artery disease underwent dobutamine echocardiography. Five were given dobutamine alone, while the other 5 were given a low intravenous dose of dipyridamole with the maximum dose of dobutamine, to see whether the sensitivity of the test could be improved. Four of the patients given both drugs experienced severe hypotension while no hypotension was seen in the control group. The conclusion was reached that this combination of drugs can be hazardous and should not be used in patients suspected of coronary heart disease.[1] Note that, although both of these drugs are commonly used in stress echocardiography, they are not given together.

1. Shaheen J, Rosenmann D, Tzivoni D. Severe hypotension induced by combination of dobutamine and dipyridamole. *Isr J Med Sci* (1996) 32, 1105–7.

Inotropes and Vasopressors; Dopamine + Phenytoin

Some limited evidence suggests that patients needing dopamine to support their blood pressure can become severely hypotensive if they are also given intravenous phenytoin.

Clinical evidence, mechanism, importance and management

Five critically ill patients treated with a number of different drugs, were given dopamine to maintain an adequate blood pressure. When seizures developed they were given intravenous phenytoin at an infusion rate of 5 to 25 mg/minute. Their previously stable blood pressures then fell rapidly, one patient became bradycardic, and 2 patients died from cardiac arrest. A similar reaction was found in *dogs* made hypovolaemic and hypotensive by bleeding, and then given dopamine followed by a phenytoin infusion.[1] However, another study in *dogs* was unable to find evidence of this serious adverse interaction,[2] and no evidence of marked hypotension occurred when a patient with cardiogenic shock was given a phenytoin infusion while receiving dopamine and dobutamine.[3]

The documentation of this adverse interaction therefore appears to be limited to this single report. However, intravenous phenytoin is known to cause hypotension if it is given rapidly, particularly in gravely ill patients. Blood pressure is doubtless being monitored in patients receiving dopamine, and should be monitored when phenytoin is given intravenously. However, more frequent monitoring may be necessary initially, as any interaction appears to develop rapidly.

1. Bivins BA, Rapp RP, Griffen WO, Blouin R, Bustrack J. Dopamine-phenytoin interaction. A cause of hypotension in the critically ill. *Arch Surg* (1978) 113, 245–9.
2. Smith RD, Lomas TE. Modification of cardiovascular responses to intravenous phenytoin by dopamine in dogs: evidence against an adverse interaction. *Toxicol Appl Pharmacol* (1978) 45, 665–73.
3. Torres E, Garcia B, Sosa P, Alba D. No interaction between dopamine and phenytoin. *Ann Pharmacother* (1995) 29, 1300–1.

Inotropes and Vasopressors; Dopamine + Selegiline

A case report describes a hypertensive reaction attributed to the concurrent use of dopamine and selegiline.

Clinical evidence, mechanism, importance and management

A 75-year-old man, who was taking selegiline 5 mg twice daily for Parkinson's disease, was given intravenous dopamine 3.5 micrograms/kg per minute because of a decline in blood pressure and urine output following a serious road traffic accident. Twenty minutes after the infusion was started his blood pressure had hardly changed, but 30 minutes later it had risen from 108/33 mmHg to 228/50 mmHg. The dopamine infusion was discontinued and the blood pressure decreased to 121/40 mmHg over the next 30 minutes. The dopamine infusion was reinstituted twice more at lower doses (1.03 and 0.9 micrograms/kg per minute), but each time similar reactions occurred. The exaggerated vasopressor response was thought to be due to inhibition of dopamine metabolism by selegiline.[1]

The authors of the report[1] and the manufacturers of selegiline recommend that dopamine should be used cautiously,[2] and only after careful risk-benefit assessment,[3] in patients who are currently taking selegiline or who have taken selegiline in the 2 weeks before dopamine is required. In addition, the manufacturers of dopamine warn that in patients who have received MAOIs within the previous 2 to 3 weeks, the initial dose of dopamine should be no greater than 10% of the usual dose.[4]

1. Rose LM, Ohlinger MJ, Mauro VF. A hypertensive reaction induced by concurrent use of selegiline and dopamine. *Ann Pharmacother* (2000) 34, 1020–4.
2. Eldepryl (Selegiline hydrochloride). Orion Pharma (UK) Ltd. UK Summary of product characteristics, February 2012.
3. Zelapar (Selegiline hydrochloride). Cephalon Ltd. UK Summary of product characteristics, March 2012.
4. Dopamine Sterile Concentrate (Dopamine hydrochloride). Hospira UK Ltd. UK Summary of product characteristics, April 2003.

Inotropes and Vasopressors; Dopamine + Tolazoline

Acute and eventually fatal hypotension occurred in a patient given dopamine and tolazoline.

Clinical evidence

A patient receiving ventilatory support following surgery was given **dopamine** on the third postoperative day. Pulmonary arterial pressure had been steadily rising since the surgery, so on day 4 he was given a slow 2-mg/kg bolus injection of tolazoline. Systemic arterial pressure immediately fell to 50/30 mmHg so the **dopamine** infusion was increased but, contrary to the expected effect, the arterial pressure then fell even further to 38/15 mmHg. The **dopamine** was stopped and ephedrine, methoxamine and fresh frozen plasma were given. Two hours later his blood pressure was 70/40 mmHg. Two further attempts were made to give **dopamine**, but the arterial pressure fell to 40/15 mmHg on the first occasion, and to 38/20 mmHg on the second, which resulted in a fatal cardiac arrest.[1]

Mechanism

The interaction between dopamine and tolazoline is not fully understood. Dopamine has both alpha (vasoconstrictor) and beta (vasodilator) activity. With the alpha effects on the systemic circulation competitively blocked by the tolazoline, its vasodilatory actions would predominate, resulting in paradoxical hypotension.

Importance and management

Information on the interaction between dopamine and tolazoline is limited but this interaction would appear to be established. The authors of this report warn that an infusion of dopamine should not be considered for several hours after even a small single dose of tolazoline has been given. They point out that impaired renal function often accompanies severe respiratory failure, which may significantly prolong the effects of tolazoline.

1. Carlon GC. Fatal association of tolazoline and dopamine. *Chest* (1979) 76, 336.

Ivabradine + CYP3A4 inducers

The manufacturers advise that patients taking CYP3A4 inducers (they specifically name barbiturates, phenytoin, and rifampicin (rifampin)) may need dose increases of ivabradine.[1] This would seem prudent as St John's wort, a known CYP3A4 inducer, reduces ivabradine levels, see 'Ivabradine + St John's wort (*Hypericum perforatum*)', p.1068. See also 'Table 1.9', p.11, for a list of known CYP3A4 inducers. Monitor the concurrent use of these drugs for ivabradine efficacy and adjust the dose as necessary. Remember to re-adjust the dose of ivabradine if concurrent use of these drugs is stopped.

1. Procoralan (Ivabradine hydrochloride). Servier Laboratories Ltd. UK Summary of product characteristics, October 2009.

Ivabradine + CYP3A4 inhibitors

Ivabradine is metabolised by CYP3A4 and its concentrations may therefore be increased significantly in the presence of inhibitors of this isoenzyme, such as some azoles, diltiazem, grapefruit juice, some macrolides, nefazodone, HIV-protease inhibitors, or verapamil.

Clinical evidence

A study found that **ketoconazole** 200 mg daily or **josamycin** 1 g twice daily increased ivabradine plasma concentrations by seven- to eightfold. Studies in healthy subjects and patients given **diltiazem** or **verapamil** have resulted in an increase in the AUC of ivabradine of two to threefold, and an additional heart rate reduction of 5 bpm.[1]

Mechanism

Ivabradine is a substrate of CYP3A4, and its metabolism is reduced by inhibitors of CYP3A4, resulting in increased plasma concentrations and increased therapeutic effects.[1]

Importance and management

The manufacturer contraindicates the use of potent inhibitors of CYP3A4 with ivabradine, (they specifically mention **clarithromycin**, **oral erythromycin**, **itraconazole**, josamycin, ketoconazole, **nefazodone**, **nelfinavir**, **ritonavir**, and **telithromycin**).The manufacturer suggests that if moderate inhibitors of CYP3A4 are given (they name **fluconazole**), ivabradine may be used, but at a lower starting dose of 2.5 mg twice daily, with consideration of heart rate monitoring.[1] Diltiazem and verapamil are also moderate inhibitors of CYP3A4, but their use is not recommended because of their effects on heart rate. Note that clinically relevant inhibitors of CYP3A4 are listed in 'Table 1.9', p.11. The manufacturers of ivabradine[1] also state that **grapefruit juice** (an inhibitor of CYP3A4 in the intestine) increases the exposure to ivabradine twofold, and they therefore recommend that the intake of grapefruit juice by patients also taking ivabradine is restricted. Note that this increase is similar to that seen with moderate inhibitors of CYP3A4, for which an ivabradine dose reduction has been suggested.

1. Procoralan (Ivabradine hydrochloride). Servier Laboratories Ltd. UK Summary of product characteristics, October 2009.

Ivabradine + Drugs that prolong the QT interval

The manufacturers advise that ivabradine should not be taken with drugs that prolong the QT interval, but also advise that if concurrent use with such drugs appears necessary, close cardiac monitoring is needed. Bradycardia is a pharmacological effect of ivabradine, and QT prolongation may be exacerbated by heart rate reductions.[1] For a list of drugs known to affect the QT interval see 'Table 9.2', p.273.

1. Procoralan (Ivabradine hydrochloride). Servier Laboratories Ltd. UK Summary of product characteristics, October 2009.

Ivabradine + Miscellaneous

The manufacturers say that in specific drug-drug interaction studies, ivabradine was also found not to interact with sildenafil, statins (simvastatin), dihydropyridine calcium-channel blockers (amlodipine, lacidipine), digoxin and warfarin. During clinical studies, ivabradine was taken with ACE inhibitors, angiotensin II receptor antagonists, diuretics, short and long acting nitrates, statins, fibrates, proton pump inhibitors, oral antidiabetics, aspirin and other antiplatelet drugs, and there was no evidence of safety concerns.[1] A specific drug interaction study in 12 healthy subjects found that omeprazole 40 mg daily or lansoprazole 60 mg daily for 5 days did not significantly affect the pharmacokinetics of a single 10-mg dose of ivabradine.[2]

1. Procoralan (Ivabradine hydrochloride). Servier Laboratories Ltd. UK Summary of product characteristics, October 2009.
2. Portolés A, Calvo A, Terleira A, Laredo L, Resplandy G, Gorostiaga C, Moreno A. Lack of pharmacokinetic interaction between omeprazole or lansoprazole and ivabradine in healthy volunteers: an open-label, randomized, crossover, pharmacokinetic interaction clinical trial. *J Clin Pharmacol* (2006) 46, 1195–203.

Ivabradine + St John's wort (*Hypericum perforatum*)

The metabolism of ivabradine is increased by St John's wort.

Clinical evidence

Twelve healthy subjects were given a single oral dose of ivabradine 10 mg 24 hours before St John's wort (*Jarsin* tablets) 300 mg three times daily was given for 14 days. On day 16, they were given a further dose of ivabradine 10 mg with a single 300-mg dose of St John's wort. The maximum levels and AUC of ivabradine were reduced by more than half by St John's wort. The maximum levels and AUC of its active metabolite were reduced by 25% and 32%, respectively. No adverse effects were reported, and the heart rate and blood pressure remained unchanged.[1] Similar findings are also reported by the manufacturers of ivabradine.[2]

Mechanism

St John's wort is a known inducer of the cytochrome P450 isoenzyme CYP3A4, by which ivabradine is metabolised. Concurrent use therefore increases the metabolism of ivabradine, which results in a reduction in its plasma levels, and a potential reduction in effects.

Importance and management

Evidence is limited to the study above, and despite the lack of change in pharmacodynamic effects seen in this study, the pharmacokinetic changes may be large enough to affect individual patients. Monitor concurrent use for ivabradine efficacy and adjust the dose as necessary. Remember to re-adjust the dose of ivabradine if the concurrent use of these drugs is stopped. The UK manufacturer suggests that the use of St John's wort should be restricted in patients taking ivabradine.[2]

1. Portolés A, Terleira A, Calvo A, Martínez I, Resplandy G. Effects of Hypericum perforatum on ivabradine pharmacokinetics in healthy volunteers: an open-label, pharmacokinetic interaction clinical trial. *J Clin Pharmacol* (2006) 46, 1188–94.
2. Procoralan (Ivabradine hydrochloride). Servier Laboratories Ltd. UK Summary of product characteristics, October 2009.

Ketanserin + Beta blockers

There is no pharmacokinetic interaction between ketanserin and propranolol, but additive hypotensive effects may occur. Very marked acute hypotension has been seen in two patients taking atenolol when they were first given ketanserin.

Clinical evidence, mechanism, importance and management

A study in 6 patients and 2 healthy subjects given ketanserin 40 mg twice daily for 3 weeks found that **propranolol** 80 mg twice daily for 6 days did not significantly alter the steady-state plasma levels of ketanserin.[1] Another study in healthy subjects, using single doses of both drugs, found that neither drug affected the pharmacokinetics of the other.[2] In a third study, **propranolol** 80 mg twice daily had no effect on the pharmacokinetics of a single 10-mg intravenous dose of ketanserin. However, ketanserin 40 mg twice daily modestly decreased the clearance of a single 160-mg dose of **propranolol** by 29% and increased its maximum serum level by 38%, although neither of these changes were statistically significant.[3] The hypotensive effects of ketanserin were slightly increased by **propranolol** in the first study,[1] and additive hypotensive effects were seen in another study in patients with essential hypertension.[4]

Acute hypotension is reported to have occurred in 2 patients taking **atenolol** within an hour of taking a 40-mg oral dose of ketanserin. One of them briefly lost consciousness.[5]

The concurrent use of ketanserin and beta blockers can be valuable and uneventful, but a few patients may experience marked hypotensive effects when first given ketanserin. Patients should be warned.

1. Trenk D, Lühr A, Radkow N, Jähnchen E. Lack of effect of propranolol on the steady-state plasma levels of ketanserin. *Arzneimittelforschung* (1985) 35, 1286–8.
2. Williams FM, Leeser JE, Rawlins MD. Pharmacodynamics and pharmacokinetics of single doses of ketanserin and propranolol alone and in combination in healthy volunteers. *Br J Clin Pharmacol* (1986) 22, 301–8.
3. Ochs HR, Greenblatt DJ, Höller M, Labedzky L. The interactions of propranolol and ketanserin. *Clin Pharmacol Ther* (1987) 41, 55–60.
4. Hedner T, Persson B. Antihypertensive properties of ketanserin in combination with β-adrenergic blocking agents. *J Cardiovasc Pharmacol* (1985) 7 (Suppl 7), S161–S163.
5. Waller PC, Cameron HA, Ramsey LE. Profound hypotension after the first dose of ketanserin. *Postgrad Med J* (1987) 63, 305–7.

Ketanserin + Diuretics

Sudden deaths, probably from cardiac arrhythmias, were markedly increased in patients taking potassium-depleting diuretics and high doses of ketanserin. No interaction occurred with low doses of ketanserin in those with normal potassium levels. Potassium-sparing diuretics do not interact in this way.

Clinical evidence

A large multi-national study[1] in 3899 patients found that a harmful and potentially fatal interaction could occur in those given ketanserin 40 mg three times daily and **potassium-depleting diuretics**. Of 249 patients taking both drugs, 35 patients (14%) died (16 suddenly) compared with only 15 patients (6%, with 5 sudden deaths) of 260 patients taking a placebo and **potassium-depleting diuretics**. No significant increase in the number of deaths occurred in those taking ketanserin and **potassium-sparing diuretics**. A further analysis of the results found that in patients given ketanserin, the relative mortality was 87% for those not taking diuretics, 76% for those taking **potassium-sparing diuretics** and 313% for those taking **potassium-depleting diuretics**.[2]

It was found that the corrected QT interval was prolonged as follows: ketanserin alone 18 milliseconds, ketanserin with **potassium-sparing diuretics** 24 milliseconds, ketanserin with **potassium-depleting diuretics** 30 milliseconds. Preliminary results of a later study in 33 patients using a smaller dose of ketanserin (20 mg twice daily) with **potassium-depleting diuretics (furosemide, thiazides)** found no evidence of a prolonged QTc interval in patients with normal potassium levels.[3] The pharmacokinetics of a single 20-mg dose of ketanserin were not altered by single 25-mg doses of **hydrochlorothiazide**.[4]

Mechanism

Potassium-depleting diuretics may cause hypokalaemia, which increases the risk of QT-prolongation and torsade de pointes, which can result in sudden death. Ketanserin also prolongs the QT interval in a dose-related way, and its effects would be expected to be additive with that of diuretic-induced hypokalaemia. See also 'Drugs that prolong the QT interval + Other drugs that prolong the QT interval', p.272.

Importance and management

The use of potassium-depleting diuretics (see 'Table 26.1', p.1117) with ketanserin 40 mg three times daily should be avoided. Lower doses of ketanserin (20 mg twice daily) have less effect on the QT interval, and can probably be used cautiously with potassium-depleting diuretics, as long as serum potassium levels are maintained. Potassium-sparing diuretics do not interact.

1. Prevention of Atherosclerotic Complications with Ketanserin Trial Group. Prevention of atherosclerotic complications: controlled trial of ketanserin. *BMJ* (1989) 298, 424–30.
2. Verstraete M. The PACK trial: morbidity and mortality effects of ketanserin. *Vasc Med* (1996) 1 135–40.
3. Van Gool R, Symoens J. Ketanserin in combination with diuretics: effect on QTc-interval. *Eur Heart J* (1990) 11 (Suppl), 57.
4. Botha JH, McFadyen ML, Leary WPP, Janssens M. No effect of single-dose hydrochlorothiazide on the pharmacokinetics of single-dose ketanserin. *Curr Ther Res* (1991) 49, 225–30.

Ketanserin + Miscellaneous

Ketanserin should not be given with certain antiarrhythmics, naftidrofuryl, or tricyclic antidepressants because of the risk of potentially fatal cardiac arrhythmias. Drowsiness and dizziness are common adverse effects, which may possibly be additive with the effects of other CNS depressants.

Clinical evidence, mechanism, importance and management

Ketanserin has weak class III antiarrhythmic activity and can prolong the QT_c interval. For safety reasons it has therefore been advised that it should be avoided in patients with existing QT_c prolongation, atrioventricular or sinoauricular block of higher degree, or severe bradycardia of less than 50 bpm.[1] For the same reason the concurrent use of drugs that affect repolarisation (**class Ia, class Ic** and **class III arrhythmics**) or drugs that cause conduction disturbances (**naftidrofuryl, tricyclic antidepressants**) should be avoided.[1] See also 'Drugs that prolong the QT interval + Other drugs that prolong the QT interval', p.272, and 'Ketanserin + Diuretics', above.

Dizziness and drowsiness are common adverse effects of ketanserin and therefore it seems likely that these will be additive with other **CNS depressants** and **alcohol**, which may possibly make driving more hazardous, but this needs confirmation.

1. Distler A. Clinical aspects during therapy with the serotonin antagonist ketanserin. *Clin Physiol Biochem* (1990) 8 (Suppl 3), 64–80.

Ketanserin + Nifedipine

Two patients experienced an increase in cardiac arrhythmias when they were given ketanserin with nifedipine.

Clinical evidence, mechanism, importance and management

A study in 20 subjects aged 60 years or more, with normal or slightly raised blood pressures, found that the concurrent use of ketanserin and nifedipine for a week did not, on average, affect their blood pressures, heart rates, or QT intervals, but two of the subjects monitored over 24 hours had a marked increase in the frequency of ectopic beats, couplets and ventricular tachycardia.[1] The reasons are not understood. The authors of this study say that their findings do not exclude the possibility that the concurrent use of these two drugs might therefore increase arrhythmia in some elderly patients.[1] Concurrent use should be monitored.

1. Alberio L, Beretta-Piccoli C, Tanzi F, Koch P, Zehender M. Kardiale Interaktionen zwischen Ketanserin und dem Calcium-Antagonisten Nifedipin. *Schweiz Med Wochenschr* (1992) 122, 1723–7.

Levosimendan + ACE inhibitors

The haemodynamic effects of levosimendan were not significantly altered by captopril in one study.

Clinical evidence, mechanism, importance and management

Captopril, in doses of up to 50 mg twice daily, did not change the haemodynamic effects of a single 1-mg or 2-mg intravenous dose of levosimendan in 24 patients with heart failure. No additional decrease in blood pressure was observed.[1] No special precautions appear to be required if levosimendan is given to patients taking captopril. Other ACE inhibitors do not appear to have been studied, but they would be expected to behave in the same way as captopril.

1. Antila S, Eha J, Heinpalu M, Lehtonen L, Loogna I, Mesikepp A, Planken U, Sandell E-P. Haemodynamic interactions of a new calcium sensitizing drug levosimendan and captopril. *Eur J Clin Pharmacol* (1996) 49, 451–8.

Levosimendan + Beta blockers

The haemodynamic effects of levosimendan were not significantly altered by carvedilol or other unnamed beta blockers.

Clinical evidence, mechanism, importance and management

In 12 healthy subjects, carvedilol 25 mg twice daily for 7 to 9 days did not alter the effects of a single 2-mg intravenous dose of levosimendan on cardiac contractility. In addition, the heart rate and diastolic blood pressure responses were not altered, but the systolic blood pressure response was blunted.[1] In a study to compare levosimendan with dobutamine in patients with severe, low-output heart failure, 33 of the 102 patients receiving levosimendan were also given unnamed beta blockers. The use of a beta blocker was found not to reduce the haemodynamic effects of levosimendan. The authors say this suggests that there may be a place for levosimendan in the management of exacerbations of heart failure not controlled by beta blockers.[2] In another study in elderly patients with acute decompensated systolic heart failure, beta blockers did not reduce the beneficial haemodynamic effects of levosimendan.[3]

1. Lehtonen L, Sundberg S. The contractility enhancing effect of the calcium sensitiser levosimendan is not attenuated by carvedilol in healthy subjects. *Eur J Clin Pharmacol* (2002) 58, 449–52.
2. Follath F, Cleland JGF, Just H, Papp JGY, Scholz H, Peuhkurinen K, Harjola VP, MItrovic V, Abdalla M, Sandell E-P, Lehtonen L, for the Steering Committee and Investigators of the Levosimendan Infusion versus Dobutamine (LIDO) Study. Efficacy and safety of intravenous levosimendan compared with dobutamine in severe low-output heart failure (the LIDO study): a randomised double-blind trial. *Lancet* (2002) 360, 196–202.
3. Kirlidis TT, Skoularigis J, Tsaknakis KT, Karayiannis G, Tsaknakis TK, Triposkiadis F. The influence of β-blockade on the hemodynamic effects of levosimendan in elderly (≥ 70 years) patients with acutely decompensated heart failure. *Int J Clin Pharmacol Ther* (2009) 47, 454–9.

Levosimendan + CYP3A4 inhibitors

Itraconazole does not alter the pharmacokinetics of levosimendan and therefore interactions with other CYP3A4 inhibitors are unlikely.

Clinical evidence, mechanism, importance and management

A study in 12 healthy subjects found that the pharmacokinetics of a single 2-mg oral dose of levosimendan were unchanged by **itraconazole** 200 mg daily for 5 days, and there was no change in heart rates or ECGs (including the QTc interval). It was concluded that because **itraconazole**, a potent inhibitor of the cytochrome P450 isoenzyme CYP3A4, does not interact significantly with levosimendan, interactions with other CYP3A4 inhibitors, by this mechanism, are unlikely.[1] For a list of CYP3A4 inhibitors, see 'Table 1.9', p.11.

1. Antila S, Honkanen T, Lehtonen L, Neuvonen PJ. The CYP3A4 inhibitor itraconazole does not affect the pharmacokinetics of a new calcium-sensitizing drug levosimendan. *Int J Clin Pharmacol Ther* (1998) 36, 446–9.

Levosimendan + Felodipine

The haemodynamic effects of levosimendan were not significantly altered by felodipine.

Clinical evidence, mechanism, importance and management

A study of the use of oral levosimendan 500 micrograms four times daily and felodipine 5 mg daily in 24 men with coronary heart disease found that concurrent use was well tolerated. Felodipine did not antagonise the positive inotropic effects of levosimendan and had no effect on exercise capacity. Both drugs increased heart rate during exercise, and there was a slight additional effect with concurrent use (5 to 8 bpm for levosimendan alone versus 6 to 10 bpm for the combination).[1] There would appear to be no reason for avoiding concurrent use.

1. Põder P, Eha J, Antila S, Heinpalu M, Planken Ü, Loogna I, Mesikepp A, Akkila J, Lehtonen L. Pharmacodynamic interactions of levosimendan and felodipine in patients with coronary heart disease. *Cardiovasc Drugs Ther* (2003) 17, 451–8.

Levosimendan + Nitrates

Orthostatic hypotension occurred when levosimendan was given with isosorbide mononitrate.

Clinical evidence, mechanism, importance and management

In 12 healthy subjects at rest, giving an infusion of levosimendan (12 micrograms/kg over 10 minutes, then 0.2 micrograms/kg per minute for 110 minutes) with a single 20-mg oral dose of **isosorbide mononitrate** had no additional effects on haemodynamic parameters (heart rate, blood pressure, leg blood flow, cardiac output) to the use of levosimendan alone. However, during an orthostatic test, the circulatory response of the combination was significantly potentiated, and three subjects were unable to remain standing for the stipulated time.[1] Care is therefore required when levosimendan and **isosorbide mononitrate**, or similar drugs, are used concurrently. Whether a similar effect occurs with oral levosimendan is unclear, but as with other drugs that cause postural hypotension, patients should be warned.

1. Sundberg S, Lehtonen L. Haemodynamic interactions between the novel calcium sensitiser levosimendan and isosorbide-5-mononitrate in healthy subjects. *Eur J Clin Pharmacol* (2000) 55, 793–9.

Methyldopa + Barbiturates

Methyldopa levels are not altered by the use of phenobarbital.

Clinical evidence, mechanism, importance and management

Indirect evidence from one study in hypertensive patients suggested that phenobarbital could reduce methyldopa levels,[1] but later work, which directly measured the plasma levels of methyldopa, did not find any evidence of a pharmacokinetic interaction.[2,3]

1. Káldor A, Juvancz P, Demeczky M, Sebestyen, Palotas J. Enhancement of methyldopa metabolism with barbiturate. *BMJ* (1971) 3, 518–19.
2. Kristensen M, Jørgensen M, Hansen T. Plasma concentration of alfamethyldopa and its main metabolite, methyldopa-O-sulphate, during long term treatment with alfamethyldopa with special reference to possible interaction with other drugs given simultaneously. *Clin Pharmacol Ther* (1973) 14, 139–40.
3. Kristensen M, Jørgensen M, Hansen T. Barbiturates and methyldopa metabolism. *BMJ* (1973) 1, 49.

Methyldopa + Bile-acid binding resins

Colestyramine and colestipol are reported to have no important effect on the absorption of methyldopa.[1]

1. Hunninghake DB, King S. Effect of cholestyramine and colestipol on the absorption of methyldopa and hydrochlorothiazide. *Pharmacologist* (1978) 20, 220.

Methyldopa + Cephalosporins

Pustular eruptions developed in two women taking methyldopa and cefradine or cefazolin. The use of methyldopa may have been coincidental.

Clinical evidence, mechanism, importance and management

A 74-year-old black woman taking methyldopa and insulin developed pruritus on her arms and legs within 2 hours of starting to take **cefradine** 250 mg every 6 hours. **Cefradine** was stopped after 7 doses. Over the next 2 days, fever and a widespread pustular eruption developed.[1] Another 65-year-old black woman taking methyldopa and furosemide experienced severe pruritus within 8 hours of starting to receive intravenous **cefazolin sodium** 1 g every 12 hours. Over the next 2 days superficial and coalescing pustules appeared on her trunk, arms and legs.[2] The authors of the first report attributed the reaction to **cefradine**.[1] The authors of the second report note that the concurrent use of methyldopa may or may not have been a contributing factor in both reports.[2] There seem to be no other reports of this reaction.

1. Kalb RE, Grossman ME. Pustular eruption following administration of cephradine. *Cutis* (1986) 38, 58–60.
2. Stough D, Guin JD, Baker GF, Haynie L. Pustular eruptions following administration of cefazolin: a possible interaction with methyldopa. *J Am Acad Dermatol* (1987) 16, 1051–2.

Methyldopa + Disulfiram

An isolated report describes a patient with hypertension, which was unresponsive to methyldopa in the presence of disulfiram.

Clinical evidence, mechanism, importance and management

An alcoholic patient taking disulfiram did not respond to moderate to high doses of intravenous methyldopa, given to control his hypertension, but responded to oral low-dose clonidine. The suggested reason for this lack of response to methyldopa is that disulfiram blocks the activity of dopamine beta-hydroxylase, the enzyme responsible for the conversion of the methyldopa to its active form.[1] The general importance of this apparent interaction is uncertain.

1. McCord RW, LaCorte WS. Hypertension refractory to methyldopa in a disulfiram-treated patient. *Clin Res* (1984) 32, 923A.

Methyldopa + Haloperidol

Two cases of marked CNS adverse effects have been attributed to the use of methyldopa and haloperidol. Another patient taking both drugs became irritable and aggressive. In a small pilot study, the concurrent use of methyldopa and haloperidol lowered blood pressure, and symptomatic hypotension occurred in one patient. The combination also caused marked sedation.

Clinical evidence

Two patients who had been taking methyldopa 1 to 1.5 g daily for hypertension, without problems, developed a dementia syndrome (cognitive disabilities, loss of memory, disorientation, etc.) within 3 days of starting to take haloperidol 6 to 8 mg daily for anxiety. The symptoms totally cleared within 72 hours of stopping the haloperidol.[1] Another patient taking haloperidol for schizophrenia, and methyldopa for hypertension, became very irritable and aggressive. When the methyldopa was replaced with hydrochlorothiazide, the patient's behaviour improved dramatically.[2]

In a pilot study of the therapeutic potential of using haloperidol 10 mg daily with methyldopa 500 mg daily for 4 weeks, in the treatment of schizophrenia, the supine diastolic blood pressure decreased significantly from 65 mmHg to 59.5 mmHg. Six of the 10 patients complained of dizziness, and one patient needed a reduction in the drug doses because of transient hypotension. Somnolence occurred in 8 of the 10 patients.[3]

Mechanism

The hypotensive effects of methyldopa and haloperidol might be expected to be additive. The CNS effects are not understood, although methyldopa can cause sedation, depression and dementia, and haloperidol can cause drowsiness, dizziness and depression.

Importance and management

Concurrent use need not be avoided, but it would be prudent to be on the alert for excessive sedation, excessive reductions in blood pressure or the development of other unexpected CNS adverse effects, particularly in the initial stages of concurrent use.

1. Thornton WE. Dementia induced by methyldopa with haloperidol. *N Engl J Med* (1976) 294, 1222.
2. Nadel I, Wallach M. Drug interaction between haloperidol and methyldopa. *Br J Psychiatry* (1979) 135, 484.
3. Chouinard G, Pinard G, Serrano M, Tetreault L. Potentiation of haloperidol by α-methyldopa in the treatment of schizophrenic patients. *Curr Ther Res* (1973) 15, 473–83.

Methyldopa + Iron compounds

The antihypertensive effects of methyldopa can be reduced by ferrous sulfate. Ferrous gluconate appears to interact similarly. Ferric chloride may also interact but iron complexes such as iron polymaltose are predicted not to interact with methyldopa.

Clinical evidence

Ferrous sulfate 325 mg three times daily was given to 5 hypertensive patients who had been taking methyldopa 250 mg to 1.5 g daily for more than a year. After 2 weeks the blood pressures of all of them had risen, and the systolic pressures of 3 of them had risen by more than 15 mmHg. Four had diastolic blood pressure rises, two of them exceeding 10 mmHg.[1] The renal excretion of unmetabolised methyldopa was reduced by 88% and 79% when methyldopa was given with **ferrous sulfate** and **ferrous gluconate**, respectively.[1] A further study found that if the **ferrous sulfate** was given 2 hours before, one hour before or with the methyldopa, its bioavailability was reduced by 42%, 55%, and 83%, respectively.[2] An *in vitro* study suggests that ferric chloride but not iron polymaltose would interact with methyldopa.[3]

Mechanism

The increase in the metabolic sulfonation of the methyldopa seems to have a part to play in the interaction. However, it appears that methyldopa chelates or complexes with the iron in the gut, reducing its absorption by about 50%.[1,4,5] It has been suggested that if iron is in the form of a complex such as iron polymaltose, it will not form complexes with methyldopa.[3]

Importance and management

Information is limited, but an interaction between methyldopa and iron compounds appears to be established and clinically important. Monitor the effects of concurrent use and increase the methyldopa dose as necessary. Separating the doses by up to 2 hours apparently only partially reduces the effects of this interaction. Ferrous gluconate appears to interact like ferrous sulfate, and all iron salts would be expected to interact similarly, but iron in the form of complexes with carbohydrates such as iron polymaltose is predicted not to interact.

1. Campbell N, Paddock V, Sundaram R. Alteration of methyldopa absorption, metabolism, and blood pressure control caused by ferrous sulfate and ferrous gluconate. *Clin Pharmacol Ther* (1988) 43, 381–6.
2. Campbell NRC, Hasinoff BB. Iron supplements: a common cause of drug interactions. *Br J Clin Pharmacol* (1991) 31, 251–55.
3. Burckhardt-Herold S, Klotz J, Funk F, Büchi R, Petrig-Schaffland J, Geisser P. Interactions between iron (III)-hydroxide polymaltose complex and commonly used drugs: simulations and *in vitro* studies. *Arzneimittelforschung* (2007) 57, 360–9.
4. Campbell NRC, Campbell RRA, Hasinoff BB. Ferrous sulfate reduces methyldopa absorption: methyldopa: iron complex formation as a likely mechanism. *Clin Invest Med* (1990) 13, 329–32.
5. Greene RJ, Hall AD, Hider RC. The interaction of orally administered iron with levodopa and methyldopa therapy. *J Pharm Pharmacol* (1990) 42, 502–4.

Methyldopa + Nasal decongestants

Phenylpropanolamine and related drugs might be expected to cause a blood pressure rise in patients taking methyldopa, and an isolated case report describes such a reaction. The mydriatic effects of ephedrine are reported to be reduced by methyldopa.

Clinical evidence, mechanism, importance and management

A man with renal hypertension, whose blood pressure was well controlled with methyldopa 250 mg twice daily and oxprenolol 160 mg three times daily, had a rise in blood pressure from under 140/80 mmHg to 200/150 mmHg within 2 days of starting to take two tablets of *Triogesic* (**phenylpropanolamine** 12.5 mg and paracetamol 500 mg) three times daily. His blood pressure fell when the *Triogesic* was withdrawn.[1]

The reason for this is uncertain. One suggestion is that the methyldopa causes the replacement of noradrenaline at adrenergic nerve endings by methylnoradrenaline, which has weaker pressor (alpha) activity but greater vasodilator (beta) activity. With the vasodilator activity blocked by the oxprenolol, the vasoconstrictor (pressor) activity of the **phenylpropanolamine** would be unopposed and exaggerated. Alternatively it could have been that he was unusually sensitive to the pressor effects of **phenylpropanolamine**.

In a study in 5 hypertensive patients taking methyldopa 2 to 3 g daily, the rise in blood pressure in response to **tyramine** was doubled.[2] In another study the pressor effect of **tyramine** was 50/16 mmHg, compared with 18/10 mmHg before methyldopa was given.[3]

Despite the information derived from the studies with tyramine and the single report cited, there seems to be nothing else in the literature to suggest that phenylpropanolamine and other indirectly-acting sympathomimetics normally cause an adverse reaction with methyldopa. One report briefly mentions that the antihypertensive effects of various drugs, including methyldopa, were not affected by **diethylpropion**.[4] In contrast, one report suggests that methyldopa may reduce the effects of other related drugs. In 9 patients with untreated hypertension, the normal mydriatic effects of **ephedrine** were reduced by 54% after they started treatment with methyldopa 500 mg to 1.5 g daily.[5] The clinical relevance of this finding is unclear.

1. McLaren EH. Severe hypertension produced by interaction of phenylpropanolamine with methyldopa and oxprenolol. *BMJ* (1976) 3, 283–4.
2. Pettinger W, Horwitz D, Spector S, Sjoerdsma A. Enhancement by methyldopa of tyramine sensitivity in man. *Nature* (1963) 200, 1107–8.
3. Dollery CT, Harington M, Hodge JV. Haemodynamic studies with methyldopa: effect on cardiac output and response to pressor amines. *Br Heart J* (1963) 25, 670–6.
4. Seedat YK, Reddy J. Diethylpropion hydrochloride (Tenuate, Dospan) in the treatment of obese hypertensive patients. *S Afr Med J* (1974) 48, 569.
5. Sneddon JM, Turner P. Ephedrine mydriasis in hypertension and the response to treatment. *Clin Pharmacol Ther* (1969) 10, 64–71.

Methyldopa + Oxazepam

A single, unsubstantiated case report suggests that blood pressure control with methyldopa may possibly be made more difficult in the presence of oxazepam.

Clinical evidence, mechanism, importance and management

A 54-year-old woman with insomnia and essential hypertension had unexplained variability in blood pressure while taking methyldopa 750 mg three times daily and a thiazide diuretic. Within a week of stopping oxazepam 60 mg at night, she developed grand mal convulsions and hypertension (190/90 mmHg standing, 240/140 mmHg lying). Her hypertension was then successfully controlled by switching to atenolol and prazosin. The authors of this report suggest that short-acting benzodiazepines such as oxazepam can cause transient hypotension after a dose, but that *hyper*tension may occur on withdrawal. These effects may complicate the management of hypertension.[1] The general importance of this possible interaction is not established, but it seems likely to be limited.

1. Stokes GS. Can short-acting benzodiazepines exacerbate essential hypertension? *Cardiovasc Rev Rep* (1989) 10, 60–1.

Methyldopa + Phenothiazines

The hypotensive adverse effects of chlorpromazine and other phenothiazines may be additive with the antihypertensive effects of methyldopa. Patients may feel faint and dizzy if they stand up quickly. An isolated report describes paradoxical hypertension in a patient given methyldopa and trifluoperazine.

Clinical evidence

In one study, 8 normotensive patients given methyldopa 500 mg to 1 g daily with **chlorpromazine** 200 to 400 mg daily for schizophrenia experienced orthostatic dizziness and had reductions in their standing systolic blood pressure.[1] In contrast, an isolated report describes a paradoxical *rise* in blood pressure in a patient with systemic lupus erythematosus and renal failure when methyldopa and **trifluoperazine** were given. When the **trifluoperazine** was stopped, the blood pressure fell.[2]

Mechanism

Simple addition of the hypotensive effects of both drugs seems to be the explanation for the increased hypotension and orthostasis. The suggested explanation for the hypertensive interaction with methyldopa and trifluoperazine is that the phenothiazine blocked the reuptake of the 'false transmitter' (alpha-methyl noradrenaline) that is produced when methyldopa is given.[2]

Importance and management

The increased hypotension and orthostasis that can occur if chlorpromazine or other phenothiazines are used with antihypertensive drugs such as methyldopa is established. Note that, of the phenothiazines, **levomepromazine** is particularly associated with postural hypotension. Warn patients that they may feel faint and dizzy particularly during the initial stages of concurrent use, and that if this occurs they should lie down, and that they should remain lying down until symptoms abate completely. Dose adjustments may be necessary.

1. Chouinard G, Pinard G, Prenoveau Y, Tetreault L. Alpha methyldopa-chlorpromazine interaction in schizophrenic patients. *Curr Ther Res* (1973) 15, 60–72.
2. Westhervelt FB, Atuk NO. Methyldopa-induced hypertension. *JAMA* (1974) 227, 557.

Methyldopa + Phenoxybenzamine

An isolated case report describes a patient who had undergone bilateral lumbar sympathectomy who developed total urinary incontinence when taking methyldopa and phenoxybenzamine.

Clinical evidence, mechanism, importance and management

A woman who had previously had bilateral lumbar sympathectomy for Raynaud's disease developed total urinary incontinence when given methyldopa 500 mg to 1.5 g daily in divided doses with phenoxybenzamine 12.5 mg daily, but not when she was taking either drug alone. This would seem to be the outcome of the additive effects of the sympathectomy and the two drugs on the sympathetic control of the bladder sphincters.[1] Stress incontinence has previously been described with these drugs alone, and therefore the general importance of this interaction is probably small.

1. Fernandez PG, Sahni S, Galway BA, Granter S, McDonald J. Urinary incontinence due to interaction of phenoxybenzamine and α-methyldopa. *Can Med Assoc J* (1981) 124, 174.

Methyldopa + Tricyclic and related antidepressants

The antihypertensive effects of methyldopa are not normally adversely affected by desipramine, but an isolated report describes hypertension, tachycardia, tremor and agitation in a man taking methyldopa and amitriptyline. The tetracyclic mianserin does not appear to interact with methyldopa to a clinically significant extent.

Clinical evidence

A man with hypertension, taking methyldopa 250 mg three times daily and a thiazide diuretic, experienced tremor, agitation, tachycardia (148 bpm) and hypertension (a rise from under 150/90 mmHg to 170/110 mmHg) within 10 days of starting to take **amitriptyline** 25 mg three times daily. A week after stopping all treatment his pulse rate was 100 bpm and his blood pressure 160/90 mmHg.[1] In contrast, a double-blind, crossover study in 5 subjects (one with mild hypertension) found that **desipramine** 25 mg three times daily for 3 days had no significant effect on the hypotensive effects of a single 750-mg dose of methyldopa.[2] Another study in 3 hypertensive patients taking methyldopa 2.5 to 3 g daily found that **desipramine** 75 mg daily for 5 to 6 days did not antagonise the action of methyldopa. In fact, the blood pressure fell slightly.[3] **Mianserin** 20 mg three times daily for 2 weeks had no effect on the control of blood pressure in 6 patients receiving methyldopa, although 2 patients developed symptomatic hypotension after the first dose of **mianserin**.[4,5]

Mechanism

Not understood. Antagonism of the antihypertensive actions of methyldopa by tricyclic antidepressants is seen in *animals* and it seems to occur within the brain.[6,7]

Importance and management

Normally no adverse interaction occurs. However, in view of the case report consider an interaction as a possible cause if a patient taking a tricyclic antidepressant appears unresponsive to methyldopa. Note that methyldopa sometimes induces depression, and so it should generally be avoided in depressed patients.

1. White AG. Methyldopa and amitriptyline. *Lancet* (1965) ii, 441.
2. Reid JL, Porsius AJ, Zamboulis C, Polak G, Hamilton CA, Dean CR. The effects of desmethylimipramine on the pharmacological actions of alpha methyldopa in man. *Eur J Clin Pharmacol* (1979) 16, 75–80.
3. Mitchell JR, Cavanaugh JH, Arias L, Oates JA. Guanethidine and related agents. III. Antagonism by drugs which inhibit the norepinephrine pump in man. *J Clin Invest* (1970) 49, 1596–1604.
4. Elliott HL, Whiting B, Reid JL. Assessment of the interaction between mianserin and centrally-acting antihypertensive drugs. *Br J Clin Pharmacol* (1983) 15, 323S–328S.
5. Elliott HL, McLean K, Sumner DJ, Reid JL. Absence of an effect of mianserin on the actions of clonidine or methyldopa in hypertensive patients. *Eur J Clin Pharmacol* (1983) 24, 15–19.
6. van Spanning HW, van Zwieten PA. The interaction between alpha-methyl-dopa and tricyclic antidepressants. *Int J Clin Pharmacol Biopharm* (1975) 11, 65–7.
7. van Zwieten PA. Interaction between centrally acting hypotensive drugs and tricyclic antidepressants. *Arch Int Pharmacodyn Ther* (1975) 214, 12–30.

Minoxidil + Glibenclamide (Glyburide)

There is some evidence that a 5-mg dose of glibenclamide, but not a 2.5-mg dose, may reduce the hypotensive effect of minoxidil.

Clinical evidence, mechanism, importance and management

A single-dose study in 9 healthy subjects found that glibenclamide 2.5 mg did not alter the hypotensive effect of oral minoxidil 5 mg. However, in a further 4 subjects a 5-mg dose of glibenclamide appeared to cause some loss in the hypotensive effect of minoxidil, but this was not statistically significant. The authors therefore suggested that this interaction may be dose-related. The suggested reason for these effects is that these two drugs have opposing effects on the potassium channels of the smooth muscle of blood vessels.[1] In this study, subjects were pre-treated with propranolol to prevent reflex tachycardia when given minoxidil, which is how minoxidil is used clinically.[1] What is not yet clear is whether any interaction occurs between minoxidil and glibenclamide in a clinical setting.

1. Stein CM, Brown N, Carlson MG, Campbell P, Wood AJJ. Coadministration of glyburide and minoxidil, drugs with opposing effects on potassium channels. *Clin Pharmacol Ther* (1997) 61, 662–8.

Minoxidil + Miscellaneous

The manufacturers of minoxidil note that excessive blood pressure reductions and possibly orthostatic hypotension may occur if minoxidil is given to patients taking guanethidine, because of the adrenergic blocking effects of guanethidine.[1,2] The UK manufacturer of oral minoxidil specifically states that guanethidine should be stopped as far in advance as possible before minoxidil is started; however, if this is not possible, they advise that minoxidil should be started in hospital with close monitoring for excessive blood pressure-lowering effects.[1] If excessive hypotension occurs with minoxidil, this should *not* be treated with adrenaline (epinephrine) or noradrenaline (norepinephrine), because this may result in excessive tachycardia. They advise that intravenous sodium chloride 0.9% should be used.[1]

Note that there is a theoretical possibility that topical minoxidil may also interact with guanethidine, see 'Minoxidil; Topical + Miscellaneous', below.

1. Loniten Tablets (Minoxidil). Pharmacia Ltd. UK Summary of product characteristics, February 2010.
2. Minoxidil. Watson Pharmaceuticals, Inc. US Prescribing information, October 2002.

Minoxidil; Topical + Miscellaneous

The absorption of topical minoxidil is increased by topical tretinoin and also possibly by topical corticosteroids, dithranol and soft paraffin. Increased minoxidil absorption could possibly potentiate the hypotensive effects of vasodilators.

Clinical evidence, mechanism, importance and management

A study in 19 healthy subjects found that the absorption of topical minoxidil was increased by almost threefold by the use of topical **tretinoin** 0.05% applied one hour before the minoxidil.[1] In another study, in 29 male patients, the use of topical minoxidil 5% with **tretinoin** 0.01% daily in 15 patients was found to be as effective and safe as the use of minoxidil 5% alone twice daily in the other 14 patients for the treatment of male pattern baldness.[2]

The manufacturer notes that *topical* drugs that alter the stratum corneum barrier, such as **corticosteroids**, **tretinoin**, **dithranol**, or **white** or **yellow soft paraffin**, could result in increased absorption of minoxidil if both drugs are applied concurrently. They suggest that, theoretically, one possible effect of minoxidil absorption would be potentiation of orthostatic hypotension caused by **vasodilators**.[3] The exact drugs are not stated but this caution would be expected to cover drugs such as the **nitrates** and **hydralazine**.

1. Ferry JJ, Forbes KK, VanderLugt JT, Szpunar GJ. Influence of tretinoin on the percutaneous absorption of minoxidil from an aqueous topical solution. *Clin Pharmacol Ther* (1990) 47, 439–46.
2. Shin HS, Won CH, Lee SH, Kwon OS, Kim KH, Eun HC. Efficacy of 5% minoxidil versus combined 5% minoxidil and 0.01% tretinoin for male pattern hair loss: a randomized, double-blind, comparative clinical trial. *Am J Clin Dermatol* (2007) 8, 285–90.
3. Regaine for Men Gel (Minoxidil). McNeil Ltd. UK Summary of product characteristics, April 2008.

Moxisylyte + Miscellaneous

There is a theoretical possibility of increased blood pressure lowering effects if moxisylyte is used with antihypertensives or tricyclic antidepressants.

Clinical evidence, mechanism, importance and management

Moxisylyte is an alpha-1, and to a lesser extent, an alpha-2 blocker, which may be used orally as a peripheral vasodilator in Raynaud's syndrome. The manufacturer suggests that if moxisylyte is used by patients taking **antihypertensives**, it may theoretically potentiate the antihypertensive effect of these drugs, although at the recommended doses this has not been reported.[1]

The manufacturer also says that **tricyclic antidepressants** might increase any hypotensive effect of moxisylyte.[1]

For further commentary on the use of two or more drugs with antihypertensive effects, see 'Antihypertensives + Other drugs that affect blood pressure', p.1054.

1. Opilon (Moxisylyte hydrochloride). Archimedes Pharma UK Ltd. UK Summary of product characteristics, October 2008.

Moxonidine + Hydrochlorothiazide

No clinically significant pharmacokinetic interaction occurs between moxonidine and hydrochlorothiazide; however, the blood pressure lowering effects of the combination is greater than that seen with either drug alone.

Clinical evidence, mechanism, importance and management

In a study in 18 healthy subjects, no clinically relevant pharmacokinetic interaction was seen at steady state between moxonidine 200 micrograms twice daily and hydrochlorothiazide 25 mg twice daily.[1] A double-blind, placebo-controlled study found that when moxonidine 400 micrograms daily was given with hydrochlorothiazide 25 mg daily an increased blood pressure lowering effect was seen, compared with either drug alone. A mean reduction of 27/16 mmHg was noted with the combination, compared with 13/9 mmHg, 20/12 mmHg, and 22/13 mmHg for placebo, moxonidine and hydrochlorothiazide, respectively.[2] No particular precautions seem necessary on concurrent use, unless the combined effect on blood pressure is greater than desired.

1. Weimann H-J, Pabst G, Weber W. Lack of pharmacokinetic interaction between moxonidine and hydrochlorothiazide. *Eur J Clin Pharmacol* (1992) 43, 209–10.
2. Frei M, Küster L, Gardosch von Krosigk PP, Koch HF, Küppers H. Moxonidine and hydrochlorothiazide in combination: a synergistic antihypertensive effect. *J Cardiovasc Pharmacol* (1994) 24, (Suppl 1), S25–S28.

Moxonidine + Miscellaneous

No clinically significant pharmacokinetic interactions occur with moxonidine and digoxin, glibenclamide (glyburide), moclobemide, or quinidine.

Clinical evidence, mechanism, importance and management

(a) Digoxin

In 15 healthy subjects, no clinically relevant pharmacokinetic interaction was seen at steady state between moxonidine 200 micrograms twice daily and digoxin 200 micrograms daily.[1]

(b) Glibenclamide (Glyburide)

In 18 healthy subjects, glibenclamide 2.5 mg daily had no effect on the steady-state pharmacokinetics of moxonidine 200 micrograms twice daily. There was a minor 12% decrease in the AUC of glibenclamide, and a 14% increase in its clearance, but these changes are unlikely to be of any clinical relevance.[2]

(c) Moclobemide

A study found no pharmacokinetic interaction occurred when healthy subjects were given moxonidine 400 micrograms daily and a single 300-mg dose of moclobemide. Moxonidine alone or with moclobemide did not significantly affect cognitive function.[3]

(d) Quinidine

In a single-dose study in 6 healthy subjects, quinidine sulfate 400 mg, given one hour before moxonidine 200 micrograms, caused a minor 11% increase in the AUC of moxonidine and decreased its clearance by 10%. These small changes are unlikely to be of any clinical relevance.[4]

1. Pabst G, Weimann H-J, Weber W. Lack of pharmacokinetic interactions between moxonidine and digoxin. *Clin Pharmacokinet* (1992) 23, 477–81.
2. Müller M, Weimann H-J, Eden G, Weber W, Michaelis K, Dilger C, Achtert G. Steady state investigation of possible pharmacokinetic interactions of moxonidine and glibenclamide. *Eur J Drug Metab Pharmacokinet* (1993) 18, 277–83.
3. Wesnes K, Simpson PM, Jansson B, Grahnén A, Wemann H-J, Küppers H. Moxonidine and cognitive function: interactions with moclobemide and lorazepam. *Eur J Clin Pharmacol* (1997) 52, 351–8.
4. Wise SD, Chan C, Schaefer HG, He MM, Pouliquen IJ, Mitchell MI. Quinidine does not affect the renal clearance of moxonidine. *Br J Clin Pharmacol* (2002) 54, 251–4.

Nicorandil + Miscellaneous

Neither cimetidine nor rifampicin had any clinically relevant effect on the pharmacokinetics of nicorandil. Nicorandil did not alter the anticoagulant effects of acenocoumarol. Although *animal* studies suggest antagonism of effects, a study in patients found no pharmacodynamic interaction between nicorandil and glibenclamide. Nicorandil may potentiate the hypotensive effects of other vasodilators, tricyclic antidepressants and alcohol. Gastrointestinal perforations have been reported during the concurrent use of nicorandil and corticosteroids.

Clinical evidence, mechanism, importance and management

(a) Acenocoumarol

Nicorandil 10 mg twice daily for 4 days then 20 mg twice daily for 7 days did not alter the INR in 11 patients stabilised on acenocoumarol.[1]

(b) Cimetidine

Cimetidine 400 mg twice daily for 7 days had no effect on the pharmacokinetics of nicorandil 20 mg twice daily for 7 days, except that the nicorandil AUC showed a minor 10% increase, which is not clinically important.[1]

(c) Corticosteroids

Gastrointestinal perforations have been reported in patients given nicorandil and corticosteroids. Therefore, the manufacturer advises caution if concurrent use is considered.[2]

(d) Glibenclamide

Studies in *animals* have indicated that there may be antagonism between nicorandil and glibenclamide. However, in a study, 8 patients with diabetes and angina taking glibenclamide, and 11 similar patients not receiving glibenclamide, were given nicorandil 15 mg daily for more than 8 weeks. In contrast to the findings in the *animal* studies, glibenclamide did not cause inhibition of the anti-anginal effects of nicorandil, nor was there any disturbance of diabetic control.[3]

(e) Miscellaneous drugs

Combined data from clinical studies in 1 152 patients taking nicorandil found no evidence of increased adverse effects or an increased number of withdrawals in patients taking unnamed **beta blockers** (210 patients), **calcium-channel blockers** (117 patients), **long-acting nitrates** (130 patients), **diltiazem** (91 patients), **verapamil** (9 patients), **amiodarone** (23 patients) or **molsidomine** (30 patients). It has also been reported that unnamed **antihypertensives**, **antidiabetic** or **lipid-regulating drugs** do not appear to interact adversely with nicorandil.[4] No adverse ECG effects have been seen (including QT or ST segment modifications) with nicorandil.[4] However, the manufacturers suggest that nicorandil may possibly potentiate the blood pressure-lowering effects of other **vasodilators**, **tricyclic antidepressants** or **alcohol**.[2] For further discussion on additive blood pressure lowering effects, consider also 'Antihypertensives + Other drugs that affect blood pressure', p.1054. For mention that phosphodiesterase inhibitors (e.g. **sildenafil**, **tadalafil**, **vardenafil**) should not be used with nicorandil, see 'Phosphodiesterase type-5 inhibitors + Nitrates', p.1545.

(f) Rifampicin

Rifampicin 600 mg daily for 5 days had no effect on the pharmacokinetics of nicorandil 20 mg twice daily for 5 days, except for a minor 17% decrease in the elimination half-life, which is not clinically important.[1]

1. Frydman A. Pharmacokinetic profile of nicorandil in humans: an overview. *J Cardiovasc Pharmacol* (1992) 20 (Suppl 3), S34–S44.
2. Ikorel (Nicorandil). Zentiva. UK Summary of product characteristics, November 2014.
3. Hata N, Takano M, Kunimi T, Kishida H, Takano T. Lack of antagonism between nicorandil and sulfonylurea in stable angina pectoris. *Int J Clin Pharmacol Res* (2001) 21, 59–63.
4. Witchitz S, Darmon J-Y. Nicorandil safety in the long-term treatment of coronary heart disease. *Cardiovasc Drugs Ther* (1995) 9, 237–43.

Pentoxifylline + Cimetidine

Cimetidine increases pentoxifylline levels to a moderate extent, which may increase the incidence of adverse effects.

Clinical evidence, mechanism, importance and management

A study in 10 healthy subjects found that the mean steady-state plasma levels of controlled-release pentoxifylline 400 mg every 8 hours were raised by about 27% when cimetidine 300 mg four times daily for 7 days was added.[1] Adverse effects such as headache, nausea, and vomiting were said to be more common and bothersome while taking the cimetidine.[1]

The reason for this interaction is not known. However, cimetidine is known to inhibit the metabolism of theophylline (see 'Theophylline + H_2-receptor antagonists', p.1445, to which pentoxifylline is structurally related.

The findings of this study suggest that this interaction may be clinically relevant. If cimetidine is required in a patient taking pentoxifylline, monitor for adverse effects, and decrease the pentoxifylline dose if problems occur.

1. Mauro VF, Mauro LS, Hageman JH. Alteration of pentoxifylline pharmacokinetics by cimetidine. *J Clin Pharmacol* (1988) 28, 649–54.

Pentoxifylline + Ciprofloxacin

Evidence from one study suggests that ciprofloxacin increases the levels of pentoxifylline, and may increase the incidence of adverse effects. In some clinical studies ciprofloxacin has been used to boost the levels of pentoxifylline.

Clinical evidence

Because patients taking pentoxifylline and ciprofloxacin often complained of headache, the possibility of a pharmacokinetic interaction was studied in 6 healthy subjects.

The study found that ciprofloxacin 500 mg daily for 3 days increased the peak serum levels of a single 400-mg dose of pentoxifylline by almost 60% (from 114.5 to 179.5 nanograms/mL), and increased the AUC by 15%. All 6 subjects complained of a frontal headache.[1]

Mechanism

The evidence suggests that ciprofloxacin inhibits the metabolism of the pentoxifylline (a xanthine derivative) by the liver. Studies in *animals* found that ciprofloxacin inhibited the cytochrome P450 isoenzyme CYP1A2 which is involved in the metabolism of pentoxifylline.[2]

Importance and management

Information on this interaction and its clinical relevance is limited. The author of the pharmacokinetic study suggests that, if the drugs need to be used together, the dose of pentoxifylline should be halved.[1] In the absence of other information, if a short-course of ciprofloxacin is required in a patient taking pentoxifylline, this may be a sensible precaution. Alternatively, because the increase in AUC was minor, it may be sufficient to recommend a reduction in pentoxifylline dose only in those who experience adverse effects (e.g. nausea, headache). Note that ciprofloxacin has been used to boost pentoxifylline levels in studies investigating the possible therapeutic value of the ability of pentoxifylline to inhibit various cytokines. For example, ciprofloxacin 500 mg twice daily was used with pentoxifylline 800 mg three times daily for up to one year in patients with myelodysplastic syndrome.[3]

1. Cleary JD. Ciprofloxacin (CIPRO) and pentoxifylline (PTF): a clinically significant drug interaction. *Pharmacotherapy* (1992) 12, 259–60.
2. Peterson TC, Peterson MR, Wornell PA, Blanchard MG, Gonzalez FJ. Role of CYP1A2 and CYP2E1 in the pentoxifylline ciprofloxacin drug interaction. *Biochem Pharmacol* (2004) 68, 395–402.
3. Raza A, Qawi H, Lisak L, Andric T, Dar S, Andrews C, Venugopal P, Gezer S, Gregory S, Loew J, Robin E, Rifkin S, Hsu W-T, Huang R-W. Patients with myelodysplastic syndromes benefit from palliative therapy with amifostine, pentoxifylline, and ciprofloxacin with or without dexamethasone. *Blood* (2000) 95, 1580–87.

Perhexiline + SSRIs

Case reports describe an increase in perhexiline levels resulting in toxicity when citalopram, fluoxetine or paroxetine were given.

Clinical evidence, mechanism, importance and management

An 86-year-old woman taking perhexiline was admitted to hospital because of ataxia, falls, lethargy, nausea, and an inability to cope at home. She had started to take **paroxetine** 20 mg daily 5 weeks earlier. Her serum perhexiline levels were 2.02 mg/L (reference range 0.15 to 0.6 mg/L).[1] Perhexiline toxicity was also seen in two other elderly women, following the use of **paroxetine** in one case, and **fluoxetine** in the other. The perhexiline serum levels fell when both drugs were stopped, but in one case the fall was very slow.[2] Another case report describes toxicity and raised perhexiline levels in an elderly man shortly after he started taking **citalopram**.[3]

The reason for the rise in perhexiline levels is not known, but it seems likely that these SSRIs can inhibit its metabolism, probably by the cytochrome P450 isoenzyme CYP2D6, although note that citalopram is usually considered to be a weak inhibitor of this isoenzyme. The general importance of these interactions is not known, but it would seem prudent to monitor the outcome of concurrent use for perhexiline toxicity and consider monitoring perhexiline levels where possible. The perhexiline dose may need to be reduced. More study is needed.

1. Alderman CP. Perhexiline-paroxetine interaction. *Aust J Hosp Pharm* (1998) 28, 254–5.
2. Alderman CP, Hundertmark JD, Soetratma TW. Interaction of serotonin re-uptake inhibitors with perhexiline. *Aust N Z J Psychiatry* (1997) 31, 601–3.
3. Nyfort-Hansen K. Perhexiline toxicity related to citalopram use. *Med J Aust* (2002) 176, 560–61.

Ranolazine + Azoles

Ketoconazole raises ranolazine levels. Other azoles are expected to interact similarly.

Clinical evidence

In a double-blind, randomised study, healthy subjects were given slow-release ranolazine 375 mg twice daily for 9 days, with ketoconazole 200 mg twice daily on days 5 to 9. The same study was repeated with ranolazine 1 g twice daily. It was found that ketoconazole increased the AUC, levels (mean, peak and trough) and half-life of ranolazine by 2.5- to 4.5-fold. The most common adverse events were headaches, dizziness and nausea. In some patients the higher dose of ranolazine with ketoconazole resulted in intolerable adverse effects.[1]

Mechanism

Ranolazine is a substrate of cytochrome P450 isoenzyme CYP3A4, of which ketoconazole is a potent inhibitor. Concurrent use therefore raises ranolazine levels. All azoles are, to a greater or lesser extent, inhibitors of this isoenzyme and may therefore interact similarly.

Importance and management

Information regarding an interaction between ranolazine and ketoconazole appears to be limited to this study, but what is known is in line with the known effects of these drugs, and is therefore established. The dose-related adverse effects of ranolazine such as nausea and dizziness are increased by ketoconazole. Further, increases in plasma levels of ranolazine may cause significant QT prolongation and the possible risk of arrhythmias (see also, 'Drugs that prolong the QT interval + Other drugs that prolong the QT interval', p.272).

The manufacturers of ranolazine contraindicate its use with ketoconazole and other potent CYP3A4 inhibitors. Others they specifically name include **itraconazole**, **posaconazole**, and **voriconazole**.[2,3]

Fluconazole is only a moderate inhibitor of CYP3A4, and therefore the US manufacturer recommends that the dose of ranolazine should be limited to 500 mg twice daily,[2] whereas the UK manufacturer recommends careful dose titration of ranolazine.[3] There appear to be no recommendations about **miconazole**; however, a large proportion of miconazole oral gel (both prescription and non-prescription doses) may be swallowed and therefore adequate systemic absorption may occur to produce an interaction. It would therefore seem prudent to monitor concurrent use closely. For systemic miconazole, similar precautions to those recommended for fluconazole would seem prudent.

1. Jerling M, Huan B-L, Leung K, Chu N, Abdallah H, Hussein Z. Studies to investigate the pharmacokinetic interactions between ranolazine and ketoconazole, diltiazem or simvastatin during combined administration in healthy subjects. J Clin Pharmacol. (2005) 45, 422–33.
2. Ranexa (Ranolazine). Gilead Sciences, Inc. US Prescribing Information, December 2011.
3. Ranexa (Ranolazine). A. Menarini Pharma UK SRL. UK Summary of product characteristics, April 2012.

Ranolazine + Calcium-channel blockers

Diltiazem and verapamil raise ranolazine levels, which increases the risk of ranolazine adverse effects. However, concurrent use may be beneficial.

Clinical evidence

(a) Diltiazem

In a placebo-controlled study in 12 healthy subjects, diltiazem 60 mg three times daily was given to 12 healthy subjects for 7 days with ranolazine 240 mg three times daily on days 4 to 7. Ranolazine did not alter the pharmacokinetics of diltiazem, but diltiazem increased the AUC and maximum plasma level of ranolazine by 85% and twofold, respectively. A further study using modified-release diltiazem 180 mg, 240 mg, and 360 mg daily, and a slow-release preparation of ranolazine 1 g twice daily, resulted in increases in the AUC of ranolazine of 52%, 93%, and 139%, respectively.[1] However, a clinical study in patients with angina who were taking diltiazem 180 mg daily, with amlodipine or atenolol, and were given ranolazine or placebo, found that ranolazine 750 mg or 1000 mg twice daily provided additional anti-anginal efficacy with minimal haemodynamic effects.[2]

(b) Verapamil

The plasma levels of ranolazine are reported to be increased twofold by the concurrent use of verapamil 120 mg three times daily.[3]

Mechanism

Ranolazine is a substrate of cytochrome P450 isoenzyme CYP3A4. Diltiazem and verapamil are moderate inhibitors of this isoenzyme, and therefore increase ranolazine levels. Ranolazine is also a substrate of P-glycoprotein and therefore verapamil, which also inhibits P-glycoprotein, may increase its levels by this mechanism as well.

Importance and management

Information regarding an interaction between ranolazine and diltiazem or verapamil is limited, but what is known is in line with the known effects of these drugs, and is therefore established. The dose-related adverse effects of ranolazine such as nausea and dizziness may be increased by concurrent use of drugs that increase its plasma levels. Further, increases in plasma levels of ranolazine may cause significant QT prolongation and the possible risk of arrhythmias (see also, 'Drugs that prolong the QT interval + Other drugs that prolong the QT interval', p.272).

The US manufacturer recommends that the dose of ranolazine should be limited to 500 mg twice daily when given to patients also taking moderate CYP3A4 inhibitors including diltiazem, verapamil.[3] The UK manufacturer recommends careful dose titration of ranolazine in patients taking diltiazem or verapamil, and suggests that lower ranolazine doses may be needed in the presence of verapamil.[4]

There appears to be no information about the use of ranolazine with other calcium-channel blockers, but as these drugs are not inhibitors of CYP3A4 or P-glycoprotein, a pharmacokinetic interaction would not be expected.

1. Jerling M, Huan B-L, Leung K, Chu N, Abdallah H, Hussein Z. Studies to investigate the pharmacokinetic interactions between ranolazine and ketoconazole, diltiazem or simvastatin during combined administration in healthy subjects. J Clin Pharmacol. (2005) 45, 422–33.
2. Chaitman BR, Pepine CJ, Parker JO, Skopal J, Chumakova G, Kuch J, Wang W, Skettino SL, Wolff AA, for the Combination Assessment of Ranolazine In Stable Angina (CARISA) investigators. Effects of ranolazine with atenolol, amlodipine, or diltiazem on exercise tolerance and angina frequency in patients with severe chronic angina: a randomized controlled trial. *JAMA* (2004) 291, 309–16.
3. Ranexa (Ranolazine). Gilead Sciences, Inc. US Prescribing Information, December 2011.
4. Ranexa (Ranolazine). A. Menarini Pharma UK SRL. UK Summary of product characteristics, April 2012.

Ranolazine + CYP2D6 inhibitors or substrates

Ranolazine increases the levels of the CYP2D6 substrate, metoprolol. Other CYP2D6 substrates are expected to be similarly affected. Paroxetine does not affect ranolazine levels to a clinically significant extent.

Clinical evidence, mechanism, importance and management

(a) CYP2D6 inhibitors

Paroxetine has been reported to increase the average steady-state plasma concentrations of ranolazine 1 g twice daily by 20%.[1,2] Ranolazine is partially metabolised by the cytochrome P450 isoenzyme CYP2D6, which **paroxetine** inhibits. Therefore, the UK manufacturer predicts that a potent inhibitor of CYP2D6, like **paroxetine**, could increase the AUC of ranolazine 500 mg twice daily (therapeutic dose) by about 62%.[1] However, as CYP2D6 is not the main route of metabolism, only very modest effects are seen, and no dose adjustment is necessary.[1,2]

(b) CYP2D6 substrates

The UK manufacturer of ranolazine reports that in a study, ranolazine 750 mg twice daily increased the plasma concentration of metoprolol by 80%, suggesting that ranolazine is a weak inhibitor of the cytochrome P450 isoenzyme CYP2D6, by which metoprolol is metabolised.[1] The manufacturers therefore predict that the levels of other drugs metabolised by CYP2D6, such as **flecainide**, **propafenone**, the **tricyclic antidepressants** and some **antipsychotics**, may be increased by ranolazine and that lower doses of these drugs may be required.[1,2]

1. Ranexa (Ranolazine). A. Menarini Pharma UK SRL. UK Summary of product characteristics, April 2012.
2. Ranexa (Ranolazine). Gilead Sciences, Inc. US Prescribing Information, December 2011.

Ranolazine + CYP3A4 inducers

Rifampicin (a CYP3A4 and P-glycoprotein inducer) markedly reduces ranolazine levels. Other CYP3A4 inducers are predicted to interact similarly.

Clinical evidence, mechanism, importance and management

Rifampicin 600 mg daily is reported to decrease the steady-state plasma levels of ranolazine 1 g twice daily by about 95%. This is due to the induction of the metabolism of ranolazine by cytochrome P450 isoenzyme CYP3A4 and possibly also by P-glycoprotein. Such a marked reduction in levels would be expected to abolish the effects of ranolazine and the manufacturers of ranolazine therefore contraindicate concurrent use.[1,2] The manufacturers recommend avoiding the concurrent use of ranolazine with other CYP3A4 inducers, including **carbamazepine**, **phenobarbital**, **phenytoin**, **rifabutin**, **rifapentine** and **St John's wort**.[1,2] In the absence of any information on the magnitude of the effect of these CYP3A4 inducers on ranolazine levels, this seems prudent.

1. Ranexa (Ranolazine). Gilead Sciences, Inc. US Prescribing Information, December 2011.
2. Ranexa (Ranolazine). A. Menarini Pharma UK SRL. UK Summary of product characteristics, April 2012.

Ranolazine + Miscellaneous

Ranolazine may increase concentrations of ciclosporin and digoxin. Ciclosporin may also increase ranolazine concentrations. In theory ranolazine may increase the concentrations of bupropion, efavirenz and cyclophosphamide. The concurrent use of ranolazine and moderate or potent inhibitors of CYP3A4, will result in increased concentrations of ranolazine, and can predispose the patient to adverse effects including QT interval prolongation. Cimetidine does not interact with ranolazine to a clinically significant extent. Ranolazine may increase the concentrations of simvastatin.

Clinical evidence, mechanism, importance and management

(a) Ciclosporin

Ranolazine inhibits P-glycoprotein and has been shown to raise digoxin concentrations (see *Digoxin*, below). However, ranolazine is also a substrate of P-glycoprotein and plasma concentrations of ranolazine are increased by inhibitors of P-glycoprotein, such as ciclosporin. The manufacturers of ranolazine therefore advise caution if it is given to patients taking ciclosporin, which is also a P-glycoprotein inhibitor [and substrate].[1,2] The dose of ranolazine should be titrated according to clinical response and down-titration may be required.[1,2] Until more is known it may also be prudent to be alert for any changes in ciclosporin concentrations.

(b) Cimetidine

The manufacturers report that in healthy subjects cimetidine 400 mg three times daily does not increase concentrations of ranolazine.[1]

(c) CYP2B6 substrates

Although the potential for ranolazine to inhibit the cytochrome P450 isoenzyme CYP2B6 has not been evaluated, the UK manufacturer advises caution if it is given with CYP2B6 substrates and they give as examples **bupropion**, **efavirenz** and **cyclophosphamide**.[2] The clinical relevance of any interaction is unknown.

(d) Digoxin

A study in healthy subjects given ranolazine 1 g twice daily and digoxin 125 micrograms found that ranolazine increased the plasma concentrations of digoxin by about 50%. Plasma concentrations of ranolazine were not significantly affected by digoxin.[1,2] Ranolazine probably raises digoxin concentrations by inhibiting P-glycoprotein. Digoxin concentrations should be monitored if ranolazine is started or stopped, and the digoxin dose may have to be adjusted.[1,2]

(e) Other drugs

Ranolazine is a substrate of the cytochrome P450 isoenzyme CYP3A4 and inhibitors of CYP3A4 increase plasma concentrations of ranolazine. Potent inhibitors of CYP3A4 such as ketoconazole (see 'Ranolazine + Azoles', p.1073) cause a three to fourfold increase in ranolazine concentrations and moderate inhibitors such as diltiazem (see 'Ranolazine + Calcium-channel blockers', p.1073) may increase concentrations about 2-fold. The dose-related adverse effects of ranolazine such as nausea and dizziness may be increased by concurrent use of drugs that increase its plasma concentrations. Further, increases in plasma concentrations of ranolazine may cause significant QT prolongation and the possible risk of arrhythmias (see also, 'Drugs that prolong the QT interval + Other drugs that prolong the QT interval', p.272).

The manufacturers of ranolazine contraindicate its use with potent CYP3A4 inhibitors. They include **clarithromycin**, **nefazodone** and the **HIV-protease inhibitors** (the US manufacturer[1] names **indinavir, nelfinavir, ritonavir** and **saquinavir**). The UK manufacturer[2] also names **telithromycin**.

The US manufacturer recommends that the dose of ranolazine should be limited to 500 mg twice daily when given to patients taking moderate CYP3A4 inhibitors, including **erythromycin**.[1] The UK manufacturer recommends careful dose titration of ranolazine in patients taking moderately potent CYP3A4 inhibitors, and name **erythromycin**.

While the UK manufacturers of ranolazine consider **grapefruit juice** to be a potent inhibitor of CYP3A4 and therefore contraindicate its use with ranolazine, the US manufacturer includes **grapefruit juice** and **grapefruit-containing products** as moderate inhibitors and recommends limiting the dose of ranolazine to 500 mg twice daily during concurrent use.[1]

Ranolazine is also a substrate of P-glycoprotein and therefore ritonavir, which inhibits P-glycoprotein may also increase ranolazine concentrations by this mechanism (see *Digoxin*, above).

1. Ranexa (Ranolazine). Gilead Sciences, Inc. US Prescribing Information, December 2011.
2. Ranexa (Ranolazine). A. Menarini Pharma UK SRL. UK Summary of product characteristics, April 2012.

Riociguat + Miscellaneous

Ketoconazole moderately increases the exposure to riociguat; other azoles and HIV protease inhibitors might act similarly. Clarithromycin slightly increased the exposure to riociguat. The moderate CYP3A4 inducer, bosentan, slightly reduces the exposure to riociguat, and potent CYP3A4 inducers might also do so, but to a greater extent. Tobacco smoking reduces riociguat concentrations. The exposure to riociguat is reduced by aluminium/magnesium hydroxide antacids and by omeprazole. Other antacids and proton pump inhibitors, and H_2-receptor antagonists, might also decrease the riociguat exposure. Food increases the maximum concentration of riociguat. Erlotinib and inhibitors of both P-glycoprotein and BCRP might increase the exposure to riociguat, and riociguat might increase the exposure to erlotinib and granisetron. Riociguat does not affect the pharmacokinetics of sildenafil. Additive hypotension might occur with glyceryl trinitrate and phosphodiesterase type-5 inhibitors. Riociguat did not affect the bleeding time or platelet aggregation when given with aspirin, and it did not alter the pharmacokinetics of midazolam.

Clinical evidence, mechanism, importance and management

(a) Aspirin

The UK and US manufacturers of riociguat briefly note that concurrent use with aspirin did not prolong the bleeding time or affect platelet aggregation.[1,2] No dose adjustment is required on concurrent use of riociguat and aspirin.[2]

(b) CYP1A1 inhibitors

The UK manufacturer of riociguat notes that concurrent use of CYP1A1 inhibitors (they name **erlotinib**) might increase riociguat exposure, and advise considering a riociguat dose reduction, with close monitoring of blood pressure, on concurrent use.[1] Erlotinib is also a substrate of CYP1A1, see *CYP1A1 substrates*, below.

(c) CYP1A1 substrates

The UK manufacturer of riociguat notes that it inhibited CYP1A1 *in vitro*, therefore they predict that an interaction with drugs which are substrates of this isoenzyme (they name **erlotinib** and **granisetron**) is possible.[1] However, note that *in vitro* findings do not always directly translate to the clinical situation.

(d) CYP3A4 inducers

The UK and US manufacturers of riociguat briefly report that **bosentan,** a moderate CYP3A4 inducer, decreased steady-state riociguat concentrations by 27%.[1,2] This slight decrease is unlikely to be clinically relevant, and the US manufacturer states that no dose adjustment is required on concurrent use with any moderate CYP3A4 inducer (see 'Table 1.9', p.11 for a list).[2] The effect of potent CYP3A4 inducers does not appear to have been studied, however, they would be expected to have a greater effect on riociguat concentrations than bosentan. Until further evidence is available, it would seem prudent to closely monitor the efficacy of riociguat on concurrent use with a potent CYP3A4 inducer, and to consider the need to increase the riociguat dose. Note that the UK manufacturer lists **St John's wort** as a potent CYP3A4 inducer but it is generally considered to be moderate. For a list of potent CYP3A4 inducers, see 'Table 1.9', p.11.

(e) CYP3A4 inhibitors

The US manufacturer of riociguat reports that **clarithromycin** (a potent CYP3A4 inhibitor) increased the AUC of riociguat about 1.5-fold, but did not increase its maximum plasma concentration.[2] This slight increase in riociguat exposure is unlikely to be clinically relevant, therefore no riociguat dose adjustment is expected to be required on concurrent use. Other potent CYP3A4 inhibitors might be expected to interact similarly (see 'Table 1.9', p.11 for a list), however the UK and US manufacturers report that the P-glycoprotein, BCRP, and potent CYP3A4 inhibitor, **ketoconazole** (400 mg once daily[1]), moderately increased the riociguat maximum concentration by 46% and increased its AUC 2.5-fold.[1,2] The UK manufacturer predicts that other drugs which inhibit multiple cytochrome P450 pathways, P-glycoprotein, and BCRP (they specifically name **azoles**, such as **itraconazole**, and the **HIV protease inhibitors**, such as **ritonavir**) are likely to act similarly. They therefore do not recommend concurrent use of such drugs.[1] In contrast, the US manufacturer advises considering a lower riociguat starting dose of 0.5 mg three times daily in patients taking cytochrome P450, P-glycoprotein, and BCRP inhibitors, with close monitoring for signs and symptoms of hypotension on initiation and during treatment.

(f) CYP3A4 substrates

The US manufacturer of riociguat briefly notes that it did not alter **midazolam** pharmacokinetics.[2] Note that midazolam can be used as a probe substrate to assess the activity of drugs on CYP3A4, and this study would suggest that riociguat is not a CYP3A4 inducer or inhibitor, and that an interaction with other CYP3A4 substrates is unlikely to occur by this mechanism.

(g) Drugs which affect gastric pH

The UK and US manufacturers of riociguat briefly report that an **aluminium/magnesium hydroxide** antacid (*Maalox*) decreased the AUC and maximum concentration of riociguat[1,2] by 34% and 56% respectively. The UK manufacturer advises taking antacids at least 2 hours before, or 1 hour after riociguat,[1] whereas the US manufacturer advises antacids should not be taken within 1 hour of taking riociguat.[2]

Concurrent use of **omeprazole** 40 mg with riociguat (dose not stated) resulted in a 26% decrease in the AUC of riociguat and a 35% decrease in its maximum concentration.[3] These decreases are unlikely to be clinically relevant, and the US manufacturer of riociguat therefore notes that no dose adjustment is required on concurrent use.[2] The UK manufacturer notes that riociguat is less soluble in a neutral pH medium than in an acid pH medium, and that the concurrent use of drugs which increase the gastric pH (this would include **antacids**, **H2-receptor antagonists**, and **proton pump inhibitors**) might reduce the bioavailability of riociguat.[1]

(h) Food

The UK manufacturer briefly notes that food slightly reduces the AUC of riociguat, and reduces its maximum concentration by 35%.[1] The US manufacturer of riociguat notes that food does not affect its bioavailability.[2] Generally riociguat can be taken without regard to food, however the UK manufacturer notes that because the maximum plasma concentration of riociguat was higher in the fasting state, compared with the fed state, patients prone to hypertension should avoid switching between taking riociguat in the fed and fasted state.[1]

(i) Nitrates

The UK and US manufacturers of riociguat note that in a study, riociguat 2.5 mg enhanced the blood pressure lowering effect of sublingual **glyceryl trinitrate** 0.4 mg, given 4 to 8 hours after the riociguat. They therefore contraindicate its use with nitrates or nitric oxide donors[1,2] such as **amyl nitrate**.[1]

(j) Phosphodiesterase type-5 inhibitors

The US manufacturer of riociguat briefly reports that it did not affect the pharmacokinetics of **sildenafil**.[2] However, the UK and US manufacturers note that in a study, the concurrent use of riociguat and sildenafil resulted in a high rate of discontinuation due to hypotension. Therefore they contraindicate its concurrent use with any phosphodiesterase type-5 inhibitor.[1,2]

(k) P-glycoprotein and BCRP inhibitors

The UK manufacturer of riociguat notes that inhibitors of both P-glycoprotein and BCRP (they name **ciclosporin**) might increase exposure to riociguat, and should be used with caution on concurrent use.[1]

(l) Tobacco

The UK and US manufacturers note that riociguat plasma concentrations are lower in smokers compared with non-smokers,[1,2] by 50 to 60%.[2] The UK manufacturer advises that smokers should stop smoking whilst taking riociguat.[1] However in those who continue to smoke, both the UK and US manufacturers recommend that a riociguat dose of 2.5 mg three times daily might be needed.[1,2] Riociguat dose adjustments should be considered if a patient starts or stops smoking during treatment with riociguat.[1]

1. Adempas (Riociguat). Bayer plc. UK Summary of product characteristics, October 2014.
2. Adempas (Riociguat). Bayer HealthCare Pharmaceuticals Inc. US Prescribing information, September 2014.
3. European Medicines Agency. CHMP assessment report for Adempas. Procedure No. EMEA/H/C/002737/0000. Available at: http://www.ema.europa.eu/docs/en_GB/document_library/EPAR_-_Public_assessment_report/human/002737/WC500165036.pdf (accessed 22/09/15).

Sodium nitroprusside + Miscellaneous

Smaller doses of sodium nitroprusside might be required in patients receiving antihypertensive drugs. Clonidine does not affect the response to nitroprusside. There is a risk of severe hypotension if phosphodiesterase type-5 inhibitors are used with sodium nitroprusside.

Clinical evidence, mechanism, importance and management

(a) Antihypertensives

The manufacturer notes that smaller doses of sodium nitroprusside might be required in patients receiving antihypertensive drugs. In any event the required dose varies considerably between patients and so should be titrated to effect.[1]

In a placebo-controlled study, patients with hypertension were given intravenous sodium nitroprusside in increasing bolus doses of 30 to 300 micrograms on the day before surgery, before induction of anaesthesia, and one and 3 hours postoperatively. Oral **clonidine** 6 micrograms/kg, was given 2 hours before surgery with a further dose of 3 micrograms/kg intravenously over the last hour of surgery. **Clonidine** did not affect the perioperative response to nitroprusside.[2]

When nitroprusside is used for controlled hypotension during anaesthesia, the hypotensive effect of other drugs, particularly anaesthetics, should be remembered.[1] The manufacturer specifically names **halothane** and **enflurane**. Consider also 'Antihypertensives + Other drugs that affect blood pressure', p.1054.

(b) Phosphodiesterase type-5 inhibitors

The use of phosphodiesterase type-5 inhibitors with sodium nitroprusside is contraindicated by the manufacturers, due to the risk of severe hypotension.[3] See also 'Phosphodiesterase type-5 inhibitors + Nitrates', p.1545 for further information. A case report describes the therapeutic use of **sildenafil** to enhance the hypotensive effect of sodium nitroprusside and other antihypertensives in a patient with a hypertensive crisis.[3]

1. Sodium Nitroprusside. Mayne Pharma plc. UK Summary of product characteristics, May 2005.
2. Parlow JL, Sagnard P, Begou G, Viale J-P, Quinin L. The effects of clonidine on sensitivity to phenylephrine and nitroprusside in patients with essential hypertension recovering from surgery. *Anesth Analg* (1999) 88, 1239–43.
3. Bahadur MM, Aggarwal VD, Mali M, Thamba A. Novel therapeutic option in hypertensive crisis: sildenafil augments nitroprusside-induced hypotension. *Nephrol Dial Transplant* (2005) 20, 1254–6.

Tirilazad + Miscellaneous

Phenobarbital and phenytoin reduce the levels of tirilazad mesilate whereas ketoconazole increases them. Finasteride inhibits the metabolism of tirilazad mesilate to its active metabolite. No pharmacokinetic interaction appears to occur between cimetidine or nimodipine and tirilazad mesilate.

Clinical evidence, mechanism, importance and management

(a) Cimetidine

A study in 16 healthy men found that cimetidine 300 mg every 6 hours for 4 days had no effect on the pharmacokinetics of a single 2-mg/kg dose of tirilazad mesilate, given by infusion over 10 minutes on day 2, nor on U-89678, its active metabolite.[1] No special precautions would seem necessary if cimetidine is given with tirilazad mesilate.

(b) Finasteride

In a study, 8 healthy men were given finasteride 5 mg daily for 10 days, with tirilazad mesilate 10 mg/kg orally or 2 mg/kg intravenously on day 7. Finasteride increased the AUCs of intravenous and oral tirilazad by 21% and 29%, respectively. Oral finasteride reduced the AUCs of the active metabolite (U-89678) by 92% when tirilazad was given intravenously and by 75% when tirilazad was given orally. Although the metabolism of tirilazad to U-89678 was inhibited there was only a moderate effect on the overall clearance of tirilazad and the interaction was considered unlikely to be of clinical significance.[2]

(c) Ketoconazole

Tirilazad mesilate, 10 mg/kg orally or 2 mg/kg intravenously, was given to 12 healthy subjects (both men and women), either alone or on day 4 of a 7-day regimen of ketoconazole 200 mg daily. The ketoconazole more than doubled the absolute bioavailability of the oral tirilazad mesilate (from 8.7% to 20.9%), apparently because its metabolism by the cytochrome P450 isoenzyme CYP3A in the gut wall and during the first pass through the liver was inhibited.[3] The clinical importance of this interaction awaits assessment.

(d) Nimodipine

In a single-dose study in 12 healthy men, there was no pharmacokinetic or pharmacodynamic interaction between intravenous tirilazad mesilate 2 mg/kg and oral nimodipine 60 mg.[4] No special precautions would seem necessary if nimodipine is given with tirilazad mesilate

(e) Phenobarbital

The pharmacokinetics of tirilazad mesilate (1.5 mg/kg as 10 minute intravenous infusions every 6 hours for 29 doses) were studied in 15 healthy subjects before and after they took phenobarbital 100 mg daily for 8 days. Phenobarbital increased the clearance of tirilazad by 25% in the male subjects and 29% in the female, and the AUC of the active metabolite of tirilazad (U-89678) was reduced by 51% in the males and 69% in the females. This was thought to occur because phenobarbital acts as an enzyme inducer, which increases the metabolism of the tirilazad.[5] The clinical importance of these pharmacokinetic changes awaits assessment, but be alert for evidence of reduced effects if both drugs are given. It is doubtful if the full enzyme-inducing effects of the phenobarbital would have been reached in this study after only one week, so anticipate a greater effect if it is given for a longer period. Note that **primidone** is metabolised to phenobarbital, and therefore it may be expected to interact similarly.

(f) Phenytoin

In a study in 12 healthy subjects, phenytoin 200 mg every 8 hours for 11 doses then 100 mg every 8 hours for 5 doses, reduced the AUC_{0-6} of tirilazad mesilate by 35%. The AUC of the active metabolite, U-89678, was reduced by 87%.[6] Another report by the same group of workers[7] found that phenytoin every 8 hours for 7 days (9 doses of 200 mg followed by 13 doses of 100 mg) reduced the clearance of tirilazad by 92% and of U-89678 by 93%. In another report the authors noted that phenytoin increased the metabolism of tirilazad and its metabolite in men and women to similar extents.[8] The clinical importance of these reductions is still to be assessed, but be alert for any evidence of reduced tirilazad effects if both drugs are given. Note that **fosphenytoin** is a prodrug of phenytoin, and may therefore be expected to interact similarly.

1. Fleishaker JC, Hulst LK, Peters GR. Lack of pharmacokinetic interaction between cimetidine and tirilazad mesylate. *Pharm Res* (1994) 11, 341–4.
2. Fleishaker JC, Pearson PG, Wienkers LC, Pearson LK, Moore TA, Peters GR. Biotransformation of tirilazad in human: 4. effect of finasteride on tirilazad clearance and reduced metabolite formation. J Pharmacol Exp Ther. (1998) 287, 591–7.
3. Fleishaker JC, Pearson PG, Wienkers LC, Pearson LK, Peters GR. Biotransformation of tirilazad in humans: 2. Effect of ketoconazole on tirilazad clearance and oral bioavailability. *J Pharmacol Exp Ther* (1996) 277, 991–8.
4. Fleishaker JC, Hulst LK, Peters GR. Lack of a pharmacokinetic/pharmacodynamic interaction between nimodipine and tirilazad mesylate in healthy volunteers. *J Clin Pharmacol* (1994) 34, 837–41.
5. Fleishaker JC, Pearson LK, Peters GR. Gender does not affect the degree of induction of tirilazad clearance by phenobarbital. *Eur J Clin Pharmacol* (1996) 50, 139–45.
6. Fleishaker JC, Hulst LK, Peters GR. The effect of phenytoin on the pharmacokinetics of tirilazad mesylate in healthy male volunteers. *Clin Pharmacol Ther* (1994) 56, 389–97.
7. Fleishaker JC, Pearson LK, Peters GR. Induction of tirilazad clearance by phenytoin. *Biopharm Drug Dispos* (1998) 19, 91–6.
8. Fleishaker JC, Pearson LK, Peters GR. Effect of gender on the degree of induction of tirilazad clearance by phenytoin. *Clin Pharmacol Ther* (1996) 59, 168.

Tolazoline + H_2-receptor antagonists

Cimetidine and ranitidine can reduce or abolish the effects of tolazoline used as a pulmonary vasodilator in children.

Clinical evidence

A newborn infant with persistent foetal circulation was given a continuous infusion of tolazoline to reduce pulmonary hypertension. The oxygenation improved but gastrointestinal bleeding occurred. When **cimetidine** was given, the condition of the child deteriorated with a decrease in oxygen saturation and arterial pO_2 values.[1] A second case report describes a similar outcome in a 2-day-old neonate, who had an initial improvement with tolazoline alone, but then developed worsening hypoxaemia when cimetidine was given.[2]

These reports are similar to another, in which the tolazoline-induced reduction in pulmonary arterial pressure in a child was reversed when **cimetidine** was given, for acute gastrointestinal haemorrhage.[3] Another study in 12 children found that intravenous **ranitidine** 3 mg/kg abolished the tolazoline-induced reduction in pulmonary and systemic vascular.[4]

Mechanism

Tolazoline dilates the pulmonary vascular system by stimulating both H_1- and H_2-receptors. Cimetidine and ranitidine block H_2-receptors so that at least part of the effects of tolazoline are abolished. It has been suggested that this interaction is confined to children.[3]

Importance and management

An established interaction. Cimetidine and ranitidine are not suitable drugs for prophylaxis of the gastrointestinal adverse effects of tolazoline in children. Other H_2-receptor antagonists would be expected to behave similarly.

1. Roll C, Hanssler L. Interaktion von Tolazolin und Cimetidin bei persistierender fetaler Zirkulation des Neugeborenen. *Monatsschr Kinderheilkd* (1993) 141, 297–9.
2. Huang C-B, Huang S-C. Caution with use of cimetidine in tolazoline induced upper gastrointestinal bleeding. Changgeng Yi Xue Za Zhi. (1996) 19, 268–71.
3. Jones ODH, Shore DF, Rigby ML, Leijala M, Scallan J, Shinebourne EA, Lincoln JCR. The use of tolazoline hydrochloride as a pulmonary vasodilator in potentially fatal episodes of pulmonary vasoconstriction after cardiac surgery in children. *Circulation* (1981) 64 (Suppl II), II-134–II-139.
4. Bush A, Busst CM, Knight WB, Shinebourne EA. Cardiovascular effects of tolazoline and ranitidine. *Arch Dis Child* (1987) 62, 241–6.

25
Digitalis glycosides

Plant extracts containing cardiac glycosides have been in use for thousands of years. The ancient Egyptians were familiar with squill (a source of **proscillaridin**), as were the Romans who used it as a heart tonic and diuretic. The foxglove was mentioned in the writings of Welsh physicians in the thirteenth century and features in 'An Account of the Foxglove and some of its Medical Uses', published by William Withering in 1785, in which he described its application in the treatment of 'dropsy' or the oedema that results from heart failure.

The most commonly used cardiac glycosides are those obtained from the members of the foxglove family, *Digitalis purpurea* and *Digitalis lanata*. The leaves of *D. lanata* are the source of a number of purified glycosides including **digoxin**, **digitoxin**, **acetyldigoxin**, **acetyldigitoxin**, **lanatoside C**, **deslanoside**, of **gitalin** (an amorphous mixture largely composed of digitoxin and digoxin), and of powdered whole leaf **digitalis lanata leaf**. *D. purpurea* is the source of **digitoxin**, **digitalis leaf**, and the standardised preparation **digitalin**. **Metildigoxin** is a semi-synthetic digitalis glycoside. Occasionally ouabain or strophanthin-K (also of plant origin) are used for particular situations, while for a number of years the Russians have exploited cardiac glycosides from lily of the valley (**convallaria**). Bufalin is a related cardioactive compound obtained from toads, and is found in a number of Chinese medicines.

Digitalisation

The cardiac glycosides have two main actions and two main applications. They reduce conductivity within the atrioventricular (AV) node, hence are used for treating supraventricular tachycardias (especially atrial fibrillation), and they have a positive inotropic effect (i.e. increase the force of contraction), and hence may be used for congestive heart failure.

Because the most commonly used glycosides are derived from digitalis, the achievement of the desired therapeutic serum concentration of any cardiac glycoside is usually referred to as digitalisation. Treatment can be started with a large loading dose so that the therapeutic concentrations are achieved reasonably quickly, but once these have been reached the amount is reduced to a maintenance dose. This has to be done carefully because there is a relatively narrow gap between therapeutic and toxic serum concentrations. Normal therapeutic levels are about one-third of those that are fatal, and serious toxic arrhythmias begin at about two-thirds of the fatal levels. The therapeutic range for digoxin levels is 0.8 to 2 nanograms/mL (or 1.02 to 2.56 nanomol/L). To convert nanograms/mL to nanomol/L multiply by 1.28, or to convert nanomol/L to nanograms/mL multiply by 0.781. Note that micrograms/L is the same as nanograms/mL.

If a patient is over-digitalised, signs of toxicity will occur, which can include loss of appetite, nausea and vomiting, and bradycardia. These symptoms are often used as clinical indicators of toxicity and a pulse rate of less than 60 bpm is usually considered to be an indication of overtreatment. Note that paroxysmal atrial tachycardia with AV block and junctional tachycardia can also occur as a result of digitalis toxicity. Other symptoms include visual disturbances, headache, drowsiness and occasionally diarrhoea. Death can result from cardiac arrhythmias. Patients given digitalis for cardiac arrhythmias can therefore demonstrate arrhythmias when they are both under- as well as over-digitalised.

Interactions of the cardiac glycosides

The pharmacological actions of these glycosides are very similar, but their rates and degree of absorption, metabolism and clearance are different. For example, digoxin is mainly renally cleared whereas digitoxin undergoes a degree of metabolism by the liver. It is therefore most important not to extrapolate a pharmacokinetic interaction seen with one cardiac glycoside and apply it uncritically to any other. Because the therapeutic ratio of the cardiac glycosides is low, a quite small change in serum levels might lead to inadequate digitalisation or to toxicity. For this reason interactions that have a relatively modest effect on serum levels can sometimes have serious consequences.

Many interactions between digoxin and other drugs are mediated by P-glycoprotein, and digoxin is often used as a probe drug in studying whether other drugs affect P-glycoprotein. Drugs that inhibit the activity of P-glycoprotein in the renal tubules reduce the elimination of digoxin in the urine and this can result in toxic serum levels. Further, the induction or inhibition of P-glycoprotein in the gut may affect the oral absorption of digoxin. See also 'Drug transporter proteins', p.13, for more information on P-glycoprotein.

Interference with digitalis glycoside assays

Some drugs might interfere with digoxin assays, but these are not routinely included in this publication because they are not drug interactions, see *What is a drug interaction*, under 'Drug interactions overview', p.1. The occasions where interference with digoxin assays is covered include situations where a drug interaction is proposed but where interference with the digoxin assay could be a relevant factor, for example spironolactone, see 'Digoxin and related drugs + Diuretics; Potassium-sparing', p.1094. Another situation is with herbal medicines, for which routine information on possible interference with assays is unlikely to be available from the assay manufacturers, and where such information might contribute to unexpected digoxin levels on monitoring.

Digoxin and related drugs + ACE inhibitors

Most ACE inhibitors do not interact with digoxin to a clinically relevant extent. Some studies in patients have found that serum digoxin levels rise by about 20 or 30% if captopril is used, while others have reported no changes. Captopril does not interact with digitoxin.

Clinical evidence

(a) Digitoxin and Captopril

A study in 12 healthy subjects given digitoxin 70 micrograms daily for up to 58 days found that the addition of captopril 25 mg daily had no effect on either the pharmacokinetics of digitoxin, or its effects on the heart.[1]

(b) Digoxin and Captopril

The serum digoxin levels of 16 patients with severe chronic congestive heart failure rose by 21% (from 1.1 nanograms/mL to 1.3 nanograms/mL), while taking captopril (average dose 93.7 mg daily). Serum digoxin levels were above the therapeutic range at 2 nanograms/mL on 3 out of 63 occasions, but no toxicity was seen. All patients had impaired renal function and were taking diuretics.[2,3] Another study[4] found a rise of about 30% in serum digoxin levels in patients with congestive heart failure (NYHA class II) given captopril, and a further study[5] found an approximate 60% rise in peak serum digoxin levels and a 39% increase in the AUC of digoxin in patients with congestive heart failure (NYHA class IV) given captopril. Conversely, a study in 31 patients with stable congestive heart failure, given captopril 25 mg three times daily, found no changes in serum digoxin levels over a 6-month period.[6] Two other studies in healthy subjects[7] and patients with congestive heart failure[8] also found no evidence of an interaction.

(c) Digoxin and Other ACE inhibitors

In general no pharmacokinetic interactions have been seen between ACE inhibitors and digoxin.

Benazepril has been reported to have had no important pharmacokinetic interaction with digoxin. The US manufacturer also reports no evidence of clinically important adverse interactions when benazepril was used with digoxin.[9]

Cilazapril 5 mg for 14 days did not alter the trough plasma digoxin levels in healthy subjects.[10]

Enalapril 20 mg daily for 30 days had no effect on the pharmacokinetics of digoxin 250 micrograms daily in 7 patients with congestive heart failure.[11]

Imidapril 10 mg daily had no effect on the serum digoxin levels of 12 healthy subjects, but reductions in levels of the active form imidaprilat and in ACE inhibition of about 15% were seen.[12]

Lisinopril 5 mg daily for 4 weeks had no effect on the serum digoxin levels of 9 patients.[13] This confirms the findings of a single-dose study.[14]

Moexipril has been reported, by the manufacturer, to have had no important pharmacokinetic interaction with digoxin in healthy subjects.[15] The manufacturer also has clinical studies that show no evidence of clinically important adverse interactions when moexipril was used with digoxin.[16]

Perindopril 2 to 4 mg daily for a month had no effect on the steady-state serum digoxin levels of 10 patients with mild chronic heart failure.[17]

Quinapril is reported not to alter the steady-state levels of digoxin in healthy subjects,[18] and patients with congestive heart failure.[19]

Ramipril 5 mg daily for 14 days had no effect on the serum digoxin levels of 12 healthy subjects.[20]

Spirapril 12 to 48 mg daily did not affect the pharmacokinetics or the steady-state serum levels of digoxin in 15 healthy subjects taking digoxin 250 micrograms twice daily.[21]

Trandolapril did not affect the plasma levels of digoxin 250 micrograms measured pre-dose and 2 hours post-dose.[22] The manufacturers also note that, in patients with left ventricular dysfunction after myocardial infarction, no clinical interactions have been found between trandolapril and digoxin.[22,23]

Mechanism

Not fully understood. It has been suggested that an interaction is only likely to occur in patients that have renal impairment because the glomerular filtration rate of these patients might be maintained by the vasoconstrictor action of angiotensin II on the post-glomerular blood vessels, which would be impaired by ACE inhibition. As a result some of the loss of digoxin through the tubules is reduced.[7]

Importance and management

The overall picture is that no clinically important adverse interaction occurs between digoxin and ACE inhibitors in patients with normal renal function, and that serum digoxin monitoring is only needed in those patients that have a high risk of reversible ACE inhibitor-induced renal failure (e.g. patients with congestive heart failure during chronic diuretic treatment, with bilateral renal artery stenosis or unilateral renal artery stenosis in a solitary kidney);[7] however, note these latter two conditions are contra-indications to the use of ACE inhibitors. The critical factor does not seem to be the particular ACE inhibitor used but the existence of abnormal renal function or conditions that increase the risk of renal impairment. This needs confirmation.

Captopril does not appear to interact with digitoxin.

1. de Mey C, Elich D, Schroeter V, Butzer R, Belz GG. Captopril does not interact with the pharmacodynamics and pharmacokinetics of digitoxin in healthy man. *Eur J Clin Pharmacol* (1992) 43, 445–7.
2. Cleland JGF, Dargie HJ, Hodsman GP, Robertson JIS, Ball SG. Interaction of digoxin and captopril. *Br J Clin Pharmacol* (1984) 17, 214P.
3. Cleland JGF, Dargie HJ, Pettigrew A, Gillen C, Robertson JIS. The effects of captopril on serum digoxin and urinary urea and digoxin clearances in patients with congestive heart failure. *Am Heart J* (1986) 112, 130–5.
4. Mazurek W, Haczyński J, Interakcja kaptoprilu i digoksyny. *Pol Tyg Lek* (1993) 48, 834–5.
5. Kirimli O, Kalkan S, Guneri S, Tuncok Y, Akdeniz B, Ozdamar M, Guven H. The effects of captopril on serum digoxin levels in patients with severe congestive heart failure. *Int J Clin Pharmacol Ther* (2001) 39, 311–14.
6. Magelli C, Bassein L, Ribani MA, Liberatore S, Ambrosioni E, Magnani B. Lack of effect of captopril on serum digoxin in congestive heart failure. *Eur J Clin Pharmacol* (1989) 36, 99–100.
7. Rossi GP, Semplicini A, Bongiovi S, Mozzato MG, Paleari CD, Pessina AC. Effect of acute captopril administration on digoxin pharmacokinetics in normal subjects. *Curr Ther Res* (1989) 46, 439–44.
8. Miyakawa T, Shionoiri H, Takasaki I, Kobayashi K, Ishii M. The effect of captopril on pharmacokinetics of digoxin in patients with mild congestive heart failure. *J Cardiovasc Pharmacol* (1991) 17, 576–80.
9. Lotensin (Benazepril hydrochloride). Novartis Pharmaceuticals Corporation. US Prescribing information, May 2011.
10. Kleinbloesem CH, van Brummelen P, Francis RJ, Wiegand U-W. Clinical pharmacology of cilazapril. *Drugs* (1991) 41 (Suppl 1), 3–10.
11. Douste-Blazy Ph, Blanc M, Montastruc JL, Conte D, Cotonat J, Galinier F. Is there any interaction between digoxin and enalapril? *Br J Clin Pharmacol* (1986) 22, 752–3.
12. Harder S, Thürmann PA. Pharmacokinetic and pharmacodynamic interaction trial after repeated oral doses of imidapril and digoxin in healthy volunteers. *Br J Clin Pharmacol* (1997) 43, 475–80.
13. Vandenburg MJ, Kelly JG, Wiseman HT, Mannering D, Long C, Glover DR. The effect of lisinopril on digoxin pharmacokinetics in patients with congestive heart failure. *Br J Clin Pharmacol* (1988) 21, 656P–657P.
14. Vandenburg MJ, Morris F, Marks C, Kelly JG, Dews IM, Stephens JD. A study of the potential pharmacokinetic interaction of lisinopril and digoxin in normal volunteers. *Xenobiotica* (1988) 18, 1179–84.
15. Perdix (Moexipril hydrochloride). UCB Pharma Ltd. UK Summary of product characteristics, August 2010.
16. Perdix (Moexipril). Schwarz Pharma. Product monograph, September 1995.
17. Vandenburg MJ, Stephens JD, Resplandy G, Dews IM, Robinson J, Desche P. Digoxin pharmacokinetics and perindopril in heart failure patients. *J Clin Pharmacol* (1993) 33, 146–9.
18. Ferry JJ, Sedman AJ, Hengy H, Vollmer KO, Dunkey A, Klotz U, Colburn WA. Concomitant multiple dose quinapril administration does not alter steady-state pharmacokinetics of digoxin. *Pharm Res* (1987) 4, S98.
19. Kromer EP, Elsner D, Riegger GAJ. Digoxin, converting-enzyme inhibition (quinapril) and the combination in patients with congestive heart failure functional class II and sinus rhythm. *J Cardiovasc Pharmacol* (1990) 16, 9–14.
20. Doering W, Maass L, Irmisch R and König E. Pharmacokinetic interaction study with ramipril and digoxin in healthy volunteers. *Am J Cardiol* (1987) 59, 60D–64D.
21. Johnson BF, Wilson J, Johnson J, Flemming J. Digoxin pharmacokinetics and spirapril, a new ACE inhibitor. *J Clin Pharmacol* (1991) 31, 527–30.
22. Mavik (Trandolapril). Abbott Laboratories. US Prescribing information, September 2011.
23. Gopten (Trandolapril). Abbott Laboratories Ltd. UK Summary of product characteristics, July 2010.

Digoxin + Acipimox

One study suggests that acipimox does not interact with digoxin.

Clinical evidence, mechanism, importance and management

In a study in 6 elderly patients, the pharmacokinetics of digoxin appeared to be unaffected by acipimox 250 mg three times daily for a week. In addition, there was no change in clinical condition, ECGs, plasma urea or electrolyte levels.[1] No digoxin dose adjustments would be expected to be necessary during the concurrent use of acipimox.

1. Chijioke PC, Pearson RM, Benedetti S. Lack of acipimox-digoxin interaction in patient volunteers. *Hum Exp Toxicol* (1992) 11, 357–9.

Digoxin + Activated factor X inhibitors

The pharmacokinetics of digoxin are not altered by edoxaban or rivaroxaban, and do not appear to be altered by apixaban. Digoxin does not alter the pharmacokinetics of edoxaban or rivaroxaban.

Clinical evidence and mechanism

(a) Apixaban

The UK manufacturer briefly reports that, in a study, apixaban 20 mg daily did not alter the AUC or maximum concentration of digoxin 250 micrograms daily.[1]

(b) Edoxaban

In a randomised study, in one group of 23 healthy subjects, edoxaban 60 mg daily for 7 days did not alter the AUC of steady-state digoxin 250 micrograms daily, but did increase its maximum concentration by 28%. In another group of 23 healthy subjects, steady-state digoxin 250 micrograms daily did not alter the AUC of edoxaban 60 mg daily for 7 days, but its maximum concentration was increased by 16%. The anticoagulant effect of edoxaban was not affected.[2]

(c) Rivaroxaban

In a randomised, crossover study in 17 healthy subjects, rivaroxaban 20 mg twice daily for 19 doses did not alter the pharmacokinetics of steady-state digoxin. In addition, digoxin did not have a clinically important effect on the AUC or maximum concentration of rivaroxaban, and the anticoagulant effect of rivaroxaban was not affected.[3]

Importance and management

No clinically important pharmacokinetic interaction occurs between apixaban, edoxaban, or rivaroxaban and digoxin, and no dose adjustments would seem necessary on concurrent use.

Note that digoxin can be used as a probe substrate to assess the activity of drugs on P-glycoprotein. These studies therefore suggest that apixaban, edoxaban, and rivaroxaban are not inhibitors or inducers of P-glycoprotein, and therefore are not expected to affect the exposure to other substrates of P-glycoprotein via this mechanism.

1. Eliquis (Apixaban). Bristol-Myers Squibb-Pfizer. UK Summary of product characteristics, July 2014.
2. Mendell J, Noveck RJ, Shi M. Pharmacokinetics of the direct Factor Xa inhibitor edoxaban and digoxin administered alone and in combination. *J Cardiovasc Pharmacol* (2012) 60, 335–41.
3. Kubitza D, Becka M, Roth A, Mueck W. Absence of clinically relevant interactions between rivaroxaban—an oral, direct Factor Xa inhibitor—and digoxin or atorvastatin in healthy subjects. J Int Med Res 2012 (40), 1688–1707.

Digoxin + Allopurinol

Allopurinol does not appear to affect digoxin levels.

Clinical evidence, mechanism, importance and management

There was no change in the serum digoxin levels of 5 healthy subjects over a 7-day period while they were taking allopurinol 300 mg daily.[1] No digoxin dose adjustments would appear to be necessary on concurrent use.

1. Havelund T, Abildtrup N, Birkebaek N, Breddam E, Rosager AM. Allopurinols effekt på koncentrationen af digoksin i serum. *Ugeskr Laeger* (1984) 146, 1209–11.

Digoxin + Alpha blockers

A rapid and marked rise in serum digoxin levels occurred in one study when prazosin was also given, whereas in another study with prazosin a decrease in digoxin levels was reported. Alfuzosin, doxazosin, silodosin, tamsulosin, and terazosin do not appear to interact with digoxin.

Clinical evidence, mechanism, importance and management

(a) Alfuzosin

The manufacturers of alfuzosin report that no pharmacodynamic or pharmacokinetic interaction[1,2] was observed in healthy subjects given alfuzosin 10 mg daily with digoxin 250 micrograms daily for 7 days.[2] Digoxin dose adjustments are not necessary when alfuzosin is given concurrently.

(b) Doxazosin

Doxazosin is highly bound to plasma proteins (98%), but the manufacturer notes that *in vitro* data in human plasma indicates that doxazosin does not affect the protein binding of digoxin.[3,4] However, note that altered protein binding of digoxin is not a mechanism for any known clinically relevant digoxin interaction. Another *in vitro* study found that doxazosin inhibited the P-glycoprotein-mediated transcellular transport of digoxin.[5] If this were to occur *in vivo*, then raised digoxin levels would be expected via inhibition of digoxin renal transport. However, the lack of any evidence of an interaction between doxazosin and digoxin suggests that no clinically relevant interaction occurs. No digoxin dose adjustment would appear necessary when it is used with doxazosin.

(c) Prazosin

In 20 patients, prazosin 2.5 mg twice daily increased the mean steady-state plasma digoxin level by 43% (from 0.94 nanograms/mL to 1.34 nanograms/mL) after one day, and by 60% (from 0.94 nanograms/mL to 1.51 nanograms/mL) after 3 days, although the individual response varied from an increase to a decrease, or no effect. Three days after prazosin was stopped, by which time it would be totally cleared from the body, the serum digoxin concentrations had fallen to their previous levels.[6] Another study found that prazosin shortened the half-life of digoxin, decreased its serum levels and increased its clearance, but did not affect digoxin bioavailability.[7]

The reason for this response is not understood. There do not appear to be any other reports in the literature, and the manufacturer notes that, in clinical experience, prazosin has been given with digoxin (and **digitalis**) without any adverse drug interaction.[8] However, bear this interaction in mind in case of an unexpected response to treatment.

(d) Silodosin

The US manufacturer of silodosin describes a study in which 16 healthy subjects were given silodosin with digoxin 250 micrograms daily for 7 days. As silodosin had no notable effect on digoxin pharmacokinetics, they state that no dose adjustments are necessary on concurrent use.[9]

(e) Tamsulosin

A placebo-controlled study in 10 healthy subjects found that tamsulosin 800 micrograms daily had no effect on the pharmacokinetics of a single 500-microgram intravenous dose of digoxin.[10] Digoxin dose adjustments are not likely to be necessary when tamsulosin is given with digoxin.

(f) Terazosin

The UK manufacturer of terazosin states that terazosin has been given with cardiac glycosides without evidence of an interaction.[11]

1. Xatral (Alfuzosin hydrochloride). Sanofi. UK Summary of product characteristics, September 2013.
2. Uroxatral (Alfuzosin hydrochloride extended-release tablets). Sanofi-Aventis US LLC. US Prescribing information, October 2011.
3. Cardura (Doxazosin mesilate). Pfizer Ltd. UK Summary of product characteristics, August 2009.
4. Cardura (Doxazosin mesylate). Pfizer Inc. US Prescribing information, November 2013.
5. Takara K, Kakumoto M, Tanigawara Y, Funakoshi J, Sakaeda T, Okumura K. Interaction of digoxin with antihypertensive drugs *via* MDR1. *Life Sci* (2002) 70, 1491–1500.
6. Çopur S, Tokgözoğlu L, Oto A, Oram E, Uğurlu Ş. Effects of oral prazosin on total plasma digoxin levels. *Fundam Clin Pharmacol* (1988) 2, 13–17.
7. Halawa B, Mazurek W. Interakcja digoksyny z dihydralazyną I prazosyną. *Pol Tyg Lek* (1986) 41, 1521–3.
8. Hypovase (Prazosin hydrochloride). Pfizer Ltd. UK Summary of product characteristics, June 2009.
9. Rapaflo (Silodosin). Watson Pharma, Inc. US Prescribing information, January 2013.
10. Miyazawa Y, Starkey LP, Forrest A, Schentag JJ, Kamimura H, Swarz H, Ito Y. Effects of the concomitant administration of tamsulosin (0.8 mg) on the pharmacokinetic and safety profile of intravenous digoxin (Lanoxin®) in normal healthy subjects: a placebo-controlled evaluation. *J Clin Pharm Ther* (2002) 27, 13–19.
11. Hytrin (Terazosin monohydrochloride dihydrate). Amdipharm Mercury Company Ltd. UK Summary of product characteristics, June 2009.

Digoxin + Alpha-glucosidase inhibitors

Some but not all studies have found that digoxin levels can be sizeably reduced by acarbose. Miglitol reduced digoxin levels in healthy subjects, but no change was seen in diabetic patients. Voglibose does not appear to interact adversely with digoxin.

Clinical evidence, mechanism, importance and management

(a) Acarbose

A woman taking digoxin 250 micrograms daily, insulin, nifedipine, isosorbide dinitrate, clorazepate and nabumetone had subtherapeutic plasma digoxin levels of 0.48 to 0.64 nanograms/mL while taking acarbose (dose not stated), even when her digoxin dose was increased by adding 125 micrograms on 2 days of the week. Later, in the absence of acarbose and with the original digoxin dose, her plasma digoxin levels were 1.9 nanograms/mL.[1,2] Similarly, another report describes 2 patients with sizeably reduced plasma digoxin levels while taking acarbose. In one case, when acarbose 50 mg three times daily was stopped, the plasma digoxin levels rose from 0.23 nanograms/mL to 1.6 nanograms/mL; in the second case, when acarbose 100 mg twice daily was stopped the plasma digoxin level rose from 0.56 nanograms/mL to 1.9 nanograms/mL.[3] Another patient with heart failure and type 2 diabetes taking digoxin and voglibose, was found to have subtherapeutic levels of digoxin when his treatment was changed from voglibose (see below) to acarbose 300 mg daily. The serum levels unexpectedly remained subtherapeutic for at least a month when treatment was switched back to voglibose.[4]

A pharmacokinetic study in 7 healthy subjects, using either a single 200-mg dose of acarbose or pretreatment with acarbose 100 mg doses three times daily, similarly found that the serum levels and AUC of a single 500-microgram dose of digoxin were reduced. Maximum digoxin serum levels were reduced by about 30 to 40% and the AUC was reduced by about 40%.[5] In contrast, in two other studies in healthy subjects, acarbose 50 mg three times daily for 12 days[6] or 300 mg daily for a week[7] had no effect on the single-dose pharmacokinetics of digoxin, except for a small 29% *increase* in the maximum digoxin level in one study.[6]

The reason for any interaction is not understood, but a reduction in the absorption of the digoxin from the gut has been suggested.[5] Just why there is an inconsistency between the findings of the controlled studies is not understood, but it would clearly be prudent to consider monitoring digoxin levels if both drugs are used together, being alert for any evidence of reduced levels.

(b) Miglitol

The US manufacturer of miglitol notes that in a study in healthy subjects, miglitol 50 mg or 100 mg three times daily reduced the average plasma concentrations of digoxin by 19% and 28%, respectively. However, in diabetic patients plasma digoxin levels were not altered by the concurrent use of miglitol 100 mg three times daily for 14 days.[8] The effects in healthy subjects are small, and the lack of effect in patients suggests that no interaction is likely, but this needs confirmation.

(c) Voglibose

A randomised, crossover study in 8 healthy subjects taking digoxin 250 micrograms daily after breakfast for 8 days found that voglibose 200 micrograms three times daily had no effect on the pharmacokinetics of the digoxin.[9] No dose adjustment of digoxin therefore seems necessary if voglibose is given.

1. Serrano JS, Jiménez CM, Serrano MI, Balboa B. A possible interaction of potential clinical interest between digoxin and acarbose. *Clin Pharmacol Ther* (1996) 60, 589–92.
2. Menchén del Cerro E. Acarbosa y digoxina. *Aten Primaria* (1995) 16, 508.
3. Ben-Ami H, Krivoy N, Nagachandran P, Roguin A, Edoute Y. An interaction between digoxin and acarbose. *Diabetes Care* (1999) 22, 860–1.
4. Nagai Y, Hayakawa T, Abe T, Nomura G. Are there different effects of acarbose and voglibose on serum levels of digoxin in a diabetic patient with congestive heart failure? *Diabetes Care* (2000) 23, 1703.
5. Miura T, Ueno K, Tanaka K, Sugiura Y, Mizutani M, Takatsu F, Takano Y, Shibakawa M. Impairment of absorption of digoxin by acarbose. *J Clin Pharmacol* (1998) 38, 654–7.
6. Cohen E, Almog S, Staruvin D, Garty M. Do therapeutic doses of acarbose alter the pharmacokinetics of digoxin? *Isr Med Assoc J* (2002) 4, 772–5.
7. Hillebrand I, Graefe KH, Bischoff H, Frank G, Raemsch KD, Berchtold P. Serum digoxin and propranolol levels during acarbose treatment. *Int Congr Ser* (1982) 594, 244–6.
8. Glyset (Miglitol). Pfizer Inc. US prescribing information, October 2010.
9. Kusumoto M, Ueno K, Fujimura Y, Kameda T, Mashimo K, Takeda K, Tatami R, Shibakawa M. Lack of kinetic interaction between digoxin and voglibose. *Eur J Clin Pharmacol* (1999) 55, 79–80.

Digoxin + 5-Alpha reductase inhibitors

Dutasteride and finasteride do not appear to affect the pharmacokinetics of digoxin.

Clinical evidence, mechanism, importance and management

In a study in 20 healthy subjects, the steady-state pharmacokinetics of digoxin were unchanged by **dutasteride** 500 micrograms daily for 3 weeks.[1] Similarly, in a study in

17 healthy subjects, **finasteride** 5 mg daily for 10 days had no effect on the single-dose pharmacokinetics of digoxin 400 micrograms.[2] No digoxin dose adjustment would be expected to be necessary on the concurrent use of either of these 5-alpha reductase inhibitors.

1. Avodart (Dutasteride). GlaxoSmithKline. US Prescribing information, October 2012.
2. Gregoire S, Williams R, Gormley G, Lin E. Effect of finasteride (MK-906) on the disposition of digoxin. *J Clin Pharmacol* (1990) 30, 847.

Digoxin + Aminoglycosides

Digoxin levels can be reduced by oral neomycin and increased by intramuscular gentamicin.

Clinical evidence

(a) Gentamicin

In a study in 12 patients with congestive heart failure taking digoxin 250 micrograms daily, the addition of gentamicin 80 mg intramuscularly twice daily for 7 days was found to increase serum digoxin levels 2.3-fold, from 0.59 nanograms/mL to 1.36 nanograms/mL. In a further 12 patients with congestive heart failure and diabetes, the same dose of gentamicin increased digoxin levels 3.1-fold, from 0.64 nanograms/mL to 2 nanograms/mL. It should be noted that serum creatinine levels were higher in both groups than those in healthy controls even before receiving gentamicin, and were further increased after gentamicin.[1]

An earlier study similarly found that gentamicin prolonged the half-life of digoxin and increased its serum levels by 47% (from 1.9 nanograms/mL to 2.8 nanograms/mL).[2]

(b) Neomycin

Neomycin 1 to 3 g orally was found to delay and reduce the absorption of a single 500-microgram dose of digoxin in healthy subjects.[3] The AUC of digoxin was reduced by 41 to 51%. Absorption was affected even when neomycin was given 3 to 6 hours before digoxin. In a steady-state study, neomycin 2 g given with digoxin 250 to 500 micrograms daily reduced the serum level of digoxin by 8 to 49% (mean 28%).[3]

Mechanism

Gentamicin impairs renal function, so decreasing digoxin clearance.[2] Higher digoxin levels and serum creatinine levels in diabetic compared with non-diabetic patients might be due to differences in renal function,[1] with concurrent gentamicin causing a further impairment of renal function and even higher digoxin levels. The reduction in digoxin toxicity is not fully understood but changes in ionic transport might be involved. The inhibition by gentamicin of Na^+/K^+ ATPase, which acts as a specific receptor for digoxin, could also be a factor.[1]

Neomycin can cause a general but reversible malabsorption syndrome, which affects the absorption of several drugs. The extent of this is probably offset in some patients, because the neomycin also reduces the breakdown of digoxin by the bacteria in the gut.[4]

Importance and management

Information is limited, but patients should be monitored for increased digoxin effects if gentamicin is given, especially those with diabetes or any other patient with renal impairment. Initially, checking pulse rate is probably adequate. All aminoglycosides have the potential to impair renal function, and as there seems to be no information about other parenteral aminoglycosides, it would seem prudent to follow the same precautions given for gentamicin on concurrent use.

Patients should be monitored for reduced digoxin effects if neomycin is given orally and suitable dose adjustments made if necessary. Separating administration of the two drugs does not prevent this interaction. Other aminoglycosides that can be given orally such as **kanamycin** and **paromomycin** might possibly interact with digoxin in a similar way to neomycin, but this requires confirmation.

1. Alkadi HO, Nooman MA, Raja'a YA. Effect of gentamicin on serum digoxin level in patients with congestive heart failure. *Pharm World Sci* (2004) 26, 107–9.
2. Halawa B. Interakcje digoksyny z cefradina (Sefril), tetracyklina (Tetracyclinum), gentamycyna (Gentamycin) i wankomycyna (Vancocin). *Pol Tyg Lek* (1984) 39, 1717–20.
3. Lindenbaum J, Maulitz RM, Butler VP. Inhibition of digoxin absorption by neomycin. *Gastroenterology* (1976) 71, 399–404.
4. Lindenbaum J, Tse-Eng D, Butler VP, Rund DG. Urinary excretion of reduced metabolites of digoxin. *Am J Med* (1981) 71, 67–74.

Digoxin + 5-Aminosalicylates

Digoxin levels can be reduced by sulfasalazine. The UK manufacturer of balsalazide suggests that it could interact similarly.

Clinical evidence, mechanism, importance and management

The observation that a patient taking **sulfasalazine** 8 g daily had low serum digoxin levels prompted a crossover study in 10 healthy subjects. In this study a single 500-microgram dose of digoxin syrup was given alone, and after the subjects had taken oral **sulfasalazine** 2 to 6 g daily for 6 days. Digoxin absorption was reduced, ranging from 0 to 50% depending on the dose of **sulfasalazine** used.[1] Serum digoxin levels were reduced accordingly.[1] The reasons for this effect are not understood, and this seems to be the only report of this interaction. Concurrent use need not be avoided, but it would be prudent to check for under-digitalisation, initially by checking symptoms and pulse rate, and then taking digoxin levels if an interaction is suspected. In the initial patient, separating the doses did not appear to prevent this interaction.[1]

Although no interaction involving digoxin and **balsalazide** has been reported, based on the information with sulfasalazine, the UK manufacturer of **balsalazide** recommends that plasma levels of digoxin should be monitored in digitalised patients starting **balsalazide**.[2]

1. Juhl RP, Summers RW, Guillory JK, Blaug SM, Cheng FH, Brown DD. Effect of sulfasalazine on digoxin bioavailability. *Clin Pharmacol Ther* (1976) 20, 387–94.
2. Colazide (Balsalazide). Almirall Ltd. UK Summary of product characteristics, January 2010.

Digoxin + Aminosalicylic acid

Aminosalicylic acid causes a small reduction in single-dose digoxin exposure.

Clinical evidence, mechanism, importance and management

In a study in 10 healthy subjects, the bioavailability of a single 750-microgram dose of digoxin, using urinary excretion as a measure, was reduced by 20% by aminosalicylic acid 2 g four times daily for 2 weeks.[1] This seems to be just another aspect of the general malabsorption caused by aminosalicylic acid. The importance of this interaction in patients is not known, but it would be expected to be small.

1. Brown DD, Juhl RP, Warner SL. Decreased bioavailability of digoxin due to hypocholesterolemic interventions. *Circulation* (1978) 58, 164–72.

Digoxin and related drugs + Amiodarone

Digoxin levels can be approximately doubled by amiodarone. Some individuals have had even greater increases. The same interaction also appears to occur with digitoxin and metildigoxin. Isolated cases of torsade de pointes have been reported in patients taking acetyldigoxin, digitoxin or digoxin when also given amiodarone, particularly at higher doses.

Clinical evidence

(a) Acetyldigoxin

Torsade de pointes developed in one patient 3 days after the amiodarone dose was increased to 600 mg daily, and beta-acetyldigoxin 100 micrograms and bisoprolol 1.25 mg daily were added, for persistent atrial fibrillation. Serum levels of digoxin and amiodarone were normal. Withdrawal of all medications and treatment with intravenous magnesium resolved the arrhythmias.[1] Similarly, the same authors later reported the case of a 62-year-old patient taking acetyldigoxin 200 micrograms daily and nebivolol who developed torsade de pointes 3 hours after he was started on a loading dose of intravenous amiodarone (190 mg given) for persistent atrial fibrillation. Amiodarone was stopped and intravenous magnesium given with no further ventricular arrhythmias.[2]

(b) Digitoxin

Two elderly patients (aged 77 years and 78 years) taking digitoxin 100 micrograms daily were given loading doses of amiodarone followed by maintenance doses of 200 to 400 mg daily. Within 2 months in one case, and within 4 months in the other, they were hospitalised because of bradycardia, dyspnoea, nausea and malaise. One of them had total AV block (38 bpm). The serum digitoxin levels of both patients were found to be elevated (54 nanograms/mL and 45 nanograms/mL, respectively) well above the therapeutic range of 9 to 30 nanograms/mL. Serum amiodarone and desethylamiodarone levels were normal. Both patients recovered when the digitoxin was stopped.[3]

Another report describes torsade de pointes in 2 patients taking digitoxin and beta blockers and given loading doses of amiodarone for persistent atrial fibrillation. In one case, QT prolongation was reported 48 hours after oral amiodarone (approximately 2.2 g given) was added to digitoxin 100 micrograms daily and torsade de pointes occurred. Amiodarone was stopped without resolution of the torsade de pointes, and an implantable cardioverter-defibrillator was fitted. In the second case, torsade de pointes was reported 24 hours after intravenous amiodarone (approximately 1 g given) was added to intravenous digitoxin 400 micrograms. Amiodarone was stopped and an implantable cardioverter-defibrillator was fitted; however, due to persistent atrial fibrillation, oral amiodarone 200 mg daily was restarted along with beta-acetyldigoxin 200 micrograms daily with no further arrhythmias.[2]

(c) Digoxin

The observation that patients taking digoxin developed digoxin toxicity when given amiodarone[4] prompted a study of this interaction. Seven patients receiving digoxin had a mean rise in their plasma digoxin levels of 69% (from 1.17 nanograms/mL to 1.98 nanograms/mL), when they were given amiodarone 200 mg three times daily. Two other patients similarly treated also had increased plasma digoxin levels.[4]

Numerous studies in patients have confirmed this interaction,[5-12] with reported increases in serum digoxin levels of 75 to 158%.[5-8] The occasional patient has had three- to fourfold increases in digoxin levels, whereas others have had little or no change,[6,9] with one group of workers stating that they observed no change in serum digoxin levels in 5 patients given amiodarone.[13,14] Children seem particularly sensitive, with threefold, and even as much as ninefold rises reported.[15] Other reports confirm that digoxin levels are increased by amiodarone and toxicity can occur,[16-20] including a case of bidirectional ventricular tachycardia.[21] The interaction has also been demonstrated in healthy subjects.[22,23] There is also a case report of a 31-year-old man with dilated cardiomyopathy who had his dose of digoxin reduced, from 250 micrograms daily to 125 micrograms daily, 4 days before starting an oral loading-dose regimen of amiodarone 600 mg daily. Before starting amiodarone, his digoxin level was 1.27 nanograms/mL, and this increased to 1.79 nanograms/mL 10 hours post-dose on day 2, and 2.93 nanograms/mL 8.4 hours post-dose on day 3. Digoxin was stopped and 15.5 hours later his digoxin level was 1.8 nanograms/mL. However, on day 4, 9.25 hours after amiodarone was given, the digoxin level had increased to 2.52 nanograms/mL. Twice daily monitoring of digoxin over the next 3 days found that levels rose and fell, with the highest levels occurring between 8 and 10 hours after amiodarone was given. The patient did not develop any signs of digoxin toxicity.[24]

Following reports of sinus arrests and sudden deaths, another study compared the mortality rate in patients taking amiodarone and digoxin with that in patients taking digoxin alone. They found that concurrent use had an unfavourable effect on survival, both in patients with atrial fibrillation and those with sinus rhythm.[25]

A review of prescribing in an Australian hospital revealed 42 patients who had taken amiodarone with digoxin; both long-term (16), either drug recently started (21), or both drugs recently started (5). Of 31 patients who had digoxin levels monitored, 12 required a change in the dose of digoxin, and in 3, digoxin was stopped.[26] It is unclear whether this was purely on the basis of serum levels, or whether patients experienced adverse effects.

In 2 patients who had been on taking digoxin and amiodarone, digoxin toxicity occurred after 8 months and 36 months, respectively. In these cases, amiodarone-induced hypothyroidism was found to be the cause of the digoxin toxicity.[27]

A 74-year-old woman taking digoxin had a cardiac arrest secondary to torsade de pointes 4 days after starting oral amiodarone 1.2 g daily for resistant atrial tachyarrhythmias.[28]

(d) Metildigoxin

Eight patients taking metildigoxin had a rise in their steady-state levels when amiodarone was started, and two of them developed symptoms of digitalis intoxication.[5]

Mechanism

Not fully understood. The rise in serum digoxin levels with amiodarone has been attributed to reductions in both the renal and non-renal excretion of digoxin.[23] Digoxin is a substrate of the efflux pump P-glycoprotein and *in vitro* studies have found that amiodarone (and possibly desethylamiodarone) inhibits the P-glycoprotein-mediated transcellular transport of digoxin.[29] This can result in raised serum digoxin levels, leading to digoxin toxicity. Other transporter mechanisms might also be involved.

Note that amiodarone can also cause hypo- or hyperthyroidism in euthyroid patients and hypothyroidism can precipitate digoxin toxicity,[27] see also 'Digoxin and related drugs + Thyroid hormones and Antithyroid drugs', p.1113

It is thought that amiodarone inhibits the metabolism of digitoxin by the liver, which would explain why digitoxin serum levels are increased on concurrent use.[3]

The cases of torsade de pointes are unexplained (this arrhythmia is not an adverse effect of digoxin and related digitalis glycosides). Amiodarone alone can cause torsade de pointes, and the risk of this may be dose related. It has been suggested that the risk might be increased by digoxin and related drugs because of digoxin-induced after-depolarisations,[28] or because of bradycardia induced by the digitalis glycosides and beta blockers.[2]

Importance and management

The pharmacokinetic interaction between **digoxin** and amiodarone is well documented, well established and of considerable clinical importance. It occurs in most patients. It is clearly evident after a few days and develops over the course of one to 4 weeks.[7] If no account is taken of this interaction the patient might develop digitalis toxicity. Reduce the digoxin dose by between one-third to one-half when amiodarone is added,[4,5,18,22] with further adjustment of the dose after a week or two, and possibly a month or more,[18] depending on digoxin levels. Particular care is needed in children, who possibly have much larger rises in digoxin levels than adults. Amiodarone has a long half-life so that the effects of this interaction will persist for several weeks after its withdrawal.[11] A synergistic effect on heart rate and atrioventricular conduction is also possible, which might result in the development of new arrhythmias. Also note that some authors suggest that concurrent use might possibly worsen the prognosis in some patients.[25,28]

Far less is known about the interaction between **digitoxin** or **metildigoxin** and amiodarone but the limited evidence available suggests that all of the precautions appropriate for digoxin should be used for these drugs as well. Note that the interaction might possibly take months to develop.

The relevance of acetyldigoxin, digitoxin or digoxin to the isolated cases of torsade de pointes on starting amiodarone is uncertain.

1. Schrickel J, Bielik H, Yang A, Schwab JO, Shlevkov N, Schimpf R, Lüderitz B, Lewalter T. Amiodarone-associated 'torsade de pointes'. *Z Kardiol* (2003) 92, 889–92.
2. Schrickel JW, Schwab JO, Yang A, Bitzen A, Lüderitz B, Lewalter T. "Torsade de pointes" in patients with structural heart disease and atrial fibrillation treated with amiodarone, β-blockers and digitalis. *Pacing Clin Electrophysiol* (2006) 29, 363–6.
3. Läer S, Scholz H, Buschmann I, Thoenes M, Meinertz T. Digitoxin intoxication during concomitant use of amiodarone. *Eur J Clin Pharmacol* (1998) 54, 95–6.
4. Moysey JO, Jaggarao NSV, Grundy EN, Chamberlain DA. Amiodarone increases plasma digoxin concentrations. *BMJ* (1981) 282, 272.
5. Fornaro G, Rossi P, Padrini R, Piovan D, Ferrari M, Fortina A, Tomassini G, Aquili C. Ricerca farmacologico-clinica sull'interazione digitale-amiodarone in pazienti cardiopatici con insufficienza cardiaca di vario grado. *G Ital Cardiol* (1984) 14, 990–8.
6. Oetgen WJ, Sobol SM, Tri TB, Heydorn WH, Rakita L. Amiodarone-digoxin interaction. Clinical and experimental observations. *Chest* (1984) 86, 75–9.
7. Vitale P, Jacono A, Gonzales y Reyero E, Zeuli L. Effect of amiodarone on serum digoxin levels in patients with atrial fibrillation. *Clin Trials J* (1984) 21, 199–206.
8. Nademanee K, Kannan R, Hendrickson J, Ookhtens M, Kay I, Singh BN. Amiodarone-digoxin interaction: clinical significance, time course of development, potential pharmacokinetic mechanisms and therapeutic implications. *J Am Coll Cardiol* (1984) 4, 111–16.
9. Nager G, Nager F. Interaktion zwischen Amiodaron und Digoxin. *Schweiz Med Wochenschr* (1983) 113, 1727–30.
10. Strocchi E, Malini PL, Graziani A, Ambrosioni E, Magnani B. L'interazione tra digossina ed amiodarone. *G Ital Cardiol* (1984) 14, 12–15.
11. Robinson K, Johnston A, Walker S, Mulrow JP, McKenna WJ, Holt DW. The digoxin-amiodarone interaction. *Cardiovasc Drugs Ther* (1989) 3, 25–28.
12. Douste-Blazy P, Montastruc JL, Bonnet B, Auriol P, Conte D, Bernadet P. Influence of amiodarone on plasma and urine digoxin concentrations. *Lancet* (1984) i, 905.
13. Achilli A, Serra N. Amiodarone increases plasma digoxin concentrations. *BMJ* (1981) 282, 1630.
14. Achilli A, Giacci M, Capezzuto A, de Luca F, Guerra R, Serra N. Interazione digossina-chinidina e digossina-amiodarone. *G Ital Cardiol* (1981) 11, 918–25.
15. Koren G, Hesslein PS, MacLeod SM. Digoxin toxicity associated with amiodarone therapy in children. *J Pediatr* (1984) 104, 467–70.
16. McQueen EG. New Zealand Committee on Adverse Drug Reactions. 17th Annual Report 1982. *N Z Med J* (1983) 96, 95–9.
17. McGovern B, Garan H, Kelly E, Ruskin JN. Adverse reactions during treatment with amiodarone hydrochloride. *BMJ* (1983) 287, 175–80.
18. Marcus FI, Fenster PE. Drug therapy. Digoxin interactions with other cardiac drugs. *J Cardiovasc Med* (1983) 8, 25–8.
19. Giordano G, Franciosini MF, Zuanetti G, Latini R. Intossicazione digitalica in presenza di epatite acuta da amiodarone. *G Ital Cardiol* (1988) 18, 862–4
20. Mingardi G. Amiodarone and plasma digoxin levels. *Lancet* (1984) i, 1238.
21. Lien W-C, Huang C-H, Chen W-J. Bidirectional ventricular tachycardia resulting from digoxin and amiodarone treatment of rapid atrial fibrillation. *Am J Emerg Med* (2004) 22, 235–6.
22. Santostasi G, Fantin M, Maragno I, Gaion RM, Basadonna O, Dalla-Volta S. Effects of amiodarone on oral and intravenous digoxin kinetics in healthy subjects. *J Cardiovasc Pharmacol* (1987) 9, 385–90.
23. Fenster PE, White NW, Hanson CD. Pharmacokinetic evaluation of the digoxin-amiodarone interaction. *J Am Coll Cardiol* (1985) 5, 108–12.
24. DeVore KJ, Hobbs RA. Plasma digoxin concentration fluctuations associated with timing of plasma sampling and amiodarone administration. *Pharmacotherapy* (2007) 27, 472–5.
25. Mortara A, Cioffi G, Opasich C, Pozzoli M, Febo O, Riccardi G, Cobelli F, Tavazzi L. Combination of amiodarone plus digoxin in chronic heart failure: an adverse effect on survival independently of the presence of sinus rhythm or atrial fibrillation. *Circulation* (1996) 94 (8 Suppl), I-21.
26. Freitag D, Bebee R, Sunderland B. Digoxin–quinidine and digoxin–amiodarone interactions: frequency of occurrence and monitoring in Australian repatriation hospitals. *J Clin Pharm Ther* (1995) 20, 179–83.
27. Ben-Chetrit E, Ackerman Z, Eliakim M. Case-report: Amiodarone-associated hypothyroidism — a possible cause of digoxin intoxication. *Am J Med Sci* (1985) 289, 114–16.
28. Bajaj BP, Baig MW, Perrins EJ. Amiodarone-induced torsades de pointes: the possible facilitatory role of digoxin. *Int J Cardiol* (1991) 33, 335–8.
29. Kakumoto M, Takara K, Sakaeda T, Tanigawara Y, Kita T, Okumura K. MDR1-mediated interaction of digoxin with antiarrhythmic or antianginal drugs. *Biol Pharm Bull* (2002) 25, 1604–7.

Digoxin + Angiotensin II receptor antagonists

Candesartan, eprosartan, irbesartan, losartan, olmesartan, and valsartan do not appear to affect the pharmacokinetics of digoxin, but telmisartan might increase serum digoxin levels.

Clinical evidence

(a) Candesartan

In a study in 12 healthy subjects there was no pharmacokinetic interaction between candesartan 16 mg daily and digoxin, given as a loading dose of 750 micrograms then 250 micrograms daily.[1]

(b) Eprosartan

A study in 12 healthy men given a single 600-microgram dose of digoxin found that eprosartan 200 mg every 12 hours for 4 days did not affect the pharmacokinetics of digoxin.[2]

(c) Irbesartan

A study in 10 healthy subjects taking digoxin for 2 weeks found no changes in the AUC or maximum serum levels of digoxin, when, during the second week, they also took irbesartan 150 mg daily.[3]

(d) Losartan

In 13 healthy subjects the pharmacokinetics of a single 500-microgram oral or intravenous dose of digoxin were not affected by losartan 50 mg daily for a week.[4]

(e) Olmesartan

In a study in 24 healthy subjects, the pharmacokinetics of digoxin 375 micrograms daily (after a loading dose of 1.125 mg on day one) were unaffected by olmesartan medoxomil 20 mg daily for 7 days.[5]

(f) Telmisartan

A study in 12 healthy subjects given a 500-microgram loading dose of digoxin followed by 250 micrograms daily found that the maximum serum concentration, the trough serum concentration and the AUC were increased by 50%, 13%, and 22%, respectively, when telmisartan 120 mg daily was given for 7 days.[6] No clinically relevant changes in vital signs or ECGs were noted.

(g) Valsartan

In a study in 12 healthy subjects there was no adverse interaction between a single 160-mg dose of valsartan and digoxin 250 micrograms.[7]

Mechanism

An *in vitro* study suggests that telmisartan, and to a lesser extent candesartan cilexetil and irbesartan (but not candesartan, losartan, olmesartan, olmesartan medoxomil, or eprosartan) inhibit the P-glycoprotein-mediated transcellular transport of digoxin.[8]

Importance and management

No particular precautions seem to be necessary when digoxin is used with candesartan, eprosartan, irbesartan, losartan, olmesartan or valsartan. However, note that information for eprosartan, losartan, and valsartan is from single-dose studies, although the authors of the eprosartan study consider that a clinically relevant interaction with multiple doses of digoxin is unlikely.[2] The small increase in trough serum digoxin level with telmisartan suggests that the dose of digoxin need not automatically be reduced when telmisartan is started, but consideration should be given to more frequent monitoring of digoxin effects (e.g. bradycardia), taking levels and adjusting the digoxin dose if necessary.

1. Jonkman JH, van Lier JJ, van Heiningen PN, Lins R, Sennewald R, Hogemann A. Pharmacokinetic drug interaction studies with candesartan cilexetil. *J Hum Hypertens* (1997) 11 (Suppl 2), S31–S35.
2. Martin DE, Tompson D, Boike SC, Tenero D, Ilson B, Citerone D, Jorkasky DK. Lack of effect of eprosartan on the single dose pharmacokinetics of orally administered digoxin in healthy male volunteers. *Br J Clin Pharmacol* (1997) 43, 661–4.
3. Marino MR, Vachharajani NN. Drug interactions with irbesartan. *Clin Pharmacokinet* (2001) 40, 605–14.
4. De Smet M, Schoors DF, De Meyer G, Verbesselt R, Goldberg MR, Fitzpatrick V, Somers G. Effect of multiple doses of losartan on the pharmacokinetics of single doses of digoxin in healthy volunteers. *Br J Clin Pharmacol* (1995) 40, 571–5.
5. Laeis P, Püchler K, Kirch W. The pharmacokinetic and metabolic profile of olmesartan medoxomil limits the risk of clinically relevant drug interaction. *J Hypertens* (2001) 19 (Suppl 1), S21–S32.
6. Stangier J, Su C-APF, Hendricks MGC, van Lier JJ, Sollie FAE, Oosterhuis B, Jonkman JHG. The effect of telmisartan on the steady-state pharmacokinetics of digoxin in healthy male volunteers. *J Clin Pharmacol* (2000) 40, 1373–9.
7. Ciba Laboratories. Data on file. Protocol 39.
8. Weiss J, Sauer A, Divac N, Herzog M, Schwedhelm E, Böger RH, Haefeli WE, Benndorf RA. Interaction of angiotensin receptor type 1 blockers with ATP-binding cassette transporters. *Biopharm Drug Dispos* (2010) 31, 150–61.

Digoxin and related drugs + Antacids

Although some studies suggest that antacids can reduce the bioavailability of digoxin, there is other evidence suggesting that no clinically relevant interactions occur. Aluminium/magnesium hydroxide does not interact with digitoxin when administration is separated.

Clinical evidence

(a) Digoxin

1. Evidence of an interaction. In a single-dose study in 10 healthy subjects given digoxin 750 micrograms simultaneously with 60 mL of either 4% **aluminium hydroxide gel**, 8% **magnesium hydroxide gel** or **magnesium trisilicate**, the cumulative 6-day urinary excretion of digoxin was reduced by 25.8% for **aluminium hydroxide**; 35.5% for **magnesium hydroxide**; and 29% for **magnesium trisilicate**.[1] In 10 healthy subjects, when digoxin was given with 30 mL of an **aluminium/magnesium hydroxide** antacid and mexiletine, the AUC of digoxin was approximately halved. As mexiletine (see 'Digoxin + Mexiletine', p.1102) does not appear to interact with digoxin the interaction was attributed to the antacid.[2]

2. Evidence of no interaction. In a study in 4 patients taking long-term digoxin 250 to 500 micrograms daily the concurrent use of **aluminium hydroxide mixture BP** 10 mL three times daily for 7 days did not reduce the bioavailability of the digoxin compared with digoxin alone, and none of the patients had any reduction in the control of their symptoms. The same results were noted in these 4 patients with the concurrent use of digoxin and **magnesium trisilicate mixture BP** 10 mL three times daily for 7 days.[3] Similarly, in a controlled study in 12 healthy subjects, 60 mL of **aluminium/magnesium hydroxide** had no effect on the AUC of digoxin, given as capsules or tablets.[4]

In a single-dose study, aluminium/magnesium hydroxide tablets did not appear to alter the AUC of **beta-acetyldigoxin**.[5]

(b) Digitoxin

A study in 10 patients with heart failure found that their steady-state serum digitoxin levels were slightly, but not statistically significantly *raised* by 11% (from 13.6 nanograms/mL to 15.1 nanograms/mL) while taking 20 mL of **aluminium/magnesium hydroxide** gel three or four times daily, separated from the digitoxin dose by at least one to 2 hours.[6]

Mechanism

Uncertain. One suggestion is that, as has been demonstrated *in vitro* for **magnesium trisilicate** in particular,[7,8] the **digoxin** can become adsorbed onto the antacid and therefore unavailable for absorption.[1,8] This has also been shown for **digitoxin** *in vitro*,[8] but not **lanatoside C**.[9] However, some clinical results are not consistent with this idea.

Importance and management

The interactions between digoxin or digitoxin and antacids are only moderately well documented, and the evidence is inconsistent. Nevertheless, the findings of most studies indicate a modest interaction, at worst, and no clearly clinically relevant interactions have been reported. Separating the doses by one to 2 hours to minimise admixture is effective in resolving the interaction with many other drugs that interact with antacids in this way, and seems to work with digitoxin. However, unless further information becomes available it seems unlikely that separating administration is necessary, although it may be worth bearing in mind if, on rare occasions, a patient experiences an interaction.

1. Brown DD, Juhl RP, Lewis K, Schrott M, Bartels B. Decreased bioavailability of digoxin due to antacids and kaolin-pectin. *N Engl J Med* (1976) 295, 1034–7.
2. Saris SD, Lowenthal DT, Affrime MB. Steady-state digoxin concentration during oral mexiletine administration. *Curr Ther Res* (1983) 34, 662–66.
3. Cooke J, Smith JA. Absence of interaction of digoxin with antacids under clinical conditions. *BMJ* (1978) 2, 1166.
4. Allen MD, Greenblatt DJ, Harmatz JS, Smith TW. Effect of magnesium-aluminum hydroxide and kaolin-pectin on the absorption of digoxin from tablets and capsules. *J Clin Pharmacol* (1981) 21, 26–30.
5. Bonelli J, Hruby K, Magometschnigg D, Hitzenberger G, Kaik G. The bioavailability of β-acetyldigoxine alone and combined with aluminium hydroxide and magnesium hydroxide (Alucol®). *Int J Clin Pharmacol* (1977) 15, 337–9.
6. Kuhlmann J. Plasmaspiegel und renale Elimination von Digitoxin bei Langzeittherapie mit Aluminium-Magnesium-Hydroxid-Gel. *Dtsch Med Wochenschr* (1984) 109, 59–61.
7. McElnay JC, Harron DWG, D'Arcy PF, Eagle MRG. Interaction of digoxin with antacid constituents. *BMJ* (1978) i, 1554.
8. Khalil SAH. The uptake of digoxin and digitoxin by some antacids. *J Pharm Pharmacol* (1974) 26, 961–7.
9. Aldous S, Thomas R. Absorption and metabolism of lanatoside C. *Clin Pharmacol Ther* (1977) 21, 647–58.

Digoxin and related drugs + Anticholinesterases; Centrally acting

Donepezil, galantamine, rivastigmine and tacrine do not alter the pharmacokinetics of digoxin. Digoxin does not appear to alter donepezil or rivastigmine pharmacokinetics. In one healthy subject, bradycardia and heart block occurred on the concurrent use of galantamine and digoxin. The concurrent use of digoxin and donepezil did not appear to increase the risk of bradycardia.

Clinical evidence

(a) Donepezil

A single-dose study in 12 healthy subjects found that the pharmacokinetics of donepezil 5 mg and digoxin 250 micrograms were not affected by concurrent use and no clinically relevant changes in cardiac conduction parameters occurred.[1] In a study in patients with Alzheimer's disease who were given donepezil for 12 weeks, the risk of bradycardia was not increased by the concurrent use of digoxin.[2] Similarly, in a case-control study of 161 patients taking cholinesterase inhibitors (mainly donepezil) admitted to hospital with a diagnosis of bradycardia, there was no increased risk in those who were also taking other drugs that slow the heart rate, including beta blockers, digoxin, diltiazem and verapamil. The odds ratio for hospitalisation for bradycardia was 2.13 for patients that had recently started a cholinesterase inhibitor and 2.34 in those also taking other drugs that slow the heart rate.[3]

(b) Galantamine

In a study in healthy subjects, galantamine 24 mg daily had no effect on the pharmacokinetics of digoxin 375 micrograms daily. However, one subject was hospitalised for second-and third-degree heart block and bradycardia.[4]

(c) Rivastigmine

The manufacturers of rivastigmine[5,6] state that no pharmacokinetic interaction was seen when oral rivastigmine was given with digoxin. In addition no cardiac conduction disturbances were noted on concurrent use.[5]

(d) Tacrine

In one study in healthy subjects given a single 500-microgram dose of digoxin, the pharmacokinetics of digoxin were unchanged by tacrine 20 mg every 6 hours.[7]

Mechanism

No pharmacokinetic interaction appears to occur. Both the centrally-acting anticholinesterases and digoxin (and indeed other **digitalis glycosides**) can slow the heart rate, and the bradycardia seen in the isolated case might simply have been due to the additive effects of both drugs.

Importance and management

No pharmacokinetic interaction appears to occur between any of the centrally-acting anticholinesterases and digoxin, and therefore, on a pharmacokinetic basis, no dose adjustments are needed on concurrent use. However, the digitalis glycosides are known to slow the heart rate, and in clinical studies of galantamine, bradycardia was reported in 1.2% of patients taking galantamine compared with less than 1% of those given placebo.[4] Therefore the UK manufacturer of galantamine[8] recommends caution based on the possibility of a pharmacodynamic interaction that might result in bradycardia. It would seem prudent to be alert for bradycardia if any of these centrally-acting anticholinesterases are given with a digitalis glycoside.

1. Tiseo PJ, Perdomo CA, Friedhoff LT. Concurrent administration of donepezil HCl and digoxin: assessment of pharmacokinetic changes. *Br J Clin Pharmacol* (1998) 46 (Suppl 1), 40–4.
2. Relkin NR, Reichman WE, Orazem J, McRae T. A large, community-based, open-label trial of donepezil in the treatment of Alzheimer's disease. *Dementia Geriatr Cogn Disord* (2003) 16, 15–24.
3. Park-Wyllie LY, Mamdani MM, Li P, Gill SS, Laupacis A, Juurlink DN. Cholinesterase inhibitors and hospitalisation for bradycardia: a population-based study. *PLoS Med* (2009) 6, e1000157.
4. Razadyne ER (Galantamine hydrobromide). Ortho-McNeil-Janssen Pharmaceuticals, Inc. US Prescribing information, July 2013.
5. Exelon (Rivastigmine hydrogen tartrate). Novartis Pharmaceuticals UK Ltd. UK Summary of product characteristics, April 2013.
6. Exelon (Rivastigmine tartrate). Novartis Pharmaceuticals Corp. US Prescribing information, July 2013.
7. deVries TM, Siedlik P, Smithers JA, Brown RR, Reece PA, Posvar EL, Sedman AJ, Koup JR, Forgue ST. Effect of multiple-dose tacrine administration on single-dose pharmacokinetics of digoxin, diazepam, and theophylline. *Pharm Res* (1993) 10 (10 Suppl), S-333.
8. Reminyl Tablets (Galantamine hydrobromide). Shire Pharmaceuticals Ltd. UK Summary of product characteristics, August 2013.

Digoxin and related drugs + Antineoplastics; Cytotoxic

Treatment with radiation and/or antineoplastic cytotoxics appears to reduce the absorption of digoxin tablets but has a negligible effect on digoxin capsules. The absorption of digitoxin does not appear to be affected by the concurrent use of antineoplastic cytotoxics.

Clinical evidence

A study in 13 patients with various forms of neoplastic disease found that radiation therapy and/or various high-dose cytotoxic regimens (including **carmustine**, **cyclophosphamide**, **melphalan**, **cytarabine** and **methotrexate**) reduced the absorption of digoxin from tablets (*Lanoxin*) by almost 46%, but the reduction was not statistically significant (15%) when the digoxin was given as capsules (*Lanoxicaps*).[1]

Other studies confirm that a 50% reduction in serum digoxin levels (using **beta-acetyldigoxin**) occurred in patients given **cyclophosphamide**, **vincristine**, **procarbazine** and prednisone (COPP); **cyclophosphamide**, **vincristine** and prednisone (COP); **cyclophosphamide**, **vincristine**, **cytarabine** and prednisone (COAP); and **doxorubicin**, **bleomycin** and prednisone (ABP). These effects disappeared about a week after cytotoxic therapy finished.[2] Radiation has a smaller effect.[3] **Digitoxin** absorption does not seem to be affected by antineoplastics.[4]

Mechanism

Damage to the intestinal epithelium caused by the antineoplastic cytotoxics is thought to cause a reduction in the absorption of digoxin on concurrent use.[5]

Importance and management

The interaction between digoxin and the antineoplastic cytotoxics appears to be established. Patients taking digoxin and receiving treatment with these antineoplastic cytotoxics (cyclophosphamide and vincristine appear to be the most frequently implicated) should be monitored for signs of under-digitalisation. The problem appears to be overcome by replacing digoxin tablets with digoxin in liquid form or in solution inside a capsule. The effects of the interaction are short-lived so that a downward readjustment seems likely to be necessary about a week after treatment is withdrawn. An alternative is to use digitoxin, which does not appear to be affected.

1. Bjornsson TD, Huang AT, Roth P, Jacob DS, Christenson R. Effects of high-dose cancer chemotherapy on the absorption of digoxin in two different formulations. *Clin Pharmacol Ther* (1986) 39, 25–8.
2. Kuhlmann J, Zilly W, Wilke J. Effects of cytostatic drugs on plasma levels and renal excretion of β-acetyldigoxin. *Clin Pharmacol Ther* (1981) 30, 518–27.
3. Sokol GH, Greenblatt DJ, Lloyd BL, Georgotas A, Allen MD, Harmatz JS, Smith TW, Shader RI. Effect of abdominal radiation therapy on drug absorption in humans. *J Clin Pharmacol* (1978) 18, 388–96.
4. Kuhlmann J, Wilke J, Rietbrock N. Cytostatic drugs are without significant effect on digitoxin plasma level and renal excretion. *Clin Pharmacol Ther* (1982) 32, 646–51.
5. Jusko WB, Conti DR, Molson A, Kuritzky P, Giller J, Schultz R. Digoxin absorption from tablets and elixir: the effect of radiation-induced malabsorption. *JAMA* (1974) 230, 1554–5.

Digoxin + Aprepitant

Aprepitant does not affect the pharmacokinetics of digoxin.

Clinical evidence, mechanism, importance and management

A placebo-controlled, randomised study in 11 healthy subjects found that the pharmacokinetics of digoxin 250 micrograms daily were not affected by aprepitant (125 mg given on day 7 and 80 mg given daily on days 8 to 11). *In vitro* evidence indicates that aprepitant is a substrate and a weak inhibitor of P-glycoprotein. However, at the doses used for the prevention of chemotherapy-induced nausea and vomiting, it appears unlikely to interact with P-glycoprotein substrates such as digoxin.[1] **Fosaprepitant** is a prodrug of aprepitant, and it would therefore be expected to behave in the same way.

1. Feuring M, Lee Y, Orlowski LH, Michiels N, De Smet M, Majumdar AK, Petty KJ, Goldberg MR, Murphy MG, Gottesdiener KM, Hesney M, Brackett LE, Wehling M. Lack of effect of aprepitant on digoxin pharmacokinetics in healthy subjects. *J Clin Pharmacol* (2003) 43, 912–17.

Digoxin + Aspirin

Aspirin, in analgesic doses, might increase digoxin levels.

Clinical evidence, mechanism, importance and management

Although aspirin can double the serum concentrations of digoxin in *dogs*, a study in 8 healthy subjects found no interaction, even when high doses of aspirin (975 mg three times daily) were given.[1] However, in another study in 9 healthy subjects given aspirin 1.5 g daily for 10 days, the serum levels of digoxin were increased by 31%.[2] A further study found a 49% increase in digoxin levels when it was given with aspirin 1.5 g daily.[3] Bearing in mind that both drugs have been in use for a very considerable number of years, the lack of reports in the literature describing problems suggests that no clinically important interaction normally occurs.

1. Fenster PE, Comess KA, Hanson CD and Finley PR. Kinetics of digoxin-aspirin combination. *Clin Pharmacol Ther* (1982) 32, 428–30.
2. Isbary J, Doering W, König E.Der Einfluβ von Tiaprofensäure auf die Digoxinkonzentration im Serum (DKS) im Vergleich zu anderen Antirheumatika (AR). *Z Rheumatol* (1982) 41, 164.
3. Halawa B, Mazurek W. Interakcja digoksyny i niektórych niesteroidowych leków przeciwzapalnych, kwasu acetylosalicylowego i nifedipiny. *Pol Tyg Lek* (1982) 37, 1475–6.

Digoxin + Azoles; Itraconazole or Ketoconazole

Itraconazole causes a sizeable increase in digoxin levels. Ketoconazole is predicted to interact similarly. Theoretically, itraconazole might also oppose the positive inotropic effects of digoxin.

Clinical evidence

In a placebo-controlled, crossover study, 10 healthy subjects taking digoxin 250 micrograms daily were given itraconazole 200 mg daily for 10 days. The serum digoxin levels increased by about 80% (from 1 nanograms/mL to 1.8 nanograms/mL). New steady-state digoxin levels were not fully achieved during the 10-day period with itraconazole, so greater rises might occur on longer-term use.[1] A study in 3 patients with congestive heart failure taking digoxin found that itraconazole decreased digoxin clearance by 50% and increased digoxin levels: ECG changes (premature ventricular contractions, AV block and ST depression) occurred.[2]

A number of cases of this interaction have been reported. A 68-year-old man taking digoxin 250 micrograms twice daily and ibuprofen developed nausea and fatigue (interpreted later as digoxin toxicity) after starting to take itraconazole 400 mg daily for an infected elbow. The symptoms disappeared when both itraconazole and ibuprofen were stopped, but returned when itraconazole was restarted. After 7 days the patient's heart rate had fallen, from 60 bpm to 40 bpm, and his digoxin level had doubled (from 1.6 nanograms/mL to 3.2 nanograms/mL). He was later satisfactorily restabilised on a quarter of the digoxin dose while taking the same dose of itraconazole.[3] Several other patients developed digoxin toxicity (a sixfold increase in serum digoxin level in one case) within 3 to 13 days of starting to take itraconazole,[4-10] and after 4 weeks in one case.[11] A possible case of digoxin toxicity has also occurred with itraconazole pulse therapy.[12] Two cases of digoxin toxicity have been reported when itraconazole was given to kidney transplant patients, but other factors could have contributed to the high levels of digoxin in these 2 patients.[13]

In contrast to all the above reports, one 75-year-old patient taking digoxin 125 micrograms daily had no change in plasma digoxin levels 8 days and 130 days after starting to take itraconazole 200 mg daily (1.1 and 1 nanograms/mL, respectively), when compared with the day before starting itraconazole (0.8 nanograms/mL).[14]

Mechanism

Digoxin is a substrate of the P-glycoprotein efflux pump. Itraconazole inhibits P-glycoprotein, which transports digoxin out of kidney tubule cells into the urine,[15-18] and therefore digoxin urinary clearance is reduced and its serum levels are increased.[5,10] Ketoconazole is also known to inhibit P-glycoprotein, and would therefore be expected to interact similarly.

Importance and management

The pharmacokinetic interaction between **itraconazole** and digoxin is established and clinically important. Monitor the effects of digoxin (e.g. bradycardia) if itraconazole is started, anticipating the need to reduce the digoxin dose. Halving the dose was suggested in one study.[2] Two of the patients cited above were restabilised with a quarter of the digoxin dose[3,4] and another with about one-third of the original digoxin dose[5] while taking itraconazole. Note also that, it has been suggested that itraconazole might possess significant negative inotropic properties, and the CSM in the UK suggests that it should be used with caution in patients at risk of heart failure.[19] This suggests that itraconazole might oppose the pharmacological effects of digoxin.

Although clinical data for **ketoconazole** are lacking, it would be expected to raise digoxin levels similarly to itraconazole (see *Mechanism*, above) and therefore, until more is known, similar precautions to those suggested for itraconazole would seem prudent.

1. Partanen J, Jalava K-M, Neuvonen PJ. Itraconazole increases serum digoxin concentration. *Pharmacol Toxicol* (1996) 79, 274–6.
2. Wagasugi H, Isizuka R, Koreeda N, Yano I, Futami T, Nohara R, Sasayoma S, Inui K. Effect of itraconazole on digoxin clearance in patients with congestive heart failure. *Yakugaku Zasshi* (2000) 120, 807–11.
3. Rex J. Itraconazole-digoxin interaction. *Ann Intern Med* (1992) 116, 525.
4. Kauffman CA, Bagnasco FA. Digoxin toxicity associated with itraconazole therapy. *Clin Infect Dis* (1992) 15, 886–7.
5. Sachs MK, Blanchard LM, Green PJ. Interaction of itraconazole and digoxin. *Clin Infect Dis* (1993) 16, 400–3.
6. Alderman CP, Jersmann HPA. Digoxin-itraconazole interaction. *Med J Aust* (1993) 159, 838–9.
7. McClean KL, Sheehan GJ. Interaction between itraconazole and digoxin. *Clin Infect Dis* (1994) 18, 259–60.
8. Meyboom RH, de Jonge K, Veentjer H, Dekens-Konter JA, de Koning GH. Potentiering van digoxine door itraconazol. *Ned Tijdschr Geneeskd* (1994) 138, 2353–6.
9. Cone LA, Himelman RB, Hirschberg JN, Hutcheson JW. Itraconazole-related amaurosis and vomiting due to digoxin toxicity. *West J Med* (1996) 165, 322.
10. Alderman CP, Allcroft PD. Digoxin-itraconazole interaction: possible mechanisms. *Ann Pharmacother* (1997) 31, 438–40.
11. Lopez F, Hancock EW. Nausea and malaise during treatment of coccidioidomycosis. *Hosp Pract* (1997) 32, 21–2.
12. Brodell RT, Elewski B. Antifungal drug Interactions. Avoidance requires more than memorization. *Postgrad Med* (2000) 107, 41–3.
13. Mathis AS, Friedman GS. Coadministration of digoxin with itraconazole in renal transplant recipients. *Am J Kidney Dis* (2001) 37, 1–8.
14. Mochizuki M, Murase S, Takahashi K, Shimada S. Serum itraconazole and hydroxyitraconazole concentrations and interaction with digoxin in a case of chronic hypertrophic pachymeningitis cause by *Aspergillus flavus*. *Nihon Ishinkin Gakkai Zasshi* (2000) 41, 33–9.
15. Ito S, Koren G. Comment: possible mechanism of digoxin-itraconazole interaction. *Ann Pharmacother* (1997) 31, 1091–2.
16. Woodland C, Ito S, Koren G. A model for the prediction of digoxin–drug interactions at the renal tubular cell level. *Ther Drug Monit* (1998) 20, 134–8.
17. Angirasa AK, Koch AZ. P-glycoprotein as the mediator of itraconazole–digoxin interaction. *J Am Podiatr Med Assoc* (2002) 92, 471–2.

18. Jalava K-M, Partanen J, Neuvonen PJ. Itraconazole decreases renal clearance of digoxin. *Ther Drug Monit* (1997) 19, 609–13.
19. Committee on Safety of Medicines/Medicines Control Agency. Cardiodepressant effects of itraconazole (Sporanox). *Current Problems* (2001) 27, 11–12.

Digoxin + Azoles; Posaconazole

Posaconazole might increase digoxin concentrations.

Clinical evidence, mechanism, importance and management

The US manufacturer of posaconazole states that increased plasma concentrations of digoxin have been found in patients taking digoxin and posaconazole, and they therefore advise monitoring during concurrent use.[1] Although the UK manufacturer of posaconazole does not mention a specific interaction between the two drugs, they do advise that digoxin concentrations should be monitored when initiating or discontinuing posaconazole, in the light of the increase in digoxin concentrations seen when it has been given with other azoles.[2] See 'Digoxin + Azoles; Itraconazole or Ketoconazole', p.1083.

1. Noxafil (Posaconazole). Merck & Co., Inc. US Prescribing information. June 2014.
2. Noxafil (Posaconazole). Merck Sharp & Dohme Ltd. UK Summary of product characteristics, September 2014.

Digoxin + Azoles; Voriconazole

Voriconazole did not affect the steady-state pharmacokinetics of digoxin in a study in healthy patients. Another study briefly mentions increased digoxin levels in two patients given voriconazole.

Clinical evidence, mechanism, importance and management

A placebo-controlled study in healthy subjects given a digoxin loading dose over 2 days, then digoxin 250 micrograms daily for 20 days, found that voriconazole 200 mg twice daily for the last 12 days had no effect on the steady-state pharmacokinetics of digoxin.[1] Unlike itraconazole (see 'Digoxin + Azoles; Itraconazole or Ketoconazole', p.1083), voriconazole does not appear to alter the P-glycoprotein-mediated transport of digoxin. However, a clinical study in severely ill patients with invasive mycosis briefly mentions that 2 patients receiving voriconazole developed high trough digoxin levels, which required digoxin to be withdrawn. One patient was symptomatic with an arrhythmia and ECG changes.[2] These cases appear to be the only ones reported; nevertheless, they introduce a note of caution, and it might be prudent to consider an interaction as a possible cause, if bradycardia or other digoxin adverse effects develop in a patient given voriconazole.

1. Purkins L, Wood N, Kleinermans D, Nichols D. Voriconazole does not affect the steady-state pharmacokinetics of digoxin. *Br J Clin Pharmacol* (2003) 56, 45–50.
2. Cesaro S, Toffolutti T, Messina C, Calore E, Alaggio R, Cusinato R, Pillon M, Zanesco L. Safety and efficacy of caspofungin and liposomal amphotericin B, followed by voriconazole in young patients affected by refractory invasive mycosis. *Eur J Haematol* (2004) 73, 50–5.

Digoxin and related drugs + Barbiturates

Digitoxin levels can be halved by phenobarbital and its effects can be expected to be reduced accordingly. However, another study found that phenobarbital did not affect digitoxin, digoxin or acetyldigitoxin pharmacokinetics.

Clinical evidence

Phenobarbital 60 mg three times daily for 12 weeks, halved the steady-state plasma levels of **digitoxin** 100 micrograms daily.[1] In associated studies the half-life of **digitoxin** decreased from 7.8 days to 4.5 days during the use of **phenobarbital**.[1] In another study[2] the rate of conversion of **digitoxin** to digoxin increased from 4% to 27% in one patient who took **phenobarbital** 96 mg daily for 13 days.

In contrast, a study in groups of 10 healthy subjects given either **digitoxin** 400 micrograms, digoxin 1 mg or **acetyldigitoxin** 800 micrograms daily did not find any changes in the serum concentrations of any of these digitalis glycosides when **phenobarbital** 100 mg was given three times daily for 7 to 9 days.[3]

Mechanism

Phenobarbital and other barbiturates are well-known potent liver enzyme inducers which, it would seem, can increase the metabolism and conversion of digitoxin to digoxin.[1,2] The lack of interaction in one study could possibly have been because the barbiturate was taken for a relatively short time.[3]

Importance and management

The interaction between digitoxin and phenobarbital is established, although its clinical importance is somewhat uncertain because there seem to be few reports of the effects of using digitoxin with phenobarbital, or of problems in practice. Nevertheless, patients taking both drugs should be monitored for possible under-digitalisation and the dose of digitoxin increased if necessary. Other barbiturates would be expected to behave like phenobarbital, but ideally this needs confirmation. It seems unlikely that digoxin will be affected by the barbiturates because it is excreted largely unchanged in the urine.

1. Solomon HM, Abrams WB. Interactions between digitoxin and other drugs in man. *Am Heart J* (1972) 83, 277–80.
2. Jelliffe RW, Blankenhorn DH. Effect of phenobarbital on digitoxin metabolism. *Clin Res* (1966) 14, 160.
3. Káldor A, Somogyi G, Debreczeni LA, Gachályi B. Interaction of heart glycosides and phenobarbital. *Int J Clin Pharmacol* (1975) 12, 403–7.

Digoxin and related drugs + Benzodiazepines and related drugs

Digoxin toxicity occurred in two elderly patients, and rises in digoxin levels have been seen in others, when they were given alprazolam. A reduction in the urinary clearance of digoxin has been described during the use of diazepam. One case-control study found a small increased risk of digoxin toxicity after starting benzodiazepines. No pharmacokinetic interaction seems to occur between digoxin and eszopiclone, zaleplon, or zolpidem.

Clinical evidence

(a) Benzodiazepines

In a case-control study in 3 144 patients who had been admitted to hospital with digoxin toxicity, patients were more likely than controls to have received a new prescription for benzodiazepines (type not stated) in the 30 days before admission (adjusted odds ratio 2.1). This was after adjusting for renal impairment and other interacting drugs. Benzodiazepines were analysed in this study because the authors considered they have no known basis for an interaction, and were therefore not expected to interact.[1] Studies and reports involving named benzodiazepines are discussed in the subsections below.

1. Alprazolam. An elderly woman taking digoxin, maprotiline, isosorbide dinitrate, furosemide and potassium chloride had signs of digoxin toxicity during the second week of taking alprazolam 1 mg daily. Her serum digoxin levels were later found to have risen almost 300% (from 1.6 to 4.3 nanograms/mL), and her apparent digoxin clearance had fallen by about 60%.[2] In a later study in 6 patients taking digoxin 250 micrograms daily, the concurrent use of alprazolam 500 micrograms twice daily increased the AUC of digoxin, particularly in those over 65 years old. One elderly man developed clinical digoxin toxicity. However, in a further 6 patients, a lower dose of alprazolam of 250 micrograms twice daily had little effect on the AUC of digoxin.[3] In contrast, a controlled study in 8 healthy subjects found no changes in the clearance of a single 1.25-mg intravenous dose of digoxin after they took alprazolam 1.5 mg daily.[4]

2. Diazepam. The observation that 3 patients developed raised digoxin levels while also taking diazepam prompted a further study in 7 healthy subjects.[5] After taking diazepam 5 mg, both with and 12 hours after a single 500-microgram dose of digoxin, all subjects had a substantial reduction in the urinary excretion of digoxin and 5 subjects had a moderate increase in the half-life of digoxin. No further details were given.[5]

3. Metaclazepam. No statistically significant interaction was seen in 9 patients taking **beta-acetyldigoxin** when they were given metaclazepam.[6]

(b) Non-benzodiazepine hypnotics

1. Eszopiclone. In a study in 12 healthy subjects, a 3-mg single dose of eszopiclone did not alter the pharmacokinetics of digoxin, given for 7 days.[7]

2. Zaleplon. Zaleplon 10 mg daily, given to 20 healthy subjects for 5 days, had no effects on the steady-state pharmacokinetics of digoxin 375 micrograms daily. There were no differences in QTc or PR intervals.[8]

3. Zolpidem. No pharmacokinetic interaction occurs between zolpidem and digoxin.[9]

Mechanism

Uncertain. It has been suggested that diazepam and some other benzodiazepines might alter the extent of the protein binding of digoxin within the plasma, which could have some influence on the renal tubular excretion.[5] However, see comments on protein binding interactions in 'Drug distribution interactions', p.3. The reason for the interaction between digoxin and alprazolam is not understood. In addition, the reason for the unexpected small increased risk of digoxin toxicity with benzodiazepines in the case-control study is unclear.[1]

Importance and management

Information on the interaction between digoxin and **alprazolam** is limited, and an interaction is not established. However, given the range of benzodiazepines available, it might be sensible to consider an alternative to alprazolam in patients taking digoxin. If concurrent use is necessary, it would seem prudent to monitor the effects of digoxin (e.g. bradycardia), taking digoxin levels and reducing the digoxin dose as necessary. What is known suggests that an adverse interaction appears to be more likely in the elderly.

The reduction in the urinary excretion of digoxin when it is given with **diazepam** seems unlikely to be clinically important, but bear the interaction in mind in case of an unexpected rise in digoxin levels.

Other benzodiazepines and digoxin have been used for a considerable time but there seem to be no other reports of adverse interactions, apart from the unexpected finding of a small increased risk of digoxin toxicity after starting benzodiazepines in one case control study, which requires confirmation. The newer **non-benzodiazepine hypnotics**, eszopiclone, zaleplon and zolpidem, do not appear to affect the pharmacokinetics of digoxin.

1. Juurlink DN, Mamdani MM, Kopp A, Herrmann N, Laupacis A. A population-based assessment of the potential interaction between serotonin-specific reuptake inhibitors and digoxin. *Br J Clin Pharmacol* (2005) 59, 102–7.
2. Tollefson G, Lesar T, Grothe D, Garvey M. Alprazolam-related digoxin toxicity. *Am J Psychiatry* (1984) 141, 1612–14.
3. Guven H, Tuncok Y, Guneri S, Cavdar C, Fowler J. Age-related digoxin-alprazolam interaction. *Clin Pharmacol Ther* (1993) 54, 42–4.
4. Ochs HR, Greenblatt DJ, Verburg-Ochs B. Effect of alprazolam on digoxin kinetics and creatinine clearance. *Clin Pharmacol Ther* (1985) 38, 595–8.
5. Castillo-Ferrando JR, Garcia M, Carmona J. Digoxin levels and diazepam. *Lancet* (1980) ii, 368.
6. Völker D, Müller R, Günther C, Bode R. Digoxin-Plasmaspiegel während der Behandlung mit Metaclazepam. *Arzneimittelforschung* (1988) 38, 923–5.
7. Caron J, Wessel T, Maier G. Evaluation of a pharmacokinetic interaction between eszopiclone and digoxin. *Sleep* (2004) 27, A55.
8. Sanchez Garcia P, Paty I, Leister CA, Guerra P, Frias J, García Pérez LE, Darwish M. Effect of zaleplon on digoxin pharmacokinetics and pharmacodynamics. *Am J Health-Syst Pharm* (2000) 57, 2267–70.
9. Salvà P, Costa J. Clinical pharmacokinetics and pharmacodynamics of zolpidem: therapeutic implications. *Clin Pharmacokinet* (1995) 29, 142–53.

Digoxin and related drugs + Beta-agonist bronchodilators

Oral salbutamol (albuterol) might reduce digoxin levels. Beta agonists can cause hypokalaemia, which could lead to the development of digitalis toxicity.

Clinical evidence, mechanism, importance and management

A study in 10 healthy subjects who had taken digoxin 500 micrograms daily for 10 days[1] found that, 3 hours after taking oral **salbutamol** (albuterol) 3 to 4 mg, their serum digoxin levels had fallen by 0.23 nanograms/mL and their serum potassium levels had fallen by 0.58 mmol/L. A follow-up study suggested that the digoxin distribution to skeletal muscle might have been increased.[2]

Note that all beta$_2$ agonists can cause a fall in serum potassium, which could possibly affect the response of patients to digoxin or other **digitalis glycosides**. The clinical importance of these changes is uncertain but concurrent use should be monitored (e.g. bradycardia). Consider monitoring potassium levels if the effects of digoxin seem excessive.

1. Edner M, Jogestrand T. Oral salbutamol decreases serum digoxin concentration. *Eur J Clin Pharmacol* (1990) 38, 195–7.
2. Edner M, Jogestrand T, Dahlqvist R. Effect of salbutamol on digoxin pharmacokinetics. *Eur J Clin Pharmacol* (1992) 42, 197–201.

Digoxin and related drugs + Beta blockers

In general there appears to be no pharmacokinetic interaction between digoxin and beta blockers, although talinolol and carvedilol appear to increase the bioavailability of digoxin. Pharmacodynamic interactions, resulting in additive bradycardia, are possible. A few cases of excessive bradycardia have been reported when propranolol was used to control digitalis-induced arrhythmias.

Clinical evidence

(a) Acebutolol

In a study in 8 healthy subjects, acebutolol 400 mg twice daily for 5 days did not affect the pharmacokinetics of a single 750-microgram dose of digoxin.[1]

(b) Atenolol

In a study in 6 healthy subjects given atenolol 100 mg daily for 10 days, there was no change in the pharmacokinetics of digoxin 20 micrograms/kg daily given on days 8 to 10. Atenolol did not affect digoxin-induced inotropism.[2]

(c) Bevantolol

In a multiple-dose study in 10 healthy subjects, bevantolol 200 mg daily did not affect the mean plasma levels of digoxin 250 micrograms daily. There was also no change in resting heart rate.[3]

(d) Bisoprolol

In 14 healthy subjects[4] the pharmacokinetics of digoxin 250 micrograms daily for 13 days (following a loading dose of digoxin 375 micrograms on day one), were unaffected by the concurrent use of bisoprolol 10 mg daily from days 2 to 14.

(e) Carvedilol

A 12-year-old boy with dilated cardiomyopathy taking digoxin 250 micrograms in the morning and 125 micrograms in the evening was subsequently given carvedilol 70 micrograms/kg twice daily. Several days later he lost his appetite and started vomiting, and his digoxin serum level was found to have increased from 1.6 to 2.3 nanograms/mL up to 4.2 nanograms/mL. Digoxin was stopped and subsequently restarted at half the original dose.[5] In one study, 8 children aged 2 weeks to 8 years were given digoxin for ventricular failure secondary to congenital heart disease. When they were also given carvedilol 0.06 to 1.06 mg/kg daily the clearance of digoxin was approximately halved and 2 children developed digoxin toxicity.[5]

A single-dose study in healthy adults given carvedilol 25 mg found that the maximum plasma levels of a 500-microgram dose of digoxin were increased by 0.97 nanograms/mL (60%) and the AUC was increased by about 20%, but the clinical effects of these changes were considered likely to be small.[6] No pharmacokinetic interaction was found in other single-dose studies in adults given carvedilol and **digitoxin**,[7] or carvedilol and intravenous digoxin.[6]

In a multiple-dose study in adult patients with hypertension, carvedilol raised the maximum serum levels and AUC of digoxin 250 micrograms daily by 32% and 14%, respectively, after 2 weeks of concurrent use.[8] In another study, in 12 male and 12 female patients taking digoxin 62.5 to 250 micrograms daily for heart failure, the addition of carvedilol 6.25 mg twice daily for 7 days increased the maximum concentration and the AUC$_{0-16}$ of digoxin by 37% and 56%, respectively, in the men, but no changes to the pharmacokinetics of digoxin were noted in the women.[9] In 14 patients with heart failure taking digoxin, the addition of carvedilol 6.25 mg twice daily, increased to 12.5 mg twice daily over two months, had no effect on serum digoxin levels when compared with control patients.[10]

(f) Esmolol

A single dose of intravenous esmolol did not affect the pharmacokinetics of multiple-dose digoxin, except that a small increase was seen in the AUC$_{0-6}$ of digoxin. There were also no changes in the pharmacodynamics of digoxin, with no changes in heart rate or blood pressure occurring.[11]

(g) Nadolol

In a placebo-controlled study of the use of nadolol in patients with chronic atrial fibrillation taking digoxin, 32 patients were randomised to take nadolol 20 mg daily (titrated up to 120 mg daily as tolerated) for 6 weeks or placebo. Nadolol had no effect on serum digoxin levels.[12] The same finding was reported in a similar crossover study.[13]

(h) Nebivolol

In 13 healthy subjects,[14] the pharmacokinetics of digoxin 250 micrograms twice daily for one day, followed by once daily for 16 days, were unaffected by the concurrent use of nebivolol 10 mg four times daily from days 8 to 17.

(i) Propranolol

Two cases, where propranolol 10 mg orally was used to treat arrhythmias associated with digoxin toxicity, are reported.[15] The first patient (who had heart failure) became bradycardic, asystolic and then died, while the second patient became bradycardic (30 bpm) but recovered after being given atropine. A further fatality was reported when intravenous propranolol was used.[16]

(j) Sotalol

In a placebo-controlled study of the use of sotalol in digitalised patients with chronic atrial fibrillation, 2 of 24 sotalol recipients withdrew due to bradycardia compared with none of 10 given placebo. However, the combination was still considered valuable.[17] In this study, the pharmacokinetics of multiple-dose digoxin were unaffected by sotalol 80 to 320 mg daily.[17]

(k) Talinolol

In healthy subjects talinolol 100 mg orally increased the bioavailability of a single 500-microgram dose of digoxin. The AUC$_{0-72}$ and the maximum serum levels of digoxin were increased by 23% and 45%, respectively.[18] Conversely, intravenous talinolol 30 mg had no effect on digoxin pharmacokinetics.[18]

(l) Timolol

A report describes marked bradycardia of 35 to 50 bpm in a 91-year-old patient taking **digoxin** and using timolol 0.25% eye drops.[19] Bradycardia persisted when **digoxin** was withdrawn, and improved only after discontinuation of the timolol as well.

(m) Miscellaneous

A prospective analysis of adverse drug reactions leading to hospital admission over a 4-year period identified 83 patients admitted with bradycardia. Of these, 62 were taking **digitalis glycosides**, and 14 were also taking a beta blocker.[20] Increased bradycardia might occur with the concurrent use of a digitalis glycoside and a beta blocker, but reports of this becoming a problem seem rare (although see *Propranolol*, *Sotalol*, and *Timolol*, above).

Mechanism

In most cases where the concurrent use of a digitalis glycoside and a beta blocker has resulted in an adverse outcome, this appears to be related to the additive effects of the two drugs on the slowing of the heart.

It has been suggested that the pharmacokinetic interaction with talinolol is due to competition with digoxin for *intestinal* P-glycoprotein, although this needs confirmation.[18] *In vitro* studies suggest that the P-glycoprotein mediated transcellular transport of digoxin is inhibited by carvedilol[21,22] and, to a lesser extent, propranolol[22] (but not atenolol,[21] metoprolol[21,22] or sotalol[22]). It is possible that P-glycoprotein inhibition by carvedilol enhances the intestinal absorption of digoxin and also decreases its renal excretion. This may explain why the interaction has greater clinical importance in children, as they have a higher renal clearance rate of digoxin than adults.[5]

Importance and management

On the whole, the concurrent use of a digitalis glycoside and a beta blocker appears to be beneficial. However, the potential for additive bradycardia should be borne in mind when considering concurrent use with *intravenous*, *oral* or *topical* beta blockers. Nevertheless, any adverse effect appears rare with digoxin, and there appear to be no reports of additive bradycardia with beta blockers and **digitoxin**, although this is perhaps due to a lack of reporting, as this is an expected effect of concurrent use. In addition, it would seem prudent to monitor digoxin levels with talinolol, and also with carvedilol, particularly in children. It has been suggested that the dose of digoxin should be reduced by at least 25% in children given carvedilol, with further adjustments as required.[5]

1. Ryan JR. Clinical pharmacology of acebutolol. *Am Heart J* (1985) 109, 1131–6.
2. Hansen PB, Buch J, Rasmussen OØ, Waldorf S, Steiness E. Influence of atenolol and nifedipine on digoxin-induced inotropism in humans. *Br J Clin Pharmacol* (1984) 18, 817–22.
3. Frishman WH, Goldberg RJ, Benfield P. Bevantolol. A preliminary review of its pharmacodynamic and pharmacokinetic properties, and therapeutic efficacy in hypertension and angina pectoris. *Drugs* (1988) 35, 1–21.
4. Vechlekar DL, Cheung WK, Pearse S, Greene DS, Dukart G, Unczowsky R, Weiss AI, Silber BM, Faulkner RD. Bisoprolol does not alter the pharmacokinetics of digoxin. *Pharm Res* (1988) 5 (Suppl), S176.
5. Ratnapalan S, Griffiths K, Costei AM, Benson L, Koren G. Digoxin-carvedilol interactions in children. *J Pediatr* (2003) 142, 572–4.
6. De Mey C, Brendel E, Enterling D. Carvedilol increases the systemic bioavailability of oral digoxin. *Br J Clin Pharmacol* (1990) 29, 486–90.
7. Harder S, Brei R, Caspary S, Merz PG. Lack of a pharmacokinetic interaction between carvedilol and digitoxin or phenprocoumon. *Eur J Clin Pharmacol* (1993) 44, 583–6.
8. Wermeling DP, Feild CJ, Smith DA, Chandler MHH, Clifton GD, Boyle DA. Effects of long-term oral carvedilol on the steady-state pharmacokinetics of oral digoxin in patients with mild to moderate hypertension. *Pharmacotherapy* (1994) 14, 600–6.
9. Baris N, Kalkan S, Güneri S, Bozdemir V, Guven H. Influence of carvedilol on serum digoxin levels in heart failure: is there any gender difference? *Eur J Clin Pharmacol* (2006) 62, 535–38.
10. Agarwal AK, Venugopalan P. Beneficial effect of carvedilol on heart rate response to exercise in digitalised patients with heart failure in atrial fibrillation due to idiopathic dilated cardiomyopathy. *Eur J Heart Fail* (2001) 3, 437–40.
11. Lowenthal DT, Porter RS, Achari R, Turlapaty P, Laddu AR and Matier WL. Esmolol-digoxin drug interaction. *J Clin Pharmacol* (1987) 27, 561–6.
12. Zoble RG, Brewington J, Olukotun AY, Gore R. Comparative effects of nadolol-digoxin combination therapy and digoxin monotherapy for chronic atrial fibrillation. *Am J Cardiol* (1987) 60, 39D–45D.
13. DiBianco R, Morganroth J, Freitag JA, Ronan JA, Lindgren KM, Donohue DJ, Larca LJ, Chadda KD, Olukotun AY. Effects of nadolol on the spontaneous and exercise-provoked heart rate of patients with chronic atrial fibrillation receiving stable dosages of digoxin. *Am Heart J* (1984) 108, 1121–127.
14. Lawrence TE, Liu S, Fischer JW, Vukic-Bugarski T, Donnelly CM, Huang MY, Rackley RJ. No interaction between nebivolol and digoxin in healthy volunteers. *Clin Pharmacol Ther* (2005) 77, P76.
15. Watt DAL. Sensitivity to propranolol after digoxin intoxication. *BMJ* (1968) 3, 413–14.
16. Schamroth L. The immediate effects of intravenous propranolol in various cardiac arrhythmias. *Am J Cardiol* (1966) 18, 438.
17. Singh S, Saini RK, DiMarco J, Kluger J, Gold R, Chen Y. Efficacy and safety of sotalol in digitalized patients with chronic atrial fibrillation. *Am J Cardiol* (1991) 68, 1227–30.
18. Westphal K, Weinbrenner A, Giessmann T, Stuhr M, Gerd F, Zschiesche M, Oertel R, Terhaag B, Kroemer HK, Siegmund W. Oral bioavailability of digoxin is enhanced by talinolol: Evidence for involvement of P-glycoprotein. *Clin Pharmacol Ther* (2000) 68, 6–12.
19. Rynne MV. Timolol toxicity: ophthalmic medication complicating systemic disease. *J Maine Med Assoc* (1980) 71, 82.
20. Haase G, Pietzsch M, Fähnrich A, Voss W, Riethling A-K. Results of a systematic adverse drug reaction (ADR)-screening concerning bradycardia caused by drug interactions in departments of internal medicine in Rostock. *Int J Clin Pharmacol Ther* (2002) 40,116–19.
21. Takara K, Kakumoto M, Tanigawara Y, Funakoshi J, Sakaeda T, Okumura K. Interaction of digoxin with antihypertensive drugs *via* MDR1. *Life Sci* (2002) 70, 1491–1500.
22. Bachmakov I, Werner U, Endress B, Auge D, Fromm MF. Characterization of β-adrenoceptor antagonists as substrates and inhibitors of the drug transporter P-glycoprotein. *Fundam Clin Pharmacol* (2006) 20, 273–82.

Digoxin and related drugs + Bufalin

Bufalin can interfere with the assay of cardiac glycosides.

Clinical evidence, mechanism, importance and management

Bufalin, a cardioactive substance of amphibian origin, and Chinese medicines such as Chan Su, Lu-Shen-Wan and Kyushin that contain bufalin, can interfere with some immunoassay methods of **digitoxin** and digoxin, particularly the fluorescence polarisation immunoassay.[1-4] The digoxin-like immunoreactivity of Kyushin was found to be equivalent to varying amounts of digoxin because of differences in the cross-reactivity of the antibody used in different immunoassays.[3] A chemiluminescent assay for **digitoxin**[2,5] and digoxin[2] did not cross-react with bufalin.

Bufalin and an extract of Chan Su displaced **digitoxin** from protein-binding sites *in vitro*.[5] Whether this would result in elevated free **digitoxin** levels and toxicity *in vivo* is not known. However, this is probably unlikely, because *in vivo* the free drug would be available for metabolism (see *Protein-binding interactions*, under 'Drug distribution interactions', p.3).

Another possibility, given the similarities between bufalin and digitalis glycosides, is that toxicity could result from additive cardiac effects. Cases of cardiotoxicity following the ingestion of bufalin (or toads) alone have been reported. In one case, the symptoms seen were very similar to those of digoxin toxicity, with nausea, vomiting, blurred vision, mental confusion, cardiopulmonary arrest and severe bradyarrhythmia. Assay for digoxin was positive (2.1 nanograms/mL) when measured by the fluorescence energy transfer immunoassay. The patient had ingested a bowl of toad soup (*Bufo melanosticus* Schneider) shortly before his symptoms developed.[6]

1. Chow L, Johnson M, Wells A, Dasgupta A. Effect of the traditional Chinese medicines Chan Su, Lu-Shen-Wan, Dan Shen, and Asian ginseng on serum digoxin measurement by Tina-quant (Roche) and Synchron LX System (Beckman) digoxin immunoassays. *J Clin Lab Anal* (2003) 17, 22–7.
2. Dasgupta A, Datta P. Rapid detection of cardioactive bufalin toxicity using fluorescence polarization immunoassay for digitoxin. *Ther Drug Monit* (1998) 20, 104–8.
3. Fushimi R, Koh T, Iyama S, Yasuhara M, Tachi J, Kohda K, Amino N, Miyai K. Digoxin-like immunoreactivity in Chinese medicine. *Ther Drug Monit* (1990) 12, 242–5.
4. Reyes MA, Actor JK, Risin SA, Dasgupta A. Effect of Chinese medicines Chan Su and Lu-Shen-Wan on serum digoxin measurement by Digoxin III, a new digoxin immunoassay. *Ther Drug Monit* (2008) 30, 95–99.
5. Datta P, Dasgupta A. Interactions between drugs and Asian medicine: displacement of digitoxin from protein binding site by bufalin, the constituent of Chinese medicines Chan Su and Lu-Shen-Wan. *Ther Drug Monit* (2000) 22, 155–9.
6. Chern M-S. Ray C-Y, Wu D. Biologic intoxication due to digitalis-like substance after ingestion of cooked toad soup. *Am J Cardiol* (1991) 67, 443–4.

Digoxin and related drugs + Calcium-channel blockers; Dihydropyridines

Felodipine, isradipine, lacidipine, lercanidipine, and nicardipine do not alter digoxin exposure, although small increases in maximum digoxin levels have been seen with some of these calcium-channel blockers. Amlodipine and nimodipine appear not to interact with digoxin. Nisoldipine might cause a minor rise in trough digoxin levels. The situation with nitrendipine is uncertain but it possibly causes only a very slight increase in digoxin exposure. Serum digoxin levels are normally unchanged or increased only to a limited extent by nifedipine; however, a few studies describe increases ranging from 45 to 66%. Nifedipine appears not to interact with digitoxin.

Clinical evidence

(a) Amlodipine

In a study in 21 healthy subjects, amlodipine 5 mg daily had no effect on the serum levels or renal clearance of digoxin 375 micrograms daily.[1]

(b) Felodipine

In a placebo-controlled study in 23 patients taking digoxin, felodipine 10 mg twice daily for 8 weeks did not affect serum digoxin levels.[2] In another study, 14 patients taking digoxin 375 micrograms daily were given felodipine 10 mg daily for a week as extended-release then plain tablets. Neither formulation altered the AUC of digoxin, but the plain tablets caused a rise in the maximum steady-state digoxin serum levels of 11%.[3] Similarly, in a third study in 12 patients given felodipine, the peak plasma digoxin levels were transiently raised by about 40%, but the AUC of digoxin was not affected.[4]

(c) Isradipine

Isradipine (given as 2.5 mg every 12 hours for 2 days, 5 mg every 12 hours for 2 days and then 5 mg three times daily for 10 days) did not affect the pharmacokinetics of a single 1-mg intravenous dose of digoxin, given to 24 healthy subjects.[5] A similar study by the same group found that the same dosage regimen of isradipine given with oral digoxin 250 micrograms twice daily caused a 25% increase in peak serum digoxin levels but no changes in its steady-state levels or AUC.[6]

(d) Lacidipine

In 12 healthy subjects,[7] a single 4-mg oral dose of lacidipine did not affect the AUC or minimum serum levels of digoxin 250 micrograms daily for 7 days, but the maximum serum levels of digoxin were increased by 34%.

(e) Lercanidipine

The maximum serum levels of digoxin rose by 33% in healthy subjects also given lercanidipine, although the AUC and renal clearance of digoxin were not affected. However, there was no evidence of a pharmacokinetic interaction in patients given **metildigoxin** with lercanidipine.[8]

(f) Nicardipine

Nicardipine 20 mg three times daily for 14 days did not affect the digoxin plasma levels of 9 patients taking digoxin 130 to 250 micrograms daily, although one other patient had a twofold increase.[9] Another 20 patients with congestive heart failure also had no changes in steady-state serum digoxin levels or AUC while taking nicardipine 30 mg three times daily for 5 days.[10] Yet another study in 9 patients confirmed the absence of an interaction.[11]

(g) Nifedipine

1. Serum digoxin levels unchanged. Studies in patients[12,13] and healthy subjects[14,15] given oral digoxin found that serum digoxin levels were not affected by nifedipine 30 to 60 mg daily. Similarly no changes in the pharmacokinetics of a single intravenous dose of digoxin were found in patients[16] or healthy subjects[17,18] taking nifedipine 40 to 90 mg daily. Furthermore, no changes in the pharmacokinetics of nifedipine were seen.[17]

Similarly, in a study in patients taking **beta-acetyldigoxin**, plasma digoxin levels were not affected by nifedipine.[19] A study in 18 subjects found that nifedipine 40 to 60 mg daily had no effect on steady-state plasma **digitoxin** levels over a 6-week period.[20] This study has also been published elsewhere.[21]

2. Serum digoxin levels increased. In 12 healthy subjects, nifedipine 30 mg increased the plasma levels of digoxin 375 micrograms daily by 45% (from 0.505 nanograms/mL to 0.734 nanograms/mL) over 14 days.[22] In a study in 7 healthy subjects, nifedipine 15 to 60 mg daily increased the levels of digoxin 250 micrograms twice daily by 15%.[23] These studies have been reported elsewhere.[24,25]

Nifedipine 20 mg twice daily increased the steady-state serum digoxin levels of 9 patients by 15% (from 0.87 nanograms/mL to 1.04 nanograms/mL).[26] A 61% increase in serum digoxin levels was found in a study involving nifedipine in daily doses of 30 mg.[27] A retrospective analysis of pharmacokinetic data suggested that clearance of digoxin could be reduced by 10% in patients also taking nifedipine.[28]

In a study in 10 patients with congestive heart failure given **metildigoxin** 200 micrograms daily for 9 days, the concurrent use of nifedipine 60 mg for a further 7 days, increased levels of digoxin by about 25%. In another 10 patients given both nifedipine 60 mg and verapamil 320 mg daily for 7 days, digoxin levels were increased by about 66%.[29]

(h) Nimodipine

In a study in 12 healthy subjects, nimodipine 30 mg twice daily caused no change in the pharmacokinetics or haemodynamic effects of **beta-acetyldigoxin**.[30]

(i) Nisoldipine

In 10 patients with heart failure nisoldipine 20 mg daily increased the trough plasma levels of digoxin by about 15%.[31,32] In 8 healthy subjects, nisoldipine 10 mg twice daily caused no changes in the pharmacokinetics or haemodynamic effects of **beta-acetyldigoxin**.[30]

(j) Nitrendipine

In a study in 8 healthy subjects taking digoxin 250 micrograms twice daily for 2 weeks, nitrendipine 10 mg daily did not affect plasma digoxin levels. A higher dose of nitrendipine of 20 mg daily very slightly increased the AUC of digoxin by 15%, increased the maximum plasma levels from 1.34 nanograms/mL to 2.1 nanograms/mL, and reduced its clearance by 13%. One subject dropped out of the study because of dizziness, nausea and vomiting, palpitations, insomnia and nervousness.[33,34] Similar, or the same results, have been reported elsewhere.[35]

Other studies in healthy subjects and patients found that nitrendipine 20 mg twice daily caused no changes in the pharmacokinetics or haemodynamic effects of digoxin[36] or **beta-acetyldigoxin**.[30,37]

Mechanism

Where an interaction occurs it is probably due to changes in the renal excretion of digoxin. An *in vitro* study found that several calcium-channel blockers including nicardipine, and to a lesser extent nisoldipine (as well as barnidipine, manidipine, nilvadipine, and verapamil) inhibited the P-glycoprotein-mediated transcellular transport of digoxin. This suggests that any interaction may occur, at least in part, by affecting digoxin renal tubular excretion. Nitrendipine only weakly inhibited the transcellular transport of digoxin.[38] Nifedipine did not affect P-glycoprotein-mediated transcellular transport of digoxin in one study,[38] but did in another.[12]

Importance and management

The extent of the information varies from drug to drug, but the concurrent use of digoxin and calcium-channel blockers can be therapeutically valuable. Most calcium-channel blockers (amlodipine, felodipine, isradipine, lacidipine, lercanidipine, nicardipine and nimodipine) either cause only minimal increases in digoxin levels, which are unlikely to be clinically important in most patients, or do not interact at all. Nevertheless, the UK manufacturer of **lercanidipine** recommends close monitoring for signs of digoxin toxicity when both drugs are given together,[8] while the UK manufacturer of **nicardipine** recommends careful monitoring of digoxin levels when patients are given both drugs together.[39] If monitoring is considered appropriate, monitor the effects of digoxin (e.g. bradycardia), and consider measuring levels if the effects of digoxin seem excessive. Reduce the digoxin dose as necessary.

For nifedipine, the weight of evidence appears to suggest that serum digoxin levels are normally unchanged or only modestly increased by **nifedipine**. Concurrent use appears normally to be safe and effective.[40] One report suggests that nifedipine has some attenuating effect on the digoxin-induced inotropism.[41] Another points out that under some circumstances (renal impairment or pre-existing digoxin overdosing) some risk of an undesirable interaction still exists.[23] If undesirable bradycardia occurs in a patient taking digoxin and nifedipine, consider measuring digoxin levels, and adjust the dose accordingly. Nifedipine does not appear to interact with digitoxin.

The situation with **nitrendipine** needs clarification, although the pharmacokinetic changes seen in one study are probably too small to be clinically important.

1. Schwartz JB. Effects of amlodipine on steady-state digoxin concentrations and renal digoxin clearance. *J Cardiovasc Pharmacol* (1988) 12, 1–5.
2. Dunselman PHJM, Scaf AHJ, Kuntze CEE, Lie KI, Wesseling H. Digoxin-felodipine interaction in patients with congestive heart failure. *Eur J Clin Pharmacol* (1988) 35, 461–5.
3. Kirch W, Laskowski M, Ohnhaus EE, Åberg J. Effects of felodipine on plasma digoxin levels and haemodynamics in patients with heart failure. *J Intern Med* (1989) 225, 237–39.
4. Rehnqvist N, Billing E, Moberg L, Lundman T, Olsson G. Pharmacokinetics of felodipine and effect on digoxin plasma levels in patients with heart failure. *Drugs* (1987) 34 (Suppl 3), 33–42.
5. Johnson BF, Wilson J, Marwaha R, Hoch K, Johnson J. The comparative effects of verapamil and a new dihydropyridine calcium channel blocker on digoxin pharmacokinetics. *Clin Pharmacol Ther* (1987) 42, 66–71.
6. Rodin SM, Johnson BF, Wilson J, Ritchie P, Johnson J. Comparative effects of verapamil and isradipine on steady-state digoxin kinetics. *Clin Pharmacol Ther* (1988) 43, 668–72.
7. Hall ST, Harding SM, Anderson DM, Ward C, Stevens LA. The effect of single 4 mg oral dose of calcium antagonist lacidipine on the pharmacokinetics of digoxin. In: Carpi C, Zanchetti A, eds. IVth Int Symp Calcium Antagonists: Pharmacology and Clinical Research. Florence, May 1989: 161.
8. Zanidip (Lercanidipine hydrochloride). Recordati Pharmaceuticals Ltd. UK Summary of product characteristics, April 2006.
9. Lessem J, Bellinetto A. Interaction between digoxin and the calcium antagonists nicardipine and tiapamil. *Clin Ther* (1983) 5, 595–602.
10. Debruyne D, Commeau Ph, Grollier G, Huret B, Scanu P, Moulin M. Nicardipine does not significantly affect serum digoxin concentrations at the steady state of patients with congestive heart failure. *Int J Clin Pharmacol Res* (1989) IX, 15–19.
11. Scanu P, Commeau P, Huret B, Gérard JL, Debruyne D, Moore N, Lamy E, Dorey H, Grolier G, Potier JC. Pharmacocinétique et effets pharmacodynamiques de la digoxine dans les myocardiopathies dilatées. Influence de la nicardipine. *Arch Mal Coeur Vaiss* (1987) 80, 1773–83.
12. Schwartz JB, Raizner A, Akers S. The effect of nifedipine on serum digoxin concentrations in patients. *Am Heart J* (1984) 107, 669–73.
13. Halawa B, Walentyna M. Interakcje digoksyny z nifedypiną i diltiazemem. *Pol Tyg Lek* (1990) 45, 467–69.
14. Schwartz JB, Migliore PJ. Effect of nifedipine on serum digoxin concentration and renal clearance. *Clin Pharmacol Ther* (1984) 36, 19–24.
15. Pedersen KE, Madsen JL, Klitgaard NA, Kjoer K, Hvidt S. Non-interaction between nifedipine and digoxin. *Dan Med Bull* (1986) 33, 109–10.
16. Garty M, Shamir E, Ilfeld D, Pitlik S, Rosenfeld JB. Non interaction of digoxin and nifedipine in cardiac patients. *J Clin Pharmacol* (1986) 26, 304–5.
17. Koren G, Zylber-Katz E, Granit L, Levy M. Pharmacokinetic studies of nifedipine and digoxin co-administration. *Int J Clin Pharmacol Ther Toxicol* (1986) 24, 39–42.
18. Pedersen KE, Dorph-Pedersen A, Hvidt S, Klitgaard NA, Kjaer K, Nielsen-Kudsk F. Effect of nifedipine on digoxin kinetics in healthy subjects. *Clin Pharmacol Ther* (1982) 32, 562–5.
19. Kuhlmann J. Effects of nifedipine and diltiazem on plasma levels and renal excretion of beta-acetyldigoxin. *Clin Pharmacol Ther* (1985) 37, 150–6.
20. Kuhlmann J. Effects of quinidine, verapamil and nifedipine on the pharmacokinetics and pharmacodynamics of digitoxin during steady-state conditions. *Arzneimittelforschung* (1987) 37, 545–8.
21. Kuhlmann J. Effects of verapamil, diltiazem, and nifedipine on plasma levels and renal excretion of digitoxin. *Clin Pharmacol Ther* (1985) 38, 667–73.
22. Belz GG, Doering W, Munkes R, Matthews J. Interaction between digoxin and calcium antagonists and antiarrhythmic drugs. *Clin Pharmacol Ther* (1983) 33, 410–17.
23. Kirch W, Hutt HJ, Dylewicz P, Gräf KJ, Ohnhaus EE. Dose-dependence of the nifedipine-digoxin interaction? *Clin Pharmacol Ther* (1986) 39, 35–9.
24. Belz GG, Aust PE, Munkes R. Digoxin plasma concentrations and nifedipine. *Lancet* (1981) i, 844–5.
25. Hutt HJ, Kirch W, Dylewicz P, Ohnhaus EE. Dose-dependence of the nifedipine/digoxin interaction? *Arch Toxicol* (1986) (Suppl 9), 209–12.
26. Kleinbloesem CH, van Brummelen P, Hillers J, Moolenaar AJ, Breimer DD. Interaction between digoxin and nifedipine at steady state in patients with atrial fibrillation. *Ther Drug Monit* (1985) 7, 372–6.
27. Halawa B, Mazurek W. Interakcja digoksyny i niektórych niesteroidowych leków przeciwzapalnych, kwasu acetylosalicylowego i nifedipiny. *Pol Tyg Lek* (1982) 37, 1475–6.
28. Suematsu F, Yukawa E, Yukawa M, Minemoto M, Ohdo S, Higuchi S, Goto Y. Pharmacoepidemiologic detection of calcium channel blocker-induced change on digoxin clearance using multiple trough screen analysis. *Biopharm Drug Dispos* (2002) 23, 173–81.
29. De Cesaris R, Balestrazzi M, Chiarappa R, Ranieri G. Aumentata attività digitalica nella somministrazione contemporanea di calcioantagonisti e digitalici. *G Ital Cardiol* (1983) 13, 188–91.
30. Ziegler R, Horstmann R, Wingender W, Kuhlmann J. Do dihydropyridines influence pharmacokinetic and hemodynamic parameters of digoxin? *J Clin Pharmacol* (1987) 27, 712.
31. Kirch W, Stenzel J, Dylewicz P, Hutt HJ, Santos SR, Ohnhaus EE. Influence of nisoldipine on haemodynamic effects and plasma levels of digoxin. *Br J Clin Pharmacol* (1986) 22, 155–9.
32. Kirch W, Stenzel J, Santos SR, Ohnhaus EE. Nisoldipine, a new calcium channel antagonist, elevates plasma levels of digoxin. *Arch Toxicol* (1987) (Suppl 11), 310–12.
33. Kirch W, Logemann C, Heidemann H, Santos SR, Ohnhaus EE. Effect of two different doses of nitrendipine on steady-state plasma digoxin levels and systolic time intervals. *Eur J Clin Pharmacol* (1986) 31, 391–5.
34. Kirch W, Logemann C, Heidemann H, Santos SR, Ohnhaus EE. Nitrendipine/digoxin interaction. *J Cardiovasc Pharmacol* (1987) 10 (Suppl 10), S74–S75.
35. Kirch W, Hutt HJ, Heidemann H, Rämsch K, Janisch HD, Ohnhaus EE. Drug interactions with nitrendipine. *J Cardiovasc Pharmacol* (1984) 6 (Suppl 7), S982–S985.
36. Debbas NMG, Johnston A, Jackson SHD, Banim SO, Camm AJ, Turner P. The effect of nitrendipine on predose digoxin serum concentration. *Br J Clin Pharmacol* (1988) 25, 151P.
37. Ziegler R, Wingender W, Boehme K, Raemsch K, Kuhlmann J. Study of pharmacokinetic and pharmacodynamic interaction between nitrendipine and digoxin. *J Cardiovasc Pharmacol* (1987) 9 (Suppl 4), S101–S106.
38. Takara K, Kakumoto M, Tanigawara Y, Funakoshi J, Sakaeda T, Okumura K. Interaction of digoxin with antihypertensive drugs *via* MDR1. *Life Sci* (2002) 70, 1491–1500.
39. Cardene (Nicardipine hydrochloride). Astellas Pharma Ltd. UK summary of product characteristics, December 2010.
40. Cantelli I, Pavesi PC, Parchi C, Naccarella F, Bracchetti D. Acute hemodynamic effects of combined therapy with digoxin and nifedipine in patients with chronic heart failure. *Am Heart J* (1983) 106, 308–15.
41. Hansen PB, Buch J, Rasmussen OØ, Waldorff S, Steiness E. Influence of atenolol and nifedipine on digoxin-induced inotropism in humans. *Br J Clin Pharmacol* (1984) 18, 817–22.

Digoxin and related drugs + Calcium-channel blockers; Diltiazem

Digoxin levels are reported to be unchanged by diltiazem in a number of studies but others describe increases in digoxin levels, with the effects highly variable between studies and individual patients. Serum digitoxin levels have also been reported to rise in some patients taking diltiazem, but the effect is small. There is a risk of additive bradycardia when digitalis glycosides are given with diltiazem.

Clinical evidence

(a) Digitoxin

Five out of 10 patients taking digitoxin had a 6 to 31% (mean 21%) rise in plasma digitoxin levels while taking diltiazem 180 mg daily for 4 to 6 weeks.[1]

(b) Digoxin

Diltiazem 30 or 60 mg four times daily had no effect on the serum levels of digoxin 250 micrograms daily in 9 patients with cardiac diseases.[2] Three similar studies in patients[3,4] and healthy subjects,[5] taking digoxin with diltiazem 120 to 360 mg daily confirmed the absence of an interaction. Two further studies in healthy subjects,[6,7] found that diltiazem 120 mg daily did not affect the pharmacokinetics of a single 1-mg intravenous dose of digoxin.

In contrast, a study in 17 Japanese patients (some with rheumatic valvular disease) taking either digoxin or **metildigoxin** found that diltiazem 60 mg three times daily for 2 weeks increased their serum digoxin levels measured at 24 hours by 36% and 51%, respectively.[8] Another study in 8 patients with chronic heart failure secondary to ischaemic disease, taking digoxin 250 micrograms daily, found that diltiazem 60 mg three times daily increased the AUC and mean steady-state serum levels of digoxin by about 50%, increased its peak serum level by 37% and prolonged its elimination half-life by 29%, but there was no evidence of any haemodynamic changes.[9]

Other studies in Western patients[10,11] and healthy subjects[12-15] have found rises of 20 to 85% in plasma digoxin levels during diltiazem use. In one case report a 143% increase was seen.[16] The authors of two of these studies noted that the effect was highly individual with some subjects having no increase and some a large increase.[11,13] Another case report describes raised serum digoxin levels and toxicity in a man taking digoxin when he was given diltiazem with or without nifedipine.[17]

In addition to these pharmacokinetic changes, a pharmacodynamic interaction has also been seen. A study in patients without sinoatrial (SA) or atrioventricular (AV) node dysfunction, found that intravenous diltiazem alone depressed SA and AV node function and slightly shortened atrial refractoriness. These effects were amplified by subsequent administration of intravenous digoxin 18 micrograms/kg. However, concurrent use did not cause any notable adverse effects in this group of patients.[18] A study identified 62 patients who had been admitted to hospital with bradycardia over a 4-year period, 18 of whom had been taking digoxin and a non-dihydropyridine calcium-channel blocker, and 12 patients who had been taking digoxin, a beta blocker and a non-dihydropyridine calcium-channel blocker. However, the specific calcium-channel blockers were not named.[19]

Mechanism

Not understood. In those individuals showing a pharmacokinetic interaction, falls in total digoxin clearance of about 25% have been described.[9,11,12,20,21] Although several calcium-channel blockers may inhibit the P-glycoprotein-mediated renal clearance of digoxin, the results of an *in vitro* study[22] suggest that this might not occur with diltiazem. A synergistic effect on heart rate and atrioventricular conduction is also possible.

Importance and management

A thoroughly investigated and well documented pharmacokinetic interaction but there is no clear explanation for the inconsistent results. All patients taking digoxin given diltiazem should be well monitored for signs of over-digitalisation (e.g. bradycardia) with digoxin levels measured as necessary. Dose reductions could be necessary. Those most at risk are patients with digoxin levels near the top end of the range. Similar precautions would appear to be necessary with **digitoxin**, although the documentation of this interaction is very limited and the expected rise in levels only small. The potential for additive bradycardia and heart block should be borne in mind when using diltiazem with any digitalis glycoside.

1. Kuhlmann J. Effects of verapamil, diltiazem, and nifedipine on plasma levels and renal excretion of digitoxin. *Clin Pharmacol Ther* (1985) 38, 667–73.
2. Elkayam U, Parikh K, Torkan B, Weber L, Cohen JL, Rahimtoola SH. Effect of diltiazem on renal clearance and serum concentration of digoxin in patients with cardiac disease. *Am J Cardiol* (1985) 55, 1393–5.
3. Schrager BR, Pina I, Frangi M, Applewhite S, Sequeira R, Chahine RA. Diltiazem, digoxin interaction? *Circulation* (1983) 68 (Suppl), III368.
4. Halawa B, Walentyna M. Interakcje digoksyny z nifedypiną i diltiazemem. *Pol Tyg Lek* (1990) 45, 467–69.
5. Boden WE, More G, Sharma S, Bough EW, Korr KS, Young PM, Shulman RS. No increase in serum digoxin concentrations with high dose diltiazem. *Am J Med* (1986) 81, 425–8.
6. Beltrami TR, May JJ, Bertino JS. Lack of effects of diltiazem on digoxin pharmacokinetics. *J Clin Pharmacol* (1985) 25, 390–392.
7. Jones WN, Kern KB, Rindone JP, Mayersohn M, Bliss M, Goldman S. Digoxin-diltiazem interaction: a pharmacokinetic evaluation. *Eur J Clin Pharmacol* (1986) 31, 351–3.
8. Oyama Y, Fujii S, Kanda K, Akino E, Kawasaki H, Nagata M, Goto K. Digoxin-diltiazem interaction. *Am J Cardiol* (1984) 53, 1480–1.
9. Mahgoub AA, El-Medany AH, Abdulatif AS. A comparison between the effects of diltiazem and isosorbide dinitrate on digoxin pharmacodynamics and kinetics in the treatment of patients with chronic ischemic heart failure. *Saudi Med J* (2002) 23, 725–31.
10. Andrejak M, Hary L, Andrjak M-Th, Lesbre J Ph. Diltiazem increases steady state digoxin serum levels in patients with cardiac disease. *J Clin Pharmacol* (1987) 27, 967–70.
11. Kuhlmann J. Effects of nifedipine and diltiazem on plasma levels and renal excretion of beta-acetyldigoxin. *Clin Pharmacol Ther* (1985) 37, 150–6.
12. Rameis H, Magometschnigg D, Ganzinger U. The diltiazem-digoxin interaction. *Clin Pharmacol Ther* (1984) 36, 183–9.
13. North DS, Mattern AL, Hiser WW. The influence of diltiazem hydrochloride on trough serum digoxin levels. *Drug Intell Clin Pharm* (1986) 20, 500–503.
14. Gallet M, Aupetit JF, Lopez M, Manchon J, Lestaevel M, Lefrancois JJ. Interaction diltiazem-digoxine. Évolution de la digoxinémie et des paramtres électrocardiographiques chez le sujet sain. *Arch Mal Coeur* (1986) 79, 1216–20.
15. Larman RC. A pharmacokinetic evaluation of the digoxin-diltiazem interaction. *J Pharm Sci* (1987) 76, S79.
16. King T, Mallet L. Diltiazem-digoxin interaction in an elderly woman: a case report. *J Geriatr Drug Ther* (1991) 5, 79–83.
17. Kasmer RJ, Jones EM. Diltiazem-nifedipine-digoxin interaction. *Drug Intell Clin Pharm* (1986) 20, 985–6.
18. Mitchell LB, Jutzy KR, Lewis S, Schroeder JS, Mason JW. Intracardiac electrophysiologic study of intravenous diltiazem and combined diltiazem-digoxin in patients. *Am Heart J* (1982) 103, 57–66.
19. Haase G, Pietzsch M, Fähnrich A, Voss W, Riethling A-K. Results of a systematic adverse drug reaction (ADR)-screening concerning bradycardia caused by drug interactions in departments of internal medicine in Rostock. *Int J Clin Pharmacol Ther* (2002) 40,116–19.
20. Yoshida A, Fujita M, Kurosawa N, Nioka M, Shichinohe T, Arakawa M, Fukuda R, Owada E, Ito K. Effects of diltiazem on plasma level and urinary excretion of digoxin in healthy subjects. *Clin Pharmacol Ther* (1984) 35, 681–5.
21. Suematsu F, Yukawa E, Yukawa M, Minemoto M, Ohdo S, Higuchi S, Goto Y. Pharmacoepidemiologic detection of calcium channel blocker-induced change on digoxin clearance using multiple trough screen analysis. *Biopharm Drug Dispos* (2002) 23, 173–81.
22. Takara K, Kakumoto M, Tanigawara Y, Funakoshi J, Sakaeda T, Okumura K. Interaction of digoxin with antihypertensive drugs *via* MDR1. *Life Sci* (2002) 70, 1491–1500.

Digoxin and related drugs + Calcium-channel blockers; Verapamil

Serum digoxin levels are increased by about 40% by verapamil 160 mg daily, and by about 70% by verapamil 240 mg daily. Digoxin toxicity can develop, and deaths have occurred. Verapamil causes a rise of about 35% in digitoxin levels. There is a risk of additive bradycardia and conduction disturbances when cardiac glycosides are given with verapamil. Gallopamil, a drug chemically related to verapamil, does not appear to affect digoxin levels to a clinically relevant extent.

Clinical evidence

(a) Digitoxin

Eight out of 10 patients had a 35% rise (range 14 to 97%) in plasma digitoxin levels over a 4 to 6 week period while taking verapamil 240 mg daily, in three divided doses. In 2 patients (and 3 other healthy subjects given a single dose of digitoxin) the pharmacokinetics of digitoxin were not affected by verapamil.[1,2]

(b) Digoxin

After 2 weeks of treatment with verapamil 240 mg daily, in three divided doses, the mean serum digoxin levels of 49 patients with chronic atrial fibrillation had risen by 72%. The rise was seen in most patients, and it occurred largely within the first 7 days. A rise of about 40% has been seen with verapamil 160 mg daily.[3,4]

Reports in a total of 21 healthy subjects,[5,6] and 54 patients[7-9] describe rises in serum digoxin levels of 22 to 147% when verapamil 240 to 360 mg daily was added to digoxin. Similar rises are reported elsewhere.[4,10-12]

A rise in digoxin levels of about 50% was seen in chronic haemodialysis patients given verapamil 120 to 240 mg daily.[13] Nine healthy subjects had a 53% rise in their digoxin levels while taking verapamil 240 mg three times daily for 2 weeks.[5] Toxicity[14] and a fatality[15] occurred in patients whose digoxin levels were sizeably increased by verapamil. Both asystole and sinus arrest have been described.[16,17] A single-dose study indicated that cirrhosis magnifies the extent of this interaction.[18]

A study identified 62 patients who had been admitted to hospital with bradycardia over a 4-year period, 18 of whom had been taking a combination of digoxin and a non-dihydropyridine calcium-channel blocker, and 12 patients who had been taking digoxin, a beta blocker and a non-dihydropyridine calcium-channel blocker. However, the specific calcium-channel blockers were not named.[19]

In a study in 10 patients with congestive heart failure given **metildigoxin** 200 micrograms daily for 9 days, the concurrent use of verapamil 320 mg for a further 7 days, increased levels of digoxin by about 35%. In another 10 patients given both verapamil 320 mg and nifedipine 60 mg daily for 7 days, digoxin levels were increased by about 66%.[20]

In 12 healthy subjects, **gallopamil** (a calcium-channel blocker that is chemically related to verapamil), in a dose of 50 mg three times daily for 2 weeks, raised the serum levels of digoxin 375 micrograms daily by 16% (from 0.58 nanograms/mL to 0.67 nanograms/mL).[21] This change would not be expected to be clinically relevant.

Mechanism

The rise in serum digoxin levels with verapamil is due to reductions in renal and especially extra-renal (biliary) clearance; a diminution in the volume of distribution also takes place.[4,9,10,22] It has been suggested that P-glycoprotein could be involved.[23] An *in vitro* study found that verapamil can inhibit the P-glycoprotein-mediated transcellular transport of digoxin,[24] which suggests that any interaction occurs, at least in part, by inhibiting the renal tubular excretion of digoxin. The increased digoxin plasma levels caused by verapamil are reported to increase both inotropism[25] and toxic effects.[26] Verapamil might enhance the digoxin-induced elevation of intracellular sodium, which could increase the risk of arrhythmias.[26,27] A synergistic effect on heart rate and atrioventricular conduction is also possible.

Impaired extra-renal excretion is suggested as the reason for the rise in serum digitoxin levels.[1]

Importance and management

The pharmacokinetic interaction between **digoxin** and verapamil is well documented, well established and occurs in most patients.[10,28] Serum digoxin levels should be well monitored and downward dose adjustments made to avoid digoxin toxicity (deaths have occurred[15]). An initial 30 to 50% dose reduction has been recommended.[29-31] The interaction develops within 2 to 7 days, approaching or reaching a maximum within 14 days or so.[3,8] The magnitude of the rise in serum digoxin is dose-dependent[32] with a significant increase if the verapamil dose is increased from 160 to 240 mg daily,[3] but with no further significant increase if the dose is raised any higher.[6] The mean rise with verapamil 160 mg daily is about 40%, and with 240 mg or more is about 60 to 80%, but the response is variable. Some patients have had rises of up to 150%. One study found that although the rise in serum digoxin levels was 60% within a week, this had lessened to about 30% five weeks later.[10] Large interpatient variability in the reduction in digoxin clearance has been reported.[31] Initial individual digoxin dose titration, regular monitoring and dose adjustments would seem to be necessary. Note that the potential for additive bradycardia and heart block should also be borne in mind.

The documentation of the **digitoxin** and verapamil interaction is limited, but the interaction appears to be established. Downward dose adjustments may be necessary, particularly in some patients.[1]

1. Kuhlmann J, Marcin S. Effects of verapamil on pharmacokinetics and pharmacodynamics of digitoxin in patients. *Am Heart J* (1985) 110, 1245–50.
2. Kuhlmann J. Effects of verapamil, diltiazem, and nifedipine on plasma levels and renal excretion of digitoxin. *Clin Pharmacol Ther* (1985) 38, 667–73.
3. Klein HO, Lang R, Weiss E, Di Segni E, Libhaber C, Guerrero J, Kaplinsky E. The influence of verapamil on serum digoxin concentration. *Circulation* (1982) 65, 998–1003.
4. Lang R, Klein HO, Weiss E, Libhaber C, Kaplinsky E. Effect of verapamil on digoxin blood level and clearance. *Chest* (1980) 78, 525.
5. Doering W. Effect of coadministration of verapamil and quinidine on serum digoxin concentration. *Eur J Clin Pharmacol* (1983) 25, 517–21.
6. Belz GG, Doering W, Munkes R, Matthews J. Interaction between digoxin and calcium antagonists and antiarrhythmic drugs. *Clin Pharmacol Ther* (1983) 33, 410–17.
7. Klein HO, Lang R, Di Segni E, Kaplinsky E. Verapamil-digoxin interaction. *N Engl J Med* (1980) 303, 160.
8. Merola P, Badin A, Paleari DC, De Petris A, Maragno I. Influenza del verapamile sui livelli plasmatici di digossina nell'uomo. *Cardiologia* (1982) 27, 683–7.
9. Hedman A, Angelin B, Arvidsson A, Beck O, Dahlqvist R, Nilsson B, Olsson M, Schenck-Gustafsson K. Digoxin-verapamil interaction: reduction of biliary but not renal digoxin clearance. *Clin Pharmacol Ther* (1991) 49, 256–62.
10. Pedersen KE, Dorph-Pedersen A, Hvidt S, Klitgaard NA, Pedersen KK. The long-term effect of verapamil on plasma digoxin concentration and renal digoxin clearance in healthy subjects. *Eur J Clin Pharmacol* (1982) 22, 123–7.
11. Klein HO, Lang R, Di Segni E, Sareli P, David D, Kaplinsky E. Oral verapamil versus digoxin in the management of chronic atrial fibrillation. *Chest* (1980) 78, 524.

12. Schwartz JB, Keefe D, Kates RE, Harrison DC. Verapamil and digoxin. Another drug-drug interaction. *Clin Res* (1981) 29, 501A.
13. Rendtorff C, Johannessen AC, Halck S, Klitgaard NA. Verapamil-digoxin interaction in chronic hemodialysis patients. *Scand J Urol Nephrol* (1990) 24, 137–9.
14. Gordon M, Goldenberg LMC. Clinical digoxin toxicity in the aged in association with co-administered verapamil. A report of two cases and a review of the literature. *J Am Geriatr Soc* (1986) 34, 659–62.
15. Zatuchni J. Verapamil-digoxin interaction. *Am Heart J* (1984) 108, 412–3.
16. Kounis NG. Asystole after verapamil and digoxin. *Br J Clin Pract* (1980) 34, 57–8.
17. Kounis NG, Mallioris C. Interactions with cardioactive drugs. *Br J Clin Pract* (1986) 40, 537–8.
18. Maragno I, Gianotti C, Tropeano PF, Rodighiero V, Gaion RM, Paleari C, Prandoni R, Menozzi L. Verapamil-induced changes in digoxin kinetics in cirrhosis. *Eur J Clin Pharmacol* (1987) 32, 309–11.
19. Haase G, Pietzsch M, Fähnrich A, Voss W, Riethling A-K. Results of a systematic adverse drug reaction (ADR)-screening concerning bradycardia caused by drug interactions in departments of internal medicine in Rostock. *Int J Clin Pharmacol Ther* (2002) 40,11619.
20. De Cesaris R, Balestrazzi M, Chiarappa R, Ranieri G. Aumentata attività digitalica nella somministrazione contemporanea di calcioantagonisti e digitalici. *G Ital Cardiol* (1983) 13, 188–91.
21. Belz GG, Doering W, Munkes R, Matthews J. Interaction between digoxin and calcium antagonists and antiarrhythmic drugs. *Clin Pharmacol Ther* (1983) 33, 410–17.
22. Pedersen KE, Dorph-Pedersen A, Hvidt S, Klitgaard NA, Nielsen-Kudsk F. Digoxin-verapamil interaction. *Clin Pharmacol Ther* (1981) 30, 311–16.
23. Verschraagen M, Koks CHW, Schellens JHM, Beijnen JH. P-glycoprotein system as a determinant of drug interactions: the case of digoxin-verapamil. *Pharmacol Res* (1999) 40, 301–6.
24. Takara K, Kakumoto M, Tanigawara Y, Funakoshi J, Sakaeda T, Okumura K. Interaction of digoxin with antihypertensive drugs *via* MDR1. *Life Sci* (2002) 70, 1491–1500.
25. Pedersen KE, Thayssen P, Klitgaard NA, Christiansen BD, Nielsen-Kudsk F. Influence of verapamil on the inotropism and pharmacokinetics of digoxin. *Eur J Clin Pharmacol* (1983) 25, 199–206.
26. Pedersen KE. The influence of calcium antagonists on plasma digoxin concentration. *Acta Med Scand* (1984) (Suppl 681), 31–6.
27. Pedersen KE, Christiansen BD, Kjaer K, Klitgaard NA, Nielsen-Kudsk F. Verapamil-induced changes in digoxin kinetics and intraerythrocytic sodium concentration. *Clin Pharmacol Ther* (1983) 34, 8–13.
28. Belz GG, Aust PE, Munkes R. Digoxin plasma concentrations and nifedipine. *Lancet* (1981) i, 844–5.
29. Marcus FI. Pharmacokinetic interactions between digoxin and other drugs. *J Am Coll Cardiol* (1985) 5, 82A–90A.
30. Klein HO, Kaplinsky E. Verapamil and digoxin: their respective effects on atrial fibrillation and their interaction. *Am J Cardiol* (1982) 50, 894–902.
31. Bauer LA, Horn JR, Pettit H. Mixed-effect modeling for detection and evaluation of drug interactions: digoxin–quinidine and digoxin–verapamil combinations. *Ther Drug Monit* (1996) 18, 46–52.
32. Schwartz JB, Keefe D, Kates RE, Kirsten E, Harrison DC. Acute and chronic pharmacodynamic interaction of verapamil and digoxin in atrial fibrillation. *Circulation* (1982) 65, 1163–70.

Digoxin and related drugs + Carbamazepine and related drugs

Eslicarbazepine does not affect the exposure to digoxin. In one report, bradycardia was tentatively attributed to the use of carbamazepine with digitalis.

Clinical evidence, mechanism, importance and management

(a) Carbamazepine

In an early clinical study, bradycardia in 3 patients taking **digitalis** and carbamazepine was tentatively attributed to their concurrent use.[1] There appear to be no other reports to confirm this interaction; therefore, it is unlikely to be of general relevance.

(b) Eslicarbazepine

In a crossover study in 12 healthy subjects, eslicarbazepine acetate 1.2 g daily for 8 days did not affect the AUC of digoxin (500 micrograms daily on days one and two, followed by 250 micrograms daily). The maximum plasma concentration of digoxin was reduced by 15%,[2] but this is not clinically relevant. No digoxin dose adjustment would therefore appear necessary if eslicarbazepine is also given.

1. Killian JM, Fromm GH. Carbamazepine in the treatment of neuralgia. Use and side effects. *Arch Neurol* (1968) 19, 129–36.
2. Vaz da Silva M, Costa R, Soares E, Maia J, Falcão A, Almeida L, Soares da Silva P. Effect of eslicarbazepine acetate on the pharmacokinetics of digoxin in healthy subjects. *Fundam Clin Pharmacol* (2009) 23, 509–14.

Digoxin and related drugs + Cephalosporins

No interaction normally occurs between digoxin and cefazolin or cefuroxime. In contrast, one early study found that cefradine increased digoxin levels.

Clinical evidence

A study found no reduction in the excretion of digoxin metabolites from the gut in 3 patients taking **cefazolin**.[1]

A case-control study using data from healthcare databases in Ontario from 1994 to 2000 identified 1 051 patients who had been admitted to hospital with digoxin toxicity. Of these, 5 patients (0.5%) had been exposed to **cefuroxime** in the preceding 3 weeks when compared with 0.3% of controls, suggesting that digoxin toxicity was not related to **cefuroxime** exposure.[2] Similar data for **cefuroxime** from this research group have been published elsewhere.[3]

In an early study, **cefradine** prolonged the half-life of digoxin and increased its serum levels from 1.8 nanograms/mL to 2.6 nanograms/mL. This effect was considered to occur as a result of reduced renal clearance.[4]

Mechanism

Up to 10% of patients receiving oral digoxin excrete it in substantial amounts in the faeces and urine as inactive metabolites (digoxin reduction products or DRPs). This metabolism seems to be due to gut flora,[5] in particular *Eubacterium lentum*, which is anaerobic and Gram positive. It was suggested that inhibition of digoxin metabolism by gut flora was responsible for any interaction, but doubt has been thrown on this theory, (see *Mechanism* under 'Digoxin and related drugs + Macrolides', p.1100).

Importance and management

The silence of the literature on adverse interactions between digoxin and cephalosporins, and the limited evidence for a plausible mechanism suggest that clinically relevant interactions are unlikely with most cephalosporins. However, an element of caution would seem sensible with cefradine, and it might be prudent to check for digoxin adverse effects, initially by checking symptoms and pulse rate, and then taking digoxin levels if an interaction is suspected.

1. Dobkin JF, Saha JR, Butler VP, Lindenbaum J. Effects of antibiotic therapy on digoxin metabolism. *Clin Res* (1982) 30, 517A.
2. Juurlink DN, Mamdani M, Kopp A, Laupacis A, Redelmeier DA. Drug-drug interactions among elderly patients hospitalized for drug toxicity. *JAMA* (2003) 289, 1652–8.
3. Gomes T, Mamdani MM, Juurlink DN. Macrolide-induced digoxin toxicity: a population-based study. *Clin Pharmacol Ther* (2009) 86, 383–86.
4. Halawa B. Interakcje digoksyny z cefradina (Sefril), tetracyklina (Tetracyclinum), gentamycyna (Gentamycin) i wankomycyna (Vancocin). *Pol Tyg Lek* (1984) 39, 1717–20.
5. Lindenbaum J, Rund DG, Butler VP, Tse-Eng D, Saha JR. Inactivation of digoxin by the gut flora: reversal by antibiotic therapy. *N Engl J Med* (1981) 305, 789–94.

Digoxin + Chloroquine and related drugs

The levels of digoxin were found to be increased by over 70% in two elderly patients when they were given hydroxychloroquine. Chloroquine might be expected to behave similarly.

Clinical evidence, mechanism, importance and management

Two women aged 65 years and 68 years who had been taking digoxin 250 micrograms daily for 2 to 3 years for arrhythmias were given hydroxychloroquine 250 mg twice daily for rheumatoid arthritis. When the hydroxychloroquine was withdrawn the plasma digoxin levels of both women fell by 70 to 75% (from 2.3 nanograms/mL to 0.5 nanograms/mL and from 2.4 nanograms/mL to 0.7 nanograms/mL, respectively). There was no evidence of toxicity during concurrent use, and one patient even claimed that the regularity of her heart rhythm had been improved.[1] The reason for this apparent interaction is not understood and, given the lack of other data suggesting any interaction, it seems unlikely to be of general relevance.

There appear to be no clinical reports of an interaction between digoxin and chloroquine, but increases in peak serum digoxin levels of about 77% have been seen in *dogs*.[2]

1. Leden I. Digoxin-hydroxychloroquine interaction? *Acta Med Scand* (1982) 211, 411–12.
2. McElnay JC, Sidahmed AM, D'Arcy PF and McQuade RD. Chloroquine-digoxin interaction. *Int J Pharmaceutics* (1985) 26, 267–74.

Digoxin + Cibenzoline (Cifenline)

Cibenzoline does not appear to affect plasma digoxin levels.

Clinical evidence, mechanism, importance and management

A study in 12 healthy subjects taking digoxin 250 to 375 micrograms daily found that cibenzoline 160 mg twice daily for 7 days had no effect on the pharmacokinetics of digoxin.[1] Similarly, a study in 22 patients taking digoxin 250 micrograms daily found that the addition of cibenzoline 65 mg or 130 mg twice daily for 4 weeks did not affect the plasma levels of digoxin. Concurrent use was well-tolerated in 16 of 21 patients available for evaluation and no important changes in vital signs occurred during the study period.[2] An *in vitro* study found that cibenzoline only slightly inhibited the P-glycoprotein-mediated transcellular transport of digoxin and therefore inhibition of the renal tubular secretion of digoxin is unlikely.[3] There appears to be no pharmacokinetic reason to adjust the dose of digoxin in patients given cibenzoline.

1. Khoo K-C, Givens SV, Parsonnet M, Massarella JW. Effect of oral cibenzoline on steady-state digoxin concentrations in healthy volunteers. *J Clin Pharmacol* (1988) 28, 29–35.
2. Garnier LF, Bine-Scheck F, Pruvost P, Wanszelbaum H, Arnaud R. Association de la cibenzoline et de la digoxine administrées par voie orale chez des patients ayant une arythmie supraventriculaire. *Ann Cardiol Angeiol (Paris)* (1992) 41, 411–17.
3. Kakumoto M, Takara K, Sakaeda T, Tanigawara Y, Kita T, Okumura K. MDR1-mediated interaction of digoxin with antiarrhythmic or antianginal drugs. *Biol Pharm Bull* (2002), 25, 1604–7.

Digoxin + Ciclosporin

Ciclosporin causes a large rise in digoxin levels in some patients.

Clinical evidence

Digoxin toxicity developed in 4 patients given ciclosporin before a heart transplant. In the two cases described in detail, ciclosporin 10 mg/kg daily was given to patients taking digoxin 375 micrograms daily. Fourfold rises in digoxin levels, from 1.2 nanograms/mL to 4.5 nanograms/mL and from 2 nanograms/mL to 8.3 nanograms/mL, were seen within 2 to 3 days. This was accompanied by rises in serum creatinine levels from 110 micromol/L to 120 micromol/L and from 84 micromol/L to 181 micromol/L, respectively, which were considered insufficient to explain the rise in digoxin levels. As a consequence of these findings, the same authors conducted a study in 4 patients given ciclosporin and digoxin. Two patients developed acute renal failure. In the other 2 patients, the volume of distribution of digoxin was decreased by 69% and 72%, while the clearance was reduced by 47% and 58%, in each of the patients, respectively.[1] In a further 7 patients, digoxin pharmacokinetics were assessed before heart transplant, then after transplantation during the use of maintenance ciclosporin.[2] The total body clearance of digoxin remained unchanged, which appeared to be at odds with the earlier results.[1] It was suggested that haemodynamic improvements brought about by a successful heart transplant could have counterbalanced any inhibitory effect ciclosporin had on renal clearance.[2]

Mechanism

Not fully understood. Digoxin is a substrate of the efflux pump, P-glycoprotein, which is involved in the intestinal absorption and renal elimination of digoxin. Ciclosporin inhibits P-glycoprotein and concurrent use can therefore lead to increased digoxin levels.

Importance and management

Information regarding an interaction between ciclosporin and digoxin seems to be limited to the studies cited. Nevertheless, the effects of concurrent use should be monitored very closely, and the digoxin dose should be adjusted as necessary.

1. Dorian P, Cardella C, Strauss M, David T, East S, Ogilvie R. Cyclosporine nephrotoxicity and cyclosporine-digoxin interaction prior to heart transplantation. *Transplant Proc* (1987) 19, 1825–7.
2. Robieux I, Dorian P, Klein J, Chung D, Zborowska-Sluis D, Ogilvie R, Koren G. The effects of cardiac transplantation and cyclosporine therapy on digoxin pharmacokinetics. *J Clin Pharmacol* (1992) 32, 338–43.

Digoxin + Clopidogrel

Clopidogrel does not alter the pharmacokinetics of digoxin, and digoxin does not appear to alter the antiplatelet response to clopidogrel.

Clinical evidence, mechanism, importance and management

In a study in 12 healthy subjects given digoxin 250 micrograms for 20 days, clopidogrel 75 mg daily (from day 11 to 20) did not alter the pharmacokinetics of digoxin. The antiplatelet response to clopidogrel in this study did not differ from historical data, suggesting that digoxin does not affect this. Therefore no additional precautions seem necessary on the concurrent use of clopidogrel and digoxin.[1]

1. Peeters PAM, Crijns HJMJ, Tamminga WJ, Jonkman JHG, Dickinson JP, Necciari J. Clopidogrel, a novel antiplatelet agent, and digoxin: absence of pharmacodynamic and pharmacokinetic interaction. *Semin Thromb Hemost* (1999) 25 (Suppl 2), 51–4.

Digoxin + Cobicistat

Cobicistat appears to increase digoxin exposure.

Clinical evidence, mechanism, importance and management

In a study in 22 healthy subjects, cobicistat 150 mg daily increased the AUC of a single 500-microgram dose of digoxin by 8% and increased its maximum plasma concentration by 41%.[1] Cobicistat inhibits P-glycoprotein, and this study, using digoxin as a probe substrate, shows that its inhibitory activity is negligible.

The increase in digoxin exposure seen is unlikely to be clinically relevant. Nevertheless, the US manufacturer of elvitegravir boosted with cobicistat (in a fixed-dose combination also including emtricitabine and tenofovir) advises caution on concurrent use and recommends monitoring plasma digoxin concentrations.[1]

1. Stribild (Elvitegravir, cobicistat, emtricitabine, tenofovir disoproxil fumarate). Gilead Sciences, Inc. US Prescribing information, August 2012.

Digoxin + Colesevelam

The absorption of a single dose of digoxin is not affected by colesevelam.

Clinical evidence, mechanism, importance and management

In a single-dose study in which 26 healthy subjects were given digoxin 250 micrograms, simultaneously with or without colesevelam 4.5 g, followed by a standardised meal, colesevelam did not affect the rate (maximum level and time to maximum level) or extent (AUC) of digoxin absorption.[1] This suggests it is unlikely to be necessary to separate digoxin and colesevelam administration.

1. Donovan JM, Stypinski D, Stiles MR, Olson TA, Burke SK. Drug interactions with colesevelam hydrochloride, a novel, potent lipid-lowering agent. *Cardiovasc Drugs Ther* (2000) 14, 681–90.

Digoxin and related drugs + Colestipol

Colestipol does not appear to interfere with the absorption of either digoxin or digitoxin if it is given at least 1.5 hours after the digitalis glycoside.

Clinical evidence

(a) Digitoxin

Four patients with digitoxin toxicity were given colestipol 10 g at once and 5 g every 6 to 8 hours thereafter to reduce their digitoxin serum levels. The average digitoxin half-life fell to 2.75 days compared with an untreated control patient in whom the digitoxin half-life was 9.3 days.

In contrast, in a comparative study in 11 patients with plasma digitoxin levels greater than 40 nanograms/mL, when the digitoxin was stopped and colestipol 5 g four times daily was given before meals, the digitoxin half-life (6.3 days) was unaffected, when compared with 11 other patients not given colestipol (6.8 days).[1] For another study in which the levels of digitoxin were not affected by colestipol when administration was separated, see under *Digoxin*, below.

(b) Digoxin

In a patient with digoxin toxicity who was given colestipol in an attempt to reduce digoxin levels, the digoxin half-life was 16 hours compared with 1.8 to 2 days in two other control patients.[2] A digoxin elimination half-life of 55 hours was reported in a second patient with digoxin toxicity who was given colestipol, and this compared with a predicted time of at least 85 hours for digoxin alone.[3] Other reports also found colestipol reduced the half-life of digoxin in patients with digoxin toxicity.[4,5]

In contrast, a study in healthy subjects found that colestipol 10 g given immediately after a single 250-microgram dose of digoxin did not reduce the absorption of digoxin.[6] Furthermore, 10 patients receiving long-term treatment with either digoxin 125 to 250 micrograms daily or **digitoxin** 100 to 200 micrograms daily were given colestipol 15 g daily or a placebo, taken 1.5 hour after the digitalis glycoside. Their serum digitalis levels were not altered over a 1-year period by the colestipol.[7]

Mechanism

Colestipol is an ion-exchange resin, which can bind to digoxin and digitoxin.[2] In cases of toxicity, colestipol might reduce serum digitalis levels because under these circumstances the excretion of digitalis in the bile increases and more becomes available for binding in the gut.[7]

Importance and management

The interaction between digoxin or digitoxin and colestipol is not well established. Giving either digoxin or digitoxin 1.5 hours before colestipol appears to avoid any possible interaction in the gut.[7] Note that it is usually recommended that other drugs are given one hour before or 4 hours after colestipol.

1. van Bever RJ, Duchateau AMJA, Pluym BFM, Merkus FWHM. The effect of colestipol on digitoxin plasma levels. *Arzneimittelforschung* (1976) 26, 1891–3.
2. Bazzano G, Bazzano GS. Digitalis intoxication. Treatment with a new steroid-binding resin. *JAMA* (1972) 220, 828–30.
3. Payne VW, Secter RA, Noback RK. Use of colestipol in a patient with digoxin intoxication. *Drug Intell Clin Pharm* (1981) 15, 902–3.
4. Hamburger S, Covinsky JO, Styczynski M, Uhrig L. Acute digoxin overdosage: potential role of colestipol therapy. *J Kans Med Soc* (1980) 81, 464.
5. Kilgore TL, Lehmann CR. Treatment of digoxin intoxication with colestipol. *South Med J* (1982) 75, 1259–60.
6. Neuvonen PJ, Kivistö K, Hirvisalo EL. Effects of resins and activated charcoal on the absorption of digoxin, carbamazepine and frusemide. *Br J Clin Pharmacol* (1988) 25, 229–33.
7. Bazzano G, Bazzano GS. Effect of digitalis-binding resins on cardiac glycosides plasma levels. *Clin Res* (1972) 20, 24.

Digoxin and related drugs + Colestyramine

The levels of both digoxin and digitoxin can be reduced by colestyramine.

Clinical evidence

(a) Digitoxin

Some studies have found that colestyramine reduces the half-life of digitoxin by 35 to 40%.[1,2] There are reports of colestyramine successfully being used in patients with digitoxin toxicity to increase its elimination.[3-6] However, not all studies and cases have found pronounced interactions with digitoxin. In one case report of digitoxin overdose, the effects of colestyramine on digitoxin appeared to be delayed for 48 hours and the reduction in half-life of digitoxin from 7.4 days to 6 days was less pronounced than noted in other studies.[7] In another study, the half-life of digitoxin is reported to have remained unchanged when colestyramine was given.[8] For another study in which the levels of digitoxin were not affected by colestyramine when administration was separated, see under *Digoxin*, below.

(b) Digoxin

A single-dose study in 12 healthy subjects given digoxin 750 micrograms found that the cumulative 6-day recovery of digoxin from the urine was reduced by almost 20% (from 40.5% to 33.1%) when colestyramine 4 g was given.[9,10] Four of the subjects in this study participated in a multiple dose study and were given digoxin 500 micrograms daily for 14 days. In this study, colestyramine 4 g once daily or 4 g four times daily reduced steady-state digoxin levels by 24% and 33%, respectively, when digoxin was given at the same time. However, when colestyramine 8 g twice daily was taken 8 hours apart from the digoxin, there was no change in digoxin level.[10] Similarly, in a study in 10 patients receiving long-term treatment with either digoxin 125 to 250 micrograms daily or **digitoxin** 100 to 200 micrograms daily who were given colestyramine 12 g daily or a placebo taken 1.5 hour after the digitalis glycoside, plasma digitalis levels were not altered by the colestyramine over a 1-year period.[11] Other studies have confirmed a modest reduction in digoxin absorption on the simultaneous administration of colestyramine[12,13] and a small increase in the loss of digoxin and its metabolites in the faeces during long-term use.[14] Another study found that giving digoxin as a solution in a capsule reduced the effects of this interaction when compared with a tablet formulation.[15]

The use of colestyramine has been tried in cases of toxic digoxin levels. For example, two patients with congestive heart failure and toxic serum levels of digoxin (3 nanograms/mL and 4 nanograms/mL) were given colestyramine 4 g every 4 hours for 4 doses. The levels of digoxin fell to therapeutic levels within 13 to 24 hours.[16]

Similarly, the half-life of digoxin fell from 75.5 hours to 19.9 hours when a 94-year-old man with a serum digoxin level of 2.63 nanograms/mL was given colestyramine 4 g every 6 hours for 4 doses.[17]

(c) Metildigoxin

In a study in 6 patients given a single dose of metildigoxin with and without colestyramine, the AUC of the digitalis glycoside was not affected by colestyramine.[18]

Mechanism

Not totally understood. Colestyramine appears to bind with digitoxin in the gut, thereby reducing its bioavailability and interfering with enterohepatic recirculation so that its half-life is shortened. Digoxin may interact similarly,[16] although the effect is modest.[13]

Importance and management

The overall picture is far from clear. Some interaction between colestyramine and digoxin or digitoxin seems possible, but the extent to which it impairs the treatment of patients receiving these drugs is uncertain. Be alert for any evidence of under-digitalisation if digoxin or, more particularly, digitoxin is given with colestyramine. The studies suggest that colestyramine should not be given less than 1.5 to 2 hours after the digitalis glycoside to minimise the possibility of an interaction.[11] Note that the standard recommendation is to give other drugs one hour before or 4 to 6 hours after colestyramine.

1. Caldwell JH, Bush CA, Greenberger NJ. Interruption of the enterohepatic circulation of digitoxin by cholestyramine. *J Clin Invest* (1971) 50, 2638–44.
2. Carruthers SG, Dujovne CA. Cholestyramine and spironolactone and their combination in digitoxin elimination. *Clin Pharmacol Ther* (1980) 27, 184–7.
3. Gilfrich HJ, Kasper W, Meinertz T, Okonek S, Bork R. Treatment of massive digitoxin overdose by charcoal haemoperfusion and cholestyramine. *Lancet* (1978) I, 505.
4. Pieroni RE, Fisher JG. Use of cholestyramine resin in digitoxin toxicity. *JAMA* (1981) 245, 1939–40.
5. Hantson P, Vandenplas O, Mahieu P, Wallemacq P, Hassoun A. Repeated doses of activated charcoal and cholestyramine for digitoxin overdose: pharmacokinetic data and urinary elimination. *J Toxicol Clin Exp* (1991) 11, 401–5.
6. Cady WJ, Rehder TL, Campbell J. Use of cholestyramine resin in the treatment of digitoxin toxicity. *Am J Hosp Pharm* (1979) 36, 92–4.
7. Baciewicz AM, Isaacson ML, Lipscomb GL. Cholestyramine resin in the treatment of digitoxin toxicity. *Drug Intell Clin Pharm* (1983) 17, 57–9.
8. Pabst J, Leopold G, Schad W, Meub R. Bioavailability of digitoxin during chronic administration and influence of food and cholestyramine on the bioavailability after a single dose. *Naunyn Schmiedebergs Arch Pharmacol* (1979) 307, R70.
9. Brown DD, Juhl RP, Warner SL. Decreased bioavailability of digoxin produced by dietary fiber and cholestyramine. *Am J Cardiol* (1977) 39, 297.
10. Brown DD, Juhl RP, Warner SL. Decreased bioavailability of digoxin due to hypocholesterolemic interventions. *Circulation* (1978) 58, 164–72.
11. Bazzano G, Bazzano GS. Effects of digitalis binding resins on cardiac glycoside plasma levels. *Clin Res* (1972) 20, 24.
12. Smith TW. New approaches to the management of digitalis intoxication, In 'Symposium on Digitalis'. *Gyldenkal Norsk Forlag* (1977) 39, 312.
13. Neuvonen PJ, Kivistö K, Hirvisalo EL. Effects of resins and activated charcoal on the absorption of digoxin, carbamazepine and frusemide. *Br J Clin Pharmacol* (1988) 25, 229–33.
14. Hall WH, Shappell SD, Doherty JE. Effect of cholestyramine on digoxin absorption and excretion in man. *Am J Cardiol* (1977) 39, 213–16.
15. Brown DD, Schmid J, Long RA, Hull JH. A steady-state evaluation of the effects of propantheline bromide and cholestyramine on the bioavailability of digoxin when administered as tablets or capsules. *J Clin Pharmacol* (1985) 25, 360–4.
16. Roberge RJ, Sorensen T. Congestive heart failure and toxic digoxin levels: role of cholestyramine. *Vet Hum Toxicol* (2000) 42, 172–3.
17. Henderson RP, Solomon CP. Use of cholestyramine in the treatment of digoxin intoxication. *Arch Intern Med* (1988) 148, 745–46.
18. Hahn K-J, Weber E. Effect of cholestyramine on absorption of drugs. In: Blondheim SH, Alkan WJ, Brunner D (eds). Frontiers of Internal Medicine, 12th International Congress of Internal Medicine, Tel Aviv, Israel, September 1974. Basel: Karger; 1975 p. 409–11.

Digoxin + Danaparoid

A single dose of danaparoid very slightly decreased digoxin exposure. The effect of danaparoid on clotting tests was not altered by digoxin.

Clinical evidence, mechanism, importance and management

In a study, 6 healthy subjects were given digoxin 250 micrograms daily for 8 days, with a single 3250 anti-Xa-unit bolus-dose of danaparoid on day 7. The AUC and average plasma concentration of digoxin were very slightly decreased by danaparoid (by 15% and 13%, respectively.) The renal clearance of digoxin was unaffected. Digoxin increased the clearance of danaparoid by 10% and reduced its elimination half-life by 20% (as measured by anti-Xa activity); however, it did not alter the effects of danaparoid on clotting tests (including aPTT).[1] The changes in the pharmacokinetics of digoxin and danaparoid reported in this study are unlikely to be clinically important and no dose adjustments would appear to be necessary on concurrent use.

1. de Boer A, Stiekema JCJ, Danhof M, Moolenaar AJ, Breimer DD. Interaction of ORG 10172, a low molecular weight heparinoid, and digoxin in healthy volunteers. *Eur J Clin Pharmacol* (1991) 41, 245–50.

Digoxin and related drugs + Danshen (*Salvia miltiorrhiza*)

Danshen can falsify the results of serum immunoassay methods for digoxin.

Clinical evidence, mechanism, importance and management

Danshen can falsify some laboratory measurements of digoxin because it contains digoxin-like immunoreactive components. A study found that a fluorescent polarization immunoassay method (Abbott Laboratories) for digoxin gave falsely high readings in the presence of danshen, whereas a microparticle enzyme immunoassay (Abbott Laboratories) gave falsely low readings. These, or similar findings have been reported elsewhere.[1] These false readings could be eliminated by monitoring the free (i.e. unbound) digoxin concentrations[2] or by choosing assay systems that are unaffected by the presence of danshen (said to be the Roche and Beckman systems[3] or an enzyme linked chemiluminescent immunosorbent digoxin assay by Bayer HealthCare[1,4]). Similarly, when assaying serum from patients taking digoxin, to which a variety of danshen extracts were added, the use of a fluorescent polarization immunoassay gave variable results, whereas the results were more consistent with a chemiluminescent assay, the EMIT 2000 digoxin assay and the Randox digoxin assay.[5] It would therefore seem prudent, wherever possible, to use a chemiluminescent assay for digoxin in patients also taking danshen.

1. Dasgupta A, Actor JK, Olsen M, Wells A, Datta P. In vivo digoxin-like immunoreactivity in mice and interference of Chinese medicine Danshen in serum digoxin measurement: elimination of interference by using a chemiluminescent assay. *Clin Chim Acta* (2002) 317, 231–4.
2. Wahed A, Dasgupta A. Positive and negative in vitro interference of Chinese medicine dan shen in serum digoxin measurement. Elimination of interference by monitoring free digoxin concentration. *Am J Clin Pathol* (2001) 116, 403–8.
3. Chow L, Johnson M, Wells A, Dasgupta A. Effect of the traditional Chinese medicines Chan Su, Lu-Shen-Wan, Dan Shen, and Asian ginseng on serum digoxin measurement by Tina-quant (Roche) and Synchron LX System (Beckman) digoxin immunoassays. *J Clin Lab Anal* (2003) 17, 22–7.
4. Dasgupta A, Kang E, Olsen M, Actor JK, Datta P. New enzyme-linked chemiluminescent immunosorbent digoxin assay is free from interference of Chinese medicine DanShen. *Ther Drug Monit* (2006) 28, 775–8.
5. Datta P, Dasgupta A. Effect of Chinese medicines Chan Su and Danshen on EMIT 2000 and Randox digoxin immunoassays: wide variation in digoxin-like immunoreactivity and magnitude of interference in digoxin measurement by different brands of the same product. *Ther Drug Monit* (2002) 24, 637–44.

Digoxin + Dasabuvir

No pharmacokinetic interaction appears to occur between dasabuvir and digoxin.

Clinical evidence, mechanism, importance and management

The UK manufacturer briefly reports that, in a study in healthy subjects given a single 500-microgram dose of digoxin with dasabuvir 250 or 400 mg twice daily (with a fixed-dose combination of ombitasvir and paritaprevir boosted with ritonavir), the pharmacokinetics of digoxin and dasabuvir were unaffected.[1] No dose adjustments are necessary on concurrent use.

Note that digoxin can be used as a probe substrate to assess the activity of drugs on P-glycoprotein. This study therefore suggests that dasabuvir might not inhibit P-glycoprotein.

1. Exviera (Dasabuvir sodium monohydrate). AbbVie Ltd. UK Summary of product characteristics, January 2015.

Digoxin + Deferasirox

Deferasirox does not affect the pharmacokinetics of digoxin.

Clinical evidence, mechanism, importance and management

In a randomised study in 15 healthy subjects,[1] the pharmacokinetics of digoxin (500 micrograms on day one, and then 250 micrograms daily on days 2 to 8) were not affected by a single 20-mg/kg oral dose of **deferasirox**, given on day 8. Therefore no digoxin dose adjustment would be expected to be necessary on concurrent use.

1. Sechaud R, Robeva A, Belleli R, Balez S. Absence of an effect of a single-dose deferasirox on the steady-state pharmacokinetics of digoxin. *Int J Clin Pharmacol Ther* (2008) 46, 519–26.

Digoxin + Dexmedetomidine

An isolated report describes bradycardia when an infant receiving digoxin was given dexmedetomidine.

Clinical evidence, mechanism, importance and management

A 5-week-old infant with an atrioventricular septal defect, taking digoxin 10 micrograms twice daily and furosemide for mild congestive heart failure, developed respiratory failure requiring intubation and mechanical ventilation. She was given dexmedetomidine for sedation and received a loading dose of 0.5 micrograms/kg over 15 minutes, followed by an infusion of 0.44 micrograms/kg per hour. During the loading dose period her heart rate decreased from 133 bpm to 116 bpm. Throughout the next 13 hours the heart rate continued to decrease to about 90 bpm, with episodes of sinus bradycardia (heart rate around 50 bpm). Within one hour of discontinuing dexmedetomidine, the heart rate increased to its baseline value and no further episodes of bradycardia were observed. The reasons for this case are not known, but the authors of the report suggested that caution is warranted if dexmedetomidine is used for sedation in patients receiving digoxin.[1]

1. Berkenbosch JW, Tobias JD. Development of bradycardia during sedation with dexmedetomidine in an infant concurrently receiving digoxin. *Pediatr Crit Care Med* (2003) 4, 203–5.

Digoxin + Dietary fibre or Laxatives

Bisacodyl reduces digoxin levels. Dietary fibre, guar gum and bulk-forming laxatives (containing carrageenan, ispaghula, or microcrystal-

line cellulose) appear to have no effect on the absorption of digoxin. Single-dose studies show that macrogol 4000, a laxative polymer, reduces digoxin levels.

Clinical evidence

(a) Bisacodyl

Bisacodyl reduced the mean serum digoxin levels of 11 healthy subjects by about 12%. When the bisacodyl was taken 2 hours before the digoxin, serum digoxin levels were slightly raised, but not to a statistically significant extent.[1] Another study in 10 patients taking **alpha-acetyldigoxin** found that bisacodyl 30 mg daily reduced plasma digoxin levels from a peak of just over 1.6 nanograms/mL, to a low of about 1.25 nanograms/mL.[2]

(b) Carrageenan

There was no change in the average 4-hour postprandial digoxin levels of 5 healthy subjects given a single 800-microgram dose of *β*-**acetyldigoxin** with carrageenan 5 g.[3]

(c) Fibre

The serum digoxin levels of 12 patients taking digoxin 125 to 250 micrograms daily 15 to 30 minutes before breakfast were unchanged over a 10-day period when they were given a diet supplemented each day with 22 g of dietary fibre. The fibre was given in this way to simulate the conditions that might be encountered clinically (for example to reduce the symptoms of diverticular disease).[4]

Wheat bran 7.5 g twice daily caused a small 10% reduction in the plasma digoxin levels of 14 geriatric patients after 2 weeks, but there was no change after 4 weeks.[5] Bran fibre 11 g caused a 6 to 7% reduction in the absorption and the steady-state serum levels of digoxin in 16 healthy subjects.[6] The cumulative urinary recovery of a single oral dose of digoxin in healthy subjects was reduced almost 20% by 5 g of fibre, whereas 0.75 g of fibre had no effect.[7] In another study there was no change in the average 4-hour postprandial digoxin levels of 5 healthy subjects given a single 800-microgram dose of *β*-**acetyldigoxin** with wheat bran 10 g or pectin 5 g.[3]

(d) Guar gum

In 10 healthy subjects *Guarem* (95% guar gum) 5 g reduced the peak serum levels of a single 500-microgram oral dose of digoxin by 21% and the AUC_{0-6} was reduced by 16%, but the amount excreted in the urine over 24 hours was only minimally reduced.[8] Guar gum 18 g with a test meal did not affect steady-state plasma digoxin levels in 11 healthy subjects given digoxin 1 mg on day one, 750 micrograms on day 2, and then 500 micrograms daily for 3 days.[9]

(e) Ispaghula

An ispaghula preparation (*Vi-Siblin S*) was found to have no effect on the serum digoxin levels of 16 geriatric patients.[5] The same lack of effect was seen in another study in 15 patients given 3.6 g of an ispaghula preparation (*Metamucil*) three times daily.[10]

(f) Macrogol 4000

A randomised, crossover study in 18 healthy subjects found that 20 g of macrogol 4000 daily over an 8-day period reduced the maximum serum levels of a single 500-microgram dose of digoxin by 40%, and reduced its AUC by 30%. Heart rate and the PR interval were unchanged.[11]

(g) Microcrystalline cellulose

There was no change in the average 4-hour postprandial digoxin levels of 5 healthy subjects given a single 800-microgram dose of *β*-**acetyldigoxin** with microcrystalline cellulose 5 g.[3]

Mechanism

Not established. Digoxin can bind to some extent to fibre within the gut.[12] However, *in vitro* studies (with bran, carrageenan, pectin, sodium pectinate, xylan and carboxymethylcellulose) have shown that most of the binding is reversible.[13]

Importance and management

Information seems to be limited to these reports. The reduction in serum digoxin levels caused by bisacodyl is small, and not expected to be of clinical importance, and apparently preventable by giving the bisacodyl 2 hours before the digoxin. Neither dietary fibre (bran), guar gum nor the two bulk-forming laxatives (*Vi-Siblin* and *Metamucil*) have a clinically important effect on serum digoxin levels. No special precautions would appear to be necessary. The importance of the interaction between digoxin and macrogol 4000 awaits further assessment, but on the available evidence it would be prudent to be alert for the need to increase the digoxin dose.

1. Wang D-J, Chu K-M, Chen J-D. Drug interaction between digoxin and bisacodyl. *J Formos Med Assoc* (1990) 89, 913, 915–9.
2. Botzler R, Ritter. Einfluß von Abführmaßnahmen auf die Serumkonzentration von Digoxin beim Menschen. *Leber Magen Darm* (1982) 12, 255–7.
3. Kasper H, Zilly W, Fassl H, Fehle F. The effect of dietary fiber on postprandial serum digoxin concentration in man. *Am J Clin Nutr* (1979) 32, 2436–38.
4. Woods MN, Ingelfinger JA. Lack of effect of bran on digoxin absorption. *Clin Pharmacol Ther* (1979) 26, 21–3.
5. Nordström M, Melander A, Robertsson E, Steen B. Influence of wheat bran and of a bulk-forming ispaghula cathartic on the bioavailability of digoxin in geriatric in-patients. *Drug Nutr Interact* (1987) 5, 67–9.
6. Johnson BF, Rodin SM, Hoch K, Shekar V. The effect of dietary fiber on the bioavailability of digoxin in capsules. *J Clin Pharmacol* (1987) 27, 487–90.
7. Brown DD, Juhl RP, Warner SL. Decreased bioavailability of digoxin due to hypocholesterolemic interventions. *Circulation* (1978) 58, 164–72.
8. Huupponen R, Seppälä P, Iisalo E. Effect of guar gum, a fibre preparation, on digoxin and penicillin absorption in man. *Eur J Clin Pharmacol* (1984) 26, 279–81.
9. Lembcke B, Häsler K, Kramer P, Caspary WF, Creuzfeldt W. Plasma digoxin concentrations during administration of dietary fibre (guar gum) in man. *Z Gastroenterol* (1982) 20, 164–7.
10. Walan A, Bergdahl B, Skoog M-L. Study of digoxin bioavailability during treatment with a bulk forming laxative (*Metamucil*). *Scand J Gastroenterol* (1977) 12 (Suppl 45), 111.
11. Ragueneau I, Poirier J-M, Radembino N, Sao AB, Funck-Brentano C, Jaillon P. Pharmacokinetic and pharmacodynamic drug interactions between digoxin and macrogol 4000, a laxative polymer, in healthy volunteers. *Br J Clin Pharmacol* (1999) 48, 453–6.
12. Floyd RA. Digoxin interaction with bran and high fiber foods. *Am J Hosp Pharm* (1978) 35, 660.
13. Hamamura J, Burros BC, Clemens RA, Smith CH. Dietary fiber and digoxin. *Fedn Proc* (1985) 44, 759.

Digoxin and related drugs + Digoxin-like herbal medicines

Some herbal medicines contain digitalis glycosides, which could in theory have additive effects with digoxin or related digitalis glycosides, or interfere with their assays. However, there appear to be few such interactions reported.

Clinical evidence, mechanism, importance and management

(a) Additive effects possible

A 26-year-old woman developed severe and unexplained chest pain, and was later noted to have a heart rate of 39 bpm and a blood pressure of 59/36 mmHg, but these rose to normal with conservative management. She was found to have a digoxin level of 0.9 nanograms/mL and was diagnosed as having digoxin toxicity, despite not taking any prescribed digoxin. The digoxin-like digitalis glycosides were thought to have come from an unnamed herbal remedy for stress, which contained **black cohosh root** (*Cimicifuga racemosa*), **cayenne pepper fruit** (*Capsicum annuum*), **hops flowers** (*Humulus lupulus*), **skullcap herb** (*Scutellaria lateriflora*), **valerian root** (*Valeriana officinalis*) and **wood betony herb** (*Pedicularis canadensis*).[1] All of these herbal constituents had previously been shown to contain small amounts of digoxin-like compounds, which were only partially detected by digoxin antibody immunoassays.[1,2] In this previous *in vitro* study, 46 commercially packaged herb teas and 78 teas prepared from herbs were assayed for digoxin-like factors by their cross-reactivity with digoxin antibody or inhibition of ouabain binding, and these values were used to give approximate equivalent daily doses of digoxin. Three packaged teas (***Breathe Easy***, **blackcurrant**, and **jasmine**) and 3 herbs (**pleurisy root**, **chaparral**, **peppermint**) were found to contain greater than 30 micrograms of digoxin equivalents per cup and were postulated to provide a therapeutic daily dose of digoxin if 5 cups a day were drunk.[2] However, note that some common teas sampled in this study (e.g. English Breakfast, Earl Grey) contained over 20 micrograms of digoxin equivalents per cup, and tea drinking has not been associated with adverse cardiovascular risk.[3] Therefore the interpretation of the findings of this study is unclear.

Theoretical interactions with herbal remedies are not always translated into practice, and there do not appear to be any cases of herbals interacting with digoxin because of their cardiac glycoside content.

(b) Effects on digoxin or digitoxin assays

A 68-year-old woman who was given a loading dose of digitoxin 750 micrograms then 100 micrograms on the second day was found to have markedly elevated levels of digitoxin (greater than 100 nanograms/mL), but no clinical signs of toxicity. Two days before admission she had ingested 90 drops of **Uzara**, a preparation from *Xysmalobium undulatum*, which contains weak digitalis glycosides. Later investigations in 4 healthy subjects given 30 drops of **Uzara** confirmed that assays for **digitoxin** (CEDIA digitoxin test, Roche Diagnostics, Germany) and digoxin (Tina-quant digoxin test, Roche Diagnostics, Germany) were markedly elevated by **Uzara** to levels well above usual therapeutic concentrations, but that there were no clinically relevant changes in heart rate and blood pressure.[4]

In an *in vitro* study, **plantain** (*Plantago major*) extract from capsules, liquid extract, or dry leaf did not affect the results of digoxin assays when using fluorescence polarization immunoassay or microparticle enzyme immunoassay.[5] Note that contamination of **plantain** with *Digitalis lanata* has been reported.[6]

1. Scheinhost ME. Digoxin toxicity in a 26-year-old woman taking a herbal dietary supplement. *J Am Osteopath Assoc* (2001), 101, 444–6.
2. Longerich L, Johnson E, Gault MH. Digoxin-like factors in herbal teas. *Clin Invest Med* (1993) 16, 210–8.
3. *Martindale. The Complete Drug Reference*, [online] London: Pharmaceutical Press. https://www.medicinescomplete.com/mc/martindale/current/3874-t.htm (accessed 19/10/15).
4. Thürmann PA, Neff A, Fleisch J. Interference of uzara glycosides in assays of digitalis glycosides. *Int J Clin Pharmacol Ther* (2004) 42, 281–4.
5. Dasgupta A, Davis B, Wells A. Effect of plantain on therapeutic drug monitoring of digoxin and thirteen other common drugs. *Ann Clin Biochem* (2006) 43, 223–5.
6. Slifman NR, Obermeyer WR, Aloi BK, Musser SM, Correll WA, Cichowicz SM, Betz JM, Love LA. Contamination of botanical dietary supplements by Digitalis lanata. *N Engl J Med* (1998) 339, 806–11.

Digoxin + Dihydroergocryptine

Dihydroergocryptine does not appear to affect the pharmacokinetics of digoxin.

Clinical evidence, mechanism, importance and management

In a randomised study in 12 healthy subjects, dihydroergocryptine 20 mg did not affect the pharmacokinetics of a single 500-microgram dose of digoxin. No changes were seen in the ability of the heart to initiate and conduct impulses, or repolarise. The slight drop in blood pressure noted during the first 2 to 4 hours after digoxin was given was more pronounced in the presence of dihydroergocryptine, but there was no evidence of impaired orthostatic blood pressure control.[1] No particular precautions would seem necessary during concurrent use.

1. Retzow A, Althaus M, de Mey C, Mazur D, Vens-Cappell B. Study on the interaction of the dopamine agonist α-dihydroergocryptine with the pharmacokinetics of digoxin. *Arzneimittelforschung* (2000) 50, 591–6.

Digoxin + Dipeptidylpeptidase-4 inhibitors

There appears to be no pharmacokinetic interaction between digoxin and alogliptin, linagliptin, saxagliptin, or vildagliptin. Sitagliptin increases digoxin exposure.

Clinical evidence

(a) Alogliptin

The US manufacturer of alogliptin briefly notes that, in clinical studies, alogliptin 25 mg daily did not meaningfully alter the pharmacokinetics of digoxin 250 micrograms daily, when both drugs were given for 10 days.[1]

(b) Linagliptin

In a crossover study, 20 healthy subjects were given digoxin 250 micrograms daily for 11 days, either alone or with linagliptin 5 mg daily from days 6 to 11. There was no change in the AUC, maximum plasma concentration, or renal clearance of digoxin.[2]

(c) Saxagliptin

In a study in 14 healthy subjects, there was no change in the pharmacokinetics of digoxin or saxagliptin when digoxin (loading dose over 2 days then 250 micrograms daily for 5 days) was given with saxagliptin 10 mg daily, when compared with either drug alone.[3]

(d) Sitagliptin

In a study in 32 healthy subjects, digoxin 250 micrograms daily was given with either sitagliptin 100 mg or 200 mg daily for 10 days. The AUC and maximum concentration of digoxin was increased by 11% and 18%, respectively.[4]

(e) Vildagliptin

In a study, 18 healthy subjects were given either vildagliptin 100 mg daily for 7 days or digoxin 500 micrograms on the first day then 250 micrograms for 6 days, and then both drugs together. No changes in the pharmacokinetics of either drug occurred.[5]

Mechanism

Unknown. Digoxin is a substrate of the efflux pump, P-glycoprotein. Sitagliptin did not inhibit P-glycoprotein mediated digoxin transport *in vitro*,[6] so the mechanism for the very slight increase in digoxin exposure is unknown.

Importance and management

The very slight rise in digoxin exposure with sitagliptin is unlikely to be clinically relevant, and no digoxin dose adjustment is needed when sitagliptin is started. However, the UK manufacturer recommends that patients at risk of digoxin toxicity should be monitored for this when sitagliptin is used,[7] which is a cautious approach.

Alogliptin, linagliptin, saxagliptin, and vildagliptin do not alter digoxin pharmacokinetics, and so no dose adjustment is required on concurrent use.

1. Nesina (Alogliptin). Takeda Pharmaceuticals America, Inc. US Prescribing information, January 2013.
2. Friedrich C, Ring A, Brand T, Sennewald R, Graefe-Mody EU, Woerle HJ. Evaluation of the pharmacokinetic interaction after multiple oral doses of linagliptin and digoxin in healthy volunteers. *Eur J Drug Metab Pharmacokinet* (2011) 36, 17–24.
3. Boulton DW, Li L, Patel CG, Komoroski BJ, Whigan D, Frevert EU, Kornhauser DM. No pharmacokinetic interaction between saxagliptin and digoxin in healthy subjects. 36th Annual Meeting of the American College of Clinical Pharmacology, San Francisco, California, 2007.
4. Miller JL, Migoya E, Talaty JE, Bergman AJ, Xu, Y, Zheng W, Gutierrez M, Wagner JA, Herman GA. The effect of MK-0431 on the pharmacokinetics of digoxin after concomitant administration for 10 days in healthy subjects. *Clin Pharmacol Ther* (2006) 79, 24.
5. He Y-L, Sabo R, Sunkara G, Bizot M-N, Riviere G-J, Leon S, Ligueros-Saylan M, Dole WP, Howard D. Evaluation of pharmacokinetic interactions between vildagliptin and digoxin in healthy volunteers. *J Clin Pharmacol* (2007) 47, 998–1004.
6. Chu XY, Bleasby K, Yabut J, Cai X, Chan GH, Hafey MJ, Xu S, Bergman AJ, Braun MP, Dean DC, Evers R. Transport of the dipeptidyl peptidase-4 inhibitor sitagliptin by human organic anion transporter 3, organic anion transporting polypeptide 4C1, and multidrug resistance P-glycoprotein. *J Pharmacol Exp Ther* (2007) 321, 673–83.
7. Januvia (Sitagliptin phosphate monohydrate). Merck Sharp & Dohme Ltd. UK Summary of product characteristics, December 2012.

Digoxin + Dipyridamole

Dipyridamole can increase the absorption of digoxin.

Clinical evidence, mechanism, importance and management

A study in 12 healthy subjects found that dipyridamole 150 mg twice daily for 5 doses increased the AUC_{0-4} and the AUC_{0-24} of a single 500-microgram oral dose of digoxin by 20% and 13%, respectively. This was attributed to an increase in digoxin absorption possibly mediated by intestinal P-glycoprotein inhibition.[1] *In vitro* studies[1,2] found that dipyridamole inhibits the P-glycoprotein-mediated transport of digoxin, but in one study this was only at dipyridamole levels higher than those achieved clinically.[2] The magnitude of the increase in digoxin exposure reported in this study is unlikely to be clinically relevant in most patients.

1. Verstuyft C, Strabach S, El Morabet H, Kerb R, Brinkmann U, Dubert L, Jaillon P, Funck-Brentano C, Trugnan G, Becquemont L. Dipyridamole enhances digoxin bioavailability via P-glycoprotein inhibition. *Clin Pharmacol Ther* (2003) 73, 51–60.
2. Kakumoto M, Takara K, Sakaeda T, Tanigawara Y, Kita T, Okumura K. MDR1-mediated interaction of digoxin with antiarrhythmic or antianginal drugs. *Biol Pharm Bull* (2002) 25, 1604–7.

Digoxin and related drugs + Disopyramide

Disopyramide does not usually affect digoxin levels. A single report describes toxicity in a patient taking digitoxin and disopyramide.

Clinical evidence, mechanism, importance and management

A number of studies have clearly shown that disopyramide causes only a very small increase or no increase at all in the serum levels of digoxin,[1-7] and the weight of evidence suggests that no clinically important interaction occurs if digoxin and disopyramide are used together. However, a very brief report describes toxicity and serious arrhythmia in one patient given **digitoxin** and disopyramide.[8] The general relevance of this isolated case is unclear.

1. Doering W. Quinidine-digoxin interaction. *N Engl J Med* (1979) 301, 400–4.
2. Leahey EB, Reiffel JA, Giardina E-GV, Bigger JT. The effect of quinidine and other oral antiarrhythmic drugs on serum digoxin: a prospective study. *Ann Intern Med* (1980) 92, 605–8.
3. Manolas EG, Hunt D, Sloman G. Effects of quinidine and disopyramide on serum digoxin concentrations. *Aust N Z J Med* (1980) 10, 426–9.
4. Wellens HJ, Gorgels AP, Braat SJ, Bär FW, Vanagt EJ, Phaf B. Effect of oral disopyramide on serum digoxin levels. A prospective study. *Am Heart J* (1980) 100, 934–5.
5. Risler T, Burk M, Peters U, Grabensee B, Seipel L. On the interaction between digoxin and disopyramide. *Clin Pharmacol Ther* (1983) 34, 176–80.
6. García-Barreto D, Groning E, González-Gómez A, Pérez A, Hernández-Cañero A, Toruncha A. Enhancement of the antiarrhythmic action of disopyramide by digoxin. *J Cardiovasc Pharmacol* (1981) 3, 1236–42.
7. Elliott HL, Kelman AW, Sumner DJ, Bryson SM, Campbell BC, Hillis WS, Whiting B. Pharmacodynamic and pharmacokinetic evaluation of the interaction between digoxin and disopyramide. *Br J Clin Pharmacol* (1982) 14, 141P.
8. Manchon ND, Bercoff E, Lemarchand P, Chassagne P, Senant J, Bourreille J. Fréquence et gravité des interactions médicamenteuses dans une population âgée: étude prospective concernant 63 malades. *Rev Med Interne* (1989) 10, 521–5.

Digoxin and related drugs + Diuretics; Potassium-depleting

The potassium loss caused by potassium-depleting diuretics increases the toxicity of the digitalis glycosides.

Clinical evidence

A comparative study[1] of the medical records of 418 patients taking digitalis over the period 1950 to 1952, and of 679 patients over the period 1964 to 1966, found that the incidence of digitalis toxicity had more than doubled. Of the earlier group 8.6% developed toxicity (58% taking diuretics, mainly of the **organomercurial type**) compared with 17.2% of the latter group (81% taking diuretics, mainly **chlorothiazides, furosemide, etacrynic acid, chlortalidone**). It was concluded that the increased toxicity was related to the increased use of potassium-depleting diuretics.

A retrospective study of over 400 patients taking digoxin found that almost one in five had some toxic reactions attributable to the use of the digoxin. Of these, 16% had demonstrable hypokalaemia (defined as serum potassium less than 3.5 mmol/L). Almost half of the patients who had toxicity were taking potassium-depleting diuretics, notably **hydrochlorothiazide** or **furosemide**.[2] Similar results were found in other studies in a considerable number of patients.[3-9] In a case-control study of 595 cases of digoxin toxicity requiring hospitalisation from 2001 to 2004, cases were 2.97 times more likely to have been prescribed **loop diuretics** in the previous month, 2.36 times more likely to have been prescribed **thiazide diuretics**, 4 times more likely to have been prescribed the combination of a **loop** and **thiazide** diuretic, and 6.85 times more likely to have been prescribed a combination of **loop, thiazide** and potassium-sparing diuretics. For the individual diuretics analysed, the odds ratios for thiazides were 4.63 for **hydrochlorothiazide** and about 2 for **indapamide** and **trichlormethiazide**. For the loop diuretics, the odds ratio was 2.97 for **furosemide**.[10]

In contrast, a retrospective study of patients who developed digitalis toxicity found that the likelihood of its development in those with potassium levels below 3.5 mmol/L was no greater than those with normal potassium levels.[11] Two other studies in a total of almost 200 patients did not detect any association between the development of digitalis toxicity and the use of diuretics or changes in potassium levels.[12,13]

A pharmacokinetic study in 6 patients found that single 50-mg and 100-mg doses of **cicletanine** had no effect on the plasma levels of digoxin 125 to 250 micrograms daily.[14] In addition there is also some evidence that **furosemide** might raise serum digoxin levels,[15] although two other studies found no evidence that **furosemide** affects the urinary excretion of digoxin.[16,17]

Mechanism

Not fully understood. The cardiac glycosides inhibit sodium-potassium ATP-ase, which is concerned with the transport of sodium and potassium ions across the membranes of the myocardial cells. This is associated with an increase in the availability of calcium ions concerned with the contraction of the cells. Potassium loss caused by these diuretics exacerbates the potassium loss from the myocardial cells, thereby increasing the activity and the toxicity of the digitalis. Some loss of magnesium could also have a part to play. The difference in risk with individual diuretics might be due to their differing potential to cause hypokalaemia.[10]

Importance and management

A direct link between the use of these potassium-depleting diuretics and the development of digitalis toxicity is not established beyond doubt, but concurrent use can result in digitalis toxicity. It is therefore important that potassium levels remain within the accepted normal range during the use of a digitalis glycoside. Potassium levels should be routinely monitored when diuretics are given and it would seem prudent to recheck levels if patients develop digitalis adverse effects (e.g. bradycardia). See 'Table 26.1', p.1117, for a list of potassium-depleting diuretics. There is some evidence that the addition of a potassium-sparing diuretic to loop and thiazide diuretics might further increase the risk of digoxin toxicity, see also 'Digoxin and related drugs + Diuretics; Potassium-sparing', below.

1. Jørgenson AW, Sørensen OH. Digitalis intoxication. A comparative study on the incidence of digitalis intoxication during the periods 1950–52 and 1964–66. *Acta Med Scand* (1970) 188, 179–83.
2. Shapiro S, Slone D, Lewis GP, Jick H. The epidemiology of digoxin. A study in three Boston Hospitals. *J Chron Dis* (1969) 22, 361–71.
3. Tawakkol AA, Nutter DO, Massumi RA. A prospective study of digitalis toxicity in a large city hospital. *Med Ann Dist Columbia* (1967) 36, 402–9.
4. Soffer A. The changing clinical picture of digitalis intoxication. *Arch Intern Med* (1961) 107, 681–8.
5. Rodensky PL, Wasserman F. Observations on digitalis intoxication. *Arch Intern Med* (1961) 108, 171–88.
6. Steiness E, Olesen KH. Cardiac arrhythmias induced by hypokalaemia and potassium loss during maintenance digoxin therapy. *Br Heart J* (1976) 38, 167–72.
7. Binnion PF. Hypokalaemia and digoxin-induced arrhythmias. *Lancet* (1975) i, 343–4.
8. Poole-Wilson PA, Hall R, Cameron IR. Hypokalaemia, digitalis, and arrhythmias. *Lancet* (1975) i, 575–6.
9. Shapiro W, Taubert K. Hypokalaemia and digoxin-induced arrhythmias. *Lancet* (1975) ii, 604–5.
10. Wang MT, Su CY, Chan ALF, Lian PW, Leu HB, Hsu YJ. Risk of digoxin intoxication in heart failure patients exposed to digoxin-diuretic interactions: a population-based study. *Br J Clin Pharmacol* (2010) 70, 258–67.
11. Ogilvie RI, Ruedy J. An educational program in digitalis therapy. *JAMA* (1972) 222, 50–55.
12. Smith TW, Haber E. Digoxin intoxication: the relationship of clinical presentation to serum digoxin concentration. *J Clin Invest* (1970) 49, 2377–86.
13. Beller GA, Smith TW, Abelmann WH, Haber E, Hood WB. Digitalis intoxication. A prospective clinical study with serum level correlations. *N Engl J Med* (1971) 284, 989–97.
14. Clement DL, Teirlynck O, Belpaire F. Lack of effect of cicletanine on plasma digoxin levels. *Int J Clin Pharmacol Res* (1988) 8, 9–11.
15. Tsutsumi E, Fujiki H, Takeda H, Fukushima H. Effect of furosemide on serum clearance and renal excretion of digoxin. *J Clin Pharmacol* (1979) 19, 200–204.
16. Malcolm AD, Leung FY, Fuchs JCA, Duarte JE. Digoxin kinetics during furosemide administration. *Clin Pharmacol Ther* (1977) 21, 567–574.
17. Brown DD, Dormois JC, Abraham GN, Lewis K, Dixon K. Effect of furosemide on the renal excretion of digoxin. *Clin Pharmacol Ther* (1976) 20, 395–400.

Digoxin and related drugs + Diuretics; Potassium-sparing

Digoxin levels might be increased by spironolactone. Eplerenone causes a negligible increase in digoxin exposure. Amiloride has little effect on digoxin levels in healthy subjects, but it might reduce its inotropic effects, and in patients with renal impairment amiloride possibly raises digoxin levels. There is some evidence suggesting an increased risk of risk of digoxin toxicity when it is given with both a potassium-sparing diuretic and a potassium-depleting diuretic.

The effects of digitoxin are reported to be both increased and decreased by spironolactone.

Clinical evidence

(a) Digitoxin

A study in 6 healthy subjects who had been taking digitoxin 100 or 150 micrograms daily for 30 days found that **spironolactone** 300 mg daily increased the digitoxin half-life by one-third (from 142 hours to 192 hours).[1] In contrast, other studies have found that the digitoxin half-life was reduced (from 256 hours to 205 hours) by **spironolactone**.[2]

(b) Digoxin

In a case-control study of 595 cases of digoxin toxicity requiring hospitalisation from 2001 to 2004, cases were 1.72 times more likely to have been prescribed potassium-sparing diuretics alone (unspecified) in the previous month, an increase which was not statistically significant. However, the combination of potassium-sparing diuretics with potassium-depleting diuretics was associated with an increase compared with potassium-depleting diuretics alone: cases were 3.79 times more likely to have been prescribed loop diuretics with potassium-sparing diuretics (2.97 for loop diuretics alone) and 6.85 times more likely to have been prescribed a combination of loop, thiazide and potassium-sparing diuretics (compared with 4 times more likely to have been prescribed the combination of a loop and a thiazide diuretic).[3] Reports regarding interactions between named diuretics and digoxin are covered in the subsections below.

1. Amiloride. In 6 healthy subjects, amiloride 5 mg twice daily for 8 days almost doubled the renal clearance of digoxin (from 1.3 mL/kg per minute to 2.4 mL/kg per minute), but reduced the extra-renal clearance (from 2.1 mL/kg per minute to 0.1 mL/kg per minute). The balance of the two effects was to cause a small fall in the total clearance and a small rise in plasma digoxin levels.[4] The positive inotropic effects of digoxin were reduced, but whether this is clinically important is uncertain. In contrast, a later study in 8 healthy subjects found that a single 75-mg (sic) oral dose of amiloride given 3 hours before an infusion of digoxin did not reduce the inotropic effects of digoxin.[5]

2. Eplerenone. In one study, the steady-state AUC of digoxin 200 micrograms daily increased by 16% (90% confidence interval: 4% to 30%) when it was given with eplerenone.[6,7]

3. Spironolactone. The plasma digoxin levels of 9 patients were increased by about 20% (from 0.8 nanograms/mL to 1 nanograms/mL) when they were given spironolactone 100 mg daily. One patient had a three- to fourfold rise in digoxin levels.[8]

The clearance of a single 750-microgram intravenous dose of digoxin was reduced by about 25% in 4 patients and 4 healthy subjects following 5 days of treatment with spironolactone 100 mg twice daily.[9] A sizeable fall in serum digoxin levels occurred in an elderly patient when spironolactone was withdrawn,[10] but the accuracy of the assay method used is uncertain (see *Importance and management* below). One study found that no clinically important reduction in digoxin clearance occurred when *Aldactazide* (spironolactone with hydrochlorothiazide) was also given.[11]

Mechanism

Not fully understood. Spironolactone inhibits the excretion of digoxin by the kidney (by 13%) but does not affect its biliary clearance.[12] *Animal* studies have suggested that spironolactone might induce P-glycoprotein expression, resulting in reduced intestinal absorption of substrates such as digoxin.[13] Spironolactone probably also causes a reduction in the volume of distribution of digoxin, with a corresponding increase in digoxin plasma levels. This increase could increase the risk of digoxin toxicity, and might add to the increased risk seen with potassium-sparing diuretics, rather than offset it.[3]

It has been suggested that amiloride might have increased the production of aldosterone, which suppressed the positive inotropic effects of digoxin.[4] Studies in patients with congestive heart failure are needed.

Importance and management

Digoxin

The pharmacokinetic interaction between digoxin and **spironolactone** appears to be established. What is known suggests that a rise in digoxin levels of up to 25% is likely to occur, although much greater increases can apparently occur in some patients.[8] Monitor concurrent use carefully for signs of over-digitalisation, initially by checking symptoms and pulse rate, and then taking digoxin levels if an interaction is suspected. Note that spironolactone or its metabolite, canrenone, can interfere with some digoxin assay methods.[14] In one report, radioimmunoassay (RIA) and affinity-column-mediated immunoassay (ACMIA) were particularly affected by spironolactone and its metabolites.[15] Conversely, falsely low digoxin readings with the AxSym MEIA assay method led to digoxin overdose and toxicity in one patient.[16] This means that monitoring is difficult unless the digoxin assay method is known to be reliable. Measurement of free digoxin levels or use of a chemiluminescent assay (CLIA) or turbidimetric immunoassay for digoxin has been reported to mostly eliminate interference from spironolactone, potassium canrenoate and canrenone;[17,18] additionally, these drugs do not appear to affect the Dimension Vista Digoxin Assay to a clinically relevant extent.[19] In clinical practice there is some evidence suggesting an increased risk of risk of digoxin toxicity when potassium-sparing diuretics are added to potassium-depleting diuretics,[3] so bear this possibility in mind.

Eplerenone also appears to cause a negligible increase in digoxin exposure. The UK manufacturers recommend that caution is warranted when digoxin is dosed near the upper limit of therapeutic range.[6] However, the US manufacturer states that the pharmacokinetic interaction is not clinically relevant.[20]

Patients with poor renal function would be expected to have a rise in digoxin levels when given **amiloride** (due to the increased reliance on renal clearance) but the clinical importance of this awaits confirmation.

Digitoxin

The situation with digitoxin and **spironolactone** is confusing because the reports are contradictory and the outcome uncertain. Concurrent use should be well monitored.

1. Carruthers SG, Dujovne CA. Cholestyramine and spironolactone and their combination in digitoxin elimination. *Clin Pharmacol Ther* (1980) 27, 184–7.
2. Wirth KE, Frölich JC, Hollifield JW, Falkner FC, Sweetman BS, Oates JA. Metabolism of digitoxin in man and its modification by spironolactone. *Eur J Clin Pharmacol* (1976) 9, 345–54.
3. Wang MT, Su CY, Chan ALF, Lian PW, Leu HB, Hsu YJ. Risk of digoxin intoxication in heart failure patients exposed to digoxin-diuretic interactions: a population-based study. *Br J Clin Pharmacol* (2010) 70, 258–67.
4. Waldorff S, Hansen PB, Kjærgård H, Buch J, Egeblad H, Steiness E. Amiloride-induced changes in digoxin dynamics and kinetics: abolition of digoxin-induced inotropism with amiloride. *Clin Pharmacol Ther* (1981) 30, 172–6.
5. Richter JP, Sommers De K, Snyman JR, Millard SM. The acute effects of amiloride and potassium canrenoate on digoxin-induced positive inotropism in healthy volunteers. *Eur J Clin Pharmacol* (1993) 45, 195–6.
6. Inspra (Eplerenone). Pfizer Ltd. UK Summary of product characteristics, October 2009.
7. Cook CS, Berry LM, Burton E. Prediction of in vivo drug interactions with eplerenone in man from in vitro metabolic inhibition data. *Xenobiotica* (2004) 34, 215–28.
8. Steiness E. Renal tubular secretion of digoxin. *Circulation* (1974) 50. 103–7.
9. Waldorff S, Andersen JD, Heebøll-Nielsen N, Nielsen OG, Moltke E, Sørensen U, Steiness E. Spironolactone-induced changes in digoxin kinetics. *Clin Pharmacol Ther* (1978) 24, 162–7.
10. Paladino JA, Davidson KH, McCall BB. Influence of spironolactone on serum digoxin concentration. *JAMA* (1984) 251, 470–1.
11. Finnegan TP, Spence JD, Cape R. Potassium-sparing diuretics: interaction with digoxin in elderly men. *J Am Geriatr Soc* (1984) 32, 129–31.
12. Hedman A, Angelin B, Arvidsson A, Dahlqvist R. Digoxin-interactions in man: spironolactone reduces renal but not biliary digoxin clearance. *Eur J Clin Pharmacol* (1992) 42, 481–5.
13. Ghanem CI, Gómez PC, Arana MC, Perassolo M, Delli Carpini G, Luquita MG, Veggi LM, Catania VA, Bengochea LA, Mottino AD. Induction of rat intestinal P-glycoprotein by spironolactone and its effect on absorption of orally administered digoxin. *J Pharmacol Exp Ther* (2006) 318, 1146–52.
14. Steimer W, Müller C, Eber B. Digoxin assays: frequent, substantial, and potentially dangerous interference by spironolactone, canrenone, and other steroids. *Clin Chem* (2002) 48, 507–16.
15. Pleasants RA, Williams DM, Porter RS, Gadsden RH. Reassessment of cross-reactivity of spironolactone metabolites with four digoxin immunoassays. *Ther Drug Monit* (1989) 11, 200–4.

16. Steimer W, Müller C, Eber B, Emmanuilidis K. Intoxication due to negative canrenone interference in digoxin drug monitoring. *Lancet* (1999) 354, 1176–7.
17. Dasgupta A, Saffer H, Wells A, Datta P. Bidirectional (positive/negative) interference of spironolactone, canrenone, and potassium canrenoate on serum digoxin measurement: elimination of interference by measuring free digoxin or using a chemiluminescent assay for digoxin. *J Clin Lab Anal* (2002) 16, 172–7.
18. Datta P, Dasgupta A. A new turbidometric digoxin immunoassay on the ADVIA 1650 analyzer is free from interference by spironolactone, potassium canrenoate, and their common metabolite canrenone. *Ther Drug Monit* (2003) 25, 478–82.
19. Dasgupta A, Johnson MJ. Effect of spironolactone, potassium canrenoate and their common metabolite canrenone on Dimension Vista Digoxin Assay. *J Clin Lab Anal* (2010) 24, 413–7.
20. Inspra (Eplerenone). Pfizer Inc. US Prescribing information, April 2008.

Digoxin + Dofetilide

Dofetilide does not affect the pharmacokinetics of digoxin.

Clinical evidence, mechanism, importance and management

In a placebo-controlled study in 13 subjects, dofetilide 250 micrograms twice daily for 5 days had no effect on the steady-state pharmacokinetics of digoxin, given at a dose of 250 micrograms daily after a loading dose.[1] No digoxin dose adjustment would be expected to be needed on the concurrent use of dofetilide.

1. Kleinermans D, Nichols DJ, Dalrymple I. Effect of dofetilide on the pharmacokinetics of digoxin. *Am J Cardiol* (2001) 87, 248–50.

Digoxin and related drugs + Drugs that affect calcium

The effects of digitalis glycosides might be increased by rises in blood calcium levels, and the use of intravenous calcium might result in the development of potentially life-threatening digitalis-induced arrhythmias. The use of digitalis glycosides in the presence of hypercalcaemia due to vitamin D administration might result in arrhythmias. Parathyroid hormones can increase calcium levels, although teriparatide appears not to affect the calcium-mediated effects of digoxin. Calcitonin might transiently decrease calcium levels and, therefore could, theoretically, reduce cardiac sensitivity to digoxin.

Clinical evidence

(a) Calcium

Two patients developed cardiac arrhythmias and died after being given digitalis intramuscularly and either **calcium chloride** or **calcium gluconate** intravenously. No absolutely certain causative relationship was established.[1]

There is some evidence that increases or decreases in blood **calcium** levels can increase or decrease, respectively, the effects of digitalis. A patient with congestive heart failure and atrial fibrillation was resistant to the actions of digoxin (serum levels of 1.5 to 3 nanograms/mL) until his serum **calcium** levels were raised from 1.68 mmol/L to about 2.13 mmol/L by oral **calcium and vitamin D**.[2] However, in a retrospective study, of 23 patients diagnosed with digoxin toxicity (those with a serum digoxin concentration greater than 2 nanograms/mL or diagnosed as 'digoxin-toxic') and also given intravenous calcium, there were no reported cases of life-threatening dysrhythmias within one hour of calcium administration. In addition, the mortality rate in the 23 patients receiving intravenous calcium (22%) was similar to that in 136 other patients with digoxin toxicity who did not receive intravenous calcium (20%).[3]

(b) Teriparatide

A placebo-controlled study in 15 healthy subjects given digoxin 500 micrograms daily, adjusted to maintain steady-state serum levels in the range 1 to 2 nanograms/mL, found that a single 20-microgram subcutaneous dose of teriparatide on day 15 or 16 did not alter the calcium-mediated effects of digoxin (systolic time interval), or heart rate. Serum calcium increased slightly, with a maximum increase of 0.05 mmol/L.[4]

Mechanism

The actions of the cardiac glycosides (even now not fully understood) are closely tied up with the movement of calcium ions into heart muscle cells. Increased concentrations of calcium outside these cells increase the inflow of calcium and this enhances the activity of the glycosides. This can lead to effective over-digitalisation and even potentially life-threatening arrhythmias. Conversely, a drop in calcium levels can attenuate the activity of the glycosides; and **disodium edetate**,[5-7] which lowers blood calcium levels, has been used successfully in the treatment of digitalis toxicity, although less toxic drugs are generally preferred.

Importance and management

The report of deaths associated with digitalis and calcium compounds (published in 1936) seems to be the only direct clinical evidence of a serious adverse interaction, although there is plenty of less direct evidence that an interaction is possible. *Intravenous* calcium should generally be avoided in patients receiving cardiac glycosides. If that is not possible, it has been suggested[8] that it should be given slowly or only in small amounts in order to avoid transient serum calcium levels higher than 7.5 mmol/L, but it seems likely that very large doses of calcium would be required to reach this level, even transiently. However, some authors have questioned the advice to avoid intravenous calcium in patients with digoxin toxicity.[3]

Vitamin D-mediated hypercalcaemia can occur with **vitamin D** or its analogues. This is one of the most common adverse effects of **alfacalcidol** and **paricalcitol**, and is reported to be a common adverse effect of **calcitriol** and **ergocalciferol**, usually occurring with excessive doses. Although calcium levels should be monitored in patients taking these drugs, it is particularly important to ensure that this is done in patients also taking cardiac glycosides.

The very slight increases in calcium levels in patients given teriparatide were considered insufficient to increase cardiac sensitivity to digoxin.[4] Nevertheless, calcium levels should routinely be monitored in patients given parathyroid hormones, and the manufacturer of teriparatide advises caution in patients taking digitalis, because of the possibility for transiently raised calcium levels.[9,10] Bear the possibility of an interaction in mind should digoxin adverse effects (such as bradycardia) occur and monitor digoxin levels if toxicity is suspected.

The UK manufacturer of calcitonin for systemic administration states that calcium levels might transiently be *decreased* following administration of **calcitonin**, and they advise that the dose of cardiac glycoside might need to be adjusted accordingly.[11] These changes are unlikely to be clinically important, but bear them in mind in case of an unexpected response to treatment. No clinically relevant interaction appears likely with intranasal calcitonin.

1. Bower JO, Mengle HAK. The additive effects of calcium and digitalis. A warning with a report of two deaths. *JAMA* (1936) 106, 1151.
2. Chopra D, Janson P, Sawin CT. Insensitivity to digoxin associated with hypocalcaemia. *N Engl J Med* (1977) 296, 917–18.
3. Levine M, Nikkanen H, Pallin DJ. The effects of intravenous calcium in patients with digoxin toxicity. *J Emerg Med* (2011) 40, 41–6.
4. Benson CT, Voelker JR. Teriparatide has no effect on the calcium-mediated pharmacodynamics of digoxin. *Clin Pharmacol Ther* (2003) 73, 87–94.
5. Jick S, Karsh R. The effect of calcium chelation on cardiac arrhythmias and conduction disturbances. *Am J Cardiol* (1959) 4, 287–93.
6. Szekely P, Wynne NA. Effects of calcium chelation on digitalis-induced cardiac arrhythmias. *Br Heart J* (1963) 25, 589–94.
7. Rosenbaum JL, Mason D, Seven MJ. The effect of disodium EDTA on digitalis intoxication. *Am J Med Sci* (1960) 240, 111–18.
8. Nola GT, Pope S, Harrison DC. Assessment of the synergistic relationship between serum calcium and digitalis. *Am Heart J* (1970) 79, 499–507.
9. Forsteo (Teriparatide). Eli Lilly and Company Ltd. UK Summary of product characteristics, July 2011.
10. Forteo (Teriparatide). Eli Lilly and Company. US Prescribing information, March 2012.
11. Miacalcic Solution for Injection and Infusion (Calcitonin) Novartis Pharmaceuticals UK Ltd. UK Summary of product characteristics. December 2011.

Digoxin and related drugs + Drugs that lower potassium concentrations

A number of drugs, including amphotericin B, carbenoxolone, and the corticosteroids, cause potassium loss, which could lead to the development of digitalis toxicity.

Clinical evidence, mechanism, importance and management

Among the well-recognised adverse effects of **amphotericin B** is hypokalaemia, which can be severe. Although there seem to be no reports of adverse interactions, it would be logical to expect that digitalis toxicity could develop in patients given both drugs if the potassium levels fall. Amiloride has been successfully used to counteract the potassium loss caused by **amphotericin B**.[1]

The adverse effects of **carbenoxolone** include an increase in blood pressure (both systolic and diastolic), fluid retention and reduced serum potassium levels. The incidence of these adverse effects is said in some reports to be as high as 50%; others quote lower figures. Hypertension and fluid retention occur early in **carbenoxolone** treatment, whereas hypokalaemia develops later and can occur in the absence of the other two adverse effects.[2-5] **Carbenoxolone** is therefore unsuitable for patients with congestive heart failure, or those taking digitalis glycosides, unless measures to avoid hypokalaemia are taken.

Systemic corticosteroids can increase the loss of potassium, particularly those that are naturally occurring (**cortisone, deoxycortone, hydrocortisone**) whereas the synthetic derivatives (**betamethasone, dexamethasone, methylprednisolone, prednisolone, prednisone, triamcinolone**) have much less mineralocorticoid activity. There is therefore the possibility of potassium depletion, particularly when corticosteroids are used long-term, which can increase the risk of digitalis toxicity. These corticosteroids also cause sodium and water retention, resulting in oedema and hypertension, which can lead to cardiac failure in some individuals.

It is therefore important to monitor the use of digoxin and any of these drugs well. Potassium levels should be routinely monitored in any patient taking **amphotericin B**, but it is particularly important in those also taking digoxin. With other drugs where potassium monitoring is not routine, it would seem prudent to watch for signs of digoxin adverse effects (e.g. bradycardia) and consider measuring potassium levels if these develop. No problems of this kind would be expected with corticosteroids used topically or by inhalation, because the amounts absorbed are likely to be relatively small.

For reports of digoxin toxicity or increased sensitivity to digoxin associated with other drugs that cause hypokalaemia, see 'Digoxin and related drugs + Diuretics; Potassium-depleting', p.1093, and 'Digoxin and related drugs + Beta-agonist bronchodilators', p.1085.

1. Smith SR, Galloway MJ, Reilly JT, Davies JM. Amiloride prevents amphotericin B related hypokalaemia in neutropenic patients. *J Clin Pathol* (1988) 41, 494–7.
2. Geismar P, Mosbech J, Myren J. A double-blind study of the effect of carbenoxolone sodium in the treatment of gastric ulcer. *Scand J Gastroenterol* (1973) 8, 251–6.
3. Turpie AGG, Thomson TJ. Carbenoxolone sodium in the treatment of gastric ulcer with special reference to side-effects. *Gut* (1965) 6, 591–4.
4. Langman MJS, Knapp DR, Wakley EJ. Treatment of chronic gastric ulcer with carbenoxolone and gefarnate: a comparative trial. *BMJ* (1973) 3, 84–6.
5. Davies GJ, Rhodes J, Calcraft BJ. Complications of carbenoxolone therapy. *BMJ* (1974) 3, 400–402.

Digoxin + Echinacea

Echinacea does not appear to affect the pharmacokinetics of digoxin.

Clinical evidence, mechanism, importance and management

In a study, 18 healthy subjects were given an extract containing *Echinacea purpurea* 195 mg and *Echinacea angustifolia* 72 mg three times daily for 14 days, with a single 250-microgram dose of digoxin before and after the course of echinacea. The pharmacokinetics of digoxin were not affected by echinacea.[1] Echinacea does not appear to interact with digoxin, and no digoxin dose adjustments would seem necessary on concurrent use.

1. Gurley BJ, Swain A, Williams DK, Barone G, Battu SK. Gauging the clinical significance of P-glycoprotein mediated herb-drug interactions: comparative effects of St John's wort, Echinacea, clarithromycin and rifampin on digoxin pharmacokinetics. *Mol Nutr Food Res* (2008) 52, 755–63.

Digoxin and related drugs + Edrophonium

Excessive bradycardia and AV-block might occur if patients taking digitalis glycosides are given edrophonium.

Clinical evidence, mechanism, importance and management

The rapid intravenous injection of edrophonium 10 mg has been used in the differentiation of cardiac arrhythmias, but in one study, 4 of 10 digitalised patients given edrophonium developed atrial tachycardia with AV block. The effect was transient, with recovery of baseline ECGs occurring 15 to 20 minutes after administration.[1] Nevertheless, the authors recommended that edrophonium should not be given to patients with atrial flutter or tachycardia who are taking **digitalis glycosides**. This recommendation is reinforced by the case of an elderly woman[2] who developed bradycardia, AV block and asystole following concurrent use. She recovered after being given atropine 1 mg.

1. Reddy RCV, Gould L, Gomprecht RF. Use of edrophonium (Tensilon) in the evaluation of cardiac arrhythmias. *Am Heart J* (1971) 82, 742–9.
2. Gould L, Zahir M, Gomprecht RF. Cardiac arrest during edrophonium administration. *Am Heart J* (1971) 81, 437–8.

Digoxin + Endothelin receptor antagonists

Ambrisentan and bosentan do not appear to affect the pharmacokinetics of digoxin.

Clinical evidence, mechanism, importance and management

(a) Ambrisentan

A study in 15 healthy subjects found that ambrisentan 10 mg daily for 9 days, with a single 500-microgram dose of digoxin on day 5, increased the maximum plasma concentration of digoxin by 29%. There was a 9% increase in the AUC of digoxin, which was within the limits for equivalence.[1] These changes are not expected to be clinically relevant and therefore no digoxin dose adjustments are needed if ambrisentan is also given.

(b) Bosentan

In a study in 18 healthy subjects, bosentan 500 mg twice daily for a week did not affect the steady-state maximum or minimum concentrations of digoxin 375 micrograms daily. There was a decrease of about 12% in the AUC of digoxin, which might have been due to induction of P-glycoprotein by bosentan. There were no changes in ECG recordings and vital signs. The results suggest that bosentan does not interact with digoxin to a clinically relevant extent, and that concurrent use need not be avoided. However, the authors of the report note that further studies over the longer term, and in patients with renal impairment, are needed to confirm this.[2]

1. Richards DB, Spence R, Mandagere A, Henderson LS, Magee MH. Effect of multiple doses of ambrisentan on the pharmacokinetics of a single dose of digoxin in healthy volunteers. *J Clin Pharmacol* (2011) 51, 102–6.
2. Weber C, Banken L, Birnboeck H, Nave S, Schulz R. The effect of bosentan on the pharmacokinetics of digoxin in healthy male subjects. *Br J Clin Pharmacol* (1999) 47, 701–6.

Digoxin and related drugs + Enoximone

Studies in patients taking digoxin or digitoxin on a long-term basis found that *oral* enoximone 100 mg three times daily for a week had no effect on the plasma levels of either of these digitalis glycosides.[1,2] Cardiac function was improved. Therefore no dose adjustments of these cardiac glycosides are expected to be necessary if enoximone is also given.

1. Glauner T, Hertrich F, Winkelmann B, Dieterich HA, Trenk D, Jähnchen E. Lack of effect of enoximone on steady-state plasma concentrations of digoxin and digitoxin. *Eur Heart J* (1988) 9 (Suppl 1), 151.
2. Trenk D, Hertrich F, Winkelmann B, Glauner T, Dieterich HA, Jähnchen E. Lack of effect of enoximone on the pharmacokinetics of digoxin in patients with congestive heart failure. *J Clin Pharmacol* (1990) 30, 235–40.

Digoxin + Etanercept

Etanercept does not appear to affect the pharmacokinetics of digoxin. Etanercept exposure might be decreased by digoxin.

Clinical evidence, mechanism, importance and management

In a study in 12 healthy subjects given an oral loading dose of digoxin (500 micrograms twice daily on day one, followed by 250 micrograms daily), subcutaneous etanercept 25 mg twice weekly reduced the AUC of digoxin by 8%. Although this difference was just statistically significant, it was still within the accepted limits of bioequivalence. The AUC of etanercept was 13% lower during concurrent use, although there was wide intersubject variability.[1] Nevertheless, none of these differences are clinically relevant. No digoxin dose adjustments would appear to be necessary on the concurrent use of etanercept.

1. Zhou H, Parks V, Patat A, Le Coz F, Simcoe D, Korth-Bradley J. Absence of a clinically relevant interaction between etanercept and digoxin. *J Clin Pharmacol* (2004) 44, 1244–51.

Digoxin + Ezetimibe

Ezetimibe does not affect the pharmacokinetics of digoxin.

Clinical evidence, mechanism, importance and management

In a study in 12 healthy subjects, ezetimibe 10 mg daily for 8 days did not alter the pharmacokinetics of a single 500-microgram dose of digoxin given on day 8. In addition, ezetimibe did not alter the ECG effects of digoxin.[1] No digoxin dose adjustment would be expected to be necessary if ezetimibe is also given.

1. Kosoglou T, Statkevich P, Bauer KS, Cutler DL, Maxwell SE, Yang B, Soni PP, Batra VK. Ezetimibe does not affect the pharmacokinetics and pharmacodynamics of digoxin. *AAPS PharmSci* (2001) 3, S1. Available at: http://aapsj.org/abstracts/AM_2001/290.htm (accessed 20/10/15).

Digoxin + Famciclovir

Famciclovir does not alter the pharmacokinetics of digoxin.

Clinical evidence, mechanism, importance and management

In a single-dose study in 12 healthy subjects, famciclovir 500 mg had no effect on the AUC of digoxin.[1] Similarly, in a further placebo-controlled multiple-dose study, the steady-state pharmacokinetics of **digoxin** 375 micrograms daily and famciclovir 500 mg three times daily were unaffected by concurrent use.[2] Therefore, no dose adjustments would seem to be necessary if digoxin is given with famciclovir.

1. Pue MA, Saporito M, Laroche J, Lua S, Bygate E, Daniels S, Broom C. An investigation of the potential interaction between digoxin and oral famciclovir in healthy male volunteers. *Br J Clin Pharmacol* (1993) 36, 177P.
2. Siederer S, Scott S, Fowles S, Haveresch L, Hust R. Lack of interaction between steady-state digoxin and famciclovir. *Intersci Conf Antimicrob Agents Chemother* (1996) 36, A33.

Digoxin + Fenoldopam

Oral fenoldopam appears to reduce plasma digoxin levels.

Clinical evidence, mechanism, importance and management

Ten patients with congestive heart failure taking digoxin long-term (doses not stated) were given *oral* fenoldopam 100 mg three times daily for 9 days. The mean AUC and steady-state plasma levels of digoxin were reduced by about 20%, but the difference was not statistically significant.[1] The magnitude of the reduction in digoxin exposure reported in the study is unlikely to be clinically relevant in most patients.

1. Strocchi E, Tartagni F, Malini PL, Valtancoli G, Ambrosioni E, Pasinelli F, Riva E, Fuccella LM. Interaction study of fenoldopam-digoxin in congestive heart failure. *Eur J Clin Pharmacol* (1989) 37, 395–7.

Digoxin + Flecainide

Digoxin levels are unchanged or only minimally increased by the use of flecainide.

Clinical evidence

The plasma digoxin levels of 10 patients with congestive heart failure were unchanged when they took flecainide 100 to 200 mg twice daily for 7 days. A similar lack of interaction was also seen in 4 patients who took both drugs over a 4-week period.[1] However, in a study in 15 healthy subjects given digoxin 250 micrograms daily, flecainide 200 mg twice daily for 5 days increased the steady-state trough and peak plasma levels of digoxin by 24% and 13%, respectively. Five subjects had a slight increase in PR interval with digoxin alone, whereas 12 subjects had transient increases during the concurrent use of flecainide.[2] Based on the results of a single-dose study, the steady-state digoxin levels were predicted to rise by about 15% during the use of flecainide 200 mg twice daily.[3]

Mechanism

Uncertain. It is suggested that any changes could be due to alterations in the volume of distribution.[3]

Importance and management

Documentation regarding an interaction between flecainide and digoxin is limited, but what is known suggests that either no interaction occurs, or any changes are small and unlikely to be clinically relevant in most patients. However, the UK manufacturers of flecainide recommend that digoxin plasma levels should be measured before or after the administration of flecainide,[4] while the US manufacturers suggest close monitoring of cardiac function on concurrent use.[5] The authors of one of the reports[2] suggest that patients with high drug levels, atrioventricular nodal dysfunction, or both, should be monitored during concurrent treatment.

1. McQuinn RL, Kvam DC, Parrish SL, Fox TL, Miller AM, Franciosa JA. Digoxin levels in patients with congestive heart failure are not altered by flecainide. *Clin Pharmacol Ther* (1988) 43, 150.
2. Weeks CE, Conard GJ, Kvam DC, Fox JM, Chang SF, Paone RP, Lewis GP. The effect of flecainide acetate, a new antiarrhythmic, on plasma digoxin levels. *J Clin Pharmacol* (1986) 26, 27–31.
3. Tjandramaga TB, Verbesselt R, Van Hecken A, Mullie A, De Schepper PJ. Oral digoxin pharmacokinetics during multiple-dose flecainide treatment. *Arch Int Pharmacodyn Ther* (1982) 260, 302–3.
4. Tambocor 50 mg Tablets (Flecainide acetate). Meda Pharmaceuticals. UK Summary of product characteristics, July 2010.
5. Tambocor (Flecainide acetate). Graceway Pharmaceuticals LLC. US Prescribing information, April 2007.

Digoxin + Fondaparinux

No pharmacokinetic interaction appears to occur between digoxin and fondaparinux.

Clinical evidence, mechanism, importance and management

In a phase I randomised study in 24 healthy subjects given digoxin 250 micrograms daily, the steady-state pharmacokinetics of digoxin were unaffected by subcutaneous fondaparinux 10 mg daily for 7 days. The pharmacokinetics of fondaparinux were not affected by digoxin.[1] No particular precautions therefore seem necessary on concurrent use.

1. Mant T, Fournié P, Ollier C, Donat F, Necciari J. Absence of interaction of fondaparinux sodium with digoxin in healthy volunteers. *Clin Pharmacokinet* (2002), 41 (Suppl 2), 39–45.

Digoxin + Ginkgo (*Ginkgo biloba*)

Ginkgo does not appear to affect the pharmacokinetics of digoxin.

Clinical evidence

A study in 8 healthy subjects found that ginkgo biloba leaf extract 80 mg three times daily had no effect on the pharmacokinetics of a single 500-microgram dose of digoxin.[1]

Mechanism

Digoxin is a P-glycoprotein substrate and *in vitro* studies[2] suggest that ginkgo might inhibit the activity of this drug transporter protein, which could lead to increased digoxin levels. However, this effect was not seen clinically.

Importance and management

The clinical study suggests that ginkgo is unlikely to alter digoxin levels in clinical use. Therefore no dose adjustment would be expected to be necessary if patients taking digoxin also wish to take ginkgo.

1. Mauro VF, Mauro LS, Kleshinski JF, Khuder SA, Wang Y, Erhardt PW. Impact of Ginkgo biloba on the pharmacokinetics of digoxin. *Am J Ther* (2003) 10, 247–51.
2. Hellum BH, Nilsen OG. *In vitro* inhibition of CYP3A4 metabolism and P-glycoprotein-mediated transport by trade herbal products. *Basic Clin Pharmacol Toxicol* (2008) 102, 466–75.

Digoxin + Ginseng

***Panax ginseng* (Asian ginseng), *Panax quinquefolius* (American ginseng) and *Eleutherococcus senticosus* (Siberian ginseng) might interfere with the results of digoxin assays.**

Clinical evidence

A 74-year-old man who had been taking digoxin for many years (serum levels normally in the range 0.9 to 2.2 nanograms/mL) was found, during a routine check, to have a digoxin level of 5.2 nanograms/mL, but without evidence of toxicity, bradycardia or any other ECG changes.[1] His levels remained high even when digoxin was stopped. It turned out he had also been taking ***Eleutherococcus senticosus* (Siberian ginseng)** capsules. When ginseng was stopped, the digoxin levels returned to his usual range, and digoxin was resumed. Later rechallenge with ginseng caused a rise in his serum digoxin levels. No digoxin or digitoxin contamination was found in the ginseng capsules, and the authors of the report also rejected the idea that the eleutherosides (chemically related to cardiac glycosides) in ginseng might have been converted *in vivo* into digoxin, or that the renal elimination of digoxin might have been impaired, as the patient showed no signs of toxicity.

Mechanism

Panax ginseng (Asian ginseng), *Panax quinquefolius* (American ginseng) and *Eleutherococcus senticosus* (Siberian ginseng) have been found to interfere with some digoxin assays, including fluorescence polarisation immunoassay (FPIA, Abbott Laboratories)[2-4] and microparticle enzyme immunoassay (MEIA, Abbott Laboratories).[2,3] The more specific monoclonal antibody-based digoxin immunoassay, Tina-quant (Roche), was unaffected by all the ginsengs,[3,4] the Beckman (Synchron LX system) monoclonal assay was unaffected by *Panax ginseng* (Asian ginseng),[4] and the ECLIA-digoxin (Bayer) and turbidimetric assay (TIA; Bayer) were unaffected by *Panax ginseng* (Asian ginseng) and *Panax quinquefolius* (American ginseng).[5] It therefore seems possible that the ginsengs affected the accuracy of the digoxin assays so that they gave false results.

Importance and management

The interference in digoxin measurements in the presence of ginseng described in the assays was not as high as that reported in the elderly patient and there is some doubt as to whether the herbal medicine taken by the patient was actually *Eleutherococcus senticosus* (Siberian ginseng).[3,6] So, whether this is clinically important, and measurement of serum digoxin levels is actually affected, is uncertain. Nevertheless it would be sensible to ask about ginseng use when interpreting unexpected digoxin levels and consider using a more specific monoclonal immunoassay.

1. McRae S. Elevated serum digoxin levels in a patient taking digoxin and Siberian ginseng. *Can Med Assoc J* (1996) 155, 293–5.
2. Dasgupta A, Wu S, Actor J, Olsen M, Wells A, Datta P. Effect of Asian and Siberian ginseng on serum digoxin measurement by five digoxin immunoassays. Significant variation in digoxin-like immunoreactivity among commercial ginsengs. *Am J Clin Pathol* (2003) 119, 298–303.
3. Dasgupta A, Reyes MA. Effect of Brazilian, Indian, Siberian, Asian, and North American ginseng on serum digoxin measurement by immunoassays and binding of digoxin-like immunoreactive components of ginseng with Fab fragment of antidigoxin antibody (Digibind). *Am J Clin Pathol* (2005) 124, 229–36.
4. Chow L, Johnson M, Wells A, Dasgupta A. Effect of the traditional Chinese medicines Chan Su, Lu-Shen-Wan, Dan Shen, and Asian ginseng on serum digoxin measurement by Tina-quant (Roche) and Synchron LX System (Beckman) digoxin immunoassays. *J Clin Lab Anal* (2003) 17, 22–7.
5. Dasgupta A, Kang E, Olsen M, Actor JK, Datta P. Interference of Asian, American, and Indian (ashwagandha) ginsengs in serum digoxin measurements by a fluorescent polarization immunoassay can be minimised by using a new enzyme-linked chemiluminescent immunosorbent or turbidimetric assay. *Arch Pathol Lab Med* (2007) 131, 619–21.
6. Awang DVC. Siberian ginseng toxicity may be case of mistaken identity. *CMAJ* (1996) 155, 1237.

Digoxin + Glucagon-like peptide-1 receptor agonists

Albiglutide and exenatide delay digoxin absorption, but do not affect its exposure. Dulaglutide, liraglutide, and lixisenatide appear to have similar effects.

Clinical evidence

(a) Albiglutide

In a study in 24 healthy subjects, albiglutide 50 mg weekly had no effect on the AUC or maximum concentration of a single 500-microgram dose of digoxin given 3 days after the last dose of albiglutide, but did increase the median time to maximum concentration by 30 minutes.[1]

(b) Dulaglutide

The UK and US manufacturers briefly report that, in a study, dulaglutide (2 doses, dose not stated) had no effect on the AUC and time to maximum concentration of digoxin at steady state (dose not stated), but did decrease the maximum concentration by up to 22%.[2,3]

(c) Exenatide

In a pharmacokinetic study, 21 healthy subjects were given digoxin (a loading dose of 500 micrograms twice daily on day one, then 250 micrograms daily for 11 days, given as tablets), with subcutaneous exenatide 10 micrograms twice daily on days 8 to 12. The median time to reach the digoxin maximum plasma concentration was increased from 1.5 hours to 4 hours, and there was a decrease of 17% in digoxin maximum concentrations. There was no change in the AUC and minimum concentrations of digoxin, and the renal clearance of digoxin was not altered.[4]

(d) Liraglutide

A preliminary report of a randomised, crossover study in 27 healthy subjects, states that steady-state liraglutide 1.8 mg daily decreased the AUC of a single 1-mg dose of digoxin, given 7 hours after the liraglutide, by 16% and decreased its maximum concentration by 31%, with a delay in time to maximum concentration of 1.12 hours.[5]

(e) Lixisenatide

The UK manufacturer briefly reports that, in a study, concurrent use of lixisenatide 20 micrograms and digoxin 250 micrograms at steady state did not alter the AUC of digoxin. The time to maximum digoxin concentration was delayed by 1.5 hours and the maximum concentration was decreased by 26%.[6]

Mechanism

The glucagon-like peptide-1 receptor agonists are all said to slow gastric emptying, although this has been seen to varying extents when given with paracetamol (acetaminophen), which can be used as a marker of gastric emptying (see 'Paracetamol (Acetaminophen) + Antidiabetics', p.202 for details). This might therefore offer some explanation for the changes in digoxin pharmacokinetics seen in the studies, although note that overall exposure was largely unaffected.

Importance and management

Evidence for an interaction between the glucagon-like peptide-1 receptor agonists and digoxin is limited, but a pharmacokinetic interaction cannot be ruled out. However concurrent use would seem unlikely to have any clinically relevant consequences. As such, no digoxin dose adjustment would seem necessary on concurrent use with any of the glucagon-like peptide-1 receptor agonists.

1. Bush M, Scott R, Watanalumlerd P, Zhi H, Lewis E. Effects of multiple doses of albiglutide on the pharmacokinetics, pharmacodynamics, and safety of digoxin, warfarin, or a low-dose oral contraceptive. *Postgrad Med* (2012) 124, 55–72.
2. Trulicity (Dulaglutide). Eli Lilly and Company Ltd. UK Summary of product characteristics, November 2014.
3. Trulicity (Dulaglutide). Eli Lilly and Company. US Prescribing information, March 2015.
4. Kothare AP, Soon DKW, Linnebjerg H, Park S, Chan C, Yeo A, Lim M, Mace KF, Wise SD. Effect of Exenatide on the steady-state pharmacokinetics of digoxin. *J Clin Pharmacol* (2005) 45, 1032–7.
5. Malm-Erjefalt M, Ekblom M, Brondsted L, Vouis J, Lennernas H, Zdravkovic M. A randomized, double-blind, cross-over trial investigating the effect of liraglutide on the absorption pharmacokinetics of concomitantly administered oral drugs in healthy subjects. *Diabetes* (2008) 57 (Suppl 1), A130.
6. Lyxumia (Lixisenatide). Sanofi. UK Summary of product characteristics, October 2014.

Digoxin + Grapefruit juice

Digoxin levels are generally unaltered or only minimally increased by grapefruit juice, but in one study two subjects had asymptomatic heart block associated with 50% increases in digoxin levels .

Clinical evidence

A crossover study in 12 healthy subjects found that when they were given either grapefruit juice 220 mL or water, 30 minutes before, and 3.5, 7.5, and 11.5 hours after, a single 500-microgram dose of digoxin (taken with 50 mL of grapefruit juice or water respectively), the AUC_{0-4} and AUC_{0-24} of digoxin were increased by about 10%. The maximum plasma levels and renal clearance of digoxin were not affected. However, in 2 subjects taking grapefruit juice, the ECGs, recorded 90 minutes after digoxin was taken, revealed asymptomatic first-degree atrioventricular block. Digoxin levels in these subjects had increased by 50%, to 2.4 nanograms/mL and 2.8 nanograms/mL, respectively.[1] Another study found that grapefruit juice decreased the rate, but not the extent, of digoxin absorption and had no effect on its AUC or renal clearance, but there was wide inter-individual variability in these findings.[2]

Mechanism

The increases in digoxin levels might be due to increased intestinal absorption of digoxin, possibly as a result of grapefruit juice inhibiting P-glycoprotein-mediated digoxin transport, although this mechanism has been questioned.[1] *In vitro*, pomelo (*Citrus grandis*) juice and grapefruit juice inhibited the transport of digoxin by P-glycoprotein.[3]

Importance and management

Although grapefruit juice appears to have little effect on the bioavailability of digoxin, it is possible that in some individuals the interaction could be of clinical importance.[2] Therefore, if a patient taking digoxin unexpectedly develops bradycardia or other adverse effects it would seem be prudent to ask about grapefruit juice intake, and consider this as a possible cause. More study is needed to identify which patients are at risk of a clinically relevant interaction.

1. Becquemont L, Verstuyft C, Kerb R, Brinkmann U, Lebot M, Jaillon P, Funck-Brentano C. Effect of grapefruit juice on digoxin pharmacokinetics in humans. *Clin Pharmacol Ther* (2001) 70, 311–6.
2. Parker RB, Yates CR, Soberman JE, Laizure SC. Effects of grapefruit juice on intestinal P-glycoprotein: evaluation using digoxin in humans. *Pharmacotherapy* (2003) 23, 979–87.
3. Xu J, Go ML, Lim L-Y. Modulation of digoxin transport across Caco-2 cell monolayers by citrus fruit juices: lime, lemon, grapefruit and pummelo. *Pharm Res* (2003) 20, 169–76.

Digoxin and other P-glycoprotein substrates + HCV-protease inhibitors

In a single-dose study, telaprevir increased the exposure to digoxin. Boceprevir, paritaprevir boosted with ritonavir given *without* dasabuvir, and simeprevir appear to have similar effects.

Clinical evidence

(a) Boceprevir

The UK and US manufacturers briefly note that, in a study in healthy subjects given boceprevir 800 mg three times daily for 10 days with a single 250-microgram dose of digoxin, the AUC and maximum concentration of digoxin were increased by 19% and 18%, respectively.[1,2]

(b) Paritaprevir

The UK and US manufacturers briefly report that, in a study in healthy subjects given paritaprevir 150 mg daily (in a fixed-dose combination with ritonavir and ombitasvir, and given with dasabuvir) and a single 500-microgram dose of digoxin, the pharmacokinetics of both drugs were unaffected.[3,4] However, the UK manufacturer also notes that when paritaprevir 150 mg daily (in a fixed-dose combination with ritonavir and ombitasvir, and given *without* dasabuvir) was given with a single 500-microgram dose of digoxin, the AUC and maximum concentration of digoxin were increased by 36% and 58%, respectively. The pharmacokinetics of paritaprevir were unaffected.[4]

(c) Simeprevir

The UK and US manufacturers briefly note that, in a study in 16 healthy subjects given simeprevir 150 mg daily for 7 days with a single 250-microgram dose of digoxin, the AUC and maximum concentration of digoxin were increased by 39% and 31%, respectively.[5,6]

(d) Telaprevir

In a study in 20 healthy subjects, telaprevir 750 mg three times daily for 11 days increased the AUC and maximum plasma concentration of a single 500-microgram dose of digoxin by 85% and 50%, respectively.[7]

Mechanism

Digoxin is a P-glycoprotein substrate and so the increase in digoxin exposure seen with boceprevir, paritaprevir boosted with ritonavir, simeprevir, and telaprevir indicates that they are inhibitors of P-glycoprotein. However, also note that ritonavir itself is a P-glycoprotein inhibitor and so the exact role of paritaprevir in the effect on digoxin is unclear.

Importance and management

A pharmacokinetic interaction between digoxin and the HCV-protease inhibitors would appear to be established and in general, would be expected to be of clinical importance. It would therefore seem prudent to monitor concurrent use of any of these HCV-protease inhibitors for digoxin adverse effects (such as bradycardia). If an interaction is suspected, digoxin concentrations should be checked, and the digoxin dose adjusted if necessary. The US manufacturer of boceprevir recommends digoxin concentrations are measured prior to and after starting boceprevir and the dose of digoxin adjusted accordingly,[1] whereas the UK manufacturer advises that no dose adjustment is required.[2] The UK and US manufacturers of telaprevir[8,9] recommend starting at the lowest possible dose of digoxin. The US manufacturer of simeprevir advises that routine monitoring of digoxin concentrations is acceptable.[6] Note that advice for paritaprevir varies, depending on whether it is given with or without dasabuvir. When given in a fixed-dose combination including ritonavir and ombitasvir, and also given with dasabuvir, no dose adjustments are necessary,[3,4] however, when given in the same fixed-dose combination, but given *without* dasabuvir, the UK manufacturer advises that the digoxin dose should be decreased by 30 to 50%, with appropriate monitoring of digoxin concentrations.[4]

Note that digoxin can be used as a probe substrate to assess the activity of drugs on P-glycoprotein. These studies therefore suggests that boceprevir, paritaprevir boosted with ritonavir, simeprevir, and telaprevir are inhibitors of P-glycoprotein, and would be predicted to increase the exposure to drugs that are substrates for this transporter. For a list of P-glycoprotein substrates see 'Table 1.12', p.14.

Dabigatran is a P-glycoprotein substrate and as such, its exposure is predicted to be increased by the UK manufacturers of boceprevir, paritaprevir boosted with ritonavir (in a fixed-dose combination including ombitasvir), and telaprevir. Caution is recommended with paritaprevir boosted with ritonavir and telaprevir,[4,8] and monitoring is recommended with boceprevir and telaprevir[2,8] (for adverse effects such as bleeding and anaemia).

1. Victrelis (Boceprevir). Merck & Co., Inc. US Prescribing information, July 2014.
2. Victrelis (Boceprevir). Merck Sharp & Dohme Ltd. UK Summary of product characteristics, August 2014.
3. Viekira Pak (Ombitasvir, paritaprevir, ritonavir co-packaged with dasabuvir sodium monohydrate). AbbVie Inc. US Prescribing information, December 2014.
4. Viekirax (Ombitasvir, paritaprevir, ritonavir). AbbVie Ltd. UK Summary of product characteristics, January 2015.
5. Olysio (Simeprevir sodium). Janssen-Cilag Ltd. UK Summary of product characteristics, May 2014.
6. Olysio (Simeprevir sodium). Janssen Products, LP. US Prescribing information, November 2014.
7. Garg V, Chandorkar G, Farmer HF, Smith F, Alves K, van Heeswijk RPG. Effect of telaprevir on the pharmacokinetics of midazolam and digoxin. *J Clin Pharmacol* (2012) 52, 1566–73.
8. Incivo (Telaprevir). Janssen-Cilag Ltd. UK Summary of product characteristics, July 2014.
9. Incivek (Telaprevir). Vertex Pharmaceuticals, Inc. US Prescribing information, October 2013.

Digoxin + HIV-protease inhibitors

A woman taking digoxin developed elevated digoxin concentrations and signs of toxicity after she was given ritonavir. Pharmacokinetic studies have shown that ritonavir and saquinavir boosted with ritonavir increase digoxin exposure.

Clinical evidence

(a) Ritonavir

A 61-year-old HIV-positive woman taking lamivudine, indinavir, stavudine, pentamidine; with warfarin and digoxin 250 micrograms daily for atrial fibrillation, presented with increasing nausea and vomiting 3 days after starting to take ritonavir 200 mg twice daily. Digoxin concentrations about 5 hours and 27 hours after her last dose were 5.6 nanograms/mL and 2.1 nanograms/mL, respectively.[1]

A study in 12 healthy subjects found that ritonavir 300 mg twice daily for 11 days increased the AUC and volume of distribution of a single 500-microgram intravenous dose of digoxin by 86% and 77%, respectively. Non-renal and renal digoxin clearance were decreased by 48% and 35%, respectively, and its half-life increased by 156%.[2] Another study found that ritonavir 200 mg twice daily for 15 days increased the AUC of a single 400-microgram oral dose of digoxin by 22%, with 9 of 12 subjects having an increase. Non-renal clearance (but not renal clearance) was reduced.[3]

(b) Saquinavir

In a crossover study in 16 healthy subjects, saquinavir boosted with ritonavir 1000/100 mg twice daily for 16 days increased the AUC and maximum concentrations of a single 500-microgram dose of digoxin given on day 14 by 49% and 27%, respectively.[4]

Mechanism

Digoxin is a substrate of the efflux pump P-glycoprotein and raised digoxin concentrations are possibly due to inhibition of the P-glycoprotein-mediated renal transport of digoxin by ritonavir and saquinavir.[1-4]

Importance and management

A pharmacokinetic interaction between ritonavir and digoxin would appear to be established, although its extent is uncertain. The study with intravenous digoxin found a marked effect, whereas the study with oral digoxin found a much smaller effect. Nevertheless, given the case report and the study with saquinavir boosted with ritonavir, it would seem prudent to closely monitor digoxin concentrations when ritonavir and/or saquinavir is started or stopped, being alert for the need to adjust the digoxin dose. There do not appear to be any reports or studies of the interaction of digoxin with other HIV-protease inhibitors; however, most HIV-protease inhibitors are inhibitors of P-glycoprotein, so it would seem likely that they could all interact, to a greater or lesser extent.

1. Phillips EJ, Rachlis AR, Ito S. Digoxin toxicity and ritonavir: a drug interaction mediated through p-glycoprotein? *AIDS* (2003) 17, 1577–8.
2. Ding R, Tayrouz Y, Riedel K-D, Burhenne J, Weiss J, Mikus G, Haefeli WE. Substantial pharmacokinetic interaction between digoxin and ritonavir in healthy volunteers. *Clin Pharmacol Ther* (2004) 76, 73–84.
3. Penzak SR, Shen JM, Alfaro RM, Remaley AT, Natarajan V, Falloon J. Ritonavir decreases the nonrenal clearance of digoxin in healthy volunteers with known MDR1 genotypes. *Ther Drug Monit* (2004) 26, 322–30.
4. Schmitt C, Kaeser B, Riek M, Bech N, Kreuzer C. Effect of saquinavir/ritonavir on P-glycoprotein activity in healthy volunteers using digoxin as a probe. *Int J Clin Pharmacol Ther* (2010) 48, 192–9.

Digoxin and related drugs + H_2-receptor antagonists

Most studies have found that cimetidine does not change the pharmacokinetics of digoxin, although one study reported a small reduction and one study reported a small increase in digoxin levels. Ranitidine does not appear to interact with metildigoxin.

Clinical evidence, mechanism, importance and management

In a study in 11 patients with congestive heart failure, **cimetidine** 300 mg every 6 or 12 hours reduced the steady-state serum digoxin levels by 25% (from 2 nanograms/mL to 1.5 nanograms/mL), but none of the patients had any ECG changes or signs that their condition had worsened.[1] However, in four other patients with stable congestive heart failure, there was no change in the pharmacokinetics of digoxin 125 to 250 micrograms daily when they were given **cimetidine** 300 mg every 6 hours.[2] Similarly, three single-dose studies in a total of 19 healthy subjects,[3,4] and 6 patients with duodenal ulcers[5] found that **cimetidine** 600 mg to 1.2 g daily had no effect on the absorption[3] or the pharmacokinetics[4,5] of digoxin. Another series of studies found a 23% increase in the AUC of single-dose digoxin and an increase in steady-state digoxin levels (33% and 15%, with digoxin 250 micrograms and 500 micrograms, respectively) in healthy subjects, but no change in the steady-state digoxin levels of 11 patients given **cimetidine** 400 mg four times daily.[6] Six patients with chronic congestive heart failure given **metildigoxin** had no changes in their serum digoxin levels when they were given **ranitidine** 150 mg twice daily for a week.[7]

No interaction of clinical importance with either cimetidine or ranitidine has been established and no particular precautions would therefore seem to be necessary if they are given with digoxin.

1. Fraley DS, Britton HL, Schwinghammer TL, Kalla R. Effect of cimetidine on steady-state serum digoxin concentrations. *Clin Pharm* (1983) 2, 163–5.
2. Mouser B, Nykamp D, Murphy JE, Krissman PH. Effect of cimetidine on oral digoxin absorption. *DICP Ann Pharmacother* (1990) 24, 286–8.
3. Jordaens L, Hoegaerts J, Belpaire F. Non-interaction of cimetidine with digoxin absorption. *Acta Clin Belg* (1981) 36, 109–10.
4. Ochs HR, Gugler R, Guthoff T, Greenblatt DJ. Effect of cimetidine on digoxin kinetics and creatinine clearance. *Am Heart J* (1984) 107, 170–2.
5. Garty M, Perry G, Shmueli H, Ilfeld D, Boner G, Pitlik S, Rosenfeld J. Effect of cimetidine on digoxin disposition in peptic ulcer patients. *Eur J Clin Pharmacol* (1986) 30, 489–91.
6. Crome P, Curl B, Holt D, Volans GN, Bennett PN, Cole DS. Digoxin and cimetidine: investigation of the potential for a drug interaction. *Hum Toxicol* (1985) 4, 391–9.
7. Enomoto N, Kurasawa T, Ichikawa M, Shimuzu T, Matsuyama T, Sakai K, Shimamura K, Oda M. Lack of interaction of β-methyldigoxin with ranitidine in patients with chronic congestive heart failure. *Eur J Clin Pharmacol* (1992) 43, 205–6.

Digoxin and related drugs + HRT

Post hoc analysis of one study found an increased rate of cardiovascular adverse events in women taking HRT who were also taking digitalis.

Clinical evidence, mechanism, importance and management

Retrospective analysis of data from a large, randomised, placebo-controlled study of HRT (conjugated estrogens 0.625 mg with medroxyprogesterone 2.5 mg, given daily) in women with coronary heart disease was conducted to see if there were any subgroups of patients who responded differently. Use of digitalis was associated with a fivefold excess rate of cardiovascular events in the first year, when women receiving HRT were compared with the control group. A lower 1.5-fold excess rate was seen over the whole duration of the study (average 4.1 years). Possible mechanisms could be a drug-drug interaction or a drug-disease effect (HRT with congestive heart failure).[1]

However, it is impossible to say whether this represents a true effect, because the number of positive sub-group analyses in this study was the same as the number predicted by chance alone. Confirmatory evidence is required.[1]

See also 'Digoxin and related drugs + Medroxyprogesterone or Megestrol', p.1102 for a report suggesting that high-dose medroxyprogesterone does not have a clinically relevant effect on digitoxin levels.

1. Furberg CD, Vittinghoff E, Davidson M, Herrington DM, Simon JA, Wenger NK, Hulley S. Subgroup interactions in the Heart and Estrogen/Progestin replacement study. Lessons learned. *Circulation* (2002) 105, 917–22.

Digoxin + Kaolin-pectin

Digoxin levels might be reduced if it is given simultaneously with kaolin-pectin.

Clinical evidence

In a study, giving kaolin-pectin suspension simultaneously with digoxin reduced the peak plasma digoxin levels of 7 patients by 36%, while the $AUC_{0\text{-}24}$ was reduced by 15%.[1] Similarly, two single-dose studies also found 42% and 62% reductions in the bioavailability of digoxin caused by kaolin-pectin.[2,3] In one of these studies, when two doses of kaolin-pectin were taken, the first 2 hours before digoxin and the other 2 hours after digoxin, no pharmacokinetic changes were seen.[1]

Another study using kaolin-pectin found an interaction with digoxin tablets but not with digoxin capsules.[4]

Mechanism

Not understood. The digoxin might become adsorbed onto the kaolin so that less is available for absorption. Another possibility is that the kaolin reduces the motility of the gut, which normally increases mixing and brings the digoxin into contact with the absorbing surface.

Importance and management

Evidence from these studies shows a variable degree of interaction between digoxin and kaolin-pectin; however, steady-state studies reflect the every-day situation much more closely than single-dose studies, and the one cited above[1] indicates that the total reduction in digoxin absorption is small (15%). This is unlikely to be of clinical importance in most patients. However, if an interaction does occur the effects can seemingly be minimised by separating the doses by 2 hours.

1. Albert KS, Elliott WJ, Abbott RD, Gilbertson TJ, Data JL. Influence of kaolin-pectin suspension on steady-state plasma digoxin levels. *J Clin Pharmacol* (1981) 21, 449–55.
2. Brown DD, Juhl RP, Lewis K, Schrott M, Bartels B. Decreased bioavailability of digoxin due to antacids and kaolin-pectin. *N Engl J Med* (1976) 295, 1034–7.
3. Albert KS, Ayres JW, Disanto AR, Weidler DJ, Sakmar E, Hallmark MR, Stoll RG, DeSante KA, Wagner JG. Influence of kaolin-pectin suspension on digoxin bioavailability. *J Pharm Sci* (1978) 67, 1582–6.
4. Allen MD, Greenblatt DJ, Harmatz JS, Smith TW. Effect of magnesium aluminum hydroxide and kaolin-pectin on absorption of digoxin from tablets and capsules. *J Clin Pharmacol* (1981) 21, 26–30.

Digoxin + Kava

A standardised kava extract did not alter the pharmacokinetics of digoxin.

Clinical evidence, mechanism, importance and management

A study in 20 healthy subjects given a single 500-microgram dose of digoxin before and on the last day of treatment with a standardised kava rhizome (*Piper methysticum*) extract 1227 mg three times daily for 14 days, found no changes in the pharmacokinetics of digoxin. The product used was standardised for kavalactone content.[1]

It was suggested that kava might alter digoxin pharmacokinetics by affecting P-glycoprotein because kavalactones are modulators of P-glycoprotein *in vitro*. However, the clinical study showed that kava does not cause clinically relevant changes in digoxin pharmacokinetics. Therefore no changes in digoxin levels would be anticipated on concurrent use, the caveat being that, as with all herbal medicines, these results might not be applicable to all kava products.[1]

1. Gurley BJ, Swain A, Barone GW, Williams DK, Breen P, Yates CR, Stuart LB, Hubbard MA, Tong Y, Cheboyina S. Effect of goldenseal (*Hydrastis canadensis*) and kava kava (*Piper methysticum*) supplementation on digoxin pharmacokinetics in humans. *Drug Metab Dispos* (2007) 35, 240–5.

Digoxin and related drugs + Ketanserin

Ketanserin does not appear to affect the pharmacokinetics of either digoxin or digitoxin.

Clinical evidence, mechanism, importance and management

In a study in healthy subjects, ketanserin 40 mg twice daily did not cause any changes in the pharmacokinetics of single doses of either digoxin 1.25 mg or **digitoxin** 1 mg, and it was concluded that ketanserin is unlikely to alter serum concentrations of either of these drugs during clinical use.[1] No dose adjustments of these cardiac glycosides would therefore appear to be necessary on concurrent use with ketanserin.

1. Ochs HR, Verburg-Ochs B, Höller M, Greenblatt DJ. Effect of ketanserin on the kinetics of digoxin and digitoxin. *J Cardiovasc Pharmacol* (1985) 7, 205–7.

Digoxin + Lanthanum

Lanthanum does not affect the pharmacokinetics of digoxin.

Clinical evidence, mechanism, importance and management

In a crossover study, 14 healthy subjects were given three doses of lanthanum 1 g on one day, followed by a fourth dose the following day. A single 500-microgram dose of digoxin was given 30 minutes after the fourth dose of lanthanum. The AUC and maximum level of digoxin were not affected by lanthanum but the half-life was increased from 11.4 hours to 14.8 hours, although this is unlikely to be clinically important.[1] The available evidence suggests that a clinically relevant interaction between digoxin and lanthanum is unlikely, and that digoxin dose adjustments would not be expected to be necessary on concurrent use.

1. Fiddler G. Fosrenol™ (lanthanum carbonate) does not affect the pharmacokinetics of concomitant treatment with digoxin. *J Am Soc Nephrol* (2002) 13, 749A.

Digoxin + Laropiprant

Laropiprant has no clinically relevant effect on the pharmacokinetics of digoxin.

Clinical evidence, mechanism, importance and management

In a randomised, crossover study, 12 healthy subjects were given laropiprant 40 mg daily for 10 days with a single 500-microgram dose of digoxin on day 6. Laropiprant decreased the AUC of digoxin by 9%, which was statistically significant, but had no effect on the maximum digoxin level.[1] The reason for this minor decrease in digoxin exposure is not known; however, it is unlikely to be clinically relevant. Digoxin dose adjustments would therefore not be expected to be necessary on the concurrent use of laropiprant. Note that, laropiprant is only available as a combination product with nicotinic acid.

1. Liu F, Vessey L, Wenning L, Connolly S, Buckland M, Johnson-Levonas AO, Denker A, Wagner JA, Lai E. Effects of laropiprant, a selective prostaglandin D_2 receptor 1 antagonist, on the steady-state pharmacokinetics of digoxin in healthy adult subjects. *J Clin Pharmacol* (2010) 50, 823–8.

Digoxin + Lasofoxifene

Lasofoxifene does not affect the pharmacokinetics of digoxin.

Clinical evidence, mechanism, importance and management

A pharmacokinetic study in 10 healthy postmenopausal women given digoxin 250 micrograms daily for 20 days, found that lasofoxifene (a 4-mg loading dose given on day 11, followed by 500 micrograms daily for 10 days) had no effect on the AUC or maximum plasma concentrations of digoxin.[1] No digoxin dose adjustments would therefore be expected to be necessary in patients also given lasofoxifene.

1. Roman D, Bramson C, Ouellet D, Randinitis E, Gardner M. Effect of lasofoxifene on the pharmacokinetics of digoxin in healthy postmenopausal women. *J Clin Pharmacol* (2005) 45, 1407–12.

Digoxin + Levetiracetam

Levetiracetam does not appear to affect the pharmacokinetics of digoxin.

Clinical evidence, mechanism, importance and management

In a placebo-controlled study, 11 healthy subjects were given an initial loading dose of digoxin 500 micrograms followed by 250 micrograms daily with levetiracetam 1 g twice daily for one week. Levetiracetam did not affect the pharmacokinetics or pharmacodynamics of digoxin.[1] No additional precautions or digoxin dose adjustment seem necessary on concurrent use.

1. Levy RH, Ragueneau-Majlessi I, Baltes E. Repeated administration of the novel antiepileptic agent levetiracetam does not alter digoxin pharmacokinetics and pharmacodynamics in healthy volunteers. *Epilepsy Res* (2001) 46, 93–9.

Digoxin + Liquorice

An isolated case of digoxin toxicity reported in an elderly patient was attributed to the use of a herbal laxative containing kanzo (liquorice).

Clinical evidence

An 84-year-old man taking digoxin 125 micrograms daily and furosemide complained of loss of appetite, fatigue and oedema of the lower extremities 5 days after starting to take a Chinese herbal laxative containing liquorice (kanzo) 400 mg and rhubarb (daio) 1.6 g three times daily. He was found to have a raised digoxin level of 2.9 nanograms/mL (previous level 1 nanogram/mL) with a pulse rate of 30 bpm, and a slightly low potassium level (2.9 mmol/L).[1]

Mechanism

The reason for the increase in digoxin levels is unclear. Digoxin inhibits the sodium-potassium ATP-ase pump, which is concerned with the transport of sodium and potassium ions across the membranes of the myocardial cells. Potassium loss, caused by a combination of the liquorice, rhubarb and diuretics, exacerbated the potassium loss from the myocardial cells, thereby enhancing the bradycardia already caused by an elevated digoxin level. Hypokalaemia also promotes the binding of digoxin to myocardial cells. Pre-existing cardiovascular disease might have predisposed the patient to enhanced digoxin effects.

Importance and management

Evidence for an interaction between digoxin and liquorice appears to be limited to one case. It is likely that the effects of the elevated digoxin levels were exacerbated by hypokalaemia, which might have been caused by the herbal laxative. The theoretical basis for an interaction between liquorice and digoxin is well established, but there are few actual cases. Any herbal preparation that can reduce potassium levels would be expected to increase the risk of digoxin toxicity. This is likely to be additive with other concurrent medications a patient may also be taking that can cause hypokalaemia, such as loop diuretics. It would be prudent to exercise caution in patients who are taking digitalis glycosides and who regularly use/abuse laxatives including liquorice and/or anthraquinone-containing substances such as rhubarb. However, note that if these laxatives are used as recommended (at a dose producing a comfortable soft-formed motion), then this interaction is probably unlikely to be important.

1. Harada T, Ohtaki E, Misu K, Sumiyoshi T, Hosoda S. Congestive heart failure caused by digitalis toxicity in an elderly man taking a licorice-containing Chinese herbal laxative. *Cardiology* (2002) 98, 218.

Digoxin + Lithium

No pharmacokinetic interaction occurs between digoxin and lithium but giving digoxin to patients taking lithium possibly has a detrimental short-term effect on the control of mania. An isolated report describes severe bradycardia in one patient given both drugs.

Clinical evidence, mechanism, importance and management

In a study in 6 healthy subjects taking lithium carbonate in doses to achieve mean steady-state serum levels of 0.76 mmol/L (range 0.4 to 1 mmol/L), the pharmacokinetics of a 750-microgram intravenous dose of digoxin were unchanged by lithium, and there was no effect on sodium pump activity or electrolyte concentrations.[1] However, in an experimental 7-day study in patients with manic-depressive psychoses, there was a greater improvement in those given lithium with placebo than in those given lithium with digoxin. This might be a reflection of changes in Na-K ATP-ase.[2] An isolated report describes tremor, confusion and severe nodal bradycardia in a patient given lithium and digoxin. The bradycardia worsened (30 bpm) even after both drugs were stopped.[3] The clinical relevance of all of these findings is uncertain. Note that one UK manufacturer of digoxin[4] lists lithium as a drug that could increase sensitivity to digoxin because it might cause hypokalaemia or intracellular potassium deficiency, but note that hypokalaemia does not appear to be a commonly accepted adverse effect of lithium.

1. Cooper SJ, Kelly JG, Johnston GD, Copeland S, King DJ, McDevitt DG. Pharmacodynamics and pharmacokinetics of digoxin in the presence of lithium. *Br J Clin Pharmacol* (1984) 18, 21–5.
2. Chambers CA, Smith AHW, Naylor GJ. The effect of digoxin on the response to lithium therapy in mania. *Psychol Med* (1982) 12, 57–60.
3. Winters WD, Ralph DD. Digoxin-lithium drug interaction. *Clin Toxicol* (1977) 10, 487–8.
4. Lanoxin (Digoxin). Aspen. UK Summary of product characteristics, November 2009.

Digoxin and related drugs + Macrolides

Clarithromycin causes a sizeable increase in digoxin levels, and numerous cases of digoxin toxicity have been reported. Increases in digoxin levels also occur with telithromycin. Cases of rapid and marked two- to fourfold increases in digoxin levels have also been reported for azithromycin, erythromycin, josamycin and roxithromycin. A similar case of toxicity has been seen with digitoxin and azithromycin.

Clinical evidence

A. Digitoxin

A man with congestive heart failure taking digitoxin 70 micrograms daily for 5 days of each week, with enalapril and furosemide, was admitted to hospital with nausea and bradycardia of 26 bpm 4 days after starting a 3-day course of **azithromycin** (dose not stated). His serum digitoxin levels were found to be raised from his usual baseline range of 9.9 to 19 nanograms/mL up to 34 nanograms/mL. His renal function was normal. Another patient receiving intravenous digitoxin 250 micrograms daily had a marked rise from his steady-state digitoxin range of 11 to 15 nanograms/mL after being given **azithromycin** 500 mg daily for 3 days. The digitoxin was withdrawn one day later, but the levels climbed to a peak of 32 nanograms/mL after a further 3 days, and remained in the toxic range for a further 3 days.[1]

B. Digoxin

(a) Azithromycin

A 31-month-old boy with Down's syndrome and tetralogy of Fallot (a congenital heart defect resulting in reduced blood flow to the lungs) was discharged from hospital after repair of his heart defect. He was taking digoxin 60 micrograms twice daily, furosemide, and potassium chloride. Eight days later, when readmitted with symptoms of heart failure, intermittent fever and wheezing, he was given azithromycin (10 mg/kg on day one, then 5 mg/kg daily for 4 days). Three days later his steady-state serum digoxin levels had risen from 1.79 nanograms/mL to 2.37 nanograms/mL and he experienced anorexia, nausea, and second degree atrioventricular block. All the symptoms resolved when the digoxin was withdrawn. Digoxin was restarted at 50 micrograms twice daily after the azithromycin course was completed, and steady-state digoxin levels of 1.42 nanograms/mL were noted.[2]

The manufacturers of azithromycin stated that, as of October 2000, there were 230 cases of the concurrent use of azithromycin and digoxin on their database. Of these, 78 cases had adverse events indicating possible digoxin toxicity. However on review, 21 cases were clearly excluded. Of the remaining cases, only 13 provided digoxin levels, and of these, high serum digoxin concentrations were reported in 6, but generally insufficient data made interpretation difficult.[3] The manufacturers concluded that the possibility that a patient might experience an increase in digoxin levels while taking azithromycin cannot be entirely excluded.[3]

In a case-control study[4] using data from healthcare databases in Ontario from 1993 to 2008, there was an increased risk of hospitalisation for digoxin toxicity in patients who had been exposed to azithromycin in the preceding 14 days (adjusted odds ratio 3.71), which was similar to the risk with *erythromycin* and much lower than that for *clarithromycin*, see below.

(b) Clarithromycin

A woman taking warfarin, heparin, carbamazepine and digoxin was admitted to hospital with syncope, vomiting and an irregular heart rhythm shortly after starting clarithromycin 1 g daily. Her serum digoxin levels were found to be raised. Her clarithromycin dose was decreased, carbamazepine and digoxin stopped, and she was treated with digoxin-specific antibody fragments (*Digibind*) and intravenous fluids. Her serum digoxin levels fell again and the digitalis toxicity disappeared.[5]

In 1995, the manufacturers of clarithromycin had a few other cases on their records of raised digoxin levels in patients following the use of clarithromycin[5] and there are many other case reports of this interaction in the literature,[6-21] including a case series of 6 patients with end-stage renal disease.[22]

A subsequent randomised, placebo-controlled study in 12 healthy subjects confirmed that clarithromycin 250 mg twice daily for 3 days increased the AUC of a single 750-microgram oral dose of digoxin by 70%. The non-glomerular renal clearance of digoxin was reduced by 40%.[23] Intravenous digoxin was much less affected.[23,24] In three further studies clarithromycin 500 mg twice daily for 7 days increased the AUC of digoxin by 57%, 46% and 35%.[25-27] Note that these three studies were designed to investigate the interaction of other drugs, and clarithromycin was being used as a positive control.

Two studies that prospectively measured digoxin levels in patients before and during the use of clarithromycin found an important increase in all patients: in one study digoxin levels were increased by 70%,[28] and in the other, digoxin levels were increased from a range of 1 to 1.6 nanograms/mL up to a range of 2.3 to greater than 4 nanograms/mL.[29] In one of these studies, there was a significant correlation between the dose of clarithromycin and the increase in digoxin serum levels.[28]

A case-control study using data from healthcare databases in Ontario from 1994 to 2000 identified 1 051 patients who had been admitted to hospital with digoxin toxicity. Of these, 55 patients (5.2%) had been exposed to clarithromycin in the preceding 3 weeks, when compared with just 0.5% of controls, which represented about a tenfold increase in risk.[30] In a further study from this database, the risk of hospitalisation for digoxin toxicity was reported to be 14.8-fold higher in those who had taken clarithromycin in the preceding 14 days, and this risk was substantially higher than for *azithromycin*, see above, or *erythromycin*, see below.[4] Yet another case-control study using data from a healthcare database in Taiwan from 2001 to 2004 identified 595 patients admitted to hospital with digoxin toxicity. After adjusting for previous hospitalisations and other interacting drugs, patients were 4.36-, 5.07- and 2.98-fold more likely to have been prescribed clarithromycin in the preceding 7, 14 or 30 days, respectively. In this study, there was some evidence that the risk was dose-related.[31]

(c) Erythromycin

An elderly woman with a prosthetic heart valve and left ventricular dysfunction, taking warfarin, furosemide, hydralazine, isosorbide dinitrate and digoxin, was given erythromycin. She took only four 250-mg doses. Four days later her serum digoxin levels were found to have risen to 2.6 nanograms/mL from a normal steady-state range of 1.4 to 1.7 nanograms/mL, and she had evidence of digitalis toxicity.[32] Another four similar cases have also been reported.[33-35]

A study in a man who was resistant to digoxin found that erythromycin 1 g daily increased the AUC of digoxin by 300%.[36] A neonate given oral digoxin 5 micrograms/kg daily developed digoxin toxicity 2 days after erythromycin (10 mg three times daily, then 17 mg three times daily) was given. Digoxin levels rose from 1.8 nanograms/mL to 16 nanograms/mL.[37]

In a case-control study[4] using data from healthcare databases in Ontario from 1993 to 2008, there was an increased risk of hospitalisation with digoxin toxicity in patients who had been exposed to erythromycin in the preceding 14 days (adjusted odds ratio 3.69), which was similar to the risk with *azithromycin* and much lower than that for *clarithromycin*, see above.

(d) Josamycin

A case report describes a premature neonate receiving digoxin, who had a 50% increase in digoxin levels (from 2 nanograms/mL to 2.95 nanograms/mL), resulting in bradycardia and sinoatrial block after being given josamycin for 4 days. This was treated with antidigitalis Fab fragments.[38]

(e) Rokitamycin

In a study in 10 subjects rokitamycin did not affect serum digoxin levels.[39]

(f) Roxithromycin

A 76-year-old woman taking digoxin and a number of other drugs (enalapril, isosorbide mononitrate, furosemide, diltiazem, glyceryl trinitrate, slow-release potassium, prednisolone, omeprazole, calcitriol) developed signs of digoxin toxicity (nausea, vomiting, first degree heart block) within 4 days of starting to take roxithromycin 150 mg twice daily. Her serum digoxin levels were raised about fourfold.[40]

(g) Telithromycin

A study in 26 healthy subjects given digoxin 500 micrograms twice daily on the first day followed by 250 micrograms twice daily found that telithromycin 800 mg daily increased the AUC of digoxin by 37% and increased its maximum blood levels by 74%. Trough plasma levels were increased by 21% and remained within the therapeutic range. No signs of digoxin toxicity were observed on ECGs.[41]

A 58-year-old woman taking digoxin 250 micrograms daily developed syncope and malaise after a 5-day course of telithromycin 800 mg daily. Her digoxin levels were 55% higher than her normal baseline level, and there were ECG changes.[42]

Mechanism

It was originally thought that the interaction between the macrolides and digoxin was due to the effect of the antibacterials on gut flora. Up to 10% of patients receiving oral digoxin excrete it in substantial amounts in the faeces and urine as inactive metabolites (digoxin reduction products or DRPs). This metabolism seems to be the responsibility of the gut flora,[33] in particular *Eubacterium lentum*, which is anaerobic and Gram positive.[35,43] In the presence of antibacterials that inhibit this organism, much more digoxin becomes available for absorption, which results in a marked rise in serum levels. At the same time the inactive metabolites derived from the gut disappear.[33,44] However, it is worth noting that most classes of antibacterials do not appear to interact with digoxin despite inhibiting *E. lentum in vitro*.[43] In addition, more recent data showing that digoxin levels are affected by clarithromycin in all, or the majority, of patients or subjects throw doubt on this theory.

A more plausible explanation for the interaction between digoxin and clarithromycin, and probably also erythromycin, is that the antibacterials inhibit the intestinal[24,45] or renal[15,28] P-glycoprotein transport of digoxin, which would increase the oral bioavailability and reduce the non-glomerular renal clearance respectively. Both mechanisms could be important.[23] Further, the increased gastric emptying due to erythromycin might also increase the bioavailability of digoxin[46] or digitoxin.[43]

Importance and management

The pharmacokinetic interaction between digoxin and **clarithromycin** is established, and likely to occur in the majority of patients. Digoxin toxicity has been commonly reported. Monitor all patients well for signs of increased digoxin effects when clarithromycin is first given (e.g. bradycardia), taking digoxin levels and reducing the digoxin dose as necessary. **Telithromycin** appears to interact similarly to clarithromycin, and so similar advice applies.

Information about **azithromycin** and **erythromycin** is limited to a relatively small number of patients, although there is some retrospective evidence suggesting that the risk of digoxin toxicity is lower with azithromycin or erythromycin than clarithromycin. There is only one report of an interaction between digoxin and **josamycin** or digoxin and **roxithromycin**. However, until more is known, it would be prudent to monitor all patients for signs of increased digoxin effects when any of these macrolide antibacterials is first given, reducing the digoxin dose as necessary. In addition, remember that azithromycin has a long serum half-life (60 hours), which means that it can continue to interact for several days after it has been withdrawn.

Rokitamycin appears not to interact with digoxin.

1. Thalhammer F, Hollenstein UM, Locker GJ, Janata K, Sunder-Plassmann G, Frass M, Burgmann H. Azithromycin-related toxic effects of digitoxin. *Br J Clin Pharmacol* (1998) 45, 91–2.
2. Ten Eick AP, Sallee D, Preminger T, Weiss A, Reed DM. Possible drug interaction between digoxin and azithromycin in a young child. *Clin Drug Invest* (2000) 20, 61–4.
3. Pfizer Ltd. Personal Communication, February 2001.
4. Gomes T, Mamdani M, Juurlink D. Macrolide-induced digoxin toxicity: a population-based study. *Clin Pharmacol Ther* (2009) 86, 383–86.
5. Abbott Labs, Personal communication 1995.
6. Midoneck SR, Etingin OR. Clarithromycin-related toxic effects of digoxin. *N Engl J Med* (1995) 333, 1505.
7. Taylor JW, Gammenthaler SA, Rape JM. Clarithromycin (Biaxin) induced digoxin toxicity. Presented at the American Society of Healthcare Pharmacists Midyear Clinical Meeting, Miami, December 1994.
8. Ford A, Crocker Smith L, Baltch AL, Smith RP. Clarithromycin-induced digoxin toxicity in a patient with AIDS. *Clin Infect Dis* (1995) 21, 1051–2.
9. Brown BA, Wallace RJ, Griffith DE, Warden R. Clarithromycin-associated digoxin toxicity in the elderly. *Clin Infect Dis* (1997) 24, 92–3.
10. Guillemet C, Alt M, Arpin-Bott MP, Imler M. Clarithromycine-digoxine: une interaction méconnue chez certains patients? *Presse Med* (1997) 26, 512.
11. Nordt S, Williams S, Manoguerra A, Clark R. Clarithromycin-induced digoxin poisoning. *J Toxicol Clin Toxicol* (1997) 35, 501–2.
12. Guerriero SE, Ehrenpreis E, Gallagher KL. Two cases of clarithromycin-induced digoxin toxicity. *Pharmacotherapy* (1997) 17, 1035–7.
13. Laberge P, Martineau P. Clarithromycin-induced digoxin intoxication. *Ann Pharmacother* (1997) 31, 999–1001.
14. Trivedi S, Hyman J, Lichstein E. Clarithromycin and digoxin toxicity. *Ann Intern Med* (1998) 128, 604.
15. Wakasugi H, Yano I, Ito T, Hashida T, Futami T, Nohara R, Sasayama S, Inui K-I. Effect of clarithromycin on renal excretion of digoxin: interaction with P-glycoprotein. *Clin Pharmacol Ther* (1998) 64, 123–8.
16. Nawarskas JJ, McCarthy DM, Spinler SA. Digoxin toxicity secondary to clarithromycin therapy. *Ann Pharmacother* (1997) 31, 864–6.
17. Nordt SP, Williams SR, Manoguerra AS, Clark RF. Clarithromycin induced digoxin toxicity. *J Accid Emerg Med* (1998) 15, 194–5.
18. Juurlink DN, Ito S. Comment: clarithromycin-digoxin interaction. *Ann Pharmacother* (1999) 33, 1375–6.
19. Kiran N, Azam S, Dhakam S. Clarithromycin induced digoxin toxicity: Case report and review. *J Pakistan Med Assoc* (2004) 54, 440–41.
20. Gooderham MJ, Bolli P, Fernandez PG. Concomitant digoxin toxicity and warfarin interaction in a patient receiving clarithromycin. *Ann Pharmacother* (1999) 33, 796–9.

21. Intoxicación digitálica secundaria a una alteración delmetabolismo intestinal de la digoxina en una pacientetratada con claritromicina. Vergara-López S, Garciá-Garciá JA, Merchante N, Mira JA. Med Clin (Barc) 2004 (123) 639.
22. Hirata S, Izumi S, Furukubo T, Ota M, Fujita M, Yamakawa T, Hasegawa I, Ohtani H, Sawada Y. Interactions between clarithromycin and digoxin in patients with end-stage renal disease. *Int J Clin Pharmacol Ther* (2005) 43, 30–36.
23. Rengelshausen J, Göggelmann C, Burhenne J, Riedel K-D, Ludwig J, Weiss J, Mikus G, Walter-Sack I, Haefeli WE. Contribution of increased oral bioavailability and reduced nonglomerular renal clearance of digoxin to the digoxin–clarithromycin interaction. *Br J Clin Pharmacol* (2003) 56, 32–8.
24. Tsutsumi K, Kotegawa T, Kuranari M, Otani Y, Morimoto T, Matsuki S, Nakano S. The effect of erythromycin and clarithromycin on the pharmacokinetics of intravenous digoxin in healthy volunteers. *J Clin Pharmacol* (2002) 42, 1159–64.
25. Gurley BJ, Swain A, Barone GW, Williams DK, Breen P, Yates CR, Stuart LB, Hubbard MA, Tong Y, Cheboyina S. Effect of goldenseal (*Hydrastis canadensis*) and kava kava (*Piper methysticum*) supplementation on digoxin pharmacokinetics in humans. *Drug Metab Dispos* (2007) 35, 240–5.
26. Gurley BJ, Swain A, Williams DK, Barone G, Battu SK. Gauging the clinical significance of P-glycoprotein-mediated herb-drug interactions: comparative effects of St. John's wort, Echinacea, clarithromycin, and rifampin on digoxin pharmacokinetics. *Mol Nutr Food Res* (2008) 52, 772–79.
27. Gurley BJ, Barone GW, Williams DK, Carrier J, Breen P, Yates CR, Song P-f, Hubbard MA, Tong Y, Cheboyina S. Effect of milk thistle (*Silybum marianum*) and black cohosh (*Cimicifuga racemosa*) supplementation on digoxin pharmacokinetics in humans. *Drug Metab Dispos* (2006) 34, 69–74.
28. Tanaka H, Matsumoto K, Ueno K, Kodama M, Yoneda K, Katayama Y, Miyatake K. Effect of clarithromycin on steady-state digoxin concentrations. *Ann Pharmacother* (2003) 37, 178–81.
29. Zapater P, Reus S, Tello A, Torrús D, Pérez-Mateo M, Horga JF. A prospective study of the clarithromycin–digoxin interaction in elderly patients. *J Antimicrob Chemother* (2002) 50, 601–6.
30. Juurlink DN, Mamdani M, Kopp A, Laupacis A, Redelmeier DA. Drug-drug interactions among elderly patients hospitalized for drug toxicity. *JAMA* (2003) 289, 1652–8.
31. Chan ALF, Wang M-T, Su C-Y, Tsai F-H. Risk of digoxin intoxication caused by clarithromycin-digoxin interactions in heart failure patients: a population-based study. *Eur J Clin Pharmacol* (2009) 65, 1237–43.
32. Friedman HS, Bonventre MV. Erythromycin-induced digoxin toxicity. *Chest* (1982) 82, 202.
33. Lindenbaum J, Rund DG, Butler VP, Tse-Eng D, Saha JR. Inactivation of digoxin by the gut flora: reversal by antibiotic therapy. *N Engl J Med* (1981) 305, 789–94.
34. Maxwell DL, Gilmour-White SK, Hall MR. Digoxin toxicity due to interaction of digoxin with erythromycin. *BMJ* (1989) 298, 572.
35. Morton MR, Cooper JW. Erythromycin-induced digoxin toxicity. *DICP Ann Pharmacother* (1989) 23, 668–70.
36. Nørregaard-Hansen K, Klitgaard NA, Pedersen KE. The significance of the enterohepatic circulation on the metabolism of digoxin in patients with the ability of intestinal conversion of the drug. *Acta Med Scand* (1986) 220, 89–92.
37. Coudray S, Janoly A, Belkacem-Kahlouli A, Bourhis Y, Bleyzac N, Bourgeois J, Putet G, Aulagner G. L'érythromycine responsable d'une intoxication sévère par la digoxine dans un service de réanimation néonatale. *J Pharm Clin* (2001) 20, 129–31.
38. Cambonie G, Sabatier E, Guillaumont S, Masson F, Charbit J, Pidoux O, Hillaire-Buys D, Picaud JC. Digoxin-Josamycin: a dangerous drug interaction in children. *Arch Pediatr* (2006) 13, 1118–20.
39. Ishioka T. Effect of a new macrolide antibiotic 3''-O-propionyl-leucomycin A_5 (Rokitamycin) on serum concentrations of theophylline and digoxin in the elderly. *Acta Ther* (1987) 13, 17–23.
40. Corallo CE, Rogers IR. Roxithromycin-induced digoxin toxicity. *Med J Aust* (1996) 165, 433–4.
41. Montay G, Shi J, Leroy B, Bhargava V. Effects of telithromycin on the pharmacokinetics of digoxin in healthy men. *Intersci Conf Antimicrob Agents Chemother* (2002) 42, 28.
42. Nenciu LM, Laberge P, Thirion DJG. Telithromycin-induced digoxin toxicity and electrocardiographic changes. *Pharmacotherapy* (2006) 26, 872–6.
43. Ten Eick AP, Reed MD. Hidden dangers of coadministration of antibiotics and digoxin in children: focus on azithromycin. *Curr Ther Res* (2000) 61, 148–60.
44. Lindenbaum J, Tse-Eng D, Butler VP, Rund DG. Urinary excretion of reduced metabolites of digoxin. *Am J Med* (1981) 71, 67–74.
45. Berndt A, Gramatté T, Kirch W. Digoxin-erythromycin interaction: in vitro evidence for competition for intestinal P-glycoprotein. *Eur J Clin Pharmacol* (1996) 50, 538.
46. Sutton A, Pilot M-A. Digoxin toxicity and erythromycin. *BMJ* (1989) 298, 1101.

Digoxin and related drugs + Medroxyprogesterone or Megestrol

Doses of medroxyprogesterone acetate or megestrol used for malignant disease appear to have minimal effects on digitoxin levels.

Clinical evidence, mechanism, importance and management

Steady-state **digitoxin** levels were monitored in 3 patients before and after 5 weeks of treatment with oral medroxyprogesterone acetate 500 mg twice daily or megestrol 160 mg daily. Only small and clinically irrelevant changes in **digitoxin** levels and clearance were seen.[1]

For the possible effect of HRT including medroxyprogesterone on digitalis glycosides (unnamed), see 'Digoxin and related drugs + HRT', p.1099.

1. Lundgren S, Kvinnsland S, Utaaker E, Bakke O, Ueland PM. Effect of oral high-dose progestins on the disposition of antipyrine, digitoxin, and warfarin in patients with advanced breast cancer. *Cancer Chemother Pharmacol* (1986) 18, 270–5.

Digoxin + Methyldopa

Methyldopa does not appear to affect digoxin levels, but marked bradycardia has been seen in two elderly women given both drugs.

Clinical evidence

In 8 healthy subjects, methyldopa 250 mg daily had no effect on the steady-state serum levels of digoxin 250 micrograms daily.[1] However, a case report describes two elderly women with hypertension and left ventricular failure, who developed marked bradycardia when they were given digoxin with methyldopa 750 mg or 3.75 g daily, but not when they were given digoxin alone. Average heart rates were 50 bpm and 48 bpm, respectively, while minimum heart rates were 32 bpm and 38 bpm, respectively. They were subsequently discharged taking digoxin and hydralazine with heart rates within the normal range.[2]

Mechanism

Uncertain. Both digoxin and methyldopa[3] can cause some bradycardia, but these effects seem to have been more than simply the sum of the individual drug effects on the autonomic nervous system.[2]

Importance and management

Information is limited; it would seem that concurrent use of digoxin and methyldopa need not be avoided, but be aware that on rare occasions undesirable bradycardia has occurred.

1. May CA, Vlasses PH, Rocci ML, Rotmensch HH, Swanson BN, Tannenbaum RP, Ferguson RK, Abrams WB. Methyldopa does not alter the disposition of digoxin. *J Clin Pharmacol* (1984) 24, 386–9.
2. Davis JC, Reiffel JA, Bigger JT. Sinus node dysfunction caused by methyldopa and digoxin. *JAMA* (1981) 245, 1241–3.
3. Lund-Johansen P. Hemodynamic changes in long term α-methyldopa therapy of essential hypertension. *Acta Med Scand* (1972) 192, 221–6.

Digoxin + Metoclopramide

Digoxin levels can be reduced if metoclopramide is given with slowly dissolving forms of digoxin. No interaction is likely with digoxin in liquid form or in fast-dissolving preparations. A case report describes bradycardia and asystole on the concurrent use of digoxin and intravenous metoclopramide.

Clinical evidence

A study in 11 patients taking slowly dissolving digoxin tablets (*Orion*) found that metoclopramide 10 mg three times daily for 10 days reduced the serum digoxin levels by 36% (from 0.72 nanograms/mL to 0.46 nanograms/mL).[1] The digoxin concentrations rose to their former levels when the metoclopramide was withdrawn. Similarly, a study in healthy subjects found that metoclopramide 10 mg three times daily caused a 19% reduction in the AUC of digoxin and a 27% reduction in peak serum digoxin levels (digoxin formulation not stated).[2] Another study in healthy subjects clearly showed that metoclopramide decreased the absorption of digoxin from tablets (*Lanoxin*) but not capsules (*Lanoxicaps*).[3]

A case report describes a 56-year-old man with extensive burns who was started on digoxin for atrial fibrillation, with intravenous metoclopramide 20 mg four times daily started 16 days later. After a further 20 days, he experienced multiple episodes of bradycardia and asystole over 48 hours: serum digoxin levels remained below 1 nanogram/mL. Both drugs were stopped and several hours later the arrhythmias stopped.[4]

Mechanism

It would seem[5-7] that metoclopramide increases the motility of the gut to such an extent that full dissolution and absorption of some digoxin formulations does not occur. The cause of the bradyarrhythmias described in one case involving intravenous metoclopramide[4] is unclear.

Importance and management

Information about an interaction between digoxin and metoclopramide is very limited, but the interaction seems to be established. It is not likely to occur with solid form, fast-dissolving digoxin preparations (e.g. liquid-filled capsules) or digoxin in liquid form, but only with those preparations which are slowly dissolving (i.e. some tablet formulations). A reduction in digoxin levels of one-third could result in under-digitalisation. Be aware of this interaction if both drugs are given. The general relevance of the case of bradycardia and asystole with digoxin and intravenous metoclopramide is uncertain. Bear it in mind in case of an unexpected response to treatment.

1. Manninen V, Apajalahti A, Melin J, Karesoja M. Altered absorption of digoxin in patients given propantheline and metoclopramide. *Lancet* (1973) i, 398–400.
2. Kirch W, Janisch HD, Santos SR, Duhrsen U, Dylewicz P, Ohnhaus EE. Effect of cisapride and metoclopramide on digoxin bioavailability. *Eur J Drug Metab Pharmacokinet* (1986) 11, 249–50.
3. Johnson BF, Bustrack JA, Urbach DR, Hull JH, Marwaha R. Effect of metoclopramide on digoxin absorption from tablets and capsules. *Clin Pharmacol Ther* (1984) 36, 724–30.
4. Schwartz BG. Metoclopramide and digoxin cause 22 episodes of bradyarrhythmias. *Am J Med* (2010) 123, e5–6.
5. Manninen V, Apajalahti A, Simonen H, Reissell P. Effect of propantheline and metoclopramide on the absorption of digoxin. *Lancet* (1973) i, 1118–9.
6. Medin S, Nyberg L. Effect of propantheline and metoclopramide on the absorption of digoxin. *Lancet* (1973) i, 1393.
7. Fraser EJ, Leach RH, Poston JW, Bold AM, Culank LS, Lipede AB. Dissolution-rates and bioavailability of digoxin tablets. *Lancet* (1973) i, 1393.

Digoxin + Mexiletine

Digoxin levels are not altered by mexiletine.

Clinical evidence, mechanism, importance and management

In 10 healthy subjects, mexiletine 200 mg every 8 hours for 4 days reduced the steady-state levels of digoxin 250 micrograms daily by 16%, from 0.32 nanograms/mL to 0.27 nanograms/mL, although this difference was not statistically significant.[1] Two other studies in a total of 17 patients[2,3] confirmed that mexiletine does not affect serum digoxin levels. No digoxin dose adjustments would appear to be necessary on concurrent use

1. Saris SD, Lowenthal DT, Affrime MB. Steady-state digoxin concentration during oral mexiletine administration. *Curr Ther Res* (1983) 34, 662–66.
2. Leahey EB, Reiffel JA, Giardina E-GV, Bigger T. The effect of quinidine and other oral antiarrhythmic drugs on serum digoxin. *Ann Intern Med* (1980) 92, 605–8.
3. Day T, Hunt D. Interaction between mexiletine and digoxin. *Med J Aust* (1983) 2, 630.

Digoxin + Mizolastine

Mizolastine does not alter digoxin exposure.

Clinical evidence, mechanism, importance and management

In a placebo-controlled, crossover study in 12 healthy subjects given digoxin 250 micrograms daily, mizolastine 10 mg daily for a week caused a 17% increase in the maximum plasma levels of digoxin and a 14% increase in the minimum plasma levels of digoxin. The AUC and half-life of digoxin were unchanged and the haemodynamic parameters measured (blood pressure, ECG) were unaltered.[1] The magnitude of the reduction in digoxin exposure reported in this study is unlikely to be clinically relevant. No digoxin dose adjustments would therefore appear to be necessary on the concurrent use of mizolastine.

1. Chaufour S, Le Coz F, Denolle T, Dubruc C, Cimarosti I, Deschamps C, Ulliac N, Delhotal-Landes B, Rosenweig P. Lack of effect of mizolastine on the safety and pharmacokinetics of digoxin administered orally in repeated doses to healthy volunteers. *Int J Clin Pharmacol Ther* (1998) 36, 286–91.

Digoxin and related drugs + Moclobemide

Moclobemide does not alter beta-acetyldigoxin levels.

Clinical evidence, mechanism, importance and management

In a study in 14 patients with decompensated heart failure, who were given an individualised dose of **beta-acetyldigoxin** for 2 weeks, moclobemide 100 mg three times daily given for 8 days did not alter plasma **beta-acetyldigoxin** levels. No adverse effects attributable to an interaction were seen.[1] No particular precautions appear to be required during the concurrent use of **acetyldigoxin** and moclobemide.

1. Amrein R, Güntert TW, Dingemanse J, Lorscheid T, Stabl M, Schmid-Burgk W. Interactions of moclobemide with concomitantly administered medication: evidence from pharmacological and clinical studies. *Psychopharmacology (Berl)* (1992) 106, S24–S31.

Digoxin + Montelukast

Montelukast does not affect the pharmacokinetics of digoxin.

Clinical evidence, mechanism, importance and management

In a randomised study in 11 healthy subjects, montelukast 10 mg was given for 12 days with a single 500-microgram dose of digoxin on day 7. It was found that the pharmacokinetic profile of digoxin was unchanged by montelukast.[1] No digoxin dose adjustments are therefore needed if montelukast is used concurrently.

1. Depre M, Van Hecken A, Verbesselt R, Wynants K, De Lelepeire I, Freeman A, Holland S, Shahane A, Gertz B, De Schepper PJ. Effect of multiple doses of montelukast, a CysLT1 receptor agonist, on digoxin pharmacokinetics in healthy volunteers. *J Clin Pharmacol* (1999) 39, 941–4.

Digoxin + Moracizine

Moracizine does not affect digoxin levels; however, some adverse conduction effects have been seen on their concurrent use.

Clinical evidence

Thirteen patients taking digoxin 125 to 250 micrograms daily had no change in their serum digoxin levels when they were given moracizine 10 mg/kg daily in three divided doses for 2 weeks. Further, 9 patients who took digoxin and moracizine for one to 6 months had no changes in their serum digoxin levels.[1]

Similarly, in a single-dose study in 9 healthy subjects, and in a study in patients receiving maintenance treatment with digoxin over a 13-day period, the pharmacokinetics of intravenous and oral digoxin were not affected by moracizine.[2,3] However, cardiac arrhythmias (AV junctional rhythm and heart block) were seen, which resolved when the moracizine was stopped.[3]

Mechanism

Not established. There does not appear to be a pharmacokinetic interaction between moracizine and digoxin; however, concurrent use can cause an increase in the PR interval and QRS duration, which can result in AV block.[4]

Importance and management

Although no clinically important changes in digoxin levels appear to occur during the concurrent use of moracizine, the occurrence of arrhythmias in a few patients indicates that good monitoring is advisable. It has been pointed out that the additive effects of both drugs on intranodal and intraventricular conduction can be excessive in some patients with heart disease.[4] More study is needed.

1. Kennedy HL, Sprague MK, Redd RM, Wiens RD, Blum RI, Buckingham TA. Serum digoxin concentrations during ethmozine antiarrhythmic therapy. *Am Heart J* (1986) 111, 667–72.
2. MacFarland RT, Moeller VR, Pieniaszek HJ, Whitney CC, Marcus FI. Assessment of the potential pharmacokinetic interaction between digoxin and ethmozine. *J Clin Pharmacol* (1985) 25, 138–43.
3. Antman EM, Arnold JMO, Friedman PL, White H, Bosak M, Smith TW. Drug interactions with cardiac glycosides: evaluation of a possible digoxin-ethmozine pharmacokinetic interaction. *J Cardiovasc Pharmacol* (1987) 9, 622–7.
4. Siddoway LA, Schwartz SL, Barbey JT, Woosley RL. Clinical pharmacokinetics of moricizine. *Am J Cardiol* (1990) 65, 21D–25D.

Digoxin + Nateglinide or Repaglinide

The pharmacokinetics of nateglinide and digoxin are not altered by concurrent use. Repaglinide does not affect the pharmacokinetics of digoxin.

Clinical evidence, mechanism, importance and management

(a) Nateglinide

A crossover study in 12 healthy subjects found that when a single 1-mg dose of digoxin was given with the first dose of nateglinide 120 mg three times daily for 2 days, there were no changes in the pharmacokinetics of either drug.[1] No digoxin dose adjustments would therefore appear to be necessary on the concurrent use of nateglinide.

(b) Repaglinide

A crossover, multiple-dose study in 14 healthy subjects found that repaglinide 2 mg three times daily before meals had no effect on the pharmacokinetics of digoxin 250 micrograms daily.[2] No digoxin dose adjustments would therefore appear to be necessary on the concurrent use of repaglinide.

1. Zhou H, Walter YH, Smith H, Devineni D, McLeod JF. Nateglinide, a new mealtime glucose regulator. Lack of pharmacokinetic interaction with digoxin in healthy volunteers. *Clin Drug Invest* (2000) 19, 465–71.
2. Hatorp V, Thomsen MS. Drug interaction studies with repaglinide: repaglinide on digoxin or theophylline pharmacokinetics and cimetidine on repaglinide pharmacokinetics. *J Clin Pharmacol* (2000) 40, 184–92.

Digoxin + Nefazodone

Nefazodone can increase digoxin levels. Digoxin does not appear to affect the pharmacokinetics of nefazodone.

Clinical evidence, mechanism, importance and management

In a study, 18 healthy subjects were given digoxin 200 micrograms daily for 8 days, then nefazodone 200 mg twice daily for 8 days, and then both drugs together for 8 days. Nefazodone increased the AUC of digoxin by 15%, and increased the peak and trough plasma levels of digoxin by 29% and 27%, respectively. However, no changes in ECG measurements occurred (PR, QRS and QT intervals), nor was the heart rate or any other vital sign altered. The pharmacokinetics of nefazodone were unchanged.[1]

Evidence appears to be limited to this study, but as it was well conducted, an interaction is probably established. However, the magnitude of the reduction in digoxin exposure reported in the study is unlikely to be clinically relevant in most patients. No digoxin dose adjustments would generally appear to be necessary on the concurrent use of nefazodone.

1. Dockens RC, Greene DS, Barbhaiya RH. Assessment of pharmacokinetic and pharmacodynamic drug interactions between nefazodone and digoxin in healthy male volunteers. *J Clin Pharmacol* (1996) 36, 160–7.

Digoxin and related drugs + Neuromuscular blockers

Serious cardiac arrhythmias can develop in patients receiving digitalis glycosides who are given suxamethonium (succinylcholine) or pancuronium.

Clinical evidence

Eight out of 17 digitalised patients (anaesthetised with thiamylal and then maintained with nitrous oxide and oxygen) developed serious ventricular arrhythmias following the intravenous injection of **suxamethonium (succinylcholine)** 40 to 100 mg. Four out of the 8 patients reverted to their previous rhythm when they were given tubocurarine 15 to 30 mg, with one patient returning to a regular nodal rhythm from ventricular tachycardia.[1] Of the other 9 patients, 3 had immediate and definite ST-T wave changes, and the remaining 6 had no demonstrable changes.[1] There are other reports of this interaction,[2-4] including one that describes sinus tachycardia and atrial flutter in 6 out of 18 patients taking digoxin after they were given **pancuronium.**[4]

Mechanism

Not understood. One possibility is that the suxamethonium (succinylcholine) might cause the rapid removal of potassium from the myocardial cells. Another idea is that it affects catecholamine-releasing cholinergic receptors.

Importance and management

Information regarding an interaction between the digitalis glycosides and the neuromuscular blockers is limited, but the interaction with suxamethonium (succinylcholine) appears to be established. Suxamethonium should be used with great caution in patients taking digitalis glycosides. Similarly, caution would seem appropriate with pancuronium.

1. Dowdy EG, Fabian LW. Ventricular arrhythmias induced by succinylcholine in digitalized patients: A preliminary report. *Anesth Analg* (1963) 42, 501–13.
2. Pérez HR. Cardiac arrhythmia after succinylcholine. *Anesth Analg* (1970) 49, 33–8.
3. Smith RB, Petrusack J. Succinylcholine, digitalis, and hypercalcaemia: a case report. *Anesth Analg* (1972) 51, 202–5.
4. Bartolone RS, Rao TLK. Dysrhythmias following muscle relaxant administration in patients receiving digitalis. *Anesthesiology* (1983) 58, 567–9.

Digoxin + NNRTIs

Etravirine causes a small increase in digoxin concentrations, and rilpivirine is predicted to interact similarly.

Clinical evidence, mechanism, importance and management

The manufacturer reports that, in a study in 16 subjects, **etravirine** increased the AUC and maximum concentration of a single 500-microgram dose of digoxin by 18% and 19%, respectively.[1,2] **Etravirine** is a weak inhibitor of P-glycoprotein,[1,2] by which digoxin is transported. This minor change in digoxin concentrations with **etravirine** would not be expected to be of clinical relevance, and no digoxin dose adjustment is needed on concurrent use. The US manufacturer states that, when starting digoxin in a patient taking **etravirine**, the lowest possible dose of digoxin should be used. If **etravirine** is started in a patient taking digoxin, they state that no dose adjustments of either drug are necessary.[2] Both the UK and US manufacturer advise monitoring of digoxin concentrations on the concurrent use of **etravirine**.[1,2]

The UK manufacturer of **rilpivirine** states that **rilpivirine** has been reported to inhibit P-glycoprotein *in vitro*. They predict that rilpivirine might increase digoxin concentrations, and therefore recommend monitoring digoxin concentrations.[3]

1. Intelence (Etravirine). Janssen-Cilag Ltd. UK Summary of product characteristics, July 2012.
2. Intelence (Etravirine). Tibotec, Inc. US Prescribing information, August 2012.
3. Edurant (Rilpivirine hydrochloride). Janssen-Cilag Ltd. UK Summary of product characteristics, November 2011.

Digoxin and other P-glycoprotein substrates + NS5A inhibitors

Daclatasvir increases the exposure to digoxin, and ledipasvir is predicted to interact similarly. Ombitasvir does not appear to interact with digoxin. The exposure to other P-glycoprotein substrates, such as dabigatran, is predicted to be increased by daclatasvir and ledipasvir.

Clinical evidence

1. Daclatasvir. The UK manufacturer briefly reports that, in a study in healthy subjects, daclatasvir 60 mg daily increased the AUC and maximum concentration of digoxin 125 micrograms daily by 27% and 65%, respectively.[1]

2. Ombitasvir. The UK manufacturer briefly reports that, in a study in healthy subjects given a single 500-microgram dose of digoxin with ombitasvir 25 mg daily (in a fixed-dose combination with paritaprevir boosted with ritonavir, and given with dasabuvir), the pharmacokinetics of ombitasvir and digoxin were unaffected.[2] The US manufacturer similarly reports no effects.[3]

Mechanism

Digoxin is a substrate of P-glycoprotein, which is inhibited by daclatasvir. Concurrent use therefore results in increased digoxin exposure.

Importance and management

Evidence for an interaction between the NS5A inhibitors and digoxin is limited. An interaction between **daclatasvir** and digoxin would seem to be established, although the clinical relevance of an increase in exposure of the magnitude seen is not known. The UK manufacturer advises caution on concurrent use, and use of the lowest digoxin dose on initiation, with careful monitoring of digoxin concentrations to guide dose titration.[1] Until more is known, this would seem prudent.

There would appear to be no pharmacokinetic interaction between **ombitasvir** (and digoxin, and hence no need for dose adjustments on concurrent use. However, note that other components of the fixed-dose preparation interact with digoxin, see 'Digoxin and other P-glycoprotein substrates + HCV-protease inhibitors', p.1098.

The UK and US manufacturers of **ledipasvir** (in a fixed-dose combination with sofosbuvir) predict that digoxin exposure might be increased by concurrent use, as ledipasvir has been shown to inhibit P-glycoprotein *in vitro*. They advise monitoring of digoxin concentrations if given together.[4,5] Until more is known, this might be prudent.

Note that digoxin can be used as a probe substrate to assess the activity of drugs on P-glycoprotein. The data here, therefore suggest that daclatasvir is an inhibitor of P-glycoprotein, but ombitasvir is not. For a list of P-glycoprotein substrates see 'Table 1.12', p.14. The UK manufacturers of daclatasvir and ledipasvir (in a fixed-dose combination with sofosbuvir) specifically predict that the exposure to **dabigatran** (a P-glycoprotein substrate) will be increased. They therefore advise monitoring (for increased dabigatran effects (such as bleeding and anaemia) if given concurrently.[1,4] Dabigatran dose adjustment might be necessary.

1. Daklinza (Daclatasvir dihydrochloride). Bristol-Myers Squibb Pharmaceutical Ltd. UK Summary of product characteristics, September 2014.
2. Viekirax (Ombitasvir, paritaprevir, ritonavir). AbbVie Ltd. UK Summary of product characteristics, January 2015.
3. Viekira Pak (Ombitasvir, paritaprevir, ritonavir co-packaged with dasabuvir sodium monohydrate). AbbVie Inc. US Prescribing information, December 2014.
4. Harvoni (Ledipasvir, sofosbuvir). Gilead Sciences Ltd. UK Summary of product characteristics, November 2014.
5. Harvoni (Ledipasvir, sofosbuvir). Gilead Sciences, Inc. US Prescribing information, March 2015.

Digoxin and related drugs + NSAIDs

Diclofenac might increase serum digoxin levels. Two studies found that ibuprofen raised serum digoxin levels, whereas another found no evidence of an interaction. Indometacin can cause potentially toxic rises in digoxin levels, particularly in neonates. The concurrent use of lornoxicam and digoxin has a small effect on the pharmacokinetics of each drug. In one study, phenylbutazone caused a small reduction in serum digoxin levels whereas in another study there was no change. Etoricoxib, fenbufen, isoxicam, ketoprofen, meloxicam, nimesulide, piroxicam, rofecoxib and tiaprofenic acid appear to have no effect on the pharmacokinetics of digoxin. Phenylbutazone appears to halve digitoxin plasma levels, whereas azapropazone does not appear to alter digitoxin exposure. Digitoxin appears to have no effect on the plasma levels of diclofenac.

Clinical evidence

A. Digitoxin

(a) Azapropazone

In 8 patients with arthritis, azapropazone 900 mg daily did not alter the AUC of a single 500-microgram intravenous dose of digitoxin. The half-life of digitoxin was increased by about 10%, and two of the patients had individual half-life increases of almost one-third, although the difference was not statistically significant.[1]

(b) Diclofenac

Digitoxin 100 micrograms had no effect on the plasma levels of diclofenac 50 mg twice daily in 8 subjects. Digitoxin levels were not reported.[2]

(c) Phenylbutazone

In 6 patients, phenylbutazone 200 or 400 mg daily halved the plasma levels of digitoxin 100 micrograms daily, on two separate occasions. Digitoxin levels returned to their former values within roughly the same period of time after phenylbutazone was withdrawn.[3] Another report describes a similar response in one patient.[4]

B. Digoxin

(a) Diclofenac

A study in 7 healthy subjects found that diclofenac 100 mg daily for 10 days increased the serum levels of digoxin by 29%.[5] Another study in 6 healthy subjects similarly found that diclofenac 50 mg three times daily raised the serum digoxin levels by about one-third.[6] A brief report describes a 77-year-old woman taking several drugs, including digoxin 250 micrograms daily, furosemide 40 mg three times a week and hydroquinine 100 mg daily, who complained of nausea, vomiting, loss of appetite and constipation when she started taking diclofenac 25 mg three times daily for 2 weeks. However, the symptoms continued when she stopped the diclofenac, and 4 weeks later her digoxin level was 2.3 nanograms/mL. Digoxin and furosemide were stopped and her symptoms disappeared.[7]

(b) Etoricoxib

In a placebo-controlled crossover study in 14 healthy subjects given digoxin 250 micrograms daily, the addition of etoricoxib 120 mg daily for 10 days did not alter the steady-state AUC of digoxin or its renal elimination, but the maximum serum digoxin levels were increased by about 33%.[8]

(c) Fenbufen

Fenbufen 900 mg daily was found to cause an insignificant rise in the serum levels of digoxin.[9]

(d) Ibuprofen

The serum digoxin levels of 12 patients were reported to have risen by about 60% after they were given at least 1.6 g of ibuprofen daily for a week. However, after a month the digoxin levels had returned to their former amount.[10] These findings are potentially unreliable because half of the patients were not satisfactorily compliant with treatment. Another study found that ibuprofen 1.2 g daily for 10 days raised the serum digoxin levels of 9 healthy subjects by 25%.[5] Yet another study found that ibuprofen 600 mg three times daily for 10 days had no effect on steady-state serum digoxin levels of 8 patients.[11]

(e) Indometacin

1. Neonates. A study in 11 premature neonates (gestational age 25 to 33 weeks) given digoxin found that when they were given indometacin (mean total dose of 320 micrograms/kg over 12 to 24 hours) for patent ductus arteriosus, their mean serum digoxin levels rose on average by 40%. Digoxin was stopped in 5 of them because serum levels were potentially toxic.[12] This confirms the observation of digitalis toxicity in 3 similarly treated premature neonates,[13] and of toxic serum digoxin levels in another neonate.[14] A further report describes very high digoxin levels (8.2 nanograms/mL) without symptoms of toxicity in a full-term neonate given indometacin.[15]

2. Adults. Indometacin 50 mg three times daily for 10 days increased steady-state digoxin levels of 10 patients by about 40% (from 0.57 nanograms/mL to 0.8 nanograms/mL), with a range of 0 to 100%.[11] Indometacin 150 mg daily for 10 days increased the serum digoxin levels of 9 healthy subjects by 25%.[5] In yet another study, a 60% increase in digoxin levels was seen with indometacin 150 mg daily.[16] This contrasts with the results of single-dose studies in two groups of 6 healthy adult subjects[17,18] who were given a 4-hour infusion of digoxin. Both studies suggested that no interaction occurs with indometacin.

(f) Isoxicam

Isoxicam 200 mg daily did not affect the steady-state plasma levels of 12 healthy subjects taking **beta-acetyldigoxin**.[19] This confirms the findings of a previous study.[20]

(g) Ketoprofen

Ketoprofen 50 mg four times daily for 4 days had no effect on the serum digoxin levels of 12 patients.[21]

(h) Lornoxicam

In 12 healthy subjects, the concurrent use of lornoxicam 4 mg twice daily for 14 days and digoxin 250 micrograms daily had only a small effect on the pharmacokinetics of each drug. The apparent clearance of the digoxin was decreased by 14% while the maximum serum level of the lornoxicam was decreased by 21% and its elimination half-life was increased by 36%.[22]

(i) Meloxicam

In 12 healthy subjects meloxicam 15 mg daily for 8 days had no effect on the pharmacokinetics of digoxin (given as **beta-acetyldigoxin**).[23]

(j) Nimesulide

Nimesulide 100 mg twice daily for 7 days did not alter steady-state digoxin levels in 9 patients with mild heart failure taking digoxin 250 micrograms daily. No change in their clinical condition occurred.[24]

(k) Phenylbutazone

Six healthy subjects had an a decrease of about 20% in their serum digoxin levels while taking phenylbutazone 200 mg three times daily for 4 days.[6] In contrast, one study found no alteration in the levels of digoxin when it was given with phenylbutazone 600 mg daily.[16]

(l) Piroxicam

In 10 patients taking digoxin for mild heart failure, piroxicam 10 or 20 mg daily for 15 days had no effect on the steady-state digoxin levels, nor were consistent effects seen on the pharmacokinetics of digoxin.[25] Piroxicam 20 mg daily for 10 days was found to have no effect on serum digoxin levels in 6 healthy subjects.[5]

(m) Rofecoxib

In a crossover study in 10 healthy subjects, rofecoxib 75 mg daily for 11 days had no effect on the plasma pharmacokinetics or renal elimination of a single 500-microgram dose of digoxin elixir.[26]

(n) Tiaprofenic acid

Tiaprofenic acid 200 mg three times daily for 10 days had no effect on the serum digoxin levels of 12 healthy subjects.[27]

Mechanism

The reasons for the altered digoxin pharmacokinetics in some of the studies are not clear. However, in the studies in neonates, the elevated digoxin levels were clearly related to an indometacin-induced deterioration in renal function.[12,14,15] It should be noted that all NSAIDs have the potential to cause renal impairment.

It is suggested that phenylbutazone lowers digitoxin levels by increasing its rate of metabolism by the liver.[3]

Importance and management

Digoxin

The interaction between digoxin and **indometacin** seems established in neonates, but documentation is limited. It has been suggested that the digoxin dose should be halved if indometacin is given to premature or full-term infants and the serum digoxin levels and urinary output monitored. Also be alert for increases in serum digoxin levels in adults if indometacin is given. In adults it is probably sufficient to monitor pulse rate (for bradycardia) and take digoxin levels if an interaction is suspected. Adjust the digoxin dose accordingly.

The interaction between digoxin and **diclofenac** is less well established and its clinical importance is somewhat uncertain as the rises in digoxin levels were mostly small. It would be prudent to monitor concurrent use (e.g. for bradycardia) and monitor digoxin levels as necessary. Adjust the digoxin dose accordingly.

The minor changes seen in digoxin pharmacokinetics on the concurrent use of etoricoxib or lornoxicam are not expected to be clinically relevant. Similarly, no digoxin dose adjustments would appear to be necessary with fenbufen, isoxicam, ketoprofen, meloxicam, nimesulide, piroxicam, rofecoxib or tiaprofenic acid. With ibuprofen, the evidence is conflicting (although note that the one study reporting a potentially clinically relevant interaction was poor). Note that all NSAIDs can cause renal impairment, which would result in reduced renal elimination of digoxin and an increased risk of digoxin toxicity.

Digitoxin

The interaction between **phenylbutazone** and digitoxin appears to be in direct contrast to that with the other NSAIDs, but documentation is limited. However, phenylbutazone has, unlike many of the other NSAIDs, been found to have clinically relevant effects on hepatic enzymes. The dose of digitoxin might need to be increased to avoid under-digitalisation if phenylbutazone is added to established treatment. Monitor concurrent use well. Azapropazone does not appear to interact with digitoxin, and digitoxin does not appear to interact with diclofenac.

1. Faust-Tinnefeldt G, Gilfrich HJ. Digitoxin-Kinetik unter antirheumatischer Therapie mit Azapropazon. *Arzneimittelforschung* (1977) 27, 2009–11.
2. Schumacher A, Faust-Tinnefeldt G, Geissler HE, Gilfrich HJ, Mutschler E. Untersuchungen potentieller Interaktionen von Diclofenac-Natrium (Voltaren) mit einem Antazidum und mit Digitoxin. *Therapiewoche* (1983) 33, 2619–25.
3. Wirth KE. Arzneimittelinteraktionen bei der Anwendung herzwirksamer Glykoside. *Med Welt* (1981) 32, 234–8.
4. Solomon HM, Reich S, Spirt N, Abrams WB. Interactions between digitoxin and other drugs *in vitro* and *in vivo*. *Ann N Y Acad Sci* (1971) 179, 362–9.
5. Isbary J, Doering W, König E. Der Einfluβ von Tiaprofensäure auf die Digoxinkonzentration im Serum (DKS) im Vergleich zu anderen Antirheumatika (AR). *Z Rheumatol* (1982) 41, 164.
6. Rau R, Georgiopoulos G, Neumann P, Gross D. Die Beeinflussung des Digoxinblutspiegels durch Antirheumatika. *Akt Rheum* (1980) 5, 349–58.
7. Mannesse CK, van der Cammen TJM. Bijwerkingen van geneesmiddelen bij 3 oudere patiënten: ook bij ongewijzigd medicatiegebruik. *Ned Tijdschr Geneeskd* (2003) 147, 585–87.
8. Schwartz JI, Agarwal NGB, Wehling M, Musser BJ, Gumbs CP, Michiels N, De Smet M, Wagner JA. Evaluation of the pharmacokinetics of digoxin in healthy subjects receiving etoricoxib. *Br J Clin Pharmacol* (2008) 66, 811–17..
9. Dunky A, Eberi R. Anti-inflammatory effects of a new anti-rheumatic drug fenbufen in rheumatoid arthritis. XIV Int Congr Rheumatology, San Francisco, 1977. Abstract No 379.
10. Quattrocchi FP, Robinson JD, Curry RW, Grieco ML, Schulman SG. The effect of ibuprofen on serum digoxin concentrations. *Drug Intell Clin Pharm* (1983) 17, 286–8.
11. Jørgensen HS, Christensen HR, Kampmann JP. Interaction between digoxin and indomethacin or ibuprofen. *Br J Clin Pharmacol* (1991) 31, 108–110.
12. Koren G, Zarfin Y, Perlman M, MacLeod SM. Effects of indomethacin on digoxin pharmacokinetics in preterm infants. *Pediatr Pharmacol* (1984) 4, 25–30.
13. Mayes LC, Boerth RC. Digoxin-indomethacin interaction. *Pediatr Res* (1980) 14, 469.
14. Schimmel MS, Inwood RL, Eidelman AI, Eylath U. Toxic digitalis levels associated with indomethacin therapy in a neonate. *Clin Pediatr (Phila)* (1980) 19, 768–9.
15. Haig GM, Brookfield EG. Increase in serum digoxin concentrations after indomethacin therapy in a full-term neonate. *Pharmacotherapy* (1992) 12, 334–6.
16. Halawa B, Mazurek W. Interakcja digoksyny i niektórych niesteroidowych leków przeciwzapalnych, kwasu acetylosalicylowego i nifedipiny. *Pol Tyg Lek* (1982) 37, 1475–6.
17. Finch MB, Johnston GD, Kelly JG, McDevitt DG. Pharmacokinetics of digoxin alone and in the presence of indomethacin therapy. *Br J Clin Pharmacol* (1984) 17, 353–5.
18. Sziegoleit W, Weiss M, Fahr A, Förster W. Are serum levels and cardiac effects of digoxin influenced by indometacin? *Pharmazie* (1986) 41, 340–2.
19. Zöller B, Engel HJ, Faust-Tinnefeldt G, Gilfrich HJ, Zimmer M. Untersuchungen zur Wechselwirkung von Isoxicam und Digoxin. *Z Rheumatol* (1984) 43, 182–4.
20. Chlud K. Zur Frage der Interaktionen in der Rheumatherapie: Untersuchungen von Isoxicam und Glibenclamid bei Diabetien mit rheumatischen Enkrankungen. *Tempo Med* (1983) 12A, 15–18.
21. Lewis GR, Jacobs SG, Vavra I. Effect of ketoprofen on serum digoxin concentrations. *Curr Ther Res* (1985) 38, 494–9.
22. Ravic M, Johnston A, Turner P. Clinical pharmacological studies of some possible interactions of lornoxicam with other drugs. *Postgrad Med J* (1990) 66 (Suppl 4), S30–S34.
23. Degner FL, Heinzel G, Narjes H, Türck D. The effect of meloxicam on the pharmacokinetics of β-acetyldigoxin. *Br J Clin Pharmacol* (1995) 40, 486–8.
24. Baggio E, Maraffi F, Montalto C, Nava ML, Torti L, Casciarri I. A clinical assessment of the potential for pharmacological interaction between nimesulide and digoxin in patients with heart failure. *Drugs* (1993) 46 (Suppl 1), 91–4.
25. Rau R. Interaction study of piroxicam with digoxin. In 'Piroxicam: A New Non-steroidal Anti-inflammatory Agent.' Proc IXth Eur Cong Rheumatol, Wiesbaden, September 1979, pp 41–6. Academy Professional Information Services, NY.
26. Schwartz JI, De Smet M, Larson PJ, Verbesselt R, Ebel DL, Lins R, Lens S, Porras AG, Gertz BJ. Effect of rofecoxib on the pharmacokinetics of digoxin in healthy volunteers. *J Clin Pharmacol* (2001) 41, 107–112.
27. Doering W, Isbary J. Der Einfluß von Tiaprofensäure auf die Digoxin-konzentration im Serum. *Arzneimittelforschung* (1983) 33, 167–8.

Digoxin + Orlistat

Orlistat does not appear to affect the pharmacokinetics of digoxin.

Clinical evidence, mechanism, importance and management

In 12 healthy subjects, orlistat 120 mg three times daily for 6 days had no effect on the pharmacokinetics of a single 400-microgram oral dose of digoxin (in soft gelatin capsules).[1] This suggests that an approximate 30% reduction in dietary fat absorption induced by orlistat does not alter digoxin absorption, and that no digoxin dose adjustments are likely to be necessary on concurrent use.

1. Melia AT, Zhi J, Koss-Twardy SG, Min BH, Smith BL, Freundlich NL, Arora S, Passe SM. The influence of reduced dietary fat absorption induced by orlistat on the pharmacokinetics of digoxin in healthy volunteers. *J Clin Pharmacol* (1995) 35, 840–3.

Digoxin + Penicillamine

Penicillamine appears to reduce the serum levels digoxin, both after oral and intravenous administration.

Clinical evidence, mechanism, importance and management

In 10 patients, penicillamine 1 g daily taken 2 hours after an oral dose of digoxin, reduced the serum digoxin levels measured 2, 4 and 6 hours later, by 13%, 20% and 39%, respectively. In 10 other patients similarly treated but given digoxin intravenously, the serum digoxin levels measured 4 and 6 hours later were reduced by 23% and 64%, respectively.[1] The same authors have also reported this interaction in children.[2]

Information seems to be limited to the reports cited, and the reason for its occurrence is unknown. Patients taking digoxin should be checked for signs of under-digitalisation if penicillamine is added. Note that one manufacturer of penicillamine states that digoxin should not be taken within 2 hours of penicillamine.[3] However, the efficacy of this approach does not appear to have been studied, and as penicillamine can reduce the levels of digoxin given intravenously, it would appear that the interaction is not entirely related to digoxin absorption. Therefore it would still seem prudent to monitor concurrent use for digoxin efficacy, even if the doses are separated.

1. Moezzi B, Fatourechi V, Khozain R, Eslami B. The effect of penicillamine on serum digoxin levels. *Jpn Heart J* (1978) 19, 366–70.
2. Moezzi B, Khozein R, Pooymehr F, Shakibi JG. Reversal of digoxin-induced changes in erythrocyte electrolyte concentrations by penicillamine in children. *Jpn Heart J* (1980) 21, 335–9.
3. Distamine (Penicillamine). Alliance Pharmaceuticals. UK Summary of product characteristics, June 2010.

Digoxin and related drugs + Penicillins

Amoxicillin, flucloxacillin, phenoxymethylpenicillin and ticarcillin with clavulanic acid do not normally alter digoxin levels. Ampicillin does not alter digitoxin pharmacokinetics.

Clinical evidence

In 6 healthy subjects, **ampicillin** 500 mg four times daily for 5 days had no effect on the pharmacokinetics of a single 1-mg dose of **digitoxin**.[1] No changes in digoxin serum concentrations were found in 16 elderly patients given **amoxicillin** (2 patients also took erythromycin and one **flucloxacillin**), and 2 patients who took **flucloxacillin** and **phenoxymethylpenicillin**. However, a few patients complained of some 'toxic' symptoms (nausea, vomiting, anorexia, headache, fatigue, blurred vision, confusion), which the authors of the report attributed to the underlying illness or the antibacterials rather than to an interaction.[2] In a study in 15 healthy subjects, **ticarcillin** with **clavulanic acid** 1 g/200 mg intramuscularly every 12 hours for one week did not affect the pharmacokinetics of digoxin.[3] In another study, there was a reduction in the excretion of digoxin metabolites from the gut in only 1 of 10 patients taking penicillins (**ampicillin** 6, **oxacillin** 3, **penicillin** 1).[4]

Mechanism

Up to 10% of patients receiving oral digoxin excrete it in substantial amounts in the faeces and urine as inactive metabolites (digoxin reduction products or DRPs). This metabolism seems to be due to gut flora,[5] in particular *Eubacterium lentum*, which is anaerobic and Gram positive. It was suggested that inhibition of digoxin metabolism by gut flora was responsible for any interaction, but doubt has been thrown on this theory (see *Mechanism* under 'Digoxin and related drugs + Macrolides', p.1100).

Importance and management

The limited evidence above suggesting a lack of pharmacokinetic interaction, along with the silence in the literature on adverse interactions between digoxin and penicillins, and the limited evidence for a plausible mechanism suggest that interactions are unlikely. No digoxin dose adjustments would be expected to be needed on the concurrent use of penicillins.

1. Lucena MI, Moreno A, Fernandez MC, Garcia-Morillas M, Andrade R. Digitoxin elimination in healthy subjects taking ampicillin. *Int J Clin Pharmacol Res* (1987) VII, 33–7.
2. Rhodes KM, Brown SN. Do the penicillin antibiotics interact with digoxin? *Eur J Clin Pharmacol* (1994) 46, 479–80.
3. Cazzola M, Matera MG, Santangelo G, Angrisani M, Loffreda A, de Prisco F, Paizis G, Rossi F. Serum digoxin levels after concomitant ticarcillin and clavulanic acid administration. *Ther Drug Monit* (1994) 16, 46–8.
4. Dobkin JF, Saha JR, Butler VP, Lindenbaum J. Effects of antibiotic therapy on digoxin metabolism. *Clin Res* (1982) 30, 517A.
5. Lindenbaum J, Rund DG, Butler VP, Tse-Eng D, Saha JR. Inactivation of digoxin by the gut flora: reversal by antibiotic therapy. *N Engl J Med* (1981) 305, 789–94.

Digoxin and related drugs + Phenytoin

Limited evidence suggests that phenytoin reduces the levels of digoxin and digitoxin. Isolated cases of bradycardia have been seen in digitalised patients given phenytoin. Phenytoin was formerly used for the treatment of digitalis-induced cardiac arrhythmias, but sudden cardiac arrest has been reported.

Clinical evidence

(a) Acetyldigoxin

A study in 6 healthy subjects given beta-acetyldigoxin 400 micrograms daily found that the half-life of digoxin was reduced by 30% (from 33.9 hours to 23.7 hours) and its AUC was reduced by 23% after they took phenytoin 200 mg twice daily for a week. Total digoxin clearance increased by 27%.[1]

(b) Digitoxin

A single report describes a patient who had a fall in his plasma levels of digitoxin on three occasions when he was given phenytoin. On the third occasion, while taking digitoxin 200 micrograms daily, the addition of phenytoin 900 mg daily caused a 60% fall in digitoxin levels (from 25 nanograms/mL to 10 nanograms/mL) over 7 to 10 days.[2]

(c) Digoxin

A patient with Down's syndrome and mitral valve insufficiency taking digoxin 250 micrograms daily developed bradycardia of 34 bpm and complete heart block when his phenytoin dose was increased from 200 mg daily to 300 mg daily.[3]

(d) Unnamed digitalis glycosides

A patient with suspected digitalis-induced cardiac arrhythmias developed bradycardia, then became asystolic and died, following an intravenous injection of phenytoin.[4] The discussion of this case briefly mentions a further 6 fatalities in patients similarly treated.[4]

Mechanism

Phenytoin has a stabilising effect on the myocardial cells so that the toxic threshold of digoxin at which arrhythmias occur is raised. However, the bradycardic effects of the digitalis glycoside are not opposed and the lethal dose is unaltered, so that the cardiac arrest reported would appear to be the result of excessive bradycardia. It seems possible that the fall in plasma digitoxin levels could be due to a phenytoin-induced increase in the metabolism of the digitoxin by the liver.[5]

Importance and management

Phenytoin was formerly used for treating digitalis-induced arrhythmias, but this use now appears to be obsolete. Intravenous phenytoin should not be used in patients with a high degree of heart block or marked bradycardia because of the risk that cardiac arrest may occur. Information about the effects of phenytoin on digitalis glycoside levels seems to be confined to these single reports, but it would seem be prudent to check that patients who are taking digitoxin (and possibly digoxin), and are subsequently given phenytoin, do not become under-digitalised.

1. Rameis H. On the interaction between phenytoin and digoxin. *Eur J Clin Pharmacol* (1985) 29, 49–53.
2. Solomon HM, Reich S, Spirt N, Abrams WB. Interactions between digitoxin and other drugs *in vitro* and *in vivo*. *Ann N Y Acad Sci* (1971) 179, 362–9.
3. Viukari NMA, Aho K. Digoxin-phenytoin interaction. *BMJ* (1970) 2, 51.
4. Zoneraich S, Zoneraich O, Siegel J. Sudden death following intravenous sodium diphenylhydantoin. *Am Heart J* (1976) 91, 375–7.
5. Rameis H. The importance of prospective planning of pharmacokinetic trials. Considerations of studies on the phenytoin-digoxin-(P-D) and phenytoin-digitoxin-(P-DT) interaction. *Int J Clin Pharmacol Ther Toxicol* (1992) 30, 528–9.

Digoxin + Phosphodiesterase type-5 inhibitors

Tadalafil and vardenafil do not alter digoxin exposure.

Clinical evidence, mechanism, importance and management

(a) Tadalafil

Tadalafil 40 mg once daily for 10 days had no effect on the steady-state pharmacokinetics of digoxin 250 micrograms daily in healthy subjects.[1] No digoxin dose adjustments would therefore be expected to be needed in patients given tadalafil.

(b) Vardenafil

In a placebo-controlled study, 19 healthy subjects were given digoxin 375 micrograms daily for 28 days, with vardenafil 20 mg daily on alternate days from day 16 to day 28. The pharmacokinetics of digoxin were not affected by vardenafil.[2] No digoxin dose adjustments would therefore be expected to be needed in patients given vardenafil.

1. Adcirca (Tadalafil). Eli Lilly and Company. US Prescribing information, April 2015.
2. Rohde G, Bauer R-J, Unger S, Ahr G, Wensing G. Vardenafil, a new selective PDE5 inhibitor, produces no interaction with digoxin. *Pharmacotherapy* (2001) 21, 1254.

Digoxin and related drugs + Pinaverium

Digoxin levels are not affected by pinaverium in patients taking digoxin, beta-acetyldigoxin or metildigoxin. Pinaverium does not alter digitoxin levels.

Clinical evidence, mechanism, importance and management

A study in 25 patients, taking either **beta-acetyldigoxin** or **metildigoxin** for congestive heart failure, found that pinaverium 50 mg three times daily for 12 days had no effect on their plasma digoxin levels.[1] Two other studies in patients taking either digoxin 125 to 250 micrograms daily or **digitoxin** 100 micrograms daily, or every other day, found that pinaverium bromide 50 mg three times daily did not affect cardiac glycoside blood levels.[2] No dose adjustments of these digitalis glycosides seem necessary on the concurrent use of pinaverium.

1. Weitzel O, Seidel G, Engelbert S, Berksoy M, Eberhardt G, Bode R. Investigation of possible interaction between pinaverium bromide and digoxin. *Curr Med Res Opin* (1983) 8, 600–2.
2. Devred C , Godeau P, Guerot C, Librez P, Mougeot G, Orsetti A, Segrestaa J-M. Investigation of drug interactions with pinaverium bromide. *Curr Med Res Opin* (1986) 10, 1–9.

Digoxin + Prasugrel

The manufacturers report that prasugrel has no clinically significant effect on the pharmacokinetics of digoxin.[1,2] Therefore no digoxin dose adjustments are likely to be needed on the concurrent use of prasugrel.

1. Efient (Prasugrel hydrochloride). Eli Lilly and Company Ltd. UK Summary of product characteristics, December 2013.
2. Effient (Prasugrel). Eli Lilly and Company. US Prescribing information, November 2013.

Digoxin + Probenecid

Probenecid does not appear to affect digoxin levels.

Clinical evidence, mechanism, importance and management

In a study in 2 healthy subjects taking digoxin 250 micrograms daily, *ColBenemid* (probenecid 500 mg with colchicine 500 micrograms) twice daily for 3 days had no effect on plasma digoxin levels.[1] In another study in 6 healthy subjects, probenecid 2 g daily for 8 days had no effect on the pharmacokinetics of digoxin.[2] No digoxin dose adjustments would appear to be necessary on the concurrent use of probenecid.

1. Jaillon P, Weissenburger J, Cheymol G, Graves P, Marcus F. Les effets du probénécide sur la concentration plasmatique à l'équilibre de digoxine. *Therapie* (1980) 35, 655–6.
2. Hedman A, Angelin B, Arvidsson A, Dahlqvist R. No effect of probenecid on the renal and biliary clearances of digoxin in man. *Br J Clin Pharmacol* (1991) 32, 63–7.

Digoxin + Procainamide

Procainamide does not appear to affect digoxin levels.

Clinical evidence, mechanism, importance and management

In a prospective study in 22 patients who had been taking digoxin for at least 7 days, procainamide (given to steady-state) did not affect serum digoxin levels.[1] This suggests that no digoxin dose adjustments are likely to be necessary on concurrent use.

1. Leahey EB, Reiffel JA, Giardina E-GV, Bigger JT. The effect of quinidine and other oral antiarrhythmic drugs on serum digoxin: a prospective study. *Ann Intern Med* (1980) 92, 605–8.

Digoxin + Propafenone

Propafenone can increase digoxin levels by 30 to 90%, and even more in children.

Clinical evidence

In 5 patients, propafenone (increasing over 6 days to 300 mg every 8 hours) increased the mean steady-state serum levels of digoxin 125 to 250 micrograms daily by 83%. Three patients continued to take both drugs for 6 months, at which point the digoxin levels were 63% higher. No digitalis toxicity was seen.[1] In another study, propafenone 600 mg daily in divided doses increased the steady-state serum digoxin levels of 10 patients by 90% (from 0.97 nanograms/mL to 1.54 nanograms/mL), and two of them developed symptoms of toxicity (nausea, vomiting).[2] An even greater increase was seen in 3 children, who had rises in their serum digoxin levels of 112 to 254% over 3 to 24 days when given propafenone 250 to 500 mg/m^2 daily.[3] The mean AUC of digoxin increased by 14% in 27 patients receiving propafenone 10 mg/kg daily in divided doses. However, there was great inter-individual variability, with 22 patients having an increase in AUC, and 5 a decrease in AUC. One patient experienced digoxin toxicity resulting in fatal ventricular fibrillation.[4]

Propafenone 450 mg daily increased the mean steady-state plasma digoxin levels of 12 healthy subjects by about 35% (from 0.58 nanograms/mL to 0.78 nanograms/mL), and the cardiac effects were increased accordingly.[5] In a study in 6 subjects[6] given a single 1-mg intravenous dose of digoxin, propafenone 150 or 300 mg every 8 hours increased the AUC of digoxin by 28% and decreased the total clearance of digoxin by 22%. A similar study with oral digoxin found a 25% increase in the AUC of digoxin when healthy subjects were given propafenone.[7]

Mechanism

Not understood. One suggestion is that propafenone increases the bioavailability of digoxin.[7] Another is that the volume of distribution and non-renal clearance of digoxin are changed by the propafenone.[6] Conversely, others reported that propafenone decreased the renal clearance of digoxin.[2,5] There is certainly some *in vitro* evidence that propafenone and its metabolite inhibit P-glycoprotein, which is concerned with digoxin secretion by the renal tubular cells.[8,9]

Importance and management

The interaction between digoxin and propafenone is very well established and of clinical importance. Monitor the effects of concurrent use and reduce the digoxin dose appropriately in order to avoid toxicity. Most patients appear to be affected and dose reductions in the range of 15 to 70% were found necessary in one of the studies cited.[2] The data available suggest that the extent of the rise might depend on the propafenone serum concentration rather than on its dose.[6,10]

1. Salerno DM, Granrud G, Sharkey P, Asinger R, Hodges M. A controlled trial of propafenone for treatment of frequent and repetitive ventricular premature complexes. *Am J Cardiol* (1984) 53, 77–83.
2. Calvo MV, Martin-Suarez A, Luengo CM, Avila C, Cascon M, Hurlé AD-G. Interaction between digoxin and propafenone. *Ther Drug Monit* (1989) 11, 10–15.
3. Zalzstein E, Koren G, Bryson SM, Freedom RM. Interaction between digoxin and propafenone in children. *J Pediatr* (1990) 116, 310–2.
4. Palumbo E, Svetoni N, Casini M, Spargi T, Biagi G, Martelli F, Lanzetta T. Interazione digoxina-propafenone: valori e limiti del dosaggio plasmatico dis due farmaci. *G Ital Cardiol* (1986) 16, 855–62.
5. Belz GG, Doering W, Munkes R, Matthews J. Interaction between digoxin and calcium antagonists and antiarrhythmic drugs. *Clin Pharmacol Ther* (1983) 33, 410–17.
6. Nolan PE, Marcus FI, Erstad BL, Hoyer GK, Furman C, Kirsten EB. Effects of coadministration of propafenone on the pharmacokinetics of digoxin in healthy volunteer subjects. *J Clin Pharmacol* (1989) 29, 46–52.
7. Cardaioli P, Compostella L, De Domenico R, Papalia D, Zeppellini R, Libardoni M, Pulido E, Cucchini F. Influenza del propafenone sulla farmacocinetica della digossina somministrata per via orale: studio su volontari sani. *G Ital Cardiol* (1986) 16, 237–40.
8. Woodland C, Verjee Z, Giesbrecht E, Koren G, Ito S. The digoxin-propafenone interaction: characterization of a mechanism using renal tubular cell monolayers. *J Pharmacol Exp Ther* (1997) 283, 39–45.
9. Bachmakov I, Rekersbrink S, Hofmann U, Eichelbaum M, Fromm MF. Characterisation of (*R/S*)-propafenone and its metabolites as substrates and inhibitors of P-glycoprotein. *Naunyn Schmiedebergs Arch Pharmacol* (2005) 371, 195–201.
10. Bigot M-C, Debruyne D, Bonnefoy L, Grollier G, Moulin M, Potier J-C. Serum digoxin levels related to plasma propafenone levels during concomitant treatment. *J Clin Pharmacol* (1991) 31, 521–6.

Digoxin + Propantheline

Digoxin levels can be increased if propantheline is given with slow-dissolving forms of digoxin tablets. However, propantheline does not appear to affect digoxin levels when digoxin is given as a liquid or in soft-gelatin capsules or in the form of fast-dissolving tablets.

Clinical evidence

The serum digoxin levels of 9 out of 13 patients rose by 30% (from 1.02 nanograms/mL to 1.33 nanograms/mL), when they took a slow-dissolving formulation of digoxin tablets (*Orion*) with propantheline 15 mg three times daily for 10 days. The serum digoxin levels stayed the same in 3 patients and fell slightly in one patient. An associated study in 4 healthy subjects given digoxin in liquid form found that serum digoxin levels were unaffected by propantheline.[1]

Another study by the same workers found that propantheline increased the digoxin serum levels of a slow-dissolving tablet formulation (*Orion*) by 40%, but had no effect on serum digoxin levels with a fast-dissolving tablet formulation (*Lanoxin*).[2] In a further study, propantheline increased the AUC of digoxin from *Lanoxin* tablets by 24%, compared with a non-statistically significant increase of 13% with digoxin in the form of a solution in a capsule (*Lanoxicaps*).[3]

Mechanism

Propantheline is an antimuscarinic, which reduces gut motility. This allows the slow-dissolving formulations of digoxin more time to pass into solution so that more is available for absorption.

Importance and management

The interaction between digoxin and propantheline appears to be established, but it is only of importance if slow-dissolving digoxin formulations are used. With slow-dissolving forms of digoxin tablets it might be necessary to reduce the digoxin dose in those also taking propantheline. No interaction is likely with liquid or liquid-filled capsule forms of digoxin.

1. Manninen V, Apajalahti A, Melin J, Karesoja M. Altered absorption of digoxin in patients given propantheline and metoclopramide. *Lancet* (1973) i, 398–400.
2. Manninen V, Apajalahti A, Simonen H, Reissell P. Effect of propantheline and metoclopramide on absorption of digoxin. *Lancet* (1973) i, 1118–19.
3. Brown DD, Schmid J, Long RA, Hull JH. A steady-state evaluation of the effects of propantheline bromide and cholestyramine on the bioavailability of digoxin when administered as tablets or capsules. *J Clin Pharmacol* (1985) 25, 360–4.

Digoxin + Prostaglandins

Epoprostenol appears to cause a small decrease in digoxin clearance in the short-term. Iloprost does not appear to affect digoxin pharmacokinetics.

Clinical evidence, mechanism, importance and management

(a) Epoprostenol

In a pharmacokinetic modelling study in patients with congestive heart failure, the clearance of digoxin was an estimated 15% lower the day after starting a continuous maintenance infusion of epoprostenol, but this effect was no longer apparent by the end of 12 weeks of concurrent use.[1] Further pharmacokinetic modelling suggested that this increase in digoxin bioavailability was attributable to an increase in gastrointestinal blood flow induced by epoprostenol.[2] The apparent initial small decrease in clearance seems unlikely to be clinically important. However, the authors of the report suggest that the possible short-term changes in patients with high trough plasma digoxin levels and those prone to digoxin toxicity should be borne in mind when using the combination.[1]

(b) Iloprost

In a study, 12 patients taking digoxin 250 micrograms daily were given a 6-hour intravenous infusion of iloprost 2 nanograms/kg per minute over a period of 20 days. The mean time to maximum digoxin levels was delayed by an hour, but overall the pharmacokinetics of the digoxin were unchanged.[3,4] No digoxin dose adjustment would be expected to be necessary if iloprost is also given.

1. Carlton LD, Patterson JH, Mattson CN, Schmith VD. The effects of epoprostenol on drug disposition I. A pilot study of the pharmacokinetics of digoxin with and without epoprostenol in patients with congestive heart failure. *J Clin Pharmacol* (1996) 36, 247–56.
2. Carlton LD, Pollack GM, Brouwer KLR. Physiologic pharmacokinetic modelling of gastrointestinal blood flow as a rate-limiting step in the oral absorption of digoxin: implications for patients with congestive heart failure receiving epoprostenol. *J Pharm Sci* (1996) 85, 473–77.
3. Cabane J, Penin I, Bouslama K, Benchouieb A, Giral Ph, Picard O, Wattiaux MJ, Cheymol G, Souvignet G, Imbert JC. Traitement par iloprost des ischémies critiques des membres inférieurs associées à une insuffisance cardiaque. *Therapie* (1991) 46, 235–40.
4. Penin E, Cheymol G, Bouslama K, Benchouieb A, Cabane J, Souvignet G. No pharmacokinetic interaction between iloprost and digoxin. *Eur J Clin Pharmacol* (1991) 41, 505–6.

Digoxin and related drugs + Proton pump inhibitors

The exposure to digoxin was negligibly to very slightly increased by omeprazole, pantoprazole and rabeprazole. One case of digoxin toxicity has been reported with omeprazole.

Clinical evidence

(a) Omeprazole

In a study in healthy subjects, omeprazole 20 mg daily for 11 days caused only minor changes in the disposition of a single 1-mg oral dose of digoxin. On average the AUC was increased by 10%, with an increase of about 30% in 2 subjects, but this was within the accepted range of bioequivalence.[1] However, a 65-year-old woman had signs of digoxin toxicity 3 months after starting to take omeprazole 20 mg daily. She was found to have a digoxin level of 3.9 nanograms/mL (previous level 1.1 nanograms/mL) and ECG changes, which resolved after she was given digoxin immune Fab. Her renal function was normal.[2]

(b) Pantoprazole

Beta-acetyldigoxin 200 micrograms twice daily was given to 18 healthy subjects, with and without pantoprazole 40 mg daily, for 5 days. Pantoprazole caused a 10% rise in the AUC of digoxin. There were no changes in the digoxin-induced height reduction in the T-wave on the ECG.[3]

(c) Rabeprazole

A preliminary report, giving few details, states that rabeprazole increased the trough levels of digoxin by about 20%, and also increased its AUC and maximum level.[4] The US manufacturer of rabeprazole states that it increases the AUC and maximum level of digoxin by 19%, and 29%, respectively.[5] However, the data on the digoxin interaction was removed from the UK manufacturers' information, because the changes in digoxin levels were thought to be within the normal limits of bioequivalence.[6] A study in 47 patients regularly taking digoxin and either **lansoprazole** or omeprazole found that changing the proton pump inhibitor to an equivalent dose of rabeprazole did not change the mean serum digoxin level, although 12 of the patients had increases of more than 15%.[7]

Mechanism

Uncertain. The increase in digoxin levels with omeprazole might be the result of a higher gastric pH, which results in less digoxin hydrolysis and an increase in digoxin absorption.[8] If this mechanism is correct, it would apply to all proton pump inhibitors. It has been suggested that non-selective digoxin assay methods are not sensitive enough to detect an interaction, whereas selective HPLC assay methods and ECG studies provide evidence that the bioavailability of digoxin might be increased by omeprazole.[8] Alternatively, an *in vitro* study found that omeprazole, pantoprazole and lansoprazole inhibit the P-glycoprotein-mediated intestinal transport of digoxin, which would increase digoxin levels.[9]

Importance and management

Although some studies suggest minor changes in digoxin pharmacokinetics might occur with omeprazole, pantoprazole and rabeprazole, these changes are unlikely to be clinically important. No digoxin dose adjustment would therefore seem to be necessary if proton pump inhibitors and digoxin are given concurrently. However, some manufacturers advise caution with the combination and state that digoxin levels might need to be monitored, particularly with high doses of the proton pump inhibitor used in the elderly.

1. Oosterhuis B, Jonkman JHG, Andersson T, Zuiderwijk PBM, Jedema JN. Minor effect of multiple dose omeprazole on the pharmacokinetics of digoxin after a single oral dose. *Br J Clin Pharmacol* (1991) 32, 569–72.
2. Kiley CA, Cragin DJ, Roth BJ. Omeprazole-associated digoxin toxicity. *South Med J* (2007) 100, 400–2.
3. Hartmann M, Huber R, Bliesath H, Steinijans VW, Koch HJ, Wurst W, Kunz K. Lack of interaction between pantoprazole and digoxin at therapeutic doses in man. *Int J Clin Pharmacol Ther* (1995) 33, 481–5.
4. Humphries TJ, Nardi RV, Lazar JD, Spanyers SA. Drug-drug interaction evaluation of rabeprazole sodium: a clean/expected slate? *Gut* (1996) 39 (Suppl 3), A47.
5. Aciphex (Rabeprazole sodium). Eisai Inc. US Prescribing information, May 2012.
6. Anon. Notice board. *Pharm J* (2003) 271, 541.
7. Le GH, Schaefer MG, Plowman BK, Morreale AP, Delattre M, Okino L, Felicio L. Assessment of potential digoxin-rabeprazole interaction after formulary conversion of proton-pump inhibitors. *Am J Health-Syst Pharm* (2003) 60, 1343–5.
8. Cohen AF, Kroon R, Schoemaker HC, Hoogkamer JFW, van Vliet-Verbeek A. Effects of gastric acidity on the bioavailability of digoxin. Evidence for a new mechanism for interactions with omeprazole. *Br J Clin Pharmacol* (1991) 31, 565P.
9. Pauli-Magnus C, Rekersbrink S, Klotz U, Fromm MF. Interaction of omeprazole, lansoprazole and pantoprazole with P-glycoprotein. *Naunyn Schmiedebergs Arch Pharmacol* (2001) 364, 551–7.

Digoxin and related drugs + Quinidine

In most patients the serum levels of digoxin are approximately doubled within five days of starting quinidine. Digitoxin levels are also increased by quinidine, but possibly to a lesser extent, and the interaction takes a longer period of time to develop.

Clinical evidence

(a) Digitoxin

Quinidine 750 mg daily increased the steady-state plasma digitoxin levels of 8 healthy subjects by 45% (from 13.6 nanograms/mL to 19.7 nanograms/mL), over 32 days.[1] In another study in healthy subjects, there was a similar 31% increase in serum digitoxin levels over just 10 days,[2] whereas yet another found a greater 115% increase in plasma levels after 70 days of use of quinidine 360 mg three times daily.[3] A further study in 5 healthy subjects found that quinidine reduced the total body clearance of digitoxin by 63%, resulting in raised serum digitoxin levels.[4]

(b) Digoxin

The observation that quinidine appeared to increase serum digoxin levels prompted a retrospective study of patient records, which revealed that 25 out of 27 patients taking digoxin had a rise in their serum digoxin levels from 1.4 nanograms/mL to 3.2 nanograms/mL when given quinidine. Of the patients who had a rise, 16 developed typical signs of digoxin toxicity (nausea, vomiting, anorexia), which resolved in 10 of them when the dose of digoxin was reduced or when digoxin was withdrawn, and in 5 when quinidine was withdrawn.[5] This is one of the first reports published in 1978 (two other groups independently reported it at a similar time[6,7]) that clearly describes this interaction, although hints of its existence can be found in papers published over the previous 50 years. Since then large numbers of research reports, both retrospective and prospective, and case studies have confirmed and established the incidence and magnitude of this interaction. It occurs in over 90% of patients and, on average, there is a 100% increase in serum digoxin levels, although there are pronounced inter-individual differences and the increase is somewhat dependent on the quinidine dose. There are numerous reports and reviews of this interaction, only a selection of which are listed here. Two reviews published in 1982 and 1983 contain valuable bibliographies.[8,9]

Mechanism

Digoxin is a substrate of the efflux pump, P-glycoprotein. Quinidine appears to reduce the renal excretion of digoxin (by 40 to 50%), as well as reducing digoxin excretion in the bile[10] and increasing the rate and extent of absorption of digoxin from the gut.[11] More recent studies show that the mechanism behind these effects on absorption and renal excretion is likely to be P-glycoprotein inhibition by quinidine.[12-14] Digoxin also appears to cause a small reduction in the renal clearance of quinidine.[15] Quinidine appears to increase digitoxin serum levels by reducing its non-renal clearance.

Importance and management

The interaction between **digoxin** and quinidine is very well-documented, well-established and of definite clinical importance. As serum digoxin levels are usually roughly doubled (up to fivefold increases have been seen[8]) and over 90% of patients are affected, digitalis toxicity seems likely to develop unless the dose of digoxin is reduced (approximately halved).[5,8,16,17] Another suggested rule-of-thumb is that if serum digoxin levels are no greater than 0.9 nanograms/mL and potassium levels are within the reference range then the addition of quinidine is unlikely to cause toxic digoxin levels, whereas with levels of 1 nanogram/mL or more, toxic concentrations can develop.[18] Monitor the effects and readjust the dose as necessary. Clinically relevant effects occur within a day of taking quinidine and reach a maximum after about 3 to 6 days (quicker or slower in some patients), but digoxin levels will only stabilise when the quinidine has reached steady-state and that depends on whether a loading dose of quinidine is given. The effects are to some extent dose-related but the correlation is not good: less than 400 to 500 mg of quinidine daily has minimal effects, and increasing doses up to 1.2 g has greater effects.[16,19] About 5 days are needed after withdrawing the quinidine before serum digoxin levels fall to their former levels. It has been recommended that patients with chronic renal failure should have their digoxin dose reduced by as much as two-thirds.[20-22] An appropriate upward readjustment will be necessary if the quinidine is subsequently withdrawn.

Far less is known about the interaction between **digitoxin** and quinidine but it appears to develop much more slowly. Similar precautions to those suggested for digoxin should be taken.

1. Kuhlmann J, Dohrmann M, Marcin S. Effects of quinidine on pharmacokinetics and pharmacodynamics of digitoxin achieving steady-state conditions. *Clin Pharmacol Ther* (1986) 39, 288–94.
2. Peters U, Risler T, Grabensee B, Falkenstein U, Kroukou J. Interaktion von Chinidin und Digitoxin beim Menschen. *Dtsch Med Wochenschr* (1980) 105, 438–42.
3. Kreutz G, Keller F, Gast D and Prokein E. Digitoxin-quinidine interaction achieving steady-state conditions for both drugs. *Naunyn Schmiedebergs Arch Pharmacol* (1982) 319, R82.
4. Garty M, Sood P, Rollins DE. Digitoxin elimination reduced during quinidine therapy. *Ann Intern Med* (1981) 94, 35–7.
5. Leahey EB, Reiffel JA, Drusin RE, Heisenbuttel RH, Lovejoy WP, Bigger JT. Interaction between quinidine and digoxin. *JAMA* (1978) 240, 533–4.
6. Ejvinsson G. Effect of quinidine on plasma concentrations of digoxin. *BMJ* (1978) i, 279–80.
7. Reid PR, Meek AG. Digoxin-quinidine interaction. *Johns Hopkins Med J* (1979) 145, 227–9.
8. Bigger JT, Leahey EB. Quinidine and digoxin. An important interaction. *Drugs* (1982) 24, 229–39.
9. Fichtl B, Doering W. The quinidine-digoxin interaction in perspective. *Clin Pharmacokinet* (1983) 8, 137–54.
10. Schenck-Gustafsson K, Angelin B, Hedman A, Arvidsson A, Dahlqvist R. Quinidine-induced reduction of the biliar excretion of digoxin in patients. *Circulation* (1985) 72 (Suppl), III-19.
11. Pedersen KE, Christiansen BD, Klitgaard NA, Nielsen-Kudsk F. Effect of quinidine on digoxin bioavailability. *Eur J Clin Pharmacol* (1983) 24, 41–7.
12. Su S-F, Huang J-D. Inhibition of the intestinal digoxin absorption and exsorption by quinidine. *Drug Metab Dispos* (1996) 24, 142–7.
13. Fromm MF, Kim RB, Stein CM, Wilkinson GR, Roden DM. Inhibition of P-glycoprotein–mediated drug transport. A unifying mechanism to explain the interaction between digoxin and quinidine. *Circulation* (1999) 99, 552–7.
14. Drescher S, Glaeser H, Mürdter T, Hitzl M, Eichelbaum M, Fromm MF. P-glycoprotein–mediated intestinal and biliary digoxin transport in humans. *Clin Pharmacol Ther* (2003) 73, 223–31.
15. Rameis H. Quinidine-digoxin interaction: are the pharmacokinetics of both drugs altered? *Int J Clin Pharmacol Ther Toxicol* (1985) 23, 145–53.
16. Doering W. Quinidine-digoxin interaction: pharmacokinetics, underlying mechanism and clinical implications. *N Engl J Med* (1979) 301, 400–4.
17. Leahey EB, Reiffel JA, Heissenbuttel RH, Drusin RE, Lovejoy WP, Bigger JT. Enhanced cardiac effect of digoxin during quinidine treatment. *Arch Intern Med* (1979) 139, 519–21.
18. Friedman HS, Chen T-S. Use of control steady-state serum digoxin levels for predicting serum digoxin concentration after quinidine administration. *Am Heart J* (1982) 104, 72–6.

19. Fenster PE, Powell JR, Hager WD, Graves PE, Conrad K, Goldman S. Onset and dose dependence of digoxin-quinidine interaction. *Am J Cardiol* (1980) 45, 413.
20. Fichtl B, Doering W, Seidel H. The quinidine-digoxin interaction in patients with impaired renal function. *Int J Clin Pharmacol Ther Toxicol* (1983) 21, 229–33.
21. Fenster PE, Hager WD, Perrier D, Powell JR, Graves PE, Michael UF. Digoxin-quinidine interaction in patients with chronic renal failure. *Circulation* (1982) 66, 1277–80.
22. Woodcock BG, Rietbrock N. Digitalis-quinidine interactions. *Trends Pharmacol Sci* (1982) 3, 118–22.

Digoxin + Quinine

In some studies, quinine raised digoxin levels, whereas no effect was reported in other studies. A case report describes digoxin toxicity in an elderly patient, which developed during the concurrent use of quinine.

Clinical evidence

After taking quinine 300 mg four times daily for a day, the steady-state digoxin levels of 4 subjects taking digoxin 250 micrograms daily rose by 63%, from 0.49 nanograms/mL to 0.8 nanograms/mL. After taking the quinine for a further 3 days the digoxin levels rose a further 11% (to 0.86 nanograms/mL). Digoxin renal clearance fell by 20%.[1]

Smaller rises in digoxin levels were seen in another study where quinine sulfate 250 mg daily for 7 days increased the mean serum digoxin levels of 7 healthy subjects by 25%, from 0.64 nanograms/mL to 0.8 nanograms/mL. When quinine sulfate 250 mg was given three times daily there was a further 8% rise. Considerable individual differences were seen; one subject had a 92% rise.[2] Another study found that quinine reduced the total clearance of intravenous digoxin by 26%, without any effect on renal clearance.[3]

In contrast, 17 patients given quinine 750 mg daily had only a small and statistically insignificant rise in mean serum digoxin levels, from 0.8 nanograms/mL to 0.91 nanograms/mL. Serum levels were virtually unaltered in 11 patients, decreased in two and sizeably increased (amount not stated) in four.[4]

An 76-year-old man with hypertension and atrial fibrillation taking digoxin 500 micrograms daily and quinine sulfate 750 mg daily as well as aspirin, candesartan and amlodipine was admitted after an episode of fainting, and an ECG detected AV block, a prolonged QTc interval of 570 milliseconds and torsade de pointes. Digoxin levels were found to be 5 nanograms/mL. The authors attributed the effect to digoxin toxicity caused by the presence of quinine.[5]

Mechanism

Not fully understood. A reduction in non-renal clearance is apparently largely responsible for the rise in serum digoxin levels with quinine.[2,3,6] This is possibly due to changes in digoxin metabolism or in its biliary excretion.[3,6]

Importance and management

The interaction between digoxin and quinine is established and clinically important, but only moderately well documented. Monitor the effects of concurrent use (e.g. for bradycardia) and reduce the digoxin dose where necessary. Some patients might have a substantial increase in serum digoxin levels; nevertheless, there appears to be only one case report of digoxin toxicity arising from this interaction.

1. Aronson JK, Carver JG. Interaction of digoxin with quinine. *Lancet* (1981) i, 1418.
2. Pedersen KE, Madsen JL, Klitgaard NA, Kjær K, Hvidt S. Effect of quinine on plasma digoxin concentration and renal digoxin clearance. *Acta Med Scand* (1985) 218, 229–32.
3. Wandell M, Powell JR, Hager WD, Fenster PE, Graves PE, Conrad KA, Goldman S. Effect of quinine on digoxin kinetics. *Clin Pharmacol Ther* (1980) 28, 425–30.
4. Doering W. Is there a clinically relevant interaction between quinine and digoxin in human beings? *Am J Cardiol* (1981) 48, 975–6.
5. Ramirez A, Galván JM. Taquicardia ventricular tipo torsades de pointes en un paciente con intoxicación digitálica en tratamiento crónico con sulfato de quinina. *Med Intensiva* (2007) 31, 106–7.
6. Hedman A, Angelin B, Arvidsson A, Dahlqvist R, Nilsson B. Interactions in the renal and biliary elimination of digoxin: stereoselective difference between quinine and quinidine. *Clin Pharmacol Ther* (1990) 47, 20–6.

Digoxin and related drugs + Quinolones

Gatifloxacin can cause a small increase in digoxin levels and a very slight increase in digoxin exposure. Levofloxacin, gemifloxacin, moxifloxacin and sparfloxacin do not affect the pharmacokinetics of digoxin. Moxifloxacin does not appear to affect the exposure to beta-acetyldigoxin or digoxin. The effects of garenoxacin on digoxin pharmacokinetics are unclear.

Clinical evidence

(a) Garenoxacin

In a study designed to look at the effects of garenoxacin on gut flora, 16 healthy subjects were given digoxin 250 micrograms every 6 hours on day one, then 250 micrograms daily to day 14, with garenoxacin 600 mg daily on days 8 to 14. Garenoxacin did not decrease (but might actually increase) the numbers of *E. lentum* in faeces (see 'Digoxin and related drugs + Macrolides', p.1100, for an explanation of the possible significance of these findings). Thus an interaction due to the effect of garenoxacin on intestinal microflora is unlikely.[1]

(b) Gatifloxacin

The vital signs of 12 healthy subjects given gatifloxacin 400 mg daily for 7 days while taking digoxin 250 micrograms daily were not altered. The AUC and steady-state levels of digoxin were increased by 19% and 12% respectively. Dose adjustments were not considered necessary.[2]

(c) Gemifloxacin

In placebo-controlled study in 14 healthy subjects, gemifloxacin 320 mg daily for 7 days did not affect the pharmacokinetics of digoxin 250 micrograms daily. No clinically important changes in vital signs or ECGs were found.[3]

(d) Levofloxacin

The pharmacokinetics of a single 400-microgram dose of digoxin were unchanged when 12 healthy subjects were given levofloxacin 500 mg twice daily for 6 days.[4]

(e) Moxifloxacin

In 14 healthy subjects, moxifloxacin 400 mg daily for 14 days did not cause any clinically relevant changes in the steady-state pharmacokinetics of digoxin 250 micrograms daily.[5] No pharmacokinetic changes were seen in another study with 12 healthy subjects given a single 600-microgram dose of **beta-acetyldigoxin** with moxifloxacin 400 mg daily for 2 days.[6]

(f) Sparfloxacin

In 24 healthy subjects, sparfloxacin, 400 mg as a loading dose, followed by 200 mg daily for 9 days did not affect the pharmacokinetics of digoxin 300 micrograms daily.[7]

Mechanism

Up to 10% of patients receiving oral digoxin excrete it in substantial amounts in the faeces and urine as inactive metabolites (digoxin reduction products or DRPs). This metabolism seems to be due to gut flora,[8] in particular *Eubacterium lentum*, which is anaerobic and Gram positive. However, there is some doubt about this as a probable mechanism and, despite *in vitro* susceptibility of *E. lentum* to a range of antibacterials including some quinolones, there is currently no information to suggest that quinolones inhibit the gut flora-mediated metabolism of digoxin.[9] For further information on the possible significance of *E. lentum*, see *Mechanism* under 'Digoxin and related drugs + Macrolides', p.1100.

Importance and management

There appears to be no clinically relevant interaction between digoxin and the quinolones studied (gatifloxacin, gemifloxacin, levofloxacin, moxifloxacin and sparfloxacin). Information about other digitalis glycosides and quinolones generally seems to be lacking. Bearing in mind their extensive use, this silence in the literature would suggest that no problems usually arise.

1. Nord CE, Meurling L, Russo RL, Bello A, Grasela DM, Gajjar DA. Effect of garenoxacin on Eubacteria in the normal intestinal microflora when administered concomitantly with digoxin. *J Chemother* (2003) 15, 244–7.
2. Olsen SJ, Uderman HD, Kaul S, Kollia GD, Birkhoffer MJ, Grasela DM. Pharmacokinetics of concomitantly administered gatifloxacin and digoxin. *Intersci Conf Antimicrob Agents Chemother* (1999) 39, 12.
3. Vousden M, Allen A, Lewis A, Ehren N. Lack of pharmacokinetic interaction between gemifloxacin and digoxin in healthy elderly volunteers. *Chemotherapy* (1999) 45, 485–90.
4. Chien S-C, Rogge MC, Williams RR, Natarajan J, Wong F, Chow AT. Absence of a pharmacokinetic interaction between digoxin and levofloxacin. *J Clin Pharm Ther* (2002) 27, 7–12.
5. Staß H, Frey R, Kubitza D, Möller J-G, Zühlsdorf M. Influence of orally administered moxifloxacin (MOX) on the steady state pharmacokinetics (PK) of digoxin (D) in healthy male volunteers. *J Antimicrob Chemother* (1999) 44 (Suppl A), 134–5.
6. Horstmann R, Delesen H, Dietrich H, Ochmann K, Sachse R, Staß H, Zuehlsdorf M, Kuhlmann J. No drug-drug interaction between moxifloxacin and β-acetyldigoxin. *Clin Invest Med* (1998) (Suppl), S20.
7. Johnson RD, Dorr MB, Hunt TL, Conway S, Talbot GH. Pharmacokinetic interaction of sparfloxacin and digoxin. *Clin Ther* (1999) 21, 368–79.
8. Lindenbaum J, Rund DG, Butler VP, Tse-Eng D, Saha JR. Inactivation of digoxin by the gut flora: reversal by antibiotic therapy. *N Engl J Med* (1981) 305, 789–94.
9. Ten Eick AP, Reed MD. Hidden dangers of coadministration of antibiotics and digoxin in children: focus on azithromycin. *Curr Ther Res* (2000) 61, 148–60.

Digoxin and related drugs + Rifampicin (Rifampin)

Digitoxin levels can be halved by rifampicin. Digoxin levels are also reduced by rifampicin.

Clinical evidence

(a) Digitoxin

A comparative study in 21 patients with tuberculosis and 19 healthy subjects taking digitoxin 100 micrograms daily found that the serum digitoxin levels of the patients taking rifampicin were about half of the levels in healthy subjects not taking rifampicin (18.4 nanograms/mL compared with 39.1 nanograms/mL).[1] The half-life of digitoxin was reduced from 8.2 days to 4.5 days by rifampicin. Case reports also suggest that rifampicin can cause sizeable reductions in serum digitoxin levels.[2,3]

(b) Digoxin

A woman hospitalised for endocarditis, taking digoxin 250 to 375 micrograms daily, furosemide, aspirin, isosorbide dinitrate and potassium chloride, had a reduction of about 80% in her serum digoxin level when she was given rifampicin 600 mg daily. Her serum digoxin level returned to its former level over the 2 weeks following rifampicin withdrawal.[4] She had only moderate renal impairment (serum creatinine 221 micromol/L).

Another report describes 2 patients undergoing renal dialysis whose digoxin dose needed to be doubled while they were taking rifampicin, and similarly reduced when the rifampicin was withdrawn.[5] This confirms an earlier report.[6]

A study in 8 healthy subjects found that the AUC and maximum plasma levels of a single 1-mg oral dose of digoxin were reduced by 30% and 52%, respectively, by rifampicin 600 mg daily for 10 days.[7] In three further studies rifampicin 300 mg twice daily for 7 days reduced the AUC of a single oral dose of digoxin by 16 to 25%, and reduced its maximum levels by 23 to 38%.[8-10] Note that these three studies were designed to investigate the interaction of other drugs, and rifampicin was being used as a positive control.

A 15% reduction in the AUC and maximum plasma levels of digoxin was seen when a single 1-mg intravenous dose of digoxin was given after pre-treatment with rifampicin 600 mg daily for 10 days.[7] Similarly, a study in 8 healthy subjects who were given a single 1-mg intravenous dose of digoxin after 14 days of treatment with rifampicin 600 mg daily found an increased excretion of digoxin into the bile, and a 27% reduction in the AUC of digoxin.[11]

A case report describes rifampicin 600 mg daily being used to increase the metabolism of digoxin (as well as propafenone and warfarin) in a case of a multiple drug overdose in a 16-year-old girl. Two hours after plasma exchange, the serum digoxin level was 3.45 nanograms/mL and this had fallen by 50% 26 hours after starting rifampicin. The usual digoxin half-life is reported to be 36 to 48 hours.[12]

Mechanism

The interaction between digitoxin and rifampicin is almost certainly due to the increase in digitoxin metabolism caused by rifampicin, which is a known enzyme inducer.[1] Digoxin is largely excreted unchanged in the urine and the interaction with rifampicin appears to be mainly due to induction of P-glycoprotein, resulting in reduced digoxin absorption from the intestine,[7,11] and increased biliary excretion.[11]

Importance and management

The interaction between **digitoxin** and rifampicin is established and clinically important. Under-digitalisation could occur unless the digitoxin dose is increased appropriately. Good monitoring is obviously advisable.

The pharmacokinetic interaction between **digoxin** and rifampicin is also established, but rifampicin causes only a small reduction in digoxin exposure, and the few case reports suggest that these changes are generally not clinically relevant. However, it would be prudent to monitor the concurrent use of these drugs, being alert for the need to increase the digoxin dose. It might be that renal impairment increases the extent of this interaction, as several of the cases cited involved patients with some degree of renal impairment.

There does not seem to be any information regarding the other rifamycins, **rifabutin** and **rifapentine**. However, the UK manufacturers and the CSM in the UK warn that rifabutin could possibly reduce the effects of digitalis (but not digoxin).[13,14]

1. Peters U, Hausamen T-U, Grosse-Brockhoff F. Einfluβ von Tuberkulostatika auf die Pharmakokinetik des Digitoxins. *Dtsch Med Wochenschr* (1974) 99, 2381–6.
2. Boman G, Eliasson K, Odarcederlöf I. Acute cardiac failure during treatment with digitoxin - an interaction with rifampicin. *Br J Clin Pharmacol* (1980) 10, 89–90.
3. Poor DM, Self TH, Davis HL. Interaction of rifampin and digitoxin. *Arch Intern Med* (1983) 143, 599.
4. Bussey HI, Merritt GJ, Hill EG. The influence of rifampin on quinidine and digoxin. *Arch Intern Med* (1984) 144, 1021–3.
5. Gault H, Longerich L, Dawe M, Fine A. Digoxin-rifampin interaction. *Clin Pharmacol Ther* (1984) 35, 750–4.
6. Novi C, Bissoli F, Simonati V, Volpini T, Baroli A, Vignati G. Rifampin and digoxin: possible drug interaction in a dialysis patient. *JAMA* (1980) 244, 2521–2.
7. Greiner B, Eichelbaum M, Fritz P, Kreichgauer H-P, von Richter O, Zundler J, Kroemer HK. The role of intestinal P-glycoprotein in the interaction of digoxin and rifampin. *J Clin Invest* (1999) 104, 147–53. Correction. ibid. (2002) 110, 571.
8. Gurley BJ, Swain A, Barone GW, Williams DK, Breen P, Yates CR, Stuart LB, Hubbard MA, Tong Y, Cheboyina S. Effect of goldenseal (*Hydrastis canadensis*) and kava kava (*Piper methysticum*) supplementation on digoxin pharmacokinetics in humans. *Drug Metab Dispos* (2007) 35, 240–5.
9. Gurley BJ, Barone GW, Williams DK, Carrier J, Breen P, Yates CR, Song P-f, Hubbard MA, Tong Y, Cheboyina S. Effect of milk thistle (*Silybum marianum*) and black cohosh (*Cimicifuga racemosa*) supplementation on digoxin pharmacokinetics in humans. *Drug Metab Dispos* (2006) 34, 69–74.
10. Gurley BJ, Swain A, Williams DK, Barone G, Battu SK. Gauging the clinical significance of P-glycoprotein mediated herb-drug interactions: comparative effects of St. John's wort, echinacea, clarithromycin, and rifampicin on digoxin pharmacokinetics. *Mol Nutr Food Res* (2008) 52, 772–9.
11. Drescher S, Glaeser H, Mürdter T, Hitzl M, Eichelbaum M, Fromm MF. P-glycoprotein-mediated intestinal and biliary digoxin transport in humans. *Clin Pharmacol Ther* (2003) 73, 223–31.
12. Unal S, Bayrakci B, Yasar U, Karagoz T. Successful treatment of propafenone, digoxin and warfarin overdosage with plasma exchange therapy and rifampicin. *Clin Drug Invest* (2007) 27, 505–8.
13. Mycobutin (Rifabutin). Pfizer Ltd. UK Summary of product characteristics, December 2013.
14. Committee on the Safety of Medicines/Medicines Control Agency. Revised indication and drug interactions of rifabutin. *Current Problems* (1997) 23, 14.

Digoxin + Roflumilast

Roflumilast does not appear to affect the pharmacokinetics of digoxin.

Clinical evidence, mechanism, importance and management

In a crossover study in 16 healthy subjects,[1] roflumilast 500 micrograms daily for 14 days did not affect the AUC of a single 250-microgram dose of digoxin given on day 14. The digoxin maximum level was increased by 15%.[1] No digoxin dose adjustment would appear necessary if roflumilast is also given.

1. Eckermann G, Lahu G, Nassr N, Bethke TD. Absence of pharmacokinetic interaction between roflumilast and digoxin in healthy adults. *J Clin Pharmacol* (2011) Epub.

Digoxin + Ropinirole

Ropinirole appears to decrease digoxin exposure

Clinical evidence, mechanism, importance and management

In a placebo-controlled study, 10 patients with Parkinson's disease were given ropinirole (initially 250 micrograms increasing to 2 mg three times daily) in addition to their usual treatment with digoxin 125 or 250 micrograms daily. Although ropinirole decreased the AUC of digoxin by 10%, and decreased its maximum plasma concentration by 25%, the digoxin minimum plasma concentration was not affected. The authors therefore reasonably concluded that no digoxin dose adjustment would be needed on concurrent use.[1]

1. Taylor A, Beerahee A, Citerone D, Davy M, Fitzpatrick K, Lopez-Gil A, Stocchi F. The effect of steady-state ropinirole on plasma concentrations of digoxin in patients with Parkinson's disease. *Br J Clin Pharmacol* (1999) 47, 219–22.

Digoxin + Sevelamer

The pharmacokinetics of a single dose of digoxin were not affected by sevelamer in one study.

Clinical evidence, mechanism, importance and management

In a randomised study, a single 1-mg oral dose of digoxin was given with or without sevelamer 2.4 g followed by a standard breakfast. Five further doses of sevelamer were given immediately before subsequent meals over the following 2 days. During this time, the pharmacokinetic profile of digoxin was not altered.[1]

Sevelamer is a non-absorbed phosphate-binding polymer with bile-acid binding properties, but it appears that it does not bind with digoxin. Ideally this finding requires confirmation in long-term studies, but the available evidence suggests that a clinically significant interaction with sevelamer is unlikely, and no digoxin dose adjustments would be necessary on concurrent use.

1. Burke S, Amin N, Incerti C, Plone M, Watson N. Sevelamer hydrochloride (Renagel®), a nonabsorbed phosphate-binding polymer, does not interfere with digoxin or warfarin pharmacokinetics. *J Clin Pharmacol* (2001) 41, 193–8.

Digoxin + Sodium-glucose co-transporter-2 inhibitors

Canagliflozin appears to very slightly increase digoxin exposure, but dapagliflozin has no effect. Empagliflozin does not affect the exposure to digoxin to a clinically relevant extent.

Clinical evidence

(a) Canagliflozin

In a randomised, crossover study, 16 healthy subjects were given canagliflozin 300 mg once daily for 7 days, with a single 500-microgram of digoxin on day one followed by digoxin 250 microgram daily for 6 days. The AUC and maximum concentration of digoxin were increased by 19% and 40%, respectively.[1]

(b) Dapagliflozin

In a randomised, crossover study, 16 healthy subjects were given dapagliflozin 20 mg on day 1 followed by 10 mg daily for 7 days, with a single 250-microgram dose of oral digoxin on day 2. The pharmacokinetics of digoxin were unaltered, compared with when it was given alone.[2]

(c) Empagliflozin

In a randomised, crossover study, 19 healthy subjects were given empagliflozin 25 mg once daily for 8 days with a single dose of digoxin 500 micrograms on day 5. The AUC and maximum concentration of digoxin were increased by 6% and 10%, respectively, when compared with digoxin alone.[3]

Mechanism

In vitro canagliflozin inhibits the drug transporter P-glycoprotein,[4] for which digoxin is a substrate. The study therefore suggests that this also occurs *in vivo*, resulting in increased exposure to digoxin. Further clinical study is needed.

Importance and management

A pharmacokinetic interaction appears to occur between canagliflozin and digoxin, but not between dapagliflozin and digoxin. Some caution on the concurrent use of digoxin with canagliflozin, and monitoring of digoxin concentrations, would seem prudent. The increase in digoxin exposure when given with empagliflozin is not considered to be clinically relevant.

1. Devineni D, Manitpisitkul P, Vaccaro N, Bernard A, Skee D, Mamidi RN, Tian H, Weiner S, Stieltjes H, Sha S, Rothenberg P. Effect of canagliflozin, a sodium glucose co-transporter 2 inhibitor, on the pharmacokinetics of oral contraceptives, warfarin, and digoxin in healthy participants. *Int J Clin Pharmacol Ther* (2015) 53, 41–53.
2. Kasichayanula S, Chang M, Liu X, Shyu W-C, Griffen SC, LaCreta FP, Boulton DW. Lack of pharmacokinetic interactions between dapagliflozin and simvastatin, valsartan, warfarin or digoxin. *Adv Therapy* (2012) 29, 163–77.
3. Macha S, Sennewald R, Rose P, Schoene K, Pinnetti S, Woerle HJ, Broedl UC. Lack of clinically relevant drug-drug interaction between empagliflozin, a sodium glucose cotransporter 2 inhibitor, and verapamil, ramipril, or digoxin in healthy volunteers. *Clin Ther* (2013) 35, 226–35.
4. Invokana (Canagliflozin). Janssen Pharmaceuticals, Inc. US Prescribing information, September 2015.

Digoxin + SSRIs

Citalopram, fluvoxamine, paroxetine, and sertraline appear not to affect the pharmacokinetics of digoxin. However, one case-control study found a small increased risk of digoxin toxicity after starting fluoxetine, fluvoxamine, paroxetine or sertraline, and two isolated reports describe

increased serum digoxin levels attributed to the use of fluoxetine or paroxetine.

Clinical evidence

In a case-control study in 3 144 patients who had been admitted to hospital with digoxin toxicity, patients were more likely than controls to have taken a new prescription for **fluoxetine**, **fluvoxamine**, **paroxetine** or **sertraline**, in the 30 days before admission (adjusted odds ratios, 2.8 to 3). This was after adjusting for renal impairment and other interacting drugs. Nevertheless, this increased risk was not statistically significantly different to that in patients taking tricyclics (1.5) or benzodiazepines (2.1), which the authors considered have no known basis for an interaction.[1] Consider also 'Digoxin and related drugs + Benzodiazepines and related drugs', p.1084. In addition, the risk was small compared with the 12-fold increased risk found by the same authors in a similar study with clarithromycin, see 'Digoxin and related drugs + Macrolides', p.1100. Furthermore, there is little evidence of an interaction in other studies, although isolated case reports do describe toxicity. These are discussed in the individual sections below.

(a) Citalopram

In a study in 11 healthy subjects,[2] citalopram 40 mg daily for 28 days did not affect the pharmacokinetics of a single 1-mg dose of digoxin taken on day 21.

(b) Fluoxetine

An isolated report describes a 93-year-old woman with congestive heart failure who developed increased serum digoxin levels on two occasions when **fluoxetine** 10 mg daily was added.[3]

(c) Fluvoxamine

After taking fluvoxamine 100 mg daily for 15 days, the pharmacokinetics of a single 1.25-mg intravenous dose of digoxin were unchanged in 8 healthy subjects.[4]

(d) Paroxetine

A study in healthy subjects found that paroxetine 30 mg daily had no effect on the pharmacokinetics of digoxin 250 micrograms daily. The pharmacokinetics of paroxetine were unaffected by digoxin.[5] However, a case report describes digoxin toxicity in a 68-year-old woman with atrial fibrillation and depression, which was attributed to the addition of paroxetine 20 mg daily. Her digoxin levels reached 5.2 nanograms/mL.[6]

(e) Sertraline

A placebo-controlled study in 19 healthy subjects found that sertraline, in an initial dose of 50 mg daily titrated to 200 mg daily, had no effect on the steady-state pharmacokinetics of digoxin, except for a decrease in time to maximum plasma levels.[7]

Mechanism

It has been suggested that paroxetine might inhibit P-glycoprotein leading to reduced renal excretion of digoxin.[6] This suggestion has been criticised by other authors who propose that the increase in levels seen in the case with paroxetine could have been due to hospital-induced compliance or renal impairment.[8,9] Moreover, the case-control study found no evidence of a notably different risk of digoxin toxicity between those SSRIs with greater P-glycoprotein inhibitory activity (sertraline and paroxetine) than those with less P-glycoprotein inhibitory activity (fluoxetine, fluvoxamine).[1]

Importance and management

The pharmacokinetic studies show that, in general, it is unlikely that SSRIs will affect the steady-state serum levels of digoxin. The excess risk seen in the case-control study was considered to be small and related to detection bias or confounding by indication,[1] although the findings do introduce a note of caution. Nevertheless, the fact that there are only isolated case reports of a possible interaction with digoxin for such a widely used class of drugs suggests that problems are rarely encountered. No digoxin dose adjustments would seem to be necessary on concurrent use.

1. Juurlink DN, Mamdani MM, Kopp A, Herrmann N, Laupacis A. A population-based assessment of the potential interaction between serotonin-specific reuptake inhibitors and digoxin. *Br J Clin Pharmacol* (2005) 59, 102–7.
2. Larsen F, Priskorn M, Overø KF. Lack of citalopram effect on oral digoxin pharmacokinetics. *J Clin Pharmacol* (2001) 41, 340–6.
3. Leibovitz A, Bilchinsky T, Gil I, Habot B. Elevated serum digoxin level associated with coadministered fluoxetine. *Arch Intern Med* (1998) 158, 1152–3.
4. Ochs HR, Greenblatt DJ, Verburg-Ochs B, Labedski L. Chronic treatment with fluvoxamine, clovoxamine and placebo: interaction with digoxin and effects on sleep and alertness. *J Clin Pharmacol* (1989) 29, 91–95.
5. Bannister SJ, Houser VP, Hulse JD, Kisicki JC, Rasmussen JGC. Evaluation of the potential for interactions of paroxetine with diazepam, cimetidine, warfarin, and digoxin. *Acta Psychiatr Scand* (1989) 80 (Suppl 350), 102–6.
6. Yasui-Furukori N, Kaneko S. Digitalis intoxication induced by paroxetine co-administration. *Lancet* (2006) 367, 788.
7. Rapeport WG, Coates PE, Dewland PM, Forster PL. Absence of a sertraline-mediated effect on digoxin pharmacokinetics and electrocardiographic findings. *J Clin Psychiatry* (1996) 57 (Suppl 1), 16–19.
8. Bateman DN, Thanacoody HKR, Waring WS. Digitalis intoxication induced by paroxetine co-administration. *Lancet* (2006) 368, 1962–3.
9. Hallberg P, Melhus H. Digitalis intoxication induced by paroxetine co-administration. *Lancet* (2006) 368, 1963.

Digoxin + St John's wort (*Hypericum perforatum*)

Digoxin toxicity occurred in a patient taking digoxin when he stopped taking St John's wort. There is good evidence that some preparations of St John's wort can reduce digoxin exposure. Preparations with low hyperforin content appear to have a smaller effect.

Clinical evidence

An 80-year-old man taking long-term digoxin and St John's wort herbal tea (2 litres daily) developed symptoms of digoxin toxicity (nodal bradycardia of 36 bpm and bigeminy) when he stopped taking the herbal tea.[1]

In a study, 13 healthy subjects were given digoxin for 5 days until steady-state had been achieved, and then St John's wort extract (*LI 160*, Lichtwer Pharma) 300 mg three times daily for a further 10 days. The AUC and trough level of digoxin decreased by 28% and 37%, respectively. When compared with a parallel group of 12 subjects taking digoxin and placebo, the St John's wort group had 26% lower maximum plasma digoxin levels, 33% lower trough digoxin levels and a 25% lower AUC.[2]

In another study, 8 healthy subjects pretreated with St John's wort 300 mg three times daily for 14 days were given a single 500-microgram dose of digoxin. St John's wort decreased the AUC_{0-7} of digoxin by 18%.[3]

Another study in 18 healthy subjects found that St John's wort 300 mg three times daily (Nature's Way, containing a daily dose of 24 mg of hyperforin) for 14 days reduced the maximum levels and AUC_{0-24} of a single 250-microgram dose of digoxin by 36% and 23%, respectively. These findings were comparable to rifampicin (an established P-glycoprotein inducer) 600 mg daily for 7 days.[4]

In a further randomised, placebo-controlled study, 93 healthy subjects were given digoxin alone for 7 days and then with one of ten St John's wort preparations for 14 days. The extract used in an earlier study (*LI 160*, *Jarsin 300*, Lichtwer Pharma) 300 mg three time daily similarly reduced the digoxin AUC, peak and trough plasma levels by 25%, 37%, and 19%, respectively. Comparable results were found with hypericum powder containing similar amounts of hyperforin (about 21 mg daily), while hypericum powder with half the hyperforin content (about 10 mg daily) reduced the AUC, peak and trough plasma levels by about 18%, 21%, and 13%, respectively. Some St John's wort products, including tea, juice, oil extract, and powder with low-dose hyperforin (all 5 mg daily or less), did not affect the pharmacokinetics of digoxin.[5] Similarly, a further study in 28 healthy subjects found no change in digoxin pharmacokinetics when another low-hyperforin (about 3.5 mg daily) St John's wort extract (*Esbericum*) 120 mg was given twice daily for 11 days to patients who had received a digoxin loading dose of 750 micrograms daily for 2 days before starting St John's wort, and then received digoxin 250 micrograms daily each day during the study.[6]

Mechanism

Digoxin is a substrate of the efflux pump, P-glycoprotein. St John's wort, and specifically hyperforin, a major active constituent, has been shown to increase the activity of the P-glycoprotein drug transporter protein in the intestines, which reduces the absorption of digoxin.[2,4,7,8]

Importance and management

An interaction between St John's wort and digoxin would appear to be established. The extent of the interaction might depend on the St John's wort preparation involved and dose used, and seems to be correlated with the dose of hyperforin.[4-6,8] Reductions in serum digoxin levels of the size seen with *LI 160* could diminish the control of arrhythmias or heart failure. Digoxin serum levels should therefore be well monitored if St John's wort is either started or stopped and appropriate dose adjustments made if necessary. The recommendation of the CSM in the UK is that St John's wort should not be used by patients taking digoxin.[9]

1. Anđelić S. Bigeminija – rezultat interakcije digoksina i kantariona. *Vojnosanit Pregl* (2003) 60, 361–4.
2. Johne A, Brockmöller J, Bauer S, Maurer A, Langheinrich M, Roots I. Pharmacokinetic interaction of digoxin with an herbal extract from St John's wort (*Hypericum perforatum*). *Clin Pharmacol Ther* (1999) 66, 338–45.
3. Dürr D, Stieger B, Kullak-Ublick GA, Rentsch KM, Steinert HC, Meier PJ, Fattinger K. St John's wort induces intestinal P-glycoprotein/MDR1 and intestinal and hepatic CYP3A4. *Clin Pharmacol Ther* (2000) 68, 598–604.
4. Gurley BJ, Swain A, Williams DK, Barone G, Battu SK. Gauging the clinical significance of P-glycoprotein-mediated herb-drug interactions: Comparative effects of St John's wort, Echinacea, clarithromycin, and rifampin on digoxin pharmacokinetics. *Mol Nutr Food Res* (2008) 52, 772–9.
5. Mueller SC, Uehleke B, Woehling H, Petzsch M, Majcher-Peszynska J, Hehl E-M, Sievers H, Frank B, Riethling A-K, Drewelow B. Effect of St John's wort dose and preparations on the pharmacokinetics of digoxin. *Clin Pharmacol Ther* (2004) 75, 546–57.
6. Arold G, Donath F, Maurer A, Diefenbach K, Bauer S, Henneicke-von Zepelin HH, Friede M, Roots I. No relevant interaction with alprazolam, caffeine, tolbutamide and digoxin by treatment with a low-hyperforin St John's wort extract. *Planta Med* (2005) 71, 331–337.
7. Dürr D, Stieger B, Kullak-Ublick GA, Rentsch KM, Steinert HC, Meier PJ, Fattinger K. St John's wort induces intestinal P-glycoprotein/MDR1 and intestinal and hepatic CYP3A4. *Clin Pharmacol Ther* (2000) 68, 598–604.
8. Tian R, Koyabu N, Morimoto S, Shoyama Y, Ohtani H, Sawada Y. Functional induction and de-induction of P-glycoprotein by St. John's wort and its ingredients in a human colon adenocarcinoma cell line. *Drug Metab Dispos* (2005) 33, 547–54.
9. Committee on the Safety of Medicines (UK). Message from Professor A Breckenridge (Chairman of CSM) and Fact Sheet for Health Care Professionals, 29th February 2000.

Digoxin and related drugs + Statins

Atorvastatin, fluvastatin and simvastatin might cause small increases in the plasma levels of digoxin. Pitavastatin, pravastatin and rosuvastatin

appear to have no effect on digoxin pharmacokinetics. One case report describes rhabdomyolysis in a patient taking simvastatin and amiodarone when he was given digitoxin.

Clinical evidence

A. Digitoxin

(a) Simvastatin

A case report describes a 62 year-old-man taking amiodarone 200 mg daily and simvastatin 40 mg daily. Two years later, he started taking digitoxin 70 micrograms daily and within a month he developed rhabdomyolysis with elevated creatinine levels. Digitoxin levels were within the reference range. Simvastatin was stopped and over several days his creatinine levels returned to normal.[1]

B. Digoxin

(a) Atorvastatin

Digoxin 250 micrograms daily was given to 24 healthy subjects for 10 days, with atorvastatin 10 or 80 mg daily for a further 10 days. The mean steady-state plasma levels of digoxin were unaffected by atorvastatin 10 mg, but atorvastatin 80 mg caused a 20% rise in the maximum levels of digoxin and a 15% rise in its AUC.[2]

(b) Fluvastatin

In a crossover study in 18 patients, fluvastatin 40 mg caused no changes in the pharmacokinetics of digoxin 100 to 375 micrograms daily.[3] Another similar study in patients found changes of up to 15% in the maximum plasma levels and clearance of digoxin.[4]

(c) Pitavastatin

In a pharmacokinetic study in healthy subjects given pitavastatin 4 mg daily and digoxin 250 micrograms daily alone and together, there was no notable change in the steady-state exposure of either drug.[5]

(d) Pravastatin

In 18 healthy subjects, pravastatin 20 mg daily for 9 days had no effect on the steady-state serum levels of digoxin 200 micrograms daily.[6]

(e) Rosuvastatin

In a randomised study, 18 healthy subjects were given rosuvastatin 40 mg daily or placebo for 12 days, with a single 500-microgram dose of digoxin on day 8. The absorption, renal excretion, AUC and maximum serum levels of digoxin were unaffected by rosuvastatin.[7]

(f) Simvastatin

Plasma digoxin levels can be slightly raised, by about 0.3 nanograms/mL, by simvastatin.[8]

Mechanism

Digoxin is a substrate of the efflux pump, P-glycoprotein. The small changes seen in digoxin levels are probably due to the inhibitory effects of these statins on P-glycoprotein. Atorvastatin and lovastatin appear to inhibit P-glycoprotein *in vitro*, while fluvastatin and rosuvastatin do not appear to interact with P-glycoprotein at clinically achievable concentrations.[9] Pravastatin does not appear to inhibit P-glycoprotein.[10]

The cause of rhabdomyolysis in one patient taking simvastatin and amiodarone when digitoxin was added is unknown. Note that amiodarone and simvastatin can increase the risk of rhabdomyolysis when given concurrently (see 'Statins + Amiodarone', p.1320.)

Importance and management

The small changes seen in digoxin levels that occur on the concurrent use of a statin seem unlikely to be clinically relevant in most patients and no digoxin dose adjustments would seem necessary on concurrent use.

The contribution of **digitoxin** to the isolated case of statin-induced rhabdomyolysis is unproven, and it is unlikely to be of general relevance.

1. Nägele H, Behrns S, Hashagen S, Azizi M. Rhabdomyolysis after addition of digitoxin to chronic simvastatin and amiodarone therapy. *Drug Metabol Drug Interact* (2007) 22, 195–200.
2. Boyd RA, Stern RH, Stewart BH, Wu X, Reyner EL, Zegarac EA, Randinitis EJ, Whitfield L. Atorvastatin coadministration may increase digoxin concentrations by inhibition of intestinal P-glycoprotein-mediated secretion. *J Clin Pharmacol* (2000) 40, 91–8.
3. Smith HT, Jokubaitis LA, Troendle AJ, Hwang DS, Robinson WT. Pharmacokinetics of fluvastatin and specific drug interactions. *Am J Hypertens* (1993) 6 (Suppl), 375S–382S.
4. Garnett WR, Venitz J, Wilkens RC, Dimenna G. Pharmacokinetic effects of fluvastatin in patients chronically receiving digoxin. *Am J Med* (1994) 96 (Suppl 6A), 84S–86S.
5. Livalo (Pitavastatin). Kowa Pharmaceuticals America, Inc. US Prescribing information, October 2013.
6. Triscari J, Swanson BN, Willard DA, Cohen AI, Devault A, Pan HY. Steady state serum concentrations of pravastatin and digoxin when given in combination. *Br J Clin Pharmacol* (1993) 36, 263–5.
7. Martin PD, Kemp J, Dane AL, Warwick MJ, Schneck DW. No effect of rosuvastatin on the pharmacokinetics of digoxin in healthy volunteers. *J Clin Pharmacol* (2002) 42, 1352–7.
8. Garnett WR. Interactions with hydroxymethylglutaryl-coenzyme A reductase inhibitors. *Am J Health-Syst Pharm* (1995) 52, 1639–45.
9. Goard CA, Mather RG, Vinepal B, Clendening JW, Martirosyan A, Boutros PC, Sharom FJ, Penn LZ. Differential interactions between statins and P-glycoprotein: implications for exploiting statins as anticancer agents. *Int J Cancer* (2010) 127, 2936–48.
10. Sakaeda T, Takara K, Kakumoto M, Ohmoto N, Nakamura T, Iwaki K, Tanigawara Y, Okumura K. Simvastatin and lovastatin, but not pravastatin, interact with MDR1. *J Pharm Pharmacol* (2002) 54, 419–23.

Digoxin + Sucralfate

Sucralfate caused a very slight reduction in the absorption of digoxin in one study, but an isolated report describes an important reduction in digoxin levels in one patient given sucralfate.

Clinical evidence

In a study in 12 healthy subjects, sucralfate 1 g four times daily for 2 days had no effect on most of the pharmacokinetic parameters of a single 750-microgram dose of digoxin; however, the AUC of digoxin was reduced by 19% and the amount of digoxin eliminated in the urine was reduced by 12%. Digoxin was also absorbed faster.[1] No interaction occurred when the digoxin was given 2 hours before the sucralfate.[1]

An elderly patient, taking several drugs including digoxin 125 micrograms daily and sucralfate 2 g twice daily, was admitted to hospital with pressure-like chest pain, shortness of breath and generalised fatigue. Her digoxin levels were found to be subtherapeutic (about 0.1 nanograms/mL), even though the doses of digoxin and sucralfate were separated by 2 hours. She was given intravenous digoxin 250 micrograms for an episode of atrial flutter on the day of admission, with a further dose the next day. Sucralfate was discontinued on day 4 as she had not had any recent gastrointestinal symptoms and, on day 5 digoxin levels were within the therapeutic range (0.9 nanograms/mL). She continued to take oral digoxin 125 micrograms daily without sucralfate and her digoxin levels remained at about the therapeutic range in the 2-week period after hospitalisation.[2]

Mechanism

Uncertain. One possibility is that the digoxin and sucralfate bind together in the gut, which reduces digoxin absorption.

Importance and management

Information regarding an interaction between digoxin and sucralfate appears to be limited to the reports cited. The magnitude of the reduction in digoxin exposure reported in the study is unlikely to be clinically relevant in most patients, but the unexplained and isolated case suggests that clinicians should at least be aware of the possibility of an interaction.

1. Giesing DH, Lanman RC, Dimmitt DC, Runser DJ. Lack of effect of sucralfate on digoxin pharmacokinetics. *Gastroenterology* (1983) 84,1165.
2. Rey AM, Gums JG. Altered absorption of digoxin, sustained-release quinidine, and warfarin with sucralfate administration. *Ann Pharmacother* (1991) 25, 745–6.

Digoxin + Surfactant excipients

Non-ionic surfactants used as pharmaceutical excipients, such as polyoxyl castor oil (*Cremophor*), might enhance the absorption of digoxin.

Clinical evidence, mechanism, importance and management

A placebo-controlled study in 12 healthy subjects found that **polyoxyl castor oil** (***Cremophor RH40***) 600 mg three times daily increased the AUC_{0-5} and peak plasma levels of a single 500-microgram oral dose of digoxin by about 22%. The absorption of digoxin was delayed. The pharmacodynamic effects of digoxin were not affected by ***Cremophor***. It was suggested that ***Cremophor*** increases digoxin plasma levels by inhibiting intestinal P-glycoprotein, or that the ***Cremophor*** prolongs the dissolution of digoxin tablets resulting in delayed absorption from the intestines.[1] Whatever the reason, the effects found were very slight, and their clinical relevance is not established.

1. Tayrouz Y, Ding R, Burhenne J, Riedel K-D, Weiss J, Hoppe-Tichy T, Haefeli WE, Mikus G. Pharmacokinetic and pharmaceutic interaction between digoxin and Cremophor RH40. *Clin Pharmacol Ther* (2003) 73, 397–405.

Digoxin + Tetracyclines

Limited early evidence suggested that tetracycline might cause a rise in digoxin levels. Tigecycline does not alter digoxin exposure.

Clinical evidence

(a) Tetracycline

A patient taking digoxin tablets 500 micrograms daily was given tetracycline 500 mg every 6 hours for 5 days. His urinary excretion of digoxin metabolites fell sharply within 2 days, and his steady-state serum digoxin levels rose by 43%.[1] Another subject had a marked fall in the excretion of digoxin metabolites from the gut after taking tetracycline.[2] In a study, tetracycline prolonged the half-life of digoxin and increased its serum levels by about 70% (from 1.7 nanograms/mL to 2.9 nanograms/mL).[3]

(b) Tigecycline

In a crossover study, 20 healthy subjects were given a single 100-mg intravenous dose of tigecycline then, after a washout period, oral digoxin 500 micrograms for one day followed by 250 micrograms daily for 12 days, with intravenous tigecycline 100 mg on day 8 followed by tigecycline 50 mg twice daily. The pharmacokinetics of tigecycline were not affected by digoxin, apart from a 46% increase in the half-life of tigecycline. The pharmacokinetics of digoxin were not affected by tigecycline, apart from a 13% decrease in the maximum plasma level of digoxin. ECG parameters were not affected by concurrent use.[4]

Mechanism

Uncertain. Up to 10% of patients taking oral digoxin excrete it in substantial amounts in the faeces and urine as inactive metabolites (digoxin reduction products or DRPs). This metabolism seems to be performed by the gut flora,[1] in particular *Eubacterium lentum*, which is anaerobic and Gram positive.[2,5] In the presence of some antibacterials, such as tetracycline, which can inhibit this organism, more digoxin becomes available for absorption, which results in a rise in serum levels. At the same time the inactive metabolites derived from the gut disappear.[2] However, doubt has been thrown on this theory, see *Mechanism* under 'Digoxin and related drugs + Macrolides', p.1100.

The increase in the half-life of tigecycline seen with digoxin was, in the absence of a change in exposure and other pharmacokinetic variables, attributed to a difference in single-dose compared with multiple-dose tigecycline pharmacokinetics.[4]

Importance and management

The interaction between digoxin and tetracycline is not well established, the evidence is very limited, and its general clinical importance is uncertain. Bear this interaction in mind in case of an unexpected response to digoxin.

The increase in tigecycline half-life in the presence of digoxin might have been affected by study design (see *Mechanism*, above), and is therefore unlikely to be of general relevance. Tigecycline does not alter digoxin exposure, and the very small change in digoxin maximum levels is not clinically relevant; therefore, no digoxin dose adjustments would appear to be necessary on concurrent use.

1. Lindenbaum J, Rund DG, Butler VP, Tse-Eng D, Saha JR. Inactivation of digoxin by the gut flora: reversal by antibiotic therapy. *N Engl J Med* (1981) 305, 789–94.
2. Dobkin JF, Saha JR, Butler VP, Lindenbaum J. Effects of antibiotic therapy on digoxin metabolism. *Clin Res* (1982) 30, 517A.
3. Halawa B. Interakcje digoksyny z cefradina (Sefril), tetracyklina (Tetracyclinum), gentamycyna (Gentamycin) i wankomycyna (Vancocin). *Pol Tyg Lek* (1984) 39, 1717–20.
4. Zimmerman JJ, Harper DM, Matschke K, Speth JL, Raible DG, Fruncillo RJ. Absence of an interaction between tigecycline and digoxin in healthy men. *Pharmacotherapy* (2007) 27, 835–44.
5. Ten Eick AP, Reed MD. Hidden dangers of coadministration of antibiotics and digoxin in children: focus on azithromycin. *Curr Ther Res* (2000) 61, 148–60.

Digoxin and related drugs + Thiazolidinediones

Pioglitazone and rosiglitazone do not affect the pharmacokinetics of digoxin, but they might adversely affect cardiac function in patients with cardiac failure.

Clinical evidence

(a) Pioglitazone

In 12 healthy subjects given digoxin 250 micrograms daily, concurrent pioglitazone 45 mg daily increased the AUC of digoxin by 15%, and increased its maximum concentration by 17%.[1,2]

(b) Rosiglitazone

A study in healthy subjects found that rosiglitazone 8 mg daily for 14 days had no effect on the steady-state pharmacokinetics of digoxin 375 micrograms daily.[3]

Mechanism

Pioglitazone and rosiglitazone can cause fluid retention, which might cause or exacerbate heart failure.

Importance and management

No pharmacokinetic interaction of any clinical relevance occurs between digoxin and pioglitazone or rosiglitazone. However, the US manufacturers caution the use of pioglitazone or rosiglitazone in those with a history of heart failure because they can cause fluid retention, which could lead to a deterioration in cardiac function.[1,4] They state that starting these drugs in those with severe heart failure (NYHA class III or IV) is contraindicated,[1,4] whereas the UK manufacturers contraindicate use in any degree of heart failure (NYHA class I to IV).[5,6] Note that rosiglitazone has been withdrawn in Europe because of its cardiovascular risk profile. If digoxin or any other **digitalis glycoside** is being used to manage cardiac failure, the use of pioglitazone or rosiglitazone would not therefore be recommended. This is not a drug-drug interaction but a drug-disease interaction.

1. Actos (Pioglitazone hydrochloride). Takeda Pharmaceutical Company Ltd. US Prescribing information, November 2013.
2. Kortboyer JM, Eckland DJA. Pioglitazone has low potential for drug interactions. *Diabetologia* (1999) 42 (Suppl 1), A228.
3. Di Cicco RA, Miller AK, Patterson S, Freed MI. Rosiglitazone does not affect the steady-state pharmacokinetics of digoxin. *J Clin Pharmacol* (2000) 40, 1516–21.
4. Avandia (Rosiglitazone maleate). GlaxoSmithKline. US Prescribing information, September 2013.
5. Actos (Pioglitazone hydrochloride). Takeda UK Ltd. UK Summary of product characteristics, November 2013.
6. Avandia (Rosiglitazone maleate). GlaxoSmithKline UK. UK Summary of product characteristics, May 2009.

Digoxin + Thrombin inhibitors

Dabigatran and argatroban do not alter the pharmacokinetics of digoxin, and digoxin does not appear to alter the pharmacokinetics or anticoagulant effect of dabigatran.

Clinical evidence, mechanism, importance and management

(a) Argatroban

A placebo-controlled, crossover study in 12 healthy subjects found that the pharmacokinetics of steady-state digoxin 375 micrograms daily were not affected by an infusion of argatroban 2 micrograms/kg per minute for 120 hours. Steady-state argatroban concentrations were obtained within 3 hours and maintained throughout the infusion. Digoxin dose adjustments should not be necessary during the concurrent use of argatroban.[1]

(b) Dabigatran

In a randomised, crossover study in 23 healthy subjects the concurrent use of dabigatran 150 mg twice daily and digoxin for 4 days had no effect on the AUC and maximum plasma concentration of either drug. The anticoagulant effect of dabigatran was also unaffected by digoxin.[2] No dose adjustments would therefore be expected to be necessary if digoxin is given with dabigatran.

1. Inglis AML, Sheth SB, Hursting MJ, Tenero DM, Graham AM, DiCicco RA. Investigation of the interaction between argatroban and acetaminophen, lidocaine, or digoxin. *Am J Health-Syst Pharm* (2002) 59, 1258–66.
2. Stangier J, Stähle H, Rathgen K, Roth W, Reseski K, Körnicke T. Pharmacokinetics and pharmacodynamics of dabigatran etexilate, an oral direct thrombin inhibitor, with coadministration of digoxin. *J Clin Pharmacol* (2012) 52, 243–50.

Digoxin and related drugs + Thyroid hormones and Antithyroid drugs

Thyrotoxic patients are relatively resistant to the effects of digitalis glycosides and could need reduced doses of these drugs as treatment with antithyroid drugs (carbimazole, thiamazole) progresses, whereas patients with hypothyroidism could need increased doses of digitalis glycosides as treatment with thyroid hormones progresses. Carbimazole has been shown to reduce digoxin levels in healthy subjects. Thiamazole does not appear to affect the pharmacokinetics of single-dose digoxin.

Clinical evidence

(a) Carbimazole

The observation of relatively low plasma digoxin levels in a patient taking carbimazole prompted a further study in 10 healthy subjects. In 9 out of the 10 subjects, steady-state peak serum digoxin levels were reduced by 23% (from 1.72 nanograms/mL to 1.33 nanograms/mL) by a single 60-mg dose of carbimazole, but in the other subject the serum digoxin levels were increased. Other pharmacokinetic parameters were unaffected.

Carbimazole abolished the systolic blood pressure decrease seen in the first 3 hours with digoxin, and also reduced the duration of the digoxin-induced diastolic blood pressure fall from 12 hours to 6 hours. The changes in heart rates, cardiac output and stroke volumes were not statistically significant, but inter-individual differences were large.[1-3]

(b) Thiamazole

In a study in 12 patients with hyperthyroidism, a single 20-mg dose of thiamazole did not affect the pharmacokinetics of a single 500-microgram dose of digoxin. Additionally, normalisation of serum T3 and thyroxine by thiamazole treatment over several weeks did not affect the pharmacokinetics of a single 500-microgram dose of digoxin. The AUC of digoxin in 28 patients with hyperthyroidism was 15% lower than in 15 healthy control subjects.[4]

Mechanism

Unclear. One explanation for the changed response to digitalis with carbimazole is that there is a direct and altered response of the heart due to the raised or lowered thyroid hormone levels. Another is that changes in glomerular filtration rate associated with hypo- or hyperthyroidism result in increased or decreased serum digoxin levels, respectively.[5] A further explanation is that, as digoxin is a substrate of the efflux pump P-glycoprotein, increased serum digoxin levels could be due to a down-regulation of renal P-glycoprotein in hypothyroidism.[6] An increase in T3 (as seen in hyperthyroidism) might also stimulate expression of P-glycoprotein in intestinal cells leading to a reduction in digoxin absorption.[7] Why carbimazole *reduced* serum digoxin levels in healthy subjects (normal thyroid status) is not known.

Importance and management

Evidence for an interaction between thyroid hormones or antithyroid drugs and digitalis glycosides is limited, but given the evidence here, and the way thyroid hormones or antithyroid drugs are known to affect other drugs, an interaction certainly seems possible. As thyroid status is returned to normal by the use of antithyroid drugs or thyroid hormones the dose of the digitalis glycosides might need to be adjusted appropriately. Hyperthyroid patients could need to have their digitalis dose gradually reduced as treatment proceeds (because initially they are relatively resistant to the effects of digitalis and start off needing higher doses). They are also relatively insensitive to the chronotropic effects of digitalis.[8,9] Hypothyroid patients, on the other hand, could need a gradually increasing dose (because initially they are relatively sensitive to digitalis).[5,8] In either of these situations, it would be prudent to monitor serum digoxin levels as treatment continues.

The modest reduction in digoxin levels caused by carbimazole in healthy subjects does not fit with the need to decrease digoxin doses when antithyroid drugs are used in patients. However, the situation in healthy subjects might not accurately reflect that in subjects with thyroid disease.

1. Petereit G, Ramesh Rao B, Siepmann M, Kirch W. Influence of carbimazole on the steady state serum levels and haemodynamic effects of digoxin in healthy subjects. *Eur J Clin Pharmacol* (1995) 49, A159.
2. Rao BR, Petereit G, Ebert U, Siepmann M, Kirch W. Influence of carbimazole on the steady state serum levels and haemodynamic effects of digoxin in healthy subjects. *Therapie* (1995) 50 (Suppl), 406.
3. Rao R, Petereit G, Ebert U, Kirch W. Influence of carbimazole on serum levels and haemodynamic effects of digoxin. *Clin Drug Invest* (1997) 13, 350–4.
4. Izbicka M, Gasińska Teresa, Dec Renata. Farmakokinetyka digoksyny u chrych z nadczynnościa tarczycy. Wpływ metimazolu. *Wiad Lek* (2010) 63, 10–16.
5. Croxson MS, Ibbertson HK. Serum digoxin in patients with thyroid disease. *BMJ* (1975) 3, 566–8.
6. Burk O, Brenner SS, Hofmann U, Tegude H, Igel S, Schwab M, Eichelbaum M, Alscher MD. The impact of thyroid disease on the regulation, expression, and function of ABCB1 (MDR1/P-glycoprotein) and consequences for the disposition of digoxin. *Clin Pharmacol Ther* (2010) 88, 685–94.
7. Nishio N, Katsura T, Inui K. Thyroid hormone regulates the expression and function of P-glycoprotein in Caco-2 cells. *Pharm Res* (2008) 25, 1037–42.
8. Lawrence JR, Sumner DJ, Kalk WJ, Ratcliffe WA, Whiting B, Gray K, Lindsay M. Digoxin kinetics in patients with thyroid dysfunction. *Clin Pharmacol Ther* (1977) 22, 7–13.
9. Huffman DH, Klaassen CD, Hartman CR. Digoxin in hyperthyroidism. *Clin Pharmacol Ther* (1977) 22, 533–8.

Digoxin + Tiagabine

Tiagabine does not alter the pharmacokinetics of digoxin.

Clinical evidence, mechanism, importance and management

In a crossover study, 13 healthy subjects were given a loading dose of digoxin 500 micrograms twice daily for one day then 250 micrograms daily for 8 days, either alone or with tiagabine 4 mg three times daily for 9 days. It was found that the pharmacokinetics of digoxin were not altered by tiagabine.[1] No digoxin dose adjustments would be expected to be needed on the concurrent use of tiagabine.

1. Snel S, Jansen JA, Pedersen PC, Jonkman JHG, van Heiningen PNM. Tiagabine, a novel antiepileptic agent: lack of pharmacokinetic interaction with digoxin. *Eur J Clin Pharmacol* (1998) 54, 355–7.

Digoxin + Ticagrelor

Ticagrelor appears to increase digoxin exposure. The pharmacokinetics of ticagrelor are not altered by digoxin.

Clinical evidence

The UK manufacturer reports that ticagrelor 400 mg daily increased the maximum plasma concentration and AUC of digoxin 250 micrograms daily by 75% and 28%, respectively. The mean digoxin minimum concentration increased by about 30%, although some individuals had up to 2-fold increases in their minimum concentrations. In addition, digoxin did not alter the pharmacokinetics of ticagrelor or its active metabolite.[1]

Mechanism

Digoxin is a substrate of P-glycoprotein, of which ticagrelor is an inhibitor.[1] Concurrent use can therefore lead to an increase in digoxin concentrations.

Importance and management

Information on the interaction between digoxin and ticagrelor is limited to the study cited. In view of the narrow therapeutic range of digoxin, the increased exposure and concentrations of digoxin seem likely to be clinically relevant and it would therefore seem prudent to be alert for digoxin adverse effects (such as bradycardia) and consider monitoring digoxin concentrations. No ticagrelor dose adjustments would appear necessary on concurrent use.

1. Brilique (Ticagrelor). AstraZeneca UK Ltd. UK Summary of product characteristics, July 2015.

Digoxin + Ticlopidine

Ticlopidine reduces digoxin exposure.

Clinical evidence, mechanism, importance and management

In a pharmacokinetic study in 15 healthy subjects, ticlopidine 250 mg twice daily for 10 days reduced the peak serum levels and AUC of digoxin by about 10%.[1] Reductions of this magnitude are unlikely to be of clinical importance and therefore no digoxin dose adjustments would appear to be necessary on the concurrent use of ticlopidine.

1. Vargas R, Reitman M, Teitelbaum P, Ryan JR, McMahon FG, Jain AK, Ryan M, Regel G. Study of the effect of ticlopidine on digoxin blood levels. *Clin Pharmacol Ther* (1988) 43, 176.

Digoxin + Tiludronate

Tiludronate does not appear to affect the pharmacokinetics of digoxin.

Clinical evidence, mechanism, importance and management

In a study in 12 healthy subjects, tiludronate 600 mg daily for 2 days then 400 mg daily for the next 10 days, had no effect on the pharmacokinetics of digoxin 250 micrograms daily.[1] No digoxin dose adjustments would appear to be needed on concurrent use.

1. Sanofi Winthrop. Data on file. June 1996.

Digoxin + Topiramate

Topiramate causes a very slight reduction in digoxin exposure.

Clinical evidence, mechanism, importance and management

In a study in 12 healthy subjects, topiramate 100 mg twice daily for 9 days reduced the maximum serum levels and AUC of digoxin by 16% and 12%, respectively, and oral digoxin clearance was increased by 13%.[1] The UK manufacturer of topiramate suggests good monitoring of serum digoxin levels if topiramate is added or withdrawn,[2] but changes in the pharmacokinetics of digoxin of this magnitude seem unlikely to be clinically relevant in most patients. Note that the US manufacturer makes no suggestion that monitoring is necessary.[3]

1. Liao S, Palmer M. Digoxin and topiramate drug interaction study in male volunteers. *Pharm Res* (1993) 10 (10 Suppl), S405.
2. Topamax (Topiramate). Janssen-Cilag Ltd. UK Summary of product characteristics, October 2012.
3. Topamax (Topiramate). Ortho-McNeil Neurologics. US Prescribing information, January 2012.

Digoxin + Tramadol

One UK manufacturer of tramadol states that digoxin toxicity has occurred rarely during the concurrent use of digoxin and tramadol.[1] There appear to be no published reports of an interaction, and in the absence of any further data, this information is of little general relevance.

1. Zamadol 24 hr 150 mg Tablets (Tramadol hydrochloride). Meda Pharmaceuticals. UK Summary of product characteristics, August 2009.

Digoxin + Trapidil

Trapidil does not alter digoxin levels, but might oppose some of its effects.

Clinical evidence, mechanism, importance and management

In 10 healthy subjects, trapidil 400 mg daily for 8 days had no effect on the steady-state serum levels of digoxin 375 micrograms daily. It was noted that the positive chronotropic effect of trapidil opposed the negative chronotropic effect of digoxin, which should be remembered when using both drugs, but overall no adverse effects that would prevent concurrent use were noted.[1]

1. Sziegoleit W, Weiss M, Fahr A, Scharfe S. Trapidil does not affect serum levels and cardiotonic action of digoxin in healthy humans. *Jpn Circ J* (1987) 51, 1305–9.

Digoxin + Trazodone

A rise in digoxin levels, accompanied by toxicity in one instance, has been seen when two patients taking digoxin were given trazodone.

Clinical evidence, mechanism, importance and management

An elderly woman taking digoxin 125 micrograms daily (and also taking quinidine, clonidine and triamterene with hydrochlorothiazide) complained of nausea and vomiting within about 2 weeks of starting to take trazodone (initially 50 mg, increasing to 300 mg daily over 11 days). Her serum digoxin levels had risen more than threefold (from 0.8 nanograms/mL to 2.8 nanograms/mL). The digoxin was stopped and then restarted at half the original dose, which maintained therapeutic levels.[1] The patient had poor renal function, but this did not notably change during this incident. Another case report also describes raised digoxin levels, apparently caused by trazodone.[2]

Direct information seems to be limited to these two reports, which is insufficient evidence to make any general recommendations; however, if a patient taking digoxin develops otherwise unexplained adverse effects, it would be prudent to consider trazodone as a possible cause.

1. Rauch PK, Jenike MA. Digoxin toxicity possibly precipitated by trazodone. *Psychosomatics* (1984) 25, 334–5.
2. Knapp JE. Mead Johnson Pharmaceutical Newsletter, 1983.

Digoxin + Trimetazidine

Trimetazidine does not appear to affect the pharmacokinetics of digoxin.

Clinical evidence, mechanism, importance and management

In 13 healthy subjects, trimetazidine 20 mg twice daily for at least 14 days did not affect the pharmacokinetics of a single 500-microgram dose of digoxin.[1] These results suggest that the dose of digoxin is unlikely to need adjusting in patients who are also given trimetazidine.

1. Edeki TI, Johnston A, Campbell DB, Ings RMJ, Brownsill R, Genissel P, Turner P. An examination of the possible pharmacokinetic interaction of trimetazidine with theophylline, digoxin and antipyrine. *Br J Clin Pharmacol* (1989) 26, 657P.

Digoxin + Trimethoprim

Digoxin levels can be increased by trimethoprim.

Clinical evidence

(a) Elderly patients

After taking trimethoprim 200 mg twice daily for 14 days, the mean serum digoxin levels in 9 elderly patients (aged 62 to 92 years) had risen by 22% (from 0.9 nanograms/mL to 1.2 nanograms/mL). A 34% increase in mean serum creatinine levels was also seen. When the trimethoprim was withdrawn, the mean serum digoxin levels returned to their previous value. Although one patient had a greater rise in serum digoxin levels from 1.25 nanograms/mL to 2.1 nanograms/mL, in this patient the levels only dropped to 1.9 nanograms/mL after stopping the trimethoprim,[1,2] suggesting that the original rise was not solely due to an interaction.

(b) Young healthy adult subjects

Trimethoprim 200 mg twice daily for 10 days did not affect the total body clearance of a single 1-mg intravenous dose of digoxin in 6 young healthy subjects (aged 24 to 31 years). Renal clearance was reduced, but this was compensated for by an increase in extra-renal clearance.[2]

Mechanism

It is suggested that trimethoprim reduces the renal excretion of digoxin.[1,2] The paradoxical finding between the elderly patients and the young healthy subjects could be the age difference: in elderly patients there might not be a compensatory increase extra-renal digoxin clearance to offset the reduced renal clearance.

Importance and management

Information on an interaction between digoxin and trimethoprim seems to be limited to the information cited. Although the rise in serum digoxin levels in the elderly patients was small, it might be prudent to monitor the effects of digoxin (e.g. bradycardia) in the elderly. Take digoxin levels and reduce the digoxin dose if necessary. Trimethoprim is contained in **co-trimoxazole** but it is not known whether prophylactic doses of co-trimoxazole (160 mg trimethoprim a day, from 960 mg co-trimoxazole) will interact to a clinically relevant extent. An interaction would seem possible with high-dose co-trimoxazole regimens, and care with any co-trimoxazole regimen is needed in the elderly.

1. Kastrup J, Bartram R, Petersen P, Hansen JM. Trimetoprims indvirkning på serum-digoksin og serum-kreatinin. *Ugeskr Laeger* (1983) 145, 2286–8.
2. Petersen P, Kastrup J, Bartram R, Hansen JM. Digoxin-trimethoprim interaction. *Acta Med Scand* (1985) 217, 423–7.

Digoxin + Urapidil

Urapidil does not appear to affect the pharmacokinetics of digoxin.

Clinical evidence, mechanism, importance and management

In 12 healthy subjects given digoxin 250 micrograms twice daily on day one, then 250 micrograms daily on days 2 to 8, the concurrent use of urapidil 60 mg twice daily for the last 4 days had no effect on the AUC or maximum serum level of digoxin.[1] No digoxin dose adjustment is therefore likely to be necessary on concurrent use.

1. Solleder P, Haerlin R, Wurst W, Klingmann I, Mosberg H. Effect of urapidil on steady-state serum digoxin concentration in healthy subjects. *Eur J Clin Pharmacol* (1989) 37, 193–4.

Digoxin + Urinary antimuscarinics

Trospium increases the absorption of digoxin elixir. Darifenacin very slightly increased the exposure to digoxin in one study. Solifenacin does not appear to alter the pharmacokinetics of digoxin, and imidafenacin does not appear to affect the exposure to digoxin or its renal clearance.

Clinical evidence, mechanism, importance and management

(a) Darifenacin

The manufacturers note that the concurrent use of digoxin 250 micrograms and darifenacin 30 mg daily (twice the recommended dose) increased the AUC and steady-state levels of digoxin by 16% and 20%, respectively.[1,2] They suggest that the increase in digoxin exposure could be due to competition between digoxin and darifenacin for P-glycoprotein.[2] This very slight increase would generally not be expected to be clinically relevant, but the UK manufacturer advises monitoring digoxin when starting or stopping darifenacin, or when changing the dose of darifenacin.[2]

(b) Imidafenacin

In a crossover study in 12 healthy subjects, imidafenacin 100 micrograms twice daily for 8 days did not affect the AUC or renal clearance of oral digoxin (250 micrograms daily for 2 days, followed by 125 micrograms daily).[3] No digoxin dose adjustment would appear necessary if imidafenacin is also given.

(c) Solifenacin

In a crossover study in 24 healthy subjects, solifenacin 10 mg daily for 10 days had no effect on the pharmacokinetics of digoxin 125 micrograms daily.[4] This study suggests that no pharmacokinetic interaction occurs, and that no digoxin dose adjustment would be expected to be needed on concurrent use.

(d) Trospium

In a study in 40 healthy subjects, trospium 20 mg twice daily for 12 days increased digoxin exposure and maximum levels by about 10% when a single 500-microgram dose of digoxin *elixir* given on day 7. There was also a delay in time to maximum level from about 39 minutes to 56 minutes.[5] Trospium does not inhibit P-glycoprotein,[5] so these minor changes might be due to its antimuscarinic effect causing a slowing of gastrointestinal transit time, and an increase in digoxin absorption.

However, such minor changes are unlikely to be clinically relevant, and no digoxin dose adjustments would appear necessary on concurrent use. Nevertheless, to be certain, it would be necessary to repeat the study with *tablet* formulations of digoxin, compare 'Digoxin + Propantheline', p.1107.

1. Enablex (Darifenacin hydrobromide). Novartis. US Prescribing information, January 2010.
2. Emselex (Darifenacin hydrobromide). Novartis Pharmaceuticals UK Ltd. UK Summary of product characteristics, December 2011.
3. Nakade S, Ohno T, Nakayama K, Kitagawa J, Hasimoto Y, Ohnishi A, Miyata Y. No effect of imidafenacin, a novel antimuscarinic drug, on digoxin pharmacokinetics in healthy subjects. *Drug Metab Pharmacokinet* (2008) 23, 95–100.
4. Smulders RA, Kuipers ME, Krauwinkel WJJ. Multiple doses of the antimuscarinic agent solifenacin do not affect the pharmacodynamics or pharmacokinetics of warfarin or the steady-state pharmacokinetics of digoxin in healthy subjects. *Br J Clin Pharmacol* (2006) 62, 210–17.
5. Sandage B, Sabounjian L, Shipley J, Profy A, Lasseter K, Fox L, Harnett M. Predictive power of an in vitro system to assess drug interactions of an antimuscarinic medication: a comparison of in vitro and in vivo drug-drug interaction studies of trospium chloride with digoxin. *J Clin Pharmacol* (2006) 46, 776–84.

Digoxin + Ursodeoxycholic acid (Ursodiol)

Ursodeoxycholic acid causes a very slight reduction in the exposure to digoxin.

Clinical evidence, mechanism, importance and management

In a study in 8 healthy subjects, ursodeoxycholic acid 13 mg/kg daily for 19 days decreased the AUC_{0-4} and the AUC_{0-72} of a single 500-microgram dose of digoxin given on day 15 by 17% and 12%, respectively, although only the early decrease was statistically significant. The pharmacokinetics of a single intravenous dose of digoxin were not affected by ursodeoxycholic acid. A modelling analysis showed that the oral bioavailability of digoxin was decreased by 9% relative to intravenous administration. It was suggested that this reduction in the absorption of oral digoxin could have occurred because ursodeoxycholic acid might induce P-glycoprotein, which is involved in the transport of digoxin.[1]

Evidence for an interaction between digoxin and ursodeoxycholic acid appears to be limited to the study cited, but an interaction would appear to be established. However, the changes seen were very slight, and seem unlikely to be clinically relevant. Therefore, based on this study, no adjustment in the dose of digoxin would seem to be necessary if ursodeoxycholic acid is also given.

1. Becquemont L, Glaeser H, Drescher S, Hitzl M, Simon N, Murdter TE, Heinkele G, Hofmann U, Schaefer C, Burk O, Verstuyft C, Eichelbaum M, Fromm MF. Effects of ursodeoxycholic acid on P-glycoprotein and cytochrome P450 3A4–dependent pharmacokinetics in humans. *Clin Pharmacol Ther* (2006) 79, 449–60.

Digoxin + Valaciclovir

Valaciclovir does not alter digoxin pharmacokinetics.

Clinical evidence, mechanism, importance and management

In a randomised study, 12 healthy subjects were given 1 g of oral valaciclovir alone, two 750-microgram doses of digoxin alone, valaciclovir 1 g after the second of two 750-microgram doses of digoxin given 12 hours apart, and finally valaciclovir 1 g three times daily for 8 days starting 12 hours before the first digoxin dose.[1] No clinically relevant changes occurred in the pharmacokinetics of either drug. It was therefore concluded that no dose adjustments of either drug are needed if they are given concurrently.[1] Valaciclovir is a prodrug of **aciclovir**: it therefore seems unlikely that an interaction will occur between **aciclovir** and digoxin.

1. Soul-Lawton JH, Weatherley BC, Posner J, Layton G, Peck RW. Lack of interaction between valaciclovir, the L-valyl ester of aciclovir and digoxin. *Br J Clin Pharmacol* (1998) 45, 87–9.

Digoxin + Valspodar

Valspodar increases digoxin exposure.

Clinical evidence

In a study, 12 healthy subjects were given digoxin 1 mg on day one, followed by 125 micrograms daily for the next 10 days. Starting on day 7 they were also given a single 400-mg dose of valspodar, followed by valspodar 200 mg twice daily for the next 4 days. The steady-state AUC of digoxin was increased by 76% after the first dose of valspodar, and by the end of valspodar dosing it had increased threefold. This was apparently due to a 73% reduction in digoxin renal clearance and a 58% reduction in non-renal clearance. No symptoms of digitalis toxicity were seen and there were no changes in blood pressure and most ECG parameters; however, there was a small increase in ventricular rate and a decrease in PR interval on concurrent use, when compared with digoxin alone.[1]

Mechanism

Valspodar is an inhibitor of the P-glycoprotein efflux pump, of which digoxin is a substrate. The reduction in digoxin clearance is possibly due to reduced tubular secretion, reduced biliary elimination, and increased intestinal absorption caused by P-glycoprotein inhibition.[1]

Importance and management

Information on an interaction between dioxin and valspodar seems to be limited, but an interaction is established. The digoxin dose should be reduced if valspodar is given. An initial 50% reduction has been suggested, with careful monitoring for signs of digoxin adverse effects[1] (e.g. bradycardia) and further dose adjustment, according to symptoms and digoxin levels, as necessary.

1. Kovarik JM, Rigaudy L, Guerret M, Gerbeau C, Rost K-L. Longitudinal assessment of a P-glycoprotein-mediated drug interaction of valspodar on digoxin. *Clin Pharmacol Ther* (1999) 66, 391–400.

Digoxin + Vancomycin

Very limited evidence suggests that vancomycin might reduce digoxin clearance.

Clinical evidence, mechanism, importance and management

In one early study, vancomycin prolonged the half-life of digoxin and increased its serum levels from 1.6 nanograms/mL to 3 nanograms/mL. It was suggested that this effect might be as a result of reduced renal clearance.[1] This appears to be the only evidence of a possible interaction, and as such, no general recommendations can be made.

1. Halawa B. Interakcje digoksyny z cefradina (Sefril), tetracylina (Tetracyclinum), gentamycyna (Gentamycin) i wankomycyna (Vancocin). *Pol Tyg Lek* (1984) 39, 1717–20.

Digoxin + Varenicline

Varenicline does not alter the pharmacokinetics of digoxin.

Clinical evidence, mechanism, importance and management

In a crossover study in 18 healthy subjects (current smokers), varenicline (500 micrograms daily for 3 days, then 500 micrograms twice daily for 4 days, then 1 mg twice daily for 7 days) had no effect on the pharmacokinetics of digoxin 200 micrograms daily.[1] Digoxin renal clearance was increased by 11%, but this is not clinically relevant. No digoxin dose adjustment would appear necessary if varenicline is also given.

1. Faessel HM, Burstein AH, Troutman MD, Willavize SA, Rohrbacher KD, Clark DJ. Lack of a pharmacokinetic interaction between a new smoking cessation therapy, varenicline, and digoxin in adult smokers. *Eur J Clin Pharmacol* (2008) 64, 1101–1109.

Digoxin + Vasodilators

Dihydralazine, sodium nitroprusside and hydralazine infusions can reduce digoxin levels. Isosorbide dinitrate did not alter digoxin pharmacokinetics in one study.

Clinical evidence, mechanism, importance and management

(a) Hydralazine or Sodium nitroprusside

An experimental study in 8 patients with congestive heart failure found that when they were given either sodium nitroprusside by infusion (7 to 425 micrograms/minute) or hydralazine by intravenous injection (5 mg every 10 to 20 minutes to a total dose of 10 to 60 mg) the total renal digoxin clearance was increased by about 50% by both drugs and the serum digoxin levels were decreased by 20% by nitroprusside and 11% by hydralazine.[1] Another study found that **dihydralazine** shortened the half-life of digoxin and reduced its serum levels, but did not affect digoxin bioavailability.[2]

It is not known whether these changes would be sustained during long-term concurrent use, but the changes in the levels seen were relatively small. A clinically important interaction seems unlikely, but ideally longer-term studies are needed to confirm this.

(b) Isosorbide dinitrate

In a crossover study in 8 patients with chronic heart failure, given digoxin 250 micrograms daily for 20 days with isosorbide dinitrate 10 mg three times daily for the last 10 days, there was no change in the mean steady-state concentration, AUC or half-life of digoxin.[3]

1. Cogan JJ, Humphreys MH, Carlson CJ, Benowitz NL, Rapaport E. Acute vasodilator therapy increases renal clearance of digoxin in patients with congestive heart failure. *Circulation* (1981) 64, 973–6.
2. Halawa B, Mazurek W. Interakcja digoksyny z dihydralazyną I prazosyną. *Pol Tyg Lek* (1986) 41, 1521–3.
3. Mahgoub AA, El-Medany AH, Abdulatif AS. A comparison between the effects of diltiazem and isosorbide dinitrate on digoxin pharmacodynamics and kinetics in the treatment of patients with chronic ischemic heart failure. *Saudi Med J* (2002) 23, 725–31.

Digoxin + Vasopressin antagonists

Conivaptan, and to a lesser extent tolvaptan, appear to increase digoxin concentrations.

Clinical evidence

The US manufacturer reports that oral **conivaptan** 40 mg twice daily increased the maximum plasma concentration and AUC of a single 500-microgram dose of digoxin by 79% and 43%, respectively.[1]

In a study in 14 healthy subjects, **tolvaptan** 60 mg daily for 5 days increased the steady-state AUC and minimum plasma concentration of digoxin 250 micrograms daily by 18% and 21%, respectively.[2]

Mechanism

Digoxin is a substrate of the drug transporter protein, P-glycoprotein, which appears to be inhibited by tolvaptan and conivaptan. Concurrent use therefore results in an increase in digoxin exposure.

Importance and management

Evidence for a pharmacokinetic interaction between digoxin and the vasopressin antagonists is limited, although given the likely mechanism the interaction would appear to be established. The increase in the digoxin concentration with **conivaptan** seems likely to be clinically relevant. It would therefore seem prudent to monitor concurrent use closely for digoxin adverse effects (such as bradycardia), monitoring digoxin concentrations and adjusting the digoxin dose, if necessary.

The small increase in the digoxin concentration with **tolvaptan** might be clinically relevant in some patients. It would seem prudent to bear the possibility of digoxin adverse effects (such as bradycardia) in mind on concurrent use, monitoring digoxin concentrations and adjusting the digoxin dose, if necessary.

1. Vaprisol (Conivaptan hydrochloride). Astellas Pharma US, Inc. US Prescribing information, February 2011.
2. Shoaf SE, Wang Z, Mallikaarjun S, Bricmont P, Bramer SL. In vitro P-glycoprotein interactions and steady-state pharmacokinetic interactions between tolvaptan and digoxin in healthy subjects. *Clin Pharmacol Ther* (2011) 51, 761.

Digoxin + Vitamin E substances

Alpha tocoferil acetate had no effect on digoxin pharmacokinetics in one study, but vitamin E formulations with polyethylene glycol might affect digoxin pharmacokinetics.

Clinical evidence, mechanism, importance and management

In a study in healthy subjects, **alpha tocoferil acetate** 400 units twice daily for 15 days did not affect the pharmacokinetics of a single 500-microgram dose of digoxin given on day 15. This was in contrast to a formulation of vitamin E containing polyethylene glycol (**alpha tocoferil acid succinate**), which altered digoxin pharmacokinetics (amount not stated) without altering its ECG effects.

It was suggested that the effect of polyethylene glycol on digoxin was via P-glycoprotein inhibition,[1] see also 'Digoxin + Surfactant excipients', p.1112. The clinical relevance of this finding is unclear as the magnitude of effect on digoxin pharmacokinetics was not stated.

1. Chan L, Humma LM, Schriever CA, Fahsingbauer BS, Dominguez CP, Baum CL. Vitamin E formulation affects digoxin absorption by inhibiting P-glycoprotein (P-GP) in humans. *Clin Pharmacol Ther* (2004) 75, P95.

Digoxin + Zileuton

Zileuton does not alter the pharmacokinetics of digoxin.

Clinical evidence, mechanism, importance and management

In a placebo-controlled study, 12 healthy subjects were given zileuton 600 mg every 6 hours for 13 days, with digoxin 250 micrograms daily from days 1 to 11. Zileuton had no effect on the steady-state pharmacokinetics of digoxin, although the time to reach maximum plasma levels was reduced from 1.43 hours to 0.95 hours.[1] This evidence suggests that no digoxin dose adjustment is necessary if zileuton is also given.

1. Awni WM, Hussein Z, Cavanaugh JH, Granneman GR, Dube LM. Assessment of the pharmacokinetic interaction between zileuton and digoxin in humans. *Clin Pharmacokinet* (1995) 29 (Suppl 2), 92–7.

26
Diuretics

The majority of the interactions of the diuretics appear to be pharmacodynamic in nature, that is, they appear to be due to the combined effects of the diuretic and the other interacting drug. Obvious examples of this would be hypotension caused by the use of a loop diuretic and a beta blocker, or hyperkalaemia caused by the use of an ACE inhibitor and a potassium-sparing diuretic. Some commonly accepted interactions appear to be sparsely documented, most probably because they are perceived to be a predictable effect of the concurrent use of two drugs with similar actions. 'Table 26.1', below, lists the major diuretic drug groups classified by their effect on potassium. Carbonic anhydrase inhibitors are included under potassium-depleting diuretics, but note that hypokalaemia caused by this type of drug is said to be transient and rarely clinically significant.

Eplerenone, a selective aldosterone antagonist similar to spironolactone, is metabolised by CYP3A4 and is therefore affected by other drugs that are inhibitors or inducers of this isoenzyme; it appears to be unique amongst the diuretics in this regard.

The interactions covered in this section are mainly those in which the diuretic is affected. There are many other interactions throughout the publication where diuretics affect the actions of other drugs.

Table 26.1 Diuretics

Group	*Drugs*
Potassium-depleting diuretics	
Carbonic anhydrase inhibitors*	Acetazolamide, Diclofenamide (Dichlorphenamide)
Loop diuretics	Bumetanide, Etacrynic acid, Furosemide, Piretanide, Torasemide
Thiazides and related diuretics	Altizide, Bemetizide, Bendroflumethiazide, Benzthiazide, Butizide, Chlorothiazide, Chlortalidone, Cicletanine, Clopamide, Cyclopenthiazide, Cyclothiazide, Epitizide, Hydrochlorothiazide, Hydroflumethiazide, Indapamide, Mefruside, Methyclothiazide, Metipamide, Metolazone, Teclothiazide, Trichlormethiazide, Xipamide
Potassium-sparing diuretics	
Aldosterone inhibitors	Eplerenone, Potassium canrenoate, Spironolactone
Other	Amiloride, Triamterene

*Note that hypokalaemia caused by this type of drug is said to be transient and rarely clinically significant

Acetazolamide + NSAIDs

A woman developed acute renal failure following retinal surgery, after the postoperative use of a total of 2 g of acetazolamide, 80 g of mannitol and 700 mg of ketoprofen over a 2-day period.[1] There appear to be no other similar case reports, and therefore the general relevance of this case is unclear. However, note that other interactions have been reported with related drugs. For instance, loop diuretics are known to increase the risk of NSAID-induced acute renal failure, see 'Loop diuretics + NSAIDs', p.1120, and a severe toxic reaction has been reported in patients receiving concurrent high-dose aspirin and acetazolamide, see 'Aspirin or other Salicylates + Carbonic anhydrase inhibitors', p.140.

1. Truc C, Rigal E, Pernot A, Vaudelin G, Boulétreau P. Anti-inflammatoires non stéroïdiens et diurétiques: une association à risque néphrotoxique. *Ann Fr Anesth Reanim* (2000) 19, 675–7.

Acetazolamide + Sodium bicarbonate

Acetazolamide is associated with the development of renal calculi and it has been claimed that sodium bicarbonate, even on alternate days, potentiates the risk of calculus formation.[1] There seem to be no case reports describing an adverse interaction, and so the general significance of this suggested interaction is unclear.

1. Rubenstein MA, Bucy JG. Acetazolamide-induced renal calculi. *J Urol (Baltimore)* (1975) 114, 610–12.

Acetazolamide + Timolol

The use of acetazolamide tablets with timolol eye drops resulted in severe mixed acidosis in a patient with chronic obstructive pulmonary disease.

Clinical evidence, mechanism, importance and management

An elderly man with severe COPD was given oral acetazolamide 750 mg daily and timolol maleate 0.5% eye drops, one drop in each eye twice daily, as premedication to reduce ocular hypertension before surgery for glaucoma. Five days later he developed progressively worsening dyspnoea and he was found to have a severe, mixed acidosis.[1] This seems to have been caused by the additive effects of acetazolamide, which blocked the excretion of hydrogen ions in the kidney, and the bronchoconstrictor effects of the timolol, which was absorbed in sufficient amounts to exacerbate the airway obstruction in this patient, and thereby reduced respiration. This isolated case emphasises the potential risks of using beta blockers, even as non-systemic preparations, such as eye drops, in patients with obstructive pulmonary disease. The manufacturers of acetazolamide note that it should be used with caution in those with pulmonary obstruction or emphysema because of the increased risk of acidosis.[2,3] This is therefore, in part, a drug-disease interaction.

1. Boada JE, Estopa R, Izquierdo J, Dorca J, Manresa F. Severe mixed acidosis by combined therapy with acetazolamide and timolol eyedrops. *Eur J Respir Dis* (1986) 68, 226–8.
2. Diamox Tablets (Acetazolamide). Goldshield plc. UK Summary of product characteristics, August 2009.
3. Acetazolamide Tablets. Taro Pharmaceuticals USA Inc. US Prescribing information, March 2005.

Diuretics + Aliskiren

Aliskiren reduces the plasma levels of furosemide, but does not appear to affect the pharmacokinetics of hydrochlorothiazide to a clinically relevant extent. Aliskiren may cause hypotension in patients receiving high doses of diuretics and may possibly increase serum potassium levels in patients receiving potassium-sparing diuretics.

Clinical evidence, mechanism, importance and management

(a) Loop diuretics

In a study, 21 healthy subjects were given furosemide 20 mg daily for 3 days followed by a 3-day washout period. They were then given aliskiren 300 mg daily for 10 days with furosemide 20 mg daily on days 8 to 10. The AUC and peak plasma levels of aliskiren were reduced by 7% and 20%, respectively, but this was not considered clinically relevant. The AUC and maximum plasma level of furosemide were reduced by 28% and 49%, respectively, by the concurrent use of aliskiren.[1] The UK manufacturer of aliskiren recommends that the effects of furosemide should be monitored when starting or adjusting therapy in patients taking aliskiren.[2] In addition, the manufacturers of aliskiren note that in patients with marked volume- and/or salt-depletion, for example those receiving high doses of diuretics, symptomatic hypotension could occur after initiation of treatment with aliskiren. Close medical supervision is required in such patients.[2,3]

(b) Potassium-sparing diuretics

Based on experience with the use of other substances that affect the renin-angiotensin system, the concurrent use of potassium-sparing diuretics and aliskiren may lead to increases in serum potassium and caution is advisable.[2]

(c) Thiazides

In a study in healthy subjects, aliskiren 300 mg daily did not have a clinically relevant effect on the pharmacokinetics of hydrochlorothiazide 25 mg daily. The AUC of aliskiren was not affected by hydrochlorothiazide, whereas its steady-state maximum plasma level was reduced by 22%; however, this was not considered to be clinically relevant. There was an increased incidence of dizziness in subjects receiving aliskiren and hydrochlorothiazide, when compared with either drug alone, but this might be expected with two effective antihypertensive drugs given to normotensive healthy subjects.[4] The concurrent use of aliskiren and hydrochlorothiazide has been widely studied for its therapeutic use. A review paper of these studies notes that in patients with mild-to-moderate hypertension, there was no difference in the rate of dizziness or the incidence of adverse effects with the combination, when compared with monotherapy.[5]

The manufacturers of aliskiren note that in patients with marked volume- and/or salt-depletion, for example those receiving high doses of diuretics, symptomatic hypotension could occur after initiation of treatment with aliskiren. Close medical supervision is required in such patients.[2,3]

1. Vaidyanthan S, Bartlett M, Dieterich HA, Yeh C-M, Antunes A, Howard D, Dole WP. Pharmacokinetic interaction of the direct renin inhibitor aliskiren with furosemide and extended-release isosorbide-5-mononitrate in healthy subjects. *Cardiovasc Ther* (2008) 26, 238–46.
2. Rasilez 300 mg Tablets (Aliskiren hemifumarate). Novartis Pharmaceuticals UK Ltd. UK Summary of product characteristics, August 2012.
3. Tekturna (Aliskiren hemifumarate). Novartis. US Prescribing information, September 2012.
4. Vaidyanathan S, Valencia J, Kemp C, Zhao C, Yeh C-M, Bizot M-N, Denouel J, Dieterich HA, Dole WP. Lack of pharmacokinetic interactions of aliskiren, a novel direct renin inhibitor for the treatment of hypertension, with the antihypertensives amlodipine, valsartan, hydrochlorothiazide (HCTZ) and ramipril in healthy volunteers. *Int J Clin Pract* (2006) 60, 1343–56.
5. Chrysant SG. Aliskiren-hydrochlorothiazide combination for the treatment of hypertension. *Expert Rev Cardiovasc Ther* (2008) 6, 305–14.

Diuretics + Liquorice

Hypokalaemia has occurred in a few subjects taking hydrochlorothiazide and liquorice. This interaction seems possible with liquorice and any potassium-depleting diuretic (i.e. thiazides or loop diuretics).

Clinical evidence, mechanism, importance and management

A 41-year-old woman who presented with hypertension was unsuccessfully treated with atenolol and candesartan. After the addition of **hydrochlorothiazide**, she developed hypokalaemia with muscle cramps and weakness, which persisted for more than 4 weeks after the hydrochlorothiazide was discontinued. The patient had denied eating liquorice sweets, but was found to have been drinking at least 3 litres of liquorice tea daily.[1]

In a study, 10 healthy subjects were given low-dose liquorice 32 g daily (in the form of confectionary) alone or with **hydrochlorothiazide** 25 mg daily for 2 weeks. There were no changes in plasma potassium, sodium, creatinine, renin activity, serum aldosterone, blood pressure or heart rate with liquorice alone, but there were weight increases of about 0.4 kg. When **hydrochlorothiazide** was also given, plasma potassium decreased by 0.32 mmol/L, plasma renin activity increased, and weight decreased by 0.9 kg. Two of the 10 subjects became hypokalaemic during the first week of concurrent use, requiring withdrawal from the study.[2]

Liquorice has mineralocorticoid-like actions, which may lower potassium levels. This effect may be additive with the effects of the potassium-depleting diuretics (i.e. thiazides or loop diuretics), which may result in clinically significant hypokalaemia. Consider this interaction in a case of otherwise unexplained hypokalaemia.

1. Brouwers AJBW, van der Meulen J. 'Drophypertensie'; ook door zoethoutthee. *Ned Tijdschr Geneeskd* (2001) 145, 744–7.
2. Hukkanen J, Okkola O, Savolainen MJ. Effects of low-dose liquorice alone or in combination with hydrochlorothiazide on the plasma potassium in healthy volunteers. *Blood Pressure* (2009) 18, 192–5.

Diuretics + Sodium phosphate or Sodium picosulfate

Seizures in two patients, which occurred after the use of either sodium phosphate or sodium picosulfate bowel preparations, were associated with hyponatraemia, which may have been potentiated by thiazides.

Clinical evidence

One patient given *Phospho-soda* (monobasic and dibasic sodium phosphate) and a second patient given *Picoprep* (sodium picosulfate with magnesium citrate) as oral bowel preparations for colonoscopy had grand mal seizures with hyponatraemia. The patient given *Phospho-soda* was also taking **cyclopenthiazide** and the patient given *Picoprep* was also taking **hydrochlorothiazide**. Neither of the patients had a history of seizures and electrolyte levels were normal 10 days before use of the bowel preparation.[1]

Mechanism

Both sodium phosphate and sodium picosulfate may cause electrolyte abnormalities, including hyponatraemia, which is associated with seizures.[1] This may be exacerbated by the concurrent use of diuretics, which can also lower sodium levels.

Importance and management

Evidence for an interaction between sodium phosphate or sodium picosulfate and the thiazides appears to be limited to these two cases, but the mechanism for an effect is consistent with the known effects of these drugs. Care is therefore advised if these bowel preparations are used in patients taking thiazides or any other diuretic, as they all have the potential to reduce sodium levels, particularly in those with a low seizure threshold.

1. Frizelle FA, Colls BM. Hyponatremia and seizures after bowel preparation: report of three cases. *Dis Colon Rectum* (2005) 48, 393–6.

Loop diuretics + Aspirin or other Salicylates

Aspirin may reduce the diuretic effect of bumetanide, furosemide, or piretanide, and reduce the venodilation produced by furosemide. The combination of aspirin and furosemide may increase the risk of acute renal failure and salicylate toxicity. The risk of ototoxicity with high doses of salicylates may theoretically be increased by loop diuretics.

Clinical evidence

(a) Bumetanide

In 8 healthy subjects aspirin 640 mg four times daily reduced the 24-hour urinary output in response to bumetanide 1 mg by 18%.[1]

(b) Furosemide

A study in 11 patients with chronic heart failure found that both aspirin 75 mg daily and aspirin 300 mg daily for 14 days reduced the venodilatory effects produced by a single 20-mg intravenous dose of furosemide (as measured by the forearm venous capacitance).[2] Six patients with cirrhosis and ascites had a reduced diuretic response to intravenous furosemide 40 mg given after a single intravenous dose of **lysine aspirin** 450 mg.[3] A further study in 6 patients found that the concurrent use of furosemide and aspirin temporarily reduced creatinine clearance in patients with chronic renal impairment.[4]

Studies in healthy subjects similarly found that intravenous aspirin or **lysine aspirin** blunted the diuresis[5,6] and sodium excretion[6] caused by intravenous furosemide, and appeared to increase potassium excretion;[6] the reduced diuretic effect seemed to correlate with an inhibition of proximal tubular secretion.[5] A similar reduction in sodium excretion was found in a study where healthy subjects were given aspirin and furosemide orally.[7]

In contrast, another study in healthy subjects found that oral aspirin 4 g daily did not influence the effects of oral furosemide 40 mg on renal sodium excretion or urinary creatinine excretion.[8]

A study in healthy subjects found that when aspirin 600 mg and furosemide 40 mg were given at the same time there was a significant reduction in the total excretion of salicylates, but when the drugs were given 30 minutes apart the total amount of salicylate excreted increased slightly.[7]

(c) Piretanide

A study in 4 healthy subjects found that intravenous **lysine aspirin** 1 g decreased the diuresis and sodium excretion caused by intravenous piretanide 12 mg.[6]

Mechanism

Uncertain. Aspirin may compete with furosemide for a common secretory mechanism in the proximal tubule.[5,7] In addition, aspirin may also inhibit renal prostaglandins, which appear to mediate the increased renal blood flow induced by loop diuretics in cirrhotics with ascites.[3] Consider also 'Loop diuretics + NSAIDs', p.1120.

Importance and management

An interaction between aspirin and loop diuretics, which results in an attenuation of the diuretic effect, is established; however, the clinical relevance of this effect does not appear to have been studied. Nevertheless, the reduction in diuretic effects seen in the studies might reasonably be expected to lead to a worsening of the condition being treated with the loop diuretic. The UK manufacturer of furosemide warns that aspirin may attenuate the action of furosemide and may cause acute renal failure in cases of pre-existing hypovolaemia or dehydration.[9] It would therefore seem prudent to avoid the use of high-dose salicylates in those taking loop diuretics, giving an alternative non-NSAID analgesic wherever possible. If concurrent use is considered essential, closely monitor for signs of a reduced diuretic effect as well as for signs of renal impairment, and reconsider the use of the salicylate or adjust the dose of the diuretic as necessary.

The manufacturers of furosemide warn that salicylate toxicity may occur on the concurrent use of furosemide and high doses of a salicylate, as in rheumatic disease, because of competition for renal excretory sites.[4,9] Furthermore, high doses of salicylates can be ototoxic, particularly if the patient is dehydrated, and the risk of ototoxicity may theoretically be increased if salicylates are given with other ototoxic drugs, including loop diuretics such as bumetanide, **etacrynic acid** or furosemide.[10,11] It would therefore seem prudent to monitor for signs of hearing impairment if patients given salicylates, including analgesic doses of aspirin, are also given loop diuretics.

There is even less evidence regarding a possible interaction between loop diuretics and antiplatelet doses of aspirin. Until more is known, it would seem prudent to bear the possibility of an interaction in mind should a patient taking low-dose aspirin have a reduced response to a loop diuretic, and adjust the dose of the diuretic accordingly. Note that the proven protective cardiovascular benefits of low-dose aspirin in patients with hypertension and/or coronary artery disease seem likely to outweigh the possible reduction in the efficacy of the loop diuretic.

1. Kaufman J, Hamburger R, Matheson J, Flamenbaum W. Bumetanide-induced diuresis and natriuresis: effect of prostaglandin synthetase inhibition. *J Clin Pharmacol* (1981) 21, 663–7.
2. Jhund PS, Davie AP, McMurray JJV. Aspirin inhibits the acute venodilator response to furosemide in patients with chronic heart failure. *J Am Coll Cardiol* (2001) 37, 1234–8.
3. Planas R, Arroyo V, Rimola A, Pérez-Ayuso RM, Rodés J. Acetylsalicylic acid suppresses the renal hemodynamic effect and reduces the diuretic action of furosemide in cirrhosis with ascites. *Gastroenterology* (1983) 84, 247–52.
4. Lasix (Furosemide). Sanofi-Aventis. US Prescribing information, July 2009.
5. Bartoli E, Arras S, Faedda R, Soggia G, Satta A, Olmeo NA. Blunting of furosemide diuresis by aspirin in man. *J Clin Pharmacol* (1980) 20, 452–8.
6. Valette H, Apoil E. Interaction between salicylate and two loop diuretics. *Br J Clin Pharmacol* (1979) 8, 592–4.
7. Oyekan AO, Laniyonu AA, Ashorobi RB. Interaction between frusemide and aspirin. *Gen Pharmacol* (1984) 15, 163–6.
8. Berg KJ. Acute effects of acetylsalicylic acid on renal function in normal man. *Eur J Clin Pharmacol* (1977) 11, 117–23.
9. Lasix (Furosemide). Sanofi-Aventis. UK Summary of product characteristics, July 2010.
10. Yorgason JG, Fayad JN, Kalinec F. Understanding drug ototoxicity: molecular insights for prevention and clinical management. *Expert Opin Drug Safety* (2006) 5, 383–99.
11. Lheureux Ph, Penaloza A. Les vertiges d'origine ototoxique. Ototoxicity-related dysequilibrium. *Rev Med Brux* (2002) 23, A356–A362.

Loop diuretics + Epoprostenol

In a study modelling data from 23 patients with heart failure, an infusion of epoprostenol did not alter the pharmacokinetics of furosemide to a clinically relevant extent.[1] Note that the concurrent use of loop diuretics with epoprostenol may lead to an enhanced hypotensive effect.

1. Carlton LD, Patterson JH, Mattson CN, Schmith VD. The effects of epoprostenol on drug disposition II: a pilot study of the pharmacokinetics of furosemide with and without epoprostenol in patients with congestive heart failure. *J Clin Pharmacol* (1996) 36, 257–64.

Loop diuretics + Food

Some studies suggest that food modestly reduces the bioavailability and slightly reduces the diuretic effects of furosemide, whereas other studies suggest that food does not affect furosemide bioavailability or the diuretic response to furosemide. Food does not appear to affect the bioavailability of bumetanide solution or torasemide tablets.

Clinical evidence

(a) Bumetanide

A study in 9 healthy subjects found that the absorption of bumetanide 2 mg, given as a *solution*, was delayed, and its peak plasma levels were reduced, by a standard breakfast. However, the bioavailability of bumetanide was not significantly reduced (75% with food and 84% fasting).[1]

(b) Furosemide

1. Solutions or standard tablets. In a study, 10 healthy subjects were given furosemide 40 mg with and without a standard breakfast. Food reduced the peak plasma levels and bioavailability of furosemide, by 55% and about 30%, respectively.[2] The results were almost identical when 5 of the subjects were given a heavy meal.[2] Furthermore, the diuresis over 10 hours was reduced by 21% (from 2072 mL to 1640 mL) and the diuresis over 24 hours was reduced by 15% (from 2668 mL to 2270 mL) when furosemide was taken with breakfast.[2]

A study in 10 patients with chronic respiratory failure found that food decreased furosemide absorption and bioavailability: the mean 24-hour urinary recovery of unchanged drug was 11.5 mg and 9.41 mg, when the furosemide was given before and after food, respectively. In addition, when the data from these patients was compared with that from 11 healthy fasted subjects, the furosemide bioavailability was found to be lower, possibly due to enhanced glucuronidation and incomplete drug absorption. The diuretic effect was also lower in patients than healthy subjects; however, when furosemide was taken after food there was no significant change in the resulting diuresis, when compared with the fasting state.[3]

A study in 8 healthy subjects found that the absorption of furosemide 40 mg, given as a *solution*, was delayed, and its peak plasma levels were reduced, by a standard breakfast.[1] Food reduced the oral bioavailability of furosemide by about one-third, from 76% to 43%. In two other studies food delayed the absorption but did not significantly alter the bioavailability of furosemide as tablets or solutions.[4,5] In one of these studies, there was no difference in diuresis between fed and fasting subjects.[5]

2. Sustained-release tablets. In a single-dose, crossover study, 28 subjects were given two different controlled-release formulations of furosemide 60 mg with and without breakfast. The absorption of one preparation (*Furix Retard*) was reduced by about 32% by the breakfast, whereas the extent of absorption of the other formulation (*Lasix Retard*) was *increased* by about 18% by the breakfast. In the fasting phase of the study, *Furix Retard* had a higher extent and rate of absorption than *Lasix Retard*. However, the differences in diuresis and total natriuresis between the formulations, and between the fed and fasted state, were minor.[6] Another study suggested that furosemide extended-release tablets, which use an erosional matrix designed to retain the preparation in the stomach and deliver furosemide to the duodenum and upper jejunum over 6 hours, should be given in the fed state to ensure that the formulation remains in the stomach for long enough for the absorption of furosemide to occur.[7]

(c) Torasemide

A study in 14 healthy subjects given torasemide 10 mg as a tablet found that administration with food decreased the absorption rate of torasemide, but did not affect the extent of absorption, when compared with the fasting state.[8]

Mechanism

Not understood.

Importance and management

Information about the effect of food on **furosemide** absorption is somewhat contradictory. Of the five studies using solutions or standard tablets, three found that the bioavailability of furosemide was modestly reduced by food (by about 30%) and the other two found no effect. Similarly, one study found a reduction in diuresis, whereas two others found no clinically relevant decrease in diuresis. It would also seem that the absorption of controlled-release formulations of furosemide may be modestly affected by food, but this may lead to increased or decreased absorption, depending on the preparation. On balance, any effect appears modest, and it would seem that furosemide can be given to most patients without regard to meal times; however, it has been suggested that in some patients, such as those with heart failure or renal impairment, reduced furosemide absorption may decrease the urinary excretion of the drug and that the diuretic threshold may not therefore be achieved. In such patients giving furosemide without food might maximise the chance of achieving a diuretic response.[9]

Food does not appear to affect the bioavailability of **bumetanide** given as solution or **torasemide** tablets and therefore they may be given without regard to meal times.

1. McCrindle JL, Li Kam Wa TC, Barron W, Prescott LF. Effect of food on the absorption of frusemide and bumetanide in man. *Br J Clin Pharmacol* (1996) 42, 743–6.
2. Beermann B, Midskov C. Reduced bioavailability and effect of furosemide given with food. *Eur J Clin Pharmacol* (1986) 29, 725–7.
3. Ogata H, Kawatsu Y, Maruyama Y, Machida K, Haga T. Bioavailability and diuretic effect of furosemide during long-term treatment of chronic respiratory failure. *Eur J Clin Pharmacol* (1985) 28, 53–9.
4. Hammarlund MM, Paalzow LK, Odlind B. Pharmacokinetics of furosemide in man after intravenous and oral administration. Application of moment analysis. *Eur J Clin Pharmacol* (1984) 26, 197–207.
5. Kelly MR, Cutler RE, Forrey AW, Kimpel BM. Pharmacokinetics of orally administered furosemide. *Clin Pharmacol Ther* (1974) 15, 178–86.
6. Paintaud G, Alván G, Eckernäs S-Å, Wakelkamp M, Grahnén A. The influence of food intake on the effect of two controlled release formulations of furosemide. *Biopharm Drug Dispos* (1995) 16, 221–32.
7. Berner B, Cowles VE. Case studies in swelling polymeric gastric retentive tablets. *Expert Opin Drug Deliv* (2006) 3, 541–8.
8. Kramer WG. Effect of food on the pharmacokinetics and pharmacodynamics of torsemide. *Am J Ther* (1995) 2, 499–503.
9. Bard RL, Bleske BE, Nicklas JM. Food: an unrecognized source of loop diuretic resistance. *Pharmacotherapy* (2004) 24, 630–7.

Loop diuretics + H_2-receptor antagonists

Ranitidine and cimetidine may cause a slight increase in the bioavailability of furosemide, but this does not appear to be clinically relevant. Cimetidine does not appear to affect the pharmacokinetics or pharmacodynamics of torasemide.

Clinical evidence, mechanism, importance and management

(a) Furosemide

In a study in 6 healthy subjects, a single 400-mg dose of **cimetidine** increased the mean AUC of furosemide by one-third, although there was wide interpatient variation. However, there were no changes in the diuretic effects of furosemide or in the pharmacokinetics of cimetidine, and an associated study using multiple doses of **cimetidine** over 5 days found no pharmacokinetic or pharmacodynamic interaction.[1] A similar study in patients with hepatic cirrhosis also found that **cimetidine** does not interact with furosemide.[2] No particular precautions therefore seem necessary on concurrent use.

Eighteen healthy subjects were given oral furosemide 40 mg one hour after intravenous **ranitidine** 50 mg or saline. **Ranitidine** increased the AUC of furosemide by 28% and increased its maximum serum levels by 37%.[3] The effects of furosemide could possibly be slightly increased by **ranitidine**, but the clinical importance of this is probably small. No particular precautions therefore seem necessary on concurrent use.

(b) Torasemide

In 11 healthy subjects **cimetidine** 300 mg four times daily for 3 days was found to have no effect on the pharmacokinetics of a single 10-mg oral dose of torasemide, nor were there any changes in the volume of urine or the excretion of sodium, potassium or chloride.[4] No particular precautions therefore seem necessary on concurrent use.

1. Rogers HJ, Morrison P, House FR, Bradbrook ID. Effect of cimetidine on the absorption and efficacy of orally administered furosemide. *Int J Clin Pharmacol Ther Toxicol* (1982) 20, 8–11.
2. Sanchis Closa A, Lambert C, du Souich P. Lack of effect of cimetidine on furosemide kinetics and dynamics in patients with hepatic cirrhosis. *Int J Clin Pharmacol Ther Toxicol* (1993) 31, 461–6.
3. Müller FO, De Vaal AC, Hundt KL, Luus HG. Intravenous ranitidine enhances furosemide bioavailability. *Klin Pharmakol Akt* (1993) 4, 26.
4. Kramer WG. Lack of effect of cimetidine on torsemide pharmacokinetics and pharmacodynamics in healthy subjects. *Int Congr Ser* (1993), 361–4.

Loop diuretics + NSAIDs

The antihypertensive and diuretic effects of the loop diuretics appear to be reduced by NSAIDs, including coxibs, although the extent of this interaction largely depends on the individual NSAID. Diuretics increase the risk of NSAID-induced acute renal failure. The concurrent use of NSAIDs with loop diuretics may exacerbate congestive heart failure and increase the risk of hospitalisation. Some NSAIDs may theoretically increase the risk of ototoxicity associated with loop diuretics.

Clinical evidence

Various large epidemiological studies and meta-analyses of clinical studies have been conducted to assess the effect of NSAIDs on blood pressure in patients taking **antihypertensives**, and the findings of these are summarised in 'Table 23.2', p.1031. In these studies, NSAIDs were not always associated with an increase in blood pressure, and the maximum increase was 6.2 mmHg. The effect has been shown for both coxibs and non-selective NSAIDs. In two meta-analyses,[1,2] the effects were evaluated by NSAID. The confidence intervals for all the NSAIDs overlapped, showing that there was no statistically significant difference between the NSAIDs, with the exception of the comparison between **indometacin** and **sulindac** in one analysis.[2] Nevertheless, an attempt was made at ranking the NSAIDs based on the means. In one analysis,[1] the effect was greatest for **piroxicam**, **indometacin**, and **ibuprofen**, intermediate for **naproxen**, and least for **sulindac** and **flurbiprofen**. In the other meta-analysis,[2] the effect was greatest for **indometacin** and **naproxen**, intermediate for **piroxicam**, and least for **ibuprofen** and **sulindac**. An attempt was also made to evaluate the effect by **antihypertensive** in one analysis.[1] The mean effect was greatest for beta blockers, intermediate for vasodilators (includes ACE inhibitors and calcium-channel blockers), and least for **diuretics**. However, the differences between the groups were not significant.

A retrospective analysis of records of patients taking **diuretics** (thiazides, loop and/or potassium-sparing) with NSAIDs found a twofold increase in the risk of hospitalisation for congestive heart failure on concurrent use. The most common NSAIDs taken by this cohort of patients were **diclofenac**, **ibuprofen**, **indometacin** and **naproxen**. The **diuretics** most often used were thiazides combined with potassium-sparing drugs and this therapy showed a significantly higher risk than the other diuretic therapies.[3]

A case-control study using the UK General Practice Research Database found that current NSAID use increased the risk of acute renal failure (relative risk 3.2 compared with no NSAID use) and this risk was further increased with concurrent **diuretic** use (relative risk 11.6).[4] Note that the risk of renal complications appear to be similar with coxibs as with non-specific NSAIDs.[5]

Individual clinical reports and clinical or pharmacological studies of the effects of specific NSAIDs on diuretics are outlined in the subsections below and in 'Table 26.2', p.1121.

A. Bumetanide

(a) Celecoxib and other Coxibs

A patient taking celecoxib with bumetanide developed moderately raised serum creatinine levels. Another patient taking an ACE inhibitor, spironolactone and bumetanide developed severely raised serum creatinine levels, hyperkalaemia, and worsening of congestive heart failure shortly after starting celecoxib.[6] A similar case occurred in another patient taking bumetanide about 8 days after **rofecoxib** was started.[6]

(b) Indometacin

In two studies, a single 100-mg dose of indometacin was found to reduce the bumetanide-induced output of urine, sodium and chloride (but not potassium) by about 25%.[7-9] There are other reports confirming this interaction between bumetanide and indometacin, including a clinical study,[10] and a report of a patient who developed heart failure as a result of this interaction.[11]

(c) Sulindac

A study in 8 healthy subjects found that a single 300-mg dose of sulindac did not reduce the diuretic response (measured by urinary volume, and urinary excretion of sodium, potassium, and chloride) to a single 1-mg dose of bumetanide.[12] However, another study in 9 healthy subjects found that pretreatment with sulindac 200 mg twice daily for 5 days reduced the diuretic effect of a single 1-mg dose of bumetanide (mean urine flow rate after 2 hours reduced by 21% and cumulative sodium excretion at 3 hours reduced by 22%).[13]

(d) Tolfenamic acid

A study in 8 healthy subjects found that tolfenamic acid 300 mg reduced the diuretic response (measured by urinary volume, and urinary excretion of sodium, potassium, and chloride) to a single 1-mg dose of bumetanide by 34% at 2 hours.[12]

B. Furosemide

A comparison of four NSAIDs with different chemical structures and different potencies for inhibiting urinary prostaglandin E_2 synthesis found that **flurbiprofen**, **indometacin**, **piroxicam** and **sulindac** were equipotent in reducing furosemide-stimulated sodium excretion and creatinine clearance.[14]

(a) Azapropazone

Ten healthy subjects had no change in their urinary excretion in response to furosemide 40 mg daily when they were also given azapropazone 600 mg twice daily. Furosemide did not antagonise the uricosuric effects of azapropazone.[15]

(b) Celecoxib and other Coxibs

In a placebo-controlled study, 7 patients with cirrhosis and ascites were given a single 40-mg intravenous dose of furosemide before and after receiving celecoxib 200 mg twice daily for 5 doses. It was found that this short-term use of celecoxib did not reduce the natriuretic or diuretic effects of furosemide.[16]

Two patients with a history of chronic heart failure, taking furosemide 40 or 80 mg daily, developed acute renal failure when they started to take celecoxib 100 or 200 mg twice daily. Neither patient showed any sign of decompensated heart failure on

Table 26.2 Summary of the interactions of diuretics and NSAIDs

NSAID	*Excretion of sodium*	*Excretion of potassium*	*Diuresis*	*Blood pressure*	*Other effects*
Bumetanide					
Celecoxib					Increased serum creatinine
Indometacin	Reduced by 25%		Reduced by 25%		Development of congestive heart failure in one case
Rofecoxib					Increased serum creatinine Worsening congestive heart failure
Sulindac	Reduced by 22%		Reduced by 21%		
Tolfenamic acid			Reduced by 34%		
Furosemide					
Azapropazone			Non-significant effect		
Celecoxib	Non-significant effect		Non-significant effect		Increased serum creatinine Acute renal failure developed in 2 cases
Diclofenac	Decreased by 38%		Non-significant effect		
Diflunisal	Decreased by 36 to 59%	No significant effect in healthy subjects Decreased by 47% in patients			
Flupirtine			Delayed		
Flurbiprofen	Decreased by 9%	Decreased by 12%	Decreased by 10%		
Ibuprofen			Decreased		Development of congestive heart failure in one case Decreased GFR
Indometacin	Decreased by 64 to 82%	Decreased by 49%	Decreased by 41 to 69%	Mean blood pressure increased by 13 mmHg	
Ketoprofen			Decreased		
Ketorolac	Decreased by 26%		Decreased by 16%		
Lornoxicam	Decreased		Decreased		
Meloxicam	Non-significant effect	Non-significant effect	Non-significant effect		
Metamizole (Dipyrone)			Non-significant effect		
Mofebutazone	Non-significant effect	Non-significant effect	Non-significant effect		
Naproxen	Decreased		Decreased by 50%		GFR decreased
Nimesulide	Decreased		Slight decrease		GFR transiently reduced
Piroxicam	No effect in healthy subjects, decreased in patients with creatinine clearance less than 60 mL/minute	No effect in healthy subjects, decreased in patients with creatinine clearance less than 60 mL/minute	No effect in healthy subjects, decreased in patients with creatinine clearance less than 60 mL/minute		
Rofecoxib					Development of acute renal failure
Sulindac	Decreased by 38 to 52%	Decreased by 8%	Decreased by 25 to 38%		
Tenoxicam	Non-significant effect			Non-significant effect	
Piretanide					
Indometacin	Decreased by 35%				
Naproxen		Decreased by 14%	Non-significant effect		
Piroxicam	Decreased				
Sulindac	Decreased at 0 to 4 hours, increased at 4 to 8 hours				

Continued

Table 26.2 Summary of the interactions of diuretics and NSAIDs (continued)

NSAID	*Excretion of sodium*	*Excretion of potassium*	*Diuresis*	*Blood pressure*	*Other effects*
Torasemide					
Indometacin	Decreased, but only if given with low sodium diet				
Altizide					
Rofecoxib					Congestive heart failure with weight gain occurred in one case
Bemetizide					
Indometacin	Decreased by 47%				
Bendroflumethiazide					
Ibuprofen				Small increase	Weight gain in 2 patients but overall the effect was non-significant
Indometacin				Increase of 17/12 mmHg	Weight gain
Sulindac				*Decreased*	
Chlortalidone					
Ibuprofen					Diabetic nephropathy reported in one case
Hydrochlorothiazide					
Diclofenac	Decreased	Non-significant effect		Non-significant effect	Weight gain
Ibuprofen				Small increase (systolic)	Weight gain
Indometacin				Transient increase of 6/3 mmHg Increase of 23/3 mmHg seen in one patient when amiloride also taken	Weight gain
Kebuzone				18 mmHg increase (systolic)	
Naproxen			Non-significant effect		Hyponatraemia reported in a patient also taking amiloride
Phenylbutazone				18 mmHg increase (systolic)	
Piroxicam				Slight increase (patients also taking amiloride)	
Rofecoxib	Decreased	Non-significant effect			
Sulindac	Decreased by 29% over 0 to 4 hours		Usually non-significant but a decrease of 35% over 0 to 4 hours has been reported	Non-significant effect Non-significant effect, or *enhanced* hypotensive effects reported when amiloride also taken	Acute renal failure reported in one case
Methyclothiazide					
Indometacin					Acute renal failure reported in one case
Metolazone					
Indometacin	Decreased by 34%	Decreased by 30%			
Sulindac	Decreased by 19%	Decreased by 16%			
Amiloride					
Indometacin					Case of hyperkalaemia in a patient also taking hydrochlorothiazide

Continued

Table 26.2 Summary of the interactions of diuretics and NSAIDs (continued)

NSAID	*Excretion of sodium*	*Excretion of potassium*	*Diuresis*	*Blood pressure*	*Other effects*
Spironolactone					
Indometacin	Decreased by 54%				
Mefenamic acid			Decreased		
Triamterene					
Diclofenac					Acute renal failure reported in one case (trichlormethiazide also taken)
Ibuprofen				Non-significant (hydrochlorothiazide also taken)	Acute renal failure reported in two cases and increased serum creatinine reported in one case (hydrochlorothiazide also taken in all cases)
Indometacin					Acute renal failure reported in six cases (hydrochlorothiazide also taken in one case) and increased serum creatinine reported in two cases; marked reduction of creatinine clearance reported in two healthy subjects

admission (which can in itself cause renal failure) and both recovered on stopping celecoxib and furosemide. One patient was also taking enalapril, and this was restarted with the furosemide without any changes in renal function.[17] The same authors also described two other patients taking furosemide who developed renal failure when they started to take **rofecoxib**.[17] Other cases have occurred in patients taking furosemide, often with ACE inhibitors, after they started **rofecoxib**.[6]

(c) Diclofenac

A study in patients with heart failure and cirrhosis found that diclofenac 150 mg daily reduced the furosemide-induced excretion of sodium by 38%, but the excretion of potassium was unaltered.[18]

(d) Diflunisal

A study in 12 healthy subjects found that diflunisal 500 mg twice daily reduced sodium excretion in response to furosemide by 59%, but potassium excretion remained unchanged.[19] In patients with heart failure and cirrhosis taking furosemide, the concurrent use of diflunisal 500 to 700 mg daily decreased the sodium excretion by 36% and the potassium excretion by 47%.[18] However, another study in healthy subjects found no interaction between diflunisal and furosemide.[20]

(e) Dipyrone (Metamizole)

A study in 9 healthy subjects found that dipyrone 3 g daily for 3 days, reduced the clearance of intravenous furosemide 20 mg from 175 to 141 mL/minute but the diuretic effects of the furosemide were unchanged.[21]

(f) Flupirtine

A study in healthy subjects found that a single 200-mg dose of flupirtine did not affect the overall furosemide diuresis, but the diuretic effect was slightly delayed.[22]

(g) Flurbiprofen

A study in 7 healthy subjects found that the increase in renal osmolal clearance of a standard water load in response to furosemide 40 mg orally or 20 mg intravenously fell from 105% to 19% and from 140% to 70%, respectively, after flurbiprofen 100 mg was given.[23] A single-dose study in 10 healthy subjects found that flurbiprofen 100 mg reduced the urinary volume, and urinary excretion of sodium and potassium, in response to oral furosemide 80 mg by 10%, 9%, and 12%, respectively.[24,25]

(h) Ibuprofen

An elderly man with heart failure taking digoxin, isosorbide dinitrate and furosemide 80 mg daily, developed symptomatic congestive heart failure with ascites when given ibuprofen 400 mg three times daily. His serum urea and creatinine levels rose and no diuresis occurred, even when the furosemide dose was doubled. Two days after withdrawing the ibuprofen, brisk diuresis took place, renal function returned to normal, and his condition improved steadily.[26] Another elderly patient similarly had a poor response to furosemide (also hydrochlorothiazide and later to metolazone as well) until she stopped taking ibuprofen 600 mg four times daily and at least two **aspirin** daily (for headache).[27] This was due to hyponatraemic hypovolaemia brought on by the drug combination.

In a small, placebo-controlled, crossover study in 8 healthy subjects, ibuprofen 400 mg and 800 mg three times daily for 3 days significantly reduced the glomerular filtration rate and the diuresis produced by a single 20-mg intravenous dose of furosemide, but did not alter sodium excretion.[28]

Loop diuretics such as furosemide have been reported to occasionally cause hearing loss and NSAIDs, including ibuprofen, have also been reported to have ototoxic effects: these effects could theoretically be additive.[29]

(i) Indometacin

A study in 4 healthy subjects and 6 patients with essential hypertension found that furosemide 80 mg three times daily reduced the mean blood pressure by 13 mmHg, but when indometacin 50 mg four times daily was also given the blood pressures returned to virtually pretreatment levels. Moreover, the normal urinary sodium loss induced by the furosemide was significantly reduced.[30]

A study in healthy subjects and patients with congestive heart failure found that indometacin 100 mg reduced the furosemide-induced urinary output by 53% and also reduced the excretion of sodium, potassium, and chloride by 64%, 49%, and 62%, respectively, in the patients with congestive heart failure. The drug interaction was much less pronounced in the healthy subjects.[31] A study in 14 patients with ascites secondary to liver cirrhosis found that indometacin 50 mg every 6 hours for two doses significantly reduced the urinary volume and the natriuretic response to furosemide, by 69% and 82%, respectively, but produced only a small reduction in creatinine clearance, which was not statistically significant.[32] Another study found that indometacin reduced the urinary output in response to furosemide by 28% in healthy subjects and by 41% in elderly patients (three with mild-to-moderate heart failure).[33] Other case reports and studies confirm the interaction between furosemide and indometacin.[28,34-40]

(j) Ketoprofen

A study in 12 healthy subjects given furosemide 40 mg daily found that ketoprofen 100 mg twice daily reduced the 6-hour urine output by 67 mL, and the 24-hour urine output by 651 mL on the first day of treatment. However no notable differences were seen after 5 days of treatment.[41]

(k) Ketorolac

Twelve healthy subjects were given oral ketorolac 30 mg four times daily, and then a single 30-mg intramuscular dose of ketorolac 30 minutes before a 40-mg intravenous dose of furosemide. No precise figures are given, but the maximum serum level of the furosemide, its diuretic effect, and the electrolyte loss were said to be significantly reduced by the ketorolac.[42] Another study in healthy elderly subjects found that when they were given oral ketorolac 120 mg, then, on the following day, intramuscular ketorolac 30 mg, followed 30 minutes later by furosemide 40 mg, the urinary output fell by 16% and the sodium output fell by 26% over the next 8 hours, when compared with furosemide alone.[43]

(l) Lornoxicam

A study in 12 healthy subjects found that lornoxicam 4 mg significantly antagonised the diuretic and natriuretic effects of furosemide, but the magnitude of this effect was not quantified.[44]

(m) Meloxicam

In a study in 12 healthy subjects, meloxicam 15 mg daily for 3 days had no clinically relevant effect on the pharmacokinetics of furosemide 40 mg. The furosemide-induced diuresis was unchanged, and although the cumulative urinary electrolyte excretion was somewhat lower, this was also not considered to be clinically significant.[45] A similar study in patients with heart failure taking an ACE inhibitor also found no clinically significant pharmacokinetic or pharmacodynamic interaction between furosemide and meloxicam.[46]

(n) Mofebutazone

A study in 10 healthy subjects found that mofebutazone 600 mg had no effect on the diuretic effects of furosemide 40 mg. The urinary volume and excretion of sodium, potassium and chloride were unchanged.[47]

(o) Naproxen

Two elderly women with congestive heart failure did not respond to treatment with furosemide and digoxin until the naproxen they were taking was withdrawn.[26] A single-dose study in patients with heart failure found that the volume of urine excreted in response to furosemide was reduced about 50% by naproxen.[33] In a placebo-controlled study, 6 patients with cirrhosis and ascites were given a single 40-mg intravenous dose of furosemide before and after naproxen 500 mg twice daily for 5 doses. It was found that this short-term use of naproxen reduced the glomerular filtration rate and the natriuretic and diuretic effects of furosemide.[16]

Loop diuretics such as furosemide have been reported to occasionally cause hearing loss and NSAIDs including naproxen have also been reported to have ototoxic effects: these effects could theoretically be additive.[29,48]

(p) Nimesulide

A study in 8 healthy subjects found that nimesulide 200 mg twice daily attenuated the effects of furosemide 40 mg twice daily. Subjects who had initially lost weight when taking furosemide regained weight, diuresis was slightly reduced, cumulative sodium excretion was decreased and the glomerular filtration rate was transiently reduced.[49]

(q) Piroxicam

A 96-year-old woman with congestive heart failure did not adequately respond to furosemide until the dose of piroxicam she was taking was reduced from 20 mg daily to 10 mg daily.[50]

In one study in 9 hypertensive patients with a creatinine clearance of less than 60 mL/minute, who were taking furosemide, the use of piroxicam 20 mg daily for 3 days reduced the natriuretic and kaliuretic effects of an additional single 40-mg dose of furosemide. However, in 13 other patients, with a creatinine clearance of greater than 60 mL/minute, who were taking a thiazide diuretic, piroxicam did not alter the effects of a single 40-mg dose of furosemide. In a third group of 8 healthy subjects, the same dose of piroxicam reduced the natriuretic effects, but not the kaliuretic effects, of a single 40-mg dose of furosemide.[51]

(r) Sulindac

A study in 5 healthy subjects found that pretreatment with two 150-mg oral doses of sulindac reduced urinary volume and urinary sodium, following an intravenous dose of furosemide 80 mg, by 25% and 38%, respectively. In patients with cirrhosis and ascites, two doses of sulindac 150 mg reduced the urinary volume, urinary sodium, and urinary potassium, following an 80-mg intravenous dose of furosemide, by 38%, 52%, and 8%, respectively.[52] In another placebo-controlled study in 15 healthy women, sulindac 200 mg twice daily for 5 days produced a similar but slightly smaller reduction in the natriuretic effect of a single 40-mg intravenous dose of furosemide, than indometacin.[39]

(s) Tenoxicam

A study in 12 patients found that tenoxicam 20 to 40 mg daily had no significant effect on the urinary excretion of sodium or chloride due to furosemide 40 mg daily, and blood pressure, heart rate and body-weight also were not affected.[53]

C. Piretanide

(a) Indometacin

A comparative study[54] into the pharmacological mechanisms underlying the way that drugs interfere with the actions of loop diuretics found that indometacin 50 mg three times daily for 2 days reduced the peak fractional and cumulative excretion of sodium in response to a single 6-mg dose of piretanide. The clinical importance of this change was not studied.

(b) Naproxen

Pretreatment of healthy subjects with naproxen 500 mg decreased the fractional potassium clearance produced by piretanide 6 mg by 14%, but no attenuation of the diuretic response was seen. Estimation of piretanide urinary clearance was not possible as naproxen interfered with the analysis.[55]

(c) Piroxicam

A comparative study into the pharmacological mechanisms underlying the way that drugs interfere with the actions of loop diuretics found that piroxicam 20 mg twice daily for 2 days did not significantly affect the peak fractional excretion of sodium in response to a single 6-mg dose of piretanide, but the cumulative excretion of sodium over 5 hours and 24 hours was reduced.[54]

(d) Sulindac

Pretreatment of healthy subjects with sulindac 200 mg decreased the fractional urinary flow rate produced by piretanide 6 mg by 15% and attenuated the natriuretic effect of piretanide over 0 to 4 hours. However, natriuresis was increased over the 4 to 8-hour period of the study.[55]

D. Torasemide

A study in healthy subjects suggested that **indometacin** did not affect the diuretic and natriuretic effects of torasemide,[56] but on the basis of a later study, the same workers suggested that pathological factors in patients may allow an interaction similar to that between furosemide and indometacin to occur. **Indometacin** was found to reduce the natriuretic actions of torasemide when the subjects were given a low sodium diet, but did not affect the natriuretic actions when they received a normal diet. The sodium balance, therefore, appeared to be a determinant of the interaction between NSAIDs and loop diuretics.[57]

Mechanism

Uncertain and complex. It is likely that a number of different mechanisms come into play. NSAIDs cause fluid and salt retention, which would be expected to antagonise the effects produced by diuretics. The sodium retentive properties of NSAIDs appear to be most noticeable in patients who already have a predisposition to sodium retention, such as those with heart disease or liver disease.[3,58] A reduction in glomerular filtration rate is sometimes observed with NSAIDs and this may reduce the natriuretic efficacy of loop diuretics, particularly in states of renal underperfusion, such as congestive heart failure, volume depletion, and liver cirrhosis.[59]

One probable mechanism involves the synthesis of renal prostaglandins, particularly prostaglandin E_2 and prostacyclin, which inhibit the reabsorption of sodium and help to maintain renal blood flow and glomerular filtration rates in the face of disease or circulatory stress, and when the loop diuretics cause sodium excretion.[60] If this synthesis is blocked by an NSAID, then renal blood flow, natriuresis and diuresis will be reduced.[59,61]

NSAIDs can also decrease renin release, leading to reduced aldosterone secretion, which results in reduced potassium secretion in the distal nephron. Patients with renal impairment or patients who are receiving other drugs that decrease potassium secretion, for example the ACE inhibitors (see 'ACE inhibitors + NSAIDs', p.38) are at increased risk of hyperkalaemia.[58] It appears that coxibs also affect renal prostaglandins and renin release and are likely to interact similarly to non-selective NSAIDs.[58,62] In addition, NSAIDs may alter the access of some diuretics to their tubular site of action by competing for transport in the proximal tubule.[59,63]

Importance and management

The antihypertensive and diuretic effects of the loop diuretics are reduced by NSAIDs. This interaction is very well documented between furosemide and indometacin, and of clinical importance, whereas less is known about the interactions with other NSAIDs. Nevertheless, the interaction should be anticipated with all of them, and it would be prudent to always consider the use of an alternative non-NSAID analgesic. However, in cases where concurrent use cannot be avoided, the dose of the loop diuretic may need to be raised (according to clinical response), with the effects on renal function and electrolytes, as well as efficacy, closely monitored. The joint American College of Cardiology and American Heart Association heart failure guidelines (2009) advise that in patients with heart failure who become unresponsive to diuretics, such as in those taking an NSAID, clinicians should consider giving the diuretic intravenously, giving an additional diuretic (they give the example of adding metolazone to furosemide), or giving a drug to increase renal blood flow (such as an inotrope).[64] Patients at greatest risk of an adverse interaction include the elderly, and patients with cirrhosis, cardiac failure and/or renal impairment: NSAIDs should usually be used with caution or avoided in these patient groups regardless of the concurrent use of diuretics.

Much less is known about the interactions of NSAIDs with **bumetanide**, and even less about **piretanide**, **torasemide**, and **etacrynic acid**, but the evidence suggests that they probably interact in the same way as furosemide. It would therefore seem prudent to be alert for a potential reduction in effect if an NSAID is given with any loop diuretic.

NSAIDs, including coxibs, can cause renal impairment, particularly in patients with hypovolaemia or dehydration and in whom prostaglandins are playing an important role in maintaining renal function. Such patients include those taking diuretics, the elderly and those with concurrent conditions, such as congestive heart failure and ascites. Hence the concurrent use of a diuretic and an NSAID might increase the nephrotoxicity of the NSAID.[4,38,65-68]

Loop diuretics, such as **etacrynic acid**[69] and furosemide,[29] can exhibit ototoxic properties, particularly if given in high doses and in renal impairment.[29,69] The risk of ototoxicity may theoretically be increased if loop diuretics are given with other ototoxic drugs such as some NSAIDs, including ibuprofen and naproxen.[29,48]

1. Johnson AG, Nguyen TV, Day RO. Do nonsteroidal anti-inflammatory drugs affect blood pressure? A meta-analysis. *Ann Intern Med* (1994) 121, 289–300.
2. Pope JE, Anderson JJ, Felson DT. A meta-analysis of the effects of nonsteroidal anti-inflammatory drugs on blood pressure. *Arch Intern Med* (1993) 153, 477–84.
3. Heerdink ER, Leufkens HG, Herings RMC, Ottervanger JP, Stricker BHC, Bakker A. NSAIDs associated with increased risk of congestive heart failure in elderly patients taking diuretics. *Arch Intern Med* (1998) 158, 1108–12.
4. Huerta C, Castellsague J, Varas-Lorenzo C, García Rodríguez LA. Nonsteroidal anti-inflammatory drugs and risk of ARF in the general population. *Am J Kidney Dis* (2005) 45, 531–9.
5. Krzesinski J-M, Piront P. Décompensation cardiaque, fonction rénale et anti-inflammatoires non stéroïdiens. *Rev Med Liege* (2002) 57, 582–6.
6. Verrico MM, Weber RJ, McKaveney TP, Ansani NT, Towers AL. Adverse drug events involving COX-2 inhibitors. *Ann Pharmacother* (2003) 37, 1203–13.
7. Aggernæs KH. Indometacinhæmning af bumetaniddiurese. *Ugeskr Laeger* (1980) 142, 691–3.
8. Brater C, Chennavasin P. Indomethacin and the response to bumetanide. *Clin Pharmacol Ther* (1980) 27, 421–5.
9. Brater DC, Fox WR, Chennavasin P. Interaction studies with bumetanide and furosemide. Effects of probenecid and of indomethacin on response to bumetanide in man. *J Clin Pharmacol* (1981) 21, 647–53.
10. Kaufman J, Hamburger R, Matheson J, Flamenbaum W. Bumetanide-induced diuresis and natriuresis: effect of prostaglandin synthetase inhibition. *J Clin Pharmacol* (1981) 21, 663–7.

11. Ahmad S. Indomethacin-bumetanide interaction: an alert. *Am J Cardiol* (1984) 54, 246–7.
12. Pentikäinen PJ, Tokola O, Vapaatalo H. Non-steroidal anti-inflammatory drugs and bumetanide response in man. Comparison of tolfenamic acid and sulindac. *Clin Pharmacol Ther* (1986) 39, 219.
13. Skinner MH, Mutterperl R, Zeitz HJ. Sulindac inhibits bumetanide-induced sodium and water excretion. *Clin Pharmacol Ther* (1987) 42, 542–6.
14. Wilkins MR, Woods KL, Kendall MJ. The effects of selective and non-selective inhibition of cyclo-oxygenase on frusemide-stimulated natriuresis. *Int J Clin Pharmacol Ther Toxicol* (1986) 24, 55–7.
15. Williamson PJ, Ene MD, Roberts CJC. A study of the potential interactions between azapropazone and frusemide in man. *Br J Clin Pharmacol* (1984) 18, 619–23.
16. Clària J, Kent JD, López-Parra M, Escolar G, Ruiz-del-Arbol L, Ginès P, Jiménez W, Vucelic B, Arroyo V. Effects of celecoxib and naproxen on renal function in nonazotemic patients with cirrhosis and ascites. *Hepatology* (2005) 41, 579–87.
17. Braden GL, O'Shea MH, Mulhern JG, Germain MJ. Acute renal failure and hyperkalaemia associated with cyclooxygenase-2 inhibitors. *Nephrol Dial Transplant* (2004) 19, 1149–53.
18. Jean G, Meregalli G, Vasilicò M, Silvani A, Scapaticci R, Della Ventura GF, Baiocchi C, Thiella G. Interazioni tra terapia diuretica e farmaci antiinfiammatori non steroidei. *Clin Ter* (1983) 105, 471–5.
19. Favre L, Glasson PH, Riondel A, Vallotton MB. Interaction of diuretics and non-steroidal anti-inflammatory drugs in man. *Clin Sci* (1983) 64, 407–15.
20. Tobert JA, Ostaszewski T, Reger B, Meisinger MAP, Cook TJ. Diflunisal-furosemide interaction. *Clin Pharmacol Ther* (1980) 27, 289–90.
21. Rosenkranz B, Lehr K-H, Mackert G, Seyberth HW. Metamizole-furosemide interaction study in healthy volunteers. *Eur J Clin Pharmacol* (1992) 42, 593–8.
22. Johnston A, Warrington SJ, Turner P, Riethmuller-Winzen H. Comparison of flupirtine and indomethacin on frusemide-induced diuresis. *Postgrad Med J* (1987) 63, 959–61.
23. Rawles JM. Antagonism between non-steroidal anti-inflammatory drugs and diuretics. *Scott Med J* (1982) 27, 37–40.
24. Symmons D, Kendall MJ. Non-steroidal anti-inflammatory drugs and frusemide-induced diuresis. *BMJ* (1981) 283, 988–9.
25. Symmons DPM, Kendall MJ, Rees JA, Hind ID. The effect of flurbiprofen on the responses to frusemide in healthy volunteers. *Int J Clin Pharmacol Ther Toxicol* (1983) 21, 350–4.
26. Laiwah ACY, Mactier RA. Antagonistic effect of non-steroidal anti-inflammatory drugs on frusemide-induced diuresis in cardiac failure. *BMJ* (1981) 283, 714.
27. Goodenough GK, Lutz LJ. Hyponatremic hypervolemia caused by a drug-drug interaction mistaken for syndrome of inappropriate ADH. *J Am Geriatr Soc* (1988) 36, 285–6.
28. Passmore AP, Copeland S, Johnston GD. A comparison of the effects of ibuprofen and indomethacin upon renal haemodynamics and electrolyte excretion in the presence and absence of frusemide. *Br J Clin Pharmacol* (1989) 27, 483–90.
29. Lheureux Ph, Penaloza A. Les vertiges d'origine ototoxique. Ototoxicity-related dysequilibrium. *Rev Med Brux* (2002) 23, A356–A362.
30. Patak RV, Mookerjee BK, Bentzel CJ, Hysert PE, Babej M, Lee JB. Antagonism of the effects of furosemide by indomethacin in normal and hypertensive man. *Prostaglandins* (1975) 10, 649–59.
31. Sörgel F, Koob R, Gluth WP, Krüger B, Lang E. The interaction of indomethacin and furosemide in patients with congestive heart failure. *Clin Pharmacol Ther* (1985) 37, 231.
32. Mirouze D, Zipser RD, Reynolds TB. Effect of inhibitors of prostaglandin synthesis on induced diuresis in cirrhosis. *Hepatology* (1983) 3, 50–5.
33. Faunch R. Non-steroidal anti-inflammatory drugs and frusemide-induced diuresis. *BMJ* (1981) 283, 989.
34. Allan SG, Knox J, Kerr F. Interaction between diuretics and indomethacin. *BMJ* (1981) 283, 1611.
35. Poe TE, Scott RB, Keith JF. Interaction of indomethacin with furosemide. *J Fam Pract* (1983) 16, 610–16.
36. Ritland S. Alvorlig interaksjon mellom indometacin og furosemid. *Tidsskr Nor Laegeforen* (1983) 103, 2003.
37. Nordrehaug JE. Alvorlig interaksjon mellom indometacin og furosemid. *Tidsskr Nor Laegeforen* (1983) 103, 1680–1.
38. Thomas MC. Diuretics, ACE inhibitors and NSAIDs—the triple whammy. *Med J Aust* (2000) 172, 184–5.
39. Roberts DG, Gerber JG, Barnes JS, Zerbe GO, Nies AS. Sulindac is not renal sparing in man. *Clin Pharmacol Ther* (1985) 38, 258–65.
40. Brater DC. Analysis of the effect of indomethacin on the response to furosemide in man: effect of dose of furosemide. *J Pharmacol Exp Ther* (1979) 210, 386–90.
41. Wa TCLK, Lawson M, Jackson SHD, Hitoglou-Makedou A, Turner P. Interaction of ketoprofen and frusemide in man. *Postgrad Med J* (1991) 67, 655–8.
42. Shah J, Bullingham R, Jonkman J, Curd J, Taylor R, Fratis A. PK-PD interaction of ketorolac and furosemide in healthy volunteers in a normovolemic state. *Clin Pharmacol Ther* (1994) 55, 198.
43. Jones RW, Notarianni LJ, Parker G. The effect of ketorolac tromethamine on the diuretic response of frusemide in healthy elderly people. *Therapie* (1995) 50 (Suppl), Abstract 98.
44. Ravic M, Johnston A, Turner P. Clinical pharmacological studies of some possible interactions of lornoxicam with other drugs. *Postgrad Med J* (1990) 66 (Suppl 4), S30–S34.
45. Müller FO, Schall R, de Vaal AC, Groenewoud G, Hundt HKL, Middle MV. Influence of meloxicam on furosemide pharmacokinetics and pharmacodynamics in healthy volunteers. *Eur J Clin Pharmacol* (1995) 48, 247–51.
46. Müller FO, Middle MV, Schall R, Terblanché J, Hundt HKL, Groenewoud G. An evaluation of the interaction of meloxicam with frusemide in patients with compensated chronic cardiac failure. *Br J Clin Pharmacol* (1997) 44, 393–8.
47. Matthei U, Grabensee B, Loew D. The interaction of mofebutazone with furosemide. *Curr Med Res Opin* (1987) 10, 638–44.
48. Yorgason JG, Fayad JN, Kalinec F. Understanding drug ototoxicity: molecular insights for prevention and clinical management. *Expert Opin Drug Safety* (2006) 5, 383–99.
49. Steinhäuslin F, Munafo A, Buclin T, Macciocchi A, Biollaz J. Renal effects of nimesulide in furosemide-treated subjects. *Drugs* (1993) 46 (Suppl 1), 257–62.
50. Baker DE. Piroxicam-furosemide drug interaction. *Drug Intell Clin Pharm* (1988) 22, 505–6.
51. Lin MS. Effects of piroxicam on natriuresis and kaliuresis in hypertensives and healthy volunteers. *Scand J Rheumatol* (1990) 19, 145–9.
52. Daskalopoulos G, Kronborg I, Katkov W, Gonzalez M, Laffi G, Zipser RD. Sulindac and indomethacin suppress the diuretic action of furosemide in patients with cirrhosis and ascites: evidence that sulindac affects renal prostaglandins. *Am J Kidney Dis* (1985) 6, 217–21.
53. Hartmann D, Kleinbloesem CH, Lücker PW, Vetter G. Study on the possible interaction between tenoxicam and furosemide. *Arzneimittelforschung* (1987) 37, 1072–6.
54. Dixey JJ, Noormohamed FH, Pawa JS, Lant AF, Brewerton DA. The influence of nonsteroidal anti-inflammatory drugs and probenecid on the renal response to and kinetics of piretanide in man. *Clin Pharmacol Ther* (1988) 44, 531–9.
55. Dixey JJ, Noormohamed FH, Lant AF, Brewerton DA. The effects of naproxen and sulindac on renal function and their interaction with hydrochlorothiazide and piretanide in man. *Br J Clin Pharmacol* (1987) 23, 55–63.
56. van Ganse E, Douchamps J, Deger F, Staroukine M, Verniory A, Herchuelz A. Failure of indomethacin to impair the diuretic and natriuretic effects of the loop diuretic torasemide in healthy volunteers. *Eur J Clin Pharmacol* (1986) 31 (Suppl), 43–7.
57. Herchuelz A, Derenne F, Deger F, Juvent M, van Ganse E, Staroukine M, Verniory A, Boeynaems JM, Douchamps J. Interaction between nonsteroidal anti-inflammatory drugs and loop diuretics: modulation by sodium balance. *J Pharmacol Exp Ther* (1989) 248, 1175–81.
58. Brater DC. Effects of nonsteroidal anti-inflammatory drugs on renal function: focus on cyclooxygenase-2–selective inhibition. *Am J Med* (1999) 107, 65S–70S. Discussion ibid., 70S–71S.
59. Sahloul MZ, al-Kiek R, Ivanovich P, Mujais SK. Nonsteroidal anti-inflammatory drugs and anti-hypertensives. Cooperative malfeasance. *Nephron* (1990) 56, 345–52.
60. Harris K. The role of prostaglandins in the control of renal function. *Br J Anaesth* (1992) 69, 233–5.
61. Passmore AP, Copeland S, Johnston GD. The effects of ibuprofen and indomethacin on renal function in the presence and absence of frusemide in healthy volunteers on a restricted sodium diet. *Br J Clin Pharmacol* (1990) 29, 311–19.
62. Stichtenoth DO, Marhauer V, Tsikas D, Gutzki F-M, Frölich JC. Effects of specific COX-2-inhibition on renin release and renal and systemic prostanoid synthesis in healthy volunteers. *Kidney Int* (2005) 68, 2197–2207.
63. Chennavasin P, Seiwell R, Brater DC. Pharmacokinetic-dynamic analysis of the indomethacin-furosemide interaction in man. *J Pharmacol Exp Ther* (1980) 215, 77–81.
64. Hunt SA, Abraham WT, Chin MH, Feldman AM, Francis GS, Ganiats TG, Jessup M, Konstam MA, Mancini DM, Michl K, Oates JA, Rahko PS, Silver MA, Stevenson LW, Yancy CW. 2009 focused update incorporated into the ACC/AHA 2005 guidelines for the diagnosis and management of heart failure in adults: a report of the American College of Cardiology Foundation/American Heart Association Task Force on Practice Guidelines developed in collaboration with the international society for heart and lung transplantation. *J Am Coll Cardiol* (2009) 53, e1–e90. Available at: http://content.onlinejacc.org/article.aspx?articleid=1136916 (accessed 21/10/15).
65. Murray MD, Brater DC, Tierney WM, Hui SL, McDonald CJ. Ibuprofen-associated renal impairment in a large general internal medicine practice. *Am J Med Sci* (1990) 299, 222–9.
66. Blackshear JL, Davidman M, Stillman MT. Identification of risk for renal insufficiency from nonsteroidal anti-inflammatory drugs. *Arch Intern Med* (1983) 143, 1130–4.
67. Menkes CJ. Renal and hepatic effects of NSAIDs in the elderly. *Scand J Rheumatol* (1989) 83 (Suppl), 11–13.
68. Ahmad SR, Kortepeter C, Brinker A, Chen M, Beitz J. Renal failure associated with the use of celecoxib and rofecoxib. *Drug Safety* (2002) 25, 537–44.
69. Edecrin (Ethacrynic acid). Aton Pharma, Inc. US Prescribing information, October 2007.

Loop diuretics + Probenecid

Probenecid decreases the renal clearance of furosemide and bumetanide and reduces the natriuretic effect of piretanide.

Clinical evidence

(a) Bumetanide

Probenecid 1 g did not affect the natriuretic or diuretic response of 8 healthy subjects to 500 micrograms or 1 mg of intravenous bumetanide.[1] Another study reported a fall in natriuresis and a reduction in the clearance of bumetanide when probenecid was given, but this was of minimal clinical importance.[2]

(b) Furosemide

The concurrent use of furosemide and probenecid has been closely studied to determine the renal pharmacological mechanisms of loop diuretics. One study in patients given furosemide 40 mg daily found that the addition of probenecid 500 mg twice daily for 3 days reduced their urinary excretion of sodium by about 36% (from 56.3 mmol daily to 35.9 mmol daily).[3] Other studies have found that probenecid causes a mild fall,[4] a rise,[5] and no change[6,7] in diuresis in response to furosemide, and causes a reduction of 35 to 80% in the renal clearance of furosemide.[4,6-9] One study found that probenecid 1 g increased the half-life of furosemide by 70% and decreased its oral clearance by 65%.[8] Similar results were found in another study.[10]

(c) Piretanide

A comparative study[11] into the pharmacological mechanisms underlying the way drugs interfere with the actions of loop diuretics found that probenecid 1 g reduced the peak fractional excretion of sodium produced by a 6-mg dose of oral piretanide by 65%. Another study confirmed that probenecid reduces the natriuretic effects of piretanide.[12] The clinical importance of these changes was not studied.

Mechanism

Loop diuretics are secreted from the blood into the urine through the organic acid transport pathway. Other organic acids such as probenecid can alter loop diuretic secretion by competing for transport in the proximal tubule.[13]

Importance and management

Probenecid appears to reduce the renal clearance of furosemide and bumetanide, but the effect on diuresis does not usually appear to be clinically relevant. Nevertheless, one manufacturer of furosemide warns that probenecid may reduce its effects.[14] Probenecid reduces the natriuretic effects of piretanide, and as the clinical effects of this have not been studied, it may be prudent to be alert for a decreased response to piretanide if probenecid is also given, increasing the diuretic dose according to response. Until more is known about other loop diuretics, such as **torasemide**, similar precautions would seem appropriate.

1. Brater DC, Chennavasin P. Effect of probenecid on response to bumetanide in man. *J Clin Pharmacol* (1981) 21, 311–15.
2. Lant AF. Effects of bumetanide on cation and anion transport. *Postgrad Med J* (1975) 51 (Suppl 6), 35–42.
3. Hsieh Y-Y, Hsieh B-S, Lien W-P, Wu T-L. Probenecid interferes with the natriuretic action of furosemide. *J Cardiovasc Pharmacol* (1987) 10, 530–4.
4. Honari J, Blair AD, Cutler RE. Effects of probenecid on furosemide kinetics and natriuresis in man. *Clin Pharmacol Ther* (1977) 22, 395–401.
5. Brater DC. Effects of probenecid on furosemide response. *Clin Pharmacol Ther* (1978) 24, 548–54.
6. Homeida M, Roberts C, Branch RA. Influence of probenecid and spironolactone on furosemide kinetics and dynamics in man. *Clin Pharmacol Ther* (1977) 22, 402–9.
7. Smith DE, Gee WL, Brater DC, Lin ET, Benet LZ. Preliminary evaluation of furosemide-probenecid interaction in humans. *J Pharm Sci* (1980) 69, 571–5.
8. Vree TB, van den Biggelaar-Martea M, Verwey-van Wissen CPWGM. Probenecid inhibits the renal clearance of frusemide and its acyl glucuronide. *Br J Clin Pharmacol* (1995) 39, 692–5.
9. Sommers DK, Meyer EC, Moncrieff J. The influence of co-administered organic acids on the kinetics and dynamics of frusemide. *Br J Clin Pharmacol* (1991) 32, 489–93.
10. Chennavasin P, Seiwell R, Brater DC, Liang WMM. Pharmacodynamic analysis of the furosemide-probenecid interaction in man. *Kidney Int* (1979) 16, 187–95.
11. Dixey JJ, Noormohamed FH, Pawa JS, Lant AF, Brewerton DA. The influence of nonsteroidal anti-inflammatory drugs and probenecid on the renal response to and kinetics of piretanide in man. *Clin Pharmacol Ther* (1988) 44, 531–9.
12. Noormohamed FH, Lant AF. Analysis of the natriuretic action of a loop diuretic, piretanide, in man. *Br J Clin Pharmacol* (1991) 31, 463–9.
13. Bard RL, Bleske BE, Nicklas JM. Food: an unrecognized source of loop diuretic resistance. *Pharmacotherapy* (2004) 24, 630–7.
14. Lasix (Furosemide). Sanofi-Aventis. UK Summary of product characteristics, July 2010.

Loop diuretics; Furosemide + Bile-acid binding resins

Colestyramine and colestipol markedly reduce the absorption and diuretic effects of furosemide.

Clinical evidence

In 6 healthy subjects **colestyramine** 8 g reduced the absorption of a single 40-mg dose of furosemide by 95%. The 4-hour diuretic response was reduced by 77% (urinary output reduced from 1510 mL to 350 mL). Similarly, **colestipol** 10 g reduced the absorption of furosemide by 80% and reduced the 4-hour diuretic response by 58% (urinary output reduced from 1510 mL to 630 mL).[1]

Mechanism

Both colestyramine and colestipol are anionic exchange resins, which can bind with furosemide in the gut, thereby reducing its absorption and its effects.

Importance and management

The interaction between furosemide and colestipol or colestyramine appears to be established, although direct evidence seems to be limited to this study. The absorption of furosemide is relatively rapid; therefore giving it 2 to 3 hours before either the colestyramine or colestipol should be an effective way of overcoming this interaction; however, this needs confirmation. Note that it is normally recommended that other drugs are given 1 hour before or 4 to 6 hours after colestyramine and 1 hour before or 4 hours after colestipol.

1. Neuvonen PJ, Kivistö K, Hirvisalo EL. Effects of resins and activated charcoal on the absorption of digoxin, carbamazepine and frusemide. *Br J Clin Pharmacol* (1988) 25, 229–33.

Loop diuretics; Furosemide + Cloral hydrate and related drugs

Intravenous furosemide, given after cloral hydrate, occasionally causes sweating, hot flushes, a variable blood pressure, and tachycardia. Dichloralphenazone and cloral betaine may interact similarly.

Clinical evidence

Six patients in a coronary care unit, given an intravenous bolus dose of furosemide 40 to 120 mg and who had received cloral hydrate during the previous 24 hours, developed sweating, hot flushes, variable blood pressure, and tachycardia. The reaction was immediate and lasted for about 15 minutes. No special treatment was given. Furosemide had not caused any problems when it was given before the cloral hydrate was started.[1]

A retrospective study of hospital records revealed that, out of 43 patients who had received both cloral hydrate and furosemide, one patient developed this reaction and two others may have done so.[2] The interaction has also been described in an 8-year-old boy.[3]

Mechanism

Not understood. One suggestion is that furosemide displaces trichloroacetic acid (the metabolite of cloral hydrate) from its protein binding sites, which in turn displaces levothyroxine or alters the serum pH. As a result, the levels of free levothyroxine rise leading to a hypermetabolic state.[1]

Importance and management

Information regarding an interaction between furosemide and cloral hydrate is limited to three reports, all involving intravenous furosemide. The incidence is uncertain but probably low. Concurrent use need not be avoided, but it would be prudent to give intravenous furosemide cautiously if cloral hydrate has been given recently. It seems possible that drugs that release cloral hydrate when metabolised (e.g. **dichloralphenazone, cloral betaine**) might interact similarly. There is no evidence that furosemide given orally or cloral hydrate given to patients already taking furosemide causes this reaction.[2]

1. Malach M, Berman N. Furosemide and chloral hydrate. Adverse drug interaction. *JAMA* (1975) 232, 638–9.
2. Pevonka MP, Yost RL, Marks RG, Howell WS, Stewart RB. Interaction of chloral hydrate and furosemide. A controlled retrospective study. *Drug Intell Clin Pharm* (1977) 11, 332–5.
3. Dean RP, Rudinsky BF, Kelleher MD. Interaction of chloral hydrate and intravenous furosemide in a child. *Clin Pharm* (1991) 10, 385–7.

Loop diuretics; Furosemide + Germanium

An isolated case report describes a man who became resistant to furosemide after he took germanium.

Clinical evidence, mechanism, importance and management

A 63-year-old man was hospitalised for hypertension and oedema 10 days after adding ginseng with germanium to his usual treatment with cyclophosphamide and furosemide. He gained almost 13 kg in weight. After treatment with intravenous furosemide he was discharged and again took ginseng with germanium. This time he gained 12 kg in weight over 14 days, despite an increase in the dose of furosemide from 80 mg twice daily to 240 mg twice daily. The weight gain and oedema again resolved when the ginseng and germanium was withdrawn and intravenous furosemide was given. The authors suggest that germanium was responsible for this interaction.[1]

This is an isolated report, and its general significance is unclear. However, note that it has been said that the use of germanium should be discouraged due to its potential to cause renal toxicity.[2]

1. Becker BN, Greene J, Evanson J, Chidsey G, Stone WJ. Ginseng-induced diuretic resistance. *JAMA* (1996) 276, 606–7.
2. *Martindale. The Complete Drug Reference*, [online] London: Pharmaceutical Press. https://www.medicinescomplete.com/mc/martindale/current/5251-b.htm (accessed 19/10/15).

Loop diuretics; Furosemide + Metolazone

The pharmacokinetics of furosemide are not affected by metolazone. Furosemide and metolazone have additive diuretic effects, possibly due to differences in their sites of action.

Clinical evidence

In a study, 8 healthy subjects were given an intravenous infusion of furosemide 4 mg/hour for 12 hours with a single 2.5-mg oral dose of metolazone at 6 hours. Diuresis and the urinary excretion of sodium and chloride increased after the addition of metolazone but the urinary excretion of calcium decreased. Metolazone had an effect on sodium and chloride excretion, independent of furosemide. Furosemide steady-state plasma levels were not affected by metolazone, and the total body clearance and renal clearance of furosemide were similar before and after metolazone use.[1]

Mechanism

The mechanism by which metolazone exerts its positive effects in patients refractory to high-dose furosemide is not clear. It may be due to the drugs having different sites of action, as furosemide exerts its effects in the ascending loop of Henle and metolazone works in both the proximal and distal segments of the nephron. As the plasma levels and clearance of furosemide are not affected by metolazone, a pharmacokinetic interaction is not likely.[1]

Importance and management

Evidence for an interaction between metolazone and furosemide appears to be limited to one study, which suggests that metolazone may potentiate the diuresis in response to furosemide. However, the manufacturers suggest that this may result in electrolyte disorders and therefore suggest monitoring electrolyte balance.[2] This seems a prudent precaution.

1. Marone C, Muggli F, Lahn W, Frey FJ. Pharmacokinetic and pharmacodynamic interaction between furosemide and metolazone in man. *Eur J Clin Invest* (1985) 15, 253–7.
2. Metenix (Metolazone). Sanofi-Aventis. UK Summary of product characteristics, September 2010.

Loop diuretics; Furosemide + Paracetamol (Acetaminophen)

In 10 healthy women, paracetamol 1 g four times daily for 2 days was found to have no effect on the diuresis or natriuresis in response to 20 mg of intravenous furosemide.[1]

1. Martin U, Prescott LF. The interaction of paracetamol with frusemide. *Br J Clin Pharmacol* (1994) 37, 464–7.

Loop diuretics; Furosemide + Phenytoin

The diuretic effects of furosemide can be reduced by as much as 50% by phenytoin.

Clinical evidence

A group of patients with epilepsy were noted to have higher than expected dependent oedema, with an apparently reduced response to diuretics: this prompted further study. In 30 patients taking phenytoin 200 to 400 mg daily with phenobarbital 60 to 180 mg daily the maximal diuresis in response to furosemide 20 or 40 mg occurred after 3 to 4 hours instead of the usual 2 hours. The total diuresis was reduced by 32% for the 20-mg dose, 49% for the 40-mg dose and 50% when intravenous furosemide 20 mg was given. Some of the patients were also taking carbamazepine, pheneturide, ethosuximide, diazepam or chlordiazepoxide.[1]

Another study, in 5 healthy subjects given phenytoin 100 mg three times daily for 10 days, found that the maximum serum levels of furosemide 20 mg, given orally or intravenously, were reduced by 50%.[2]

Mechanism

Not understood. One suggestion is that phenytoin causes changes in the jejunal sodium pump activity, which reduces the absorption of furosemide,[2] but this is not the whole story because an interaction also occurs when furosemide is given intravenously.[1] Other suggestions, based on *in vitro* or *animal* evidence, are that phenytoin generates a ‘liquid membrane,’ which blocks the transport of furosemide to its active site,[3] or that phenytoin antagonises the diuretic effect of furosemide by interfering with the renal tubular sodium pump mechanism.[4]

Importance and management

Information regarding an interaction between furosemide and phenytoin is limited, but the available evidence suggests that a reduced diuretic response to furosemide is possible in the presence of phenytoin. It seems unlikely that this interaction will be of clinical relevance if furosemide is given to a patient already taking phenytoin, as the dose will be titrated to effect. If the diuretic response to furosemide appears to be diminished in a patient given phenytoin, consider increasing the diuretic dose.

1. Ahmad S. Renal insensitivity to frusemide caused by chronic anticonvulsant therapy. *BMJ* (1974) 3, 657–9.
2. Fine A, Henderson IS, Morgan DR, Tilstone WJ. Malabsorption of frusemide caused by phenytoin. *BMJ* (1977) 2, 1061–2.
3. Srivastava RC, Bhise SB, Sood R, Rao MNA. On the reduced furosemide response in the presence of diphenylhydantoin. *Colloids and Surfaces* (1986) 19, 83–8.
4. Tongia SK. Antagonism of frusemide diuresis by diphenylhydantoin sodium. *Indian J Med Res* (1981) 74, 572–4.

Loop diuretics; Furosemide + Sevelamer

Sevelamer abolished the diuretic effect of furosemide in a haemodialysis patient.

Clinical evidence, mechanism, importance and management

A haemodialysis patient taking furosemide 250 mg twice daily found that her urine output reduced from 950 mL/day to zero when she started taking sevelamer, 800 mg at breakfast and lunchtime, and 1.6 g with dinner. Urine output returned to the previous level within 24 hours of stopping the sevelamer. This effect also occurred on rechallenge. The dose times were adjusted so that she took furosemide 500 mg in the morning and sevelamer 1.6 g at lunch and dinner, and her urine output was unaffected and remained stable.[1]

The authors suggest that furosemide became bound to sevelamer in the gut, and this prevented its absorption.

This appears to be the only case report of an interaction between these drugs; however, it is worth bearing this case in mind should a similar situation arise in other patients. Note that the manufacturers of sevelamer[2,3] suggest that, when giving any other oral drug for which a reduction in the bioavailability could have a clinically significant effect on safety or efficacy, the drug should be given at least one hour before or 3 hours after sevelamer.

1. Fleuren HWHA, Kho Y, Schuurmans MMJ, Vollaard EJ. Drug interaction between sevelamer and furosemide. *Nephrol Dial Transplant* (2005) 20, 2288–9.
2. Renagel (Sevelamer hydrochloride). Sanofi. UK Summary of product characteristics, February 2015.
3. Renvela (Sevelamer carbonate). Genzyme. US Prescribing information, May 2011.

Loop diuretics; Furosemide + Sucralfate

The manufacturer of furosemide notes that sucralfate decreases the absorption of furosemide from the intestine and states that its effects are therefore reduced.[1] Presumably on this basis, some manufacturers state that oral furosemide and sucralfate must not be taken within 2 hours of each other.[1-3] However, the only available evidence appears to be a study in *animals*, which showed that the amount of furosemide excreted in the urine was not affected by the concurrent use of oral sucralfate, and the excretion of sodium and potassium in response to furosemide was not altered.[4] The outcome of concurrent use is therefore unclear.

1. Lasix (Furosemide). Sanofi-Aventis. UK Summary of product characteristics, July 2010.
2. Lasix (Furosemide). Sanofi-Aventis. US Prescribing information, July 2009.
3. Frusol (Furosemide). Rosemont Pharmaceuticals Ltd. UK Summary of product characteristics, April 2009.
4. Hikal AH, Walker LA, Ramachandran T. *In vitro* and *in vivo* interactions of furosemide and sucralfate. *Pharm Res* (1987) 4, 171–2.

Potassium-sparing diuretics + H_2-receptor antagonists

Although the H_2-receptor antagonists appear to cause some slight changes in the pharmacokinetics of amiloride and triamterene, none of these have been shown to be of clinical significance.

Clinical evidence, mechanism, importance and management

(a) Amiloride

A study in 8 healthy subjects given amiloride 5 mg daily found that **cimetidine** 400 mg twice daily for 12 days reduced the renal clearance of amiloride by 17% and reduced its urinary excretion from 65% to 53%. Amiloride also reduced the excretion of **cimetidine** from 43% to 32%, and its AUC was reduced by 14%.[1] No changes in the diuretic effects (urinary volume, sodium or potassium excretion) occurred. It seems that each drug reduces the gastrointestinal absorption of the other drug by as yet unidentified mechanisms. The overall plasma levels of the amiloride remain unchanged because the reduced absorption is offset by a reduction in its renal excretion. These mutual interactions do not seem to be clinically significant.

(b) Triamterene

A study in 6 healthy subjects given triamterene 100 mg daily for 4 days found that **cimetidine** 400 mg twice daily increased the AUC of triamterene by 22%, reduced its metabolism (hydroxylation) by 32%, and reduced its renal clearance by 28%. There also appeared to be a reduction in the absorption of triamterene. However, the loss of sodium in the urine was not significantly changed, and the potassium-sparing effects of triamterene were not altered.[2] Because the diuretic effects of triamterene are minimally changed, this interaction is unlikely to be clinically important.[2]

In 8 healthy subjects, **ranitidine** 150 mg twice daily for 4 days roughly halved the absorption (as measured by renal clearance) of triamterene 100 mg daily. Its metabolism was also reduced, with the total effect being a 21% reduction in the AUC. As a result of the reduced plasma triamterene levels, the urinary sodium loss was reduced to some extent but potassium excretion remained unchanged.[3] Overall the diuretic effects of triamterene were only mildly affected. Another study found that a 22% reduction in the AUC of triamterene is unlikely to result in a significant change in its diuretic effects.[2] No clinically significant interaction is therefore anticipated.

1. Somogyi AA, Hovens CM, Muirhead MR, Bochner F. Renal tubular secretion of amiloride and its inhibition by cimetidine in humans and in an animal model. *Drug Metab Dispos* (1989) 17, 190–6.
2. Muirhead MR, Somogyi AA, Rolan PE, Bochner F. Effect of cimetidine on renal and hepatic drug elimination: studies with triamterene. *Clin Pharmacol Ther* (1986) 40, 400–7.
3. Muirhead M, Bochner F, Somogyi A. Pharmacokinetic drug interactions between triamterene and ranitidine in humans: alterations in renal and hepatic clearances and gastrointestinal absorption. *J Pharmacol Exp Ther* (1988) 244, 734–9.

Potassium-sparing diuretics + NSAIDs

The concurrent use of triamterene (with or without a thiazide) and an NSAID has, in several cases, rapidly led to acute renal failure. NSAIDs may possibly antagonise the antihypertensive and/or diuretic effects of potassium-sparing diuretics and may also increase the risk of hyperkalaemia. There may be an increased risk of gastrointestinal events (e.g. gastrointestinal bleeding) with spironolactone and NSAIDs.

Clinical evidence

A retrospective analysis of records of patients taking diuretics (thiazides, loop and/or potassium-sparing) and NSAIDs found a twofold increase in the risk of hospitalisation for congestive heart failure on concurrent use, although the relative risk (1.4) with potassium-sparing diuretics was less than that when combined with a thiazide (2.9). The most common NSAIDs taken by this cohort of patients were **diclofenac**, **ibuprofen**, **indometacin** and **naproxen**.[1] The use of an NSAID, for example indometacin, with potassium-sparing diuretics has been associated with severe hyperkalaemia, particularly in patients with renal impairment.[2-5] NSAIDs can reduce the diuretic, natriuretic and antihypertensive effects of diuretics in some patients.[2-5] Various large epidemiological studies and meta-analyses of clinical studies have been conducted to assess the effect of NSAIDs on blood pressure in patients taking antihypertensives, including diuretics, and the findings of these are summarised in 'Table 23.2', p.1031. Individual clinical reports and clinical or pharmacological studies of the effects of specific NSAIDs on diuretics are outlined in the subsections below and in 'Table 26.2', p.1121.

A. Amiloride

A 78-year-old woman, who had been receiving **indometacin** 100 mg twice daily as suppositories and furosemide 40 mg every other day, experienced progressive weakness after furosemide was discontinued and amiloride 5 mg with hydrochlorothiazide 50 mg daily started She was found to have severe hyperkalaemia (serum potassium 6.8 mmol/L), which resolved after the drugs were discontinued. On rechallenge neither **indometacin** nor amiloride with hydrochlorothiazide, given alone, significantly changed her serum potassium levels, but giving indometacin with amiloride subsequently resulted in hyperkalaemia.[6] For further mention of interactions between amiloride with hydrochlorothiazide and indometacin or other NSAIDs, see 'Thiazide diuretics + NSAIDs', p.1132.

B. Spironolactone

(a) Indometacin

A study in healthy subjects found that indometacin 150 mg daily reduced the natriuretic effect of spironolactone 300 mg daily by 54%.[7]

(b) Mefenamic acid

The UK manufacturer of spironolactone reports that mefenamic acid has been shown to attenuate the diuretic effect of spironolactone.[8]

(c) Rofecoxib

For a report of heart failure in an elderly woman taking spironolactone, altizide and other drugs, when rofecoxib was added to her treatment, see 'Thiazide diuretics + NSAIDs', p.1132.

(d) Unspecified NSAIDs

A retrospective, population based case-control study suggested that the current use of spironolactone was associated with a 2.7-fold increased risk of a gastrointestinal event. This association was stronger as the dose increased and was more pronounced when spironolactone was given with ulcerogenic drugs including NSAIDs. Increasing the dose of other diuretics including **amiloride** or loop diuretics was not associated with upper gastrointestinal bleeding.[9] However, note that this study has been criticised because of, among other things, the use of unmatched controls.[10,11]

C. Triamterene

(a) Diclofenac

A patient receiving triamterene 100 mg and **trichlormethiazide** 2 mg daily was given intramuscular diclofenac 75 mg before admission to hospital with breast pain. On admission serum creatinine was 91 micromol/L and after 2 days it had increased to 248 micromol/L, but it returned to normal over 2 weeks. The subsequent use of oral diclofenac produced no adverse effects. The observed deterioration in renal function was attributed to an interaction between triamterene and diclofenac.[12]

(b) Diflunisal

Diflunisal had no effects on the pharmacokinetics of triamterene in healthy subjects, but the plasma AUC of an active metabolite, *p*-hydroxytriamterene was increased more than fourfold.[13]

(c) Ibuprofen

A 37-year-old man who had regularly taken ibuprofen 800 mg one to three times daily and hydrochlorothiazide 50 mg with triamterene 75 mg daily, developed acute renal failure after strenuous exercise. A renal biopsy showed acute tubular necrosis. The patient had taken the ibuprofen and diuretics 2 hours before exercise and it was suggested that peak anti-prostaglandin effects of the ibuprofen probably coincided with maximal exercise-induced renal vasoconstriction. Other factors such as diuretic use, hypertension and hypertensive nephrosclerosis may also have predisposed the patient to ischaemic tubular damage.[14] See also *Indometacin*, below for a further case of renal impairment involving the use of ibuprofen and triamterene.

(d) Indometacin

A study in 4 healthy subjects found that indometacin 150 mg daily given with triamterene 200 mg daily over a 3-day period reduced the creatinine clearance in 2 subjects by 62% and 72%, respectively. Renal function returned to normal after a month. Indometacin alone caused an average 10% fall in creatinine clearance, but triamterene alone caused no consistent change in renal function. No adverse reactions were seen in 18 other subjects given indometacin with other diuretics (furosemide, hydrochlorothiazide or spironolactone).[15,16]

A patient with systemic lupus erythematosus and membranous glomerulopathy who was taking triamterene 50 mg with hydrochlorothiazide 25 mg daily developed raised serum creatinine after taking **ibuprofen** 600 mg daily for 35 days. One day after changing to a high dose of indometacin (50 mg three times daily by mouth and 100 mg at night as a suppository) the patient developed acute renal failure with oliguria and slight hypertension.[17] Five patients are reported to have rapidly developed acute renal failure after receiving indometacin and triamterene, either concurrently or sequentially.[18-21]

Mechanism

Uncertain. One suggestion is that triamterene causes renal ischaemia, for which the kidney compensates by increasing prostaglandin production, thereby preserving renal blood flow. Indometacin opposes this by inhibiting prostaglandin synthesis, so that the damaging effects of triamterene on the kidney continue unchecked. As renal production of prostaglandins helps to maintain renal blood flow and renal vasodilatation during volume depletion, other NSAIDs might also be expected to affect this compensatory mechanism when diuretics are used. Prostaglandins may also contribute to the natriuretic effects of spironolactone and therefore the NSAIDs may reduce the diuretic effects of spironolactone by blocking prostaglandin synthesis.

Increases in the pharmacologically active metabolites of triamterene may occur due to competition for renal excretory pathways.

Importance and management

Information regarding an interaction between indometacin and **triamterene** is limited to these reports, but the increased risk of renal impairment is established, although the incidence is uncertain. Acute renal failure can apparently develop unpredictably and very rapidly, and therefore it would seem prudent to use triamterene with indometacin cautiously, or avoid their concurrent use altogether. The manufacturer of triamterene[22] and the authors of the report with diclofenac[12] suggest that any NSAID should be used cautiously in a patient taking triamterene. Strenuous exercise can reduce renal blood flow, and the author of the case report with ibuprofen notes that although renal failure secondary to this is rare, patients taking medication that reduces renal blood flow are more at risk of this complication.[14] The manufacturers of **amiloride**[4] and **eplerenone**[23] also warn about the possibility of hyperkalaemia and acute renal failure in patients also taking NSAIDs, and recommend that these patients should be adequately hydrated and have their renal function monitored.[23]

The joint American College of Cardiology/American Heart Association guidelines (2009) on the management of chronic heart failure recommend that NSAIDs, including coxibs, should be avoided, if possible, with aldosterone antagonists [such as **eplerenone** or spironolactone], as this increases the risk of developing hyperkalaemia and renal failure.[24]

1. Heerdink ER, Leufkens HG, Herings RMC, Ottervanger JP, Stricker BHC, Bakker A. NSAIDs associated with increased risk of congestive heart failure in elderly patients taking diuretics. *Arch Intern Med* (1998) 158, 1108–12.
2. Aldactone (Spironolactone). G.D. Searle LLC. US Prescribing information, January 2008.
3. Inspra (Eplerenone). Pfizer Inc. US Prescribing information, April 2008.
4. Amilamont (Amiloride hydrochloride). Rosemont Pharmaceuticals Ltd. UK Summary of product characteristics, March 2011.
5. Amiloride hydrochloride tablets USP. Paddock Laboratories, Inc. US Prescribing information, November 2008.
6. Mor R, Pitlik S, Rosenfeld JB. Indomethacin- and Moduretic®-induced hyperkalemia. *Isr J Med Sci* (1983) 19, 535–7.
7. Hofmann LM, Garcia HA. Interaction of spironolactone and indomethacin at the renal level. *Proc Soc Exp Biol Med* (1972) 141, 353–5.
8. Aldactone (Spironolactone). Pharmacia Ltd. UK Summary of product characteristics, May 2007.
9. Verhamme K, Mosis G, Dieleman J, Stricker B, Sturkenboom M. Spironolactone and risk of upper gastrointestinal events: population based case-control study. *BMJ* (2006) 333, 330–3.
10. Campbell E, Shonde A, Foley S. Spironolactone and risk of upper gastrointestinal events: spironolactone may not be guilty. *BMJ* (2006) 333, 500.
11. Dawwas MF. Spironolactone and risk of upper gastrointestinal events: association is unproved. *BMJ* (2006) 333, 501.
12. Härkönen M, Ekblom-Kullberg S. Reversible deterioration of renal function after diclofenac in patient receiving triamterene. *BMJ* (1986) 293, 698–9.
13. Jacob SS, Franklin ME, Dickinson RG, Hooper WD. The effect of diflunisal on the elimination of triamterene in human volunteers. *Drug Metabol Drug Interact* (2000) 16, 159–71.
14. Sanders LR. Exercise-induced acute renal failure associated with ibuprofen, hydrochlorothiazide, and triamterene. *J Am Soc Nephrol* (1995) 5, 2020–3.
15. Favre L, Glasson P, Vallotton MB. Reversible acute renal failure from combined triamterene and indomethacin. A study in healthy subjects. *Ann Intern Med* (1982) 96, 317–20.
16. Favre L, Glasson PH, Riondel A, Vallotton MB. Interaction of diuretics and non-steroidal anti-inflammatory drugs in man. *Clin Sci* (1983) 64, 407–15.
17. ter Borg EJ, de Jong PE, Meyer S, van Rijswijk MH, Kallenberg CGM. Indomethacin and ibuprofen-induced reversible acute renal failure in a patient with systemic lupus erythematosus. *Neth J Med* (1987) 30, 181–6.
18. McCarthy JT, Torres VE, Romero JC, Wochos DN, Velosa JA. Acute intrinsic renal failure induced by indomethacin: role of prostaglandin synthetase inhibition. *Mayo Clin Proc* (1982) 57, 289–96.
19. McCarthy JT. Drug-induced renal failure. *Mayo Clin Proc* (1982) 57, 463.
20. Weinberg MS, Quigg RJ, Salant DJ, Bernard DB. Anuric renal failure precipitated by indomethacin and triamterene. *Nephron* (1985) 40, 216–18.
21. Mathews A, Bailie GR. Acute renal failure and hyperkalemia associated with triamterene and indomethacin. *Vet Hum Toxicol* (1986) 28, 224–5.
22. Dyrenium (Triamterene). WellSpring Pharmaceutical Corp. US Prescribing information, March 2009.
23. Inspra (Eplerenone). Pfizer Ltd. UK Summary of product characteristics, October 2009.
24. Hunt SA, Abraham WT, Chin MH, Feldman AM, Francis GS, Ganiats TG, Jessup M, Konstam MA, Mancini DM, Michl K, Oates JA, Rahko PS, Silver MA, Stevenson LW, Yancy CW. 2009 focused update incorporated into the ACC/AHA 2005 guidelines for the diagnosis and management of heart failure in adults: a report of the American College of Cardiology Foundation/American Heart Association Task Force on Practice Guidelines developed in collaboration with the international society for heart and lung transplantation. *J Am Coll Cardiol* (2009) 53, e1–e90. Available at: http://content.onlinejacc.org/article.aspx?articleID=1139601 (accessed 22/10/15).

Potassium-sparing diuretics + Potassium compounds

The concurrent use of spironolactone or triamterene with a potassium supplement can result in severe and even life-threatening hyperkalaemia. Amiloride and eplerenone are expected to interact similarly. Potassium-containing salt substitutes can be as hazardous as potassium supplements.

Clinical evidence

(a) Spironolactone

In a retrospective analysis of hospitalised patients who had received spironolactone, hyperkalaemia had developed in 5.7% of patients taking spironolactone alone and in 15.4% of those also taking spironolactone with **potassium chloride**. The incidence of hyperkalaemia was 42% in those with severe azotaemia (a high blood level of urea or nitrogen compounds) given spironolactone with **potassium chloride**.[1] A retrospective survey of another group of 25 patients taking spironolactone and oral **potassium chloride** found that half of the patients had developed hyperkalaemia.[2]

A patient developed severe hyperkalaemia and cardiotoxicity as a result of taking spironolactone and a **potassium supplement**.[3] Three patients taking furosemide and spironolactone became hyperkalaemic[4,5] because they took **potassium-containing salt substitutes** (*No Salt* in one case[4]): two developed cardiac arrhythmias.[5]

(b) Triamterene

A case report describes the failure of a pacemaker in a patient, which was attributed to hyperkalaemia caused by the concurrent use of triamterene with hydrochlorothiazide and **potassium chloride**.[6]

Mechanism

The effects of the potassium-sparing diuretics and potassium compounds are additive, which can result in hyperkalaemia.

Importance and management

The interaction between spironolactone and potassium compounds is established and the hyperkalaemia that results is of clinical importance. A case has also been reported with triamterene: **amiloride** and **eplerenone** would be expected to behave similarly. Avoid potassium compounds in patients taking potassium-sparing diuretics except in cases of marked potassium depletion, where the effects can be closely monitored. Warn patients about the risks of salt substitutes containing potassium, which may increase the potassium intake by 50 to 60 mmol daily.[5] The signs and symptoms of hyperkalaemia include muscular weakness, fatigue, paraesthesia, flaccid paralysis of the extremities, bradycardia, shock and ECG abnormalities, which may develop slowly and insidiously. Note that the manufacturers of eplerenone[7,8] specifically contraindicate the concurrent use of potassium supplements, but in the US, this contraindication is only in patients given eplerenone for hypertension.

1. Greenblatt DJ, Koch-Weser J. Adverse reactions to spironolactone. A report from the Boston Collaborative Drug Surveillance Program. *Clin Pharmacol Ther* (1973) 14, 136–7.
2. Simborg DN. Medication prescribing on a university medical service — the incidence of drug combinations with potential adverse interactions. *Johns Hopkins Med J* (1976) 139, 23–6.
3. Kalbian VV. Iatrogenic hyperkalemic paralysis with electrocardiographic changes. *South Med J* (1974) 67, 342–5.
4. McCaughan D. Hazards of non-prescription potassium supplements. *Lancet* (1984) i, 513–14.
5. Yap V, Patel A, Thomsen J. Hyperkalemia with cardiac arrhythmia. Induction by salt substitutes, spironolactone, and azotemia. *JAMA* (1976) 236, 2775–6.
6. O'Reilly MV, Murnaghan DP, Williams MB. Transvenous pacemaker failure induced by hyperkalemia. *JAMA* (1974) 228, 336–7.
7. Inspra (Eplerenone). Pfizer Ltd. UK Summary of product characteristics, October 2009.
8. Inspra (Eplerenone). Pfizer Inc. US Prescribing information, April 2008.

Potassium-sparing diuretics + Total parenteral nutrition

Two patients receiving total parenteral nutrition developed metabolic acidosis associated with the concurrent use of triamterene or amiloride. The cases were complicated by a number of pathological and other factors, but it was suggested that the major reason for the acidosis was because the diuretics prevented the kidneys from responding normally to the acid load from the TPN. The authors of the report advise caution during concurrent use.[1]

1. Kushner RF, Sitrin MD. Metabolic acidosis. Development in two patients receiving a potassium-sparing diuretic and total parenteral nutrition. *Arch Intern Med* (1986) 146, 343–5.

Potassium-sparing with and without thiazide diuretics + Co-trimoxazole or Trimethoprim

Two studies in elderly patients suggest that the concurrent use of spironolactone and co-trimoxazole might increase the risk of hospitalisation for hyperkalaemia and/or sudden death. Case reports describe hyperkalaemia in patients taking spironolactone and co-trimoxazole. Excessively low sodium concentrations have been seen in a few patients taking hydrochlorothiazide with amiloride or triamterene when they were given trimethoprim or co-trimoxazole.

Clinical evidence

(a) Hydrochlorothiazide

A 75-year-old woman with multiple medical conditions taking methyldopa, levothyroxine, and hydrochlorothiazide with **amiloride** developed nausea and anorexia, and was found to have hyponatraemia (sodium 107 mmol/L), within 4 days of starting to take trimethoprim 200 mg twice daily. The problem resolved when the diuretics and trimethoprim were stopped. When she was rechallenged 4 months later with trimethoprim, hyponatraemia did not occur, but it developed rapidly when hydrochlorothiazide with amiloride was also restarted.[1] The authors report several other patients who developed hyponatraemia within 4 to 12 days of starting trimethoprim or co-trimoxazole (trimethoprim with sulfamethoxazole), all of whom were elderly and all but one of whom were taking a diuretic (unnamed).[1]

Another report describes 2 patients taking hydrochlorothiazide with **amiloride** or **triamterene** who developed hyponatraemia after co-trimoxazole was also given.[2]

(b) Spironolactone

A case-control study of patients aged 66 years and over and taking spironolactone, found that of 6 903 admissions to hospital for hyperkalaemia during the 18-year study period, 306 admissions occurred within 14 days of antibacterial exposure (co-trimoxazole, norfloxacin, nitrofurantoin, or amoxicillin). Using matched controls, the risk of admission due to hyperkalaemia was found to be 12-fold higher if they had taken co-trimoxazole, than if they had taken **amoxicillin**. The risk with **nitrofurantoin** was 2.4-fold higher than with amoxicillin, but there was no increased risk with **norfloxacin**.[3] In a similar study by the same authors, of 11 968 sudden deaths while taking spironolactone during the 17-year study period, 328 occurred within 14 days of antibacterial exposure (co-trimoxazole, ciprofloxacin, norfloxacin, nitrofurantoin, or amoxicillin). Using matched controls, the risk of sudden death was found to be 2.5-fold higher if they had taken co-trimoxazole, than if they had taken **amoxicillin**. The risk with **ciprofloxacin** was 1.6-fold, and that with **nitrofurantoin** was 1.7-fold higher, when compared with amoxicillin. There was no increased risk with **norfloxacin**.[4] A retrospective analysis of medical records for patients who received co-trimoxazole during a 5-year period, found that of 6 162 patients there were 91 cases of hyperkalaemia. Of the cases of hyperkalaemia, 4.4% were also taking spironolactone compared with 0.9% in the 6 071 patients who did not develop hyperkalaemia.[5]

Several case reports describe hyperkalaemia in elderly patients (66 to 85-years-old) taking spironolactone after co-trimoxazole was added. All patients recovered a few days after the drugs were stopped and treatment for hyperkalaemia was given.[6-8] In one of the cases the patient was also taking enalapril,[7] and in another, they were also taking valsartan,[8] both of which could also have been implicated (see 'ACE inhibitors or Angiotensin II receptor antagonists + Co-trimoxazole or Trimethoprim', p.27), although timescales for the effects seen suggest that the combination of spironolactone and co-trimoxazole was a major contributory factor.

Mechanism

Not established, although it would seem likely that the hyponatraemia and hyperkalaemia seen are due to additive adverse effects, based on the known effects of all of these drugs: thiazide diuretics given with potassium-sparing diuretics are said to be particularly liable to cause hyponatraemia;[9] trimethoprim can cause hyponatraemia and/or hyperkalaemia[10,11] by blocking amiloride-sensitive sodium channels in the collecting duct (this produces a similar effect to that of a potassium-sparing diuretic); and a well-known adverse effect of potassium sparing diuretics is hyperkalaemia.

Importance and management

Evidence for an interaction between potassium-sparing diuretics with and without thiazides, and co-trimoxazole or trimethoprim is limited. However, the case-control studies in elderly patients taking spironolactone and co-trimoxazole suggest that the risk of hyperkalaemia might be greatly increased by this combination, and the authors suggest that the increased risk of sudden death seen in one of the studies[4] might have been a result of additive hyperkalaemia caused by the combination, although this is only a hypothesis and requires specific study to verify. Clinical cases of hyperkalaemia in patients taking this combination suggest that this could be an important interaction, although perhaps more so in elderly patients whose ability to regulate potassium concentrations is already diminished. It would therefore seem sensible to carefully monitor potassium concentrations in patients receiving spironolactone and co-trimoxazole, and particularly in those who might be more susceptible to electrolyte imbalances. Some consideration should be given to adjusting the dose of spironolactone, or choosing an alternative antibacterial. A similar effect might be expected with trimethoprim alone, and with **eplerenone**, and similar precautions would seem sensible with these drugs.

The case reports of hyponatraemia with potassium-sparing diuretics with thiazides and co-trimoxazole or trimethoprim suggest that it would be prudent to be on the alert for any signs of hyponatraemia (such as nausea or anorexia) in any patient taking these drugs.

1. Eastell R, Edmonds CJ. Hyponatraemia associated with trimethoprim and a diuretic. *BMJ* (1984) 289, 1658–9.
2. Hart TL, Johnston LJ, Edmonds MW, Brownscombe L. Hyponatremia secondary to thiazide-trimethoprim interaction. *Can J Hosp Pharm* (1989) 42, 243–6.
3. Antoniou T, Gomes T, Mamdani MM, Yao Z, Hellings C, Garg AX, Weir MA, Juurlink DN. Trimethoprim-sulfamethoxazole induced hyperkalaemia in elderly patients receiving spironolactone: nested case-control study. *BMJ* (2011) 343, d5228.
4. Antoniou T, Hollands S, Macdonald EM, Gomes T, Mamdani MM, Juurlink DN. Trimethoprim-sulfamethoxazole and risk of sudden death among patients taking spironolactone. *CMAJ* (2015) 187, E138–43.
5. Gentry CA, Nguyen AT. An evaluation of hyperkalemia and serum creatinine elevation associated with different dosage levels of outpatient trimethoprim-sulfamethoxazole with and without concomitant medications. *Ann Pharmacother* (2013) 47, 1618–26.
6. Marinella MA. Severe hyperkalaemia associated with trimethoprim-sulfamethoxazole and spironolactone. *Infect Dis Clin Pract* (1997) 256–8.
7. Martin J, Mourton S, Nicholls G. Severe hyperkalaemia with prescription of potassium-retaining agents in an elderly patient. *N Z Med J* (2003) 116, U542.
8. Juvet T, Gourineni VC, Ravi S, Zarich SW. Life-threatening hyperkalaemia: a potentially lethal drug combination. *Conn Med* (2013) 77, 491–3.
9. Hornick P. Severe hyponatraemia in elderly patients: cause for concern. *Ann R Coll Surg Engl* (1996) 78, 230–1.
10. Perazella MA. Trimethoprim-induced hyperkalaemia. Clinical data, mechanism, prevention and management. *Drug Safety* (2000) 22, 227–36.
11. Mori H, Kuroda Y, Imamura S, Toyoda A, Yoshida I, Kawakami M, Tabei K. Hyponatremia and/or hyperkalemia in patients treated with the standard dose of trimethoprim-sulfamethoxazole. *Intern Med* (2003) 42, 665–9.

Potassium-sparing diuretics; Eplerenone + CYP3A4 inducers

St John's wort, a CYP3A4 inducer, slightly decreases the AUC of eplerenone. Other stronger inducers of CYP3A4, such as rifampicin (rifampin), are predicted to interact to a greater extent.

Clinical evidence, mechanism, importance and management

St John's wort (*Hypericum perforatum*) caused a slight 30% decrease in the AUC of a single 100-mg dose of eplerenone.[1,2] Eplerenone is metabolised by CYP3A4, and therefore inducers of this isoenzyme, such as **St John's wort**, would be expected to decrease its levels. In the UK, the manufacturer predicts that a more pronounced decrease in the AUC of eplerenone might occur with stronger CYP3A4 inducers, such as **rifampicin (rifampin)**.[1] Because of the possibility of decreased efficacy, they do not recommend the concurrent use of potent CYP3A4 inducers with eplerenone, and they specifically name **carbamazepine**, **phenytoin** [and therefore probably fosphenytoin], **phenobarbital** [and therefore probably primidone], **rifampicin**, and **St John's wort**.[1] However, it is unlikely that the decrease seen with **St John's wort** is clinically relevant. Further study of the other potential interactions is needed to demonstrate their clinical significance.

1. Inspra (Eplerenone). Pfizer Ltd. UK Summary of product characteristics, October 2009.
2. Inspra (Eplerenone). Pfizer Inc. US Prescribing information, April 2008.

Potassium-sparing diuretics; Eplerenone + CYP3A4 inhibitors

Ketoconazole, a potent CYP3A4 inhibitor, markedly increases the bioavailability of eplerenone. Other potent inhibitors of CYP3A4 are expected to interact similarly. Less potent inhibitors of CYP3A4 (including diltiazem, fluconazole, saquinavir and verapamil) moderately increase the AUC of eplerenone. Grapefruit juice had a small but unimportant effect on the AUC of eplerenone.

Clinical evidence

(a) Azoles

Ketoconazole 200 mg twice daily for 7 days increased the AUC of a single 100-mg dose of eplerenone 5.4-fold in 18 healthy subjects.[1,2] The manufacturers predict that **itraconazole** will have a similar effect to **ketoconazole**.[1,3] **Fluconazole** 200 mg daily for 7 days increased the AUC of eplerenone 2.2-fold in 18 healthy subjects.[2] A case report describes the development of hypotension when intravenous **voriconazole** was started in a patient stable taking eplerenone 50 mg daily and nifedipine 40 mg daily. A complete resolution was achieved by stopping the eplerenone and halving the daily dose of nifedipine.[4] However, it is unclear to what extent the eplerenone contributed to the hypotensive effects seen, as nifedipine concentrations can, in theory, also be raised by **voriconazole**, see 'Calcium-channel blockers + Azoles', p.1033.

(b) Calcium-channel blockers

In 24 healthy subjects the steady-state AUC of eplerenone 100 mg daily was increased about twofold by **verapamil** 240 mg daily for 7 days.[2] **Diltiazem** has caused similar increases in the AUC of eplerenone.[3]

(c) Grapefruit juice

Grapefruit juice caused only a slight 25% increase in the AUC of eplerenone 100 mg.[1]

(d) HIV-protease inhibitors

In 24 healthy subjects, **saquinavir** 1.2 g three times daily caused a 2.1-fold increase in the steady-state AUC of eplerenone 100 mg daily.[2] The manufacturers predict that **ritonavir** and **nelfinavir** will have a greater effect.[1,3] Eplerenone reduced the maximum concentration of **saquinavir** by 30%, and the AUC by 21%,[2] but the clinical relevance of this has not been assessed.

(e) Macrolides

In 24 healthy subjects **erythromycin** 500 mg twice daily caused a 2.9-fold increase in the steady-state AUC of eplerenone 100 mg daily.[2] The manufacturers predict that **clarithromycin**[1,3] and **telithromycin**[3] will have a greater effect. Eplerenone reduced the AUC of **erythromycin** by 14%, which was not considered clinically relevant.[2]

Mechanism

Eplerenone is primarily metabolised by CYP3A4, and therefore inhibitors of this isoenzyme will increase its bioavailability.

Importance and management

The pharmacokinetic interactions between eplerenone and CYP3A4 inhibitors are established. Although the clinical relevance of the increase in eplerenone exposure has not been assessed, it is known that the risk of hyperkalaemia with eplerenone is related to its dose.[3] As the increase in the AUC of eplerenone with ketoconazole is so great, the manufacturers contraindicate concurrent use.[1,3] They also contraindicate the concurrent use of other potent inhibitors of CYP3A4, and they name drugs including clarithromycin, itraconazole, **nefazodone**, nelfinavir, ritonavir,[1,3] and telithromycin.[3]

In the UK, the manufacturer recommends that the dose of eplerenone should not exceed 25 mg daily in patients taking less potent CYP3A4 inhibitors, such as **amiodarone**, diltiazem, erythromycin, fluconazole, saquinavir and verapamil.[3] In the US, the manufacturer recommends that the starting dose of eplerenone for hypertension should be reduced to 25 mg daily for patients taking these drugs.[1] This seems a sensible precaution. However, note that erythromycin sometimes appears to be as potent an inhibitor of CYP3A4 as clarithromycin and so additional caution (e.g. increased monitoring of potassium concentrations) is probably warranted with on concurrent use.

1. Inspra (Eplerenone). Pfizer Inc. US Prescribing information, April 2008.
2. Cook CS, Berry LM, Burton E. Prediction of *in vivo* drug interactions with eplerenone in man from *in vitro* metabolic inhibition data. *Xenobiotica* (2004) 34, 215–28.
3. Inspra (Eplerenone). Pfizer Ltd. UK Summary of product characteristics, October 2009.
4. Kato J, Mori T, Nakamura Y, Sakurai M, Aisa Y, Ikeda Y, Okamoto S. Hypotension due to the drug interaction of voriconazole with eplerenone and nifedipine. *Eur J Clin Pharmacol* (2009) 65, 323–4.

Potassium-sparing diuretics; Eplerenone + Miscellaneous

Corticosteroids or tetracosactide may potentially reduce the antihypertensive effect of eplerenone, whereas alpha blockers, antipsychotics, amifostine, baclofen, and tricyclic antidepressants may increase its antihypertensive effects. Antacids have no effect on eplerenone pharmacokinetics, and no pharmacokinetic interaction has been seen between eplerenone and midazolam. In addition, eplerenone has no important effect on warfarin or contraceptive steroid pharmacokinetics.

Clinical evidence, mechanism, importance and management

(a) Antacids

The US manufacturer notes that **aluminium/magnesium**-containing antacids had no effect on the pharmacokinetics of eplerenone.[1]

(b) Combined hormonal contraceptives

Eplerenone 100 mg daily was given to 24 healthy subjects on days 1 to 11 of a 28-day cycle of a combined hormonal contraceptive (**ethinylestradiol** 35 micrograms with **norethisterone** 1 mg). There was no change in the **ethinylestradiol** AUC, but there was a small 17% increase in the **norethisterone** AUC, which is unlikely to be clinically relevant.[2]

For comment that drospirenone may increase the risk of hyperkalaemia if it is given with eplerenone or other potassium-sparing diuretics, see 'Drospirenone-containing contraceptives or HRT + Potassium-sparing drugs', p.1191.

(c) Corticosteroids or Tetracosactide (Cosyntropin)

Corticosteroids or tetracosactide can cause fluid and sodium retention and therefore their concurrent use with eplerenone may potentially reduce its antihypertensive effect.[3] Bear the possibility of an interaction in mind if a patient has a reduced antihypertensive response to eplerenone.

(d) Drugs that may cause postural hypotension

The manufacturer suggests that there is a risk of increased hypotensive effects and/or postural hypotension if eplerenone is given with **alpha blockers** (e.g. **alfuzosin**, **prazosin**), **tricyclic antidepressants**, **antipsychotics**, **amifostine** and **baclofen**.[3] Increased monitoring would seem prudent.

(e) Midazolam

The manufacturers state that a pharmacokinetic study has shown no interaction between midazolam (a CYP3A4 substrate) and eplerenone.[1,3]

(f) Warfarin

Eplerenone did not alter the pharmacokinetics of warfarin to a clinically relevant extent.[1,3] However, the UK manufacturer still recommends caution when the warfarin dose is near the upper limit of the therapeutic range.[3]

1. Inspra (Eplerenone). Pfizer Inc. US Prescribing information, April 2008.
2. Cook CS, Berry LM, Burton E. Prediction of *in vivo* drug interactions with eplerenone in man from *in vitro* metabolic inhibition data. *Xenobiotica* (2004) 34, 215–28.
3. Inspra (Eplerenone). Pfizer Ltd. UK Summary of product characteristics, October 2009.

Potassium-sparing diuretics; Spironolactone + Aspirin

Although aspirin reduces the spironolactone-induced loss of sodium in the urine it does not appear to alter the antihypertensive effects of spironolactone. A single case report describes the development of gynaecomastia and a rash when a man taking spironolactone was given aspirin, and several other drugs.

Clinical evidence

(a) Effects on blood pressure

In a crossover study, 5 patients with low-renin essential hypertension, well-controlled for 4 months or more with spironolactone 100 to 300 mg daily, were given aspirin 2.4 to 4.8 g daily over 6-week periods. The addition of aspirin did not affect blood pressure, serum electrolytes, body-weight, blood-urea-nitrogen or plasma renin activity.[1]

(b) Effects on natriuresis

A study in 10 healthy subjects given single 25-, 50- and 100-mg doses of spironolactone, found that a single 600-mg dose of aspirin reduced the urinary excretion of sodium in response to spironolactone.[2] In a further study in 7 of these subjects, the effectiveness of the spironolactone was reduced by 70%, and the overnight sodium excretion was reduced by one-third when they were given spironolactone 25 mg four times daily for one week followed by a single 600-mg dose of aspirin.[2] Reductions in sodium excretion are described in other studies of this interaction.[3,4] In one of these, the sodium excretion brought about by spironolactone was completely abolished when aspirin was given 90 minutes after the spironolactone, but when the drugs were given in the reverse order, the inhibition of sodium excretion that was caused by aspirin was not completely reversed by spironolactone.[4]

In another study in 7 patients with ascites due to liver cirrhosis, pretreatment with two doses of aspirin 900 mg reduced the natriuretic effect of spironolactone 300 mg daily by 33%. However, there was no significant change in urinary output.[5]

(c) Gynaecomastia

A patient who had been taking spironolactone uneventfully for 4 years developed swollen, tender breasts and a rash on his chest and neck a fortnight after starting to take *Darvon Compound* (**dextropropoxyphene**, aspirin, **phenacetin** and **caffeine**). The problem disappeared when both drugs were withdrawn but the rash reappeared when the *Darvon Compound* alone was given and disappeared when it was withdrawn. No problems occurred when the spironolactone was given alone, but both the rash and the gynaecomastia recurred when the *Darvon Compound* was again added.[6] Consequently the authors attributed the reaction to an interaction with *Darvon Compound*, but noted that they cannot be sure which of the components is responsible.

Mechanism

Uncertain. There is evidence that the active secretion of canrenone (the active metabolite of spironolactone) is blocked by aspirin, but the significance of this is not entirely clear.[3] The reasons for the development of gynaecomastia are not understood. Gynaecomastia is a known adverse effect of spironolactone (incidence 1.2%), but the authors considered it unlikely that it should spontaneously develop after so many years of treatment.

Importance and management

The interaction between spironolactone and aspirin is adequately but not extensively documented. Despite the results of the studies showing a reduced natriuretic effect, the small study in hypertensive patients suggests that the effects of spironolactone on reducing blood pressure might not be affected by anti-inflammatory doses of aspirin. In general, concurrent use need not be avoided, but if the diuretic response to spironolactone is less than expected consider this interaction as a cause.

None of these studies looked at the effects of low-dose aspirin on spironolactone Nevertheless, the proven protective cardiovascular benefits of low-dose aspirin in patients with hypertension and/or coronary artery disease seem likely to outweigh the possible reduction in the efficacy of spironolactone. Nevertheless it may still be prudent to consider the possibility of an interaction if the diuretic response to spironolactone is reduced.

The isolated case of gynaecomastia seems unlikely to be of general relevance.

1. Hollifield JW. Failure of aspirin to antagonize the antihypertensive effect of spironolactone in low-renin hypertension. *South Med J* (1976) 69, 1034–6.
2. Tweeddale MG, Ogilvie RI. Antagonism of spironolactone-induced natriuresis by aspirin in man. *N Engl J Med* (1973) 289, 198–200.
3. Ramsay LE, Harrison IR, Shelton JR, Vose CW. Influence of acetylsalicylic acid on the renal handling of a spironolactone metabolite in healthy subjects. *Eur J Clin Pharmacol* (1976) 10, 43–8.
4. Elliott HC. Reduced adrenocortical steroid excretion rates in man following aspirin administration. *Metabolism* (1962) 11, 1015–18.
5. Mirouze D, Zipser RD, Reynolds TB. Effect of inhibitors of prostaglandin synthesis on induced diuresis in cirrhosis. *Hepatology* (1983) 3, 50–5.
6. Licata AA, Bartter FC. Spironolactone-induced gynaecomastia related to allergic reaction to 'Darvon Compound'. *Lancet* (1976) ii, 905.

Potassium-sparing diuretics; Spironolactone + Colestyramine

A few case reports have described hyperchloraemic metabolic acidosis, which was associated with the use of colestyramine and spironolactone.

Clinical evidence

Four case reports describe the development of hyperchloraemic metabolic acidosis in patients with liver cirrhosis taking colestyramine (up to about 25 g daily), who were also taking spironolactone 75 mg or 100 mg daily.[1-4] One patient developed significant hyperkalaemia (potassium 8 mmol/L),[4] and 2 patients developed mild renal impairment.[1,3] One patient had recently recovered from a respiratory tract infection, which the authors suggested may have contributed to the acidosis.[1] Acidosis resolved when colestyramine was stopped.

Mechanism

Bicarbonate has been shown to compete *in vitro* with bile acids for binding sites on the colestyramine resin.[1,3] The chloride ions in the colestyramine resin may cause an anion exchange of not only the bile salts, as is the intention, but also bicarbonate in the small bowel. This removal of bicarbonate from the body can predispose to the development of a hyperchloraemic metabolic acidosis and hyperkalaemia. This might be exacerbated by the bicarbonate-losing and hyperkalaemic effects of spironolactone.[1-4]

Importance and management

Evidence for an interaction between colestyramine and spironolactone is sparse, and any interaction may be restricted to patients with predisposing conditions. In healthy subjects with normal renal function, acidosis does not usually occur, as the kidneys can correct it by increasing the excretion of chloride and production of bicarbonate.[1-4] However, it may occur in patients with renal impairment, volume depletion (e.g. secondary to diuretics or diarrhoea) or concurrent conditions that predispose to acidosis (such as a respiratory tract infection). It has been suggested that electrolytes should be closely monitored when patients who are at risk of an interaction are taking colestyramine and spironolactone,[1] although note, even in predisposed patients, the interaction appears to be rare.

1. Eaves ER, Korman MG. Cholestyramine induced hyperchloremic metabolic acidosis. *Aust N Z J Med* (1984) 14, 670–2.
2. Clouston WM, Lloyd HM. Cholestyramine induced hyperchloremic metabolic acidosis. *Aust N Z J Med* (1985) 15, 271.
3. Scheel PJ, Whelton A, Rossiter K, Watson A. Cholestyramine-induced hyperchloremic metabolic acidosis. *J Clin Pharmacol* (1992) 32, 536–8.
4. Zapater P, Alba D. Acidosis and extreme hyperkalemia associated with cholestyramine and spironolactone. *Ann Pharmacother* (1995) 29, 199–200.

Potassium-sparing diuretics; Spironolactone + Food

Food may increase the plasma levels of spironolactone, but this did not alter its antihypertensive efficacy in one long-term study.

Clinical evidence, mechanism, importance and management

In a study in 7 healthy subjects, food increased the AUC of canrenone (the major active metabolite of spironolactone) by about 30% after a single 100-mg dose of spironolactone, when compared with the fasted state.[1] However, a 60-day study in 10 healthy subjects by the same research group subsequently found that steady-state canrenone levels did not differ when spironolactone 100 mg daily was taken at least 30 minutes before eating, compared with immediately after eating. Furthermore, in a crossover study in 10 hypertensive patients, the antihypertensive efficacy of spironolactone was not altered by food. It was suggested that the difference is due to a more specific drug assay in the second study.[2] Other authors have also found that, in healthy subjects, food increased the AUC of a single dose of spironolactone by 71%, and also increased the AUC of three of its metabolites (including canrenone) by 32%, but they did not assess whether this altered the hypotensive effects of spironolactone.[3] It appears from the long-term study, that food does not alter the antihypertensive efficacy of spironolactone. However, note that it has been recommended that spironolactone should be taken with food to try to reduce the gastric irritant effects of the drug.[2]

1. Melander A, Danielson K, Scherstén B, Thulin T, Wåhlin E. Enhancement by food of canrenone bioavailability from spironolactone. *Clin Pharmacol Ther* (1977) 22, 100–3.
2. Thulin T, Wåhlin-Boll E, Liedholm H, Lindholm L, Melander A. Influence of food intake on antihypertensive drugs: spironolactone. *Drug Nutr Interact* (1983) 2, 169–73.
3. Overdiek HWPM, Merkus FWHM. Influence of food on the bioavailability of spironolactone. *Clin Pharmacol Ther* (1986) 40, 531–6.

Thiazide diuretics + Bile-acid binding resins

The absorption of hydrochlorothiazide can be reduced by more than one-third if colestipol is given concurrently. Chlorothiazide appears to interact similarly. Colestyramine also reduces the absorption of hydrochlorothiazide by more than two-thirds.

Clinical evidence

In 6 healthy subjects, the plasma levels of **hydrochlorothiazide** were reduced by about two-thirds by **colestyramine** 8 g, taken 2 minutes before, 6 hours after and 12 hours after a single 75-mg oral dose of **hydrochlorothiazide**. The total urinary excretion of **hydrochlorothiazide** was reduced by 83%. In a parallel study with **colestipol** 10 g, the blood levels of **hydrochlorothiazide** were reduced by about 14% and the total urinary excretion was reduced by 31%.[1] A further study found that giving **colestyramine** 4 hours after **hydrochlorothiazide** reduced the effects of the interaction but **hydrochlorothiazide** absorption was still reduced by one-third.[2] In another study **colestipol**, given simultaneously or one hour after **chlorothiazide**, reduced the urinary excretion of **chlorothiazide** by 58% and 54%, respectively.[3]

Mechanism

Hydrochlorothiazide becomes bound to colestyramine and colestipol within the gut, and less is available for absorption.

Importance and management

The interactions between colestipol or colestyramine and hydrochlorothiazide are established and of clinical importance. It is normally recommended that other drugs are given 1 hour before or 4 to 6 hours after colestyramine to avoid interactions, but one study found that even giving hydrochlorothiazide 4 hours before colestyramine (to minimise mixing in the gut) resulted in a one-third reduction in hydrochlorothiazide absorption.[2] It would therefore seem prudent to separate administration by as much as possible in order to minimise the interaction and remain aware that a reduction in the effects of hydrochlorothiazide may still be possible. The optimum time-interval with colestipol has not been investigated but it would be reasonable to take similar precautions.

1. Hunninghake DB, King S, La Croix K. The effect of cholestyramine and colestipol on the absorption of hydrochlorothiazide. *Int J Clin Pharmacol Ther Toxicol* (1982) 20, 151–4.
2. Hunninghake DB, Hibbard DM. Influence of time intervals for cholestyramine dosing on the absorption of hydrochlorothiazide. *Clin Pharmacol Ther* (1986) 39, 329–34.
3. Kauffman RE, Azarnoff DL. Effect of colestipol on gastrointestinal absorption of chlorothiazide in man. *Clin Pharmacol Ther* (1973) 14, 886–90.

Thiazide diuretics + Calcium and/or Vitamin D

Hypercalcaemia and possibly metabolic alkalosis can develop in patients who are given fairly high doses of vitamin D and/or moderately large amounts of calcium if they are also given a thiazide. The oral vitamin D analogue, paricalcitol, is predicted to interact similarly. One case of hypercalcaemia has been reported in a patient using a high-strength topical tacalcitol with a thiazide.

Clinical evidence

(a) Calcium and vitamin D

An elderly woman taking **hydrochlorothiazide** 25 mg and triamterene 50 mg daily became confused, disorientated and dehydrated 6 months after starting to take vitamin D_2 50 000 units and calcium 1.5 g daily (as calcium carbonate) for osteoporosis. Her serum calcium level had risen to about 3.5 mmol/L (reference range about 2 to 2.6 mmol/L).[1]

A young woman with osteoporosis taking 3 mg of vitamin D_2 and calcium 2 g daily (as lactate) became hypercalcaemic 3 days after starting to take **chlorothiazide** 500 mg every 6 hours.[2]

(b) Calcium carbonate

A 47-year-old man was admitted to hospital complaining of dizziness and general weakness, which had begun 2 months previously. He was taking **chlorothiazide** 500 mg daily for hypertension, 'thyroid' 120 mg daily for hypothyroidism and calcium carbonate 7.5 to 10 g daily for heartburn. On examination he was found to have metabolic alkalosis with respiratory compensation, a total serum calcium concentration of 3.4 mmol/L (reference range given as 2.15 to 2.6 mmol/L) and an abnormal ECG. He was diagnosed as having the milk-alkali syndrome. Recovery was rapid when the thiazide and calcium carbonate were withdrawn, and a sodium chloride infusion, furosemide and oral phosphates given.[3]

An elderly woman with normal renal function taking **hydrochlorothiazide** 50 mg daily developed hypercalcaemia about 3 weeks after increasing her dose of calcium carbonate from 2.5 g daily to 7.5 g daily.[4] Another case describes hypercalcaemic alkalosis in an 87-year-old woman who had been prescribed **hydrochlorothiazide** with amiloride, but was also regularly self-medicating with a calcium-containing antacid (calcium/magnesium carbonate).[5]

In all three cases the thiazide was thought to be implicated as the levels of calcium ingestion, although moderately high, were in the region of the normally recommended doses.

(c) Oral vitamin D

In a group of 12 patients treated for hypoparathyroidism with vitamin D (**dihydrotachysterol** or **ergocalciferol**), 5 patients became hypercalcaemic when they took

bendroflumethiazide or **methyclothiazide**.[6] A significant rise in plasma calcium levels occurred in 7 patients given vitamin D and **methyclothiazide** or **chlorothiazide**, and hypercalcaemia developed in 3 of them.[7] A study in 12 children taking **calcitriol** 31 nanograms/kg daily found that the addition of **hydrochlorothiazide** 1 to 2 micrograms/kg daily reduced the urinary excretion of calcium caused by calcitriol.[8] Another study in 7 patients with vitamin D-induced calciuria found that the addition of **hydrochlorothiazide** and amiloride reduced the urinary excretion of calcium due to **calcitriol** to a greater extent than **hydrochlorothiazide** alone. Moreover, the addition of amiloride helped to prevent adverse effects associated with the use of **hydrochlorothiazide**, such as hypokalaemia and alkalosis.[9]

(d) Topical vitamin D analogues

A case of asymptomatic hypercalcaemia has been reported in a patient taking **trichlormethiazide** 6 mg daily and applying about 10 g of a high-strength topical **tacalcitol** ointment (equivalent to about 200 micrograms of tacalcitol daily) for psoriasis, as part of a clinical study. His calcium level reached a peak of 3.55 mmol/L 28 days after starting the **tacalcitol** ointment and it fell back to within the normal range within 7 days of stopping the ointment.[10]

Mechanism

The thiazides can cause calcium retention by reducing the urinary excretion of calcium. This, added to an increased intake of calcium, can result in excessive calcium levels. Alkalosis (the milk-alkali syndrome, associated with hypercalcaemia, alkalosis, and renal impairment) may also occur in some individuals because the thiazide limits the excretion of bicarbonate. Note that loop diuretics such as furosemide increase the urinary excretion of calcium.

Importance and management

The interaction between thiazides and **calcium compounds and/or vitamin D** is established. The incidence is unknown but the reports cited[6,7] suggest that it can be considerable if the intake of vitamin D and calcium are high. Concurrent use need not be avoided (thiazides have been used clinically to aid in the treatment of hypocalcaemia, by reducing urinary calcium excretion,[11] and to reduce vitamin-D induced hypercalciuria[8,9]) but the serum calcium levels should be regularly monitored to ensure that they do not become excessive. Patients should be warned about the ingestion of very large amounts of calcium carbonate (readily available without prescription) if they are taking a thiazide. The manufacturer of **paricalcitol** suggests that a similar interaction is possible;[12] however, calcium levels should be routinely monitored in patients taking this drug, and so further precautions are unlikely to be necessary in patients also taking thiazides.

The case of hypercalcaemia with the use of a topical vitamin D analogue is rare and the strength of the preparation of tacalcitol used was fivefold higher than the current licensed preparation of 4 micrograms/g (*Curatoderm*). However, severe hypercalcaemia may develop when ointments containing **tacalcitol, calcipotriol** or **maxacalcitol** are abundantly applied to patients with psoriasis because the drugs can be easily absorbed through the skin lesions,[13] and it would seem reasonable to assume that this effect may be exacerbated by the concurrent use of a thiazide. It may therefore be worth bearing this interaction in mind if a topical vitamin D analogue and a thiazide are given.

1. Drinka PJ, Nolten WE. Hazards of treating osteoporosis and hypertension concurrently with calcium, vitamin D, and distal diuretics. *J Am Geriatr Soc* (1984) 32, 405–7.
2. Parfitt AM. Chlorothiazide-induced hypercalcemia in juvenile osteoporosis and hyperparathyroidism. *N Engl J Med* (1969) 281, 55–9.
3. Gora ML, Seth SK, Bay WH, Visconti JA. Milk-alkali syndrome associated with use of chlorothiazide and calcium carbonate. *Clin Pharm* (1989) 8, 227–9.
4. Hakim R, Tolis G, Goltzman D, Meltzer S, Friedman R. Severe hypercalcemia associated with hydrochlorothiazide and calcium carbonate therapy. *Can Med Assoc J* (1979) 121, 591–4.
5. Crowe M, Wollner L, Griffiths RA. Hypercalcaemia following vitamin D and thiazide therapy in the elderly. *Practitioner* (1984) 228, 312–13.
6. Parfitt AM. Thiazide-induced hypercalcemia in vitamin D-treated hypoparathyroidism. *Ann Intern Med* (1972) 77, 557–63.
7. Parfitt AM. The interactions of thiazide diuretics with parathyroid hormone and vitamin D. Studies in patients with hypoparathyroidism. *J Clin Invest* (1972) 51, 1879–88.
8. Santos F, Smith MJV, Chan JCM. Hypercalciuria associated with long-term administration of calcitriol (1,25-dihydroxyvitamin D_3). Action of hydrochlorothiazide. *Am J Dis Child* (1986) 140, 139–42.
9. Alon U, Costanzo LS, Chan JCM. Additive hypocalciuric effects of amiloride and hydrochlorothiazide in patients treated with calcitriol. *Miner Electrolyte Metab* (1984) 10, 379–86.
10. Kawaguchi M, Mitsuhashi Y, Kondo S. Iatrogenic hypercalcemia due to vitamin D_3 ointment (1,24(OH)$_2D_3$) combined with thiazide diuretics in a case of psoriasis. *J Dermatol* (2003) 30, 801–4.
11. Sato K, Hasegawa Y, Nakae J, Nanao K, Takahashi I, Tajima T, Shinohara N, Fujieda K. Hydrochlorothiazide effectively reduces urinary calcium excretion in two Japanese patients with gain-of-function mutations of the calcium-sensing receptor gene. *J Clin Endocrinol Metab* (2002) 87, 3068–73.
12. Zemplar Soft Capsules (Paricalcitol). Abbott Laboratories Ltd. UK Summary of product characteristics, January 2012.
13. Sato K. Drug-induced hypercalcemia. *Clin Calcium* (2006) 16, 67–72.

Thiazide diuretics + NSAIDs

There is evidence that most NSAIDs can increase blood pressure in patients taking antihypertensives, including diuretics, although some studies have not found the increase to be clinically relevant. The concurrent use of NSAIDs with thiazide diuretics may exacerbate congestive heart failure and increase the risk of hospitalisation. Diuretics may increase the risk of NSAID-induced acute renal failure.

Clinical evidence

Various large epidemiological studies and meta-analyses of clinical studies have been conducted to assess the effect of NSAIDs on blood pressure in patients taking **antihypertensives**, and the findings of these are summarised in 'Table 23.2', p.1031. In these studies, NSAIDs were not always associated with an increase in blood pressure, and the maximum increase was 6.2 mmHg. The effect has been shown for both coxibs and non-selective NSAIDs. In two meta-analyses,[1,2] the effects were evaluated by NSAID. The confidence intervals for all the NSAIDs overlapped, showing that there was no statistically significant difference between the NSAIDs, with the exception of the comparison between **indometacin** and **sulindac** in one analysis.[2] Nevertheless, an attempt was made at ranking the NSAIDs based on the means. In one analysis,[1] the effect was greatest for **piroxicam, indometacin,** and **ibuprofen**, intermediate for **naproxen**, and least for **sulindac** and **flurbiprofen**. In the other meta-analysis,[2] the effect was greatest for **indometacin** and **naproxen**, intermediate for **piroxicam**, and least for **ibuprofen** and **sulindac**. An attempt was also made to evaluate the effect by **antihypertensive** in one analysis.[1] The mean effect was greatest for beta blockers, intermediate for vasodilators (includes ACE inhibitors and calcium-channel blockers), and least for **diuretics**. However, the differences between the groups were not significant.

A retrospective analysis of records of patients taking **diuretics** (thiazides, loop and/or potassium-sparing) with NSAIDs found a twofold increase in the risk of hospitalisation for congestive heart failure on concurrent use. The most common NSAIDs taken by this cohort of patients were **diclofenac, ibuprofen, indometacin** and **naproxen**. The **diuretics** most often used were thiazides combined with potassium-sparing drugs and this therapy showed a significantly higher risk than the other diuretic therapies.[3]

A case-control study using the UK General Practice Research Database found that current NSAID use increased the risk of acute renal failure (relative risk 3.2 compared with no NSAID use) and this risk was further increased with concurrent **diuretic** use (relative risk 11.6).[4] Note that the risk of renal complications appear to be similar with coxibs and non-specific NSAIDs.[5]

Individual clinical reports and clinical or pharmacological studies of the effects of specific NSAIDs on diuretics are outlined in the subsections below and in 'Table 26.2', p.1121.

A. Altizide

An 80-year-old woman who had been successfully treated with altizide, **spironolactone**, bisoprolol and aspirin for 5 years experienced symptoms of progressive breathlessness, weight gain and nocturnal orthopnoea about 4 days after starting to take **rofecoxib** for arthritis. About 10 days later, she was admitted to hospital with heart failure and started to recover over the next 2 to 5 days following discontinuation of the **rofecoxib** and replacement of the beta blocker and diuretics with furosemide.[5]

B. Bemetizide

In a study in healthy subjects **indometacin** 100 mg was found to reduce the urinary excretion of sodium and chloride caused by bemetizide, by 47% and 44%, respectively.[6]

C. Bendroflumethiazide

(a) Ibuprofen

In a randomised, placebo-controlled study, 7 hypertensive patients taking bendroflumethiazide 5 to 10 mg daily were also given ibuprofen 400 mg four times daily for 2 weeks. Although some small increases in blood pressure occurred, the diastolic blood pressure of all patients remained below 90 mmHg throughout the ibuprofen phase. Overall no statistically significant weight gain was noted, although 2 patients gained more than 2 kg.[7]

(b) Indometacin

A controlled study in 5 hypertensive patients taking bendroflumethiazide 5 or 10 mg daily found that indometacin 100 mg daily for 3 weeks raised their blood pressure by 17/12 mmHg when lying or standing. Body-weight increased by 1.2 kg.[8] Indometacin also attenuated the hypotensive effect of bendroflumethiazide in another study.[9]

(c) Sulindac

A brief report suggested that sulindac *enhanced* the hypotensive effects of bendroflumethiazide in 5 hypertensive patients.[9]

D. Chlortalidone

A 61-year-old man with a history of mild diabetes and hypertension, who was taking chlortalidone 25 mg daily, developed diabetic nephropathy after starting **ibuprofen**.[10]

E. Hydrochlorothiazide

(a) Coxibs

A study in healthy subjects found that a single 25-mg oral dose of **rofecoxib** reduced the natriuretic effect of hydrochlorothiazide 25 mg, but potassium excretion was unaltered.[11]

(b) Diclofenac

Diclofenac 25 mg three times daily was given to 8 patients with essential hypertension who were taking hydrochlorothiazide. Blood pressure was not significantly altered after the addition of diclofenac, but a weight gain of about 1 to 2 kg was noted, which was thought to have been caused by the sodium retaining effects of diclofenac.[12] In another study in hypertensive black women, diclofenac 75 mg twice daily for one month did not alter the antihypertensive effect of the combination of hydrochlorothiazide 25 mg daily and lisinopril 10 to 40 mg daily.[13] A further study, in healthy subjects, found that diclofenac 50 mg reduced the natriuretic effect of hydrochlorothiazide, but potassium excretion was unchanged.[11]

(c) Diflunisal

Diflunisal 375 mg twice daily increased the plasma levels of hydrochlorothiazide by 25 to 30%, but this does not appear to be clinically relevant.[14] Diflunisal also has uricosuric activity, which may counteract the uric acid retention that occurs with hydrochlorothiazide.

(d) Ibuprofen

In two studies, ibuprofen 400 or 600 mg three times daily for 4 weeks caused a small rise in systolic but not in diastolic blood pressure in patients taking hydrochlorothiazide.[12,15] However, a weight gain of about 1 to 2 kg was noted in one of the studies.[12] Another study found that ibuprofen 400 mg three times daily had no effect on blood pressure controlled by **triamterene** with hydrochlorothiazide, although one patient had a marked reduction in renal function.[16] Ibuprofen 800 mg four times daily for a week had little effect on blood pressure controlled with hydrochlorothiazide in yet another study.[17] In two further studies, ibuprofen 800 mg three times daily for one month did not alter the antihypertensive effect of the combinations of hydrochlorothiazide 25 mg daily with fosinopril 10 to 40 mg daily[18] or lisinopril 10 to 40 mg daily.[13]

An 88-year-old patient taking multiple drugs developed severe hyponatraemia when hydrochlorothiazide was given with **furosemide** and ibuprofen. The authors comment that the use of thiazides is sometimes overlooked when other drugs that may affect serum sodium, such as NSAIDs, are prescribed.[19]

For a report of acute renal failure after strenuous exercise, in a patient taking ibuprofen and hydrochlorothiazide with triamterene, see 'Potassium-sparing diuretics + NSAIDs', p.1127.

(e) Indometacin

A controlled study including 2 patients with hypertension taking **amiloride** 5 mg with hydrochlorothiazide 50 mg or amiloride 10 mg with hydrochlorothiazide 100 mg, found that indometacin 100 mg daily for 3 weeks resulted in only slight changes in their blood pressure, except for the patient taking the higher dose of diuretic, whose standing blood pressure was increased by 23/3 mmHg. Body-weight increased by 0.6 and 0.8 kg, respectively.[8] A later study in 10 hypertensive patients taking hydrochlorothiazide 50 mg daily found a 6/3 mmHg blood pressure rise after they took indometacin 50 mg twice daily for 2 weeks, but this had gone after 4 weeks.[20] A blood pressure rise of only 5/1 mmHg was seen in another study in hypertensive patients taking hydrochlorothiazide 50 mg daily with indometacin 100 mg daily.[21] Indometacin also attenuated the hypotensive effect of hydrochlorothiazide (given with **amiloride**) in another study.[9]

In other studies indometacin had no effect on the sodium excretion caused by hydrochlorothiazide,[22] and did not affect the pharmacokinetics of hydrochlorothiazide.[22,23] However, in one of these studies indometacin did attenuate the hydrochlorothiazide-induced decreases in body-weight and plasma potassium levels.[23]

For a report of hyperkalaemia in a patient taking indometacin and hydrochlorothiazide with amiloride, and a report of acute renal failure in a patient taking indometacin and hydrochlorothiazide with triamterene, see 'Potassium-sparing diuretics + NSAIDs', p.1127.

(f) Kebuzone

A mean systolic blood pressure rise of 18 mmHg (from 171 mmHg to 189 mmHg) occurred in 15 patients taking hydrochlorothiazide 50 mg daily, when they were given kebuzone 750 mg daily. This rise represents about a 35% reduction in the antihypertensive effect of hydrochlorothiazide.[24]

(g) Naproxen

One study found that naproxen had no clinically relevant interaction with hydrochlorothiazide.[20] In another study, in healthy subjects, naproxen had a similar lack of influence on the diuretic response to hydrochlorothiazide.[25] In a further study, in hypertensive patients, naproxen attenuated the antihypertensive efficacy of hydrochlorothiazide taken with **amiloride** and timolol, but how much of the attenuation was due to an interaction with the diuretic was unclear.[26]

A case report describes severe hyponatraemia resulting from the use of hydrochlorothiazide with **amiloride** and naproxen.[27]

(h) Phenylbutazone

A mean systolic blood pressure rise of 18 mmHg (from 171 mmHg to 189 mmHg) occurred in 15 patients taking hydrochlorothiazide 50 mg daily, when they were given phenylbutazone 750 mg daily. This rise represents about a 35% reduction in the antihypertensive effect of hydrochlorothiazide.[24]

(i) Piroxicam

One study found that piroxicam attenuated the antihypertensive efficacy of hydrochlorothiazide taken with **amiloride** and timolol, but how much of the attenuation is due to an interaction with the diuretic is unclear.[26]

(j) Sulindac

One study in healthy subjects found that pretreatment with sulindac 200 mg decreased the fractional urinary flow rate, produced by hydrochlorothiazide 100 mg alone, by 35%; and attenuated the natriuretic effect of hydrochlorothiazide, over 0 to 4 hours, by 29%. However, beyond 4 hours, sulindac pretreatment did not affect these renal responses to hydrochlorothiazide.[25] Sulindac does not usually appear to reduce either the hypotensive or diuretic effects of hydrochlorothiazide,[12,20,21] and may even slightly *enhance* the antihypertensive effects of hydrochlorothiazide with **amiloride**, given with[26] or without,[9] timolol. Another study found that sulindac did not alter the antihypertensive efficacy of hydrochlorothiazide with **amiloride**, given with beta blockers.[28] Similarly, sulindac 200 mg twice daily for one month did not alter the antihypertensive effect of the combinations of hydrochlorothiazide 25 mg daily with fosinopril 10 to 40 mg daily,[18] or lisinopril 10 to 40 mg daily.[13]

An 81-year-old woman who was taking hydrochlorothiazide, digoxin, methyldopa and potassium was admitted to hospital with pseudogout and was prescribed sulindac 400 mg followed by 200 mg twice daily for 2 days. She received 800 mg of sulindac within the first 22 hours and developed renal impairment over the next 4 days. The sulindac was discontinued and her renal function improved.[10]

F. Methyclothiazide

A 68-year-old woman with long-standing hypertension and diabetes who was receiving methyclothiazide, insulin, quinidine and nitrates was admitted to hospital with pericarditis. Renal impairment developed within 4 days of starting **indometacin** 25 mg three times daily and improved on discontinuation of the indometacin.[10]

G. Metolazone

(a) Indometacin

Indometacin was found to reduce the urinary sodium excretion in response to metolazone by 34% in 6 healthy subjects.[29] The excretion of total potassium fell by 30%.

(b) Sulindac

Sulindac was found to reduce the urinary sodium excretion in response to metolazone by 19% in 6 healthy subjects.[29] The excretion of total potassium fell by 16%.

H. Trichlormethiazide

For a report of raised serum creatinine levels when a patient receiving triamterene and trichlormethiazide was given diclofenac, see 'Potassium-sparing diuretics + NSAIDs', p.1127.

I. Unspecified

In a randomised study, **ibuprofen** 400 mg every 8 hours caused a mean increase in blood pressure of about 5 to 7 mmHg in 12 hypertensive patients taking thiazides with beta blockers or centrally-acting antihypertensives.[30]

Mechanism

Not understood. NSAIDs, including coxibs, can affect renal function and cause salt and water retention, which antagonises the effects of diuretics.[31] Prostaglandins have a role to play in renal function and drugs such as the NSAIDs, which inhibit prostaglandin synthesis, would therefore be expected to have some effect on the actions of diuretics, whose venodilatory effects also depend on the activity of the prostaglandins.

The attenuation of the antihypertensive effect of thiazides by NSAIDs has not been uniformly observed; for example sulindac has been found to enhance the antihypertensive effect in some, but not all, studies, and ibuprofen and indometacin have been found to have variable effects.[32] It has been suggested that, in some cases, differences in the metabolism of NSAIDs may possibly affect renal prostaglandins, for example sulindac may have less effect because its active metabolite is highly protein bound and does not appear in the urine in appreciable amounts,[9,26] but currently there appears to be insufficient data to distinguish between the NSAIDs. NSAIDs suppress diuretic-stimulated renin secretion and dietary salt intake may also alter the effect by varying endogenous renin activity.[32] A study in *rats* suggested that indometacin may oppose the effects of the thiazides by reducing chloride delivery to the site of thiazide action in the distal tubule.[33]

Importance and management

Overall, the evidence suggests that some patients taking a thiazide can have a rise in blood pressure, and sometimes associated weight gain,[32] when given an NSAID, but this may not always be clinically relevant. Furthermore the concurrent use of an NSAID and a diuretic may increase the risk of acute renal failure. Some consider that the use of NSAIDs should be kept to a minimum in patients taking antihypertensives.[34] The effects may be greater in the elderly and in those with blood pressures that are relatively high, as well as in those with salt imbalance such as in cardiac failure or liver disease.[31,34] However, others consider that the clinical importance of an interaction between NSAIDs and antihypertensives is less than has previously been suggested.[35] While their findings do not rule out a 2/1 mmHg increase in blood pressure with NSAIDs in treated hypertensives, they suggest that if patients in primary care have inadequate control of blood pressure, other reasons (e.g. poor compliance or 'white-coat' hypertension) may be more likely than any effect of concurrent NSAIDs.[35] There is insufficient data at present to clearly differentiate between NSAIDs, although there is some evidence that the effects of indometacin are greatest and sulindac least.

Thiazide diuretics may be used in patients with heart failure and associated hypertension; or in conjunction with a loop diuretic. In these patients, where exacerbation of fluid retention in response to an NSAID might reduce the effectiveness of the diuretic and worsen the condition for which the diuretic is being given, the use of an alternative non-NSAID analgesic should always be considered. However, in cases where concurrent use cannot be avoided, monitor for adverse effects on renal function, electrolytes and disease control, and, if necessary, consider increasing the dose of the thiazide. The joint American College of Cardiology and American Heart Association heart failure guidelines (2009) advise that in patients with heart failure who become unresponsive to diuretics, such as in those taking an NSAID, clinicians should consider giving the diuretic intravenously, giving an additional diuretic (they give the example of adding metolazone to furosemide), or giving a drug to increase renal blood flow (such as an inotrope).[36]

For the effects of NSAIDs on other antihypertensive drug classes see 'ACE inhibitors + NSAIDs', p.38, 'Beta blockers + Aspirin or NSAIDs', p.1003, 'Calcium-channel blockers + Aspirin or NSAIDs', p.1030, and 'Loop diuretics + NSAIDs', p.1120.

1. Johnson AG, Nguyen TV, Day RO. Do nonsteroidal anti-inflammatory drugs affect blood pressure? A meta-analysis. *Ann Intern Med* (1994) 121, 289–300.

2. Pope JE, Anderson JJ, Felson DT. A meta-analysis of the effects of nonsteroidal anti-inflammatory drugs on blood pressure. *Arch Intern Med* (1993) 153, 477–84.
3. Heerdink ER, Leufkens HG, Herings RMC, Ottervanger JP, Stricker BHC, Bakker A. NSAIDs associated with increased risk of congestive heart failure in elderly patients taking diuretics. *Arch Intern Med* (1998) 158, 1108–12.
4. Huerta C, Castellsague J, Varas-Lorenzo C, García Rodríguez LA. Nonsteroidal anti-inflammatory drugs and risk of ARF in the general population. *Am J Kidney Dis* (2005) 45, 531–9.
5. Krzesinski J-M, Piront P. Décompensation cardiaque, fonction rénale et anti-inflammatoires non stéroïdiens. *Rev Med Liege* (2002) 57, 582–6.
6. Düsing R, Nicolas V, Glatte B, Glänzer K, Kipnowski J, Kramer HJ. Interaction of bemetizide and indomethacin in the kidney. *Br J Clin Pharmacol* (1983) 16, 377–84.
7. Davies JG, Rawlins DC, Busson M. Effect of ibuprofen on blood pressure control by propranolol and bendrofluazide. *J Int Med Res* (1988) 16, 173–81.
8. Watkins J, Abbott EC, Hensby CN, Webster J, Dollery CT. Attenuation of hypotensive effect of propranolol and thiazide diuretics by indomethacin. *BMJ* (1980) 281, 702–5.
9. Steiness E, Waldorff S. Different interactions of indomethacin and sulindac with thiazides in hypertension. *BMJ* (1982) 285, 1702–3.
10. Blackshear JL, Davidman M, Stillman MT. Identification of risk for renal insufficiency from nonsteroidal anti-inflammatory drugs. *Arch Intern Med* (1983) 143, 1130–4.
11. Knauf H, Bailey MA, Hasenfuss G, Mutschler E. The influence of cardiovascular and antiinflammatory drugs on thiazide-induced hemodynamic and saluretic effects. *Eur J Clin Pharmacol* (2006) 62, 885–92.
12. Koopmans PP, Thien Th, Gribnau FWJ. The influence of ibuprofen, diclofenac and sulindac on the blood pressure lowering effect of hydrochlorothiazide. *Eur J Clin Pharmacol* (1987) 31, 553–7.
13. Bhagat K. Effects of non-steroidal anti-inflammatory drugs on hypertension control using angiotensin converting enzyme inhibitors and thiazide diuretics. *East Afr Med J* (2001) 78, 507–9.
14. Tempero KF, Cirillo VJ, Steelman SL. Diflunisal: a review of the pharmacokinetic and pharmacodynamic properties, drug interactions and special tolerability studies in humans. *Br J Clin Pharmacol* (1977) 4, 31S–36S.
15. Gurwitz JH, Everitt DE, Monane M, Glynn RJ, Choodnovskiy I, Beaudet MP, Avorn J. The impact of ibuprofen on the efficacy of antihypertensive treatment with hydrochlorothiazide in elderly persons. *J Gerontol* (1996) 51A, M74–M79.
16. Gehr TWB, Sica DA, Steiger BW, Marshall C. Interaction of triamterene-hydrochlorothiazide and ibuprofen. *Clin Pharmacol Ther* (1990) 47, 200.
17. Wright JT, McKenney JM, Lehany AM, Bryan DL, Cooper LW, Lambert CM. The effect of high-dose short-term ibuprofen on antihypertensive control with hydrochlorothiazide. *Clin Pharmacol Ther* (1989) 46, 440–4.
18. Thakur V, Cook ME, Wallin JD. Antihypertensive effect of the combination of fosinopril and HCTZ is resistant to interference by nonsteroidal antiinflammatory drugs. *Am J Hypertens* (1999) 12, 925–8.
19. Kalksma R, Leemhuis MP. Hyponatriëmie bij gebruik van thiazidediuretica: let op combinaties van geneesmiddelen die dit effect versterken. *Ned Tijdschr Geneeskd* (2002) 146, 1521–5.
20. Koopmans PP, Thien Th, Gribnau FWJ. Influence of non-steroidal anti-inflammatory drugs on diuretic treatment of mild to moderate essential hypertension. *BMJ* (1984) 289, 1492–4.
21. Koopmans PP, Thien Th, Thomas CMG, van den Berg RJ, Gribnau FWJ. The effects of sulindac and indomethacin on the antihypertensive and diuretic action of hydrochlorothiazide in patients with mild to moderate essential hypertension. *Br J Clin Pharmacol* (1986) 21, 417–23.
22. Williams RL, Davies RO, Berman RS, Holmes GI, Huber P, Gee WL, Lin ET, Benet LZ. Hydrochlorothiazide pharmacokinetics and pharmacologic effect: the influence of indomethacin. *J Clin Pharmacol* (1982) 22, 32–41.
23. Koopmans PP, Kateman WGPM, Tan Y, van Ginneken CAM, Gribnau FWJ. Effects of indomethacin and sulindac on hydrochlorothiazide kinetics. *Clin Pharmacol Ther* (1985) 37, 625–8.
24. Polak F. Die hemmende Wirkung von Phenylbutazon auf die durch einige Antihypertonika hervorgerufene Blutdrucksenkung bei Hypertonikern. *Z Gesamte Inn Med* (1967) 22, 375–6.
25. Dixey JJ, Noormohamed FH, Lant AF, Brewerton DA. The effects of naproxen and sulindac on renal function and their interaction with hydrochlorothiazide and piretanide in man. *Br J Clin Pharmacol* (1987) 23, 55–63.
26. Wong DG, Spence JD, Lamki L, Freeman D, McDonald JWD. Effect of non-steroidal anti-inflammatory drugs on control of hypertension by beta-blockers and diuretics. *Lancet* (1986) 3, 997–1001.
27. Aaseth JO, Tangen MK, Beitnes JO. Hyponatremisk krise—alvorlig diuretikabivirkning hos eldre. *Tidsskr Nor Laegeforen* (2001) 121, 921–3.
28. Stokes GS, Brooks PM, Johnston HJ, Monaghan JC, Okoro EO, Kelly D. The effects of sulindac and diclofenac in essential hypertension controlled by treatment with a beta blocker and/or diuretic. *Clin Exp Hypertens A* (1991) 13, 1169–78.
29. Ripley EBD, Gehr TWB, Wallace H, Wade J, Kish C, Sica DA. The effect of nonsteroidal agents (NSAIDs) on the pharmacokinetics and pharmacodynamics of metolazone. *Int J Clin Pharmacol Ther* (1994) 32, 12–18.
30. Radack KL, Deck CC, Bloomfield SS. Ibuprofen interferes with the efficacy of antihypertensive drugs. A Randomized, double-blind, placebo-controlled trial of ibuprofen compared with acetaminophen. *Ann Intern Med* (1987) 107, 628–35.
31. Brater DC. Effects of nonsteroidal anti-inflammatory drugs on renal function: focus on cyclooxygenase-2-selective inhibition. *Am J Med* (1999) 107, 65S–70S. Discussion ibid., 70S–71S.
32. Sahloul MZ, al-Kiek R, Ivanovich P, Mujais SK. Nonsteroidal anti-inflammatory drugs and antihypertensives. Cooperative malfeasance. *Nephron* (1990) 56, 345–52.
33. Kirchner KA, Brandon S, Mueller RA, Smith MJ, Bower JD. Mechanism of attenuated hydrochlorothiazide response during indomethacin administration. *Kidney Int* (1987) 31, 1097–1103.
34. Johnson AG. NSAIDs and blood pressure. Clinical importance for older patients. *Drugs Aging* (1998) 12, 17–27.
35. Sheridan R, Montgomery AA, Fahey T. NSAID use and BP in treated hypertensives: a retrospective controlled observational study. *J Hum Hypertens* (2005) 19, 445–50.
36. Hunt SA, Abraham WT, Chin MH, Feldman AM, Francis GS, Ganiats TG, Jessup M, Konstam MA, Mancini DM, Michl K, Oates JA, Rahko PS, Silver MA, Stevenson LW, Yancy CW. 2009 focused update incorporated into the ACC/AHA 2005 guidelines for the diagnosis and management of heart failure in adults: a report of the American College of Cardiology Foundation/American Heart Association Task Force on Practice Guidelines developed in collaboration with the international society for heart and lung transplantation. *J Am Coll Cardiol* (2009) 53, e1–e90. Available at: http://content.onlinejacc.org/article.aspx?articleid=1139601 (accessed 22/10/15).

Thiazide diuretics; Chlorothiazide + Fluoxetine

In one study fluoxetine 30 mg daily for 8 days did not affect the pharmacokinetics of a single 500-mg dose of chlorothiazide.[1] No chlorothiazide dose adjustments would therefore seem necessary on concurrent use.

1. Lemberger L, Bergstrom RF, Wolen RL, Farid NA, Enas GG, Aronoff GR. Fluoxetine: clinical pharmacology and physiologic disposition. *J Clin Psychiatry* (1985) 46, 14–19.

Thiazide diuretics; Hydrochlorothiazide + Phenytoin

A study in 7 healthy subjects found that pretreatment with phenytoin 100 mg three times daily for 6 days did not influence the pharmacokinetics of a single 75-mg oral dose of hydrochlorothiazide.[1] No hydrochlorothiazide dose adjustment is therefore needed on concurrent use with phenytoin.

1. Keller E, Sulzer U, Brennes M, Schollmeyer P, Hoppe-Seyler G. Disposition of hydrochlorothiazide (Hct) during phenytoin (Ph) treatment. *Klin Wochenschr* (1981) 59, 1223–4.

Thiazide diuretics; Hydrochlorothiazide + Propantheline

Propantheline can slightly increase the absorption of hydrochlorothiazide.

Clinical evidence, mechanism, importance and management

In 6 healthy fasting subjects, the absorption of hydrochlorothiazide 75 mg was delayed and increased (AUC increased by 23% and urinary recovery increased by 36%) by propantheline 60 mg. It was suggested that this occurs because propantheline slows the delivery of hydrochlorothiazide to its areas of absorption.[1] This slight increase is unlikely to be clinically important.

1. Beermann B, Groschinsky-Grind M. Enhancement of the gastrointestinal absorption of hydrochlorothiazide by propantheline. *Eur J Clin Pharmacol* (1978) 13, 385–7.

27

Gastrointestinal drugs

The various gastrointestinal drug groups covered in this section are listed in 'Table 27.1', below. Some of the interactions of these drugs occur by causing alterations in the absorption of other drugs, and these are covered under the affected drug. The section 'Drug absorption interactions', p.3, discusses how these interactions occur and contains more detailed information on some of the mechanisms.

Interactions of H_2-receptor antagonists

Cimetidine is a non-specific weak inhibitor of a number of the cytochrome P450 isoenzymes, including CYP1A2, CYP2C19, CYP2D6 and CYP3A4, and therefore inhibits the metabolism of many drugs, increasing their plasma levels and/or bioavailability. These interactions are most likely to be clinically significant for drugs with a narrow therapeutic index. Famotidine, nizatidine and ranitidine do not inhibit cytochrome P450 to a clinically relevant extent and are therefore less likely than cimetidine to be involved in interactions that occur by this mechanism. However, it should be noted that the absorption of some drugs may be affected by the changes in gastric pH, which can be produced by any of the H_2-receptor antagonists. Furthermore, drug interactions may also occur because of inhibition of renal tubular secretion: cimetidine, famotidine and ranitidine have all been implicated in this type of interaction, which occurs via renal organic cation transporters.

Interactions of 5-HT_3 receptor antagonists

Many 5-HT_3 receptor antagonists (dolasetron, ondansetron, palonosetron and tropisetron) are metabolised in part by CYP2D6.[1] This isoenzyme is subject to genetic polymorphism (see 'Genetic factors in drug metabolism', p.8, for a further explanation of polymorphism). Granisetron is not metabolised by CYP2D6, and is principally metabolised by CYP3A; and alosetron is primarily metabolised by CYP1A2. The available 5-HT_3 receptor antagonists appear to have little effect on the metabolism of other drugs by cytochrome P450.

Interactions of neurokinin receptor antagonists

Aprepitant and its prodrug fosaprepitant are currently the only available drugs in this class. Aprepitant is metabolised by CYP3A4, and may interact with drugs that inhibit or induce this isoenzyme. Aprepitant is unusual in that in the short term it acts as a dose-dependent, weak to moderate inhibitor of CYP3A4, but this is followed by a period of induction of CYP3A4, CYP2C9 and glucuronidation after treatment is stopped. It can therefore both increase and/or decrease the levels of drugs that are metabolised by these isoenzymes, such as midazolam (see 'Benzodiazepines + Aprepitant', p.813), warfarin (see 'Coumarins + Aprepitant', p.404), and the combined hormonal contraceptives (see 'Combined hormonal contraceptives + Aprepitant', p.1167).

Interactions of proton pump inhibitors

The cytochrome P450 isoenzyme CYP2C19 is the main route of metabolism of esomeprazole, lansoprazole, omeprazole, pantoprazole, and is also involved in the metabolism of rabeprazole. This isoenzyme is subject to genetic polymorphism[1] (see 'Genetic factors in drug metabolism', p.4, for a further explanation of polymorphism). The poor metaboliser phenotype for CYP2C19 (that is, those lacking or deficient in this isoenzyme) is found in approximately 1 to 6% of Caucasians, 1 to 7.5% of Blacks and 12 to 23% of Oriental and Indian Asians.[2] Most patients are extensive CYP2C19 metabolisers (that is, they have normal levels of this isoenzyme), and their major route for the metabolism of these proton pump inhibitors will be through this isoenzyme. As a consequence,[2] the levels of the proton pump inhibitors in these patients are likely to be affected by drugs that inhibit or induce CYP2C19, such as fluvoxamine (see 'Proton pump inhibitors + SSRIs', p.1154). Patients of the extensive metaboliser phenotype have also been shown in some studies to have a poorer clinical outcome, when compared with poor metabolisers e.g. in the eradication of *H. pylori*, as they tend to have lower therapeutic levels of proton pump inhibitors.[2-4]

Poor metabolisers, who lack CYP2C19 metabolising capacity, use alternative pathways to metabolise proton pump inhibitors, and this is mainly CYP3A4. Because poor metabolisers are more dependent on CYP3A4 for

Table 27.1 Gastrointestinal drugs

Group	*Drugs*
5-Aminosalicylates	Balsalazide, Mesalazine, Olsalazine, Sulfasalazine
Antacids	Aluminium hydroxide, Aluminium-magnesium complexes, Bismuth salicylate, Bismuth subnitrate, Magnesium carbonate, Magnesium hydroxide, Magesium trisilicate
Antidiarrhoeals	Crofelemer, Loperamide
Antiemetics	
Antihistamines, p.628	Cinnarizine, Cyclizine, Promethazine
Cannabinoids	Dronabinol, Nabilone
Dopamine antagonists	Domperidone, Metoclopramide
5-HT_3-receptor antagonists	Alosetron, Dolasetron, Granisetron, Ondansetron, Palonosetron, Tropisetron
Neurokinin-1 receptor antagonists	Aprepitant, Fosaprepitant
Phenothiazines	Prochlorperazine
Antisecretory drugs	
H_2-receptor antagonists	Cimetidine, Famotidine, Nizatidine, Ranitidine, Roxatidine
Prostaglandin analogues	Misoprostol
Proton pump inhibitors	Esomeprazole, Dexlansoprazole, Lansoprazole, Omeprazole, Pantoprazole, Rabeprazole
Antispasmodics	
Antimuscarinics	Dicycloverine, Hyoscine, Propantheline
Other antispasmodics	Alverine, Mebeverine
Laxatives	
Bulk-forming	Ispaghula, Methycellulose, Sterculia
Osmotic	Lactulose, Macrogols, Magnesium hydroxide, Phosphates, Sodium citrate
Peripheral opioid antagonists	Alvimopan, Methylnaltrexone
Stimulants	Bisacodyl, Dantron, Docusate sodium, Glycerol, Senna, Sodium picosulfate
Mucosal protectants	
Bismuth compounds	Bismuth subcitrate potassium, Tripotassium dicitratobismuthate
Other mucosal protectants	Carbenoxolone, Liquorice, Sucralfate
Prokinetic drugs (motility stimulants)	
Chloride-channel activator	Lubiprostone
Dopamine antagonists	Domperidone, Metoclopramide
Guanylate cyclase-C agonist	Linaclotide
5-HT_4-receptor agonists	Cisapride, Mosapride, Prucalopride

metabolism of the proton pump inhibitors the levels of proton pump inhibitors may be more significantly raised in these patients, when compared with extensive metabolisers, when they are given CYP3A4 inhibitors, such as ketoconazole, see 'Azoles + Proton pump inhibitors', p.238.

Omeprazole and esomeprazole are potent inhibitors of CYP2C19, and therefore they may increase the levels of drugs that are metabolised by this isoenzyme, such as diazepam.[1,2] Omeprazole is a very weak inducer of CYP1A2, but this is probably not clinically relevant.

In vitro study suggests that some proton pump inhibitors, including omeprazole, lansoprazole and pantoprazole, may possibly be P-glycoprotein substrates and inhibitors, and this may be a factor in some of their interactions.[5] A possible example of this is the increase in levels of these proton pump inhibitors caused by the P-glycoprotein inhibitor clarithromycin, see 'Proton pump inhibitors + Macrolides', p.1153.

1. Robinson M, Horn J. Clinical pharmacology of proton pump inhibitors. What the practising physician needs to know. *Drugs* (2003) 63, 2739–54.
2. Desta Z, Zhao X, Shin JG, Flockhart DA. Clinical significance of the cytochrome P450 2C19 genetic polymorphism. *Clin Pharmacokinet* (2002) 41, 913–58.
3. Furuta T, Shirai N, Sugimoto M, Nakamura A, Hishida A, Ishizaki T. Influence of CYP2C19 pharmacogenetic polymorphism on proton pump inhibitor-based therapies. *Drug Metab Pharmacokinet* (2005) 20, 153–67.
4. Klotz U. Pharmacokinetic considerations in the eradication of *Helicobacter pylori*. *Clin Pharmacokinet* (2000) 38, 243–70.
5. Pauli-Magnus C, Rekersbrink S, Klotz U, Fromm MF. Interaction of omeprazole, lansoprazole and pantoprazole with P-glycoprotein. *Naunyn Schmiedebergs Arch Pharmacol* (2001) 364, 551–7.

Aluminium hydroxide + Ascorbic acid (Vitamin C) or Citrates

Patients with renal failure given aluminium compounds and oral citrates can develop a potentially fatal encephalopathy due to a very marked rise in blood-aluminium levels. There is also some evidence that aluminium compounds and ascorbic acid (vitamin C) may interact similarly.

Clinical evidence

(a) Ascorbic acid

A study in 13 healthy subjects given aluminium hydroxide 900 mg three times daily found that ascorbic acid 2 g daily increased the urinary excretion of aluminium threefold.[1]

(b) Citrates

Four patients with advanced chronic renal impairment taking aluminium hydroxide and citrate (Shohl's) solution died due to hyperaluminaemia.[2] When these cases were compared with another 34 renal patients, it was found that the fatalities had occurred in patients who had taken more aluminium hydroxide, more citrate, and who were older. When both groups were considered together, increased serum aluminium levels were found to be correlated with increased citrate intake.[3]

In a study in 5 healthy subjects given aluminium hydroxide with or without citrate solution, aluminium levels were found to be 11 micrograms/L at baseline, 44 micrograms/L when aluminium hydroxide was given, and 98 micrograms/L when citrate was given with the aluminium hydroxide. Aluminium clearance also dramatically increased in the presence of citrate.[3] Another report describes this interaction in 2 patients with renal impairment, and in a possible further 6 patients with renal failure, all of whom died.[4] In a further single-dose study in 6 patients with end-stage renal disease, sodium citrate with citric acid 30 mL markedly increased the AUC of aluminium (from a 30-mL dose of aluminium hydroxide gel) 4.6-fold.[5] A haemodialysis patient given effervescent co-codamol had a tenfold increase in serum aluminium levels. This was attributed to sodium citrate in the formulation, which is used to produce the effervescence.[6]

A number of other studies, mainly in healthy subjects, have confirmed that citrate markedly increases aluminium absorption, see *Mechanism*, below.

Mechanism

Studies in healthy subjects clearly demonstrate that citrate markedly increases the absorption of aluminium from the gut,[3,7,8] and one study in 20 adults with end-stage renal failure receiving chronic haemodialysis found that the administration of calcium citrate gave rise to enhanced aluminium absorption.[9] The absorption of aluminium is increased threefold if it is taken with **lemon juice**,[10] eight- to tenfold if it is taken with **orange juice**,[11,12] and five- to 50-fold if it is taken with citrate,[3,7,8,11] but the reason for this is not understood. It could be that a highly soluble aluminium citrate complex is formed.[4,7]

Importance and management

The interaction between aluminium compounds and citrates in patients with renal impairment is established and clinically important as it is potentially fatal. Concurrent use should be strictly avoided. Remember that some effervescent and dispersible tablets (including many proprietary non-prescription analgesics, indigestion and hang-over remedies such as *Alka-Seltzer*) contain citric acid or citrates,[6,13] and they may also occur in soft drinks.[13] Haemodialysis patients should be strongly warned about these products as aluminium is not dialysed and will accumulate in this patient group.

The interaction between aluminium compounds and ascorbic acid is not yet well established, but the information available so far suggests that this combination should also be avoided by patients with renal impairment. It is not clear whether orange juice is also unsafe but the available evidence suggests that concurrent administration is probably best avoided.

The importance of the interaction between aluminium and citrates in subjects with normal renal function is by no means clear because it is still not known whether increased aluminium absorption results in aluminium accumulation over the long-term in those with normal renal function.[12] Some authors have recommended that food or drinks containing citric acid (citrus fruits and fruit juices) should not be taken at the same time as aluminium-containing medicines, and that their ingestion should be separated by 2 to 3 hours.[12] However, one study in healthy subjects reported significantly raised aluminium levels when a citric acid solution and an aluminium hydroxide antacid were taken 2 hours apart.[14]

1. Domingo JL, Gomez M, Llobet JM, Richart C. Effect of ascorbic acid on gastrointestinal aluminium absorption. *Lancet* (1991) 338, 1467.
2. Bakir AA, Hryhorczuk DO, Berman E, Dunea G. Acute fatal hyperaluminemic encephalopathy in undialyzed and recently dialyzed uremic patients. *Trans Am Soc Artif Intern Organs* (1986) 32, 171–6.
3. Bakir AA, Hryhorczuk DO, Ahmed S, Hessl SM, Levy PS, Spengler R, Dunea G. Hyperaluminemia in renal failure: the influence of age and citrate intake. *Clin Nephrol* (1989) 31, 40–4.
4. Kirschbaum HB, Schoolwerth AC. Acute aluminum toxicity associated with oral citrate and aluminum-containing antacids. *Am J Med Sci* (1989) 297, 9–11.
5. Rudy D, Sica DA, Comstock T, Davis J, Savory J, Schoolwerth AC. Aluminum-citrate interaction in end-stage renal disease. *Int J Artif Organs* (1991) 14, 625–9.
6. Main J, Ward MK. Potentiation of aluminium absorption by effervescent analgesic tablets in a haemodialysis patient. *BMJ* (1992) 304, 1686.
7. Coburn JW, Mischel MG, Goodman WG, Salusky IB. Calcium citrate markedly enhances aluminum absorption from aluminium hydroxide. *Am J Kidney Dis* (1991) 17, 708–11.
8. Walker JA, Sherman RA, Cody RP. The effect of oral bases on enteral aluminum absorption. *Arch Intern Med* (1990) 150, 2037–9.
9. Lindberg JS, Copley JB, Koenig KG, Cushner HM. Effect of citrate on serum aluminum concentrations in hemodialysis patients: a prospective study. *South Med J* (1993) 86, 1385–8.
10. Slanina P, Frech W, Ekström L-G, Lööf L, Slorach S, Cedergren A. Dietary citric acid enhances absorption of aluminum in antacids. *Clin Chem* (1986) 32, 539–41.
11. Weberg R, Berstad A. Gastrointestinal absorption of aluminium from single doses of aluminium containing antacids in man. *Eur J Clin Invest* (1986) 16, 428–32.
12. Fairweather-Tait S, Hickson K, McGaw B, Reid M. Orange juice enhances aluminium absorption from antacid preparation. *Eur J Clin Nutr* (1994) 48, 71–3.
13. Dorhout Mees EJ, Başçi A. Citric acid in calcium effervescent tablets may favour aluminium intoxication. *Nephron* (1991) 59, 322.
14. Mauro LS, Kuhl DA, Kirchhoff JR, Mauro VF, Hamilton RW. Impact of oral bases on aluminium absorption. *Am J Ther* (2001) 8, 21–5.

Alvimopan + Miscellaneous

The gastrointestinal adverse effects of alvimopan are expected to be greater in those who have recently taken opioids. Alvimopan does not appear to alter the pharmacokinetics of intravenous morphine. Antibacterials that affect gut flora and drugs that inhibit gastric acid secretion appear to reduce the formation of the metabolite of alvimopan. Theoretically, potent P-glycoprotein inhibitors may interact with alvimopan.

Clinical evidence, mechanism, importance and management

(a) Antibacterials

In a drug interaction study, 42 healthy subjects were given alvimopan 6 mg twice daily for 30 days, with **ciprofloxacin** 500 mg twice daily on days 11 to 20. **Ciprofloxacin** almost totally abolished the plasma levels of the metabolite of alvimopan, and this effect partially persisted in some subjects 10 days after **ciprofloxacin** was stopped. The AUC of alvimopan was unchanged by **ciprofloxacin**.[1]

In a population pharmacokinetic analysis, the pharmacokinetics of alvimopan were not affected by the preoperative use of oral antibacterials (not specified), but the plasma concentration of its metabolite was reduced by 81%.[2]

Alvimopan is metabolised by intestinal flora to a metabolite that is slightly less active than the parent molecule. Any antibacterial that reduces intestinal flora may therefore reduce the formation of this metabolite. However, the manufacturer notes that as this metabolite is not required for efficacy, no alvimopan dose adjustment is needed if antibacterials are also given.[2]

(b) Cytochrome P450 isoenzyme inhibitors, inducers and substrates

Alvimopan is not a substrate of the cytochrome P450 isoenzyme system, and therefore drugs that are inhibitors or inducers of these isoenzymes are not expected to alter the pharmacokinetics of alvimopan by this mechanism.[2]

Alvimopan is not an inhibitor or inducer of any of the key cytochrome P450 isoenzymes, and would therefore not be expected to alter the pharmacokinetics of drugs that are substrates of these isoenzymes by this mechanism.[2]

(c) Drugs that inhibit gastric acid secretion

The manufacturer of alvimopan notes that, in a population pharmacokinetic analysis, the pharmacokinetics of alvimopan were not affected by 'acid blockers' (not specified), but the pharmacokinetics of its metabolite were reduced by 49%.[2] However, the manufacturer notes that as the metabolite is not required for efficacy, no alvimopan dose adjustment is needed if these drugs are also given.[2]

(d) Opioids

The manufacturer of alvimopan briefly states that alvimopan had no clinically relevant effect on the pharmacokinetics of intravenous **morphine** or its 6-glucuronide metabolite. Therefore, no dose adjustment of intravenous **morphine** is likely to be needed on concurrent use.[2] However, as alvimopan is a peripheral μ-opioid receptor antagonist, it may antagonise the peripheral effects of opioids, such as **morphine**, on gastrointestinal motility without reversing their central analgesic effects.[2] Patients who have been taking opioids in the week before starting alvimopan are expected to be more sensitive to alvimopan, and may experience more gastrointestinal adverse effects (abdominal pain, nausea and vomiting, diarrhoea).[2] Alvimopan should therefore be used with caution in these patients.[2]

(e) P-glycoprotein inhibitors and substrates

Alvimopan and its metabolite are both substrates for P-glycoprotein *in vitro*.[2] However, the manufacturer briefly states that, in a population pharmacokinetic analysis, there was no evidence that the pharmacokinetics of alvimopan and its metabolite were altered by mild to moderate P-glycoprotein inhibitors (not specified).[2] Nevertheless, they state that no clinical studies have been conducted on the effect of potent P-glycoprotein inhibitors on alvimopan[2] and until more is known, some caution might be prudent with these drugs (they name **amiodarone**, **ciclosporin (cyclosporine)**, **diltiazem**, **itraconazole**, **quinidine**, **quinine**, **spironolactone**, and **verapamil**).

Alvimopan does not inhibit P-glycoprotein, and would therefore not be expected to alter the pharmacokinetics of drugs that are P-glycoprotein substrates.[2]

1. Schmith VD, Johnson BM, Vasist LS, Kelleher DL, Hewens DA, Young MA, Ameen V, Dukes GE. The effects of short courses of antibiotics on alvimopan metabolite pharmacokinetics. *J Clin Pharmacol* (2010) 50, 338–349.
2. Entereg (Alvimopan). GlaxoSmithKline. US Prescribing information, November 2009.

Antacids + Calcium compounds

Hypercalcaemia, alkalosis and renal impairment (milk-alkali syndrome) can develop in patients taking antacids with calcium-containing sub-

stances, including dairy products. Note that excess calcium carbonate alone can cause this syndrome.

Clinical evidence

Milk-alkali syndrome was a common cause of hypercalcaemia when milk plus antacids was the standard therapy for peptic ulcer disease, and reports for this are not cited here. Nevertheless, occasionally, cases of milk-alkali syndrome are still reported in patients taking antacids and milk to excess. For example, a man presented with nausea, vomiting, constipation, polyuria and polydipsia, which was diagnosed as milk-alkali syndrome, due to daily treatment with 6 tablets of *Caved-S* and about 2 litres (3.5 pints) of milk, for dyspepsia related to a peptic ulcer.[1] This dose of *Caved-S* meant he was taking 600 mg of **aluminium hydroxide**, 1.2 g of **magnesium carbonate**, 600 mg of **sodium bicarbonate** and 2.28 g of **deglycyrrhizinised liquorice** daily.[1]

The most common cause of milk-alkali syndrome is now the use of calcium carbonate alone for osteoporosis or as an antacid. Note that calcium carbonate is both a source of calcium and of alkali. These cases tend to occur when the doses used are excessive, or when there are other risk factors for hypercalcaemia such as renal impairment. The many reports for this are not cited here as they are not an interaction. Two cases are cited in patients taking large amounts of *Rennies* antacid (**calcium/magnesium carbonate**) for which milk consumption may have contributed.[2,3]

Mechanism

High intake and absorption of calcium can suppress the parathyroid hormone, which leads to bicarbonate retention by the kidneys, leading to metabolic and respiratory alkalosis. The alkalosis also causes reduced excretion of calcium by the kidneys. Hypermagnesaemia may also have a part to play.

Importance and management

While taking antacids, even well within the recommended dose range, as in the first case, it is still possible to develop a serious and potentially life-threatening reaction (known as milk-alkali syndrome) if the intake of calcium is high. The milk-alkali syndrome was a common adverse effect of antacid use when the concurrent use of milk and antacids was the primary treatment of peptic ulcer disease, and chronic milk-alkali syndrome can lead to the formation of calcification and kidney damage, which may be irreversible. The quantity of calcium ingested does not appear to be directly correlated to either the development or severity of milk-alkali syndrome, which has been reported with an intake of between 4 g to 60 g of calcium carbonate.[3] However, milk-alkali syndrome as a result of an interaction has become very uncommon with the advent of H_2-receptor antagonists and proton pump inhibitors and now the principal cause of the 'milk-alkali' syndrome would appear to be the use of calcium carbonate alone (for osteoporosis or as an antacid), as this is both a source of calcium and a source of alkali. Although the risk of this might also be higher in patients also taking calcium from milk, the milk is not necessary for the syndrome, so many of the cases are probably not actually interactions at all. Nevertheless, consider the possibility of an interaction in patients who take medications containing calcium, such as antacids or supplements for the prophylaxis of osteoporosis, and also consume large quantities of dairy products in their diet. Note that many calcium-containing antacids are freely available without prescription.

1. Gibbs CJ, Lee HA. Milk-alkali syndrome due to Caved-S. *J R Soc Med* (1992) 85, 498–9.
2. Verburg FA, van Zanten RAA, Brouwer RML, Woittiez AJJ, Veneman TF. Een man met een ernstig klassiek melk-alkalisyndroom en een maagcarcinoom. *Ned Tijdschr Geneeskd* (2006) 150, 1624–7.
3. Gordon MV, Hamblin PS, McMahon LP. Life-threatening milk-alkali syndrome resulting from antacid ingestion during pregnancy. *Med J Aust* (2005) 182, 350–351

Aprepitant + CYP3A4 substrates

Aprepitant (and therefore probably fosaprepitant) can increase the exposure to CYP3A4 substrates in the short-term, then reduce their exposure within 2 weeks. Any effect is likely to be important with drugs that have a narrow therapeutic range (e.g. ciclosporin) and be most important with drugs associated with significant toxicity with increased concentrations (e.g. pimozide).

Clinical evidence, mechanism, importance and management

In the first few days of use, aprepitant (125 mg on day one followed by 80 mg daily for 4 days) moderately increases the exposure to oral midazolam, a probe substrate for CYP3A4. The effect of aprepitant appears to diminish over 2 weeks, see 'Benzodiazepines + Aprepitant', p.813, for the full details. This effect was not seen with an aprepitant dose regimen of 40 mg on day one followed by 25 mg daily for 4 days. Aprepitant is therefore both a dose-dependent inhibitor and an inducer of CYP3A4.

Because of this, aprepitant is expected to increase the exposure to other CYP3A4 substrates up to about 3-fold, and the UK and US manufacturers recommend caution if aprepitant is given with CYP3A4 substrates.[1,2] The UK manufacturer of aprepitant specifically recommends caution with CYP3A4 substrates that have a narrow therapeutic range including some immunosuppressants (**ciclosporin, everolimus**), **ergot derivatives, alfentanil, fentanyl,** and **quinidine**.[1] For details of recommended everolimus dose reductions on the concurrent use of CYP3A4 inhibitors such as aprepitant, see 'Everolimus + Ketoconazole and other CYP3A4 inhibitors or P-glycoprotein inhibitors', p.1262. Note that the manufacturers specifically contraindicate the concurrent use of aprepitant with some CYP3A4 substrates, including **pimozide**,[1,2] because of the risk of life-threatening torsade de pointes with increased concentrations of these drugs. As **fosaprepitant** is rapidly converted to aprepitant, it would be expected to interact in the same way as aprepitant.

For a list of CYP3A4 substrates, see 'Table 1.10', p.12. Within 2 weeks of aprepitant use, the exposure to CYP3A4 substrates might be reduced, and caution is also advised during this time.

For recommendations regarding antineoplastics that are CYP3A4 substrates, see 'Antineoplastics + Aprepitant', p.656.

1. EMEND (Aprepitant). Merck Sharp & Dohme Ltd. UK Summary of product characteristics, December 2013.
2. EMEND Capsules (Aprepitant). Merck & Co., Inc. US Prescribing information, August 2014.

Aprepitant + Ketoconazole and other CYP3A4 inhibitors

Ketoconazole (a potent CYP3A4 inhibitor) markedly increases aprepitant concentrations, and would also be expected to increase the concentrations of aprepitant derived from fosaprepitant. Other potent inhibitors of CYP3A4 are predicted to interact in a similar way to ketoconazole.

Clinical evidence, mechanism, importance and management

The manufacturers note that when a single 125-mg dose of aprepitant was given on day 5 of a 10-day course of ketoconazole 400 mg daily, the AUC of aprepitant was increased by about 5-fold, and the half-life by about 3-fold.[1,2]

Ketoconazole is an inhibitor of the cytochrome P450 isoenzyme CYP3A4, by which aprepitant is metabolised, and concurrent use therefore raises aprepitant concentrations. Although the clinical outcome of these increases has not been assessed, such marked increases in concentrations could increase the risk of aprepitant adverse effects. The manufacturers recommend caution when aprepitant is given with ketoconazole or other drugs that are potent inhibitors of CYP3A4 (see 'Table 1.9', p.11 for a list). They additionally name the **nefazodone** and **posaconazole**, but these are generally considered to be moderate inhibitors of CYP3A4.[1,2] Until more is known it would seem prudent to consider using the lowest dose of aprepitant possible, and monitor for an increase in aprepitant adverse effects (such as hiccups, fatigue, constipation, headache) on the concurrent use of these drugs.

Fosaprepitant is rapidly metabolised to aprepitant and would therefore be expected to be similarly affected by the concurrent use of potent CYP3A4 inhibitors.

For the effect of **diltiazem** (a moderate CYP3A4 inhibitor), see 'Calcium-channel blockers + Aprepitant', p.1030. Other inhibitors of CYP3A4 are listed in 'Table 1.9', p.11.

1. EMEND (Aprepitant). Merck Sharp & Dohme Ltd. UK Summary of product characteristics, December 2013.
2. EMEND Capsules (Aprepitant). Merck & Co., Inc. US Prescribing information, August 2014.

Aprepitant + Phenytoin and other CYP2C9 substrates

Aprepitant is predicted to decrease the levels of phenytoin, a CYP2C9 substrate and phenytoin is predicted to decrease aprepitant levels and efficacy. Aprepitant is also predicted to reduce the levels of other CYP2C9 substrates.

Both aprepitant and phenytoin are available as prodrugs: fosaprepitant would be expected to interact in the same way as aprepitant and fosphenytoin would be expected to interact in the same way as phenytoin.

Clinical evidence, mechanism, importance and management

Aprepitant is an inducer of the cytochrome P450 isoenzyme CYP2C9, and slightly reduces the plasma levels of substrates of this isoenzyme such as warfarin (see 'Coumarins + Aprepitant', p.404) and tolbutamide (see 'Sulfonylureas + Aprepitant', p.542). The manufacturers therefore recommend caution when aprepitant is given with other drugs that are known to be metabolised by CYP2C9, because of the possibility that their plasma levels may be reduced. They specifically name phenytoin.[1,2] However, phenytoin is also an inducer of CYP3A4 and the manufacturers[1,2] predict that it will decrease the levels of aprepitant, and might reduce its efficacy, see 'Aprepitant + Rifampicin (Rifampin) and other CYP3A4 inducers', p.1138. Consequently, the UK manufacturers advise avoiding the concurrent use of aprepitant and phenytoin.[1]

The manufacturers of aprepitant[1,2] recommend caution when aprepitant is given with other drugs that are known to be metabolised by CYP2C9, because of the possibility that their levels may be reduced. See 'Table 1.5', p.7, for a list of CYP2C9 substrates.

Fosaprepitant, the prodrug of aprepitant, is expected to interact in the same way as aprepitant, and as **fosphenytoin** is a prodrug of phenytoin, it would be expected to interact in the same way as phenytoin.

1. EMEND (Aprepitant). Merck Sharp & Dohme Ltd. UK Summary of product characteristics, December 2013.
2. EMEND Capsules (Aprepitant). Merck & Co., Inc. US Prescribing information, August 2014.

Aprepitant + Rifampicin (Rifampin) and other CYP3A4 inducers

Rifampicin (an inducer of CYP3A4) markedly reduces the AUC of aprepitant, and other potent inducers of CYP3A4 may also interact

with aprepitant in this way. Fosaprepitant would be expected to be affected in the same way as aprepitant.

Clinical evidence, mechanism, importance and management

The manufacturers of aprepitant note that when a single 375-mg dose of aprepitant was given on day 9 of a 14-day course of rifampicin 600 mg daily, the AUC of aprepitant was decreased by 91% and the half-life was decreased by 68%.[1,2]

Rifampicin is an inducer of the cytochrome P450 isoenzyme CYP3A4, by which aprepitant is metabolised. Concurrent use therefore decreases aprepitant levels. Fosaprepitant is rapidly metabolised to aprepitant and would therefore be expected to be similarly affected. Although not assessed, this marked reduction in aprepitant levels is likely to result in reduced efficacy.

In the UK, the manufacturer states that the concurrent use of aprepitant or fosaprepitant with potent inducers of CYP3A4, such as rifampicin, should be avoided.[1,3] For a list of potent CYP3A4 inducers see 'Table 1.9', p.11. See also 'Aprepitant + Phenytoin and other CYP2C9 substrates', p.1138. They also state that concurrent use of **St John's wort** (a moderate CYP3A4 inducer) is not recommended.[1,3]

1. EMEND (Aprepitant). Merck Sharp & Dohme Ltd. UK Summary of product characteristics, December 2013.
2. EMEND Capsules (Aprepitant). Merck & Co., Inc. US Prescribing information, August 2014.
3. IVEMEND (Fosaprepitant dimeglumine). Merck Sharp & Dohme Ltd. UK Summary of product characteristics, December 2011.

Aprepitant + Tyrosine kinase inhibitors

An isolated case report describes increased erlotinib concentrations after aprepitant was given. Other tyrosine kinase inhibitors metabolised by CYP3A4 are predicted to be affected in the same way and fosaprepitant, a prodrug of aprepitant, would be expected to similarly increase the concentrations of these tyrosine kinase inhibitors.

Clinical evidence

A 54-year-old patient with lung cancer who developed **erlotinib**-induced pruritus, was given aprepitant 80 mg daily as an unlicensed treatment for the pruritus. At days 0, 7, and 14, the **erlotinib** minimum concentrations were 1210 nanograms/mL, 2455 nanograms/mL, and 2440 nanograms/mL, respectively, but no toxic effects were reported. The pruritus improved over 8 days and the patient was continued on the combination.[1]

Mechanism

In the short-term, aprepitant is an inhibitor of CYP3A4, by which erlotinib is metabolised. It might therefore increase their concentrations and hence their toxicity. There is some evidence (with midazolam) that aprepitant has a greater effect on CYP3A4 substrates when they are given orally rather than intravenously (see 'Benzodiazepines + Aprepitant', p.813).

Importance and management

Evidence for an interaction between erlotinib and aprepitant is very limited, and although not established the proposed mechanism is consistent with the known metabolism of erlotinib and the potential effects of aprepitant on CYP3A4. Bear this interaction in mind if aprepitant is to be given with erlotinib. Other tyrosine kinase inhibitors that are metabolised by CYP3A4 could be similarly affected (see 'Table 1.10', p.12), with larger effects on sensitive substrates and smaller effects on minor substrates.

1. Mir O, Blanchet B, Goldwasser F. More on aprepitant for erlotinib-induced pruritus. *N Engl J Med* (2011) 364, 487.

Bismuth compounds + Food

Food may reduce the absorption of bismuth from some, but not all, bismuth compounds.

Clinical evidence, mechanism, importance and management

(a) Bismuth carbonate

In a single-dose study in healthy subjects, **bismuth carbonate** (equivalent to 160 mg of bismuth) produced very low systemic levels of bismuth (no subject had a level greater than 2.7 micrograms/L) and food did not significantly affect its absorption.[1] It therefore appears that bismuth carbonate may be taken without regard to food.

(b) Bismuth subcitrate potassium

In one study, food reduced the bioavailability of a single tablet containing a combination of **bismuth subcitrate potassium**, metronidazole and tetracycline. However, the efficacy of this combined preparation for eradication of *Helicobacter pylori* did not seem to be affected (eradication rates reported at nearly 90%) and the authors suggested that this prolonged local exposure in the stomach may be clinically beneficial.[2]

The manufacturer notes that the reduced absorption of bismuth in the presence of food is not considered clinically relevant and they recommend that **bismuth subcitrate potassium** (*Pylera*) should be given after meals and at bedtime.[3]

(c) Ranitidine bismuth citrate

The manufacturer of **ranitidine bismuth citrate** (*Pylorid*) noted that food causes a decrease in bismuth absorption which is not of clinical relevance. However, because of limited data that suggest increased ulcer healing when **ranitidine bismuth citrate** is given with food, they noted that it should preferably be taken with food.[4]

(d) Tripotassium dicitratobismuthate

In a study in healthy subjects given **tripotassium dicitratobismuthate** (containing about 216 mg of bismuth) 2 hours before a standard breakfast, peak plasma levels of bismuth were found to be on average 64 micrograms/L around 30 minutes later; one subject had a bismuth level of 232 micrograms/L and ten others had a level greater than 50 micrograms/L. However, when the same bismuth compound was taken immediately after a standard breakfast, the bismuth levels were found to be lower (an average of 10.9 micrograms/mL, one subject levels were 120 micrograms/mL).[1] The authors note that levels achieved in the fasted state are within the range associated with bismuth toxicity.[1] As bismuth is thought to have a local effect, there is no advantage in it being absorbed. Nevertheless, the manufacturers recommend that **tripotassium dicitratobismuthate** (*De-Noltab*, containing 120 mg of bismuth oxide per tablet, usual dose of up to 4 tablets daily) should be taken half an hour before each of the three main meals of the day and 2 hours after the last meal of the day or taken twice daily, half-an-hour before both breakfast and the evening meal.[5]

1. Madaus S, Schulte-Frohlinde E, Scherer C, Kämmereit A, Schusdziarra V, Classen M. Comparison of plasma bismuth levels after oral dosing with basic bismuth carbonate or tripotassium dicitrato bismuthate. *Aliment Pharmacol Ther* (1992) 6, 241–9.
2. Spénard J, Aumais C, Massicotte J, Brunet J-S, Tremblay C, Grace M, Lefebvre M. Effects of food and formulation on the relative bioavailability of bismuth biskalcitrate, metronidazole, and tetracycline given for *Helicobacter pylori* eradication. *Br J Clin Pharmacol* (2005) 60, 374–7.
3. Pylera (Bismuth subcitrate potassium, metronidazole, and tetracycline hydrochloride). Axcan Pharma Inc. US Prescribing information, May 2007.
4. Pylorid Tablets (Ranitidine bismuth citrate). GlaxoSmithKline UK. UK Summary of product characteristics, December 2005.
5. De-Noltab (Tripotassium dictratobismuthate). Astellas Pharma Ltd. UK Summary of product characteristics, July 2008.

Bismuth compounds + H_2-receptor antagonists

Ranitidine possibly causes an increase in the absorption of bismuth from tripotassium dicitratobismuthate, but not bismuth salicylate or bismuth subnitrate. Other H_2-receptor antagonists would be expected to interact similarly.

Clinical evidence, mechanism, importance and management

In a study in 12 healthy subjects, the AUC of a single 240-mg dose of **tripotassium dicitratobismuthate** (*De Noltab*) was increased fourfold by two 300-mg doses of ranitidine (taken the night before and 2 hours before the bismuth compound). The maximum serum levels of bismuth were approximately doubled by ranitidine. In contrast, the same regimen of ranitidine had no significant effect on the absorption of bismuth from **bismuth salicylate** (*Pepto-Bismol*) or **bismuth subnitrate** (*Roter* tablets).[1]

The authors suggest that the reduction in gastric acidity maintains **tripotassium dicitratobismuthate** in its colloidal form, which is more likely to be absorbed, and that this may result in increased bismuth toxicity.[1] Therefore other H_2-receptor antagonists would be expected to interact similarly. However, the manufacturers of **tripotassium dicitratobismuthate** state that the toxic range of bismuth is arbitrary and a small increase in absorption is not clinically relevant, except perhaps in patients with renal failure, in whom this bismuth compound should be avoided in any case.[2] No clinically relevant effect would be expected with recommended short courses for *H. pylori* eradication; however, some caution might be appropriate with longer term use of H_2-receptor antagonists and bismuth compounds.

1. Nwokolo CU, Prewett EJ, Sawyerr AM, Hudson M, Pounder RE. The effect of histamine H_2-receptor blockade on bismuth absorption from three ulcer-healing compounds. *Gastroenterology* (1991) 101, 889–94.
2. Yamanouchi Pharma Ltd. Personal communication, November 1994.

Bismuth compounds + Proton pump inhibitors

Omeprazole markedly increases the absorption and bioavailability of bismuth from bismuth subcitrate potassium and tripotassium dicitratobismuthate. Other proton pump inhibitors are expected to interact similarly.

Clinical evidence

In a randomised study, 34 healthy subjects were given a triple therapy capsule *Helizide* (containing **bismuth subcitrate potassium** 140 mg, metronidazole 125 mg, and tetracycline 125 mg) at a dose of three capsules four times daily, with or without omeprazole 20 mg twice daily for 6 days. Omeprazole increased the maximum plasma levels and AUC of bismuth about threefold. However, the maximum plasma level achieved was 25.5 micrograms/L, which was still well below 50 micrograms/L, a bismuth level reported to be highly unlikely to cause toxicity.[1] The authors also state that in clinical studies in which *Helizide* was given with omeprazole for 10 days to several hundred patients,[2] no patient showed signs of encephalopathy, a notable toxic adverse effect of bismuth.[1]

In an earlier single-dose study in 6 healthy subjects, a single 240-mg dose of **tripotassium dicitratobismuthate** was taken one hour after the last dose of a one-week course of omeprazole 40 mg daily. Omeprazole increased the AUC of bismuth fourfold, and increased its maximum plasma levels from 36.7 micrograms/L to 86.7 micrograms/L, which the authors pointed out approaches the considered 'toxic range' for bismuth (100 micrograms/L and above).[3]

Mechanism

The solubility and absorption of some bismuth compounds are known to be increased by decreased acidity of the stomach, which increases the risk of bismuth toxicity.[1]

Importance and management

The authors of the single-dose study recommended that the dose of tripotassium dicitratobismuthate should be halved if it is given with omeprazole because of the possibility of systemic bismuth toxicity.[3] However, the manufacturers of tripotassium dicitratobismuthate say that the toxic range of bismuth is arbitrary and the small increase in absorption is not clinically relevant, except perhaps in patients with renal failure, in whom this bismuth compound should be avoided in any case.[4] No clinically relevant effect would be expected if the use of omeprazole and either of these two bismuth salts is limited to the recommended 2-week regimen for resistant *Helicobacter pylori* infection. However, some caution might be appropriate with the longer term use of omeprazole and bismuth compounds.

There appear to be no studies with bismuth compounds and other proton pump inhibitors, but as this interaction is due to changes in gastric pH, all proton pump inhibitors would be expected to interact similarly.

1. Spénard J, Aumais C, Massicotte J, Tremblay C, Lefebvre M. Influence of omeprazole on bioavailability of bismuth following administration of a triple capsule of bismuth biskalcitrate, metronidazole, and tetracycline. *J Clin Pharmacol* (2004) 44, 640–5.
2. O'Morain C, Borody T, Farley A, De Boer WA, Dallaire C, Schuman R, Piotrowski J, Fallone CA, Tytgat G, Mégraud F, Spénard J. Efficacy and safety of single-triple capsules of bismuth biskalcitrate, metronidazole and tetracycline, given with omeprazole, for the eradication of Helicobacter pylori: an international multicentre study. *Aliment Pharmacol Ther* (2003) 17, 415–20.
3. Treiber G, Walker S, Klotz U. Omeprazole-induced increase in the absorption of bismuth from tripotassium dicitrato bismuthate. *Clin Pharmacol Ther* (1994) 55, 486–91.
4. Yamanouchi Pharma Ltd. Personal communication, November 1994.

Cisapride + Miscellaneous

In many countries cisapride has been withdrawn from the market, or is only available for restricted use because of its potential to cause torsade de pointes, especially when cisapride levels are elevated.[1] This can lead to cardiac arrest and sudden death. Cisapride is known to be metabolised by CYP3A4, and the manufacturers of many drugs known to inhibit this isoenzyme, even weakly, often still include contraindications for the concurrent use of cisapride because of the possible risk of torsade de pointes. For a list of clinically relevant CYP3A4 inhibitors, see 'Table 1.9', p.11, but note that this list may not include every drug contraindicated for use with cisapride. Also, see 'Drugs that prolong the QT interval + Other drugs that prolong the QT interval', p.272, for a further discussion on the concurrent use of drugs that prolong the QT interval.

Studies and reports of interactions with cisapride and their importance and management are summarised in 'Table 27.2', p.1141.

1. Ahmad SR, Wolfe SM. Cisapride and torsades de pointes. *Lancet* (1995) 345, 508.

Crofelemer + Miscellaneous

Crofelemer does not have a clinically relevant effect on the exposure to nelfinavir, zidovudine, or lamivudine. The exposure to crofelemer is not affected by food.

Clinical evidence, mechanism, importance and management

(a) Food

In a clinical study in healthy subjects, giving a single 500-mg dose of crofelemer half an hour before a high-fat meal did not affect its exposure.[1] Crofelemer can therefore be given with or without a meal.

(b) Other drugs

A crossover study in healthy subjects found that crofelemer 500 mg four times daily for 5 days had no effect on the exposure to single doses of **zidovudine** and **nelfinavir**. In the same study, crofelemer caused a 20% decrease in the exposure to **lamivudine**, but this was not considered to be clinically important.[1] Dose adjustments of these antivirals would therefore not be expected to be necessary in patients also taking crofelemer.

1. Fulyzaq (Crofelemer). Salix Pharmaceuticals Inc. US Prescribing information January 2013.

Domperidone + CYP3A4 inhibitors

Ketoconazole and erythromycin moderately increase domperidone exposure and further increase the QT prolongation seen with domperidone alone. Other CYP3A4 inhibitors might be expected to interact similarly.

Clinical evidence

(a) Erythromycin

The UK manufacturer of domperidone briefly reports that, in a study, healthy subjects were given domperidone 10 mg four times daily and erythromycin 500 mg three times daily, alone and in combination. The maximum plasma concentration and AUC of domperidone were increased about 3-fold by erythromycin. In this study, domperidone and erythromycin alone were found to increase the QTc interval by 2.5 milliseconds and 4.9 milliseconds, respectively, whereas the mean increase in the QTc interval on concurrent use was 9.9 milliseconds.[1]

(b) Ketoconazole

In a crossover study, 22 healthy subjects were given domperidone 10 mg four times daily and ketoconazole 200 mg twice daily, alone and in combination, each for 7 days. Ketoconazole increased the AUC of domperidone 3-fold. In the 12 male subjects, domperidone and ketoconazole alone increased the QTc interval by 4.2 milliseconds and 9.2 milliseconds, respectively, and the combination increased the QTc interval by 15.9 milliseconds. In the 10 female subjects, there was no notable difference in the QTc interval for either drug when taken separately, or together.[2] The UK manufacturer of domperidone briefly reports that, in a similar study the maximum plasma concentration and AUC of domperidone were increased about 3-fold by ketoconazole. In this study, domperidone and ketoconazole alone were found to increase the QTc interval by 1.6 milliseconds and 3.8 milliseconds, respectively, whereas the mean increase in the QTc interval on concurrent use was 9.8 milliseconds.[1]

Mechanism

Domperidone is metabolised by CYP3A4, which is inhibited by erythromycin and ketoconazole (albeit to varying extents). Concurrent use therefore increases domperidone exposure, which increases its effects on the QT interval after oral administration. Giving erythromycin or ketoconazole with domperidone has more than additive effects on the QT interval, since the increases in QTc interval seen with the combinations in the studies, were greater than the additive effects of each drug when given alone.

Importance and management

Evidence for an interaction between domperidone and CYP3A4 inhibitors is limited to that with erythromycin or ketoconazole. This suggests that the increase in the QT interval due to increased domperidone exposure caused by CYP3A4 inhibition alone would probably not be clinically relevant, however when added to the increase in QT interval seen with erythromycin or ketoconazole alone, the overall increase might reach a level at which some concern is warranted (see 'Drugs that prolong the QT interval + Other drugs that prolong the QT interval', p.272). Other CYP3A4 inhibitors (see 'Table 1.9', p.11) would also be expected to increase the exposure to domperidone, but this is probably only of concern for those CYP3A4 inhibitors that also prolong the QT interval. Due to a higher risk of serious cardiac drug reactions, including QTc prolongation, the MHRA in the UK and the European Medicines Agency contraindicate the concurrent use of domperidone with other drugs that prolong the QT interval (see 'Table 9.2', p.273, for examples) or with potent CYP3A4 inhibitors (see 'Table 1.9', p.11 for a list).[3,4]

1. Motilium Tablets (Domperidone maleate). Zentiva. UK Summary of product characteristics, September 2013.
2. Boyce MJ, Baisley KJ, Warrington SJ. Pharmacokinetic interaction between domperidone and ketoconazole leads to QT prolongation in healthy volunteers: a randomized, placebo-controlled, double-blind, crossover study. *Br J Clin Pharmacol* (2012) 73, 411–21.
3. Medicines and Healthcare Products Regulatory Agency and the Commission on Human Medicines. Domperidone: risks of cardiac side effects – indication restricted to nausea and vomiting, new contraindications, and reduced dose and duration of use. *Drug Safety Update* (2014) 7, A1. Available at: http://webarchive.nationalarchives.gov.uk/20141205150130/http://www.mhra.gov.uk/home/groups/dsu/documents/publication/con418529.pdf (accessed 20/10/15).
4. European Medicines Agency. CMDh confirms recommendations on restricting use of domperidone-containing medicines, April 2014. Available at: http://www.ema.europa.eu/docs/en_GB/document_library/Referrals_document/Domperidone_31/Position_provided_by_CMDh/WC500165647.pdf (accessed 20/10/15).

Domperidone + Proton pump inhibitors

Omeprazole does not alter the pharmacokinetics of domperidone. An isolated case describes myopathy and rhabdomyolysis in a patient taking rabeprazole and domperidone.

Clinical evidence

In a crossover study in 10 healthy subjects, **omeprazole** 20 mg twice daily was given for 5 doses, with a single 10-mg dose of domperidone (as the free base or the maleate) given 4 hours after the last dose of **omeprazole**. **Omeprazole** had no effect on the AUC of domperidone given as either the maleate or the free base, and slightly decreased the rate of absorption of the free base (maximum level decreased by 16%).[1]

A single case report describes the development of myopathy and rhabdomyolysis in a patient 2 days after **rabeprazole** 20 mg daily and domperidone 6 tablets daily (strength not specified) were started. The patient had a creatine kinase level of 12 700 units/L (range 15 to 100 units/L) and a myoglobin level of 650 micrograms/L (level usually less than 90 micrograms/L). The patient had no significant medical history and the domperidone and **rabeprazole** were prescribed to treat epigastric pain post-hysterectomy.[2]

Mechanism

Rhabdomyolysis has rarely been reported with proton pump inhibitors,[3] and the authors considered that rabeprazole itself, rather than the concurrent use of domperidone, was the likely cause in this particular case.[2]

Importance and management

Omeprazole does not appear to cause a clinically relevant change in the pharmacokinetics of domperidone, and so no dose adjustment of domperidone is needed on

Table 27.2 Summary of the interactions of cisapride

Interacting drugs	*Reported effects*	*Action*	*Refs*
Alcohol	Cisapride increases gastric emptying and can modestly increase serum alcohol levels. A modest 22% increase in the AUC of cisapride seen in one study.	Unlikely to be significant, however the sedative effects might be accelerated. Unknown significance; monitor patient for sedation.	1-5
Antacids Aluminium [hydr]oxide and magnesium hydroxide	No effect on cisapride absorption seen.	None.	6
Antiepileptics e.g. Phenytoin	Increase in gastrointestinal motility caused by cisapride may affect the rate and/or extent of absorption, which may be important for some drugs with a narrow therapeutic index, such as some antiepileptics. However, no available case reports to suggest this is a problem, and one case reporting no interaction.	Uncertain. Monitor antiepileptic drug levels as usual practice. Advise the patient to report any increase in adverse effects.	1, 7
Antimuscarinics e.g. Disopyramide	Cisapride increases gastric emptying but antimuscarinics slow gastric emptying. Disopyramide absorption and serum levels were increased by cisapride in one study.	The clinical outcome is uncertain but caution is warranted if increased levels of the other drug likely to be significant e.g. Disopyramide is contraindicated as it can prolong the QT interval.	8
Butyrophenones Bromperidol Haloperidol	Increased psychotic symptoms and bromperidol levels occurred in one case report. No significant pharmacokinetic interaction between cisapride and either bromperidol or haloperidol in a study in schizophrenic patients, but possible worsening of psychotic symptoms seen when cisapride was given with haloperidol.	Significance uncertain, but probably small.	9, 10
Ciclosporin	An increase in AUC and serum levels of ciclosporin has been reported.	Monitor ciclosporin levels more frequently.	11
CYP3A4 inhibitors: **Macrolides** e.g. Clarithromycin, Erythromycin **Azoles** e.g. Ketoconazole **HIV-protease inhibitors** **Nefazodone** **Diltiazem** **Cimetidine** See also Table 1.4, p.6	Increased levels of cisapride result in an increase in the risk of QT prolongation and life-threatening ventricular arrhythmias e.g. *torsade de pointes*.	Avoid.	1, 12-22
Diazepam	Accelerated absorption of diazepam reported. Transient increase in sedation possible.	Monitor the patient and advise that sedation may occur more quickly.	1, 23
Digoxin	Small reduction in the AUC and serum levels of digoxin seen in one study.	Unlikely to be clinically significant.	24
Diltiazem	A case of syncope and prolonged QT interval reported – see also CYP3A4 inhibitors above.	See CYP3A4 inhibitors above.	25
Drugs that prolong the QT interval	Increased risk of QT prolongation and life-threatening ventricular arrhythmias.	Avoid. Should not be used with other drugs that prolong the QT interval, p.272.	1, 16
Eplerenone	Manufacturers report no pharmacokinetic interaction.	No action needed.	26
Fluoxetine	No effect on the QT interval seen.	None.	27
Grapefruit juice	Significant increases in cisapride levels seen but high inter-subject variability occurred. No QT interval changes were seen.	May be of more significance in patients taking higher doses of cisapride or also taking other interacting drugs. Avoid concurrent use if possible.	28-30
H_2-receptor antagonists Cimetidine Ranitidine	Increase in cisapride levels and reduction in cimetidine and ranitidine bioavailability seen.	Unlikely to be clinically significant. For cimetidine, see also CYP3A4 inhibitors, above.	1, 31-35
Morphine	An increase in peak morphine serum levels was seen but with no increase in the adverse effects of morphine.	Uncertain but be aware in case of increased morphine adverse effects.	36
Nifedipine	An increase in nifedipine levels with increased nifedipine effects seen, probably due to increased absorption.	Monitor patient and adjust the nifedipine dose accordingly.	37
Paracetamol	No significant effect on the pharmacokinetics of paracetamol was found in one study but another small study found that the metabolism of paracetamol was reduced.	Unlikely to be clinically significant.	38, 39
Propranolol	No change in levels or effect of propranolol.	None.	40
Proton pump inhibitors Esomeprazole Pantoprazole	An increase in AUC and elimination half-life of cisapride reported with esomeprazole, but no increase in cisapride levels or QT-prolonging effects seen. Small reduction in cisapride levels and no effects on the QT interval seen with pantoprazole.	Unlikely to be clinically significant.	1, 41, 42

Continued

Table 27.2 Summary of the interactions of cisapride (continued)

Interacting drugs	*Reported effects*	*Action*	*Refs*
Red wine	Minor changes in cisapride levels seen in one single-dose study.	Significance is unclear.	30
Simvastatin	Slightly increased cisapride levels and reduced simvastatin levels.	Unlikely to be generally significant although it may be prudent to check that simvastatin remains effective.	43
Warfarin and related anticoagulants	**Warfarin**: A small but insignificant increase in INR was seen in healthy subjects, but one case report describes a large rise in INR. **Acenocoumarol**: Increased anticoagulant effect reported, which resolved when cisapride stopped. **Phenoprocoumon**: No significant change in anticoagulant effects.	It seems prudent to monitor patients taking anticoagulants who are given cisapride until their INR is stable.	1, 44-47

1. Prepulsid (Cisapride). Janssen Pharmaceuticals. ABPI Compendium of Datasheets and Summaries of Product Characteristics 1999–2000, p 655–6.
2. Janssen Pharmaceuticals. An evaluation of possible interactions between ethanol and cisapride. Data on file (Unpublished report, N 49087), 1986.
3. Roine R, Heikkonen E, Salaspuro M. Cisapride enhances alcohol absorption and leads to high blood alcohol levels. *Gastroenterology* (1992) 102, A507.
4. Dziekan G, Contesse J, Werth B, Schwarzer G, Reinhardt WH. Cisapride increases peak plasma and saliva ethanol levels under fasting conditions. *J Intern Med* (1997) 242, 479–82.
5. Kechagias S, Jönsson K-Å, Jones AW. Impact of gastric emptying on the pharmacokinetics of ethanol as influenced by cisapride. *Br J Clin Pharmacol* (1999) 48, 728–32.
6. Janssen Pharmaceuticals. Unaltered oral absorption of cisapride on coadministration of antacids. Data on file (Study R 51 619/69), 1986.
7. Roberts GW, Kowalski SR, Calabretto JP. Lack of effect of cisapride on phenytoin free fraction. *Ann Pharmacother* (1992) 26, 1016–17.
8. Kuroda T, Yoshihara Y, Nakamura H, Azumi T, Inatome T, Fukuzaki H, Takanashi H, Yogo K, Akima M. Effects of cisapride on gastrointestinal motor activity and gastric emptying of disopyramide. *J Pharmacobiodyn* (1992) 15, 395–402.
9. Ishida M, Iotani K, Yasui N, Inoue Y, Kaneko S. Possible interaction between cisapride and bromperidol. *Prog Neuropsychopharmacol Biol Psychiatry* (1997) 21, 235–8.
10. Mihara K, Otani K, Yasui N, Ishida M, Kondo T, Suzuki A, Furukori H, Nagashima U, Kaneko S, Inoue Y. No pharmacokinetic but pharmacodynamic interactions between cisapride and bromperidol or haloperidol. *Ther Drug Monit* (1999) 21, 297–300.
11. Finet L, Westeel PF, Hary G, Maurel M, Andrejak M, Dupas JL. Effects of cisapride on the intestinal absorption of cyclosporine in renal transplant recipients. *Gastroenterology* (1991) 100, A209.
12. Ahmad SR, Wolfe SM. Cisapride and torsades de pointes. *Lancet* (1995) 345, 508.
13. van Haarst AD, van't Klooster GEA, van Gerven JMA, Schoemaker RC, van Oene JC, Burggraaf J, Coene M-C, Cohen AF. The influence of cisapride and clarithromycin on QT intervals in healthy volunteers. *Clin Pharmacol Ther* (1998) 64, 542–6.
14. Sekkarie MA. Torsades de pointes in two chronic renal failure patients treated with cisapride and clarithromycin. *Am J Kidney Dis* (1997) 30, 437–9.
15. Gray VS. Syncopal episodes associated with cisapride and concurrent drugs. *Ann Pharmacother* (1998) 32, 648–51.
16. Janssen-Cilag Ltd. Dear Doctor letter, November 1995.
17. Janssen-Cilag UK Ltd. Confidential Report from Medical Information Department and Drug Safety Unit, December 18th 1995.
18. Jenkins IR, Gibson J. Cisapride, erythromycin and arrhythmia. *Anaesth Intensive Care* (1996) 24, 728.
19. Wysowski DK, Bacsanyi J. Cisapride and fatal arrhythmia. *N Engl J Med* (1996) 335, 290–1.
20. Janssen-Cilag Ltd. Personal communication, April 1995.
21. Committee on Safety of Medicines/Medicines Control Agency. Cisapride (Prepulsid): Risk of arrhythmias. Current Problems (1998) 24, 11.
22. Kyrmizakis DE, Chimona TS, Kanoupakis EM, Papadakis CE, Velegrakis GA, Helidonis ES. QT prolongation and torsades de pointes associated with concurrent use of cisapride and erythromycin. *Am J tolaryngol* (2002) 23, 303–7.
23. Bateman DN. The action of cisapride on gastric emptying and the pharmacodynamics and pharmacokinetics of oral diazepam. *Eur J Clin Pharmacol* (1986) 30, 205–8.
24. Kirch W, Janisch HD, Santos SR, Duhrsen U, Dylewicz P, Ohnhaus EE. Effect of cisapride and metoclopramide on digoxin bioavailability. *Eur J Drug Metab Pharmacokinet* (1986) 11, 249–50.
25. Thomas AR, Chan L-N, Bauman JL, Olopade CO. Prolongation of the QT interval related to cisapride-diltiazem interaction. *Pharmacotherapy* (1998) 18, 381–5.
26. Inspra (Eplerenone). Pfizer Inc. US Prescribing information, April 2008.
27. Zhao Q, Wojcik MA, Parier J-L, Pesco-Koplowitz L. Influence of coadministration of fluoxetine on cisapride pharmacokinetics and QTc intervals in healthy volunteers. *Pharmacotherapy* (2001) 21, 149–57.
28. Gross AS, Goh YD, Addison RS, Shenfield GM. Influence of grapefruit juice on cisapride pharmacokinetics. *Clin Pharmacol Ther* (1999) 65, 395–401.
29. Kivistö KT, Lilja JJ, Backman JT, Neuvonen PJ. Repeated consumption of grapefruit juice considerably increases plasma concentrations of cisapride. *Clin Pharmacol Ther* (1999) 66, 448–53.
30. Offman EM, Freeman DJ, Dresser GK, Munoz C, Bend JR, Bailey DG. Red wine–cisapride interaction: comparison with grapefruit juice. *Clin Pharmacol Ther* (2001) 70, 17–23.
31. Kirch W, Janisch HD, Ohnhaus EE, van Peer A. Cisapride-cimetidine interaction: enhanced cisapride bioavailability and accelerated cimetidine absorption. *Ther Drug Monit* (1989) 11, 411–14.
32. Milligan KA, McHugh P, Rowbotham DJ. Effects of concomitant administration of cisapride and ranitidine on plasma concentrations in volunteers. *Br J Anaesth* (1989) 63, 628P.
33. Janssen Pharmaceuticals. Cisapride-ranitidine interaction. Data on file (Study R 51 619/74), 1986.
34. Valdes L, Champel V, Olivier C, Jonville-Bera AP, Autret E. Malaise avec allongement de l'espace QT chez un nourrisson de 39 jours traité par cisapride. *Arch Pediatr* (1997) 4, 535–7.
35. Rowbotham DJ, Milligan K, McHugh P. Effect of single doses of cisapride and ranitidine administered simultaneously on plasma concentrations of cisapride and ranitidine. *Br J Anaesth* (1991) 67, 302–5.
36. Rowbotham DJ, Milligan K, McHugh P. Effect of cisapride on morphine absorption after oral administration of sustained-release morphine. *Br J Anaesth* (1991) 67, 421–5.
37. Satoh C, Sakai T, Kashiwagi H, Hongo K, Aizawa O, Watanabe H, Mochizuki S, Okamura T. Influence of cisapride on the pharmacokinetics and antihypertensive effect of sustained-release nifedipine. *Int Med* (1996) 35, 941–5.
38. Rowbotham DJ, Parnacott S, Nimmo WS. No effect of cisapride on paracetamol absorption after oral simultaneous administration. *Eur J Clin Pharmacol* (1992) 42, 235–6.
39. Itoh H, Nagano T, Takeyama M. Cisapride raises the bioavailability of paracetamol by inhibiting its glucuronidation in man. *J Pharm Pharmacol* (2001) 53, 1041-45.
40. Janssen Pharmaceuticals. Effect of cisapride on the plasma concentrations of a delayed formulation of propranolol and on its clinical effects on blood pressure in mildly hypertensive patients. Data on file (Study R 51619/23-NL), 1986.
41. Nexium (Esomeprazole). AstraZeneca UK Ltd. UK Summary of product characteristics, October 2004.
42. Ferron GM, Paul JC, Fruncillo RJ, Martin PT, Yacoub L, Mayer PR. Lack of pharmacokinetic interaction between oral pantoprazole and cisapride in healthy adults. *J Clin Pharmacol* (1999) 39, 945–50.
43. Simard C, O'Hara GE, Prévost J, Guilbaud R, Massé R, Turgeon J. Study of the drug-drug interaction between simvastatin and cisapride in man. *Eur J Clin Pharmacol* (2001) 57, 229–34.
44. Janssen Pharmaceutica (Jonker JJC). Effect of cisapride on anticoagulant treatment with acenocoumarol. Data on file (Clinical Research Report, R 51619-NL), August 1985.
45. Wesemeyer D, Mönig H, Gaska T, Masuch S, Seiler KU, Huss H, Bruhn HD. Der Einfluß von Cisaprid und Metoclopramid auf die Bioverfügbarkeit von Phenprocoumon. *Hamostaseologie* (1991) 11, 95–102.
46. Daneshmend TK, Mahida YR, Bhaskar NK, Hawkey CJ. Does cisapride alter the anticoagulant effect of warfarin? A pharmacodynamic assessment. British Society of Gastroenterology Spring Meeting, 12–14 April 1989.
47. Darlington MR. Hypoprothrombinemia induced by warfarin sodium and cisapride. *Am J Health-Syst Pharm* (1997) 54, 320–1.

concurrent use. The case of rhabdomyolysis with rabeprazole and domperidone is likely to be due to the proton pump inhibitor alone, and is not therefore an interaction.

1. Zhang YF, Chen XY, Dai XJ, Zhang YN, Liu QZ, Yu HL, Zhong DF. Influence of omeprazole on pharmacokinetics of domperidone given as free base and maleate salt in healthy Chinese patients. *Acta Pharmacol Sin* (2007) 28, 1243–6.
2. Bourlon S, Veyrac G, Armand C, Lambert O, Bourin M, Jolliet P. Rhabdomyolyse lors d'un traitement par rabéprazole (Pariet®), un inhibiteur de la pompe à protons associé à la dompéridone (Peridys®). *Therapie* (2002) 57, 597–600.
3. Clark DWJ, Strandell J. Myopathy including polymyositis: a likely class adverse effect of proton pump inhibitors? *Eur J Clin Pharmacol* (2006) 62, 473–9.

Enteral feeds + Aluminium compounds and/or Sucralfate

Aluminium-containing antacids and sucralfate can interact with high-protein liquid enteral feeds to produce an obstructive plug.

Clinical evidence

(a) Aluminium-containing antacids

Three patients, who were being fed with a liquid high-protein nutrient (*Fresubin liquid*) through an enteral tube, developed an obstructing protein-aluminium-complex oesophageal plug when intermittently given an aluminium/magnesium hydroxide antacid (*Alucol-Gel*).[1] Another report also describes the blockage of a nasogastric tube in a patient given aluminium hydroxide (*Aludrox*) with an enteral feed (*Nutrison*).[2]

(b) Sucralfate alone or with aluminium-containing antacids

A number of reports describe the development of hard putty-like or creamy precipitations and encrustations that have blocked the oesophagus or stomach of patients given sucralfate with enteral feeds (*Ensure Plus*,[3] *Fresubin plus F*,[4] *Glucerna*,[5] *Jevity*,[5] or *Osmolite*[6]). Another patient developed this precipitate when given an enteral feed (*Isocal*) and sucralfate with aluminium/magnesium hydroxide.[7] Similarly, a patient receiving a nasogastric feed (*Pulmocare*), sucralfate and aluminium hydroxide gel also developed an oesophageal bezoar, which was analysed and found to contain components of both the drugs and the enteral feed.[8]

Data from the French Pharmacovigilance system database found 16 adults and 5 newborn babies who developed bezoars while taking sucralfate; nasogastric feeding was identified as a risk factor.[9]

Mechanism

It seems that a bezoar (a relatively insoluble complex) forms between the protein in the enteral feeds, and the aluminium from the antacids or sucralfate (sucralfate is about 18% aluminium). It thickens when the pH falls.[3]

Importance and management

An established and clinically important interaction that can result in the blockage of enteral or nasogastric tubes. The authors of one report state that high molecular protein solutions should not be mixed with antacids or followed by antacids: if an antacid is needed, it should be given some time after the nutrients and the tube should be vigorously flushed beforehand.[1] The authors of another report state that they feed for 18 hours daily and then give the sucralfate overnight without problems.[2] The manufacturer of sucralfate recommends separating the administration of sucralfate suspension and enteral feeds given by nasogastric tube by one hour.[10]

1. Valli C, Schulthess H-K, Asper R, Escher F, Häcki WH. Interaction of nutrients with antacids: a complication during enteral tube feeding. *Lancet* (1986) i, 747–8.
2. Tomlin ME, Dixon S. Aluminium and nasogastric feeds. *Pharm J* (1996) 256, 40.
3. Rowbottom SJ, Wilson J, Samuel L, Grant IS. Total oesophageal obstruction in association with combined enteral feed and sucralfate therapy. *Anaesth Intensive Care* (1993) 21, 372–4.
4. Vohra SB, Strang TI. Sucralfate therapy - a caution. *Br J Intensive Care* (1994) 4, 114.
5. García-Luna PP, García E, Pereira JL, Garrido M, Parejo J, Migens V, Serrano P, Romero H, Gómez-Cía T, Murillo F. Esophageal obstruction by solidification of the enteral feed: a complication to be prevented. *Intensive Care Med* (1997) 23, 790–2.
6. Anderson W. Esophageal medication bezoar in a patient receiving enteral feedings and sucralfate. *Am J Gastroenterol* (1989) 84, 205–6.
7. Algozzine GJ, Hill G, Scoggins WG, Marr MA. Sucralfate bezoar. *N Engl J Med* (1983) 309, 1387.
8. Krupp KB, Johns P, Troncoso V. Esophageal bezoar formation in a tude-fed patient receiving sucralfate and antacid therapy: a case report. *Gastroenterol Nurs* (1995) 18, 46–8.
9. Guy C, Ollagnier M. Sucralfate et bézoard: bilan de l'enquête officielle de pharmacovigilance et revue de la littérature. *Therapie* (1999) 54, 55–8.
10. Antepsin Suspension (Sucralfate). Chugai Pharma UK Ltd. UK Summary of product characteristics, September 2013.

H_2-receptor antagonists + Antacids

The absorption of cimetidine, famotidine, nizatidine, and ranitidine may be reduced to some extent by antacids, whereas roxatidine absorption does not appear to be affected. Cimetidine does not appear to interfere with the effectiveness of *Gaviscon* (sodium alginate compound).

Clinical evidence

(a) Cimetidine

When 12 healthy subjects were given oral cimetidine 300 mg four times daily for 5 doses, with and without 30 mL of *Mylanta II* (**aluminium/magnesium hydroxide** mixture), the absorption of cimetidine was unaffected.[1] No interaction was found with cimetidine in single-dose studies using **aluminium phosphate**[2,3] or **aluminium/magnesium** hydroxide.[4,5]

In contrast, a number of other single-dose studies indicated that antacids modestly reduce the absorption of cimetidine. The AUCs of 200- to 800-mg doses of cimetidine were reduced by an average of 19 to 34% by 10 to 45 mL doses of a variety of **aluminium/magnesium**-containing antacids.[6-10] When the antacids were given one to 3 hours after cimetidine, minor or statistically insignificant reductions occurred in the AUCs.[7,11,12]

A study in 12 healthy subjects, designed to find out if an H_2-receptor antagonist would alter the effectiveness of *Liquid Gaviscon* (sodium **alginate** compound), found that cimetidine 400 mg four times daily for 7 days caused some slight changes in gastric emptying, but the distribution of *Gaviscon* in the fundus of the stomach was not altered.[13]

In a study in 11 healthy subjects, the pharmacokinetics of a 200-mg dose of cimetidine were not significantly changed by **[simeticone]** 2.25 g.[14]

(b) Famotidine

In a study, *Mylanta II* (**aluminium/magnesium hydroxide** mixture) 30 mL reduced the AUC and peak plasma levels of famotidine by about one-third when both drugs were taken simultaneously: no significant interaction occurred when the antacid was taken 2 hours after famotidine.[15] Another study, in 17 healthy subjects, also found that *Mylanta II* reduced the maximum plasma levels of famotidine by about 25%.[16] *Mylanta Double Strength* (**aluminium/magnesium hydroxide** with **simeticone**) was found to reduce the absorption of famotidine by 19%, a difference that was considered unimportant.[10]

In contrast, a study in 18 healthy subjects found that two chewable tablets of *Mylanta II* had no effect on the pharmacokinetics or pharmacodynamics of a single 10-mg or 20-mg dose of famotidine.[17]

In a single-dose study in 12 healthy subjects, **calcium carbonate** 800 mg and **magnesium hydroxide** 165 mg had no effect on the pharmacokinetics of famotidine (all drugs given together as a combined formulation), when compared with famotidine alone.[18]

(c) Nizatidine

In a study, *Mylanta Double Strength* (**aluminium/magnesium hydroxide** with **simeticone**) reduced the absorption of nizatidine by 12%, which was not considered clinically relevant.[10] Another study, in 11 healthy subjects, found that a single 30-mL dose of *Gelusil* (**aluminium/magnesium hydroxide** with **simeticone**) reduced the mean AUC and maximum serum levels of nizatidine (given simultaneously) by 13% and 17%, respectively.[19] Another study found that the pharmacokinetics of nizatidine were not affected by *Maalox* (**aluminium/magnesium hydroxide**), although an increase in the time to peak effect of nizatidine was seen.[20]

(d) Ranitidine

In 6 healthy subjects, *Mylanta II* (**aluminium/magnesium hydroxide** mixture) 30 mL reduced the peak plasma levels and AUC of a single 150-mg dose of ranitidine by about one-third.[21] *Mylanta Double Strength* (**aluminium/magnesium hydroxide** with **simeticone**) reduced the absorption of ranitidine by 26%, which was not thought to be clinically significant.[10] Another study found that **aluminium/magnesium**-containing antacids reduced the absorption of ranitidine by up to almost 60%.[9] Yet another study found that **aluminium phosphate** reduced the bioavailability of ranitidine by 30%.[22] In contrast, one study found no significant changes in the pharmacokinetics of ranitidine given with *Maalox* (**aluminium/magnesium hydroxide**).[20]

(e) Roxatidine

In a crossover study in 24 healthy subjects, 10 mL of *Maalox* (**aluminium/magnesium hydroxide**) four times daily had no clinically relevant effect on the pharmacokinetics of a single 150-mg dose of roxatidine.[23]

Mechanism

Not fully understood. Changes in gastric pH caused by the antacid, and retarded gastric motility have been suggested as potential mechanisms for the reduced absorption of these H_2-receptor antagonists. An *in vitro* study showed that adsorption of cimetidine by **aluminium/magnesium hydroxide** antacids is unlikely to be a contributing factor.[5]

Gaviscon (sodium alginate with an antacid) is an anti-reflux preparation that needs a small amount of gastric acid to be present in order for the alginic acid 'raft' to form. Theoretically, an H_2-receptor antagonist would be predicted to reduce this effect; however, the study with cimetidine suggests that this is not the case.

Importance and management

A modest reduction in the bioavailability of cimetidine, famotidine, nizatidine and ranitidine can occur with some antacids, although this appears to be more likely when larger doses of antacids are used. None of these interactions are well established and evidence that there is a clinically relevant reduction in the effects of the H_2-receptor antagonists seems to be lacking. If antacids are given one to 2 hours before or after an H_2-receptor antagonist (if fasting), or one hour after (if the H_2-receptor antagonist is taken with food), no reduction in absorption should occur.[7,15,16,24]

Given the evidence available it seems unlikely that a clinically relevant interaction will occur between any H_2-receptor antagonist and standard doses of an antacid, including alginate-based preparations.

1. Shelly DW, Doering PL, Russell WL, Guild RT, Lopez LM, Perrin J. Effect of concomitant antacid administration on plasma cimetidine concentrations during repetitive dosing. *Drug Intell Clin Pharm* (1986) 20, 792–5.
2. Albin H, Vinçon G, Pehoucq F, Dangoumau J. Influence d'un antacide sur la biodisponibilité de la cimétidine. *Therapie* (1982) 37, 563–6.

3. Albin H, Vinçon G, Demotes-Mainard F, Begaud B, Bedjaoui A. Effect of aluminium phosphate on the bioavailability of cimetidine and prednisolone. *Eur J Clin Pharmacol* (1984) 26, 271–3.
4. Burland WL, Darkin DW, Mills MW. Effect of antacids on absorption of cimetidine. *Lancet* (1976) 308, 965.
5. Allgayer H, Röllinghoff W, Paumgartner G. Absence of in vivo and in vitro interactions of an aluminium hydroxide, magnesium hydroxide containing antacid with cimetidine in patients with peptic ulcer. *Z Gastroenterol* (1983) 21, 351–4.
6. Bodemar G, Norlander B, Walan A. Diminished absorption of cimetidine caused by antacids. *Lancet* (1979) 313, 444–5.
7. Steinberg WM, Lewis JH, Katz DM. Antacids inhibit absorption of cimetidine. *N Engl J Med* (1982) 307, 400–4.
8. Gugler R, Brand M, Somogyi A. Impaired cimetidine absorption due to antacids and metoclopramide. *Eur J Clin Pharmacol* (1981) 20, 225–8.
9. Desmond PV, Harman PJ, Gannoulis N, Kamm M, Mashford ML. The effect of an antacid and food on the absorption of cimetidine and ranitidine. *J Pharm Pharmacol* (1990) 42, 352–4.
10. Sullivan TJ, Reese JH, Jauregui L, Miller K, Levine L, Bachmann KA. Short report: a comparative study of the interaction between antacid and H_2-receptor antagonists. *Aliment Pharmacol Ther* (1994) 8, 123–6.
11. Russell WL, Lopez LM, Normann SA, Doering PL, Guild RT. Effect of antacids on predicted steady-state cimetidine concentrations. *Dig Dis Sci* (1984) 29, 385–9.
12. Barzaghi N, Crema F, Mescoli G, Perucca E. Effects on cimetidine bioavailability of metoclopramide and antacids given two hours apart. *Eur J Clin Pharmacol* (1989) 37, 409–10.
13. Washington N, Wilson CG, Williams DL, Robertson C. An investigation into the effect of cimetidine pre-treatment on raft formation of an anti-reflux agent. *Aliment Pharmacol Ther* (1993) 7, 553–9.
14. Boismare F, Flipo JL, Moore N, Chanteclair G. Etude de l'effet du diméticone sur la biodisponibilité de la cimétidine. *Therapie* (1987) 42, 9–11.
15. Barzaghi N, Gatti G, Crema F, Perucca E. Impaired bioavailability of famotidine given concurrently with a potent antacid. *J Clin Pharmacol* (1989) 29, 670–2.
16. Lin JH, Chremos AN, Kanovsky SM, Schwartz S, Yeh KC, Kann J. Effects of antacids and food on absorption of famotidine. *Br J Clin Pharmacol* (1987) 24, 551–3.
17. Schwartz JI, Yeh KC, Bolognese J, Laskin OL, Patterson PM, Shamblen EC, Han R, Lasseter KC. Lack of effect of chewable antacid on famotidine pharmacodynamics and pharmacokinetics. *Pharmacotherapy* (1994) 14, 375.
18. Zhai Q, Fu J, Huang X, Xu B, Yuan Y-Z, Jiang T, Rong Z-X, Chen H-Z. Clinical study on the influence of a fixed-dose combination of famotidine with calcium carbonate and magnesium hydroxide on the bioavailability of famotidine. *Arzneimittelforschung* (2008) 58, 581–4.
19. Knadler MP, Bergstrom RF, Callaghan JT, Obermeyer BD, Rubin A. Absorption studies of the H_2-blocker nizatidine. *Clin Pharmacol Ther* (1987) 42, 514–20.
20. Desager JP, Harvengt C. Oral bioavailability of nizatidine and ranitidine concurrently administered with antacid. *J Int Med Res* (1989) 17, 62–7.
21. Mihaly GW, Marino AT, Webster LK, Jones DB, Louis WJ, Smallwood RA. High dose of antacid (Mylanta II) reduces the bioavailability of ranitidine. *BMJ* (1982) 285, 998–9.
22. Albin H, Vinçon G, Begaud B, Bistue C, Perez P. Effect of aluminum phosphate on the bioavailability of ranitidine. *Eur J Clin Pharmacol* (1987) 32, 97–99.
23. Labs RA. Interaction of roxatidine acetate with antacids, food and other drugs. *Drugs* (1988) 35 (Suppl 3), 82–9.
24. Frislid K, Berstad A. High dose of antacid reduces bioavailability of ranitidine. *BMJ* (1983) 286, 1358.

H_2-receptor antagonists + Metoclopramide

Metoclopramide slightly reduces the bioavailability of cimetidine. Ranitidine may cause a minor increase in the bioavailability and half-life of metoclopramide whereas metoclopramide has no clinically relevant effect on the pharmacokinetics of ranitidine.

Clinical evidence

(a) Cimetidine

In a study in 8 healthy subjects, the AUC of a single 200-mg dose of **cimetidine** was reduced by about 30% by a single 20-mg dose of metoclopramide.[1] In another study in 8 healthy subjects, a 14-mg dose of a liquid formulation of metoclopramide (given as two 7-mg doses, 10 minutes before and 30 minutes after cimetidine) reduced the bioavailability of **cimetidine** by 22%, although this result did not reach statistical significance.[2] A further study, in 9 healthy subjects, found that **cimetidine** bioavailability was not significantly affected when it was given 2 hours before metoclopramide.[3]

(b) Ranitidine

In a single-dose study in 6 healthy subjects given ranitidine 300 mg and metoclopramide 10 mg, the time to maximum serum levels of ranitidine was reduced from 2.3 hours to 1.4 hours by metoclopramide; however, the AUC and maximum serum level of ranitidine were not significantly decreased.[4]

In a study in 14 healthy subjects, ranitidine 150 mg twice daily for 5 days increased the AUC of a single 20-mg dose of metoclopramide by about 13% and increased its half-life from 5.6 hours to 6.7 hours.[5]

Mechanism

The reduction in cimetidine bioavailability may have been due to the reduced gastrointestinal transit time caused by metoclopramide.[1] Similarly, the shortened time to maximum ranitidine levels may be due to accelerated gastric emptying caused by metoclopramide.[4]

Importance and management

The minor pharmacokinetic changes reported on the concurrent use of cimetidine or ranitidine and metoclopramide are unlikely to be clinically relevant and there appear to be no reports of H_2-receptor antagonist treatment failure when metoclopramide has also been taken. Therefore no additional precautions appear to be needed on concurrent use.

1. Kanto J, Allonen H, Jalonen H, Mäntylä R. The effect of metoclopramide and propantheline on the gastrointestinal absorption of cimetidine. *Br J Clin Pharmacol* (1981) 11, 629–31.
2. Gugler R, Brand M, Somogyi A. Impaired cimetidine absorption due to antacids and metoclopramide. *Eur J Clin Pharmacol* (1981) 20, 225–8.
3. Barzaghi N, Crema F, Mescoli G, Perucca E. Effects on cimetidine bioavailability of metoclopramide and antacids given two hours apart. *Eur J Clin Pharmacol* (1989) 37, 409–10.
4. Lee H-T, Lee Y-J, Chung S-J, Shim C-K. Effect of prokinetic agents, cisapride and metoclopramide, on the bioavailability in humans and intestinal permeability in rats of ranitidine, and intestinal charcoal transit in rats. *Res Commun Mol Pathol Pharmacol* (2000) 108, 311–23.
5. Leucuţa A, Vlase L, Farcău D, Nanulescu M. Pharmacokinetic interaction study between ranitidine and metoclopramide. *Rom J Gastroenterol* (2004) 13, 211–14.

H_2-receptor antagonists + Probenecid

Probenecid decreases the renal clearance of famotidine and cimetidine.

Clinical evidence, mechanism, importance and management

In a randomised, crossover study, 6 healthy subjects were given probenecid 500 mg every 6 hours for 13 doses, with a single 300-mg intravenous dose of **cimetidine** 3 hours after the last dose of probenecid. Probenecid reduced the renal clearance of **cimetidine** by 22%, without affecting its overall clearance or plasma pharmacokinetics.[1] In another study, in 8 healthy subjects, probenecid 1.5 g increased the AUC of a single 20-mg dose of **famotidine** by 81% and reduced its renal tubular clearance by 89%.[2]

It has been suggested that probenecid inhibits the renal secretion of **cimetidine** and **famotidine**, thereby reducing their renal clearance. This is consistent with the way that probenecid affects some other drugs.

The increase in exposure to **famotidine** is unlikely to be clinically relevant, as it has a wide therapeutic margin. Similarly, the minor reduction in **cimetidine** renal clearance is not clinically relevant. There would therefore seem to be no reason to avoid the concurrent use of probenecid and these H_2-receptor antagonists. Nevertheless the UK manufacturer of famotidine advises avoiding the concurrent use of **famotidine** and probenecid.[3]

Other H_2-receptor antagonists are also renally excreted and therefore their levels may be increased by probenecid, but this does not appear to have been studied; however, any change would not be expected to be clinically relevant.

1. Gisclon LG, Boyd RA, Williams RL, Giacomini KM. The effect of probenecid on the renal elimination of cimetidine. *Clin Pharmacol Ther* (1989) 45, 444–52.
2. Inotsume N, Nishimura M, Nakano M, Fujiyama S, Sato T. The inhibitory effect of probenecid on renal excretion of famotidine in young, healthy volunteers. *J Clin Pharmacol* (1990) 30, 50–56.
3. Pepcid Tablets (Famotidine). Merck Sharp & Dohme Ltd. UK Summary of product characteristics, January 2010.

H_2-receptor antagonists + Rifampicin (Rifampin)

Rifampicin appears to decrease the exposure to oral ranitidine, but has no clinically relevant effect on the clearance of intravenous cimetidine. Ranitidine has no effect on the urinary excretion of rifampicin.

Clinical evidence

(a) Cimetidine

In a study, a single 300-mg dose of intravenous cimetidine was given to a control group of 13 healthy subjects, and to 12 patients who were also given rifampicin 8 mg/kg daily, isoniazid 8 mg/kg daily and ethambutol 25 mg/kg daily for at least 14 days. In the patients given the antimycobacterials, the non-renal clearance of cimetidine was 52% higher, but the total clearance and volume of distribution were unchanged, when compared with the control subjects.[1]

(b) Ranitidine

In a controlled study, 112 patients with pulmonary tuberculosis starting rifampicin 10 mg/kg, isoniazid 300 mg and ethambutol 20 mg/kg were randomised to also receive oral ranitidine 150 mg twice daily or placebo. The pharmacokinetics of rifampicin (as measured by the total and unchanged urinary excretion) were not affected by ranitidine. No changes occurred in the incidence of hepatic adverse effects, while gastrointestinal adverse effects were reduced.[2]

In a crossover study in 12 healthy subjects, oral rifampicin 600 mg daily for 7 days approximately halved the AUC and maximum level of a single 150-mg oral dose of ranitidine. The renal clearance of ranitidine was not altered.[3]

Mechanism

It was suggested that rifampicin increased the metabolism of intravenous cimetidine resulting in greater non-renal clearance.[1] Rifampicin probably reduced the bioavailability of oral ranitidine by inducing intestinal P-glycoprotein.[3]

Importance and management

Rifampicin has no clinically relevant effect on the clearance of intravenous cimetidine, but the possibility of an effect on the pharmacokinetics of *oral* cimetidine was not studied. The clinical significance of the reduction in the bioavailability of oral ranitidine with rifampicin is unclear; however, there appear to be no reports of treatment failure on concurrent use. There would seem to be no reason to avoid the concurrent use of ranitidine or intravenous cimetidine in patients taking rifampicin. However, consider the potential for a decrease in the bioavailability of ranitidine or cimetidine after oral administration should any unexplained reduction in efficacy occur.

1. Keller E, Schollmeyer P, Brandenstein U, Hoppe-Seyler G. Increased nonrenal clearance of cimetidine during antituberculous therapy. *Int J Clin Pharmacol Ther Toxicol* (1984) 22, 307–11.
2. Purohit SD, Johri SC, Gupta PR, Mehta YR, Bhatnagar M. Ranitidine-rifampicin interaction. *J Assoc Physicians India* (1992) 40, 308–10.
3. Machavaram KK, Gundu J, Yamsani MR. Effect of ketoconazole and rifampicin on the pharmacokinetics of ranitidine in healthy human volunteers: a possible role of P-glycoprotein. *Drug Metabol Drug Interact* (2006) 22, 47–65.

H_2-receptor antagonists + Sucralfate

Sucralfate does not appear to have a clinically relevant effect on the absorption of cimetidine, roxatidine or ranitidine.

Clinical evidence, mechanism, importance and management

Most clinical pharmacokinetic studies have found that sucralfate does not affect the absorption of either **cimetidine**[1-3] or **roxatidine**.[4] A similar lack of interaction has been found with **ranitidine** and sucralfate,[5] and although two other studies found modest 22 to 29% reductions in **ranitidine** bioavailability,[6,7] these changes would not be expected to be clinically significant. There is therefore no clear reason for avoiding the concurrent use of sucralfate and these H_2-receptor antagonists.

There appears to be no evidence regarding an interaction between **famotidine** and sucralfate, and based on the way other H_2-receptor antagonists, a clinically relevant interaction would not be expected. Nevertheless, one manufacturer states that the sucralfate should not be given within 2 hours of **famotidine**.[8]

1. Albin H, Vincon G, Lalague MC, Couzigou P, Amouretti M. Effect of sucralfate on the bioavailability of cimetidine. *Eur J Clin Pharmacol* (1986) 30, 493–4.
2. D'Angio R, Mayersohn M, Conrad KA, Bliss M. Cimetidine absorption in humans during sucralfate coadministration. *Br J Clin Pharmacol* (1986) 21, 515–20.
3. Beck CL, Dietz AJ, Carlson JD, Letendre PW. Evaluation of potential cimetidine sucralfate interaction. *Clin Pharmacol Ther* (1987) 41, 168.
4. Seibert-Grafe M, Pidgen A. Lack of effect of multiple dose sucralfate on the pharmacokinetics of roxatidine acetate. *Eur J Clin Pharmacol* (1991) 40, 637–8.
5. Mullersman G, Gotz VP, Russell WL, Derendorf H. Lack of clinically significant in vitro and in vivo interactions between ranitidine and sucralfate. *J Pharm Sci* (1986) 75, 995–8.
6. Maconochie JG, Thomas M, Michael MF, Jenner WR, Tanner RJN. Ranitidine sucralfate interaction study. *Clin Pharmacol Ther* (1987) 41, 205.
7. Kimura K, Sakai H, Yoshida Y, Kasano T, Hirose M. Effects of concomitant drugs on the blood concentration of a histamine H_2 antagonist (the 2nd report) - concomitant or time lag administration of ranitidine and sucralfate. *Nippon Shokakibyo Gakkai Zasshi* (1986) 83, 603–7.
8. Pepcid Tablets (Famotidine). Merck Sharp & Dohme Ltd. UK Summary of product characteristics, January 2010.

H_2-receptor antagonists + Tobacco or Nicotine

Smoking does not appear to have a clinically significant effect on the pharmacokinetics of cimetidine, famotidine or ranitidine. Cimetidine, and to a lesser extent ranitidine, reduce the clearance of nicotine in non-smokers, but there is some evidence to suggest that cimetidine has no effect on nicotine clearance in smokers.

Clinical evidence

(a) Nicotine

In a study in 6 healthy, non-smokers, **cimetidine** 600 mg twice daily for one day, given before nicotine (1 microgram/kg per minute given intravenously for 30 minutes), reduced the clearance of nicotine by 27 to 30%. **Ranitidine** 300 mg twice daily, taken for one day, reduced the clearance of nicotine by about 7 to 10%.[1] See also *Tobacco*, below.

(b) Tobacco

In a study, tobacco smokers were given single oral doses of either **ranitidine** 150 mg or **cimetidine** 200 mg on two separate days. On one of the days they were allowed to smoke as normal and on the other they were not allowed to smoke. Peak levels of ranitidine and cimetidine occurred sooner and were slightly higher on the smoking day than on the non-smoking day, whereas the plasma levels at 3 hours were slightly lower, but there was no change in the AUC of the two drugs. No effect was seen when intravenous **cimetidine** or **ranitidine** were given.[2]

A study in heavy smokers (more than 20 cigarettes per day for at least one year) given **cimetidine** 400 mg three times daily for 2 weeks found no reduction in the clearance of **nicotine** or in the number of cigarettes smoked, when compared with placebo.[3]

Another study found that there was no difference in the pharmacokinetics and gastric acid-lowering effect of **famotidine** between 12 healthy smokers and 8 non-smokers.[4]

Mechanism

The authors of one of the above studies[3] noted that tobacco smoking induces nicotine metabolism. This may at least partially explain the lack of effect of cimetidine on nicotine clearance seen in the study in non-smokers.[1]

Importance and management

Evidence is limited, but on balance it appears that cimetidine and the other H_2-receptor antagonists probably have little effect on nicotine replacement therapy or tobacco smoking. However, the healing of duodenal ulcers in patients taking H_2-receptor antagonists such as cimetidine,[5,6] famotidine,[7] **nizatidine**[8] and ranitidine[6,7] is slower, and ulcer recurrence is more common, in smokers than in non-smokers. It is quite possible that this is due to smoking being a risk factor for the occurrence of duodenal ulcers[5,7-9] rather than a significant interaction between smoking and H_2-receptor antagonists.

1. Bendayan R, Sullivan JT, Shaw C, Frecker RC, Sellers EM. Effect of cimetidine and ranitidine on the hepatic and renal elimination of nicotine in humans. *Eur J Clin Pharmacol* (1990) 38, 165–9.
2. Boyd EJS, Johnston DA, Wormsley KG, Jenner WN, Salanson X. The effects of cigarette smoking on plasma concentrations of gastric antisecretory drugs. *Aliment Pharmacol Ther* (1987) 1, 57–65.
3. Bendayan R, Kennedy G, Frecker RC, Sellers EM. Lack of effect of cimetidine on cigarette smoking. *Eur J Clin Pharmacol* (1993) 44, 51–55.
4. Baak LC, Ganesh S, Jansen JBMJ, Lamers CBHW. Does smoking influence the pharmacokinetics and pharmacodynamics of the H_2-receptor antagonist famotidine. *Br J Clin Pharmacol* (1992) 33, 193–6.
5. Hetzel DJ, Korman MG, Hansky J, Shearman DJ, Eaves ER, Schmidt GT, Hecker R, Fitch RJ. The influence of smoking on the healing of duodenal ulcer treated with oxmetidine or cimetidine. *Aust N Z J Med* (1983) 13, 587–90.
6. Korman MG, Hansky J, Merrett AC, Schmidt GT. Ranitidine in duodenal ulcer: incidence of healing and effect of smoking. *Dig Dis Sci* (1982) 27, 712–15.
7. Reynolds JC, Schoen RE, Maislin G, Zangari GG. Risk factors for delayed healing of duodenal ulcers treated with famotidine and ranitidine. *Am J Gastroenterol* (1994) 89, 571–80.
8. Battaglia G. Risk factors of relapse in gastric ulcer: a one-year, double-blind comparative study of nizatidine versus placebo. *Ital J Gastroenterol* (1994) 26 (1 Suppl 1), 19–22.
9. Boyd EJS, Wilson JA, Wormsley KG. Smoking impairs therapeutic gastric inhibition. *Lancet* (1983) 321, 95–7.

H_2-receptor antagonists; Cimetidine + Mannitol

Oral mannitol reduces the bioavailability of cimetidine.

Clinical evidence, mechanism, importance and management

In a crossover study in 7 healthy, fasting subjects, a single 200-mg dose of cimetidine was given in four ways; as a chewable tablet or a 200 mL aqueous solution; with either 2.264 g of mannitol or sucrose. When compared with sucrose, the concurrent use of mannitol in either the tablet or the aqueous solution reduced the AUC and maximum plasma concentration of cimetidine by about 30% and 50%, respectively. Mannitol in aqueous solution decreased the small intestinal transit time of cimetidine by about 20%.[1]

A reduction in small intestinal transit time, and a solvent drag effect (the holding of water in the small bowel, rather than letting it pass into the plasma) resulting from the osmotic properties of mannitol, were both considered to have contributed to the reduction in cimetidine bioavailability.[1] However, this effect is likely to be of limited clinical relevance as the bioavailability of cimetidine was only modestly reduced. Mannitol given intravenously would not be expected to interact.

1. Adkin DA, Davis SS, Sparrow RA, Huckle PD, Wilding IR. The effect of mannitol on the oral bioavailability of cimetidine. *J Pharm Sci* (1995) 84, 1405–9.

H_2-receptor antagonists; Cimetidine + Phenobarbital

Phenobarbital does not appear to have a clinically relevant effect on the pharmacokinetics of cimetidine.

Clinical evidence, mechanism, importance and management

In 8 healthy subjects, phenobarbital 100 mg daily for 3 weeks reduced the AUC of a single 400-mg oral dose of cimetidine by 15%, and the time during which the plasma concentrations of the cimetidine exceeded 0.5 micrograms/mL (regarded as therapeutically desirable) was reduced by 11%.[1]

Phenobarbital apparently induces the enzymes in the gut wall so that the metabolism of the cimetidine is increased. Thus the amount of cimetidine absorbed and released into the circulation is reduced.

Direct information is very limited, but the effect of phenobarbital on cimetidine levels is small and unlikely to be clinically important. Therefore, the dose of cimetidine is unlikely to need adjusting on the concurrent use of phenobarbital.

1. Somogyi A, Thielscher S, Gugler R. Influence of phenobarbital treatment on cimetidine kinetics. *Eur J Clin Pharmacol* (1981) 19, 343–7.

H_2-receptor antagonists; Cimetidine + Propantheline

Propantheline slightly reduces the bioavailability of cimetidine.

Clinical evidence, mechanism, importance and management

In a single-dose study in 8 healthy subjects, propantheline 30 mg reduced the AUC and peak plasma levels of cimetidine 200 mg by about 22% and 33%, respectively. It was suggested that the reduced bioavailability of cimetidine was possibly due to delayed gastric emptying, decreased gastrointestinal motility, and reduced mixing of intestinal contents caused by the propantheline.[1] Reductions of this magnitude are unlikely to be clinically relevant.

1. Kanto J, Allonen H, Jalonen H, Mäntylä R. The effect of metoclopramide and propantheline on the gastrointestinal absorption of cimetidine. *Br J Clin Pharmacol* (1981) 11, 629–31.

5-HT_3-receptor antagonists + Antacids

The absorption of ondansetron is not affected by an aluminium/magnesium hydroxide antacid.

In a study in 12 healthy subjects, the bioavailability of a single 8-mg tablet of ondansetron was not affected when it was taken 5 minutes after a 30-mL dose of an **aluminium/magnesium hydroxide** antacid (*Maalox*).[1]

1. Bozigian HP, Pritchard JF, Gooding AE, Pakes GE. Ondansetron absorption in adults: effect of dosage form, food, and antacids. *J Pharm Sci* (1994) 83, 1011–13.

5-HT$_3$-receptor antagonists + Aprepitant

Aprepitant appears to have no clinically relevant effect on the pharmacokinetics of dolasetron, granisetron, ondansetron or palonosetron.

Clinical evidence and mechanism

(a) Dolasetron

In a study in 12 healthy subjects, aprepitant 125 mg on day one, then 80 mg on days 2 and 3 had no effect on the pharmacokinetics of a single 100-mg oral dose of dolasetron given on day one.[1]

(b) Granisetron

In a study in 17 healthy subjects, aprepitant 125 mg on day one, then 80 mg on days 2 and 3 had no effect on the pharmacokinetics of oral granisetron 2 mg given on day one.[2]

(c) Ondansetron

In a study in 15 healthy subjects, aprepitant 375 mg on day one, then 250 mg on days 2 to 5 caused a minor 15% increase in the AUC of intravenous ondansetron 32 mg given on day one.[2]

(d) Palonosetron

Aprepitant 125 mg on day one, then 80 mg on days 2 and 3 had no effect on the pharmacokinetics of a single 250-microgram intravenous dose of palonosetron given to 12 healthy subjects on day one.[3]

Importance and management

Aprepitant does not appear to have an important effect on the pharmacokinetics of single doses of dolasetron, granisetron, ondansetron, or palonosetron and therefore, no dose adjustment is required if aprepitant is given with one of these 5-HT$_3$-receptor antagonists. **Fosaprepitant**, a prodrug of aprepitant, would be expected to behave in the same way as aprepitant.

1. Li SX, Pequignot E, Panebianco D, Lupinacci P, Majumdar A, Rosen L, Ahmed T, Royalty JE, Rushmore TH, Murphy MG, Petty KJ. Lack of effect of aprepitant on hydrodolasetron pharmacokinetics in CYP2D6 extensive and poor metabolizers. *J Clin Pharmacol* (2006) 46, 792–801.
2. Blum RA, Majumdar A, McCrea J, Busillo J, Orlowski LH, Panebianco D, Hesney M, Petty KJ, Goldberg MR, Murphy MG, Gottesdiener KM, Hustad CM, Lates C, Kraft WK, Van Buren S, Waldman SA, Greenberg HE. Effects of aprepitant on the pharmacokinetics of ondansetron and granisetron in healthy subjects. *Clin Ther* (2003) 25, 1407–19.
3. Shah AK, Hunt TL, Gallagher SC, Cullen MT. Pharmacokinetics of palonosetron in combination with aprepitant in healthy volunteers. *Curr Med Res Opin* (2005) 21, 595–601.

5-HT$_3$-receptor antagonists + Cimetidine

Cimetidine has no clinically significant effect on the pharmacokinetics of dolasetron or granisetron, whereas it is predicted to increase alosetron exposure.

Clinical evidence, mechanism, importance and management

(a) Alosetron

Fluvoxamine, a potent CYP1A2 inhibitor, increases the AUC of alosetron levels 6-fold (see 'SSRIs + 5-HT$_3$-receptor antagonists', p.1488) The manufacturer therefore predicts that cimetidine, which they consider to be a moderate CYP1A2 inhibitor, will also increase alosetron exposure, and, because of a lack of data, they state that concurrent use should be avoided.[1] However, note that cimetidine is usually considered to be a weak enzyme inhibitor. If concurrent use is considered necessary it might be prudent to monitor for alosetron adverse effects (e.g. constipation, abdominal discomfort, nausea) and reduce the alosetron dose accordingly.

(b) Dolasetron

A study in 18 healthy subjects given dolasetron 200 mg daily found that cimetidine 300 mg four times daily for 7 days increased the AUC and maximum plasma level of the active metabolite of dolasetron, hydrodolasetron, by 24% and 15%, respectively, probably due to the inhibitory effect of cimetidine on the dolasetron by cytochrome P450. As 400-mg oral doses of dolasetron have been shown to be well tolerated (the usual oral dose is up to 200 mg) these changes were not considered to be clinically significant.[2] Therefore no dolasetron dose adjustments appear to be necessary on the concurrent use of cimetidine.

(c) Granisetron

In a study in 12 healthy subjects,[3] pretreatment with oral cimetidine 200 mg four times daily for 8 days had no effect on the pharmacokinetics of a single 40-microgram/kg intravenous dose of granisetron given on day 8. Therefore, no granisetron dose adjustments are likely to be necessary if cimetidine is given.

1. Lotronex (Alosetron hydrochloride). Prometheus Laboratories, Inc. US Prescribing information, March 2014.
2. Dimmitt DC, Cramer MB, Keung A, Arumugham T, Weir SJ. Pharmacokinetics of dolasetron with coadministration of cimetidine or rifampin in healthy subjects. *Cancer Chemother Pharmacol* (1999) 43, 126–32.
3. Youlten L. The effect of repeat dosing with cimetidine on the pharmacokinetics of intravenous granisetron in healthy volunteers. *J Pharm Pharmacol* (2004) 56, 169–75.

5-HT$_3$-receptor antagonists + Drugs that prolong the QT interval

The 5-HT$_3$-receptor antagonists granisetron, palonosetron, and tropisetron have been rarely reported to cause prolongation of the QTc interval, which, theoretically, could be additive with other drugs that prolong the QT interval. However, in well-controlled studies in healthy subjects, granisetron and palonosetron were not found to increase the QT interval. A study in patients similarly found no effect with tropisetron.

Clinical evidence, mechanism, importance and management

Two controlled studies in healthy subjects given intravenous **granisetron** found no effect on QT interval when compared with baseline. In both studies, moxifloxacin was used as a positive control.[1,2] In a study in 221 healthy subjects, intravenous **palonosetron** 250 micrograms, 750 micrograms, and 2.25 mg had no effect on the QT interval, when compared with that of moxifloxacin used as a positive control.[3] Similarly, several clinical studies in cancer patients have also found no increase in the QT interval after **palonosetron** administration.[4-6] In an uncontrolled study in 55 cancer patients given a single 5-mg dose of intravenous **tropisetron**, there was no change in the QT interval measured 30 minutes after administration when compared with baseline.[7]

It is generally considered that the 5-HT$_3$-receptor antagonists as a class have the propensity to increase the QT interval, which could theoretically be additive with the effects of other drugs that also prolong the QT interval (see 'Table 9.2', p.273 for a list), but the evidence is variable. **Dolasetron** and **ondansetron** are both known to prolong the QT interval, see 'Table 9.2', p.273, however studies have found that **granisetron**, **palonosetron**, and **tropisetron** did not increase the QT interval. Nevertheless, the manufacturers of the 5-HT$_3$-receptor antagonists note that they have been associated with QT prolongation, either specifically or as a class, and they give differing guidance about the concurrent use of the 5-HT$_3$-receptor antagonists with other QT prolonging drugs:

- **Granisetron**: both the UK and the US manufacturers advise caution with other drugs known to cause QT prolongation.[8,9]
- **Palonosetron**: The UK manufacturer recommends caution with **antiarrhythmics** and other drugs that increase the QT interval, or cause electrolyte abnormalities.[3]
- **Tropisetron**: the Australian manufacturer recommends care when it is used with other drugs that are likely to prolong the QT interval.[10]

For further information about drug interactions involving the QT interval see 'Drugs that prolong the QT interval + Other drugs that prolong the QT interval', p.272.

1. Mason JW, Selness DS, Moon TE, O'Mahony B, Donachie P, Howell J. Pharmacokinetics and repolarization effects of intravenous and transdermal granisetron. *Clin Cancer Res* (2012) 18, 2913–21.
2. Mason JW, Moon TE, O'Boyle E, Dietz A. A randomized, placebo-controlled, four-period crossover, definitive QT study of the effects of APF530 exposure, high-dose intravenous granisetron, and moxifloxacin on QTc prolongation. *Cancer Manag Res* (2014) 6, 181–90.
3. Aloxi Soft Capsules (Palonosetron hydrochloride). Sinclair IS Pharma. UK Summary of product characteristics, May 2013.
4. Dogan U, Yavas G, Tekinalp M, Yavas C, Ata OY, Ozdemir K. Evaluation of the acute effect of palonosetron on transmural dispersion of myocardial repolarization. *Eur Rev Med Pharmacol Sci* (2012) 16, 462–8.
5. Yavas C, Dogan U, Yavas G, Araz M, Ata OY. Acute effect of palonosetron on electrocardiographic parameters in cancer patients: a prospective study. *Support Care Cancer* (2012) 20, 2343–7.
6. Gonullu G, Demircan S, Demirag MK, Erdem D, Yucel I. Electrocardiographic findings of palonosetron in cancer patients. *Support Care Cancer* (2012) 20, 1435–9.
7. Yavas O, Yazici M, Eren O, Boruban C, Artac M, Genc M. The acute effect of tropisetron on ECG parameters in cancer patients. *Support Care Cancer* (2008) 16, 1011–5.
8. Kytril Tablets (Granisetron hydrochloride). Roche Products Ltd. UK Summary of product characteristics, October 2013.
9. Kytril Injection (Granisetron hydrochloride). Genentech USA, Inc. US Prescribing information, April 2011.
10. Navoban (Tropisetron hydrochloride). Novartis Pharmaceuticals Australia Pty Ltd. Australian Prescribing information, March 2008.

5-HT$_3$-receptor antagonists + Food

Food has no clinically relevant effect on the absorption of alosetron, dolasetron, granisetron, ondansetron, palonosetron or tropisetron.

Clinical evidence, mechanism, importance and management

(a) Alosetron

The US manufacturer of alosetron states that food reduces the absorption of alosetron by about 25% and increases the time to maximum concentration by 15 minutes.[1] However, these changes would not be expected to be clinically relevant and alosetron may be taken without regard to meals.

(b) Dolasetron

In a single-dose study, 23 healthy subjects were given a 200 mg tablet of dolasetron orally either alone, or following a **high-fat breakfast** (containing fat 55 g, protein 33 g and carbohydrate 58 g). Although there was a slight delay in absorption, dosing with a meal and dosing without a meal were considered to be bioequivalent.[2] Dolasetron may therefore be taken without regard to meals.

(c) Granisetron

The UK manufacturer of granisetron states that its oral bioavailability is not generally affected by food,[3] therefore it can be taken without regard to meals.

(d) Ondansetron

In a study in 12 healthy subjects, taking a single 8-mg tablet of ondansetron 5 minutes after a meal slightly increased the AUC of ondansetron by 17%.[4] Ondansetron may therefore be taken without regard to meals.

(e) Palonosetron

The UK manufacturer reports that a high-fat meal had no significant effect on the AUC or maximum concentration of oral palonosetron. They therefore state that palonosetron may be taken without regard to meals.[5]

(f) Tropisetron

The Australian manufacturer of tropisetron notes that food slightly increases the bioavailability of tropisetron capsules by about one-third (from 60% to 80%).[6] This change would not be expected to be clinically relevant.

1. Lotronex (Alosetron hydrochloride). Prometheus Laboratories, Inc. US Prescribing information, March 2014.
2. Lippert C, Keung A, Arumugham T, Eller M, Hahne W, Weir S. The effect of food on the bioavailability of dolasetron mesylate tablets. *Biopharm Drug Dispos* (1998) 19, 17–19.
3. Kytril Tablets (Granisetron hydrochloride) Roche Products Ltd. UK Summary of product characteristics, October 2013.
4. Bozigian HP, Pritchard JF, Gooding AE, Pakes GE. Ondansetron absorption in adults: effect of dosage form, food, and antacids. *J Pharm Sci* (1994) 83, 1011–13.
5. Aloxi Soft Capsules (Palonosetron hydrochloride). Sinclair IS Pharma. UK Summary of product characteristics, May 2013.
6. Navoban (Tropisetron hydrochloride). Novartis Pharmaceuticals Australia Pty Ltd. Australian Prescribing information, March 2008.

5-HT$_3$-receptor antagonists + Rifampicin (Rifampin) and other CYP3A4 inducers

Rifampicin causes a minor reduction in dolasetron levels and a modest to marked reduction in ondansetron levels. Rifampicin may affect granisetron and tropisetron similarly, but does not appear to alter palonosetron levels. Phenobarbital causes a minor reduction in the levels of granisetron: primidone, which is metabolised to phenobarbital, may interact similarly.

Clinical evidence, mechanism, importance and management

(a) Dolasetron

In a study in 17 healthy subjects given dolasetron 200 mg daily, rifampicin 600 mg daily for 7 days decreased the AUC and maximum plasma level of the active metabolite of dolasetron, hydrodolasetron, by 28% and 17%, respectively, probably due to induction of hydrodolasetron metabolism by rifampicin.[1] These changes were not considered to be clinically relevant and therefore no dose adjustments appear necessary if rifampicin and dolasetron are used concurrently.

(b) Granisetron

The US manufacturer notes that, in a pharmacokinetic study, **phenobarbital** increased the clearance of intravenous granisetron by 25%. They state that the relevance of this change is unknown,[2] but such a modest change is unlikely to be clinically important. **Primidone**, which is metabolised to phenobarbital, would be expected to interact similarly.

(c) Ondansetron

In a study in 10 healthy subjects, pretreatment with rifampicin 600 mg daily for 5 days markedly decreased the AUC of a single 8-mg dose of ondansetron by 65% when it was given orally and by 48% when it was given intravenously. This is most likely due to the induction of the metabolism of ondansetron by the cytochrome P450 isoenzyme CYP3A4 by rifampicin. The authors concluded that oral ondansetron in particular may not be as effective if given to patients taking rifampicin.[3]

The preliminary report of another controlled study, describes subjects receiving long-term treatment with either carbamazepine or phenytoin, who received a single 8-mg oral dose of ondansetron. There was a marked reduction in the AUC and maximum levels of ondansetron in the presence of carbamazepine (69% and 67%, respectively), and phenytoin (78% and 67%, respectively), when compared with control subjects.[4] Nevertheless, the US manufacturer states that, although the potent CYP3A4 inducers **phenytoin** [and therefore probably its prodrug **fosphenytoin**], **carbamazepine**, and rifampicin increase ondansetron clearance, on the basis of the available data, no ondansetron dose adjustment is recommended for patients taking these drugs.[5] Nevertheless, it may be prudent to monitor the outcome of concurrent use to assess ondansetron efficacy, and consider increasing the ondansetron dose if necessary.

(d) Palonosetron

The UK manufacturer notes that, in a population pharmacokinetic analysis, **dexamethasone** and rifampicin had no effect on palonosetron clearance.[6] The US manufacturer notes that, in healthy subjects, there was no pharmacokinetic interaction between intravenous palonosetron 250 micrograms and intravenous **dexamethasone** 20 mg.[7] Therefore, no palonosetron dose adjustment is likely to be necessary when it is given with these drugs.

(e) Tropisetron

The Australian manufacturer states that drugs known to induce hepatic enzymes, such as **rifampicin** and **phenobarbital**, lower tropisetron plasma concentrations. They advise that this requires an increase in the dose of tropisetron in patients of extensive metaboliser status[8] (for the cytochrome P450 isoenzyme CYP2D6). Note that metaboliser status is generally unknown. Therefore, for patients taken these enzyme inducers, consider increasing the tropisetron dose if it is not adequately effective. **Primidone** is metabolised to phenobarbital, and would be expected to interact similarly

1. Dimmitt DC, Cramer MB, Keung A, Arumugham T, Weir SJ. Pharmacokinetics of dolasetron with coadministration of cimetidine or rifampin in healthy subjects. *Cancer Chemother Pharmacol* (1999) 43, 126–32.
2. Kytril Injection (Granisetron hydrochloride). Genentech USA, Inc. US Prescribing information, April 2011.
3. Villikka K, Kivistö KT, Neuvonen PJ. The effect of rifampin on the pharmacokinetics of oral and intravenous ondansetron. *Clin Pharmacol Ther* (1999) 65, 377–81.
4. Britto MR, Hussey EK, Mydlow P, Powell JR, Brouwer KLR. Effect of enzyme inducers on ondansetron (OND) metabolism in humans. *Clin Pharmacol Ther* (1997) 61, 228.
5. Zofran (Ondansetron hydrochloride). GlaxoSmithKline. US Prescribing information, September 2011.
6. Aloxi Soft Capsules (Palonosetron hydrochloride). Sinclair IS Pharma. UK Summary of product characteristics, May 2013.
7. Aloxi Injection (Palonosetron hydrochloride). Eisai Inc. US Prescribing information, September 2008.
8. Navoban (Tropisetron hydrochloride). Novartis Pharmaceuticals Pty Ltd. Australian Summary of product characteristics, March 2008.

5-HT$_3$-receptor antagonists; Dolasetron + Miscellaneous

Dolasetron can prolong the QRS and PR interval, and this could be additive with the effects of other drugs that also prolong the QRS and/or PR interval (e.g. flecainide, quinidine and verapamil). Atenolol slightly reduced the clearance of the active metabolite of dolasetron, but ACE inhibitors, diltiazem, furosemide, glibenclamide (glyburide), nifedipine, propranolol and verapamil had no effect on dolasetron clearance.

Clinical evidence, mechanism, importance and management

(a) Beta blockers

The US manufacturer notes that **atenolol** reduced the clearance of the active metabolite of dolasetron, hydrodolasetron, by 27%, whereas **propranolol** had no effect.[1] The slight change with **atenolol** is not expected to be clinically relevant.

(b) Calcium-channel blockers

The US manufacturer reports that in patients taking **diltiazem**, **nifedipine**, or **verapamil**, the clearance of hydrodolasetron (the active metabolite of dolasetron) was unchanged.[1] Therefore no dose adjustment of dolasetron appears to be needed on the concurrent use of these calcium-channel blockers. However, note that dolasetron can prolong the PR interval and this might be additive with the PR prolonging effects of **verapamil**, see under *Drugs that prolong the QRS and/or PR interval*, below.

(c) Drugs that prolong the QRS and/or PR interval

The US manufacturer reports that dolasetron can cause a dose-dependent prolongation of the PR and QRS interval. Cases of second and third degree atrioventricular block, cardiac arrest and ventricular arrhythmias (including fatalities) have also been reported. They therefore advise caution if dolasetron is given to patients taking other drugs known to prolong the PR and QRS interval, and they name **flecainide**, **quinidine** and **verapamil**.[1] If concurrent use is necessary, patients should have their ECG checked more frequently and should be closely monitored for adverse cardiac effects. Note that the elderly, patients with underlying structural heart disease, conduction system abnormalities, sick sinus syndrome, myocardial ischaemia, and patients with atrial fibrillation with a slow ventricular response are at increased risk of developing PR and/or QRS interval prolongation with dolasetron, and it would seem prudent to avoid the concurrent use of dolasetron and other drugs that prolong the QRS and PR interval, if possible, in these patients.

Note that both dolasetron and **quinidine** can have additive effects on the QT interval, see '5-HT$_3$-receptor antagonists + Drugs that prolong the QT interval', p.1146.

(d) Miscellaneous

The US manufacturer briefly notes that in patients taking **furosemide**, **ACE inhibitors**, **glibenclamide (glyburide)**, and various chemotherapy agents, no effect was shown on the clearance of hydrodolasetron.[1]

1. Anzemet Tablets (Dolasetron mesylate). Sanofi-Aventis US LCC. US Prescribing information, September 2011.

5-HT$_3$-receptor antagonists; Palonosetron + Metoclopramide

The US manufacturer of palonosetron reports that, in a study in healthy subjects, no significant pharmacokinetic interaction occurred between oral metoclopramide 10 mg four times daily and a single 750-microgram intravenous dose of palonosetron.[1] Therefore, no dose adjustments of either drug appear to be necessary on the concurrent use of metoclopramide and palonosetron.

1. Aloxi Injection (Palonosetron hydrochloride). Eisai Inc. US Prescribing information, September 2008.

Linaclotide + Miscellaneous

Linaclotide taken immediately after a high-fat meal resulted in more gastrointestinal adverse effects compared with the fasting state. Severe or prolonged linaclotide-induced diarrhoea is predicted to reduce the efficacy of oral combined hormonal contraceptives. Taking linaclotide with NSAIDs or proton pump inhibitors might increase the risk of diarrhoea.

Clinical evidence, mechanism, importance and management

(a) Food

The UK and US manufacturers of linaclotide note that, in a crossover study in 18 healthy subjects, taking a 290-microgram dose of linaclotide immediately after a high-fat breakfast caused more gastrointestinal adverse events, and looser, more frequent stools when compared with the fasted state. Linaclotide should therefore be taken 30 minutes before a meal on an empty stomach.[1,2]

(b) Combined hormonal contraceptives

The UK manufacturer of linaclotide states that because it can cause severe diarrhoea, linaclotide might reduce the efficacy of oral combined hormonal contraceptives.[1] They therefore recommend the use of an additional contraceptive method (such as a barrier method) in case patients develop severe or prolonged diarrhoea.

(c) Other drugs

The UK manufacturer of linaclotide advises that concurrent use of **NSAIDs** or **proton pump inhibitors** might increase the risk of diarrhoea with linaclotide alone,[1] and that this might reduce the efficacy of other drugs absorbed in the intestinal tract, especially those with a narrow therapeutic range, such as **levothyroxine**.

1. Constella (Linaclotide). Almirall Ltd. UK Summary of product characteristics, March 2014.
2. Linzess (Linaclotide). Forest Laboratories, Inc. US Prescribing information, July 2014.

Loperamide + Colestyramine

An isolated report, supported by an *in vitro* study, indicates that the effects of loperamide can be reduced by colestyramine.

Clinical evidence, mechanism, importance and management

A man who had undergone extensive surgery to the gut, with the creation of an ileostomy, needed treatment for excessive fluid loss. His fluid loss was observed to be substantially less when he took loperamide 2 mg every 6 hours alone, than when he took loperamide with colestyramine 2 g every 4 hours.[1] The probable reason for this effect is that colestyramine binds to loperamide in the gut, thereby reducing its activity. This suggestion is supported by an *in vitro* study using 50 mL of simulated gastric fluid, which found that 64% of a 5.5-mg dose of loperamide was bound by 4 g of colestyramine.[1]

Direct information about the interaction between loperamide and colestyramine is limited to one case report, but what occurred is consistent with the way colestyramine interacts with other drugs. It has been suggested that administration of the two drugs should be separated by as much as possible to prevent mixing in the gut, or that the loperamide dose should be increased.[1] Note that it is generally recommended that other drugs should be given one hour before or 4 to 6 hours after colestyramine.

1. Ti TY, Giles HG, Sellers EM. Probable interaction of loperamide and cholestyramine. *Can Med Assoc J* (1978) 119, 607–8.

Loperamide + Co-trimoxazole

Co-trimoxazole moderately increases the levels of loperamide.

Clinical evidence

In a study, healthy subjects were given co-trimoxazole (sulfamethoxazole with trimethoprim) 960 mg twice daily, for 24 hours before and then 48 hours after they took a single 4-mg dose of loperamide (12 subjects) or loperamide oxide (a prodrug of loperamide, 10 subjects). Co-trimoxazole increased the AUC of loperamide by 89% and doubled its maximum plasma levels. Co-trimoxazole also increased the AUC and maximum plasma levels of loperamide from loperamide oxide by 54% and 41%, respectively.[1]

Mechanism

Loperamide is metabolised by the cytochrome P450 isoenzymes CYP2C8 and CYP3A4. Therefore, it is possible that trimethoprim, a known CYP2C8 inhibitor and component of co-trimoxazole, inhibited the metabolism of loperamide by this isoenzyme.

Importance and management

Co-trimoxazole moderately increases loperamide exposure. However, as loperamide has a very wide margin of safety, it is thought unlikely that any loperamide dose reductions are needed. Note that, if the suggested mechanism of this interaction is correct, **trimethoprim** alone would be expected to interact similarly.

1. Kamali F, Huang ML. Increased systemic availability of loperamide after oral administration of loperamide and loperamide oxide with cotrimoxazole. *Br J Clin Pharmacol* (1996) 41, 125–8.

Loperamide + Gemfibrozil and/or Itraconazole

Gemfibrozil and itraconazole alone markedly increase the bioavailability of loperamide. However, the combination of gemfibrozil and itraconazole very markedly increases loperamide bioavailability.

Clinical evidence

In a placebo-controlled, crossover study, 12 healthy subjects were given a single 4-mg dose of loperamide on day 4 of taking either itraconazole 200 mg then 100 mg twice daily, gemfibrozil 600 mg twice daily, or both drugs together, each for 5 days. Itraconazole alone increased the AUC and peak levels of loperamide by 3.8-fold and 2.9-fold, respectively, and increased its half-life from 11.9 to 18.7 hours. Gemfibrozil alone increased the AUC and peak levels of loperamide by 2.2-fold and 1.6-fold, respectively, and increased its half-life from 11.9 to 16.7 hours. Itraconazole plus gemfibrozil synergistically increased the AUC and peak levels of loperamide by 12.6-fold and 4.2-fold, respectively, and increased its half-life from 11.9 to 36.9 hours.[1]

Despite the large increases in loperamide bioavailability produced by gemfibrozil and/or itraconazole, no changes in drowsiness or psychomotor test results for loperamide were reported during concurrent treatment.[1]

Mechanism

Loperamide is thought to be metabolised by both the cytochrome P450 isoenzymes CYP3A4 and CYP2C8, and is also a substrate for P-glycoprotein. Therefore, the large increases in loperamide levels are thought to be due to CYP2C8 inhibition by gemfibrozil and CYP3A4 inhibition by itraconazole, and inhibition of P-glycoprotein in the gut by itraconazole resulting in increased oral bioavailability.[1] Loperamide is thought to lack CNS effects because it is a substrate for P-glycoprotein, which transports drugs out of the cells at the blood-brain barrier, thereby restricting its CNS penetration. The lack of effect of itraconazole on the CNS effects of loperamide in this study suggests that itraconazole might not inhibit P-glycoprotein at the blood-brain barrier.

Importance and management

From the study above, it appears that the concurrent use of a single 4-mg dose of loperamide with gemfibrozil or itraconazole does not increase the risk of clinically significant CNS adverse effects, despite the large increases in loperamide levels. Therefore, no loperamide dose reduction would appear to be necessary if a single 4-mg dose of loperamide is given with these drugs. However, the increased exposure to loperamide with both gemfibrozil and itraconazole together was so marked in this study that, although no increase in drowsiness was seen, adverse effects cannot be excluded with repeated use. Some caution would therefore seem prudent if multiple-doses of loperamide are given with gemfibrozil and/or itraconazole.

A similar interaction would be predicted to occur if multiple doses of loperamide are given with the combination of other potent CYP3A4 inhibitors (see 'Table 1.9', p.11, for a list) and CYP2C8 inhibitors (see 'Table 1.4', p.6, for a list). Until further information is available, it would seem prudent to apply similar caution if loperamide is given with potent inhibitors of these isoenzymes.

1. Niemi M, Tornio A, Pasanen MK, Fredrikson H, Neuvonen PJ, Backman JT. Itraconazole, gemfibrozil and their combination markedly raise the plasma concentrations of loperamide. *Eur J Clin Pharmacol* (2006) 62, 463–72.

Loperamide + HIV-protease inhibitors

Loperamide reduces the bioavailability of saquinavir by about 50%. Ritonavir increases the plasma concentrations of loperamide without increasing its CNS adverse effects, and saquinavir similarly increases the bioavailability of loperamide. Conversely, tipranavir alone and tipranavir boosted with ritonavir reduce the bioavailability and plasma concentrations of loperamide and its metabolites.

Clinical evidence

(a) Ritonavir

In a single-dose study, 12 healthy subjects were given a 600-mg dose of ritonavir with either loperamide 16 mg or placebo. Ritonavir increased the AUC and maximum plasma concentrations of loperamide threefold and 17%, respectively; however, no additional CNS adverse effects were seen.[1] In another study, ritonavir 200 mg twice daily for 9 doses increased the maximum concentration and AUC of a single 16-mg dose of loperamide (given one hour after the final dose of ritonavir) by 83% and 121%, respectively.[2]

For the contrasting effect of ritonavir given as a pharmacokinetic booster with tipranavir, see *Tipranavir*, below.

(b) Saquinavir

In a placebo-controlled study, 12 healthy subjects were given single doses of either saquinavir 600 mg, loperamide 16 mg, or both drugs together. Loperamide reduced the AUC of saquinavir by about 54%. The maximum plasma concentration of saquinavir was also reduced by loperamide although this was not statistically significant. Saquinavir increased the AUC of loperamide by 40% and also produced a non-significant increase in the maximum concentration of loperamide.[3]

(c) Tipranavir

In a study, 20 healthy subjects were given a single 16-mg dose of loperamide taken with either tipranavir 750 mg twice daily, ritonavir 200 mg twice daily or both drugs together. Tipranavir alone *reduced* the maximum concentration and AUC of loperamide by 58% and 63%, respectively. Tipranavir boosted with ritonavir resulted in a net reduction in the maximum concentration and AUC of loperamide of 61% and 51%, respectively, similar to the effect seen with tipranavir alone. The maximum concentration and AUC of the metabolites of loperamide were also reduced. There were no clinically significant loperamide adverse effects on respiration or pupil contractility with either ritonavir or tipranavir alone, or in combination.[2]

Mechanism

Loperamide is primarily metabolised by the cytochrome P450 isoenzyme CYP3A4, and is thought to lack CNS effects because it is a substrate for P-glycoprotein, which transports drugs out of the cells at the blood-brain barrier, thereby restricting CNS penetration.[2]

The increase in loperamide concentrations with ritonavir alone is thought to be due to ritonavir inhibiting its metabolism by CYP3A4, and possibly also increasing its bioavailability by inhibiting gastrointestinal P-glycoprotein. The lack of an increase in loperamide CNS effects suggests that ritonavir alone does not inhibit P-glycoprotein at the blood-brain barrier.[1,2]

Saquinavir probably also inhibits the CYP3A4-mediated metabolism of loperamide. Loperamide reduces gastrointestinal motility and therefore may affect the absorption of some drugs. It is thought that this therapeutic action may have reduced the absorption of saquinavir leading to the reduction in its bioavailability.[3]

The reduction in loperamide concentrations with tipranavir alone or tipranavir with ritonavir is thought to be due to induction of gastrointestinal P-glycoprotein by tipranavir, resulting in a decrease in the systemic bioavailability of loperamide.[2]

Importance and management

The reduced concentrations of saquinavir seen in the single-dose study suggest that loperamide may reduce the antiviral efficacy of saquinavir. Although the evidence is limited to this study and only a single, low-dose of unboosted saquinavir was given, it may be prudent to monitor patients taking loperamide with saquinavir to ensure that the antiviral efficacy of saquinavir is maintained. Whether loperamide would cause as large a reduction in saquinavir concentrations with higher doses of saquinavir boosted with ritonavir (as is usual practice) is unclear. Further study is needed. Pharmacokinetic information about other HIV-protease inhibitors appears to be lacking. However, one efficacy study reported that the viral load and CD4 count were maintained in patients taking loperamide for **nelfinavir**-induced diarrhoea.[4]

Despite the increases in loperamide plasma concentrations seen in both studies with ritonavir alone, there was no evidence of an increase in loperamide central opioid effects (such as pupillary constriction, respiratory depression and also analgesic effects). This suggests that loperamide is potentially a safe antidiarrhoeal to give with ritonavir during episodes of HIV-protease inhibitor-induced diarrhoea.[1] The increases in loperamide bioavailability seen with the single dose of unboosted saquinavir are also not thought to be clinically significant, although the dose of saquinavir used in this study were much smaller than that commonly used in HIV regimens.[3] It would appear from the results of these studies that use of saquinavir boosted with ritonavir and loperamide is also unlikely to lead to a clinically relevant increase in loperamide adverse effects.

The clinical relevance of the decrease in loperamide bioavailability with tipranavir alone or tipranavir boosted with ritonavir is unknown, but may not be important because loperamide is thought to have a local action in the gut.[2] Note that the dose of tipranavir given in this study is higher than the usual dose of 500 mg twice daily when boosted with ritonavir.

1. Tayrouz Y, Ganssmann B, Ding R, Klingmann A, Aderjan R, Burhenne J, Haefeli WE, Mikus G. Ritonavir increases loperamide plasma concentrations without evidence for P-glycoprotein involvement. *Clin Pharmacol Ther* (2001) 70, 405–14.
2. Mukwaya G, MacGregor T, Hoelscher D, Heming T, Legg D, Kavanaugh K, Johnson P, Sabo JP, McCallister S. Interaction of ritonavir-boosted tipranavir with loperamide does not result in loperamide-associated neurologic side effects in healthy volunteers. *Antimicrob Agents Chemother* (2005) 49, 4903–10.
3. Mikus G, Schmidt L, Burhenne J, Ding R, Riedel K-D, Tayrouz Y, Weiss J, Haefeli WE. Reduction of saquinavir exposure by coadministration of loperamide; a two-way pharmacokinetic interaction. *Clin Pharmacokinet* (2004) 43, 1015–24.
4. Rachlis A, Gill J, Baril J-G, LeBlanc RP, Trottier B, MacLeod J, Walmsley S, Van der Vliet W, Belsky G, Burgoyne R. Effectiveness of step-wise intervention plan for managing nelfinavir-associated diarrhea: a pilot study. *HIV Clin Trials* (2005) 6, 203–12.

Loperamide + Quinidine

Quinidine increases the penetration of loperamide into the brain, which results in respiratory depression.

Clinical evidence

In a study in 8 healthy subjects, a single 600-mg dose of quinidine increased the AUC of loperamide and its metabolite by 148% and 94%, respectively. Loperamide alone did not produce respiratory depression, but when given with quinidine, respiratory depression occurred, as measured by the ventilatory response of the subjects to increasing carbon dioxide concentrations.[1]

Mechanism

Loperamide is mainly metabolised by the cytochrome P450 isoenzyme CYP3A4, and is thought to lack CNS effects because it is also a substrate for P-glycoprotein, which transports drugs out of the cells at the blood-brain barrier, thereby restricting CNS penetration. The central opioid adverse effects of loperamide that occurred in the study appear to be due to inhibition of CNS P-glycoprotein by quinidine, resulting in increased loperamide penetration into the brain, and respiratory depression.[1]

Importance and management

Although information is limited, it would seem prudent to be alert for CNS adverse effects, such as drowsiness, if quinidine is given to a patient taking loperamide. If adverse effects are troublesome consider reducing the dose of loperamide.

1. Sadeque AJM, Wandel C, He H, Shah S, Wood AJJ. Increased drug delivery to the brain by P-glycoprotein inhibition. *Clin Pharmacol Ther* (2000) 68, 231–7.

Lubiprostone + Miscellaneous

A high-fat meal decreased the maximum concentration, but not the exposure, to lubiprostone. The efficacy of lubiprostone might theoretically be reduced by methadone, in a dose-dependent manner.

Clinical evidence, mechanism, importance and management

(a) Food

The UK and US manufacturers of lubiprostone note that when given following a high fat meal, the maximum concentration of a single 72-microgram dose of lubiprostone was decreased by 55%, but the AUC was unchanged.[1,2] The clinical relevance of this finding is unclear.[2]

(b) Methadone

The US manufacturer of lubiprostone notes that in an *in vitro* study, the activation of chloride channels in the gastrointestinal tract by lubiprostone has been shown to be reduced by methadone in a dose-dependent manner. The manufacturer therefore states that it is possible that this might also occur *in vivo*.[2] Further research is needed, however it would seem prudent to be aware of the possibility of a reduction in the efficacy of lubiprostone in patients taking methadone.

1. Amitiza (Lubiprostone). Sucampo Pharma Europe Ltd. UK Summary of product information, October 2013.
2. Amitiza (Lubiprostone). Sucampo Pharma Americas, LLC. US Prescribing information, April 2013.

Mesalazine (Mesalamine) + Laxatives

Ispaghula husk and lactulose do not appear to affect the bioavailability of mesalazine from a delayed-release preparation (*Asacol*).

Clinical evidence

In a study in 10 patients with quiescent ulcerative colitis taking delayed-release mesalazine (*Asacol*), colonic acidification by **ispaghula** husk (*Fybogel*) did not appear to affect the release of mesalazine because the 24-hour faecal and urinary excretion of the metabolites of mesalazine were unchanged.[1] Similarly, another study in 14 healthy subjects given delayed-release mesalazine (*Asacol*) 400 mg three times daily, found that **lactulose** (15 mL twice daily for 8 days, then increased to 30 mL twice daily for 8 days) did not affect the urinary or faecal excretion of mesalazine and its metabolites.[2]

Mechanism

Some preparations of mesalazine are coated with an acrylic-based resin (*Eudragit*) that disintegrates above pH 6 or 7 and thereby releases the mesalazine into the terminal ileum and colon.[3-5] The pH in the colon can be lowered by lactulose and lactitol, which are metabolised by gut bacteria to a number of acids (e.g. acetic, butyric, propionic, and lactic acid).[6] In healthy subjects, lactulose 30 to 80 g daily has been found to cause slight falls in colonic pH (from about 6 to 5 in the right colon and from 7 to 6.7 in the left colon).[6,7] Lactitol 40 to 180 g daily can cause similar falls in colonic pH.[6] Ispaghula can also lower colonic pH (from 6.5 to 5.8 in the right colon, and from 7.3 to 6.6 in the left colon).[8] Theoretically, lowering the pH of the colon with these drugs may impair the release of mesalazine from pH-dependent preparations, although this has not been shown in the above studies. It is also possible that decreasing gastrointestinal transit time with laxatives might reduce the release of mesalazine from some preparations.[9]

Importance and management

Although on theoretical grounds ispaghula husk and lactulose might be expected to reduce the release of mesalazine from some preparations and thereby reduce its efficacy, the studies above suggest that no interaction of clinical importance would be expected to occur, and there have been no published reports as yet of any interaction with either ispaghula husk, lactulose or **lactitol**. Nevertheless, the UK manufacturers of *Asacol*,[3] *Ipocol*[5] and *Salofalk* granules[10] (but not tablets[4]) recommend avoiding the concurrent use of preparations that can lower stool pH. However, note that this interaction is not mentioned by the US manufacturers of *Asacol*,[11] nor by the UK manufacturers of *Mesren MR*.[12]

1. Riley SA, Tavares IA, Bishai PM, Bennett A, Mani V. Mesalazine release from coated tablets: effect of dietary fibre. *Br J Clin Pharmacol* (1991) 32, 248–50.
2. Hussain FN, Ajjan RA, Moustafa M, Weir NW, Riley SA. Mesalazine release from a pH dependent formulation: effects of omeprazole and lactulose co-administration. *Br J Clin Pharmacol* (1998) 46, 173–5.

3. Asacol Tablets (Mesalazine). Warner Chilcott UK Ltd. UK Summary of product characteristics, May 2010.
4. Salofalk Tablets (Mesalazine). Dr. Falk Pharma UK. UK Summary of product characteristics, September 2010.
5. Ipocol (Mesalazine). Sandoz Ltd. UK Summary of product characteristics, October 2009.
6. Patil DH, Westaby D, Mahida YR, Palmer KR, Rees R, Clark ML, Dawson AM, Silk DBA. Comparative modes of action of lactitol and lactulose in the treatment of hepatic encephalopathy. *Gut* (1987) 28, 255–9.
7. Bown RL, Gibson JA, Sladen GE, Hicks B, Dawson AM. Effects of lactulose and other laxatives on ileal and colonic pH as measured by a radiotelemetry device. *Gut* (1974) 15, 999–1004.
8. Evans DF, Crompton J, Pye G, Hardcastle JD. The role of dietary fibre on acidification of the colon in man. *Gastroenterology* (1988) 94, A118.
9. Rijk MC, van Hogezand RA, van Schaik A, van Tongeren JHM. Disposition of 5-aminosalicylic acid from 5-aminosalicylic acid-delivering drugs during accelerated intestinal transit in healthy volunteers. *Scand J Gastroenterol* (1989) 24, 1179–85.
10. Salofalk Gastro-resistant Prolonged-release Granules (Mesalazine). Dr. Falk Pharma UK. UK Summary of product characteristics, May 2010.
11. Asacol (Mesalamine). Warner Chilcott. US Prescribing information, May 2010.
12. Mesren MR (Mesalazine). Norton Healthcare Ltd. UK Summary of product characteristics, August 2008.

Mesalazine (Mesalamine) + Proton pump inhibitors

Omeprazole does not affect the release of mesalazine from a delayed-release preparation (*Asacol*).

Clinical evidence, mechanism, importance and management

Asacol is a preparation of mesalazine coated with an acrylic-based resin (*Eudragit S*) that disintegrates above pH 7 and thereby releases the mesalazine into the terminal ileum and colon. The release is rapid at pH values of 7 and above, but it can also occur between pH 6 and 7. As the proton pump inhibitors can raise the pH in the stomach to 6 and above, the potential exists for the premature release of mesalazine from *Asacol*. However, a study in 6 healthy subjects given *Asacol* 400 mg three times daily for 3 weeks found that when they were also given **omeprazole** 20 mg daily during the second week, and **omeprazole** 40 mg daily during the third week, the steady-state pharmacokinetics of mesalazine remained unchanged.[1] Had mesalazine been released earlier, the absorption characteristics would have changed. There would therefore appear to be no reason for avoiding the concurrent use of *Asacol* and **omeprazole** in doses of up to 40 mg daily. On the basis of this study, it seems likely that other proton pump inhibitors will behave similarly, at equivalent doses.

1. Hussain FN, Ajjan RA, Moustafa M, Weir NW, Riley SA. Mesalazine release from a pH dependent formulation: effects of omeprazole and lactulose co-administration. *Br J Clin Pharmacol* (1998) 46, 173–5.

Methylnaltrexone + Miscellaneous

Cimetidine does not have a clinically relevant effect on the pharmacokinetics of methylnaltrexone. The pharmacokinetics of dextromethorphan are not affected by methylnaltrexone.

Clinical evidence, mechanism, importance and management

(a) Cimetidine

The UK manufacturer of methylnaltrexone notes that, in a study in 18 healthy subjects, multiple 400-mg doses of cimetidine did not cause any clinically relevant changes in the AUC or maximum plasma levels of a single dose of methylnaltrexone. However, there was a 42% reduction in the renal clearance of methylnaltrexone, and a small 11% reduction in its total clearance.[1]

The reduction in methylnaltrexone renal clearance is thought to be due to inhibition of organic cation transporters by cimetidine, but these changes are not thought to be clinically relevant.[1] Therefore, no dose adjustment of methylnaltrexone is expected to be needed if cimetidine is also given.

(b) Dextromethorphan

The manufacturers of methylnaltrexone briefly report that, in a study in healthy male subjects, the metabolism of dextromethorphan was unaffected by a subcutaneous 300-microgram/kg dose of methylnaltrexone bromide.[1,2]

This study was conducted because, *in vitro* methylnaltrexone was found to be a weak inhibitor of the cytochrome P450 isoenzyme CYP2D6, for which dextromethorphan is a substrate. However, the study suggests that methylnaltrexone causes no clinically relevant inhibition of this isoenzyme.

1. Relistor (Methylnaltrexone bromide). Wyeth Pharmaceuticals. UK Summary of product characteristics, December 2009.
2. Relistor (Methylnaltrexone bromide). Wyeth Pharmaceuticals Inc. US Prescribing information, June 2009.

Mosapride + Macrolides

In one study, erythromycin increased the levels and prolonged the half-life of mosapride, but no QT prolongation was seen. It seems likely that some other macrolides may interact similarly.

Clinical evidence, mechanism, importance and management

In a study, 10 healthy subjects were given mosapride 5 mg three times daily for 14 days, with **erythromycin** stearate 300 mg four times daily on the last 7 days. **Erythromycin** increased the peak plasma levels and AUC of mosapride by about 60% and 84%, respectively, and increased its half-life from 1.6 hours to 2.4 hours. Mosapride, either alone or with erythromycin did not have any adverse changes on the ECG, including the QT interval.[1]

It was suggested that these pharmacokinetic changes occurred because erythromycin inhibited the metabolism of mosapride by the cytochrome P450 isoenzyme CYP3A4.

The clinical relevance of the increased exposure to mosapride seen with erythromycin is uncertain. Nevertheless, it may be prudent to monitor concurrent use for an increase in mosapride adverse effects (e.g. on the gastrointestinal system). Although other macrolides do not appear to have been studied, if the suggested mechanism is correct, other macrolides that inhibit CYP3A4 (e.g. **clarithromycin, telithromycin**) would be expected to interact similarly. If these macrolides are given with mosapride, it may therefore be prudent to follow the same precautions advised for the concurrent use of erythromycin.

1. Katoh T, Saitoh H, Ohno N, Tateno M, Nakamura T, Dendo I, Kobayashi S, Nagasawa K. Drug interaction between mosapride and erythromycin without electrocardiographic changes. *Jpn Heart J* (2003) 44, 225–34.

Proton pump inhibitors + Antacids

Antacids may cause a slight reduction in the bioavailability of lansoprazole. Aluminium/magnesium hydroxide-containing antacids do not appear to alter the pharmacokinetics of omeprazole, pantoprazole or rabeprazole to a clinically relevant extent and no interaction appears to occur between sodium alginate and omeprazole.

Clinical evidence, mechanism, importance and management

(a) Lansoprazole

In a study in 12 healthy subjects a single 30-mL dose of *Maalox* (**aluminium/magnesium hydroxide**) slightly reduced the AUC of a 30-mg dose of lansoprazole by 13% (not statistically significant), and reduced its maximum plasma level by 27%. However, no changes were seen when the lansoprazole was given one hour after the antacid.[1] Note that in this study, the bioavailability of lansoprazole was highly variable between subjects (the AUC varied by a factor of 6). In another study, **magaldrate** had no effect on the AUC of lansoprazole, but slightly reduced its maximum level by 28%; however, this change was not considered clinically relevant.[2]

Despite these findings, one UK manufacturer of lansoprazole suggests that it should not be taken until at least one hour after a dose of antacid,[3] but on the basis of the evidence above, this seems to be an over-cautious recommendation. Furthermore, the US manufacturer makes no such recommendation, and notes that, in clinical studies, there was no evidence of a change in the efficacy of lansoprazole when it was given with antacids.[4]

(b) Omeprazole

Two single-dose studies have shown that *Maalox* suspension (**aluminium/magnesium hydroxide**) did not affect the absorption or disposition of omeprazole from an enteric-coated formulation.[5,6] Similar findings were reported for *Maalox* suspension in another single-dose study, although in contrast, this study found that *Maalox* granules reduced the AUC of omeprazole enteric-coated tablets by 74% and significantly reduced its plasma levels.[7]

A randomised, crossover study in healthy subjects given omeprazole capsules 20 mg daily for 3 days, with two *Gaviscon* tablets (**aluminium hydroxide, magnesium trisilicate** and **sodium alginate**) on day 3, found that omeprazole did not significantly affect the alginate raft formation or the length of time the raft stayed in the stomach.[8] In another study in healthy subjects, the concurrent use of *Gaviscon Advance* (**sodium alginate**) 10 mL four times daily and omeprazole (*Losec MUPS*) 20 mg daily for 3 days did not affect the pharmacokinetics of omeprazole.[9] No additional precautions appear to be necessary if omeprazole is given with these antacids.

(c) Pantoprazole

In a study in 24 healthy subjects, pantoprazole 40 mg daily was given alone and with a 10-mL dose of *Maalox* (**aluminium/magnesium hydroxide**). The AUC, maximum serum levels, and the half-life of pantoprazole were unchanged by the antacid.[10] Therefore, no additional precautions would seem to be necessary if pantoprazole is given with **aluminium/magnesium hydroxide**-containing antacids.

(d) Rabeprazole

In a single-dose study, 12 healthy subjects were, on separate occasions, given 20 mg of rabeprazole alone, with, and one hour after a dose of an **aluminium/magnesium hydroxide** antacid (*Maalox*).[11] The antacid had no effect on the pharmacokinetics of rabeprazole, and therefore no additional precautions would seem to be necessary on concurrent use.

1. Delhotal-Landes B, Cournot A, Vermerie N, Dellatolas F, Benoit M, Flouvat B. The effect of food and antacids on lansoprazole absorption and disposition. *Eur J Drug Metab Pharmacokinet* (1991), Spec No 3, 315–20.
2. Gerloff J, Barth H, Mignot A, Fuchs W, Heintze K. Does the proton pump inhibitor lansoprazole interact with antacids? *Naunyn Schmiedebergs Arch Pharmacol* (1993) 347, R31.
3. Lansoprazole Gastro-resistant Capsules. Zentiva. UK Summary of product characteristics, April 2015.
4. Prevacid (Lansoprazole). Takeda Pharmaceuticals America, Inc. US Prescribing information, August 2010.
5. Tuynman HARE, Festern HPM, Röhss K, Meuwissen SGM. Lack of effect of antacids on plasma concentrations of omeprazole given as enteric-coated granules. *Br J Clin Pharmacol* (1987) 24, 833–5.
6. Howden CW, Reid JL. The effect of antacids and metoclopramide on omeprazole absorption and disposition. *Br J Clin Pharmacol* (1988) 25, 779–80.

7. Iwao K, Saitoh H, Takeda K, Azuumi Y, Takada M. Decreased plasma levels of omeprazole after coadministration with magnesium-aluminium hydroxide dry suspension granules. *Yakugaku Zasshi* (1999) 119, 221–8.
8. Dettmar PW, Little SL, Baxter T. The effect of omeprazole pre-treatment on rafts formed by reflux suppressant tablets containing alginate. *J Int Med Res* (2005) 33, 301–8.
9. Dettmar PW, Hampson FC, Jain A, Choubey S, Little SL, Baxter T. Administration of an alginate based gastric reflux suppressant on the bioavailability of omeprazole. *Indian J Med Res* (2006) 123, 517–24.
10. Hartmann M, Bliesath H, Huber R, Koch H, Steinijans VW, Wurst W. Lack of influence of antacids on the pharmacokinetics of the new gastric H^+/K^+-ATPase inhibitor pantoprazole. *Gastroenterology* (1994) 106 (Suppl), A91.
11. Yasuda S, Higashi S, Murakami M, Tomono Y, Kawaguchi M. Antacids have no influence on the pharmacokinetics of rabeprazole, a new proton pump inhibitor, in healthy volunteers. *Int J Clin Pharmacol Ther* (1999) 37, 249–53.

Proton pump inhibitors + Artemisinin

Artemisinin increases the metabolism of omeprazole resulting in a modest reduction in its exposure.

Clinical evidence

A study in 9 healthy subjects found that artemisinin 250 mg twice daily for 7 days reduced the AUC of a single 20-mg dose of omeprazole by 35%. The pharmacokinetics of the omeprazole metabolites were unchanged, but the ratio of hydroxyomeprazole to omeprazole increased 2.2-fold in those who were extensive CYP2C19 metabolisers (that is, those with normal levels of CYP2C19).[1] As part of the same study, it was found that a single 250-mg dose of artemisinin had no effect on the pharmacokinetics of omeprazole.[1]

A subsequent study in 8 healthy subjects who were extensive CYP2C19 metabolisers similarly found that artemisinin 500 mg daily for 7 days decreased the AUC of both the *S*- and *R*-enantiomers of a single 20-mg dose of omeprazole to the same extent, and increased the oral clearance of both enantiomers about threefold.[2]

Mechanism

The data suggest that artemisinin affects the pharmacokinetics of omeprazole by inducing its metabolism by the cytochrome P450 isoenzyme CYP2C19, although other isoenzymes may also be involved.

Importance and management

Evidence for an interaction between artemisinin and omeprazole is limited, and the clinical relevance of this interaction is unclear; however, as the reduction in omeprazole exposure is modest, and artemisinin is only used short-term, it is probably unlikely to be clinically important.

There appears to be no direct information about other proton pump inhibitors; however, one study found that the effects on the *R*- and *S*-enantiomers of omeprazole were similar, which suggests that **esomeprazole** is likely to behave in the same way as omeprazole.

1. Svensson USH, Ashton M, Hai TN, Bertilsson L, Huong DX, Huong NV, Niêu NT, Sy ND, Lykkesfeldt J, Công LD. Artemisinin induces omeprazole metabolism in human beings. *Clin Pharmacol Ther* (1998) 64, 160–67.
2. Mihara K, Svensson USH, Tybring G, Hai TN, Bertilsson L, Ashton M. Stereospecific analysis of omeprazole supports artemisinin as a potent inducer of CYP2C19. *Fundam Clin Pharmacol* (1999) 13, 671–5.

Proton pump inhibitors + Calcium-channel blockers

The concurrent use of nifedipine and omeprazole appears to slightly reduce the clearance of both drugs. Pantoprazole does not affect the pharmacokinetics of nifedipine, and verapamil does not appear to affect the pharmacokinetics of rabeprazole to a clinically relevant extent.

Clinical evidence, mechanism, importance and management

(a) Omeprazole

In a study in 10 healthy subjects, omeprazole 20 mg daily for 7 days reduced the clearance of **nifedipine** by 21%. In the same subjects, the clearance of a 40-mg intravenous dose of omeprazole was reduced by 14% by **nifedipine** 10 mg three times daily for 5 days.[1] In a related study, the same group of workers found that omeprazole 20 mg daily for 8 days increased the AUC of a single 10-mg dose of **nifedipine** by 26%, but blood pressure and heart rate were unchanged.[2] These changes are minor and would not be expected to be clinically relevant.

(b) Pantoprazole

In a randomised, crossover study, 24 healthy subjects were given pantoprazole 40 mg daily for 10 days, with sustained-release **nifedipine** 20 mg twice daily from day 6 to 10. The pharmacokinetics of **nifedipine** were unchanged by pantoprazole,[3] and therefore, no nifedipine dose adjustment appears to be necessary on the concurrent use of pantoprazole.

(c) Rabeprazole

A study in 19 healthy subjects found that **verapamil** 120 mg twice daily for 6 days did not significantly affect the pharmacokinetics of a single 20-mg dose of rabeprazole, although the AUC of the inactive thioether metabolite was increased about twofold.[4]

The main metabolic pathway of rabeprazole is non-enzymatic reduction to an inactive thioether metabolite, with the cytochrome P450 isoenzymes CYP3A4 and CYP2C19 involved only to a minor extent. The results of this study indicate that verapamil does not appear to affect the metabolism of rabeprazole by CYP3A4, although it may affect the metabolic clearance of the inactive metabolite, rabeprazole thioether.[4] Nevertheless, the available evidence suggests that the dose of rabeprazole will not need adjusting if verapamil is also given.

1. Danhof M, Soons PA, van den Berg G, Van Brummelen P, Jansen JBMJ. Interactions between nifedipine and omeprazole. *Eur J Clin Pharmacol* (1989) 36 (Suppl), A258.
2. Soons PA, van den Berg G, Danhof M, van Brummelen P, Jansen JBMJ, Lamers CBHW, Breimer DD. Influence of single- and multiple-dose omeprazole treatment on nifedipine pharmacokinetics and effects in healthy subjects. *Eur J Clin Pharmacol* (1992) 42, 319–24.
3. Bliesath H, Huber R, Steinijans VW, Koch HJ, Kunz K, Wurst W. Pantoprazole does not interact with nifedipine in man under steady-state conditions. *Int J Clin Pharmacol Ther* (1996) 34, 51–5.
4. Shimizu M, Uno T, Yasui-Furukori N, Sugawara K, Tateishi T. Effects of clarithromycin and verapamil on rabeprazole pharmacokinetics between CYP2C19 genotypes. *Eur J Clin Pharmacol* (2006) 62, 597–603.

Proton pump inhibitors + Drugs that lower magnesium concentrations

Proton pump inhibitors can cause hypomagnesaemia and are predicted to interact with diuretics and other drugs that can cause hypomagnesaemia (e.g. some antineoplastics and antibacterials).

Clinical evidence, mechanism, importance and management

A case series describes 10 patients taking proton pump inhibitors for at least 2 years who developed hypomagnesaemia, severe enough to require emergency hospital admissions: notably 8 of the patients were also taking diuretics.[1] The authors of the study commented on the difficulty correcting the hypomagnesaemia, both oral and intravenous magnesium were reported relatively ineffective; however, stopping the proton pump inhibitor resolved the problem within 2 weeks in 5 patients.[1]

Both proton pump inhibitors and diuretics can cause hypomagnesaemia. These effects appear to be additive when they are used together. Some other drugs that may cause hypomagnesaemia include the aminoglycosides, amphotericin B, carboplatin, cetuximab, ciclosporin, cisplatin, erlotinib, foscarnet, pentamidine, sirolimus, and tacrolimus.[2]

The MHRA in the UK and the FDA in the US have given guidance on this potential interaction, stating that consideration should be given to monitoring magnesium concentrations before starting and intermittently during treatment if a proton pump inhibitor is to be used long term with diuretics or other drugs that can cause hypomagnesaemia.[3,4]. Note that hypomagnesaemia developed after more than one year in most of the cases reviewed by the regulatory authorities, and the authors of the case series advise monitoring annually, or in response to symptoms. It would also be prudent to advise patients to visit their doctor if they experience symptoms of hypomagnesaemia, such as muscle twitching or cramps, tremors, vomiting, tiredness, or loss of appetite.[2,3] In those patients who develop hypomagnesaemia, oral and parenteral magnesium supplements might not be as effective as anticipated. Stopping the proton pump inhibitor (where possible) might be necessary.

1. Mackay JD, Bladon PT. Hypomagnesaemia due to proton-pump inhibitor therapy: a clinical case series. *Q J Med* (2010) 103, 387–95.
2. Lameris AL, Monnens LA, Bindels RJ, Hoenderop JGJ. Drug-induced alterations in Mg2+ homeostasis. *Clin Sci* (2012) 123, 1–14.
3. Medicines and Healthcare Products Regulatory Agency. Proton pump inhibitors in long-term use: reports of hypomagnesaemia. *Drug Safety Update* (2012) 5, 9. Available at: https://www.gov.uk/drug-safety-update/proton-pump-inhibitors-in-long-term-use-reports-of-hypomagnesaemia (accessed 21/10/15).
4. FDA. Drug Safety Communication: Low magnesium levels can be associated with long-term use of proton pump inhibitor drugs (PPIs). March 2, 2011. Available at: www.fda.gov/drugs/drugsafety/ucm245011.htm (accessed 21/10/15).

Proton pump inhibitors + Food

Food modestly to markedly reduces the bioavailability of lansoprazole and esomeprazole, but slightly increases that of dexlansoprazole. Food appears to have no effect on the absorption of omeprazole, pantoprazole, or rabeprazole. Small amounts of foods such as apple sauce, or apple or orange juice, or yoghurt do not seem to significantly affect the bioavailability of esomeprazole, lansoprazole or omeprazole from the contents of the capsules.

Clinical evidence, mechanism, importance and management

(a) Dexlansoprazole

1. Meals. In a single-dose, crossover study in 46 healthy subjects, the AUC of dexlansoprazole was slightly increased by 15%, 21% and 21% when delayed-release dexlansoprazole 90 mg was taken 30 minutes before, 5 minutes before or 30 minutes after a high-fat breakfast, respectively, when compared with the fasted state. There was little difference in pantoprazole effects on intragastric pH between the different administration regimens, although the time spent with a pH greater than 4 was 8% lower when the drug was taken 30 minutes after a meal, when compared with the fasted state, presumably because of the delay in absorption (time to maximum level was delayed by 2 hours).[1]

The increase in exposure to dexlansoprazole and slight delay in absorption seen in this study are unlikely to be of any clinical relevance, and delayed-release dexlansoprazole can be taken without regard to meals.[1,2]

2. Soft foods and beverages. The US manufacturer states that delayed-release dexlansoprazole capsules can be opened and the contents taken with one tablespoon of apple sauce.[2]

(b) Esomeprazole

1. Meals. The AUC of esomeprazole can be reduced by 43 to 53% by food. Because of this, the US manufacturer recommends that esomeprazole *capsules* and *oral suspension* should be taken at least one hour before meals.[3] However, the UK manufacturer notes that, although food delays and decreases the absorption of esomeprazole, this does not appreciably alter the effect of esomeprazole on gastric acidity.[4,5] They therefore make no recommendations about the timing of esomeprazole administration in relation to meals.[4,5]

2. Soft food and beverages. In a crossover study in fasting, healthy subjects, the bioavailability of the contents of an esomeprazole capsule mixed with one tablespoonful of apple sauce were similar to those of an intact esomeprazole capsule taken with water. Apple sauce was chosen because it is acidic and would therefore be unlikely to affect the enteric coating of the esomeprazole granules from the capsule.[6] An *in vitro* study found that esomeprazole enteric-coated granules from an opened capsule were stable when mixed with 100 mL tap water, yoghurt, orange juice or apple juice.[7] The authors suggest that it is likely that esomeprazole could be mixed with these juices or other soft acidic foods in patients who cannot swallow a capsule.[6,7]

On the basis of the clinical study, the US manufacturer permits administration of the contents of the esomeprazole *capsule* with one tablespoonful of apple sauce.[3] However, they still recommend that the *granules for oral suspension* be mixed with 5 to 15 mL of water, depending on the dose.[3] The UK manufacturer recommends dispersing esomeprazole *tablets*[4] or *granules for oral suspension*[5] only in non-carbonated water to avoid dissolving the enteric coating.

(c) Lansoprazole

1. Meals. A study in 12 healthy subjects found that food (a standard meal) reduced lansoprazole bioavailability by 27%.[8] Another study in 12 healthy subjects found a 50% reduction in the bioavailability of a lansoprazole capsule when it was given with food (a standard breakfast).[9] The US manufacturer notes that maximum plasma levels and AUC of lansoprazole were reduced by 50 to 70% when it was given 30 minutes after food, but that no significant effect was found when lansoprazole was given before meals.[10] However, in one study, the efficacy of lansoprazole, measured by intra-gastric pH, seemed to be greater when it was given 15 minutes before breakfast compared with the fasted state. In this study in healthy subjects, gastric pH remained greater than 4 for longer when either lansoprazole or **omeprazole** were taken 15 minutes before breakfast than when they were taken without breakfast (just water), with the next meal being lunch time (median 81% versus 71%, after accounting for the possible effect of the breakfast *per se*). There was no statistically significant difference in findings between those taking lansoprazole and those taking omeprazole, so the results were pooled.[11] In another study, there was no difference in intragastric pH over 24 hours when lansoprazole 15 mg was taken 30 minutes after breakfast, when compared with 60 minutes before dinner.[12]

Nevertheless, some manufacturers recommend that, to achieve optimal efficacy, lansoprazole should be given at least 30 minutes before food, and in the morning if it is to be given once daily.[13,14]

2. Soft food and beverages. In crossover studies in fasting healthy subjects, the bioavailability of enteric-coated granules (removed from a capsule of lansoprazole 30 mg) mixed with either orange juice, tomato juice, or with one tablespoonful of strained pear, yoghurt, cottage cheese, or *Ensure* pudding was comparable to that of an intact capsule given with water.[15,16] These studies suggest that for patients who are unable to swallow or who have difficulty swallowing, mixing the capsule contents with these specific juices or soft foods is acceptable. The US manufacturer permits the intact contents of the *delayed-release capsules* to be mixed in with a small volume (60 mL) of a number of foods or fruit juices including apple sauce, *Ensure* pudding, cottage cheese, or yoghurt. However, they say the *soluble tablets* may be dispersed only in water.[10] One UK manufacturer of lansoprazole recommends that the *gastro-resistant capsules* should be swallowed whole with liquid.[14]

(d) Omeprazole

1. Meals. In a study in 12 healthy subjects, giving a single 20-mg dose of omeprazole as enteric-coated granules with breakfast delayed omeprazole absorption, but did not affect the total amount absorbed.[17] Similarly, in another study in healthy subjects, a standardised breakfast did not affect the bioavailability or maximum plasma level of omeprazole (given as enteric-coated tablets), when compared with the fasting state, or when taken immediately before a meal, although the time to reach the maximum plasma level was increased.[18] Omeprazole may therefore be taken without regard to meals.

For a study suggesting that the effect of omeprazole on intra-gastric pH might be improved by taking it 15 minutes before breakfast, when compared with fasting, see under *Lansoprazole*, above.

2. Soft foods and beverages. For patients unable to swallow the capsule, the manufacturers recommend mixing the intact contents of the opened capsule with non-carbonated water, fruit juice, or apple sauce.[19,20]

(e) Pantoprazole

The manufacturers state that food delays the absorption of pantoprazole from the *tablets* (by 2 hours or more[21]), but has no effect on the total amount absorbed (AUC).[21,22] The US manufacturer recommends that pantoprazole *tablets* are swallowed whole with water, with or without food.[21] However, the UK manufacturer advises taking pantoprazole *tablets* before a meal.[22]

The delayed-release *granules for oral suspension* should be taken 30 minutes before food and should be mixed only with apple juice or one teaspoonful of apple sauce. This is because apple provides an appropriate pH for stability of the granules.[21]

(f) Rabeprazole

A study in healthy subjects found that, although a standard breakfast delayed the absorption of rabeprazole, its AUC and maximum plasma level were not significantly affected.[23] The US manufacturer also reports that a high-fat meal may delay the absorption of rabeprazole without altering its AUC and maximum serum levels.[24] In another study, there was no difference in intragastric pH over 24 hours when rabeprazole 10 mg was taken 30 minutes after breakfast, when compared with 60 minutes before dinner.[12]

Therefore the manufacturers say that rabeprazole tablets may be taken with or without food.[24,25] The UK manufacturer notes that, although food has no effect on the activity of rabeprazole, for once daily regimens they recommend taking it in the morning, before breakfast, to aid compliance.[25]

1. Lee RD, Vakily M, Mulford D, Wu J, Atkinson SN. Clinical trial: the effect and timing of food on the pharmacokinetics and pharmacodynamics of dexlansoprazole MR, a novel dual delayed release formulation of a proton pump inhibitor – evidence for dosing flexibility. *Aliment Pharmacol Ther* (2009) 29, 824–33.
2. Dexilant (Dexlansoprazole). Takeda Pharmaceuticals America, Inc. US Prescribing information, August 2010.
3. Nexium (Esomeprazole magnesium). AstraZeneca Pharmaceuticals LP. US Prescribing information, November 2012.
4. Nexium Tablets (Esomeprazole magnesium trihydrate). AstraZeneca UK Ltd. UK Summary of product characteristics, August2013.
5. Nexium Gastro-resistant Granules (Esomeprazole magnesium trihydrate). AstraZeneca UK Ltd. UK Summary of product characteristics, September 2009.
6. Andersson T, Magner D, Patel J, Rogers P, Levine JG. Esomeprazole 40 mg capsules are bioequivalent when administered intact or as the contents mixed with applesauce. *Clin Drug Invest* (2001) 21, 67–71.
7. Johnson DA, Roach AC, Carlsson AS, Karlsson AAS, Behr DE. Stability of esomeprazole capsule contents after in vitro suspension in common soft foods and beverages. *Pharmacotherapy* (2003) 23, 731–4.
8. Delhotal-Landes B, Cournot A, Vermerie N, Dellatolas F, Benoit M, Flouvat B. The effect of food and antacids on lansoprazole absorption and disposition. *Eur J Drug Metab Pharmacokinet* (1991), Spec No 3, 315–20.
9. Bergstrand R, Grind M, Nyberg G, Olofsson B. Decreased oral bioavailability of lansoprazole in healthy volunteers when given with a standardised breakfast. *Clin Drug Invest* (1995) 9, 67–71.
10. Prevacid (Lansoprazole). Takeda Pharmaceuticals America, Inc. US Prescribing information, August 2010.
11. Hatlebakk JG, Katz PO, Camacho-Lobato L, Castell DO. Proton pump inhibitors: better acid suppression when taken before a meal than without a meal. *Aliment Pharmacol Ther* (2000) 14, 1267–72.
12. Miki M, Adachi K, Azumi T, Koshino K, Furuta K, Kinoshita Y. A comparative study of intragastric acidity during post-breakfast and pre-dinner administration of low-dose proton pump inhibitors: a randomized three-way crossover study. *Aliment Pharmacol Ther* (2006) 24, 1445–51.
13. Zoton (Lansoprazole). Pfizer Ltd. UK Summary of product characteristics, June 2012.
14. Lansoprazole Gastro-resistant Capsules. Zentiva. UK Summary of product characteristics, April 2015.
15. Chun AHC, Erdman K, Chiu YL, Pilmer BL, Achari R, Cavanaugh JH. Bioavailability of lansoprazole granules administered in juice or soft food compared to the intact capsule formulation. *Clin Ther* (2002) 24, 1322–31.
16. Chun AHC, Erdman K, Zhang Y, Achari R, Cavanaugh JH. Effects of bioavailability of admixing the contents of lansoprazole capsules with selected soft foods. *Clin Ther* (2000) 22, 231–6.
17. Röhss K, Andrén K, Heggelund A, Lagerström P-O, Lundborg P. Bioavailability of omeprazole given in conjunction with food. III World Conf Clin Pharmacol Ther, Stockholm July-Aug 1986. *Acta Pharmacol Toxicol (Copenh)* (1986) 85 (Suppl 5), Abstract 207.
18. Thomson ABR, Sinclair P, Matisko A, Rosen E, Andersson T, Olofsson B. Influence of food on the bioavailability of an enteric-coated tablet formulation of omeprazole under repeated dose conditions. *Can J Gastroenterol* (1997) 11, 663–7.
19. Losec Capsules (Omeprazole). AstraZeneca UK Ltd. UK Summary of product characteristics, May 2013.
20. Prilosec (Omeprazole). AstraZeneca. US Prescribing information, March 2010.
21. Protonix (Pantoprazole sodium). Wyeth Pharmaceuticals Inc. US Prescribing information, December 2014.
22. Pantoprazole Gastro-Resistant Tablets (Pantoprazole sodium sesquihydrate). Sandoz Ltd. UK Summary of product characteristics, September 2013.
23. Yasuda S, Ohnishi A, Ogawa T, Tomono Y, Hasegawa J, Nakai H, Shimamura Y, Morishita N. Pharmacokinetic properties of E3810, a new proton pump inhibitor, in healthy male volunteers. *Int J Clin Pharmacol Ther* (1994) 32, 466–73).
24. Aciphex (Rabeprazole sodium). Eisai Inc. US Prescribing information, May 2012.
25. Pariet (Rabeprazole sodium). Eisai Ltd. UK Summary of product characteristics, March 2013.

Proton pump inhibitors + Ginkgo (*Ginkgo biloba*)

Ginkgo induces the metabolism of omeprazole, and this might result in reduced efficacy. Other proton pump inhibitors might be similarly affected.

Clinical evidence

In one study, 18 healthy Chinese subjects were given a single 40-mg dose of omeprazole before and after a 12-day course of a standardised extract of ginkgo 140 mg twice daily. The subjects were divided into three groups: homozygous extensive CYP2C19 metabolisers (6 subjects), heterozygous extensive CYP2C19 metabolisers (5 subjects) and poor CYP2C19 metabolisers (7 subjects). The AUC of omeprazole was modestly decreased by 42%, 27% and 40%, in the homozygous extensive, heterozygous extensive and poor metabolisers, respectively, and the AUC of the sulfone metabolite was reduced by 41%, 36% and 36% in the three groups, respectively. The ratio of the AUC of omeprazole to the sulfone metabolite was therefore not significantly altered by ginkgo. Conversely, the AUC of the inactive metabolite, hydroxyomeprazole, was increased by 38%, 100%, and 232% in the three groups, respectively, resulting in a decrease in the ratio of the AUC of omeprazole to hydroxyomeprazole. Ginkgo also reduced the renal clearance of hydroxyomeprazole. The ginkgo product used in this study contained 22.9% flavonol glycosides and 6.8% terpene lactones (ginkgolides).[1]

Mechanism

It has been suggested that ginkgo might increase the metabolism of omeprazole by inducing its hydroxylation by the cytochrome P450 isoenzyme CYP2C19, although this is not certain, as the effect also occurred in poor CYP2C19 metabolisers (that is, those lacking or with low levels of CYP2C19). Ginkgo does not appear to alter the metabolism of omeprazole to the sulphone by CYP3A4.[1]

Importance and management

This appears to be the only study examining the effects of ginkgo on proton pump inhibitors. However, the reduction seen in the AUC of omeprazole (about 40%) suggest that there is a possibility that omeprazole will be less effective in patients taking ginkgo. As all proton pump inhibitors are metabolised by CYP2C19 to varying extents, it is possible that the effects of ginkgo seen in these studies will be similar with other proton pump inhibitors, although note that the mechanism is not established.

There is insufficient evidence to generally recommend that ginkgo should be avoided in patients taking proton pump inhibitors. However, the potential reduction in the efficacy of the proton pump inhibitor should be borne in mind, particular where the consequences may be serious, such as in patients with healing ulcers.

1. Yin OQP, Tomlinson B, Waye MMY, Chow AHL, Chow MSS. Pharmacogenetics and herb–drug interactions: experience with Ginkgo biloba and omeprazole. *Pharmacogenetics* (2004) 14, 841–50.

Proton pump inhibitors + Grapefruit juice

Grapefruit juice has no clinically relevant effect on the AUC of lansoprazole or omeprazole or their sulfone metabolites.

Clinical evidence

(a) Lansoprazole

In a randomised, crossover study, 21 healthy subjects were given a single 60-mg dose of lansoprazole with either 200 mL of water or freshly-squeezed grapefruit juice. Grapefruit juice slightly increased the AUC of lansoprazole (by 18%) and reduced the formation of its sulfone metabolite. Metabolism to the hydroxyl metabolite was not significantly affected.[1] In another similar study, grapefruit juice had no effect on the pharmacokinetics of either of the enantiomers of lansoprazole (analysed separately).[2]

(b) Omeprazole

In a single-dose study in 12 healthy subjects, grapefruit juice 300 mL had no significant effect on the AUC or half-life of omeprazole 20 mg. However, there was a slight 20% reduction in AUC of omeprazole sulfone.[3]

Mechanism

From the studies above[1,3] it appears that grapefruit juice may have a minor inhibitory effect on the intestinal metabolism of omeprazole and lansoprazole by the cytochrome P450 isoenzyme CYP3A4 (which results in the formation of the sulfone metabolites). Grapefruit juice does not affect the hydroxylation of the proton pump inhibitors by CYP2C19.

Importance and management

Evidence for an interaction between grapefruit juice and the proton pump inhibitors appears to be limited to the studies cited. However, the minor changes in the pharmacokinetics of lansoprazole and omeprazole are not clinically relevant, so it appears that they may be taken with grapefruit juice without the need for any particular precautions.

See also 'Proton pump inhibitors + Food', p.1151, for the finding that other fruit juices had no effect on esomeprazole, lansoprazole or omeprazole bioavailability from gastro-resistant granules.

1. Uno T, Yasui-Furukori N, Takahata T, Sugawara K, Tateishi T. Lack of significant effect of grapefruit juice on the pharmacokinetics of lansoprazole and its metabolites in subjects with different CYP2C19 genotypes. *J Clin Pharmacol* (2005) 45, 690–4.
2. Miura M, Kagaya H, Tada H, Uno T, Yasui-Furukori N, Tateishi T, Suzuki T. Intestinal CYP3A4 is not involved in the enantioselective disposition of lansoprazole. *Xenobiotica* (2006) 36, 95–102.
3. Tassaneeyakul W, Tassaneeyakul W, Vannaprasaht S, Yamazoe Y. Formation of omeprazole sulphone but not 5-hydroxyomeprazole is inhibited by grapefruit juice. *Br J Clin Pharmacol* (2000) 49, 139–44.

Proton pump inhibitors + Macrolides

Clarithromycin increases the levels of esomeprazole, lansoprazole and omeprazole, but has no significant effect on the pharmacokinetics of pantoprazole or rabeprazole. Esomeprazole, lansoprazole, omeprazole and rabeprazole may cause a small rise in the serum levels of clarithromycin and/or its active metabolite.

Limited evidence indicates that erythromycin raises omeprazole levels. Lansoprazole and omeprazole do not appear to alter the pharmacokinetics of roxithromycin.

Clinical evidence

(a) Clarithromycin

See also 'Proton pump inhibitors + Penicillins', p.1154, which describes case reports of glossitis, stomatitis and a black tongue when lansoprazole was given with antibacterial regimens including clarithromycin.

1. Esomeprazole. In a study in 18 healthy subjects, the AUC, maximum serum levels and half-life of esomeprazole 40 mg daily, taken for 7 days, were increased by 70%, 18% and 35%, respectively, when clarithromycin 500 mg twice daily and amoxicillin 1 g twice daily for 7 days were also taken. When the study was repeated in 19 healthy subjects who were extensive CYP2C19 metabolisers (that is, those with normal levels of CYP2C19), clarithromycin increased the AUC, maximum serum levels and half-life of esomeprazole by 127%, 39% and 50%, respectively. Similar increases in esomeprazole levels (e.g. AUC doubled) were seen when a further 6 subjects who were poor CYP2C19 metabolisers (that is, those lacking or with low levels of CYP2C19) were given clarithromycin.[1] In these studies, esomeprazole did not alter clarithromycin levels,[1] but the manufacturer notes that the AUC of the active hydroxyclarithromycin metabolite was slightly increased, by about 20%.[2]

2. Lansoprazole. In a crossover study in healthy subjects,[3] the AUC of a single 60-mg dose of lansoprazole was raised by 55 to 80% by clarithromycin 500 mg twice daily for 6 days in both extensive CYP2C19 metabolisers and poor CYP2C19 metabolisers (that is, those with normal levels and those lacking or with low levels of CYP2C19, respectively). In another crossover study in healthy subjects, the AUC of lansoprazole 30 mg twice daily was increased by 25% by clarithromycin 500 mg twice daily and amoxicillin 1 g twice daily for 4 days. The AUC of the hydroxyl metabolite of clarithromycin was also increased, by about 25%.[4] Conversely, a study found that lansoprazole 60 mg daily for 5 days slightly reduced the AUC of clarithromycin by 10% and 30% in healthy subjects and *H. pylori*-positive subjects, respectively. In this study, the AUC of the hydroxyl metabolite of clarithromycin was not measured.[5] Another study generally reflects these findings.[6]

3. Omeprazole. When 11 healthy subjects taking omeprazole 40 mg daily were also given clarithromycin 500 mg every 8 hours for 5 days, the maximum plasma levels of omeprazole rose by 30% and its AUC_{0-24} rose by 89%, but the effect of omeprazole on gastric pH was unchanged. The clarithromycin and 4-hydroxyclarithromycin AUC_{0-8} were increased by 15% and 48%, respectively, and there was a marked increase in levels in the gastric mucus.[7] In a similar study, approximately twofold increases in the AUC of omeprazole were reported irrespective of CYP2C19 metaboliser status.[8] In another study in 8 subjects (all extensive CYP2C19 metabolisers), clarithromycin 500 mg twice daily for 7 days caused a similar twofold increase in the AUC of omeprazole 20 mg twice daily. However, in this study the levels of clarithromycin were not affected by the proton pump inhibitor.[9]

In yet another study, omeprazole 20 mg daily for 7 days also had no effect on the plasma pharmacokinetics of clarithromycin. However, this study found that omeprazole caused a twofold increase in intragastric levels (AUC_{0-2}).[10] However, a further study found that omeprazole 40 mg twice daily for 5 days did not alter the pharmacokinetics of a single 500-mg dose of intravenous clarithromycin in either gastric juice, or plasma.[11]

4. Pantoprazole. In a study in 8 subjects, clarithromycin 500 mg twice daily for 7 days did not affect the AUC of pantoprazole 40 mg twice daily. The levels of clarithromycin were not affected by pantoprazole. The subjects in this study were all extensive CYP2C19 metabolisers (that is, they had normal levels of CYP2C19).[9]

5. Rabeprazole. A study in 19 healthy subjects found that clarithromycin 400 mg twice daily for 6 days did not significantly affect the pharmacokinetics of a single 20-mg dose of rabeprazole, irrespective of CYP2C19 metaboliser status, although levels of the inactive thioether were increased.[12]

The US manufacturer reports that, in a crossover study in 16 healthy subjects, rabeprazole had no effect on the AUC of clarithromycin, but increased the AUC of its 4-hydroxyclarithromycin metabolite by about 40%. The AUC and maximum plasma level of rabeprazole were also increased, by 11% and 34%, respectively, by clarithromycin.[13]

(b) Erythromycin

A study in one patient found that erythromycin base 500 mg daily and **omeprazole** 20 mg daily for 8 weeks increased the AUC of **omeprazole** almost fourfold. The AUC of the sulfone metabolite of **omeprazole** was undetectable.[14]

(c) Roxithromycin

In a study, when roxithromycin 300 mg twice daily was given with **omeprazole** 20 mg twice daily or **lansoprazole** 30 mg twice daily for 6 days, the pharmacokinetics of roxithromycin were unchanged.[15]

Mechanism

Clarithromycin appears to inhibit the metabolism of esomeprazole, lansoprazole and omeprazole by the cytochrome P450 isoenzyme CYP3A4, one of the isoenzymes involved in their metabolism, although inhibition of P-glycoprotein might also be involved.[3] Pantoprazole appears not to be affected. The main metabolic pathway of rabeprazole is non-enzymatic reduction to an inactive thioether metabolite, with CYP3A4 and CYP2C19 involved only to a minor extent. Therefore, clarithromycin has only minor effects on the metabolism of rabeprazole.

Erythromycin interacts in a similar way to clarithromycin.

Importance and management

The pharmacokinetic interactions between clarithromycin and omeprazole, esomeprazole and lansoprazole are established. However, none of the changes reported represents an adverse interaction, but they may help to explain why concurrent use is valuable in the eradication of *Helicobacter pylori*. Erythromycin is likely to interact similarly, whereas roxithromycin does not appear to interact.

No clinically significant interaction appears to occur between rabeprazole or pantoprazole and clarithromycin.

1. Hassan-Alin M, Andersson T, Niazi M, Liljeblad M, Persson BA, Röhss K. Studies on drug interactions between esomeprazole, amoxicillin and clarithromycin in healthy subjects. *Int J Clin Pharmacol Ther* (2006) 44, 119–27.

2. Nexium (Esomeprazole magnesium). AstraZeneca Pharmaceuticals LP. US Prescribing information, November 2012.
3. Saito M, Yasui-Furukori N, Uno T, Takahata T, Sugawara K, Munakata A, Tateishi T. Effects of clarithromycin on lansoprazole pharmacokinetics between CYP2C19 genotypes. *Br J Clin Pharmacol* (2005) 59, 302–9.
4. Mainz D, Borner K, Koeppe P, Kotwas J, Lode H. Pharmacokinetics of lansoprazole, amoxicillin and clarithromycin after simultaneous and single administration. *J Antimicrob Chemother* (2002) 50, 699–706.
5. Ortiz RAM, Calafatti SA, Moraes LA, Deguer M, Ecclissato CC, Marchioretto MAM, Ribeiro ML, Bernasconi G, Pedrazzoli J. Effect of *Helicobacter pylori* infection and acid blockade by lansoprazole on clarithromycin bioavailability. *Braz J Med Biol Res* (2007) 40, 383–9.
6. Ushiama H, Echizen H, Nachi S, Ohnishi A. Dose-dependent inhibition of CYP3A activity by clarithromycin during *Helicobacter pylori* eradication therapy assessed by changes in plasma lansoprazole levels and partial cortisol clearance to 6β-hydrocortisol. *Clin Pharmacol Ther* (2002) 72, 33–43.
7. Gustavson LE, Kaiser JF, Edmonds AL, Locke CS, DeBartolo ML, Schneck DW. Effect of omeprazole on concentrations of clarithromycin in plasma and gastric tissue at steady state. *Antimicrob Agents Chemother* (1995) 39, 2078–83.
8. Furuta T, Ohashi K, Kobayashi K, Iida I, Yoshida H, Shirai N, Takashima M, Kosuge K, Hanai H, Chiba K, Ishizaki T, Kaneko E. Effects of clarithromycin on the metabolism of omeprazole in relation to CYP2C19 genotype status in humans. *Clin Pharmacol Ther* (1999) 66, 265–74.
9. Calabresi L, Pazzucconi F, Ferrara S, di Paolo A, Del Tacca M, Sirtori C. Pharmacokinetic interactions between omeprazole/pantoprazole and clarithromycin in healthy volunteers. *Pharmacol Res* (2004) 49, 493–9.
10. Pedrazzoli J, Calafatti SA, Ortiz RAM, Dias FE, Deguer M, Mendes FD, Bento AP, Pereira AA, Piovesana H, Ferraz JGP, Lerner F, de Nucci G. Transfer of clarithromycin to gastric juice is enhanced by omeprazole in *Helicobacter pylori*-infected individuals. *Scand J Gastroenterol* (2001) 36, 1248–53.
11. Goddard AF, Jessa MJ, Barrett DA, Shaw PN, Idström J-P, Cederberg C, Spiller RC. Effect of omeprazole on the distribution of metronidazole, amoxicillin, and clarithromycin in human gastric juice. *Gastroenterology* (1996) 111, 358–67.
12. Shimizu M, Uno T, Yasui-Furukori N, Sugawara K, Tateishi T. Effects of clarithromycin and verapamil on rabeprazole pharmacokinetics between CYP2C19 genotypes. *Eur J Clin Pharmacol* (2006) 62, 597–603.
13. Aciphex (Rabeprazole sodium). Eisai Inc. US Prescribing information, May 2012.
14. Salcedo JA, Benjamin SB, Maher KA, Sukhova N. Erythromycin inhibits the metabolism of omeprazole. *Gastroenterology* (1997) 112 (4 Suppl), A277.
15. Kees F, Holstege A, Ittner KP, Zimmermann M, Lock G, Schölmerich J, Grobecker H. Pharmacokinetic interaction between proton pump inhibitors and roxithromycin in volunteers. *Aliment Pharmacol Ther* (2000) 14, 407–12.

Proton pump inhibitors + Mosapride

Mosapride moderately increases the absorption of omeprazole and rabeprazole.

Clinical evidence, mechanism, importance and management

In a study, 9 healthy subjects were given a single 20-mg dose of **omeprazole** alone or one hour before a single 5-mg dose of mosapride. The peak levels and AUC of omeprazole were increased by 45% and 65%, respectively, when given with mosapride. It was suggested that mosapride increased **omeprazole** absorption by increasing gastric emptying.[1]

In a single-dose study in 9 healthy subjects, **rabeprazole** 20 mg was given alone or with mosapride 5 mg. Mosapride increased the AUC and maximum concentration of **rabeprazole** by 47% and 57%, respectively.[2]

The clinical relevance of these interactions have not been studied; however, the increases reported are modest and as the proton pump inhibitors generally have a wide therapeutic margin. Therefore an increase in adverse effects would not be expected, and the interaction might in fact be beneficial.[2]

1. Takeuchi Y, Watanabe H, Imawari M. Mosapride citrate, a serotonin HT4 selective agonist, beneficially [sic] affects pharmacokinetics of proton pump inhibitor. *Gastroenterology* (2005) 128 (Suppl 2), A-531.
2. Arai K, Takeuchi Y, Watanabe H, Tsukurimichi A, Uchida N, Imawari M. Prokinetics influence the pharmacokinetics of rabeprazole. *Digestion* (2008) 78, 67–71.

Proton pump inhibitors + Penicillins

Esomeprazole, lansoprazole and omeprazole do not alter the pharmacokinetics of amoxicillin, and omeprazole does not alter ampicillin or bacampicillin bioavailability.

Isolated reports describe glossitis, stomatitis and/or black tongue in a small number of patients given lansoprazole and antibacterials, which included amoxicillin, clarithromycin and metronidazole.

Clinical evidence

(a) Pharmacokinetic interactions

1. Amoxicillin. A study in 12 healthy subjects found no significant changes in the pharmacokinetics of amoxicillin 1 g twice daily when it was given with **lansoprazole** 30 mg twice daily and clarithromycin 500 mg twice daily for 4 days.[1]

Other randomised, crossover studies in a total of 36 healthy subjects also found no changes in the oral bioavailability or half-life of amoxicillin 1 g twice daily when it was given with clarithromycin 500 mg twice daily and **esomeprazole**, either 20 mg twice daily or 40 mg once daily for 7 days.[2] Similarly, in another study, **omeprazole** 40 mg twice daily for 5 days did not alter the pharmacokinetics of amoxicillin 750 mg twice daily for 5 days, although the mean serum level of **omeprazole** was 12% lower and intragastric pH was slightly lower with the combination, than with omeprazole alone. This was felt to be partly due to suppression of *H. pylori.*[3] In a placebo-controlled study in 12 patients with non-ulcer dyspepsia, serum levels of a single 1-g oral dose of amoxicillin were not affected by pre-treatment with **omeprazole** 20 mg twice daily for one week.[4]

Other studies have confirmed the lack of effect of **omeprazole** on the AUC of amoxicillin pharmacokinetics.[5-7] In one of these studies, amoxicillin levels were detected in gastric juice after intravenous dosing, and were higher during **omeprazole** administration,[6] but, conversely, in another study, no amoxicillin was detected in gastric juice after intravenous administration, either when given alone or with **omeprazole.**[7] Gastric mucosa levels of amoxicillin have been reported to be unaffected by **omeprazole.**[4,8]

2. Ampicillin. In a crossover study in 28 healthy subjects, oral omeprazole 20 mg daily for 7 days had no effect on the plasma AUC of a single 1-g intravenous dose of ampicillin. No ampicillin was detected in gastric juice either when given alone or with omeprazole. There was no difference in findings between *H. pylori* infected individuals and those not infected with *H. pylori.*[7]

3. Bacampicillin. In a study in healthy subjects, **omeprazole** 20 mg daily for a week slightly delayed the absorption of a single oral dose of **bacampicillin**, as indicated by a reduction of about 10% in the maximum level and increase in time to maximum level, but the total amount absorbed (AUC) was not reduced.[5]

(b) Stomatitis and similar adverse effects

Six cases of glossitis, stomatitis and/or black tongue were reported to the Sicilian Regional Pharmacovigilance Centre in patients taking **lansoprazole** and antibacterials used to treat *H. pylori* infections. All 6 patients had been given daily doses of **lansoprazole** 60 mg with clarithromycin 1 g and either metronidazole 1 g (3 patients) or **amoxicillin** 2 g (3 patients) for one week, after which the antibacterials were stopped. The **lansoprazole** was continued at 30 mg daily for periods of up to 3 weeks. The glossitis (1 patient), black tongue (3 patients) and stomatitis (2 patients) developed between days 2 and 19 of the courses of treatment.[9] In one small randomised study, 9 cases of glossitis occurred when **lansoprazole** was given with **amoxicillin** but none occurred with **lansoprazole** alone.[10]

Mechanism

Unknown.

Importance and management

Cases of glossitis, stomatitis and black tongue reported with lansoprazole and antibacterials appear to be rare. No new cases appear to have been published since these reports, even though these drug combinations are commonly used for the eradication of *H. pylori*. Just why these drugs cause these adverse effects, and whether they are due to just one drug or to an interaction is not understood. Note that the CSM in the UK have received reports of stomatitis, glossitis and a black, hairy tongue or discoloration with each of the reported drugs individually, but these are also rare effects.[11]

The pharmacokinetics of amoxicillin do not appear to be affected by the concurrent use of esomeprazole, lansoprazole and omeprazole, and omeprazole pharmacokinetics were not affected by amoxicillin.

1. Mainz D, Borner K, Koeppe P, Kotwas J, Lode H. Pharmacokinetics of lansoprazole, amoxicillin and clarithromycin after simultaneous and single administration. *J Antimicrob Chemother* (2002) 50, 699–706.
2. Hassan-Alin M, Andersson T, Niazi M, Liljeblad M, Persson BA, Röhss K. Studies on drug interactions between esomeprazole, amoxicillin and clarithromycin in healthy subjects. *Int J Clin Pharmacol Ther* (2006) 44, 119–27.
3. Pommerien W, Braun M, Idström JP, Wrangstadh M, Londong W. Pharmacokinetic and pharmacodynamic interactions between omeprazole and amoxycillin in Helicobacter pylori-positive healthy subjects. *Aliment Pharmacol Ther* (1996) 10, 295–301.
4. Wittayalertpanya S, Wannachai N, Thongnopnua P, Mahachai V. Effect of omeprazole on gastric mucosa and serum levels of amoxicillin in patients with non-ulcer dyspepsia. *J Med Assoc Thai* (2000) 83, 611–8.
5. Paulsen O, Högland P, Walder M. No effect of omeprazole-induced hypoacidity on the bioavailability of amoxycillin and bacampicillin. *Scand J Infect Dis* (1989) 21, 219–23.
6. Goddard AF, Jessa MJ, Barrett DA, Shaw PN, Idström J-P, Wason C, Wrangstadh M, Spiller RC. Effect of omeprazole on the distribution of antibiotics in gastric juice. *Gastroenterology* (1995) 108 (Suppl), A102.
7. Ortiz RAM, Calafatti SA, Corazzi A, Souza JM, Deguer M, De Souza CAF, Marchioretto MAM, Bernasconi G, Ferraz JGP, Pedrazzoli J. Amoxicillin and ampicillin are not transferred to gastric juice irrespective of Helicobacter pylori status or acid blockade by omeprazole. *Aliment Pharmacol Ther* (2002) 16, 1163–70.
8. Cardaci G, Lambert JR, Aranda-Michel J, Underwood B. Omeprazole has no effect on the gastric mucosal bioavailability of amoxycillin. *Gut* (1995) 37 (Suppl 1), A90.
9. Greco S, Mazzaglia G, Caputi AP, Pagliaro L. Glossitis, stomatitis and black tongue with lansoprazole plus clarithromycin and other antibiotics. *Ann Pharmacother* (1997) 31, 1548.
10. Hatlebakk JG, Nesje LB, Hausken T, Bang CJ, Berstad A. Lansoprazole capsules and amoxicillin oral suspension in the treatment of peptic ulcer disease. *Scand J Gastroenterol* (1995) 30, 1053–7.
11. Drug analysis prints (Amoxicillin, clarithromycin, lansoprazole and metronidazole). Medicines and Healthcare Regulatory Agency, UK. Available at: http://www.mhra.gov.uk/drug-analysis-prints/ (accessed 21/10/15).

Proton pump inhibitors + SSRIs

Fluvoxamine moderately to markedly increases the exposure to the proton pump inhibitors lansoprazole, omeprazole, and rabeprazole in most patients. Theoretically, other proton pump inhibitors might be similarly affected. Omeprazole slightly to moderately increases the exposure to citalopram and escitalopram. A case report suggests that esomeprazole might affect escitalopram similarly, and concurrent use resulted in serotonin syndrome. Pantoprazole does not appear to alter the pharmacokinetics of vilazodone.

Clinical evidence

(a) Citalopram

In a crossover study, 9 healthy subjects (all CYP2C19 extensive metabolisers) were given **omeprazole** 20 mg daily for 18 days, with a single 20-mg dose of citalopram on day 8. **Omeprazole** increased the mean AUC of *S*-citalopram 2.2-fold, without affecting the AUC of *R*-citalopram to a statistically significant extent.[1] In a prospective study in 201 elderly patients, the QTcF interval (Fridericia's correction) was 30.2 milliseconds longer in 23 patients taking citalopram 10 mg daily with **ome-**

prazole 20 mg daily, than in 129 control patients not taking either of these drugs. Further, it was estimated that the risk of developing a QTcF interval greater than 450 milliseconds was almost 3-fold higher in those taking both these drugs.[2]

(b) Escitalopram

In a study in healthy subjects, **omeprazole** 30 mg daily for 6 days increased the AUC of a single 20-mg dose of escitalopram, given on day 5, by 50%.[3]

A case report describes serotonin syndrome in a 46-year-old woman who had been taking escitalopram 10 mg twice daily for 5 years and was started on **esomeprazole** 40 mg daily. Symptoms developed about one week later and the escitalopram was stopped. Twelve hours later, her escitalopram serum concentration was supratherapeutic (695 nanomol/L). Her escitalopram serum concentration had been therapeutic (52 nanomol/L) 3 days before starting esomeprazole, but 2 days after starting esomeprazole the concentration had increased to 619 nanomol/L. The patient was also found to be a CYP2C19 and CYP2D6 poor metaboliser, that is she had lower than normal activity of both of these isoenzymes.[4]

(c) Fluoxetine

In a study in 18 healthy subjects, fluoxetine 60 mg daily for 8 days increased the AUC and maximum concentration of a single 30-mg dose of **lansoprazole** 2.6-fold and by 68%, respectively.[5]

(d) Fluvoxamine

Several studies in healthy subjects have investigated the effects of fluvoxamine (a CYP2C19 inhibitor) on the metabolism of proton pump inhibitors. In these studies, fluvoxamine 25 mg twice daily for 6 days altered the pharmacokinetics of three different proton pump inhibitors in patients who were extensive CYP2C19 metabolisers (that is, those with normal activity of CYP2C19) as follows:

- **Lansoprazole**: fluvoxamine increased the AUC and elimination half-life of a single 40-mg dose of lansoprazole 3.8-fold and 3-fold, respectively;[6]
- **Omeprazole**: fluvoxamine increased the AUC, half-life, and maximum plasma concentration of a single 40-mg dose of omeprazole 6-fold, 2.6-fold, and 3.7-fold, respectively;[7]
- **Rabeprazole**: fluvoxamine increased the AUC, elimination half-life, and maximum plasma concentration of a single 20-mg dose of rabeprazole 2.8-fold, 2.4-fold, and 2-fold, respectively.[8]

These pharmacokinetic changes essentially had the effect of turning the extensive metabolisers into poor metabolisers[6-8] (that is, those with lower than normal activity of CYP2C19). In contrast, in patients who were CYP2C19 poor metabolisers, fluvoxamine did not have any effect on the pharmacokinetics of these three proton pump inhibitors.[6-8]

In an earlier study, 12 healthy subjects (7 CYP2C19 extensive metabolisers and 5 CYP2C19 poor metabolisers) were given fluvoxamine 10 to 50 mg daily for 7 days, with a single 20-mg dose of **omeprazole** on day 7. The AUC of **omeprazole** was increased nearly 3-fold by fluvoxamine 10 to 20 mg and over 4-fold by fluvoxamine 25 to 50 mg (all subjects combined).[9]

(e) Vilazodone

The US manufacturer of vilazodone briefly notes that **pantoprazole** does not alter the pharmacokinetics of vilazodone.[10]

Mechanism

All proton pump inhibitors are primarily metabolised by CYP2C19, which is subject to genetic polymorphism, see *Interactions of proton pump inhibitors*, under 'Gastrointestinal drugs', p.1135. As fluvoxamine inhibits CYP2C19, it can increase the exposure to the proton pump inhibitors in patients who are CYP2C19 extensive metabolisers, but does not affect the pharmacokinetics of proton pump inhibitors in patients who are CYP2C19 poor metabolisers. Fluoxetine is not known to inhibit CYP2C19 to a clinically relevant extent, and therefore the mechanism behind the increased exposure of lansoprazole is not known.

Omeprazole is also an inhibitor of CYP2C19, and therefore increases the exposure of the SSRIs, citalopram and escitalopram, which are metabolised by this route. Esomeprazole inhibits CYP2C19 and this, together with the poor CYP2C19 metaboliser status of the patient in the case report,[4] most likely led to the greatly increased escitalopram concentrations and serotonin syndrome.

Importance and management

The interaction between **fluvoxamine** with the proton pump inhibitors appears to be established. However, the increased exposure to these proton pump inhibitors seen in CYP2C19 extensive metabolisers taking fluvoxamine is similar to that seen in CYP2C19 poor metabolisers not taking fluvoxamine, and is unlikely to lead to an increase in adverse effects because of the wide therapeutic margin of proton pump inhibitors. Nevertheless, at least one UK manufacturer of lansoprazole suggests considering decreasing the dose of the proton pump inhibitor in patients taking fluvoxamine.[11] The moderate increase in lansoprazole exposure seen in the study with **fluoxetine** appears to occur via an as yet unknown mechanism, and given the apparent lack of other studies and case reports demonstrating a clinically important interaction between these two well-used drugs, the general clinical importance of this would seem limited. Further study is required to establish the mechanism behind this effect.

Omeprazole causes a slight to moderate increase in the exposure to the active *S*-enantiomer of **citalopram** and to **escitalopram**. As **citalopram** is known to cause a dose-dependent increase in the QT interval, in 2012 the FDA advised that the maximum dose of citalopram in patients taking a CYP2C19 inhibitor [which would include omeprazole] should be 20 mg daily because concurrent use can lead to increased citalopram concentrations and increase the risk of QT interval prolongation and Torsade de pointes.[12] See 'Table 1.6', p.8 for a list of other CYP2C19 inhibitors. However, the UK manufacturer of citalopram[13] suggests caution, and that a dose adjustment of citalopram might be needed. The clinical relevance of the finding with **escitalopram** is unclear, and the UK manufacturer[14] gives the same advice as that for citalopram. The case report describing serotonin syndrome in a patient taking escitalopram and esomeprazole also suggests some caution with this combination. Until more is known, be alert for an increase in citalopram or escitalopram adverse effects (such as dry mouth, increased sweating, insomnia) if omeprazole or esomeprazole is also given, decreasing the dose of the SSRI if these become troublesome.

The pharmacokinetics of **vilazodone** were not affected by **pantoprazole** and so no vilazodone dose adjustment is required on concurrent use.[10]

1. Rocha, A, Coelho EB, Sampaio SA, Lanchote VL. Omeprazole preferentially inhibits the metabolism of (+)-(S)-citalopram in healthy volunteers. *Br J Clin Pharmacol* (2010) 70, 43–51.
2. Lozano R, Bibian C, Quilez RM, Gil J, Constante Y, Garcia-Arilla E. Clinical relevance of the (S)-citalopram-omeprazole interaction in geriatric patients. *Br J Clin Pharmacol* (2013) 77, 1086–7.
3. Malling D, Poulsen MN, Søgaard B. The effect of cimetidine or omeprazole on the pharmacokinetics of escitalopram in healthy subjects. *Br J Clin Pharmacol* (2005) 60, 287–90.
4. Lorenzini KI, Calmy A, Ambrosioni J, Assouline B, Daali Y, Fathi M, Rebsamen M, Desmeules J, Samer CF, Serotonin syndrome following drug-drug interactions and CYP2D6 and CYP2C19 genetic polymorphisms in an HIV-infected patient. *AIDS* (2012) 26, 2417–8.
5. Vlase L, Popa A, Neag M, Muntean D, Leucuta SE. Effect of fluoxetine on the pharmacokinetics of lansoprazole. A two-treatment period study in healthy male subjects. *Clin Drug Investig* (2011) 31, 727–33.
6. Yasui-Furukori N, Saito M, Uno T, Takahata T, Sugawara K, Tateishi T. Effects of fluvoxamine on lansoprazole pharmacokinetics in relation to CYP2C19 genotypes. *J Clin Pharmacol* (2004) 44, 1223–9.
7. Yasui-Furukori N, Takahata T, Nakagami T, Yoshiya G, Inoue Y, Kaneko S, Tateishi T. Different inhibitory effect of fluvoxamine on omeprazole metabolism between CYP2C19 genotypes. *Br J Clin Pharmacol* (2004) 57, 487–94.
8. Uno T, Shimizu M, Yasui-Furukori N, Sugawara K, Tateishi T. Different effects of fluvoxamine on rabeprazole pharmacokinetics in relation to CYP2C19 genotype status. *Br J Clin Pharmacol* (2006) 61, 309–14.
9. Christensen M, Tybring G, Mihara K, Yasui-Furokori N, Carrillo JA, Ramos SI, Andersson K, Dahl M-L, Bertilsson L. Low daily 10-mg and 20-mg doses of fluvoxamine inhibit the metabolism of both caffeine (cytochrome P4501A2) and omeprazole (cytochrome P4502C19). *Clin Pharmacol Ther* (2002) 71, 141–52.
10. Viibryd (Vilazodone hydrochloride). Forest Pharmaceuticals, Inc. US Prescribing information, March 2015.
11. Lansoprazole Gastro-resistant Capsules. Zentiva. UK Summary of product characteristics, April 2015.
12. FDA. Drug safety communication: Revised recommendations for Celexa (citalopram hydrochloride) related to a potential risk of abnormal heart rhythms with high doses. March 28, 2012. Available at: http://www.fda.gov/Drugs/DrugSafety/ucm297391.htm (accessed 06/10/15).
13. Cipramil Tablets (Citalopram hydrobromide). Lundbeck Ltd. UK Summary of product characteristics, July 2015.
14. Cipralex Tablets (Escitalopram oxalate). Lundbeck Ltd. UK Summary of product characteristics, September 2013.

Proton pump inhibitors + St John's wort (*Hypericum perforatum*)

St John's wort induces the metabolism of omeprazole, and this might result in reduced efficacy. Other proton pump inhibitors are likely to be similarly affected.

Clinical evidence

In a crossover study, 12 healthy subjects were given St John's wort 300 mg three times daily or placebo for 14 days, followed by a single 20-mg dose of omeprazole on day 15. Six of the subjects in this study were CYP2C19 extensive metabolisers (that is, they had normal levels of this isoenzyme) and 6 were poor CYP2C19 metabolisers (that is, those lacking or with low levels of CYP2C19). St John's wort modestly decreased the AUC of omeprazole in all subjects (by 49% in extensive metabolisers and 41% in poor metabolisers), and also increased the plasma levels of the inactive metabolite, hydroxyomeprazole by 35%, only in those who were extensive metabolisers. It also markedly increased the levels of the inactive sulfone metabolite of omeprazole in both extensive and poor metabolisers (about 2.5-fold and 2.3-fold, respectively). The St John's wort product used in this study contained 0.3% total hypericin and a minimum of 4% hyperforin.[1]

Mechanism

St John's wort increases the metabolism of omeprazole by inducing both its hydroxylation by the cytochrome P450 isoenzyme CYP2C19 and, to a greater extent, its sulfoxidation by CYP3A4.[1]

Importance and management

This appears to be the only study examining the effects of St John's wort on the proton pump inhibitors. However, the reduction seen in the AUC of omeprazole (about 40%) suggests that there is a possibility that omeprazole will be less effective in patients taking St John's wort. As all proton pump inhibitors are, to varying extents, metabolised by CYP2C19 and CYP3A4, it is likely that the effects of St John's wort seen in these studies will be similar with other proton pump inhibitors.

There is insufficient evidence to suggest that St John's wort should be avoided in patients taking proton pump inhibitors. However, the potential reduction in the efficacy of the proton pump inhibitor should be borne in mind, particular where the consequences may be serious, such as in patients with healing ulcers.

1. Wang LS, Zhou G, Zhu B, Wu J, Wang JG, Abd El-Aty AM, Li T, Liu J, Yang TL, Wang D, Zhong XY, Zhou HH. St John's wort induces both cytochrome P450 3A4–catalyzed sulfoxidation and 2C19–dependent hydroxylation of omeprazole. *Clin Pharmacol Ther* (2004) 75, 191–7.

Proton pump inhibitors + Sucralfate

Sucralfate causes a minor reduction in the bioavailability of lansoprazole and omeprazole.

Clinical evidence, mechanism, importance and management

In a single-dose, crossover study, sucralfate 1 g delayed the absorption of **lansoprazole** 30 mg and **omeprazole** 20 mg and reduced their bioavailability by 17% and 16%, respectively.[1]

The minor reduction in the bioavailability of **lansoprazole** and **omeprazole** in the presence of sucralfate is unlikely to be clinically relevant. Nevertheless, at least one UK manufacturer of **lansoprazole** recommends that it should be taken at least one hour after sucralfate,[2] and the US manufacturer recommends that **lansoprazole** should be taken at least 30 minutes before sucralfate.[1] This seems very cautious.

1. Prevacid (Lansoprazole). Takeda Pharmaceuticals America, Inc. US Prescribing information, August 2010.
2. Zoton (Lansoprazole). Pfizer Ltd. UK Summary of product characteristics, June 2012.

Proton pump inhibitors + Ticlopidine

Ticlopidine markedly decreases the clearance and increases the bioavailability of omeprazole in most patients. Theoretically other proton pump inhibitors may be similarly affected.

Clinical evidence

In a study, 6 healthy subjects were given ticlopidine 100 mg three times daily with a single 40-mg dose of **omeprazole** on day 7. Ticlopidine increased the AUC_{0-8} of **omeprazole** by about 76%, and reduced its clearance in 5 out of the 6 subjects. In this study, all of the subjects were extensive CYP2C19 metabolisers (that is, they had normal levels of CYP2C19).[1] In another study, 18 healthy subjects were given ticlopidine 200 mg daily with **omeprazole** 20 mg taken on day 8. Ticlopidine markedly increased the AUC of **omeprazole** in the 12 subjects that were extensive CYP2C19 metabolisers about five- to sixfold, but did not alter **omeprazole** levels in the poor CYP2C19 metaboliser group (that is, those patients lacking or with low levels of CYP2C19). The AUC of omeprazole in the extensive metabolisers given ticlopidine was similar to that in poor metabolisers (with or without ticlopidine). No adverse effects due to either **omeprazole** or ticlopidine were reported.[2]

Mechanism

Omeprazole is principally metabolised by the cytochrome P450 isoenzyme CYP2C19 to 5-hydroxyomeprazole. Poor CYP2C19 metabolisers (that is those lacking or with low levels of this isoenzyme) have higher levels of omeprazole than extensive CYP2C19 metabolisers. When extensive CYP2C19 metabolisers are given ticlopidine, a CYP2C19 inhibitor, they are effectively changed in to poor metabolisers, with a corresponding increase in omeprazole levels.

Other proton pump inhibitors that are metabolised by CYP2C19, see *Interactions of proton pump inhibitors*, under 'Gastrointestinal drugs', p.1135, would be expected to be similarly affected.

Importance and management

An interaction between omeprazole and ticlopidine is established; however, the increase in omeprazole levels reported is unlikely to be clinically relevant as omeprazole has a wide safety margin. Therefore, no additional precautions or omeprazole dose adjustments appear to be necessary on the concurrent use of ticlopidine.

1. Tateishi T, Kumai T, Watanabe M, Nakura H, Tanaka M, Kobayashi S. Ticlopidine decreases the *in vivo* activity of CYP2C19 as measured by omeprazole metabolism. *Br J Clin Pharmacol* (1999) 47, 454–7.
2. Leiri I, Kimura M, Irie S, Urae A, Otsubo K, Ishizaki T. Interaction magnitude, pharmacokinetics and pharmacodynamics of ticlopidine in relation to CYP2C19 genotypic status. *Pharmacogenet Genomics* (2005) 15, 851–9.

Proton pump inhibitors; Omeprazole + Disulfiram

An isolated case describes a catatonic reaction in a patient given omeprazole and disulfiram.

Clinical evidence, mechanism, importance and management

A patient who had been taking omeprazole 40 mg daily for 7 months was also given disulfiram 500 mg daily. Six days later he gradually developed confusion, which progressed to a catatonic state, with muscle rigidity and trismus (spasm of the muscles used to chew food) after 15 days. Both drugs were withdrawn and he gradually recovered. Some months later while taking disulfiram 250 mg daily, he again developed confusion, disorientation and nightmares within 72 hours of starting to take omeprazole 40 mg each morning. Again he recovered when both drugs were stopped.[1]

The reason for this reaction is not understood, but the authors of the report suggest that omeprazole may have allowed the accumulation of one of the metabolites of disulfiram, carbon disulfide, which could have been responsible for the toxic effects.[1]

This is the first and only report of a possible interaction between omeprazole and disulfiram. Other patients given both drugs are said not to have shown adverse effects.[2] The general relevance of this adverse interaction is therefore uncertain, but it seems likely to be limited.

1. Hajela R, Cunningham G M, Kapur B M, Peachey J E, Devenyi P. Catatonic reaction to omeprazole and disulfiram in a patient with alcohol dependence. *Can Med Assoc J* (1990) 143, 1207–8.
2. Astra Pharmaceuticals Ltd. Personal communication, May 1991.

Proton pump inhibitors; Omeprazole + Fexofenadine

Fexofenadine does not affect the pharmacokinetics of omeprazole and its metabolites.

Clinical evidence, mechanism, importance and management

In a study in 8 healthy subjects, fexofenadine 60 mg twice daily for 6 days had no effect on the pharmacokinetics of a single 40-mg dose of omeprazole. The pharmacokinetics of the metabolites of omeprazole (5-hydroxyomeprazole and omeprazole sulfone) were similarly unaffected by fexofenadine. The study had been devised to investigate the possibility that fexofenadine, which is a P-glycoprotein substrate, might compete with omeprazole for P-glycoprotein-mediated absorption. It was suggested that the lack of an interaction could be due to a limited contribution of P-glycoprotein to omeprazole absorption, or the involvement of other transport systems.[1] This study suggests that no omeprazole dose adjustments are necessary if both drugs are given.

1. Takahata T, Yasui-Furukori N, Yoshiya G, Uno T, Sugawara K, Tateishi T. Fexofenadine does not affect omeprazole pharmacokinetics; both are putative P-glycoprotein substrates. *Basic Clin Pharmacol Toxicol* (2004) 94, 252–6.

Proton pump inhibitors; Omeprazole + Finasteride

Finasteride has no clinically relevant effect on the pharmacokinetics of omeprazole.

Clinical evidence, mechanism, importance and management

In a crossover study, 24 healthy subjects were given finasteride 1 mg daily for 3 days with a single 20-mg dose of omeprazole on day 3. In 12 of the subjects who were extensive CYP2C19 metabolisers (that is, those with normal levels of this isoenzyme) the AUC of omeprazole was increased by a minor 13%. In the other 12 subjects, who were poor CYP2C19 metabolisers (that is, those lacking or with low levels of this isoenzyme), there was little change in the AUC of omeprazole.[1]

In vitro, finasteride is an inhibitor of the cytochrome P450 isoenzyme CYP2C19, by which omeprazole is metabolised.[1] However, this clinical study shows that low-dose finasteride 1 mg daily has no clinically relevant effect on the pharmacokinetics of omeprazole. Usual therapeutic doses of finasteride, such as 5 mg daily, might be expected to have a greater effect, although this would still not be expected to be clinically important for omeprazole as it has a wide therapeutic margin.

1. Yasumori T, Narita H, Matsuda T, Takubo T, Ogawa M, Ishii M, Hara K, Ishii Y, Okuyama K, Fujimoto G, Ochiai H, Kano A, Hasegawa S, Sato K, Taniguchi T. Finasteride 1 mg has no inhibitory effect on omeprazole metabolism in extensive and poor metabolizers for CYP2C19 in Japanese. *Eur J Clin Pharmacol* (2006) 62, 939–46.

Proton pump inhibitors; Omeprazole + Ranitidine

Ranitidine slightly increases the AUC of omeprazole.

Clinical evidence, mechanism, importance and management

In a study in 14 healthy subjects, omeprazole 40 mg (as two 20-mg capsules containing gastro-resistant pellets) was given either alone or after ranitidine 150 mg twice daily for 5 days. The AUC and peak plasma levels of omeprazole were increased by 20% and 10%, respectively, after pre-treatment with ranitidine.[1] These changes are small and therefore unlikely to be clinically relevant.

1. Leucuta A, Vlase L, Farcau D, Nanulescu M. A pharmacokinetic interaction study between omeprazole and the H_2-receptor antagonist ranitidine. *Drug Metabol Drug Interact* (2004) 20, 273–81.

Prucalopride + Miscellaneous

Ketoconazole slightly increases the exposure to prucalopride, probably by inhibiting P-glycoprotein: other P-glycoprotein inhibitors are predicted to interact similarly. Prucalopride causes a small increase in erythromycin exposure. Antimuscarinics are predicted to antagonise the prokinetic effect of prucalopride.

Cimetidine, probenecid, and paroxetine do not appear to alter the pharmacokinetics of prucalopride, and prucalopride does not alter the pharmacokinetics of alcohol, digoxin, paroxetine or warfarin.

Clinical evidence, mechanism, importance and management

(a) Antimuscarinics

Theoretically, **antimuscarinics** (such as **atropine**) are likely to antagonise the prokinetic effect of prucalopride because the 5-HT_4-receptor agonist effect of prucalopride results in the release of acetylcholine.[1] Until more is known, it would seem prudent to bear the potential for an interaction in mind should a patient have any otherwise unexplained change in their response to prucalopride while taking these drugs.

(b) Erythromycin

The Canadian manufacturer reports that the concurrent use of prucalopride and erythromycin increased the maximum concentration and AUC of erythromycin by 40% and 28%, respectively. They note that although the mechanism for this increase is uncertain, it is most likely due to the interindividual variability in the pharmacokinetics of erythromycin, rather than an interaction with prucalopride.[1] Either way, a 28% increase in erythromycin exposure is unlikely to be clinically relevant. However, erythromycin, particularly if given intravenously, can prolong the QT interval, and the small increase in erythromycin maximum concentrations seen with prucalopride might further increase this risk. Erythromycin did not alter the pharmacokinetics of prucalopride.[1,2]

(c) Food

Food had no effect on the pharmacokinetics of prucalopride and therefore, it might be taken without regard to food.[2]

(d) P-glycoprotein inhibitors

The Canadian and UK manufacturers of prucalopride report that **ketoconazole** 200 mg twice daily increased the AUC of prucalopride by 40%. This is likely to be due to inhibition of renal P-glycoprotein, of which prucalopride is a weak substrate, by **ketoconazole**.[1,2] The manufacturers note that other potent inhibitors of P-glycoprotein would be expected to interact similarly, and they name **verapamil**, **ciclosporin**, and **quinidine**.[1,2] However, this increase in prucalopride exposure seems unlikely to be clinically relevant.[2] No prucalopride dose adjustment is expected to be needed on the concurrent use of these drugs but until more is known consider an interaction if prucalopride adverse effects (nausea, fatigue, dizziness) are increased.

(e) Other drugs

The Canadian and UK manufacturers briefly note that in studies in healthy subjects, prucalopride had no clinically relevant effect on the pharmacokinetics of **alcohol**, **digoxin**, **paroxetine** or **warfarin**.[1,2] They also state that **paroxetine** did not alter the pharmacokinetics of prucalopride.[1,2]

Prucalopride is mainly renally excreted. However, the manufacturers report that **probenecid** and **cimetidine** do not alter the pharmacokinetics of prucalopride,[1,2] which suggests that the renal anion and cation transporters are not involved in the active secretion of prucalopride.

1. Resotran (Prucalopride succinate). Janssen Inc. Canadian product monograph, August 2014.
2. Resolor (Prucalopride succinate). Shire Pharmaceuticals Ltd. UK Summary of product characteristics, July 2014.

Sulfasalazine + Antibacterials

Ampicillin moderately reduces, and rifampicin (rifampin), given with ethambutol, markedly reduces, the colonic release of 5-aminosalicylic acid (the active drug) from sulfasalazine. No pharmacokinetic interaction appears to occur between sulfasalazine and metronidazole.

Clinical evidence

(a) Ampicillin

In a study in 5 healthy subjects, ampicillin 250 mg four times daily for 5 days reduced the conversion and release of the active metabolite of sulfasalazine, 5-aminosalicylic acid, from a single 2-g dose of sulfasalazine by one-third.[1]

(b) Metronidazole

A study in 10 patients (7 with Crohn's disease and 5 with ulcerative colitis) taking long-term sulfasalazine 2 to 4 g daily found that no statistically significant changes in the serum levels of sulfapyridine (derived from sulfasalazine) occurred while they were also taking metronidazole 400 mg twice daily for 8 to 14 days.[2] A study in 6 patients found that sulfasalazine 1 g twice daily had no significant effect on the pharmacokinetics of metronidazole 250 mg twice daily, when both drugs were given concurrently for 6 days.[3]

(c) Rifampicin (Rifampin)

A crossover study in 11 patients with Crohn's disease receiving long-term treatment with sulfasalazine found that rifampicin 10 mg/kg daily and **ethambutol** 15 mg/kg daily reduced the plasma levels of both 5-aminosalicylic acid and sulfapyridine (derived from sulfasalazine) by about 60%.[4] A similar study in patients taking sulfasalazine 1.5 g to 4 g daily found that the plasma sulfapyridine levels were reduced by 57% when patients were taking rifampicin 10 mg/kg and ethambutol 15 mg/kg daily, when compared with placebo. They also noted an increase in the erythrocyte sedimentation rate (ESR) during antibacterial treatment.[5]

Mechanism

The azo link of sulfasalazine is split by anaerobic bacteria in the colon to release sulfapyridine and 5-aminosalicylic acid, the latter being the active metabolite that acts locally in the treatment of inflammatory bowel disease. Antibacterials that are active against gut flora can apparently reduce this conversion and this is reflected in lower plasma levels.[4,5]

Importance and management

Information is limited, but the interactions between sulfasalazine and ampicillin or rifampicin (rifampin) given with ethambutol appear to be established. The extent to which these antibacterials actually reduce the effectiveness of sulfasalazine in the treatment of Crohn's disease or ulcerative colitis seems not to have been assessed, but the studies do not suggest that the outcome is worse in patients given these antibacterials while taking sulfasalazine; however, the increase in ESR with rifampicin does add a note of caution.

Metronidazole does not appear to interact with sulfasalazine. Information about other antibacterials appears to be lacking, but **neomycin**, which also affects the activity of the gut microflora, has been seen to interact similarly in *animal* studies.[6]

1. Houston JB, Day J, Walker J. Azo reduction of sulphasalazine in healthy volunteers. *Br J Clin Pharmacol* (1982) 14, 395–8.
2. Shaffer JL, Kershaw A, Houston JB. Disposition of metronidazole and its effects on sulphasalazine metabolism in patients with inflammatory bowel disease. *Br J Clin Pharmacol* (1986) 21, 431–5.
3. Eradiri O, Jamali F, Thomson ABR. Interaction of metronidazole with phenobarbital, cimetidine, prednisone, and sulfasalazine in Crohn's disease. *Biopharm Drug Dispos* (1988) 9, 219–277.
4. Shaffer JL, Houston JB. The effect of rifampicin on sulphapyridine plasma concentrations following sulphasalazine administration. *Br J Clin Pharmacol* (1985) 19, 526–8.
5. Shaffer JL, Hughes S, Linaker BD, Baker RD, Turnberg LA. Controlled trial of rifampicin and ethambutol in Crohn's disease. *Gut* (1984) 25, 203–5.
6. Peppercorn MA, Goldman P. The role of intestinal bacteria in the metabolism of salicylazosulfapyridine. *J Pharmacol Exp Ther* (1972) 181, 555–62.

Sulfasalazine + Colestyramine

***Animal* studies show that colestyramine can bind with sulfasalazine in the gut, thereby reducing its activity, but it is not known if this also occurs in clinical use.**

Clinical evidence, mechanism, importance and management

A study in *rats* found that colestyramine binds with sulfasalazine so that the azo-bond is protected against attack by the bacteria within the gut. As a result the active 5-aminosalicylic acid is not released and the faecal excretion of intact sulfasalazine increases 30-fold.[1] It seems possible that this interaction could also occur in humans, but confirmation of this is lacking. Separating the drug doses to prevent their admixture in the gut has proved effective with other drugs that bind with colestyramine. Standard advice is to avoid other drugs for one hour before, and 4 to 6 hours after taking colestyramine.

1. Pieniaszek HJ, Bates TR. Cholestyramine-induced inhibition of salicylazosulfapyridine (sulfasalazine) metabolism by rat intestinal microflora. *J Pharmacol Exp Ther* (1976) 198, 240–5.

Sulfasalazine + H_2-receptor antagonists

Cimetidine and famotidine do not appear to alter the pharmacokinetics of sulfasalazine.

Clinical evidence

(a) Cimetidine

In a study, 5 patients with rheumatoid arthritis were given sulfasalazine alone, and another 9 patients were given cimetidine 400 mg three times daily for 18 weeks as well as their usual sulfasalazine. On comparing the two groups, it was found that cimetidine did not affect the plasma or urinary concentrations of sulfasalazine and there were no changes in blood cell counts or haemoglobin levels.[1]

(b) Famotidine

In a single-dose study in 36 healthy subjects, simultaneous administration of famotidine 40 mg had no effect on the plasma pharmacokinetics, or urinary recovery, of sulfasalazine (given as enteric-coated sulfasalazine 500 mg). There was also no change in the plasma pharmacokinetics of sulfapyridine or 5-aminosalicylic acid, or the urinary recovery of sulfapyridine.[2]

Mechanism

Sulfasalazine efficacy is based on its intact delivery to the colon, where it is cleaved by intestinal bacteria to the active 5-aminosalicylic acid and inactive sulfapyridine. Administration of cimetidine or famotidine does not appear to alter this process. Blood dyscrasias are an adverse effect of sulfasalazine and also a rare adverse effect of H_2-receptor antagonists such as cimetidine; therefore, hypothetically, the risk could be additive or synergistic.

Importance and management

No clinically important pharmacokinetic interaction occurs when cimetidine or famotidine are given with sulfasalazine, and therefore none would be anticipated with other H_2-receptor antagonists. The study with cimetidine and sulfasalazine is too small to conclude that there will not be an increase in the risk of blood dyscrasias with the concurrent use of these drugs since this adverse effect is rare.

1. Pirmohamed M, Coleman MD, Galvani D, Bucknall RC, Breckenridge AM, Park BK. Lack of interaction between sulphasalazine and cimetidine in patients with rheumatoid arthritis. *Br J Rheumatol* (1993) 32, 222–6.
2. Adkison KK, Vaidya SS, Lee DY, Koo SH, Li L, Mehta AA, Gross AS, Polli JW, Humphreys JE, Lou Y, Lee EJ. Oral sulfasalazine as a clinical BCRP probe substrate: pharmacokinetic effects of genetic variation (C421A) and pantoprazole coadministration. *J Pharm Sci* (2010) 99, 1046–62.

Sulfasalazine + Iron compounds

Sulfasalazine and iron appear to bind together in the gut but the absorption of sulfapyridine (derived from sulfasalazine) does not appear to be affected.

Clinical evidence, mechanism, importance and management

An *in vitro* study found that **ferrous sulfate** formed a precipitate with sulfasalazine suggesting it could possibly interfere with sulfasalazine absorption. However, in a study in 5 healthy subjects, although **ferrous sulfate** 400 mg (containing iron 80 mg) reduced the absorption of sulfasalazine from a single 50-mg/kg dose of sulfasalazine (by up to 40%), it had no effect on the absorption of sulfapyridine (derived from sulfasalazine).[1] It therefore seems unlikely that the chelation of sulfasalazine by ferrous sulfate will affect the ability of the intestinal bacteria to split sulfasalazine and release its locally active metabolite, 5-aminosalicylic acid. Consequently the effect of this interaction on the clinical response to sulfasalazine would appear to be limited.

1. Das KM, Eastwood MA. Effect of iron and calcium on salicylazosulphapyridine metabolism. *Scott Med J* (1973) 18, 45–50.

Sulfasalazine + Pantoprazole

In a single-dose study, pantoprazole did not alter the pharmacokinetics of sulfasalazine.

Clinical evidence

In a single-dose study in 36 healthy subjects, simultaneous administration of pantoprazole 40 mg had no effect on the plasma pharmacokinetics, or urinary recovery of sulfasalazine (given as enteric-coated sulfasalazine 500 mg), irrespective of the genotype of the drug transporter protein BCRP. There was also no change in the plasma pharmacokinetics of sulfapyridine or 5-aminosalicylic acid, or the urinary recovery of sulfapyridine.[1]

Mechanism

Sulfasalazine is poorly absorbed from the gastrointestinal tract (10 to 20%), and this is thought to be because it is a substrate of BCRP, which pumps the drug back into the intestinal lumen. Pantoprazole is a known inhibitor of BCRP, and it was therefore hypothesised that pantoprazole would increase absorption of sulfasalazine.[1] Clinically, sulfasalazine efficacy is based on its intact delivery to the colon (hence the enteric coating), where it is cleaved by intestinal bacteria to the active 5-aminosalicylic acid and inactive sulfapyridine. Any drug that appreciably increases the absorption of intact sulfasalazine might therefore decrease its efficacy.

Importance and management

Evidence of an interaction between sulfasalazine and pantoprazole is limited to this one study, but the results indicate that pantoprazole has no clinically relevant effect on the pharmacokinetics of sulfasalazine. No sulfasalazine dose adjustment is therefore necessary on concurrent use.

1. Adkison KK, Vaidya SS, Lee DY, Koo SH, Li L, Mehta AA, Gross AS, Polli JW, Humphreys JE, Lou Y, Lee EJ. Oral sulfasalazine as a clinical BCRP probe substrate: pharmacokinetic effects of genetic variation (C421A) and pantoprazole coadministration. *J Pharm Sci* (2010) 99, 1046–62.

Sulfasalazine + Zileuton

The pharmacokinetics of sulfasalazine and zileuton do not appear to be affected by concurrent use.

Clinical evidence, mechanism, importance and management

In a randomised study, 14 healthy subjects were given sulfasalazine 1 g every 12 hours for 8 days, with zileuton 800 mg or a placebo every 12 hours on days 3 to 8. It was found that the pharmacokinetics of sulfasalazine and its metabolites (sulfapyridine and *N*-acetylsulfapyridine) were not significantly changed. This study did not directly look at the pharmacokinetics of zileuton but, when compared with a previous study, the pharmacokinetics of zileuton appeared unchanged.[1] There would seem to be no reason for additional precautions if both drugs are used.

1. Awni WM, Braeckman RA, Locke CS, Dubé LM, Granneman GR. The influence of multiple oral doses of zileuton on the steady-state pharmacokinetics of sulfasalazine and its metabolites, sulfapyridine and N-acetylsulfapyridine. *Clin Pharmacokinet* (1995) 29 (Suppl 2), 98–104.

Teduglutide + Miscellaneous

Teduglutide might increase the absorption of other drugs given concurrently, although evidence for this appears limited to an association with altered mental status in patients also taking benzodiazepines.

Clinical evidence

In clinical studies, patients taking benzodiazepines while receiving teduglutide were noted to have an altered mental status. One patient taking **prazepam** experienced a dramatic deterioration in mental status, resulting in coma, during the first week of treatment with teduglutide 50 micrograms/kg per day. Teduglutide and **prazepam** were stopped and coma resolved over 5 days.[1]

Mechanism

Teduglutide is an analogue of human glucagon-like peptide-2, used in the treatment of short bowel syndrome, which increases intestinal and portal blood flow and inhibits gastric acid secretion. The manufacturers state that this action might result in an increase in the absorption of oral drugs.

Importance and management

Evidence for teduglutide affecting the absorption of other drugs appears to be limited to the association with altered mental status in patients taking benzodiazepines, and an interaction is not established. Nevertheless, the manufacturers state that the possibility of this effect should be considered, particularly for those drugs a narrow therapeutic range or where the dose is titrated against effect (they specifically name the benzodiazepines and phenothiazines), as dose adjustments might be required. Until more is known it would seem prudent to consider the possibility of an interaction if the adverse effects of these drugs increase in patients given teduglutide.

1. Gattex (Teduglutide). NPS Pharmaceuticals. US Prescribing information, December 2012.

28

Hormonal contraceptives and Sex hormones

The hormonal contraceptives are of two main types: the **combined hormonal contraceptives** containing both an oestrogen and a progestogen, which are available as tablets, a patch or a vaginal ring; and the **progestogen-only contraceptives**, which are available as tablets (sometimes called 'mini' pills), parenteral preparations (implants, depot injections) and intrauterine devices.

The oestrogen most commonly used in combined hormonal contraceptives is ethinylestradiol, in a usual daily dose of 20 micrograms (low-dose) or 30 or 35 micrograms (standard dose), although higher doses of ethinylestradiol may be used with liver enzyme-inducing drugs, such as rifampicin (rifampin). Mestranol (a pro-drug of ethinylestradiol) is used only rarely (daily dose of 50 micrograms, equivalent to about 35 micrograms of ethinylestradiol). A combined hormonal contraceptive containing the natural oestrogen, estradiol valerate, is also available, in doses of 1 to 3 mg daily.

The progestogens used in both oral combined and progestogen-only contraceptives are commonly those derived from 19-nortestosterone and can be subdivided into first generation (e.g. etynodiol diacetate, lynestrenol, norethisterone), second generation (levonorgestrel, norgestrel) and third generation (e.g. desogestrel, drospirenone, gestodene, norgestimate). Note that drospirenone is an analogue of spironolactone and also has anti-androgenic and antimineralocorticoid effects. A patch containing ethinylestradiol and norelgestromin (the active metabolite of norgestimate) and a vaginal ring containing ethinylestradiol and etonogestrel (the active metabolite of desogestrel) are also available. The progestogens used in parenteral progestogen-only contraceptives are either 19-nortestosterone derivatives (e.g. etonogestrel, norethisterone) or derived from progesterone (e.g. medroxyprogesterone acetate). Those in intrauterine devices are 19-nortestosterone derivatives (e.g. levonorgestrel).

Combined hormonal contraceptives are most usually taken cyclically for 21 days, followed by a period of 7 days during which withdrawal bleeding occurs. Some of them include 7 inert tablets to be taken at this time so that the daily routine of taking a tablet is not broken. The daily doses of both the oestrogen and progestogen can be the same (monophasic preparations), or the dose of the progestogen can vary (biphasic or triphasic). Sometimes the dose of oestrogen is also varied (sequential). The combined hormonal contraceptive patch is applied weekly for 3 weeks followed by a patch-free week. The vaginal ring is inserted for 3 weeks, followed by a one-week break before inserting a new ring. The oestrogenic and progestogenic components of these contraceptives act together to consistently suppress ovulation.

The oral progestogen-only contraceptives are taken continuously; the implants, injections or intra-uterine devices slowly release the progestogen over an extended period of time. They vary in their ability to inhibit ovulation, and not all reliably inhibit ovulation in all cycles; they probably act mainly by increasing the viscosity of the cervical mucus so that the movement of the sperm is retarded. They may also cause changes in the endometrium, which inhibit successful implantation.

Interactions

(a) Combined hormonal contraceptives

1. Altered metabolism. Almost all of the information on interactions of the hormonal contraceptives involve the oral combined hormonal contraceptives. Most of the clinically important interactions with these contraceptives involve increased metabolism. The major route for hepatic metabolism of ethinylestradiol is hydroxylation (about 30% of a dose) principally by CYP3A4 and also by CYP2C9. Progestogens are also substrates for CYP3A4. Ethinylestradiol and its metabolites also undergo conjugation by sulfation and glucuronidation (via UGT1A1). Thus, enzyme inducers can increase the clearance of the contraceptive steroids and possibly increase breakthrough bleeding and decrease contraceptive efficacy (see 'Combined hormonal contraceptives + Barbiturates or Phenytoin', p.1169). The drugs that have been shown to induce the metabolism of hormonal contraceptives and/or reduce their ovulation suppressant effects are listed in 'Table 28.1', p.1160. Intuitively, low-dose combined hormonal contraceptives might be expected to be more susceptible to these types of drug interactions than standard-dose or high-dose preparations, but evidence to support this is scant. Conversely, inhibitors of CYP3A4 (such as some azoles, see 'Combined hormonal contraceptives + Azoles', p.1168) or inhibitors of conjugation enzymes (such as some coxibs, see 'Combined hormonal contraceptives + Coxibs', p.1172) reduce the clearance of contraceptive steroids, and, although there is no good evidence for this, may increase the incidence of adverse effects such as nausea, breast tenderness, headaches, and potentially more serious complications such as thromboembolic events.

2. Enterohepatic recirculation. Some of the conjugated metabolites of ethinylestradiol undergo enterohepatic recirculation, and certain antibacterials were formerly postulated to reduce this by inhibiting gut flora, thereby possibly decreasing contraceptive efficacy, although this seems unlikely, see 'Combined hormonal contraceptives + Antibacterials', p.1162.

3. Interaction studies. In drug interaction studies, in addition to assessing the effect on the pharmacokinetics of the contraceptive steroids, ovulation parameters are also often assessed to confirm the absence of ovulation. When evaluating drug interactions with combined hormonal contraceptives, it is important to bear in mind that they are usually given cyclically, and that levels of the contraceptive steroids increase to steady state between about day 10 and 21 and decrease to zero in the seven-day drug-free interval. In reducing contraceptive steroid levels, enzyme-inducing drugs may therefore increase the length of the pill-free interval, as well as reducing the levels at steady-state. If an interacting drug is to be used continuously, such as rifampicin (rifampin) for tuberculosis, it needs to be taken with the contraceptive for at least one full cycle to assess the full effect of the drug on ovulation.

4. Other drugs affected. Increasing information is accumulating to show that hormonal contraceptives can cause clinically relevant pharmacokinetic interactions with other drugs. Ethinylestradiol appears to be a weak to moderate inhibitor of the CYP1A2 (see 'Tizanidine + CYP1A2 inhibitors', p.1588) and an inducer of glucuronidation (see 'Combined hormonal contraceptives + Lamotrigine', p.1178), and might also have some inhibitory effect on CYP2C19 (see 'Hormonal contraceptives + Proton pump inhibitors', p.1193). Because of the usual cyclical administration of combined hormonal contraceptives, these interactions with other drugs will be cyclical (greatest at steady state, and least on the last day of the pill free interval), as has been demonstrated with lamotrigine (see 'Combined hormonal contraceptives + Lamotrigine', p.1178), and this complicates their management. Continuous use of a monophasic oral combined hormonal contraceptive (without any break) would eliminate the cyclical nature of the interaction,

(b) Progestogen-only contraceptives

There is very little direct information about interactions with the progestogen-only contraceptives (oral, parenteral, and intrauterine). It is unwise to uncritically assume that interactions known to occur with the combined hormonal contraceptives also occur with these contraceptives. However, it seems probable that an increased risk of failure with the oral and parenteral progestogen-only contraceptives is likely with drugs that cause enzyme induction (listed in 'Table 28.1', p.1160), which results in an increased clearance of the progestogen, with an accompanying loss of efficacy. The progestogen-releasing intrauterine system is thought to have a primarily local effect, and may not be affected by enzyme-inducers (see 'Progestogen-only contraceptives; Intra-uterine system + Enzyme inducers', p.1200). However, much more study is needed to clarify the situation.

Table 28.1 Enzyme-inducing drugs shown to increase the metabolism of combined hormonal contraceptives and reduce their ovulation suppressant effect

Group	*Drugs*	*Decrease in exposure (AUC)*	
		Ethinylestradiol	Progestogen
Antibacterials*	Rifampicin (Rifampin), p.1184	63%	55% Norethisterone
	Rifabutin, p.1184	35%	17% Norethisterone
Antiepileptics	Phenytoin†, p.1169	49%	42% Levonorgestrel
	Oxcarbazepine, p.1172	47%	36% to 47% Levonorgestrel
	Carbamazepine, p.1172	42% to 45%	58% Norethisterone 40% to 46% Levonorgestrel
	Eslicarbazepine, p.1172	42%	37% Levonorgestrel
	Rufinamide, p.1185	22%	14% Norethisterone
	Topiramate, p.1188	0% to 18% (50 to 200 mg daily) 21% (400 mg daily) 30% (800 mg daily)	No change Norethisterone
	Perampanel, p.589	No change	40% Levonorgestrel
	Phenobarbital‡	No AUC data	No AUC data
HIV-protease inhibitors**	**Unboosted HIV-protease inhibitors**		
	Nelfinavir, p.1177	47%	18% Norethisterone
	Ritonavir, p.1177	41%	No data
	HIV-protease inhibitors boosted with ritonavir, p.1177		
	Atazanavir	19%	*(85% increase Norgestimate)*
	Darunavir	44%	14% Norethisterone
	Fosamprenavir	37%	34% Norethisterone
	Lopinavir	42%	17% Norethisterone *(83% increase Norelgestromin)*
	Tipranavir	43% to 48%	*(14% to 27% increase Norethisterone)*
NNRTIs	Efavirenz, p.1181	No change	64% Norgestimate
	Nevirapine, p.1181	29%	19% Norethisterone
Other drugs	Aprepitant†, p.1167	19% to 43%	8% Norethisterone 10% Norgestimate
	Bosentan, p.1173	31%	14% Norethisterone
	Modafinil†, p.1180	18%	No data
	St John's wort (*Hypericum perforatum*), p.1185	No change, 16%, 24%	40% Desogestrel 10%, 13% Norethisterone

*__Rifapentine__ — although there are no data, based on its known enzyme-inducing properties, rifapentine would be predicted to have an effect greater than that of rifabutin but less than that of rifampicin.
†Data for the prodrugs or isomers of these drugs (**fosphenytoin, fosaprepitant, armodafinil**) are lacking, but they would be expected to have similar effects on the contraceptive steroids.
‡**Primidone** is metabolised to phenobarbital and would be expected to interact similarly, but direct data for this are lacking. Many other **barbiturates** have similar enzyme-inducing effects to phenobarbital and so it would be prudent to consider the possibility of an interaction with all of them.
**HIV-protease inhibitors are usually inhibitors of CYP3A4 by which ethinylestradiol is partially metabolised. However, some, including ritonavir, appear to induce glucuronidation and thereby reduce ethinylestradiol exposure.

(c) Emergency hormonal contraceptives

It is not known whether interacting drugs are likely to affect the emergency hormonal contraceptives, although it is common practice that women taking enzyme-inducing drugs (see 'Table 28.1', above) are given an increased dose to accommodate the increased rate of metabolism by the liver (see 'Emergency hormonal contraceptives + Enzyme inducers', p.1192). Note that a more recently available emergency contraceptive contains **ulipristal** (a progesterone receptor antagonist), the metabolism of which may also be increased by enzyme inducers, see 'Ulipristal + Miscellaneous', p.1201.

The efficacy of progestogen-only emergency hormonal contraceptives is not affected by antibacterials that do not induce liver enzymes (see 'Emergency hormonal contraceptives + Antibacterials', p.1191).

(d) Hormone replacement therapy (HRT)

The preparations used for HRT contain oestrogens, either alone or combined with progestogens. They differ from the hormonal contraceptives as the most commonly used oestrogens in HRT are natural oestrogens, such as estradiol, and conjugated oestrogens, and their doses are generally lower than equivalent doses of ethinylestradiol used in combined hormonal contraceptives. There are only a few reports of interactions with HRT preparations, but generally they are expected to behave very much like the oral combined hormonal contraceptives.

(e) Other preparations

Cyproterone acetate combined with ethinylestradiol (co-cyprindiol) is intended for use in women with androgen-dependent skin conditions, but it also acts as an oral contraceptive and is therefore predicted to interact like conventional oestrogen-containing oral contraceptives (see 'Co-cyprindiol (Cyproterone with Ethinylestradiol) + Miscellaneous', p.1161).

1. Shader RI, Oesterheld JR. Contraceptive effectiveness: cytochromes and induction. *J Clin Psychopharmacol* (2000) 20, 119–121.
2. Shader RI, Greenblatt DJ. More on oral contraceptives, drug interactions, herbal medicines, and hormone replacement therapy. *J Clin Psychopharmacol* (2000) 20, 397–8.
3. Elliman A. Interactions with hormonal contraception. *Br J Fam Plann* (2000) 26, 109–11.
4. Zhang H, Cui D, Wang B, Han Y-H, Balimane P, Yang Z, Sinz M, Rodrigues AD. Pharmacokinetic drug interactions involving 17α-ethinylestradiol: a new look at an old drug. *Clin Pharmacokinet* (2007) 46, 133–57.

Co-cyprindiol (Cyproterone with Ethinylestradiol) + Miscellaneous

Co-cyprindiol is expected to interact with enzyme inducing drugs in a similar manner to the combined hormonal contraceptives, and therefore the risk of contraceptive failure is increased. There is some evidence that co-cyprindiol also interacts with minocycline to increase facial pigmentation.

Clinical evidence, mechanism, importance and management

Co-cyprindiol is a mixture of the anti-androgenic progestogen, cyproterone acetate 2 mg, with ethinylestradiol 35 micrograms. It is used for the treatment of acne and moderately severe hirsutism in women who might also wish to use it as a contraceptive.

(a) Antibacterials

1. Short-term use. In their November 2010 product information the UK manufacturer of co-cyprindiol stated that women receiving short courses of broad-spectrum antibacterials should use additional, non-hormonal (except rhythm or temperature method) contraceptive precautions, both during concurrent use and for 7 days after stopping the antibacterial.[1] This advice regarding short courses of antibacterials with combined hormonal contraceptives was traditionally given in the UK; however, having reviewed all the evidence, in 2011, the UK Faculty of Sexual and Reproductive Healthcare changed their guidance to recommend that no additional contraceptive precautions are necessary with non-enzyme-inducing antibacterials, including the tetracyclines, see 'Combined hormonal contraceptives + Antibacterials', p.1162. Additional contraceptive precautions would not therefore seem necessary when antibacterials are used with co-cyprindiol.

2. Long-term use. There are anecdotal reports of contraceptive failure when long-term antibacterials, including tetracycline, have been used for the treatment of acne, although there is also evidence that the failure rate does not differ from that seen generally with oral contraceptives, and that no real interaction occurs, see 'Combined hormonal contraceptives + Antibacterials', p.1162. Moreover, additional contraceptive precautions for long-term use of antibacterials (after 3 weeks) have never been recommended in the UK. Although the manufacturer of co-cyprindiol also notes that oral **tetracyclines** have not actually been shown to reduce the contraceptive efficacy of co-cyprindiol, they nevertheless state that when **tetracyclines** are being taken it is advisable to use additional non-hormonal methods of contraception (except the rhythm or temperature methods) as an extremely high degree of contraceptive protection must be provided during co-cyprindiol use due to the theoretical risk of cyproterone causing feminisation of a male foetus. However, if an extremely high degree of contraceptive protection is required, then co-cyprindiol on its own may not be suitable for all women because oral combined hormonal contraceptives have a stated failure rate of up to 8% in typical use (where users may forget to take occasional doses).

Co-cyprindiol may also possibly interact with **minocycline** to accentuate facial pigmentation (see 'Tetracyclines; Minocycline + Ethinylestradiol', p.363).

(b) Enzyme-inducing drugs

The contraceptive efficacy of co-cyprindiol is expected to be reduced by the same enzyme inducers that interact with conventional oral combined hormonal contraceptives.[1] The UK Faculty of Sexual and Reproductive Healthcare (FSRH) have issued guidance on the concurrent use of drugs that induce liver enzymes and combined hormonal contraceptives, and these are discussed in detail under 'Combined hormonal contraceptives + Barbiturates or Phenytoin', p.1169. The precautions described in this section for these contraceptives for the *short-term* use of any of the various enzyme-inducing drugs listed in 'Table 28.1', p.1160, should therefore be followed for co-cyprindiol namely, tricycling of the co-cyprindiol with a shortened 4-day pill free interval, and use of additional non-hormonal contraception.

For *long-term* use of an enzyme-inducing drug, the FSRH advice is to use an alternative [non-hormonal] method of contraception that is not affected by enzyme-inducers and this should be followed for co-cyprindiol, which should also be continued for its non-contraceptive indication. The alternative FSRH advice, to increase the dose of ethinylestradiol to 50 micrograms daily, would generally not be appropriate for co-cyprindiol because doubling the dose of co-cyprindiol would give an ethinylestradiol dose of 70 micrograms daily. Although a maximum ethinylestradiol dose of 70 micrograms is permitted in cases of poor cycle control, it is unlikely to be appropriate for all women taking co-cyprindiol. Combining co-cyprindiol with a low-dose, oral combined hormonal contraceptive is not appropriate because none contain cyproterone acetate, and the progestogens contained in these products may oppose the benefits of cyproterone, see also *Other hormonal contraceptives*, below.

Note that the manufacturer of co-cyprindiol includes **griseofulvin** and **phenylbutazone** in their list of enzyme inducing drugs; however, griseofulvin is not an established enzyme inducer, see 'Hormonal contraceptives + Griseofulvin', p.1192, and phenylbutazone is not a known enzyme inducer.

Note that the efficacy of co-cyprindiol in the treatment of acne and hirsutism might also be expected to be reduced by these enzyme-inducing drugs.

(c) Other hormonal contraceptives

The manufacturer states that other hormonal contraceptives must not be taken with co-cyprindiol.[1] To do this would be analogous to increasing the dose of the contraceptive steroids with a consequent increased risk of adverse effects. In addition, some of the progestogens in combined hormonal contraceptives have weak androgenic effects, which could oppose the benefits of cyproterone.

1. Dianette (Cyproterone acetate with Ethinylestradiol). Bayer plc. UK Summary of product characteristics, November 2010.

Combined hormonal contraceptives + Alosetron

Alosetron does not alter the pharmacokinetics or the suppression of ovulation of an oral combined hormonal contraceptive containing ethinylestradiol with levonorgestrel.

Clinical evidence, mechanism, importance and management

In a crossover study in 18 healthy women taking an oral combined hormonal contraceptive (**ethinylestradiol** 20 micrograms with **levonorgestrel** 100 micrograms), alosetron 1 mg twice daily (given alone for 7 days beginning on day 22 of one cycle and with the contraceptive from day one until day 21 of the next cycle) had no effect on the AUC of **ethinylestradiol** or **levonorgestrel**. In addition, there was no change in progesterone, FSH and LH levels, and no evidence of ovulation based on follicle size.[1] This study suggests that alosetron is unlikely to alter the efficacy of combined hormonal contraceptives, and no additional contraceptive precautions would appear to be necessary when it is used with any combined hormonal contraceptive (tablet, patch or vaginal ring)..

1. Koch K, Campanella C, Baidoo CA, Manzo JA, Ameen VZ, Kersey KEE. Pharmacodynamics and pharmacokinetics of oral contraceptives co-administered with alosetron (Lotronex). *Dig Dis Sci* (2004) 49, 1244–9.

Combined hormonal contraceptives + Antacids

Despite *in vitro* evidence that some antacids might reduce the availability of norethisterone acetate, evidence from healthy women indicates that no pharmacokinetic interaction occurs between antacids and oral combined hormonal contraceptives containing norethisterone or levonorgestrel.

Clinical evidence, mechanism, importance and management

An *in vitro* study found that a 1% suspension of **magnesium trisilicate** in water adsorbed about 80% of **mestranol** and 50% of **norethisterone**, but minimal amounts of **ethinylestradiol**.[1,2] Similarly, another *in vitro* study reported reduced dissolution of **norethisterone acetate** from oral combined hormonal contraceptive tablets in the presence of **magnesium trisilicate**, **kaolin mixture**, and **aluminium hydroxide**.[3]

In contrast, a single-dose study in 12 healthy women given an oral combined hormonal contraceptive (**ethinylestradiol** 30 micrograms and either **norethisterone acetate** 1 mg or **levonorgestrel** 150 micrograms) with **magnesium trisilicate** 500 mg and **aluminium hydroxide** 250 mg, found that the AUC and peak levels of all three steroids were unchanged.[4] This is in line with common experience. There do not appear to be any reports of contraceptive failure with antacids and **norethisterone acetate** or **mestranol**-containing oral combined hormonal contraceptives. No particular precautions therefore seem to be necessary on concurrent use.

1. Khalil SAH, Iwuagwu M. The in vitro uptake of some oral contraceptive steroids by magnesium trisilicate. *J Pharm Pharmacol* (1976) 28 (Suppl), 47P.
2. Khalil SAH, Iwuagwu M. *In vitro* uptake of oral contraceptive steroids by magnesium trisilicate. *J Pharm Sci* (1978) 67, 287–9.
3. Fadel H, Abd Elbary A, Nour El-Din E, Kassem AA. Availability of norethisterone acetate from combined oral contraceptive tablets. *Pharmazie* (1979) 34, 49–50.
4. Joshi JV, Sankolli GM, Shah RS, Joshi UM. Antacid does not reduce the bioavailability of oral contraceptive steroids in women. *Int J Clin Pharmacol Ther Toxicol* (1986) 24, 192–5.

Combined hormonal contraceptives + Anthelmintics

Praziquantel and metrifonate do not appear to alter the pharmacokinetics of oral combined hormonal contraceptives containing ethinylestradiol and levonorgestrel.

Clinical evidence, mechanism, importance and management

A study in 25 women with early active schistosomiasis (*S. haematobium* or *S. mansoni*) without signs of liver disease and 6 healthy women found that neither the disease itself nor the concurrent use of **praziquantel**, given as a single 40-mg/kg dose, or **metrifonate**, in three doses of 10 mg/kg given at two-weekly intervals, had any effect on the plasma levels of steroids from an oral combined hormonal contraceptive (**ethinylestradiol** 50 micrograms with **levonorgestrel** 500 micrograms).[1] Moreover, in other studies there was no evidence that women with early active schistosomiasis without signs of liver disease[2] or with liver fibrosis with normal liver function[3] were at any greater risk of hepatic impairment while taking oral combined hormonal contraceptives. No particular precautions would therefore appear to be necessary in women with schistosomiasis taking oral combined hormonal contraceptives and **praziquantel** or **metrifonate**. Note that the use of a combined hormonal contraceptive (any form) is usually considered contraindicated in schistosomiasis with liver involvement when there is cirrhosis, especially if this is severe (decompensated).

1. El-Raghy I, Back DJ, Osman F, Orme ML'E, Fathalla M. Contraceptive steroid concentrations in women with early active schistosomiasis: lack of effect of antischistosomal drugs. *Contraception* (1986) 33, 373–7.

2. Shaaban MM, Hammad WA, Fathalla MF, Ghaneimah SA, El-Sharkawy MM, Salim TH, Liao WC, Smith SC. Effects of oral contraception on liver function tests and serum proteins in women with active schistosomiasis. *Contraception* (1982) 26, 75–82.
3. Tagy AHEI, Saker ME, Moussa AA, Kolgah A. The effect of low-dose combined oral contraceptive pills versus injectable contraceptive (Depot Provera) on liver function tests of women with compensated bilharzial liver fibrosis. *Contraception* (2001) 64, 173–6.

Combined hormonal contraceptives + Antibacterials

In anecdotal cases, the failure of oral combined hormonal contraceptives has been attributed to antibacterials, including cephalosporins, co-trimoxazole, erythromycin, metronidazole, penicillins, tetracyclines and various miscellaneous antibacterials (chloramphenicol, fusidic acid, nitrofurantoin). However, controlled studies have not shown any reduction in contraceptive steroid levels and the suppression of ovulation in women given any antibacterial with a variety of combined hormonal contraceptives (oral, patch, or vaginal ring). Moreover, increases in contraceptive steroid levels have been seen with erythromycin, clarithromycin and co-trimoxazole.

Clinical evidence

A. Effect on contraceptives

(a) Case reports of contraceptive failure

Over a 16-year period from 1968 to 1984, the CSM in the UK received reports of a total of 63 pregnancies in women taking oral contraceptives who also received antibacterials. These included **penicillins** (32 reports), **tetracyclines** (12), **co-trimoxazole (trimethoprim** with **sulfamethoxazole** (5)), **metronidazole** (3), **cephalosporins** (2), **trimethoprim** (2) **erythromycin** (2), **sulphonamides** (1), **fusidic acid** (1) and unspecified (2). Apart from erythromycin (where the number of cases was lower relative to frequency of use of the antibacterial), these figures were broadly in line with the estimated number of prescriptions dispensed, demonstrating that no one antibacterial was associated with a higher incidence of failure. Where specified, these occurred with oral combined hormonal contraceptives containing **ethinylestradiol** 50 micrograms (12 cases), 30 micrograms (33 cases) and 20 micrograms (3 cases).[1] A case report briefly mentions that, in the Netherlands, over the 10-year period from 1980 to 1989, 6 cases of contraceptive failure had been reported (two with **doxycycline** and one each with **nifurtoinol, nitrofurantoin, nitrofurantoin** with **trimethoprim**, and **co-trimoxazole**).[2]

The individual published case reports of contraceptive failure are covered in the following subsections.

1. Cefalexin. One case of contraceptive failure (resulting in an ectopic pregnancy) has been attributed to the concurrent use of cefalexin 3 g daily for 2 weeks with an oral combined hormonal contraceptive (**ethinylestradiol** 30 micrograms with **levonorgestrel** 150 micrograms).[3]

2. Chloramphenicol. One woman taking an oral combined hormonal contraceptive was briefly reported to have developed breakthrough bleeding and to have become pregnant while also taking chloramphenicol.[4,5]

3. Penicillins. A case report describes 3 women taking an oral contraceptive who became pregnant when given **ampicillin**.[6] One woman had two unwanted pregnancies while taking an oral combined hormonal contraceptive (**ethinylestradiol** with **norethisterone**). On both occasions conception occurred when she was taking **ampicillin** for tonsillitis.[7] Another woman taking **ethinylestradiol** with **norethisterone** for 5 years with no history of breakthrough bleeding, lost a quantity of blood similar to a normal period loss within a day of starting to take **ampicillin** (exact dose unknown). There was no evidence of diarrhoea or vomiting in either case.[7] Two other case reports attributed oral combined hormonal contraceptive failure to **oxacillin**,[8] and to an intramuscular injection of **benethamine penicillin, procaine penicillin** and **benzylpenicillin**.[9]

4. Spiramycin. One case of oral contraceptive failure has been attributed to the concurrent use of spiramycin.[10]

5. Sulfonamides. One woman taking an oral combined hormonal contraceptive is briefly reported to have developed breakthrough bleeding and to have become pregnant while taking **sulfamethoxypyridazine**.[4,5]

6. Tetracyclines. A woman taking an oral combined hormonal contraceptive (**ethinylestradiol** with **levonorgestrel**) became pregnant, the evidence indicating that she had conceived during or in the week after taking **tetracycline** 500 mg every 6 hours for 3 days and then 250 mg every 6 hours for 2 days. There was no evidence of either nausea or vomiting, which might have been an alternative explanation for the contraceptive failure.[11] A case of breakthrough bleeding attributed to the concurrent use of **tetracycline** was also mentioned in this report.[11] Two other case reports describe pregnancies in women taking an oral combined hormonal contraceptive and long-term **tetracycline** 500 mg daily[12] or long-term **minocycline** 100 mg daily.[2]

(b) Controlled studies

The available studies of the effect of various antibacterials (non-enzyme inducing) on the pharmacokinetics and/or ovulatory suppressant effects of combined hormonal contraceptives (oral, patch or vaginal ring) are summarised in 'Table 28.2', p.1163. None of these studies showed that any of these antibacterials reduced **ethinylestradiol** exposure (AUC), with the exception of a tiny, clinically irrelevant, 7.6% decrease with **dirithromycin**. Indeed, some of these antibacterials (such as **co-trimoxazole, clarithromycin** and **erythromycin**) have been reported to *increase* the levels of contraceptive steroids or their active metabolites. The pharmacokinetic study with the best design is for a combined hormonal contraceptive given as a vaginal ring: in this study, there was no difference in the AUC of **ethinylestradiol** for the first 12 hours, on day 10, on days 1 to 11 (duration of the antibacterial) and on days 1 to 22 (duration of use of the ring) between a cycle where **amoxicillin** was given for the first 10 days, a cycle were **doxycycline** was given for the first 10 days, and a cycle where no antibacterial was given.

Moreover, none of the studies have shown a reduction in ovulation suppression (as measured by FSH and LH levels) or ovulation (indicated by a progesterone level of greater than 4 nanograms/mL) with any of the antibacterials studied. The only exception is one study with **metronidazole**, where a few women possibly ovulated, both in the control period and with the antibacterial; however, another study with metronidazole found no change in progesterone levels, suggesting that ovulation did not occur.

In the best designed studies, where no contraceptive was used in the first cycle to confirm ovulation, then the contraceptive was given alone for one cycle to confirm suppression of ovulation, and then the contraceptive was given with the antibacterial during another cycle, neither **roxithromycin** or **telithromycin** altered the suppression of ovulation. Moreover, **co-trimoxazole** and **clarithromycin** actually decreased levels of FSH, suggesting *increased* suppression of ovulation.

Antibacterials can cause vomiting and/or diarrhoea, which can reduce the absorption of oral contraceptives. Of the controlled studies mentioning drug-related adverse events, vomiting and/or diarrhoea did not occur in most. However, in one of the **doxycycline** studies, one of 24 subjects vomited on day one of antibacterial use (day 14 of cycle) and was found to have an 80% lower **ethinylestradiol** level and a 67% lower **norethisterone** level in that cycle (day 18).[13] Similarly, in the **dirithromycin** study, one subject withdrew because of gastrointestinal intolerance (moderate to severe diarrhoea, nausea and vomiting) after taking 6 days of the antibacterial. Her ethinylestradiol AUC, taken 8 days later on the day when she should have finished the 14-day course of dirithromycin (day 8 of cycle), was 32% lower.[14] Two subjects had moderate diarrhoea while receiving **ciprofloxacin** in one study, but their ethinylestradiol levels were not reported separately: there was no change for the group as a whole.[15]

(c) Observational studies

1. Surveys with no controls. Various surveys have been conducted in women after failure of their oral contraceptive to establish possible risk factors for this; however, the value of these data are limited by recall-bias and by the absence of control data, which would allow for a comparison of outcomes with women who did not have contraceptive failure while taking antibacterials. In one of these surveys, in women who had undergone pregnancy termination over a 4-year period from 1981 to 1985, the 60% of cases for which unreliable pill-taking was considered a factor were excluded, and, in the remaining 163 cases, antibacterials had been taken by 37 women. In these 37 women, the known antibacterials used were **amoxicillin** (16 cases), other penicillins (**flucloxacillin, phenoxymethylpenicillin, pivampicillin**, 5 cases), tetracyclines (**doxycycline, lymecycline, minocycline**, 6 cases), **co-trimoxazole** or **trimethoprim** (3 cases), **amoxicillin** with **phenoxymethylpenicillin** (one case), **doxycycline** with **metronidazole** (one case). However, vomiting and/or diarrhoea had occurred in 56 cases, and it was not stated whether there was any overlap between the group taking antibacterials and those who developed diarrhoea and/or vomiting.[16] A similar, later analysis by the same research group, for a 3-year period from 1985 to 1988, identified 23 out of 137 women who became pregnant while taking oral contraceptives and who had been taking antibacterials; although it was stated that, in most cases, there were other contributing factors (note that smoking was found to be a factor for contraceptive failure in this analysis, but see 'Hormonal contraceptives + Tobacco or Nicotine', p.1195). Where known, the antibacterials taken were **amoxicillin** (9 cases), **tetracycline** (3 cases), **trimethoprim** (1 case), **co-trimoxazole** (2 cases) and **penicillins** (1 case).[17] Similarly, in another survey of unplanned pregnancy over 8 months from 1985 to 1986, 48 of 209 women taking oral contraceptives and who became pregnant reported taking an antibacterial. Where specified these were **amoxicillin** (17 cases), **penicillin** (5 cases), **co-trimoxazole** (3 cases), **tetracycline** (2 cases), and one case each for **erythromycin** and **metronidazole**. In this survey, 56 women reported diarrhoea or vomiting,[18] but it was not stated whether there was an overlap between the group taking antibacterials and those who developed diarrhoea and/or vomiting. In a follow-up survey for 7 months in 1990, 26 of 113 women who had unplanned pregnancies while taking oral contraceptives reported also taking antibacterials (**amoxicillin, co-trimoxazole, tetracycline, doxycycline, penicillin, metronidazole**), and 32 women reported diarrhoea and/or vomiting.[19]

In a small survey of an obstetrics and gynaecology practice over a 2-year period, 13 women recalled taking an antibacterial around the suspected time of conception: five cases occurred with **ampicillin** and three with **'penicillin'**, often in combination with 'cold remedies', two cases occurred with **sulfafurazole (sulfisoxazole)**, and one case each with **cefalexin**, a **sulphonamide** (unspecified), and **tetracycline**.[20]

In an early review of the concurrent use of antibacterials and contraceptives, 79 cases were identified, but no pregnancies occurred. However, the authors reported that intermenstrual bleeding occurred in 14 cases, which they considered to be a high incidence.[21]

2. Surveys with controls. After publishing an uncontrolled survey of contraceptive failure for 7 months in 1990 (discussed above[19]), a subsequent survey was conducted in a similar number of non-pregnant users of oral contraceptives, during 9 months in 1991, to assess the prevalence of factors such as use of antibacterials, to allow for comparison with the results of the previous survey in users of oral contraceptives who became pregnant.[22] In the 109 non-pregnant users, 60 (55%) stated that they had taken antibacterials [not specified] in the previous 12 months, which is much higher than the 26 of 113 women (23%) who experienced contraceptive failure in the previous survey. Of the 60 non-pregnant subjects who had taken antibacterials in the previous

Table 28.2 Summary of the controlled studies of the effect of antibacterials on the pharmacokinetics and/or pharmacodynamics of combined hormonal contraceptives

Study details	*Number of healthy subjects (unless otherwise indicated)*	*Antibacterial*	*Contraceptive*	*Effect on contraceptive steroids*	*Effect on measures of ovulation*	*Refs*
Macrolides						
One cycle with contraceptive alone, one cycle with contraceptive and antibacterial	10	**Clarithromycin** 250 mg twice daily, days 1 to 7 of the cycle	Oral phasic; ethinylestradiol 30 micrograms with levonorgestrel or desogestrel	Ethinylestradiol* AUC unchanged on days 5, 6, 7 or 8 Levonorgestrel AUC unchanged 3-keto desogestrel AUC increased 2.3-fold	Decreased FSH and LH levels, no change in progesterone levels	1
One cycle with contraceptive alone, one cycle with contraceptive and antibacterial	15	**Dirithromycin** 500 mg daily for 14 days from day 21 of the cycle	Oral triphasic; ethinylestradiol 35 micrograms with norethisterone	Ethinylestradiol AUC decreased by 8% on day 8	No change in estradiol or progesterone levels, ovulation not detected by ultrasound	2
Day before antibacterial compared with during antibacterial	24	**Erythromycin** 500 mg three times daily, day 8 to 14 of the cycle	Oral; estradiol 2 mg with dienogest 3 mg for 14 days	Estradiol AUC increased by 33% on day 14 Dienogest AUC increased by 62%		3
Cycle with no contraceptive, cycle with contraceptive alone, cycle with contraceptive and antibacterial	21	**Roxithromycin** 150 mg twice daily for complete cycle	Oral triphasic; ethinylestradiol 30 to 40 micrograms with levonorgestrel		No change in progesterone levels, ovulation not detected by ultrasound	4
Cycle with no contraceptive, cycle with contraceptive alone, cycle with contraceptive and antibacterial	38	**Telithromycin** 800 mg daily, day 3 to 12 of the cycle	Oral triphasic; ethinylestradiol with levonorgestrel	Ethinylestradiol AUC unchanged on days 9, 10 or 11 Levonorgestrel AUC increased by 50%	No change in progesterone levels	5,6
Metronidazole						
Day before antibacterial compared with during antibacterial	10	**Metronidazole** 400 mg three times daily for 6 to 8 days from day 6 or 7 of the cycle	Oral; ethinylestradiol 30 micrograms with norethisterone 1 mg	Ethinylestradiol AUC unchanged on the last day of antibacterial use Norethisterone AUC unchanged	Increased progesterone levels seen in 2 subjects	7
One cycle with contraceptive alone, one cycle with contraceptive and antibacterial	11	**Metronidazole** 400 mg three times daily, day 5 to 15 of the cycle	Oral; ethinylestradiol 30 micrograms with norethisterone 1 mg		No change in progesterone levels	8
Penicillins						
One cycle with contraceptive alone, one cycle with contraceptive and antibacterial Crossover	16	**Amoxicillin** 875 mg twice daily, day 1 to 10 of the cycle	Vaginal ring; ethinylestradiol with etonogestrel	Ethinylestradiol AUC unchanged on day 1, 10, and days 1 to 11 and 1 to 22 Etonogestrel AUC unchanged		9
One cycle with contraceptive alone, one cycle with contraceptive and antibacterial Placebo-controlled	11	**Ampicillin** 250 mg four times daily, day 1 to 16 of the cycle	Oral; ethinylestradiol 50 micrograms with etynodiol 1 mg		No change in FSH, LH or progesterone levels	10
One cycle with contraceptive alone, one cycle with contraceptive and antibacterial	7 patients	**Ampicillin** 500 mg three times daily for 8 days	Oral; ethinylestradiol 30 or 50 micrograms with levonorgestrel or norethisterone	Ethinylestradiol* AUC unchanged on days 5, 6, 7 or 8‡ Levonorgestrel AUC unchanged Norethisterone AUC unchanged	No change in FSH or progesterone levels	11
One cycle with contraceptive alone, one cycle with contraceptive and antibacterial	6	**Ampicillin** 500 mg three times daily, day 9 to 16 of the cycle	Oral; ethinylestradiol 30 micrograms with levonorgestrel	Ethinylestradiol* AUC unchanged on days 5, 6, 7 or 8 Levonorgestrel AUC unchanged	No change in FSH or progesterone levels	11

* Plasma concentration at 10 to 12 hours after taking the contraceptive
† Plasma concentration at 24 hours after taking the contraceptive
‡ Two patients had lower ethinylestradiol levels during ampicillin, but neither ovulated

Continued

Table 28.2 Summary of the controlled studies of the effect of antibacterials on the pharmacokinetics and/or pharmacodynamics of combined hormonal contraceptives (continued)

Study details	*Number of healthy subjects (unless otherwise indicated)*	*Antibacterial*	*Contraceptive*	*Effect on contraceptive steroids*	*Effect on measures of ovulation*	*Refs*
Day before antibacterial compared with during antibacterial	6	**Ampicillin** 500 mg twice daily for 6 to 8 days	Ethinylestradiol 30 micrograms with norethisterone 1 mg	Ethinylestradiol AUC unchanged Norethisterone AUC unchanged	No change in progesterone levels	7
Quinolones						
One cycle with contraceptive alone, one cycle with contraceptive and antibacterial Double-blind, placebo-controlled, crossover	10	**Ciprofloxacin** 500 mg twice daily, day 1 to 7 of the cycle	Oral; ethinylestradiol 30 micrograms with desogestrel, gestodene or levonorgestrel		No change in FSH, LH or estradiol levels	12
One cycle with contraceptive alone, one cycle with contraceptive and antibacterial Double-blind, placebo-controlled, crossover	24	**Ciprofloxacin** 500 mg twice daily, day 1 to 10 of the cycle	Oral; ethinylestradiol 30 micrograms with desogestrel	Ethinylestradiol AUC unchanged on days 11 and 16	No change in progesterone or estradiol levels	13
One cycle with contraceptive alone, one cycle with contraceptive and antibacterial Double-blind, placebo-controlled, crossover	29	**Moxifloxacin** 400 mg daily, day 1 to 7 of the cycle	Oral; ethinylestradiol 30 micrograms with levonorgestrel	Ethinylestradiol AUC unchanged on day 7 Levonorgestrel AUC unchanged	No change in FSH, LH, progesterone or estradiol levels	14
Two cycles with contraceptive alone, two cycles with contraceptive and antibacterial Double-blind, placebo-controlled, crossover	19	**Ofloxacin** 200 mg twice daily, day 1 to 7 of the cycle for 2 consecutive cycles	Oral; ethinylestradiol 30 micrograms with levonorgestrel		No change in FSH, progesterone or estradiol levels, ovulation not detected by ultrasound	15
Sulfonamides and Trimethoprim						
One cycle with contraceptive alone, one cycle with contraceptive and antibacterial	9	**Co-trimoxazole** (sulfamethoxazole with trimethoprim) 960 mg twice daily, day 10 to 17 of the cycle	Oral triphasic; ethinylestradiol 30 to 40 micrograms with levonorgestrel	Ethinylestradiol AUC increased by 30%* and 50%† on days 13, 14, 15 and 16 Levonorgestrel AUC unchanged	FSH levels decreased, progesterone levels unchanged	16
Tetracyclines						
One cycle with contraceptive alone, one cycle with contraceptive and antibacterial Crossover	16	**Doxycycline** 200 mg then 100 mg daily, day 1 to 10 of the cycle	Vaginal ring; ethinylestradiol with etonogestrel	Ethinylestradiol AUC unchanged Etonogestrel AUC unchanged		9
One cycle with contraceptive alone, one cycle with contraceptive and antibacterial	23	**Doxycycline** 100 mg twice daily, day 14 to 20 of the cycle	Oral; ethinylestradiol 35 micrograms with norethisterone 1 mg	Ethinylestradiol* AUC unchanged on days 18 to 20 Norethisterone AUC unchanged	Progesterone levels unchanged	17
Day before antibacterial compared with during antibacterial	6	**Tetracycline** 500 mg four times daily for 10 days	Oral; ethinylestradiol 35 micrograms with norethisterone 1 mg	Ethinylestradiol AUC unchanged on day 1 and days 5 to 10 Norethisterone AUC increased		18
One cycle with contraceptive alone, one cycle with contraceptive and antibacterial Crossover	24	**Tetracycline** 500 mg four times daily for 10 days starting 3 days before patch	Transdermal patch; ethinylestradiol with norelgestromin for 7 days	Ethinylestradiol AUC unchanged on days 0 to 10 Norelgestromin AUC unchanged		19, 20

* Plasma concentration at 10 to 12 hours after taking the contraceptive
† Plasma concentration at 24 hours after taking the contraceptive
‡ Two patients had lower ethinylestradiol levels during ampicillin, but neither ovulated

1. Back DJ, Tjia J, Martin C, Millar E, Salmon P, Orme M. The interaction between clarithromycin and combined oral-contraceptive steroids. *J Pharm Med* (1991) 2, 81–7.
2. Wermeling DP, Chandler MHH, Sides GD, Collins D, Muse KN. Dirithromycin increases ethinyl estradiol clearance without allowing ovulation. *Obstet Gynecol* (1995) 86, 78–84.
3. Blode H, Schott, B, Rohde B, Knuz M, Zeun S. Effects of CYP3A4 induction and inhibition on the pharmacokinetics of estradiol valerate/dienogest. *11th World Congress on Controversies in Obstetrics and Gynecology & Infertility*, Paris, November 2008, 68A.

Continued

Table 28.2 Summary of the controlled studies of the effect of antibacterials on the pharmacokinetics and/or pharmacodynamics of combined hormonal contraceptives (continued)

4. Meyer BH, Müller FO, Wessels P, Maree J. A model to detect interactions between roxithromycin and oral contraceptives. *Clin Pharmacol Ther* (1990) 47, 671–4.
5. Scholtz HE, Sultan E, Wessels D, Hundt AF, Passot V, Renouz A, van Neikerk N. HMR 3647, a new ketolide antimicrobial, does not affect the reliability of low-dose, triphasic oral contraceptives. *Intersci Conf Antimicrob Agents Chemother* (1999) 39, 3.
6. Ketek (Telithromycin). Sanofi-aventis. US Prescribing information, December 2010.
7. Joshi JV, Joshi UM, Sankholi GM, Krishna U, Mandlekar A, Chowdhury V, Hazari K, Gupta K, Sheth UK, Saxena BN. A study of interaction of low-dose combination oral contraceptive with ampicillin and metronidazole. *Contraception* (1980) 22, 643–52.
8. Viswanathan MK, Govindarajulu P. Metronidazole therapy on the efficacy of oral contraceptive steroid pills. *J Reprod Biol Comp Endocrinol* (1985) 5, 69–72.
9. Dogterom P, van den Heuvel MW, Thomsen T. Absence of pharmacokinetic interactions of the combined contraceptive vaginal ring NuvaRing® with oral amoxicillin or doxycycline in two randomised trials. *Clin Pharmacokinet* (2005) 44, 429–38.
10. Friedman CI, Huneke AL, Kim MH, Powell J. The effect of ampicillin on oral contraceptive effectiveness. *Obstet Gynecol* (1980) 55, 33–7.
11. Back DJ, Breckenridge AM, MacIver M, Orme M, Rowe PH, Staiger C, Thomas E, Tjia J. The effects of ampicillin on oral contraceptive steroids in women. *Br J Clin Pharmacol* (1982) 14, 43–8.
12. Maggiolo F, Puricelli G, Dottorini M, Caprioli S, Bianchi W, Suter F. The effect of ciprofloxacin on oral contraceptive steroid treatments. *Drugs Exp Clin Res* (1991) 17, 451–4.
13. Scholten PC, Droppert RM, Zwinkels MGJ, Moesker HL, Nauta JJP, Hoepelman IM. No interaction between ciprofloxacin and an oral contraceptive. *Antimicrob Agents Chemother* (1998) 42, 3266–8.
14. Staß H, Sachse R, Heinig R, Zühlsdorf M, Horstmann R. Pharmacokinetics (PK) of steroid hormones in oral contraceptives (OC) are not altered by oral moxifloxacin (MOX). *J Antimicrob Chemother* (1999) 44 (Suppl A) 138–9.
15. Csemiczky G, Alvendal C, Landgren B-M. Risk for ovulation in women taking a low-dose oral contraceptive (Microgynon) when receiving antibacterial treatment with a fluoroquinolone (ofloxacin). *Adv Contracept* (1996) 12, 101–9.
16. Grimmer SFM, Allen WL, Back DJ, Breckenridge AM, Orme M, Tjia J. The effect of cotrimoxazole on oral contraceptive steroids in women. *Contraception* (1983) 28, 53–9.
17. Neely JL, Abate M, Swinker M, D'Angio R. The effect of doxycycline on serum levels of ethinyl estradiol, norethindrone, and endogenous progesterone. *Obstet Gynecol* (1991) 77, 416–20.
18. Murphy AA, Zacur HA, Charache P, Burkman RT. The effect of tetracycline on levels of oral contraceptives. *Am J Obstet Gynecol* (1991) 164, 28–33.
19. Abrams LS, Skee D, Natarajan J, Hutman W, Wong F. Tetracycline HCl does not affect the pharmacokinetics of a contraceptive patch. *Int J Gynaecol Obstet* (2000) 70, 57–8.
20. Abrams LS, Skee D, Natarajan J, Wong FA. Pharmacokinetic overview of Ortho Evra/Evra. *Fertil Steril* (2002) 77 (2 Suppl 2), S3–S12.

12 months, 73% had taken them once or twice, and 27% had taken them more than three times. In the same group, 25% stated that they never used secondary contraceptive precautions while taking the antibacterial, and about 17% rarely used secondary contraceptive precautions, whereas about 20% usually used, and 38% always used secondary contraceptive precautions while taking antibacterials.[22] Use of secondary contraceptive precautions was not assessed in the original survey. The only differences between the groups of women in the two surveys were age distribution (five times as many teenagers in the pregnant group) and a higher incidence of smoking (60% higher).[22]

3. Case-control and cohort studies. In a dermatological practice, of 124 women taking an oral contraceptive with an antibacterial (**tetracyclines**, 58, **erythromycin**, 54, **co-trimoxazole**, 8, **clindamycin**, 2, **trimethoprim** 1, **amoxicillin** 1), two became pregnant, with a calculated contraceptive failure rate of 1.2%. One patient was taking long-term **minocycline** and **ethinylestradiol** with **norethisterone**, and one had taken a 5-day course of **oxytetracycline** while taking **ethinylestradiol** with **levonorgestrel**. This contraceptive failure rate was reported to be sixfold higher than the accepted failure rate of 0.2%.[23] However, a rate of 0.2% represents perfect rather than typical use of oral combined hormonal contraceptives. In a similar analysis, one of 34 women who had taken antibacterials (**erythromycin**, 20, **tetracycline**, 17, **minocycline**, 5, and/or **co-trimoxazole**, 3) became pregnant after taking long-term **tetracycline** and **ethinylestradiol** with **norethisterone**. This contraceptive failure rate of 1.4% was not considered to be significantly different from an accepted failure rate of 0.27%.[24]

In a larger, better-designed, case-control study, 356 women who had received oral hormonal contraceptives and antibacterials (said to be **cephalosporins**, **penicillins**, **tetracyclines**) were identified over a 5-year period in three dermatological practices. The contraceptive failure rate in these women (1.6% per year; 2 pregnancies occurred in women taking a **cephalosporin** and 3 in women taking **minocycline**) was indistinguishable from the failure rate seen in control patients taking oral hormonal contraceptives and no antibacterials (1% per year). All of these five cases occurred after the antibacterial had been taken for at least 3 months,[25] a period when additional contraceptive precautions have never been recommended.

B. Effect on the antibacterial

In a study in 10 healthy women taking an oral combined hormonal contraceptive (containing **ethinylestradiol** 50 micrograms), there was no difference in the pharmacokinetics of a single 500-mg dose of **ampicillin** when it was given on day 21 of a cycle (steady-state contraceptive steroids) compared with day 28 (anticipated zero levels of contraceptive steroids, at the end of the pill-free interval).[26]

In a non-randomised study looking at the effects of oral combined hormonal contraceptives (unspecified) on the pharmacokinetics of a single 400-mg dose of **moxifloxacin**, the total oral clearance of moxifloxacin was 20% greater and its AUC and maximum plasma concentrations were 15% lower in the 15 women taking oral combined hormonal contraceptives, when compared with 15 women using non-hormonal methods of contraception.[27] The authors considered that these changes might be clinically important if a pathogen has only borderline sensitivity to the antibacterial.[27] However, note that changes of the magnitude seen in this study are not generally considered to be clinically relevant, and the non-randomised nature of this study means that the change could just reflect differences between the two groups rather than an effect of the contraceptive.

Mechanism

The ethinylestradiol component of the combined hormonal contraceptive undergoes enterohepatic recirculation (i.e. it is repeatedly secreted in the bile as sulfate and glucuronide conjugates, which are hydrolysed by the gut bacteria before being reabsorbed). One early idea to explain why contraceptive failure might occur is that if these bacteria are suppressed by the use of an antibacterial, the steroid conjugates are not hydrolysed and are therefore only poorly reabsorbed, resulting in lower than normal concentrations of circulating ethinylestradiol in some women. This may result in inadequate suppression of ovulation.[28] However, increasing evidence points to the conclusion that the enterohepatic recirculation of ethinylestradiol is not clinically important for the following reasons:

- although reduced enterohepatic recirculation of ethinylestradiol with antibacterials has been shown in *animals*,[29] and the penicillins reduce *urinary* oestriol secretion in pregnant women,[30-34] no relevant decreases in ethinylestradiol exposure have been found in controlled studies in women taking an oral combined hormonal contraceptive with any of the antibacterials that have been studied. Indeed, some of the antibacterials that have been implicated in cases of contraceptive failure, have been reported to *increase* ethinylestradiol exposure (such as co-trimoxazole).
- fluoroquinolones are very active against intestinal flora, and yet, they do not alter ethinylestradiol exposure, and they have not been implicated in any published cases of contraceptive failure.
- women with an ileostomy after lower bowel surgery, in which enterohepatic recirculation of ethinylestradiol would not occur, have been reported to have normal serum contraceptive steroid levels while taking oral combined hormonal contraceptives.[35]
- as gut bacteria rapidly become resistant to the antibacterial, any effect should not be apparent on continued use; however, a number of contraceptive failures have been reported with long-term antibacterials used for acne.
- one early hypothesis to explain the lack of an interaction in available, small, controlled studies, was that there may be a very small proportion of women, not yet identified, who are unable to hydroxylate ethinylestradiol and therefore in these subjects enterohepatic recirculation would be important.[29] However, it is now known that ethinylestradiol is principally hydroxylated by CYP3A4, which does not show clinically relevant genetic polymorphism (i.e. there are no population groups who lack active CYP3A4), therefore, this hypothesis seems unlikely.

Additionally, almost all of the evidence suggesting that antibacterials might cause contraceptive failure stems from a period when ethinylestradiol doses were higher than those currently used. If 20 micrograms of ethinylestradiol is considered sufficient for effective contraception, then it seems unlikely that a theoretical small reduction in ethinylestradiol levels when using a 30 to 50 microgram preparation would be sufficient to result in contraceptive failure.

Note that the progestogens do not undergo enterohepatic recirculation in their active forms, see also 'Progestogen-only contraceptives + Antibacterials', p.1197, so the progestogen component of the contraceptive would remain effective.

Alternative possibilities as to why antibacterials may be associated with oral hormonal contraceptive failure include vomiting and/or diarrhoea induced by the antibacterial (and/or the illness being treated), or failure to take the contraceptive properly because of the illness. Combined hormonal contraceptives are not 100% effective, even with perfect use, and contraceptive failure with no obvious reason does occur. As contraceptives and antibacterials are widely co-prescribed, it could equally be that some cases of contraceptive failure with antibacterial use are simply coincidental and represent a chance association rather than a drug interaction.

Importance and management

The interaction between combined hormonal contraceptives and antibacterials is not established. Almost all of the evidence suggesting that antibacterials might cause combined hormonal contraceptive failure is anecdotal with no controls, and the very limited evidence with controls shows no increase in risk. Moreover, data from over 20 studies have not shown any clinically important pharmacokinetic interaction or reduction in the suppression of ovulation by the contraceptive. The total number of contraceptive failures is extremely small, when viewed against the number of women worldwide using combined hormonal contraceptives, and it seems likely that the anecdotal cases of contraceptive failure with broad-spectrum antibacterials are indistinguishable from the accepted contraceptive failure rate.

Nevertheless, despite the limited evidence, a cautious approach has traditionally been adopted in, for example, the UK, where it has generally been recommended that an additional contraceptive should be used during short courses of antibacterials and for 7 days after stopping them. In addition, if fewer than 7 active pills were left in the pack after the antibacterial had been stopped, the new packet should be started without a pill-free break, omitting any of the inactive tablets. In 1999, the UK Family Planning Association recommended these precautions particularly for penicillins and tetracyclines, but excluded erythromycin, co-trimoxazole and sulphonamides, because of evidence to suggest that no interaction occurs.[36] In 2005, for simplicity, and on pragmatic grounds, the first guidance on drug interactions from the UK Faculty of Family Planning and Reproductive Health Care (FFPRHC) Clinical Effectiveness Unit extended the recommendation to short courses of *any antibacterial* (non-enzyme inducing).[37] Note that these precautions have never been applied to the longer-term use of antibacterials, despite there being similar anecdotal cases of contraceptive failure during the long-term use of various antibacterials for acne. In addition, note that it has been suggested that these sorts of precautions may confuse patients, and complicate pill taking, and could have the opposite effect of increasing the failure rate of hormonal contraceptives.[38]

The recommendation for additional contraceptive precautions with antibacterials has never been universally adopted. For example, the WHO does not recommend any additional contraceptive precautions while taking any antibacterials with combined hormonal contraceptives given orally, as the patch, or as the vaginal ring.[39] The exception is the concurrent use of enzyme-inducing antibacterials, such as rifampicin (rifampin) and rifabutin, see 'Combined hormonal contraceptives + Rifamycins', p.1184.

After a review of all the evidence, in 2011 the UK Faculty of Sexual and Reproductive Healthcare (FSRH, formerly the FFPRHC) updated their guidance on hormonal contraceptives and drug interactions, to advise that additional contraceptive precautions are not required during or after short courses of antibacterials (non-enzyme inducing). They note that, should the antibacterials and/or the illness cause vomiting or diarrhoea, then the usual additional precautions relating to these conditions should be observed.[40] This approach is the one most readily justified from the available evidence.

1. Back DJ, Grimmer SFM, Orme ML'E, Proudlove C, Mann RD, Breckenridge AM. Evaluation of Committee on Safety of Medicines yellow card reports on oral contraceptive-drug interactions with anticonvulsants and antibiotics. *Br J Clin Pharmacol* (1988) 25, 527–32.
2. de Groot AC, Eshuis H, Stricker BHC. Ineffectiviteit van orale anticonceptie tijdens gebruik van minocycline. *Ned Tijdschr Geneeskd* (1990) 134, 1227–9.
3. Friedman M, Divon M, Peretz BA. Cephalexin and Microgynon-30 do not go well together. *J Obstet Gynaecol* (1982) 2, 195–6.
4. Hempel E, Böhm W, Carol W, Klinger G. Medikamentöse enzyminduktion und hormonale kontrazeption. *Zentralbl Gynakol* (1973) 95, 1451–7.
5. Hempel E. Personal communication, 1975.
6. Dossetor J. Drug interactions with oral contraceptives. *BMJ* (1975) 4, 467–8.
7. Dossetor J. Personal communication, 1975.
8. Silber TJ. Apparent oral contraceptive failure associated with antibiotic administration. *J Adolesc Health Care* (1983) 4, 287–9.
9. Bainton R. Interaction between antibiotic therapy and contraceptive medication. *Oral Surg Oral Med Oral Pathol* (1986) 61, 453–5.
10. Pedretti E, Brunenghi GM, Morali GC. Interazione tra antibiotici e contraccettivi orali: la spiramicina. *Quad Clin Ostet Ginecol* (1991) 46, 153–4.
11. Bacon JF, Shenfield GM. Pregnancy attributable to interaction between tetracycline and oral contraceptives. *BMJ* (1980) 1, 293.
12. Lequeux A. Grossesse sous contraceptif oral après prise de tétracycline. *Louvain Med* (1980) 99, 413–14.
13. Neely JL, Abate M, Swinker M, D'Angio R. The effect of doxycycline on serum levels of ethinyl estradiol, norethindrone, and endogenous progesterone. *Obstet Gynecol* (1991) 77, 416–20.
14. Wermeling DP, Chandler MHH, Sides GD, Collins D, Muse KN. Dirithromycin increases ethinyl estradiol clearance without allowing ovulation. *Obstet Gynecol* (1995) 86, 78–84.
15. Scholten PC, Droppert RM, Zwinkels MGJ, Moesker HL, Nauta JJP, Hoepelman IM. No interaction between ciprofloxacin and an oral contraceptive. *Antimicrob Agents Chemother* (1998) 42, 3266–8.
16. Sparrow MJ. Pill method failures. *N Z Med J* (1987) 100, 102–5.
17. Sparrow MJ. Pregnancies in reliable pill takers. *N Z Med J* (1989) 102, 575–7.
18. Kovacs GT, Riddoch G, Duncombe P, Welberry L, Chick P, Weisberg E, Leavesley GM, Baker HWG. Inadvertent pregnancies in oral contraceptive users. *Med J Aust* (1989) 150, 549–51.
19. Kakouris H, Kovacs GT. Pill failure and non-use of secondary precautions. *Br J Fam Plann* (1992) 18, 41–4.
20. DeSano EA, Hurley SC. Possible interactions of antihistamines and antibiotics with oral contraceptive effectiveness. *Fertil Steril* (1982) 37, 853–4.
21. Hetényi G. Possible interactions between antibiotics and oral contraceptives. *Ther Hung* (1989) 37, 86–9.
22. Kakouris H, Kovacs GT. How common are predisposing factors to pill failure among pill users? *Br J Fam Plann* (1994) 20, 33–35.
23. Hughes BR, Cunliffe WJ. Interactions between the oral contraceptive pill and antibiotics. *Br J Dermatol* (1990) 122, 717–8.
24. London BM, Lookingbill DP. Frequency of pregnancy in acne patients taking oral antibiotics and oral contraceptives. *Arch Dermatol* (1994) 130, 392–3.
25. Helms SE, Bredle DL, Zajic J, Jarjoura D, Brodell RT, Krishnarao I. Oral contraceptive failure rates and oral antibiotics. *J Am Acad Dermatol* (1997) 36, 705–10.
26. Philipson A. Plasma and urine levels produced by an oral dose of ampicillin 0.5 g administered to women taking oral contraceptives. *Acta Obstet Gynecol Scand* (1979) 58, 69–71.
27. Shain CS, Whitaker A-M, Amsden GW. Effects of oral contraceptives on the pharmacokinetics of moxifloxacin in premenopausal women. *Clin Drug Invest* (2002) 22, 429–34.
28. Back DJ, Breckenridge AM, Crawford FE, MacIver M, Orme ML'E, Rowe PH. Interindividual variation and drug interactions with hormonal steroid contraceptives. *Drugs* (1981) 21, 46–61.
29. Orme M, Back DJ. Oral contraceptive steroids – pharmacological issues of interest to the prescribing physician. *Adv Contracept* (1991) 7, 325–31.
30. Willman K, Pulkkinen MO. Reduced maternal plasma and urinary estriol during ampicillin treatment. *Am J Obstet Gynecol* (1971) 109, 893–6.
31. Tikkanen MJ, Aldercreutz H, Pulkkinen MO. Effect of antibiotics on oestrogen metabolism. *BMJ* (1973) 1, 369.
32. Pulkkinen MO, Willman K. Maternal oestrogen levels during penicillin treatment. *BMJ* (1971) 4, 48.
33. Sybulski S, Maughan GB. Effect of ampicillin administration on estradiol, estriol, and cortisol levels in maternal plasma and on estriol levels in urine. *Am J Obstet Gynecol* (1976) 124, 379–81.
34. Trybuchowski H. Effect of ampicillin on the urinary output of steroidal hormones in pregnant and non-pregnant women. *Clin Chim Acta* (1973) 45, 9–18.
35. Grimmer SFM, Back DJ, Orme MLE, Cowie A, Gilmore I, Tjia J. The bioavailability of ethinyloestradiol and levonorgestrel in patients with an ileostomy. *Contraception* (1986) 33, 51–9.
36. Belfield T, ed. FPA Contraceptive Handbook: a guide for family planning and other health professionals. 3rd ed. London: Family Planning Association, 1999.
37. Faculty of Family Planning and Reproductive Health Care Clinical Effectiveness Unit. FFPRHC Guidance (April 2005): Drug interactions with hormonal contraception. *J Fam Plann Reprod Health Care* (2005) 31, 139–51.
38. Weaver K, Glasier A. Interaction between broad-spectrum antibiotics and the combined oral contraceptive pill. *Contraception* (1999) 59, 71–8.
39. Reproductive Health and Research, World Health Organization. Medical eligibility criteria for contraceptive use. 5th edition. Geneva, WHO; 2015. Available at: https://extranet.who.int/iris/restricted/bitstream/10665/181468/1/9789241549158_eng.pdf (accessed 22/10/15).
40. Faculty of Sexual and Reproductive Healthcare Guidance. Drug interactions with hormonal contraception: Clinical Effectiveness Unit, January 2011. Available at: http://www.fsrh.org/pdfs/CEUGuidanceDrugInteractionsHormonal.pdf (accessed 22/10/15).

Combined hormonal contraceptives or HRT + Antibacterials; Troleandomycin

Severe pruritus and jaundice have been seen in women taking oral combined hormonal contraceptives shortly after starting treatment with troleandomycin. One case has also been reported with oestrogens for HRT.

Clinical evidence

A report describes 10 cases of cholestatic jaundice and pruritus in women taking oral [combined] hormonal contraceptives and troleandomycin. All had been using the contraceptive for 7 to 48 months and were given the antibacterial in daily doses of 1 to 3 g. The pruritus was intense, and started within 2 to 24 days of the first dose of troleandomycin, and preceded the jaundice. In 8 of the patients the pruritus and jaundice persisted for over a month.[1] A later report and letter by the same authors describes a total of 24 cases of this reaction with oral combined hormonal contraceptives containing **ethinylestradiol** 30 or 50 micrograms.[2,3]

There are numerous other reports of this adverse reaction in a total of over 40 other women.[4-12] The adverse reactions (fatigue, anorexia, severe itching, jaundice) can begin very rapidly, sometimes even within 2 days of starting troleandomycin, and may last up to 14 weeks or more.[3,4,12]

One report also describes a similar reaction in a 48-year-old woman taking oestrogens for HRT.[4]

Mechanism

Uncertain. Hepatotoxicity has been associated with the use of both types of drug, but it is not common. The reaction suggests that their damaging effects on the liver may be additive or synergistic.[10,11] Troleandomycin may cause an increase in the levels of contraceptive steroids, as it is a liver enzyme inhibitor.[12,13]

Importance and management

The interaction between troleandomycin and contraceptive steroids is well established, well documented and clinically important. The incidence is unknown. Concurrent use should be avoided. Other macrolides may be suitable alternatives. See also, 'Combined hormonal contraceptives + Antibacterials', p.1162.

1. Miguet JP, Monange C, Vuitton D, Allemand H, Hirsch JP, Carayon P, Gisselbrecht H. Ictère cholestatique survenu après administration de triacétyloléandomycine: interférence avec les contraceptifs oraux? Dix observations. *Nouv Presse Med* (1978) 7, 4304.
2. Miguet J-P, Vuitton D, Pessayre D, Allemand H, Metreau J-M, Poupon R, Capron J-P, Blanc F. Jaundice from troleandomycin and oral contraceptives. *Ann Intern Med* (1980) 92, 434.
3. Miguet J-P, Vuitton D, Allemand H, Pessayre D, Monange C, Hirsch J-P, Metreau J-M, Poupon R, Capron J-P, Blanc F. Une épidémie d'ictères due a l'association troléandomycine – contraceptifs oraux. *Gastroenterol Clin Biol* (1980) 4, 420–4.
4. Perol R, Hincky J, Desnos M. Hépatites cholestatiques lors de la prise de troléandomycine chez deux femmes prenant des estrogènes. *Nouv Presse Med* (1978) 7, 4302.
5. Goldfain D, Chauveinc L, Guillan J, Verduron J. Ictère cholestatique chez des femmes prenant simultanément de la triacétyloléandomycine et des contraceptifs oraux. *Nouv Presse Med* (1979) 8, 1099.
6. Rollux R, Plottin F, Mingat J, Bessard G. Ictère apres association estroprogestatif-troléandomycine. Trois observations. *Nouv Presse Med* (1979) 8, 1694.
7. Haber I, Hubens H. Cholestatic jaundice after triacetyloleandomycin and oral contraceptives. The diagnostic value of gamma-glutamyl transpeptidase. *Acta Gastroenterol Belg* (1980) 43, 475–82.
8. Descotes J, Evreux JC, Foyatier N, Gaumer R, Girard D, Savoye B. Trois nouvelles observations d'ictère après estroprogestatifs et troléandomycine. *Nouv Presse Med* (1979) 8, 1182–3.
9. Belgian Centre for Drug Supervison. Levertoxiciteit van troleandomycine en oestrogen. *Folia Pharmaceutica (Brussels)* (1979) 6, 64.
10. Dellas JA, Hugues FC, Roussel G, Marche J. Contraception orale et troléandomycine. Un nouveau cas d'ictère. *Therapie* (1982) 37, 443–6.
11. Girard D, Pillon M, Bel A, Petigny A, Savoye B. Hepatite au decours d'un traitment a la triacetyloleandomycine chez les jeunes femmes sous estro-progestatifs. *Lyon Mediterr Med Med Sud Est* (1980) 16, 2335–44.
12. Fevery J, Van Steenbergen W, Desmet V, Deruyttere M, De Groote J. Severe intrahepatic cholestasis due to the combined intake of oral contraceptives and triacetyloleandomycin. *Acta Clin Belg* (1983) 38, 242–5.
13. Claudel S, Euvrard P, Bory R, Chavaillon A, Paliard P. Cholestase intra-hépatique après association triacétyloléandomycine-estroprogestatif. *Nouv Presse Med* (1979) 8, 1182.

Combined hormonal contraceptives + Antihistamines

The pharmacokinetics of single doses of doxylamine and diphenhydramine do not appear to be altered by oral combined hormonal contraceptives. Isolated cases of contraceptive failure have been reported with doxylamine and chlorphenamine and with unnamed antihistamines.

Clinical evidence, mechanism, importance and management

In a study, the pharmacokinetics of a single 25-mg dose of **doxylamine** in 13 women and the pharmacokinetics of a single 50-mg dose of **diphenhydramine** in 10 women were not significantly altered by the use of oral combined hormonal contraceptives.[1] In one report, three cases of oral contraceptive failure were attributed to the use of **doxylamine** or **chlorphenamine** used in conjunction with penicillins (see also 'Combined hormonal contraceptives + Antibacterials', p.1162) and one case with unnamed antihistamines for hayfever.[2] It seems likely that these represent coincidental cases, especially as no other cases appear to have been reported. Although the effect of the antihistamines on the pharmacokinetics and pharmacodynamics of contraceptive steroids appear not to have been studied, there is no theoretical reason to predict an interaction. No particular contraceptive precautions would seem necessary during concurrent use.

1. Luna BG, Scavone JM, Greenblatt DJ. Doxylamine and diphenhydramine pharmacokinetics in women on low-dose estrogen oral contraceptives. *J Clin Pharmacol* (1989) 29, 257–60.
2. DeSano EA, Hurley SC. Possible interactions of antihistamines and antibiotics with oral contraceptive effectiveness. *Fertil Steril* (1982) 37, 853–4.

Combined hormonal contraceptives + Antimalarials

Chloroquine and primaquine do not appear to have a clinically relevant effect on the pharmacokinetics of ethinylestradiol or norethisterone from an oral combined hormonal contraceptive. In addition, chloroquine does not appear to affect the suppression of ovulation caused by oral combined hormonal contraceptives.

Oral contraceptives do not appear to alter the pharmacokinetics or antimalarial effects of mefloquine or the pharmacokinetics of quinine. However, there is some evidence to suggest that an oral combined hormonal contraceptive modestly reduced the conversion of proguanil to its active metabolite, cycloguanil.

Clinical evidence and mechanism

(a) Chloroquine

A pharmacokinetic study in 12 healthy women taking an oral combined hormonal contraceptive (**ethinylestradiol** 30 micrograms with **norethisterone** 1 mg) found that the prophylactic use of chloroquine phosphate 500 mg once weekly for 4 weeks caused a small 15% increase in the AUC of **ethinylestradiol**, and no change in the levels of **norethisterone**. Chloroquine did not alter the inhibition of ovulation caused by the contraceptive, as assessed by mid-luteal progesterone levels and the lack of breakthrough spotting and bleeding. In a further group of 7 women, the same oral combined hormonal contraceptive did not alter the pharmacokinetics of a single 500-mg dose of chloroquine phosphate.[1] Another study in 6 healthy women given a single dose of an oral combined hormonal contraceptive (**ethinylestradiol** 30 micrograms with **levonorgestrel** 150 micrograms) confirmed that a single 300-mg dose of chloroquine had no effect on the pharmacokinetics of either the oestrogen or the progestogen.[2]

(b) Mefloquine

In a study in 12 Thai women with falciparum malaria, 6 of whom were taking unnamed oral contraceptives, the response to mefloquine (parasite and fever clearance) was not affected by oral contraceptives. Similarly, the pharmacokinetics of mefloquine 750 mg did not differ between the patients taking oral contraceptives and those not taking oral contraceptives.[3]

(c) Primaquine

A study in 6 healthy women given a single dose of an oral combined hormonal contraceptive (**ethinylestradiol** 30 micrograms with **levonorgestrel** 150 micrograms) found that a single 45-mg dose of primaquine had no significant effect on the pharmacokinetics of either the oestrogen or the progestogen.[2]

(d) Proguanil

In a study in women who were CYP2C19 extensive metabolisers (that is, those with normal levels of this isoenzyme), the use of an oral combined hormonal contraceptive (**ethinylestradiol** with **levonorgestrel**) reduced the levels of cycloguanil (the active metabolite of proguanil) by 34% after 3 weeks, when compared with the cycloguanil levels before starting the contraceptive.[4] It was suggested that ethinylestradiol might have inhibited the metabolism of proguanil by CYP2C19. However, inhibition of CYP2C19 essentially turns extensive metabolisers into poor metabolisers (that is, those lacking or deficient in this isoenzyme), and there is some evidence that CYP2C19 poor metaboliser status does not reduce the efficacy of proguanil for prophylaxis or treatment of malaria, see 'Proguanil + Fluvoxamine', p.254.

(e) Quinine

A controlled study in Thai women found that the pharmacokinetics of a single 600-mg dose of quinine sulfate in 7 women taking oral contraceptives were not notably different from those in 7 other women not taking contraceptives. The contraceptives being used were oral combined hormonal contraceptives in 6 women (**ethinylestradiol** with **levonorgestrel** or **norgestrel**) and a progestogen-only oral contraceptive in one (**norethisterone**).[5]

Importance and management

Chloroquine had no clinically relevant effect on the pharmacokinetics or ovulation suppressant effect of an oral combined hormonal contraceptive and oral contraceptives possibly do not alter chloroquine efficacy. Limited data suggest that **primaquine** does not alter the pharmacokinetics of an oral combined hormonal contraceptive. Oral contraceptives do not appear to alter the pharmacokinetics of **quinine** or **mefloquine**, nor do they appear to alter mefloquine efficacy. There would seem to be no reason for avoiding the concurrent use of these antimalarials and oral contraceptives.

The production of the active metabolite of **proguanil** appeared to be modestly decreased by oral combined hormonal contraceptives in one study, and the authors of the study recommended that the dose of proguanil should be increased by 50% in women taking these contraceptives.[4] However, there is evidence that this pharmacokinetic interaction may not be clinically relevant, see 'Proguanil + Fluvoxamine', p.254.

1. Gupta KC, Joshi JV, Desai NK, Sankolli GM, Chowdhary VN, Joshi UM, Chitalange S, Satoskar RS. Kinetics of chloroquine and contraceptive steroids in oral contraceptive users during concurrent chloroquine prophylaxis. *Indian J Med Res* (1984) 80, 658–62.
2. Back DJ, Breckenridge AM, Grimmer SFM, Orme ML'E, Purba HS. Pharmacokinetics of oral contraceptive steroids following the administration of the antimalarial drugs primaquine and chloroquine. *Contraception* (1984) 30, 289–95.
3. Karbwang J, Looareesuwan S, Back DJ, Migasana S, Bunnag D, Breckenridge AM. Effect of oral contraceptive steroids on the clinical course of malaria infection and on the pharmacokinetics of mefloquine in Thai women. *Bull WHO* (1988) 66, 763–7.
4. McGready R, Stepniewska K, Seaton E, Cho T, Cho D, Ginsberg A, Edstein MD, Ashley E, Looareesuwan S, White NJ, Nosten F. Pregnancy and use of oral contraceptives reduces the biotransformation of proguanil to cycloguanil. *Eur J Clin Pharmacol* (2003) 59, 553–7.
5. Wanwimolruk S, Kaewvichit S, Tanthayaphinant O, Suwannarach C, Oranratnachai A. Lack of effect of oral contraceptive use on the pharmacokinetics of quinine. *Br J Clin Pharmacol* (1991) 31,179–81.

Combined hormonal contraceptives + Antimycobacterials; Miscellaneous

The concurrent use of aminosalicylic acid, isoniazid and streptomycin does not appear to affect the pharmacokinetics or ovulation suppressant effect of oral combined hormonal contraceptives. Isoniazid has been listed as an antibacterial used in two cases of oral contraceptive failure.

Clinical evidence, mechanism, importance and management

In a study of contraceptives and antimycobacterials, none of 8 women taking **aminosalicylic acid** 4 g twice daily, **isoniazid** 125 mg twice daily and **streptomycin** 0.75 g daily for tuberculosis ovulated while taking an oral combined hormonal contraceptive (**ethinylestradiol** 30 micrograms with **norethisterone** 1 mg). In addition, there was no difference in the AUC of ethinylestradiol or norethisterone between these 8 women and 10 women in the control group given the same contraceptive alone.[1] In a list of oral contraceptive failures reported to the CSM in the UK in women taking antibacterials, **isoniazid** was listed for one case.[2] Similarly, isoniazid was mentioned for one case in a survey of women with oral contraceptive failure.[3]

Isoniazid is not a broad-spectrum antibacterial, and would therefore not have been anticipated to interact with ethinylestradiol in the way formerly hypothesised for some antibacterials, see 'Combined hormonal contraceptives + Antibacterials', p.1162. No additional contraceptive precautions would be expected to be required in women taking combined hormonal contraceptives and requiring isoniazid.

Note that rifampicin (rifampin) is an enzyme inducer and is known to reduce contraceptive steroid exposure and the ovulation suppressant effect of combined hormonal contraceptives; therefore if rifampicin is also taken, see 'Combined hormonal contraceptives + Rifamycins', p.1184, for guidance on managing this important interaction.

1. Joshi JV, Joshi UM, Sankolli GM, Gupta K, Rao AP, Hazari K, Sheth UK, Saxena BN. A study of interaction of low-dose combination oral contraceptive with anti-tubercular drugs. *Contraception* (1980) 21, 617–29.
2. Back DJ, Breckenridge AM, Crawford FE, MacIver M, Orme ML'E, Rowe PH. Interindividual variation and drug interactions with hormonal steroid contraceptives. *Drugs* (1981) 21, 46–61.
3. Kovacs GT, Riddoch G, Duncombe P, Welberry L, Chick P, Weisberg E, Leavesley GM, Baker HWG. Inadvertent pregnancies in oral contraceptive users. *Med J Aust* (1989) 150, 549–51.

Combined hormonal contraceptives + Aprepitant

Aprepitant reduces ethinylestradiol exposure from an oral combined hormonal contraceptive. Fosaprepitant, a prodrug of aprepitant, is expected to interact similarly.

Clinical evidence

The manufacturer notes that aprepitant 100 mg daily for 14 days given with an oral combined hormonal contraceptive (**ethinylestradiol** 35 micrograms with **norethisterone** 1 mg) decreased the AUC of **ethinylestradiol** and **norethisterone** by 43% and 8%, respectively.[1] Reduced contraceptive steroid levels were reported in another study using a recommended antiemetic regimen including aprepitant (125 mg on the first day, then 80 mg daily for 2 days with dexamethasone 12 mg on the first day, then 8 mg daily for 3 days and ondansetron 32 mg on the first day), which was started on day 8 of a 21-day cycle of an oral combined hormonal contraceptive (**ethinylestradiol** with **norethisterone**).[1] Within 2 days of starting the antiemetics (day 10) the **ethinylestradiol** AUC was reduced by 19% and the **norethisterone** level was unchanged.[1] However, the trough level of **ethinylestradiol** was reduced by as much as 64% and the trough level of **norethisterone** was reduced by 60% during days 9 to 21.[1,2]

In yet another study, a single 40-mg dose of aprepitant was given on day 8 of a 21-day cycle of an oral combined hormonal contraceptive (**ethinylestradiol** with **norgestimate**). The AUC of **ethinylestradiol** decreased by 4% and 29% on day 8 and day 12, respectively, while the AUC of norelgestromin (the metabolite of **norgestimate**) increased by 18% on day 8 and decreased by 10% on day 12.[1]

Mechanism

During the first few days of use, aprepitant is an inhibitor of CYP3A4 and therefore it would be expected to *increase* the levels of the contraceptive steroids. However, aprepitant then becomes an inducer of CYP3A4 (which usually becomes apparent after the end of a standard 3-day course), reaching a maximal inductive effect within 3 to 5 days of stopping aprepitant, and hence reduces the levels of the contraceptive steroids. This effect lasts only a few days and then reduces to become clinically irrelevant within 2 weeks of stopping aprepitant.[2]

Importance and management

The pharmacokinetic interaction between aprepitant and combined hormonal contraceptives would appear to be established. Although the effects of the reduced contraceptive steroid exposure on ovulation were not assessed, it is likely that they could result in a reduction in the efficacy of any combined hormonal contraceptive (tablets, patch or vaginal ring). The manufacturer therefore recommends that alternative or additional contraceptive methods should be used during, and for 2 months (UK advice)[2] or one month (US advice)[1] after, aprepitant use. The same advice is given for **fosaprepitant**, which is a prodrug of aprepitant, for intravenous use.[3,4] This seems a sensible precaution. In the UK, the Faculty of Sexual and Reproductive Healthcare 2011 guideline on hormonal contraception and drug interactions includes aprepitant in their list of enzyme-inducing drugs that reduce contraceptive hormone levels.[5] As aprepitant is generally given as a single dose or a short course, the FSRH guidance on the *short-term* use of enzyme-inducers with combined hormonal contraceptives should be followed; see 'Combined hormonal contraceptives + Barbiturates or Phenytoin', p.1169, for further details of this guidance.

In addition to the possibility of a pharmacokinetic interaction leading to decreased contraceptive efficacy, the clinical situation in which aprepitant is used (such as chemotherapy-induced nausea and vomiting) may also need consideration in terms of an appropriate choice of contraceptive: vomiting decreases the efficacy of oral contraceptives, and cytotoxic chemotherapy and/or cancer *per se* are associated with an increased risk of venous thromboembolic disease).

1. EMEND Capsules (Aprepitant). Merck & Co., Inc. US prescribing information, March 2011.
2. EMEND (Aprepitant). Merck Sharp & Dohme Ltd. UK Summary of product characteristics, December 2013.
3. IVEMEND (Fosaprepitant dimeglumine). Merck Sharp & Dohme Ltd. UK Summary of product characteristics, December 2011.
4. EMEND for Injection (Fosaprepitant dimeglumine). Merck & Co., Inc. US prescribing information, March 2011.
5. Faculty of Sexual and Reproductive Healthcare Guidance. Drug interactions with hormonal contraception: Clinical Effectiveness Unit, January 2011. Available at: http://www.fsrh.org/pdfs/CEUGuidanceDrugInteractionsHormonal.pdf (accessed 21/10/15).

Combined hormonal contraceptives + Ascorbic acid (Vitamin C)

Ascorbic acid does not alter ethinylestradiol or levonorgestrel exposure from oral combined hormonal contraceptives. There are a few unconfirmed anecdotal reports of contraceptive failure associated with ascorbic acid.

Clinical evidence

In one study in 5 women taking oral combined hormonal contraceptives, ascorbic acid 1 g *raised* serum **ethinylestradiol** levels by 16% at 6 hours post-dose and by 48% at 24 hours post-dose.[1] However, a later well-controlled study found that ascorbic acid 1 g daily caused no changes in **ethinylestradiol** AUC in 37 women taking an oral combined hormonal contraceptive (**ethinylestradiol** 30 micrograms with **levonorgestrel** 150 micrograms) nor did it alter ethinylestradiol sulfate levels.[2] A similar study by the same workers found that ascorbic acid 1 g did not affect the pharmacokinetics of **levonorgestrel**.[3]

A single case report describes a woman taking an oral combined hormonal contraceptive (**ethinylestradiol** with **levonorgestrel**) who experienced heavy breakthrough bleeding in three cycles within 2 to 3 days of stopping ascorbic acid 1 g daily. This did not occur in three other cycles when no ascorbic acid was taken. It was suggested that this was due to a fall in **ethinylestradiol** levels when the vitamin C was stopped, which could increase the risk of contraceptive failure.[4] One report attributed contraceptive failure in one case to ascorbic acid and multivitamins.[5] Another two studies of pregnancies in oral contraceptive users found that vitamin C had been taken in 44 of 209 cases[6] and 15 of 137 cases,[7] although other drugs and/or factors may possibly have been involved in some of these cases.

Mechanism

Both ascorbic acid and ethinylestradiol undergo sulfate conjugation. It was suggested that large doses of ascorbic acid might compete for the metabolism of ethinylestradiol to the sulfate, and therefore increase its levels;[1] however, this was not found to occur.[2] In addition, if raised ethinylestradiol levels did occur, this would be expected to increase the efficacy of the hormonal contraceptive. However, some have suggested that enhanced levels could be followed by rebound ovulation,[4] but there is no evidence to support this.

Importance and management

Despite the initial reported interaction of raised ethinylestradiol levels in patients taking ascorbic acid, later well-controlled studies have found that ascorbic acid does not alter the pharmacokinetics of contraceptive steroids. The isolated reports of contraceptive failure are unexplained, and might simply be coincidental, reflecting the usual expected failure rate of the contraceptives used. Therefore, from the point of view of contraceptive reliability, there seems to be little reason for avoiding the use of combined hormonal contraceptives and ascorbic acid, and no additional contraceptive precautions are required on concurrent use.

1. Back DJ, Breckenridge AM, MacIver M, Orme ML'E, Purba H, Rowe PH. Interaction of ethinyloestradiol with ascorbic acid in man. *BMJ* (1981) 282, 1516.
2. Zamah NM, Hümpel M, Kuhnz W, Louton T, Rafferty J, Back DJ. Absence of an effect of high vitamin C dosage on the systemic availability of ethinyl estradiol in women using a combination oral contraceptive. *Contraception* (1993) 48, 377–91.
3. Kuhnz W, Louton T, Hümpel M, Back DJ, Zamah NM. Influence of high doses of vitamin C on the bioavailability and the serum protein binding of levonorgestrel in women using a combination oral contraceptive. *Contraception* (1995) 51, 111–16.
4. Morris JC, Beeley L, Ballantine N. Interaction of ethinyloestradiol with ascorbic acid in man. *BMJ* (1981) 283, 503.
5. DeSano EA, Hurley SC. Possible interactions of antihistamines and antibiotics with oral contraceptive effectiveness. *Fertil Steril* (1982) 37, 853–4.
6. Kovacs GT, Riddoch G, Duncombe P, Welberry L, Chick P, Weisberg E, Leavesley GM, Baker HWG. Inadvertent pregnancies in oral contraceptive users. *Med J Aust* (1989) 150, 549–51.
7. Sparrow MJ. Pregnancies in reliable pill takers. *N Z Med J* (1989) 102, 575–7.

Combined hormonal contraceptives + Azoles

There are isolated reports of breakthrough bleeding and failure of oral combined hormonal contraceptives in women taking fluconazole (including single 150 mg doses), itraconazole and ketoconazole. However, fluconazole, itraconazole and voriconazole have been shown to *increase* contraceptive steroid exposure. Similarly, ketoconazole increased estradiol and dienogest exposure. Intravaginal miconazole very slightly increases ethinylestradiol and etonogestrel exposure during the use of an intravaginal contraceptive ring. Oral combined hormonal contraceptives modestly increase voriconazole exposure.

Clinical evidence

(a) Fluconazole

Up to 1990 the UK manufacturer of fluconazole had received 11 reports of menstrual disorders possibly associated with single-dose fluconazole 150 mg. Eight of these were in women taking an oral contraceptive (unspecified) who developed breakthrough bleeding (5 cases), no withdrawal bleeding (one case), and unintended pregnancies (2 cases).[1] Three other cases of unintended pregnancy have been very briefly mentioned elsewhere.[2] However, some pharmacokinetic studies have reported an *increase* in contraceptive steroid levels on concurrent use. One study found that a single 150-mg dose of fluconazole increased the AUC of **ethinylestradiol** by 29% in women taking an oral combined hormonal contraceptive (**ethinylestradiol** with **norethisterone** or **levonorgestrel**).[3] Similarly, fluconazole 300 mg once weekly for 4 weeks caused a 24% increase in the AUC of **ethinylestradiol** and a 13% increase in the AUC of **norethisterone**.[4] Moreover, in a study in 25 healthy women, fluconazole 200 mg daily for 10 days raised the AUC of **ethinylestradiol** by about 40% and of **levonorgestrel** by about 25% (given as a single dose of an oral combined hormonal contraceptive on day 10).[5,6] In contrast, in a study in 10 healthy women, a lower dose of fluconazole (a single 50-mg dose or 50 mg of fluconazole daily for 10 days), had no effect on the pharmacokinetics of **ethinylestradiol** and **norgestrel** (given as an oral combined hormonal contraceptive).[7]

One other study in 10 women taking oral combined hormonal contraceptives found no changes in progesterone levels (suggesting no ovulation occurred) and no menstrual disorders while they were taking fluconazole 50 mg daily.[8] Furthermore, during clinical studies in which single 150-mg doses of fluconazole were used by over 700 women taking oral contraceptives (unspecified), no clinical evidence of an interaction was seen.[9] For mention that fluconazole has no effect on the AUC of desogestrel, see 'Progestogen-only contraceptives + Azoles', p.1198.

(b) Itraconazole

A 25-year-old woman who had been taking an oral combined hormonal contraceptive (**ethinylestradiol** 30 micrograms with **levonorgestrel** 150 micrograms) for a year, without problems, became pregnant when she was given itraconazole 200 mg daily for 3 months for a fungal infection. The patient was said to be compliant, had suffered no gastrointestinal upset, and was not taking any other drugs that might have accounted for the failure of the contraceptive.[2]

The Netherlands Pharmacovigilance Foundation (LAREB) have 9 cases of menstrual changes on their records in women taking an oral combined hormonal contraceptive (**ethinylestradiol** with either **desogestrel** or **levonorgestrel**) during or after taking itraconazole 100 to 400 mg daily for one to 4 weeks. Seven women reported delayed withdrawal bleeding (2 to 5 days). In 2 of them the menstrual flow was decreased and one transiently had a positive pregnancy test after having previously experienced an intermenstrual blood loss. The remaining two reports were of amenorrhoea during one cycle, and breakthrough bleeding.[10] A later extension of this report from LAREB, covering the period 1991 to 1997, describes 12 women taking oral combined hormonal contraceptives containing **ethinylestradiol** with **desogestrel**, whose withdrawal bleeding was either delayed or did not occur at all while taking itraconazole. Three other women taking **ethinylestradiol** with **levonorgestrel** had breakthrough bleeding, and yet another taking **ethinylestradiol** with **cyproterone** became pregnant while taking itraconazole.[11]

However, the manufacturer has data on file of a study showing that itraconazole 200 mg daily for 15 days had no effect on the pharmacokinetics of **ethinylestradiol**, and *increased* the bioavailability of **norethisterone** by about 40%. In this study, a single dose of an oral combined hormonal contraceptive (**ethinylestradiol** with **norethisterone**) was given before the first dose and with the last dose of itraconazole.[12] Similarly, for mention that itraconazole increases the AUC of desogestrel, see 'Progestogen-only contraceptives + Azoles', p.1198.

(c) Ketoconazole

An early report described 7 out of 147 women taking oral combined hormonal contraceptives (**ethinylestradiol** with **norgestrel**) who experienced breakthrough bleeding or spotting within 2 to 5 days of starting a 5-day course of ketoconazole 400 mg daily. No pregnancies occurred.[13] One unintended pregnancy attributed to contraceptive failure due to ketoconazole has been very briefly mentioned elsewhere.[2]

In one controlled study in postmenopausal women given an oral combined hormonal contraceptive (**estradiol** 2 mg with **dienogest** 3 mg) for 14 days, ketoconazole 400 mg daily for 7 days increased the steady-state AUC of **estradiol** by up to 65% and that of **dienogest** by 186%.[14-16]

(d) Miconazole

A study found that both single and multiple-dose intravaginal regimens of miconazole pessaries or cream very slightly increased the AUC of **ethinylestradiol** and **etonogestrel** during the use of an intravaginal ring (*NuvaRing*). The AUC over days 8 to 21 was increased by 16% for **ethinylestradiol** and 17% for **etonogestrel** with a single vaginal dose of miconazole 1.2 g given on day 8.[17]

(e) Voriconazole

In a pharmacokinetic study in 15 healthy subjects (given an oral combined hormonal contraceptive (ethinylestradiol 35 micrograms with norethisterone 1 mg) for 2 menstrual cycles, the steady-state AUC of **ethinylestradiol** and **norethisterone** were increased by 61% and 53%, respectively, by the concurrent use of voriconazole for 4 days (400 mg twice daily on day one, then 200 mg twice daily). Moreover, the maximum levels and AUC of voriconazole were increased by 14% and 46%, respectively, by the contraceptive, when compared with voriconazole given alone. Voriconazole alone did not cause irregular uterine bleeding (metrorrhagia), but this occurred with the contraceptive alone and with the contraceptive plus voriconazole (incidence not stated).[18]

Mechanism

The azoles are, to varying degrees, inhibitors of CYP3A4, by which contraceptive steroids are partially metabolised. They would therefore be expected to increase the levels of the contraceptive steroids to varying extents, as has been shown for fluconazole, itraconazole, ketoconazole, intravaginal miconazole and voriconazole. Therefore the azoles would *not* be expected to increase the incidence of breakthrough bleeding or contraceptive failure when given with combined hormonal contraceptives. It should be noted that the manufacturers list menstrual irregularities as adverse effects of itraconazole, ketoconazole and **posaconazole**, irrespective of the use of hormonal contraceptives,[19-21] and menstrual disorders have also been reported with fluconazole alone.[1]

The increase in voriconazole levels was expected to be due to inhibition of CYP2C19 by ethinylestradiol.[18]

Importance and management

The picture presented by these reports is somewhat confusing and contradictory. The anecdotal reports of contraceptive failure and the cases of breakthrough bleeding would suggest that these azoles can, rarely, make oral contraception less reliable in some individuals. However, the problem with this interpretation is that the pharmacokinetic data suggest that, if anything, an *enhanced* effect of oral combined hormonal contraceptives is likely. Note that, of all the drugs proven to decrease the efficacy of oral combined hormonal contraceptives, all have also been shown to decrease the steroid levels. Menstrual disorders have been reported with the azoles alone, and may not be indicative of reduced contraceptive efficacy. As there are so few reports of pregnancy, it could just be that they fall within the accepted failure rate of oral combined hormonal contraceptives, and it was just coincidental they occurred when the azole was being taken. Note that the manufacturers do not advise any additional precautions when taking hormonal contraceptives and these azoles.[5,19,22] However, some authors have considered that the data warrant consideration being given to the use of additional contraceptive measures.[11] The theoretical teratogenic risk[5,19-22] from these azoles may have a bearing on this, and the UK manufacturers of a number of the azoles recommend using effective contraception (unspecified) in women of child-bearing age taking an azole because of this.[5,19,21,22]

The main concern regarding the increased ethinylestradiol or progestogen exposure is whether this would increase the risk of adverse effects of these contraceptive steroids; however, there are no data on the effect of these 24 to 61% increases in steroid levels on adverse effects. It could be argued that a 40% increase for ethinylestradiol might turn a standard-strength oral combined hormonal contraceptive (35 micrograms) into a high-dose oral combined hormonal contraceptive (50 micrograms), and, indeed, in one study, the AUC of ethinylestradiol 35 micrograms with voriconazole was comparable to that seen in earlier studies with a 50-microgram dose of ethinylestradiol.[18] Bear this in mind if an increase in adverse effects, such as nausea and breast tenderness, is seen on concurrent use. Further study is needed.

There is also the potential for a slight increase in voriconazole exposure on the concurrent use of an oral combined hormonal contraceptive; however, this would not be expected to be clinically relevant.

1. Pfizer Ltd. Data on file. Summary of unpublished reports: female reproductive disorders possibly associated with Diflucan (Ref DIFLU:diflu41.1). 1990.
2. Pillans PI, Sparrow MJ. Pregnancy associated with a combined oral contraceptive and itraconazole. *N Z Med J* (1993) 106, 436.
3. Sinofsky FE, Pasquale SA. The effect of fluconazole on circulating ethinyl estradiol levels in women taking oral contraceptives. *Am J Obstet Gynecol* (1998) 178, 300–4.
4. Hilbert J, Messig M, Kuye O, Friedman H. Evaluation of interaction between fluconazole and an oral contraceptive in healthy women. *Obstet Gynecol* (2001) 98, 218–23.
5. Diflucan (Fluconazole). Pfizer Ltd. UK Summary of product characteristics, June 2009.
6. Diflucan (Fluconazole). Pfizer Inc. US Prescribing information, June 2011.
7. Lazar JD, Wilner KD. Drug interactions with fluconazole. *Rev Infect Dis* (1990) 12, Suppl 3, S327–S333.
8. Devenport MH, Crook D, Wynn V, Lees LJ. Metabolic effects of low-dose fluconazole in healthy female users and non-users of oral contraceptives. *Br J Clin Pharmacol* (1989) 27, 851–9.
9. Dodd GK (Pfizer Ltd). Personal communication, 1990.
10. Meyboom RHB, van Puijenbroek EP, Vinks MHAM, Lastdrager CJ. Disturbance of withdrawal bleeding during concomitant use of itraconazole and oral contraceptives. *N Z Med J* (1997) 110, 300.
11. van Puijenbroek EP, Feenstra J, Meyboom RHB. Verstoring van de pilcyclus tijdens het gelijktijdig gebruik van itraconazol en orale anticonceptiva. *Ned Tijdschr Geneeskd* (1998) 142, 146–9.
12. Jones AR (Janssen). Personal communication, 1994.
13. Kovács I, Somos P, Hámori M. Examination of the potential interaction between ketoconazole (Nizoral) and oral contraceptives with special regard to products of low hormone content (Rigevidon, Anteovin). *Ther Hung* (1986) 34, 167–70.
14. Qlaira (Estradiol valerate and Estradiol valerate with dienogest). Bayer plc. UK Summary of product characteristics, November 2010.
15. Blode H, Schott, B, Rohde B, Kunz M, Zeun S. Effects of CYP3A4 induction and inhibition on the pharmacokinetics of estradiol valerate/dienogest. 11th World Congress on Controversies in Obstetrics and Gynecology & Infertility, Paris, November 2008, 68A.
16. Natazia (Estradiol valerate and Estradiol valerate with Dienogest). Bayer HealthCare Pharmaceuticals, Inc. US Prescribing information, May 2010.
17. Verhoeven CHJ, van den Heuvel MW, Mulders TMT, Dieben TOM. The contraceptive vaginal ring, NuvaRing®, and antimycotic co-medication. *Contraception* (2004) 69, 129–32.
18. Andrews E, Damle BD, Fang A, Foster G, Crownover P, LaBadie R, Glue P. Pharmacokinetics and tolerability of voriconazole and a combination oral contraceptive co-administered in healthy female subjects. *Br J Clin Pharmacol* (2008) 65, 531–9.
19. Sporanox Capsules (Itraconazole). Janssen-Cilag Ltd. UK Summary of product characteristics, October 2011.
20. Nizoral Tablets (Ketoconazole). Janssen-Cilag Ltd. UK Summary of product characteristics, June 2010.
21. Noxafil (Posaconazole). Merck Sharp & Dohme Ltd. UK Summary of product characteristics, September 2014.
22. VFEND (Voriconazole). Pfizer Ltd. UK Summary of product characteristics, October 2014.

Combined hormonal contraceptives + Barbiturates or Phenytoin

Combined hormonal contraceptives are less reliable during the use of phenytoin, and barbiturates such as phenobarbital and primidone. Intermenstrual breakthrough bleeding and spotting can take place, and unintended pregnancies have occurred. Controlled studies have found that phenytoin and phenobarbital reduce contraceptive steroid levels.

Clinical evidence

(a) Case reports of contraceptive failure

A woman with epilepsy taking phenytoin 200 mg and sultiame 50 mg daily (with ferrous gluconate and folic acid) became pregnant despite the regular use of an oral combined hormonal contraceptive (**ethinylestradiol** 50 micrograms with **norethisterone** 3 mg).[1] Since this first report in 1972, at least 33 pregnancies have been reported in the literature in women taking a range of oral hormonal contraceptives (mostly combined) and a barbiturate (such as **phenobarbital** or **primidone**) and/or phenytoin (see 'Table 28.3', p.1170). Note that most of these cases were with an oral combined hormonal contraceptive containing at least 50 micrograms of **ethinylestradiol**. In addition, between the years 1968 to 1984, the CSM in the UK received reports of a further 39 pregnancies in women using an oral combined hormonal contraceptive while taking phenytoin (20 users) and/or **phenobarbital** (25 users) and/or **primidone** (7 users), with or without other antiepileptics.[2] In this report, over half the cases of contraceptive failure with antiepileptics related to high-dose contraceptives (50 micrograms of ethinylestradiol).[2]

(b) Studies of breakthrough bleeding

In one study, breakthrough bleeding (which was regarded as loss of reliability of the contraceptive) occurred in 30 of 51 women taking an oral combined hormonal contraceptive (**ethinylestradiol** with **norethisterone** or **mestranol** with **chlormadinone**) given **phenobarbital**.[3] In another study, 7 out of 11 patients taking **phenobarbital** and one of 2 patients taking phenytoin had breakthrough bleeding.[4] The incidence of breakthrough bleeding was 90% with preparations containing **ethinylestradiol** 30 micrograms and 29% with preparations containing **ethinylestradiol** 75 micrograms. Similarly, with preparations containing **ethinylestradiol** 50 micrograms, decreasing the dose of **norgestrel** from 500 micrograms to 125 micrograms increased breakthrough bleeding from 50% to 62%.[4]

(c) Pharmacokinetic studies

A pharmacokinetic study in 6 women given a single dose of an oral combined hormonal contraceptive (**ethinylestradiol** 50 micrograms with **levonorgestrel** 250 micrograms) found that the AUCs of **ethinylestradiol** and **levonorgestrel** were 49% and 42% lower, respectively, after taking phenytoin 200 to 300 mg daily for 8 to 12 weeks, when compared with before starting phenytoin.[5] In another study in 4 women taking an oral combined hormonal contraceptive (**ethinylestradiol** with **norethisterone** or **norgestrel**), 2 of the women had 54% and 60% reductions in their **ethinylestradiol** levels (measured at 10 to 12 hours after a dose at steady state) in the 2 cycles after starting **phenobarbital** 30 mg twice daily. These 2 women had breakthrough bleeding, but the suppression of ovulation was maintained. However, the other 2 women had no decrease in their **ethinylestradiol** levels.[6]

Mechanism

The likeliest explanation for the unreliability and failure of combined hormonal contraceptives is that phenytoin and the barbiturates, which are known potent liver enzyme inducers, increase the metabolism and clearance of the contraceptive steroids

Table 28.3 Case reports of pregnancies in women taking combined oral contraceptives with barbiturates and/or phenytoin

Antiepileptic	*Oestrogen*	*Progestogen*	*Number of cases*	*Refs*
Phenytoin + Sultiame	Ethinylestradiol 50 micrograms	Norethisterone 3 mg	1	1
Phenytoin + Primidone, Phenobarbital or Methylphenobarbital	Not stated	Not stated	7	2,3
Primidone	Ethinylestradiol 50 or 100 micrograms	Norgestrel 500 micrograms or Megestrol 1 mg	2	4,5
Phenytoin + Primidone or Phenobarbital	Ethinylestradiol 50 micrograms	Norgestrel 250 or 500 micrograms or Norethisterone 1 mg	3	4,5
Phenytoin + Primidone or Phenobarbital + Other	Ethinylestradiol 50 micrograms	Norgestrel 500 micrograms	2	4,5
Phenytoin + Carbamazepine	Ethinylestradiol 50 micrograms	Norgestrel 250 micrograms	1	4,5
Primidone or Phenobarbital	Ethinylestradiol	Norgestrel	3	6
Phenobarbital or Butobarbital	Ethinylestradiol or Mestranol	Norethisterone	3	7
Phenytoin	Ethinylestradiol 100 micrograms	Dimethisterone 25 mg	1	8
Phenobarbital or Methylphenobarbital	Ethinylestradiol 50 micrograms or Mestranol 80 micrograms	Etynodiol 1 mg or Chlormadinone 2 mg	2	8
Phenytoin + Phenobarbital	Mestranol 100 micrograms	Noretynodrel 2.5 mg	1	8
Phenobarbital	Ethinylestradiol 50 micrograms	Desogestrel 75 mg	1	9
Phenytoin + Phenobarbital	Ethinylestradiol	Levonorgestrel	1	10
Phenytoin then Carbamazepine	Ethinylestradiol	Lynestrol	1	10
Phenytoin and/or phenobarbital or primidone (with or without other antiepileptics)	Ethinylestradiol 30 or 50 micrograms or Mestranol 50 micrograms	Megestrol, Norethisterone, Etynodiol, Norgestrel or Levonorgestrel	39	11
Phenytoin	Ethinylestradiol 50 micrograms	Not stated	1	12
Phenytoin	Ethinylestradiol less than 50 micrograms	Not stated	2	13
Phenobarbital	Ethinylestradiol 35 micrograms ('back up' contraception also used)	Norgestimate 180 to 250 micrograms	1*	14

*This same woman previously became pregnant while using the levonorgestrel implant, see progestogen-only contraceptives, p.1199

1. Kenyon IE. Unplanned pregnancy in an epileptic. *BMJ* (1972) 1, 686–7.
2. Hempel E, Böhm W, Carol W, Klinger G. Medikamentöse Enzyminduktion und hormonale Kontrazeption. *Zentralbl Gynakol* (1973) 95, 1451–7.
3. Hempel E, Klinger W. Drug stimulated biotransformation of hormonal steroid contraceptives: clinical implications. *Drugs* (1976) 12, 442–8.
4. Janz D, Schmidt D. Anti-epileptic drugs and failure of oral contraceptives. *Lancet* (1974) i, 1113.
5. Janz D, Schmidt D. Antiepileptika und die Sicherheit oraler Kontrazeptiva. *Bibl Psychiatr* (1975) 151, 82–5.
6. Belaisch J, Driguez P, Janaud A. Influence de certains médicaments sur l'action des pilules contraceptives. *Nouv Presse Med* (1976) 5, 1645–6.
7. Gagnaire JC, Tchertchian J, Revol A, Rochet Y. Grossesses sous contraceptifs oraux chez les patientes recevant des barbituriques. *Nouv Presse Med* (1975) 4, 3008.
8. Coulam CB, Annegers JF. Do anticonvulsants reduce the efficacy of oral contraceptives? *Epilepsia* (1979) 20, 519–26.
9. Fanøe E. P-pillesvigt – antagelig på grund af interaktion med fenemal. *Ugeskr Laeger* (1977) 139, 1485.
10. Sparrow MJ. Pill method failures. *N Z Med J* (1987) 100, 102–5.
11. Back DJ, Grimmer FM, Orme ML'E, Proudlove C, Mann RD, Breckenridge AM. Evaluation of Committee on Safety of Medicines yellow card reports on oral contraceptive-drug interactions with anticonvulsants and antibiotics. *Br J Clin Pharmacol* (1988) 25, 527–32.
12. Kovacs GT, Riddoch G, Duncombe P, Welberry L, Chick P, Weisberg E, Leavesley GM, Baker HWG. Inadvertent pregnancies in oral contraceptive users. *Med J Aust* (1989) 150, 549–51.
13. van der Graaf WT, van Loon AJ, Postmus PE, Sleijfer DT. Twee patiënten met hersenmetastasen die zwanger werden tijdens fenytoïnegebruik. *Ned Tijdschr Geneeskd* (1992) 136, 2236–8.
14. Shane-McWhorter L, Cerveny JD, MacFarlane LL, Osborn C. Enhanced metabolism of levonorgestrel during phenobarbital treatment and resultant pregnancy. *Pharmacotherapy* (1998) 18, 1360–4.

from the body, thereby reducing their effects, and in some instances, allowing ovulation to occur.

Importance and management

The interactions between the oral combined hormonal contraceptives and phenobarbital or phenytoin are clinically important and fairly well documented, with pharmacokinetic data showing that ethinylestradiol exposure is halved by phenytoin. Primidone is metabolised to phenobarbital and appears to interact similarly. The risk of breakthrough bleeding and spotting is high (bleeding disturbances are usually regarded as an indication of reduced efficacy if cycles were previously regular[7]). However, the actual incidence of contraceptive failure when oral combined hormonal contraceptives are given with these drugs is unknown. It appears that the incidence of unintended pregnancies is quite small: in one cohort, a failure rate of 3.1 per 100 woman years was calculated for women taking antiepileptics, compared with an expected 0.7 per 100 woman years.[8] Note that, although this is about a fourfold increase in failure rate, the absolute failure rate seen is still less than that seen with barrier methods, such as condoms. Direct evidence regarding an interaction between combined hormonal contraceptives and **fosphenytoin** is lacking, but as it is a prodrug of phenytoin, it has the potential to interact in the same way as phenytoin.

General considerations

As the personal and ethical consequences of an unplanned pregnancy can be very serious, it is important to take the necessary practical steps to reduce any increased risk. Moreover, pregnancy in women with epilepsy should ideally be planned so that therapy can be reviewed to minimise the risks of foetal malformation.[9] In this regard, it is of concern that some surveys have shown a lack of knowledge of these interactions and their management among prescribers,[10] and the frequent use of enzyme-inducing antiepileptics with oral combined hormonal contraceptives containing less than 50 micrograms of ethinylestradiol.[11]

Contraceptive doses required to suppress ovulation

In most patients taking enzyme-inducing antiepileptics ovulation suppression and/or suppression of breakthrough bleeding was achievable with oral combined hormonal contraceptives containing ethinylestradiol 50 to 80 micrograms daily, although some patients may need 100 micrograms daily.[4,9,12] If these larger doses are required for good cycle control, there should be no increase in adverse effects because the enzyme-inducing effects of the antiepileptics reduce the blood levels of the steroids. However, note that many of the early cases of unintended pregnancies cited were with products containing 50 micrograms of ethinylestradiol or more, and, conversely, one review of contraceptive interactions suggested that women taking standard-dose oestrogen-containing contraceptives may not be at a greater risk of an interaction.[13] However, in a recent well-designed study of a low-dose oral combined hormonal contraceptive (ethinylestradiol 20 micrograms), there was a marked increase in ovulation when the contraceptive was given with the enzyme-inducing antiepileptic, carbamazepine, see 'Combined hormonal contraceptives + Carbamazepine and related drugs', p.1172.

Guidelines

In the UK, the Faculty of Sexual and Reproductive Healthcare (FSRH) have issued guidance on the use of drugs that induce liver enzymes, including phenytoin, phenobarbital and primidone, with combined hormonal contraceptives (oral, patch and vaginal ring). In their 2011 guidance,[14] they recommend that women taking these drugs should preferably change to a contraceptive method unaffected by enzyme-inducing drugs (that is, copper IUDs, the 'levonorgestrel-releasing intrauterine system', p.1200, or 'depot progestogen-only injections', p.1199). Alternatively, for women who wish to use a combined hormonal contraceptive, they provide advice for both the short-term and the long-term concurrent use of enzyme-inducing drugs.

Short-term use (less than 2 months). The FSRH recommend that women can continue to use the combined hormonal contraceptive (patch, vaginal ring, and standard-strength tablet containing at least 30 micrograms of ethinylestradiol), but that they should use additional contraceptive precautions, such as condoms, while taking the enzyme-inducing drug and for 28 days after it has been stopped. In addition, to minimise the risk of contraceptive failure, they recommend an extended or tricycling regimen with a shortened hormone-free interval of 3 to 4 days. In women taking a short-term course of enzyme-inducing drugs and who do not wish to use additional contraceptive precautions, they advise the same ethinylestradiol dose adjustments as recommended for the long-term use of enzyme-inducing drugs, see below. For a list of enzyme-inducing drugs that affect the metabolism of combined hormonal contraceptives and/or reduce their ovulatory suppressant effects, see 'Table 28.1', p.1160.

Long-term use (greater than 2 months). The FSRH recommend that women should take an oral combined hormonal contraceptive with an ethinylestradiol dose of at least 50 micrograms daily (either by using two tablets of a 30-microgram preparation or one tablet of a 20-microgram preparation with one tablet of a 30-microgram preparation) during the concurrent use of an enzyme-inducing drug, and for 28 days after it has been stopped. They also recommend that this preparation should be used in an extended or tricycling regimen, with a shortened pill-free interval of 4 days.[14] If breakthrough bleeding occurs, and other causes such as chlamydia are excluded, then the dose of ethinylestradiol may be increased in 10 microgram increments up to a maximum of 70 micrograms daily (two tablets of a 35-microgram preparation).[14] Alternatively, additional precautions can be used, or the contraceptive can be switched to one unaffected by enzyme-inducing drugs. The combined hormonal contraceptives in the form of the **transdermal patch** and **vaginal ring** are not suitable for use with enzyme-inducing drugs long-term because use of two patches or two rings is not recommended. For potent enzyme-inducing drugs such as phenytoin and carbamazepine and related drugs (see 'Table 28.1', p.1160), this guidance seems prudent.

The WHO guidance includes similar advice for certain antiepileptics (they specifically list phenytoin, carbamazepine, barbiturates, primidone, topiramate and oxcarbazepine). They advise that the use of these enzyme-inducing drugs with combined hormonal contraceptives (tablet, patch and vaginal ring) is not usually recommended, unless other more appropriate methods are not available or acceptable, and the use of other contraceptives should be encouraged for women who are long-term users of any of these drugs. They also advise that, when an oral combined hormonal contraceptive is chosen, a preparation containing a minimum of 30 micrograms of ethinylestradiol should be used;[15] however, this is lower than the FSRH guidelines of 50 micrograms. Although a 30-microgram dose of ethinylestradiol would seem adequate for weak enzyme inducers, such as topiramate, it is probably not sufficient for potent inducers, such as phenytoin or carbamazepine and related drugs.

Note that, in some situations, the use of a non-interacting antiepileptic drug might be an appropriate consideration: 'ethosuximide', p.1174, 'gabapentin', p.1174, 'levetiracetam', p.1180, 'sodium valproate', p.1190, 'tiagabine', p.1188, and 'vigabatrin', p.1190 do not appear to interact with the hormonal contraceptives.

Pill-free intervals. There are no studies to show whether omitting or reducing the pill-free interval reduces the risk of ovulation with liver enzyme inducers. However, enzyme-inducing drugs are likely to increase the length of the pill-free interval (see *Interaction studies* under 'Hormonal contraceptives and Sex hormones', p.1159), and this might contribute to their effects in reducing contraceptive efficacy. Some (including the FSRH[14]) therefore recommend that, in women using a combined hormonal contraceptive with an enzyme-inducing antiepileptic, in addition to increasing the ethinylestradiol dose, the usual 7-day pill-free interval every fourth week should be avoided, and that the pill should be taken in a tricycling regimen (i.e. a monophasic preparation continuously for 3 or 4 packets, then a short pill-free interval of 4 days).[16] Others contend that it is actually the progestogen dose that is more important in inhibiting ovulation in combined hormonal contraceptives, and that continuous use (without any pill-free interval) of an oral combined hormonal contraceptive containing a high dose of progestogen should be used in a woman taking an enzyme-inducing antiepileptic. However, they say that additional protection may still be worthwhile as contraceptive efficacy cannot be guaranteed.[17]

1. Kenyon IE. Unplanned pregnancy in an epileptic. *BMJ* (1972) 1, 686–7.
2. Back DJ, Grimmer FM, Orme ML'E, Proudlove C, Mann RD, Breckenridge AM. Evaluation of Committee on Safety of Medicines yellow card reports on oral contraceptive-drug interactions with anticonvulsants and antibiotics. *Br J Clin Pharmacol* (1988) 25, 527–32.
3. Hempel E, Böhm W, Carol W, Klinger G. Medikamentöse Enzyminduktion und hormonale Kontrazeption. *Zentralbl Gynakol* (1973) 95, 1451–7.
4. Sonnen AEH. Sodium valproate and the pill. In: Akimoto H, Kazamatsuri H, Seino M, Ward A, Eds. Advances in Epileptology. New York: Raven Press, 1982: 429–32.
5. Crawford P, Chadwick DJ, Martin C, Tjia J, Back DJ, Orme M. The interaction of phenytoin and carbamazepine with combined oral contraceptive steroids. *Br J Clin Pharmacol* (1990) 30, 892–6.
6. Back DJ, Bates M, Bowden A, Breckenridge AM, Hall MJ, Jones H, MacIver M, Orme M, Perucca E, Richens A, Rowe PH, Smith E. The interaction of phenobarbital and other anticonvulsants with oral contraceptive steroid therapy. *Contraception* (1980) 22, 495–503.
7. Hempel E, Klinger W. Drug stimulated biotransformation of hormonal steroid contraceptives: clinical implications. *Drugs* (1976) 12, 442–8.
8. Coulam CB, Annegers JF. Do anticonvulsants reduce the efficacy of oral contraceptives? *Epilepsia* (1979) 20, 519–26.
9. O'Brien MD, Gilmour-White S. Epilepsy and pregnancy. *BMJ* (1993) 307, 492–5.
10. Krauss GL, Brandt J, Campbell M, Plate C, Summerfield M. Antiepileptic medication and oral contraceptive interactions: a national survey of neurologists and obstetricians. *Neurology* (1996) 46, 1534–9.
11. Shorvon SD, Tallis RC, Wallace HK. Antiepileptic drugs: coprescription of proconvulsant drugs and oral contraceptives: a national study of antiepileptic drug prescribing practice. *J Neurol Neurosurg Psychiatry* (2002) 72, 114–15.
12. Orme M, Back DJ. Oral contraceptive steroids – pharmacological issues of interest to the prescribing physician. *Adv Contracept* (1991) 7, 325–31.
13. Szoka PR, Edgren RA. Drug interactions with oral contraceptives: compilation and analysis of an adverse experience report database. *Fertil Steril* (1988) 49 (Suppl), S31–S38.
14. Faculty of Sexual and Reproductive Healthcare Guidance. Drug interactions with hormonal contraception: Clinical Effectiveness Unit, January 2011. Available at: http://www.fsrh.org/pdfs/CEUGuidanceDrugInteractionsHormonal.pdf (accessed 20/10/15).
15. Reproductive Health and Research, World Health Organization. Medical eligibility criteria for contraceptive use. 5th ed. Geneva, WHO; 2015. Available at: http://www.who.int/reproductivehealth/publications/family_planning/MEC-5/en/(accessed 20/10/15).
16. O'Brien MD, Guillebaud J. Contraception for women with epilepsy. Epilepsia. (2006) 47, 1419–22.
17. Schwenkhagen AM, Stodieck SRG. Which contraception for women with epilepsy? *Seizure* (2008) 17, 145–50.

Combined hormonal contraceptives + Bile-acid binding resins

Colesevelam, given at the same time as an oral combined hormonal contraceptive, reduces the absorption of ethinylestradiol, but has less effect when given 4 hours after the contraceptive. Colestipol and colestyramine might be expected to interact similarly.

Clinical evidence

(a) Colesevelam

In a single-dose pharmacokinetic study in 35 healthy women, colesevelam 3.75 g, taken at the same time as an oral combined hormonal contraceptive (**ethinylestradiol** 35 micrograms with **norethisterone** 1 mg), reduced the AUC of **ethinylestradiol** by 24%. Giving the contraceptive one hour before the colesevelam reduced the AUC of ethinylestradiol by 18%, but the 90% confidence interval was still outside the 80 to 125% bounds for no effect.[1] In a further study in 32 women, giving the contraceptive 4 hours before the colesevelam reduced the AUC of ethinylestradiol by 12%, which was within the bounds of no effect. Colesevelam had no effect on the pharmacokinetics of norethisterone at any of the above administration times.[1]

(b) Colestyramine

A brief review of the drug interactions of contraceptives reported that the half-life of **ethinylestradiol** was reduced from 8.2 hours to 4.8 hours in a healthy subject taking 4 g of colestyramine three times daily (duration of treatment not stated).[2]

Mechanism

Colestyramine, colestipol, and colesevelam are bile-acid binding resins, intended to bind to bile acids within the gut, but they can also bind with some drugs thereby reducing the amount available for absorption. As ethinylestradiol undergoes enterohepatic circulation (i.e. after absorption it is excreted in the bile and reabsorbed), it has been suggested that its reabsorption may be reduced by these bile-acid binding resins.[2] However, separation of administration would not normally be expected to minimise the effect on enterohepatic recirculation, and, in any case, the importance of enterohepatic recirculation of ethinylestradiol to its efficacy is not established.

Importance and management

The reduction in exposure to ethinylestradiol is small when taken at the same time as **colesevelam**, but may be of clinically relevance in some women. Note that the reduction in ethinylestradiol exposure is similar to that seen with some weak enzyme inducers, see 'Table 28.1', p.1160. On the basis of these results, the manufacturers of colesevelam recommend taking oral contraceptives [presumably oral combined hormonal contraceptives] at least 4 hours before colesevelam.[3,4] This would seem to be a prudent precaution.

There appears to be no specific data relating to an interaction between combined hormonal contraceptives and **colestipol**, and only the report in one subject for **colestyramine**. However, as both of these drugs are known to affect the absorption of many drugs, it may be prudent to apply the standard recommendation of taking other oral drugs at least one hour before or 4 hours after colestipol, and one hour before or 4 to 6 hours after colestyramine, to minimise the risk of an interaction.

1. Brown KS, Armstrong IC, Wang A, Walker JR, Noveck RJ, Swearingen D, Allison M, Kissling JC, Kisicki J, Salazar DE. Effect of the bile acid sequestrant colesevelam on the pharmacokinetics of pioglitazone, repaglinide, estrogen estradiol, norethindrone, levothyroxine, and glyburide. *J Clin Pharmacol* (2010) 50, 554–65.
2. Bolt HM. Interactions between clinically used drugs and oral contraceptives. *Environ Health Perspect* (1994) 102 (Suppl 9), 35–8.
3. Welchol (Colesevelam hydrochloride). Daiichi Sankyo, Inc. US Prescribing information, January 2014.
4. Cholestagel (Colesevelam hydrochloride). Sanofi. UK Summary of product characteristics, December 2014.

Combined hormonal contraceptives + Candesartan

Candesartan does not alter the pharmacokinetics or ovulation suppressant effect of an oral combined hormonal contraceptive containing ethinylestradiol with levonorgestrel.

Clinical evidence, mechanism, importance and management

In a placebo-controlled study in 12 healthy women given an oral combined hormonal contraceptive for 2 cycles, candesartan cilexetil 8 mg daily for 21 days had no effect on the pharmacokinetics of **ethinylestradiol** and **levonorgestrel**, and no ovulation occurred during concurrent use.[1] No reduction in contraceptive efficacy would therefore be expected if candesartan is used with any oral combined hormonal contraceptive, or with the patch or vaginal ring.

Consider also 'Drospirenone-containing contraceptives or HRT + Potassium-sparing drugs', p.1191, for a possible interaction between angiotensin II receptor antagonists and drospirenone, and 'Antihypertensives + Hormonal contraceptives', p.1053, for a discussion of the effect of combined hormonal contraceptives on blood pressure.

1. Jonkman JHG, van Lier JJ, van Heiningen PNM, Lins R, Sennewald R, Högemann A. Pharmacokinetic drug interaction studies with candesartan cilexetil. *J Hum Hypertens* (1997) 11 (Suppl 2), S31–S35.

Combined hormonal contraceptives + Carbamazepine and related drugs

Oral combined hormonal contraceptives are less reliable during treatment with carbamazepine: breakthrough bleeding and spotting can take place, and unintended pregnancies have occurred. Controlled studies have shown that carbamazepine, eslicarbazepine and oxcarbazepine reduce contraceptive steroid exposure, all to a similar extent, and that carbamazepine reduces the ovulation suppressant effect of a low-dose oral combined hormonal contraceptive.

Clinical evidence

(a) Carbamazepine

1. Pharmacological studies. In a well-designed study, 24 women were given a low-dose oral combined hormonal contraceptive (**ethinylestradiol** 20 micrograms with **levonorgestrel** 100 micrograms) with carbamazepine 600 mg daily for 2 months and with a placebo for 2 months. In the 10 women who completed the study, carbamazepine reduced the ethinylestradiol AUC by 45% and the levonorgestrel AUC by 46%. In addition, ovulation occurred in 5 of 10 carbamazepine cycles compared with one of 10 placebo cycles, and 3 or more days of breakthrough bleeding occurred during 7 of 10 carbamazepine cycles compared with 2 of 10 placebo cycles.[1]

Similar pharmacokinetic findings were reported in an earlier study of carbamazepine with a standard-dose oral combined hormonal contraceptive (**ethinylestradiol** 35 micrograms with **norethisterone** 1 mg). In the 10 patients who received carbamazepine (600 mg daily from day one to 21 of a cycle), the AUC of **ethinylestradiol** and **norethisterone** were reduced by 42% and 58%, respectively, on day 20 of the cycle, when compared with an earlier cycle when they took the contraceptive alone.[2] Similarly, in another study, the AUC of **ethinylestradiol** was reduced by 42% and the AUC of **levonorgestrel** was reduced by 40% in 4 women given a single dose of an oral combined hormonal contraceptive (**ethinylestradiol** 50 micrograms with **levonorgestrel** 250 micrograms) before and after 8 to 12 weeks of carbamazepine 300 to 600 mg daily.[3]

In an early study, 6 of 12 women taking an oral combined hormonal contraceptive (**ethinylestradiol** with **norethisterone**) developed spotting or breakthrough bleeding while taking carbamazepine (this is regarded as a possible loss of reliability of the contraceptive.[4] A similar study also reported breakthrough bleeding in 4 of 6 patients taking carbamazepine and an oral combined hormonal contraceptive,[5] and the same author later briefly reported 37 out of 59 patients had breakthrough bleeding while taking this combination.[6]

2. Case reports of contraceptive failure. One woman taking a low-dose oral combined hormonal contraceptive (not specified) conceived 6 weeks after starting carbamazepine, initially 200 mg daily then 600 mg daily.[7] In another case, the failure of an oral combined hormonal contraceptive containing **ethinylestradiol** 30 micrograms was attributed to carbamazepine.[8] Six pregnancies were identified in women who took carbamazepine and an oral contraceptive (unspecified) in the adverse reactions register of the CSM in the UK for the years 1968 to 1984. However, it is unclear how many of these 6 women were taking carbamazepine alone, as the authors note that some women were taking multiple antiepileptics.[9] Two further pregnancies have been reported in women taking oral combined hormonal contraceptives and antiepileptics including carbamazepine and phenytoin,[10] and one in a woman who was switched from phenytoin to carbamazepine.[11]

(b) Eslicarbazepine

The manufacturer briefly notes that, in women taking an oral combined hormonal contraceptive, eslicarbazepine 1.2 g daily decreased the AUC of **ethinylestradiol** and **levonorgestrel** by 42% and 37%, respectively.[12]

(c) Oxcarbazepine

In a pharmacokinetic study in 10 healthy women taking an oral triphasic contraceptive, oxcarbazepine 300 mg three times daily for 4 weeks reduced the AUCs of **ethinylestradiol** and **levonorgestrel** by 47% and 36%, respectively. Three women had menstrual bleeding disturbances.[13] Similar results (a 47% reduction in AUC of both ethinylestradiol and levonorgestrel) were reported in a later placebo-controlled study with oxcarbazepine 1.2 g daily and an oral combined hormonal contraceptive (**ethinylestradiol** 50 micrograms with **levonorgestrel** 250 micrograms).[14]

Preliminary observations in another report revealed that 4 out of 6 women taking oxcarbazepine had breakthrough bleeding when they were given an oral combined hormonal contraceptive containing **ethinylestradiol** 30 micrograms. This resolved in two women when they took double the dose of **ethinylestradiol**.[6] No cases of unintended pregnancy appear to have been published.

Mechanism

The most likely explanation for these interactions is that carbamazepine, oxcarbazepine and eslicarbazepine (the main active metabolite of oxcarbazepine) reduce the levels of the contraceptive steroids, presumably by inducing their metabolism. This may result in loss of contraceptive efficacy.

Importance and management

The reduction in contraceptive steroid levels caused by carbamazepine, oxcarbazepine, and eslicarbazepine is established, with ethinylestradiol exposure being reduced to a similar extent (42 to 47%) by all three drugs. However, the actual incidence of contraceptive failure when oral combined hormonal contraceptives are given with these drugs is unknown. Given the few published reports, it appears that unintended pregnancies with carbamazepine are rare, and still less frequent than that seen with barrier methods, such as condoms. There appear to be no published reports of pregnancies in patients taking an oral combined hormonal contraceptive and oxcarbazepine, or the much newer eslicarbazepine. Nevertheless, given the personal and ethical consequences of an unwanted pregnancy, the level of reduction in contraceptive steroid levels seen with carbamazepine and related drugs, and the marked increase in ovulation seen on the concurrent of carbamazepine and a low-dose oral combined hormonal contraceptive for 2 months, is of real concern. The ovulation data suggests that low-dose preparations, in particular, are not suitable for use in women taking carbamazepine. Standard or low-dose combined hormonal contraceptives should not be used with carbamazepine, oxcarbazepine or eslicarbazepine without additional contraceptive precautions or dose modification. The specific recommendations of the UK Faculty of Sexual and Reproductive Healthcare, to ensure effective contraception in women taking liver enzyme inducers, such as carbamazepine, eslicarbazepine or oxcarbazepine, are discussed in detail under 'Combined hormonal contraceptives + Barbiturates or Phenytoin', p.1169, and these should be followed.

1. Davis AR, Westhoff CL, Stanczyk FZ. Carbamazepine coadministration with an oral contraceptive: Effects on steroid pharmacokinetics, ovulation, and bleeding. *Epilepsia* (2011) 52, 243–7.
2. Doose DR, Wang S-S, Padmanabhan M, Schwabe S, Jacobs D, Bialer M. Effect of topiramate or carbamazepine on the pharmacokinetics of an oral contraceptive containing norethindrone and ethinyl estradiol in healthy obese and nonobese female subjects. *Epilepsia* (2003) 44, 540–9.
3. Crawford P, Chadwick DJ, Martin C, Tjia J, Back DJ, Orme M. The interaction of phenytoin and carbamazepine with combined oral contraceptive steroids. *Br J Clin Pharmacol* (1990) 30, 892–6.
4. Hempel E, Klinger W. Drug stimulated biotransformation of hormonal steroid contraceptives: clinical implications. *Drugs* (1976) 12, 442–8.
5. Sonnen AEH. Sodium valproate and the pill. In: Akimoto H, Kazamatsuri H, Seino M, Ward A, Eds. Advances in Epileptology. New York: Raven Press, 1982: 429–32.
6. Sonnen AEH. Oxcarbazepine and oral contraceptives. *Acta Neurol Scand* (1990) 82 (Suppl 133) 37.
7. Rapport DJ, Calabrese JR. Interactions between carbamazepine and birth control pills. *Psychosomatics* (1989) 30, 462–4.
8. Kovacs GT, Riddoch G, Duncombe P, Welberry L, Chick P, Weisberg E, Leavesley GM, Baker HWG. Inadvertent pregnancies in oral contraceptive users. *Med J Aust* (1989) 150, 549–51.
9. Back DJ, Grimmer FM, Orme ML'E, Proudlove C, Mann RD, Breckenridge AM. Evaluation of Committee on Safety of Medicines yellow card reports on oral contraceptive-drug interactions with anticonvulsants and antibiotics. *Br J Clin Pharmacol* (1988) 25, 527–32.
10. Janz D, Schmidt D. Antiepileptika und die Sicherheit oraler Kontrazeptiva. *Bibl Psychiatr* (1975) 151, 82–5.
11. Sparrow MJ. Pill method failures. *N Z Med J* (1987) 100, 102–5.
12. Zebinix (Eslicarbazepine acetate). Eisai Ltd. UK Summary of product characteristics, August 2012.
13. Klosterskov Jensen P, Saano V, Haring P, Svenstrup B, Menge GP. Possible interaction between oxcarbazepine and an oral contraceptive. *Epilepsia* (1992) 33, 1149–52.
14. Fattore C, Cipolla G, Gatti G, Limido GL, Sturm Y, Bernasconi C, Perucca E. Induction of ethinylestradiol and levonorgestrel metabolism by oxcarbazepine in healthy women. *Epilepsia* (1999) 40, 783–7.

Combined hormonal contraceptives + Coxibs

High-dose etoricoxib raises ethinylestradiol exposure by 50 to 60%. Rofecoxib increases contraceptive steroid exposure to a small extent, whereas celecoxib does not appear to affect the pharmacokinetics of an oral combined hormonal contraceptive containing ethinylestradiol with norethisterone. One case of pulmonary embolism has been reported in a patient taking valdecoxib with an oral combined hormonal contraceptive.

Clinical evidence

(a) Celecoxib

The UK manufacturer briefly notes that celecoxib had no clinically relevant effects on the pharmacokinetics of an oral combined hormonal contraceptive containing **ethinylestradiol** 35 micrograms with **norethisterone** 1 mg.[1]

(b) Etoricoxib

In a placebo-controlled, crossover study in women taking an oral triphasic combined hormonal contraceptive (**ethinylestradiol** 35 micrograms with **norethisterone** 0.5 to 1 mg) for 21 days, the addition of etoricoxib 120 mg daily taken at the same time or 12 hours after the contraceptive increased the AUC of **ethinylestradiol** by 50% and 60%, respectively.[2] The **norethisterone** AUC showed minimal changes (9% and 22% increase). In a further study, a lower dose of etoricoxib 60 mg daily taken with the same contraceptive increased the AUC of **ethinylestradiol** by 37% with a non-statistically significant 11% increase in the AUC of **norethisterone.**[2]

(c) Rofecoxib

In a placebo-controlled, crossover study in 18 healthy women taking an oral combined hormonal contraceptive (**ethinylestradiol** 35 micrograms with **norethisterone** 1 mg), rofecoxib 175 mg daily for 2 weeks raised the AUCs of **ethinylestradiol** and **nor-**

ethisterone by 13% and 18%, respectively. No abnormal menstrual bleeding was reported.[3]

(d) Valdecoxib

A single case of left iliac vein thrombosis and bilateral multiple pulmonary emboli has been reported in a 25-year-old woman taking an oral combined hormonal contraceptive (**ethinylestradiol** with **norgestimate**), which developed within a month of starting valdecoxib 20 mg twice daily. The patient had been taking the same contraceptive (containing ethinylestradiol doses of 35 micrograms and then 25 micrograms) for 3 years before taking valdecoxib with no adverse effects. No risk factors were identified apart from prolonged stasis (a 6-hour car journey) and hormonal contraceptive use.[4]

Mechanism

It is thought that etoricoxib increases ethinylestradiol levels because it inhibits sulfotransferase activity thereby inhibiting ethinylestradiol metabolism. Rofecoxib possibly interacts similarly, although to a lesser extent, and celecoxib appears not to interact. Coxibs as a class and some non-selective NSAIDs appear to be associated with a small increased risk of rare thrombotic events (especially myocardial infarction and stroke). Combined hormonal contraceptives are also associated with a small increased risk of rare thrombotic events. It is possible that these effects could be additive or synergistic.

Importance and management

The increase in ethinylestradiol levels with etoricoxib 120 mg daily would be expected to be similar to switching from a standard-dose oral combined hormonal contraceptive (ethinylestradiol 30 micrograms) to a high-dose preparation (50 micrograms), and could therefore have clinical consequences. The manufacturer suggests that this increase in ethinylestradiol levels should be considered when choosing a contraceptive because of the possible increased risk of adverse events, such as venous thromboembolism.[5] It may therefore be appropriate to use an oral combined hormonal contraceptive with a low 20 microgram dose of ethinylestradiol or the vaginal ring if etoricoxib is required regularly, particularly at higher doses, and especially as coxibs themselves are associated with an increased risk of thrombotic events. Celecoxib does not appear to affect the pharmacokinetics of oral combined hormonal contraceptives.

The small changes in ethinylestradiol exposure seen with rofecoxib (now withdrawn), although statistically significant, are modest, and unlikely to be clinically important.

The general relevance of the one case of pulmonary embolism with valdecoxib (now withdrawn) and an oral combined hormonal contraceptive is unclear. However, it cannot be excluded that combined use of these two products contributed to this rare adverse effect. Note that risk factors for venous thromboembolism and cardiovascular disease should be taken into account when prescribing any combined hormonal contraceptive (tablets, patch or vaginal ring) alone, or a coxib alone, and therefore it may be prudent to re-evaluate these risks when a coxib is required in a woman using a combined hormonal contraceptive, and vice versa.

1. Celebrex (Celecoxib). Pfizer Ltd. UK Summary of product characteristics, January 2013.
2. Schwartz J, Hunt T, Smith WB, Wong P, Larson P, Crumley T, Mehta A, Gottesdiener K, Agrawal N. The effect of etoricoxib on the pharmacokinetics of oral contraceptives in healthy participants. *J Clin Pharmacol* (2009) 49, 807–15.
3. Schwartz JI, Wong PH, Porras AG, Ebel DL, Hunt TR, Gertz BJ. Effect of rofecoxib on the pharmacokinetics of chronically administered oral contraceptives in healthy female volunteers. *J Clin Pharmacol* (2002) 42, 215–21.
4. Westgate EJ, Fitzgerald GA. Pulmonary embolism in a woman taking oral contraceptives and valdecoxib. *PLoS Med* (2005) 2, e197.
5. Arcoxia (Etoricoxib). Merck Sharp & Dohme Ltd. UK Summary of product characteristics, May 2012.

Combined hormonal contraceptives + Dipeptidylpeptidase-4 inhibitors

Linagliptin does not alter the pharmacokinetics of oral combined hormonal contraceptives containing ethinylestradiol with levonorgestrel. Alogliptin and sitagliptin do not alter the pharmacokinetics of oral combined hormonal contraceptives containing ethinylestradiol with norethisterone.

Clinical evidence and mechanism

(a) Alogliptin

The US manufacturer of alogliptin briefly notes that, in clinical studies, the pharmacokinetics of both **ethinylestradiol** 35 micrograms and **norethisterone** 1 mg were not meaningfully altered when they were given with alogliptin 25 mg daily for 21 days of a cycle.[1]

(b) Linagliptin

In a study in 18 healthy women taking an oral combined hormonal contraceptive (**ethinylestradiol** 30 micrograms with **levonorgestrel** 150 micrograms), linagliptin 5 mg once daily for 7 days of a cycle, beginning on day 15, did not alter the steady-state pharmacokinetics of **ethinylestradiol** and negligibly increased the AUC of **levonorgestrel** by 8%.[2]

(c) Sitagliptin

In a study in 18 healthy women taking an oral triphasic combined hormonal contraceptive (**ethinylestradiol** 35 micrograms with **norethisterone** 0.5 to 1 mg), sitagliptin 200 mg once daily for 21 days of a cycle did not alter the steady-state pharmacokinetics of **ethinylestradiol** or **norethisterone**.[3]

Importance and management

The evidence suggests that alogliptin, linagliptin, and sitagliptin do not affect the pharmacokinetics of oral combined hormonal contraceptives. Therefore, no additional contraceptive precautions seem necessary if these antidiabetic drugs are given to women taking any combined hormonal contraceptive (tablets, patch, or vaginal ring).

For the possible adverse effect of hormonal contraceptives on diabetic control, and for the general precautions for the use of these contraceptives in diabetes, see 'Antidiabetics + Hormonal contraceptives', p.510.

1. Nesina (Alogliptin). Takeda Pharmaceuticals America, Inc. US Prescribing information, January 2013.
2. Friedrich C, Port A, Ring A, Graefe-Mody U, Giessmann T, Iovino M, Woerle H-J. Effect of multiple oral doses of linagliptin on the steady-state pharmacokinetics of a combination oral contraceptive in healthy female adults: an open-label, two-period, fixed-sequence, multiple-dose study. *Clin Drug Investig* (2011) 31, 643–53.
3. Migoya E, Larson P, Bergman A, Miller J, Johnson-Levonas AO, Lasseter KC, Wagner JA. Sitagliptin, a dipeptidyl peptidase-4 inhibitor, does not affect the pharmacokinetics of ethinyl estradiol or norethindrone in healthy female subjects. *J Clin Pharmacol* (2011) 51, 1319–25.

Combined hormonal contraceptives + Endothelin receptor antagonists

Bosentan decreases ethinylestradiol and norethisterone exposure from an oral combined hormonal contraceptive, and is likely to decrease contraceptive efficacy. Ambrisentan has minor effects on the pharmacokinetics of contraceptive steroids. Macitentan is not expected to affect the pharmacokinetics of hormonal contraceptives.

Clinical evidence

(a) Ambrisentan

In a pharmacokinetic study in 28 healthy women, ambrisentan 10 mg daily for 16 days decreased the AUC of **ethinylestradiol** by 4% (not statistically significant) and increased the AUC of **norethisterone** by 14% when a single dose of an oral combined hormonal contraceptive (ethinylestradiol 35 micrograms with norethisterone 1 mg) was given on day 12.[1]

(b) Bosentan

In a randomised, crossover study in 19 healthy women, a single dose of an oral combined hormonal contraceptive (**ethinylestradiol** 35 micrograms with **norethisterone** 1 mg) was given alone and on the last day of bosentan 125 mg twice daily for one week. Bosentan reduced the mean AUC of norethisterone by 14% (maximum reduction 56%) and the mean AUC of ethinylestradiol by 31% (maximum reduction 66%), with marked inter-individual variability. The maximum concentration and half-life of both contraceptive steroids were not affected.[2]

Mechanism

The contraceptive steroids are partially metabolised by CYP3A4, and it was thought that the changes in their pharmacokinetics might have been caused by induction of CYP3A4 by bosentan. However, other mechanisms could not be excluded.[2]

Importance and management

The clinical relevance of the decrease in contraceptive steroid exposure seen with **bosentan** is not certain: it was less than that seen with some potent enzyme inducers (such as carbamazepine, see 'Table 28.1', p.1160), but greater than that seen with some weak enzyme inducers (such as rufinamide). Nevertheless, a 31% decrease in ethinylestradiol exposure might be equivalent to changing a 30 microgram preparation to a 20 microgram preparation, and greater reductions were seen in some patients. The risk of contraceptive failure might therefore be increased in some patients, particularly those taking low-dose 20 microgram preparations. This is of particular importance because bosentan is potentially teratogenic, and pregnancy is contraindicated in pulmonary hypertension (for which bosentan is used), due to a high risk of mortality.[3] The UK manufacturer therefore recommends that additional or alternative methods to hormonal contraceptives (of any form) are used.[4] Similarly, the US manufacturer recommends that hormonal contraceptives (oral, injectable, implants, transdermal) should not be used as the sole form of contraception (with the exception of the levonorgestrel intra-uterine system, which can be used alone).[5] In the UK, the Faculty of Sexual and Reproductive Healthcare include bosentan in their 2011 guidance on the use of enzyme inducers with combined hormonal contraceptives, see 'Combined hormonal contraceptives + Barbiturates or Phenytoin', p.1169, for details of this guidance.

Ambrisentan has no clinically relevant effect on the pharmacokinetics of oral combined hormonal contraceptives, and so no decrease in contraceptive efficacy would be expected on concurrent use. Similarly, the UK manufacturer of **macitentan** states that it is not expected to reduce hormonal contraceptive efficacy on the basis that it did not alter the pharmacokinetics of another CYP3A4 substrate, sildenafil (see 'Phosphodiesterase type-5 inhibitors + Endothelin receptor antagonists', p.1541). However, ambrisentan and macitentan are both potentially teratogenic and so effective contraception during use is essential,[6,7] as it is in pulmonary hypertension in general, given the high risk of mortality associated with pregnancy in this patient population. The advice of the US manufacturers of ambrisentan and macitentan is to use an additional barrier method of contraception, if a combined hormonal contraceptive is used.[8,9]

1. Spence R, Mandagere A, Walker G, Dufton C, Boinpally R. Effect of steady-state ambrisentan on the pharmacokinetics of a single dose of the oral contraceptive norethindrone (norethisterone) 1 mg/ethinylestradiol 35 μg in healthy subjects: an open-label, single-sequence, single-centre study. *Clin Drug Investig* (2010) 30, 313–24.
2. Van Giersbergen PLM, Halabi A, Dingemanse J. Pharmacokinetic interaction between bosentan and the oral contraceptives norethisterone and ethinyl estradiol. *Int J Clin Pharmacol Ther* (2006) 44, 113–18.
3. Heng EL. Pulmonary hypertension in pregnancy: a risky business. British Cardiovascular Society Editorial, September 2013. Available at: http://www.bcs.com/pages/news_full.asp?NewsID=19792170 (accessed 21/10/15).
4. Tracleer (Bosentan monohydrate). Actelion Pharmaceuticals UK Ltd. UK Summary of product characteristics, September 2013.
5. Tracleer (Bosentan). Actelion Pharmaceuticals US, Inc. US Prescribing information, October 2012.
6. Volibris (Ambrisentan). GlaxoSmithKline UK. UK Summary of product characteristics, September 2014.
7. Opsumit (Macitentan). Actelion Pharmaceuticals UK Ltd. UK Summary of product characteristics, May 2014.
8. Letairis (Ambrisentan). Gilead Sciences, Inc. US Prescribing information, May 2014.
9. Opsumit (Macitentan). Actelion Pharmaceuticals US, Inc. US Prescribing information, October 2013.

Combined hormonal contraceptives + Ethosuximide

Ethosuximide probably does not alter the efficacy of oral combined hormonal contraceptives.

Clinical evidence, mechanism, importance and management

Four pregnancies were identified in women who took ethosuximide and an oral contraceptive (unspecified) in the adverse reactions register of the CSM in the UK for the years 1968 to 1984. However, the authors note that ethosuximide was the sole antiepileptic prescribed in only one of the cases reported.[1] As ethosuximide is not an inducer of hepatic enzymes, it is likely that this one case is a chance association. Another case describes pregnancy in a woman who had been taking ethosuximide, phenytoin, and phenobarbital, with an oral combined hormonal contraceptive for 6 years.[2] If indeed this case does represent an interaction, the known enzyme-inducers phenytoin and phenobarbital are more likely to be implicated than ethosuximide (see 'Combined hormonal contraceptives + Barbiturates or Phenytoin', p.1169). There do not appear to have been any pharmacokinetic or pharmacodynamic studies of the use of ethosuximide with oral combined hormonal contraceptives and no further case reports have been published. No additional contraceptive precautions appear to be necessary on the concurrent use of ethosuximide with any combined hormonal contraceptives (tablet, patch or vaginal ring).

1. Back DJ, Grimmer FM, Orme ML'E, Proudlove C, Mann RD, Breckenridge AM. Evaluation of Committee on Safety of Medicines yellow card reports on oral contraceptive-drug interactions with anticonvulsants and antibiotics. *Br J Clin Pharmacol* (1988) 25, 527–32.
2. Janz D, Schmidt D. Anti-epileptic drugs and failure of oral contraceptives. *Lancet* (1974) i, 1113.

Combined hormonal contraceptives + Ezetimibe

Ezetimibe does not alter the pharmacokinetics of an oral combined hormonal contraceptive containing ethinylestradiol with norgestrel.

Clinical evidence, mechanism, importance and management

In a randomised, crossover study, 18 healthy women who had been taking a triphasic oral combined hormonal contraceptive (containing **ethinylestradiol** with **norgestrel**) were also given ezetimibe 10 mg daily or placebo for 7 days from days 8 to 14 of two consecutive contraceptive cycles. Ezetimibe did not affect the pharmacokinetics of **ethinylestradiol** or **norgestrel**.[1] Therefore, no additional contraceptive precautions seem necessary if ezetimibe is given to women taking any combined hormonal contraceptive (tablets, patch or vaginal ring). Bear in mind that the indications for ezetimibe may be a contraindication to the use of any form of combined hormonal contraceptive if other risk factors for arterial disease are present. This is because these contraceptives can have adverse effects on serum lipids.

1. Keung ACF, Kosoglou T, Statkevich P, Anderson L, Boutros T, Cutler DL, Batra V, Sellers EM. Ezetimibe does not affect the pharmacokinetics of oral contraceptives. *Clin Pharmacol Ther* (2001) 69, P55.

Combined hormonal contraceptives + Felbamate

Felbamate appears to increase the clearance of gestodene from an oral combined hormonal contraceptive, without altering ovulation suppression.

Clinical evidence, mechanism, importance and management

In a randomised, placebo-controlled study, 23 healthy women were given an oral combined hormonal contraceptive (**ethinylestradiol** 30 micrograms with **gestodene** 75 micrograms) for 3 months or more. During months one and 2 they were also given either felbamate in a dose of up to 2.4 g daily, or a placebo, from day 15 of month one to day 14 of month 2. None of the women showed any evidence of ovulation during the entire 3 months, although one had intermenstrual spotting. However, felbamate reduced the **gestodene** AUC by 42% and the **ethinylestradiol** AUC by 13%.[1] The reasons for this effect are not understood. The change in ethinylestradiol exposure is not clinically important, but it cannot be ruled out that the reduction in gestodene exposure might be; therefore, some reduction in contraceptive efficacy seems possible with gestodene-containing oral combined hormonal contraceptives. More study is needed to assess the clinical relevance, and to see whether other progestogens are similarly affected.

1. Saano V, Glue P, Banfield CR, Reidenberg P, Colucci RD, Meehan JW, Haring P, Radwanski E, Nomeir A, Lin C-C, Jensen PK, Affrime MB. Effects of felbamate on the pharmacokinetics of a low-dose combination oral contraceptive. *Clin Pharmacol Ther* (1995) 58, 523–31.

Combined hormonal contraceptives + Gabapentin

Gabapentin does not alter ethinylestradiol or norethisterone exposure from an oral combined hormonal contraceptive.

Clinical evidence, mechanism, importance and management

In 13 healthy women taking an oral combined hormonal contraceptive (**ethinylestradiol** 50 micrograms with **norethisterone** 2.5 mg) gabapentin 400 mg every 8 hours for 7 days had no effect on the AUC of **ethinylestradiol** or **norethisterone**. Ovulation suppression was not assessed.[1] It appears unlikely that gabapentin will alter the efficacy of combined hormonal contraceptives (tablet, patch or vaginal ring).

1. Eldon MA, Underwood BA, Randinitis EJ, Sedman AJ. Gabapentin does not interact with a contraceptive regimen of norethindrone acetate and ethinyl estradiol. *Neurology* (1998) 50, 1146–8.

Combined hormonal contraceptives + Glucagon-like peptide-1 receptor agonists

Exenatide delays the absorption of an oral combined hormonal contraceptive containing ethinylestradiol with levonorgestrel, unless administration is separated. Liraglutide delays the absorption of ethinylestradiol and levonorgestrel from a single dose of a combined hormonal contraceptive, and lixisenatide appears to have the same effect. Dulaglutide appears to delay the absorption of ethinylestradiol and norgestimate from a combined hormonal contraceptive. Albiglutide had no clinically relevant effect on the pharmacokinetics of an oral combined hormonal contraceptive containing ethinylestradiol with norethisterone.

Clinical evidence

(a) Albiglutide

In a study in 18 healthy women taking an oral combined hormonal contraceptive (**ethinylestradiol** 35 micrograms with **norethisterone** 500 micrograms), albiglutide 50 mg weekly on days 5, 12, and 19 had no clinically relevant effect on the pharmacokinetics of either of the contraceptive steroids. Similarly, the concentrations of FSH, LH and progesterone were unaffected.[1]

(b) Dulaglutide

The UK and US manufacturers briefly report that, in a study, concurrent administration of dulaglutide with a combined hormonal contraceptive containing **ethinylestradiol** 25 micrograms with **norgestimate** 180 micrograms, had no effect on the AUC of ethinylestradiol or norelgestromin (the principal active metabolite of norgestimate). However, the maximum concentrations were decreased by 13% and 26%, and the time to maximum concentrations was delayed by 18 minutes and 2 hours, respectively.[2,3]

(c) Exenatide

In a study in healthy women taking an oral combined hormonal contraceptive (**ethinylestradiol** 30 micrograms with **levonorgestrel** 150 micrograms), when the contraceptive was taken one hour before exenatide 10 micrograms twice daily the steady-state AUC and minimum concentrations of the contraceptive steroids were unaffected, with only a 15% decrease in the maximum concentration of **ethinylestradiol**. However, giving the contraceptive 30 minutes after exenatide delayed the time to maximum concentration by about 3 hours and decreased the maximum concentration of **ethinylestradiol** and **levonorgestrel** by 45% and 27%, respectively. Further, the minimum concentration of **ethinylestradiol** was increased by 20%, but without any effect on the overall extent of absorption (AUC). In this study, exenatide was given by subcutaneous injection 15 minutes before the morning and evening meals.[4]

(d) Liraglutide

In a randomised, crossover study, 21 postmenopausal women were given liraglutide increasing to 1.8 mg daily over 3 weeks (steady-state) with a single dose of an oral combined hormonal contraceptive (containing **ethinylestradiol** 30 micrograms with **levonorgestrel** 150 micrograms) 7 hours after liraglutide on day 19. The exposure (AUC) of **ethinylestradiol** was unaffected, but there was an 18% increase in the AUC of levonorgestrel. There was a decrease in the maximum concentration of **ethinylestradiol** and **levonorgestrel**, of 12% and 13%, respectively, and the time to maximum concentration was delayed by 1.5 hours.[5]

(e) Lixisenatide

The UK manufacturer briefly reports that, in a study, giving a single dose of an oral contraceptive (containing **ethinylestradiol** 30 micrograms with **levonorgestrel** 150 micrograms) 1 hour before, or 11 hours after, lixisenatide 10 micrograms, did not result in any changes to the pharmacokinetics of either of the contraceptive steroids. However, when the contraceptive was given 1 hour or 4 hours after the lixisenatide, the maximum concentration of **ethinylestradiol** was decreased by 52% and 39%, respectively, and the maximum concentration of **levonorgestrel** was decreased by 46% and 20%, respectively. The median time to maximum concentrations was delayed by between 1 and 3 hours, but the overall exposure (AUC) of each contraceptive steroid was unaffected.[6]

Mechanism

Albiglutide, dulaglutide, exenatide, liraglutide, and lixisenatide are all said to delay gastric emptying, although this has been seen to varying extents when given with paracetamol (acetaminophen), which can be used as a marker of gastric emptying (see 'Paracetamol (Acetaminophen) + Antidiabetics', p.202 for details). These glucagon-like peptide-1 receptor agonists therefore delay the absorption of the contraceptive steroids, but this does not alter the overall extent of absorption.

Importance and management

The pharmacokinetic interaction between these glucagon-like peptide-1 receptor agonists and oral combined hormonal contraceptives is established, but unlikely to be clinically important. Contraceptive exposure (the overall extent of absorption) is the clinically important factor for contraceptive steroids, and this was unchanged by any of these drugs. The authors of the exenatide study discuss the evidence for a similar decrease in the maximum concentrations of contraceptive steroids when taken with food, and note that oral combined hormonal contraceptives are taken without regard to timing of meals.[4] However, there was no pharmacokinetic interaction if the contraceptive was taken one hour before exenatide, and the US manufacturer of exenatide recommends that administration is separated this way.[7] The UK manufacturer of exenatide states that no adjustment of contraceptive dosing is needed.[8] Note that this interaction would not apply to non-oral routes of administration of combined hormonal contraceptives (patch or vaginal ring).

No clinically relevant interaction is anticipated between albiglutide, dulaglutide, liraglutide, or lixisenatide and combined hormonal contraceptives, therefore no dose adjustment would appear necessary with any of these drugs.

For the possible adverse effect of hormonal contraceptives on diabetic control, and for the general precautions for the use of these contraceptives in diabetes, see 'Antidiabetics + Hormonal contraceptives', p.510.

1. Bush M, Scott R, Watanalumlerd P, Zhi H, Lewis E. Effects of multiple doses of albiglutide on the pharmacokinetics, pharmacodynamics, and safety of digoxin, warfarin, or a low-dose oral contraceptive. *Postgrad Med* (2012) 124, 55–72.
2. Trulicity (Dulaglutide). Eli Lilly and Company Ltd. UK Summary of product characteristics, November 2014.
3. Trulicity (Dulaglutide). Eli Lilly and Company. US Prescribing information, March 2015.
4. Kothare PA, Seger ME, Northrup J, Mace K, Mitchell MI, Linnebjerg H. Effect of exenatide on the pharmacokinetics of a combination oral contraceptive in healthy women: an open-label, randomised, crossover trial. *BMC Clin Pharmacol* (2012) 12, 8.
5. Jacobsen LV, Vouis J, Hindsberger C, Zdravkovic M. Treatment with liraglutide – a once-daily GLP-1 analog – does not reduce the bioavailability of ethinyl estradiol/levonorgestrel taken as an oral combination contraceptive drug. *J Clin Pharmacol* (2011) 51, 1696–703.
6. Lyxumia (Lixisenatide). Sanofi. UK Summary of product characteristics, October 2014.
7. Byetta (Exenatide). AstraZeneca Pharmaceuticals LP. US Prescribing information, February 2015.
8. Byetta (Exenatide). AstraZeneca UK Ltd. UK Summary of product characteristics, January 2015.

Combined hormonal contraceptives + Grapefruit juice

Large amounts of grapefruit juice slightly increase the levels of a single dose of ethinylestradiol. A case report describes a deep vein thrombosis in a woman taking an oral combined hormonal contraceptive, for which grapefruit consumption was suggested as a contributing factor.

Clinical evidence

In 13 healthy young women given a single 50-microgram dose of ethinylestradiol, grapefruit juice increased the mean maximum plasma level and AUC_{0-8} of **ethinylestradiol** by 37% and 30%, respectively, when compared with a control drink (herb tea). The mean 28% rise in the AUC_{0-24} was not statistically significant, but there was wide intersubject variation. The subjects drank grapefruit juice 100 mL or herb tea 30 minutes before the **ethinylestradiol**, a further 100 mL with the **ethinylestradiol**, and then 200 mL every 3 hours for 12 hours after taking the **ethinylestradiol**.[1] The herbal tea used was not specified.

A 42-year-old woman who had been taking an oral combined hormonal contraceptive (**ethinylestradiol** with **drospirenone**) for a year and levothyroxine for 4 years developed a deep vein thrombosis in her left leg, consistent with May-Turner syndrome. Three days earlier she had begun an aggressive weight-loss diet including 225 g of grapefruit every morning. Her only other risk factors were a 1.5-hour car journey and factor V Leiden mutation (detected on a subsequent screen). She was only slightly overweight and did not smoke.[2]

Mechanism

It is thought that the increase in ethinylestradiol bioavailability probably occurs because grapefruit juice inhibits intestinal CYP3A4, by which ethinylestradiol is partially metabolised.[1]

Deep vein thrombosis is a rare adverse effect of combined hormonal contraceptives, the risk of which appears to be higher with higher doses, and with some progestogens and in those with factor V Leiden (a type of thrombophilia). It was suggested that grapefruit may have increased ethinylestradiol levels in this patient, which enhanced hypercoagulability. This, coupled with the stasis of blood flow as a result of compression of the stenosed iliac vein, thought to be caused by hip flexion during the car journey, resulted in an acute thrombosis.[2]

Importance and management

The study suggests that drinking a litre of grapefruit juice over 12 hours might slightly increase ethinylestradiol levels, but the clinical relevance of this is uncertain, and seems unlikely to be important. Moreover, whether the findings can be directly extrapolated to daily consumption of one glass of grapefruit juice at a similar time to the combined hormonal contraceptive is also uncertain. Further study is needed. The authors suggest that diet may be a factor in the known inter-individual variability of contraceptive steroid levels.[1]

It is possible that whole grapefruit consumption may have been a contributing factor in the case of venous thrombosis, but it is more likely that it was just coincidental as this patient had several other established risk factors. This isolated case is therefore unlikely to be of general relevance.

1. Weber A, Jäger R, Börner A, Klinger G, Vollanth R, Matthey K, Balogh A. Can grapefruit juice influence ethinylestradiol bioavailability? *Contraception* (1996) 53, 41–7.
2. Grande LA, Mendez RD, Krug RT, Verschuyl E-J. Attention—grapefruit. *Lancet* (2009) 373, 1222.

Combined hormonal contraceptives + HCV-protease inhibitors

Boceprevir and telaprevir slightly reduce the exposure to ethinylestradiol, when given as an oral combined hormonal contraceptive. Simeprevir does not appear to alter the exposure to ethinylestradiol. Boceprevir appears to increase the exposure to drospirenone. Paritaprevir boosted with ritonavir appears to moderately increase norelgestromin and norgestrel exposure, and concurrent use of ethinylestradiol greatly increases the incidence of increased ALT concentrations.

Clinical evidence

(a) Boceprevir

In a study, 20 healthy subjects received an oral combined hormonal contraceptive containing **ethinylestradiol** 35 micrograms and **norethisterone** 1 mg for 21 days of a 28 day cycle, for 3 cycles, with boceprevir 800 mg three times daily on day one to day 28 of the third cycle of the oral contraceptive. Boceprevir *decreased* the maximum concentration of norethisterone by 17%, but did not affect the AUC. The AUC and maximum concentration of ethinylestradiol were *decreased* by 26% and 21%, respectively. Despite these changes, concentrations of LH, FSH, and progesterone were not affected, indicating that ovulation had still been suppressed.[1] The UK and US manufacturers also briefly report that, in a study, boceprevir 800 mg three times daily for 7 days increased the AUC and maximum plasma concentration of **drospirenone** 3 mg daily by 99% and 57%, respectively, when taken with **ethinylestradiol** 20 micrograms daily as a combined hormonal contraceptive for 14 days. Boceprevir *decreased* the AUC of ethinylestradiol by 24%, but had no effect on its maximum plasma concentration.[2,3]

(b) Paritaprevir

The UK and US manufacturers briefly report that, in a study in healthy subjects given an oral combined hormonal contraceptive containing **ethinylestradiol** 35 micrograms and **norgestimate** 250 micrograms daily with paritaprevir 150 mg daily (in a fixed-dose combination with ombitasvir and ritonavir, given with and without dasabuvir) the pharmacokinetics of ethinylestradiol and paritaprevir were unaffected. However, the AUC and maximum concentrations of norelgestromin and norgestrel (the active metabolites of norgestimate) were increased 2.6- and 2-fold, and 2.5- and 2.3-fold, respectively. Furthermore, in clinical trials with paritaprevir (in a fixed-dose combination with ombitasvir and ritonavir, and given with dasabuvir), increases in ALT concentrations greater than 5 times the upper limit of normal were seen in 1% of all patients, but were considerably more frequent in female subjects taking ethinylestradiol-containing contraceptives (oral combined hormonal contraceptives, contraceptive patches, or contraceptive vaginal rings).[4,5]

(c) Simeprevir

The UK and US manufacturers briefly report that, in a study in 16 healthy subjects given an oral combined hormonal contraceptive containing **ethinylestradiol** 35 micrograms and **norethisterone** 1 mg for 21 days with simeprevir 150 mg daily for 10 days, the AUC of ethinylestradiol was unaffected, but the maximum concentration was increased by 18%. The AUC and maximum concentration of norethisterone were unaffected.[6,7]

(d) Telaprevir

In a study, 24 healthy subjects who had been taking an oral combined hormonal contraceptive containing **ethinylestradiol** 35 micrograms and **norethisterone** 0.5 mg for at least 3 months were given telaprevir 750 mg every 8 hours on day one to day 28 of the second cycle of the oral contraceptive. Telaprevir *decreased* the AUC and minimum plasma concentration of **ethinylestradiol** by 28% and 33%, respectively, but had no effect on the pharmacokinetics of **norethisterone**. Furthermore, although concentrations of progesterone were decreased, concentrations of LH and FSH were increased, suggesting that ovulation might not be suppressed. The pharmacokinetics of telaprevir were similarly unaffected.[8]

Mechanism

Unknown. Boceprevir and telaprevir are known to *inhibit* CYP3A4, by which ethinylestradiol is partially metabolised, and would be expected to *increase* the exposure to ethinylestradiol, the opposite of the results of the above studies. It has been suggested that telaprevir might affect drug transporters in the gastrointestinal tract, thereby reducing the absorption of ethinylestradiol.[8] Simeprevir also inhibits CYP3A4, although perhaps not to a clinically relevant extent, but did cause a small increase in the ethinylestradiol maximum concentration in the study cited. The reason for the increase in norelgestromin exposure seen with paritaprevir (in a fixed-dose combination with ombitasvir and ritonavir, and given with dasabuvir), is unclear, but the involvement of ritonavir in this combination (which is used as a pharmacokinetic enhancer) cannot be ruled out, since some HIV-protease inhibitors boosted with ritonavir have been shown to have a similar effect on norelgestromin (see 'Combined hormonal contraceptives + HIV-protease inhibitors', p.1177 for details).

Importance and management

Evidence for a pharmacokinetic interaction between combined hormonal contraceptives and the HCV-protease inhibitors is limited, and in the cases of boceprevir and telaprevir, unexpected, based on the known disposition and interactions of these drugs. The slight decrease in ethinylestradiol exposure caused by both boceprevir and telaprevir and might not be expected to affect contraceptive effectiveness, as suggested in one study with boceprevir,[1] however, this is in contrast to the study with telaprevir where ovulation was possibly not suppressed.[8] Therefore, it cannot be ruled out that this decreased exposure would be sufficient to cause the failure of combined hormonal contraceptives in very rare cases. Until more is known, it would seem reasonable to avoid the use of oral combined hormonal contraceptives with a low 20-microgram dose of ethinylestradiol in patients also taking boceprevir or telaprevir. Note that as boceprevir, simeprevir, and telaprevir are used as part of triple therapy with ribavirin and interferon, contraceptive restrictions apply to the duration of the triple therapy and a period afterwards, as a result of the teratogenic potential of ribavirin. The advice included below refers specifically to the relevant HCV-protease inhibitor without ribavirin. The UK and US manufacturers of **telaprevir** advise that two non-hormonal methods of contraception (such as barrier methods and IUDs) should be used during, and for 2 months (UK manufacturer[9]), or 2 weeks (US manufacturer[10]), after stopping telaprevir. In contrast, the UK and US manufacturers of **boceprevir** advise that concurrent use with a combined hormonal contraceptive containing ethinylestradiol and at least 1 mg of norethisterone is unlikely to alter the effectiveness of the contraceptive.[2,3] The US manufacturer specifically states that during triple therapy including boceprevir, one of the required effective methods of contraception can be a combined hormonal contraceptive containing at least 1 mg of norethisterone.[3] The UK and US manufacturers of **simeprevir** simply advise that no dose adjustment of ethinylestradiol with norethisterone is required on concurrent use.[6,7]

Based on the above data, the UK and US manufacturers of boceprevir and telaprevir extend their advice to oestrogen-containing **HRT**, predicting that this too might be affected, and they advise monitoring for signs of oestrogen deficiency.[2,3,9,10] Note that this effect would be most noticeable where HRT is prescribed for menopausal vasomotor symptoms, but might be difficult to detect where the indication is osteoporosis. Any interaction might be expected to be less likely with transdermal HRT. However, the clinical relevance of any interaction between HRT and telaprevir is as yet unclear.

Drospirenone is an aldosterone antagonist, and the increase in its plasma concentration seen with boceprevir might increase the risk of adverse effects, in particular hyperkalaemia. The US manufacturer of boceprevir therefore contraindicates concurrent use with drospirenone,[3] but the UK manufacturer advises caution in patients who are at high risk of developing hyperkalaemia, such as those taking potassium-sparing diuretics or patients with conditions that predispose them to hyperkalaemia [such as renal impairment], and recommends that alternative contraceptives should be considered in these patients.[2] Consider also 'Drospirenone-containing contraceptives or HRT + Potassium-sparing drugs', p.1191, for further information on the use of drospirenone in patients taking potassium-sparing drugs.

The moderate increase in the exposure to norelgestromin and norgestrel seen with **paritaprevir** boosted with ritonavir (in a fixed-dose combination with ombitasvir, and given with or without dasabuvir) might result in increased progestogen-related adverse effects (such as spotting and acne) and result in reduced contraceptive compliance. Furthermore, because of the greatly increased incidence of increased ALT concentrations in women taking ethinylestradiol-containing contraceptives, the UK and US manufacturers contraindicate the concurrent use of such contraceptives, and state that they must be discontinued prior to starting treatment,[4,5] but can be restarted about 2 weeks after treatment has stopped.[4] Alternative methods of contraception must be used during treatment, such as progestogen-only contraceptives or non-hormonal methods.[4,5] For information on the concurrent use of the progestogen-only contraceptive, norethisterone and paritaprevir, see 'HCV-protease inhibitors; Paritaprevir + Miscellaneous', p.909.

1. Lin WH, Feng HP, Shadle CR, O'Reilly T, Wagner JA, Butterton JR. Pharmacokinetic and pharmacodynamic interactions between the hepatitis C virus protease inhibitor, boceprevir, and the oral contraceptive ethinyl estradiol/norethindrone. *Eur J Clin Pharmacol* (2014) 70, 1107–13.
2. Victrelis (Boceprevir). Merck Sharp & Dohme Ltd. UK Summary of product characteristics, August 2014.
3. Victrelis (Boceprevir). Merck & Co., Inc. US Prescribing information, July 2014.
4. Viekira Pak (Ombitasvir, paritaprevir, ritonavir co-packaged with dasabuvir sodium monohydrate). AbbVie Inc. US Prescribing information, December 2014.
5. Viekirax (Ombitasvir, paritaprevir, ritonavir). AbbVie Ltd. UK Summary of product characteristics, January 2015.
6. Olysio (Simeprevir sodium). Janssen-Cilag Ltd. UK Summary of product characteristics, May 2014.
7. Olysio (Simeprevir sodium). Janssen Products, LP. US Prescribing information, November 2014.
8. Garg V, van Heeswijk R, Yang Y, Kauffman R, Smith F, Adda N. The pharmacokinetic interaction between an oral contraceptive containing ethinyl estradiol and norethindrone and the HCV protease inhibitor telaprevir. *J Clin Pharmacol* (2012) 52, 1574–83.
9. Incivo (Telaprevir). Janssen-Cilag Ltd. UK Summary of product characteristics, July 2014.
10. Incivek (Telaprevir). Vertex Pharmaceuticals, Inc. US Prescribing information, October 2013.

Combined hormonal contraceptives + HIV-integrase inhibitors

Elvitegravir boosted with cobicistat decreases ethinylestradiol exposure, and increases the exposure to norelgestromin (the active metabolite of norgestimate) from an oral combined hormonal contraceptive, whereas raltegravir and dolutegravir have no effect.

Clinical evidence

(a) Dolutegravir

In a study in 15 healthy women given an oral combined hormonal contraceptive (**ethinylestradiol** 35 micrograms with **norgestimate** 250 micrograms) and dolutegravir 50 mg twice daily for 10 days, the pharmacokinetics of ethinylestradiol and norelgestromin (the main active metabolite of norgestimate) were unaffected.[1] There was also no effect on the pharmacokinetics of dolutegravir, and no effect on LH, FSH, or progesterone concentrations.[1]

(b) Elvitegravir

In a study in 15 healthy women, elvitegravir boosted with cobicistat 150/150 mg daily (in a fixed-dose combination also including emtricitabine and tenofovir disoproxil fumarate) was given for the last 10 days of a cycle (days 12 to 21) of an oral combined hormonal contraceptive (**ethinylestradiol** 25 micrograms with **norgestimate** 180 to 250 micrograms). When compared with the contraceptive alone, concurrent use of the antiretrovirals decreased the AUC of ethinylestradiol by 25% and increased the AUC and maximum plasma concentration of norelgestromin (the active metabolite of norgestimate) about 2-fold. The ovulation suppressant effect of the contraceptive (as measured by progesterone concentrations and suppression of FSH or LH) was unaffected;[2] however, the antiretroviral was taken for just 10 days of the cycle (it is necessary to give drugs for a complete cycle or longer to reliably assess effects on ovulation).

(c) Raltegravir

In a study in 19 healthy women taking an oral combined hormonal contraceptive (**ethinylestradiol** 35 micrograms with **norgestimate** 180 to 250 micrograms), raltegravir 400 mg twice daily on days 1 to 21 of a cycle did not alter ethinylestradiol exposure and increased norelgestromin (the main active metabolite of norgestimate) exposure by 14%.[3]

Mechanism

The reason why elvitegravir boosted with cobicistat decreases ethinylestradiol exposure and increases norgestimate active metabolite exposure is not known. Tenofovir does not alter ethinylestradiol and norgestimate exposure, and emtricitabine is predicted not to interact, see 'Hormonal contraceptives + NRTIs', p.1193. However, some involvement of cobicistat, an analogue of ritonavir which has a similar interaction profile, cannot be ruled out (see 'Combined hormonal contraceptives + HIV-protease inhibitors', p.1177), but requires study.

Importance and management

The clinical relevance of the changes in the exposure to ethinylestradiol and the active metabolite of norgestimate on concurrent use of **elvitegravir** boosted with cobicistat are unknown. The decrease in ethinylestradiol exposure is small, but is of some concern. Although the increase in the exposure to the active metabolite of norgestimate might compensate for the small reduction in ethinylestradiol exposure, it might also result in increased progestogen-related adverse effects (such as acne and an increased risk of insulin resistance and venous thrombosis). The authors of the study suggest that a contraceptive with a dose of at least 30 micrograms of ethinylestradiol should be used,[2] and, until more is known, this seems prudent. The effect of elvitegravir boosted with cobicistat on other progestogens in oral combined hormonal contraceptives, or on other hormonal contraceptives (e.g. the vaginal ring and patch) is unknown and requires study. Until more is known, other non-hormonal methods of contraception are preferable. In addition, as the risk of progestogen-related adverse effects is not known, it would be prudent to bear this in mind on concurrent use, and advise and monitor patients accordingly. The US manufacturer of elvitegravir boosted with cobicistat (in a fixed-dose combination also including emtricitabine and tenofovir disoproxil fumarate) adds that this is particularly important in individuals with risk factors.[4] On the basis of the data with cobicistat, the UK manufacturer of elvitegravir licensed for use with an HIV-protease inhibitor boosted with ritonavir, gives the same advice as above.[5] However, the US manufacturer advises that alternative methods of non-hormonal contraception should be used.[6] Similarly, the UK and US manufacturers of **cobicistat** licensed for use with atazanavir or darunavir, advise that due to a lack of data, non-hormonal contraception should be used.[7,8]

Dolutegravir does not appear to alter the exposure to, or efficacy of, oral combined hormonal contraceptives, and **raltegravir** is also unlikely to alter the efficacy of oral combined hormonal contraceptives, by a pharmacokinetic mechanism. For both these HIV-integrase inhibitors, this can probably also be extended to include the patch and vaginal ring. No dose adjustments or additional contraceptive precautions appear to be necessary on concurrent use.

Note that regardless of the methods of contraception being used, barrier methods are always advisable to reduce the risk of HIV transmission.

1. Song IH, Borland J, Chen S, Wajima T, Peppercorn AF, Piscitelli SC. Dolutegravir has no effect on the pharmacokinetics of oral contraceptives with norgestimate and ethinyl estradiol. *Ann Pharmacother* (2015) 49, 784–9.

2. German P, Wang M, Warren D, Kearney PB. Pharmacokinetic interaction between norgestimate/ethinyl estradiol and EVG/COB/FTC/TDF single tablet regimen. 12th International Workshop on Clinical Pharmacology of HIV Therapy, Miami, 2011, Abstract 17.
3. Anderson MS, Hanley WD, Moreau AR, Jin B, Bieberdorf FA, Kost JT, Wenning LA, Stone JA, Wagner JA, Iwamoto M. Effect of raltegravir on estradiol and norgestimate plasma pharmacokinetics following oral contraceptive administration in healthy women. *Br J Clin Pharmacol* (2011) 71, 616–20.
4. Stribild (Elvitegravir, cobicistat, emtricitabine, tenofovir disoproxil fumarate). Gilead Sciences, Inc. US Prescribing information, December 2014.
5. Vitekta (Elvitegravir). Gilead Sciences Ltd. UK Summary of product characteristics, March 2014.
6. Vitekta (Elvitegravir). Gilead Sciences, Inc. US Prescribing information, September 2014.
7. Tybost (Cobicistat). Gilead Sciences Ltd. UK Summary of product characteristics, October 2014.
8. Tybost (Cobicistat). Gilead Sciences, Inc. US Prescribing information, September 2014.

Combined hormonal contraceptives + HIV-protease inhibitors

Ritonavir and nelfinavir, given alone, *reduce* the exposure of ethinylestradiol given as an oral combined hormonal contraceptive. Similarly, most HIV-protease inhibitors boosted with ritonavir studied (darunavir, fosamprenavir, lopinavir and tipranavir) also *reduce* ethinylestradiol exposure to a similar extent, and this might result in reduced contraceptive efficacy, although atazanavir boosted with ritonavir had less effect. Conversely, atazanavir, indinavir or amprenavir alone *increase* the exposure of ethinylestradiol and norethisterone. The changes in norethisterone exposure with these HIV-protease inhibitors have been minor, but greater increases in norgestimate and norelgestromin exposure have been seen.

An oral combined hormonal contraceptive did not alter the exposure of amprenavir (derived from fosamprenavir) or saquinavir, and other limited evidence suggests that hormonal contraceptives do not alter antiretroviral activity of HAART (mostly HIV-protease inhibitor based) regimens.

Clinical evidence

A. Unboosted HIV-protease inhibitors

(a) Amprenavir

The UK manufacturer briefly noted that amprenavir *increased* the minimum plasma concentrations of **ethinylestradiol** and **norethisterone**, given as an oral combined hormonal contraceptive, by 32% and 45%, respectively. Conversely, the amprenavir minimum concentration and AUC were *decreased* by 20% and 22%, respectively.[1] Note that amprenavir has generally been superseded by its pro-drug, fosamprenavir; for information on the interactions of this drug with combined hormonal contraceptives, see under *HIV-protease inhibitors boosted with ritonavir*, below.

(b) Atazanavir

In a study in 22 healthy women given an oral combined hormonal contraceptive (**ethinylestradiol** with **norethisterone**), atazanavir 400 mg daily for the first 2 weeks of a cycle *increased* the AUC of **ethinylestradiol** by 48% and *increased* the AUC of **norethisterone** by about 110%.[2] Note that, atazanavir with ritonavir decreased ethinylestradiol concentrations, see under *HIV-protease inhibitors boosted with ritonavir*, below.

(c) Indinavir

The manufacturers briefly report that indinavir 800 mg three times daily given with an oral combined hormonal contraceptive (**ethinylestradiol** 35 micrograms with **norethisterone** 1 mg) for 8 days caused a modest 22% and 26% *increase* in the AUCs of **ethinylestradiol** and **norethisterone**, respectively.[3,4] In a retrospective study there were no reports of contraceptive failure in 9 patients taking indinavir (overall there were 8 contraceptive failures out of 33 women taking HIV-protease inhibitors). However, medication adherence could not be confirmed.[5]

(d) Nelfinavir

The manufacturer briefly notes that in a study in 12 women taking an oral combined hormonal contraceptive (**ethinylestradiol** 35 micrograms with **norethisterone** 400 micrograms) for 15 days, nelfinavir 750 mg three times daily for one week *decreased* the AUCs of **ethinylestradiol** and **norethisterone** by 47% and 18%, respectively.[6,7] In a retrospective study, 7 of 21 women taking nelfinavir experienced contraceptive failure, which was the highest rate of failure of the HIV-protease inhibitors being taken (overall there were 8 contraceptive failures out of 33 women taking HIV-protease inhibitors). However, medication adherence could not be confirmed.[5]

(e) Ritonavir

In a study in 23 healthy women, ritonavir 500 mg every 12 hours for 16 days *decreased* the AUC of **ethinylestradiol** by 41% and decreased its elimination half-life from 17 hours to 13 hours. The women received a single dose of an oral combined hormonal contraceptive (**ethinylestradiol** 50 micrograms with **etynodiol** 1 mg), 14 days before the ritonavir and on day 15 of ritonavir.[8] In a retrospective study there were no reports of contraceptive failure in 6 women taking ritonavir (overall there were 8 contraceptive failures out of 33 women taking HIV-protease inhibitors). However, medication adherence could not be confirmed.[5]

(f) Saquinavir

A study in 8 healthy women found that the pharmacokinetics of a single 600-mg dose of saquinavir were not affected by an oral combined hormonal contraceptive containing **ethinylestradiol** 30 micrograms with **gestodene** 75 micrograms taken for 21 days.[9] Similarly, in a clinical study of the use of saquinavir soft capsules in HIV-positive patients, there was no evidence that the pharmacokinetics of saquinavir were altered by oral contraceptives [unspecified].[10] In a retrospective study there was one report of contraceptive failure out of 5 women taking saquinavir (overall there were 8 contraceptive failures out of 33 women taking HIV-protease inhibitors). However, medication adherence could not be confirmed.[5]

B. HIV-protease inhibitors boosted with ritonavir

(a) Atazanavir

The manufacturer notes that when atazanavir boosted with ritonavir 300/100 mg daily was given with an oral combined hormonal contraceptive (**ethinylestradiol** with **norgestimate**) for 14 days, there was a 19% *decrease* in the AUC of ethinylestradiol and an 85% *increase* in the AUC of the active metabolite of norgestimate.[11,12] This is in contrast to the increase in AUC of ethinylestradiol seen after unboosted atazanavir, see *Atazanavir*, above.

(b) Darunavir

In a study in healthy women taking an oral combined hormonal contraceptive (**ethinylestradiol** with **norethisterone**), darunavir boosted with ritonavir 600/100 mg twice daily for the first 2 weeks of a cycle *decreased* the concentration of **ethinylestradiol** by 44% and *decreased* the AUC of **norethisterone** by 14%.[13]

(c) Fosamprenavir

In a study in 25 women, when fosamprenavir boosted with ritonavir 700/100 mg twice daily was given with an oral combined hormonal contraceptive containing **ethinylestradiol** 35 micrograms with **norethisterone** 500 micrograms daily for 21 days the AUC of ethinylestradiol was *decreased* by 37% and the AUC of norethisterone *decreased* by 34%.[14,15] The pharmacokinetics of amprenavir (derived from fosamprenavir) were not affected; however, the AUC and maximum concentration of **ritonavir** were 45% and 63% higher, respectively, when compared with historical data in female subjects taking fosamprenavir and ritonavir alone.[14] In this study, clinically significant increases in liver transaminases occurred in some healthy subjects.[14]

(d) Lopinavir

A study in 12 healthy subjects found that lopinavir boosted with ritonavir 400/100 mg twice daily for 14 days *decreased* the AUC of **ethinylestradiol** and **norethisterone** (given as an oral combined hormonal contraceptive for 21 days) by 42% and 17%, respectively.[16] Similarly, in another study in 8-HIV positive women using a combined hormonal contraceptive patch (**ethinylestradiol** with **norelgestromin**), the AUC of ethinylestradiol was 45% lower in those taking lopinavir boosted with ritonavir 400/100 mg twice daily (4 patients available to be assessed) than in 15 control women not taking antiretrovirals. However, the AUC of norelgestromin was 83% higher in the women taking lopinavir boosted with ritonavir (7 patients assessed). In addition, when these women were given a single dose of an oral combined hormonal contraceptive before patch placement, the AUC of ethinylestradiol was 55% lower in the women taking lopinavir boosted with ritonavir (5 patients assessed) than in the control group. The ovulation suppressant effect of the contraceptive patch appeared to be unaffected by this short-term use of lopinavir boosted with ritonavir (as measured by progesterone concentrations).[17] However, it is necessary to give drugs for a complete cycle or longer to reliably assess effects on ovulation.

(e) Tipranavir

The manufacturer reports that in a study, tipranavir boosted with ritonavir 500/100 mg twice daily or 750/200 mg twice daily for 10 days *decreased* the AUC of **ethinylestradiol** by 48% and 43%, respectively, and *increased* the AUC of **norethisterone** by 14% and 27%, respectively, when these contraceptive steroids were given as a single dose of an oral combined hormonal contraceptive.[18,19] In this study, 33% of women developed a rash, which is a higher incidence than is usually seen in patients given tipranavir boosted with ritonavir.[18]

Mechanism

Ritonavir more commonly *inhibits* CYP3A4, by which ethinylestradiol is partially metabolised, and the results for ritonavir are the opposite of those originally predicted based on *in vitro* data showing *inhibition* of ethinylestradiol metabolism (2-hydroxylation, mediated by the cytochrome P450 subfamily CYP3A).[20] However, ethinylestradiol is also substantially metabolised by conjugation, and the clinical findings suggest that ritonavir induces glucuronyltransferase (UGT) activity, thereby reducing ethinylestradiol exposure.[8] The finding in one study that a combined hormonal contraceptive patch appeared to be affected to the same extent as an oral preparation suggests that ritonavir is not acting to inhibit first pass metabolism in the gut.[17]

Nelfinavir probably interacts similarly to ritonavir. The effect of ritonavir appears so strong that it is apparent with all HIV-protease inhibitors boosted with ritonavir studied (atazanavir, darunavir, fosamprenavir, lopinavir and tipranavir). Atazanavir alone may increase ethinylestradiol concentrations by inhibition of UGT, and this partially offsets the effect of ritonavir.[12] Indinavir also slightly increases contraceptive steroid concentrations, but the mechanism is uncertain. Ritonavir and HIV-protease inhibitors boosted with ritonavir appear to cause a minor reduction in norethisterone exposure, but atazanavir and lopinavir, both boosted with ritonavir, increased the exposure of norgestimate and norelgestromin (the active metabolite of norgestimate), which suggests that it is metabolised differently to norethisterone.

Importance and management

The reduced exposure to the ethinylestradiol component of combined hormonal contraceptives with **nelfinavir** or **ritonavir** and most **HIV-protease inhibitors boosted with ritonavir** so far studied (darunavir, fosamprenavir, lopinavir and tipranavir) appears to be established and is likely to be clinically important. Similar *decreases* in the concentrations of ethinylestradiol caused by potent enzyme-inducing drugs (see 'Table 28.1', p.1160) have resulted in a reduced efficacy and reliability of oral combined hormonal contraceptives, and one retrospective report suggests that this has occurred with nelfinavir.[5]

In the UK, the Faculty of Sexual and Reproductive Healthcare (FSRH) Clinical Effectiveness Unit include ritonavir and HIV-protease inhibitors boosted with ritonavir in their 2011 guidance on the use of enzyme inducers with hormonal contraceptives.[21] For the short-term use of enzyme-inducers (which could include use of HIV-protease inhibitors for post-exposure prophylaxis) in those who choose a combined hormonal contraceptive, the advice is to use a standard-strength preparation (30 or 35 micrograms of ethinylestradiol), with additional contraceptive precautions such as condoms, see 'Combined hormonal contraceptives + Barbiturates or Phenytoin', p.1169, for further details of this guidance. This advice would also seem to be most relevant to the long-term use of HIV-protease inhibitors, where oral combined hormonal contraceptives are the preferred method of contraception, because whatever other methods of contraception are being used, barrier methods are always advisable to reduce the risk of HIV transmission. In the absence of barrier methods, standard-strength preparations might not be sufficiently effective given the reductions in ethinylestradiol exposure that occur, and at least 50 micrograms (as advised by the FSRH) is likely to be necessary. Note that the manufacturers of fosamprenavir actually advise alternative non-hormonal methods of contraception because of the risk of increased liver enzymes and the decrease in hormone exposure seen in the oral combined hormonal contraceptive study.[14,15] The manufacturers of tipranavir specifically note that women using oestrogens with tipranavir might also have an increased risk of non-serious rash.[18,19]

The situation for **atazanavir boosted with ritonavir** is less clear cut. Although there is a 19% decrease in ethinylestradiol exposure, this is about half that seen with the other HIV-protease inhibitors boosted with ritonavir mentioned above. In addition, unlike the majority of other studies, this study used a norgestimate-containing contraceptive, and there was an 85% increase in norgestimate exposure.[12] Although this might compensate for the small reduction in ethinylestradiol concentrations, it may also result in increased progestogen-related adverse effects (such as spotting and acne) which may reduce contraceptive compliance. While noting that the increase in norgestimate exposure might increase adverse effects, the manufacturer recommends that, for atazanavir boosted with ritonavir, an oral combined hormonal contraceptive with at least 30 micrograms[12] or 35 micrograms[11] of ethinylestradiol should be used. In addition, they state that because there is no information on the concurrent use of other progestogens, preparations with progestogens other than norgestimate should be avoided.[12] Where atazanavir is used *without ritonavir*, the increases in norethisterone and ethinylestradiol exposure suggest some caution is appropriate. The US manufacturer recommends that, for unboosted atazanavir, an oral combined hormonal contraceptive with no more than 30 micrograms of ethinylestradiol be used.[11]

The only data for the **combined hormonal contraceptive patch** are for lopinavir boosted with ritonavir. This appears to reduce ethinylestradiol exposure to a similar extent to oral combined hormonal contraceptives; however, it also increased the exposure to the progestogen component, norelgestromin. It has been suggested that the balance of these effects would maintain contraceptive efficacy,[17] but further study is needed to assess this.

Note that the increases in contraceptive steroid concentrations with **indinavir** alone are unlikely to be clinically relevant, and the manufacturers state that there is no need to adjust the dose of oral combined hormonal contraceptives containing ethinylestradiol 35 micrograms with norethisterone 1 mg when used with unboosted indinavir.[3] There are no data for indinavir used with ritonavir, but as with the other HIV-protease inhibitors boosted with ritonavir, the effects of ritonavir, resulting in a reduction in ethinylestradiol exposure, might be predicted to predominate.

Amprenavir concentrations are decreased by combined hormonal contraceptives, but the effects are modest. There is some evidence to suggest that hormonal contraceptives (including oral combined hormonal contraceptives) do not alter the antiretroviral efficacy of HAART (mostly HIV-protease-inhibitor based),[22] but evidence is preliminary and more study is needed.

1. Agenerase (Amprenavir). GlaxoSmithKline UK. UK Summary of product characteristics, February 2007.
2. Tackett D, Child M, Agarwala S, Geiger M, Geraldes M, Laura B, O'Mara E. Atazanavir: A summary of two pharmacokinetic drug interaction studies in healthy subjects. 10th Conference on Retroviruses and Opportunistic Infections, Boston, MA, 2003, abstract 543.
3. Crixivan (Indinavir sulphate). Merck Sharp & Dohme Ltd. UK Summary of product characteristics, February 2012.
4. Crixivan (Indinavir sulfate). Merck & Co., Inc. US Prescribing information, April 2012.
5. Clark RA, Theall K. Population-based study evaluating association between selected antiretroviral therapies and potential oral contraceptive failure. *J Acquir Immune Defic Syndr* (2004) 37, 1219–20.
6. Viracept (Nelfinavir mesilate). Roche Products Ltd. UK Summary of product characteristics, June 2012.
7. Viracept (Nelfinavir mesylate). Agouron Pharmaceuticals, Inc. US Prescribing information, May 2013.
8. Ouellet D, Hsu A, Qian J, Locke CS, Eason CJ, Cavanaugh JH, Leonard JM, Granneman GR. Effect of ritonavir on the pharmacokinetics of ethinyl oestradiol in healthy female volunteers. *Br J Clin Pharmacol* (1998) 46, 111–16.
9. Fröhlich M, Burhenne J, Martin-Facklam M, Weiss J, von Wolff M, Strowitzki T, Walter-Sack I, Haefeli WE. Oral contraception does not alter single dose saquinavir pharmacokinetics in women. *Br J Clin Pharmacol* (2004) 57, 244–52.
10. Mayer K, Poblete R, Hathaway B, Palic B, Pilson R, Siemon-Hryczyk P, de Caprariis P. Efficacy, effect of oral contraceptives, and adherence in HIV infected women receiving Fortovase (saquinavir) soft gel capsule (SQV-SGC) thrice (TID) and twice (BID) daily regimens. *Int Conf AIDS* (2000) 13, abstract no. TuPeB3226.
11. Reyataz (Atazanavir sulfate). Bristol-Myers Squibb. US Prescribing information, March 2012.
12. Reyataz (Atazanavir sulfate). Bristol-Myers Squibb Pharmaceuticals Ltd. UK Summary of product characteristics, August 2012.
13. Sekar VJ, Lefebvre E, Guzman SS, Felicione E, De Pauw M, Vangeneugden T, Hoetelmans RMW. Pharmacokinetic interaction between ethinyl estradiol, norethindrone and darunavir with low-dose ritonavir in healthy women. *Antivir Ther* (2008) 13, 563–9.
14. Telzir (Fosamprenavir calcium). ViiV Healthcare UK Ltd. UK Summary of product characteristics, May 2011.
15. ViiV Healthcare. US Prescribing information. April 2013.
16. Bertz R, Hsu A, Lam W, Williams L, Renz C, Karol M, Dutta S, Carr R, Zhang Y, Wang Q, Schweitzer S, Foit C, Andre A, Bernstein B, Granneman GR, Sun E. Pharmacokinetic interaction between lopinavir/ritonavir (ABT-378r) and other non-HIV drugs (P291). *AIDS* (2000) 14 (Suppl 4), S100.
17. Vogler MA, Patterson K, Kamemoto L, Park J-G, Watts H, Aweeka F, Klingman KL, Cohn SE. Contraceptive efficacy of oral and transdermal hormones when co-administered with protease inhibitors in HIV-1-infected women: pharmacokinetic results of ACTG trial A5188. *J Acquir Immune Defic Syndr* (2010) 55, 473–82.
18. Aptivus Soft Capsules (Tipranavir). Boehringer Ingelheim Ltd. UK Summary of product characteristics, December 2011.
19. Aptivus (Tipranavir). Boehringer Ingelheim Pharmaceuticals, Inc. US Prescribing information, April 2012.
20. Kumar GN, Rodrigues AD, Buko AM, Denissen JF. Cytochrome P450-mediated metabolism of the HIV-1 protease inhibitor ritonavir (ABT-538) in human liver microsomes. *J Pharmacol Exp Ther* (1996) 277, 423–31.
21. Faculty of Sexual and Reproductive Healthcare Guidance. Drug interactions with hormonal contraception: Clinical Effectiveness Unit, January 2011. Available at: http://www.fsrh.org/pdfs/CEUGuidanceDrugInteractionsHormonal.pdf (accessed 21/10/15).
22. Chu JH, Gange SJ, Anastos K, Minkoff H, Cejtin H, Bacon M, Levine A, Greenblatt RM. Hormonal contraceptive use and the effectiveness of highly active antiretroviral therapy. *Am J Epidemiol* (2005) 161, 881–90.

Combined hormonal contraceptives + Lacosamide

Lacosamide does not alter the pharmacokinetics or the ovulation suppressant effect of an oral combined hormonal contraceptive containing ethinylestradiol with levonorgestrel.

Clinical evidence, mechanism, importance and management

In a study in healthy women, the pharmacokinetics of an oral combined hormonal contraceptive (**ethinylestradiol** 30 micrograms with **levonorgestrel** 150 micrograms) were not affected by lacosamide 400 mg daily (except for a minor 20% increase in the **ethinylestradiol** maximum level),[1,2] and the suppression of ovulation was not altered (there were no changes in progesterone levels).[2] These findings indicate that no additional contraceptive precautions are needed if lacosamide is used concurrently with any combined hormonal contraceptive (tablet, patch or vaginal ring).

1. Vimpat (Lacosamide). UCB, Inc. US Prescribing information, February 2012.
2. Vimpat (Lacosamide). UCB Pharma Ltd. UK Summary of product characteristics, July 2012.

Combined hormonal contraceptives + Lamotrigine

In one study, lamotrigine for two weeks did not alter the mean plasma levels of ethinylestradiol and levonorgestrel or the suppression of ovulation in women taking an oral combined hormonal contraceptive. However, another study of six weeks' use found a very slight reduction in levonorgestrel exposure, and some loss of FSH and LH suppression, but no evidence of ovulation.

Combined hormonal contraceptives moderately reduce lamotrigine exposure, which can lead to a decrease in seizure control during the active hormone phase, and, conversely, an increase in lamotrigine exposure with a risk of toxicity during the hormone free week.

Clinical evidence

(a) Contraceptive efficacy

The preliminary results of a study in women taking an oral combined hormonal contraceptive (**ethinylestradiol** 30 micrograms with **levonorgestrel** 150 micrograms), suggested that lamotrigine 150 mg daily for 10 to 14 days had no statistically significant effect on the mean plasma levels of **ethinylestradiol** (11% decrease) and **levonorgestrel** (no change). No ovulation occurred (assessed by progesterone levels) and no changes in menstrual pattern were observed. Furthermore, lamotrigine did not induce hepatic enzymes (assessed by 6-β-hydroxycortisol excretion).[1] Nevertheless, another study by the manufacturer, in 16 healthy women taking an oral combined hormonal contraceptive (**ethinylestradiol** 30 micrograms with **levonorgestrel** 150 micrograms) and given lamotrigine for 6 weeks (titrated to 300 mg daily), found a very slight reduction in the AUC of **levonorgestrel** of 19%, compared with hormone levels before starting lamotrigine. The AUC of **ethinylestradiol** was minimally affected (7% reduction). There was a 4.7-fold increase in FSH and a 3.4-fold increase in LH; however, there was no increase in the levels of progesterone, indicating that ovulation did not occur. Intermenstrual bleeding was reported in 32% of subjects when they were taking lamotrigine, and no bleeding was reported when they were not taking lamotrigine.[2]

(b) Lamotrigine efficacy

In 2001, a case series described 6 women with epilepsy in whom lamotrigine plasma levels were decreased by 41 to 64% by an oral combined hormonal contraceptive (**ethinylestradiol** with **desogestrel** or **norethisterone**). Five had an increase in seizure frequency or a recurrence of seizures after starting an oral hormonal contraceptive, and one had lamotrigine adverse effects on stopping the contraceptive.[3] In a subsequent study comparing lamotrigine levels in 22 women taking combined hormonal contraceptives with those in 30 women not taking contraceptives, lamotrigine levels were

54% lower in the women taking contraceptives.[4] Three further similar studies have confirmed this finding of lower lamotrigine levels in users of oral combined hormonal contraceptives than in non-users.[5-7] Moreover, other studies in women with epilepsy have found that lamotrigine plasma concentrations varied with combined hormonal contraceptive monthly cycles.[8,9] In one, the median lamotrigine plasma level was 15% higher during the hormonal contraceptive washout week than during the phase of hormonal contraceptive intake, although there was a wide interpatient variability.[8] In another, reductions in lamotrigine levels were seen within one to 3 days of starting the combined hormonal contraceptive (oral or vaginal ring), were maximal at 21 days, and increased to within 80 to 100% of baseline levels in the contraceptive-free week.[9]

In a controlled study in 16 healthy women, the maximum serum level and AUC of lamotrigine were decreased by about 39% and 52%, respectively while they were taking an oral combined hormonal contraceptive (**ethinylestradiol** 30 micrograms with **levonorgestrel** 150 micrograms) when compared with a 3-week period when they received lamotrigine 300 mg daily alone.[2] Similarly, in a crossover study in 7 women with epilepsy, taking lamotrigine and an oral combined hormonal contraceptive (**ethinylestradiol** 35 micrograms with **norgestimate** 250 micrograms) or placebo, lamotrigine plasma levels were 84% higher during the placebo phase, when compared with the contraceptive phase. Three patients experienced seizures while taking the contraceptive; two were given an increased dose of lamotrigine, and one was given clobazam.[10]

In a study in women taking lamotrigine with sodium valproate, lamotrigine dose concentration ratios did not differ between women also taking oral combined hormonal contraceptives (7) and those not taking these contraceptives (15).[11]

Mechanism

The reason for the reduction in levonorgestrel levels with lamotrigine is unknown, and this on its own is unlikely to be clinically important. Nevertheless, the increase in FSH and LH levels and increase in intermenstrual bleeding suggest some reduction in the suppression of ovulation. Ethinylestradiol increases the glucuronidation of lamotrigine, thereby increasing its clearance. This effect is cyclical when combined hormonal contraceptives are taken cyclically (usual practice). It is suggested that, when lamotrigine glucuronidation is strongly inhibited by valproate (see 'Lamotrigine + Valproate', p.587), ethinylestradiol does not appear to have any effect.

Importance and management

Effects on contraceptive efficacy

The above studies show that there is some concern regarding the efficacy of oral combined hormonal contraceptives while taking lamotrigine. Based on the small reduction in levonorgestrel levels, and the rises in FSH and LH levels, the manufacturer of lamotrigine suggests that the possibility of decreased contraceptive efficacy cannot be ruled out.[12,13] If an oral combined hormonal contraceptive is used as the only form of contraception, they advise that women should be alert for signs of breakthrough bleeding, which may be a sign of reduced contraceptive efficacy.[12,13] This advice should probably also be applied to the combined hormonal contraceptive patch and vaginal ring. On the basis of the available evidence, the UK Faculty of Sexual and Reproductive Healthcare (FSRH) 2011 guideline on drug interactions with hormonal contraceptives does not advise the use of additional contraception when combined hormonal contraceptives [any form] are used with lamotrigine. However, the effects of these contraceptives on lamotrigine levels should also be considered, see below.

Effects on lamotrigine levels

There is good evidence that combined hormonal contraceptives reduce lamotrigine exposure and efficacy, in a cyclical manner, which may increase the risk of seizures during concurrent use and toxicity during the hormone-free days. Most of the data relates to oral use of these contraceptives, but one study suggested the vaginal ring interacts similarly. The UK Faculty of Sexual and Reproductive Healthcare (FSRH) 2011 guideline on drug interactions with hormonal contraceptives does not usually recommend the use of combined hormonal contraceptives with lamotrigine monotherapy because of the cyclical effect of the contraceptive on lamotrigine exposure.[14] However, if concurrent use is necessary and a combined hormonal contraceptive (oral, patch or vaginal ring) is started in women already taking lamotrigine (as monotherapy or with other drugs that are *not* strong inducers or inhibitors of lamotrigine glucuronidation), the maintenance dose of lamotrigine may need to be increased as much as twofold (according to clinical response). If this group of patients stop taking a combined hormonal contraceptive, the lamotrigine dose should be reviewed (and may need to be decreased by as much as 50%) to reduce the risk of lamotrigine adverse effects, such as dizziness, ataxia, and diplopia.[12,13] It has been suggested that the cyclical nature of the interaction could be overcome by using a combined hormonal contraceptive as an extended regimen or continuously without a hormone-free (e.g. a pill-free) interval.[12,14,15] This advice seems sensible, and there are preparations that are licensed for extended or continuous use in some countries.

The situation is somewhat different in women already taking lamotrigine with a drug that strongly alters lamotrigine metabolism. In this case, the modest effect of ethinylestradiol is unlikely to be apparent. Therefore, in those already taking lamotrigine with strong inducers of lamotrigine glucuronidation, such as phenytoin and carbamazepine, changes in the dose of lamotrigine are unlikely to be necessary when starting combined hormonal contraceptives;[12] however, remember that these enzyme inducers might reduce the efficacy of combined hormonal contraceptives (see 'Table 28.1', p.1160). Changes in lamotrigine doses also appear unlikely to be needed in those already taking lamotrigine with valproate, which is a strong inhibitor of lamotrigine glucuronidation.

Consider also 'Progestogen-only contraceptives + Lamotrigine', p.1198.

1. Holdich T, Whiteman P, Orme M, Back D, Ward S. Effect of lamotrigine on the pharmacology of the combined oral contraceptive pill. *Epilepsia* (1991) 32 (Suppl 1), 96.
2. Sidhu J, Job S, Singh S, Philipson R. The pharmacokinetic and pharmacodynamic consequences of the co-administration of lamotrigine and a combined oral contraceptive in healthy female subjects. *Br J Clin Pharmacol* (2006) 61, 191–9.
3. Sabers A, Buchholt JM, Uldall P, Hansen EL. Lamotrigine plasma levels reduced by oral contraceptives. *Epilepsy Res* (2001) 47, 151–4.
4. Sabers A, Öhman I, Christensen J, Tomson T. Oral contraceptives reduce lamotrigine plasma levels. *Neurology* (2003) 61, 570–1.
5. Reimers A, Helde G, Brodtkorb E. Ethinyl estradiol, not progestogens, reduces lamotrigine serum concentrations. *Epilepsia* (2005) 46, 1414–17.
6. Öhman I, Luef G, Tomson T. Effects of pregnancy and contraception on lamotrigine disposition: new insights through analysis of lamotrigine metabolites. *Seizure* (2008) 17, 199–202.
7. Herzog AG, Blum AS, Farina EL, Maestri XE, Newman J, Garcia E, Krishnamurthy KB, Hoch DB, Replansky S, Fowler KM, Smithson SD, Dworetzky BA, Bromfield EB. Valproate and lamotrigine level variation with menstrual cycle phase and oral contraceptive use. *Neurology* (2009) 72, 911–14.
8. Contin M, Albani F. Ambrosetto G, Avoni P, Bisulli F, Riva R, Tinuper P, Baruzzi A. Variation in lamotrigine plasma concentrations with hormonal contraceptive monthly cycles in patients with epilepsy. *Epilepsia* (2006) 47, 1573–5.
9. Stodieck SRG, Schwenkhagen AM. Lamotrigine plasma levels and combined monophasic oral contraceptives or a contraceptive vaginal ring. A prospective evaluation in 30 women. *Epilepsia* (2004) 45 (Suppl. 7), 187.
10. Christensen J, Petrenaite V, Atterman J, Sidenius P, Öhman I, Tomson T, Sabers A. Oral contraceptives induce lamotrigine metabolism: evidence from a double-blind, placebo-controlled trial. *Epilepsia* (2007) 48, 484–9.
11. Tomson T, Luef G, Sabers A, Pittschieler S, Öhman I. Valproate effects on kinetics of lamotrigine in pregnancy and treatment with oral contraceptives. *Neurology* (2006) 67, 1297–9.
12. Lamictal (Lamotrigine). GlaxoSmithKline UK. UK Summary of product characteristics, July 2012.
13. Lamictal XR (Lamotrigine). GlaxoSmithKline. US Prescribing information, January 2011.
14. Faculty of Sexual and Reproductive Heathcare Clinical Guidance. Drug interactions with hormonal contraception: Clinical Effectiveness Unit, January 2011. Available at: http://www.fsrh.org/pdfs/CEU-GuidanceDrugInteractionsHormonal.pdf (accessed 22/10/15).
15. Schwenkhagen AM, Stodieck SRG. Which contraception for women with epilepsy? *Seizure* (2008) 17, 145–50.

Combined hormonal contraceptives + Laropiprant

Laropiprant has no clinically relevant effect on the pharmacokinetics of an oral combined hormonal contraceptive containing ethinylestradiol and norgestimate.

Clinical evidence, mechanism, importance and management

In a randomised, placebo-controlled study, 16 healthy women taking a combined hormonal contraceptive (**ethinylestradiol** with **norgestimate**) were given laropiprant 40 mg daily for 21 days starting on day one of a cycle. Laropiprant did not alter the pharmacokinetics of norelgestromin, the major metabolite of **norgestimate**. In addition, laropiprant had no effect on the exposure to **ethinylestradiol**, whereas the maximum plasma level was increased by about 16%;[1] however, this is unlikely to be clinically relevant. Therefore, laropiprant would not be expected to alter the efficacy of combined hormonal contraceptives, and no additional contraceptive precautions would seem to be necessary on concurrent use.

Note that laropiprant is only available as a combination product with nicotinic acid for the treatment of dyslipidaemias, an indication that is a contraindication to the use of any form of combined hormonal contraceptive when other risk factors for arterial disease are present. This is because these contraceptives can have adverse effects on serum lipids.

1. Schwartz JI, Liu F, Wang Y-H, Pramanik B, Johnson-Levonas AO, Gutierrez MJ, Lai E, Wagner JA. Effect of laropiprant, a PGD_2 receptor 1 antagonist, on estradiol and norgestimate pharmacokinetics after oral contraceptive administration in women. *Am J Ther* (2009) 16, 487–95.

Combined hormonal contraceptives + Leflunomide or Teriflunomide

Leflunomide does not alter the ovulation suppressant effect of an oral combined hormonal contraceptive containing ethinylestradiol with levonorgestrel. Teriflunomide appears to cause small increases in the exposure to ethinylestradiol and levonorgestrel.

Clinical evidence, mechanism, importance and management

In a study in 32 healthy women taking a triphasic oral combined hormonal contraceptive (**ethinylestradiol** with **levonorgestrel**), leflunomide 100 mg daily for 3 days, then 20 mg daily for 17 days, did not reduce ovulation suppression (as assessed by progesterone concentration). In addition, the pharmacokinetics of teriflunomide (the active metabolite of leflunomide) were as expected, suggesting that the contraceptive steroid had no effect on this metabolite.[1,2] However, in another study, after repeated doses of teriflunomide the maximum concentration and AUC of **ethinylestradiol** were increased by 58% and 54%, respectively. The maximum concentration and AUC of **levonorgestrel** were also increased, by 33% and 41%, respectively.[3,4]

It appears that leflunomide and teriflunomide are unlikely to alter the efficacy of combined hormonal contraceptives (tablets, patch, or vaginal ring). However the manufacturers of teriflunomide advise that some consideration should be given to the choice or dose of oral contraceptive if used concurrently with teriflunomide.[3,4]

Note that teriflunomide is potentially teratogenic and therefore reliable contraception is required in women of child-bearing age both during, and after, the use of leflunomide (the parent drug) and teriflunomide. As the concentration of teriflunomide can remain elevated for prolonged periods, in the UK, reliable contraception is mandated for up to 2 years after leflunomide and teriflunomide treatment has stopped, unless a washout procedure is undertaken.[1,3] In the US, once leflunomide or teriflunomide treatment has stopped, it is recommended that all women of child-bearing potential undergo a washout procedure.[4,5] In all cases, the concentration of teriflunomide must be checked at least twice in order to confirm that it is sufficiently low as to not pose a risk should pregnancy occur.[1,3-5]

1. Arava (Leflunomide). Sanofi. UK Summary of product characteristics, September 2014.
2. Sanofi-Aventis. Personal communication. September 2009.
3. Aubagio (Teriflunomide). Genzyme Therapeutics. UK Summary of product characteristics, September 2014.
4. Aubagio (Teriflunomide). Genzyme Corp. US Prescribing information, October 2014.
5. Arava (Leflunomide). Sanofi-Aventis US, LLC. US Prescribing information, August 2014.

Combined hormonal contraceptives + Leukotriene antagonists

Montelukast and zafirlukast do not alter the pharmacokinetics of contraceptive steroids from an oral combined hormonal contraceptive, and ovulation suppression is not altered by zafirlukast.

Clinical evidence

(a) Montelukast

The manufacturers state that the recommended clinical dose of montelukast did not have a clinically relevant effect on the pharmacokinetics of an oral combined hormonal contraceptive (**ethinylestradiol** 35 micrograms with **norethisterone** 1 mg).[1,2]

(b) Zafirlukast

The US manufacturer briefly mentions that, in a study in 39 healthy women taking oral combined hormonal contraceptives, zafirlukast 40 mg twice daily had no effect on the serum levels of **ethinylestradiol** nor on its ovulation suppressant effect.[3].

Mechanism, importance and management

The available data suggest that neither montelukast nor zafirlukast are likely to affect the pharmacokinetics or efficacy of oral combined hormonal contraceptives, and an interaction with the patch and vaginal ring also seems unlikely. No additional contraceptive precautions would seem necessary on concurrent use.

1. Singulair (Montelukast sodium). Merck Sharp & Dohme Ltd. UK Summary of product characteristics, June 2010.
2. Singulair (Montelukast sodium). Merck & Co., Inc. US Prescribing information, July 2010.
3. Accolate (Zafirlukast). AstraZeneca Pharmaceuticals LP. US Prescribing information, February 2011.

Combined hormonal contraceptives + Levetiracetam

Levetiracetam does not alter the pharmacokinetics or the ovulation suppressant effect of an oral combined hormonal contraceptive containing ethinylestradiol with levonorgestrel.

Clinical evidence, mechanism, importance and management

In a placebo-controlled, crossover study in 18 healthy women given an oral combined hormonal contraceptive (**ethinylestradiol** 30 micrograms with **levonorgestrel** 150 micrograms) with levetiracetam 500 mg twice daily for one cycle, levetiracetam did not alter the steady-state pharmacokinetics of either steroid, or the ovulation suppressant effect, as measured by progesterone and LH levels.[1,2] These findings indicate that levetiracetam is unlikely to alter the efficacy of any combined hormonal contraceptives (tablet, patch or vaginal ring), and no additional contraceptive precautions are needed on concurrent use.

1. Giuliano RA, Hiersemenzel R, Baltes E, Johnscher G, Janik F, Weber W. Influence of a new antiepileptic drug (Levetiracetam, ucb L059) on the pharmacokinetics and pharmacodynamics of oral contraceptives. *Epilepsia* (1996) 37, 90.
2. Ragueneau-Majlessi I, Levy RH, Janik F. Levetiracetam does not alter the pharmacokinetics of an oral contraceptive in healthy women. *Epilepsia* (2002) 43, 697–702.

Combined hormonal contraceptives + Maraviroc

Maraviroc does not alter the pharmacokinetics of ethinylestradiol or levonorgestrel, given as an oral combined hormonal contraceptive.

Clinical evidence, mechanism, importance and management

In a study in healthy women given an oral combined hormonal contraceptive (**ethinylestradiol** 30 micrograms with **levonorgestrel** 150 micrograms) for 7 days, a low dose of maraviroc 100 mg twice daily for 10 days starting 3 days before the contraceptive had no effect on the AUC of the contraceptive steroids when compared with a placebo.[1]

This study suggests that maraviroc is unlikely to alter the efficacy of oral combined hormonal contraceptives, and therefore probably also the patch and vaginal ring, by a pharmacokinetic mechanism. No additional contraceptive precautions appear to be necessary on concurrent use. However, note that regardless of the methods of contraception being used, barrier methods are always advisable to reduce the risk of HIV transmission.

1. Abel S, Russell D, Whitlock LA, Ridgway CE, Muirhead GJ. Effect of maraviroc on the pharmacokinetics of midazolam, lamivudine/zidovudine, and ethinyloestradiol/levonorgestrel in healthy volunteers. *Br J Clin Pharmacol* (2008) 65 (Suppl 1), 19–26.

Combined hormonal contraceptives + Moclobemide

Moclobemide did not alter the ovulation suppressant effect of an oral combined hormonal contraceptive.

Clinical evidence, mechanism, importance and management

In a study in 7 women taking oral combined hormonal contraceptives (unspecified), estradiol, progesterone, FSH, and LH levels were similar when they took moclobemide 200 mg three times daily for one cycle compared with a cycle without moclobemide, which suggests that ovulation did not occur.[1] Therefore the contraceptive efficacy of oral combined hormonal contraceptives seems unlikely to be affected on the concurrent use of moclobemide.

1. Amrein R, Güntert TW, Dingemanse J, Lorscheid T, Stabl M, Schmid-Burgk W. Interactions of moclobemide with concomitantly administered medication: evidence from pharmacological and clinical studies. *Psychopharmacology (Berl)* (1992) 106, S24–S31.

Combined hormonal contraceptives + Modafinil

Modafinil very slightly reduces ethinylestradiol exposure from an oral combined hormonal contraceptive. Armodafinil, the *R*-isomer of modafinil, would be expected to interact similarly.

Clinical evidence

In 16 healthy women taking an oral combined hormonal contraceptive (**ethinylestradiol** 35 micrograms with **norgestimate**), modafinil 200 mg daily for 7 days followed by 400 mg daily for 21 days decreased the AUC of **ethinylestradiol** by 18%. Minor increases in plasma FSH and LH of about 0.4 mIU/L occurred, which were not statistically significant nor of any clinical relevance.[1]

Mechanism

Modafinil and its *R*-isomer, armodafinil, are weak inducers of CYP3A4, which is partially responsible for the metabolism of ethinylestradiol.

Importance and management

The very small changes seen in ethinylestradiol exposure in the presence of **modafinil** are lower than those seen with other enzyme inducers known to reduce the reliability of combined hormonal contraceptives (see 'Table 28.1', p.1160). However, it cannot be ruled out that they would be sufficient to cause the failure of combined hormonal contraceptives in very rare cases. It would seem reasonable to avoid the use of oral combined hormonal contraceptives with a low 20-micrograms dose of ethinylestradiol, but a standard-dose preparation (30 or 35 micrograms) would probably be adequate. However, the manufacturer recommends that additional or alternative methods of contraception to hormonal contraceptives [presumably all forms] should be used during and for one month[2] or 2 months after stopping modafinil.[3] This advice seems overly cautious, and, use of alternative methods is likely to increase the risk of pregnancy because most reversible, non-hormonal methods of contraception are less reliable than hormonal methods; and this needs to be considered in light of the potential teratogenicity of modafinil. In the UK, the Faculty of Sexual and Reproductive Healthcare (FSRH) Clinical Effectiveness Unit include modafinil in their guidance on the use of enzyme inducers with combined hormonal contraceptives.[4] For long-term use, where oral combined hormonal contraceptives are the preferred method, they recommend a minimum of 50 micrograms of ethinylestradiol for all enzyme-inducers, see 'Combined hormonal contraceptives + Barbiturates or Phenytoin', p.1169, for further details of this guidance.

Although direct evidence regarding **armodafinil**, the *R*-isomer of modafinil appears lacking, it would be expected to interact in the same way as modafinil. The US manufacturers of armodafinil give the same advice as for modafinil, namely that additional or alternative methods of contraception to hormonal contraceptives [presumably all forms] should be used during and for one month after stopping armodafinil.[5]

1. Robertson P, Hellriegel ET, Arora S, Nelson M. Effect of modafinil on the pharmacokinetics of ethinyl estradiol and triazolam in healthy volunteers. *Clin Pharmacol Ther* (2002) 71, 46–56.
2. Provigil (Modafinil). Cephalon, Inc. US Prescribing information, October 2010.
3. Provigil (Modafinil). Cephalon (UK) Ltd. UK Summary of product characteristics, August 2013.
4. Faculty of Sexual and Reproductive Healthcare Guidance. Drug interactions with hormonal contraception: Clinical Effectiveness Unit, January 2011. Available at: http://www.fsrh.org/pdfs/CEUGuidanceDrugInteractionsHormonal.pdf (accessed 21/10/15).
5. Nuvigil (Armodafinil). Cephalon, Inc. US Prescribing information, June 2013.

Combined hormonal contraceptives + Mycophenolate

Mycophenolate mofetil does not alter the pharmacokinetics or the ovulation suppressant effect of oral combined hormonal contraceptives.

Clinical evidence, mechanism, importance and management

The manufacturer states that no pharmacokinetic interaction was seen in a single-dose study in 15 healthy women taking mycophenolate mofetil and an oral combined hormonal contraceptive (**ethinylestradiol** 35 micrograms with **norethisterone** 1 mg).[1]

In a study in 18 women with psoriasis taking oral combined hormonal contraceptives (**ethinylestradiol** 20 to 40 micrograms with either **levonorgestrel** 50 to 200 micrograms, **desogestrel** 150 micrograms or **gestodene** 50 to 100 micrograms) and who had not previously taken immunosuppressants, mycophenolate mofetil 1 g twice daily over 3 consecutive menstrual cycles had no clinically relevant influence on the suppression of ovulation.[2,3] The AUC of **ethinylestradiol** and **desogestrel** were not changed, but the mean **levonorgestrel** AUC was decreased by about 15%. Note that large interpatient variability was seen in AUCs, especially for **ethinylestradiol**.[3]

Mycophenolate mofetil is unlikely to reduce the contraceptive efficacy of oral combined hormonal contraceptives, or the patch or vaginal ring. The small 15% decrease in levonorgestrel levels seen is unlikely to be clinically relevant.

Note that, because mycophenolate is associated with an increased risk of pregnancy loss and of congenital malformations, the manufacturers of mycophenolate mofetil and mycophenolate sodium state that effective contraception must be used before during, and for 6 weeks after, mycophenolate has been stopped.[2-5] In this regard, the US manufacturers specifically advise that oral contraceptives should be used with caution, and additional birth control methods used.[3,5]

1. Syntex. Data on file. A single-dose pharmacokinetic drug interaction study of oral mycophenolate mofetil and an oral contraceptive in normal subjects (Study No. MYCS2308). 1994.
2. CellCept Tablets (Mycophenolate mofetil). Roche Products Ltd. UK Summary of product characteristics, July 2013.
3. CellCept (Mycophenolate mofetil). Genentech USA, Inc. US Prescribing information, September 2013.
4. Myfortic (Mycophenolate sodium). Novartis Pharmaceuticals UK Ltd. UK Summary of product characteristics, November 2012.
5. Myfortic (Mycophenolate sodium). Novartis. US Prescribing information, September 2013.

Combined hormonal contraceptives + Nefazodone

A woman experienced increased combined oral contraceptive adverse effects while taking nefazodone.

Clinical evidence, mechanism, importance and management

Within a week of starting to take nefazodone 50 mg twice daily, a woman taking a low-dose combined oral contraceptive (**ethinylestradiol** 20 micrograms with **desogestrel** 150 micrograms) reported breast tenderness, bloating, weight gain, and increased premenstrual irritability. She had previously experienced identical symptoms while taking a combined oral contraceptive with a higher dose of oestrogen. Nefazodone was discontinued after 6 weeks, and within 24 hours the adverse effects resolved.[1] Nefazodone is a known inhibitor of CYP3A4, by which **ethinylestradiol** is partially metabolised, and might therefore be expected to increase **ethinylestradiol** levels. However, the general importance of this isolated case is unknown. Note that nefazodone has generally been withdrawn due to adverse hepatic effects.

1. Adson DE, Kotlyar M. A probable interaction between a very low-dose oral contraceptive and the antidepressant nefazodone: a case report. *J Clin Psychopharmacol* (2001) 21, 618–19.

Combined hormonal contraceptives + NNRTIs

Efavirenz increased the exposure to ethinylestradiol from a single-dose of an oral combined hormonal contraceptive in one study, but did not affect the pharmacokinetics of ethinylestradiol at steady-state in two other studies. Efavirenz moderately to markedly decreased the exposure of the active metabolites of norgestimate from an oral combined hormonal contraceptive. Efavirenz also appears to moderately decrease concentrations of the active metabolite of desogestrel (etonogestrel) from an oral combined hormonal contraceptive. Single-dose ethinylestradiol had no effect on efavirenz exposure in one study, but in another an oral combined hormonal contraceptive containing ethinylestradiol and desogestrel decreased efavirenz concentrations. Potential contraceptive failures have been reported in women taking efavirenz, but a low incidence of contraceptive failure was noted in one study.

Nevirapine appears to slightly reduce ethinylestradiol and norethisterone exposure, however, in one study ethinylestradiol and levonorgestrel concentrations were increased. An oral combined hormonal contraceptive containing ethinylestradiol and desogestrel did not alter nevirapine plasma concentrations. Nevirapine does not appear to affect the suppression of ovulation by oral combined hormonal contraceptives. Etravirine increased ethinylestradiol exposure and did not change norethisterone exposure or the suppression of ovulation in women taking an oral combined hormonal contraceptive. Rilpivirine had negligible effects on ethinylestradiol and norethisterone exposure from an oral combined hormonal contraceptive, and the contraceptive did not appear to alter rilpivirine pharmacokinetics. Delavirdine is predicted to increase ethinylestradiol exposure.

Clinical evidence

(a) Efavirenz

1. Contraceptive efficacy. A study in 16 HIV-positive women taking a combined hormonal contraceptive (**ethinylestradiol** 30 micrograms with **desogestrel** 150 micrograms) with an antiretroviral regimen including efavirenz, found that serum progesterone concentrations in 3 out of the 16 subjects were greater than 3 nanograms/mL, which might indicate that ovulation was not suppressed, and therefore there could potentially result in contraceptive failure.[1]

A retrospective review identified 22 women who were prescribed an oral contraceptive while taking an NNRTI. Two of the 16 women taking efavirenz experienced contraceptive failure. However, medication adherence could not be confirmed.[2]

As part of a 6-month clinical study in West Africa, 548 women received efavirenz with two NRTIs for HIV infection. At each month of the study the percentage of women using contraceptives was 58%, 70%, 77%, 79%, 80%, and 80% (about two-thirds were using an **intramuscular progestogen** and one-third an oral combined hormonal contraceptive). There were just 7 pregnancies in the study, giving an overall incidence of 2.6/100 person-years.[3] The paper did not mention which, if any, contraceptives these 7 women were using at the time of conception. However, even if all of these 7 pregnancies constituted failure of an oral combined hormonal contraceptive, this is still only 7 pregnancies in about 140 women over 6 months. Nevertheless, the authors note that it is possible that these women had low fertility related to their disease, and that fertility might increase over time with effective treatment.[3]

2. Pharmacokinetics. In a study in 13 women, efavirenz 400 mg daily for 10 days *increased* the AUC of a single dose of **ethinylestradiol** by 37%, while its maximum plasma concentration remained unchanged. **Ethinylestradiol** had no effect on the AUC or maximum plasma concentration of efavirenz.[4] However, in a later multiple-dose study in 19 healthy women taking a triphasic oral combined hormonal contraceptive (**ethinylestradiol** with **norgestimate**), efavirenz 600 mg daily for the first 14 days of the third contraceptive cycle, had no effect on the AUC of **ethinylestradiol** and *decreased* the AUC of **norelgestromin** (the principal active metabolite of norgestimate) by 64%. A sub-analysis in 6 of these women found that the AUC of **levonorgestrel** (a secondary active metabolite) was decreased by 83%.[5] Analysis of data from a study found that in 16 HIV-positive women taking an oral combined hormonal contraceptive (**ethinylestradiol** 30 micrograms with **desogestrel** 150 micrograms) and an antiretroviral regimen including efavirenz, the steady-state **etonogestrel** concentrations (the active metabolite of desogestrel) were 61% lower, when compared with 14 HIV-negative women taking the contraceptive alone. **Ethinylestradiol** concentrations did not differ between the 2 groups of women.[6] The initial report from the same study stated that, in the 16 HIV positive women, efavirenz plasma concentrations were decreased by 18% when compared with those prior to starting the combined hormonal contraceptive. In 3 of the 16 subjects the efavirenz plasma concentrations were less than 1 mg/L, which could lead to loss of efficacy.[1]

(b) Etravirine

In a study in 16 women taking an oral combined hormonal contraceptive (**ethinylestradiol** 35 micrograms with **norethisterone** 1 mg), etravirine 200 mg twice daily (from day one to 15 of a cycle) increased the AUC of **ethinylestradiol** by 22% and did not change the AUC of **norethisterone**, when compared with a cycle without etravirine. In addition, the suppression of ovulation, as measured by FSH, LH, and, progesterone concentrations, was not altered.[7]

(c) Nevirapine

1. Contraceptive efficacy. In a study in HIV-positive women given a low-dose oral combined hormonal contraceptive (**ethinylestradiol** 35 micrograms with **norgestrel** 75 micrograms), the ovulation and pregnancy rates in 172 women also taking an antiretroviral regimen including nevirapine, did not differ from those in another group of 178 women not taking antiretrovirals.[8] Similarly, a study in 18 HIV-positive women taking an oral combined hormonal contraceptive (**ethinylestradiol** 30 micrograms with **desogestrel** 150 micrograms) with an antiretroviral regimen including nevirapine found that serum progesterone concentrations in all 18 subjects indicated that ovulation was suppressed.[1] In another study, 3 HIV-positive women taking antiretrovirals (nevirapine 200 mg, stavudine 30 mg, and lamivudine 150 mg twice daily) and a combined hormonal contraceptive (**ethinylestradiol** 30 micrograms with **norgestrel** 300 micrograms), progesterone concentrations indicated the successful suppression of ovulation.[9] A retrospective study identified 22 women who were prescribed oral contraceptives while taking an NNRTI. None of the 6 women taking nevirapine experienced contraceptive failure.[2]

2. Pharmacokinetics. In a study, 10 HIV-positive women were given a single dose of an oral combined hormonal contraceptive (**ethinylestradiol** 35 micrograms with **norethisterone** 1 mg) 2 days before and on the last day of nevirapine 200 mg daily for 2 weeks then twice daily for a further 2 weeks. The women were already taking an antiretroviral regimen (commonly 3 drugs, including nelfinavir or indinavir), which had been unchanged for at least 4 weeks. The median AUC and elimination half-life of **ethinylestradiol** were decreased by 29% and 31%, respectively, and the median AUC of **norethisterone** was decreased by 19%.[10] Analysis of data from another study in 18 HIV-positive women taking an oral combined hormonal contraceptive (**ethinylestradiol** 30 micrograms with **desogestrel** 150 micrograms), found that an antiretroviral regimen including nevirapine resulted in steady-state ethinylestradiol concentrations that were 58% lower than in 14 HIV-negative women taking the contraceptive alone. **Etonogestrel** concentrations (the active metabolite of desogestrel) did not differ between the two groups of women.[6] In contrast, a study in women taking an oral combined hormonal contraceptive (**ethinylestradiol** 30 micrograms with norgestrel 300 micrograms) compared the contraceptive concentrations in 3 HIV-positive women taking an antiretroviral regimen including nevirapine, 3 HIV-positive women not taking antiretrovirals, and 3 HIV-negative women. **Ethinylestradiol** and **levonorgestrel** concentrations were *higher* in all the HIV-positive women, including those taking antiretrovirals, than in the 3 HIV-negative women. A study in 18 HIV-positive women taking an antiretroviral regimen including nevirapine, found that a combined hormonal contraceptive (**ethinylestradiol** 30 micrograms with **desogestrel** 150 micrograms) did not alter nevirapine plasma concentrations when compared with those prior to starting the contraceptive.[1]

(d) Rilpivirine

A study in 15 healthy subjects given an oral combined hormonal contraceptive (**ethinylestradiol** 35 micrograms with **norethisterone** 1 mg) for three cycles, with rilpivirine 25 mg daily on days 1 to 15 of the third cycle, found that rilpivirine increased the maximum concentration of ethinylestradiol by 17%, but its AUC was not affected. There was no change in the AUC or maximum plasma concentration of norethisterone. Rilpivirine pharmacokinetics were similar to those of healthy subjects in other studies who took rilpivirine 25 mg alone.[11]

Mechanism

Both efavirenz and nevirapine are established inducers of CYP3A4, whereas etravirine is a weak inducer of CYP3A4, the isoenzyme by which ethinylestradiol is partially metabolised. As such these NNRTIs might be expected to decrease contraceptive steroid exposure, as has been shown for nevirapine. For efavirenz, the finding of *increased* ethinylestradiol exposure after a single ethinylestradiol dose and no change after multiple doses, is unexpected, but the decrease in norgestimate metabolites and in etonogestrel concentrations fits with the enzyme-inducing properties. For etravirine, the finding of an *increase* in ethinylestradiol exposure with no change in norethisterone exposure is also unexpected, and the mechanism for this effect is uncertain.

Importance and management

The original finding that **efavirenz** increased ethinylestradiol exposure (after a single dose) suggested that efavirenz might not adversely alter the efficacy of oral combined hormonal contraceptives. Nevertheless, in later studies in women using these contraceptives, although efavirenz had no effect on ethinylestradiol exposure, it did moderately to markedly decrease exposure to the active metabolites of norgestimate, and decrease concentrations of the active metabolite of norgestrel, which suggests that a reduction in the activity of the contraceptive is possible. Furthermore the failure of the etonogestrel implant has been attributed to efavirenz, see 'Progestogen-only contraceptives; Implants + Enzyme inducers', p.1199. Data regarding the pharmacokinetic interaction of **nevirapine** with oral combined hormonal contraceptives is limited and conflicting. Two studies suggest that nevirapine decreases contraceptive exposure as would be predicted. In contrast, another very small study, found an increase in contraceptive concentrations. Despite this, a number of studies suggest that the suppression of ovulation might not be affected in patients taking antiretroviral treatment containing nevirapine. However, until further evidence is available it would seem prudent to assume that nevirapine could affect contraceptive exposure and reduce the ovulation suppressant effect of the oral combined hormonal contraceptive. Therefore, the possibility of reduced efficacy of any combined hormonal contraceptive (oral, patch, or vaginal ring) with both nevirapine and efavirenz should be considered. In the UK, the Faculty of Sexual and Reproductive Healthcare include both efavirenz and nevirapine in their 2011 guidance on the use of enzyme inducers with hormonal contraceptives.[12] They recommend that their general guidance on hormonal contraceptives and liver enzyme inducers is followed for these drugs, see 'Combined hormonal contraceptives + Barbiturates or Phenytoin', p.1169, for the full details of this guidance. For short-term use of enzyme-inducers in those who choose an oral combined hormonal contraceptive, their advice is to use a standard-strength preparation (30 or 35 micrograms of ethinylestradiol), with additional contraceptive precautions such as condoms. This advice would also seem to be most relevant to the situation of long-term use of efavirenz or nevirapine, when oral combined hormonal contraceptives are the preferred method, because whatever other methods of contraception are being used, barrier methods are always advisable to reduce the risk of HIV transmission. In the absence of barrier methods, they recommend a preparation with at least 50 micrograms of ethinylestradiol.[12]

For **etravirine** and for **rilpivirine**, based on the available data, no reduction in contraceptive efficacy would be expected when using an oral combined hormonal contraceptive containing ethinylestradiol and norethisterone. The slight increase in ethinylestradiol exposure seen with etravirine, and the negligible increase in the ethinylestradiol maximum concentration seen with rilpivirine are unlikely to be clinically relevant.

The US manufacturer of **delavirdine** notes that it might increase the concentrations of ethinylestradiol, but further study is needed to confirm and quantify this.[13] Until more is known, some caution is prudent, being aware of the possibility of increased adverse effects.

1. Landolt NK, Phanuphak N, Ubolyam S, Pinyakorn S, Kriengsinyot R, Ahluwalia J, Thongpaeng P, Gorowara M, Thammajaruk N, Chaithongwongwatthana S, Lange JMA, Ananworanich J. Efavirenz, in contrast to nevirapine, is associated with unfavourable progesterone and antiretroviral levels when coadministered with combined oral contraceptives. *J Acquir Immune Defic Syndr* (2013) 62, 534–39.
2. Clark RA, Theall K. Population-based study evaluating association between selected antiretroviral therapies and potential oral contraceptive failure. *J Acquir Immune Defic Syndr* (2004) 37, 1219–20.
3. Danel C, Moh R, Anzian A, Abo Y, Chenal H, Guehi C, Gabillard D, Sorho S, Rouet F, Eholié S, Anglaret X. Tolerance and acceptability of an efavirenz-based regimen in 740 adults (predominantly women) in West Africa. *J Acquir Immune Defic Syndr* (2006) 42, 29–35.
4. Joshi AS, Fiske WD, Benedek IH, White SJ, Joseph JL, Kornhauser DM. Lack of a pharmacokinetic interaction between efavirenz (DMP 266) and ethinyl estradiol in healthy female volunteers. The 5th Conference on Retroviruses and Opportunistic Infections, Chicago, IL, February 1998.
5. Sevinsky H, Eley T, Persson A, Garner D, Yones C, Nettles R, Krantz K, Bertz R, Zhang J. The effect of efavirenz on the pharmacokinetics of an oral contraceptive containing ethinyl estradiol and norgestimate in healthy HIV-negative women. *Antivir Ther* (2011) 16, 149–56.
6. Landolt NK, Phanuphak N, Ubolyam S, Pinyakorn S, Kerr S, Ahluwalia J, Thongpaeng P, Thammajaruk N, Cremers S, Thomas T, Chaithongwongwatthana S, Lange JMA, Ananworanich J. Significant decrease of ethinylestradiol with nevirapine, and of etonogestrel with efavirenz in HIV-positive women. *J Acquir Immune Defic Syndr* (2014) 66, e50–2.
7. Schöller-Gyüre M, Kakuda TN, Woodfall B, Aharchi F, Peeters M, Vandermeulen K, Hoetelmans RMW. Effect of steady-state etravirine on the pharmacokinetics and pharmacodynamics of ethinylestradiol and norethindrone. *Contraception* (2009) 80, 44–52.
8. Nanda K, Delany-Moretlwe S, Dubé K, Lendvay A, Kwok C, Molife L, Nakubulwa S, Edward VA, Mpairwe B, Mirembe FM. Nevirapine-based antiretroviral therapy does not reduce oral contraceptive effectiveness. *AIDS* (2013) 27 (Suppl 1), S17–S25.
9. Stuart GS, Moses A, Corbett A, Phiri G, Kumwenda W, Mkandawire N, Chintedze J, Malunga G, Hosseinipour M, Cohen MS, Stanczyk FZ, Kashuba A. Pharmacokinetics and pharmacodynamics of a combined oral contraceptive and a generic combined formulation antiretroviral in Malawi. *J Acquir Immune Defic Syndr* (2011) 58, e40–e43.
10. Mildvan D, Yarrish R, Marshak A, Hutman HW, McDonough M, Lamson M, Robinson P. Pharmacokinetic interaction between nevirapine and ethinyl estradiol/norethindrone when administered concurrently to HIV-infected women. *J Acquir Immune Defic Syndr* (2002) 29, 471–7.
11. Crauwels HM, van Heeswijk RPG, Buelens A, Stevens M, Hoetelmans RMW. Lack of an effect of rilpivirine on the pharmacokinetics of ethinylestradiol and norethindrone in healthy volunteers. *Int J Clin Pharmacol Ther* (2014) 52, 118–28.
12. Faculty of Sexual and Reproductive Healthcare Guidance. Drug interactions with hormonal contraception: Clinical Effectiveness Unit, January 2011. Available at: http://www.fsrh.org/pdfs/CEUGuidanceDrugInteractionsHormonal.pdf (accessed 22/10/15).
13. Rescriptor (Delavirdine mesylate). ViiV Healthcare. US Prescribing information, August 2012.

Combined hormonal contraceptives + NS5A inhibitors

The pharmacokinetics of ethinylestradiol and norgestimate in a combined hormonal contraceptive are not altered by daclatasvir or ledipasvir. The pharmacokinetics of ombitasvir do not appear to be affected by a combined hormonal contraceptive containing ethinylestradiol and norgestimate, but concurrent use of ethinylestradiol greatly increases the incidence of elevated ALT concentrations.

Clinical evidence, mechanism, importance and management

(a) Daclatasvir

In a study, 18 healthy subjects received a triphasic oral combined hormonal contraceptive containing **ethinylestradiol** 35 micrograms and **norgestimate** 180 to 250 micrograms for 21 days of a 28 day cycle, for 3 cycles, with daclatasvir 60 mg daily for 10 days of the third cycle of the oral contraceptive. The pharmacokinetics of ethinylestradiol and norelgestromin (the active metabolite of norgestimate) were not altered by daclatasvir.[1] The UK manufacturer of daclatasvir states that if an oral contraceptive is required, one containing ethinylestradiol 35 micrograms and norgestimate 180 to 250 micrograms is recommended, and that concurrent use of other oral contraceptives have not been studied. Note that daclatasvir should not be used in women of child bearing potential who are not using contraception. Furthermore, adequate contraception must be continued for 5 weeks after daclatasvir has been stopped.[2]

(b) Ledipasvir

In a study, 15 healthy subjects received an oral combined hormonal contraceptive containing **ethinylestradiol** 25 micrograms and **norgestimate** 180 to 250 micrograms for 21 days of a 28 day cycle, for 3 cycles, with ledipasvir 90 mg daily for 14 days of the third cycle of the oral contraceptive. Ledipasvir increased the maximum concentration of ethinylestradiol by 40%, but had no effect on the pharmacokinetics of norelgestromin. Concentrations of FSH, LH, and progesterone were monitored, suggesting that no loss of contraceptive efficacy would be expected with concurrent use of ledipasvir.[3] No dose adjustments are necessary on concurrent use.

(c) Ombitasvir

The UK and US manufacturers briefly report that, in a study in healthy subjects given an oral combined hormonal contraceptive containing **ethinylestradiol** 35 micrograms and **norgestimate** 250 micrograms daily, and ombitasvir 25 mg daily (in a fixed-dose combination with paritaprevir boosted with ritonavir, given with or without dasabuvir) the pharmacokinetics of ethinylestradiol and ombitasvir were unaffected. The AUC of the norgestimate metabolites norgestrel and norelgestromin were increased about 2.5-fold and the maximum and minimum concentrations increased around 2-fold and 3-fold, respectively. In clinical trials with the fixed-dose combination and dasabuvir, increases in ALT concentrations greater than 5 times the upper limit of normal were seen in 1% of all patients, but was considerably more frequent in female subjects taking ethinylestradiol-containing contraceptives (oral combined hormonal contraceptives, contraceptive patches, or contraceptive vaginal rings). The concurrent use of such contraceptives is therefore contraindicated, and they must be discontinued prior to starting treatment,[4,5] but can be restarted about 2 weeks after treatment has stopped.[4] Alternative methods of contraception must be used during treatment, such as progestogen-only contraceptives or non-hormonal methods.[4,5]

1. Bifano M, Sevinsky H, Hwang C, Kandoussi H, Jiang H, Grasela D, Bertz R. Effect of the coadministration of daclatasvir on the pharmacokinetics of a combined oral contraceptive containing ethinyl estradiol and norgestimate. *Antivir Ther* (2014) 19, 511–9.
2. Daklinza (Daclatasvir dihydrochloride). Bristol-Myers Squibb Pharmaceutical Ltd. UK Summary of product characteristics, September 2014.
3. German P, Moorehead L, Pang P, Vimal M, Mathias A. Lack of a clinically important pharmacokinetic interaction between sofosbuvir or ledipasvir and hormonal oral contraceptives norgestimate/ethinyl estradiol in HCV-uninfected female subjects. *J Clin Pharmacol* (2014) 54, 1290–8.
4. Viekira Pak (Ombitasvir, paritaprevir, ritonavir co-packaged with dasabuvir sodium monohydrate). AbbVie Inc. US Prescribing information, December 2014.
5. Viekirax (Ombitasvir, paritaprevir, ritonavir). AbbVie Ltd. UK Summary of product characteristics, January 2015.

Combined hormonal contraceptives + NS5B inhibitors

Dasabuvir might increase the exposure to norgestimate metabolites in a combined hormonal contraceptive, but appears not to affect the pharmacokinetics of ethinylestradiol. The pharmacokinetics of dasabuvir, do not appear to be affected by a combined hormonal contraceptive con-

taining ethinylestradiol and norgestimate, but concurrent use of ethinylestradiol greatly increases the incidence of elevated ALT concentrations. The pharmacokinetics of ethinylestradiol and norgestimate in a combined hormonal contraceptive are not altered by sofosbuvir.

Clinical evidence, mechanism, importance and management

(a) Dasabuvir

The UK and US manufacturers briefly reports that, in a study in healthy subjects given an oral combined hormonal contraceptive containing **ethinylestradiol** 35 micrograms and **norgestimate** 250 micrograms daily, and dasabuvir 250 or 400 mg twice daily (with a fixed-dose combination of ombitasvir and paritaprevir boosted with ritonavir) the pharmacokinetics of ethinylestradiol and dasabuvir were unaffected. The AUC of the norgestimate metabolites norgestrel and norelgestromin were increased about 2.5-fold and the maximum and minimum concentrations increased around 2-fold and 3-fold, respectively. In clinical trials with this combination, increases in ALT concentrations greater than 5 times the upper limit of normal were seen in 1% of all patients, but were considerably more frequent in female subjects taking ethinylestradiol-containing contraceptives (oral combined hormonal contraceptives, contraceptive patches, or contraceptive vaginal rings). The concurrent use of such contraceptives is therefore contraindicated, and they must be discontinued prior to starting treatment,[1] but can be restarted about 2 weeks after treatment has stopped.[2] Alternative methods of contraception must be used during treatment, such as progestogen-only contraceptives or non-hormonal methods.[1,2]

(b) Sofosbuvir

In a study, 15 healthy subjects received a triphasic oral combined hormonal contraceptive containing **ethinylestradiol** 25 micrograms and **norgestimate** 180 to 250 micrograms for 21 days of a 28 day cycle, for 3 cycles, with sofosbuvir 400 mg daily for 7 days of the second cycle of the oral contraceptive. There were no changes in the pharmacokinetics of ethinylestradiol or norelgestromin. Concentrations of FSH, LH, and progesterone were monitored, and although slightly lower than the reference ranges, it was considered that no loss of contraceptive efficacy would be expected with concurrent sofosbuvir.[3] No dose adjustments are necessary on concurrent use.

1. Exviera (Dasabuvir sodium monohydrate). AbbVie Ltd. UK Summary of product characteristics, January 2015.
2. Viekira Pak (Ombitasvir, paritaprevir, ritonavir co-packaged with dasabuvir sodium monohydrate). AbbVie Inc. US Prescribing information, December 2014.
3. German P, Moorehead L, Pang P, Vimal M, Mathias A. Lack of a clinically important pharmacokinetic interaction between sofosbuvir or ledipasvir and hormonal oral contraceptives norgestimate/ethinyl estradiol in HCV-uninfected female subjects. *J Clin Pharmacol* (2014) 54, 1290–8.

Combined hormonal contraceptives + Phosphodiesterase type-5 inhibitors

No pharmacokinetic interaction appears to occur between sildenafil and an oral combined hormonal contraceptive containing ethinylestradiol with levonorgestrel. Tadalafil slightly increases the exposure of ethinylestradiol from an oral combined hormonal contraceptive, without altering the ovulation suppressant effect.

Clinical evidence, mechanism, importance and management

(a) Sildenafil

The pharmacokinetics of sildenafil were not altered by the concurrent use of an oral combined hormonal contraceptive (**ethinylestradiol** 30 micrograms with **levonorgestrel** 150 micrograms), and the plasma levels of these contraceptive steroids were not altered by sildenafil.[1,2] This suggests that sildenafil is unlikely to alter the efficacy of any combined hormonal contraceptives (tablets, patch or vaginal ring), and no additional contraceptive precautions are required on concurrent use.

(b) Tadalafil

The concurrent use of tadalafil 10 mg with an oral combined hormonal contraceptive (**ethinylestradiol** with **levonorgestrel**) increased the steady-state AUC of **ethinylestradiol** by 18% and increased its maximum level by 53%, with no change in its systemic clearance.[3] The pharmacokinetics of **levonorgestrel** were not affected and there were no changes in levels of LH, FSH, and progesterone,[3] indicating that ovulation suppression was maintained. Similarly, in a further study, tadalafil 40 mg daily at steady state increased the AUC of **ethinylestradiol** (given as an oral combined hormonal contraceptive) by 26% and increased its maximum concentration by 70%, with no change in **levonorgestrel** exposure.[4,5] The mechanism for the increase in **ethinylestradiol** exposure is unknown, however, the slight increase seen is unlikely to be clinically relevant. No particular precautions are likely to be required on concurrent use.

1. Revatio Tablets (Sildenafil citrate). Pfizer Ltd. UK Summary of product characteristics, April 2015.
2. Revatio (Sildenafil citrate). Pfizer Inc. US Prescribing information, April 2015.
3. Eli Lilly. Personal communication, March 2008.
4. Adcirca (Tadalafil). Eli Lilly and Company. US Prescribing information, April 2015.
5. Adcirca (Tadalafil). Eli Lilly and Company Ltd. UK Summary of product characteristics, May 2013.

Combined hormonal contraceptives + Pregabalin

Pregabalin does not alter the pharmacokinetics or the ovulation suppressant effect of an oral combined hormonal contraceptive containing ethinylestradiol with norethisterone.

Clinical evidence, mechanism, importance and management

In 16 healthy women given an oral combined hormonal contraceptive, pregabalin 200 mg every 8 hours for 21 days had no effect on the steady-state pharmacokinetics of **ethinylestradiol** or **norethisterone**. In addition, the ovulation suppressant effect of the contraceptive was not reduced, as measured by progesterone levels. The pharmacokinetics of pregabalin did not appear to be affected by the contraceptive [when compared with historical data].[1] This suggests that pregabalin is unlikely to alter the efficacy of combined hormonal contraceptives (tablet, patch or vaginal ring).

1. Bockbrader HN, Posvar EL, Hunt T, Randinitis EJ. Pharmacokinetics of pregabalin and a concomitantly administered oral contraceptive show no-drug drug interaction. *Epilepsia* (2004) 45 (Suppl 3), 153.

Combined hormonal contraceptives + Prucalopride

Prucalopride does not appear to alter the pharmacokinetics of ethinylestradiol or norethisterone. Severe prucalopride-induced diarrhoea is predicted to reduce the efficacy of oral combined hormonal contraceptives.

Clinical evidence, mechanism, importance and management

In a randomised, crossover study in 12 healthy women, prucalopride 2 mg daily was given with an oral combined hormonal contraceptive, containing ethinylestradiol 35 micrograms and norethisterone 1 mg, once daily for 5 days. The AUC and maximum concentrations of ethinylestradiol and norethisterone were not altered.[1] No dose adjustments would appear necessary with concurrent use, however, the concurrent use of prucalopride and combined hormonal contraceptives has not been studied long-term.

Note that the Canadian and UK manufacturers of prucalopride state that because it can cause severe diarrhoea, prucalopride might reduce the efficacy of oral combined hormonal contraceptives.[2,3] They therefore recommend the use of an additional contraceptive method (such as a barrier method) in case patients develop severe diarrhoea.

1. Van de Velde V, Vandeplassche L, Hoppenbrouwers M, Boterman M, Ausma J. Effect of prucalopride on the pharmacokinetics of oral contraceptives in healthy women. *Drugs R D* (2013) 13, 43–51.
2. Resolor (Prucalopride succinate). Shire Pharmaceuticals Ltd. UK Summary of product characteristics, July 2014.
3. Resotran (Prucalopride succinate). Janssen Inc. Canadian product monograph, August 2014.

Combined hormonal contraceptives + Remacemide

Remacemide appears not to alter the pharmacokinetics or ovulation suppressant effect of oral combined hormonal contraceptives.

Clinical evidence, mechanism, importance and management

The preliminary results of a study suggested that remacemide 200 mg twice daily for 14 days had no effect on the pharmacokinetics of **ethinylestradiol, desogestrel**, or **levonorgestrel**, when compared with placebo, in women taking an oral combined hormonal contraceptive (**ethinylestradiol** 30 micrograms with **levonorgestrel** 150 micrograms or **desogestrel** 150 micrograms). Inhibition of ovulation was maintained (assessed by measurement of progesterone, FSH, and LH levels).[1] It appears that no particular contraceptive precautions are needed during concurrent use.

1. Blakey GE, Lockton JA, Corfield J, Oliver SD, Back D. Absence of interaction of remacemide with oral contraceptives. *Epilepsia* (1999) 40 (Suppl 2), 95.

Combined hormonal contraceptives + Repaglinide

The pharmacokinetics of repaglinide and an oral combined hormonal contraceptive containing ethinylestradiol with levonorgestrel are unaffected by concurrent use.

Clinical evidence, mechanism, importance and management

A crossover study in healthy subjects found that 5 days of concurrent use of an oral combined hormonal contraceptive (**ethinylestradiol** 30 micrograms with **levonorgestrel** 150 micrograms) increased the maximum plasma concentration of repaglinide 2 mg three times daily by 17%, although the AUC of repaglinide was not altered.[1] Repaglinide did not alter the pharmacokinetics of **ethinylestradiol** or **levonorgestrel**.[1] No additional contraceptive precautions therefore seem necessary if repaglinide is given to women taking any combined hormonal contraceptive (tablets, patch, or vaginal ring).

Although the pharmacokinetic interaction would suggest that the dose of repaglinide need not be altered on concurrent use, hormonal contraceptives can have adverse effects on diabetic control. For the general precautions for the use of these contraceptives in diabetes, see 'Antidiabetics + Hormonal contraceptives', p.510.

1. Hatorp V, Hansen KT, Thomsen MS. Influence of drugs interacting with CYP3A4 on the pharmacokinetics, pharmacodynamics, and safety of the prandial glucose regulator repaglinide. *J Clin Pharmacol* (2003) 43, 649–60.

Combined hormonal contraceptives + Retigabine (Ezogabine)

Retigabine does not appear to alter the pharmacokinetics of ethinylestradiol and norgestrel from an oral combined hormonal contraceptive.

Clinical evidence, mechanism, importance and management

The preliminary results of a study suggested that retigabine 150 mg three times daily from day 10 to 13 of a cycle had no effect on the pharmacokinetics of **ethinylestradiol** or **norgestrel** in women taking an oral combined hormonal contraceptive (**ethinylestradiol** 30 micrograms with **norgestrel** 300 micrograms).[1] This suggests that no additional contraceptive precautions are needed on the concurrent use of retigabine and any combined hormonal contraceptives (tablet, patch or vaginal ring).

1. Paul J, Ferron GM, Richards L, Getsy J, Troy SM. Retigabine does not alter the pharmacokinetics of a low-dose oral contraceptive in women. *Neurology* (2001) 56 (Suppl 3), A335–A336.

Combined hormonal contraceptives + Rifamycins

Rifampicin (rifampin) reduces contraceptive steroid exposure and reduces the ovulation suppressant effect of oral combined hormonal contraceptives. Combined hormonal contraceptives are less reliable during treatment with rifampicin: breakthrough bleeding and spotting commonly occur, and cases of contraceptive failure have been reported. Rifabutin also reduces contraceptive steroid exposure and the ovulation suppressant effect of oral combined hormonal contraceptives, although it interacts to a lesser extent than rifampicin. Rifapentine is predicted to interact in a similar way to these other rifamycins, whereas oral rifaximin appears not to alter the pharmacokinetics of contraceptive steroids.

Clinical evidence

(a) Rifabutin

In two studies,[1,2] rifabutin 300 mg daily for only 10 or 14 days reduced **ethinylestradiol** and **norethisterone** exposure in women taking an oral combined hormonal contraceptive, but to about half the extent of rifampicin (rifampin). In both studies, the AUC of **ethinylestradiol** decreased by about 35%, and the AUC of **norethisterone** decreased by 17%. In one of the studies, spotting occurred in 21.7% of women when they took rifabutin (compared with 3.7% in the control cycle and 36% with rifampicin).[1] Ovulation did not occur with rifabutin or rifampicin in either study,[1,2] although in one study an increase in FSH and LH occurred with rifabutin, which was less than that seen with rifampicin.[1] It is probable that the use of rifabutin for a complete cycle or longer would have a greater effect on ovulation parameters, as contraceptive steroid levels would be reduced for the whole cycle.

(b) Rifampicin (Rifampin)

1. Estradiol-containing contraceptives. In one controlled study in 16 postmenopausal women given an oral combined hormonal contraceptive (**estradiol** valerate 2 mg with **dienogest** 3 mg) for 17 days, rifampicin 600 mg daily for only 5 days from day 12 to 16 decreased the steady-state AUC of **estradiol** by 44% and decreased the steady-state AUC of **dienogest** by 83%.[3-5]

2. Ethinylestradiol-containing contraceptives. A report in 1971 noted a marked increase in the frequency of intermenstrual breakthrough bleeding (regarded as loss of reliability of the contraceptive) in women taking an oral combined hormonal contraceptive and rifampicin.[6] In a later report by the same researchers, 62 out of 88 women taking an oral combined hormonal contraceptive had menstrual cycle disorders of various kinds (spotting, bleeding, failure to menstruate) while taking a rifampicin-based regimen for tuberculosis, compared with only one of 26 women given a streptomycin-based regimen. In addition, 5 pregnancies occurred in women taking the rifampicin-based regimen.[7,8] Other early case reports have confirmed this interaction, and there have been a total of at least 11 other pregnancies reported.[9-16] Oral combined hormonal contraceptives commonly mentioned in these reports include **ethinylestradiol** with **norgestrel** or **norethisterone**.[10,12-16] A more recent report described two cases of contraceptive failure in women taking oral combined hormonal contraceptives (**ethinylestradiol** 30 micrograms with **levonorgestrel** or **desogestrel**) that occurred within 2 months of starting rifampicin 600 mg with isoniazid 300 mg (*Rifinah*), which was prescribed for tuberculosis prophylaxis during treatment with tumour necrosis factor antibodies (infliximab, adalimumab).[17]

There are four pharmacodynamic studies of the effects of rifampicin on oral combined hormonal contraceptives that assessed measures of ovulation (FSH, LH, progesterone),[1,2,18,19] three of which also assessed the contraceptive steroid pharmacokinetics.[1,2,19] One of these studies was in patients requiring antimycobacterials, and 2 out of the 7 patients taking an oral combined hormonal contraceptive (**ethinylestradiol** 30 micrograms with **norethisterone** 1 mg) ovulated one month after starting rifampicin 8 to 10 mg/kg (started on day 23 of a cycle and ovulation assessed on day 19 to 23 of the next cycle). In addition, rifampicin reduced the AUC of **norethisterone** by 30% and reduced the AUC of **ethinylestradiol** by 12% (which was not statistically significant), although there was wide variation.[19] Similarly, in a randomised drug interaction study, where rifampicin was used as a control, 11 out of 21 women taking an oral triphasic contraceptive (**ethinylestradiol** 30 to 40 micrograms with **levonorgestrel** 50 to 125 micrograms) ovulated (assessed by increased progesterone levels of above 10 nanomol/L and presence of a follicle) while taking rifampicin 300 mg daily for 21 days, and 8 had intermenstrual bleeding.[18] Conversely, two other well-controlled studies did not detect ovulation in 34 women taking an oral combined hormonal contraceptive (**ethinylestradiol** 35 micrograms with **norethisterone** 1 mg) and rifampicin 300 or 600 mg daily,[1,2] although in these studies, the rifampicin was given for shorter periods (for only 10 or 14 days from day 1 or day 7 of the cycle). Nevertheless, both studies reported some increase in LH and FSH levels with rifampicin, and an increased incidence of spotting was noted in one of these studies (36% versus 3.7% in the control cycle).[1] Furthermore, both of these studies found that rifampicin 300 mg daily for 10 days or 600 mg daily for 14 days considerably reduced the AUCs of **ethinylestradiol** and **norethisterone** by about 63% and 55%, respectively. These pharmacokinetic results confirm the findings of earlier studies using single doses of contraceptive steroids.[20,21]

Rifampicin plasma levels[22] and efficacy[6] are reported to be unchanged by oral combined hormonal contraceptives.

(c) Rifaximin

In a crossover study in 26 healthy women, rifaximin 200 mg every 8 hours for 3 days had no effect on the pharmacokinetics of **ethinylestradiol, norgestrel** or **deacetylnorgestimate** after administration of a single dose of two tablets of an oral combined hormonal contraceptive (**ethinylestradiol** 35 micrograms with **norgestimate** 250 micrograms).[23]

Mechanism

Rifampicin (rifampin) is a potent non-specific enzyme inducer, which has been shown to increase the hydroxylation of ethinylestradiol fourfold in an *in vitro* study,[24,25] and twofold in an *in vivo* study.[26] Another study found that the metabolism of ethinylestradiol derived from mestranol was similarly affected.[27] As a result, the reduced steroid levels may be insufficient to prevent the re-establishment of a normal menstrual cycle with ovulation, which would explain the breakthrough bleeding and pregnancies that have occurred. Rifabutin similarly acts as an enzyme inducer, but it is less potent than rifampicin (about half as potent in reducing contraceptive steroid levels).[2] **Rifapentine** is stated to be less potent an enzyme inducer than rifampicin but more potent than rifabutin.[22] Rifaximin is also an inducer of cytochrome P450 isoenzymes, but its oral absorption is minimal (0.4%) and it therefore appears to have no effect on the metabolism of the contraceptive steroids.

Importance and management

The interaction between the oral combined hormonal contraceptives and **rifampicin (rifampin)** is well documented, well established and clinically important. Menstrual cycle disturbances of 36 to 70%,[1,6,7] and an ovulation rate of 29 to 52% when used for 21 days or more[18,19] have been reported.

Long-term use

In the UK, for long-term (greater than 2 months) use of rifampicin, the Faculty of Sexual and Reproductive Healthcare (FSRH)[28] recommend that women receiving combined hormonal contraceptives (tablets, patch or vaginal ring) should use an alternative form of contraception that is unaffected by enzyme-inducing drugs (that is, **copper IUDs** or the **levonorgestrel-releasing intra-uterine system**, see 'Progestogen-only contraceptives; Intra-uterine system + Enzyme inducers', p.1200, and depot progestogen-only injections, see 'Progestogen-only contraceptives; Injections + Enzyme inducers', p.1199), both during and for 28 days after the withdrawal of the interacting drug.

Short-term use

For *short-term* (less than 2 months) use of rifampicin, the UK Faculty of Sexual and Reproductive Healthcare (FSRH) give the same advice as for long-term use (see above); however, they advise that if a woman using a combined hormonal contraceptive does not wish to change method, she may continue to use the combined patch, ring or standard-strength combined pill (containing at least 30 micrograms of ethinylestradiol), and use additional contraceptive precautions (e.g. condoms) while taking rifampicin, both during and for 28 days after its withdrawal. The FSRH also recommends that the oral combined hormonal contraceptive is taken as an extended or tricycling regimen with a shortened 3 to 4 day pill-free interval.[28] See also 'Combined hormonal contraceptives + Barbiturates or Phenytoin', p.1169, for more general discussion of the interaction between enzyme-inducing drugs and combined hormonal contraceptives. In the absence of any information on very short courses of rifampicin, such as those used for the prophylaxis of meningococcal meningitis (2 days) or *Haemophilus influenza* type b (4 days), it would be prudent to adopt the same precautions, because rifampicin is such a potent enzyme-inducer.

Direct information about the interaction between combined hormonal contraceptives and **rifabutin** seems to be limited to the studies cited, but they are supported by the well-recognised enzyme-inducing properties of rifabutin. It would clearly be prudent for women receiving rifabutin to take the same precautions recommended for rifampicin with any combined hormonal contraceptive,[28] although the risks are probably somewhat lower because rifabutin is a less potent enzyme inducer. See also 'Table 28.1', p.1160, for a comparison of the effects of various enzyme-inducers on contraceptive steroid exposure.

Similarly, although there are no data regarding the effect of **rifapentine** on combined hormonal contraceptives, based on its known enzyme-inducing properties (see under *Mechanism*, above), it would be prudent for women receiving rifapentine to take the same precautions recommenced for rifampicin with any combined hormonal contraceptive.

Oral **rifaximin** does not appear to alter the pharmacokinetics of contraceptive steroids and would therefore not be expected to alter contraceptive efficacy of combined hormonal contraceptives.

1. LeBel M, Masson E, Guilbert E, Colborn D, Paquet F, Allard S, Vallée F, Narang PK. Effects of rifabutin and rifampicin on the pharmacokinetics of ethinylestradiol and norethindrone. *J Clin Pharmacol* (1998) 38, 1042–50.
2. Barditch-Crovo P, Braun Trapnell C, Ette E, Zacur HA, Coresh J, Rocco LE, Hendrix CW, Flexner C. The effects of rifampin and rifabutin on the pharmacokinetics and pharmacodynamics of a combination oral contraceptive. *Clin Pharmacol Ther* (1999) 65, 428–38.
3. Qlaira (Estradiol valerate and Estradiol valerate with Dienogest). Bayer plc. UK Summary of product characteristics, November 2010.
4. Blode H, Schott, B, Rohde B, Knuz M, Zeun S. Effects of CYP3A4 induction and inhibition on the pharmacokinetics of estradiol valerate/dienogest. 11th World Congress on Controversies in Obstetrics and Gynecology & Infertility, Paris, November 2008, 68A.
5. Natazia (Estradiol valerate and Estradiol valerate with Dienogest). Bayer HeathCare Pharmaceuticals, Inc. US Prescribing information, May 2010.
6. Reimers D, Ježek A. Rifampicin und andere Antituberkulotika bei gleichzeitiger oraler Kontrazeption. *Prax Pneumol* (1971) 25, 255–62.
7. Nocke-Finck L, Breuer H, Reimers D. Wirkung von Rifampicin auf den Menstruationszyklus und die Östrogenausscheidung bei Einnahme oraler Kontrazeptiva. *Dtsch Med Wochenschr* (1973) 98, 1521–3.
8. Reimers D, Nocke-Finck L, Breuer H. Rifampicin causes a lowering in efficacy of oral contraceptives by influencing oestrogen excretion. Reports on Rifampicin: XXII International Tuberculosis Conference, Tokyo, September 1973, 87–9.
9. Kropp R. Rifampicin und Ovulationshemmer. *Prax Pneumol* (1974) 28, 270–2.
10. Bessot J-C, Vandevenne A, Petitjean R, Burghard G. Effets opposés de la rifampicine et de l'isoniazide sur le métabolisme des contraceptifs oraux? *Nouv Presse Med* (1977) 6, 1568.
11. Hirsch A. Pilules endormies. *Nouv Presse Med* (1973) 2, 2957.
12. Piguet B, Muglioni JF, Chaline G. Contraception orale et rifampicine. *Nouv Presse Med* (1975) 4, 115–16.
13. Skolnick JL, Stoler BS, Katz DB, Anderson WH. Rifampicin, oral contraceptives and pregnancy. *JAMA* (1976) 236, 1382.
14. Gupta KC, Ali MY. Failure of oral contraceptive with rifampicin. *Med J Zambia* (1980/81) 15, 23.
15. Hirsch A, Tillement JP, Chrétein J. Effects contrariants de la rifampicine sur les contraceptifs oraux: a propos de trois grossesses non désirées observées chez deux malades. *Rev Fr Mal Respir* (1975) 3, 174–82.
16. Lafaix Ch, Cadoz M, Richard A, Patouillard P. L'effect "antipilule" de la rifampicine. *Med Hyg (Geneve)* (1976) 1181, 181–2.
17. Wibaux C, Andrei I, Paccou J, Philippe P, Biver E, Duquesnoy B, Flipo RM. Pregnancy during TNFalpha antagonist therapy: beware the rifampin-oral contraceptive interaction. Report of two cases. *Joint Bone Spine* (2010) 77, 268–70.
18. Meyer B, Müller F, Wessels P, Maree J. A model to detect interactions between roxithromycin and oral contraceptives. *Clin Pharmacol Ther* (1990) 47, 671–4.
19. Joshi JV, Joshi UM, Sankolli GM, Gupta K, Rao AP, Hazari K, Sheth UK, Saxena BN. A study of interaction of low-dose combination oral contraceptive with anti-tubercular drugs. *Contraception* (1980) 21, 617–29.
20. Back DJ, Breckenridge AM, Crawford F, MacIver M, Orme ML'E, Park BK, Rowe PH, Smith E. The effect of rifampicin on norethisterone pharmacokinetics. *Eur J Clin Pharmacol* (1979) 15, 193–7.
21. Back DJ, Breckenridge AM, Crawford FE, Hall JM, MacIver M, Orme ML'E, Rowe PH, Smith E, Watts MJ. The effect of rifampicin on the pharmacokinetics of ethynylestradiol in women. *Contraception* (1980) 21, 135–43.
22. Gupta KC, Joshi JV, Anklesaria PS, Shah RS, Satoskar RS. Plasma rifampicin levels during oral contraception. *J Assoc Physicians India* (1988) 36, 365–6.
23. Trapnell CB, Connolly M, Pentikis H, Forbes WP, Bettenhausen DK. Absence of effect of oral rifaximin on the pharmacokinetics of ethinylestradiol/norgestimate in healthy females. *Ann Pharmacother* (2007) 41, 222–8.
24. Bolt HM, Kappus H, Bolt M. Rifampicin and oral contraception. *Lancet* (1974) i, 1280–1.
25. Bolt HM, Kappus H, Bolt M. Effect of rifampicin treatment on the metabolism of oestradiol and 17α-ethinyloestradiol by human liver microsomes. *Eur J Clin Pharmacol* (1975) 8, 301–7.
26. Bolt HM, Bolt M, Kappus H. Interaction of rifampicin treatment with pharmacokinetics and metabolism of ethinyloestradiol in man. *Acta Endocrinol (Copenh)* (1977) 85, 189–97.
27. Gelbke HP, Gethmann U, Knuppen R. Influence of rifampicin treatment on the metabolic fate of [4-^{14}C] mestranol in women. *Horm Metab Res* (1977) 9, 415–19.
28. Faculty of Sexual and Reproductive Healthcare Guidance. Drug interactions with hormonal contraception: Clinical Effectiveness Unit, January 2011. Available at: http://www.fsrh.org/pdfs/CEUGuidanceDrugInteractionsHormonal.pdf (accessed 22/10/15).

Combined hormonal contraceptives + Rotigotine

Transdermal rotigotine does not alter the pharmacokinetics or the ovulation suppressant effect of an oral combined hormonal contraceptive containing ethinylestradiol with levonorgestrel.

Clinical evidence, mechanism, importance and management

In a crossover study, 37 healthy women taking an oral combined hormonal contraceptive (**ethinylestradiol** 30 micrograms with **levonorgestrel** 150 micrograms) applied transdermal rotigotine 2 mg daily for 3 days, then 3 mg daily for 10 days, or matching placebo patches, starting on the first day of the contraceptive cycle. Transdermal rotigotine had no effect on the steady-state AUC of ethinylestradiol or levonorgestrel. There was one subject who had high ethinylestradiol levels (but not levonorgestrel levels) during rotigotine use but not during placebo use. This subject had rotigotine levels that were lower than the mean for the group, and the reason for the high ethinylestradiol levels was not identified. No subject ovulated as determined by LH, FSH and mid-luteal progesterone levels.[1]

The findings of this study indicate that transdermal rotigotine is unlikely to alter efficacy of combined hormonal contraceptives (tablets, patch or vaginal ring).

1. Braun M, Elshoff J-P, Andreas J-O, Müller LI, Horstmann R. Influence of transdermal rotigotine on ovulation suppression by a combined oral contraceptive. *Br J Clin Pharmacol* (2009) 68, 386–94.

Combined hormonal contraceptives + Rufinamide

Rufinamide caused a very slight decrease in ethinylestradiol and norethisterone exposure from an oral combined hormonal contraceptive.

Clinical evidence

The preliminary results of a study in 18 healthy women taking an oral combined hormonal contraceptive (**ethinylestradiol** 35 micrograms with **norethisterone** 1 mg) suggest that rufinamide 800 mg twice daily for 14 days, from day 22 of cycle one to day 7 of cycle two, decreased the AUC of **ethinylestradiol** by 22% and decreased the AUC of **norethisterone** by 14%, measured on day 7 of cycle two. Inhibition of ovulation was not assessed.[1]

Mechanism

Rufinamide is a weak inducer of CYP3A4,[2] by which the contraceptive steroids are partially metabolised.

Importance and management

The reductions in exposure to the contraceptive hormones caused by rufinamide are similar to those seen with other weak enzyme inducers (such as topiramate), and less than those seen with more potent enzyme inducers (such carbamazepine, see 'Table 28.1', p.1160'), and their clinical relevance is unknown. However, given these findings, low-dose oral combined hormonal contraceptives (**ethinylestradiol** 20 micrograms) should probably be considered unsuitable for use with rufinamide. Nevertheless, the manufacturers recommend that additional effective forms of contraception are also used,[2,3] although note that the UK manufacturer also advises that the prescriber should use clinical judgement when assessing whether oral hormonal contraceptives, or the doses of the contraceptive steroids, are adequate, based on the individual patients clinical situation.[2] In the UK, the Faculty of Sexual and Reproductive Healthcare include rufinamide in their 2011 guidance on the use of enzyme inducers with hormonal contraceptives.[4] For long-term use, when combined oral contraceptives are the preferred method, they recommend a minimum of 50 micrograms of ethinylestradiol for all enzyme-inducers, see 'Combined hormonal contraceptives + Barbiturates or Phenytoin', p.1169, for further details of this guidance.

1. Svendsen KD, Choi L, Chen B-L, Karolchyk MA. Single-center, open-label, multiple-dose pharmacokinetic trial investigating the effect of rufinamide administration on Ortho-Novum 1/35 in healthy women. *Epilepsia* (1998) 39 (Suppl 6), 59.
2. Inovelon (Rufinamide). Eisai Ltd. UK Summary of product characteristics, October 2009.
3. Banzel (Rufinamide). Eisai Inc. US Prescribing information, March 2011.
4. Faculty of Sexual and Reproductive Healthcare Guidance. Drug interactions with hormonal contraception: Clinical Effectiveness Unit, January 2011. Available at: http://www.fsrh.org/pdfs/CEUGuidanceDrugInteractionsHormonal.pdf (accessed 21/10/15).

Combined hormonal contraceptives + Sirolimus

Sirolimus did not alter the pharmacokinetics of ethinylestradiol or norgestrel from a single dose of an oral combined hormonal contraceptive.

Clinical evidence, mechanism, importance and management

In a single-dose study, the pharmacokinetics of an oral combined hormonal contraceptive (**ethinylestradiol** 30 micrograms with **norgestrel** 300 micrograms) were unaffected by sirolimus,[1,2] and sirolimus whole blood exposure was unaffected by the contraceptive.[2] This suggests that the efficacy of the contraceptive is unlikely to be changed by sirolimus. Nevertheless, the UK manufacturer cautiously points out that the effects of long-term sirolimus on oral contraception are unknown. Note that as sirolimus has been found to cause reproductive toxicity in *animals*, the UK manufacturer advises that effective contraception should be used during, and for 12 weeks after sirolimus is stopped.[1]

1. Rapamune (Sirolimus). Pfizer Ltd. UK Summary of product characteristics, August 2013.
2. Zimmerman JJ. Exposure-response relationships and drug interactions of sirolimus. *AAPS J* (2004) 6, e28.

Combined hormonal contraceptives + Spermicides

Nonoxinol 9 does not affect the absorption of ethinylestradiol or etonogestrel from the combined hormonal contraceptive vaginal ring.

Clinical evidence, mechanism, importance and management

In a placebo-controlled study in healthy women using the combined hormonal contraceptive vaginal ring (**ethinylestradiol** with **etonogestrel**), a single dose of a vaginal gel spermicide (4% **nonoxinol 9**) given on day 8 of a cycle had no effect on the AUC of **ethinylestradiol** or **etonogestrel** measured over three time periods (day 8 to 9, day 8 to 10 and day 8 to 21).[1] This study suggests that **nonoxinol 9** is unlikely to alter the efficacy of the combined hormonal contraceptive ring.

1. Haring T, Mulders TMT. The combined contraceptive ring NuvaRing® and spermicide co-medication. *Contraception* (2003) 67, 271–2.

Combined hormonal contraceptives + St John's wort (*Hypericum perforatum*)

St John's wort might cause small decreases in the concentrations of desogestrel, ethinylestradiol, and norethisterone from oral combined hormonal contraceptives, although there is some evidence that an extract with low hyperforin content might not interact. Both breakthrough bleeding and, rarely, contraceptive failure have been reported in women also taking St John's wort.

Clinical evidence

(a) Controlled studies

1. Hypericin 0.3%. In a crossover study in 17 healthy women given an oral combined hormonal contraceptive (**ethinylestradiol** 20 micrograms with **desogestrel**

150 micrograms), St John's wort (300 mg two, then three, times daily for a complete cycle) did not affect the AUC or maximum concentration of **ethinylestradiol**. However, the AUC and maximum concentration of the active metabolite of **desogestrel** were decreased, by about 40% and 20%, respectively. There was no evidence that ovulation occurred. However, the frequency of breakthrough bleeding increased considerably from 35% to around 80%. The St John's wort preparation (*Jarsin*) used in this study contained a methanolic extract (LI160).[1]

Similarly, another study in 12 healthy women taking an oral combined hormonal contraceptive (**ethinylestradiol** 35 micrograms with **norethisterone** 1 mg) found that St John's wort 300 mg three times daily for 8 weeks caused some changes to the pharmacokinetics of the contraceptive steroids (a 24% decrease in the AUC of ethinylestradiol and a 10% decrease in the AUC of norethisterone), but the only statistically significant changes were a 15% increase in the oral clearance of **norethisterone** and a 48% decrease in the half-life of **ethinylestradiol**. Nevertheless, ovulation did not occur, as indicated by unaffected serum concentrations of LH, FSH, and progesterone. However, there was an increase in breakthrough bleeding (7 subjects reported breakthrough bleeding while taking St John's wort compared with 2 subjects in the control phase). A sample of the St John's wort capsules in this study (Rexall-Sundown Pharmaceuticals) were analysed and found to contain 0.37% hypericin and 3% hyperforin.[2]

A crossover study in 16 subjects also found very small reductions in the concentrations of low-dose **ethinylestradiol** 20 micrograms with **norethisterone** 1 mg (median reductions in AUC of 16% and 13%, respectively) while they were taking St John's wort 300 mg three times daily. Furthermore, they found increased progesterone concentrations of more than 3 nanograms/mL (an indication that ovulation occurred) in 3 patients taking St John's wort compared with one subject taking placebo. The incidence of breakthrough bleeding was also increased (56% versus 31%). This study used an alcoholic St John's Wort extract standardised to 0.3% hypericin, which contained 3.7% hyperforin.[3] In a secondary analysis of this study, the anti-androgenic effects of **ethinylestradiol** with **norethisterone**, utilised in the treatment of hirsutism and acne, were not affected by St John's wort.[4]

2. Hypericin 0.2% with low hyperforin. In a study, 16 healthy women took an oral combined hormonal contraceptive (**ethinylestradiol** 20 micrograms with **desogestrel** 150 micrograms) with an extract of St John's wort (with a low hyperforin content of less than 0.2%, Ze117, standardised to 0.2% hypericin), 250 mg twice daily for 14 days from day 7 of the cycle. In contrast to the studies above, the AUCs of **ethinylestradiol** and the active metabolite of **desogestrel** were not altered by St John's wort (day 7 compared with day 14). None of the women experienced any breakthrough bleeding or spotting, and measurements of plasma hormone concentrations indicated that the contraceptive efficacy was unchanged.[5] However, this study would have been more conclusive if the extract had been given for a whole cycle and the pharmacokinetics of the contraceptive steroids had been compared on the same day of each cycle.

(b) Contraceptive failure and breakthrough bleeding

The Adverse Drug Reactions Database of the Swedish Medical Products Agency has on record 2 cases of pregnancy due to the failure of an oral combined hormonal contraceptive, which was attributed to the use of products containing St John's wort (*Esbericum* and *Kira*). One woman was taking **ethinylestradiol** and **norethisterone** and the other was taking **ethinylestradiol** and **levonorgestrel**.[6] This follows an earlier report from the Swedish Medical Products Agency of 8 cases of breakthrough bleeding in women aged 23 to 31 years taking long-term oral hormonal contraceptives and St John's wort. Breakthrough bleeding occurred within about a week of starting St John's wort in 5 of the cases, and was known to have resolved in 3 cases when the St John's wort was stopped.[7]

The MHRA in the UK has on record a further 11 cases of pregnancy in women taking St John's wort and oral hormonal contraceptives between 2000 and the last quarter of 2013, and 4 cases of breakthrough bleeding without pregnancies.[8] Six of these women were taking combined hormonal contraceptives (**ethinylestradiol** with **desogestrel**, **levonorgestrel**, **norethisterone** or **norgestimate**), generally for at least 7 months before starting St John's wort. Preparations were standard dose in 5 cases (**ethinylestradiol** 30 or 35 micrograms) and low dose (20 micrograms) in one case. The unplanned pregnancies occurred after they had been taking the St John's wort for an average of about 4 months (one to 9 months).[9] A single case of pregnancy has also been reported in a patient taking St John's wort and **ethinylestradiol** with **dienogest**.[10] The German Federal Institute for Drugs and Medical Devices has received a total of 8 case reports of contraceptive failure in women also taking St John's wort.[11]

Another earlier brief report describes 3 women taking an oral combined hormonal contraceptive (**ethinylestradiol** 30 micrograms with **desogestrel** 150 micrograms) who developed breakthrough bleeding one week (2 cases) and 3 months (one case) after starting to take St John's wort.[12] Controlled studies have found that the frequency of breakthrough bleeding in women taking combined hormonal contraceptives increased considerably when St John's wort was taken, see under *Hypericin 0.3%*, above.

Mechanism

St John's wort is an inducer of CYP3A4, by which contraceptive steroids are partially metabolised.[2] This can lead to breakthrough bleeding and it appears, in some cases, to contraceptive failure. This is consistent with the way St John's wort appears to lower the concentrations of some other drugs. Note that St John's wort is a herbal preparation, and the specific constituents responsible for enzyme induction are currently unknown, although there is some evidence that hyperforin might be responsible. Also, the concentrations of individual constituents can vary between different preparations of the herb. However, it is also possible that some of the cases of contraceptive failure on concurrent use are coincidental.

Importance and management

The interaction between oral combined hormonal contraceptives and St John's wort is established, although the effect on contraceptive steroid concentrations appears to be very small, and therefore probably not relevant in many women. Its incidence is not known, but the evidence so far suggests that breakthrough bleeding might be a problem (and might be a sign of reduced efficacy), although pregnancy resulting from this interaction appears to be rare. However, as it is not known which patients are particularly likely to be at risk, women taking oral hormonal contraceptives should generally avoid St John's wort (the recommendation of the MHRA in the UK[8]). Given that there are many established antidepressants that do not interact with contraceptives, this would seem prudent advice. Note that the combined hormonal contraceptive patch and vaginal ring might also be affected (the 2014 MHRA advice extends to all hormonal contraceptives, except IUDs[8]). If concurrent use is considered essential, in the UK, the Faculty of Sexual and Reproductive Healthcare include St John's wort in their 2011 guidance on the use of enzyme inducers with combined hormonal contraceptives.[13] See 'Combined hormonal contraceptives + Barbiturates or Phenytoin', p.1169, for further details of this guidance.

Although the considerable worldwide popularity of St John's wort is fairly recent, its use has been widespread in Germany and it has been used for very many years in both Germany and Austria. Nevertheless, there seems to be no published evidence that oral hormonal contraceptive failure in those countries is more frequent than anywhere else. This would seem to suggest that contraceptive failure leading to pregnancy occurring as a result of this interaction is very uncommon, although it is always possible that it has failed to be identified as a possible cause. Further study is needed to confirm whether St John's wort extracts with a low hyperforin content (0.2% as opposed to about 3%) do not interact with hormonal contraceptives, as these might be an alternative.

1. Pfrunder A, Schiesser M, Gerber S, Haschke M, Bitzer J, Drewe J. Interaction of St John's wort with low-dose oral contraceptive therapy: a randomized controlled trial. *Br J Clin Pharmacol* (2003) 56, 683–90.
2. Hall SD, Wang Z, Huang S-M, Hamman MA, Vasavada N, Adigun AQ, Hilligoss JK, Miller M, Gorski JC. The interaction between St John's wort and an oral contraceptive. *Clin Pharmacol Ther* (2003) 74, 525–35.
3. Murphy PA, Kern SE, Stanczyk FZ, Westhoff CL. Interaction of St John's wort with oral contraceptives: effects on the pharmacokinetics of norethindrone and ethinyl estradiol, ovarian activity and breakthrough bleeding. *Contraception* (2005) 71, 402–8.
4. Fogle RH, Murphy PA, Westhoff CL, Stanczyk FZ. Does St. John's Wort interfere with the antiandrogenic effect of oral contraceptive pills? *Contraception* (2006) 74, 245–8.
5. Will-Shahab L, Bauer S, Kunter U, Roots I, Brattström A. St John's wort extract (Ze 117) does not alter the pharmacokinetics of a low-dose oral contraceptive. *Eur J Clin Pharmacol* (2009) 65, 287–94. Erratum: *ibid.* 541.
6. Swedish Medical Products Agency. Data on file. St John's wort may influence other medication. 2002.
7. Yue Q-Y, Bergquist C, Gerdén B. Safety of St John's wort (Hypericum perforatum). *Lancet* (2000) 355, 576–7.
8. Medicines and Healthcare Products Regulatory Agency and the Commission on Human Medicines. St John's wort: interaction with hormonal contraceptives, including implants – reduced contraceptive effect. *Drug Safety Update* (2014) 7, A2. Available at: http://webarchive.nationalarchives.gov.uk/20141205150130/http://www.mhra.gov.uk/home/groups/dsu/documents/publication/con392897.pdf (accessed 21/10/15).
9. Henderson L, Yue QY, Bergquist C, Gerden B, Arlett P. St John's wort (Hypericum perforatum): drug interactions and clinical outcomes. *Br J Clin Pharmacol* (2002) 54, 349–56.
10. Schwarz UI, Büschel B, Kirch W. Unwanted pregnancy on self-medication with St John's wort despite hormonal contraception. *Br J Clin Pharmacol* (2003) 55, 112–13.
11. Bundesinstitut für Arzneimittel und Medizinprodukte. Personal communication, March 2007.
12. Bon S, Hartmann K, Kuhn M. Johanniskraut: Ein Enzyminduktor? *Schweiz Apothekerzeitung* (1999) 16, 535–6.
13. Faculty of Sexual and Reproductive Healthcare Guidance. Drug interactions with hormonal contraception: Clinical Effectiveness Unit, January 2011 (Updated January 2012). Available at: http://www.fsrh.org/pdfs/CEUGuidanceDrugInteractionsHormonal.pdf (accessed 21/10/15).

Combined hormonal contraceptives + Statins

Atorvastatin and rosuvastatin may slightly increase oral combined hormonal contraceptive exposure, and rosuvastatin did not alter the ovulation suppressant effect of an oral combined hormonal contraceptive. The pharmacokinetics of a single dose of pravastatin appear to be unaffected by oral combined hormonal contraceptives. Lovastatin and simvastatin may prevent some of the adverse effects of oral combined hormonal contraceptives on lipids.

Clinical evidence

(a) Atorvastatin

In a study in 12 healthy women taking an oral combined hormonal contraceptive (**ethinylestradiol** 35 micrograms with **norethisterone** 1 mg), atorvastatin 40 mg daily increased the AUC of **ethinylestradiol** and **norethisterone** by about 19% and 28%, respectively.[1]

(b) Lovastatin

In a study, 60 women were randomised to take a triphasic oral combined hormonal contraceptive (**ethinylestradiol** 30 to 40 micrograms with **levonorgestrel** 50 to 125 micrograms) alone or with lovastatin 20 mg daily for 3 months. Serum triglycerides were increased in those receiving the contraceptive alone (from 90 to 157 mg/dL), but showed little change in those also given lovastatin (105 to 113 mg/dL). LDL-cholesterol did not change in those given the contraceptive alone, but tended to decrease in those also receiving lovastatin.[2] The effects of lovastatin alone were not assessed in this study, so it is not possible to say whether the contraceptive attenuated any of the benefits of lovastatin.

(c) Pravastatin

The pharmacokinetics of a single 20-mg dose of pravastatin did not differ between 15 young women taking oral combined hormonal contraceptives (**ethinylestradiol** with **norethisterone**, **norgestrel** or **levonorgestrel**) and a control group of similar women not taking contraceptives.[3]

(d) Rosuvastatin

In a study in 18 healthy women taking a triphasic oral combined hormonal contraceptive (**ethinylestradiol** 35 micrograms with **norgestimate** 180 to 250 micrograms), the addition of rosuvastatin 40 mg daily for one cycle increased the AUC of **ethinylestradiol** by 26% and increased that of norgestrel, an active metabolite of norgestimate, by 34%, when compared with placebo. The ovulation suppressant activity was unchanged as measured by FSH, LH and progesterone levels.[4] The pharmacokinetics and lipid-lowering effects of rosuvastatin were consistent with those seen in historical controls.[4]

(e) Simvastatin

In a crossover study, 48 women with polycystic ovary syndrome received an oral combined hormonal contraceptive (**ethinylestradiol** 20 micrograms with **desogestrel** 150 micrograms) alone for 12 weeks and with simvastatin 20 mg daily for 12 weeks. Simvastatin prevented the contraceptive-induced 20% increase in triglycerides, and decreased LDL-cholesterol (the contraceptive alone increased this).[5] The effects of simvastatin alone were not assessed in this study, so it is not possible to say whether the contraceptive attenuated any of the benefits of simvastatin.

Mechanism

It is not known why atorvastatin and rosuvastatin increase contraceptive steroid exposure, but this is unlikely to be via CYP3A4 inhibition, because these statins are not inhibitors of this isoenzyme.

Oral combined hormonal contraceptives are known to be associated with some adverse effects on plasma lipids, which can depend on the progestogen used. Those containing an androgenic progestogen probably have the greatest effects whereas non-androgenic (third generation) progestogens (e.g. desogestrel, gestodene, norgestimate) have less detrimental effects on lipids. Statins appear to attenuate some of the adverse effects of oral combined hormonal contraceptives on plasma lipids.

Importance and management

The increases in exposure of ethinylestradiol and progestogens seen with atorvastatin and rosuvastatin are only slight and unlikely to be clinically important, but some manufacturers state that they should be considered when selecting an appropriate oral combined hormonal contraceptive dose for women given these statins.[6,7] If adverse effects, such as nausea and breast tenderness, become troublesome, it may be appropriate to try a lower dose oral combined hormonal contraceptive.

Note that statins are potentially teratogenic and therefore reliable contraception is required if they are used in women of child-bearing age. However, bear in mind also that the indications for statins may be a contraindication to the use of any form of combined hormonal contraceptive, if other risk factors for arterial disease are present. This is because these contraceptives can have adverse effects on serum lipids. Statins may attenuate some of these effects.

1. Yang B-B, Siedlik PH, Smithers JA, Sedman AJ, Stern RH. Atorvastatin pharmacokinetic interactions with other CYP3A4 substrates: erythromycin and ethinyl estradiol. *Pharm Res* (1996) 13 (9 Suppl), S-437.
2. Colakoglu M, Kodama H, Tanaka T. The effect of combined medication of triphasic oral contraceptive with an anti-lipid agent, lovastatin, on plasma lipid levels. *Jpn J Fertil Steril* (1996) 41, 317–20.
3. Pan HY, Waclawski AP, Funke PT, Whigan D. Pharmacokinetics of pravastatin in elderly versus young men and women. *Ann Pharmacother* (1993) 27, 1029–33.
4. Simonson SG, Martin PD, Warwick MJ, Mitchell PD, Schneck DW. The effect of rosuvastatin on oestrogen & progestin pharmacokinetics in healthy women taking an oral contraceptive. *Br J Clin Pharmacol* (2004) 57, 279–86.
5. Banaszewska B, Pawelczyk L, Spaczynski RZ, Dziura J, Duleba AJ. Effects of simvastatin and oral contraceptive agent on polycystic ovary syndrome: prospective, randomized, crossover trial. *J Clin Endocrinol Metab* (2007) 92, 456–61.
6. Lipitor (Atorvastatin calcium). Pfizer Inc. US Prescribing information, March 2015.
7. Crestor (Rosuvastatin calcium). AstraZeneca UK Ltd. UK Summary of product characteristics, May 2013.

Combined hormonal contraceptives + Sucrose polyesters

Sucrose polyester did not alter the pharmacokinetics or ovulation suppressant effect of an oral combined hormonal contraceptive containing ethinylestradiol with norgestrel.

Clinical evidence, mechanism, importance and management

When 28 healthy women took 18 g of sucrose polyester (*Olestra*) daily for 28 days, with an oral combined hormonal contraceptive (**ethinylestradiol** 30 micrograms with **norgestrel** 300 micrograms), the pharmacokinetics of the contraceptive steroids were unchanged. Serum progesterone levels also remained unaltered, suggesting no ovulation occurred.[1] This agrees with the findings of earlier single-dose studies, which found that sucrose polyester had no effect on the bioavailability of single doses of **ethinylestradiol** or **norethisterone**.[2] No additional contraceptive precautions appear to be necessary with oral combined hormonal contraceptives used in the presence of sucrose polyesters.

1. Miller KW, Williams DS, Carter SB, Jones MB, Mishell DR. The effect of olestra on systemic levels of oral contraceptives. *Clin Pharmacol Ther* (1990) 48, 34–40.
2. Roberts RJ, Leff RD. Influence of absorbable and nonabsorbable lipids and lipidlike substances on drug availability. *Clin Pharmacol Ther* (1989) 45, 299–304.

Combined hormonal contraceptives + Tacrolimus

Limited evidence suggests that ethinylestradiol increases tacrolimus concentrations. However, a vaginal ring formulation of a combined hormonal contraceptive had no effect on tacrolimus concentrations. Theoretically, tacrolimus might increase hormonal contraceptive exposure.

Clinical evidence, mechanism, importance and management

The UK manufacturer of tacrolimus states that, during clinical use, **ethinylestradiol** has been shown to increase tacrolimus concentrations to a minor extent. They also note that, *in vitro*, **gestodene** and **norethisterone** are potential inhibitors of tacrolimus metabolism.[1] The mechanism for any pharmacokinetic interaction is unclear as these contraceptive steroids do not inhibit CYP3A4, by which tacrolimus is principally metabolised. Furthermore, in a study of 17 women with renal or liver transplants taking tacrolimus or low-dose ciclosporin with prednisone, the use of a vaginal ring formulation of a combined hormonal contraceptive (releasing **ethinylestradiol** 15 micrograms and **etonogestrel** 120 micrograms daily) for 12 cycles did not require any change in immunosuppressive therapy to maintain concentrations of ciclosporin or tacrolimus within the therapeutic range.[2]

In addition, the UK manufacturer notes that tacrolimus is an inhibitor of CYP3A4, by which contraceptive steroids are partially metabolised. They therefore predict that tacrolimus could reduce the clearance of hormonal contraceptives, leading to increased hormone exposure.[1] The extent of any interaction does not appear to have been studied, but, given the limited effect of potent CYP3A4 inhibitors, such as some of the azoles, on the metabolism of contraceptive steroids (see 'Combined hormonal contraceptives + Azoles', p.1168) a clinically relevant increase with tacrolimus seems unlikely. Nevertheless, the UK manufacturer states that care should be taken when deciding upon contraceptive measures in patients also given tacrolimus.[1]

1. Prograf (Tacrolimus monohydrate). Astellas Pharma Ltd. UK Summary of product characteristics, November 2014.
2. Paternoster DM, Riboni F, Bertolino M, Garofalo G, Lazzarich E, Surico N, Stratta P. The contraceptive vaginal ring in women with renal and liver transplantation: analysis of preliminary results. *Transplant Proc* (2010) 42, 1162–5.

Combined hormonal contraceptives + Terbinafine

Terbinafine appears unlikely to alter the efficacy of combined hormonal contraceptives.

Clinical evidence, mechanism, importance and management

An *in vitro* study in human liver microsomes found that high levels of terbinafine had little inhibitory effect on the hydroxylation of **ethinylestradiol**,[1] indicating that, in clinical use, it is unlikely to alter the pharmacokinetics of ethinylestradiol-containing combined hormonal contraceptives (oral, patch, or vaginal ring) by this mechanism.

The UK manufacturer of terbinafine notes that some cases of menstrual disturbances (breakthrough bleeding and irregular cycle) have been reported in patients taking both oral contraceptives (type not stated) and terbinafine.[2] Nevertheless, in a post-marketing survey that included 314 patients taking both oral contraceptives (type not stated) and terbinafine, the rate of menstrual disorders (4.5%) was within the rate reported in the literature for patients taking oral contraceptives alone.[3] It seems unlikely that terbinafine will alter the efficacy of oral contraceptives.

1. Back DJ, Stevenson P, Tjia JF. Comparative effects of two antimycotic agents, ketoconazole and terbinafine, on the metabolism of tolbutamide, ethinyloestradiol, cyclosporin and ethoxycoumarin by human liver microsomes *in vitro*. *Br J Clin Pharmacol* (1989) 28, 166–70.
2. Lamisil Tablets (Terbinafine hydrochloride). Novartis Pharmaceuticals UK Ltd. UK Summary of product characteristics, March 2012.
3. O'Sullivan DP, Needham CA, Bangs A, Atkin K, Kendall FD. Postmarketing surveillance of oral terbinafine in the UK: report of a large cohort study. *Br J Clin Pharmacol* (1996) 42, 559–65.

Combined hormonal contraceptives + Thiazolidinediones

Pioglitazone causes a negligible decrease in the exposure to ethinylestradiol from an oral combined hormonal contraceptive whereas rosiglitazone does not alter the pharmacokinetics of an oral hormonal contraceptive containing ethinylestradiol with norethisterone.

Clinical evidence

(a) Pioglitazone

In a study in 35 healthy women given an oral combined hormonal contraceptive (**ethinylestradiol** 35 micrograms with **norethisterone** 1 mg) with pioglitazone 45 mg daily for 21 days, pioglitazone reduced the AUC of **ethinylestradiol** by 11%, but had no effect on the AUC of **norethisterone**, when compared with placebo.[1] Similar results were reported in another study.[2]

(b) Rosiglitazone

Rosiglitazone 8 mg daily, given for the first 2 weeks of two cycles in 32 women taking an oral combined hormonal contraceptive (**ethinylestradiol** 35 micrograms with **norethisterone** 35 micrograms), had no effect on the pharmacokinetics of either contraceptive steroid.[3]

Mechanism

Unknown.

Importance and management

Evidence for an interaction between the thiazolidinediones and combined hormonal contraceptives comes from two studies. An 11% decrease in ethinylestradiol exposure with pioglitazone is unlikely to be clinically important, especially as norethisterone exposure was unaltered. However, it would have been useful if the study had also measured ovulation suppression to confirm the likely continued efficacy of the contraceptive. Rosiglitazone had no effect on contraceptive steroid pharmacokinetics, but note that marketing of this drug has been suspended or restricted in some countries because of possible adverse cardiovascular effects.

For the possible adverse effect of hormonal contraceptives on diabetic control, and for the general precautions for the use of these contraceptives in diabetes, see 'Antidiabetics + Hormonal contraceptives', p.510.

1. Karim A, Schwartz L, Perez A, Cao C. Lack of clinically significant drug interaction in the coadministration of pioglitazone with ethinyl estradiol and norethindrone. *Diabetes* (2003) 52 (Suppl 1) A123.
2. Carey RA, Liu Y. Pioglitazone does not markedly alter oral contraceptive or hormone replacement therapy pharmacokinetics. *Diabetes* (2000) 49 (Suppl 1), A100.
3. Inglis AML, Miller AK, Culkin KT, Finnerty D, Patterson SD, Jorkasky DK, Freed MI. Lack of effect of rosiglitazone on the pharmacokinetics of oral contraceptives in healthy female volunteers. *J Clin Pharmacol* (2001) 41, 683–90.

Combined hormonal contraceptives + Tiagabine

Tiagabine did not alter the pharmacokinetics or the ovulation suppressant effect of oral combined hormonal contraceptives containing ethinylestradiol with levonorgestrel or desogestrel.

Clinical evidence, mechanism, importance and management

In a study in 10 healthy women, tiagabine 2 mg four times daily, from day 24 of one cycle to day 7 of the next cycle, had no effect on the mean plasma levels of any of the steroids in two oral combined hormonal contraceptives (**ethinylestradiol** 30 micrograms with **levonorgestrel** 150 micrograms or **desogestrel** 150 micrograms). There was no evidence that the suppression of ovulation was altered in any way (no significant changes in the plasma concentrations of progesterone, FSH, or LH were seen between the first and second cycles, and progesterone levels remained in the non-ovulatory range). Tiagabine did not induce hepatic enzymes, as assessed by 6β-hydroxycortisol excretion. Two women did develop breakthrough bleeding, but given the above findings, this was not thought to represent a reduction in the efficacy of the contraceptive.[1] There would therefore appear to be no reason for any additional contraceptive precautions on the concurrent use of tiagabine and any combined hormonal contraceptives (tablet, patch or vaginal ring).

1. Mengel HB, Houston A, Back DJ. An evaluation of the interaction between tiagabine and oral contraceptives in female volunteers. *J Pharm Med* (1994) 4, 141–50.

Combined hormonal contraceptives + Ticagrelor

Ticagrelor slightly increases the exposure to ethinylestradiol and does not affect the suppression of ovulation in response to the contraceptive.

Clinical evidence

In a crossover study, 22 healthy women taking **ethinylestradiol** 30 micrograms with **levonorgestrel** 150 micrograms daily were given ticagrelor 90 mg or placebo, twice daily for 21 days. Ticagrelor increased the AUC and maximum plasma concentration of **ethinylestradiol** by 20% and 31%, respectively. **Levonorgestrel** pharmacokinetics were not affected by ticagrelor. Estradiol, progesterone, FSH, and LH concentrations were similar in the presence of ticagrelor and placebo indicating that the effects of the contraceptive were not altered by ticagrelor.[1]

Mechanism

Ticagrelor is a weak inhibitor of CYP3A4 and therefore very slightly increases the exposure to ethinylestradiol, which is metabolised by this isoenzyme.

Importance and management

Evidence for an interaction between ticagrelor and contraceptives appears to be limited to this one study, which found that ticagrelor has only very slight effects on ethinylestradiol exposure and does not alter the effects of the combined hormonal contraceptive. Therefore the contraceptive efficacy of oral combined hormonal contraceptives seems unlikely to be affected on the concurrent use of ticagrelor.

1. Butler K, Teng R. Effect of ticagrelor on the pharmacokinetics of ethinyl oestradiol and levonorgestrel in healthy volunteers. *Curr Med Res Opin* (2011) 27, 1585–93.

Combined hormonal contraceptives + Topiramate

Ethinylestradiol exposure may be reduced by high-dose topiramate, increasing the risk of breakthrough bleeding in women taking oral combined hormonal contraceptives.

Clinical evidence

In a study, 11 women with epilepsy taking sodium valproate and an oral combined hormonal contraceptive (**ethinylestradiol** 35 micrograms with **norethisterone** 1 mg) were also given three escalating doses of topiramate 200 mg, 400 mg and 800 mg daily (as two divided doses) for 28-day periods. The mean AUC of the **ethinylestradiol** fell by 18%, 21%, and 30%, with the three doses respectively. No statistically significant changes were found in the **norethisterone** AUC. No ovulation occurred, as assessed by progestogen levels, but one patient had breakthrough bleeding.[1] A follow-up study evaluated the effect of lower doses of topiramate on the pharmacokinetics of the same oral combined hormonal contraceptive in healthy subjects. Subjects were randomised to take daily doses of topiramate of 50 mg (11 subjects), 100 mg (10 subjects) or 200 mg (2 groups of 12 subjects). This study found minor changes in the pharmacokinetics of both **ethinylestradiol** and **norethisterone**, which were not dose-related and were not statistically significant. Moreover, the pharmacokinetic changes were further reduced when the data from 2 subjects were excluded due to compliance issues (maximum decrease of 12% in the **ethinylestradiol** AUC).[2]

Mechanism

Not understood. It is suggested that high-dose topiramate weakly induces drug-metabolising enzymes [specific isoenzymes unknown], which increases the metabolism of the ethinylestradiol.[1,2]

Importance and management

The pharmacokinetic interaction between topiramate and the oral combined hormonal contraceptives appears to be established. The authors of one study noted that the difference between the two studies was due to the difference in the doses of topiramate used, as topiramate is a weak liver enzyme-inducer, and this effect is only apparent at higher doses.[2] The very small changes in the pharmacokinetics of the oral combined hormonal contraceptive with lower therapeutic doses of topiramate (50 to 100 mg daily) are much lower than those seen with other enzyme-inducing antiepileptics (such as carbamazepine and phenytoin, see 'Table 28.1', p.1160), and would generally not be considered clinically relevant. However, with higher doses of topiramate, the possibility that an interaction would be sufficient to cause contraceptive failure in some women cannot be excluded. The authors of one study considered that an oral combined hormonal contraceptive containing at least 35 micrograms of ethinylestradiol would be suitable for women taking topiramate.[1] In the UK, the Faculty of Sexual and Reproductive Healthcare 2011 guidance on the concurrent use of liver enzyme inducers with combined hormonal contraceptives includes topiramate in their list of enzyme-inducing drugs that reduce contraceptive hormone levels, but only at doses of 200 mg daily or more.[3] Note that, for long-term use of topiramate in doses of 200 mg daily or more, they recommend a minimum of 50 micrograms of ethinylestradiol. See also, 'Combined hormonal contraceptives + Barbiturates or Phenytoin', p.1169, for the details of this guidance, and for guidance on the short-term use of enzyme-inducers.

Bear in mind that, as topiramate is teratogenic, the manufacturers state that the concurrent use of adequate contraception (not specified) is required in women of child-bearing age.[4,5]

1. Rosenfeld WE, Doose DR, Walker SA, Nayak RK. Effect of topiramate on the pharmacokinetics of an oral contraceptive containing norethindrone and ethinyl estradiol in patients with epilepsy. *Epilepsia* (1997) 38, 317–23.
2. Doose DR, Wang S-S, Padmanabhan M, Schwabe S, Jacobs D, Bialer M. Effect of topiramate or carbamazepine on the pharmacokinetics of an oral contraceptive containing norethindrone and ethinyl estradiol in healthy obese and nonobese female subjects. *Epilepsia* (2003) 44, 540–9.
3. Faculty of Sexual and Reproductive Healthcare Guidance. Drug interactions with hormonal contraception: Clinical Effectiveness Unit, January 2011. Available at: http://www.fsrh.org/pdfs/CEUGuidanceDrugInteractionsHormonal.pdf (accessed 21/10/15).
4. Topamax (Topiramate). Janssen-Cilag Ltd. UK Summary of product characteristics, October 2012.
5. Topamax (Topiramate). Ortho-McNeil Neurologics. US Prescribing information, January 2012.

Combined hormonal contraceptives + Triptans

Oral combined hormonal contraceptives appear to slightly raise frovatriptan, naratriptan and zolmitriptan exposure, and negligibly increase sumatriptan exposure, but might not affect eletriptan exposure. Almotriptan, rizatriptan and sumatriptan do not alter the pharmacokinetics of contraceptive steroids.

Clinical evidence

(a) Almotriptan

In a well-controlled study in 21 women, a single 12.5-mg dose of almotriptan given between days 8 and 12 of a cycle had no effect on the pharmacokinetics of an oral combined hormonal contraceptive (**ethinylestradiol** 30 micrograms with **desogestrel** 150 micrograms) taken for two cycles.[1]

(b) Eletriptan

The UK manufacturer notes that population pharmacokinetic analysis of clinical studies has suggested that oestrogen-containing oral contraceptives [combined hormonal contraceptives] are unlikely to have an effect on the pharmacokinetic properties of eletriptan.[2]

(c) Frovatriptan

In a retrospective analysis of pharmacokinetic data from phase I studies, the mean maximum concentration and AUC of frovatriptan were 25% and 30% higher, respectively, in women taking oral contraceptives (unspecified) than in women not taking these contraceptives.[3]

(d) Naratriptan

The US manufacturer notes that the clearance of naratriptan was reduced by 32% by oral contraceptives (unspecified) leading to a slightly higher level of naratriptan.[4] A case of ischaemic colitis has been reported in a 42-year-old woman who had been taking an oral combined hormonal contraceptive (**ethinylestradiol** 30 micrograms with **drospirenone** 3 mg) for 3 years, naratriptan 2.5 mg as needed for 18 months (maximum dose of one tablet in a day and 9 tablets in a month), and topiramate 25 mg twice daily for 4 months.[5]

(e) Rizatriptan

In a placebo-controlled study in 20 healthy young women taking an oral combined hormonal contraceptive (**ethinylestradiol** 35 micrograms with **norethisterone** 1 mg), the concurrent use of rizatriptan (6 days of 10 mg daily followed by 2 days of 10 mg every 4 hours to a total of 3 doses daily) did not alter the pharmacokinetics of either contraceptive steroid. Blood pressure, heart rate and temperature were unaffected and adverse effects were similar to those seen with placebo.[6]

(f) Sumatriptan

A study was designed to investigate the effects of an oral combined hormonal contraceptive (**ethinylestradiol** 35 micrograms with **norethisterone** 1 mg) on the pharmacokinetics of sumatriptan in 26 women who had been taking this contraceptive for at least 3 months. A single 50-mg oral dose of sumatriptan was given once after 21 days of active treatment with the contraceptive, and again after 7 days of placebo (day 28). A 16% higher AUC and a 17% higher maximum concentration of sumatriptan was noted on day 21, compared with day 29. There was an 18% reduction in the maximum concentration of **norethisterone** when it was given with sumatriptan, but no change in its AUC. Similarly, there was no change in the AUC or maximum concentration of **ethinylestradiol** when it was given with sumatriptan.[7]

In a large prospective study of subcutaneous sumatriptan, there was no difference in the incidence of cardiovascular adverse events between 1 188 patients taking oral contraceptives (types not stated) and 11 151 patients who were not taking contraceptives. Two cardiovascular adverse events occurred within 24 hours of sumatriptan use in women also using oral contraceptives. One 44-year-old women experienced angina, and the other had palpitations.[8]

(g) Zolmitriptan

The US manufacturer states that, in a retrospective analysis of pharmacokinetic data from several studies, the mean maximum concentration and AUC of zolmitriptan were 30% and 50% higher, respectively, in women taking oral contraceptives (types not stated) than in women not taking these contraceptives.[9] The effects of zolmitriptan on oral contraceptive steroids have not been studied.[9]

Mechanism

Uncertain, but ethinylestradiol is known to be an inhibitor of CYP1A2, by which a number of these triptans (particularly frovatriptan and zolmitriptan) are at least partially metabolised.

Importance and management

Although the data are limited, the slight possible increases in frovatriptan, naratriptan, sumatriptan and zolmitriptan exposure on the concurrent use of an oral combined hormonal contraceptive are not likely to produce clinically relevant adverse effects. Almotriptan, rizatriptan and sumatriptan do not have any clinically important effect on the pharmacokinetics of contraceptive steroids, and so no additional contraceptive precautions would appear to be necessary on concurrent use.

The general relevance of the single case report of ischaemic colitis associated with the concurrent use of naratriptan and an oral combined hormonal contraceptive is unclear. Note that ischaemic colitis has, rarely, been reported with naratriptan alone.[10] The manufacturers have found no cases of ischaemic colitis in approximately 450 women taking oral contraceptives (type not stated) and naratriptan, for prophylaxis for 5 to 6 days.[10]

More importantly, the use of combined hormonal contraceptives in women who suffer from migraine increases the risk of stroke.[11] Migraine with aura (which indicates ischaemia) is generally thought to be a greater risk for stroke. As a result, migraine, and the type of migraine that occurs, should be taken into account when considering whether or not to use any form of combined hormonal contraceptive (tablets, patch or vaginal ring). In the UK, the Faculty of Sexual and Reproductive Healthcare (FSRH) guidance includes information on the use of combined hormonal contraceptives in migraine, and alternative contraceptive choices.[12]

1. Cabarrocas X, Macher J-P. Lack of a pharmacokinetic interaction between almotriptan and oral contraceptives: a double-blind, placebo-controlled, crossover study in healthy female volunteers. *Cephalalgia* (2003) 23, 716.
2. Replax (Eletriptan). Pfizer Ltd. UK Summary of product characteristics, February 2008.
3. Buchan P. Effects of alcohol, smoking and oral contraceptives on the pharmacokinetics of frovatriptan. *Eur J Neurol* (2000) 7 (Suppl 3), 86–7.
4. Amerge (Naratriptan hydrochloride). GlaxoSmithKline. US Prescribing information, February 2010.
5. Charles JA, Pullicino PM, Stoopack PM, Shroff Y. Ischemic colitis associated with naratriptan and oral contraceptive use. *Headache* (2005) 45, 386–9.
6. Shadle CR, Liu G, Goldberg MR. A double-blind, placebo-controlled evaluation of the effect of oral doses of rizatriptan 10 mg on oral contraceptive pharmacokinetics in healthy female volunteers. *J Clin Pharmacol* (2000) 40, 309–15.
7. Moore KHP, McNeal S, Britto MR, Bye C, Sale M, Richardson MS. The pharmacokinetics of sumatriptan when administered with norethindrone 1 mg/ethinyl estradiol 0.035 mg in healthy volunteers. *Clin Ther* (2002) 24, 1887–1901.
8. Putnam GP, O'Quinn S, Bolden-Watson CP, Davis RL, Gutteman DL, Fox AW. Migraine polypharmacy and the tolerability of sumatriptan: a large-scale, prospective study. *Cephalalgia* (1999) 19, 668–75.
9. Zomig (Zolmitriptan). AstraZeneca Pharmaceuticals LP. US Prescribing information, October 2008.
10. Malone TD, Kori SH. Ischemic colitis associated with naratriptan and oral contraceptive use: A response. *Headache* (2005) 45, 1419–20.
11. Curtis KM, Mohllajee AP, Peterson HB. Use of combined oral contraceptives among women with migraine and nonmigrainous headaches: a systematic review. *Contraception* (2006) 73, 189–4.
12. Faculty of Sexual and Reproductive Healthcare (FSRH) of the Royal College of Obstetricians & Gynaecologists. UK Medical eligibility criteria for contraceptive use (UKMEC), 2009. Available at: http://www.fsrh.org/pdfs/UKMEC2009.pdf / (accessed 21/10/15).

Combined hormonal contraceptives + Tyrosine kinase inhibitors

A woman taking an oral combined hormonal contraceptive developed gallstones after starting imatinib. Tofacitinib appears to have no effect on the pharmacokinetics of ethinylestradiol or levonorgestrel.

Clinical evidence, mechanism, importance and management

(a) Imatinib

A 31-year-old woman taking a low-dose oral combined hormonal contraceptive developed nausea and abdominal pain after taking imatinib 400 mg daily for 4 months. Ultrasound showed multiple gallstones and increased gallbladder wall thickness. The contraceptive was stopped, and the imatinib temporarily stopped, and the gallstones remained stable in size on periodic monitoring.[1]

Imatinib is an inhibitor of CYP3A4, by which oestrogens are partially metabolised. The authors suggested that an increase in oestrogen concentrations could possibly lead to increased cholesterol excretion, reduced bile salt excretion, and gallstone development. However, this needs confirmation. The clinical relevance of this isolated case report is unclear.

(b) Tofacitinib

The US manufacturer of tofacitinib briefly notes that in a study, it had no clinically important effect on the pharmacokinetics of oral **ethinylestradiol** or oral **levonorgestrel**; no contraceptive dose adjustments are therefore necessary on concurrent use.[2]

1. Breccia M, D'Andrea M, Alimena G. Can nifedipine and estrogen interaction with imatinib be responsible for gallbladder stone development? *Eur J Haematol* (2005) 75, 89–90.
2. Xeljanz (Tofacitinib citrate). Pfizer Inc. US Prescribing information, November 2012.

Combined hormonal contraceptives + Urinary antimuscarinics

Darifenacin, fesoterodine, solifenacin and tolterodine do not alter the pharmacokinetics of an oral combined hormonal contraceptive containing ethinylestradiol with levonorgestrel. In addition, fesoterodine, solifenacin and tolterodine do not alter the ovulation suppressant effects of this contraceptive. Hormonal contraceptives do not appear to alter the pharmacokinetics of oxybutynin.

Clinical evidence and mechanism

(a) Darifenacin

The manufacturers note that, in a study in 22 healthy women, steady-state darifenacin 10 mg three times daily had no effect on the pharmacokinetics of an oral combined hormonal contraceptive (**ethinylestradiol** with **levonorgestrel**).[1,2]

(b) Fesoterodine

In a randomised, crossover study in 26 healthy women, fesoterodine 8 mg daily for 14 days, beginning on day one of a cycle, had no effect on the pharmacokinetics of an oral combined hormonal contraceptive (**ethinylestradiol** 30 micrograms with **levonorgestrel** 150 micrograms). Fesoterodine did not alter suppression of ovulation assessed by progesterone, LH and FSH levels.[3]

(c) Oxybutynin

The pharmacokinetics of a single 10-mg dose of oxybutynin as a controlled-release tablet did not differ between women taking contraceptive steroids (type not stated), women not taking contraceptive steroids, and men.[4]

(d) Solifenacin

In a randomised, crossover study in healthy women, solifenacin 10 mg daily for 10 days, beginning on day 12 of a cycle, had no effect on the pharmacokinetics of an oral combined hormonal contraceptive (**ethinylestradiol** 30 micrograms with **levonorgestrel** 150 micrograms). Solifenacin did not alter suppression of LH or FSH.[5]

(e) Tolterodine

A randomised, crossover study in 24 women found that tolterodine 2 mg twice daily on days one to 14 of two 28-day contraceptive cycles had no effect on the pharmacokinetics of an oral combined hormonal contraceptive (**ethinylestradiol** 30 micrograms with **levonorgestrel** 150 micrograms). The serum levels of estradiol and progesterone indicated that suppression of ovulation continued during both periods of treatment. The pharmacokinetics of tolterodine were consistent with previous studies, so do not appear to be altered by the contraceptive.[6]

Importance and management

The evidence from these controlled studies suggests that these urinary antimuscarinics (darifenacin, fesoterodine, solifenacin and tolterodine) are unlikely to alter the efficacy of oral combined hormonal contraceptives. No additional contraceptive precautions

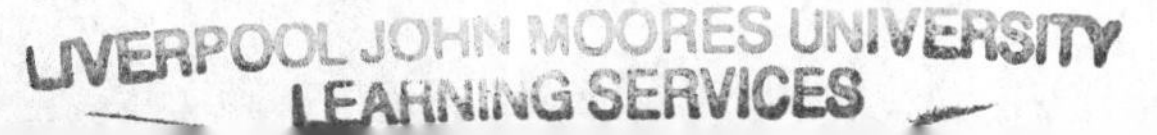

would therefore seem to be needed if these drugs are used concurrently with any combined hormonal contraceptive (tablets, patch or vaginal ring).

1. Enablex (Darifenacin hydrobromide). Novartis. US Prescribing information, January 2010.
2. Skerjanec A. The clinical pharmacokinetics of darifenacin. *Clin Pharmacokinet* (2006) 45, 325–50.
3. Malhotra B, Sachse R, Wood N. Evaluation of drug-drug interactions with fesoterodine. *Eur J Clin Pharmacol* (2009) 65, 551–60.
4. Lukkari E, Hakonen T, Neuvonen PJ. The pharmacokinetics of oxybutynin is unaffected by gender and contraceptive steroids. *Eur J Clin Pharmacol* (1998) 53, 351–4.
5. Taekema-Roelvink MEJ, Swart PJ, Kuipers ME, Krauwinkel WJJ, Visser N, Smulders RA. Pharmacokinetic interaction of solifenacin with an oral contraceptive containing ethinyl estradiol and levonorgestrel in healthy women: a double-blind, placebo-controlled study. *Clin Ther* (2005) 27, 1403–10.
6. Olsson B, Landgren B-M. The effect of tolterodine on the pharmacokinetics and pharmacodynamics of a combination oral contraceptive containing ethinyl estradiol and levonorgestrel. *Clin Ther* (2001) 23, 1876–88.

Combined hormonal contraceptives or Oestrogens + Ursodeoxycholic acid (Ursodiol)

Ursodeoxycholic acid does not affect the exposure to ethinylestradiol. However, oestrogens are predicted to decrease the effectiveness of ursodeoxycholic acid.

Clinical evidence, mechanism, importance and management

In a placebo-controlled study, 8 healthy women were given an oral hormonal contraceptive (**ethinylestradiol** 30 micrograms with gestodene 75 micrograms daily) with ursodeoxycholic acid 8 to 10 mg/kg daily for 21 days. Ursodeoxycholic acid did not affect the AUC of **ethinylestradiol**. Mean serum triglyceride levels increased from 58.3 mg/dL at the start of the study, to 91.4 mg/dL and 88.6 mg/dL, during **ethinylestradiol** treatment, with placebo and ursodeoxycholic acid, respectively.[1]

The study indicates that contraceptive efficacy is unlikely to be affected by ursodeoxycholic acid, although further study is required to evaluate the combination in patients with cholestatic liver disease, as there is some evidence to suggest that these patients may metabolise bile salt acids differently.[1] However, note that one UK manufacturer of ursodeoxycholic acid recommends that drugs such as **oestrogens** including combined hormonal contraceptives, which increase cholesterol elimination in the bile and thereby can promote gallstone formation, should not be taken with ursodeoxycholic acid[2] as they might reduce its effectiveness.[3]

1. Baisini O, Benini F, Petraglia F, Kuhnz W, Scalia S, Marschall HU, Brunetti G, Tauschel HD, Lanzini A. Ursodeoxycholic acid does not affect ethinylestradiol bioavailability in women taking oral contraceptives. *Eur J Clin Pharmacol* (2004) 60, 481–7.
2. Destolit (Ursodeoxycholic acid). Norgine Ltd. UK Summary of product characteristics, December 2010.
3. Urso 250/Urso Forte (Ursodeoxycholic acid). Axcan Pharma US, Inc. US Prescribing information, November 2009.

Combined hormonal contraceptives + Valproate

Sodium valproate does not appear to alter the efficacy of oral combined hormonal contraceptives. In one single-dose study, sodium valproate did not alter ethinylestradiol or levonorgestrel exposure. Ethinylestradiol may modestly reduce valproate levels, an effect which is cyclical. There is one published case where this resulted in an increase in seizure frequency.

Clinical evidence

(a) Contraceptive efficacy

In a series of 32 patients taking an oral hormonal contraceptive, none of 7 patients taking sodium valproate 600 mg to 1.8 g daily had breakthrough bleeding, whereas about two-thirds of those taking carbamazepine or phenobarbital had breakthrough bleeding (a sign of possible reduced contraceptive efficacy). Most of the 7 patients taking valproate were taking oral combined hormonal contraceptives containing 50 micrograms of **ethinylestradiol**; one was taking less than 50 micrograms, and one was using an oral **progestogen-only contraceptive**. One of the 7 patients had previously experienced breakthrough bleeding while taking phenobarbital, but this stopped when it was replaced with sodium valproate. Two further patients did not have breakthrough bleeding while taking sodium valproate and benzodiazepines, but breakthrough bleeding started when phenytoin was also given.[1]

In a pharmacokinetic study, sodium valproate 200 mg twice daily had no effect on the AUC of a single dose of an oral combined hormonal contraceptive (**ethinylestradiol** 50 micrograms with **levonorgestrel** 250 micrograms) given to women with epilepsy 8 to 16 weeks after they started sodium valproate. However, a 50% *increase* in the peak plasma levels of **ethinylestradiol** was noted.[2]

Conversely, one pregnancy was identified in a woman who took sodium valproate and an oral hormonal contraceptive (unspecified) in the adverse reactions register of the CSM in the UK for the years 1968 to 1984. However, the authors consider this one case to be a chance association.[3]

(b) Valproate efficacy

In 9 women with epilepsy taking valproic acid 500 mg to 1.5 g daily, the serum levels of total and unbound valproic acid were 21% and 41% lower, respectively, during combined hormonal contraceptive intake compared with the pill-free period. These women were taking oral combined hormonal contraceptives containing **ethinylestradiol** and either **gestodene** (5 women) or **drospirenone** (2 women), or the transdermal patch containing **ethinylestradiol** and **norelgestromin** (2 women). The pill-free interval was 7 days in seven women and 4 days in two women.[4] In another study in 12 women taking valproate monotherapy, a very similar median 23.4% lower serum valproate level was seen during the third week of an oral combined hormonal contraceptive cycle when compared with the fourth pill-free week. These women were taking **ethinylestradiol** with either **norethisterone**, **levonorgestrel** or **norgestimate**.[5]

In one case report, lower valproate levels and more frequent seizures occurred in a woman taking an oral combined hormonal contraceptive (**ethinylestradiol** 35 micrograms with **ethynodiol** 1 mg) during the active pill phase, when compared with the inactive 7-day period. Specifically, over a 5-month period, she had 12 seizures during 105 days of active pill use and none during the 35 days of inactive pill use, and total and unbound valproate levels were 36% and 46% lower, respectively, during active pill use.[6] No further cases appear to have been published.

Mechanism

Valproate is metabolised by glucuronide conjugation, and therefore its levels may be reduced due to induction of glucuronosyltransferases by ethinylestradiol. Valproate is an inhibitor of glucuronidation, and might therefore be expected to increase ethinylestradiol levels, but only an increase in maximum levels and not the AUC was seen in the one single-dose study available.

Importance and management

Although specific data are limited, it appears that valproate is unlikely to reduce the efficacy of oral combined hormonal contraceptives. No additional contraceptive precautions are required during concurrent use of valproate and any combined hormonal contraceptives (tablet, patch or vaginal ring). The general relevance of the modest cyclical reduction in valproate levels during active pill taking, and the case report of an increase in seizure frequency is unclear, and further study is needed. However, bear the possibility of this interaction in mind.

1. Sonnen AEH. Sodium valproate and the pill. In: Akimoto H, Kazamatsuri H, Seino M, Ward A, Eds. Advances in Epileptology. New York: Raven Press, 1982: 429–32.
2. Crawford P, Chadwick D, Cleland P, Tjia J, Cowie A, Back DJ, Orme ML'E. The lack of effect of sodium valproate on the pharmacokinetics of oral contraceptive steroids. *Contraception* (1986) 33, 23–9.
3. Back DJ, Grimmer SFM, Orme L'E, Proudlove C, Mann RD, Breckenridge AM. Evaluation of Committee on Safety of Medicines yellow card reports on oral contraceptive-drug interactions with anticonvulsants and antibiotics. *Br J Clin Pharmacol* (1988) 25, 527–32.
4. Galimberti CA, Mazzucchelli I, Arbasino C, Canevini MP, Fattore C, Perucca E. Increased apparent oral clearance of valproic acid during intake of combined contraceptive steroids in women with epilepsy. *Epilepsia* (2006) 47, 1569–72.
5. Herzog AG, Blum AS, Farina EL, Maestri XE, Newman J, Garcia E, Krishnamurthy KB, Hoch DB, Replansky S, Fowler KM, Smithson SD, Dworetzky BA, Bromfield EB. Valproate and lamotrigine level variation with menstrual cycle phase and oral contraceptive use. *Neurology* (2009) 72, 911–14.
6. Herzog AG, Farina EL, Blum AS. Serum valproate levels with oral contraceptive use. *Epilepsia* (2005) 46, 970–1.

Combined hormonal contraceptives + Vigabatrin

Vigabatrin does not appear to alter the pharmacokinetics of ethinylestradiol or levonorgestrel given as an oral combined hormonal contraceptive.

Clinical evidence, mechanism, importance and management

Vigabatrin 3 g daily had no statistically significant effect on the pharmacokinetics of **ethinylestradiol** and **levonorgestrel** in 13 healthy women given a single dose of an oral combined hormonal contraceptive (**ethinylestradiol** 30 micrograms with **levonorgestrel** 150 micrograms); although 2 of the women had a 39% and a 50% fall in the AUC of **ethinylestradiol**. Vigabatrin did not induce hepatic enzymes as assessed by antipyrine clearance and 6β-hydroxycortisol excretion.[1]

This study would seem to confirm the lack of reports of an interaction between combined hormonal contraceptives and vigabatrin; however, the authors of the report introduced a small note of caution because it is not clear whether the reduced **ethinylestradiol** AUCs seen in two of the women resulted from an interaction or were simply normal individual variations.[1] The latter now seems most likely given the lack of subsequent reports of any interaction. No additional contraceptive precautions would seem to be necessary on concurrent use of vigabatrin with any combined hormonal contraceptives (tablet, patch or vaginal ring).

1. Bartoli A, Gatti G, Cipolla G, Barzaghi N, Veliz G, Fattore C, Mumford J, Perucca E. A double-blind, placebo-controlled study on the effect of vigabatrin on in vivo parameters of hepatic microsomal enzyme induction and on the kinetics of steroid oral contraceptives in healthy female volunteers. *Epilepsia* (1997) 38, 702–7.

Combined hormonal contraceptives + Vortioxetine

Vortioxetine does not alter the pharmacokinetics of ethinylestradiol or levonorgestrel when given as an oral combined hormonal contraceptive.

Clinical evidence, mechanism, importance and management

A crossover study in healthy women taking an oral combined hormonal contraceptive (**ethinylestradiol** 30 micrograms with **levonorgestrel** 150 micrograms) and vortioxetine 10 mg daily for 21 days, found that the pharmacokinetics of **ethinylestradiol** and **levonorgestrel** were not altered by vortioxetine.[1]

No dose adjustments would seem necessary on concurrent use of vortioxetine and combined hormonal contraceptives containing ethinylestradiol and levonorgestrel.

1. 1. Chen G, Lee R, Højer AM, Buchbjerg JK, Serenko M, Zhao Z. Pharmacokinetic drug interactions involving vortioxetine (Lu AA21004), a multimodal antidepressant. *Clin Drug Investig* (2013) 33, 727–36.

Combined hormonal contraceptives + Ziprasidone

Ziprasidone does not alter the pharmacokinetics of an oral combined hormonal contraceptive containing ethinylestradiol with levonorgestrel.

Clinical evidence, mechanism, importance and management

In a placebo-controlled, crossover study, 18 healthy women taking an oral combined hormonal contraceptive (**ethinylestradiol** 30 micrograms with **levonorgestrel** 150 micrograms) for at least 3 cycles were also given ziprasidone 20 mg twice daily for 8 days, from day 8 to 15 of a cycle. The only pharmacokinetic change was an increase of about 30 minutes in the time to maximum plasma concentration of **levonorgestrel**, but this is not clinically relevant. On the basis of this pharmacokinetic study, ziprasidone appears unlikely to affect the efficacy of oral combined hormonal contraceptives.[1]

1. Muirhead GJ, Harness J, Holt PR, Oliver S, Anziano RJ. Ziprasidone and the pharmacokinetics of a combined oral contraceptive. *Br J Clin Pharmacol* (2000) 49 (Suppl 1), 49S–56S.

Combined hormonal contraceptives + Zonisamide

Zonisamide does not alter the pharmacokinetics or the ovulation suppressant effect of an oral combined hormonal contraceptive containing ethinylestradiol with norethisterone.

Clinical evidence, mechanism, importance and management

In a study in healthy women taking an oral combined hormonal contraceptive (**ethinylestradiol** 35 micrograms with **norethisterone** 1 mg), zonisamide 100 mg daily titrated to 200 to 400 mg daily taken from day 15 of a cycle to day 13 of the following cycle had no effect on the pharmacokinetics of **ethinylestradiol** or **norethisterone**. There was no change in FSH and LH levels, and the levels of progesterone indicated the absence of ovulation.[1] This suggests that no additional contraceptive precautions are needed during concurrent use of zonisamide and any combined hormonal contraceptive (tablet, patch or vaginal ring).

1. Griffith SG, Dai Y. Effect of zonisamide on the pharmacokinetics and pharmacodynamics of a combination ethinyl estradiol-norethindrone oral contraceptive in healthy women. *Clin Ther* (2004) 26, 2056–65.

Drospirenone-containing contraceptives or HRT + Potassium-sparing drugs

Drospirenone, which is given as the progestogen component of oral combined hormonal contraceptives or HRT, can raise potassium levels, and this effect might be additive with that of other potassium-sparing drugs.

Clinical evidence

(a) Drospirenone in combined hormonal contraceptives

In a small study in 27 women with acne taking a drospirenone-containing oral combined hormonal contraceptive (**ethinylestradiol** 30 micrograms with drospirenone 3 mg) and **spironolactone** 100 mg daily, serum potassium levels remained normal 4 to 6 weeks after starting the contraceptive. Although this study was non-comparative, it does provide some useful evidence about the effect of concurrent use on potassium levels.[1]

In a matched cohort study, there was no difference in the rate of diagnosed hyperkalaemia between 22 429 women who started to take a drospirenone-containing oral combined hormonal contraceptive (**ethinylestradiol** with drospirenone) and 44 858 women who started other oral contraceptives [unspecified] (one versus 4) over an average follow-up of 7.6 months. In addition, there was no difference in the rate of clinical outcomes that could be related to hyperkalaemia.[2]

(b) Drospirenone in HRT

In a controlled study in 24 postmenopausal women taking **enalapril** 10 mg twice daily there was no change in serum potassium levels after taking HRT (**estradiol** 1 mg with drospirenone 3 mg daily) for 14 days, when compared with placebo. In addition, no subject developed hyperkalaemia (defined as a serum potassium greater than 5.5 mmol/L).[3] Similarly, in a larger study in postmenopausal women taking an **ACE inhibitor** or an **angiotensin II receptor antagonist**, there was no statistically significant difference in incidence of hyperkalaemia (potassium level 5.5 mmol/L or more) between those receiving **estradiol** 1 mg with drospirenone 3 mg daily for 28 days and placebo (7.3% versus 2.6%). This study included women with diabetes, women without diabetes, and women without diabetes who were also given a 5-day course of **ibuprofen** 400 mg three times daily.[4] Nevertheless, the UK manufacturer notes that the concurrent use of all three types of medications together (drospirenone in HRT with an **NSAID** and an **ACE inhibitor** or **angiotensin II receptor antagonist**) may cause a small increase in serum potassium, which is more pronounced in diabetic women.[5]

In yet another study in 33 healthy postmenopausal women, there was no difference in the potassium levels between the concurrent use of **estradiol** 1 mg with drospirenone 3 mg daily for 17 days and **indometacin** 50 mg three times daily for the last 5 days, and **indometacin** alone. In addition there was no difference in the incidence of hyperkalaemia (5 women versus 3 women). However, in 14 women, at least one potassium level above 4.4 mmol/L was seen both during combined treatment and with indometacin alone. Of the other women, 12 had raised potassium levels only during the combined treatment, whereas just one woman had a raised potassium level during the use of indometacin alone,[6] which seems to suggest some additive effect.

The US manufacturer also notes a study of the effect of drospirenone 3 mg daily on serum potassium levels in women with normal renal function (11 women) and mild renal impairment (10 women) or moderate renal impairment (7 women). During the study, 7 patients continued to use **potassium-sparing drugs** (not specified). Drospirenone had no significant effect on potassium levels and no hyperkalaemia occurred. However, in 5 of the 7 patients also taking **potassium-sparing drugs**, there was a rise in potassium level of up to 0.33 mmol/L.[7]

Mechanism

Drospirenone, an analogue of spironolactone, has weak antimineralocorticoid and potassium-sparing effects, and therefore may increase the risk of hyperkalaemia if it is given with other drugs that can increase potassium levels. Drospirenone 3 mg is said to have a hyperkalaemic effect similar to that of spironolactone 25 mg.[8]

Importance and management

The risk of hyperkalaemia developing in women taking an oral combined hormonal contraceptive or HRT containing drospirenone with other drugs that can increase potassium levels appears to be low, especially if renal function is normal. In the US, it is recommended that consideration be given to monitoring potassium levels during the first cycle in women [with normal renal function] who regularly take any drugs that increase serum potassium: ACE inhibitors, **aldosterone antagonists**, angiotensin II receptor antagonists, **heparin**, NSAIDs, **potassium-sparing diuretics** and **potassium supplements** are named.[7,8] However, the UK advice for women without renal impairment is to monitor potassium during the first treatment cycle if they are also taking another aldosterone antagonist (e.g. spironolactone and **eplerenone**) or a potassium-sparing diuretic, but there is no requirement for monitoring with ACE inhibitors or NSAIDs.[9] In the UK, if a woman has mild or moderate renal impairment, it is recommended that the potassium level is measured during the first cycle or month of treatment, especially if they are also taking any other drugs that increase serum potassium.[5,9] Note that in the UK, the manufacturers[5,9] contraindicate the use of drospirenone-containing contraceptives in women with severe renal impairment, whereas, in the US,[7,8] its use in renal impairment [to any degree] is contraindicated. However, note that in one survey of 58 US physicians, only 40% of 466 women starting a drospirenone-containing contraceptive and taking concurrent potassium-sparing drugs had a potassium test. Physicians who did not do the test were more likely to disagree with the need for it in patients taking ACE inhibitors, angiotensin II receptor antagonists, heparin and NSAIDs.[10]

For the drospirenone-containing HRT preparation, the UK manufacturer notes that the concurrent use of more than one drug that can raise potassium levels (an NSAID with an ACE inhibitor or angiotensin II receptor antagonist) may cause a small increase in potassium levels, which is more pronounced in diabetic women.[5]

For mention of the risks of hypertension with combined hormonal contraceptives, and the fact that drospirenone-containing HRT appears to slightly decrease blood pressure, see 'Antihypertensives + Hormonal contraceptives', p.1053.

1. Krunic A, Ciurea A, Scheman A. Efficacy and tolerance of acne treatment using both spironolactone and a combined contraceptive containing drospirenone. *J Am Acad Dermatol* (2008) 58, 60–2.
2. Loughlin J, Seeger JD, Eng PM, Foegh M, Clifford CR, Cutone J, Walker AM. Risk of hyperkalemia in women taking ethinylestradiol/drospirenone and other oral contraceptives. *Contraception* (2008) 78, 377–83.
3. Karara AH, Zhang P, Blode H, Schuermann R, Preston R. Effect of drospirenone/estradiol combination product on the serum potassium of mildly hypertensive postmenopausal women maintained on enalapril maleate [Abstract 45]. *J Clin Pharmacol* (2001) 41, 1024.
4. Preston RA, White WB, Pitt B, Bakris G, Norris PM, Hanes V. Effects of drospirenone/17-beta estradiol on blood pressure and potassium balance in hypertensive postmenopausal women. *Am J Hypertens* (2005) 18, 797–804.
5. Angeliq (Drospirenone with Estradiol). Bayer plc. UK Summary of product characteristics, December 2011.
6. Schütt B, Kunz M, Blode H. Coadministration of estradiol/drospirenone and indomethacin does not cause hyperkalemia in healthy postmenopausal women: a randomized open-label crossover study. *J Clin Pharmacol* (2007) 47, 774–81.
7. Angeliq (Drospirenone with Estradiol). Bayer HealthCare Pharmaceuticals, Inc. US Prescribing information, February 2012.
8. Yasmin (Drospirenone with Ethinylestradiol). Bayer HealthCare Pharmaceuticals, Inc. US Prescribing information, April 2010.
9. Yasmin (Drospirenone with Ethinylestradiol). Bayer plc. UK Summary of product characteristics, April 2010.
10. Mona Eng P, Seeger JD, Loughlin J, Oh K, Walker AM. Serum potassium monitoring for users of ethinyl estradiol/drospirenone taking medications predisposing to hyperkalemia: physician compliance and survey of knowledge and attitudes. *Contraception* (2007) 75, 101–7.

Emergency hormonal contraceptives + Antibacterials

The efficacy of levonorgestrel alone given for emergency contraception is not likely to be affected by antibacterials that do not induce liver enzymes. Similarly, the emergency contraceptive efficacy of oral combined hormonal preparations such as norgestrel with ethinylestradiol is also unlikely to be affected by these antibacterials.

Clinical evidence, mechanism, importance and management

(a) Oral combined hormonal preparations

The UK manufacturer of *Schering PC4* has previously stated that the efficacy of **norgestrel** with **ethinylestradiol** may be reduced by **ampicillin** and other antibacterials.[1] This is presumably an extrapolation from the rare cases of combined hormonal contraceptive failure seen with various other antibacterials that do not induce liver enzymes. It was suggested that this could be due to reduced enterohepatic recycling of **ethinylestradiol**; however, this seems unlikely, see 'Combined hormonal contraceptives + Antibacterials', p.1162). Moreover, it has been suggested that it is likely that sufficient hormone is absorbed initially for the emergency contraceptive to be effective[2] (it is taken as 2 doses within 12 hours of each other). No change in recommended dose would therefore be needed if an oral combined hormonal preparation is used for emergency contraception in a woman currently taking antibacterials. However, if the antibacterial and/or the disease being treated causes vomiting, then the usual advice for vomiting should be followed.

Note that rifampicin (rifampin) and rifabutin are likely to reduce the efficacy of oral combined hormonal contraceptives used for emergency contraception, as they induce the metabolism of oestrogens and progestogens, see 'Emergency hormonal contraceptives + Enzyme inducers', below.

Note that the use of an oestrogen with a progestogen as an emergency contraceptive has generally been superseded by a progestogen-only preparation (see below), as the latter is associated with a higher efficacy and less oestrogen-related adverse effects.

(b) Oral progestogen-only preparations

Levonorgestrel is metabolised to inactive substances before it is conjugated,[3] and does not undergo enterohepatic recycling of the active moiety. Therefore, there is no reason to expect that its efficacy as an emergency contraceptive would be affected by antibacterials that alter gut flora and do not induce liver enzymes, see also 'Progestogen-only contraceptives + Antibacterials', p.1197. No particular precautions are necessary with these antibacterials. However, rifampicin (rifampin) and rifabutin are likely to reduce the efficacy of levonorgestrel given as an emergency contraceptive, as they induce the metabolism of progestogens, see 'Emergency hormonal contraceptives + Enzyme inducers', p.1192.

1. Schering PC4 (Norgestrel/ethinylestradiol). Schering Health Care Ltd. UK Summary of product characteristics, July 1995.
2. Elliman A. Interactions with hormonal contraception. *Br J Fam Plann* (2000) 26, 109–11.
3. Levonelle One Step (Levonorgestrel). Bayer plc. UK Summary of product characteristics, March 2010.

Emergency hormonal contraceptives + Enzyme inducers

Two cases of pregnancy, despite the use of emergency hormonal contraception, were attributed to the use of St John's wort. The efficacy of emergency contraception (both levonorgestrel and oral combined hormonal preparations) is likely to be reduced by enzyme inducers that have been shown to affect oral combined hormonal contraceptives, such as rifampicin (rifampin), the enzyme-inducing antiepileptics, and some antiretrovirals.

Clinical evidence, mechanism, importance and management

Between 2000 and 2002 the CSM in the UK had received reports of 2 women taking **St John's wort** who became pregnant despite taking emergency hormonal contraception.[1] One of them had also been taking an oral combined hormonal contraceptive and took *Levonelle-2* (**levonorgestrel**).[1,2]

Various enzyme inducers have specifically been shown to decrease the concentrations of contraceptive steroids and/or reduce their effects on the suppression of ovulation when used as components of combined hormonal contraceptives (see 'Table 28.1', p.1160). This would also be expected when **ethinylestradiol** with **norgestrel**, or **levonorgestrel** alone, are used as emergency hormonal contraceptives. It would be easy to specifically evaluate the pharmacokinetic changes that occur with single doses of emergency hormonal contraceptive products when given with enzyme-inducing drugs, although no such studies appear to have been published. However, it is difficult to envisage a practical study design that would show to what extent this reduced metabolism results in reduced efficacy of emergency contraception.

In the UK, in 2011 the Faculty of Sexual and Reproductive Healthcare guidelines on drug interactions and hormonal contraceptives recommended that, in women requiring emergency contraception while taking enzyme-inducing drugs or within 28 days of stopping them, a **copper IUD** is the most effective method. In women who decline or who are not eligible for a copper IUD, 3 mg of **levonorgestrel** should be given as a single dose (double the usual dose).[3] For a list of drugs that induce the metabolism of contraceptive steroids, to which this advice should be applied, see 'Table 28.1', p.1160. Further, the MHRA in the UK specifically advises that all patients taking hormonal contraceptives for prevention of pregnancy (except IUDs, but probably including emergency hormonal contraceptives) should not take herbal products that contain **St John's wort**.[4] In some countries it is possible to buy emergency hormonal contraception without a prescription; however, in the UK it has been advised that patients taking enzyme inducers should not be supplied the emergency hormonal contraceptive but should be referred to a doctor or family planning service.[5] Given the potential consequences of an unwanted pregnancy, these seem sensible precautions.

For information on the potential for ulipristal, a progesterone receptor modulator used as an emergency contraceptive, to be affected by enzyme inducers, see 'Ulipristal + Miscellaneous', p.1201.

1. Committee on Safety of Medicines. Personal communication, February 15th, 2002.
2. Henderson L, Yue QY, Bergquist C, Gerden B, Arlett P. St John's wort (*Hypericum perforatum*): drug interactions and clinical outcomes. *Br J Clin Pharmacol* (2002) 54, 349–56.
3. Faculty of Sexual and Reproductive Heathcare Guidance. Drug interactions with hormonal contraception: Clinical Effectiveness Unit, January 2011. (Updated January 2012) Available at: http://www.fsrh.org/pdfs/CEUGuidanceDrugInteractionsHormonal.pdf (accessed 20/10/15).
4. Medicines and Healthcare Products Regulatory Agency and the Commission on Human Medicines. St John's wort: interaction with hormonal contraceptives, including implants – reduced contraceptive effect. *Drug Safety Update* (2014) 7, A2. Available at: http://webarchive.nationalarchives.gov.uk/20141205150130/http://www.mhra.gov.uk/home/groups/dsu/documents/publication/con392897.pdf (accessed 20/10/15).
5. Royal Pharmaceutical Society of Great Britain. Practice guidance on the supply of emergency hormonal contraception as a pharmacy medicine. September 2004.

Gestrinone + Enzyme inducers

The manufacturer states that rifampicin (rifampin) and some antiepileptics may reduce the effects of gestrinone.

Clinical evidence, mechanism, importance and management

The manufacturer states that **rifampicin (rifampin)** and **antiepileptics** [not named, but by implication those that are enzyme inducers, see 'Table 28.1', p.1160] may accelerate the metabolism of gestrinone.[1] Be aware that gestrinone may not be as effective if any of these drugs are given concurrently.

1. Dimetriose (Gestrinone). Sanofi-Aventis. UK Summary of product characteristics, February 2008.

Hormonal contraceptives + Danazol or Gestrinone

There is a theoretical risk that the effects of danazol or gestrinone and hormonal contraceptives might be altered or reduced on concurrent use.

Clinical evidence, mechanism, importance and management

(a) Danazol

The manufacturer states that there is a theoretical risk that danazol and exogenously administered oestrogens and/or progestogens, including oral contraceptives, might possibly compete for the same oestrogen, progestogen, and androgen receptors, thereby altering the effects of both drugs.[1] This would also apply to other non-oral forms of hormonal contraceptives, such as progestogen-only implants and injections. As yet there appears to be no direct evidence that any interaction by this mechanism actually occurs. However, as danazol can cause virilisation of a female foetus, the manufacturer advises that reliable non-hormonal contraceptive methods should be used while taking danazol,[2] and, by inference, the avoidance of hormonal contraceptives. Note that although danazol inhibits ovulation, it is not considered reliable enough to be used as a hormonal contraceptive alone.[1,3,4]

(b) Gestrinone

The manufacturer states that the effects of gestrinone may possibly be modified by the concurrent use of oral contraceptives.[5] As yet there appears to be no direct evidence that any interaction by this mechanism actually occurs. However, because of this and because high doses of gestrinone have been shown to be embryotoxic in some *animal* species, they strongly emphasise the importance of using barrier methods of contraception while taking gestrinone,[5] and, by inference, the avoidance of hormonal contraceptives. Note that although gestrinone inhibits ovulation in some women, it is not considered reliable enough to be used as a hormonal contraceptive alone.[5]

1. Sterling-Winthrop, Personal communication 1990.
2. Danol (Danazol). Sanofi. UK Summary of product characteristics, May 2012.
3. Greenblatt RB, Oettinger M, Borenstein R, Bohler CS-S. Influence of danazol (100 mg) on conception and contraception. *J Reprod Med* (1974) 13, 201–3.
4. Colle ML, Greenblatt RB. Contraceptive properties of danazol. *J Reprod Med* (1976) 17, 98–102.
5. Dimetriose (Gestrinone). Sanofi-Aventis. UK Summary of product characteristics, February 2008.

Hormonal contraceptives + Griseofulvin

The effects of the oral contraceptives (unspecified) may possibly be disturbed (either intermenstrual bleeding or amenorrhoea) if griseofulvin is also given. A few isolated reports describe women taking oral contraceptives (combined or unspecified) who became pregnant while taking griseofulvin.

Clinical evidence

In 1984, regulatory authorities in the UK and the Netherlands noted that they had received a total of 22 reports of possible interactions between oral contraceptives and griseofulvin. These included 15 reports of transient intermenstrual bleeding and 5 of amenorrhoea, occurring during the first or second cycle, after griseofulvin 500 mg to 1 g daily was started. Four of these patients were rechallenged with griseofulvin (2 with intermenstrual bleeding and 2 with amenorrhoea) and all developed their original reactions. The other two women were reported to have become pregnant while taking griseofulvin and a sulfonamide (co-trimoxazole in one instance and an unknown sulfonamide in the other, see also 'Combined hormonal contraceptives + Antibacterials', p.1162).[1] Another case of contraceptive failure on concurrent use of griseofulvin has been reported from an analysis of the database of the CSM in the UK from 1968 to 1984,[2] but note this case may be included in the two already reported.[1] One other case report describes a woman taking an oral, triphasic combined hormonal contraceptive who became pregnant about 2 months after she started to take griseofulvin 330 mg twice daily,[3] and another report describes a woman taking an oral contraceptive who became pregnant 6 weeks after starting to take griseofulvin 500 mg daily for 3 months and a 7-day course of erythromycin,[4] see also 'Combined hormonal contraceptives + Antibacterials', p.1162. Irregular menses and reduced menstrual flow have been described in another woman taking an oral combined hormonal contraceptive (**ethinylestradiol** 35 micrograms with **norethisterone** 500 micrograms to 1 mg) with griseofulvin 250 to 500 mg daily. When the contraceptive was substituted with another with a higher oestrogen dose (**ethinylestradiol** 50 micrograms with **norgestrel** 500 micrograms), the menstrual cycle became normal again.[5]

Mechanism

Not understood. Early evidence led to the suggestion that griseofulvin may possibly induce the activity of the liver enzymes concerned with the metabolism of the contraceptive steroids, thereby reducing their effects.[1] For this reason, griseofulvin has often been classified as an enzyme inducer. However, there is no clinical evidence to support this. The apparent lack of interactions of griseofulvin with many other drugs that are substrates of liver enzymes suggests that griseofulvin is not a clinically important enzyme inducer, although this can only be confirmed by a controlled clinical study.

Importance and management

Information about an interaction between griseofulvin and oral contraceptives is very limited, but there is some evidence to suggest that menstrual disturbances might occur. The risk of contraceptive failure is uncertain but probably very small. However, it is important to ensure adequate contraception during and for one month after taking griseofulvin because it can induce aneuploidy (abnormal segregation of chromosomes during cell division), which carries the potential risk of teratogenicity.[6] Therefore, for maximal contraceptive protection, additional contraceptive measures (such as a barrier method) should be used routinely with oral combined hormonal contraceptives or oral progestogen-only contraceptives while taking griseofulvin and for one month afterwards.

It has been suggested that **oral progestogen-only contraceptives** are not the contraceptive of choice in those taking griseofulvin, not because of reduced efficacy, but because of increased menstrual irregularities.[7]

1. van Dijke CPH, Weber JCP. Interaction between oral contraceptives and griseofulvin. *BMJ* (1984) 288, 1125–6.
2. Back DJ, Grimmer SFM, Orme ML'E, Proudlove C, Mann RD, Breckenridge AM. Evaluation of Committee on Safety of Medicines yellow card reports on oral contraceptive-drug interactions with anticonvulsants and antibiotics. *Br J Clin Pharmacol* (1988) 25, 527–32.
3. Côté J. Interaction of griseofulvin and oral contraceptives. *J Am Acad Dermatol* (1990) 22, 124–5.
4. Bollen M. Use of antibiotics when taking the oral contraceptive pill. *Aust Fam Physician* (1995) 24, 928–9.
5. McDaniel PA, Caldroney RD. Oral contraceptives and griseofulvin interaction. *Drug Intell Clin Pharm* (1986) 20, 384.
6. Committee on Safety of Medicines/Medicines Control Agency. Griseofulvin (Fulcin, Grisovin): contraceptive precautions. *Current Problems* (1996) 22, 8.
7. McCann MF, Potter LS. Progestin-only contraception: a comprehensive review. *Contraception* (1994) 50 (Suppl 1), S1–S198.

Hormonal contraceptives + NRTIs

Tenofovir does not alter the pharmacokinetics of ethinylestradiol or norgestimate from an oral combined hormonal contraceptive. Hormonal contraception (oral combined hormonal contraceptives or depot medroxyprogesterone acetate) does not alter the pharmacokinetics of zidovudine.

Clinical evidence and mechanism

(a) Tenofovir

In a study in 20 women taking an oral combined hormonal contraceptive (**ethinylestradiol** with **norgestimate**), tenofovir disoproxil fumarate 300 mg daily for 7 days from day 15 of a cycle had no effect on the pharmacokinetics of **ethinylestradiol** or the active metabolite of **norgestimate**. The pharmacokinetics of tenofovir in this study did not differ from historical data suggesting that the contraceptive does not alter tenofovir pharmacokinetics.[1]

(b) Zidovudine

In a study in 14 women, there was no difference in the AUCs of either plasma zidovudine or intracellular zidovudine phosphorylates when zidovudine 200 mg three times daily for 7 days was given before or after starting hormonal contraception. One dose of the zidovudine was given intravenously. There was a modest 40% increase in the AUC ratio of glucuronidated zidovudine to zidovudine after intravenous administration only; however, this was not statistically significant. Six women were given an oral combined hormonal contraceptive (**ethinylestradiol** 35 micrograms with **norethisterone** 1 mg) and 8 women were given depot **medroxyprogesterone acetate**. There were no differences in any of the pharmacokinetic parameters between the two types of contraceptive, although note that the study was insufficiently powered to reliably assess this.[2] It had been expected that contraception would increase the zidovudine AUC because an *in vitro* study found that **ethinylestradiol** inhibited the glucuronidation of zidovudine by 50% or more.[3] Although the clinical study included only a small number of women taking a oral combined hormonal contraceptive, it does discount a marked effect of this on zidovudine exposure. Note also that other drugs that had a similar effect *in vitro* did not alter zidovudine pharmacokinetics in subsequent clinical studies, see 'NRTIs; Zidovudine + Drugs that inhibit glucuronidation', p.985.

Importance and management

Tenofovir does not alter the pharmacokinetics of oral combined hormonal contraceptives, and would not therefore be expected to alter their efficacy by this mechanism. Oral combined hormonal contraceptives and depot medroxyprogesterone acetate do not appear to alter zidovudine exposure. There appears to be no published evidence at present of any clinically relevant interactions between the other NRTIs (**abacavir, didanosine, emtricitabine, lamivudine, stavudine,** and **zalcitabine**) and hormonal contraceptives, and note that no pharmacokinetic interaction would be expected. A study[4] found no evidence to suggest that hormonal contraceptives (mostly oral combined hormonal contraceptives or depot medroxyprogesterone acetate) affect the efficacy of HAART. The specific HAART drugs were not named; however, most patients were noted to be on a regimen containing an NRTI and a HIV-protease inhibitor, but no NNRTI.

Note that whatever other methods of contraception are being used, barrier methods are also advisable to reduce the risk of HIV transmission.

1. Kearney BP, Mathias A. Lack of effect of tenofovir disoproxil fumarate on pharmacokinetics of hormonal contraceptives. *Pharmacotherapy* (2009) 29, 924–9.
2. Aweeka FT, Rosenkranz SL, Segal Y, Coombs RW, Bardeguez A, Thevanayagam L, Lizak P, Aberg J, Watts DH; NIAID AIDS Clinical Trials Group. The impact of sex and contraceptive therapy on the plasma and intracellular pharmacokinetics of zidovudine. *AIDS* (2006) 20, 1833–41.
3. Sim SM, Back DJ, Breckenridge AM. The effect of various drugs on the glucuronidation of zidovudine (azidothymidine, AZT) by human liver microsomes. *Br J Clin Pharmacol* (1991) 32, 17–21.
4. Chu JH, Gange SJ, Anastos K, Minkoff H, Cejtin H, Bacon M, Levine A, Greenblatt RM. Hormonal contraceptive use and the effectiveness of highly active antiretroviral therapy. *Am J Epidemiol* (2005) 161, 881–90.

Hormonal contraceptives + Orlistat

Orlistat does not alter the suppression of ovulation in women taking oral combined hormonal contraceptives. However, an isolated pregnancy has been reported in a woman taking an oral combined hormonal contraceptive with orlistat. Severe orlistat-induced diarrhoea is predicted to reduce the bioavailability of contraceptive steroids.

Clinical evidence

In a crossover study, 20 healthy women taking an oral combined hormonal contraceptive were given **orlistat** 120 mg three times daily or a placebo on days one to 23 of two menstrual cycles. Orlistat had no effect on ovulation (measured by LH and progesterone levels). The contraceptives used by all subjects contained **ethinylestradiol** [dose not stated], but the progestogens differed: 10 contained **desogestrel,** 4 **levonorgestrel**, 3 **gestodene**, 2 **cyproterone acetate** and one **lynestrenol**.[1]

However, there is a brief published case of a woman who had been taking a low-dose oral combined hormonal contraceptive (**ethinylestradiol** 20 micrograms with **desogestrel** 150 micrograms) for 2 years who was found to be pregnant within 9 weeks of starting to take orlistat 120 mg three times daily.[2]

Mechanism

The UK manufacturer states that orlistat may indirectly reduce the bioavailability of oral contraceptives (as it can cause severe diarrhoea), and that this may lead to unexpected pregnancies in individual cases.[3] The one published case does not mention to what extent the woman had orlistat-induced diarrhoea.

Importance and management

It seems feasible that if orlistat causes appreciable diarrhoea this could increase the risk of contraceptive failure with **oral contraceptives**, whether combined or progestogen-only. Therefore, the UK manufacturer recommends using an additional contraceptive method in case patients develop severe diarrhoea.[3] Note that the contraceptive effect of the combined hormonal contraceptive given as a **patch** is said not to be affected by diarrhoea.

1. Hartmann D, Güzelhan C, Zuiderwijk PBM, Odink J. Lack of interaction between orlistat and oral contraceptives. *Eur J Clin Pharmacol* (1996) 50, 421–4.
2. Peleg R. Caution when using oral contraceptive pills with orlistat. *Isr Med Assoc J* (2000) 2, 712.
3. Xenical (Orlistat). Roche Products Ltd. UK Summary of product characteristics, April 2014.

Hormonal contraceptives + Proton pump inhibitors

Lansoprazole and pantoprazole do not alter the ovulation suppressant effect, and lansoprazole does not alter the pharmacokinetics, of oral combined hormonal contraceptives containing ethinylestradiol with levonorgestrel. Oral combined hormonal contraceptives slightly inhibit the metabolism of omeprazole, but the levonorgestrel oral progestogen-only contraceptive appears to have no effect.

Clinical evidence

(a) Lansoprazole

In a placebo-controlled, crossover study, 24 healthy women were given an oral combined hormonal contraceptive (**ethinylestradiol** 30 micrograms with **levonorgestrel** 150 micrograms) for two monthly cycles, with lansoprazole 60 mg daily and placebo for one cycle each. The AUC of the contraceptive steroids were not altered by lansoprazole, and levels of FSH, LH and progesterone where unchanged, indicating that ovulation did not occur.[1] The manufacturer has information about three other unpublished studies in a total of 59 women, which have also found no evidence to suggest that lansoprazole interacts with oral contraceptives in any way which would affect their reliability.[2]

(b) Omeprazole

A study in 10 healthy women given an oral combined hormonal contraceptive (**ethinylestradiol** 40 micrograms with **levonorgestrel** 75 micrograms) for 10 days found that the contraceptive increased the AUC of a single 40-mg dose of omeprazole (*Losec MUPS*) by 38%. This increase was not seen when the subjects were given

levonorgestrel 60 micrograms daily alone for 10 days, taken as two tablets of a progestogen-only oral contraceptive.[3] Similarly, in a pharmacokinetic probe study in 10 women, an oral combined hormonal contraceptive (**ethinylestradiol** 35 micrograms with **norgestimate** 180 to 250 micrograms) caused about a 50% increase in the ratio of omeprazole to its metabolite 5-hydroxyomeprazole, which indicates an inhibition of CYP2C19-mediated omeprazole metabolism.[4] This confirms earlier similar findings of a higher omeprazole to hydroxyomeprazole ratio in women taking oral contraceptives when compared with non-users of these contraceptives.[5]

(c) Pantoprazole

A study over four menstrual cycles was completed by 64 women. The women were confirmed to be ovulating before taking a low-dose triphasic oral combined hormonal contraceptive (**ethinylestradiol** with **levonorgestrel**), and not ovulating during contraceptive use. They continued not ovulating during a cycle when pantoprazole 40 mg daily was also given, indicating that pantoprazole did not affect the ovulation suppressant effect of the oral combined hormonal contraceptive.[6]

Mechanism

Ethinylestradiol appears to be a weak inhibitor of CYP2C19, by which omeprazole is principally metabolised.[4,5] As this is also the main route of metabolism of most of the other proton pump inhibitors (see 'Gastrointestinal drugs', p.1135), they might be similarly affected. Levonorgestrel does not have this effect.

Importance and management

The proton pump inhibitors studied (lansoprazole, pantoprazole) do not alter the suppression of ovulation in women taking oral combined hormonal contraceptives, and would therefore not be expected to alter their reliability. There is nothing to suggest that omeprazole will be any different. No additional contraceptive precautions would therefore be required with any combined hormonal contraceptive (tablets, patch or vaginal ring) on the concurrent use of these proton pump inhibitors.

Oral combined hormonal contraceptives increase omeprazole exposure (and might similarly affect some other proton pump inhibitors), but the effect is slight and therefore not clinically relevant. Omeprazole is used as a probe substrate to assess the activity of drugs on CYP2C19. This study therefore suggests that ethinylestradiol is a weak inhibitor of CYP2C19. The oral progestogen-only contraceptive containing levonorgestrel does not have this effect.

1. Fuchs W, Sennewald R, Klotz U. Lansoprazole does not affect the bioavailability of oral contraceptives. *Br J Clin Pharmacol* (1994) 38, 376–80.
2. Wyeth, Personal communication, February 1998.
3. Palovaara S, Tybring G, Laine K. The effect of ethinyloestradiol and levonorgestrel on the CYP2C19-mediated metabolism of omeprazole in healthy female subjects. *Br J Clin Pharmacol* (2003) 56, 232–7.
4. Shelepova T, Nafziger AN, Victory J, Kashuba ADM, Rowland E, Zhang Y, Sellers E, Kearns G, Leeder JS, Gaedigk A, Bertino JS. Effect of a triphasic oral contraceptive on drug-metabolizing enzyme activity as measured by the validated Cooperstown 5+1 cocktail. *J Clin Pharmacol* (2005) 45, 1413–21.
5. Laine K, Tybring G, Bertilsson L. No sex-related differences but significant inhibition by oral contraceptives of CYP2C19 activity as measured by the probe drugs mephenytoin and omeprazole in healthy Swedish white subjects. *Clin Pharmacol Ther* (2000) 68, 151–9.
6. Middle MV, Müller FO, Schall R, Hundt HKL, Mogilnicka EM, Beneke PC. Effect of pantoprazole on ovulation suppression by a low-dose hormonal contraceptive. *Clin Drug Invest* (1995) 9, 54–6.

Hormonal contraceptives + Retinoids

The pharmacokinetics and/or ovulation suppressant effect of oral combined hormonal contraceptives are not affected by acitretin, alitretinoin, etretinate, isotretinoin or tazarotene, all given orally. A woman taking an oral progestogen-only contraceptive had raised progestogen levels after starting acitretin. The adverse effects of isotretinoin on lipids may be additive with those of oral contraceptives.

Clinical evidence

(a) Combined hormonal contraceptives

1. Acitretin. Eight women taking an oral combined hormonal contraceptive (**ethinylestradiol** with **levonorgestrel**) were given acitretin 25 to 40 mg daily for at least two cycles. The suppression of ovulation in response to the contraceptive was not affected by acitretin, as assessed by plasma progesterone levels.[1]

2. Alitretinoin. In a study in 14 women taking an oral combined hormonal contraceptive (**ethinylestradiol** with **norgestimate**), the use of alitretinoin 40 mg daily for one cycle did not alter the pharmacokinetics of ethinylestradiol. There was a negligible 12% reduction in the AUC of main metabolite of norgestimate. No women ovulated in the two cycles without concurrent alitretinoin, but one subject was presumed to have ovulated during the cycle they took alitretinoin, as assessed by progestogen levels. This rate of ovulation was considered consistent with the expected rate of 'escape' ovulations for oral combined hormonal contraceptives. The AUC of alitretinoin was a negligible 14% lower when given with the contraceptive when compared with alitretinoin alone.[2]

3. Etretinate. In a study in 12 women taking an oral combined hormonal contraceptive (**ethinylestradiol** with **levonorgestrel**, **norethisterone**, **norgestrel**, or **cyproterone**) the use of **etretinate** 0.7 to 1 mg/kg did not affect the suppression of ovulation in response to the contraceptive.[3]

4. Isotretinoin. In a pharmacokinetic study in 9 women taking an oral combined hormonal contraceptive, the mean plasma levels of **ethinylestradiol** and **levonorgestrel** were not changed in the first and third cycle after starting isotretinoin 500 micrograms/kg when compared with before starting the retinoid. Suppression of ovulation was maintained.[4] In another study in 26 women taking a triphasic, oral combined hormonal contraceptive (**ethinylestradiol** 35 micrograms with **norethisterone** 500 micrograms to 1 mg), the pharmacokinetics of the contraceptive steroids were almost identical when isotretinoin 1 mg/kg daily was also given. The only changes were a 9% decrease in the ethinylestradiol AUC on day 6 (but not day 20), and an 11% decrease in the maximum level of norethisterone on day 20. FSH showed a significant 44% decline (day 20) after starting isotretinoin, suggesting a greater suppression of ovulation, and there were no changes in LH or progesterone. However large inter-patient variability in the results was noted and 2 patients had increases in progesterone levels, possibly indicating that ovulation had occurred, one of these in the phase before isotretinoin treatment (noted to be non-compliant), and one during isotretinoin.[5]

The US manufacturer noted that pregnancies have occurred in women taking isotretinoin while using combined hormonal contraceptives, given orally, as the patch, or as the vaginal ring, and that these reports are more frequent in women using only one form of contraception.[6]

The adverse effects of isotretinoin and any combined hormonal contraceptives on plasma lipids may be additive. A case-control study found that women who had hypertriglyceridaemia and/or hypercholesterolaemia while taking isotretinoin were 2 to 12 times as likely to be also taking an oral contraceptive (unspecified).[7]

5. Tazarotene. In a study in 27 healthy women taking an oral combined hormonal contraceptive (**ethinylestradiol** 35 micrograms with **norethisterone** 1 mg), *oral* tazarotene 1.1 mg daily for 27 days did not alter the AUC of ethinylestradiol or norethisterone. In addition, measurements of FSH and LH suggested that ovulation suppression was maintained.[8] Similar findings were presented in an almost identical study using a higher 6 mg daily dose of *oral* tazarotene.[8]

(b) Progestogen-only contraceptives

One woman taking an oral progestogen-only contraceptive (**levonorgestrel** 30 micrograms) had a significant increase in her progesterone levels after 3 cycles while taking **acitretin** 400 micrograms/kg daily. Plasma progesterone levels rose from 2.15 nanograms/mL before taking the **acitretin** to 3.87 to 13.46 nanograms/mL with **acitretin**. This rise in progesterone levels was taken as evidence that ovulation had occurred.[1]

The US manufacturer noted that pregnancies have occurred in women taking **isotretinoin** while using contraceptive implants or injections.[6]

Mechanism, importance and management

The available data suggest that these *oral* retinoids do not alter the pharmacokinetics or ovulation suppressant effects of oral combined hormonal contraceptives, and are therefore unlikely to alter their contraceptive efficacy. The very small reduction in ethinylestradiol exposure seen in one study with isotretinoin on one day is not clinically relevant, and the rate of one women in 14 who was presumed to have ovulated while taking alitretinoin was considered to be consistent with the expected rate of escape ovulations for oral combined hormonal contraceptives. The case with acitretin suggests that it might reduce the efficacy of progestogen-only oral contraceptives. However, note that oral progestogen-only contraceptives do not reliably suppress ovulation in all cycles, and that this is not considered their primary mechanism of action (see 'Hormonal contraceptives and Sex hormones', p.1159). The single report cannot therefore be taken as proof that acitretin reduces the efficacy of progestogen-only contraceptives.

Also note that because the retinoids are established human teratogens, it is very important that women taking them systemically do not become pregnant. For this reason, oral progestogen-only contraceptives are generally not considered suitable for use with oral retinoids.[9] Unless contraindicated, oral combined hormonal contraceptives are considered appropriate contraceptives for use with systemic retinoids.[9,10] The oral combined hormonal contraceptive should be started one month before the oral retinoid is given, and continued for one month after stopping alitretinoin,[11] isotretinoin,[10] and **tretinoin**,[12] for 2 years after stopping etretinate,[9] and for at least 2 years (UK manufacturer[13]) or 3 years (US manufacturer[14] and British Association of Dermatologists[15]) after stopping acitretin. In the US, it is standard practice to mandate that a second form of contraception, such as a barrier method, should also be used,[6,14] and this is also advised by the British Association of Dermatologists for isotretinoin,[10] and is also preferred by the UK manufacturers of alitretinoin,[11] and isotretinoin.[16] This is because, even though oral combined hormonal methods of contraception are highly effective, they do, on rare occasions, fail.[17] Because of the very small reduction in ethinylestradiol exposure in one study with isotretinoin and the wide variability in hormonal levels, the authors state that their results reinforce the advice of using two forms of contraception.[5] Note that an oral combined hormonal contraceptive containing a non-androgenic (third generation) progestogen (e.g. desogestrel, gestodene, norgestimate) is preferred, as these have less detrimental effects on lipids,[9] and some favour the use of the anti-androgen cyproterone.[18] Some UK authors consider that, given the continuing rare cases of contraceptive failure in women prescribed isotretinoin and using oral combined hormonal contraceptives, that parenteral progestogen-only contraceptives (depot injections, implants, the levonorgestrel-releasing intra-uterine system) might be preferable as these are more effective contraceptives than oral combined hormonal contraceptives.[19]

The currently available formulations of **tazarotene** are for topical use, and, on the basis of the data for *oral* tazarotene, these would not be expected to interact with combined hormonal contraceptives. The manufacturers advise that women of child bearing age should use adequate contraception while using topical tazarotene, because of the theoretical teratogenic risk.[20,21]

1. Berbis Ph, Bun H, Geiger JM, Rognin C, Durand A, Serradimigni A, Hartmann D, Privat Y. Acitretin (RO10-1670) and oral contraceptives: interaction study. *Arch Dermatol Res* (1988) 280, 388–9.

2. Schmitt-Hoffman AH, Roos B, Sauer J, Schleimer M, Schoetzau A, Leese PT, Weidekamm E, Maares J. Influence of alitretinoin on the pharmacokinetics of the oral contraceptive ethinyl estradiol/norgestimate. *Clin Exp Dermatol* (2011) 36 (Suppl 2), 4–11.
3. Berbis P, Bounameaux Y, Rognin C, Hartmann D, Privat Y. Study on the influence of etretinate on biologic activity of oral contraceptives. *J Am Acad Dermatol* (1987) 17, 302–3.
4. Orme M, Back DJ, Shaw MA, Allen WL, Tjia J, Cunliffe WJ, Jones DH. Isotretinoin and contraception. *Lancet* (1984) ii, 752–3.
5. Hendrix CW, Jackson KA, Whitmore E, Guidos A, Kretzer R, Liss CM, Shah LP, Khoo K-C, McLane J, Trapnell CB. The effect of isotretinoin on the pharmacokinetics and pharmacodynamics of ethinyl estradiol and norethindrone. *Clin Pharmacol Ther* (2004) 75, 464–75.
6. Accutane (Isotretinoin). Roche Laboratories Inc. US Prescribing information, November 2008.
7. Chen Y, Xue S, Dai W, LaBraico J. Evaluation of serum triglyceride and cholesterol levels from isotretinoin therapy with concomitant oral contraceptives. *Pharmacoepidemiol Drug Safety* (1995) 4, 91–6.
8. Yu Z, Yu D, Walker PS, Tang-Liu DD-S. Tazarotene does not affect the pharmacokinetics and efficacy of a norethindrone/ethinylestradiol oral contraceptive. *Clin Pharmacokinet* (2004) 43, 673–84.
9. Ceyrac DL, Serfaty D, Lefrancq H. Retinoids and contraception. *Dermatology* (1992) 184, 161–70.
10. Goodfield MJD, Cox NH, Bowser A, McMillan JC, Millard LG, Simpson NB, Ormerod AD. Advice on the safe introduction and continued use of isotretinoin in the UK 2010. *Br J Dermatol* (2010) 162, 1172–9. Available at: http://www.bad.org.uk/healthcare-professionals/clinical-standards/clinical-guidelines (accessed (21/10/15).
11. Toctino (Alitretinoin). Basilea Pharmaceutica. UK Summary of product characteristics, July 2014.
12. Vesanoid (Tretinoin). Roche Products Ltd. UK Summary of product characteristics, May 2015.
13. Neotigason (Acitretin). Actavis UK Ltd. UK Summary of product characteristics, February 2015.
14. Soriatane (Acitretin). Stiefel Labs, Inc. US Prescribing information, May 2015.
15. Ormerod AD, Campalani E, Goodfield MJD. British Association of Dermatologists guidelines on the efficacy and use of acitretin in dermatology. *Br J Dermatol* (2010) 162, 952–63. Available at: http://www.bad.org.uk/healthcare-professionals/clinical-standards/clinical-guidelines (accessed 21/10/15).
16. Roaccutane (Isotretinoin). Roche Products Ltd. UK Summary of product characteristics, January 2012.
17. Perlman SE, Leach EE, Dominguez L, Ruszkowski AM, Rudy SJ. "Be smart, be safe, be sure". The revised pregnancy prevention program for women on isotretinoin. *J Reprod Med* (2001), 46 (Suppl), 179–85.
18. Holmes SC, Bankowska U, Mackie RM. The prescription of isotretinoin to women: is every precaution taken? *Br J Dermatol* (1998) 138, 450–5.
19. Kanelleas AI, Thornton S, Berth-Jones J. Suggestions for effective contraception in isotretinoin therapy. *Br J Clin Pharmacol* (2009) 67, 137–8.
20. Zorac (Tazarotene). Allergan Ltd. UK Summary of product characteristics, May 2009.
21. Tazorac Gel (Tazarotene). Allergan, Inc. US Prescribing information, March 2011.

Hormonal contraceptives + Thalidomide and related drugs

The pharmacokinetics of ethinylestradiol and norethisterone, given as an oral combined hormonal contraceptive, are not affected by thalidomide. The concurrent use of combined hormonal contraceptives with thalidomide, or the related drugs lenalidomide and pomalidomide, are associated with a theoretical increased risk of thromboembolic events.

Clinical evidence

In studies in 10 women who had undergone surgical sterilisation and 10 postmenopausal women, the pharmacokinetics of single doses of an oral combined hormonal contraceptive (**ethinylestradiol** 70 micrograms with **norethisterone** 2 mg) were not affected by pretreatment with thalidomide 200 mg daily for 3 weeks.[1,2]

Mechanism

No pharmacokinetic interaction would be anticipated. Thalidomide and the related drugs lenalidomide and pomalidomide are known to cause venous and arterial thrombosis, and this is also a rare adverse effect of combined hormonal contraceptives and HRT. Therefore, the risk of thrombotic events might be additive when these drugs are used together.

Importance and management

These studies indicate that thalidomide is unlikely to have a pharmacokinetic interaction with combined hormonal contraceptives (tablets, patch or vaginal ring), and would not therefore reduce the efficacy of these contraceptives via that mechanism.

Note that thalidomide, and its structurally related drugs **lenalidomide** and **pomalidomide** are powerful teratogens, and therefore it is essential that women of child-bearing age use reliable contraception while taking these drugs. The UK manufacturers of thalidomide, lenalidomide, and pomalidomide advise using one reliable contraceptive method for at least 4 weeks before starting these drugs, during their use, and for 4 weeks after stopping.[3-5] In the US, the manufacturers of thalidomide, lenalidomide, and pomalidomide both mandate the use of two methods of contraception, which must include one highly effective method (they include all hormonal methods of contraception) with an additional contraceptive method, such as a barrier method.[6-8] However, the UK manufacturers of thalidomide, lenalidomide, and pomalidomide advise against the concurrent use of combined hormonal contraceptives, as they consider that the increased risk of thromboembolic events in patients receiving thalidomide, lenalidomide, or pomalidomide for multiple myeloma might be further increased.[3-5] They state that, if a hormonal contraceptive is used, progestogen-only contraceptives should be used, and they specifically recommend implants, depot injections, the levonorgestrel-containing intra-uterine system or an oral progestogen that inhibits ovulation (oral desogestrel).[3-5] In contrast, the US manufacturers make no mention of the theoretical increased risk of thrombosis specifically with combined hormonal contraceptives, and do not exclude their use (in conjunction with another form of contraception).[6-8]

It must also be borne in mind in women taking thalidomide, lenalidomide, or pomalidomide, that the reliability of some hormonal contraceptives might be compromised by the concurrent use of other drugs. For example, the UK manufacturer of lenalidomide[4] suggests that, as lenalidomide should be taken with dexamethasone, the possibility that the contraceptive efficacy of oral contraceptives might be reduced cannot be excluded. This is because they state that dexamethasone is a weak to moderate inducer of CYP3A4, by which contraceptive steroids are metabolised. However, there appears to be no evidence that dexamethasone interacts to clinically relevant extent with any drugs by this mechanism, and the manufacturer does not suggest any changes in their recommended hormonal contraceptives on the basis of this interaction.

1. Trapnell CB, Donahue SR, Collins JM, Flockhart DA, Thacker D, Abernethy DR. Thalidomide does not alter the pharmacokinetics of ethinyl estradiol and norethindrone. *Clin Pharmacol Ther* (1998) 64, 597–602.
2. Scheffler MR, Colburn W, Kook KA, Thomas SD. Thalidomide does not alter estrogen-progesterone hormone single dose pharmacokinetics. *Clin Pharmacol Ther* (1999) 65, 483–90.
3. Thalidomide Celgene (Thalidomide). Celgene Ltd. UK Summary of product characteristics, June 2014.
4. Revlimid (Lenalidomide). Celgene Ltd. UK Summary of product characteristics, March 2015.
5. Imnovid (Pomalidomide). Celgene Ltd. UK Summary of product characteristics, May 2015.
6. Thalomid (Thalidomide). Celgene Corporation. US Prescribing information, June 2014.
7. Revlimid (Lenalidomide). Celgene Corp. US Prescribing information, February 2015.
8. Pomalyst (Pomalidomide). Celgene Corporation. US Prescribing information, April 2015.

Hormonal contraceptives + Tobacco or Nicotine

There is some evidence that smoking tobacco increases the risk of breakthrough bleeding with oral combined hormonal contraceptives, although smoking appears not to alter contraceptive steroid levels. The risk of cardiovascular disease in women taking oral combined hormonal contraceptives is greatly increased if they smoke, particularly in the older age group. Oral combined hormonal contraceptives may slightly increase nicotine metabolism.

Clinical evidence

(a) Cardiovascular effects

Early after the introduction of **oral combined hormonal contraceptives** it was realised that they increase the risk of cardiovascular disease, such as thromboembolism, myocardial infarction, and stroke, and that the risks were substantially increased in women who also smoked.[1-5] For example, one of these studies found a relative risk of non-fatal myocardial infarction in women taking an oral contraceptive (unspecified) of 39 in heavy smokers compared with 4.5 in non-smokers.[4] Another study found a relative risk of subarachnoid haemorrhage in women taking oral contraceptives (unspecified) of 22 for smokers compared with 6.5 for non-smokers.[5] Heavy smokers (who smoke more than 15 cigarettes daily) have a threefold increased risk of myocardial infarction and a twofold increase in the risk of stroke compared with non-smokers, and these risks are further increased by the use of oral combined hormonal contraceptives.[6] A study involving 17 032 women aged 25 to 39 years at entry, who had used oral contraceptives (mainly combined preparations containing 50 micrograms of oestrogen), a diaphragm, or an intrauterine device, found that the risk of death from ischaemic heart disease was slightly, but not statistically significantly, raised in all oral contraceptive users. However, smoking had a substantial effect on mortality from ischaemic heart disease: in heavy smokers (more that 15 cigarettes daily) the mortality rate ratios for oral hormonal contraceptive use for 48 months or less, for 49 to 96 months, and for 97 months or more compared with non-use were 2.4, 4.8, and 2.8, respectively.[7]

(b) Contraceptive efficacy

An analysis of data from three large clinical studies in a total of 2 956 women found that smoking was associated with an increased incidence of spotting and bleeding in users of **oral combined hormonal contraceptives**. The relative risk was 1.3 during the first cycle of use and increased to 1.9 by the sixth cycle.[8] Similarly, in a study of women who became pregnant while taking oral contraceptives, smokers were more likely to have menstrual disturbances, and smokers taking an oral combined hormonal contraceptive had a 20% greater pill failure rate than expected.[9] This association was not noted for **oral progestogen-only contraceptive** failure.[9] Conversely, in a large cohort study in the UK, the failure rate of oral contraceptives (unspecified) was not increased in smokers.[10]

In one study in 311 women taking oral contraceptives, the plasma levels of **ethinylestradiol** and **norgestrel** were similar in smokers and non-smokers.[11] In another study in healthy women, there was no difference in levonorgestrel clearance between smokers and non-smokers, and variable evidence for an increase or decrease in **ethinylestradiol** clearance in smokers compared with non-smokers (45% decrease in ethinylestradiol clearance with a single dose of an oral combined hormonal contraceptive and a 54% increase in ethinylestradiol clearance with steady-state oral combined hormonal contraceptive).[12]

(c) Nicotine metabolism

In a non-randomised comparison, the metabolism of nicotine after a single intravenous infusion was slightly faster in 53 women using oral contraceptives than in 153 women not using these contraceptives. This was demonstrated by a 28% faster clearance and a 19% shorter half-life of nicotine. In the 50 women using **oral combined hormonal contraceptives**, nicotine clearance was 30% faster, whereas in the just 3 women who were taking a **progestogen-only contraceptive**, nicotine clearance appeared to be 12% slower. Nevertheless, there was no difference in mean daily cigarette consumption between women using oral contraceptives and those not.[13] Another study presented similar findings that nicotine metabolism was faster in girls using hormonal contraception than those not using these contraceptives.[14]

Mechanism

The cardiovascular effects reported do not appear to be attributable to any effect of smoking on the metabolism of contraceptives steroids (see below). Rather, the adverse effects of oral combined hormonal contraceptives on cardiovascular risk factors, such as plasma lipids and coagulation parameters, appear to be additive or synergistic with those of smoking.

Smoking does not appear to alter the levels of contraceptive steroids to a clinically relevant extent. Nicotine is metabolised by CYP2A6 to cotinine, and the limited available evidence suggests that this may be slightly induced by oral combined hormonal contraceptives.

Importance and management

The cardiovascular interaction between smoking and **oral combined hormonal contraceptives** is well established. In the UK, the Faculty of Sexual and Reproductive Healthcare (FSRH) Clinical Effectiveness Unit guidelines on criteria for the use of contraceptives recommend that combined hormonal contraceptives (tablets, patch or vaginal ring) should not be used in women aged over 35 years who are current heavy smokers (greater than 15 cigarettes daily), and should also generally not be used in women of this age group who smoke less than 15 cigarettes daily or who stopped smoking less than one year ago as the risks, particularly of cardiovascular disease, usually outweigh the benefits.[6,15] Women over the age of 35 years with no additional risk factors (such as diabetes, hypertension etc.) and who stopped smoking more than one year ago may consider using a combined hormonal contraceptive.[6,15] This is because the risk of cardiovascular disease decreases within 1 to 5 years of smoking cessation.[15] They consider that women aged under 35 years who smoke and have no other associated risk factors may use a combined hormonal contraceptive, but should be informed about the increased risk of cardiovascular disease.[15] Conversely, the BNF in the UK states that women who smoke 40 or more cigarettes a day should not receive combined hormonal contraceptives.[16] Any woman with multiple risk factors for cardiovascular disease (older age, smoking, diabetes, hypertension, obesity, family history of arterial disease, migraine) should not use any form of combined hormonal contraceptive.[6,15,16] In women who smoke, for whom a combined hormonal contraceptive is not contraindicated, ones with the lowest doses of ethinylestradiol may be safer.[17] In the UK, **progestogen-only contraceptives** (implants, injections, levonorgestrel-containing intra-uterine system, and tablets) are considered suitable for women who are heavy smokers.[15]

Smoking may increase the incidence of breakthrough bleeding, decreasing the acceptability of the oral contraceptive, and this may lead to the use of less effective contraceptive methods.[8] However, this also raises the question of whether smoking increases the failure rate of oral contraceptives. The only evidence that this may occur is anecdotal and further study is needed.

Oral combined hormonal contraceptives might slightly increase nicotine metabolism, but the relevance of this to **nicotine replacement therapy**, if any, remains to be determined, and seems likely to be minor.

1. Arntzenius AC, van Gent CM, van der Voort H, Stegerhoek CI, Styblo K. Reduced high-density lipoprotein in women aged 40–41 using oral contraceptives. *Lancet* (1978) i, 1221–3.
2. Frederiksen H, Ravenholt RT. Thromboembolism, oral contraceptives and cigarettes. *Public Health Rep* (1970) 85, 197–205.
3. Collaborative Group for the study of stroke in young women. Oral contraceptives and stroke in young women: associated risk factors. *JAMA* (1975) 231, 718–22.
4. Shapiro S, Slone D, Rosenberg L, Kaufman DW, Stolley PD, Miettinen OS. Oral-contraceptive use in relation to myocardial infarction. *Lancet* (1979) i, 743–7.
5. Petitti DB, Wingerd J. Use of oral contraceptives, cigarette smoking, and risk of subarachnoid haemorrhage. *Lancet* (1978) ii, 234–6.
6. Faculty of Sexual and Reproductive Healthcare Clinical Effectiveness Unit Guidance: Contraception for women aged over 40 years, July 2010. Available at: http://www.ffprhc.org.uk/pdfs/ContraceptionOver40-July10.pdf (accessed 20/10/15).
7. Vessey M, Painter R, Yeates D. Mortality in relation to oral contraceptive use and cigarette smoking. *Lancet* (2003) 362, 185–91.
8. Rosenberg MJ, Waugh MS, Stevens CM. Smoking and cycle control among oral contraceptive users. *Am J Obstet Gynecol* (1996) 174, 628–32.
9. Sparrow MJ. Pregnancies in reliable pill takers. *N Z Med J* (1989) 102, 575–7.
10. Vessey MP, Villard-Mackintosh L, Jacobs HS. Anti-estrogenic effect of cigarette smoking. *N Engl J Med* (1987) 317, 769–70.
11. Crawford FE, Back DJ, Orme ML'E, Breckenridge AM. Oral contraceptive steroid plasma concentrations in smokers and non-smokers. *BMJ* (1981) 282, 1829–30.
12. Kanarkowski R, Tornatore KM, D'Ambrosio R, Gardner MJ, Jusko WJ. Pharmacokinetics of single and multiple doses of ethinyl estradiol and levonorgestrel in relation to smoking. *Clin Pharmacol Ther* (1988) 43, 23–31.
13. Benowitz NL, Lessov-Schlaggar CN, Swan GE, Jacob P. Female sex and oral contraceptive use accelerate nicotine metabolism. *Clin Pharmacol Ther* (2006) 79, 480–8.
14. Berlin I, Gasior MJ, Moolchan ET. Sex-based and hormonal contraception effects on the metabolism of nicotine among adolescent tobacco-dependent smokers. *Nicotin Tob Res* (2007) 9, 493–8.
15. Faculty of Sexual and Reproductive Healthcare of the Royal College of Obstetricians and Gynaecologists. UK Medical eligibility criteria for contraceptive use (UKMEC 2009). Available at: http://www.ffprhc.org.uk/pdfs/UKMEC2009.pdf (accessed 20/10/15).
16. Joint Formulary Committee. *British National Formulary*. 70 ed. London: BMJ Group and Pharmaceutical Press; 2015. p.684.
17. Schiff I, Bell WR, Davis V, Kessler CM, Meyers C, Nakajima S, Sexton BJ. Oral contraceptives and smoking, current considerations: recommendations of a consensus panel. *Am J Obstet Gynecol* (1999) 180 (Part 2) S383–S384.

HRT + Ascorbic acid (Vitamin C)

There is some limited evidence that ascorbic acid might somewhat increase estradiol levels in women receiving HRT.

Clinical evidence

In 25 postmenopausal women receiving *transdermal* **estradiol** HRT, ascorbic acid 500 mg twice daily for one month caused a 21% increase in plasma **estradiol** levels, which was not statistically significant. However, in the 9 women with initially low **estradiol** levels, ascorbic acid doubled the **estradiol** levels, and this was statistically significant.[1]

Mechanism

Ascorbic acid may reverse the oxidation of oestrogens.[1]

Importance and management

Evidence for an interaction between ascorbic acid and HRT appears to be limited to this one study. The authors state that their findings do not support the general use of ascorbic acid as an adjuvant to HRT, but that further study is needed. Until more data is available, no routine precautions appear to be needed on concurrent use.

1. Vihtamäki T, Parantainen J, Koivisto A-M, Metsä-Ketelä T, Tuimala R. Oral ascorbic acid increases plasma oestradiol during postmenopausal hormone replacement therapy. *Maturitas* (2002) 42, 129–35.

HRT + Azoles

Ketoconazole very slightly increases the levels of estrone, a metabolite of estradiol.

Clinical evidence, mechanism, importance and management

In a study in 6 postmenopausal women given a single 2-mg dose of **estradiol** after **ketoconazole** 100 mg twice daily for 4 days, there was an increase in the AUC and maximum plasma levels of **estrone** (a metabolite of estradiol) of 16% and 30%, respectively.[1] These increases are unlikely to be clinically relevant.[1] For mention that ketoconazole increased estradiol exposure when given as part of an oral combined hormonal contraceptive, see 'Combined hormonal contraceptives + Azoles', p.1168.

1. Annas A, Carlström K, Alván G, AL-Shurbaji A. The effect of ketoconazole and diltiazem on oestrogen metabolism in postmenopausal women after single dose oestradiol treatment. *Br J Clin Pharmacol* (2003) 56, 334–6.

HRT + Enzyme inducers

Enzyme-inducing drugs that increase the metabolism of contraceptive steroids might also be expected to reduce the efficacy of HRT. An isolated case describes reduced efficacy of oral conjugated oestrogens in a patient taking phenytoin.

Clinical evidence, mechanism, importance and management

A report describes a 28-year-old woman taking oral **conjugated oestrogens** (*Premarin*) 1.25 mg daily after hysterectomy and ovariectomy, who had a dramatic increase in the incidence of hot flushes when she began to take **phenytoin** 300 mg daily. Her estrone and estradiol levels were found to be very low, and they subsequently increased four- to sixfold after the **phenytoin** was stopped, at which point the incidence of hot flushes decreased.[1] This seems to be the only report of this interaction, and there do not appear to be any pharmacokinetic drug interaction studies of HRT preparations with enzyme-inducing drugs. Nevertheless, **rifampicin (rifampin)** caused a 44% reduction in the AUC of **estradiol** used as the oestrogen component of an oral combined hormonal contraceptive, which is similar to its interaction with ethinylestradiol, see 'Combined hormonal contraceptives + Rifamycins', p.1184. Therefore, it is not unreasonable to assume that other enzyme inducers that increase the metabolism of contraceptive steroids (see 'Table 28.1', p.1160, for a list) would also increase the metabolism of oestrogens used for HRT. These drugs may therefore reduce the efficacy of HRT preparations. This would be most likely to be noticed where HRT is prescribed for menopausal vasomotor symptoms, but might be difficult to detect where the indication is osteoporosis. The interaction is not relevant to HRT applied locally for menopausal vaginitis. Further study is needed to confirm the clinical importance of this possible interaction.

1. Notelovitz M, Tjapkes J, Ware M. Interaction between estrogen and Dilantin in a menopausal woman. *N Engl J Med* (1981) 304, 788–9.

HRT + Grapefruit juice

Grapefruit juice caused a slight increase in estrogen exposure after a single oral dose of estradiol. One epidemiological study found that the consumption of whole grapefruit caused a minor increased risk for breast cancer, and that this was additive with the effect of HRT, whereas another similar study did not confirm this.

Clinical evidence

In a study in 8 women given a single 2-mg dose of **estradiol**, simultaneous administration of 200 mL of **grapefruit juice** produced a 16% increase in the AUC of estrone, a metabolite of **estradiol**, and a 40% increase (not statistically significant) in the AUC of **estradiol**.[1]

In a large cohort study, eating more than a quarter of a **whole grapefruit** per day increased the relative risk of breast cancer in current users of HRT by about one-third (relative risk 2.55 versus 2.01 in users of oestrogen and progestogen, and 2.12 versus 1.56 in users of oestrogen alone). A similar increased risk of breast cancer with grapefruit was seen in women not using HRT (1.44 versus 1). This study was unable to assess the effect of **grapefruit juice**, because the original dietary questionnaire had combined this with orange juice.[2] In contrast, a later very similar study did not find an association between eating the same amount of whole grapefruit daily and breast cancer, including in women taking HRT.[3]

Mechanism

It appears that grapefruit juice has some minor inhibitory effect on the metabolism of estradiol (see also 'Combined hormonal contraceptives + Grapefruit juice', p.1175). Increasing oestrogen exposure may increase the risk of adverse effects, including estrogen-associated breast cancer.

Importance and management

The small pharmacokinetic study provides some reassurance that grapefruit juice has only a minor effect on oestrogen levels after estradiol administration. However, a larger study is needed to provide a more conclusive picture. One epidemiological study found that the daily consumption of whole grapefruit caused a minor increase in the risk of breast cancer, which was additive with the effect of menopausal HRT. However, the effect was very much smaller than the increased risk with HRT alone. Moreover, another study did not find an association between grapefruit and increased breast cancer risk. Interpretation of these studies is complicated by the fact they did not control for grapefruit juice consumption.

1. Schubert W, Cullberg G, Edgar B, Hedner T. Inhibition of 17β-estradiol metabolism by grapefruit juice in ovariectomized women. *Maturitas* (1994) 20, 155–63.
2. Monroe KR, Murphy SP, Kolonel LN, Pike MC. Prospective study of grapefruit intake and risk of breast cancer in postmenopausal women: the Multiethnic Cohort Study. *Br J Cancer* (2007) 97, 440–5.
3. Spencer EA, Key TJ, Appleby PN, van Gils CH, Olsen A, Tjønneland A, Clavel-Chapelon F, Boutron-Ruault M-C, Touillaud M, Sánchez M-J, Bingham S, Khaw KT, Slimani N, Kaaks R, Riboli E. Prospective study of the association between grapefruit intake and risk of breast cancer in the European Prospective Investigation into Cancer and Nutrition (EPIC). *Cancer Causes Control* (2009) 20, 803–9.

HRT + NSAIDs

Etoricoxib appears to increase the exposure to conjugated oestrogens from HRT. The findings of one observational study raise the possibility that the risk of myocardial infarction might be higher with the concurrent use of NSAIDs and HRT.

Clinical evidence

The UK manufacturer reports that, high-dose **etoricoxib** 120 mg daily for 28 days taken with HRT containing 0.625 mg of conjugated oestrogens (*Premarin*) increased the AUC of unconjugated estrone, equilin and 17-β estradiol by 41%, 76%, and 22%, respectively.[1]

In a large population-based epidemiological study, the odds ratio of a myocardial infarction was increased in women taking HRT with an NSAID (1.7), was lower in women taking HRT without an NSAID (0.64) and unchanged in women taking an NSAID with no HRT (1.02), relative to women not taking HRT or an NSAID. In this study, the three most widely used NSAIDs, **diclofenac**, **ibuprofen**, and **naproxen**, accounted for 75% of NSAID use.[2]

Mechanism

Etoricoxib inhibits the conjugation of oestrogens by sulfation (see also 'Combined hormonal contraceptives + Coxibs', p.1172). It is possible that the rare adverse cardiovascular effects of HRT and NSAIDs could be additive or synergistic.

Importance and management

The increased oestrogen exposure seen with high-dose etoricoxib is less than half that seen with twice the dose of conjugated oestrogens (1.25 mg) taken alone.[1] The effects of usual recommended lower doses of etoricoxib have not been studied. The manufacturers state that these increases should be taken into account when selecting HRT in patients taking etoricoxib, because of the possible increased risk of HRT adverse effects.[1]

The findings of the epidemiological study suggest that the concurrent use of HRT and NSAIDs might have adverse cardiovascular effects. The authors suggested that this showed that NSAIDs possibly inhibit the beneficial effects of HRT,[2] but subsequent randomised studies have not shown HRT to have beneficial cardiovascular effects, and may possibly even cause an increase in cardiovascular events in the first year of use. An alternative hypothesis is that the rare adverse cardiovascular effects of HRT could be additive or synergistic with the small increased risk of rare thrombotic events (in particular myocardial infarction and stroke) seen with coxibs and some NSAIDs. Further study is needed.

1. Arcoxia (Etoricoxib). Merck Sharp & Dohme Ltd. UK Summary of product characteristics, May 2012.
2. García Rodríguez LA, Egan K, FitzGerald GA. Traditional nonsteroidal anti-inflammatory drugs and postmenopausal hormone therapy: a drug-drug interaction? *PLoS Med* (2007) 4, e157.

HRT + Senna

Senna does not appear to affect the pharmacokinetics of estradiol.

Clinical evidence

In a clinical study in 19 women, the maximum daily tolerated dose of senna tablets (*Senokot*) was taken for 10 to 12 days with a single 1.5-mg dose of **estradiol glucuronide** given 4 days before the end of the assessment period. Senna had no significant effect on the median AUC of estradiol or estrone.[1]

Mechanism

It was thought that reducing intestinal transit time with senna might lead to reduced levels of estradiol.

Importance and management

This limited evidence suggests that anthraquinone-containing laxatives such as senna are unlikely to have a clinically relevant effect on the pharmacokinetics of estradiol.

1. Lewis SJ, Oakey RE, Heaton KW. Intestinal absorption of oestrogen: the effect of altering transit-time. *Eur J Gastroenterol Hepatol* (1998) 10, 33–9.

HRT + Thalidomide and related drugs

The UK manufacturers of thalidomide and lenalidomide advise that the concurrent use of hormone replacement therapy may increase the risk of venous thromboembolism, and they therefore advise caution on their concurrent use.[1,2]

1. Thalidomide Celgene (Thalidomide). Celgene Ltd. UK Summary of product characteristics, June 2014.
2. Revlimid (Lenalidomide). Celgene Ltd. UK Summary of product characteristics, March 2015.

HRT + Triptans

The manufacturer of naratriptan briefly notes that HRT did not appear to affect the pharmacokinetics of naratriptan.[1]

1. Amerge (Naratriptan hydrochloride). GlaxoSmithKline. US Prescribing information, February 2010.

IUDs; Copper + Anti-inflammatory drugs

There are a few early reports suggesting that the very occasional contraceptive failure of a copper IUD may have been due to an interaction with a corticosteroid, aspirin or an NSAID.

Clinical evidence, mechanism, importance and management

The cases of 4 women who each had two successive pregnancies, despite being fitted with copper IUDs, have been reported. Two were taking **corticosteroids** regularly and the other two often took **aspirin** for migraine.[1,2] Unwanted pregnancies have also been reported in 3 women with copper IUDs who were taking **corticosteroids**,[3-5] in 2 women taking NSAIDs (**indometacin** and **naproxen**),[5] and in 2 renal transplant recipients taking **prednisolone** and **azathioprine**.[6] A later case-control study found that **aspirin** and **NSAIDs** were used more frequently in 717 women who became pregnant while using IUDs than in 717 non-pregnant IUD users (the majority of IUDs were copper). The difference was significant only for **aspirin** (102 IUD failures, 59 control failures). It is possible that this finding could have resulted from bias in recall or reporting.[2] The suggested mechanism for any interaction was that part of the efficacy of copper IUDs may be based on local inflammatory effects, and that anti-inflammatory drugs might reduce this.

The evidence for this possible interaction is very slim and inconclusive, and there appear to be no further reports of any problems. Modern copper-containing IUDs are one of the most effective methods of contraception. Also, intermittent use of anti-inflammatory drugs such as NSAIDs is widespread. A recent Cochrane Database Systematic Review of studies on the use of NSAIDs to reduce pain and/or bleeding with IUDs recommends the use of NSAIDs as first-line drugs to reduce these adverse effects.[7] One manufacturer of copper IUDs states that the evidence does not justify general precautions.[8] No additional contraceptive precautions therefore appear to be necessary.

1. Buhler M, Papiernik E. Successive pregnancies in women fitted with intrauterine devices who take anti-inflammatory drugs. *Lancet* (1983) 1, 483.
2. Papiernik R, Rozenbaum H, Amblard P, Dephot N, de Mouzon J. Intra-uterine device failure: relation with drug use. *Eur J Obstet Gynecol Reprod Biol* (1989) 32, 205–12.
3. Inkeles DM, Hansen RI. Unexpected pregnancy in a woman using an intrauterine device and receiving steroid therapy. *Ann Ophthalmol* (1982) 14, 975.
4. Zerner J, Miller AB, Festino MJ. Failure of an intrauterine device concurrent with administration of corticosteroids. *Fertil Steril* (1976) 27, 1467–8.
5. Thomas P-R, Stérilet et anti-inflammatoires: à propos de quatre observations. *Concours Med* (1977) 45, 7095–6.
6. Zerner J, Doil KL, Drewry J, Leeber DA. Intrauterine contraceptive device failures in renal transplant patients. *J Reprod Med* (1981) 26, 99–102.
7. Grimes DA, Hubacher D, Lopez LM, Schulz KF. Non-steroidal anti-inflammatory drugs for heavy bleeding or pain associated with intrauterine-device use. Available in The Cochrane Database of Systematic Reviews; Issue 2. Chichester: John Wiley; 2006.
8. NOVA T 380 (copper containing intrauterine contraceptive device). Schering Health Care Limited. Technical data sheet, May 2003.

Progestogen-only contraceptives + Antibacterials

The reliability of progestogen-only methods of hormonal contraception is probably not affected by antibacterials that do not induce liver enzymes, such as the penicillins and tetracyclines.

Clinical evidence

In the records of the CSM in the UK for 1968 to 1984, four of the 63 contraceptive failures attributed to the use of antibacterials occurred with a progestogen-only contraceptive (unspecified).[1] In another study, 2 of 37 cases of contraceptive failure attributed to the use of antibacterials occurred with a progestogen-only contraceptive (unspecified).[2]

The available controlled studies of the effect of various antibacterials (non-enzyme inducing) on the pharmacokinetics and/or ovulatory suppressant effects of *combined* hormonal contraceptives (oral, patch or vaginal ring) are summarised in 'Table 28.2', p.1163. These studies show that the progestogen component (**levonorgestrel**, **norethi-**

sterone) of oral combined hormonal contraceptives is not affected by **ampicillin**,[3,4] **clarithromycin**,[5] **co-trimoxazole** (**sulfamethoxazole** with **trimethoprim**),[6] **doxycycline**,[7] **metronidazole**,[4] **moxifloxacin**,[8] or **tetracycline**.[9] Moreover, **desogestrel** exposure was moderately increased by **clarithromycin**,[5] **dienogest** exposure was slightly increased by **erythromycin**,[10] and **levonorgestrel** exposure was slightly increased by **telithromycin**.[11] The progestogen component of the vaginal ring (**etonogestrel**) was not affected by **ampicillin** or **doxycycline**,[12] and the progestogen component of the transdermal patch (**norelgestromin**) was not affected by **tetracycline**.[13,14]

Mechanism

The mechanism behind the rare cases of failure of oral combined hormonal contraceptives seen with various non-enzyme-inducing antibacterials was postulated to be reduced enterohepatic recycling of ethinylestradiol (see 'Combined hormonal contraceptives + Antibacterials', p.1162). As progestogens are largely metabolised to inactive substances before they are conjugated, they do not undergo enterohepatic recycling of the active substance. Progestogens are partially metabolised by CYP3A4, so antibacterials that inhibit this isoenzyme, such as some of the macrolides, may actually increase progestogen exposure. A reduction in the contraceptive efficacy of these progestogen-only contraceptives therefore seems highly unlikely.

Importance and management

There is no reason to expect that the contraceptive efficacy of the various progestogen-only contraceptive methods (tablets, implants, injections, IUDs) would be affected by antibacterials that alter gut flora and do not induce liver enzymes.

It is generally accepted that no interaction occurs,[15] and it is likely that the few cases seen with progestogen-only contraceptives are chance associations.[1] No additional contraceptive precautions are required on the concurrent use of progestogen-only contraceptives and antibacterials (non-enzyme inducing); however, if the antibacterial and/or the illness being treated causes vomiting and/or persistent severe diarrhoea, the usual recommendations for diarrhoea and vomiting should be followed. However, note that rifampicin (rifampin) and rifabutin are likely to reduce the efficacy of some forms of progestogen-only contraceptives, as they induce the metabolism of progestogens, see 'Progestogen-only contraceptives; Oral + Enzyme inducers', p.1200.

1. Back DJ, Grimmer SFM, Orme ML'E, Proudlove C, Mann RD, Breckenridge AM. Evaluation of Committee on Safety of Medicines yellow card reports on oral contraceptive-drug interactions with anticonvulsants and antibiotics. *Br J Clin Pharmacol* (1988) 25, 527–32.
2. Sparrow MJ. Pill method failures. *N Z Med J* (1987) 100, 102–5.
3. Back DJ, Breckenridge AM, MacIver M, Orme M, Rowe PH, Staiger Ch, Thomas E, Tjia J. The effects of ampicillin on oral contraceptive steroids in women. *Br J Clin Pharmacol* (1982) 14, 43–8.
4. Joshi JV, Joshi UM, Sankholi GM, Krishna U, Mandlekar A, Chowdhury V, Hazari K, Gupta K, Sheth UK, Saxena BN. A study of interaction of low-dose combination oral contraceptive with ampicillin and metronidazole. *Contraception* (1980) 22, 643–52.
5. Back DJ, Tjia J, Martin C, Millar E, Salmon P, Orme M. The interaction between clarithromycin and combined oral-contraceptive steroids. *J Pharm Med* (1991) 2, 81–7.
6. Grimmer SFM, Allen WL, Back DJ, Breckenridge AM, Orme M, Tjia J. The effect of cotrimoxazole on oral contraceptive steroids in women. *Contraception* (1983) 28, 53–9.
7. Neely JL, Abate M, Swinker M, D'Angio R. The effect of doxycycline on serum levels of ethinyl estradiol, norethindrone, and endogenous progesterone. *Obstet Gynecol* (1991) 77, 416–20.
8. Staß H, Sachse R, Heinig R, Zühlsdorf M, Horstmann R. Pharmacokinetics (PK) of steroid hormones in oral contraceptives (OC) are not altered by oral moxifloxacin (MOX). *J Antimicrob Chemother* (1999) 44 (Suppl A) 138–9.
9. Murphy AA, Zacur HA, Charache P, Burkman RT. The effect of tetracycline on levels of oral contraceptives. *Am J Obstet Gynecol* (1991) 164, 28–33.
10. Blode H, Schott, B, Rohde B, Knuz M, Zeun S. Effects of CYP3A4 induction and inhibition on the pharmacokinetics of estradiol valerate/dienogest. 11th World Congress on Controversies in Obstetrics and Gynecology & Infertility, Paris, November 2008, 68A.
11. Scholtz HE, Sultan E, Wessels D, Hundt AF, Passot V, Renouz A, van Neikerk N. HMR 3647, a new ketolide antimicrobial, does not affect the reliability of low-dose, triphasic oral contraceptives. *Intersci Conf Antimicrob Agents Chemother* (1999) 39, 3.
12. Dogterom P, van den Heuvel MW, Thomsen T. Absence of pharmacokinetic interactions of the combined contraceptive vaginal ring NuvaRing® with oral amoxicillin or doxycycline in two randomised trials. *Clin Pharmacokinet* (2005) 44, 429–38.
13. Abrams LS, Skee D, Natarajan J, Hutman W, Wong F. Tetracycline HCl does not affect the pharmacokinetics of a contraceptive patch. *Int J Gynaecol Obstet* (2000) 70, 57–8.
14. Abrams LS, Skee D, Natarajan J, Wong FA. Pharmacokinetic overview of Ortho Evra/Evra. *Fertil Steril* (2002) 77, (2 Suppl 2), S3–S12.
15. McCann MF, Potter LS. Progestin-only contraception: a comprehensive review. *Contraception* (1994) 50, S1–S198.

Progestogen-only contraceptives + Azoles

Itraconazole increases exposure to the active metabolite of desogestrel, whereas fluconazole has no effect on this metabolite.

Clinical evidence

In a crossover study in 11 healthy women, **itraconazole** 200 mg daily for 4 days increased the AUC of 3-keto-desogestrel (etonogestrel) by about 72% after a single 150-microgram oral dose of **desogestrel** was given one hour after the last itraconazole dose. There was no change in the maximum level of 3-keto-desogestrel or its elimination half-life. Conversely, **fluconazole** 200 mg daily for 4 days had no effect on the pharmacokinetics of 3-keto-desogestrel.[1]

Note that, pharmacokinetic data show that the AUC of **norethisterone** (given as the progestogen component of an oral *combined* hormonal contraceptive) is increased by **voriconazole** (53%)[2] and **itraconazole** (40%),[3] but only minimally by **fluconazole** (13%).[4] Similarly, **levonorgestrel** was only slightly affected by **fluconazole** (24%)[5] and systemic exposure to **etonogestrel** (given as the progestogen component of the vaginal ring form of a *combined* hormonal contraceptive) was only minimally affected by vaginal **miconazole** (17%).[6]

Mechanism

Itraconazole is principally a potent inhibitor of the CYP3A4, whereas fluconazole is a moderate inhibitor of CYP2C9 and CYP3A4. The data here suggest that the active metabolite of desogestrel, 3-keto-desogestrel (etonogestrel) is partially metabolised by CYP3A4.

Importance and management

Although based on a single-dose study, the available information suggests that fluconazole and itraconazole are unlikely to reduce the efficacy of desogestrel-containing progestogen-only contraception by a pharmacokinetic mechanism. However, the increase in exposure to the active metabolite of desogestrel (etonogestrel) with itraconazole suggests that itraconazole (and other potent CYP3A4 inhibitors) might increase the incidence of adverse effects of desogestrel. It is possible that the same pharmacokinetic interaction might occur if itraconazole is given with other hormonal contraceptives containing either desogestrel (oral combined hormonal contraceptives) or etonogestrel (combined vaginal ring or progestogen-only implant). Further study is needed.

Note that itraconazole and voriconazole have also been reported to increase norethisterone exposure when given as part of a *combined* hormonal contraceptive. This suggests that they might also be expected to increase norethisterone exposure from a progestogen-only contraceptive. Data from the use of other combined hormonal contraceptives suggest that levonorgestrel and etonogestrel are, at worst, only minimally affected by fluconazole and vaginal miconazole, respectively.

1. Korhonen T, Tolonen A, Uusitalo J, Lundgren S, Jalonen J, Laine K. The role of CYP2C and CYP3A in the disposition of 3-keto-desogestrel after administration of desogestrel. *Br J Clin Pharmacol* (2005) 60, 69–75.
2. Andrews E, Damle BD, Fang A, Foster G, Crownover P, LaBadie R, Glue P. Pharmacokinetics and tolerability of voriconazole and a combination oral contraceptive co-administered in healthy female subjects. *Br J Clin Pharmacol* (2008) 65, 531–9.
3. Jones AR (Janssen). Personal communication, 1994.
4. Hilbert J, Messig M, Kuye O, Friedman H. Evaluation of interaction between fluconazole and an oral contraceptive in healthy women. *Obstet Gynecol* (2001) 98, 218–23.
5. Diflucan (Fluconazole). Pfizer Ltd. UK Summary of product characteristics, June 2009.
6. Verhoeven CHJ, van den Heuvel MW, Mulders TMT, Dieben TOM. The contraceptive vaginal ring, NuvaRing®, and antimycotic co-medication. *Contraception* (2004) 69, 129–32.

Progestogen-only contraceptives + Lamotrigine

Preliminary evidence suggests that desogestrel might increase lamotrigine levels and adverse effects. However, there was no difference in lamotrigine levels between non-users of hormonal contraceptives and users of the levonorgestrel-containing intra-uterine system, or a variety of other progestogen-only contraceptives in two other studies.

Clinical evidence

In a preliminary report[1] of one study in 10 women stable taking lamotrigine, an oral progestogen-only contraceptive, **desogestrel** 75 micrograms daily for 12 weeks, caused a 20 to 100% increase in lamotrigine levels in 7 out of the 10 women. The increase in maximum levels was said to be greater than the increase in trough levels, and some women (number not stated) had dose-dependent increases in lamotrigine adverse effects about 30 minutes to 3 hours after their lamotrigine dose. The increase in lamotrigine levels occurred about 2 weeks after starting desogestrel, and increased up to weeks 8 to 12.

In another study which compared lamotrigine levels in 16 women taking progestogen-only contraceptives with those in 18 women not using hormonal contraceptives, the lamotrigine serum-concentration to dose ratio did not differ between the two groups. The progestogen-only contraceptives used included oral **desogestrel** (3 women), oral **norethisterone** (one woman), **etonogestrel** implant (7 women), **levonorgestrel** implant (one woman), depot **medroxyprogesterone acetate** (one woman) or the **levonorgestrel**-containing intra-uterine system (3 women). There were no obvious differences between these contraceptives, although the number of women in each group is too limited to be certain.[2] In another similar study, there was no difference in the lamotrigine serum-concentration to dose ratio between 12 women with a **levonorgestrel**-containing intra-uterine system and 20 women not using hormonal contraception.[3]

Mechanism

Unknown. In contrast to the finding here for continuous desogestrel alone, a combined hormonal contraceptive containing ethinylestradiol and desogestrel caused a reduction in lamotrigine levels, see 'Combined hormonal contraceptives + Lamotrigine', p.1178.

Importance and management

There are very limited data on the effect of using progestogen-only contraceptives with lamotrigine. Available data suggest that the levonorgestrel-containing intra-uterine system has no effect on lamotrigine levels, but that desogestrel might increase lamotrigine levels in some women. This is in contrast to the effects of combined hormonal contraceptives, which are known to decrease lamotrigine levels, as a result of the ethinylestradiol component (see 'Combined hormonal contraceptives + Lamotrigine', p.1178). Until more is known, it may be prudent to increase monitoring of lamotrigine levels and adverse effects (such as such as dizziness, ataxia, and diplopia) when desogestrel is started or stopped. Further study is needed.

There are no data on whether the efficacy of progestogen-only contraceptives is altered by lamotrigine. In one study with an *oral combined hormonal contraceptive* there was a very slight reduction in levonorgestrel exposure, with an increase in FSH and LH levels and an increase in intermenstrual bleeding, which suggests some reduction in the suppression of the hypothalamic-pituitary-ovarian axis. However, in that study no ovulation occurred, and the oral combined hormonal contraceptive is generally considered to remain effective when used with lamotrigine, see 'Combined hormonal contraceptives + Lamotrigine', p.1178. Nevertheless, it is less certain whether this applies to the situation when smaller doses of levonorgestrel are used alone as an oral progestogen-only contraceptive, particularly as these are generally less effective contraceptives than oral combined hormonal contraceptives. There is insufficient evidence to make a specific recommendation, but bear this information in mind when making contraceptive choices in women taking lamotrigine. The data seen with oral contraceptives suggest that the efficacy of long-acting forms of progestogen-only contraceptives (implants, injections and the levonorgestrel-containing intrauterine system) would not be expected to be reduced by lamotrigine.

1. Schwenkhagen AM, Stodieck SRG. Interaction between lamotrigine and a progestin-only contraceptive pill containing desogestrel 75-μg (Cerazette®). *Epilepsia* (2004) 45 (Suppl 7) 144.
2. Reimers A, Helde G, Brodtkorb E. Ethinyl estradiol, not progestogens, reduces lamotrigine serum concentrations. *Epilepsia* (2005) 46, 1414–17.
3. Öhman I, Luef G, Tomson T. Effects of pregnancy and contraception on lamotrigine disposition: new insights through analysis of lamotrigine metabolites. *Seizure* (2008) 17, 199–202.

Progestogen-only contraceptives; Implants + Enzyme inducers

There are a number of reports of pregnancies in women using levonorgestrel implants or etonogestrel implants with a potent enzyme-inducing antiepileptic, rifampicin (rifampin), efavirenz or St. John's wort. In addition, there is limited evidence of lower levonorgestrel concentrations when the implant was used with potent enzyme-inducing antiepileptics.

Clinical evidence

(a) Etonogestrel

There are 4 published case reports of pregnancy in women using the etonogestrel implant (*Implanon*) with enzyme-inducing drugs. One case occurred in a patient taking **carbamazepine** 600 mg daily, one month after insertion of the implant.[1] A pregnancy (ectopic) that occurred in a woman who had received the implant was considered to be due to the use of **rifampicin (rifampin)**.[2] Another pregnancy occurred in a woman who had been fitted with this implant for approximately 2 years, about 6 months after starting **rifampicin** 300 mg twice daily for hidradenitis suppurativa.[3] There is also a case of contraceptive failure (ectopic pregnancy) in a woman taking **efavirenz**, lamivudine, and zidovudine, which occurred 2.5 years after insertion of the etonogestrel implant.[4] Similarly, 2 women taking **efavirenz**, lamivudine, and zidovudine experienced contraceptive failure (with one patient found to have an ectopic pregnancy) around 28 months[5] and 23 months[6] after insertion of an etonogestrel implant. Similarly, a woman taking tenofovir with emtricitabine and efavirenz was found to be pregnant 27 months after insertion of an etonogestrel implant.[6]

In addition, to these case reports, an Australian post-marketing report for the 3 years from May 2001 describes 8 other cases of contraceptive failure with the etonogestrel implant in patients who were taking enzyme-inducing antiepileptics (7 of the 8 were taking **carbamazepine**).[7] An updated report in 2007 identified 32 pregnancies in users of the etonogestrel implant possibly related to other medicines (26 with **carbamazepine**, 4 with **phenytoin**, one with **methylphenobarbital**, and one with **rifampicin**).[8] Yet another report mentions that, up to August 2010, there have been 32 cases of possible contraceptive failure in women using the etonogestrel implant with **carbamazepine**.[9] The MHRA in the UK reports that since 2000, it has received 4 reports of suspected interactions between **St John's wort** and contraceptive implants (from a total of 19 reports with St John's wort and hormonal contraceptives), all of which resulted in unplanned pregnancies. Two of these were reported in the last quarter of 2013, in women with etonogestrel implants and who had started taking St John's wort.[10]

(b) Levonorgestrel

In a study, a levonorgestrel implant (*Norplant*) was inserted in 8 women taking enzyme-inducing antiepileptics (**phenytoin** and/or **carbamazepine**) and 10 women taking no other drugs. At 3, 6, and 9 months after insertion, plasma levonorgestrel concentrations were 38% lower in the 6 women taking **phenytoin** alone, or in combination with **carbamazepine** or valproate, than in the women not taking these enzyme inducers. Low levonorgestrel concentrations were also seen in the two women taking **carbamazepine** alone. Two of the 8 women became pregnant (one taking **phenytoin** 250 mg daily, occurring about 11 months after insertion of the implant, and one taking **phenytoin** 400 mg daily with **carbamazepine** 400 mg daily, occurring 20 months after insertion of the implant).[11]

In three other cases, women using levonorgestrel implants with enzyme-inducing antiepileptics became pregnant.[12-14] In one, a woman taking **phenytoin** 300 mg daily became pregnant 9 months after the insertion of the implant. Levonorgestrel concentrations increased by 50% after **phenytoin** was stopped, and progesterone concentrations decreased, suggesting greater suppression of ovulation.[12] Similarly, one woman taking **phenobarbital** 210 mg daily became pregnant about 17 months after the insertion of a levonorgestrel implant (this woman subsequently also became pregnant while using an oral combined hormonal contraceptive containing 35 micrograms of ethinylestradiol and a back up method).[13] Another report[14] briefly mentions that one woman taking enzyme-inducing antiepileptics became pregnant while using a levonorgestrel implant, and mentions that, as of 1995, the manufacturer had 30 other similar cases on file.

Mechanism

Enzyme-inducing drugs increase the metabolism of hormonal contraceptives, including levonorgestrel and probably etonogestrel. When formulated as implants, there is a slow controlled-release of the progestogen over a number of years, and the dose is very low. For example, the etonogestrel implant releases 60 to 70 micrograms daily initially reducing to 25 to 30 micrograms daily by the end of the third year,[15] which is comparable to the doses of some progestogens used in oral progestogen-only contraceptives. Reduced progestogen concentrations might therefore result in reduced contraceptive efficacy.

Importance and management

Evidence for an interaction between progestogen implants (both levonorgestrel and etonogestrel) and enzyme inducers is largely limited to case reports, although there are a reasonable number of these, which taken together, show that contraceptive failure can occur with concurrent use. However, progestogen implants are the most effective form of hormonal contraceptive (even more effective than perfect use of oral combined hormonal contraceptives), and the question therefore is, to what extent do enzyme-inducing drugs reduce their efficacy? Very limited evidence from the one study with the levonorgestrel implant suggests that the incidence might be high (2 out of 8 women), and, on this basis the use of progestogen implants with enzyme-inducing drugs is, generally, not recommended. For example, in the UK, the Faculty of Sexual and Reproductive Healthcare 2011 guideline on hormonal contraception and drug interactions[16] recommends that women with progestogen-only implants requiring *short courses* (less than 2 months) of enzyme inducers, should use additional contraceptive methods (such as condoms) during and for at least 28 days after the enzyme-inducing drug is stopped. Alternatively, they state that women could be offered a one-off injection of medroxyprogesterone acetate to cover the period of risk. They also recommend that alternatives to the progestogen-only implant should be considered when enzyme inducers are required *long-term* (more than 2 months), such as progestogen-only injections (see 'Progestogen-only contraceptives; Injections + Enzyme inducers', p.1199), the copper IUD or the levonorgestrel intra-uterine system (see, 'Progestogen-only contraceptives; Intra-uterine system + Enzyme inducers', p.1200). Conversely, while the WHO acknowledge that enzyme-inducing antiepileptics might decrease the efficacy of progestogen implants, and that the use of other contraceptives should be encouraged, they advise that progestogen-only implants containing levonorgestrel or etonogestrel can generally be used (category 2) in women taking enzyme inducers.[17] A list of enzyme inducers can be found in 'Table 28.1', p.1160. Further, in the UK the MHRA specifically advises that women using hormonal contraceptives, including implants, should not take herbal products that contain **St John's wort** due to the risk of unplanned pregnancy.[10]

Further study is needed to better define the increased risk of contraceptive failure when these progestogen implants are used with enzyme-inducing drugs.

1. Schindlbeck C, Janni W, Friese K. Failure of Implanon contraception in a patient taking carbamazepin for epilepsia. *Arch Gynecol Obstet* (2006) 273, 255–6.
2. Patni S, Kevelighan E, Bibby J, Ebden P. Ectopic pregnancy with Implanon®. *J Fam Plann Reprod Health Care* (2006) 32, 115.
3. Bacon L, Mina M. Unintended pregnancies with Implanon. *Contraception* (2006) 73, 111.
4. Matiluko AA, Soundararjan L, Hogston P. Early contraceptive failure of Implanon® in an HIV-seropositive patient on triple antiretroviral therapy with zidovudine, lamivudine and efavirenz. *J Fam Plann Reprod Health Care* (2007) 33, 277–8.
5. McCarty EJ, Keane H, Quinn K, Quah S. Implanon® failure in an HIV-positive woman on antiretroviral therapy resulting in two ectopic pregnancies. *Int J STD AIDS* (2011) 22, 413–14.
6. Leticee N, Viard J-P, Yamgnane A, Karmochkine M, Benachi A. Contraceptive failure of etonogestrel implant in patients treated with antiretrovirals including efavirenz. *Contraception* (2012) 85, 425–7.
7. Harrison-Woolrych M, Hill R. Unintended pregnancies with the etonogestrel implant (Implanon): a case series from postmarketing experience in Australia. *Contraception* (2005) 71, 306–8.
8. Implanon: interactions and failure of contraception. *Aust Adverse Drug React Bull* (2007) 26, 14–15.
9. Medicines Safety Update. Unintended pregnancy due to interaction between etonogestrel implant (Implanon) and carbamazepine. *Aust Prescriber* (2010) 33, 185.
10. Medicines and Healthcare Products Regulatory Agency and the Commission on Human Medicines. St John's wort: interaction with hormonal contraceptives, including implants – reduced contraceptive effect. *Drug Safety Update* (2014) 7, A2. Available at: http://www.mhra.gov.uk/home/groups/dsu/documents/publication/con392897.pdf (accessed 21/05/14).
11. Haukkamaa M. Contraception by Norplant® subdermal capsules is not reliable in epileptic patients on anticonvulsant treatment. *Contraception* (1986) 33, 559–65.
12. Odlind V, Olsson S-E. Enhanced metabolism of levonorgestrel during phenytoin treatment in a woman with Norplant® implants. *Contraception* (1986) 33, 257–61.
13. Shane-McWhorter L, Cerveny JD, MacFarlane LL, Osborn C. Enhanced metabolism of levonorgestrel during phenobarbital treatment and resultant pregnancy. *Pharmacotherapy* (1998) 18, 1360–4.
14. Krauss GL, Brandt J, Campbell M, Plate C, Summerfield M. Antiepileptic medication and oral contraceptive interactions: a national survey of neurologists and obstetricians. *Neurology* (1996) 46, 1534–9.
15. Nexplanon (Etonogestrel). Organon Laboratories Ltd. UK Summary of product characteristics, November 2013.
16. Faculty of Sexual and Reproductive Healthcare Guidance. Drug interactions with hormonal contraception: Clinical Effectiveness Unit, January 2011 (Updated January 2012). Available at: http://www.fsrh.org/pdfs/CEUGuidanceDrugInteractionsHormonal.pdf (accessed 20/10/15).
17. Reproductive Health and Research, World Health Organization. Medical eligibility criteria for contraceptive use. 5th ed. Geneva, WHO; 2015. Available at: http://www.who.int/reproductivehealth/publications/family_planning/MEC-5/en/(accessed 20/10/15).

Progestogen-only contraceptives; Injections + Enzyme inducers

The efficacy of the medroxyprogesterone depot injection might not be affected by enzyme inducers, and no pharmacokinetic interaction has been seen with this contraceptive and efavirenz, nevirapine or nelfinavir. Similarly, the contraceptive reliability of the norethisterone depot injection is unlikely to be affected by enzyme inducers.

Clinical evidence

In a study in women taking NRTIs with **efavirenz** (17), **nevirapine** (16), or **nelfinavir** (21), there was no difference in the pharmacokinetics of depot **medroxyprogesterone acetate** 150 mg, when compared with 16 women not taking any antiretrovirals or taking just NRTIs. Suppression of ovulation was maintained. Furthermore, viral load and CD4 counts were not altered.[1,2] In another similar study, there was no difference in the pharmacokinetics of depot **medroxyprogesterone acetate** between 15 women taking **efavirenz** plus two NRTIs (lamivudine and zidovudine) compared with 15 women not taking any antiretrovirals. No ovulation occurred in the women taking the antiretrovirals.[3] For mention of another study that found a low incidence of pregnancy in women taking an **efavirenz**-based regimen and using an intramuscular progestogen or an oral combined hormonal contraceptive, see 'Combined hormonal contraceptives + NNRTIs', p.1181.

Mechanism

The UK manufacturer states that the clearance of medroxyprogesterone acetate is about equal to hepatic blood flow, and as such, would not be expected to be affected by drugs that alter hepatic enzyme activity,[4] whereas the US manufacturer considers that enzyme inducers might decrease medroxyprogesterone concentrations.[5] The limited available evidence here for antiretrovirals (which have been shown to reduce concentrations of oral combined hormonal contraceptives, see 'Table 28.1', p.1160), suggests that they do not affect medroxyprogesterone acetate concentrations.

There are no data for the effect of enzyme inducers on the concentrations of norethisterone from the depot injection, although there are data showing that some rifamycins and carbamazepine can reduce the plasma concentrations of norethisterone when it is used as a component of an oral combined hormonal contraceptive, see 'Table 28.1', p.1160, so a reduction is theoretically possible.

For both depot preparations, if an enzyme-inducing drug increased the metabolism of the contraceptive steroid, one possibility is that there might be a faster release from the depot maintaining similar plasma concentrations, but with the possibility of a shorter duration of action of the depot. Alternatively, if the release from the depot is unchanged, and enzyme-inducing drugs lower plasma concentrations, because both depot preparations provide high doses of the hormones (higher than that used in other forms of hormonal contraceptives) it is also possible that concentrations may remain sufficient for effective contraception.[6]

Importance and management

The limited data with the antiretrovirals and the lack of published case reports of contraceptive failure with enzyme inducers, seems to support a lack of an interaction between these drugs and the **medroxyprogesterone acetate depot** contraceptive. The UK manufacturer states that no dose adjustment is needed,[4] and this is also the advice given by the UK Faculty of Sexual and Reproductive Healthcare,[7] although some have recommended giving the injection more frequently,[8] see also *Mechanism*, above. Conversely, the US manufacturer recommends additional contraceptive precautions or switching to an alternative method of contraception;[5] however, given the lack of reported contraceptive failures, and the fact that this depot has generally been recommended as suitable for use with enzyme inducers, this approach seems overly cautious. Note also, that the UK Faculty of Sexual and Reproductive Healthcare advises that a one-off dose of medroxyprogesterone acetate depot can be used to cover the short-term concurrent use of enzyme inducers in women taking combined or progestogen-only contraceptives.[7]

Although a pharmacokinetic interaction between the **norethisterone enantate depot** contraceptive and enzyme inducers is theoretically possible, and the manufacturer considers that its efficacy might be reduced,[9] they have had no reports of contraceptive failure relating to the concurrent use of enzyme-inducing drugs.[10] The dose of norethisterone provided by the depot injection is much higher than that provided by oral combined hormonal contraceptives, and it is therefore possible that it might remain effective even in women taking enzyme-inducing drugs.[6] In the UK, the 2011 guidance from the Faculty of Sexual and Reproductive Healthcare states that no additional contraceptive precautions are required when the norethisterone enantate depot is used in women taking enzyme inducers,[7] which seems sensible. They also state that it can be used with no dose adjustment or change in the normal injection schedule, and can be used to cover the short-term concurrent use of enzyme inducers in women taking progestogen-only contraceptives.[7] However, some have recommended giving the injection more frequently,[8] see also *Mechanism*, above.

In contrast, the MHRA in the UK specifically advises that women taking hormonal contraceptives for pregnancy prevention (except IUDs) should not take herbal products containing **St John's wort**, due to the risk of unplanned pregnancy.[11] However, note that the UK Faculty of Sexual and Reproductive Healthcare 2011 guidance does cover St John's wort.[7]

1. Cohn SE, Park J-G, Watts DH, Stek A, Hitti J, Clax PA, Yu S, Lertora JJL, for the ACTG A5093 Protocol Team. Depo-medroxyprogesterone in women on antiretroviral therapy: effective contraception and lack of clinically significant interactions. *Clin Pharmacol Ther* (2007) 81, 222–7.
2. Watts DH, Park J-G, Cohn SE, Yu S, Hitti J, Stek A, Clax PA, Muderspach L, Lertora JJL. Safety and tolerability of depot medroxyprogesterone acetate among HIV-infected women on antiretroviral therapy: ACTG A5093. *Contraception* (2008) 77, 84–90.
3. Nanda K, Amaral E, Hays M, Viscola MAM, Mehta N, Bahamondes L. Pharmacokinetic interactions between depot medroxyprogesterone acetate and combination antiretroviral therapy. *Fertil Steril* (2008) 90, 965–71.
4. Depo-Provera (Medroxyprogesterone acetate). Pfizer Ltd. UK Summary of product characteristics, September 2012.
5. Depo-Provera (Medroxyprogesterone acetate). Pharmacia & Upjohn Company. US Prescribing information, April 2012.
6. Schwenkhagen AM, Stodieck SR. Which contraception for women with epilepsy? *Seizure* (2008) 17, 145–50.
7. Faculty of Sexual and Reproductive Healthcare Guidance. Drug interactions with hormonal contraception: Clinical Effectiveness Unit, January 2011 (Updated January 2012). Available at: http://www.fsrh.org/pdfs/CEUGuidanceDrugInteractionsHormonal.pdf (accessed 20/10/15).
8. Crawford P. Interactions between antiepileptic drugs and hormonal contraception. *CNS Drugs* (2002) 16, 263–72.
9. Noristerat (Norethisterone enantate). Bayer plc. UK Summary of product characteristics, May 2013.
10. Bayer HealthCare. Personal communication. May 2010.
11. Medicines and Healthcare Products Regulatory Agency and the Commission on Human Medicines. St John's wort: interaction with hormonal contraceptives, including implants – reduced contraceptive effect. *Drug Safety Update* (2014) 7, A2. Available at: http://webarchive.nationalarchives.gov.uk/20141205150130/http://www.mhra.gov.uk/home/groups/dsu/documents/publication/con392897.pdf (accessed 20/10/15).

Progestogen-only contraceptives; Intra-uterine system + Enzyme inducers

The contraceptive reliability of the levonorgestrel-releasing intrauterine system does not appear to be appreciably affected by enzyme inducers.

Clinical evidence

In a pilot study in 47 women (most with epilepsy) using a **levonorgestrel** intra-uterine system with at least one enzyme-inducing drug, there was only one apparent contraceptive failure for 1075 months of use for contraception. This occurred 2 years after insertion of the intra-uterine system in a 42-year-old woman taking **primidone** 500 mg daily and **phenytoin** 300 mg daily. In this study, enzyme-inducing drugs being taken were **carbamazepine**, **efavirenz**, **nevirapine**, **phenytoin**, **phenobarbital**, **primidone**, **rifabutin**, **ritonavir** and **topiramate**. The failure rate calculated was 1.1 per 100 women-years, whereas the usual quoted failure rate of the levonorgestrel intra-uterine system is 0.2 per 100 women-years.[1]

Mechanism

Some enzyme inducers have specifically been shown to increase the metabolism of levonorgestrel when used as a component of oral combined hormonal contraceptives (see 'Table 28.1', p.1160). Although there are no data, these drugs might be expected to reduce the systemic exposure to levonorgestrel from the intra-uterine system. Nevertheless, the overall efficacy of the intra-uterine system is thought to be mainly via local hormonal and non-hormonal effects,[2] and might not be dependent on the extent of systemic exposure to levonorgestrel.

Importance and management

From the limited published evidence, the rate of contraceptive failure when a levonorgestrel-containing intra-uterine system is used with enzyme-inducing drugs appears low. The systemic absorption of levonorgestrel from the intra-uterine system leads to lower blood levels than are seen with standard oral progestogen-only contraceptives, and many women using a levonorgestrel intra-uterine system continue to ovulate. Thus, the contraceptive effects of this product are thought to be mainly local,[2] and it might therefore not be as susceptible to enzyme-inducing drugs.[3] Nevertheless, the manufacturer has said that they cannot be sure that the foreign body effect (i.e. the effect whereby the presence of the intra-uterine system prevents implantation) and/or locally acting hormone will provide reliable contraception when systemic hormone levels and suppression of ovaries are reduced by drug interactions.[4] However, this appears to be overly cautious. Furthermore, the manufacturer also includes **griseofulvin** in their list of enzyme-inducers;[2] however, griseofulvin is not an established enzyme inducer, see 'Hormonal contraceptives + Griseofulvin', p.1192.

In the UK, the Faculty of Sexual and Reproductive Healthcare 2011 guideline on hormonal contraceptives and drug interactions considers that the levonorgestrel-releasing intra-uterine system is unlikely to be affected by enzyme inducers, and recommends that no additional contraceptive protection is required.[5] It is therefore considered a suitable hormonal contraceptive for women taking enzyme-inducing drugs.

1. Bounds W, Guillebaud J. Observational series on women using the contraceptive Mirena concurrently with anti-epileptic and other enzyme-inducing drugs. *J Fam Plann Reprod Health Care* (2002) 28, 78–80.
2. Mirena (Levonorgestrel Intrauterine System). Bayer plc. UK Summary of product characteristics, July 2010.
3. Schwenkhagen AM, Stodieck SR. Which contraception for women with epilepsy? *Seizure* (2008) 17, 145–50.
4. Personal communication. Schering Health Care Limited. April 2001.
5. Faculty of Sexual and Reproductive Healthcare Guidelines. Drug interactions with hormonal contraception: Clinical Effectiveness Unit, January 2011 (Updated January 2012). Available at: http://www.fsrh.org/pdfs/CEUGuidanceDrugInteractionsHormonal.pdf (accessed 21/10/15).

Progestogen-only contraceptives; Oral + Enzyme inducers

The contraceptive efficacy of oral progestogen-only contraceptives is probably reduced by enzyme-inducing drugs, and there are isolated reports of pregnancies in women given these contraceptives with an enzyme-inducing antiepileptic or St John's wort.

Clinical evidence

In a review of pregnancies reported to the CSM in the UK between the years 1968 to 1984 in women taking antiepileptics and oral contraceptives, 3 cases were identified in women taking progestogen-only pills (progestogen not stated). The antiepileptics used in these specific cases were not stated, but most of the women were taking enzyme-inducing antiepileptics, such as **phenytoin**, **phenobarbital**, **primidone**, and **carbamazepine** (alone or as combinations).[1] In 2002, the UK regulatory authority had one case on record of an unplanned pregnancy that occurred 4 months after starting **St John's wort** in a woman who had been taking **norethisterone** for 2 years.[2]

Mechanism

There do not appear to have been any clinical pharmacokinetic studies of enzyme inducers with any of the oral progestogen-only contraceptives (desogestrel, levonorgestrel, norethisterone). Nevertheless, various enzyme inducers have specifically been shown to decrease the concentrations of levonorgestrel and norethisterone when used as components of oral combined hormonal contraceptives (see 'Table 28.1', p.1160).

Importance and management

Information on a possible interaction between enzyme inducers and oral progestogen-only contraceptives is very limited, and there do not appear to have been any clinical pharmacokinetic studies of enzyme inducers with any of these progestogens (desogestrel, levonorgestrel, norethisterone). Nevertheless, based on pharmacokinetic considerations and data from oral combined hormonal contraceptives it can be assumed that there is also a risk of contraceptive failure if oral progestogen-only contraceptives are given with enzyme-inducing drugs.[3] This is of particular concern as oral progestogen-only contraceptives are not as effective as oral combined hormonal contraceptives, especially the **levonorgestrel** and **norethisterone** preparations, which are given in very low doses that do not consistently inhibit ovulation. Some have suggested at least doubling the dose of the oral progestogen-only contraceptive to manage any interaction.[4] However, others consider that this is not an option as higher doses of progestogen tend to increase the rate of irregular bleeding (a common adverse effect of these contraceptives). They consider that oral progestogen-only contraceptives are not suitable for use in women taking enzyme-inducing antiepileptics,[3,5] and this is the view taken by the UK Faculty of Sexual and Reproductive Healthcare,[6] and by the WHO.[7] Both these organisations extend this advice to other drugs which are enzyme inducers.[6,7] For a list of drugs that induce the metabolism of contraceptive steroids, to which this advice should be applied, see 'Table 28.1', p.1160. Further, the MHRA in the UK specifically advises that women using hormonal contraceptives, including progestogen-only contraceptives, should not take herbal products that contain **St John's wort** due to the risk of unplanned pregnancy.[8] Alternative progestogen-only contraceptive methods might be suitable in women taking enzyme-inducing drugs, see 'Progestogen-only contraceptives; Intra-uterine system + Enzyme inducers', p.1200, 'Progestogen-only contraceptives; Injections + Enzyme inducers', p.1199.

1. Back DJ, Grimmer SFM, Orme ML'E, Proudlove C, Mann RD, Breckenridge AM. Evaluation of Committee on Safety of Medicines yellow card reports on oral contraceptive-drug interactions with anticonvulsants and antibiotics. *Br J Clin Pharmacol* (1988) 25, 527–32.
2. Henderson L, Yue QY, Bergquist C, Gerden B, Arlett P. St John's wort (*Hypericum perforatum*): drug interactions and clinical outcomes. *Br J Clin Pharmacol* (2002) 54, 349–56.
3. McCann MF, Potter LS. Progestin-only contraception: a comprehensive review. *Contraception* (1994) 50 (Suppl 1), S1–S198.
4. O'Brien MD, Gilmour-White S. Epilepsy and pregnancy. *BMJ* (1993) 307, 492–5.
5. Schwenkhagen AM, Stodieck SR. Which contraception for women with epilepsy? *Seizure* (2008) 17, 145–50.
6. Faculty of Sexual and Reproductive Healthcare Guidance. Drug interactions with hormonal contraception: Clinical Effectiveness Unit, January 2011. (Updated January 2012) Available at: http://www.fsrh.org/pdfs/CEUGuidanceDrugInteractionsHormonal.pdf (accessed 20/10/15).
7. Reproductive Health and Research, World Health Organization. Medical eligibility criteria for contraceptive use. 5th ed. Geneva, WHO; 2015. Available at: http://www.who.int/reproductivehealth/publications/family_planning/MEC-5/en/ (accessed 20/10/15).
8. Medicines and Healthcare Products Regulatory Agency and the Commission on Human Medicines. St John's wort: interaction with hormonal contraceptives, including implants – reduced contraceptive effect. *Drug Safety Update* (2014) 7, A2. Available at: http://webarchive.nationalarchives.gov.uk/20141205150130/http://www.mhra.gov.uk/home/groups/dsu/documents/publication/con392897.pdf (accessed 20/10/15).

Tibolone + St John's wort (*Hypericum perforatum*)

An isolated report describes acute hepatitis in a patient taking tibolone, after a 10 week course of St John's wort.

Clinical evidence, mechanism, importance and management

A case report describes a 57-year-old woman taking tibolone 2.5 mg daily for 2 years with no adverse effects, who developed jaundice, severe pruritis, dark urine, fatigue, and reduced appetite after 10 weeks of St John's wort (given as 2 g infusions). Her ALT and AST concentrations were greatly increased, and a liver specimen showed a lack of bile ducts. Both tibolone and St John's wort were stopped and she was treated with ursodeoxycholic acid. She slowly improved, with her liver function tests returning to normal after about a year. The authors suggested that this case was most likely due to an interaction between tibolone and St John's wort, although the mechanism was unknown,[1] however, both drugs can affect liver function alone. This is an isolated report, and as such its general clinical relevance is not known. If symptoms of liver toxicity (nausea, vomiting, dark urine) become apparent on concurrent use, consider an interaction as a possible cause.

1. Etogo-Asse F et al. Acute hepatitis with prolonged cholestasis and disappearance of interlobular bile ducts following tibolone and Hypericum perforatum (St. John's wort). Case of drug interaction? *Acta Gastroenterol Belg* (2008) 71, 36–8.

Ulipristal + CYP3A4 Inhibitors

Erythromycin appears to moderately increase the exposure to ulipristal, and ketoconazole appears to have a marked effect. Other moderate and potent inhibitors of CYP3A4 are predicted to interact similarly.

Clinical evidence

(a) Erythromycin

In a study in 18 healthy female subjects, a single 20-mg dose of ulipristal was given alone, and on day 5, of a 9-day course of erythromycin 500 mg twice daily. The ulipristal maximum concentration was increased by 24% and the AUC was increased 3.3-fold.[1]

(b) Ketoconazole

One UK manufacturer briefly notes that, in a study in healthy subjects ketoconazole 400 mg twice daily for 7 days increased the maximum concentration and AUC of ulipristal 2-fold and 5.9-fold, respectively.[2]

Mechanism

In vitro,[3] ulipristal is metabolised by CYP3A4, which is inhibited by erythromycin and ketoconazole, albeit to varying extents. Concurrent use therefore results in increased exposure to ulipristal.

Importance and management

An interaction between ulipristal and CYP3A4 inhibitors appears to be established, and the magnitude of the increases in ulipristal exposure with erythromycin (moderate increase) and ketoconazole (marked increase) might be clinically important. Therefore the UK manufacturer of ulipristal for the symptomatic management of fibroids does not recommend its concurrent use with moderate and potent CYP3A4 inhibitors[2] (see 'Table 1.9', p.11 for a list). Note that they specifically mention nefazodone as a potent CYP3A4 inhibitor, but it is generally considered to be a moderate inhibitor, and they specifically mention grapefruit juice as a moderate CYP3A4 inhibitor, but it is generally considered to be a weak inhibitor. Further, they say that no dose adjustment is required with the concurrent use of weak CYP3A4 inhibitors.[2]

On the basis of the evidence here, the UK manufacturer of ulipristal for emergency contraception states that CYP3A4 inhibitors are unlikely to have any clinically relevant effects.[3]

1. Pohl O, Osterloh I, Gotteland JP. Effects of erythromycin at steady-state concentrations on the pharmacokinetics of ulipristal acetate. *J Clin Pharm Ther* (2013) 38, 512–7.
2. Esmya (Ulipristal acetate). Gedeon Richter (UK) Ltd. UK Summary of product characteristics, December 2013.
3. ellaOne (Ulipristal acetate). HRA Pharma UK and Ireland Ltd. UK Summary of product characteristics, January 2014.

Ulipristal + Drugs that affect gastric pH

Esomeprazole does not appear to affect the exposure to ulipristal.

Clinical evidence, mechanism, importance and management

In a study in 18 healthy female subjects, a single 10-mg dose of ulipristal was given alone and on day 5 of a 6-day course of **esomeprazole** 20 mg daily. The ulipristal maximum concentration was decreased by 65% and the AUC was increased by 15%. In addition, the time to reach maximum concentration was increased from 0.75 hours to 1 hour. These changes were not considered to be clinically relevant,[1] however, the UK manufacturer of ulipristal for emergency contraception, states that the clinical relevance in this scenario is not known.[2] The UK manufacturer of ulipristal for the management of fibroids states that no clinically relevant effect would be expected if given with drugs that increase gastric pH.[3] This would be expected to include other **proton pump inhibitors**, **antacids**, and **H_2-receptor antagonists**.

1. Pohl O, Osterloh I, Lecomte V, Gotteland JP. Changes in gastric pH and in pharmacokinetics of ulipristal acetate - a drug-drug interaction study using the proton pump inhibitor esomeprazole. *Int J Clin Pharmacol Ther* (2013) 51, 26–33.
2. ellaOne (Ulipristal acetate). HRA Pharma UK and Ireland Ltd. UK Summary of product characteristics, January 2014.
3. Esmya (Ulipristal acetate). Gedeon Richter (UK) Ltd. UK Summary of product characteristics, December 2013.

Ulipristal + Miscellaneous

The efficacy of ulipristal is expected to be reduced by enzyme-inducing drugs. Ulipristal has the potential to reduce the efficacy of hormonal contraceptives, and hormonal contraceptives might reduce the efficacy of ulipristal. Ulipristal did not alter the pharmacokinetics of fexofenadine when given 1.5 hours before.

Clinical evidence, mechanism, importance and management

(a) Contraceptive steroids

The UK manufacturers note that ulipristal acetate binds to the progesterone receptor with high affinity, and therefore could theoretically interfere with the action of progestogen-containing products,[1,2] and the action of ulipristal could be affected.[2] They state that it might reduce the efficacy of **combined hormonal contraceptives**, **progestogen-only contraceptives**,[1,2] and **progestogens** used for any other indication.[2] One US manufacturer simply advises that it might reduce the contraceptive action of regular contraceptive methods.[3] One UK manufacturer additionally states that the efficacy of ulipristal might be reduced by hormonal contraceptives and progestogens.[2] When ulipristal is given as emergency contraception, the UK and US manufacturers recommend that a reliable barrier method of contraception should be used until the next menstrual period starts.[1,3] In addition, the UK manufacturer specifically states that the concurrent use of ulipristal acetate and emergency hormonal contraception containing **levonorgestrel** is not recommended.[1] When ulipristal is given for the symptomatic management of fibroids, the UK manufacturer advises that concurrent use of ulipristal with any progestogen-containing products is not recommended, and such products should not be taken within 12 days of stopping ulipristal.[2]

(b) Enzyme inducers

The UK manufacturers of ulipristal briefly note that, in a study in healthy subjects, **rifampicin** (**rifampin**) 300 mg twice daily for 9 days decreased the maximum concentration and AUC of ulipristal by about 90%.[1,2] They therefore advise that ulipristal should not be used for emergency contraception or the symptomatic management of fibroids, in women taking CYP3A4 inducers.[1,2] One manufacturer specifically notes that the effect on ulipristal is still possible even if the inducer has been stopped within the last 2 to 3 weeks, and therefore does not recommend giving ulipristal to women who have stopped taking an enzyme inducer within the last 2 to 3 weeks.[1] Until more is known, this advice seems prudent, and should be applied to all drugs listed in 'Table 28.1', p.1160. Because ulipristal is a synthetic steroid derivative, it is possible that it will undergo similar interactions to combined hormonal contraceptives. Note that the MHRA in the UK specifically advises that women taking hormonal contraceptives for pregnancy prevention (except IUDs, but probably including emergency hormonal contraceptives) should not take herbal products containing **St John's wort**.[4]

The US manufacturer of ulipristal for emergency contraception states that enzyme inducers might reduce the effectiveness of ulipristal, but gives no advice.[3] Note also, that in addition to naming some of the drugs listed in 'Table 28.1', p.1160, they include **griseofulvin** and **felbamate** in their list of enzyme inducers; however, griseofulvin is not an established enzyme inducer, see 'Hormonal contraceptives + Griseofulvin', p.1192, and nor is felbamate, see 'Combined hormonal contraceptives + Felbamate', p.1174.

(c) P-glycoprotein substrates

The UK and US manufacturers briefly note that ulipristal appears to inhibit P-glycoprotein *in vitro*.[1-3] However, one UK manufacturer notes that, when a single 10-mg dose of ulipristal was given 1.5 hours before a single 60-mg dose of **fexofenadine**, the pharmacokinetics of fexofenadine were unaltered. They suggest that administration of ulipristal and P-glycoprotein substrates should be separated by at least 1.5 hours.[2] Simultaneous administration has not been studied. In contrast, the US manufacturer predicts that on the basis of the *in vitro* data, ulipristal might increase the concentrations of P-glycoprotein substrates.[3] For a list of P-glycoprotein substrates, see 'Table 1.12', p.14.

1. ellaOne (Ulipristal acetate). HRA Pharma UK and Ireland Ltd. UK Summary of product characteristics, January 2014.
2. Esmya (Ulipristal acetate). Gedeon Richter (UK) Ltd. UK Summary of product characteristics, December 2013.
3. ella (Ulipristal acetate). Afaxys Inc. US Prescribing information, February 2014.
4. Medicines and Healthcare Products Regulatory Agency and the Commission on Human Medicines. St John's wort: interaction with hormonal contraceptives, including implants – reduced contraceptive effect. *Drug Safety Update* (2014) 7, A2. Available at: http://webarchive.nationalarchives.gov.uk/20141205150130/http://www.mhra.gov.uk/home/groups/dsu/documents/publication/con392897.pdf (accessed 21/10/15).

29

Immunosuppressants

The immunosuppressants dealt with in this section are principally used for diseases considered to have an auto-immune component or in organ and tissue transplantation. They include the corticosteroids, calcineurin inhibitors (ciclosporin and tacrolimus), monoclonal antibodies (e.g. basiliximab), cytokine modulators (e.g. etanercept and infliximab) and various others, as classified in 'Table 29.1', below. When any of these drugs acts as the interacting agent the relevant monograph is categorised in the section dealing with the drug whose effects are changed. The cytotoxic drugs that are also used for immunosuppression (e.g. azathioprine, cyclophosphamide and methotrexate) are found in the section on antineoplastic drugs.

Immunosuppressant interactions

A. Pharmacological interactions

The most important pharmacological interactions of these drugs relate to their immunosuppressant effects. These will be additive with other immunosuppressants and, for example, increases the risk of infection. The risk of this sort of interaction obviously depends on the potency of the immunosuppressant and the duration of use. The additive risk can be such that certain combinations should be avoided, e.g. anakinra with TNF antagonists such as etanercept (see 'Etanercept + Miscellaneous', p.1261). Similarly, the use of live vaccines is not usually recommended in patients receiving immunosuppressants, see 'Immunosuppressants + Vaccines', p.1264.

B. Pharmacokinetic interactions

Many of the potent immunosuppressants discussed in this section have their doses titrated carefully to a given pharmacological effect or therapeutic range. For this reason, the use of drugs that cause a modest pharmacokinetic interaction may have clinically relevant consequences.

(a) Calcineurin inhibitors

1. Ciclosporin. Ciclosporin undergoes extensive metabolism, principally by the hepatic cytochrome P450 isoenzyme CYP3A4. The primary route of its excretion is biliary. Hence, drugs may alter ciclosporin concentrations by inhibiting or inducing its metabolism or altering its biliary secretion. An important dose-related adverse effect of ciclosporin is nephrotoxicity (raised serum creatinine and urea concentrations). In the transplant setting, the ciclosporin dose adjustments are usually based on the monitoring of its concentrations and serum creatinine. In general, minimum concentrations (pre-dose concentrations, C_0) are measured in whole blood. More recently, there has been interest in the use of monitoring ciclosporin concentrations 2 hours post dose (C_2 concentrations). With the lower doses of ciclosporin used in various autoimmune disorders, the dose is usually titrated to efficacy, and ciclosporin concentrations are not necessarily routinely monitored.

Ciclosporin is itself an inhibitor of P-glycoprotein and also a modest inhibitor of CYP3A4. It may therefore have pharmacokinetic interactions with other drugs (covered in other sections). More recently, it has been found that ciclosporin may also interacts with some drugs via inhibition of drug transporter proteins.

2. Tacrolimus. Tacrolimus is a substrate of CYP3A4 and P-glycoprotein, principally in the intestine. This is demonstrated by the fact that inhibitors or inducers of this isoenzymes and drug transporter increase or decrease the oral bioavailability of tacrolimus to a greater extent than they alter its clearance. In general, interactions of tacrolimus are similar to those of ciclosporin. Tacrolimus doses are adjusted on the basis of therapeutic drug monitoring. Tacrolimus is itself a modest inhibitor of CYP3A4.

(b) Corticosteroids

Some corticosteroids such as methylprednisolone are substrates for the cytochrome P450 isoenzyme CYP3A4 and therefore may interact with CYP3A4 inhibitors or inducers e.g. 'azoles', p.1246, 'macrolides', p.1254, or 'rifampicin (rifampin)', p.1258. Inhaled corticosteroids e.g. fluticasone may, in certain circumstances, also interact, see 'Corticosteroids + HIV-protease inhibitors', p.1252.

(c) Monoclonal antibodies

Monoclonal antibodies generally have few reported interactions, partly because studies can be difficult to design due to long elimination half-lives, and also because metabolising enzymes are generally not involved in monoclonal antibody elimination.

(d) Mycophenolate

Mycophenolate is rapidly hydrolysed to the active mycophenolic acid, which is subsequently metabolised by glucuronidation by glucuronyltransferases (UGT enzymes). Drugs that induce or inhibit glucuronidation may interact with mycophenolate. The glucuronide metabolite undergoes enterohepatic recycling being cleaved by gut bacteria to mycophenolic acid, which is then reabsorbed leading to a second peak in plasma concentrations. Drugs that interfere with this process, such as bile acid sequestrants and some antibacterials, may reduce this enterohepatic recycling. Mycophenolate is not metabolised by the cytochrome P450 isoenzyme system, so is not subject to interactions via this system. Note that blood concentrations of mycophenolic acid are not routinely monitored.

(e) Sirolimus and related drugs

Sirolimus (previously known as rapamycin) is a substrate of CYP3A4 and P-glycoprotein, principally in the intestine. It is therefore subject to drug interactions similar to those of tacrolimus. Its doses are adjusted on the basis of therapeutic drug monitoring. **Everolimus** is an analogue of sirolimus that was developed to improve the oral bioavailability of sirolimus. **Temsirolimus** is an ester prodrug of sirolimus. They therefore interact similarly to sirolimus.

Table 29.1 Immunosuppressant drugs†

Group	*Drugs*
Corticosteroids	
Glucocorticoids	Beclometasone, Budesonide, Ciclesonide, Deflazacort, Dexamethasone, Fluticasone, Hydrocortisone, Methylprednisolone, Prednisolone, Prednisone, Triamcinolone
Mineralocorticoids	Aldosterone, Fludrocortisone, Liquorice
Monoclonal antibodies	
Tumour necrosis factor (TNF) antagonists	Adalimumab, Certolizumab pegol, Golimumab, Infliximab
Miscellaneous	Abatacept, Anakinra, Basiliximab, Daclizumab, Muromonab-CD3, Natalizumab, Rituximab, Tocilizumab
Other immunosuppressants	
Calcineurin inhibitors	Ciclosporin (Cyclosporine), Tacrolimus
Tumour necrosis factor (TNF) antagonists	Etanercept
Miscellaneous	Everolimus, Leflunomide (DMARD), Mycophenolate, Sirolimus, Teriflunomide

†For other immunosuppressants that may also be used as cytotoxics, such as azathioprine, cyclophosphamide, methotrexate and mercaptopurine, see under Antineoplastics.

Abatacept + Miscellaneous

An increased risk of serious infection is reported if abatacept is given with tumour necrosis factor antagonists. Abatacept does not appear to affect the clearance of methotrexate, NSAIDs or corticosteroids. Live vaccines should not been given to patients taking abatacept.

Clinical evidence, mechanism, importance and management

(a) Anakinra

The US manufacturer recommends that anakinra is not given with abatacept because of insufficient information regarding the safety and efficacy of using these two drugs together.[1]

(b) Tumour necrosis factor antagonists

In clinical studies it was noted that tumour necrosis factor antagonists did not alter the clearance of abatacept.[1,2] However, patients who received treatment with abatacept and unnamed tumour necrosis factor antagonists [e.g. infliximab, adalimumab] experienced a higher incidence of infections and serious infections, 63% and 4.4%, respectively, when compared with treatment with tumour necrosis factor antagonists alone, 43% and 0.8%, respectively.[1] The manufacturers say that concurrent use is not recommended.[1,2]

(c) Vaccines

As no data are available on the use of live vaccines in patients receiving abatacept, the manufacturers recommend that live vaccines should not be given concurrently or within 3 months of discontinuation of abatacept. The response to some vaccines may be reduced.[1,2]

(d) Other drugs

The manufacturers note that population pharmacokinetic data suggests that the clearance of abatacept is not affected by **corticosteroids**, **methotrexate**, or **NSAIDs**.[1,2] There were no safety issues noted when abatacept was given with **sulfasalazine**, **hydroxychloroquine** or **leflunomide**.[2]

1. Orencia (Abatacept). Bristol-Myers Squibb. US Prescribing information, April 2008.
2. Orencia (Abatacept). Bristol-Myers Squibb Pharmaceuticals Ltd. UK Summary of product characteristics, May 2009.

Anakinra + Miscellaneous

Live vaccines should not be given with anakinra. No interaction has been reported between anakinra and corticosteroids, NSAIDs or other antirheumatics.

Clinical evidence, mechanism, importance and management

(a) Methotrexate

The manufacturers note that, in studies in *rats* concurrent use of methotrexate with anakinra did not affect the clearance of either drug or result in an increase in their adverse effects.[1,2] The clinical safety and efficacy of the combined use of anakinra and methotrexate has been proven in clinical studies,[2] and concurrent use is licensed.[1,2]

(b) Vaccines

The manufacturer states that live vaccines should not be given to patients receiving anakinra as the clinical safety of concurrent use has not been established. Patients may be at risk of developing generalised infections. The manufacturers also note that vaccination may be less effective in patients receiving anakinra.[1,2]

(c) Other drugs

The manufacturers state that no interaction has been reported between anakinra and **corticosteroids**, **NSAIDs** or other disease-modifying anti-rheumatic drugs (DMARDs).[2] **Infliximab** inhibits the activity of tumour necrosis factor (TNFα). In clinical studies the use of anakinra with another TNFα inhibitor, etanercept, has been associated with an increased risk of serious infection and neutropenia and no additional benefit, when compared to the use of these drugs alone.[3,4] As a result of this the manufacturers of **infliximab** note that similar toxicity may occur if anakinra is given with **infliximab** and therefore advise against concurrent use.[3,4]

1. Kineret (Anakinra). Amgen. US Prescribing information.
2. Kineret (Anakinra). Swedish Orphan Biovitrum Ltd. UK Summary of product characteristics, November 2013.
3. Remicade (Infliximab). Schering-Plough Ltd. UK Summary of product characteristics, March 2009.
4. Remicade (Infliximab). Janssen Biotech, Inc. US Prescribing information, November 2013.

Ciclosporin + ACE inhibitors or Angiotensin II receptor antagonists

Acute renal failure developed in four kidney transplant patients taking ciclosporin when they were given enalapril. Oliguria was seen in another patient taking ciclosporin with captopril. Other studies have found no significant changes in renal function with candesartan, losartan, valsartan, or enalapril. Hyperkalaemia can develop in patients taking ACE inhibitors or angiotensin II receptor antagonists with ciclosporin.

Clinical evidence

(a) ACE inhibitors

Two kidney transplant patients taking ciclosporin developed acute renal failure 10 to 42 days after starting to take **enalapril** 5 to 10 mg twice daily. Recovery was complete when the **enalapril** was stopped in one of the patients, and when both **enalapril** and ciclosporin were stopped in the other. The latter patient had no problems when ciclosporin was restarted. In both cases renal function had recovered after 10 to 30 days. Neither had any previous evidence of renal artery stenosis or chronic rejection, which are conditions known to predispose to renal failure during the use of an ACE inhibitor. Two other patients appeared to tolerate concurrent use well.[1] Two further kidney transplant patients developed acute renal failure when given **enalapril**. Neither had renal arterial stenosis or acute rejection.[2] The manufacturer briefly mentions that transient oliguria was seen in a kidney transplant patient given ciclosporin and **captopril**.[3]

A study in 13 kidney transplant patients taking ciclosporin found that concurrent treatment with **enalapril** 5 or 10 mg daily for 3 weeks caused a larger increase in potassium concentrations (mean increase of 0.5 mmol/L) than in those patients given **losartan** 50 mg daily (mean increase of 0.2 mmol/L). Potassium concentrations were not increased to above 5.5 mmol/L in any of the patients studied. Uric acid concentrations were also increased by **enalapril** but decreased by **losartan**, although this was not statistically significant. No changes in ciclosporin minimum concentrations were seen during the study and the serum creatinine concentrations remained stable.[4] Another study in kidney transplant patients taking ciclosporin with either **enalapril** (33 patients) or **enalapril** with amlodipine (32 patients) found that the potassium and serum creatinine concentrations did not increase in the group given **enalapril** and amlodipine whereas they increased by 0.2 mmol/L and 9 micromol/L, respectively, in the group given **enalapril** alone. Ciclosporin concentrations remained stable in all patients.[5]

(b) Angiotensin II receptor antagonists

A study in kidney transplant patients taking ciclosporin with **losartan** found that the serum creatinine concentration was only slightly and non-significantly increased in 5 patients. Losartan was stopped in 3 patients because of an increase in creatinine concentrations. Transient hyperkalaemia (potassium above 5.5 mmol/L) developed in 4 patients but the potassium had decreased to less than 5.5 mmol/L by week 12 in all patients. Ciclosporin concentrations remained stable during the study and no significant dose changes were made, although one patient was withdrawn from the study due to ciclosporin toxicity which the authors state was not related to the use of losartan.[6] Another study in 14 kidney transplant patients taking ciclosporin with **losartan** 50 to 100 mg daily for 8 weeks found serum creatinine, potassium, and ciclosporin concentrations were unaffected.[7]

A study in 41 kidney transplant patients with proteinuria taking ciclosporin found that the addition of **candesartan** 4 to 12 mg daily had no clinically significant effects on the creatinine clearance or ciclosporin concentrations.[8] A randomised study in 75 kidney transplant patients taking ciclosporin (with mycophenolate mofetil and prednisolone), found that **valsartan** 80 mg daily given for 24 weeks did not affect ciclosporin plasma concentrations.[9]

Mechanism

Not understood. One suggestion is that ciclosporin reduces renal blood flow and reduces perfusion through the glomerulus, which is worsened when angiotensin II is inhibited by the ACE inhibitor.[1] One study suggested that the larger increase in potassium concentrations might be related to changes in aldosterone concentrations seen with enalapril.[4]

Importance and management

There have been few specific case reports of renal failure and hyperkalaemia with ciclosporin and ACE inhibitors or angiotensin II receptor antagonists. Data from the few examples of efficacy studies cited above, suggest that the incidence of renal failure and hyperkalaemia is low, nevertheless care and good monitoring are needed if ACE inhibitors or angiotensin II receptor antagonists and ciclosporin are used concurrently. Monitor potassium concentrations more closely in the initial weeks of concurrent use, bearing in mind that an increase in potassium concentrations might be due to worsening renal function as well as the use of these drugs.

1. Murray BM, Venuto RC, Kohli R, Cunningham EE. Enalapril-associated renal failure in renal transplants: possible role of cyclosporine. *Am J Kidney Dis* (1990) 16, 66–9.
2. Garcia TM, da Costa JA, Costa RS, Ferraz AS. Acute tubular necrosis in kidney transplant patients treated with enalapril. *Ren Fail* (1994) 16, 419–23.
3. Cockburn I. Cyclosporine A: a clinical evaluation of drug interactions. *Transplant Proc* (1986) 18 (Suppl 5), 50–5.
4. Schmidt A, Gruber U, Böhmig G, Köller E, Mayer G. The effect of ACE inhibitor and angiotensin II receptor antagonist therapy on serum uric acid levels and potassium homeostasis in hypertensive renal transplant recipients treated with CsA. *Nephrol Dial Transplant* (2001) 16, 1034–7.
5. Halimi JM, Giraudeau B, Buchler M, Al-Najjar A, Etienne I, Laouad I, Bruyere F, Lebranchu Y. Enalapril/amlodipine combination in cyclosporine-treated renal transplant recipients: a prospective randomized trial. *Clin Transplant* (2007) 21, 277–84.
6. del Castillo D, Campistol JM, Guirado L, Capdevilla L, Martínez JG, Pereira P, Bravo J, Pérez R. Efficacy and safety of losartan in the treatment of hypertension in renal transplant patients. *Kidney Int* (1998) 54, (Suppl 68) S135–S139.
7. Tylicki L, Biedunkiewicz B, Chamienia A, Wojnarowski K, Zdrojewski Z, Rutkowski B. Randomized placebo-controlled study on the effects of losartan and carvedilol on albuminuria in renal transplant recipients. *Transplantation* (2006) 81, 52–6.
8. Omoto K, Tanabe K, Tokumoto T, Shimmura H, Ishida H, Toma H. Use of candesartan cilexetil decreases proteinuria in renal transplant patients with chronic allograft dysfunction. *Transplantation* (2003) 76, 1170–4.

9. Cai J, Huang Z, Yang G, Cheng K, Ye Q, Ming Y, Zuo X, Zhou P, Yuan H. Comparing antihypertensive effect and plasma ciclosporin concentration between amlodipine and valsartan regimens in hypertensive renal transplant patients receiving ciclosporin therapy. *Am J Cardiovasc Drugs* (2011) 11, 401–9.

Ciclosporin + Acetazolamide

There is some limited evidence to suggest that oral acetazolamide can cause a large and rapid increase in ciclosporin concentrations, possibly accompanied by renal toxicity.

Clinical evidence, mechanism, importance and management

A study in 3 men found that 72 hours after they started taking acetazolamide (dose not stated), their minimum serum ciclosporin concentrations increased more than 6-fold, from a range of 54 to 270 nanograms/mL up to a range of 517 to 1827 nanograms/mL.[1] Another man with a heart transplant had a 5-fold increase in his serum ciclosporin concentrations, marked renal impairment, and neurotoxicity when he was given oral acetazolamide for increased intra-ocular pressure secondary to panuveitis.[2] The increase in ciclosporin serum concentrations has also been seen in *animal* studies.[3]

Information seems to be limited to these reports but it seems that the concurrent use of ciclosporin and acetazolamide should be closely monitored, being alert of the need to reduce the ciclosporin dose. The interaction can apparently develop very rapidly.

1. Tabbara KF, Al-Faisal Z, Al-Rashed W. Interaction between acetazolamide and cyclosporine. *Arch Ophthalmol* (1998) 116, 832–3.
2. Keogh A, Esmore D, Spratt P, Savdie E, McClusky P, Chang V. Acetazolamide and cyclosporine. *Transplantation* (1988) 46, 478–9.
3. El-Sayed YM, Tabbara KF, Gouda MW. Effect of acetazolamide on the pharmacokinetics of cyclosporin in rabbits. *Int J Pharmaceutics* (1995) 121, 181–6.

Ciclosporin + Aciclovir and related drugs

Aciclovir does not normally seem to affect ciclosporin concentrations or worsen renal function on concurrent use, but cases of nephrotoxicity and increased ciclosporin concentrations have been reported. Valaciclovir, a prodrug of aciclovir, is expected to interact similarly.

Limited evidence suggests ganciclovir does not affect ciclosporin concentrations or worsen renal function on concurrent use. However, four patients given ciclosporin and ganciclovir developed an acute but reversible eye movement disorder.

Clinical evidence

(a) Aciclovir

A retrospective study in kidney transplant patients taking ciclosporin (serum concentrations in the range 100 to 250 nanograms/mL) found that in 12 patients, oral aciclovir 800 mg four times daily for 3 months had no effect on their ciclosporin serum concentrations or on nephrotoxicity when compared with 9 control subjects.[1] No notable changes in renal function were seen in 11 patients taking ciclosporin when they were given intravenous aciclovir 750 to 1500 mg/m^2 daily for at least 7 days to treat herpes infections.[2] No notable changes in serum creatinine or ciclosporin concentrations were seen during the 14 days following kidney transplant in 17 patients given aciclovir 800 mg daily.[3] Fifty-three kidney transplant patients were given ciclosporin and aciclovir 800 mg to 3.2 g daily for 12 weeks. The aciclovir was withdrawn from 2 patients because of unexplained and temporary increases in serum creatinine concentrations. The serum ciclosporin concentrations were not reported.[4] Five patients (2 adults and 3 children) taking ciclosporin, prednisone, and azathioprine were given aciclovir 200 mg five times daily for 6 days for herpes zoster or chicken pox. Ciclosporin serum concentrations remained unchanged and renal function improved.[5]

In contrast to the cases cited above, 3 of 7 bone marrow transplant patients given ciclosporin and intravenous aciclovir 500 mg/m^2 every 8 or 12 hours (depending on renal function) developed nephrotoxicity, which was fatal in one case. Histological evidence suggested ciclosporin nephrotoxicity.[6] The manufacturer briefly notes that an increase in serum creatinine was seen in patients taking ciclosporin in one report, and increased aciclovir concentrations accompanied by reversible acute tubular necrosis were seen in another.[7] Yet another report describes a 3-fold increase in ciclosporin serum concentrations, which occurred when a child with a heart transplant was given intravenous aciclovir.[8]

(b) Ganciclovir

In a retrospective analysis, 7 patients taking ciclosporin with ganciclovir 3 mg/kg every 12 hours for 5 to 7 days during antirejection therapy with antithymocyte globulin or muromonab-CD3 had no significant change in their ciclosporin concentrations (increase of 7.8%) and the ciclosporin dose was not altered. In these patients, serum creatinine concentrations remained stable.[9]

Another retrospective study identified 582 allogeneic bone marrow transplant patients taking ciclosporin and about 45% of whom were given ganciclovir at some time during the first 3 months after the transplant. Four patients (0.7%) developed an acute eye movement disorder (unilateral or bilateral sixth nerve palsies) within 4 to 34 days of starting ganciclovir. Three of the four patients also had bilateral ptosis, which resolved 24 to 48 hours after withdrawal of both drugs from 3 patients and after the withdrawal of just ciclosporin from the other patient. Objective eye movement abnormality with diplopia recurred in one patient when both drugs were restarted, but not when ciclosporin alone was given.[10]

Mechanism

The renal toxicity of aciclovir and related drugs might occasionally be additive or synergistic with that of ciclosporin. The reason for the eye movement disorders with ganciclovir is not known but the authors of the report suggest an interaction as eye movement disorders are not known to occur with either drug alone.[10]

Importance and management

The evidence available indicates that ciclosporin concentrations and renal function are usually unaltered by the concurrent use of aciclovir, but the handful of cases where problems have arisen introduce a note of caution. One group of workers suggest that aciclovir, in doses of 250 mg/m^2 by slow infusion, does not adversely affect renal function in well-hydrated patients taking ciclosporin if their ciclosporin concentrations are carefully monitored.[2] Similar precautions should be used with **valaciclovir**, a prodrug of aciclovir. Note that the manufacturers recommend that renal function is closely monitored if valaciclovir,[11] or aciclovir infusion,[12] are given with drugs that affect renal function, such as ciclosporin.

Limited evidence suggests that ganciclovir does not alter ciclosporin concentrations or renal function, but, like aciclovir, ganciclovir can cause increases in serum creatinine concentrations and accumulates in renal impairment, so some caution is warranted on concurrent use. The same advice would appear to apply to **valganciclovir**, the prodrug of ganciclovir.

The report of eye movement disorders with ganciclovir cited here seems to be the only report of this interaction; therefore its general relevance is uncertain.

1. Dugandzic RM, Sketris IS, Belitsky P, Schlech WF, Givner ML. Effect of coadministration of acyclovir and cyclosporine on kidney function and cyclosporine concentrations in renal transplant patients. *DICP Ann Pharmacother* (1991) 25, 316–7.
2. Johnson PC, Kumor K, Welsh MS, Woo J, Kahan BD. Effects of coadministration of cyclosporine and acyclovir on renal function of renal allograft recipients. *Transplantation* (1987) 44, 329–31.
3. Stoffel M, Squifflet JP, Pirson Y, Lamy M, Alexandre GPJ. Effectiveness of oral acyclovir prophylaxis in renal transplant recipients. *Transplant Proc* (1987) 19, 2190–3.
4. Balfour HH, Chace BA, Stapleton JT, Simmons RL, Fryd DS. A randomized, placebo-controlled trial of oral acyclovir for the prevention of cytomegalovirus disease in recipients of renal allografts. *N Engl J Med* (1989) 320, 1381–7.
5. Hayes K, Shakuntala V, Pingle A, Dhawan IK, Masri MA. Safe use of acyclovir (Zovirax) in renal transplant patients on cyclosporine A therapy: case reports. *Transplant Proc* (1992) 24, 1926.
6. Shepp DH, Dandliker PS, Meyers JD. Treatment of varicella-zoster virus infection in severely immunocompromised patients: a randomized comparison of acyclovir and vidarabine. *N Engl J Med* (1986) 314, 208–12.
7. Cockburn I. Cyclosporine A: a clinical evaluation of drug interactions. *Transplant Proc* (1986) 18 (Suppl 5), 50–5.
8. Boardman M, Yodur Purdy C. Cyclosporine and aciclovir; report of a drug interaction. Am Soc Hosp Pharmacists Midyear Clinical Meeting, Dallas, Texas. December 1988, Abstract SP-16.
9. Cantarovich M, Latter D. Effect of prophylactic ganciclovir on renal function and cyclosporine levels after heart transplantation. *Transplant Proc* (1994) 26, 2747–8.
10. Openshaw H, Slatkin NE, Smith E. Eye movement disorders in bone marrow transplant patients on cyclosporin and ganciclovir. *Bone Marrow Transplant* (1997) 19, 503–5.
11. Valtrex (Valaciclovir hydrochloride). GlaxoSmithKline UK. UK Summary of product characteristics, April 2014.
12. Aciclovir sterile concentrate. Hospira UK Ltd. UK Summary of product characteristics, February 2008.

Ciclosporin + Alcohol

An isolated report describes a increase in serum ciclosporin concentrations in a patient after an episode of binge drinking, but a subsequent study found that moderate, single doses of alcohol in other patients had no such effect. A large amount of red wine, taken concurrently with ciclosporin in the fasted state, decreased ciclosporin bioavailability in one study.

Clinical evidence

The serum ciclosporin concentrations of a kidney transplant patient doubled, from 101 to 205 nanograms/mL, and remained high for about 4 days after he went on a 2-day alcohol binge. However, a subsequent study in 8 other patients with kidney transplants found no changes in serum ciclosporin or creatinine concentrations when they took their regular dose of ciclosporin followed by 50 mL of 100% alcohol in orange juice consumed over a one-hour period (about equivalent to about 120 mL (4 oz) of whisky).[1]

A crossover study in 12 fasted, healthy subjects given a single 8 mg/kg dose of ciclosporin (*Sandimmun*) with water or 350 mL (12 oz) of Californian red wine found that red wine caused a 50% increase in the oral clearance of ciclosporin. The ciclosporin AUC was reduced by 30% and the maximum blood concentrations were reduced by 38% (from 1258 to 779 micrograms/L), but there was no change in elimination half-life. There was a high degree of variability, with increases in oral clearance ranging from 1.5 to 129%, with Caucasians experiencing a greater degree of change than Asians. In this study, half of the wine was consumed 15 minutes before the ciclosporin, and the other half was consumed at the same time as taking ciclosporin and in the 15 minutes afterwards. In their discussion the authors briefly note that, in a separate study of theirs, white wine did not have an effect on ciclosporin clearance.[2]

Mechanism

The mechanism by which red wine decreases ciclosporin absorption is not known. White wine[2] and pure alcohol[1] do not appear to affect ciclosporin pharmacokinetics, so the interaction is not believed to be an effect of alcohol itself. Antioxidants in red wine such as resveratrol might inactivate CYP3A4, but this would be expected to increase ciclosporin concentrations. The solubility of ciclosporin is decreased in red wine, and it is possible that substances in red wine bind ciclosporin in the gastrointestinal tract and reduce its bioavailability.[2] Another study by the same authors suggested that ciclosporin absorption is possibly impaired by P-glycoprotein induction by red wine.[3]

Importance and management

The evidence for an interaction between ciclosporin and alcohol consumption is relatively limited. The authors of the first study[1] state that they currently advise their kidney transplant patients to avoid heavy drinking, but that an occasional drink probably does not affect ciclosporin concentrations. The second study[2] suggests that it might be wise to avoid red wine close to a ciclosporin dose. However, this finding does not imply that an interaction would occur with an occasional single glass of red wine taken with a meal and separate from ciclosporin dosing. Note that patients might be advised to avoid alcohol if they are taking ciclosporin after transplantation.

1. Paul MD, Parfrey PS, Smart M, Gault H. The effect of ethanol on serum cyclosporine A levels in renal transplant patients. *Am J Kidney Dis* (1987) 10, 133–5.
2. Tsunoda SM, Harris RZ, Christians U, Velez RL, Freeman RB, Benet LZ, Warshaw A. Red wine decreases cyclosporine bioavailability. *Clin Pharmacol Ther* (2001) 70, 462–7.
3. Tsunoda SM, Christians U, Velez RL, Benet LZ, Harris RZ. Red wine (RW) effects on cyclosporine (CyA) metabolites. *Clin Pharmacol Ther* (2000) 67, 150.

Ciclosporin + Alfalfa (*Medicago sativa*) and Black cohosh (*Cimicifuga racemosa*)

An isolated report describes acute rejection and vasculitis after a renal transplant patient taking ciclosporin started supplements containing black cohosh and alfalfa.

Clinical evidence

A stable kidney transplant patient taking **azathioprine** 50 mg daily and ciclosporin 75 mg twice daily began to take alfalfa and black cohosh supplements (specific products not stated) on medical advice for severe menopausal symptoms. Her serum creatinine concentration increased from between about 97 to 124 micromol/L up to 168 micromol/L after 4 weeks and, to 256 micromol/L after 6 weeks with no associated change in her ciclosporin concentrations. Biopsy revealed severe acute rejection with vasculitis and she was treated with corticosteroids and anti-T lymphocyte immunoglobulin with partial improvement in renal function.[1]

Mechanism

Alfalfa has been reported to cause worsening of lupus and immunostimulation and it was suggested that immunostimulation might have contributed to the acute rejection in this patient.[1]

Importance and management

The evidence for an interaction between alfalfa and/or black cohosh and immunosuppressants is limited, with the mechanism suggesting that alfalfa is the more likely culprit, although an effect of black cohosh cannot be ruled out. As the effects in the case were so severe, it would seem prudent to avoid the use of alfalfa supplements in patients receiving immunosuppressants for serious indications, such as organ or tissue transplantation. Similarly, it would seem prudent to avoid the use of alfalfa supplements in those taking immunosuppressants for indications such as eczema, psoriasis, or rheumatoid arthritis; however, if these patients particularly wish to take alfalfa a short-term trial of concurrent use is likely to be less hazardous. Nevertheless, patients should be counselled about the possible risks (i.e. loss of disease control).

1. Light TD, Light JA. Acute renal transplant rejection possibly related to herbal medications. *Am J Transplant* (2003) 3, 1608–9.

Ciclosporin + Allopurinol

Isolated case reports describe large increases in ciclosporin concentrations in patients given standard doses of allopurinol for the treatment of gout. However, in two clinical studies, a trend towards lower ciclosporin concentrations with low-dose allopurinol has been seen.

Clinical evidence, mechanism, importance and management

The ciclosporin concentrations of a kidney transplant patient increased approximately 3-fold, accompanied by an increase in serum creatinine from 124 to 194 micromol/L, after allopurinol 100 mg daily was taken for 12 days for the treatment of gout.[1] Another previously stable kidney transplant patient had a 2- to 3-fold increase in her ciclosporin concentrations when allopurinol 200 mg daily was given for gout. Her serum creatinine remained unchanged throughout.[2] The general importance of these two reports of increased ciclosporin concentrations is unknown, although increases in ciclosporin concentrations are associated with increased risk of nephrotoxicity.

Two clinical studies in kidney transplant patients taking ciclosporin, azathioprine, and prednisolone, with low-dose allopurinol 25 mg daily or on alternate days to improve the efficacy of azathioprine, found a reduction in ciclosporin concentrations (32% in one group), as well as a beneficial reduction in the acute rejection rate.[3] Note that azathioprine concentrations can be increased by allopurinol, usually requiring a dose reduction, see 'Thiopurines + Allopurinol', p.720.

The case reports above and the clinical studies are probably insufficient to recommend increased monitoring of ciclosporin concentrations in all patients given allopurinol, but bear them in mind in the event of an unexpected response to treatment.

1. Stevens SL, Goldman MH. Cyclosporine toxicity associated with allopurinol. *South Med J* (1992) 85, 1265–6.
2. Gorrie M, Beaman M, Nicholls A, Backwell P. Allopurinol interaction with cyclosporine. *BMJ* (1994) 308, 113.
3. Chocair PR, Duley JA, Cameron JS, Arap S, Ianhez L, Sabbaga E, Simmonds HA. Does low-dose allopurinol, with azathioprine, cyclosporin and prednisolone, improve renal transplant immunosuppression? *Adv Exp Med Biol* (1994) 370, 205–8.

Ciclosporin + Alpha blockers

Preliminary studies found that prazosin caused a small reduction in the glomerular filtration rate in kidney transplant patients taking ciclosporin. Ciclosporin is predicted to increase silodosin exposure.

Clinical evidence, mechanism, importance and management

(a) Prazosin

A study in 8 kidney transplant patients found that prazosin 1 mg twice daily for one week did not alter their ciclosporin blood concentrations, and arterial blood pressures and renal vascular resistance were reduced. However, the glomerular filtration rate (GFR) was reduced by about 10% (from 47 to 42 mL/minute).[1] Previous studies in kidney transplant patients taking azathioprine, prednisone, and prazosin found no reduction in GFR.[2] There would seem to be no strong reason for avoiding prazosin in patients taking ciclosporin, but the authors of the report point out that the fall in GFR makes prazosin a less attractive antihypertensive than a calcium-channel blocker.

(b) Silodosin

The US manufacturer of silodosin[3] states that *in vitro* studies suggest that silodosin is a P-glycoprotein substrate. They therefore suggest that P-glycoprotein inhibitors (ciclosporin is named) will increase silodosin exposure and concentrations. Concurrent use is not recommended; however, if both drugs are given it would seem prudent to be alert for any evidence of silodosin adverse effects (e.g. dizziness, diarrhoea, and orthostatic hypotension). If these become troublesome consider reducing the dose of silodosin or withdrawing the drug as necessary.

1. Kiberd BA. Effects of prazosin therapy in renal allograft recipients receiving cyclosporine. *Transplantation* (1990) 49, 1200–1.
2. Curtis JR, Bateman FJA. Use of prazosin in management of hypertension in patients with chronic renal failure and in renal transplant recipients. *BMJ* (1975) 4, 432.
3. Rapaflo (Silodosin). Watson Pharma, Inc. US Prescribing information, January 2013.

Ciclosporin + Amiodarone

Increased ciclosporin serum concentrations have been reported in patients starting amiodarone, and nephrotoxicity has occurred as a result of these increased concentrations. Conversely, one report describes a small decrease in ciclosporin concentrations and increased amiodarone concentrations on their concurrent use.

A case report describes pulmonary toxicity in patients stopping amiodarone and starting ciclosporin.

Clinical evidence

Eight patients with heart transplants and 3 patients with heart-lung transplants taking ciclosporin were also given amiodarone (dose not stated) for atrial flutter or fibrillation. Their serum ciclosporin concentrations increased by 9% despite a 13 to 14% reduction in the ciclosporin dose, serum creatinine concentrations increased by 38% (from 157 to 216 micromol/L), and blood urea nitrogen increased by 30%.[1] In another report, one patient is said to have had a 50% decrease in the clearance of ciclosporin when given amiodarone (1 g, then 600 mg daily for 5 days, then 400 mg daily).[2] Eight other patients with heart or heart-lung transplants were effectively treated with amiodarone (dose not stated) for atrial flutter and/or atrial fibrillation, but they had a 31% increase in their serum ciclosporin concentration, from 248 to 325 nanograms/mL despite a 44% reduction in the ciclosporin dose (from 6.2 to 3.5 mg/kg daily). Serum creatinine concentrations increased by 39%.[3] The serum ciclosporin concentration of a kidney transplant patient doubled when amiodarone 600 mg twice daily was given.[4]

In contrast, in 5 heart transplant patients in whom amiodarone was stopped and ciclosporin subsequently started, the metabolism of ciclosporin appeared to be increased for 4 to 5 weeks compared with patients who had not received amiodarone (total plasma metabolites 1437 nanograms/mL and 720 nanograms/mL, respectively). The maintenance ciclosporin concentration was reduced by only a small amount in those who had received amiodarone compared with those who had not been given amiodarone (225 nanograms/mL and 240 nanograms/mL, respectively).[5] In this study, 2 patients had amiodarone concentrations monitored, and it was found that the plasma concentrations of amiodarone and its main metabolite, desethylamiodarone were increased over 4 to 5 weeks. During this period increased adverse effects, including pulmonary toxicity in one patient, were seen.[5]

Mechanism

Uncertain. Ciclosporin is metabolised by CYP3A4 an isoenzyme thought to be inhibited by amiodarone. Concurrent use could therefore increase ciclosporin concentrations. It has also been suggested that amiodarone might inhibit P-glycoprotein, a drug transporter protein known to affect ciclosporin disposition.

Importance and management

The increase in ciclosporin concentrations on starting amiodarone would appear to be an established and clinically important interaction. Concurrent use need not be avoided but close monitoring is needed and ciclosporin dose reductions might also be required to minimise the potential nephrotoxicity. Remember to re-adjust the ciclosporin dose if the amiodarone is stopped, bearing in mind that it may take weeks before amiodarone is totally cleared from the body.

The general significance of the increase in amiodarone concentrations, apparent decrease in ciclosporin concentrations and the occurrence of pulmonary toxicity in patients who had stopped amiodarone and started ciclosporin is unclear. It would seem prudent to consider an interaction as a possible cause if amiodarone adverse effects are increased.

1. Egami J, Mullins PA, Mamprin F, Chauhan A, Large SR, Wallwork J, Schofield PM. Increase in cyclosporine levels due to amiodarone therapy after heart and heart-lung transplantation. *J Am Coll Cardiol* (1993) 21, 141A.
2. Nicolau DP, Uber WE, Crumbley AJ, Strange C. Amiodarone-cyclosporine interaction in a heart transplant patient. *J Heart Lung Transplant* (1992) 11, 564–8.
3. Mamprin F, Mullins P, Graham T, Kendall S, Biocine B, Large S, Wallwork J, Schofield P. Amiodarone-cyclosporine interaction in cardiac transplantation. *Am Heart J* (1992) 123, 1725–6.
4. Chitwood KK, Abdul-Haqq AJ, Heim-Duthoy KL. Cyclosporine-amiodarone interaction. *Ann Pharmacother* (1993) 27, 569–71.
5. Preuner JG, Lehle K, Keyser A, Merk J, Rupprecht L, Goebels R. Development of severe adverse effects after discontinuing amiodarone therapy in human heart transplant recipients. *Transplant Proc* (1998) 30, 3943–4.

Ciclosporin + Amphotericin B

There is some good evidence to suggest that the risk of nephrotoxicity is increased if ciclosporin and amphotericin B are used concurrently. However, other limited evidence suggests that the concurrent use of a liposomal form of amphotericin B (*AmBisome*) with ciclosporin does not increase nephrotoxicity or hepatotoxicity. Ciclosporin blood concentrations might be increased or decreased by amphotericin B.

Clinical evidence

(a) Ciclosporin concentrations

A retrospective analysis in allogeneic bone marrow transplant patients found that those patients taking high-dose prednisone with a continuous infusion of ciclosporin and prophylactic amphotericin B 5 to 10 mg daily had 13 to 23% lower plasma concentrations of ciclosporin in the first 4 weeks post-transplant, when compared with those given the same GVHD (graft-versus-host-disease) prophylactic regimen who did not receive amphotericin B. No obvious dose reductions or changes in renal function were noted in these patients. It was also noted in this study that patients with ciclosporin plasma concentrations of 500 nanograms/mL had a 2.2-fold increased risk of developing GVHD when compared with patients with levels of 1000 nanograms/mL.[1] Similarly, a 23-year-old man taking oral ciclosporin had a reduction in his blood concentration of ciclosporin from about 100 to 50 nanograms/mL within 10 days of starting intravenous amphotericin B.[2]

In contrast, a study in 187 transplant patients given an average dose of ciclosporin 10 mg/kg daily found that ciclosporin blood concentrations increased significantly from 275 to 328 nanograms/mL during the use of liposomal amphotericin B (*AmBisome*) and decreased to 242 nanograms/mL one week after amphotericin B was stopped.[3] A retrospective study in 22 patients who had undergone allogeneic stem cell transplants found a non-significant increase in ciclosporin blood concentrations (from 259 to 296 nanograms/mL) when given amphotericin B (0.6 to 2 mg/kg daily for 3 to 112 days). However, a lower ciclosporin maximum blood concentration of 775 nanograms/mL was seen in those patients who received amphotericin B compared with 1240 nanograms/mL in 62 patients receiving ciclosporin without amphotericin B, although again the difference was not statistically significant.[4]

(b) Toxic effects

1. Nephrotoxicity. The concurrent use of ciclosporin and amphotericin B increased the incidence of nephrotoxicity in 47 patients with bone marrow transplants. Out of 10 patients who had received both drugs, 5 doubled and 3 tripled their serum creatinine concentration within 5 days. In contrast, only 8 out of 21 (38%) taking ciclosporin alone, and 3 out of 16 (19%) taking methotrexate and amphotericin B, doubled their serum creatinine within 14 to 30 days and 5 days, respectively.[5] Similarly, in a retrospective study, 14 potential drug-drug interactions were identified in patients given both ciclosporin and amphotericin B, and of these, 7 resulted in a clinically significant interaction (increased creatinine concentrations in all cases, with one patient developing nephrotoxicity).[6]

Two studies of the risk factors associated with amphotericin B identified the concurrent use of ciclosporin as posing a particularly significant risk for the development of the moderate to severe nephrotoxicity seen in 8 to 12% of patients given amphotericin B.[7,8] Two other studies in bone marrow transplant patients taking ciclosporin found that amphotericin B contributed significantly to nephrotoxicity and renal failure.[9,10] Renal impairment can apparently develop even after amphotericin B has been withdrawn.[9] Marked nephrotoxicity is described in one patient in another report.[11] A retrospective study of patients taking ciclosporin also found an increase in creatinine concentrations during the concurrent use of a continuous infusion of amphotericin B (*Fungizone*) in 22 patients (compared with 62 patients taking ciclosporin alone); however, large reductions in renal function (creatinine clearance less than 30 mL/minute) were not found.[4] A study including 8 severely ill infants undergoing bone marrow transplantation for severe immunodeficiency, found no evidence of significant nephrotoxicity or hepatotoxicity when liposomal amphotericin B (*AmBisome*) was given with ciclosporin. The average course of treatment lasted for 29 days.[12]

2. Neurotoxicity. An isolated case report described severe tremors, later becoming myoclonic, attributed to the concurrent use of liposomal amphotericin B (*AmBisome*) and oral ciclosporin. Serum ciclosporin concentrations were unaltered and creatinine concentrations only increased slightly.[13] This alleged neurotoxicity was challenged in a letter citing 187 transplant patients who had received ciclosporin and *AmBisome*, none of whom developed neurotoxicity attributable to an interaction.[14]

3. Other adverse effects. In a retrospective analysis in bone marrow transplant patients, renal tubular acidosis and hypomagnesaemia were noted to be the most common adverse effects of the concurrent use of low-dose amphotericin B 5 to 10 mg daily with ciclosporin.[1]

Mechanism

Amphotericin B and ciclosporin are both nephrotoxic, and their adverse effects on the kidneys might be additive. The mechanism of the effects of amphotericin B on ciclosporin blood concentrations is not understood, especially as contrasting effects have been noted. However, in one *animal* study, amphotericin B decreased ciclosporin bioavailability by inducing the cytochrome P450 subfamily CYP3A and P-glycoprotein.[2]

Importance and management

The increased nephrotoxicity associated with ciclosporin and amphotericin B appears to be established and clinically important. The authors of one report[5] suggest that, in patients needing amphotericin B, renal toxicity can be decreased without losing the immunosuppressant effect of ciclosporin by withholding ciclosporin until the serum concentration is less than about 150 nanograms/mL.

The reports supporting a lack of significant nephrotoxicity all used liposomal amphotericin B, a formulation that is recommended when amphotericin toxicity (particularly nephrotoxicity) is considered to be a significant risk. This would seem to suggest that in patients taking ciclosporin, the less nephrotoxic forms of amphotericin B are advisable. Renal function should be closely monitored during concurrent use.

The changes in ciclosporin blood concentrations reported with amphotericin B are inconsistent. However, these studies should be borne in mind when using both drugs, and ciclosporin concentrations as well as renal function and electrolytes should be closely monitored.

1. O'Donnell MR, Schmidt GM, Tegtmeier BR, Faucett C, Fahey JL, Ito J, Nademanee A, Niland J, Parker P, Smith EP, Snyder DS, Stein AS, Blume KG, Forman SJ. Prediction of systemic fungal infection in allogeneic marrow recipients: impact of amphotericin prophylaxis in high-risk patients. *J Clin Oncol* (1994) 12, 827–34.
2. Ishizaki J, Ito S, Jin M, Shimada T, Ishigaki T, Harasawa Y, Yokogawa K, Takami A, Nakao S, Miyamoto K. Mechanism of decrease of oral bioavailability of cyclosporin A during immunotherapy upon coadministration of amphotericin B. *Biopharm Drug Dispos* (2008) 29,195–203.
3. Ringdén O, Andström E, Remberger M, Svahn B-M, Tollemar J. Safety of liposomal amphotericin B (AmBisome) in 187 transplant recipients treated with ciclosporin. *Bone Marrow Transplant* (1994) 14, (Suppl 5) S10–S14.
4. Furrer K, Schaffner A, Vavricka SR, Halter J, Imhof A, Schanz U. Nephrotoxicity of cyclosporine A and amphotericin B-deoxycholate as continuous infusion in allogeneic stem cell transplantation. *Swiss Med Wkly* (2002) 132, 316–20.
5. Kennedy MS, Deeg HJ, Siegel M, Crowley JJ, Storb R, Thomas ED. Acute renal toxicity with combined use of amphotericin B and cyclosporine after bone marrow transplantation. *Transplantation* (1983) 35, 211–15.
6. Depont F, Vargas F, Dutronc H, Giauque E, Ragnaud J-M, Galpérine T, Abouelfath A, Valentino R, Dupon M, Hérbert G, Moore N. Drug-drug interactions with systemic antifungals in clinical practice. *Pharmacoepidemiol Drug Safety* (2007) 16, 1227–33.
7. Luber AD, Maa L, Lam M, Guglielmo BJ. Risk factors for amphotericin B- induced nephrotoxicity. *J Antimicrob Chemother* (1999) 43, 267–71.
8. Harbarth S, Pestotnik SL, Lloyd JF, Burke JP, Samore MH. The epidemiology of nephrotoxicity associated with conventional amphotericin B therapy. *Am J Med* (2001) 111, 528–34.
9. Tutschka PJ, Beschorner WE, Hess AD, Santos GW. Cyclosporin-A to prevent graft-versus-host-disease: a pilot study in 22 patients receiving allogeneic marrow transplants. *Blood* (1983) 61, 318–25.
10. Miller KB, Schenkein DP, Comenzo R, Erban JK, Fogaren T, Hirsch CA, Berkman E, Rabson A. Adjusted-dose continuous-infusion cyclosporin A to prevent graft-versus-host disease following allogeneic bone marrow transplantation. *Ann Hematol* (1994) 68, 15–20.
11. Conti DJ, Tolkoff-Rubin NE, Baker GP, Doran M, Cosimi AB, Delmonico F, Auchincloss H, Russell PS, Rubin RH. Successful treatment of invasive fungal infection with fluconazole in organ transplant recipients. *Transplantation* (1989) 48, 692–5.
12. Pasic S, Flannagan L, Cant AJ. Liposomal amphotericin (AmBisome) is safe in bone marrow transplantation for primary immunodeficiency. *Bone Marrow Transplant* (1997) 19, 1229–32.
13. Ellis ME, Spence D, Ernst P, Meunier F. Is cyclosporin neurotoxicity enhanced in the presence of liposomal amphotericin B? *J Infect* (1994) 29, 106–7.
14. Ringdén O, Andström EE, Remberger M, Svahn B-M, Tollemar J. No increase in cyclosporin neurotoxicity in transplant recipients treated with liposomal amphotericin B. *Infection* (1996) 24, 269.

Ciclosporin + Anabolic steroids or Androgens

The ciclosporin concentrations of two patients were increased when they were also given methyltestosterone. Hepatotoxicity has been seen in three patients given ciclosporin and norethandrolone.

Clinical evidence

(a) Methyltestosterone

A man with a kidney transplant who had been stable taking ciclosporin, prednisolone, and azathioprine for 23 months was given methyltestosterone 5 mg three times daily for impotence. After 4 weeks he developed anorexia and pruritus. He was found to have an increased bilirubin concentration and his ciclosporin concentration had increased from 70 to 252 nanograms/mL, with an accompanying decrease in his renal function. Methyltestosterone was withdrawn and he was later restabilised.[1] Another case describes abnormally high ciclosporin concentrations (in excess of 2000 nanograms/mL) when a patient taking methyltestosterone was given ciclosporin 15 mg/kg daily.[2]

(b) Norethandrolone

Three out of four patients with bone marrow aplasia taking ciclosporin and prednisone developed liver toxicity. The adverse effects developed in 2 of them when norethandrolone was added. No toxicity occurred when they were given either of the drugs alone.[3] A 14-year-old girl developed jaundice associated with toxic hepatitis during the post-transplant period, which was attributed to the concurrent use of ciclosporin and norethandrolone.[4]

Mechanism

Uncertain. In the first case, the increase in ciclosporin concentrations was attributed to cholestatic jaundice brought on by the methyltestosterone.[1] Both norethandrolone and ciclosporin are known to be hepatotoxic, so additive hepatotoxicity could occur.

Importance and management

Information is limited; however, it would seem prudent to avoid the use of androgens or anabolic steroids in patients taking ciclosporin wherever possible. If no alternative is available, it might be prudent to increase the frequency of liver function monitoring.

1. Goffin E, Pirson Y, Geubel A, van Ypersele de Strihou C. Cyclosporine-methyltestosterone interaction. *Nephron* (1991) 59, 174–5.
2. Møller BB, Ekelund B. Toxicity of cyclosporine during treatment with androgens. *N Engl J Med* (1985) 313, 1416.
3. Sahnoun Z, Frikha M, Zeghal KM, Souissi T. Toxicité hépatique de la ciclosporine et interaction médicamenteuse avec les androgènes. *Sem Hop Paris* (1993) 69, 26–8.
4. Vinot O, Cochat P, Dubourg-Derain L, Bouvier R, Vial T, Philippe N. Jaundice associated with concomitant use of norethandrolone and cyclosporine. *Transplantation* (1993) 56, 470–1.

Ciclosporin + Antibacterials; Aminoglycosides

Studies indicate that nephrotoxicity might be increased by the concurrent use of ciclosporin and gentamicin. Similar effects are expected with other aminoglycosides and nephrotoxicity or renal impairment has been seen with ciclosporin and amikacin, gentamicin, and tobramycin.

Clinical evidence

A comparative study in patients given **gentamicin** 30 mg with lincomycin just before kidney transplantation found that the concurrent use of ciclosporin increased the incidence of nephrotoxicity from 5% to 67%.[1] When **gentamicin** and lincomycin were replaced with ampicillin, ceftazidime, and lincomycin the incidence of nephrotoxicity was 10%.[1] Another study describes increased nephrotoxicity associated with the concurrent use of ciclosporin and **tobramycin** in bone marrow transplant recipients.[2,3]

One case report describes reversible acute worsening of renal function in a kidney transplant patient receiving ciclosporin with **gentamicin**,[4] and another case report describes impaired renal function in a heart transplant patient taking ciclosporin and given **amikacin**.[5]

A retrospective analysis of the medical records of bone marrow transplant patients suggested that aminoglycosides can be safely given with a continuous infusion of ciclosporin without excessive nephrotoxicity, if the patient is carefully monitored.[6]

Mechanism

Uncertain. As both ciclosporin and the aminoglycosides can individually be nephrotoxic, it seems that their toxicities can be additive.

Importance and management

The interaction between ciclosporin and the aminoglycosides is established and clinically important. In general the concurrent use of two drugs with nephrotoxic potential should be avoided; however, the concurrent use of ciclosporin and aminoglycosides is clinically valuable. Renal function should be monitored with either drug alone, but if concurrent use is undertaken then it would seem prudent to increase the frequency of this monitoring.

1. Termeer A, Hoitsma AJ, Koene RAP. Severe nephrotoxicity caused by the combined use of gentamicin and cyclosporine in renal allograft recipients. *Transplantation* (1986) 42, 220–1.
2. Hows JM, Chipping PM, Fairhead S, Smith J, Baughan A, Gordon-Smith EC. Nephrotoxicity in bone marrow transplant recipients treated with cyclosporin A. *Br J Haematol* (1983) 54, 69–78.
3. Hows JM, Palmer S, Want S, Dearden C, Gordon-Smith EC. Serum levels of cyclosporin A and nephrotoxicity in bone marrow transplant patients. *Lancet* (1981) ii, 145–6.
4. Morales JM, Andres A, Prieto C, Diaz Rolòn JA, Rodicio JL. Reversible acute renal toxicity by toxic sinergic effect between gentamicin and cyclosporine. *Clin Nephrol* (1988) 29, 272.
5. Thaler F, Gotainer B, Teodori G, Dubois C, Loirat Ph. Mediastinitis due to *Nocardia asteroides* after cardiac transplantation. *Intensive Care Med* (1992) 18, 127–8.
6. Chandrasekar PH, Cronin SM. Nephrotoxicity in bone marrow transplant recipients receiving aminoglycoside plus cyclosporine or aminoglycoside alone. *J Antimicrob Chemother* (1991) 27, 845–9.

Ciclosporin + Antibacterials; Aztreonam

Aztreonam does not appear to alter ciclosporin concentrations.

Clinical evidence, mechanism, importance and management

A study in 20 kidney transplant patients taking ciclosporin found that when aztreonam (dose not stated) was added for the treatment of various infections the ciclosporin blood concentrations were not significantly changed. The ciclosporin blood concentrations before, during, and after aztreonam treatment were 517 nanograms/mL, 534 nanograms/mL, and 592 nanograms/mL, respectively.[1] On the basis of this study it appears that no ciclosporin dose adjustment is needed on the concurrent use of aztreonam.

1. Alonso Hernández A. Effects of aztreonam on cyclosporine levels in kidney transplant patients. *Transplantology J Cell Organ Transplant* (1993) 4, 85–6.

Ciclosporin + Antibacterials; Cephalosporins

Isolated case reports suggest that ceftazidime, ceftriaxone, and latamoxef might increase ciclosporin concentrations, whereas one report suggests ceftazidime, ceftriaxone, and cefuroxime do not, although ceftazidime caused deterioration in some measures of renal function.

Clinical evidence, mechanism, importance and management

Two kidney transplant patients had 2- to 4-fold increases in ciclosporin blood concentrations within 2 to 3 days of starting **ceftriaxone** 1 g twice daily. Concentrations decreased when the antibacterial was stopped.[1] In contrast, a report of 51 kidney transplant patients stated that **ceftriaxone** and **cefuroxime** had no effect on ciclosporin blood concentrations and also that they were not nephrotoxic. This report similarly stated that **ceftazidime** did not affect ciclosporin blood concentrations; however, it did increase blood urea nitrogen and creatinine concentrations, indicating that it was nephrotoxic.[2] A report briefly mentions that **ceftazidime** and **latamoxef** have also been implicated in an increase in ciclosporin blood concentrations.[3] A study in 28 bone marrow transplant patients taking ciclosporin found no evidence that **ceftazidime** 2 g three times daily worsened renal function.[4]

Information about these cephalosporins is very limited indeed. Although two reports suggest that ceftazidime might be nephrotoxic this is not generally an effect associated with this drug at recommended doses.[5] The general relevance of these reports is therefore uncertain, but it is probably limited.

1. Soto Alvarez J, Sacristán Del Castillo JA, Alsar Ortiz MJ. Interaction between ciclosporin and ceftriaxone. *Nephron* (1991) 59, 681–2.
2. Xu F, Wu Z, Zou H. Effects on renal function and cyclosporine blood concentration by combination with three cephalosporins in renal transplant patients. *Zhongguo Kang Sheng Su Za Zhi* (1997) 22, 223–5.
3. Cockburn I. Cyclosporin A: a clinical evaluation of drug interactions. *Transplant Proc* (1986) 18 (Suppl 5), 50–5.
4. Verhagen C, de Pauw BE, de Witte T, Holdrinet RSG, Janssen JTP, Williams KJ. Ceftazidime does not enhance cyclosporin-A nephrotoxicity in febrile bone marrow transplantation patients. *Blut* (1986) 53, 333–9.
5. Fortum Injection (Ceftazidime pentahydrate). GlaxoSmithKline UK. UK Summary of product characteristics, June 2013.

Ciclosporin + Antibacterials; Chloramphenicol

Increased ciclosporin concentrations have been reported in patients who have also been given intravenous or oral chloramphenicol.

Clinical evidence

A retrospective study identified 3 transplant patients taking ciclosporin who had received a total of 6 courses of intravenous chloramphenicol, each lasting for at least 12 days. By day 4 of concurrent use, ciclosporin blood concentrations had increased on average by about 40%. Ciclosporin doses tended to be somewhat reduced over the course of treatment, and by day 10, ciclosporin concentrations were about 31% below baseline.[1]

A woman with a heart-lung transplant and with a ciclosporin minimum concentration of 84 nanograms/mL started to take oral chloramphenicol (dose not stated) to treat an infection with *Xanthomonas maltophilia*. On the next day ciclosporin concentrations had increased to 240 micrograms/L. Chloramphenicol was continued and the ciclosporin dose was reduced from 300 to 225 mg daily. By day 8, the ciclosporin concentrations were back within the therapeutic range.[2]

Two kidney transplant patients had large increases in ciclosporin blood concentrations (almost doubled in one case) when they were given chloramphenicol for urinary tract infections.[3] Another report describes a similar interaction, but the case is greatly complicated by the presence of ciprofloxacin, vancomycin, ceftazidime, and a recent course of rifampicin (rifampin) taken by the patient.[4]

Mechanism

Uncertain. The authors suggest that chloramphenicol might reduce the metabolism of ciclosporin by the liver.[4]

Importance and management

Information regarding an interaction between chloramphenicol and ciclosporin seems to be limited to these reports, so although the interaction appears to be established, its incidence is uncertain. It would be prudent to monitor ciclosporin concentrations if systemic chloramphenicol is added, being alert for the need to reduce the ciclosporin dose. The retrospective study highlights the need to monitor concentrations closely throughout the whole chloramphenicol course,[1] as ciclosporin concentrations might alter as treatment progresses. It seems doubtful that there would be enough chloramphenicol absorbed from eye drops to interact with ciclosporin, but this ideally needs confirmation.

1. Mathis AS, Shah N, Knipp GT, Friedman GS. Interaction of chloramphenicol and the calcineurin inhibitors in renal transplant recipients. *Transpl Infect Dis* (2002) 4, 169–74.
2. Steinfort CL, McConachy KA. Cyclosporin-chloramphenicol drug interaction in a heart-lung transplant recipient. *Med J Aust* (1994) 161, 455.
3. Zawadzki J, Prokurat S, Smirska E, Jelonek A. Interaction between cyclosporine A and chloramphenicol after kidney transplantation. *Pediatr Nephrol* (1991) 5, C49.
4. Bui LL, Huang DD. Possible interaction between cyclosporine and chloramphenicol. *Ann Pharmacother* (1999) 33, 252–3.

Ciclosporin + Antibacterials; Clindamycin

Two patients had a large reduction in their serum ciclosporin concentrations when they took clindamycin.

Clinical evidence, mechanism, importance and management

A lung transplant patient taking ciclosporin in a dose to maintain concentrations of 100 to 150 nanograms/mL, required ciclosporin dose increases to achieve this concentration when clindamycin 600 mg three times daily was given. Initially the concentrations were almost halved by the addition of clindamycin. Ciclosporin was reduced to the original dose when the clindamycin was stopped.[1] In a second lung transplant patient, the use of clindamycin 600 mg three times daily necessitated ciclosporin dose increases from 325 mg daily to 1.1 g daily over 4 weeks to maintain serum concentrations of about 200 nanograms/mL.

The reasons for the interaction are not understood, but the authors suggest close monitoring of ciclosporin concentrations to prevent under-dosing if clindamycin is given;[1] however, this seems exceptionally cautious as these two cases appear to be all that have been reported.

1. Thurnheer R, Laube I, Speich R. Possible interaction between clindamycin and cyclosporin. *BMJ* (1999) 319, 163.

Ciclosporin + Antibacterials; Imipenem with Cilastatin

Several transplant patients with impaired renal function have experienced adverse CNS effects (including convulsions and tremors) while taking imipenem with cilastatin and ciclosporin. Imipenem with cilastatin appears to decrease the nephrotoxicity of ciclosporin, but its effect on ciclosporin concentrations is uncertain.

Clinical evidence

(a) Ciclosporin concentrations

In one heart transplant patient, the dose of ciclosporin required to maintain a therapeutic concentration needed to be reduced from 240 mg to 180 mg daily when imipenem with cilastatin was given for mediastinitis.[1] Another patient had an increase in ciclosporin blood concentrations, from about 400 to 1000 nanograms/mL, in the 4 days after receiving two doses of imipenem with cilastatin.[2] This patient also developed CNS toxicity, see *CNS effects and seizures*, below.

Conversely, in a randomised, controlled study of the use of imipenem with cilastatin to reduce ciclosporin nephrotoxicity, there was no difference in the ciclosporin concentrations or dose between the 10 patients who were given imipenem with cilastatin, and the 10 patients who were given placebo.[3] Similar findings were reported in another study.[4] However, in a retrospective analysis, ciclosporin concentrations were *lower* in 64 patients given imipenem with cilastatin (208 nanograms/mL) than in the 40 patients who were not given imipenem with cilastatin (265 nanograms/mL). Nevertheless, no difference in the incidence of graft versus host disease was found between the two groups.[5]

(b) CNS effects and seizures

A kidney transplant patient taking ciclosporin developed a urinary-tract infection for which she was given imipenem with cilastatin 500 mg intravenously every 12 hours (dose adjusted for renal function). About 20 minutes after the second dose she became confused, disorientated, agitated, and developed motor aphasia and intense tremor. This was interpreted as being a combination of the adverse CNS effects of both drugs. The imipenem and cilastatin was not given again, and the effects subsided over the next few days.[2] This patient also developed increased ciclosporin concentrations, see *Ciclosporin concentrations*, above.

Similarly, 4 transplant patients who were taking ciclosporin developed seizures when they were given imipenem with cilastatin 1 g daily, and a fifth patient developed myoclonia. These patients all had chronic renal impairment.[6] Moreover, in one randomised study of the use of imipenem with cilastatin to reduce ciclosporin nephrotoxicity, 2 patients were withdrawn from the study because of seizures.[3]

In contrast, in an analysis of the incidence of seizure in patients who had been given ciclosporin and imipenem with cilastatin or either drug alone, there was no difference between the groups. Three of 77 patients (3.8%) given ciclosporin alone, and 2 of 45 patients (4.4%) who were given ciclosporin and imipenem with cilastatin, had seizures, whereas none of the 44 patients who received imipenem with cilastatin alone had seizures.[7]

(c) Reduction in nephrotoxicity

Various randomised prospective and retrospective studies have been published suggesting that serum creatinine concentrations are lower, and the risk of acute renal failure is reduced, in patients given ciclosporin and imipenem with cilastatin. In a meta-analysis of the data, the odds ratio for developing acute renal failure was 0.24 with the combination compared with ciclosporin alone.[8]

Mechanism

Focal tremors, myoclonus, and convulsions are known adverse effects of imipenem with cilastatin and are most likely to occur in patients with renal impairment. Ciclosporin can also cause tremor, and rarely, convulsions, hence the effects of both drugs might be additive.

Cilastatin might reduce the nephrotoxicity of ciclosporin because of its effect as an inhibitor of dehydropeptidase I, an enzyme found in the brush border of the renal tubules. Alternatively, it has been suggested it might reduce nephrotoxicity by reducing the concentrations of ciclosporin by altering ciclosporin metabolism,[9,10] but evidence for reduced ciclosporin concentrations is not conclusive.

Importance and management

An interaction between imipenem with cilastatin and ciclosporin leading to an increase in CNS adverse effects is not established. What occurred could simply represent the increased risk of seizures when imipenem with cilastatin is used in patients with renal impairment. The manufacturers of imipenem with cilastatin recommend that patients who develop focal tremors, myoclonus, and convulsions while receiving the antibacterial should be started on an antiepileptic drug. If symptoms persist the dose should be reduced, or the drug withdrawn.[11,12]

The effect of imipenem with cilastatin on ciclosporin concentrations is uncertain, but bear these reports in mind if unexpected effects are seen on their concurrent use.

Note that the risk of nephrotoxicity is possibly reduced if patients taking ciclosporin are given cilastatin, although the use of imipenem with cilastatin for this purpose is investigational.

1. Thaler F, Gotainer B, Teodori G, Dubois C, Loirat Ph. Mediastinitis due to *Nocardia asteroides* after cardiac transplantation. *Intensive Care Med* (1992) 18, 127–8.
2. Zazgornik J, Schein W, Heimberger K, Shaheen FAM, Stockenhuber F. Potentiation of neurotoxic side effects by coadministration of imipenem to cyclosporine therapy in a kidney transplant recipient–synergism of side effects or drug interaction? *Clin Nephrol* (1986) 26, 265–6.
3. Markewitz A, Hammer C, Pfeiffer M, Zahn S, Drechsel J, Reichenspurner H, Reichart B. Reduction of cyclosporine-induced nephrotoxicity by cilastatin following clinical heart transplantation. *Transplantation* (1994) 57, 865–70.
4. Carmellini M, Frosini F, Filipponi F, Boggi U, Mosca F. Effect of cilastatin on cyclosporine-induced acute nephrotoxicity in kidney transplant recipients. *Transplantation* (1997) 64,164–6..
5. Gruss E, Tomás JF, Bernis C, Rodriguez F, Traver JA, Fernández-Rañada JM. Nephroprotective effect of cilastatin in allogeneic bone marrow transplantation. Results from a retrospective analysis. *Bone Marrow Transplant* (1996) 18, 761–5.
6. Bösmüller C, Steurer W, Königsrainer A, Willeit J, Margreiter R. Increased risk of central nervous system toxicity in patients treated with ciclosporin and imipenem/cilastatin. *Nephron* (1991) 58, 362–4.
7. Turhal NS. Cyclosporin A and imipenem associated seizure activity in allogeneic bone marrow transplantation patients. *J Chemother* (1999) 11, 410–13.
8. Tejedor A, Torres AM, Castilla M, Lazaro JA, de Lucas C, Caramelo C. Cilastatin protection against cyclosporin A-induced nephrotoxicity: clinical evidence. *Curr Med Res Opin* (2007) 23, 505–13.
9. Mraz W, Sido B, Knedel M, Hammer C. Concomitant immunosuppressive and antibiotic therapy-reduction of cyclosporine A blood levels due to treatment with imipenem/cilastatin. *Transplant Proc* (1987) 19, 4017–20.
10. Mraz W, Modic PK, Hammer C. Impact of imipenem/cilastatin on cyclosporine metabolism and excretion. *Transplant Proc* (1992) 24, 1704–8.
11. Primaxin IV Injection (Imipenem monohydrate/Cilastatin sodium). Merck Sharp & Dohme Ltd. UK Summary of product characteristics, October 2013.
12. Primaxin IV Injection (Imipenem monohydrate/Cilastatin sodium). Merck & Co. Inc. US Prescribing information, April 2012.

Ciclosporin + Antibacterials; Macrolides

Ciclosporin concentrations can be greatly increased by clarithromycin, erythromycin, josamycin, pristinamycin, and possibly midecamycin. Rokitamycin and telithromycin are predicted to interact similarly. Roxithromycin appears to interact minimally, while no interaction is normally seen with azithromycin, dirithromycin, or spiramycin, although there are two isolated reports of an interaction with azithromycin.

Clinical evidence

(a) Azithromycin

In a study in 8 healthy subjects, ciclosporin 3.75 to 7.5 mg/kg was given alone and after taking azithromycin 500 mg initially then 250 mg daily for 4 days. Azithromycin did not alter ciclosporin concentrations.[1] Similarly, in another controlled study in 8 patients with kidney transplants stabilised on ciclosporin, there was no clinically relevant change in ciclosporin exposure after azithromycin 500 mg daily for 3 days (7% increase in AUC).[2] A number of other studies have also found no evidence of a clinically important interaction between ciclosporin and azithromycin used for respiratory tract infections (dose not stated)[3] or for ciclosporin-induced gingival overgrowth (500 mg daily for 3 days).[4,5] However, there are two isolated reports describing large increases in ciclosporin concentrations in 2 patients, which were attributed to the use of azithromycin (500 mg on day one, then 250 mg daily for 4 days;[6] and 500 mg daily for 9 days[7]).

(b) Clarithromycin

In a study in 8 healthy subjects, ciclosporin 3.75 to 7.5 mg/kg was given alone and after clarithromycin 250 mg every 12 hours for 7 days. The maximum ciclosporin concentrations were increased by 50% by clarithromycin. In another study, a mean 30% reduction in the dose of ciclosporin was needed in 6 transplant patients also given clarithromycin.[8] Clarithromycin 500 mg twice daily as part of a *Helicobacter pylori* eradication regimen caused a 2- to 3-fold increase in ciclosporin concentrations in 27 kidney transplant patients.[9,10] The ciclosporin concentrations in 4 renal transplant patients with stable renal function increased by about 72% when clarithromycin 250 mg twice daily for 6 days was added to treat gingival hyperplasia. Ciclosporin concentrations returned to baseline within 7 days of stopping clarithromycin. Only two patients required a ciclosporin dose reduction.[11]

Numerous case reports also describe this interaction: the AUC or concentrations of ciclosporin have been increased 2- to 3-fold,[12-15] with changes being seen within 3 to 6 days of clarithromycin 250 or 500 mg twice daily being started.[12,15] Another patient had a 7- to 12-fold increase in ciclosporin serum concentrations and acute renal failure within 3 weeks of starting to take clarithromycin 1 g daily.[16] Another case report, describing a heart transplant patient taking ciclosporin, found that the addition of rifampicin (rifampin) to clarithromycin negated the increase in ciclosporin concentrations seen with clarithromycin alone, and the ciclosporin dose requirement with both clarithromycin and rifampicin was similar to that before clarithromycin or rifampicin were started.[17]

(c) Dirithromycin

In a study in 8 healthy subjects, dirithromycin 500 mg daily for 14 days did not affect the pharmacokinetics of a single 15-mg/kg oral dose of ciclosporin.[18]

(d) Erythromycin

A study in 9 transplant patients taking ciclosporin found that erythromycin increased the minimum serum concentrations of 3 kidney transplant patients 7-fold (from 147 to 1125 nanograms/mL), and of 6 heart transplant patients 4- to 5-fold (from 185 to 815 nanograms/mL). Acute nephrotoxicity occurred in all 9 patients, and 7 had mild to severe hepatotoxicity caused by the increased ciclosporin concentrations.[19]

Greatly increased ciclosporin blood concentrations and/or toxicity have been described in a number of other studies and case reports with erythromycin given orally or intravenously to about 50 other patients.[20-35] The interaction has also been demonstrated in controlled studies in healthy subjects.[1,36] Oral erythromycin might possibly have a greater effect than intravenous erythromycin.[31,37]

Erythromycin-related ototoxicity, possibly associated with the use of ciclosporin, has been reported in liver transplant patients.[38]

(e) Josamycin

A kidney transplant patient who was taking azathioprine, prednisone, and ciclosporin 330 mg daily, had an almost 7-fold increase in his plasma ciclosporin concentrations (from about 90 to 600 nanograms/mL) when he took josamycin 2 g daily for 5 days. He responded in the same way when later rechallenged with josamycin. Another patient also reacted in the same way.[39] Increases in ciclosporin concentrations of 2- to 4-fold have been seen in 9 other patients given josamycin 2 to 3 g (50 mg/kg) daily.[40-42] Another patient had a 40% increase in ciclosporin concentrations when given josamycin 500 mg twice daily.[43]

(f) Midecamycin

The steady-state ciclosporin blood concentrations of 10 kidney transplant patients were roughly doubled when they took midecamycin 800 mg twice daily.[44] A 43-year-old kidney transplant patient taking ciclosporin, azathioprine, and prednisone, began further treatment on day 27 after the transplant, with midecamycin diacetate 600 mg twice daily and co-trimoxazole three times daily for pneumonia. By day 33 the concentration-to-dose ratio of ciclosporin had doubled, and ciclosporin concentrations had reached 700 nanograms/mL, accompanied by an increase in serum creatinine concentrations. When the midecamycin was replaced by cefuroxime, the concentrations of both ciclosporin and creatinine returned to baseline within 3 days.[45] Ciclosporin concentrations in another kidney transplant patient taking ciclosporin 120 mg twice daily increased from 95 to 380 nanograms/mL 3 days after starting midecamycin 800 mg twice daily.[46] In a further kidney transplant patient, blood concentrations of ciclosporin increased from 97 to 203 nanograms/mL 4 days after starting midecamycin diacetate 600 mg twice daily.[47]

(g) Pristinamycin

A kidney transplant patient had a 10-fold increase in plasma ciclosporin concentrations (from 30 to 290 nanograms/mL) after taking pristinamycin 2 g daily for 8 days. Blood creatinine concentrations increased from 75 to 120 micromol/L. Another patient given pristinamycin 1.25 g had a increase in ciclosporin concentrations from 78 to 855 nanograms/mL after 6 days. Ciclosporin and creatinine concentrations returned to normal within 2 days of stopping both drugs.[48]

In a study in 10 patients, pristinamycin 50 mg/kg daily increased the ciclosporin blood concentrations by 65% (from 560 to 925 nanograms/mL). Ciclosporin concentrations decreased when the pristinamycin was stopped.[49] Within 5 days of starting to take pristinamycin 4 g daily the ciclosporin concentrations of another patient more than doubled. His serum creatinine concentrations also increased. Both decreased back to baseline within 3 days of stopping the antibacterial.[50]

(h) Roxithromycin

Eight patients with heart transplants taking ciclosporin 8 mg/kg daily, prednisolone, and azathioprine for at least one month, were given roxithromycin 150 mg twice daily for 11 days. A 38% increase in plasma ciclosporin concentrations occurred at the time the roxithromycin was given, and a 60% increase occurred 4 hours later. Ciclosporin concentrations decreased again when roxithromycin was stopped. A small (10%) increase in serum creatinine concentrations occurred, but there was no evidence of a deterioration in renal function.[51] One study in kidney transplant patients taking ciclosporin found that the half-life of roxithromycin was doubled, from 17 to 34.4 hours.[52]

(i) Spiramycin

The ciclosporin plasma concentrations of 6 heart transplant patients taking corticosteroids, azathioprine, and ciclosporin remained unchanged when they were given spiramycin 3 million units twice daily for 10 days.[53] Similarly, no interaction was found between ciclosporin and spiramycin in other studies in patients with kidney transplants.[54-57]

Mechanism

In vitro studies with human liver microsomes have found that clarithromycin, erythromycin, josamycin, rokitamycin, roxithromycin, and troleandomycin (but not spiramycin) inhibit ciclosporin metabolism, which is catalysed by the cytochrome P450 subfamily CYP3A.[16,58] This would be expected to result in increased ciclosporin concentrations. Telithromycin is also an inhibitor of CYP3A4 and might increase ciclosporin concentrations. Erythromycin[31,35] and clarithromycin[14] also possibly increase the absorption of ciclosporin from the gut by inhibiting CYP3A4 in the gut wall, or by increasing uptake via inhibition of P-glycoprotein.

In one of the case reports with azithromycin, intravenous azithromycin was thought to have increased ciclosporin concentrations through P-glycoprotein inhibition and/or competition for biliary excretion.[7]

Importance and management

The interaction between ciclosporin and **erythromycin** or **clarithromycin** is well documented, well established, and potentially serious. If concurrent use is thought appropriate, monitor ciclosporin concentrations closely and reduce the dose as required: a reduction of about 35% might be needed.[33] The effect of intravenous erythromycin is less than oral erythromycin so if the route of administration is changed, be alert for the need to change the ciclosporin dose.[31,37]

Information about the interaction with **josamycin**, **midecamycin**, and **pristinamycin** is much more limited, but as they appear to behave like erythromycin, the same precautions should be taken. There seems to be no direct clinical information about **telithromycin**, **troleandomycin**, and **rokitamycin** but they would also be expected to interact like erythromycin.

Dirithromycin and **spiramycin** do not appear to interact with ciclosporin, and **roxithromycin** appears only to interact very minimally. However, bear in mind that roxithromycin serum concentrations might be increased.

Most evidence indicates that **azithromycin** does not affect ciclosporin concentrations, although some authors[7] recommend increased monitoring because of the isolated reports of increased ciclosporin concentrations. Bear the case reports in mind should an unexplained increase in ciclosporin concentrations occur on concurrent use.

1. Bottorff MB, Marien ML, Clendening C. Macrolide antibiotics and inhibition of CYP3A isozymes: differences in cyclosporin pharmacokinetics. *Clin Pharmacol Ther* (1997) 56, 224.
2. Bachmann K, Jauregui L, Chandra R, Thakker K. Influence of a 3-day regimen of azithromycin on the disposition kinetics of cyclosporine A in stable renal transplant patients. *Pharmacol Res* (2003) 47, 549–54.
3. Bubic-Filipi Lj, Puretic Z, Thune S, Glavas-Boras S, Pasini J, Marekovic Z. Influence of azithromycin on cyclosporin levels in patients with a kidney transplant. *Nephrol Dial Transplant* (1998) 13, A276.
4. Gómez E, Sánchez JE, Aguado S, Alvarez Grande J. Interaction between azithromycin and cyclosporin? *Nephron* (1996) 73, 724.
5. Palomar R, Belart M, Soy D, Oppenheimer F, Campistol JM. Effectiveness and safety of azithromycin on the treatment of cyclosporine-induced gingival overgrowth. *Nephron* (1998) 79, 101–2.
6. Ljutic D, Rumboldt Z. Possible interaction between azithromycin and cyclosporine: a case report. *Nephron* (1995) 70, 130.
7. Page RL, Ruscin JM, Fish D, LaPointe M. Possible interaction between intravenous azithromycin and oral cyclosporine. *Pharmacotherapy* (2001) 21, 1436–43.
8. Sádaba B, López De Ocáriz A, Azanza JR, Quiroga J, Cienfuegos JA. Concurrent clarithromycin and cyclosporin A treatment. *J Antimicrob Chemother* (1998) 42, 393–5.
9. Skálová P, Marečková O, Skála I, Lácha J, Teplan V, Vítko Š, Petrásek R. Eradication of *Helicobacter pylori* with clarithromycin: danger of toxic levels of cyclosporin A. *Gut* (1998) 43 (Suppl 2), A109.
10. Skalova P, Mareckova O, Skala I, Lacha J, Teplan V, Vitko S, Petrasek R. Toxic levels of cyclosporin A after renal transplantation on clarithromycin therapy. *Nephrol Dial Transplant* (1998) 13, A256.
11. Sánchez-Nuñez ML, Gómez E, Sánchez JE, Portal C, Alvarez-Grande J. Clarithromycin in the treatment of cyclosporin-associated gingival hyperplasia. *Nephrol Dial Transplant* (1997) 12, 2040–1.
12. Gersema LM, Porter CB, Russell EH. Suspected drug interaction between cyclosporine and clarithromycin. *J Heart Lung Transplant* (1994) 13, 343–5.
13. Ferrari SL, Goffin E, Mourad M, Wallemacq P, Squifflet J-P, Pirson Y. The interaction between clarithromycin and cyclosporine in kidney transplant recipients. *Transplantation* (1994) 58, 725–7.
14. Sketris IS, Wright MR, West ML. Possible role of intestinal P-450 enzyme system in a cyclosporine-clarithromycin interaction. *Pharmacotherapy* (1996) 16, 301–5.
15. Treille S, Quoidbach A, Demol H, Vereerstraeten P, Abramowicz D. Kidney graft dysfunction after drug interaction between clarithromycin and cyclosporin. *Nephrol Dial Transplant* (1996) 11, 1192–3.
16. Spicer ST, Liddle C, Chapman JR, Barclay P, Nankivell BJ, Thomas P, O'Connell PJ. The mechanism of cyclosporine toxicity induced by clarithromycin. *Br J Clin Pharmacol* (1997) 43, 194–6.
17. Plemmons RM, McAllister CK, Garces MC, Ward RL. Osteomyelitis due to *Mycobacterium haemophilum* in a cardiac transplant patient: case report and analysis of interactions among clarithromycin, rifampin, and cyclosporine. *Clin Infect Dis* (1997) 24, 995–7.
18. Bachmann K, Sullivan TJ, Resse JH, Miller K, Scott M, Jauregui L, Sides G. The pharmacokinetics of oral cyclosporine A are not affected by dirithromycin. *Intersci Conf Antimicrob Agents Chemother* (1994) 34, 4.
19. Jensen CWB, Flechner SM, Van Buren CT, Frazier OH, Cooley DA, Lorber MI, Kahan BD. Exacerbation of cyclosporine toxicity by concomitant administration of erythromycin. *Transplantation* (1987) 43, 263–70.
20. Kohan DE. Possible interaction between cyclosporine and erythromycin. *N Engl J Med* (1986), 314, 448.
21. Hourmant M, Le Bigot JF, Vernillet L, Sagniez G, Remi JP, Soulillou JP. Coadministration of erythromycin results in an increase of blood cyclosporine to toxic levels. *Transplant Proc* (1985) 17, 2723–7.
22. Wadhwa NK, Schroeder TJ, O'Flaherty E, Pesce AJ, Myre SA, Munda R, First MR. Interaction between erythromycin and cyclosporine in a kidney and pancreas allograft recipient. *Ther Drug Monit* (1987) 9, 123–5.
23. Murray BM, Edwards L, Morse GD, Kohli RR, Venuto RC. Clinically important interaction of cyclosporine and erythromycin. *Transplantation* (1987) 43, 602–4.
24. Griño JM, Sabate I, Castelao AM, Guardia M, Seron D, Alsina J. Erythromycin and cyclosporine. *Ann Intern Med* (1986) 105, 467–8.
25. Gonwa TA, Nghiem DD, Schulak JA, Corry RJ. Erythromycin and cyclosporine. *Transplantation* (1986) 41, 797–9.
26. Harnett JD, Parfrey PS, Paul MD, Gault MH. Erythromycin-cyclosporine interaction in renal transplant patients. *Transplantation* (1987) 43, 316–18.
27. Kessler M, Louis J, Renoult E, Vigneron B, Netter P. Interaction between cyclosporin and erythromycin in a kidney transplant patient. *Eur J Clin Pharmacol* (1986) 30, 633–4.
28. Godin JRP, Sketris IS, Belitsky P. Erythromycin-cyclosporine interaction. *Drug Intell Clin Pharm* (1986) 20, 504–5.
29. Martell R, Heinrichs D, Stiller CR, Jenner M, Keown PA, Dupre J. The effects of erythromycin in patients treated with cyclosporine. *Ann Intern Med* (1986) 104, 660–1.
30. Ptachcinski PJ, Carpenter BJ, Burckart GJ, Venkataramanan R, Rosenthal JT. Effect of erythromycin on cyclosporine levels. *N Engl J Med* (1985) 313, 1416–17.
31. Gupta SK, Bakran A, Johnson RWG, Rowland M. Erythromycin enhances the absorption of cyclosporin. *Br J Clin Pharmacol* (1988) 25, 401–2.
32. Morales JM, Andres A, Prieto C, Arenas J, Ortuño B, Praga M, Ruilope LM, Rodicio JL. Severe reversible cyclosporine-induced acute renal failure. A role for urinary PGE_2 deficiency? *Transplantation* (1988) 46, 163–5.
33. Vereerstraeten P, Thiry P, Kinnaert P, Toussaint C. Influence of erythromycin on cyclosporine pharmacokinetics. *Transplantation* (1987) 44, 155–6.
34. Ben-Ari J, Eisenstein B, Davidovits M, Shmueli D, Shapira Z, Stark H. Effect of erythromycin on blood cyclosporine concentrations in kidney transplant patients. *J Pediatr* (1988) 112, 992–3.

35. Gupta SK, Bakran A, Johnson RWG, Rowland M. Cyclosporin-erythromycin interaction in renal transplant patients. *Br J Clin Pharmacol* (1989) 27, 475–81.
36. Freeman DJ, Martell R, Carruthers SG, Heinrichs D, Keown PA, Stiller CR. Cyclosporin-erythromycin interaction in normal subjects. *Br J Clin Pharmacol* (1987) 23, 776–8.
37. Zylber-Katz E. Multiple drug interactions with cyclosporine in a heart transplant patient. *Ann Pharmacother* (1995) 29, 127–31. Correction. ibid. 790.
38. Moral A, Navasa M, Rimola A, García-Valdecasas JC, Grande L, Visa J, Rodés J. Erythromycin ototoxicity in liver transplant patients. *Transpl Int* (1994) 7, 62–4.
39. Kreft-Jais C, Billaud EM, Gaudry C, Bedrossian J. Effect of josamycin on plasma cyclosporine levels. *Eur J Clin Pharmacol* (1987) 32, 327–8.
40. Azanza JR, Catalán M, Alvarez MP, Sádaba B, Honorato J, Llorens R, Harreros J. Possible interaction between cyclosporine and josamycin: a description of three cases. *Clin Pharmacol Ther* (1992) 51, 572–5.
41. Torregrosa JV, Campistol JM, Franco A, Andreu J. Interaction of josamycin with cyclosporin A. *Nephron* (1993) 65, 476–7.
42. Azanza J, Catalán M, Alvarez P, Honorato J, Herreros J, Llorens R. Possible interaction between cyclosporine and josamycin. *J Heart Transplant* (1990) 9, 265–6.
43. Capone D, Aiello C, Santoro GA, Gentile A, Stanziale P, D'Alessandro R, Imperatore P, Basile V. Drug interaction between cyclosporine and two antimicrobial agents, josamycin and rifampicin, in organ-transplanted patients. *Int J Clin Pharmacol Res* (1996) 16, 73–6.
44. Couet W, Istin B, Seniuta P, Morel D, Potaux L, Fourtillan JB. Effect of ponsinomycin on cyclosporin pharmacokinetics. *Eur J Clin Pharmacol* (1990) 39, 165–7.
45. Alfonso I, Alcalde G, Garcia-Sáiz M, de Cos MA, Mediavilla A. Interaction between cyclosporine a and midecamycin. *Eur J Clin Pharmacol* (1997) 52, 79–80.
46. Finielz P, Mondon J-M, Chuet C, Guiserix J. Drug interaction between midecamycin and cyclosporin. *Nephron* (1995) 70, 136.
47. Treille S, Quoidbach A, Demol H, Juvenois A, Dehout F, Abramowicz D. Kidney graft dysfunction after drug interaction between miocamycin and cyclosporin. *Transpl Int* (1999) 12, 157.
48. Gagnadoux MF, Loirat C, Pillion G, Bertheleme JP, Pouliquen M, Guest G, Broyer M. Néphrotoxicité due à l'interaction pristinamycine-cyclosporine chez le transplanté rénal. *Presse Med* (1987) 16, 1761.
49. Herbrecht R, Garcia J-J, Bergerat J-P, Oberling F. Effect of pristinamycin on cyclosporin levels in bone marrow transplant recipients. *Bone Marrow Transplant* (1989) 4, 457–8.
50. Garraffo R, Monnier B, Lapalus P, Duplay H. Pristinamycin increases cyclosporin blood levels. *Med Sci Res* (1987) 15, 461.
51. Billaud E M, Guillemain R, Fortineau N, Kitzis M-D, Dreyfus G, Amrein C, Kreft-Jaïs C, Husson J-M, Chrétien P. Interaction between roxithromycin and cyclosporin in heart transplant patients. *Clin Pharmacokinet* (1990) 19, 499–502.
52. Morávek J, Matoušovic K, Prát V, Šedivý J. Pharmacokinetics of roxithromycin in kidney grafted patients under cyclosporin A or azathioprine immunosuppression and in healthy volunteers. *Int J Clin Pharmacol Ther Toxicol* (1990) 28, 262–7.
53. Guillemain R, Billaud E, Dreyfus G, Amrein C, Kitzis M, Jebara VA and Kreft-Jais C. The effects of spiramycin on plasma cyclosporin A concentrations in heart transplant patients. *Eur J Clin Pharmacol* (1989) 36, 97–8.
54. Kessler M, Netter P, Zerrouki M, Renoult E, Trechot P, Dousset B, Jonon B, Mur JM. Spiramycin does not increase plasma cyclosporin concentrations in renal transplant patients. *Eur J Clin Pharmacol* (1988) 35, 331–2.
55. Vernillet L, Bertault-Peres P, Berland Y, Barradas J, Durand A, Olmer M. Lack of effect of spiramycin on cyclosporin pharmacokinetics. *Br J Clin Pharmacol* (1989) 27, 789–94.
56. Birmele B, Lebranchu Y, Beliveau F, Rateau H, Furet Y, Nivet H, Bagros PH. Absence of interaction between cyclosporine and spiramycin. *Transplantation* (1989) 47, 927–8.
57. Kessler M, Netter P, Renoult E, Trechot P, Dousset B, Bannwarth B. Lack of effect of spiramycin on cyclosporin pharmacokinetics. *Br J Clin Pharmacol* (1990) 29, 370–1.
58. Marre R, de Sousa G, Orloff AM, Rahmani R. *In vitro* interaction between cyclosporin A and macrolide antibiotics. *Br J Clin Pharmacol* (1993) 35, 447–8.

Ciclosporin + Antibacterials; Metronidazole

Three reports describe an increase in ciclosporin concentrations in patients given metronidazole.

Clinical evidence

The ciclosporin blood concentrations of a kidney transplant patient increased from 850 to 1930 nanograms/mL when metronidazole 2.25 g daily and cimetidine 800 mg daily were started. Ciclosporin concentrations then decreased to about 1500 nanograms/mL when the metronidazole dose was halved and cimetidine was stopped. Because the concentrations of ciclosporin were still so high, the dose of ciclosporin was reduced from 7.1 to 5.7 mg/kg daily, which resulted in a further decrease in the ciclosporin concentration to a range of about 1200 to 1380 nanograms/mL. When metronidazole was stopped, the ciclosporin concentrations decreased to a range of 501 to 885 nanograms/mL.[1]

Another kidney transplant patient developed an increased serum creatinine concentration (from 223 to 304 micromol/L) with virtually doubled ciclosporin blood concentrations when metronidazole 1.5 g daily was given.[2]

Ciclosporin concentrations in yet another kidney transplant patient doubled (from 134 to 264 micrograms/L) accompanied by a modest elevation in serum creatinine concentrations when metronidazole 400 mg three times daily was also given. The concentrations decreased when metronidazole was stopped.[3]

These three cases appear to be the only reports of an interaction, one of which is confused by the presence of cimetidine (see also 'Ciclosporin + H_2-receptor antagonists', p.1230).

Mechanism

Uncertain. It was suggested that metronidazole might have increased ciclosporin concentrations by inhibiting CYP3A4. However, some pharmacokinetic studies have found that metronidazole is not an inhibitor of CYP3A4/5, and conclude that increases in plasma concentrations of CYP3A4 substrates in the presence of metronidazole are not the result of CYP3A4 inhibition.[4]

Importance and management

An interaction between ciclosporin and metronidazole is not established and there is insufficient evidence to advocate monitoring every patient given the combination, but it would be prudent to at least bear this interaction in mind on their concurrent use.

1. Zylber-Katz E, Rubinger D and Berlatzky Y. Cyclosporine interactions with metronidazole and cimetidine. *Drug Intell Clin Pharm* (1988) 22, 504–5.
2. Vincent F, Glotz D, Kreft-Jais C, Boudjeltia S, Duboust A, Bariety J. Insuffisance rénale aiguë chez un transplanté rénal traité par cyclosporine A et métronidazole. *Therapie* (1994) 49, 155.
3. Herzig K, Johnson DW. Marked elevation of blood cyclosporin and tacrolimus levels due to concurrent metronidazole therapy. *Nephrol Dial Transplant* (1999) 14, 521–3.
4. Roedler R, Neuhauser MM, Penzak SR. Does metronidazole interact with CYP3A substrates by inhibiting their metabolism through this metabolic pathway? Or should other mechanisms be considered? *Ann Pharmacother* (2007) 41, 653–8.

Ciclosporin + Antibacterials; Penicillins

In general, the penicillins do not appear to affect ciclosporin concentrations, although not all combinations have been studied. Limited evidence suggests that intravenous flucloxacillin might decrease ciclosporin concentrations and the concurrent use of nafcillin and ciclosporin might result in increased nephrotoxicity, although reduced ciclosporin concentrations have been seen in one patient.

Clinical evidence

(a) Ampicillin

Seventy-one kidney transplant patients taking ciclosporin had no changes in serum urea, creatinine, or ciclosporin concentrations when ampicillin was given.[1]

(b) Flucloxacillin

In a retrospective study in 7 kidney transplant recipients, it was noted that the use of intravenous flucloxacillin for septicaemia reduced ciclosporin minimum concentrations by 55%. The ciclosporin dose needed to be increased 2.2-fold, but despite this, biopsy-proven rejection occurred in 3 patients within 10 days of starting flucloxacillin. Ciclosporin minimum concentrations returned to normal within about 2 days of stopping the flucloxacillin.[2]

(c) Nafcillin

A retrospective study of 19 lung transplant patients taking ciclosporin found that those given nafcillin for one week as prophylaxis against staphylococci had a greater degree of renal impairment than those not taking nafcillin. Serum creatinine concentrations increased steadily over 6 days until nafcillin was stopped, whereas patients not taking nafcillin had no changes in creatinine concentrations. Three of the nafcillin group temporarily needed haemodialysis. Ciclosporin doses in the nafcillin group were higher but the blood concentrations in both groups were not notably different. The incidence of viral infections was also greater in the nafcillin group.[3]

A kidney transplant patient taking ciclosporin and prednisone experienced a large decrease in her serum ciclosporin concentrations on two occasions when given nafcillin 2 g every 6 hours. Minimum blood concentrations fell from 229 to 119 nanograms/mL after 3 days, and then to 68 nanograms/mL after 7 days of nafcillin and increased when nafcillin was stopped. On the second occasion ciclosporin concentrations decreased from 272 to 42 nanograms/mL after 9 days of treatment with nafcillin.[4]

(d) Ticarcillin

A patient had an increase in his plasma ciclosporin concentrations from 90 to 230 nanograms/mL within 5 days, and from 120 to 300 nanograms/mL within 10 days, of starting ticarcillin 10 g daily.[5]

Mechanism

The authors of the study using nafcillin[3] suggest that it could have interfered with the ciclosporin assay, resulting in an underestimate of the actual concentrations, so that the nephrotoxicity was simply due to higher ciclosporin concentrations.[3] The reduction in ciclosporin concentrations in the individual patient taking nafcillin[4] is not understood, although nafcillin has been said to possess enzyme-inducing potential. The increase in concentrations seen in the patient taking ticarcillin is also not understood.[5] *In vitro* evidence[6] suggests that flucloxacillin at high concentrations might act as an inducer of CYP3A4 and P-glycoprotein, both of which are involved in the metabolism of ciclosporin. However, in clinical use, there is little evidence to suggest that flucloxacillin interacts in this way.

Importance and management

Information regarding an interaction between the penicillins and ciclosporin seems to be limited to the studies and cases cited. Nafcillin is possibly associated with renal impairment but the case report of a reduction in ciclosporin concentrations is not proven. Nevertheless, it would seem prudent to monitor ciclosporin concentrations and renal function more closely in the presence of nafcillin.

The general importance of the interaction with flucloxacillin, resulting in decreased ciclosporin concentrations, is uncertain, although the 3 patients developing rejection introduce a note of caution. Given that flucloxacillin is not generally considered to affect the metabolism of other drugs and the single retrospective study cited appears to be the only documented report of an interaction it seems likely that if an interaction exists it will be managed by routine monitoring: it would be prudent to confirm that this is being undertaken.

The isolated report with ticarcillin is of unknown general significance. No special precautions would seem necessary if patients taking ciclosporin are given ampicillin.

1. Xu F, Shi XH. Interaction between ampicillin, norfloxacin and cyclosporine in renal transplant recipients. *Zhongguo Kang Sheng Su Za Zhi* (1992) 17, 290–2.
2. Cynke E, Binet I, Haefeli WE, Thiel G. Flucloxacillin & cyclosporine A: an unrecognised but relevant interaction in renal transplant recipients. *Kidney Int* (1999) 55, 1156–7.
3. Jahansouz F, Kriett JM, Smith CM, Jamieson SW. Potentiation of cyclosporin nephrotoxicity by nafcillin in lung transplant recipients. *Transplantation* (1993) 55, 1045–8.

4. Veremis SA, Maddux MS, Pollak R, Mozes MF. Subtherapeutic cyclosporine concentrations during nafcillin therapy. *Transplantation* (1987) 43, 913–5.
5. Lambert C, Pointet P, Ducret F. Interaction ciclosporine-ticarcilline chez un transplanté rénal. *Presse Med* (1989) 18, 230.
6. Huwyler J, Wright MB, Gutmann H, Drewe J. Induction of cytochrome P450 3A4 and P-glycoprotein by the isoxazolyl-penicillin antibiotic flucloxacillin. *Curr Drug Metab* (2006) 7, 119–26.

Ciclosporin + Antibacterials; Quinolones

Ciclosporin concentrations are normally unchanged by ciprofloxacin, but increased concentrations and nephrotoxicity might occur in a small number of patients. Some evidence suggests increased ciclosporin concentrations might develop in patients given norfloxacin or levofloxacin, but other studies found no change. Enoxacin, moxifloxacin, ofloxacin, pefloxacin, and trovafloxacin do not appear to affect the pharmacokinetics of ciclosporin to a clinically relevant extent.

Clinical evidence

(a) Ciprofloxacin

A single-dose study in 10 healthy subjects found that after taking ciprofloxacin 500 mg twice daily for 7 days the pharmacokinetics of oral ciclosporin 5 mg/kg were unchanged.[1] Five other studies confirm the lack of a pharmacokinetic interaction in:

- kidney transplant patients taking ciprofloxacin 750 mg twice daily for 13 days;[2]
- kidney transplant patients taking ciprofloxacin 500 mg twice daily for 7 days;[3]
- bone marrow transplant patients taking ciprofloxacin 500 mg twice daily for 4 days;[4]
- heart transplant patients taking ciprofloxacin 250 to 500 mg for 7 to 140 days;[5]
- heart transplant patients taking ciprofloxacin 800 mg to 1.5 g daily.[6]

There were no changes in the serum concentrations of ciclosporin or evidence of nephrotoxicity.

In contrast, case reports describe renal adverse effects on the concurrent use of ciclosporin and ciprofloxacin, including nephrotoxicity,[7-9] acute renal failure,[10] decreased renal function,[7] and acute interstitial nephritis.[11-13] Furthermore, the ciclosporin concentrations of a patient taking ciclosporin for red cell aplasia increased from 120 nanograms/mL to 297 nanograms/mL, requiring a dose reduction from 250 mg to 200 mg daily, when intravenous ciprofloxacin 200 mg two or three times daily (exact dose unclear) was started. A ciclosporin dose increase back to 250 mg daily was required when the ciprofloxacin course was finished.[8] In addition, a case-control study in 42 kidney transplant patients suggested that the proportion of cases experiencing at least one episode of biopsy-proved rejection within one to 3 months of receiving a transplant were greater in those who had taken ciprofloxacin (45%) than in those who had not (19%). There was also an increase in the incidence of rejection associated with ciprofloxacin use (29%) compared with the controls (2%).[14]

(b) Enoxacin

In a study in 10 healthy subjects, enoxacin 400 mg twice daily for 5 days had little effect on either the blood or plasma concentrations of single doses of ciclosporin.[15]

(c) Levofloxacin

In a study in 12 healthy subjects, levofloxacin 500 mg twice daily for 6 days had no effect on the pharmacokinetics of ciclosporin when a single dose of the oral solution (*Sandimmune*) was given on day 5.[16] A case report describes a patient taking oral ciclosporin 250 mg daily (as the emulsion formulation) whose ciclosporin concentrations were unaffected when he was given intravenous levofloxacin 500 mg daily for 9 days.[8]

In a study in 5 kidney transplant patients taking ciclosporin (microemulsion formulation), the AUC of ciclosporin was increased by 26% and the minimum concentration was increased by 36% when levofloxacin 500 mg twice daily for 6 days was taken for a urinary-tract infection. The authors concluded that this interaction might be clinically relevant, and warned about extrapolating the results from single-dose studies in healthy subjects to patients with transplants.[17]

(d) Moxifloxacin

A study in 11 patients taking ciclosporin after a kidney transplant found that moxifloxacin 400 mg daily for 7 days, taken for a urinary-tract infection, did not affect the pharmacokinetics of ciclosporin.[18] Similarly, a study in 9 patients stable taking ciclosporin 150 to 380 mg daily after bone marrow or kidney transplants and given moxifloxacin 400 mg daily for 7 days found that the pharmacokinetics of ciclosporin and its metabolites were unaffected. Furthermore, when compared with historical controls, the pharmacokinetics of moxifloxacin appeared to be unaffected by ciclosporin.[19]

(e) Norfloxacin

In a retrospective analysis, 6 kidney transplant patients given norfloxacin 400 mg twice daily for 3 to 23 days for urinary-tract infections,[20] and 4 heart transplant patients given norfloxacin 400 mg for 7 to 140 days had no changes in their serum concentrations of ciclosporin.[5] However, two reports describe increases, one sizeable, in the serum concentrations of ciclosporin in a heart transplant patient and a kidney transplant patient given norfloxacin.[21] Similarly, a retrospective study of paediatric kidney transplant patients, found that the ciclosporin dose at discharge was lower in 5 children who were also taking norfloxacin 5 to 10 mg/kg daily, when compared with a control group of 6 children not taking norfloxacin (4.5 mg/kg versus 7.4 mg/kg daily).[22]

(f) Ofloxacin

Thirty-nine patients with kidney transplants taking ciclosporin and prednisolone had no evidence of nephrotoxicity nor of any other adverse interaction when they were given ofloxacin 100 to 400 mg daily for periods of 3 to 500 days.[23]

(g) Pefloxacin

A study in kidney transplant patients taking corticosteroids, azathioprine, and ciclosporin found that the pharmacokinetics of ciclosporin appeared to be unaffected by pefloxacin 400 mg twice daily for 4 days.[24]

(h) Trovafloxacin

A placebo-controlled crossover study in 7 stable kidney transplant patients taking ciclosporin (*Sandimmune*) found that trovafloxacin 200 mg daily for 7 days had no statistically significant effect on the pharmacokinetics of ciclosporin.[25]

Mechanism

Uncertain. On the basis of *in vitro* analysis, it was suggested that norfloxacin inhibits CYP3A4, which would result in a reduction in ciclosporin metabolism.[22] However, there is no direct evidence from controlled studies to suggest that norfloxacin increases ciclosporin concentrations, and norfloxacin is not known as a clinically important inhibitor of CYP3A4, so further study is needed to establish the mechanism behind the modest interaction reported in one study.

The interaction between ciclosporin and ciprofloxacin resulting in increased rejection episodes, might possibly be due to some antagonism by ciprofloxacin of the ciclosporin-dependent inhibition of interleukin-2, which thereby opposes its immunosuppressant action.[14]

Importance and management

Information regarding an interaction between the quinolones and ciclosporin is variable. Evidence for an interaction with levofloxacin or norfloxacin is sparse and a clinically significant pharmacokinetic interaction seems generally unlikely. However, as some changes in ciclosporin concentrations have been reported, it would be prudent to bear the possibility of an interaction in mind should any unexplained change in ciclosporin concentrations occur in patients taking either of these quinolones. No pharmacokinetic interaction usually occurs between ciclosporin and ciprofloxacin but very occasionally and unpredictably an increase in ciclosporin serum concentrations and/or nephrotoxicity occurs. There is also some evidence that the immunosuppressant effects of ciclosporin might be reduced,[14] although this is not established. Bear these interactions in mind if both drugs are given.

There seem to be no reports of problems on the concurrent use of ciclosporin and enoxacin, moxifloxacin, ofloxacin, pefloxacin, or trovafloxacin.

1. Tan KKC, Trull AK, Shawket S. Co-administration of ciprofloxacin and cyclosporin: lack of evidence for a pharmacokinetic interaction. *Br J Clin Pharmacol* (1989) 28, 185–7.
2. Lang J, Finaz de Villaine J, Garraffo R, Touraine J-L. Cyclosporine (cyclosporin A) pharmacokinetics in renal transplant patients receiving ciprofloxacin. *Am J Med* (1989) 87 (Suppl 5A), 82S–85S.
3. Van Buren DH, Koestner J, Adedoyin A, McCune T, MacDonell R, Johnson HK, Carroll J, Nylander W, Richie RE. Effect of ciprofloxacin on cyclosporine pharmacokinetics. *Transplantation* (1990) 50, 888–9.
4. Krüger HU, Schuler U, Proksch B, Göbel M, Ehninger G. Investigation of potential interaction of ciprofloxacin with cyclosporine in bone marrow transplant recipients. *Antimicrob Agents Chemother* (1990) 34, 1048–52.
5. Robinson JA, Venezio FR, Costanzo-Nordin MR, Pifarre R, O'Keefe PJ. Patients receiving quinolones and cyclosporine after heart transplantation. *J Heart Transplant* (1990) 9, 30–1.
6. Hooper TL, Gould FK, Swinburn CR, Featherstone G, Odom NJ, Corris PA, Freeman R, McGregor CGA. Ciprofloxacin: a preferred treatment for legionella infections in patients receiving cyclosporin A. *J Antimicrob Chemother* (1988) 22, 952–3.
7. Nasir M, Rotellar C, Hand M, Kulczycki L, Alijani MR, Winchester JF. Interaction between ciclosporin and ciprofloxacin. *Nephron* (1991) 57, 245–6.
8. Borrás-Blasco J, Conesa-García V, Navarro-Ruiz A, Marín-Jiménez F, González-Delgado M, Gomez-Corrons A. Ciprofloxacin, but not levofloxacin, affects cyclosporine blood levels in a patient with pure red blood cell aplasia. *Am J Med Sci* (2005) 330, 144–6.
9. Elston RA, Taylor J. Possible interaction of ciprofloxacin with cyclosporine A. *J Antimicrob Chemother* (1988) 21, 679–80.
10. Avent CK, Krinsky JK, Kirklin JK, Bourge RC, Figg WD. Synergistic nephrotoxicity due to ciprofloxacin and cyclosporine. *Am J Med* (1988) 85, 452–3.
11. Rosado LJ, Siskind MS, Copeland JG. Acute interstitial nephritis in a cardiac transplant patient receiving ciprofloxacin. *J Thorac Cardiovasc Surg* (1994) 107, 1364.
12. Bourge RC. Invited letter concerning: acute interstitial nephritis in a cardiac transplant recipients receiving ciprofloxacin. *J Thorac Cardiovasc Surg* (1994) 107, 1364–5.
13. Rosado LJ, Siskind MS, Nolan PE, Copeland JG. Invited letter concerning: acute interstitial nephritis in a cardiac transplant recipients receiving ciprofloxacin. *J Thorac Cardiovasc Surg* (1994) 107, 1365–6.
14. Wrishko RE, Levine M, Primmett DRN, Kim S, Partovi N, Lewis S, Landsberg D, Keown PA. Investigation of a possible interaction between ciprofloxacin and cyclosporine in renal transplant patients. *Transplantation* (1997) 64, 996–999.
15. Ryerson BA, Toothaker RD, Posvar EL, Sedman AJ, Koup JR. Effect of enoxacin on cyclosporine pharmacokinetics in healthy subjects. *Intersci Conf Antimicrob Agents Chemother* (1991) 31, 198.
16. Doose DR, Walker SA, Chien SC, Williams RR, Nayak RK. Levofloxacin does not alter cyclosporine disposition. *J Clin Pharmacol* (1998) 38, 90–3.
17. Federico S, Carrano R, Capone D, Gentile A, Palmiero G, Basile V. Pharmacokinetic interaction between levofloxacin and ciclosporin or tacrolimus in kidney transplant recipients. *Clin Pharmacokinet* (2006) 45, 169–75.
18. Capone D, Tarantino G, Polichetti G, Kadilli I, Sabbatini M, Basile V, Carrano R, Nappi R, Federico S. Absence of pharmacokinetic interference of moxifloxacin on cyclosporine and tacrolimus in kidney transplant recipients. *J Clin Pharmacol* (2010) 50, 576–80.
19. Stass H, Delesen H, Kubitza D, Mai I, Bauer S, Roots I. Moxifloxacin does not alter ciclosporin pharmacokinetics in transplant patients: a multiple-dose, uncontrolled, single-centre study. *Clin Drug Investig* (2010) 30, 279–87.
20. Jadoul M, Pirson Y, van Ypersele de Strihou C. Norfloxacin and cyclosporine-a safe combination. *Transplantation* (1989) 47, 747–8.
21. Thomson DJ, Menkis AH, McKenzie FN. Norfloxacin-cyclosporine interaction. *Transplantation* (1988) 46, 312–13.

22. McLellan RA, Drobitch RK, McLellan DH, Acott PD, Crocker JFS, Renton KW. Norfloxacin interferes with cyclosporine disposition in pediatric patients undergoing renal transplantation. *Clin Pharmacol Ther* (1995) 58, 322–7.
23. Vogt P, Schorn T, Frei U. Ofloxacin in the treatment of urinary tract infection in renal transplant recipients. *Infection* (1988) 16, 175–8.
24. Lang J, Finaz de Villaine J, Guemei A, Touraine JL, Faucon C. Absence of pharmacokinetic interaction between pefloxacin and cyclosporin A in patients with renal transplants. *Rev Infect Dis* (1989) 11 (Suppl 5), S1094.
25. Johnson HJ, Swan SK, Heim-Duthoy KL, Pelletier SM, Teng R, Vincent J. The effect of trovafloxacin on steady-state pharmacokinetics of cyclosporine (CSA) in stable renal transplant patients. *Pharm Res* (1997) 14 (11 Suppl), S-509.

Ciclosporin + Antibacterials; Quinupristin with Dalfopristin

Quinupristin with dalfopristin increased single-dose ciclosporin concentrations in healthy subjects: an isolated case report supports these findings. There is limited evidence suggesting that ciclosporin might increase the risk of myalgia and/or arthralgia in patients taking quinupristin with dalfopristin.

Clinical evidence

(a) Ciclosporin concentrations

In a study, 24 subjects were given a single 300-mg dose of ciclosporin, taken 1.5 hours before the fourth of 9 infusions of quinupristin with dalfopristin (7.5 mg/kg given at intervals of 8 hours). Quinupristin with dalfopristin increased the AUC and maximum blood concentrations of ciclosporin by 63% and 30%, respectively, and decreased ciclosporin clearance by 34%.[1]

A kidney transplant patient, taking ciclosporin with minimum blood concentrations of between 80 and 105 nanograms/mL, developed a vancomycin-resistant enterococcal infection. After a series of antibacterials had failed to clear the infection, she was given intravenous quinupristin with dalfopristin 300 mg every 8 hours. After 3 days her ciclosporin minimum concentration increased to almost 300 nanograms/mL. A ciclosporin dose reduction from 75 to 50 mg twice daily returned her concentrations to baseline. However, 2 days after the antibacterials were discontinued she was found to have a ciclosporin minimum concentration of only 34 nanograms/mL. She was subsequently restabilised on her original dose of ciclosporin.[2]

(b) Myalgias or arthralgias

In a case-control study[3] of 50 patients receiving quinupristin with dalfopristin 7.5 mg/kg every 8 hours, 10 of the 25 patients who experienced arthralgia or myalgia were also taking ciclosporin, and the risk of these adverse effects with concurrent use was associated with an odds ratio of 3.8.

Mechanism

Quinupristin with dalfopristin inhibits CYP3A4, by which ciclosporin is metabolised.[4] Myalgias and/or arthralgias are common in patients receiving quinupristin with dalfopristin and their aetiology is uncertain.[4]

Importance and management

The available evidence suggests that quinupristin with dalfopristin is likely to increase ciclosporin concentrations. It would therefore seem prudent to monitor ciclosporin concentrations being aware that ciclosporin dose reductions might be necessary. Furthermore, consider the possibility that ciclosporin use might increase the risk of myalgias and/or arthralgias in patients taking quinupristin with dalfopristin. The US manufacturer notes that improvement has been noted in some patients with this adverse effect when the quinupristin with dalfopristin dose frequency has been extended.[4]

1. Nordic Pharma UK. Data on file. Randomized, crossover, phase I study of the interaction between quinupristin/dalfopristin (RP 59500) at steady state and cyclosporine in healthy volunteers (Ref-Syn-0188).
2. Stamatakis MK, Richards JG. Interaction between quinupristin/dalfopristin and cyclosporine. *Ann Pharmacother* (1997) 31, 576–8.
3. Carver PL, Whang E, VandenBussche HL, Kauffman CA, Malani PN. Risk factors for arthralgias or myalgias associated with quinupristin-dalfopristin therapy. *Pharmacotherapy* (2003) 23, 159–64.
4. Synercid (Quinupristin/Dalfopristin). Pfizer Injectables. US Prescribing information, October 2013.

Ciclosporin + Antibacterials; Sulfonamides and/or Trimethoprim

Co-trimoxazole increases serum creatinine concentrations in kidney transplant patients taking ciclosporin. Isolated reports have shown a similar effect with trimethoprim. Isolated cases involving sulfadiazine given orally or sulfadimidine given intravenously with trimethoprim describe a reduction in ciclosporin concentrations. Sulfametoxydiazine possibly caused a minor reduction in ciclosporin concentrations in one case.

Clinical evidence

(a) Co-trimoxazole

A large-scale study in 132 kidney transplant patients taking ciclosporin encompassing 33 876 patient days found that the concurrent use of co-trimoxazole was effective and well tolerated. Ciclosporin pharmacokinetics remained unchanged. A 15% increase in serum creatinine concentrations occurred, which reversed when the co-trimoxazole was stopped. This increase was not interpreted as a sign of nephrotoxicity but appeared to be due to inhibition of the tubular excretion of creatinine by the co-trimoxazole.[1]

Other reports describe a few patients given ciclosporin with co-trimoxazole who developed increases in creatinine concentrations (interpreted as evidence of nephrotoxicity),[2-5] interstitial nephritis,[6] granulocytopenia, and thrombocytopenia.[7,8]

(b) Sulfadiazine or Sulfametoxydiazine

Three heart transplant patients treated for toxoplasmosis had a reduction in their ciclosporin concentrations when they were given sulfadiazine 4 or 6 g daily. Their ciclosporin dose-to-concentration ratios rose by 58%, 82%, and 29%. Two had previously been given sulfametoxydiazine and this had caused a minor reduction in ciclosporin concentrations in one of them.[9]

(c) Sulfadimidine with Trimethoprim

A heart transplant patient taking ciclosporin and prednisolone, developed undetectable serum ciclosporin concentrations 7 days after starting intravenous sulfadimidine 2 g four times daily and **trimethoprim** 300 to 500 mg twice daily. Doubling the ciclosporin dose had little effect and evidence of transplant rejection was seen. Within 10 days of starting to take the antibacterials orally instead of intravenously the serum ciclosporin concentrations returned to roughly their former levels and the rejection problems disappeared.[10]

Another report by some of the same authors describes a similar large reduction in serum ciclosporin concentrations in 5 heart transplant patients (one of them the same as the report already cited[10]) when given sulfadimidine and **trimethoprim** intravenously.[11]

(d) Trimethoprim

In 4 kidney transplant patients taking ciclosporin, serum creatinine concentrations increased during the use of trimethoprim. Renal function deteriorated within 2 to 3 days of starting trimethoprim and returned to normal within a week of stopping this antibacterial.[12]

Mechanism

Uncertain. Co-trimoxazole and trimethoprim can increase serum creatinine concentrations, possibly due to inhibition of creatinine secretion by the renal tubules.[13] The reduction in serum ciclosporin concentrations apparently caused by the sulfonamides is not understood.

Importance and management

The documentation supporting an interaction between ciclosporin and the sulfonamides and trimethoprim is only moderate, and these interactions are not firmly established. Be aware that intravenous sulfadimidine with trimethoprim might cause a large decrease in serum ciclosporin concentrations with accompanying inadequate immunosuppression. Sulfadiazine might also decrease ciclosporin concentrations. The available evidence suggests that oral sulfadimidine with trimethoprim, sulfametoxydiazine, and co-trimoxazole do not interact adversely and are normally safe and effective, although toxicity can apparently occur in a small number of patients.

Until more information is available it would be prudent to monitor ciclosporin concentrations if any sulphonamide is added to established treatment with ciclosporin. The US manufacturer of ciclosporin recommends close monitoring of renal function when it is used with co-trimoxazole[14] and this available evidence suggests that this is a prudent precaution, both with co-trimoxazole and trimethoprim alone.

1. Maki DG, Fox BC, Kuntz J, Sollinger HW, Belzer FO. A prospective, randomized, double-blind study of trimethoprim-sulfamethoxazole for prophylaxis of infection in renal transplantation. Side effects of trimethoprim-sulfamethoxazole interaction with cyclosporine. *J Lab Clin Med* (1992) 119, 11–24.
2. Thompson JF, Chalmers DHK, Hunnisett AGW, Wood RFM, Morris PJ. Nephrotoxicity of trimethoprim and cotrimoxazole in renal allograft recipients treated with cyclosporine. *Transplantation* (1983) 36, 204–6.
3. Ringdén O, Myrenfors P, Klintmalm G, Tydén G, Öst L. Nephrotoxicity by co-trimoxazole and cyclosporin in transplanted patients. *Lancet* (1984) i, 1016–17.
4. Klintmalm G, Säwe J, Ringdén O, von Bahr C, Magnusson A. Cyclosporine plasma levels in renal transplant patients. Association with renal toxicity and allograft rejection. *Transplantation* (1985) 39, 132–7.
5. Klintmalm G, Ringdén O, Groth CG. Clinical and laboratory signs in nephrotoxicity and rejection in cyclosporine treated renal allograft recipients. *Transplant Proc* (1983) 15 (Suppl 1), 2815–20.
6. Smith EJ, Light JA, Filo RS, Yum MN. Interstitial nephritis caused by trimethoprim-sulfamethoxazole in renal transplant recipients. *JAMA* (1980) 244, 360–1.
7. Bradley PP, Warden GD, Maxwell JG, Rothstein G. Neutropenia and thrombocytopenia in renal allograft recipients treated with trimethoprim-sulfamethoxazole. *Ann Intern Med* (1980) 93, 560–2.
8. Hulme B, Reeves DS. Leucopenia associated with trimethoprim-sulfamethoxazole after renal transplantation. *BMJ* (1971) 3, 610–12.
9. Spes CH, Angermann CE, Stempfle HU, Wenke K, Theisen K. Sulfadiazine therapy for toxoplasmosis in heart transplant recipients decreases cyclosporine concentration. *Clin Investig* (1992) 70, 752–4.
10. Wallwork J, McGregor CGA, Wells FC, Cory-Pearce R, English TAH. Cyclosporin and intravenous sulphadimidine and trimethoprim therapy. *Lancet* (1983) i, 336–7.
11. Jones DK, Hakim M, Wallwork J, Higenbottam TW, White DJG. Serious interaction between cyclosporin A and sulphadimidine. *BMJ* (1986) 292, 728–9.
12. Nyberg G, Gäbel H, Althoff P, Bjoörk S, Herlitz H, Brynger H. Adverse effect of trimethoprim on kidney function in renal transplant patients. *Lancet* (1984) i, 394–5.
13. Berg KJ, Gjellestad A, Norby G, Rootwelt K, Djøseland O, Fauchald P, Mehl A, Narverud J, Talseth T. Renal effects of trimethoprim in ciclosporin- and azathioprine-treated kidney-allografted patients. *Nephron* (1989) 53, 218–22.
14. Neoral (Ciclosporin). Novartis Pharmaceuticals Corporation. US Prescribing information, May 2013.

Ciclosporin + Antibacterials; Vancomycin

Vancomycin appears to increase the risk of nephrotoxicity when it is given with ciclosporin.

Clinical evidence, mechanism, importance and management

In a subgroup analysis of bone marrow transplant patients who were taking ciclosporin, there was a 42% decrease in creatinine clearance in those receiving intravenous vancomycin 15 mg/kg every 12 hours compared with a 15% decrease in those receiving teicoplanin. All patients also received tobramycin and piperacillin.[1]

Both vancomycin and ciclosporin can individually be nephrotoxic, and this study provides some evidence that their toxicities can be additive. Bear in mind the possibility of increased nephrotoxicity if vancomycin is required in a patient taking ciclosporin.

1. Kureishi A, Jewesson PJ, Rubinger M, Cole CD, Reece DE, Phillips GL, Smith JA, Chow AW. Double-blind comparison of teicoplanin versus vancomycin in febrile neutropenic patients receiving concomitant tobramycin and piperacillin: effect on cyclosporin A-associated nephrotoxicity. *Antimicrob Agents Chemother* (1991) 35, 2246–52.

Ciclosporin + Antidiabetics; Repaglinide

A single-dose study found that ciclosporin increased repaglinide bioavailability, but not all studies have found this effect.

Clinical evidence

A placebo-controlled study in 12 healthy subjects given ciclosporin 100 mg twice daily for two doses, with a single 250-microgram dose of repaglinide on day 2, found that ciclosporin significantly increased the maximum plasma concentration and AUC of repaglinide 2.75-fold and 3.44-fold, respectively.[1,2]

In a study in kidney transplant patients stabilised on immunosuppressants, 7 patients taking ciclosporin had no notable changes in ciclosporin blood concentrations and no dose changes were required on starting repaglinide 1 to 3 mg daily (mostly as monotherapy, but in a few cases given with either metformin or rosiglitazone).[3] Six of the 7 patients had a successful outcome. This success rate was higher than that seen with tacrolimus (8 of 14), and others have suggested that this might have been due to the pharmacokinetic interaction, which results in increased repaglinide concentrations.[2] However, commenting further, the authors noted that they were unable to demonstrate a consistent, increased blood glucose-lowering effect with the concurrent use of repaglinide and ciclosporin when compared with tacrolimus and repaglinide, and that there was no obvious difference in the median repaglinide dose.[4] It is therefore difficult to draw any significant conclusions from this study.

Mechanism

It was suggested that ciclosporin inhibited the metabolism of repaglinide by CYP3A4 as well as affecting the hepatic uptake of repaglinide by organic anion transporters.[1,2]

Importance and Management

Data for an interaction between repaglinide and ciclosporin is inconclusive.

The large increases in repaglinide concentrations seen in the single-dose study in healthy subjects might well be clinically relevant in some patients. Because of this, the possibility of an increased blood-glucose-lowering effect should be borne in mind if ciclosporin is added to the established use of repaglinide. Patients should be advised to report any adverse effects, particularly an increase in the number of hypoglycaemic events.

In the clinical study where repaglinide was given to patients stabilised on ciclosporin, ciclosporin concentrations were unaffected. However, note that, in this study repaglinide was started at a low dose and titrated upwards as necessary.[4] It might therefore be prudent to introduce repaglinide in this way.

1. Kajosaari LI, Niemi M, Neuvonen M, Laitila J, Neuvonen PJ, Backman JT. Cyclosporine markedly raises the plasma concentrations of repaglinide. *Clin Pharmacol Ther* (2005) 78, 388–99.
2. Backman JT, Kajosaari LI, Niemi M, Neuvonen PJ. Cyclosporine A increases plasma concentrations and effects of repaglinide. *Am J Transplant* (2006) 6, 2221–2.
3. Türk T, Peitruck F, Dolff S, Kribben A, Janssen OE, Mann K, Philipp T, Heemann U, Witzke O. Repaglinide in the management of new-onset diabetes mellitus after renal transplantation. *Am J Transplant* (2006) 6, 842–6.
4. Türk T, Witzke O. Pharmacological interaction between cyclosporine A and repaglinide. Is it clinically relevant? *Am J Transplant* (2006) 6, 2223.

Ciclosporin + Antidiabetics; Sulphonylureas

Some preliminary evidence suggests that glibenclamide (glyburide) can increase ciclosporin concentrations. Glipizide approximately doubled ciclosporin concentrations in 2 patients, but one study found no interaction.

Clinical evidence, mechanism, importance and management

A review of 6 post-transplant patients with diabetes, taking ciclosporin found that their steady-state plasma ciclosporin concentrations rose by 57% when they were given **glibenclamide (glyburide)**. Hepatic and renal function were unchanged. The reason for this reaction is not known, but it was suggested that **glibenclamide** possibly inhibits the CYP3A4, the major isoenzyme involved in the metabolism of ciclosporin, resulting in a reduction in its clearance.[1] However, glibenclamide is not known to be a CYP3A4 inhibitor.

Ciclosporin blood concentrations in 2 patients were more than doubled, and they needed reductions of 20 to 30% in their ciclosporin dose when they were also given **glipizide** 10 mg daily.[2] In contrast, a study in 11 post-transplant patients with diabetes found no significant alterations in ciclosporin pharmacokinetics when **glipizide** was given.[3]

These interactions are unconfirmed and of uncertain clinical significance. There is insufficient evidence to recommend increased monitoring, but be aware of the potential for an interaction in the case of an unexpected response to treatment. Information about other sulfonylureas appears not to be available. However, note that one of the rare adverse effects of ciclosporin is hyperglycaemia, and therefore, even in the absence of a pharmacokinetic interaction, ciclosporin might interfere with diabetic control. Nevertheless, the effect is rare, and does not justify an increase in monitoring all patients.

1. Islam SI, Masuda QN, Bolaji OO, Shaheen FM, Sheikh IA. Possible interaction between cyclosporine and glibenclamide in posttransplant diabetic patients. *Ther Drug Monit* (1996) 18, 624–6.
2. Chidester PD, Connito DJ. Interaction between glipizide and cyclosporine: report of two cases. *Transplant Proc* (1993) 25, 2136–7.
3. Sagedal S, Åsberg A, Hartmann A, Bergan S, Berg KJ. Glipizide treatment of post-transplant diabetes does not interfere with cyclosporine pharmacokinetics in renal allograft recipients. *Clin Transplant* (1998) 12, 553–6.

Ciclosporin + Antiepileptics

Ciclosporin concentrations are greatly reduced by carbamazepine, phenobarbital, and phenytoin. Oxcarbazepine similarly appears to cause a decrease in ciclosporin concentrations. Valproate does not appear to affect ciclosporin concentrations, but two case reports suggest that it might damage renal grafts and cause hepatotoxicity in patients taking ciclosporin. Levetiracetam might not alter ciclosporin concentrations.

Clinical evidence

(a) Carbamazepine

The ciclosporin serum concentrations of a kidney transplant patient decreased from 346 to 64 nanograms/mL, within 3 days of starting to take carbamazepine 200 mg three times daily. A week later serum concentrations had further decreased to 37 nanograms/mL. They increased when the carbamazepine was stopped but decreased once more when it was restarted, and the ciclosporin dose was increased to keep the concentrations within the therapeutic range.[1]

The steady-state blood concentrations of ciclosporin (adjusted for dose) in a group of 3 children with kidney transplants taking carbamazepine were 50% lower than in 3 other matched patients not taking carbamazepine.[2] This interaction has also been described in four other individual patients.[3-5] One needed her ciclosporin dose to be doubled in order to maintain adequate blood concentrations while taking carbamazepine 800 mg daily.[3] When the carbamazepine was replaced by sodium valproate in 3 patients, the ciclosporin doses could be reduced.[3,4]

(b) Oxcarbazepine

A kidney transplant patient taking ciclosporin 270 mg daily and valproate, gabapentin, prednisone, doxepin, allopurinol, levothyroxine, and pravastatin was also given oxcarbazepine. Fourteen days later, with the dose of oxcarbazepine at 750 mg daily, the ciclosporin minimum concentration was below 100 nanograms/mL and after a further 2 days was 87 nanograms/mL. The ciclosporin dose was increased to 290 mg daily and the oxcarbazepine dose reduced to 600 mg daily. The ciclosporin concentration then remained stable above 100 nanograms/mL and seizure frequency was reduced by 95%.[6] Another case report describes a 14-year-old girl taking ciclosporin 310 mg daily after a heart transplant whose ciclosporin concentration became subtherapeutic after oxcarbazepine was started (and titrated up to 750 mg daily). Despite increasing the ciclosporin dose to 600 mg daily her ciclosporin concentration remained subtherapeutic. Oxcarbazepine was switched to **levetiracetam** 750 mg twice daily and a therapeutic ciclosporin concentration was subsequently achieved with a ciclosporin dose of 340 mg daily.[7]

(c) Phenobarbital

A 4-year-old child with a bone marrow transplant who was receiving phenobarbital 50 mg twice daily had a ciclosporin serum concentration of less than 60 nanograms/mL even after increasing the ciclosporin dose to 18 mg/kg daily. When the phenobarbital dose was reduced to 25% of the original dose the ciclosporin minimum serum concentration increased to 205 nanograms/mL.[8] Another report describes a patient whose ciclosporin concentration increased from 512 to 810 nanograms/mL after phenytoin and phenobarbital were replaced by sodium valproate.[9]

A 3-fold increase in ciclosporin clearance was seen in a child with a kidney transplant while taking phenobarbital.[10] Reductions in ciclosporin concentrations due to phenobarbital have been described in other patients.[11-14]

(d) Phenytoin

The observation that patients taking ciclosporin needed large dose increases while taking phenytoin[15] prompted a further controlled study in 6 healthy subjects.[16] Phenytoin 300 or 400 mg daily reduced the ciclosporin maximum blood concentration and AUC by 37% (from 1325 to 831 micrograms/L) and 47%, respectively.[16]

Other reports describe patients who needed 2- to 4-fold increases in their ciclosporin doses when they were given phenytoin,[17-20] and one patient who had a variable ciclosporin concentration and a rejection episode in the first 10 days after a kidney transplant while taking phenytoin.[21]

Another report describes a patient who had an increase in ciclosporin concentration, from 512 to 810 nanograms/mL, after phenytoin and phenobarbital were replaced by sodium valproate.[9]

A subgroup analysis of results from a retrospective study in liver transplant patients, observed that 30 days or more after discharge, the average dose of ciclosporin required to maintain therapeutic concentrations in patients taking concurrent phenytoin, was more than double that required in patients taking **levetiracetam**.[22] However note that deficiencies in study design and small patient numbers limit the interpretation of this observation.

A report of severe gingival overgrowth in a kidney transplant patient was attributed to the additive adverse effects of ciclosporin and phenytoin. Ciclosporin was replaced by tacrolimus, which might have fewer oral adverse effects, and almost complete reversal of gingival overgrowth was achieved within 6 months.[23]

(e) Sodium valproate

In four cases an interacting antiepileptic was successfully replaced by sodium valproate,[3,4,9] see *Carbamazepine, Phenobarbital*, and *Phenytoin*, above. However, sodium valproate might not always be without problems because interstitial nephritis was suspected in one patient with a renal graft taking ciclosporin and valproate,[11] and fatal valproate-induced hepatotoxicity occurred in another patient taking ciclosporin.[24]

Mechanism

It is thought that phenytoin,[15,16] carbamazepine,[1,2] and phenobarbital[8,12] increase the metabolism of ciclosporin by cytochrome P450 isoenzymes in the liver (most probably via CYP3A4) thereby decreasing its serum concentration. Oxcarbazepine produced a decrease in ciclosporin concentrations in two cases, and is known to produce clinically important effects on other drugs also metabolised by CYP3A4. Phenytoin also possibly reduces the absorption of ciclosporin.[25]

Importance and management

Evidence for an interaction between ciclosporin and antiepileptics is not extensive and largely limited to case reports or a few small studies. Nevertheless, all the effects described appear to be of clinical importance, and serum ciclosporin concentrations should be well monitored if carbamazepine, phenobarbital, or phenytoin are added and the ciclosporin dose increased appropriately. **Primidone** is metabolised to phenobarbital, and **fosphenytoin** is a prodrug of phenytoin, and they would therefore also be expected to decrease ciclosporin concentrations. Information about oxcarbazepine is limited but similar precautions to those described for the other enzyme-inducing antiepileptics would seem prudent. Note that the effects of the interaction could persist for a week or more after the antiepileptic is withdrawn. Sodium valproate seems not to alter ciclosporin concentrations, but the case reports of nephritis and hepatotoxicity suggest some caution is warranted. Similarly, levetiracetam might not alter ciclosporin concentrations, but evidence is limited and further study is required in order to draw more general conclusions.

1. Lele P, Peterson P, Yang S, Jarell B, Burke JF. Cyclosporine and tegretol — another drug interaction. *Kidney Int* (1985) 27, 344.
2. Cooney GF, Mochon M, Kaiser B, Dunn SP, Goldsmith B. Effects of carbamazepine on cyclosporine metabolism in pediatric renal transplant recipients. *Pharmacotherapy* (1995) 15, 353–6.
3. Hillebrand G, Castro LA, van Scheidt W, Beukelmann D, Land W, Schmidt D. Valproate for epilepsy in renal transplant recipients receiving cyclosporine. *Transplantation* (1987) 43, 915–16.
4. Schofield OMV, Camp RDR, Levene GM. Cyclosporin A in psoriasis: interaction with carbamazepine. *Br J Dermatol* (1990) 122, 425–6.
5. Alvarez JS, Del Castillo JAC, Ortiz MJA. Effect of carbamazepine on ciclosporin blood level. *Nephron* (1991) 58, 235–6.
6. Rösche J, Fröscher W, Abendroth D, Liebel J. Possible oxcarbazepine interaction with cyclosporine serum levels: a single case study. *Clin Neuropharmacol* (2001) 24, 113–16.
7. Franzoni E, Sarajlija J, Garone C, Malaspina E, Marchiani V. No kinetic interaction between levetiracetam and cyclosporine: a case report. *J Child Neurol* (2007) 22, 440–2.
8. Carstensen H, Jacobsen N, Dieperink H. Interaction between cyclosporin A and phenobarbitone. *Br J Clin Pharmacol* (1986) 21, 550–1.
9. Noguchi M, Kiuchi C, Akiyama H, Sakamaki H, Onozawa Y. Interaction between cyclosporin A and anticonvulsants. *Bone Marrow Transplant* (1992) 9, 391.
10. Burckart GJ, Venkataramanan R, Starzl T, Ptachcinski JR, Gartner JC, Rosenthal T. Cyclosporine clearance in children following organ transplantation. *J Clin Pharmacol* (1984) 24, 412.
11. Kramer G, Dillmann U, Tettenborn B. Cyclosporine-phenobarbital interaction. *Epilepsia* (1989) 30, 701.
12. Beierle FA, Bailey L. Cyclosporine metabolism impeded/blocked by co-administration of phenobarbital. *Clin Chem* (1989) 35, 1160.
13. Wideman CA. Pharmacokinetic monitoring of cyclosporine. *Transplant Proc* (1983) 15 (Suppl 1), 3168–75.
14. Nishioka T, Ikegami M, Imanishi M, Ishii T, Uemura T, Kunikata S, Kanda H, Matsuura T, Akiyama T, Kurita T. Interaction between phenobarbital and ciclosporin following renal transplantation: a case report. *Hinyokika Kiyo* (1990) 36, 447–50.
15. Keown PA, Laupacis A, Carruthers G, Stawecki M, Koegler J, McKenzie FN, Wall W, Stiller CR. Interaction between phenytoin and cyclosporine following organ transplantation. *Transplantation* (1984) 38, 304–6.
16. Freeman DJ, Laupacis A, Keown PA, Stiller CR, Carruthers SG. Evaluation of cyclosporin-phenytoin interaction with observations on cyclosporin metabolites. *Br J Clin Pharmacol* (1984) 18, 887–93.
17. Grigg-Damberger MM, Costanzo-Nordin R, Kelly MA, Bahamon-Dussan JE, Silver M, Zucker MJ, Celesia GG. Phenytoin may compromise efficacy of cyclosporine immunosuppression in cardiac transplant patients. *Epilepsia* (1988) 29, 693.
18. Schmidt H, Naumann R, Jaschonek K, Einsele H, Dopfer R, Ehninger G. Drug interaction between cyclosporin and phenytoin in allogeneic bone marrow transplantation. *Bone Marrow Transplant* (1989) 4, 212–13.
19. Schweitzer EJ, Canafax DM, Gillingham KJ, Najarian JS, Matas AJ. Phenytoin administration in kidney recipients on CSA immunosuppression. *J Am Soc Nephrol* (1991) 2, 816.
20. Castelao AM. Cyclosporine A – drug interactions. 2nd Int Conf Therapeutic Drug Monitoring Toxicology, Barcelona, Spain 1992. 203–9.
21. Formea CM, Evans CG, Karlix JL. Altered cytochrome P450 metabolism of calcineurin inhibitors: case report and review of the literature. *Pharmacotherapy* (2005) 25, 1021–9.
22. Glass GA, Stankiewicz J, Mithoefer A, Freeman R, Bergethon PR. Levetiracetam for seizures after liver transplantation. *Neurology* (2005) 64, 1084–5.
23. Hernandez G, Arriba L, Lucas M, de Andres A. Reduction of severe gingival overgrowth in a kidney transplant patient by replacing cyclosporin A with tacrolimus. *J Periodontol* (2000) 71, 1630–6.
24. Fischman MA, Hull D, Bartus SA, Schweizer RT. Valproate for epilepsy in renal transplant recipients receiving cyclosporine. *Transplantation* (1989) 48, 542.
25. Rowland M, Gupta SK. Cyclosporin-phenytoin interaction: re-evaluation using metabolite data. *Br J Clin Pharmacol* (1987) 24, 329–34.

Ciclosporin + Azoles; Fluconazole

Fluconazole can increase ciclosporin concentrations.

Clinical evidence

Oral fluconazole 200 mg daily for 14 days roughly doubled the ciclosporin minimum blood concentrations of 8 kidney transplant patients stabilised on oral ciclosporin, from 27 to 58 nanograms/mL. The AUC increased by 80% but serum creatinine concentrations were unchanged.[1,2]

Other reports describe 2- to 3-fold increases in ciclosporin blood concentrations in kidney transplant patients within 6 to 11 days of starting treatment with fluconazole 100 to 300 mg daily.[3-9] One patient developed nephrotoxicity, which resolved when the doses of both drugs were reduced.[10]

In contrast, some patients have had little or no changes in serum ciclosporin or creatinine concentrations when fluconazole was given.[7,8,11-15] It has been suggested that the interaction is dose-dependent.[8] In addition, the route of administration might influence the interaction. For example, in one study there was only a 20% increase in ciclosporin concentrations when intravenous ciclosporin was given with high-dose intravenous fluconazole, which was not considered clinically relevant.[16] In a retrospective study in patients receiving intravenous ciclosporin, there was a small increase in ciclosporin blood concentration (from 362 to 394 nanograms/mL) when intravenous fluconazole was switched to oral fluconazole.[17] One study found a lack of interaction in females and African-American patients, suggesting that gender and ethnicity might also be factors.[18]

Mechanism

Fluconazole inhibits hepatic CYP3A4, by which ciclosporin is metabolised, and as a result ciclosporin blood concentrations increase. Some evidence suggests that fluconazole also appears to inhibit the metabolism of ciclosporin in the gut wall.[16]

Importance and management

Information about the use of ciclosporin with fluconazole is reasonably well documented, although much of the evidence comes from case reports. Concurrent use should be closely monitored, being alert for the need to reduce the ciclosporin dose, in some cases by up to 50% or more, although some patients might demonstrate no major changes in ciclosporin concentrations. There is also some evidence that the interaction possibly depends on its dose,[8] gender and ethnicity,[18] and the route of ciclosporin[16] or fluconazole[17] administration.

1. Canafax DM, Graves NM, Hilligoss DM, Carleton BC, Gardner MJ, Matas AJ. Interaction between cyclosporine and fluconazole in renal allograft recipients. *Transplantation* (1991) 51, 1014–18.
2. Canafax DM, Graves NM, Hilligoss DM, Carleton BC, Gardner MJ, Matas AJ. Increased cyclosporine levels as a result of simultaneous fluconazole and cyclosporine therapy in renal transplant recipients: a double-blind, randomized pharmacokinetic and safety study. *Transplant Proc* (1991) 23, 1041–2.
3. Torregrosa V, De la Torre M, Campistol JM, Oppenheimer F, Ricart MJ, Vilardell J, Andreu J. Interaction of fluconazole with ciclosporin A. *Nephron* (1992) 60, 125–6.
4. Sugar AM, Saunders C, Idelson BA, Bernard DB. Interaction of fluconazole and cyclosporine. *Ann Intern Med* (1989) 110, 844.
5. Barbara JAJ, Clarkson AR, LaBrooy J, McNeil JD, Woodroffe AJ. Candida albicans arthritis in a renal allograft recipient with an interaction between cyclosporin and fluconazole. *Nephrol Dial Transplant* (1993) 8, 263–6.
6. Tett S, Carey D, Lee H-S. Drug interactions with fluconazole. *Med J Aust* (1992) 156, 365.
7. Koselj M, Bren A, Kandus A, Kovac D. Drug interactions between cyclosporine and rifampicin, erythromycin, and azoles in kidney recipients with opportunistic infections. *Transplant Proc* (1994) 26, 2823–4.
8. López-Gil JA. Fluconazole-cyclosporine interaction: a dose-dependent effect? *Ann Pharmacother* (1993) 27, 427–30.
9. Sud K, Singh B, Krishna VS, Thennarasu K, Kohli HS, Jha V, Gupta KL, Sakhuja V. Unpredictable cyclosporin-fluconazole interaction in renal transplant recipients. *Nephrol Dial Transplant* (1999) 14, 1698–1703.
10. Collignon P, Hurley B, Mitchell D. Interaction of fluconazole with cyclosporin. *Lancet* (1989) i, 1262.
11. Ehninger G, Jaschonek K, Schuler U, Krüger HU. Interaction of fluconazole with cyclosporin. *Lancet* (1989) ii, 104–5.
12. Krüger HU, Schuler U, Zimmermann R, Ehninger G. Absence of significant interaction of fluconazole with cyclosporin. *J Antimicrob Chemother* (1989) 24, 781–6.
13. Conti DJ, Tolkoff-Rubin NE, Baker GP, Doran M, Cosimi AB, Delmonico F, Auchincloss H, Russell PS, Rubin RH. Successful treatment of invasive fungal infection with fluconazole in organ transplant recipients. *Transplantation* (1989) 48, 692–5.
14. Rubin RH, Debruin MF, Knirsch AK. Fluconazole therapy for patients with serious *Candida* infections who have failed standard therapies. *Intersci Conf Antimicrob Agents Chemother* (1989), 112.
15. Lumbreras C, Cuervas-Mons V, Jara P, del Palacio A, Turrión VS, Barrios C, Moreno E, Noriega AR, Paya CV. Randomized trial of fluconazole versus nystatin for the prophylaxis of *Candida* infection following liver transplantation. *J Infect Dis* (1996) 174, 583–8.
16. Osowski CL, Dix SP, Lin LS, Mullins RE, Geller RB, Wingard JR. Evaluation of the drug interaction between intravenous high-dose fluconazole and cyclosporine or tacrolimus in bone marrow transplant patients. *Transplantation* (1996) 61, 1268–72.
17. Mihara A, Mori T, Aisa Y, Yamazaki R, Iketani O, Tanigawara Y, Ikeda Y, Okamoto S. Greater impact of oral fluconazole on drug interaction with intravenous calcineurin inhibitors as compared with intravenous fluconazole. *Eur J Clin Pharmacol* (2008) 64, 89–91.
18. Mathis AS, DiRenzo T, Friedman GS, Kaplan B, Adamson R. Sex and ethnicity may chiefly influence the interaction of fluconazole with calcineurin inhibitors. *Transplantation* (2001) 71, 1069–75.

Ciclosporin + Azoles; Itraconazole

Itraconazole can increase ciclosporin concentrations. Rhabdomyolysis has been reported with the combination of ciclosporin and itraconazole, but four of these cases were complicated by the presence of statins.

Clinical evidence

In 4 heart-lung, 2 heart, and one lung transplant patients an average 56% reduction (range 33 to 84%) in the ciclosporin doses were needed when itraconazole (dose not stated) was given. Serum creatinine concentrations increased temporarily until the ciclosporin dose had been readjusted.[1] Increases in ciclosporin concentrations of 2- to 3-fold were seen in another 2 patients given itraconazole 200 mg daily,[2,3] and in one case the increased concentrations persisted for more than 4 weeks after the itraconazole was stopped.[3] In a study in 8 patients given intravenous ciclosporin, intravenous itraconazole 200 mg twice daily for 2 days then 200 mg daily caused a mean 80% increase in the concentrations of ciclosporin.[4] In another study, the concentration-to-dose ratio of ciclosporin was increased about 2-fold (range 37% to 221%) when itraconazole oral solution was also given.[5] In one study, 7 patients taking ciclosporin and given itraconazole 100 mg twice daily for 3 months required a 94% increase in their ciclosporin dose when itraconazole was stopped.[6]

Other case reports and studies suggest that dose reductions of about 50 to 80% (where stated) were needed when patients taking ciclosporin were given itraconazole.[7-11] Enhanced itraconazole absorption in the presence of a carbonated drink that increased stomach acidity was found to allow decreases in the ciclosporin dose and increases in its dose interval.[12]

These reports contrast with another describing 14 bone marrow transplant patients taking ciclosporin. Those given itraconazole 100 mg twice daily had no notable changes in ciclosporin or creatinine serum concentrations.[13] Another patient required only a 10% reduction in ciclosporin dose when given itraconazole 400 mg daily for 40 days.[14]

Rhabdomyolysis has been reported in 3 lung transplant patients[7,15] and 2 heart transplant patients[16,17] when itraconazole was given with ciclosporin. However, in three of these cases the concurrent use of simvastatin and in one case concurrent simvastatin and gemfibrozil would also have been factors,[7,15-17] as both ciclosporin and itraconazole can increase simvastatin concentrations (see 'Statins + Ciclosporin', p.1327, and also 'Statins + Azoles', p.1322).

In a pharmacokinetic study in patients undergoing stem cell transplantation, the AUC of itraconazole after a single 200-mg intravenous dose did not differ before and after patients were stabilised on ciclosporin. However, the median AUC of the main active itraconazole metabolite, hydroxyitraconazole, was increased by 49%. This is probably not clinically relevant, but might have a bearing in situations when itraconazole concentrations are monitored.[18]

Mechanism

Itraconazole is a potent inhibitor of CYP3A4, by which ciclosporin is metabolised, and as a result ciclosporin blood concentrations increase.

Importance and management

Information about the use of ciclosporin with itraconazole is not extensive, but that which exists suggests that large increases in ciclosporin concentrations might result, and sizeable decreases in ciclosporin dose might be necessary. As such, concurrent use should be closely monitored, being alert for the need to reduce the ciclosporin dose, perhaps by up to 50% or more, although note that some patients might demonstrate no major changes at all. Ciclosporin can increase the concentrations of the hydroxy metabolite of itraconazole, but the relevance of this is uncertain.

1. Kramer MR, Marshall SE, Denning DW, Keogh AM, Tucker RM, Galgiani JN, Lewiston NJ, Stevens DA, Theodore J. Cyclosporine and itraconazole interaction in heart and lung transplant recipients. *Ann Intern Med* (1990) 113, 327–9.
2. Kwan JT C, Foxall PJD, Davidson DGC, Bending MR, Eisinger AJ. Interaction of cyclosporin and itraconazole. *Lancet* (1987) ii, 282.
3. Trenk D, Brett W, Jähnchen E, Birnbaum D. Time course of cyclosporin/itraconazole interaction. *Lancet* (1987) ii, 1335–6.
4. Leather H, Boyette RM, Tian L, Wingard JR. Pharmacokinetic evaluation of the drug interaction between intravenous itraconazole and intravenous tacrolimus or intravenous cyclosporin A in allogeneic hematopoietic stem cell transplant recipients. *Biol Blood Marrow Transplant* (2006) 12, 325–34.
5. Mori T, Aisa Y, Kato J, Nakamura Y, Ikeda Y, Okamoto S. Drug interaction between oral solution itraconazole and calcineurin inhibitors in allogeneic hematopoietic stem cell transplantation recipients: an association with bioavailability of oral solution itraconazole. *Int J Hematol* (2009) 90, 103–7.
6. Kramer MR, Merin G, Rudis E, Bar I, Nesher T, Bublil M, Milgalter E. Dose adjustment and cost of itraconazole prophylaxis in lung transplant recipients receiving cyclosporine and tacrolimus (FK 506). *Transplant Proc* (1997) 29, 2657–9.
7. Malouf MA, Bicknell M, Glanville AR. Rhabdomyolysis after lung transplantation. *Aust N Z J Med* (1997) 27, 186.
8. Faggian G, Livi U, Bortolotti U, Mazzucco A, Stellin G, Chiominto B, Viviani MA, Gallucci V. Itraconazole therapy for acute invasive pulmonary aspergillosis in heart transplantation. *Transplant Proc* (1989) 21, 2506–7.
9. Florea NR, Capitano B, Nightingale CH, Hull D, Leitz GJ, Nicolau DP. Beneficial pharmacokinetic interaction between cyclosporine and itraconazole in renal transplant recipients. *Transplant Proc* (2003) 35, 2873–7.
10. McLachlan AJ, Tett SE. Effect of metabolic inhibitors on cyclosporine pharmacokinetics using a population approach. *Ther Drug Monit* (1998) 20, 390–5.
11. Linthoudt H, Van Raemdonck D, Lerut T, Demedts M, Verleden G. The association of itraconazole and methylprednisolone may give rise to important steroid-related side effects. *J Heart Lung Transplant* (1996) 15, 1165.
12. Wimberley SL, Haug MT 3rd, Shermock KM, Qu A, Maurer JR, Mehta AC, Schilz RJ, Gordon SM. Enhanced cyclosporine-itraconazole interaction with cola in lung transplant recipients. *Clin Transplant* (2001) 15, 116–22.
13. Nováková I, Donnelly P, de Witte T, de Pauw B, Boezeman J, Veltman G. Itraconazole and cyclosporin nephrotoxicity. *Lancet* (1987) ii, 920–1.
14. Koselj M, Bren A, Kandus A, Kovac D. Drug interactions between cyclosporine and rifampicin, erythromycin, and azoles in kidney recipients with opportunistic infections. *Transplant Proc* (1994) 26, 2823–4.
15. Cohen E, Kramer MR, Maoz C, Ben-Dayan D, Garty M. Cyclosporin drug-interaction-induced rhabdomyolysis. A report of two cases in lung transplant recipients. *Transplantation* (2000) 70, 119–22.
16. Vlahakos DV, Manginas A, Childou D, Zamanika C, Alivizatos PA. Itraconazole-induced rhabdomyolysis and acute renal failure in a heart transplant recipient treated with simvastatin and cyclosporine. *Transplantation* (2002) 73, 1962–4.
17. Maxa JL, Melton LB, Ogu CC, Sills MN, Limanni A. Rhabdomyolysis after concomitant use of cyclosporine, simvastatin, gemfibrozil, and itraconazole. *Ann Pharmacother* (2002) 36, 820–2.
18. Timmers GJ, Kessels LW, Wilhelm AJ, Veldkamp AI, Bosch TM, Beijnen JH, Huijgens PC. Effects of cyclosporine A on single-dose pharmacokinetics of intravenous itraconazole in patients with hematologic malignancies. *Ther Drug Monit* (2008) 30, 301–5.

Ciclosporin + Azoles; Ketoconazole

Ketoconazole can cause a large, rapid increase in ciclosporin concentrations.

Clinical evidence

Ketoconazole 200 mg daily caused a large and rapid increase in the ciclosporin blood concentrations of 36 renal transplant patients. On the basis of experience with previous patients, the ciclosporin dose was reduced by 70% when ketoconazole was started, and after a year the dose reduction was 85% (from 420 to 66 mg daily). Minimal nephrotoxicity was seen.[1-3] A study in children with nephrotic syndrome found the addition of ketoconazole allowed a ciclosporin dose reduction of about 37%. They also found that those given ketoconazole (153 patients) had a lower frequency of renal impairment, were more likely to be able to stop taking steroids and had a better chance of staying in remission than those not given ketoconazole (54 patients).[4] Another similar study by this same research group found comparable results.[5]

Other reports[6-20] describe essentially similar increases in ciclosporin concentrations during the concurrent use of ketoconazole. The effects of ketoconazole on ciclosporin were found to be increased (from 80 to 85% or from 77 to 84%) when diltiazem was also given.[21,22]

In a retrospective study an increased incidence of severe liver toxicity was seen in patients also taking ketoconazole when the method of monitoring ciclosporin concentrations was switched from minimum concentrations (C_0) to concentrations 2 hours post dose (C_2). Liver toxicity developed in 26% of patients monitored solely using C_2 concentrations compared with no patients monitored using C_0 and C_2 concentrations.[23]

For mention of a report of seizures occurring when ketoconazole was added to ciclosporin and high-dose methylprednisolone, see 'Ciclosporin + Corticosteroids', p.1224.

Mechanism

Ketoconazole is an inhibitor of hepatic CYP3A4, by which ciclosporin is metabolised, and as a result ciclosporin blood concentrations increase. Ketoconazole also appears to inhibit the metabolism of ciclosporin in the gut wall.[18]

Importance and management

The interaction between ciclosporin and ketoconazole is very well established and clinically important. Ciclosporin blood concentrations increase rapidly and sharply, but they can be controlled by reducing the ciclosporin dose by about 70 to 80%.[1,6,9,19] A ciclosporin dose reduction of 68 to 89% was required over a 13-month period in one study, with no adverse changes in immunosuppressive activity, resulting in a total cost saving of about 65%, partially offset because of the need for more frequent patient follow-up and the cost of the ketoconazole.[1,2] Other studies have also suggested that this interaction can be exploited to make cost savings.[19,24,25] Reviews of the pros and cons of concurrent use have been published.[3,26] Ketoconazole might have a kidney protective effect.[1,2] A study in kidney transplant patients suggested that variability in absorption and in the response to metabolic inhibition by ketoconazole made the ciclosporin blood concentration response difficult to predict and monitor.[27] There are also other confounding factors. For example, a patient who was given ketoconazole to increase ciclosporin concentrations was subsequently given famotidine. The famotidine increased gastric pH, which resulted in a reduction in the ketoconazole absorption, and the ciclosporin concentrations consequently decreased.[28] Also bear in mind the possibility that, in patients taking ketoconazole, monitoring the use of ciclosporin with ciclosporin concentrations taken 2 hours post-dose might not be the best method.[23,29]

1. First MR, Schroeder TJ, Weiskittel P, Myre SA, Alexander JW, Pesce AJ. Concomitant administration of cyclosporin and ketoconazole in renal transplant patients. *Lancet* (1989) ii, 1198–1201.
2. First MR, Schroeder TJ, Alexander JW, Stephens GW, Weiskittel P, Myre SA, Pesce AJ. Cyclosporine dose reduction by ketoconazole administration in renal transplant recipients. *Transplantation* (1991) 51, 365–70.
3. First MR, Schroeder TJ, Michael A, Hariharan S, Weiskittel P, Alexander JW. Cyclosporin-ketoconazole interaction. Long-term follow-up and preliminary results of a randomized trial. *Transplantation* (1993) 55, 1000–4.
4. El-Husseini A, El-Basuony F, Donia A, Mahmoud I, Hassan N, Sayed-Ahmad N, Sobh M. Concomitant administration of cyclosporine and ketoconazole in idiopathic nephrotic syndrome. *Nephrol Dial Transplant* (2004) 19, 2266–71.
5. El-Husseini A, El-Basuony F, Mahmoud I, Donia A, Sheashaa H, Sabry A, Hassan N, Sayed-Ahmad N, Sobh M. Impact of the cyclosporine-ketoconazole interaction in children with steroid-dependent idiopathic nephrotic syndrome. *Eur J Clin Pharmacol* (2006) 62, 3–8.
6. Koselj M, Bren A, Kandus A, Kovac D. Drug interactions between cyclosporine and rifampicin, erythromycin, and azoles in kidney recipients with opportunistic infections. *Transplant Proc* (1994) 26, 2823–4.
7. Ferguson RM, Sutherland DER, Simmons RL, Najarian JS. Ketoconazole, cyclosporin metabolism and renal transplantation. *Lancet* (1982) ii, 882–3.
8. Morgenstern GR, Powles R, Robinson B, McElwain TJ. Cyclosporin interaction with ketoconazole and melphalan. *Lancet* (1982) ii, 1342.
9. Dieperink H, Møller J. Ketoconazole and cyclosporin. *Lancet* (1982) ii, 1217.
10. Gluckman E, Devergie A, Lokiec F, Poirier O, Baumelou A. Nephrotoxicity of cyclosporin in bone-marrow transplantation. *Lancet* (1981) ii, 144–5.
11. Shepard JH, Canafax DM, Simmons RL, Najarian JS. Cyclosporine-ketoconazole: a potentially dangerous drug-drug interaction. *Clin Pharm* (1986) 5, 468.
12. Schroeder TJ, Melvin DB, Clardy CW, Wadhwa NK, Myre SA, Reising JM, Wolf RK, Collins JA, Pesce AJ, First MR. Use of cyclosporine and ketoconazole without nephrotoxicity in two heart transplant recipients. *J Heart Transplant* (1987) 6, 84–9.
13. Girardet RE, Melo JC, Fox MS, Whalen C, Lusk R, Masri ZH, Lansing AM. Concomitant administration of cyclosporine and ketoconazole for three and a half years in one heart transplant recipient. *Transplantation* (1989) 48, 887–90.
14. Schroeder TJ, Weiskittel P, Pesce AJ, Myre SA, Alexander JW, First MR. Cyclosporine pharmacokinetics with concomitant ketoconazole therapy. *Clin Chem* (1989) 35, 1176–7.
15. Charles BG, Ravenscroft PJ, Rigby RJ. The ketoconazole-cyclosporin interaction in an elderly renal transplant patient. *Aust N Z J Med* (1989) 19, 292–3.

16. Veraldi S, Menni S. Severe gingival hyperplasia following cyclosporin and ketoconazole therapy. *Int J Dermatol* (1988) 27, 730.
17. Kiss D, Thiel G. Glucose-intolerance and prolonged renal-transplant insufficiency due to ketoconazole-cyclosporin A interaction. *Clin Nephrol* (1990) 33, 207–8.
18. Gomez DY, Wacher VJ, Tomlanovich SJ, Hebert MF, Benet LZ. The effects of ketoconazole on the intestinal metabolism and bioavailability of cyclosporine. *Clin Pharmacol Ther* (1995) 58, 15–9.
19. Butman SM, Wild JC, Nolan PE, Fagan TC, Finley PR, Hicks MJ, Mackie MJ, Copeland JG. Prospective study of the safety and financial benefit of ketoconazole as adjunctive therapy to cyclosporine after heart transplantation. *J Heart Lung Transplant* (1991) 10, 351–8.
20. Foradori A, Mezzano S, Videla C, Pefaur J, Elberg A. Modification of the pharmacokinetics of cyclosporine A and metabolites by the concomitant use of Neoral and diltiazem or ketoconazol in stable adult kidney transplants. *Transplant Proc* (1998) 30, 1685–7.
21. McLachlan AJ, Tett SE. Effect of metabolic inhibitors on cyclosporine pharmacokinetics using a population approach. *Ther Drug Monit* (1998) 20, 390–5.
22. Hariharan S, Schroeder T, First MR. The effect of diltiazem on cyclosporin A (CYA) bioavailability in patients treated with CYA and ketoconazole. *J Am Soc Nephrol* (1992) 3, 861.
23. Videla C, Vega J, Borja H. Hepatotoxicity associated with cyclosporine monitoring using C_2 recommendations in adults renal recipients receiving ketoconazole. *Transplant Proc* (2005) 37, 1574–6.
24. Kriett JM, Jahansouz F, Smith CM, Hayden AM, Fox KJ, Kapelanski DP, Jamieson SW. The cyclosporine-ketoconazole interaction: safety and economic impact in lung transplantation. *J Heart Lung Transplant* (1994) 13, S43.
25. Keogh A, Spratt P, McCosker C, Macdonald P, Mundy J, Kaan A. Ketoconazole to reduce the need for cyclosporine after cardiac transplantation. *N Engl J Med* (1995) 333, 628–33.
26. Albengres E, Tillement JP. Cyclosporin and ketoconazole, drug interaction or therapeutic association? *Int J Clin Pharmacol Ther Toxicol* (1992) 30, 555–70.
27. Sorenson AL, Lovdahl M, Hewitt JM, Granger DK, Almond PS, Russlie HQ, Barber D, Matas AJ, Canafax DM. Effects of ketoconazole on cyclosporine metabolism in renal allograft recipients. *Transplant Proc* (1994) 26, 2822.
28. Karlix JL, Cheng MA, Brunson ME, Ramos EL, Howard RJ, Peterson JC, Patton PR, Pfaff WW. Decreased cyclosporine concentrations with the addition of an H_2-receptor antagonist in a patient on ketoconazole. *Transplantation* (1993) 56, 1554–5.
29. Ray JE, Keogh AM, McLachlan AJ. Decision support tool to individualize cyclosporine dose in stable, long-term heart transplant recipients receiving metabolic inhibitors: overcoming limitations of cyclosporine C_2 monitoring. *J Heart Lung Transplant* (2006) 25, 1223–9.

Ciclosporin + Azoles; Miconazole

A case report suggests that intravenous miconazole increases ciclosporin concentrations and, in theory, miconazole oral gel might also interact.

Clinical evidence

A single case report describes an increase of about 65% in ciclosporin serum concentrations within 3 days of intravenous miconazole 1 g every 8 hours being started. Ciclosporin concentrations increased again during subsequent treatment with miconazole.[1]

Mechanism

Miconazole is an inhibitor of CYP3A4, by which ciclosporin is metabolised, and as a result ciclosporin blood concentrations increase.

Importance and management

Evidence for an interaction between ciclosporin and miconazole is limited to one case report of *intravenous* miconazole administration, but it supports the outcome that would be predicted based on the enzyme-inhibiting capability of miconazole. The interaction is potentially serious and of clinical importance and it would seem prudent to closely monitor ciclosporin concentrations if intravenous miconazole is also given.

There is no evidence of an interaction with other forms of miconazole. However, a large proportion of miconazole *oral* gel (both prescription and non-prescription doses) might be swallowed and therefore adequate systemic absorption can occur for interactions with other medications. The UK manufacturers of miconazole oral gel recommend close monitoring and possible dose reduction of ciclosporin if given concurrently.[2] An interaction with *intravaginal* miconazole would not normally be expected because its systemic absorption is usually very low (less than 2%) in healthy women of child-bearing age.[3] Similarly, an interaction with topical miconazole creams would also not be expected.

1. Horton CM, Freeman CD, Nolan PE, Copeland JG. Cyclosporine interactions with miconazole and other azole-antimycotics: a case report and review of the literature. *J Heart Lung Transplant* (1992) 11, 1127–32.
2. Daktarin Oral Gel (Miconazole). Janssen-Cilag Ltd. UK Summary of product characteristics, December 2014.
3. Daneshmend TK. Systemic absorption of miconazole from the vagina. *J Antimicrob Chemother* (1986) 18, 507–11.

Ciclosporin + Azoles; Posaconazole

Posaconazole can increase ciclosporin concentrations. Concurrent use has been reported to result in cases of ciclosporin toxicity.

Clinical evidence

Posaconazole 200 mg daily for 10 days was given to 4 heart transplant patients receiving stable doses of ciclosporin. Three of the 4 patients required dose reductions of between 14 and 29% to maintain ciclosporin concentrations.[1] In a 30-day study, 41 bone marrow transplant patients with steady-state ciclosporin concentrations, were given posaconazole oral solution 200 mg three times daily post-transplantation. In order to maintain ciclosporin concentrations within the desired therapeutic range (125 to 300 nanograms/mL), the ciclosporin dose had to be almost halved, from 3.09 to 1.58 mg/kg daily.[2] In another report, increased ciclosporin concentrations occurred in just one of 12 transplant patients given posaconazole 800 mg daily. In this patient, the ciclosporin dose was decreased by 45% on starting posaconazole, and the ciclosporin concentration was normal (193 nanograms/mL) 17 days later at discharge. However, 7 days later the patient had altered mental status and very high ciclosporin concentrations. She had thrombotic thrombocytopenic purpura and pancytopenia and eventually died. The authors stated that it was not clear if this case represents a patient medication error, or an interaction.[3] The UK manufacturer also reports cases of ciclosporin toxicity that resulted in serious adverse effects, including nephrotoxicity and one fatal case of leukoencephalopathy, which occurred in posaconazole efficacy studies.[4]

Mechanism

Posaconazole is a moderate inhibitor of CYP3A4, by which ciclosporin is metabolised, and as a result ciclosporin blood concentrations increase.

Importance and management

Evidence for an interaction between ciclosporin and posaconazole is limited, with the majority of the data suggesting that any increase in ciclosporin concentrations is often modest and slow to develop. However, the reports of toxicity add a note of caution. The UK and US manufacturers of posaconazole recommend that the dose of ciclosporin should be reduced by about 25% when posaconazole is started, with careful monitoring of ciclosporin concentrations and further dose adjustment as needed.[4,5] However, the authors of one review state that pre-emptive ciclosporin dose reductions when starting azoles are not standard practice among transplant clinicians, because of the concern of an increased risk of rejection[6] (due to subtherapeutic ciclosporin concentrations). A study specifically addressing the requirement for pre-emptive dose reductions also suggested that it was unnecessary to pre-emptively reduce the dose of ciclosporin, providing adequate therapeutic drug monitoring was undertaken. In this study, dose adjustments were most frequently required between 7 and 14 days after starting posaconazole.[2] If both drugs are given, monitor ciclosporin concentrations (possibly as frequently as three times weekly), making dose adjustments if necessary. Note also, that the UK manufacturer of posaconazole predicts that its concentrations will be increased by ciclosporin as a result of P-glycoprotein inhibition.[4] Although clinical evidence for this appears to be lacking, it would seem prudent to be aware of the possibility of increased posaconazole adverse effects on concurrent use.

1. Sansone-Parsons A, Krishna G, Martinho M, Kantesaria B, Gelone S, Mant TG. Effect of oral posaconazole on the pharmacokinetics of cyclosporine and tacrolimus. *Pharmacotherapy* (2007) 27, 825–34.
2. Sánchez-Ortega I, Vázquez L, Montes C, Patiño B, Arnan M, Bermúdez A, Yáñez L, Caballero T, Duarte RF. Effect of posaconazole on cyclosporine blood levels and dose adjustment in allogeneic blood and marrow transplant recipients. *Antimicrob Agents Chemother* (2012) 56, 6422–4.
3. Alexander BD, Perfect JR, Daly JS, Restrepo A, Tobón AM, Patino H, Hardalo CJ, Graybill JR. Posaconazole as salvage therapy in patients with invasive fungal infections after solid organ transplant. *Transplantation* (2008) 86, 791–6.
4. Noxafil (Posaconazole). Merck Sharp & Dohme Ltd. UK Summary of product characteristics, September 2014.
5. Noxafil (Posaconazole). Merck & Co., Inc. US Prescribing information, June 2014.
6. Saad AH, DePestel DD, Carver PL. Factors influencing the magnitude and clinical significance of drug interactions between azole antifungals and select immunosuppressants. *Pharmacotherapy* (2006) 26, 1730–44.

Ciclosporin + Azoles; Voriconazole

Voriconazole can increase ciclosporin concentrations.

Clinical evidence

In a placebo-controlled, crossover study, 14 kidney transplant patients receiving stable doses of ciclosporin were given voriconazole 200 mg every 12 hours for 15 doses. Of the 14 patients, 7 stopped ciclosporin during the voriconazole phase due to adverse effects: 4 due to increased ciclosporin concentrations (mean 2.48-fold), one due to increased liver function [tests], one due to asthenia, dyspnoea, and oedema, and one due to an underlying condition unrelated to the voriconazole. In the remaining 7 patients voriconazole increased the AUC of ciclosporin by 70%.[1] In another study in 10 stem cell transplant recipients receiving stable doses of ciclosporin, oral voriconazole (300 mg twice daily for two doses followed by 200 mg twice daily, 7 patients) or intravenous voriconazole (6 mg/kg twice daily for 2 doses followed by 4 mg/kg twice daily, 3 patients) resulted in a median increase in the ciclosporin concentration-to-dose ratio of 82%. The route of voriconazole administration had no effect on the result, but there was wide interindividual variability.[2] A case report describes an 18-year-old stem cell transplant patient admitted with dizziness, headaches, and blurred vision lasting 2 days. Two hours after admission, she deteriorated and developed convulsions of her limbs and epileptiform seizures which were controlled with diazepam and phenobarbital. She had been stable on ciclosporin 100 mg twice daily for several months (as part of triple immunosuppressive therapy with mycophenolate and methylprednisolone), but had started voriconazole (400 mg twice daily for two doses followed by 200 mg twice daily) one week prior to admission. On day 2 of admission her ciclosporin concentration had increased by 64%. On day 4 she was diagnosed with leucoencephalopathy, which was attributed to the increase in ciclosporin blood concentrations which were felt to be the result of an interaction with voriconazole.[3] Another case describes a pre-emptive ciclosporin dose reduction from 150 mg twice daily to 25 mg twice daily in a kidney transplant patient, when voriconazole 200 mg daily was started for aspergillosis. The minimum ciclosporin concentration was maintained between 3.2 and 27.9 nanograms/mL for 3 months of concurrent treatment, during which time the patient's respiratory symptoms improved, her serum creatinine concentration was satisfactorily maintained, and good allograft function was achieved.[4] Ciclosporin concentrations were considerably *reduced* in a bone marrow transplant patient, from a range of 150 to 184 nanograms/mL to 56 to 111 nanograms/mL, when prophylactic voriconazole was *stopped* due to abnormal liver function tests. The concentrations returned to range when the voriconazole was restarted.[5]

Mechanism

Voriconazole is a potent inhibitor of CYP3A4, by which ciclosporin is metabolised, and as a result ciclosporin blood concentrations increase.

Importance and management

Evidence for an interaction between ciclosporin and voriconazole is limited, but the effects seen are consistent with the known interactions of both of these drugs, and are likely to be clinically important. Close monitoring of ciclosporin concentrations on concurrent use, and alertness to the need to adjust ciclosporin doses would seem sensible. Further, the UK and US manufacturers of voriconazole suggest that the dose of ciclosporin should be halved when initiating voriconazole.[6,7]

1. Romero AJ, Le Pogamp P, Nilsson L-G, Wood N. Effect of voriconazole on the pharmacokinetics of cyclosporine in renal transplant patients. *Clin Pharmacol Ther* (2002) 71, 226–34.
2. Mori T, Aisa Y, Kato J, Nakamura Y, Ikeda Y, Okamoto S. Drug interaction between voriconazole and calcineurin inhibitors in allogeneic hematopoietic stem cell transplant recipients. *Bone Marrow Transplant* (2009) 44, 371–4.
3. Caihong Q, Weimin L, Jieming Z. Elevation of blood ciclosporin levels by voriconazole leading to leukoencephalopathy. *J Pharmacol Pharmacother* (2013) 4, 294–7.
4. Park SJ, Song IS, Kang SW, Joo H, Kim TH, Yoon YC, Kim E, Choi YL, Shin JG, Son JH, Kim YH. Pharmacokinetic effect of voriconazole on cyclosporine in the treatment of aspergillosis after renal transplantation. *Clin Nephrol* (2012) 78, 412–7.
5. Groll AH, Kolve H, Ehlert K, Paulussen M, Vormoor J. Pharmacokinetic interaction between voriconazole and ciclosporin following allogeneic bone marrow transplantation. *J Antimicrob Chemother* (2004) 53, 113–4.
6. VFEND (Voriconazole). Pfizer Ltd. UK Summary of product characteristics, October 2014.
7. VFEND (Voriconazole). Pfizer Inc. US Prescribing information, February 2014.

Ciclosporin + Basiliximab

Ciclosporin concentrations and adverse effects might be altered by basiliximab.

Clinical evidence, mechanism, importance and management

A study in 39 paediatric kidney transplant patients taking ciclosporin found that, in 24 patients who were also given basiliximab 10 or 20 mg on days 0 and 4 after transplantation, lower doses of ciclosporin resulted in higher ciclosporin minimum concentrations and some evidence of early ciclosporin toxicity within the first 10 days. At days 28 to 50, ciclosporin concentrations declined and 20% higher doses were required to maintain adequate minimum concentrations in the basiliximab group.[1] Another study, in 54 paediatric liver transplant patients, found that the addition of basiliximab to ciclosporin and corticosteroids did not notably alter the overall ciclosporin dose requirements. However, 9 patients given basiliximab experienced acute rejection at 21 to 28 days after transplantation, and this was associated with low ciclosporin minimum concentrations, requiring an increased ciclosporin dose in 6 of the 9 patients.[2] It was suggested that the effect on ciclosporin was due to an interleukin-2 receptor mediated alteration of the cytochrome P450 enzyme system.[1] This was considered to only play a minor role in the liver transplant patients because of significantly lower target minimum concentrations in these patients.[2] However, a further study found no increase in rejection rates between days 28 to 50 in kidney transplant patients given basiliximab and ciclosporin.[3]

The authors of the first study[1] recommend that the initial dose of ciclosporin should be limited to 400 mg/m^2 in children receiving kidney transplants who are also given basiliximab. Dose reductions were not considered necessary by other authors, but close monitoring was recommended.[2,3]

A retrospective analysis of kidney transplant patients compared the rates of acute rejection within 6 months in patients given ciclosporin, mycophenolate mofetil and prednisone, with or without basiliximab. Overall the rates of acute rejection were 11% and 23% in the basiliximab and no-basiliximab groups, respectively. In 74 patients not given basiliximab, low therapeutic ciclosporin exposure on day 3 was associated with increased acute rejection within the first 6 months post-transplantation (45% with ciclosporin AUC less than 4400 nanogram.h/mL compared with 15% with a ciclosporin AUC of greater than 4400 nanogram.h/mL). In 93 patients given basiliximab, rates of acute rejection were similar (about 10%) in patients with low or therapeutic ciclosporin exposure at day 3. It was suggested that achieving early ciclosporin therapeutic targets might not be required if basiliximab is also used.[4]

1. Strehlau J, Pape L, Offner G, Nashan B, Ehrich JHH. Interleukin-2 receptor antibody-induced alterations of ciclosporin dose requirements in paediatric transplant recipients. *Lancet* (2000) 356, 1327–8.
2. Ganschow R, Grabhorn E, Burdelski M. Basiliximab in paediatric liver-transplant recipients. *Lancet* (2001) 357, 388.
3. Vester U, Kranz B, Treichel U, Hoyer PF. Basiliximab in paediatric liver-transplant recipients. *Lancet* (2001) 357, 388–9.
4. Balbontin FG, Kiberd B, Singh D, Fraser A, Belitsky P, Lawen J. Basiliximab lowers the therapeutic threshold for cyclosporine exposure in the early post kidney transplant period. *J Am Soc Nephrol* (2003) 14, 650A.

Ciclosporin + Benzbromarone

Benzbromarone does not appear to interact with ciclosporin.

Clinical evidence, mechanism, importance and management

Twenty-five kidney transplant patients taking ciclosporin were given benzbromarone 100 mg daily to treat hyperuricaemia. The plasma uric acid concentrations decreased from 579 to 313 micromol/L and the 24-hour urinary uric acid secretion increased from 2082 to 3233 micromol after 4 weeks of treatment. The plasma uric acid concentrations normalised in 21 of the patients who had a creatinine clearance of over 25 mL/minute. No significant adverse effects developed and the ciclosporin serum concentrations remained unchanged. The authors of the report emphasise the advantages of benzbromarone over allopurinol because of its efficacy, lack of significant adverse effects and because, unlike allopurinol, it does not interact with azathioprine, which often accompanies ciclosporin treatment.[1]

1. Zürcher RM, Bock HA, Thiel G. Excellent uricosuric efficacy of benzbromarone in cyclosporin-A-treated renal transplant patients. A prospective study. *Nephrol Dial Transplant* (1994) 9, 548–51.

Ciclosporin + Berberine

Berberine appears to increase the bioavailability and minimum blood concentrations of ciclosporin.

Clinical evidence, mechanism, importance and management

A study in 6 kidney transplant patients looked at the effects of berberine on the pharmacokinetics of ciclosporin. The patients were taking ciclosporin 3 mg/kg twice daily for an average of 12 days before berberine 200 mg three times daily for 12 days was added. The AUC and minimum blood concentrations of ciclosporin were increased by 35% and 88%, respectively. The maximum ciclosporin concentration was decreased but this was not statistically significant.[1] A clinical study by the same authors in 52 kidney transplant patients stable taking ciclosporin and given berberine 200 mg three times daily for 3 months found that the ciclosporin minimum concentrations were increased by about 24% when the berberine-treated group was compared with 52 similar patients taking ciclosporin without berberine. The ciclosporin concentrations in 8 patients decreased after berberine was stopped. Creatinine clearance was not significantly altered, and no serious adverse effects were reported.[1] A similar increase in ciclosporin concentrations was found in a study in Chinese heart transplant patients taking ciclosporin with berberine.[2]

A single-dose study in healthy subjects found conflicting results. Six subjects given a single 6-mg/kg dose of ciclosporin daily found that berberine 300 mg twice daily, taken for 10 days before the dose of ciclosporin, had no significant effects on the pharmacokinetics of ciclosporin. However, a separate study in another 6 subjects given a single 3-mg/kg dose of ciclosporin found that a single 300-mg dose of berberine increased the AUC of ciclosporin by 19%. No adverse events were reported in this study.[3]

Mechanism

The mechanism for the increase in ciclosporin concentrations seen in the clinical studies is unclear, although it has been suggested that it might be due to inhibition of CYP3A by berberine.

Animal studies[4,5] suggest that ciclosporin might also affect the handling of berberine possibly by inhibiting P-glycoprotein, therefore affecting its intestinal absorption and distribution into the bile and liver.

Importance and management

Although the increase in ciclosporin concentrations is not sufficiently severe to suggest that the concurrent use of berberine should be avoided, it could make ciclosporin concentrations less stable. If concurrent use is undertaken, ciclosporin concentrations should be well monitored, and the dose of ciclosporin adjusted accordingly, or the berberine stopped.

1. Wu X, Li Q, Xin H, Yu A, Zhong M. Effects of berberine on the blood concentration of cyclosporin A in renal transplanted recipients: clinical and pharmacokinetic study. *Eur J Clin Pharmacol* (2005) 61, 567–72.
2. Huang XS, Yang GF, Pan YC. Effect of berberin hydrochloride on blood concentration of cyclosporine A in cardiac transplanted recipients. *Zhongguo Zhong Xi Yi Jie He Za Zhi* (2008) 28, 702–4.
3. Xin HW, Wu XC, Li Q, Yu AR, Zhong MY, Liu YY. The effects of berberine on the pharmacokinetics of cyclosporin A in healthy volunteers. *Methods Find Exp Clin Pharmacol* (2006) 28, 25–9.
4. Tsai P-L, Tsai T-H. Hepatobiliary excretion of berberine. *Drug Metab Dispos* (2004) 32, 405–12.
5. Pan G-Y, Wang G-J, Liu X-D, Fawcett JP, Xie Y-Y. The involvement of P-glycoprotein in berberine absorption. *Pharmacol Toxicol* (2002) 91, 193–7.

Ciclosporin + Beta blockers

Carvedilol might modestly increase ciclosporin concentrations in some patients. In general, atenolol, and metoprolol do not appear to interact with ciclosporin.

Clinical evidence

A study in 21 kidney transplant patients found that when **atenolol** was gradually replaced by **carvedilol** in a stepwise manner, starting with **carvedilol** 6.25 mg daily, gradually increasing to 50 mg daily, the ciclosporin dose had to be gradually reduced. At 90 days the ciclosporin dose had been reduced by 20% (from 3.7 to 3 mg/kg daily) to maintain concentrations within the therapeutic range but considerable inter-individual variations were seen.[1] A retrospective study in 12 heart transplant patients found that **carvedilol** increased the ciclosporin concentration in 10 patients from a mean of 257 to 380 nanograms/mL. This required a mean dose reduction of 31 mg daily (10%). In the same study, 20 patients taking **metoprolol** were also assessed. Twelve patients had a decrease, and 8 patients an increase, in their ciclosporin concentration, although the overall mean change was only 1 nanogram/mL. However, in one case, metoprolol appears to have increased the ciclosporin concentration from about 300 to

900 nanograms/mL, but insufficient detail is given to be able to assess this finding. None of these changes with **metoprolol** required any notable ciclosporin dose alterations (mean dose alteration 0.03%).[2] A study in 30 kidney transplant patients found no change in the ciclosporin concentrations of those taking **atenolol** 25 to 100 mg daily.[3]

Mechanism

Carvedilol appears to increase ciclosporin concentrations by inhibiting P-glycoprotein.[4]

Importance and management

The modest interaction of carvedilol with ciclosporin would appear to be established. The available data suggest that ciclosporin dose reductions of 10 to 20% might be necessary to maintain ciclosporin concentrations at the target level. It would therefore be prudent to monitor ciclosporin concentrations being aware that any change appears to be gradual and that it could take some months for the full extent of the effect to become clear.

In general it appears that no ciclosporin dose adjustment would be expected to be needed in patients taking metoprolol or atenolol.

1. Kaijser M, Johnsson C, Zezina L, Backman U, Dimeny E, Fellstrom B. Elevation of cyclosporin A blood levels during carvedilol treatment in renal transplant patients. *Clin Transplant* (1997) 11, 577–81.
2. Bader FM, Hagan ME, Crompton JA, Gilbert EM. The effect of β-blocker use on cyclosporine level in cardiac transplant recipients. *J Heart Lung Transplant* (2005) 24, 2144–7.
3. Hausberg M, Barenbrock M, Hohage H, Müller S, Heidenreich S, Rahn K-H. ACE inhibitor versus β-blocker for the treatment of hypertension in renal allograft recipients. *Hypertension* (1999) 33, 862–8.
4. Amioka K, Kuzuya T, Kushihara H, Ejiri M, Nitta A, Nabeshima T. Carvedilol increases ciclosporin bioavailability by inhibiting P-glycoprotein-mediated transport. *J Pharm Pharmacol* (2007) 59, 1383–7.

Ciclosporin + Bifendate

Two case reports suggest that bifendate can cause a gradual decrease in the serum concentrations of ciclosporin, and a modest decrease in ciclosporin concentrations was seen in one study in healthy subjects.

Clinical evidence

Two kidney transplant patients were successfully treated with ciclosporin and prednisolone for 30 months and 36 months. When they were given bifendate 75 mg daily for the treatment of chronic hepatitis, both of them had a gradual decrease in their serum ciclosporin minimum concentrations. The ciclosporin concentration of the first patient decreased from 97.7 to 78 nanograms/mL at 4 weeks, and decreased further, to 49 nanograms/mL, at 6 weeks. The ciclosporin concentration of the other patient also decreased, from 127.5 to 70.5 nanograms/mL at 8 weeks and to 45 nanograms/mL at 16 weeks. The ciclosporin doses remained unchanged throughout, and despite the low serum concentrations that occurred, no graft rejection was seen. When the bifendate was stopped, ciclosporin concentrations gradually increased again, at about the same rate as their decline, to roughly their former concentrations.[1] In a subsequent placebo-controlled study in 18 healthy subjects given a single oral dose of ciclosporin, bifendate 15 mg three times daily for 14 days decreased the AUC of ciclosporin by 10 to 38% and increased its oral clearance by 10 to 32%.[2]

Mechanism

The reasons for this interaction are not understood. It is possible that bifendate is an inducer of CYP3A4,[2] which is involved in ciclosporin metabolism.

Importance and management

The available information suggests that a modest interaction might occur between bifendate and ciclosporin, and therefore it would seem prudent to monitor the outcome, being alert for the need to increase the ciclosporin dose if bifendate is used. Bifendate is derived from *Schisandra* therefore, until more is known, it might be wise to extend this caution to all herbal preparations containing *Schisandra*. However, in contrast to the above data, an extract from *Schisandra sphenanthera increased* the concentrations of tacrolimus, which is also a substrate of CYP3A4, see 'Tacrolimus + Schisandra', p.1305. Therefore the exact outcome of concurrent use is far from clear.

1. Kim YS, Kim DH, Kim DO, Lee BK, Kim KW, Park JN, Lee JC, Choi YS, Rim H. The effect of diphenyl-dimethyl-dicarboxylate on cyclosporine-A blood level in kidney transplants with chronic hepatitis. *Korean J Intern Med* (1997) 12, 67–9.
2. Zeng Y, He YJ, He FY, Fan L, Zhou HH. Effect of bifendate on the pharmacokinetics of cyclosporine in relation to the CYP3A4*18B genotype in healthy subjects. *Acta Pharmacol Sin* (2009) 30, 478–84.

Ciclosporin + Bile acids or Ursodeoxycholic acid (Ursodiol)

Ursodeoxycholic acid unpredictably increases both the absorption and concentrations of ciclosporin in some, but not all, patients. Bile acids (cholic and dehydrocholic acids) appear not to interact with ciclosporin.

Clinical evidence

(a) Bile acids

In a study, 11 healthy subjects were given a single oral dose of ciclosporin on three occasions: while fasting, with breakfast, and with breakfast plus bile acid tablets (**cholic acid** 400 mg, **dehydrocholic acid** 100 mg). The mean ciclosporin AUCs were 7283 nanograms/mL, 7453 nanograms/mL, and 9078 nanograms/mL, respectively, indicating that the bile acids increased the absorption of ciclosporin by 22%.[1] However, a related study in 19 transplant patients found that their 12-hour ciclosporin minimum serum concentrations were unchanged by the concurrent use of this dose of bile acids over an 8-day period.[1]

(b) Ursodeoxycholic acid (Ursodiol)

When a heart transplant patient, who had previously had his entire ileum removed and about one metre of the residual jejunum anastomosed to the transverse colon, started taking ursodeoxycholic acid 1 to 2 g daily, it was possible to reduce his ciclosporin dose from 1.6 to 1.2 g daily. However, when the ursodeoxycholic acid was stopped, his ciclosporin serum concentrations became subtherapeutic and severe acute rejection developed. The ciclosporin concentrations increased when ursodeoxycholic acid was restarted, and the ciclosporin AUC was increased by more than 3-fold.[2] Similarly, the serum ciclosporin minimum concentrations of a patient with chronic active hepatitis C increased from 150 to 500 nanograms/mL when he was given ursodeoxycholic acid, and it was necessary to halve his daily ciclosporin dose to keep the ciclosporin concentrations at 150 nanograms/mL.[3]

In contrast, various other studies[4-6] and one case report[7] have shown little or no effect of ursodeoxycholic acid on ciclosporin concentrations. In one of these in liver transplant patients, there was no difference in ciclosporin (*Sandimmun*) dose requirements between 17 patients given ursodeoxycholic acid 15 mg/kg daily for 3 months and 16 patients given placebo.[6] Similarly, in 7 liver transplant patients there were no statistically significant changes in ciclosporin concentrations when a single 600-mg dose of ursodeoxycholic acid was given at the same time as the ciclosporin (*Sandimmun*).[4] Yet another study in 12 liver transplant patients, 6 of whom were cholestatic, found that ciclosporin (*Sandimmun*) was absorbed more rapidly after a single dose of ursodeoxycholic acid in 8 patients, but, although 7 patients had some increase in their AUC, the 24-hour AUC was not significantly changed. There was no consistent improvement in ciclosporin pharmacokinetics in the cholestatic patients.[5]

Furthermore, variable effects were seen in another study using the microemulsion formulation of ciclosporin (*Neoral*) in liver transplant recipients. Ursodeoxycholic acid appeared to *reduce* the absorption rate and bioavailability of ciclosporin in 9 patients without cholestasis, but increased the absorption rate and bioavailability in 3 cholestatic patients.[8]

Mechanism

When an interaction occurs it is thought to do so because the ursodeoxycholic acid improves micellation of the oil-containing oral ciclosporin formulation so that its absorption is increased.[2]

Importance and management

Information is limited but bile acids do not appear to interact with ciclosporin. However, the effects of the interaction with ursodeoxycholic acid appears to be variable and unpredictable. It would therefore be prudent to monitor the effects of starting or stopping ursodeoxycholic acid in any patient taking ciclosporin, being alert for the need to adjust the ciclosporin dose.

1. Lindholm A, Henricsson S, Dahlqvist R. The effect of food and bile acid administration on the relative bioavailability of cyclosporin. *Br J Clin Pharmacol* (1990) 29, 541–8.
2. Gutzler F, Zimmermann R, Ring GH, Sauer P, Stiehl A. Ursodeoxycholic acid enhances the absorption of cyclosporine in a heart transplant patient with short bowel syndrome. *Transplant Proc* (1992) 24, 2620–1.
3. Sharobeem R, Bacq Y, Furet Y, Grezard O, Nivet H, Breteau M, Bagros P, Lebranchu Y. Cyclosporine A and ursodeoxycholic acid interaction. *Clin Transplant* (1993) 7, 223–6.
4. Maboundou CW, Paintaud G, Vanlemmens C, Magnette J, Bresson-Hadni S, Mantion G, Miguet JP, Bechtel PR. A single dose of ursodiol does not affect cyclosporine absorption in liver transplant patients. *Eur J Clin Pharmacol* (1996) 50, 335–7.
5. Al-Quaiz MN, O'Grady JG, Tredger JM, Williams R. Variable effect of ursodeoxycholic acid on cyclosporin absorption after orthotopic liver transplantation. *Transpl Int* (1994) 7, 190–4.
6. Söderdahl G, Nowak G, Duraj F, Wang FH, Einarsson C, Ericzon BG. Ursodeoxycholic acid increased bile flow and affects bile composition in the early postoperative phase following liver transplantation. *Transpl Int* (1998)11 (Suppl 1), S231–S238.
7. Kino KJ, Wittkowsky AK. Influence of bile acid replacement on cyclosporine absorption in a patient with jejunoileal bypass. *Pharmacotherapy* (1995) 15, 350–2.
8. Caroli-Bosc FX, Iliadis A, Salmon L, Macheras P, Montet AM, Bourgeon A, Garraffo R, Delmont JP, Montet JC. Ursodeoxycholic acid modulates cyclosporin A oral absorption in liver transplant recipients. *Fundam Clin Pharmacol* (2000) 14, 601–9.

Ciclosporin + Bupropion

An isolated case describes a large decrease in ciclosporin concentrations when a 10-year-old boy was given bupropion.

Clinical evidence, mechanism, importance and management

A 10-year-old boy, who had received a heart transplant 6 years previously, started taking bupropion 75 mg twice daily in addition to his usual transplant medication, which included ciclosporin. After taking bupropion for 22 days, his ciclosporin concentration was found to be only 39 nanograms/mL. The last concentration measured before bupropion treatment had been 197 nanograms/mL. Despite an increase in his ciclosporin dose from 420 to 500 mg daily, the ciclosporin concentration decreased further, to 27 nanograms/mL. The ciclosporin dose was then increased to 550 mg daily and bupropion was stopped.[1]

The reason for this probable interaction is unclear, although an interaction via CYP3A4 is a possibility. This appears to be the only reported case of an interaction between ciclosporin and bupropion, and its general importance is unknown.

1. Lewis BR, Aoun SL, Bernstein GA, Crow SJ. Pharmacokinetic interactions between cyclosporin and bupropion or methylphenidate. *J Child Adolesc Psychopharmacol* (2001) 11, 193–8.

Ciclosporin + Calcium-channel blockers

Diltiazem, nicardipine and verapamil greatly increase ciclosporin concentrations, but also appear to possess kidney protective effects. Nifedipine normally appears not to interact, but increases and decreases in ciclosporin concentrations have been seen in a few patients. Amlodipine has modestly increased ciclosporin concentrations in some studies, but not in others, and it might also have kidney protective properties. A single case describes elevated ciclosporin concentrations caused by nisoldipine. Felodipine, isradipine, lacidipine, and nitrendipine normally appear not to increase ciclosporin concentrations. Ciclosporin has been seen to greatly increase lercanidipine concentrations, and increase felodipine concentrations. The concurrent use of calcium-channel blockers and ciclosporin increases the risk of gingival overgrowth.

Clinical evidence

(a) Ciclosporin concentrations and nephrotoxicity

1. Amlodipine. Ten hypertensive patients with kidney transplants taking ciclosporin (3 of them also taking azathioprine) were given amlodipine 5 to 10 mg daily for 4 weeks. The hypertension was well controlled, the drugs were well tolerated, and the pharmacokinetics of ciclosporin were unaltered by amlodipine.[1] However, another study in 11 hypertensive kidney transplant patients found that amlodipine, given for 7 weeks, increased the ciclosporin concentrations by 40%, without affecting creatinine concentrations.[2] Similarly, in a study in 75 kidney transplant patients taking ciclosporin (with mycophenolate mofetil and prednisolone), amlodipine 5 mg daily for 24 weeks increased the ciclosporin plasma concentration 2 hours post dose by about 19%, when compared with a group given valsartan 80 mg daily (where there was no difference).[3] A review identified two other studies that have found increases in ciclosporin concentrations of 23% and 43% with amlodipine, whereas four studies have found no change.[4] Amlodipine is reported to reduce ciclosporin-associated nephrotoxicity in a study in patients with psoriasis,[5] and in a review of kidney transplant recipients.[4]

2. Diltiazem. A pharmacokinetic study in 9 patients taking ciclosporin found that the addition of diltiazem 180 mg daily increased the minimum blood concentration, maximum blood concentration, and half-life of ciclosporin by 112%, 37%, and 43%, respectively.[6] Sixty-five kidney transplant patients taking ciclosporin and diltiazem were found to need less ciclosporin when compared with 63 control patients not given diltiazem (7.3 mg/kg daily compared with 9 mg/kg daily). There were considerable individual differences in dose requirements.[7] Other studies clearly confirm that diltiazem can increase ciclosporin blood concentrations.[8-34] In some cases, the ciclosporin blood concentrations were not only controlled by reducing the ciclosporin dose by 10 to 60%, but it appeared that diltiazem had a kidney protective role (reduced nephrotoxicity, fewer rejection episodes and haemodialysis sessions).[12,23,34-39] Another study found that a reduction in ciclosporin dose of about 21% was required for both men and women during the long-term use of diltiazem 90 mg twice daily, despite reports of higher activity of CYP3A4 in women than in men.[40]

3. Felodipine. Thirteen kidney transplant patients had no changes in their serum ciclosporin concentrations when they took felodipine 2.5 to 10 mg daily; serum creatinine concentrations were also unchanged. Mean blood pressures fell from 161/100 mmHg to 152/90 mmHg.[41] Another study found no changes in ciclosporin concentrations in patients also given felodipine.[42] A single 10-mg dose of felodipine was found to have beneficial effects on blood pressure, renal haemodynamics, and renal tubular sodium and water handling in kidney transplant patients taking ciclosporin. The effects of long-term use were not studied.[43] A single-dose study in 12 healthy subjects found that the maximum serum concentrations of ciclosporin 5 mg/kg were increased by 16% by felodipine 10 mg, while the AUC and maximum plasma concentration of felodipine were increased by 58% and 151%, respectively, but blood pressures were unchanged.[44] The same group of researchers also briefly described acute and short-term studies in groups of kidney transplant patients and dermatological patients, which found that felodipine 5 to 10 mg reduced blood pressure and opposed ciclosporin nephrotoxicity.[45] A study in heart transplant patients taking ciclosporin found that felodipine attenuated the hypertrophic effects of ciclosporin on transplanted hearts.[46]

4. Isradipine. Twelve kidney transplant patients had no changes in their ciclosporin concentrations over 4 weeks while taking up to 2.5 mg of isradipine twice daily.[47] Similar findings are noted in another study.[42] Three other studies in 31 kidney transplant patients confirmed that ciclosporin blood concentrations are unchanged by isradipine and blood pressures are reduced.[48-50]

5. Lacidipine. Ten kidney transplant patients taking ciclosporin, prednisone and azathioprine started taking lacidipine 4 mg daily. A very small increase in the minimum blood concentrations (6%) and AUC (14%) of the ciclosporin occurred. The blood pressures fell from 142/93 mmHg to 125/79 mmHg, and the 14-hour urinary output increased from 1401 mL to 2050 mL.[51]

6. Lercanidipine. The UK manufacturer of lercanidipine notes that, in healthy subjects given lercanidipine and ciclosporin simultaneously, the plasma concentrations of lercanidipine were increased 3-fold by ciclosporin, and the ciclosporin AUC was increased by 21% by lercanidipine. When the ciclosporin was given 3 hours after the lercanidipine, the concentrations of lercanidipine did not change, and the AUC of ciclosporin increased by 27%.[52]

7. Nicardipine. In a study in 9 patients, nicardipine 20 mg three times daily increased the ciclosporin blood concentrations by 110% (from 226 to 430 nanograms/mL, range 24 to 341%). Their serum creatinine concentrations increased from 136 micromol/L to 147 micromol/L.[53] Other studies have found increases in serum ciclosporin concentrations, in some cases as much as 2- to 3-fold, when nicardipine was given.[54-60]

8. Nifedipine. Five of 9 patients who had an increase in ciclosporin concentrations with nicardipine (see *Nicardipine*, above) had no interaction when they were given nifedipine.[53] No changes in ciclosporin concentrations were seen in other studies,[38,61-65] but increased[18,21] and reduced concentrations[66] have been reported in others. Two studies found that nifedipine appeared to protect patients against ciclosporin-induced nephrotoxicity.[67,68] However, there is some evidence that the adverse effects of nifedipine such as flushing and rash might be increased.[69] For a discussion of gingival overgrowth, see under *Gingival overgrowth*, below.

9. Nisoldipine. A 46-year-old man taking azathioprine, prednisolone, and ciclosporin after a kidney transplant 18 months previously was given nisoldipine 5 mg twice daily. During the following month his ciclosporin concentrations increased from a range of 100 to 150 micrograms/L up to 200 micrograms/L and an increase in serum creatinine concentrations occurred. His ciclosporin dose was gradually reduced from 325 to 250 mg daily, and his ciclosporin and creatinine concentrations returned to the acceptable range.[70]

10. Nitrendipine. Nitrendipine 20 mg daily for 3 weeks had no effect on the ciclosporin blood concentrations of 16 kidney transplant patients.[71]

11. Verapamil. Twenty-two kidney transplant patients given ciclosporin and verapamil had ciclosporin blood concentrations that were 50 to 70% higher than in 18 other patients not given verapamil, despite similar ciclosporin doses in both groups. Serum creatinine concentrations were lower in those taking verapamil. Moreover, only 3 of the 22 patients had rejection episodes within 4 weeks compared with 10 out of 18 patients not given verapamil.[72]

Other studies have found that verapamil 120 to 320 mg daily can increase, double or even triple ciclosporin blood concentrations in individual patients with kidney or heart transplants.[25,42,64,66,73-77]

(b) Gingival overgrowth

Both ciclosporin and calcium-channel blockers are well-known to be associated with gingival overgrowth in transplant recipients, and there is evidence that concurrent use exacerbates this effect. In a randomised, controlled study, **nifedipine** increased the frequency and severity of gingival overgrowth seen with ciclosporin. After 3 months of treatment, 0 of 15 patients taking ciclosporin (17 mg/kg daily gradually reduced to 7 mg/kg daily) had moderate to severe overgrowth (grade 3 or 4) compared with 9 of 17 patients receiving the same ciclosporin regimen with **nifedipine**.[78] Many other cohort studies (two are cited as examples[79,80]) but by no means all (one is cited as an example[81]) have reported similar findings for **nifedipine**.

There are fewer data on other individual calcium-channel blockers. In one cohort study in patients taking ciclosporin, there was a higher incidence of gingival overgrowth in those receiving **amlodipine** than in those receiving **nifedipine** (72% versus 53%).[82] Conversely, in another cohort study, the incidence of gingival overgrowth was higher with **nifedipine** (86%) than **amlodipine** (47%) or **verapamil** (35%).[83] In one study of **verapamil**, patients taking the combination had a slightly higher incidence and severity of gingival overgrowth than ciclosporin alone, but this was not statistically significant.[84] In another study, **diltiazem** did not increase gingival overgrowth, but neither did **nifedipine**.[81]

Various other cohort studies have found that calcium-channel blockers as a class (individual drugs not specified) are associated with an increased risk of gingival overgrowth when used with ciclosporin. One is cited as an example.[85]

Mechanism

The increased ciclosporin concentrations are largely due to inhibition of ciclosporin metabolism by CYP3A4 in the liver. Diltiazem and verapamil are moderate CYP3A4 inhibitors, however other calcium-channel blockers do not generally cause clinically relevant inhibition of CYP3A4 (with the possible exception of nicardipine), see 'Calcium-channel blockers', p.1029. One study suggests that CYP3A5 metaboliser status might have affected the interaction between amlodipine and ciclosporin.[3] Diltiazem also appears to reduce ischaemia-induced renal tubular necrosis.[86] Other calcium-channel blockers also seem to have a kidney-protective effect. The increased felodipine and lercanidipine concentrations are possibly due to competitive inhibition by ciclosporin of intestinal and liver metabolism (by CYP3A4), or inhibition of P-glycoprotein. Whether ciclosporin affects other calcium-channel blockers similarly does not appear to have been studied.

Both ciclosporin and calcium-channel blockers can cause gingival overgrowth, and this effect is probably additive.

Importance and management

The pharmacokinetic interactions of ciclosporin with diltiazem, nicardipine, and verapamil are established and relatively well documented. Concurrent use need not be avoided, but ciclosporin concentrations should be monitored closely and dose reductions made as necessary. Even though ciclosporin blood concentrations are increased, these calcium-channel blockers appear to have a kidney protective effect. One study[87] noted that, although calcium-channel blockers increase ciclosporin blood concentrations, this is of no harm to the patient, as no changes in renal function were observed. With diltiazem and verapamil, the ciclosporin dose can apparently be reduced by about 25 to 50% and possibly more with nicardipine. One case suggests that this is also true with nisoldipine. Several studies suggest that substantial cost savings can be made by giving either diltiazem[14,88,89] or verapamil[25] with ciclosporin. Take care not to substitute one diltiazem product for another after the patient has been stabilised because there is evidence that differences in their bioequivalence can alter the extent of the interaction.[28,90] The situation with nifedipine is not totally clear (no effect or decreases or increases), but it appears to have a kidney protective effect,[65] as does felodipine. The situation with amlodipine is also uncertain, but isradipine, lacidipine, and nitrendipine appear to be non-interacting alternatives.

Many of the calcium-channel blockers have a kidney protective effect. The increase in lercanidipine concentrations by ciclosporin is such that the UK manufacturer contraindicates concurrent use,[52] and the UK manufacturer of ciclosporin recommends caution.[91] Ciclosporin modestly increases felodipine concentrations, which would not be expected to be clinically relevant, and its effect on the concentrations of other calcium-channel blockers does not appear to have been studied.

The increased risk of gingival overgrowth when calcium-channel blockers are used with ciclosporin also appears to be established, with most data relating to nifedipine. Note that the UK manufacturer of ciclosporin specifically recommends avoiding nifedipine in patients who develop gingival overgrowth whilst taking ciclosporin.[91] It might be prudent to apply this to all calcium-channel blockers, when possible. Note that tacrolimus has been suggested as an alternative to ciclosporin, although it is not entirely free from gingival adverse effects (see 'Tacrolimus + Calcium-channel blockers', p.1291). The association between sirolimus and calcium-channel blocker use and gingival overgrowth is less-well documented, but concurrent use might result in additive effects, albeit less so than with ciclosporin or tacrolimus (see 'Sirolimus + Calcium-channel blockers', p.1282). The ACE inhibitors might be suitable alternatives to the calcium-channel blockers, but they are not entirely free of problems when used with ciclosporin (see 'Ciclosporin + ACE inhibitors or Angiotensin II receptor antagonists', p.1204). Note that a useful paper about minimising the risk of gingival overgrowth and its management has been published.[92]

1. Toupance O, Lavaud S, Canivet E, Bernaud C, Hotton J-M, Chanard J. Antihypertensive effect of amlodipine and lack of interference with cyclosporine metabolism in renal transplant recipients. *Hypertension* (1994) 24, 297–300.
2. Pesavento TE, Jones PA, Julian BA, Curtis JJ. Amlodipine increases cyclosporine levels in hypertensive renal transplant patients: results of a prospective study. *J Am Soc Nephrol* (1996) 7, 831–5.
3. Cai J, Huang Z, Yang G, Cheng K, Ye Q, Ming Y, Zuo X, Zhou P, Yuan H. Comparing antihypertensive effect and plasma ciclosporin concentration between amlodipine and valsartan regimens in hypertensive renal transplant patients receiving ciclosporin therapy. *Am J Cardiovasc Drugs* (2011) 11, 401–9.
4. Schrama YC, Koomans HA. Interactions of cyclosporin A and amlodipine: blood cyclosporin A levels, hypertension and kidney function. *J Hypertens* (1998) 16 (Suppl 4), S33–S38.
5. Raman GV, Campbell SK, Farrer A, Albano JDM, Cook J. Modifying effects of amlodipine on cyclosporin A-induced changes in renal function in patients with psoriasis. *J Hypertens* (1998) 16 (Suppl 4), S39–S41.
6. Foradori A, Mezzano S, Videla C, Pefaur J, Elberg A. Modification of the pharmacokinetics of cyclosporine A and metabolites by the concomitant use of Neoral and diltiazem or ketoconazole in stable adult kidney transplants. *Transplant Proc* (1998) 30, 1685–7.
7. Kohlhaw K, Wonigeit K, Frei U, Oldhafer K, Neumann K, Pichlmayr R. Effect of calcium channel blocker diltiazem on cyclosporine A blood levels and dose requirements. *Transplant Proc* (1988) 20 (Suppl 2), 572–4.
8. Pochet JM, Pirson Y. Cyclosporin-diltiazem interaction. *Lancet* (1986) i, 979.
9. Griño JM, Sabate I, Castelao AM, Alsina J. Influence of diltiazem on cyclosporin clearance. *Lancet* (1986) i, 1387.
10. Kunzendorf U, Walz G, Neumayer H-H, Wagner K, Keller F, Offermann G. Einfluss von Diltiazem auf die Ciclosporin-Blutspiegel. *Klin Wochenschr* (1987) 65, 1101–3.
11. Sabaté I, Griñó JM, Castelao AM, Huguet J, Serón D, Blanco A. Cyclosporin-diltiazem interaction: comparison of cyclosporin levels measured with two monoclonal antibodies. *Transplant Proc* (1989) 21, 1460–1.
12. Choi KC, Kang YJ, Kim SK, Ryu SB. Effects of the calcium channel blocker diltiazem on the blood and serum levels of cyclosporin A. *Chonnam J Med Sci* (1989) 2, 131–6.
13. Campistol JM, Oppenheimer F, Vilardell J, Ricart MJ, Alcaraz A, Ponz E, Andreu J. Interaction between ciclosporin and diltiazem in renal transplant patients. *Nephron* (1991) 57, 241–2.
14. Valantine H, Keogh A, McIntosh N, Hunt S, Oyer P, Schroeder J. Cost containment: Coadministration of diltiazem with cyclosporine after heart transplantation. *J Heart Lung Transplant* (1992) 11, 1–8.
15. Bourge RC, Kirklin JK, Naftel DC, Figg WD, White-Williams C, Ketchum C. Diltiazem-cyclosporine interaction in cardiac transplant recipients: impact on cyclosporine dose and medication costs. *Am J Med* (1991) 90, 402–4.
16. Maddux MS, Veremis SA, Bauma WD, Pollak R. Significant drug interactions with cyclosporine. *Hosp Ther* (1987) 12, 56–70.
17. Brockmöller J, Neumayer H-H, Wagner K, Weber W, Heinemeyer G, Kewitz H, Roots I. Pharmacokinetic interaction between cyclosporin and diltiazem. *Eur J Clin Pharmacol* (1990) 38, 237–42.
18. Diaz C, Gillum DM. Interaction of diltiazem and nifedipine with cyclosporine in renal transplant recipients. *Kidney Int* (1989) 35, 513.
19. Wagner K, Albrecht S, Neumayer H-H. Prevention of posttransplant acute tubular necrosis by the calcium antagonist diltiazem: a prospective randomized study. *Am J Nephrol* (1987) 7, 287–91.
20. McCauley J, Ptachcinski RJ, Shapiro R. The cyclosporine-sparing effects of diltiazem in renal transplantation. *Transplant Proc* (1989) 21, 3955–7.
21. Castelao AM. Cyclosporine A - drug interactions. 2nd Int Conf Therapeutic Drug Monitoring Toxicology, Barcelona, Spain, 1992. 203–9.
22. Shennib H, Auger J-L. Diltiazem improves cyclosporine dosage in cystic fibrosis lung transplant recipients. *J Heart Lung Transplant* (1994) 13, 292–6.
23. Macdonald P, Keogh A, Connell J, Harvison A, Richens D, Spratt P. Diltiazem co-administration reduces cylosporine toxicity after heart transplantation: a prospective randomised study. *Transplant Proc* (1992) 24, 2259–62.
24. Masri MA, Shakuntala V, Shanwaz M, Zaher M, Dhawan I, Yasin I, Pingle A. Pharmacokinetics of cyclosporine in renal transplant patients on diltiazem. *Transplant Proc* (1994) 26, 1921.
25. Sketris IS, Methot ME, Nicol D, Belitsky P, Knox MG. Effect of calcium-channel blockers on cyclosporine clearance and use in renal transplant patients. *Ann Pharmacother* (1994) 28, 1227–31.
26. Bleck JS, Thiesemann C, Kliem V, Christians U, Hecker H, Repp H, Frei U, Westhoff-Bleck M, Manns M, Sewing KF. Diltiazem increases blood concentrations of cyclized cyclosporine metabolites resulting in different cyclosporine metabolite patterns in stable male and female renal allograft recipients. *Br J Clin Pharmacol* (1996) 41, 551–6.
27. Morris RG, Jones TE. Diltiazem disposition and metabolism in recipients of renal transplants. *Ther Drug Monit* (1998) 20, 365–70.
28. Jones TE, Morris RG, Mathew TH. Formulation of diltiazem affects cyclosporin-sparing activity. *Eur J Clin Pharmacol* (1997) 52, 55–8.
29. Jones TE, Morris RG, Mathew TH. Diltiazem-cyclosporin pharmacokinetic interaction — dose-response relationship. *Br J Clin Pharmacol* (1997) 44, 499–504.
30. Sharma A, Bell L, Drolet D, Drouin E, Gaul M, Girardin P, Goodyer P, Schreiber R. Cyclosporine (CSA) Neoral kinetics in children treated with diltiazem. *J Am Soc Nephrol* (1996) 7, 1923.
31. Wagner C, Sperschneider H, Korn A, Christians U. Influence of diltiazem on cyclosporine metabolites in renal graft recipients treated with Sandimmun® and Neoral®. *J Am Soc Nephrol* (1997) 8, 707A.
32. Asberg A, Christensen H, Hartmann A, Carlson E, Molden E, Berg KJ. Pharmacokinetic interactions between microemulsion formulated cyclosporine A and diltiazem in renal transplant recipients. *Eur J Clin Pharmacol* (1999) 55, 383–7.
33. Kumana CR, Tong MKL, Li C-S, Lauder IJ, Lee JSK, Kou M, Walley T, Haycox A, Chan TM. Diltiazem co-treatment in renal transplant patients receiving microemulsion cyclosporin. *Br J Clin Pharmacol* (2003) 56, 670–8.
34. Xue W, Ding X, Tian P, Pan X, Yan H, Hou J, Feng X, Xiang H, Tian X. Long-term follow-up of co-administration of diltiazem and cyclosporine in Chinese kidney transplant recipients. *Ren Fail* (2010) 32, 314–9.
35. Neumayer H-H, Wagner K. Diltiazem and economic use of cyclosporin. *Lancet* (1986) ii, 523.
36. Wagner K, Albrecht S, Neumayer H-H. Prevention of delayed graft function in cadaveric kidney transplantation by a calcium antagonist. Preliminary results of two prospective randomized trials. *Transplant Proc* (1986) 18, 510–15.
37. Wagner K, Albrecht S, Neumayer H-H. Prevention of delayed graft function by a calcium antagonist- a randomized trial in renal graft recipients on cyclosporine A. *Transplant Proc* (1986) 18, 1269–71.
38. Wagner K, Philipp T, Heinemeyer G, Brockmüller F, Roots I, Neumayer HH. Interaction of cyclosporin and calcium antagonists. *Transplant Proc* (1989) 21, 1453–6.
39. Neumayer H-H, Kunzendorf U, Schreiber M. Protective effects of calcium antagonists in human renal transplantation. *Kidney Int* (1992) 41 (Suppl 36), S87–S93.
40. Aros CA, Ardiles LG, Schneider HO, Flores CA, Alruiz PA, Jerez VR, Mezzano SA. No gender-associated differences of cyclosporine pharmacokinetics in stable renal transplant patients treated with diltiazem. *Transplant Proc* (2005) 37, 3364–6.
41. Cohen DJ, Teng S-N, Valeri A, Appel GB. Influence of oral felodipine on serum cyclosporine concentrations in renal transplant patients. *J Am Soc Nephrol* (1993) 4, 929.
42. Yildiz A, Sever MŞ, Türkmen A, Ecder T, Türk S, Akkaya V, Ark E. Interaction between cyclosporin A and verapamil, felodipine, and isradipine. *Nephron* (1999) 81, 117–18.
43. Pedersen EB, Sørensen SS, Eiskjær H, Skovbon H, Thomsen K. Interaction between cyclosporine and felodipine in renal transplant recipients. *Kidney Int* (1992) 41 (Suppl 36), S82–S86.
44. Madsen JK, Jensen JD, Jensen LW, Pedersen EB. Pharmacokinetic interaction between cyclosporine and the dihydropyridine calcium antagonist felodipine. *Eur J Clin Pharmacol* (1996) 50, 203–8.
45. Madsen JK, Kornerup HJ, Sørensen SS, Zachariae H, Pedersen EB. Ciclosporine nephrotoxicity can be counteracted by a calcium antagonist (felodipine) in acute and short-term studies. *J Am Soc Nephrol* (1995) 6, 1102.
46. Schwitter J, DeMarco T, Globits S, Sakuma H, Klinski C, Chatterjee K, Parmley WW, Higgins CB. Influence of felodipine on left ventricular hypertrophy and systolic function in orthoptic heart transplant recipients: possible interaction with cyclosporine medication. *J Heart Lung Transplant* (1999) 18, 1003–13.
47. Endresen L, Bergan S, Holdaas H, Pran T, Sinding-Larsen B, Berg KJ. Lack of effect of the calcium antagonist isradipine on cyclosporine pharmacokinetics in renal transplant patients. *Ther Drug Monit* (1991) 13, 490–5.
48. Martinez F, Pirson Y, Wallemacq P, van Ypersele de Strihou C. No clinically significant interaction between ciclosporin and isradipine. *Nephron* (1991) 59, 658–9.
49. Vernillet L, Bourbigot B, Codet JP, Le Saux L, Moal MC, Morin JF. Lack of effect of isradipine on cyclosporin pharmacokinetics. *Fundam Clin Pharmacol* (1992) 6, 367–74.
50. Ahmed K, Michael B, Burke JF. Effects of isradipine on renal hemodynamics in renal transplant patients treated with cyclosporine. *Clin Nephrol* (1997) 48, 307–10.
51. Ruggenenti P, Perico N, Mosconi L, Gaspari F, Benigni A, Amuchastegui CS, Bruzzi I, Remuzzi G. Calcium channel blockers protect transplant patients from cyclosporine-induced daily renal hypoperfusion. *Kidney Int* (1993) 43, 706–11.
52. Zanidip (Lercanidipine hydrochloride). Recordati Pharmaceuticals Ltd. UK Summary of product characteristics, April 2006.
53. Bourbigot B, Guiserix J, Airiau J, Bressollette L, Morin JF, Cledes J. Nicardipine increases cyclosporin blood levels. *Lancet* (1986) i, 1447.
54. Cantarovich M, Hiesse C, Lockiec F, Charpentier B, Fries D. Confirmation of the interaction between cyclosporine and the calcium channel blocker nicardipine in renal transplant patients. *Clin Nephrol* (1987) 28, 190–3.
55. Kessler M, Renoult E, Jonon B, Vigneron B, Huu TC, Netter P. Interaction ciclosporine-nicardipine chez le transplanté rénal. *Therapie* (1987) 42, 273–5.
56. Deray G, Aupetit B, Martinez F, Baumelou A, Worcel A, Benhmida M, Legrand JC, Jacobs C. Cyclosporin-nicardipine interaction. *Am J Nephrol* (1989) 9, 349.
57. Kessler M, Netter P, Renoult E, Jonon B, Mur JM, Trechot P, Dousset B. Influence of nicardipine on renal function and plasma cyclosporin in renal transplant patients. *Eur J Clin Pharmacol* (1989) 36, 637–8.
58. Todd P, Garioch JJ, Rademaker M, Thomson J. Nicardipine interacts with cyclosporin. *Br J Dermatol* (1989) 121, 820.
59. Bouquet S, Chapelle G, Barrier L, Boutaud P, Menu P, Courtois P Interactions ciclosporine-nicardipine chez un transplanté cardiaque, adaptation posologique. *J Pharm Clin* (1992) 11, 59.
60. Mabin D, Fourquet I, Richard P, Esnault S, Islam MS, Bourbigot B. Leucoencéphalopathie régressive au cours d'un surdosage en cyclosporine A. *Rev Neurol (Paris)* (1993) 149, 576–8.
61. McNally P, Mistry N, Idle J, Walls J, Feehally J. Calcium channel blockers and cyclosporine metabolism. *Transplantation* (1989) 48, 1071.
62. Rossi SJ, Hariharan S, Schroeder TJ, First MR. Cyclosporine dosing and blood levels in renal transplants receiving Procardia XL. *Clin Pharmacol Ther* (1993) 53, 238.
63. Rossi SJ, Hariharan S, Schroeder TJ, First MR. Cyclosporine dosing and blood levels in renal transplant recipients receiving Procardia XL. *J Am Soc Nephrol* (1992) 3, 877.
64. Ogborn MR, Crocker JFS, Grimm PC. Nifedipine, verapamil and cyclosporin A pharmacokinetics in children. *Pediatr Nephrol* (1989) 3, 314–16.
65. Propper DJ, Whiting PH, Power DA, Edward N, Catto GRD. The effect of nifedipine on graft function in renal allograft recipients treated with cyclosporin A. *Clin Nephrol* (1989) 32, 62–7.
66. Howard RL, Shapiro JI, Babcock S, Chan L. The effect of calcium channel blockers on the cyclosporine dose requirement in renal transplant recipients. *Ren Fail* (1990) 12, 89–92.
67. Feehally J, Walls J, Mistry N, Horsburgh T, Taylor J, Veitch PS, Bell PRF. Does nifedipine ameliorate cyclosporin A nephrotoxicity? *BMJ* (1987) 295, 310.
68. Morales JM, Andrés A, Alvarez C, Prieto C, Ortuño B, Ortuño T, Paternina ER, Hernandez Poblete G, Praga M, Ruilope LM, Rodicio JL. Calcium channel blockers and early cyclosporine nephrotoxicity after renal transplantation: a prospective randomized study. *Transplant Proc* (1990) 22, 1733–5.
69. McFadden JP, Pontin JE, Powles AV, Fry L, Idle JR. Cyclosporin decreases nifedipine metabolism. *BMJ* (1989) 299, 1224.
70. Fourtounas C, Kopelias I, Kiriaki D, Agroyannis B. Increased cyclosporine blood levels after nisoldipine administration in a renal transplant recipient. *Transpl Int* (2002) 15, 586–8.
71. Çopur MS, Tasdemir I, Turgan Ç, Yasavul Ü, Çaglar S. Effects of nitrendipine on blood pressure and blood ciclosporin A level in patients with posttransplant hypertension. *Nephron* (1989) 52, 227–30.
72. Dawidson I, Rooth P, Fry WR, Sandor Z, Willms C, Coorpender L, Alway C, Reisch J. Prevention of acute cyclosporine-induced renal blood flow inhibition and improved immunosuppression with verapamil. *Transplantation* (1989) 48, 575–80.
73. Lindholm A, Henricsson S. Verapamil inhibits cyclosporin metabolism. *Lancet* (1987) i, 1262–3.
74. Hampton EM, Stewart CF, Herrod HG, Valenski WR. Augmentation of in- vitro immunosuppressive effects of cyclosporin by verapamil. *Clin Pharmacol Ther* (1987) 41, 169.
75. Robson RA, Fraenkel M, Barratt LJ, Birkett DJ. Cyclosporin-verapamil interaction. *Br J Clin Pharmacol* (1988) 25, 402–3.
76. Angermann CE, Spes CH, Anthuber M, Kemkes BM, Theisen K. Verapamil increases cyclosporin-A blood trough levels in cardiac recipients. *J Am Coll Cardiol* (1988) 11, 206A.
77. Sabaté I, Griñó JM, Castelao AM, Ortolá J. Evaluation of cyclosporin-verapamil interaction, with observations on parent cyclosporin and metabolites. *Clin Chem* (1988) 34, 2151.
78. Morgan JDT, Swarbrick MJ, Edwards CM, Donnelly PK. Cyclosporin, nifedipine and gingival hyperplasia: a randomized controlled study. *Transpl Int* (1994) 7 (Suppl 1), S320–S321.
79. Thomason JM, Seymour RA, Rice N. The prevalence and severity of cyclosporin and nifedipine-induced gingival overgrowth. *J Clin Periodontol* (1993) 20, 37–40.
80. Khoori AH, Einollahi B, Ansari G, Moozeh MB. The effect of cyclosporine with and without nifedipine on gingival overgrowth in renal transplant patients. *J Can Dent Assoc* (2003) 69, 236–41.

81. King GN, Fullinfaw R, Higgins TJ, Walker RG, Francis DM, Wiesenfeld D. Gingival hyperplasia in renal allograft recipients receiving cyclosporin-A and calcium antagonists. *J Clin Periodontol* (1993) 20, 286–93.
82. James JA, Marley JJ, Jamal S, Campbell BA, Short CD, Johnson RW, Hull PS, Spratt H, Irwin CR, Boomer S, Maxwell AP, Linden GJ. The calcium channel blocker used with cyclosporin has an effect on gingival overgrowth. *J Clin Periodontol* (2000) 27, 109–15.
83. Radwan-Oczko M, Boratyńska M, Klinger M, Zietek M. Risk factors of gingival overgrowth in kidney transplant recipients treated with cyclosporine A. *Ann Transplant* (2003) 8, 57–62.
84. Cebeci I, Kantarci A, Firatli E, Çarin M, Tuncer Ö. The effect of verapamil on the prevalence and severity of cyclosporine-induced gingival overgrowth in renal allograft recipients. *J Periodontol* (1996) 67, 1201–5.
85. Greenberg KV, Armitage GC, Shiboski CH. Gingival enlargement among renal transplant recipients in the era of new-generation immunosuppressants. *J Periodontol* (2008) 79, 453–60.
86. Oppenheimer F, Alcaraz A, Mañalich M, Ricart MJ, Vilardell J, Campistol JM, Andreu J, Talbot-Wright R, Fernandez-Cruz L. Influence of the calcium blocker diltiazem on the prevention of acute renal failure after renal transplantation. *Transplant Proc* (1992) 24, 50–1.
87. Wagner K, Henkel M, Heinemeyer G, Neumayer H-H. Interaction of calcium blockers and cyclosporine. *Transplant Proc* (1988) 20 (Suppl 2), 561–8.
88. Smith CL, Hampton EM, Pederson JA, Pennington LR, Bourne DWA. Clinical and medicoeconomic impact of the cyclosporine-diltiazem interaction in renal transplant recipients. *Pharmacotherapy* (1994) 14, 471–81.
89. Iqbal S, Holland D, Toffelmire EB. Diltiazem inhibition of cyclosporin metabolism provides cost effective therapy. *Clin Pharmacol Ther* (1995) 57, 219.
90. Cooke CE. Nontherapeutic cyclosporine levels. Sustained-release diltiazem products are not the same. *Transplantation* (1994) 57, 1687.
91. Neoral (Ciclosporin). Novartis Pharmaceuticals UK Ltd. UK Summary of product characteristics, February 2012.
92. Hood KA. Drug-induced gingival hyperplasia in transplant recipients. *Prog Transplant* (2002) 12, 17–23.

Ciclosporin + Chlorambucil

An isolated report describes a reduction in ciclosporin concentrations in a patient given chlorambucil.

Clinical evidence, mechanism, importance and management

A woman with B-chronic lymphocytic leukaemia and autoimmune haemolytic anaemia controlled with ciclosporin started taking chlorambucil 5 mg daily because of disease progression. When she reached a total cumulative dose of chlorambucil of 200 mg she suddenly relapsed, and her serum ciclosporin concentrations were found to have dropped to 60 nanograms/mL from a range of 200 to 400 nanograms/mL. The ciclosporin concentration remained low despite a doubling of the ciclosporin dose and withdrawal of the chlorambucil. Only after one month did the anaemia respond and the ciclosporin concentration increase again.[1] This appears to be an isolated report so the general significance of this interaction is unclear.

1. Emilia G, Messora C. Interaction between cyclosporin and chlorambucil. *Eur J Haematol* (1993) 51, 179.

Ciclosporin + Chloroquine and related drugs

Three transplant patients had rapid increases in ciclosporin concentrations, with evidence of nephrotoxicity in two of them, when they were given chloroquine. Neither chloroquine nor hydroxychloroquine altered the incidence of increased creatinine concentrations seen with low-dose ciclosporin in rheumatoid arthritis.

Clinical evidence

(a) Chloroquine

A kidney transplant patient taking ciclosporin, azathioprine, and prednisolone had a 3-fold increase in ciclosporin blood concentrations, from 148 to 420 nanograms/mL, accompanied by an increase in serum creatinine concentrations within 48 hours of starting chloroquine 900 mg daily for suspected malarial fever. On days 2 and 3 the chloroquine dose was reduced to 300 mg daily. The ciclosporin and creatinine returned to their former concentrations 7 days after the chloroquine was stopped.[1]

When another kidney transplant patient taking ciclosporin, azathioprine, and prednisolone was given chloroquine 100 mg daily for 6 days, his ciclosporin serum concentration increased from 105 to 470 nanograms/mL and his serum creatinine concentration increased from 200 to 234 micromol/L, accompanied by an increase in blood pressure from 130/80 to 160/100 mmHg. These changes reversed when the chloroquine was stopped, and occurred again when chloroquine was restarted.[2] The ciclosporin serum concentration of another patient was doubled by chloroquine 100 mg daily.[3]

A randomised, controlled study in 88 patients with recent onset rheumatoid arthritis found that the addition of ciclosporin (1.25 or 2.5 mg/kg daily) to chloroquine 100 mg daily was moderately effective, but changes in serum creatinine concentrations occurred. In the presence of chloroquine, the creatinine concentration was not significantly altered by placebo or ciclosporin 1.25 mg/kg, but was increased by 10 micromol/L by ciclosporin 2.5 mg/kg, indicating that some renal effects can occur.[4] As there was no group given ciclosporin alone, it is not possible to be certain if the renal effects were due to an interaction with chloroquine, or just due to ciclosporin alone. However, the results of a further study suggest that the findings were probably due to ciclosporin alone: there was no difference in the incidence of increased creatinine concentrations between rheumatoid arthritis patients taking ciclosporin 2.5 mg/kg daily alone or the same dose of ciclosporin with chloroquine 150 mg daily. Note that in this study, there was no advantage to using the combination.[5]

(b) Hydroxychloroquine

In a randomised study in rheumatoid arthritis patients receiving ciclosporin 3 mg/kg daily alone or the same dose of ciclosporin with hydroxychloroquine 400 mg daily, there was no difference in incidence of renal impairment or in temporary or permanent reductions in ciclosporin dose between the groups. Note that in this study, there was no advantage to using the combination.[6]

Mechanism

The reason for the increased ciclosporin concentrations in these few cases is not understood.

Importance and management

Information is limited, but it would be prudent to monitor for increases in serum ciclosporin concentrations when chloroquine is given to patients receiving high doses of ciclosporin. In the setting of the use of low doses of ciclosporin in rheumatoid arthritis, neither chloroquine nor hydroxychloroquine appear to contribute to the known adverse effects of ciclosporin on creatinine and renal function.

1. Nampoory MRN, Nessim J, Gupta RK, Johny KV. Drug interaction of chloroquine and ciclosporin. *Nephron* (1992) 62, 108–9.
2. Finielz P, Gendoo Z, Chuet C, Guiserix J. Interaction between cyclosporin and chloroquine. *Nephron* (1993) 65, 333.
3. Guiserix J, Aizel A. Interactions ciclosporine-chloroquine. *Presse Med* (1996) 25, 1214.
4. van den Borne BEEM, Landewé RBM, Goei The HS, Rietveld JH, Zwinderman AH, Bruyn GAW, Breedveld FC, Dijkmans BAC. Combination therapy in recent onset rheumatoid arthritis: a randomized double blind trial of the addition of low dose cyclosporine to patients treated with low dose chloroquine. *J Rheumatol* (1998) 25, 1493–8.
5. Miranda JM, Alvarez-Nemegyei J, Saavedra MA, Terán L, Galván-Villegas F, García-Figueroa J, Jara LJ, Barile L; GRECIA Group. A randomized, double-blind, multicenter, controlled clinical trial of cyclosporine plus chloroquine vs. cyclosporine plus placebo in early-onset rheumatoid arthritis. *Arch Med Res* (2004) 35, 36–42.
6. Sarzi-Puttini P, D'Ingianna E, Fumagalli M, Scarpellini M, Fiorini T, Chérié-Lignière EL, Panni B, Fiorentini F, Corbelli V, Beyene NB, Mastaglio C, Severi C, Locati M, Cazzola M, Menozzi G, Monti G, Saccardo F, Alfieri G, Atzeni F. An open, randomized comparison study of cyclosporine A, cyclosporine A + methotrexate and cyclosporine A + hydroxychloroquine in the treatment of early severe rheumatoid arthritis. *Rheumatol Int* (2005) 25, 15–22.

Ciclosporin + Cinacalcet

Cinacalcet does not appear to affect ciclosporin minimum concentrations. In one study it has caused a small decrease in renal function in patients taking ciclosporin.

Clinical evidence

In a pharmacokinetic study in 8 kidney transplant patients taking ciclosporin, cinacalcet 30 mg daily for 6 days had no effect on the pharmacokinetics of ciclosporin, but there was a minor 9% increase in the AM19 metabolite of ciclosporin. The increase in this metabolite correlated with a small decrease in renal function (from 78 to 72 mL/minute).[1]

In clinical use, no changes in ciclosporin minimum concentrations have been seen. For example, in one 3-month study in 13 transplant patients, there was no change in ciclosporin minimum concentrations after one, 2, and 3 months use of cinacalcet 30 mg daily.[2] In two other reports, no change in ciclosporin dose was needed in patients when they were given cinacalcet, initially 30 mg daily then titrated to effect, for 6 months.[3,4] One of these studies did find a decrease in glomerular filtration rate and a modest increase in serum creatinine concentrations (from 140 micromol/L; to 153 micromol/L at 2 months and 148 micromol/L at 3 months).[2] Another found that serum creatinine and creatinine clearance were stable during 6 months use of cinacalcet.[3]

Mechanism

The small impairment in renal function in patients taking ciclosporin might be due to cinacalcet increasing concentrations of the ciclosporin AM19 metabolite, but the mechanism for this is unclear.

Importance and management

Cinacalcet does not appear to alter ciclosporin concentrations, and so no ciclosporin dose adjustment is likely to be necessary with concurrent use. Further study is needed to establish any possible impairment of renal function when cinacalcet is used with ciclosporin and to assess its clinical relevance. Until more is known, bear the possibility of adverse renal effects in mind.

1. Falck P, Vethe NT, Åsberg A, Midtvedt K, Bergan S, Reubsaet JL, Holdaas H. Cinacalcet's effect on the pharmacokinetics of tacrolimus, cyclosporine and mycophenolate in renal transplant recipients. *Nephrol Dial Transplant* (2008) 23, 1048–53.
2. Kruse AE, Eisenberger U, Frey FJ, Mohaupt MG. The calcimimetic cinacalcet normalizes serum calcium in renal transplant patients with persistent hyperparathyroidism. *Nephrol Dial Transplant* (2005) 20, 1311–14.
3. Serra AL, Savoca R, Huber AR, Hepp U, Delsignore A, Hersberger M, Wüthrich RP. Effective control of persistent hyperparathyroidism with cinacalcet in renal allograft recipients. *Nephrol Dial Transplant* (2007) 22, 577–83.
4. Szwarc I, Argilés À, Garrigue V, Delmas S, Chong G, Deleuze S, Mourad G. Cinacalcet chloride is efficient and safe in renal transplant recipients with posttransplant hyperparathyroidism. *Transplantation* (2006) 82, 675–80.

Ciclosporin + Clodronate

Clodronate does not appear to alter ciclosporin blood concentrations.

Clinical evidence, mechanism, importance and management

Ten heart transplant patients taking ciclosporin, azathioprine, and diltiazem were also given clodronate 800 mg daily for one week (timing of clodronate and ciclosporin administration not stated). No statistically significant differences were seen in their ciclosporin blood concentrations or AUCs. Three of them were also taking simvastatin, two were taking ranitidine, and one was taking propafenone, furosemide, and cyclophosphamide. There would seem to be no reason for avoiding concurrent use; however, the authors of the report suggest that longer-term use of clodronate should be well monitored.[1] Note that the UK manufacturer of sodium clodronate recommends doses of clodronate should be taken at least two hours after and one hour before other oral medications.[2] There seems to be no information about other bisphosphonates.

1. Baraldo M, Furlanut M, Puricelli C. No effect of clodronate on cyclosporin A blood levels in heart transplant patients simultaneously treated with diltiazem and azathioprine. *Ther Drug Monit* (1994) 16, 435.
2. Bonefos Capsules (Sodium clodronate). Schering Health Care Ltd. UK Summary of product characteristics, June 2013.

Ciclosporin + Clonidine

A child taking ciclosporin had a large increase in his ciclosporin blood concentrations when clonidine was also given.

Clinical evidence, mechanism, importance and management

A 3-year-old kidney transplant patient taking ciclosporin, azathioprine, and prednisone was given a combination of propranolol, hydralazine, furosemide, and nifedipine postoperatively in an attempt to control his blood pressure. Minoxidil was added, but was considered unacceptable because of adverse cosmetic effects. When it was replaced with clonidine, the ciclosporin concentration increased about 3-fold to 927 nanograms/mL, despite a ciclosporin dose reduction. Ciclosporin concentrations returned to the patient's normal range of 150 to 300 nanograms/mL when the clonidine was withdrawn, and blood pressure was controlled by the addition of an ACE inhibitor. It was suggested that clonidine inhibited the metabolism of ciclosporin by cytochrome P450.[1]

As this appears to be the only report of an interaction, there is insufficient evidence to recommend routinely increasing the monitoring of ciclosporin concentrations in every patient taking these drugs. However, the possibility of an interaction should still be considered if both drugs are given.

1. Gilbert RD, Kahn D, Cassidy M. Interaction between clonidine and cyclosporine A. *Nephron* (1995) 71, 105.

Ciclosporin + Codergocrine mesilate (Ergoloid mesylates)

Codergocrine does not appear to affect ciclosporin exposure.

Clinical evidence, mechanism, importance and management

In 5 healthy male subjects given codergocrine mesilate 6 mg daily for 6 days, there was no clinically relevant change in the AUC of a single oral 15 mg/kg dose of ciclosporin.[1] No ciclosporin dose adjustment would therefore seem necessary on concurrent use.

1. Heinrichs DA, Martell R, Stiller CR, Freeman D, Carruthers G. The effects of co-dergocrine on cyclosporin A pharmacokinetics and pharmacodynamics. *Br J Clin Pharmacol* (1987) 24, 117–8.

Ciclosporin + Coenzyme Q_{10} (Ubidecarenone)

Coenzyme Q_{10} did not alter ciclosporin concentrations in a clinical study.

Clinical evidence, mechanism, importance and management

In a study in 11 renal transplant patients, coenzyme Q_{10} 30 mg three times daily for 4 weeks did not alter the serum concentrations of creatinine or ciclosporin (137 to 155 nanograms/mL). This suggests no ciclosporin dose adjustment is likely to be needed on the concurrent use of coenzyme Q_{10}.[1]

1. Długosz A, Kuźniar J, Sawicka E, Marchewka Z, Lembas-Bogaczyk J, Sajewicz W, Boratyńska M. Oxidative stress and coenzyme Q10 supplementation in renal transplant recipients. *Int Urol Nephrol* (2004) 36, 253–8.

Ciclosporin + Colchicine

In single-dose studies, ciclosporin has increased the exposure to colchicine. A number of cases of serious muscle disorders (myopathy, rhabdomyolysis), some with multiple organ failure, have been seen when colchicine and ciclosporin were given concurrently. Ciclosporin toxicity has, rarely, also been seen.

Clinical evidence

In a single-dose, pharmacokinetic study in 23 healthy subjects, ciclosporin 100 mg increased the AUC and maximum concentration of colchicine 600 micrograms about 3.2-fold.[1] This data has also been published elsewhere.[2]

A large number of case reports describe myopathy (muscle weakness, myalgia), rhabdomyolysis, or neuromyopathy,[3-21] on the concurrent use of ciclosporin and colchicine, some with multiple organ failure[15,18] or impairment.[16,21] For example, a patient taking ciclosporin, azathioprine, prednisone, and colchicine 1.2 mg daily immediately after a renal transplant developed colchicine neuromyopathy (possibly rhabdomyolysis), ciclosporin nephrotoxicity, and liver function abnormalities within 31 days.[3] Further, an increase in gastrointestinal adverse effects (nausea, diarrhoea, abdominal pain), as well as myopathy, was seen when ciclosporin was started in patients stable taking colchicine 1 mg daily for amyloidosis due to familial Mediterranean fever.[19] The onset of symptoms has occurred after just a few days of taking colchicine[8,18,20,21] or after many months of concurrent use.[11,14] At the time of the development of toxicity, ciclosporin concentrations were normal in many cases,[6,8,12,16,17,20] but increased in some.[11] Increased creatine kinase concentrations have been a feature of some[14,17,21] but not all cases. The incidence of myopathy might be high. For example, in one retrospective study, 5 of 10 kidney transplant patients who had received colchicine with ciclosporin experienced muscular symptoms after a mean of 12 months of colchicine use. This improved after colchicine withdrawal.[10] In another study in four kidney transplant patients with familial Mediterranean fever taking colchicine, an attempt to replace azathioprine with ciclosporin failed after 3 weeks because of pronounced adverse effects even before achieving therapeutic concentrations of ciclosporin. These included elevations in serum creatinine, liver enzymes, and bilirubin, and one patient was hospitalised for general muscle weakness and severe myalgia.[6]

Another kidney transplant patient had a transient increase (lasting 2 to 3 days) in serum creatinine, and an increase in ciclosporin blood concentrations, from a range of 100 to 200 nanograms/mL up to 1519 nanograms/mL, one day after receiving a total of 4 mg of colchicine.[22]

Mechanism

Myotoxicity is a known adverse effect of colchicine alone, which is more common in renal impairment due to a reduction in colchicine excretion. Myopathy has also occurred with ciclosporin alone.[4,23] The myotoxic effects of both ciclosporin and colchicine might be additive or synergistic.[24] In addition, patients taking ciclosporin who develop ciclosporin-impaired renal function are likely to accumulate colchicine and be at greater risk of colchicine toxicity.[24] Moreover, ciclosporin might directly increase colchicine concentrations, because it inhibits P-glycoprotein and might thereby impair colchicine excretion.[12,21,25]

Importance and management

Evidence for an interaction between ciclosporin and colchicine is limited to two single-dose pharmacokinetic studies, but it appears that ciclosporin slightly to moderately increases the exposure to colchicine. In addition, numerous case reports suggest that the risk of colchicine-induced muscle toxicity can be increased on concurrent use.

If both colchicine and ciclosporin are thought to be necessary, patients should be very closely monitored for signs of colchicine toxicity (such as nausea, vomiting, myopathy, and pancytopenia) because the outcome can be serious. The manufacturers of colchicine state that in patients with normal renal or hepatic function, who are also taking P-glycoprotein inhibitors, such as ciclosporin, the colchicine dose should be reduced or treatment interrupted.[25,26] The US manufacturer gives the following specific advice for colchicine dose reductions in patients taking **P-glycoprotein inhibitors** (they name ciclosporin; but also see 'Table 1.12', p.14, for a list) or if they have stopped taking them within 2 weeks of starting colchicine:

- For the treatment of gout, the dose of colchicine should be reduced to a single dose of 600 micrograms. The dose should not be repeated within 3 days.
- For gout prophylaxis, the dose of colchicine should be reduced to 300 micrograms daily (if the initial dose was 600 micrograms twice daily) or 300 micrograms on alternate days (if the initial dose was 600 micrograms daily).
- For familial Mediterranean fever, a maximum total daily dose of colchicine 600 micrograms (which can be given as 300 micrograms twice daily) is recommended.[25]

Patients should be reminded to report any unexplained muscle pain, tenderness or weakness, or dark urine. Note that the manufacturers of colchicine contraindicate the concurrent use of ciclosporin in patients with renal or hepatic impairment.[25,26]

1. Wason S, DiGiacinto JL, Davis MW. Effect of cyclosporine on the pharmacokinetics of colchicine in healthy subjects. *Postgrad Med* (2012) 124, 189–96.
2. Terkeltaub RA, Furst DE, DiGiacinto JL, Kook KA, Davis MW. Novel evidence-based colchicine dose-reduction algorithm to predict and prevent colchicine toxicity in the presence of cytochrome P450 3A4/P-glycoprotein inhibitors. *Arthritis Rheum* (2011) 63, 226. Erratum ibid. (2011) 63, 3521.
3. Rieger EH, Halasz NA, Wahlstrom HE. Colchicine neuromyopathy after renal transplantation. *Transplantation* (1990) 49, 1196–8.
4. Arellano F, Krupp P. Muscular disorders associated with cyclosporin. *Lancet* (1991), 337, 915.
5. Shibata K, Takeuchi M, Kikuchi M, Kobayashi I, Maruyama S. A case of Behçet's disease associated with myopathy during cyclosporin treatment. *Rinsho Shinkeigaku* (1991) 31, 847–52.
6. Yussim A, Bar-Nathan N, Lustig S, Shaharabani E, Geier E, Shmuely D, Nakache R, Shapira Z. Gastrointestinal, hepatorenal, and neuromuscular toxicity caused by cyclosporine-colchicine interaction in renal transplantation. *Transplant Proc* (1994) 26, 2825–6.
7. Tapal MF. Colchicine myopathy. *Scand J Rheumatol* (1996) 5, 105–6.
8. Lee BI, Shin SJ, Yoon SN, Choi YJ, Yang CW, Bang BK. Acute myopathy induced by colchicine in a cyclosporine-treated renal recipient. A case report and review of the literature. *J Korean Med Sci* (1997) 12, 160–1.
9. Jagose JT, Bailey RR. Muscle weakness due to colchicine in a renal transplant recipient. *N Z Med J* (1997) 110, 343.
10. Ducloux D, Schuller V, Bresson-Vautrin C, Chalopin J-M. Colchicine myopathy in renal transplant recipients on cyclosporin. *Nephrol Dial Transplant* (1997) 12, 2389–92.
11. Rana SS, Giuliani MJ, Oddis CV, Lacomis D. Acute onset of colchicine myoneuropathy in cardiac transplant recipients: case studies of three patients. *Clin Neurol Neurosurg* (1997) 99, 266–70.
12. Gruberg L, Har-Zahav Y, Agranat O, Freimark D. Acute myopathy induced by colchicine in a cyclosporine treated heart transplant recipient: possible role of the multidrug resistance transporter. *Transplant Proc* (1999) 31, 2157–8.
13. Dupont P, Hunt I, Goldberg L, Warrens A. Colchicine myoneuropathy in a renal transplant patient. *Transpl Int* (2002) 15, 374–6.
14. Çağlar K, Safali M, Yavuz I, OdabaŞi Z, Yenicesu M, Vural A. Colchicine-induced myopathy with normal creatinine phosphokinase level in a renal transplant patient. *Nephron* (2002) 92, 922–4.
15. Minetti EE, Minetti L. Multiple organ failure in a kidney transplant patient receiving both colchicine and cyclosporine. *J Nephrol* (2003) 16, 421–5.
16. Jonsson J, Gelpi JR, Light JA, Aquino A, Maszaros S. Colchicine-induced myoneuropathy in a renal transplant patient. *Transplantation* (1992) 53, 1369–71..

17. Cook M, Ramos E, Peterson J, Croker B. Colchicine neuromyopathy in a renal transplant patient with normal muscle enzyme levels. *Clin Nephrol* (1994) 42, 67–8.
18. Eleftheriou G, Bacis G, Fiocchi R, Sebastiano R. Colchicine-induced toxicity in a heart transplant patient with chronic renal failure. *Clin Toxicol* (2008) 46, 827–30.
19. Cohen SL, Boner G, Shmueli D, Yusim A, Rosenfeld J, Shapira Z. Cyclosporin: poorly tolerated in familial Mediterranean fever. *Nephrol Dial Transplant* (1989) 4, 201–4.
20. Bouquié R, Deslandes G, Renaud C, Dailly E, Haloun A, Jolliet P. Colchicine-induced rhabdomyolysis in a heart/lung transplant patient with concurrent use of cyclosporin, pravastatin, and azithromycin. *J Clin Rheumatol* (2011) 17, 28–30.
21. Garrouste C, Philipponnet C, Kaysi S, Enache I, Tiple A, Heng AE. Severe colchicine intoxication in a renal transplant recipient on cyclosporine. *Transplant Proc* (2012) 44, 2851–2.
22. Menta R, Rossi E, Guariglia A, David S, Cambi V. Reversible acute cyclosporin nephrotoxicity induced by colchicine administration. *Nephrol Dial Transplant* (1987) 2, 380–1.
23. Noppen M, Velkeniers B, Dierckx R, Bruyland M, Vanhaelst L. Cyclosporine and myopathy. *Ann Intern Med* (1987) 107, 945–6.
24. Rumpf KW, Henning HV. Is myopathy in renal transplant patients induced by cyclosporin or colchicine? *Lancet* (1990) 335, 800–1.
25. Colcrys (Colchicine). Takeda Pharmaceuticals America, Inc. US Prescribing information, November 2012.
26. Colchicine. Wockhardt UK Ltd. UK Summary of product characteristics, June 2010.

Ciclosporin + Colestyramine

Colestyramine does not appear to alter ciclosporin concentrations.

Clinical evidence, mechanism, importance and management

Five transplant patients taking ciclosporin and colestyramine had their colestyramine suspended for one week. It was then restarted for one week, and given simultaneously with ciclosporin on the day of testing. There was no difference in the maximum and minimum concentrations of ciclosporin and a non-significant average increase of 6% in the AUC of ciclosporin, but one patient had a 55% increase, and another a 23% decrease, in the AUC of ciclosporin.[1] In another pharmacokinetic study in 6 kidney transplant patients, colestyramine 4 g daily caused no notable change in the ciclosporin AUC, maximum, and minimum concentrations.[2] Ciclosporin was given at 8 am and 8 pm, with colestyramine taken at noon. Similarly, in a 12-month efficacy study, 18 heart transplant patients taking ciclosporin were randomised to receive colestyramine 4 g twice daily taken one to 2 hours after ciclosporin. Colestyramine had no effect on ciclosporin concentrations.[3]

In general, it appears that colestyramine has little effect on ciclosporin absorption. However, the occasional patient might be affected, and therefore, because of the clinical consequences of the loss of ciclosporin efficacy, it would seem prudent to separate the administration of colestyramine and ciclosporin. It is usually advised that colestyramine is given one hour before, or 4 to 6 hours after, other drugs.

1. Keogh A, Day R, Critchley L, Duggin G, Baron D. The effect of food and cholestyramine on the absorption of cyclosporine in cardiac transplant patients. *Transplant Proc* (1988) 20, 27–30.
2. Jensen RA, Lal SM, Diaz-Arias A, James-Kracke M, Van Stone JC, Ross G. Does cholestyramine interfere with cyclosporine absorption? A prospective study in renal transplant patients. *ASAIO J* (1995) 41, M704–M706.
3. Pflugfelder PW, Huff M, Oskalns R, Rudas L, Kostuk WJ. Cholesterol-lowering therapy after heart transplantation: a 12-month randomized trial. *J Heart Lung Transplant* (1995) 14, 613–22.

Ciclosporin + Corticosteroids

Some evidence suggests that ciclosporin concentrations might be increased by high-dose methylprednisolone or reduced by prednisone. Ciclosporin can reduce the clearance of the corticosteroids. Convulsions have been described during the concurrent use of ciclosporin and high-dose methylprednisolone, and the incidence of diabetes mellitus might also be increased. One case of osteonecrosis has been reported with high-dose topical betamethasone and ciclosporin.

Clinical evidence

(a) Betamethasone

A patient with psoriasis taking ciclosporin and applying an average of betamethasone 30 mg daily (as 15 g to 150 g of topical betamethasone 0.05% cream or ointment) developed avascular osteonecrosis of the femoral heads of both hip joints.[1]

(b) Methylprednisolone

A study found that the pharmacokinetics of methylprednisolone in patients taking ciclosporin and azathioprine varied widely between individual kidney transplant patients, but the mean values were similar to those found in healthy subjects.[2] Another later study by the same research group found that ciclosporin did not appear to affect methylprednisolone pharmacokinetics.[3]

The ciclosporin plasma concentrations of 22 out of 33 patients were reported to be more than doubled by intravenous methylprednisolone used for acute graft rejection, and the ciclosporin dose needed to be reduced in 6 patients.[4,5] Others have similarly observed that high doses of methylprednisolone increased or more than doubled ciclosporin concentrations.[6-8] However, a study found that ciclosporin minimum concentrations were unchanged when an intravenous dose of ciclosporin was given with high-dose intravenous methylprednisolone, although the clearance of ciclosporin was slightly increased (by 20%) in 8 out of 9 patients.[9] In another analysis of the use of methylprednisolone in 17 rejection episodes in 13 patients, there was no change in ciclosporin concentrations before, during, and after methylprednisolone in most cases. Increases in ciclosporin concentrations occurred only in 3 rejection episodes in 3 patients, and these were not attributed to an interaction.[10] Similarly, a further study into the use of methylprednisolone in 14 rejection episodes, found that ciclosporin concentrations were increased in 2 of the episodes, when the same definition of an increase was used.[11] A retrospective study into the effects of decreasing methylprednisolone doses on the bioavailability of ciclosporin during the first year after kidney transplantation, found no effect on ciclosporin.[12]

A report describes 4 young patients (aged 10, 12, 13, and 18 years) who had undergone bone marrow transplants for severe aplastic anaemia and who developed convulsions when given high-dose methylprednisolone (5 to 20 mg/kg daily) and ciclosporin.[13] Convulsions also occurred in a 25-year-old woman given ciclosporin with high-dose methylprednisolone.[14] In another report, seizures occurred in 3 patients taking ciclosporin and high-dose methylprednisolone, but only after ketoconazole was added to permit a reduction in ciclosporin dose.[15]

A study of 314 kidney transplant patients during the period 1979 to 1987 found that the incidence of diabetes mellitus in those given ciclosporin and methylprednisolone was twice that of other patients given azathioprine and methylprednisolone. The diabetes developed within less than 2 months.[16]

(c) Prednisolone or Prednisone

A pharmacokinetic study in 40 patients found that the clearance of prednisolone was about 30% lower in those taking ciclosporin when compared with those taking azathioprine.[17] Another study in patients with kidney transplants by the same group of researchers reported a 25% lower clearance of prednisolone in the presence of ciclosporin.[18] A further study in kidney, liver and lung transplant patients receiving ciclosporin, found that the prednisolone dose-normalised AUC was 1.6- to 2.4-fold higher than in healthy controls.[19]

Other studies confirm that the clearance of prednisolone is about one-third lower in patients also taking ciclosporin and that it is lower at 3 to 6 months than at 2 to 4 weeks.[4,20] As a result, some patients develop signs of corticosteroid toxicity (cushingoid symptoms and impaired glucose metabolism).[4] In contrast, these studies have all been questioned by the authors of another study, who found that the metabolism of prednisolone after an oral and intravenous dose did not differ between patients taking ciclosporin and those taking azathioprine.[21] Similarly, another study found no change in the pharmacokinetics of intravenous prednisolone before and after starting ciclosporin.[22]

A comparative study over a year, in two groups of kidney transplant patients taking ciclosporin and azathioprine, one group with, and the other without, prednisone, found that those taking prednisone had lower ciclosporin minimum concentrations (about 10 to 20%) despite using the same or higher doses of ciclosporin.[23] Other evidence suggests that low-dose prednisolone does not increase the immunosuppression of ciclosporin, but it can reduce ciclosporin nephrotoxicity.[24]

Mechanism

Uncertain. Some evidence suggests that ciclosporin reduces the metabolism of the corticosteroids by the liver thereby raising their concentrations,[4] but not all studies have found an interaction. *In vitro*, methylprednisolone inhibited the metabolism of ciclosporin.[25] There is some evidence that prednisolone-induced changes in lipoproteins might correlate with the changes in ciclosporin concentrations.[26] Corticosteroids are known to cause osteonecrosis and ciclosporin can depress bone resorption as well as bone remodelling.[1]

Importance and management

None of these adverse interactions between ciclosporin and the corticosteroids are well established. Concurrent use is common and advantageous but be alert for any evidence of increased ciclosporin and corticosteroid adverse effects.

It is not clear whether or not high-dose corticosteroids cause an increase in ciclosporin concentrations. If they do, the authors of one report point out that this interaction could possibly lead to a misinterpretation of clinical data as an increase in serum creatinine concentrations in patients with kidney transplants is assumed to be due to rejection, unless proven otherwise. If a corticosteroid is then given, this could lead to increased ciclosporin concentrations, which might lead to the rejection episode being re-interpreted as ciclosporin nephrotoxicity.[5] It has been suggested that ciclosporin concentrations measured by [the non-specific] RIA (radioimmunoassay) method should be interpreted with caution in patients taking high-dose corticosteroids as the concentrations of ciclosporin metabolites, which can interfere with the test, might be altered.[9] However, a study using both the RIA method and HPLC did not find a difference in the interaction between the two methods.[10]

The contribution of ciclosporin and high-dose *topical* corticosteroid to the development of osteonecrosis in the isolated case report is not known.

1. Reichert-Pénétrat S, Tréchot P, Barbaud A, Gillet P, Schmutz J-L. Bilateral femoral avascular necrosis in a man with psoriasis: responsibility of topical corticosteroids and role of cyclosporine. *Dermatology* (2001) 203, 356–7.
2. Tornatore KM, Morse GD, Jusko WJ, Walshe JJ. Methylprednisolone disposition in renal transplant recipients receiving triple-drug immunosuppression. *Transplantation* (1989) 48, 962–5.
3. Tornatore KM, Walshe JJ, Reed KA, Holdsworth MT, Venuto RC. Comparative methylprednisolone pharmacokinetics in renal transplant patients receiving double- or triple-drug immunosuppression. *Ann Pharmacother* (1993) 27, 545–9.
4. Öst L, Klintmalm G, Ringdén O. Mutual interaction between prednisolone and cyclosporine in renal transplant patients. *Transplant Proc* (1985) 17, 1252–5.
5. Klintmalm G, Säwe J. High dose methylprednisolone increases plasma cyclosporin levels in renal transplant recipients. *Lancet* (1984) i, 731.
6. Klintmalm G, Säwe J, Ringdéen O, von Bahr C, Magnusson A. Cyclosporine plasma levels in renal transplant patients. Association with renal toxicity and allograft rejection. *Transplantation* (1985) 39, 132–7.
7. Hall TG. Effect of methylprednisolone on cyclosporine blood levels. *Pharmacotherapy* (1990) 10, 248.
8. Rogerson ME, Marsden JT, Reid KE, Bewick M, Holt DW. Cyclosporine blood concentrations in the management of renal transplant recipients. *Transplantation* (1986) 41, 276–8.
9. Ptachcinski RJ, Venkataramanan R, Burckart GJ, Hakala TR, Rosenthal JT, Carpenter BJ, Taylor RJ. Cyclosporine–high-dose steroid interaction in renal transplant recipients: assessment by HPLC. *Transplant Proc* (1987) 19, 1728–9.

10. Ubhi CS, Woodhouse L, Giles GR. Interaction of intravenous methylprednisolone with oral cyclosporin. *Nephrol Dial Transplant* (1990) 5, 376–8.
11. Huisman RM, van Son WJ, Tegzess AM. Interaction of intravenous methylprednisolone with oral CsA. *Nephrol Dial Transplant* (1990) 5, 905–6.
12. Lemahieu WPD, Maes BD, Vanrenterghem Y. Different evolution of trough and dose levels during the first year after transplantation for tacrolimus versus cyclosporine. *Transplant Proc* (2005) 37, 2051–3.
13. Durrant S, Chipping PM, Palmer S, Gordon-Smith EC. Cyclosporin A, methylprednisolone and convulsions. *Lancet* (1982) ii, 829–30.
14. Boogaerts MA, Zachee P, Verwilghen RL. Cyclosporin, methylprednisolone and convulsions. *Lancet* (1982) ii, 1216–17.
15. Hwang W-L, Gau J-P, Young J-H, Chia L-G. Ketoconazole and high-dose methylprednisolone predisposing to cyclosporine-induced seizures: report of 3 cases. *Acta Haematol (Basel)* (1992) 88, 139–41.
16. Roth D, Milgrom M, Esquenazi V, Fuller L, Burke G, Miller J. Posttransplant hyperglycaemia. Increased incidence in cyclosporine-treated renal allograft recipients. *Transplantation* (1989) 47, 278–81.
17. Langhoff E, Madsen S, Olgaard K, Ladefoged J. Clinical results and cyclosporine effect on prednisolone metabolism. *Kidney Int* (1984) 26, 642.
18. Langhoff E, Madsen S, Flachs H, Olgaard K, Ladefoged J, Hvidberg EF. Inhibition of prednisolone metabolism by cyclosporine in kidney-transplanted patients. *Transplantation* (1985) 39, 107–9.
19. Jeng S, Chanchairujira T, Jusko W, Steiner R. Prednisone metabolism in recipients of kidney or liver transplants and in lung recipients receiving ketoconazole. *Transplantation* (2003) 75, 792–5.
20. Öst L. Impairment of prednisolone metabolism by cyclosporine treatment in renal graft recipients. *Transplantation* (1987) 44, 533–35.
21. Frey FJ, Schnetzer A, Horber FF, Frey BM. Evidence that cyclosporine does not affect the metabolism of prednisolone after renal transplantation. *Transplantation* (1987) 43, 494–8.
22. Rocci ML Jr, Tietze KJ, Lee J, Harris H, Danzeisen J, Burke JF. The effect of cyclosporine on the pharmacokinetics of prednisolone in renal transplant patients. *Transplantation* (1988) 45, 656–60.
23. Hricik DE, Moritz C, Mayes JT, Schulak JA. Association of the absence of steroid therapy with increased cyclosporine blood levels in renal transplant recipients. *Transplantation* (1990) 49, 221–3.
24. Nott D, Griffin PJA, Salaman JR. Low-dose steroids do not augment cyclosporine immunosuppression but do diminish cyclosporine nephrotoxicity. *Transplant Proc* (1985) 17, 1289–90.
25. Henricsson S, Lindholm A, Aravoglou M. Cyclosporin metabolism in human liver microsomes and its inhibition by other drugs. *Pharmacol Toxicol* (1990) 66, 49–52.
26. Sugioka N, Kokuhu T, Okamoto M, Yoshimura N, Ito Y, Shibata N, Takada K. Effect of plasma lipid on pharmacokinetics of ciclosporin and its relationship with plasma prednisolone level in renal transplant patients. *J Pharm Pharmacol* (2006) 58, 1193–200.

Ciclosporin + Coumarins

A case report describes reduced ciclosporin concentrations and reduced warfarin efficacy in patients given both drugs concurrently. A further report describes an increase in serum ciclosporin concentrations when an unnamed anticoagulant was given. Other reports describe increased or decreased acenocoumarol effects and decreased ciclosporin concentrations in two patients given both drugs.

Clinical evidence

(a) Acenocoumarol

The anticoagulant dose of a patient taking acenocoumarol needed to be *reduced* by about half to maintain a therapeutic INR when he was given ciclosporin after a kidney transplant. The required dose of ciclosporin slightly decreased.[1] A patient taking acenocoumarol 32 mg per week was given ciclosporin for nephrotic syndrome. After 10 days his acenocoumarol dose needed to be *increased* to maintain a therapeutic INR, and the ciclosporin concentration was considered too low so the dose was increased from 100 to 150 mg daily. However, a further 10 days later (after the increase in the acenocoumarol dose) the ciclosporin concentration was even lower. Eventually the patient achieved therapeutic concentrations in the presence of acenocoumarol with a ciclosporin dose of 200 mg daily.[2]

(b) Warfarin

A man with erythrocyte aplasia effectively treated with ciclosporin for 18 months, relapsed within a week of starting warfarin. His ciclosporin concentrations had decreased from a range of 300 to 350 nanograms/mL down to 170 nanograms/mL. He responded well when the ciclosporin dose was increased from 3 to 7 mg/kg daily, but his prothrombin activity rose from 17 to 64% and he needed an increase in the warfarin dose to achieve satisfactory anticoagulation.[3] The patient was also taking phenobarbital. A woman with angioimmunoblastic T-cell lymphoma receiving chemotherapy developed a deep vein thrombosis and was therefore given heparin and later warfarin. When ciclosporin 300 mg daily was added, her INR decreased by about 40% and she needed a progressive warfarin dose increase from 18.75 to 27.5 mg per week.[4] Another report briefly states that the serum ciclosporin concentrations increased in a patient given a warfarin derivative.[5]

Mechanism

Unknown. Neither drug is known to affect drug transporters or cytochrome P450 isoenzymes important to the distribution or metabolism of the other drug.

Importance and management

Information about the interactions of the coumarins and ciclosporin seems to be limited to these few reports. Because of the many other factors influencing anticoagulant control, it is not possible to reliably ascribe a change in INR specifically to a drug interaction in a single case report without other supporting evidence. Consider these cases in the event of an unexpected response to treatment.

1. Campistol JM, Maragall D, Andreu J. Interaction between cyclosporin A and sintrom. *Nephron* (1989) 53, 291–2.
2. Borrás-Blasco J, Enriquez R, Navarro-Ruiz A, Martinez-Ramirez M, Cabezuelo JB, Gonzalez-Delgado M. Interaction between cyclosporine and acenocoumarol in a patient with nephrotic syndrome. *Clin Nephrol* (2001) 55, 338–40.
3. Snyder DS. Interaction between cyclosporine and warfarin. *Ann Intern Med* (1988) 108, 311.
4. Turri D, Lannitto E, Caracciolo C, Mariani G. Oral anticoagulants and cyclosporin A. *Haematologica* (2000) 85, 893–4.
5. Cockburn I. Cyclosporin A: a clinical evaluation of drug interactions. *Transplant Proc* (1986) 18 (Suppl 5), 50–5.

Ciclosporin + Cyclophosphamide

Cyclophosphamide was found to reduce ciclosporin concentrations in a retrospective study.

Clinical evidence, mechanism, importance and management

A retrospective study in stem cell transplant patients found that the ciclosporin concentrations in 47 patients whose pre-transplant conditioning regimens contained cyclophosphamide were lower (149.7 nanograms/mL) than those in 56 patients whose regimens did not contain cyclophosphamide (217.3 nanograms/mL). However, there was no difference in the incidence of acute graft versus host disease of grade 2 or higher.[1] The reason for this possible interaction is not understood, and its clinical relevance is uncertain. Further study is needed.

1. Nagamura F, Takahashi T, Takeuchi M, Iseki T, Ooi J, Tomonari A, Uchimaru K, Takahashi S, Tojo A, Tani K, Asano S. Effect of cyclophosphamide on serum cyclosporine levels at the conditioning of hematopoietic stem cell transplantation. *Bone Marrow Transplant* (2003) 32, 1051–8.

Ciclosporin + Danazol

Large increases in ciclosporin concentrations have been reported in patients taking danazol.

Clinical evidence

A 15-year-old girl, one-year post kidney transplant, taking ciclosporin and prednisone, had a large increase in her serum ciclosporin concentrations over about 2 weeks (from a range of 250 to 325 micromol/L up to 680 to 860 micromol/L) when she was given danazol 200 mg twice daily, even though the ciclosporin dose was reduced from 350 to 250 mg daily.[1]

Similar increased ciclosporin concentrations were seen in another patient, from about 400 to 600 nanograms/mL on one occasion, and from 150 to about 450 nanograms/mL on another occasion, over about a 6-week period when danazol 400 mg daily and later 600 mg daily was given.[2] A 12-year-old boy needed a reduction in his ciclosporin dose from 10 to 2 mg/kg daily when danazol 400 mg twice daily was added.[3] A large increase in ciclosporin blood concentrations has been described in 2 other patients when given danazol 200 mg three or four times daily.[4,5]

A pharmacokinetic study in one kidney transplant patient found that danazol 200 mg three times daily given with ciclosporin 120 mg twice daily, reduced the ciclosporin clearance by 50%, prolonged its half-life by 66%, and increased its AUC by 65% when compared with a 20% higher ciclosporin dose of 150 mg twice daily.[6]

A patient with aplastic anaemia taking ciclosporin was given danazol 200 mg daily for pancytopenia and endometriosis. Within 4 days the patient had epigastric pain, and elevated serum ciclosporin and creatinine concentrations. Danazol was stopped and the ciclosporin dose was halved. Two weeks later abrupt severe hepatic injury occurred and the patient died of liver failure, although this was thought to be due to danazol toxicity rather than the interaction.[7]

Mechanism

Uncertain. It has been suggested that danazol increases ciclosporin concentrations by inhibiting its metabolism, possibly by CYP3A4.[3] However, further study is needed to confirm this suggestion.

Importance and management

Although the information seems to be limited to these few reports an interaction between ciclosporin and danazol seems likely. It would therefore seem prudent to monitor the ciclosporin concentration of any patient who is given danazol, with dose adjustments made as necessary.

1. Ross WB, Roberts D, Griffin PJA and Salaman JR. Cyclosporin interaction with danazol and norethisterone. *Lancet* (1986) i, 330.
2. Schröder O, Schmitz N, Kayser W, Euler HH, Löffler H. Erhöhte Ciclosporin-A-spiegel bei gleichzeitiger Therapie mit Danazol. *Dtsch Med Wochenschr* (1986) 111, 602–3.
3. Blatt J, Howrie D, Orlando S. Burckart G. Interaction between cyclosporine and danazol in a pediatric patient. *J Pediatr Hematol Oncol* (1996) 18, 95.
4. Borrás-Blasco J, Rosique-Robles JD, Peris-Marti J, Navarro-Ruiz J, Gonzalez-Delgado M, Conesa-Garcia V. Possible cyclosporin-danazol interaction in a patient with aplastic anaemia. *Am J Hematol* (1999) 62, 63–4.
5. Koneru B, Hartner C, Iwatsuki S, Starzl TE. Effect of danazol on cyclosporine pharmacokinetics. *Transplantation* (1988) 45, 1001.
6. Passfall J, Schuller I, Keller F. Pharmacokinetics of cyclosporin during administration of danazol. *Nephrol Dial Transplant* (1994) 9, 1807–8.
7. Hayashi T, Takahashi T, Minami T, Akaike J, Kasahara K, Adachi M, Hinoda Y, Takahashi S, Hirayama T, Imai K. Fatal acute hepatic failure induced by danazol in a patient with endometriosis and aplastic anemia. *J Gastroenterol* (2001) 36, 783–6.

Ciclosporin + Disopyramide

An isolated report describes the development of nephrotoxicity, which was attributed to an interaction between ciclosporin and disopyramide.

Clinical evidence, mechanism, importance and management

Ten months after receiving a kidney transplant, a 40-year-old woman taking ciclosporin and methylprednisolone developed premature ventricular beats and was given oxprenolol. After 2 months she had shown no improvement so she started taking disopyramide 100 mg three times daily. Over the next week her serum creatinine increased from 88 micromol/L to 159 micromol/L, at which point the disopyramide was stopped, and her renal function returned to normal over the next week. As she had previously been stable taking ciclosporin, and, as nephrotoxicity had not been reported with disopyramide, an interaction was suspected.[1]

This interaction is unconfirmed and of uncertain clinical significance. There is insufficient evidence to recommend increased monitoring, but be aware of the potential for an interaction in the case of an unexpected response to treatment.

1. Nanni G, Magalini SC, Serino F, Castagneto M. Effect of disopyramide in a cyclosporine-treated patient. *Transplantation* (1988) 45, 257.

Ciclosporin + Diuretics

Isolated cases of nephrotoxicity have been described when patients taking ciclosporin were given either amiloride with hydrochlorothiazide, metolazone, or mannitol. The concurrent use of ciclosporin with thiazides, but not loop diuretics, might increase magnesium concentrations. The concurrent use of ciclosporin with potassium-sparing diuretics can cause hyperkalaemia. Eplerenone does not appear to affect the pharmacokinetics of ciclosporin. The use of both ciclosporin and diuretics might increase the risk of hyperuricaemia and gout.

Clinical evidence, mechanism, importance and management

(a) Nephrotoxicity

A 39-year-old man taking ciclosporin, whose second kidney transplant functioned subnormally, and who required treatment for hypertension with atenolol and minoxidil, developed ankle oedema, which was resistant to **furosemide**, despite doses of up to 750 mg daily. When **metolazone** 2.5 mg daily was added for 2 weeks his serum creatinine concentration more than doubled (from 193 to 449 micromol/L). When **metolazone** was stopped the creatinine concentration decreased. His ciclosporin serum concentration was unchanged and neither graft rejection nor hypovolaemia occurred.[1]

The kidney transplant of another patient taking ciclosporin almost ceased to function when **mannitol** was given, and a biopsy indicated severe ciclosporin nephrotoxicity. Transplant function recovered when the **mannitol** was stopped.[2]

A woman taking ciclosporin had an increase in her serum creatinine concentration from 121 to 171 micromol/L three weeks after she started to take *Moduretic* (**amiloride** with **[hydro]chlorothiazide**). Ciclosporin minimum concentrations were unchanged.[3]

One clinical study suggested that furosemide may have a protective effect against ciclosporin-induced nephrotoxicity.[4] These cases appear to be isolated, and their general relevance is unclear.

(b) Magnesium wasting

Although ciclosporin and **loop diuretics** are both known to cause magnesium wasting, a review of magnesium serum concentrations, magnesium replacement doses and diuretic use in 50 heart transplant recipients indicated that magnesium requirements were not altered by the use of ciclosporin with **loop diuretics**. However, the use of **thiazides** with ciclosporin resulted in *increases* in serum magnesium concentrations and decreases in magnesium replacement.[5] Electrolytes, including magnesium, should be monitored as a matter of routine in patients taking ciclosporin with loop or thiazide diuretics.

(c) Hyperkalaemia

No clinically significant pharmacokinetic interaction was noted when **eplerenone** was given with ciclosporin.[6] It has been suggested that aldosterone receptor blockade with **eplerenone** might reduce ciclosporin nephrotoxicity by reducing aldosterone-mediated renal vasoconstriction.[7]

Note that ciclosporin alone can cause hyperkalaemia, especially if renal function is impaired, and the risk might be additive with potassium-sparing drugs. Because of this, the US manufacturers suggest that ciclosporin should not be used with **potassium-sparing diuretics**,[8] whereas the UK manufacturers suggest that caution is required on concurrent use, with close control of potassium concentrations.[9] Very careful monitoring would appear prudent if concurrent use is considered essential.

(d) Hyperuricaemia

Hyperuricaemia is a common adverse effect associated with ciclosporin use.[8,9] A number of studies suggest that the risk of hyperuricaemia might be further increased by the concurrent use of diuretics (only a selection are cited here to illustrate to the risk). One study reported that 90% of kidney transplant patients developed hyperuricaemia when taking ciclosporin in addition to a diuretic, compared with 60% of those taking ciclosporin without a diuretic.[10] Another report found that uric acid levels were 30% higher in kidney transplant patients taking ciclosporin with diuretics (both **loop** and **thiazide diuretics**) compared with those taking ciclosporin without diuretics. Ciclosporin alone increased uric acid concentrations, but only patients taking the combination of diuretics and ciclosporin developed clinical symptoms of gout.[11] These findings demonstrate that the risk of gout is probably increased by the concurrent use of diuretics and ciclosporin and it has been suggested that, in patients at high risk of gout, the continued use of diuretics after the initial stages of transplantation, should be carefully evaluated.[12]

1. Christensen P, Leski M. Nephrotoxic drug interaction between metolazone and cyclosporin. *BMJ* (1987) 294, 578.
2. Brunner FP, Hermle M, Mihatsch MJ, Thiel G. Mannitol potentiates cyclosporine nephrotoxicity. *Clin Nephrol* (1986) 25 (Suppl 1), S130–S136.
3. Deray G, Baumelou B, Le Hoang P, Aupetit B, Girard B, Baumelou A, Legrand JC, Jacobs C. Enhancement of cyclosporin nephrotoxicity by diuretic therapy. *Clin Nephrol* (1989) 32, 47.
4. Driscoll DF, Pinson CW, Jenkins RL, Bistrian BR. Potential protective effects of furosemide against early cyclosporine-induced renal injury in hepatic transplant recipients. *Transplant Proc* (1989) 21, 3549–50.
5. Arthur JM, Shamin S. Interaction of cyclosporine and FK506 with diuretics in transplant patients. *Kidney Int* (2000) 58, 325–30.
6. Cook CS, Berry LM, Burton E. Prediction of in vivo drug interactions with eplerenone in man from in vitro metabolic inhibition data. *Xenobiotica* (2004) 34, 215–28.
7. Pérez-Rojas JM, Bobadilla NA. Acción novedosa de la aldosterona en la nefrotoxicidad por ciclosporina. *Rev Invest Clin* (2005) 57, 147–55.
8. Neoral (Ciclosporin). Novartis Pharmaceuticals Corporation. US Prescribing information, May 2013.
9. Neoral (Ciclosporin). Novartis Pharmaceuticals UK Ltd. UK Summary of product characteristics, February 2012.
10. Lin HY, Rocher LL, McQuillan MA, Schmaltz S, Palella TD, Fox IH. Cyclosporine-induced hyperuricemia and gout. *N Engl J Med* (1989) 321, 287–92.
11. Tiller DJ, Hall BM, Horvarth JS, Duggin GG, Thompson JF, Sheil AGR. Gout and hyperuricaemia in patients on cyclosporin and diuretics. *Lancet* (1985) 1, 453.
12. Stamp L, Ha L, Searle M, O'Donnell J, Frampton C, Chapman P. Gout in renal transplant recipients. *Nephrology (Carlton)* (2006) 11, 367–71.

Ciclosporin + Echinocandins

Ciclosporin appears to slightly increase the exposure to caspofungin, and concurrent use might result in increased liver enzymes. Ciclosporin very slightly increased the exposure to anidulafungin in one study.

Caspofungin does not affect the plasma concentration of ciclosporin. No pharmacokinetic interaction appears to occur between micafungin and ciclosporin.

Clinical evidence, mechanism, importance and management

(a) Anidulafungin

Intravenous anidulafungin 200 mg on day one, then 100 mg daily for 7 days was given to 12 healthy subjects with oral ciclosporin solution (*Neoral*) 1.25 mg/kg twice daily on the last 4 days. Ciclosporin caused a 22% increase in the steady-state AUC of anidulafungin, which was not considered to be clinically relevant. No dose-limiting toxicities or serious adverse events were noted. One subject had a mild increase in liver enzymes on day 6 (after 2 days of concurrent use), and the study drugs were withdrawn at this point.[1]

Anidulafungin is not expected to alter the plasma concentration of ciclosporin, based on an *in vitro* study where anidulafungin had no effect on the metabolism of ciclosporin.[1]

The UK and US manufacturers state that no dose adjustment of either drug is needed on concurrent use.[2,3]

(b) Caspofungin

The UK and US manufacturers report that in two studies in healthy subjects, ciclosporin (a single 4-mg/kg dose or two 3-mg/kg doses 12 hours apart) increased the AUC of caspofungin by 35%. Moreover, 5 of 12 subjects had increases in AST and ALT of up to 3-fold. The liver enzymes returned to normal on discontinuation of both drugs, and during concurrent use the plasma concentration of ciclosporin was not affected.[4-6] These findings led to the exclusion of patients receiving ciclosporin from phase II/III studies of caspofungin.[6] Note that elevated liver enzymes (typically mild and rarely leading to discontinuation) are a common adverse effect of caspofungin alone.[4] More recently, several studies have reported retrospective analyses of the clinical use of caspofungin in more than 100 patients taking ciclosporin.[7-12] No serious hepatic adverse events were found, and some of these studies reported no clinically relevant elevations of liver enzymes;[7,9-11] however, one study found 2 of 40 patients had discontinued treatment because of abnormalities in hepatic enzymes, possibly related to caspofungin and/or ciclosporin.[8] Another study also noted that the elevations observed fell after caspofungin was discontinued.[12] Another retrospective review of 54 patients with invasive aspergillosis found that the concurrent use of caspofungin with ciclosporin for more than 7 days was an independent risk factor for elevated liver enzymes.[13]

Further analysis of the pharmacokinetic data from 7 of 14 patients in one of the above studies[7] additionally found no effect of caspofungin on the pharmacokinetics of ciclosporin. The effect of ciclosporin on the plasma concentration of caspofungin was not studied.[14] Similarly, a study in heart-lung transplant patients found that ciclosporin concentrations in 3 patients did not change during caspofungin treatment.[15] In another study in 12 transplant patients taking ciclosporin, only one required a ciclosporin dose adjustment (no details given) when also given caspofungin.[16]

The UK and US manufacturers of caspofungin state that ciclosporin and caspofungin can be used together if the potential benefit outweighs the risk. If they are used together, close monitoring of liver enzymes is recommended.[4,5]

(c) Micafungin

In a study in 27 healthy subjects, a single 5-mg/kg dose of oral ciclosporin (*Neoral*) was given alone, with a single 100-mg dose of intravenous micafungin, and on the last day of a 5-day course of intravenous micafungin 100 mg daily. Micafungin (at steady state) increased the AUC and half-life of ciclosporin and decreased the mean oral clearance by about 10%. However in five subjects, oral ciclosporin clearance was decreased by about 25% (up to about 60% in two patients with steady-state micafungin).[17] The UK and US manufacturers of micafungin briefly note that in studies in healthy subjects, ciclosporin did not alter the pharmacokinetics of micafungin,[18,19] and the US manufacturer states that single and multiple doses of micafungin did not alter the pharmacokinetics of ciclosporin.[18] No dose adjustments are likely to be necessary on concurrent use.

1. Dowell JA, Stogniew M, Krause D, Henkel T, Weston IE. Assessment of the safety and pharmacokinetics of anidulafungin when administered with cyclosporine. *J Clin Pharmacol* (2005) 45, 227–33.
2. Eraxis (Anidulafungin). Pfizer Injectables. US Prescribing information, November 2013.
3. Ecalta (Anidulafungin). Pfizer Ltd. UK Summary of product characteristics, August 2014.
4. Cancidas (Caspofungin acetate). Merck Sharp & Dohme Ltd. UK Summary of product characteristics, June 2014.
5. Cancidas (Caspofungin acetate). Merck & Co., Inc. US Prescribing information, August 2013.
6. Sable CA, Nguyen B-YT, Chodakewitz JA, DiNubile MJ. Safety and tolerability of caspofungin acetate in the treatment of fungal infections. *Transpl Infect Dis* (2002) 4, 25–30.
7. Sanz-Rodriguez C, Lopez-Duarte M, Jurado M, Lopez J, Arranz R, Cisneros JM, Martino ML, Garcia-Sanchez PJ, Morales P, Olive T, Rovira M, Solano C. Safety of the concomitant use of caspofungin and cyclosporin A in patients with invasive fungal infections. *Bone Marrow Transplant* (2004) 34, 13–20.
8. Marr KA, Hachem R, Papanicolaou G, Somani J, Arduino JM, Lipka CJ, Ngai AL, Kartsonis N, Chodakewitz J, Sable C. Retrospective study of the hepatic safety profile of patients concomitantly treated with caspofungin and cyclosporin A. *Transpl Infect Dis* (2004) 6, 110–16.
9. Glasmacher A, Cornely OA, Orlopp K, Reuter S, Blaschke S, Eichel M, Silling G, Simons B, Egerer G, Siemann M, Florek M, Schnitzler R, Ebeling P, Ritter J, Reinel H, Schutt P, Fischer H, Hahn C, Just-Nuebling G. Caspofungin treatment in severely ill, immunocompromised patients: a case-documentation study of 118 patients. *J Antimicrob Chemother* (2006) 57, 127–34.
10. Saner F, Gensicke J, Rath P, Fruhauf N, Gu Y, Paul A, Radtke A, Malagó M, Broelsch C. Safety profile of concomitant use of caspofungin and cyclosporine or tacrolimus in liver transplant patients. *Infection* (2006) 34, 328–32..
11. Candoni A, Mestroni R, Damiani D, Tiribelli M, Michelutti A, Silvestri F, Castelli M, Viale P, Fanin R. Caspofungin as first line therapy of pulmonary invasive fungal infections in 32 immunocompromised patients with hematological malignancies. *Eur J Haematol* (2006) 75, 227–33.
12. Christopeit M, Eikam M, Behre G. Comedication of caspofungin acetate and cyclosporine A after allogenic haematologic stem cell transplantation leads to negligible hepatotoxicity. *Mycoses* (2008) 51 (Suppl 1), 19–24.
13. Morrissey CO, Slavin MA, O'Reilly MA, Daffy JR, Seymour JF, Schwarer AP, Szer J. Caspofungin as salvage monotherapy for invasive aspergillosis in patients with haematological malignancies or following allogeneic stem cell transplant: efficacy and concomitant cyclosporin A. *Mycoses* (2007) 50 (Suppl 1), 24–37.
14. Sanz-Rodriguez C, Arranz R, Cisneros J-M, Garcia-Sanchez PJ, Jurado M, Lopez J, Olivé T, Solano C. Absence of clinically relevant effect of caspofungin on cyclosporin pharmacokinetics. *Swiss Med Wkly* (2005) 135, 658–9.
15. Groetzner J, Kaczmarek I, Wittwer T, Strauch J, Meiser B, Wahlers T, Daebritz S, Reichart B. Caspofungin as first-line therapy for the treatment of invasive aspergillosis after thoracic organ transplantation. *J Heart Lung Transplant* (2008) 27, 1–6.
16. Veroux M, Macarone M, Fiamingo P, Cappello D, Gagliano M, Di Mare M, Vizcarra D, Spataro M, Giuffrida G, Sorbello M, Severino V, Veroux P. Caspofungin in the treatment of azole-refractory esophageal candidiasis in kidney transplant recipients. *Transplant Proc* (2006) 38, 1037–9.
17. Hebert MF, Townsend RW, Austin S, Balan G, Blough DK, Buell D, Keirns J, Bekersky I. Concomitant cyclosporine and micafungin pharmacokinetics in healthy volunteers. *J Clin Pharmacol* (2005) 45, 954–60.
18. Mycamine (Micafungin sodium). Astellas Pharma US, Inc. US Prescribing information, June 2013.
19. Mycamine (Micafungin sodium). Astellas Pharma Ltd. UK Summary of product characteristics, December 2013.

Ciclosporin + Endothelin receptor antagonists

Bosentan decreases ciclosporin exposure. Ciclosporin greatly increases bosentan exposure, and moderately increases ambrisentan exposure. Ciclosporin has no clinically relevant effect on macitentan exposure. Ambrisentan has no clinically relevant effect on ciclosporin exposure.

Clinical evidence

(a) Ambrisentan

In a study in 28 healthy male subjects, ambrisentan 5 mg daily was given for 14 days, with ciclosporin 100 to 150 mg twice daily on days 6 to 14. Ciclosporin increased the AUC and maximum serum concentration of ambrisentan 2.2-fold and 48%, respectively. In a separate parallel study by the same group, 16 healthy male subjects were given ciclosporin 100 to 150 mg twice daily for 14 days, with the same dose of ambrisentan on days 9 to 14. Ambrisentan increased the AUC and maximum serum concentration of ciclosporin by 10% and 12%, respectively.[1]

(b) Bosentan

In a crossover study designed to assess the effects of bosentan on ciclosporin renal toxicity, 7 healthy male subjects were given bosentan 500 mg and ciclosporin 300 mg, both twice daily, for 7 days. Bosentan did maintain renal plasma flow, which is decreased by ciclosporin. However, bosentan was calculated to have decreased the AUC of ciclosporin by about 50%. In addition, bosentan had no effect on the ciclosporin-induced increase in blood pressure, and headache, nausea, and, vomiting were a problem with the combination. Moreover, the steady-state AUC of bosentan was increased by 70%, when compared with the AUC of a single dose of bosentan.[2]

It should be noted that bosentan induces its own metabolism, and after 7 days, plasma concentrations are about 50 to 65% of those seen after a single dose.[3] Therefore, the effect of ciclosporin on the AUC of bosentan might be twice that described in this study (i.e. up to a 4-fold increase in the AUC of bosentan). The UK and US manufacturers of bosentan state that when bosentan is given with ciclosporin, its plasma concentration is greatly increased (30-fold after a single dose and 3- to 4-fold at steady state).[3,4]

(c) Macitentan

In a crossover study, 10 healthy male subjects were given macitentan 30 mg on day 1 followed by 10 mg daily, with ciclosporin 200 mg daily from day 6 to 17. The minimum plasma concentration and AUC of macitentan were increased by 38% and 10%, respectively.[5]

Mechanism

Uncertain. Bosentan probably decreases ciclosporin concentrations because it is an inducer of CYP3A4, by which ciclosporin is metabolised. Ciclosporin is not a clinically relevant inhibitor of CYP3A4, by which bosentan is partly metabolised, and therefore another mechanism must be involved. *In vitro* study shows that ciclosporin inhibits the hepatic uptake of bosentan by the organic anion transporting polypeptides (OATPs), and this might explain the interaction.[6] The UK manufacturer lists ciclosporin as an example of a drug, like bosentan, that inhibits the bile salt export pump, and is therefore expected to increase the risk of liver toxicity when used with bosentan.[3]

Importance and management

Although the data are limited, a pharmacokinetic interaction between **bosentan** and ciclosporin would appear to be established, resulting in decreased ciclosporin concentrations, and greatly increased bosentan concentrations. Because of this, the UK and US manufacturers of bosentan contraindicate concurrent use.[3,4] In addition, the UK manufacturer of bosentan also states that the concurrent use of ciclosporin might increase the risk of liver toxicity.[3]

Other endothelin receptor antagonists are less well studied, but the UK and US manufacturers of **ambrisentan** state that the dose of ambrisentan should be limited to 5 mg daily in patients also given ciclosporin and that patients should be closely monitored.[7,8] Ciclosporin dose adjustments do not appear to be necessary. The negligible increase in **macitentan** exposure is unlikely to be clinically important and no dose adjustment is necessary on concurrent use with ciclosporin.

1. Spence R, Mandagere A, Richards DB, Magee MH, Dufton C, Boinpally R. Potential for pharmacokinetic interactions between ambrisentan and cyclosporine. *Clin Pharmacol Ther* (2010) 88, 513–20.
2. Binet I, Wallnöfer A, Weber C, Jones R, Thiel G. Renal hemodynamics and pharmacokinetics of bosentan with and without cyclosporine A. *Kidney Int* (2000) 57, 224–31.
3. Tracleer (Bosentan monohydrate). Actelion Pharmaceuticals UK Ltd. UK Summary of product characteristics, September 2013.
4. Tracleer (Bosentan). Actelion Pharmaceuticals US, Inc. US Prescribing information, October 2012.
5. Bruderer S, Äänismaa P, Homery MC, Häusler S, Landskroner K, Sidharta PN, Treiber A, Dingemanse J. Effect of cyclosporine and rifampin on the pharmacokinetics of macitentan, a tissue-targeting dual endothelin receptor antagonist. *AAPS J* (2012) 14, 68–78.
6. Treiber A, Schneiter R, Häusler S, Stieger B. Bosentan is a substrate of human OATP1B1 and OATP1B3: inhibition of hepatic uptake as the common mechanism of its interactions with cyclosporin A, rifampicin, and sildenafil. *Drug Metab Dispos* (2007) 35, 1400–7.
7. Volibris (Ambrisentan). GlaxoSmithKline UK. UK Summary of product characteristics, September 2014.
8. Letairis (Ambrisentan). Gilead Sciences, Inc. US Prescribing information, May 2014.

Ciclosporin + Epoetins

It has been suggested that epoetin alfa might alter ciclosporin concentrations.

Clinical evidence, mechanism, importance and management

Some UK manufacturers of epoetin alfa state that, because ciclosporin is bound by red blood cells, there is potential for a drug interaction. They recommend that if epoetin alfa is given, ciclosporin concentrations should be monitored and the ciclosporin dose adjusted as the haematocrit increases.[1,2]

This is a theoretical interaction, and there does not appear to be any published data to suggest that an interaction occurs in practice, and the manufacturers of other epoetins make no mention of such an interaction. Furthermore, it seems likely that any increase in the haematocrit will be sufficiently slow that any interaction would be picked up by routine ciclosporin monitoring.

1. Eprex Pre-filled Syringe (Epoetin alfa). Janssen-Cilag Ltd. UK Summary of product characteristics, November 2012.
2. Binocrit (Epoetin alfa). Sandoz Ltd. UK Summary of product characteristics, July 2013.

Ciclosporin + Ethambutol

Some case reports suggest that ethambutol does not interact with ciclosporin whereas others, usually also involving other drugs, have described alterations in ciclosporin concentrations.

Clinical evidence, mechanism, importance and management

Case reports describe the uneventful use of ethambutol (with isoniazid and/or a range of other antitubercular drugs) for the treatment of tuberculosis in patients taking ciclosporin after heart transplants.[1,2] Successful treatment of tuberculosis in heart and kidney transplant patients has also been reported using isoniazid, ethambutol, pyrazinamide, and streptomycin, see 'Ciclosporin + Pyrazinamide', p.1239. However, one case report describes a patient who had a gradual increase in ciclosporin serum concentrations (from 250 to 400 micrograms/L) when isoniazid and ethambutol were stopped.[3]

Evidence regarding an interaction between ethambutol and ciclosporin is very limited and the picture is often masked by the presence of other drugs. On balance, an interaction between ethambutol and ciclosporin seems unlikely.

1. Aguado JM, Herrero JA, Gavaldá J, Torre-Cisneros J, Blanes M, Rufí G, Moreno A, Gurguí A, Hayek M, Lumbreras C and the Spanish Transplantation Infection Study Group, GESITRA. Clinical presentation and outcome of tuberculosis in kidney, liver, and heart transplant recipients in Spain. *Transplantation* (1997) 63, 1276–86.
2. Muñoz P, Palomo J, Muños R, Rodríguez-Creixéms M, Pelaez T, Bouza E. Tuberculosis in heart transplant recipients. *Clin Infect Dis* (1995) 21, 398–402.
3. Leimenstoll G, Schlegelberger T, Fulde R, Niedermayer W. Interaktion von Ciclosporin und Ethambutol-Isoniazid. *Dtsch Med Wochenschr* (1988) 113, 514–15.

Ciclosporin + Fibrates

The use of bezafibrate with ciclosporin has resulted in significantly increased serum creatinine concentrations. Reductions, no change, or increased ciclosporin concentrations have also been seen. The use of fenofibrate has also been associated with reduced renal function and possibly reduced ciclosporin concentrations. Three studies found no pharmacokinetic interaction between ciclosporin and gemfibrozil while a fourth found gemfibrozil caused a reduction in ciclosporin concentrations and an increase in serum creatinine in some patients.

Clinical evidence

(a) Bezafibrate

A kidney transplant patient had an increase in his previously stable ciclosporin blood concentrations from a range of 150 to 200 nanograms/mL to about 340 nanograms/mL over a 6-week period after bezafibrate 200 mg twice daily was given. The increase was accompanied by increases in blood urea nitrogen and creatinine concentrations. Renal biopsy found evidence of possible ciclosporin toxicity, and rejection. The patient recovered when the bezafibrate was stopped.[1]

Two other transplant patients (one kidney and the other heart) had a reversible deterioration in renal function when they were given bezafibrate. This was severe in one, and it occurred on two occasions in the other patient. Neither had any changes in ciclosporin blood concentrations.[2,3] Two other similar cases have been reported, one of whom was subsequently given gemfibrozil without problems.[4]

Another study over 3 months in 40 heart transplant patients taking ciclosporin found that bezafibrate was associated with an increase in serum creatinine concentrations, although none of the patients had to be withdrawn from the study. The ciclosporin concentration tended to be lower (198 nanograms/mL at baseline, compared with 144 nanograms/mL after 3 months).[5]

(b) Fenofibrate

In a study in 10 heart transplant patients, fenofibrate 200 mg daily for 2 weeks effectively reduced the blood cholesterol concentrations from 7.7 to 6.5 mmol/L without particularly altering ciclosporin blood concentrations over a 2-week period. The only possible adverse effect was an increase in creatinine concentrations from 145 to 157 mmol/L, suggesting some possible nephrotoxicity. No other clinically adverse effects were seen. However, the authors of this study suggested that longer follow-up studies were needed to confirm the safety of using these drugs together.[6] They followed this up with a one-year study[7] in 43 heart transplant patients, only 14 of whom completed the study (67% withdrew for various reasons). Fourteen patients had an increase in blood creatinine concentrations and a decrease in renal function, which improved when the fenofibrate was stopped. There was also some evidence of a reduction in ciclosporin concentrations in 5 patients, who developed rejection, and 14 patients, who had to stop fenofibrate because ciclosporin concentrations could not be maintained without adversely affecting renal function.

(c) Gemfibrozil

Forty kidney transplant patients taking ciclosporin had a reduction in hypertriglyceridaemia when gemfibrozil 900 mg daily for 6 months or 600 mg twice daily for 4 months was added, and their ciclosporin blood concentrations and serum creatinine concentrations remained unaltered.[8] Two other studies similarly found that gemfibrozil did not affect ciclosporin blood concentrations.[9,10]

In contrast to these findings, another study in 7 kidney transplant patients with hyperlipidaemia found that gemfibrozil 450 mg once or twice daily was associated with a decline in minimum ciclosporin concentrations. Concentrations decreased from 93 to 76 nanograms/mL after 6 weeks of concurrent use, and after dose increases in 3 patients, the concentration at 3 months was 88 nanograms/mL. In 8 similar patients not given gemfibrozil, and with the same ciclosporin dose throughout, minimum concentrations changed from 99 to 98 nanograms/mL at 6 weeks and to 123 nanograms/mL at 3 months. In 2 patients there was a significant increase in serum creatinine, and biopsy revealed chronic rejection in one and ciclosporin toxicity in the other. The study was stopped at 6 months because a drug interaction was suspected.[11]

Mechanism

The mechanism of the interaction between ciclosporin and the fibrates is not known, but changes in distribution of lipoproteins during treatment with fibrates might cause changes in the free fraction of ciclosporin. Ciclosporin absorption might also be reduced.

Importance and management

Neither the incidence nor the reasons for the interactions between ciclosporin and the fibrates are known, but because the outcome is uncertain and potentially serious, closely monitor the effects of adding a fibrate, particularly bezafibrate or fenofibrate, to ciclosporin in any patient. The UK and US manufacturers of ciclosporin suggest close monitoring of renal function during concurrent use, and a dose reduction or withdrawal of the fibrate should significant impairment occur.[12,13]

1. Hirai M, Tatuso E, Sakurai M, Ichikawa M, Matsuya F, Saito Y. Elevated blood concentrations of cyclosporine and kidney failure after bezafibrate in renal graft recipient. *Ann Pharmacother* (1996) 30, 883–4.
2. Lipkin GW, Tomson CRV. Severe reversible renal failure with bezafibrate. *Lancet* (1993) 341, 371.
3. Jespersen B, Tvedegaard E. Bezafibrate induced reduction of renal function in a renal transplant recipient. *Nephrol Dial Transplant* (1995) 10, 702–3.
4. Devuyst O, Goffin E, Pirson Y, van Ypersele de Strihou C. Creatinine rise after fibrate therapy in renal graft recipients. *Lancet* (1993) 341, 840.
5. Barbir M, Hunt B, Kushwaha S, Kehely A, Prescot R, Thompson GR, Mitchell A, Yacoub M. Maxepa versus bezafibrate in hyperlipidemic cardiac transplant recipients. *Am J Cardiol* (1992) 70, 1596–1601.
6. deLorgeril M, Boissonnat P, Bizollon CA, Guidollet J, Faucon G, Guichard JP, Levy-Prades-Sauron R, Renaud S, Dureau G. Pharmacokinetics of cyclosporine in hyperlipidaemic long-term survivors of heart transplantation. Lack of interaction with the lipid-lowering agent, fenofibrate. *Eur J Clin Pharmacol* (1992) 43, 161–5.
7. Boissonnat P, Salen P, Guidollet J, Ferrara R, Dureau G, Ninet J, Renaud S, de Lorgeril M. The long-term effects of the lipid-lowering agent fenofibrate in hyperlipidemic heart transplant recipients. *Transplantation* (1994) 58, 245–7.
8. Pisanti N, Stanziale P, Imperatore P, D'Alessandro R, De Marino V, Capone D, De Marino V. Lack of effect of gemfibrozil on cyclosporine blood concentrations in kidney-transplanted patients. *Am J Nephrol* (1998) 18, 199–203.
9. Valino RN, Reiss WG, Hanes D, White M, Hoehn-Saric E, Klassen D, Bartlett S, Weir MR. Examination of the potential interaction between HMG-CoA reductase inhibitors and cyclosporine in transplant patients. *Pharmacotherapy* (1996) 16, 511.
10. Pflugfelder PW, Huff M, Oskalns R, Rudas L, Kostuk WJ. Cholesterol-lowering therapy after heart transplantation: a 12-month randomized trial. *J Heart Lung Transplant* (1995) 14, 613–22.
11. Fehrman-Ekholm I, Jogestrand T, Angelin B. Decreased cyclosporine levels during gemfibrozil treatment of hyperlipidemia after kidney transplantation. *Nephron* (1996) 72, 483.
12. Neoral (Ciclosporin). Novartis Pharmaceuticals UK Ltd. UK Summary of product characteristics, February 2012.
13. Neoral (Ciclosporin). Novartis Pharmaceuticals Corporation. US Prescribing information, May 2013.

Ciclosporin + Food

Food can slightly decrease the bioavailability of ciclosporin from the *Neoral* formulation and slightly increase the bioavailability of ciclosporin from the *Cicloral* formulation. Lipid admixtures for parenteral nutrition appear not to affect intravenous ciclosporin pharmacokinetics.

Clinical evidence

(a) Oral ciclosporin

1. Food or Milk. In early studies with oral ciclosporin,[1] presumably the *Sandimmun* formulation, food and milk increased its bioavailability. For example, patients taking ciclosporin with milk had a 39% higher AUC after food and 23% higher AUC when fasting, compared with other patients taking ciclosporin with orange juice (which is known not to interact, see 'Ciclosporin + Grapefruit and other fruit juices', p.1229). In another study, food more than doubled the AUC of ciclosporin (bioavailability increased from about 21% to 79%).[2] Similarly, when 18 patients with kidney transplants were given ciclosporin mixed with 240 mL of chocolate milk and taken with a standard hospital breakfast, their ciclosporin maximum concentrations increased by 31% (from 1120 to 1465 nanograms/mL), minimum blood concentrations increased by 17% (from 228 to 267 nanograms/mL), and the AUC increased by 45%. Very considerable individual variations occurred.[3]

The *Neoral* formulation was developed to increase ciclosporin bioavailability and reduce variability in absorption,[4] and has now replaced the oral *Sandimmun* formulation. The *Neoral* formulation is less affected by food,[4] and this has been demonstrated in a study in healthy subjects that found that a high-fat meal decreased the AUC of ciclosporin by a very slight 15% and decreased its maximum concentration by 26%, when compared with fasting conditions.[5] Another study, in patients with psoriasis given *Neoral*, found that the AUC and maximum concentration of ciclosporin were 57% and 74% lower when given after food and the pharmacokinetics across the group showed greater variability, when compared with dosing before food.[6] However, a small study examining the effect of fat content on ciclosporin exposure in kidney transplant patients taking *Neoral* found only minor, statistically insignificant effects.[7]

Other ciclosporin formulations also show improved pharmacokinetics in relation to food, with a study in 12 healthy subjects taking the *Cicloral* formulation finding that the AUC and maximum concentration of ciclosporin were increased by only 21% and 32% when the capsules were taken immediately after a fat-rich breakfast when compared with the fasting state.[8]

Other studies, in which the formulation of ciclosporin was not stated, found little clinically relevant difference in ciclosporin exposure in those given high-fat or low-fat diets[9] and in those given a low-cholesterol, normal-protein diet or a low-cholesterol, high-protein diet.[10]

2. Soft drinks. A lung transplant patient taking ciclosporin had large variations in his ciclosporin concentrations, which ranged between 319 and 761 nanograms/mL, on discharge from hospital, which were unexplained by changes in his current medication or ciclosporin dose changes. It was found that on the days when the ciclosporin concentrations were increased, the patient had drunk a citrus soft drink (*Sun Drop*) at breakfast. These fluctuations resolved when he stopped drinking the soft drink.[11] However, a subsequent pharmacokinetic study in 12 healthy subjects found that neither *Sun Drop* nor another citrus soft drink, *Fresca*, had any significant effects on the pharmacokinetics of a single 2.5-mg/kg dose of ciclosporin. Both *Sun Drop* and *Fresca* were tested, and found to contain bergamottin 0.078 and 6.5 mg/L, respectively (note that grapefruit contains about 5.6 mg/L). The authors note that factors such as genetic and disease-related variability in ciclosporin metabolism as well as changes in the bergamottin content between batches of the drinks may account for the contrasting results.[12] For more discussion about the effects of grapefruit and other fruit juices see also 'Ciclosporin + Grapefruit and other fruit juices', p.1229.

(b) Intravenous ciclosporin

A study in 10 patients undergoing bone-marrow transplantation and given isocaloric and isonitrogenous parenteral nutrition with or without lipids found that ciclosporin pharmacokinetics after intravenous administration were not affected by lipid-enriched admixtures.[13]

Mechanism

The *Neoral* formulation of ciclosporin contains ethanol as a volatile cosolvent, and undergoes a microemulsification process with fluid in the gastrointestinal tract; therefore, its absorption is less affected by food than the old oral *Sandimmun* formulation.[4] The authors of the report of an interaction with a citrus soda drink confirmed with the manufacturers that it contained furanocoumarins such as bergamottin which are thought to inhibit CYP3A4,[11,12] the major isoenzyme involved in the metabolism of ciclosporin. Compare also 'Ciclosporin + Grapefruit and other fruit juices', below.

Importance and management

Food has a minor effect on the extent of absorption of ciclosporin from the *Neoral* formulation although the timing of administration in relation to food can still result in a variability in its pharmacokinetics. The US the manufacturer recommends that ciclosporin should be taken on a consistent schedule in relation to time of day and meals,[14] and there is some evidence to support this suggestion. However, in the UK the manufacturer makes no reference to timing in relation to meals.[4] Similarly, the effect of absorption of ciclosporin from the *Cicloral* formulation is minimal, but the authors of the study suggest that it should be taken on a consistent schedule in relation to time of day and meals.[8]

Lipid admixtures in parenteral nutrition do not appear to affect ciclosporin pharmacokinetics and it is speculated that they might protect against ciclosporin-induced nephrotoxicity. Close supervision and monitoring is required. There is insufficient evidence to allow extrapolation of the results to bone-marrow transplant recipients with risk factors such as dyslipidaemia, or liver or renal impairment.[13]

The isolated report[11] of an interaction between a citrus soft drink (containing furanocoumarins) and ciclosporin was not confirmed by a subsequent single-dose pharmacokinetic study in healthy subjects[12] and therefore its significance is unclear. The case does highlight the influence diet can have on ciclosporin and it should be borne in mind should any unexpected changes in ciclosporin concentrations occur.

1. Keogh A, Day R, Critchley L, Duggin G, Baron D. The effect of food and cholestyramine on the absorption of cyclosporine in cardiac transplant recipients. *Transplant Proc* (1988) 20, 27–30.
2. Gupta SK, Manfro RC, Tomlanovich SJ, Gambertoglio JG, Garovoy MR, Benet LZ. Effect of food on the pharmacokinetics of cyclosporine in healthy subjects following oral and intravenous administration. *J Clin Pharmacol* (1990) 30. 643–53.
3. Ptachcinski RJ, Venkataramanan R, Rosenthal JT, Burckart GJ, Taylor RJ, Hakala TR. The effect of food on cyclosporine absorption. *Transplantation* (1985) 40, 174–6.
4. Neoral (Ciclosporin). Novartis Pharmaceuticals UK Ltd. UK Summary of product characteristics, February 2012.
5. Mueller EA, Kovarik JM, van Bree JB, Grevel J, Lücker PW, Kutz K. Influence of a fat-rich meal on the pharmacokinetics of a new oral formulation of cyclosporine in a crossover comparison with the market formulation. *Pharm Res* (1994) 11 151–5.
6. Umezawa Y, Mabuchi T, Ozawa A. Preprandial vs. postprandial pharmacokinetics of cyclosporine in patients with psoriasis. *Int J Dermatol* (2007) 46 880–82.
7. Klauser RM, Irschik H, Kletzmayr J, Sturm I, Brunner W, Woloszczuk W, Kovarik J. Pharmacokinetic cyclosporine A profiles under long-term Neoral treatment in renal transplant recipients: does fat intake still matter? *Transplant Proc* (1997) 29, 3137–40.
8. Kees F, Mair G, Dittmar M, Bucher M. Cicloral versus Neoral: a bioequivalence study in healthy volunteers on the influence of a fat-rich meal on the bioavailability of Cicloral. *Transplant Proc* (2004) 36, 3234–8.
9. Tan KKC, Trull AK, Uttridge JA, Metcalfe S, Heyes CS, Facey S, Evans DB. Effect of dietary fat on the pharmacokinetics and pharmacodynamics of cyclosporine in kidney transplant recipients. *Clin Pharmacol Ther* (1995) 57, 425–33.
10. Borges W, González Caraballo Z, Santiago Delpín EA, Morales Otero L. Chronic effect of a high-protein low-fat diet in transplant patients. *Transplant Proc* (1996) 28, 3400–3401.
11. Johnston PE, Milstone A. Probable interaction of bergamottin and cyclosporine in a lung transplant recipient. *Transplantation* (2005) 79, 746.
12. Schwarz UI, Johnston PE, Bailey DG, Kim RB, Mayo G, Milstone A. Impact of citrus soft drinks relative to grapefruit juice on ciclosporin disposition. *Br J Clin Pharmacol* (2006) 62, 485–91.
13. Santos P, Lourenço R, Camilo ME, Oliveira AG, Figueira I, Pereira ME, Ferreira B, Carmo JA, Lacerda JMF. Parenteral nutrition and cyclosporine: do lipids make a difference? A prospective randomized crossover trial. *Clin Nutr* (2001) 20, 31–6.
14. Neoral (Ciclosporin). Novartis Pharmaceuticals Corporation. US Prescribing information, May 2013.

Ciclosporin + Foscarnet

Acute but reversible renal failure occurred in two transplant patients when foscarnet was given with ciclosporin.

Clinical evidence

A man with a kidney transplant taking corticosteroids and ciclosporin developed a cytomegalovirus infection that was treated with foscarnet 85 mg/kg daily. Despite efforts to minimise the nephrotoxic effects of foscarnet (hydration with 2.5 litres of isotonic saline daily and nifedipine 80 mg the day before and during treatment) the patient developed non-oliguric worsening of his renal function after 8 days. Nine days after stopping foscarnet, the former renal function was restored.[1]

A liver transplant patient taking steroids, azathioprine, and ciclosporin was given foscarnet 180 mg/kg daily for a hepatitis B infection. Acute renal failure occurred 5 days after the foscarnet was started, and renal function was restored 10 days after the foscarnet was stopped. The ciclosporin blood concentrations were therapeutic and not significantly altered at any time in either patient.[1]

Mechanism

Not understood. It seems that the nephrotoxic effects of ciclosporin and foscarnet could be additive.

Importance and management

Direct information appears to be limited to this report, but it is consistent with the known potential toxicity of both ciclosporin and foscarnet. Acute renal failure can clearly occur despite the preventative measures taken. The authors of this report[1] state that monitoring of renal function is mandatory when both drugs are given.

1. Morales JM, Muñoz MA, Fernández Zatarain G, Garcia Cantón C, García Rubiales MA, Andrés A, Aguado JM, Pinto IG. Reversible acute renal failure caused by the combined use of foscarnet and cyclosporin in organ transplanted patients. *Nephrol Dial Transplant* (1995) 10, 882–3.

Ciclosporin + *Geum chiloense*

A single case report describes a large, rapid increase in the ciclosporin concentrations of a man after he drank an infusion of *Geum chiloense*.

Clinical evidence, mechanism, importance and management

A 54-year-old kidney transplant patient taking ciclosporin, prednisone, azathioprine, diltiazem, and nifedipine had a sudden, large increase in his ciclosporin concentrations from his usual range of 60 to 90 [nanograms/mL] up to a range of 469 to 600 [nanograms/mL]. He had been taking ciclosporin 2 to 3 mg/kg daily for 15 months since the transplant. His serum creatinine concentration was found to be 115 micromol/L. It eventually turned out that about 2 weeks earlier he had started to drink an infusion of *Geum chiloense* (or *Geum quellyon*), a herbal remedy claimed to increase virility and to treat prostatism. When the herbal remedy was stopped, his serum ciclosporin concentrations rapidly returned to their usual values. The reasons for this apparent interaction are not known.[1]

This appears to be the only case on record but it serves, along with reports about other herbs, to emphasise that herbal remedies may not be safe just because they are 'natural'. In this instance the herbal remedy greatly increased the potential nephrotoxicity of the ciclosporin. Patients should be warned.

1. Duclos J, Goecke H. "Hierba del clavo" *(Geum chiloense)* interfiere niveles de ciclosporin: potencial riesgo para trasplantados. *Rev Med Chil* (2001) 129, 789–90.

Ciclosporin + Grapefruit and other fruit juices

Grapefruit juice, and possibly pomelo juice, but not cranberry or orange juices, can increase the bioavailability of oral ciclosporin. Purple grape juice reduced the bioavailability of ciclosporin in one study.

Clinical evidence

(a) Cranberry juice

In a single-dose study in healthy subjects, cranberry juice 240 mL did not have any effects on ciclosporin pharmacokinetics when given at the same time as ciclosporin (*Neoral*).[1]

(b) Grapefruit juice

Many single and multiple-dose pharmacokinetic studies in healthy subjects,[2-5] transplant recipients,[6-11] and other patients with autoimmune diseases[12,13] have shown that if oral ciclosporin is taken at the same time as 150 to 250 mL (5 to 8 ozs) of grapefruit juice, the minimum and maximum blood concentrations and the bioavailability of ciclosporin can be greatly increased. The increases reported vary considerably: increases in minimum blood concentrations range from about 15 to 85%,[6,8-11,13] increases in maximum blood concentrations range from 4 to 43%,[2-4,7-11,13] and increases in AUCs range from about 15 to 59%.[2-4,7-11,13,14] In one other study where grapefruit juice was given every 3 hours for 30 hours, with a dose of ciclosporin given at 7.5 hours, separated by 1.5 hours from the grapefruit juice, the maximum concentrations of ciclosporin increased by 22% and the AUC by just 7% (not statistically significant).[15] Where stated, these studies were with the original *Sandimmun* formulation of ciclosporin.

A few studies have looked at the effect of grapefruit juice on the microemulsion formulation of ciclosporin (*Neoral*) in healthy subjects[14,16] or transplant patients.[17,18] In these studies, when grapefruit juice was taken at the same time as ciclosporin, the AUC was increased by 25 to 47% and the maximum concentrations were largely unchanged (2 to 10% increase). In one study using an intravenous control, grapefruit juice increased the bioavailability of ciclosporin from 38% to 55%.[14] A further study found a greater effect in African-American subjects: the maximum concentrations and AUC were increased by 39% and 60%, respectively, compared with smaller increases of 8% and 44% in Caucasian subjects.[16]

In a study comparing two oral liquid formulations in 6 paediatric kidney transplant patients, giving ciclosporin oral solution (*Sandimmun*) simultaneously with grapefruit juice produced a large increase (109%) in the 12-hour minimum concentration although the AUC was not changed. When ciclosporin was given as the microemulsion (*Neoral*), grapefruit juice did not affect the pharmacokinetics of ciclosporin.[19]

Grapefruit juice has no effect on ciclosporin concentrations when the ciclosporin is given *intravenously*.[3]

(c) Orange juices

In single-dose studies in healthy subjects, ciclosporin concentrations and/or exposure were unaffected by simultaneous administration of orange juice,[2,5,20,21] tangerine juice,[20,22] or Seville (bitter) orange juice.[4]

(d) Pomelo juice

In a single-dose study in 12 healthy subjects, pomelo juice 240 mL increased the AUC and maximum concentration of ciclosporin by about 19% and 12%, respectively, when given at the same time as the ciclosporin (*Neoral*).[1]

(e) Purple grape juice

In a single-dose study in 12 healthy subjects, 200-mL of purple grape juice (pasteurised juice from 3 varieties of *Vitis labrusca*) decreased the AUC and maximum concentration of a single 200-mg dose of ciclosporin by 30% and 28%, respectively, but did not alter its half-life, when taken at the same time as the ciclosporin.[23]

Mechanism

Grapefruit juice inhibits intestinal CYP3A4. Ciclosporin is primarily metabolised by CYP3A4 and so its bioavailability increases; however, because grapefruit juice has minor effects on hepatic CYP3A4 this effect is not seen with intravenous use of ciclosporin. A number of active constituents of grapefruit juice have been suggested, but it is probably the furanocoumarins (which include bergamottin and 6',7'-dihydroxybergamottin) that are responsible for this interaction because a furanocoumarin-free grapefruit juice did not interact.[5] Another *in vitro* study suggested that 6',7'-dihydroxybergamottin is not responsible.[4] More study is needed.

Pomelo is related to grapefruit and therefore potentially interacts by the same mechanism. The effect of purple grape juice is the opposite of that seen with grapefruit juice, and the exact mechanism is not known. The authors of the study suggest that the effect is due to reduced absorption rather than an effect on metabolism, and suggest that induction of CYP3A4 and/or P-glycoprotein in the gut, possibly by polyphenolic compounds found in the juice, might have been involved.[23] See also 'Ciclosporin + Alcohol', p.1205, for discussion of a similar effect seen with *red wine*.

Importance and management

The interaction between grapefruit juice and ciclosporin is established and clinically important, and results in increases in the bioavailability of oral ciclosporin. Patients taking ciclosporin should be warned about drinking grapefruit juice because increased ciclosporin concentrations are associated with increased nephrotoxicity. In general, grapefruit juice should be avoided. It has been suggested that separation of administration could minimise this interaction. However, apart from one study,[15] all the data relate to drinking grapefruit juice around the same time as taking the ciclosporin dose. The study that separated administration (by 1.5 hours) still found a minor interaction. However, in this study a large quantity of grapefruit juice was consumed over 30 hours, and the study did not test simultaneous administration for comparison. It is therefore unclear if separation of administration would reduce or negate the effect of grapefruit juice on ciclosporin.

It has been suggested[2] that the interaction between grapefruit juice and ciclosporin could be exploited to save money. One group of authors has suggested that grapefruit juice is roughly as effective as diltiazem in increasing ciclosporin blood concentrations, and has the advantage of being inexpensive, nutritious, and lacking the systemic effects of diltiazem and ketoconazole which have been used in this way. However, it has also been pointed out that it might be risky to try to exploit this interaction because the increases appear to be so variable and difficult, if not impossible, to control. This is because batches of grapefruit juice vary so much, and also considerable patient variation occurs with this interaction.[24-26] Grapefruit juice has been used to improve ciclosporin efficacy in two patients with psoriasis[27] and four patients with autoimmune haematological disorders.[4]

The US manufacturer suggests that patients taking ciclosporin should avoid **whole grapefruit**, as well as the juice.[28]

The general importance of the single report of the small increases in ciclosporin bioavailability and blood concentrations seen with pomelo juice in healthy subjects is unclear.[1] However, a similar interaction has been seen in a kidney transplant patient taking tacrolimus, see 'Tacrolimus + Grapefruit and other fruit juices', p.1296. There is insufficient evidence to recommend avoiding pomelo juice or pomelo fruit when taking ciclosporin but bear this potential interaction in mind. More study is needed. Similarly, the importance of the *reduction* in bioavailability of ciclosporin seen with purple grape juice in one study is also unclear. The authors suggest that subtherapeutic ciclosporin concentrations could occur as a result of this interaction and so concurrent use should be discouraged, adding that an interval of at least 2 hours should be observed between ciclosporin dosing and purple grape juice intake.[23] However, there is insufficient evidence to support this suggestion. Until more is known, it would be prudent to bear this potential interaction in mind.

Both cranberry juice and orange juices do not appear to interact with ciclosporin.

1. Grenier J, Fradette C, Morelli G, Merritt GJ, Vranderick M, Ducharme MP. Pomelo juice, but not cranberry juice, affects the pharmacokinetics of cyclosporine in humans. *Clin Pharmacol Ther* (2006) 79, 255–62.
2. Yee GC, Stanley DL, Pessa LJ, Costa TD, Beltz SE, Ruiz J, Lowenthal DT. Effect of grapefruit juice on blood cyclosporine concentration. *Lancet* (1995) 345, 955–6.
3. Ducharme MP, Warbasse LH, Edwards DJ. Disposition of intravenous and oral cyclosporine after administration with grapefruit juice. *Clin Pharmacol Ther* (1995) 57, 485–91.
4. Edwards DJ, Fitzsimmons ME, Schuetz EG, Yasuda K, Ducharme MP, Warbasse LH, Woster PM, Schuetz JD, Watkins P. 6',7'-dihydroxybergamottin in grapefruit juice and Seville orange juice: effects on cyclosporine disposition, enterocyte CYP3A4, and P-glycoprotein. *Clin Pharmacol Ther* (1999) 65, 237–44.
5. Paine MF, Widmer WW, Pusek SN, Beavers KL, Criss AB, Snyder J, Watkins PB. Further characterization of a furanocoumarin-free grapefruit juice on drug disposition: studies with cyclosporine. *Am J Clin Nutr* (2008) 87, 863–71.
6. Ducharme MP, Provenzano R, Dehoorne-Smith M, Edwards DJ. Trough concentrations of cyclosporine in blood following administration with grapefruit juice. *Br J Clin Pharmacol* (1993) 36, 457–9.
7. Herlitz H, Edgar B, Hedner T, Lidman K, Karlberg I. Grapefruit juice: a possible source of variability in blood concentration of cyclosporin A. *Nephrol Dial Transplant* (1993) 8, 375.
8. Proppe DG, Hoch OD, McLean AJ, Visser KE. Influence of chronic ingestion of grapefruit juice on steady-state blood concentrations of cyclosporine A in renal transplant patients with stable graft function. *Br J Clin Pharmacol* (1995) 39, 337–8.
9. Min DI, Ku Y-M, Perry PJ, Ukah FO, Ashton K, Martin MF, Hunsicker LG. Effect of grapefruit juice on cyclosporine pharmacokinetics in renal transplant patients. *Transplantation* (1996) 62, 123–5.
10. Brunner L, Munar MY, Vallian J, Wolfson M, Stennett DJ, Meyer MM, Bennett WM. Interaction between cyclosporine and grapefruit juice requires long-term ingestion in stable renal transplant recipients. *Pharmacotherapy* (1998) 18, 23–9.
11. Mehrsai AR, Pourmand G, Mansour D, Zand S, Rezaali A. Effect of grapefruit juice on serum concentration of cyclosporine in Iranian renal transplant patients. *Transplant Proc* (2003) 35, 2739–41.
12. Emilia G, Longo G, Bertesi M, Gandini G, Ferrara L, Valenti C. Clinical interaction between grapefruit juice and cyclosporine: is there any interest for the hematologists? *Blood* (1998) 91, 362–3.
13. Ioannides-Demos LL, Christophidis N, Ryan P, Angelis P, Liolios L, McLean AJ. Dosing implications of a clinical interaction between grapefruit juice and cyclosporine and metabolite concentrations in patients with autoimmune diseases. *J Rheumatol* (1997) 24, 49–54.
14. Ku Y-M, Min DI, Flanigan M. Effect of grapefruit juice on the pharmacokinetics of microemulsion cyclosporine and its metabolite in healthy volunteers: does the formulation difference matter? *J Clin Pharmacol* (1998) 38, 959–65.
15. Hollander AAMJ, van Rooij J, Lentjes EGWM, Arbouw F, van Bree JB, Schoemaker RC, van Es LA, van der Woude FJ, Cohen AF. The effect of grapefruit juice on cyclosporine and prednisone metabolism in transplant patients. *Clin Pharmacol Ther* (1995) 57, 318–24.
16. Lee M, Min DI, Ku Y-M, Flanigan M. Effect of grapefruit juice on pharmacokinetics of microemulsion cyclosporine in African American subjects compared with Caucasian subjects: does ethnic difference matter? *J Clin Pharmacol* (2001) 41, 317–23.
17. Bistrup C, Nielsen FT, Jeppesen UE, Dieperink H. Effect of grapefruit juice on Sandimmun Neoral® absorption among stable renal allograft recipients. *Nephrol Dial Transplant* (2001) 16, 373–7.
18. Hermann M, Asberg A, Reubsaet JL, Sæther S, Berg KJ, Christensen H. Intake of grapefruit juice alters the metabolic pattern of cyclosporin A in renal transplant recipients. *Int J Clin Pharmacol Ther* (2002) 40, 451–6.
19. Brunner LJ, Pai K-S, Munar MY, Lande MB, Olyaei AJ, Mowry JA. Effect of grapefruit juice on cyclosporin A pharmacokinetics in pediatric renal transplant patients. *Pediatr Transplant* (2000) 4, 313–21.
20. Sorkhi H, Oliaei F, Moghadamnia AA, Pouramin M, Firoozjahi AR. Effect of orange and tangerine juice on cyclosporine levels in renal transplant recipients. *Transplant Proc* (2007) 39, 1228–30.
21. Sorkhi H, Moghadamnia AA, Oaliaee F, PourAmir M, Firoozjahi AR, Pasha AA, Goodarzi MR. Serum cyclosporine level and orange juice in pediatric renal-transplanted patients. *Pediatr Transplant* (2009) 13, 411–3.
22. Sorkhi H, Moghadamnia AA, Oaliaee F, PourAmir M, Firoozjahi AR, Pasha AA, Goodarzi MR. Effect of tangerine juice on cyclosporine levels in renal transplant children. *Pediatr Nephrol* (2008) 23, 499–501.
23. Oliveira-Freitas VL, Dalla Costa T, Manfro RC, Cruz LB, Schwartsmann G. Influence of purple grape juice in cyclosporine bioavailability. *J Ren Nutr* (2010) 20, 309–13.
24. Johnston A, Holt DW. Effect of grapefruit juice on blood cyclosporin concentration. *Lancet* (1995) 346, 122–3.
25. Hollander AAMJ, van der Woude FJ, Cohen AF. Effect of grapefruit juice on blood cyclosporin concentration. *Lancet* (1995) 346, 123.
26. Yee GC, Lowenthal DT. Effect of grapefruit juice on blood cyclosporin concentration. *Lancet* (1995) 346, 123–4.
27. Taniguchi S, Kobayashi H, Ishii M. Treatment of psoriasis by cyclosporine and grapefruit juice. *Arch Dermatol* (1996) 132, 1249.
28. Neoral (Ciclosporin). Novartis Pharmaceuticals Corporation. US Prescribing information, May 2013.

Ciclosporin + Griseofulvin

An isolated report describes decreased ciclosporin concentrations in a patient given griseofulvin, whereas another report found no interaction.

Clinical evidence, mechanism, importance and management

A 57-year-old-man, who had been stable for almost one year taking ciclosporin, azathioprine, and prednisolone following a kidney transplant, was given griseofulvin 500 mg daily for onychomycosis. Two weeks later his minimum ciclosporin concentration had decreased from 90 to 50 nanograms/mL and remained low, despite an increase in his ciclosporin dose from 2.8 to 4.8 mg/kg. When griseofulvin was later stopped, his ciclosporin concentration increased to over 200 nanograms/mL and his dose of ciclosporin was readjusted.[1] In contrast, the authors of another report noted that there was no appreciable interaction when griseofulvin 1 g daily for 8 weeks was used to treat tinea capitis in a kidney transplant patient taking ciclosporin, and graft function remained stable.[2]

The first case appears to be the only report of an interaction with griseofulvin, and its general significance is unclear.

1. Abu-Romeh SH, Rashed A. Ciclosporin A and griseofulvin: another drug interaction. *Nephron* (1991) 58, 237.
2. Chen CH, Wen MC, Cheng CH, Wu MJ, Yu TM, Chuang YW, Shu KH. Infectious alopecia in a dog breeder after renal transplantation. *J Chin Med Assoc* (2008) 71, 477–80.

Ciclosporin + H_2-receptor antagonists

Reports are inconsistent. Cimetidine has been reported to increase ciclosporin concentrations in some studies, whereas others found no interaction. Ranitidine, and probably famotidine, do not appear to affect ciclosporin concentrations. Both cimetidine and ranitidine have been reported to cause an increase in serum creatinine concentrations, in some but not all studies. Isolated cases of thrombocytopenia and hepatotoxicity have been reported with ranitidine and ciclosporin.

Clinical evidence

(a) Cimetidine

A study in 5 liver transplant patients taking ciclosporin found that cimetidine 800 mg given every 12 hours for 3 doses increased maximum ciclosporin concentrations, but no changes in minimum concentrations were seen after 4 hours. Similarly, no change in minimum ciclosporin concentrations were seen in 2 patients who received cimetidine 400 mg four times daily for 4 weeks, and the conclusion was reached that it was safe to use cimetidine over at least a 4-week period.[1] However, a retrospective study reported that heart transplant patients taking cimetidine found the dose of ciclosporin required to give a specific concentration was 55% lower in 22 patients taking cimetidine (dose not stated), when compared with 140 patients not taking cimetidine.[2] Similarly, a study in 6 healthy subjects found a 30% increase in the AUC of ciclosporin 300 mg given after a 3-day course of cimetidine 400 mg daily.[3] Increased ciclosporin blood concentrations have also been seen in a patient given cimetidine and metronidazole[4] (see 'Ciclosporin + Antibacterials; Metronidazole', p.1211).

Cimetidine or **ranitidine** increased the mean serum creatinine concentrations in 7 kidney transplant patients taking ciclosporin by 41% (from 202 to 285 micromol/L). All of the patients had an increase, whereas only 2 out of 5 other patients with heart transplants had an increase in their serum creatinine concentrations when given either cimetidine or **ranitidine**, nevertheless the increase was 37% (from 152 to 209 micromol/L). Ciclosporin concentrations were not altered.[5] Another study in 7 kidney transplant patients given cimetidine 400 mg daily for 7 days reported a transient minor increase in creatinine serum concentrations at days 2 and 5, which was not statistically significant. Again ciclosporin concentrations were not altered.[6] Similarly, in two studies in healthy subjects, cimetidine did not alter ciclosporin blood concentrations.[7,8]

(b) Famotidine

Several studies have reported that famotidine does not affect ciclosporin blood concentrations.[9-11] No significant changes in the pharmacokinetics of ciclosporin were seen in a single-dose study in 8 healthy subjects[8] and no changes in serum creatinine or BUN concentrations were seen in 7 kidney transplant patients.[11] However, a retrospective study of heart transplant patients given famotidine, found the dose of ciclosporin required to give a specific concentration was 29% lower in 38 patients taking famotidine (dose not stated), when compared with 66 patients not taking famotidine.[2]

(c) Ranitidine

One report (see *Cimetidine* above), where the effects of cimetidine and ranitidine were examined together, suggests that ranitidine increases creatinine concentrations in patients taking ciclosporin, without affecting ciclosporin concentrations.[5] Similarly, several other reports suggest that ranitidine does not alter ciclosporin blood concentrations.[6,12-15] Two also note that ranitidine does not alter creatinine concentrations[6,13] or inulin clearance.[13]

A report describes thrombocytopenia in a man taking ciclosporin after a kidney transplant who was given ranitidine.[16] Another patient experienced hepatotoxicity while taking ciclosporin with ranitidine.[17]

Mechanism

It has been suggested that any increase in serum creatinine concentrations could simply be because these H_2-receptor antagonists compete with creatinine for secretion by the kidney tubules, and therefore increases are not an indicator of nephrotoxicity[18,19]

Importance and management

Information about the possible interaction of ciclosporin and cimetidine are inconsistent, but there appear to be very few reports of confirmed toxicity. Most of the evidence suggests that famotidine does not affect ciclosporin concentrations, and ranitidine does not appear to affect ciclosporin concentrations. The reported increases in serum creatinine concentrations seen with the H_2-receptor antagonists might not be a reflection of increased nephrotoxicity (see *Mechanism*). Thus there is little to suggest that concurrent use should be avoided, but good initial monitoring is possibly advisable with cimetidine.

1. Puff MR, Carey WD. The effect of cimetidine on cyclosporine A levels in liver transplant recipients: a preliminary report. *Am J Gastroenterol* (1992) 87, 287–91.
2. Reichenspurner H, Meiser BM, Muschiol F, Nolltert G, Überfuhr P, Markewitz A, Wagner F, Pfeiffer M, Reichart B. The influence of gastrointestinal agents on resorption and metabolism of cyclosporine after heart transplantation: experimental and clinical results. *J Heart Lung Transplant* (1993) 12, 987–92.
3. Choi J-S, Choi I, Min DI. Effect of cimetidine on pharmacokinetics of cyclosporine in healthy volunteers. *Pharmacotherapy* (1997) 17, 1120.
4. Zylber-Katz E, Rubinger D, Berlatzky Y. Cyclosporine interactions with metronidazole and cimetidine. *Drug Intell Clin Pharm* (1988) 22, 504–5.
5. Jarowenko MV, Van Buren CT, Kramer WG, Lorber MI, Flechner SM, Kahan BD. Ranitidine, cimetidine, and the cyclosporine-treated recipient. *Transplantation* (1986) 42, 311–12.
6. Barri YM, Ramos EL, Balagtas RS, Peterson JC, Karlix JL. Cimetidine or ranitidine in renal transplant patients receiving cyclosporine. *Clin Transplant* (1996) 10, 34–8.
7. Freeman DJ, Laupacis A, Keown P, Stiller C, Carruthers G. The effect of agents that alter drug metabolizing enzyme activity on the pharmacokinetics of cyclosporine. *Ann R Coll Physicians Surg Can* (1984) 17, 301.
8. Shaefer MS, Rossi SJ, McGuire TR, Schaaf LJ, Collier DS, Stratta RJ. Evaluation of the pharmacokinetic interaction between cimetidine or famotidine and cyclosporine in healthy men. *Ann Pharmacother* (1995) 29, 1088–91.
9. Schütz A, Kemkes BM. Ciclosporinspiegel unter Gabe von Famotidin. *Fortschr Med* (1990) 23, 457–8.
10. Morel D, Bannwarth B, Vinçon G, Penouil F, Elouaer-Blanc L, Aparicio M, Potaux L. Effect of famotidine on renal transplant patients treated with ciclosporine A. *Fundam Clin Pharmacol* (1993) 7, 167–70.
11. Inoue S, Sugimoto H, Nagao T, Akiyama N. Does H_2-receptor antagonist alter the renal function of cyclosporine-treated kidney grafts? *Jpn J Surg* (1990) 20, 553–8.
12. Zazgornik J, Schindler J, Gremmel F, Balcke P, Kopsa H, Derfler K, Minar E. Ranitidine does not influence the blood ciclosporin levels in renal transplant patients (RTP). *Kidney Int* (1985) 28, 401.
13. Jadoul M, Hené RJ. Ranitidine and the cyclosporine-treated recipient. *Transplantation* (1989) 48, 359.
14. Popovic J, Cameron JS. Effects of ranitidine on renal function in transplant recipients. *Nephrol Dial Transplant* (1990) 5, 980–1.
15. Tsang VT, Johnston A, Heritier F, Leaver N, Hodson ME, Yacoub M. Cyclosporin pharmacokinetics in heart-lung transplant recipients with cystic fibrosis. *Eur J Clin Pharmacol* (1994) 46, 261–5.
16. Bailey RR, Walker RJ, Swainson CP. Some new problems with cyclosporin A? *N Z Med J* (1985) 98, 915–6.
17. Hiesse C, Cantarovich M, Santelli C, Francais P, Charpentier B, Fries D, Buffet C. Ranitidine hepatotoxicity in a renal transplant patient. *Lancet* (1985) i, 1280.
18. Pachon J, Lorber MI, Bia MJ. Effects of H_2-receptor antagonists on renal function in cyclosporine-treated renal transplant patients. *Transplantation* (1989) 47, 254–9.
19. Lewis SM, McClosky WW. Potentiation of nephrotoxicity by H_2-antagonists in patients receiving cyclosporine. *Ann Pharmacother* (1997) 31, 363–5.

Ciclosporin + HCV-protease inhibitors

Paritaprevir boosted with ritonavir markedly to moderately increases the exposure to ciclosporin, depending on whether it is given with, or without, dasabuvir. Boceprevir and telaprevir moderately increase the exposure to ciclosporin, but simeprevir appears to cause only a very slight increase. Ciclosporin appears to markedly increase simeprevir exposure, but only slightly increases that of paritaprevir.

Clinical evidence

(a) Boceprevir

In a study in 10 healthy subjects, boceprevir 800 mg three times daily for 7 days increased the AUC and maximum plasma concentration of a single 100-mg dose of ciclosporin (taken on day 6) 2.7-fold and 2-fold, respectively. In a single-dose study by the same authors, ciclosporin 100 mg caused a 16% increase in the AUC of boceprevir 800 mg and had no effect on its maximum plasma concentration.[1] In another study in 18 liver transplant patients with HCV recurrence and given boceprevir 800 mg three times daily, 12 were already taking ciclosporin. After a pre-emptive ciclosporin dose reduction when boceprevir was started, further dose reductions (36%) were required during the first week after concurrent treatment in order to maintain concentrations within the target range of 50 to 150 nanograms/mL.[2] Similarly, in three liver transplant patients taking ciclosporin, and started on boceprevir 800 mg three times daily, the oral clearance of ciclosporin decreased by about 50% during the first week, and ciclosporin dose reductions were required in 2 of the 3 patients in order to maintain a minimum concentration within the target range of 50 to 150 nanograms/mL.[3]

(b) Paritaprevir

The UK and US manufacturers briefly report that, in a study in 10 healthy subjects, a single 30-mg dose of ciclosporin increased the AUC and maximum concentration of paritaprevir 150 mg daily (in a fixed-dose combination with ritonavir and ombitasvir, given with dasabuvir) by 72% and 44%, respectively. The dose-normalised AUC of ciclosporin was increased 5.8-fold but there was no effect on the maximum concentration. The minimum concentration was increased almost 16-fold.[4,5] The UK manufacturer also reports that when paritaprevir 150 mg daily (in a fixed-dose combination with ritonavir and ombitasvir, and given *without* dasabuvir) was given with a single 10-mg dose of ciclosporin, the AUC and maximum concentration of paritaprevir were increased by 46% and 39%, respectively. The dose-normalised AUC of ciclosporin was increased 4.3-fold and the minimum concentration was increased almost 13-fold.[5]

(c) Simeprevir

The UK and US manufacturers briefly note that, in a study in 14 healthy subjects given simeprevir 150 mg daily for 7 days with a single 100-mg dose of ciclosporin, the AUC and maximum concentration of ciclosporin were increased by 19% and 16%, respectively.[6,7] Further, the US manufacturer also reports that in a study in 9 patients taking ciclosporin (individualised dose) and given simeprevir 150 mg daily for 14 days, the AUC and maximum concentration of simeprevir were about 6-fold and 5-fold higher, respectively, than in historical controls.[7] Note that this study involved use of an unstated investigational drug.

(d) Telaprevir

In a study, 9 healthy subjects were given a single 100-mg dose of ciclosporin (as an oral solution) alone, followed 8 days later, by a single 10-mg dose of ciclosporin on day one and day 8 of an 11-day course of telaprevir 750 mg three times daily. Steady-state telaprevir (day 8) increased the dose-normalised AUC and maximum plasma concentration of ciclosporin 4.6-fold and 32%, respectively. Similar increases in ciclosporin exposure were also seen after a single 750 mg-dose of telaprevir.[8] In another study in 19 liver transplant patients with HCV recurrence and given telaprevir 750 mg three times daily,10 were already taking ciclosporin. After a pre-emptive ciclosporin dose reduction when telaprevir was started, further dose reductions (46%) were required during the first week after concurrent treatment in order to maintain concentrations within the target range of 50 to 150 nanograms/mL.[2] Similarly, a retrospective study of 4 liver transplant patients with HCV recurrence requiring telaprevir-based triple therapy and taking ciclosporin, found that ciclosporin dose reductions of about 60% were required to maintain minimum concentrations within the target range of 70 to 100 nanograms/mL. This equated to an average daily dose of 48.5 mg.[9] Another study describes one patient who required a ciclosporin dose reduction of about 70% during 12 weeks of triple therapy with telaprevir, pegylated interferon, and ribavirin for HCV recurrence after liver transplantation.[10]

Mechanism

Boceprevir, simeprevir, and telaprevir inhibit CYP3A4 (albeit to varying extents), the main isoenzyme by which ciclosporin is metabolised, and P-glycoprotein, of which ciclosporin is also a substrate, resulting in an increase in its exposure. Paritaprevir does not appear to affect CYP3A4 itself, but it is given with ritonavir as a pharmacokinetic enhancer, and as this is a well-known potent inhibitor of CYP3A4, the effects on ciclosporin seen when given as part of a fixed-dose combination would seem to be most likely due to the ritonavir. The US manufacturer suggests that the effect on simeprevir is due to inhibition of CYP3A4, P-glycoprotein, and the organic anion transporting polypeptide, OATP1B1, by ciclosporin,[7] however further study is warranted and a contributory effect by the unnamed investigational drug cannot be ruled.

The increase in paritaprevir exposure is suggested to be possibly due to inhibition of OATP, BCRP, or P-glycoprotein by ciclosporin[5] but this also needs confirmation.

Importance and management

A pharmacokinetic interaction between the HCV-protease inhibitors and ciclosporin is established, resulting in very slight (simeprevir), moderate (boceprevir, paritaprevir boosted with ritonavir in a fixed dose combination including ombitasvir and given *without* dasabuvir, and telaprevir), or marked (paritaprevir boosted with ritonavir in a fixed dose combination including ombitasvir and given *with* dasabuvir) increases in ciclosporin exposure. Except for simeprevir, these increases would be expected to be clinically important. If telaprevir or boceprevir is required in patients taking ciclosporin, increase the frequency of monitoring ciclosporin concentrations and monitor for its adverse effects (such as effect on renal function), anticipating the need to reduce the ciclosporin dose: given the increase in ciclosporin exposure seen, ciclosporin dose adjustments and/or extended dosing intervals seem likely to be needed. It might also be prudent to consider a pre-emptive ciclosporin dose reduction when either drug is started, although note that further dose reductions during concurrent use might also be necessary. One group of authors also note the need for close monitoring of ciclosporin concentrations when boceprevir or telaprevir are discontinued, and in particular recommend increasing the ciclosporin dose the day immediately following their discontinuation, together with 48-hourly monitoring until steady state is achieved.[2] The UK and US manufacturers of paritaprevir boosted with ritonavir (in a fixed-dose combination with ombitasvir, and given with or without dasabuvir) recommend that on starting concurrent treatment with ciclosporin, the ciclosporin dose should be reduced to one-fifth of the patients current dose. Ciclosporin concentrations should be monitored throughout treatment and the dose adjusted accordingly, including when treatment is stopped.[4,5] Renal function[4] and ciclosporin-related adverse effects should be monitored.[4,5] The slight increase in paritaprevir exposure is not likely to be clinically important and no paritaprevir dose adjustment is necessary on concurrent use with ciclosporin.

The very slight increase in ciclosporin exposure seen with simeprevir would not be expected to be clinically important and as such, the UK manufacturer advises that no ciclosporin dose adjustment is necessary, but does advise monitoring ciclosporin concentrations.[6] However, because ciclosporin appeared to markedly increase simeprevir exposure, the US manufacturer states that concurrent use is not recommended.[7]

1. Hulskotte E, Gupta S, Xuan F, van Zutven M, O'Mara E, Feng HP, Wagner J, Butterton J. Pharmacokinetic interaction between the hepatitis C virus protease inhibitor boceprevir and cyclosporine and tacrolimus in healthy volunteers. *Hepatology* (2012) 56, 1622–30.
2. Coilly A, Roche B, Dumortier J, Leroy V, Botta-Fridlund D, Radenne S, Pageaux GP, Si-Ahmed SN, Guillaud O, Antonini TM, Haïm-Boukobza S, Roque-Afonso AM, Samuel D, Duclos-Vallée JC. Safety and efficacy of protease inhibitors to treat hepatitis C after liver transplantation: a multicenter experience. *J Hepatol* (2014) 60, 78-86.
3. Coilly A, Furlan V, Roche B, Barau C, Noël C, Bonhomme-Faivre L, Antonini TM, Roque-Afonso AM, Samuel D, Taburet AM, Duclos-Vallée JC. Practical management of boceprevir and immunosuppressive therapy in liver transplant recipients with hepatitis C virus recurrence. *Antimicrob Agents Chemother* (2012) 56, 5728–34.
4. Viekira Pak (Ombitasvir, paritaprevir, ritonavir co-packaged with dasabuvir sodium monohydrate). AbbVie Inc. US Prescribing information, December 2014.
5. Viekirax (Ombitasvir, paritaprevir, ritonavir). AbbVie Ltd. UK Summary of product characteristics, January 2015.
6. Olysio (Simeprevir sodium). Janssen-Cilag Ltd. UK Summary of product characteristics, May 2014.
7. Olysio (Simeprevir sodium). Janssen Products, LP. US Prescribing information, November 2014.
8. Garg V, van Heeswijck R, Lee JE, Alves K, Nadkarni P, Luo X. Effect of telaprevir on the pharmacokinetics of cyclosporine and tacrolimus. *Hepatology* (2011) 54, 20–7.
9. Werner CR, Egetemeyr DP, Lauer UM, Nadalin S, Königsrainer A, Malek NP, Berg CP. Telaprevir-based triple therapy in liver transplant patients with hepatitis C virus: a 12-week pilot study providing safety and efficacy data. *Liver Transpl* (2012) 18, 1464–70.
10. Herzer K, Papadopoulos-Köhn A, Timm J, Paul A, Jochum C, Gerken G. HCV-reinfektion nach lebertransplantation - management und erste ergebnisse mit der telaprevir-basierten triple-therapie. *Dtsch Med Wochenschr* (2013) 138, 1759–64.

Ciclosporin + HIV-protease inhibitors

HIV-protease inhibitors can greatly increase the concentrations of ciclosporin. This has been demonstrated for unboosted fosamprenavir, indinavir, nelfinavir, saquinavir, and amprenavir, and also indinavir and lopinavir when boosted with ritonavir. Some evidence suggests that ciclosporin might increase indinavir, nelfinavir, and saquinavir concentrations, but in one study, this effect was not sustained.

Clinical evidence

(a) Fosamprenavir

An HIV-positive patient taking ciclosporin 250 to 350 mg twice daily (to maintain a therapeutic ciclosporin minimum concentration of 300 to 400 nanograms/mL) was restarted on his usual HAART regimen of tenofovir, lamivudine, and fosamprenavir 1.4 g twice daily on day 12 post-liver transplantation. Within 2 days, the ciclosporin concentration had increased to 600 nanograms/mL, requiring a ciclosporin dose reduction of about 70%, to 100 mg twice daily.[1]

(b) Nelfinavir

A pilot study in 7 HIV-positive subjects taking nelfinavir 1.25 g twice daily found that a single 4-mg/kg oral dose of ciclosporin increased the time to maximum serum concentration for nelfinavir from 2.6 to 3.2 hours. The AUC of nelfinavir was increased by 55%, but this was not statistically significant. In the same study, a single 2-mg/kg intravenous dose of ciclosporin given over 2.5 hours had little effect on the pharmacokinetics of oral nelfinavir. The pharmacokinetics of oral ciclosporin in this study did not appear to differ from that seen in healthy subjects in other studies, but there was high inter-individual variability.[2] However, in another study by the same research group, when ciclosporin was added to established antiretroviral therapy after liver or kidney transplantation in 35 HIV-positive patients, those taking HIV-protease inhibitor-based regimens (not specified) required a large reduction in ciclosporin dose and about a 50% increase in dosing interval at week 2 when compared with those taking an NNRTI-based regimen.[3] Furthermore, the same authors reported the results of the first 18 patients recruited into this study in an earlier paper, and showed that in 5 patients taking nelfinavir or **indinavir**-based antiretroviral regimens, the required ciclosporin dose decreased by 85% from 1.3 mg/kg to just 0.2 mg/kg in the 2 years after transplantation. The AUC of the HIV-protease inhibitor generally increased in the first few weeks after starting ciclosporin, but by week 28 had gradually returned to baseline.[4]

(c) Ritonavir-boosted regimens

Three HIV-positive patients who had undergone liver transplantation required reductions in their ciclosporin doses when they started taking HAART that included **lopinavir** boosted with ritonavir. One patient taking ciclosporin 150 mg twice daily had an increase in his ciclosporin concentration to 900 nanograms/mL when HAART was started, and needed a dose reduction of 95% to maintain a usual ciclosporin minimum concentration of 75 to 150 nanograms/mL. A second patient also required a similar reduction. The third patient needed a dose reduction of 80% when taking **lopinavir** boosted with ritonavir, but no further ciclosporin dose alteration was needed when his treatment was changed to **indinavir** boosted with ritonavir.[5] In a similar case, a reduction in ciclosporin dose from 200 to 350 mg twice daily to just 25 mg twice daily was required on restarting an **amprenavir** boosted with ritonavir-containing regimen (about a 90% reduction).[1] Likewise, a study in 35 HIV-positive patients given ciclosporin post-transplant, found a greater reduction in ciclosporin dose requirements when ritonavir was given with HIV-protease inhibitors (not specified) than when the HIV-protease inhibitors were given alone (25 mg twice daily compared with 57 to 75 mg twice daily).[3]

(d) Saquinavir

An HIV-positive patient taking lamivudine and zidovudine, and ciclosporin for a kidney transplant, started taking saquinavir 1.2 g three times daily. Within 2 days he started to complain of fatigue, headache, and gastrointestinal discomfort. On investigation his ciclosporin concentration was found to have increased from a range of 150 to 200 nanograms/mL up to 580 nanograms/mL, and his saquinavir AUC was increased 4.3-fold (by comparison with subjects not taking ciclosporin). His ciclosporin dose was reduced by 50% from 150 mg twice daily to 75 mg twice daily, and his saquinavir dose was reduced to 600 mg three times daily, which resulted in a ciclosporin concentration similar to that achieved previously.[6]

Mechanism

All HIV-protease inhibitors can inhibit CYP3A4 to varying degrees, and as ciclosporin is metabolised by CYP3A4, any inhibition of this isoenzyme is likely to increase ciclosporin concentrations. Ciclosporin can also inhibit P-glycoprotein, which might explain the increased nelfinavir and saquinavir concentrations.

Importance and management

An interaction between the HIV-protease inhibitors and ciclosporin is established. The inhibition of ciclosporin metabolism by HIV-protease inhibitors might lead to large increases in ciclosporin concentrations. Therefore ciclosporin concentrations should be carefully monitored and the dose adjusted accordingly during concurrent use, bearing in mind that large dose reductions might be required in some patients. The dose reductions needed in the various case reports have been 80 to 95% for regimens boosted with ritonavir, 85% for nelfinavir or indinavir, 67% for fosamprenavir, and 50% for saquinavir. The clinical importance of the effects of ciclosporin on saquinavir or nelfinavir pharmacokinetics is unclear, but in one study the effect was not sustained.

1. Guaraldi G, Cocchi S, Codeluppi M, Di Benedetto F, Bonora S, Motta A, Luzi K, Pecorari M, Gennari W, Masetti M, Gerunda GE, Esposito R. Pharmacokinetic interaction between amprenavir/ritonavir and fosamprenavir on cyclosporine in two patients with human immunodeficiency virus infection undergoing orthotopic liver transplantation. *Transplant Proc* (2006) 38, 1138–40.
2. Frassetto L, Tahi T, Aggarwal AM, Bucher P, Jacobsen W, Christians U, Benet LZ, Floren LC. Pharmacokinetic interactions between cyclosporine and protease inhibitors in HIV+ subjects. *Drug Metab Pharmacokinet* (2003) 18, 114–20.
3. Frassetto LA, Browne M, Cheng A, Wolfe AR, Roland ME, Stock PG, Carlson L, Benet LZ. Immunosuppressant pharmacokinetics and dosing modifications in HIV-1 infected liver and kidney transplant recipients. *Am J Transplant* (2007) 7, 2816–20.
4. Frassetto L, Baluom M, Jacobsen W, Christians U, Roland ME, Stock PG, Carlson L, Benet LZ. Cyclosporine pharmacokinetics and dosing modifications in human immunodeficiency virus-infected liver and kidney transplant recipients. *Transplantation* (2005) 80, 13–17.
5. Vogel M, Voight E, Michaelis H-C, Sudhop T, Wolff M, Türler A, Sauerbruch T, Rockstroh JK, Spengler U. Management of drug-to-drug interactions between cyclosporine A and the protease-inhibitor lopinavir/ritonavir in liver-transplanted HIV-infected patients. *Liver Transpl* (2004) 10, 939–44.
6. Brinkman K, Huysmans F, Burger DM. Pharmacokinetic interaction between saquinavir and cyclosporine. *Ann Intern Med* (1998) 129, 914–15.

Ciclosporin + Hormonal contraceptives and Progestogens

Isolated reports describe hepatotoxicity and increased ciclosporin concentrations in two patients taking ciclosporin when given oral combined hormonal contraceptives. However, a vaginal ring formulation of a combined hormonal contraceptive had no effect on ciclosporin concentrations. A couple of reports describe some increase in ciclosporin

concentrations with norethisterone, but one found no change in ciclosporin concentrations.

Clinical evidence

(a) Combined hormonal contraceptives

A woman with uveitis taking ciclosporin 5 mg/kg daily had an increase in her ciclosporin minimum plasma concentration (roughly doubled) on two occasions within 8 to 10 days of starting an oral combined hormonal contraceptive (**ethinylestradiol** 30 micrograms with **levonorgestrel** 150 micrograms). She also experienced nausea, vomiting, and hepatic pain, and had evidence of severe hepatotoxicity (increases in AST and ALT, serum bilirubin, and alkaline phosphatase).The woman had previously taken this oral contraceptive for 5 years without problems.[1]

Another report describes hepatotoxicity in a patient taking ciclosporin 2 weeks after she started an oral combined hormonal contraceptive (**ethinylestradiol** 30 micrograms with **desogestrel** 150 micrograms). The contraceptive was stopped, and liver enzyme concentrations promptly started to decrease, but ciclosporin concentrations continued to increase, and peaked about 10 days later, at a concentration about 3-fold higher than they had been.[2]

In a study of 17 women with renal or liver transplants taking tacrolimus or low-dose ciclosporin with prednisone, the use of a vaginal ring formulation of a combined hormonal contraceptive (releasing **ethinylestradiol** 15 micrograms and **etonogestrel** 120 micrograms daily) for 12 cycles did not require any change in immunosuppressive therapy to maintain concentrations of ciclosporin or tacrolimus within the therapeutic range.[3]

(b) Norethisterone

A 15-year-old girl taking ciclosporin who had a large increase in ciclosporin serum concentrations when she was given danazol (see 'Ciclosporin + Danazol', p.1225), continued to have elevated concentrations, but not as high, when danazol was replaced by norethisterone 5 mg three times daily. The concentrations returned to her previous normal range when norethisterone was stopped.[4] Two women had a minor increase in ciclosporin concentrations with no changes in serum creatinine when they were given norethisterone 10 mg daily for 10 days.[5] No changes in ciclosporin concentrations were seen in another patient who was intermittently given norethisterone.[6]

Mechanism

Combined hormonal contraceptives are not known to have clinically relevant effects on CYP3A4, which is important in ciclosporin metabolism. The mechanism of the hepatotoxicity is not understood, but in some cases it seems that it occurs simply as a rare adverse effect of the sex hormone.

Importance and management

The interaction between ciclosporin and oral combined hormonal contraceptives or norethisterone is unconfirmed and of uncertain clinical relevance. There is insufficient evidence to recommend a general increase in monitoring, but be aware of the potential for an interaction in the case of an unexpected response to treatment. Note that there is limited evidence from one clinical study that a vaginal combined hormonal contraceptive does not alter ciclosporin concentrations. Note that, aside from the pharmacokinetic implications, there are drug-disease precautions (such as adverse cardiovascular effects) to consider when making the decision to use a hormonal contraceptive in a patient with an organ transplant taking ciclosporin.

1. Deray G, le Hoang P, Cacoub P, Assogba U, Grippon P, Baumelou A. Oral contraceptive interaction with cyclosporin. *Lancet* (1987) i, 158–9.
2. Leimenstoll G, Jessen P, Zabel P, Niedermayer W. Arzneimittelschaädigung der leber bei kombination von cyclosporin A und einem antikonzeptivum. *Dtsch Med Wochenschr* (1984) 109, 1989–90.
3. Paternoster DM, Riboni F, Bertolino M, Garofalo G, Lazzarich E, Surico N, Stratta P. The contraceptive vaginal ring in women with renal and liver transplantation: analysis of preliminary results. *Transplant Proc* (2010) 42, 1162–5.
4. Ross WB, Roberts D, Griffin PJA and Salaman JR. Cyclosporin interaction with danazol and norethisterone. *Lancet* (1986) i, 330.
5. Castelao AM. Cyclosporine A — drug interactions. 2nd Int Conf Therapeutic Drug Monitoring Toxicology, Barcelona, Spain, 1992. 203–9.
6. Koneru B, Hartner C, Iwatsuki S, Starzl TE. Effect of danazol on cyclosporine pharmacokinetics. *Transplantation* (1988) 45, 1001.

Ciclosporin + Isoniazid

Isoniazid does not generally appear to interact with ciclosporin, although case reports have described alterations in ciclosporin concentrations.

Clinical evidence, mechanism, importance and management

In a small study, 7 kidney transplant patients taking ciclosporin were also given isoniazid 300 mg daily. Ciclosporin concentrations assessed after 14 days were unchanged from those measured before isoniazid was started.[1] In addition, case reports and a case series of 22 patients describe the uneventful use of isoniazid (sometimes with ethambutol and/or a range of other antitubercular drugs) for the treatment of tuberculosis in patients taking ciclosporin after heart or kidney transplants.[2-4] Successful treatment of tuberculosis in heart and kidney transplant patients has also been reported using isoniazid, ethambutol, pyrazinamide, and streptomycin, see 'Ciclosporin + Pyrazinamide', p.1239. However, there is one case report describing a patient who had a gradual increase in ciclosporin serum concentrations when isoniazid and ethambutol were stopped,[5] and another which attributed a sizeable increase in ciclosporin concentrations to the use of isoniazid.[6]

Evidence regarding an interaction between ethambutol and ciclosporin is limited but what is known suggests that isoniazid does not affect the pharmacokinetics of ciclosporin. No ciclosporin dose adjustments would therefore be expected to be necessary on their concurrent use.

1. Sud K, Muthukumar T, Singh B, Garg SK, Kohli HS, Jha V, Gupta KL, Sakhuja V. Isoniazid does not affect bioavailability of cyclosporine in renal transplant recipients. *Methods Find Exp Clin Pharmacol* (2000) 22, 647–9.
2. Aguado JM, Herrero JA, Gavaldá J, Torre-Cisneros J, Blanes M, Rufí G, Moreno A, Gurguí A, Hayek M, Lumbreras C and the Spanish Transplantation Infection Study Group, GESITRA. Clinical prese ntation and outcome of tuberculosis in kidney, liver, and heart transplant recipients in Spain. *Transplantation* (1997) 63, 1276–86.
3. Muñoz P, Palomo J, Muños R, Rodríguez-Creixéms M, Pelaez T, Bouza E. Tuberculosis in heart transplant recipients. *Clin Infect Dis* (1995) 21, 398–402.
4. Jurewicz WA, Gunson BK, Ismail T, Angrisani L, McMaster P. Cyclosporin and antituberculous therapy. *Lancet* (1985) i, 1343.
5. Leimenstoll G, Schlegelberger T, Fulde R, Niedermayer W. Interaktion von Ciclosporin und Ethambutol-Isoniazid. *Dtsch Med Wochenschr* (1988) 113, 514–15.
6. Diaz Couselo FA, Porato F, Turin M, Etchegoyen FP, Diez RA. Interacciones de la ciclosporina en transplantados renales. *Medicina (B Aires)* (1992) 52, 296–302.

Ciclosporin + Lamivudine

Lamivudine did not alter ciclosporin concentrations in one study in kidney transplant patients.

Clinical evidence, mechanism, importance and management

In a study, the ciclosporin concentrations of 4 kidney transplant patients were unchanged when lamivudine 100 to 150 mg daily was started for chronic hepatitis B. Normal graft function was maintained.[1] Another study in 15 kidney transplant patients also found that lamivudine 50 to 100 mg daily for 4 to 29 months did not affect ciclosporin concentrations and no acute rejection was seen.[2] Therefore, no ciclosporin dose adjustment seems to be necessary on the concurrent use of lamivudine.

1. Jung YO, Lee YS, Yang WS, Han DJ, Park JS, Park S-K. Treatment of chronic hepatitis B with lamivudine in renal transplant recipients. *Transplantation* (1998) 66, 733–7.
2. Mouquet C, Bernard B, Poynard T, Thibault V, Opolon P, Coriat P, Bitker MO. Chronic hepatitis B treatment with lamivudine in kidney transplant patients. *Transplant Proc* (2000) 32, 2762.

Ciclosporin + Melphalan

Melphalan might increase the nephrotoxic effects of ciclosporin.

Clinical evidence, mechanism, importance and management

A comparative study found that 13 out of 17 patients receiving bone marrow transplants and given ciclosporin 12.5 mg/kg daily with high-dose melphalan (single injection of 140 to 250 mg/m^2) developed renal failure, compared with no cases of renal failure in 7 other patients given melphalan but no ciclosporin.[1] In another study, one out of 4 patients given both drugs developed nephrotoxicity.[2] Renal function should be monitored closely on concurrent use. Note that melphalan is an established part of conditioning regimens given before bone marrow transplantation, for which ciclosporin is used to prevent graft-versus-host disease.

1. Morgenstern GR, Powles R, Robinson B, McElwain TJ. Cyclosporin interaction with ketoconazole and melphalan. *Lancet* (1982) ii, 1342.
2. Dale BM, Sage RE, Norman JE, Barber S, Kotasek D. Bone marrow transplantation following treatment with high-dose melphalan. *Transplant Proc* (1985) 17, 1711–13.

Ciclosporin + Methotrexate

Previous or concurrent treatment with methotrexate might increase the risk of liver and other toxicity in those given ciclosporin. Ciclosporin might cause a modest rise in serum methotrexate concentrations, but methotrexate does not appear to affect the pharmacokinetics of ciclosporin.

Clinical evidence

(a) Bone marrow transplant

In a pilot study of the use of reduced-dose ciclosporin and methotrexate for the control of acute graft-versus-host disease in bone marrow transplant patients, a 50% lower ciclosporin dose (1.5 mg/kg per day) appeared to be as effective and associated with reduced hepatotoxicity. The methotrexate doses were 10 to 15 mg/m^2 on days 1, 3, 6, and 11 after grafting.[1] Another study in three bone marrow transplant patients found that low-dose methotrexate (15 mg/m^2 on day 1, and 10 mg/m^2 on days 3, 6 and 11) given with ciclosporin did not significantly affect clinical care and no interaction of clinical significance was seen.[2] Nevertheless, in a large retrospective study of kidney function impairment post-haematopoietic stem cell transplantation, the main cause of acute renal failure was found to be ciclosporin use. The concurrent use of methotrexate in patients taking ciclosporin was also found to be associated with an increased risk of acute renal failure in the first 100 days (hazard ratio 1.9).[3]

(b) Psoriasis

A limited comparative study in patients with chronic plaque psoriasis suggested that the previous use of methotrexate, which can cause liver damage, possibly increases the risk of ciclosporin toxicity (higher ciclosporin blood and serum creatinine concentrations, hypertension).[4] This was confirmed by another study in 4 patients with resistant psoriasis taking ciclosporin 2.5 to 5 mg/kg daily in whom the addition of methotrexate 2.5 mg every 12 hours for three doses at weekly intervals increased creatinine concentrations and liver enzymes (AST, ALT), which resulted in the study being stopped.[5] Nevertheless, successful concurrent use has been described. In one such study in patients with poorly controlled disease on maximum tolerated doses of ciclosporin or methotrexate alone, concurrent use allowed the reduction in dose of the established drug with better control of psoriasis. However, in 6 of 12 patients receiving both drugs for longer than a year, renal impairment developed, which responded to a reduction in the ciclosporin dose in 3 patients, remained stable in 2 patients, and resulted in the withdrawal of ciclosporin in one patient. There was no evidence of impaired liver function.[6]

(c) Rheumatoid arthritis

An open-label pharmacokinetic study in 26 patients with rheumatoid arthritis taking methotrexate 7.5 to 22.5 mg weekly with ciclosporin 1.5 mg/kg every 12 hours for 14 days, found that the AUC of the weekly dose of methotrexate increased by 26%, whereas the plasma concentrations of its major metabolite (7-hydroxymethotrexate), which is much less active and potentially associated with toxicity, were reduced by 80%.[7] Another study in patients with rheumatoid arthritis found that the pharmacokinetics of ciclosporin after the first dose did not differ between those who had been receiving intramuscular methotrexate 10 mg each week for 6 months and those not receiving methotrexate.[8]

A number of efficacy studies have evaluated the concurrent use of methotrexate and ciclosporin in rheumatoid arthritis. In one, there was no difference in the incidence of renal impairment, or patient withdrawals between patients taking ciclosporin 3 mg/kg daily alone or the same dose of ciclosporin with methotrexate 7.5 to 10 mg weekly. However, there was a tendency for more patients to require dose modification when they were given both drugs (56% versus 28%).[9] In another study, there was no difference in ciclosporin dose between 60 patients receiving ciclosporin alone and 60 patients receiving ciclosporin with methotrexate. However, hypertension or an increase in serum creatinine, or both, were more often a reason for discontinuation in the group given both drugs (9 patients versus 2 patients).[10]

Mechanism

The mechanism by which this interaction occurs is not understood. For the renal adverse effects, additive nephrotoxicity has been proposed.

Importance and management

The reports cited here give an inconsistent picture. Patients receiving ciclosporin should routinely be monitored for renal adverse effects, and those receiving methotrexate routinely monitored for hepatotoxicity. If both drugs are used concurrently it could be worth increasing the frequency of this monitoring to aid rapid detection of any adverse effects. Note that the US manufacturer of ciclosporin states that ciclosporin and methotrexate can be used concurrently in patients with rheumatoid arthritis who do not respond to treatment with methotrexate alone, whereas in patients with psoriasis, they contraindicate concurrent use due to a link between these drugs and increased malignancies in this condition.[11]

1. Stockschlaeder M, Storb R, Pepe M, Longton G, McDonald G, Anasetti C, Appelbaum F, Doney K, Martin P, Sullivan K, Witherspoon R. A pilot study of low-dose cyclosporin for graft-versus-host prophylaxis in marrow transplantation. *Br J Haematol* (1991) 80, 49–54.
2. Dix S, Devine SM, Geller RB, Wingard JR. Re: severe interaction between methotrexate and a macrolide antibiotic. *J Natl Cancer Inst* (1995) 87, 1641–2.
3. Piñana JL, Valcárcel D, Martino R, Barba P, Moreno E, Sureda A, Vega M, Delgado J, Briones J, Brunet S, Sierra J. Study of kidney function impairment after reduced-intensity conditioning allogeneic hematopoietic stem cell transplantation. A single-center experience. *Biol Blood Marrow Transplant* (2009) 15, 21–9.
4. Powles AV, Baker BS, Fry L, Valdimarsson H. Cyclosporin toxicity. *Lancet* (1990) 335, 610.
5. Korstanje MJ, van Breda Vriesman CJP, van de Staak WJBM. Cyclosporine and methotrexate: a dangerous combination. *J Am Acad Dermatol* (1990) 23, 320–1.
6. Clark CM, Kirby B, Morris AD, Davison S, Zaki I, Emerson R, Saihan EM, Chalmers RJ, Barker JN, Allen BR, Griffiths CE. Combination treatment with methotrexate and cyclosporin for severe recalcitrant psoriasis. *Br J Dermatol* (1999) 141, 279–82.
7. Fox RI, Morgan SL, Smith HT, Robbins BA, Choc MG, Baggott JE. Combined oral cyclosporin and methotrexate therapy in patients with rheumatoid arthritis elevates methotrexate levels and reduces 7-hydroxymethotrexate levels when compared with methotrexate alone. *Rheumatology (Oxford)* (2003) 42, 989–94.
8. Baraldo M, Ferracioli G, Pea F, Gremese E, Furlanut M. Cyclosporine A pharmacokinetics in rheumatoid arthritis patients after 6 months of methotrexate therapy. *Pharm Res* (1999) 40, 483–6.
9. Sarzi-Puttini P, D'Ingianna E, Fumagalli M, Scarpellini M, Fiorini T, Chérié-Lignière EL, Panni B, Fiorentini F, Corbelli V, Beyene NB, Mastaglio C, Severi C, Locati M, Cazzola M, Menozzi G, Monti G, Saccardo F, Alfieri G, Atzeni F. An open, randomized comparison study of cyclosporine A, cyclosporine A + methotrexate and cyclosporine A + hydroxychloroquine in the treatment of early severe rheumatoid arthritis. *Rheumatol Int* (2005) 25, 15–22.
10. Gerards AH, Landewé RB, Prins AP, Bruyn GA, Goei Thé HS, Laan RF, Dijkmans BA. Cyclosporin A monotherapy versus cyclosporin A and methotrexate combination therapy in patients with early rheumatoid arthritis: a double blind randomised placebo controlled trial. *Ann Rheum Dis* (2003) 62, 291–6.
11. Neoral (Ciclosporin). Novartis Pharmaceuticals Corporation. US Prescribing information, May 2013.

Ciclosporin + Methoxsalen

In a single-dose study, oral methoxsalen slightly increased the exposure to ciclosporin.

Clinical evidence, mechanism, importance and management

In a single-dose study in 12 healthy subjects, oral methoxsalen 40 mg increased the AUC and maximum plasma concentration of ciclosporin 200 mg by about 14% and 8%, respectively, when given at the same time. In two subjects the ciclosporin AUCs increased by 80% and 2.7-fold, respectively. The half-life and time to maximum concentrations were not affected. As methoxsalen absorption is subject to high interindividual variation, this particular study was unable to detect a statistically significant difference in methoxsalen pharmacokinetics, although ciclosporin tended to reduce the AUC and maximum concentration of methoxsalen by 25% and 35%, respectively.[1]

Methoxsalen might interact by increasing the absorption of ciclosporin. Further study is required to see if this interaction is clinically significant. Until more is known, bear this interaction in mind in patients taking ciclosporin if its concentrations are increased.

1. Rheeders M, Bouwer M, Goosen TC. Drug-drug interaction after single oral doses of the furanocoumarin methoxsalen and cyclosporine. *J Clin Pharmacol* (2006) 46, 768–75.

Ciclosporin + Methylphenidate

In an isolated case, the ciclosporin concentrations of a 10-year-old-boy were increased after he started to take methylphenidate.

Clinical evidence, mechanism, importance and management

A 10-year-old boy who had received a heart transplant 6 years previously, started taking methylphenidate 5 mg twice daily in addition to his transplant medication, which included ciclosporin. After 4 days his ciclosporin concentration was found to have increased, from 195 to 302 nanograms/mL. His ciclosporin dose was therefore reduced from 550 to 500 mg daily, and at the same time the methylphenidate was increased to 7.5 mg twice daily. As the next ciclosporin concentration was still increased, at 251 nanograms/mL, the ciclosporin dose was further reduced to 450 mg daily. The boy then remained on this dose of ciclosporin with acceptable concentrations, despite further dose increases in the methylphenidate to an eventual dose of 20 mg daily.[1]

The reason for this probable interaction is unclear. This appears to be the only reported case of an interaction between ciclosporin and methylphenidate, and its general importance is unknown.

1. Lewis BR, Aoun SL, Bernstein GA, Crow SJ. Pharmacokinetic interactions between cyclosporin and bupropion or methylphenidate. *J Child Adolesc Psychopharmacol* (2001) 11, 193–8.

Ciclosporin + Metoclopramide

Metoclopramide very slightly increases the exposure to ciclosporin and increases its blood concentrations.

Clinical evidence, mechanism, importance and management

When 14 kidney transplant patients were given metoclopramide their ciclosporin maximum blood concentrations were increased by 46% (from 388 to 567 nanograms/mL) and the ciclosporin AUC was increased by 22%. The dose of metoclopramide, by mouth, was 10 mg 30 minutes before, 5 mg with, and 5 mg 30 minutes after the morning dose of ciclosporin, which was given after breakfast.[1] Ciclosporin is largely absorbed by the small intestine so the likely mechanism for this interaction is increased absorption of ciclosporin as a result of metoclopramide hastening gastric emptying.

The clinical importance of this interaction is uncertain. The very slight increase in ciclosporin exposure seems unlikely to be generally relevant; however, the increase in ciclosporin maximum concentrations might increase adverse effects. If adverse effects become troublesome, consider monitoring ciclosporin maximum concentrations.

1. Wadhwa NK, Schroeder TJ, O'Flaherty E, Pesce AJ, Myre SA, First MR. The effect of oral metoclopramide on the absorption of cyclosporine. *Transplant Proc* (1987) 19, 1730–3.

Ciclosporin + Minoxidil

The concurrent use of ciclosporin and minoxidil can cause excessive hairiness (hypertrichosis).

Clinical evidence, mechanism, importance and management

Six male kidney transplant patients taking ciclosporin (blood concentrations of 100 to 200 nanograms/mL) were given methyldopa, a diuretic, and minoxidil 15 to 40 mg daily for intractable hypertension. After 4 weeks of treatment all of them complained of severe and unpleasant hypertrichosis (excessive hairiness). Two months after stopping minoxidil, the hypertrichosis had significantly improved.[1] Both ciclosporin and minoxidil cause hypertrichosis and it would seem that their effects might be additive. The authors of the report point out that this is not a life-threatening problem, but it limits the concurrent use of these drugs in both men and women.[1]

1. Sever MS, Sonmez YE, Kocak N. Limited use of minoxidil in renal transplant recipients because of the additive side-effects of cyclosporine on hypertrichosis. *Transplantation* (1990) 50, 536.

Ciclosporin + Modafinil

Ciclosporin concentrations were reported to be reduced by modafinil in one patient. Armodafinil would be expected to interact with ciclosporin in a similar way to modafinil.

Clinical evidence, mechanism, importance and management

A kidney transplant patient, stable for 9 years taking ciclosporin 200 mg daily, developed Gélineau's syndrome (narcoleptic syndrome) and was given modafinil

200 mg daily. Within a few weeks her ciclosporin blood concentrations were noted to have decreased, and it was necessary to increase her ciclosporin dose stepwise to 300 mg daily before her blood concentrations were back to their former values.[1]

Modafinil is a known weak inducer of CYP3A4, a major isoenzyme involved in the metabolism of ciclosporin. Concurrent use therefore increases ciclosporin metabolism and decreases its concentrations.

Evidence is limited to this single case report, but, on the basis of the proposed mechanism, a clinically relevant interaction seems possible, as ciclosporin has a narrow therapeutic range. It would seem prudent to anticipate a reduction in ciclosporin concentrations if modafinil is used, although as the effects would generally be expected to be slight, ciclosporin dose adjustments might not always be necessary. There seems to be no direct evidence regarding an interaction between ciclosporin and **armodafinil**, the *R*-isomer of modafinil; however, it is also known to be an inducer of CYP3A4, and therefore, until more is known, it would seem prudent to follow the same precautions given for modafinil.

1. Le Cacheux Ph, Charasse C, Mourtada R, Muh Ph, Boulahrouz R, Simon P. Syndrome de Gélineau chez une transplantée rénale. Mise en évidence d'une interaction cyclosporine-modafinil. *Presse Med* (1997) 26, 466.

Ciclosporin + Nefazodone

Four cases of increased ciclosporin concentrations have been seen in patients taking nefazodone and ciclosporin, one with increased creatinine concentrations and tremor, and one with increased liver enzymes.

Clinical evidence

A kidney transplant patient had a 70% increase in minimum serum ciclosporin concentrations within 3 days of starting to take nefazodone 25 mg twice daily.[1] Another kidney transplant patient had a 2- to 3-fold increase in ciclosporin concentrations associated with increased creatinine concentrations and marked generalised tremors after starting nefazodone 100 mg twice daily. The patient was eventually stabilised on a 50% lower dose of ciclosporin.[2] Similarly, a heart transplant patient taking ciclosporin had a 10-fold increase in ciclosporin concentrations shortly after the addition of nefazodone 150 mg twice daily. Concentrations returned to baseline over 6 days after nefazodone was stopped.[3] A patient taking nefazodone developed greatly increased liver enzymes (AST and ALT) one month after kidney transplantation. His ciclosporin concentration was high, at 614 nanograms/mL, and both ciclosporin and nefazodone were stopped. He had previously taken nefazodone uneventfully, and subsequently took ciclosporin uneventfully, so the increased liver enzymes were attributed to a pharmacokinetic interaction between the two drugs.[4]

Mechanism

Nefazodone is a moderate inhibitor of CYP3A4, the main isoenzyme by which ciclosporin is metabolised. Concurrent use can therefore lead to increased ciclosporin concentrations.

Importance and management

Although the evidence is limited, it appears that nefazodone can cause a large increase in ciclosporin concentrations, with an increase in adverse effects. Alternative antidepressants should probably be given, or concurrent use very well monitored. Note that nefazodone has generally been withdrawn due to its adverse effects on the liver.

1. Helms-Smith KM, Curtis SL, Hatton RC. Apparent interaction between nefazodone and cyclosporine. *Ann Intern Med* (1996) 125, 424.
2. Vella JP, Sayegh MH. Interactions between cyclosporine and newer antidepressant medications. *Am J Kidney Dis* (1998) 31, 320–3.
3. Wright DH, Lake KD, Bruhn PS, Emery RW. Nefazodone and cyclosporine drug-drug interaction. *J Heart Lung Transplant* (1999) 18, 913–15.
4. Garton T, Nefazodone and CYP450 3A4 interactions with cyclosporine and tacrolimus. *Transplantation* (2002) 74, 745.

Ciclosporin + NNRTIs

Efavirenz, and to a lesser extent nevirapine, appear to decrease the concentration of ciclosporin. The ciclosporin concentration of one patient dramatically decreased following the addition of efavirenz. Etravirine is also predicted to interact in this way. In contrast, delavirdine is predicted to inhibit the metabolism of ciclosporin and increase its concentration.

Clinical evidence

A patient was diagnosed as HIV-positive 3 years after a kidney transplant, for which he was taking ciclosporin. He was started on **efavirenz** 600 mg daily, lamivudine, and zidovudine, and 7 days later, after an initial increase, his ciclosporin concentration dropped from about 203 to 80 nanograms/mL. A nadir of 50 nanograms/mL was reached one month later.[1] Several reports of a study conducted by the same research group, describe the effects of **efavirenz** and **nevirapine** on ciclosporin pharmacokinetics in HIV-positive patients after kidney or liver transplantation, at different time points or in various subsets of patients.[2-4] The most comprehensive of these, in 47 patients, reports that the median dose of ciclosporin in patients taking **efavirenz** was much greater than in those patients taking **nevirapine** between weeks 2 and 12 (4.03 mg/kg compared with 2.21 mg/kg), and was similar to the dose requirement in transplant patients not infected with HIV. The ciclosporin AUC was about 55% lower in those taking efavirenz than in those taking nevirapine. The difference during weeks 28 to 104 was much smaller (1.74 mg/kg with efavirenz compared with 1.47 mg/kg with nevirapine).[4] A separate report of results from weeks 2 to 12 in 35 patients (the majority of whom were taking ciclosporin), similarly reports that those patients taking **efavirenz** required much higher ciclosporin doses than those taking **nevirapine** (275 mg twice daily compared to 189 mg twice daily at week 2 and 279 mg twice daily compared to 147 mg twice daily at week 12). Additionally patients taking **nevirapine** had similar ciclosporin concentrations and dose requirements to patients not infected with HIV taking ciclosporin. Dose requirements in the **efavirenz** patients were also much higher than those in patients taking any other antiretroviral (HIV-protease inhibitors with or without ritonavir). Ciclosporin concentrations were about 30% lower with **efavirenz** than with **nevirapine** (91 nanograms/mL compared with 130 nanograms/mL at week 2, and 84 nanograms/mL compared with 116 nanograms/mL at week 12).[2] The results of the first 18 patients recruited into this study have also been reported separately. This report additionally noted that there were minimal changes in the pharmacokinetics of the NNRTIs during the study.[3]

Mechanism

Efavirenz, etravirine, and nevirapine induce CYP3A4 (although perhaps to varying extents). Ciclosporin is extensively metabolised by CYP3A4, so concurrent use would be expected to decrease ciclosporin concentrations. Note that delavirdine *inhibits* CYP3A4 and is predicted to *increase* ciclosporin concentrations.[5]

Importance and management

The available evidence suggests that **efavirenz** decreases ciclosporin concentrations and increases the ciclosporin dose requirements. **Nevirapine** might also affect ciclosporin concentrations but it appears that its effects are much less than those of efavirenz. The effect of **etravirine** on ciclosporin metabolism has not been studied, but based on its effects on other CYP3A4 substrates it might be expected to decrease ciclosporin concentrations; albeit to a lesser degree than efavirenz or nevirapine. As subtherapeutic concentrations of ciclosporin might have important consequences, including transplant rejection, it would be prudent to monitor ciclosporin concentrations closely in patients given efavirenz, etravirine, or nevirapine, and be alert to the need to alter ciclosporin doses accordingly.

In contrast, **delavirdine** is predicted to increase ciclosporin concentrations and so a dose reduction of ciclosporin might be needed. As increased concentrations could lead to toxicity, it would be prudent to monitor ciclosporin concentrations and renal function closely in patients also given delavirdine.

1. Tseng A, Nguyen ME, Cardella C, Humar A, Conly J. Probable interaction between efavirenz and cyclosporine. *AIDS* (2002) 16, 505–6.
2. Frassetto LA, Browne M, Cheng A, Wolfe AR, Roland ME, Stock PG, Carlson L, Benet LZ. Immunosuppressant pharmacokinetics and dosing modifications in HIV-1 infected liver and kidney transplant recipients. *Am J Transplant* (2007) 7, 2816–20.
3. Frassetto L, Baluom M, Jacobsen W, Christians U, Roland ME, Stock PG, Carlson L, Benet LZ. Cyclosporine pharmacokinetics and dosing modifications in human immunodeficiency virus-infected liver and kidney transplant recipients. *Transplantation* (2005) 80, 13–17.
4. Frassetto L, Floren L, Barin B, Browne M, Wolfe A, Roland M, Stock P, Carlson L, Christians U, Benet L. Changes in clearance, volume and bioavailability of immunosuppressants when given with HAART in HIV-1 infected liver and kidney transplant recipients. *Biopharm Drug Dispos* (2013) 34, 442–51.
5. Rescriptor (Delavirdine mesylate). ViiV Healthcare. US Prescribing information, August 2012.

Ciclosporin + NS5A inhibitors

No interaction appears to occur between daclatasvir and ciclosporin, and ciclosporin does not appear to alter the pharmacokinetics of ombitasvir. No clinically relevant interaction is predicted between ledipasvir and ciclosporin.

Clinical evidence, mechanism, importance and management

(a) Daclatasvir

The UK manufacturer briefly reports that, in a study in healthy subjects given a single 400-mg dose of ciclosporin with daclatasvir 60 mg daily, the pharmacokinetics of both drugs were unaffected.[1] No dose adjustments are therefore necessary on concurrent use.

(b) Ledipasvir

The UK manufacturer of ledipasvir (in a fixed-dose combination with sofosbuvir) predicts that ledipasvir exposure might be increased when given with ciclosporin, and that ciclosporin exposure will be unaffected.[2] The US manufacturer states that no change was seen in the pharmacokinetics of ciclosporin when given with ledipasvir.[3] They advise that no dose adjustments are necessary on concurrent use.[2,3]

(c) Ombitasvir

The UK and US manufacturers briefly report that, in a study in 10 healthy subjects, a single 30-mg dose of ciclosporin had no effect on the pharmacokinetics of ombitasvir 25 mg daily (in a fixed-dose combination with paritaprevir boosted with ritonavir, given with and without dasabuvir). No ombitasvir dose adjustment is necessary on concurrent use.[4,5] Note that other components of the fixed-dose preparation do affect the exposure of ciclosporin, see 'Ciclosporin + HCV-protease inhibitors', p.1231 and 'Ciclosporin + HIV-protease inhibitors', p.1232 for details.

1. Daklinza (Daclatasvir dihydrochloride). Bristol-Myers Squibb Pharmaceutical Ltd. UK Summary of product characteristics, September 2014.
2. Harvoni (Ledipasvir, sofosbuvir). Gilead Sciences Ltd. UK Summary of product characteristics, November 2014.

3. Harvoni (Ledipasvir, sofosbuvir). Gilead Sciences, Inc. US Prescribing information, March 2015.
4. Viekira Pak (Ombitasvir, paritaprevir, ritonavir co-packaged with dasabuvir sodium monohydrate). AbbVie Inc. US Prescribing information, December 2014.
5. Viekirax (Ombitasvir, paritaprevir, ritonavir). AbbVie Ltd. UK Summary of product characteristics, January 2015.

Ciclosporin + NSAIDs and Aspirin

NSAIDs sometimes reduce renal function in individual patients, which is reflected in increases in serum creatinine concentrations and possibly in changes in ciclosporin concentrations, but concurrent use can also be uneventful. Diclofenac concentrations can be doubled by ciclosporin. There is an isolated report of colitis in a child taking ciclosporin and diclofenac or indometacin.

Clinical evidence

(a) Aspirin

In a study in healthy subjects, no pharmacokinetic interaction was found when ciclosporin was given with aspirin 960 mg three times daily.[1]

(b) Diclofenac

A study in 20 patients with rheumatoid arthritis given ciclosporin and diclofenac found that 7 of them had a high probability of an interaction (increases in serum creatinine concentrations and blood pressures), and 9 possibly had an interaction.[2] A kidney transplant patient taking ciclosporin, digoxin, furosemide, prednisolone, and spironolactone had a notable increase in serum creatinine concentrations immediately after starting to take diclofenac 25 mg three times daily. A decrease in serum ciclosporin concentration from 409 to 285 nanograms/mL also occurred.[3] Increased nephrotoxicity was seen in another patient taking ciclosporin for idiopathic uveitis when diclofenac 150 mg daily was given.[4]

A 6-month study in 20 patients with severe rheumatoid arthritis given diclofenac 100 to 200 mg with ciclosporin 3 mg/kg daily found that the AUC of diclofenac was doubled and serum creatinine concentrations increased from 71 to 88.4 micromol/L. The overall pattern of adverse events and laboratory abnormalities were similar to those in patients with rheumatoid arthritis taking ciclosporin and other NSAIDs. It was suggested that it would be prudent to start with low doses of diclofenac and to monitor well.[5] A study in 24 healthy subjects found that diclofenac 50 mg every 8 hours for 8 days caused no changes in the pharmacokinetics of ciclosporin, but there was some inconclusive evidence that diclofenac serum concentrations were increased.[6]

A child with rheumatoid arthritis taking ciclosporin 10 mg/kg daily developed colitis when diclofenac was given. The NSAID was stopped and her symptoms resolved while the ciclosporin was continued.[7]

(c) Dipyrone (Metamizole sodium)

A placebo-controlled, crossover study in 6 kidney and 2 heart transplant patients taking ciclosporin, found that while they were taking dipyrone 500 mg three times daily for 4 days the pharmacokinetics of ciclosporin (AUC, minimum and maximum blood concentrations, elimination half-life) were unchanged, but the time to reach maximum blood concentrations was slightly prolonged, from 2.1 hours to 3.8 hours. It is not known what the effects of more prolonged use might be.[8]

(d) Indometacin

A study in 16 healthy subjects found that indometacin 100 mg twice daily for 9 days reduced the maximum blood concentrations of a single 300-mg dose of ciclosporin by 18% and slowed its absorption (time to maximum concentration increased by 30 minutes) but the extent of absorption was not changed, indicating the absence of a clinically relevant pharmacokinetic interaction. Further, the pharmacokinetics of indometacin were not affected by ciclosporin.[9] A study in rheumatoid arthritis patients taking ciclosporin 2.5 mg/kg daily, found that creatinine clearances were reduced by 6% in those taking indometacin 50 mg four times daily, but this was not considered to be clinically important.[10] An experimental study in healthy subjects found that ciclosporin 10 mg/kg twice daily for 4 days had no effect on effective renal plasma flow or the glomerular filtration rate, but when indometacin 50 mg twice daily was added the effective renal plasma flow decreased by 32% and the glomerular filtration rate fell by 37%.[11]

A child with rheumatoid arthritis taking ciclosporin 10 mg/kg daily developed colitis when indometacin was given. The NSAID was stopped and her symptoms resolved while the ciclosporin was continued.[7]

(e) Ketoprofen

A study in rheumatoid arthritis patients taking ciclosporin 2.5 mg/kg daily, found that creatinine clearances were reduced by 2.3% in those taking ketoprofen 50 mg four times daily, but this was not considered to be clinically important.[10] Another report describes increased serum creatinine concentrations in a patient with rheumatoid arthritis who took ciclosporin and ketoprofen.[12]

(f) Mefenamic acid

The ciclosporin blood concentrations in a renal transplant patient doubled, accompanied by a rise in creatinine concentrations from 113 to 168 micromol/L, within a day of starting to take mefenamic acid. Concentrations returned to normal within a week of stopping the mefenamic acid.[13]

(g) Naproxen

When 11 patients with rheumatoid arthritis taking ciclosporin were given naproxen and sulindac, their serum creatinine concentrations increased by 24% and renal function was reduced (glomerular filtration rate reduced from 98 mL/minute at baseline to 67 mL/minute).[14]

(h) Piroxicam

Piroxicam is reported to have increased the serum creatinine concentrations of a patient with rheumatoid arthritis by an unknown amount (but classed as a significant adverse event). This resolved when the piroxicam was withdrawn.[12] A study in healthy subjects given piroxicam 20 mg daily for 11 days and a single 300-mg dose of ciclosporin on day 10 found no clinically relevant pharmacokinetic interaction.[9]

(i) Sulindac

A study in rheumatoid arthritis patients taking ciclosporin 2.5 mg/kg daily, found that the creatinine clearance was reduced by 2.6% in those taking sulindac 100 mg four times daily, but this was not considered to be clinically important.[10]

A kidney transplant patient had an increase in serum creatinine concentrations when sulindac was used. Ciclosporin blood concentrations decreased and increased again when the sulindac was stopped.[3] Another report states that the ciclosporin concentrations of a woman with a kidney transplant were more than doubled within 3 days of her starting to take sulindac 150 mg twice daily.[15] When 11 patients with rheumatoid arthritis taking ciclosporin were given sulindac and naproxen their serum creatinine concentrations increased by 24% and renal function was reduced (glomerular filtration rate reduced from 98 mL/minute at baseline to 67 mL/minute).[14]

Another report describes a patient with rheumatoid arthritis taking ciclosporin who developed increased serum creatinine concentrations when given ketoprofen, but not when given sulindac.[12]

Mechanism

Uncertain. One idea is that intact kidney prostacyclin synthesis is needed to maintain the glomerular filtration rate and renal blood flow in patients given ciclosporin, which may possibly protect the kidney from the development of ciclosporin-induced nephrotoxicity. If NSAIDs that inhibit prostaglandin production in the kidney are given, the nephrotoxic effects of the ciclosporin manifest themselves, possibly independently of changes in serum ciclosporin concentrations.[3] A study in *rats* found that indometacin and ciclosporin together can cause rises in serum creatinine concentrations that are much greater than with either drug alone.[16]

Ciclosporin may decrease the first-pass metabolism of NSAIDs that are metabolised in this way, such as diclofenac.[17]

The occurrence of colitis in a child receiving ciclosporin and either diclofenac or indometacin appeared to be independent of changes in ciclosporin concentrations and could be a result of additive effects of both drugs.[7]

Importance and management

Information about the individual NSAIDs listed here is sparse, but when viewed as a group, the overall picture appears to be that concurrent use in rheumatoid arthritis need not be avoided but renal function should be very well monitored. The UK manufacturer of ciclosporin also specifically recommends that patients with rheumatoid arthritis taking ciclosporin and an NSAID should have their liver function measured as well as renal function, because hepatotoxicity is a potential adverse effect of both drugs.[17] It has been suggested that gastrointestinal symptoms should also be carefully evaluated.[7] It is clearly difficult to generalise about what will or will not happen if any particular NSAID is given, but in the case of diclofenac, as its serum concentrations can be doubled by ciclosporin, it has been recommended that doses at the lower end of the range should be used initially.[5] The UK manufacturer recommends halving the diclofenac dose, and using lower than usual doses of other NSAIDs known to undergo first-pass metabolism in patients also taking ciclosporin.[17]

Evidence is even more limited for aspirin, but what is known suggests that analgesic-dose aspirin will not affect ciclosporin pharmacokinetics and therefore smaller antiplatelet doses would also not be expected to affect ciclosporin pharmacokinetics.

1. Kovarik JM, Mueller EA, Gaber M, Johnston A, Jähnchen E. Pharmacokinetics of cyclosporine and steady-state aspirin during coadministration. *J Clin Pharmacol* (1993) 33, 513–21.
2. Branthwaite JP, Nicholls A. Cyclosporin and diclofenac interaction in rheumatoid arthritis. *Lancet* (1991) 337, 252.
3. Harris KP, Jenkins D, Walls J. Nonsteroidal antiinflammatory drugs and cyclosporine. A potentially serious adverse interaction. *Transplantation* (1988) 46, 598–9.
4. Deray G, Le Hoang P, Aupetit B, Achour A, Rottembourg J, Baumelou A. Enhancement of cyclosporine A nephrotoxicity by diclofenac. *Clin Nephrol* (1987) 27, 213–14.
5. Kovarik JM, Kurki P, Mueller E, Guerret M, Markert E, Alten R, Zeidler H, Genth-Stolzenburg S. Diclofenac combined with cyclosporine in treatment of refractory rheumatoid arthritis: longitudinal safety assessment and evidence of a pharmacokinetic/dynamic interaction. *J Rheumatol* (1996) 23, 2033–8.
6. Mueller EA, Kovarik JM, Koelle EU, Merdjan H, Johnston A, Hitzenberger G. Pharmacokinetics of cyclosporine and multiple-dose diclofenac during coadministration. *J Clin Pharmacol* (1993) 33, 936–43.
7. Constantopoulos A. Colitis induced by interaction of cyclosporine A and non-steroidal anti-inflammatory drugs. *Pediatr Int* (1999) 41, 184–6.
8. Caraco Y, Zylber-Katz E, Fridlander M, Admon D, Levy M. The effect of short-term dipyrone administration on cyclosporin pharmacokinetics. *Eur J Clin Pharmacol* (1999) 55, 475–8.
9. Kovarik JM, Mueller EA, Gerbeau C, Tarral A, Francheteau P, Guerret M. Cyclosporine and nonsteroidal antiinflammatory drugs: exploring potential drug interactions and their implications for the treatment of rheumatoid arthritis. *J Clin Pharmacol* (1997) 37, 336–43.
10. Tugwell P, Ludwin D, Gent M, Roberts R, Bensen W, Grace E, Baker P. Interaction between cyclosporin A and nonsteroidal antiinflammatory drugs. *J Rheumatol* (1997) 24, 1122–5.
11. Sturrock NDC, Lang CC, Struthers AD. Indomethacin and cyclosporin together produce marked renal vasoconstriction in humans. *J Hypertens* (1994) 12, 919–24.
12. Ludwin D, Bennett KJ, Grace EM, Buchanan WA, Bensen W, Bombardier C, Tugwell PX. Nephrotoxicity in patients with rheumatoid arthritis treated with cyclosporine. *Transplant Proc* (1988) 20 (Suppl 4), 367–70.
13. Agar JWMacD. Cyclosporin A and mefenamic acid in a renal transplant patient. *Aust N Z J Med* (1991) 21, 784–5.
14. Altman RD, Perez GO, Sfakianakis GN. Interaction of cyclosporine A and nonsteroidal anti-inflammatory drugs on renal function in patients with rheumatoid arthritis. *Am J Med* (1992) 93, 396–402.

15. Sesin GP, O'Keefe E, Roberto P. Sulindac-induced elevation of serum cyclosporine concentration. *Clin Pharm* (1989) 8, 445–6.
16. Whiting PH, Burke MD, Thomson AW. Drug interactions with cyclosporine. Implications from animal studies. *Transplant Proc* (1986) 18 (Suppl 5), 56–70.
17. Neoral (Ciclosporin). Novartis Pharmaceuticals UK Ltd. UK Summary of product characteristics, February 2012.

Ciclosporin + Opioids

An isolated report describes neuropsychosis in a patient who was given intravenous ciclosporin and morphine. A single case report describes a patient taking ciclosporin who developed opioid withdrawal after stopping low-dose, transdermal fentanyl.

Clinical evidence, mechanism, importance and management

A patient who underwent kidney transplantation was given ciclosporin 6 mg/kg daily by intravenous infusion over 2 hours and intravenous methylprednisolone postoperatively. He also received patient-controlled analgesia (PCA) as bolus doses of **morphine** 0.5 mg to a total dose of 13 mg on the first day and 11 mg on the second day. On the third day he developed insomnia, anxiety, amnesia, aphasia, and severe confusion. The morphine was discontinued and the symptoms subsided after treatment with propofol, diazepam, and haloperidol. It was suggested that ciclosporin might have decreased the excitation threshold of neuronal cells, which potentiated the dysphoric effects of **morphine**.[1]

A patient taking ciclosporin following a stem cell transplant developed opioid withdrawal symptoms when transdermal **fentanyl** 25 micrograms/hour was discontinued. The authors suggested that, as withdrawal symptoms are not usual at this dose of fentanyl, ciclosporin might have increased **fentanyl** concentrations by inhibiting CYP3A4. However, they also note that other factors could have played a role, such as the physical and mental status of the patient after the stem cell transplant.[2]

These appear to be isolated cases and almost certainly not of general importance.

1. Lee P-C, Hung C-J, Lei H-Y, Tsai Y-C. Suspected acute post-transplant neuropsychosis due to interaction of morphine and cyclosporin after a renal transplant. *Anaesthesia* (2000) 55, 827–8.
2. Tsutsumi Y, Kanamori H, Tanaka J, Asaka M, Imamura M, Masauzi N. Withdrawal symptoms from transdermal fentanyl (TDF) after an allogeneic blood stem cell transplant. *Pain Med* (2006) 7, 164–5.

Ciclosporin + Orlistat

The absorption of ciclosporin is markedly reduced by orlistat, and cases of low concentrations have been reported with both the microemulsion formulation (*Neoral*) and the oil formulation (*Sandimmun*), including an episode of acute graft rejection.

Clinical evidence

In the first year after orlistat approval in the US, the FDA in the US noted that they had received six reports of transplant recipients who developed subtherapeutic ciclosporin minimum concentrations (formulation not mentioned) soon after starting to take orlistat.[1] A number of reports have also been published, both with the *Sandimmun* and *Neoral* formulations, as outlined below.

(a) Neoral formulation

In a pharmacokinetic study in healthy subjects given low-dose ciclosporin 50 mg twice daily, orlistat 120 mg three times daily with meals reduced the minimum concentration and AUC of ciclosporin by 27% and 34%, respectively, when ciclosporin was also taken with meals. When ciclosporin was taken 3 hours after meals, the reduction in ciclosporin minimum concentrations was similar.[2]

A heart transplant patient taking ciclosporin had an unexpected non-significant acute rejection episode noted on routine endocardial biopsy, with a very low ciclosporin minimum concentration of 38 nanograms/mL, 24 days after starting to take orlistat. The ciclosporin minimum concentration returned to previous levels of between 90 to 110 nanograms/mL when the orlistat was stopped, suggesting that orlistat had caused about a 60% drop in the ciclosporin concentration.[3] Another similar report describes one patient who was found to have about a 50% reduction in ciclosporin concentration 44 days after starting orlistat 120 mg twice daily (lunch and dinner), and another who had a 45% reduction in ciclosporin concentration, noted 6 days after starting orlistat 120 mg three times daily.[4] One patient who was unable to achieve a therapeutic ciclosporin concentration after starting orlistat 360 mg daily while taking the *Sandimmun* formulation (see below) was subsequently stabilised on the *Neoral* formulation at a 50% higher dose than his original *Sandimmun* dose.[5] Another case report attributes very low ciclosporin concentrations post-transplant to the pre-operative use of orlistat. Ciclosporin concentrations remained low 7 days after the orlistat was stopped, even after the use of very high ciclosporin doses of 30 mg/kg daily, and it was suggested that orlistat had persisted in the gastrointestinal tract as the patient had no bowel movements over these 7 days.[6]

(b) Sandimmun formulation

In a heart transplant patient taking ciclosporin, orlistat 120 mg three times daily for 2 weeks was found to have reduced the minimum blood concentration of ciclosporin by 50%, to 50 nanograms/mL. A subsequent pharmacokinetic study in this patient confirmed that orlistat reduced the maximum and minimum concentrations, and the AUC of ciclosporin by 47%, 86%, and 75%, respectively.[7] In a further patient taking ciclosporin 250 mg daily, orlistat 360 mg daily reduced the ciclosporin concentration by 67% (from 150 to 50 nanograms/mL). Increasing the dose of ciclosporin did not result in an increased ciclosporin concentration, so the patient was given *Neoral* instead (see above).[5] Another heart transplant patient had a progressive reduction in her ciclosporin concentration when she started to take orlistat 120 mg three times daily (28% reduction at 5 days and 46% reduction at 10 days), despite taking orlistat 2 hours before ciclosporin. Stopping the breakfast dose of orlistat did not result in an increased ciclosporin concentration, but the concentration did return to normal when orlistat was stopped. Note that this patient was also reported to have severe diarrhoea secondary to poor adherence to a low-fat diet when taking orlistat, which could have contributed to the low ciclosporin concentrations seen.[8]

Mechanism

Orlistat inhibits pancreatic lipase and prevents the absorption of dietary fat and lipophilic molecules such as ciclosporin. Absorption of ciclosporin from the oil suspension formulation (*Sandimmun*) is more dependent on the lipid absorption stage and thus is likely to be more affected by orlistat than the microemulsion form (*Neoral*).[5]

Importance and management

The interaction between ciclosporin and orlistat is established, and has the potential to be clinically important. It has been suggested that the effects of the interaction can be reduced by using the microemulsion formulation of ciclosporin (*Neoral*),[5] which has generally replaced the corn oil suspension (*Sandimmun*). However, close monitoring is required if the two drugs are used together, either in the standard or microemulsion form, because there is still a risk of subtherapeutic concentrations. Some authors recommend avoidance of the combination.[4,7] The UK manufacturer of orlistat does not recommend concurrent use, but notes that if it is unavoidable more frequent ciclosporin monitoring is recommended.[9] The US manufacturer also advises against concurrent use. They recommend taking ciclosporin at least 3 hours after orlistat to reduce the chance of an interaction, and that ciclosporin concentrations should be monitored more frequently.[10] However, there is evidence to suggest that separating the doses does not avoid the interaction.[2,8]

1. Colman E, Fossler M. Reduction in blood cyclosporine concentrations by orlistat. *N Engl J Med* (2000) 342, 1141–2.
2. Zhi J, Moore R, Kanitra L, Mulligan TE. Pharmacokinetic evaluation of the possible interaction between selected concomitant medications and orlistat at steady state in healthy subjects. *J Clin Pharmacol* (2002) 42, 1011–9.
3. Schnetzler B, Kondo-Oestreicher M, Vala D, Khatchatourian G, Faidutti B. Orlistat decreases the plasma level of cyclosporine and may be responsible for the development of acute rejection episodes. *Transplantation* (2000) 70, 1540–1.
4. Errasti P, García I, Lavilla J, Ballester B, Manrique J, Purroy A. Reduction in blood cyclosporine concentration by orlistat in two renal transplant patients. *Transplant Proc* (2002) 34, 137–9.
5. Le Beller C, Bezie Y, Chabatte C, Guillemain R, Amrein C, Billaud EM. Co-administration of orlistat and cyclosporine in a heart transplant recipient. *Transplantation* (2000) 70, 1541–2.
6. Evans S, Michael R, Wells H, MacLean D, Gordon I, Taylor J, Goldsmith D. Drug interaction in a renal transplant patient: cyclosporin-Neoral and orlistat. *Am J Kidney Dis* (2003) 41, 493–6.
7. Nägele H, Petersen B, Bonacker U, Rödiger W. Effect of orlistat on blood cyclosporin concentration in an obese heart transplant patient. *Eur J Clin Pharmacol* (1999) 55, 667–9.
8. Barbaro D, Orsini P, Pallini S, Piazza F, Pasquini C. Obesity in transplant patients: case report showing interference of orlistat with absorption of cyclosporine and review of literature. *Endocr Pract* (2002) 8, 124–6.
9. Xenical (Orlistat). Roche Products Ltd. UK Summary of product characteristics, April 2014.
10. Xenical (Orlistat). Roche Pharmaceuticals. US Prescribing information, December 2013.

Ciclosporin + Oxybutynin

Oxybutynin did not appear to affect ciclosporin concentrations in two children.

Clinical evidence, mechanism, importance and management

In a retrospective analysis, one child with a kidney transplant taking ciclosporin had no change in his ciclosporin concentration and dose over the 2 months before, and the 2 months after, he started taking oxybutynin 2 mg twice daily. Another patient had no change in ciclosporin concentrations and dose over the 3 months before, and 3 months after, stopping oxybutynin 5 mg twice daily.[1]

Although the evidence is limited, it suggests that oxybutynin is unlikely to have an important effect on ciclosporin concentrations.

1. Springate JE. Oxybutynin does not affect cyclosporin blood levels. *Ther Drug Monit* (2001) 23, 155–6.

Ciclosporin + Pancreatic enzymes

Pancreatic enzyme extracts do not appear to increase the bioavailability of ciclosporin in cystic fibrosis patients.

Clinical evidence, mechanism, importance and management

A study in 7 heart-lung transplant patients with cystic fibrosis found that they needed almost five times the oral dose of ciclosporin compared to patients without heart-lung transplants or cystic fibrosis, confirming other studies that had found a very much reduced bioavailability of oral ciclosporin in patients with cystic fibrosis. This is probably a reflection of the generally poor digestion and absorption in cystic fibrosis patients. The addition of pancreatic enzymes (*Creon*) was not found to improve this poor ciclosporin bioavailability. No adverse effects were reported.[1]

1. Tsang VT, Johnston A, Heritier F, Leaver N, Hodson ME, Yacoub M. Cyclosporin pharmacokinetics in heart-lung transplant recipients with cystic fibrosis. Effects of pancreatic enzymes and ranitidine. *Eur J Clin Pharmacol* (1994) 46, 261–5.

Ciclosporin + Paracetamol (Acetaminophen)

Limited evidence suggests that paracetamol can be used as an analgesic in patients taking ciclosporin.

Clinical evidence, mechanism, importance and management

A study in rheumatoid arthritis patients taking ciclosporin 2.5 mg/kg daily, found that creatinine clearances were reduced by 3.5% in those taking paracetamol 650 mg four times daily, but this was not considered to be clinically important.[1] It was concluded that paracetamol could be used as an analgesic in patients receiving ciclosporin.

1. Tugwell P, Ludwin D, Gent M, Roberts R, Bensen W, Grace E, Baker P. Interaction between cyclosporin A and nonsteroidal antiinflammatory drugs. *J Rheumatol* (1997) 24, 1122–5.

Ciclosporin + Phosphodiesterase type-5 inhibitors

Sildenafil and vardenafil do not affect ciclosporin concentrations.

Clinical evidence

(a) Sildenafil

In a clinical study in kidney transplant recipients, sildenafil 25 to 100 mg in repeated doses had no effect on the AUC, and minimum or maximum concentrations of ciclosporin over 8 weeks in a group of 5 patients selected for this analysis.[1] Similarly, in other clinical studies, repeated doses of sildenafil 50 or 100 mg given for 72 hours had no effect on ciclosporin minimum concentrations.[2,3] A further study which gave repeated sildenafil doses during a 4-week period, suggests that ciclosporin concentrations were not affected, but specific details are lacking.[4]

(b) Vardenafil

In a study in 14 kidney transplant patients, vardenafil 10 or 20 mg (maximum frequency of once in 24 hours) in repeated doses during a 4-week period had no effect on the concentrations or required dose of ciclosporin and no change in renal function was reported.[5]

Mechanism

None.

Importance and management

No pharmacokinetic interaction appears to occur between ciclosporin and sildenafil or vardenafil. Therefore, no ciclosporin dose adjustment would be expected to be necessary in patients taking these drugs. Information for other phosphodiesterase type-5 inhibitors appears to be lacking.

1. Sharma RK, Prasad N, Gupta A, Kapoor R. Treatment of erectile dysfunction with sildenafil citrate in renal allograft recipients: a randomized, double-blind, placebo-controlled, crossover trial. *Am J Kidney Dis* (2006) 48, 128–33.
2. Cofán F, Gutiérrez R, Beardo P, Campistol JM, Oppenheimer F, Alcover J. Interacción entre sildenafilo y los inhibidores de la calcineurina en trasplantados renales con disfunción eréctil. *Nefrologia* (2002) 22, 470–6.
3. Zhang Y, Guan DL, Ou TW, Wang Y, Chen X, Xing NZ, Zhang XD, Yang Y. Sildenafil citrate treatment for erectile dysfunction after kidney transplantation. *Transplant Proc* (2005) 37, 2100–3.
4. Russo D, Musone D, Alteri V, Cindolo L, Lanzillo B, Federico S, Andreucci VE. Erectile dysfunction in kidney transplanted patients: efficacy of sildenafil. *J Nephrol* (2004) 17, 291–5.
5. Demir E, Balal M, Paydas S, Sertdemir Y, Erken U. Efficacy and safety of vardenafil in renal transplant recipients with erectile dysfunction. *Transplant Proc* (2006) 38, 1379–81.

Ciclosporin or Tacrolimus + Potassium compounds

Ciclosporin and tacrolimus alone can cause or worsen pre-existing hyperkalaemia, and the concurrent use of potassium compounds might exacerbate this.

Clinical evidence, mechanism, importance and management

Both ciclosporin and tacrolimus can cause hyperkalaemia.[1,2] Hyperkalaemia can itself be a sign of worsening renal function but might be exacerbated by ciclosporin or tacrolimus. This can be worsened further by the use of potassium supplements.

Note that potassium concentrations are usually routinely monitored during the use of ciclosporin and tacrolimus, and this monitoring should probably be increased if other drugs that affect potassium concentrations, such as potassium supplements, are also given. The UK manufacturer of tacrolimus recommends that patients should avoid a high potassium intake,[1] such as that in supplements.

1. Prograf (Tacrolimus monohydrate). Astellas Pharma Ltd. UK Summary of product characteristics, November 2014.
2. Neoral (Ciclosporin). Novartis Pharmaceuticals UK Ltd. UK Summary of product characteristics, November 2013.

Ciclosporin + Probucol

Probucol slightly reduces ciclosporin exposure.

Clinical evidence

A study in 6 heart transplant patients taking ciclosporin found that the concurrent use of probucol 500 mg every 12 hours decreased the ciclosporin whole blood minimum concentration by 42%, from 139 to 81 nanograms/mL, and reduced the AUC_{0-9} by 28%. The clearance was increased by 60% and volume of distribution also increased.[1] Another study similarly found that 9 out 10 kidney transplant patients had a reduction in their ciclosporin minimum blood concentrations while taking probucol.[2]

In 5 patients with nephrotic syndrome, probucol 250 to 500 mg daily decreased ciclosporin minimum concentrations by 36 to 56%.[3] Although not specified, it is assumed that these studies used the original *Sandimmun* formulation. The same group of workers found that in 4 patients with nephrotic syndrome taking ciclosporin (*Neoral*), probucol 500 mg daily decreased the ciclosporin minimum concentrations by 17 to 30%.[4]

Mechanism

Not understood. Probucol appears to reduce the absorption of ciclosporin. Evidence from *in vitro* and *animal* studies found that probucol does not affect ciclosporin absorption via P-glycoprotein-mediated transport.[5]

Importance and management

Information regarding an interaction between probucol and ciclosporin is limited to these studies, but the available evidence suggests that probucol slightly decreases ciclosporin exposure. The majority of the evidence appears to come from studies with the *Sandimmun* formulation of ciclosporin, and one group of researchers consider that *Neoral* is less affected than *Sandimmun*.[4] It would therefore appear that, when using oral ciclosporin as *Neoral* the risk of a clinically relevant interaction is low. Nevertheless, for patients in which the ciclosporin concentration is critical, it would seem prudent to be aware of the potential for a reduction in ciclosporin minimum concentrations and monitor concurrent use accordingly.

1. Sundararajan V, Cooper DKC, Muchmore J, Manion CV, Liguori C, Zuhdi N, Novitzky D, Chen P-N, Bourne DWA, Corder CN. Interaction of cyclosporine and probucol in heart transplant patients. *Transplant Proc* (1991) 23, 2028–32.
2. Gallego C, Sánchez P, Planells C, Sánchez S, Monte E, Romá E, Sánchez J, Pallardó LM. Interaction between probucol and cyclosporine in renal transplant patients. *Ann Pharmacother* (1994) 28, 940–2.
3. Wakasugi H, Yoshimoto M, Aoki M, Osawa R, Futami T, Ono T, Muso E, Inui K. Effect of probucol on the concentration of cyclosporin A in patients with nephrotic syndrome. *Nippon Jinzo Gakkai Shi* (2001) 43, 595–9.
4. Wakasugi H, Yoshimoto M, Ono T, Muso E, Inui K. Effect of probucol on the blood concentration of cyclosporin A in patients with nephrotic syndrome: a case study with a microemulsion formulation (Neoral). *Nippon Jinzo Gakkai Shi* (2002) 44, 792–7.
5. Sugimoto K-I, Sudoh T, Tsuruoka S, Yamamoto Y, Maezono S, Watanabe Y, Fujimura A. Effect of probucol on oral bioavailability of cyclosporine A. *Eur J Pharm Sci* (2004) 22, 71–7.

Ciclosporin + Propafenone

In an isolated report, propafenone caused a 60% increase in the ciclosporin concentrations of a patient.

Clinical evidence, mechanism, importance and management

A heart transplant patient taking ciclosporin, azathioprine, and prednisolone developed ventricular tachycardia 9 months after transplantation, for which he was given propafenone 600 or 750 mg daily. After the first day, his ciclosporin concentration had increased from about 160 to 190 nanograms/mL, and after 5 days the concentration had reached around 260 nanograms/mL. Over the same time period his serum creatinine concentration increased from 168 to 212 micromol/L. His ciclosporin dose was reduced from 240 mg daily to a final dose of 200 mg daily after which his renal function and ciclosporin concentrations were re-established at about the level before propafenone was started.[1] The authors suggest that propafenone interferes with the metabolism of ciclosporin by affecting hepatic cytochrome P450, or that propafenone might enhance the absorption of ciclosporin. Information appears to be limited to this one report, the general importance of which is unknown. Nevertheless, the UK manufacturer of propafenone advises caution on concurrent use and a reduction of the ciclosporin dose if ciclosporin toxicity occurs.[2]

1. Spes CH, Angermann CE, Horn K, Strasser T, Mudra H, Landgraf R, Theisen K. Ciclosporin-propafenone interaction. *Klin Wochenschr* (1990) 68, 872.
2. Arythmol (Propafenone hydrochloride). Abbott Laboratories Ltd. UK Summary of product characteristics, November 2012.

Ciclosporin + Proton pump inhibitors

Omeprazole does not usually appear to affect ciclosporin concentrations, but there is an isolated report of increased ciclosporin concentrations in one patient, and, conversely, decreased ciclosporin concentrations in another. Pantoprazole does not appear to affect ciclosporin concentrations.

Clinical evidence

(a) Omeprazole

In a placebo-controlled study in 10 kidney transplant patients the minimum ciclosporin concentration was not affected by the concurrent use of omeprazole 20 mg daily for 2 weeks.[1] Similarly, 8 kidney transplant patients given omeprazole 20 mg daily for 6 days had no notable change in their ciclosporin concentrations, when compared with control patients not taking omeprazole.[2] In addition, there were no notable changes in ciclosporin concentrations in another kidney transplant patient given omeprazole 20 mg daily for 8 weeks.[3]

In contrast, in one retrospective analysis, the dose of ciclosporin required to give a specific concentration was 28% lower in 21 patients taking omeprazole (dose not stated), when compared with 139 patients not taking omeprazole.[4] A case report also describes a liver transplant patient whose ciclosporin blood concentration roughly doubled (from a range of 187 to 261 nanograms/mL up to 510 nanograms/mL) about 2 weeks after omeprazole 40 mg daily was started. His ciclosporin concentration was readjusted by reducing the dose from 130 to 80 mg twice daily. The ciclosporin concentration then remained steady at about 171 nanograms/mL for the following 4 months.[5] In contrast, the serum ciclosporin concentration of a bone marrow transplant patient fell from 254 nanograms/mL to about 100 nanograms/mL over 14 days in the presence of omeprazole 40 mg daily. The ciclosporin concentration increased rapidly when omeprazole was stopped.[6]

(b) Pantoprazole

Two studies in kidney transplant patients found that pantoprazole 40 mg daily did not affect ciclosporin blood concentrations when given in the evening,[7] or when both drugs were given together in the morning.[8]

Mechanism

Not understood.

Importance and management

There is good evidence that omeprazole 20 mg daily does not alter ciclosporin concentrations, but there is no explanation for the opposite findings (an increase or decrease in ciclosporin concentrations) from the two isolated case reports in patients given omeprazole 40 mg daily. The concurrent use of ciclosporin and omeprazole need not be avoided, but it would be prudent to consider the possibility of an interaction if patients taking higher doses of omeprazole have otherwise unexplained changes in ciclosporin concentrations. Pantoprazole does not appear to interact with ciclosporin and might therefore be an alternative to omeprazole in some patients.

1. Blohmé I, Idström J-P, Andersson T. A study of the interaction between omeprazole and cyclosporine in renal transplant patients. *Br J Clin Pharmacol* (1993) 35, 156–60.
2. Kahn D, Manas D, Hamilton H, Pascoe MD, Pontin AR. The effect of omeprazole on cyclosporine metabolism in renal transplant recipients. *S Afr Med J* (1993) 83, 785.
3. Castellote E, Bonet J, Lauzurica R, Pastor C, Cofan F, Caralps A. Does interaction between omeprazole and cyclosporin exist? *Nephron* (1993) 65, 478.
4. Reichenspurner H, Meiser BM, Muschiol F, Nollert G, Überfuhr P, Markewitz A, Wagner F, Pfeiffer M, Reichart B. The influence of gastrointestinal agents on resorption and metabolism of cyclosporine after heart transplantation: experimental and clinical results. *J Heart Lung Transplant* (1993) 12, 987–92.
5. Schouler L, Dumas F, Couzigou P, Janvier G, Winnock S, Saric J. Omeprazole-cyclosporin interaction. *Am J Gastroenterol* (1991) 86, 1097.
6. Arranz R, Yañez E, Franceschi JL, Fernandez-Rañada JM. More about omeprazole-cyclosporine interaction. *Am J Gastroenterol* (1993) 88, 154–5.
7. Lorf T, Ramadori G, Ringe B, Schwörer H. Pantoprazole does not affect cyclosporin A blood concentration in kidney-transplant patients. *Eur J Clin Pharmacol* (2000) 55, 733–5.
8. Lorf T, Ramadori G, Ringe B, Schwörer H. The effect of pantoprazole on tacrolimus and cyclosporin A blood concentration in transplant patients. *Eur J Clin Pharmacol* (2000) 56, 439–40.

Ciclosporin + Pyrazinamide

Pyrazinamide does not normally appear to interact with ciclosporin, but one isolated report suggests that it might have contributed to the effects of rifampicin in one patient, which resulted in lowered ciclosporin concentrations. Another patient developed toxic myopathy, which was attributed to the use of pyrazinamide with ciclosporin.

Clinical evidence, mechanism, importance and management

A number of reports mention that anti-tuberculosis regimens containing pyrazinamide and without rifampicin, do not appear to alter ciclosporin concentrations in kidney transplant patients, and some are cited as examples.[1-4] These regimens frequently consisted of combinations of pyrazinamide, ethambutol, isoniazid and streptomycin.

In one early report, a 12-year-old girl with a kidney transplant taking ciclosporin and prednisolone had a rejection episode while taking rifampicin and isoniazid, apparently due to the decrease in serum ciclosporin concentrations caused by the rifampicin. The rejection settled when the rifampicin was replaced by pyrazinamide.[1] However, an anecdotal report suggested that when pyrazinamide was given with rifampicin and isoniazid it appeared to add to the effects of the rifampicin causing an additional reduction in ciclosporin blood concentrations.[5] Another report attributed the development of toxic myopathy in a kidney transplant patient to the concurrent use of pyrazinamide and ciclosporin.[6]

There would seem to be no reason for avoiding pyrazinamide in patients taking ciclosporin, but be aware of these rare complications.

1. Coward RA, Raftery AT, Brown CB. Cyclosporin and antituberculous therapy. *Lancet* (1985) i, 1342–3.
2. Aguado JM, Herrero JA, Gavaldá J, Torre-Cisneros J, Blanes M, Rufí G, Moreno A, Gurguí A, Hayek M, Lumbreras C and the Spanish Transplantation Infection Study Group, GESITRA. Clinical presentation and outcome of tuberculosis in kidney, liver, and heart transplant recipients in Spain. *Transplantation* (1997) 63, 1276–86.
3. Vachharajani TJ, Oza UG, Phadke AG, Kirpalani AL. Tuberculosis in renal transplant recipients: rifampicin sparing treatment protocol. *Int Urol Nephrol* (2002) 34, 551–3.
4. Sakhuja V, Jha V, Varma PP, Joshi K, Chugh KS. The high incidence of tuberculosis among renal transplant recipients in India. *Transplantation* (1996) 61, 211–15.
5. Jiménez del Cerro LA, Hernández FR. Effect of pyrazinamide on ciclosporin levels. *Nephron* (1992) 62, 113.
6. Fernández-Solà J, Campistol JM, Miró Ó, Garcés N, Soy D, Grau JM. Acute toxic myopathy due to pyrazinamide in a patient with renal transplantation and cyclosporine therapy. *Nephrol Dial Transplant* (1996) 11, 1850–2.

Ciclosporin + Quinine

An isolated case suggests that quinine reduces ciclosporin concentrations.

Clinical evidence, mechanism, importance and management

A man with a kidney transplant and mild cerebral falciparum malaria had a gradual decrease in his ciclosporin blood concentrations, from 328 to 107 nanograms/mL over 7 days, when he was given quinine 600 mg every 8 hours. A gradual increase in the ciclosporin concentrations occurred when the quinine was stopped.[1]

The reason for this apparently isolated report is unclear and its general importance is unknown. There is insufficient evidence to recommend increased monitoring, but be aware of the potential for an interaction in the case of an unexpected response to treatment. The effects of lower quinine doses used for cramps are unclear.

1. Tan HW, Ch'ng SL. Drug interaction between cyclosporine A and quinine in a renal transplant patient with malaria. *Singapore Med J* (1991) 32, 189–90.

Ciclosporin or Tacrolimus + Raltegravir

Raltegravir does not appear to alter ciclosporin or tacrolimus concentrations, and raltegravir concentrations appear not to be altered by ciclosporin or tacrolimus.

Clinical evidence, mechanism, importance and management

A retrospective study reviewed 13 HIV-positive liver or kidney transplant patients who were switched from HIV-protease inhibitor-based HAART to raltegravir with two NRTIs (out of abacavir, emtricitabine, enfuvirtide, lamivudine, and tenofovir), either at the time of transplantation (6 patients, all taking tacrolimus) or at a median of 21 months post-transplant (7 patients; 4 taking tacrolimus and 3 taking ciclosporin). In those patients who were switched at the time of transplantation, tacrolimus concentrations within the target range were achieved promptly and with standard doses. In those patients who were switched post-transplantation, the ciclosporin and tacrolimus doses were increased 5 to 15-fold to maintain therapeutic concentrations. The pharmacokinetics of raltegravir did not appear to be affected by the concurrent use of ciclosporin or tacrolimus.[1] A case report describes an HIV-positive kidney transplant patient given tacrolimus 1.5 mg twice daily, whose dose was stopped at day 5 post-transplant due to elevated tacrolimus concentrations. She had been receiving atazanavir boosted with ritonavir, which was changed to raltegravir on day 8. Tacrolimus was withheld for 13 days, and within 5 days of restarting her tacrolimus concentrations were within the target range and remained so at 1 year follow-up.[2] Another report describes 2 patients treated with tacrolimus and raltegravir without the need for dose adjustments.[3] The first patient was an HIV-positive liver transplant patient with hepatitis B, who was taking tacrolimus 1 mg twice daily with tenofovir, lamivudine, and zidovudine, and had stable tacrolimus concentrations within the desired range for 30 months. His tenofovir was then changed to raltegravir 400 mg twice daily due to suspected nephrotoxicity, and during the following 12 months his tacrolimus dose and blood concentrations remained stable.[3] The second was a HIV-positive patient with Crohn's disease was started on tacrolimus 2 mg twice daily while taking raltegravir 400 mg (with tenofovir and emtricitabine once daily), who achieved stable tacrolimus blood concentrations within the desired range. Raltegravir concentrations were within the expected range in both patients.[3] In another case, a 40-year-old HIV-positive man, who underwent a simultaneous pancreas-kidney transplant, was successfully treated with tacrolimus and raltegravir (with lamivudine and tenofovir for 1 month, and then lamivudine with abacavir).[4]

Evidence for an interaction between ciclosporin or tacrolimus, and raltegravir is limited, but that which is available suggests that no interaction occurs. This is in agreement with the apparent lack of effect of raltegravir on cytochrome P450 isoenzymes (in particular CYP3A4, by which ciclosporin and tacrolimus are metabolised) and P-glycoprotein.[5] No dose adjustments would seem necessary on concurrent use. Furthermore, ciclosporin and tacrolimus concentrations are monitored routinely so that should any alterations occur, they will be identified and can be managed accordingly.

1. Tricot L, Teicher E, Peytavin G, Zucman D, Conti F, Calmus Y, Barrou B, Duvivier C, Fontaine C, Welker Y, Billy C, de Truchis P, Delahousse M, Vittecoq D, Salomn-Céron D. Safety and efficacy of raltegravir in HIV-infected transplant patients co treated with immunosuppressive drugs. *Am J Transplant* (2009) 9, 1946–52.
2. Cousins D, Topping K, Lee V, Sweeney J, Lawton M. Successful tacrolimus treatment following renal transplant in a HIV-infected patient with raltegravir previously treated with a protease inhibitor based regimen. *Drug Metabol Drug Interact* (2011) 26, 139–41.
3. Bickel M, Anadol E, Vogel M, Hofmann WP, von Hentig N, Kuetscher J, Kurowski M, Moench C, Lennemann T, Lutz T, Bechstein WO, Brodt HR, Rockstroh J. Daily dosing of tacrolimus in patients treated with HIV-1 therapy containing a ritonavir-boosted protease inhibitor or raltegravir. *J Antimicrob Chemother* (2010) 65, 999–1004.
4. Miro JM, Ricart MJ, Trullas JC, Cofan F, Cervera M, Brunet M, Tuset C, Manzardo C, Oppenheimer F, Moreno A. Simultaneous pancreas-kidney transplantation in HIV-infected patients: a case report and literature review. *Transplant Proc* (2010) 42, 3887–91.
5. Isentress (Raltegravir potassium). Merck Sharp and Dohme Ltd. UK Summary of product characteristics, November 2014.

Ciclosporin + Red yeast rice (*Monascus purpureus*)

Red yeast rice has been reported to cause rhabdomyolysis in a kidney transplant patient taking ciclosporin.

Clinical evidence, mechanism, importance and management

A kidney transplant patient taking ciclosporin 300 mg daily developed asymptomatic rhabdomyolysis when she started to take a herbal preparation of red yeast rice containing rice fermented with red yeast, beta-sitosterol, danshen root (*Salvia miltiorrhiza*), and garlic bulb (*Allium sativum*). Two months later, her creatine phosphokinase increased to 1050 units/L but decreased to 600 units/L 2 weeks after stopping the herbal preparation. It is thought that a component of the red yeast rice called monacolin K (identical to lovastatin) probably caused the muscle toxicity.[1] Although this appears to be an isolated case it would be expected to be generally significant as ciclosporin is well known to interact with the statins, and this interaction appeared to be mediated by a statin-like component. Concurrent use need not be avoided, but it would seem prudent to discuss the potential effects with patients and describe the symptoms of myopathy. Patients should report any unexplained muscle pain, tenderness or weakness.

1. Prasad GVR, Wong T, Meliton G, Bhaloo S. Rhabdomyolysis due to red yeast rice (*Monascus purpureus*) in a renal transplant recipient. *Transplantation* (2002) 74, 1200–1.

Ciclosporin + Retinoids

An increase in ciclosporin blood concentrations in one patient was attributed, in part, to starting etretinate. Two patients had an increase in their ciclosporin concentrations while taking isotretinoin, although in neither case was this attributed to an interaction. Another patient taking both drugs had no alteration in ciclosporin concentrations. No pharmacokinetic interaction appears to occur between alitretinoin and ciclosporin.

Clinical evidence

(a) Alitretinoin

In a study in 16 healthy subjects, both a single 30-mg dose of alitretinoin and alitretinoin 30 mg daily for 12 days were found to have no effect on the pharmacokinetics of a single 300-mg dose of ciclosporin. In addition, ciclosporin did not affect the pharmacokinetics of alitretinoin.[1]

(b) Etretinate

In one case, a woman with generalised pustular psoriasis taking ciclosporin 200 mg daily had a considerable increase in her ciclosporin blood concentration, from 176 to 540 micrograms/L, 7 days after the ciclosporin dose was increased to 300 mg daily and 3 days after etretinate 50 mg daily was added. An interaction was suspected as contributing to this effect because it was found possible to reduce the ciclosporin dose gradually to 150 mg daily (accompanied by a decrease in the minimum ciclosporin blood concentration, to 168 micrograms/L), without any loss in the control of the disease.[2] In small studies or case reports, etretinate has been considered to have a ciclosporin-sparing effect,[3-5] or to have modest or no additional benefit.[6,7]

(c) Isotretinoin

A 27-year old man taking ciclosporin following a heart transplant was given isotretinoin 40 mg daily for 2 months, then 80 mg daily up to 20 weeks. His ciclosporin minimum concentration remained within the recommended range, and there was no evidence of graft rejection.[8] Another man taking ciclosporin following a heart transplant received isotretinoin 1 mg/kg daily for 4 months. His daily ciclosporin dose was reduced from 7 to 6 mg/kg one month after starting isotretinoin because of an increased ciclosporin concentration of 587 nanograms/mL. However, it was noted that this might have had nothing to do with the isotretinoin, because the patient required alterations in ciclosporin dose in three instances before isotretinoin was started. No laboratory abnormalities or ciclosporin toxicity were seen, and the heart transplant function remained satisfactory.[9] A 13-year-old girl with aplastic anaemia, who was taking ciclosporin, was given isotretinoin 40 mg daily for 20 weeks. She had a 3-fold increase in her ciclosporin minimum concentration at week 17, which was considered probably unrelated to isotretinoin, and was managed by reducing her ciclosporin dose. Serum lipids did not change during concurrent use.[10]

Mechanism

Uncertain. An *in vitro* study using human liver microsomes found that concentrations of 100 micromols of acitretin, etretinate, and isotretinoin inhibited the total ciclosporin metabolism and total primary ciclosporin metabolite production to the same extent (32 to 45%).[2] These figures suggest that the retinoids might inhibit ciclosporin metabolism. However, another *in vitro* study using human liver microsomes did not find that etretinate inhibits the metabolism of ciclosporin.[11]

Importance and management

From the one published case, it is unclear if etretinate has any effect on ciclosporin concentrations. Similarly, from the cases presented, it is also unclear if isotretinoin alters ciclosporin concentrations. However, the potential for an interaction cannot entirely be dismissed. Note, that it has been suggested that serum lipids should be monitored if isotretinoin is given with ciclosporin because both drugs can cause an increase in lipids.[8]

No pharmacokinetic interaction appears to occur between alitretinoin and ciclosporin.

1. Schmitt-Hoffmann AH, Roos B, Sauer J, Spickermann J, Maares J, Schoetzau A, Meyer I. Pharmacokinetic interactions between alitretinoin and ketoconazole or simvastatin or ciclosporin A. *Clin Exp Dermatol* (2011) 36 (Suppl 2), 24–8.
2. Shah IA, Whiting PH, Omar G, Ormerod AD, Burke MD. The effects of retinoids and terbinafine on the human hepatic microsomal metabolism of cyclosporin. *Br J Dermatol* (1993) 129, 395–8.
3. Korstanje MJ, Bessems PJMJ, van de Staak WJBM. Combination therapy cyclosporin-etretinate effective in erythrodermic psoriasis. *Dermatologica* (1989) 179, 94.
4. Brechtel B, Wellenreuther U, Toppe E, Czarnetzki BM. Combination of etretinate with cyclosporine in the treatment of severe recalcitrant psoriasis. *J Am Acad Dermatol* (1994) 30, 1023–4.
5. Kokelj F, Plozzer C, Torsello P, Trevisan G. Efficacy of cyclosporine plus etretinate in the treatment of erythrodermic psoriasis (three case reports). *J Eur Acad Dermatol Venereol* (1998) 11, 177–9.
6. Meinardi MMHM, Bos JD. Cyclosporine maintenance therapy in psoriasis. *Transplant Proc* (1988) 20 (Suppl 4), 42–9.
7. Korstanje MJ, van de Staak WJBM. Combination-therapy cyclosporin-A-etretinate for psoriasis. *Clin Exp Dermatol* (1990) 15, 172–3.
8. Abel EA. Isotretinoin treatment of severe cystic acne in a heart transplant patient receiving cyclosporine: consideration of drug interactions. *J Am Acad Dermatol* (1991) 24, 511.
9. Bunker CB, Rustin MHA, Dowd PM. Isotretinoin treatment of severe acne in posttransplant patients taking cyclosporine. *J Am Acad Dermatol* (1990) 22, 693–4.
10. Hazen PE, Walker AE, Stewart JJ, Carney JF, Engstrom CW, Turgeon KL, Shurin S. Successful use of isotretinoin in a patient on cyclosporine: apparent lack of toxicity. *Int J Dermatol* (1993) 32, 466–7.
11. Webber IR, Back DJ. Effect of etretinate on cyclosporin metabolism *in vitro*. *Br J Dermatol* (1993) 128, 42–4.

Ciclosporin + Rifamycins

Ciclosporin concentrations are greatly reduced by rifampicin (rifampin) and transplant rejection can rapidly develop. One case report suggests that rifabutin interacts similarly, although to a lesser extent, and rifapentine might also interact similarly. Topical rifamycin has been reported to reduce ciclosporin concentrations in one patient.

Clinical evidence

(a) Rifabutin

The clearance of ciclosporin in a patient with a kidney transplant doubled when isoniazid, ethambutol, pyridoxine, and rifampicin 600 mg daily were given. When these drugs were replaced by rifabutin 150 mg and clofazimine 100 mg daily, the ciclosporin clearance returned to about its former level, but after about 3 weeks the clearance was about 20% greater than before the antimycobacterial drugs were given.[1]

(b) Rifampicin (Rifampin)

A study in 39 kidney transplant patients taking ciclosporin at a mean dose of 158 mg daily found that the ciclosporin dose needed to be increased by between 150 to 525 mg daily (an average dose of 469 mg daily) when rifampicin 450 to 600 mg daily was taken as part of a regimen for tuberculosis. An increased incidence of acute rejection occurred during treatment with ciclosporin and rifampicin, and 16 patients had kidney graft failure and needed to go back on haemodialysis because of this interaction.[2]

A heart transplant patient taking ciclosporin started taking rifampicin 600 mg daily with amphotericin B for the treatment of an *Aspergillus fumigatus* infection. Within 11 days her ciclosporin serum concentration had decreased from 473 nanograms/mL to less than 31 nanograms/mL and severe acute graft rejection occurred. The dose of ciclosporin was increased stepwise and the concentration increased and reached a plateau before suddenly decreasing again. The dose had to be increased to more than 30 mg/kg daily to achieve ciclosporin serum concentrations in the range of 100 to 300 nanograms/mL.[3]

A considerable number of other reports about individual patients, both adult and paediatric, confirm that a very large reduction in ciclosporin serum concentrations occurs, often to undetectable levels, accompanied by transplantation rejection in many instances, if rifampicin is given either intravenously or orally without increasing the ciclosporin dose.[1,4-28] Ciclosporin concentrations become toxic within 2 weeks of stopping rifampicin unless the previously adjusted ciclosporin dose is reduced.[4,6]

Three patients needed increases in the dose of ciclosporin when given rifampicin, despite the additional use of erythromycin, which normally reduces ciclosporin requirements.[19,29,30] Another patient whose ciclosporin concentration had been increased by clarithromycin had a reduction in the ciclosporin concentration when rifampicin was added.[31] For further information on the effects of the macrolides on ciclosporin, see 'Ciclosporin + Antibacterials; Macrolides', p.1209.

(c) Rifamycin sodium

Rifamycin sodium used to irrigate a wound has been reported to reduce the serum concentration of ciclosporin in a kidney transplant patient.[32]

Mechanism

Rifampicin (rifampin) is a potent inducer of CYP3A4, by which ciclosporin is metabolised and so concurrent use results in a large increase in ciclosporin clearance. The drug transporter protein P-glycoprotein might also be involved in this interaction. Rifabutin has some enzyme-inducing effects but these are smaller than those of rifampicin and thus the extent of the interaction is more limited.

Importance and management

The interaction between ciclosporin and rifampicin (rifampin) is very well documented, well established, and clinically important, and transplant rejection can occur unless the ciclosporin dose is increased. In one study 27% of patients taking rifampicin lost grafts due to rejection, and this was directly attributed to the interaction.[22] The interaction develops within a few days (within a single day in one case[20]). If the concurrent use of rifampicin is essential, monitor the effects closely and increase the ciclosporin dose appropriately: 3- to 5-fold dose increases (sometimes increasing the dose frequency from two to three times daily) have proven to be effective, with daily monitoring.

The authors of one large study concluded that it is better to avoid rifampicin in patients taking ciclosporin and to use other antimycobacterials instead.[22] They found that the use of three antitubercular drugs (not including rifampicin) for at least 9 months reduced mortality. Other reports similarly found that regimens without rifampicin were suitable for the treatment of tuberculosis in transplant patients.[23,33] Other rifamycins might also be an option; limited evidence from one case suggests that **rifabutin** interacts minimally. However, the manufacturer of rifabutin[34] and the CSM in the UK[35] warn about the possibility of an interaction, and close monitoring of ciclosporin concentrations would still be advisable. Until more is known, this would also seem prudent with **rifapentine**, which is also an enzyme inducer.

Topical rifamycin interacted like rifampicin in one patient when it was applied to a wound but the general relevance of this is unclear.

1. Vandevelde C, Chang A, Andrews D, Riggs W, Jewesson P. Rifampin and ansamycin interactions with cyclosporine after renal transplantation. *Pharmacotherapy* (1991) 11, 88–9.
2. El-Agroudy AE, Refaie AF, Moussa OM, Ghoneim MA. Tuberculosis in Egyptian kidney transplant recipients: study of clinical course and outcome. *J Nephrol* (2003) 16, 404–11.
3. Modry DL, Stinson EB, Oyer PE, Jamieson SW, Baldwin JC, Shumway NE. Acute rejection and massive cyclosporine requirements in heart transplant recipients treated with rifampin. *Transplantation* (1985) 39, 313–14.
4. Langhoff E, Madsen S. Rapid metabolism of cyclosporin and prednisone in kidney transplant patients on tuberculostatic treatment. *Lancet* (1983) ii, 1303.
5. Cassidy MJD, Van Zyl-Smit R, Pascoe MD, Swanepoel CR, Jacobson JE. Effect of rifampicin on cyclosporin A blood levels in a renal transplant recipient. *Nephron* (1985) 41, 207–8.
6. Coward RA, Raferty AT, Brown CB. Cyclosporin and antituberculous therapy. *Lancet* (1985) i, 1342–3.
7. Howard P, Bixler TJ, Gill B. Cyclosporine-rifampin drug interaction. *Drug Intell Clin Pharm* (1985) 19, 763–4.
8. Van Buren D, Wideman CA, Ried M, Gibbons S, Van Buren CT, Jarowenko M, Flechner SM, Frazier OH, Cooley DA, Kahan BD. The antagonistic effect of rifampin upon cyclosporine bioavailability. *Transplant Proc* (1984) 16, 1642–5.
9. Allen RDM, Hunnisett AG, Morris PJ. Cyclosporin and rifampicin in renal transplantation. *Lancet* (1985) i, 980.
10. Langhoff E, Madsen S. Rapid metabolism of cyclosporin and prednisone in kidney transplant patient receiving tuberculostatic treatment. *Lancet* (1983) ii, 1031.
11. Offermann G, Keller F, Molzahn M. Low cyclosporin A blood levels and acute graft rejection in a renal transplant recipient during rifampin treatment. *Am J Nephrol* (1985) 5, 385–7.
12. Jurewicz WA, Gunson BK, Ismail T, Angrisani L, McMaster P. Cyclosporin and antituberculous therapy. *Lancet* (1985) i, 1343.
13. Daniels NJ, Dover JS, Schachter RK. Interaction between cyclosporin and rifampicin. *Lancet* (1984) ii, 639.
14. Leimenstoll G, Schlegelberger T, Fulde R, Niedermayer W. Interaktion von Ciclosporin und Ethambutol-Isoniazid. *Dtsch Med Wochenschr* (1988) 113, 514–15.
15. Prado A, Ramirez M, Aguirre EC, Martin RS, Zucchini A. Interaccion entre ciclosporina y rifampicina en un caso de transplante renal. *Medicina (B Aires)* (1987) 47, 521–4.
16. Al-Sulaiman MH, Dhar JM, Al-Khader AA. Successful use of rifampicin in the treatment of tuberculosis in renal transplant patients immunosuppressed with cyclosporine. *Transplantation* (1990) 50, 597–8.
17. Sánchez DM, Rincón LC, Asensio JM, Serna AB. Interacción entre ciclosporina y rifampicina. *Rev Clin Esp* (1988) 183, 217.
18. Peschke B, Ernst W, Gossmann J, Kachel HG, Schoeppe W, Scheuermann EH. Antituberculous drugs in kidney transplant recipients treated with cyclosporine. *Transplantation* (1993) 56, 236–8.
19. Zylber-Katz E. Multiple drug interactions with cyclosporine in a heart transplant patient. *Ann Pharmacother* (1995) 29, 127–31. Correction. ibid. 790.
20. Wandel C, Böhrer H, Böcker R. Rifampicin and cyclosporine dosing in heart transplant patients. *J Cardiothorac Vasc Anesth* (1995) 9, 621–2.
21. Capone D, Aiello C, Santoro GA, Gentile A, Stanziale P, D'Alessandro R, Imperatore P, Basile V. Drug interaction between cyclosporine and two antimicrobial agents, josamycin and rifampicin, in organ-transplanted patients. *Int J Clin Pharmacol Res* (1996) 16, 73–6.
22. Aguado JM, Herrero JA, Gavaldá J, Torre-Cisneros J, Blanes M, Rufí G, Moreno A, Gurguí A, Hayek M, Lumbreras C and the Spanish Transplantation Infection Study Group, GESITRA. Clinical presentation and outcome of tuberculosis in kidney, liver, and heart transplant recipients in Spain. *Transplantation* (1997) 63, 1276–86.
23. Muñoz P, Palomo J, Muños R, Rodríguez-Creixéms M, Pelaez T, Bouza E. Tuberculosis in heart transplant recipients. *Clin Infect Dis* (1995) 21, 398–402.
24. Freitag VL, Skifton RD, Lake KD. Effect of short-term rifampin on stable cyclosporine concentration. *Ann Pharmacother* (1999) 33, 871–2.
25. Almeida RV, Carvalho JGR, Mulinari A, Hauck P. Tuberculosis in renal transplant recipients. *J Am Soc Nephrol* (1997) 8, 709A.
26. Kim YH, Yoon YR, Kim YW, Shin JG, Cha IJ. Effects of rifampin on cyclosporine disposition in kidney recipients with tuberculosis. *Transplant Proc* (1998) 30, 3570–2.
27. Zelunka EJ. Intravenous cyclosporine-rifampin interaction in a pediatric bone marrow transplant recipient. *Pharmacotherapy* (2002) 22, 387–90.
28. Koselj M, Bren A, Kandus A, Kovac D. Drug interactions between cyclosporine and rifampicin, erythromycin, and azoles in kidney recipients with opportunistic infections. *Transplant Proc* (1994) 26, 2823–4.
29. Hooper TL, Gould FK, Swinburne CR, Featherstone G, Odom NJ, Corris PA, Freeman R, McGregor CGA. Ciprofloxacin: a preferred treatment for legionella infections in patients receiving cyclosporin A. *J Antimicrob Chemother* (1988) 22, 952–3.
30. Soto J, Sacristan JA, Alsar MJ. Effect of the simultaneous administration of rifampicin and erythromycin on the metabolism of cyclosporine. *Clin Transplant* (1992) 6, 312–14.
31. Plemmons RM, McAllister CK, Garces MC, Ward RL. Osteomyelitis due to *Mycobacterium haemophilum* in a cardiac transplant patient: case report and analysis of interactions among clarithromycin, rifampin and cyclosporine. *Clin Infect Dis* (1997) 24, 995–7.
32. Renoult E, Hubert J, Trechot Ph, Hestin D, Kessler M, L'Hermite J. Effect of topical rifamycin SV treatment on cyclosporin A blood levels in a renal transplant patient. *Eur J Clin Pharmacol* (1991) 40, 433–4.
33. Vachharajani TJ, Oza UG, Phadke AG, Kirpalani AL. Tuberculosis in renal transplant recipients: rifampicin sparing treatment protocol. *Int Urol Nephrol* (2002) 34, 551–3.
34. Mycobutin (Rifabutin). Pfizer Ltd. UK Summary of product characteristics, December 2013.
35. Committee on the Safety of Medicines/Medicines Control Agency. Revised indication and drug interactions of rifabutin. *Current Problems* (1997) 23, 14.

Ciclosporin + Sevelamer

Sevelamer did not appear to alter ciclosporin concentrations in one study; however, a case report describes a large reduction in ciclosporin concentrations within 6 days of starting sevelamer.

Clinical evidence

In a study in 18 kidney transplant patients taking ciclosporin (with 9 patients also taking mycophenolate), the pharmacokinetics of ciclosporin were unchanged; both after they took sevelamer as a single 1.6- or 1.2-g dose, and when this dose of sevelamer was given three times daily for 4 days.[1] Eight of the patients were children (average age 12 years). The largest change was a 9% decrease in the ciclosporin AUC after 4 days of sevelamer use, but this was not statistically significant. The AUC of one metabolite of ciclosporin, AM1, was reduced by about 30%. In this study, ciclosporin was taken at the same time as sevelamer.[1] In contrast, a transplant patient taking ciclosporin 60 mg daily needed a dose increase to 85 mg daily to maintain ciclosporin concentrations within about 6 days of starting sevelamer 806 mg three times daily. Her minimum ciclosporin concentration decreased from about 79 to 62 nanograms/mL on day one, to 42 nanograms/mL on day 3, and then to 35 nanograms/mL on day 6 (figures taken from a graph). When the sevelamer was stopped after 50 days because of gastrointestinal intolerance, ciclosporin concentrations increased, but decreased again on restarting sevelamer.[2]

Mechanism

Sevelamer can bind with ciclosporin in the gut preventing ciclosporin absorption.[2,3] It might also bind with the ciclosporin metabolite AM1 secreted in the bile, so preventing its reabsorption.[1]

Importance and management

The first study did not find a clinically relevant interaction between sevelamer and ciclosporin with 4 days of sevelamer use, but the case report adds a note of caution. The manufacturers of sevelamer recommend that drugs for which a reduction in bioavailability could be clinically important should be taken at least one hour before, or 3 hours after, sevelamer, or consideration should be given to monitoring blood concentrations of these drugs.[4,5] The UK manufacturer specifically names ciclosporin and recommends that close monitoring should be considered both on concurrent use and when sevelamer is stopped.[4] Until more is known, this would appear to be prudent. Further study is required with longer-term administration and to evaluate whether separating doses minimises the extent of the interaction.

1. Pieper A-K, Buhle F, Bauer S, Mai I, Budde K, Haffner D, Neumayer H-H, Querfeld U. The effect of sevelamer on the pharmacokinetics of cyclosporin A and mycophenolate mofetil in patients following renal transplantation. *Nephrol Dial Transplant* (2004) 19, 2630–3.
2. Guillen-Ananya M-A, Jadoul M. Drug interaction between sevelamer and cyclosporin. *Nephrol Dial Transplant* (2004) 19, 515.
3. Wauters J-P, Uelinger D, Marti H-P. Drug interaction between sevelamer and cyclosporin. *Nephrol Dial Transplant* (2005) 20, 660–1.
4. Renagel (Sevelamer hydrochloride). Sanofi. UK Summary of product characteristics, February 2015.
5. Renvela (Sevelamer carbonate). Genzyme. US Prescribing information, May 2011.

Ciclosporin + Sibutramine

One case report describes an increase in ciclosporin concentrations when orlistat was stopped and sibutramine started. Ciclosporin is predicted to increase sibutramine concentrations.

Clinical evidence

A kidney transplant patient taking ciclosporin 100 mg twice daily was changed from orlistat to sibutramine 10 mg daily, as orlistat for 27 months had been unsuccessful. One week later her minimum ciclosporin concentration had increased from 79 to 152 nanograms/mL and her ciclosporin daily dose was reduced by 25 mg. Her ciclosporin concentration was still raised one week later (at 162 nanograms/mL) and her ciclosporin daily dose was again reduced by 25 mg. No increase in blood pressure or serum creatinine occurred, and the ciclosporin minimum concentrations remained stable over the following 10 months.[1]

Mechanism

Unknown. The authors propose a mechanism via inhibition of CYP3A4;[1] however, sibutramine is not an inhibitor of this isoenzyme.[2] Note that the UK manufacturer of sibutramine predicted that ciclosporin could lead to an increase in concentrations of the active metabolites of sibutramine, by inhibiting CYP3A4,[2] although note that ciclosporin is not known to be a clinically relevant inhibitor of this isoenzyme.

Importance and management

This appears to be the only case report of an increase in ciclosporin concentrations with sibutramine, and therefore its general relevance is uncertain. The fact that the patient had previously been taking orlistat, which can reduce ciclosporin concentrations, raises the possibility that the increase in ciclosporin concentrations in this case was due to stopping orlistat rather than starting sibutramine, but insufficient information was presented to evaluate this possibility. For further information on the interaction of orlistat with ciclosporin, see 'Ciclosporin + Orlistat', p.1237.

1. Clerbaux G, Goffin E, Pirson Y. Interaction between sibutramine and cyclosporine. *Am J Transplant* (2003) 3, 906.
2. Reductil (Sibutramine hydrochloride monohydrate). Abbott Laboratories Ltd. UK Summary of product characteristics, December 2009.

Ciclosporin + Somatostatin analogues

Octreotide causes a reduction in ciclosporin concentrations and inadequate immunosuppression might result. Lanreotide is predicted to interact similarly.

Clinical evidence

A diabetic man with kidney and pancreatic segment transplants was successfully immunosuppressed with azathioprine, methylprednisolone, and ciclosporin. When he was also given subcutaneous **octreotide** 100 micrograms twice daily to reduce fluid collection around the pancreatic graft, his ciclosporin minimum blood concentrations decreased to below the assay detection limit of 50 nanograms/mL. Serum creatinine increased dramatically, which was interpreted as a selective rejection episode of the kidney transplant. Nine other patients with diabetes similarly treated with **octreotide** for peripancreatic fluid collection and fistulas after pancreatic transplantation also had significant decreases in their ciclosporin blood concentrations within 24 to 48 hours of starting the **octreotide**, in 3 of them to undetectable concentrations.[1] A similar interaction was seen in another patient.[2]

Mechanism

Uncertain. A suggestion is that the octreotide reduces the intestinal absorption of ciclosporin.[1,2]

Importance and management

The interaction between octreotide and ciclosporin is established and clinically important, although the documentation is limited. The authors of one report recommend that before giving octreotide the oral dose of ciclosporin should be increased on average by 50% and the serum concentrations monitored daily.[1] The UK manufacturer of **lanreotide** states that, as with other somatostatin analogues, it might reduce the absorption of ciclosporin from the gut.[3] As yet there appear to be no reports of this interaction in practice; however, it would be prudent to monitor the outcome of the use of lanreotide with ciclosporin, following the same advice given for octreotide.

1. Landgraf R, Landgraf-Leurs MMC, Nusser J, Hillebrand G, Illner W-D, Abendroth D, Land W. Effect of somatostatin analogue (SMS 201–995) on cyclosporine levels. *Transplantation* (1987) 44, 724–5.
2. Rosenberg L, Dafoe DC, Schwartz R, Campbell DA, Turcotte JG, Tsai S-T, Vinik A. Administration of somatostatin analog (SMS 201–995) in the treatment of a fistula occurring after pancreas transplantation. Interference with cyclosporine suppression. *Transplantation* (1987) 43, 764–6.
3. Somatuline LA (Lanreotide acetate). Ipsen Ltd. UK Summary of product characteristics, July 2010.

Ciclosporin + SSRIs or SNRIs

A small study found no evidence of an interaction between fluoxetine and ciclosporin although one case of doubled ciclosporin concentrations has been seen. One case of increased ciclosporin concentrations with an increase in serum creatinine has been reported with fluvoxamine. Limited evidence suggests that citalopram, paroxetine, and sertraline do not interact with ciclosporin. Serotonin syndrome has been seen in one patient taking ciclosporin and sertraline, one taking ciclosporin and escitalopram, and another taking ciclosporin and venlafaxine.

Clinical evidence

(a) Citalopram

In 5 transplant patients, citalopram 10 to 20 mg daily did not have a clinically or statistically significant effect on the pharmacokinetics of ciclosporin.[1]

(b) Escitalopram

An 84-year-old kidney transplant patient taking ciclosporin developed delirium associated with hyperthermia, 6 months after escitalopram was started and titrated up to 15 mg daily. Her condition improved rapidly after stopping escitalopram and the case was attributed to serotonin syndrome.[2]

(c) Fluoxetine

A small, retrospective study in 9 liver transplant and 4 heart transplant patients found no evidence that fluoxetine 5 to 20 mg daily increased ciclosporin blood concentrations.[3] Another patient had just a minimal 7% increase in ciclosporin concentration after starting fluoxetine 20 mg daily.[4] However, the ciclosporin blood concentration of a heart transplant patient was doubled by fluoxetine 20 mg daily for 10 days. It decreased when the ciclosporin dose was reduced and needed to be increased again when fluoxetine was stopped.[5]

(d) Fluvoxamine

A kidney transplant patient had an approximate 60% increase in ciclosporin blood concentration, an increase in serum creatinine concentration, and fine tremor 2 weeks after starting fluvoxamine 100 mg daily. The ciclosporin dose was subsequently reduced by 33%.[6]

(e) Paroxetine

Two patients had minimal changes in ciclosporin concentrations (7.5% decrease and a 23% increase) after starting paroxetine 20 mg daily.[4]

(f) Sertraline

A 53-year-old man taking ciclosporin following a kidney transplant developed serotonin syndrome 5 days after starting sertraline 50 mg daily. His symptoms resolved after stopping the sertraline.[7]

Three patients had just minimal changes in ciclosporin concentrations (11.5% increase, 10 to 12% decrease, 9 to 17% decrease) after starting sertraline (25 mg daily, 50 to 100 mg daily, 50 mg daily, respectively).[4] One report briefly mentions that a patient taking ciclosporin had her antidepressant medication switched from nefazodone to sertraline, because sertraline did not affect ciclosporin concentrations.[8]

(g) Venlafaxine

A report describes a 33-year-old lung transplant patient taking ciclosporin who developed serotonin syndrome during the 4 days after venlafaxine was started and titrated up to 150 mg daily. Ciclosporin and venlafaxine concentrations were within the normal range, but desmethylvenlafaxine concentrations were over twice the upper limit of normal. Venlafaxine was stopped, and the symptoms resolved within the following 24 to 36 hours.[9] The patient was taking tacrolimus and desvenlafaxine prior to this hospitalisation. Tacrolimus was switched to ciclosporin on the day of admission, and desvenlafaxine had been stopped about 2 weeks earlier. For details of a case of serotonin syndrome in a patient taking tacrolimus and venlafaxine, see 'Tacrolimus + SSRIs or SNRIs and related antidepressants', p.1306.

Mechanism

Fluvoxamine appears to be a weak inhibitor of CYP3A4, the main isoenzyme by which ciclosporin is metabolised. Concurrent use might therefore lead to small increases in ciclosporin concentrations. Fluoxetine is not a notable inhibitor of CYP3A4; nevertheless it has been suggested that it might possibly increase ciclosporin concentrations by this mechanism. Citalopram, paroxetine, and sertraline do not usually inhibit CYP3A4, and would therefore not be expected to interact.

Serotonin syndrome is a rare adverse effect, usually, but not always, associated with the use of more than one serotonergic drug. For more information on serotonin syndrome and its management, see 'Drugs that cause serotonin syndrome + Other drugs that cause serotonin syndrome', p.1471. On the basis that ciclosporin has been reported to increase serotonin turnover within the brain in *mice*, the reaction was attributed to an interaction between the SSRIs and ciclosporin in one of the cases described.[7] The authors of the case reporting serotonin syndrome with ciclosporin and venlafaxine suggest that inhibition of P-glycoprotein by ciclosporin might have resulted in an increase in the venlafaxine metabolite, desmethylvenlafaxine.[4] Further research is needed to confirm this theory. However, note that serotonin syndrome has occurred with SSRIs alone, so ciclosporin might not have played any role in these cases.

Importance and management

Evidence is limited. The case report involving **fluvoxamine** suggests that, in some patients at least, this SSRI might cause a clinically relevant increase in ciclosporin concentrations, resulting in an increase in adverse effects. Fluvoxamine is known to be a weak inhibitor of the isoenzyme by which ciclosporin is metabolised and therefore it would seem prudent to be aware of the possibility of an interaction if using both drugs. Consider monitoring ciclosporin concentrations or choose a non-interacting antidepressant.

Fluoxetine has been used with ciclosporin without interaction, but in one case, ciclosporin concentrations were doubled. However, fluoxetine is not known to inhibit the metabolism of ciclosporin and so in general an interaction would not be expected. **Citalopram**, **paroxetine**, and **sertraline** do not appear to affect ciclosporin concentrations to a clinically relevant extent, and could therefore be suitable alternatives. Escitalopram, the *S*-isomer of citalopram, would also not be expected to interact. The relevance of ciclosporin to the occurrence of serotonin syndrome with escitalopram, sertraline, and venlafaxine in the cases cited is uncertain.

1. Liston HL, Markowitz JS, Hunt N, DeVane CL, Boulton DW, Ashcraft E. Lack of citalopram effect on the pharmacokinetics of cyclosporine. *Psychosomatics* (2001) 42, 370–2.
2. Lang PO, Hasso Y, Hilleret H, Vogt-Ferrier N. Serotonin syndrome as a result of escitalopram and cyclosporin combination in an 84-year-old woman. *Rev Med Interne* (2008) 29, 583–6.
3. Strouse TB, Fairbanks LA, Skotzko CE, Fawzy FI. Fluoxetine and cyclosporine in organ transplantation: failure to detect significant drug interactions or adverse clinical events in depressed organ recipients. *Psychosomatics* (1996) 37, 23–30.
4. Markowitz JS, Gill HS, Hunt NM, Monroe RR Jr, DeVane CL. Lack of antidepressant-cyclosporine pharmacokinetic interactions. *J Clin Psychopharmacol* (1998) 18, 91–3.
5. Horton RC, Bonser RS. Interaction between cyclosporin and fluoxetine. *BMJ* (1995) 311, 422.
6. Vella JP, Sayegh MH. Interactions between cyclosporine and newer antidepressant medications. *Am J Kidney Dis* (1998) 31, 320–3.
7. Wong EH, Chan NN, Sze KH, Or KH. Serotonin syndrome in a renal transplant patient. *J R Soc Med* (2002) 95, 304–5.
8. Wright DH, Lake KD, Bruhn PS, Emery RW. Nefazodone and cyclosporine drug-drug interaction. *J Heart Lung Transplant* (1999) 18, 913–15.
9. Newey CR, Khawam E, Coffman K. Two cases of serotonin syndrome with venlafaxine and calcineurin inhibitors. *Psychosomatics* (2011) 52, 286–90.

Ciclosporin + St John's wort (*Hypericum perforatum*)

Large reductions in ciclosporin blood concentrations and transplant rejection can occur within a few weeks of starting St John's wort.

Clinical evidence

A large decrease in ciclosporin blood concentrations in one kidney transplant patient was identified as being due to the addition of St John's wort extract 300 mg three times daily. When the St John's wort was stopped the ciclosporin concentration increased. The authors of this report identified another 35 kidney and 10 liver transplant patients whose ciclosporin concentrations had decreased by an average of 49% (range 30 to 64%) after starting St John's wort. Two of them had rejection episodes.[1,2] In addition, subtherapeutic ciclosporin concentrations in 8 kidney transplant patients,[3-8] one liver transplant patient,[9] and 6 heart transplant patients[10-12] have been attributed to the concurrent use of St John's wort, often as self-medication without the knowledge of the clinician. Acute graft rejection episodes occurred in 7 cases,[3,5,7,9,10,12] and one patient subsequently developed chronic rejection, requiring a return to dialysis.[5] Another case of subtherapeutic ciclosporin concentrations occurred in a kidney transplant patient during the concurrent use of a herbal tea containing St John's wort. The patient's ciclosporin concentrations remained subtherapeutic despite a ciclosporin dose increase from 150 to 250 mg daily. The concentrations recovered within 5 days of stopping the herbal tea and the ciclosporin dose was reduced to 175 mg daily.[13]

These case reports are supported by a small study in which 11 kidney transplant patients, with stable dose requirements for ciclosporin, were given St John's wort extract (*Jarsin 300*) 600 mg daily for 14 days. Pharmacokinetic changes were noted

3 days after the St John's wort was added. By day 10 the ciclosporin dose had to be increased from an average of 2.7 to 4.2 mg/kg daily in an attempt to keep ciclosporin concentrations within the therapeutic range. Two weeks after the St John's wort was stopped, only 3 patients had been successfully re-stabilised on their baseline ciclosporin dose. Additionally, the pharmacokinetics of various ciclosporin metabolites were substantially altered.[14]

Another study in 10 kidney transplant patients stable taking ciclosporin found that the content of hyperforin in the St John's wort affected the extent of the interaction with ciclosporin. In patients taking St John's wort with a high hyperforin content (hyperforin 7 mg; hypericin 0.45 mg) the reduction in the AUC_{0-12} of ciclosporin was 45% greater than that in patients taking St John's wort with a low hyperforin content (hyperforin 0.1 mg; hypericin 0.45 mg). The blood ciclosporin maximum concentration and the ciclosporin minimum concentration were also reduced by 36% and 45%, respectively, in the patients taking the higher hyperforin-containing St John's wort preparation, when compared with the patients taking the preparation with a lower hyperforin content. The patients taking the high-hyperforin preparation required a mean ciclosporin dose increase of 65% whereas the patients taking the low-hyperforin preparation did not require any ciclosporin dose alterations.[15]

Mechanism

St John's wort is a known inducer of CYP3A4 by which ciclosporin is metabolised. Concurrent use therefore reduces ciclosporin concentrations. It has also been suggested that St John's wort affects ciclosporin reabsorption by inducing the drug transporter protein, P-glycoprotein, in the intestine.[10,14]

Importance and management

An established and clinically important interaction. The incidence is not known, but all transplant patients taking ciclosporin should avoid St John's wort because of the potential severity of this interaction. Transplant rejection can develop within 3 to 4 weeks. It is possible to accommodate this interaction by increasing the ciclosporin dose[12] (possibly about doubled) but this raises the costs of an already expensive drug. Also, the varying content of natural products would make this hard to monitor. The advice of the CSM in the UK is that patients receiving ciclosporin should avoid or stop taking St John's wort. In the latter situation, ciclosporin blood concentrations should be well monitored and the dose adjusted as necessary.[16] One of the studies described above suggests that increased monitoring will be needed for at least 2 weeks after the St John's wort is stopped.[14]

There appears to be no information on the clinical relevance of this interaction in patients taking ciclosporin for reasons other than immunosuppression following transplantation. Nevertheless, because of the large reduction in ciclosporin concentrations seen, treatment failure seems likely, and therefore it would also seem prudent for these patients to avoid the use of St John's wort.

1. Breidenbach Th, Hoffmann MW, Becker Th, Schlitt H, Klempnauer J. Drug interaction of St John's wort with ciclosporin. *Lancet* (2000) 355, 1912.
2. Breidenbach T, Kliem V, Burg M, Radermacher J, Hoffmann MW, Klempnauer J. Profound drop of cyclosporin A whole blood trough levels caused by St John's wort (Hypericum perforatum). *Transplantation* (2000) 69, 2229–30.
3. Barone GW, Gurley BJ, Ketel BL, Abul-Ezz SR. Herbal supplements: a potential for drug interactions in transplant recipients. *Transplantation* (2001) 71, 239–41.
4. Mai I, Kreuger H, Budde K, Johne A, Brockmoeller J, Neumayer H-H, Roots I. Hazardous pharmacokinetic interaction of Saint John's wort (Hypericum perforatum) with the immunosuppressant cyclosporin. *Int J Clin Pharmacol Ther* (2000) 38, 500–2.
5. Barone GW, Gurley BJ, Ketel BL, Lightfoot ML, Abul-Ezz SR. Drug interaction between St John's wort and cyclosporine. *Ann Pharmacother* (2000) 34, 1013–16.
6. Moschella PA-C, Jaber BL. Interaction between cyclosporine and Hypericum perforatum (St John's wort) after organ transplantation. *Am J Kidney Dis* (2001) 38, 1105–7.
7. Turton-Weeks SM, Barone GW, Gurley BJ, Ketel BL, Lightfoot ML, Abul-Ezz SR. St John's wort: a hidden risk for transplant patients. *Prog Transplant* (2001) 11, 116–20.
8. Nowack R, Ballé C, Birnkammer F, Koch W, Sessler R, Birck R. Impact of food and herbal medication on calcineurin inhibitor dose in renal transplant patients: a cross-sectional study. *J Med Food* (2011) 14, 756–60.
9. Karliova M, Treichel U, Malagò M, Frilling A, Gerken G, Broelsch CE. Interaction of *hypericum perforatum* (St John's wort) with cyclosporin A metabolism in a patient after liver transplantation. *J Hepatol* (2000) 33, 853–5.
10. Ruschitzka F, Meier PJ, Turina M, Lüscher TF, Noll G. Acute heart transplant rejection due to Saint John's wort. *Lancet* (2000) 355, 548–9.
11. Ahmed SM, Banner NR, Dubrey SW. Low cyclosporin-A level due to Saint-John's-wort in heart-transplant patients. *J Heart Lung Transplant* (2001) 20, 795.
12. Bon S, Hartmann K, Kuhn M. Johanniskraut: ein enzyminduktor? *Schweiz Apothekerzeitung* (1999) 16, 535–6.
13. Alscher DM, Klotz U. Drug interaction of herbal tea containing St. John's wort with cyclosporine. *Transpl Int* (2003) 16, 543–4.
14. Bauer S, Störmer E, Johne A, Krüger H, Budde K, Neumayer H-H, Roots I, Mai I. Alterations in cyclosporin A pharmacokinetics and metabolism during treatment with St John's wort in renal transplant patients. *Br J Clin Pharmacol* (2003) 55, 203–11.
15. Mai I, Bauer S, Perloff ES, Johne A, Uehleke B, Frank B, Budde K, Roots I. Hyperforin content determines the magnitude of the St John's wort–cyclosporine drug interaction. *Clin Pharmacol Ther* (2004) 76, 330–40.
16. Committee on Safety of Medicines (UK). Message from Professor A Breckenridge (Chairman of CSM) and Fact Sheet for Health Care Professionals, 29th February 2000.

Ciclosporin + Sucrose polyesters

Sucrose polyesters (e.g. *Olestra*) might very slightly reduce the exposure to ciclosporin.

Clinical evidence, mechanism, importance and management

In a study in 7 kidney transplant patients aged 9 to 18 years, a single 0.35-g/kg dose (maximum of 16 g) of sucrose polyesters (*Olestra*), reduced the AUC and maximum concentration of ciclosporin by 19% and 27%, respectively, when taken at the same time as the usual dose of ciclosporin (*Neoral*). Ciclosporin minimum concentrations and elimination rate were not affected by sucrose polyesters.[1] The reduced bioavailability was thought to be due to sucrose polyesters reducing the absorption of ciclosporin. Sucrose polyesters (*Olestra*) is marketed as a non-absorbable, non-calorific fat ingredient in snack foods. The authors note that it is mainly consumed by children and adolescents, with the age group of 13 to 17-year-olds being reported to eat 16.2 g of *Olestra* per snack, and therefore this interaction could be of particular significance for young transplant patients taking ciclosporin.[1] However, note that changes in the AUC of ciclosporin of this size are very slight and would not generally be expected to be of clinical relevance.

1. Terrill CJ, Lill J, Somerville KT, Sherbotie JR. Modifications in cyclosporine (CsA) microemulsion blood concentrations by Olestra. *J Ren Nutr* (2003) 13, 26–30.

Ciclosporin + Sulfasalazine

An isolated report describes increased ciclosporin concentrations in a kidney transplant patient that developed when sulfasalazine was stopped.

Clinical evidence, mechanism, importance and management

A patient with a kidney transplant was taking azathioprine, ciclosporin, prednisone, and sulfasalazine 1.5 g daily. After initial adjustments, the dose of ciclosporin remained at 480 mg daily for 8 months. The dose of prednisone was reduced and treatment stopped at 8 months, and azathioprine was stopped at 12 months, without any need to adjust the ciclosporin dose. However, when sulfasalazine was stopped 13.5 months after transplantation, the mean ciclosporin concentration increased from 205 nanograms/mL to 360 nanograms/mL within 5 days, and to 389 nanograms/mL after 10 days. The ciclosporin dose was reduced over the following 2 months from 9.6 to 5.6 mg/kg to maintain blood concentrations at about 200 nanograms/mL.[1] The mechanism for this interaction is not understood, although the time course of the interaction, noted after 5 days, probably excludes decreased absorption.

Information appears to be limited to this isolated case report. There is insufficient evidence to recommend increased monitoring in all patients, but be aware of the potential for an interaction in the case of an unexpected response to treatment.

1. Du Cheyron D, Debruyne D, Lobbedez T, Richer C, Ryckelynck J-P, Hurault de Ligny B. Effect of sulfasalazine on cyclosporin blood concentration. *Eur J Clin Pharmacol* (1999) 55, 227–8..

Ciclosporin + Sulfinpyrazone

Sulfinpyrazone can reduce ciclosporin concentrations, and episodes of transplant rejection have occurred as a result of this interaction.

Clinical evidence

A study in 120 heart transplant patients found that sulfinpyrazone 200 mg daily was effective in the treatment of hyperuricaemia. The mean uricaemia over 4 to 8 months decreased by 22% (from 0.51 to 0.4 mmol/L), but unexpectedly the minimum ciclosporin concentrations decreased by 39% (from 183 to 121 micrograms/L) despite a 7.7% increase in the ciclosporin daily dose. Two of the patients developed rejection: one after 4 months of taking sulphinpyrazone, when the ciclosporin concentrations decreased to 50 micrograms/L, and the other after 7 months of taking sulfinpyrazone, when the ciclosporin concentrations decreased to 20 micrograms/L.[1]

Another report describes a patient who needed unusually high doses of ciclosporin while taking sulfinpyrazone,[2] while yet another report describes *increased* ciclosporin concentrations in a patient taking sulfinpyrazone. In this latter case there is the possibility that the findings might have been an artefact due to interference with the assay method.[3]

Mechanism

Not understood.

Importance and management

Information appears to be limited to these reports, but the interaction would seem to be established and clinically important. If sulfinpyrazone is added to established treatment with ciclosporin, be alert for the need to increase the ciclosporin dose. The decrease in minimum concentrations of ciclosporin seen in the major study cited was 39%.[1] This study does comment on how quickly this interaction develops, but the two cases of transplant rejection occurred after 4 months and 7 months, which implies that it can possibly be slow. Long-term monitoring would therefore be a prudent precaution.

1. Caforio ALP, Gambino A, Tona F, Feltrin G, Marchini F, Pompei E, Testolin L, Angelini A, Dalla Volta S, Casarotto D. Sulfinpyrazone reduces cyclosporine levels: a new drug interaction in heart transplant recipients. *J Heart Lung Transplant* (2000) 19, 1205–8.
2. Dossetor JB, Kovithavongs T, Salkie M, Preiksaitis J. Cyclosporine-associated lymphoproliferation, despite controlled cyclosporine blood concentrations, in a renal allograft recipient. *Proc Eur Dial Transplant Assoc Eur Ren Assoc* (1985) 21, 1021–6.
3. Cockburn I. Cyclosporin A: a clinical evaluation of drug interactions. *Transplant Proc* (1986) 18 (Suppl 5), 50–5.

Ciclosporin + Terbinafine

Terbinafine does not usually have a clinically relevant effect on ciclosporin concentrations.

Clinical evidence

In a study in 20 healthy subjects, terbinafine 250 mg daily for 6 to 7 days decreased the AUC of a single 300-mg dose of ciclosporin by 13% and decreased its maximum blood concentration by 14%. It was suggested that as the *Sandimmun* formulation was used in the study, inter- and intra-individual variations in ciclosporin absorption caused these differences, rather than any drug interaction.[1] This study has been briefly reported elsewhere.[2] Another study in 11 patients with kidney, heart, or lung transplants found that terbinafine 250 mg daily for 12 weeks caused a small but clinically irrelevant decrease in serum ciclosporin concentrations.[3] Similarly, another study in 30 kidney transplant patients taking ciclosporin and given terbinafine 250 mg daily for 6 to 12 weeks found no significant interaction and none of the patients required ciclosporin dose changes.[4] However, the ciclosporin concentrations of 4 other kidney transplant patients were decreased when they were given terbinafine 250 mg daily for fungal skin and nail infections. In 3 of the patients, ciclosporin concentrations remained within the therapeutic range and therefore no dose adjustment was needed. In the remaining patient, an increase in the ciclosporin dose was required to maintain concentrations within the therapeutic range, and then a reduction in the ciclosporin dose was needed on stopping terbinafine.[5]

Mechanism

These studies broadly confirm previous *in vitro* work with human liver microsomal enzymes, which found that terbinafine either does not inhibit or causes only modest inhibition of ciclosporin metabolism.[6-8]

Importance and management

In general, the changes in the pharmacokinetics of ciclosporin seen with terbinafine are not clinically important. However, it might be prudent to bear the possibility of an interaction in mind, in the event of otherwise unexplained decreases in ciclosporin concentrations.

1. Long CC, Hill SA, Thomas RC, Johnston A, Smith SG, Kendall F, Finlay AY. Effect of terbinafine on the pharmacokinetics of cyclosporin in humans. *J Invest Dermatol* (1994) 102, 740–3.
2. Long CC, Hill SA, Thomas RC, Holt DW, Finlay AY. The effect of terbinafine on the pharmacokinetics of cyclosporin in vivo. *Skin Pharmacol* (1992) 5, 200–1.
3. Jensen P, Lehne G, Fauchald P, Simonsen S. Effect of oral terbinafine treatment on cyclosporin pharmacokinetics in organ transplant recipients with dermatophyte nail infection. *Acta Derm Venereol (Stockh)* (1996) 76, 280–1.
4. Lee KH, Kim YS, Kim MS, Chung HS, Park K. Study of the efficacy and tolerability of oral terbinafine in the treatment of onychomycosis in renal transplant patients. *Transplant Proc* (1996) 28, 1488–9.
5. Lo ACY, Lui S-L, Lo W-K, Chan DTM, Cheng IKP. The interaction of terbinafine and cyclosporine A in renal transplant patients. *Br J Clin Pharmacol* (1997) 43, 340–1.
6. Back DJ, Stevenson P, Tjia JF. Comparative effects of two antimycotic agents, ketoconazole and terbinafine, on the metabolism of tolbutamide, ethinyloestradiol, cyclosporin and ethoxycoumarin by human liver microsomes *in vitro*. *Br J Clin Pharmacol* (1989) 28, 166–70.
7. Shah IA, Whiting PH, Omar G, Ormerod AD, Burke MD. The effects of retinoids and terbinafine on the human hepatic microsomal metabolism of cyclosporin. *Br J Dermatol* (1993) 129, 395–8.
8. Back DJ, Tjia JF, Abel SM. Azoles, allylamines and drug metabolism. *Br J Dermatol* (1992) 126 (Suppl 39), 14–18.

Ciclosporin + Ticlopidine

Three case reports describe decreases in ciclosporin concentrations, and one study noted that minimum ciclosporin concentrations were halved by ticlopidine. However, the interaction was not confirmed in a later randomised, controlled study.

Clinical evidence

The ciclosporin blood concentrations of a patient with nephrotic syndrome were roughly halved on two occasions when he was given ticlopidine 500 mg daily.[1] Another two patients with kidney transplants had similar decreases (one patient on two occasions) when ticlopidine 250 mg or 500 mg daily was given.[2,3] In one of these cases, there was a progressive decrease in ciclosporin concentrations during 4 months of ticlopidine use, requiring an progressive increase in the ciclosporin dose after 2 months of concurrent use. When aspirin was substituted for ticlopidine, ciclosporin concentrations increased, and the ciclosporin dose was reduced.[3] Similar findings were reported in an uncontrolled study in 12 heart transplant patients taking ciclosporin, who were given ticlopidine 250 mg twice daily. After 3 months, the mean whole blood minimum ciclosporin concentrations were noted to be halved from 136 to 72 nanograms/mL, without a change in the mean ciclosporin dose. One case of acute rejection occurred, with a ciclosporin concentration of 74 nanograms/mL.[4] However, in a randomised, placebo-controlled study by the same group in 20 heart transplant patients, the pharmacokinetics of ciclosporin were not altered by ticlopidine at the lower dose of 250 mg daily for 14 days. The mean decrease in minimum concentration and AUC of ciclosporin were 20% and 14%, respectively, which was not statistically significant. Nevertheless, one patient was withdrawn from the study after 3 days because of a 60% decrease in ciclosporin concentrations.[5]

Mechanism

Not understood.

Importance and management

Information appears to be limited to the reports cited, and the reason for the difference between the controlled study and the other study and reports is not certain. However, the controlled study used a low dose of ticlopidine and just 2 weeks of concurrent use, whereas in the other study and reports the interaction was noted after a few months of concurrent use. For this reason, it would be prudent to closely monitor ciclosporin concentrations, both when ticlopidine is first added, and for the first few months of concurrent use.

1. Birmelé B, Lebranchu Y, Bagros Ph, Nivet H, Furet Y, Pengloan J. Interaction of cyclosporin and ticlopidine. *Nephrol Dial Transplant* (1991) 6, 150–1.
2. Verdejo A, de Cos MA, Zubimendi JA. Probable interaction between cyclosporin A and low dose ticlopidine. *BMJ* (2000) 320, 1037.
3. Feriozzi S, Massimetti C, Anacarani E. Treatment with ticlopidine is associated with reduction of cyclosporin A blood levels. *Nephron* (2002) 92, 249–50.
4. de Lorgeril M, Boissonnat P, Dureau G, Guidollet J, Renaud S. Evaluation of ticlopidine, a novel inhibitor of platelet aggregation, in heart transplant recipients. *Transplantation* (1993) 55, 1195–6.
5. Boissonat P, de Lorgeril M, Perroux V, Salen P, Batt AM, Barthelemy JC, Brouard R, Serres E, Delaye J. A drug interaction study between ticlopidine and cyclosporin in heart transplant recipients. *Eur J Clin Pharmacol* (1997) 53, 39–45.

Ciclosporin + Tigecycline

The ciclosporin concentrations of one patient increased after tigecycline was started.

Clinical evidence

A case report describes a 61-year-old kidney transplant patient taking ciclosporin 120 mg daily, whose serum ciclosporin concentrations doubled (from about 300 nanograms/mL to a peak of around 600 nanograms/mL) within 4 days of starting intravenous tigecycline (dose not stated). Her ciclosporin dose was reduced to 60 mg daily and her serum ciclosporin concentration decreased to below 200 nanograms/mL. The ciclosporin dose was gradually increased and returned to the initial dose of 120 mg daily, 3 days after tigecycline was stopped.[1]

Mechanism

Not understood. Ciclosporin is metabolised by CYP3A4, but any interaction is unlikely to occur as a result of CYP3A inhibition, as *in vitro*, tigecycline has been shown not to affect this subfamily of isoenzymes.[2] Involvement of the drug transporter protein P-glycoprotein, for which ciclosporin is a substrate, has been suggested[1] but this requires further study.

Importance and management

Evidence for an interaction between ciclosporin and tigecycline is limited to this isolated case and as such its general importance is unclear. Nevertheless, given the potential implications of greatly increased ciclosporin concentrations, until more is known, consider increasing the frequency at which ciclosporin concentrations are monitored if tigecycline is given and adjust the ciclosporin dose if necessary.

1. Stumpf AN, Schmidt C, Hiddemann W, Gerbitz A. High serum concentrations of ciclosporin related to administration of tigecycline. *Eur J Clin Pharmacol* (2009) 65, 101–3.
2. Tygacil (Tigecycline). Pfizer Ltd. UK Summary of product characteristics, December 2013.

Ciclosporin + Trimetazidine

Trimetazidine does not appear to alter the pharmacokinetics or immunosuppressive effects of ciclosporin.

Clinical evidence, mechanism, importance and management

In a study in 12 kidney transplant patients taking ciclosporin, trimetazidine 40 mg twice daily for 5 days caused no changes in the pharmacokinetics of ciclosporin, and there were no alterations in interleukin-2 concentrations or soluble interleukin-2 receptors.[1] An associated study by the same group of workers using two models (the lymphoproliferative response of normal human lymphocytes to phytohaemagglutinin and a delayed *mouse* hypersensitivity model), similarly found that trimetazidine did not interfere with the effects of ciclosporin.[2] It was concluded on the basis of these two studies that the concurrent use of ciclosporin and trimetazidine need not be avoided.

1. Simon N, Brunet P, Roumenov D, Dussol B, Barre J, Duche JC, Albengres E, D'Athis Ph, Crevat A, Berland Y, Tillement JP. The effects of trimetazidine-cyclosporin A coadministration on interleukin 2 and cyclosporin A blood levels in renal transplant patients. *Therapie* (1995) 50 (Suppl), 498.
2. Albengres E, Tillement JP, d'Athis P, Salducci D, Chauvet-Monges AM, Crevat A. Lack of pharmacodynamic interaction between trimetazidine and cyclosporin A in human lymphoproliferative and mouse delayed hypersensitivity response models. *Fundam Clin Pharmacol* (1996) 10, 264–8.

Ciclosporin + Tyrosine kinase inhibitors

Ciclosporin appears to slightly increase tofacitinib exposure. Tyrosine kinase inhibitors are predicted to increase ciclosporin concentrations.

Clinical evidence, mechanism, importance and management

A preliminary report of a pharmacokinetic study in 12 healthy subjects given ciclosporin 200 mg twice daily for 5 days followed by a single 10-mg dose of **tofacitinib** with a final 200 mg dose of ciclosporin on day 6, describes a 73% increase in the AUC of **tofacitinib** and a 17% decrease in the maximum concentration.[1] This slight increase in tofacitinib exposure may be clinically important, such that a tofacitinib dose reduction may be necessary on concurrent use. Note that the manufacturer warns of the risk of increased immunosuppression if these drugs are given together.[2] Some caution would seem prudent, with consideration given to reducing the dose if increased adverse effects are seen (such as diarrhoea and headache) and monitoring for signs of excessive immunosuppression, such as infection.

Evidence with other tyrosine kinase inhibitors is lacking, but note that some inhibit CYP3A4 (see 'Table 1.9', p.11) by which ciclosporin is metabolised, and might therefore be expected to increase its concentrations. It would therefore seem prudent to monitor ciclosporin concentrations on starting or stopping any tyrosine kinase inhibitor that inhibits CYP3A4.

1. Lamba M, Redifer P, Wang R, Alvey C, Krishnaswami S, Chan G. Effect of co-administration of multiple-dose tacrolimus and cyclosporine on the pharmacokinetics of tasocitinib (CP-690,550) in healthy volunteers. *Clin Pharmacol Ther* (2011) 89 (Suppl 1), S22.
2. Xeljanz (Tofacitinib citrate). Pfizer Inc. US Prescribing information, November 2012.

Ciclosporin + Vitamins

In two studies, ciclosporin concentrations were increased by vitamin E in a water-soluble formulation, while in another study vitamin E modestly decreased the ciclosporin AUC. Other studies have also found modestly reduced ciclosporin concentrations with vitamin E combined with vitamin C, with or without betacarotene.

Clinical evidence

(a) Vitamin E alone

Ten healthy subjects were given a single 10-mg/kg oral dose of ciclosporin (*Sandimmun* formulation) with and without a 0.1-mL/kg oral dose of vitamin E (d-alpha tocopheryl polyethylene glucose 1000 succinate; *Liqui-E*). The AUC of the ciclosporin increased by 60%.[1] In a further study in liver transplant patients, this same formulation of vitamin E (*Liqui-E*) decreased the required dose of oral ciclosporin [probably the *Sandimmun* formulation] by 28% in 19 adults and 32% in 7 children.[2] A similar study in children (age not stated), given both oral and intravenous ciclosporin, found that ciclosporin concentrations at 48 hours were 83% higher in the 8 children also given 10 units/kg of a water soluble formulation of vitamin E (D-α-tocopherol-polyethylene-glycol-1000 succinate; TPGS), when compared with 18 children given ciclosporin alone.[3]

In contrast, another study in 12 healthy subjects found that vitamin E (ACO, Sweden) 800 units daily for 6 weeks modestly reduced the AUC of a single 5-mg/kg dose of ciclosporin (*Neoral* formulation) by 21%. In this study, vitamin E did not significantly attenuate the transient reduction in renal plasma flow and glomerular filtration rate (GFR) seen with ciclosporin.[4]

(b) Vitamin E with Vitamin C

A study in 10 kidney transplant patients taking ciclosporin found that the addition of an antioxidant vitamin supplement (product not specified) for 6 months containing vitamin C 500 mg, vitamin E 400 units and **betacarotene** (vitamin A precursor) 6 mg daily reduced the ciclosporin blood concentration by 24%. An associated improvement in renal function, indicated by an increase in glomerular filtration rate of 17%, was also seen and might have been associated with reduced ciclosporin concentrations.[5] In a placebo-controlled study in 56 kidney transplant patients taking ciclosporin with vitamin C 1 g daily and vitamin E 300 mg daily, ciclosporin minimum concentrations were decreased in the group given vitamins, when compared with the placebo group (14 micrograms/L decrease compared with 10 micrograms/L increase, respectively, from baseline values). A reduction in serum creatinine was also seen.[6] Similarly, in a retrospective study of 22 heart transplant patients, vitamin E 400 units twice daily with vitamin C 500 mg twice daily taken at the same time as ciclosporin, decreased ciclosporin minimum concentrations by about 28%. The reduction in concentrations was more marked in the 6 patients taking the *Sandimmun* preparation than in the 16 patients taking the *Neoral* preparation, but the difference was not statistically significant (42% versus 25%).[7]

Mechanism

Unknown. The formulation of the vitamin E and of the ciclosporin appears to affect the interaction, suggesting that reduction in concentrations occurs as a result of altered absorption.

Importance and management

The clinical significance of these studies is unclear, and there appear to be no published case reports of any adverse effects due to this interaction. However, in some patients, changes in ciclosporin concentrations might significantly affect immunosuppression, and dose modification might be required. If vitamin E and C are used in transplant patients taking ciclosporin, ciclosporin concentrations should be well monitored. In addition, it might be prudent to question patients about their intake of vitamin supplements before starting or when taking ciclosporin, particularly if a sudden or unexplained reduction in stable ciclosporin concentrations occurs. More study is needed, particularly with regard to the concurrent use of standard, commercially available multivitamin preparations, which generally contain much lower doses of vitamin C and E than described here.

1. Chang T, Benet LZ, Hebert MF. The effect of water-soluble vitamin E on cyclosporine pharmacokinetics in healthy volunteers. *Clin Pharmacol Ther* (1996) 59, 297–303.
2. Pan SH, Lopez RR Jr, Sher LS, Hoffman AL, Podesta LG, Makowka L, Rosenthal P. Enhanced oral cyclosporine absorption with water-soluble vitamin E early after liver transplantation. *Pharmacotherapy* (1996) 16, 59–65.
3. Boudreaux JP, Hayes DH, Mizrahi S, Maggiore P, Blazek J, Dick D. Use of water-soluble liquid vitamin E to enhance cyclosporine absorption in children after liver transplant. *Transplant Proc* (1993) 25 1875.
4. Bárány P, Stenvinkel P, Ottosson-Seeberger A, Alvestrand A, Morrow J, Roberts JJ, Salahudeen AK. Effect of 6 weeks of vitamin E administration on renal haemodynamic alterations following a single dose of neoral in healthy volunteers. *Nephrol Dial Transplant* (2001) 16, 580–4.
5. Blackhall ML, Fassett RG, Sharman JE, Geraghty DP, Coombes JS. Effects of antioxidant supplementation on blood cyclosporin A and glomerular filtration rate in renal transplant recipients. *Nephrol Dial Transplant* (2005) 20, 1970–75.
6. de Vries APJ, Oterdoom LH, Gans ROB, Bakker SJL. Supplementation with anti-oxidants vitamin C and E decreases cyclosporine A trough-levels in renal transplant recipients. *Nephrol Dial Transplant* (2006) 21, 231–2.
7. Lake KD, Aaronson KD, Gorman LE, Pagani FD, Koelling TM. Effect of oral vitamin E and C therapy on calcineurin inhibitor levels in heart transplant recipients. *J Heart Lung Transplant* (2005) 24, 990–4.

Corticosteroids + Aminoglutethimide

The effects of dexamethasone, but not hydrocortisone, can be reduced or abolished by aminoglutethimide.

Clinical evidence

(a) Dexamethasone

In a study in 6 patients, aminoglutethimide 500 to 750 mg daily reduced the half-life of dexamethasone 1 mg from 264 to 120 minutes.[1] In another 22 patients it was found that larger doses of dexamethasone (1.5 to 3 mg daily) compensated for the increased dexamethasone metabolism caused by aminoglutethimide and complete adrenal suppression was achieved over a prolonged period.[1] Another study found a fourfold increase in dexamethasone clearance in 10 patients taking aminoglutethimide 1 g daily.[2]

A patient, dependent on dexamethasone due to brain oedema caused by a tumour, deteriorated rapidly, with headache and lethargy, when aminoglutethimide was also given. The problem was solved by withdrawing the aminoglutethimide and temporarily increasing the dexamethasone dosage from 6 to 16 mg daily.[3]

(b) Hydrocortisone

One study found that aminoglutethimide did not affect the response to hydrocortisone, and that hydrocortisone 40 mg was adequate replacement therapy in patients taking aminoglutethimide 1 g daily. In this study, aminoglutethimide did not affect the half-life of ^{3}H-cortisol, which suggests that it does not affect hydrocortisone metabolism.[2] Hydrocortisone 30 mg daily is normally adequate replacement in patients taking aminoglutethimide.[4]

Mechanism

Aminoglutethimide is an enzyme inducer and it seems likely that it interacts with dexamethasone by increasing its hepatic metabolism and clearance, thereby reducing its effects.[5]

Importance and management

Information is limited but the interaction between dexamethasone and aminoglutethimide is established. The reduction in the serum corticosteroid levels can be enough to reduce or even abolish the effects of corticosteroid replacement therapy,[1] or to cause the loss of control of a disease condition.[3] This has been successfully accommodated by increasing the dosage of the dexamethasone. Hydrocortisone is routinely used with aminoglutethimide as replacement therapy, and would seem to be a suitable alternative to dexamethasone, where clinically appropriate. Other synthetic corticosteroids are predicted to interact in the same way as dexamethasone, but this needs confirmation.

1. Santen RJ, Lipton A, Kendall J. Successful medical adrenalectomy with amino-glutethimide. Role of altered drug metabolism. *JAMA* (1974) 230, 1661–5.
2. Santen RJ, Wells SA, Runić S, Gupta C, Kendall J, Rudy EB, Samojlik E. Adrenal suppression with aminoglutethimide. I. Differential effects of aminoglutethimide on glucocorticoid metabolism as a rationale for use of hydrocortisone. *J Clin Endocrinol Metab* (1977) 45, 469–79.
3. Halpern J, Catane R, Baerwald H. A call for caution in the use of aminoglutethimide: negative interactions with dexamethasone and beta blocker treatment. *J Med* (1984) 15, 59–63.
4. Cytadren (Aminoglutethimide). Novartis Pharmaceuticals Corporation. US Prescribing information, March 2002.
5. Santen RJ, Brodie AMH. Suppression of oestrogen production as treatment of breast carcinoma: pharmacological and clinical studies with aromatase inhibitors. *Clin Oncol* (1982) 1, 77–130.

Corticosteroids + Antacids

The absorption of prednisone, and probably prednisolone, can be reduced by large doses of aluminium/magnesium hydroxide antacids; small doses of antacid do not appear to interact. Dexamethasone absorption is reduced by magnesium trisilicate.

Clinical evidence

(a) Dexamethasone

In 6 healthy subjects, **magnesium trisilicate** 5 g in 100 mL of water considerably reduced the bioavailability of a single 1-mg oral dose of dexamethasone. Using the urinary excretion of 11-hydroxycorticosteroids as a measure, the reduction in bioavailability was about 75%.[1]

(b) Prednisolone

A study in 8 healthy subjects given a single 20-mg dose of prednisolone found that 30 mL of **Magnesium Trisilicate Mixture BP** or *Aludrox* (**aluminium hydroxide gel**) caused small changes in peak prednisolone levels and absorption, but these did not reach statistical significance. However, one subject given **magnesium trisilicate** had considerably reduced prednisolone levels.[2] **Aluminium phosphate** has also been found not to affect prednisolone absorption.[3,4]

(c) Prednisone

In a study in 5 patients and 2 healthy subjects, *Gastrogel* (**aluminium/magnesium hydroxide** and **magnesium trisilicate**) 20 mL had no significant effect on the serum levels, half-life or AUC of prednisone 10 or 20 mg.[5] In contrast, another study in healthy subjects and patients given 60 mL of *Aldrox* or *Melox* (both containing **aluminium/magnesium hydroxide**) found that the bioavailability of prednisone 10 mg was reduced by 30% on average, and even by 40% in some individuals.[6]

Mechanism

The reduction in dexamethasone absorption is attributed to adsorption onto the surface of the magnesium trisilicate.[1,7]

Importance and management

Information seems to be limited to these studies. The indication is that large doses of some antacids can reduce the bioavailability of corticosteroids, but small doses do not, although this needs confirmation. Nevertheless, it might be prudent to consider separating administration, and in other similar antacid interactions 2 to 3 hours is usually sufficient. Concurrent use should be monitored to confirm that the therapeutic response is adequate. Information about the interaction of other corticosteroids and antacids is lacking.

1. Naggar VF, Khalil SA, Gouda MW. Effect of concomitant administration of magnesium trisilicate on GI absorption of dexamethasone in humans. *J Pharm Sci* (1978) 67, 1029–30.
2. Lee DAH, Taylor GM, Walker JG, James VHT. The effect of concurrent administration of antacids on prednisolone absorption. *Br J Clin Pharmacol* (1979) 8, 92–4.
3. Albin H, Vinçon G, Demotes-Mainard F, Begaud B, Bedjaoui A. Effects of aluminium phosphate on the bioavailability of cimetidine and prednisolone. *Eur J Clin Pharmacol* (1984) 26, 271–3.
4. Albin H, Vinçon G, Pehourcq F, Lecorre C, Fleury B, Conri C. Influence d'un anti-acide sur la biodisponibilité de la prednisolone. *Therapie* (1983) 38, 61–5.
5. Tanner AR, Caffin JA, Halliday JW, Powell LW. Concurrent administration of antacids and prednisone: effect on serum levels of prednisolone. *Br J Clin Pharmacol* (1979) 7, 397–400.
6. Uribe M, Casian C, Rojas S, Sierra JG, Go VLW, Muñoz RM, Gil S. Decreased bioavailability of prednisone due to antacids in patients with chronic active liver disease and in healthy volunteers. *Gastroenterology* (1981) 80, 661–5.
7. Prakash A, Verma RK. *In vitro* adsorption of dexamethasone and betamethasone on antacids. *Indian J Pharm Sci* (1984) Jan-Feb, 55–6.

Corticosteroids + Antithyroid drugs

Prednisolone clearance is increased by the use of carbimazole or thiamazole.

Clinical evidence

A comparative study was conducted in three groups of euthyroid women:

Group 1 – eight women taking **levothyroxine** with **thiamazole** 2.5 mg daily or **carbimazole** 5 mg daily for Graves' ophthalmology,

Group 2 – six women taking **levothyroxine** who had undergone subtotal thyroidectomy for Graves' disease, and

Group 3 – six healthy women.

It was found that the clearance of a 540-microgram/kg dose of intravenous **prednisolone** in those in group 1 was much greater than in groups 2 and 3 (0.37, 0.24 and 0.2 L/h.kg, respectively). After 6 hours the plasma **prednisolone** levels in group 1 were only about 10% of those in the healthy women (group 3) and were undetectable after 8 hours, whereas total and unbound **prednisolone** levels were much higher and measurable over the 10 hour study period in those women who had not taken **thiamazole** or **carbimazole**.[1] In another group of previously hyperthyroid patients, now euthyroid because of **carbimazole** treatment, the total **prednisolone** clearance was 0.4 L/hour.[1]

Mechanism

Not established. It seems possible that thiamazole and carbimazole increase the metabolism of prednisolone by the liver microsomal enzymes, thereby increasing its clearance.

Importance and management

Direct information seems to be limited to this study, although the authors point out that there is a clinical impression that higher doses of prednisolone are needed in patients with Graves' disease. Be alert for the need to use higher doses of prednisolone in patients taking either thiamazole or carbimazole. Also note that a hypothyroid state may increase corticosteroid effects, and thus corticosteroids are cautioned in hypothyroid patients.

1. Legler UF. Impairment of prednisolone disposition in patients with Graves' disease taking methimazole. *J Clin Endocrinol Metab* (1988) 66, 221–3.

Corticosteroids + Aprepitant

In the short term, aprepitant (and therefore fosaprepitant) increases the plasma levels of dexamethasone and methylprednisolone.

Clinical evidence

(a) Dexamethasone

In a crossover study in 20 healthy subjects, aprepitant 125 mg on day one and 80 mg on days 2 to 5, given with a standard dexamethasone regimen (20 mg on day one, and 8 mg on days 2 to 5) increased the dexamethasone AUC 2.2-fold. When the same dose of aprepitant was given with a reduced-dose dexamethasone regimen (12 mg on day one, and 4 mg on days 2 to 5), the AUC of dexamethasone was similar to that seen with the standard dexamethasone regimen given alone. All regimens in this study also included intravenous ondansetron 32 mg, given on day one.[1]

(b) Methylprednisolone

In a crossover study in 10 healthy subjects, aprepitant 125 mg on day one and 80 mg on days 2 and 3, given with a methylprednisolone regimen (125 mg intravenously on day one, and 40 mg orally on days 2 and 3), increased the AUC of methylprednisolone 1.3-fold on day one and 2.5-fold on day 3.[1]

Mechanism

Aprepitant is a moderate inhibitor of the cytochrome P450 isoenzyme CYP3A4, and probably raises levels of these corticosteroids in the short term, by inhibiting their metabolism via CYP3A4. However, aprepitant is also a mild inducer of CYP3A4 with a transient effect that may only become apparent after the end of treatment with aprepitant. The maximal effect is seen 3 to 5 days after stopping treatment and is clinically insignificant within 2 weeks, see 'Benzodiazepines + Aprepitant', p.813.

Importance and management

An established interaction of clinical importance. The manufacturers[2,3] recommend that the usual dose of dexamethasone should be reduced by about 50% when given with aprepitant (although note that the dose given in the manufacturer's dexamethasone/aprepitant antiemetic regimen accounts for the interaction). The manufacturers also recommend that the usual dose of intravenous methylprednisolone should be reduced by approximately 25%, and the usual oral dose by approximately 50%, when given with aprepitant. However, the UK manufacturer[2] also notes that during continuous treatment with methylprednisolone, corticosteroid levels may be expected to *decrease* at later time points within 2 weeks of starting aprepitant and the effect is expected to be greater if methylprednisolone is given orally rather than intravenously.

Fosaprepitant is a prodrug of aprepitant, and therefore similar precautions are appropriate in the presence of these corticosteroids.

1. McCrea JB, Majumdar AK, Goldberg MR, Iwamoto M, Gargano C, Panebianco DL, Hesney M, Lines CR, Petty KJ, Deutsch PJ, Murphy MG, Gottesdiener KM, Goldwater DR, Blum RA. Effects of the neurokinin1 receptor antagonist aprepitant on the pharmacokinetics of dexamethasone and methylprednisolone. *Clin Pharmacol Ther* (2003) 74, 17–24.
2. EMEND (Aprepitant). Merck Sharp & Dohme Ltd. UK Summary of product characteristics, December 2013.
3. EMEND Capsules (Aprepitant). Merck & Co., Inc. US Prescribing information, August 2014.

Corticosteroids + Azathioprine

In a study in 11 subjects, a single dose of azathioprine did not appear to affect the pharmacokinetics of prednisolone given as a single oral dose of prednisone.[1]

1. Frey FJ, Lozada F, Guentert T, Frey BM. A single dose of azathioprine does not affect the pharmacokinetics of prednisolone following oral prednisone. *Eur J Clin Pharmacol* (1981) 19, 209–12.

Corticosteroids + Azoles; Itraconazole

There is some evidence to suggest that itraconazole can increase the exposure to, and/or the effects of, inhaled budesonide, inhaled fluticasone, deflazacort, dexamethasone, and methylprednisolone, and, to a lesser extent, prednisolone and prednisone. Inhaled beclometasone and ciclesonide might interact similarly. A few case reports describe the development of secondary Cushing's syndrome in patients taking itraconazole with budesonide, fluticasone, or deflazacort.

Clinical evidence

(a) Budesonide

In a double-blind, randomised, crossover study, 10 healthy subjects were given 1 mg of inhaled budesonide over a period of 2 minutes after taking itraconazole 200 mg daily for 5 days. The AUC of budesonide was increased 4.2-fold by itraconazole, and the plasma cortisol concentrations of the patients were suppressed, indicating an increased budesonide effect.[1] Another study compared the results of the ACTH (tetracosactide) test in 25 patients taking itraconazole 400 to 600 mg daily and high-dose inhaled budesonide 800 micrograms to 1.6 mg daily with patients receiving either drug alone. Adrenal insufficiency was detected in 44% of those taking both drugs, but in none of the patients taking itraconazole or budesonide alone.[2]

A 70-year-old patient receiving long-term treatment for asthma, which included inhaled budesonide 1.2 to 1.6 mg daily, developed Cushing's syndrome after taking itraconazole 200 mg twice daily for 8 weeks for a fungal infection of the skin and subcutaneous tissues. Corticosteroid exposure might already have been increased as the patient was also taking diltiazem (see 'Corticosteroids + Calcium-channel blockers; Diltiazem or Verapamil', p.1249), with the effects becoming more pronounced after starting itraconazole. Budesonide and itraconazole were discontinued but the patient subsequently required long-term oral hydrocortisone for secondary adrenal insufficiency.[3]

Two other reports describe the development of Cushing's syndrome in patients with cystic fibrosis given inhaled budesonide, and then itraconazole for bronchopulmonary aspergillosis.[4] One patient was also taking clarithromycin, which could have contributed to the increased budesonide effects (see 'Corticosteroids + Macrolides', p.1254). The other patient was a 4-year-old boy who developed Cushing's syndrome 2 weeks after starting to take itraconazole 200 mg daily and inhaled budesonide 400 micrograms daily.[5]

An analysis of 46 cases of adrenal insufficiency in users of inhaled corticosteroids from a retrospective study, found that 15 of these cases were possibly due to an interaction In two of these cases, the patients were taking itraconazole with inhaled budesonide (1 mg to 1.6 mg daily). No other details are given.[6]

(b) Deflazacort

A patient with cystic fibrosis taking deflazacort 15 mg daily developed Cushing's syndrome within 2 months of starting to take itraconazole 200 mg twice daily. The patient recovered within 4 months of stopping the itraconazole and reducing the dose of deflazacort to 12 mg daily.[7]

(c) Dexamethasone

A study in 8 healthy subjects found that itraconazole 200 mg daily for 4 days increased the AUC, maximum plasma concentration, and elimination half-life of a single 4.5-mg dose of dexamethasone 3.7-fold, 1.7-fold, and 2.8-fold, respectively. In another phase of the study, itraconazole decreased the systemic clearance of intravenous dexamethasone 5 mg by 68%, and increased the AUC and elimination half-life 3.3-fold and 3.2-fold, respectively. The adrenal-suppressant effects of dexamethasone were enhanced by itraconazole.[8]

(d) Fluticasone

A case report describes profound adrenal suppression with secondary Cushing's syndrome in a patient with cystic fibrosis given itraconazole 200 mg twice daily and low-dose inhaled fluticasone 250 micrograms daily.[9] Another report describes a patient with asthma who had been taking inhaled fluticasone 1 to 1.5 mg twice daily for 2 years who developed secondary Cushing's syndrome and adrenal suppression 6 weeks after starting to take itraconazole (initially 100 mg daily then 200 mg daily).[10] An analysis of 46 cases of adrenal insufficiency in users of inhaled corticosteroids from a retrospective study, found that 15 of these cases were possibly due to an interaction. In 4 of these, the patients were also taking itraconazole with inhaled fluticasone (500 micrograms to 1 mg daily). In two cases, the patients (one of which was an adolescent) were reported to have developed Cushing's syndrome, and the other two patients were reported to have developed adrenal insufficiency. No other details are given.[6]

(e) Methylprednisolone

A study in 14 healthy subjects found that itraconazole 400 mg for one day followed by 200 mg daily for the next 3 days, increased the AUC of a single 48-mg dose of oral methylprednisolone more than 2.5-fold.[11] Other studies in healthy subjects have found that itraconazole decreases the clearance, increases the elimination half-life, and increases the AUC of both oral and intravenous methylprednisolone. Enhanced adrenal suppression also occurred.[12,13]

A man with a lung transplant taking methylprednisolone, ciclosporin, and azathioprine was given itraconazole 200 mg twice daily to treat a suspected *Aspergillus fumigatus* infection. Three weeks later signs of corticosteroid toxicity developed, namely myopathy (confirmed by electromyography) and diabetes mellitus. Ten days after stopping the itraconazole, the muscle force had improved and his daily dose of insulin had decreased from 120 units to 20 units.[14]

(f) Prednisolone or Prednisone

Six patients with allergic bronchopulmonary aspergillosis (3 with underlying cystic fibrosis and 3 with severe asthma) were given itraconazole 200 mg twice daily for one to six months. Four of the patients, who were also taking systemic prednisone, were able to reduce the corticosteroid dose by 44% (from 43 mg daily to 24 mg daily) without any clinical deterioration.[15] Another study in healthy subjects found no clinically important pharmacokinetic interaction between itraconazole (400 mg on day one, then 200 mg daily for 3 days) and a single 60-mg dose of prednisone.[11]

A study in 10 healthy subjects found that itraconazole 200 mg daily for 4 days increased the AUC of a single 20-mg oral dose of prednisolone by 24%, but this was considered to be of limited clinical importance.[16]

Mechanism

It seems probable that itraconazole inhibits the metabolism of these corticosteroids by CYP3A4 leading to increased exposure and therefore increased effects. The active metabolite of ciclesonide is also metabolised by CYP3A4.[17] Prednisolone is less likely than methylprednisolone to interact with CYP3A4 inhibitors.[16]

Importance and management

The interactions between these corticosteroids and itraconazole appear to be established. There is currently too little data to assess the incidence, but it would be prudent to monitor the outcome of giving itraconazole with **deflazacort**, **dexamethasone**, or **methylprednisolone**, being alert for the need to reduce the steroid dose. Adrenal function should also be monitored in patients receiving inhaled **budesonide** or **fluticasone** who are also given itraconazole, as Cushing's syndrome has been reported in a number of patients taking these combinations. One US manufacturer of inhaled budesonide advises caution on the long-term concurrent use of itraconazole due to the risk of increased adverse effects.[18] However, the UK manufacturers of oral and inhaled budesonide advise avoiding concurrent use itraconazole. If this is not possible, they state that the time interval between giving the interacting drugs should be as long as possible, and that a reduction in the dose of budesonide should also be considered.[19-21] Similar advice is given for intranasal budesonide,[22] and the UK manufacturer of budesonide rectal foam also advises avoiding the concurrent use of itraconazole.[23] In addition, some UK manufacturers of inhaled and intranasal budesonide state that the increase in budesonide exposure is of little clinical importance for short-term use (1 to 2 weeks), but should be taken into account for long-term use.[19,22] Similarly, the UK manufacturer of inhaled[24] and intranasal[25] fluticasone recommends caution, and, if possible, long-term concurrent use with itraconazole should be avoided. One UK manufacturer of inhaled **beclometasone** also predicts that, despite low systemic absorption, drugs that inhibit CYP3A4, such as itraconazole, might theoretically increase the systemic exposure to beclometasone, and they therefore advise caution on concurrent use.[26]

Itraconazole appears to interact with **prednisone** and **prednisolone** to a lesser extent, but the effects might still be clinically important in some patients: consider this interaction as a possible cause if corticosteroid adverse effects develop on concurrent use.

Ketoconazole has been reported to increase the exposure to the active metabolite of **ciclesonide**, see 'Corticosteroids + Azoles; Ketoconazole', p.1247. The UK manufacturer of **ciclesonide** predicts that itraconazole might interact similarly, increasing the risk of systemic adverse effects, and they suggest that it should not be used concurrently with itraconazole unless the benefits outweigh the risks.[17]

General advice

Information about other corticosteroids is lacking but it would seem prudent to bear this possible interaction in mind if itraconazole is given to patients receiving any systemic or inhaled corticosteroid as most are metabolised, at least in part, by CYP3A4. Patients should be warned to be alert for any evidence of increased corticosteroid effects (such as moon face, weight gain, hyperglycaemia) and to seek medical advice if these occur.

1. Raaska K, Niemi M, Neuvonen M, Neuvonen PJ, Kivistö KT. Plasma concentrations of inhaled budesonide and its effects on plasma cortisol are increased by the cytochrome P4503A4 inhibitor itraconazole. *Clin Pharmacol Ther* (2002) 72, 362–9.
2. Skov M, Main KM, Sillesen IB, Müller J, Koch C, Lanng S. Iatrogenic adrenal insufficiency as a side-effect of combined treatment of itraconazole and budesonide. *Eur Respir J* (2002) 20,127–33.
3. Bolland MJ, Bagg W, Thomas MG, Lucas JA, Ticehurst R, Black PN. Cushing's syndrome due to interaction between inhaled corticosteroids and itraconazole. *Ann Pharmacother* (2004) 38, 46–9.
4. Main KM, Skov M, Sillesen IB, Dige-Petersen H, Müller J, Koch C, Lanng S. Cushing's syndrome due to pharmacological interaction in a cystic fibrosis patient. *Acta Paediatr* (2002) 91, 1008–11.
5. De Wachter E, Malfroot A, De Schutter I, Vanbesien J, De Schepper J. Inhaled budesonide induced Cushing's syndrome in cystic fibrosis patients, due to drug inhibition of cytochrome P450. *J Cyst Fibros* (2003) 2, 72–5.
6. Daveluy A, Raignoux C, Miremont-Salamé G, Girodet P-O, Moore N, Haramburu F, Molimard M. Drug interactions between inhaled corticosteroids and enzymatic inhibitors. *Eur J Clin Pharmacol* (2009) 65, 743–5.
7. Sauty A, Héritier F, Leuenberger Ph, Fitting J-W. Cushing's syndrome in a patient with cystic fibrosis treated with itraconazole and deflazacort for allergic bronchopulmonary aspergillosis. *Eur Respir J* (1995) 8 (Suppl 19), 441S.
8. Varis T, Kivistö KT, Backman JT, Neuvonen PJ. The cytochrome P450 3A4 inhibitor itraconazole markedly increases the plasma concentrations of dexamethasone and enhances its adrenal-suppressant effect. *Clin Pharmacol Ther* (2000) 68, 487–94.
9. Parmar JS, Howell T, Kelly J, Bilton D. Profound adrenal suppression secondary to treatment with low dose inhaled steroids and itraconazole in allergic bronchopulmonary aspergillosis in cystic fibrosis. *Thorax* (2002) 57, 749–50.
10. Woods DR, Arun CS, Corris PA, Perros P. Cushing's syndrome without excess cortisol. *BMJ* (2006) 332, 469–70.
11. Lebrun-Vignes B, Corbrion Archer V, Diquet B, Levron JC, Chosidow O, Puech AJ, Warot D. Effect of itraconazole on the pharmacokinetics of prednisolone and methylprednisolone and cortisol secretion in healthy subjects. *Br J Clin Pharmacol* (2001) 51, 443–50.
12. Varis T, Kaukonen K-M, Kivistö KT, Neuvonen PJ. Plasma concentrations and effects of oral methylprednisolone are considerably increased by itraconazole. *Clin Pharmacol Ther* (1998) 64, 363–8.
13. Varis T, Kivistö KT, Backman JT, Neuvonen PJ. Itraconazole decreases the clearance and enhances the effects of intravenously administered methylprednisolone in healthy volunteers. *Pharmacol Toxicol* (1999) 85, 29–32.
14. Linthoudt H, Van Raemdonck D, Lerut T, Demedts M, Verleden G. The association of itraconazole and methylprednisolone may give rise to important steroid-related side effects. *J Heart Lung Transplant* (1996) 15, 1165.
15. Denning DW, Van Wye JE, Lewiston NJ, Stevens DA. Adjunctive therapy of allergic bronchopulmonary aspergillosis with itraconazole. *Chest* (1991) 100, 813–9.
16. Varis T, Kivistö KT, Neuvonen PJ. The effect of itraconazole on the pharmacokinetics and pharmacodynamics of oral prednisolone. *Eur J Clin Pharmacol* (2000) 56, 57–60.
17. Alvesco (Ciclesonide). Nycomed UK Ltd. UK Summary of product characteristics, May 2011.
18. Pulmicort Respules (Budesonide). AstraZeneca LP. US Prescribing information, July 2010.
19. Easyhaler (Budesonide). Orion Pharma (UK) Ltd. UK Summary of product characteristics, July 2011.
20. Entocort CR Capsules (Budesonide). AstraZeneca UK Ltd. UK Summary of product characteristics, April 2012.
21. Pulmicort Turbohaler (Budesonide). AstraZeneca UK Ltd. UK Summary of product characteristics, April 2012.
22. Rhinocort Aqua Nasal Spray (Budesonide). AstraZeneca UK Ltd. UK Summary of product characteristics, July 2012.
23. Budenofalk Rectal Foam (Budesonide). Dr. Falk Pharma UK Ltd. UK Summary of product characteristics, November 2011.
24. Flixotide Evohaler (Fluticasone propionate). Allen & Hanburys Ltd. UK Summary of product characteristics, August 2011.
25. Flixonase Aqueous Nasal Spray (Fluticasone propionate). Allen & Hanburys Ltd. UK Summary of product characteristics, September 2011.
26. Pulvinal (Beclometasone dipropionate). Chiesi Ltd. UK Summary of product characteristics, April 2011.

Corticosteroids + Azoles; Ketoconazole

Ketoconazole reduces the metabolism and clearance of methylprednisolone and might increase the exposure to the active metabolite of ciclesonide. Ketoconazole increases the systemic effects of inhaled budesonide and possibly fluticasone, and markedly increases the exposure to oral budesonide. Inhaled beclometasone might be similarly affected. The situation with prednisone and prednisolone is uncertain: studies have shown some pharmacokinetic effects, but this does not appear to alter the action of either drug.

Clinical evidence

(a) Budesonide

In a study, 16 healthy subjects were given a single 1-mg dose of inhaled budesonide after taking ketoconazole 200 mg daily for 2 days. Plasma cortisol concentrations and urinary cortisol excretion were used as a measure of how much budesonide was absorbed systemically. Ketoconazole was found to cause a 37% decrease in the AUC_{0-24} of cortisol, which suggests an increase in systemic budesonide exposure.[1]

Another study, in 8 healthy subjects, found that the AUC of a single 3-mg oral dose of budesonide was increased 6.5-fold when it was given with the last dose of ketoconazole 200 mg daily for 4 days. When budesonide was given 12 hours before the last dose of ketoconazole, the AUC was increased 3.8-fold.[2] One UK manufacturer of inhaled budesonide also briefly reports that in a study, ketoconazole 100 mg twice daily increased the plasma concentration of a single 10-mg dose of *oral* budesonide 7.8-fold.[3]

(b) Ciclesonide

The UK manufacturer briefly notes that, in an interaction study, ketoconazole increased the exposure to the active M1 metabolite of ciclesonide about 3.5-fold, but did not alter ciclesonide exposure.[4]

(c) Fluticasone

In a study, 16 healthy subjects were given a single 500-microgram dose of inhaled fluticasone after taking ketoconazole 200 mg daily for 2 days. Plasma cortisol concentrations and urinary cortisol excretion were used as a measure of how much fluticasone was absorbed systemically, and it was found that ketoconazole had no effect on fluticasone absorption.[1] However, the UK manufacturer of fluticasone cites a study in which the exposure to fluticasone was increased 2.5-fold by ketoconazole, which resulted in a reduction in the plasma cortisol concentration.[5]

(d) Methylprednisolone

In a study in 6 healthy subjects, ketoconazole 200 mg daily for 6 days increased the mean AUC of a single 20-mg intravenous dose of methylprednisolone 2.4-fold and decreased its clearance by 60%. The 24-hour cortisol AUC was reduced by 44%.[6] These findings were confirmed in another study by the same group of workers.[7]

(e) Prednisolone or Prednisone

In a study in 10 healthy subjects, ketoconazole 200 mg daily for 6 to 7 days caused a 50% increase in the plasma concentrations of both total and unbound prednisolone, following a dose of either oral prednisone (which is metabolised to prednisolone) or intravenous prednisolone.[8] In contrast, two other studies found that ketoconazole 200 mg daily for 6 days did not affect either the pharmacokinetics or the pharmacodynamics of prednisolone, as measured by the suppressive effects on serum cortisol, blood basophil, and helper T-lymphocyte values of prednisolone.[9,10]

Mechanism

Ketoconazole inhibits CYP3A4 in the intestinal wall and liver so that the metabolism of corticosteroids metabolised by this isoenzyme (such as budesonide, fluticasone, and methylprednisolone) is reduced and therefore their exposure is increased. The active metabolite of ciclesonide is also metabolised by CYP3A4,[4] and it might therefore be similarly affected. Prednisolone is less dependent on CYP3A4 for metabolism, and is therefore affected to a lesser extent.

Importance and management

The interaction between **methylprednisolone** and ketoconazole appears to be established and clinically important. A 50% reduction in the dose of methylprednisolone was recommended by the authors of one study.[7] It has been noted that increased corticosteroid serum concentrations have an increased immunosuppressive effect, which would be undesirable in those with a fungal infection needing treatment with ketoconazole.[8] The situation with **prednisone** and **prednisolone** is as yet uncertain,[11,12] and more study is needed.

The study using inhaled **budesonide** indicates that ketoconazole increases its systemic effects. One US manufacturer of inhaled budesonide advises caution on the long-term concurrent use of ketoconazole due to the risk of increased adverse effects.[13] However, because of the large increase in exposure seen with oral budesonide, some UK manufacturers of inhaled budesonide advise avoiding concurrent use with ketoconazole. If this is not possible, they state that the time interval between giving the two drugs should be as long as possible, and that a reduction in the budesonide dose should be considered.[3,14] Similar advice is given for intranasal budesonide,[15] and the UK manufacturer of budesonide rectal foam also advises avoiding the concurrent use of ketoconazole.[16] In addition, some UK manufacturers of inhaled and intranasal budesonide state that the increase in budesonide exposure is of little clinical importance for short-term use (1 to 2 weeks), but should be taken into account for long-term use.[14,15] An important interaction is likely to occur with the concurrent use of ketoconazole and oral budesonide; however, the effects of ketoconazole on budesonide appear to be reduced by about half by separating the administration of the two drugs by 12 hours.[2] One UK manufacturer of oral budesonide recommends that, if concurrent use cannot be avoided, the interval between giving the two drugs should be as great as possible; a reduction in the dose of budesonide should also be considered.[17]

The situation with inhaled **fluticasone** is less clear, with one study finding an effect and another finding no effect. The UK manufacturer of inhaled[5] and intranasal[18] fluticasone suggests that caution is warranted and, where possible, long-term concurrent use should be avoided. Similarly, the UK manufacturer of **ciclesonide** suggests that it should not be used with ketoconazole unless the benefits outweigh the risks.[4]

One UK manufacturer of inhaled **beclometasone** states that, although the systemic absorption is low, drugs that inhibit CYP3A4, such as ketoconazole, might theoretically increase the systemic exposure to beclometasone, and they therefore advise caution on concurrent use.[19]

General advice

Information about an interaction between ketoconazole and other corticosteroids is lacking but it would seem prudent to bear this possible interaction in mind if ketoconazole is given to patients receiving any systemic or inhaled corticosteroid as most are metabolised, at least in part, by CYP3A4. Patients should be warned to be alert for any evidence of increased corticosteroid effects (such as moon face, weight gain, hyperglycaemia) and to seek medical advice if these occur.

1. Falcoz C, Lawlor C, Hefting NR, Borgstein NG, Smeets FWM, Wemer J, Jonkman JHG, House F. Effects of CYP450 3A inhibition by ketoconazole on systemic activity of inhaled fluticasone propionate and budesonide. *Eur Respir J* (1997) 10 (Suppl 25), 175S–176S.
2. Seidegård J. Reduction of the inhibitory effect of ketoconazole on budesonide pharmacokinetics by separation of their time of administration. *Clin Pharmacol Ther* (2000) 68, 13–17.
3. Pulmicort Turbohaler (Budesonide). AstraZeneca UK Ltd. UK Summary of product characteristics, April 2012.
4. Alvesco (Ciclesonide). Nycomed UK Ltd. UK Summary of product characteristics, May 2011.
5. Flixotide Evohaler (Fluticasone propionate). Allen & Hanburys Ltd. UK Summary of product characteristics, August 2011.
6. Glynn AM, Slaughter RL, Brass C, D'Ambrosio R, Jusko WJ. Effects of ketoconazole on methylprednisolone pharmacokinetics and cortisol secretion. *Clin Pharmacol Ther* (1986) 39, 654–9.
7. Kandrotas RJ, Slaughter RL, Brass C, Jusko WJ. Ketoconazole effects on methylprednisolone disposition and their joint suppression of endogenous cortisol. *Clin Pharmacol Ther* (1987) 42, 465–70.
8. Zürcher RM, Frey BM, Frey FJ. Impact of ketoconazole on the metabolism of prednisolone. *Clin Pharmacol Ther* (1989) 45, 366–72.
9. Yamashita SK, Ludwig EA, Middleton E, Jusko WJ. Lack of pharmacokinetic and pharmacodynamic interactions between ketoconazole and prednisolone. *Clin Pharmacol Ther* (1991) 49, 558–70.
10. Ludwig EA, Slaughter RL, Savliwala M, Brass C, Jusko WJ. Steroid-specific effects of ketoconazole on corticosteroid disposition: unaltered prednisolone elimination. *Drug Intell Clin Pharm* (1989) 23, 858–61.
11. Jusko WJ. Ketoconazole effects on corticosteroid disposition. *Clin Pharmacol Ther* (1990) 47, 418–19.
12. Zürcher RM, Frey BM, Frey FJ. Ketoconazole effects on corticosteroid disposition. *Clin Pharmacol Ther* (1990) 47, 419–21.
13. Pulmicort Respules (Budesonide). AstraZeneca LP. US Prescribing information, July 2010.
14. Easyhaler (Budesonide). Orion Pharma (UK) Ltd. UK Summary of product characteristics, July 2011.
15. Rhinocort Aqua Nasal Spray (Budesonide). AstraZeneca UK Ltd. UK Summary of product characteristics, July 2012.
16. Budenofalk Rectal Foam (Budesonide). Dr. Falk Pharma UK Ltd. UK Summary of product characteristics, November 2011.
17. Entocort CR Capsules (Budesonide). AstraZeneca UK Ltd. UK Summary of product characteristics, April 2012.
18. Flixonase Aqueous Nasal Spray (Fluticasone propionate). Allen & Hanburys Ltd. UK Summary of product characteristics, September 2011.
19. Pulvinal (Beclometasone dipropionate). Chiesi Ltd. UK Summary of product characteristics, April 2011.

Corticosteroids + Azoles; Voriconazole

Voriconazole increases the plasma concentrations of prednisolone but not to a clinically relevant extent. A case report notes that voriconazole appears not to interact with oral hydrocortisone. Voriconazole is predicted to increase budesonide concentrations.

Clinical evidence

In healthy subjects, voriconazole 200 mg twice daily for 30 days increased the maximum plasma concentration and AUC of a single 60-mg dose of **prednisolone** by 11% and 34%, respectively.[1,2]

A patient who developed Cushing's syndrome and secondary adrenal insufficiency during treatment with itraconazole and inhaled budesonide was given oral **hydrocortisone** replacement. The patient was then also given voriconazole 200 mg twice daily for 3 months without any apparent effects on the **hydrocortisone**.[3]

Mechanism

Voriconazole is a potent inhibitor of CYP3A4, the isoenzyme by which many of the corticosteroids are, at least in part metabolised, and so concurrent use is likely to increase the concentrations of these drugs.

Importance and management

Evidence for an interaction between voriconazole and the corticosteroids is limited, However, given the magnitude of the effect, no dose adjustment of prednisolone is likely to be necessary if voriconazole is also given,[1,2] and this also appears to be the case if voriconazole is given with hydrocortisone.[3]

The effects of voriconazole on other corticosteroids do not appear to have been studied; however, other azoles, which are also potent CYP3A4 inhibitors have increased the plasma concentrations of a number of corticosteroids, see (see 'Corticosteroids + Azoles; Itraconazole', p.1246). It would seem prudent to monitor concurrent use closely for signs of adrenal suppression (such as moon-face, flushing, increased bruising, and acne), adjusting the corticosteroid dose if necessary.

1. VFEND (Voriconazole). Pfizer Ltd. UK Summary of product characteristics, October 2014.
2. VFEND (Voriconazole). Pfizer Inc. US Prescribing information, February 2014.
3. Bolland MJ, Bagg W, Thomas MG, Lucas JA, Ticehurst R, Black PN. Cushing's syndrome due to interaction between inhaled corticosteroids and itraconazole. *Ann Pharmacother* (2004) 38, 46–9.

Corticosteroids + Barbiturates

The therapeutic effects of systemic dexamethasone, methylprednisolone, prednisone and prednisolone are decreased by phenobarbital. Other

barbiturates, including primidone, and some other corticosteroids probably interact similarly.

Clinical evidence

(a) Dexamethasone

A 14-year-old girl with congenital adrenal hyperplasia taking dexamethasone rapidly became over-treated (weight gain, signs of hypercortisolism) when **primidone** 250 mg twice daily was withdrawn over a month. Satisfactory control was only achieved when the dexamethasone dosage was reduced threefold.[1] A reduction in the effects of dexamethasone has been described when another patient with congenital adrenal hyperplasia was given **primidone** for petit mal seizures.[2] A patient with pemphigus vulgaris failed to respond to large doses of corticosteroids including **prednisolone** 100 mg daily or dexamethasone 30 mg daily when he was given **phenobarbital** and phenytoin. Dramatic improvement occurred following gradual discontinuation of the antiepileptic drugs.[3]

(b) Methylprednisolone

Phenobarbital increased the clearance of intravenous methylprednisolone in asthmatic children by 209%, but had no significant effect on the bioavailability of oral methylprednisolone.[4]

(c) Prednisolone

Phenobarbital increased the clearance of intravenous prednisolone in asthmatic children by 41%, but had no significant effect on the bioavailability of oral prednisolone.[4] Another study, in renal transplant patients, found that prednisolone elimination is increased by **phenobarbital**.[5]

Nine patients with rheumatoid arthritis taking prednisolone 8 to 15 mg daily had strong evidence of clinical deterioration (worsening joint tenderness, pain, morning stiffness, fall in grip strength) when they took **phenobarbital** for 2 weeks (plasma levels 0 to 86.2 micromol/L). The prednisolone half-life fell by 25%.[6]

For mention of a patient with pemphigus vulgaris, who was unresponsive to prednisolone following antiepileptic treatment including phenobarbital, see under *Dexamethasone*, above.

(d) Prednisone

In a group of 75 children with kidney transplants taking azathioprine and prednisone, the incidence of graft failure was increased in 11 epileptic children taking **phenobarbital** 60 to 120 mg daily. Two of the 11 children were also taking phenytoin 100 mg daily.[7] Three prednisone-dependent patients with bronchial asthma taking prednisone 10 to 40 mg daily had a marked worsening of their symptoms within a few days of starting to take **phenobarbital** 120 mg daily. There was a deterioration in pulmonary function tests (FEV_1, degree of bronchospasm) and a rise in eosinophil counts, all of which improved when the **phenobarbital** was stopped. The prednisone clearance was increased by the **phenobarbital**.[8] In contrast, the prednisone requirements of asthmatic children were unaltered when they took a compound preparation containing **phenobarbital** 24 mg daily.[9]

Mechanism

Phenobarbital is a recognised potent liver enzyme inducer that increases the metabolism of corticosteroids, thereby reducing their effects. Pharmacokinetic studies have shown that phenobarbital reduces the half-lives of these corticosteroids and increases their clearances by 40 to 209%.[4,8,10] Primidone interacts in a similar way because it is metabolised in the body to phenobarbital.[1]

Importance and management

The interaction between the corticosteroids and phenobarbital is well documented, well established and clinically important. Concurrent use need not be avoided but the outcome should be monitored. Increase the corticosteroid dosage as necessary. The extent of the increase is variable, but dexamethasone,[8] **hydrocortisone**,[11] methylprednisolone,[4,10] prednisone[7,8] and prednisolone[4,6] are all known to be affected. Prednisolone is less affected than methylprednisolone and may therefore be preferred in some situations. Be alert for the same interaction with other corticosteroids and other barbiturates, which also are enzyme-inducers, although direct evidence seems to be lacking. The dexamethasone adrenal suppression test may be expected to be unreliable in those taking phenobarbital, just as it is with phenytoin, another potent enzyme-inducer. See 'Corticosteroids + Phenytoin', p.1257.

1. Young MC, Hughes IA. Loss of therapeutic control in congenital adrenal hyperplasia due to interaction between dexamethasone and primidone. *Acta Paediatr Scand* (1991) 80, 120–4.
2. Primidone/dexamethasone interaction. *Lancet* (1978) ii, 97–8.
3. Sehgal VN, Srivastava G. Corticosteroid-unresponsive pemphigus vulgaris following antiepileptic therapy. *Int J Dermatol* (1988) 27, 258.
4. Bartoszek M, Brenner AM, Szefler SJ. Prednisolone and methylprednisolone kinetics in children receiving anticonvulsant therapy. *Clin Pharmacol Ther* (1987) 42, 424–32.
5. Gambertoglio JG, Holford NHG, Kapusnik JE, Nishikawa R, Saltiel M, Stanik-Lizak P, Birnbaum JL, Hau T, Amend WJC. Disposition of total and unbound prednisolone in renal transplant patients receiving anticonvulsants. *Kidney Int* (1984) 25, 119–23.
6. Brooks PM, Buchanan WW, Grove M, Downie WW. Effects of enzyme induction on metabolism of prednisolone. Clinical and laboratory study. *Ann Rheum Dis* (1976) 35, 339–43.
7. Wassner SJ, Pennisi AJ, Malekzadeh MH, Fine RN. The adverse effect of anticonvulsant therapy on renal allograft survival. *J Pediatr* (1976) 88, 134–7.
8. Brooks SM, Werk EE, Ackerman SJ, Sullivan I, Thrasher K. Adverse effects of phenobarbital on corticosteroid metabolism in patients with bronchial asthma. *N Engl J Med* (1972) 286, 1125–8.
9. Falliers CJ. Corticosteroids and phenobarbital in asthma. *N Engl J Med* (1972) 287, 201.
10. Stjernholm MR, Katz FH. Effects of diphenylhydantoin, phenobarbital, and diazepam on the metabolism of methylprednisolone and its sodium succinate. *J Clin Endocrinol Metab* (1975) 41, 887–93.
11. Burstein S, Klaiber EL. Phenobarbital-induced increase in 6-*β*-hydroxycortisol excretion: clue to its significance in human urine. *J Clin Endocrinol Metab* (1965) 25, 293–6.

Corticosteroids + Bile-acid binding resins

Colestyramine and possibly colestipol reduce the absorption of oral hydrocortisone. Some other corticosteroids may possibly be affected, although colestyramine does not appear to affect prednisolone absorption.

Clinical evidence

(a) Colestipol

A man with hypopituitarism taking **hydrocortisone** 20 mg each morning and 10 mg each evening became lethargic, ataxic, and developed headaches (all signs of **hydrocortisone** insufficiency) within 4 days of starting to take colestipol 15 g three times daily for hypercholesterolaemia. He responded rapidly when given intravenous **hydrocortisone** 100 mg, and was discharged with the colestipol replaced by a statin.[1]

(b) Colestyramine

In 10 healthy subjects, colestyramine 4 g reduced the AUC of a 50-mg oral dose of **hydrocortisone** by 43%. Peak **hydrocortisone** levels were reduced and delayed (by about 50 minutes).[2] Two of the subjects were given both 4 g and 8 g of colestyramine, and their AUCs were reduced by 47% and 59% by the 4-g dose and by 97% and 86% by the 8-g dose.[2]

In contrast, an 8-g dose of colestyramine did not affect the bioavailability of **prednisolone** in 2 patients receiving long-term **prednisolone**.[3]

Mechanism

It seems that hydrocortisone can become bound to colestyramine or colestipol in the gut, thereby reducing its absorption.[2,4]

Importance and management

Information is limited, but the interactions of colestipol and colestyramine with hydrocortisone appear to be established (they are consistent with the interactions of both of these bile-acid resins with other drugs). Separate the administration of the drugs as much as possible to minimise admixture in the gut, although the authors of one report warn that this may not necessarily avoid this interaction because their data show that the colestyramine may remain in the gut for a considerable time.[2] The usual recommendation is to give other drugs one hour before or 4 to 6 hours after taking colestyramine, and one hour before or 4 hours after taking colestipol. Monitor the effects and increase the hydrocortisone dosage, or use an alternative to colestyramine, if necessary. Some manufacturers of other corticosteroids including **budesonide** and **dexamethasone** have suggested that colestyramine may potentially reduce the absorption of the corticosteroid,[5,6] and it would therefore be prudent to separate administration. One manufacturer advises taking oral budesonide and colestyramine at least 2 hours apart.[5] Prednisolone may be a non-interacting alternative, but the evidence for this is extremely limited.

1. Nekl KE, Aron DC. Hydrocortisone-colestipol interaction. *Ann Pharmacother* (1993) 27, 980–1.
2. Johansson C, Adamsson U, Stierner U, Lindsten T. Interaction by cholestyramine on the uptake of hydrocortisone in the gastrointestinal tract. *Acta Med Scand* (1978) 204, 509–12.
3. Audétat V, Paumgartner G, Bircher J. Beeinträchtigt Cholestyramin die biologische Verfügbarkeit von Prednisolon? *Schweiz Med Wochenschr* (1977) 107, 527–8.
4. Ware AJ, Combes B. Influence of sodium taurocholate, cholestyramine, and Mylanta on the intestinal absorption of glucocorticoids in the rat. *Gastroenterology* (1973) 64, 1150–5.
5. Budenofalk Gastro-resistant Capsules (Budesonide). Dr. Falk Pharma UK Ltd. UK Summary of product characteristics, September 2010.
6. Dexsol Oral Solution (Dexamethasone sodium phosphate). Rosemont Pharmaceuticals Ltd. UK Summary of product characteristics, March 2008.

Corticosteroids + Calcium-channel blockers; Diltiazem or Verapamil

Diltiazem increases the exposure to intravenous and oral methylprednisolone. The metabolism of oral prednisone is also reduced by diltiazem. Cases of adrenal insufficiency have been described on the concurrent use of diltiazem with inhaled budesonide, and verapamil with inhaled fluticasone.

Clinical evidence

(a) Diltiazem

In a study, 5 healthy subjects were given diltiazem 180 mg daily for 4 days, with and without *intravenous* **methylprednisolone** 300 micrograms/kg (based on ideal bodyweight) on day 5. Diltiazem increased the AUC of **methylprednisolone** by 50%, prolonged its half-life by 37%, and reduced its clearance by 33%. Although the morning cortisol concentration was only 12% of that during the placebo phase, overall the suppressive effects of **methylprednisolone** on cortisol excretion were unchanged.[1] Another similar study in which patients were given diltiazem and a single 16-mg oral dose of **methylprednisolone** found much larger effects: the AUC of **methylprednisolone** was increased 2.6-fold, and the morning cortisol excretion was only 12% of that in the absence of diltiazem,[2] suggesting an enhanced effect.

Another study in healthy subjects found that diltiazem 180 mg daily for 3 days inhibited the metabolism of a single 15-mg oral dose of **prednisone**; the AUC of **prednisolone** (the major active metabolite of prednisone) was increased by 21%.[3]

An analysis of 46 cases of adrenal insufficiency in users of inhaled corticosteroids from a retrospective study, found that 15 of these cases were possibly due to an interaction. In two of these cases, the patients were taking diltiazem with inhaled **budesonide** (1.6 mg daily and 2 mg daily). No other details are given.[4]

(b) Verapamil

An analysis of 46 cases of adrenal insufficiency in users of inhaled corticosteroids from a retrospective study, found that 15 of these cases were possibly due to an interaction. In two of these cases, the patients were taking verapamil with inhaled **fluticasone**. In one case, the dose of fluticasone was 1.5 mg daily but in the other, the dose of fluticasone was not stated. The patient in the first case was reported to have developed Cushing's syndrome and the patient in the second case was reported to have developed adrenal insufficiency. No other details are given.[4]

Mechanism

Diltiazem and verapamil are both moderate inhibitors of CYP3A4. As methylprednisolone is mainly metabolised by CYP3A4, any inhibition of its activity would be expected to increase its exposure.[1,2] Fluticasone and budesonide are also mainly metabolised by CYP3A4, and therefore appear to interact similarly. Prednisolone is less dependent on CYP3A4 for its metabolism, and is therefore affected to a lesser degree. It has been suggested that P-glycoprotein might also play a role in the interaction with methylprednisolone.[1,2] Inhibition of intestinal and hepatic CYP3A4 might increase the oral bioavailability of methylprednisolone, which could contribute to the pharmacokinetic differences seen in the interaction when methylprednisolone is given orally rather than intravenously.

Importance and management

Evidence for an interaction between the corticosteroids and diltiazem or verapamil is limited, but is in line with the known metabolism of the corticosteroids described, and the known CYP3A4 inhibitory effects of diltiazem and verapamil. Information about the interaction between diltiazem and **methylprednisolone** comes from only two studies; however, the effect of concurrent use is clear, although the clinical importance of the increased exposure to methylprednisolone has not yet been established. It would seem prudent to monitor the concurrent use of diltiazem or verapamil and methylprednisolone for an increase in corticosteroid adverse effects.

There appears to be no published pharmacokinetic studies regarding the possible interaction between diltiazem and verapamil and the inhaled corticosteroids, **budesonide** and **fluticasone**; nevertheless the case studies describing adrenal insufficiency are in line with the way these drugs might be predicted to interact. Until more is known, monitor the effects of the concurrent use of diltiazem or verapamil with inhaled fluticasone or budesonide on adrenal function for any signs of excessive corticosteroid effects. Similar precautions would seem sensible in patients taking oral budesonide with these calcium-channel blockers. Patients should be warned to be alert for any evidence of increased corticosteroid effects (such as moon face, weight gain, hyperglycaemia) and to seek medical advice if these occur. There appears to be no published data regarding a possible interaction with other routes of administration for budesonide or fluticasone, such as intranasal or rectal; however, until more is known, it would seem prudent to bear the possibility of an interaction in mind should any otherwise unexplained increase in corticosteroid adverse effects occur. Note that one UK manufacturer of inhaled budesonide states that the increase in the plasma concentration of budesonide seen with other more potent CYP3A4 inhibitors is of little clinical importance for short-term concurrent use (1 to 2 weeks), but should be taken into account for longer term use.[5]

It appears that prednisone/prednisolone bioavailability might possibly be affected by diltiazem but the effect is negligible, and therefore unlikely to be clinically relevant.

1. Booker BM, Magee MH, Blum RA, Lates CD, Jusko WJ. Pharmacokinetic and pharmacodynamic interactions between diltiazem and methylprednisolone in healthy volunteers. *Clin Pharmacol Ther* (2002) 72, 370–82.
2. Varis T, Backman JT, Kivistö KT, Neuvonen PJ. Diltiazem and mibefradil increase the plasma concentrations and greatly enhance the adrenal-suppressant effect of oral methylprednisolone. *Clin Pharmacol Ther* (2000) 67, 215–21.
3. Imani S, Jusko WJ, Steiner R. Diltiazem retards the metabolism of oral prednisone with effects on T-cell markers. *Pediatr Transplant* (1999) 3, 126–30.
4. Daveluy A, Raignoux C, Miremont-Salamé G, Girodet P-O, Moore N, Haramburu F, Molimard M. Drug interactions between inhaled corticosteroids and enzymatic inhibitors. *Eur J Clin Pharmacol* (2009) 65, 743–5.
5. Easyhaler (Budesonide). Orion Pharma (UK) Ltd. UK Summary of product characteristics, July 2011.

Corticosteroids + Carbamazepine

The clearance of dexamethasone, methylprednisolone, prednisolone, and probably some other corticosteroids, can be increased in patients taking carbamazepine. The results of the dexamethasone suppression test may be invalid in those taking carbamazepine.

Clinical evidence

(a) Dexamethasone

A study in 8 healthy subjects found that, in the presence of carbamazepine 800 mg daily, the dosage of dexamethasone needed to suppress cortisol secretion (as part of the dexamethasone adrenal suppression test) was increased two- to fourfold.[1] A further study found that it took 2 to 13 days for false-positive results to occur after carbamazepine was started, and 3 to 12 days to recover when the carbamazepine was stopped.[2] A report describes two patients suspected of having Cushing's syndrome because the overnight suppression test with dexamethasone 1 mg had not suppressed their cortisol levels. Further investigation found no clinical evidence of Cushing's syndrome and the false-positive test results were attributed to the fact that both patients were taking carbamazepine 400 mg three times daily at the time of the test. The test was repeated in one of the patients 3 weeks after carbamazepine was stopped and it indicated normal cortisol suppression.[3]

(b) Prednisolone

A study in 8 patients receiving long-term treatment with carbamazepine found that the elimination half-life of prednisolone was about 45 minutes shorter, and its clearance was 42% higher, than in 9 healthy subjects not taking carbamazepine.[4]

A study in asthmatic children found that carbamazepine increased the clearance of intravenous prednisolone by 79% and increased the clearance of intravenous **methylprednisolone** by 342%.[5] A patient taking carbamazepine and valproate required high-dose prednisolone (20 to 60 mg daily) for polymyalgia rheumatica. It was noted that when carbamazepine was discontinued her response to prednisolone improved, allowing the dose to be reduced to 20 mg then 10 mg daily.[6]

Mechanism

Carbamazepine induces liver enzymes, which results in the increased metabolism of the corticosteroids.

Importance and management

Information is limited but the interaction appears to be established. Patients taking carbamazepine are likely to need increased doses of dexamethasone, methylprednisolone or prednisolone. Prednisolone is less affected than methylprednisolone and may therefore be preferred in some situations. The same interaction seems likely with other corticosteroids but more study is needed to confirm this. Note that **hydrocortisone** and **prednisone** are affected by another potent enzyme inducer, phenobarbital (see 'Corticosteroids + Barbiturates', p.1248), and would therefore also be expected to interact with carbamazepine.

1. Köbberling J, v zur Mühlen A. The influence of diphenylhydantoin and carbamazepine on the circadian rhythm of free urinary corticoids and on the suppressibility of the basal and the 'impulsive' activity by dexamethasone. *Acta Endocrinol (Copenh)* (1973) 72, 308–18.
2. Privitera MR, Greden JF, Gardner RW, Ritchie JC, Carroll BJ. Interference by carbamazepine with the dexamethasone suppression test. *Biol Psychiatry* (1982) 17, 611–20.
3. Ma RCW, Chan WB, So WY, Tong PCY, Chan JCN, Chow CC. Carbamazepine and false positive dexamethasone suppression tests for Cushing's syndrome. *BMJ* (2005) 330, 299–300.
4. Olivesi A. Modified elimination of prednisolone in epileptic patients on carbamazepine monotherapy, and in women using low-dose oral contraceptives. *Biomed Pharmacother* (1986) 40, 301–8.
5. Bartoszek M, Brenner AM, Szefler SJ. Prednisolone and methylprednisolone kinetics in children receiving anticonvulsant therapy. *Clin Pharmacol Ther* (1987) 42, 424–32.
6. Sato A, Katada S, Sato M, Kobayashi H. A case of polymyalgia rheumatica with improved steroid-responsibility after discontinuing carbamazepine. *No To Shinkei* (2004) 56, 61–3.

Corticosteroids + Diuretics; Potassium-depleting

Both corticosteroids and the loop or thiazide diuretics can cause potassium loss, severe depletion is therefore possible if they are used together.

Clinical evidence, mechanism, importance and management

There seem to be no formal clinical studies about the extent of the additive potassium depletion that can occur when potassium-depleting diuretics and corticosteroids are given together, but an exaggeration of the potassium loss undoubtedly occurs (e.g. seen with **hydrocortisone** and **furosemide**[1]). One study looking at hypokalaemia with potassium-depleting diuretics found that corticosteroids were a significant risk factor for hypokalaemic events; 20% of patients taking a potassium-depleting diuretic developed hypokalaemia, whereas 31% of patients taking a potassium-depleting diuretic and a corticosteroid developed hypokalaemia.[2] Hypokalaemia in patients taking potassium-depleting diuretics should be corrected before a corticosteroid is started. Concurrent use should be well monitored and the potassium intake increased as appropriate to balance this loss.

The greatest potassium loss occurs with the naturally occurring corticosteroids such as **cortisone** and **hydrocortisone**. **Corticotropin (ACTH)**, which is a pituitary hormone, and **tetracosactrin** (a synthetic polypeptide) stimulate corticosteroid secretion by the adrenal cortex and can thereby indirectly cause potassium loss. **Fludrocortisone** also causes potassium loss. The synthetic corticosteroids (glucocorticoids) have a less marked potassium-depleting effect and are therefore less likely to cause problems. These include **betamethasone**, **dexamethasone**, **prednisolone**, **prednisone** and **triamcinolone**.

The potassium-depleting diuretics (i.e. **loop diuretics** or **thiazide** and related diuretics) are listed in 'Table 26.1', p.1117. **Acetazolamide**, a weak diuretic, has also been predicted to cause hypokalaemia in the presence of corticosteroids. However, hypokalaemia seen with **acetazolamide** is rarely clinically significant, and therefore any risk is lower.

1. Manchon ND, Bercoff E, Lemarchand P, Chassagne P, Senant J, Bourreille J. Fréquence et gravité des interactions médicamenteuses dans une population âgée: étude prospective concernant 639 malades. *Rev Med Interne* (1989) 10, 521–5.
2. Widmer P, Maibach R, Künzi UP, Capaul R, Mueller U, Galeazzi R, Hoigné R. Diuretic-related hypokalaemia: the role of diuretics, potassium supplements, glucocorticoids and β_2-adrenoceptor agonists. *Eur J Clin Pharmacol* (1995) 49, 31–6.

Corticosteroids + Ephedrine

Ephedrine increases the clearance of dexamethasone.

Clinical evidence, mechanism, importance and management

Nine asthmatic patients had a 40% increase in the clearance and a similar reduction in the half-life of **dexamethasone** when they were given ephedrine 100 mg daily for 3 weeks.[1] This would be expected to reduce the overall effects of **dexamethasone**, but this requires confirmation. Be alert for any evidence that the **dexamethasone** effects are reduced if both drugs are given; an increase in the dexamethasone dose might be necessary. It is not clear whether other corticosteroids behave similarly.

1. Brooks SM, Sholiton LJ, Werk EE, Altenau P. The effects of ephedrine and theophylline on dexamethasone metabolism in bronchial asthma. *J Clin Pharmacol* (1977) 17, 308–18.

Corticosteroids + Fluoxetine

Fluoxetine does not affect the pharmacokinetics of prednisolone or its effects on cortisol suppression.

Clinical evidence, mechanism, importance and management

In healthy subjects, fluoxetine 20 mg daily for 5 days then 60 mg daily for 9 days did not significantly affect the pharmacokinetics of a single 40-mg dose of **prednisolone succinate**, given as an intravenous bolus, or the duration of cortisol suppression in response to the **prednisolone**.[1] Although fluoxetine has some inhibitory effect on the cytochrome P450 isoenzyme CYP3A4, and thus may inhibit the metabolism of corticosteroids that are CYP3A4 substrates, its effects are weak and not usually clinically relevant. Furthermore, **prednisolone** is only partly metabolised by this route.[2] No clinically important interaction is likely if **prednisolone** and fluoxetine are given concurrently. The situation with other corticosteroids that may be more likely to interact (e.g. **methylprednisolone**, which is mainly metabolised by CYP3A4) is not known.

1. Carson SW, Letrent KJ, Kotlyar M, Foose G, Tancer ME. Lack of fluoxetine effect on prednisolone disposition and cortisol suppression. *Pharmacotherapy* (2004) 24, 482–7.
2. Varis T, Kivistö KT, Neuvonen PJ. The effect of itraconazole on the pharmacokinetics and pharmacodynamics of oral prednisolone. *Eur J Clin Pharmacol* (2000) 56, 57–60.

Corticosteroids + Grapefruit juice

Grapefruit juice increases the plasma concentrations of budesonide and methylprednisolone. Grapefruit juice does not affect the pharmacokinetics of prednisolone or prednisone.

Clinical evidence, mechanism, importance and management

(a) Budesonide

In a study in 8 healthy subjects, giving oral enteric-coated budesonide with concentrated grapefruit juice resulted in a 2-fold increase in the bioavailability of budesonide, compared with oral enteric-coated budesonide alone. Similar results were obtained with a non-enteric-coated oral formulation, but the clearance, volume of distribution, and half-life of budesonide given intravenously were not altered by grapefruit juice. These results suggest that grapefruit juice increases the systemic availability of oral budesonide due to inhibition of intestinal CYP3A4 activity.[1] These results have been confirmed by another similar study.[2] One UK manufacturer of budesonide therefore states that regular ingestion of grapefruit or grapefruit juice should be avoided in connection with budesonide administration, but if this is not possible, the time interval between ingestion of grapefruit (or its juice) and taking oral budesonide should be as long as possible, and a reduction of the budesonide dose should be considered.[3] Another UK manufacturer of oral and rectal budesonide also recommends avoiding concurrent use.[4,5]

(b) Methylprednisolone

In a crossover study, 10 healthy subjects were given either double-strength grapefruit juice 200 mL or water three times daily for 2 days. On day 3, grapefruit juice 200 mL or water was given at the same time, 30 minutes after, and 90 minutes after a single 16-mg dose of methylprednisolone. Grapefruit juice increased the AUC and maximum plasma concentration of methylprednisolone by 75% and 27%, respectively. The time to reach the maximum plasma concentration was increased from 2 to 3 hours and the elimination half-life was increased by 35%. Plasma cortisol concentrations after methylprednisolone was given with grapefruit juice, or water, were no different, although grapefruit juice caused a small decrease in plasma cortisol concentrations before the morning dose of methylprednisolone. As the effects on plasma cortisol concentrations were minimal, this interaction is unlikely to be of clinical importance in most patients, although the authors note that in some sensitive subjects large amounts of grapefruit juice might enhance the effects of oral methylprednisolone.[6]

(c) Prednisolone or Prednisone

A study in 12 kidney transplant patients taking ciclosporin and corticosteroids found that grapefruit juice, given every 3 hours for 30 hours, increased the plasma concentration of ciclosporin, but had no effect on the AUC of prednisolone or prednisone.[7] No particular precautions are therefore needed if patients drink grapefruit juice while taking these corticosteroids.

1. Edsbäcker S, Andersson T. Pharmacokinetics of budesonide (Entocort™ EC) capsules for Crohn's disease. *Clin Pharmacokinet* (2004) 43, 803–21.
2. Seidegård J, Randvall G, Nyberg L, Borgå O. Grapefruit juice interaction with oral budesonide: equal effect on immediate-release and delayed-release formulations. *Pharmazie* (2009) 64, 461–5.
3. Entocort CR Capsules (Budesonide). AstraZeneca UK Ltd. UK Summary of product characteristics, April 2012.
4. Budenofalk Gastro-resistant Capsules (Budesonide). Dr. Falk Pharma UK Ltd. UK Summary of product characteristics, September 2010.
5. Budenofalk Rectal Foam (Budesonide). Dr. Falk Pharma UK Ltd. UK Summary of product characteristics, November 2011.
6. Varis T, Kivistö KT, Neuvonen PJ. Grapefruit juice can increase the plasma concentrations of oral methylprednisolone. *Eur J Clin Pharmacol* (2000) 56, 489–93.
7. Hollander AA, van Rooij J, Lentjes EGWM, Arbouw F, van Bree JB, Schoemaker RC, van Es LA, van der Woude FJ, Cohen AF. The effect of grapefruit juice on cyclosporine and prednisone metabolism in transplant patients. *Clin Pharmacol Ther* (1995) 57, 318–24.

Corticosteroids + H_2-receptor antagonists

Cimetidine does not appear to interact with budesonide, dexamethasone prednisolone, or prednisone, and ranitidine does not interact with prednisone.

Clinical evidence, mechanism, importance and management

A double-blind crossover study in 9 healthy subjects found that **cimetidine** 300 mg every 6 hours or **ranitidine** 150 mg twice daily for 4 days did not significantly alter the pharmacokinetics of prednisolone after a single 40-mg oral dose of **prednisone**.[1] **Prednisone** is a pro-drug, which must be converted to prednisolone within the body to become active.

Another double-blind, crossover study found that **cimetidine** 1 g daily only caused minor changes in plasma **prednisolone** levels following a 10-mg dose of enteric-coated **prednisolone**.[2] Similarly, **cimetidine** has been reported to have a slight but clinically insignificant effect on the pharmacokinetics of oral **budesonide**.[3] Another study found that **cimetidine** 600 mg twice daily for 7 days had no effect on the pharmacokinetics of a single 8-mg intravenous dose of **dexamethasone sodium phosphate**.[4]

Dosage adjustments therefore seem unlikely to be necessary if any of these corticosteroids are given with cimetidine or other H_2-receptor antagonists.

Drugs such as cimetidine, which inhibit the cytochrome P450 isoenzyme CYP3A4, might be expected to decrease the rate of metabolism of corticosteroids, such as **methylprednisolone**, that are largely metabolised by this route. However, information appears to be lacking, and cimetidine has only weak to modest effects on this isoenzyme. Therefore no clinically significant interaction is anticipated.

1. Sirgo MA, Rocci ML, Ferguson RK, Eshelman FN, Vlasses PH. Effects of cimetidine and ranitidine on the conversion of prednisone to prednisolone. *Clin Pharmacol Ther* (1985) 37, 534–8.
2. Morrison PJ, Rogers HJ, Bradbrook ID, Parsons C. Concurrent administration of cimetidine and enteric-coated prednisolone: effect on plasma levels of prednisolone. *Br J Clin Pharmacol* (1980) 10, 87–9.
3. Edsbäcker S, Andersson T. Pharmacokinetics of budesonide (Entocort™ EC) capsules for Crohn's disease. *Clin Pharmacokinet* (2004) 43, 803–21.
4. Peden NR, Rewhorn I, Champion MC, Mussani R, Ooi TC. Cortisol and dexamethasone elimination during treatment with cimetidine. *Br J Clin Pharmacol* (1984) 18, 101–3.

Corticosteroids + HCV-protease inhibitors

Boceprevir does not alter exposure to prednisolone or prednisone to a clinically relevant extent. Boceprevir and telaprevir are predicted to increase the concentrations of inhaled and/or intranasal budesonide and fluticasone. Telaprevir is also predicted to increase the concentrations of methylprednisolone and prednisolone. Paritaprevir boosted with ritonavir is predicted to increase the concentration of inhaled and/or intranasal fluticasone, or other similarly metabolised corticosteroids. Simeprevir is not expected to interact with budesonide, fluticasone, methylprednisolone or prednisone. The plasma concentrations of boceprevir, simeprevir, and telaprevir are predicted to be decreased by dexamethasone.

Clinical evidence

(a) Budesonide

The UK and US manufacturers of **telaprevir**[1,2] and the US manufacturer of **boceprevir**[3] predict that they will increase the systemic concentrations of inhaled[1-3] or intranasal[1,2] budesonide, which could result in a reduction in cortisol concentrations.

(b) Fluticasone

The UK and US manufacturers of **telaprevir**[1,2] and **paritaprevir** boosted with ritonavir (in a fixed-dose combination),[4,5] and the US manufacturer of **boceprevir**[3] predict that they will increase the systemic concentrations of inhaled[1-5] or intranasal[1,2,5] fluticasone, which could result in a reduction in cortisol concentrations.

(c) Methylprednisolone, prednisolone, or prednisone

The preliminary report of a crossover study in 12 healthy subjects given a single 40-mg dose of prednisone, alone, and with **boceprevir** 800 mg three times daily for 6 days, notes that boceprevir increased the AUC of prednisone and of prednisolone by 22% and 37%, respectively.[6]

The US manufacturer of **telaprevir** predicts that it will increase the plasma concentrations of prednisolone and methylprednisolone.[2]

Mechanism

Boceprevir and telaprevir are both potent inhibitors of CYP3A4, by which budesonide, fluticasone, and methylprednisolone are metabolised. Concurrent use could therefore result in increased exposure to these corticosteroids. Prednisone is less dependent on CYP3A4 for its metabolism and is generally less affected by CYP3A4 inhibitors. Paritaprevir does not appear to affect CYP3A4 itself, but it is given with ritonavir as a pharmacokinetic enhancer, and as this is a well-known potent inhibitor of CYP3A4, the predicted effect on fluticasone, would be due to the activity of ritonavir.

Importance and management

Evidence for an interaction between corticosteroids and HCV-protease inhibitors is limited to a study between boceprevir and prednisone. The minimal effect of boceprevir on the exposure to prednisone and prednisolone in this study, would not be expected to be clinically important, and no prednisone or prednisolone dose reductions would seem necessary on concurrent use. However, the use of inhaled[1-3] or intranasal[1,2] **budesonide** and **fluticasone** is not recommended by the UK and US manufacturers of telaprevir[1,2] and the US manufacturer of boceprevir (if possible, and particularly long-term)[3], unless the benefits outweigh the risks.[1,2] In addition, the US manufacturer of telaprevir does not recommend concurrent use with **prednisolone** and **methylprednisolone**.[2] However, if concurrent use of any of these corticosteroids is essential, it would seem prudent to monitor for an increase in corticosteroid adverse effects (such as moon face, weight gain, hyperglycaemia), adjusting the corticosteroid dose if necessary. Note that topical corticosteroids were used in clinical trials to provide symptomatic relief from telaprevir-induced rash,[1,2] but the use of systemic corticosteroids for this purpose is not recommended by the US manufacturer.[2]

The UK manufacturer of **paritaprevir** boosted with ritonavir (in a fixed-dose combination with ombitasvir, and given with or without dasabuvir) advises that inhaled fluticasone (or other corticosteroids similarly metabolised by CYP3A4), particularly for long-term use, should only be given concurrently if the potential benefits of treatment outweigh the risks of systemic corticosteroid effects (such as Cushing's syndrome and adrenal suppression seen with other ritonavir-containing regimens).[4] The US manufacturer advises that alternative corticosteroids should be considered instead of inhaled or intranasal fluticasone, especially if long-term use is required.[5] Caution would seem prudent given the effects of HIV-protease inhibitors boosted with ritonavir (which are also all potent CYP3A4 inhibitors) in patients receiving various corticosteroids, see 'Corticosteroids + HIV-protease inhibitors', below for details.

The UK and US manufacturers of **simeprevir** note that no interaction is expected with budesonide, fluticasone, methylprednisolone, or prednisone,[7,8] and no dose adjustments are therefore necessary on concurrent use.

Boceprevir, simeprevir, and telaprevir are themselves metabolised by CYP3A4 (boceprevir only partly). The US manufacturers of boceprevir[3] and the UK and US manufacturers of simeprevir,[7,8] and telaprevir,[1,2] predict that **dexamethasone** could reduce their plasma concentrations and possibly reduce their antiviral efficacy by induction of this isoenzyme. For this reason, they recommend avoiding dexamethasone,[1-3,7,8] or if this is not possible they advise caution on concurrent use.[2,3] However, note that dexamethasone rarely appears to cause clinically relevant interactions by inducing CYP3A4.

1. Incivo (Telaprevir). Janssen-Cilag Ltd. UK Summary of product characteristics, July 2014.
2. Incivek (Telaprevir). Vertex Pharmaceuticals, Inc. US Prescribing information, October 2013.
3. Victrelis (Boceprevir). Merck & Co., Inc. US Prescribing information, July 2014.
4. Viekirax (Ombitasvir, paritaprevir, ritonavir). AbbVie Ltd. UK Summary of product characteristics, January 2015.
5. Viekira Pak (Ombitasvir, paritaprevir, ritonavir co-packaged with dasabuvir sodium monohydrate). AbbVie Inc. US Prescribing information, December 2014.
6. Jumes P, Feng HP, Chatterjee M, Xuan F, Connolly SM, Wagner JA, Butterton JR. Pharmacokinetic interaction between the HCV protease inhibitor boceprevir and prednisone in healthy volunteers (Abstract 1896). *Hepatology* (2012) 56, (Suppl 1) 1076A.
7. Olysio (Simeprevir sodium). Janssen-Cilag Ltd. UK Summary of product characteristics, May 2014.
8. Olysio (Simeprevir sodium). Janssen Products, LP. US Prescribing information, November 2014.

Corticosteroids + HIV-protease inhibitors

Numerous cases of Cushing's syndrome have been seen in patients given inhaled or intranasal fluticasone with ritonavir, and several cases have been reported with inhaled, intranasal, and oral budesonide. In healthy subjects given fluticasone propionate intranasally, ritonavir increased fluticasone propionate plasma concentrations several hundred fold, resulting in markedly reduced serum cortisol concentrations. Ritonavir might reduce the clearance of prednisone, prednisolone, and some other corticosteroids. Ritonavir and nelfinavir might increase the exposure to the active metabolite of ciclesonide and possibly beclometasone. Several cases of cushingoid adverse effects and adrenal suppression have been reported in patients taking HIV-protease inhibitors boosted with ritonavir, such as atazanavir, indinavir, and lopinavir, when they were also given epidural, intra-articular, or intramuscular injections of triamcinolone.

Dexamethasone is predicted reduce the plasma concentrations of indinavir, saquinavir, and possibly darunavir.

Clinical evidence

(a) Budesonide

Three HIV-positive children receiving **ritonavir** alone, or with **lopinavir** developed adrenal suppression and Cushing's syndrome after inhaled budesonide (and intranasal in one case) was added. In one 4-year-old, symptoms developed 3 months after inhaled and intranasal budesonide were started, and in another 4-year-old given inhaled budesonide only, the symptoms took 2 years to develop. In the 7-year-old, symptoms had developed while receiving fluticasone (see below) and had not resolved one month after fluticasone was switched to budesonide.[1] Another case of Cushing's syndrome has been described in a 37-year-old woman taking **lopinavir** boosted with **ritonavir** 800/200 mg twice daily, which initially developed after she received inhaled fluticasone (see under *Fluticasone*, below) for asthma, and resolved within 2 months of stopping, but returned after starting inhaled budesonide. No improvement occurred after reducing the ritonavir dose (by changing to **fosamprenavir boosted with ritonavir** 1400/100 mg daily), but the symptoms resolved again within weeks of stopping the budesonide.[2] A further case describes a 75-year-old HIV-positive patient taking **atazanavir boosted with ritonavir** 300/100 mg daily who developed Cushing's syndrome 12 days after oral budesonide 3 mg three times daily was started for lymphocytic colitis.[3]

(b) Fluticasone

1. Case reports of adverse effects. A HIV-positive 32-year-old man who had been using intranasal fluticasone 200 micrograms twice daily for 3 years for allergic rhinitis, developed a cushingoid face and gained 6.5 kg in weight within 5 months of starting to take **ritonavir**, zidovudine, and lamivudine.[4] Another HIV-positive man receiving inhaled beclometasone 400 to 800 micrograms daily for asthma and intranasal fluticasone 800 micrograms daily for allergic rhinitis was also given **ritonavir**, **saquinavir**, stavudine, and nevirapine, after which he developed mild cushingoid facial changes. Both patients had high plasma concentrations of fluticasone. The problems resolved when the fluticasone was withdrawn. A third HIV-positive patient receiving inhaled beclometasone and intranasal fluticasone as well as **ritonavir**, zidovudine, and lamivudine, had an increased fluticasone plasma concentration, but no signs of Cushing's syndrome.[4]

A further 6 HIV-positive patients with HIV-lipodystrophy and taking HIV-protease inhibitors, including low doses of **ritonavir**, developed symptomatic Cushing's syndrome when given inhaled fluticasone. All had adrenal suppression, and after withdrawal of fluticasone, 3 patients required oral corticosteroids for several months. Exacerbation of pre-existing diabetes mellitus occurred in one patient and 4 patients had osteoporosis (one with fractures). Diagnosis was made more difficult by the lipodystrophy masking the Cushingoid features.[5] Another report describes exacerbation of AIDS-associated Kaposi sarcoma together with iatrogenic Cushing syndrome in a patient receiving **atazanavir boosted with ritonavir** and fluticasone. Discontinuation of the fluticasone resulted in resolution of the cutaneous Kaposi sarcoma.[6]

There are numerous reports of other patients, including children or adolescents,[1,7-11] who have developed Cushing's syndrome within 2 weeks to 5 months of using inhaled[1,2,7-17] or intranasal[18] fluticasone with **ritonavir alone**[9,18] or with the following **ritonavir**-boosted HIV-protease inhibitors: **amprenavir**,[12,16] **atazanavir**,[10,17] **fosamprenavir**,[11] **indinavir**,[16] **lopinavir**,[1,2,7,8,10,14] **saquinavir**,[13] or **lopinavir** with **saquinavir**.[15] The interaction was confirmed in one patient by replacing **ritonavir** with nevirapine for 3 weeks and then restarting **ritonavir**.[18]

2. Pharmacokinetic studies. In a crossover study in 18 healthy subjects, fluticasone propionate nasal spray 200 micrograms was given daily for 7 days. Plasma fluticasone propionate concentrations were undetectable in most subjects, and when they were detectable, maximum concentrations averaged 11.9 picograms/mL. After the addition of **ritonavir** 100 mg twice daily for 7 days, the maximum plasma concentration of fluticasone propionate increased to 318 picograms/mL, and the AUC increased approximately 370-fold. The serum cortisol AUC decreased by 86%.[19]

(c) Prednisolone or Prednisone

A study in healthy subjects found that the AUC of a single 20-mg dose of prednisone, given before and on days 4 and 14 of a 14.5-day course of **ritonavir** 200 mg twice daily, was increased by about 30% by **ritonavir**. The apparent oral clearance of prednisolone was reduced from 8.84 L/hour, to 6.45 L/hour and 6.88 L/hour on days 4 and 14, respectively.[20] A further study in HIV-positive subjects found that **lopinavir boosted with ritonavir** increased the AUC of a single 20-mg dose of prednisolone, when compared with the AUC in subjects not receiving antiretroviral medications, although this was not statistically significant.[21]

(d) Triamcinolone

A 41 year-old HIV-positive man taking emtricitabine 200 mg, tenofovir 300 mg, and **atazanavir boosted with ritonavir** 300/100 mg daily developed cushingoid adverse effects (hypertension, weight gain, abdominal striae) and adrenal suppression after two separate transforaminal epidural injections of triamcinolone acetonide 80 mg in the previous 3 months. His triamcinolone acetate blood concentration was found to have increased to 98.9 mmol/L (normal upper limit of 6.9 mmol/L).[22] Similarly, a 42 year-old HIV-positive woman taking the same antiretroviral regimen also developed adrenal suppression with cushingoid adverse effects (including weight gain, palpitations, hypertension) following a subacromial injection of triamcinolone acetonide 40 mg in the previous 2 weeks. Six months previously she had no reported problems when given a transforaminal epidural injection of **betamethasone** acetate.[22]

A number of other case results also describe corticosteroid adverse effects and or adrenal suppression in patients taking:

- **Atazanavir boosted with ritonavir** and given single doses of intra-articular (80 mg), intramuscular (60 mg), or epidural triamcinolone acetonide[23-25] in one case the symptoms developed within 3 days of the triamcinolone dose.[23]
- **Lopinavir boosted with ritonavir**,[26,27]
- **Indinavir boosted with ritonavir**,[26]
- Unnamed HIV-protease inhibitors[28] within one to 2 weeks of receiving single or multiple intra-articular injections or root infiltration of triamcinolone acetonide 40 mg to 80 mg.

In one case all antiretrovirals were stopped temporarily[23] and in 2 cases[27,28] only ritonavir was stopped.

Mechanism

Ritonavir, and all HIV-protease inhibitors, inhibit CYP3A4. Fluticasone and budesonide, and probably triamcinolone, are metabolised by this isoenzyme and therefore the HIV-protease inhibitors cause their plasma concentrations to rise. The active metabolite of ciclesonide is also metabolised by CYP3A4,[29] and is therefore similarly affected. Prednisolone is less dependent on CYP3A4 for metabolism, and is therefore affected to a lesser extent.

Importance and management

The interaction between ritonavir and **budesonide**, **fluticasone**, and **triamcinolone** is established and clinically important. The incidence is not known, but any patient using combinations of these drugs should be very closely monitored for any signs of corticosteroid overdose. The problem can take months to manifest itself. It has been suggested that if an inhaled corticosteroid is required by a patient taking ritonavir, a corticosteroid that is not a substrate for CYP3A4 (e.g. beclometasone),[30] or one with less systemic availability, should be given at the lowest effective dose.[31] However, note that one UK manufacturer of inhaled **beclometasone** states that, despite low systemic absorption, drugs that inhibit CYP3A4, such as ritonavir or nelfinavir, might theoretically increase the systemic exposure of beclometasone, and they therefore advise caution on concurrent use.[32]

The UK and US manufacturers of inhaled[19,33] and intranasal[34,35] **fluticasone** advise against their concurrent use with ritonavir unless the potential benefit is considered to outweigh the risk of systemic corticosteroid adverse effects; similar advice has been given by the manufacturers of HIV-protease inhibitors boosted with ritonavir. The UK manufacturers of **budesonide** nasal spray,[36] oral capsules,[37] and rectal foam[38] advise avoiding the concurrent use of potent CYP3A4 inhibitors. If this is not possible, the time interval between giving the interacting drugs should be as long as possible and a reduction in the dose of budesonide should also be considered.[36,37] One UK manufacturer of inhaled budesonide[39] and the UK manufacturer of budesonide oral capsules[37] state that the increase in budesonide exposure is of little clinical importance for short-term use (1 to 2 weeks), but should be taken into account for long term use. In the US, the manufacturer of budesonide respules, oral capsules, and nasal spray simply advise caution on long-term use due to the risk of increased budesonide adverse effects.[40-42]

Ritonavir might also increase the exposure to **prednisone** and **prednisolone** and some UK manufacturers of **dexamethasone**[43,44] predict a similar interaction. As a result, concurrent use is not generally recommended due to the increased risk of systemic adverse effects of corticosteroids, but if the combination is essential, careful monitoring would be prudent. The need for dose reduction of the corticosteroid should be borne in mind. The UK manufacturer of **ciclesonide** advises against concurrent use with ritonavir, unless the benefit outweighs the increased risk of corticosteroid systemic adverse effects.[29]

The UK manufacturers of **dexamethasone** also state that it reduces the plasma concentrations of indinavir and saquinavir,[44] presumably by inducing CYP3A4; however, note that no clinically relevant interactions with dexamethasone as a result of this mechanism appear to have been reported. Similar warnings are given by the UK manufacturer of **darunavir**.[30] The clinical outcome of this predicted effect is unknown, but until more is known, it would seem prudent to monitor antiviral efficacy if these combinations are used.

1. Gray D, Roux P, Carrihill M, Klein M. Adrenal suppression and Cushing's syndrome secondary to ritonavir and budesonide. *S Afr Med J* (2010) 100, 296–7.
2. Kedem E, Shahar E, Hassoun G, Pollack S. Iatrogenic Cushing's syndrome due to coadministration of ritonavir and inhaled budesonide in an asthmatic human immunodeficiency virus infected patient. *J Asthma* (2010) 47, 830–1.
3. Frankel JK, Packer CD. Cushing's syndrome due to antiretroviral-budesonide interaction. *Ann Pharmacother* (2011) 45, 823–4.
4. Chen F, Kearney T, Robinson S, Daley-Yates PT, Waldron S, Churchill DR. Cushing's syndrome and severe adrenal suppression in patients treated with ritonavir and inhaled nasal fluticasone. *Sex Transm Infect* (1999) 75, 274.
5. Samaras K, Pett S, Gowers A, McMurchie M, Cooper DA. Iatrogenic Cushing's syndrome with osteoporosis and secondary adrenal failure in human immunodeficiency virus-infected patients receiving inhaled corticosteroids and ritonavir-boosted protease inhibitors: six cases. *J Clin Endocrinol Metab* (2005) 90, 4394–8.
6. Jinno S, Goshima C. Progression of Kaposi sarcoma associated with iatrogenic Cushing syndrome in a person with HIV/AIDS. *AIDS Read* (2008) 18, 102–4.
7. Johnson SR, Marion AA, Vrchoticky T, Emmanuel PJ, Lujan-Zilbermann J. Cushing syndrome with secondary adrenal insufficiency from concomitant therapy with ritonavir and fluticasone. *J Pediatr* (2006) 148, 386–8.
8. Bhumbra NA, Sahloff EG, Oehrtman SJ, Horner JM. Exogenous Cushing syndrome with inhaled fluticasone in a child receiving lopinavir/ritonavir. *Ann Pharmacother* (2007) 41, 1306–9.
9. Pessanha TM, Campos JMS, Barros ACM, Pone MVS, Garrido JR, Pone SM. Iatrogenic Cushing's syndrome in a adolescent with AIDSs on ritonavir and inhaled fluticasone. Case report and literature review. *AIDS* (2007) 21, 529–32.
10. St. Germain RM, Yigit S, Wells L, Girotto JE, Salazar JC. Cushing syndrome and severe adrenal suppression caused by fluticasone and protease inhibitor combination in an HIV-infected adolescent. *AIDS Patient Care STDS* (2007) 21, 373–7.
11. Daveluy A, Raignoux C, Miremont-Salamé G, Girodet P-O, Moore N, Haramburu F, Molimard M. Drug interactions between inhaled corticosteroids and enzymatic inhibitors. *Eur J Clin Pharmacol* (2009) 65, 743–5.
12. Clevenbergh P, Corcostegui M, Gérard D, Hieronimus S, Mondain V, Chichmanian RM, Sadoul JL, Dellamonica P. Iatrogenic Cushing's syndrome in an HIV-infected patient treated with inhaled corticosteroids (fluticasone propionate) and low dose ritonavir enhanced PI containing regimen. *J Infect* (2002) 44, 194–5.
13. Gupta SK, Dubé MP. Exogenous Cushing syndrome mimicking human immunodeficiency virus lipodystrophy. *Clin Infect Dis* (2002) 35, e69–e71.
14. Rouanet I, Peyrière H, Mauboussin JM, Vincent D. Cushing's syndrome in a patient treated by ritonavir/lopinavir and inhaled fluticasone. *HIV Med* (2003) 4, 149–50.
15. Gillett MJ, Cameron PU, Nguyen HV, Hurley DM, Mallal SA. Iatrogenic Cushing's syndrome in an HIV-infected patient treated with ritonavir and inhaled fluticasone. *AIDS* (2005) 19, 740–1.
16. Soldatos G, Sztal-Mazer S, Woolley I, Stockigt J. Exogenous glucocorticoid excess as a result of ritonavir-fluticasone interaction. *Intern Med J* (2005) 35, 67–8.
17. Bouldouyre M-A, Moachon L, Guillevin L, Launay O. Syndrome de Cushing iatrogène chez une patiente infectée par le VIH: attention à l'interaction corticoïdes inhalés-ritonavir. *Presse Med* (2008) 37, 1834–5.
18. Hillebrand-Haverkort ME, Prummel MF, ten Veen JH. Ritonavir-induced Cushing's syndrome in a patient treated with nasal fluticasone. *AIDS* (1999) 13, 1803.
19. Flovent HFA Inhalation Aerosol (Fluticasone propionate). GlaxoSmithKline. US Prescribing information, January 2012.
20. Penzak SR, Formentini E, Alfaro RM, Long M, Natarajan V, Kovacs J. Prednisolone pharmacokinetics in the presence and absence of ritonavir after oral prednisone administration to healthy volunteers. *J Acquir Immune Defic Syndr* (2005) 40, 573–80.
21. Busse KH, Formentini E, Alfaro RM, Kovacs JA, Penzak SR. Influence of antiretroviral drugs on the pharmacokinetics of prednisolone in HIV-infected individuals. *J Acquir Immune Defic Syndr* (2008) 48, 561–6.
22. Dort K, Padia S, Wispelwey B, Moore CC. Adrenal suppression due to an interaction between ritonavir and injected triamcinolone: a case report. *AIDS Res Ther* (2009) 6, 10.
23. Danaher PJ, Salsbury TL, Delmar JA. Metabolic derangement after injection of triamcinolone into the hip of an HIV-infected patient receiving ritonavir. *Orthopedics* (2009) 32, 450.
24. Levine D, Ananthakrishnan S, Garg A. Iatrogenic Cushing syndrome after a single intramuscular corticosteroid injection and concomitant protease inhibitor therapy. *J Am Acad Dermatol* (2011) 65, 877–8.
25. Grierson MJ, Harrast MA. Iatrogenic Cushing syndrome after epidural steroid injections for lumbar radiculopathy in an HIV-infected patient treated with ritonavir: a case report highlighting drug interactions for spine interventionalists. *PM R* (2012) 4, 234–7.
26. Yombi JC, Maiter D, Belkhir L, Nzeusseu A, Vandercam B. Iatrogenic Cushing's syndrome and secondary adrenal insufficiency after a single intra-articular administration of triamcinolone acetonide in HIV-infected patients treated with ritonavir. *Clin Rheumatol* (2008) 27, S79–S82.
27. Ramanathan R, Pau AK, Busse KH, Zemskova M, Nieman L, Kwan R, Hammer JH, Mican JM, Maldarelli F. Iatrogenic cushing syndrome after epidural triamcinolone injections in an HIV type 1-infected patient receiving therapy with ritonavir-lopinavir. *Clin Infect Dis* (2008) 47, e97–e99.
28. Herold MA, Günthard HF. Cushing-syndrom nach steroid-infiltration bei zwei behandelten HIV-infizierten patienten. *Praxis (Bern 1994)* (2010) 99, 863–5.
29. Alvesco (Ciclesonide). Nycomed UK Ltd. UK Summary of product characteristics, May 2011.
30. Prezista (Darunavir ethanolate). Janssen-Cilag Ltd. UK Summary of product characteristics, June 2012.
31. Li AM. Ritonavir and fluticasone: beware of this potentially fatal combination. *J Pediatr* (2006) 148, 294–5.
32. Pulvinal (Beclometasone dipropionate). Chiesi Ltd. UK Summary of product characteristics, April 2011.
33. Flixotide Evohaler (Fluticasone propionate). Allen & Hanburys Ltd. UK Summary of product characteristics, August 2011.
34. Flixonase Aqueous Nasal Spray (Fluticasone propionate). Allen & Hanburys Ltd. UK Summary of product characteristics, September 2011.
35. Flonase Nasal Spray (Fluticasone propionate). GlaxoSmithKline. US Prescribing information, August 2007.
36. Rhinocort Aqua Nasal Spray (Budesonide). AstraZeneca UK Ltd. UK Summary of product characteristics, July 2012.
37. Entocort CR Capsules (Budesonide). AstraZeneca UK Ltd. UK Summary of product characteristics, April 2012.
38. Budenofalk Rectal Foam (Budesonide). Dr. Falk Pharma UK Ltd. UK Summary of product characteristics, November 2011.
39. Easyhaler (Budesonide). Orion Pharma (UK) Ltd. UK Summary of product characteristics, July 2011.
40. Entocort EC (Budesonide). AstraZeneca LP. US Prescribing information, December 2011.
41. Pulmicort Respules (Budesonide). AstraZeneca LP. US Prescribing information, July 2010.
42. Rhinocort Aqua Nasal Spray (Budesonide). AstraZeneca LP. US Prescribing information, December 2010.
43. Dexsol Oral Solution (Dexamethasone sodium phosphate). Rosemont Pharmaceuticals Ltd. UK Summary of product characteristics, March 2008.
44. Dexamethasone Tablets. Merck Sharp & Dohme Ltd. UK Summary of product characteristics, January 2011.

Corticosteroids + Hormonal contraceptives or Sex hormones

The serum levels of cloprednol, methylprednisolone, prednisolone, prednisone, and possibly other corticosteroids are increased by combined hormonal contraceptives. In theory, both the therapeutic and toxic effects would be expected to be increased, but in practice it is uncertain whether these changes are important. Total serum cortisol levels may also be increased by hormonal contraceptives. Fluocortolone and oral budesonide levels were not affected by oral contraceptives. Prasterone did not affect the pharmacokinetics of prednisone or the effects of its metabolite, prednisolone, on cortisol secretion. Progesterone appears not to affect the metabolism of prednisolone.

Clinical evidence

(a) Hormonal contraceptives

1. Budesonide. The plasma levels of oral budesonide 4.5 mg daily for 7 days, and cortisol suppression were no different in 20 women taking an oral contraceptive (**ethinylestradiol/desogestrel**) when compared with 20 women not taking an oral contraceptive.[1]

2. Cloprednol. The clearance of cloprednol 20 mg was decreased by about one-third in 7 women taking an oral contraceptive (**ethinylestradiol/norethisterone**), when compared with women not taking an oral contraceptive.[2]

3. Corticotropin. In a study in 11 healthy women who were not taking hormonal contraceptives, the mean basal concentration of total serum cortisol was 454 nanomol/L, but when the women took combined hormonal contraceptives orally for 3 months the cortisol level increased to 861 nanomol/L. After a low-dose (1 microgram) corticotropin (ACTH) test, using **tetracosactide** (*Synacthen*), the mean serum cortisol level at 30 minutes increased to 652 nanomol/L and 1374 nanomol/L before and after hormonal contraceptive use, respectively. The basal plasma concentration of corticotropin also increased from 17.2 to 38.2 nanograms/L after hormonal contraceptive use. However, the basal and corticotropin-stimulated salivary cortisol was not significantly different between the baseline period and the hormonal contraceptive period.[3]

4. Fluocortolone. A study in 7 women found that the pharmacokinetics of fluocortolone 20 mg were unaffected by an oral contraceptive (**ethinylestradiol/norethisterone**).[4]

5. Methylprednisolone. A study in two groups of 6 patients found that the clearance of methylprednisolone was decreased to about half in the group taking oral contraceptives (**ethinylestradiol/levonorgestrel**), when compared with the group not taking oral contraceptives. The oral contraceptive group were less sensitive to the suppressive effects of methylprednisolone on the secretion of cortisol, and had more suppression of basophils, but no changes in the T-helper cell response patterns.[5]

6. Prednisolone. In a placebo-controlled study, 20 healthy women took an oral contraceptive (**ethinylestradiol/desogestrel** 30/150 micrograms) for at least 4 months before being given prednisolone 20 mg daily for 7 days. The prednisolone AUC and steady-state levels were 2.3-fold higher, when compared with those in 20 women not taking oral contraceptives.[1] Several other studies have found similar results, with the prednisolone AUC increasing 1.6- to 6-fold,[6,7] and the clearance reducing by about 35 to 85% in the presence of oral contraceptives containing **ethinylestradiol** or **mestranol** and various progestogens such as **levonorgestrel**, **norgestrel** and **norethisterone**.[6-11] Similarly, a 2.3-fold increase in the AUC of prednisolone and a 45% decrease in its clearance was seen when **prednisone** was given to 10 women (9 taking an oral combined hormonal contraceptive and one taking ethinylestradiol).[12]

(b) Prasterone

In a study in 14 healthy women, prasterone 200 mg daily for one menstrual cycle (approximately 28 days) did not affect the pharmacokinetics of a single 20-mg dose of **prednisone** or its inhibition of cortisol secretion.[13]

(c) Progesterone

Intravenous and oral **prednisolone** were given to 6 post-menopausal women before and after they took progesterone 5 mg for 2 months. The pharmacokinetics of **prednisolone** were not significantly altered by progesterone.[14]

Mechanism

Not fully understood. The possibilities include a change in the metabolism of the corticosteroids, or in their binding to serum proteins.[12] The absence of an interaction with progesterone suggests that the oestrogenic component of the oral contraceptive is possibly responsible for any interaction.[14] Endogenous and synthetic oestrogens appear to cause an increase in the plasma concentration of cortisol binding globulin, which results in an elevation of the total cortisol level.[3]

Importance and management

It is established that the pharmacokinetics of some corticosteroids are affected by combined hormonal contraceptives, but the clinical importance of any such changes is not known. The therapeutic and adverse effects would be expected to be increased but there appear to be no clinical reports of adverse reactions arising from concurrent use. In fact the authors of one study[5] concluded that women can be dosed similarly with methylprednisolone irrespective of contraceptive use.

However, until more is known it would be prudent to bear this interaction in mind when using any corticosteroid and combined hormonal contraceptive together. Only prednisone, prednisolone, cloprednol and methylprednisolone have been reported to interact although some other corticosteroids possibly behave similarly, the exceptions apparently being fluocortolone and oral budesonide.

Total serum cortisol levels may be increased by hormonal contraceptives, but the unbound fraction of cortisol appears to be unaffected.[3]

Progesterone appears not to interact with prednisolone.

1. Seidegård J, Simonsson M, Edsbäcker S. Effect of an oral contraceptive on the plasma levels of budesonide and prednisolone and the influence on plasma cortisol. *Clin Pharmacol Ther* (2000) 67, 373–81.
2. Legler UF. Altered cloprednol disposition in oral contraceptive users. *Clin Pharmacol Ther* (1987) 41, 237.
3. Šim<u-ANGSTROM>nková K, Stárka L, Hill M, K<r-CZ/V>íž L, Hampl R, Vondra K. Comparison of total and salivary cortisol in a low-dose ACTH (Synacthen) test: influence of three-month oral contraceptives administration to healthy women. *Physiol Res* (2008) 57 (Suppl 1), S193–S199.
4. Legler UF. Lack of impairment of fluocortolone disposition in oral contraceptive users. *Eur J Clin Pharmacol* (1988) 35, 101–3.
5. Slayter KL, Ludwig EA, Lew KH, Middleton E, Ferry JJ, Jusko WJ. Oral contraceptive effects on methylprednisolone pharmacokinetics and pharmacodynamics. *Clin Pharmacol Ther* (1996) 59, 312–21.
6. Legler UF, Benet LZ. Marked alterations in prednisolone elimination for women taking oral contraceptives. *Clin Pharmacol Ther* (1982) 31, 243.
7. Olivesi A. Modified elimination of prednisolone in epileptic patients on carbamazepine monotherapy, and in women using low-dose oral contraceptives. *Biomed Pharmacother* (1986) 40, 301–8.
8. Boekenoogen SJ, Szefler SJ, Jusko WJ. Prednisolone disposition and protein binding in oral contraceptive users. *J Clin Endocrinol Metab* (1983) 56, 702–9.
9. Kozower M, Veatch L, Kaplan MM. Decreased clearance of prednisolone, a factor in the development of corticosteroid side effects. *J Clin Endocrinol Metab* (1974) 38, 407–12.
10. Legler UF, Benet LZ. Marked alterations in dose-dependent prednisolone kinetics in women taking oral contraceptives. *Clin Pharmacol Ther* (1986) 39, 425–9.
11. Meffin PJ, Wing LMH, Sallustio BC, Brooks PM. Alterations in prednisolone disposition as a result of oral contraceptive use and dose. *Br J Clin Pharmacol* (1984) 17, 655–64.
12. Frey BM, Schaad HJ, Frey FJ. Pharmacokinetic interaction of contraceptive steroids with prednisone and prednisolone. *Eur J Clin Pharmacol* (1984) 26, 505–11.
13. Meno-Tetang GML, Blum RA, Schwartz KE, Jusko WJ. Effects of oral prasterone (dehydroepiandrosterone) on single-dose pharmacokinetics of oral prednisone and cortisol suppression in normal women. *J Clin Pharmacol* (2001) 41, 1195–1205.
14. Tsunoda SM, Harris RZ, Mroczkowski PJ, Hebert MF, Benet LZ. Oral progesterone therapy does not affect the pharmacokinetics of prednisolone and erythromycin in post-menopausal women. *Clin Pharmacol Ther* (1995) 57, 182.

Corticosteroids + Liquorice

Liquorice can delay the clearance of prednisolone and hydrocortisone. Dexamethasone may attenuate the mineralocorticoid effects of glycyrrhizin. Liquorice, if given in large quantities with corticosteroids, may cause additive hypokalaemia.

Clinical evidence

Liquorice has a great number of active compounds of different classes that act in different ways. The most important constituent is usually considered to be glycyrrhizin (glycyrrhizic or glycyrrhizinic acid).

(a) Dexamethasone

In a parallel group study, 6 patients were given **glycyrrhizin** 225 mg daily for 7 days, and 6 patients were given the same dose of **glycyrrhizin** and dexamethasone 1.5 mg daily for 7 days. The mineralocorticoid effects of **glycyrrhizin** were significantly reduced by dexamethasone; cortisol plasma concentrations and urinary excretions were reduced by up to 70%.[1]

(b) Hydrocortisone

Glycyrrhizin slightly increased the AUC of cortisol by 14% in 4 patients with adrenocorticol insufficiency taking oral hydrocortisone 20 to 40 mg daily. Note that **glycyrrhizin** had no effect on endogenous cortisol levels in 7 control subjects without adrenal insufficiency.[2] In a study in 23 healthy subjects, topical **glycyrrhetinic acid** markedly potentiated the activity of topical hydrocortisone, as assessed by cutaneous vasoconstrictor effect.[3]

(c) Prednisolone

A study in 6 healthy subjects found that after taking four 50-mg oral doses of **glycyrrhizin** at 8-hourly intervals, followed by a bolus injection of prednisolone hemisuccinate 96 micrograms/kg, the AUC of total prednisolone was increased by 50% and the AUC of free prednisolone was increased by 55%.[4] This confirms previous findings with **glycyrrhizin** 200 mg given by intravenous infusion.[5]

Glycyrrhizin slightly increased the AUC of prednisolone by about 16 to 20% in 12 patients who had been taking oral prednisolone 10 to 30 mg daily for at least 3 months.[2]

Mechanism

Inhibition of 11 β-hydroxysteroid dehydrogenase by glycyrrhetinic acid may slightly delay the clearance of hydrocortisone and prednisolone and thereby enhance their effects. However, note that whether a mineralocorticoid or glucocorticoid is a substrate for this enzyme system depends on its chemical structure. Therefore, it cannot be assumed that liquorice will inhibit the inactivation of all corticosteroids.

Dexamethasone appears to attenuate the mineralocorticoid effects of glycyrrhizin because it suppresses endogenous cortisol secretion (causes adrenal suppression). Other corticosteroids would be expected to interact similarly if given in adrenal-suppressant doses.

Deglycyrrhizinated liquorice would not have these effects.

Importance and management

The clinical importance of these observations is uncertain. Doses of corticosteroids sufficient to cause adrenal suppression would be expected to reduce the mineralocorticoid activity of liquorice, but mineralocorticoid activity might still occur. Glycyrrhizin (an active constituent of liquorice) and its metabolite glycyrrhetinic acid slightly increased the plasma levels of hydrocortisone and prednisolone and markedly potentiated the cutaneous effects of hydrocortisone. This suggests that liquorice will slightly potentiate the effects of these steroids. However, this might not apply to other corticosteroids (see *Mechanism*, above). Nevertheless, it might be prudent to monitor the concurrent use of liquorice and corticosteroids, especially if liquorice ingestion is prolonged or if large doses are taken, as additive effects on water and sodium retention, and potassium depletion may occur.

Note that several manufacturers of corticosteroids comment that the hypokalaemic effects of **carbenoxolone**, a synthetic derivative of glycyrrhizic acid, may be enhanced by corticosteroids.

1. Kageyama Y, Suzuki H, Saruta T. Glycyrrhizin induces mineralocorticoid activity through alterations in cortisol metabolism in the human kidney. *J Endocrinol* (1992) 135, 147–52.
2. Ojima M, Satoh K, Gomibuchi T, Itoh N, Kin S, Fukuchi S, Miyachi Y. The inhibitory effects of glycyrrhizin and glycyrrhetinic acid on the metabolism of cortisol and prednisolone — in vivo and in vitro studies. *Nippon Naibunpi Gakkai Zasshi* (1990) 66, 584–96.
3. Teelucksingh S, Mackie ADR, Burt D, McIntyre MA, Brett L, Edwards CRW. Potentiation of hydrocortisone activity in skin by glycyrrhetinic acid. *Lancet* (1990) 335, 1060–1063.
4. Chen M-F, Shimada F, Kato H, Yano S, Kanaoka M. Effect of oral administration of glycyrrhizin on the pharmacokinetics of prednisolone. *Endocrinol Jpn* (1991) 38, 167–74.
5. Chen M-F, Shimada F, Kato H, Yano S, Kanaoka M. Effect of glycyrrhizin on the pharmacokinetics of prednisolone following low dosage of prednisolone hemisuccinate. *Endocrinol Jpn* (1990) 37, 331–41.

Corticosteroids + Macrolides

Clarithromycin and erythromycin can reduce the clearance of methylprednisolone, thereby increasing both its therapeutic and adverse effects. Azithromycin does not appear to affect the pharmacokinetics of methylprednisolone. A patient receiving long-term clarithromycin developed Cushing's syndrome after using inhaled budesonide. There appears to be no pharmacokinetic interaction between erythromycin and inhaled ciclesonide or fluticasone. Similarly,the pharmacokinetics of prednisolone do not appear to be affected by macrolides, except possibly in those patients also taking enzyme-inducers such as phenobarbital. Isolated case reports describe the development of acute mania and psychosis in two patients, apparently due to an interaction between prednisone and clarithromycin.

Clinical evidence

(a) Budesonide

A 40-year-old woman with cystic fibrosis given **clarithromycin** 500 mg twice daily for 4 years for a *Mycobacterium abscessus* infection developed Cushing's syndrome with adrenal suppression 6 weeks after starting to use inhaled budesonide 400 micrograms daily. A slow increase in her morning free cortisol serum concentration was found 4 weeks after stopping budesonide.[1]

(b) Ciclesonide

In a crossover study, healthy subjects were given a single 500-mg dose of **erythromycin** and inhaled ciclesonide 640 micrograms, alone or together. Concurrent use did not alter the pharmacokinetics of either drug.[2]

(c) Fluticasone

In a multiple-dose study, giving **erythromycin** 333 mg three times daily did not affect the pharmacokinetics of inhaled fluticasone propionate 500 micrograms twice daily.[3]

(d) Methylprednisolone

1. Azithromycin. A review by the manufacturers of azithromycin briefly mentions that azithromycin does not alter the pharmacokinetics of methylprednisolone.[4]

2. Clarithromycin. A study in 6 patients with asthma found that clarithromycin 500 mg twice daily for 9 days reduced the clearance of a single dose of methylprednisolone by 65% and resulted in considerably higher plasma methylprednisolone concentrations.[5]

3. Erythromycin. A study in 9 patients with asthma aged 9 to 18 years found that after taking erythromycin 250 mg four times daily for a week, the clearance of methylprednisolone was decreased by 46% (range 28 to 61%) and the half-life was increased by 47%, from 2.3 to 3.5 hours.[6]

4. Troleandomycin. A pharmacokinetic study in 4 children and 6 adult corticosteroid-dependent asthmatics found that troleandomycin 14 mg/kg daily for one week increased the half-life of methylprednisolone by 88%, from 2.46 to 4.63 hours, and reduced the total body clearance by 64%. All 10 subjects had cushingoid symptoms (moon face and weight gain), which resolved when the methylprednisolone dose was reduced, without any loss in the control of the asthma.[7] Another study found that the dose of methylprednisolone could be reduced by 50% in the presence of troleandomycin, without loss of disease control.[8] Other studies have found similar effects.[9-14] However, a randomised, placebo-controlled, 2-year study found that although troleandomycin modestly reduced the required dose of methylprednisolone, this did not reduce corticosteroid-related adverse effects.[14] A case report describes a fatal varicella infection attributed to the potentiation of steroid effects by troleandomycin.[15]

(e) Prednisolone or Prednisone

1. Clarithromycin. A 30-year-old woman with no history of mental illness was treated for acute sinusitis with prednisone 20 mg daily for 2 days, followed by 40 mg daily for a further 2 days and clarithromycin 1 g daily. After 5 days she stopped taking both drugs (for unknown reasons), but a further 5 days later she was hospitalised with acute mania (disorganised thoughts and behaviour, pressured speech, increased energy, reduced need for sleep, and labile effect). She spontaneously recovered after a further 5 days and had no evidence of psychiatric illness 4 months later.[16] A 50-year-old man with emphysema was given prednisone 20 mg daily to improve dyspnoea. After about 2 weeks he was also given clarithromycin 500 mg twice daily for purulent bronchitis. Shortly afterwards his family noticed psychiatric symptoms characterised by paranoia, delusions, and what was described as dangerous behaviour. He recovered following treatment with low-dose olanzapine, a gradual reduction of the prednisone dose, and discontinuation of the clarithromycin. An interaction was suspected as the patient had previously received prednisone on a number of occasions without the development of psychosis.[17]

A study in 6 patients with asthma found that clarithromycin 500 mg twice daily for 9 days had no effect on prednisone pharmacokinetics.[5]

2. Troleandomycin. A study found that prednisolone clearance was not affected by troleandomycin in 3 patients, but was reduced by about 50% by troleandomycin in one patient who was also taking **phenobarbital**, which is an enzyme inducer.[9]

Mechanism

Some macrolides (particularly clarithromycin, telithromycin, and also erythromycin) are known to inhibit CYP3A4. Budesonide, fluticasone, and methylprednisolone are all metabolised by this isoenzyme and so the exposure to, and the effects of, macrolides would be expected to increase on their concurrent use. However, the magnitude of the increase is likely to vary depending on the potency of inhibition and the degree to which the corticosteroid is metabolised by CYP3A4. For example, prednisolone is less dependent on CYP3A4 for its metabolism, and was not affected by clarithromycin.

Azithromycin does not generally interact by this mechanism, and this can be seen by its lack of effect on methylprednisolone. The active metabolite of ciclesonide is metabolised by CYP3A4, but the pharmacokinetics of ciclesonide itself were not affected by erythromycin.

Importance and management

Information about the interaction between clarithromycin or erythromycin and **methylprednisolone** is much more limited than information about the interaction between troleandomycin and methylprednisolone, but they all appear to be established interactions of clinical importance. The effect should be taken into account on concurrent use and appropriate methylprednisolone dose reductions made to avoid the development of corticosteroid adverse effects. The authors of one study[7] suggest that this reduction should be empirical, based primarily on clinical symptoms. Another group found that a 68% reduction in methylprednisolone dose was possible within 2 weeks.[11]

Prednisolone seems less likely to interact and it might therefore be a non-interacting alternative to methylprednisolone, except possibly in those taking enzyme-inducers (such as phenobarbital). Nevertheless, one UK manufacturer of prednisolone advises caution on the concurrent use of CYP3A4 inhibitors [which would be expected to include clarithromycin, telithromycin, and erythromycin], and states that the doses of the corticosteroid might need to be decreased.[18]

The evidence for the interaction leading to psychosis between prednisone and clarithromycin is limited and its general importance is uncertain, but prescribers should be aware of the reports of psychosis if both drugs are used together. Note that psychosis is a rare adverse effect of high-dose corticosteroids given alone.

One case report indicates that clarithromycin might enhance the effects of inhaled **budesonide** and although the authors suggest that prolonged use of clarithromycin and the terminal condition of the patient might have been factors, they advise close monitoring if the combination is used.[1] Several UK and US manufacturers of inhaled,[19,20] intranasal,[21] oral,[22] and rectal[23] budesonide advise that potent inhibitors of CYP3A4 should be avoided: some specifically name clarithromycin[19,20] and **telithromycin**.[20] However, given the evidence available, this seems a very cautious approach.

Some other manufacturers of corticosteroids, including **dexamethasone** and **hydrocortisone** have also mentioned the potential for increased plasma concentrations of corticosteroids with macrolides such as erythromycin. In general the concurrent use of these corticosteroids and CYP3A4-inhibiting macrolides need not be avoided, but it would seem prudent to monitor for corticosteroid adverse effects (such as moon face, weight gain, hyperglycaemia) and suspect an interaction if symptoms occur. Patients should be warned to be alert for any evidence of increased corticosteroid effects (such as moon face, weight gain, hyperglycaemia) and to seek medical advice if these occur. In most cases the interaction should be manageable by reducing the dose of the corticosteroid until the macrolide is withdrawn.

1. De Wachter E, Malfroot A, De Schutter I, Vanbesien J, De Schepper J. Inhaled budesonide induced Cushing's syndrome in cystic fibrosis patients, due to drug inhibition of cytochrome P450. *J Cyst Fibros* (2003) 2, 72–5.
2. Nave R, Drollmann A, Steinijans VW, Zech K, Bethke TD. Lack of pharmacokinetic drug-drug interaction between ciclesonide and erythromycin. *Int J Clin Pharmacol Ther* (2005) 43, 264–70.
3. Flovent HFA Inhalation Aerosol (Fluticasone propionate). GlaxoSmithKline. US Prescribing information, January 2012.
4. Hopkins S. Clinical toleration and safety of azithromycin. *Am J Med* (1991) 91 (Suppl 3A), 40S–45S.
5. Fost DA, Leung DYM, Martin RJ, Brown EE, Szefler SJ, Spahn JD. Inhibition of methylprednisolone elimination in the presence of clarithromycin therapy. *J Allergy Clin Immunol* (1999) 103, 1031–5.
6. LaForce CF, Szefler SJ, Miller MF, Ebling W, Brenner M. Inhibition of methylprednisolone elimination in the presence of erythromycin therapy. *J Allergy Clin Immunol* (1983) 72, 34–9.
7. Szefler SJ, Rose JQ, Ellis EF, Spector SL, Green AW, Jusko WJ. The effect of troleandomycin on methylprednisolone elimination. *J Allergy Clin Immunol* (1980) 66, 447–51.
8. Ball BD, Hill M, Brenner M, Sanks R, Szefler SJ. Critical assessment of troleandomycin in severe steroid-requiring asthmatic children. *Ann Allergy* (1988) 60, 155.
9. Szefler SJ, Ellis EF, Brenner M, Rose JQ, Spector SL, Yurchak AM, Andrews F, Jusko WJ. Steroid-specific and anticonvulsant interaction aspects of troleandomycin-steroid therapy. *J Allergy Clin Immunol* (1982) 69, 455–60.
10. Itkin IH, Menzel M. The use of macrolide antibiotic substances in the treatment of asthma. *J Allergy* (1970) 45, 146–62.
11. Wald JA, Friedman BF, Farr RS. An improved protocol for the use of troleandomycin (TAO) in the treatment of steroid-requiring asthma. *J Allergy Clin Immunol* (1986) 78, 36–43.
12. Zeiger RS, Schatz M, Sperling W, Simon RA, Stevenson DD. Efficacy of troleandomycin in outpatients with severe, corticosteroid-dependent asthma. *J Allergy Clin Immunol* (1980) 66, 438–46.
13. Kamada AK, Hill MR, Brenner AM, Szefler SJ. Glucocorticoid reduction with troleandomycin in chronic, severe asthmatic children: implications for future trials and clinical application. *J Allergy Clin Immunol* (1992) 89, 285.
14. Nelson HS, Hamilos DL, Corsello PR, Levesque NV, Buchmeier AD, Bucher BL. A double-blind study of troleandomycin and methylprednisolone in asthmatic subjects who require daily corticosteroids. *Am Rev Respir Dis* (1993) 147, 398–404.
15. Lantner R, Rockoff JB, DeMasi J, Boran-Ragotzy R, Middleton E. Fatal varicella in a corticosteroid-dependent asthmatic receiving troleandomycin. *Allergy Proc* (1990) 11, 83–7.
16. Finkenbine R, Gill HS. Case of mania due to prednisone-clarithromycin interaction. *Can J Psychiatry* (1997) 42, 778.
17. Finkenbine RD, Frye MD. Case of psychosis due to prednisone-clarithromycin interaction. *Gen Hosp Psychiatry* (1998) 20, 325–6.
18. Deltacortril Gastro-resistant Tablets (Prednisolone). Alliance Pharmaceuticals. UK Summary of product characteristics, May 2012.
19. Budenofalk Rectal Foam (Budesonide). Dr. Falk Pharma UK Ltd. UK Summary of product characteristics, November 2011.
20. Pulmicort Respules (Budesonide). AstraZeneca LP. US Prescribing information, July 2010.
21. Rhinocort Aqua Nasal Spray (Budesonide). AstraZeneca UK Ltd. UK Summary of product characteristics, July 2012.
22. Entocort CR Capsules (Budesonide). AstraZeneca UK Ltd. UK Summary of product characteristics, April 2012.
23. Pulmicort Turbohaler (Budesonide). AstraZeneca UK Ltd. UK Summary of product characteristics, April 2012.

Corticosteroids + Mifepristone

The UK manufacturer of mifepristone says that, due to the anti-glucocorticoid activity of mifepristone, the efficacy of long-term corticosteroids (including inhaled corticosteroids) may be decreased during the 3 to 4 days following intake of mifepristone.[1] Patients taking corticosteroids should be monitored during this time, and consideration given to increasing the corticosteroid dose. However, the US manufacturer contraindicates the use of mifepristone in patients receiving long-term corticosteroid therapy.[2]

1. Mifegyne (Mifepristone). Exelgyn Laboratories. UK Summary of product characteristics, May 2008.
2. Mifeprex (Mifepristone). Danco Laboratories, LLC. US Prescribing information, April 2009.

Corticosteroids + Nefazodone

Nefazodone moderately increases the exposure to intravenous methylprednisolone and prolongs its effects on cortisol suppression. A case of Cushing's syndrome and adrenal insufficiency has been described in a patient taking nefazodone after receiving triamcinolone injections.

Clinical evidence

In a study in healthy subjects, nefazodone (initial dose of 100 mg, increased to 150 mg, then 200 mg, twice daily, for a total of 9 days) increased the AUC of a single 600-microgram/kg intravenous dose of **methylprednisolone** 2-fold and increased its half-life from 2.3 hours to 3.3 hours. **Methylprednisolone** clearance was decreased by about 50%. The duration of cortisol suppression after **methylprednisolone** alone was 23.3 hours, but was increased to more than 32 hours when nefazodone was also given.[1]

A case report describes a 43-year-old woman taking nefazodone 600 mg daily, who developed symptoms of Cushing's syndrome about one month after receiving the second of two 20 mg **triamcinolone** injections, which were given about 3 to 4 weeks apart. A cortisol stimulation test revealed a baseline cortisol concentration of less than 1 microgram/dL and her baseline ACTH concentration was undetectable. Secondary adrenal insufficiency was diagnosed and hydrocortisone replacement therapy was started, but after about one month, her serum cortisol concentration was still less than 1 microgram/dL. Nefazodone was stopped and over the course of the following 8 months her pituitary-adrenal axis recovered. Note that **triamcinolone** was still detectable in the serum (0.26 microgram/dL, lower limit 0.03 microgram/dL), about two and a half months after the last injection.[2]

Mechanism

Nefazodone probably inhibits the metabolism of methylprednisolone[1] and triamcinolone[2] by CYP3A4.

Importance and management

At clinically relevant doses, nefazodone decreases methylprednisolone clearance and greatly prolongs methylprednisolone-induced cortisol suppression. Patients should be warned to be alert for any evidence of increased corticosteroid adverse effects (such as moon face, weight gain, or hyperglycaemia) on concurrent use and to seek medical advice if these occur. Note that many other corticosteroids are metabolised, at least in part, by the same route as methylprednisolone, and might therefore also be expected to interact with nefazodone to some extent. The case report with triamcinolone, although isolated, seems to confirm this theory, but confirmation is needed for other corticosteroids metabolised by CYP3A4. Note also that nefazodone has been generally withdrawn from the market because of adverse hepatic effects.

1. Kotlyar M, Brewer ER, Golding M, Carson SW. Nefazodone inhibits methylprednisolone disposition and enhances its adrenal-suppressant effect. *J Clin Psychopharmacol* (2003) 23, 652–6.
2. Hagan JB, Erickson D, Singh RJ. Triamcinolone acetonide induced secondary adrenal insufficiency related to impaired CYP3A4 metabolism by coadministration of nefazodone. *Pain Med* (2010) 11, 1132–5.

Corticosteroids + NNRTIs

Efavirenz appears to slightly decrease prednisolone exposure, and might be predicted to decrease the concentrations of some other corticosteroids such as dexamethasone. Nevirapine would be expected to interact similarly, whereas delavirdine is predicted to increase the concentrations of dexamethasone and possibly other corticosteroids.

Dexamethasone is predicted to decrease the plasma concentrations of delavirdine, etravirine and rilpivirine. Prednisone might increase the incidence and severity of rash associated with the use of nevirapine.

Clinical evidence, mechanism, importance and management

(a) Delavirdine

The manufacturer of delavirdine states that it should be used with caution with **dexamethasone** because delavirdine might be less effective due to decreased plasma concentrations.[1] This is presumably because delavirdine is primarily metabolised by CYP3A4,[1] which is said to be induced by **dexamethasone**.[2] However, evidence of **dexamethasone** having clinically relevant interactions as a result of this mechanism is generally lacking. The concentrations of **dexamethasone** might be increased by delavirdine, due to inhibition of CYP3A4.[2] There appears to be little information about other corticosteroids and delavirdine, but many corticosteroids (particularly **methylprednisolone**) are metabolised, at least in part, by CYP3A4 and therefore their plasma concentrations could also be increased to some extent by delavirdine. Be alert for increased corticosteroid adverse effects.

(b) Efavirenz or Nevirapine

A study in HIV-positive subjects given a single 20-mg dose of **prednisone**, found that efavirenz, as part of antiretroviral medication, decreased the AUC of **prednisolone** by about 20%, when compared with similar patients who were not taking antiretrovirals; however, this was not statistically significant. When the patients taking efavirenz were compared with patients receiving lopinavir boosted with ritonavir, there was a 40% reduction in the AUC of **prednisolone**. This indicates that **prednisolone** exposure might fluctuate widely when HIV-positive individuals established on efavirenz change to lopinavir boosted with ritonavir or *vice versa*.[3] However, note that the apparent slight reduction in prednisolone exposure with efavirenz would not be expected to be clinically relevant. There appears to be little information about other corticosteroids and efavirenz or nevirapine, but many corticosteroids (particularly **methylprednisolone** and also **dexamethasone**[2]) are metabolised, at least in part, by CYP3A4. It is possible that their exposure might be decreased if efavirenz or nevirapine are used. Bear this possibility in mind.

Corticosteroids can be used to treat rash associated with efavirenz.[4] However, the manufacturers of nevirapine state that **prednisone** 40 mg daily for the first 14 days of nevirapine use has not been shown to reduce the incidence of nevirapine-associated rash and might be associated with an increase in incidence and severity of rash during the first 6 weeks of nevirapine use.[5,6] The US manufacturer therefore states that the use of **prednisone** to prevent nevirapine-associated rash is not recommended.[6]

(c) Etravirine

The manufacturer of etravirine states that it should be used with caution with **dexamethasone** because etravirine might be less effective due to decreased plasma concentrations. They advise that alternatives to dexamethasone should be considered if possible, particularly for long-term use.[7,8] This is presumably because etravirine is metabolised by CYP3A4,[1] which is said to be induced by **dexamethasone**.[2] However, evidence of **dexamethasone** having clinically relevant interactions as a result of this mechanism is generally lacking.

(d) Rilpivirine

The manufacturers of rilpivirine state that **dexamethasone** might reduce rilpivirine concentrations by inducing CYP3A4, and contraindicate the concurrent use of rilpivirine with multiple-dose dexamethasone.[9,10] However, evidence of **dexamethasone** having clinically relevant interactions as a result of this mechanism is generally lacking.

1. Rescriptor (Delavirdine mesylate). ViiV Healthcare. US Prescribing information, August 2012.
2. de Maat MMR, Ekhart GC, Huitema ADR, Koks CHW, Mulder JW, Beijnen JH. Drug interactions between antiretroviral drugs and comedicated agents. *Clin Pharmacokinet* (2003) 42, 223–82.
3. Busse KH, Formentini E, Alfaro RM, Kovacs JA, Penzak SR. Influence of antiretroviral drugs on the pharmacokinetics of prednisolone in HIV-infected individuals. *J Acquir Immune Defic Syndr* (2008) 48, 561–6.
4. Sustiva Film-coated Tablets (Efavirenz). Bristol-Myers Squibb Pharmaceutical Ltd. UK Summary of product characteristics, March 2014.
5. Viramune (Nevirapine). Boehringer Ingelheim Ltd. UK Summary of product characteristics, January 2012.
6. Viramune (Nevirapine). Boehringer Ingelheim Pharmaceuticals, Inc. US Prescribing information, November 2011.
7. Intelence (Etravirine). Janssen-Cilag Ltd. UK Summary of product characteristics, July 2012.
8. Intelence (Etravirine). Tibotec, Inc. US Prescribing information, August 2012.
9. Edurant (Rilpivirine hydrochloride). Janssen-Cilag Ltd. UK Summary of product characteristics, November 2011.
10. Edurant (Rilpivirine hydrochloride). Tibotec Pharmaceuticals. US Prescribing information, August 2012.

Corticosteroids + NSAIDs

Corticosteroids or NSAIDs alone may be risk factors for gastrointestinal bleeding and ulceration. The concurrent use of NSAIDs and corticosteroids increases the risk of gastrointestinal bleeding and probably ulceration.

Ibuprofen, indometacin and naproxen may increase the levels of free prednisolone, and the plasma levels of diclofenac are modestly increased by triamcinolone. Dexamethasone and prednisone do not appear to affect the levels of oxyphenbutazone.

Clinical evidence, mechanism, importance and management

(a) Gastrointestinal bleeding and ulceration

A retrospective study of about 20 000 patients who had taken corticosteroids found that the incidence of upper gastrointestinal bleeding resulting in hospitalisation was very low in outpatients taking corticosteroids for dermatitis and asthma. Bleeding occurred in only 45 (0.23%) of the patients. However, the risk of bleeding was increased if the patients were also taking aspirin or other NSAIDs (incidence rate of 5.1 per 10 000 person-months, compared with 2.2 per 10 000 person-months in those who did not take NSAIDs).[1] This is consistent with the results of another study in patients taking **prednisone** and **indometacin**.[2]

A case-control study reviewed 1415 patients aged 65 years or older, hospitalised between 1984 and 1986 for peptic ulcer or upper gastrointestinal haemorrhage of unknown cause, and 7063 control patients. The relative risk for the development of peptic ulcer disease was estimated to be 2 in those taking oral corticosteroids; however, for those corticosteroid users not receiving NSAIDs it was 1.1 and the estimated risk was only increased in those taking corticosteroids with NSAIDs (relative risk 4.4). It was estimated that patients taking corticosteroids with NSAIDs have an approximately 15-fold greater risk for peptic ulcer disease than patients taking neither drug.[3]

Another study compared 1121 patients aged 60 years or over who were admitted to hospital with bleeding peptic ulcers, with 989 control patients, to investigate factors other than NSAIDs that may have contributed to the risk of bleeding.[4] The risk (calculated as odds ratio) was about threefold greater for the use of corticosteroids alone, but when corticosteroids were used with NSAIDs, the risk was ninefold greater.[4]

NSAIDs alone increase the risk of gastrointestinal adverse effects.[5-8] Most patients with NSAID-associated ulcers are elderly: this is because there is a greater prevalence of ulcer disease in the elderly, and they are more likely to be taking NSAIDs and to be sensitive to them.[7] A history of ulcer disease is a further risk factor.[7] Corticosteroids alone are reported not to be a risk factor in some studies,[1,9] while other studies found they were a risk factor for gastrointestinal adverse effects.[4,10] However, several studies have found that the risk of gastrointestinal adverse effects is increased by the combined use of corticosteroids and NSAIDs[3,4,11,12] and caution with concurrent use has been suggested.[3] It may be prudent to consider the use of gastroprotection in patients taking NSAIDs and corticosteroids, especially if they are elderly.

(b) Pharmacokinetic interactions

A patient with rheumatoid arthritis taking **prednisolone** 5 to 10 mg daily with the intermittent use of an NSAID (aspirin 700 mg to 2.8 g daily, **ibuprofen** 400 mg to 1.2 g daily, or **naproxen** 250 to 500 mg daily), developed osteonecrosis of the upper third of the femoral head, which was attributed to increased free levels of **prednisolone** due to protein-binding displacement by the NSAID.[13] A study in 11 patients with stable rheumatoid disease regularly taking a corticosteroid found that **indometacin** 75 mg or **naproxen** 250 mg twice daily for 2 weeks did not alter the total plasma levels of a single 7.5-mg dose of **prednisolone** but the amount of unbound (free) **prednisolone** increased by 30 to 60%.[14] The probable reason for this effect is that these NSAIDs displace both administered and endogenous corticosteroids from their plasma protein binding sites. In a double-blind, crossover study 12 healthy subjects were given **rofecoxib** 250 mg daily or placebo for 14 days, with a single 30-mg dose of either intravenous **prednisolone** or oral **prednisone** on days 10 and 14. **Rofecoxib** did not affect the pharmacokinetics of the corticosteroids, even at a dose 10 times greater than that used clinically.[15]

In a double-blind, crossover study in healthy subjects given a single intramuscular dose of **diclofenac** 75 mg, the use of **triamcinolone** 40 mg increased the maximum plasma levels of **diclofenac** by 24%. This was possibly due to an increased rate of absorption. Other pharmacokinetic parameters of **diclofenac** were not significantly changed.[16] In another study, neither **prednisone** 5 mg nor **dexamethasone** 1.5 mg daily were found to affect **oxyphenbutazone** levels.[17]

The majority of these pharmacokinetic interactions seem unlikely to be of clinical significance, but they may well contribute to the adverse effects of both drugs, particularly the corticosteroids. No particular action appears to be necessary to account for these pharmacokinetic effects.

1. Carson JL, Strom BL, Schinnar R, Duff A, Sim E. The low risk of upper gastrointestinal bleeding in patients dispensed corticosteroids. *Am J Med* (1991) 91, 223–8.
2. Emmanuel JH, Montgomery RD. Gastric ulcer and anti-arthritic drugs. *Postgrad Med J* (1971) 47, 227–32.
3. Piper JM, Ray WA, Daugherty JR, Griffin MR. Corticosteroid use and peptic ulcer disease: role of nonsteroidal anti-inflammatory drugs. *Ann Intern Med* (1991) 114, 735–40.
4. Weil J, Langman MJS, Wainwright P, Lawson DH, Rawlins M, Logan RFA, Brown TP, Vessey MP, Murphy M, Colin-Jones DG. Peptic ulcer bleeding: accessory risk factors and interactions with non-steroidal anti-inflammatory drugs. *Gut* (2000) 46, 27–31.
5. Langman MJS, Weil J, Wainwright P, Lawson DH, Rawlins MD, Logan RFA, Murphy M, Vessey MP, Colin-Jones DG. Risks of bleeding peptic ulcer associated with individual non-steroidal anti-inflammatory drugs. *Lancet* (1994) 343, 1075–9.
6. Weil J, Colin-Jones D, Langman M, Lawson D, Logan R, Murphy M, Rawlins M, Vessey M, Wainwright P. Prophylactic aspirin and risk of peptic ulcer bleeding. *BMJ* (1995) 310, 827–30.
7. Seager JM, Hawkey CJ. ABC of the upper gastrointestinal tract: indigestion and non-steroidal anti-inflammatory drugs. *BMJ* (2001) 323, 1236–9.
8. CSM/MCA. Non-steroidal anti-inflammatory drugs (NSAIDs) and gastrointestinal (GI) safety. *Current Problems* (2002) 28, 5.
9. Conn HO, Blitzer BL. Nonassociation of adrenocorticosteroid therapy and peptic ulcer. *N Engl J Med* (1976) 294, 473–9.
10. Messer J, Reitman D, Sacks HS, Smith H, Chalmers TC. Association of adrenocorticosteroid therapy and peptic-ulcer disease. *N Engl J Med* (1983) 309, 21–4.
11. Gabriel SE, Jaakkimainen L, Bombardier C. Risk for serious gastrointestinal complications related to use of nonsteroidal anti-inflammatory drugs. A meta-analysis. *Ann Intern Med* (1991) 115, 787–96.
12. Gutthann SP, García Rodríguez LA, Raiford DS. Individual nonsteroidal antiinflammatory drugs and other risk factors for upper gastrointestinal bleeding and perforation. *Epidemiology* (1997) 8, 18–24.
13. Patial RK, Bansal SK, Kashyap S, Negi A. Drug interaction–induced osteonecrosis of femoral head. *J Assoc Physicians India* (1990) 38, 446–7.
14. Rae SA, Williams IA, English J, Baylis EM. Alteration of plasma prednisolone levels by indomethacin and naproxen. *Br J Clin Pharmacol* (1982) 14, 459–61.
15. Schwartz JI, Mukhopadhyay S, Porras AG, Viswanathan-Aiyer K-J, Adcock S, Ebel DL, Gertz BJ. Effect of rofecoxib on prednisolone and prednisone pharmacokinetics in healthy subjects. *J Clin Pharmacol* (2003) 43, 187–92.
16. Derendorf H, Mullersman G, Barth J, Grüner A, Möllmann H. Pharmacokinetics of diclofenac sodium after intramuscular administration in combination with triamcinolone acetate. *Eur J Clin Pharmacol* (1986) 31, 363–5.
17. Weiner M, Siddiqui AA, Shahani RT, Dayton PG. Effect of steroids on disposition of oxyphenbutazone in man. *Proc Soc Exp Biol Med* (1967) 124, 1170–3.

Corticosteroids + Phenytoin

The therapeutic effects of dexamethasone, fludrocortisone, methylprednisolone, prednisolone, prednisone, and probably other corticosteroids, can be greatly reduced by phenytoin. One study suggested that dexamethasone might modestly increase phenytoin serum concentrations, but another study and two case reports of patients with brain metastases suggest that a *decrease* can occur. The results of the dexamethasone adrenal suppression test might prove to be unreliable in those taking phenytoin.

Clinical evidence

Several studies suggest that phenytoin can affect the half-life and clearance of a number of corticosteroids. These are shown in 'Table 29.2', p.1258. Other information regarding specific corticosteroids is given in the sections below.

(a) Dexamethasone

1. Dexamethasone concentration/response. A comparative pharmacokinetic study in 6 neurological or neurosurgical patients taking oral dexamethasone and phenytoin found that the average amount of dexamethasone that reached the general circulation was a quarter of that observed in 9 other patients taking dexamethasone alone (mean oral bioavailability fractions of 0.21 and 0.84, respectively).[1] Another report describes patients who needed increased doses of dexamethasone while taking phenytoin,[2] and a patient with pemphigus vulgaris did not respond to large doses of corticosteroids including **prednisolone** 100 mg daily or dexamethasone 30 mg daily when he took phenytoin and phenobarbital. Dramatic improvement occurred following gradual discontinuation of the antiepileptic drugs.[3]

A study in 7 patients found that phenytoin 300 to 400 mg daily reduced the plasma cortisol concentration in response to dexamethasone from 220 microgram/L to 190 microgram/L, compared with a reduction from 180 microgram/L to 40 microgram/L in the absence of phenytoin.[4] Other studies confirmed that, in patients taking long-term phenytoin, plasma cortisol and urinary 17-hydroxycorticosteroid concentrations were suppressed far less than might be expected with small doses of dexamethasone (500 micrograms every 6 hours for 8 doses), but with larger doses (2 mg every 6 hours for 8 doses) suppression was normal.[5] However, one case describes a patient in whom even 16 mg of dexamethasone did not cause cortisol depression while she was taking phenytoin, but when she was re-tested in the absence of phenytoin only 1 mg of dexamethasone was needed to elicit a response.[6]

2. Phenytoin concentrations. A study into epilepsy prophylaxis post-trauma found that the phenytoin serum concentration in those taking dexamethasone 16 to 150 mg (mean 63.6 mg) were 40% higher than in those taking phenytoin alone (17.3 micrograms/mL compared with 12.5 micrograms/mL). The phenytoin was given as a loading dose of 11 mg/kg intravenously and then 13 mg/kg intramuscularly.[7] Conversely, a retrospective study of 40 patient records (diagnosis unspecified) indicated that dexamethasone reduced phenytoin serum concentrations: the phenytoin serum concentration of 6 patients receiving fixed doses of phenytoin were halved by dexamethasone.[8] Another report describes a patient with brain metastases who required over 8 mg/kg of phenytoin (600 mg) to achieve a therapeutic phenytoin concentration in the presence of dexamethasone 16 mg. When the dexamethasone was increased to 28 mg daily he experienced seizures, and an increase in his phenytoin dose from 600 mg to 1 g only resulted in an increase in his phenytoin concentration from 13.9 micrograms/mL to 16.4 micrograms/mL.[9] Another patient, also with a brain metastasis, needed a large dose of phenytoin (greater than 10 mg/kg) while taking dexamethasone. He had an almost 4-fold rise in his phenytoin serum concentration when dexamethasone was stopped.[10]

(b) Other corticosteroids

The **fludrocortisone** doses of two patients required 4-fold and 10- to 20-fold increases, respectively, in the presence of phenytoin.[11] A case report describes a 14-year-old boy whose **hydrocortisone** dose was doubled after phenytoin was added. Even this increased dose was unable to fully control his Addison's disease, with episodes of hyponatraemia, vomiting, and fatigue reported. When phenytoin was replaced with levetiracetam, the **hydrocortisone** dose was reduced without any further episodes of hyponatraemia and vomiting.[12]

Renal allograft survival is decreased in patients taking **prednisone** and phenytoin, due (it is believed) to a reduction in the immunosuppressant effects of the corticosteroid.[13] For mention of a patient with pemphigus vulgaris who did not respond to corticosteroids including **prednisolone** when he was also given a number of drugs including phenytoin, see under *Dexamethasone*, above.

Mechanism

Phenytoin is a potent liver enzyme inducer that increases the metabolism of the corticosteroids, probably by CYP3A4, so that they are cleared more quickly, reducing both their therapeutic and adrenal suppressant effects.

Importance and management

The reduction in corticosteroid serum concentrations seen with the concurrent use of phenytoin is established and of clinical importance in systemic treatment, but it seems unlikely to affect the response to steroids given topically or by inhalation, intra-articular injection or enema.[14] The interaction can be accommodated in several ways:

- Increase the corticosteroid dose proportionately to the increase in clearance (see 'Table 29.2', p.1258). With prednisolone an average increase of 100% (range 58 to 260% in 5 subjects) proved effective.[14] A 4-fold increase might be necessary with dexamethasone,[1] and much greater increases have been required with fludrocortisone.[11]

- Switch the corticosteroid for another that is less affected (see 'Table 29.2', p.1258). A comparative study in children found that **methylprednisolone** was more affected than prednisolone.[15] In another case the exchange of dexamethasone 16 mg daily for prednisone 100 mg daily was successful.[16]

- Switch phenytoin for another antiepileptic: barbiturates (including primidone[17]) and carbamazepine, are also enzyme-inducers, but valproate is a possible non-interacting alternative,[2] where clinically appropriate. However, remember that corticosteroids should only be given to patients with epilepsy with caution and good monitoring because of the risk that they will exacerbate the disease condition.

The effects of phenytoin on the dexamethasone adrenal suppression test can apparently be accommodated by using larger than usual doses of dexamethasone (2 mg every 6 hours for 8 doses)[5] or by an overnight test using 50 mg of hydrocortisone.[18]

Table 29.2 A comparison of the effects of phenytoin on the pharmacokinetics of different corticosteroids (after Petereit and colleagues[1])

Corticosteroid	*Daily dosage of phenytoin (mg)*	*Half-life without phenytoin (minutes)*	*Decreased half-life with phenytoin (%)*	*Increased mean clearance rate with phenytoin (%)*	*Refs*
Dexamethasone	300	250	51	140	2
Hydrocortisone	300 to 400	60 to 90	15	25	3
Methylprednisolone	300	165	56	130	4
Prednisolone	300	190 to 240	45	77	3
Prednisone	Prednisolone is the biologically active metabolite of prednisone so that the values for prednisone and prednisolone should be similar				5

1. Petereit LB, Meikle AW. Effectiveness of prednisolone during phenytoin therapy. *Clin Pharmacol Ther* (1977) 22, 912–16.
2. Haque N, Thrasher K, Werk EE, Knowles HC, Sholiton LJ. Studies on dexamethasone metabolism in man. Effect of diphenylhydantoin. *J Clin Endocrinol Metab* (1972) 34, 44–50.
3. Choi Y, Thrasher K, Werk EE, Sholiton LJ, Olinger C. Effect of diphenylhydantoin on cortisol kinetics in humans. *J Pharmacol Exp Ther* (1971) 176, 27–34.
4. Stjernholm MR, Katz FH. Effects of diphenylhydantoin, phenobarbital, and diazepam on the metabolism of methylprednisolone and its sodium succinate. *J Clin Endocrinol Metab* (1975) 41, 887–93.
5. Meikle AW, Weed JA, Tyler FH. Kinetics and interconversion of prednisolone and prednisone studied with new radioimmunoassays. *J Clin Endocrinol Metab* (1975) 41, 717–21.

The reports on the changes in phenytoin serum concentrations are inconsistent (both increases and decreases have been reported). The effects of concurrent use should be closely monitored.

1. Chalk JB, Ridgeway K, Brophy TRO'R, Yelland JDN, Eadie MJ. Phenytoin impairs the bioavailability of dexamethasone in neurological and neurosurgical patients. *J Neurol Neurosurg Psychiatry* (1984) 47, 1087–90.
2. McLelland J, Jack W. Phenytoin/dexamethasone interaction: a clinical problem. *Lancet* (1978) i, 1096–7.
3. Sehgal VN, Srivastava G. Corticosteroid-unresponsive pemphigus vulgaris following antiepileptic therapy. *Int J Dermatol* (1988) 27, 258.
4. Werk EE, Choi Y, Sholiton L, Olinger C, Haque N. Interference in the effect of dexamethasone by diphenylhydantoin. *N Engl J Med* (1969) 281, 32–4.
5. Jubiz W, Meikle AW, Levinson RA, Mizutani S, West CD, Tyler FH. Effect of diphenylhydantoin on the metabolism of dexamethasone. *N Engl J Med* (1970) 283, 11–14.
6. Debrunner J, Schmid C, Schneemann M. Falsely positive dexamethasone suppression test in a patient treated with phenytoin to prevent seizures due to nocardia brain abscesses. *Swiss Med Wkly* (2002) 132, 267.
7. Lawson LA, Blouin RA, Smith RB, Rapp RP, Young AB. Phenytoin-dexamethasone interaction: a previously unreported observation. *Surg Neurol* (1981) 16, 23–4.
8. Wong DD, Longenecker RG, Liepman M, Baker S, LaVergne M. Phenytoin-dexamethasone: a possible drug-drug interaction. *JAMA* (1985) 254, 2062–3.
9. Recuenco I, Espinosa E, García B, Carcas A. Effect of dexamethasone on the decrease of serum phenytoin concentrations. *Ann Pharmacother* (1995) 29, 935.
10. Lackner TE. Interaction of dexamethasone with phenytoin. *Pharmacotherapy* (1991) 11, 344–7.
11. Keilholz U, Guthrie GP. Case report: adverse effect of phenytoin on mineralocorticoid replacement with fludrocortisone in adrenal insufficiency. *Am J Med Sci* (1986) 291, 280–3.
12. Kara C, Ucaktürk A, Aydin ÖF, Aydin M. Adverse effect of phenytoin on glucocorticoid replacement in a child with adrenal insufficiency. *J Pediatr Endocrinol Metab* (2010) 23, 963–6.
13. Wassner SJ, Pennisi AJ, Malekzadeh MH, Fine RN. The adverse effect of anticonvulsant therapy on renal allograft survival. *J Pediatr* (1976) 88, 134–7.
14. Petereit LB, Meikle AW. Effectiveness of prednisolone during phenytoin therapy. *Clin Pharmacol Ther* (1977) 22, 912–6.
15. Bartoszek M, Brenner AM, Szefler SJ. Prednisolone and methylprednisolone kinetics in children receiving anticonvulsant therapy. *Clin Pharmacol Ther* (1987) 42, 424–32.
16. Boylan JJ, Owen DS, Chin JB. Phenytoin interference with dexamethasone. *JAMA* (1976) 235, 803–4.
17. Hancock KW, Levell MJ. Primidone/dexamethasone interaction. *Lancet* (1978) ii, 97–8.
18. Meikle AW, Stanchfield JB, West CD, Tyler FH. Hydrocortisone suppression test for Cushing syndrome: therapy with anticonvulsants. *Arch Intern Med* (1974) 134, 1068–71.

Corticosteroids + Proton pump inhibitors

Lansoprazole appears to have no effect on the pharmacokinetics of prednisolone following a single dose of prednisone. Omeprazole has no effect on oral budesonide or prednisone pharmacokinetics in healthy subjects, but an isolated and unexplained report describes a reduction in the effects of prednisone in a patient taking omeprazole.

Clinical evidence, mechanism, importance and management

(a) Lansoprazole

A placebo-controlled, randomised study in 18 healthy subjects found that lansoprazole 30 mg daily had no effect on the absorption of a single 40-mg oral dose of **prednisone**. Furthermore, the biotransformation of prednisone to **prednisolone**, and the pharmacokinetics of prednisolone were not affected.[1]

(b) Omeprazole

A placebo-controlled, randomised study in 18 healthy subjects found that omeprazole 40 mg daily had no effect on the pharmacokinetics of **prednisolone** after a single 40-mg dose of **prednisone**.[1] This contrasts with an isolated and unexplained report of a patient suffering from pemphigus who was given **prednisone** 1 mg/kg daily with, a week later, ranitidine 200 mg daily for a gastric ulcer. Four weeks later, when the skin lesions were well controlled, it was decided to replace the ranitidine with omeprazole 40 mg daily. Within 4 days the skin lesions began to worsen progressively, although the **prednisone** dosage remained unchanged. After 3 weeks it was decided to stop the omeprazole and restart the ranitidine because an adverse interaction between the **prednisone** and the omeprazole was suspected. Within about a week, the skin condition had begun to improve.[2] The suggested explanation for the interaction is that the omeprazole inhibited the liver enzyme (11β-hydroxylase) that normally converts **prednisone** into its active form (prednisolone) resulting in inadequate treatment of the pemphigus.[2]

A placebo-controlled, randomised study in 11 healthy subjects found that omeprazole 20 mg daily for 5 days had no effect on the pharmacokinetics of a single 9-mg dose of **budesonide** (*Entocort CR* capsules).[3]

It would seem that adverse interactions between oral **budesonide** or **prednisone** and omeprazole are unlikely, but the isolated case should be borne in mind in the event of an unexpected response to treatment.

1. Cavanaugh JH, Karol MD. Lack of pharmacokinetic interaction after administration of lansoprazole or omeprazole with prednisone. *J Clin Pharmacol* (1996) 36, 1064–71.
2. Joly P, Chosidow O, Laurent-Puig P, Delchier J-C, Roujeau J-C, Revuz J. Possible interaction prednisone-oméprazole dans la pemphigoïde bulleuse. *Gastroenterol Clin Biol* (1990) 14, 682–3.
3. Edsbäcker S, Larsson P, Bergstrand M. Pharmacokinetics of budesonide controlled-release capsules when taken with omeprazole. *Aliment Pharmacol Ther* (2003) 17, 403–8.

Corticosteroids + Rifampicin (Rifampin)

The effects of systemic cortisone, dexamethasone, fludrocortisone, hydrocortisone, methylprednisolone, prednisone and prednisolone can be markedly reduced by rifampicin, but aldosterone appears not to be affected. Rifabutin and rifapentine are predicted to interact similarly, all be it to a lesser extent.

Clinical evidence

(a) Aldosterone

In 7 patients with Addison's disease due to tuberculosis, there were no changes in the pharmacokinetics of intravenous aldosterone after they were also given rifampicin 600 mg daily for 6 days.[1]

(b) Cortisone and Fludrocortisone

A patient with Addison's disease taking cortisone and fludrocortisone had typical signs of corticosteroid overdosage when the rifampicin he was taking was replaced by ethambutol,[2] suggesting that the rifampicin had reduced the levels of these corticosteroids. Another Addisonian patient needed an increase in her dosage of cortisone from 37.5 mg daily to 50 mg daily, and fludrocortisone 100 micrograms daily, when rifampicin 450 mg daily was started.[3] A patient had an Addisonian crisis when rifampicin was added to treatment with **dexamethasone** and fludrocortisone.[4]

(c) Dexamethasone

Rifampicin markedly increases the clearance of dexamethasone.[5,6] A patient had an Addisonian crisis when rifampicin was added to treatment with dexamethasone and **fludrocortisone**.[4]

(d) Hydrocortisone

A metabolic study in an Addisonian patient taking hydrocortisone found that rifampicin shortened its half-life and reduced its AUC.[7]

(e) Other corticosteroids

A child with nephrotic syndrome taking **prednisolone**, and accidentally given a BCG vaccine, was given rifampicin and isoniazid to prevent possible dissemination of the vaccine. When the nephrotic condition did not respond, the prednisolone dosage was raised from 2 to 3 mg/kg daily without any evidence of corticosteroid overdosage. Later when the rifampicin and isoniazid were withdrawn, remission of the nephrotic condition was achieved with the original dosage of prednisolone.[8] A number of other reports describe a reduction in the response to **prednisone**, **prednisolone** or **methylprednisolone** in patients given rifampicin.[4,9-17] Pharmacokinetic studies in patients have shown that the AUC of **prednisolone** is reduced by about 60% by rifampicin, and its half-life is decreased by 40% to 60%.[11,15,18]

Mechanism

Rifampicin is a potent liver enzyme inducer, which increases the metabolism of the corticosteroids by the liver,[10] thereby decreasing their levels and reducing their effects.

Importance and management

The interactions between the corticosteroids and rifampicin are established, well documented and clinically important. The need to increase the dosages of cortisone, dexamethasone, fludrocortisone, hydrocortisone, methylprednisolone, prednisolone and prednisone should be expected if rifampicin is given. It has been suggested that as an initial adjustment the dosage of prednisolone should be increased two- to threefold, and reduced proportionately if the rifampicin is withdrawn.[10,11,18,19] In the case of prednisolone the interaction develops maximally by 14 days and disappears about 14 days after withdrawal of the rifampicin.[20]

There seems to be no direct information about corticosteroids other than those mentioned here, but be alert for them to be similarly affected. Systemic corticosteroids are usually considered as contraindicated, or only to be used with great care, in patients with active or quiescent tuberculosis.

It is not clear whether any of the topically applied corticosteroids will interact with rifampicin, but any clinically significant interaction would be expected to be very rare.

There does not seem to be any information regarding the other rifamycins, **rifabutin** (a weak enzyme inducer) and **rifapentine** (a moderate enzyme inducer). However, the UK manufacturers and the CSM in the UK warn that rifabutin may possibly reduce the effects of a number of drugs,[21,22] including corticosteroids,[21] and therefore some caution is probably prudent.

1. Schulte HM, Mönig H, Benker G, Pagel H, Reinwein D, Ohnhaus EE. Pharmacokinetics of aldosterone in patients with Addison's disease: effect of rifampicin treatment on glucocorticoid and mineralocorticoid metabolism. *Clin Endocrinol (Oxf)* (1987) 27, 655–62.
2. Edwards OM, Courtenay-Evans RJ, Galley JM, Hunter J, Tait AD. Changes in cortisol metabolism following rifampicin therapy. *Lancet* (1974) ii, 549–51.
3. Maisey DN, Brown RC, Day JL. Rifampicin and cortisone replacement therapy. *Lancet* (1974) ii, 896–7.
4. Kyriazopoulou V, Parparousi O, Vagenakis AG. Rifampicin-induced adrenal crisis in Addisonian patients receiving corticosteroid replacement therapy. *J Clin Endocrinol Metab* (1984) 59, 1204–6.
5. Ediger SK, Isley WL. Rifampicin-induced adrenal insufficiency in the acquired immunodeficiency syndrome: difficulties in diagnosis and treatment. *Postgrad Med J* (1988) 64, 405–6.
6. Kawai S. A comparative study of the accelerated metabolism of cortisol, prednisolone and dexamethasone in patients under rifampicin therapy. *Nippon Naibunpi Gakkai Zasshi* (1985) 61, 145–61.
7. Wang YH, Shi YF, Xiang HD. Effect of rifampin on the metabolism of glucocorticoids in Addison's disease. *Zhonghua Nei Ke Za Zhi* (1990) 29, 108–11,127.
8. Hendrickse W, McKiernan J, Pickup M, Lowe J. Rifampicin-induced non-responsiveness to corticosteroid treatment in nephrotic syndrome. *BMJ* (1979) i, 306.
9. van Marle W, Woods KL, Beeley L. Concurrent steroid and rifampicin therapy. *BMJ* (1979) i, 1020.
10. Buffington GA, Dominguez JH, Piering WF, Hebert LA, Kauffman HM, Lemann J. Interaction of rifampin and glucocorticoids. Adverse effect on renal allograft function. *JAMA* (1976) 236, 1958–60.
11. McAllister WAC, Thompson PJ, Al-Habet SM, Rogers HJ. Rifampicin reduces effectiveness and bioavailability of prednisolone. *BMJ* (1983) 286, 923–5.
12. Powell-Jackson PR, Gray BJ, Heaton RW, Costello JF, Williams R, English J. Adverse effect of rifampicin administration on steroid-dependent asthma. *Am Rev Respir Dis* (1983) 128, 307–10.
13. Bitaudeau Ph, Clément S, Chartier JPh, Papapietro PM, Bonnafoux A, Arnaud M, Trèves R, Desproges-Gotteron R. Interaction rifampicine-prednisolone. A propos de deux cas au cours d'une maladie de Horton. *Rev Rhum Mal Osteoartic* (1989) 56, 87–8.
14. Kawai S, Ichikawa Y. Drug interactions between glucocorticoids and other drugs. *Nippon Rinsho* (1994) 52, 773–8.
15. Carrie F, Roblot P, Bouquet S, Delon A, Roblot F, Becq-Giraudon B. Rifampin-induced nonresponsiveness of giant cell arteritis to prednisone treatment. *Arch Intern Med* (1994) 154, 1521–4.
16. Verma M, Singh T, Chhatwal J, Saini V, Pawar B. Rifampicin induced steroid unresponsiveness in nephrotic syndrome. *Indian Pediatr* (1994) 31, 1437.
17. Lin FL. Rifampin-induced deterioration in steroid-dependent asthma. *J Allergy Clin Immunol* (1996) 98, 1125.
18. Bergrem H, Refvem OK. Altered prednisolone pharmacokinetics in patients treated with rifampicin. *Acta Med Scand* (1983) 213, 339–43.
19. Löfdahl C-G, Mellstrand T, Svedmyr N, Wåhlén P. Increased metabolism of prednisolone and rifampicin after rifampicin treatment. *Am Rev Respir Dis* (1984) 129, A201.
20. Lee KH, Shin JG, Chong WS, Kim S, Lee JS, Jang IJ, Shin SG. Time course of the changes in prednisolone pharmacokinetics after co-administration or discontinuation of rifampin. *Eur J Clin Pharmacol* (1993) 45, 287–89.
21. Mycobutin (Rifabutin). Pfizer Ltd. UK Summary of product characteristics, December 2013.
22. Committee on the Safety of Medicines/Medicines Control Agency. Revised indication and drug interactions of rifabutin. *Current Problems* (1997) 23, 14.

Corticosteroids + Somatropin

Corticosteroid doses may possibly require increasing if somatropin is also given. Corticosteroid replacement therapy may attenuate the growth promoting effects of somatropin.

Clinical evidence, mechanism, importance and management

One manufacturer of somatropin says that it inhibits 11β-hydroxysteroid dehydrogenase type 1 (11βHSD-1) in adipose and hepatic tissue and may affect the metabolism of cortisol and cortisone.[1] Limited *in vitro*[2] and *in vivo*[3] data also indicate that somatropin may be an inducer of cytochrome P450 isoenzymes and that it may increase the clearance of drugs that are metabolised by CYP3A4 enzymes, including a number of corticosteroids.[1-4] The clinical significance of this is unknown, but careful monitoring is advisable. Somatropin has been reported to induce a modest reduction of serum cortisol levels in growth hormone deficient patients receiving adrenal substitution treatment.[2] Therefore, patients receiving corticosteroid replacement therapy may require an increase in their maintenance or stress doses of corticosteroid if they are given somatropin;[1,2] this may be especially true for patients taking **cortisone acetate** and **prednisone** since conversion of these drugs to their biologically active metabolites is dependent on the activity of the 11βHSD-1 enzyme.[1]

In addition, glucocorticoid therapy may attenuate the growth promoting effects of somatropin.[1,2,4] Therefore, glucocorticoid replacement therapy should be carefully adjusted in patients with growth hormone and glucocorticoid deficiency to avoid both hypoadrenalism and an inhibitory effect on growth.[1]

1. Omnitrope (Somatropin). Sandoz Inc. US Prescribing information, March 2009.
2. Saizen (Somatropin). Merck Serono. UK Summary of product characteristics, April 2009.
3. Genotropin (Somatropin). Pharmacia Ltd. UK Summary of product characteristics, March 2009.
4. Zomacton (Somatropin). Ferring Pharmaceuticals Ltd. UK Summary of product characteristics, November 2008.

Corticosteroids + St John's wort (*Hypericum perforatum*)

St John's wort does not appear to affect the pharmacokinetics of prednisone or its metabolite, prednisolone.

Clinical evidence

In a pharmacokinetic study, 8 healthy subjects were given a single 20-mg oral dose of **prednisone** before, and at the end, of a 28-day course of St John's wort 300 mg three times daily. The pharmacokinetics of **prednisone**, and its metabolite **prednisolone**, were not significantly affected by St John's wort. The St John's wort extract was standardised to contain hypericin 0.3% and a minimum of 4% hyperforin.[1]

Mechanism

It was thought that St John's wort, a known inducer of the cytochrome P450 isoenzyme CYP3A4, would increase the metabolism of prednisone and prednisolone and reduce their levels. While prednisone and prednisolone are substrates of CYP3A4, it is not a major metabolic pathway as they have been shown to be only modestly affected by potent CYP3A4 inhibitors in healthy subjects.

Importance and management

St John's wort does not appear to induce the metabolism of a single dose of prednisone, or its metabolite prednisolone, in healthy subjects; however, further study is needed to clarify significance of this in patients receiving long-term prednisone.

1. Bell EC, Ravis WR, Chan HM, Lin Y-J. Lack of pharmacokinetic interaction between St. John's wort and prednisone. *Ann Pharmacother* (2007) 41, 1819–24.

Corticosteroids + Sucralfate

Sucralfate does not appear to affect the pharmacokinetics of prednisone to a clinically relevant extent.

Clinical evidence, mechanism, importance and management

In 12 healthy subjects, sucralfate 1 g every 6 hours had no significant effect on the pharmacokinetics of a single 20-mg dose of **prednisone**; however, the peak plasma levels were delayed by about 45 minutes when the drugs were given at the same time, but not when the sucralfate was given 2 hours after the **prednisone**.[1] No particular precautions are likely to be needed in patients given both drugs. Information about other corticosteroids is lacking.

1. Gambertoglio JG, Romac DR, Yong C-L, Birnbaum J, Lizak P, Amend WJC. Lack of effect of sucralfate on prednisone bioavailability. *Am J Gastroenterol* (1987) 82, 42–5.

Corticosteroids + Tobacco

The pharmacokinetics of dexamethasone, prednisone and prednisolone do not appear to be affected by smoking. Cigarette smoking in asthma is associated with a reduced sensitivity to corticosteroids.

Clinical evidence, mechanism, importance and management

Studies have shown that cigarette smoking impairs the efficacy of inhaled corticosteroids,[1-4] including **beclometasone**,[1,2] **budesonide**[3] and **fluticasone**.[4] One study showed that smokers with mild persistent asthma were insensitive to the therapeutic effect of low-doses of inhaled corticosteroids, although some benefit was observed with high-doses of inhaled corticosteroids.[2] However, another study found that neither lung function nor eosinophil markers changed in smokers, even when high doses of inhaled corticosteroids were given.[3]

Active smoking also impairs the therapeutic response to short-term oral corticosteroids in chronic asthma. In a study in asthmatic patients, **prednisolone** 40 mg daily for 14 days significantly improved FEV_1 in patients who had never smoked, but had no effect on smokers, when compared with placebo.[5] Ex-smokers who had stopped smoking for more than one year showed a trend towards improvement in asthma control after **prednisolone** treatment.[5] However, in another study there was no change in airway corticosteroid responses in patients who had only stopped smoking for 6 weeks, although baseline lung function had improved.[6]

In addition, the insensitivity to corticosteroids in smokers with asthma appears to affect tissue sites other than the airways; the cutaneous vasoconstrictor response to topical **beclometasone** is reduced in smokers with asthma, when compared with patients with asthma who have never smoked.[7] In a study in asthmatic patients who smoked, the vasoconstrictor response to topical **beclometasone** improved in those who had stopped smoking for 6 weeks, compared with those who continued to smoke.[6]

A study involving 18 healthy subjects, half of whom were smokers, found that smoking had no overall effect on the pharmacokinetics of oral or intravenous **dexamethasone**, oral **prednisone**, or intravenous **prednisolone**.[8]

Cigarette smoking is an important factor associated with corticosteroid resistance in asthmatics. The mechanism behind the reduced sensitivity to corticosteroids in smokers is not fully understood, but may possibly be due to increased oxidative stress resulting in reduced histone deacetylase activity, airway inflammation, and/or impaired glucocorticoid receptor function. There is some evidence that smoking cessation may at least partially restore corticosteroid responsiveness.[9-11] These findings reinforce the need for those with airways disease, including asthma, to give up smoking tobacco.

1. Lazarus SC, Chinchilli VM, Rollings NJ, Boushey HA, Cherniack R, Craig TJ, Deykin A, DiMango E, Fish JE, Ford JG, Israel E, Kiley J, Kraft M, Lemanske RF, Leone FT, Martin RJ, Pesola GR, Peters SP, Sorkness CA, Szefler SJ, Wechsler ME, Fahy JV, for the National Heart, Lung, and Blood Institute's Asthma Clinical Research Network. Smoking affects response to inhaled corticosteroids or leukotriene receptor antagonists in asthma. *Am J Respir Crit Care Med* (2007) 175, 783–90.
2. Tomlinson JEM, McMahon AD, Chaudhuri R, Thompson JM, Wood SF, Thomson NC. Efficacy of low and high dose inhaled corticosteroid in smokers versus non-smokers with mild asthma. *Thorax* (2005) 60, 282–7.
3. Pedersen B, Dahl R, Karlström R, Peterson CGB, Venge P. Eosinophil and neutrophil activity in asthma in a one-year trial with inhaled budesonide. The impact of smoking. *Am J Respir Crit Care Med* (1996) 153, 1519–29.
4. Chalmers GW, Macleod KJ, Little SA, Thomson LJ, McSharry CP, Thomson NC. Influence of cigarette smoking on inhaled corticosteroid treatment in mild asthma. *Thorax* (2002) 57, 226–30.
5. Chaudhuri R, Livingston E, McMahon AD, Thomson L, Borland W, Thomson NC. Cigarette smoking impairs the therapeutic response to oral corticosteroids in chronic asthma. *Am J Respir Crit Care Med* (2003) 168, 1308–11.
6. Chaudhuri R, Livingston E, McMahon AD, Lafferty J, Fraser I, Spears M, McSharry CP, Thomson NC. Effects of smoking cessation on lung function and airway inflammation in smokers with asthma. *Am J Respir Crit Care Med* (2006) 174, 127–33.
7. Livingston E, Chaudhuri R, McMahon AD, Fraser I, McSharry CP, Thomson NC. Systemic sensitivity to corticosteroids in smokers with asthma. *Eur Respir J* (2007) 29, 64–70.
8. Rose JQ, Yurchak AM, Meikle AW, Jusko WJ. Effect of smoking on prednisone, prednisolone, and dexamethasone pharmacokinetics. *J Pharmacokinet Biopharm* (1981) 9, 1–14.
9. Livingston E, Thomson NC, Chalmers GW. Impact of smoking on asthma therapy: a critical review of clinical evidence. *Drugs* (2005) 65, 1521–36.
10. Thomson NC, Chaudhuri R. Asthma in smokers: challenges and opportunities. *Curr Opin Pulm Med* (2009) 15, 39–45.
11. Ahmad T, Barnes PJ, Adcock IM. Overcoming steroid insensitivity in smoking asthmatics. *Curr Opin Investig Drugs* (2008) 9, 470–7.

Corticosteroids + Vaccines

Patients who are immunised with live vaccines while receiving immunosuppressive doses of corticosteroids may develop generalised, possibly life-threatening, infections. Corticosteroids may attenuate the response to vaccination.

Clinical evidence, mechanism, importance and management

The use of corticosteroids can reduce the number of circulating lymphocytes and suppress the normal immune response, so that concurrent immunisation with live vaccines can lead to generalised infection. It has been suggested that **prednisone** in doses of greater than 10 to 15 mg daily will suppress the immune response, whereas doses of up to 40 to 60 mg on alternate days probably will not,[1] although this is debated.

A patient with lymphosarcoma and hypogammaglobulinaemia, taking **prednisone** 15 mg daily, developed a generalised vaccinial infection when she was given **smallpox vaccine**.[2] A fatal vaccinial infection developed following **smallpox vaccination** in another patient taking **cortisone**.[3] This type of problem can be controlled with immunoglobulin to give cover against a general infection while immunity develops, and this has been successfully used in steroid-dependent patients needing **smallpox vaccination**.[4]

The principles applied to **smallpox** may be generally applicable to other live attenuated vaccines (e.g. **measles**, **mumps**, **rubella**, **poliomyelitis**, **BCG**), but no studies seem to have been done to establish what is safe.[1]

It is generally accepted that patients taking immunosuppressants should not be given live vaccines. Problems with topical or inhaled steroids in normal dosages seem unlikely because the amounts absorbed are relatively small.[1] However, this needs confirmation. The UK Department of Health contraindicates the use of live vaccines in all patients receiving systemic high-dose steroids, until at least 3 months after treatment has been stopped.[5] This includes children who receive **prednisolone**, orally or rectally, at a daily dose (or its equivalent) of 2 mg/kg per day for at least one week, or 1 mg/kg per day for one month. For adults, immunosuppression should be considered in those who receive at least 40 mg of **prednisolone** per day for more than one week.

Note that immunosuppression caused by corticosteroids may also attenuate the response to other vaccines. In one study patients given a higher dose of **prednisolone** per kg had a reduced antibody response to **influenza vaccine**, and those given a daily dose had a reduced response, when compared with those given an alternate day schedule.[6] Consider also 'Immunosuppressants + Vaccines', p.1264.

1. Shapiro L. Questions and Answers. Live virus vaccine and corticosteroid therapy: answered by Fauci AS, Bellanti JA, Polk IJ, Cherry JD. *JAMA* (1981) 246, 2075–6.
2. Rosenbaum EH, Cohen RA, Glatstein HR. Vaccination of a patient receiving immunosuppressive therapy for lymphosarcoma. *JAMA* (1966) 198, 737–40.
3. Olansky S, Smith JG, Hansen-Pruss OCE. Fatal vaccinia associated with cortisone therapy. *JAMA* (1956) 162, 887–8.
4. Joseph MR. Vaccination of patients on steroid therapy. *Med J Aust* (1974) 2, 181.
5. Department of Health. Immunisation Against Infectious Disease (updated 11th September 2013): "The Green Book". Available at: https://www.gov.uk/government/publications/green-book-the-complete-current-edition (accessed 25/09/13).
6. Mack DR, Chartrand SA, Ruby EI, Antonson DL, Shaw BW, Heffron TG. Influenza vaccination following liver transplantation in children. *Liver Transpl Surg* (1996) 2, 431–7.

Corticosteroids + Zileuton

No clinically relevant pharmacokinetic interaction occurs between prednisone and zileuton.

Clinical evidence, mechanism, importance and management

In a randomised, crossover study, 16 healthy subjects were given zileuton 600 mg every 6 hours for a week, with either a 40-mg dose of **prednisone** or placebo on day 6. The pharmacokinetics of both drugs were slightly altered but this was not considered to be clinically relevant. The half-life of **prednisolone** (derived from **prednisone**) increased from 2.8 to 2.9 hours, while the zileuton AUC and the time to achieve maximum serum levels were decreased by 13% and 26%, respectively. It was concluded that concurrent use carries a minimal risk of a clinically important pharmacokinetic interaction.[1] No special precautions would appear to be needed if both drugs are given.

1. Awni WM, Cavanaugh JH, Tzeng T-B, Witt G, Granneman GR, Dubé LM. Pharmacokinetic interactions between zileuton and prednisone. *Clin Pharmacokinet* (1995) 29 (Suppl 2), 105–111.

Corticosteroids; Dexamethasone + Asparaginase

Recent treatment with asparaginase may reduce dexamethasone clearance.

Clinical evidence, mechanism, importance and management

A study in 214 children with acute lymphoblastic leukaemia found that there was considerable inter- and intrapatient variability in the pharmacokinetics of dexamethasone 8 mg/m^2 daily on days 1 and 8 of an 8-day re-induction course of dexamethasone: more than a tenfold variability in systemic exposure to the drug was found. Much of the variability in dexamethasone clearance was accounted for by variability in serum albumin concentrations, which in turn were affected by the intensity of previous asparaginase treatment. Hypoalbuminaemia, a biomarker of asparaginase activity, was associated with a low dexamethasone apparent clearance, whilst higher apparent clearance of dexamethasone was associated with a greater serum albumin concentration and also with younger children (who tended to be treated in the low-risk group).[1] The authors of the report suggest that this interaction may be, at least in part, responsible for the variability in response to dexamethasone in this patient group. More study is needed.

1. Yang L, Panetta JC, Cai X, Yang W, Pei D, Cheng C, Kornegay N, Pui C-H, Relling MV. Asparaginase may influence dexamethasone pharmacokinetics in acute lymphoblastic leukemia. *J Clin Oncol* (2008) 26, 1932–9.

Corticosteroids; Dexamethasone + Caffeine

The results of the dexamethasone suppression test can be falsified by the acute ingestion of caffeine but long-term caffeine use does not appear to have an effect.

Clinical evidence, mechanism, importance and management

In a placebo-controlled study, 22 healthy subjects and 6 depressed patients were given a single 480-mg dose of caffeine at 2 pm, following a single 1-mg dose of dexamethasone given at 11 pm the previous evening. Caffeine significantly increased the cortisol levels following the dexamethasone dose: cortisol levels taken at 4 pm were about 146 nanomol/L with caffeine, compared with about 64 nanomol/L with placebo.[1] Thus the equivalent of about 4 to 5 cups of coffee may effectively falsify the results of the dexamethasone suppression test. However, in a study in 121 patients with depression, there was no correlation between long-term low to high intake of caffeine (6 mg to 2.3 g daily) and cortisol levels at 8 am, 4 pm or 11 pm on the day after a 1-mg dose of dexamethasone was given (at 11 pm the previous evening). It was suggested that long-term caffeine intake produces tolerance to the effects of acute caffeine on the hypothalamic-pituitary adrenal (HPA) axis.[2]

1. Uhde TW, Bierer LM, Post RM. Caffeine-induced escape from dexamethasone suppression. *Arch Gen Psychiatry* (1985) 42, 737–8.
2. Lee MA, Flegel P, Cameron OG, Greden JF. Chronic caffeine consumption and the dexamethasone suppression test in depression. *Psychiatry Res* (1988) 24, 61–5.

Corticosteroids; Dexamethasone + Valspodar

Dexamethasone does not affect the pharmacokinetics of valspodar. Valspodar modestly increases the AUC of dexamethasone.

Clinical evidence, mechanism, importance and management

In a crossover study, healthy fasting subjects were given single doses of dexamethasone 8 mg and valspodar 400 mg either alone or together. Dexamethasone had no effect on the pharmacokinetics of valspodar. The AUC of dexamethasone was increased by 24% by valspodar. This change is modest and therefore dosage alterations are probably not required if concurrent use is of a short duration.[1]

1. Kovarik JM, Purba HS, Pongowski M, Gerbeau C, Humbert H, Mueller EA. Pharmacokinetics of dexamethasone and valspodar, a P-glycoprotein (*mdr1*) modulator: implications for coadministration. *Pharmacotherapy* (1998) 18, 1230–6.

Corticosteroids; Fluticasone + Azoles; Fluconazole

Cushing's syndrome and adrenal insufficiency have been reported in two patients receiving inhaled fluticasone (with intranasal fluticasone in one) after taking fluconazole.

Clinical evidence

A case report describes a 9-year-old patient with cystic fibrosis receiving inhaled fluticasone 880 micrograms daily, who developed intense thirst and frequent urination, with a blood glucose level greater than 600 mg/dL, just 3 days after starting a

5-day course of fluconazole 100 mg daily. The child was subsequently diagnosed with cystic fibrosis-related diabetes, which was managed with insulin. During the weeks following this diagnosis, the child gained weight in a central distribution, bruised easily, and developed a round face, hirsutism, and violet-coloured striae. The child's serum cortisol concentration was found to be less than 0.2 micrograms/dL, and she was diagnosed with Cushing's syndrome and adrenal insufficiency. The fluticasone was stopped and a 9-week prednisone replacement course was started, during which the dose of insulin was gradually reduced and then stopped. Two weeks after completion of the prednisone course, her cortisol concentration was 6.4 micrograms/dL and she responded well to a cortisol stimulation test.[1]

An HIV-positive patient taking stable doses of atazanavir boosted with ritonavir and efavirenz together with inhaled fluticasone 250 micrograms twice daily for chronic bronchitis, developed dyspnoea, wheezing, and nasal congestion. His fluticasone dose was increased to 500 micrograms twice daily and he started to use intranasal fluticasone 0.05% [dose not stated]. Two months later he developed candidiasis and was given oral fluconazole 400 mg daily for 7 days and advised to stop the fluticasone. After 2 days he developed Cushing's syndrome with secondary adrenal insufficiency associated with a low adrenocorticotrophic hormone (ACTH) concentration of 5 picograms/mL.[2]

Mechanism

It seems probable that fluconazole inhibits the metabolism of fluticasone by CYP3A4 in the liver leading to an increase in the concentrations and effects of fluticasone. Note that fluconazole is a moderate inhibitor of CYP3A4, and this inhibition generally occurs with doses greater than 200 mg daily. However, the authors of the second case suggest that inhibition of adrenal steroidogenesis by fluconazole, rather than CYP3A4 inhibition, contributed to the rapid onset of Cushing's syndrome in this patient and the severity of the symptoms seen.[2]

Importance and management

The reports describing an interaction between fluconazole and inhaled fluticasone are isolated and their general importance is unclear, although it is in line with the known CYP3A4-inhibitory effects of fluconazole, particularly at high doses. However, the authors of the first case report note that this patient had impaired liver function which might have contributed to the effects seen by reducing fluticasone metabolism.[1] Furthermore, the patient in the second case was taking atazanavir boosted with ritonavir, which is also known to inhibit fluticasone metabolism. This might mean that the effect of fluconazole on fluticasone is limited to patients with other factors that influence systemic corticosteroid concentrations. Further study regarding the mechanism and general clinical relevance of this interaction is needed. Until more is known, it would seem prudent to bear this interaction in mind in cases of otherwise unexplained corticosteroid adverse effects in patients also given fluconazole.

The effects of fluconazole on other corticosteroids has not been documented, but note that most of them are also metabolised, in part, by CYP3A4 and might be expected to be similarly affected, although, as with fluticasone, perhaps only if other factors are also present.

1. Hoover WC, Britton LJ, Gardner J, Jackson T, Gutierrez H. Rapid onset of iatrogenic adrenal insufficiency in a patient with cystic fibrosis-related liver disease treated with inhaled corticosteroids and a moderate CYP3A4 inhibitor. *Ann Pharmacother* (2011) 45, e38.
2. St Clair K, Maguire JD. Role of fluconazole in a case of rapid onset ritonavir and inhaled fluticasone-associated secondary adrenal insufficiency. *Int J STD AIDS* (2012) 23, 371.

Etanercept + Methotrexate

Methotrexate does not appear to alter the pharmacokinetics of etanercept.

Clinical evidence, mechanism, importance and management

A double-blind study in 98 patients with rheumatoid arthritis receiving subcutaneous etanercept 25 mg twice weekly, or etanercept with oral methotrexate (median weekly dose of 20 mg) found that the pharmacokinetics of etanercept were not altered by methotrexate.[1] No particular precautions or dosage adjustments appear to be necessary on concurrent use.

1. Zhou H, Mayer PR, Wajdula J, Fatenejad S. Unaltered etanercept pharmacokinetics with concurrent methotrexate in patients with rheumatoid arthritis. *J Clin Pharmacol* (2004) 44, 1235–43.

Etanercept + Miscellaneous

A higher incidence of malignancies has been reported in patients with Wegener's granulomatosis when given both cyclophosphamide and etanercept. A reduced neutrophil count may occur in patients taking etanercept with sulfasalazine. No interactions have been found when etanercept was given with salicylates other than sulfasalazine, corticosteroids, or NSAIDs.

Clinical evidence, mechanism, importance and management

(a) Cyclophosphamide

The US manufacturer says that etanercept is not recommended in patients receiving cyclophosphamide. They state that in a study in patients with Wegener's granulomatosis, the addition of etanercept to standard treatment, including cyclophosphamide, was associated with a higher incidence of non-cutaneous solid malignancies.[1]

(b) Sulfasalazine

A study in patients taking sulfasalazine found that when etanercept was also given, patients had a decrease in neutrophil counts, when compared to other groups of patients receiving either drug alone. The clinical significance of this finding is not known.[1,2]

(c) Other drugs

The UK manufacturer notes that no interactions have been found when etanercept was given with **corticosteroids**, **salicylates** (except *sulfasalazine*, see above), **NSAIDs** or other analgesics.[2]

1. Enbrel (Etanercept). Amgen Inc. & Wyeth Pharmaceuticals. US Prescribing information, April 2009.
2. Enbrel (Etanercept). Wyeth Pharmaceuticals. UK Summary of product characteristics, October 2013.

Everolimus + Calcium-channel blockers

Increased concentrations of both everolimus and verapamil can occur on concurrent use. Diltiazem increased everolimus concentrations in lung transplant patients, but there was no clear evidence of an interaction in a population model. In this model, there was also no evidence of an interaction between everolimus and amlodipine, isradipine, or nifedipine.

Clinical evidence

A study in 16 healthy subjects given a single 2-mg dose of everolimus before and on day 2 of a 6-day course of **verapamil** 80 mg three times daily found that verapamil increased the AUC and maximum blood concentration of everolimus 3.5-fold and 2.3-fold, respectively. Everolimus also increased the plasma concentration of verapamil 2.3-fold.[1] In another study in 65 lung transplant patients, 30 of whom were also taking **diltiazem**, the dose-corrected everolimus minimum concentration was almost 2-fold higher than in 35 patients not taking diltiazem.[2]

In a pharmacokinetic modelling study, the difference in everolimus clearance in 5 patients taking **verapamil** was not statistically significant. In addition, there was no clear evidence of an effect on everolimus clearance for **diltiazem** in 22 patients or the dihydropyridines, **amlodipine**, **isradipine**, or **nifedipine**, in 267 patients.[3] These suggested findings require confirmation.

Mechanism

Verapamil is an inhibitor of CYP3A4, and also inhibits P-glycoprotein, by which everolimus is metabolised and transported, respectively. Therefore concurrent use reduces its metabolism, and increases its uptake, resulting in increased everolimus exposure. Diltiazem is also an inhibitor of CYP3A4 and so might be expected to interact similarly, although data are conflicting. Note also, that diltiazem does not inhibit P-glycoprotein. Further study is needed.

It is not known exactly why verapamil concentrations are increased.

Importance and management

Evidence for an interaction between everolimus and calcium-channel blockers is limited, but suggests that verapamil and diltiazem might increase everolimus concentrations. If either of these calcium-channel blockers are given with everolimus, it would seem prudent to monitor everolimus blood concentrations as well as monitoring for calcium-channel blocker adverse effects (such as hypotension, flushing, and oedema), and to adjust the doses of both drugs as needed. One UK manufacturer of everolimus licensed for use in various malignancies, recommends an everolimus dose reduction to 5 or 2.5 mg daily on concurrent use with moderate CYP3A4 inhibitors, such as verapamil or diltiazem. However, they state that this dose decrease is a prediction and therefore good monitoring is still required.[4] The US manufacturer of a similarly licensed product advises an everolimus dose reduction to 2.5 mg daily, with an increase to 5 mg daily considered based on tolerability.[5] The UK and US manufacturers of everolimus products licensed for astrocytoma, recommend a 50% dose reduction on the concurrent use of verapamil or diltiazem, with monitoring of minimum concentrations about every 2 weeks and further advise that these should be used to guide subsequent dosing.[5,6] One US manufacturer of everolimus licensed for use in organ transplant, advises monitoring everolimus plasma concentrations and adjusting the dose accordingly if given concurrently with verapamil, and predicts that diltiazem might also increase everolimus concentrations.[7]

One Australian manufacturer[8] suggests that **nicardipine** might increase everolimus concentrations, but note that nicardipine is not an established CYP3A4 inhibitor.

Amlodipine, isradipine, and nifedipine do not appear to interact with everolimus, although this ideally needs confirmation in formal pharmacokinetic studies.

1. Kovarik JM, Beyer D, Bizot MN, Jiang Q, Allison MJ, Schmouder RL. Pharmacokinetic interaction between verapamil and everolimus. *Br J Clin Pharmacol* (2005) 60, 434–7.
2. Schoeppler KE, Aquilante CL, Kiser TH, Fish DN, Zamora MR. The impact of genetic polymorphisms, diltiazem, and demographic variables on everolimus trough concentrations in lung transplant recipients. *Clin Transplant* (2014) 28, 590–7.
3. Kovarik JM, Hsu C-H, McMahon L, Berthier S, Rordorf C. Population pharmacokinetics of everolimus in de novo renal transplant patients: impact of ethnicity and comedications. *Clin Pharmacol Ther* (2001) 70, 247–54.
4. Afinitor (Everolimus). Novartis Pharmaceuticals UK Ltd. UK Summary of product characteristics, December 2014.
5. Afinitor (Everolimus). Novartis. US Prescribing information, January 2015.
6. Votubia (Everolimus). Novartis Pharmaceuticals UK Ltd. UK Summary of product characteristics, July 2014.
7. Zortress (Everolimus). Novartis. US Prescribing information, February 2013.
8. Certican (Everolimus). Novartis Pharmaceuticals Australia Pty Ltd. Australian product information, August 2013.

Everolimus + Ciclosporin

Ciclosporin weakly to moderately increases the exposure to everolimus. Although everolimus appears to have no clinically relevant effects on ciclosporin concentrations, concurrent use might potentiate ciclosporin-induced renal toxicity.

Clinical evidence

(a) Effect on ciclosporin

In a phase I pharmacokinetic study in 7 patients with kidney transplants stabilised on ciclosporin, there was no change in ciclosporin pharmacokinetics when they were given a single dose of everolimus, ranging from 0.25 to 15 mg.[1] Similarly, in a placebo-controlled study in 54 kidney transplant patients taking ciclosporin (93% also taking prednisone), everolimus 0.75 to 10 mg daily in single or divided doses had no clinically relevant effect on ciclosporin concentrations in 44 patients, when compared with the 10 patients given placebo. However, because of wide interpatient variability, this study could not entirely rule out an interaction.[2] Another study in 101 kidney transplant patients taking ciclosporin and prednisone with everolimus 0.5 to 2 mg twice daily for one year also found no evidence that everolimus affected ciclosporin pharmacokinetics.[3] However, in a randomised study in patients, those given everolimus 0.75 or 1.5 mg daily needed a 15% or 20% lower dose of ciclosporin, respectively, to achieve the same ciclosporin minimum plasma concentration as those given azathioprine with ciclosporin.[4]

(b) Effect on everolimus

In a crossover study, 24 healthy subjects were given a single 2-mg dose of everolimus alone and with single doses of ciclosporin (either *Neoral* (microemulsion) 175 mg or *Sandimmun* (corn oil suspension) 300 mg). *Neoral* increased the maximum blood concentration and AUC of everolimus by 82% and 2.7-fold, respectively. *Sandimmun* did not affect the maximum blood concentration of everolimus but increased its AUC by 74%.[5] Similarly, in a randomised study in 56 patients with kidney transplants, the addition of ciclosporin increased the minimum plasma concentration of everolimus 2.9-fold. However, further analysis in 10 of these patients found there was wide inter-patient variability, ranging from no increase to a 5.6-fold increase in the minimum plasma concentration.[6]

In a pharmacokinetic study in 6 heart transplant recipients taking everolimus, minimum concentrations of everolimus were almost halved from 4.2 to 2.3 micrograms/L when ciclosporin was stopped and tacrolimus was started. The AUC of everolimus was also decreased by about 50% and its maximum concentration was decreased by 35%.[7]

Mechanism

Not fully understood. Ciclosporin inhibits P-glycoprotein of which everolimus is a substrate, which might at least in part explain the increased everolimus exposure. Some have also suggested a role for CYP3A4, although this is not established.

Importance and management

Evidence for a pharmacokinetic interaction between everolimus and ciclosporin appears to be limited; however, the weak to moderate increases in everolimus concentrations seen are likely to be clinically relevant. Therefore, it would be prudent to monitor everolimus on the concurrent use of these drugs, and adjust the everolimus dose as necessary. One UK manufacturer of everolimus licensed for use in various malignancies, recommends that, in patients also taking ciclosporin, an everolimus dose reduction to 5 or 2.5 mg daily should be considered. However, they state that this dose decrease is a prediction and therefore good monitoring is still required.[8] The UK manufacturer of everolimus licensed for astrocytoma, recommends a 50% dose reduction on the concurrent use of ciclosporin, with monitoring of minimum concentrations about every 2 weeks and further advise that these should be used to guide subsequent dosing.[9]

It would appear that, in general, everolimus has no clinically important effects on the pharmacokinetics of ciclosporin. However, concurrent use might potentiate the renal toxicity of ciclosporin and, in kidney transplant patients, everolimus is licensed for use with reduced-dose ciclosporin.[10] Another manufacturer advises reducing the dose of ciclosporin over time, based on ciclosporin concentrations and tolerability, to reduce nephrotoxicity in both kidney and heart transplant patients.[11] Even with these precautions, renal function should still be monitored and a reduction in the ciclosporin dose should be considered in patients with an increased serum creatinine concentration.[11]

1. Kirchner GI, Winkler M, Mueller L, Vidal C, Jacobsen W, Franzke A, Wagner S, Blick S, Manns MP, Sewing K-F. Pharmacokinetics of SDZ RAD and cyclosporin including their metabolites in seven kidney graft patients after the first dose of SDZ RAD. *Br J Clin Pharmacol* (2000) 50, 449–54.
2. Budde K, Lehne G, Winkler M, Renders L, Lison A, Fritsche L, Soulillou J-P, Fauchald P, Neumayer H-H, Dantal J and RADW 102 Renal Transplant Study Group. Influence of everolimus on steady-state pharmacokinetics of cyclosporine in maintenance renal transplant patients. *J Clin Pharmacol* (2005) 45, 781–91.
3. Kovarik JM, Kahan BD, Kaplan B, Lorber M, Winkler M, Rouilly M, Gerbeau C, Cambon N, Boger R, Rordorf C on behalf of the Everolimus Phase II Study Group. Longitudinal assessment of everolimus in de novo renal transplant recipients over the first post-transplant year: pharmacokinetics, exposure-response relationships, and influence of cyclosporine. *Clin Pharmacol Ther* (2001). 69, 48–56.
4. Kovarik JM, Eisen H, Dorent R, Mancini D, Vigano M, Rouilly M, Hsu C-H, Rordorf C. Everolimus in de novo cardiac transplantation: pharmacokinetics, therapeutic range, and influence on cyclosporine exposure. *J Heart Lung Transplant* (2003) 22, 1117–25.
5. Kovarik JM, Kalbag J, Figueiredo J, Rouilly M, O'Bannon LF, Rordorf C. Differential influence of two cyclosporine formulations on everolimus pharmacokinetics: a clinically relevant pharmacokinetic interaction. *J Clin Pharmacol* (2002) 42, 95–9.
6. Kovarik JM, Dantal J, Civati G, Rizzo G, Rouilly M, Bettoni-Ristic O, Rordorf C. Influence of delayed initiation of cyclosporine on everolimus pharmacokinetics in *de novo* renal transplant patients. *Am J Transplant* (2003) 3, 1576–80.
7. Brandhorst G, Tenderich G, Zittermann A, Oezpeker C, Koerfer R, Oellerich M, Armstrong VW. Everolimus exposure in cardiac transplant recipients is influenced by concomitant calcineurin inhibitor. *Ther Drug Monit* (2008) 30, 113–16.
8. Afinitor (Everolimus). Novartis Pharmaceuticals UK Ltd. UK Summary of product characteristics, December 2014.
9. Votubia (Everolimus). Novartis Pharmaceuticals UK Ltd. UK Summary of product characteristics, July 2014.
10. Zortress (Everolimus). Novartis. US Prescribing information, February 2013.
11. Certican (Everolimus). Novartis Pharmaceuticals Australia Pty Ltd. Australian product information, August 2013.

Everolimus + Food

A high-fat meal minimally reduces the exposure to everolimus.

Clinical evidence

In a single-dose study in 24 healthy subjects, giving everolimus 2 mg tablets with a high-fat breakfast reduced the maximum concentration of everolimus by 60% and delayed the time to maximum concentration by about 1.25 hours when compared with the fasting state.[1] However, the AUC of everolimus was reduced by just 16%. Similarly, in a study in 6 transplant patients taking ciclosporin and everolimus 2.5 mg daily, giving everolimus with a high-fat meal reduced the maximum concentration and AUC of everolimus by 53% and 21%, respectively, without altering the minimum concentration.[1]

Mechanism

Unknown.

Importance and management

Evidence for an interaction between everolimus and food is limited to one study, but this suggests that food has little effect on the exposure to everolimus. Nevertheless, the authors of the study suggest that everolimus should be taken consistently either with or without food, to minimise variability in exposure.[1]

1. Kovarik JM, Hartmann S, Figueiredo J, Rordorf C, Golor G, Lison A, Budde K, Neumayer HH. Effect of food on everolimus absorption: quantification in healthy subjects and a confirmatory screening in patients with renal transplants. *Pharmacotherapy* (2002) 22, 154–9.

Everolimus + Ketoconazole and other CYP3A4 inhibitors or P-glycoprotein inhibitors

Ketoconazole very markedly increases the exposure to everolimus. A report describes reduced everolimus clearance in a patient also given itraconazole, and another patient required a greatly reduced everolimus dose while receiving voriconazole. Posaconazole also increased everolimus concentrations in one patient, but to a lesser extent than voriconazole. A reduced everolimus dose was required in a patient taking fluconazole. Other inhibitors of CYP3A4 and/or P-glycoprotein are predicted to increase everolimus concentrations.

Clinical evidence

In a study, 12 healthy subjects were given a single 1-mg dose of everolimus on day 4 of an 8-day course of **ketoconazole** 200 mg twice daily. Ketoconazole increased the AUC, maximum blood concentration, and half-life of everolimus by 15-fold, 3.9-fold, and 1.9-fold, respectively.[1]

Similarly, in a pharmacokinetic modelling study, a patient taking **itraconazole** with everolimus, ciclosporin, and prednisone had a 74% lower everolimus clearance. However, everolimus clearance was reduced by a non-significant 7% in 16 patients who were also taking **fluconazole**.[2] In one severely-ill patient receiving intravenous **fluconazole**, the authors stated that everolimus was started at about a 50 to 75% lower dose than usual (0.75 mg twice daily), and this maintained everolimus concentrations within the desired range.[3] However, note that the starting dose of 0.75 mg twice daily used in this case is the recommended initial dose in kidney and heart transplant patients. When fluconazole was switched to **voriconazole**, the everolimus dose was reduced to just 0.25 mg daily, with everolimus concentrations remaining within the therapeutic range, although the concentration-to-dose ratio suggested that 0.25 mg twice daily might have been more appropriate.[3] In a 54-year-old kidney transplant patient taking everolimus 1.5 mg twice daily, oral **voriconazole** 400 mg for 2 doses followed by 200 mg twice daily, started on day 14 post-transplant, resulted in a 7.5-fold increase in the everolimus minimum blood concentrations, requiring a dose reduction to 0.25 mg twice daily. Hepatotoxicity occurred after one month of concurrent use, and so voriconazole was stopped, with the everolimus dose readjusted to 1 mg twice daily (to maintain an everolimus minimum concentration of 10 nanograms/mL). One month later, **posaconazole** was started, resulting in a 3.8-fold increase in everolimus minimum blood concentrations requiring an everolimus dose reduction to 0.5 mg twice daily.[4]

Mechanism

Everolimus, a derivative of sirolimus, is a substrate of CYP3A4 and P-glycoprotein. The azoles inhibit CYP3A4 and P-glycoprotein, albeit to varying degrees, and therefore decrease everolimus metabolism and increasing its uptake, leading to an increase in everolimus exposure.

Importance and management

The pharmacokinetic interaction between everolimus and ketoconazole is established and likely to be clinically important. One group recommends that, given the magnitude of the interaction, ketoconazole should be avoided if possible in patients taking everolimus,[5] and this seems prudent advice. If concurrent use cannot be avoided it is likely that the dose of everolimus will need to be greatly reduced. With everolimus used in organ transplantation, it would be prudent to monitor everolimus concentrations and adjust the dose accordingly, considering a pre-emptive dose decrease. Similar precautions might be advisable with everolimus used for malignancy. This advice should also be extended to other potent CYP3A4 inhibitors; for a list see 'Table 1.9', p.11.

Moderate CYP3A4 inhibitors are also expected to increase everolimus concentrations, and the dosing recommendations as stated for erythromycin under 'Everolimus + Macrolides', below, apply. For a list of known moderate CYP3A4 inhibitors, see 'Table 1.9', p.11.

It is also important to note that drugs that are potent or moderate inhibitors of CYP3A4, might also inhibit P-glycoprotein, and that drugs that solely inhibit P-glycoprotein might also increase exposure to everolimus. See 'Table 1.12', p.14 for a list of P-glycoprotein inhibitors.

The concurrent use of **grapefruit juice** is not recommended with everolimus because the effect of the expected increases in everolimus exposure varies widely.[6-9] The US manufacturers also extend this recommendation to patients eating whole grapefruit.[6,9] However, grapefruit juice is generally considered a weak CYP3A4 inhibitor and might therefore not be expected to have an important effect. Nevertheless, given the difficulties of standardising grapefruit juice, and the possible implications of increased everolimus concentrations, this advice would seem prudent and patients should be advised of the potential risk.

For further information about the CYP3A4 inhibitors, clarithromycin, erythromycin, and telithromycin, see 'Everolimus + Macrolides', below, and for diltiazem and verapamil, see 'Everolimus + Calcium-channel blockers', p.1261.

1. Kovarik JM, Beyer D, Bizot MN, Jiang Q, Shenouda M, Schmouder RL. Blood concentrations of everolimus are markedly increased by ketoconazole. *J Clin Pharmacol* (2005) 45, 514–8.
2. Kovarik JM, Hsu C-H, McMahon L, Berthier S, Rordorf C. Population pharmacokinetics of everolimus in de novo renal transplant patients: impact of ethnicity and comedications. *Clin Pharmacol Ther* (2001) 70, 247–54.
3. Pea F, Baccarani U, Tavio M, Cojutti P, Adani GL, Londero A, Baraldo M, Franceschi L, Furlanut M, Viale P. Pharmacokinetic interaction between everolimus and antifungal triazoles in a liver transplant patient. *Ann Pharmacother* (2008) 42, 1711–16.
4. Billaud EM, Antoine C, Berge M, Abboud I, Lefeuvre S, Benammar M, Glotz D. Management of metabolic cytochrome P450 3A4 drug-drug interaction between everolimus and azole antifungals in a renal transplant patient. *Clin Drug Investig* (2009) 29, 481–6.
5. Rothenburger M, Zuckermann A, Bara C, Hummel M, Strüber M, Hirt S, Lehmkuhl H; Certican Consensus Study Group. Recommendations for the use of everolimus (Certican) in heart transplantation: results from the second German-Austrian Certican Consensus Conference. *J Heart Lung Transplant* (2007) 26, 305–11.
6. Afinitor (Everolimus). Novartis. US Prescribing information, January 2015.
7. Afinitor (Everolimus). Novartis Pharmaceuticals UK Ltd. UK Summary of product characteristics, December 2014.
8. Votubia (Everolimus). Novartis Pharmaceuticals UK Ltd. UK Summary of product characteristics, July 2014.
9. Zortress (Everolimus). Novartis. US Prescribing information, February 2013.

Everolimus + Macrolides

Erythromycin moderately increased everolimus concentrations in one study. Other macrolides are predicted to interact similarly, but perhaps to varying extents.

Clinical evidence

In a study, 16 healthy subjects were given a single 4-mg dose of everolimus before and on day 5 of a 9-day course of **erythromycin** 500 mg three times daily. The maximum blood concentration and AUC of everolimus were increased 2-fold and 4.4-fold, respectively, and its half-life was prolonged by 39%.[1] In a pharmacokinetic modelling study, 9 patients were identified who had received a macrolide antibacterial. Those patients receiving **erythromycin** had a 22% lower clearance of everolimus, and those receiving **azithromycin** had an 18% lower clearance, than patients not receiving a macrolide.[2]

Mechanism

Erythromycin is an inhibitor of CYP3A4 and P-glycoprotein, by which everolimus is metabolised and transported, respectively. This reduces the metabolism, and increases the uptake, of everolimus leading to increased exposure. Other macrolides are also CYP3A4 inhibitors (to varying extents, although azithromycin does not generally inhibit this isoenzyme to any clinically relevant extent) and inhibit P-glycoprotein, and so would be predicted to interact similarly.

Importance and management

The interaction between everolimus with erythromycin is consistent with the known mechanisms of both of these drugs, and is likely to be clinically relevant. The authors recommend that appropriate everolimus dose reductions based on frequently monitored blood concentrations should be made when patients are given erythromycin.[1] One UK manufacturer of everolimus licensed for use in various malignancies, recommends an everolimus dose reduction to 5 or 2.5 mg daily with moderate CYP3A4 inhibitors, such as erythromycin. However, they state that this dose decrease is a prediction and therefore good monitoring is still required.[3] The US manufacturer of a similarly licensed product, advises an everolimus dose reduction to 2.5 mg daily on concurrent use with erythromycin, with an increase to 5 mg daily considered based on tolerability.[4] The UK and US manufacturers of everolimus products licensed for astrocytoma, recommend a 50% dose reduction on the concurrent use of erythromycin, with monitoring of minimum concentrations about every 2 weeks and further advise that these should be used to guide subsequent dosing.[4,5] One US manufacturer of everolimus licensed for use in organ transplant, advises monitoring everolimus blood concentrations and adjusting the dose accordingly.[6]

As other macrolides inhibit CYP3A4 and/or P-glycoprotein to varying extents (see 'Table 1.9', p.11 and 'Table 1.12', p.14, respectively), their effects can vary. Therefore if concurrent use with everolimus is considered necessary, everolimus concentrations should also be closely monitored and the dose adjusted as required. Note that the UK and US manufacturers either do not recommend, or advise avoiding, the concurrent use of **clarithromycin** and **telithromycin** (both potent CYP3A4 inhibitors).[3-6]

1. Kovarik JM, Beyer D, Bizot MN, Jiang Q, Shenouda M, Schmouder R. Effect of multiple-dose erythromycin on everolimus pharmacokinetics. *Eur J Clin Pharmacol* (2005) 61, 35–8.
2. Kovarik JM, Hsu C-H, McMahon L, Berthier S, Rordorf C. Population pharmacokinetics of everolimus in de novo renal transplant patients: impact of ethnicity and comedications. *Clin Pharmacol Ther* (2001) 70, 247–54.
3. Afinitor (Everolimus). Novartis Pharmaceuticals UK Ltd. UK Summary of product characteristics, December 2014.
4. Afinitor (Everolimus). Novartis. US Prescribing information, January 2015.
5. Votubia (Everolimus). Novartis Pharmaceuticals UK Ltd. UK Summary of product characteristics, July 2014.
6. Zortress (Everolimus). Novartis. US Prescribing information, February 2013.

Everolimus + Rifamycins and other CYP3A4 inducers

Rifampicin moderately decreases the exposure to everolimus, and increases its clearance. A case report describes the successful switch from rifampicin to rifabutin in a patient with greatly decreased everolimus concentrations. Other inducers of CYP3A4 and P-glycoprotein are predicted to interact similarly.

Clinical evidence

In a study, 12 healthy subjects were given a single 4-mg dose of everolimus before and after taking **rifampicin** 600 mg daily for 7 days. **Rifampicin** increased the clearance of everolimus 2.7-fold, and decreased its AUC and maximum blood concentration by 63% and 58%, respectively, although there was large interindividual variation in the AUC.[1] A case report describes a 72-year-old kidney transplant patient stable taking everolimus for basal cell carcinoma (with an everolimus blood concentration of about 9 nanograms/mL) who was diagnosed with tuberculosis. **Rifampicin** 600 mg daily (with pyrazinamide) was started, and his everolimus dose had to be increased by 75% (from 2 mg daily to 3.5 mg daily) to give an everolimus blood concentration of about 5 nanograms/mL.[2] Another case report describes the successful management of this interaction by switching from rifampicin to rifabutin: a 63-year-old liver transplant patient taking everolimus 1 mg daily had his dose increased 24-fold (to 24 mg daily) after starting **rifampicin** 600 mg daily as part of tuberculosis treatment, due to a low everolimus minimum blood concentration . Despite this large increase, his everolimus minimum blood concentration was still less than 5 nanograms/mL. On day 45, the rifampicin was switched to **rifabutin** 450 mg daily and within a few days his everolimus minimum blood concentration increased, and his dose was gradually reduced over the following 30 days to 5.25 mg daily which achieved a therapeutic minimum blood concentration of 10.3 nanograms/mL.[3]

Mechanism

Everolimus is metabolised by CYP3A4 and is a substrate for P-glycoprotein. Rifampicin is a well-known inducer of both CYP3A4 and P-glycoprotein, therefore it increases the metabolism and decreases the uptake of everolimus, resulting in decreased exposure. Rifabutin also induces CYP3A4, although to a lesser extent than rifampicin.

Importance and management

The moderate decrease in everolimus exposure on the concurrent use of **rifampicin** is clinically important, and could lead to treatment failure. If concurrent use is necessary, it would be prudent to increase the dose of everolimus and monitor blood concentrations very closely. One group has suggested a 2- to 3-fold increase in everolimus dose when given with rifampicin.[4] The authors of the case report with **rifabutin** suggest that this might be a suitable alternative to rifampicin in everolimus patients requiring treatment for tuberculosis, and allows easy management of the interaction through therapeutic drug monitoring.[3] However, the UK and US manufacturers of everolimus state that the concurrent use of rifampicin should be avoided where possible,[5-8] and some extend this to other CYP3A4 inducers, which would include rifabutin. For a list of known, clinically important CYP3A4 inducers, see 'Table 1.9', p.11. While some manufacturers list **dexamethasone**, **prednisone**, and **prednisolone** as CYP3A4 inducers, the clinical importance of these drugs as inducers of CYP3A4 is not established.[5,6,8]

Some manufacturers of everolimus licensed for various malignancies, recommend that an everolimus dose increase, from 10 mg daily to 20 mg daily, in steps of 5 mg or less (starting on day 4 of concurrent use[6]), should be considered.[5,6] When licensed for astrocytoma, the UK manufacturer advises titrating the dose to achieve minimum concentrations of 5 to 15 micrograms/L. If the concentrations are lower than this target range, they state that the daily dose can be increased by 2.5 mg every 2 weeks.[8]

However, in the US, the advice for this same indication is to double the everolimus dose and, after 2 weeks, monitor blood concentrations and adjust the dose to maintain a minimum concentration of 5 to 15 nanograms/mL, where necessary.[5] Any dose adjustments should be based on tolerability and continued monitoring is advisable. In contrast, the US manufacturer of everolimus licensed for use in organ transplantation, simply advises monitoring everolimus concentrations.[7]

1. Kovarik JM, Hartmann S, Figueiredo J, Rouilly M, Port A, Rordorf C. Effect of rifampicin on apparent clearance of everolimus. *Ann Pharmacother* (2002) 36, 981–5.
2. Fijalkowska-Morawska JB, Jagodzińska M, Nowicki M. Pulmonary embolism and reactivation of tuberculosis during everolimus therapy in a kidney transplant recipient. *Ann Transplant* (2011) 16, 107–10.
3. Lefeuvre S, Rebaudet S, Billaud EM, Wyplosz B. Management of rifamycins-everolimus drug-drug interactions in a liver-transplant patient with pulmonary tuberculosis. *Transpl Int* (2012) 25, e120–2.
4. Rothenburger M, Zuckermann A, Bara C, Hummel M, Strüber M, Hirt S, Lehmkuhl H; Certican Consensus Study Group. Recommendations for the use of everolimus (Certican) in heart transplantation: results from the second German-Austrian Certican Consensus Conference. *J Heart Lung Transplant* (2007) 26, 305–11.
5. Afinitor (Everolimus). Novartis. US Prescribing information, January 2015.
6. Afinitor (Everolimus). Novartis Pharmaceuticals UK Ltd. UK Summary of product characteristics, December 2014.
7. Zortress (Everolimus). Novartis. US Prescribing information, February 2013.
8. Votubia (Everolimus). Novartis Pharmaceuticals UK Ltd. UK Summary of product characteristics, July 2014.

Everolimus + Tacrolimus

No pharmacokinetic interaction appears to occur between everolimus and tacrolimus, but in one study increased tacrolimus doses were required to achieve target concentrations in the presence of everolimus.

Clinical evidence

(a) Effect on everolimus

In one study, 8 kidney transplant patients taking tacrolimus were switched from mycophenolate to everolimus 1.5 mg twice daily. After everolimus had been taken for 10 days, the tacrolimus dose was halved. There was no difference in the pharmacokinetics of everolimus between the full-dose tacrolimus and half-dose tacrolimus periods (minimum concentration 3.3 nanograms/mL compared with 3 nanograms/mL). In addition, the everolimus minimum concentration and AUC were about 2.5-fold lower than in a previous study of patients taking the same dose of everolimus with ciclosporin, which is known to increase everolimus concentrations.[1] Similarly, a pharmacokinetic sub-study of 46 kidney transplant patients included in the ASSET trial found that everolimus pharmacokinetics were no different between those patients taking low-dose tacrolimus (to achieve a minimum concentration of 4 to 7 nanograms/mL, 20 patients) and those taking very low-dose tacrolimus (to achieve a minimum concentration of 1.5 to 3 nanograms/mL, 26 patients). When compared with data from a separate study in which patients received everolimus with ciclosporin, the mean dose of everolimus required to achieve the same exposure as with tacrolimus was about 1.5-fold higher.[2] In another study, minimum concentrations of everolimus were almost halved (from 4.2 to 2.3 nanograms/mL) when ciclosporin was stopped and tacrolimus was started in 6 heart transplant recipients taking everolimus. The AUC of everolimus was decreased by about 50% and its maximum concentration was decreased by 35%.[3]

(b) Effect on tacrolimus

In a study in 8 kidney transplant patients taking tacrolimus, there was no statistically significant change in the tacrolimus minimum concentration (7.9 nanograms/mL compared with 8.4 nanograms/mL) or its AUC when mycophenolate was replaced with everolimus 1.5 mg twice a day.[1] Similarly, there was no change in tacrolimus pharmacokinetics in 6 heart transplant patients taking tacrolimus when azathioprine was replaced with everolimus 1.5 mg twice daily.[3] In a pharmacokinetic study in 20 kidney transplant patients taking tacrolimus with everolimus 1.5 mg or 3 mg daily, the pharmacokinetics of tacrolimus were no different between the groups, but higher tacrolimus doses were required to achieve target concentrations in the group taking everolimus 3 mg daily.[4]

Mechanism

Unclear.

Importance and management

The limited available data suggest that there is no clinically relevant pharmacokinetic interaction between tacrolimus and everolimus. The consequence of this is that higher everolimus doses are likely to be required in patients taking tacrolimus than in those patients taking ciclosporin. For further discussion on the effect of ciclosporin on everolimus concentrations, see 'Everolimus + Ciclosporin', p.1262. However, there is limited evidence that everolimus might affect the dose of tacrolimus required to achieve target concentrations, but as tacrolimus is given as individualised doses based on blood concentrations, any change in the dose required to achieve target concentrations should be identified with routine monitoring.

1. Kovarik JM, Curtis JJ, Hricik DE, Prescovitz MD, Scantlebury V, Vasquez A. Differential pharmacokinetic interaction of tacrolimus and cyclosporine on everolimus. *Transplant Proc* (2006) 38, 3456–8.
2. Rostaing L, Christiaans MH, Kovarik JM, Pascual J. The pharmacokinetics of everolimus in de novo kidney transplant patients receiving tacrolimus: an analysis from the randomized ASSET study. *Ann Transplant* (2014) 19, 337–45.
3. Brandhorst G, Tenderich G, Zittermann A, Oezpeker C, Koerfer R, Oellerich M, Armstrong VW. Everolimus exposure in cardiac transplant recipients is influenced by concomitant calcineurin inhibitor. *Ther Drug Monit* (2008) 30, 113–16.
4. Pascual J, del Castillo D, Cabello M, Pallardó L, Grinyó JM, Fernández AM, Brunet M. Interaction between everolimus and tacrolimus in renal transplant recipients: a pharmacokinetic controlled trial. *Transplantation* (2010) 89, 994–1000.

Immunosuppressants + Vaccines

The body's immune response is suppressed by immunosuppressants such as ciclosporin, mycophenolate, sirolimus, and tacrolimus. The antibody response to vaccines might be reduced, although even partial protection might be of benefit.

Clinical evidence

(a) Diphtheria, tetanus, and inactivated polio or pertussis vaccines

In a case-control review, organ transplant recipients taking immunosuppressants, tetanus vaccines,[1,2] and inactivated polio vaccines[1] produced protective antibody titres. The response to diphtheria vaccine was lower than in healthy controls[1] and the antibody titre had decreased below the protective concentration by 12 months in 38% of patients in one study,[1] and 24% in another.[2] In a study in 67 preterm infants receiving **dexamethasone** for chronic lung disease, the immune response to the combined diptheria, tetanus, and pertussis vaccine was slightly impaired when compared to the response in 26 preterm infants not receiving dexamethasone.[3] Note that live polio vaccines are not recommended in immunosuppressed patients (see *Live vaccines*, below).

(b) Hepatitis vaccines

The antibody response to **hepatitis B vaccine** is generally poor in patients taking immunosuppressants after organ transplantation,[4,5] although one research group reported a sustained antibody response in half of their patients,[6] and an overall 85% seroconversion rate was seen in one study in children (aged between 4 and 16 years).[7] In this latter study,[7] children receiving **ciclosporin** monotherapy had a higher seroconversion rate (100%) than those receiving **ciclosporin** and **corticosteroids** (84%) and those receiving **ciclosporin**, **azathioprine**, and **corticosteroids** (66%). The antibody response to **hepatitis A vaccine** in patients taking immunosuppressants after organ transplantation is variable,[8-10] and declines quicker than in healthy controls.[10] In kidney transplant recipients, there is some evidence that the response is inversely related to the number of immunosuppressant drugs.[9]

(c) Influenza vaccine

A number of studies have been published on the efficacy of influenza vaccination in organ transplant recipients taking immunosuppressants. Some have found a reduction in the proportion of patients developing a protective antibody titre compared with healthy control subjects,[11-13] whereas others have found no reduction.[14] A few studies have looked at the effects of specific immunosuppressant drugs. In one comparative study in 59 kidney transplant patients, 21 patients taking **ciclosporin** and **prednisone** had a considerably lower immune response to influenza vaccine (inactivated trivalent) than 38 patients taking **azathioprine** and **prednisone** or 29 healthy subjects taking no drugs. All of the immune response measurements were reduced by 20 to 30% in those taking **ciclosporin**.[15] In another study, 13 patients taking **mycophenolate**, **ciclosporin**, and **prednisolone** had a reduction in antibody response to influenza vaccine, when compared with 25 patients taking **ciclosporin**, **azathioprine**, and **prednisolone**.[16] In yet another study, patients taking **ciclosporin** had lower antibody responses when compared with patients taking **tacrolimus**.[17] Confirmation of the practical importance of the reduced antibody titre in some patients is described in a case report of a heart transplant patient taking **ciclosporin** who did not respond to influenza vaccination while taking **ciclosporin** and **prednisone**. He had two episodes of influenza, one serologically confirmed, and it was later shown that vaccination had not resulted in seroconversion.[18] Similarly, a patient taking **tacrolimus** after a liver transplant developed influenza A myocarditis despite prophylactic vaccination.[19] In 82 patients taking immunosuppressants for rheumatoid arthritis, influenza vaccination led to fewer seroconversions when compared to 30 healthy controls. This response was not affected by the use of **prednisone** or DMARDs (including **etanercept**, **infliximab**, and **leflunomide**).[20] A study in 56 patients with systemic lupus erythematosus (SLE) found that influenza vaccination led to fewer seroconversions than in 18 healthy controls, and that the concurrent use of **azathioprine** was associated with fewer seroconversions than the concurrent use of **hydroxychloroquine** or **prednisone**.[21]

(d) Live vaccines

The use of live vaccines in patients receiving **corticosteroids** has caused generalised infection, see 'Corticosteroids + Vaccines', p.1260. Similarly, the use of live vaccines in patients taking other immunosuppressants is not recommended: probably as a consequence of this there are few published reports about the use of live vaccines with immunosuppressants. One study found that **measles vaccine** was effective in 7 of 18 children under 3 years old after liver transplantation, and that there were no complications directly attributable to the vaccine.[22]

(e) Measles, mumps, and rubella vaccines

A small study in 10 children with juvenile idiopathic arthritis found that low-dose **methotrexate** or methotrexate with **etanercept** 400 micrograms/kg twice weekly for at least 6 months before measles, mumps, and rubella (MMR) revaccination did not interfere with the immune response to revaccination to a clinically relevant extent, when compared with healthy children. Neither vaccine failure nor occurrence of overt measles, mumps, and rubella or secondary severe infections was observed within 6 months of MMR revaccination. However, further studies are needed to provide a safety basis for the use of MMR vaccine in juvenile idiopathic arthritis.[23]

(f) Meningococcal vaccines

A study in 121 children with atopic dermatitis found that the use of topical **tacrolimus** 0.03% ointment did not alter the immune response to vaccination with meningitis C vaccine compared with the response in 44 healthy controls.[24]

(g) Pneumococcal vaccines

Good responses to pneumococcal vaccines have been seen in patients taking immunosuppressant drugs after organ transplantation,[11,25,26] and in patients taking **etanercept** or **infliximab** for arthritis.[27,28] However, it has been suggested that protective antibody titres might not persist as long as in renal transplant patients compared with healthy subjects.[29,30] In contrast, a study in heart transplant patients (taking **daclizumab, prednisolone, mycophenolate mofetil**, and either **ciclosporin** or **tacrolimus**),[31] and another in rheumatoid arthritis patients taking **methotrexate**,[28] found that the immune response was impaired. In 23 children with atopic dermatitis, the topical use of **tacrolimus** 0.03% ointment did not impair the response to pneumococcal vaccination.[32]

Mechanism

Immunosuppression by these drugs diminishes the ability of the body to respond immunologically both to transplants and to vaccination.

Importance and management

These are established and clinically important interactions. Public Health England[33] recommends that live vaccines should not be used in the following individuals:

- Patients who have received a solid organ transplant and are currently on immunosuppressive treatment.
- Patients who have received a bone marrow transplant, until at least 12 months after finishing all immunosuppressive treatment.
- Patients taking immunosuppressive drugs such as azathioprine, ciclosporin, methotrexate, cyclophosphamide, leflunomide, and cytokine inhibitors [presumably including etanercept] should not be given live vaccines during or for at least 6 months after treatment has stopped.
- Patients taking systemic high dose steroids, until at least 3 months after treatment has stopped (see 'Corticosteroids + Vaccines', p.1260).

They recommend that immunosuppressed patients be given inactivated vaccines in accordance with national recommendations, bearing in mind that they might not achieve as good an antibody response.

They state that, in individuals about to start immunosuppressive treatments, inactivated vaccines should ideally be given at least 2 weeks before immunosuppressive therapy is started, and in the case of live vaccines, a longer period before immunosuppression commences might be desirable.

The proportion of patients developing protective antibody titres to vaccines is often reduced in patients taking immunosuppressants. Nevertheless, for many vaccines, the reduced response seen is still considered clinically useful, and, for example, in the case of kidney transplant patients,[33] and in patients who are immunosuppressed (either by drugs or disease), influenza vaccination is actively recommended.[33] Pneumococcal vaccine should also be given to these patients.[33] If a vaccine is given, it might be prudent to monitor the response, so that alternative prophylactic measures can be considered where it is deemed inadequate. Note that, even where effective antibody titres are produced, these might not persist as long as in healthy subjects, and more frequent booster doses might be required.

1. Huzly D, Neifer S, Reinke P, Schröder K, Schönfeld C, Hofmann T, Bienzle U. Routine immunizations in adult renal transplant recipients. *Transplantation* (1997) 63, 839–45.
2. Enke BU, Bökenkamp A, Offner G, Bartmann P, Brodehl J. Response to diphtheria and tetanus booster vaccination in pediatric renal transplant recipients. *Transplantation* (1997) 64, 237–41.
3. Robinson MJ, Heal C, Gardener E, Powell P, Sims DG. Antibody response to diphtheria-tetanus-pertussis immunization in preterm infants who receive dexamethasone for chronic lung disease. *Pediatrics* (2004) 113, 733–7.
4. Angelico M, Di Paolo D, Trinito MO, Petrolati A, Araco A, Zazza S, Lionetti R, Casciani CU, Tisone G. Failure of a reinforced triple course of hepatitis B vaccination in patients transplanted for HBV-related cirrhosis. *Hepatology* (2002) 35, 176–81.
5. Loinaz C, Ramón de Juanes J, Moreno Gonzalez E, López A, Lumbreras C, Gómez R, Gonzalez-Pinto I, Jiménez C, Garcia I, Fuertes A. Hepatitis B vaccination results in 140 liver transplant recipients. *Hepatogastroenterology* (1997) 44, 235–8.
6. Bienzle U, Günther M, Neuhaus R, Neuhaus P. Successful hepatitis B vaccination in patients who underwent transplantation for hepatitis B virus-related cirrhosis: preliminary results. *Liver Transpl* (2002) 8, 562–4.
7. Duca P, Del Pont JM, D'Agostino D. Successful immune response to a recombinant hepatitis B vaccine in children after liver transplantation. *J Pediatr Gastroenterol Nutr* (2001) 32, 168–70.
8. Arslan M, Wiesner RH, Poterucha JJ, Zein NN. Safety and efficacy of hepatitis A vaccination in liver transplantation recipients. *Transplantation* (2001) 72, 272–6.
9. Stark K, Günther M, Neuhaus R, Reinke P, Schröder K, Linnig S, Bienzle U. Immunogenicity and safety of hepatitis A vaccine in liver and renal transplant recipients. *J Infect Dis* (1999) 180, 2014–17.
10. Günther M, Stark K, Neuhaus R, Reinke P, Schröder K, Bienzle U. Rapid decline of antibodies after hepatitis A immunization in liver and renal transplant recipients. *Transplantation* (2001) 71, 477–90.
11. Dengler TJ, Strnad N, Buhring I, Zimmermann R, Girgsdies O, Kubler WE, Zielen S. Differential immune response to influenza and pneumococcal vaccination in immunosuppressed patients after heart transplantation. *Transplantation* (1998) 66, 1340–47.
12. Soesman NMR, Rimmelzwaan GF, Nieuwkoop NJ, Beyer WEP, Tilanus HW, Kemmeren MH, Metselaar HJ, de Man RA, Osterhaus ADME. Efficacy of influenza vaccination in adult liver transplant recipients. *J Med Virol* (2000) 61, 85–93.
13. Sanchez-Fructuoso AI, Prats D, Naranjo P, Fernández-Pérez C, González MJ, Mariano A, González J, Figueredo MA, Martin JM, Paniagua V, Fereres J, Gómez de la Concha E, Barrientos A. Influenza virus immunization effectivity in kidney transplant patients subjected to two different triple-drug therapy immunosuppressant protocols. *Transplantation* (2000) 69, 436–9.
14. Edvardsson VO, Flynn JT, Deforest A, Kaiser BA, Schulman SL, Bradley A, Palmer J, Polinsky MS, Baluarte HJ. Effective immunization against influenza in pediatric renal transplant recipients. *Clin Transplant* (1996) 10, 556–60.
15. Versluis DJ, Beyer WEP, Masurel N, Wenting GJ, Weimar W. Impairment of the immune response to influenza vaccination in renal transplant recipients by cyclosporine, but not azathioprine. *Transplantation* (1986) 42, 376–9.
16. Smith KGC, Isbel NM, Catton MG, Leydon JA, Becker GJ, Walker RG. Suppression of the humoral immune response by mycophenolate mofetil. *Nephrol Dial Transplant* (1998) 13, 160–4.
17. Mazzone PJ, Mossad SB, Mawhorter SD, Mehta AC, Schilz RJ, Maurer JR. The humoral immune response to influenza vaccination in lung transplant patients. *Eur Respir J* (2001) 18, 971–6.
18. Beyer WEP, Diepersloot RJA, Masurel N, Simoons ML, Weimar W. Double failure of influenza vaccination in a heart transplant patient. *Transplantation* (1987) 43, 319.
19. Vilchez RA, Fung JJ, Kusne S, Influenza A myocarditis developing in an adult liver transplant recipient despite vaccination: a case report and review of the literature. *Transplantation* (2000) 70, 543–5.
20. Fomin I, Caspi D, Levy V, Varsano N, Shalev Y, Paran D, Levartovsky D, Litinsky I, Kaufman I, Wigler I, Mendelson E, Elkayam O. Vaccination against influenza in rheumatoid arthritis: the effect of disease modifying drugs, including TNFα blockers. *Ann Rheum Dis* (2006) 65, 191–4.
21. Holvast A, Huckriede A, Wilschut J, Horst G, De Vries JJ, Benne CA, Kallenberg CG, Bijl M. Safety and efficacy of influenza vaccination in systemic lupus erythematosus patients with quiescent disease. *Ann Rheum Dis* (2006) 913–9.
22. Rand EB, McCarthy CA, Whitington PF. Measles vaccination after orthotopic liver transplantation. *J Pediatr* (1993) 123, 87–9.
23. Borte S, Liebert UG, Borte M, Sack U. Efficacy of measles, mumps and rubella revaccination in children with juvenile idiopathic arthritis treated with methotrexate and etanercept. *Rheumatology (Oxford)* (2009) 48, 144–8.
24. Hofman T, Cranswick N, Kuna P, Bozananski A, Latos T, Gold M, Murrell DF, Gebauer K, Behre U, Machura E, Ólafsson J, Szalai Z. Tacrolimus ointment does not affect the immediate response to vaccination, the generation of immune memory, or humoral and cell-mediated immunity in children. *Arch Dis Child* (2006) 91, 905–10.
25. Kazancioğlu R, Sever MŞ, Yüksel-Önel D, Eraksoy H, Yildiz A, Çelik AV, Kauacan SM, Badur S. Immunization of renal transplant recipients with pneumococcal polysaccharide vaccine. *Clin Transplant* (2000) 14, 61–5.
26. Silberman H, Overturf GD, Field RJ, Butler J, Berne TV, Witt R. Response of renal allograft recipients to pneumococcal vaccine. *Ann Surg* (1980) 192, 199–201.
27. Mease PJ, Ritchlin CT, Martin RW, Gottlieb AB, Baumgartner SW, Burge DJ, Whitmore JB. Pneumococcal vaccine response in psoriatic arthritis patients during treatment with etanercept. *J Rheumatol* (2004) 31, 1356–61.
28. Kapetanovic MC, Saxne T, Sjöholm A, Truedsson L, Jönsson G, Geborek P. Influence of methotrexate, TNF blockers and prednisolone on antibody responses to pneumococcal polysaccharide vaccine in patients with rheumatoid arthritis. *Rheumatology (Oxford)* (2006) 45, 106–11.
29. Linnemann CC, First MR, Schiffman G. Revaccination of renal transplant and hemodialysis recipients with pneumococcal vaccine. *Arch Intern Med* (1986) 146, 1554–6.
30. Kumar D, Welsh B, Siegal D, Hong Chen M, Humar A. Immunogenicity of pneumococcal vaccine in renal transplant recipients - three year follow-up of a randomized trial. *Am J Transplant* (2007) 7, 633–8.
31. Sarmiento E, Rodríguez-Hernández C, Rodríguez-Molina J, Fernández-Yánez J, Palomo J, Anguita J, Pérez JL, Lanio N, Fernández-Cruz E, Carbone J. Impaired anti-pneumococcal infection following heart transplant. *Int Immunopharmacol* (2006) 2027–30.
32. Stiehm ER, Roberts RL, Kaplan MS, Corren J, Jaracz E, Rico MJ. Pneumococcal seroconversion after vaccination for children with atopic dermatitis treated with tacrolimus ointment. *J Am Acad Dermatol* (2005) 53, S206–13.
33. Public Health England. Immunisation Against Infectious Disease (updated 2nd September 2014): "The Green Book". Available at: https://www.gov.uk/government/collections/immunisation-against-infectious-disease-the-green-book (accessed 08/04/15).

Leflunomide + Infliximab

An isolated report describes a delayed hypersensitivity reaction in a boy receiving leflunomide and infliximab. However, one study suggests that concurrent use does not increase the rate of adverse effects.

Clinical evidence, mechanism, importance and management

In a 30-week study, 72 patients with active rheumatoid arthritis who had received oral leflunomide for at least 16 weeks were given infliximab 3 mg/kg intravenously at weeks 0, 2, 6, 14, and 22. Serious adverse events occurred in 16 patients (22%), but the combination did not appear to increase the rate of toxicities or result in unexpected adverse events.[1] However, a 17-year-old boy with refractory psoriatic arthritis developed a unique cutaneous hypersensitivity reaction, manifesting as a vasculitic-like skin rash, after he had been receiving infliximab and leflunomide for 9 months. The rash cleared within 2 months of discontinuing treatment.[2] The general relevance of this isolated case is unclear.

1. Kalden JR, Nüßlein HG, Wollenhaupt J, Burmester GR, Krüger K, Antoni C. Combination treatment with infliximab and leflunomide in patients with active rheumatoid arthritis: safety and efficacy in an open-label clinical trial. *Clin Exp Rheumatol* (2008) 26, 834–40.
2. Vesel T, Luzar B, Calonje E, Avčin T. Syringotropic hypersensitivity reaction associated with infliximab and leflunomide combination therapy in a child with psoriatic arthritis. *J Cutan Pathol* (2008) 36, 991–4..

Leflunomide + Itraconazole

A case of fatal fulminant hepatic failure has been reported in a patient taking leflunomide and itraconazole.

Clinical evidence, mechanism, importance and management

A 68-year-old woman who had been taking leflunomide 10 mg daily for about 4 months started taking itraconazole 300 mg daily for a fungal infection. About one month later her leflunomide dose was increased to 20 mg daily, and liver function tests were normal. The following month, she developed abdominal pain, vomiting, and weakness. Despite symptomatic treatment and washout with colestyramine, fatal fulminant hepatic failure occurred. The authors of the report attribute the reaction to additive hepatotoxicity between the leflunomide and itraconazole.[1] This interaction serves to highlight the cautions about the use of leflunomide with other hepatotoxic drugs, see *Alcohol* under 'Leflunomide or Teriflunomide + Miscellaneous', p.1266, and 'Leflunomide + Methotrexate', p.1266.

1. Legras A, Bergemer-Fouquet A-M, Jonville-Bera A-P. Fatal hepatitis with leflunomide and itraconazole. *Am J Med* (2002) 113, 352–3.

Leflunomide + Methotrexate

Methotrexate may increase leflunomide hepatotoxicity and haematotoxicity.

Clinical evidence, mechanism, importance and management

No pharmacokinetic interaction was seen in patients taking methotrexate (mean dose 17.2 mg per week) with leflunomide (100 mg daily for 2 days as a loading dose followed by 10 to 20 mg daily).[1] However, elevated liver enzyme levels have been seen following concurrent use.[2,3] By March 2001, the EMEA was aware of 129 cases of serious hepatic reactions in patients taking leflunomide, and 78% of these were in patients also taking other hepatotoxic medications. In patients with elevated liver function tests, 58% were also taking methotrexate and/or NSAIDs.[4]

Pancytopenia has also been associated with the use of leflunomide with methotrexate.[5,6] The Australian Adverse Drug Reactions Advisory Committee (ADRAC) received 11 reports of pancytopenia associated with the use of leflunomide during its first 31 months of marketing and in 9 of these cases, the patients were also taking methotrexate. In 2 cases, methotrexate was added to leflunomide and in the other 7 cases methotrexate use preceded leflunomide use. In 5 of these cases methotrexate had been taken in weekly doses for a mean of 336 weeks (range 103 to 650 weeks) without the development of pancytopenia; however, when leflunomide was added the blood dyscrasia developed within 6 to 78 weeks. Of the total 394 reports describing any type of adverse reaction associated with leflunomide over the 31-month study period, 128 reports (32.5%) also recorded methotrexate being taken concurrently.[6] Another report describes 5 cases of severe pancytopenia occurring within 23 days to 4 years of starting leflunomide and methotrexate.[7]

Due to the possible risks of additive or synergistic liver toxicity or haematotoxicity, particularly when used long-term, the UK manufacturer says that the concurrent use of methotrexate is not advisable.[2] The US manufacturer says that if concurrent use is undertaken, long-term monitoring should be increased to monthly intervals.[3] Close liver enzyme and haematological monitoring is also recommended if switching between these drugs, and colestyramine or activated charcoal washout is recommended as it may decrease the risk of toxicity when switching from leflunomide to methotrexate.[2,3]

1. Weinblatt ME, Kremer JM, Coblyn JS, Maier AL, Helfgott SM, Morrell M, Byrne VM, Kaymakcian MV, Strand V. Pharmacokinetics, safety, and efficacy of combination treatment with methotrexate and leflunomide in patients with active rheumatoid arthritis. *Arthritis Rheum* (1999) 42, 1322–8.
2. Arava (Leflunomide). Sanofi. UK Summary of product characteristics, September 2014.
3. Arava (Leflunomide). Sanofi-Aventis US LLC. US Prescribing information, August 2014.
4. EMEA. EMEA public statement on leflunomide (Arava) - severe and serious hepatic reactions. London, 12 March 2001. Available at: http://www.ema.europa.eu/docs/en_GB/document_library/Public_statement/2009/12/WC500018389.pdf (accessed 21/10/15).
5. Hill RL, Topliss DJ, Purcell PM. Pancytopenia associated with leflunomide and methotrexate. *Ann Pharmacother* (2003) 37, 149.
6. McEwen J, Purcell PM, Hill RL, Calcino LJ, Riley CG. The incidence of pancytopenia in patients taking leflunomide alone or with methotrexate. *Pharmacoepidemiol Drug Safety* (2007) 16, 65–73.
7. Chan J, Sanders DC, Du L, Pillans PI. Leflunomide-associated pancytopenia with or without methotrexate. *Ann Pharmacother* (2004) 38, 1206–11.

Leflunomide or Teriflunomide + Miscellaneous

The serum concentrations of the active metabolite of leflunomide (teriflunomide) are reduced by activated charcoal and colestyramine. The manufacturers predict interactions between leflunomide or teriflunomide and CYP1A2 substrates, CYP2C8 substrates, and substrates of the drug transporter proteins BCRP, OAT, and OATP. The effect of rifampicin (rifampin) on teriflunomide is not conclusive. Concurrent use of leflunomide with other DMARDs (other than methotrexate) has not been studied, but there might be an increased risk of serious adverse reactions. No clinically relevant interaction occurs between leflunomide or teriflunomide and cimetidine, corticosteroids, NSAIDs, or tolbutamide.

Clinical evidence, mechanism, importance and management

(a) Charcoal or Colestyramine

Studies in healthy subjects found that colestyramine 8 g three times daily for 24 hours reduced the plasma concentration of the active metabolite of leflunomide (teriflunomide) by 40% after 24 hours and by 49 to 65% after 48 hours.[1,2]

Treatment with activated charcoal 50 g every 6 hours for 24 hours, either orally or by nasogastric tube, reduced teriflunomide concentrations by 37% after 24 hours and by 48% after 48 hours.[1,2]

These drugs are thought to bind with teriflunomide in the gut, reducing plasma concentrations by a gastrointestinal dialysis mechanism and/or by interrupting the enterohepatic cycle.[1] Patients should therefore not be given either colestyramine or activated charcoal with leflunomide[1] or teriflunomide,[3] unless the intention is to remove either drug from the body more quickly (see also *DMARDs*, below).

(b) Cimetidine

The UK manufacturer of leflunomide briefly notes that cimetidine had no clinically relevant effect on the exposure of its active metabolite, teriflunomide.[1] For discussion of the potential for teriflunomide to alter the exposure to cimetidine, via OAT3, see *Drug transporter proteins*, below.

(c) Corticosteroids

The UK and US manufacturers of leflunomide state that corticosteroids can continue to be used if leflunomide is given.[1,2]

(d) CYP1A2 substrates

The manufacturers of leflunomide[1] and teriflunomide[3,4] briefly note that, in a study, repeated doses of teriflunomide decreased the maximum concentration and AUC of the CYP1A2 substrate, **caffeine**, by 18% and 55%, respectively. They recommend that drugs that are CYP1A2 substrates should be used with caution due to the potential for reduced efficacy,[1,3] or that their use should be monitored and the dose adjusted as necessary.[4] Note that caffeine can be used as a probe substrate to assess the activity of CYP1A2. This study therefore suggests that teriflunomide (and hence leflunomide) is a moderate inducer of CYP1A2. For a list of CYP1A2 substrates see 'Table 1.2', p.5.

(e) CYP2C8 substrates

The manufacturers of leflunomide[1] and teriflunomide[3,4] briefly note that, in a study, repeated doses of teriflunomide increased the maximum concentration and AUC of the CYP2C8 substrate, **repaglinide**, by 70% and 2.4-fold, respectively. They recommend that drugs that are CYP2C8 substrates should be used with caution,[1,3] or that their use should be monitored and the dose adjusted as necessary.[4] The US manufacturer of teriflunomide also notes that the increase in exposure to CYP2C8 substrates in patients could be higher at the recommended dose of repaglinide (only a single 0.25 mg dose was used in the study).[4] Note that repaglinide can be used as a probe substrate to assess the activity of CYP2C8. This study therefore suggests that teriflunomide (and hence leflunomide) is a moderate inhibitor of CYP2C8. For a list of CYP2C8 substrates see 'Table 1.4', p.6.

(f) DMARDs

The UK and US manufacturers state that the concurrent use of leflunomide and other DMARDs (they list **azathioprine**, **chloroquine**, **hydroxychloroquine**, intramuscular or oral **gold**, and **penicillamine**) has not yet been studied,[1,2] but the UK manufacturer states that combined use is not advisable because of the increased risk of serious adverse reactions (haemo- or hepatotoxicity).[1] As teriflunomide, the active metabolite of leflunomide, has a long half-life of 1 to 4 weeks, a washout with colestyramine or activated charcoal is recommended and the manufacturers state that this might decrease the risk of toxicity if patients are to be given other DMARDs.[1,2]

See also 'Leflunomide + Methotrexate', above.

(g) Drug transporter proteins

The manufacturers of leflunomide[1] and teriflunomide[3,4] briefly note that, in a study, repeated doses of teriflunomide increased the maximum concentration and AUC of **cefaclor**, by 43% and 54%, respectively. They suggest that teriflunomide (and hence leflunomide) is an inhibitor of organic anion transporter-3 (OAT3) and recommend that drugs that are OAT3 substrates should be used with caution,[1,3] or that their use should be monitored and the dose adjusted as necessary.[4] They specifically name **benzylpenicillin**, **cefaclor**, **cimetidine**, **ciprofloxacin**, **furosemide**, **ketoprofen**, **methotrexate**, and **zidovudine**.[1,3,4] The UK manufacturers additionally list **indometacin**.[1,3]

Similarly, the manufacturers briefly note that, in another study, repeated doses of teriflunomide increased the maximum concentration and AUC of **rosuvastatin** 2.7- and 2.5-fold, respectively.[1,3,4] The UK manufacturers also note that the increase in rosuvastatin exposure did not result in an increase in the effect on HMG-CoA reductase activity.[1,3] The UK manufacturers of teriflunomide[3] recommend that the dose of rosuvastatin should be reduced by 50% on concurrent use. The US manufacturer of teriflunomide, and the UK manufacturer of leflunomide[1], recommend that the dose of rosuvastatin be restricted to a maximum of 10 mg daily on concurrent use.[4] For other drugs that are substrates of breast cancer resistance protein (BCRP) or the organic anion transporting polypeptide (OATP) family (in particular, the **statins**), they advise some caution, and suggest that patients should be closely monitored for signs and symptoms of excessive exposure, with consideration given to reducing the dose of these drugs on concurrent use.[1,3,4] The manufacturers specifically name **daunorubicin**, **doxorubicin**, **methotrexate**, **sulfasalazine**, **topotecan**,[1,3] and **mitoxantrone**[4] as substrates of BCRP, and **atorvastatin**, **methotrexate**, **nateglinide**, **pravastatin**, **repaglinide**, **rifampicin (rifampin)**, and **simvastatin**,[1,3,4] as substrates of OATP.

(h) Food

The manufacturers briefly note that food does not have clinically relevant effects on the pharmacokinetics of either leflunomide[1] or teriflunomide.[3,4]

(i) NSAIDs

The US manufacturer of leflunomide states that its active metabolite, teriflunomide, inhibits the activity of CYP2C9 *in vitro*, and might therefore be expected to increase the serum concentrations of NSAIDs that are metabolised by this isoenzyme.[2] In addition, it is extensively bound to protein and might displace other highly protein-bound drugs, and both the UK and US manufacturers of leflunomide briefly note that, *in vitro* teriflunomide displaced **diclofenac** and **ibuprofen**. However, as the unbound fraction only increased between 10 and 50%, the effect was not considered to be clinically relevant,[1,2] and no safety problems were seen in clinical studies when leflunomide was used extensively with NSAIDs.[2] Therefore, the use of NSAIDs can be continued with leflunomide.[1,2]

(j) Rifampicin (Rifampin)

When a single dose of leflunomide was given to subjects after taking multiple-dose rifampicin, the maximum concentration of its active metabolite, teriflunomide, increased by 40% but the AUC was unchanged.[1,2] There would seem to be no reason for avoiding concurrent use of leflunomide and rifampicin, but note that the US manufacturer advises caution as metabolite concentrations could increase with multiple dosing.[2] It might therefore be prudent to increase the frequency of leflunomide monitoring if these two drugs are used together.

In contrast, when a high single 70-mg dose of teriflunomide was given after rifampicin 600 mg once daily for 22 days, the teriflunomide AUC was decreased by 40%.[3] However, the US manufacturer states that rifampicin does not affect the pharmacokinetics of teriflunomide.[4] The UK manufacturer of teriflunomide advises caution if rifampicin or other potent inducers of cytochrome P450 isoenzymes or transporters, they name **carbamazepine**, **phenobarbital** (and therefore **primidone**), **phenytoin** (and therefore **fosphenytoin**), and **St John's wort**, are given concurrently.[3]

(k) Tolbutamide

Teriflunomide (the active metabolite of leflunomide) is extensively bound to protein and might displace other highly protein-bound drugs. The UK and US manufacturers of leflunomide briefly note that, *in vitro*, teriflunomide displaced tolbutamide, but the unbound fraction of tolbutamide only increased between 10 and 50%.[1,2] However, the unbound fraction of teriflunomide increased 2- to 3-fold in the presence of tolbutamide.[1] Neither of these changes are considered clinically relevant.[1] Tolbutamide is also a substrate for CYP2C9, which is inhibited by teriflunomide *in vitro*, however the clinical importance of this is not known, as teriflunomide has been shown not to affect the metabolism of the CYP2C9 probe substrate *S*-warfarin. Nevertheless changes in INR have been seen clinically, see 'Coumarins + Leflunomide or Teriflunomide', p.443.

(l) Other CYP substrates

The US manufacturer of teriflunomide briefly notes that it has no effect on the pharmacokinetics of **bupropion** (a CYP2B6 substrate), **omeprazole** (a CYP2C19 substrate), **metoprolol** (a CYP2D6 substrate), or **midazolam** (a CYP3A4 substrate).[4] The US manufacturer of leflunomide also notes that because teriflunomide (its active metabolite) inhibits CYP2C9 *in vitro*, it has the potential to affect the pharmacokinetics of **phenytoin** which is metabolised by this isoenzyme, but they state that the clinical importance of this is not known.[2] Note that teriflunomide has been shown not to affect the metabolism of the CYP2C9 probe substrate *S*-warfarin. Nevertheless changes in INR have been seen clinically, see 'Coumarins + Leflunomide or Teriflunomide', p.443.

1. Arava (Leflunomide). Sanofi. UK Summary of product characteristics, September 2014.
2. Arava (Leflunomide). Sanofi-Aventis US LLC. US Prescribing information, August 2014.
3. Aubagio (Teriflunomide). Genzyme Therapeutics. UK Summary of product characteristics, September 2014.
4. Aubagio (Teriflunomide). Genzyme Corp. US Prescribing information, October 2014.

Leflunomide + Tegafur with Uracil

A case of peripheral neuropathy has been reported in a patient taking leflunomide and tegafur with uracil.

Clinical evidence, mechanism, importance and management

A 75-year-old man with rectal cancer was given a 28-day course of tegafur 200 mg three times daily (with uracil) and calcium folinate 30 mg daily. Treatment was withheld because of an episode of minor duodenal bleeding and 3 months later he was given leflunomide 100 mg daily for 3 days followed by 20 mg daily to treat rheumatoid arthritis. A further two courses of tegafur and uracil (separated by 7 days) were given because of tumour progression, after which the patient had increasing numbness of the lower extremities, diagnosed as polyneuropathy. He also had severe diarrhoea and hand-foot syndrome. These symptoms had not occurred when tegafur and uracil had been given without leflunomide, and hence an interaction was suspected.

Tegafur is a prodrug of fluorouracil, which is given with uracil to prevent fluorouracil degradation (by inhibiting dihydropyrimidine dehydrogenase). Both tegafur with uracil and leflunomide may cause neurotoxicity and therefore the effects seen may have occurred as a result of simple additive toxicity. The authors suggested that leflunomide may increase fluorouracil toxicity by increasing its conversion to fluorouracil monophosphate, or by enhancing the effect of uracil by additional inhibition of dihydropyrimidine dehydrogenase.[1] This is an isolated case and its general importance is unclear.

1. Kopp H-G, Kanz L, Hartmann JT, Moerike K. Leflunomide and peripheral neuropathy: a potential interaction between uracil/tegafur and leflunomide. *Clin Pharmacol Ther* (2005) 78, 89–90.

Monoclonal antibodies + Azathioprine or Mercaptopurine

Infliximab can increase serum concentrations of azathioprine metabolites, and giving azathioprine and mercaptopurine with infliximab might be associated with higher minimum concentrations of infliximab. Adalimumab clearance is not affected by azathioprine or mercaptopurine, and basiliximab clearance is only slightly affected by azathioprine.

A rare T-cell lymphoma has been reported in adolescents and young adults given infliximab and azathioprine or mercaptopurine, and serious infection might be associated with the concurrent use of natalizumab and azathioprine or mercaptopurine.

Clinical evidence, mechanism, importance and management

(a) Adalimumab

In a study of the pharmacokinetics of adalimumab, the concurrent use of either azathioprine (36 patients) or mercaptopurine (23 patients) slightly lowered or had no impact on adalimumab clearance.[1] Therefore, no adalimumab dose adjustment would appear to be necessary on concurrent use. However, the manufacturers of adalimumab state that cases of hepatosplenic T-cell lymphoma have been reported in patients with ulcerative colitis or Crohn's disease and given adalimumab with azathioprine or mercaptopurine, although a causative link is not established.[2,3] Until more is known, it would seem prudent to bear this possible risk in mind if concurrent use is necessary.

(b) Basiliximab

Azathioprine, added to regimens including basiliximab, ciclosporin microemulsion, and corticosteroids, reduced the clearance of basiliximab by 22%.[4-6] However, the use of basiliximab in triple regimens with azathioprine did not increase adverse effects or infections.[4,5] No dose adjustment is considered necessary if basiliximab is added to triple-immunosuppression regimens including ciclosporin, corticosteroids, and azathioprine.[5,6]

(c) Infliximab

In 32 patients with Crohn's disease taking azathioprine (mean dose 2.81 mg/kg) and with stable concentrations of 6-tioguanine nucleotides (the active metabolites of azathioprine), an infusion of infliximab 5 mg/kg over 2 hours resulted in a considerable increase in 6-tioguanine nucleotide concentrations in 21 patients after 1 to 3 weeks, when compared with pre-infusion concentrations. The leucocyte count was decreased and mean corpuscular volume increased. Increases in 6-tioguanine nucleotides were associated with good tolerance and a favourable response to infliximab. These changes were transient even in patients who received two additional infusions of infliximab over the following 6 weeks: concentrations returned to normal 3 months after the first infusion.[7]

The manufacturers state that rare post-marketing cases of an aggressive and usually fatal hepatosplenic T-cell lymphoma have been reported in adolescent and young adult patients with Crohn's disease who were given infliximab. All cases occurred in patients also receiving azathioprine or mercaptopurine, either with or immediately before the use of infliximab. A causal relationship is unclear.[8,9] Up until October 2006, the Adverse Event Reporting System (AERS) database of the FDA in the US had received 8 case reports of hepatosplenic T-cell lymphoma associated with infliximab use in young patients being treated for Crohn's disease or ulcerative colitis; all had received concurrent azathioprine and/or mercaptopurine.[10] Further study has suggested that, in patients with Crohn's disease, continuing azathioprine or mercaptopurine with infliximab beyond 6 months offers no clear benefit over infliximab monotherapy, but is associated with a higher median infliximab minimum concentration and a decreased C-reactive protein concentration.[11]

No infliximab dose adjustments appear to be necessary on the concurrent use of azathioprine or mercaptopurine, but the long-term benefits of treatment need further study.

(d) Natalizumab

In clinical studies in patients with Crohn's disease, the concurrent use of natalizumab with long-term mercaptopurine and azathioprine did not result in an increase in overall infections, when compared with natalizumab alone.[12] Nevertheless, for patients with Crohn's disease, the manufacturer states that natalizumab should not be used with azathioprine or mercaptopurine because of the potential for increased risk of progressive multifocal leukoencephalopathy and other infections.[12]

1. Garimella TS, Peng JZ, Beck K, Noertersheuser PA, Lomax KG, Paulson SK, Pollack PF. Pharmacokinetics of adalimumab in a long-term investigation of the induction and maintenance of remission in patients with Crohn's disease (CLASSIC I and CLASSIC II). *Gastroenterology* (2006) 130 (Suppl 2), A481.
2. Humira (Adalimumab). AbbVie Ltd. UK Summary of product characteristics, August 2012.
3. Humira (Adalimumab). Abbott Laboratories. US Prescribing information, May 2014.
4. Simulect (Basiliximab). Novartis Pharmaceuticals UK Ltd. UK Summary of product characteristics, October 2008.
5. Simulect (Basiliximab). Novartis Pharmaceuticals Corporation. US Prescribing information, September 2005.
6. Kovarik JM, Pescovitz MD, Sollinger HW, Kaplan B, Legendre C, Salmela K, Book BK, Gerbeau C, Girault D, Somberg K; on behalf of the Simulect Phase IV Study Group. Differential influence of azathioprine and mycophenolate mofetil on the disposition of basiliximab in renal transplant patients. *Clin Transplant* (2001) 15, 123–30.
7. Roblin X, Serre-Debeauvais F, Phelip J-M, Bessard G, Bonaz B. Drug interaction between infliximab and azathioprine in patients with Crohn's disease. *Aliment Pharmacol Ther* (2003) 18, 917–25.
8. Remicade (Infliximab). Schering-Plough Ltd. UK Summary of product characteristics, March 2009.
9. Remicade (Infliximab). Janssen Biotech, Inc. US Prescribing information, November 2013.
10. Mackey AC, Green L, Liang L-c, Dinndorf P, Avigan M. Hepatosplenic T cell lymphoma associated with infliximab use in young patients treated for inflammatory bowel disease. *J Pediatr Gastroenterol Nutr* (2007) 44, 265–7.
11. Van Assche G, Magdelaine-Beuzelin C, D'Haens G, Baert F, Noman M, Vermeire S, Ternant D, Watier H, Paintaud G, Rutgeerts P. Withdrawal of immunosuppression in Crohn's disease treated with scheduled infliximab maintenance: a randomized trial. *Gastroenterology* (2008) 134, 1861–8.
12. Tysabri (Natalizumab). Biogen Idec Inc. US Prescribing information, October 2008.

Monoclonal antibodies + Cytochrome P450 substrates

Although the manufacturers of anakinra, adalimumab, golimumab, and infliximab predict that they might interact with substrates of the cytochrome P450 isoenzyme system, clinical data to confirm this is lacking.

Clinical evidence, mechanism, importance and management

The UK manufacturer of **anakinra**,[1] and the US manufacturers of **adalimumab**,[2] **golimumab**,[3] and **infliximab**[4] note that they might reverse the suppression of cytochrome P450 isoenzymes caused by the cytokines which monoclonal antibodies antagonise, and thus could increase the production of cytochrome P450 isoenzymes. They therefore advise that patients taking drugs metabolised by cytochrome P450 isoenzymes, that have a narrow therapeutic window (they name **ciclosporin**,[2-4] **phenytoin**,[1] **theophylline**,[2-4] and **warfarin**[1-4]) should be monitored when any of these monoclonal antibodies are started or stopped, as they might require a dose adjustment.[1] At present there appears to be no *in vitro* or clinical data to confirm these predicted interactions. Furthermore, infliximab does not appear to have these effects in practice.

For details of the effects of tocilizumab on cytochrome P450 substrates, see 'Monoclonal antibodies; Tocilizumab + Cytochrome P450 substrates', below and 'Statins + Monoclonal antibodies; Tocilizumab', p.1351.

1. Kineret (Anakinra). Swedish Orphan Biovitrum Ltd. UK Summary of product characteristics, November 2013.
2. Humira (Adalimumab). AbbVie Inc. US Prescribing information, May 2014.
3. Simponi (Golimumab). Janssen Biotech Inc. US Prescribing information, January 2014.
4. Remicade (Infliximab). Janssen Biotech, Inc. US Prescribing information, November 2013.

Monoclonal antibodies; Tocilizumab + Cytochrome P450 substrates

Tocilizumab appears to slightly reduce omeprazole exposure, but its effects on dextromethorphan were minimal. It is predicted that it might interact similarly with other substrates of cytochrome P450 isoenzymes.

Clinical evidence

(a) Dextromethorphan

The US manufacturer briefly notes that in a study in 13 rheumatoid arthritis patients, a single infusion of tocilizumab 8-mg/kg given 1 week after dextromethorphan 30 mg, reduced the AUC of dextromethorphan and its active metabolite, dextrorphan, by 5% and 29% , respectively.[1]

(b) Omeprazole

The US manufacturer briefly notes that in a study in rheumatoid arthritis patients, a single infusion of tocilizumab 8-mg/kg given 1 week after omeprazole 10 mg reduced the AUC of omeprazole by 28%.[1]

Mechanism

Cytokines, such as interleukin-6, which is found at increased concentrations in patients with rheumatoid arthritis, can suppress the expression of cytochrome P450 enzymes. *In vitro* studies have shown that tocilizumab, an interleukin-6 inhibitor, can reverse the suppression of cytochrome P450 isoenzymes caused by interleukin. As a result, the activity of CYP1A2, CYP2B6, CYP2C9, CYP2C19, CYP2D6, and CYP3A4 might return to normal, and their metabolic capacity could increase.[1,2] Results from the studies in patients demonstrate this for CYP2C19 (using omeprazole) and CYP2D6 (using dextromethorphan). Further study is required to confirm the effect on other isoenzymes.

Importance and management

Evidence for interactions between tocilizumab and cytochrome P450 substrates is limited. However, from that available it seems that tocilizumab does slightly reduce omeprazole exposure, but as omeprazole has a wide therapeutic range, a change of this magnitude is unlikely to be of clinical importance. The reduction in dextromethorphan exposure seen is too small to be of any clinical importance. For drugs with a narrow therapeutic range, changes in pharmacokinetics as a result of the concurrent use of tocilizumab could be important. As such, the UK manufacturer therefore advises that patients taking drugs metabolised by these isoenzymes (they name **theophylline** (CYP1A2), **warfarin** (CYP2C9), **phenytoin** (CYP2C19), **benzodiazepines** [e.g. midazolam], **calcium-channel blockers**, and **ciclosporin** (CYP3A4)) should be monitored as they might require a dose adjustment on concurrent use with tocilizumab to ensure efficacy.[2] The US manufacturer offers the same advice, but limits this to **ciclosporin**, **theophylline**, and **warfarin**. However, it also advises caution with drugs where a decrease in effectiveness is undesirable, such as **oral contraceptives**.[1] Until more is known, it would be prudent to consider the possibility of an interaction if clinical symptoms suggest that the concentrations of these drugs have been reduced. Note that as tocilizumab has a long half-life, any clinically relevant effect on cytochrome P450 isoenzymes is likely to persist for up to several weeks after it has been stopped.[2]

For information on an interaction between tocilizumab and simvastatin (a CYP3A4 substrate), see 'Statins + Monoclonal antibodies; Tocilizumab', p.1351.

1. Actemra (Tocilizumab). Genentech, Inc. US Prescribing information, October 2013.
2. RoActemra (Tocilizumab). Roche Products Ltd. Summary of product characteristics, April 2014.

Monoclonal antibodies + Methotrexate

The clearance of adalimumab may be decreased by methotrexate. Concurrent use may decrease antibody formation and result in elevations in liver enzymes. The concurrent use of methotrexate with natalizumab is predicted to increase the risk of developing infections, some of which may be severe. Several other monoclonal antibodies do not appear to interact with methotrexate, and some are specifically licensed for concurrent use.

Clinical evidence, mechanism, importance and management

(a) Adalimumab

In 45 patients with rheumatoid arthritis taking stable doses of methotrexate for at least 3 months, the mean clearance of a single intravenous dose of adalimumab was decreased by approximately 22%, when compared with 89 similar patients who did not receive methotrexate.[1] Another study found that giving adalimumab to patients taking methotrexate had no statistically significant effect on the pharmacokinetics of methotrexate.[2] No dose adjustment of either adalimumab or methotrexate is considered necessary when they are given concurrently.[3]

The manufacturers say that giving adalimumab in the absence of methotrexate resulted in increased formation of antibodies, increased clearance and reduced efficacy of adalimumab.[3,4] Elevations in liver enzymes have been observed with adalimumab alone, but appear to be more frequent in patients who have received both adalimumab and methotrexate.[3,4] It may therefore be prudent to increase the frequency of liver enzyme monitoring if both drugs are given.

(b) Rituximab

A study in 38 patients with highly active rheumatoid arthritis found that the pharmacokinetics of rituximab were not altered by the concurrent use of methotrexate.[5]

(c) Tocilizumab

The manufacturer reports that a single 10 mg/kg dose of tocilizumab had no clinically relevant effect on the overall exposure to methotrexate (given weekly at a dose of 10 to 25 mg weekly). They also state that, in population pharmacokinetic analyses, methotrexate had no significant effect on the clearance of tocilizumab. Therefore, no dose adjustments appear to be necessary should tocilizumab be given with weekly methotrexate. Note that it is licensed for concurrent use with methotrexate.[6]

(d) Other monoclonal antibodies

Although specific interaction studies appear to be lacking certolizumab pegol[7] and golimumab[8] have been safely given with methotrexate in clinical studies. Note that certolizumab pegol and golimumab are specifically licensed for use with methotrexate.

In clinical studies, the concurrent use of natalizumab with methotrexate did not increase the risk of infection when compared with natalizumab alone. However, the US manufacturer specifically advises against the concurrent use of natalizumab with methotrexate due to the risk of progressive multifocal leukoencephalopathy (a viral infection that can lead to severe disability and death) and other infections, which have been associated with the use of natalizumab in immunosuppressed patients.[9]

1. Velagapudi RB, Noertersheuser PA, Awni WM, Fischkoff SA, Kupper H, Granneman RG, van de Putte LBA, Keystone EC. Effect of methotrexate coadministration on the pharmacokinetics of adalimumab (Humira, Abbott) following a single intravenous injection. *Arthritis Rheum* (2003) 48 (Suppl), S141.
2. Weisman MH, Moreland LW, Furst DE, Weinblatt ME, Keystone EC, Paulus HE, Teoh LS, Velagapudi RB, Noertersheuser PA, Granneman GR, Fischkoff SA, Chartash EK. Efficacy, pharmacokinetic, and safety assessment of adalimumab, a fully human anti-tumor necrosis factor-alpha monoclonal antibody, in adults with rheumatoid arthritis receiving concomitant methotrexate: a pilot study. *Clin Ther* (2003) 25, 1700–21.
3. Humira (Adalimumab). Abbott Laboratories. US Prescribing information, May 2014.
4. Humira (Adalimumab). AbbVie Ltd. UK Summary of product characteristics, August 2012.
5. Davies B, Shaw T. Rituximab pharmacokinetic characteristics are not influenced by combination with methotrexate or cyclophosphamide. *Ann Rheum Dis* (2004) 63, FRI0128.
6. RoActemra (Tocilizumab). Roche Products Ltd. Summary of product characteristics, April 2014.
7. Cimzia (Certolizumab pegol). UCB Inc. US Prescribing information, December 2008.
8. Simponi (Golimumab). Janssen Biotech Inc. US Prescribing information, January 2014.
9. Tysabri (Natalizumab). Biogen Idec Inc. US Prescribing information, October 2008.

Monoclonal antibodies; Infliximab + Methotrexate

The concurrent use of methotrexate has been reported to result in higher infliximab concentrations in some indications (e.g. rheumatoid arthritis), when compared with infliximab alone, but not others (e.g. ankylosing spondylitis).

Clinical evidence

In a clinical study in patients with rheumatoid arthritis, those given a low dose of infliximab 1 mg/kg alone (15 patients) had substantially lower infliximab minimum concentrations (0.1 micrograms/L, the lower limit of the assay), than 14 patients also given methotrexate 7.5 mg weekly (about 2 micrograms/L). However, no difference was found with higher infliximab doses (3 mg/kg and 10 mg/kg).[1] A cohort study in patients with Crohn's disease found that the 50 patients given methotrexate (15 mg weekly, either subcutaneously or intramuscularly) with infliximab (dose not stated) tended to have higher maximum infliximab concentrations (31 micrograms/mL) 4-weeks after the infliximab infusion, than the 59 patients given infliximab alone (21 micrograms/mL).[2] In a later prospective population pharmacokinetic study, 26 patients with axial ankylosing spondylitis were given either infliximab 5 mg/kg at weeks 0, 2, 6, 12, and 18 (14 patients), or the same dose of infliximab with methotrexate 10 mg weekly (12 patients). The AUC_{0-18} and the efficacy of infliximab were no different between the two groups.[3]

Mechanism

Uncertain. The authors of the studies showing lower infliximab concentrations alone than with concurrent methotrexate, suggest that this might possibly be due to the effect of methotrexate on infliximab antibody production. The development of infliximab antibodies might be reduced by methotrexate, thereby decreasing infliximab immunogenicity and improving infliximab pharmacokinetics.[1,2]

Table 29.3 Drugs that are not expected to interact with monoclonal antibodies as listed by the manufacturers

	Adalimumab[1]	*Basiliximab*[2,3]	*Infliximab*[4,5]	*Tocilizumab*[6]
Aminosalicylates	May be continued during treatment with adalimumab.		Infliximab levels unaffected by baseline aminosalicylate use.	
Analgesics		No increase in adverse effects with unspecified analgesics.	Infliximab clearance not affected by NSAIDs (population pharmacokinetic data).	Tocilizumab clearance not affected by NSAIDs (population pharmacokinetic data).
Antibacterials		No increase in adverse effects with unspecified antibacterials.	Infliximab levels unaffected by baseline ciprofloxacin or metronidazole use.	
Antifungals		No increase in adverse effects with unspecified antifungals.		
Antivirals		No increase in adverse effects with unspecified antivirals.		
Beta blockers		No increase in adverse effects with unspecified beta blockers.		
Calcium-channel blockers		No increase in adverse effects with unspecified calcium-channel blockers.		
Corticosteroids	May be continued during treatment with adalimumab.		Infliximab levels unaffected by baseline prednisolone use.	Tocilizumab clearance not affected (population pharmacokinetic data).
Diuretics		No increase in adverse effects with unspecified diuretics.		
PPIs			Infliximab clearance not affected by omeprazole (population pharmacokinetic data).	

1. Humira (Adalimumab). Abbott Laboratories. US Prescribing information, November 2009.
2. Simulect (Basiliximab). Novartis Pharmaceuticals UK Ltd. UK Summary of product characteristics, October 2008.
3. Simulect (Basiliximab). Novartis Pharmaceuticals Corporation. US Prescribing information, September 2005.
4. Remicade (Infliximab). Centocor Ortho Biotech, Inc. US Prescribing information, November 2009.
5. Xu Z, Seitz K, Fasanmade A, Ford J, Williamson P, Xu W, Davis HM, Zhou H. Population pharmacokinetics of infliximab in patients with ankylosing spondylitis. *J Clin Pharmacol* (2008) 48, 681–95.
6. RoActemra (Tocilizumab). Roche Products Ltd. UK Summary of product characteristics, November 2009.

The contrasting results seen in the population pharmacokinetic study, might be due to disease specific differences in tumour necrosis factor-alpha (TNF-α), which might limit the possible effects of methotrexate on infliximab pharmacokinetics in different patients.[3]

Importance and management

Evidence for a pharmacokinetic interaction between infliximab and methotrexate is limited and conflicting and so an interaction is not established. The effects seen in two of the studies[1,2] might possibly be due to the effect of methotrexate on infliximab antibody production rather than a direct effect of methotrexate on infliximab metabolism. The influence of disease cannot be ruled out and it appears that if any interaction occurs, it might be beneficial in some conditions and it might improve or maintain infliximab efficacy. It would seem that no additional precautions are necessary on the concurrent use of infliximab and methotrexate. Note that concurrent use is licensed for some conditions (e.g. rheumatoid arthritis).

1. Maini RN, Breedveld FC, Kalden JR, Smolen JS, Davis D, MacFarlane JD, Antoni C, Leeb B, Elliott MJ, Woody JN, Schaible TF, Feldmann M. Therapeutic efficacy of multiple intravenous infusions of anti-tumor necrosis factor α monoclonal antibody combined with low-dose weekly methotrexate in rheumatoid arthritis. *Arthritis Rheum* (1998) 41, 1552–63.
2. Vermeire S, Noman M, Van Assche G, Baert F, D'Haens G, Rutgeerts P. Effectiveness of concomitant immunosuppressive therapy in suppressing the formation of antibodies to infliximab in Crohn's disease. *Gut* (2007) 56, 1226–31.
3. Ternant D, Mulleman D, Lauféron F, Vignault C, Ducourau E, Wendling D, Goupille P, Paintaud G. Influence of methotrexate on infliximab pharmacokinetics and pharmacodynamics in ankylosing spondylitis. *Br J Clin Pharmacol* (2012) 73, 55–65.

Monoclonal antibodies + Miscellaneous

Monoclonal antibodies appear to increase the risk of infection in patients receiving drugs that are known to alter immune function (e.g. antineoplastics, immunosuppressants). They may also increase the risk of malignancy in predisposed individuals (e.g. tobacco smokers).

Clinical evidence, mechanism, importance and management

For a list of drugs that are not expected to interact with monoclonal antibodies, see 'Table 29.3', above.

(a) Antineoplastics

A study in 37 patients with highly active rheumatoid arthritis found that the pharmacokinetics of **rituximab** were not altered by the concurrent use of **cyclophosphamide**.[1]

The UK manufacturer of **natalizumab** contraindicates the concurrent use of immunosuppressant drugs, or other drugs that modulate the immune response, due to the increased risk of opportunistic infections, particularly progressive multifocal leukoencephalopathy (PML). They specifically name **cyclophosphamide** and **mitoxantrone**.[2] However, PML has developed in 2 patients taking **natalizumab** as monotherapy[3] and the US manufacturer says that the number of cases is too low to suggest that concurrent use of immunosuppressant drugs increases the risk of PML. Nevertheless, they suggest that concurrent use should be avoided wherever possible.[4] See also 'Monoclonal antibodies + Methotrexate', p.1268, and 'Monoclonal antibodies + Azathioprine or Mercaptopurine', p.1267.

(b) Corticosteroids

In clinical studies in patients with multiple sclerosis, short courses of corticosteroids were not associated with an increased rate of infection and therefore can be used in combination with **natalizumab**.[2,4] Furthermore, in clinical studies in patients with Crohn's disease, the concurrent use of natalizumab with long-term corticosteroids did not result in an increase in overall infections, when compared with **natalizumab** alone.[4] Nevertheless, it has been advised that care should be taken with patients who have previously received immunosuppressants, to allow sufficient time for immune function recovery to occur.[2,5]

(c) Glatiramer acetate

The UK manufacturer of **natalizumab** contraindicates its concurrent use with the immunomodulator glatiramer acetate,[2] because of the potential for an increase in the risk of infections.

(d) Muromonab-CD3

The manufacturers of **basiliximab** say that patients in phase 3 studies received **basiliximab** with muromonab-CD3 for episodes of rejection, with no increase in adverse events or infections. Human antimurine antibody responses were reported in 2 of 138 patients receiving basiliximab and 4 of 34 patients receiving both **basiliximab** and muromonab-CD3. Therefore, the manufacturers say that if **basiliximab** has been given, muromonab-CD3 or other murine antilymphocytic antibody preparations can still subsequently be given.[6,7]

In a clinical study in heart transplant patients taking ciclosporin, mycophenolate mofetil, and corticosteroids, the use of **daclizumab** was associated with an increase in infection-related deaths. Furthermore, concurrent use of another antilymphocyte (such as muromonab-CD3 or antithymocyte immunoglobulin) appeared to be associated with a higher incidence of fatal infection: 8 of 40 patients died, compared with 2 of 37 who received an antilymphocyte and placebo. The manufacturer suggested that the concurrent use of **daclizumab** with another antilymphocyte antibody in patients receiving intensive immunosuppression may be a factor leading to fatal infection.[8] Caution may be warranted.

(e) Mycophenolate

Mycophenolate mofetil, added to regimens including **basiliximab**, ciclosporin microemulsion and corticosteroids, reduced the clearance of **basiliximab** by 51%.[6,7,9] However, the use of basiliximab in triple regimens with mycophenolate did not increase adverse effects or infections.[6,7] No dose adjustment is considered necessary if **basiliximab** is added to triple-immunosuppression regimens including ciclosporin, corticosteroids and mycophenolate mofetil.[7,9]

A study in 75 renal transplant recipients given immunosuppressants, including mycophenolate mofetil, found that **daclizumab** had no effect on the pharmacokinetics of its active metabolite, mycophenolic acid. The pharmacokinetics of **daclizumab** were comparable with historical data, suggesting that mycophenolate mofetil did not affect the clearance of **daclizumab**. The addition of **daclizumab** to immunosuppressant treatment including mycophenolate mofetil did not appear to result in any increase in adverse events.[10] However, in one clinical study in heart transplant patients taking ciclosporin, mycophenolate mofetil, and corticosteroids, the use of **daclizumab** was associated with an increase in infection-related deaths.[8]

(f) Tobacco

In a study in patients with moderate to severe chronic obstructive pulmonary disease (COPD), more malignancies were reported in patients given **infliximab** than in control patients: all patients had a history of heavy smoking. The manufacturer suggests caution when considering the use of **infliximab** in patients with an increased risk for malignancy due to heavy smoking.[11] Furthermore, because of these findings, the manufacturer of **adalimumab** suggests caution in patients with COPD, as well as in patients with increased risk for malignancy due to heavy smoking.[12] Note that both **infliximab** and **adalimumab** are both tumour necrosis factor antibodies.

1. Davies B, Shaw T. Rituximab pharmacokinetic characteristics are not influenced by combination with methotrexate or cyclophosphamide. *Ann Rheum Dis* (2004) 63, FRI0128.
2. Tysabri (Natalizumab). Biogen Idec Ltd. UK Summary of product characteristics, January 2009.
3. Food and Drug Administration. Natalizumab (marketed as Tysabri) information. FDA Alert, August 2008. Available at: http://www.fda.gov/Drugs/DrugSafety/PostmarketDrugSafetyInformationforPatientsandProviders/ucm126592.htm (accessed 21/10/15).
4. Tysabri (Natalizumab). Biogen Idec Inc. US Prescribing information, October 2008.
5. Ilanjian H, Shane R. Washout period for immune-modifying drugs before natalizumab therapy. *Am J Health-Syst Pharm* (2008) 65, 18–19.
6. Simulect (Basiliximab). Novartis Pharmaceuticals UK Ltd. UK Summary of product characteristics, October 2008.
7. Simulect (Basiliximab). Novartis Pharmaceuticals Corporation. US Prescribing information, September 2005.
8. Zenapax (Daclizumab). Roche Pharmaceuticals. US Prescribing information, September 2005.
9. Kovarik JM, Pescovitz MD, Sollinger HW, Kaplan B, Legendre C, Salmela K, Book BK, Gerbeau C, Girault D, Somberg K; on behalf of the Simulect Phase IV Study Group. Differential influence of azathioprine and mycophenolate mofetil on the disposition of basiliximab in renal transplant patients. *Clin Transplant* (2001) 15, 123–30.
10. Pescovitz MD, Bumgardner G, Gaston RS, Kirkman RL, Light S, Patel IH, Nieforth K, Vincenti F. Pharmacokinetics of daclizumab and mycophenolate mofetil with cyclosporine and steroids in renal transplantation. *Clin Transplant* (2003) 17, 511–17.
11. Remicade (Infliximab). Schering-Plough Ltd. UK Summary of product characteristics, March 2009.
12. Humira (Adalimumab). AbbVie Ltd. UK Summary of product characteristics, August 2012.

Monoclonal antibodies + Tumour necrosis factor antagonists

The use of tumour necrosis factor antagonists with monoclonal antibodies can increase the incidence of neutropenia and severe infections.

Clinical evidence, mechanism, importance and management

A short-term study in patients with active Crohn's disease receiving **infliximab**, found that addition of **natalizumab** did not result in any significant safety concerns and the proportion of patients who experienced adverse effects associated with infection was comparable with patients who received infliximab alone.[1]

Despite one study suggesting safe effective use, it is generally recommended that the concurrent use of tumour necrosis factor antagonists should be avoided with monoclonal antibodies, because of the increased risk of neutropenia and severe infections.

1. Sands BE, Kozarek R, Spainhour J, Barish CF, Becker S, Goldberg L, Katz S, Goldblum R, Harrigan R, Hilton D, Hanauer SB. Safety and tolerability of concurrent natalizumab treatment for patients with Crohn's disease not in remission while receiving infliximab. *Inflamm Bowel Dis* (2007) 13, 2–11.

Monoclonal antibodies + Vaccines

Live vaccines should not be given to patients receiving monoclonal antibodies.

Clinical evidence, mechanism, importance and management

In general, there is little experience of the concurrent use of live vaccines with monoclonal antibodies. Therefore, many manufacturers of monoclonal antibodies (such as **adalimumab, certolizumab, golimumab, infliximab, tocilizumab**) recommend that live vaccines are not given to patients receiving a monoclonal antibody, because of the risk of generalised infection. Information about the use of other vaccines with monoclonal antibodies is similarly sparse. The manufacturer of **adalimumab** reports that, in a study in 226 patients with rheumatoid arthritis, the antibody response to **pneumococcal vaccine** and **influenza trivalent vaccine** did not differ between patients given adalimumab and patients given placebo.[1] Similarly, in a study in patients, **golimumab** had no significant effect on the response to **pneumococcal vaccine**. The fact that patients who also received methotrexate had a lower response to vaccination acted as a positive control.[2] The manufacturers advise that vaccines, other than live vaccines, may be given to patients receiving **adalimumab**[1] or **golimumab**.[2] However, it is also recommended that, if possible, patients with juvenile idiopathic arthritis are brought up-to-date with all standard scheduled immunisations before starting **adalimumab**.[1]

1. Humira (Adalimumab). AbbVie Ltd. UK Summary of product characteristics, August 2012.
2. Simponi (Golimumab). Janssen Biotech Inc. US Prescribing information, January 2014.

Monoclonal antibodies; Muromonab-CD3 + Indometacin

One report suggested that indometacin may possibly increase the incidence of encephalopathy and psychosis in patients given muromonab-CD3.

Clinical evidence, mechanism, importance and management

A study of patient records found that 4 out of a total of 55 kidney transplant patients (7.3%) given muromonab-CD3 and indometacin 50 mg orally or rectally every 6 to 8 hours for 48 to 72 hours developed serious encephalopathy and psychosis, compared with only 2 out of 173 patients (1.2%) who had received muromonab-CD3 without indometacin.[1]

This appears to be an isolated report, and its general significance is unknown. Indometacin has been used to reduce the adverse effects of muromonab-CD3, and in one analysis, concurrent use was associated with reduced fever, headache, and gastrointestinal disturbances.[2] Muromonab-CD3 alone is associated with encephalopathy and other CNS adverse effects, and the manufacturer warns that patients should be closely monitored for these effects.[3]

1. Chan GL, Weinstein SS, Wright CE, Bowers VD, Alveranga DY, Shires DL, Ackermann JR, LeFor WW, Kahana L. Encephalopathy associated with OKT3 administration. Possible interaction with indomethacin. *Transplantation* (1991) 52, 148–50.
2. Gaughan WJ, Francos BB, Dunn SR, Francos GC, Burke JF. A retrospective analysis of indomethacin on adverse reactions to orthoclone OKT3 in the therapy of acute renal allograft rejection. *Am J Kidney Dis* (1994) 24, 486–90.
3. Orthoclone OKT3 (Muromonab-CD3). Ortho Biotech. US Prescribing information, November 2004.

Monoclonal antibodies; Natalizumab + Interferon beta

Two cases of progressive multifocal leukoencephalopathy occurred in patients receiving natalizumab with interferon beta. Concurrent use does not cause a clinically relevant change in the pharmacokinetics of either drug.

Clinical evidence, mechanism, importance and management

In a study in 38 patients with multiple sclerosis who were receiving interferon beta-1a 30 micrograms weekly, 15 patients were given a single 3-mg/kg dose of natalizumab and 21 patients were given a single 6-mg/kg dose of natalizumab. There was no significant change in the pharmacokinetics of interferon beta, although there were large variations in interferon beta levels between patients. Using historical control data interferon beta did not cause a clinically significant increase in the exposure to natalizumab 6 mg, when compared with natalizumab alone.[1]

Two cases of progressive multifocal leukoencephalopathy (PML) occurred in patients with relapsing multiple sclerosis who were receiving natalizumab with interferon beta-1a.[2] The use of natalizumab has been associated with an increased risk of PML[3,4] but no causal link has been confirmed with the concurrent use interferon beta; however, the UK manufacturer contraindicates the use of natalizumab with beta interferons.[3]

1. Vollmer TL, Phillips JT, Goodman AD, Agius MA, Libonati MA, Giacchino JL, Grundy JS. An open-label safety and drug interaction study of natalizumab (Antegren™) in combination with interferon-beta (Avonex®) in patients with multiple sclerosis. *Multiple Sclerosis* (2004) 10, 511–20.
2. Rudick RA, Stuart WH, Calabresi PA, Confavreux C, Galetta SL, Radue E-W, Lublin FD, Weinstock-Guttman B, Wynn DR, Lynn F, Panzara MA, Sandrock AW, for the SENTINEL Investigators. Natalizumab plus interferon beta-1a for relapsing multiple sclerosis. *N Engl J Med* (2006) 354, 911–23.
3. Tysabri (Natalizumab). Biogen Idec Ltd. UK Summary of product characteristics, January 2009.
4. Tysabri (Natalizumab). Biogen Idec Inc. US Prescribing information, October 2008.

Mycophenolate + Aciclovir and related drugs

The concurrent use of aciclovir or ganciclovir and mycophenolate mofetil does not appear to alter the pharmacokinetics of either drug. There are reports of haematological toxicity in patients taking mycophenolate with valaciclovir, ganciclovir, or valganciclovir.

Clinical evidence

(a) Aciclovir or Valaciclovir

In a crossover study, healthy subjects were given single-doses of oral aciclovir 800 mg and mycophenolate mofetil 1 g, together and alone. The renal clearances of both drugs were not altered by concurrent use, but the AUC of aciclovir was increased by about 17% (not statistically significant), that of mycophenolic acid was increased by about 9% (not statistically significant), and that of the glucuronide metabolite of mycophenolate was increased by about 9%.[1,2] In another single-dose study in healthy subjects, the AUC of aciclovir was increased by 31% when it was given with mycophenolate mofetil, but there were no changes to mycophenolic acid pharmacokinetics. The concurrent use of valaciclovir 2 g with mycophenolate mofetil 1 g did not alter aciclovir pharmacokinetics, and the only change in mycophenolate pharmacokinetics was a 12% decrease in AUC of its glucuronide metabolite.[3]

A case report describes a kidney transplant patient taking mycophenolate mofetil 1 g twice daily (with a number of other drugs), who developed neutropenia after starting valaciclovir 6 g daily for prophylactic treatment of a cytomegalovirus infection, following successful treatment with ganciclovir. The neutropenia resolved on stopping the valaciclovir.[4]

(b) Ganciclovir or Valganciclovir

A crossover study in 12 transplant patients found no pharmacokinetic interaction between a single 1.5-g oral dose of mycophenolate mofetil and intravenous ganciclovir 5 mg/kg, but the renal clearance of ganciclovir was reduced, by 12%.[5]

Five cases of neutrophil dysplasia in transplant patients appeared to be related to the concurrent use of ganciclovir and mycophenolate, rather than to the use of mycophenolate alone.[6] A case report describes a kidney transplant patient who developed leucopenia which was attributed to the use of mycophenolate and valganciclovir,[7] and, in three retrospective analyses, the use of valganciclovir with mycophenolate appeared to be associated with an increased risk of myelotoxicity.[8-10] In one study, there was some evidence that this was more frequent with higher dose valganciclovir (900 mg versus 450 mg daily).[10]

Mechanism

The UK and US manufacturers of mycophenolate state that there might be competition for tubular secretion if it is given with aciclovir (or valaciclovir) or ganciclovir (or valganciclovir), and that increases in the concentrations of all these drugs, and the glucuronide metabolite of mycophenolate could occur. This might be of greatest importance in renal impairment.[11,12] Neutropenia is a rare adverse effect of valaciclovir alone, and the authors of the case report suggested that mycophenolate might increase the haematotoxicity of valaciclovir, especially at high doses.[4] Both mycophenolate mofetil and ganciclovir have the potential to cause neutropenia and leucopenia, therefore additive toxicity is possible on concurrent use.

Importance and management

Evidence for an interaction between mycophenolate and aciclovir and related drugs indicates that in general no clinically important interaction occurs, but in patients with impaired renal function clinically important changes in the pharmacokinetics of **aciclovir** (or **valaciclovir**), **ganciclovir** (or **valganciclovir**), or the glucuronide metabolite of mycophenolate might occur. It would seem prudent to monitor patients for adverse effects on concurrent use, if renal impairment is present.

The isolated case of neutropenia with mycophenolate and **valaciclovir**, suggests that it would be prudent to bear the possibility of an interaction in mind should neutropenia occur with the combination. Similarly, the cases of haematological toxicity with mycophenolate and **ganciclovir** or **valganciclovir** add a note of caution, and these combinations warrant monitoring for toxicity.

1. Shah J, Juan D, Bullingham R, Wong B, Wong R, Fu C. A single dose drug interaction study of mycophenolate mofetil and acyclovir in normal subjects. *J Clin Pharmacol* (1994) 34, 1029.
2. Syntex. Data on file. A single-dose, pharmacokinetic drug interaction study of oral mycophenolate mofetil and oral acyclovir in normal subjects. 1994.
3. Gimenez F, Foeillet E, Bourdon O, Weller S, Garret C, Bidault R, Singlas E. Evaluation of pharmacokinetic interactions after oral administration of mycophenolate mofetil and valaciclovir or aciclovir to healthy subjects. *Clin Pharmacokinet* (2004) 43, 685–92.
4. Royer B, Zanetta G, Bérard M, Davani S, Tanter Y, Rifle G, Kantelip J-P. A neutropenia suggesting an interaction between valacyclovir and mycophenolate mofetil. *Clin Transplant* (2003) 17, 158–61.
5. Wolfe EJ, Mathur V, Tomlanovich S, Jung D, Wong R, Griffy K, Aweeka FT. Pharmacokinetics of mycophenolate mofetil and intravenous ganciclovir alone and in combination in renal transplant recipients. *Pharmacotherapy* (1997) 17, 591–8.
6. Kennedy GA, Kay TD, Johnson DW, Hawley CM, Campbell SB, Isbel NM, Marlton P, Cobcroft R, Gill D, Cull G. Neutrophil dysplasia characterised by a pseudo-Pelger–Huet anomaly occurring with the use of mycophenolate mofetil and ganciclovir following renal transplantation: a report of five cases. *Pathology* (2002) 34, 263–6.
7. Izquierdo MJ, Rodrigo E, de Cos MA, Arias M. Leucopenia en el trasplantado renal consecuencia de la interacción entre el micofenolato mofetil y el valganciclovir. *Nefrologia* (2007) 27, 232–3.
8. Rerolle JP, Szelag JC, Le Meur Y. Unexpected rate of severe leucopenia with the association of mycophenolate mofetil and valganciclovir in kidney transplant recipients. *Nephrol Dial Transplant* (2007) 22, 671–2.
9. Manuel O, Venetz JP, Fellay J, Wasserfallen JB, Sturzenegger N, Fontana M, Matter M, Meylan PR, Pascual M. Efficacy and safety of universal valganciclovir prophylaxis combined with a tacrolimus/mycophenolate-based regimen in kidney transplantation. *Swiss Med Wkly* (2007) 137, 669–76.
10. Brum S, Nolasco F, Sousa J, Ferreira A, Possante M, Pinto JR, Barroso E, Santos JR. Leukopenia in kidney transplant patients with the association of valganciclovir and mycophenolate mofetil. *Transplant Proc* (2008) 40, 752–4.
11. CellCept Tablets (Mycophenolate mofetil). Roche Products Ltd. UK Summary of product characteristics, July 2013.
12. CellCept (Mycophenolate mofetil). Genentech USA, Inc. US Prescribing information, September 2013.

Mycophenolate + Allopurinol

No clinically relevant interactions have been seen between mycophenolate mofetil and allopurinol.

Clinical evidence, mechanism, importance and management

A study in 5 kidney transplant patients with gouty arthritis, who were switched from azathioprine to mycophenolate mofetil 2 g daily (to avoid the risk of an interaction between azathioprine and allopurinol), found that no adverse effects occurred when they were given allopurinol 100 or 200 mg daily. On average, 10 weeks after the switch had taken place, uricaemia had fallen by 21%, mean serum creatinine concentrations were only slightly increased (by 12%,) and white cell counts were unchanged.[1] Another study in 19 kidney transplant patients taking mycophenolate 2 g daily, ciclosporin, and prednisolone also found a reduction in uricaemia without any adverse effects on white cell count, after allopurinol 100 mg daily was also taken for 60 days.[2]

No particular precautions would therefore seem necessary if allopurinol is used with mycophenolate, although the authors of both studies suggest that long-term randomised studies are ideally needed to confirm safety.

1. Jacobs F, Mamzer-Bruneel MF, Skhiri H, Thervet E, Legendre Ch, Kreis H. Safety of the mycophenolate mofetil-allopurinol combination in kidney transplant recipients with gout. *Transplantation* (1997) 64, 1087–8.
2. Navascués RA, Gómez E, Rodriguez M, Laures AS, Baltar J, Grande JA. Safety of the allopurinol-mycophenolate mofetil combination in the treatment of hyperuricemia of kidney transplant patients. *Nephron* (2002) 91, 173–4.

Mycophenolate + Angiotensin II receptor antagonists

Telmisartan appears to decrease mycophenolic acid exposure, whereas candesartan and valsartan do not appear to affect mycophenolate pharmacokinetics.

Clinical evidence

In a study, 40 kidney transplant patients taking tacrolimus, corticosteroids, and mycophenolate mofetil were divided into four groups, and given telmisartan 40 mg daily, valsartan 80 mg daily, candesartan 8 mg daily, or no additional treatment, for at least 6 months. Candesartan and valsartan had no effect on the pharmacokinetics of mycophenolic acid, the active metabolite of mycophenolate, when compared with the control group, whereas the dose-adjusted AUC of mycophenolic acid was 29% lower in the telmisartan group than the control group.[1]

Mechanism

Unknown. The authors suggest that induction of glucuronidation by telmisartan might have some part to play.[1]

Importance and management

Evidence for an interaction between mycophenolate mofetil and the angiotensin II receptor antagonists appears to be limited to this study. Nevertheless, the reduction in mycophenolic acid exposure might be relevant in some patients and therefore it would appear prudent to consider the contribution of telmisartan if mycophenolic acid exposure declines over time or is less than desirable. If mycophenolic acid therapeutic drug monitoring is not being routinely undertaken, it might be prudent to consider periodic monitoring. Candesartan and valsartan do not appear to interact with mycophenolate mofetil.

1. Miura M, Satoh S, Kagaya H, Saito M, Inoue T, Ohkubo T, Habuchi T, Suzuki T. Effect of telmisartan, valsartan and candesartan on mycophenolate mofetil pharmacokinetics in Japanese renal transplant recipients. *J Clin Pharm Ther* (2009) 34, 68392.

Mycophenolate + Antacids

Aluminium/magnesium hydroxide antacids reduce the exposure to mycophenolate mofetil and mycophenolate sodium.

Clinical evidence, mechanism, importance and management

In a study in 10 patients, 10 mL of an **aluminium/magnesium hydroxide**-containing antacid (*Maalox TC*) taken four times daily with a single 2-g dose of mycophenolate mofetil, reduced the AUC of mycophenolic acid (the active form of the drug) by 17% and reduced its maximum plasma concentration by 38%.[1] Similarly, the UK and US manufacturers of mycophenolate sodium note that a single 30-mL dose of an **aluminium/magnesium hydroxide**-containing antacid reduced the AUC and maximum concentration of mycophenolic acid by about 37% and 25%, respectively.[2,3] However, the preliminary report of a retrospective study in 137 kidney transplant patients taking mycophenolate mofetil notes that, over a 20-week period, there was no difference in the AUC of mycophenolic acid in patients who also took an antacid (type not stated, 41 patients) when compared with those who did not (96 patients).[4]

The overall reduction in mycophenolate exposure seen when given with an **aluminium/magnesium hydroxide**-containing antacid is small, however the reductions in plasma concentration might be clinically important. The US manufacturer of mycophenolate mofetil states that **aluminium/magnesium**-containing antacids can be used in patients taking mycophenolate, but that they should not be given simultaneously.[5] With many other (but not all) antacid interactions, a 2-hour separation is usually sufficient to avoid an interaction. Similarly, the US manufacturer of mycophenolate sodium states that simultaneous administration of antacids should be avoided.[3] The UK manufacturer of mycophenolate mofetil states that **aluminium/magnesium**-containing antacids can be used intermittently for the treatment of occasional dyspepsia. However their long-term daily use with mycophenolate sodium is not recommended due to the potential for decreased mycophenolic acid exposure and reduced efficacy.[2] It would seem prudent to separate administration and check that the immunosuppressant effects of mycophenolate remain adequate in the presence of **aluminium/magnesium**-containing antacids. No general recommendations can be made based on the preliminary report, as it is not known what types of antacids were taken.

1. Bullingham R, Shah J, Goldblum R, Schiff M. Effects of food and antacid on the pharmacokinetics of single doses of mycophenolate mofetil in rheumatoid arthritis patients. *Br J Clin Pharmacol* (1996) 41, 513–16.
2. Myfortic (Mycophenolate sodium). Novartis Pharmaceuticals UK Ltd. UK Summary of product characteristics, November 2012.
3. Myfortic (Mycophenolate sodium). Novartis. US Prescribing information, September 2013.
4. van Gelder T, Pescovitz MD, Elzein H, Hamzeh F. The effect of gastric pH modulators on the pharmacokinetics of mycophenolate mofetil (MMF) in de novo renal transplant patients. *Transplantation* (2004) 78, P230.
5. CellCept (Mycophenolate mofetil). Genentech USA, Inc. US Prescribing information, September 2013.

Mycophenolate + Antibacterials

Amoxicillin with clavulanic acid, ciprofloxacin, metronidazole (alone and with norfloxacin), and a selective bowel decontamination regimen of nystatin, tobramycin, and cefuroxime have all modestly reduced mycophenolate minimum concentrations. No interaction appears to occur between mycophenolate and co-trimoxazole.

Clinical evidence

(a) Co-trimoxazole (Sulfamethoxazole with Trimethoprim)

In a study in healthy subjects,[1] co-trimoxazole 960 mg twice daily for 10 days had no effect on the AUC or maximum concentration of mycophenolic acid, when a single-dose of mycophenolate mofetil 1.5 g was given on day 8.

(b) Metronidazole

A study in 9 healthy subjects found that metronidazole 500 mg three times daily for 5 days reduced the AUC of a single 1-g oral dose of mycophenolate mofetil, given 2 hours after metronidazole on day 4, by 19%. The AUC of the glucuronide metabolite was also reduced, by 27%. When norfloxacin 400 mg twice daily was also given, the AUC of mycophenolate and its glucuronide metabolite were reduced by 33% and 41%, respectively.[2] A study analysing mycophenolic acid concentrations 12-hours post-dose in patients who had recently undergone kidney transplantation suggested that the use of metronidazole was associated with a 37% reduction in mycophenolic acid concentrations.[3]

(c) Penicillins

In a study in kidney transplant patients taking mycophenolate, mycophenolic acid minimum concentrations were monitored in patients receiving **amoxicillin** with **clavulanic acid** 375 mg three times daily for 7 days (20 patients) or for 14 days or more (17 patients). In both groups the minimum concentrations of mycophenolic acid were about 50% lower 3 days after starting the antibacterial, and they were still at this level on day 7. Three days after stopping the antibacterial in the 7-day group, the minimum concentration had returned to baseline. On day 14 in the longer-term group, the minimum concentrations had *increased*, and were just 19% lower than baseline.[4] A study analysing mycophenolic acid concentrations 12-hours post-dose in patients who had recently undergone kidney transplantation suggested that the use of **amoxicillin** with **clavulanic acid** was associated with a 53% reduction in mycophenolic acid concentrations.[3] A case report describes two kidney transplant patients who had a reduction in the AUC of mycophenolic acid after starting to take **amoxicillin** with **clavulanic acid**. In the first patient the AUC of mycophenolic acid, measured after 7 days of concurrent use, had decreased by about 40%. In the second patient the AUC of mycophenolic acid, measured after 10 days of concurrent use, was considered low (no baseline available for comparison): 5 days after **amoxicillin** with **clavulanic acid** was stopped the AUC had increased by 91%.[5]

(d) Quinolones

A study in 11 healthy subjects found that **norfloxacin** 400 mg twice daily reduced the AUC of a single 1-g oral dose of mycophenolate mofetil, given 2 hours after the antibacterial on day 4, by 10%. The AUC of the glucuronide metabolite was also reduced by 10%. When metronidazole 400 mg twice daily was also given, the AUC of mycophenolate and its glucuronide metabolite were reduced by 33% and 41%, respectively.[2]

In a study in kidney transplant patients taking mycophenolate, mycophenolic acid minimum concentrations were monitored in patients taking **ciprofloxacin** 500 mg twice daily for 7 days (24 patients) or for 14 days or more (21 patients). In both groups the minimum concentrations were about 35 to 40% lower 3 days after starting **ciprofloxacin**, and they were still at this level on day 7. Three days after stopping **ciprofloxacin** in the 7-day group, the minimum concentration had returned to baseline. On day 14 in the longer-term group, the minimum concentration had *increased*, and was just 17% lower than baseline.[4] A study analysing mycophenolic acid concentrations 12-hours post-dose in patients who had recently undergone kidney transplantation suggested that the use of **ciprofloxacin** was associated with a 46% reduction in mycophenolic acid concentrations.[3]

(e) Rifampicin (Rifampin)

For the effect of rifampicin on the pharmacokinetics of mycophenolate, see 'Mycophenolate + Rifampicin (Rifampin)', p.1276.

(f) Selective bowel decontamination

Six liver transplant patients were given a regimen for selective bowel decontamination for 21 days after the transplant, which consisted of **nystatin**, **tobramycin**, and **cefuroxime** and also took mycophenolate mofetil 1 g twice daily. The AUC of mycophenolic acid was measured when the patients were taking the antibacterials (one measurement between day 17 and 20, at which time mycophenolate had been given for at least 10 days) and then again after stopping the antibacterials (one measurement between day 23 and 29). The AUC was 31% lower while taking the antibacterials, although this did not reach statistical significance. However, the reduction in AUC_{6-12} of 57% was statistically significant.[6]

Mechanism

Mycophenolic acid is metabolised to the glucuronide conjugate, which is excreted in bile and urine. Gut bacteria that express the beta-glucuronidase enzyme (mostly Gram-negative anaerobes) cleave the glucuronide conjugate allowing free mycophenolic acid to be reabsorbed (enterohepatic recirculation). Antibacterials that decimate gut bacteria can reduce this enterohepatic recirculation leading to lower concentrations of mycophenolic acid.[2,4] However, the effect might lessen over time as the bowel flora recover even with continued use of the antibacterial.[4]

Importance and management

The available evidence suggests that antibacterials that can decimate gut bacteria might reduce mycophenolic acid minimum concentrations by up to one-third or one-half. In the study with ciprofloxacin, assessing the time course of this effect during an antibacterial course, the effect was rapid, occurring within 3 days of starting the antibacterial and recovering within 3 days of stopping it. Also, interestingly, the effect lessened with continued use of the antibacterial beyond 7 days.

The clinical relevance of these reductions has not been assessed. One UK manufacturer considers that a change in the dose of mycophenolate should not normally be necessary, in the absence of clinical evidence of graft dysfunction, if amoxicillin with clavulanic acid or ciprofloxacin are also given. However, close clinical monitoring is advisable during the concurrent use of the antibacterial, and shortly after it is stopped.[7] The available evidence suggests that this advice should be applied to any antibacterial that affects gut flora. Note that the US manufacturer considers that the combination of metronidazole and norfloxacin should not be used with mycophenolate mofetil.[1]

1. CellCept (Mycophenolate mofetil). Genentech USA, Inc. US Prescribing information, September 2013.
2. Naderer OJ, Dupuis RE, Heinzen EL, Wiwattanawongsa MS, Johnson MW, Smith PC. The influence of norfloxacin and metronidazole on the disposition of mycophenolate mofetil. *J Clin Pharmacol* (2005) 45, 219–26.
3. Borrows R, Chusney G, James A, Stichbury J, Van Tromp J, Cairns T, Griffith M, Hakim N, McLean A, Palmer A, Papalois V, Taube D. Determinants of mycophenolic acid levels after renal transplantation. Ther Drug Monit. (2005) 27,442–50.
4. Borrows R, Chusney G, Loucaidou M, James A, Van Tromp J, Cairns T, Griffith M, Hakim N, McLean A, Palmer A, Papalois V, Taube D. The magnitude and time course of changes in mycophenolic acid 12-hour predose levels during antibiotic therapy in mycophenolate mofetil-based renal transplantation. *Ther Drug Monit* (2007) 29, 122–6.
5. Ratna P, Mathew BS, Annapandian VM, Saravanakumar K, Basu G, Tamilarasi V, Fleming DH. Pharmacokinetic drug interaction of mycophenolate with co-amoxiclav in renal transplant patients. *Transplantation* (2011) 91, e36–e38.
6. Schmidt LE, Rasmussen A, Nørrelykke MR, Poulsen HE, Hansen BA. The effect of selective bowel decontamination on the pharmacokinetics of mycophenolate mofetil in liver transplant recipients. *Liver Transpl* (2001) 7, 739–42.
7. CellCept Tablets (Mycophenolate mofetil). Roche Products Ltd. UK Summary of product characteristics, July 2013.

Mycophenolate + Azathioprine

The UK and US manufacturers of mycophenolate have recommended that it should not be given with azathioprine because they state that concurrent use has not been studied,[1–4] and as both drugs inhibit purine metabolism,[4] they have the potential to cause bone marrow suppression.[1]

1. CellCept (Mycophenolate mofetil). Genentech USA, Inc. US Prescribing information, September 2013.
2. CellCept Tablets (Mycophenolate mofetil). Roche Products Ltd. UK Summary of product characteristics, July 2013.
3. Myfortic (Mycophenolate sodium). Novartis Pharmaceuticals UK Ltd. UK Summary of product characteristics, November 2012.
4. Myfortic (Mycophenolate sodium). Novartis. US Prescribing information, September 2013.

Mycophenolate + Ciclosporin

Ciclosporin reduces the concentrations of mycophenolic acid. Some evidence from a study in children suggests that mycophenolate might reduce the exposure to ciclosporin.

Clinical evidence

(a) Effect on ciclosporin

A study, in 33 children taking ciclosporin with prednisolone and 15 children additionally taking mycophenolate mofetil, found that ciclosporin concentrations taken 2 hours after the ciclosporin dose were lower in those patients taking mycophenolate.[1] Another study in children found similar results.[2]

(b) Effect on mycophenolate

1. Comparisons with everolimus. A study in 24 kidney transplant patients taking mycophenolate sodium with ciclosporin, found that after switching from ciclosporin to everolimus after 28 days, the AUC of mycophenolic acid was 43% higher, but the AUCs of the glucuronide metabolites of mycophenolate were about 30% lower.[3]

2. Comparisons with sirolimus. A study in 21 kidney transplant patients taking mycophenolate mofetil 500 mg once or twice daily with ciclosporin or sirolimus, found no difference in the maximum concentrations of mycophenolic acid between the groups. However, the minimum concentrations of mycophenolic acid in the patients also taking sirolimus were 4.4-fold higher than in those also taking ciclosporin, and the AUC was about 1.8-fold higher.[4]

3. Comparisons with tacrolimus. A study in 78 kidney transplant patients taking corticosteroids with mycophenolate 1 g two or three times daily, and also taking either ciclosporin (68 patients) or tacrolimus (10 patients), found lower minimum concentrations of the active metabolite, mycophenolic acid, and higher concentrations of the glucuronide metabolite in patients taking ciclosporin during the first 3 months post-transplant, when compared with those taking tacrolimus. Of interest, of the 11 patients that switched from ciclosporin to tacrolimus during the study, 5 patients subsequently required mycophenolate dose reductions because of adverse effects.[5] Another study found that despite a higher dose of mycophenolate, patients also taking ciclosporin had a 50% lower minimum concentration of mycophenolic acid when compared with those taking mycophenolate with tacrolimus.[6] Other studies have found similar results.[7-10] In another study, 12 stable kidney transplant patients taking ciclosporin were given enteric-coated mycophenolate sodium 720 mg twice daily for 14 days. After pharmacokinetic assessment, they were then switched to tacrolimus with the same dose and formulation of mycophenolate sodium. This study found that when tacrolimus was given the AUC of mycophenolic acid was 20% greater than with ciclosporin, whereas the maximum concentration of mycophenolic acid was 24% greater with ciclosporin than with tacrolimus.[11] In a 3-month pharmacokinetic sub-study, 67 kidney transplant patients were given standard-dose ciclosporin, mycophenolate 2 g daily, and corticosteroids or daclizumab induction, followed by mycophenolate 2 g daily and corticosteroids with low-dose ciclosporin or low-dose tacrolimus. The study found that patients receiving low-dose tacrolimus had a higher mycophenolic acid AUC at day 7 and month one than those receiving standard-dose ciclosporin (2.1-fold and 60% higher, respectively). The AUC of the glucuronide metabolite was 43% lower in the low-dose tacrolimus group than the standard-dose ciclosporin group at month one. Mycophenolic acid minimum concentrations did not differ between the groups at any time.[12] In contrast, a study in liver transplant patients receiving a fixed 2 g daily dose of mycophenolate with low-dose ciclosporin or low-dose tacrolimus, found that although there was wide interindividual variability in the pharmacokinetic parameters for mycophenolic acid and its metabolites, there were no differences between the two groups.[13]

4. Comparisons with baseline. There are reports that the minimum concentration of the active metabolite of mycophenolate, mycophenolic acid, might be reduced in the presence of ciclosporin.[14] In a study, 52 kidney transplant patients were given mycophenolate mofetil 1 g twice daily with ciclosporin and prednisone. Six months after transplantation 19 patients continued triple therapy, 19 discontinued ciclosporin, and 14 discontinued prednisone. Three months later, patients in whom ciclosporin had been discontinued had higher mycophenolic acid minimum concentrations compared with the other groups of patients. Discontinuing ciclosporin resulted in almost a doubling of mycophenolic acid minimum concentrations.[15] Other studies note similar effects on mycophenolic acid concentrations in adult[16,17] and paediatric patients,[18-20] although note that one study found inadequate immunosuppression in the ciclosporin withdrawal group.[17] In contrast, a study in 22 kidney transplant patients taking mycophenolate found that ciclosporin (13 patients) did not affect the plasma concentrations of mycophenolic acid, but concentrations of the glucuronide metabolite were increased.[21] Similarly, a study in 35 kidney transplant patients taking mycophenolate mofetil (1 or 2 g daily) with ciclosporin (150 to 640 mg daily), and prednisolone over a period of almost 6 months, found no effect on mycophenolic acid concentrations or on those of the glucuronide metabolite, and there was no correlation between ciclosporin and mycophenolic acid minimum concentrations.[22]

Mechanism

Mycophenolate is hydrolysed to form an active metabolite, mycophenolic acid. This then undergoes glucuronidation by glucuronosyltransferases (UGT) to form an inactive glucuronide metabolite. This metabolite is then either excreted in urine or undergoes enterohepatic recirculation, where it is converted back into the active form, mycophenolic acid. Ciclosporin inhibits the enterohepatic conversion of the glucuronide metabolite back to the active metabolite, mycophenolic acid, leading to lower concentrations of mycophenolic acid.[17,23]

Importance and management

The addition of mycophenolate to ciclosporin has been found to reduce the incidence of rejection episodes in kidney transplant patients[24] and it is licensed for concurrent use.[25] From the studies above, ciclosporin appears to reduce the concentrations of the active metabolite, mycophenolic acid, and increase the concentrations of the glucuronide metabolite (which is associated with mycophenolate adverse effects). One UK manufacturer of mycophenolate states that as efficacy studies were conducted in patients taking ciclosporin, mycophenolate, and corticosteroids, the finding that ciclosporin reduces the AUC of mycophenolic acid by about 20% does not affect the recommended dose requirements.[26]

Evidence for an effect on ciclosporin is conflicting, with studies in children[1,2] suggesting that ciclosporin concentrations are reduced by mycophenolate, whereas the manufacturers state that ciclosporin pharmacokinetics are not affected.[25,26] It has also been observed that the use of triple therapy with corticosteroids, ciclosporin, and mycophenolate mofetil rather than with azathioprine makes it possible to use a lower dose of ciclosporin.[27] However, other studies have noted that adjusting ciclosporin doses affects mycophenolic acid concentrations, and therefore the overall effect on immunosuppression needs careful monitoring.[18]

Note that there are inherent problems in interpretation of the results of studies comparing ciclosporin with everolimus,[3] sirolimus,[4] and tacrolimus.[6,8,28,29] The authors of one study with tacrolimus, suggest that the changes in mycophenolic acid minimum concentrations are because *tacrolimus* increases mycophenolic acid concentrations.[8] However, a growing body of evidence (see 'Mycophenolate + Tacrolimus', p.1278) suggests that another more likely interpretation might be that the differences in mycophenolic acid minimum concentrations and exposure are because ciclosporin decreases mycophenolic acid exposure.[28] The picture with everolimus and sirolimus (see 'Mycophenolate + Sirolimus', p.1277) is even less clear.

Patients taking ciclosporin with mycophenolate should have their immunosuppressive response closely monitored, particularly if changing from ciclosporin to everolimus, sirolimus, or tacrolimus, or *vice versa*. Dose adjustment of mycophenolate should be considered if patients develop mycophenolate-related adverse effects (such as diarrhoea, vomiting, and leucopenia) on switching from ciclosporin.

1. Pape L, Froede K, Strehlau J, Ehrich JHH, Offner G. Alterations of cyclosporin A metabolism induced by mycophenolate mofetil. *Pediatr Transplant* (2003) 7, 302–4.
2. Filler G, Drug interactions between mycophenolate and cyclosporine. *Pediatr Transplant* (2004) 8, 201–4.
3. Tedesco-Silva H, Felipe CR, Slade A, Schmouder RL, Medina Pestana JO. Chronopharmacokinetics of mycophenolic acid and its glucuronide and acyl glucuronide metabolites in kidney transplant recipients converted from cyclosporine to everolimus. *Ther Drug Monit* (2012) 34, 652–9.
4. Cattaneo D, Merlini S, Zenoni S, Baldelli S, Gotti E, Remuzzi G, Perico N. Influence of co-medication with sirolimus or cyclosporine on mycophenolic acid pharmacokinetics in kidney transplantation. *Am J Transplant* (2005) 5, 2937–44.
5. Mandla R, Midtvedt K, Line P-D, Hartmann A, Bergan S. Mycophenolic acid clinical pharmacokinetics influenced by a cyclosporine C2 based immunosuppressive regimen in renal allograft recipients. *Transpl Int* (2006) 19, 44–53.
6. Gerbase MW, Fathi M, Spiliopoulos A, Rochat T, Nicod LP. Pharmacokinetics of mycophenolic acid associated with calcineurin inhibitors: long-term monitoring in stable lung recipients with and without cystic fibrosis. *J Heart Lung Transplant* (2003) 22, 587–90.
7. Pou L, Brunet M, Cantarell C, Vidal E, Oppenheimer F, Monforte V, Vilardell J, Roman A, Martorell J, Capdevila L. Mycophenolic acid plasma concentrations: influence of co-medication. *Ther Drug Monit* (2001) 23, 35–8.
8. Hübner GI, Eismann R, Sziegoleit W. Drug interaction between mycophenolate mofetil and tacrolimus detectable within therapeutic mycophenolic acid monitoring in renal transplant patients. *Ther Drug Monit* (1999) 21, 536–9.
9. Vidal E, Cantarell C, Capdevila L, Monforte V, Roman A, Pou L. Mycophenolate mofetil pharmacokinetics in transplant patients receiving cyclosporine or tacrolimus in combination therapy. *Pharmacol Toxicol* (2000) 87, 182–4.
10. Naito T, Mino Y, Otsuka A, Ushiyama T, Ito T, Ozono S, Kagawa Y, Kawakami J. Impact of calcineurin inhibitors on urinary excretion of mycophenolic acid and its glucuronide in kidney transplant recipients. *J Clin Pharmacol* (2009) 49, 710–8.
11. Kaplan B, Meier-Kriesche H-U, Minnick P, Bastien M-C, Sechaud R, Yeh C-M, Balez S, Picard F, Schmouder R. Pharmacokinetics (PK) of enteric-coated mycophenolate sodium (EC-MPS, *Myfortic*) in stable renal transplant patients with Neoral or tacrolimus. *J Am Soc Nephrol* (2003) 14, 910A.
12. Grinyó JM, Ekberg H, Mamelok RD, Oppenheimer F, Sánchez-Plumed J, Gentil MA, Hernandez D, Kuypers DR, Brunet M. The pharmacokinetics of mycophenolate mofetil in renal transplant recipients receiving standard-dose or low-dose cyclosporine, low-dose tacrolimus or low-dose sirolimus: the Symphony pharmacokinetic substudy. *Nephrol Dial Transplant* (2009) 24, 2269–76.
13. Beckebaum S, Armstrong VW, Cicinnati VR, Streit F, Klein CG, Gerken G, Paul A, Oellerich M. Pharmacokinetics of mycophenolic acid and its glucuronide metabolites in stable adult liver transplant recipients with renal dysfunction on a low-dose calcineurin inhibitor regimen and mycophenolate mofetil. *Ther Drug Monit* (2009) 31, 205–10.
14. Weber SW, Keller F. Low mycophenolate predose levels with cyclosporine co-medication. *Kidney Blood Press Res* (1999) 22, 390.
15. Smak Gregoor PJH, de Sévaux RGL, Hené RJ, Hesse CJ, Hilbrands LB, Vos P, van Gelder T, Hoitsma AJ, Weimar W. Effect of cyclosporine on mycophenolic acid trough levels in kidney transplant recipients. *Transplantation* (1999) 68, 1603–6.
16. Smak Gregoor PJH, van Gelder T, Hesse CJ, van der Mast BJ, van Besouw NM, Weimar W. Mycophenolic acid plasma concentrations in kidney allograft recipients with or without cyclosporin: a cross-sectional study. *Nephrol Dial Transplant* (1999) 14, 706–8.
17. Kuypers DR, Ekberg H, Grinyó J, Nashan B, Vincenti F, Snell P, Mamelok RD, Bouw RM. Mycophenolic acid exposure after administration of mycophenolate mofetil in the presence and absence of ciclosporin in renal transplant recipients. *Clin Pharmacokinet* (2009) 48, 329–41.
18. Filler G, Lepage N, Delisle B, Mai I. Effect of cyclosporine on mycophenolic acid area under the concentration-time curve in pediatric kidney transplant recipients. *Ther Drug Monit* (2001) 23, 514–19.
19. Ghio L, Ferraresso M, Viganò SM, Ginevri F, Perfumo F, Gianoglio B, Murer L, Zacchello G, Dello Strologo L, Cardillo M, Tirelli S, Valente U, Edefonti A. Mycophenolate mofetil pharmacokinetic monitoring in pediatric kidney transplant recipients. *Transplant Proc* (2005) 37, 856–8.
20. Ghio L, Ferraresso M, Zacchello G, Murer L, Ginevri F, Belingheri M, Peruzzi L, Zanon F, Perfumo F, Berardinelli L, Tirelli S, Dello Strologo L, Fontana I, Valente U, Cardillo M, Edefonti A. Longitudinal evaluation of mycophenolic acid pharmacokinetics in pediatric kidney transplant recipients. The role of post-transplant clinical and therapeutic variables. *Clin Transplant* (2009) 23, 264–70.
21. Naito T, Shinno K, Maeda T, Kagawa Y, Hashimoto H, Otsuka A, Takayama T, Ushiyama T, Suzuki K, Ozono S. Effects of calcineurin inhibitors on pharmacokinetics of mycophenolic acid and its glucuronide metabolite during the maintenance period following renal transplantation. *Biol Pharm Bull* (2006) 29, 275–80.
22. Merkel U, Lindner S, Vollandt R, Sperschneider H, Balogh A. Trough levels of mycophenolic acid and its glucuronidated metabolite in renal transplant recipients. *Int J Clin Pharmacol Ther* (2005) 43, 379–88.
23. Yau W-P, Vathsala A, Lou H-X, Zhou S, Chan E. Mechanism-based enterohepatic circulation model of mycophenolic acid and its glucuronide metabolite: assessment of impact of cyclosporine dose in Asian renal transplant patients. *J Clin Pharmacol* (2009) 49, 684–99.
24. Sollinger HW. Mycophenolate mofetil for the prevention of acute rejection in primary care cadaveric renal allograft recipients. *Transplantation* (1995) 60, 225–32.
25. CellCept Tablets (Mycophenolate mofetil). Roche Products Ltd. UK Summary of product characteristics, July 2013.
26. Myfortic (Mycophenolate sodium). Novartis Pharmaceuticals UK Ltd. UK Summary of product characteristics, November 2012.
27. Sanz Moreno C, Gomez Sanchez M, Fdez Fdez J, Botella J. Cyclosporine A (CsA) needs are reduced with substitution of azathioprine (Aza) by mycophenolate mofetil (MMF). *Nephrol Dial Transplant* (1998) 13, A260.
28. van Gelder T, Smak Gregoor PJH, Weimar W. Letter to the editor. *Ther Drug Monit* (2000) 22, 639.
29. Hübner GI, Sziegoleit W. Response to letter from van Gelder. *Ther Drug Monit* (2000) 22, 498–9.

Mycophenolate + Cinacalcet

Cinacalcet does not appear to affect the pharmacokinetics of mycophenolic acid or mycophenolate.

Clinical evidence, mechanism, importance and management

In a pharmacokinetic study in 10 kidney transplant patients taking mycophenolate, cinacalcet 30 mg daily for 7 days had no effect on the pharmacokinetics of mycophenolic acid.[1] In another study, no change in mycophenolate mofetil dose was needed in 9 patients when they were given cinacalcet 30 mg daily then titrated to effect for 6 months.[2] Although limited to two small studies, the evidence suggests that no mycophenolate dose adjustment is likely to be needed with concurrent use of cinacalcet.

1. Falck P, Vethe NT, Asberg A, Midtvedt K, Bergan S, Reubsaet JL, Holdaas H. Cinacalcet's effect on the pharmacokinetics of tacrolimus, cyclosporine and mycophenolate in renal transplant recipients. *Nephrol Dial Transplant* (2008) 23, 1048–53.
2. Serra AL, Savoca R, Huber AR, Hepp U, Delsignore A, Hersberger M, Wüthrich RP. Effective control of persistent hyperparathyroidism with cinacalcet in renal allograft recipients. *Nephrol Dial Transplant* (2007) 22, 577–83.

Mycophenolate + Colestyramine

Colestyramine slightly reduces the exposure to mycophenolic acid, an active metabolite of mycophenolate.

Clinical evidence

In a study in healthy subjects, colestyramine 4 g three times daily for 4 days reduced the AUC of mycophenolic acid, given as a single 1.5-g oral dose of mycophenolate mofetil one hour after the first colestyramine dose on day 2, by 37% (range 10 to 61%).[1,2] There was no difference in the maximum concentration of mycophenolic acid, but its concentration decreased from 6 hours onwards.[2]

Mechanism

Mycophenolic acid is metabolised to the glucuronide conjugate, which is excreted in bile and urine. Gut bacteria cleave the glucuronide conjugate allowing free mycophenolic acid to be reabsorbed (enterohepatic recirculation). Colestyramine appears to reduce the enterohepatic recirculation of mycophenolate.[2]

Importance and management

The clinical importance of the slight decrease in mycophenolic acid exposure that occurs after the concurrent use of colestyramine has not been assessed; however, enterohepatic recirculation of mycophenolic acid varies widely between individuals,[2] and therefore this interaction could be clinically relevant in some patients. If colestyramine is considered essential, it would seem prudent to confirm that the immunosuppressant effects of mycophenolate remain adequate. Separating the administration of colestyramine and mycophenolate is not likely to eliminate this interaction. Note that the US manufacturers of mycophenolate advise avoiding the concurrent use of colestyramine[1,3] and other drugs that bind to bile acids, such as **bile-acid binding resins**.[3]

1. CellCept (Mycophenolate mofetil). Genentech USA, Inc. US Prescribing information, September 2013.
2. Bullingham RE, Nicholls AJ, Kamm BR. Clinical pharmacokinetics of mycophenolate mofetil. *Clin Pharmacokinet* (1998) 34, 429–55.
3. Myfortic (Mycophenolate sodium). Novartis. US Prescribing information, September 2013.

Mycophenolate + Corticosteroids

One study suggests that methylprednisolone might slightly decrease mycophenolate exposure, but a similar study suggests that it does not. In another study, prednisone did not alter mycophenolic acid concentrations.

Clinical evidence

(a) Methylprednisolone

In a study in kidney transplant patients taking mycophenolate, ciclosporin, and methylprednisolone, the dose-normalised AUC of mycophenolic acid was 35% lower in the first month when patients were taking higher doses of methylprednisolone (about 16 mg daily) than at 6 months when lower maintenance doses of methylprednisolone (8 mg daily) were being used. In addition, plasma concentrations of the glucuronide metabolite were 2.7-fold higher in the first month than at 6 months. Moreover, in those patients in whom methylprednisolone was tapered and discontinued, there was a 56% and 31% increase in the minimum concentration and AUC of mycophenolic acid, respectively. This difference was apparent even when controlling for ciclosporin exposure[1] (see 'Mycophenolate + Ciclosporin', p.1272).

In contrast, in another very similar study, the authors reported that methylprednisolone dose reductions or withdrawal had no effect on the mycophenolic acid minimum concentration or AUC.[2]

(b) Prednisone

In a study in patients taking triple therapy (mycophenolate, ciclosporin, and prednisone), mycophenolic acid minimum concentrations did not differ between 19 patients who continued this therapy and 14 patients who stopped taking prednisone.[3]

Mechanism

Corticosteroids might induce the glucuronidation of mycophenolic acid, thereby decreasing its concentrations.[1]

Importance and management

It is unclear from these studies whether corticosteroids can alter mycophenolate exposure, but the extent was only slight in the one study that did find a decrease, and is therefore probably of limited clinical relevance. The combination is in general clinical use.

1. Cattaneo D, Perico N, Gaspari F, Gotti E, Remuzzi G. Glucocorticoids interfere with mycophenolate mofetil bioavailability in kidney transplantation. *Kidney Int* (2002) 62, 1060–7.
2. Kuypers DR, Claes K, Evenepoel P, Maes B, Coosemans W, Pirenne J, Vanrenterghem Y. Long-term changes in mycophenolic acid exposure in combination with tacrolimus and corticosteroids are dose dependent and not reflected by trough plasma concentration: a prospective study in 100 de novo renal allograft recipients. *J Clin Pharmacol* (2003) 43, 866–80.
3. Smak Gregoor PJH, de Sévaux RGL, Hené RJ, Hesse CJ, Hilbrands LB, Vos P, van Gelder T, Hoitsma AJ, Weimar W. Effect of cyclosporine on mycophenolic acid trough levels in kidney transplant recipients. *Transplantation* (1999) 68, 1603–6.

Mycophenolate + Diltiazem

Diltiazem appeared to minimally decrease the concentration of mycophenolic acid.

Clinical evidence, mechanism, importance and management

In a study, 29 kidney transplant patients were taking mycophenolate mofetil 2 g daily (with ciclosporin and prednisolone) and diltiazem 30 to 360 mg daily over a period of almost 6 months. In 12 patients taking diltiazem doses between 240 and 360 mg daily, the concentrations of mycophenolic acid and the glucuronide metabolite were 54% and 28% lower, respectively, than in 17 patients taking diltiazem doses between 30 and 120 mg daily. However, when creatinine concentration was taken into account, the differences between the two groups were no longer statistically significant.[1] This is an isolated, small study, and given the small differences seen, the results are unlikely to be of general clinical importance.

1. Merkel U, Lindner S, Vollandt R, Sperschneider H, Balogh A. Trough levels of mycophenolic acid and its glucuronidated metabolite in renal transplant recipients. *Int J Clin Pharmacol Ther* (2005) 43, 379–88.

Mycophenolate + Diuretics

Xipamide, but not furosemide, appeared to increase mycophenolic acid concentrations in a small study.

Clinical evidence, mechanism, importance and management

A study in 32 kidney transplant patients taking mycophenolate mofetil 2 g daily (with ciclosporin and prednisolone) over a period of almost 6 months, found that concurrent use of **furosemide** (10 to 80 mg daily) had no effect on mycophenolic acid concentrations or those of the glucuronide metabolite. In contrast, in 7 patients taking **xipamide** (10 to 40 mg daily) the concentrations of mycophenolic acid and the glucuronide metabolite were almost 2-fold higher than in those patients not taking xipamide. However there was a trend towards higher creatinine concentrations in the xipamide group, and when this was taken into account the differences between the two groups were no longer statistically significant.[1] This is an isolated, small study, the results of which might be explained by alterations in renal function rather than an interaction and as such its general clinical importance is likely to be limited.

1. Merkel U, Lindner S, Vollandt R, Sperschneider H, Balogh A. Trough levels of mycophenolic acid and its glucuronidated metabolite in renal transplant recipients. *Int J Clin Pharmacol Ther* (2005) 43, 379–88.

Mycophenolate + Echinocandins

There appear to be no pharmacokinetic interactions between mycophenolate and caspofungin or micafungin.

Clinical evidence, mechanism, importance and management

The UK and US manufacturers of caspofungin briefly note that, in clinical studies in healthy subjects, the pharmacokinetics of **caspofungin** and mycophenolate were not altered by concurrent use.[1,2] Similarly the manufacturers of **micafungin** briefly note that no pharmacokinetic interaction between micafungin and mycophenolate was seen in studies in healthy subjects.[3,4] No additional precautions would appear to be needed on the concurrent use of either **caspofungin** or **micafungin** with mycophenolate.

1. Cancidas (Caspofungin acetate). Merck Sharp & Dohme Ltd. UK Summary of product characteristics, June 2014.
2. Cancidas (Caspofungin acetate). Merck & Co., Inc. US Prescribing information, August 2013.
3. Mycamine (Micafungin sodium). Astellas Pharma US, Inc. US Prescribing information, June 2013.
4. Mycamine (Micafungin sodium). Astellas Pharma Ltd. UK Summary of product characteristics, December 2013.

Mycophenolate + Food

Food had no effect on the extent of absorption of mycophenolate mofetil or mycophenolate sodium, but notably delayed the absorption of mycophenolate sodium.

Clinical evidence, mechanism, importance and management

(a) Mycophenolate mofetil

In a study in 10 rheumatoid arthritis patients, there was no difference in the AUC of mycophenolic acid when a single 2-g dose of mycophenolate mofetil was given in the fasting state or immediately after a high-fat breakfast. The time to maximum concentration was delayed from one to two hours and there was a 24% reduction in the maximum concentration, suggesting some delay in absorption. There was also a 14% increase in the AUC of the glucuronide metabolite.[1] Similarly, the UK and US manufacturers report that, in a further study in kidney transplant patients, there was no change in extent of absorption (AUC), but there was a 40% reduction in maximum concentrations.[2,3] It is doubtful if this is clinically relevant, but note that the US manufacturer recommends that mycophenolate mofetil is taken on an empty stomach. They state that, in stable kidney transplant patients, mycophenolate mofetil can be taken with food if necessary.[2]

(b) Mycophenolate sodium

The UK and US manufacturers report that no difference was seen in the AUC of mycophenolic acid when a single dose of mycophenolate sodium was given in the fasting state or immediately after a high-fat meal. However, there was a 33% decrease in the maximum concentration and a 5-hour delay in the time to maximum concentration, suggesting a notable delay in absorption.[4,5] Some patients had a time to maximum concentration of greater than 15 hours, which can lead to an absorption overlap from one dose interval to the next.[4] Because of this, the UK manufacturer recommends that patients take mycophenolate sodium consistently, either with or without food.[4] However, the US manufacturer advises that, to avoid the variability in absorption between doses, mycophenolate sodium should be taken on an empty stomach, one hour before or 2 hours after food intake.[5]

1. Bullingham R, Shah J, Goldblum R, Schiff M. Effects of food and antacid on the pharmacokinetics of single doses of mycophenolate mofetil in rheumatoid arthritis patients. *Br J Clin Pharmacol* (1996) 41, 513–6.
2. CellCept (Mycophenolate mofetil). Genentech USA, Inc. US Prescribing information, September 2013.
3. CellCept Tablets (Mycophenolate mofetil). Roche Products Ltd. UK Summary of product characteristics, July 2013.
4. Myfortic (Mycophenolate sodium). Novartis Pharmaceuticals UK Ltd. UK Summary of product characteristics, November 2012.
5. Myfortic (Mycophenolate sodium). Novartis. US Prescribing information, September 2013.

Mycophenolate + H_2-receptor antagonists

H_2-receptor antagonists do not appear to alter the exposure to mycophenolic acid.

Clinical evidence, mechanism, importance and management

The preliminary report of a retrospective study in 141 kidney transplant patients taking mycophenolate mofetil, notes that, over a 20-week period, there was no difference in the AUC of mycophenolic acid in patients who also took H_2-receptor antagonists (drugs not stated, 104 patients), when compared with those who did not (37 patients).[1] Data are limited to this study, but no dose adjustment on concurrent use would appear necessary.

1. van Gelder T, Pescovitz MD, Elzein H, Hamzeh F. The effect of gastric pH modulators on the pharmacokinetics of mycophenolate mofetil (MMF) in de novo renal transplant patients. *Transplantation* (2004) 78, P230.

Mycophenolate + Iron compounds

Most studies have found that oral iron has no effect on the absorption of mycophenolate mofetil.

Clinical evidence, mechanism, importance and management

In a study in 7 healthy, fasting subjects, a single 1050-mg dose of sustained-release **ferrous sulfate** (210 mg of elemental iron) reduced the AUC and maximum concentrations of mycophenolic acid by more than 90% when given at the same time as a single 1-g dose of mycophenolate mofetil.[1] However, this finding was not replicated in an identical study in which 16 healthy fasting subjects were given a single 1-g dose of mycophenolate mofetil with sustained-release **ferrous sulfate** (210 mg elemental iron). There was no change in the AUC of mycophenolic acid.[2]

Moreover, three studies in kidney transplant patients taking mycophenolate have also not identified an interaction.[3-5] In one study in 10 kidney transplant patients taking mycophenolate mofetil 1 g daily, a single 105-mg dose of elemental iron (as **ferrous sulfate**) had no effect on the absorption of mycophenolate in the fasted state, either when given at the same time, or 4 hours apart.[3] Similarly, another study in 40 kidney transplant patients found that two sustained-release tablets of **ferrous sulfate** (dose not stated) daily, given either at the same time or 4 hours after the morning dose of mycophenolate (for 5 days after kidney transplantation), had no effect on the absorption of mycophenolate 1 g twice daily, when compared with patients not given an iron supplement. In addition, the groups appeared comparable in terms of incidence of rejection and adverse effects, although the study was not large enough to properly assess this.[4] A further study in 5 transplant patients, found no change in the AUC of mycophenolic acid when slow-release **ferrous sulfate** (dose not stated) was given daily for 7 days, either at the same time as the morning dose of mycophenolate mofetil or 2 hours afterwards. Furthermore, with a **polysaccharide iron complex** (dose not stated), the mean AUC of mycophenolic acid was *increased* by 22% when it was given 2 hours after mycophenolate mofetil, with no change when given at the same time.[5]

The reason why the first study had such a different finding to all the others is unknown, but it has been suggested that there could have been a problem with the assay.[2]

On balance, it would appear that oral iron compounds do not alter the pharmacokinetics of mycophenolic acid, and that no special precautions are required if an iron supplement is needed in a patient taking mycophenolate.

1. Morii M, Ueno K, Ogawa A, Kato R, Yoshimura H, Wada K, Hashimoto H, Takeda M, Tanaka K, Nakatani T, Shibakawa M. Impairment of mycophenolate mofetil absorption by iron ion. *Clin Pharmacol Ther* (2000) 68, 613–16.
2. Ducray PS, Banken L, Gerber M, Boutouyrie B, Zandt H. Absence of an interaction between iron and mycophenolate mofetil absorption. *Br J Clin Pharmacol* (2006) 62, 492–5.
3. Lorenz M, Wolzt M, Wiegel G, Puttinger H, Horl WH, Fodinger M, Speiser W, Sunder-Plassmann G. Ferrous sulfate does not affect mycophenolic acid pharmacokinetics in kidney transplant patients. *Am J Kidney Dis* (2004) 43, 1098–103.
4. Mudge DW, Atcheson B, Taylor PJ, Sturtevant JM, Hawley CM, Campbell SB, Isbel NM, Nicol DL, Pillans PI, Johnson DW. The effect of oral iron administration on mycophenolate mofetil absorption in renal transplant recipients: a randomized, controlled trial. *Transplantation* (2004) 77, 206–9.
5. Gelone DK, Park JM, Lake KD. Lack of an effect of oral iron administration on mycophenolic acid pharmacokinetics in stable renal transplant recipients. *Pharmacotherapy* (2007) 27, 1272–8.

Mycophenolate + Methotrexate

A study in patients with rheumatoid arthritis found that the concurrent use of methotrexate and mycophenolate mofetil was well tolerated and there were no pharmacokinetic interactions.[1] There would appear to be no need for dose adjustments if both drugs are given for rheumatoid arthritis.

1. Yocum D, Kremer J, Blackburn W, Caldwell J, Furst D, Nunez M, Zuzga J, Zeig S, Gutierrez M, Merrill J, Dumont E, B Leishman. Cellcept® (mycophenolate mofetil - MMF) and methotrexate (MTX) safety and pharmacokinetic (PK) interaction study in rheumatoid arthritis patients. *Arthritis Rheum* (1999) 42 (9 Suppl), S83.

Mycophenolate + Polycarbophil calcium

Polycarbophil calcium reduced the exposure to mycophenolate in one study in healthy subjects.

Clinical evidence, mechanism, importance and management

A study in 5 healthy subjects given a single 1-g dose of mycophenolate alone or with polycarbophil calcium 2.4 g found that the AUC and maximum serum concentrations of mycophenolic acid were reduced by about 51% and 69%, respectively. The authors suggest that this interaction was probably the result of reduced absorption due to chelate-complex formation between mycophenolate and the calcium ions, which they also demonstrated in an *in vitro* study. It was concluded that mycophenolate and polycarbophil calcium should not be taken at the same time.[1] A suitable interval was not specified, but a separation of 2 hours has been suggested with antacids, which might interact by a similar mechanism (see 'Mycophenolate + Antacids', p.1271). Further study is needed, especially as this study used the same assay method as that in a study with iron, the validity of which has been questioned.

1. Kato R, Ooi K, Ikura-Morii M, Tsuchishita Y, Hashimoto H, Yoshimura H, Uenishi K, Kawai M, Tanaka K, Ueno K. Impairment of mycophenolate mofetil absorption by calcium polycarbophil. *J Clin Pharmacol* (2002) 42, 1275–80.

Mycophenolate + Probenecid

Probenecid might increase mycophenolic acid exposure.

Clinical evidence, mechanism, importance and management

In *animals*, probenecid increased the AUC of mycophenolic acid 2-fold and the AUC of its glucuronide metabolite 3-fold.[1] This was thought to be because probenecid competitively inhibits the renal excretion of the glucuronide metabolite of mycophenolate.[1] The UK and US manufacturers warn that other drugs that affect renal tubular secretion could interact similarly.[1,2] However, note that co-trimoxazole which is known to affect renal tubular secretion, was found not to affect the pharmacokinetics of mycophenolate (see 'Mycophenolate + Antibacterials', p.1272). As there appear to be no clinical reports of an interaction between mycophenolate and probenecid, the clinical relevance of the effects seen in *animals* is unclear. Further study is needed to determine if an interaction occurs *in vivo*.

1. CellCept (Mycophenolate mofetil). Genentech USA, Inc. US Prescribing information, September 2013.
2. CellCept Tablets (Mycophenolate mofetil). Roche Products Ltd. UK Summary of product characteristics, July 2013.

Mycophenolate + Proton pump inhibitors

Lansoprazole, omeprazole, and pantoprazole might reduce mycophenolic acid concentrations from mycophenolate mofetil; however, some data with pantoprazole suggest that mycophenolate sodium might not be affected.

One study suggests that low doses of rabeprazole do not affect mycophenolic acid concentrations.

Clinical evidence

(a) Lansoprazole

In a retrospective study in 22 kidney transplant patients taking mycophenolate mofetil, tacrolimus, and lansoprazole 30 mg daily, the dose-adjusted maximum and minimum concentrations of mycophenolic acid were 32% and 45% lower, respectively, when compared with 22 control patients not taking a proton pump inhibitor. The dose-adjusted AUC of mycophenolic acid was 25% lower, but this was not statistically significant. The interaction tended to be greater in intermediate CYP2C19 metabolisers than in extensive metabolisers (that is, the interaction was greater in those with lower activity of this isoenzyme).[1]

(b) Omeprazole

In a study in 12 healthy subjects, omeprazole 20 mg twice daily for 4 days reduced the AUC_{0-12} and maximum plasma concentration of mycophenolic acid from a 1-g dose of mycophenolate mofetil by 22% and 51%, respectively. In contrast, the pharmacokinetics of mycophenolic acid following a 720-mg dose of enteric-coated mycophenolate sodium were unchanged.[2] A retrospective analysis of mycophenolic acid pharmacokinetic data from 72 patients taking mycophenolate mofetil, found that at day 7 post-transplant, the mycophenolic acid AUC_{0-12} and maximum concentration were lower (about 17.6% and 18%, respectively) in those patients who were taking omeprazole than in those who did not. The use of tacrolimus or ciclosporin as adjunctive immunosuppression did not affect the outcome. The reduced mycophenolic acid exposure with omeprazole was maintained throughout the first year post-transplant. The clinical relevance of the reduced exposure was reviewed, and felt to be greatest within the first 7 days post-transplant because the AUC_{0-12}.was at the lower end of its therapeutic range at this point[3]

(c) Pantoprazole

In a study, 23 patients with various autoimmune disorders taking mycophenolate mofetil 1 to 2 g daily for at least 4 months were given pantoprazole 40 mg daily. When compared with a control group of 13 patients not taking a proton pump inhibitor or antacids, the pre-dose (C_0) plasma concentration and the AUC of mycophenolic acid, were found to be about 40% lower, suggesting that pantoprazole reduced the exposure to mycophenolic acid. Furthermore, there was some evidence that the immunosuppressive effect of mycophenolic acid was reduced in the presence of pantoprazole.[4]

A prospective study in 22 heart transplant recipients taking tacrolimus and mycophenolate mofetil 2 g daily found that when patients were given pantoprazole 40 mg daily, the pre-dose (C_0) plasma concentration of mycophenolic acid was reduced by 24%, although this was not statistically significant. However, the AUC and maximum plasma concentration of mycophenolic acid were 25% and 41% lower, respectively, than when the patients were not taking pantoprazole.[5] Similar results were found in another study.[6] A study in 12 healthy subjects found that pantoprazole 40 mg twice daily for 4 days reduced the AUC and maximum plasma concentration of mycophenolic acid from a 1-g dose of mycophenolate mofetil by 10% and 57%, respectively.[7] Furthermore, another study found that the concurrent use of pantoprazole and mycophenolate mofetil led to a trend for more acute transplant rejection episodes and transplant vasculopathy, although this did not reach statistical significance.[8]

In contrast, in a study in 12 healthy subjects, the pharmacokinetics of mycophenolic acid following a 720-mg dose of enteric-coated mycophenolate sodium, were unchanged by pantoprazole 40 mg twice daily for 4 days.[7] Similarly, in a prospective study in 21 heart or lung transplant recipients taking tacrolimus, enteric-coated mycophenolate sodium, and pantoprazole 40 mg daily, the pharmacokinetics of mycophenolic acid were unchanged when pantoprazole was stopped.[9]

(d) Rabeprazole

In a retrospective study in 17 kidney transplant patients taking mycophenolate mofetil and tacrolimus, rabeprazole 10 mg daily had no effect on the pharmacokinetics of mycophenolic acid, when compared with a control group of 22 patients not taking a proton pump inhibitor.[1]

(e) Various proton pump inhibitors

In a randomised study, 126 kidney transplant patients taking tacrolimus and prednisone were given either mycophenolate mofetil 1.5 g twice daily for 5 days followed by 1 g twice daily, or mycophenolate mofetil 1 g twice daily. Of these patients, 73 were also taking a proton pump inhibitor: pantoprazole (32), omeprazole (28), rabeprazole (12), lansoprazole (5), and esomeprazole (2). On day 5 post-transplant, there was no difference in mycophenolate mofetil concentrations in patients taking mycophenolate mofetil 3 g daily with, or without, a proton pump inhibitor. In patients taking mycophenolate mofetil 2 g daily, 2-hour post-dose mycophenolate concentrations were lower in patients taking a proton pump inhibitor (4.4 micrograms/mL) than in those not taking a proton pump inhibitor (7.6 micrograms/mL). However, there was no difference in mycophenolate concentrations at 12 hours post-dose.[10] The preliminary report of a retrospective study in 141 kidney transplant patients taking mycophenolate mofetil, notes that, over a 20-week period, there was no difference in the AUC of mycophenolic acid in patients who also took proton pump inhibitors (drugs not stated, 28 patients), when compared with those who did not (113 patients). However, time to maximum concentration was longer among proton pump inhibitor users than those taking H_2-receptor antagonists or antacids, from day 11 onwards (75 minutes v 40 minutes).[11]

Mechanism

The reduction in the bioavailability of mycophenolate mofetil appears to be related to the acid-suppressant effects of the proton pump inhibitors, which leads to incomplete gastric dissolution of mycophenolate mofetil and a subsequent reduction in its absorption. This effect was not seen with an enteric-coated tablet formulation of mycophenolate sodium, which was said to be due to differences in its dissolution.[2]

Importance and management

An interaction between mycophenolate mofetil and **pantoprazole** appears to be established; however, its clinical relevance is unclear. It seems possible that the decrease in mycophenolate mofetil exposure seen in patients given pantoprazole could lead to a higher risk of treatment failure, although this is not established. Nevertheless, until more is known it would seem prudent to be aware of the possibility of reduced mycophenolic acid exposure in patients taking pantoprazole. Two studies suggest that mycophenolate sodium enteric-coated tablets might not interact in the same way.

Evidence for an interaction between mycophenolate mofetil and other proton pump inhibitors is more limited and suggests that **lansoprazole** and **omeprazole** might interact in the same way as pantoprazole, whereas **rabeprazole** did not interact. However, the differences seen between the effects of the various proton pump inhibitors could be due to the differing acid-suppressant effects of the doses studied. Although the effects seen with lansoprazole and omeprazole were small, and their clinical relevance was generally not studied, they were of a similar magnitude to those seen with pantoprazole where there was limited evidence of reduced efficacy. The authors of the retrospective study with omeprazole concluded that mycophenolate mofetil doses should be increased during the first 7 days of concurrent use. Further, they say that the time-dependent increase in mycophenolic acid absorption after this time negates the effect of omeprazole.[3] This requires confirmation and therefore, until more is known it would be prudent to be aware of the possibility of reduced mycophenolate mofetil exposure with any proton pump inhibitor.

1. Miura M, Satoh S, Inoue K, Kagaya H, Saito M, Suzuki T, Habuchi T. Influence of lansoprazole and rabeprazole on mycophenolic acid pharmacokinetics one year after renal transplantation. *Ther Drug Monit* (2008) 30, 46–51.
2. Kees MG, Steinke T, Moritz S, Rupprecht K, Paulus EM, Kees F, Bucher M, Faerber L. Omeprazole impairs the absorption of mycophenolate mofetil but not of enteric-coated mycophenolate sodium in healthy volunteers. *J Clin Pharmacol* (2012) 52, 1265–72.
3. David-Neto E, Takaki KM, Agena F, Romano P, Sumita NM, Mendes ME, Neri LAL, Nahas WC. Diminished mycophenolic acid exposure caused by omeprazole may be clinically relevant in the first week posttransplantation. *Ther Drug Monit* (2012) 34, 331–6.
4. Schaier M, Scholl C, Scharpf D, Hug F, Bönisch-Schmidt S, Dikow R, Schmitt WH, Schwenger V, Zeier M, Sommerer C. Proton pump inhibitors interfere with the immunosuppressive potency of mycophenolate mofetil. *Rheumatology (Oxford)* (2010) 49, 2061–7.
5. Kofler S, Shvets N, Bigdeli AK, König MA, Kaczmarek P, Deutsch M-A, Vogeser M, Steinbeck G, Reichart B, Kaczmarek I. Proton pump inhibitors reduce mycophenolate exposure in heart transplant recipients – a prospective case-controlled study. *Am J Transplant* (2009) 9, 1650–6.
6. Doesch AO, Mueller S, Konstandin M, Celik S, Erbel C, Kristen A, Frankenstein L, Koch A, Ehlermann P, Zugck C, Katus HA. Proton pump inhibitor co-medication reduces active drug exposure in heart transplant recipients receiving mycophenolate mofetil. *Transplant Proc* (2010) 42, 4243–6.
7. Rupprecht K, Schmidt C, Raspé A, Schweda F, Shipkova M, Fischer W, Bucher M, Kees F, Faerber L. Bioavailability of mycophenolate mofetil and enteric-coated mycophenolate sodium is differentially affected by pantoprazole in healthy volunteers. *J Clin Pharmacol* (2009) 49, 1196–1201.
8. Kofler S, Deutsch M-A, Bigdeli AK, Shvets N, Vogeser M, Mueller TH, Meiser B, Steinbeck G, Reichart B, Kaczmarek I. Proton pump inhibitor co-medication reduces mycophenolate acid drug exposure in heart transplant recipients. *J Heart Lung Transplant* (2009) 28, 605–11.
9. Kofler S, Wolf C, Shvets N, Sisic Z, Müller T, Behr J, Sohn HY, Vogeser M, Shipkova M, Meiser B, Steinbeck G, Reichart B, Kaczmarek I. The proton pump inhibitor pantoprazole and its interaction with enteric-coated mycophenolate sodium in transplant recipients. *J Heart Lung Transplant* (2011) 30, 565–71.
10. Kiberd BA, Wrobel M, Dandavino R, Keown P, Gourishankar S. The role of proton pump inhibitors on early mycophenolic acid exposure in kidney transplantation: evidence from the CLEAR study. *Ther Drug Monit* (2011) 33, 120–3.
11. van Gelder T, Pescovitz MD, Elzein H, Hamzeh F. The effect of gastric pH modulators on the pharmacokinetics of mycophenolate mofetil (MMF) in de novo renal transplant patients. *Transplantation* (2004) 78, P230.

Mycophenolate + Rifampicin (Rifampin)

In a controlled study, rifampicin caused a small reduction in the concentrations of mycophenolic acid (the active metabolite of mycophenolate) and a large increase in the concentrations of the acyl-glucuronide metabolite. Cases reports describe greatly increased mycophenolate dose requirements in patients taking rifampicin.

Clinical evidence

A 57-year-old kidney transplant patient taking mycophenolate 1.5 g daily was diagnosed with tuberculosis and started taking rifampicin (dose not stated). Due to a slight elevation in his creatinine concentration, rifampicin was stopped, and one week later his mycophenolic acid exposure was assessed and found to be almost 75% lower than 2 months before. Two weeks later the mycophenolic acid exposure was reassessed and was found to still be low, at only 65% of the baseline value.[1]

A heart-lung transplant patient, taking tacrolimus 7 mg twice daily and mycophenolate mofetil 1 g twice daily, was given rifampicin 600 mg daily, pyrazinamide 1 g daily, isoniazid 300 mg daily, and pyridoxine 250 mg weekly for a suspected mycobacterial infection. As expected, the tacrolimus dose needed to be substantially increased when rifampicin was started, and the rifampicin dose was reduced to 450 mg daily to try to minimise the interaction. However, the mycophenolate mofetil dose also needed to be increased 3-fold, to 6 g daily, without achieving an adequate concentration (target minimum plasma concentration of 2.5 micrograms/mL). Rifampicin was then stopped and the patient continued taking isoniazid and pyrazinamide. Pharmacokinetic analysis of mycophenolate before, and 13 days after, rifampicin was stopped, found that the dose-corrected minimum concentration of mycophenolic acid increased 18-fold and the AUC_{0-12} increased 3-fold after stopping rifampicin.[2] A subsequent study by the same authors in 8 kidney transplant patients taking mycophenolate 750 mg to 1 g twice daily found that rifampicin 600 mg daily for 8 days decreased the AUC_{0-12} and maximum concentration of mycophenolic acid by 18% and 19%, respectively. The AUC_{0-12} of the inactive 7-*O*-glucuronide metabolite was increased by 34%, and the AUC_{0-12} and maximum concentration of the acyl-glucuronide metabolite were increased by about 2.9-fold and 2.2-fold, respectively. The acyl-glucuronide metabolite has been associated with an increase in mycophenolate adverse effects, but this was not seen in this study.[3]

A study designed to identify the optimum dosing regimen of mycophenolate in paediatric liver transplant patients identified 2 patients also taking rifampicin 40 mg or

50 mg daily for cholestatic pruritus. The exposure to mycophenolic acid in these 2 patients was less than half of that seen in the 13 patients not taking rifampicin, despite them receiving double the dose of mycophenolate.[4]

Mechanism

The exact mechanism of this interaction is unknown. Mycophenolate is a prodrug and is metabolised to its active form, mycophenolic acid, which undergoes glucuronidation by glucuronosyltransferases (UGTs) in the liver, kidney, and intestine to its inactive 7-*O*-glucuronide metabolite. The authors of one of the case reports and a study suggest that rifampicin induces intestinal, renal, and hepatic glucuronidation of mycophenolic acid by UGT and reduces its enterohepatic recirculation and absorption.[2,3] Other mechanisms might also be involved.

Importance and management

The available evidence supports a pharmacokinetic interaction between rifampicin and mycophenolate but the exact mechanism is unknown, and information about its clinical relevance is limited. However, the effects of reduced mycophenolic acid concentrations could be important in terms of acute graft rejection. Also the increases in the concentrations of the acyl-glucuronide metabolite could theoretically put the patient at greater risk of adverse effects. Mycophenolate should be monitored closely during the concurrent use of rifampicin and the dose adjusted as required. However, note that the authors of one report[4] suggested that concurrent use should be avoided.

1. Annapandian VM, Fleming DH, Mathew BS, John GT. Mycophenolic acid area under the curve recovery time following rifampicin withdrawal. *Indian J Nephrol* (2010) 20, 51–3.
2. Kuypers DRJ, Verleden G, Naesens M, Vanrenterghem Y. Drug interaction between mycophenolate mofetil and rifampin: possible induction of uridine diphosphate-glucuronosyltransferase. *Clin Pharmacol Ther* (2005) 78, 81–8.
3. Naesens M, Kuypers DRJ, Streit F, Armstrong VW, Oellerich M, Verbeke K, Vanrenterghem Y. Rifampin induces alterations in mycophenolic acid glucuronidation and elimination: implications for drug exposure in renal allograft recipients. *Clin Pharmacol Ther* (2006) 80, 509–21.
4. Barau C, Barrail-Tran A, Hemerziu B, Habes D, Taburet A-M, Debray D, Furlan V. Optimization of the dosing regimen of mycophenolate mofetil in pediatric liver transplant recipients. *Liver Transpl* (2011) 17, 1152–8.

Mycophenolate + Rosiglitazone

A case report describes anaemia and increased mycophenolic acid exposure which was attributed to the use of rosiglitazone in a patient taking mycophenolate.

Clinical evidence, mechanism, importance and management

A 47-year-old man taking mycophenolate mofetil 1 g twice daily and ciclosporin, as well as numerous other drugs, after a kidney transplant, was given rosiglitazone 4 mg daily. At this point his mycophenolate dose was halved, to 500 mg twice daily, as his mycophenolic acid AUC was considered high, which was felt to be contributing to his anaemia, and ramipril was also started to further control his blood pressure. Over the 3 months after starting rosiglitazone his red cell count progressively declined (despite treatment with epoetins), his haemoglobin and haematocrit were also decreased from baseline, and his mycophenolic acid AUC was more than twice that seen with the higher dose of mycophenolate. Rosiglitazone was stopped, and over 2 months his red cell count, haemoglobin, and haematocrit improved, and his mycophenolic acid AUC decreased by 32%.[1]

Evidence for an interaction between mycophenolate and rosiglitazone appears to be limited to this isolated case and therefore an interaction is not established. Nevertheless, if a patient taking mycophenolate and rosiglitazone develops otherwise unexplained anaemia, consider monitoring the mycophenolic acid AUC. If this is increased, it would seem prudent to consider the potential for an interaction and adjust treatment accordingly.

1. Cattaneo D, Bitto A, Baldelli S, Cortinovis M, Gotti E, Perico N, Remuzzi G. Pharmacokinetic/pharmacodynamic drug interaction between rosiglitazone and mycophenolate mofetil in kidney transplantation: a case report. *Transplantation* (2008) 85, 921–2.

Mycophenolate + Sevelamer

The short-term use of sevelamer resulted in a small decrease in mycophenolic acid exposure in kidney transplant patients.

Clinical evidence

In a pharmacokinetic study, 3 adult and 6 paediatric kidney transplant patients taking mycophenolate and ciclosporin were given sevelamer (at the same time), either as a single 1.6-g dose in the adults, or a single 1.2-g dose in the children, or for 4 days (same dose given three times daily). The average age of the children was 12 years. The single dose of sevelamer decreased the AUC of mycophenolic acid by 23%, and multiple-dosing of sevelamer reduced the AUC by 26%. The maximum concentration of mycophenolic acid was not altered by single- or multiple-dosing, but the time to reach maximum concentration was increased by 40 minutes after multiple-dosing.[1] The UK manufacturer notes that no graft rejection occurred in this study.[2]

Mechanism

Sevelamer is a non-absorbed phosphate-binding polymer with bile-acid binding properties, and mycophenolate undergoes enterohepatic recirculation. The authors of the study suggested that the decreased exposure seen was due to sevelamer interfering with the absorption of mycophenolate.[1]

Importance and management

The clinical importance of this small decrease in mycophenolate exposure on concurrent use of sevelamer is unclear. However, until more is known, it would seem prudent to confirm that the immunosuppressant effects of mycophenolate remain adequate in any patient given sevelamer. The UK manufacturer of mycophenolate mofetil recommends that it should be taken at least one hour before, or three hours after, taking sevelamer,[2] and one US manufacturer advises taking mycophenolate 2 hours before sevelamer.[3] However, note that separating administration in this way does not usually eliminate interactions involving enterohepatic recirculation. Further study is therefore required to evaluate if separation of doses is an effective way of reducing the interaction, and to evaluate the effects of longer-term administration of sevelamer.

1. Pieper A-K, Buhle F, Bauer S, Mai I, Budde K, Haffner D, Neumayer H-H, Querfeld U. The effect of sevelamer on pharmacokinetics of cyclosporin A and mycophenolate-mofetil after renal transplantation. *Nephrol Dial Transplant* (2004) 19, 2630–3.
2. CellCept Tablets (Mycophenolate mofetil). Roche Products Ltd. UK Summary of product characteristics, July 2013.
3. CellCept (Mycophenolate mofetil). Genentech USA, Inc. US Prescribing information, September 2013.

Mycophenolate + Sirolimus

Higher concentrations of mycophenolic acid have been seen in kidney transplant patients taking mycophenolate with sirolimus, when compared with similar patients taking mycophenolate with ciclosporin. Both lower mycophenolic acid concentrations, and no differences, have been seen in kidney transplant patients when mycophenolate was taken with sirolimus, when compared with patients taking mycophenolate with tacrolimus.

Clinical evidence

1. Comparisons with ciclosporin. Various studies in kidney transplant patients taking mycophenolate 1 g twice daily[1-4] or 500 mg once or twice daily[5] with sirolimus, have found that the AUC and minimum concentrations of the active metabolite of mycophenolate, mycophenolic acid, were higher when compared with similar groups of patients taking ciclosporin instead of sirolimus. The mycophenolic acid AUCs seen were between 37% and about 1.9-fold higher,[1-5] with minimum concentrations between 70% and 4.4-fold higher,[2,3,5] than in the patients taking ciclosporin. In a study comparing the effects of sirolimus on different mycophenolate doses, the use of sirolimus with a dose of mycophenolate 750 mg twice daily resulted in a mycophenolic acid AUC and minimum concentration that were comparable to those seen with the concurrent use of mycophenolate 1 g twice daily and ciclosporin (which is known to reduce mycophenolic acid concentrations). Further, the use of sirolimus with a mycophenolate dose of 500 mg twice daily resulted in a *lower* mycophenolic acid AUC and minimum concentration (38 and 16% lower, respectively) than those seen with the concurrent use of mycophenolate 1 g twice daily and ciclosporin.[3] Other pharmacokinetic parameters have been noted in some studies, with one finding similar mycophenolic acid maximum concentrations in the presence or absence of sirolimus,[2] and another finding reduced exposure to the glucuronide metabolite of mycophenolic acid in the sirolimus group.[4]

Mycophenolate dose reductions were required in one study; in 2 patients in the first month, another 3 patients in the second month and 6 patients in the third month (total of 11 patients), compared with the ciclosporin group where only 5 patients needed mycophenolate dose reductions.[2]

A higher incidence of leucopenia at months one and two after transplantation was reported in patients taking sirolimus, rather than ciclosporin, with mycophenolate in one study,[2] and biopsy proven rejection was higher in the sirolimus group of another study when compared with the ciclosporin group (40% versus 13.3%).[4]

2. Comparisons with tacrolimus. A study in 23 kidney transplant patients taking mycophenolate mofetil with sirolimus (9 patients) or tacrolimus (14 patients), found that the AUC of mycophenolic acid was 54% lower in those taking sirolimus than in those taking tacrolimus. The maximum and minimum concentrations of mycophenolic acid were also much lower (41% and 60%, respectively) in the sirolimus patients. The pharmacokinetics of the glucuronide metabolite of mycophenolic acid were no different between the groups.[6] In contrast, a study in 70 kidney transplant patients taking mycophenolate mofetil with sirolimus (42 patients) or tacrolimus (28 patients) found that there were no differences in the dose-corrected AUC or minimum and maximum concentrations of either mycophenolic acid or its glucuronide metabolite.[7]

Mechanism

Ciclosporin is known to inhibit the enterohepatic conversion of the glucuronide metabolite back to the active metabolite of mycophenolate (mycophenolic acid), producing lower concentrations of mycophenolic acid, see 'Mycophenolate + Ciclosporin', p.1272. Tacrolimus might inhibit the metabolism of mycophenolic acid, see 'Mycophenolate + Tacrolimus', p.1278, but whether sirolimus specifically increases mycophenolic acid concentrations compared with mycophenolate taken on its own is unclear.

Importance and management

Evidence for an interaction between sirolimus and mycophenolate is limited to comparisons with the effects of ciclosporin or tacrolimus. However, increased mycophenolic acid concentrations have been associated with an increased risk of adverse effects.[1,2,5] The authors of one of the studies suggest that the mycophenolate dose should be reduced from 1 g to 750 mg twice daily in patients taking sirolimus, as this produced comparable mycophenolic acid concentrations to the recommended dose of mycophenolate 1 g twice daily with ciclosporin.[3]

Until further information is available, patients taking mycophenolate who are switched from ciclosporin to sirolimus should be closely monitored for mycophenolate adverse effects (such as diarrhoea, vomiting, and leucopenia), and the dose of mycophenolate reduced accordingly. The situation with those switched from tacrolimus to sirolimus is less clear, but potentially higher mycophenolate doses will be required.

1. Picard, N, Prémaud, Rousseau A, Le Meur Y, Marquet P. A comparison of the effect of ciclosporin and sirolimus on the pharmacokinetics of mycophenolate in renal transplant patients. *Br J Clin Pharmacol* (2006) 62, 477–84.
2. Büchler M, Lebranchu Y, Bénéton M, Le Meur Y, Heng AE, Westeel PF, le Guellec C, Libert F, Hary L, Marquet P, Paintaud G. Higher exposure to mycophenolic acid with sirolimus than with cyclosporine cotreatment. *Clin Pharmacol Ther* (2005) 78, 34–42.
3. El Haggan W, Ficheux M, Debruyne D, Rognant N, Lobbedez T, Allard C, Coquerel A, Ryckelynck JP, Hurault de Ligny B, Pharmacokinetics of mycophenolic acid in kidney transplant patients receiving sirolimus versus cyclosporine. *Transplant Proc* (2005) 37, 864–6.
4. Pescovitz MD, Vincenti F, Hart M, Melton L, Whelchel J, Mulgaonkar S, McKay D, Leung M, Calleja E, Bouw MR. Pharmacokinetics, safety, and efficacy of mycophenolate mofetil in combination with sirolimus or ciclosporin in renal transplant patients. *Br J Clin Pharmacol* (2007) 64, 758–71.
5. Cattaneo D, Merlini S, Zenoni S, Baldelli S, Gotti E, Remuzzi G, Perico N. Influence of co-medication with sirolimus or cyclosporine on mycophenolic acid pharmacokinetics in kidney transplantation. *Am J Transplant* (2005) 5, 2937–44.
6. Braun F, Schöcklmann H, Ziegler E, Kunzendorf U, Armstrong, Renders L. Increased mycophenolic acid exposure in stable kidney transplant recipients on tacrolimus as compared with those on sirolimus: implications for pharmacokinetics. *Clin Pharmacol Ther* (2009) 86, 411–5.
7. Picard N, Yee SW, Woillard J-B, Lebranchu Y, Le Meur Y, Giacomini KM, Marquet P. The role of organic anion-transporting polypeptides and their common genetic variants in mycophenolic acid pharmacokinetics. *Clin Pharmacol Ther* (2010) 87, 100–8.

Mycophenolate + St John's wort (*Hypericum perforatum*)

St John's wort does not appear to alter the pharmacokinetics of mycophenolate.

Clinical evidence

In a pharmacokinetic study, 8 stable kidney transplant patients taking mycophenolate 1 to 2 g daily and tacrolimus were given 600 mg of St John's wort extract (*Jarsin 300*) daily for 14 days. The concentrations of mycophenolic acid, the main metabolite of mycophenolate, were measured before St John's wort was started, on day 14, and two weeks after St John's wort was stopped. The pharmacokinetics of mycophenolic acid were unchanged throughout the study, and no dosage adjustments were needed in any of the 8 patients.[1]

Mechanism

No mechanism. St John's wort is an inducer of CYP3A4, and P-glycoprotein. As mycophenolate is not metabolised or transported by these routes, an interaction would not be expected.

Importance and management

St John's wort does not appear to affect the pharmacokinetics of mycophenolate, and therefore no additional precautions seem necessary on concurrent use.

1. Mai I, Störmer E, Bauer S, Krüger H, Budde K, Roots I. Impact of St John's wort treatment on the pharmacokinetics of tacrolimus and mycophenolic acid in renal transplant patients. *Nephrol Dial Transplant* (2003) 18, 819–22.

Mycophenolate + Tacrolimus

Tacrolimus does not appear to affect the pharmacokinetics of mycophenolic acid. However, some evidence from one study suggests that mycophenolate might increase the exposure to tacrolimus.

Clinical evidence

(a) Effect on mycophenolate

1. Comparisons with ciclosporin. For details of the studies showing the effect of tacrolimus on mycophenolate compared with ciclosporin, see 'Mycophenolate + Ciclosporin', p.1272.

2. Comparisons with sirolimus. A study in 23 kidney transplant patients taking mycophenolate mofetil with tacrolimus (14 patients) or sirolimus (9 patients), found that the AUC of mycophenolic acid was 2.2-fold higher in those taking tacrolimus than in those taking sirolimus. The maximum and minimum concentrations of mycophenolic acid were also much higher (1.7-fold and 2.5-fold, respectively) in the tacrolimus patients. The pharmacokinetics of the glucuronide metabolite of mycophenolic acid were no different between the groups.[1] In contrast, a study in 70 kidney transplant patients taking mycophenolate mofetil with tacrolimus (28 patients) or sirolimus (42 patients) found that there were no differences in the dose-corrected AUC or minimum and maximum concentrations of either mycophenolic acid or its glucuronide metabolite.[2]

3. Comparisons with baseline. A study in 22 kidney transplant patients taking mycophenolate found that tacrolimus (9 patients) did not affect the plasma concentrations of mycophenolic acid or its glucuronide metabolite.[3] Similarly, two studies in kidney transplant patients found no association between the pharmacokinetics of tacrolimus and mycophenolic acid.[4,5] In one, the dose-corrected AUC of tacrolimus did not correlate with the dose-corrected AUC of mycophenolic acid. These patients were also taking reducing doses of prednisone.[4] In the other, tacrolimus did not affect the AUC or minimum and maximum concentrations of mycophenolate.[5] In another study comparing the effect of standard-dose and low-dose tacrolimus on mycophenolate pharmacokinetics in liver transplant patients, there was no difference in the maximum plasma concentrations or AUC of mycophenolic acid between the two groups. There was also no relationship between the minimum concentrations or AUC of tacrolimus and the AUC of mycophenolic acid; and safety and efficacy were similar between groups.[6] Another study in 100 kidney transplant patients found that mycophenolic acid pharmacokinetics were not affected by tacrolimus.[7]

(b) Effect on tacrolimus

A study in kidney transplant patients taking tacrolimus long-term found that the addition of mycophenolate mofetil resulted in an increase in the tacrolimus AUC, but this was not statistically significant.[8] Another study in kidney transplant patients found no change in tacrolimus concentrations when mycophenolate was given.[9] Similarly, two studies in kidney transplant patients found no association between the pharmacokinetics of mycophenolic acid and tacrolimus.[4,5] In one, the dose-corrected AUC of mycophenolic acid did not correlate with the dose-corrected AUC of tacrolimus. These patients were also taking reducing doses of prednisone.[4] In the other, mycophenolate did not affect the AUC or minimum and maximum concentrations of tacrolimus.[5] However, a 20% increase in tacrolimus concentrations has been reported in a study in liver transplant patients given mycophenolate 1.5 g twice daily.[9]

Mechanism

Tacrolimus might inhibit glucuronosyltransferases (UGTs) which metabolise mycophenolic acid to the glucuronide metabolite.[3,10]

Importance and management

Evidence for an interaction between mycophenolate and tacrolimus is limited to comparative studies. Although tacrolimus does not appear to affect the pharmacokinetics of mycophenolic acid, changes in mycophenolic acid concentrations have been reported in studies comparing the effects of tacrolimus with *ciclosporin* (see 'Mycophenolate + Ciclosporin', p.1272) and with *sirolimus* (see 'Mycophenolate + Sirolimus', p.1277). The reasons for the differences seen are unclear. However, in relation to ciclosporin, it has been suggested that tacrolimus increases mycophenolic acid concentrations;[11] although, another more likely interpretation might be that the differences in mycophenolic acid pharmacokinetics occur because *ciclosporin decreases* mycophenolic acid exposure.[12]

Evidence for an effect on tacrolimus pharmacokinetics is conflicting, with most studies suggesting that tacrolimus concentrations are not affected by mycophenolate, and one study reporting an increase in tacrolimus exposure.

The UK manufacturers of mycophenolate note that the benefit of concurrent use with tacrolimus has not been established.[9,13] Patients taking tacrolimus with mycophenolate should have their immunosuppressive response closely monitored, particularly if changing from ciclosporin to tacrolimus or *vice versa*, and dose adjustment of mycophenolate should be considered if patients develop mycophenolate-related adverse effects (such as diarrhoea, vomiting, and leucopenia) on switching from ciclosporin to tacrolimus.

1. Braun F, Schöcklmann H, Ziegler E, Kunzendorf U, Armstrong, Renders L. Increased mycophenolic acid exposure in stable kidney transplant recipients on tacrolimus as compared with those on sirolimus: implications for pharmacokinetics. *Clin Pharmacol Ther* (2009) 86, 411–5.
2. Picard N, Yee SW, Woillard J-B, Lebranchu Y, Le Meur Y, Giacomini KM, Marquet P. The role of organic anion-transporting polypeptides and their common genetic variants in mycophenolic acid pharmacokinetics. *Clin Pharmacol Ther* (2010) 87, 100–8.
3. Naito T, Shinno K, Maeda T, Kagawa Y, Hashimoto H, Otsuka A, Takayama T, Ushiyama T, Suzuki K, Ozono S. Effects of calcineurin inhibitors on pharmacokinetics of mycophenolic acid and its glucuronide metabolite during the maintenance period following renal transplantation. *Biol Pharm Bull* (2006) 29, 275–80.
4. Park S-I, Felipe CR, Pinheiro-Machado PG, Garcia R, Fernandes FB, Casarini DE, Tedesco-Silva H, Medina-Pestana JO. Tacrolimus pharmacokinetic drug interactions: effect of prednisone, mycophenolic acid or sirolimus. *Fundam Clin Pharmacol* (2009) 23, 137–45.
5. Kagaya H, Miura M, Satoh S, Inoue K, Saito M, Inoue T, Habuchi T, Suzuki T. No pharmacokinetic interactions between mycophenolic acid and tacrolimus in renal transplant recipients. *J Clin Pharm Ther* (2008) 33, 193–201.
6. Nashan B, Saliba F, Durand F, Barcéna R, Herrero JI, Mentha G, Neuhaus P, Bowles M, Patch D, Bernardos A, Klempnauer J, Bouw R, Ives J, Mamelok R, McKay D, Truman M, Marotta P. Pharmacokinetics, efficacy, and safety of mycophenolate mofetil in combination with standard-dose or reduced-dose tacrolimus in liver transplant recipients. *Liver Transpl* (2009) 15, 136–47.
7. Kuypers DR, Claes K, Evenepoel P, Maes B, Coosemans W, Pirenne J, Vanrenterghem Y. Long-term changes in mycophenolic acid exposure in combination with tacrolimus and corticosteroids are dose dependent and not reflected by trough plasma concentration: a prospective study in 100 de novo renal allograft recipients. *J Clin Pharmacol* (2003) 43, 866–80.
8. Pirsch J, Bekersky I, Vincenti F, Boswell G, Woodle ES, Alak A, Kruelle M, Fass N, Facklam D, Mekki Q. Coadministration of tacrolimus and mycophenolate mofetil in stable kidney transplant patients: pharmacokinetics and tolerability. *J Clin Pharmacol* (2000) 40, 527–32.
9. CellCept Tablets (Mycophenolate mofetil). Roche Products Ltd. UK Summary of product characteristics, July 2013.
10. Mandla R, Midtvedt K, Line P-D, Hartmann A, Bergan S. Mycophenolic acid clinical pharmacokinetics influenced by a cyclosporine C2 based immunosuppressive regimen in renal allograft recipients. *Transpl Int* (2006) 19, 44–53.
11. Hübner GI, Eismann R, Sziegoleit W. Drug interaction between mycophenolate mofetil and tacrolimus detectable within therapeutic mycophenolic acid monitoring in renal transplant patients. *Ther Drug Monit* (1999) 21, 536–9.
12. van Gelder T, Smak Gregoor PJH, Weimar W. Letter to the editor. *Ther Drug Monit* (2000) 22, 639.
13. Myfortic (Mycophenolate sodium). Novartis Pharmaceuticals UK Ltd. UK Summary of product characteristics, November 2012.

Mycophenolate + Tyrosine kinase inhibitors; Tofacitinib

Tofacitinib does not appear to alter the concentrations of mycophenolic acid in kidney transplant patients.

Clinical evidence, mechanism, importance and management

A retrospective, population pharmacokinetic analysis of kidney transplant patients who received mycophenolate with tacrolimus (9 patients) or tofacitinib (8 patients), compared the pharmacokinetics of mycophenolic acid in both groups. The analysis found no apparent differences in the minimum concentrations of mycophenolic acid between those patients given tofacitinib and those given tacrolimus. Because of previous reports that tacrolimus does not affect the pharmacokinetics of mycophenolic acid, the authors concluded that tofacitinib does not alter the systemic exposure to mycophenolic acid in kidney transplant patients.[1] See 'Mycophenolate + Tacrolimus', p.1278, for discussion of the effects of tacrolimus on mycophenolic acid pharmacokinetics.

On the basis of this study, a mycophenolate dose reduction would not appear necessary on concurrent use with tofacitinib, but further study is needed to establish this effect as the available data is only comparative. Note that the US manufacturer of tofacitinib states that there is a risk of increased immunosuppression if it is given with potent immunosuppressants,[2] which would be expected to include mycophenolate. Some caution would therefore seem prudent on concurrent use.

1. Lamba M, Tafti B, Melcher M, Chan G, Krishnaswami S, Busque S. Population pharmacokinetic analysis of mycophenolic acid coadministered with either tasocitinib (CP-690,550) or tacrolimus in adult renal allograft recipients. *Ther Drug Monit* (2010) 32, 778–81.
2. Xeljanz (Tofacitinib citrate). Pfizer Inc. US Prescribing information, November 2012.

Mycophenolate + Voriconazole

Voriconazole does not alter the pharmacokinetics of mycophenolate.

Clinical evidence, mechanism, importance and management

In a study, voriconazole had no effect on the pharmacokinetics of a single 1-g dose of mycophenolate.[1] Similarly, the AUC, minimum concentration, and maximum concentration, of mycophenolic acid did not change in a kidney transplant patient 7 days after stopping a 3-month course of voriconazole.[2] Mycophenolate is not metabolised by the cytochrome P450 system and is not a substrate for P-glycoprotein, so it would not be expected to be affected by drugs that affect this isoenzyme and drug transporter, such as voriconazole.

No pharmacokinetic interaction occurs, so no dose adjustment of mycophenolate should be necessary on concurrent use.

1. Wood N, Abel, Fielding A, Nichols DJ, Bygrave E. Voriconazole does not affect the pharmacokinetics of mycophenolic acid. *Intersci Conf Antimicrob Agents Chemother* (2001) 41, 3.
2. Kuypers DR, Claes K, Evenepoel P, Vanrenterghem Y. Clinically relevant drug interaction between voriconazole and tacrolimus in a primary renal allograft recipient. *Transplantation* (2006) 81, 1750–2.

Sirolimus and related drugs + ACE inhibitors or Angiotensin II receptor antagonists

Angioedema has been reported in patients taking everolimus, sirolimus, or temsirolimus with ACE inhibitors. Cases have also been reported in patients given everolimus or sirolimus with losartan.

Clinical evidence

(a) Everolimus

One report described 6 cases of tongue angioedema in 114 patients given everolimus, all of whom were taking an ACE inhibitor (**enalapril**, **ramipril**) or angiotensin II receptor antagonist (**losartan**). All 6 required hospitalisation. In 5 patients, concurrent use was continued and there had been no recurrences (15 to 126 days follow-up). One patient had two recurrences (day 42 and 67) and everolimus was discontinued.[1] Another report describes a 58-year-old woman taking **lisinopril** for 1 year without adverse effects, who developed facial angioedema 1 month after everolimus was added. Both drugs were stopped and the patient was given corticosteroids, after which the angioedema rapidly resolved. Everolimus was restarted with amlodipine and no recurrence occurred.[2] Two other similar cases were briefly mentioned in a consensus conference report.[3]

(b) Sirolimus

A study in 52 kidney transplant patients taking sirolimus 2 to 5 mg daily with **ramipril** 2.5 to 5 mg daily found that 5 of these patients developed non-life threatening tongue oedema within one month of starting ramipril. All of these patients had taken ramipril before their transplant without any adverse effects or signs of angioedema. The tongue oedema resolved within 2 weeks of stopping ramipril. The authors noted that at that time all 5 patients were taking sirolimus 5 mg daily and ramipril 5 mg daily, with their sirolimus concentrations in the higher end of the range 16 to 20 nanograms/mL. Three months after their transplant, when sirolimus had been stabilised at a lower dose of 2 to 4 mg daily, resulting in blood concentrations of 8 to 12 nanograms/mL, ramipril was restarted at 2.5 mg daily with no adverse effects.[4] A retrospective analysis of 80 kidney transplant patients taking sirolimus, found that 12 of these had developed angioedema, either of the face (10 patients), arm (1 patient), or leg (1 patient). The angioedema was life-threatening in 1 patient. Of these 12 patients, 5 were also taking **enalapril** (1 with tacrolimus) and 2 were taking **losartan**.[5]

A kidney transplant patient taking sirolimus 9 mg daily developed non-pitting oedema of the eyelid, cheek, and lips when he started to take **ramipril** (dose not specified).[6] Another kidney transplant patient who had taken **enalapril** 2.5 mg daily for 2 months developed erythematous skin lesions with non-pitting oedema of the neck, face, and chest 9 days after she was switched from tacrolimus to sirolimus 2 mg daily. Symptoms resolved in both patients when the ACE inhibitor was stopped and corticosteroid therapy was increased.[6]

(c) Temsirolimus

The UK and US manufacturers of temsirolimus note that angioneurotic oedema-type reactions (including delayed reactions occurring 2 months following initiation of therapy) have been observed in some patients who were given temsirolimus with ACE inhibitors.[7,8]

Mechanism

ACE inhibitors alone can cause angioedema, and this has also been reported for sirolimus (rarely[9]) and everolimus (common with ACE inhibitors[10]). It is therefore possible that the risk of angioedema might be increased by the concurrent use of ACE inhibitors. Although angioedema is not specifically listed as an adverse effect of temsirolimus, facial oedema is common,[7,8] and as temsirolimus is a pro-drug of sirolimus, the risk of angioedema cannot be ruled out.

Importance and management

Evidence for an interaction between sirolimus and related drugs and ACE inhibitors or angiotensin II receptor antagonists is limited to reports of angioedema on concurrent use. These reports suggest that it would be prudent to be more alert to the possibility of angioedema when either starting an ACE inhibitor in a patient already taking everolimus, sirolimus, or temsirolimus, or when starting these immunosuppressants in a patient taking an ACE inhibitor. The effect might be dose-related, with higher doses of both drugs potentially posing a greater risk. Although there appear to be fewer reports with angiotensin II receptor antagonists, and given the potential consequences of angioedema, the same precautions as with ACE inhibitors would be prudent.

1. Fuchs U, Zittermann A, Berthold HK, Tenderich G, Deyerling KW, Minami K, Koerfer R. Immunosuppressive therapy with everolimus can be associated with potentially life-threatening lingual angioedema. *Transplantation* (2005) 79, 981–3.
2. Rothermundt C, Gillessen S. Angioedema in a patient with renal cell cancer treated with everolimus in combination with an angiotensin-converting enzyme inhibitor. *J Clin Oncol* (2013) 31, e57–e58.
3. Rothenburger M, Zuckermann A, Bara C, Hummel M, Strüber M, Hirt S, Lehmkuhl H; Certican Consensus Study Group. Recommendations for the use of everolimus (Certican) in heart transplantation: results from the second German-Austrian Certican Consensus Conference. *J Heart Lung Transplant* (2007) 26, 305–11.
4. Stallone G, Infante B, Di Paolo S, Schena A, Grandaliano G, Gesualdo L, Schena FP. Sirolimus and angiotensin-converting enzyme inhibitors together induce tongue oedema in renal transplant recipients. *Nephrol Dial Transplant* (2004) 19, 2906–8.
5. Mahé E, Morelon E, Lechaton S, Kreis H, de Prost Y, Bodemer C. Angioedema in renal transplant recipients on sirolimus. *Dermatology* (2007) 214, 205–9.
6. Burdese M, Rossetti M, Guarena C, Consiglio V, Mezza E, Soragna G, Gai M, Segoloni GP, Piccoli GB. Sirolimus and ACE-inhibitors: a note of caution. *Transplantation* (2005) 79, 251–2.
7. Torisel (Temsirolimus). Pfizer Ltd. UK Summary of product characteristics, October 2013.
8. Torisel (Temsirolimus). Wyeth Pharmaceuticals Inc. US Prescribing information, October 2014.
9. Rapamune (Sirolimus). Pfizer Ltd. UK Summary of product characteristics, August 2013.
10. Certican (Everolimus). Novartis Pharmaceuticals Australia Pty Ltd. Australian product information, August 2013.

Sirolimus or Tacrolimus + Amiodarone

Increased sirolimus and tacrolimus concentrations in a paediatric patient and greatly elevated tacrolimus concentrations in an adult were both associated with the concurrent use of amiodarone. A case of QTc interval prolongation was attributed to an interaction between amiodarone and tacrolimus.

Clinical evidence

A 2-year-old heart transplant patient taking tacrolimus 20 micrograms/kg daily was given amiodarone to control ventricular arrhythmias. Her tacrolimus minimum concentration was reported to be within the target range of 8 to 10 micrograms/L on both day one and day 3 after starting amiodarone. She was then switched from tacrolimus to sirolimus 60 micrograms/kg daily, increased to 120 micrograms/kg after 2 days, with tacrolimus continued until a therapeutic sirolimus concentration was achieved. The sirolimus and tacrolimus concentrations 9 days after starting amiodarone were found to be 53 and 13 micrograms/L, respectively. Subsequent sirolimus doses were put on hold and tacrolimus was stopped. The sirolimus concentration was increased for a further 14 days. Sirolimus was restarted at a lower dose (30 micrograms/kg daily) but the concentration remained above 10 micrograms/L and the sirolimus dose was reduced further to 20 micrograms/kg daily.[1]

A 73-year-old kidney transplant patient, who had been taking ciclosporin and amiodarone long-term, had the ciclosporin switched to tacrolimus 7 mg daily. About 3 months later he was found to have a greatly increased tacrolimus concentration of 63 nanograms/mL. The tacrolimus dose was reduced to 2 mg daily, with a resulting concentration of 12.9 nanograms/mL.[2]

Another case report describes QTc prolongation (from 440 milliseconds to 535 milliseconds) in a 65-year-old man taking amiodarone 200 mg daily, one day after starting tacrolimus 3 mg twice daily as part of an immunosuppression regime post kidney transplant. The QTc prolongation did not respond adequately to treatment and so on the following day the amiodarone was stopped. Over the following few days his QTc interval decreased and was 493 milliseconds on day 5 post-transplant, when he was discharged on tacrolimus 1.5 mg twice daily with his tacrolimus concentration maintained within the range of 12.3 to 14.9 nanograms/mL.[3]

Mechanism

The elevated concentrations of tacrolimus and sirolimus were attributed to an interaction with amiodarone, which can inhibit CYP3A4 and P-glycoprotein, and are involved in the metabolism and transport of sirolimus and tacrolimus.[1]

Importance and management

Evidence for an interaction between sirolimus or tacrolimus and amiodarone is very limited, and confined to individual case reports. The authors of the first report advise that, because of the long half-life of sirolimus, and the difficulty in reducing elevated concentrations quickly, prescribers should consider reducing sirolimus and tacrolimus doses before starting amiodarone[1] rather than waiting for the interaction to occur. They also advise more frequent monitoring of sirolimus and tacrolimus concentrations if amiodarone is also given. Although there are limited data, given that a similar interaction has been reported with ciclosporin (see 'Ciclosporin + Amiodarone', p.1206), which is metabolised in a similar way to sirolimus and tacrolimus, this would seem prudent.

The report of QTc prolongation after tacrolimus was added to amiodarone should be interpreted with caution given the long-half life of amiodarone and the rapid resolution of the QTc prolongation after amiodarone was stopped (within 3 days). Note that tacrolimus is associated with QT prolongation, and amiodarone is known to prolong the QT interval. See 'Drugs that prolong the QT interval + Other drugs that prolong the QT interval', p.272 for further information on the concurrent use of two or more drugs that prolong the QT interval.

1. Nalli N, Stewart-Texeira L, Dipchand AI. Amiodarone-sirolimus/tacrolimus interaction in a pediatric heart transplant patient. *Pediatr Transplant* (2006) 10, 736–9.
2. Kisters K, Cziborra M, Funke C, Brylak S, Hausberg M. Amiodarone-tacrolimus interaction in kidney transplantation. *Clin Nephrol* (2008) 70, 563.
3. Burger CI, Clase CM, Gangji AS. Case report: drug interaction between tacrolimus and amiodarone with QT prolongation. *Transplantation* (2010) 89, 1166–7.

Sirolimus + Antiepileptics; Enzyme-inducing

Several case reports describe increased sirolimus dose requirements in the presence of phenytoin. Other enzyme-inducing antiepileptics would be expected to interact similarly.

Clinical evidence

An 11-year-old girl with a kidney transplant taking **phenytoin** started taking sirolimus 30 micrograms/kg twice daily following an episode of acute rejection. The dose of sirolimus was increased 10-fold over the next few weeks in an attempt to achieve the target minimum concentration of 10 to 20 nanograms/mL, and two further episodes of acute rejection occurred. About one month after the sirolimus had been started, tacrolimus was added, and her phenytoin was stopped. Over the next few weeks her sirolimus concentration increased to about 40 nanograms/mL. The patient subsequently recovered.[1]

A 62-year-old woman started taking **phenytoin** 100 mg twice daily because she developed a seizure disorder following a liver transplant. At this time she was taking ciclosporin, but it was decided to start sirolimus because of neurological complications. The initial sirolimus dose of 5 mg daily produced a subtherapeutic sirolimus concentration. She was subsequently stabilised taking sirolimus 15 mg daily, with a minimum concentration of less than 5 nanograms/mL. Phenytoin was stopped, and about 5 days later her minimum sirolimus concentration was found to be around 15 to 20 nanograms/mL. After a further 5 days, the sirolimus dose was reduced to 10 mg daily.[2]

A 68-year-old man stable taking sirolimus 2 mg daily for the previous 5 years (along with a large number of other drugs) was started on **carbamazepine** 200 mg twice daily, increased to 400 mg twice daily after 48 hours, for focal seizures. On day 5 he experienced a further seizure, and **phenytoin** was added (500 mg intravenous loading dose followed by 100 mg three times daily). On day 6 his carbamazepine concentration was 65 micromols/L (normal range 20 to 50 micromols/L) and so this was discontinued gradually over the following 10 days. Phenytoin was continued and, over the following 3 weeks, the sirolimus dose needed to be increased 4-fold, to 8 mg daily, in order to maintain a therapeutic concentration with increasing doses of phenytoin. Phenytoin was then switched to **levetiracetam** due to lack of seizure control, and during the following few months, the sirolimus dose needed to be decreased back to the original dose of 2 mg daily.[3]

Mechanism

Sirolimus is extensively metabolised by CYP3A4 in the intestinal wall and is a substrate for P-glycoprotein. Phenytoin and other antiepileptics that induce the activity of this isoenzyme and transporter protein would be expected to decrease sirolimus concentrations.

Importance and management

Evidence for an interaction between sirolimus and the enzyme-inducing antiepileptics appears to be limited to the reports with **phenytoin**, but they are consistent with the way both drugs are known to interact. It would therefore seem prudent to closely monitor sirolimus concentrations in any patient in whom phenytoin is started or withdrawn, and to adjust the sirolimus dose as necessary. This advice would also seem sensible for patients taking **carbamazepine**, **fosphenytoin** (the prodrug of phenytoin), and **phenobarbital** (and its parent drug **primidone**) as these drugs would be expected to interact in a similar way to phenytoin.

1. Hodges CB, Maxwell H, Beattie TJ, Murphy AV, Jindal RM. Use of rapamycin in a transplant patient who developed ciclosporin neurotoxicity. *Pediatr Nephrol* (2001) 16, 777–8.
2. Fridell JA, Jain AKB, Patel K, Virji M, Rao KN, Fung JJ, Venkataramanan R. Phenytoin decreases the blood concentrations of sirolimus in a liver transplant recipient: a case report. *Ther Drug Monit* (2003) 25, 117–19.
3. Bates D, Burak KW, Coffin CS, Ying T, Enns EM. Phenytoin-induced reduction in sirolimus levels. *Can J Hosp Pharm* (2011) 64, 271–4.

Sirolimus or Tacrolimus + Aprepitant

Sirolimus concentrations appear to be greatly increased by aprepitant. Tacrolimus concentrations might be expected to be similarly affected, but in one study they appeared to be only minimally increased by concurrent use.

Clinical evidence

In a retrospective study, 85 patients undergoing hematopoietic stem cell transplantation were given sirolimus 12 mg as a loading dose, followed by 4 mg daily, with tacrolimus 0.02 mg/kg daily intravenously. Doses of both drugs were subsequently adjusted to maintain a serum concentration between 5 and 10 nanograms/mL. In those also given aprepitant 125 mg on day 1 followed by 80 mg on days 2 and 3 (14 patients), the serum concentration of sirolimus was 2.2-fold higher than in those not given aprepitant (71 patients). Sirolimus doses were decreased in response to the higher concentrations. In contrast, the serum concentration of tacrolimus did not differ between those given aprepitant and those not.[1] In another retrospective study, 26 patients undergoing hematopoietic stem cell transplantation were given intravenous tacrolimus 0.03 mg/kg daily starting 6 days prior to transplant (and then adjusted to maintain a minimum blood concentration between 5 and 20 nanograms/mL), with aprepitant 125 mg on day 1 followed by 80 mg on days 2 and 3 starting one day after transplant. The concentration of tacrolimus during aprepitant treatment (defined as days 1 to 7 post-transplant) was 43% higher than that before (defined as 6 days prior to transplant until day 1 post-transplant). The tacrolimus concentration remained at a similarly higher level between day 7 post-transplant and conversion to oral tacrolimus (mean day 11).[2] No pharmacokinetic data were collected for oral tacrolimus. It is important to note that patients received phenytoin for 4 days during the conditioning regimen prior to transplantation (from days 10 to 7 pre-transplant).

Mechanism

Sirolimus and tacrolimus are both metabolised by CYP3A4, which is inhibited (in a dose-dependent manner) and induced by aprepitant (albeit perhaps transiently). Concentrations of drugs that are substrates of CYP3A4 are therefore expected to increase on concurrent use.

Importance and management

Evidence for an interaction between sirolimus or tacrolimus and aprepitant is limited to retrospective studies. However, the study with sirolimus suggests that the increase in concentrations when aprepitant is given is likely to be large and clinically important. Concurrent use should therefore be undertaken with caution, with close monitoring of sirolimus concentrations, adjusting the dose as required and awareness of signs of toxicity. The study with tacrolimus found only a small effect on concentrations, however residual inducing effects from the use of phenytoin (a CYP3A4 inducer) prior to transplant cannot be ruled out, and thus the true effect could be greater. The same cautions and monitoring on concurrent use as with sirolimus would also seem prudent with tacrolimus and aprepitant use.

1. Shayani S, Palmer JM, Stiller T, Chan H, Keuylian S, Parker P, Thomas S, Pullarkat V, Nademance A, Forman SJ, Nakamura R. Aprepitant (Emend) significantly increases sirolimus levels in patients undergoing allogeneic hematopoietic SCT. *Bone Marrow Transplant* (2012) 47, 291–3.
2. Ibrahim RB, Abidi MH, Ayash LJ, Cronin SM, Cadotte C, Mulawa J, Jacobson PA, Smith DW, Uberti JP, Edwards DJ. Effect of aprepitant on intravenous tacrolimus disposition in reduced intensity hematopoietic stem cell transplantation. *J Oncol Pharm Pract* (2008) 14, 113–21.

Sirolimus + Azoles

Sirolimus concentrations are greatly increased by ketoconazole, posaconazole, and voriconazole. Itraconazole appears to interact similarly, and fluconazole has also caused large increases in sirolimus concentrations. Clotrimazole and miconazole oral gel are predicted to interact similarly.

Clinical evidence

(a) Fluconazole

A study in 33 paediatric bone marrow transplant patients taking sirolimus, found that the minimum sirolimus concentrations in 22 patients given fluconazole (intravenous in 16 patients and oral in 6 patients, with a mean dose of 201 mg daily) were 67% higher than in 11 patients who did not receive fluconazole.[1] A kidney transplant patient taking sirolimus was given fluconazole 200 mg daily for oesophageal candidiasis. As an interaction was anticipated, the sirolimus dose was reduced from 4 mg daily to 3 mg daily. After 4 days, the sirolimus concentration had increased from about 10 to 22.8 micrograms/L. The dose of sirolimus was then reduced to 2 mg daily, but by the seventh day of fluconazole, the sirolimus concentration had reached

35 micrograms/L, after which it began to decrease. The patient then had a hyperkalaemic arrest and died.[2] The sirolimus concentration of another kidney transplant patient increased almost 5-fold about 3 weeks after she started to take fluconazole.[3]

(b) Itraconazole

A heart transplant patient needed only half of his normal sirolimus dose to maintain about the same minimum concentration when he took itraconazole 400 mg daily for a year.[3] A kidney transplant patient taking sirolimus 5 mg daily was given an initial dose of itraconazole 600 mg daily on day 10 post-transplant followed by 400 mg daily. The sirolimus minimum concentration was subtherapeutic at 6.8 nanograms/mL one day after starting itraconazole so the sirolimus dose was increased to 10 mg daily. However, the sirolimus concentration then increased rapidly and reached a concentration of 82.5 nanograms/mL 6 days later.[4] A haematopoietic stem cell transplant patient taking itraconazole 200 mg twice daily was changed from tacrolimus to sirolimus 7 mg daily. The sirolimus dose was reduced to 5 mg daily 6 days later because the sirolimus concentration was 17.5 nanograms/mL (therapeutic range 5 to 15 nanograms/mL). As the sirolimus concentration was found to be 35.6 nanograms/mL two days later, sirolimus was stopped until the concentration had decreased to within the therapeutic range. Sirolimus was subsequently restarted, with the dose adjusted to between 0.5 mg and 2 mg daily according to concentrations.[5]

(c) Ketoconazole

A pharmacokinetic study in 23 healthy subjects found that while taking ketoconazole 200 mg daily for 10 days, the maximum serum concentration and AUC of a single 5-mg dose of sirolimus were increased 4.3- and 10.9-fold, respectively.[6] In a study in 6 kidney transplant patients, ciclosporin was stopped because of toxicity or rejection episodes, and sirolimus was started. The subjects were given about a 75 to 87% lower than recommended dose of sirolimus (250 to 500 micrograms daily) along with ketoconazole 100 to 200 mg daily, adjusted to maintain sirolimus concentrations within the therapeutic range. The serum creatinine concentrations of the patients improved, reducing from 230 to 194 micromol/L.[7]

In a phase I study, patients with advanced cancer were given increasing weekly doses of sirolimus, starting at 1 mg and adjusted to finally achieve a similar sirolimus AUC to temsirolimus 25 mg (3810 ng-h/mL). When sirolimus was given alone in week one, a sirolimus dose of 90 mg was required to achieve this exposure. When ketoconazole 200 mg twice daily for one day followed by 200 mg daily for 3 days was given with each increasing sirolimus dose in week 2, the final dose of sirolimus required to achieve this exposure or higher was 16 mg (5007 ng-h/mL). Ketoconazole increased the AUC of sirolimus between 3.4- and 6.4-fold for each dose increment between 1 mg and 16 mg, when compared with sirolimus alone.[8]

(d) Posaconazole

In a study in 12 healthy subjects, posaconazole 400 mg given orally twice daily for 16 days increased the maximum serum concentration and AUC of a single 2-mg dose of sirolimus, taken on day 7, 6.7-fold and 8.9-fold, respectively.[9] In a retrospective study, 15 stem cell transplant patients taking sirolimus 1 to 3 mg daily were found to have also taken posaconazole for a median of 78 days (range 6 to 503 days). The median reduction in the sirolimus dose when posaconazole was started was 50%, and 7 days later, the required median dose reduction was 33%, although one patient required a 50% *increase* in their sirolimus dose. The sirolimus minimum concentration of one patient increased from 4.1 to 19.5 nanograms/mL, despite a 30% reduction in his sirolimus dose, when posaconazole was started, and one week later, he developed a suspected thrombotic microangiopathy.[10] A case report describes the successful use of posaconazole 400 mg twice daily for a soft tissue infection in a liver transplant patient taking sirolimus. On starting the posaconazole, the sirolimus dose was decreased from 2 mg daily to 1 mg daily, and then further to 1 mg on alternate days with close monitoring of sirolimus concentrations, which were stable between 3.6 and 5.3 micrograms/L. The patient completed a 6-month course of posaconazole.[11]

(e) Voriconazole

The UK and US manufacturers of both sirolimus and voriconazole report that voriconazole 400 mg twice daily for one day, then 200 mg twice daily for 8 days, increased the maximum serum concentration and AUC of a single 2-mg dose of sirolimus about 7- and 11-fold, respectively.[12,13] In a retrospective study of allogeneic haematopoietic stem cell transplant patients, 11 patients were found to have received both sirolimus and voriconazole for a median of 33 days (range 3 to 100 days). Three patients had an increased minimum sirolimus concentration of between 10 and 19 nanograms/mL and serious toxicity occurred in 2 of them. The other 8 patients had their sirolimus dose reduced by 90% when voriconazole was started, in anticipation of the interaction, and in these patients, minimum sirolimus concentrations were similar to those before voriconazole was started: no serious toxicity from either drug occurred.[14] In a retrospective chart review, 23 patients were found to have received concurrent sirolimus and voriconazole within a 24-hour period. No cases of increased sirolimus concentrations (greater than 20 nanograms/mL) occurred in 4 patients already taking voriconazole who were given a low dose of sirolimus (0.5 to 1 mg daily), or in 7 patients already taking sirolimus 0.5 to 2 mg daily (with a baseline sirolimus concentration of 13.2 nanograms/mL or less) and given voriconazole. Increased sirolimus concentrations were seen in some (but not all) patients given sirolimus doses of 4 mg daily or higher and/or who had a baseline sirolimus concentration of 12 nanograms/mL or more, regardless of whether they were given voriconazole before or after starting sirolimus.[15]

A patient taking sirolimus, who had large increases in sirolimus concentrations with itraconazole, was given voriconazole, and the sirolimus dose was decreased from 1.5 mg daily to 0.5 mg daily in anticipation of a similar interaction. The sirolimus minimum concentration was 6.4 nanograms/mL (about the patients' usual range) two days after starting voriconazole.[5]

A case report describes a heart transplant patient who was given two doses of voriconazole 400 mg then 200 mg twice daily for 16 days. When sirolimus was started, a dose of 1 mg gave a sirolimus minimum concentration of 12.8 nanograms/mL, but after voriconazole was stopped, a dose of 3 mg only gave a minimum sirolimus concentration of 7.4 nanograms/mL.[3] Voriconazole has been reported to cause large increases in sirolimus concentrations in a number of other patients.[3,16]

Mechanism

Sirolimus is metabolised by CYP3A4 and is a substrate for P-glycoprotein. Ketoconazole, itraconazole, posaconazole, and voriconazole are known inhibitors of CYP3A4, although to varying extents (see 'Table 1.9', p.11), and some also inhibit intestinal P-glycoprotein, leading to an increase in sirolimus concentrations. Fluconazole and miconazole also inhibit CYP3A4, but are less potent than ketoconazole, and so sirolimus concentrations increase when fluconazole is given, but this is not as great as that seen with other azoles.

Importance and management

The interactions between the azoles and sirolimus are established and of clinical importance. The increases in sirolimus concentration caused by **voriconazole** might be too large to be easily accommodated by reducing the dose of the sirolimus, although one study found that an initial empiric reduction in the sirolimus dose of 90% when voriconazole was started was adequate. However, more study is required to confirm the safety of such regimens.[14] Another study suggests that the sirolimus dose and its minimum concentration might also be an important factor in this interaction. Patients given lower doses or with lower concentrations appear to be less at risk of adverse increases in their sirolimus concentrations.[15] Note that the concurrent use of sirolimus is contraindicated by the manufacturers of **voriconazole**,[12,17] and not recommended by the manufacturers of sirolimus.[13,18]

The increases in sirolimus concentrations with **ketoconazole** and **posaconazole** are of a similar magnitude to those seen with voriconazole, and, although data are more limited, **itraconazole** also appears to interact to the same extent. If these azoles are required in a patient taking sirolimus, a pre-emptive sirolimus dose reduction would appear to be prudent, and minimum sirolimus concentrations should be very closely monitored both during use and after they are stopped. About an 80% reduction in sirolimus dose was used in one study with ketoconazole.[7] However, note that the manufacturers of sirolimus state that the concurrent use of sirolimus with ketoconazole or itraconazole is not recommended.[13,18] Similar advice is also given by the manufacturers of **posaconazole**.[19,20] If the combination is unavoidable, the UK manufacturer advises aiming for minimum sirolimus concentrations in the upper part of the therapeutic range. This is because there is a change in the disposition of sirolimus which means that lower concentrations, even within the therapeutic range, might be subtherapeutic.[19]

Fluconazole, although a weaker inhibitor of CYP3A4 than ketoconazole, voriconazole, or itraconazole, has been reported to interact, and a retrospective study suggests that an initial sirolimus dose reduction of about 50 to 75% should be considered if fluconazole is required.[21] However, note that this was a small study and further study is required to validate this suggestion.

Clotrimazole[13,18] (presumably systemic clotrimazole) might also interact similarly. Sirolimus plasma concentrations should be closely monitored during treatment with and following the withdrawal of both of these antifungals.

There appear to be no reports of an interaction between **miconazole** and sirolimus. However, a large proportion of miconazole oral gel (both prescription and non-prescription doses) might be swallowed and therefore adequate systemic absorption might occur to produce an interaction. The UK manufacturer of miconazole oral gel recommends close monitoring and possible dose reduction of sirolimus if both drugs are given.[22] An interaction with intravaginal miconazole would not normally be expected because its systemic absorption is usually very low (less than 2%).[23]

1. Goyal RK, Han K, Wall DA, Pulsipher MA, Bunin N, Grupp SA, Mada SR, Venkataramanan R. Sirolimus pharmacokinetics in early postmyeloablative pediatric blood and marrow transplantation. *Biol Blood Marrow Transplant* (2013) 19, 569–75.
2. Cervelli MJ. Fluconazole-sirolimus drug interaction. *Transplantation* (2002) 74, 1477–8.
3. Sádaba B, Campanero MA, Quetglas EG, Azanza JR. Clinical relevance of sirolimus drug interactions in transplant patients. *Transplant Proc* (2004) 36, 3226–8.
4. Kuypers DR, Claes K, Evenepoel P, Maes B, Vandecasteele S, Vanrenterghem Y, Van Damme B, Desmet K. Drug interaction between itraconazole and sirolimus in a primary renal allograft recipient. *Transplantation* (2005) 79, 737.
5. Said A, Garnick JJ, Dieterle N, Peres E, Abidi MH, Ibrahim RB. Sirolimus-itraconazole interaction in a hematopoietic stem cell transplant recipient. *Pharmacotherapy* (2006) 26, 289–95.
6. Floren LC, Christians U, Zimmerman JJ, Neefe L, Schorer R, Rushowrth D, Harper D, Renz J, Benet LZ. Sirolimus oral bioavailability increases ten-fold with concomitant ketoconazole. *Clin Pharmacol Ther* (1999) 65, 159.
7. Thomas PP, Manivannan J, John GT, Jacob CK. Sirolimus and ketoconazole co-prescription in renal transplant recipients. *Transplantation* (2004) 77, 474–5.
8. Cohen EEW, Wu K, Hartford C, Kocherginsky M, Eaton KN, Zha Y, Nallari A, Maitland ML, Fox-Kay K, Moshier K, House L, Ramirez J, Undevia SD, Fleming GF, Gajewski TF, Ratain MJ. Phase I studies of sirolimus alone or in combination with pharmacokinetic modulators in advanced cancer patients. *Clin Cancer Res* (2012) Epub.
9. Moton A, Ma L, Krishna G, Martinho M, Seiberling M, McLeod J. Effects of oral posaconazole on the pharmacokinetics of sirolimus. *Curr Med Res Opin* (2009) 25, 701–7.
10. Kubiak DW, Koo S, Hammond SP, Armand P, Baden LR, Antin JH, Marty FM. Safety of posaconazole and sirolimus coadministration in allogeneic hematopoietic stem cell transplants. *Biol Blood Marrow Transplant* (2012) 18, 1462–5.
11. Dahlan R, Patel A, Haider S. Successful use of posaconazole to treat invasive cutaneous fungal infection in a liver transplant patient on sirolimus. *Can J Infect Dis Med Microbiol* (2012) 23, e44–e47.
12. VFEND (Voriconazole). Pfizer Inc. US Prescribing information, February 2014.
13. Rapamune (Sirolimus). Pfizer Ltd. UK Summary of product characteristics, August 2013.
14. Marty FM, Lowry CM, Cutler CS, Campbell BJ, Fiumara K, Baden LR, Antin JH. Voriconazole and sirolimus coadministration after allogeneic hematopoietic stem cell transplantation. *Biol Blood Marrow Transplant* (2006) 12, 552–9.
15. Surowiec D, DePestel DD, Carver PL. Concurrent administration of sirolimus and voriconazole: a pilot study assessing safety and approaches to appropriate management. *Pharmacotherapy* (2008) 28, 719–29.

16. Mathis AS, Shah NK, Friedman GS. Combined use of sirolimus and voriconazole in renal transplantation: a report of two cases. *Transplant Proc* (2004) 36, 2708–9.
17. VFEND (Voriconazole). Pfizer Ltd. UK Summary of product characteristics, October 2014.
18. Rapamune (Sirolimus). Wyeth Pharmaceuticals Inc. US Prescribing information, December 2012.
19. Noxafil (Posaconazole). Merck Sharp & Dohme Ltd. UK Summary of product characteristics, September 2014.
20. Noxafil (Posaconazole). Merck & Co., Inc. US Prescribing information, June 2014.
21. Peksa GD, Schultz K, Fung HC. Dosing algorithm for concomitant administration of sirolimus, tacrolimus, and an azole after allogeneic hematopoietic stem cell transplantation. *J Oncol Pharm Pract* (2014) Epub.
22. Daktarin Oral Gel (Miconazole). Janssen-Cilag Ltd. UK Summary of product characteristics, December 2014.
23. Daneshmend TK. Systemic absorption of miconazole from the vagina. *J Antimicrob Chemother* (1986) 18, 507–11.

Sirolimus + Calcium-channel blockers

Sirolimus caused a small increase in verapamil concentrations in one study, but did not appear to affect diltiazem concentrations in another. Diltiazem and verapamil increase sirolimus concentrations. Nicardipine is predicted to interact similarly. Nifedipine appears not to interact with sirolimus. The concurrent use of sirolimus and calcium-channel blockers might be associated with gingival overgrowth.

Clinical evidence

(a) Sirolimus concentrations

1. Diltiazem. A crossover study in 18 healthy subjects found that a single 120-mg oral dose of diltiazem increased the AUC and the maximum serum concentration of a single 10-mg oral dose of sirolimus by 60% and 43%, respectively. The pharmacokinetics of diltiazem and its metabolites were unchanged.[1] Similarly, in a study in 76 patients given sirolimus 2 mg daily alone for 28 days then with diltiazem 180 mg daily after coronary stenting, blood concentrations of sirolimus were increased by 50%, from 6.2 to 9.3 nanograms/mL.[2]

2. Nifedipine. In a study comparing 16 patients taking nifedipine and sirolimus with 10 patients taking sirolimus alone, there were no differences in sirolimus pharmacokinetics between the two groups.[3] Similarly, in a study in healthy subjects, there was no pharmacokinetic interaction between nifedipine and sirolimus.[4]

3. Verapamil. The UK and US manufacturers of sirolimus briefly note, that in 26 healthy subjects, the concurrent use of sirolimus oral solution 2 mg daily and verapamil 180 mg every 12 hours to steady-state, resulted in an increase in the sirolimus maximum concentration and AUC of 2.3- and 2.2-fold, respectively. In addition, there was a 50% increase in the maximum concentration and the AUC of the active *S*-verapamil isomer.[5,6]

(b) Gingival overgrowth

Calcium-channel blockers are well-known to be associated with gingival overgrowth in transplant patients, but the association with sirolimus is less well established. In a study of 144 kidney transplant patients taking sirolimus for at least 2 months post-transplant, the incidence of gingival overgrowth was found to be 20.8%, although no cases were defined as clinically significant. A greater number of patients experiencing gingival overgrowth were also taking a calcium-channel blocker than in those patients who did not experience gingival overgrowth (50% vs 23.7%).[7] A follow-up study in 35 of these same patients over a period of 44-months, found that the incidence of gingival overgrowth decreased to zero in all patients, including those taking calcium channel blockers (14.3%).[8] Another study found that the incidence of gingival overgrowth among sirolimus-treated kidney transplant patients was 15.6%, and this was associated with calcium-channel blocker use.[9]

Mechanism

Diltiazem and verapamil inhibit CYP3A4 in the intestinal wall and liver, which is the primary route of sirolimus metabolism. Verapamil also inhibits P-glycoprotein activity, which leads to increased sirolimus absorption. It is not known why verapamil concentrations were increased. Nifedipine is not an inhibitor of CYP3A4 or P-glycoprotein. The concurrent use of sirolimus and calcium-channel blockers might cause additive gingival overgrowth.

Importance and management

The pharmacokinetic interactions between sirolimus and diltiazem or verapamil would appear to be established. The UK and US manufacturers recommend whole blood monitoring and a possible sirolimus dose reduction (based on sirolimus concentrations) if diltiazem or verapamil are used concurrently.[5,6] The clinical relevance of the modest increase in verapamil concentrations is uncertain, but bear it in mind in the event of an increase in adverse effects due to verapamil, such as hypotension, flushing, and oedema. The manufacturers note that other calcium-channel blockers that inhibit CYP3A4 might interact similarly, and they specifically name **nicardipine**,[5,6] although note that other calcium-channel blockers do not usually act as CYP3A4 inhibitors.

The association between sirolimus and calcium-channel blocker use, and gingival overgrowth is less-well documented than with ciclosporin or tacrolimus and calcium-channel blockers (see 'Ciclosporin + Calcium-channel blockers', p.1220 and 'Tacrolimus + Calcium-channel blockers', p.1291), but concurrent use might result in additive effects, albeit less so than with ciclosporin or tacrolimus.[9] It would seem prudent to aware of the possibility of gingival overgrowth occurring if a calcium-channel blocker is required, particularly if gingival overgrowth has occurred while taking sirolimus.

1. Böttiger Y, Säwe J, Brattström C, Tollemar J, Burke JT, Häss G, Zimmerman JJ. Pharmacokinetic interaction between single oral doses of diltiazem and sirolimus in healthy volunteers. *Clin Pharmacol Ther* (2001) 69, 32–40.
2. Rodríguez AE, Rodríguez Alemparte M, Vigo CF, Fernández Pereira C, Llauradó C, Vetcher D, Pocovi A, Ambrose J. Role of oral rapamycin to prevent restenosis in patients with de novo lesions undergoing coronary stenting: results of the Argentina single centre study (ORAR trial). *Heart* (2005) 91, 1433–7.
3. Zimmerman JJ, Kahan BD. Pharmacokinetics of sirolimus in stable renal transplant patients after multiple oral dose administration. *J Clin Pharmacol* (1997) 37, 405–15.
4. Zimmerman JJ. Exposure-response relationships and drug interactions of sirolimus. *AAPS J* (2004) 6, 1–12.
5. Rapamune (Sirolimus). Wyeth Pharmaceuticals Inc. US Prescribing information, December 2012.
6. Rapamune (Sirolimus). Pfizer Ltd. UK Summary of product characteristics, August 2013.
7. Cota LO, Oliveira AP, Costa JE, Cortelli SC, Costa FO. Gingival status of Brazilian renal transplant recipients under sirolimus-based regimens. *J Periodontol* (2008) 79, 2060–8.
8. Costa LC, Costa FO, Cortelli SC, Cortelli JR, Cota LC. Gingival overgrowth in renal transplant subjects: a 44-month follow-up study. *Transplantation* (2013) 96, 890–6.
9. Cota LO, Aquino DR, Franco GC, Cortelli JR, Cortelli SC, Costa FO. Gingival overgrowth in subjects under immunosuppressive regimens based on cyclosporine, tacrolimus, or sirolimus. *J Clin Periodontol* (2010) 37, 894–902.

Sirolimus + Ciclosporin

Ciclosporin greatly increases sirolimus concentrations. Concurrent use for longer than 3 to 4 months possibly increases renal toxicity. Sirolimus does not appear to alter ciclosporin blood concentrations in the short-term.

Clinical evidence

(a) Effect on ciclosporin

In a placebo-controlled study in kidney transplant patients, when sirolimus was added to a regimen including ciclosporin and a corticosteroid for 2 weeks, the steady-state ciclosporin concentrations remained unchanged. Blood pressure, glomerular filtration rate, creatinine concentrations, triglyceride concentrations, and liver enzymes (ALT, AST) were unchanged.[1] Similarly, in a 2-week pharmacokinetic study in 40 kidney transplant patients, sirolimus 0.5 to 6.5 mg/m^2 given twice daily did not affect the pharmacokinetics of ciclosporin 75 to 400 mg twice daily. The patients were also taking prednisone.[2] In a related study in kidney transplant patients, a single dose of sirolimus had no effect on the pharmacokinetics of ciclosporin.[3] Similarly, in another study in healthy subjects, single doses of sirolimus did not affect the pharmacokinetics of a single dose of ciclosporin when given either at the same time or 4 hours apart.[4] A multiple-dose study in kidney transplant patients also found that the pharmacokinetics of ciclosporin were not altered by simultaneous administration or when the doses were given 4 hours apart.[5]

In contrast, a study in kidney transplant patients found that the AUC of ciclosporin was higher, and the dose required to achieve target whole blood concentrations was lower, in patients also taking sirolimus than in those also taking azathioprine, despite separating the doses by 4 hours.[6] Similar results were found when the comparison was made against placebo.[7]

An isolated report describes a kidney transplant patient who had a large increase in ciclosporin concentration shortly after starting sirolimus 2 mg daily. Within 2 weeks of starting the sirolimus, she was readmitted to hospital with signs of ciclosporin toxicity, including increased creatinine and urea concentrations, high blood pressure, and an increased ciclosporin concentration (536 nanograms/mL). The ciclosporin dose was reduced from 400 to 300 mg daily, sirolimus was continued, and her ciclosporin concentration decreased to 276 nanograms/mL. The sirolimus concentration remained within the therapeutic range, at 5.2 to 10.6 nanograms/mL.[8]

(b) Effect on sirolimus

In a multiple-dose study in kidney transplant patients, giving ciclosporin at the same time as sirolimus resulted in higher sirolimus maximum and minimum plasma concentrations (72% and 49%, respectively), and a higher sirolimus AUC (45%), than when ciclosporin was given 4 hours before sirolimus.[5] Similarly, in a single-dose study in healthy subjects, ciclosporin, given 4 hours before sirolimus, increased the maximum serum concentration of sirolimus by 40% and increased its AUC by 80%. When the drugs were given at the same time, the effect was even greater, with a 2.2-fold increase in the sirolimus maximum concentration and 3.3-fold increase in its AUC.[4] Another study found a 40% increase in all the pharmacokinetic parameters of sirolimus when it was given 6 hours after ciclosporin.[9] When sirolimus was taken at the same time or 2 hours after ciclosporin, the AUC of sirolimus increased 2.8- and 2.4-fold, respectively, but when sirolimus was given 2 hours before ciclosporin there was no effect on its AUC or maximum plasma concentration.[10] The US manufacturer of sirolimus also presents data showing that ciclosporin oral solution (*Sandimmune*) given at the same time as sirolimus, increased the sirolimus minimum concentration by 67 to 86% in 150 patients with psoriasis.[11] In a retrospective study of 210 kidney transplant recipients, the dose-normalised sirolimus minimum concentration was 27% higher in the 165 patients also taking ciclosporin, than in the 45 patients also taking mycophenolate.[12] A case report describes an increased sirolimus concentration in a 3-year-old liver transplant patient after tacrolimus was switched to ciclosporin. His sirolimus concentration while also taking tacrolimus was 8 nanograms/mL (range 6 to 10.1 nanograms/mL) but increased to 16.2 nanograms/mL (range 9.6 to 27 nanograms/mL) after the ciclosporin was started.[13]

(c) Renal toxicity

The manufacturers note that, in clinical studies in patients with kidney transplants, the concurrent use of ciclosporin and sirolimus for more than 6 months and up to

36 months was associated with an increase in serum creatinine concentrations and a decrease in glomerular filtration rate when compared with patients given ciclosporin and placebo.[10,11] The difference in glomerular filtration rate was about 5.5 mL/minute (10%) at 12 and 36 months.[11] In patients in whom ciclosporin was successfully withdrawn, glomerular filtration rates were higher than in those maintained on ciclosporin.[10,11]

Mechanism

It has been suggested that ciclosporin inhibits the metabolism of sirolimus by CYP3A4 in the intestine and liver leading to increased sirolimus concentrations[4,10,11] and inhibits P-glycoprotein leading to increased sirolimus absorption. There is some experimental evidence to suggest that sirolimus might increase ciclosporin renal toxicity by increasing intracellular ciclosporin concentrations in the renal epithelial cells by inhibiting P-glycoprotein.[14]

Importance and management

The interaction between ciclosporin and sirolimus leading to increased sirolimus concentrations is established. The UK and US manufacturers recommend that, to minimise the interaction, sirolimus should be given 4 hours after ciclosporin micro-emulsion, and consistently, either with or without food.[10,11] Despite this, it might still be necessary to reduce the sirolimus dose,[4] and the blood concentration of sirolimus should be monitored and the dose adjusted to maintain a concentration of 4 to 12 nanograms/mL.[10] Renal function should be closely monitored, and if the serum creatinine concentration increases, consider stopping sirolimus or ciclosporin.[11] Moreover, the manufacturers do not recommend continued use of the combination long-term, because higher serum creatinine concentrations and lower glomerular filtration rates have been seen.[10,11] Ciclosporin should be gradually discontinued over 4 to 8 weeks, increasing the sirolimus dose to obtain a higher sirolimus minimum concentration of 12 to 20 nanograms/mL.[10] In general, the sirolimus dose will need to be increased 4-fold to take into account the absence of the interaction (2-fold increase) and the need for increased immunosuppression (2-fold increase).[10]

The UK manufacturer of sirolimus does not recommend its use with ciclosporin in patients at high-immunological risk of graft rejection as insufficient numbers of this type of patient were studied in clinical trials.[10] However, the US manufacturer of sirolimus states that it can be used in combination with ciclosporin in such patients for up to one year.[11]

The concurrent use of both drugs increases the risk of developing calcineurin inhibitor-induced haemolytic uraemic syndrome, thrombotic thrombocytopenic purpura, and thrombotic microangiopathy.[10,11] An increased risk of hepatic artery thrombosis, leading to graft loss and/or death in most cases, has also been seen in clinical studies in *de novo* liver transplant patients taking sirolimus with ciclosporin.[10,11]

1. Murgia MG, Jordan S, Kahan BD. The side effect profile of sirolimus: a phase I study in quiescent cyclosporine-prednisone-treated renal transplant patients. *Kidney Int* (1996) 49, 209–16.
2. Zimmerman JJ, Kahan BD. Pharmacokinetics of sirolimus in stable renal transplant patients after multiple oral dose administration. *J Clin Pharmacol* (1997) 37, 405–15.
3. Ferron GM, Mishina EV, Zimmerman JJ, Jusko WJ. Population pharmacokinetics of sirolimus in kidney transplant patients. *Clin Pharmacol Ther* (1997) 61, 416–28.
4. Zimmerman JJ, Harper D, Getsy J, Jusko WJ. Pharmacokinetic interactions between sirolimus and microemulsion cyclosporine when orally administered jointly and 4 hours apart in healthy volunteers. *J Clin Pharmacol* (2003) 42, 1168–76.
5. Kaplan B, Meier-Kriesche H-U, Napoli KL, Kahan BD. The effects of relative timing of sirolimus and cyclosporine microemulsion formulation coadministration on the pharmacokinetics of each agent. *Clin Pharmacol Ther* (1998) 63, 48–53.
6. Kahan BD; the Rapamune US Study Group. Efficacy of sirolimus compared with azathioprine for reduction of acute renal allograft rejection: a randomised multicentre study. *Lancet* (2000) 356, 194–202.
7. Wyeth Pharmaceuticals. Data on file. Study GMR-32348.
8. Dąbrowska-Zamojcin E, Pawlik A, Domański L, Różański J, Droździk M. Cyclosporine and sirolimus interaction in a kidney transplant patient. *Transplant Proc* (2005) 37, 2317–19.
9. Wu FLL, Tsai M-K, Chen RR-L, Sun S-W, Huang J-D, Hu R-H, Chen K-H, Lee P-H. Effects of calcineurin inhibitors on sirolimus pharmacokinetics during staggered administration in renal transplant recipients. *Pharmacotherapy* (2005) 25, 646–53.
10. Rapamune (Sirolimus). Pfizer Ltd. UK Summary of product characteristics, August 2013.
11. Rapamune (Sirolimus). Wyeth Pharmaceuticals Inc. US Prescribing information, December 2012.
12. Cattaneo D, Merlini S, Pellegrino M, Carrara F, Zenoni S, Murgia S, Baldelli S, Gaspari F, Remuzzi G, Perico N. Therapeutic drug monitoring of sirolimus: effect of concomitant immunosuppressive therapy and optimization of drug dosing. *Am J Transplant* (2004) 4, 1345–51.
13. Shinke H, Hashi S, Kinoshita R, Taniguchi R, Sugimoto M, Matsubara K, Ogawa E, Sonoda M, Takada N, Yoshizawa A, Ogawa K, Okamoto S, Uemoto S, Masuda S. Effectiveness of sirolimus in combination with cyclosporine against chronic rejection in a pediatric liver transplant patient. *Biol Pharm Bull* (2013) 36, 1221–5.
14. Anglicheau D, Pallet N, Rabant M, Marquet P, Cassinat B, Méria P, Beaune P, Legendre C, Thervet E. Role of P-glycoprotein in cyclosporine cytotoxicity in the cyclosporine-sirolimus interaction. *Kidney Int* (2006) 70, 1019–25.

Sirolimus + Corticosteroids

Intravenous methylprednisolone appears to have no effect on sirolimus minimum concentrations. Sirolimus minimally increases prednisolone concentrations (derived from prednisone).

Clinical evidence, mechanism, importance and management

(a) Methylprednisolone

When 14 kidney transplant patients taking sirolimus (and also taking either azathioprine or mycophenolate) were given methylprednisolone as a daily intravenous bolus for one to 5 days (total dose of between 500 mg and 3 g) the sirolimus minimum concentration was not altered.[1] No sirolimus dose adjustment appears to be necessary on concurrent use.[1]

(b) Prednisolone or Prednisone

In a study in kidney transplant patients taking ciclosporin and prednisone 5 to 20 mg daily, only small changes occurred in the pharmacokinetics of the metabolite, prednisolone, when sirolimus 6 to 13 mg/m² daily was given for 2 weeks.[2] The maximum plasma concentration of prednisolone was increased by 14%, and the AUC was increased by 18%. These findings seem unlikely to be clinically relevant.

(c) Unspecified corticosteroids

In a retrospective study of 386 kidney transplant patients, the inclusion of steroids (exact drugs not specified) to a regimen containing sirolimus and ciclosporin, resulted in a 15% lower dose-normalised sirolimus minimum concentration than with sirolimus and ciclosporin alone.[3] The clinical importance of this small change is not known, but it seems likely to be minor.

1. Bäckman L, Kreis H, Morales JM, Wilczek H, Taylor R, Burke JT. Sirolimus steady-state trough concentrations are not affected by bolus methylprednisolone therapy in renal allograft recipients. *Br J Clin Pharmacol* (2002) 54, 65–8.
2. Jusko WJ, Ferron GM, SM Mis, Kahan BD, Zimmerman JJ. Pharmacokinetics of prednisolone during administration of sirolimus in patients with renal transplants. *J Clin Pharmacol* (1996) 36, 1100–6.
3. Cattaneo D, Merlini S, Pellegrino M, Carrara F, Zenoni S, Murgia S, Baldelli S, Gaspari F, Remuzzi G, Perico N. Therapeutic drug monitoring of sirolimus: effect of concomitant immunosuppressive therapy and optimization of drug dosing. *Am J Transplant* (2004) 4, 1345–51.

Sirolimus + Co-trimoxazole

A single dose of co-trimoxazole did not alter sirolimus concentrations in one study.

Clinical evidence, mechanism, importance and management

In a study in 15 kidney transplant patients who had started sirolimus one week previously, there was no change in the AUC and maximum concentration of sirolimus after the first daily dose of oral co-trimoxazole (sulfamethoxazole with trimethoprim) 480 mg when compared with the day before.[1] There was also no change in serum creatinine concentrations between these two days, although a 4.3% increase was seen in 9 of the 15 patients on the following day.

The evidence suggests that co-trimoxazole does not have an important effect on the pharmacokinetics of sirolimus and that no sirolimus dose adjustment is likely to be needed with concurrent use. However, the authors note that it does not rule out the possibility that longer-term concurrent use might lead to increases in sirolimus concentrations, particularly if renal function is impaired leading to co-trimoxazole accumulation.[1]

1. Böttiger Y, Brattström C, Bäckman L, Claesson K, Burke JT. Trimethoprim-sulphamethoxazole does not affect the pharmacokinetics of sirolimus in renal transplant recipients. *Br J Clin Pharmacol* (2005) 60, 566–9.

Sirolimus and related drugs or Tacrolimus + Dronedarone

Dronedarone increased the sirolimus concentration of a patient. Everolimus, temsirolimus, and tacrolimus are predicted to be similarly affected.

Clinical evidence

A 67-year-old kidney transplant patient stable taking **sirolimus** 5 mg daily was given dronedarone 400 mg twice daily following electrical cardioversion for atrial fibrillation. Three days later his minimum sirolimus concentration was 38.6 nanograms/mL and sirolimus was stopped; concentrations over the previous year had not exceeded 13.5 nanograms/mL. The minimum sirolimus concentration peaked the following day at 45.2 nanograms/mL. Sirolimus was restarted, about a week after it had been stopped, at a lower dose of 2 mg daily, which was subsequently further titrated down to 1 mg daily to keep the minimum concentration within the therapeutic range.[1]

Mechanism

Dronedarone is an inhibitor of CYP3A4 and P-glycoprotein by which sirolimus is extensively metabolised and transported, respectively. Concurrent use therefore causes sirolimus concentrations to increase.

Importance and management

Evidence for an interaction between dronedarone and **sirolimus** is limited to one case report, but what is known is in line with the way these drugs would be expected to interact, and therefore an interaction would appear to be established. It would seem prudent to increase the frequency of monitoring the concentration of sirolimus if dronedarone is started, adjusting the dose accordingly.

The sirolimus analogues, **everolimus** and **temsirolimus**, and **tacrolimus** are also substrates of CYP3A4 and P-glycoprotein and so would be expected to be affected similarly to sirolimus. Therefore it would seem prudent to follow the same precautions with any of these drugs, as those described for sirolimus.

Note that dronedarone can prolong the QT interval and increase the risk of torsade de pointes, and tacrolimus is also associated with an increased risk of QT-interval prolongation. See 'Drugs that prolong the QT interval + Other drugs that prolong the QT interval', p.272, for further information on the concurrent use of two or more drugs that prolong the QT interval.

1. 1. Tichy EM, Medwid AJ, Mills EA, Formica RN, Kulkarni S. Significant sirolimus and dronedarone interaction in a kidney transplant recipient. *Ann Pharmacother* (2010) 44, 1338–41.

Sirolimus + Fish oils

Fish oils might increase sirolimus concentrations.

Clinical evidence

A retrospective analysis of sirolimus pharmacokinetic data in patients who received low-dose sirolimus and omega-3 fatty acids and those who did not, found that dose-adjusted sirolimus minimum concentrations in patients receiving omega-3 fatty acids were 50% higher after the omega-3 fatty acids were started. In addition, the dose-adjusted AUC of sirolimus was 24% higher in those patients who received omega-3 fatty acids than in those who did not. A corresponding dose adjustment was required in patients receiving omega-3 fatty acids in order to achieve sirolimus minimum concentrations and AUC comparable to those patients not receiving omega-3 fatty acids.[1]

Mechanism

Sirolimus is metabolised by CYP3A4, which might be inhibited by the omega-3 fatty acid, docosahexaenoic acid (DHA), present in fish oils, and this could have been the cause of the increased minimum concentrations seen. However the US manufacturer of omega-3- acid ethyl esters states that *in vitro* study has indicated that clinically significant inhibition of cytochrome P450 isoenzymes by a combination of eicosapentaenoic acid and docosahexaenoic acid is not expected to occur in humans;[2] another mechanism could therefore be involved. Further study is needed.

Importance and management

Evidence for an interaction between omega-3 fatty acids and sirolimus is limited to this retrospective study, and the general clinical importance of the increase in sirolimus minimum concentrations and exposure seen is not clear. The clinical importance of the CYP3A4 inhibition exerted by docosahexaenoic acid in fish oils is not known, as clinical evidence of an effect appears to be limited to this study which suggests that it might only be a very weak inhibitor of CYP3A4. Until more is known, some caution might be appropriate with concurrent use, and an interaction suspected if an unexpected increase in sirolimus minimum concentrations occurs after starting omega-3 fatty acid-containing supplements.

1. Cortinovis M, Gotti E, Remuzzi G, Perico N, Cattaneo D, Baldelli S. Omega-3 polyunsaturated fatty acids affect sirolimus exposure in kidney transplant recipients on calcineurin inhibitor-free regimen. *Transplantation* (2010) 89, 126–7.
2. Lovaza (Omega-3- acid ethyl esters). GlaxoSmithKline. US Prescribing information, September 2013.

Sirolimus + Food

A high-fat meal slightly increases the exposure to sirolimus.

Clinical evidence, mechanism, importance and management

In a single-dose study in healthy subjects, giving a non-aqueous solution of sirolimus with a high-fat breakfast reduced the maximum sirolimus concentration by 34%, delayed the time to maximum concentration by about 2 hours, and increased the AUC by 34%, when compared with the fasting state. There was no change in the elimination half-life of sirolimus.[1] In a similar study using sirolimus tablets, the maximum concentration and AUC of sirolimus were increased by 65% and 23%, respectively, by a high-fat meal.[2] The extent of this interaction was considered minor when compared with the large variability in sirolimus concentrations between subjects.[1] Nevertheless, the UK and US manufacturers recommend that sirolimus solution or tablets should be taken consistently either with or without food, to minimise variability.[2,3]

1. Zimmerman JJ, Ferron GM, Lim HK, Parker V. The effect of a high-fat meal on the oral bioavailability of the immunosuppressant sirolimus (rapamycin). *J Clin Pharmacol* (1999) 39, 1155–61.
2. Rapamune (Sirolimus). Pfizer Ltd. UK Summary of product characteristics, August 2013.
3. Rapamune (Sirolimus). Wyeth Pharmaceuticals Inc. US Prescribing information, December 2012.

Sirolimus + Grapefruit juice

Grapefruit juice appears to increase the exposure to oral sirolimus.

Clinical evidence

In a phase I study, patients with advanced cancer were given increasing weekly doses of oral sirolimus, starting at 1 mg and adjusted to achieve a specific AUC (intended to match the equivalent of intravenous temsirolimus 25 mg weekly). When sirolimus was given alone, a sirolimus dose of 90 mg weekly was required to achieve the required AUC. When 240-mL of grapefruit juice (as a frozen concentrate with a consistent concentration of furanocoumarins between batches) was given daily with sirolimus, a similar AUC was achieved with sirolimus 15 mg weekly (one-sixth of the previous dose).[1]

Mechanism

Grapefruit juice inhibits intestinal CYP3A4, the isoenzyme that is at least partly responsible for the metabolism of sirolimus, leading to an increase in its exposure.

Importance and management

Although the evidence for an interaction between sirolimus and grapefruit juice is limited to the study above, given the likely mechanism, it would appear to be established and of clinical importance. The authors of this study suggest that the interaction between grapefruit juice and sirolimus could be exploited to save money. However, this could be risky because the concentrations of the constituents of grapefruit vary between batches of grapefruit juice, which could make any increases in sirolimus exposure variable and difficult to control. The UK and US manufacturers of sirolimus recommend that patients should avoid grapefruit juice.[2,3] Furthermore the US manufacturer states that grapefruit juice should not be used for the dilution of sirolimus oral solution.[3] Given the large increases in sirolimus exposure reported, this advice would seem sensible.

1. Cohen EEW, Wu K, Hartford C, Kocherginsky M, Eaton KN, Zha Y, Nallari A, Maitland ML, Fox-Kay K, Moshier K, House L, Ramirez J, Undevia SD, Fleming GF, Gajewski TF, Ratain MJ. Phase I studies of sirolimus alone or in combination with pharmacokinetic modulators in advanced cancer patients. *Clin Cancer Res* (2012) Epub.
2. Rapamune (Sirolimus). Pfizer Ltd. UK Summary of product characteristics, August 2013.
3. Rapamune (Sirolimus). Wyeth Pharmaceuticals Inc. US Prescribing information, December 2012.

Sirolimus + HCV-Protease inhibitors

Telaprevir very markedly increases sirolimus exposure, and boceprevir has a marked effect. Simeprevir might increase or decrease sirolimus exposure. Boceprevir exposure does not appear to be affected by sirolimus.

Clinical evidence

(a) Boceprevir

The UK manufacturer briefly notes that, in a study in healthy subjects given a single 2-mg dose of sirolimus with boceprevir 800 mg three times daily, the maximum sirolimus concentration and AUC were increased 4.8- and 8-fold, respectively. The AUC and maximum plasma concentration of boceprevir were not affected to a clinically relevant extent.[1]

(b) Telaprevir

A report describes 10 liver transplant patients (7 of whom were taking mycophenolate), given sirolimus 0.5 mg initially and then adjusted according to plasma concentrations, who were treated with telaprevir 1125 mg twice daily (with ribavirin and interferon alpha) for recurrent hepatitis C infection. The dose-corrected maximum sirolimus concentration and AUC were 3- and 26-fold higher, respectively, than historical data. The average dose of sirolimus during the first 4 weeks of telaprevir treatment was just 7.6% of that prior to telaprevir being started.[2]

Mechanism

Boceprevir and telaprevir are both potent CYP3A4 inhibitors, by which sirolimus is metabolised. Concurrent use therefore results in increased sirolimus exposure.

Importance and management

Evidence for an interaction between sirolimus and the HCV-protease inhibitors is limited, but is consistent with the known disposition and interactions of these drugs. The marked and very marked increases in exposure seen with boceprevir and telaprevir, respectively, are clinically important, and will require large reductions in the sirolimus dose, and/or prolongation of the dosing interval in order to maintain concentrations within the therapeutic range. To avoid toxicity, sirolimus concentrations, adverse effects, and renal function should be closely monitored on concurrent use.

The effects of **simeprevir** do not appear to have been studied, but the UK and US manufacturers predict that increases or decreases in sirolimus exposure might occur on concurrent use, and recommend monitoring of sirolimus concentrations.[3,4] The US manufacturer suggests that routine monitoring is sufficient.[4]

1. Victrelis (Boceprevir). Merck Sharp & Dohme Ltd. UK Summary of product characteristics, August 2014.
2. O'Leary JG, McKenna GJ, Klintmalm GB, Davis GL. et al. Effect of telaprevir on the pharmacokinetics of sirolimus in liver transplant recipients. *Liver Transpl* (2013) 19, 463–5.
3. Olysio (Simeprevir sodium). Janssen-Cilag Ltd. UK Summary of product characteristics, May 2014.
4. Olysio (Simeprevir sodium). Janssen Products, LP. US Prescribing information, November 2014.

Sirolimus + HIV-protease inhibitors

Nelfinavir greatly increased the concentrations of sirolimus in one patient. The concurrent use of sirolimus with fosamprenavir boosted with ritonavir resulted in a lower sirolimus dose being necessary to maintain therapeutic sirolimus concentrations. Other HIV-protease inhibitors are predicted to interact similarly.

Clinical evidence

(a) Fosamprenavir

An HIV-positive kidney transplant patient stable taking tacrolimus and fosamprenavir boosted with ritonavir 700/100 mg (with lamivudine and zidovudine) was switched from tacrolimus to sirolimus 1 mg, 11 months post-transplant due to the development of Kaposi's sarcoma. The sirolimus concentration was maintained between 5 and 9.5 nanograms/mL during 40 days of sirolimus 1 mg weekly and the eventual steady-state dose of sirolimus was 1.5 mg weekly.[1]

(b) Nelfinavir

An HIV-positive, liver transplant patient taking sirolimus 5 mg daily was given nelfinavir 250 mg twice daily (one-fifth of the normal dose), lamivudine, and zidovudine. Three weeks later, because of a reduced full blood count, her sirolimus blood concentration was checked, and found to be 24.7 nanograms/mL. Her sirolimus dose was reduced to 3 mg daily and then 2 mg daily and her concentration rechecked 5 days later. The minimum sirolimus concentration was found to be 4.6 nanograms/mL, which was almost 5-fold higher than the minimum concentrations of 3 control patients taking sirolimus 5 to 7 mg daily but not taking nelfinavir. The maximum concentration and AUC of sirolimus were also much higher in the patient taking nelfinavir.[2]

Mechanism

Sirolimus is a substrate for both CYP3A4 and P-glycoprotein. The HIV-protease inhibitors inhibit CYP3A4 and P-glycoprotein, leading to an increase in sirolimus concentrations.

Importance and management

Evidence for a pharmacokinetic interaction between sirolimus and the HIV-protease inhibitors is limited to the cases above, but suggests that large reductions in the dose of sirolimus are required on concurrent use to maintain therapeutic concentrations and avoid toxicity. On the basis of the interaction with ketoconazole (see 'Sirolimus + Azoles', p.1280), the UK and US manufacturers[3,4] of sirolimus advise against the concurrent use of potent inhibitors of CYP3A4. This would generally be expected to include the HIV-protease inhibitors (see 'Table 1.9', p.11). Given the known potent CYP3A4 inhibitory effects of the HIV-protease inhibitors, their clinically relevant effects on other CYP3A4 substrates (in particular, those also with a narrow therapeutic range), and the risk of serious adverse effects (such as nephrotoxicity) with greatly increased sirolimus concentrations, very close monitoring of sirolimus concentrations on the concurrent use of sirolimus and HIV-protease inhibitors would seem essential. In addition, it would seem sensible to consider a pre-emptive sirolimus dose reduction or increasing its dose interval, with close monitoring of sirolimus concentrations and further dose adjustments as necessary. However, note that this has not been formerly studied and the extent of the pre-emptive dose reduction that might be required is not known.

1. Barau C, Blouin P, Creput C, Taburet AM, Durrbach A, Furlan V. Effect of coadministered HIV-protease inhibitors on tacrolimus and sirolimus blood concentrations in a kidney transplant recipients [sic]. *Fundam Clin Pharmacol* (2009) 23, 423–5.
2. Jain AKB, Venkataramanan R, Fridell JA, Gadomski M, Shaw LM, Ragni M, Korecka M, Fung J. Nelfinavir, a protease inhibitor, increases sirolimus levels in a liver transplantation patient: a case report. *Liver Transpl* (2002) 8, 838–40.
3. Rapamune (Sirolimus). Wyeth Pharmaceuticals Inc. US Prescribing information, December 2012.
4. Rapamune (Sirolimus). Pfizer Ltd. UK Summary of product characteristics, August 2013.

Sirolimus + Macrolides

Erythromycin moderately increased sirolimus exposure in healthy subjects, and there is a report of two patients who had large elevations in their sirolimus concentrations when they were given erythromycin. Similarly, there is a case report of clarithromycin causing a sizeable increase in sirolimus concentrations and renal impairment. Telithromycin is expected to interact similarly.

Clinical evidence

(a) Clarithromycin

A kidney transplant patient taking sirolimus 2 mg daily and with stable, but poor, renal function (creatinine clearance 14 mL/minute) was given clarithromycin 250 mg twice daily for a week. At the end of the week, her minimum sirolimus concentration was found to have increased 8.4-fold (from 6.2 to 52.2 nanograms/mL) and there was a sharp decrease in her creatinine clearance to 6.8 mL/minute. Sirolimus was temporarily stopped until her minimum concentration decreased to 4.9 nanograms/mL (8 days), and the creatinine clearance gradually improved.[1]

(b) Erythromycin

The UK and US manufacturers of sirolimus report that, in 24 healthy subjects, the concurrent use of erythromycin 800 mg three times daily with sirolimus oral solution 2 mg daily resulted in 4.2- and 4.4-fold increases in the maximum blood concentration and AUC of sirolimus, respectively. The maximum plasma concentration and AUC of erythromycin were also increased, by 60% and 70%, respectively.[2,3]

A case report describes 2 patients taking sirolimus who were also given erythromycin 1 g three times daily for suspected Legionella pneumonia. Despite large reductions in the sirolimus dose (actual reductions not stated), the sirolimus concentrations of both patients increased 5-fold.[4]

Mechanism

Erythromycin and clarithromycin are inhibitors of CYP3A4 and P-glycoprotein, which are involved in the metabolism and transport of sirolimus. Exposure to sirolimus is therefore increased on concurrent use. The mechanism behind sirolimus increasing erythromycin concentrations is uncertain.

Importance and management

Evidence for a pharmacokinetic interaction between clarithromycin, or erythromycin, and sirolimus is limited, but given the known interactions of these drugs an interaction would appear to be established and the resulting increase in sirolimus exposure would be expected to be of clinical importance. The moderate increase in sirolimus exposure seen in healthy subjects given **erythromycin** would suggest that concurrent use need not be avoided, but should be carefully monitored and sirolimus doses adjusted accordingly. However, note that the US manufacturer states that concurrent erythromycin is not recommended[3] [based on their classification of erythromycin as a potent CYP3A4 inhibitor, but note that it is generally considered to be a moderate inhibitor]. The effect of **clarithromycin** would appear to be greater (which is consistent with its classification as a potent inhibitor of CYP3A4) and concurrent use in patients taking sirolimus is not recommended.[2,3] **Telithromycin** is also a potent CYP3A4 inhibitor and so would be predicted to have the same effect, and is similarly not recommended.[2,3]

The increase in erythromycin exposure seen was slight and is probably of little clinical relevance. Nevertheless, the UK manufacturer advises that the erythromycin dose might need to be reduced on concurrent use.[2]

1. Capone D, Palmiero G, Gentile A, Basile V, Federico S, Sabbatini M, Potenza M, Perfetti A, Pieri M, Tarantino G. A pharmacokinetic interaction between clarithromycin and sirolimus in kidney transplant recipient. *Curr Drug Metab* (2007) 8, 379–81.
2. Rapamune (Sirolimus). Pfizer Ltd. UK Summary of product characteristics, August 2013.
3. Rapamune (Sirolimus). Wyeth Pharmaceuticals Inc. US Prescribing information, December 2012.
4. Claesson K, Brattström C, Burke JT. Sirolimus and erythromycin interaction: two cases. *Transplant Proc* (2001) 33, 2136.

Sirolimus and related drugs + Miscellaneous

It has been suggested that bromocriptine, cimetidine, danazol, and metoclopramide might interact with everolimus and sirolimus. Temsirolimus, a prodrug of sirolimus, might interact similarly. No pharmacokinetic interaction appears to occur between sirolimus and aciclovir, digoxin, or glibenclamide (glyburide).

Clinical evidence, mechanism, importance and management

(a) Aciclovir

In a study in healthy subjects, there was no pharmacokinetic interaction between aciclovir and sirolimus.[1]

(b) Digoxin

In a study in healthy subjects, there was no pharmacokinetic interaction between digoxin and sirolimus.[1]

(c) Glibenclamide (Glyburide)

In a study in healthy subjects, there was no pharmacokinetic interaction between glibenclamide and sirolimus.[1]

(d) Prokinetic drugs

The UK and US manufacturers of sirolimus note that **metoclopramide** might increase sirolimus concentrations,[2,3] although there do not appear to be any published reports of this interaction. The Australian manufacturer of **everolimus** also lists **metoclopramide** as potentially interacting.[4]

(e) Other drugs

The manufacturers of **everolimus** and sirolimus list **bromocriptine**, **cimetidine**, and **danazol** as drugs that might increase sirolimus concentrations,[2-4] on the basis of these drugs being inhibitors of CYP3A4.[2,4] However an important interaction with **bromocriptine** would not generally be expected as it is not usually considered to be a clinically relevant CYP3A4 inhibitor. Further, **cimetidine** is a non-specific inhibitor of cytochrome P450, and would be expected to cause only a minor interaction via this mechanism. Nevertheless, until more is known, some caution might be appropriate if cimetidine is given with sirolimus, **temsirolimus** (a prodrug of sirolimus), or **everolimus**. The effect of **danazol** on CYP3A4 is not established, but as it appears to have an effect on ciclosporin concentrations, possibly through inhibition of CYP3A4 (see 'Ciclosporin + Danazol', p.1225), an effect on sirolimus, **temsirolimus**, or **everolimus** cannot be ruled out.

1. Zimmerman JJ. Exposure-response relationships and drug interactions of sirolimus. *AAPS J* (2004) 6, 1–12.
2. Rapamune (Sirolimus). Pfizer Ltd. UK Summary of product characteristics, August 2013.
3. Rapamune (Sirolimus). Wyeth Pharmaceuticals Inc. US Prescribing information, December 2012.
4. Certican (Everolimus). Novartis Pharmaceuticals Australia Pty Ltd. Australian product information, August 2013.

Sirolimus + Repaglinide

Repaglinide does not appear to alter sirolimus concentrations.

Clinical evidence, mechanism, importance and management

In a study in kidney transplant patients stabilised on immunosuppressants, the concurrent use of repaglinide in the 5 patients taking sirolimus caused no notable changes in sirolimus blood concentrations and no sirolimus dose changes were required on starting repaglinide 1 to 3 mg daily (mostly as monotherapy but a few patients were also given either metformin or rosiglitazone).[1] It would appear from the limited data from this observational study, that a clinically important pharmacokinetic interaction between sirolimus and repaglinide does not occur, however this ideally needs confirmation in a pharmacokinetic study.

1. Türk T, Peitruck F, Dolff S, Kribben A, Janssen OE, Mann K, Philipp T, Heemann U, Witzke O. Repaglinide in the management of new-onset diabetes mellitus after renal transplantation. *Am J Transplant* (2006) 6, 842–6.

Sirolimus + Rifampicin (Rifampin) and other CYP3A4 inducers

Rifampicin greatly decreases sirolimus concentrations. Other CYP3A4 inducers are predicted to interact similarly.

Clinical evidence

A clinical study in 14 healthy subjects found that rifampicin 600 mg daily for 6 days increased the clearance of a single 10-mg oral dose of sirolimus 5.5-fold, and reduced the AUC and maximum serum concentration of sirolimus by 82% and 71%, respectively.[1,2]

A case report describes 2 patients taking sirolimus after kidney transplants who were given rifampicin after being diagnosed with tuberculosis. The first, a 60-year-old man, had his sirolimus dose increased from 4 mg daily to 30 mg daily in order to maintain his target sirolimus concentration. The second, a 28-year-old man, was taking sirolimus 4 to 6 mg daily and needed a sirolimus dose increase to 25 mg daily to maintain an adequate sirolimus concentration.[3]

Mechanism

Sirolimus is extensively metabolised by CYP3A4 in the intestine and liver, and is also a substrate for the drug transporter protein P-glycoprotein. Drugs such as rifampicin that induce the activity of this isoenzyme and drug transporter would be expected to lower sirolimus concentrations.[1,2]

Importance and management

Evidence for an interaction between sirolimus and rifampicin comes from one study, but the findings are consistent with what would be expected based on the known disposition of these drugs. Rifampicin is therefore very likely to greatly reduce sirolimus minimum concentrations and efficacy. The UK and US manufacturers of sirolimus state that concurrent use is not recommended, and that alternatives to rifampicin should be used.[1,2] However, note that **rifabutin** and **rifapentine** also induce CYP3A4, albeit perhaps to a lesser extent than rifampicin, and so might also interact. The concurrent use of **rifabutin** in particular is not recommended.[1,2]

On the basis of the interaction with rifampicin, the UK and US manufacturers of sirolimus state that the concurrent use of potent CYP3A4 inducers should be avoided, and advise caution with the use of other CYP3A4 inducers.[1,2] For a list of CYP3A4 inducers, see 'Table 1.9', p.11.

The UK manufacturer of **etravirine** predicts that it will induce the metabolism of sirolimus by CYP3A4 and thus reduce sirolimus concentrations, and they advise caution on concurrent use.[4] However, note that etravirine is perhaps only a weak inducer of this isoenzyme and might only have a minimal effect. Nevertheless, until more is known close monitoring of sirolimus concentrations would seem prudent.

1. Rapamune (Sirolimus). Pfizer Ltd. UK Summary of product characteristics, August 2013.
2. Rapamune (Sirolimus). Wyeth Pharmaceuticals Inc. US Prescribing information, December 2012.
3. Ngo BT, Pascoe M, Khan D. Drug interaction between rifampicin and sirolimus in transplant patients. *Saudi J Kidney Dis Transpl* (2011) 22, 112–15.
4. Intelence (Etravirine). Janssen-Cilag Ltd. UK Summary of product characteristics, May 2014.

Sirolimus and related drugs + Tyrosine kinase inhibitors

The exposure to sirolimus was increased in one phase I study with sorafenib, but the maximum concentration of sirolimus was decreased in another. Exposure to sunitinib was increased in a phase I study with sirolimus. Everolimus with sunitinib, sirolimus with sorafenib, and temsirolimus with sorafenib were all associated with clinically important toxicities in phase I studies. The pharmacokinetics of gefitinib and sorafenib were not affected by everolimus, and the exposure to everolimus was minimally affected by gefitinib in a phase I study. Imatinib is predicted to increase the plasma concentration of sirolimus. Unexpected dose-limiting toxicity was seen in a phase I study in which temsirolimus was given with sunitinib.

Clinical evidence

(a) Everolimus

1. Gefitinib. In a phase I study, patients with advanced non-small cell lung cancer were given a single 5- or 10-mg dose of everolimus on day 1, followed by gefitinib 250 mg daily from day 8, with everolimus 5 or 10 mg daily from day 22. At day 28, the everolimus AUC_{0-8} was reduced by 5% in the 5 mg group (5 patients) and increased by 12% in the 10 mg group (3 patients), but there was wide interindividual variability among the groups. The gefitinib AUC_{0-8} on day 22 was not affected by a single 5- or 10-mg dose of everolimus (9 patients).[1]

2. Sorafenib. In a phase I study of 20 patients with renal cell carcinoma, 14 patients were given everolimus 2.5 mg or 5 mg daily with sorafenib 400 mg twice daily. The pharmacokinetics of sorafenib were not altered by everolimus.[2]

3. Sunitinib. In a phase I study in 13 patients with metastatic renal cell carcinoma given everolimus (dose-normalised to 20 mg weekly) and sunitinib (dose-normalised to 37.5 mg daily), there were no changes in the pharmacokinetics of everolimus, sunitinib, or the N-desethyl metabolite of sunitinib.[3]

(b) Sirolimus

1. Sorafenib. A pharmacokinetic study in 12 patients with advanced malignancies given sirolimus 3 mg daily or sorafenib 400 mg twice daily for 14 days alone, and then together from day 15 to day 28, found that the maximum concentration of sirolimus was increased by 3.9% and its AUC was increased by 43.7%. The pharmacokinetics of sorafenib were unchanged.[4] In a phase I study in patients with advanced solid cancer given sirolimus as single 1- or 2-mg doses with sorafenib 200 mg twice daily, or sirolimus 1 mg daily with sorafenib 400 mg twice daily, the pharmacokinetics of sorafenib were unaltered, compared with administration alone. However, the maximum concentration of sirolimus was reduced by 55% when sirolimus was administered either as a single 2-mg dose with sorafenib 200 mg twice daily, or a single 1-mg dose with sorafenib 400 mg twice daily.[5]

2. Sunitinib. A pharmacokinetic study in 15 patients with advanced malignancies given sirolimus 4 mg daily or sunitinib 25 mg daily for 14 days alone, and then together from day 15 to day 28, found that the pharmacokinetics of sirolimus were unaltered. The AUC of sunitinib was increased by 54%, but the maximum concentration was unaltered.[4]

(c) Temsirolimus

1. Sorafenib. A phase I study in patients with metastatic melanoma, given temsirolimus and sorafenib in escalating doses, found that the maximum concentrations of sorafenib were similar to historical values when used alone.[6]

2. Sunitinib. In a phase I study, two of the first 3 patients who received treatment with intravenous temsirolimus 15 mg weekly and oral sunitinib 25 mg daily for 19 to 21 days of a 4 week course, experienced dose-limiting toxicities (including erythematous rash, thrombocytopenia, gout and cellulitis requiring hospitalisation).[7] The study was terminated early because of the toxicity seen at these low starting doses of both drugs..

Mechanism

The reasons for the pharmacokinetic changes seen are unknown.

Importance and management

Evidence is limited and where pharmacokinetic changes have been seen, the reason for these is unexplained. Although the magnitude of the pharmacokinetic changes would not seem likely to be clinically important, clinically important toxicity was noted in several of the studies,[3,5,6] and this in itself will limit the use of such combinations. Note also that a temsirolimus and sunitinib combination study was stopped early due to unacceptable toxicities, and the authors concluded that this regimen should not be used.[7]

On the basis of its effect on tacrolimus (see 'Tacrolimus + Tyrosine kinase inhibitors', p.1307), imatinib is predicted to similarly increase the plasma concentration of sirolimus.

1. Milton DT, Riely GJ, Azzoli CG, Gomez JE, Heelan RT, Kris MG, Krug LM, Pao W, Pizzo B, Rizvi NA, Miller VA. Phase I trial of everolimus and gefitinib in patients with advanced nonsmall-cell lung cancer. *Cancer* (2007) 110, 599–605.
2. Harzstark AL, Small EJ, Weinberg VK, Sun J, Ryan CJ, Lin AM, Fong L, Brocks DR, Rosenberg JE. A phase I study of everolimus and sorafenib for metastatic clear cell renal cell carcinoma. *Cancer* (2011) 117, 4194–200.
3. Molina AM, Feldman DR, Voss MH, Ginsberg MS, Baum MS, Brocks DR, Fischer PM, Trinos MJ, Patil S, Motzer RJ. Phase I trial of everolimus plus sunitinib in patients with metastatic renal cell carcinoma. *Cancer* (2012) 118, 1868–76.
4. Gangadhar TC, Cohen EE, Wu K, Janisch L, Geary D, Kocherginsky M, House LK, Ramirez J, Undevia SD, Maitland ML, Fleming GF, Ratain MJ. Two drug interaction studies of sirolimus in combination with sorafenib or sunitinib in patients with advanced malignancies. *Clin Cancer Res* (2011) 17, 1956–63.
5. Desar IM, Timmer-Bonte JN, Burger DM, van der Graaf WT, van Herpen CM. A phase I dose-escalation study to evaluate safety and tolerability of sorafenib combined with sirolimus in patients with advanced solid cancer. *Br J Cancer* (2010) 103, 1637–43.
6. Davies MA, Fox PS, Papadopoulos NE, Bedikian AY, Hwu W-J, Lazar AJ, Prieto VG, Culotta KS, Madden TL, Xu Q, Huang S, Deng W, Ng CS, Gupta S, Liu W, Dancey JE, Wright JJ, Bassett RL, Hwu P, Kim KB. Phase I study of the combination of sorafenib and temsirolimus in patients with metastatic melanoma. *Clin Cancer Res* (2012) 18, 1120–8.
7. Patel PH, Senico PL, Curiel RE, Motzer RJ. Phase I study combining treatment with temsirolimus and sunitinib malate in patients with advanced renal cell carcinoma. *Clin Genitourin Cancer* (2009) 7, 24–7.

Tacrolimus + ACE inhibitors or Angiotensin II receptor antagonists

Candesartan and losartan do not appear to affect the pharmacokinetics of tacrolimus, although concurrent use might increase the risk of hyperkalaemia.

Clinical evidence

A study in 12 kidney transplant patients taking tacrolimus twice daily for 12 days with **candesartan** (2 mg daily for 3 days, then 4 mg daily for 3 days, and then 16 mg daily for 3 days) found that the pharmacokinetics of tacrolimus were unchanged. Renal function remained stable and unchanged, and no adverse effects were reported.[1]

Another study in a group of 21 kidney transplant patients taking tacrolimus found no notable change in serum creatinine or tacrolimus concentrations when they also took **candesartan** 4 to 12 mg daily for one year. Serum potassium concentrations were reported to have increased by an average of 0.34 mmol/L, although it is unclear from the study if this was specifically in the tacrolimus group or also included another group taking candesartan and ciclosporin.[2]

A study in kidney transplant patients taking tacrolimus and given **losartan** 50 mg daily for 12 weeks (some receiving 100 mg daily from week 8) for hypertension found no notable changes in tacrolimus concentrations. Transient hyperkalaemia occurred in 4 of the 67 patients.[3]

Mechanism

Both ACE inhibitors and angiotensin II receptor antagonists can increase potassium concentrations, and this effect might be additive with that of tacrolimus.

Importance and management

No pharmacokinetic interaction appears to occur between tacrolimus and angiotensin II receptor antagonists, and none would be anticipated with ACE inhibitors. However, as tacrolimus might cause nephrotoxicity and hyperkalaemia, bear in mind the possibility of additive effects if ACE inhibitors or angiotensin II receptor antagonists are also given.

1. Pietruck F, Kiel G, Birkel M, Stahlheber-Dilg B, Philipp T. Evaluation of the effect of candesartan cilexetil on the steady-state pharmacokinetics of tacrolimus in renal transplant patients. *Biopharm Drug Dispos* (2005) 26, 135–41.
2. Omoto K, Tanabe K, Tokumoto T, Shimmura H, Ishida H, Toma H. Use of candesartan cilexetil decreases proteinuria in renal transplant patients with chronic allograft dysfunction. *Transplantation* (2003) 76, 117–4.
3. del Castillo D, Campistol JM, Guirado L, Capdevilla L, Martínez JG, Pereira P, Bravo J, Pérez R. Efficacy and safety of losartan in the treatment of hypertension in renal transplant patients. *Kidney Int* (1998) (Suppl 68) 54, S-135–S-139.

Tacrolimus + Antacids

Aluminium/magnesium hydroxide caused a minor increase in tacrolimus concentrations in one study. There is some evidence to suggest that sodium bicarbonate might possibly reduce the tacrolimus concentrations.

Clinical evidence

(a) Aluminium/magnesium antacids

In an early *in vitro* study, **aluminium hydroxide** gel and **magnesium oxide** caused a notable reduction in tacrolimus concentrations due to pH-mediated degradation, leading to the suggestion that the administration of antacids and tacrolimus should be separated until data from clinical studies became available.[1] However, in a cross-over study in healthy subjects, a single dose of **aluminium/magnesium hydroxide** *increased* the AUC of tacrolimus by 21% and decreased the maximum concentration of tacrolimus by 10%.[2] Moreover, a retrospective study in 18 kidney transplant patients found that the concurrent use of antacid medications (H_2-receptor antagonists, **magnesium oxide**, sodium bicarbonate, or proton pump inhibitors) did not reduce tacrolimus blood concentrations, and no patients required a tacrolimus dose increase,[3] although interpretation of this study is limited by the broad range of drugs considered together.

(b) Sodium bicarbonate

A review very briefly states that widely variable tacrolimus minimum plasma concentrations have been seen in patients taking sodium bicarbonate close to the time when the tacrolimus was given, and that the use of sodium bicarbonate results in lower blood concentrations of tacrolimus. No details were given.[4] It was suggested that their administration should be separated by at least 2 hours[4] However, a retrospective study in 18 renal transplant patients found that the concurrent use of antacid medications (H_2-receptor antagonists, magnesium oxide, sodium bicarbonate, or proton pump inhibitors) did not reduce tacrolimus blood concentrations, and no patient required a tacrolimus dose increase,[3] although interpretation of this study is limited by the broad range of drugs considered together.

Mechanism

Unknown.

Importance and management

Evidence for an interaction between tacrolimus and antacids is very limited. As such, more study is needed to confirm and assess the extent and clinical importance of these interactions, but the best available evidence suggests that aluminium/magnesium hydroxide might cause a minor increase in tacrolimus concentrations, which is probably unlikely to be clinically relevant. Nevertheless, it would seem prudent to bear this in mind if tacrolimus is given with any antacids, and be alert for the need to separate the doses by at least 2 hours.

1. Steeves M, Abdallah HY, Venkataramanan R, Burckart GT, Ptachcinski RJ, Abu-Elmagd K, Jain AK, Fung F, Todo S, Starzl TE. In-vitro interaction of a novel immunosuppressant, FK506, and antacids. *J Pharm Pharmacol* (1991) 43, 574–7.
2. Prograf (Tacrolimus). Astellas Pharma US Inc. US Prescribing information, September 2013.
3. Chisholm MA, Mulloy LL, Jagadeesan M, DiPiro JT. Coadministration of tacrolimus with anti-acid drugs. *Transplantation* (2003) 76, 665–6.
4. Venkataramanan R, Swaminathan A, Prasad T, Jain A, Zuckerman S, Warty V, McMichael J, Lever J, Burckart G, Starzl T. Clinical pharmacokinetics of tacrolimus. *Clin Pharmacokinet* (1995) 29, 404–30.

Tacrolimus + Antiepileptics; Enzyme-inducing

An isolated report describes an increase in phenytoin concentrations attributed to the use of tacrolimus. Phenytoin decreased tacrolimus concentrations in three cases, and has been used to reduce tacrolimus concentrations after an overdose. Phenobarbital has also been used to reduce tacrolimus concentrations after an overdose and reduced tacrolimus concentrations to below the therapeutic range in one patient. Carbamazepine also reduced tacrolimus concentrations in one patient.

Clinical evidence

(a) Carbamazepine

A 40-year-old heart transplant patient taking tacrolimus had decreased minimum tacrolimus concentrations within 7 days of starting carbamazepine 200 mg daily. Her tacrolimus dose was increased by 30 to 40% in order to maintain adequate tacrolimus serum concentrations. At 11 days after starting carbamazepine, her tacrolimus AUC-to-dose ratio was 50% lower than before carbamazepine was started. Despite a dose increase of about 50%, her tacrolimus AUC-to-dose ratio remained low (40% lower 3 months after carbamazepine had been started). Her tacrolimus serum concentrations were also reduced by the carbamazepine but were restored to therapeutic concentrations by the tacrolimus dose increase.[1] Sub-therapeutic tacrolimus serum concentrations have also been seen in a transplant patient taking carbamazepine and phenobarbital, see under *Phenobarbital*, below.

(b) Phenobarbital

In a 4-month-old liver transplant recipient with tacrolimus toxicity, intravenous phenobarbital 5 mg/kg was used to try to increase tacrolimus clearance. The half-life of tacrolimus was calculated as 70 to 235 hours before phenobarbital was given, and 13 to 30 hours during phenobarbital use.[2] Two other infants were similarly treated, resulting in about 3- to 5-fold decreases in the half-life of tacrolimus.[3] A kidney transplant patient had sub-therapeutic tacrolimus concentrations while taking carbamazepine and phenobarbital, which only reached the desired range after tacrolimus dose increases from 3 mg twice daily to 15 mg twice daily, stopping carbamazepine (3 days after transplant) and the gradual reduction of the phenobarbital dose from 64.8 mg twice daily to 16.2 mg twice daily during the 11 days following transplant. Phenobarbital was stopped completely 37 days post-transplant and 4 days later, a tacrolimus dose reduction to 13 mg twice daily was necessary.[4]

(c) Phenytoin

1. Effect on phenytoin. A kidney transplant patient taking phenytoin 500 and 600 mg on alternate days (and also taking azathioprine, bumetanide, digoxin, diltiazem, heparin, insulin, and prednisone) had his immunosuppressant changed from ciclosporin, to tacrolimus 14 to 16 mg daily. About 7 weeks later, he presented to hospital because of a fainting episode and his phenytoin concentration was found to have increased from 18.4 to 36.2 micrograms/mL. Phenytoin was temporarily stopped until his serum concentrations had decreased, and he was discharged on a reduced phenytoin dose of 400 and 500 mg on alternate days with no further problems.[5] The presumption is that the fainting episode was due to the increased phenytoin serum concentrations.

2. Effect on tacrolimus. In one kidney transplant patient taking phenytoin, tacrolimus 250 micrograms/kg daily was needed to give a tacrolimus blood concentration of 9 nanograms/mL. Three months later phenytoin was gradually stopped, with gradual tapering of the tacrolimus dose. The patient was eventually stabilised with a tacrolimus dose of 160 micrograms/kg daily giving a blood concentration of 11 nanograms/mL.[6] Similarly, in two other cases, tacrolimus requirements were increased 2- to 3-fold when phenytoin 200 mg daily was taken. The tacrolimus requirements decreased when phenytoin was stopped.[7] In another patient, variable tacrolimus doses and concentrations were seen in the post-transplant period while taking phenytoin, and phenytoin was eventually tapered and replaced with oxcarbazepine.[8]

Another report describes the use of an intravenous phenytoin infusion to treat acute tacrolimus overdoses in 2 patients, with the aim of enhancing tacrolimus metabolism.[9]

3. Gingival overgrowth. A case report describes almost complete reversal of gingival overgrowth, which occurred in a kidney transplant patient taking ciclosporin and phenytoin, 6 months after the ciclosporin was switched to tacrolimus 7 mg daily.[10] Phenytoin and ciclosporin are both known to cause gingival overgrowth and this case was considered to be an additive effect of the two drugs. Tacrolimus might be associated with less oral adverse effects and so this was chosen as a replacement for the ciclosporin.

Mechanism

Tacrolimus is extensively metabolised by CYP3A4, which is known to be induced by carbamazepine, phenytoin, and phenobarbital, and these enzyme-inducing antiepileptics therefore decrease tacrolimus concentrations. In the case of increased phenytoin concentrations, it was suggested that tacrolimus might have inhibited the metabolism of phenytoin, although other factors could have had some part to play.[5]

Importance and management

Information about an interaction between the enzyme-inducing antiepileptics and tacrolimus is limited, but based on the known metabolic effects of these drugs, it would be prudent to monitor tacrolimus concentrations in all patients given carbamazepine, phenytoin, or phenobarbital. It would therefore also be prudent to monitor tacrolimus concentrations if any of the enzyme-inducing antiepileptics (including the prodrug of phenytoin, **fosphenytoin**; and **primidone**, which is metabolised to phenobarbital) are given and adjust the dose accordingly. The isolated case report of improvement in gingival overgrowth after ciclosporin was switched to tacrolimus in a patient also taking phenytoin suggests that tacrolimus might be an alternative if this effect is severe, but this requires confirmation. Note that a review of the management of drug-induced gingival overgrowth also suggests that tacrolimus could be an alternative to ciclosporin.[11] Information for oxcarbazepine is limited to one case report which suggests that it might not interact in the same way, but further study is needed to establish this. Similarly, until more is known, based on the single case of phenytoin toxicity, it might also be advisable to monitor phenytoin concentrations in patients taking tacrolimus.

1. Wada K, Takada M, Sakai M, Ochi H, Kotake T, Okade H, Morishita H, Oda N, Mano A, Kato TS, Komamura K, Nakatani T. Drug interaction between tacrolimus and carbamazepine in a Japanese heart transplant recipient: a case report. *J Heart Lung Transplant* (2009) 28, 409–11.
2. McLaughlin GE, Rossique-Gonzalez M, Gelman B, Kato T. Use of phenobarbital in the management of acute tacrolimus toxicity: a case report. *Transplant Proc* (2000) 32, 665–8.
3. Quirós-Tejeira RE, Chang I-F, Bristow LJ, Karpen SJ, Goss JA. Treatment of acute tacrolimus whole-blood elevation with phenobarbital in the pediatric liver transplant recipient. *Pediatr Transplant* (2005) 9, 792–6.
4. Siddiqi N, Marfo K. Clinically significant drug-drug interaction between tacrolimus and phenobarbital: the price we pay. *J Pharm Pract* (2010) 23, 585–9.
5. Thompson PA, Mosley CA. Tacrolimus-phenytoin interaction. *Ann Pharmacother* (1996) 30, 544.
6. Moreno M, Latorre C, Manzanares C, Morales E, Herrero JC, Dominguez-Gil B, Carreño A, Cubas A, Delgado M, Andres A, Morales JM. Clinical management of tacrolimus drug interactions in renal transplant patients. *Transplant Proc* (1999) 31, 2252–3.
7. Wada K, Takada M, Ueda T, Ochi H, Kotake T, Morishita H, Hanatani A, Nakatani T. Drug interactions between tacrolimus and phenytoin in Japanese heart transplant recipients: 2 case reports. *Int J Clin Pharmacol Ther* (2007) 45, 524–8.
8. Formea CM, Evans CG, Karlix JL. Altered cytochrome P450 metabolism of calcineurin inhibitors: case report and review of the literature. *Pharmacotherapy* (2005) 25, 1021–9.
9. Karasu Z, Gurakar A, Carlson J, Pennington S, Kerwin B, Wright H, Nour B, Sebastian A. Acute tacrolimus overdose and treatment with phenytoin in liver transplant recipients. *J Okla State Med Assoc* (2001) 94, 121–3.
10. Hernandez G, Arriba L, Lucas M, de Andres A. Reduction of severe gingival overgrowth in a kidney transplant patient by replacing cyclosporin A with tacrolimus. *J Periodontol* (2000) 71, 1630–6.
11. Hood KA. Drug-induced gingival hyperplasia in transplant recipients. *Prog Transplant* (2002) 12, 17–21.

Tacrolimus + Azoles; Fluconazole

Fluconazole increases tacrolimus concentrations and increases the risk of nephrotoxicity. Intravenous tacrolimus appears not to interact.

Clinical evidence

(a) Oral tacrolimus

Twenty organ transplant patients (11 liver, 6 kidney, 2 heart, and one bone marrow) taking tacrolimus were also given fluconazole 100 mg or 200 mg daily for various fungal infections. On day one, the median minimum plasma concentrations of tacrolimus in those patients given fluconazole 100 mg increased by 40%, and in those taking 200 mg, increased 3.1-fold. The dose of tacrolimus was reduced to accommodate this increase: the median dose reduction was 56% (range 0 to 88%). The highest tacrolimus concentration was seen within 3 days. A pharmacokinetic study in one patient found that when fluconazole 100 mg daily was stopped, the AUC of tacrolimus decreased by about 60%.[1] In two other studies, patients given fluconazole required a tacrolimus dose reduction of 40% or 47% (increased to 65% at 3 months) to achieve similar minimum concentrations.[2,3] Even greater reductions in the tacrolimus dose were required in a study in paediatric thoracic organ transplant patients given fluconazole or itraconazole, with tacrolimus dose reductions of 33% on day one, 42% on day 2, and 55% on day 4 resulting in a mean 15 to 38% increase in tacrolimus concentrations. The mean decrease in the tacrolimus dose 30 days after fluconazole was started was 61%.[4] This was similar to the dose reductions required with *itraconazole*, see 'Tacrolimus + Azoles; Itraconazole', below.

Other studies in adult[5] and paediatric patients[6] and case reports[7-9] have confirmed that tacrolimus concentrations are increased by oral fluconazole, increasing the risk of nephrotoxicity.[6-8] A bone-marrow transplant patient taking tacrolimus and given fluconazole for oral candidiasis experienced headache and was found to have glycosuria, increased serum creatinine concentrations, and Pelger-Huet anomaly of granulocytes, which disappeared after tacrolimus was discontinued. The effects were thought to be due to tacrolimus toxicity due to an interaction with fluconazole.[10] In yet another study in patients taking oral tacrolimus, both oral and intravenous fluconazole appeared to increase tacrolimus minimum concentrations to a similar extent,[11] but other studies suggest that an interaction with intravenous tacrolimus might be smaller than with oral tacrolimus, see *Intravenous tacrolimus*, below. Further, there is some evidence from a study in 29 kidney transplant patients taking tacrolimus who had received fluconazole, that CYP3A5 genotype might influence the extent of the effect of fluconazole, such that CYP3A5 non-expressers (that is those with non-functioning CYP3A5) might be at greater risk of higher tacrolimus concentrations than CYP3A5 expressers. In this study, the increase in tacrolimus minimum concentrations was about 2.5-fold greater in CYP3A5 non-expressers than in CYP3A5 expressers.[12]

(b) Intravenous tacrolimus

When intravenous tacrolimus was given with intravenous fluconazole 400 mg, the steady-state concentrations of tacrolimus were increased by about 16%, which was considered to be clinically unimportant.[13] In a retrospective study in patients receiving intravenous tacrolimus, there was a small increase in tacrolimus blood concentration (from 17.4 to 18.8 nanograms/mL) when they were switched from intravenous to oral fluconazole.[14]

Mechanism

Fluconazole is an inhibitor of CYP3A4 (by which tacrolimus is metabolised) in the gut wall and/or liver, and so tacrolimus concentrations increase. Intravenous tacrolimus is less affected as it does not undergo first-pass metabolism in the gut.[13]

Importance and management

The evidence suggests that the interaction between tacrolimus and fluconazole is established, clinically important, and can develop rapidly (within 3 days). The authors of one of the reports state that up to 200 mg of oral fluconazole daily can be used safely and effectively provided that the tacrolimus dose is reduced by half;[1] however, note that clinically relevant, although less dramatic increases, do occur with lower fluconazole doses. Concurrent use should be closely monitored and the tacrolimus dose adjusted as required. One study specifically examining dose adjustments suggested that fluconazole can be safely used if 60% of the original tacrolimus dose is given.[2] If tacrolimus is given intravenously, no clinically important interaction appears to occur.[13] The clinical relevance of the effect of CYP3A5 genotype on the interaction is unclear, and a patient's genotype is rarely known in clinical practice. Further study into the importance of this is needed.

1. Mañez R, Martin M, Raman V, Silverman D, Jain A, Warty V, Gonzalez-Pinto I, Kusne S, Starzl TE. Fluconazole therapy in transplant recipients receiving FK506. *Transplantation* (1994) 57, 1521–23.
2. Toda F, Tanabe K, Ito S, Shinmura H, Tokumoto T, Ishida H, Toma H. Tacrolimus trough level adjustment after administration of fluconazole to kidney recipients. *Transplant Proc* (2002) 34, 1733–5.
3. Lumlertgul D, Noppakun K, Rojanasthien N, Kanchanarattanakorn K, Jittikanont S, Manoyot A, Bunnachak D, Ophascharoensuk V. Pharmacokinetic study of the combination of tacrolimus and fluconazole in renal transplant patients. *J Med Assoc Thai* (2006) 89 (Suppl 2), S73–S78.
4. Mahnke CB, Sutton RM, Venkataramanan R, Michaels M, Kurland G, Boyle GJ, Law YM, Miller SA, Pigula FA, Gandhi S, Webber SA. Tacrolimus dosage requirements after initiation of azole antifungal therapy in pediatric thoracic organ transplantation. *Pediatr Transplant* (2003) 7, 474–8.
5. Toy S, Tata P, Jain A, Patsy K, Lever J, Burckart G, Warty V, Kusne S, Abu-Elmagd K, Fung J, Starzi T, Venkataramanan R. A pharmacokinetic interaction between tacrolimus and fluconazole. *Pharm Res* (1996) 13 (9 Suppl), S435.
6. Vincent I, Furlan V, Debray D, Jacquemin E, Taburet AM. Effects of antifungal agents on the pharmacokinetics and nephrotoxicity of FK506 in paediatric liver transplant recipients. *Intersci Conf Antimicrob Agents Chemother* (1995) 35, 5.
7. Assan R, Fredj G, Larger E, Feutren G, Bismuth H. FK 506/fluconazole interaction enhances FK506 nephrotoxicity. *Diabete Metab* (1994) 20, 49–52.
8. Chamorey E, Nouveau B, Viard L, Garcia-Credoz F, Durand A, Pisano P. Interaction tacrolimus-fluconazole chez un enfant transplanté coeur-poumons. A propos d'un cas clinique. *J Pharm Clin* (1998) 17, 51–3.
9. Hairhara Y, Makuuchi M, Kawarasaki H, Takayama T, Kubota K, Ito M, Tanaka H, Yoshino H, Hirata M, Kita Y, Kusaka K, Sano K, Saiura A, Ijichi M, Matsukura A, Watanabe M, Hashizume K, Nakatsuka T. Effect of fluconazole on blood levels of tacrolimus. *Transplant Proc* (1999) 31, 2767.
10. Gondo H, Okamura C, Osaki K, Shimoda K, Asano Y, Okamura T. Acquired Pelger-Huet anomaly in association with concomitant tacrolimus and fluconazole therapy following allogenic bone marrow transplantation. *Bone Marrow Transplant* (2000) 26, 1255–7.
11. Mathis AS, DiRenzo T, Friedman GS, Kaplan B, Adamson R. Sex and ethnicity may chiefly influence the interaction of fluconazole with calcineurin inhibitors. *Transplantation* (2001) 71, 1069–75.
12. Kuypers DR, de Jonge H, Naesens M, Vanrenterghem Y. Effects of CYP3A5 and MDR1 single nucleotide polymorphisms on drug interactions between tacrolimus and fluconazole in renal allograft recipients. *Pharmacogenet Genomics* (2008) 18, 861–8.
13. Osowski CL, Dix SP, Lin LS, Mullins RE, Geller RB, Wingard JR. Evaluation of the drug interaction between intravenous high-dose fluconazole and cyclosporine or tacrolimus in bone marrow transplant patients. *Transplantation* (1996) 61, 1268–72.
14. Mihara A, Mori T, Aisa Y, Yamazaki R, Iketani O, Tanigawara Y, Ikeda Y, Okamoto S. Greater impact of oral fluconazole on drug interaction with intravenous calcineurin inhibitors as compared with intravenous fluconazole. *Eur J Clin Pharmacol* (2008) 64, 89–91.

Tacrolimus + Azoles; Itraconazole

Itraconazole can greatly increase tacrolimus concentrations.

Clinical evidence

A study in 40 lung transplant patients taking tacrolimus with prophylactic itraconazole 200 mg twice daily for 6 months found that when itraconazole was stopped the tacrolimus dose needed to maintain therapeutic concentrations increased by 76% (to 5.74 mg daily). The adverse effects and rejection rate were not affected by itraconazole.[1] Similar findings were reported in two other studies in heart and lung transplant patients, who required about one-third of the tacrolimus dose while taking itraconazole.[2,3] Even greater reductions in tacrolimus dose were required in a study in paediatric thoracic organ transplant patients also given fluconazole or itraconazole, with tacrolimus dose reductions of 33% on day one, 42% on day 2, and 55% on day 4 resulting in a 15 to 38% increase in tacrolimus concentrations. The decrease in the tacrolimus dose 30 days after itraconazole was started was 68%.[4] This was similar to the dose reductions required with *fluconazole*, see 'Tacrolimus + Azoles; Fluconazole', above. In another study, the concentration-to-dose ratio of tacrolimus was increased 2.4-fold (range 43% to 4.3-fold) when itraconazole oral solution was also given.[5] In one study, 3 patients taking tacrolimus and given itraconazole 100 mg twice daily for 3 months required a 2.9-fold increase in their tacrolimus dose when itraconazole was stopped.[6] In a study in 9 patients, intravenous itraconazole 200 mg twice daily for 2 days then 200 mg daily caused a mean 83% increase in the concentrations of *intravenous* tacrolimus.[7]

Various cases of this interaction have also been reported. The minimum blood concentrations of tacrolimus in a heart-lung transplant patient increased 3-fold (from 16 to 57 nanograms/mL) and serum creatinine concentrations also increased after she was given itraconazole 200 mg daily.[8] A kidney transplant patient taking tacrolimus 6 mg daily was given itraconazole 100 mg twice daily for a urinary candida infection. Within a day, the tacrolimus minimum concentration increased from 12.6 to 21 nanograms/mL, and the tacrolimus dose needed to be progressively reduced to 3 mg daily. Four days after itraconazole was stopped, tacrolimus had to be gradually increased back to its initial dose.[9] Another kidney transplant patient taking tacrolimus 4 mg in the morning and 3 mg in the evening, had a substantial increase in his tacrolimus concentration from 7 to 46.6 micrograms/L, requiring a 94% tacrolimus dose reduction over a period of time to 400 micrograms daily. The patient was restabilised on 3 mg twice daily, to give a tacrolimus concentration between 5 and 10 micrograms/L, after itraconazole was stopped.[10] The interaction has been reported in other transplant recipients.[3,11-14]

Mechanism

Itraconazole is an inhibitor of CYP3A4 (by which tacrolimus is metabolised) in the gut wall and/or liver, and so tacrolimus concentrations increase. Itraconazole is a known inhibitor of P-glycoprotein and might also inhibit the transport of tacrolimus by this route. Intravenous tacrolimus is less affected as it does not undergo first-pass metabolism in the gut.[15]

Importance and management

The interaction between tacrolimus and itraconazole is established and the risk of an increase in tacrolimus concentrations is clinically important. The UK manufacturer of tacrolimus states that nearly all patients will require tacrolimus dose reductions when given with itraconazole.[16] Pre-emptive tacrolimus dose reductions when starting azoles have been successful in maintaining tacrolimus concentrations within the therapeutic range;[17] however the authors of one review state that this is not standard practice among transplant clinicians, because of the concern of an increased risk of rejection[18] (due to subtherapeutic tacrolimus concentrations). Similarly, the authors of some studies also suggest that a pre-emptive tacrolimus dose reduction might not be appropriate because of the wide variability in the increase in tacrolimus concentrations between patients.[19,20] Whatever is done, close monitoring of tacrolimus concentrations, with appropriate tacrolimus dose adjustments, is essential.

1. Kramer MR, Amital A, Fuks L, Shitrit D. Voriconazole and itraconazole in lung transplant recipients receiving tacrolimus (FK 506): efficacy and drug interaction. *Clin Transplant* (2011) Epub.
2. Banerjee R, Leaver N, Lyster H, Banner NR. Coadministration of itraconazole and tacrolimus after thoracic organ transplantation. *Transplant Proc* (2001) 33, 1600–2.
3. Billaud EM, Guillemain R, Tacco F, Chevalier P. Evidence for a pharmacokinetic interaction between itraconazole and tacrolimus in organ transplant patients. *Br J Clin Pharmacol* (1998) 46, 271–2.
4. Mahnke CB, Sutton RM, Venkataramanan R, Michaels M, Kurland G, Boyle GJ, Law YM, Miller SA, Pigula FA, Gandhi S, Webber SA. Tacrolimus dosage requirements after initiation of azole antifungal therapy in pediatric thoracic organ transplantation. *Pediatr Transplant* (2003) 7, 474–8.
5. Mori T, Aisa Y, Kato J, Nakamura Y, Ikeda Y, Okamoto S. Drug interaction between oral solution itraconazole and calcineurin inhibitors in allogeneic hematopoietic stem cell transplantation recipients: an association with bioavailability of oral solution itraconazole. *Int J Hematol* (2009) 90, 103–7.
6. Kramer MR, Merin G, Rudis E, Bar I, Nesher T, Bublil M, Milgalter E. Dose adjustment and cost of itraconazole prophylaxis in lung transplant recipients receiving cyclosporine and tacrolimus (FK 506). *Transplant Proc* (1997) 29, 2657–9.
7. Leather H, Boyette RM, Tian L, Wingard JR. Pharmacokinetic evaluation of the drug interaction between intravenous itraconazole and intravenous tacrolimus or intravenous cyclosporin A in allogeneic hematopoietic stem cell transplant recipients. *Biol Blood Marrow Transplant* (2006) 12, 325–34.
8. Furlan V, Parquin F, Penaud JF, Cerrina J, Le Roy Ladurie F, Dartevelle P, Taburet AM. Interaction between tacrolimus and itraconazole in a heart-lung transplant recipient. *Transplant Proc* (1998) 30, 187–8.
9. Capone D, Gentile A, Imperatore P, Palmiero G, Basile V. Effects of itraconazole on tacrolimus blood concentrations in a renal transplant recipient. *Ann Pharmacother* (1999) 33, 1124–5.
10. Cervelli MJ, Russ GR. Itraconazole-tacrolimus drug interaction. *Ther Drug Monit* (2003) 25, 483–4.
11. Katari SR, Magnone M, Shapiro R, Jordan M, Scantlebury V, Vivas C, Gritsch A, McCauley J, Demetris AJ, Randhawa PS. Clinical features of acute reversible tacrolimus (FK506) nephrotoxicity in kidney transplant recipients. *Clin Transplant* (1997) 11, 237–42.
12. Outeda Macías M, Salvador P, Hurtado JL, Martín I. Tacrolimus-itraconazole interaction in a kidney transplant patient. *Ann Pharmacother* (2000) 34, 536.
13. Ideura T, Muramatsu T, Higuchi M, Tachibana N, Hora K, Kiyosawa K. Tacrolimus/itraconazole interactions: a case report of ABO-incompatible living-related renal transplantation. *Nephrol Dial Transplant* (2000) 15, 1721–3.
14. Nara M, Takahashi N, Miura M, Saitoh H, Kagaya H, Sawada K. Effect of oral itraconazole on the pharmacokinetics of tacrolimus in a hematopoietic stem cell transplant recipient with CYP3A5*3/*3. *Am J Hematol* (2010) 85, 634–5.
15. Osowski CL, Dix SP, Lin LS, Mullins RE, Geller RB, Wingard JR. Evaluation of the drug interaction between intravenous high-dose fluconazole and cyclosporine or tacrolimus in bone marrow transplant patients. *Transplantation* (1996) 61, 1268–72.
16. Prograf (Tacrolimus monohydrate). Astellas Pharma Ltd. UK Summary of product characteristics, November 2014.
17. Trifilio SM, Scheetz MH, Pi J, Mehta J. Tacrolimus use in adult allogeneic stem cell transplant recipients receiving voriconazole: preemptive dose modification and therapeutic drug monitoring. *Bone Marrow Transplant* (2010) 45, 1352–6.
18. Saad AH, DePestel DD, Carver PL. Factors influencing the magnitude and clinical significance of drug interactions between azole antifungals and select immunosuppressants. *Pharmacotherapy* (2006) 26, 1730–44.
19. Mori T, Aisa Y, Kato J, Nakamura Y, Ikeda Y, Okamoto S. Drug interaction between voriconazole and calcineurin inhibitors in allogeneic hematopoietic stem cell transplant recipients. *Bone Marrow Transplant* (2009) 44, 371–4.
20. Mori T, Kato J, Yamane A, Sakurai M, Kohashi S, Kikuchi T, Ono Y, Okamoto S. Drug interaction between voriconazole and tacrolimus and its association with the bioavailability of oral voriconazole in recipients of allogeneic hematopoietic stem cell transplantation. *Int J Hematol* (2012) 95, 564–9.

Tacrolimus + Azoles; Ketoconazole

Ketoconazole can greatly increase tacrolimus concentrations. There is some evidence that, after intravenous administration of tacrolimus, the concentration of tacrolimus is less affected by ketoconazole.

Clinical evidence

In a kidney transplant patient taking tacrolimus and prednisone, the addition of ketoconazole 200 mg daily resulted in an increase in tacrolimus blood concentrations from 11.1 to 27.9 nanograms/mL, despite a 45% decrease in the dose of tacrolimus. Eventually the dose of tacrolimus had to be reduced by 80% to keep the concentration within the therapeutic range. The tacrolimus concentration decreased to 5.8 nanograms/mL within one week of stopping ketoconazole and so the dose was increased.[1] Similarly, in a study in 11 kidney transplant patients taking tacrolimus, the concurrent use of ketoconazole 87 mg daily allowed a reduction in the tacrolimus dose of about 75 to 80%.[2] In another similar study, a reduction in the tacrolimus dose of about 50% was needed with ketoconazole 100 mg daily.[3] A pharmacokinetic study in 6 healthy subjects found that ketoconazole 200 mg orally at bedtime for 12 days increased the bioavailability of a single 100-microgram/kg dose of oral tacrolimus from 14 to 30%.[4] The US manufacturer of tacrolimus notes that the clearance of *intravenous* tacrolimus was not significantly changed by ketoconazole, although it was highly variable between patients.[5] There is some evidence from a study in 79 kidney transplant patients taking tacrolimus and ketoconazole that CYP3A5 genotype might influence the extent of the effect of ketoconazole, such that CYP3A5 non-expressers (that is those with non-functioning CYP3A5) might be at greater risk of higher tacrolimus concentrations than CYP3A5 expressers. In this study, the increase in tacrolimus minimum concentrations was 30% greater in CYP3A5 non-expressers, and they required larger dose reductions, than CYP3A5 expressers.[6]

Mechanism

Ketoconazole is an inhibitor of CYP3A4 (by which tacrolimus is metabolised) in the gut wall and/or liver, and so tacrolimus concentrations increase. Ketoconazole is also a known inhibitor of P-glycoprotein and so might also inhibit the transport of tacrolimus by this route. Intravenous tacrolimus is less affected as it does not undergo first-pass metabolism in the gut.[7]

Importance and management

The evidence suggests that the interaction between tacrolimus and ketoconazole is established, and can result in clinically important increases in tacrolimus concentrations. The UK manufacturer of tacrolimus states that nearly all patients will require tacrolimus dose reductions when given with ketoconazole.[8] Pre-emptive tacrolimus dose reductions when starting azoles have been successful in maintaining tacrolimus concentrations within the therapeutic range;[9] however the authors of one review state that this is not standard practice among transplant clinicians, because of the concern of an increased risk of rejection[10] (due to subtherapeutic tacrolimus concentrations). Similarly, the authors of some studies also suggest that a pre-emptive tacrolimus dose reduction might not be appropriate because of the wide variability in the increase in tacrolimus concentrations between patients.[11,12] Whatever is done, close monitoring of tacrolimus concentrations, with appropriate tacrolimus dose adjustments, is essential.

The clinical relevance of the effect of CYP3A5 genotype on this interaction is unclear, and a patient's genotype is rarely known in clinical practice. Further study into the importance of this is needed.

1. Moreno M, Latorre C, Manzanares C, Morales E, Herrero JC, Dominguez-Gil B, Carreño A, Cubas A, Delgado M, Andres A, Morales JM. Clinical management of tacrolimus drug interactions in renal transplant patients. *Transplant Proc* (1999) 31, 2252–3.
2. Soltero L, Carbajal H, Rodríguez-Montalvo C, Valdés A. Coadministration of tacrolimus and ketoconazole in renal transplant recipients: cost analysis and review of metabolic effects. *Transplant Proc* (2003) 35, 1319–21.
3. El-Dahshan KF, Bakr MA, Donia AF, El-Sayed Badr A, Sobh MAK. Ketoconazole-tacrolimus coadministration in kidney transplant recipients: two-year results of a prospective randomized study. *Am J Nephrol* (2006) 26, 293–8.
4. Floren LC, Bekersky I, Benet LZ, Mekki Q, Dressler D, Lee JW, Roberts JP, Hebert MF. Tacrolimus oral bioavailability doubles with coadministration of ketoconazole. *Clin Pharmacol Ther* (1997) 62, 41–9.
5. Prograf (Tacrolimus). Astellas Pharma US Inc. US Prescribing information, September 2013.
6. Chandel N, Aggarwal PK, Minz M, Sakhuja V, Kohli KK, Jha V. CYP3A5*1/*3 genotype influences the blood concentration of tacrolimus in response to metabolic inhibition by ketoconazole. Pharmacogenet Genomics. (2009) 19, 458–63.
7. Osowski CL, Dix SP, Lin LS, Mullins RE, Geller RB, Wingard JR. Evaluation of the drug interaction between intravenous high-dose fluconazole and cyclosporine or tacrolimus in bone marrow transplant patients. *Transplantation* (1996) 61, 1268–72.
8. Prograf (Tacrolimus monohydrate). Astellas Pharma Ltd. UK Summary of product characteristics, November 2014.
9. Trifilio SM, Scheetz MH, Pi J, Mehta J. Tacrolimus use in adult allogeneic stem cell transplant recipients receiving voriconazole: preemptive dose modification and therapeutic drug monitoring. *Bone Marrow Transplant* (2010) 45, 1352–6.
10. Saad AH, DePestel DD, Carver PL. Factors influencing the magnitude and clinical significance of drug interactions between azole antifungals and select immunosuppressants. *Pharmacotherapy* (2006) 26, 1730–44.
11. Mori T, Aisa Y, Kato J, Nakamura Y, Ikeda Y, Okamoto S. Drug interaction between voriconazole and calcineurin inhibitors in allogeneic hematopoietic stem cell transplant recipients. *Bone Marrow Transplant* (2009) 44, 371–4.
12. Mori T, Kato J, Yamane A, Sakurai M, Kohashi S, Kikuchi T, Ono Y, Okamoto S. Drug interaction between voriconazole and tacrolimus and its association with the bioavailability of oral voriconazole in recipients of allogeneic hematopoietic stem cell transplantation. *Int J Hematol* (2012) 95, 564–9.

Tacrolimus + Azoles; Miscellaneous

Oral clotrimazole lozenges increase tacrolimus concentrations. Miconazole oral gel is predicted to interact similarly. No interaction is expected between tacrolimus and topical clotrimazole (e.g. pessaries or cream).

Clinical evidence

In a study in 35 kidney transplant patients taking tacrolimus 150 micrograms/kg twice daily, patients were randomised to receive either **clotrimazole** lozenges 10 mg three times daily (17 patients) or nystatin oral suspension (control group, 18 patients). **Clotrimazole** increased tacrolimus minimum blood concentrations from a mean of about 15 nanograms/mL up to 53 nanograms/mL at day 5, whereas tacrolimus concentrations were not affected by nystatin. By day 7, patients in the **clotrimazole** group were found to require considerably lower tacrolimus doses than those in the nystatin group.[1] In a further pharmacokinetic study in 6 patients by this research group, a 5-day course of **clotrimazole** lozenges increased the AUC and minimum concentrations of tacrolimus about 2.5-fold.[2]

Similarly, in a liver transplant patient the minimum plasma concentration of tacrolimus 6 mg daily increased from 3.5 to 5.6 nanograms/mL within one day of **clotrimazole** 10 mg four times daily being started, and reached more than 9 nanograms/mL within 8 days. Later studies and rechallenge confirmed that **clotrimazole** was responsible for the increase in tacrolimus concentration. The AUC of tacrolimus was nearly doubled.[3] In a kidney transplant patient taking tacrolimus 5 mg twice daily, the tacrolimus minimum concentration decreased from

13.7 to 5.4 nanograms/mL over 6 days when prophylactic **clotrimazole** lozenges (10 mg four times daily), given for one month post-transplant, were stopped. When **clotrimazole** was restarted with an increased tacrolimus dose of 6 mg twice daily, the tacrolimus minimum concentration increased to 19.2 nanograms/mL. Tacrolimus doses were further reduced until a dose of tacrolimus 4 mg twice daily gave a tacrolimus minimum concentration of 11 to 12 nanograms/mL.[4]

Mechanism

Clotrimazole can inhibit CYP3A4 by which tacrolimus is metabolised, albeit perhaps only weakly, leading to an increase in tacrolimus concentrations.

Importance and management

Evidence for an interaction between oral **clotrimazole** and tacrolimus is limited, but is consistent with the known interactions of these drugs. On the basis of the case reports and studies cited, it would be prudent to monitor tacrolimus concentrations, and adjust the tacrolimus dose as necessary. No interaction would generally be expected with clotrimazole used *topically* (e.g. pessaries or cream), as the systemic absorption is usually low.

In vitro studies with human liver microsomes have shown that **miconazole**[5] also inhibits CYP3A4, and it seems possible that it might interact with tacrolimus in a similar way, but this needs confirmation. Although there appear to be no clinical reports of an interaction between miconazole and tacrolimus, a large proportion of miconazole oral gel (both prescription and non-prescription doses) can be swallowed, and therefore adequate systemic absorption might occur, which could cause an interaction. The UK manufacturer of miconazole oral gel recommends close monitoring and a possible dose reduction of tacrolimus if both drugs are given concurrently.[6] An interaction with *intravaginal* miconazole would not normally be expected because its systemic absorption is usually very low (less than 2%) in healthy women of child-bearing age.[7] No interaction would be expected if miconazole is applied to the skin.

1. Vasquez EM, Pollak R, Benedetti E. Clotrimazole increases tacrolimus blood levels: a drug interaction in kidney transplant patients. *Clin Transplant* (2001) 15, 95–9.
2. Vasquez EM, Shin GP, Sifontis N, Benedetti E. Concomitant clotrimazole therapy more than doubles the relative oral bioavailability of tacrolimus. *Ther Drug Monit* (2005) 27, 587–91.
3. Mieles L, Venkataramanan R, Yokoyama I, Warty VJ, Starzl TE. Interaction between FK506 and clotrimazole in a liver transplant recipient. *Transplantation* (1991) 52, 1086–7.
4. Choy M. Tacrolimus interaction with clotrimazole: a concise case report and literature review. *P T* (2010) 35, 568–9.
5. Christians U, Schmidt G, Bader A, Lampen A, Schottmann R, Linck A, Sewing K-F. Identification of drugs inhibiting the *in vitro* metabolism of tacrolimus by human liver microsomes. *Br J Clin Pharmacol* (1996) 41, 187–90.
6. Daktarin Oral Gel (Miconazole). Janssen-Cilag Ltd. UK Summary of product characteristics, December 2014.
7. Daneshmend TK. Systemic absorption of miconazole from the vagina. *J Antimicrob Chemother* (1986) 18, 507–11.

Tacrolimus + Azoles; Posaconazole

Posaconazole can greatly increase tacrolimus concentrations.

Clinical evidence

In a study in healthy subjects, the maximum blood concentration and AUC of a single 50 microgram/kg dose of tacrolimus were increased 2.2-fold and 4.6-fold, respectively, when posaconazole 400 mg twice daily was given for 7 days.[1]

In a study in 12 patients with lung transplants, the tacrolimus dose required to maintain therapeutic tacrolimus concentrations was 75% lower when posaconazole was added, when compared with patients not taking an azole. Five patients were switched from another azole to posaconazole: 3 of these required no tacrolimus dose adjustment when changed from voriconazole to posaconazole, whereas 2 patients changed from itraconazole to posaconazole required a tacrolimus dose increase of 500 micrograms.[2] In another report, increased tacrolimus concentrations occurred in just 2 of 10 transplant patients given posaconazole 800 mg daily, occurring after 17 days and 39 days of concurrent use. One of these patients had acute renal impairment.[3] The UK manufacturer of posaconazole notes that, in clinical efficacy studies, clinically important interactions with tacrolimus, resulting in hospitalisation and/or posaconazole discontinuation, have been reported.[4]

Mechanism

Posaconazole is an inhibitor of CYP3A4 (by which tacrolimus is metabolised) in the gut wall and/or liver, and so tacrolimus concentrations increase. Intravenous tacrolimus would be predicted to be less affected as it does not undergo first-pass metabolism in the gut.[5]

Importance and management

The evidence suggests that an interaction between tacrolimus and posaconazole is established, and concurrent use can greatly increase tacrolimus concentrations. The UK and US manufacturers of posaconazole and the US manufacturer of tacrolimus recommend that the tacrolimus dose is initially reduced (they suggest by about two-thirds) in patients given posaconazole, with further dose adjustments made as required on the basis of close monitoring of tacrolimus concentrations both during concurrent use and after the antifungal is stopped.[4,6,7]

Pre-emptive tacrolimus dose reductions when starting azoles have been successful in maintaining tacrolimus concentrations within the therapeutic range;[8] however the authors of one review state that this is not standard practice among transplant clinicians, because of the concern of an increased risk of rejection[9] (due to subtherapeutic tacrolimus concentrations). Similarly, the authors of some studies also suggest that a pre-emptive tacrolimus dose reduction might not be appropriate because of the wide variability in the increase in tacrolimus concentrations between patients.[10,11] Whatever is done, close monitoring of tacrolimus concentrations, with appropriate tacrolimus dose adjustments, is essential.

1. Sansone-Parsons A, Krishna G, Martinho M, Kantesaria B, Gelone S, Mant TG. Effect of oral posaconazole on the pharmacokinetics of cyclosporine and tacrolimus. *Pharmacotherapy* (2007) 27, 825–34.
2. Berge M, Chevalier P, Benammar M, Guillemain R, Amrein C, Lefeuvre S, Boussaud V, Billaud EM. Safe management of tacrolimus together with posaconazole in lung transplant patients with cystic fibrosis. *Ther Drug Monit* (2009) 31,396–9.
3. Alexander BD, Perfect JR, Daly JS, Restrepo A, Tobón AM, Patino H, Hardalo CJ, Graybill JR. Posaconazole as salvage therapy in patients with invasive fungal infections after solid organ transplant. *Transplantation* (2008) 86, 791–6.
4. Noxafil (Posaconazole). Merck Sharp & Dohme Ltd. UK Summary of product characteristics, September 2014.
5. Osowski CL, Dix SP, Lin LS, Mullins RE, Geller RB, Wingard JR. Evaluation of the drug interaction between intravenous high-dose fluconazole and cyclosporine or tacrolimus in bone marrow transplant patients. *Transplantation* (1996) 61, 1268–72.
6. Prograf (Tacrolimus). Astellas Pharma US Inc. US Prescribing information, September 2013.
7. Noxafil (Posaconazole). Merck & Co., Inc. US Prescribing information, June 2014.
8. Trifilio SM, Scheetz MH, Pi J, Mehta J. Tacrolimus use in adult allogeneic stem cell transplant recipients receiving voriconazole: preemptive dose modification and therapeutic drug monitoring. *Bone Marrow Transplant* (2010) 45, 1352–6.
9. Saad AH, DePestel DD, Carver PL. Factors influencing the magnitude and clinical significance of drug interactions between azole antifungals and select immunosuppressants. *Pharmacotherapy* (2006) 26, 1730–44.
10. Mori T, Aisa Y, Kato J, Nakamura Y, Ikeda Y, Okamoto S. Drug interaction between voriconazole and calcineurin inhibitors in allogeneic hematopoietic stem cell transplant recipients. *Bone Marrow Transplant* (2009) 44, 371–4.
11. Mori T, Kato J, Yamane A, Sakurai M, Kohashi S, Kikuchi T, Ono Y, Okamoto S. Drug interaction between voriconazole and tacrolimus and its association with the bioavailability of oral voriconazole in recipients of allogeneic hematopoietic stem cell transplantation. *Int J Hematol* (2012) 95, 564–9.

Tacrolimus + Azoles; Voriconazole

Voriconazole can greatly increase tacrolimus concentrations.

Clinical evidence

In a retrospective study, 20 patients with lung transplants taking tacrolimus were given voriconazole 200 mg twice daily for aspergillosis for one to 3 months. When voriconazole was stopped, the tacrolimus dose required to maintain therapeutic concentrations increased by 64%. The adverse effects and transplant rejection rate were not affected by voriconazole.[1] In a study in 11 stem cell transplant patients taking stable doses of tacrolimus, a 2.2-fold (range 25% to 4.1-fold) increase in the concentration-to-dose ratio of tacrolimus was seen when oral voriconazole (300 mg twice daily for two doses followed by 200 mg twice daily, 4 patients) or intravenous voriconazole (6 mg/kg twice daily for 2 doses followed by 4 mg/kg twice, 7 patients) was started. The route of voriconazole administration had no effect on the findings, but there was wide interindividual variability, which might have diminished the ability of the study to detect a difference.[2] In another study in 25 allogeneic haematopoietic stem cell transplant recipients, the concentration-to-dose ratio of oral tacrolimus was 2.4-fold higher (range 32% lower to 7.9-fold higher) 7 to 10 days after oral voriconazole 400 mg daily was started. The plasma concentration of voriconazole did not correlate with the increase in the tacrolimus concentration-to-dose ratio.[3] The tacrolimus concentrations of a liver transplant patient also taking voriconazole 200 mg twice daily were nearly 10-fold higher than those in another liver transplant patient taking tacrolimus but not taking voriconazole. These results come from a study originally designed as a larger study that was stopped after the finding in these initial two subjects.[4]

A study in 14 healthy subjects found that voriconazole 400 mg twice daily on day one, followed by 200 mg twice daily for 6 days, increased the AUC and maximum plasma concentration of a single 100 microgram/kg dose of tacrolimus 3.2-fold and 2.3-fold, respectively.[5]

A liver transplant patient taking tacrolimus was hospitalised with multiple complaints, and was found to have a high tacrolimus concentration. Tacrolimus was withheld and later restarted at 3 mg daily and then gradually reduced to 1.5 mg daily. When voriconazole 400 mg twice daily was started, the tacrolimus dose was reduced by one-third to 500 micrograms daily, but eventually needed to be reduced to 150 micrograms daily (a 90% reduction in the overall dose) as a result of increasing tacrolimus concentrations.[6] A kidney transplant patient taking tacrolimus 2 mg daily had an increase in tacrolimus concentrations from less than 12 to 25 nanograms/mL when voriconazole 4 mg/kg twice daily was added. His renal function also worsened. The tacrolimus dose was eventually reduced to 500 micrograms on alternate days, with an improvement in his renal function.[7] Other similar cases have been reported.[8-10]

A brief report describes a 4-fold increase in tacrolimus plasma concentrations in a patient when the route of administration of both tacrolimus and voriconazole was changed from *intravenous* to *oral*,[11] and another describes a 66% increase in tacrolimus concentrations when *intravenous* voriconazole was changed to an *oral* formulation.[12] A stem cell transplant patient had a 4.9-fold increase in the tacrolimus concentration-to-dose ratio when oral fluconazole 200 mg daily was changed to intravenous voriconazole. Similarly, the tacrolimus concentration-to-dose ratio of another patient taking the same dose of oral fluconazole was increased 3.2-fold by the same dose of intravenous voriconazole, and 4.5-fold by oral voriconazole 200 to 300 mg.[13] A case of thrombotic microangiopathy and severe leukoencephalopathy was attributed to tacrolimus toxicity in a patient who had no tacrolimus dose reduction when given voriconazole.[14] Painful neuromuscular disorders occurred in 9 of 27 patients taking tacrolimus who were also treated with voriconazole. Tacrolimus concentrations were maintained within the therapeutic range. At the time of onset of the symptoms, minimum voriconazole concentrations were higher than in the patients without symptoms. Patients completely recovered when voriconazole was stopped. It was suggested that tacrolimus triggered voriconazole neurotoxicity, and that this does not appear to occur if voriconazole doses are adjusted to maintain voriconazole minimum concentrations below 1.5 mg/mL.[15]

Mechanism

Voriconazole is an inhibitor of CYP3A4 (by which tacrolimus is metabolised) in the gut wall and/or liver, and so tacrolimus concentrations increase. Intravenous tacrolimus would be predicted to be less affected as it does not undergo first-pass metabolism in the gut.[16]

Importance and management

The evidence suggests that an interaction between tacrolimus and voriconazole is established and can greatly increase tacrolimus concentrations. The UK manufacturer of tacrolimus states that nearly all patients will require tacrolimus dose reductions when given with voriconazole.[17]

The UK and US manufacturers of voriconazole and the US manufacturer of tacrolimus advise reducing the tacrolimus dose by two-thirds when starting voriconazole, closely monitoring tacrolimus concentrations throughout, and increasing the tacrolimus dose in response to concentrations obtained when voriconazole is stopped.[18-20] Note that greater reductions in the dose of tacrolimus might be needed in some patients.[4,6] Pre-emptive tacrolimus dose reductions when starting azoles have been successful in maintaining tacrolimus concentrations within the therapeutic range;[21] however the authors of one review state that this is not standard practice among transplant clinicians, because of the concern of an increased risk of rejection[22] (due to subtherapeutic tacrolimus concentrations). Similarly, the authors of some studies also suggest that a pre-emptive tacrolimus dose reduction might not be appropriate because of the wide variability in the increase in tacrolimus concentrations between patients.[2,3] Whatever is done, close monitoring of tacrolimus concentrations, with appropriate tacrolimus dose adjustments, is essential.

1. Kramer MR, Amital A, Fuks L, Shitrit D. Voriconazole and itraconazole in lung transplant recipients receiving tacrolimus (FK 506): efficacy and drug interaction. *Clin Transplant* (2011) Epub.
2. Mori T, Aisa Y, Kato J, Nakamura Y, Ikeda Y, Okamoto S. Drug interaction between voriconazole and calcineurin inhibitors in allogeneic hematopoietic stem cell transplant recipients. *Bone Marrow Transplant* (2009) 44, 371–4.
3. Mori T, Kato J, Yamane A, Sakurai M, Kohashi S, Kikuchi T, Ono Y, Okamoto S. Drug interaction between voriconazole and tacrolimus and its association with the bioavailability of oral voriconazole in recipients of allogeneic hematopoietic stem cell transplantation. *Int J Hematol* (2012) 95, 564–9.
4. Venkataramanan R, Zang S, Gayowski T, Singh N. Voriconazole inhibition of the metabolism of tacrolimus in a liver transplant recipient and in human liver microsomes. *Antimicrob Agents Chemother* (2002) 46, 3091–3.
5. Wood N, Tan K, Allan R, Fielding A, Nichols DJ. Effect of voriconazole on the pharmacokinetics of tacrolimus. *Intersci Conf Antimicrob Agents Chemother* (2001) 41, 2.
6. Pai MP, Allen S. Voriconazole inhibition of tacrolimus metabolism. *Clin Infect Dis* (2003) 36, 1089–91.
7. Tintillier M, Kirch L, Goffin E, Cuvelier C, Pochet J-M. Interaction between voriconazole and tacrolimus in a kidney-transplanted patient. *Nephrol Dial Transplant* (2005) 20, 664–5.
8. Kuypers DR, Claes K, Evenepoel P, Vanrenterghem Y. Clinically relevant drug interaction between voriconazole and tacrolimus in a primary renal allograft recipient. *Transplantation* (2006) 81, 1750–2.
9. Chang H-H, Lee N-Y, Ko W-C, Lee H-C, Yang Y-HK, Wu C-J, Chang C-M. Voriconazole inhibition of tacrolimus metabolism in a kidney transplant recipient with fluconazole-resistant cryptococcal meningitis. *Int J Infect Dis* (2010) 14, e348–50.
10. Capone D, Tarantino G, Gentile A, Sabbatini M, Polichetti G, Santagelo M, Nappi R, Ciotola A, D'Alessandro V, Renda A, Basile V, Federico S. Effects of voriconazole on tacrolimus metabolism in a kidney transplant recipient. *J Clin Pharm Ther* (2010) 35, 121–4.
11. Inoue Y, Saito T, Takimoto M, Ogawa K, Shibuya Y, Suzuki Y, Kato M, Takahashi M, Miura I, Hatta Y, Takeuchi J. Highly activated oral bioavailability of tacrolimus on coadministration of oral voriconazole. *Int J Clin Pharmacol Ther* (2011) 49, 291–2.
12. Spriet I, Grootaert V, Meyfroidt G, Debaveye Y, Willems L. Switching from intravenous to oral tacrolimus and voriconazole leads to a more pronounced drug-drug interaction. *Eur J Clin Pharmacol* (2012) Epub.
13. Kawazoe H, Takiguchi Y, Tanaka H, Fukuoka N, Ohnishi H, Ishida T, Houchi H. Change of the blood concentration of tacrolimus after the switch from fluconazole to voriconazole in patients receiving allogeneic hematopoietic stem cell transplantation. *Biol Pharm Bull* (2006) 29, 2528–31.
14. Marty FM, Lowry CM, Cutler CS, Campbell BJ, Fiumara K, Baden LR, Antin JH. Voriconazole and sirolimus coadministration after allogeneic hematopoietic stem cell transplantation. *Biol Blood Marrow Transplant* (2006) 12, 552–9.
15. Boussaud V, Daudet N, Billaud EM, Lillo-Le Louet A, Chevalier P, Amrein C, Bergé MM, Guillemain R, Le Beller C. Neuromuscular painful disorders: a rare side effect of voriconazole in lung transplant patients under tacrolimus. *J Heart Lung Transplant* (2008) 27, 229–32.
16. Osowski CL, Dix SP, Lin LS, Mullins RE, Geller RB, Wingard JR. Evaluation of the drug interaction between intravenous high-dose fluconazole and cyclosporine or tacrolimus in bone marrow transplant patients. *Transplantation* (1996) 61, 1268–72.
17. Prograf (Tacrolimus monohydrate). Astellas Pharma Ltd. UK Summary of product characteristics, November 2014.
18. Prograf (Tacrolimus). Astellas Pharma US Inc. US Prescribing information, September 2013.
19. VFEND (Voriconazole). Pfizer Ltd. UK Summary of product characteristics, October 2014.
20. VFEND (Voriconazole). Pfizer Inc. US Prescribing information, February 2014.
21. Trifilio SM, Scheetz MH, Pi J, Mehta J. Tacrolimus use in adult allogeneic stem cell transplant recipients receiving voriconazole: preemptive dose modification and therapeutic drug monitoring. *Bone Marrow Transplant* (2010) 45, 1352–6.
22. Saad AH, DePestel DD, Carver PL. Factors influencing the magnitude and clinical significance of drug interactions between azole antifungals and select immunosuppressants. *Pharmacotherapy* (2006) 26, 1730–44.

Tacrolimus + Basiliximab

There is limited evidence suggesting that basiliximab might increase tacrolimus concentrations.

Clinical evidence, mechanism, importance and management

A retrospective analysis of 12 kidney transplant patients receiving tacrolimus, with basiliximab on day 1 and day 4, found that minimum tacrolimus concentrations on day 3 were 63% higher than in 8 patients receiving tacrolimus with antithymocyte globulin daily from day 1 to day 7 (control group). Half of the patients in the basiliximab group had minimum tacrolimus concentrations above the upper limit of the target range of 15 to 20 ng/mL, compared with only 2 in the control group. Three of the 6 patients in the basiliximab group who had elevated tacrolimus minimum concentrations developed acute tubular necrosis, compared with none in the control group. Tacrolimus dose requirements were lower in the group receiving basiliximab throughout the 60-day study period, when compared with the control group.[1] Despite the differences observed, it is important to note that the minimum tacrolimus concentrations did not differ between the 2 groups during the 60-day period.

The reason for this effect is not known, but the authors suggested that it might be due to an interleukin-2-mediated down-regulation of CYP3A4 activity.[1] This could lead to decreased tacrolimus metabolism, and hence increased exposure. On the basis of this one small study, no additional monitoring, over and above that normally undertaken immediately post-transplant, would seem necessary on concurrent use, but it would seem prudent to be alert for the need to adjust tacrolimus doses more than might be expected. Also bear in mind, that due to the half-life of basiliximab, its effects might persist for several weeks after it is discontinued.

1. Sifontis NM, Benedetti E, Vasquez EM. Clinically significant drug interaction between basiliximab and tacrolimus in renal transplant recipients. *Transplant Proc* (2002) 34, 1730–2.

Tacrolimus + Berberine

An isolated case report suggests that berberine might increase tacrolimus concentrations.

Clinical evidence

A case report describes a 16-year-old girl with nephrotic syndrome taking tacrolimus 6.5 mg twice daily who was started on berberine 200 mg three times daily for diarrhoea. Her tacrolimus minimum concentration increased from 8 to 22 nanograms/mL, and her creatinine concentration also increased (from 62 to 109 micromols/L. The tacrolimus dose was decreased to 3 mg daily and after 5 days her tacrolimus minimum concentration was 12 nanograms/mL, and her creatinine concentration had similarly decreased (to 84 micromols/L).[1]

Mechanism

Uncertain, but it is suggested that berberine inhibits CYP3A4, by which tacrolimus is metabolised. Concurrent use could therefore increase tacrolimus concentrations. A similar effect has been seen with ciclosporin, which is also a CYP3A4 substrate (see 'Ciclosporin + Berberine', p.1218).

Importance and management

Evidence for an interaction between tacrolimus and berberine is limited to an isolated case report, but an increase in tacrolimus minimum concentration of the magnitude seen, could be clinically important. Until more is known, if the combination is used, careful monitoring of the tacrolimus concentration and for adverse effects, with appropriate dose adjustments where required, would seem a sensible approach. Consideration should be given to stopping the berberine if tacrolimus concentrations cannot be adequately maintained with dose adjustments.

1. Hou Q, Han W, Fu X. Pharmacokinetic interaction between tacrolimus and berberine in a child with idiopathic nephrotic syndrome. *Eur J Clin Pharmacol* (2013) 69, 1861–2.

Tacrolimus + Calcium-channel blockers

Nifedipine can cause a small increase in tacrolimus concentrations and also appears to be kidney protective. Large increases in tacrolimus concentrations have been reported in a few cases with diltiazem, although one study found no interaction. Cases of increased tacrolimus concentrations have been reported on the concurrent use of amlodipine, felodipine, and nicardipine. Verapamil, and possibly nilvadipine, are predicted to interact similarly. The concurrent use of tacrolimus and calcium-channel blockers appears to be associated with gingival overgrowth.

Clinical evidence

(a) Tacrolimus concentrations

1. Amlodipine. A brief report describes a 4-year-old boy taking prolonged-release tacrolimus 2.5 mg daily following a kidney transplant, who had an increase in his tacrolimus minimum concentration from 3.7 to 12.2 nanograms/mL, with an increase in his serum creatinine, when amlodipine 500 micrograms/kg daily (with enalapril) was started. His tacrolimus dose was reduced to 2 mg daily, and 3 days later, his tacrolimus minimum concentration was 9.4 nanograms/mL.[1]

A report describes a 19-year-old kidney transplant patient taking tacrolimus 9 mg daily and amlodipine 5 mg daily who experienced tenderness and heaviness in both breasts, with nipple discharge. Her tacrolimus minimum concentration was found to be 12.1 nanograms/mL, and the dose was reduced over the following 4 weeks to achieve a tacrolimus minimum concentration of 7.2 nanograms/mL. When amlodipine was changed to metoprolol, her symptoms resolved within 5 days, but recurred on rechallenge with the amlodipine.[2] There is some evidence from a crossover study in healthy subjects taking a single 5-mg dose of tacrolimus alone, and with a single 5-mg dose of amlodipine, that CYP3A5 genotype might influence the interaction with amlodipine, such that CYP3A5 expressers (that is those with functioning CYP3A5) require lower doses of tacrolimus if also taking amlodipine, than non-expressers of

CYP3A5 (that is those with non-functioning CYP3A5). In the study, the AUC of tacrolimus was increased 2.3-fold by amlodipine in CYP3A5 expressers but was unaffected in non-expressers.[3] Further study is required to confirm the importance of this finding.

2. Diltiazem. A liver transplant patient taking tacrolimus 8 mg twice daily had an increase in his tacrolimus minimum blood concentration from 12.9 to 55 nanograms/mL within 3 days of starting diltiazem (initially 5 to 10 mg/hour intravenously for one day, then 30 mg orally every 8 hours). The patient became delirious, confused, and agitated. Both drugs were stopped, and over the next 3 days his mental state improved and his tacrolimus concentration decreased to 6.7 nanograms/mL. Tacrolimus was then restarted, gradually increasing to a dose of 5 mg twice daily, which produced concentrations of 9 to 10 nanograms/mL.[4] Another report briefly mentions that one kidney transplant patient with acute tacrolimus nephrotoxicity required a 66% tacrolimus dose reduction after starting diltiazem.[5] Diltiazem was thought to have contributed to a case of a very high tacrolimus concentration in a patient also taking HIV-protease inhibitors (see 'Tacrolimus + HIV-protease inhibitors', p.1297), but ritonavir alone could equally have been responsible.

Similarly, a study in 2 liver and 2 kidney transplant patients found that diltiazem increased the AUC of tacrolimus. In the kidney transplant patients, the increase appeared to be dose-related: a 20 mg dose of diltiazem caused a 26% and 67% increase, while a 180 mg dose caused a 48% and 2.8-fold increase in each patient, respectively. The liver transplant patients did not have any alteration in the AUC of tacrolimus until they were given higher doses of diltiazem: one patient had an 18% increase following a 120 mg dose, the other a 22% increase following a 180 mg dose.[6] In contrast, in a study in liver transplant patients given tacrolimus, there was no difference in the required tacrolimus dose at day 3, day 7, month one, and month 3 in 7 patients also given modified-release diltiazem 90 mg daily, when compared with 7 patients not given diltiazem.[7] The authors of the other study[6] suggested that this lack of effect might have been because only 90 mg of diltiazem was used. However, a case report describes a kidney transplant patient stable taking tacrolimus (dose not stated) and diltiazem 240 mg for years without evidence of interaction, until ranolazine was added (see 'Tacrolimus + Ranolazine', p.1303 for details).[8]

There is some evidence from studies in transplant patients that CYP3A5 genotype might influence the extent of the effect of diltiazem, such that expressers of CYP3A5 (that is those with non-functioning CYP3A5) might have higher tacrolimus concentrations than CYP3A5 non-expressers.[9,10] Further study is required to confirm the importance of this finding.

3. Felodipine. A 13-year-old boy taking tacrolimus 4 mg twice daily was given felodipine 2.5 mg daily 15 days after receiving a kidney transplant. Two weeks later his tacrolimus concentration was reported as greater than 30 nanograms/mL (previous concentrations ranged from 10.6 to 20 nanograms/mL), and despite a reduction in the dose of tacrolimus to 3 mg twice daily, a subsequent tacrolimus concentration was 53.9 nanograms/mL. He was eventually stabilised at the original tacrolimus concentration with 500 micrograms twice daily. When felodipine was stopped several months later, his tacrolimus dose needed to be increased to maintain therapeutic concentrations.[11]

4. Nicardipine. In a study, 12 patients with kidney transplants taking tacrolimus were given continuous intravenous infusions of nicardipine 2 micrograms/kg per minute for a mean of 43 hours. Their tacrolimus minimum concentrations increased from a target range of 10 to 20 nanograms/mL to 22 nanograms/mL within 48 hours. Further analysis showed that the tacrolimus minimum concentration was outside the target range (greater than 20 nanograms/mL) only in those patients who were CYP3A5 non-expressers.[12]

Two case reports describe altered tacrolimus minimum concentrations when nicardipine was also given in kidney transplant patients. In the first patient, tacrolimus 5 mg twice daily was started immediately post-transplant. As he was hypertensive immediately post-transplant, he was given intravenous nicardipine 1 microgram/kg per minute, rapidly increased to 3 micrograms/kg per minute, with extended-release nifedipine 60 mg and labetalol overnight. His minimum tacrolimus concentration on day one post-transplant was 16.3 nanograms/mL (target range 12 to 18 nanograms/mL), and he was continued on nicardipine and nifedipine. His tacrolimus dose was reduced to 2.5 mg that evening with a 4 mg dose the following morning. His urine output decreased abruptly despite a positive fluid balance. Nicardipine was stopped, and his 12-hour minimum tacrolimus concentration was 50 nanograms/mL with a minimum tacrolimus concentration that evening of 84.8 nanograms/mL. Tacrolimus was withheld until its concentration had dropped to 9.6 nanograms/mL 3 days later, and was restarted at 2 mg twice daily. His urine output had improved and 2 days later his tacrolimus dose needed to be increased to 6 mg twice daily to achieve a 12-hour minimum concentration of about 10 nanograms/mL, and he continued to take extended-release nifedipine 120 mg twice daily. In the second patient, less dramatic increases in the tacrolimus minimum concentration were seen (up to 18 nanograms/mL) while receiving intravenous nicardipine and oral extended-release nifedipine 120 mg twice daily, followed by a low tacrolimus concentration requiring dose increases after nicardipine was stopped.[13] See also *Nifedipine*, below.

5. Nifedipine. A one-year retrospective study of two groups of liver transplant patients found that in the 22 patients taking nifedipine 30 or 60 mg daily there was a 55% increase in the tacrolimus blood concentrations after one month. By 6 months, the tacrolimus dose had been reduced by a total of 25.5% in the nifedipine group, and by 12 months by 31.4%, when compared with the group not taking nifedipine. The nifedipine group also had improved renal function (decreased serum creatinine).[14]

(b) Gingival overgrowth

Calcium-channel blockers are well known to be associated with gingival overgrowth in transplant patients, however results from studies assessing the association between tacrolimus and gingival overgrowth are not entirely conclusive, with some studies finding no association (three are cited as examples[15-17]) and others finding that there is an association (one is cited as an example[18]). Overall, the prevalence of gingival overgrowth in tacrolimus patients appears to be 0 to 30%.[19] Further, some studies[20,21] have found that the occurrence with tacrolimus is less than that with ciclosporin, which is well-known to be associated with this effect (with a prevalence of about 15% to 81%[19]). Another study suggests that tacrolimus might ameliorate the risk of oral diseases (including gingival hyperplasia) in renal transplant patients.[22]

There is some evidence that the concurrent use of tacrolimus with calcium-channel blockers increases the occurrence of gingival overgrowth.[20,22,23] For example, in a study in 45 kidney transplant patients taking tacrolimus, 13 developed gingival overgrowth, and 9 of these were also taking a calcium-channel blocker (not specified). Of the remaining 32 patients who did not develop gingival overgrowth, 5 were also taking a calcium-channel blocker (not specified).[23]

Other studies have found that switching from ciclosporin to tacrolimus leads to improvement in gingival overgrowth.[24-26]

Mechanism

Diltiazem is an inhibitor of CYP3A4, by which tacrolimus is metabolised, and therefore decreases the metabolism of tacrolimus, leading to increased blood concentrations. It has been suggested that nicardipine can also inhibit CYP3A4, but nifedipine and felodipine are not known to act as inhibitors of drug metabolism, therefore the reasons for the potential interactions described with these two calcium-channel blockers are unclear. However, an early *in vitro* study using human liver microsomes did find inhibition of tacrolimus metabolism by nifedipine and nilvadipine,[27] although there is some doubt about the clinical relevance of these findings. The role of CYP3A5 genotype in the interaction between the calcium channel blockers and tacrolimus is unclear, with some variable evidence, but it might be involved in the interaction with amlodipine, diltiazem, and nicardipine.

Both tacrolimus and calcium-channel blockers can cause gingival overgrowth, which might be additive on concurrent use.

Importance and management

Information about an interaction between tacrolimus and **diltiazem** is limited. However, given that diltiazem is known to affect one of the main routes of tacrolimus metabolism and that large increases in tacrolimus concentrations have been seen in some patients, it would seem wise to closely monitor tacrolimus concentrations when diltiazem is started or stopped. **Verapamil** inhibits CYP3A4 like diltiazem, and also inhibits P-glycoprotein which is involved in the transport of tacrolimus, and so would also be expected to interact with tacrolimus in a similar way. Similar precautions to those advised for diltiazem would be prudent on concurrent use.

Limited evidence from one retrospective study suggests that **nifedipine** might interact with tacrolimus. However, the increase seems slow, and it seems likely that any decrease in the dose requirements of tacrolimus will be detected by routine monitoring.

There is only one isolated case report with **felodipine**, and no interaction is established; however, the UK and US manufacturers of felodipine advise monitoring tacrolimus concentrations if felodipine is given, and adjusting the tacrolimus dose as required.[28,29]

The study and two case reports with **nicardipine** are consistent with the known CYP3A4 inhibitory activity of nicardipine, and monitoring of tacrolimus concentrations might also be prudent on concurrent use.

The general importance of the isolated case reports[1,2] with **amlodipine** is unclear. Published information about other calcium-channel blockers appears to be lacking, but the UK manufacturer of tacrolimus suggests that **nilvadipine** might interact similarly, based on *in vitro* data.[30] The clinical relevance of the effect of CYP3A5 genotype on the interactions of tacrolimus with amlodipine, diltiazem, and nicardipine is unclear as a patient's genotype is rarely known in clinical practice.

The association between gingival overgrowth and tacrolimus use is the subject of some debate, but there does appear to be some evidence that it does occur in transplant patients taking tacrolimus, but less so than with ciclosporin (see 'Ciclosporin + Calcium-channel blockers', p.1220 for details) and possibly more so that with sirolimus (see 'Sirolimus + Calcium-channel blockers', p.1282). Concurrent calcium-channel blocker use does also seem to be a risk factor. It would seem prudent to aware of the possibility of gingival overgrowth occurring if a calcium-channel blocker is required, particularly if gingival overgrowth has occurred while taking tacrolimus. Note that a useful paper about minimising the risk of gingival overgrowth and its management has been published.[31]

1. Zhao W, Baudouin V, Fakhoury M, Storme T, Deschênes G, Jacqz-Aigrain E. Pharmacokinetic interaction between tacrolimus and amlodipine in a renal transplant child. *Transplantation* (2012) 93, e29–e30.
2. Khaira A, Rathi OP, Gupta A, Mahajan S, Bhowmik, D, Agarwal S, Tiwari SC. Galactorrhoea and mastalgia in a renal transplant recipient on tacrolimus and amlodipine. *Nephrology (Carlton)* (2009) 14, 700–1.
3. Zuo XC, Zhou YN, Zhang BK, Yang GP, Cheng ZN, Yuan H, Ouyang DS, Liu SK, Barrett JS, Li PJ, Liu Z, Tan HY, Guo R, Zhou LY, Xie YL, Li ZJ, Li J, Wang CJ, Wang JL. Effect of CYP3A5*3 polymorphism on pharmacokinetic drug interaction between tacrolimus and amlodipine. *Drug Metab Pharmacokinet* (2013) 28, 398–405.
4. Hebert MF, Lam AY. Diltiazem increases tacrolimus concentrations. *Ann Pharmacother* (1999) 33, 680–2.
5. Katari SR, Magnone M, Shapiro R, Jordan M, Scantlebury V, Vivas C, Gritsch A, McCauley J, Starzl T, Demetris J, Randhawa PS. Clinical features of acute reversible tacrolimus (FK 506) nephrotoxicity in kidney transplant recipients. *Clin Transplant* (1997) 11, 237–42.
6. Jones TE, Morris RG. Pharmacokinetic interaction between tacrolimus and diltiazem: dose-response relationship in kidney and liver transplant recipients. *Clin Pharmacokinet* (2002) 41, 381–8.
7. Teperman L, Turgut S, Negron C, John D, Diflo T, Morgan G, Tobias H. Diltiazem is a safe drug in transplant patients on Prograf and does not affect Prograf levels. *Hepatology* (1996) 24, 180A.

8. Patni H, Gitman M, Hazzan A, Jhaveri KD. Ranolazine, tacrolimus, and diltiazem might be a hazardous combination in a transplant patient. *Ren Fail* (2012) 34, 251–3.
9. Li JL, Wang XD, Chen SY, Liu LS, Fu Q, Chen X, Teng LC, Wang CX, Huang M. Effects of diltiazem on pharmacokinetics of tacrolimus in relation to CYP3A5 genotype status in renal recipients: from retrospective to prospective. *Pharmacogenomics J* (2011) 11, 300–6.
10. Chen SY, Li JL, Meng FH, Wang XD, Liu T, Li J, Liu LS, Fu Q, Huang M, Wang CX. Individualization of tacrolimus dosage basing on cytochrome P450 3A5 polymorphism - a prospective, randomized, controlled study. *Clin Transplant* (2013) 27, E272–81.
11. Butani L, Berg G, Makker SP. Effect of felodipine on tacrolimus pharmacokinetics in a renal transplant recipient. *Transplantation* (2002) 73, 159.
12. Hooper DK, Fukuda T, Gardiner R, Logan B, Roy-Chaudhury A, Kirby CL, Vinks AA, Goebel J. Risk of tacrolimus toxicity in CYP3A5 nonexpressors treated with intravenous nicardipine after kidney transplantation. *Transplantation* (2012) 93, 806–12.
13. Hooper DK, Carle AC, Schuchter J, Goebel J. Interaction between tacrolimus and intravenous nicardipine in the treatment of post-kidney transplant hypertension at pediatric hospitals. *Pediatr Transplant* (2011) 15, 88–95.
14. Seifeldin RA, Marcos-Alvarez A, Gordon FD, Lewis WD, Jenkins RL. Nifedipine interaction with tacrolimus in liver transplant recipients. *Ann Pharmacother* (1997) 31, 571–5.
15. Shiboski CH, Krishnan S, Besten PD, Golinveaux M, Kawada P, Tornabene A, Rosenthal P, Mathias R. Gingival enlargement in pediatric organ transplant recipients in relation to tacrolimus-based immunosuppressive regimens. *Pediatr Dent* (2009) 31, 38–46.
16. McKaig SJ, Kelly D, Shaw L. Investigation of the effect of FK506 (tacrolimus) and cyclosporin on gingival overgrowth following paediatric liver transplantation. *Int J Paediatr Dent* (2002) 12, 398–403.
17. Greenberg KV, Armitage GC, Shiboski CH. Gingival enlargement among renal transplant recipients in the era of new-generation immunosuppressants. *J Periodontol* (2008) 79, 453–60.
18. Cezário ES, Cota LO, Ferreira SD, Siqueira FM, Soares RV, Zenóbio EG, Costa FO. Gingival overgrowth in renal transplant subjects medicated with tacrolimus in the absence of calcium channel blockers. *Transplantation* (2008) 85, 232–6.
19. Costa LC, Costa FO, Cortelli SC, Cortelli JR, Cota LC. Gingival overgrowth in renal transplant subjects: a 44-month follow-up study. *Transplantation* (2013) 96, 890–6.
20. de Oliveira Costa F, Diniz Ferreira S, de Miranda Cota LO, da Costa JE, Aguiar MA. Prevalence, severity, and risk variables associated with gingival overgrowth in renal transplant subjects treated under tacrolimus or ciclosporin regimens. *J Periodontol* (2006) 77, 969–75.
21. Lima RB, Benini V, Sens YA. Gingival overgrowth in renal transplant recipients: a study concerning prevalence, severity, periodontal, and predisposing factors. *Transplant Proc* (2008) 40, 1425–8.
22. Spolidorio LC, Spolidorio DM, Massucato EM, Neppelenbroek KH, Campanha NH, Sanches MH. Oral health in renal transplant recipients administered cyclosporin A or tacrolimus. *Oral Dis* (2006) 12, 309–14.
23. Cota LO, Aquino DR, Franco GC, Cortelli JR, Cortelli SC, Costa FO. Gingival overgrowth in subjects under immunosuppressive regimens based on cyclosporine, tacrolimus, or sirolimus. *J Clin Periodontol* (2010) 37, 894–902.
24. Párraga-Linares L, Almendros-Marqués N, Berini-Aytés L, Gay-Escoda C. Effectiveness of substituting cyclosporin A with tacrolimus in reducing gingival overgrowth in renal transplant patients. *Med Oral Patol Oral Cir Bucal* (2009) 14, e429–33.
25. Zadrazil J, Horak P, Zahalkova J, Strebl P, Horcicka V, Krejci K, Bachleda P, Dedochova J, Valkovsky I. Improvement of cardiovascular risk factors and cosmetic side effects in kidney transplant recipients after conversion to tacrolimus. *Biomed Pap Med Fac Univ Palacky Olomouc Czech Repub* (2009) 153, 67–73.
26. Rostaing L, Sánchez-Fructuoso A, Franco A, Glyda M, Kuypers DR, Jaray J. Conversion to tacrolimus once-daily from ciclosporin in stable kidney transplant recipients: a multicenter study. *Transpl Int* (2012) 25, 391–400.
27. Iwasaki K, Matsuda H, Nagase K, Shiraga T, Tokuma Y, Uchida K. Effects of twenty-three drugs on the metabolism of FK506 by human liver microsomes. *Res Commun Chem Pathol Pharmacol* (1993) 82, 209–16.
28. Plendil (Felodipine). AstraZeneca UK Ltd. UK Summary of product characteristics, July 2013.
29. Plendil (Felodipine). AstraZeneca. US Prescribing information, October 2012.
30. Prograf (Tacrolimus monohydrate). Astellas Pharma Ltd. UK Summary of product characteristics, November 2014.
31. Hood KA. Drug-induced gingival hyperplasia in transplant recipients. *Prog Transplant* (2002) 12, 17–23.

Tacrolimus + Ceftriaxone

An isolated report describes an increase in tacrolimus plasma concentration in a patient given intravenous azithromycin and ceftriaxone.

Clinical evidence, mechanism, importance and management

A case report describes a 54-year old woman with a heart transplant, stable taking tacrolimus 4 mg in the morning and 5 mg in the evening, whose tacrolimus concentration was increased when she was given intravenous azithromycin 500 mg daily and a single 1-g dose of intravenous ceftriaxone, followed by 2 g daily for 2 days, for pneumonia. On admission, her tacrolimus plasma concentration was 9.2 nanograms/mL, which increased to 37.2 nanograms/mL on day 2 and then 30.2 nanograms/mL on day 3. The ceftriaxone was stopped on day 3, the next two doses of tacrolimus were withheld, and the tacrolimus concentrations normalised, with subsequent tacrolimus doses adjusted according to the plasma concentration. Azithromycin was continued orally for a further 12 days. No changes in tacrolimus concentration had been reported when she had previously taken a 4-day course of oral azithromycin the week before her hospital admission; however, the authors state that an interaction with *intravenous* azithromycin cannot be ruled out. They advise that patients should be closely monitored on the concurrent use of intravenous azithromycin and/or ceftriaxone in patients also taking tacrolimus.[1] This is an isolated case report, the mechanism for which is unclear, and its general relevance is therefore unknown.

1. Shullo MA, Schonder K, Teuteberg JJ. Elevated tacrolimus levels associated with intravenous azithromycin and ceftriaxone: a case report. *Transplant Proc* (2010) 42, 1870–2.

Tacrolimus + Chloramphenicol

A large increase in tacrolimus minimum concentrations has been reported in several patients who were given systemic chloramphenicol.

Clinical evidence

A retrospective study identified 3 patients taking tacrolimus who had received a total of 5 courses of intravenous chloramphenicol, each lasting for at least 12 days. Tacrolimus minimum blood concentrations were doubled by day 2, and had increased by about 3-fold at their peak, on day 6. The tacrolimus dose had been decreased by about one-third by day 12, and the tacrolimus concentrations returned to around the baseline value.[1]

An adolescent patient with a kidney transplant developed a toxic tacrolimus concentration on the second day of starting chloramphenicol for a vancomycin-resistant enterococcal infection. The tacrolimus dose had to be reduced by 83% to achieve a safe serum concentration, and it was found that the dose-adjusted tacrolimus AUC was 7.5-fold greater in the presence of chloramphenicol.[2] Another report describes a similar interaction in a liver transplant patient taking tacrolimus 4 mg twice daily. The patient was given intravenous chloramphenicol, but at the unintentionally high dose of 1850 mg every 6 hours. After about 3 days the patient complained of lethargy, fatigue, headaches, and tremors, so both drugs were stopped. His tacrolimus minimum concentration had increased from a range of 9 to 11 nanograms/mL to more than 60 nanograms/mL. Seven days after chloramphenicol had been stopped his tacrolimus concentration was 8.2 nanograms/mL and his symptoms had resolved.[3] Another case report in a kidney-pancreas transplant patient taking tacrolimus 4 mg twice daily found that the addition of oral chloramphenicol 750 mg four times daily increased the tacrolimus minimum blood concentration to more than 30 micrograms/L within 3 days. After 10 days, the dose of tacrolimus was reduced to 1.5 mg twice daily and the tacrolimus concentration decreased to between 18 and 25 micrograms/L. Chloramphenicol was stopped 5 days later and the tacrolimus dose was increased to 3 mg twice daily. However, the tacrolimus concentration decreased to below 5 micrograms/L for several days leading to an episode of acute organ rejection. The tacrolimus concentration then returned to within the therapeutic range and the patient stabilised.[4]

Mechanism

The authors of one report suggest that chloramphenicol increased tacrolimus concentrations by rapidly inhibiting its metabolism.[2] Chloramphenicol has been shown to inhibit CYP3A4 (the isoenzyme by which tacrolimus is metabolised) in an *in vitro* study with human liver microsomes,[5] but *in vitro* predictions do not always mirror what happens in clinical use, and therefore further study is needed to establish an effect.

Importance and management

Evidence for an interaction between tacrolimus and chloramphenicol appears to be limited to these case reports, but they suggest that an interaction is established, albeit of uncertain incidence. However, it would seem prudent to monitor the outcome closely if systemic chloramphenicol is given to any patient taking tacrolimus, being alert for the need to reduce the tacrolimus dose. It seems doubtful if a clinically relevant interaction will occur with topical chloramphenicol because both the dose and systemic absorption are small, but this ideally needs confirmation.

1. Mathis AS, Shah N, Knipp GT, Friedman GS. Interaction of chloramphenicol and the calcineurin inhibitors in renal transplant recipients. *Transpl Infect Dis* (2002) 4, 169–74.
2. Schulman SL, Shaw LM, Jabs K, Leonard MB, Brayman KL. Interaction between tacrolimus and chloramphenicol in a renal transplant recipient. *Transplantation* (1998) 65, 1397–8.
3. Taber DJ, Dupuis RE, Hollar KD, Strzalka AL, Johnson MW. Drug-drug interaction between chloramphenicol and tacrolimus in a liver transplant recipient. *Transplant Proc* (2000) 32, 660–62.
4. Bakri R, Breen C, Maclean D, Taylor J, Goldsmith D. Serious interaction between tacrolimus FK506 and chloramphenicol in a kidney-pancreas transplant recipient. *Transpl Int* (2003) 16, 441–3.
5. Park J-Y, Kim K-A, Kim S-L. Chloramphenicol is a potent inhibitor of cytochrome P450 isoforms CYP2C19 and CYP3A4 in human liver microsomes. *Antimicrob Agents Chemother* (2003) 47, 3464–9.

Tacrolimus + Ciclosporin

The concurrent use of tacrolimus and ciclosporin appears to increase the risk of nephrotoxicity.

Clinical evidence, mechanism, importance and management

One study found that, in patients with normal bilirubin concentrations, the half-life of ciclosporin was prolonged from a range of 6 to 15 hours up to 26 to 74 hours, and the ciclosporin serum concentration, measured by a fluorescent polarisation immunoassay, was increased by tacrolimus.[1] However, another study found no changes in the pharmacokinetics of ciclosporin, as measured by HPLC, in patients given tacrolimus, but creatinine concentrations were almost doubled (suggesting kidney damage),[2] which confirmed a previous report suggesting that severe renal impairment might develop when both drugs are given.[3] In addition, tacrolimus concentrations might be increased by ciclosporin.[4]

The UK and US manufacturers of tacrolimus state that it should not be given with ciclosporin because of the risk of additive/synergistic nephrotoxicity, and, if ciclosporin is being replaced by tacrolimus, 12 to 24 hours should elapse between stopping one drug and starting the other. If ciclosporin concentrations are increased, the introduction of tacrolimus should be further delayed.[4,5]

1. Venkataramanan R, Jain A, Cadoff E, Warty V, Iwasaki K, Nagase K, Krajack A, Imventarza O, Todo S, Fung JJ, Starzl TE. Pharmacokinetics of FK 506: preclinical and clinical studies. *Transplant Proc* (1990) 22 (Suppl 1), 52–6.
2. Jain AB, Venkataramanan R, Fung J, Burckart G, Emeigh J, Diven W, Warty V, Abu-Elmagd K, Todo S, Alessiani M, Starzl TE. Pharmacokinetics of cyclosporine and nephrotoxicity in orthoptic liver transplant patients rescued with FK 506. *Transplant Proc* (1991) 23, 2777–9.
3. McCauley J, Fung J, Jain A, Todo S, Starzl TE. The effects of FK506 on renal function after liver transplantation. *Transplant Proc* (1990) 22 (Suppl 1), 17–20.
4. Prograf (Tacrolimus monohydrate). Astellas Pharma Ltd. UK Summary of product characteristics, November 2014.
5. Prograf (Tacrolimus). Astellas Pharma US Inc. US Prescribing information, September 2013.

Tacrolimus + Cinacalcet

In a controlled study, cinacalcet had little effect on the pharmacokinetics of tacrolimus. However, a case report describes a large decrease in tacrolimus concentration in a patient who started to take cinacalcet.

Clinical evidence

In a pharmacokinetic study in 6 kidney transplant patients taking tacrolimus, cinacalcet 30 mg daily for 7 days had minimal effects on the pharmacokinetics of tacrolimus. There was an average 14% reduction in the AUC of tacrolimus, with no change in the minimum concentration and no change in renal function.[1]

In clinical studies, no change in tacrolimus dose was needed in 5 patients when they were given cinacalcet, 30 mg daily then titrated to effect, for 6 months.[2,3]

However, there is one case report of a woman taking tacrolimus 4 mg twice daily whose tacrolimus concentration decreased by about 60% (from 6.3 to 2.6 micrograms/L) one week after starting to take cinacalcet 30 mg daily. Increasing the dose of tacrolimus to 6 mg twice daily resulted in a concentration within the therapeutic range once again. Because of an increase in serum creatinine, cinacalcet was withdrawn and her tacrolimus concentration increased from 6.6 to 8 micrograms/L. No further tacrolimus dose adjustment was required.[4]

Mechanism

Cinacalcet is not an inhibitor of CYP3A4, by which tacrolimus is principally metabolised, and therefore the reason for the slight reduction in tacrolimus exposure seen in the pharmacokinetic study, and the larger reduction seen in the case report, is unknown.

Importance and management

Evidence for an interaction between tacrolimus and cinacalcet is limited and inconclusive. The minor reduction in tacrolimus concentration in the pharmacokinetic study is unlikely to be clinically relevant, and this seems to be supported by data from the few patients in clinical studies taking tacrolimus who were given cinacalcet for 6 months. However, the case report of a large reduction in tacrolimus concentration introduces a note of caution. Until further clinical experience is gained, it would be prudent to monitor tacrolimus concentrations more closely with concurrent use of cinacalcet.

1. Falck P, Vethe NT, Åsberg A, Midtvedt K, Bergan S, Reubsaet JL, Holdaas H. Cinacalcet's effect on the pharmacokinetics of tacrolimus, cyclosporine and mycophenolate in renal transplant recipients. *Nephrol Dial Transplant* (2008) 23, 1048–53.
2. Serra AL, Savoca R, Huber AR, Hepp U, Delsignore A, Hersberger M, Wüthrich RP. Effective control of persistent hyperparathyroidism with cinacalcet in renal allograft recipients. *Nephrol Dial Transplant* (2007) 22, 577–83.
3. Szwarc I, Argilés A, Garrigue V, Delmas S, Chong G, Deleuze S, Mourad G. Cinacalcet chloride is efficient and safe in renal transplant recipients with posttransplant hyperparathyroidism. *Transplantation* (2006) 82, 675–80.
4. Maass E, Mueller GA, Heller T, Koziolek MJ. Decrease in serum tacrolimus level and rise in serum creatinine under late addition of cinacalcet in a renal transplant recipient with hyperparathyroidism: a case report. *Transplant Proc* (2007) 39, 3468–70.

Tacrolimus + Corticosteroids

The concurrent use of tacrolimus and corticosteroids is very common, but some evidence suggests that methylprednisolone, prednisolone, and prednisone might alter tacrolimus pharmacokinetics.

Clinical evidence

(a) Methylprednisolone

A prospective pharmacokinetic study in 100 *de novo* kidney transplant patients receiving tacrolimus 200 micrograms/kg daily with mycophenolate and oral methylprednisolone 12 to 20 mg daily (decreasing to 4 mg daily or stopping from 5-months post-transplant), found a positive correlation between decreasing tacrolimus dose requirements and decreasing methylprednisolone doses during the first year after transplantation. However, there was a negative correlation between tacrolimus minimum concentrations and methylprednisolone dose in the 6 to 12 months post-transplant.[1] In another prospective study, 10 liver transplant patients were given tacrolimus 50 micrograms/kg daily, either with (6 patients), or without (4 patients) methylprednisolone 1 g intraoperatively, followed by 200 mg daily on day one, tapered to 20 mg daily at day 7. Tacrolimus minimum concentrations on day 2 were 59% higher in those patients taking steroids than in those not taking steroids, but on day 10 there was no difference between the groups.[2] Further, a retrospective study into the effect of decreasing methylprednisolone doses on tacrolimus bioavailability during the 12 months after kidney transplant, found that the bioavailability of tacrolimus increased in parallel to decreasing the methylprednisolone dose.[3]

A case report describes a 20-year-old liver transplant patient taking tacrolimus, whose tacrolimus minimum blood concentration dramatically reduced after a 3-day course of intravenous methylprednisolone 625 mg daily. During the 11 days following the last dose of methylprednisolone the minimum blood concentration reached a low of 2.8 nanograms/mL before returning to the previously maintained range of 8 to 12 nanograms/mL.[4]

(b) Prednisolone or Prednisone

An analysis of data from retrospective and prospective evaluations of kidney transplant patients taking tacrolimus-based immunosuppression for at least 3 months, found that tacrolimus dose-normalised minimum blood concentrations increased by 12% (not statistically significant) and 14% after withdrawal of prednisolone 5 mg daily. A greater effect was seen after withdrawal of prednisolone 10 mg daily, with increases in tacrolimus dose-normalised minimum blood concentrations of 33% and 36%. In the same study, pharmacokinetic data from 8 patients showed that the AUC of tacrolimus increased by 18% and its oral clearance decreased by 10%, after withdrawal of prednisolone 5 mg daily, but maximum concentrations and time to reach maximum concentrations were not altered.[5] A population pharmacokinetic analysis of data from 31 kidney transplant patients found that a dose of prednisolone of more than 10 mg daily decreased tacrolimus bioavailability by 15% when compared with lower prednisolone doses.[6] In a randomised study conducted over 3 months, 31 patients receiving tacrolimus, mycophenolate, and daclizumab were compared with 34 patients taking tacrolimus, mycophenolate, and prednisone. Higher tacrolimus doses were required to maintain therapeutic tacrolimus concentrations in the prednisone group. This reached a maximum after one month, when a 30% larger tacrolimus dose was necessary.[7] A further study found that patients taking higher doses of prednisone (more than 0.25 mg/kg daily) also needed larger doses of tacrolimus to maintain therapeutic minimum blood concentrations.[8] In another study in 12 kidney transplant patients, a prednisolone dose reduction resulted in about a 50% increase in the dose-corrected AUC of tacrolimus in patients also taking sirolimus, but had no effect in those also taking mycophenolate.[9]

(c) Unspecified corticosteroids

A study in 30 paediatric kidney transplant patients investigated the effect of corticosteroid use (methylprednisolone or prednisone) on tacrolimus pharmacokinetics. The AUC of tacrolimus was found to be 41% higher in 9 patients who did not receive corticosteroids than in 21 who did. The tacrolimus maximum plasma concentration tended to be higher in those who did not receive corticosteroids, but this was not statistically significant. Tacrolimus minimum concentrations did not differ between the groups.[10]

Mechanism

Uncertain. The authors of one study considered that the higher doses of tacrolimus required with increasing doses of prednisone, were possibly due to induction of CYP3A4, which is involved in the metabolism of tacrolimus, by prednisone.[8] The authors of another study suggest that the involvement of P-glycoprotein is unlikely.[5]

Importance and management

The effects of corticosteroids on the pharmacokinetics of tacrolimus are not well established, but there is some evidence that they can be clinically important. The concurrent use of tacrolimus and corticosteroids is common and advantageous but be alert for any evidence of altered tacrolimus effects. The authors of one study recommend that tacrolimus concentrations should be closely monitored and adjusted according to any changes in corticosteroid dose.[8] Another group of authors warns that increased tacrolimus exposure, resulting from steroid withdrawal, might result in a corresponding increase in creatinine concentrations that could be misinterpreted as rejection, and monitoring of tacrolimus minimum concentrations after steroid withdrawal is advisable, with dose reductions if necessary.[5] Increased monitoring of tacrolimus concentrations when corticosteroid doses are altered would seem to be a prudent measure.

1. Kuypers DRJ, Claes K, Evenepoel P, Maes B, Coosemans W, Pirenne J, Vanrenterghem Y. Time-related clinical determinants of long-term tacrolimus pharmacokinetics in combination therapy with mycophenolic acid and corticosteroids: a prospective study in one hundred *de novo* renal transplant recipients. *Clin Pharmacokinet* (2004) 43, 741–62.
2. Charco R, Rimola A, García-Valdecasas JC, Fuster J, Fondevila C, Navasa M, Julian M, Forta V, Brunet M. Steroids and living liver donation increase tacrolimus blood levels in living donor liver transplantation. *Transplant Proc* (2005) 37, 3930–1.
3. Lemahieu WPD, Maes BD, Vanrenterghem Y. Different evolution of trough and dose levels during the first year after transplantation for tacrolimus versus cyclosporine. *Transplant Proc* (2005) 37, 2051–3.
4. Shimada T, Terada A, Yokogawa K, Kaneko H, Nomura M, Kaji K, Kaneko S, Kobayashi KI, Miyamoto KI. Lowered blood concentration of tacrolimus and its recovery with changes in expression of CYP3A and P-glycoprotein after high-dose steroid therapy. *Transplantation* (2002) 74, 1419–24.
5. van Duijnhoven EM, Boots JMM, Christiaans MHL, Stolk LML, Undre NA, van Hooff JP. Increase in tacrolimus trough levels after steroid withdrawal. *Transpl Int* (2003) 16, 721–5.
6. Press RR, Ploeger BA, den Hartigh J, van der Straaten T, van Pelt J, Danhof M, de Fijter JW, Guchelaar H-J. Explaining variability in tacrolimus pharmacokinetics to optimize early exposure in adult kidney transplant recipients. *Ther Drug Monit* (2009) 31, 187–97.
7. Hesselink DA, Ngyuen H, Wabbijn M, Smak Gregoor PJH, Steyerberg EW, van Riemsdijk IC, Weimar W, van Gelder T. Tacrolimus dose requirement in renal transplant recipients is significantly higher when used in combination with corticosteroids. *Br J Clin Pharmacol* (2003) 56, 327–30.
8. Anglicheau D, Flamant M, Schlageter MH, Martinez F, Cassinat B, Beaune P, Legendre C, Thervet E. Pharmacokinetic interaction between corticosteroids and tacrolimus after renal transplantation. *Nephrol Dial Transplant* (2003) 18, 2409–14.
9. Park S-I, Felipe CR, Pinheiro-Machado PG, Garcia R, Fernandes FB, Casarini DE, Tedesco-Silva Jr H, Medina-Pestana JO. Tacrolimus pharmacokinetic drug interactions: effect of prednisone, mycophenolic acid or sirolimus. *Fundam Clin Pharmacol* (2009) 23, 137–45.
10. Kim JS, Aviles DH, Silverstein DM, Leblanc PL, Vehaskari VM. Effect of age, ethnicity, and glucocorticoid use on tacrolimus pharmacokinetics in pediatric renal transplant patients. *Pediatr Transplant* (2005) 9, 162–9.

Tacrolimus + Danazol

An isolated report describes an increase in tacrolimus concentration in a patient given danazol.

Clinical evidence, mechanism, importance and management

In a kidney transplant patient, the minimum serum concentration of tacrolimus 10 mg daily increased from 0.7 to 2.7 nanograms/mL within 4 days of danazol 400 mg to

1.2 g daily being started. Despite a reduction in the danazol dose to 600 mg and then 400 mg daily, her tacrolimus and serum creatinine concentrations remained high for one month until the danazol was withdrawn.[1]

The reason for this effect is not known, but the authors suggest that danazol possibly inhibits the metabolism of tacrolimus by the liver so that it is cleared from the body more slowly.[1]

This is an isolated case, but as danazol has been seen to affect ciclosporin concentrations similarly (see 'Ciclosporin + Danazol', p.1225), it seems possible that an interaction with tacrolimus could be of more general importance. However, there is insufficient direct evidence to recommend monitoring in all patients given danazol and tacrolimus, but it would seem prudent to bear the possibility of an interaction in mind in cases of otherwise unexplained increases in tacrolimus concentrations or adverse effects.

1. Shapiro R, Venkataramanan R, Warty VS, Scantlebury VP, Rybka W, McCauley J, Fung JJ, Starzl TE. FK 506 interaction with danazol. *Lancet* (1993) 341, 1344–5.

Tacrolimus + Echinocandins

Caspofungin might decrease tacrolimus concentrations. Anidulafungin and micafungin do not appear to affect tacrolimus pharmacokinetics, and tacrolimus does not affect the pharmacokinetics of anidulafungin, caspofungin, or micafungin.

Clinical evidence, mechanism, importance and management

(a) Anidulafungin

Thirty-five healthy subjects were given a single 5-mg oral dose of tacrolimus 3 days before and on day 10 of a course of intravenous anidulafungin (200 mg loading dose and then 100 mg daily). Anidulafungin did not have any effect on the pharmacokinetics of tacrolimus and no serious adverse effects were reported. The pharmacokinetics of anidulafungin were not affected by tacrolimus.[1] No additional monitoring would seem to be required with this combination; however, bear in mind that the study above was a single-dose study in healthy subjects. Ideally, more study is required in patients taking long-term tacrolimus.

(b) Caspofungin

The preliminary results of one study in healthy subjects suggest that caspofungin reduces the AUC of tacrolimus by 20%,[2] and reduces the minimum tacrolimus concentrations by 26%.[3] Tacrolimus did not alter the pharmacokinetics of caspofungin.[2] However, in another study in 17 transplant patients taking tacrolimus, just 3 required a tacrolimus dose adjustment (no details given) when also given caspofungin.[4] Similarly, a study including 9 transplant patients taking tacrolimus found no change in tacrolimus minimum concentrations while taking concurrent caspofungin.[5] In a small retrospective study of liver transplant patients, the concurrent use of tacrolimus and caspofungin did not appear to be associated with elevations of liver enzymes.[6]

The UK and US manufacturers of caspofungin advise that standard monitoring of tacrolimus concentrations should be undertaken if caspofungin is given, and the tacrolimus dose should be adjusted as appropriate.[3,7]

(c) Micafungin

Twenty-six healthy subjects were given single 5-mg doses of tacrolimus alone, after intravenous micafungin 100 mg, and one day after intravenous micafungin 100 mg daily for 5 days. The pharmacokinetics of tacrolimus were not affected by micafungin, and single-dose tacrolimus had no effect on the pharmacokinetics of micafungin.[8] Similarly, in a clinical study of patients given micafungin, there was no difference in micafungin blood concentrations, bilirubin, or creatinine clearance between 7 patients taking tacrolimus (14 samples) and 22 patients not taking tacrolimus (26 samples).[9] Further, a study in 6 stem cell transplant patients also found no difference in tacrolimus concentrations when taken with and without micafungin.[10] No additional monitoring would seem to be required with this combination.

1. Dowell JA, Stogniew M, Krause D, Henkel T, Damle B. Lack of pharmacokinetic interaction between anidulafungin and tacrolimus. *J Clin Pharmacol* (2007) 47, 305–14.
2. Stone J, Holland S, Wickersham P, Deutsch P, Winchell G, Hesney M, Miller R, Freeman A, Dilzer S, Lasseter K. Drug interactions between caspofungin and tacrolimus. *Intersci Conf Antimicrob Agents Chemother* (2001) 41, 1.
3. Cancidas (Caspofungin acetate). Merck Sharp & Dohme Ltd. UK Summary of product characteristics, June 2014.
4. Veroux M, Macarone M, Fiamingo P, Cappello D, Gagliano M, Di Mare M, Vizcarra D, Spataro M, Giuffrida G, Sorbello M, Severino V, Veroux P. Caspofungin in the treatment of azole-refractory esophageal candidiasis in kidney transplant recipients. *Transplant Proc* (2006) 38, 1037–9.
5. Groetzner J, Kaczmarek I, Wittwer T, Strauch J, Meiser B, Wahlers T, Daebritz S, Reichart B. Caspofungin as first-line therapy for the treatment of invasive aspergillosis after thoracic organ transplantation. *J Heart Lung Transplant* (2008) 27, 1–6.
6. Saner F, Gensicke J, Rath P, Fruhauf N, Gu Y, Paul A, Radtke A, Malagó M, Broelsch C. Safety profile of concomitant use of caspofungin and cyclosporine or tacrolimus in liver transplant patients. *Infection* (2006) 34, 328–32.
7. Cancidas (Caspofungin acetate). Merck & Co., Inc. US Prescribing information, August 2013.
8. Hebert MF, Blough DK, Townsend RW, Allison M, Buell D, Keirns J, Bekersky I. Concomitant tacrolimus and micafungin pharmacokinetics in healthy volunteers. *J Clin Pharmacol* (2005) 45, 1018–23.
9. Shimoeda S, Ohta S, Kobayashi H, Saitou H, Kubota A, Yamato S, Shimada K, Sasaki M, Kawano K. Analysis of the blood level of micafungin involving patients with hematological diseases: new findings regarding combination therapy with tacrolimus. *Biol Pharm Bull* (2005) 28, 477–80.
10. Fukuoka N, Imataki O, Ohnishi H, Kitanaka A, Kubota Y, Ishida T, Tanaka T. Micafungin does not influence the concentration of tacrolimus in patients after allogeneic hematopoietic stem cell transplantation. *Transplant Proc* (2010) 42, 2725–30.

Tacrolimus + Ezetimibe

The concurrent use of single doses of ezetimibe and tacrolimus does not appear to affect the pharmacokinetics of tacrolimus, but might result in a small increase in the maximum plasma concentration of ezetimibe.

Clinical evidence

In a randomised, crossover, single-dose study, 24 healthy subjects were given ezetimibe 10 mg, tacrolimus 5 mg, or both drugs together. The pharmacokinetics of tacrolimus were not altered by ezetimibe. Tacrolimus increased the maximum plasma concentration of ezetimibe by 33%, but the AUC of ezetimibe, and the pharmacokinetics of the glucuronide metabolite of ezetimibe, were not affected.[1] This finding is supported by several clinical efficacy studies in liver[2] and kidney[3-6] transplant patients which reported that ezetimibe did not alter tacrolimus concentrations and that no pharmacodynamic interaction occurred on concurrent use.

Mechanism

In vitro evidence suggests that tacrolimus inhibits intestinal P-glycoprotein, of which ezetimibe is a substrate, leading to an increase in ezetimibe absorption.

Importance and management

Evidence for an interaction between tacrolimus and ezetimibe is limited to one pharmacokinetic study and analysis from clinical use. The small increase in single-dose ezetimibe concentrations caused by tacrolimus would not be expected to be of clinical importance, although ideally this would be confirmed in multiple-dose studies. The lack of effect of ezetimibe on tacrolimus concentrations is supported by the lack of a clinically relevant interaction in clinical studies. No dose adjustment of either drug therefore appears to be necessary on concurrent use.

1. Oswald S, Nassif A, Modess C, Keiser M, Ulrich A, Runge D, Hanke U, Lütjohann D, Engel A, Weitschies W, Siegmund W. Drug interactions between the immunosuppressant tacrolimus and the cholesterol absorption inhibitor ezetimibe in healthy volunteers. *Clin Pharmacol Ther* (2011) 89, 524–8.
2. Almutairi F, Peterson TC, Molinari M, Walsh MJ, Alwayn I, Peltekian KM. Safety and effectiveness of ezetimibe in liver transplant recipients with hypercholesterolemia. *Liver Transpl* (2009) 15, 504–8.
3. Kohnle M, Pietruck F, Kribben A, Philipp T, Heemann U, Witzke O. Ezetimibe for the treatment of uncontrolled hypercholesterolemia in patients with high-dose statin therapy after renal transplantation. *Am J Transplant* (2006) 6, 205–8.
4. Buchanan C, Smith L, Corbett J, Nelson E, Shihab F. A retrospective analysis of ezetimibe treatment in renal transplant recipients. *Am J Transplant* (2006) 6, 770–4.
5. Savvidaki E, Koukoulaki M, Benou A, Roumeliotou M, Fourtounas C, Kalliakmani P, Papachristou E, Vlachojannis JG, Goumenos D. Ezetimibe is effective in the treatment of persistent hyperlipidemia of renal allograft recipients. *Clin Nephrol* (2011) 75, 107–12.
6. Puthenparumpil JJ, Keough-Ryan T, Kiberd M, Lawen J, Kiberd BA. Treatment of hypercholesterolemia with ezetimibe in the kidney transplant population. *Transplant Proc* (2005), 37, 1033–5.

Tacrolimus + Food

Food decreases the rate and extent of tacrolimus absorption.

Clinical evidence

In a single-dose study in healthy subjects, giving tacrolimus capsules with a high-fat breakfast reduced the maximum tacrolimus concentration by 77%, delayed the time to maximum concentration by about 5 hours, and decreased the AUC by 33%, when compared with the fasting state. There was no change in the elimination half-life.[1] Smaller decreases were noted with a low-fat, high carbohydrate breakfast: a 65% and 26% decrease in maximum concentration and AUC, respectively, and about a 2 hour delay in time to maximum concentration.[1]

In another study in healthy subjects, taking tacrolimus 1.5 hours after a meal resulted in the same reduction in the AUC as when it was given immediately after a meal (39%), but the decrease in maximum concentration was less (63% versus 71%).[2]

The UK and US manufacturers report that, in a study in 11 liver transplant patients, taking tacrolimus 15 minutes after a high-fat breakfast resulted in a 27% decrease in the AUC and a 50% decrease in maximum concentrations when compared with the fasted state.[2,3] However, the effect was less pronounced in a study in kidney transplant patients given tacrolimus immediately after a continental breakfast, the AUC of tacrolimus was reduced by 2 to 12% and its maximum concentration was reduced by 15 to 38%.[3] In a study in kidney transplant patients, the maximum concentration of tacrolimus in 17 patients who took oral tacrolimus one hour before breakfast was 82% higher than in 16 patients who took oral tacrolimus one hour after breakfast. The time to maximum concentration was 2.5-times slower in those who took the tacrolimus after breakfast, but the AUC was no different between the two groups.[4]

Mechanism

Unknown.

Importance and management

Evidence for an interaction between tacrolimus and food is limited to a few studies, but these do suggest that the presence of food in the gastrointestinal tract reduces the extent and rate of absorption of oral tacrolimus, and this is likely to be clinically relevant.[1] The UK manufacturer advises that tacrolimus is taken on an empty stomach at least one hour before or 2 to 3 hours after a meal to optimise absorption.[3]

1. Bekersky I, Dressler D, Mekki QA. Effect of low- and high-fat meals on tacrolimus absorption following 5 mg single oral doses to healthy human subjects. *J Clin Pharmacol* (2001) 41, 176–82.
2. Prograf (Tacrolimus). Astellas Pharma US Inc. US Prescribing information, September 2013.

3. Prograf (Tacrolimus monohydrate). Astellas Pharma Ltd. UK Summary of product characteristics, November 2014.
4. Kimikawa M, Kamoya K, Toma H, Teraoka S. Effective oral administration of tacrolimus in renal transplant recipients. *Clin Transplant* (2001) 15, 324–9.

Tacrolimus + Grapefruit and other fruit juices

Grapefruit juice can greatly increase the concentrations of tacrolimus. Pomelo might interact similarly. An isolated case describes an increase in the tacrolimus blood concentration of a patient who had eaten grapefruit marmalade.

Clinical evidence

(a) Grapefruit juice

In a randomised study, 24 liver transplant patients taking tacrolimus were given either unprocessed grapefruit juice 250 mL twice daily, grapefruit juice diluted 1:8 (with preservatives added) 250 mL twice daily, or no grapefruit juice. After one week, the tacrolimus blood concentration in the patients given pure grapefruit juice was 2.1-fold higher than in those not given any grapefruit juice, and in 5 of these patients the tacrolimus dose had to be halved in order to maintain therapeutic tacrolimus concentrations. There was no difference in tacrolimus plasma concentrations between those patients given diluted grapefruit juice and those not given any grapefruit juice.[1] In another study, 8 liver transplant patients were given 12 oz (about 360 mL) of grapefruit juice twice daily, which they drank within 45 minutes of taking their dose of tacrolimus. After one week the 12-hour minimum concentration of tacrolimus, and the one- and 4-hour post-dose tacrolimus concentrations were increased 4-fold, almost 3-fold, and 5-fold, respectively. Two patients had headaches, one had diarrhoea, and one had an increased creatinine concentration that resolved, but none developed irreversible toxicity. Two of the patients continued to drink the grapefruit juice and it was possible to halve their tacrolimus dose.[2] Similarly, 6 kidney transplant patients had their dose of tacrolimus reduced by an average of 40% after drinking 100 mL of grapefruit juice daily for 5 days.[3]

A hospitalised liver transplant patient was advised to drink grapefruit juice in an effort to increase her minimum blood concentrations of tacrolimus, which were subtherapeutic (below 5 nanograms/mL) despite a dose of tacrolimus 10 mg daily. She drank 250 mL of grapefruit juice four times over 3 days during which time the blood concentration of tacrolimus did not increase. However, one week after she stopped the grapefruit juice the blood concentration of tacrolimus was found to have increased to 37 nanograms/mL.[4]

(b) Other grapefruit products

A 52-year-old man with a liver transplant, stabilised on tacrolimus 3 mg twice daily, began to feel anxious and febrile with continued trembling and blurred vision. Within 5 days he deteriorated and developed severe left chest pain. His tacrolimus whole blood concentration was found to be greatly increased to 55.4 nanograms/mL from a previous therapeutic concentration (between 8 and 13 nanograms/mL), and he had renal impairment (serum creatinine concentration of 174 micromols/L). It transpired that during the week preceding the onset of symptoms he had eaten more than 1.5 kg of a home-made marmalade, which was made with more than 50% grapefruit.[5]

(c) Pomelo

A case report describes a kidney transplant patient taking tacrolimus whose blood concentration of tacrolimus increased from a range of 8 to 10 nanograms/mL up to 25.2 nanograms/mL after he ate about 100 g of pomelo (*Citrus grandis*, a fruit related to grapefruit).[6]

Mechanism

Grapefruit juice inhibits the activity of CYP3A4, mainly in the gut wall. Tacrolimus is primarily metabolised by CYP3A4 and so its bioavailability increases. Pomelo is related to grapefruit and therefore potentially interacts by the same mechanism. *In vitro*, pomelo juice and grapefruit juice extracts inhibited CYP3A4, and had a lesser effect on P-glycoprotein (pomelo weaker than grapefruit).[7] However, the reason for the delayed increase in tacrolimus concentrations in the liver transplant patient is unclear.[4]

Importance and management

A pharmacokinetic interaction between tacrolimus and grapefruit juice appears to be established and of clinical importance. In practical terms the authors of two of the reports[1,2] suggest that this interaction means that the dose of tacrolimus can possibly be reduced, but there is a clear need to monitor the effects closely, not only because of the inter-individual factors affecting tacrolimus dosing, but also because of the difficulties in standardising grapefruit juice. The UK and US manufacturers of tacrolimus suggest that the combination should be avoided,[8,9] and the US manufacturer includes whole grapefruit as well as the juice.[8] This advice would appear prudent, and patients should be informed of the potential risk of this interaction.

The case report with grapefruit marmalade appears to be isolated. As such, it requires confirmation by further study. Note that in this case, the patient consumed an unusually large amount of marmalade (estimated 14 dessert spoonfuls (15 g) daily). More modest consumption (1 dessert spoonful of about 15 g daily) would appear unlikely to interact.

1. Liu C, Shang Y-F, Zhang X-F, Zhang X-G, Wang B, Wu Z, Liu X-M, Yu L, Ma F, Lv Y. Co-administration of grapefruit juice increases bioavailability of tacrolimus in liver transplant patients: a prospective study. *Eur J Clin Pharmacol* (2009) 65, 881–5.
2. Westveer MK, Farquhar ML, George P, Mayes JT. Co-administration of grapefruit juice increases tacrolimus levels in liver transplant patients. Proceedings of the 15th Annual Meeting of the American Society of Transplant Physicians 1996. Abstract P-115.
3. Michelangelo V, Piero D, Elisa C, Enrico S, Mauro B, Pietro B. Grapefruit juice and kinetics of tacrolimus. *J Am Soc Nephrol* (2001) 12, 862A.
4. Fukatsu S, Fukudo M, Masuda S, Yano I, Katsura T, Ogura Y, Oike F, Takada Y, Inui K-I. Delayed effect of grapefruit juice on pharmacokinetics and pharmacodynamics of tacrolimus in a living-donor liver transplant recipient. *Drug Metab Pharmacokinet* (2006) 21, 122–5.
5. Peynaud D, Charpiat B, Vial T, Gallavardin M, Ducerf C. Tacrolimus severe overdosage after intake of masked grapefruit in orange marmalade. *Eur J Clin Pharmacol* (2007) 63, 721–2.
6. Egashira K, Fukuda E, Onga T, Yogi Y, Matsuya F, Koyabu N, Ohtani H, Sawada Y. Pomelo-induced increase in the blood level of tacrolimus in a renal transplant patient. *Transplantation* (2003) 75, 1057.
7. Egashira K, Ohtani H, Itoh S, Koyabu N, Tsujimoto M, Murakami H, Sawada Y. Inhibitory effects of pomelo on the metabolism of tacrolimus and the activities of CYP3A4 and P-glycoprotein. *Drug Metab Dispos* (2004) 32, 828–33.
8. Prograf (Tacrolimus). Astellas Pharma US Inc. US Prescribing information, September 2013.
9. Prograf (Tacrolimus monohydrate). Astellas Pharma Ltd. UK Summary of product characteristics, November 2014.

Tacrolimus + H_2-receptor antagonists

Cimetidine might cause small increases in tacrolimus concentrations, but famotidine and ranitidine do not appear to interact.

Clinical evidence

(a) Cimetidine

In a retrospective study in 48 kidney transplant patients, patients switched from cimetidine 400 mg daily to omeprazole 20 mg daily had a 15% decrease in their dose to weight-normalised tacrolimus minimum concentrations.[1]

(b) Famotidine

In a transplant patient taking tacrolimus 8 mg daily with lansoprazole, a tacrolimus concentration of 12 to 15.4 nanograms/mL was achieved. However, when lansoprazole was replaced by famotidine, the tacrolimus concentration was decreased to 8 nanograms/mL.[2,3] Another similar case has been reported.[4] In another patient, a small decrease in tacrolimus concentration (from a range of 8.3 to 8.5 nanograms/mL down to a range of 6.2 to 8.4 nanograms/mL) was seen when rabeprazole was switched to famotidine.[3]

(c) Ranitidine

In one case report, a large increase in tacrolimus concentration occurred when ranitidine was switched to omeprazole.[5]

Mechanism

Cimetidine is a known weak inhibitor of various cytochrome P450 isoenzymes, including CYP3A4 by which tacrolimus is metabolised, and so might be expected to cause small increases in tacrolimus concentrations. The *decreased* tacrolimus concentrations in one study when stopping cimetidine and starting omeprazole would seem to support this suggestion (although the authors concluded that omeprazole might have induced tacrolimus metabolism, this would be unexpected for omeprazole, see 'Tacrolimus + Proton pump inhibitors', p.1302). Other H_2-receptor antagonists do not inhibit any cytochrome P450 isoenzymes.

Importance and management

There is very little information available regarding an interaction between tacrolimus and the H_2-receptor antagonists. Cimetidine might cause small increases in tacrolimus concentrations, although this would be expected to be of little general relevance. Other H_2-receptor antagonists are not expected to interact to a clinically relevant extent. The studies above found that when a proton pump inhibitor was substituted with ranitidine or famotidine, the increased tacrolimus concentrations caused by the proton pump inhibitor were not sustained by the H_2-receptor antagonist, supporting this predicted lack of an interaction. For more information on the modest interaction of the proton pump inhibitors with tacrolimus, see 'Tacrolimus + Proton pump inhibitors', p.1302.

1. Lemahieu WPD, Maes BD, Verbeke K, Vanrenterghem Y. Impact of gastric acid suppressants on cytochrome P450 3A4 and P-glycoprotein: consequences for FK506 assimilation. *Kidney Int* (2005) 67, 1152–60.
2. Homma M, Itagaki F, Yuzawa K, Fukao K, Kohda Y. Effects of lansoprazole and rabeprazole on tacrolimus blood concentration: case of a renal transplant recipient with CYP2C19 gene mutation. *Transplantation* (2002) 73, 303–4.
3. Itagaki F, Homma M, Yuzawa K, Fukao K, Kohda Y. Drug interaction of tacrolimus and proton pump inhibitors in renal transplant recipients with CYP2C19 gene mutation. *Transplant Proc* (2002) 34, 2777–8.
4. Takahashi K, Motohashi H, Yonezawa A, Okuda M, Ito N, Yamamoto S, Ogawa O, Inui K. Lansoprazole-tacrolimus interaction in Japanese transplant recipient with CYP2C19 polymorphism. *Ann Pharmacother* (2004) 38, 791–4.
5. Takahashi K, Yano I, Fukuhara Y, Katsura T, Takahashi T, Ito N, Yamamoto S, Ogawa O, Inui K. Distinct effects of omeprazole and rabeprazole on the tacrolimus blood concentration in a kidney transplant recipient. *Drug Metab Pharmacokinet* (2007) 22, 441–4.

Tacrolimus + HCV-protease inhibitors

Boceprevir, paritaprevir boosted with ritonavir (in a fixed-dose combination), and telaprevir very markedly increase the exposure to tacrolimus. No clinically relevant interaction appears to occur between simeprevir and tacrolimus.

Clinical evidence

(a) Boceprevir

In a study in 12 healthy subjects, boceprevir 800 mg three times daily for 11 days increased the AUC and maximum plasma concentration of a single 500-microgram dose of tacrolimus (taken on day 6) 17-fold and 9.9-fold, respectively. In a separate single-dose study by the same authors in 10 healthy subjects, tacrolimus 500 micrograms had no effect on the pharmacokinetics of boceprevir 800 mg.[1] In a 12-week study, two liver transplant patients taking tacrolimus were started on boceprevir 800 mg three times daily. The oral clearance of tacrolimus decreased by up to 80% during the first week, and tacrolimus dose reductions were required in both patients in order to maintain a tacrolimus concentration within the target range of 5 to 10 nanograms/mL.[2] In a separate study by the same authors, of 18 liver transplant patients with HCV recurrence and given boceprevir 800 mg three times daily, 6 were already taking tacrolimus. After a pre-emptive tacrolimus dose reduction when boceprevir was started, further dose reductions (of 78%) were required during the first week after concurrent use in order to maintain tacrolimus concentrations within the target range of 5 to 10 nanograms/mL.[3]

(b) Paritaprevir

The UK and US manufacturers briefly report that, in a study in 12 healthy subjects, paritaprevir 150 mg daily (in a fixed-dose combination with ritonavir and ombitasvir, given with dasabuvir) increased the dose-normalised AUC and maximum concentration of a single 2-mg dose of tacrolimus 57-fold and 4-fold, respectively. The AUC and maximum concentration of paritaprevir were decreased by 34% and 43%, respectively.[4,5] The UK manufacturer also notes that when the combination was given without dasabuvir, the dose normalised AUC of a single 500-microgram dose of tacrolimus was increased 86-fold, but the effect on paritaprevir was similar.[5]

(c) Simeprevir

The UK and US manufacturers briefly report that, in a study in 14 healthy subjects, given simeprevir 150 mg daily for 7 days with a single 2-mg dose of tacrolimus, the maximum concentration of tacrolimus was decreased by 24%, but the AUC was unaffected.[6,7] Further, the US manufacturer also reports that in a study in 11 patients taking tacrolimus (individualised dose) and given simeprevir 150 mg daily for 14 days, the AUC and maximum concentration of simeprevir were 85% and 79% higher, respectively, than in historical controls.[7] Note that this study involved use of an unstated investigational drug.

(d) Telaprevir

In a study, 9 healthy subjects were given a single 2-mg dose of tacrolimus alone followed, 14-days later, by a single 500-microgram dose of tacrolimus on day 8 of a 13-day course of telaprevir 750 mg three times daily. Steady-state telaprevir increased the dose-normalised AUC and maximum plasma concentration of tacrolimus 70.3-fold and 9.4-fold, respectively.[8] In a study in 19 liver transplant patients with HCV recurrence and given telaprevir 750 mg three times daily, 9 were already taking tacrolimus. After a pre-emptive tacrolimus dose reduction when telaprevir was started, further dose reductions (of 95%) were required during the first week after concurrent use in order to maintain tacrolimus concentrations within the target range of 5 to 10 nanograms/mL.[3] Similarly, a retrospective study of 4 liver transplant patients with HCV recurrence requiring telaprevir-based triple therapy and taking tacrolimus, found that tacrolimus dose reductions of about 95% were required to maintain minimum concentrations within the target range of 5 to 7 nanograms/mL. This equated to an average daily dose of just 50 micrograms (given as a single weekly dose).[9] Similarly, another study describes 12 patients who required a tacrolimus dose reduction of about 97% during 12 weeks of triple therapy with telaprevir, pegylated interferon, and ribavirin, for HCV recurrence after liver transplantation.[10]

Mechanism

Boceprevir and telaprevir inhibit both CYP3A4, the main isoenzyme by which tacrolimus is metabolised, and P-glycoprotein, of which tacrolimus is a substrate, resulting in a very marked increase in its exposure. Paritaprevir does not appear to affect CYP3A4 itself, but it is given with ritonavir as a pharmacokinetic enhancer, and as this is a well-known potent inhibitor of CYP3A4, the effects on tacrolimus seen on concurrent use would seem to be most likely due to the ritonavir. The reason for the *decrease* in the tacrolimus maximum concentration seen with simeprevir is unknown.

Importance and management

A pharmacokinetic interaction between boceprevir, paritaprevir boosted with ritonavir (in a fixed-dose combination), or telaprevir and tacrolimus is established, resulting in very marked increases in tacrolimus exposure which will be clinically important. The greatest body of clinical evidence is with **boceprevir** and **telaprevir**, which indicates that it is highly likely that this interaction will be difficult to manage, with some studies suggesting that large tacrolimus dose decreases (perhaps as much as 95% with telaprevir), and probably extended dosing intervals, are necessary to maintain tacrolimus concentrations within desired ranges. If the concurrent use of telaprevir or boceprevir is essential, it would seem prudent to consider a pre-emptive dose decrease as well as increasing the monitoring of tacrolimus concentrations and monitoring for its adverse effects (such as effects on renal function), with further dose reductions during concurrent treatment as necessary. One group of authors also note the need for close monitoring of tacrolimus concentrations when boceprevir or telaprevir are discontinued, and in particular recommend increasing the tacrolimus dose the day immediately following their discontinuation, together with 48-hourly monitoring until steady state is achieved.[3]

Clinical experience with **paritaprevir** boosted with ritonavir (in a fixed-dose combination with ombitasvir, and given with or without dasabuvir) is lacking, but the very marked increase in tacrolimus exposure seen in the studies cited by the manufacturers suggests that care is required on concurrent use. As a result they advise that the dose of tacrolimus should be reduced: in the UK, to 500 micrograms every 7 days,[5] and in the US, according to tacrolimus concentrations, but typically to 500 micrograms every 7 days.[4] Further, the US manufacturer advises that tacrolimus should be given the day following initiation of the combination and not the same day.[4] Tacrolimus concentrations should be monitored throughout treatment and the dose adjusted accordingly,[4,5] including when treatment is stopped.[4] Renal function[4] and tacrolimus-related adverse effects should be monitored.[4,5]

The slight decrease in the maximum concentration of tacrolimus seen with **simeprevir** seems unlikely to be clinically relevant, particularly given that the tacrolimus exposure was unaffected. The relevance of the slight increase in simeprevir concentrations when simeprevir was given with tacrolimus compared with those of historical controls is unclear. The US manufacturer notes that no dose adjustments are needed on concurrent use.[7] The UK manufacturer of simeprevir does advise monitoring tacrolimus concentrations,[6] but monitoring over and above that usually undertaken in tacrolimus patients is probably not necessary.

Note that the concurrent use of boceprevir or telaprevir and tacrolimus is predicted to increase the risk of QT prolongation, see 'Drugs that prolong the QT interval + Other drugs that prolong the QT interval', p.272, for more information on this effect.

1. Hulskotte E, Gupta S, Xuan F, van Zutven M, O'Mara E, Feng H-P, Wagner J, Butterton J. Pharmacokinetic interaction between the hepatitis C virus protease inhibitor boceprevir and cyclosporine and tacrolimus in healthy volunteers. *Hepatology* (2012) 56, 1622–30.
2. Coilly A, Furlan V, Roche B, Barau C, Noël C, Bonhomme-Faivre L, Antonini TM, Roque-Afonso AM, Samuel D, Taburet AM, Duclos-Vallée JC. Practical management of boceprevir and immunosuppressive therapy in liver transplant recipients with hepatitis C virus recurrence. *Antimicrob Agents Chemother* (2012) 56, 5728–34.
3. Coilly A, Roche B, Dumortier J, Leroy V, Botta-Fridlund D, Radenne S, Pageaux GP, Si-Ahmed SN, Guillaud O, Antonini TM, Haïm-Boukobza S, Roque-Afonso AM, Samuel D, Duclos-Vallée JC. Safety and efficacy of protease inhibitors to treat hepatitis C after liver transplantation: a multicenter experience. *J Hepatol* (2014) 60, 78–86.
4. Viekira Pak (Ombitasvir, paritaprevir, ritonavir co-packaged with dasabuvir sodium monohydrate). AbbVie Inc. US Prescribing information, December 2014.
5. Viekirax (Ombitasvir, paritaprevir, ritonavir). AbbVie Ltd. UK Summary of product characteristics, January 2015.
6. Olysio (Simeprevir sodium). Janssen-Cilag Ltd. UK Summary of product characteristics, May 2014.
7. Olysio (Simeprevir sodium). Janssen Products, LP. US Prescribing information, November 2014.
8. Garg V, van Heeswijck R, Lee JE, Alves K, Nadkarni P, Luo X. Effect of telaprevir on the pharmacokinetics of cyclosporine and tacrolimus. *Hepatology* (2011) 54, 20–7.
9. Werner CR, Egetemeyr DP, Lauer UM, Nadalin S, Königsrainer A, Malek NP, Berg CP. Telaprevir-based triple therapy in liver transplant patients with hepatitis C virus: a 12-week pilot study providing safety and efficacy data. *Liver Transpl* (2012) 18, 1464–70.
10. Herzer K, Papadopoulos-Köhn A, Timm J, Paul A, Jochum C, Gerken G. HCV-Reinfektion nach lebertransplantation—management und erste ergebnisse mit der telaprevir-basierten triple-therapie. *Dtsch Med Wochenschr* (2013) 138, 1759–64.

Tacrolimus + HIV-protease inhibitors

HIV-protease inhibitors greatly increase tacrolimus concentrations. The available evidence suggests the effect is most apparent with ritonavir-boosted regimens.

Clinical evidence

Preliminary data from a study in HIV-positive transplant patients taking a HIV-protease inhibitor-based regimen and started on tacrolimus, shows that the tacrolimus dose needed to be reduced by 80% (to 700 micrograms) and the dosing interval increased to just once every 80 hours.[1] Additional data from the same study and published separately, shows that required tacrolimus doses were considerably lower than in transplant patients treated with HIV-protease inhibitors compared with 44 transplant patients without HIV (7 micrograms/kg (8 patients) compared with 100 micrograms/kg, respectively, at weeks 2 to 12, and 3 micrograms/kg (3 patients) compared with 150 micrograms/kg, respectively at weeks 28 to 104). Tacrolimus clearance was about 90% lower in transplant patients taking HIV-protease inhibitors than in those without HIV.[2] This effect was attenuated somewhat when NNRTIs were additionally given (see 'Tacrolimus + NNRTIs', p.1300). In another case series, the average tacrolimus dose was 1 to 3 mg *weekly* in patients taking a HIV-protease inhibitor (mostly nelfinavir).[3] Another report briefly mentions that 4 HIV-positive kidney transplant patients taking an HIV-protease inhibitor (not specified) required a dramatic tacrolimus dose reduction, and 3 of them needed a change from an HIV-protease inhibitor to an NNRTI.[4]

(a) Unboosted HIV-protease inhibitors

1. Atazanavir. A HIV-positive man taking atazanavir 400 mg daily with abacavir and lamivudine who was given a kidney transplant, was started on a single 500-microgram dose of tacrolimus 2 days after transplantation with a target minimum tacrolimus concentration of 8 to 10 nanograms/mL. His tacrolimus concentration, measured 48 hours later, was less than 2 nanograms/mL. Over the following few days his tacrolimus dose and frequency was adjusted to achieve appropriate minimum concentrations and he was eventually stabilised on 1.5 mg twice daily. At 3 months his minimum tacrolimus concentration was 8.8 nanograms/mL.[5]

2. Fosamprenavir. Four transplant patients needed an average 3-fold increase in the dose of tacrolimus (from about 290 to 880 micrograms daily) when their HIV-protease inhibitor was changed from nelfinavir to fosamprenavir.[6]

3. Nelfinavir. A HIV-positive patient, with hepatitis C following a liver transplant, was given stavudine, lamivudine, and nelfinavir 500 mg three times daily. Tacrolimus 6 mg daily was started postoperatively, but high blood concentrations were observed and the dose was reduced over the next 3 months to a maintenance dose of 500 micrograms *weekly*, which achieved concentrations of 7 to 25.9 nanograms/mL.[7] In one case series, the required dose of tacrolimus varied between 500 micrograms once every 5 days and 1 mg every other day in 4 patients taking nelfinavir-based antiretroviral regimens.[8,9] Similar decreased tacrolimus dose requirements have been noted in other patients given nelfinavir (500 micrograms every 3 days[10] or weekly,[11] or a 75 to 93% reduction in daily dose[12]).

A brief report describes petit mal seizures brought on by high tacrolimus concentrations, which were thought to be due to an interaction with nelfinavir.[13] One report mentions a patient who developed acute cellular rejection progressing to chronic rejection due to low tacrolimus concentrations when nelfinavir was stopped without an increase in the tacrolimus dose.[3]

(b) HIV-protease inhibitors boosted with ritonavir

1. Atazanavir. A report describes a greatly elevated tacrolimus concentration (to a value outside the range of the assay) and renal failure in a HIV-positive patient taking atazanavir boosted with ritonavir (dose not stated), after tacrolimus 1.5 mg twice daily was started post-kidney transplant. On day 8, atazanavir and ritonavir were changed to raltegravir.[14]

2. Darunavir. A HIV-positive kidney transplant patient experienced a dramatic increase in his tacrolimus concentration, despite a pre-emptive tacrolimus dose reduction from 8 to 7 mg daily, after a new antiretroviral regimen was started, which included raltegravir, etravirine, tenofovir, and darunavir boosted with ritonavir (dose not stated). Within three days his tacrolimus minimum concentration increased from 8.7 to 106 nanograms/mL. Tacrolimus was immediately stopped, but his tacrolimus concentration reduced slowly (to 64 nanograms/mL in 8 days). His creatinine concentration almost doubled, so darunavir and ritonavir were replaced with enfuvirtide, and tenofovir was stopped. His tacrolimus concentration subsequently decreased from 64 to 4.6 nanograms/mL within 6 days and he was later maintained on tacrolimus 1 mg twice daily. Due to painful injection site reactions from enfuvirtide, darunavir boosted with ritonavir was re-started and the tacrolimus dose was reduced by 50% to 500 micrograms twice daily. Again his tacrolimus concentration increased, from 6.2 nanograms/mL to a maximum of 22.4 nanograms/mL within 5 days. In the following weeks, he was eventually stabilised on a tacrolimus dose of 500 micrograms *weekly* which achieved a minimum concentration of 6 to 7 nanograms/mL.[15] A HIV-positive liver transplant patient, taking 20 micrograms of tacrolimus twice daily, was switched from saquinavir and lopinavir boosted with ritonavir, to darunavir boosted with ritonavir (600/100 mg twice daily), due to adverse effects. His tacrolimus dose was reduced to 10 micrograms in the morning and 20 micrograms in the evening, and his tacrolimus blood concentration remained stable. His darunvair and ritonavir exposure were within acceptable ranges.[16]

3. Fosamprenavir. A HIV-positive patient taking fosamprenavir boosted with ritonavir 700/100 mg twice daily (with lamivudine and zidovudine) underwent a kidney transplant and tacrolimus was started on day 3 at a dose of 500 micrograms twice daily. Three days later, his tacrolimus concentration had increased to 37 nanograms/mL, and the tacrolimus was stopped. When his tacrolimus concentration had decreased to 15 nanograms/mL, tacrolimus was reintroduced. A tacrolimus concentration of 10 nanograms/mL was achieved with a dose of 500 micrograms every 4 days.[17] A liver transplant patient taking tacrolimus 3 mg daily, and started on fosamprenavir boosted with ritonavir (700/100 mg twice daily) required a tacrolimus dose reduction to 80 micrograms daily to maintain an acceptable tacrolimus concentration, after increases up to 140 nanograms/mL.[16]

4. Lopinavir. A liver transplant patient taking tacrolimus 5 mg twice daily (to give a tacrolimus minimum blood concentration of 10.6 nanograms/mL) had a large increase in their tacrolimus concentration to 78.5 nanograms/mL when lopinavir boosted with ritonavir was started, despite a tacrolimus dose reduction to 6 mg daily. Tacrolimus neurotoxicity developed, but no nephrotoxicity was seen. The patient was eventually stabilised taking tacrolimus 500 micrograms *weekly* while taking lopinavir boosted with ritonavir.[11] Three other patients taking lopinavir boosted with ritonavir developed increased tacrolimus concentrations and were eventually stabilised on tacrolimus doses of 500 micrograms to 1 mg weekly,[11,18] and another required a dose of 500 micrograms every 2 weeks.[19] A further patient was unable to tolerate tacrolimus and lopinavir boosted with ritonavir, and was switched to nelfinavir.[11] In a liver transplant patient taking lopinavir boosted with ritonavir (400/100 mg twice daily), saquinavir, lamivudine, and tenofovir, and given tacrolimus 500 micrograms every 9 to 21 days, the blood concentration of tacrolimus and the AUC of lopinavir were increased, but the AUC of saquinavir was lower than expected. He required a tacrolimus dose reduction to just 60 micrograms daily in order to maintain satisfactory tacrolimus, lopinavir, and saquinavir concentrations.[16] In seven liver transplant patients taking tacrolimus, the tacrolimus dose needed to be reduced by 99% (to about 20 to 250 micrograms daily) when lopinavir boosted with ritonavir was started. Maintenance doses of tacrolimus in these patients varied from 500 micrograms to 1.5 mg, given between once weekly and just once every 25 days.[12] Another case report describes a kidney transplant patient taking extended-release oral tacrolimus 200 micrograms/kg daily and lopinavir boosted with ritonavir (600/150 mg twice daily), lamivudine, raltegravir, and nevirapine, who required a tacrolimus dose reduction by day 3 post-transplant due to the tacrolimus minimum concentration exceeding 30 ng/mL. Tacrolimus was completely stopped by day 7, and restarted 40 days later when the tacrolimus minimum concentration was 8.6 nanograms/mL, with a single dose of 500-micrograms. The tacrolimus concentration increased to 13.3 nanograms/mL as a result, and over the following weeks was eventually maintained between 6 and 8 nanograms/mL with a dose of 500 micrograms every 8 days. The patient also took a 10-day course of oral fluconazole from day 15 post-transplant which might have further increased tacrolimus concentrations.[20]

5. Saquinavir. A case report describes a HIV-positive patient taking saquinavir boosted with ritonavir (800/100 mg twice daily), who developed a very high tacrolimus concentration (200 micrograms/L) 5 days after starting tacrolimus 5 mg twice daily after a kidney transplant. The tacrolimus dose was reduced by 90% to 500 micrograms twice daily, and by 15 months post-transplant he was stabilised on just 500 micrograms *weekly*.[21] In another case, a patient had a tacrolimus concentration of 10.9 nanograms/mL while taking tacrolimus 4 mg twice daily without antiretrovirals. When he was given saquinavir boosted with ritonavir, a reduced dose of tacrolimus 1 mg twice daily resulted in a tacrolimus concentration in excess of 120 nanograms/mL, with severe and prolonged toxicity.[10] For another case of a liver transplant patient taking tacrolimus with saquinavir boosted with ritonavir and lopinavir, see under *Lopinavir*, above.[16]

Mechanism

All HIV-protease inhibitors are inhibitors of CYP3A4, by which tacrolimus is metabolised. It therefore seems likely that the HIV-protease inhibitors reduced tacrolimus metabolism resulting in the extremely high concentrations seen. The HIV-protease inhibitors also inhibit P-glycoprotein, of which tacrolimus is a substrate. It has been suggested that this could lead to increased concentrations of unmetabolised tacrolimus in the bile which might be reabsorbed through the enterohepatic circulation system, thus further increasing tacrolimus concentrations.[11] The reason for the changes in the exposure to lopinavir and saquinavir seen are not known.

Importance and management

The interaction between tacrolimus and the HIV-protease inhibitors is established and clinically important. The HIV-protease inhibitors, particularly ritonavir, are potent CYP3A4 inhibitors, and therefore when given to patients taking tacrolimus, a substantial reduction in the dose of tacrolimus is required, with close and frequent monitoring of tacrolimus concentrations. One centre found that the average tacrolimus dose needed was just 1 to 3 mg *weekly* in patients taking an HIV-protease inhibitor-based HAART regimen (mostly nelfinavir-based).[3] In another centre, the average tacrolimus dose required was 700 micrograms every 80 hours (3.3 days).[1] In yet another centre, in patients specifically taking lopinavir boosted with ritonavir, the required tacrolimus dose was just 0.5 to 1.5 mg given between once *weekly* and just once every 25 days.[12] The effect of fosamprenavir appears to be less than that of nelfinavir.[6] However, when fosamprenavir is boosted with ritonavir a much greater effect is seen. This is also the case with darunavir boosted with ritonavir.

Note that saquinavir boosted with ritonavir can prolong the QT interval, and tacrolimus is associated with an increased risk of QT interval prolongation. See 'Drugs that prolong the QT interval + Other drugs that prolong the QT interval', p.272, for further information on the concurrent use of two or more drugs that prolong the QT interval.

1. Frassetto LA, Browne M, Cheng A, Wolfe AR, Roland ME, Stock PG, Carlson L, Benet LZ. Immunosuppressant pharmacokinetics and dosing modifications in HIV-1 infected liver and kidney transplant recipients. *Am J Transplant* (2007) 7, 2816–20.
2. Frassetto L, Floren L, Barin B, Browne M, Wolfe A, Roland M, Stock P, Carlson L, Christians U, Benet L. Changes in clearance, volume and bioavailability of immunosuppressants when given with HAART in HIV-1 infected liver and kidney transplant recipients. *Biopharm Drug Dispos* (2013) 34, 442–51.
3. Neff GW, Bonham A, Tzakis AG, Ragni M, Jayaweera D, Schiff ER, Shakil O, Fung JJ. Orthoptic liver transplantation in patients with human immunodeficiency virus and end-stage liver disease. *Liver Transpl* (2003) 9, 239–47.
4. Mazuecos A, Pascual J, Gómez E, Sola E, Cofán F, López F, Puig-Hooper CE, Baltar JM, González-Molina M, Oppenheimer F, Marcén R, Rivero M. Renal transplantation in HIV-infected patients in Spain. *Nefrologia* (2006) 26, 113–20.
5. Tsapepas DS, Webber AB, Aull MJ, Figueiro JM, Saal SD. Managing the atazanavir-tacrolimus drug interaction in a renal transplant recipient. *Am J Health-Syst Pharm* (2011) 68, 138–42.
6. Pea F, Tavio M, Pavan F, Londero A, Bresadola V, Adani GL, Furlanut M, Viale P. Drop in trough blood concentrations of tacrolimus after switching from nelfinavir to fosamprenavir in four HIV-infected liver transplant patients. *Antivir Ther* (2008)13, 739–42.
7. Schvarcz R, Rudbeck G, Söderdahl G, Ståhle L. Interaction between nelfinavir and tacrolimus after orthoptic liver transplantation in a patient coinfected with HIV and hepatitis C virus (HCV). *Transplantation* (2000) 69, 2194–5.
8. Jain AK, Venkataramanan R, Shapiro R, Scantlebury VP, Potdar S, Bonham CA, Pokharna R, Rohal S, Ragni M, Fung JJ. Interaction between tacrolimus and antiretroviral agents in human immunodeficiency virus-positive liver and kidney transplantation patients. *Transplant Proc* (2002) 34, 1540–1.
9. Jain AK, Venkataramanan R, Shapiro R, Scantlebury VP, Potdar S, Bonham CA, Ragni M, Fung JJ. The interaction between antiretroviral agents and tacrolimus in liver and kidney transplant patients. *Liver Transpl* (2002) 8, 841–5.
10. Sheikh AM, Wolf DC, Lebovics E, Goldberg R, Horowitz HW. Concomitant human immunodeficiency virus protease inhibitor therapy markedly reduces tacrolimus metabolism and increases blood levels. *Transplantation* (1999) 68, 307–9.
11. Jain AB, Venkataramanan R, Eghtesad B, Marcos A, Ragni M, Shapiro R, Rafail AB, Fung JJ. Effect of coadministered lopinavir and ritonavir (Kaletra) on tacrolimus blood concentration in liver transplanted patients. *Liver Transpl* (2003) 9, 954–60.
12. Teicher E, Vincent I, Bonhomme-Faivre L, Abbara C, Barrail A, Boissonnas A, Duclos-Vallée JC, Taburet AM, Samuel D, Vittecoq D. Effect of highly active antiretroviral therapy on tacrolimus pharmacokinetics in hepatitis C virus and HIV co-infected liver transplant recipients in the ANRS HC-08 study. *Clin Pharmacokinet* (2007) 46, 941–52.
13. Ragni M, Dodson SF, Hunt SC, Bontempo FA, Fung JJ. Liver transplantation in a hemophilia patient with acquired immunodeficiency syndrome. *Blood* (1999) 93, 1113–14.
14. Cousins D, Topping K, Lee V, Sweeney J, Lawton M. Successful tacrolimus treatment following renal transplant in a HIV-infected patient with raltegravir previously treated with a protease inhibitor based regimen. *Drug Metabol Drug Interact* (2011) 26, 139–41.
15. Mertz D, Battegay M, Marzolini C, Mayr M. Drug-drug interaction in a kidney transplant recipient receiving HIV salvage therapy and tacrolimus. *Am J Kidney Dis* (2009) 54, e1–4.
16. Bickel M, Anadol E, Vogel M, Hofmann WP, von Hentig N, Kuetscher J, Kurowski M, Moench C, Lennemann T, Lutz T, Bechstein WO, Brodt HR, Rockstroh J. Daily dosing of tacrolimus in patients treated with HIV-1 therapy containing a ritonavir-boosted protease inhibitor or raltegravir. *J Antimicrob Chemother* (2010) 65, 999–1004.
17. Barau C, Blouin P, Creput C, Taburet AM, Durrbach A, Furlan V. Effect of coadministered HIV-protease inhibitors on tacrolimus and sirolimus blood concentrations in a kidney transplant recipients [sic]. *Fundam Clin Pharmacol* (2009) 23, 423–5.
18. Schonder KS, Shullo MA, Okusanya O. Tacrolimus and lopinavir/ritonavir interaction in liver transplantation. *Ann Pharmacother* (2003) 37, 1793–6.
19. Guaraldi G, Cocchi S, Codeluppi M, Di Benedetto F, Bonora S, Pecorari M, Gennari W, Cautero N, Pinna AD, Gerunda GE, Esposito R. Role of therapeutic drug monitoring in a patient with human immunodeficiency virus infection and end-stage liver disease undergoing orthotopic liver transplantation. *Transplant Proc* (2005) 37, 2609–10.
20. Morelle J, Goffin E, Wallemacq P, De Meyer M, Yombi J-C, Mourad M, Kanaan N. Extended release tacrolimus and antiretroviral therapy in a renal transplant recipient: so extended. *Transpl Int* (2010) 23, 1065–7.
21. Hardy G, Stanke-Labesque F, Contamin C, Serre-Debeauvais F, Bayle F, Zaoui P, Bessard G. Protease inhibitors and diltiazem increase tacrolimus blood concentration in a patient with renal transplantation: a case report. *Eur J Clin Pharmacol* (2004) 60, 603–5.

Tacrolimus + Macrolides

Large increases in tacrolimus concentrations accompanied by evidence of renal toxicity or haemolytic uraemic syndrome have been seen in patients also given erythromycin or clarithromycin. Josamycin is predicted to interact similarly. An isolated case report describes an increase in tacrolimus concentrations when azithromycin was also given.

Clinical evidence

(a) Azithromycin

A case report describes a patient who had been given intravenous tacrolimus 20 micrograms/kg and had an increase in her tacrolimus concentration from a range of 15.8 to 17.5 nanograms/mL to greater than 30 nanograms/mL, 3 days after azithromycin 500 mg daily was started.[1] However, one report briefly describes a patient taking tacrolimus following a bone marrow transplant who took a 10-day course of azithromycin (dose not stated) without any notable alteration in his serum creatinine or minimum tacrolimus concentrations.[2] For details of a patient who experienced an increased tacrolimus concentration while receiving intravenous azithromycin and ceftriaxone, but which resolved after ceftriaxone was stopped and azithromycin was switched to oral, see 'Tacrolimus + Ceftriaxone', p.1293.

(b) Clarithromycin

A woman with a kidney transplant taking tacrolimus, prednisone, and azathioprine was given clarithromycin 500 mg twice daily for 4 days, then 250 mg daily to treat a severe *Mycoplasma pneumoniae* infection. Despite a 64% reduction in the dose of the tacrolimus, her minimum tacrolimus concentration increased sharply, from 2.8 to 36.1 nanograms/mL by day 6, and her creatinine concentration increased from 309 to 442 micromol/L. The tacrolimus dose was further reduced and then stopped, and not restarted until clarithromycin treatment was completed.[3] In another 2 kidney transplant patients, tacrolimus concentrations increased 2.5-fold and 2.3-fold, following 9 doses of clarithromycin 250 mg. Creatinine concentrations increased by 91% and 30%, respectively.[4] Similarly, the tacrolimus concentration of a bone marrow transplant patient increased from below 1.1 to 10.1 nanograms/mL after he took clarithromycin 500 mg twice daily for about 4 days.[2] Similar increases in tacrolimus concentrations have been reported in a heart transplant patient, despite an initial 33% reduction in the tacrolimus dose in anticipation of the interaction,[5] in another kidney transplant patient[6] and in a lung transplant patient who developed haemolytic uraemic syndrome.[7]

(c) Erythromycin

A liver transplant patient taking tacrolimus 6 mg twice daily for one year had a large increase in his serum tacrolimus concentration from about 1.4 to 6.5 nanomol/L when intravenous ampicillin with sulbactam 3 g every 6 hours and oral erythromycin 250 mg every 6 hours were given for 4 days to treat pneumonia. Renal toxicity, demonstrated by increased blood urea and creatinine concentrations, also occurred. Erythromycin was stopped, and the next day tacrolimus was also stopped. Over the next week the tacrolimus plasma concentration, creatinine concentration, and blood urea nitrogen concentration decreased.[8] A case of haemolytic uraemic syndrome has been described in a 48-year old lung transplant patient after erythromycin (dose not stated) was started for a chest infection. Her tacrolimus concentration increased to 21 nanograms/mL (from a range of 5 to 15 nanograms/mL).[7] A kidney transplant patient had an increase in his plasma tacrolimus concentration from 1.3 to 8.5 nanograms/mL 4 days after starting erythromycin 400 mg four times daily. His serum creatinine concentration almost doubled.[9] A man with a kidney transplant had a 6-fold increase in tacrolimus blood concentration when he took erythromycin.[10] Another similar case has been described.[11] Two children aged 3 years and 7 years also had increases in tacrolimus blood concentrations, which were accompanied by renal toxicity when erythromycin was added.[12]

Mechanism

Erythromycin and clarithromycin are inhibitors of CYP3A4 (moderate and potent, respectively), and P-glycoprotein, which are involved in the metabolism and transport of tacrolimus, respectively. Concurrent use therefore results in increased tacrolimus concentrations. Azithromycin does not inhibit CYP3A4 to any clinically relevant extent, but does inhibit P-glycoprotein, meaning an interaction with tacrolimus via this mechanism cannot be entirely ruled out.

Importance and management

Direct information about an interaction between tacrolimus and the macrolides seems to be limited to these case reports. However, what is known is in line with the way both tacrolimus and these macrolides are known to interact with other drugs. It would therefore be prudent to closely monitor the effects of adding clarithromycin or erythromycin in any patient taking tacrolimus, being alert for the need to reduce the tacrolimus dose to avoid nephrotoxicity. Remember to readjust the tacrolimus dose when the macrolide is stopped. Most other macrolides would also be expected to interact, although they do not all behave identically; the UK manufacturer of tacrolimus names **josamycin**.[13,14] Similar precautions would also be prudent with **telithromycin**, a potent inhibitor of CYP3A4.

Azithromycin would appear less likely to interact, but the case reports of increased tacrolimus concentrations should be borne in mind.

Note that some macrolides and tacrolimus are associated with an increased risk of QT interval prolongation, see 'Drugs that prolong the QT interval + Other drugs that prolong the QT interval', p.272, for further information on the concurrent use of two or more drugs that prolong the QT interval.

1. Mori T, Aisa Y, Nakazato T, Yamazaki R, Ikeda Y, Okamoto S. Tacrolimus-azithromycin interaction in a recipient of allogeneic bone marrow transplantation. *Transpl Int* (2005) 18, 757–8.
2. Ibrahim RB, Abella EM, Chandrasekar PH. Tacrolimus-clarithromycin interaction in a patient receiving bone marrow transplantation. *Ann Pharmacother* (2002) 36, 1971–2.
3. Wolter K, Wagner K, Philipp T, Fritschka E. Interaction between FK 506 and clarithromycin in a renal transplant patient. *Eur J Clin Pharmacol* (1994) 47, 207–8.
4. Gómez G, Álvarez ML, Errasti P, Lavilla FJ, García N, Ballester B, García I, Purroy A. Acute tacrolimus nephrotoxicity in renal transplant patients treated with clarithromycin. *Transplant Proc* (1999) 31, 2250–1.
5. Kunicki PW, Sobieszczańska-Malek M. Pharmacokinetic interaction between tacrolimus and clarithromycin in a heart transplant patient. *Ther Drug Monit* (2005) 27, 107–8.
6. Katari SR, Magnone M, Shapiro R, Jordan M, Scantlebury V, Vivas C, Gritsch A, McCauley J, Starzl T, Demetris J, Randhawa PS. Clinical features of acute reversible tacrolimus (FK 506) nephrotoxicity in kidney transplant recipients. *Clin Transplant* (1997) 11, 237–42.
7. Parissis H, Gould K, Dark J. Dangerous drug interactions leading to hemolytic uremic syndrome following lung transplantation. *J Cardiothorac Surg* (2010) 5, 70.
8. Shaeffer MS, Collier D, Sorrell MF. Interaction between FK506 and erythromycin. *Ann Pharmacother* (1994) 28, 280–1.
9. Jensen C, Jordan M, Shapiro R, Scantelbury V, Hakala T, Fung J, Stasrzl T, Venkataramanan R. Interaction between tacrolimus and erythromycin. *Lancet* (1994) 344, 825.
10. Padhi ID, Long P, Basha M, Anandan JV. Interaction between tacrolimus and erythromycin. *Ther Drug Monit* (1997) 19, 120–2.
11. Moreno M, Latorre C, Manzanares C, Morales E, Herrero JC, Dominguez-Gil B, Carreño A, Cubas A, Delgado M, Andres A, Morales JM. Clinical management of tacrolimus drug interactions in renal transplant patients. *Transplant Proc* (1999) 31, 2252–3.
12. Furlan V, Perello L, Jacquemin E, Debray D, Taburet A-M. Interactions between FK506 and rifampicin or erythromycin in pediatric liver recipients. *Transplantation* (1995) 59, 1217–18.
13. Prograf (Tacrolimus monohydrate). Astellas Pharma Ltd. UK Summary of product characteristics, November 2014.
14. Prograf (Tacrolimus). Astellas Pharma US Inc. US Prescribing information, September 2013.

Tacrolimus + Metoclopramide

In an isolated case, metoclopramide might have increased tacrolimus concentrations, resulting in tacrolimus toxicity and acute renal failure.

Clinical evidence, mechanism, importance and management

A case report describes a liver transplant patient taking tacrolimus up to 28 mg twice daily (and several other drugs), whose subtherapeutic tacrolimus concentrations were increased when she took metoclopramide for gastric dysmotility (initially 10 mg four times daily, then 20 mg four times daily). Her tacrolimus minimum concentrations increased from less than 2 nanograms/mL to greater than 30 nanograms/mL within 5 to 6 days, and she developed tremor, weakness, nausea, vomiting, diarrhoea, and acute renal failure. The authors considered that the increase in tacrolimus concentrations was due to metoclopramide, possibly due to its effects in increasing gut motility and hence, tacrolimus absorption. However, several other factors might have contributed, such as diarrhoea, and the use of cimetidine and ketoconazole, both of which can inhibit the metabolism of tacrolimus and increase its concentrations.[1]

This appears to be the only reported case of tacrolimus toxicity with metoclopramide, and because of the number of complicating factors, an interaction is by no means established. Its general clinical relevance is uncertain.

1. Prescott WA, Callahan BL, Park JM. Tacrolimus toxicity associated with concomitant metoclopramide therapy. *Pharmacotherapy* (2004) 24, 532–7.

Tacrolimus + Metronidazole

Two case reports describe increases in tacrolimus concentrations in patients also given metronidazole.

Clinical evidence

A kidney transplant patient taking tacrolimus 3 mg twice daily had a 3-fold increase in his tacrolimus concentrations when he was given metronidazole 500 mg four times daily for 14 days. His minimum concentration increased from 9.2 to 26.3 nanograms/mL within 4 days of starting the metronidazole, requiring a tacrolimus dose reduction to 1 mg twice daily. Five days after stopping the metronidazole his minimum concentration had returned to 9.2 nanograms/mL and his dose was increased back up to 2 mg twice daily.[1] A similar increase in tacrolimus minimum concentrations was seen in a kidney transplant patient taking tacrolimus 3 mg in the morning and 2 mg at night. His tacrolimus concentration increased from 9 to nearly 18 nanograms/mL when he started taking metronidazole 400 mg three times daily for a *C. difficile* infection. The tacrolimus dose was reduced to 1 mg twice daily and the tacrolimus concentration decreased to 8.1 nanograms/mL. When the metronidazole was stopped, his tacrolimus concentration decreased further, to 5.2 nanograms/mL, and his tacrolimus dose needed to be increased to 2 mg twice daily.[2]

Mechanism

Unknown. It was suggested that metronidazole might have increased tacrolimus concentrations by inhibiting CYP3A4, by which tacrolimus is metabolised.[1] However, some pharmacokinetic studies have found that metronidazole is not an inhibitor of CYP3A4/5, and conclude that increases in plasma concentrations of CYP3A4 substrates in the presence of metronidazole are not the result of CYP3A4 inhibition.[3]

Importance and management

These two cases appear to be the only reports of a possible interaction between tacrolimus and metronidazole. There is therefore insufficient evidence to advocate monitoring in every patient given the combination, but it would be prudent to at least bear this interaction in mind if using metronidazole in patients taking tacrolimus.

1. Page RL, Klem PM, Rogers C. Potential elevation of tacrolimus trough concentrations with concomitant metronidazole therapy. *Ann Pharmacother* (2005) 39, 1109–13.
2. Herzig K, Johnson DW. Marked elevation of blood cyclosporin and tacrolimus levels due to concurrent metronidazole therapy. *Nephrol Dial Transplant* (1999) 14, 521–3.
3. Roedler R, Neuhauser MM, Penzak SR. Does metronidazole interact with CYP3A substrates by inhibiting their metabolism through this metabolic pathway? Or should other mechanisms be considered? *Ann Pharmacother* (2007) 41, 653–8.

Tacrolimus + Mirtazapine

An isolated report describes asymptomatic hypotension in a kidney transplant patient taking tacrolimus and mirtazapine.

Clinical evidence, mechanism, importance and management

A report describes a 68-year-old woman with depression stable taking mirtazapine 30 mg daily who was given extended-release tacrolimus 200 micrograms/kg daily, with basiliximab, mycophenolate mofetil, and a single dose of corticosteroids, following a kidney transplant. Mirtazapine had been stopped before surgery but was restarted 4 days post-operatively, at which point her blood pressure dropped from around 130/70 to 92/52 mmHg, 2 hours after the dose, and further to 88/54 mmHg, 7 hours after the dose. Her blood pressure started to recover 12-hours post-dose, and the mirtazapine dose was reduced over the following 2 days until it was stopped, but with the same hypotensive response after each dose. She had no further episodes of hypotension in the 5 days after the mirtazapine had been stopped.[1]

It was noted that, during the first 7 days post-transplant, her tacrolimus serum concentrations were higher than 15 nanograms/mL, and the tacrolimus dose was reduced. The authors suggest that the high tacrolimus concentrations inhibited CYP3A4, by which mirtazapine is partially metabolised, and thus increased mirtazapine concentrations leading to the enhanced hypotensive effect of mirtazapine.[1] However, note that hypotension is a common adverse effect of mirtazapine alone and there appears to be little evidence to support the suggestion that tacrolimus is a clinically relevant CYP3A4 inhibitor.

This appears to be an isolated report and its general relevance is therefore unclear.

1. Fraile P, Garcia-Cosmes P, Garcia T, Corbacho L, Alvarez M, Tabernero JM. Hypotension, as consequence of the interaction between tacrolimus and mirtazapine, in a patient with renal transplant. *Nephrol Dial Transplant* (2009) 24, 1999–2001.

Tacrolimus + Miscellaneous

The UK and US manufacturers advise caution on the concurrent use of tacrolimus with anticoagulants, antidiabetics, nephrotoxic and neurotoxic drugs, and also with various drugs that might alter tacrolimus metabolism.

Clinical evidence, mechanism, importance and management

(a) Isoniazid

The UK manufacturer of tacrolimus states that isoniazid has the potential to decrease tacrolimus concentrations.[1] However, note that there is little to suggest that isoniazid has any enzyme-inducing effects.

(b) Neurotoxicity or nephrotoxicity

The manufacturers of tacrolimus predict that there might be additive neuro- or nephrotoxicity on the concurrent use of **aciclovir**,[1] **aminoglycosides**,[1,2] **co-trimoxazole**,[1] **ganciclovir**,[1] **gyrase inhibitors**,[1] **NSAIDs**[1] (see 'Tacrolimus + NSAIDs', p.1301), or **vancomycin**.[1] They also note that nephrotoxicity has been seen when **amphotericin B** was given with tacrolimus.[1]

(c) Protein-binding interactions

Because tacrolimus is extensively bound to plasma proteins, the UK manufacturer mentions the possibility of protein-binding interactions with oral **anticoagulants** or **antidiabetics**,[1] but this has largely been discredited as a mechanism, see 'Protein-binding interactions', p.3.

(d) Other drugs

On the basis of *in vitro* studies, the UK manufacturer of tacrolimus suggests that **bromocriptine, dapsone, ergotamine, lidocaine, midazolam, quinidine,** and **tamoxifen** might inhibit tacrolimus metabolism.[1] The US manufacturer mentions **bromocriptine** might increase tacrolimus concentrations.[2] These predictions are as yet unconfirmed, and note that these drugs are not generally considered to be associated with clinically relevant interactions by inhibition of the CYP3A4, which is the main isoenzyme involved in tacrolimus metabolism.

1. Prograf (Tacrolimus monohydrate). Astellas Pharma Ltd. UK Summary of product characteristics, November 2014.
2. Prograf (Tacrolimus). Astellas Pharma US Inc. US Prescribing information, September 2013.

Tacrolimus + Moxifloxacin

Moxifloxacin does not appear to affect the pharmacokinetics of tacrolimus.

Clinical evidence, mechanism, importance and management

A study in 11 patients taking tacrolimus after a kidney transplant found that moxifloxacin 400 mg daily for 7 days, taken for a urinary-tract infection, did not affect the pharmacokinetics of tacrolimus.[1] No tacrolimus dose adjustments would therefore be expected to be necessary on the concurrent use of moxifloxacin.

Note that moxifloxacin can prolong the QT interval and tacrolimus is associated with an increased risk of QT interval prolongation; see 'Drugs that prolong the QT interval + Other drugs that prolong the QT interval', p.272, for further information on the concurrent use of two or more drugs that prolong the QT interval.

1. Capone D, Tarantino G, Polichetti G, Kadilli I, Sabbatini M, Basile V, Carrano R, Nappi R, Federico S. Absence of pharmacokinetic interference of moxifloxacin on cyclosporine and tacrolimus in kidney transplant recipients. *J Clin Pharmacol* (2010) 50, 576–80.

Tacrolimus + NNRTIs

Limited evidence from case reports suggests that efavirenz increases tacrolimus clearance. Nevirapine possibly has less of an effect. Etravirine is predicted to interact similarly, whereas delavirdine is predicted to decrease tacrolimus clearance.

Clinical evidence

(a) Efavirenz

A kidney transplant patient taking efavirenz 600 mg daily and two nucleoside analogues needed a much larger than expected tacrolimus dose of 24 mg daily to maintain a tacrolimus concentration of 12.5 nanograms/mL.[1,2] In 4 transplant patients taking stable doses of tacrolimus and various other drugs including fluconazole, the addition of efavirenz and two nucleoside analogues had little effect on the required dose of tacrolimus, but the calculated oral clearance of tacrolimus was almost doubled. In two of these patients for whom a detailed pharmacokinetic analysis was available, one had a 51% decrease in tacrolimus minimum concentration (from 16.1 to 7.9 nanograms/mL) and the other just a 12% decrease in the tacrolimus minimum concentration.[3]

(b) Nevirapine

One case report mentions that a liver transplant patient taking nevirapine and dual nucleoside analogues was maintained on tacrolimus 1 mg daily.[4] In another report, two kidney transplant patients taking nevirapine and dual nucleoside analogues were maintained on tacrolimus 4 mg daily.[1,2]

(c) NNRTIs with HIV-protease inhibitors

Adding an NNRTI (efavirenz or nevirapine) to a HIV-protease inhibitor required a 40% increase in the tacrolimus dose to 1 mg, and a large decrease in the dosing interval (every 12 hours instead of once every 80 hours).[5]

Mechanism

Efavirenz, etravirine, and nevirapine generally act as inducers of CYP3A4 by which tacrolimus is metabolised (although perhaps to varying extents). As such, they would be expected to decrease tacrolimus concentrations. The effect of efavirenz in one study might have been attenuated by fluconazole (which inhibits CYP3A4). NNRTIs slightly attenuated the inhibitory effect of HIV-protease inhibitors on tacrolimus metabolism.

Note that delavirdine *inhibits* CYP3A4 and would be expected to *increase* tacrolimus concentrations.

Importance and management

Evidence for an interaction between tacrolimus and the NNRTIs is variable in both quantity and conclusions. There is some evidence that efavirenz increases the clearance of tacrolimus and necessitates an increase in the required dose, whereas there is more limited evidence with nevirapine, but this suggests that it has little effect on the required dose. However, until further data becomes available, it would seem prudent to closely monitor tacrolimus concentrations in any patient given efavirenz or nevirapine, because of the possibility they might decrease tacrolimus concentrations, and be alert to the need to adjust the dose accordingly. The effect of etravirine on tacrolimus metabolism has not been studied, but based on its effects on other CYP3A4 substrates it might be expected to decrease tacrolimus concentrations; albeit to a lesser degree than efavirenz or nevirapine. Until more is known, similar precautions on concurrent use would seem sensible.

In contrast, delavirdine is predicted to increase tacrolimus concentrations and so might necessitate tacrolimus dose reductions. Until further information is available, it would be prudent to monitor tacrolimus concentrations closely in patients also given delavirdine, and to be alert to the need to adjust the dose accordingly.

1. Jain AK, Venkataramanan R, Shapiro R, Scantlebury VP, Potdar S, Bonham CA, Pokharna R, Rohal S, Ragni M, Fung JJ. Interaction between tacrolimus and antiretroviral agents in human immunodeficiency virus-positive liver and kidney transplantation patients. *Transplant Proc* (2002) 34, 1540–1.
2. Jain AK, Venkataramanan R, Shapiro R, Scantlebury VP, Potdar S, Bonham CA, Ragni M, Fung JJ. The interaction between antiretroviral agents and tacrolimus in liver and kidney transplant patients. *Liver Transpl* (2002) 8, 841–5.

3. Teicher E, Vincent I, Bonhomme-Faivre L, Abbara C, Barrail A, Boissonnas A, Duclos-Vallée JC, Taburet AM, Samuel D, Vittecoq D. Effect of highly active antiretroviral therapy on tacrolimus pharmacokinetics in hepatitis C virus and HIV co-infected liver transplant recipients in the ANRS HC-08 study. *Clin Pharmacokinet* (2007) 46, 941–52.
4. Gow PJ, Mutimer D. Liver transplantation for an HIV-positive patient in the era of highly active antiretroviral therapy. *AIDS* (2001) 15, 291–2.
5. Frassetto LA, Browne M, Cheng A, Wolfe AR, Roland ME, Stock PG, Carlson L, Benet LZ. Immunosuppressant pharmacokinetics and dosing modifications in HIV-1 infected liver and kidney transplant recipients. *Am J Transplant* (2007) 7, 2816–20.

Tacrolimus + NS5A inhibitors

No interaction appears to occur between daclatasvir and tacrolimus, and tacrolimus does not appear to alter the pharmacokinetics of ombitasvir. No interaction is predicted to occur between ledipasvir and tacrolimus.

Clinical evidence, mechanism, importance and management

(a) Daclatasvir

The UK manufacturer briefly reports that, in a study in healthy subjects given a single 5-mg dose of tacrolimus with daclatasvir 60 mg daily, the pharmacokinetics of both drugs were unaffected.[1] No dose adjustments are therefore necessary on concurrent use.

(b) Ledipasvir

The UK manufacturer of ledipasvir (in a fixed-dose combination with sofosbuvir) predicts that ledipasvir exposure will be unaffected when given with tacrolimus.[2] The US manufacturer states that no interaction occurs.[3] No dose adjustments are necessary on concurrent use.

(c) Ombitasvir

The UK and US manufacturers briefly report that, in a study in 12 healthy subjects, a single 2-mg dose of tacrolimus had no effect on the pharmacokinetics of ombitasvir 25 mg daily (in a fixed-dose combination with paritaprevir boosted with ritonavir, given with and without dasabuvir).[4,5] No ombitasvir dose adjustment is necessary on concurrent use. Note that other components of the fixed-dose preparation do affect the exposure of tacrolimus, see 'Tacrolimus + HCV-protease inhibitors', p.1296 and 'Tacrolimus + HIV-protease inhibitors', p.1297 for details.

1. Daklinza (Daclatasvir dihydrochloride). Bristol-Myers Squibb Pharmaceutical Ltd. UK Summary of product characteristics, September 2014.
2. Harvoni (Ledipasvir, sofosbuvir). Gilead Sciences Ltd. UK Summary of product characteristics, November 2014.
3. Harvoni (Ledipasvir, sofosbuvir). Gilead Sciences, Inc. US Prescribing information, March 2015.
4. Viekira Pak (Ombitasvir, paritaprevir, ritonavir co-packaged with dasabuvir sodium monohydrate). AbbVie Inc. US Prescribing information, December 2014.
5. Viekirax (Ombitasvir, paritaprevir, ritonavir). AbbVie Ltd. UK Summary of product characteristics, January 2015.

Tacrolimus + NS5B inhibitors

No interaction appears to occur between sofosbuvir and tacrolimus, and tacrolimus does not appear to alter the pharmacokinetics of dasabuvir.

Clinical evidence, mechanism, importance and management

(a) Dasabuvir

The UK and US manufacturers briefly reports that, in a study in 12 healthy subjects, a single 2-mg dose of tacrolimus had no effect on the pharmacokinetics of dasabuvir 250 or 400 mg twice daily (with a fixed-dose combination of ombitasvir and paritaprevir boosted with ritonavir).[1,2] No dasabuvir dose adjustment is necessary on concurrent use. Note that other components of the fixed-dose preparation do affect the exposure of tacrolimus, see 'Tacrolimus + HCV-protease inhibitors', p.1296 and 'Tacrolimus + HIV-protease inhibitors', p.1297 for details.

(b) Sofosbuvir

The UK and US manufacturers briefly report that, in a single-dose study in 16 healthy subjects given tacrolimus 5-mg and sofosbuvir 400-mg, the AUC of tacrolimus was unaffected, by the maximum concentration was decreased by 27%. The pharmacokinetics of sofosbuvir and its major inactive metabolite were unaffected.[3,4] No dose adjustments are therefore necessary of concurrent use.

1. Exviera (Dasabuvir sodium monohydrate). AbbVie Ltd. UK Summary of product characteristics, January 2015.
2. Viekira Pak (Ombitasvir, paritaprevir, ritonavir co-packaged with dasabuvir sodium monohydrate). AbbVie Inc. US Prescribing information, December 2014.
3. Sovaldi (Sofosbuvir). Gilead Sciences Ltd. UK Summary of product characteristics, January 2015.
4. Sovaldi (Sofosbuvir). Gilead Sciences, Inc. US Prescribing information, March 2015.

Tacrolimus + NSAIDs

Two liver transplant patients taking tacrolimus developed acute renal failure after also taking ibuprofen. However, the concurrent use of an NSAID did not appear to be a contributor to tacrolimus renal toxicity in a study in rheumatoid arthritis patients.

Clinical evidence

Two patients with liver transplants taking tacrolimus developed acute but reversible renal failure, one after taking four **ibuprofen** tablets (strength not stated), and the other after taking three 400 mg tablets of **ibuprofen** over 24 hours. Both had stable renal function before taking **ibuprofen**.[1]

However, in a study of the use of tacrolimus in patients with rheumatoid arthritis, the concurrent use of an NSAID did not appear to influence the renal toxicity of tacrolimus. In this study, increases in creatinine concentrations of 40% or more above baseline occurred in 9% of patients receiving tacrolimus 1 mg daily, 19% of patients receiving 3 mg daily, and 28% of patients receiving 5 mg daily, and required tacrolimus discontinuation in 2 patients taking 3 mg daily and 7 patients taking 5 mg daily. Stable NSAID therapy (specific drugs not stated) was used in 68 to 81% of patients. The frequency of NSAID use was not higher in patients who developed creatinine elevations, nor was it higher in those who discontinued tacrolimus because of creatinine elevations (about half of the patients who discontinued tacrolimus were taking NSAIDs).[2]

Mechanism

NSAIDs are known to inhibit prostaglandin synthesis and as a result might decrease renal blood flow, which in certain circumstances can lead to renal failure. Further, renal impairment is more likely to occur in the presence of renal vasoconstrictors, and as tacrolimus is known to cause renal vasoconstriction, the combined effects of ibuprofen and tacrolimus might have led to acute renal failure. Both patients described in the case report also had a degree of liver impairment, which the authors suggest might have potentiated the toxicity of tacrolimus with ibuprofen.[1]

Importance and management

No pharmacokinetic interaction between tacrolimus and NSAIDs would be expected. However, renal impairment with tacrolimus is well known but whether NSAIDs can exacerbate this is uncertain. In general, renal function should be routinely monitored during tacrolimus use, and it should be noted that the risk of renal impairment might be increased by other nephrotoxic drugs, which would include NSAIDs. Some caution would seem appropriate with concurrent use, taking into account the usual precautions for both NSAIDs and tacrolimus in renal impairment.

1. Sheiner PA, Mor E, Chodoff L, Glabman S, Emre S, Schwartz ME, Miller CM. Acute renal failure associated with the use of ibuprofen in two liver transplant recipients on FK506. *Transplantation* (1994) 57, 1132–3.
2. Furst DE, Saag K, Fleischmann MR, Sherrer Y, Block JA, Schnitzer T, Rutstein J, Baldassare A, Kaine J, Calabrese L, Dietz F, Sack M, Senter RG, Wiesenhutter C, Schiff M, Stein CM, Satoi Y, Matsumoto A, Caldwell J, Harris RE, Moreland LW, Hurd E, Yocum D, Stamler DA. Efficacy of tacrolimus in rheumatoid arthritis patients who have been treated unsuccessfully with methotrexate: a six-month, double-blind, randomized, dose-ranging study. *Arthritis Rheum* (2002) 46, 2020–8.

Tacrolimus + Nystatin

Nystatin oral suspension did not appear to alter tacrolimus concentrations in one study.

Clinical evidence, mechanism, importance and management

In a randomised study, 18 kidney transplant patients taking tacrolimus 150 micrograms/kg twice daily were given nystatin oral suspension 5 mL four times daily for the prophylaxis of oral thrush immediately following transplantation. Tacrolimus minimum concentrations measured on days 1, 3, 5, and 7 post-transplant did not vary, and were all within the desired range of 15 to 20 nanograms/mL.[1] The nystatin in this study was used as a control for the effect of clotrimazole and therefore the conclusions that can be drawn from this study are limited. However, it would appear that nystatin has no effect on the absorption of tacrolimus, and therefore no tacrolimus dose adjustment would seem to be necessary on concurrent use.

1. Vasquez EM, Pollak R, Benedetti E. Clotrimazole increases tacrolimus blood levels: a drug interaction in kidney transplant patients. *Clin Transplant* (2001) 15, 95–9.

Tacrolimus + Orlistat

In patients adhering to recommended dietary fat intake, orlistat does not appear to affect the pharmacokinetics of tacrolimus, although small dose adjustments might be needed in some patients.

Clinical evidence, mechanism, importance and management

In a study in 12 liver transplant patients taking tacrolimus with orlistat 120 mg three times daily for 6 months, there was no statistically significant difference in the tacrolimus dose or minimum concentration-to-daily dose ratio at any time point. However, 4 patients required a reduction, and 2 required an increase, in their tacrolimus dose, although these adjustments were only minor. No elevations in liver enzymes were seen, and no episodes of rejection occurred. No diarrhoea was reported by the patients in this study, which suggests that the patients adhered well to the dietary advice regarding fat intake. In this study, patients took their morning tacrolimus dose 30 minutes before orlistat, and then ate breakfast after a further 30 minutes. In the evening the patients took orlistat 30 minutes before dinner, and took their evening dose of tacrolimus 2 hours later.[1] The authors concluded that orlistat could be safely used in patients taking tacrolimus, provided that tacrolimus concentrations are carefully monitored. They do however caution that there is a possibility that transplant patients who do not follow dietary fat advice and develop diarrhoea or steatorrhoea when taking orlistat might require a greater adjustment of their tacrolimus dose.[1]

1. Cassiman D, Roelants M, Vandenplas G, Van der Merwe SW, Mertens A, Libbrecht L, Verslype C, Fevery J, Aerts R, Pirenne J, Muls E, Nevens F. Orlistat treatment is safe in overweight and obese liver transplant recipients: a prospective, open label trial. *Transpl Int* (2006) 19, 1000–5.

Tacrolimus + Phosphodiesterase type-5 inhibitors

Sildenafil does not affect the pharmacokinetics of tacrolimus. The concentrations of sildenafil were reported to be higher in patients taking tacrolimus than in healthy subjects. A marked decrease in blood pressure occurred when both drugs were given in one study, and two patients required modification of their antihypertensives in another. Vardenafil does not appear to affect tacrolimus concentrations.

Clinical evidence

(a) Sildenafil

In 10 men with erectile dysfunction taking tacrolimus after a kidney transplant, a single 50-mg dose of sildenafil did not affect the pharmacokinetics of tacrolimus. When the pharmacokinetics of sildenafil were compared with those quoted by the manufacturer for healthy subjects, it was found that the maximum plasma concentration and AUC of sildenafil were 44% and 90% higher, respectively, in the patients taking tacrolimus. The AUC of the sildenafil metabolite was also higher. It was also noted that the mean blood pressure dropped by 27/20 mmHg after sildenafil was given.[1] A subsequent study by the same authors in 9 men with erectile dysfunction taking tacrolimus after a kidney transplant, found that sildenafil 25 mg daily for 9 days had no effect on the minimum concentrations or half-life of tacrolimus. Mean arterial blood pressure was reduced (by 1 to 7 mmHg, but this was not statistically significant), and 2 patients required a reduction in dose of their antihypertensives.[2]

Another study in 4 patients taking tacrolimus found that sildenafil 50 or 100 mg did not affect tacrolimus minimum concentrations.[3]

(b) Vardenafil

In a study in kidney transplant patients, vardenafil 10 or 20 mg (maximum frequency of once in 24 hours) in repeated doses during a 4-week period had no effect on the concentration, or required dose, of tacrolimus, and no change in renal function was reported.[4]

Mechanism

There are several possible reasons for the apparent increase in sildenafil concentrations in transplant patients other than a direct effect of tacrolimus. The pharmacokinetic data quoted by the manufacturer are from healthy subjects, not patients, and the patients in the study were taking a multitude of other drugs, some of which could have affected sildenafil.

Importance and management

It would appear that sildenafil does not affect tacrolimus concentrations; however, given the reduction in blood pressure seen in two studies,[1,2] it might be prudent to start patients on a 25-mg dose of sildenafil, as the authors of one study[1] advise, and increase the dose according to efficacy and tolerability. Vardenafil also does not appear to affect tacrolimus concentrations, but the effects on blood pressure do not appear to have been studied.

Note that both tacrolimus and some phosphodiesterase type-5 inhibitors are associated with an increased risk of QT interval prolongation. See 'Drugs that prolong the QT interval + Other drugs that prolong the QT interval', p.272, for further information on the concurrent use of two or more drugs that prolong the QT interval.

1. Christ B, Brockmeier D, Hauck EW, Friemann S. Interactions of sildenafil and tacrolimus in men with erectile dysfunction after kidney transplantation. *Urology* (2001) 58, 589–93.
2. Christ B, Brockmeier D, Hauck EW, Kamali-Ernst S. Investigation on interaction between tacrolimus and sildenafil in kidney-transplanted patients with erectile dysfunction. *Int J Clin Pharmacol Ther* (2004) 42, 149–56.
3. Cofán F, Gutiérrez R, Beardo P, Campistol JM, Oppenheimer F, Alcover J. Interacción entre sildenafilo y los inhibidores de la calcineurina en trasplantados renales con disfunción eréctile. *Nefrologia* (2002) 22, 470–6.
4. Demir E, Balal M, Paydas S, Sertdemir Y, Erken U. Efficacy and safety of vardenafil in renal transplant recipients with erectile dysfunction. *Transplant Proc* (2006) 38, 1379–81.

Tacrolimus + Potassium-sparing diuretics

The concurrent use of tacrolimus and potassium-sparing diuretics might cause hyperkalaemia.

Clinical evidence, mechanism, importance and management

Tacrolimus alone can cause hyperkalaemia, especially if renal function is impaired, and the risk might be additive with potassium-sparing drugs. Because of this, the UK and US manufacturers suggest that tacrolimus should not be used with potassium-sparing diuretics,[1,2] such as **amiloride**, **triamterene**, and **spironolactone**.[2] **Eplerenone** might also cause hyperkalaemia, therefore similar precaution would seem appropriate. It would be prudent to closely monitor potassium concentrations and renal function if the concurrent use of tacrolimus with any of these diuretics is considered essential.

1. Prograf (Tacrolimus). Astellas Pharma US Inc. US Prescribing information, September 2013.
2. Prograf (Tacrolimus monohydrate). Astellas Pharma Ltd. UK Summary of product characteristics, November 2014.

Tacrolimus + Proton pump inhibitors

Lansoprazole and omeprazole might increase tacrolimus concentrations but the outcome of concurrent use, particularly with omeprazole is variable. Case reports suggest that esomeprazole might interact with tacrolimus similarly, whereas pantoprazole and rabeprazole do not appear to interact with tacrolimus.

Clinical evidence

(a) Esomeprazole

An 18-year-old woman taking tacrolimus 6 mg daily following a renal transplant had her proton pump inhibitor changed from lansoprazole to esomeprazole 40 mg daily, 8 months post-transplant. One month later, her tacrolimus minimum concentration had increased from a range of 5 to 8 nanograms/mL up to 27.4 nanograms/mL. Tacrolimus was stopped for 24 hours, and then the dose was reduced to 4 mg daily. The following morning, her tacrolimus minimum concentration had decreased to 9.6 nanograms/mL. However, 10 days later, she reported nausea and vomiting over the previous few days, and her tacrolimus minimum concentration was 13.7 nanograms/mL. Tacrolimus was stopped until the target range was achieved, then restarted at a dose of 4 mg daily and esomeprazole was changed to omeprazole. Her tacrolimus minimum concentration became elevated again, and she was ultimately restabilised taking lansoprazole.[1]

(b) Lansoprazole

A 57-year-old woman taking tacrolimus following a kidney transplant started taking lansoprazole 30 mg daily, 19 days after her transplant, because of a peptic ulcer. After 3 days, her tacrolimus minimum concentration increased from a range of 16.3 to 17.6 nanograms/mL up to 26.7 nanograms/mL. The tacrolimus dose was reduced, and tacrolimus concentrations of 12 to 15.4 nanograms/mL were achieved. When lansoprazole was replaced by famotidine, the tacrolimus concentrations decreased to 8 nanograms/mL.[2,3] Two other very similar cases have been reported in Japanese transplant patients,[4,5] and in all these cases the patients were CYP2C19 poor metabolisers (that is, those with little or no activity of this isoenzyme). In contrast, one case report suggests that lansoprazole did not affect tacrolimus concentrations, see under *Esomeprazole*, above.

In a pharmacokinetic study in 19 healthy Japanese subjects, lansoprazole 30 mg daily for 4 days increased the AUC_{0-8} of a single 2-mg dose of tacrolimus given on day 4 by 48% and decreased its clearance by 31%. When the subjects were grouped by CYP2C19 metaboliser status, the increase in AUC was 52% greater in the 11 intermediate or poor metabolisers, than in the 8 extensive metabolisers (that is, those with normal isoenzyme activity), although there was wide variability between subjects.[6] However, in another study in 40 transplant patients taking tacrolimus and lansoprazole 30 mg daily, the degree of the interaction appeared to be influenced more by CYP3A5 genetic polymorphisms than CYP2C19 genetic polymorphisms.[7] Similarly, a study in 54 Japanese liver transplant patients taking tacrolimus and lansoprazole 30 mg daily found that the concentration-to-dose ratio of tacrolimus was not influenced by CYP2C19 polymorphisms in either the donor liver or the recipient intestine.[8]

(c) Omeprazole

In a study in 51 kidney transplant patients taking tacrolimus and omeprazole 20 mg daily for 6 months after transplantation, there was no difference in the tacrolimus concentration-to-dose ratio in the 3 months before stopping omeprazole and the 3 months after stopping omeprazole.[9] Similarly, in a study, 12 kidney transplant patients (CYP3A5 non-expressers) taking tacrolimus twice daily were given omeprazole 20 mg daily for more than 10 weeks. Omeprazole had no effect on the pharmacokinetics of tacrolimus.[10]

In contrast, a retrospective study in 48 kidney transplant patients found that when patients switched from cimetidine 400 mg daily to omeprazole 20 mg daily there was a 15% decrease in the dose to weight-normalised tacrolimus minimum concentration.[11] A study in 35 Japanese liver transplant patients taking tacrolimus and omeprazole 20 mg daily found that the concentration-to-dose ratio of tacrolimus was increased in CYP2C19 poor metabolisers compared with extensive or intermediate metabolisers (in either the donor liver or the recipient intestine.)[8] A 17-year-old kidney transplant patient, identified as a CYP2C19 poor metaboliser, had a minimum tacrolimus concentration of 29.2 ng/mL on day 4 post-transplant, which necessitated a decrease in tacrolimus dose from 9 mg twice daily to 7 mg twice daily on day 5. On the same day, omeprazole 40 mg daily was started and by day 6 her minimum tacrolimus concentration was 92 ng/mL.[12] Another case report describes a 13-year-old transplant patient whose tacrolimus minimum concentration increased from about 10 nanograms/mL up to 28 nanograms/mL when omeprazole 20 mg daily was started. This resolved on stopping the omeprazole. This patient was not a CYP2C19 poor metaboliser.[13] Another similar case is reported (genetic status unknown),[14] and a further case report also suggests that omeprazole might increase tacrolimus concentrations, see under *Esomeprazole*, above.

(d) Pantoprazole

A study in 6 transplant patients taking tacrolimus found that pantoprazole 40 mg daily for 5 days did not affect the minimum concentration of tacrolimus.[15] Similarly, in a pharmacokinetic study, when 21 heart transplant recipients taking mycophenolate mofetil and tacrolimus were given pantoprazole 40 mg daily there was no change in tacrolimus concentrations.[16] A brief report describes 12 transplant patients given tacrolimus (4 to 7 mg twice daily) and pantoprazole 40 mg in the morning for 5 days. Pantoprazole had no effect on the tacrolimus minimum concentration.[17]

(e) Rabeprazole

In a pharmacokinetic study in 15 healthy Japanese subjects, rabeprazole 10 mg daily for 4 days increased the AUC_{0-8} of tacrolimus by 18% when a single-dose of tacrolimus 2 mg was given with rabeprazole on day 4, but this change was not statistically significant.[6] Similarly, a case-control study in 17 Japanese patients with liver transplants, rabeprazole 10 mg daily had no effect on the tacrolimus concentration-to-dose ratio, regardless of CYP2C19 or CYP3A5 metaboliser status.[18]

Several case studies have also described a lack of interaction between rabeprazole and tacrolimus.[2,3,5,14]

Mechanism

Uncertain. In some of the cases and one study, the interaction with lansoprazole was greatest in patients with decreased activity of CYP2C19, by which lansoprazole (and also esomeprazole, omeprazole, and pantoprazole) is mainly metabolised. When activity of this isoenzyme is low, lansoprazole concentrations are much higher, and it has been suggested that this might be sufficient to inhibit tacrolimus metabolism by CYP3A4 and/or affect transport by P-glycoprotein (which is inhibited to some extent by all the proton pump inhibitors).[6] If this is the mechanism, then esomeprazole, omeprazole, and pantoprazole would be expected to interact similarly. Nevertheless, one study suggested that CYP3A5 metaboliser status was more important than CYP2C19 metaboliser status or P-glycoprotein.[7] Rabeprazole is principally metabolised non-enzymatically and seems less likely to interact,[2,3,6] although one study found no difference between rabeprazole and lansoprazole.[7]

The *decreased* tacrolimus concentrations in one study with omeprazole were thought to be due to induction of CYP3A4 by omeprazole,[11] but might have been more to do with stopping the cimetidine (a known enzyme inhibitor) than an effect of omeprazole. Further study is required.

Importance and management

There is a reasonable body of evidence investigating a possible interaction between tacrolimus and the proton pump inhibitors, but the evidence is somewhat conflicting and genetic factors in drug metabolism might play a large part in the outcome. There is some evidence that an interaction with lansoprazole is most likely in those with decreased CYP2C19 activity,[6] although not all evidence supports this.[7,13] The effect with omeprazole appears particularly variable, with tacrolimus concentrations reported as increased, decreased, or unaffected. No pharmacokinetic interaction has been seen with pantoprazole, although if the mechanism proposed for lansoprazole and omeprazole is correct, an interaction might be possible in some patients. The evidence suggests that rabeprazole is unlikely to interact, and this is supported by the proposed mechanism, and therefore rabeprazole might be a suitable alternative. Nevertheless, further detailed pharmacokinetic study is required for all proton pump inhibitors. Until more is known, bear the possibility of an interaction in mind and give consideration to increasing the monitoring of tacrolimus concentrations when any of these drugs are started or stopped, taking into account the relevance of a potential increase in concentrations to the individual patient. Note that one study suggests that the metaboliser status of both the donor and the recipient might be relevant to the metabolism of tacrolimus in liver transplant recipients given a proton pump inhibitor.[8]

1. Maguire M, Franz T, Hains DS. A clinically significant interaction between tacrolimus and multiple proton pump inhibitors in a kidney transplant recipient. *Pediatr Transplant* (2012) 16, E217–E220.
2. Homma M, Itagaki F, Yuzawa K, Fukao K, Kohda Y. Effects of lansoprazole and rabeprazole on tacrolimus blood concentration: case of a renal transplant recipient with CYP2C19 gene mutation. *Transplantation* (2002) 73, 303–4.
3. Itagaki F, Homma M, Yuzawa K, Fukao K, Kohda Y. Drug interaction of tacrolimus and proton pump inhibitors in renal transplant recipients with CYP2C19 gene mutation. *Transplant Proc* (2002) 34, 2777–8.
4. Takahashi K, Motohashi H, Yonezawa A, Okuda M, Ito N, Yamamoto S, Ogawa O, Inui K. Lansoprazole-tacrolimus interaction in Japanese transplant recipient with CYP2C19 polymorphism. *Ann Pharmacother* (2004) 38, 791–4.
5. Hosohata K, Masuda S, Ogura Y, Oike F, Takada Y, Katsura T, Uemoto S, Inui K. Interaction between tacrolimus and lansoprazole, but not rabeprazole in living-donor liver transplant patients with defects of CYP2C19 and CYP3A5. *Drug Metab Pharmacokinet* (2008) 23, 134–8.
6. Itagaki F, Homma M, Yuzawa K, Nishimura M, Naito S, Ueda N, Ohkochchi N, Kohda Y. Effect of lansoprazole and rabeprazole on tacrolimus pharmacokinetics in healthy volunteers with CYP2C19 mutations. *J Pharm Pharmacol* (2004) 56, 1055–9.
7. Miura M, Inoue K, Kagaya H, Satoh S, Tada H, Sagae Y, Habuchi T, Suzuki T. Influence of rabeprazole and lansoprazole on the pharmacokinetics of tacrolimus in relation to CYP2C19, CYP3A5 and MDR1 polymorphisms in renal transplant recipients. *Biopharm Drug Dispos* (2007) 28, 167–75.
8. Hosohata K, Masuda S, Katsura T, Takada Y, Kaido T, Ogura Y, Oike F, Egawa H, Uemoto S, Inui K. Impact of intestinal CYP2C19 genotypes on the interaction between tacrolimus and omeprazole, but not lansoprazole, in adult living-donor liver transplant patients. *Drug Metab Dispos* (2009) 37, 821–6.
9. Pascual J, Marcén R, Orea OE, Navarro M, Alarcón MC, Ocaña J, Villafruela JJ, Burgos FJ, Ortuño J. Interaction between omeprazole and tacrolimus in renal allograft recipients: a clinical-analytical study. *Transplant Proc* (2005) 37, 3752–3.
10. Katsakiori PF, Papapetrou EP, Goumenos DS, Nikiforidis GC, Flordellis CS. Investigation of clinical interaction between omeprazole and tacrolimus in CYP3A5 non-expressors, renal transplant recipients. *Ther Clin Risk Manag* (2010) 6, 265–9.
11. Lemahieu WPD, Maes BD, Verbeke K, Vanrenterghem Y. Impact of gastric acid suppressants on cytochrome P450 3A4 and P-glycoprotein: consequences for FK506 assimilation. *Kidney Int* (2005) 67, 1152–60.
12. Zhao W, Fakhoury M, Maisin A, Baudouin V, Storme T, Deschênes G, Jacqz-Aigrain E. Pharmacogenetic determinant of the drug interaction between tacrolimus and omeprazole. *Ther Drug Monit* (2012) 34, 739–41.
13. Moreau C, Taburet AM, Furlan V, Debray D, Loriot MA. Interaction between tacrolimus and omeprazole in a pediatric liver transplant recipient. *Transplantation* (2006) 81, 487–8. Erratum ibid.82, 1382.
14. Takahashi K, Yano I, Fukuhara Y, Katsura T, Takahashi T, Ito N, Yamamoto S, Ogawa O, Inui K. Distinct effects of omeprazole and rabeprazole on the tacrolimus blood concentration in a kidney transplant recipient. *Drug Metab Pharmacokinet* (2007) 22, 441–4.
15. Lorf T, Ramadori G, Ringe B, Schwörer H. The effect of pantoprazole on tacrolimus and cyclosporin A blood concentration in transplant recipients. *Eur J Clin Pharmacol* (2000) 56, 439–40.
16. Kofler S, Deutsch M-A, Bigdeli AK, Shvets N, Vogeser M, Mueller TH, Meiser B, Steinbeck G, Reichart B, Kaczmarek I. Proton pump inhibitor co-medication reduces mycophenolate acid drug exposure in heart transplant recipients. *J Heart Lung Transplant* (2009) 28, 605–11.
17. Lorf T, Ramdori G, Ringe B, Schwörer H. The effect of pantoprazole on tacrolimus and cyclosporin A blood concentration in transplant recipients. *Eur J Clin Pharmacol* (2000) 56, 439–40.
18. Hosohata K, Masuda S, Yonezawa A, Sugimoto M, Takada Y, Kaido T, Ogura Y, Oike F, Uemoto S, Inui K. Absence of influence of concomitant administration of rabeprazole on the pharmacokinetics of tacrolimus in adult living donor liver transplant patients: a case-control study. *Drug Metab Pharmacokinet* (2009) 24, 458–63.

Tacrolimus + Quinolones; Levofloxacin

Levofloxacin caused a small increase in tacrolimus exposure in one study.

Clinical evidence, mechanism, importance and management

A study in 5 kidney transplant patients found that levofloxacin 500 mg twice daily for 5 days increased the AUC_{0-12} of tacrolimus by about 27%.[1] The authors concluded that levofloxacin inhibits the metabolism of tacrolimus, however levofloxacin is not a known inhibitor of CYP3A4 or P-glycoprotein which are involved in the metabolism and transport, respectively, of tacrolimus.

Although this study suggests a small increase in tacrolimus exposure might occur in patients given levofloxacin, and the authors suggest that close monitoring would be appropriate if this combination is given,[1] evidence from clinical practice appears to be lacking which suggests that this is probably not likely to be clinically relevant for a short course of the antibacterial.

1. Federico S, Carrano R, Capone D, Gentile A, Palmiero G, Basile V. Pharmacokinetic interaction between levofloxacin and ciclosporin or tacrolimus in kidney transplant recipients: ciclosporin, tacrolimus and levofloxacin in renal transplantation. *Clin Pharmacokinet* (2006) 45, 169–75.

Tacrolimus + Quinupristin with Dalfopristin

Quinupristin with dalfopristin might slightly increase tacrolimus concentrations. There is limited evidence suggesting that tacrolimus might increase the risk of myalgia and/or arthralgia in patients taking quinupristin with dalfopristin.

Clinical evidence

When available in the UK, the manufacturer of quinupristin with dalfopristin stated that concurrent use with tacrolimus had been reported to increase the minimum concentrations of tacrolimus by 15%.[1]

In an analysis of myalgia and/or arthralgia in patients with cancer taking quinupristin with dalfopristin, the use of tacrolimus within the month preceding treatment was associated with a higher risk. Seven (35%) of the patients experiencing myalgia and/or arthralgia had received tacrolimus compared with 4 (11%) of those not experiencing myalgia and/or arthralgia.[2]

Mechanism

Quinupristin with dalfopristin inhibits CYP3A4, by which tacrolimus is metabolised.[1,3] Concurrent use might therefore lead to decreased tacrolimus metabolism and increased concentrations.

Myalgia and/or arthralgia are common in patients receiving quinupristin with dalfopristin and their aetiology is uncertain. It was suggested that tacrolimus-induced impairment in biliary function/cholestasis might predispose patients to develop myalgia and/or arthralgia while taking quinupristin with dalfopristin.[2]

Importance and management

Evidence for an interaction between quinupristin with dalfopristin and tacrolimus is limited, and suggests that minimum tacrolimus concentrations might be slightly increased on concurrent use. The US manufacturer of quinupristin with dalfopristin advises caution and monitoring of drugs with narrow therapeutic ranges that are CYP3A4 substrates [such as tacrolimus] during concurrent use.[3] This seems a little over cautious given the available evidence, but it would seem prudent to bear the possibility of an interaction in mind in cases of otherwise unexplained increases in tacrolimus concentrations or adverse effects. Likewise, bear in mind the possibility that tacrolimus use might increase the risk of myalgia and/or arthralgia in patients taking quinupristin with dalfopristin. The US manufacturer of quinupristin with dalfopristin notes that improvement has been noted in some patients with this adverse effect when the dose frequency has been extended.[3]

1. Synercid (Quinupristin/Dalfopristin). Monarch Pharmaceuticals Ireland Ltd. UK Summary of product characteristics, March 2005.
2. Raad I, Hachem R, Hanna H. Relationship between myalgias/arthralgias occurring in patients receiving quinupristin/dalfopristin and biliary dysfunction. *J Antimicrob Chemother* (2004) 53, 1105–8.
3. Synercid (Quinupristin/Dalfopristin). Pfizer Injectables. US Prescribing information, October 2013.

Tacrolimus + Ranolazine

Three patients taking tacrolimus developed increased tacrolimus concentrations after ranolazine was started.

Clinical evidence

A 64-year-old kidney transplant patient who had been taking tacrolimus 10 mg twice daily for 5 months, started taking ranolazine 500 mg twice daily for worsening of her chronic angina. The following day, her minimum tacrolimus concentration had doubled (from 8.1 to 17.8 nanograms/mL) and increased further to 18.9 nanograms/mL after she had been taking ranolazine for 2 days. Tacrolimus was withheld for 2 days and then titrated down to 2 mg twice daily over the following 10 days, which achieved a minimum concentration of 6.1 nanograms/mL and the patient was discharged. The patient was readmitted 12 days later and during this admission her minimum tacrolimus concentration was 3.1 to 3.5 nanograms/mL and her tacrolimus dose was increased to 3 mg twice daily. Three months later the patient was readmitted, ranolazine was stopped, and the tacrolimus dose had to be increased from 3 mg twice daily to 4.5 mg twice daily to maintain a tacrolimus minimum concentration within the desired therapeutic range.[1] Note that this case is complicated by a number of factors, including acute-on-chronic renal failure, and the addition of a 5-day course of fluconazole 50 mg daily during her first admission, which could have contributed to the interaction, see 'Tacrolimus + Azoles; Fluconazole', p.1288. Another case report describes a 62-year-old kidney transplant patient stable taking tacrolimus (dose not stated) with prednisone, enalapril, and diltiazem, who was started on ranolazine 500 mg twice daily, increased to 1000 mg twice daily, for ischaemic heart disease. Two weeks later he was admitted with decreased appetite, tremors, fatigue, and decreased urine output, and his minimum tacrolimus concentration was 14 nanograms/mL (compared with about 9 nanograms/mL measured 2 months previously). The ranolazine was stopped, and three days later the minimum concentration of tacrolimus had decreased to 7 nanograms/mL, without changing the dose of tacrolimus.[2] In a further case, a 54-year-old kidney transplant patient stable taking tacrolimus 3 mg twice daily for 5 years, started taking ranolazine 375 mg twice daily for recurrent episodes of angina. During the following 5 weeks, his serum creatinine concentration gradually increased, and his tacrolimus concentration approximately doubled from 5 to 10.9 ng/mL. Ranolazine was stopped about 5 weeks after it was started, resulting in reversal of the renal failure, and his tacrolimus concentration decreased to 3.6 ng/mL.[3]

Mechanism

Uncertain. Ranolazine inhibits CYP3A4 and it has been suggested that it also inhibits P-glycoprotein. As tacrolimus is metabolised by CYP3A4 and is also a substrate of P-glycoprotein, one or both of these mechanisms seem likely to be involved in this interaction. Further study is needed.

Importance and management

Evidence for an interaction between tacrolimus and ranolazine is limited to these reports, however they suggest that ranolazine can increase tacrolimus concentrations to a clinically important extent in some patients. There would seem to be insufficient evidence to advocate increased monitoring in all patients given this combination. Nevertheless, given the suggested mechanism for this interaction and the potential implications of sharp increases in tacrolimus concentrations, it would seem prudent to be aware of the potential for an interaction with ranolazine in cases of otherwise unexplained increases in tacrolimus concentrations or adverse effects, adjusting the tacrolimus dose if necessary.

Ranolazine can prolong the QT interval and tacrolimus is associated with an increased risk of QT interval prolongation; see 'Drugs that prolong the QT interval + Other drugs that prolong the QT interval', p.272, for further information on the concurrent use of two or more drugs that prolong the QT interval.

1. Pierce DA, Reeves-Daniel AM. Ranolazine-tacrolimus interaction. *Ann Pharmacother* (2010) 44, 1844–49.
2. Patni H, Gitman M, Hazzan A, Jhaveri KD. Ranolazine, tacrolimus, and diltiazem might be a hazardous combination in a transplant patient. *Ren Fail* (2012) 34, 251–3.
3. Seck S, Bellantoni M, Zoccali C, Enia G. Ranolazine can markedly increase tacrolimus blood levels. *NDT Plus* (2011) 4, 44–5.

Tacrolimus + Repaglinide

Repaglinide does not appear to alter tacrolimus concentrations.

Clinical evidence, mechanism, importance and management

In a study in kidney transplant patients stabilised on immunosuppressants, 14 patients taking tacrolimus had no notable changes in tacrolimus blood concentrations, and no tacrolimus dose changes were required, on starting repaglinide 1 to 3 mg daily (mostly as monotherapy, but a few patients were also given either metformin or rosiglitazone).[1] It would appear from the limited data from this observational study, that repaglinide does not affect the pharmacokinetics of tacrolimus; however, this ideally needs confirmation in a pharmacokinetic study. Note also that in this study repaglinide was started at a low dose and titrated upwards as necessary.[1] It might therefore be prudent to introduce repaglinide in this way in those already taking tacrolimus.

1. Türk T, Peitruck F, Dolff S, Kribben A, Janssen OE, Mann K, Philipp T, Heemann U, Witzke O. Repaglinide in the management of new-onset diabetes mellitus after renal transplantation. *Am J Transplant* (2006) 6, 842–6.

Tacrolimus + Rifamycins

A pharmacokinetic study found that rifampicin (rifampin) decreases tacrolimus exposure after oral and intravenous administration. A number of liver transplant patients have needed greatly increased tacrolimus doses when rifampicin was added. One case report demonstrates that rifabutin does not interact to the same extent as rifampicin.

Clinical evidence

(a) Rifabutin

A kidney transplant patient developed low tacrolimus concentrations (3.7 to 5.5 nanograms/mL) despite an increase in dose from 16 to 60 mg daily while taking rifampicin (rifampin) 600 mg daily. When rifabutin was substituted for rifampicin, the tacrolimus dose was gradually reduced to 20 mg daily, with tacrolimus serum concentrations between 10 and 15 nanograms/mL.[1]

(b) Rifampicin (Rifampin)

In a controlled study in 6 healthy subjects, pre-treatment with rifampicin 600 mg daily decreased the AUC of tacrolimus after both a single 100-micrograms/kg oral dose, and a 25-micrograms/kg intravenous dose given over 4 hours, by 68% and 35%, respectively. The clearance of tacrolimus was increased by 47%.[2]

Similar effects have also been seen in a number of case reports.[1,3-9] For example, in one case the tacrolimus minimum blood concentration of a 10-year-old boy with a liver transplant was decreased from 10 nanograms/mL to an undetectable concentration within 2 days of rifampicin 150 mg twice daily being started. His tacrolimus dose was therefore doubled from 4 to 8 mg twice daily. When rifampicin was later stopped, the tacrolimus dose had to be reduced to 3 mg twice daily to keep the blood concentrations in the region of 10 nanograms/mL.[3] In another case, a 10-fold increase in the tacrolimus dose was needed to keep minimum blood concentrations within the target range when rifampicin was started. However, despite concentrations within the acceptable range, a biopsy showed suspected tacrolimus nephrotoxicity, which it was suggested might have been due to the cumulative tacrolimus dose, or to high concentrations of tacrolimus metabolites (which were not measured).[6] A decrease in tacrolimus concentrations from 9.2 to 1.4 nanograms/mL occurred in another case, just 2 days after starting rifampicin. Rifampicin was stopped and replaced by pyrazinamide, with a gradual return to the baseline tacrolimus concentrations.[7] In one patient, where rifampicin 300 mg daily decreased the tacrolimus minimum blood concentration from 5.5 nanograms/mL to an undetectable concentration, the addition of itraconazole oral solution 200 mg daily resulted in the tacrolimus minimum blood concentration increasing to 5.7 nanograms/mL.[10] In yet another case, the effect of rifampicin was so great that the use of either fluconazole or clarithromycin, both known inhibitors of tacrolimus metabolism (see 'Tacrolimus + Azoles; Fluconazole', p.1288, and 'Tacrolimus + Macrolides', p.1299), did not increase tacrolimus concentrations.[8]

Conversely, one case report describes increased tacrolimus concentrations, requiring a dose decrease from 7 mg daily to 0.5 mg on alternate days, when rifampicin, isoniazid, ethambutol, and pyrazinamide were started for tuberculosis. The increase in tacrolimus concentrations was thought to be due to worsening of chronic diarrhoea, possibly exacerbated by rifampicin, and appeared to overcome the expected decrease in tacrolimus concentrations by the enzyme-inducing effects of rifampicin.[11]

Mechanism

Tacrolimus is metabolised by CYP3A4 and is also a P-glycoprotein substrate. Rifampicin (rifampin) is a potent inducer of CYP3A4 and it also induces P-glycoprotein, therefore concurrent use decreases tacrolimus concentrations. Rifabutin is a less potent enzyme inducer than rifampicin, and therefore has less effect on tacrolimus metabolism.

Importance and management

The interaction between tacrolimus and rifampicin (rifampin) is established and clinically important. Monitor tacrolimus concentrations closely, and anticipate the need to increase the dose of tacrolimus, sometimes greatly, if rifampicin is also given. Note that if the interaction is not managed well in patients given tacrolimus post-transplant, there is a risk of transplant rejection.

The one case report with rifabutin suggests that any interaction with tacrolimus is much less pronounced than with rifampicin. Nevertheless, until the situation is more clear, it would be prudent to closely monitor tacrolimus concentrations on concurrent use with rifabutin and other rifamycins (for example, **rifapentine**, which is a moderate CYP3A4 inducer), being alert for the need to increase the tacrolimus dose.

1. López-Montes A, Gallego E, López E, Pérez J, Lorenzo I, Llamas F, Serrano A, Andrés E, Illescas L, Gómez C. Treatment of tuberculosis with rifabutin in a renal transplant recipient. *Am J Kidney Dis* (2004) 44, e59–e63.
2. Hebert MF, Fisher RM, Marsh CL, Dressler D, Bekersky I. Effects of rifampin on tacrolimus pharmacokinetics in healthy volunteers. *J Clin Pharmacol* (1999) 39, 91–6.
3. Furlan V, Perello L, Jacquemin E, Debray D, Taburet A-M. Interactions between FK506 and rifampicin or erythromycin in pediatric liver recipients. *Transplantation* (1995) 59, 1217–18.
4. Kiuchi T, Inomata Y, Uemoto S, Satomura K, Egawa H, Okajima H, Yamaoka Y, Tanaka K. A hepatic graft tuberculosis transmitted from a living-related donor. *Transplantation* (1997) 63, 905–7.
5. Kiuchi T, Tanaka K, Inomata Y, Uemoto S, Satomura K, Egawa H, Uyama S, Sano K, Okajima H, Yamaoka Y. Experience of tacrolimus-based immunosuppression in a living-related liver transplantation complicated with graft tuberculosis: interaction with rifampicin and side effects. *Transplant Proc* (1996) 28, 3171–2.
6. Chenhsu R-Y, Loong C-C, Chou M-H, Lin M-F, Yang W-C. Renal allograft dysfunction associated with rifampin-tacrolimus interaction. *Ann Pharmacother* (2000) 34, 27–31.
7. Moreno M, Latorre C, Manzanares C, Morales E, Herrero JC, Dominguez-Gil B, Carreño A, Cubas A, Delgado M, Andres A, Morales JM. Clinical management of tacrolimus drug interactions in renal transplant patients. *Transplant Proc* (1999) 31, 2252–3.
8. Bhaloo S, Prasad GV. Severe reduction in tacrolimus levels with rifampin despite multiple cytochrome P450 inhibitors: a case report. *Transplant Proc* (2003) 35, 2449–51.
9. Hartmann A, Halvorsen CE, Jenssen T, Bjørneklett A, Brekke IB, Bakke SJ, Hirschberg H, Tønjum T, Gaustad P. Intracerebral abscess caused by *Nocardia otitidiscaviarum* in a renal transplant patient- cured by evacuation plus antibiotic therapy. Nephron. (2000) 86, 79–83.

10. Mori T, Aisa Y, Kato J, Nakamura Y, Shimizu T, Okamoto S. Overcoming the effect of rifampin on the tacrolimus metabolism by itraconazole administration in an allogeneic hematopoietic stem cell transplant recipient. *Int J Hematol* (2010) 91, 553–4.
11. Abdel Halim M, Al-Otaibi T, Gheith O, El-Kholy O, Abdel Tawab K, Said T, Nair P, Nampoory MRN. Toxic tacrolimus blood levels with rifampin administration in a renal transplant recipient. *Ann Transplant* (2010) 15, 57–60.

Tacrolimus + Schisandra

Schisandra greatly increases the exposure to tacrolimus and its adverse effects.

Clinical evidence

In a pharmacokinetic study, 12 healthy subjects were given an extract of *Schisandra sphenanthera* (containing 33.75 mg schisandrin) twice daily for 14 days, with a single 2-mg oral dose of tacrolimus on day 14. The AUC and maximum plasma concentration of tacrolimus were increased 2.6-fold and 3.3-fold, respectively, but its half-life was not altered. Six subjects experienced indigestion, and burning hands and feet, one hour after both medicines were given. These symptoms resolved over 10 hours.[1]

Mechanism

Not established. P-glycoprotein is involved in the intestinal absorption of tacrolimus. It is therefore possible that the inhibition of P-glycoprotein by schisandrin, and possibly other related compounds, might have resulted in increased absorption of tacrolimus. The authors also suggest that the metabolism of tacrolimus, which is a substrate of CYP3A4, might have been inhibited by schisandra. However, one *animal* study suggests that this effect on CYP3A4 might not be clinically relevant.[2]

Importance and management

An interaction between schisandra and tacrolimus seems fairly well established, although the mechanism is not fully established. Concurrent use appears to result in a large increase in the exposure to tacrolimus, accompanied by an increase in tacrolimus adverse effects. If the use of both medicines is considered desirable it would seem prudent to monitor the outcome of concurrent use closely, adjusting the dose of tacrolimus as necessary. It is important to note that, although the schisandra product used in the study was standardised for schisandrin content, this constituent has not been established as the cause of the interaction. Therefore the extent of the interaction might vary between different schisandra products, and different batches of the same schisandra product. This might make this interaction difficult to standardise for, and therefore it would be prudent to avoid concurrent use where blood concentrations of tacrolimus are critical, such as in organ transplantation.

1. Xin H-W, Wu X-C, Li Q, Yu A-R, Zhu M, Shen Y, Su D, Xiong L. Effects of Schisandra sphenanthera extract on the pharmacokinetics of tacrolimus in healthy volunteers. *Br J Clin Pharmacol* (2007) 64, 469–75.
2. Makino T, Mizuno F, Mizukami H. Does a Kampo medicine containing schisandra fruit affect pharmacokinetics of nifedipine like grapefruit juice? *Biol Pharm Bull* (2006) 29, 2065–9.

Tacrolimus + Sevelamer

Sevelamer might reduce the absorption of tacrolimus.

Clinical evidence

A kidney transplant patient had a progressive reduction in his tacrolimus concentration, requiring an increase in his tacrolimus dose, after he started to take sevelamer 800 mg three times daily. A pharmacokinetic study in the same patient found that the maximum tacrolimus concentration was increased from 9.9 to 13.1 nanograms/mL, and the AUC_{0-7} was increased 2.4-fold, three days after sevelamer was stopped.[1]

Mechanism

Sevelamer can bind with drugs in the gut and prevent their absorption, and this might have lead to the reduction in tacrolimus concentration seen.

Importance and management

Evidence for an interaction between tacrolimus and sevelamer appears to be limited to this one case report, but sevelamer has been seen to have similar effects on the absorption of a number of other drugs. It is recommended that any drug for which a reduction in the bioavailability might be clinically important should be taken at least one hour before, or 3 hours after, sevelamer, and/or their concentrations should be monitored.[2,3] This would therefore apply to tacrolimus, and as such its concentrations should be closely monitored and the dose adjusted as needed if concurrent use is required, or if sevelamer is stopped.

1. Merkle M, Wornle M, Rupprecht HD. The effect of sevelamer on tacrolimus target levels. *Transplantation* (2005) 80, 707.
2. Renagel (Sevelamer hydrochloride). Sanofi. UK Summary of product characteristics, February 2015.
3. Renvela (Sevelamer carbonate). Genzyme. US Prescribing information, May 2011.

Tacrolimus + Sirolimus

No pharmacokinetic interaction occurred between tacrolimus and sirolimus in a study in healthy subjects, but evidence from clinical use suggests that sirolimus might reduce tacrolimus blood concentrations. Tacrolimus does not appear to alter sirolimus concentrations, although one study did find an increase in sirolimus exposure.

Clinical evidence

(a) No pharmacokinetic effects

A crossover study in 27 healthy male subjects given single doses of sirolimus (15 mg) and tacrolimus (10 mg) alone, simultaneously, and 4 hours apart, found that there was no difference in the AUC of either drug when administered simultaneously, or 4 hours apart.[1] Similarly, a study in 18 liver transplant and 7 kidney-pancreas transplant patients taking tacrolimus and sirolimus found no difference in the pharmacokinetics of either drug when they were taken either simultaneously or 4 hours apart. No nephrotoxicity was seen.[2] Another study in 28 kidney transplant patients taking tacrolimus and given sirolimus 500 micrograms, 1 mg, or 2 mg daily found that tacrolimus did not appear to alter sirolimus concentrations, when compared with historical data from studies with sirolimus alone.[3] For the effect on tacrolimus, see below.

(b) Effect on sirolimus

In contrast to the lack of effect seen in the studies described above, one study in 12 adult kidney transplant recipients receiving tacrolimus, found that a 3-fold increase in the dose-corrected AUC of tacrolimus was associated with a 71% increase in the dose-corrected AUC of sirolimus.[4]

(c) Effect on tacrolimus

In contrast to the lack of effect seen in the studies above, other studies have found decreases in tacrolimus concentrations due to the concurrent use of sirolimus. A study in 7 children with kidney transplants taking tacrolimus and prednisone found that the addition of sirolimus to treat chronic allograft nephropathy resulted in a decrease in the dose-normalised tacrolimus minimum blood concentrations from 0.14 kg/L to 0.1 kg/L on day 3 and to 0.08 kg/L on day 28. All patients required a tacrolimus dose increase, with a mean increase of about 70% (range 22 to 245%) in order to keep the tacrolimus blood concentrations above 3 nanograms/mL.[5] Another study in 28 kidney transplant patients taking tacrolimus and given sirolimus 500 micrograms, 1 mg, or 2 mg daily also found an initial reduction in the tacrolimus concentration with the first dose. The tacrolimus concentrations recovered, but a trend towards reduced tacrolimus concentrations was seen with continued dosing.[3] A further study in 16 adult kidney transplant patients taking tacrolimus and fixed-dose sirolimus 500 micrograms or 2 mg daily found a dose-dependent increase in the AUC of tacrolimus of 16% and 31%, respectively, and an increase in the maximum concentrations of tacrolimus of 19% and 33%, respectively, when sirolimus was *stopped*.[6] Another study in 12 adult kidney transplant patients found that the AUC of tacrolimus increased by 59% in patients also taking sirolimus during the first 6 months after transplantation.[4]

(d) Renal toxicity

A retrospective study in adult kidney transplant patients taking tacrolimus and sirolimus found that concurrent use might be associated with extensive tubular cell injury and a unique form of cast nephropathy.[7]

Mechanism

Unclear. The authors of one study suggest that the reduced tacrolimus concentrations seen were due to a reduction in the bioavailability of tacrolimus rather than increased excretion.[5]

Importance and management

Evidence for an interaction between tacrolimus and sirolimus is somewhat conflicting. One controlled pharmacokinetic study found that no interaction occurs between tacrolimus and sirolimus; however, there is clinical evidence of increased tacrolimus dose requirements after starting sirolimus, and one study shows increased sirolimus exposure in patients also taking tacrolimus. As both tacrolimus and sirolimus are given as individualised doses based on target blood concentrations, any change in required dose on concurrent use should be identified with routine monitoring.

The manufacturers of sirolimus[8,9] and tacrolimus,[10] note that clinical studies in *de novo* liver transplant patients have found an increased risk of hepatic artery thrombosis, leading to graft loss and/or death in most cases, when tacrolimus was also given. As such, the US manufacturer of tacrolimus states that concurrent use with sirolimus in this patient group is not recommended.[10] Moreover, the US manufacturer of tacrolimus notes that the use of full-dose tacrolimus with sirolimus 2 mg daily in heart transplant recipients was associated with an increased risk of wound healing complications, impaired renal function, and post-transplant insulin-dependent diabetes mellitus, and is not recommended.[10]

More generally, the concurrent use of both drugs increases the risk of developing calcineurin inhibitor-induced haemolytic uraemic syndrome, thrombotic thrombocytopenic purpura, and thrombotic microangiopathy.[8,9]

1. Tortorici MA, Parks V, Matschke K, Korth-Bradley J, Patat A. The evaluation of potential pharmacokinetic interaction between sirolimus and tacrolimus in healthy volunteers. *Eur J Clin Pharmacol* (2013) 69, 835–42.
2. McAlister VC, Mahalati K, Peltekian KM, Fraser A, MacDonald AS. A clinical pharmacokinetic study of tacrolimus and sirolimus combination immunosuppression comparing simultaneous to separated administration. *Ther Drug Monit* (2002) 24, 346–50.
3. Undre NA. Pharmacokinetics of tacrolimus-based combination therapies. *Nephrol Dial Transplant* (2003) 18 (Suppl 1), i12–i15.
4. Park S-I, Felipe CR, Pinheiro-Machado PG, Garcia R, Fernandes FB, Casarini DE, Tedesco-Silva Jr H, Medina-Pestana JO. Tacrolimus pharmacokinetic drug interactions: effect of prednisone, mycophenolic acid or sirolimus. *Fundam Clin Pharmacol* (2009) 23, 137–45.
5. Filler G, Womiloju T, Feber J, Lepage N, Christians U. Adding sirolimus to tacrolimus-based immunosuppression in pediatric renal transplant recipients reduces tacrolimus exposure. *Am J Transplant* (2005) 5, 2005–10.

6. Baldan N, Rigotti P, Furian L, Margani G, Ekser B, Frison L, De Martin S, Palatini P. Co-administration of sirolimus alters tacrolimus pharmacokinetics in a dose-dependent manner in adult renal transplant recipients. *Pharmacol Res* (2006) 54, 181–5.
7. Smith KD, Wrenshall LE, Nicosia RF, Pichler R, Marsh CL, Alpers CE, Polissar N, Davis CL. Delayed graft function and cast nephropathy associated with tacrolimus plus rapamycin use. *J Am Soc Nephrol* (2003) 14, 1037–45.
8. Rapamune (Sirolimus). Pfizer Ltd. UK Summary of product characteristics, August 2013.
9. Rapamune (Sirolimus). Wyeth Pharmaceuticals Inc. US Prescribing information, December 2012.
10. Prograf (Tacrolimus). Astellas Pharma US Inc. US Prescribing information, September 2013.

Tacrolimus + SSRIs or SNRIs and related antidepressants

Increases in tacrolimus concentrations and toxicity were observed when three patients were also given nefazodone. Paroxetine and sertraline do not appear to interact with tacrolimus. Of the other SSRIs, fluvoxamine is predicted to increase tacrolimus concentrations. A report describes serotonin syndrome in a patient taking tacrolimus with venlafaxine.

Clinical evidence

A kidney transplant patient taking tacrolimus 5 mg daily developed delirium and renal failure 4 weeks after starting **nefazodone** 150 mg daily. Three months earlier, his tacrolimus concentration had been 9.4 nanograms/mL whilst taking tacrolimus 6 mg daily, but in the presence of **nefazodone** the tacrolimus concentration increased to 46.4 nanograms/mL with a tacrolimus dose of 5 mg daily, and his serum creatinine had doubled. Within 2 days of the tacrolimus dose being reduced to 3 mg daily, the tacrolimus concentration decreased to 29.6 nanograms/mL. **Nefazodone** was then replaced by **paroxetine** 20 mg daily. After 3 days, the tacrolimus dose was increased to 5 mg daily and a satisfactory concentration of 12.4 nanograms/mL was achieved.[1]

A kidney transplant patient taking prednisone, azathioprine, and tacrolimus 5 mg daily for 2 years experienced headache, confusion, and 'grey areas' in her vision within one week of starting **nefazodone** 50 mg twice daily in place of **sertraline**. Her serum creatinine had increased from 132 to 195 micromol/L and her minimum tacrolimus concentration was greater than 30 nanograms/mL. **Nefazodone** was replaced by **sertraline**, and tacrolimus was withheld for 4 days. Signs of tacrolimus-induced neurotoxicity disappeared within 36 hours, and the serum creatinine and tacrolimus concentrations returned to those seen before **nefazodone** was started, within 2 weeks.[2]

Another patient developed increased liver enzymes and tacrolimus concentrations after taking **nefazodone** and tacrolimus for 2 weeks. When the **nefazodone** was stopped his liver enzymes normalised over the next 5 days, and his tacrolimus concentration decreased from 23 to 9.5 nanograms/mL over 10 days.[3]

A report describes a case of serotonin syndrome in a 61-year-old kidney-pancreas transplant patient taking tacrolimus and **venlafaxine** when the venlafaxine dose was increased from 37.5 mg to 75 mg daily, about 5 weeks post-transplant. Her tacrolimus concentration was within the therapeutic range, and symptoms of serotonin syndrome resolved during the days after venlafaxine was stopped.[4]

Mechanism

Tacrolimus is metabolised by CYP3A4, which is inhibited by nefazodone. Concurrent use therefore results in increased concentrations of tacrolimus. Paroxetine and sertraline do not affect CYP3A4 and are therefore not expected to interact with tacrolimus, as seen in the cases. The authors of the case reporting serotonin syndrome with tacrolimus and venlafaxine suggest that inhibition of P-glycoprotein by tacrolimus might have resulted in an increase in desmethylvenlafaxine concentrations.[4] However desmethylvenlafaxine concentrations were not reported for this patient and further research is needed to confirm this theory.

Importance and management

Evidence for an interaction between tacrolimus and nefazodone is limited to case reports, but when taken together, they indicate that tacrolimus concentrations, or at least signs of tacrolimus toxicity, should be closely monitored if nefazodone is also given. In view of the narrow therapeutic index of tacrolimus, it might be advisable to avoid nefazodone. Note that nefazodone has widely been withdrawn due to adverse hepatic effects.

Of the SSRIs, **citalopram**, **fluoxetine**, **paroxetine**, and **sertraline** are not known to affect CYP3A4 activity, and so would not be expected to affect tacrolimus metabolism. They might therefore be suitable alternative antidepressants in patients taking tacrolimus, but until more is known it might be prudent to monitor patients accordingly. **Fluvoxamine**, however, is a weak inhibitor of CYP3A4 and so theoretically could affect the metabolism of tacrolimus. Close monitoring of tacrolimus concentrations would therefore be prudent on concurrent use.

The general relevance of the case of serotonin syndrome with tacrolimus and venlafaxine is unclear, but note that venlafaxine used alone can cause serotonin syndrome and this case might simply be an adverse effect. For more information on serotonin syndrome and its management, see 'Drugs that cause serotonin syndrome + Other drugs that cause serotonin syndrome', p.1471.

1. Campo JV, Smith C, Perel JM. Tacrolimus toxic reaction associated with the use of nefazodone: paroxetine as an alternative agent. *Arch Gen Psychiatry* (1998) 55, 1050–2.
2. Olyaei AJ, deMattos AM, Norman DJ, Bennett WM. Interaction between tacrolimus and nefazodone in a stable renal transplant recipient. *Pharmacotherapy* (1998) 18, 1356–9.
3. Garton T, Nefazodone and CYP450 3A4 interactions with cyclosporine and tacrolimus. *Transplantation* (2002) 74, 745.
4. Newey CR, Khawam E, Coffman K. Two cases of serotonin syndrome with venlafaxine and calcineurin inhibitors. *Psychosomatics* (2011) 52, 286–90.

Tacrolimus + St John's wort (*Hypericum perforatum*)

St John's wort decreases tacrolimus concentrations.

Clinical evidence

In a clinical study, 10 healthy subjects were given a single 100-microgram/kg dose of tacrolimus alone, or after they took St John's wort 300 mg three times daily for 14 days. On average St John's wort decreased the maximum blood concentration of tacrolimus by 65% and decreased its AUC by 32%. However, the decrease in AUC ranged from 15 to 64%, with one patient having a 31% *increase* in AUC.[1] Similar results have been found in a study in 10 kidney transplant patients given St John's wort (*Jarsin 300*) 600 mg daily for 2 weeks. In order to achieve target concentrations, the dose of tacrolimus was increased in all patients, from a median of 4.5 mg daily to 8 mg daily. Two weeks after stopping St John's wort, tacrolimus doses were reduced to a median of 6.5 mg daily, and then to the original dose of 4.5 mg daily after about 4 weeks.[2]

A case report describes a 65-year-old patient taking tacrolimus following a kidney transplant. The patient started to take St John's wort (*Neuroplant*) 600 mg daily, and after one month the minimum blood concentration of tacrolimus had decreased from a range of 6 to 10 nanograms/mL to 1.6 nanograms/mL, with an unexpected improvement in creatinine concentrations. When the St John's wort was stopped, the concentrations of tacrolimus and creatinine returned to the previous range. Subsequently a lower target range of tacrolimus was set.[3]

Mechanism

St John's wort induces CYP3A4 and P-glycoprotein, which are involved in the metabolism and transport of tacrolimus. An increase in their effects would be expected to result in a decrease in tacrolimus concentrations.

Importance and management

Although the evidence seems limited to these reports, the interaction between tacrolimus and St John's wort is consistent with the known disposition and interactions of these drugs. Given the unpredictability of the interaction (and the variability in content of St John's wort products) it would seem prudent to avoid St John's wort in transplant patients, and possibly other patients taking tacrolimus. If St John's wort is started or stopped, monitor tacrolimus concentrations and adjust the dose accordingly.

1. Hebert MF, Park JM, Chen Y-L, Akhtar S, Larson AM. Effects of St John's wort (Hypericum perforatum) on tacrolimus pharmacokinetics in healthy volunteers. *J Clin Pharmacol* (2004) 44, 89–94.
2. Mai I, Störmer E, Bauer S, Krüger H, Budde K, Roots I. Impact of St John's wort treatment on the pharmacokinetics of tacrolimus and mycophenolic acid in renal transplant patients. *Nephrol Dial Transplant* (2003) 18, 819–22.
3. Bolley R, Zülke C, Kammerl M, Fischereder M, Krämer BK. Tacrolimus-induced nephrotoxicity unmasked by induction of the CYP3A4 system with St John's wort. *Transplantation* (2002) 73, 1009.

Tacrolimus + Theophylline

An isolated report suggests that theophylline might increase tacrolimus concentrations.

Clinical evidence

A kidney transplant patient taking tacrolimus 7 mg daily was given theophylline 600 mg daily to treat post-transplant erythrocytosis. After one month, serum creatinine concentrations increased from 110 to 145 micromol/L and the tacrolimus minimum blood concentration increased to 16 nanograms/mL, from within the normal range of 5 to 15 nanograms/mL. The theophylline dose was reduced to 300 mg daily on 4 days of each week, and one month later the serum creatinine concentration was 175 micromol/L and the minimum tacrolimus concentration was 48.5 nanograms/mL. Theophylline was discontinued and the renal function and minimum tacrolimus concentrations rapidly returned to normal. Subsequently, the erythrocytosis was still uncontrolled and theophylline was tried again. This time the pharmacokinetics of tacrolimus were assessed, and theophylline 125 mg daily for 4 days was associated with an increase in the maximum tacrolimus blood concentrations from 19.3 to 37.4 nanograms/mL, but the renal function remained stable.[1]

Mechanism

Unknown.

Importance and management

Evidence regarding an interaction between tacrolimus and theophylline is limited to this single case report. As such it is of uncertain clinical importance. There is insufficient evidence to recommend increased monitoring of tacrolimus in every patient, but be aware of the potential for an interaction in cases of an unexpected increase in tacrolimus adverse effects.

1. Boubenider S, Vincent I, Lambotte O, Roy S, Hiesse C, Taburet A-M, Charpentier B. Interaction between theophylline and tacrolimus in a renal transplant patient. *Nephrol Dial Transplant* (2000) 15, 1066–8.

Tacrolimus + Tigecycline

An isolated case report describes a large increase in the concentration of tacrolimus in a patient after starting tigecycline.

Clinical evidence

A brief report describes a 51-year-old kidney transplant patient taking tacrolimus (dose not stated), whose tacrolimus concentration increased about 5-fold, within a day of starting intravenous tigecycline (dose not stated). The tacrolimus dose was reduced and tigecycline continued for a total of 6 days, during which time the tacrolimus concentration returned to baseline. When tigecycline was stopped, her tacrolimus concentration became subtherapeutic and a corresponding increase in the tacrolimus dose was required to return the concentration to within the therapeutic range.[1]

Mechanism

Not understood. The authors suggest that tigecycline might have inhibited CYP3A4, the isoenzyme involved in the metabolism of tacrolimus; however, *in vitro* tigecycline has been shown not to affect this isoenzyme.[2] Further study is needed.

Importance and management

Evidence for an interaction between tacrolimus and tigecycline is limited to this isolated case and as such its general importance is unclear. However, given the potential implications of such large variations in tacrolimus concentrations, it would seem prudent to increase the frequency of monitoring tacrolimus concentrations on concurrent use, and adjust the tacrolimus dose if necessary.

1. Pavan M, Chaudhari AP, Ranganth R. Altered bioavailability of tacrolimus following intravenous administration of tigecycline. *Am J Kidney Dis* (2011) 57, 354.
2. Tygacil (Tigecycline). Pfizer Ltd. UK Summary of product characteristics, November 2013.

Tacrolimus + Tyrosine kinase inhibitors

Imatinib increases tacrolimus concentrations. Tacrolimus very slightly increases tofacitinib exposure.

Clinical evidence

(a) Imatinib

One study, in patients with leukaemia who had undergone stem cell transplantation, found that the concentrations of tacrolimus were increased by 25 to 33% within 72 hours of starting imatinib. An empiric tacrolimus dose reduction of 25% at the start of imatinib treatment was found to prevent further serum concentration fluctuations.[1]

(b) Tofacitinib

A preliminary report of a pharmacokinetic study in 12 healthy subjects given tacrolimus 5 mg twice daily for 8 days followed by a single 10-mg dose of tofacitinib with a final 5 mg dose of tacrolimus on day 9, describes a 21% increase in the AUC of tofacitinib and a 9% decrease in the maximum concentration.[2]

Mechanism

Imatinib is an inhibitor of CYP3A4, by which tacrolimus is metabolised, and it would therefore be expected to increase its concentrations.

Importance and management

Evidence for a pharmacokinetic interaction between imatinib and tacrolimus is limited to this one study, but based on the likely mechanism and the increase in concentrations reported when imatinib was taken with the sensitive CYP3A4 substrate, simvastatin (see 'Statins + Tyrosine kinase inhibitors', p.1357), it would be prudent to monitor tacrolimus concentrations on starting or stopping imatinib. Evidence with other tyrosine kinase inhibitors is lacking, but note that some also inhibit CYP3A4 (see 'Table 1.9', p.11) and might be predicted to interact similarly. Similar precautions with these drugs would seem prudent.

The very slight increase in tofacitinib exposure suggests that no clinically important pharmacokinetic interaction occurs between tacrolimus and tofacitinib, such that no tofacitinib dose adjustment would seem necessary on concurrent use. Note that the US manufacturer warns of the risk of increased immunosuppression if these drugs are given together.[3] Some caution would seem prudent.

1. Sheth SR, Hicks K, Ippoliti C, Giralt , Champlin RE, Anderlini P. Safety, tolerability, and drug interactions of adjuvant imatinib mesylate (Gleevec) within the first 100 days following stem cell transplantation (SCT) in patients with Ph+ CML and PH+ ALL at high risk for recurrence. *Blood* (2002) 100, Abstract 2500.
2. Lamba M, Redifer P, Wang R, Alvey C, Krishnaswami S, Chan G. Effect of co-administration of multiple-dose tacrolimus and cyclosporine on the pharmacokinetics of tasocitinib (CP-690,550) in healthy volunteers. *Clin Pharmacol Ther* (2011) 89 (Suppl 1), S22.
3. Xeljanz (Tofacitinib citrate). Pfizer Inc. US Prescribing information, November 2012.

Temsirolimus + Ketoconazole and other CYP3A4 inhibitors

Ketoconazole greatly increases the concentrations of temsirolimus and its active metabolite, sirolimus. Other potent CYP3A4 inhibitors are expected to interact similarly.

Clinical evidence

To determine the effect of ketoconazole on the pharmacokinetics of temsirolimus, 14 healthy subjects were given a single 5 mg intravenous dose of temsirolimus alone, or 2 hours after the first dose of ketoconazole 400 mg daily for 7 days. There were no changes in the pharmacokinetics of temsirolimus, but the maximum plasma concentration and AUC of the active metabolite, sirolimus, were increased 2.2-fold and 3.2-fold, respectively.[1] In a study of *oral* temsirolimus (not the clinically used route of administration), the AUC of a 2-mg dose, given on day 5 of a 10-day course of ketoconazole 200 mg daily, was increased 7-fold and the AUC of the sirolimus metabolite was increased 9-fold.[2]

Mechanism

Ketoconazole is a potent inhibitor of CYP3A4 and also inhibits P-glycoprotein. Temsirolimus is metabolised by CYP3A4 to sirolimus, which is the major metabolite after intravenous administration, and is equipotent to temsirolimus.[3] Sirolimus is itself also metabolised by CYP3A4, and appears to be more sensitive to CYP3A4 inhibition than temsirolimus. Both sirolimus and temsirolimus are also substrates of P-glycoprotein. Ketoconazole had a much greater effect on oral temsirolimus than intravenous temsirolimus suggesting that intravenous administration bypasses significant gastrointestinal metabolism.

Importance and management

Although the evidence is limited, based on the likely mechanisms and large increases seen in the studies above, an interaction between ketoconazole and temsirolimus would appear to be established. As all of the azoles inhibit CYP3A4 to varying degrees, see *Azoles*, under 'Anthelmintics, Antifungals, and Antiprotozoals', p.225, they would be expected to interact similarly. Note that the intravenous study used a very low dose of temsirolimus, and it is possible that increased exposure to sirolimus with the clinically recommended doses of intravenous temsirolimus would give rise to greater increases in toxicity. The authors suggest reducing the temsirolimus dose by half if they are also given potent inhibitors of CYP3A4. They also advise, that if the CYP3A4 inhibitor is stopped, a one week washout period should be allowed before increasing temsirolimus back up to the original dose.[1] The UK and US manufacturers of temsirolimus predict that other potent inhibitors of CYP3A4 will interact similarly;[3,4] see 'Table 1.9', p.11 for a list of known clinically important CYP3A4 inhibitors. Note that in addition to those drugs listed in this table, the manufacturers include nefazodone as a potent CYP3A4 inhibitor, but this is generally considered a moderate inhibitor of CYP3A4 (see below for relevant advice). The UK manufacturer advises avoiding concurrent use with such drugs, whereas the US manufacturer suggests considering halving the temsirolimus dose if concurrent use is considered essential.[4]

The UK manufacturer[3] also suggests that the concurrent use of temsirolimus and moderate inhibitors of CYP3A4 should be used with caution in patients taking temsirolimus 25 mg [weekly], and should be avoided in patients taking doses of greater than 25 mg weekly. 'Table 1.9', p.11 includes a list of known clinically important moderate CYP3A4 inhibitors. Note that in addition to the drugs listed in this table, they also include amiodarone, clarithromycin, and grapefruit juice as moderate CYP3A4 inhibitors. However, amiodarone is not considered a clinically relevant inhibitor of CYP3A4, and clarithromycin is a potent inhibitor (see above for relevant advice). The US manufacturer recommends avoiding grapefruit juice,[4] but note that grapefruit juice is considered to be a weak CYP3A4 inhibitor and as the main interactions of grapefruit juice are with orally administered drugs (temsirolimus bypasses gastrointestinal metabolism because it is used intravenously), it would not be expected to have any relevant effect. Aprepitant has both a moderate *inhibiting* effect and a weak (albeit transient) *inducing* effect on CYP3A4, which usually occurs 3 to 5 days after it has been stopped.

1. Boni JP, Leister C, Burns J, Hug B. Differential effects of ketoconazole on exposure to temsirolimus following intravenous infusion of temsirolimus. *Br J Cancer* (2008) 98, 1797–1802.
2. Shu C, Afsharvand M, Raible D, Zhou J. Effect of ketoconazole on the temsirolimus pharmacokinetic profile in healthy subjects. *Clin Pharmacol Ther* (2005) P34.
3. Torisel (Temsirolimus). Pfizer Ltd. UK Summary of product characteristics, October 2013.
4. Torisel (Temsirolimus). Wyeth Pharmaceuticals Inc. US Prescribing information, October 2014.

Temsirolimus + Rifampicin (Rifampin) and other CYP3A4 inducers

Rifampicin, phenytoin, and carbamazepine greatly reduce the concentrations of the active metabolite of temsirolimus, sirolimus, after administration of intravenous temsirolimus. Other potent CYP3A4 inducers are expected to interact similarly.

Clinical evidence

(a) Antiepileptics

In a study in patients with malignant gliomas, the maximum tolerated dose of intravenous temsirolimus was 250 mg in patients taking enzyme-inducing antiepileptics, compared with 170 mg in patients taking non-enzyme-inducing antiepileptics. The sum of the AUC of temsirolimus and sirolimus was 50% lower in the patients taking enzyme-inducing antiepileptics, despite taking a higher temsirolimus dose. At comparable doses, the AUC for temsirolimus did not differ between the groups, but that for sirolimus was 53% lower in the enzyme-inducing antiepileptic group. The majority of the patients in the enzyme-inducing antiepileptics group were taking **phenytoin** (47%); other drugs used being **carbamazepine, oxcarbazepine, fosphenytoin, phenobarbital**, and **primidone**.[1]

In another similar study, the AUC of sirolimus was 43% lower in 11 patients receiving **carbamazepine** or **phenytoin** than in 14 patients not receiving enzyme inducers. The AUC of temsirolimus was 15% lower (not statistically significant).[2]

(b) Rifampicin

In a study in healthy subjects, a single dose of oral or intravenous temsirolimus was given on the sixth day of rifampicin 600 mg daily for 14 days. With *intravenous* temsirolimus, rifampicin reduced the maximum plasma concentration and AUC of sirolimus by 65% and 56%, respectively, but had no effect on the pharmacokinetics of temsirolimus. With *oral* temsirolimus, rifampicin had a similar effect on sirolimus pharmacokinetics (63% and 60% reduction in maximum concentration and AUC, respectively) and also reduced the temsirolimus maximum concentration and AUC, by 41% and 30%, respectively.[2]

Mechanism

Rifampicin and some antiepileptics (carbamazepine, phenytoin, phenobarbital, primidone) are all known inducers of CYP3A4, and rifampicin and carbamazepine are also known to induce P-glycoprotein. Temsirolimus is metabolised by CYP3A4 to sirolimus, which is the major metabolite after intravenous administration, and is equipotent to temsirolimus.[3] Concurrent use with these CYP3A4 inducers therefore results in decreased concentrations. Sirolimus is itself metabolised by CYP3A4, and appears to be more sensitive to CYP3A4 induction than temsirolimus. Both sirolimus and temsirolimus are also substrates of P-glycoprotein, and some involvement of this mechanism in the effects seen with rifampicin or carbamazepine cannot be ruled out. Rifampicin had a much greater effect on oral temsirolimus than intravenous, suggesting that intravenous administration bypasses significant gastrointestinal metabolism.

Importance and management

Evidence is limited, but an interaction between rifampicin, or enzyme-inducing antiepileptics, and temsirolimus would seem to be established. The reductions seen in the concentrations of the active metabolite of temsirolimus after intravenous administration (the usual clinical route) with these drugs are less than after oral temsirolimus, but could well be clinically important. The UK and US manufacturers generally advise avoiding other drugs that are potent inducers of CYP3A4;[3,4] see 'Table 1.9', p.11 for a list of known clinically important CYP3A4 inducers. However, in the UK, specific advice is given according to the indication for the temsirolimus, as follows: for renal cell cancer, avoidance is recommended only if the CYP3A4 inducer is continued beyond an initial 5 to 7 days, and for mantle cell lymphoma, concurrent use is not recommended because of the higher dose of temsirolimus used for this condition.[3] In the US, if treatment with a potent CYP3A4 inducer is essential, the manufacturer recommends that the dose of temsirolimus in patients with renal cell cancer should be doubled while the CYP3A4 inducer is being taken, and readjusted when the inducer is stopped.[4] In addition to the drugs listed in the table, the US manufacturer includes rifabutin and dexamethasone, and the UK manufacturer includes St John's wort. However, note that clinically important interactions with dexamethasone as a result of this mechanism appear to be rare. Further, rifabutin and St John's wort generally behave as moderate inducers, and so their effects would be expected to be less. However, the use of St John's wort is not recommended by the manufacturers.[3,4]

It is important to remember that the extent of the inducing effects of these drugs is not identical, so that large effects like those observed with rifampicin might not occur with other inducers; nevertheless the interaction might still be clinically important.

1. Kuhn JG, Chang SM, Wen PY, Cloughesy TF, Greenberg H, Schiff D, Conrad C, Fink KL, Robins HI, Mehta M, DeAngelis L, Raizer J, Hess K, Lamborn KR, Dancey J, Prados MD; North American Brain Tumor Consortium and the National Cancer Institute. Pharmacokinetic and tumor distribution characteristics of temsirolimus in patients with recurrent malignant glioma. *Clin Cancer Res* (2007) 13, 7401–6.
2. Boni J, Leister C, Burns J, Cincotta M, Hug B, Moore L. Pharmacokinetic profile of temsirolimus with concomitant administration of cytochrome p450-inducing medications. *J Clin Pharmacol* (2007) 47, 1430–9.
3. Torisel (Temsirolimus). Pfizer Ltd. UK Summary of product characteristics, October 2013.
4. Torisel (Temsirolimus). Wyeth Pharmaceuticals Inc. US Prescribing information, October 2014.

30

Lipid regulating drugs

This section is concerned with the drugs that are used for dyslipidaemias (i.e. disturbed concentrations of lipids in the blood). In the very broadest of terms (and ideally) they lower the blood concentrations of cholesterol and low-density lipoprotein (LDL), and raise those of high-density lipoprotein (HDL); however, none have this ideal profile. Lipid lowering drugs include the statins (more properly known as HMG-CoA (hydroxymethylglutaryl-coenzyme A) reductase inhibitors), fibrates, ezetimibe, bile-acid binding resins (e.g. colestipol, colestyramine) and nicotinic acid (niacin) and related drugs. These are listed in 'Table 30.1', below. Bile acids (e.g. ursodeoxycholic acid), which affect cholesterol concentrations in the bile are also included in this chapter. Where lipid regulating drugs or bile acids affect other drugs, the interactions are covered elsewhere.

Table 30.1 Lipid regulating drugs

Group	*Drugs*
Apolipoprotein B inhibitors	Mipomersen
Bile-acid binding resins	Colesevelam, Colestilan, Colestipol, Colestyramine
CETP inhibitors	Anacetrapib, Dalcetrapib
Cholesterol absorption inhibitors	Ezetimibe
Fibrates	Bezafibrate, Ciprofibrate, Clofibrate, Fenofibrate, Gemfibrozil
Nicotinic acid group	Acipimox, Nicotinic acid (Niacin)
Omega-3 fatty acids	Omega-3 acid ethyl esters, Omega-3 marine triglycerides
Statins	Atorvastatin, Fluvastatin, Lovastatin, Pitavastatin, Pravastatin, Rosuvastatin, Simvastatin
Miscellaneous	Lomitapide, Policosanol

A. Statins

(a) Muscle and liver toxicity

Statins are generally well tolerated, although they have two major but relatively uncommon adverse effects. They raise liver enzymes, and can cause skeletal muscle disorders (e.g. myalgia, myopathy and rhabdomyolysis). Rhabdomyolysis is a rare syndrome resulting from skeletal muscle injury, which results in the release of the enzyme creatine kinase (among other things) into the circulation. Creatine kinase (CK) is also known as creatine phosphokinase (CPK). Both terms are used throughout the text, the choice being dependent on the term used in the source quoted. Reports of muscle disorders associated with statins have not always been consistent in their definitions, although the generally accepted definition of myopathy is myalgia (muscle pain or soreness), weakness, and/or cramps plus a CK concentration greater than 10 times the upper limit of normal; rhabdomyolysis has been defined as a CK concentration of greater than 10 000 units/L or a CK concentration greater than 10 times the upper concentration or normal with worsening renal function and/or a requirement for medical intervention with intravenous hydration.[1] As well as elevated creatine kinase concentrations, signs and symptoms of rhabdomyolysis include muscle pain and weakness and reddish-brown urine (myoglobinuria).[2]

Just how statins cause muscle disorders is as yet unclear, although it is thought to be connected to elevated statin concentrations[3] and might vary with individual statins, due to lipophilicity and pharmacokinetic differences. Similarly, elevated hepatic transaminases are dose dependent, although progression to liver failure is exceedingly rare.[4] Any pharmacokinetic interaction that results in a marked rise in statin concentrations is therefore to be regarded seriously.

One of the ways blood statin concentrations can become elevated is if the interacting drug inhibits the metabolism of the statin, with the result that it is cleared more slowly and it begins to accumulate (see pharmacokinetics below). The overall risk of myopathy with the statins at standard therapeutic doses is quite low and commonly quoted as 0.01 to 0.1%, although in clinical studies involving patients taking statins, muscle symptoms have been reported to occur in 1.5 to 3% of patients.[1] A further report[5] puts the incidence of mild myopathies with a statin alone as up to 7%, while another observational study found mild to moderate muscular symptoms occurred in 10.5% of patients given a high dose of a statin.[6] However, it has been estimated that for every 15 million prescriptions there is only one occurrence of severe muscle damage.[7] The incidence seems to rise markedly if other interacting drugs are being taken concurrently. Thus a literature review of published reports for the period 1985 to 2000 found 15 cases of rhabdomyolysis with statins alone, but 54 cases when then statin was given with potentially interacting drugs.[3] Similarly, in a review of adverse reactions to statins in the Swedish Adverse Drug Reactions Advisory Committee until September 2006, the incidence of confirmed rhabdomyolysis was sixfold higher in cases with concurrent interacting drugs than in those without.[8] Other patient-related risk factors for myopathy include:[4]

- Advanced age (especially greater than 70 to 80 years),
- Frailty,
- Multisystem disease (e.g. chronic renal impairment, especially due to diabetes),
- The perioperative period,
- Hypothyroidism,
- Alcohol abuse,
- Female sex.

In order to reduce the risk of myopathy the CSM in the UK have advised that statins should be used with care in patients who are at increased risk of this adverse effect. Among other risk factors, they mention the concurrent use of fibrates such as gemfibrozil (see 'Statins + Fibrates; Gemfibrozil', p.1338), ciclosporin (see 'Statins + Ciclosporin', p.1327), macrolides (see 'Statins + Macrolides', p.1348), azoles (see 'Statins + Azoles', p.1322), and HIV-protease inhibitors (see 'Statins + HIV-protease inhibitors', p.1345). They also recommend that patients should be made aware of the risks of myopathy and rhabdomyolysis, and asked to promptly report muscle pain, tenderness, or weakness, especially if this is accompanied by malaise, fever, or dark urine.[9] The American College of Cardiology/American Heart Association/National Heart, Lung and Blood Institute (ACC/AHA/NHLBI) Clinical Advisory on Statins[4] and the National Lipid Association Safety Assessment Task Force[1] give some important safety recommendations, which are useful in the context of interactions:

- Routine monitoring of creatine kinase is of little value in the absence of clinical symptoms.
- If a patient has intolerable muscle symptoms or a creatine kinase value 10 times the upper limit of normal, and is symptomatic, statin treatment should be immediately discontinued.
- If a patient has symptoms of muscle pain with a creatine kinase of up to 10 times the upper limit of normal they should be monitored closely. The statin may be continued at the same or reduced doses and symptoms and creatine kinase concentrations can be used as the clinical guide to stop or continue treatment.

- If progressive creatine kinase elevations occur consider a dose reduction or temporary discontinuation of the statin.
- Liver transaminase concentrations should be obtained during routine general evaluation of patients being considered for a statin.
- Liver enzyme values of up to 3 times the upper limit of normal do not represent a contraindication to treatment but patients should be carefully monitored.

In June 2011, the FDA in the US restricted the use of the highest approved dose of simvastatin (80 mg daily) because of the increased risk of muscle injury with this dose relative to lower doses. They state that simvastatin 80 mg daily should no longer be used, except in patients who have already been established on this dose for more than 12 months without any evidence of muscle injury.[10] This advice was principally based on evidence from the SEARCH study[11] in which the incidence of myopathy was 0.9% in those receiving simvastatin 80 mg daily compared with just 0.03% in those receiving simvastatin 20 mg daily. In addition, 0.1% of subjects taking the high dose of simvastatin were diagnosed with rhabdomyolysis, compared with no subjects taking the low simvastatin dose. A genetic variant of the gene encoding the OAT1B1 transporter (see *Organic anion uptake transporters*, below) appeared to be associated with an increased risk of myopathy with simvastatin.[11]

(b) Pharmacokinetics

1. Cytochrome P450 isoenzymes. Lovastatin and simvastatin are extensively metabolised by CYP3A4, and drugs that inhibit this isoenzyme can cause marked rises in blood statin concentrations. Atorvastatin is also metabolised by CYP3A4, but to a lesser extent than lovastatin or simvastatin. Some of the statins are not metabolised by this isoenzyme so they interact differently. Fluvastatin is metabolised primarily by CYP2C9 (with a minor contribution from other isoenzymes, including CYP3A4), only 10% of rosuvastatin is metabolised, and the isoenzymes involved appear to be CYP2C9 and CYP2C19, while the cytochrome P450 system is minimally involved in the metabolism of pravastatin and pitavastatin.[12,13] Fluvastatin is a weak inhibitor of CYP2C9, see, for example, 'Coumarins and related drugs + Statins', p.471.

2. Organic anion uptake transporters. Hepatic uptake and biliary excretion are also important in statin elimination, and multiple uptake transporters including the organic anion transporting polypeptide (OATP) 1B1 (also known as OATP-C, OATP2, and LST-1) play an important role in the clearance of statins. Atorvastatin, pitavastatin, pravastatin and rosuvastatin have all been reported to be OATP1B1 substrates,[13] (see also 'Statins + Ciclosporin', p.1327), and there is increasing evidence that genetic polymorphisms in the gene encoding this transporter, *SLCO1B1*, are related to the risk of statin-induced myopathy.[14]

3. P-glycoprotein. The statins are also P-glycoprotein substrates, and inhibitors of this carrier might therefore interact resulting in altered oral bioavailability.[12] However, *in vitro* study has suggested that, due to the low affinity of atorvastatin and simvastatin for P-glycoprotein this is unlikely to be a clinically relevant cause of statin drug interactions.[15] Atorvastatin, fluvastatin and simvastatin have been shown to minimally inhibit P-glycoprotein, while pravastatin and rosuvastatin seem to have no effect, see 'Digoxin and related drugs + Statins', p.1111.

B. Bile-acid binding resins

Bile-acid binding resins lower cholesterol by binding with bile acids in the gastrointestinal tract to form an insoluble complex that is excreted in the faeces. This reduces enterohepatic recirculation of the bile acids resulting in increased oxidation of cholesterol to form more bile acids to replace them, thus reducing cholesterol concentrations. These resins can cause interactions by binding with other drugs in the same way as they do with bile acids, which prevents absorption or local action of the affected drug. A new bile-acid binding resin, colesevelam, is supposed to be devoid of clinically relevant drug-binding interactions.[16]

C. CETP inhibitors

Cholesteryl ester transfer protein (CETP) inhibitors are a newer class of drugs that raise HDL-cholesterol concentrations. Anacetrapib and dalcetrapib do not appear to alter the activity of cytochrome P450 isoenzymes. Anacetrapib is a CYP3A4 substrate, and its absorption is sensitive to food effects.

D. Ezetimibe

Ezetimibe is a cholesterol absorption inhibitor: it and its major metabolite, ezetimibe glucuronide, impair the intestinal absorption of cholesterol, both from the diet and cholesterol secreted in the bile.[17] The absorption of other fats is not affected. Ezetimibe has not been found to have important effects on cytochrome P450, suggesting it is unlikely to interact with other drugs by this mechanism.

E. Fibrates

Fibrates differ in their metabolism, although most are excreted renally often conjugated with glucuronide. Up to half of a dose of bezafibrate is excreted unchanged in the urine with 20% as the glucuronide conjugate. Fenofibrate undergoes metabolism to the active acid form by esterases, and is then conjugated with glucuronide and excreted in the urine. Gemfibrozil is metabolised by oxidation to inactive metabolites (enzymes involved not known), and subsequently, conjugated to the glucuronide, which is then excreted in urine. Fibrates are highly protein bound, and although protein binding contributes to their interactions, this mechanism alone does not usually lead to clinically important interactions. Fibrates are not generally recognised as inhibitors or inducers of cytochrome P450 isoenzymes, although gemfibrozil is a clinically important inhibitor of CYP2C8. In addition, gemfibrozil inhibits the transport protein OATP1B1, and seems to increase the plasma concentrations of most statins (see 'Statins + Fibrates; Gemfibrozil', p.1338), whereas bezafibrate and fenofibrate have less effect on statin bioavailability. As with the statins (see above), fibrates are also recognised as causing myopathies, and the risk of this appears to be greatly increased when they are given with statins, see 'Statins + Fibrates; Miscellaneous', p.1339.

F. Nicotinic acid (Niacin)

Nicotinic acid has little effect on cytochrome P450 isoenzymes and is therefore unlikely to cause pharmacokinetic interactions via this mechanism. It might possibly increase the risk of myopathies when given with statins, see 'Statins + Nicotinic acid (Niacin)', p.1351. **Acipimox** is an analogue of nicotinic acid, and might therefore be expected to share its interactions.

1. McKenney JM, Davidson MH, Jacobson TA, Guyton JR. Final conclusions and recommendations of the National Lipid Association Statin Safety Assessment Task Force. *Am J Cardiol* (2006) 97 (Suppl), 89C–94C.
2. Allison RC, Bedsole DL. The other medical causes of rhabdomyolysis. *Am J Med Sci* (2003) 326, 79–88.
3. Omar MA, Wilson JP, Cox TS. Rhabdomyolysis and HMG-CoA reductase inhibitors. *Ann Pharmacother* (2001) 35, 1096–1107.
4. Pasternak RC, Smith SC, Bairey-Merz CN, Grundy SM, Cleeman JI, Lenfant C. ACC/AHA/NHLBI clinical advisory on the use and safety of statins. *J Am Coll Cardiol* (2002) 40, 567–72.
5. Ucar M, Mjörndal T, Dahlqvist R, HMG-CoA reductase inhibitors and myotoxicity. *Drug Safety* (2000) 22, 441–57.
6. Bruckert E, Hayem G, Dejager S, Yau C, Bégaud B. Mild to moderate muscular symptoms with high-dosage statin therapy in hyperlipidemic patients—the PRIMO study. *Cardiovasc Drugs Ther* (2005) 19, 403–14.
7. Thompson, PD, Clarkson PM, Rosenson RS; the National Lipid Association's Muscle Safety Expert Panel. An Assessment of statin safety by muscle experts. *Am J Cardiol* (2006) 97 (Suppl), 69C–76C.
8. Hedenmalm K, Alvan G, Öhagen P, Dahl M-L. Muscle toxicity with statins. *Pharmacoepidemiol Drug Safety* (2010) 19, 223–31.
9. Committee on Safety of Medicines/Medicines Control Agency. HMG CoA reductase inhibitors (statins) and myopathy. *Current Problems* (2002) 28, 8–9.
10. FDA safety communication: new restrictions, contraindications, and dose limitations for Zocor (simvastatin) to reduce the risk of muscle injury, June 8, 2011. Available at: http://www.fda.gov/Drugs/DrugSafety/ucm256581.htm (accessed 22/10/15).
11. Study of the Effectiveness of Additional Reductions in Cholesterol and Homocysteine (SEARCH) collaborative group, Armitage J, Bowman L, Wallendszus K, Bulbulia R, Rahimi K, Haynes R, Parish S, Peto R, Collins R. Intensive lowering of LDL cholesterol with 80 mg versus 20 mg simvastatin daily in 12 064 survivors of myocardial infarction: a double-blind randomised trial. *Lancet* (2010) 376, 1658–69. Erratum in: ibid. (2011) 377, 126.
12. Williams D, Feely J. Pharmacokinetic-pharmacodynamic drug interactions with HMG-CoA reductase inhibitors. *Clin Pharmacokinet* (2002) 41, 343–70.
13. Shitara Y, Sugiyama Y. Pharmacokinetic and pharmacodynamic alterations of 3-hydroxy-3-methylglutaryl coenzyme A (HMG-CoA) reductase inhibitors: drug-drug interactions and interindividual differences in transporter and metabolic enzyme functions. *Pharmacol Ther* (2006) 112, 71–105.
14. Romaine SPR, Bailey KM, Hall AS, Balmforth AJ. The influence of *SLCO1B1* (OATP1B1) gene polymorphisms on response to statin therapy. *Pharmacogenomics J* (2010) 10, 1–11.
15. Hochman JH, Pudvah N, Qiu J, Yamazaki M, Tang C, Lin JH, Prueksaritanont T. Interactions of human P-glycoprotein with simvastatin, simvastatin acid, and atorvastatin. *Pharm Res* (2004) 21, 1686–91.
16. Donovan JM, Stypinski D, Stiles MR, Olson TA, Burke SK. Drug interactions with colesevelam hydrochloride, a novel, potent lipid-lowering agent. *Cardiovasc Drugs Ther* (2000) 14, 681–90.
17. Simard C, Turgeon J. The pharmacokinetics of ezetimibe. *Can J Clin Pharmacol* (2003) 10 (Suppl A), 13A–20A.

Acipimox + Colestyramine

Colestyramine does not appear to alter the pharmacokinetics of acipimox.

Clinical evidence, mechanism, importance and management

In a controlled study, 7 healthy subjects were given colestyramine 4 g eight-hourly for 2 days with a single 150-mg dose of acipimox given simultaneously with the first colestyramine dose on the second day. The pharmacokinetics of acipimox were not altered by colestyramine except for a slight delay in absorption (time to maximum level delayed from 1.7 hours to 2.4 hours), which is not clinically relevant.[1] There would seem to be no need to separate administration during concurrent use.

1. de Paolis C, Farina R, Pianezzola E, Valzelli G, Celotti F, Pontiroli AE. Lack of pharmacokinetic interaction between cholestyramine and acipimox, a new lipid lowering agent. *Br J Clin Pharmacol* (1986) 22, 496–7.

CETP inhibitors + Cytochrome P450 substrates

Neither anacetrapib nor dalcetrapib alter midazolam pharmacokinetics. Dalcetrapib does not alter the pharmacokinetics of caffeine, dextromethorphan, omeprazole, rosiglitazone, or warfarin, and anacetrapib similarly appears to lack pharmacokinetic effects on these drugs.

Clinical evidence, mechanism, importance and management

(a) Caffeine

In a pharmacokinetic probe study in 18 healthy subjects,[1] **dalcetrapib** 900 mg daily for 8 days reduced the metabolite to parent urinary clearance ratio of caffeine by about 20%. Caffeine is a probe substrate for CYP1A2, and this study was conducted, because **dalcetrapib** inhibited CYP1A2 *in vitro*. However, the findings show that, at higher than clinically anticipated doses, **dalcetrapib** has no clinically relevant effect on CYP1A2.

Anacetrapib has no effect on CYP1A2 *in vitro*,[2] and would not therefore interact by this mechanism clinically.

Anacetrapib and **dalcetrapib** are therefore not expected to affect the pharmacokinetics of drugs that are substrates for CYP1A2 by this mechanism. See 'Table 1.2', p.5, for a list of CYP1A2 substrates.

(b) Dextromethorphan

In a pharmacokinetic probe study in 18 healthy subjects,[1] **dalcetrapib** 900 mg daily for 8 days had no effect on the metabolite to parent urinary clearance ratio of dextromethorphan. Dextromethorphan is a probe substrate of CYP2D6, and this study was conducted because **dalcetrapib** inhibited CYP2D6 *in vitro*. However, the findings show that, at higher than clinically anticipated doses, **dalcetrapib** has no effect on CYP2D6.

Anacetrapib has no effect on CYP2D6 *in vitro*,[2] and would not therefore interact by this mechanism clinically.

Anacetrapib and **dalcetrapib** are therefore not expected to affect the pharmacokinetics of drugs that are substrates for CYP2D6 by this mechanism. See 'Table 1.7', p.9, for a list of CYP2D6 substrates.

(c) Midazolam

In a pharmacokinetic study in 8 healthy subjects, **anacetrapib** 150 mg daily for 14 days had no effect on the pharmacokinetics of midazolam when a single 2-mg dose was given on the last day.[2] Similarly, in a pharmacokinetic probe study in healthy subjects, **dalcetrapib** 900 mg daily for 8 days had no effect on the AUC of midazolam.[1] Midazolam is a sensitive probe substrate for CYP3A4; therefore, these studies show that neither **anacetrapib** nor **dalcetrapib** have any effect on CYP3A4.

Anacetrapib and **dalcetrapib** are therefore not expected to affect the pharmacokinetics of drugs that are substrates for CYP3A4 by this mechanism. See 'Table 1.10', p.12, for a list of CYP3A4 substrates.

(d) Omeprazole

In a pharmacokinetic probe study in 18 healthy subjects,[1] **dalcetrapib** 900 mg daily for 8 days had no effect on the AUC metabolite-to-parent ratio of omeprazole. Omeprazole is a probe substrate for CYP2C19, and this study was conducted because **dalcetrapib** inhibited CYP2C19 *in vitro*. However, the findings show that, at higher than clinically anticipated doses, **dalcetrapib** has no effect on CYP2C19.

Anacetrapib has no effect on CYP2C19 *in vitro*,[2] and would not therefore interact by this mechanism clinically.

Anacetrapib and **dalcetrapib** are therefore not expected to affect the pharmacokinetics of drugs that are substrates for CYP2C19 by this mechanism. See 'Table 1.6', p.8, for a list of CYP2C19 substrates.

(e) Rosiglitazone

In a pharmacokinetic study in 18 healthy subjects,[1] **dalcetrapib** 900 mg daily for 8 days had no effect on the AUC of rosiglitazone when a single 4-mg dose was given 2 hours after **dalcetrapib** on day 8. Rosiglitazone is metabolised by CYP2C8, and this study was conducted because **dalcetrapib** inhibited CYP2C8 *in vitro*. However, the findings show that, at higher than clinically anticipated doses, **dalcetrapib** has no effect on CYP2C8.

Anacetrapib has no effect on CYP2C8 *in vitro*,[2] and would not therefore interact by this mechanism clinically.

Anacetrapib and **dalcetrapib** are therefore not expected to affect the pharmacokinetics of drugs that are substrates for CYP2C8 by this mechanism. See 'Table 1.4', p.6, for a list of CYP2C8 substrates.

(f) Warfarin

In a pharmacokinetic probe study in 18 healthy subjects,[1] **dalcetrapib** 900 mg daily for 8 days decreased the AUC of *S*-warfarin by 14% when a single 5-mg dose of warfarin was given on day 8. Warfarin is a probe substrate for CYP2C9, and this study was conducted because **dalcetrapib** inhibited CYP2C9 *in vitro*, but, the findings show that, at higher than clinically anticipated doses, **dalcetrapib** has no effect on CYP2C9.

Anacetrapib has no effect on CYP2C9 *in vitro*,[2] and clinically this has been confirmed *in vivo*. In a randomised study in 11 healthy subjects,[3] anacetrapib 100 mg daily for 21 days did not alter the pharmacokinetics of a single 30-mg dose of warfarin given on day 15. No warfarin dose adjustment would seem necessary on concurrent use.

Anacetrapib and **dalcetrapib** are therefore not expected to affect the pharmacokinetics of drugs that are substrates for CYP2C9 by this mechanism. See 'Table 1.5', p.7, for a list of CYP2C9 substrates.

1. Derks M, Fowler S, Kuhlmann O. *In vitro* and *in vivo* assessment of the effect of dalcetrapib on a panel of CYP substrates. *Curr Med Res Opin* (2009) 25, 891–902.
2. Krishna R, Bergman AJ, Jin B, Garg A, Roadcap B, Chiou R, Dru J, Cote J, Laethem T, Wang RW, Didolkar V, Vets E, Gottesdiener K, Wagner JA. Assessment of the CYP3A-mediated drug interaction potential of anacetrapib, a potent cholesteryl ester transfer protein (CETP) inhibitor, in healthy volunteers. *J Clin Pharmacol* (2009) 49, 80–7.
3. Krishna R, Stypinski D, Ali M, Garg A, Cote J, Maes A, DeGroot B, Liu Y, Li S, Connolly SM, Wagner JA, Stoch SA. Lack of a meaningful effect of anacetrapib on the pharmacokinetics and pharmacodynamics of warfarin in healthy subjects. *Br J Clin Pharmacol* (2012) 74, 116–24.

CETP inhibitors + Ketoconazole and other CYP3A4 inhibitors

Diltiazem slightly increases anacetrapib exposure. Ketoconazole moderately increases anacetrapib exposure, but has a much smaller effect on dalcetrapib exposure.

Clinical evidence

(a) Anacetrapib

1. Diltiazem. In a pharmacokinetic study, 10 healthy subjects were given diltiazem 240 mg daily for 11 days with a single 25-mg dose of anacetrapib given on day 5 in the fasting state. Diltiazem slightly increased the AUC of anacetrapib, by 95%.[1]

2. Ketoconazole. In a pharmacokinetic study in 8 healthy subjects, ketoconazole 400 mg daily for 15 days moderately increased the AUC of anacetrapib 4.6-fold when a single 25-mg dose of anacetrapib was given on day 5 in the fasting state. The anacetrapib elimination half-life was halved.[2]

(b) Dalcetrapib

In a pharmacokinetic study in healthy subjects, ketoconazole 400 mg daily for 6 days had no effect on the pharmacokinetics of dalcetrapib when a single 600-mg dose was given on day 6 with the last dose of ketoconazole.[3] In another study, when the same daily dose of ketoconazole was given with a single 900-mg dose of dalcetrapib on day 6, the steady-state AUC of dalcetrapib was negligibly reduced (by 18%), with a slight increase (of 67%) in the AUC of the inactive *S*-methyl metabolite.[3]

Mechanism

Ketoconazole is a potent inhibitor, and diltiazem is a moderate inhibitor, of CYP3A4, by which anacetrapib is metabolised. The reason for the slight change in dalcetrapib pharmacokinetics is not known: it does not appear to be mediated by CYP3A4.

Importance and management

The clinical relevance of the moderate, almost fivefold increase in anacetrapib exposure with ketoconazole has not been assessed. Nevertheless, the authors of the study consider that this increase in exposure is within the extent of variability of anacetrapib exposure seen with food;[2] see also 'CETP inhibitors; Anacetrapib + Food', p.1312. Further study of the importance of this needed. Until more is known, some caution would seem to be appropriate on the concurrent use of ketoconazole and other potent CYP3A4 inhibitors, see 'Table 1.9', p.11, for a list. Consider monitoring for anacetrapib adverse effects and adjust the dose accordingly.

The almost twofold increase in anacetrapib exposure with the moderate CYP3A4 inhibitor diltiazem is unlikely to be clinically relevant as anacetrapib appears to have a wide safety margin.

The negligible to slight changes in dalcetrapib pharmacokinetics that occur with ketoconazole are not clinically relevant, and no dalcetrapib dose adjustment would be expected to be needed on their concurrent use.

1. Garg A, Maes A, Corr C, Jin B, Wadhwa T, Handa N, Van Dyck K, De Lepeleire I, Shah J, Wagner JA, Krishna R. Effect of diltiazem, a moderate CYP3A inhibitor, on the pharmacokinetics of anacetrapib, a potent cholesteryl ester transfer protein inhibitor, in healthy subjects. *J Clin Pharmacol* (2011) 51, 436–9.
2. Krishna R, Bergman AJ, Jin B, Garg A, Roadcap B, Chiou R, Dru J, Cote J, Laethem T, Wang RW, Didolkar V, Vets E, Gottesdiener K, Wagner JA. Assessment of the CYP3A-mediated drug interaction potential of anacetrapib, a potent cholesteryl ester transfer protein (CETP) inhibitor, in healthy volunteers. *J Clin Pharmacol* (2009) 49, 80–7.
3. Derks M, Fowler S, Kuhlmann O. A single-center, open-label, one-sequence study of dalcetrapib coadministered with ketoconazole, and an in vitro study of the *S*-methyl metabolite of dalcetrapib. *Clin Ther* (2009) 31, 586–99.

CETP inhibitors; Anacetrapib + Food

Anacetrapib exposure is markedly increased by a high-fat meal and moderately increased by a low-fat meal.

Clinical evidence, mechanism, importance and management

In a single-dose pharmacokinetic study in 6 healthy subjects, giving anacetrapib 125 mg with a high-fat meal markedly increased the AUC of anacetrapib about sixfold, whereas giving it with a low-fat meal moderately increased its AUC 2.25-fold, when compared with the fasting state.[1]

Anacetrapib is a hydrophobic compound and is formulated as a liquid-filled capsule with a surfactant to aid absorption. Presumably, the higher the fat content of a meal the greater the absorption.

The almost sixfold difference in anacetrapib exposure with a high-fat meal compared with the fasting state is marked, and, although its clinical relevance has not been assessed, it is probably clinically important. The authors of the report note that, as a result of these data, anacetrapib was given with a meal (type not stated) in dose-finding clinical studies.[1]

1. Krishna R, Garg A, Panebianco D, Cote J, Bergman AJ, Van Hoydonck P, Laethem T, Van Dyck K, Chen J, Chavez-Eng C, Archer L, Lutz R, Hilliard D, Snyder K, Jin B, Van Bortel L, Lasseter KC, Al-Huniti N, Dykstra K, Gottesdiener K, Wagner JA. Single-dose pharmacokinetics and pharmacodynamics of anacetrapib, a potent cholesteryl ester transfer protein (CETP) inhibitor, in healthy subjects. *Br J Clin Pharmacol* (2009) 68, 535–45.

Colestyramine + Food

A study in 10 patients with type IIA hyperlipoproteinaemia found that the efficacy of colestyramine in controlling total cholesterol and low density lipoprotein levels was unaltered whether the colestyramine was taken with or before meals.[1]

1. Sirtori M, Pazzucconi F, Gianfranceschi G, Sirtori CR. Efficacy of cholestyramine does not vary when taken before or during meals. *Atherosclerosis* (1991) 88, 249–52.

Ezetimibe + Antacids

The bioavailability of ezetimibe does not appear to be affected by aluminium/magnesium hydroxide-containing antacids.

Clinical evidence, mechanism, importance and management

In a single-dose study in 12 healthy subjects, giving ezetimibe 10 mg with 20 mL of an **aluminium/magnesium hydroxide**-containing antacid (*Supralox*) did not affect the AUC of ezetimibe or conjugated ezetimibe metabolites, although the mean maximum plasma concentration of total ezetimibe (ezetimibe plus conjugated ezetimibe) decreased by about 30% and the time to maximum plasma concentration of ezetimibe increased from 1.5 to 3 hours.[1] This indicates that the antacid slightly reduced the rate of absorption of ezetimibe without affecting the extent of absorption. These changes would not be expected to be clinically relevant, and therefore ezetimibe may be given without regard to the timing of aluminium/magnesium hydroxide-containing antacids.

1. Courtney RD, Kosoglou T, Statkevich P, Boutros T, Maxwell SE, Pember L, Batra VK. Effect of antacid on the pharmacokinetics of ezetimibe. *Clin Pharmacol Ther* (2002) 71, P80.

Ezetimibe + Bile-acid binding resins

Colestyramine moderately reduces ezetimibe exposure.

Clinical evidence

In a parallel-group study, 8 otherwise healthy hypercholesterolaemic subjects were given ezetimibe 10 mg daily for 14 days with **colestyramine** 4 g twice daily taken one hour and 13 hours after the ezetimibe: another 8 subjects were given ezetimibe alone; and a further 8 were given **colestyramine** alone. The AUC of total ezetimibe (ezetimibe plus glucuronide metabolite) was 56% lower in those also given **colestyramine**.[1,2] In addition, there was a reduction in the presence of multiple peaks in the plasma concentration-time profile of ezetimibe, indicating reduced enterohepatic recycling in the presence of **colestyramine**.[2] The combination showed a trend towards a greater reduction in LDL-cholesterol compared with **colestyramine** alone.[2]

Mechanism

Colestyramine appears to bind ezetimibe in the gut reducing its absorption and enterohepatic recycling.

Importance and management

The pharmacokinetic interaction between colestyramine and ezetimibe might reduce the expected additive effects of ezetimibe and colestyramine on LDL-cholesterol reduction. To minimise any interaction, the manufacturer of ezetimibe recommends that it should be taken at least 2 hours before or 4 hours after bile-acid binding resins.[3,4] This seems prudent for colestyramine, but note that because ezetimibe undergoes enterohepatic recirculation, separating administration might not fully resolve this interaction. For **colesevelam**, note that the UK manufacturer states that colesevelam and ezetimibe can be taken together or dosed apart,[5] although, also note that, in the published placebo-controlled studies of the efficacy of the combination of colesevelam and ezetimibe, they were taken separately; with meals and at bedtime, respectively.[6,7]

1. Kosoglou T, Statkevich P, Reyderman L, Pember LJC, Maxwell SE, Courtney R, Krishna G, Cutler DL. Effects of selected drugs on exposure to ezetimibe. *Eur Heart J* (2003) 24 (Suppl), 462.
2. Kosoglou T, Statkevich P, Johnson-Levonas AO, Paolini JF, Bergman AJ, Alton KB. Ezetimibe: a review of its metabolism, pharmacokinetics and drug interactions. *Clin Pharmacokinet* (2005) 44, 467–94.
3. Zetia (Ezetimibe). Merck/Schering-Plough Pharmaceuticals. US Prescribing information, August 2013.
4. Ezetrol (Ezetimibe). MSD-SP Ltd. UK Summary of product characteristics, September 2010.
5. Cholestagel (Colesevelam hydrochloride). Sanofi. UK Summary of product characteristics, December 2014.
6. Knopp RH, Tsunehara C, Retzlaff BM, Fish B, Nguyen H, Anderson S, Nguyen T. Lipoprotein effects of combined ezetimibe and colesevelam hydrochloride versus ezetimibe alone in hypercholesterolemic subjects: a pilot study. *Metabolism* (2006) 55, 1697–703.
7. Bays H, Rhyne J, Abby S, Lai Y-L, Jones M. Lipid-lowering effects of colesevelam HCl in combination with ezetimibe. *Curr Med Res Opin* (2006) 22, 2191–200.

Ezetimibe + Ciclosporin

Exposure to ezetimibe is moderately increased by ciclosporin, although one patient with renal impairment had a much larger increase in ezetimibe exposure. Ezetimibe very slightly increases ciclosporin exposure, but patient studies have shown no change in the minimum concentration of ciclosporin.

Clinical evidence

(a) Effect on ciclosporin

A randomised, crossover study in 12 healthy subjects found that ezetimibe 20 mg daily for 8 days very slightly increased the AUC of a single 100-mg dose of ciclosporin given on day 7 by 15%.[1] In a randomised placebo-controlled study in 59 patients with cardiac transplants receiving ciclosporin, there was no difference in the minimum concentration of ciclosporin between those given ezetimibe 10 mg daily or placebo at 1, 3, and 6 months.[2] Similarly, other efficacy studies in renal and liver transplant patients have reported that ezetimibe 10 mg daily had no effect on ciclosporin minimum concentrations.[3-6]

(b) Effect on ezetimibe

A renal transplant patient, with severe renal impairment taking multiple drugs including ciclosporin, had an ezetimibe AUC that was 12-fold higher, when compared with that in healthy subjects.[7-9] This finding prompted a study in 8 stable renal transplant patients with normal renal function taking ciclosporin to determine the pharmacokinetics of a single 10-mg dose of ezetimibe. When compared with historical data from healthy subjects taking ezetimibe alone, the AUC of ezetimibe was found to be 3.4-fold higher in the patients taking ciclosporin, and its maximum concentration was about 4-fold higher.[7]

A case report describes an excessive reduction in LDL-cholesterol in a heart transplant patient taking ciclosporin 100 mg twice daily with atorvastatin 40 mg daily when given ezetimibe 10 mg daily. His LDL-cholesterol decreased from 126 mg/dL to 51 mg/dL (target less than 100 mg/dL), and so his dose of ezetimibe was decreased to 5 mg daily.[10] The authors of this case report noted that only about 50% of heart transplant patients are able to achieve LDL-cholesterol of less than 100 mg/dL and attributed the effects seen in their patients to an interaction. However, the validity of any interaction has been debated,[11,12] and various efficacy studies in which transplant patients taking ciclosporin and a statin were given ezetimibe 10 mg daily noted an enhanced but not excessive effect on lipids.[2,4,5]

Mechanism

The reason why ciclosporin might increase exposure to ezetimibe is unknown, but it could be due to inhibition of P-glycoprotein or other drug transporter proteins.

Importance and management

The interaction between ezetimibe and ciclosporin, resulting in a very slight increase in ciclosporin exposure, would appear to be established. However, a 15% increase in the AUC of a narrow therapeutic index drug like ciclosporin is not usually considered to be clinically relevant, as confirmed in the clinical studies. Nevertheless, the UK and US manufacturers of ezetimibe recommend monitoring ciclosporin concentrations in patients given ezetimibe.[8,9]

The true effect of ciclosporin on ezetimibe exposure is uncertain, but it might range from a 3-fold increase in those with normal renal function to higher increases in those with severe renal impairment. On the basis of tolerability studies, a 3-fold increase is unlikely to be clinically relevant,[7] but the effect of greater increases is uncertain. The US manufacturer of ezetimibe states that, in patients taking ciclosporin, the potential effects of the increased exposure to ezetimibe should be carefully weighed against the benefits of alterations in lipid concentrations by ezetimibe.[9] The authors of one case report suggested that, in patients taking ciclosporin, ezetimibe should be started at a reduced dose of 5 mg daily or less, with careful monitoring of lipid concentrations if the dose is increased.[12]

1. Bergman AJ, Burke J, Larson P, Johnson-Levonas AO, Reyderman L, Statkevich P, Kosoglou T, Greenberg HE, Kraft WK, Frick G, Murphy G, Gottesdiener K, Paolini JF. Effects of ezetimibe on cyclosporine pharmacokinetics in healthy subjects. *J Clin Pharmacol* (2006) 46, 321–7.
2. Shaw SM, Chaggar P, Ritchie J, Shah MKH, Baynes AC, O'Neill N, Fildes JE, Yonan N, Williams SG. The efficacy and tolerability of ezetimibe in cardiac transplant recipients taking cyclosporin. *Transplantation* (2009) 87, 771–5.
3. Buchanan C, Smith L, Corbett J, Nelson E, Shihab F. A retrospective analysis of ezetimibe treatment in renal transplant recipients. *Am J Transplant* (2006) 6, 770–4.
4. Kohnle M, Pietruck F, Kribben A, Philipp T, Heemann U, Witzke O. Ezetimibe for the treatment of uncontrolled hypercholesterolemia in patients with high-dose statin therapy after renal transplantation. *Am J Transplant* (2006) 205–8.

5. Almutairi F, Peterson TC, Molinari M, Walsh MJ, Alwayn I, Peltekian KM. Safety and effectiveness of ezetimibe in liver transplant recipients with hypercholesterolemia. *Liver Transpl* (2009) 15, 504–8.
6. Savvidaki E, Koukoulaki M, Benou A, Roumeliotou M, Fourtounas C, Kalliakmani P, Papachristou E, Vlachojannis JG, Goumenos D. Ezetimibe is effective in the treatment of persistent hyperlipidemia of renal allograft recipients. *Clin Nephrol* (2011) 75, 107–12.
7. Bergman AJ, Burke J, Larson P, Johnson-Levonas AO, Reyderman L, Statkevich P, Maxwell SE, Kosoglou T, Murphy G, Gottesdiener K, Robson R, Paolini JF. Interaction of single-dose ezetimibe and steady-state cyclosporine in renal transplant patients. *J Clin Pharmacol* (2006) 46, 328–36.
8. Ezetrol (Ezetimibe). MSD-SP Ltd. UK Summary of product characteristics, September 2010.
9. Zetia (Ezetimibe). Merck/Schering-Plough Pharmaceuticals. US Prescribing information, August 2013.
10. Koshman SL, Lalonde LD, Burton I, Tymchak WJ, Pearson GJ. Supratherapeutic response to ezetimibe administered with cyclosporine. *Ann Pharmacother* (2005) 39, 1561–5.
11. Ito MK. Comment: supratherapeutic response to ezetimibe administered with cyclosporine. *Ann Pharmacother* (2005) 39, 2141.
12. Pearson GJ, Koshman SL, Lalonde LD, Burton I, Tymchak WJ. Comment: supratherapeutic response to ezetimibe administered with cyclosporine. Author's reply. *Ann Pharmacother* (2005) 39, 2142.

Ezetimibe + Cimetidine

Cimetidine does not alter the bioavailability of ezetimibe.

Clinical evidence, mechanism, importance and management

In a study in 12 healthy subjects, cimetidine 400 mg twice daily for 7 days caused a small increase (no greater than 22%) in the peak plasma level of ezetimibe 10 mg daily, but the overall bioavailability (AUC of total ezetimibe) was not affected.[1,2] No ezetimibe dose adjustments are therefore necessary on concurrent use.

1. Krishna G, Kosoglou T, Ezzet F, Pember L, Statkevich P, Boutros T, Maxwell SE, Basso L, Batra VK. Effect of cimetidine on the pharmacokinetics of ezetimibe. *AAPS PharmSci* (2001) 3; 3.
2. Kosoglou T, Statkevich P, Johnson-Levonas AO, Paolini JF, Bergman AJ, Alton KB. Ezetimibe: a review of its metabolism, pharmacokinetics and drug interactions. *Clin Pharmacokinet* (2005) 44, 467–94.

Ezetimibe + Cytochrome P450 substrates

Ezetimibe does not affect the pharmacokinetics of caffeine, dapsone, dextromethorphan, midazolam, and tolbutamide, and is not anticipated to affect the pharmacokinetics of other drugs that are similarly metabolised.

Clinical evidence, mechanism, importance and management

In a drug interaction study in 12 healthy subjects, using probe substrates for common cytochrome P450 isoenzymes, ezetimibe 20 mg daily for 8 days had no effect on the AUC of **caffeine** (CYP1A2 substrate) or intravenous **midazolam** (hepatic CYP3A4); or on the urinary metabolite ratios of **tolbutamide** (CYP2C9) or **dextromethorphan** (CYP2D6) when compared with placebo. Similarly, it had no effect on the AUC of **dapsone** (*N*-acetyltransferase substrate).[1]

This indicates that ezetimibe does not alter the activity of these enzymes, and it is therefore not anticipated to affect the pharmacokinetics of drugs that are substrates of these enzymes via this mechanism.

1. Zhu Y, Statkevich P, Kosoglou T, Zambas D, Patrick J, Cayen MN, Batra V. Effect of SCH 58235 on the activity of drug metabolizing enzymes in vivo. *Clin Pharmacol Ther* (2000) 67, 152.

Ezetimibe + Dalcetrapib

Ezetimibe does not alter dalcetrapib exposure. Dalcetrapib slightly reduces ezetimibe exposure.

Clinical evidence, mechanism, importance and management

In a pharmacokinetic study in 22 healthy subjects given **dalcetrapib** 900 mg daily alone for 7 days, ezetimibe 10 mg daily alone for 7 days and both drugs together, there was no change in the AUC of **dalcetrapib** and a slight 20% decrease in the AUC of ezetimibe. The effects of each drug on lipid levels were not reduced by concurrent use. The reason for the small change in ezetimibe exposure is unknown, but it is not sufficient to be clinically important.[1] No dose adjustment of either drug would be expected to be needed on concurrent use.

1. Derks M, Abt M, Phelan M. Lack of clinically relevant drug-drug interactions when dalcetrapib is co-administered with ezetimibe. *Br J Clin Pharmacol* (2010) 70, 825–33.

Ezetimibe + Everolimus or Sirolimus

Sirolimus appears to slightly increase the initial exposure to ezetimibe without altering its overall exposure. Ezetimibe does not appear to alter the exposure to sirolimus. In small efficacy studies, ezetimibe did not appear to alter everolimus or sirolimus concentrations.

Clinical evidence

(a) Everolimus

In a retrospective study in renal transplant patients stable taking everolimus, the addition of ezetimibe 10 mg daily did not alter the blood concentrations of everolimus in 9 patients.[1]

(b) Sirolimus

In a single-dose, pharmacokinetic study in 24 healthy subjects, sirolimus 5 mg increased the AUC_{0-6} of ezetimibe 10 mg by 42%, but did not affect the overall exposure to sirolimus. Ezetimibe did not alter the pharmacokinetics of sirolimus.[2] In a small cohort of renal transplant patients stable taking sirolimus, the addition of ezetimibe 10 mg daily did not alter the blood concentrations of sirolimus in 12 patients.[3]

Mechanism

It seems likely that sirolimus increases the initial exposure to ezetimibe by inhibiting the intestinal transporter P-glycoprotein.[2]

Importance and management

The changes in ezetimibe pharmacokinetics with single-dose sirolimus are unlikely to be clinically relevant; however, this needs confirmation in a steady-state study. Ezetimibe does not appear to alter sirolimus concentrations. Until more is known, no sirolimus or ezetimibe dose adjustments appear to be necessary on concurrent use. Similarly, no everolimus dose adjustment is expected to be necessary in patients also given ezetimibe.

1. Savvidaki E, Koukoulaki M, Benou A, Roumeliotou M, Fourtounas C, Kalliakmani P, Papachristou E, Vlachojannis JG, Goumenos D. Ezetimibe is effective in the treatment of persistent hyperlipidemia of renal allograft recipients. *Clin Nephrol* (2011) 75, 107–12.
2. Oswald S, Nassif A, Modess C, Keiser M, Hanke U, Engel A, Lütjohann D, Weitschies W, Siegmund W. Pharmacokinetic and pharmacodynamic interactions between the immunosuppressant sirolimus and the lipid-lowering drug ezetimibe in healthy volunteers. *Clin Pharmacol Ther* (2010) 87, 663–7.
3. Almutairi F, Peterson TC, Molinari M, Walsh MJ, Alwayn I, Peltekian KM. Safety and effectiveness of ezetimibe in liver transplant recipients with hypercholesterolemia. *Liver Transpl* (2009) 15, 504–8.

Ezetimibe + Food

The bioavailability of ezetimibe is not affected by food.

Clinical evidence, mechanism, importance and management

A study in 18 healthy subjects found that the AUC of a single 10-mg dose of ezetimibe was not affected by a high-fat or non-fat meal, when compared with the fasting state. The maximum plasma concentration of ezetimibe was increased by about 40% by the high-fat meal and slightly reduced by the non-fat meal (with high variability), but there was no change in maximum level of total ezetimibe (ezetimibe plus its glucuronide). These changes are not clinically relevant. Ezetimibe can therefore be given without regard to meals.[1]

1. Courtney RD, Kosoglou T, Statkevich P, Boutros T, Maxwell SE, Batra VK. Effect of food on the oral bioavailability of ezetimibe. *Clin Pharmacol Ther* (2002) 71, P80.

Ezetimibe + HIV-protease inhibitors

Limited evidence suggests that ezetimibe does not alter lopinavir or ritonavir concentrations, and that the lipid-lowering effects of ezetimibe are not altered by HIV-protease inhibitor-based antiretroviral therapy.

Clinical evidence, mechanism, importance and management

In a study, 10 HIV-positive patients receiving stable HIV-protease inhibitor-based therapy (**lopinavir boosted with ritonavir** in 8, **nelfinavir** in 1 and **atazanavir boosted with ritonavir** in 1) who had poorly controlled antiretroviral-associated dyslipidaemia despite the use of pravastatin 20 mg daily, were also given ezetimibe 10 mg daily. After 6, 12, or 24 weeks of concurrent use, LDL-cholesterol concentrations were lower than baseline values. No differences were observed in **lopinavir** minimum plasma concentrations measured just before and 12 weeks after ezetimibe introduction. The addition of ezetimibe appeared to be well tolerated.[1]

In another similar study in 20 patients taking HIV-protease inhibitor-based HAART, 13 of whom were taking **lopinavir boosted with ritonavir**, the addition of ezetimibe 10 mg daily to low-dose statin use lowered LDL-cholesterol and did not appear to alter trough **lopinavir** or **ritonavir** concentrations.[2]

These studies suggest that these antiretrovirals do not alter the efficacy of ezetimibe and that ezetimibe does not alter the pharmacokinetics of **lopinavir**. Concurrent use appears to be beneficial.

1. Negredo E, Moltó J, Puig J, Cinquegrana D, Bonjoch A, Pérez-Álvarez N, López-Blázquez R, Blanco A, Clotet B, Rey-Joly C. Ezetimibe, a promising lipid-lowering agent for the treatment of dyslipidaemia in HIV-infected patients with poor response to statins. *AIDS* (2006) 20, 2159–64.
2. van den Berg-Wolf M, Klibanov OM, Gaughan JP, Tedaldi EM. Ezetimibe combined with low-dose statin effectively lowers LDL in protease inhibitor-treated patients. *AIDS Patient Care STDS* (2008) 22, 483–8.

Ezetimibe + Lomitapide

Lomitapide does not appear to affect the pharmacokinetics of ezetimibe.

Clinical evidence, mechanism, importance and management

In a prospective study in healthy subjects, lomitapide 10 mg daily for 7 days had no effect on the pharmacokinetics of a single 10-mg dose of ezetimibe.[1] No ezetimibe dose adjustment is therefore required on concurrent use with lomitapide.

1. Tuteja S, Duffy D, Dunbar RL, Movva R, Gadi R, Bloedon LT, Cuchel M. Pharmacokinetic interactions of the microsomal triglyceride transfer protein inhibitor, lomitapide, with drugs commonly used in the management of hypercholesterolemia. *Pharmacotherapy* (2014) 34, 227–39.

Ezetimibe + Mipomersen

The concurrent use of ezetimibe and mipomersen does not alter the pharmacokinetics of either drug.

Clinical evidence, mechanism, importance and management

In a pharmacokinetic study in 10 healthy subjects, a single 10-mg dose of ezetimibe was given alone and then with the last dose of intravenous mipomersen (200 mg over 2 hours every 2 days for 4 doses). There was no difference in the AUC of mipomersen when given alone or with ezetimibe. In addition, there was no difference in the AUCs of ezetimibe or total ezetimibe (ezetimibe plus its glucuronide) when given alone or with mipomersen, although there was a 45% reduction in the maximum level of ezetimibe.[1]

This study demonstrates that no clinically relevant pharmacokinetic drug interaction would be expected if mipomersen and ezetimibe are given concurrently.

1. Yu RZ, Geary RS, Flaim JD, Riley GC, Tribble DL, vanVliet AA, Wedel MK. Lack of pharmacokinetic interaction of mipomersen sodium (ISIS 301012), a 2'-*O*-methoxyethyl modified antisense oligonucleotide targeting apolipoprotein B-100 messenger RNA, with simvastatin and ezetimibe. *Clin Pharmacokinet* (2009) 48, 39–50.

Ezetimibe + NNRTIs

Efavirenz does not appear to alter the pharmacokinetics of ezetimibe to a clinically relevant extent. Limited evidence suggests that ezetimibe does not alter nevirapine levels, and that the lipid-lowering effects of ezetimibe were not altered by NNRTI-based antiretroviral therapy.

Clinical evidence

(a) Efavirenz

In a study in 12 healthy subjects, the steady-state pharmacokinetics of ezetimibe 10 mg daily were assessed alone, after a single 400-mg dose of efavirenz and after multiple doses of efavirenz 400 mg daily for 8 days. The single dose of efavirenz slightly increased the AUC of ezetimibe by 36% and negligibly reduced the AUC of its glucuronide metabolite by 12%. Multiple dose efavirenz had no effect on the serum levels of ezetimibe and slightly decreased the AUC of its glucuronide metabolite by 30%.[1]

(b) Nevirapine

In a study, 8 HIV-positive patients receiving stable NNRTI-based therapy (nevirapine in 7 and **efavirenz** in 1) who had poorly controlled antiretroviral-associated dyslipidaemia despite the use of pravastatin 20 mg daily, were also given ezetimibe 10 mg daily. After 6, 12, or 24 weeks of concurrent use, LDL-cholesterol levels were lower than baseline values. No differences were observed in nevirapine minimum plasma levels measured just before and 12 weeks after ezetimibe introduction. The addition of ezetimibe appeared to be well tolerated.[2]

Mechanism

It was suggested that efavirenz might alter ezetimibe pharmacokinetics by inhibiting intestinal P-glycoprotein and inhibiting glucuronidation.[1]

Importance and management

The ezetimibe pharmacokinetic changes seen with efavirenz were at most, slight, and unlikely to be clinically relevant. The findings of the clinical study suggest that NNRTIs do not alter the efficacy of ezetimibe, and that ezetimibe does not alter the pharmacokinetics of nevirapine. Concurrent use appears to be beneficial.

1. Oswald S, Meyer zu Schwabedissen H, Nassif A, Modess C, Luetjohann D, Desta Z, Kroemer HK, Siegmund W. Drug interactions between ezetimibe and efavirenz in healthy subjects. *Clin Pharmacol Ther* (2010) 87 (Suppl 1) 59.
2. Negredo E, Moltó J, Puig J, Cinquegrana D, Bonjoch A, Pérez-Álvarez N, López-Blázquez R, Blanco A, Clotet B, Rey-Joly C. Ezetimibe, a promising lipid-lowering agent for the treatment of dyslipidaemia in HIV-infected patients with poor response to statins. *AIDS* (2006) 20, 2159–64.

Ezetimibe + Rifampicin (Rifampin)

Simultaneous single-doses of rifampicin increase ezetimibe levels without altering its overall effects on sterols, whereas multiple doses of rifampicin decrease single-dose ezetimibe levels and almost totally abolish its effects when administration is separated.

Clinical evidence

In a single-dose study investigating the disposition of ezetimibe, 8 healthy subjects were given ezetimibe 20 mg *simultaneously* with rifampicin 600 mg. Rifampicin increased the ezetimibe maximum serum levels about 2.5-fold, without affecting the AUC. The maximum serum levels of ezetimibe glucuronide (the major metabolite of ezetimibe, which contributes to its pharmacological activity) were similarly increased, and its AUC was increased about twofold. The sterol-lowering effects of ezetimibe were also more rapid in the presence of rifampicin, but the overall effect was unchanged, possibly because ezetimibe and its glucuronide were excreted more rapidly.[1]

In another study by the same researchers, subjects were given rifampicin 600 mg daily for 8 days, with a single 20-mg dose of ezetimibe given *12 hours after* the last dose of rifampicin. Both the AUCs and maximum serum levels of ezetimibe and its glucuronide were *decreased* (AUCs decreased by more than 50%) and the effect of ezetimibe on sterols was almost completely abolished.[2]

Mechanism

The raised ezetimibe levels seen in the single-dose study of simultaneous administration are thought to occur because rifampicin enhances the absorption of ezetimibe, probably by inhibiting intestinal P-glycoprotein, and another transporter protein, MRP2. However, inhibition of MRP2 also appears to reduce enterohepatic circulation, which is needed for the long duration of ezetimibe effects, and therefore might shorten the duration of the sterol-lowering effects of ezetimibe.[1] This effect is less likely if ezetimibe is given 12 hours after rifampicin.[2] When rifampicin is given longer-term it induces ezetimibe glucuronidation, which leads to a reduction in the exposure of both ezetimibe and its glucuronide thereby reducing the effects of ezetimibe. Other factors are possibly also involved.[2] The outcome of simultaneous administration of long-term rifampicin and ezetimibe is unclear because it will depend on the balance of the effect of rifampicin on drug transporters and its effects on glucuronidation.

Importance and management

Information about the interaction between ezetimibe and rifampicin appears to be limited to these studies, which were primarily designed to investigate ezetimibe disposition. However, it seems possible that the effects of ezetimibe will be reduced in patients who are also given rifampicin long-term, particularly if administration is separated. If both drugs are given it would be prudent to closely monitor the effects on lipid levels.

1. Oswald S, Giessmann T, Luetjohann D, Wegner D, Rosskopf D, Weitschies W, Siegmund W. Disposition and sterol-lowering effect of ezetimibe are influenced by single-dose coadministration of rifampin, an inhibitor of multidrug transport proteins. *Clin Pharmacol Ther* (2006) 80, 477–85.
2. Oswald S, Haenisch S, Fricke C, Sudhop T, Remmler C, Giessmann T, Jedlitschky G, Adam U, Dazert E, Warzok R, Wacke W, Cascorbi I, Kroemer HK, Weitschies W, von Bergmann K, Siegmund W. Intestinal expression of P-glycoprotein (*ABCB1*), multidrug resistance associated protein 2 (*ABCC2*), and uridine diphosphate–glucuronosyltransferase 1A1 predicts the disposition and modulates the effects of the cholesterol absorption inhibitor ezetimibe in humans. *Clin Pharmacol Ther* (2006) 79, 206–17.

Fibrates + Bile-acid binding resins

Colestipol and colesevelam do not alter the pharmacokinetics of fenofibrate. Colestipol can slightly reduce the absorption of gemfibrozil if both drugs are given at the same time, but not if they are given 2 hours apart. A similar interaction is predicted to occur between bezafibrate and bile-acid binding resins.

Clinical evidence, mechanism, importance and management

(a) Bezafibrate

The manufacturer of bezafibrate recommends that there should be a 2-hour interval between giving an ion-exchange resin [such as the bile-acid binding resins] and bezafibrate, as the absorption of bezafibrate might otherwise be impaired.[1] In the absence of any other information, this seems prudent.

(b) Fenofibrate

In a 6-day study in 6 healthy subjects the pharmacokinetics of fenofibrate were not altered when **colestipol** 10 g daily was given at the same time as fenofibrate 200 mg in the morning, and **colestipol** 5 g daily was given at the same time as fenofibrate 100 mg in the evening.[2] In a single-dose, crossover study, 27 healthy subjects took fenofibrate 160 mg at the same time as **colesevelam** 3.75 g, four hours before **colesevelam**, or alone. **Colesevelam** did not alter the AUC of the active metabolite of fenofibrate, fenofibric acid, when both drugs were given at the same time or 4 hours apart, but decreased the maximum plasma level by just 20% when given at the same time.[3] These studies show that there is no need to separate the administration of fenofibrate from **colestipol** or **colesevelam**.

(c) Gemfibrozil

A study in 10 patients with raised serum cholesterol and triglyceride levels found that if gemfibrozil 600 mg was given alone, 2 hours before or 2 hours after **colestipol** 5 g, the AUCs of gemfibrozil were similar. However, when both drugs were given at the same time, the AUC of gemfibrozil was reduced by about one-third.[4] Another study found that giving gemfibrozil at the same time as **colestipol** enhanced the LDL-lowering effects of both drugs, but tended to mitigate the HDL-raising effects of the gemfibrozil.[5] Combined use is effective, and information is very limited about the clinical importance of the slight reduction in exposure to gemfibrozil. However, the interaction can be avoided by separating the administration of the two drugs by at least 2 hours.

1. Bezalip Tablets (Bezafibrate). Actavis UK Ltd. UK Summary of product characteristics, October 2009.
2. Harvengt C, Desager JP. Lack of pharmacokinetic interaction of colestipol and fenofibrate in volunteers. *Eur J Clin Pharmacol* (1980) 17, 459–63.
3. Jones MR, Baker BA, Mathew P. Effect of colesevelam HCl on single-dose fenofibrate pharmacokinetics. *Clin Pharmacokinet* (2004) 43, 943–50.
4. Forland SC, Feng Y, Cutler RE. Apparent reduced absorption of gemfibrozil when given with colestipol. *J Clin Pharmacol* (1990) 30, 29–32.
5. East C, Bilheimer DW, Grundy SM. Combination drug therapy for familial combined hyperlipidemia. *Ann Intern Med* (1988) 109, 25–32.

Fibrates + Colchicine

Isolated case reports suggest that the concurrent use of a fibrate and colchicine can result in rhabdomyolysis or neuromyopathy.

Clinical evidence

A 40-year-old man, with chronic hepatitis and nephrotic syndrome, who had been taking colchicine 500 micrograms three times daily uneventfully for 2 to 3 years, started taking **gemfibrozil** 600 mg twice daily. About one month later he presented with muscle pain and dark brown urine, and had an elevated serum creatine kinase level of 3 559 units/L, and he was diagnosed as having rhabdomyolysis. Both drugs were stopped, and he recovered over the following 9 days.[1] Another case report describes neuromyopathy (creatine kinase level 15 084 units/L), in a patient who had been taking **bezafibrate** 400 mg daily with colchicine 3 mg daily for 14 days.[2] This patient was known to have renal impairment.

Mechanism

Colchicine alone can, rarely, cause myopathy. However, it is more common in those given colchicine long term (as in the case with gemfibrozil), in high dose, or in the presence or renal impairment (as in the case with bezafibrate).[2] As the fibrates can also, rarely, cause myopathy, an additive or synergistic effect seems possible.

Importance and management

Although information about an interaction between the fibrates and colchicine seems limited to these two cases, the effects seen are known to be associated with both colchicine and the fibrates alone, and so an interaction, all be it rare, seems possible. It would be prudent to suspect this interaction in any patient presenting with muscle pain or a raised creatine kinase level. See *Muscle and liver toxicity,* under 'Lipid regulating drugs', p.1309, for further guidance on the risk factors for muscle toxicity. It would seem prudent to be aware of these when colchicine is taken with a fibrate, as both patients in the cases above had other risk factors for rhabdomyolysis.

1. Atmaca H, Sayarlioğlu H, Külah E, Demircan N, Akpolat T. Rhabdomyolysis associated with gemfibrozil-colchicine therapy. *Ann Pharmacother* (2002) 36, 1719–21.
2. Sugie M, Kuriki A, Arai D, Ichikawa H, Kawamura M. A case report of acute neuromyopathy induced by concomitant use of colchicine and bezafibrate. *No To Shinkei* (2005) 57, 785–90.

Fibrates + Ezetimibe

Fenofibrate and gemfibrozil might slightly increase exposure to ezetimibe, but ezetimibe does not alter fenofibrate or gemfibrozil pharmacokinetics. The concurrent use of ezetimibe and a fibrate is predicted to increase cholesterol excretion into the bile, which increases the risk of gallstone formation.

Clinical evidence

(a) Fenofibrate

In a randomised, crossover study, 18 healthy subjects were given ezetimibe 10 mg daily with fenofibrate 145 mg daily for 10 days, or either drug alone. Ezetimibe did not affect the AUC of fenofibrate, but fenofibrate increased the total AUC of ezetimibe and its metabolite, ezetimibe glucuronide, by 50%.[1] Similar findings were reported in a randomised, placebo-controlled study in 32 otherwise healthy patients with hypercholesterolaemia who were given fenofibrate 200 mg daily, ezetimibe 10 mg daily, both drugs in combination, or placebo daily; each for 14 days. Concurrent use had no effect on the pharmacokinetics of fenofibrate, whereas the AUCs of ezetimibe and ezetimibe glucuronide were slightly increased by about 50%. The combination resulted in a greater reduction in LDL-cholesterol than that achieved by either ezetimibe or fenofibrate alone.[2]

A further efficacy and safety study, in 172 patients with mixed hyperlipidaemia taking ezetimibe 10 mg daily with fenofibrate 160 mg daily for 12 weeks, found that the concurrent use of fenofibrate with ezetimibe did not seem to influence the adverse effects beyond those noted with fenofibrate alone and no cases of rhabdomyolysis or myopathy were recorded. However, both drugs were discontinued in one patient because of cholelithiasis, which was managed with a cholecystectomy, although this was not thought to be due to the study medications.[3] In a 48-week extension phase of this study, the combination of fenofibrate and ezetimibe was more efficacious than fenofibrate alone.[4]

(b) Gemfibrozil

In a randomised, crossover study, 12 healthy subjects were given ezetimibe 10 mg daily with gemfibrozil 600 mg twice daily for 7 days, or either drug alone. Ezetimibe did not affect the AUC of gemfibrozil, but gemfibrozil slightly increased the total AUC of ezetimibe and it metabolite, ezetimibe glucuronide, by about 70%.[5]

Mechanism

The increase in total ezetimibe exposure with fenofibrate and gemfibrozil was thought to be due to increased bioavailability, perhaps because of the surfactant in the fibrate formulations, rather than inhibition of glucuronidation.[6] Fibrates can increase cholesterol excretion into the bile, leading to cholelithiasis. In *animal* studies, ezetimibe sometimes increased cholesterol in the gallbladder bile, therefore the possibility of gallstone formation associated with ezetimibe cannot be ruled out.[7] The concurrent use of fibrates and ezetimibe might further increase this risk.

Importance and management

Information regarding the possible interaction between ezetimibe and fibrates appears to be restricted to fenofibrate and gemfibrozil. The slight increases in ezetimibe exposure when given with these fibrates is probably not clinically important because ezetimibe has not shown dose-related increases in adverse effects.[6] Despite the seemingly favourable results on plasma lipids, the manufacturers of ezetimibe state that the safety of its concurrent use with fibrates is not yet established[7,8] and the US manufacturer further states that the concurrent use of ezetimibe and fibrates (other than fenofibrate) is not recommended.[8] This is because both fibrates and ezetimibe can increase cholesterol excretion into the bile, which could promote the production of gallstones,[7,8] as was possibly seen in one patient taking fenofibrate and ezetimibe. The manufacturers recommend that if gallstones or gall bladder disease is suspected in a patient receiving ezetimibe and fenofibrate then the combination should be discontinued.[7,8]

1. Gustavson LE, Schweitzer SM, Burt DA, Achari R, Rieser MJ, Edeki T, Chira T, Yannicelli HD, Kelly MT. Evaluation of the potential for pharmacokinetic interaction between fenofibrate and ezetimibe: a phase I, open-label, multiple-dose, three-period crossover study in healthy subjects. *Clin Ther* (2006) 28, 373–87.
2. Kosoglou T, Statkevich P, Fruchart J-C, Pember LJC, Reyderman L, Cutler DL, Guillaume M, Maxwell SE, Veltri EP. Pharmacodynamic and pharmacokinetic interaction between fenofibrate and ezetimibe. *Curr Med Res Opin* (2004) 20, 1197–1207.
3. Farnier M, Freeman MW, Macdonell G, Perevozskaya I, Davies MJ, Mitchel YB, Gumbiner B, for the Ezetimibe Study Group. Efficacy and safety of the coadministration of ezetimibe with fenofibrate in patients with mixed hyperlipidaemia. *Eur Heart J* (2005) 26, 897–905.
4. McKenney JM, Farnier M, Lo K-W, Bays HE, Perevozkaya I, Carlson G, Davies MJ, Mitchel YB, Gumbiner B. Safety and efficacy of long-term co-administration of fenofibrate and ezetimibe in patients with mixed hyperlipidemia. *J Am Coll Cardiol* (2006) 47, 1584–7.
5. Reyderman L, Kosoglou T, Statkevich P, Pember L, Boutros T, Maxwell SE, Affrime M, Batra V. Assessment of a multiple-dose drug interaction between ezetimibe, a novel selective cholesterol absorption inhibitor and gemfibrozil. *Int J Clin Pharmacol Ther* (2004) 42, 512–18.
6. Kosoglou T, Statkevich P, Johnson-Levonas AO, Paolini JF, Bergman AJ, Alton KB. Ezetimibe: a review of its metabolism, pharmacokinetics and drug interactions. *Clin Pharmacokinet* (2005) 44, 467–94.
7. Ezetrol (Ezetimibe). MSD-SP Ltd. UK Summary of product characteristics, September 2010.
8. Zetia (Ezetimibe). Merck/Schering-Plough Pharmaceuticals. US Prescribing information, August 2013.

Fibrates + Ibuprofen

Gemfibrozil slightly increases ibuprofen exposure. An isolated report describes a patient taking ciprofibrate who developed acute renal failure and rhabdomyolysis, which was, in part, attributed to the use of ibuprofen.

Clinical evidence

(a) Ciprofibrate

A 29-year-old man with type M hyperlipidaemia[1] who had been taking ciprofibrate for 6 months (current dose 200 mg daily, normal creatine kinase 3 weeks previously) began to take ibuprofen 200 mg and then 400 mg (frequency not stated) for a painful heel. The pain became general, his urine turned 'muddy' and he complained of having a 'stiff body'. Two days after a dose of a contrast medium to rule out renal colic he developed acute renal failure. His serum creatinine concentration was found to be 647 micromol/L and his creatine kinase was 13 740 units/L. He subsequently made a full recovery (treatment not stated).[1]

(b) Gemfibrozil

In a pharmacokinetic study, 10 healthy subjects were given a single 400-mg dose of ibuprofen alone and then on the third day of gemfibrozil 600 mg twice daily for 3 days. Gemfibrozil increased the AUC of *R*-ibuprofen by 34% and increased its elimination half-life by 54%, but there were minimal changes in the pharmacokinetic of *S*-ibuprofen except for a 34% increase in its half-life.[2]

Mechanism

Gemfibrozil is a known inhibitor of CYP2C8, which is involved in the metabolism of *R*-ibuprofen but not *S*-ibuprofen. Concurrent use therefore results in increased *R*-ibuprofen exposure. The slight increase in the half-life of *S*-ibuprofen is due to subsequent inversion of *R*-ibuprofen to *S*-ibuprofen.[2]

The reasons for the case of rhabdomyolysis are not known, but the authors of the report suggest that ibuprofen displaced ciprofibrate from its binding sites, thereby turning a safe dose into a toxic one.[1] However, it should be noted that this mechanism of interaction is rarely important on its own, so it seems likely that some other factors might have contributed to what happened, including the use of the contrast medium. The authors also note that, during the time this patient was treated, the recommended dose of ciprofibrate was reduced from 200 mg daily to 100 mg daily, due to a high incidence of rhabdomyolysis, so this high dose might have also been a contributing factor. Ibuprofen is also a cause of acute renal failure.

Importance and management

Evidence for an interaction between gemfibrozil and ibuprofen appears limited to the study cited. It seems unlikely that the slight increase in *R*-ibuprofen levels and conversion to *S*-ibuprofen that occurred will be clinically relevant, even on repeated dosing.

The case of rhabdomyolysis with ciprofibrate is isolated, and an interaction is by no means established. It therefore seems unlikely to be of general relevance.

1. Ramachandran S, Giles PD, Hartland A. Acute renal failure due to rhabdomyolysis in presence of concurrent ciprofibrate and ibuprofen treatment. *BMJ* (1997) 314, 1593.
2. Tornio A, Niemi M, Neuvonen PJ, Backman JT. Stereoselective interaction between the CYP2C8 inhibitor gemfibrozil and racemic ibuprofen. *Eur J Clin Pharmacol* (2007) 63, 463–9.

Fibrates; Bezafibrate + Furosemide

An isolated report describes rhabdomyolysis in a patient taking bezafibrate and furosemide.

Clinical evidence, mechanism, importance and management

An isolated report attributed a case of acute renal failure and rhabdomyolysis to treatment with bezafibrate 400 mg daily and furosemide 25 mg on alternate days.[1]

The reason for the rhabdomyolysis is unknown. This is an isolated case and therefore no general conclusions can be drawn.

1. Venzano C, Cordì GC, Corsi L, Dapelo M, De Micheli A, Grimaldi GP. Un caso di rabdomiolisi acuta con insufficienza renale acuta da assunzione contemporanea di furosemide e bezafibrato. *Minerva Med* (1990) 81, 909–11.

Fibrates; Bezafibrate + Nifedipine

It has been suggested that three cases of rhabdomyolysis occurred because of an interaction between bezafibrate and nifedipine, but it seems more likely that the dose of bezafibrate was too high.

Clinical evidence, mechanism, importance and management

Rhabdomyolysis developed in 4 of 5 patients undergoing CAPD, who were given bezafibrate 200 to 400 mg daily for raised cholesterol and triglyceride levels. Of these, 2 patients were also taking nifedipine, and one patient was also taking nifedipine and lovastatin. Raised creatine kinase levels developed within 8 to 16 days of concurrent use, and resolved within 48 hours of stopping the bezafibrate. The authors suggest that nifedipine might have competed with bezafibrate for metabolism by CYP3A4. They therefore stated that patients with renal failure needing a fibrate should avoid taking CYP3A4 substrates, especially dihydropyridines.[1] However, note that there appear to be no interactions reported for bezafibrate as a result of CYP3A4 inhibition, and nifedipine does not cause interactions via CYP3A4. Furthermore, the generally recommended dose for bezafibrate in dialysis patients is 200 mg every 72 hours with careful monitoring to avoid overdose.[2] It therefore appears likely that the high dose, and not an interaction, was responsible for the rhabdomyolysis.

1. Weissgarten J, Zaidenstein R, Fishman S, Dishi V, Michovitz-Koren M, Averbukh Z, Golik A. Rhabdomyolysis due to bezafibrate in CAPD patients. A role for dihydropyridine drugs? *Perit Dial Int* (1999) 19, 180–2.
2. Bezalip Tablets (Bezafibrate). Actavis UK Ltd. UK Summary of product characteristics, October 2009.

Fibrates; Fenofibrate + Cytochrome P450 substrates

Fenofibrate might inhibit the metabolism of drugs that are substrates of CYP2C9.

Clinical evidence, mechanism, importance and management

One UK and US manufacturer notes that *in vitro* studies using human liver microsomes indicate that fenofibrate and fenofibric acid are not inhibitors of CYP3A4, CYP2D6, CYP2E1, or CYP1A2. However, at concentrations achieved therapeutically, they are weak inhibitors of CYP2C19 and mild to moderate inhibitors of CYP2C9.[1,2] They are also weak inhibitors of CYP2A6,[1,2] but at present, there are no known drug substrates for this isoenzyme.

The UK manufacturer recommends that patients taking fenofibrate and drugs with a narrow therapeutic index that are metabolised by CYP2C19 or particularly CYP2C9 should be carefully monitored and the dose of these drugs adjusted, if necessary.[1] Given that there are cases of increased warfarin effects (a CYP2C9 substrate) with fenofibrate (see 'Coumarins and related drugs + Fibrates', p.426), the precaution with CYP2C9 substrates with a narrow therapeutic range seems prudent. For a list of CYP2C9 substrates, see 'Table 1.5', p.7. There do not appear to be any interactions reported for fenofibrate with CYP2C19 substrates.

1. Suralip (Fenofibrate). Abbott Healthcare Products Ltd. UK Summary of product characteristics, March 2011.
2. Tricor (Fenofibrate). Abbott Laboratories. US Prescribing information, October 2010.

Fibrates; Fenofibrate + Donepezil

An isolated case describes dropped head syndrome in a patient given donepezil and fenofibrate.

Clinical evidence, mechanism, importance and management

A 77-year-old patient who had been taking fenofibrate 300 mg daily for 10 years presented with a 'dropped head' 6 months after starting to also take donepezil 10 mg daily. Clinical examination showed muscle weakness and pain with swallowing difficulties, and serum muscle enzymes were increased. Donepezil and fenofibrate were discontinued and the symptoms disappeared with slow normalisation of creatine kinase. It was suggested that this effect occurred because both drugs have a potential action on muscle fibres through different mechanisms.[1] This appears to be an isolated case report and its general relevance is unknown.

1. Polivka M, Ducros A, Perchaud V, Guittard M, Amarenco P, Mikol J. Drop head syndrome during a combined treatment by donepezil and fenofibrate. *Brain Pathol* (2000) 10, 545.

Fibrates; Fenofibrate + Lomitapide

Lomitapide does not appear to affect the pharmacokinetics of fenofibrate.

Clinical evidence, mechanism, importance and management

In a prospective study in healthy subjects, lomitapide 10 mg daily for 7 days had no effect on the AUC of a single 145-mg dose of fenofibrate, but did decrease its maximum concentration by 30%.[1] Such a small effect on maximum concentration is not likely to be clinically relevant and therefore no fenofibrate dose adjustment is required on concurrent use with lomitapide.

1. Tuteja S, Duffy D, Dunbar RL, Movva R, Gadi R, Bloedon LT, Cuchel M. Pharmacokinetic interactions of the microsomal triglyceride transfer protein inhibitor, lomitapide, with drugs commonly used in the management of hypercholesterolemia. *Pharmacotherapy* (2014) 34, 227–39.

Fibrates; Gemfibrozil + Antacids

Aluminium-containing antacids can reduce the exposure to gemfibrozil.

Clinical evidence, mechanism, importance and management

A study in patients with kidney and liver disease found that the concurrent use of antacids (**aluminium hydroxide, aluminium magnesium silica hydrate**) reduced the maximum plasma levels of gemfibrozil by about 50 to 70%, and slightly to moderately reduced its AUC by about 30 to 60%. The precise values are not given in the text. The reasons for these reductions are not known, but it was suggested that gemfibrozil is adsorbed onto the antacids in the gut. The authors recommend that gemfibrozil is given 1 to 2 hours before antacids.[1] More study is needed to confirm these findings.

1. Knauf H, Kölle EU, Mutschler E. Gemfibrozil absorption and elimination in kidney and liver disease. *Klin Wochenschr* (1990) 68, 692–8.

Fibrates; Gemfibrozil + HIV-protease inhibitors

Lopinavir boosted with ritonavir slightly decreases gemfibrozil exposure.

Clinical evidence, mechanism, importance and management

In a pharmacokinetic study in 15 healthy subjects, **lopinavir boosted with ritonavir** 400/100 mg twice daily for 2 weeks slightly reduced the AUC of a single 600-mg dose of gemfibrozil by 41%, without changing its elimination half-life. **Ritonavir** is a known inducer of glucuronidation, by which gemfibrozil is metabolised; however, the authors discounted this mechanism because of the lack of change in the elimination half-life of gemfibrozil. They suggested that **lopinavir boosted with ritonavir** might have reduced gemfibrozil absorption via effects on intestinal transport proteins.[1] Whatever the mechanism, it appears that **lopinavir boosted with ritonavir** reduces gemfibrozil exposure, and might therefore be anticipated to reduce its clinical efficacy. Bear this possibility in mind on the concurrent use of these drugs.

1. Busse KH, Hadigan C, Chairez C, Alfaro RM, Formentini E, Kovacs JA, Penzak SR. Gemfibrozil concentrations are significantly decreased in the presence of lopinavir/ritonavir. *J Acquir Immune Defic Syndr* (2009) 52, 235–9.

Fibrates; Gemfibrozil + Interferon alfa

Isolated reports describe raised liver enzymes potentially due to an interaction between interferon alfa and gemfibrozil.

Clinical evidence

A 43-year-old man receiving interferon alfa-2b and a melanoma vaccine (melanoma theraccine) for malignant melanoma was given gemfibrozil 600 mg twice daily for interferon-induced hypertriglyceridaemia. About one month later, he developed severe gastrointestinal symptoms, consisting of nausea and decreased appetite, and raised liver enzymes. The dose of gemfibrozil was reduced to 300 mg daily and, 3 weeks later, his symptoms and liver enzyme levels had significantly improved. The patient had been receiving the same dose of interferon alfa for 6 months without any adverse effects.[1] Another similar case report describes a woman with melanoma who developed signs and symptoms of hepatitis within days of starting to take gemfibrozil 600 mg daily for interferon-induced hypertriglyceridaemia.[2]

Mechanism

Unknown. The adverse effects seen are known to occur with both gemfibrozil and interferon alfa alone, so it was suggested that what occurred was due to the additive effects of both drugs. However, an effect of gemfibrozil alone, and in one case an interaction involving the melanoma vaccine, was not ruled out. Furthermore, the potential for a pharmacokinetic interaction was not examined.[1]

Importance and management

Evidence for an interaction between interferon alfa and gemfibrozil appears to be limited to these case reports, and is not established. Nevertheless, as gastrointestinal adverse effects and raised liver enzymes are known adverse effects of both drugs it would be prudent to use some caution on their concurrent use. It seems likely that any interaction would be detected by the routine monitoring associated with the use of interferon alfa, but consider increasing the frequency of monitoring in stabilised patients if gemfibrozil is started.

1. Wong S-F, Jakowatz JG, Taheri R. Potential drug-drug interaction between interferon alfa-2b and gemfibrozil in a patient with malignant melanoma. *Clin Ther* (2005) 27, 1942–8.
2. Grubišić-Čabo F, Vrdoljak E. Drug-induced hepatitis in a patient with malignant melanoma treated with interferon alfa 2b adjuvantly who had been administered gemfibrozil in therapy. *Med Oncol* (2006) 23, 121–4.

Fibrates; Gemfibrozil + Ispaghula (Psyllium)

Psyllium (ispaghula) had no clinically relevant effect on gemfibrozil exposure in one study.

Clinical evidence, mechanism, importance and management

When 10 healthy subjects took gemfibrozil 600 mg with, or 2 hours after, psyllium (ispaghula) 3 g in 240 mL of water, the AUC of gemfibrozil was reduced by about 10%.[1] This reduction is too small to be clinically relevant.

1. Forland SC, Cutler RE. The effect of psyllium on the pharmacokinetics of gemfibrozil. *Clin Res* (1990) 38, 94A.

Fibrates; Gemfibrozil + Rifampicin (Rifampin)

Rifampicin does not affect the pharmacokinetics of gemfibrozil.

Clinical evidence, mechanism, importance and management

In a study in 10 healthy subjects, rifampicin 600 mg daily for 6 days did not alter the pharmacokinetics of a single 600-mg dose of gemfibrozil.[1] No gemfibrozil dose adjustment therefore seems necessary if both drugs are given.

1. Forland SC, Feng Y, Cutler RE. The effect of rifampin on the pharmacokinetics of gemfibrozil. *J Clin Pharmacol* (1988) 28, 930.

Lipid regulating drugs + Antioxidants and Vitamins

Supplementation with antioxidants (betacarotene, selenium, vitamin C, plus vitamin E) attenuated the beneficial effect of the combination of statins and nicotinic acid on HDL-cholesterol and on coronary artery stenosis in one study. This attenuation appeared to occur with betacarotene and vitamin A given alone, vitamin E given with vitamin C; but not with selenium given alone. In another study, vitamin E alone also adversely affected HDL-cholesterol in patients taking statins; however, yet another study found it did not, and, in a third outcome study, there was a beneficial effect for the combination of a statin and vitamin E in patients thought to be at high risk of oxidative stress because of their genotype.

A multivitamin and mineral supplement with additional vitamin D and calcium appeared to reduce atorvastatin levels, but, conversely, reduced LDL-cholesterol.

Clinical evidence

(a) Betacarotene, selenium, vitamin C and vitamin E

In a randomised, placebo-controlled coronary artery disease intervention study (The HDL-Atherosclerosis Treatment Study; HATS), over the first 12 months, patients taking antioxidants (vitamin E, vitamin C, betacarotene and selenium) in combination with **simvastatin** and **nicotinic acid** (niacin) were found to have a smaller increase in beneficial HDL-cholesterol when compared with those receiving the statin with **nicotinic acid** but no antioxidants. In particular, large HDL-cholesterol (HDL2) did not increase in the group given the antioxidants with lipid regulating drugs when compared with a 42% increase in the group given the lipid lowering drugs alone. There was no difference between the two groups in the reduction in LDL-cholesterol. The antioxidant combination alone actually reduced HDL2-cholesterol.[1] Similar findings were reported in the final 3-year results of this study. In addition, coronary artery stenosis *progressed* by 3.9% with placebo, 1.8% with the antioxidants, 0.7% with **simvastatin, nicotinic acid** and antioxidants, and *regressed* by 0.4% with **simvastatin** with **nicotinic acid** but no antioxidants. Thus the benefit of regression of coronary stenosis seen with **simvastatin** and **nicotinic acid** was lost when antioxidants were also given.[2] In this study, the antioxidant supplement was given at a dose of betacarotene 12.5 mg twice daily, vitamin C 500 mg twice daily, vitamin E 400 units twice daily (given as *d*-alpha-tocopherol) and selenium 50 micrograms twice daily. Simvastatin was started at a dose of 10 to 20 mg daily and titrated to 20 to 40 mg daily based on target LDL-cholesterol reductions. Nicotinic acid was started at a dose of 1 g twice daily of a slow-release preparation and titrated up to 4 g daily as an immediate-release preparation based on target HDL-cholesterol increases.[1,2]

In a later smaller study, in 44 of the patients who completed the HATs study (included in a review by the authors[3]), the same lipid lowering therapy was given for 3 months with vitamin A alone, betacarotene alone, vitamin E with vitamin C, selenium alone, the original antioxidant combination, or placebo. Each of the vitamin groups appeared to attenuate the benefit of the lipid lowering therapy on HDL-cholesterol to a similar extent to the original antioxidant combination. However, selenium alone appeared to enhance the beneficial effects on HDL-cholesterol.

(b) Multivitamins plus vitamin D and calcium

In a study in 16 patients taking stable doses of **atorvastatin**, lipid and **atorvastatin** levels were measured after taking a multivitamin containing vitamin D with additional vitamin D and calcium daily for 6 weeks and then again after 6 weeks without supplemental vitamin D or multivitamins. After taking the vitamins, the levels of total active **atorvastatin** (measured as $AUC_{0.5\text{-}10}$) were 45% lower, when compared with taking no vitamin supplements. However, unexpectedly, there was a 14.4% reduction in LDL-cholesterol after taking the vitamins (with no change in HDL-cholesterol). Three subjects continued to take calcium supplements while not taking vitamin D or multivitamins, and they still had a reduction in **atorvastatin** levels, suggesting the calcium had no effect. The daily dose of vitamin D given in this study was 800 units given as two tablets of vitamin D (colecalciferol) 200 units plus calcium carbonate 500 mg, and one multivitamin tablet containing vitamin D (ergocalciferol) 400 units. The multivitamin used was *Therapeutic-M* tablets (Goldline Laboratories), which, in addition to vitamin D, included supplemental doses of **vitamins A, C,** and **E** (30 units) and the **vitamin B substances** and about 11 **minerals** including **selenium** 10 micrograms.[4]

(c) Vitamin E substances alone

In a placebo-controlled study, vitamin E supplementation 400 units daily (given as *d*-alpha-tocopherol acetate) for 8 weeks did not affect total or LDL-cholesterol levels in hypercholesterolaemic patients taking stable doses of **lovastatin** or **simvastatin**. However, there was a small 6% decrease in HDL-cholesterol levels during vitamin E supplementation, which was apparent after 2 weeks, although it was not sufficient to change the ratio of total cholesterol to HDL–cholesterol (a measure of cardiac risk).[5] However, in another placebo-controlled study in 90 patients, of whom about 80 were taking statins, high-dose vitamin E 1200 units daily (given as *d*-alpha-tocopherol) for 2 years did not alter total HDL-cholesterol or HDL2-cholesterol.[6] Moreover, in a controlled clinical study in patients with diabetes mellitus taking statins (not specified) and with the haptoglobin 2-2-genotype (lack of an antioxidant protein), vitamin E reduced cardiovascular adverse events compared with placebo.[7]

Mechanism

It was anticipated that antioxidants would inhibit LDL-cholesterol oxidation and slow atherogenesis. However, unexpectedly, the combination of antioxidants used in the HATS study actually reduced HDL-cholesterol when used alone, and some, but not other, studies, have found that vitamin E alone has this effect. A reduction in HDL-cholesterol is detrimental and could reduce the benefit of nicotinic acid on this lipoprotein.

It was suggested that vitamin D would reduce atorvastatin levels because it increases the expression of CYP3A4, by which atorvastatin is partially metabolised.[4] However, there is no other clinical evidence to suggest that vitamin D causes drug interactions with CYP3A4 substrates. It was also suggested that vitamin D alone would have beneficial effects on cholesterol levels.[4]

Importance and management

The available evidence is not entirely consistent, but suggests that some types of antioxidants might decrease the response to lipid regulating drugs, such as statins and nicotinic acid (niacin), by reducing the beneficial HDL-cholesterol levels. More study is needed to confirm the suitability of different types and doses of antioxidant supplementation, but, until more is known, it might be prudent for patients requiring lipid regulating therapy to generally avoid the long-term use of antioxidant supplements, including higher doses of vitamin E or vitamin C. If vitamin E or C is considered essential, it might be prudent to monitor lipids to confirm no detrimental effects occur. In addition, given the data on the use of multivitamins with vitamin D, the effect of these antioxidant supplements on statin levels should be determined.

Conversely, a multivitamin supplement with minerals and additional vitamin D appeared to have additional benefits on lipid levels when given with atorvastatin, despite an apparent reduction in atorvastatin levels. This needs further study with vitamin D alone, as an effect of the supplement cannot be ruled out from this study. Also, the pharmacokinetic interaction requires further study, because, if confirmed, it has much wider implications for drug interactions.

1. Cheung MC, Zhao X-Q, Chait A, Albers JJ, Brown BG. Antioxidant supplements block the response of HDL to simvastatin-niacin therapy in patients with coronary artery disease and low HDL. *Arterioscler Thromb Vasc Biol* (2001) 21, 1320–6.
2. Brown BG, Zhao X-Q, Chait A, Fisher LD, Cheung MC, Morse JS, Dowdy AA, Marino EK, Bolson EL, Alaupovic P, Frohlich J, Serafini L, Huss-Frechette E, Wang S, DeAngelis D, Dodek A, Albers JJ. Simvastatin and niacin, antioxidant vitamins, or the combination for the prevention of coronary disease. *N Engl J Med* (2001) 345, 1583–92.
3. Brown BG, Cheung MC, Lee AC, Zhao X-Q, Chait A. Antioxidant vitamins and lipid therapy: end of a long romance? *Arterioscler Thromb Vasc Biol* (2002) 22, 1535–46.
4. Schwartz JB. Effects of vitamin D supplementation in atorvastatin-treated patients: a new drug interaction with an unexpected consequence. *Clin Pharmacol Ther* (2009) 85, 198–203.
5. Leonard SW, Joss JD, Mustacich DJ, Blatt DH, Lee YS, Traber MG. Effects of vitamin E on cholesterol levels of hypercholesterolemic patients receiving statins. *Am J Health-Syst Pharm* (2007) 64, 2257–66.
6. Singh U, Otvos J, Dasgupta A, de Lemos JA, Devaraj S, Jialal I. High-dose α-tocopherol therapy does not affect HDL subfractions in patients with coronary artery disease on statin therapy. *Clin Chem* (2007) 53, 525–8.
7. Blum S, Milman U, Shapira C, Miller-Lotan R, Bennett L, Kostenko M, Landau M, Keidar S, Levy Y, Khemlin A, Radan A, Levy AP. Dual therapy with statins and antioxidants is superior to statins alone in decreasing the risk of cardiovascular disease in a subgroup of middle-aged individuals with both diabetes mellitus and the haptoglobin 2-2 genotype. *Arterioscler Thromb Vasc Biol* (2008) 28, e18–e20.

Lomitapide + Hormonal contraceptives

Ethinylestradiol and norgestimate (given as a combined hormonal contraceptive) slightly increase lomitapide exposure when given simultaneously. Lomitapide does not appear to affect the pharmacokinetics of ethinylestradiol or norgestimate.

Clinical evidence, mechanism, importance and management

In a randomised study in 32 healthy female subjects, a combined hormonal contraceptive (containing **ethinylestradiol** 35 micrograms and **norgestimate** 250 micrograms) for 21 days increased the exposure of a single 20-mg dose of lomitapide by 32% when given simultaneously, but had no effect when the doses were separated by 12 hours. The maximum concentration of lomitapide was increased by 41% and 25%, respectively.[1] The US manufacturer of lomitapide also briefly notes that, in cross-study comparisons, its exposure was increased about 2-fold by oral hormonal contraceptives.[2] The UK and US manufacturers also briefly note that in a study, lomitapide 50 mg daily for 8 days had no effect on the pharmacokinetics of **ethinylestradiol** 35 micrograms or **norgestimate** 250 micrograms, when given as a daily combined hormonal contraceptive for 28 days.[2,3]

The authors of the study,[1] and the manufacturers[2,3] state that hormonal contraceptives are weak inhibitors of CYP3A4, by which lomitapide is metabolised, and therefore combined use increases its exposure. However, hormonal contraceptives are not usually considered to be CYP3A4 inhibitors, as they do not affect midazolam exposure (see 'Benzodiazepines and related drugs + Hormonal contraceptives', p.826). It therefore seems possible that another mechanism could be at play. Note also, that the increase in lomitapide exposure seen in the study was only slight, and only occurred when given simultaneously rather than 12 hours apart. Although such a small change in lomitapide exposure would seem unlikely to be clinically relevant, the UK manufacturer advises that the doses with oral hormonal contraceptives should be separated by 12 hours.[3] In contrast, the US manufacturer states that the dose of lomitapide should not exceed 30 mg daily in patients also taking oral hormonal contraceptives.[2] Further, because effective contraception is essential for lomitapide use, and lomitapide is associated with adverse gastrointestinal effects, the manufacturers advise that if vomiting or diarrhoea occurs while taking lomitapide, the absorption of oral hormonal contraceptives might be reduced, and additional contraceptive methods are required.[2,3] The UK manufacturer specifically advises that such measures are necessary in cases of protracted or severe diarrhoea and/or vomiting lasting more than 2 days, and that additional contraceptive methods should be used for 7 days after resolution of symptoms.[3]

1. Patel G, King A, Dutta S, Korb S, Wade JR, Foulds P, Sumeray M. Evaluation of the effects of the weak CYP3A inhibitors atorvastatin and ethinyl estradiol/norgestimate on lomitapide pharmacokinetics in healthy subjects. *J Clin Pharmacol* (2015) Epub.
2. Juxtapid (Lomitapide mesylate). Aegerion Pharmaceuticals Inc. US Prescribing information, April 2015.
3. Lojuxta (Lomitapide mesylate). Aegerion Pharmaceuticals Ltd. UK Summary of product characteristics, March 2015.

Lomitapide + Miscellaneous

Ketoconazole appears to very markedly increase lomitapide exposure, other CYP3A4 inhibitors are predicted to interact similarly, although to varying extents. Similarly, CYP3A4 inducers would be predicted to decrease lomitapide exposure. Food appears to slightly increase the exposure to lomitapide. Bile-acid binding resins might decrease the absorption of lomitapide, and lomitapide might decrease the absorption of fat soluble vitamins and nutrients.

Lomitapide appears to increase the exposure to warfarin, and is predicted to increase the exposure to P-glycoprotein substrates. Additive hepatotoxicity might occur if lomitapide is given with other hepatotoxic drugs.

Clinical evidence, mechanism, importance and management

(a) Bile-acid binding resins

The UK and US manufacturers of lomitapide note that although not studied, because bile-acid binding resins (such as **colesevelam** and **colestyramine**) can reduce the absorption of oral medicines, concurrent use should be separated by at least 4 hours.[1,2]

(b) CYP3A4 inducers

No studies appear to have been undertaken to investigate the effect of CYP3A4 inducers on lomitapide exposure. However, the interaction with ketoconazole (see under *CYP3A4 inhibitors*, below) demonstrates that lomitapide is a sensitive CYP3A4 substrate and it is therefore likely that the concurrent use of CYP3A4 inducers would considerably decrease its exposure and reduce its efficacy. Therefore the UK manufacturer of lomitapide recommends increasing the frequency of LDL cholesterol monitoring, and considering increasing the lomitapide dose to ensure adequate efficacy if long-term use of such an inducer is necessary.[2] For a list of clinically relevant CYP3A4 inducers, see 'Table 1.9', p.11. Note that the manufacturer additionally names **aminoglutethimide**, **glucocorticoids**, **pioglitazone**, and **nafcillin** as inducers of this isoenzyme.

(c) CYP3A4 inhibitors

1. Moderate or potent CYP3A4 inhibitors. The UK and US manufacturers of lomitapide briefly note that, in a drug interaction study, ketoconazole 200 mg twice daily for 9 days increased the AUC and maximum concentration of lomitapide 60 mg daily 27-fold and 15-fold, respectively.[1,2] Ketoconazole is a potent CYP3A4 inhibitor, and its effect on lomitapide exposure demonstrates that lomitapide is a sensitive substrate of CYP3A4. Because of this very marked increase in lomitapide exposure, the manufacturers contraindicate its concurrent use with potent and moderate CYP3A4 inhibitors. If a moderate or potent CYP3A4 inhibitor is essential, they state that the use of lomitapide should be temporarily suspended.[1,2] For a list of clinically relevant CYP3A4 inhibitors, see 'Table 1.9', p.11. Note that they name **ciprofloxacin**, **crizotinib**, **dronedarone**, and **mibefradil** as moderate or potent CYP3A4 inhibitors, but evidence for clinically relevant interactions with these drugs by this mechanism is lacking or inconclusive. **Grapefruit juice** is listed as a moderate CYP3A4 inhibitor but it is generally considered as weak, see advice for *weak CYP3A4 inhibitors* below.

2. Weak CYP3A4 inhibitors. Based on the effects of atorvastatin and of hormonal contraceptives on lomitapide exposure (see 'Statins + Lomitapide', p.1348 and 'Lomitapide + Hormonal contraceptives', above), the UK and US manufacturers advise caution on the concurrent use of lomitapide with weak CYP3A4 inhibitors. Specifically, the US manufacturer states that the dose of lomitapide should be restricted to 30 mg daily in patients also taking weak CYP3A4 inhibitors,[1] whereas the UK manufacturer advises that doses of the inhibitor and lomitapide should be given at least 12 hours apart.[2] For a list of weak CYP3A4 inhibitors see 'Table 1.9', p.11. The manufacturers additionally name **alprazolam**, **amiodarone**, **amlodipine**, **azithromycin**, **bicalutamide**, **cilostazol**, **ciclosporin**, **clotrimazole**, **fluoxetine**, **ginkgo** (*Ginkgo biloba*), **goldenseal** (*Hydrastis*), **isoniazid**, **ivacaftor**, **lacidipine**, **lapatinib**, **linagliptin**, **nilotinib**, **pazopanib**, **peppermint oil**, **propiverine**, **ranitidine**, **Seville oranges**, **tacrolimus**, **ticagrelor**, **tolvaptan**, and **zileuton**.[1,2] However, this list should be viewed with caution, as some drugs (such as ranitidine) are not known to be clinically relevant CYP3A4 inhibitors.

Grapefruit juice is a weak CYP3A4 inhibitor, although its effects are considered moderate by the manufacturers and they therefore state that patients taking lomitapide must avoid grapefruit juice.[1,2] It should be noted that the effects of grapefruit juice can be variable (see *Grapefruit juice*, under 'Drug-food interactions', p.16).

(d) Fat soluble vitamins and nutrients

The UK and US manufacturers of lomitapide advise that, based on its mechanism of action in the small intestine, it might decrease the absorption of fat soluble vitamins, such as **vitamin E**, and other fat soluble nutrients, such as fatty acids (e.g. **linoleic acid**). They recommend that patients should therefore be given daily supplements containing vitamin E 400 units, linoleic acid 200 mg, alpha-linoleic acid 210 mg, eicosapentaenoic acid (EPA) 110 mg, and docosahexaenoic acid (DHA) 80 mg.[1,2]

(e) Food

The UK manufacturer briefly notes that high-fat and low-fat meals increased the AUC and maximum concentration of lomitapide by 77% and 70%, and 58% and 28%, respectively.[2] Furthermore, both they and the US manufacturer, state that administration with food can adversely affect the gastrointestinal tolerability of lomitapide and therefore advise that it should be taken at least 2 hours after an evening meal.[1,2]

(f) Hepatotoxic drugs

Lomitapide is associated with liver toxicity and as a result, the UK and US manufacturers advise caution on its concurrent use with other drugs known to cause hepatotoxicity, and they advise possibly increasing monitoring of liver function. They specifically name, **amiodarone**, **isotretinoin**, **methotrexate**, **paracetamol (acetaminophen)** (at doses greater than 4 g daily for at least 3 days per week) **tetracyclines**, and **tamoxifen**.[1,2]

(g) P-glycoprotein substrates

In vitro, lomitapide has been shown to inhibit P-glycoprotein.[1,2] The UK and US manufacturers therefore predict that lomitapide might increase the absorption of P-glycoprotein substrates and recommend that a reduction in the dose of these drugs should be considered on concurrent use.[1,2] For a list of drugs that are known to be clinically relevant substrates of P-glycoprotein, see 'Table 1.12', p.14. The manufacturers additionally name **ambrisentan**, **imatinib**, **lapatinib**, **maraviroc**, **nilotinib**, **posaconazole**, **ranolazine**, **saxagliptin**, **sitagliptin**, and **tolvaptan**.[1,2] Until more is known, it would be prudent to monitor for an increase in adverse effects if lomitapide is given with these drugs, and/or consider more frequent therapeutic drug monitoring, reducing the dose if necessary (particularly for those drugs with a narrow therapeutic index, such as **digoxin**).

(h) Warfarin

The UK and US manufacturers briefly note that, lomitapide 60 mg daily for 12 days increased the INR in response to a single 10-mg dose of warfarin by 22 to 26%, and increased the AUC of both *R*-warfarin and *S*-warfarin by 25 to 30%.[1,2] The mechanism for this interaction is unclear, particularly as lomitapide is not thought to be an inhibitor of CYP2C9, the isoenzyme predominantly responsible for *S*-warfarin metabolism. Although this increase in warfarin exposure is slight, and the effect on the INR small, the manufacturers recommend regular monitoring of the INR and adjustment of the warfarin dose, particularly when initiating, stopping, or adjusting the lomitapide dose.[1,2]

1. Juxtapid (Lomitapide mesylate). Aegerion Pharmaceuticals Inc. US Prescribing information, April 2015.
2. Lojuxta (Lomitapide mesylate). Aegerion Pharmaceuticals Ltd. UK Summary of product characteristics, March 2015.

Nicotinic acid (Niacin) + Aspirin

Aspirin reduces the flushing reaction that often occurs with nicotinic acid, but there is some evidence that it can also increase nicotinic acid plasma levels.

Clinical evidence, mechanism, importance and management

Nicotinic acid (as a 70 to 100 micrograms/kg per minute infusion over 6 hours) was given to 6 healthy subjects. Two hours after the infusion was started, oral aspirin 1 g was also given. The plasma nicotinic acid levels rose, and its clearance was reduced by 30 to 54%.[1] It was thought that the salicylate competes with nicotinic acid for metabolism by glycine conjugation in the liver so that the clearance of nicotinic acid is reduced, resulting in a rise in its levels. The clinical importance of this effect when aspirin is given to reduce the annoying nicotinic acid flushing reaction[2] is not known. However, as nicotinic acid is titrated upwards, according to efficacy and tolerability, any increase in its levels caused by aspirin is probably naturally accounted for.

1. Ding RW, Kolbe K, Merz B, de Vries J, Weber E, Benet LZ. Pharmacokinetics of nicotinic acid-salicylic acid interaction. *Clin Pharmacol Ther* (1989) 46, 642–7.
2. Jungnickel PW, Maloley PA, Vander Tuin EL, Peddicord TE, Campbell JR. Effect of two aspirin pretreatment regimens on niacin-induced cutaneous reactions. *J Gen Intern Med* (1997) 12, 591–6.

Nicotinic acid (Niacin) + Bile-acid binding resins

Colestipol and colestyramine are predicted to reduce the bioavailability of nicotinic acid.

Clinical evidence, mechanism, importance and management

On the basis of *in vitro* data suggesting that colestipol, and to a lesser extent colestyramine, have high nicotinic acid binding capacity (98% and 10 to 30%, respectively),[1] the manufacturers of nicotinic acid predict that bile-acid binding resins might reduce the bioavailability of nicotinic acid.[1-3] They therefore recommend that nicotinic acid is given at least one hour before or 4 hours to 6 hours after taking a bile-acid binding resin.[1,3] In the absence of further information, this seems prudent.

1. Niaspan (Niacin). Abbott Laboratories. US Prescribing information, April 2015.
2. Niaspan (Nicotinic acid). Abbott Laboratories Ltd. UK Summary of product characteristics, December 2010.
3. Tredaptive (Nicotinic acid with Laropiprant). Merck Sharp & Dohme, Ltd. UK Summary of product characteristics, April 2012.

Nicotinic acid (Niacin) + Enfuvirtide

An isolated case report describes extreme redness, oedema and swelling at injection sites when nicotinic acid was given to a patient receiving enfuvirtide.

Clinical evidence, mechanism, importance and management

A case report describes a 47-year-old HIV-positive man newly started on subcutaneous enfuvirtide 90 mg twice daily as part of an antiretroviral regimen. He started taking extended-release nicotinic acid 500 mg daily 6 days later, and complained of extreme redness, swelling and oedema at the enfuvirtide injection sites after one week of concurrent use. The symptoms were similar to the flushing sensation the patient experienced about 30 minutes after taking the nicotinic acid. Both drugs were stopped, and when enfuvirtide was restarted, no adverse effects occurred. The authors suggest an immunological basis for this reaction.[1]

Evidence for an interaction between nicotinic acid and enfuvirtide is limited to this isolated case and as such its general importance is unclear. If nicotinic acid and enfuvirtide are given concurrently, bear the case report in mind should any unexpected adverse effects occur.

1. Oates E, Dzintars K. Interaction between enfuvirtide, an injectable fusion inhibitor, and niacin in an HIV-infected patient. *Ann Pharmacother* (2010) 44, 2014–17.

Nicotinic acid (Niacin) + Lomitapide

Lomitapide does not appear to affect the pharmacokinetics of nicotinic acid.

Clinical evidence, mechanism, importance and management

In a prospective study in healthy subjects, lomitapide 10 mg daily for 7 days increased the AUC and maximum concentration of a single 1-g dose of extended-release nicotinic acid by about 10%. However, the range of effects includes the possibility that these increases occurred by chance, and it also shows great variability.[1] Despite the lack of reliability of the result, if true, such small changes would not be clinically relevant. In the absence of additional data, and based on the known metabolism of nicotinic acid, no dose adjustment would seem to be required on concurrent use with lomitapide.

1. Tuteja S, Duffy D, Dunbar RL, Movva R, Gadi R, Bloedon LT, Cuchel M. Pharmacokinetic interactions of the microsomal triglyceride transfer protein inhibitor, lomitapide, with drugs commonly used in the management of hypercholesterolemia. *Pharmacotherapy* (2014) 34, 227–39.

Nicotinic acid (Niacin) + Nicotine

An isolated report describes an unpleasant flushing reaction that developed when a woman taking nicotinic acid started to use nicotine transdermal patches.

Clinical evidence, mechanism, importance and management

A case report describes a woman who had taken nicotinic acid 250 mg twice daily for 3 years without problems, as well as nifedipine, ranitidine, colestyramine and ferrous sulfate. Following laryngectomy for cancer of the larynx, she restarted all of the drugs except the colestyramine and began to use nicotine transdermal patches 21 mg daily to try to give up smoking. On several occasions, shortly after taking the nicotinic acid, she developed unpleasant flushing episodes lasting about 30 minutes. No further episodes developed when the nicotinic acid was stopped.[1] The reasons are not understood, but flushing is a very common adverse effect of nicotinic acid, and it would seem that in this case the nicotine patch might have been responsible for its emergence. A comment on this report suggests that this reaction could possibly have an immunological basis.[2] Either way, this reaction is more unpleasant than serious.

1. Rockwell KA. Potential interaction between niacin and transdermal nicotine. *Ann Pharmacother* (1993) 27, 1283–4.
2. Sudan BJL. Comment: niacin, nicotine, and flushing. *Ann Pharmacother* (1994) 28, 1113.

Statins + ACE inhibitors

In general the statins do not appear to interact adversely with the ACE inhibitors. The concurrent use of pitavastatin and enalapril does not affect the pharmacokinetics of either drug, and simvastatin does not alter ramipril pharmacokinetics. An isolated report describes severe hyperkalaemia in a diabetic given lisinopril with lovastatin, and acute pancreatitis has been attributed to the use of lisinopril with atorvastatin.

Clinical evidence

(a) Atorvastatin

An isolated case report describes the development of acute pancreatitis in a patient who had been taking **lisinopril** 10 mg daily with atorvastatin 20 mg daily for 9 months. No other cause for the pancreatitis was identified.[1,2]

(b) Fluvastatin

Retrospective analysis of clinical study data found no evidence that the safety or efficacy of fluvastatin was altered by the use of unspecified ACE inhibitors.[3]

(c) Lovastatin

A retrospective analysis of clinical study data found no evidence that the safety of lovastatin was altered by the use of unspecified ACE inhibitors in 142 patients.[4] Likewise, another study found that the addition of lovastatin 20 mg daily to **lisinopril**, for 6 weeks, was well tolerated and there was a substantial reduction in serum cholesterol levels without any clinically relevant effect on the antihypertensive efficacy of **lisinopril**.[5] However, one study in 70 patients taking **enalapril** or **lisinopril** found that the addition of lovastatin or **pravastatin** caused a greater reduction in blood pressure compared with the use of the ACE inhibitor alone.[6]

An isolated report describes a 33-year-old patients with type 1 diabetes (receiving insulin) with hypertension and familial hypercholesterolaemia who developed myopathy and severe hyperkalaemia (serum potassium 8.4 mmol/L) when given lovastatin 20 to 40 mg daily with **lisinopril** 50 mg daily. His serum potassium returned to about 5.5 mmol/L after lovastatin was stopped and the dose of **lisinopril** lowered (to 20 mg daily). About 3 months later, lovastatin was restarted, but after only 2 doses he again developed severe myopathy and hyperkalaemia, which resolved after the lovastatin was stopped.[7]

(d) Pitavastatin

The manufacturer of pitavastatin notes that concurrent use of pitavastatin 4 mg daily and **enalapril** 20 mg daily for 5 days had a negligible effect on the pharmacokinetics of both drugs (the AUC of pitavastatin was increased by 6% and its maximum concentration was reduced by 7%, and the AUC and maximum concentration of **enalapril** were increased by 12% whereas those for its active metabolite, enalaprilat, were unchanged).[8]

(e) Simvastatin

In a study in healthy subjects, simvastatin had no effect on the pharmacokinetics or ACE-inhibitory effects of **ramipril** or its metabolites.[9] Similarly, in a single-dose study in subjects given **ramipril** 5 mg alone or simvastatin 20 mg alone or both in a combined tablet with hydrochlorothiazide 12.5 mg, atenolol 50 mg and aspirin 100 mg, there was no difference in **ramipril** or ramiprilat pharmacokinetics between the combined tablet and **ramipril** alone. However the AUC of simvastatin was 24% lower with the combined tablet whereas the AUC of active simvastatin acid was 44% higher compared with simvastatin alone.[10] The clinical relevance of the apparent difference is also unclear, but the authors note that in an efficacy study, the combined tablet caused a slightly smaller reduction in cholesterol than simvastatin alone.[11]

A woman taking a variety of drugs, including conjugated oestrogens, developed pancreatitis about 3 months after starting both **lisinopril** 40 mg daily and simvastatin 20 mg daily. However, in this case, the patient had subsequently restarted taking conjugated oestrogens and simvastatin without a reappearance of the pancreatitis, so the **lisinopril** alone was implicated.[2]

Mechanism

It was suggested that the case of hyperkalaemia with lisinopril and lovastatin resulted from a combination of the potassium-sparing effects of lisinopril, the release of intracellular potassium into the blood stream associated with myopathy, and a predisposition to hyperkalaemia due to the diabetes and mild renal impairment.[7]

The case of pancreatitis with lisinopril and atorvastatin is unexplained, but both ACE inhibitors and statins alone have, rarely, been associated with the development of pancreatitis.[1,2]

The reason for the apparent difference in simvastatin pharmacokinetics with the multi-ingredient preparation containing ramipril is unclear, but it seems unlikely to be due to a pharmacokinetic interaction between any of the drugs and simvastatin.[10]

Importance and management

In general, no clinically relevant pharmacokinetic interaction would be expected between the statins and the ACE inhibitors, and the limited pharmacokinetic data available supports this suggestion. Further, the concurrent use of statins and ACE inhibitors appears to be generally well tolerated; however, isolated case reports have described hyperkalaemia and pancreatitis following the use of lisinopril with lovastatin and lisinopril with atorvastatin, respectively. Given the widespread concurrent use of drugs from these classes, they seem unlikely to be of general importance. However, one UK manufacturer of lisinopril (with hydrochlorothiazide) states that the concurrent use of lovastatin and ACE inhibitors increases the risk of hyperkalaemia.[12]

1. Kanbay M, Sekuk H, Yilmaz U, Gur G, Boyacioglu S. Acute pancreatitis associated with combined lisinopril and atorvastatin therapy. *Dig Dis* (2005) 23, 92–4.
2. Miller LG, Tan G. Drug-induced pancreatitis (lisinopril). *J Am Board Fam Pract* (1999) 12, 150–3.
3. Peters TK, Jewitt-Harris J, Mehra M, Muratti EN. Safety and tolerability of fluvastatin with concomitant use of antihypertensive agents. An analysis of a clinical trial database. *Am J Hypertens* (1993) 6, 346S–352S.
4. Pool JL, Shear CL, Downton M, Schnaper H, Stinnett S, Dujovne C, Bradford RH, Chremos AN. Lovastatin and coadministered antihypertensive/cardiovascular agents. *Hypertension* (1992) 19, 242–8.
5. Os I, Bratland B, Dahlöf B, Gisholt K, Syvertsen J-O, Tretli S. Effect and tolerability of combining lovastatin with nifedipine or lisinopril. *Am J Hypertens* (1993) 6, 688–92.
6. Spósito AC, Mansur AP, Coelho OR, Nicolau JC, Ramires JAF. Additional reduction in blood pressure after cholesterol-lowering treatment by statins (lovastatin or pravastatin) in hypercholesterolemic patients using angiotensin-converting enzyme inhibitors (enalapril or lisinopril). *Am J Cardiol* (1999) 83, 1497–9.
7. Edelman S, Witztum JL. Hyperkalemia during treatment with HMG-CoA reductase inhibitor. *N Engl J Med* (1989) 320, 1219–20.
8. Livalo (Pitavastatin). Kowa Pharmaceuticals America, Inc. US Prescribing information, October 2013.
9. Meyer BH, Scholtz HE, Müller FO, Luus HG, de la Rey N, Seibert-Grafe M, Eckert HG, Metzger H. Lack of interaction between ramipril and simvastatin. *Eur J Clin Pharmacol* (1994) 47, 373–5.
10. Patel A, Shah T, Shah G, Jha V, Ghosh C, Desai J, Khamar B, Chakraborty BS. Preservation of bioavailability of ingredients and lack of drug-drug interactions in a novel five-ingredient polypill (Polycap): a five-arm phase I crossover trial in healthy volunteers. *Am J Cardiovasc Drugs* (2010) 10, 95–103.
11. Indian Polycap Study (TIPS), Yusuf S, Pais P, Afzal R, Xavier D, Teo K, Eikelboom J, Sigamani A, Mohan V, Gupta R, Thomas N. Effects of a polypill (Polycap) on risk factors in middle-aged individuals without cardiovascular disease (TIPS): a phase II, double-blind, randomised trial. *Lancet* (2009) 373, 1341–51.
12. Zestoretic (Lisinopril with Hydrochlorothiazide). AstraZeneca UK Ltd. UK Summary of product characteristics, November 2010.

Statins + Amiodarone

Amiodarone increases simvastatin exposure, and there is some evidence of a higher incidence of myopathy when amiodarone is given with high doses of simvastatin: cases of myopathy and rhabdomyolysis have been reported in patients taking amiodarone and simvastatin. One case of raised liver enzyme levels has been reported with amiodarone and rosuvastatin. Amiodarone has no clinically relevant effect on pravastatin exposure.

Clinical evidence

(a) Atorvastatin

An analysis of reports to the FDA in the US suggested that the concurrent use of **simvastatin** or atorvastatin with amiodarone is associated with a higher incidence of muscle toxicity than pravastatin with amiodarone. The percentage of reports of muscle, liver, pancreas, and bone marrow toxicity associated with the concurrent use of statins and amiodarone was 1% for **simvastatin**, 0.7% for atorvastatin, and 0.4% for **pravastatin**.[1]

(b) Pravastatin

A study in 12 healthy subjects found that amiodarone 400 mg daily for 3 days decreased the AUC of a single 40-mg dose of pravastatin by just 10%.[2] For mention that the use of pravastatin with amiodarone appeared to be associated with a lower incidence of toxicity than atorvastatin or simvastatin, see *Atorvastatin*, above

(c) Rosuvastatin

Asymptomatic elevated liver enzymes (serum transaminases), which were attributed to an interaction between rosuvastatin 5 mg daily and amiodarone 200 mg daily, have been reported in a 73-year-old woman with diabetes and hypothyroidism who had recently undergone surgery.[3]

(d) Simvastatin

A study in 12 healthy subjects found that amiodarone 400 mg daily for 3 days increased the bioavailability of a single 40-mg dose of simvastatin; the AUC of simvastatin and simvastatin acid were increased by 73% and 78%, respectively. Because amiodarone has such a long half-life, and because its steady-state concentrations would be expected to be markedly higher than those achieved in this study, it would be expected that longer term amiodarone would have a greater effect.[2]

In the SEARCH study comparing simvastatin 80 mg daily with simvastatin 20 mg daily, an increased risk of myopathy was found when simvastatin 80 mg daily was used with amiodarone (based on 8 cases). Therefore, all patients taking amiodarone were subsequently given simvastatin 20 mg daily irrespective of their original study allocation.[4] The UK manufacturers of simvastatin also note that in a clinical study, myopathy (muscle pain, tenderness or weakness with a creatine kinase concentration at least 10 times the upper limit of normal) was reported in 6% of patients receiving high-dose simvastatin 80 mg daily with amiodarone.[5] This compares with a usual incidence of about 0.9% for high-dose simvastatin 80 mg daily and of just 0.02% for simvastatin 20 mg daily from a review of data from the SEARCH study.[5-7] The FDA in the US noted that in the 5 years from January 2003 (when the US prescribing information first contained information about the increased risk of myopathy when amiodarone is taken with simvastatin), 52 additional reports of rhabdomyolysis associated with concurrent use were received. Of these 52 reports, 26 were with high-dose simvastatin 80 mg daily, 13 were with 40 mg, four were with 20 mg, and, for 8, the dose was unknown. Other potentially interacting drugs were being taken in about 17 cases. Symptoms of rhabdomyolysis developed within a mean of 5 months (median 2 months) of concurrent use. Almost all the cases required hospitalisation, and 15 were considered life-threatening, with one death.[8]

For mention that the use of simvastatin with amiodarone appeared to be associated with a higher incidence of toxicity than pravastatin, see *Atorvastatin*, above

A few individual case reports of myopathy and rhabdomyolysis have been reported in patients taking amiodarone and simvastatin. A 63-year-old man with diabetes developed diffuse muscle pain with generalised muscular weakness 4 weeks after starting to take simvastatin 40 mg daily, and about 2 weeks after starting to take amiodarone (1 g daily for 10 days, then 200 mg daily thereafter). There was a marked increase in creatine kinase, which normalised after stopping both drugs.[9] A 77-year-old man taking multiple medications including amiodarone 100 mg daily and simvastatin 20 mg daily, developed increasing lower-extremity pain and darkening of his urine 3 weeks after his simvastatin dose was increased to 40 mg daily. He was diagnosed with rhabdomyolysis secondary to simvastatin use,[10] although a later comment suggested that amiodarone could have contributed.[11] Two other cases of rhabdomyolysis in patients taking amiodarone with simvastatin 40 mg and 80 mg[12,13] (one involving clarithromycin)[13] have also been reported. One of these patients had pneumonia,[13] and the other diabetes,[12] both of which have been suggested as risk factors for rhabdomyolysis. Another case with simvastatin 40 mg, amiodarone and also verapamil was briefly mentioned in a case series of patients with statin myopathy.[14]

For a case report of rhabdomyolysis in a 72-year-old HIV-positive man taking atazanavir and delavirdine shortly after switching from atorvastatin 40 mg daily to high-dose simvastatin 80 mg daily and shortly after starting amiodarone, see 'Statins + HIV-protease inhibitors', p.1345.

Mechanism

Amiodarone is an inhibitor of various cytochrome P450 isoenzymes including CYP3A4 and CYP2C9, and might therefore increase simvastatin exposure by inhibiting the metabolism of simvastatin by CYP3A4. Other extensively metabolised statins, such as **lovastatin**, would be expected to be similarly affected, and this might increase the risk of muscle toxicity. Amiodarone alone sometimes causes myopathy. Amiodarone did not appear to appreciably alter the pharmacokinetics of pravastatin, and would not therefore be expected to interact with rosuvastatin, which is also minimally metabolised by cytochrome P450 isoenzymes.

Importance and management

A pharmacokinetic interaction between **simvastatin** and amiodarone appears to be established, as does the increased risk of myopathy with the combination. The manufacturers of simvastatin recommend reducing the maximum dose of simvastatin to 20 mg daily in patients also taking amiodarone, unless the clinical benefit is likely to outweigh the increased risk of myopathy and rhabdomyolysis.[5,15] **Lovastatin** is metabolised in the same way as simvastatin, and shares many of its interactions: the manufacturer of lovastatin suggests a maximum dose of 40 mg daily when lovastatin is taken with amiodarone.[16] **Atorvastatin** is also metabolised (at least in part) by CYP3A4 inhibitors and the UK manufacturer of atorvastatin suggests that, although interaction studies have not been conducted, amiodarone might result in increased atorvastatin exposure and state that lower maximum atorvastatin doses should be considered, with appropriate clinical monitoring.[17] The US manufacturer of amiodarone includes similar information;[18] however, note that the UK manufacturer of amiodarone actually recommends that when a statin is required with amiodarone, one that is *not* metabolised by CYP3A4 should be used.[19]

As a general rule, any patient given simvastatin, lovastatin or atorvastatin with amiodarone should be told to report any signs of myopathy and possible rhabdomyolysis (i.e. otherwise unexplained muscle pain, tenderness or weakness or dark coloured urine). If myopathy does occur, the statin should be stopped immediately. See also *Muscle and liver toxicity*, under 'Lipid regulating drugs', p.1309, for further guidance on monitoring and risk factors for muscle toxicity.

The lack of a clinically relevant pharmacokinetic interaction with **pravastatin** and the apparent lower incidence of toxicity on concurrent use suggests that amiodarone does not interact with pravastatin.

The isolated case of raised liver enzymes with **rosuvastatin** is probably not of general relevance.

There are no data for **fluvastatin** with amiodarone. However, theoretically, amiodarone might be expected to increase fluvastatin concentrations because amiodarone is an inhibitor of CYP2C9 by which fluvastatin is metabolised. Until more is known, bear the possibility of an interaction in mind when both drugs are given.

1. Alsheikh-Ali AA, Karas RH. Adverse events with concomitant amiodarone and statin therapy. *Prev Cardiol* (2005) 8, 95–7.

2. Becquemont L, Neuvonen M, Verstuyft C, Jaillon P, Letierce A, Neuvonen PJ, Funck-Brentano C. Amiodarone interacts with simvastatin but not with pravastatin disposition kinetics. *Clin Pharmacol Ther* (2007) 81, 679–84.
3. Merz T, Fuller SH. Elevated serum transaminase levels resulting from concomitant use of rosuvastatin and amiodarone. *Am J Health-Syst Pharm* (2007) 64, 1818–21.
4. Study of the Effectiveness of Additional Reductions in Cholesterol and Homocysteine (SEARCH) Collaborative Group, Armitage J, Bowman L, Wallendszus K, Bulbulia R, Rahimi K, Haynes R, Parish S, Peto R, Collins R. Intensive lowering of LDL cholesterol with 80 mg versus 20 mg simvastatin daily in 12,064 survivors of myocardial infarction: a double-blind randomised trial. *Lancet* (2010) 376, 1658–69. Erratum in: ibid. (2011) 377, 126.
5. Zocor (Simvastatin). Merck Sharp & Dohme Ltd. UK Summary of product characteristics, June 2015.
6. Medicines Healthcare products Regulatory Agency and the Commission on Human Medicines. Simvastatin: increased risk of myopathy at high dose (80 mg). *Drug Safety Update* (2010) 3, 7–8.
7. FDA. Drug Safety Communication: ongoing safety review of high-dose Zocor (simvastatin) and increased risk of muscle injury. March 19, 2010. Available at: http://www.fda.gov/Drugs/DrugSafety/PostmarketDrugSafetyInformationforPatientsandProviders/ucm204882.htm (accessed 21/10/15).
8. FDA. Interaction between amiodarone (marketed as Cordarone and Pacerone) and simvastatin (marketed as Zocor and generics) or simvastatin-combination products (marketed as Vytorin and Simcor): amiodarone potentiates the risk for simvastatin-associated rhabdomyolysis. *FDA Drug Safety Newsletter* (2008) 1, 46–8. Available at: http://www.fda.gov/downloads/Drugs/DrugSafety/DrugSafetyNewsletter/ucm109178.pdf. (accessed 21/10/15).
9. Roten L, Schoenenberger RA, Krähenbühl S, Schlienger RG. Rhabdomyolysis in association with simvastatin and amiodarone. *Ann Pharmacother* (2004) 38, 978–81.
10. Wratchford P, Ponte CD. High-dose simvastatin and rhabdomyolysis. *Am J Health-Syst Pharm* (2003) 60, 698–700.
11. de Denus S, Spinler SA. Amiodarone's role in simvastatin-associated rhabdomyolysis. *Am J Health-Syst Pharm* (2003) 60, 1791.
12. Ricuarte B, Guirguis A, Taylor HC, Zabriskie D. Simvastatin–amiodarone interaction resulting in rhabdomyolysis, azotemia, and possible hepatotoxicity. *Ann Pharmacother* (2006) 40, 753–7.
13. Chouhan UM, Chakrabarti S, Millward LJ. Simvastatin interaction with clarithromycin and amiodarone causing myositis. *Ann Pharmacother* (2005) 39, 1760–1.
14. McKelvie PA, Dennett X. Myopathy associated with HMG-CoA reductase inhibitors (statins): a series of 10 patients and review of the literature. *J Clin Neuromusc Dis* (2002) 3, 143–8.
15. Zocor (Simvastatin). Merck & Co., Inc. US Prescribing information, March 2015.
16. Mevacor (Lovastatin). Merck & Co., Inc. US Prescribing information, February 2014.
17. Lipitor (Atorvastatin calcium trihydrate). Pfizer Ltd. UK Summary of product characteristics, March 2015.
18. Cordarone (Amiodarone hydrochloride). Wyeth Pharmaceuticals Inc. US Prescribing information, December 2014.
19. Cordarone X (Amiodarone hydrochloride). Zentiva. UK Summary of product characteristics, April 2014.

Statins + Angiotensin II receptor antagonists

Irbesartan, telmisartan and valsartan have no clinically relevant effect on the pharmacokinetics of simvastatin, and simvastatin does not affect the pharmacokinetics of valsartan. Fluvastatin does not alter the pharmacokinetics of losartan or its active metabolite, and olmesartan does not alter the pharmacokinetics of pravastatin.

Clinical evidence, mechanism, importance and management

(a) Fluvastatin

In a crossover study, 12 healthy subjects were given **losartan** 50 mg in the morning for 7 days, followed by fluvastatin 40 mg at bedtime for 7 days, and then both drugs together for another 7 days. It was found that the steady-state pharmacokinetics of **losartan** and its active metabolite, E-3174, were not altered by fluvastatin. It had been anticipated that fluvastatin would increase the levels of losartan and reduce the levels of E-3174 by inhibiting CYP2C9;[1] however, fluvastatin is only a weak CYP2C9 inhibitor. The findings of this study indicate that a clinically relevant pharmacokinetic interaction is unlikely, and no **losartan** dose adjustment is required on concurrent use.

(b) Pravastatin

In a study in 10 healthy subjects, **olmesartan medoxomil** 10 mg daily for 4 days did not alter the pharmacokinetics of pravastatin or its metabolite, RMS-416, after a single 10-mg dose.[2]

(c) Simvastatin

In a single-dose study in 12 healthy subjects, **irbesartan** 300 mg had no effect on the pharmacokinetics of simvastatin 40 mg, or its metabolite simvastatin acid.[3]

The US manufacturer briefly notes that no clinically relevant interaction was noted when **telmisartan** was given with simvastatin.[4]

In a crossover study, 18 healthy subjects were given **valsartan** 160 mg daily and simvastatin 40 mg daily for 7 days alone, and then together. Simvastatin had no effect on the pharmacokinetics of valsartan. Valsartan caused a 40% increase in the AUC of simvastatin, a 20% decrease in its maximum level, and a doubling of the time to maximum level; however, there was no change in AUC and maximum level of the active metabolite simvastatin acid. These changes suggest that the absorption of simvastatin is slower when it is given with valsartan, but because there was no change in exposure to the active metabolite this interaction is not considered to be clinically relevant.[5]

1. Meadowcroft AM, Williamson KM, Patterson JH, Hinderliter AL, Pieper JA. The effects of fluvastatin, a CYP2C9 inhibitor, on losartan pharmacokinetics in healthy volunteers. *J Clin Pharmacol* (1999) 39, 418–24.
2. Suwannakul S, Ieiri I, Kimura M, Kawabata K, Kusuhara H, Hirota T, Irie S, Sugiyama Y, Higuchi S. Pharmacokinetic interaction between pravastatin and olmesartan in relation to *SLCO1B1* polymorphism. *Hum Genet* (2008) 53, 899–904.
3. Marino MR, Vachharajani NN, Hadjilambris OW. Irbesartan does not affect the pharmacokinetics of simvastatin in healthy subjects. *J Clin Pharmacol* (2000) 40, 875–9.
4. Micardis (Telmisartan). Boehringer Ingelheim Pharmaceuticals Inc. US Prescribing information, October 2012.
5. Sunkara G, Reynolds CV, Pommier F, Humbert H, Yeh CM, Prasad P. Evaluation of a pharmacokinetic interaction between valsartan and simvastatin in healthy subjects. *Curr Med Res Opin* (2007) 23, 631–40.

Statins + Antacids

Aluminium/magnesium hydroxide-containing antacids cause a slight to moderate reduction in the bioavailability of atorvastatin, pravastatin, and rosuvastatin.

Clinical evidence, mechanism, importance and management

(a) Atorvastatin

In a multiple-dose study, 18 patients were given atorvastatin 10 mg daily for 15 days with 30 mL of an **aluminium/magnesium hydroxide** antacid *(Maalox TC)* four times daily for a further 17 days. The maximum plasma levels and AUC of atorvastatin were both reduced by 34%, and the absorption rate was also reduced by the antacid. However, the LDL-cholesterol reduction remained the same.[1] It was not stated whether the daily atorvastatin dose was given at the same time or separately from the antacid. However, the slight reduction in atorvastatin exposure seen with the antacid is not clinically relevant.

(b) Pravastatin

In a study, giving an **aluminium/magnesium hydroxide** antacid *(Maalox TC)* 15 mL four times daily for 3 days with a single 20-mg dose of pravastatin one hour after the first antacid dose on the third day, reduced the AUC of pravastatin by 28%. This change was less than that seen with food, which did not alter pravastatin efficacy.[2] It is possible that simultaneous administration of pravastatin and the antacid might have had a greater effect. However, the slight reduction in pravastatin exposure seen with the antacid is not clinically relevant.

(c) Rosuvastatin

In a crossover study, 14 healthy subjects were given a single 40-mg dose of rosuvastatin alone, with, or 2 hours before a single 20-mL dose of an **aluminium/magnesium hydroxide** antacid (*Maalox*). The antacid reduced the AUC of rosuvastatin by 54% when it was given simultaneously, and by 22% when it was given 2 hours after rosuvastatin.[3] On this basis, the authors concluded that antacids should be given at least 2 hours after rosuvastatin: this seems prudent.

1. Yang B-B, Smithers JA, Abel RB, Stern RH, Sedman AJ, Olson SC. Effects of Maalox TC® on pharmacokinetics and pharmacodynamics of atorvastatin. *Pharm Res* (1996) 13 (9 Suppl), S437.
2. ER Squibb. Data on file. A report on the comparative pharmacokinetics of pravastatin in the presence and absence of cimetidine or antacids in healthy male subjects (Protocol No 27, 201-43). 1988.
3. Martin PD, Schneck DW, Dane AL, Warwick MJ. The effect of a combination antacid preparation containing aluminium hydroxide and magnesium hydroxide on rosuvastatin pharmacokinetics. *Curr Med Res Opin* (2008) 24, 1231–5.

Statins + Aspirin

No pharmacokinetic interaction occurs between low-dose aspirin and atorvastatin, and aspirin does not alter pravastatin pharmacokinetics. An isolated report describes pancreatitis with the long-term concurrent use of low-dose aspirin and atorvastatin.

Clinical evidence, mechanism, importance and management

(a) Atorvastatin

In a pharmacokinetic study in healthy subjects, aspirin 100 mg daily and atorvastatin 80 mg daily were given alone and then together for 7 days. Concurrent use did not alter atorvastatin or aspirin pharmacokinetics, except for a16% increase in the AUC of aspirin.[1] This change is not clinically relevant.

An isolated report describes acute pancreatitis possibly associated with the long-term use of aspirin 100 mg daily (10 years) and atorvastatin 40 mg daily (5 years).[2] This case is not expected to be of general relevance.

(b) Pravastatin

In a single-dose study in healthy subjects, aspirin 324 mg did not affect the pharmacokinetics of pravastatin 20 mg.[3]

(c) Simvastatin

In a single-dose study in subjects given aspirin 100 mg alone, simvastatin 20 mg alone or both in a combined tablet with hydrochlorothiazide 12.5 mg, atenolol 50 mg and ramipril 5 mg, there was no difference in aspirin pharmacokinetics between the combined tablet and aspirin alone. However, the AUC of simvastatin was 24% lower with the combined tablet, whereas the AUC of active simvastatin acid was 44% higher, compared with simvastatin alone. The reason for this apparent difference is unclear, but it seems unlikely to be due to a pharmacokinetic interaction between any of the drugs and simvastatin.[4] The clinical relevance of the apparent difference is also unclear, but the authors note that in an efficacy study, the combined tablet caused a slightly smaller reduction in cholesterol than simvastatin alone.[5]

1. Cho H, Cho D, Yeo C, Bae S, Shon J, Park S, Kim E, Shin J. Evaluation of the potential for steady-state pharmacokinetic interaction between atorvastatin and aspirin in healthy subjects. *Clin Pharmacol Ther* (2010) 87 (Suppl 1), S95.
2. Miltiadous G, Anthopoulou A, Elisaf M. Acute pancreatitis possibly associated with combined salicylate and atorvastatin therapy. *JOP* (2003) 4, 20–21.
3. ER Squibb. Data on file. A report on the effect of nicotinic acid alone and in the presence of aspirin on the bioavailability of SQ 31,000 in healthy male subjects (Protocol No 27, 201-6). 1987.
4. Patel A, Shah T, Shah G, Jha V, Ghosh C, Desai J, Khamar B, Chakraborty BS. Preservation of bioavailability of ingredients and lack of drug-drug interactions in a novel five-ingredient polypill (Polycap): a five-arm phase I crossover trial in healthy volunteers. *Am J Cardiovasc Drugs* (2010) 10, 95–103.
5. Indian Polycap Study (TIPS), Yusuf S, Pais P, Afzal R, Xavier D, Teo K, Eikelboom J, Sigamani A, Mohan V, Gupta R, Thomas N. Effects of a polypill (Polycap) on risk factors in middle-aged individuals without cardiovascular disease (TIPS): a phase II, double-blind, randomised trial. *Lancet* (2009) 373, 1341–51.

Statins + Azoles

Fluconazole slightly increases fluvastatin and pravastatin exposure, but has only negligible effects on rosuvastatin exposure. Miconazole would be expected to interact with these statins in a similar way to fluconazole.

Itraconazole causes a very marked increase in lovastatin and simvastatin exposure, a moderate increase in atorvastatin exposure, a slight increase in rosuvastatin exposure, no change to a slight increase in pravastatin exposure, no change in fluvastatin exposure, and, conversely, a very slight *decrease* in pitavastatin exposure. Posaconazole causes a marked to very marked increase in simvastatin exposure. Ketoconazole does not affect rosuvastatin exposure and would be expected to interact similarly to itraconazole with other statins, whereas voriconazole would be expected to interact similarly to both fluconazole and itraconazole.

Case reports describe rhabdomyolysis associated with the use of atorvastatin, lovastatin, or simvastatin and an azole.

Clinical evidence

(a) Atorvastatin

1. Fluconazole. A case report describes a 76-year-old man taking multiple medications, including long-term fluconazole 150 mg daily, who had his treatment with pravastatin 80 mg daily changed to atorvastatin 40 mg daily because of a lack of response. Within one week he began to feel tired, and 3 weeks later he was admitted to hospital with dyspnoea, myopathy, rhabdomyolysis and renal failure. Although both drugs were stopped he later died of multi-organ failure. The authors considered an interaction between atorvastatin and fluconazole as the most likely explanation for the rhabdomyolysis.[1]

2. Itraconazole. Ten healthy subjects were given itraconazole 200 mg daily for 5 days with a single 40-mg dose of atorvastatin on day 4. Itraconazole increased the AUC of atorvastatin acid and atorvastatin lactone 4-fold and 3-fold, respectively, and increased their half-lives 3-fold and 2-fold, respectively. Correspondingly, the AUC of the principal hydroxylated metabolite of atorvastatin, which is active, was reduced. Overall, the AUCs of active and total HMG-CoA reductase inhibitors were increased by 60% and 70%, respectively.[2] Raised atorvastatin concentrations have been seen in other studies with itraconazole.[3,4]

3. Unspecified azoles. In a review of the FDA spontaneous reports of statin-associated rhabdomyolysis covering the period November 1997 to March 2000, an azole (not specified) was potentially implicated in 2 cases of rhabdomyolysis involving atorvastatin.[5]

(b) Fluvastatin

1. Fluconazole. A randomised study in 12 healthy subjects found that fluconazole (400 mg on day 1 followed by 200 mg daily for 3 days) increased the AUC of a single 40-mg dose of fluvastatin by 84% and increased its maximum plasma concentration by 44%. The pharmacokinetics of fluconazole were unaffected.[6]

2. Itraconazole. In a randomised study, itraconazole 100 mg daily for 4 days did not affect the pharmacokinetics of fluvastatin, apart from a small increase in its half-life.[7]

(c) Lovastatin

1. Itraconazole. In a placebo-controlled, crossover study, 12 healthy subjects were given itraconazole 200 mg daily for 4 days with a single 40-mg dose of lovastatin on day 4. On average the peak plasma concentration and the AUC of lovastatin were very markedly increased, more than 20-fold. The peak plasma concentration of the active metabolite of lovastatin, lovastatin acid, was also very markedly increased (13-fold increase, range 10- to 23-fold) and its AUC was increased 20-fold. The creatine kinase activity of one subject increased 10-fold, but in the other 11 subjects it remained unchanged.[8] Another study with lovastatin and itraconazole also found similar pharmacokinetic changes.[7]

One case report describes rhabdomyolysis in a patient with familial hypercholesterolaemia taking lovastatin 80 mg daily and nicotinic acid 3 g daily two weeks after starting itraconazole 100 mg twice daily.[9] The authors of one of the pharmacokinetic studies briefly mention another case of severe rhabdomyolysis in a patient taking lovastatin and itraconazole.[8]

2. Ketoconazole. A patient who had received lovastatin for several years was diagnosed with hepatitis and rhabdomyolysis about 4 weeks after ketoconazole 400 mg three times daily was started.[10]

3. Unspecified azoles. In a review of the FDA spontaneous reports of statin-associated rhabdomyolysis covering the period November 1997 to March 2000, an azole (not specified) was potentially implicated in 6 cases of rhabdomyolysis involving lovastatin.[5]

(d) Pitavastatin

The US manufacturer notes that in a study in healthy subjects, **itraconazole** 200 mg daily for 5 days reduced the AUC and maximum concentration of pitavastatin by 23% and 22%, respectively, when a single 4-mg dose of pitavastatin was given on day 4.[11]

(e) Pravastatin

1. Fluconazole. A randomised, double-blind study in 12 healthy subjects found that fluconazole (400 mg on day 1 followed by 200 mg daily for 3 days) increased the AUC of a single 40-mg dose of pravastatin by 36%, but this was not statistically significant.[6]

2. Itraconazole. In a study in 10 healthy subjects, the AUC of a single 40-mg dose of pravastatin was increased by 71% by itraconazole 200 mg daily for 4 days, although this did not reach statistical significance.[12] In a similar study, the same dose of itraconazole caused a slight 51% increase in the AUC of pravastatin.[3] In contrast, another study in healthy subjects found that itraconazole 200 mg daily for 30 days had no effect on steady-state pravastatin pharmacokinetics.[4]

(f) Rosuvastatin

1. Fluconazole. In a study in 14 healthy subjects, fluconazole 200 mg daily for 11 days increased the AUC and maximum plasma concentration of a single 80-mg dose of rosuvastatin (given on day 8) by 14% and 9%, respectively. The proportion of circulating active HMG-CoA reductase inhibitors was not affected by fluconazole.[13]

2. Itraconazole. In a study, itraconazole 200 mg daily caused a slight 28% to 39% increase in the AUC of rosuvastatin.[14]

3. Ketoconazole. In a study, ketoconazole 200 mg daily did not alter the pharmacokinetics of rosuvastatin.[15]

(g) Simvastatin

1. Fluconazole. An 83-year-old man who had been taking multiple medications including simvastatin 40 mg daily for 2 years was given fluconazole 400 mg daily as part of a prophylactic regimen against chemotherapy-induced neutropenic sepsis. After one week he developed generalised muscle weakness and was found to have brown urine and an elevated serum creatine kinase. His medication was stopped, and he was treated with hydration and diuretics, after which his symptoms resolved.[16] Two similar cases of rhabdomyolysis have been reported, one in a patient taking simvastatin 40 mg daily shortly after finishing a course of high-dose fluconazole 800 mg daily for 3 weeks,[17] and another in a patient taking simvastatin and fluconazole (dose not stated).[18]

2. Itraconazole. In a two-phase crossover study, 10 healthy subjects were given itraconazole 200 mg daily or a placebo for 4 days, with a single 40-mg dose of simvastatin on day 4. The maximum serum concentrations of total simvastatin acid (simvastatin acid plus simvastatin lactone) were very markedly increased 17-fold and the AUC was increased 19-fold. The maximum serum concentrations and the AUC of total HMG-CoA reductase inhibitors increased about 3-fold and 5-fold, respectively.[12]

An otherwise healthy subject with hypercholesterolaemia had an increase in simvastatin serum concentrations, from 0.5 to 6.5 nanograms/mL within a day of starting itraconazole 200 mg daily.[19] Six case reports describe rhabdomyolysis in patients taking simvastatin 20 to 40 mg daily after starting itraconazole (200 mg or 400 mg daily, where stated).[19-24] Symptoms started within 2 to 3 weeks of concurrent use.[19,20] Four of these cases were complicated by the presence of ciclosporin, which might also cause rhabdomyolysis with simvastatin (see 'Statins + Ciclosporin', p.1327). Gemfibrozil was also taken in one of these cases.[23]

3. Ketoconazole. Five cases of rhabdomyolysis have been reported in patients taking simvastatin (20 or 40 mg daily, where stated[25,26]), which developed between 7 days and 4 weeks after starting ketoconazole.[25-28]

4. Posaconazole. The US manufacturer of posaconazole notes that posaconazole 100 mg or 200 mg daily for 13 days markedly increased the AUC of a single 40-mg dose of simvastatin and its active metabolite, simvastatin acid, about 10-fold and 7-fold, respectively.[29]

5. Unspecified azoles. In a review of the FDA spontaneous reports of statin-associated rhabdomyolysis covering the period November 1997 to March 2000, an azole (not specified) was potentially implicated in 4 cases of rhabdomyolysis involving simvastatin.[5]

Mechanism

Fluconazole inhibits CYP2C9 and has a moderate inhibitory effect on CYP3A4, whereas itraconazole, ketoconazole and posaconazole are potent inhibitors of CYP3A4. Consequently they interact differently with the various statins depending on which isoenzymes are involved in the metabolism of the statin in question: this has been shown in several studies.[3,6,7] In addition, the more dependent the statin is on metabolism by an isoenzyme, the greater its interaction in the presence of an inhibitor of this isoenzyme. Thus, itraconazole has a greater effect on simvastatin than atorvastatin, and has less effect on fluvastatin than fluconazole. See 'Lipid regulating drugs', p.1309, for further discussion on the metabolism of the statins. **Miconazole** is an inhibitor of CYP2C9 and would be expected to interact like fluconazole whereas **voriconazole** is an inhibitor of both CYP2C9 and CYP3A4, and would therefore be expected to interact similarly to both fluconazole and itraconazole. Raised statin concentrations are known to be associated with the development of myopathy and rhabdomyolysis.

Importance and management

The interaction between the azoles and the statins is established and of clinical importance, but the outcome of concurrent use differs depending on the drug pair used. The differing risks and management of the various drug pairs are discussed below. See also *Muscle and liver toxicity* under 'Lipid regulating drugs', p.1309, for further guidance on monitoring, and risk factors for muscle toxicity.

Lovastatin or Simvastatin

The very marked increases in lovastatin and simvastatin exposure that can occur with itraconazole, and the very marked increases in simvastatin exposure that can occur with posaconazole, considerably increase the risk of severe muscle damage and therefore the use of these statins with **itraconazole**, **ketoconazole**, or **posaconazole** is contraindicated. If a short course of an azole is considered essential, the statin manufacturers suggest temporary withdrawal of the statin.[30-33] Based on its interaction profile, **voriconazole** would be expected to interact similarly, and for this reason the US manufacturer[32] of simvastatin contraindicates concurrent use; however, in contrast, the manufacturers of voriconazole recommend frequent monitoring for toxicity and consideration of a dose adjustment [reduction] of the statin on concurrent use.[34,35] **Fluconazole**, particularly at high doses (greater than 200 mg daily), and oral **miconazole** (including the oral gel, which can be absorbed sufficiently to have enzyme-inhibitory effects), have the potential to interact similarly, but probably to a lesser extent. Nevertheless, cases of rhabdomyolysis have been reported with fluconazole and therefore it would be prudent to monitor for muscle toxicity. Note that the UK manufacturers of miconazole contraindicate the concurrent use of simvastatin or lovastatin with the oral gel,[36] and advise caution with vaginal preparations.[37,38]

Atorvastatin

Although the increase in atorvastatin exposure with itraconazole is not as great as those with lovastatin or simvastatin, it is still likely to be clinically important. The UK manufacturer advises that the use of azoles that are potent inhibitors of CYP3A4 (**itraconazole**, **ketoconazole**, **posaconazole**, **voriconazole**) with atorvastatin should be avoided if possible.[39] If an azole is required, lower starting doses and reduced maximum doses of atorvastatin should be considered, with appropriate clinical monitoring for toxicity.[39,40] For itraconazole specifically, caution and clinical monitoring is recommended for atorvastatin doses greater than 40 mg daily in the UK[39] and the dose should be limited to 20 mg daily in the US.[40] As a general rule, any patient given atorvastatin with an azole should be specifically reminded to report any signs of myopathy and possible rhabdomyolysis (i.e. otherwise unexplained muscle pain, tenderness or weakness or dark coloured urine). If myopathy does occur, the statin should be stopped immediately. Note that the UK manufacturer of posaconazole[33] states that atorvastatin should be stopped during posaconazole treatment and contraindicates concurrent use.

Fluconazole, particularly at high doses (greater than 200 mg daily), and **miconazole** (including the oral gel, which can be absorbed sufficiently to have enzyme-inhibitory effects), have the potential to interact similarly, but probably to a lesser extent. Nevertheless, a case of rhabdomyolysis has been reported with fluconazole and therefore it might be prudent to monitor for muscle toxicity. The UK manufacturer of atorvastatin recommends lower maximum doses with appropriate clinical monitoring [for toxicity] if fluconazole is used concurrently.[39]

Fluvastatin

The clinical relevance of the modest changes in fluvastatin concentrations with **fluconazole** is unclear. Note that, in a review of the FDA spontaneous reports of statin-associated rhabdomyolysis for the period November 1997 to March 2000, azoles were not identified as a potentially interacting drug in any of the reports for fluvastatin.[5] However, fluconazole, **miconazole** (and **voriconazole**) are inhibitors of CYP2C9 by which fluvastatin is metabolised and so a degree of caution seems warranted. The US manufacturer limits the dose of fluvastatin to 20 mg twice daily in the presence of fluconazole.[41] Any patient given fluvastatin and one of these azoles (including miconazole in preparations such as the oral gel, which is can be absorbed in sufficient quantities to have enzyme-inhibitory effects) should be specifically reminded to report any signs of myopathy and possible rhabdomyolysis (i.e. otherwise unexplained muscle pain, tenderness or weakness or dark coloured urine). If myopathy does occur, the statin should be stopped immediately. Other azoles would not be expected to interact with fluvastatin.

Other statins

The clinical relevance of the slight changes in **pravastatin** concentrations with different azoles seems likely to be small, and a clinically relevant interaction would not be expected. Note that in a review of the FDA spontaneous reports of statin-associated rhabdomyolysis for the period November 1997 to March 2000, azoles were not identified as a potentially interacting drug in any of the reports for pravastatin.[5] Similarly, the small increase in **rosuvastatin** concentrations with fluconazole and itraconazole is not considered to be clinically relevant. Other azoles would not be expected to interact with rosuvastatin. The small *decrease* in **pitavastatin** concentrations with itraconazole is not considered clinically relevant.

1. Kahri J, Valkonen M, Bäcklund T, Vuoristo M, Kivistö KT. Rhabdomyolysis in a patient receiving atorvastatin and fluconazole. *Eur J Clin Pharmacol* (2005) 60, 905–7.
2. Kantola T, Kivistö KT, Neuvonen PJ. Effect of itraconazole on the pharmacokinetics of atorvastatin. *Clin Pharmacol Ther* (1998) 64, 58–65.
3. Mazzu AL, Lasseter KC, Shamblen E, Cooper BS, Agarwal V, Lettieri J, Sundaresen P. Itraconazole alters the pharmacokinetics of atorvastatin to a greater extent than either cerivastatin or pravastatin. *Clin Pharmacol Ther* (2000) 68, 391–400.
4. Jacobson TA. Comparative pharmacokinetic interaction profiles of pravastatin, simvastatin, and atorvastatin when coadministered with cytochrome P450 inhibitors. *Am J Cardiol* (2004) 94, 1140–6.
5. Omar MA, Wilson JP. FDA adverse event reports on statin-associated rhabdomyolysis. *Ann Pharmacother* (2002) 36, 288–95.
6. Kantola T, Backman JT, Niemi M, Kivistö KT, Neuvonen PJ. Effect of fluconazole on plasma fluvastatin and pravastatin concentrations. *Eur J Clin Pharmacol* (2000) 56, 225–9.
7. Kivistö KT, Kantola T, Neuvonen PJ. Different effects of itraconazole on the pharmacokinetics of fluvastatin and lovastatin. *Br J Clin Pharmacol* (1998) 46, 49–53.
8. Neuvonen PJ, Jalava K-M. Itraconazole drastically increases plasma concentrations of lovastatin and lovastatin acid. *Clin Pharmacol Ther* (1996) 60, 54–61.
9. Lees RS, Lees AM. Rhabdomyolysis from the coadministration of lovastatin and the antifungal agent itraconazole. *N Engl J Med* (1995) 333, 664–5.
10. Stein CA, Goel S, Ghavamian R. Hepatitis and rhabdomyolysis in a patient with hormone refractory prostate cancer on ketoconazole and concurrent lovastatin therapy. *Invest New Drugs* (2007) 25, 277–8.
11. Livalo (Pitavastatin). Kowa Pharmaceuticals America, Inc. US Prescribing information, October 2013.
12. Neuvonen PJ, Kantola T, Kivistö KT. Simvastatin but not pravastatin is very susceptible to interaction with CYP3A4 inhibitor itraconazole. *Clin Pharmacol Ther* (1998) 332–41.
13. Cooper KJ, Martin PD, Dane AL, Warwick MJ, Schneck DW, Cantarini MV. The effect of fluconazole on the pharmacokinetics of rosuvastatin. *Eur J Clin Pharmacol* (2002) 58, 527–31.
14. Cooper KJ, Martin PD, Dane AL, Warwick MJ, Schneck DW, Cantarini MV. Effect of itraconazole on the pharmacokinetics of rosuvastatin. *Clin Pharmacol Ther* (2003) 73, 322–9.
15. Cooper KJ, Martin PD, Dane AL, Warwick MJ, Raza A, Schneck DW. Lack of effect of ketoconazole on the pharmacokinetics of rosuvastatin in healthy subjects. *Br J Clin Pharmacol* (2003) 55, 94–9.
16. Shaukat A, Benekli M, Vladutiu GD, Slack JL, Wetzler M, Baer MR. Simvastatin–fluconazole causing rhabdomyolysis. *Ann Pharmacother* (2003) 37, 1032–5.
17. Findling O, Meier N, Sellner J, Nedeltchev K, Arnold M. Clinical reasoning: rhabdomyolysis after combined treatment with simvastatin and fluconazole. *Neurology* (2008) 71, e34-e37.
18. Hazin R, Abuzetun JY, Suker M, Porter J. Rhabdomyolysis induced by simvastatin-fluconazole combination. *J Natl Med Assoc* (2008) 100, 444–6.
19. Segaert MF, De Soete C, Vandewiele I, Verbanck J. Drug-interaction-induced rhabdomyolysis. *Nephrol Dial Transplant* (1996) 11, 1846–7.
20. Horn M. Coadministration of itraconazole with hypolipidemic agents may induce rhabdomyolysis in healthy individuals. *Arch Dermatol* (1996) 132, 1254.
21. Malouf MA, Bicknell M, Glanville AR. Rhabdomyolysis after lung transplantation. *Aust N Z J Med* (1997) 27, 186.
22. Vlahakos DV, Manginas A, Chilidou D, Zamanika C, Alivizatos PA. Itraconazole-induced rhabdomyolysis and acute renal failure in a heart transplant recipient treated with simvastatin and cyclosporine. *Transplantation* (2002) 73, 1962–4.
23. Maxa JL, Melton LB, Ogu CC, Sills MN, Limanni A. Rhabdomyolysis after concomitant use of cyclosporine, simvastatin, gemfibrozil, and itraconazole. *Ann Pharmacother* (2002) 36, 820–23.
24. Tiessen RG, Lagerwey HJG, Jager GJ, Sprenger HG. Geneesmiddelinteractie door communicatieproblemen. Rabdomyolyse door de combinatie van itraconazol en simvastatine. *Ned Tijdschr Geneeskd* (2010) 154, A762.
25. Gilad R, Lampl Y. Rhabdomyolysis induced by simvastatin and ketoconazole treatment. *Clin Neuropharmacol* (1999) 22, 295–7.
26. Akram K, Rao S, Parker M. A lesson for everyone in drug-drug interactions. *Int J Cardiol* (2007) 118, e19–e20.
27. Itakura H, Vaughn D, Haller DG, O'Dwyer PJ. Rhabdomyolysis from cytochrome P-450 interaction of ketoconazole and simvastatin in prostate cancer. *J Urol (Baltimore)* (2003) 169, 613.
28. McKelvie PA, Dennett X. Myopathy associated with HMG-CoA reductase inhibitors (statins): a series of 10 patients and review of the literature. *J Clin Neuromusc Dis* (2002) 3,143–8.
29. Noxafil (Posaconazole). Merck & Co., Inc. US Prescribing information, June 2014.
30. Mevacor (Lovastatin). Merck & Co., Inc. US Prescribing information, February 2014.
31. Zocor (Simvastatin). Merck Sharp & Dohme Ltd. UK Summary of product characteristics, June 2015.
32. Zocor (Simvastatin). Merck & Co., Inc. US Prescribing information, March 2015.
33. Noxafil (Posaconazole). Merck Sharp & Dohme Ltd. UK Summary of product characteristics, September 2014.
34. VFEND (Voriconazole). Pfizer Ltd. UK Summary of product characteristics, October 2014.
35. VFEND (Voriconazole). Pfizer Inc. US Prescribing information, February 2014.
36. Daktarin Oral Gel (Miconazole). Janssen-Cilag Ltd. UK Summary of product characteristics, December 2014.
37. Gyno-Daktarin Cream (Miconazole nitrate). Janssen-Cilag Ltd. UK Summary of product characteristics, July 2009.
38. Gyno-Daktarin Vaginal Capsules (Miconazole nitrate). Janssen-Cilag Ltd. UK Summary of product characteristics, July 2009.
39. Lipitor (Atorvastatin calcium trihydrate). Pfizer Ltd. UK Summary of product characteristics, March 2015.
40. Lipitor (Atorvastatin calcium). Pfizer Inc. US Prescribing information, March 2015.
41. Lescol (Fluvastatin sodium). Novartis Pharmaceuticals Corp. US Prescribing information, October 2012.

Statins + Beta blockers

Propranolol does not cause any clinically relevant changes to the pharmacokinetics of fluvastatin, lovastatin or pravastatin. The concurrent use of simvastatin and talinolol does not affect the pharmacokinetics of either drug. In clinical studies, the safety and efficacy of statins were not altered by the concurrent use of beta blockers as a class.

Clinical evidence

(a) Pharmacokinetic studies

1. Atenolol. In a single-dose study in subjects given atenolol 50 mg alone, **simvastatin** 20 mg alone or both (formulated as a tablet also including hydrochlorothiazide 12.5 mg, ramipril 5 mg and aspirin 100 mg), the pharmacokinetics of atenolol did not differ between the combined tablet and atenolol alone. However, the AUC of **simvastatin** was 24% lower with the combined tablet, whereas the AUC of active simvastatin acid was 44% higher, when compared with simvastatin alone. The reason for this apparent difference is unclear, but it seems unlikely to be due to a pharmacokinetic interaction between any of the drugs and **simvastatin**.[1] The clinical relevance of the apparent difference is also unclear, but the authors note that in an efficacy study, the combined tablet caused a slightly smaller reduction in cholesterol than **simvastatin** alone.[2]

2. Propranolol. In a study in 24 healthy subjects, the pharmacokinetics of a single 40-mg dose of **fluvastatin** was not affected by the concurrent use of propranolol 40 mg every 12 hours for 3 days.[3] Similarly, propranolol 40 mg every 12 hours reduced the AUC of **lovastatin** 20 mg and its metabolites by less than 18%, and very slightly reduced the AUC of **pravastatin** 20 mg and its metabolites by 16 to 23%.[4]

3. Talinolol. In a study in healthy subjects the pharmacokinetics of **simvastatin** and talinolol were not affected during the concurrent use of these drugs.[5]

(b) Efficacy studies

In an early retrospective analysis of clinical study data, there was no evidence that the safety or efficacy of **fluvastatin** were altered by the use of beta blockers (unspecified).[6] Similarly, in another early analysis, there was no evidence that the safety or efficacy of **lovastatin** were altered by cardioselective beta blockers (primarily **atenolol, metoprolol** and **labetalol**) or non-selective beta blockers (primarily **propranolol, nadolol** and **timolol**).[7] Conversely, in the Anglo-Scandinavian Cardiac Outcomes Trial (ASCOT), a primary prevention study, patients with high-cholesterol randomised to receive **atorvastatin** 10 mg daily had a greater reduction in coronary heart disease (non-fatal and fatal CHD events) if they were in the group randomised to receive an amlodipine-based antihypertensive regimen compared with the group receiving an **atenolol**-based antihypertensive regimen (53% versus 16%). This difference was only of borderline statistical significance, and could therefore be due to chance.[8] However, in a later prospective cohort study in patients with a myocardial infarct, those receiving beta blockers (**metoprolol** or **propranolol**) alone or with **simvastatin** appeared to have no reduction in C-reactive protein when compared with patients receiving simvastatin alone,[9] suggesting that there might be a pharmacodynamic mechanism for the finding seen in the ASCOT study, but see *Mechanism*, below. In contrast to the ASCOT findings, various other retrospective analyses have found no adverse interaction between beta blockers and statins. For example, the use of a statin alone or with a beta blocker was associated with a reduction in long-term mortality after vascular surgery,[10] and a reduction in all-cause mortality in patients with ischaemic heart disease.[11] Similarly, a favourable interaction between statins and **bisoprolol** was found in patients with chronic heart failure.[12]

Mechanism

Based on currently known mechanisms, no pharmacokinetic interactions would be expected between statins and beta blockers. It has been suggested that beta blockers might attenuate the reduction in C-reactive protein seen with statins,[9] but the relevance of C-reactive protein as a cardiovascular risk factor is not established, and is controversial.[13] Alternatively, it might be that statins act synergistically with calcium-channel blockers,[14] rather than they have an adverse interaction with beta blockers.

Importance and management

No pharmacokinetic interaction occurs between any of the pairs of beta blockers and statins studied. Furthermore, there is no clear evidence of any adverse clinical interaction between the beta blockers and the statins, and these drugs are very widely used together. No particular precautions are therefore necessary if a beta blocker is given concurrently with a statin.

1. Patel A, Shah T, Shah G, Jha V, Ghosh C, Desai J, Khamar B, Chakraborty BS. Preservation of bioavailability of ingredients and lack of drug-drug interactions in a novel five-ingredient polypill (Polycap): a five-arm phase I crossover trial in healthy volunteers. *Am J Cardiovasc Drugs* (2010) 10, 95–103.
2. Indian Polycap Study (TIPS), Yusuf S, Pais P, Afzal R, Xavier D, Teo K, Eikelboom J, Sigamani A, Mohan V, Gupta R, Thomas N. Effects of a polypill (Polycap) on risk factors in middle-aged individuals without cardiovascular disease (TIPS): a phase II, double-blind, randomised trial. *Lancet* (2009) 373, 1341–51.
3. Smith HT, Jokubaitis LA, Troendle AJ, Hwang DS, Robinson WT. Pharmacokinetics of fluvastatin and specific drug interactions. *Am J Hypertens* (1993) 6, 375S–382S.
4. Pan HY, Triscari J, DeVault AR, Smith SA, Wang-Iverson D, Swanson BN, Willard DA. Pharmacokinetic interaction between propranolol and the HMG-CoA reductase inhibitors pravastatin and lovastatin. *Br J Clin Pharmacol* (1991) 31, 665–70.
5. Bernsdorf A, Giessmann T, Modess C, Wegner D, Igelbrink S, Hecker U, Haenisch S, Cascorbi I, Terhaag B, Siegmund W. Simvastatin does not influence the intestinal P-glycoprotein and MPR2, and the disposition of talinolol after chronic medication in healthy subjects genotyped for the ABCB1, ABCC2 and SLCO1B1 polymorphisms. *Br J Clin Pharmacol* (2006) 61, 440–50.
6. Peters TK, Jewitt-Harris J, Mehra M, Muratti EN. Safety and tolerability of fluvastatin with concomitant use of antihypertensive agents. An analysis of a clinical trial database. *Am J Hypertens* (1993) 6, 346S–352S.
7. Pool JL, Shear CL, Downton M, Schnaper H, Stinnett S, Dujovne C, Bradford RH, Chremos AN. Lovastatin and coadministered antihypertensive/cardiovascular agents. *Hypertension* (1992) 19, 242–8.
8. Sever P, Dahlöf B, Poulter N, Wedel H, Beevers G, Caulfield M, Collins R,Kjeldsen S, Kristinsson A, McInnes G, Mehlsen J, Nieminem M, O'Brien E, Ostergren J; ASCOT Steering Committee Members. Potential synergy between lipid-lowering and blood-pressure-lowering in the Anglo-Scandinavian Cardiac Outcomes Trial. *Eur Heart J* (2006) 27, 2982–8.
9. Quinaglia e Silva JC, Munhoz DB, Morato TN, Gurgel A, Macedo ACT, Sever P, Sposito AC; Brasilia Heart Study Group. Effect of beta blockers (metoprolol or propranolol) on effect of simvastatin in lowering C-reactive protein in acute myocardial infarction. *Am J Cardiol* (2009) 103, 461–3.
10. Barrett TW, Mori M, De Boer D. Association of ambulatory use of statins and beta-blockers with long-term mortality after vascular surgery. *J Hosp Med* (2007) 2, 241–52.
11. Hippisley-Cox J, Coupland C. Effect of combinations of drugs on all cause mortality in patients with ischaemic heart disease: nested case-control analysis. *BMJ* (2005) 330, 1059–63.
12. Krum H, Bailey M, Meyer W, Verkenne P, Dargie H, Lechat P, Anker S. Impact of statin therapy on clinical outcomes in chronic heart failure patients according to beta-blocker use: results of CIBIS II. *Cardiology* (2007)108, 28–34.
13. Després JP. CRP: star trekking the galaxy of risk markers. *Lancet* (2011) 377, 441–2.
14. Clunn GF, Sever PS, Hughes AD. Calcium channel regulation in vascular smooth muscle cells: synergistic effects of statins and calcium channel blockers. *Int J Cardiol* (2010) 139, 2–6.

Statins + Bexarotene

Atorvastatin exposure appears to be halved by bexarotene, whereas atorvastatin does not appear to alter bexarotene exposure. Simvastatin and lovastatin might be similarly affected.

Clinical evidence, mechanism, importance and management

In a pharmacokinetic analysis as part of a phase III study in patients with non-small cell lung cancer, oral bexarotene 400 mg/m^2 daily given with antineoplastic chemotherapy reduced the dose-corrected AUC of atorvastatin by nearly 50%.[1] The antineoplastics given were either carboplatin with paclitaxel or cisplatin with vinorelbine, and there was no difference in the decrease in AUC of atorvastatin between these antineoplastics. The UK and US manufacturers of bexarotene note that in a population pharmacokinetic analysis, bexarotene concentrations were not affected by **atorvastatin**.[2,3] There is some evidence that bexarotene is an enzyme inducer, and the US manufacturer[3] suggests the interaction with atorvastatin might be due to induction of CYP3A4. Atorvastatin dose increases might be necessary in patients given bexarotene to accommodate the pharmacokinetic interaction seen. In the study cited, atorvastatin doses ranged from 10 to 100 mg daily, and dose escalation was quicker than usual.[1] If this mechanism is correct, then **simvastatin** and **lovastatin** would also be expected to be affected to a similar or greater extent. Until more is known, bear in mind the possibility of an interaction between bexarotene and these statins.

1. Wakelee HA, Takimoto CH, Lopez-Anaya A, Chu Q, Middleton G, Dunlop D, Ramlau R, Leighl N, Rowinsky EK, Hao D, Zatloukal P, Jacobs CD, Rodon J. The effect of bexarotene on atorvastatin pharmacokinetics: results from a phase I trial of bexarotene plus chemotherapy in patients with advanced non-small cell lung cancer. *Cancer Chemother Pharmacol* (2012) 69, 563–71.
2. Targretin Capsules (Bexarotene). Eisai Ltd. UK Summary of product characteristics, April 2009.
3. Targretin Capsules (Bexarotene). Eisai Inc. US Prescribing information, November 2011.

Statins + Bile-acid binding resins

Colestyramine markedly reduces fluvastatin exposure when given at the same time. The interaction is lessened by separating administration, and, when administration is separated, the overall total lipid-lowering effect is increased by concurrent use. Colestyramine and colestipol slightly reduce pravastatin exposure when given at the same time, and have minimal effects when administration is separated. Colestipol appears to have minimal effect on atorvastatin levels. Colesevelam appears not to interact with lovastatin given at the same time.

Clinical evidence

(a) Colesevelam

A crossover study in 22 healthy subjects found that the pharmacokinetics of **lovastatin** 20 mg given with a meal were not affected when colesevelam 2.25 g was given at the same time.[1]

(b) Colestipol

The manufacturer notes that, in an efficacy study in which **atorvastatin** 40 mg daily and colestipol 10 mg twice daily were given concurrently for 28 weeks, although the levels of atorvastatin were reduced by about 25%, the total reduction in the LDL-cholesterol levels was greater than when each drug was given alone.[2,3] They did not state if the daily statin dose was given at the same time as colestipol or separately, and they note that the AUC of atorvastatin was not calculated.[3]

In a study in 18 subjects, colestipol reduced the AUC of **pravastatin** by about 50% when given at the same time in the fasting state, but no reduction in AUC was seen when pravastatin was given one hour before colestipol and a meal.[4]

(c) Colestyramine

1. Fluvastatin. In a study in 19 healthy subjects, colestyramine 8 g given at the same time as fluvastatin 20 mg decreased the AUC and the maximum plasma levels of fluvastatin by 89% and 96%, respectively. When the fluvastatin was given 2 hours after the colestyramine, the AUC and the maximum plasma levels of fluvastatin were reduced by just over 50%.[5] In another study in 20 healthy subjects, the AUC and maximum plasma levels of fluvastatin were reduced by 51% and 82%, respectively, when fluvastatin was taken 4 hours after colestyramine 8 g and a meal.[5]

Despite these marked reductions in fluvastatin bioavailability, other studies in large numbers of hypercholesterolaemic patients have found that the concurrent use of colestyramine and fluvastatin actually has additive lipid-lowering effects.[5,6] In the first of these studies, fluvastatin was given 4 hours after colestyramine,[5] but the other study did not indicate whether or not doses were separated.[6]

2. Pravastatin. In a randomised study, 33 patients with primary hypercholesterolaemia were given pravastatin 5, 10, or 20 mg twice daily before their morning and evening meals for 4 weeks, and then for a further 4 weeks they also took colestyramine 24 g daily. Colestyramine was taken at least an hour after the pravastatin. Despite the fact that colestyramine reduced the bioavailability of pravastatin by 18 to 49%, the reduction in blood lipid levels was enhanced by concurrent use.[7] A related study in 18 subjects found that colestyramine reduced the AUC of pravastatin by about 40% when given at the same time, but only small and clinically irrelevant pharmacokinetic changes occurred when the pravastatin was given one hour before, or 4 hours after the colestyramine.[4] Similarly, a multicentre study in 311 patients found that the concurrent use of pravastatin 40 mg daily and colestyramine 12 g daily was highly effective in the treatment of hypercholesterolaemia. Colestyramine was taken at least one hour after pravastatin.[8]

Mechanism

It seems probable that colestyramine and colestipol bind with fluvastatin, and to a lesser extent pravastatin, in the gut and thereby reduce the amount available for absorption. Colesevelam probably has less effect.

Importance and management

The interactions of **colestipol** and **colestyramine** with the statins are established, but of only relatively minor importance if administration is separated. The slight reduction in atorvastatin levels that occurs on the concurrent use of colestipol is of limited clinical relevance, and it appears that atorvastatin can be used with bile acid-binding resins for additive effect. Similarly, despite the slight to moderate reduction in the bioavailability of pravastatin caused by colestyramine or colestipol, the overall lipid-lowering effect is increased by concurrent use.[7,8] The effects of the interaction can be minimised by separating their administration as described above. This can be achieved by taking colestyramine or colestipol with meals, and pravastatin at bedtime. Likewise, although the interaction between fluvastatin and colestyramine is marked, it can be minimised by taking fluvastatin at least one hour before or 4 hours after colestyramine, and separated use appears to be beneficial.

There would appear to be no reason for avoiding the simultaneous use of lovastatin and **colesevelam**. The manufacturer of colesevelam states that its concurrent use with a statin in clinical studies shows that colesevelam can be dosed at the same time as the statin or separately.[9]

1. Donovan JM, Kisicki JC, Stiles MR, Tracewell WG, Burke SK. Effect of colesevelam on lovastatin pharmacokinetics. *Ann Pharmacother* (2002) 36, 392–7.
2. Lipitor (Atorvastatin calcium trihydrate). Pfizer Ltd. UK Summary of product characteristics, March 2015.
3. Lipitor (Atorvastatin calcium). Pfizer Inc. US Prescribing information, March 2015.
4. Pan HY, DeVault AR, Ivashkiv E, Whigan D, Brennan JJ, Willard DA. Pharmacokinetic interaction studies of pravastatin with bile-acid-binding resins. 8th International Symposium on Atherosclerosis, Rome, October 9-13, 1988, p. 711.
5. Smith HT, Jokubaitis LA, Troendle AJ, Hwang DS, Robinson WT. Pharmacokinetics of fluvastatin and specific drug interactions. *Am J Hypertens* (1993) 6, 375S–382S.
6. Hagen E, Istad H, Ose L, Bodd E, Eriksen H-M, Selvig V, Bard JM, Fruchart JC, Borge M, Wolf M-C, Pfister P. Fluvastatin efficacy and tolerability in comparison and in combination with cholestyramine. *Eur J Clin Pharmacol* (1994) 46, 445–9.
7. Pan HY, DeVault AR, Swites BJ, Whigan D, Ivashkiv E, Willard DA, Brescia D. Pharmacokinetics and pharmacodynamics of pravastatin alone and with cholestyramine in hypercholesterolemia. *Clin Pharmacol Ther* (1990) 48, 201–7.
8. Pravastatin Multicenter Study Group II. Comparative efficacy and safety of pravastatin and cholestyramine alone and combined in patients with hypercholesterolemia. *Arch Intern Med* (1993) 153, 1321–9.
9. Cholestagel (Colesevelam hydrochloride). Sanofi. UK Summary of product characteristics, December 2014.

Statins + Calcium-channel blockers; Dihydropyridines

Steady-state amlodipine, lacidipine and lercanidipine slightly increase simvastatin exposure. In single-dose studies, amlodipine had a negligible effect on atorvastatin exposure, lercanidipine appeared to have a negligible effect on fluvastatin exposure, and fluvastatin appeared to slightly decreased lercanidipine exposure. Limited evidence suggests isradipine might slightly reduce lovastatin exposure. There do not appear to be any reports of myopathy attributed to the concurrent use of statins and dihydropyridine calcium-channel blockers.

Clinical evidence

(a) Atorvastatin

The US manufacturer[1] briefly reports that, in a single-dose study, the concurrent use of **amlodipine** 10 mg and atorvastatin 80 mg increased the AUC of atorvastatin by just 15%, and the UK manufacturer[2] states an increase in the AUC of atorvastatin of 18%.

In a randomised study involving 1 660 patients with hypertension and dyslipidaemia, over the 8-week study period various combinations of **amlodipine** 5 or 10 mg, atorvastatin 10, 20, 40, or 80 mg or placebo were well tolerated and without any adverse pharmacodynamic interaction. Atorvastatin did not modify the effect of amlodipine on systolic blood pressure, and amlodipine did not adversely affect the overall lipid-lowering capacity of atorvastatin. In addition, the occurrence of adverse effects or laboratory abnormalities was similar in patients given both drugs and patients taking either amlodipine or atorvastatin alone.[3]

(b) Fluvastatin

In a single-dose pharmacokinetic study in 8 healthy subjects, concurrent administration of fluvastatin 40 mg and **lercanidipine** 20 mg decreased the median AUC of lercanidipine by about 40% (a similar 40% decrease in the mean was not statistically significant), but caused little change in the AUC of fluvastatin (median 9% decrease in the (–) enantiomer, and median 13% increase or mean 39% increase in the (+) enantiomer).[4]

A retrospective study of the effects of antihypertensives on the efficacy of fluvastatin found that the concurrent use of unspecified calcium-channel blockers did not affect the safety or lipid-lowering effects of fluvastatin to a statistically significant extent, although there was a trend towards enhanced lowering of triglycerides.[5]

(c) Lovastatin

In a study in 12 healthy subjects, lovastatin 20 mg and **isradipine** 5 mg were given alone or together for 5 days, and the pharmacokinetics were measured on day one (single-dose) and day 5 (steady state). **Isradipine** had no effect on the AUC of lovastatin after a single dose, but appeared to reduce the steady-state AUC of lovastatin by 40% in males and also to decrease it in females, although the difference in females was not statistically significant.[6]

The use of lovastatin 20 mg daily with **nifedipine** for 6 weeks did not have any impact on the antihypertensive efficacy of nifedipine when compared with placebo.[7]

(d) Pravastatin

In an analysis of reports of myopathy submitted to the FDA in the US up to October 1997, the use of any calcium-channel blocker (unspecified, but including diltiazem and verapamil) with pravastatin was not associated with an increased incidence of myopathy.[8]

(e) Simvastatin

1. Amlodipine. In a study in 8 patients taking simvastatin 5 mg daily, the addition of amlodipine 5 mg daily for 4 weeks increased the maximum levels and AUC of simvastatin HMG-CoA reductase inhibitor activity by 40% and 30%, respectively, without affecting the lipid profiles of the patients.[9] The US manufacturer reports a study in which amlodipine 10 mg daily for 10 days increased the AUC of simvastatin by 77% and that of simvastatin acid by 58% when a single 80-mg dose of simvastatin was given on day 10.[10]

In another parallel study in patients taking amlodipine 5 mg daily with simvastatin 20 mg daily for 6 weeks, the steady-state AUC of simvastatin acid was 34% lower in 7 patients taking the amlodipine 4 hours after the simvastatin compared with 8 patients taking the drugs at the same time, although this difference was not statistically significant.[11] Interpretation of this study is hampered because of the between group comparison, the lack of a placebo group, and the non-statistically significant findings (i.e. it is impossible to say if the attenuation of the interaction is real, and what the true extent of the attenuation might be).

2. Lacidipine. In a randomised, crossover study, simvastatin 40 mg daily was given for 8 days, with or without lacidipine 4 mg daily. Lacidipine raised the AUC of simvastatin acid by 35%.[12]

3. Lercanidipine. The manufacturer of lercanidipine notes that the concurrent use of lercanidipine 20 mg daily and simvastatin 40 mg daily increased the steady-state AUC of simvastatin by 56% and of simvastatin acid by 28%. The lercanidipine AUC was not altered by simvastatin.[13] They predict that no interaction will occur if lercanidipine is given in the morning and simvastatin is given in the evening, on the basis of the data for amlodipine and simvastatin,[13,14] but see also *Amlodipine*, above.

4. Unspecified. In two simvastatin megatrials (the 4S study in 2 221 patients given simvastatin 20 to 40 mg daily, and the Heart Protection study in 10 269 patients given simvastatin 40 mg daily), about 30% of patients were taking a calcium-channel blocker (unspecified) at randomisation, and, of the 3 patients who developed myopathy while taking a statin, none were taking a dihydropyridine calcium-channel blocker.[8] In an analysis of reports of myopathy submitted to the FDA in the US up to October 1997, the use of any calcium-channel blocker (unspecified, but including diltiazem and verapamil) with simvastatin was not associated with an increased incidence of myopathy.[8]

Mechanism

The reason for the increases in lovastatin and simvastatin levels with amlodipine, lacidipine and lercanidipine is not known. These calcium-channel blockers are not inhibitors of CYP3A4, by which lovastatin and simvastatin are principally metabolised. Similarly, the mechanism for the apparent slight reduction in lercanidipine exposure with fluvastatin is unknown.

Importance and management

For **amlodipine**, the negligible increase in atorvastatin exposure seen is not clinically important, although, note that the findings were from a single-dose study, and a different effect with multiple doses cannot be ruled out, especially as the mechanism for the effect seen has not been established. It also seems unlikely that the slight increases in steady-state simvastatin exposure with amlodipine will be clinically important. In addition, statins are widely used with dihydropyridine calcium-channel blockers such as amlodipine and there are no published reports of adverse interactions attributed to concurrent use. Nevertheless, the manufacturers of simvastatin consider that the risk of myopathy will be increased by its use with amlodipine at higher simvastatin doses, and they recommend that the maximum daily dose of simvastatin be restricted to 20 mg in patients taking amlodipine.[10,15] There is no clear evidence that separating administration attenuates the pharmacokinetic interaction, and further study of this is needed.

The slight increases in steady-state simvastatin exposure with **lacidipine** and **lercanidipine** are not clinically important. The clinical relevance of the apparent slight decrease in lercanidipine exposure with fluvastatin, as seen in the single-dose study, remains to be established. Whether **isradipine** causes a decrease in lovastatin exposure and the clinical relevance of this also remains to be established.

1. Lipitor (Atorvastatin calcium). Pfizer Inc. US Prescribing information, March 2015.
2. Lipitor (Atorvastatin calcium trihydrate). Pfizer Ltd. UK Summary of product characteristics, March 2015.
3. Preston RA, Harvey P, Herfert O, Dykstra G, Jukema JW, Sun F, Gillen D. A randomised, placebo-controlled trial to evaluate the efficacy, safety, and pharmacodynamic interaction of coadministered amlodipine and atorvastatin in 1660 patients with concomitant hypertension and dyslipidemia: the Respond trial. *J Clin Pharmacol* (2007) 47, 1555–69.
4. Boralli VB, Coelho EB, Sampaio SA, Marques MP, Lanchote VL. Enantioselectivity in the pharmacokinetic interaction between fluvastatin and lercanidipine in healthy volunteers. *J Clin Pharmacol* (2009) 49, 205–11.
5. Peters TK, Jewitt-Harris J, Mehra M, Muratti EN. Safety and tolerability of fluvastatin with concomitant use of antihypertensive agents. An analysis of a clinical trial database. *Am J Hypertens* (1993) 6, 346S–352S.
6. Zhou L-X, Finley DK, Hassell AE, Holtzman JL. Pharmacokinetic interaction between isradipine and lovastatin in normal, female and male volunteers. *J Pharmacol Exp Ther* (1995) 273, 121–7.
7. Os I, Bratland B, Dahlöf B, Gisholt K, Syvertsen J-O, Tretli S. Effect and tolerability of combining lovastatin with nifedipine or lisinopril. *Am J Hypertens* (1993) 6, 688–92.
8. Gruer PJK, Vega JM, Mercuri MF, Dobrinska MR, Tobert JA. Concomitant use of cytochrome P450 3A4 inhibitors and simvastatin. *Am J Cardiol* (1999) 84, 811–15.
9. Nishio S, Watanabe H, Kosuge K, Uchida S, Hayashi H, Ohashi K. Interaction between amlodipine and simvastatin in patients with hypercholesterolemia and hypertension. *Hypertens Res* (2005) 28, 223–7.
10. Zocor (Simvastatin). Merck & Co., Inc. US Prescribing information, March 2015.
11. Park CG, Lee H, Choi JW, Lee SJ, Kim SH, Lim HE. Non-concurrent dosing attenuates the pharmacokinetic interaction between amlodipine and simvastatin. *Int J Clin Pharmacol Ther* (2010) 48, 497–503.
12. Ziviani L, Da Ros L, Squassante L, Milleri S, Cugola M, Iavarone LE. The effects of lacidipine on the steady/state plasma concentrations of simvastatin in healthy subjects. *Br J Clin Pharmacol* (2001) 51, 147–52.
13. Zanidip (Lercanidipine hydrochloride). Recordati Pharmaceuticals Ltd. UK Summary of product characteristics, April 2006.
14. Recordati Ltd. Personal Communication. January 2011.
15. Zocor (Simvastatin). Merck Sharp & Dohme Ltd. UK Summary of product characteristics, June 2015.

Statins + Calcium-channel blockers; Diltiazem or Verapamil

Diltiazem moderately increases lovastatin and simvastatin exposure, and verapamil moderately increases simvastatin exposure. Isolated cases of rhabdomyolysis have occurred as a result of these interactions. Diltiazem

slightly to moderately increases atorvastatin exposure, and there are isolated cases of rhabdomyolysis with the combination. Also, single-dose atorvastatin slightly increases verapamil exposure. Diltiazem and verapamil do not alter pravastatin pharmacokinetics or the risk of myopathy with this statin.

Clinical evidence

(a) Atorvastatin

The manufacturers report that diltiazem 240 mg daily for 28 days increased the AUC of a single 40-mg dose of atorvastatin by 51% without changing its maximum level.[1,2] A 60-year-old man taking atorvastatin 20 mg daily developed rhabdomyolysis 3 weeks after diltiazem 180 mg twice daily was started.[3] Another similar case has also been reported.[4]

In a single-dose study in 12 healthy subjects, atorvastatin 40 mg increased the AUC of verapamil 60 mg by 43%, without affecting the AUC of the metabolite norverapamil. The effect of verapamil on atorvastatin was not assessed.[5]

(b) Lovastatin

In a retrospective analysis of the effects of antihypertensive medication on lovastatin 20 to 80 mg daily, calcium-channel blockers (diltiazem, nifedipine or verapamil) did not attenuate the lipid-lowering effect of lovastatin but actually slightly enhanced it (there was an additional 3 to 5% lowering in the LDL-cholesterol), although this difference was not statistically significant.[6]

In a pharmacokinetic study in 10 healthy subjects, sustained-release oral diltiazem 120 mg twice daily for 2 weeks increased the AUC and maximum serum levels of a single 20-mg dose of lovastatin about fourfold without affecting its elimination half-life.[7] Conversely, an intravenous infusion of diltiazem (20-mg loading dose then 10 mg/hour over 13 hours) had no effect on the AUC of a single 20-mg dose of lovastatin.[8]

(c) Pravastatin

A study in 10 healthy subjects found that sustained-release diltiazem 120 mg twice daily for 2 weeks had no effect on the pharmacokinetics of a single 20-mg dose of pravastatin.[7] Similarly, a study in 15 healthy subjects found that extended-release verapamil 480 mg daily for 3 days did not affect the pharmacokinetics of a single 40-mg dose of pravastatin.[9]

In an analysis of reports of myopathy submitted to the FDA in the US up to October 1997, the use of diltiazem with pravastatin was not associated with an increased incidence of myopathy. Similarly, there was no increased risk of myopathy with concurrent use of verapamil.[10]

(d) Simvastatin

1. Diltiazem. In a pharmacokinetic study, 10 healthy subjects were given sustained-release diltiazem 120 mg twice daily for 2 weeks followed by a single 20-mg dose of simvastatin. Diltiazem caused a 4.8-fold increase in the AUC of simvastatin, a fourfold increase in its maximum serum levels, and a 2.5-fold increase in its half-life.[11] The manufacturer notes that diltiazem 120 mg twice daily for 10 days increased the AUC of simvastatin 3.1-fold and increased the AUC of active simvastatin acid 2.7-fold when a single 80-mg dose of simvastatin was given on day 10.[12,13] In a further study in 11 patients, the concurrent use of simvastatin 5 mg daily and diltiazem 30 mg three times daily for 4 weeks resulted in a twofold increase in the AUC and maximum plasma level of simvastatin HMG-CoA reductase inhibitor activity, and a 20% decrease in the AUC and maximum plasma level of diltiazem, when compared with either drug alone.[14]

In a clinical efficacy study, 30 patients received simvastatin 20 mg daily alone and with diltiazem 60 mg three times daily, both for 4 weeks. Simvastatin reduced the LDL-cholesterol levels by 41.7%, and the addition of diltiazem reduced these by just a further 1.7%, a difference that was not statistically significant.[15]

A 53-year-old man developed rhabdomyolysis 3 months after diltiazem 30 mg four times daily was added to established treatment with simvastatin 40 mg daily. Both drugs were discontinued and he recovered over the following 10 days.[16] Other similar cases have also been reported (simvastatin dose 40 to 80 mg daily).[4,17,18] For another case of rhabdomyolysis with simvastatin, in which diltiazem and ranolazine might have been contributing factors, see 'Statins + Ranolazine', p.1355. In the 4S simvastatin mega study, of the 2 221 patients given simvastatin 20 to 40 mg daily about 30% of patients were taking a calcium-channel blocker (unspecified) at randomisation, and just one of these (taking diltiazem) developed myopathy after 4 years of taking simvastatin 20 mg daily.[16]

In an analysis of reports of myopathy submitted to the FDA in the US up to October 1997, the use of diltiazem with simvastatin was not associated with an increased incidence of myopathy (proportional concomitant use ratio 0.91).[10] However, in an FDA review of data from the SEARCH study, it was briefly mentioned that the risk of myopathy was approximately doubled in patients taking a calcium-channel blocker, in particular diltiazem.[19] In addition, the UK manufacturer notes that the risk of myopathy and rhabdomyolysis was increased by the use of diltiazem with simvastatin 80 mg daily.[12]

2. Verapamil. In a study in 12 healthy subjects given verapamil 80 mg three times daily for 2 days, and a single 40-mg dose of simvastatin on the second day, there was a 4.6-fold increase in the AUC of simvastatin and a 2.8-fold increase in the AUC of simvastatin acid (the active metabolite of simvastatin). In addition, there was a 2.6-fold increase in the maximum serum levels of simvastatin, and about a twofold increase in its half-life.[20] Similarly, a study in 12 healthy subjects found that extended-release verapamil 480 mg daily for 3 days caused a 5-fold increase in the maximum serum levels of simvastatin 40 mg, and about a 4-fold increase in its AUC.[9] The manufacturer reports yet another study in which a single 80-mg dose of simvastatin was given after verapamil 240 mg daily for 7 days then 240 mg twice daily for 3 days. The AUC of simvastatin was increased 2.5-fold and that of simvastatin acid was increased 2.3-fold.[12,13]

A 63-year-old man developed rhabdomyolysis about one month after extended-release verapamil 240 mg daily was added to established treatment with simvastatin 40 mg daily and ciclosporin. Verapamil and simvastatin were discontinued and he recovered over the following 14 days.[21] Yet another case has been reported in a patient who had received ciclosporin and a statin (fluvastatin then pravastatin, doses not stated) for several years. Onset of muscle pain occurred about 2 months after simvastatin (dose not stated) was substituted for pravastatin and 2 weeks after verapamil was added to his treatment: the effect was attributed to multiple drug interactions.[22] Another case of myopathy with simvastatin 40 mg, verapamil and amiodarone was briefly mentioned in a case series of patients with statin myopathy.[23]

In an analysis of reports of myopathy submitted to the FDA in the US up to October 1997, the use of verapamil with simvastatin tended to be associated with an increased incidence of myopathy, but this increase was not statistically significant.[10] The UK manufacturer notes that the risk of myopathy and rhabdomyolysis was increased by the use of verapamil with both simvastatin 40 mg and 80 mg daily.[12]

Mechanism

Diltiazem and verapamil are moderate inhibitors of CYP3A4, the isoenzyme that is responsible for the metabolism of lovastatin, simvastatin and to a lesser extent, atorvastatin. Therefore concurrent use of these drugs results in an increase in the levels of the statin. As oral, but not intravenous, diltiazem interacts, it appears that CYP3A4 in the gut wall is the site of the interaction for lovastatin.[7,8] Note that fluvastatin, pravastatin and **rosuvastatin** are not significantly metabolised by CYP3A4, and so are less likely to interact with diltiazem or verapamil by this mechanism. See 'Lipid regulating drugs', p.1309, for more information about the way these groups of drugs are metabolised.

Atorvastatin appears to inhibit P-glycoprotein thereby increasing the absorption of verapamil.[24]

Importance and management

The moderate pharmacokinetic interactions between **simvastatin** or **lovastatin** and diltiazem or verapamil are established, but reports of serious myopathy on their concurrent use appear to be rare. The UK manufacturer suggests this risk is increased just with higher doses of simvastatin (80 mg for diltiazem, and 40 mg and 80 mg for verapamil).[12] However, a number of the cases reported with diltiazem have been with simvastatin 40 mg. Therefore, although concurrent use need not be avoided, the benefits of using simvastatin or lovastatin with diltiazem or verapamil should be carefully weighed against the risks in each individual, and the statin should be used at the lowest possible dose. In patients already taking statins, the dose of the statin might need to be considerably reduced if diltiazem or verapamil are started.

The manufacturers of simvastatin and lovastatin recommend the following dose restrictions:

- maximum daily dose of simvastatin of 20 mg (UK)[12] or 10 mg (US)[13] in the presence of either diltiazem or verapamil.
- a starting dose of lovastatin 10 mg and a maximum daily dose of lovastatin 20 mg in the presence of diltiazem or verapamil.[25]

The increase in the levels of **atorvastatin** with diltiazem is only slight and not nearly as great as those with lovastatin or simvastatin. However, there are a couple of reports of myopathy on concurrent use, suggesting that some caution might be appropriate on their concurrent use. There are no data for the effect of verapamil on atorvastatin. The UK manufacturer recommends that a lower maximum dose of atorvastatin should be considered with diltiazem or verapamil, with appropriate clinical monitoring,[1] which seems prudent. The clinical relevance of the slight rise in verapamil levels with atorvastatin in a single-dose study is uncertain, and whether it occurs with multiple doses remains to be determined.

Pravastatin appears unlikely to interact with diltiazem or verapamil, and it would be predicted that **fluvastatin** and **rosuvastatin** are similarly unlikely to interact. See also *Muscle and liver toxicity,* under 'Lipid regulating drugs', p.1309, for further guidance on monitoring and risk factors for muscle toxicity.

1. Lipitor (Atorvastatin calcium trihydrate). Pfizer Ltd. UK Summary of product characteristics, March 2015.
2. Lipitor (Atorvastatin calcium). Pfizer Inc. US Prescribing information, March 2015.
3. Lewin JJ, Nappi JM, Taylor MH. Rhabdomyolysis with concurrent atorvastatin and diltiazem. *Ann Pharmacother* (2002) 36, 1546–9.
4. Gladding P, Pilmore H, Edwards C. Potentially fatal interaction between diltiazem and statins. *Ann Intern Med* (2004) 140, W31.
5. Choi D-H, Shin W-G, Choi J-S. Drug interaction between oral atorvastatin and verapamil in healthy subjects: effects of atorvastatin on the pharmacokinetics of verapamil and norverapamil. *Eur J Clin Pharmacol* (2008) 64, 445–9.
6. Pool JL, Shear CL, Downton M, Schnaper H, Stinnett S, Dujovne C, Bradford RH, Chremos AN. Lovastatin and coadministered antihypertensive/cardiovascular agents. *Hypertension* (1992) 19, 242–8.
7. Azie NE, Brater DC, Becker PA, Jones DR, Hall SD. The interaction of diltiazem with lovastatin and pravastatin. *Clin Pharmacol Ther* (1998) 64, 369–77.
8. Masica AL, Azie NE, Brater DC, Hall SD, Jones DR. Intravenous diltiazem and CYP3A-mediated metabolism. *Br J Clin Pharmacol* (2000) 50, 273–6.
9. Jacobson TA. Comparative pharmacokinetic interaction profiles of pravastatin, simvastatin, and atorvastatin when coadministered with cytochrome P450 inhibitors. *Am J Cardiol* (2004) 94, 1140–6.
10. Gruer PJK, Vega JM, Mercuri MF, Dobrinska MR, Tobert JA. Concomitant use of cytochrome P450 3A4 inhibitors and simvastatin. *Am J Cardiol* (1999) 84, 811–15.
11. Mousa O, Brater DC, Sundblad KJ, Hall SD. The interaction of diltiazem with simvastatin. *Clin Pharmacol Ther* (2000) 67, 267–74.
12. Zocor (Simvastatin). Merck Sharp & Dohme Ltd. UK Summary of product characteristics, June 2015.
13. Zocor (Simvastatin). Merck & Co., Inc. US Prescribing information, March 2015.
14. Watanabe H, Kosuge K, Nishio S, Yamada H, Uchida S, Satoh H, Hayashi H, Ishizaki T, Ohashi K. Pharmacokinetic and pharmacodynamic interactions between simvastatin and diltiazem in patients with hypercholesterolemia and hypertension. *Life Sci* (2004) 76, 281–92.

15. You JHS, Chan WKY, Chung PFP, Hu M, Tomlinson B. Effects of concomitant therapy with diltiazem on the lipid responses to simvastatin in Chinese subjects. *J Clin Pharmacol* (2010) 50, 1151–8.
16. Kanathur N, Mathai MG, Byrd RP, Fields CL, Roy TM. Simvastatin-diltiazem drug interaction resulting in rhabdomyolysis and hepatitis. *Tenn Med* (2001) 94, 339–41.
17. Peces R, Pobes A. Rhabdomyolysis associated with concurrent use of simvastatin and diltiazem. *Nephron* (2001) 89, 117–18.
18. Molden E, Westergren T. Interaksjonsrisiko ved statinbytte. *Tidsskr Nor Laegeforen* (2007) 127, 428–31.
19. FDA Drug safety communication: new restrictions, contraindications, and dose limitations for Zocor (simvastatin) to reduce the risk of muscle injury. July 8, 2011. Available at: http://www.fda.gov/Drugs/DrugSafety/ucm256581.htm (accessed 22/10/15).
20. Kantola T, Kivistö KT, Neuvonen PJ. Erythromycin and verapamil considerably increase serum simvastatin and simvastatin acid concentrations. *Clin Pharmacol Ther* (1998) 64, 177–82.
21. Chiffoleau A, Trochu J-N, Veyrac G, Petit T, Abadie P, Bourin M, Jolliet P. Rhabdomyolyse liée à l'ajout du vérapamil à un traitement par simvastatine et cyclosporine chez un patient transplanté cardiaque. *Therapie* (2003) 58, 168–70.
22. Kusus M, Stapleton DD, Lertora JJL, Simon EE, Dreisbach AW. Rhabdomyolysis and acute renal failure in a cardiac transplant recipient due to multiple drug interactions. *Am J Med Sci* (2000) 320, 394–7.
23. McKelvie PA, Dennett X. Myopathy associated with HMG-CoA reductase inhibitors (statins): a series of 10 patients and review of the literature. *J Clin Neuromusc Dis* (2002) 3, 143–8.
24. Peters TK, Jewitt-Harris J, Mehra M, Muratti EN. Safety and tolerability of fluvastatin with concomitant use of antihypertensive agents. An analysis of a clinical trial database. *Am J Hypertens* (1993) 6, 346S–352S.
25. Mevacor (Lovastatin). Merck & Co., Inc. US Prescribing information, February 2014.

Statins + Carbamazepine and related drugs

Carbamazepine and eslicarbazepine moderately reduce simvastatin exposure. Oxcarbazepine might interact similarly. Other statins metabolised in the same way as simvastatin might also be similarly affected.

Clinical evidence

(a) Carbamazepine

In a randomised, crossover study, 12 healthy subjects were given carbamazepine 200 mg daily for 2 days, then 300 mg twice daily for 12 days, with a single 80-mg dose of **simvastatin** 12 hours after the last dose of carbamazepine. The AUC and maximum serum concentration of **simvastatin** were reduced by 75% and 68%, respectively, and the AUC and maximum serum concentration of simvastatin acid (the active metabolite of **simvastatin**) were reduced by 82% and 69%, respectively.[1]

(b) Eslicarbazepine

The manufacturer of eslicarbazepine briefly notes that, in a study in healthy subjects, eslicarbazepine 800 mg daily caused a 50% decrease in exposure to **simvastatin**.[2]

Mechanism

Carbamazepine is a potent inducer of CYP3A4, by which simvastatin is principally metabolised. Carbamazepine therefore increases simvastatin metabolism, leading to reduced exposure. Eslicarbazepine also induces CYP3A4.

Importance and management

Evidence for an interaction between **carbamazepine** and simvastatin is limited to one study, but the effects of concurrent use are consistent with both the way carbamazepine interacts with many other CYP3A4 substrates and the way simvastatin interacts with other CYP3A4 inducers. The effects of simvastatin are likely to be greatly reduced by concurrent use and a dose increase seems likely to be necessary. Monitor concurrent use to check simvastatin is effective.

Evidence for an interaction between **eslicarbazepine** and simvastatin is similarly limited to one study, but is also consistent with what is known about the enzyme-inducing effects of eslicarbazepine. Until more is known, similar precautions to those advised for carbamazepine would be prudent.

Evidence for an interaction between **oxcarbazepine** and simvastatin is lacking, but on the basis of its effects on hormonal contraceptives (see 'Combined hormonal contraceptives + Carbamazepine and related drugs', p.1172) and tyrosine kinase inhibitors (see 'Tyrosine kinase inhibitors + Antiepileptics; Enzyme-inducing', p.727), and until more is known, it might be expected to reduce simvastatin exposure. Until more is known, similar precautions to those advised for carbamazepine would be prudent.

Statins principally metabolised by the same route as simvastatin (namely **lovastatin**) would also be expected to have their exposure reduced by carbamazepine (and perhaps eslicarbazepine and oxcarbazepine), and statins partially metabolised by CYP3A4 (namely **atorvastatin**) might also have their exposure reduced, although to a lesser extent. In contrast, it seems unlikely that statins that are not metabolised by CYP3A4, will interact, and they might therefore be preferable. However, this needs confirmation. See *Statins*, under 'Lipid regulating drugs', p.1309, for more information on the metabolism of the various statins.

1. Ucar M, Neuvonen M, Luurila H, Dahlqvist R, Neuvonen PJ, Mjörndal T. Carbamazepine markedly reduces serum concentrations of simvastatin and simvastatin acid. *Eur J Clin Pharmacol* (2004) 59, 879–82.
2. Zebinix (Eslicarbazepine acetate). Eisai Ltd. UK Summary of product characteristics, August 2012.

Statins + CETP inhibitors

Anacetrapib slightly increases simvastatin exposure. Dalcetrapib slightly reduces pravastatin and simvastatin exposure, but has no effect on rosuvastatin exposure. Dalcetrapib exposure is slightly reduced by rosuvastatin and simvastatin and unchanged by pravastatin.

Clinical evidence

(a) Pravastatin

In a pharmacokinetic study, 28 healthy subjects were given pravastatin 40 mg daily for 8 days alone, **dalcetrapib** 900 mg daily for 8 days alone, and then both drugs together. The AUC of the pravastatin metabolite was slightly reduced by 21%, and the maximal HMG-CoA reductase activity was reduced by 28%. There was no change in the AUC of **dalcetrapib** or its CETP inhibitory activity.[1]

(b) Rosuvastatin

In a pharmacokinetic study, 28 healthy subjects were given rosuvastatin 40 mg daily for 8 days alone, **dalcetrapib** 900 mg daily for 8 days alone, and then both drugs together. The AUC of rosuvastatin was unchanged, its maximum levels were slightly increased, by 27%, but HMG-CoA-reductase activity was not affected. Rosuvastatin slightly reduced the AUC of **dalcetrapib** by 33%, but there was no change in its CETP inhibitory activity.[1]

(c) Simvastatin

In a pharmacokinetic study in 11 healthy subjects given simvastatin 40 mg daily for 14 days in the morning, alone and concurrently with **anacetrapib** 150 mg daily for 14 days, **anacetrapib** slightly increased the AUCs of simvastatin and simvastatin acid, by 30% and 36%, respectively.[2]

In a pharmacokinetic study, 22 healthy subjects were given simvastatin 40 mg daily for 5 days alone, **dalcetrapib** 900 mg daily for 8 days alone, and then both drugs together. The AUC of simvastatin was reduced by 42% by **dalcetrapib**, but there was no change in the AUC of the active acid metabolite. Simvastatin caused a slight 23% reduction in the AUC of **dalcetrapib**, but its CETP inhibitory activity was unchanged.[1]

Mechanism

The reasons for the pharmacokinetic changes in these studies are unknown. Anacetrapib is not an inhibitor of CYP3A4, as shown by its lack of interaction with midazolam (see 'CETP inhibitors + Cytochrome P450 substrates', p.1311), so the slight increase in simvastatin and simvastatin acid exposure is not likely to be due to this mechanism. Similarly, dalcetrapib does not alter CYP3A4 activity, so the reduction in simvastatin exposure, without an alteration in simvastatin acid exposure, is not due to this mechanism. How dalcetrapib exposure is slightly reduced by rosuvastatin and simvastatin is also unknown.

Importance and management

The potential interaction of dalcetrapib and statins appears to be fairly well studied, although not all statins have been investigated. Dalcetrapib slightly reduces pravastatin and simvastatin exposure and has minimal effect on the pharmacokinetics of rosuvastatin; none of the changes described are clinically relevant. Dalcetrapib exposure is slightly reduced by rosuvastatin and simvastatin, and unchanged by pravastatin, and these changes are also unlikely to be clinically relevant.

Anacetrapib slightly increases simvastatin exposure, an effect that is unlikely to be clinically important.

1. Derks M, Abt M, Phelan M, Turnbull L, Meneses-Lorente G, Bech N, White A-M, Parr G. Coadministration of dalcetrapib with pravastatin, rosuvastatin, or simvastatin: no clinically relevant drug-drug interactions. *J Clin Pharmacol* (2010) 50, 1188–201.
2. Krishna R, Garg A, Jin B, Keshavarz SS, Bieberdorf FA, Chodakewitz J, Wagner JA. Assessment of a pharmacokinetic and pharmacodynamic interaction between simvastatin and anacetrapib, a potent cholesteryl ester transfer protein (CETP) inhibitor, in healthy subjects. *Br J Clin Pharmacol* (2009) 67, 520–6.

Statins + Ciclosporin

Ciclosporin appears to markedly or very markedly increase the exposure to atorvastatin, lovastatin, pravastatin, rosuvastatin, and simvastatin, and appears to moderately increase the exposure to fluvastatin and pitavastatin. For many of the statins there are case reports of serious myopathy (rhabdomyolysis) and renal failure in patients also taking ciclosporin. Ciclosporin concentrations appear not to be affected by fluvastatin, lovastatin, pravastatin, or rosuvastatin, but some very slight changes in ciclosporin concentrations have been seen when atorvastatin or simvastatin were given.

Clinical evidence

(a) Atorvastatin

1. Effect on ciclosporin. In various studies in patients taking ciclosporin, atorvastatin caused minor increases or decreases in the AUC or concentrations of ciclosporin, but a few patients required ciclosporin dose adjustments. For example, in a study of 10 patients taking ciclosporin following a kidney transplant, 4 had increases in their minimum ciclosporin concentrations of between 26 and 54% when atorvastatin 10 mg was added, necessitating a dose reduction of ciclosporin. No changes were seen in the 6 other patients, and the incidence of adverse effects was no greater than in a control transplant group not given atorvastatin.[1] Similarly, when atorvastatin 10 mg daily was given to 21 renal transplant patients taking ciclosporin, the AUC and maximum serum concentrations of ciclosporin generally decreased (by a mean of 9.5% and 13.5%, respectively). However, 4 patients needed a *decrease* in their ciclosporin dose and one patient needed an increase.[2] A further analysis of blood samples from this study suggested that atorvastatin does not, on average, affect the AUC of ciclosporin (5% decrease) in renal transplant patients, although the influence of atorvastatin on the ratio between ciclosporin and a major metabolite (AM9) showed large interindividual variability.[3] In another study, atorvastatin 10 mg daily caused a very slight 9% increase in the AUC of ciclosporin in 6 liver transplant patients.[4]

2. Effect on atorvastatin. In a pharmacokinetic study in 13 healthy subjects given atorvastatin 40 mg daily for 8 days, the short-term use of ciclosporin 2.5 mg/kg (2 doses 12 hours apart) increased the AUC of atorvastatin acid 15-fold.[5] In an open study in 21 renal transplant patients taking ciclosporin and given atorvastatin 10 mg daily for 4 weeks, total plasma HMG-CoA reductase inhibitory activity was more than 7-fold higher than in historical controls not taking ciclosporin.[2] A further analysis of this study has been reported elsewhere,[6] which found the AUC of atorvastatin acid was 8.7-fold higher in patients taking ciclosporin than in healthy subjects not given ciclosporin.

A case of rhabdomyolysis has been described in a woman who had been taking various drugs including ciclosporin 125 mg daily and diltiazem 240 mg daily for several years, which occurred 2 months after she began taking atorvastatin 10 mg daily.[7] In a review of the FDA spontaneous reports of statin-associated rhabdomyolysis covering the period November 1997 to March 2000, ciclosporin was potentially implicated in 5 cases of rhabdomyolysis involving atorvastatin.[8]

(b) Fluvastatin

1. Effect on ciclosporin. In various studies in patients taking ciclosporin, fluvastatin did not alter ciclosporin minimum concentrations or exposure. For example, when fluvastatin 20 mg daily for 4 weeks was given to 16 patients taking stable doses of ciclosporin after renal transplantation, no changes were seen in their weekly minimum ciclosporin concentrations when compared with placebo.[9,10] Similar results were seen in another study using fluvastatin 20 mg once daily increased to 20 mg twice daily in 14 ciclosporin-treated patients.[11] In a pharmacokinetic study in 17 renal transplant recipients taking ciclosporin and given extended-release fluvastatin 80 mg daily for 7 days, fluvastatin had no effect on the AUC of ciclosporin.[12]

2. Effect on fluvastatin. In uncontrolled studies, when compared with historical data, ciclosporin appeared to increase fluvastatin exposure 2- to 3-fold. For example, in 20 renal transplant patients taking ciclosporin and given fluvastatin 20 mg daily, the AUC of fluvastatin was almost 2-fold higher than in historical control patients not taking ciclosporin.[13] Similarly, in another study in renal transplant patients taking ciclosporin and given fluvastatin 80 mg, there was a 2-fold increase in the AUC of fluvastatin, when compared with historical data.[12] Similarly, in a third study, the AUC of fluvastatin after taking 40 mg daily for 4 weeks was 3-fold greater in heart transplant patients taking ciclosporin than in healthy subjects not given ciclosporin.[14]

In one of these studies, 2 patients had mild myalgia without creatine phosphokinase rises, and a patient had asymptomatic elevated creatine phosphokinase.[13] However, in other studies there were no increases in creatine phosphokinase or additional adverse effects.[9-11,14] In a further double-blind efficacy study in heart transplant patients taking ciclosporin and given fluvastatin 40 mg daily for one year (52 patients), or placebo (27 patients), 7 patients given fluvastatin and one patient taking placebo had increases in their creatine phosphokinase concentrations, but the maximum recorded concentration was just 4.5 times normal, which did not require cessation of the fluvastatin and normalised without intervention. There was a difference in the reported rate of myalgia between fluvastatin and placebo recipients (12% versus 8%, respectively).[15]

The UK manufacturer of fluvastatin notes that isolated cases of myopathy have been reported post-marketing in patients taking fluvastatin and ciclosporin.[16]

(c) Lovastatin

1. Effect on ciclosporin. Minimum ciclosporin concentrations were not statistically significantly changed in 6 renal transplant patients taking ciclosporin and also given lovastatin (10 mg for 8 weeks, then 20 mg for 12 weeks).[17] Similar results were found in another study.[18] In a pharmacokinetic study in patients taking ciclosporin, lovastatin 20 mg daily for 28 days had no effect on the AUC of ciclosporin.[19]

2. Effect on lovastatin. In uncontrolled studies, ciclosporin appeared to increase lovastatin exposure 5- to 8-fold, and perhaps up to 20-fold. For example, in a study in patients given lovastatin 10 mg daily for 10 days, the AUC of lovastatin was five times greater in patients taking ciclosporin (11 transplant patients and 5 psoriasis patients) than in patients not taking ciclosporin (5 transplant patients and 8 non-transplant patients with hypercholesterolaemia). This suggests the difference was due to ciclosporin and not related to whether the patients had received a transplant or were receiving other immunosuppressants.[20] In another study in 6 transplant patients taking ciclosporin, the maximum and minimum plasma concentrations of lovastatin 10 to 20 mg daily were about the same as those seen in healthy subjects taking lovastatin 40 mg alone.[17] In another 21 renal transplant patients taking ciclosporin, the AUC of lovastatin 20 mg daily was 47% higher, after 28 days of concurrent use than on day one (suggesting accumulation) and was estimated to be 20-fold higher than values reported in healthy subjects not taking ciclosporin.[19] In yet another study, HMG-CoA reductase inhibitor activity in 6 transplant patients taking lovastatin was 4.2 to 7.8 times higher than in healthy subjects.[21]

There are at least 9 documented cases of rhabdomyolysis, often associated with acute renal failure, in patients taking ciclosporin and lovastatin.[21-25] In each of these cases the patient was taking lovastatin 40 to 80 mg daily. Several other studies suggest that this interaction might be dose-related. In one study, 15 patients taking ciclosporin were given lovastatin 20 mg daily without problem, but 4 of 5 other patients, who were given lovastatin 40 to 80 mg daily developed rhabdomyolysis, which was associated with renal failure in two of them.[26] In a further study, 24 patients were given lovastatin 10 or 20 mg daily in addition to ciclosporin. Of the 12 receiving the 20-mg dose, 7 developed either myalgia and muscle weakness or an increase in creatine phosphokinase concentrations, but only one patient from the 10-mg group did.[27] Based on clinical study data up to 1987, the manufacturer estimated that the incidence of myopathies with lovastatin was about 0.2%, but in the presence of ciclosporin the incidence appeared to be about 30%.[28]

(d) Pitavastatin

In a pharmacokinetic study in subjects given pitavastatin 2 mg daily for 6 days, a single 2-mg/kg dose of ciclosporin increased the AUC of pitavastatin 4.6-fold and the maximum plasma concentration 6.6-fold.[29]

(e) Pravastatin

1. Effect on ciclosporin. In several studies in patients taking ciclosporin, pravastatin has not altered ciclosporin concentrations or exposure. For example, in a pharmacokinetic study in patients taking ciclosporin, pravastatin 20 mg daily for 28 days had no effect on the AUC of ciclosporin.[19] In 16 patients taking ciclosporin, pravastatin 20 mg daily for 9 months had no effect on trough ciclosporin concentrations.[30] In yet another study, the AUC of ciclosporin did not differ between 20 cardiac transplant patients receiving pravastatin 20 mg daily and 17 transplant patients not receiving the statin.[31]

2. Effect on pravastatin. In uncontrolled studies, ciclosporin appeared to increase pravastatin exposure 5- to 23-fold. For example, in a study in 19 paediatric and adolescent cardiac transplant patients (mean age 12.1 years) taking triple immunosuppressant therapy (17 patients taking ciclosporin) and given a single 10-mg dose of pravastatin, the AUC of pravastatin was about 10-fold higher than in control subjects not receiving immunosuppressants. There was extremely large intersubject variation in the pravastatin AUC and maximum concentrations.[32] Similarly, in other studies in adults, the pravastatin AUC was about 12-fold,[33] 23-fold,[34] or 5- to 7-fold higher than in patients not taking ciclosporin.[19] Nevertheless, several of these studies[32,33] and other studies[30,35-37] have shown no increases in creatine phosphokinase concentrations[31,35,36] when pravastatin in doses of 10 to 40 mg daily was given with ciclosporin.

A report describes asymptomatic rhabdomyolysis in a heart transplant patient taking ciclosporin, who had taken pravastatin 40 mg daily for more than 3 years.[38] In an analysis of reports of myopathy submitted to the FDA in the US up to October 1997, the use of ciclosporin with pravastatin was associated with a notably increased incidence of myopathy.[39] In a review of the FDA spontaneous reports of statin-associated rhabdomyolysis covering the period November 1997 to March 2000, ciclosporin was potentially implicated in 2 cases of rhabdomyolysis involving pravastatin.[8]

(f) Rosuvastatin

In an open-label study 10 stable heart transplant patients taking ciclosporin were given rosuvastatin 10 mg daily for 10 days. When compared with healthy historical controls, the AUC of rosuvastatin was 7.1-fold higher. Rosuvastatin had no effect on the AUC of ciclosporin.[40]

(g) Simvastatin

1. Effect on ciclosporin. In a single-dose pharmacokinetic study in 7 healthy subjects, simultaneous administration of simvastatin 10 mg and ciclosporin 100 mg very slightly increased the AUC of ciclosporin by 13% when compared with ciclosporin alone.[41] However, in one retrospective study, the mean ciclosporin concentrations of 32 heart transplant patients decreased from 334 microgram/L to 235 micrograms/L after simvastatin 5 to 15 mg daily was added.[42] Conversely, in other studies, there was no change in minimum ciclosporin concentrations in 15 renal transplant patients given simvastatin 10 mg daily for 9 months,[30] or in 20 heart transplant patients given simvastatin 10 mg daily for 4 months,[43] or in 12 heart transplant patients given simvastatin 10 mg daily for 8 months.[44]

2. Effect on simvastatin. In a group of 20 heart transplant patients taking ciclosporin who were given simvastatin 10 mg daily for 4 months, the plasma concentrations of simvastatin acid 3 hours after a dose were at least six times higher in 7 patients taking ciclosporin than in 7 control patients not taking ciclosporin.[43] In another study, comparing 5 renal transplant patients taking ciclosporin with 5 renal transplant patients not taking ciclosporin, all given a single 20-mg dose of simvastatin, the AUC of HMG-CoA reductase inhibitory activity was 2.7-fold greater in the patients taking ciclosporin.[45] Creatine phosphokinase concentrations were not altered by simvastatin,[30,44] or were slightly increased (not statistically significant).[43]

There are at least 7 documented cases of rhabdomyolysis,[46-51] one of which was fatal,[47] mostly in transplant patients taking ciclosporin and given simvastatin 20 mg daily, but also in one patient taking simvastatin 80 mg daily and given ciclosporin 250 mg daily for uveitis.[50] A further case of rhabdomyolysis occurred in a patient taking ciclosporin and amlodipine about 2 months after his statin was changed from atorvastatin 20 mg daily to simvastatin 40 mg daily.[52] For mention of other cases of rhabdomyolysis in patients taking ciclosporin and simvastatin, to which verapamil probably contributed, see 'Statins + Calcium-channel blockers; Diltiazem or Verapamil', p.1325.

In an analysis of reports of myopathy submitted to the FDA in the US up to October 1997, the use of ciclosporin with simvastatin was associated with a notable increased incidence of myopathy.[39] In a review of the FDA spontaneous reports of statin-associated rhabdomyolysis covering the period November 1997 to March 2000, ciclosporin was potentially implicated in 31 cases of rhabdomyolysis involving simvastatin.[8] In a review of adverse reactions to statins in the Swedish Adverse Drug Reactions Advisory Committee until September 2006, six cases of confirmed rhabdomyolysis occurred in patients taking simvastatin and ciclosporin.[53]

Mechanism

Complex and not fully understood. Ciclosporin has often been considered to be an inhibitor of CYP3A4, by which simvastatin and lovastatin are principally metabolised.

However, ciclosporin appears to cause a moderate to very marked increase in the systemic exposure to statins regardless of whether they are metabolised by CYP3A4 or not. Increasing evidence shows that ciclosporin is an inhibitor of a number of transporter proteins including the organic anion transporting polypeptide (OATP) 1B1, and most statins are substrates of this transporter, see 'Lipid regulating drugs', p.1309, for more information. The reason for the very slight changes in ciclosporin concentrations when atorvastatin or simvastatin were given is not known.

Importance and management

Although most data are from uncontrolled studies, the effect of ciclosporin on the statins is well documented, well established and clinically important. Concurrent use need not be avoided, but the risks and benefits should be carefully evaluated, and it should be very well monitored, starting the statin at the lowest daily dose available.

For patients taking ciclosporin the specific recommendations of the manufacturers of the various statins are as follows:

- maximum daily dose of **atorvastatin** of 10 mg in the UK[54] but avoid concurrent use in the US[55]
- maximum daily dose of **fluvastatin** of 20 mg in the US[56]
- avoid the concurrent use of **lovastatin**[57]
- the concurrent use of **pitavastatin** is contraindicated[29]
- a starting dose of **pravastatin** of 20 mg daily, titrated to 40 mg daily with caution in the UK,[58] and of 10 mg daily with a maximum daily dose of 20 mg in the US[59]
- maximum daily dose of **rosuvastatin** of 5 mg daily (the lowest available dose) in the US,[60] but concurrent use is contraindicated in the UK[61]
- the concurrent use of **simvastatin** is contraindicated.[62,63]

Any patient given ciclosporin with a statin should be told to report any signs of myopathy and possible rhabdomyolysis (i.e. otherwise unexplained muscle pain, tenderness or weakness or dark coloured urine). If myopathy does occur, the statin should be stopped immediately. See also *Muscle and liver toxicity* under 'Lipid regulating drugs', p.1309, for further guidance on monitoring and risk factors for muscle toxicity.

The statins do not appear to alter ciclosporin exposure and concentrations, although simvastatin and atorvastatin have been reported to possibly have very slight or slight effects. However, as ciclosporin has a narrow therapeutic range, it might be prudent to increase in the frequency of ciclosporin monitoring when a statin is started, particularly atorvastatin or simvastatin.

1. Renders L, Mayer-Kadner I, Koch C, Schärffe S, Burkhardt K, Veelken R, Schmieder RE, Hauser IA. Efficacy and drug interactions of the new HMG-CoA reductase inhibitors cerivastatin and atorvastatin in CsA-treated renal transplant recipients. *Nephrol Dial Transplant* (2001) 16, 141–6.
2. Åsberg A, Hartmann A, Fjeldså E, Bergan S, Holdaas H. Bilateral pharmacokinetic interaction between cyclosporine A and atorvastatin in renal transplant recipients. *Am J Transplant* (2001) 1, 382–6.
3. Hermann M, Åsberg A, Christensen H, Reubsaet JLE, Holdaas H, Hartmann A. Atorvastatin does not affect the pharmacokinetics of cyclosporine in renal transplant recipients. *Eur J Clin Pharmacol* (2005) 61, 59–62.
4. Taylor PJ, Kubler PA, Lynch SV, Allen J, Butler M, Pillans PI. Effect of atorvastatin on cyclosporine pharmacokinetics in liver transplant recipients. *Ann Pharmacother* (2004) 38, 205–8.
5. Lemahieu WPD, Hermann M, Asberg A, Verbeke K, Holdaas H, Vanrenterghem Y, Maes BD. Combined therapy with atorvastatin and calcineurin inhibitors: no interactions with tacrolimus. *Am J Transplant* (2005) 5, 2236–43.
6. Hermann M, Åsberg A, Christensen H, Holdaas H, Hartmann A, Reubsaet JLE. Substantially elevated levels of atorvastatin and metabolites in cyclosporine-treated renal transplant recipients. *Clin Pharmacol Ther* (2004) 76, 388–91.
7. Maltz HC, Balog DL, Cheigh JS. Rhabdomyolysis associated with concomitant use of atorvastatin and cyclosporine. *Ann Pharmacother* (1999) 33, 1176–9.
8. Omar MA, Wilson JP. FDA adverse event reports on statin-associated rhabdomyolysis. *Ann Pharmacother* (2002) 36, 288–95.
9. Li PKT, Mak TWL, Wang AYM, Lee YT, Leung CB, Lui SF, Lam CWK, Lai KN. The interaction of fluvastatin and cyclosporin A in renal transplant patients. *Int J Clin Pharmacol Ther* (1995) 33, 246–8.
10. Li PKT, Mak TWL, Chan TH, Wang A, Lam CWK, Lai KN. Effect of fluvastatin on lipoprotein profiles in treating renal transplant recipients with dyslipoproteinemia. *Transplantation* (1995) 60, 652–6.
11. Holdaas H, Hartmann A, Stenstrøm J, Dahl KJ, Borge M, Pfister P. Effect of fluvastatin for safely lowering atherogenic lipids in renal transplant patients receiving cyclosporine. *Am J Cardiol* (1995) 76, 102A–106A.
12. Holdaas H, Hagen E, Åsberg A, Lund K, Hartman A, Vaidyanathan S, Prasad P, He Y-L, Yeh C-M, Bigler H, Rouilly M, Denouel J. Evaluation of the pharmacokinetic interaction between fluvastatin XL and cyclosporine in renal transplant recipients. *Int J Clin Pharmacol Ther* (2006) 44, 163–71.
13. Goldberg R, Roth D. Evaluation of fluvastatin in the treatment of hypercholesterolemia in renal transplant recipients taking cyclosporine. *Transplantation* (1996) 62, 1559–64.
14. Park J-W, Siekmeier R, Lattke P, Merz M, Mix C, Schüler S, Jaross W. Pharmacokinetics and pharmacodynamics of fluvastatin in heart transplant recipients taking cyclosporine A. *J Cardiovasc Pharmacol Ther* (2001) 6, 351–61.
15. O'Rourke B, Barbir M, Mitchell AG, Yacoub MH, Banner NR. Efficacy and safety of fluvastatin therapy for hypercholesterolemia after heart transplantation. Results of a randomised double blind placebo controlled study. *Int J Cardiol* (2004) 94, 235–40.
16. Lescol (Fluvastatin sodium). Novartis Pharmaceuticals UK Ltd. UK Summary of product characteristics, November 2013.
17. Cheung AK, DeVault GA, Gregory MC. A prospective study on treatment of hypercholesterolemia with lovastatin in renal transplant patients receiving cyclosporine. *J Am Soc Nephrol* (1993) 3, 1884–91.
18. Castelao AM, Griñó JM, Andrés E, Gilvernet S, Serón D, Castiñeiras MJ, Roca M, Galcerán JM, González MT, Alsina J. HMGCoA reductase inhibitors lovastatin and simvastatin in the treatment of hypercholesterolemia after renal transplantation. *Transplant Proc* (1993) 25, 1043–6.
19. Olbricht C, Wanner C, Eisenhauer T, Kliem V, Doll R, Boddaert M, O'Grady P, Krekler M, Mangold B, Christians U. Accumulation of lovastatin, but not pravastatin, in the blood of cyclosporine-treated kidney graft patients after multiple doses. *Clin Pharmacol Ther* (1997) 62, 311–21.
20. Gullestad L, Nordal KP, Berg KJ, Cheng H, Schwartz MS, Simonsen S. Interaction between lovastatin and cyclosporine A after heart and kidney transplantation. *Transplant Proc* (1999) 31, 2163–5.
21. Kobashigawa JA, Murphy FL, Stevenson LW, Moriguchi JD, Kawata N, Kamjoo P, Brownfield E, Wilmarth J, Leonard L, Chuck C, Drinkwater D, Laks H. Low-dose lovastatin safely lowers cholesterol after cardiac transplantation. *Circulation* (1990) 82 (Suppl IV), IV-281–IV-283.
22. Alejandro DSJ, Petersen J. Myoglobinuric acute renal failure in a cardiac transplant patient taking lovastatin and cyclosporine. *J Am Soc Nephrol* (1994) 5, 153–160.
23. Corpier CL, Jones PH, Suki WN, Lederer ED, Quinones MA, Schmidt SW, Young JB. Rhabdomyolysis and renal injury with lovastatin use. Report of two cases in cardiac transplant recipients. *JAMA* (1988) 260, 239–41.
24. East C, Alivizatos PA, Grundy SM, Jones PH, Farmer JA. Rhabdomyolysis in patients receiving lovastatin after cardiac transplantation. *N Engl J Med* (1988) 318, 47–8.
25. Norman DJ, Illingworth DR, Munson J, Hosenpud J. Myolysis and acute renal failure in a heart-transplant recipient receiving lovastatin. *N Engl J Med* (1988) 318, 46–7.
26. Ballantyne CM, Radovancevic B, Farmer JA, Frazier OH, Chandler L, Payton-Ross C, Cocanougher B, Jones PH, Young JB, Gotto AM. Hyperlipidemia after heart transplantation: report of a 6-year experience, with treatment recommendations. *J Am Coll Cardiol* (1992) 19, 1315–21.
27. Heroux AL, Thompson JA, Katz S, Hastillo AK, Katz M, Quigg RJ, Hess ML. Elimination of the lovastatin-cyclosporine adverse interaction in heart transplant patients. *Circulation* (1989) 80, II-641.
28. Tobert JA. Rhabdomyolysis in patients receiving lovastatin after cardiac transplantation. *N Engl J Med* (1988) 318, 48.
29. Livalo (Pitavastatin). Kowa Pharmaceuticals America, Inc. US Prescribing information, October 2013.
30. Capone D, Stanziale P, Gentile A, Imperatore P, Pellegrino T, Basile V. Effects of simvastatin and pravastatin on hyperlipidemia and cyclosporin blood levels in renal transplant recipients. *Am J Nephrol* (1999) 19, 411–15.
31. Cassem JD, Hamilton MA, Albanese E, Sabad A, Kobashigawa JA. Does pravastatin affect cyclosporine pharmacokinetics in cardiac transplant recipients. *J Investig Med* (1997) 45, 139A.
32. Hedman M, Neuvonen PJ, Neuvonen M, Holmberg C, Antikainen M. Pharmacokinetics and pharmacodynamics of pravastatin in pediatric and adolescent cardiac transplant recipients on a regimen of triple immunosuppression. *Clin Pharmacol Ther* (2004) 75, 101–109.
33. Park J-W, Siekmeier R, Merz M, Krell B, Harder S, März W, Seidel D, Schüler S, Groß W. Pharmacokinetics of pravastatin in heart-transplant patients taking cyclosporin A. *Int J Clin Pharmacol Ther* (2002) 40, 439–50.
34. Regazzi MB, Iacona I, Campana C, Raddato V, Lesi C, Perani G, Gavazzi A, Viganò M. Altered disposition of pravastatin following concomitant drug therapy with cyclosporin A in transplant recipients. *Transplant Proc* (1993) 25, 2732–4.
35. Yoshimura N, Oka T, Okamoto M, Ohmori Y. The effects of pravastatin on hyperlipidemia in renal transplant recipients. *Transplantation* (1992) 53, 94–9.
36. Muhlmeister HF, Hamilton MA, Cogert GA, Cassem JD, Sabad A, Kobashigawa JA. Long-term HMG-CoA reductase inhibition appears safe and effective after cardiac transplantation. *J Investig Med* (1997) 45, 139A.
37. Kobashigawa JA, Brownfield ED, Stevenson LW, Gleeson MP, Moriguchi JD, Kawata N, Hamilton MA, Hage AS, Minkley R, Salamandra J, Ruzevich S, Drinkwater DC, Laks H. Effects of pravastatin for hypercholesterolemia in cardiac transplant recipients. *J Am Coll Cardiol* (1993) 21, 141A.
38. Schindler C, Thoms M, Matschke K, Tugtekin SM, Kirch W. Asymptomatic statin-induced rhabdomyolysis after long-term therapy with the hydrophilic drug pravastatin. *Clin Ther* (2007) 29, 172–6.
39. Gruer PJK, Vega JM, Mercuri MF, Dobrinska MR, Tobert JA. Concomitant use of cytochrome P450 3A4 inhibitors and simvastatin. *Am J Cardiol* (1999) 84, 811–15.
40. Simonson SG, Raza A, Martin PD, Mitchell PD, Jarcho JA, Brown CDA, Windass AS, Schneck DW. Rosuvastatin pharmacokinetics in heart transplant recipients administered an antirejection regimen including cyclosporine. *Clin Pharmacol Ther* (2004) 76, 167–77.
41. Xu F, Wu Z-H, Zhang Z-Y, Zou H-Q. Delay of metabolism rate of ciclosporin by simvastatin in 7 Chinese healthy men. *Acta Pharmacol Sin* (1998) 19, 443–4.
42. Akhlaghi F, McLachlan AJ, Keogh AM, Brown KF. Effect of simvastatin on cyclosporine unbound fraction and apparent blood clearance in heart transplant recipients. *Br J Clin Pharmacol* (1997) 44, 537–42.
43. Campana C, Iacona I, Regazzi MB, Gavazzi A, Perani G, Raddato V, Montemartini C, Viganò M. Efficacy and pharmacokinetics of simvastatin in heart transplant recipients. *Ann Pharmacother* (1995) 29, 235–9.
44. Barbir M, Rose M, Kushwaha S, Akl S, Mitchell A, Yacoub M. Low-dose simvastatin for the treatment of hypercholesterolaemia in recipients of cardiac transplantation. *Int J Cardiol* (1991) 33, 241–6.
45. Arnadottir M, Eriksson L-O, Thysell H, Karkas JD. Plasma concentration profiles of simvastatin 3-hydroxy-3-methyl-glutaryl-coenzyme A reductase inhibitory activity in kidney transplant recipients with and without ciclosporin. *Nephron* (1993) 65, 410–13.
46. Blaison G, Weber JC, Sachs D, Korganow AS, Martin T, Kretz JG, Pasquali JL. Rhabdomyolyse causée par la simvastatine chez un transplanté cardiaque sous ciclosporine. *Rev Med Interne* (1992) 13, 61–3.
47. Weise WJ, Possidente CJ. Fatal rhabdomyolysis associated with simvastatin in a renal transplant patient. *Am J Med* (2000) 108, 351–2.
48. Meier C, Stey C, Brack T, Maggiorini M, Risti B, Krahenbuhl S. Rhabdomyolyse bei mit Simvastatin und Ciclosporin behandelten Patienten: Rolle der aktivitat des Cytochrom-P450-Enzymsystems der Leber. *Schweiz Med Wochenschr* (1995) 125, 1342–6.
49. Gumprecht J, Zychma M, Grzeszczak W, Kuźniewicz R, Burak W, Żywiec J, Karasek D, Otulski I, Mosur M. Simvastatin-induced rhabdomyolysis in a CsA-treated renal transplant recipient. *Med Sci Monit* (2003) 9, CS89–CS91.
50. Lasocki A, Vote B, Fassett R, Zamir E. Simvastatin-induced rhabdomyolysis following cyclosporine treatment for uveitis. *Ocul Immunol Inflamm* (2007) 15, 345–6.
51. Yang WH, Zeng ZS, Ren XW, Li YP, Shang WJ, Feng GW, Zhang LR. Simvastatin-induced myopathy with concomitant use of cyclosporine: a case report. *Int J Clin Pharmacol Ther* (2011) 49, 772–7.
52. Schreiber DH, Anderson TR. Statin-induced rhabdomyolysis. *J Emerg Med* (2006) 31, 177–80.
53. Hedenmalm K, Alvan G, Öhagen P, Dahl M-L. Muscle toxicity with statins. *Pharmacoepidemiol Drug Safety* (2010) 19, 223–31.
54. Lipitor (Atorvastatin calcium trihydrate). Pfizer Ltd. UK Summary of product characteristics, March 2015.
55. Lipitor (Atorvastatin calcium). Pfizer Inc. US Prescribing information, March 2015.
56. Lescol (Fluvastatin sodium). Novartis Pharmaceuticals Corp. US Prescribing information, October 2012.
57. Mevacor (Lovastatin). Merck & Co., Inc. US Prescribing information, February 2014.
58. Lipostat (Pravastatin sodium). Bristol-Myers Squibb Pharmaceutical Ltd. UK Summary of product characteristics, April 2013.
59. Pravachol (Pravastatin sodium). Bristol-Myers Squibb Company. US Prescribing information, August 2013.
60. Crestor (Rosuvastatin calcium). AstraZeneca. US Prescribing information, August 2013.
61. Crestor (Rosuvastatin calcium). AstraZeneca UK Ltd. UK Summary of product characteristics, May 2013.
62. Zocor (Simvastatin). Merck & Co., Inc. US Prescribing information, March 2015.
63. Zocor (Simvastatin). Merck Sharp & Dohme Ltd. UK Summary of product characteristics, June 2015.

Statins + Cilostazol

Cilostazol moderately increases the exposure to lovastatin: simvastatin would be expected to be similarly affected.

Clinical evidence

In a study in 13 healthy subjects, a single 80-mg oral dose of **lovastatin** was given before, and then on the final day of cilostazol 100 mg twice daily for 7 days. The AUCs of **lovastatin** and its beta-hydroxy acid metabolite were increased by about 60% and 70%, respectively, by cilostazol, but the maximum plasma levels were unaffected.[1] At the end of this study (day 9), 12 subjects were given **lovastatin** 80 mg with a larger 150-mg dose of cilostazol. It was found that the maximum level and the AUC of the metabolite of **lovastatin** were increased twofold, suggesting that larger cilostazol doses might have a greater effect.[1] Lovastatin decreased the absorption of cilostazol by about 15%.[1]

Mechanism

Lovastatin is principally metabolised by CYP3A4 and it would appear that cilostazol can inhibit this isoenzyme. **Simvastatin** is also metabolised by CYP3A4 and might therefore be expected to interact similarly.

Importance and management

Evidence for an interaction between cilostazol and the statins appears to be limited to this one study with lovastatin. The increase in lovastatin exposure described here is lower than that seen with moderate CYP3A4 inhibitors (e.g. see 'Statins + Calcium-channel blockers; Diltiazem or Verapamil', p.1325), and, although the authors of the study suggest that the dose of lovastatin might need to be reduced if cilostazol is also taken, the US manufacturer of cilostazol more reasonably states that a clinically relevant interaction is unlikely.[2] Although **simvastatin** would be expected to interact with cilostazol to a similar extent to lovastatin, the UK manufacturer[3] of cilostazol advises caution on concurrent use: this appears over-cautious. Nevertheless, it may be prudent to remind patients taking these statins with cilostazol to report any signs of myopathy and possible rhabdomyolysis (i.e. otherwise unexplained muscle pain, tenderness or weakness or dark coloured urine), particularly if other risk factors are present. If myopathy does occur, the statin should be stopped immediately. See *Muscle and liver toxicity,* under 'Lipid regulating drugs', p.1309, for further guidance on monitoring, and risk factors for muscle toxicity.

The slight decrease in cilostazol levels with lovastatin is not clinically relevant.

1. Bramer SL, Brisson J, Corey AE, Mallikaarjun S. Effect of multiple cilostazol doses on single dose lovastatin pharmacokinetics in healthy volunteers. *Clin Pharmacokinet* (1999) 37 (Suppl 2), 69–77.
2. Pletal (Cilostazol). Otsuka America Pharmaceutical, Inc. US Prescribing information, May 2007.
3. Pletal (Cilostazol). Otsuka Pharmaceuticals (UK) Ltd. UK Summary of product characteristics, October 2013.

Statins + Cobicistat with elvitegravir

Cobicistat (given with elvitegravir) slightly increases the exposure to single-dose rosuvastatin; single-dose rosuvastatin did not affect the pharmacokinetics of cobicistat or elvitegravir. Cobicistat is predicted to increase the plasma concentrations of statins by CYP3A4, such as simvastatin, lovastatin, and to a lesser extent, atorvastatin. Cobicistat is predicted not to interact with fluvastatin, pitavastatin, and pravastatin.

Clinical evidence

In a study in 10 healthy subjects, cobicistat 150 mg once daily (given as a pharmacokinetic enhancer with elvitegravir 150 mg once daily) increased the AUC of a single 10-mg dose of **rosuvastatin** by 38%, and increased its maximum plasma concentration by 89%. The pharmacokinetics of cobicistat and elvitegravir were unaffected.[1]

Mechanism

Rosuvastatin is a substrate for the organic anion transporting polypeptide OATP1B1, which was inhibited by both cobicistat and elvitegravir *in vitro*.[1] The increase in rosuvastatin exposure seen might therefore be a result of OATP1B1 inhibition by cobicistat and/or elvitegravir. Further study is required to confirm this. Cobicistat is also an inhibitor of CYP3A4, but rosuvastatin is not a substrate of this isoenzyme.

Importance and management

Evidence for an interaction between the statins and cobicistat with elvitegravir is limited to that with rosuvastatin. The increase in rosuvastatin exposure was only slight, and is probably unlikely to be clinically important. As such, no rosuvastatin dose adjustment would seem necessary on concurrent use.

The effects on other statins do not appear to have been studied, but based on the known metabolism of these drugs, predictions about their potential effects are possible. **Simvastatin** and **lovastatin** are primarily metabolised by CYP3A4, and as cobicistat is a potent inhibitor of this isoenzyme, concurrent use of these statins with cobicistat is contraindicated.

Atorvastatin is partially metabolised by CYP3A4 and is a substrate of OATP1B1, and its plasma concentration is likely to be increased by elvitegravir boosted with cobicistat. The US manufacturer of elvitegravir with cobicistat (in a fixed-dose combination also including emtricitabine and tenofovir disoproxil fumarate) and US manufacturer of cobicistat (for use with atazanavir or darunavir), recommends starting with the lowest atorvastatin dose on concurrent use, and titrating carefully while monitoring for safety.[2,3] The same advice is given by the UK manufacturers (if atorvastatin is considered strictly necessary),[4,5] otherwise concurrent use is not recommended.[1,5]

Pravastatin and **pitavastatin** are not metabolised by CYP3A4, but are substrates of OATP1B1 and so might be expected to be affected in a similar way to rosuvastatin, and hence do not require dose adjustment. **Fluvastatin** is not a substrate for CYP3A4 or OATP1B1 and no dose adjustment would seem necessary on concurrent use.

It is important to note, that as both cobicistat and elvitegravir are licensed for use in various combinations with other antiretrovirals (some of which might exert their own effects, particularly the HIV-protease inhibitors, see 'Statins + HIV-protease inhibitors', p.1345), the effects might not be entirely predictable and advice from manufacturers varies. It would therefore seem prudent, that if a statin is not contra-indicated and is to be given concurrently with elvitegravir or cobicistat in any combination, the patient should be told to report any signs of myopathy and possible rhabdomyolysis (i.e. otherwise unexplained muscle pain, tenderness, or weakness or dark coloured urine). If myopathy does occur, the statin should be stopped immediately.

Note too that separating administration should minimise any interaction by OATP1B1.

1. Custodio JM, Wang H, Hao J, Lepist EI, Ray AS, Andrews J, Ling KH, Cheng A, Kearney BP, Ramanathan S. Pharmacokinetics of cobicistat boosted-elvitegravir administered in combination with rosuvastatin. *J Clin Pharmacol* (2014) 54, 649–56.
2. Stribild (Elvitegravir, cobicistat, emtricitabine, tenofovir disoproxil fumarate). Gilead Sciences, Inc. US Prescribing information, December 2014.
3. Tybost (Cobicistat). Gilead Sciences, Inc. US Prescribing information, September 2014.
4. Stribild (Cobicistat, emtricitabine, elvitegravir, tenofovir disoproxil fumarate). Gilead Sciences Ltd. UK Summary of product characteristics, July 2014.
5. Tybost (Cobicistat). Gilead Sciences Ltd. UK Summary of product characteristics, October 2014.

Statins + Colchicine

Atorvastatin appears to slightly increase the exposure to colchicine. Several case reports describe myopathy or rhabdomyolysis in patients given colchicine with atorvastatin, fluvastatin, lovastatin, pravastatin, or simvastatin.

Clinical evidence

(a) Atorvastatin

In a study in 23 healthy subjects, atorvastatin 40 mg daily for 14 days increased the AUC and maximum concentration of a single 600-microgram dose of colchicine by about 25% and 30%, respectively.[1] Three cases describe acute myopathy in patients taking established long-term colchicine shortly after starting atorvastatin. In the first, a 45-year-old man with nephrotic syndrome with normal renal function who had been taking colchicine 1.5 mg daily for 3 years without adverse effects, began to experience lower extremity weakness, muscle pain, and gait instability about 2 weeks after he started taking low-dose atorvastatin 10 mg daily. Two weeks later rhabdomyolysis was diagnosed, with acute renal failure and an elevated creatine kinase concentration of more than 50 times the reference values. After withdrawal of colchicine and atorvastatin, his creatine kinase concentration and muscle strength improved, but he then developed septic shock as a result of hospital-acquired pneumonia and died.[2] Another report describes two other similar cases of myopathy developing 2 to 3 weeks after starting atorvastatin 10 or 20 mg daily in patients taking long-term colchicine for amyloid A amyloidosis secondary to familial Mediterranean fever. In both these patients the myopathy resolved on stopping atorvastatin and colchicine, and colchicine was subsequently successfully restarted and increased to the original dose.[3]

One case report describes rhabdomyolysis in a kidney transplant patient taking ciclosporin and atorvastatin 20 mg daily which occurred 2 months after starting colchicine 500 micrograms twice daily for gout.[4] Note that the total dose of colchicine taken by this patient exceeds that generally recommended for an acute attack of gout.

(b) Fluvastatin

A 70-year-old man with normal renal function who had been taking fluvastatin 80 mg daily for 2 years started taking colchicine 1.5 mg daily for an attack of gouty arthritis. Within 3 days he felt nauseous and began to develop muscle pains and weakness. On admission to hospital 10 days after starting the colchicine he was found to have acute renal failure and a high creatine kinase concentration, and was diagnosed with rhabdomyolysis. Both drugs were stopped and he recovered over 19 days. He was eventually restabilised on fluvastatin without incident.[5] Another similar case describes a 77-year-old man with chronic renal failure taking fluvastatin 80 mg daily for 4 years, who developed severe pain and weakness in his arms and legs, 14 days after starting to take colchicine 1 mg daily for acute gouty arthritis. His creatine kinase concentration was high, but this returned to normal range 16 days after fluvastatin and colchicine were stopped and treatment was given. He was restarted on fluvastatin and 6 months later he was still symptom free.[6] Note that the total dose of colchicine taken by these patients exceeds that generally recommended for an acute attack of gout.

(c) Lovastatin

A 74-year-old man with normal renal function taking prophylactic colchicine for gout [dose not stated], developed myopathy 2 weeks after starting lovastatin [dose not stated].[7]

(d) Pravastatin

A 65-year-old woman with mild renal impairment who had been taking pravastatin 20 mg daily for 6 years was given colchicine 1.5 mg daily for an episode of gout. Within 20 days she had developed muscle weakness in the legs and had a slightly high creatine kinase concentration. A diagnosis of myopathy was made and so both colchicine and pravastatin were stopped. The weakness resolved over the following week. Colchicine was subsequently given alone at a dose of 1 mg daily when the patient had another attack of gout, and myopathy did not occur.[8] Note that the total dose of colchicine taken by this patient exceeds that generally recommended for an acute attack of gout.

A heart and lung transplant patient who was taking pravastatin 20 mg daily, developed multi-organ failure and rhabdomyolysis 8 days after he finished a course of colchicine 1 mg three times daily on day one, 1 mg twice daily on day 2, and 1 mg daily for 6 days, for acute gout.[9] He was also taking ciclosporin and azithromycin which may have contributed to the interaction, see 'Ciclosporin + Colchicine', p.1223, and 'Colchicine + Macrolides', p.1562.

(e) Simvastatin

Several case reports describe acute myopathy in patients with renal impairment taking simvastatin and given colchicine for acute gout. In the first, a 70-year-old man with chronic renal failure who had been taking simvastatin (dose not stated) for 2 years was given colchicine 500 micrograms twice daily for gout. Within 2 weeks he developed muscle weakness, which was diagnosed as myopathy. Both drugs were stopped and the symptoms resolved.[10] Rhabdomyolysis in a 61-year-old woman with mild renal impairment taking simvastatin 40 mg daily occurred 3 weeks after she started to take colchicine 600 micrograms twice daily and 2 weeks after the dose of simvastatin was doubled, to 80 mg daily. Both drugs were discontinued and within 2 weeks the muscle weakness had resolved and the creatine kinase concentration had returned to the expected range. Simvastatin was restarted at 80 mg daily and allopurinol initiated; 6 months later, she was asymptomatic with a normal creatine kinase concentration.[11] Other reports similarly describe rhabdomyolysis or myopathy in patients taking simvastatin 40 mg daily: a 79-year-old man with mild, chronic renal impairment developed rhabdomyolysis within 8 days of starting colchicine (initially 600 micrograms daily, increased to twice daily after 4 days),[12] and an 84-year-old man developed myopathy during the 3 weeks following the addition of colchicine (initially 1 mg daily for 3 days and then 500 micrograms daily).[13] Note that the total dose of colchicine taken in these cases exceeds that generally recommended for an acute attack of gout.

In another complicated case, a patient taking ciclosporin developed progressive muscle weakness over 4 months after his simvastatin dose was doubled from 30 mg daily to 60 mg daily and colchicine 1.2 mg daily was started for gout. His creatine kinase concentration decreased on stopping colchicine and simvastatin, but it greatly increased on starting propofol sedation and high-dose methylprednisolone (while continuing ciclosporin), and fatal rhabdomyolysis occurred.[14]

Another report describes one case of myopathy which developed 3 weeks after a patient taking long-term colchicine 1.5 mg daily for amyloid A amyloidosis secondary to familial Mediterranean fever started taking simvastatin 20 mg daily. The myopathy resolved on stopping the simvastatin and colchicine, and colchicine was subsequently successfully restarted and increased to the original dose.[3]

A further case describes a patient with chronic renal impairment who had been taking colchicine 500 micrograms daily for one year and simvastatin 20 mg daily for 3 months, who developed neuromyopathy a few days after completing a 10-day course of clarithromycin (dose not stated).[15] Note that the clarithromycin could have contributed to the interaction, see 'Colchicine + Macrolides', p.1562.

Mechanism

Colchicine alone can, rarely, cause myopathy especially in those given colchicine long term, in high dose, or in the presence of renal impairment.[8] As the statins can also cause myopathy, an additive or synergistic effect seems possible.[5] It is also possible that pharmacokinetic interactions might occur and contribute, although the mechanism (s) is not known. Note that, an interaction involving CYP3A4 (of which colchicine and some of the statins are substrates) seems unlikely because neither colchicine nor the statins are known inhibitors of CYP3A4. The authors of the pharmacokinetic study suggest that possible inhibition of P-glycoprotein by atorvastatin lead to the increased colchicine exposure seen.[1] However, evidence for this is limited (see 'Digoxin and related drugs + Statins', p.1111 for the effect of atorvastatin on this P-glycoprotein probe substrate).

Importance and management

An interaction between the statins and colchicine is not established, but one pharmacokinetic study suggests that a pharmacokinetic interaction between atorvastatin and colchicine might occur. The mechanism behind this is not clear, and the clinical importance of the slight increase in colchicine exposure seen is not known. However, a number of cases exist which describe myopathy and/or rhabdomyolysis when colchicine and a statin have been taken together. Note that, in many of the cases described in patients with acute gout, the dose of colchicine exceeded that generally recommended, and patients had other risk factors for cumulative colchicine toxicity, such as renal impairment or old age. Nevertheless, statins are also rarely known to be associated with myopathy, and an additive or synergistic effect can also not be excluded. Further study into the mechanism behind the effects seen is needed.

Given the evidence available, it would be prudent to be aware that there might be an increased risk of myopathy with any statin used concurrently with colchicine. The US manufacturer of colchicine advises weighing the potential benefits and risks of concurrent use, and carefully monitoring patients for symptoms of muscle pain, tenderness and weakness, although they note that monitoring creatine [phospho]kinase concentrations might not prevent severe myopathy.[16] All patients taking statins should be warned about the symptoms of myopathy and told to report muscle pain or weakness, and it would be prudent to reinforce this advice if colchicine is taken with a statin. See also *Muscle and liver toxicity*, under 'Lipid regulating drugs', p.1309, for further guidance on monitoring and risk factors for muscle toxicity.

1. Davis MW, Wason S. Effect of steady-state atorvastatin on the pharmacokinetics of a single dose of colchicine in healthy adults under fasted conditions. *Clin Drug Investig* (2014) 34, 259–67.
2. Tufan A, Dede DS, Cavus S, Altintas ND, Iskit AB, Topeli A. Rhabdomyolysis in a patient treated with colchicine and atorvastatin. *Ann Pharmacother* (2006) 40, 1466–9.
3. Sahin G, Korkmaz C, Yalcin AU. Which statin should be used together with colchicine? Clinical experience in three patients with nephrotic syndrome due to AA type amyloidosis. *Rheumatol Int* (2008) 28, 289–91.
4. Phanish MK, Krishnamurthy S, Bloodworth LLO. Colchicine-induced rhabdomyolysis. *Am J Med* (2003) 114, 166–7.
5. Atasoyu EM, Evrenkaya TR, Solmazgul E. Possible colchicine rhabdomyolysis in a fluvastatin-treated patient. *Ann Pharmacother* (2005) 39, 1368–9.
6. Sarullo FM, Americo L, Di Franco A, Di Pasquale P. Rhabdomyolysis induced by co-administration of fluvastatin and colchicine. *Monaldi Arch Chest Dis* (2010) 74, 147–9.
7. Torgovnick J, Sethi N, Arsura E. Colchicine and HMG Co-A reductase inhibitors induced myopathy-a case report. *Neurotoxicology* (2006) 27, 1126–7.
8. Alayli G, Cengiz K, Cantürk F, Durmuş D, Akyol Y, Menekşe EB. Acute myopathy in a patient with concomitant use of pravastatin and colchicine. *Ann Pharmacother* (2005) 39, 1358–61.
9. Bouquié R, Deslandes G, Renaud C, Dailly E, Haloun A, Jolliet P. Colchicine-induced rhabdomyolysis in a heart/lung transplant patient with concurrent use of ciclosporin, pravastatin, and azithromycin. *J Clin Rheumatol* (2011) 17, 28–30.
10. Hsu W-C, Chen W-H, Chang M-T, Chiu H-C. Colchicine-induced acute myopathy in a patient with concomitant use of simvastatin. *Clin Neuropharmacol* (2002) 25, 266–8.
11. Justiniano M, Dold S, Espinoza LR. Rapid onset of muscle weakness (rhabdomyolysis) associated with the combined use of simvastatin and colchicine. *J Clin Rheumatol* (2007) 13, 266–8.
12. Baker SK, Goodwin S, Sur M, Tarnopolsky MA. Cytoskeletal myotoxicity from simvastatin and colchicine. *Muscle Nerve* (2004) 30, 799–802.
13. Oh DH, Chan SQ, Wilson AM. Myopathy and possible intestinal dysfunction in a patient treated with colchicine and simvastatin. *Med J Aust* (2012) 197, 332–3.
14. Francis L, Bonilla E, Soforo E, Neupane H, Nakhla H, Fuller C, Perl A. Fatal toxic myopathy attributed to propofol, methylprednisolone, and cyclosporine after prior exposure to colchicine and simvastatin. *Clin Rheumatol* (2008) 27, 129–31.
15. van der Velden W, Huussen J, ter Laak H, de Sévaux R. Colchicine-induced neuromyopathy in a patient with chronic renal failure: the role of clarithromycin. *Neth J Med* (2008) 66, 204–6.
16. Colcrys (Colchicine). Takeda Pharmaceuticals America, Inc. US Prescribing information, November 2012.

Statins + Danazol

Severe rhabdomyolysis and myoglobinuria developed in a man taking lovastatin about two months after danazol was added. Similar cases have been reported with danazol in other patients taking lovastatin or simvastatin.

Clinical evidence

(a) Lovastatin

A 72-year-old man taking atenolol, aspirin, dipyridamole and lovastatin 20 mg twice daily was admitted to hospital after complaining of myalgia over the last 12 days, and brown urine over the last 5 days. He was diagnosed with severe rhabdomyolysis and myoglobinuria. About 2 months previously he had started taking danazol 200 mg three times daily and prednisone, and one month previously he had received a 10-day course of doxycycline 100 mg twice daily. The aspirin and lovastatin were stopped (danazol was stopped 4 days before admission and the doxycycline was stopped 5 days before the onset of symptoms), and all the symptoms resolved. Laboratory tests were normal within 2 weeks.[1] A similar case of muscle toxicity has been reported in a woman with end-stage renal disease who had been taking lovastatin 40 mg daily for 7 weeks and danazol 600 mg daily for about 5 weeks before admission. The authors note that both drugs had been previously tolerated when given alone, but it should be noted that the lovastatin had been given in a lower dose of 20 mg daily.[2] A further similar case occurred in a patient taking danazol 400 mg daily, two months after the statin was switched from atorvastatin 10 mg daily to lovastatin 40 mg daily.[3]

(b) Simvastatin

A 68-year-old man who had been taking simvastatin 40 mg daily long-term without problem developed rhabdomyolysis (progressive muscle pain and weakness, tea-coloured urine, renal impairment, and a raised creatine phosphokinase) within 3 weeks of starting to take danazol 200 mg three times daily. He was given haemodialysis and subsequently recovered.[4] Another case of fatal rhabdomyolysis has been described in a patient taking simvastatin and danazol. He had been taking the danazol for 4 months, then 5 weeks before the occurrence of the rhabdomyolysis the dose of simvastatin had been increased from 20 mg to 40 mg daily and the danazol from 200 mg to 600 mg daily.[5]

Mechanism

It has been suggested that danazol is an inhibitor of CYP3A4 by which simvastatin and lovastatin are metabolised. This could result in raised statin levels, and therefore myopathy and rhabdomyolysis.[1,4]

Importance and management

Evidence for an interaction between danazol and the statins appears to be limited to the cases cited, all involving lovastatin or simvastatin, but the pharmacokinetic basis of the interaction appears logical, and therefore some caution would seem prudent with any statin principally metabolised by CYP3A4 (i.e. lovastatin and simvastatin). The benefits of giving lovastatin or simvastatin with danazol should be weighed against the potential risks and low doses should be used. The US manufacturer of **lovastatin**[6] states that the dose should be started at 10 mg daily, and should not exceed 20 mg daily in the presence of danazol. The UK and US manufacturers of **simvastatin** contraindicate the concurrent use of danazol.[7,8] It would seem prudent to monitor for symptoms of myopathy and tell patients to report any unexplained muscle pain, tenderness or weakness. The authors of one of the reports[1] point out that severe lovastatin muscle toxicity can be very slow to develop. See also *Muscle and liver toxicity*, under 'Lipid regulating drugs', p.1309, for further guidance on monitoring, and risk factors for muscle toxicity.

The risk of muscle toxicity on the concurrent use of danazol and **atorvastatin** would be expected to be lower, as atorvastatin is less dependent than simvastatin and lovastatin on CYP3A4 for metabolism (although note that this mechanism needs confirmation), and no cases of an interaction with danazol appear to have been reported for this statin. Nevertheless, some caution might be prudent.

Similarly, if the mechanism is confirmed, the statins that are not significantly metabolised by CYP3A4 would not be expected to interact.

1. Dallaire M, Chamberland M, Rhabdomyolyse sévère chez un patient recevant lovastatine, danazol et doxycycline. *Can Med Assoc J* (1994) 150, 1991–4.
2. Hsieh C-Y, Chen C-H. Rhabdomyolysis and pancreatitis associated with coadministration of danazol 600 mg/d and lovastatin 40 mg/d. *Clin Ther* (2008) 30, 1330–5.
3. Khanna S, Mundell WC. Rhabdomyolysis [sic] associated with co-administration of danazol and lovastatin. *Br J Clin Pharmacol* (2011) 72, 166–7.
4. Andreou ER, Ledger S. Potential drug interaction between simvastatin and danazol causing rhabdomyolysis. *Can J Clin Pharmacol* (2003) 10, 172–4.

5. Stankovic I, Vlahovic-Stipac A, Putnikovic B, Cvetkovic Z, Neskovic AN. Concomitant administration of simvastatin and danazol associated with fatal rhabdomyolysis. *Clin Ther* (2010) 32, 909–14.
6. Mevacor (Lovastatin). Merck & Co., Inc. US Prescribing information, February 2014.
7. Zocor (Simvastatin). Merck & Co., Inc. US Prescribing information, March 2015.
8. Zocor (Simvastatin). Merck Sharp & Dohme Ltd. UK Summary of product characteristics, June 2015.

Statins + Dasabuvir

Dasabuvir appears to moderately increase the exposure to rosuvastatin. Fluvastatin exposure is expected to be increased by dasabuvir (with a fixed-dose combination of ombitasvir and paritaprevir boosted with ritonavir), but dasabuvir exposure is not predicted to be affected. Rosuvastatin and pravastatin do not appear to alter the pharmacokinetics of dasabuvir.

Clinical evidence

The UK manufacturer briefly reports that, in a study in healthy subjects given **rosuvastatin** 5 mg daily and dasabuvir 250 or 400 mg twice daily (given with a fixed-dose combination of ombitasvir and paritaprevir boosted with ritonavir), the AUC and maximum concentration of rosuvastatin were increased 2.6-fold and 7-fold, respectively. The pharmacokinetics of dasabuvir were unaffected.[1] They also report that in a study with **pravastatin** 10 mg once daily, the pharmacokinetics of dasabuvir were unaffected.[1]

Mechanism

Multiple uptake transporters such as organic anion transporting polypeptide OATP1B1, breast cancer resistance protein (BCRP), and P-glycoprotein are involved in the clearance of statins; rosuvastatin is a substrate for BCRP which is said to be inhibited by dasabuvir,[1] and hence concurrent use results in increased rosuvastatin exposure. Note that other components of the dasabuvir combination can also affect uptake transporters and involvement of these in this interaction is possible.

Importance and management

Evidence for an interaction between the statins and dasabuvir is limited to that with rosuvastatin, but an interaction between these two drugs would seem to be established. Dasabuvir (with a fixed-dose combination of ombitasvir and paritaprevir boosted with ritonavir) appears to cause a moderate increase in rosuvastatin exposure, which could be clinically important. As such, the UK manufacturer advises that the maximum dose of rosuvastatin should be 5 mg daily when given concurrently.[1] Rosuvastatin and pravastatin do not appear to alter the pharmacokinetics of dasabuvir, and no dasabuvir dose adjustment is necessary on concurrent use.

Fluvastatin is predicted to have no effect on the pharmacokinetics of dasabuvir, and no dasabuvir dose adjustment is necessary on concurrent use.[1] However, note that the UK manufacturer predicts that when dasabuvir is given with a fixed-dose combination of ombitasvir and paritaprevir boosted with ritonavir, fluvastatin concentrations are expected to be increased due to inhibition of OATP1B1 and BCRP by paritaprevir.[1] A contributory effect due to inhibition of BCRP by dasabuvir cannot therefore be ruled out and concurrent use of fluvastatin and dasabuvir with a fixed-dose combination of ombitasvir and paritaprevir boosted with ritonavir is contra-indicated.[1]

Note that, as a general rule, patients taking statins should be specifically reminded to report any signs of myopathy and possible rhabdomyolysis (such as otherwise unexplained muscle pain, tenderness, or weakness, or dark coloured urine). If myopathy does occur, the statin should be stopped immediately.

1. Exviera (Dasabuvir sodium monohydrate). AbbVie Ltd. UK Summary of product characteristics, January 2015.

Statins + Dipeptidylpeptidase-4 inhibitors

Linagliptin, saxagliptin, sitagliptin, and vildagliptin do not alter the pharmacokinetics of simvastatin to a clinically relevant extent. Sitagliptin use was considered a possible contributing factor to two cases of statin-induced rhabdomyolysis (one with lovastatin and one with simvastatin). Simvastatin does not alter the pharmacokinetics of saxagliptin or vildagliptin. Alogliptin does not affect the pharmacokinetics of atorvastatin, and atorvastatin does not affect the pharmacokinetics of alogliptin.

Clinical evidence

(a) Atorvastatin

The US manufacturer of **alogliptin** briefly notes that, in clinical studies, the pharmacokinetics of both drugs were not meaningfully altered when alogliptin 25 mg daily was given with atorvastatin 80 mg daily, for 7 days.[1]

(b) Lovastatin

A case report describes a 75-year-old woman with normal renal function who had been taking lovastatin 40 mg daily for 12 years and diltiazem 240 mg daily (last dose adjustment 10 months previously) who presented with weakness and was diagnosed with rhabdomyolysis secondary to statin use. Twenty-five days earlier rosiglitazone had been switched to pioglitazone, which was given for just one week then replaced with **sitagliptin** 100 mg daily, then, after another 14 days this was replaced with glimepiride 1 mg daily, which she took for 5 days before the diagnosis. The patient had numerous medical conditions including hypothyroidism and had undergone back surgery 4 weeks previously.[2]

(c) Simvastatin

1. Linagliptin. In a study, 20 healthy subjects were given simvastatin 40 mg daily for 12 days with linagliptin 10 mg daily given on days 6 to 12. Linagliptin increased the AUC and maximum concentration of simvastatin by 34% and 10%, respectively. Linagliptin also increased the AUC and maximum concentration of its active acid metabolite, simvastatin acid, by 33% and 21%, respectively. The effects of linagliptin on the AUC of simvastatin and its acid metabolite decreased and were minimal by day 20, with the exception of the simvastatin maximum concentration, which increased again by 27% by day 16, and 39% and on day 20. The AUC and maximum concentration of linagliptin did not appear to be affected by simvastatin, when compared with historic values.[3]

2. Saxagliptin. In a study in 23 healthy subjects, when saxagliptin 10 mg daily and simvastatin 40 mg daily were given together for 4 days there was no change in the pharmacokinetics of simvastatin, when compared with simvastatin alone. In addition, there was a negligible 12% increase in the AUC of saxagliptin, and just a small 21% increase in the saxagliptin maximum concentration, when compared with saxagliptin alone.[4]

3. Sitagliptin. In a study in 12 healthy subjects, sitagliptin 200 mg daily for 5 days did not alter the pharmacokinetics of simvastatin acid or simvastatin lactone when a single 20-mg dose of simvastatin was given on day 5. In addition, there was no alteration in the plasma inhibition of HMG-CoA reductase.[5]

Two cases of possible interactions have been reported.[2,6] In one, a 76-year-old man with chronic renal impairment and numerous other medical conditions was admitted with rhabdomyolysis and acute renal failure. His medications included antihypertensives, amiodarone, simvastatin, ezetimibe, and sitagliptin. Four months previously, his simvastatin dose had been increased from 40 mg daily to 80 mg daily and ezetimibe 10 mg daily added. Six weeks previously, he had started sitagliptin 50 mg daily, which was increased to 100 mg daily 3 weeks later. Various medications were stopped including sitagliptin, simvastatin and ezetimibe, and he made a full recovery. He was later given **lovastatin** 10 mg daily, see also *Lovastatin*, above.[6]

4. Vildagliptin. In a study in 24 healthy subjects, vildagliptin 100 mg daily and simvastatin 80 mg daily were given together for 7 days. There was no change in the pharmacokinetics of vildagliptin, simvastatin or its active metabolite, compared with either drug given alone.[7]

Mechanism

Saxagliptin, sitagliptin, and vildagliptin do not affect CYP3A4, by which simvastatin is principally metabolised, therefore no pharmacokinetic interaction was expected, and the controlled studies available confirm this. It was suggested that linagliptin might have increased simvastatin exposure by slightly inhibiting CYP3A4.[3] In the case of rhabdomyolysis with simvastatin, it was suggested that too high a dose of sitagliptin for the degree of renal impairment possibly contributed to a further deterioration in renal function, which reduced simvastatin clearance.[6] However, it is also possible that the effect was due to using too high a dose of simvastatin with amiodarone.[8] In the second case with lovastatin; diltiazem could have caused this interaction, but the authors discounted this on the basis of the time frame since the diltiazem dose increase. Hypothyroidism and the perioperative period are also risk factors for myopathy, but the authors also discounted these,[2] although it is possible they were contributing factors. For more information on the interactions of amiodarone and diltiazem with the statins, see 'Statins + Amiodarone', p.1320, and 'Statins + Calcium-channel blockers; Diltiazem or Verapamil', p.1325. Alogliptin does not affect CYP3A4, by which atorvastatin is metabolised, therefore no pharmacokinetic interaction is expected.

Importance and management

It appears that saxagliptin, sitagliptin, and vildagliptin have no effect on the pharmacokinetics of simvastatin, and no interaction as a result of altered exposure would therefore be expected. Similarly, linagliptin has no clinically relevant effect on simvastatin pharmacokinetics and no dose adjustment is necessary on concurrent use. No dose adjustments are required on concurrent use of atorvastatin and alogliptin. However, two possible cases of rhabdomyolysis with sitagliptin and a statin have been reported, both of which were complicated by a number of other factors. These cases are insufficient evidence to issue a general caution, but bear them in mind in the event of an unexpected response to treatment.

1. Nesina (Alogliptin). Takeda Pharmaceuticals America, Inc. US Prescribing information, January 2013.
2. DiGregorio RV, Pasikhova Y. Rhabdomyolysis caused by a potential sitagliptin-lovastatin interaction. *Pharmacotherapy* (2009) 29, 352–6.
3. Graefe-Mody U, Huettner S, Stähle H, Ring A, Dugi KA. Effect of linagliptin (BI 1356) on the steady-state pharmacokinetics of simvastatin. *Int J Clin Pharmacol Ther* (2010) 48, 367–74.
4. Girgis S, You X, Maurer C, Whigan D, Boulton DW. Effect of simvastatin on the pharmacokinetics of saxagliptin in healthy subjects. 36th Annual Meeting of the American College of Clinical Pharmacology, San Francisco, California, 2007.
5. Bergman AJ, Cote J, Maes A, Zhao JJ, Roadcap BA, Sun L, Valesky RJ, Yang A, Keymeulen B, Mathijs Z, De Smet M, Laethem T, Davies MJ, Wagner JA, Herman GA. Effect of sitagliptin on the pharmacokinetics of simvastatin. *J Clin Pharmacol* (2009) 49, 483–8.
6. Kao DP, Kohrt HE, Kugler J. Renal failure and rhabdomyolysis associated with sitagliptin and simvastatin use. *Diabet Med* (2008) 25, 1229–30.
7. Ayalasomayajula SP, Dole K, He Y-L, Ligueros-Saylan M, Wang Y, Campestrini J, Humbert H, Sunkara G. Evaluation of the potential for steady-state pharmacokinetic interaction between vildagliptin and simvastatin in healthy subjects. *Curr Med Res Opin* (2007) 23, 2913–20.
8. Boucher BJ. Renal failure and rhabdomyolysis associated with sitagliptin and simvastatin use. But what about the amiodarone? *Diabet Med* (2009) 26, 192–3.

Statins + Distigmine

An isolated case report describes rhabdomyolysis associated with the use of pravastatin and distigmine.

Clinical evidence, mechanism, importance and management

An isolated report describes a 70-year-old woman taking **pravastatin**, colestyramine and distigmine 10 mg daily who was admitted to hospital with symptoms including reduced urine output and muscle weakness. She was found to have a creatine kinase level of 4 069 units/L (reference range 45 to 163 units/L) and was diagnosed with rhabdomyolysis, which was thought to have been due to the pravastatin and colestyramine. These drugs were discontinued immediately, but 2 days later the patient's creatine kinase level remained elevated, and so distigmine was also discontinued. After 3 days the creatine kinase levels had fallen, and had returned to the expected range after a further 8 days.[1] The authors of the report attributed the rhabdomyolysis to distigmine, with a possible contribution from pravastatin, based on the fall in the creatine kinase levels after its discontinuation, and recommend caution if distigmine is given with any statin. However, the patient had seemingly taken both drugs uneventfully for more than 18 months, distigmine is not normally associated with myopathy, it is unknown whether the creatine kinase levels would have dropped without the withdrawal of the distigmine, and the dose of pravastatin was not stated. Therefore an interaction is far from established. The current evidence is too slim to warrant any particular action if both drugs are taken.

1. Tsutsumi Y, Tanaka J, Miura T, Yamato H, Kanamori H, Kawamura T, Obara S, Asaka M, Imamura M, Masauzi N. Rhabdomyolysis caused by distigmine bromide. *Intern Med* (2003) 11, 1156.

Statins + Diuretics

In clinical studies, the safety and efficacy of statins did not appear to be altered by the concurrent use of diuretics. An isolated report describes reversible diabetes mellitus in a woman taking cyclothiazide with triamterene when she was also given pravastatin. No clinically relevant pharmacokinetic interaction occurs between simvastatin and eplerenone.

Clinical evidence, mechanism, importance and management

(a) Fluvastatin

Retrospective analysis of clinical study data found no evidence that the safety or efficacy of fluvastatin was altered by the use of unspecified diuretics.[1]

(b) Lovastatin

Retrospective analysis of clinical study data from the EXCEL study (8 245 patients) found no evidence that the safety or efficacy of lovastatin was altered by the use of **potassium-sparing diuretics** (hydrochlorothiazide with **triamterene** or **amiloride**) in 187 patients, or **thiazide diuretics** (mostly **hydrochlorothiazide**) in 126 patients.[2] Another retrospective study of 19 patients found that the addition of lovastatin to diuretic treatment caused an initial 30% fall in total serum cholesterol levels for one month, followed by a rise of about 20%. In a further 13 patients, the addition of a diuretic to lovastatin caused a 20% fall in total serum cholesterol for one month followed by a 20% rise back to baseline values. The diuretics used were **furosemide** (16 patients), **triamterene** with **hydrochlorothiazide** (7), **hydrochlorothiazide** (8), and **indapamide** (1). The fall and subsequent rise in serum cholesterol levels occurred in all of the patients except just the one taking **indapamide**.[3] The reason for this initial fall in cholesterol, particularly when the diuretic was added to the statin, is unknown, and the findings of this small uncontrolled study are difficult to interpret.

(c) Pravastatin

A 63-year-old woman who had been taking **cyclothiazide** with **triamterene**, and acebutolol, for 4 years, developed polyuria and polydipsia, which gradually worsened, within 3 weeks of starting to take pravastatin 20 mg daily. After another 4 months she was hospitalised with hyperglycaemia, which was treated with insulin and later glibenclamide (glyburide). The **cyclothiazide** with **triamterene** and pravastatin were stopped and gradually the diabetic symptoms began to abate. Five weeks after admission she was discharged without the need for any antidiabetic treatment with the diabetes fully resolved.[4] The detailed reasons for this reaction are not understood, but it would seem that the pravastatin increased the potential of the thiazide diuretic to raise blood glucose levels to the point where frank diabetes developed. This is an isolated case and its general importance is likely to be small. Indeed, a study involving dyslipidaemic, hypertensive patients found that captopril, **hydrochlorothiazide** and pravastatin were effective and well tolerated by the 128 patients taking this combination, and there was no clinically relevant change in glucose levels.[5]

(d) Simvastatin

In 18 healthy subjects, simvastatin 40 mg daily had no effect on the pharmacokinetics of **eplerenone** 100 mg daily. The maximum level and AUC of simvastatin were decreased by 32% and 14%, respectively, but this was not considered to be clinically relevant.[6,7]

In a single-dose study in subjects given **hydrochlorothiazide** 12.5 mg alone, simvastatin 20 mg alone or both in a combined tablet with atenolol 50 mg, ramipril 5 mg and aspirin 100 mg, the pharmacokinetics of **hydrochlorothiazide** did not differ between the combined tablet and hydrochlorothiazide alone. However, the AUC of simvastatin was 24% lower with the combined tablet, whereas the AUC of active simvastatin acid was 44% higher compared with simvastatin alone. The reason for this apparent difference is unclear, but it seems unlikely to be due to a pharmacokinetic interaction between any of the drugs and simvastatin.[8] The clinical relevance of the apparent difference is also unclear, but the authors note that in an efficacy study, the combined tablet caused a slightly smaller reduction in cholesterol than simvastatin alone.[9]

1. Peters TK, Jewitt-Harris J, Mehra M, Muratti EN. Safety and tolerability of fluvastatin with concomitant use of antihypertensive agents. An analysis of a clinical trial database. *Am J Hypertens* (1993) 6, 346S–352S.
2. Pool JL, Shear CL, Downton M, Schnaper H, Stinnett S, Dujovne C, Bradford RH, Chremos AN. Lovastatin and coadministered antihypertensive/cardiovascular agents. *Hypertension* (1992) 19, 242–8.
3. Aruna AS, Akula SK, Sarpong DF. Interaction between potassium-depleting diuretics and lovastatin in hypercholesterolemic ambulatory care patients. *J Pharm Technol* (1997) 13, 21–6.
4. Jonville-Bera A-P, Zakian A, Bera FJ, Carré P, Autret E. Possible pravastatin and diuretics-induced diabetes mellitus. *Ann Pharmacother* (1994) 28, 964–5.
5. Waeber B, Greminger P, Riesen W, Darioli R, Simeon-Dubach D, Wunderlin R. Combined treatment with captopril, hydrochlorothiazide and pravastatin in dyslipidemic hypertensive patients. *Blood Pressure* (1995) 4, 358–62.
6. Inspra (Eplerenone). Pfizer Inc. US Prescribing information, April 2008.
7. Cook CS, Berry LM, Burton E. Prediction of *in vivo* drug interactions with eplerenone in man from *in vitro* metabolic inhibition data. *Xenobiotica* (2004) 34, 215–28.
8. Patel A, Shah T, Shah G, Jha V, Ghosh C, Desai J, Khamar B, Chakraborty BS. Preservation of bioavailability of ingredients and lack of drug-drug interactions in a novel five-ingredient polypill (Polycap): a five-arm phase I crossover trial in healthy volunteers. *Am J Cardiovasc Drugs* (2010) 10, 95–103.
9. Indian Polycap Study (TIPS), Yusuf S, Pais P, Afzal R, Xavier D, Teo K, Eikelboom J, Sigamani A, Mohan V, Gupta R, Thomas N. Effects of a polypill (Polycap) on risk factors in middle-aged individuals without cardiovascular disease (TIPS): a phase II, double-blind, randomised trial. *Lancet* (2009) 373, 1341–51.

Statins + Dronedarone

Dronedarone moderately increases simvastatin exposure and slightly increases that of atorvastatin and rosuvastatin. Other statins metabolised similarly are predicted to interact in the same way when given with dronedarone.

Clinical evidence

The UK and US manufacturers of dronedarone briefly state that in a study, dronedarone 400 mg twice daily increased the exposure to **simvastatin** 40 mg once daily and its active metabolite, simvastatin acid, 4-fold and 2-fold, respectively.[1,2] They also report that dronedarone increased the exposure to **atorvastatin** 40 mg once daily by 70%, and **rosuvastatin** 10 mg once daily by 40%.[1,2]

Mechanism

Dronedarone is an inhibitor of CYP3A4, by which simvastatin is extensively metabolised. Concurrent use therefore increases its exposure. Atorvastatin is less dependent on CYP3A4 metabolism, and so its exposure is increased to a lesser extent. The exact mechanism behind the increase in rosuvastatin exposure is not clear as it is not metabolised by CYP3A4. However, *in vitro*[1] data suggest that dronedarone might also inhibit the organic anion transporting polypeptide, OATP1B1, by which rosuvastatin is transported, possibly resulting in increased exposure. Atorvastatin is also a substrate for OATP1B1. Further study into this possible mechanism is required. For more information on the metabolism of statins, see 'Lipid regulating drugs', p.1309.

Importance and management

Evidence for an interaction between the statins and dronedarone is limited, but is consistent with the way these drugs would be predicted to interact. The moderate increase in simvastatin exposure is likely to be clinically important, and as such the US manufacturer of dronedarone advises avoiding simvastatin doses greater than 10 mg daily in patients taking dronedarone,[1] and the UK manufacturer states that lower starting and maintenance doses of the statin should be considered.[2] The slight increases in atorvastatin and rosuvastatin exposure are unlikely to be clinically important, but until more is known some caution on their concurrent use with dronedarone would seem prudent. Likewise, similar precautions would seem warranted for **lovastatin**, which is metabolised in the same way as simvastatin. If dronedarone is given with any statin, the advice to report any symptoms suggestive of myopathy and rhabdomyolysis (i.e. otherwise unexplained muscle pain, tenderness, or weakness or dark coloured urine) should be specifically reinforced.

1. Multaq (Dronedarone). Sanofi-Aventis U.S. LLC. US Prescribing information, March 2014.
2. Multaq (Dronedarone hydrochloride). Sanofi. UK Summary of product characteristics, November 2013.

Statins + Drugs that affect gastric pH

Fluvastatin exposure is slightly increased by cimetidine, but is not affected to a clinically relevant extent by ranitidine and omeprazole. Pravastatin exposure is slightly increased by cimetidine, whereas atorvastatin exposure is not affected by cimetidine. An isolated case describes rhabdomyolysis in a patient taking atorvastatin given esomeprazole and then clarithromycin.

Clinical evidence

(a) Atorvastatin

In a crossover study, 12 healthy subjects were given atorvastatin for 15 days with and without **cimetidine** 300 mg four times daily. **Cimetidine** had no effect on the maximum serum levels or AUC of atorvastatin. **Cimetidine** had little effect on the lipid-lowering effects of atorvastatin, except that the reduction in triglycerides was slightly less, but this difference was considered to be of little clinical relevance.[1]

AV block secondary to rhabdomyolysis was diagnosed in a 51-year-old woman who had been taking atorvastatin 10 mg daily for over a year, **esomeprazole** 20 mg daily for 6 to 8 weeks and just 3 doses of clarithromycin 500 mg twice daily. She described symptoms of increased fatigue, mild chest pain and shortness of breath, beginning soon after starting **esomeprazole**. All drugs were stopped and she eventually recovered, needing a permanent pacemaker.[2] It is possible that clarithromycin also had a role in this case see 'Statins + Macrolides', p.1348.

(b) Fluvastatin

The US manufacturer of fluvastatin states that its exposure is increased by **cimetidine** 400 mg twice daily for 5 days (AUC increased by 30%), **omeprazole** 40 mg daily for 6 days (20%), and **ranitidine** 150 mg twice daily for 5 days (10%).[3]

(c) Pravastatin

Cimetidine 300 mg four times daily for 3 days increased the exposure of a single 20-mg dose of pravastatin by 58%. The dose of pravastatin was given on day 3, one hour after the first dose of **cimetidine**.[4]

(d) Unspecified statins

In March 2005, an analysis of the WHO adverse drug reaction database identified 292 spontaneous case reports of increases in creatine phosphokinase, muscle weakness, myopathy, myositis, polymyositis and rhabdomyolysis with proton pump inhibitors (**omeprazole**, **pantoprazole**, **lansoprazole**, **esomeprazole** and **rabeprazole**). In 34 of these reports a statin (unspecified) had been used concurrently, and in one third of these cases the proton pump inhibitor was the only drug given. Of 35 cases of rhabdomyolysis, 12 cases involved the concurrent use of a statin.[5] In another retrospective analysis of 37 cases of chronic muscle disease, 15 patients had been treated with a statin at the onset of their symptoms, which was 2.7-fold higher than the use of a statin in the controls. In addition, 6 of the patients were taking a proton pump inhibitor, and there was a positive interaction between a statin and proton pump inhibitor (odds ratio 3.3).[6]

Mechanism

The similar increase in exposure to fluvastatin with both H_2-receptor antagonists and proton pump inhibitors is likely to be due to increased absorption because of the effect of these drugs on gastric acidity.

It was suggested that esomeprazole might alter atorvastatin levels via inhibition of P-glycoprotein,[2] or that proton pump inhibitors might increase the levels of the statins via inhibition of CYP3A4,[5] but any pharmacokinetic interaction seems likely to be minor. Note that proton pump inhibitors alone have rarely been associated with myopathy and rhabdomyolysis,[5] and the case described could have been due to an additive effect of the proton pump inhibitor and the atorvastatin.

Importance and management

None of the pharmacokinetic interactions between the statins and the proton pump inhibitors described here are likely to be of any clinical relevance. No statin dose adjustment is likely to be needed with these H_2-receptor antagonists or proton pump inhibitors.

It is unclear whether the concurrent use of a proton pump inhibitor and a statin contributes to the risk of myopathy. Bear the possibility in mind.

1. Stern RH, Gibson DM, Whitfield LR. Cimetidine does not alter atorvastatin pharmacokinetics or LDL-cholesterol reduction. *Eur J Clin Pharmacol* (1998) 53, 475–8.
2. Sipe BE, Jones RJ, Bokhart GH. Rhabdomyolysis causing AV blockade due to possible atorvastatin, esomeprazole, and clarithromycin interaction. *Ann Pharmacother* (2003) 37, 808–11.
3. Lescol (Fluvastatin sodium). Novartis Pharmaceuticals Corp. US Prescribing information, October 2012.
4. ER Squibb. Data on file. A report on the comparative pharmacokinetics of pravastatin in the presence and absence of cimetidine or antacids in healthy male subjects (Protocol No 27, 201-43). 1988.
5. Clark DWJ, Strandell J. Myopathy including polymyositis: a likely class adverse effect of proton pump inhibitors? *Eur J Clin Pharmacol* (2006) 62, 473–9.
6. Sailler L, Pereira C, Bagheri A, Uro-Coste E, Roussel B, Adoue D, Fournie B, Laroche M, Zabraniecki L, Cintas P, Arlet P, Lapeyre-Mestre M, Montastruc JL. Increased exposure to statins in patients developing chronic muscle diseases: a 2-year retrospective study. *Ann Rheum Dis* (2008) 67, 614–19.

Statins + Eltrombopag

Eltrombopag slightly to moderately increases rosuvastatin exposure. Other statins are predicted to be affected similarly.

Clinical evidence

In a study, 39 healthy subjects were given a single 10-mg dose of **rosuvastatin** before and with the last dose of eltrombopag 75 mg daily for 5 days. Eltrombopag increased the maximum concentration of rosuvastatin twofold (103%) and increased its AUC by 55%. The increase in exposure was higher in those of non-Asian origin (88%) when compared with Asian subjects (32%), who are known to have an increased systemic exposure to rosuvastatin when compared with non-Asian subjects.[1]

Mechanism

Eltrombopag is an *in vitro* inhibitor of the organic anion transporter (OATP1B1) and breast cancer resistance protein (BCRP), of which rosuvastatin is a substrate.

Importance and management

The pharmacokinetic interaction between rosuvastatin and eltrombopag is established, and could apply to other statins. The UK manufacturer of eltrombopag[2] states that interactions are also expected with **pravastatin**, **simvastatin** and **lovastatin**, but that a clinically relevant interaction between eltrombopag and **atorvastatin** or **fluvastatin** would not be expected. In contrast, the US manufacturer suggests that **atorvastatin**, **fluvastatin** and **pravastatin** might also interact with eltrombopag.[3] The manufacturers of eltrombopag state that consideration should be given to reducing the dose of the statin if it is given with eltrombopag,[2,3] and, until more is known, it would be prudent to apply this to the use of any statin. The US manufacturer notes that in clinical studies, a 50% dose reduction of rosuvastatin was recommended.[3] They recommend that patients should be monitored closely for statin adverse effects, and in practice this probably means monitoring for muscle toxicity and rhabdomyolysis (see *Muscle and liver toxicity*, under 'Lipid regulating drugs', p.1309, for further guidance on monitoring and the risk factors for muscle toxicity with statins).

Note that patients taking statins should routinely be made aware of the risks of myopathy and rhabdomyolysis, and asked to promptly report muscle pain, tenderness, or weakness, and it may be prudent to reinforce this advice if eltrombopag is given.

1. Allred AJ, Bowen CJ, Park JW, Peng B, Williams DD, Wire MB, Lee E. Eltrombopag increases plasma rosuvastatin exposure in healthy volunteers. *Br J Clin Pharmacol* (2011) 72, 321–9.
2. Revolade (Eltrombopag olamine). Novartis Pharmaceuticals UK Ltd. UK Summary of product characteristics, May 2015.
3. Promacta (Eltrombopag olamine). GlaxoSmithKline. US Prescribing Information, December 2011.

Statins + Endothelin receptor antagonists; Bosentan

Bosentan slightly decreases the exposure to simvastatin and its active metabolite, but simvastatin had no effect on bosentan pharmacokinetics. Other statins metabolised by the same route as simvastatin could be similarly affected by bosentan.

Clinical evidence

In a three-way, crossover study, 9 healthy subjects were given either bosentan 125 mg twice daily for 5.5 days, **simvastatin** 40 mg daily for 6 days, or both treatments together. **Simvastatin** had no effect on the pharmacokinetics of bosentan, but bosentan decreased the AUC of **simvastatin** and its active metabolite, simvastatin acid, by 34% and 46%, respectively.[1]

Mechanism

Bosentan is known to be a weak inducer of CYP3A4, which is involved in the metabolism of simvastatin. Induction of simvastatin metabolism might have led to the decreased exposure seen.

Importance and management

Evidence for an interaction between bosentan and simvastatin is limited to this study, but the interaction found is consistent with the way both drugs would be expected to interact. A slight decrease in the exposure to simvastatin is potentially clinically relevant. If bosentan and simvastatin are used concurrently, it would seem prudent to monitor the outcome to ensure that simvastatin is effective. Other statins, such as **lovastatin**, that are metabolised by the same route as simvastatin (that is, predominantly by CYP3A4) are likely to interact similarly, and the same precautions described for simvastatin would seem appropriate. **Atorvastatin** seems unlikely to be affected to the same extent as simvastatin, but bear this interaction in mind if lipid-lowering targets are not met.

1. Dingemanse J, Schaarschmidt D, van Giersbergen PLM. Investigation of the mutual pharmacokinetic interactions between bosentan, a dual endothelin receptor antagonist, and simvastatin. *Clin Pharmacokinet* (2003) 42, 293–301.

Statins + Everolimus

In a single-dose study, there was no clinically relevant pharmacokinetic interaction between everolimus and atorvastatin or pravastatin.

Clinical evidence

In a single-dose study in 24 healthy subjects, everolimus 2 mg did not cause a clinically relevant alteration in the pharmacokinetics or HMG-CoA reductase activity of atorvastatin 20 mg or pravastatin 20 mg. The only changes were an 11% increase in atorvastatin maximum levels (no change in AUC); and a 10% decrease in pravastatin maximum levels and a 5% decrease in its AUC. Everolimus pharmacokinetics were unaltered by the statins (a negligible 5 to 6% decrease in AUC).[1]

Mechanism

It was thought that everolimus might increase atorvastatin levels by inhibiting CYP3A4, and that pravastatin would not be affected.[1] However, single-dose simultaneous administration studies are not generally sufficient to maximise inhibition of cytochrome P450 isoenzymes, so the study design does not exclude an interaction via this mechanism.

Importance and management

Evidence from this single-dose study suggests that no clinically relevant pharmacokinetic interaction would be anticipated between everolimus and either atorvastatin or pravastatin. However, a multiple-dose study is required to completely exclude such an interaction. Nevertheless, note that there is a multiple-dose study showing that the related drug sirolimus did not alter atorvastatin levels, see 'Statins + Sirolimus', p.1356, which further adds to the suggestion that no clinically relevant interaction is likely.

1. Kovarik JM, Hartmann S, Hubert M, Berthier S, Schneider W, Rosenkranz B, Rordorf C. Pharmacokinetic and pharmacodynamic assessments of HMG-CoA reductase inhibitors when coadministered with everolimus. *J Clin Pharmacol* (2002) 42, 222–8.

Statins + Ezetimibe

Ezetimibe does not appear to have adverse pharmacokinetic interactions with atorvastatin, fluvastatin, lovastatin, pitavastatin, rosuvastatin or simvastatin, and available evidence suggests there is no increased risk of myopathy when ezetimibe is used statins compared with statins alone. Isolated reports describe myopathy on concurrent use of ezetimibe with atorvastatin, and of raised creatine kinase with fluvastatin.

Clinical evidence

(a) Atorvastatin

In a study in otherwise healthy hypercholesterolaemic subjects, there was no change in the pharmacokinetics of either ezetimibe or atorvastatin when ezetimibe 10 mg daily was given with atorvastatin 10 mg daily for 14 days compared with either drug alone (8 subjects per treatment).[1,2]

In a 12-week efficacy study in patients with hypercholesterolaemia, ezetimibe did not worsen statin intolerance or toxicity when it was given with atorvastatin 10 to 80 mg daily (255 patients) compared with atorvastatin alone (248 patients). In this study, one patient taking atorvastatin 40 mg daily and ezetimibe developed elevated creatine kinase levels and myalgia.[3] See also, *Unnamed statins*, below.

However, a case report describes a 43-year-old man taking high-dose atorvastatin 80 mg daily who developed severe muscle pain with elevated creatine kinase levels 3 weeks after he started taking ezetimibe 10 mg daily. Symptoms resolved when both drugs were withdrawn and he later restarted the atorvastatin 80 mg daily without problems.[4] Other similar cases have also been reported, in patients taking ezetimibe 10 mg daily and atorvastatin 40 mg or 80 mg daily.[5-7]

(b) Fluvastatin

In a randomised study in otherwise healthy subjects with hypercholesterolaemia, there was no change in the pharmacokinetics of ezetimibe when ezetimibe 10 mg daily was given with fluvastatin 20 mg daily for 14 days compared with ezetimibe alone. However, ezetimibe appeared to modestly decrease the AUC of fluvastatin by 51%, although this was not statistically significant because of high intersubject variability in fluvastatin pharmacokinetics. The combination resulted in an enhanced lowering of LDL-cholesterol.[8]

In a placebo-controlled study, 199 patients with a history of muscle-related adverse effects with other statins were randomised to receive prolonged-release fluvastatin 80 mg daily alone, ezetimibe 10 mg daily alone or both drugs together for 12 weeks. The incidence of muscle-related adverse effects were 17%, 24%, and 14%, respectively, and there were no cases of creatine kinase levels greater than 10 times the upper limit of normal.[9] See also, *Unnamed statins,* below.

However, a case report describes a 52-year-old man taking fluvastatin 80 mg daily who was found to have asymptomatic elevated creatine kinase levels (2.5 times normal) 8 weeks after ezetimibe 10 mg daily was added. His creatine kinase levels returned to normal 4 weeks after the ezetimibe was withdrawn while continuing the fluvastatin at the same dose.[4]

(c) Lovastatin

In a study in otherwise healthy hypercholesterolaemic subjects, the AUC of lovastatin was 25 to 47% lower when lovastatin 20 mg daily was given concurrently with ezetimibe 5 to 20 mg daily, although this was not dose-related, and was considered to be due to small sample size, large intersubject variability, and parallel-group design.[10] A later randomised, crossover study, in 18 healthy subjects given ezetimibe 10 mg daily, lovastatin 20 mg daily and both drugs together for 7 days, confirmed that ezetimibe does not alter the pharmacokinetics of lovastatin, and lovastatin does not alter the pharmacokinetics of ezetimibe.[11] See also, *Unspecified statins*, below.

(d) Pitavastatin

A review of ezetimibe[2] cites an unpublished study in which 18 healthy subjects were given ezetimibe 10 mg and pitavastatin 2 mg, alone and together for 7 days. Concurrent use did not affect the pharmacokinetics of either drug.

(e) Pravastatin

A review of ezetimibe[2] cites an unpublished study in which hypercholesterolaemic subjects were given either ezetimibe 10 mg daily, pravastatin 20 mg daily, or both drugs together. Concurrent use did not affect the pharmacokinetics of either drug. See also, *Unnamed statins*, below.

(f) Rosuvastatin

In a placebo-controlled study, otherwise healthy subjects with hypercholesterolaemia were given ezetimibe 10 mg daily (8 subjects), rosuvastatin 10 mg daily (12 subjects) or both drugs together (12 subjects) for 14 days. Concurrent use did not affect the pharmacokinetics of either drug, and an enhanced lowering of LDL-cholesterol was noted.[12]

(g) Simvastatin

In a study in otherwise healthy subjects with hypercholesterolaemia, ezetimibe 0.25 mg, 1 mg or 10 mg daily had no effect on the pharmacokinetics of simvastatin 10 mg daily, when both drugs were given concurrently for 14 days, when compared with simvastatin alone. The combination was associated with enhanced lowering of LDL-cholesterol.[13]

In a clinical study in patients with primary hypercholesterolaemia, there was a similar safety profile between simvastatin 10, 20, 40 or 80 mg daily taken as monotherapy (560 subjects) and as a combination tablet with ezetimibe 10 mg daily (544 subjects) for up to 6 months.[14] Similarly, a retrospective analysis of 17 studies found that overall, muscle related adverse effects, including myopathy, were no more common in patients taking ezetimibe with simvastatin than in those taking simvastatin alone. The incidence of myopathy was 0.08% (2 of 2563) in those taking simvastatin alone and 0.04% (2 of 4558) in those taking ezetimibe with simvastatin. In addition, the proportion of patients who discontinued treatment because of myalgia did not differ between those taking simvastatin with ezetimibe compared with simvastatin alone.[15] In a later 48-week extension study of ezetimibe 10 mg with simvastatin 10, 20, 40 or 80 mg in a total of 786 patients, there was no evidence of an increased incidence of elevated creatine kinase levels for the combination, and the only case of myopathy was thought to be due to excessive fitness training. However, for the combination, there was a higher incidence of raised liver transaminase levels for the higher simvastatin doses when compared with simvastatin alone.[16] See also, *Unnamed statins*, below.

(h) Unspecified statins

In a meta-analysis of 18 randomised clinical studies in a total of 14 471 patients, there was no increased risk of myalgias, raised creatine kinase levels or rhabdomyolysis, or raised hepatic transaminase levels, and no increased risk of discontinuation because of adverse events, when ezetimibe was added to a statin (**atorvastatin** 4 studies, **lovastatin** 1 study, **pravastatin** 1 study, **simvastatin** 10 studies, or varying statins 2 studies).[17] The manufacturers of ezetimibe note that, in controlled clinical studies, the incidence of consecutive elevations (3 or more times the upper limit of normal) in hepatic transaminase levels was 1.3% for patients taking a statin with ezetimibe, 0.4% for patients taking statins alone and 0.5% for ezetimibe alone. These elevations in transaminases were generally asymptomatic, and resolved spontaneously, either with continued treatment or after the drugs were stopped.[18,19] Creatine phosphokinase levels greater than 10 times the upper limit of normal were not increased by the addition of ezetimibe to a statin: they were reported in 1 of 917 (0.1%) patients given ezetimibe and a statin, 4 of 1674 (0.2%) patients given ezetimibe alone, and 4 of 929 (0.4%) patients given a statin alone.[18,19]

Mechanism

Ezetimibe is not known to alter the pharmacokinetics of drugs metabolised by cytochrome P450 isoenzymes and would not be expected to alter the pharmacokinetics of statins metabolised by this route, such as simvastatin. The isolated reports of myopathy with ezetimibe and atorvastatin could just be coincidental. Alternatively, because ezetimibe has very rarely been associated with myopathy, it might add to the known risk with statins.

Importance and management

The available evidence suggests that the concurrent use of a statin with ezetimibe does not result in clinically relevant changes in the pharmacokinetics of either drug. In addition, available evidence suggests that concurrent use does not increase the risk of myopathy compared with statins alone. Nevertheless, there are isolated published reports of myopathy when ezetimibe was given to patients taking atorvastatin, and ezetimibe alone has very rarely been associated with myopathy.[5,18] However, no extra precautions are needed on the concurrent use of ezetimibe and a statin compared with those recommended for either drug alone. The manufacturers recommend that any patient given ezetimibe should be told to report any signs of myopathy and possible rhabdomyolysis (i.e. otherwise unexplained muscle pain, tenderness or weakness or dark coloured urine).[18] See also *Muscle and liver toxicity*, under 'Lipid regulating drugs', p.1309, for further guidance on monitoring, and risk factors for muscle toxicity. Note that a combination preparation containing simvastatin and ezetimibe is widely available.

1. Zhu Y, Statkevich P, Kosoglou T, Maxwell SE, Anderson L, Patrick JE, Batra V. Lack of a pharmacokinetic interaction between ezetimibe and atorvastatin. *Clin Pharmacol Ther* (2001) 69, P68.
2. Kosoglou T, Statkevich P, Johnson-Levonas AO, Paolini JF, Bergman AJ, Alton KB. Ezetimibe: a review of its metabolism, pharmacokinetics and drug interactions. *Clin Pharmacokinet* (2005) 44, 467–94.
3. Ballantyne CM, Houri J, Notarbartolo A, Melani L, Lipka LJ, Suresh R, Sun S, LeBeaut AP, Sager PT, Veltri EP for the Ezetimibe Study Group. Effect of ezetimibe coadministered with atorvastatin in 628 patients with primary hypercholesterolemia: A prospective, randomised, double-blind trial. *Circulation* (2003) 107, 2409–15.
4. Fux R, Mörike K, Gundel U-F, Hartmann R, Gleiter CH. Ezetimibe and statin-associated myopathy. *Ann Intern Med* (2004) 140, 671–2.
5. Simard C, Poirier P. Ezetimibe-associated myopathy in monotherapy and in combination with a 3-hydroxy-3-methylglutaryl coenzyme A reductase inhibitor. *Can J Cardiol* (2006) 22, 141–44.
6. Weffald LA, Flach LA. Myopathy associated with atorvastatin-ezetimibe combination therapy. *Pharmacotherapy* (2007) 27, 309–11.
7. Piedra León M, García Unzueta MT, Otero Martínez M, Amado Señaris JA. Rabdomiolisis asociada a tratamiento combinado ezetimibe-estatina. *Rev Clin Esp* (2007) 207, 425–6.
8. Reyderman L, Kosoglou T, Cutler DL, Maxwell S, Statkevich P. The effect of fluvastatin on the pharmacokinetics and pharmacodynamics of ezetimibe. *Curr Med Res Opin* (2005) 21, 1171–9.
9. Stein EA, Ballantyne CM, Windler E, Sirnes PA, Sussekov A, Yigit Z, Seper C, Gimpelewicz CR. Efficacy and tolerability of fluvastatin XL 80 mg alone, ezetimibe alone, and the combination of fluvastatin XL 80 mg with ezetimibe in patients with a history of muscle-related side effects with other statins. *Am J Cardiol* (2008) 101, 490–6.
10. Kosoglou T, Statkevich P, Meyer I, Cutler DL, Musiol B, Yang B, Zhu Y, Maxwell SE, Veltri EP. Effects of ezetimibe on the pharmacodynamics and pharmacokinetics of lovastatin. *Curr Med Res Opin* (2004) 20, 955–65.
11. Reyderman L, Kosoglou T, Boutros T, Seiberling M, Statkevich P. Pharmacokinetic interaction between ezetimibe and lovastatin in healthy volunteers. *Curr Med Res Opin* (2004) 20, 1493–1500.
12. Kosoglou T, Statkevich P, Yang B, Suresh R, Zhu Y, Boutros T, Maxwell SE, Tiessen R, Cutler DL. Pharmacodynamic interaction between ezetimibe and rosuvastatin. *Curr Med Res Opin* (2004) 20, 1185–95.

13. Kosoglou T, Meyer I, Veltri EP, Statkevich P, Yang B, Zhu Y, Mellars L, Maxwell SE, Patrick JE, Cutler DL, Batra VK, Affrime MB. Pharmacodynamic interaction between the new selective cholesterol absorption inhibitor ezetimibe and simvastatin. *Br J Clin Pharmacol* (2002) 54, 309–19.
14. Ose L, Johnson-Levonas A, Reyes R, Lin J, Shah A, Tribble D, Musliner T, for the Vytorin Extension Study Group. A multi-centre, randomised, double-blind 14-week extension study examining the long-term safety and efficacy profile of the ezetimibe/simvastatin combination tablet. *Int J Clin Pract* (2007) 61, 1469–80.
15. Davidson MH, Maccubbin D, Stepanavage M, Strony J, Musliner T. Striated muscle safety of ezetimibe/simvastatin (Vytorin). *Am J Cardiol* (2006) 97, 223–8.
16. Bays H, Sapre A, Taggart W, Liu J, Capece R, Tershakovec A. Long-term (48-week) safety of ezetimibe 10 mg/day coadministered with simvastatin compared to simvastatin alone in patients with primary hypercholesterolemia. *Curr Med Res Opin* (2008) 24, 2953–66.
17. Kashani A, Sallam T, Bheemreddy S, Mann DL, Wang Y, Foody JM. Review of side-effect profile of combination ezetimibe and statin therapy in randomized clinical trials. *Am J Cardiol* (2008) 101, 1606–13.
18. Ezetrol (Ezetimibe). MSD-SP Ltd. UK Summary of product characteristics, September 2010.
19. Zetia (Ezetimibe). Merck/Schering-Plough Pharmaceuticals. US Prescribing information, August 2013.

Statins + Fibrates; Fenofibrate

Fenofibrate can alter the exposure to a number of statins: with pravastatin there is a slight increase, with simvastatin acid there is a slight decrease, whereas with atorvastatin, fluvastatin, pitavastatin or rosuvastatin there is either no effect, or only a negligible effect. Both statins and fibrates are known to rarely cause myopathy and rhabdomyolysis, and their concurrent use increases the risk of this reaction, although there is some evidence that this is minimal for fenofibrate: isolated cases of myopathy and rhabdomyolysis have been reported with the concurrent use of fenofibrate and the statins

Clinical evidence

The pharmacokinetic studies of the effects of fibrates on statins are summarised in 'Table 30.2', p.1337.

(a) Atorvastatin

Fenofibrate did not alter the exposure to atorvastatin and had a negligible effect on its metabolites in a study in healthy subjects, see 'Table 30.2', p.1337. In a single-dose study, atorvastatin had no effect on fenofibrate exposure.[1]

A 58-year-old man who had been taking atorvastatin 10 mg daily for 4 months developed rhabdomyolysis-induced acute renal failure one month after starting to take fenofibrate 200 mg daily. He recovered within a month, after treatment with diuretics and haemodialysis.[2] In a cohort analysis, for atorvastatin alone there were 7 cases of rhabdomyolysis for 129 367 person years of use and for atorvastatin given with a fibrate, there was one case (with fenofibrate) for 2 664 person years of use.[3] In an extension study in patients who had completed a 12-week controlled study, of 86 patients taking fenofibrate 135 mg daily with atorvastatin 40 mg daily for 2 years or more, one developed creatine phosphokinase levels greater than 10 times the upper limit of normal, but did not have myalgia.[4]

(b) Fluvastatin

Fenofibrate had a negligible effect on the exposure of fluvastatin or its metabolites in a study in healthy subjects, see 'Table 30.2', p.1337.

In a pooled analysis of clinical study data, the frequency of creatine kinase elevations was low and was not statistically significantly different between 1 897 patients receiving fluvastatin alone (0.3%) and 1 017 receiving fluvastatin and a fibrate (0.5%). The fibrates used were bezafibrate (493 subjects), fenofibrate (158 subjects), and gemfibrozil (366 subjects).[5]

(c) Pitavastatin

Fenofibrate had a negligible effect on the steady-state pharmacokinetics of pitavastatin in a study in healthy subjects, see 'Table 30.2', p.1337.

(d) Pravastatin

Fenofibrate slightly increases steady-state pravastatin exposure, see 'Table 30.2', p.1337. A case report describes a patient taking fenofibrate 300 mg daily, who developed rhabdomyolysis after starting to take pravastatin 10 mg daily.[6] In another report, a 56-year-old woman who had taken pravastatin 20 mg daily for 12 years, developed severe rhabdomyolysis-induced acute renal failure about 2 months after starting to take fenofibrate 200 mg daily. She recovered in about 2 weeks, after treatment with diuretics and haemodialysis.[2]

(e) Rosuvastatin

Fenofibrate had a negligible effect on rosuvastatin exposure in two studies in healthy subjects, see 'Table 30.2', p.1337, and rosuvastatin did not alter fenofibric acid exposure in a pharmacokinetic study.[7] In an extension study in patients who had completed a 12-week controlled study, of 174 patients taking fenofibrate 135 mg daily with rosuvastatin 20 mg daily for 2 years or more, three developed creatine phosphokinase levels greater than 10 times the upper limit of normal, one with myalgia, although none of these patients discontinued treatment. Two other patients discontinued fenofibrate with rosuvastatin because of myalgia.[4] A 68-year-old man taking rosuvastatin 10 mg daily developed myopathy about 3 weeks after fenofibrate 160 mg was added. Rhabdomyolysis was diagnosed and both drugs were stopped, resulting in marked clinical improvement within 24 hours.[8] Other cases of muscle toxicity have been described shortly after both rosuvastatin 10 mg daily and fenofibrate 250 mg daily were started,[9] and shortly after the dose of rosuvastatin was increased from 10 to 20 mg daily, with the addition of fenofibrate 160 mg daily.[10]

(f) Simvastatin

Fenofibrate slightly reduced the exposure to simvastatin acid in a study in healthy subjects, see 'Table 30.2', p.1337, and the AUC of HMG-CoA reductase inhibitor activity was reduced by 12% on concurrent use. The pharmacokinetics of fenofibric acid was unchanged by concurrent use.[11]

In various clinical studies, no increased risk for myopathy has been seen in patients given fenofibrate with simvastatin. For example, an 18-week, placebo-controlled study (SAFARI) investigated the efficacy and tolerability of simvastatin 20 mg and fenofibrate 160 mg daily compared with simvastatin alone. In the 411 patients who received both drugs concurrently and in the 207 patients receiving simvastatin alone, no drug-related serious adverse events were observed and there were no instances of clinical myopathy or severe abnormalities in liver function.[12] The Action to Control Cardiovascular Risk in Diabetes (ACCORD) study randomised 5 518 patients given simvastatin (average daily dose about 22 mg daily, maximum 40 mg daily) to receive an initial dose of fenofibrate 160 mg daily (2 765 subjects) or placebo (2 753 subjects) for a mean duration of 4.7 years. There was no difference between the two groups in incidence of muscular adverse events: out of the ordinary severe muscle aches/pains not associated with known activities occurred in 40.1% of fenofibrate recipients and 40.5% of placebo recipients; creatine phosphokinase greater than 10 times the upper limit of normal occurred in 10 (0.4%) of fenofibrate recipients and 9 (0.3%) of placebo recipients; and any myopathy, myositis or rhabdomyolysis occurred in 4 (0.1%) of fenofibrate recipients and 4 (0.1%) of placebo recipients.[13,14] The UK manufacturer of simvastatin states that when simvastatin and fenofibrate are given concurrently, there is no evidence that the risk of myopathy exceeds the sum of the individual risks of each drug.[15]

A 70-year-old man with diabetes and hypothyroidism (known risk factors for myopathy), who was taking medication including simvastatin 40 mg, developed bilateral leg myalgia 2 weeks after fenofibrate 160 mg was started. Two weeks later he was found to have raised creatinine and creatine phosphokinase levels and rhabdomyolysis was diagnosed. The fenofibrate and simvastatin were discontinued and, with hydration, the myalgia resolved; his creatinine levels returned to baseline over the next week and the serum creatine phosphokinase level returned to baseline within 4 weeks.[16] In another case, in a 63-year-old woman taking simvastatin 20 mg daily and fenofibrate 200 mg daily for 4 months; previously undiagnosed hypothyroidism, was found to be a contributing factor.[17]

(g) Unspecified statins

A review using data from the adverse event reporting system of the FDA in the US concluded that the concurrent use of fenofibrate with a statin results in fewer reports of rhabdomyolysis than the concurrent use of **gemfibrozil** and a statin (0.58 cases per million prescriptions and 8.6 cases per million prescriptions, respectively).[18]

Mechanism

Complex and not fully understood. Myopathy can occur with statins and fibrates alone and their effects could therefore be additive or synergistic. The mechanisms for the slight increases in pravastatin exposure and decreases in simvastatin acid exposure when given with fenofibrate are unknown

Importance and management

The available evidence suggests that there are no clinically important pharmacokinetic interactions between fenofibrate and any statin (in contrast to the situation with gemfibrozil, see 'Statins + Fibrates; Gemfibrozil', p.1338). There is likely to be a pharmacodynamic interaction resulting in an increased risk of myopathy and rhabdomyolysis. However, although the actual increased incidence of these rare effects on the concurrent use of fenofibrate and a statin, compared with either drug alone, is unknown, on the basis of the large simvastatin with fenofibrate ACCORD study it appears to be minimal. In addition, there is limited evidence to suggest that the risk of myopathy might be lower with fenofibrate and a statin than with gemfibrozil and a statin. Nevertheless, in general, it is considered that concurrent use of a statin and fenofibrate should be undertaken only if the benefits of treatment outweigh the risks (the UK manufacturer of fenofibrate specifies patients with severe combined dyslipidaemia and high cardiovascular risk without any history of muscular disease[19]). Some statin manufacturers give statin dose recommendations for the concurrent use of any fibrate, which would therefore apply to fenofibrate, as follows:

- lower starting dose for **atorvastatin** (UK advice);[20]
- avoid 40 mg daily for **rosuvastatin** (UK advice).[21]

In contrast, fenofibrate has been specifically *excluded* from the UK maximum recommended dose of **simvastatin** to be used with fibrates.[15] As a general rule, for any patient given a statin and fenofibrate, the advice to report any signs of myopathy and possible rhabdomyolysis (i.e. otherwise unexplained muscle pain, tenderness or weakness or dark coloured urine) should be specifically reinforced. If myopathy does occur, the fibrate and statin should be stopped immediately. See also *Muscle and liver toxicity*, under 'Lipid regulating drugs', p.1309, for further guidance on monitoring and risk factors for muscle toxicity.

1. Penn R, Williams RX, Guha-Ray DK, Sawyers WG, Braun SL, Rains KT. An open-label, crossover study of the pharmacokinetics of insoluble drug delivery-microparticle fenofibrate in combination with atorvastatin, simvastatin, and extended-release niacin in healthy volunteers. *Clin Ther* (2006) 28, 45–54.
2. Unal A, Torun E, Sipahioglu MH, Tokgoz B, Kaya MG, Oymak O, Utas C. Fenofibrate-induced acute renal failure due to massive rhabdomyolysis after coadministration of statin in two patients. *Intern Med* (2008) 47, 1017–19.
3. Graham DJ, Staffa JA, Shatin D, Andrade SE, Schech SD, La Grenade L, Gurwitz JH, Chan KA, Goodman MJ, Platt R. Incidence of hospitalized rhabdomyolysis in patients treated with lipid-lowering drugs. *JAMA* (2004) 292, 2585–90.

Table 30.2 Pharmacokinetic studies of the effect of fibrates on statins

Statin	*Statin dose*	*Fibrate dose*	*Change in statin exposure (AUC)*	*Refs*
Bezafibrate, p.1339				
Fluvastatin	20 mg daily	200 mg three times daily	53% increase	1, 2
Lovastatin	40 mg single dose on day 3	400 mg daily for 3 days	No change	3
Ciprofibrate, p.1339				
Fluvastatin	Not stated	Not stated	No change	1
Fenofibrate, p.1336				
Atorvastatin	40 mg single dose on day 5	160 mg daily for 7 days	No change 18% increase 4-hydroxy lactone	4
Fluvastatin	40 mg single dose	160 mg single dose	15% increase	5
Pitavastatin	4 mg daily for 7 days	160 mg daily for 7 days	18% increase	6
Pravastatin	40 mg single dose	201 mg single dose	No change 26% increase metabolite	7
	40 mg daily for 16 days	160 mg daily for 10 days	30% increase 37% increase metabolite	8
Rosuvastatin	10 mg daily for 7 days	67 mg three times daily for 7 days	7% increase	9
	40 mg daily for 10 days	135 mg daily for 10 days (choline fenofibrate)	No change	10
Simvastatin	80 mg daily for 7 days	160 mg daily for 7 days	7% decrease 37% decrease acid	11
Gemfibrozil, p.1338				
Atorvastatin	20 mg single dose on day 3	600 mg twice daily for 5 days	24% increase 51% increase acid	12
	40 mg single dose on day 5	600 mg twice daily for 7 days	35% increase 28 to 69% increase hydroxy metabolites	4
Fluvastatin	20 mg twice daily for 2 weeks	600 mg twice daily for 2 weeks	No change	13
Lovastatin	40 mg single dose on day 3	600 mg twice daily for 3 days	No change Moderate 2.8-fold increase acid	3
Pitavastatin	4 mg daily for 7 days	600 mg twice daily for 7 days	45% increase	6
Pravastatin	20 mg single dose	600 mg single dose	No change 96% increase metabolite	14
	40 mg single dose on day 3	600 mg twice daily for 3 days	Twofold increase	15
Rosuvastatin	80 mg single dose on day 4	600 mg twice daily for 7 days	88% increase	16
Simvastatin	40 mg single dose on day 3	600 mg twice daily for 3 days	44% increase 2.9-fold increase acid	17

1. Lescol (Fluvastatin sodium). Novartis Pharmaceuticals UK Ltd. UK Summary of product characteristics, March 2009.
2. Novartis Pharmaceuticals Ltd. Personal communication. 28 February 2011.
3. Kyrklund C, Backman JT, Kivistö KT, Neuvonen M, Laitila J, Neuvonen PJ. Plasma concentrations of active lovastatin acid are markedly increased by gemfibrozil but not by bezafibrate. *Clin Pharmacol Ther* (2001) 69, 340–5.
4. Whitfield LR, Porcari AR, Alvey C, Abel R, Bullen W, Hartman D. Effect of gemfibrozil and fenofibrate on the pharmacokinetics of atorvastatin. *J Clin Pharmacol* (2011) 51, 378–8.
5. Gustavson L, Schweitzer S, Burt D, Chira T, Achari R, Rieser M, Yannicelli D. Lack of a significant pharmacokinetic drug interaction between fenofibrate and fluvastatin. *AAPS PharmSci* (2005) 7, (S2). Available at: http://www.aapsj.org/abstracts/AM_2005/AAPS2005-000081.pdf, p. (accessed 20/10/15).
6. Mathew P, Cuddy T, Tracewell WG, Salazar D. An open-label study on the pharmacokinetics (PK) of pitavastatin (NK-104) when administered concomitantly with fenofibrate or gemfibrozil in healthy volunteers. *Clin Pharmacol Ther* (2004) 75, P33.
7. Pan W-J, Gustavson LE, Achari R, Rieser MJ, Ye X, Gutterman C, Wallin BA. Lack of a clinically significant pharmacokinetic interaction between fenofibrate and pravastatin in healthy volunteers. *J Clin Pharmacol* (2000) 40, 316–23.
8. Gustavson LE, Schweitzer SM, Koehne-Voss S, Achari R, Chira TO, Esslinger H-U, Yannicelli HD. The effects of multiple doses of fenofibrate on the pharmacokinetics of pravastatin and its 3α-hydroxy isomeric metabolite. *J Clin Pharmacol* (2005) 45, 947–53.
9. Martin PD, Dane AL, Schneck DW, Warwick MJ. An open-label, randomized, three-way crossover trial of the effect of coadministration of rosuvastatin and fenofibrate on the pharmacokinetic properties of rosuvastatin and fenofibric acid in healthy male volunteers. *Clin Ther* (2003) 25, 459–71.
10. Zhu T, Awni WM, Hosmane B, Kelly MT, Sleep DJ, Stolzenbach JC, Wan K, Chira TO, Pradhan RS. ABT-335, the choline salt of fenofibric acid, does not have a clinically significant pharmacokinetic interaction with rosuvastatin in humans. *J Clin Pharmacol* (2009) 49, 63–71.
11. Bergman AJ, Murphy G, Burke J, Zhao JJ, Valesky R, Liu L, Lasseter KC, He W, Prueksaritanont T, Qiu Y, Hartford A, Vega JM, Paolini JF. Simvastatin does not have a clinically significant pharmacokinetic interaction with fenofibrate in humans. *J Clin Pharmacol* (2004) 44, 1054–62.
12. Backman JT, Luurila H, Neuvonen M, Neuvonen PJ. Rifampin markedly decreases and gemfibrozil increases the plasma concentrations of atorvastatin and its metabolites. *Clin Pharmacol Ther* (2005) 78, 154–67.
13. Spence JD, Munoz CE, Hendricks L, Latchinian L, Khouri HE. Pharmacokinetics of the combination of fluvastatin and gemfibrozil. *Am J Cardiol* (1995) 76, 80A–83A.
14. ER Squibb. Data on file. A report on the bioavailability of pravastatin in the presence and absence of gemfibrozil or probucol in healthy male subjects (Protocol No 27, 201-18). 1988.
15. Kyrklund C, Backman JT, Neuvonen M, Neuvonen PJ. Gemfibrozil increases plasma pravastatin concentrations and reduces pravastatin renal clearance. *Clin Pharmacol Ther* (2003) 73, 538–44.
16. Schneck DW, Birmingham BK, Zalikowski JA, Mitchell PD, Wang Y, Martin PD, Lasseter KC, Brown CDA, Windass AS, Raza A. The effect of gemfibrozil on the pharmacokinetics of rosuvastatin. *Clin Pharmacol Ther* (2004) 75, 455–63.
17. Backman JT, Kyrklund C, Kivistö KT, Wang J-S, Neuvonen PJ. Plasma concentrations of active simvastatin acid are increased by gemfibrozil. *Clin Pharmacol Ther* (2001) 68, 122–9.

4. Kipnes MS, Roth EM, Rhyne JM, Setze CM, Lele A, Kelly MT, Sleep DJ, Stolzenbach JC. Year two assessment of fenofibric acid and moderate-dose statin combination: a phase 3, open-label, extension study. *Clin Drug Investig* (2010) 30, 51–61.
5. Farnier M, Bortolini M, Salko T, Freudenreich M-O, Isaacsohn JL, Troendle AJ, Gonasun L. Frequency of creatine kinase elevation during treatment with fluvastatin in combination with fibrates (bezafibrate, fenofibrate, or gemfibrozil). *Am J Cardiol* (2003) 91, 238–40.
6. Raimondeau J, Le Marec H, Chevallier JC, Bouhour JB. Myolyse biologique survenue à l'occasion d'un relais thérapeutique fénofibrate-pravastatine. *Presse Med* (1992) 21, 663–4.
7. Martin PD, Dane AL, Schneck DW, Warwick MJ. An open-label, randomized, three-way crossover trial of the effect of coadministration of rosuvastatin and fenofibrate on the pharmacokinetic properties of rosuvastatin and fenofibric acid in healthy male volunteers. *Clin Ther* (2003) 25, 459–71.
8. Dedhia V, Munsi SC. Myopathy caused by a combination rosuvastatin and fenofibrate. *J Assoc Physicians India* (2007) 55, 152–3.
9. Buyukhatipoglu H, Sezen Y, Guntekin U, Kirhan I, Dag OF. Acute renal failure with the combined use of rosuvastatin and fenofibrate. *Ren Fail* (2010) 32, 633–5.
10. Ireland JHE, Eggert CH, Arendt CJ, Williams AW. Rhabdomyolysis with cardiac involvement and acute renal failure in a patient taking rosuvastatin and fenofibrate. *Ann Intern Med* (2005) 142, 949–50.
11. Bergman AJ, Murphy G, Burke J, Zhao JJ, Valesky R, Liu L, Lasseter KC, He W, Prueksaritanont T, Qiu Y, Hartford A, Vega JM, Paolini JF. Simvastatin does not have a clinically significant pharmacokinetic interaction with fenofibrate in humans. *J Clin Pharmacol* (2004) 44, 1054–62.
12. Grundy SM, Vega GL, Yuan Z, Battisti WP, Brady WE, Palmisano J. Effectiveness and tolerability of simvastatin plus fenofibrate for combined hyperlipidemia (the SAFARI trial). *Am J Cardiol* (2005) 95, 462–8.
13. ACCORD Study Group, Ginsberg HN, Elam MB, Lovato LC, Crouse JR 3rd, Leiter LA, Linz P, Friedewald WT, Buse JB, Gerstein HC, Probstfield J, Grimm RH, Ismail-Beigi F, Bigger JT, Goff DC Jr, Cushman WC, Simons-Morton DG, Byington RP. Effects of combination lipid therapy in type 2 diabetes mellitus. *N Engl J Med* (2010) 362, 1563–74. Erratum in: N Engl J Med. *ibid.* 1748.
14. Supplementary Appendix 1 to the ACCORD study. Section 13: results–follow-up period adverse events and laboratory measures. Page 20. Available at: http://www.nejm.org/doi/suppl/10.1056/NEJMoa1001282/suppl_file/nejm_accord_1563sa1.pdf (accessed 22/10/15).
15. Zocor (Simvastatin). Merck Sharp & Dohme Ltd. UK Summary of product characteristics, June 2015.
16. Jacob SS, Jacob S, Williams C, Deeg MA. Simvastatin, fenofibrate, and rhabdomyolysis. *Diabetes Care* (2005) 28, 1258.
17. Kursat S, Alici T, Colak HB. A case of rhabdomyolysis induced acute renal failure secondary to statin-fibrate-derivative combination and occult hypothyroidism. *Clin Nephrol* (2005) 64, 391–3.
18. Jones PH, Davidson MH. Reporting rate of rhabdomyolysis with fenofibrate + statin versus gemfibrozil + any statin. *Am J Cardiol* (2005) 95, 120–2.
19. Lipantil (Fenofibrate). Abbott Healthcare Products Ltd. UK Summary of product characteristics, June 2011.
20. Lipitor (Atorvastatin calcium trihydrate). Pfizer Ltd. UK Summary of product characteristics, March 2015.
21. Crestor (Rosuvastatin calcium). AstraZeneca UK Ltd. UK Summary of product characteristics, May 2013.

Statins + Fibrates; Gemfibrozil

Gemfibrozil moderately increases lovastatin, pravastatin and simvastatin exposure; slightly increases atorvastatin, pitavastatin and rosuvastatin exposure; and has no effect on fluvastatin exposure. Both statins and fibrates are known to rarely cause myopathy and rhabdomyolysis, and their concurrent use increases the risk of this reaction, especially if plasma levels of the statin are also raised. Many cases of myopathy and rhabdomyolysis have been reported with the concurrent use of gemfibrozil and lovastatin or simvastatin

Clinical evidence

The pharmacokinetic studies of the effects of fibrates on statins are summarised in 'Table 30.2', p.1337.

(a) Atorvastatin

Gemfibrozil slightly increased the exposure to atorvastatin and its metabolites in pharmacokinetic studies in healthy subjects, see 'Table 30.2', p.1337.

A 43-year-old woman with multiple medical problems was taking gemfibrozil 600 mg twice daily. After a recurrent attack of pancreatitis, atorvastatin 10 mg and glibenclamide (glyburide) 2.5 mg, both twice daily, were added. About 3 weeks later she developed brown and turbid urine (suggesting urinary myoglobin), creatine kinase levels of 4633 units/L and had myalgia: she was diagnosed as having rhabdomyolysis. Her serum creatine kinase levels rapidly fell when the atorvastatin and gemfibrozil were withdrawn.[1]

In a case series of 10 patients taking a statin who experienced myopathy and presented for muscle biopsy, one patient taking gemfibrozil developed gradual onset of weakness over a 3-month period after his dose of atorvastatin was increased from 10 mg to 20 mg daily.[2] In an analysis of reports of rhabdomyolysis to the FDA in the US up until the end of July 2001, atorvastatin alone was associated with 45 cases and atorvastatin with gemfibrozil was associated with 6 cases. Based on estimated dispensed prescriptions, this gave a crude reporting rate of just 0.03 per 100 000 prescriptions for atorvastatin alone and of 0.50 for atorvastatin with gemfibrozil,[3] which suggests about a 17-fold increase in risk.

(b) Fluvastatin

Gemfibrozil had no effect on the steady-state exposure to fluvastatin in healthy subjects, see 'Table 30.2', p.1337, and the pharmacokinetics of gemfibrozil were also unchanged by concurrent use.[4]

In a pooled analysis of clinical study data, the frequency of creatine kinase elevations was low and was not statistically significantly different between 1 897 patients taking fluvastatin alone (0.3%) and 1 017 taking fluvastatin and a fibrate (0.5%). The fibrates taken were bezafibrate (493 subjects), fenofibrate (158 subjects), and gemfibrozil (366 subjects).[5]

A case report describes a patient, who developed serious hepatocellular injury and rhabdomyolysis causing acute renal failure, one month after she started to take both fluvastatin 80 mg daily and gemfibrozil 1.2 g daily; she was not taking any other medications.[6] In an analysis of reports of rhabdomyolysis to the FDA in the US up until the end of July 2001, fluvastatin alone was associated with just one case and there were no cases for fluvastatin with gemfibrozil. Based on estimated dispensed prescriptions, this gave a crude reporting rate of zero per 100 000 prescriptions for fluvastatin alone and for fluvastatin with gemfibrozil,[3] which suggests no increase in risk.

(c) Lovastatin

Gemfibrozil moderately increased the exposure to lovastatin acid, the active metabolite of lovastatin, in a single-dose pharmacokinetic study in healthy subjects, see 'Table 30.2', p.1337.

By 1990 the FDA in the US had documented 12 case reports of severe myopathy or rhabdomyolysis associated with the concurrent use of lovastatin and gemfibrozil. The mean serum creatine kinase levels of the patients reached 15 250 units/L. Four of those tested had myoglobinuria and five had acute renal failure.[7] Other cases of rhabdomyolysis associated with the concurrent use of these drugs have been reported,[8-14] five involving renal failure.[8-10,12] Further cases of rhabdomyolysis have been seen in patients taking lovastatin and gemfibrozil and other interacting drugs such as ciclosporin,[15,16] nicotinic acid (niacin);[17] or clarithromycin, see 'Statins + Macrolides', p.1348.

In four early studies of the concurrent use of lovastatin and gemfibrozil in 179 patients, muscle symptoms occurred in 9 patients and 2 patients had elevations in creatine kinase levels of greater than 3 times normal.[18-21] In an analysis of reports of rhabdomyolysis to the FDA in the US up until the end of July 2001, lovastatin alone was associated with 120 cases and lovastatin with gemfibrozil was associated with 60 cases. Based on estimated dispensed prescriptions, this gave a crude reporting rate of 0.12 per 100 000 prescriptions for lovastatin alone and of 2.84 for lovastatin with gemfibrozil,[3] which suggests about a 24-fold increase in risk.

(d) Pitavastatin

Gemfibrozil slightly increased the steady-state exposure to pitavastatin in healthy subjects, see 'Table 30.2', p.1337.

(e) Pravastatin

Gemfibrozil moderately increased exposure to single-dose pravastatin in a pharmacokinetic study in healthy subjects, and slightly to moderately increased the exposure to the metabolite in an earlier study, see 'Table 30.2', p.1337.

In one early 12-week study of pravastatin 40 mg daily and gemfibrozil 600 mg twice daily, marked abnormalities in creatine kinase levels (four times the pretreatment values) occurred in 1 of 71 patients taking pravastatin alone, 1 of 73 patients taking placebo, 2 of 72 patients taking gemfibrozil alone, and 4 of 75 patients taking gemfibrozil with pravastatin. The differences between treatments were not statistically significant. Two patients taking gemfibrozil with pravastatin had these drugs withdrawn because of asymptomatic creatine kinase elevations. Severe myopathy or rhabdomyolysis was not seen in any patient, although 14 patients had musculoskeletal pain, but in most cases this was not considered to be related to treatment.[22] In an analysis of reports of rhabdomyolysis to the FDA in the US up until the end of July 2001, pravastatin alone was associated with just 17 cases and pravastatin with gemfibrozil was associated with 2 cases. Based on estimated dispensed prescriptions, this gave a crude reporting rate of just 0.02 per 100 000 prescriptions for pravastatin alone and of 0.14 for pravastatin with gemfibrozil,[3] which suggests about a 7-fold increase in risk.

(f) Rosuvastatin

Gemfibrozil slightly increased the exposure to single doses of rosuvastatin in a pharmacokinetic study in healthy subjects, see 'Table 30.2', p.1337. Three subjects had asymptomatic increases in ALT levels (less than 2.5 times upper limit of normal).[23]

(g) Simvastatin

Gemfibrozil slightly increased the exposure to single doses of simvastatin and moderately increased the exposure to the active simvastatin acid metabolite in a pharmacokinetic study in healthy subjects, see 'Table 30.2', p.1337.

A 62-year-old man with diabetes taking simvastatin 20 mg daily and gemfibrozil 600 mg daily (as well as acenocoumarol, glibenclamide (glyburide) and diclofenac) was hospitalised because of melaena, generalised myalgia, malaise and brown urine. Laboratory tests confirmed the diagnosis of rhabdomyolysis. He recovered when the simvastatin and gemfibrozil were stopped.[24] Another diabetic patient had been taking simvastatin and gemfibrozil 600 mg daily for two and a half years (as well as felodipine, indapamide, calcium carbonate, bumetanide, psyllium, acenocoumarol and insulin). She complained of tiredness, generalised myalgia and anuria 3 months after her dose of simvastatin had been increased to 80 mg daily. Rhabdomyolysis with renal impairment were diagnosed and confirmed. She recovered when the simvastatin and gemfibrozil were stopped.[24] Five further cases of rhabdomyolysis have been reported with the combination: three in patients taking simvastatin 40 or 80 mg daily, 3 to 4 weeks after starting gemfibrozil;[25-27] one in a patient taking gemfibrozil 3 months after starting simvastatin 10 mg daily;[28] and one 5 weeks after switching from pravastatin with fenofibrate to simvastatin 80 mg daily with gemfibrozil.[29] One of these cases was fatal.[25]

In a case series of 10 patients taking a statin who experienced myopathy and presented for muscle biopsy, two patients taking gemfibrozil gradually developed myopathy while also taking simvastatin 80 mg daily.[2] In an analysis of reports of rhabdomyolysis to the FDA in the US up until the end of July 2001, simvastatin alone was associated with 136 cases and simvastatin with gemfibrozil was associated with 37 cases. Based on estimated dispensed prescriptions, this gave a crude reporting rate of 0.08 per 100 000 prescriptions for simvastatin alone and of 3.85 for simvastatin with gemfibrozil,[3] which suggests about a 48-fold increase in risk. In a cohort analysis, for simvastatin alone there were two cases of rhabdomyolysis for 40 940 person years of use and for simvastatin given with a fibrate, there was one case (with gemfibrozil) for 552 person-years of use.[30] In a review of adverse reactions to statins in the Swedish Adverse Drug Reactions Advisory Committee until September 2006, nine cases of confirmed rhabdomyolysis occurred in patients taking simvastatin and gemfibrozil.[31]

(h) Unspecified statins

A review using data from the adverse event reporting system of the FDA in the US concluded that the concurrent use of **fenofibrate** with a statin results in fewer reports of rhabdomyolysis than the concurrent use of gemfibrozil and a statin (0.58 cases per million prescriptions and 8.6 cases per million prescriptions, respectively).[32]

Mechanism

Complex and not fully understood. Myopathy can occur with statins and fibrates alone and their effects might therefore be additive or synergistic. More recent evidence suggests that gemfibrozil increases the levels of these statins by inhibiting the drug transporter protein, organic anion transporting polypeptide OATP1B1 (also known as OATP2 and OATP-C),[33,34] with the extent of the interaction varying between the statins. There is also some evidence that gemfibrozil might inhibit the glucuronidation of simvastatin and atorvastatin metabolites.[35] With the exception of cerivastatin (now withdrawn), inhibition of cytochrome P450 isoenzymes is not involved in the pharmacokinetic interaction of gemfibrozil with statins.

Importance and management

The pharmacokinetic interaction of gemfibrozil with most statins is well established and likely to contribute to the general increased risk of myopathy that occurs when fibrates are used with statins. The pharmacokinetic interaction is greatest for simvastatin, lovastatin and pravastatin, intermediate for rosuvastatin, atorvastatin and pitavastatin, and does not occur with fluvastatin. The concurrent use of statins with gemfibrozil is generally contraindicated or should be avoided, but, if the benefits are considered to outweigh the risks, a low dose of the statin should be used with appropriate clinical monitoring for toxicity. The manufacturers of **rosuvastatin** recommend a starting dose of **rosuvastatin** of 5 mg daily on concurrent use with gemfibrozil, with a maximum daily dose of 10 mg in the US.[36] whereas, in the UK, a starting dose of 5 mg daily is recommended, with the 40 mg dose being contraindicated.[37]

Monitoring of creatine kinase has been suggested in patients taking a statin with a fibrate, but this will not necessarily identify all cases of developing rhabdomyolysis. As a general rule, for any patient given a statin and a fibrate the advice to report any signs of myopathy and possible rhabdomyolysis (i.e. otherwise unexplained muscle pain, tenderness or weakness or dark coloured urine) should be specifically reinforced. If myopathy does occur, both the statin and the fibrate should be stopped immediately. See also *Muscle and liver toxicity*, under 'Lipid regulating drugs', p.1309, for further guidance on monitoring and risk factors for muscle toxicity. If the concurrent use of gemfibrozil and a statin is required, limited evidence suggests that the increased risk of myopathy might be lower with fluvastatin. There is also evidence to suggest that the risk of myopathy might be lower with fenofibrate and a statin than gemfibrozil and a statin.

1. Duell PB, Connor WE, Illingworth DR. Rhabdomyolysis after taking atorvastatin with gemfibrozil. *Am J Cardiol* (1998) 81, 368–9.
2. McKelvie PA, Dennett X. Myopathy associated with HMG-CoA reductase inhibitors (statins): a series of 10 patients and review of the literature. *J Clin Neuromusc Dis* (2002) 3,143–8.
3. Chang JT, Staffa JA, Parks M, Green L. Rhabdomyolysis with HMG-CoA reductase inhibitors and gemfibrozil combination therapy. *Pharmacoepidemiol Drug Safety* (2004) 13, 417–26.
4. Spence JD, Munoz CE, Hendricks L, Latchinian L, Khouri HE. Pharmacokinetics of the combination of fluvastatin and gemfibrozil. *Am J Cardiol* (1995) 76, 80A–83A.
5. Farnier M, Bortolini M, Salko T, Freudenreich M-O, Isaacsohn JL, Troendle AJ, Gonasun L. Frequency of creatine kinase elevation during treatment with fluvastatin in combination with fibrates (bezafibrate, fenofibrate, or gemfibrozil). *Am J Cardiol* (2003) 91, 238–40.
6. Akoglu H, Yilmaz R, Kirkpantur A, Arici M, Altun B, Turgan C. Combined organ failure with combination antihyperlipidemic treatment: a case of hepatic injury and acute renal failure. *Ann Pharmacother* (2007) 41, 143–7.
7. Pierce LR, Wysowski DK, Gross TP. Myopathy and rhabdomyolysis associated with lovastatin-gemfibrozil combination therapy. *JAMA* (1990) 264, 71–5.
8. Tobert JA. Myolysis and acute renal failure in a heart-transplant recipient receiving lovastatin. *N Engl J Med* (1988) 318, 48.
9. Marais GE, Larson KK. Rhabdomyolysis and acute renal failure induced by combination lovastatin and gemfibrozil therapy. *Ann Intern Med* (1990) 112, 228–30.
10. Manoukian AA, Bhagavan NV, Hayashi T, Nestor TA, Rios C, Scottolini AG. Rhabdomyolysis secondary to lovastatin therapy. *Clin Chem* (1990) 36, 2145–7.
11. Kogan AD, Orenstein S. Lovastatin-induced acute rhabdomyolysis. *Postgrad Med J* (1990) 66, 294–6.
12. Goldman JA, Fishman AB, Lee JE, Johnson RJ. The role of cholesterol-lowering agents in drug-induced rhabdomyolysis and polymyositis. *Arthritis Rheum* (1989) 32, 358–9.
13. Abdul-Ghaffar NUAMA, El-Sonbaty MR. Pancreatitis and rhabdomyolysis associated with lovastatin-gemfibrozil therapy. *J Clin Gastroenterol* (1995) 21, 340–1.
14. Chucrallah A, De Girolami U, Freeman R, Federman M. Lovastatin/gemfibrozil myopathy: a clinical, histochemical, and ultrastructural study. *Eur Neurol* (1992) 32, 293–6.
15. East C, Alivizatos PA, Grundy SM, Jones PH, Farmer JA. Rhabdomyolysis in patients receiving lovastatin after cardiac transplantation. *N Engl J Med* (1988) 318, 47–8.
16. de Alava E, Sola JJ, Lozano MD, Pardo-Mindán FJ. Rhabdomyolysis and acute renal failure in a heart transplant recipient treated with hypolipemiants. *Nephron* (1994) 66, 242–3.
17. Knoll RW, Ciafone R, Galen M. Rhabdomyolysis and renal failure secondary to combination therapy of hyperlipidemia with lovastatin and gemfibrozil. *Conn Med* (1993) 57, 593–4.
18. Illingworth DR, Bacon S. Influence of lovastatin plus gemfibrozil on plasma lipids and lipoproteins in patients with heterozygous familial hypercholesterolemia. *Circulation* (1989) 79, 590–6.
19. Glueck CJ, Oakes N, Speirs J, Tracy T, Lang J. Gemfibrozil-lovastatin therapy for primary hyperlipoproteinemias. *Am J Cardiol* (1992) 70, 1–9.
20. East C, Bilheimer DW, Grundy SM. Combination drug therapy for familial combined hyperlipidemia. *Ann Intern Med* (1988) 109, 25–32.
21. Wirebaugh SR, Shapiro ML, McIntyre TH, Whitney EJ. A retrospective review of the use of lipid-lowering agents in combination, specifically, gemfibrozil and lovastatin. *Pharmacotherapy* (1992) 12, 445–50.
22. Wiklund O, Angelin B, Bergman M, Berglund L, Bondjers G, Carlsson A, Lindén T, Miettinen T, Ödman B, Olofsson S-O, Saarinen I, Sipilä R, Sjöström P, Kron B, Vanhanen H, Wright I. Pravastatin and gemfibrozil alone and in combination for the treatment of hypercholesterolemia. *Am J Med* (1993) 94, 13–20.
23. Schneck DW, Birmingham BK, Zalikowski JA, Mitchell PD, Wang Y, Martin PD, Lasseter KC, Brown CDA, Windass AS, Raza A. The effect of gemfibrozil on the pharmacokinetics of rosuvastatin. *Clin Pharmacol Ther* (2004) 75, 455–63.
24. Van Puijenbroek EP, Du Buf-Vereijken PWG, Spooren PFMJ, Van Doormaal JJ. Possible increased risk of rhabdomyolysis during concomitant use of simvastatin and gemfibrozil. *J Intern Med* (1996) 240, 403–4.
25. Federman DG, Hussain F, Walters JB. Fatal rhabdomyolysis caused by lipid-lowering therapy. *South Med J* (2001) 94, 1023–6.
26. Tal A, Rajeshawari M, Isley W. Rhabdomyolysis associated with simvastatin-gemfibrozil therapy. *South Med J* (1997) 90, 546–7.
27. Cummins D, Mackey M, Baker E. Recovery time in a case of gemfibrozil and simvastatin-associated rhabdomyolysis. *South Med J* (2009) 102, 858–60.
28. Berland Y, Vacher Coponat H, Durand C, Baz M, Laugier R, Musso JL. Rhabdomyolysis with simvastatin use. *Nephron* (1991) 57, 365–6.
29. Oldemeyer JB, Lund RJ, Koch M, Meares AJ, Dunlay R. Rhabdomyolysis and acute renal failure after changing statin-fibrate combinations. *Cardiology* (2000) 94, 127–8.
30. Graham DJ, Staffa JA, Shatin D, Andrade SE, Schech SD, La Grenade L, Gurwitz JH, Chan KA, Goodman MJ, Platt R. Incidence of hospitalized rhabdomyolysis in patients treated with lipid-lowering drugs. *JAMA* (2004) 292, 2585–90.
31. Hedenmalm K, Alvan G, Öhagen P, Dahl M-L. Muscle toxicity with statins. *Pharmacoepidemiol Drug Safety* (2010) 19, 223–31.
32. Jones PH, Davidson MH. Reporting rate of rhabdomyolysis with fenofibrate [plus] statin versus gemfibrozil [plus] any statin. *Am J Cardiol* (2005) 95, 120–2.
33. Neuvonen PJ, Niemi M, Backman JT. Drug interactions with lipid-lowering drugs: mechanisms and clinical relevance. *Clin Pharmacol Ther* (2006) 80, 565–81.
34. Nakagomi-Hagihara R, Nakai D, Tokui T, Abe T, Ikeda T. Gemfibrozil and its glucuronide inhibit the hepatic uptake of pravastatin mediated by OATP1B1. *Xenobiotica* (2007) 37, 474–86.
35. Prueksaritanont T, Zhao JJ, Ma B, Roadcap BA, Tang C, Qui Y, Liu L, Lin JH, Pearson PG, Baillie TA. Mechanistic studies on metabolic interactions between gemfibrozil and statins. *J Pharmacol Exp Ther* (2002) 301, 1042–51.
36. Crestor (Rosuvastatin calcium). AstraZeneca. US Prescribing information, August 2013.
37. Crestor (Rosuvastatin calcium). AstraZeneca UK Ltd. UK Summary of product characteristics, May 2013.

Statins + Fibrates; Miscellaneous

Exposure to fluvastatin is slightly increased by bezafibrate, but not affected by ciprofibrate. Bezafibrate has no effect on the bioavailability of lovastatin. There is one case of rhabdomyolysis in a patient taking ciprofibrate and simvastatin. Both statins and fibrates are known to rarely cause myopathy and rhabdomyolysis, and their concurrent use increases the risk of this reaction, especially if plasma levels of the statin are also raised.

Clinical evidence

(a) Bezafibrate

In pharmacokinetic study in healthy subjects, bezafibrate slightly increased the exposure to **fluvastatin** and did not affect the exposure to **lovastatin** or its metabolite, lovastatin acid, see 'Table 30.2', p.1337. Bezafibrate pharmacokinetics were not affected by **fluvastatin**.[1,2] In a pooled analysis of clinical study data, the frequency of creatine kinase elevations was low and was not statistically significantly different between 1897 patients receiving **fluvastatin** alone (0.3%) and 1017 receiving **fluvastatin** and a fibrate (0.5%) (bezafibrate, 493; fenofibrate, 158; gemfibrozil, 366).[3]

(b) Ciprofibrate

In a retrospective review of the UK General Practice Research Database, one case of rhabdomyolysis was identified in a 63-year-old man who had been taking stable doses [not stated] of ciprofibrate and **simvastatin** concurrently for more than 3 years. No change in other drug therapy had occurred in the 6 months before diagnosis. He later resumed taking simvastatin without problems. Note that 2935 concurrent users of statins and fibrates were identified in this database.[4]

The UK manufacturer of **fluvastatin** briefly reports that the concurrent use of ciprofibrate has no clinically relevant effect on the bioavailability of **fluvastatin**.[1]

(c) Unspecified fibrates

In a review[5] of the FDA spontaneous reports of statin-associated rhabdomyolysis covering the period November 1997 to March 2000, fibrates (unspecified) were potentially implicated in 10 of 73 cases of rhabdomyolysis seen with **atorvastatin**, 4 of 10 cases with **fluvastatin**, 5 of 40 cases with **lovastatin**, 6 of 71 cases with **pravastatin**, and 33 of 215 cases with **simvastatin**.

Mechanism

Complex and not fully understood. Myopathy can occur with statins and fibrates alone and their effects might therefore be additive or synergistic. Pharmacokinetic interactions might contribute to the increased risk.

Importance and management

Data on the specific interaction of bezafibrate or ciprofibrate with statins are limited, but there are data for fibrates in general, and particularly with gemfibrozil (see 'Statins + Fibrates; Gemfibrozil', p.1338), to suggest an increased risk of myopathy and rhabdomyolysis on their concurrent use with statins. Consequently, in general, the concurrent use of a statin and any fibrate, including bezafibrate and ciprofibrate, should be undertaken only if the benefits of treatment outweigh the risks, using the lowest effective doses and with careful monitoring for toxicity. The UK manufacturer of bezafibrate specifically contraindicates the concurrent use of a statin if patients have predisposing risk factors for myopathy (such as renal impairment and hypothyroidism).[6] Some statin manufacturers give statin dose recommendations for the concurrent use of any fibrate, which would therefore apply to bezafibrate and ciprofibrate, as follows: for **simvastatin** maximum 10 mg daily (UK advice);[7] for **rosuvastatin** 5 mg daily starting dose, with the 40 mg daily dose contraindicated (UK advice).[8] As a general rule, for any patient given a statin and a fibrate, the advice to report any signs of myopathy and possible rhabdomyolysis (i.e. otherwise unexplained muscle pain, tenderness or weakness or dark coloured urine) should be specifically reinforced. If myopathy does occur, the fibrate and statin should be stopped immediately. See also *Muscle and liver toxicity* under 'Lipid regulating drugs', p.1309, for further guidance on monitoring and risk factors for muscle toxicity.

1. Lescol (Fluvastatin sodium). Novartis Pharmaceuticals UK Ltd. UK Summary of product characteristics, November 2013.
2. Novartis Pharmaceuticals Ltd. Personal communication. 28 February 2011.
3. Farnier M, Bortolini M, Salko T, Freudenreich M-O, Isaacsohn JL, Troendle AJ, Gonasun L. Frequency of creatine kinase elevation during treatment with fluvastatin in combination with fibrates (bezafibrate, fenofibrate, or gemfibrozil). *Am J Cardiol* (2003) 91, 238–40.
4. Black C, Jick H. Etiology and frequency of rhabdomyolysis. *Pharmacotherapy* (2002) 22, 1524–6.
5. Omar MA, Wilson JP. FDA adverse event reports on statin-associated rhabdomyolysis. *Ann Pharmacother* (2002) 36, 288–95.
6. Bezalip Mono (Bezafibrate). Actavis UK Ltd. UK Summary of product characteristics, December 2009.
7. Zocor (Simvastatin). Merck Sharp & Dohme Ltd. UK Summary of product characteristics, June 2015.
8. Crestor (Rosuvastatin calcium). AstraZeneca UK Ltd. UK Summary of product characteristics, May 2013.

Statins + Fish oils

Omega-3 marine triglycerides do not alter the pharmacokinetics of atorvastatin, rosuvastatin, or simvastatin.

Clinical evidence, mechanism, importance and management

In a randomised, crossover study in 23 subjects, omega-3-acid ethyl esters (*Omacor*) 4 g daily did not alter the steady-state pharmacokinetics of **simvastatin** 80 mg daily when both drugs were given together for 14 days, compared with when simvastatin was given alone.[1] In two very similar studies, omega-3-acid ethyl esters (*Lovaza* formerly marketed as *Omacor*) 4 g daily did not alter the steady-state pharmacokinetics of **atorvastatin** 80 mg daily[2] or **rosuvastatin** 40 mg daily[3] compared with either drug alone.

No adjustments to the doses of these statins would appear to be necessary on the concurrent use of omega-3-acid ethyl esters.

1. McKenney JM, Swearingen D, Di Spirito M, Doyle R, Pantaleon C, Kling D, Shalwitz RA. Study of the pharmacokinetic interaction between simvastatin and prescription omega-3-acid ethyl esters. *J Clin Pharmacol* (2006) 46, 785–91.
2. Di Spirito M, Morelli G, Doyle RT, Johnson J, McKenney J. Effect of omega-3-acid ethyl esters on steady-state plasma pharmacokinetics of atorvastatin in healthy adults. *Expert Opin Pharmacother* (2008) 9, 2939–45.
3. Gosai P, Liu J, Doyle RT, Johnson J, Carter R, Sica D, McKenney JM. Effect of omega-3-acid ethyl esters on the steady-state plasma pharmacokinetics of rosuvastatin in healthy adults. *Expert Opin Pharmacother* (2008) 9, 2947–53.

Statins + Fusidic acid

Myopathy or rhabdomyolysis has been described in a number of patients taking atorvastatin, rosuvastatin, or simvastatin and given fusidic acid; some have been fatal.

Clinical evidence

Numerous case reports describe myopathy or rhabdomyolysis, sometimes fatal, with the use of fusidic acid and **atorvastatin**, **rosuvastatin**, and **simvastatin**. The details are summarised in 'Table 30.3', p.1341. Of these three statins, the effect has been most commonly reported with atorvastatin. In one of the **atorvastatin** cases,[1] the patient was also prescribed ciprofloxacin, which was reported to result in rhabdomyolysis when given to a patient taking simvastatin (see 'Statins; Simvastatin + Ciprofloxacin', p.1359). Note also that one of the **simvastatin** cases[2] included use of clarithromycin 2 weeks prior to starting fusidic acid (see also, 'Statins + Macrolides', p.1348), and a fatal **rosuvastatin** case[3] describes the use of rifampicin (see also, 'Statins + Rifampicin (Rifampin)', p.1355).

For a case where simvastatin was originally considered to be interacting with tacrolimus rather than fusidic acid, see 'Statins + Tacrolimus', p.1357.

Mechanism

Unknown. Fusidic acid is not a known inhibitor of any of the enzymes or transporter proteins known to affect atorvastatin, rosuvastatin, or simvastatin metabolism (CYP3A4, OATP1B1). There are no studies on the effect of fusidic acid on the pharmacokinetics of these statins.

Importance and management

Evidence for an interaction between fusidic acid and the statins is limited to case reports, but they are numerous, given the fact that fusidic acid is not a commonly used antibacterial. An interaction is not established, but taken together they add a note of caution on their concurrent use, and a role for fusidic acid in these cases cannot be ruled out in the absence of other information. Further study is needed to establish the mechanism and incidence. Note also that generally the cases described had other risk factors for myopathy or rhabdomyolysis. If fusidic acid is required in a patient taking **atorvastatin**, **rosuvastatin**, or **simvastatin**, the advice to report any symptoms suggestive of myopathy and rhabdomyolysis (i.e. otherwise unexplained muscle pain, tenderness, or weakness or dark coloured urine) should be specifically reinforced. If myopathy does occur, the statin should be stopped immediately.

Note that, in September 2011, the MHRA stated that systemic fusidic acid (tablets, suspension, and intravenous infusion) should not be given with **any statin** (on the basis that the mechanism is unknown). They recommended that if fusidic acid is essential, the statin be temporarily discontinued until 7 days after the last dose of the fusidic acid.[4] However, bear in mind that fusidic acid might be required long-term because of the nature of the infections it is used to treat. The MHRA also stated that the need for the concurrent use of a statin and fusidic acid in case of prolonged treatment should be considered on an individual basis with close medical supervision.[4] However, in August 2012, updated guidance specifically for **simvastatin**, advised that the concurrent use of fusidic acid should be closely monitored, and prescribers should consider temporarily stopping the statin.[5]

The authors of one case series[2] suggest that creatine kinase concentrations should be regularly monitored in any patient with diabetes taking a statin if fusidic acid is required for longer than 2 weeks; however, routine monitoring of creatine kinase in the absence of clinical signs of myopathy has been reported to be of little clinical value, see *Muscle and liver toxicity*, under 'Lipid regulating drugs', p.1309, for this and for further general guidance on monitoring, and risk factors for muscle toxicity.

This guidance would not apply to topical use of fusidic acid as creams and eye drops.

1. Nwaejike N, Sidhu P. A note to cardiothoracic surgeons: Statins can interact with ciprofloxacin and fusidic acid to cause rhabdomyolysis and myoglobinuric renal failure. *Internet J Thorac Cardiovasc Surg* (2006). Available at: http://ispub.com/IJTCVS/8/2/8615 (accessed 25/10/15).
2. Collidge TA, Razvi S, Nolan C, Whittle M, Stirling C, Russell AJC, Mann AC, Deighan CJ. Severe statin-induced rhabdomyolysis mimicking Guillain-Barré syndrome in four patients with diabetes mellitus treated with fusidic acid. *Diabet Med* (2010) 27, 696–700.
3. Cowan R, Johnson PD, Urbancic K, Grayson ML. A timely reminder about the concomitant use of fusidic acid with statins. *Clin Infect Dis* (2013) 57, 329–30.
4. Medicines and Healthcare Products Regulatory Agency and the Commission on Human Medicines. Systemic fusidic acid and interaction with statins: risk of rhabdomyolysis. *Drug Safety Update* (2011) 5, A1. Available at: https://www.gov.uk/drug-safety-update/systemic-fusidic-acid-and-interaction-with-statins (accessed 20/10/15).
5. Medicines and Healthcare Products Regulatory Agency and the Commission on Human Medicines. Simvastatin: updated advice on drug interactions - updated contraindications. *Drug Safety Update* (2012) 6, S1. Available at: https://www.gov.uk/drug-safety-update/simvastatin-updated-advice-on-drug-interactions (accessed 20/10/15).

Statins + Garlic

A garlic extract did not affect the pharmacokinetics of single doses of simvastatin or pravastatin in one study. Garlic oil with black seed enhanced the lipid-lowering effects of simvastatin in another study.

Clinical evidence

In a randomised, crossover study in 10 healthy subjects, garlic extract (Garlipure caplets) 600 mg twice daily for 21 days had no effect on the pharmacokinetics of single 20-mg doses of **pravastatin** or **simvastatin**.[1] In another randomised study, 258 hyperlipidaemic patients were given **simvastatin** 10 mg daily with placebo, or with black seed (*Nigella sativa*) 500 mg daily and garlic oil 250 mg daily, for 8 weeks. Patients taking simvastatin with black seed and garlic showed much greater decreases in concentrations of triglycerides, LDL-cholesterol, HDL-cholesterol, total cholesterol, and non-HDL-cholesterol than those patients who took simvastatin and placebo (18.9 to 29.4% decreases vs 6.9 to 10.8%, respectively).[2]

Mechanism

In one of the studies[1] subjects were tested for CYP3A4 activity. Garlic extract was found not to affect CYP3A4 in either the liver or the intestine. Simvastatin is metabolised by CYP3A4 and therefore the concurrent use of garlic extract did not affect simvastatin pharmacokinetics. Garlic and black seed are said to have lipid-lowering properties and therefore the authors of the study in hyperlipidaemic patients suggest an additive effect with simvastatin,[2] although the contribution of garlic cannot be ascertained from this study design.

Importance and management

Evidence for an interaction between garlic extract and statins appears to be limited to the two studies cited. The results of the single-dose study using simvastatin and pravastatin, suggest no interaction. The results of the study in hyperlipidaema patients suggest an additive effect of garlic (and black seed) on the cholesterol-lowering capacity of simvastatin, but further study with garlic alone would be needed to determine its effect. Therefore, the results of these studies together with what is known about the metabolism of statins, and the effects of garlic extract on drug metabolising enzymes, suggest that no pharmacokinetic interaction would be expected, but an additive pharmacodynamic effect of garlic cannot be ruled out.

1. Hajda J, Rentsch KM, Gubler C, Steinert H, Steiger B, Fattinger K. Garlic extract induces intestinal P-glycoprotein, but exhibits no effect on intestinal and hepatic CYP3A4 in humans. *Eur J Pharm Sci* (2010) 41, 729–35.
2. Ahmad Alobaidi AH. Effect of Nigella sativa and Allium sativum coadministered with simvastatin in dyslipidemia patients: a prospective, randomized, double-blind trial. *Antiinflamm Antiallergy Agents Med Chem* (2014) 13, 68–74.

Statins + Ginkgo (*Ginkgo biloba*)

Ginkgo slightly decreased the exposure to simvastatin and negligibly decreased that of atorvastatin.

Clinical evidence

In a crossover study in 14 healthy subjects, ginkgo tablets 120 mg daily (containing 40 mg of standardised *Ginkgo biloba* extract) decreased the AUC and maximum

Table 30.3 Case reports of myopathy or rhabdomyolysis with statins and fusidic acid

Patient(s)	*Fusidic acid dose*	*Statin dose*	*Notes*	*Refs*
Atorvastatin				
66-year-old	1.5 g daily	10 mg daily	Two weeks after starting the combination, the patient was admitted with progressive muscle weakness and pain in both legs. His serum creatine kinase was 3550 units/L and he had increased myoglobin concentrations. Both continued to increase for 5 days after the atorvastatin and fusidic acid were stopped, and then gradually returned to normal over one week. Serum concentrations of both fusidic acid and atorvastatin were higher than expected.	1
74-year-old	500 mg three times daily	40 mg daily	Rhabdomyolysis developed 6 weeks after starting fusidic acid and flucloxacillin 500 mg three times daily for osteomyelitis of the foot.	2
4 patients	1.5 g daily	20 or 40 mg daily	3 cases of fatal rhabdomyolysis when fusidic acid added for osteomyelitis or septic arthritis. Two patients had renal failure.	3
65-year-old	500 mg three times daily	40 mg daily	Rhabdomyolysis diagnosed after fusidic acid being taken with atorvastatin for one month. Diagnosis was delayed due to similarity of symptoms with Guillain-Barré syndrome.	4
69-year-old	2.25 g daily	40 mg daily	Muscle weakness, greatly increased creatine kinase (21 652 units/L) and deranged liver function tests were observed in a patient with multi-organ failure about 10 days after flucloxacillin 2 g daily and fusidic acid were added to atorvastatin. The patient was also taking ezetimibe. Four days after atorvastatin, ezetimibe, and fusidic acid were stopped the patient was able to walk, but remained on dialysis for a further 10 days. Two months after diagnosis his creatine kinase concentration was within normal range and he had regained his muscle power.	5
68-year-old	500 mg three times daily	80 mg daily	Muscle weakness and rhabdomyolysis occurred in a patient taking atorvastatin 7 months after fusidic acid was started. His creatine kinase was 74 000units/L and both drugs were stopped. After a few days his creatine kinase was normalising and he was mobile again.	6
5 patients	Not stated	20 to 60 mg daily	Muscle weakness and rhabdomyolysis developed 2 to 5 weeks after fusidic acid was started. One patient died, and the other 4 were all independent on discharge.	7
58-year-old	500 mg three times daily	40 mg daily	Weakness and fatigue developed one week after starting fusidic acid and ciprofloxacin 500 mg twice daily. His creatine kinase was 56 500 units/L and atorvastatin, fusidic acid and ciprofloxacin were stopped.	8
48-year-old	500 mg three times daily	40 mg daily	Two weeks after fusidic acid with linezolid 600 mg twice daily were added to atorvastatin the patient reported nausea and vomiting. His creatine kinase was 759 units/L, and his liver transaminase concentrations were increased. Acute hepatitis and rhabdomyolysis (creatine kinase 214 260 units/L) were diagnosed 5 days later and all drugs were stopped. After 3 weeks of treatment his creatine kinase and liver transaminase concentrations were within normal ranges and he regained his mobility.	9
Rosuvastatin				
1 patient	Not stated	20 mg daily	Muscle weakness and rhabdomyolysis developed 2 weeks after fusidic acid was started. The patient was independently mobile on discharge.	7
83-year-old	500 mg twice daily	Not stated	Post hip surgery, the patient was started on rifampicin and fusidic acid for lifelong suppressive treatment of *Staphylococcus aureus* infection of the hip, and his atorvastatin was changed to rosuvastatin to avoid an interaction with rifampicin. After 2 weeks, the patient was urgently readmitted with delirium, deteriorating renal function, and severe rhabdomyolysis (creatine kinase 11 627 units/L). All medication was stopped, renal replacement therapy was started, but on day 12 active treatment was withdrawn and the patient died.	10
Simvastatin				
78-year-old		10 mg daily	Rhabdomyolysis developed 15 days after starting fusidic acid, having been taking simvastatin for 10 months. The patient recovered after stopping both drugs.	11
71-year-old 63-year-old	Not stated	40 mg daily	Rhabdomyolysis and acute renal failure developed postoperatively after about 4 weeks of fusidic acid for resistant infections.	12,13
3 patients	500 mg three times daily	20 or 40 mg daily	Painless, severe, flaccid paralysis suggestive of Guillain-Barré syndrome, ultimately diagnosed as rhabdomyolysis, occurred in 3 diabetic patients, 18 to 28 days after starting fusidic acid. One had also received clarithromycin 250 mg twice daily for 7 days, completed 2 weeks before starting the fusidic acid. Two were treated with immunoglobulin for suspected Guillain-Barré syndrome.	4
2 patients	Not stated	40 mg daily	Muscle weakness and rhabdomyolysis developed 2 to 3 weeks after fusidic acid was started. One patient died, and the other was not considered independent on discharge.	7

Continued

Table 30.3 Case reports of myopathy or rhabdomyolysis with statins and fusidic acid (continued)

Patient(s)	*Fusidic acid dose*	*Statin dose*	*Notes*	*Refs*
68-year-old	500 mg three times daily	40 mg daily	Extensive muscle pains developed within a few weeks of fusidic acid and flucloxacillin 500 mg four times daily being added to simvastatin. Creatine kinase was 168 351 units/L and his liver function tests were abnormal. Fluids were started and the following day fusidic acid and simvastatin were stopped due to a suspected interaction. His creatine kinase peaked on day 2 and 3 months later was still higher than normal, and he still had mild muscle pains.	14

1. Wenisch C, Krause R, Fladerer P, El Menjawi I, Pohanka E. Acute rhabdomyolysis after atorvastatin and fusidic acid therapy. *Am J Med* (2000) 109, 78.
2. O'Mahony C, Campbell VL, Al-Khayatt MS, Brull DJ. Rhabdomyolysis with atorvastatin and fusidic acid. *Postgrad Med J* (2008) 84, 325–7.
3. Magee CN, Medani SA, Leavey SF, Conlon PJ, Clarkson MR. Severe rhabdomyolysis as a consequence of the interaction of fusidic acid and atorvastatin. *Am J Kidney Dis* (2010) 56, e11–e15.
4. Collidge TA, Razvi S, Nolan C, Whittle M, Stirling C, Russell AJC, Mann AC, Deighan CJ. Severe statin-induced rhabdomyolysis mimicking Guillain-Barré syndrome in four patients with diabetes mellitus treated with fusidic acid. *Diabet Med* (2010) 27, 696–700.
5. Teckchandani S, Robertson S, Almond A, Donaldson K, Isles C. Rhadomyolysis following co-prescription of fusidic acid and atorvastatin. *J R Coll Physicians Edinb* (2010) 40, 33–6.
6. Gabignon C, Zeller V, Le Guyader N, Desplaces N, Lidove O, Ziza JM. Interaction atorvastatine et acide fusidique: une cause de rhabdomyloyse severe. *Rev Med Interne* (2013) 34, 39–41.
7. Kearney S, Carr AS, McConville J, McCarron MO. Rhabdomyolysis after co-prescription of statin and fusidic acid. *BMJ* (2012) 345, e6562.
8. Nwaejike N, Sidhu P. A note to cardiothoracic surgeons: Statins can interact with ciprofloxacin and fusidic acid to cause rhabdomyolysis and myolobinuric renal failure. *Internet J Thorac Cardiovasc Surg* (2006). Available at: http://ispub.com/IJTCVS/8/2/8615, p. (accessed 13/08/15).
9. Saeed NTM, Azam M. Rhabdomyolysis secondary to interaction between atorvastatin and fusidic acid. *BMJ Case Rep* (2009) 2040.
10. Cowan R, Johnson PDR, Urbancic K, Grayson ML. A timely reminder about the concomitant use of fusidic acid with statins. *Clin Infect Dis* (2013) 57, 329–30.
11. Dromer C, Vedrenne C, Billey T, Pages M, Fournié B, Fournié A. Rhabdomyolyse à la simvastatine: a propos d'un cas avec revue de la littérature. *Rev Rhum Mal Osteoartic* (1992) 59, 281–3.
12. Yuen SLS, McGarity B. Rhabdomyolysis secondary to interaction of fusidic acid and simvastatin. *Med J Aust* (2003) 179, 172.
13. Burtenshaw AJ, Sellors G, Downing R. Presumed interaction of fusidic acid with simvastatin. *Anaesthesia* (2008) 63, 656–8.
14. Herring R, Caldwell G, Wade S. Rhabdomyolysis caused by an interaction of simvastatin and fusidic acid. *BMJ Case Rep* (2009) 1722.

concentration of **simvastatin** 40 mg daily (both given for 14 days) by 39% and 32%, respectively. There was no change in the pharmacokinetics of the simvastatin metabolite, simvastatin acid. These pharmacokinetic changes did not alter the lipid-lowering effects of simvastatin.[1] Another study in 16 healthy subjects found that ginkgo tablets 120 mg three times daily for 14 days, decreased the AUC and maximum concentration of a single 40-mg dose of **atorvastatin** given on day 15 by about 12% and 29%, respectively. The pharmacokinetics of atorvastatin metabolites were not altered, and neither was the efficacy of atorvastatin.[2]

Mechanism

Simvastatin and to a lesser extent, atorvastatin, are metabolised by CYP3A4. The results of these studies therefore suggest that ginkgo might induce CYP3A4, however this was not confirmed with the usual CYP3A4 probe substrate, midazolam, (see 'Benzodiazepines + Ginkgo (*Ginkgo biloba*)', p.821). The authors of the atorvastatin study[2] suggest possible involvement of the organic anion transporting polypeptide, OATP1B1, which is important in the transportation of atorvastatin into the liver. Further study is needed to establish the mechanism involved.

Importance and management

Evidence for an interaction between the statins and ginkgo is limited to studies with simvastatin and atorvastatin, which found slight and negligible decreases, respectively, in their exposures. However, such changes are unlikely to be clinically important and the efficacy of these statins is unlikely to be affected; this was demonstrated in the studies, although note that they were conducted in healthy subjects and not patients with hyperlipidaemia. Other statins would also seem unlikely to be affected given the similarities in their metabolism to simvastatin and atorvastatin (see 'Lipid regulating drugs', p.1309 for details). No statin dose adjustments would seem necessary on concurrent use with ginkgo.

1. Dai LL, Fan L, Wu HZ, Tan ZR, Chen Y, Peng XD, Shen MX, Yang GP, Zhou HH. Assessment of a pharmacokinetic and pharmacodynamic interaction between simvastatin and Ginkgo biloba extracts in healthy subjects. *Xenobiotica* (2013) 43, 862–7.
2. Guo CX, Pei Q, Yin JY, Peng XD, Zhou BT, Zhao YC, Wu LX, Meng XG, Wang G, Li Q, Ouyang DS, Liu ZQ, Zhang W, Zhou HH. Effects of Ginkgo biloba extracts on pharmacokinetics and efficacy of atorvastatin based plasma indices. *Xenobiotica* (2012) 42, 784–90.

Statins + Glucagon-like peptide-1 receptor agonists

Exenatide slightly decreased the exposure to lovastatin, but no clear pattern of altered efficacy of statins was noted in exenatide clinical studies. Liraglutide and dulaglutide appear to have no effect on the exposure to atorvastatin. Albiglutide appears to slightly decrease the exposure to simvastatin. Taking lixisenatide at the same time as atorvastatin had no effect on atorvastatin exposure, but separating their administration slightly increased atorvastatin exposure.

Clinical evidence, mechanism, importance and management

(a) Albiglutide

The US manufacturer briefly reports that, in a study, albiglutide 50 mg weekly for 5 weeks decreased the AUC of a single 80-mg dose of **simvastatin** by 40%, and increased that of its active metabolite, simvastatin acid, by 36%. The maximum concentration of simvastatin was increased by 18%, and that of simvastatin acid, by 98%. They comment that the clinical relevance of such changes has not been established.[1] However, such slight increases in exposure would not be expected to be clinically relevant, although note that the effect on multiple-dose simvastatin is not known.

(b) Dulaglutide

The UK and US manufacturers briefly report that, in a study, dulaglutide (dose not stated) decreased the AUC and maximum concentration of **atorvastatin** (dose not stated) by about 21% and 70%, respectively. They note that such a decrease is not clinically relevant, and that no atorvastatin dose adjustment is necessary on concurrent use.[2,3]

(c) Exenatide

In a crossover study in healthy subjects, exenatide 10 micrograms twice daily for 3 days decreased the AUC of a single 40-mg dose of **lovastatin** given on day 2 by 40%, decreased its maximum concentration by 28%, and increased the median time to its maximum concentration by 4 hours.[4] In a retrospective analysis of three phase III clinical studies of exenatide in patients with type 2 diabetes, the use of exenatide for 30 weeks in the subset of 348 patients already taking statins (51% **atorvastatin**, 31% **simvastatin**, 11% **pravastatin**, 5% **lovastatin**, 3% **fluvastatin**) was not associated with consistent changes in lipid profiles or statin doses when compared with placebo.[4]

The clinical effect of the slight decrease in lovastatin exposure with exenatide is unclear, but experience from clinical studies suggests that it is unlikely to be clinically relevant.

(d) Liraglutide

A preliminary report of a randomised, crossover study in 42 healthy subjects, states that steady-state liraglutide 1.8 mg daily decreased the maximum concentration of a single 40-mg dose of **atorvastatin**, given 5 hours after the liraglutide, by 38%. Its median time to maximum concentration was delayed by 1.25 hours, but there was no change in the overall exposure (AUC).[5]

The small delay in the rate of absorption of atorvastatin and the lack of effect on its exposure with concurrent use of liraglutide are unlikely to have clinically relevant adverse effects. Therefore, no adjustment of the atorvastatin dose is likely to be needed in patients also given liraglutide.

(e) Lixisenatide

The UK manufacturer briefly reports that, in a study, when lixisenatide 20 micrograms and **atorvastatin** 40 mg were given together in the morning for 6 days, the atorvastatin AUC was not altered, but the maximum concentration was decreased by 31% and the time to maximum concentration was delayed by about 3 hours. No increase in time to maximum concentration was seen when the lixisenatide was given in the morning and the atorvastatin in the evening, but the atorvastatin AUC and maximum concentration were increased by 27% and 66%, respectively. These changes are not considered clinically relevant and no atorvastatin dose adjustment is necessary.[6]

1. Tanzeum (Albiglutide). GlaxoSmithKline LLC. US Prescribing information, May 2015.
2. Trulicity (Dulaglutide). Eli Lilly and Company Ltd. UK Summary of product characteristics, November 2014.
3. Trulicity (Dulaglutide). Eli Lilly and Company. US Prescribing information, March 2015.
4. Kothare PA, Linnebjerg H, Skrivanek Z, Reddy S, Mace K, Pena A, Han J, Fineman M, Mitchell M. Exenatide effects on statin pharmacokinetics and lipid response. *Int J Clin Pharmacol Ther* (2007) 45, 114–20.
5. Malm-Erjefalt M, Ekblom M, Brondsted L, Vouis J, Lennernas H, Zdravkovic M. A randomized, double-blind, cross-over trial investigating the effect of liraglutide on the absorption pharmacokinetics of concomitantly administered oral drugs in healthy subjects. *Diabetes* (2008) 57 (Suppl 1), A130.
6. Lyxumia (Lixisenatide). Sanofi. UK Summary of product characteristics, October 2014.

Statins + Glucosamine

Glucosamine does not appear to alter the effects of statins and is unlikely to have additive effects.

Clinical evidence

In a crossover study in patients taking **atorvastatin** (13 patients) or **simvastatin** (21 patients), the addition of *Artrox* (glucosamine hydrochloride 750 mg) twice daily for 4 weeks had no effect on HDL, LDL, total cholesterol, or triglyceride concentrations.[1] However, note that the atorvastatin group did not contain enough patients for statistical power. In another study in patients not taking statins, glucosamine (as glucosamine sulphate 1.5 g daily) did not alter HDL, LDL, total cholesterol, or triglyceride concentrations.[2]

Mechanism

Glucosamine is not known to affect CYP3A4 by which simvastatin and (to a lesser extent) atorvastatin are metabolised, and so would not be expected to interact via this mechanism. No additive effects with statins would be expected as glucosamine alone does not appear to alter lipid concentrations.

Importance and management

Evidence is very limited, but that which exists suggests that glucosamine does not alter the effects of statins, and it is not likely to have additive effects if taken with a statin. No special precautions would seem necessary on concurrent use.

1. Eggertsen R, Andreasson A, Andrén L. No changes of cholesterol levels with a commercially available glucosamine product in patients treated with lipid lowering drugs: a controlled, randomised, open cross-over trial. *BMC Pharmacol Toxicol* (2012) Epub.
2. Østergaard K, Hviid T, Hyllested-Winge JL. The effect of glucosamine sulphate on the blood levels of cholesterol or triglycerides-a clinical study. *Ugeskr Laeger* (2007) 169, 407–10.

Statins + Grapefruit and other fruit juices

When taken at the same time, large amounts of grapefruit juice markedly to very markedly increase lovastatin and simvastatin exposure, and also moderately increase atorvastatin exposure. Smaller amounts of grapefruit juice and separating administration by 12 hours have lesser effect. Pitavastatin and pravastatin seem not to be affected by grapefruit juice, but orange juice appears to slightly increase the absorption of pravastatin. An isolated case describes rhabdomyolysis in a patient taking simvastatin after starting to eat grapefruit, and another case occurred in a patient taking rosuvastatin after starting to drink pomegranate juice.

Clinical evidence

(a) Atorvastatin

Twelve healthy subjects were given 200 mL of *double-strength* grapefruit juice three times daily for 5 days. On day 3 they were given a single 40-mg dose of atorvastatin with the grapefruit juice then two more 200-mL doses of grapefruit juice, one after 30 minutes and the other after 90 minutes. The AUC of atorvastatin lactone (inactive) and atorvastatin acid (active) were increased 3.3-fold and 2.5-fold, respectively, and the AUC of 2-hydroxyatorvastatin (active) decreased slightly by 26%. Overall, the AUC of active HMG-CoA reductase inhibitors was increased by about 30%.[1] Other similar studies, using 250 mL of *single-strength* grapefruit three times a day, have found smaller increases in atorvastatin acid levels of 40% and 83%.[2,3] Similarly, the manufacturers report that one 240-mL glass of grapefruit juice has a more modest effect, causing an increase of only 37% in the AUC of atorvastatin and a 20% decrease in the AUC of 2-hydroxyatorvastatin.[4]

(b) Lovastatin

Ten healthy subjects were given 200 mL of *double-strength* grapefruit juice three times daily for 3 days. On day 3 they took lovastatin 80 mg with 200 mL of grapefruit juice, then two more 200-mL doses of grapefruit juice, one after 30 minutes and the other after 90 minutes. The mean peak serum levels of the lovastatin and its active metabolite, lovastatin acid, were increased 12-fold and fourfold, respectively, and the mean AUCs were increased 15-fold and fivefold, respectively.[5] However, in another study in which lovastatin 40 mg was given in the evening and *single-strength* grapefruit juice was taken with breakfast daily for 3 days, the AUC and maximum serum level of lovastatin were approximately doubled, and the AUC and maximum serum level of lovastatin acid were only increased by 60%. The AUC of active HMG-CoA reductase inhibitors was increased by about 35%.[6] It has been suggested that if the grapefruit juice had been given at the same time as the lovastatin in the latter study[6] then much greater increases in the AUC and maximum serum levels would have been found.[7]

(c) Pitavastatin

A study in 8 healthy subjects found that 250 mL of *single-strength* grapefruit juice three times daily for 4 days had a minimal effect on the pharmacokinetics of a single dose of pitavastatin 4 mg taken simultaneously with the first 250 mL of juice given on day 4. The AUC of pitavastatin acid was increased by 13% and that of pitavastatin lactone by 30%.[3]

(d) Pravastatin

Grapefruit juice did not affect the pharmacokinetics of a single 40-mg dose of pravastatin in healthy subjects. In this study, 200 mL of *double-strength* grapefruit juice was given three times daily for 2 days, and then on the third day 200 mL was given with the pravastatin and again after 30 and 90 minutes.[1] A further study using 10 mg of pravastatin similarly found that *single-strength* grapefruit juice did not affect pravastatin pharmacokinetics.[2]

In a study in 14 healthy subjects a total of 800 mL of **orange juice**, was given over about 3 hours, starting 15 minutes before a 10-mg dose of pravastatin. **Orange juice** increased the AUC_{0-4} of pravastatin by 50%, without affecting the maximum pravastatin levels or elimination half-life.[8]

(e) Rosuvastatin

A case report describes a 48-year-old man taking ezetimibe 10 mg daily, and rosuvastatin 5 mg on alternate days, who developed rhabdomyolysis within 3 weeks of starting to drink 200 mL of **pomegranate juice** twice weekly. Although the patient had been stable taking ezetimibe with rosuvastatin for 15 months he had a history of myopathy with statins and had an elevated creatine kinase before statin treatment was started.[9]

(f) Simvastatin

Ten healthy subjects were given 200 mL of *double-strength* grapefruit juice three times daily for 2 days. On day 3 they took 60 mg of simvastatin with 200 mL of grapefruit juice, then two more 200-mL doses of grapefruit juice, one after 30 minutes and the other after 90 minutes. The mean peak serum levels of the simvastatin and simvastatin acid were increased ninefold and sevenfold, respectively, and the mean AUCs were increased 16-fold and sevenfold, respectively. Overall, the AUC of active HMG-CoA reductase inhibitors was increased about 2.4-fold.[10] In a further study by the same research group using an identical grapefruit juice regimen, the AUC of 40 mg of simvastatin was increased 13.5-fold and the AUC of simvastatin acid 4.5-fold. However, when the simvastatin was given 24 hours after the last dose of grapefruit juice (same dosage regimen) the AUC of simvastatin and simvastatin acid were increased 2.1-fold and by 70%. When simvastatin was given 3 days after the last dose of grapefruit juice, the simvastatin AUC was increased 40% and there was no change in AUC of simvastatin acid. At 7 days there was no change.[11] The manufacturers of simvastatin note a slightly lower effect when drinking 240 mL of *single-strength* grapefruit juice in the morning and taking 20 mg of simvastatin in the evening: the AUC of simvastatin increased by 90% and that of simvastatin acid by 30%.[12,13] Another study found as little as 200 mL of *single-strength* grapefruit juice daily for 3 days could increase the AUC of a single 40-mg dose of simvastatin taken simultaneously with the juice on day 3, 3.6-fold, and its metabolite, simvastatin acid, 3.3-fold.[14]

A case report describes a 40-year-old patient with familial hypercholesterolaemia (otherwise healthy) taking simvastatin 80 mg daily (dose increased 6 months before presentation), who presented with rhabdomyolysis 14 days after she started to eat one fresh grapefruit a day (she did not eat the peel and drank no additional grapefruit juice). Symptoms of muscle weakness and myalgia appeared within 4 days of starting the grapefruit, and gradually increased.[15]

Mechanism

Some components of grapefruit juice (including furanocoumarin derivatives and flavonoids such as naringenin), inhibit the activity of CYP3A4 in the gut wall, thereby reducing the metabolism of the affected statins (lovastatin and simvastatin, and to a lesser extent atorvastatin) as they are absorbed, and allowing more to pass into the body (see 'Lipid regulating drugs', p.1309, for more information about the metabolism of the statins). This interaction is most marked when the grapefruit juice and statin are taken simultaneously.

The reason for the increased absorption of pravastatin with orange juice is unclear, but may involve an effect on organic anion transporter proteins (OATPs), and is not via CYP3A4. In a study in *animals*, orange juice increased pravastatin bioavailability and did not affect simvastatin bioavailability.[8]

Although pomegranate juice has been shown to inhibit CYP3A4,[9] rosuvastatin is not metabolised by this route, so there is no known pharmacokinetic mechanism to explain the case of rhabdomyolysis with this combination.

Importance and management

Information about the interaction of statins and grapefruit juice seems to be mainly limited to pharmacokinetic reports (i.e. few adverse case reports) but they are consistent with the way other CYP3A4 inhibitors interact with the statins. The moderate increases in **lovastatin** and **simvastatin** exposure seen with usual doses of grapefruit juice are potentially hazardous because elevated statin levels carry the risk of toxicity (muscle damage and the possible development of rhabdomyolysis). On the basis of the available data, lovastatin or simvastatin should not be taken simultaneously with grapefruit juice. The interaction can be minimised, but not eliminated, if these statins are taken in the evening (as recommended), and a small quantity of grapefruit juice is taken at breakfast time. However, as even small quantities of grapefruit juice taken in the morning can still affect simvastatin levels, the UK and US manufacturers of simvastatin and the US manufacturer of lovastatin state that concurrent use should be avoided.[12,13,16] See also *Muscle and liver toxicity,* under 'Lipid regulating drugs', p.1309, for further guidance on monitoring and risk factors for muscle toxicity. The interaction with grapefruit juice is not usually applied to eating grapefruit, but the case report with simvastatin and grapefruit suggests some caution might be warranted. Bear the possibility of an interaction in mind.

The moderate increase in **atorvastatin** exposure when taken with usual doses of grapefruit juice seems less likely to be clinically relevant, but the UK manufacturer suggests that large quantities of grapefruit juice (greater than 1.2 litres daily) are not recommended.[4] In general, the occasional glass of grapefruit juice would not appear to be a problem. **Pitavastatin** and **pravastatin** seem not to interact with grapefruit juice. Information about other statins appears to be lacking, but no interaction would be expected with **fluvastatin** or **rosuvastatin**, as these statins are not appreciably metabolised by CYP3A4.

The interaction of pravastatin with **orange juice** would be expected to be of little clinical relevance, but this needs confirmation.

The isolated case of rhabdomyolysis in a patient taking **pomegranate juice** with rosuvastatin and ezetimibe is clouded by other possible contributory factors, and no firm conclusions can be drawn from this case.

1. Lilja JJ, Kivistö KT, Neuvonen PJ. Grapefruit juice increases serum concentrations of atorvastatin and has no effect on pravastatin. *Clin Pharmacol Ther* (1999) 66, 118–27.
2. Fukazawa I, Uchida N, Uchida E, Yasuhara H. Effects of grapefruit juice on pharmacokinetics of atorvastatin and pravastatin in Japanese. *Br J Clin Pharmacol* (2004) 57, 448–55.
3. Ando H, Tsuruoka S, Yanagihara H, Sugimoto K, Miyata M, Yamazoe Y, Takamura T, Kaneko S, Fujimura A. Effects of grapefruit juice on the pharmacokinetics of pitavastatin and atorvastatin. *Br J Clin Pharmacol* (2005) 60, 494–7.
4. Lipitor (Atorvastatin calcium trihydrate). Pfizer Ltd. UK Summary of product characteristics, March2015.
5. Kantola T, Kivistö KT, Neuvonen PJ. Grapefruit juice greatly increases serum concentrations of lovastatin and lovastatin acid. *Clin Pharmacol Ther* (1998) 63, 397–402.
6. Rogers JD, Zhao J, Liu L, Amin RD, Gagliano KD, Porras AG, Blum RA, Wilson MF, Stepanavage M, Vega JM. Grapefruit juice has minimal effects on plasma concentrations of lovastatin-derived 3-hydroxy-3-methylglutaryl coenzyme A reductase inhibitors. *Clin Pharmacol Ther* (1999) 66, 358–66.
7. Bailey DG, Dresser GK. Grapefruit juice-lovastatin interaction. *Clin Pharmacol Ther* (2000) 67, 690.
8. Koitabashi Y, Kumai T, Matsumoto N, Watanabe M, Sekine S, Yanagida Y, Kobayashi S. Orange juice increased the bioavailability of pravastatin, 3-hydroxy-3-methylglutaryl CoA reductase inhibitor, in rats and healthy human subjects. *Life Sci* (2006) 78, 2852–9.
9. Sorokin AV, Duncan B, Panetta R, Thompson PD. Rhabdomyolysis associated with pomegranate juice consumption. *Am J Cardiol* (2006) 98, 705–6.
10. Lilja JJ, Kivistö KT, Neuvonen PJ. Grapefruit juice-simvastatin interaction: effect on serum concentrations of simvastatin, simvastatin acid, and HMG-CoA reductase inhibitors. *Clin Pharmacol Ther* (1998) 64, 477–83.
11. Lilja JJ, Kivistö KT, Neuvonen PJ. Duration of effect of grapefruit juice on the pharmacokinetics of the CYP3A4 substrate simvastatin. *Clin Pharmacol Ther* (2000) 68, 384–90.
12. Zocor (Simvastatin). Merck & Co., Inc. US Prescribing information, March 2015.
13. Zocor (Simvastatin). Merck Sharp & Dohme Ltd. UK Summary of product characteristics, June 2015.
14. Lilja JJ, Neuvonen M, Neuvonen PJ. Effects of regular consumption of grapefruit juice on the pharmacokinetics of simvastatin. *Br J Clin Pharmacol* (2004) 58, 56–60.
15. Dreier JP, Endres M. Statin-associated rhabdomyolysis triggered by grapefruit consumption. *Neurology* (2004) 62, 670.
16. Mevacor (Lovastatin). Merck & Co., Inc. US Prescribing information, February 2014.

Statins + HCV-protease inhibitors

Telaprevir markedly increases, and boceprevir and simeprevir moderately increase, the exposure to atorvastatin. Simeprevir moderately increases the exposure to rosuvastatin, and paritaprevir boosted with ritonavir (in a fixed-dose combination) appears to slightly to moderately increase rosuvastatin exposure. Boceprevir slightly increases pravastatin exposure, and paritaprevir boosted with ritonavir (in a fixed-dose combination) appears to have a similar effect. Simvastatin exposure is slightly increased by simeprevir, and rhabdomyolysis has been reported with the concurrent use of telaprevir and simvastatin. Simvastatin exposure would also be expected to be increased by both boceprevir and telaprevir. Other statins, would be expected to be affected by the HCV-protease inhibitors to differing extents, depending on their metabolism and transport mechanisms.

Clinical evidence

(a) Atorvastatin

1. Boceprevir. In a crossover study in 10 healthy subjects, boceprevir 800 mg three times daily for 6 days increased the AUC and maximum plasma concentration of a single 40-mg dose of atorvastatin 2.3-fold and 2.7-fold, respectively. The pharmacokinetics of boceprevir were not affected.[1]

2. Simeprevir. The UK and US manufacturers briefly note that, in a study in 18 healthy subjects simeprevir 150 mg daily for 10 days increased the AUC and maximum concentration of a single 40-mg dose of atorvastatin about 2-fold and by 70%, respectively. In addition, the AUC and maximum plasma concentration of the hydroxy metabolite of atorvastatin were increased 2.3-fold and almost 2-fold, respectively.[2,3]

3. Telaprevir. In a study in 19 subjects, telaprevir 750 mg three times daily, taken for 6 days, increased the AUC and maximum plasma concentration of a single 20-mg dose of atorvastatin (given with amlodipine 5 mg) about 10-fold and 8-fold, respectively. The AUC and maximum plasma concentration of the active *ortho* hydroxy metabolite of atorvastatin tended to be lower after telaprevir administration, but limitations with the data meant it was not possible to analyse these results fully.[4]

(b) Pravastatin

1. Boceprevir. In a crossover study in 9 healthy subjects, boceprevir 800 mg three times daily for 6 days increased the AUC and maximum plasma concentration of a single 40-mg dose of pravastatin by 63% and 49%, respectively.[1]

2. Paritaprevir. The UK and US manufacturers briefly report that, in a study in 12 healthy subjects, pravastatin 10 mg daily had no effect on the pharmacokinetics of paritaprevir 150 mg daily (in a fixed-dose combination with ritonavir and ombitasvir, and given with dasabuvir). The AUC and maximum concentration of pravastatin were increased by 82% and 37%, respectively.[5,6] The UK manufacturer also reports that when paritaprevir 150 mg daily (in a fixed-dose combination with ritonavir and ombitasvir, and given *without* dasabuvir) was given with pravastatin 10 mg daily, the AUC and maximum concentration of paritaprevir were increased by 33% and 44%, respectively. The AUC and maximum concentration of pravastatin were increased by a similar magnitude to that seen when paritaprevir (in a fixed-dose combination) was given with dasabuvir.[5]

(c) Rosuvastatin

1. Paritaprevir. The UK and US manufacturers briefly report that, in a study in 11 healthy subjects, rosuvastatin 5 mg daily increased the AUC and maximum concentration of paritaprevir 150 mg daily (in a fixed-dose combination with ritonavir and ombitasvir, and given with dasabuvir) by 52% and 59%, respectively. The AUC and maximum concentration of rosuvastatin were increased 2.6-fold and 7-fold, respectively.[5,6] The UK manufacturer also reports that when paritaprevir 150 mg daily (in a fixed-dose combination with ritonavir and ombitasvir, and given *without* dasabuvir) was given with rosuvastatin 5 mg daily, the maximum concentration of paritaprevir was increased by 40%, but the AUC was unaffected. The AUC and maximum concentration of rosuvastatin were increased by 33% and 2.6-fold, respectively.[5]

2. Simeprevir. The UK and US manufacturers briefly note that, in a study in 16 healthy subjects simeprevir 150 mg daily for 7 days increased the AUC and maximum concentration of a single 10-mg dose of rosuvastatin 2.8-fold and 3.2-fold, respectively.[2,3]

(d) Simvastatin

1. Simeprevir. The UK and US manufacturers briefly note that, in a study in 18 healthy subjects simeprevir 150 mg daily for 10 days increased the AUC and maximum concentration of a single 40-mg dose of simvastatin by about 50%. In addition, the AUC and maximum concentration of the metabolite, simvastatin acid were increased by 88% and 3-fold, respectively.[2,3]

2. Telaprevir. A case report describes a 46-year-old man taking simvastatin 80 mg daily who developed muscle weakness in his legs and hands, trembling legs on walking, pain in his back and shoulders, and dyspnoea on exertion, a few weeks after starting therapy for hepatitis C infection, which included telaprevir 750 mg three times daily. He was hospitalised and simvastatin and telaprevir were stopped. His creatine kinase concentration on admission was 34 010 units/L, and Rhabdomyolysis was diagnosed. His creatine kinase concentration peaked at 62 246 units/L 3 days after admission, but then rapidly decreased, and at discharge on day 14 it was 230 units/L.[7]

Mechanism

Boceprevir, simeprevir, and telaprevir are all inhibitors of CYP3A4 (although simeprevir might not have clinically relevant effects), by which some of the statins are metabolised. The degree to which the statins are affected depends on the extent of their metabolism by CYP3A4, so that those predominantly metabolised by CYP3A4, such as simvastatin, would be expected to be greatly affected, and those such as atorvastatin, that is partially metabolised by CYP3A4, would be expected to be affected to a lesser extent. The increase in exposure of atorvastatin and simvastatin in the studies cited, might therefore be a result of CYP3A4 inhibition. However, the organic anion transporting polypeptide, OATP1B1 is also important in the metabolism of some statins, such as atorvastatin, pravastatin, and rosuvastatin. The HCV-protease inhibitors all inhibit OATP1B1, and therefore involvement of this transporter in the interactions seen with these drugs cannot be ruled out. For example, this might explain the differences in the effect of simeprevir on the exposure of atorvastatin and simvastatin. Involvement of this transporter in this interaction warrants further study. Also note that ritonavir (used as a pharmacokinetic enhancer with paritaprevir) and other components of the combination inhibit OATP1B1 and/or other transporters and their involvement in the effects seen with rosuvastatin and pravastatin is unclear.

Importance and management

Evidence for an interaction between the statins and the HCV-protease inhibitors is limited to the studies cited; however, the effects of concurrent use are consistent with that of other CYP3A4 inhibitors on statins, although the role of drug transporters cannot be ruled out and is likely to be an important factor in the interactions seen with paritaprevir boosted with ritonavir (in a fixed-dose combination), see below.

Atorvastatin

The marked increase in atorvastatin exposure reported with **telaprevir** is likely to be clinically important, and could increase the risk of serious adverse effects, such as myopathy and rhabdomyolysis. The UK manufacturer[8] of telaprevir therefore contra-indicates the concurrent use of atorvastatin, whereas the US manufacturer advises avoiding concurrent use.[9] **Boceprevir** moderately increases the exposure to atorvastatin and as a result, the UK manufacturer of boceprevir advises that when concurrent use is required, the lowest possible starting dose of atorvastatin should be considered, and the dose titrated to the desired clinical effect while monitoring for safety. The dose of atorvastatin should not exceed 20 mg daily when given with boceprevir.[10] The US manufacturer advises giving the lowest effective dose of atorvastatin, and further, states that an atorvastatin daily dose exceeding 40 mg should not be given with boceprevir.[11] **Simeprevir** appears to moderately increase exposure to atorvastatin and the UK and US manufacturers therefore advise that the lowest dose possible of atorvastatin should be used if given concurrently.[2,3] The US manufacturer limits this to 40 mg daily,[3] while the UK manufacturer advises careful dose titration and monitoring for safety.[2] Concurrent use of **paritaprevir** boosted with ritonavir (in a fixed-dose combination) with atorvastatin.[5]

Simvastatin

As simvastatin is metabolised by CYP3A4 to a greater extent than atorvastatin, both **boceprevir** and **telaprevir** (which are potent CYP3A4 inhibitors) would be expected to increase its exposure by at least a similar, and probably a greater, extent than that seen with atorvastatin, increasing the risk of serious adverse effects. A single case report of rhabdomyolysis with simvastatin and telaprevir would appear to support this. For this reason, the UK and US manufacturers of boceprevir and telaprevir contra-indicate concurrent use with simvastatin.[8-11] The effect of **simeprevir** on simvastatin exposure appears to be only slight, perhaps because simeprevir does not seem to inhibit CYP3A4 to a clinically relevant extent, and the UK and US manufacturers advise that simvastatin doses should be carefully titrated on concurrent use and the lowest dose possible should be given, with monitoring for safety.[2,3] Concurrent use of **paritaprevir** boosted with ritonavir (in a fixed-dose combination) with simvastatin is contraindicated.[5,6]

Pravastatin

The increase in pravastatin exposure seen with **boceprevir** is slight and would not be expected to be clinically relevant: no pravastatin dose adjustment is likely to be necessary on concurrent use. The UK and US manufacturers of boceprevir state that pravastatin can be initiated at the recommended dose in patients taking boceprevir, but close clinical monitoring is warranted.[10,11] The manufacturers of **telaprevir** advise caution and clinical monitoring on concurrent use with pravastatin,[8,9] and the manufacturers of **simeprevir** advise that pravastatin doses should be carefully titrated on concurrent use and the lowest dose possible should be given, with monitoring for safety.[2,3] For **paritaprevir** boosted with ritonavir (in a fixed-dose combination), advice regarding managing the increases in exposure to pravastatin varies between the UK and the US. When given *with dasabuvir*, in the US, the pravastatin dose should not exceed 40 mg daily,[6] but in the UK the pravastatin dose should be reduced by 50%.[5] When given *without dasabuvir* (UK only), the **pravastatin** dose should be reduced by 50%.[5]

Rosuvastatin

The exposure to rosuvastatin is increased by **simeprevir**, and the UK and US manufacturers advise that rosuvastatin doses should be carefully titrated on concurrent use and the lowest dose possible should be given, with monitoring for safety.[2,3] **Telaprevir** would be expected to have a similar effect, and the UK and US manufacturers advise caution and clinical monitoring on concurrent use with rosuvastatin.[8,9] For **paritaprevir** boosted with ritonavir (in a fixed-dose combination), advice regarding managing the increases in exposure to rosuvastatin varies between the UK and the US, and also varies according to whether it is given with or without dasabuvir. When given *with dasabuvir*, the US manufacturer advises that the dose of rosuvastatin should not exceed 10 mg daily,[6] whereas the UK manufacturer advises that the dose of rosuvastatin should not exceed 5 mg daily.[5] When given *without dasabuvir* (UK only), the **rosuvastatin** dose should not exceed 10 mg daily.[5]

Other statins

Fluvastatin is not appreciably metabolised by CYP3A4, and in general does not appear to be associated with the same types of interactions as other statins. An interaction with the HCV-protease inhibitors would therefore not be expected, and accordingly the UK and US manufacturers of **simeprevir** advise that no dose adjustment is necessary on concurrent use.[2,3] In contrast, the manufacturers of **telaprevir** give the same advice as for use with pravastatin and rosuvastatin, above.

In the UK, **paritaprevir** boosted with ritonavir (in a fixed-dose combination with ombitasvir, and given with or without dasabuvir) is predicted to increase the exposure to fluvastatin, such that concurrent use is not recommended. Fluvastatin should be temporarily suspended for the duration of treatment, but if a statin is required rosuvastatin or pravastatin, at the doses stated above, should be used instead.[5]

As **lovastatin** is metabolised similarly to simvastatin, its use with **boceprevir**, **telaprevir**, and **paritaprevir** boosted with ritonavir (in a fixed-dose combination) is contraindicated,[5,6,8-11] and the same advice as for simvastatin (see above) is given for concurrent use of lovastatin with **simeprevir**.[2,3]

The exposure to **pitavastatin** would be expected to be increased by **simeprevir** and **telaprevir** in a similar way to pravastatin. The UK and US manufacturers of simeprevir advise that pitavastatin doses should be carefully titrated on concurrent use and the lowest dose possible should be given, with monitoring for safety.[2,3] The UK and US manufacturers of telaprevir advise caution and clinical monitoring on concurrent use with pitavastatin.[8,9] and the manufacturers of simeprevir and telaprevir give the same advice. **Paritaprevir** boosted with ritonavir (in a fixed-dose combination with ombitasvir, and given with or without dasabuvir) is predicted to increase the exposure to pitavastatin, such that concurrent use is not recommended. Pitavastatin should be temporarily suspended for the duration of treatment, but if a statin is required rosuvastatin or pravastatin, at the doses stated above, should be used instead.[5]

Note that, as a general rule, patients taking statins should be specifically reminded to report any signs of myopathy and possible rhabdomyolysis (such as otherwise unexplained muscle pain, tenderness, or weakness or dark coloured urine). If myopathy does occur, the statin should be stopped immediately.

1. Hulskotte EG, Feng HP, Xuan F, Gupta S, van Zutven MG, O'Mara E, Wagner JA, Butterton JR. Pharmacokinetic evaluation of the interaction between hepatitis C virus protease inhibitor boceprevir and 3- Hydroxy-3-methylglutaryl coenzyme A reductase inhibitors atorvastatin and pravastatin. *Antimicrob Agents Chemother* (2013) 57, 2582–8.
2. Olysio (Simeprevir sodium). Janssen-Cilag Ltd. UK Summary of product characteristics, May 2014.
3. Olysio (Simeprevir sodium). Janssen Products, LP. US Prescribing information, November 2014.
4. Lee JE, van Heeswijck R, Alves K, Smith F, Garg V. Effect of the hepatitis C protease inhibitor telaprevir on the pharmacokinetics of amlodipine and atorvastatin. *Antimicrob Agents Chemother* (2011) 55, 4569–74.
5. Viekirax (Ombitasvir, paritaprevir, ritonavir). AbbVie Ltd. UK Summary of product characteristics, January 2015.
6. Viekira Pak (Ombitasvir, paritaprevir, ritonavir co-packaged with dasabuvir sodium monohydrate). AbbVie Inc. US Prescribing information, December 2014.
7. de Kanter CT, van Luin M, Solas C, Burger DM, Vrolijk JM. Rhabdomyolysis in a hepatitis C virus infected patient treated with telaprevir and simvastatin. *Ann Hepatol* (2014) 13, 452–5.
8. Incivo (Telaprevir). Janssen-Cilag Ltd. UK Summary of product characteristics, July 2014.
9. Incivek (Telaprevir). Vertex Pharmaceuticals, Inc. US Prescribing information, October 2013.
10. Victrelis (Boceprevir). Merck Sharp & Dohme Ltd. UK Summary of product characteristics, August 2014.
11. Victrelis (Boceprevir). Merck & Co., Inc. US Prescribing information, July 2014.

Statins + HIV-protease inhibitors

Simvastatin exposure is markedly increased by nelfinavir alone and very markedly increased by saquinavir with ritonavir, and several cases of rhabdomyolysis with simvastatin have been attributed to interactions with HIV-protease inhibitors. Lovastatin would be expected to interact similarly. Atorvastatin exposure is moderately to markedly increased by darunavir, lopinavir, fosamprenavir and tipranavir, all boosted with ritonavir, and moderately increased by saquinavir with ritonavir. Rosuvastatin exposure appears to be slightly to moderately increased by some HIV-protease inhibitors, and pravastatin exposure is usually only slightly increased or decreased, although there can be large interindividual variations. One case of rhabdomyolysis has been reported with high-dose pravastatin and atazanavir boosted with ritonavir.

Clinical evidence

(a) Atorvastatin

The pharmacokinetic studies of the effect of HIV-protease inhibitors on atorvastatin are summarised in 'Table 30.4', p.1346. These show that **nelfinavir** alone increased atorvastatin exposure by 74% and 2.8-fold, whereas the increases in atorvastatin exposure tended to be greater with HIV-protease inhibitors boosted with **ritonavir** (about 2.5-fold for **fosamprenavir**, 3- to 4-fold for **darunavir**, about 6-fold for **lopinavir**, 9- to 10-fold for **tipranavir**, and 4-fold for **ritonavir** with **saquinavir**). The almost 6-fold increase in atorvastatin exposure with lopinavir boosted with ritonavir resulted in a 2.5-fold increase in HMG-CoA reductase activity,[1] and the almost 10-fold increase in atorvastatin exposure with **tipranavir boosted with ritonavir** resulted in about a 4-fold increase in HMG-CoA reductase activity.[2] Atorvastatin, given for 4 days did not alter the pharmacokinetics of **amprenavir** (given as fosamprenavir with ritonavir),[3] or the pharmacokinetics of both **lopinavir** and **ritonavir** (given together);[1] and a single-dose of atorvastatin did not alter the pharmacokinetics of **tipranavir boosted with ritonavir**.[2]

For a case of rhabdomyolysis in a patient who had been taking atorvastatin 40 mg daily and **lopinavir boosted with ritonavir** for about a year, that occurred shortly after starting clarithromycin, see 'Statins + Macrolides', p.1348.

(b) Fluvastatin

As part of a clinical study, four patients taking an **indinavir**-based antiretroviral regimen were given fluvastatin for hyperlipidaemia. Fluvastatin did not appear to alter **indinavir** plasma concentrations in these patients.[4] There seems to be no data on the effect of HIV-protease inhibitors on fluvastatin concentrations.

(c) Pitavastatin

Unboosted **atazanavir** slightly increased the steady-state exposure of pitavastatin, whereas **lopinavir boosted with ritonavir** very slightly decreased it, see 'Table 30.4', p.1346.

(d) Pravastatin

The pharmacokinetic studies of the effect of HIV-protease inhibitors on pravastatin are summarised in 'Table 30.4', p.1346. These show that **nelfinavir** alone slightly *decreased* pravastatin exposure (by 35% or 46%). Similarly, **ritonavir** with **saquinavir** slightly to moderately decreased pravastatin exposure (by 50%). Conversely, **lopinavir** and **darunavir**, both boosted with ritonavir, slightly *increased* pravastatin exposure (30% for **lopinavir**, 81% for **darunavir**), although the increase with **darunavir** was variable, with a subset of subjects having a 5-fold increase.

Pravastatin 40 mg daily for 4 days did not alter **nelfinavir** pharmacokinetics in healthy subjects.[5] Similarly, pravastatin did not appear to alter **indinavir** concentrations in four patients taking an indinavir-based antiretroviral regimen.[4] Pravastatin did not alter the minimum and post-dose concentrations of **indinavir** (5 patients), **ritonavir** (8 patients), or **saquinavir** (6 patients) at 12 or 24 weeks, nor was virological efficacy affected.[6] Conversely, in another study, pravastatin decreased the minimum HIV-protease inhibitor concentrations, with a 28% decrease in **lopinavir** concentrations when compared with placebo. However, there was no change in the maximum lopinavir concentrations, and no difference in virological efficacy.[7]

One case of rhabdomyolysis has been published in a patient taking **atazanavir boosted with ritonavir**, emtricitabine and tenofovir, which occurred 4 months after his dose of pravastatin was increased from 40 to 80 mg daily.[8]

(e) Rosuvastatin

The pharmacokinetic studies of the effect of HIV-protease inhibitors on rosuvastatin are summarised in 'Table 30.4', p.1346. These show that HIV-protease inhibitors boosted with **ritonavir** have variable effects on rosuvastatin exposure: **fosamprenavir** and **tipranavir** had either a slight effect or no effect whereas **atazanavir** and **lopinavir** increased exposure 3-fold and 2-fold, respectively. In the **lopinavir boosted with ritonavir** study, one subject had an asymptomatic rise in creatine phosphokinase to 17 times the upper limit of normal. Nevertheless, the decrease in LDL-cholesterol seen with rosuvastatin was lower than expected, and appeared to be attenuated by the

Table 30.4 Pharmacokinetic studies of the effect of HIV-protease inhibitors on statins

HIV-protease inhibitor	*HIV-protease inhibitor dose*	*Statin dose*	*Change in statin exposure (AUC)*	*Refs*
Atorvastatin				
Fosamprenavir	1400 mg twice daily for 14 days	10 mg daily for 4 days	2.3-fold increase	1
Nelfinavir	1.25 g twice daily for 14 days 750 mg three times daily for 9 days	10 mg daily for 28 days 40 mg daily for 5 days	74% increase 2.8-fold increase	2 3
Darunavir boosted with ritonavir	300/100 mg twice daily	10 mg daily	3- to 4-fold increase	4
Fosamprenavir boosted with ritonavir	700/100 mg twice daily for 14 days	10 mg daily for 4 days	2.5-fold increase	1, 5
Lopinavir boosted with ritonavir	400/100 mg twice daily for 14 days	20 mg daily for 4 days	5.9-fold increase	6
Saquinavir boosted with ritonavir	400/300 mg twice daily for 3 days then 400/400 mg twice daily for 11 days	40 mg daily for 4 days	Median 3.9-fold increase 73% increase total active drug	7
Tipranavir boosted with ritonavir	500/200 mg twice daily for 8 days	10 mg single dose	9.4-fold increase 80 to 90% decrease, hydroxy metabolites	8
Pitavastatin				
Atazanavir	300 mg daily for 5 days	4 mg daily for 5 days	30% increase	9
Lopinavir boosted with ritonavir	400/100 mg twice daily for 16 days	4 mg daily for 5 days	20% decrease	9
Pravastatin				
Nelfinavir	750 mg three times daily for 9 days 1.25 mg twice daily for 9 days	40 mg daily for 5 days 40 mg daily for 3 days	35% decrease Median 47% decrease	3 10
Darunavir boosted with ritonavir	600/100 mg twice daily	40 mg single dose	81% increase, but a few subjects had 5-fold increase	4, 11
Lopinavir boosted with ritonavir	400/100 mg twice daily for 14 days	20 mg daily for 4 days	30% increase	6
Saquinavir boosted with ritonavir	400/300 mg twice daily for 3 days then 400/400 mg twice daily for 11 days	40 mg daily for 4 days	Median 50% decrease	7
Rosuvastatin				
Atazanavir boosted with ritonavir	300/100 mg daily for 7 days	10 mg single dose	3-fold increase 63% increase, lactone	12
Darunavir boosted with ritonavir	600/100 mg twice daily for 7 days	10 mg daily for 7 days	48% increase	13
Fosamprenavir boosted with ritonavir	700/100 mg twice daily for 7 days	10 mg single dose	No change 76% increase, lactone	12
Lopinavir boosted with ritonavir	400/100 mg twice daily for 17 days	20 mg daily for 7 days	2-fold increase	14
Tipranavir boosted with ritonavir	500/200 mg twice daily for 12 days	10 mg single dose	37% increase	8
Simvastatin				
Nelfinavir	1.25 g twice daily for 14 days	20 mg daily for 28 days	6-fold increase	2
Saquinavir boosted with ritonavir	400/300 mg twice daily for 3 days then 400/400 mg twice daily for 11 days	40 mg daily for 4 days	Median 32-fold increase, acid metabolite	7

1. Lexiva (Fosamprenavir calcium). ViiV Healthcare. US Prescribing information, May 2011.
2. Hsyu P-H, Schultz-Smith MD, Lillibridge JH, Lewis RH, Kerr BM. Pharmacokinetic interactions between nelfinavir and 3-hydroxy-methylglutaryl coenzyme A reductase inhibitors atorvastatin and simvastatin. *Antimicrob Agents Chemother* (2001) 45, 3445–50.
3. Barry M, Belz G, Roll S, O'Grady P, Swaminathan A, Geraldes M, Mangold B. Interaction of nelfinavir with atorvastatin and pravastatin in normal healthy volunteers. *AIDS* (2000) 14 (Suppl 4), S90.
4. Prezista (Darunavir ethanolate). Janssen-Cilag Ltd. UK Summary of product characteristics, July 2011.
5. Telzir (Fosamprenavir calcium). ViiV Healthcare UK Ltd. UK Summary of product characteristics, May 2011.
6. Carr RA, Andre AK, Bertz RJ, Hsu A, Lam W, Chang M, Chen P, Williams L, Bernstein B, Sun E. Concomitant administration of ABT-378/ritonavir results in a clinically important pharmacokinetic interaction with atorvastatin but not pravastatin. *Intersci Conf Antimicrob Agents Chemother* (2000) 40, 334.
7. Fichtenbaum CJ, Gerber JG, Rosenkranz SL, Segal Y, Aberg JA, Blaschke T, Alston B, Fang F, Kosel B, Aweeka F, and the NIAID AIDS Clinical Trials Group. Pharmacokinetic interactions between protease inhibitors and statins in HIV seronegative volunteers: ACTG study A5047. *AIDS* (2002) 16, 569–77.
8. Pham PA, la Porte CJ, Lee LS, van Heeswijk R, Sabo JP, Elgadi MM, Piliero PJ, Barditch-Crovo P, Fuchs E, Flexner C, Cameron DW. Differential effects of tipranavir plus ritonavir on atorvastatin or rosuvastatin pharmacokinetics in healthy volunteers. *Antimicrob Agents Chemother* (2009) 53, 4385–92.
9. Livalo (Pitavastatin). Kowa Pharmaceuticals America, Inc. US Prescribing information, August 2011.
10. Aberg JA, Rosenkranz SL, Fichtenbaum CJ, Alston BL, Brobst SW, Segal Y, Gerber JG, for the ACTG A5108 team. Pharmacokinetic interaction between nelfinavir and pravastatin in HIV-seronegative volunteers: ACTG study A5108. *AIDS* (2006) 20, 725–9.
11. Prezista (Darunavir ethanolate). Tibotec, Inc. US Prescribing information, October 2011.
12. Busti AJ, Bain AM, Hall RG 2nd, Bedimo RG, Leff RD, Meek C, Mehvar R. Effects of atazanavir/ritonavir or fosamprenavir/ritonavir on the pharmacokinetics of rosuvastatin. *J Cardiovasc Pharmacol* (2008) 51, 605–10.
13. Samineni D, Desai PB, Sallans L, Fichtenbaum CJ. Steady-state pharmacokinetic interactions of darunavir/ritonavir with lipid-lowering agent rosuvastatin. *J Clin Pharmacol* (2012) 52, 922–31.
14. Kiser JJ, Gerber JG, Predhomme JA, Wolfe P, Flynn DM, Hoody DW. Drug/drug interaction between lopinavir/ritonavir and rosuvastatin in healthy volunteers. *J Acquir Immune Defic Syndr* (2008) 47, 570–8.

HIV-protease inhibitors.[9] Similarly, another study found that, although rosuvastatin 10 or 20 mg was effective in lowering lipid parameters in HIV-positive patients (84% taking unnamed HIV-protease inhibitors), the lipid changes were smaller than those found in subjects not infected with HIV.[10] Nevertheless, in other randomised clinical studies, rosuvastatin 10 mg daily was more effective than pravastatin 40 mg daily[11,12] or atorvastatin 10 mg daily[11] in patients taking HIV-protease inhibitors.

In a study in 22 HIV-positive patients, **lopinavir boosted with ritonavir** concentrations were not affected by rosuvastatin 10 to 40 mg daily over a 12-week period, but rosuvastatin concentrations appeared to be increased by about 60%, when compared with data from healthy subjects.[13] A single-dose of rosuvastatin did not alter the pharmacokinetics of **tipranavir** when given with ritonavir.[2]

(f) Simvastatin

The pharmacokinetic studies of the effect of HIV-protease inhibitors on simvastatin are summarised in 'Table 30.4', p.1346. These show that **nelfinavir** alone markedly increased simvastatin exposure (6-fold), and **saquinavir** with **ritonavir** very markedly increased exposure (32-fold). Nevertheless, in these short-term studies there were no consistent increases in creatine phosphokinase concentrations.[5,14]

A few cases of rhabdomyolysis have been reported in patients taking simvastatin and HIV-protease inhibitors. In one, a 72-year-old HIV-positive man with coronary artery disease taking multiple medications including **atazanavir** 400 mg daily and delavirdine 600 mg twice daily presented with muscle pain, fatigue and dark orange urine. He had been taking **atorvastatin** 40 mg daily for 2 years without any adverse effects, but 27 days earlier had been switched to high-dose simvastatin 80 mg daily. Furthermore, amiodarone (400 mg daily for 7 days then 200 mg daily) had also been started 19 days earlier. The patient was diagnosed with rhabdomyolysis and acute renal failure probably due to an interaction between simvastatin and atazanavir and/or amiodarone,[15] see also 'Statins + Amiodarone', p.1320. Note that delavirdine may also increase simvastatin plasma concentrations, see 'Statins + NNRTIs', p.1352. In another case report, a 70-year-old HIV-positive man taking **nelfinavir** developed rhabdomyolysis and died, about 3 weeks after having his statin switched to high-dose simvastatin 80 mg daily. He had previously tolerated low-dose simvastatin 10 mg daily then **pravastatin** 40 mg daily.[16] A further case report describes a 51-year-old woman, who was admitted to hospital with a 4-day history of muscular aches and weakness. Among other drugs, she had been taking zidovudine, lamivudine, **indinavir** 800 mg twice daily, and simvastatin 20 mg twice daily for 2 years. **Ritonavir** 100 mg twice daily had been added to her usual regimen 2 weeks previously. The rhabdomyolysis was therefore attributed to an interaction between ritonavir and simvastatin.[17] Another similar case has also been reported.[18]

Mechanism

Many HIV-protease inhibitors, especially ritonavir, are known to be potent inhibitors of CYP3A4. The concentrations of statins metabolised by this isoenzyme (notably simvastatin, lovastatin, and to some extent atorvastatin) are therefore increased by concurrent use. The exact mechanism of the interaction with rosuvastatin (which is not appreciably metabolised by cytochrome P450 isoenzymes) is unknown, but it could be the result of inhibition of the OATP1B1 transporter protein. Pravastatin is also a substrate of OATP1B1, but both decreased and increased concentrations were seen, which are unexplained. There are no data on the pharmacokinetics of fluvastatin with HIV-protease inhibitors, although an interaction involving cytochrome P450 would not be anticipated, and an interaction involving OATP1B1 might also not occur (based on the lack of interaction with gemfibrozil, see 'Statins + Fibrates; Gemfibrozil', p.1338). However, given the unexplained effects seen with pravastatin, an interaction cannot be excluded.

Importance and management

The marked pharmacokinetic interactions of the HIV-protease inhibitors and simvastatin appear to be established, and are supported by a few case reports of myopathy and rhabdomyolysis. **Simvastatin**, and **lovastatin**, which is similarly metabolised, are generally contraindicated in patients taking any HIV-protease inhibitor, and this seems prudent.

The pharmacokinetic interactions of **atorvastatin** with HIV-protease inhibitors are also established, leading to moderate to marked increases in atorvastatin exposure. In general, atorvastatin should be not be used with most HIV-protease inhibitors: concurrent use should only be undertaken if the benefits outweigh the risks, and atorvastatin should be used in low initial doses with appropriate clinical monitoring for toxicity. The UK manufacturers of atorvastatin give specific dose advice if concurrent use is necessary as follows: for tipranavir, the maximum dose of atorvastatin should not exceed 10 mg daily; for lopinavir, it should only exceed 20 mg daily with clinical monitoring; and for darunavir, fosamprenavir, fosamprenavir boosted with ritonavir, and saquinavir, it should only exceed 40 mg daily with clinical monitoring.[19]

Rosuvastatin exposure appears to be slightly to moderately increased by HIV-protease inhibitors boosted with ritonavir, depending on the combination. The manufacturers of rosuvastatin recommend a starting dose of rosuvastatin 5 mg daily in patients taking atazanavir or lopinavir, both boosted with ritonavir,[20,21] with a maximum dose of 10 mg daily in the US.[20] The UK manufacturer recommends adjusting the dose of rosuvastatin on concurrent use with these HIV-protease inhibitors so that the rosuvastatin exposure is not greater than if a 40 mg dose was given without an interacting drug. They suggest a rosuvastatin dose of 10 mg when given with atazanavir boosted with ritonavir.[21] For fosamprenavir and tipranavir, both boosted with ritonavir, no clinically relevant pharmacokinetic interaction occurs, although the UK manufacturer of tipranavir still recommends starting with the lowest rosuvastatin dose (i.e. 5 mg daily).[22] The effect of HIV-protease inhibitors on **pravastatin** exposure is varied. A 50% reduction in pravastatin exposure occurred with nelfinavir, and saquinavir with ritonavir, which could be clinically important and result in reduced lipid-lowering efficacy. Conversely, a small subset of subjects had a marked *increase* in pravastatin exposure when they were given darunavir boosted with ritonavir, which could increase the risk of myopathy, and one case of rhabdomyolysis possibly due to the concurrent use of pravastatin and atazanavir boosted with ritonavir has been reported. Until more is known, it would seem prudent to initiate the concurrent use of pravastatin and a HIV-protease inhibitor at the lowest dose of pravastatin.

There are no pharmacokinetic data on the effect of HIV-protease inhibitors on **fluvastatin** exposure, and, because an interaction cannot be definitively excluded, some caution seems appropriate.

For **pitavastatin**, the available data are for atazanavir alone and lopinavir boosted with ritonavir, which showed no clinically relevant pharmacokinetic interaction.

In a 2003 guideline on the treatment of dyslipidaemias in patients being treated with antiretrovirals (which was developed before rosuvastatin became available), it was recommended that patients taking HIV-protease inhibitors be started on low doses of statins titrated upwards, with **pravastatin** and **atorvastatin** being the initial choice, and **fluvastatin** as an alternative.[23] The 2014 US guidelines on the treatment of HIV infection suggest that **fluvastatin**, **pitavastatin**, and **pravastatin** are alternatives to lovastatin and simvastatin as they have the least potential for interactions (except pravastatin and darunavir boosted with ritonavir). They suggest that **atorvastatin** and **rosuvastatin** should be used with caution, starting with the lowest dose possible, titrating according to tolerance and lipid-lowering effects.[24] Based on the available data, **rosuvastatin** might be preferable to **atorvastatin** because its pharmacokinetic interactions with fosamprenavir, lopinavir, and tipranavir (all boosted with ritonavir) are less than those of atorvastatin. Bear in mind that limited data suggest that the cholesterol-lowering effects of statins in patients taking HIV-protease inhibitors is modest, and that many patients do not achieve target cholesterol goals.[23] A retrospective cohort study investigating the effectiveness and toxicity of statins in 700 HIV-positive patients with hyperlipidaemias found that patients taking **atorvastatin** 10 to 20 mg or **rosuvastatin** 5 to 10 mg had greater reductions in cholesterol than those taking **pravastatin** 20 to 40 mg; toxicity rates were similar with all three statins.[25]

As a general rule, any patient given a statin and an HIV-protease inhibitor should be told to report any signs of myopathy and possible rhabdomyolysis (i.e. otherwise unexplained muscle pain, tenderness or weakness or dark coloured urine). If myopathy does occur, the statin should be stopped immediately. See also *Muscle and liver toxicity*, under 'Lipid regulating drugs', p.1309, for further guidance on monitoring, and risk factors for muscle toxicity.

1. Carr RA, Andre AK, Bertz RJ, Hsu A, Lam W, Chang M, Chen P, Williams L, Bernstein B, Sun E. Concomitant administration of ABT-378/ritonavir results in a clinically important pharmacokinetic interaction with atorvastatin but not pravastatin. *Intersci Conf Antimicrob Agents Chemother* (2000) 40, 334.
2. Pham PA, la Porte CJL, Lee LS, van Heeswijk R, Sabo JP, Elgadi MM, Piliero PJ, Barditch-Crovo P, Fuchs E, Flexner C, Cameron DW. Differential effects of tipranavir plus ritonavir on atorvastatin or rosuvastatin pharmacokinetics in healthy volunteers. *Antimicrob Agents Chemother* (2009) 53, 4385–92.
3. Lexiva (Fosamprenavir calcium). ViiV Healthcare. US Prescribing information, April 2013.
4. Benesic A, Zilly M, Kluge F, Weißbrich B, Winzer R, Klinker H, Langmann P. Lipid lowering therapy with fluvastatin and pravastatin in patients with HIV infection and antiretroviral therapy: comparison of efficacy and interaction with indinavir. *Infection* (2004) 32, 229–33.
5. Fichtenbaum CJ, Gerber JG, Rosenkranz SL, Segal Y, Aberg JA, Blaschke T, Alston B, Fang F, Kosel B, Aweeka F, and the NIAID AIDS Clinical Trials Group. Pharmacokinetic interactions between protease inhibitors and statins in HIV seronegative volunteers: ACTG study A5047. *AIDS* (2002) 16, 569–77.
6. Moyle GJ, Buss NE, Gazzard BG. Pravastatin does not alter protease inhibitor exposure or virologic efficacy during a 24-week period of therapy. *J Acquir Immune Defic Syndr* (2002) 30, 460–2.
7. Bonnet F, Aurillac-Lavignolle V, Breilh D, Thiébaut R, Peuchant E, Bernard N, Lacoste D, Dabis F, Beylot J, Chêne G, Morlat P; GECSA. Pravastatin in HIV-infected patients treated with protease inhibitors: a placebo-controlled randomized study. *HIV Clin Trials* (2007) 8, 53–60.
8. Mikhail N, Iskander E, Cope D. Rhabdomyolysis in an HIV-infected patient on anti-retroviral therapy precipitated by high-dose pravastatin. *Curr Drug Saf* (2009) 4, 121–2.
9. Kiser JJ, Gerber JG, Predhomme JA, Wolfe P, Flynn DM, Hoody DW. Drug/drug interaction between lopinavir/ritonavir and rosuvastatin in healthy volunteers. *J Acquir Immune Defic Syndr* (2008) 47, 570–8.
10. Johns KW, Bennett MT, Bondy GP. Are HIV positive patients resistant to statin therapy? *Lipids Health Dis* (2007) 6, 27.
11. Calza L, Manfredi R, Colangeli V, Pocaterra D, Pavoni M, Chiodo F. Rosuvastatin, pravastatin, and atorvastatin for the treatment of hypercholesterolaemia in HIV-infected patients receiving protease inhibitors. *Curr HIV Res* (2008) 6, 572–8.
12. Aslangul E, Assoumou L, Bittar R, Valantin M-A, Kalmykova O, Peytavin G, Fiévet M-H, Boccara F, Bonnefont-Rousselot D, Melchior J-C, Giral P, Costagliola D. Rosuvastatin versus pravastatin in dyslipidemic HIV-1-infected patients receiving protease inhibitors: a randomized trial. *AIDS* (2010) 24, 77–83.
13. Van der Lee M, Sankatsing R, Schippers E, Vogel M, Fätkenheuer G, van der Ven A, Kroon F, Rockstroh J, Wyen C, Bäumer A, de Groot E, Koopmans P, Stroes E, Reiss P, Burger D. Pharmacokinetics and pharmacodynamics of combined use of lopinavir/ritonavir and rosuvastatin in HIV-infected patients. *Antivir Ther* (2007) 12, 1127–32.
14. Hsyu P-H, Schultz-Smith MD, Lillibridge JH, Lewis RH, Kerr BM. Pharmacokinetic interactions between nelfinavir and 3-hydroxy-methylglutaryl coenzyme A reductase inhibitors atorvastatin and simvastatin. *Antimicrob Agents Chemother* (2001) 45, 3445–50.
15. Schmidt GA, Hoehns JD, Purcell JL, Friedman RL, Elhawi Y. Severe rhabdomyolysis and acute renal failure secondary to concomitant use of simvastatin, amiodarone, and atazanavir. *J Am Board Fam Med* (2007) 20, 411–16.
16. Hare CB, Vu MP, Grunfeld C, Lampiris HW. Simvastatin-nelfinavir interaction implicated in rhabdomyolysis and death. *Clin Infect Dis* (2002) 35, e111–e112.
17. Cheng CH, Miller C, Lowe C, Pearson VE. Rhabdomyolysis due to probable interaction between simvastatin and ritonavir. *Am J Health-Syst Pharm* (2002) 59, 728–30.
18. Martin CM, Hoffman V, Berggren RE. Rhabdomyolysis in a patient receiving simvastatin concurrently with highly active antiretroviral therapy. *Intersci Conf Antimicrob Agents Chemother* (2000) 40, 316.
19. Lipitor (Atorvastatin calcium trihydrate). Pfizer Ltd. UK Summary of product characteristics, March 2015.
20. Crestor (Rosuvastatin calcium). AstraZeneca. US Prescribing information, August 2013.
21. Crestor (Rosuvastatin calcium). AstraZeneca UK Ltd. UK Summary of product characteristics, May 2013.
22. Aptivus Soft Capsules (Tipranavir). Boehringer Ingelheim Ltd. UK Summary of product characteristics, December 2011.
23. Dubé MP, Stein JH, Aberg JA, Fichtenbaum CJ, Gerber JG, Tashima KT, Henry WK, Currier JS, Sprecher D, Glesby MJ; Adult AIDS Clinical Trials Group Cardiovascular Subcommittee; HIV Medical Association of the Infectious Disease Society of America. Guidelines for the evaluation and management of dyslipidemia in human immunodeficiency virus (HIV)-infected adults receiving antiretroviral therapy: recommendations of the HIV Medical Association of the Infectious Disease Society of America and the Adult AIDS Clinical Trials Group. *Clin Infect Dis* (2003) 37, 613–27.
24. Panel on Antiretroviral Guidelines for Adults and Adolescents. Guidelines for the use of antiretroviral agents in HIV-1-infected adults and adolescents. US Department of Health and Human Services (April

2015). 1–288. Available at: https://aidsinfo.nih.gov/contentfiles/lvguidelines/adultandadolescentgl.pdf (accessed 20/09/15).
25. Singh S, Willig JH, Mugavero MJ, Crane PK, Harrington RD, Knopp RH, Kosel BW, Saag MS, Kitahata MM, Crane HM. Comparative effectiveness and toxicity of statins among HIV-infected patients. *Clin Infect Dis* (2011) 52, 387–95.

Statins + Ispaghula (Psyllium) and other bulk-forming agents

Limited evidence suggests that pectin and oat bran might reduce the cholesterol-lowering effects of lovastatin. However, ispaghula had additional cholesterol-lowering effects when used with lovastatin or simvastatin.

Clinical evidence

The serum LDL-cholesterol levels of 3 patients taking **lovastatin** 80 mg daily showed a 42% rise from 4.48 mmol/L to 6.36 mmol/L when they were also given pectin 15 g daily. One patient had a 59% rise in LDL-cholesterol.[1] Two other patients taking **lovastatin** had a rise in LDL-cholesterol from 5.03 mmol/L to 6.54 mmol/L when they were also given **oat bran** 50 to 100 g daily. One patient had a 41% rise in LDL-cholesterol. When the pectin and **oat bran** were stopped, the serum levels of the LDL-cholesterol fell.[1]

In contrast to this anecdotal report, two randomised clinical studies found that the addition of ispaghula 10 g daily to **lovastatin** 20 mg daily[2] or *Metamucil* 18 g (containing ispaghula husk and soluble fibre) three times daily to **simvastatin** 10 mg daily[3] resulted in greater reductions in LDL-cholesterol than either the ispaghula or statin alone.

Mechanism

It was presumed that both pectin and oat bran reduced the absorption of lovastatin from the gut.[1] However, the studies with ispaghula suggest that no marked reduction in statin absorption is likely to occur. Nevertheless, a pharmacokinetic study would be needed to confirm if statin absorption is affected by any of these bulk-forming agents or not. Note that food actually slightly increases the absorption of lovastatin.[4]

Importance and management

Evidence for an interaction between oat bran or pectin and lovastatin is anecdotal, and limited to the one report. Other evidence suggests that ispaghula might have a beneficial effect when given with statins. This suggests that the cases with oat bran in particular might be of limited general relevance. Nevertheless, bear the possibility of an interaction in mind if a patient taking statins has a poor response to treatment while taking bulk-forming agents such as bran or pectin.

1. Richter WO, Jacob BG, Schwandt P. Interaction between fibre and lovastatin. *Lancet* (1991) 338, 706.
2. Agrawal AR Tandon M, Sharma PL. Effect of combining viscous fibre with lovastatin on serum lipids in normal human subjects. *Int J Clin Pract* (2007) 61, 1812–18.
3. Moreyra AE, Wilson AC, Koraym A. Effect of combining psyllium fiber with simvastatin in lowering cholesterol. *Arch Intern Med* (2005) 23, 1161–6.
4. Mevacor (Lovastatin). Merck & Co., Inc. US Prescribing information, February 2014.

Statins + Lomitapide

Lomitapide slightly increases exposure to atorvastatin, simvastatin and rosuvastatin. Lovastatin is predicted to be similarly affected. Atorvastatin slightly increases lomitapide exposure when given simultaneously.

Clinical evidence

In a prospective study, 16 healthy subjects were given lomitapide 60 mg daily for 7 days with a single 40-mg dose of **simvastatin** on day 8. The AUC and maximum concentration of simvastatin acid (the active metabolite of simvastatin) were increased by 68% and 57%, respectively. In another 15 subjects, given lomitapide 10 mg daily for 7 days of a single 20-mg dose of **simvastatin** on day 8, the AUC and maximum concentration of simvastatin acid increased by 39% and 35%, respectively.[1] In other studies in healthy subjects, lomitapide 60 mg daily for 7 days increased the AUC and maximum concentration of atorvastatin acid (the active metabolite of atorvastatin) after administration of a single 20-mg dose of **atorvastatin** by 52% and 63%, respectively, and increased the AUC of a single 20-mg dose of **rosuvastatin** by 32%. In contrast, lomitapide 10 mg daily for 7 days had no effect on the pharmacokinetics of either of these statins when given in the same doses.[1]

In another randomised study in 32 healthy subjects, **atorvastatin** 80 mg daily for 5 days increased the exposure of a single 20-mg dose of lomitapide by 90% and 30%, when given simultaneously and when the doses were separated by 12 hours, respectively. The maximum concentration of lomitapide was increased about 2-fold and by 25%, respectively.[2]

Mechanism

In vitro,[3,4] lomitapide inhibits CYP3A4. Simvastatin (and to a lesser extent, atorvastatin) is metabolised by CYP3A4 and therefore the increases in exposure seen in the study confirm the *in vitro* findings. Rosuvastatin is minimally metabolised by CYP3A4 and therefore its exposure is also increased by lomitapide.

The authors of the atorvastatin study[2] suggest that it is a weak CYP3A4 inhibitor, and that as a result it increases the exposure to lomitapide, which is a substrate for this isoenzyme. Note however that atorvastatin is not generally considered a clinically relevant inhibitor of CYP3A4, based on its minimal effect on the probe substrate, midazolam (see 'Benzodiazepines + Statins', p.840).

Importance and management

Evidence for a pharmacokinetic interaction between lomitapide and the statins leading to increased statin exposure is limited, but would seem to be established. The clinical relevance of these findings does not appear to have been studied, but statin adverse effects, such as myopathy and rhabdomyolysis, are known to be related to exposure and so would be expected to be increased if lomitapide is given to patients taking a statin. The UK manufacturer of lomitapide contraindicates doses of simvastatin greater than 40 mg daily when given concurrently.[4] The US manufacturer advises halving the dose of simvastatin when lomitapide is started and limiting the simvastatin dose to 20 mg daily (or 40 mg daily for patients who have tolerated simvastatin 80 mg daily for at least a year without muscle toxicity) while taking lomitapide.[3] Although not studied, lovastatin is metabolised in a similar way to simvastatin and would therefore be expected to interact with lomitapide in the same way, and similar precautions are warranted. Dose adjustments of atorvastatin or rosuvastatin are not necessary on the concurrent use of lomitapide,[3,4] but it would be prudent to advise all patients given lomitapide and a statin of the possible increased risk of adverse effects and told to promptly report any unexplained muscle pain, tenderness, or weakness. Although a mechanism for the increase in lomitapide exposure seen with atorvastatin is yet to be established, the slight increase seen with simultaneous administration has led the UK manufacturer to advise separating administration by 12 hours, or decreasing the lomitapide dose by half.[4] In contrast, the US manufacturer advises that the lomitapide dose should not exceed 30 mg daily if given concurrently.[3]

1. Tuteja S, Duffy D, Dunbar RL, Movva R, Gadi R, Bloedon LT, Cuchel M. Pharmacokinetic interactions of the microsomal triglyceride transfer protein inhibitor, lomitapide, with drugs commonly used in the management of hypercholesterolemia. *Pharmacotherapy* (2014) 34, 227–39.
2. Patel G, King A, Dutta S, Korb S, Wade JR, Foulds P, Sumeray M. Evaluation of the effects of the weak CYP3A inhibitors atorvastatin and ethinyl estradiol/norgestimate on lomitapide pharmacokinetics in healthy subjects. *J Clin Pharmacol* (2015) Epub.
3. Juxtapid (Lomitapide mesylate). Aegerion Pharmaceuticals Inc. US Prescribing information, April 2015.
4. Lojuxta (Lomitapide mesylate). Aegerion Pharmaceuticals Ltd. UK Summary of product characteristics, March 2015.

Statins + Macrolides

Pharmacokinetic studies show that clarithromycin, erythromycin, and/or telithromycin markedly increase lovastatin and simvastatin exposure, slightly to moderately increase atorvastatin, pitavastatin, and pravastatin exposure, and have little effect on fluvastatin or rosuvastatin exposure. A number of cases of acute rhabdomyolysis have been reported when clarithromycin or erythromycin were used with either lovastatin or simvastatin. Cases have also been reported for atorvastatin with clarithromycin, lovastatin with azithromycin, and simvastatin with roxithromycin. Macrolides have also been potentially implicated in cases of rhabdomyolysis with pravastatin, and azithromycin has been potentially implicated in cases of rhabdomyolysis with statins.

In one study, azithromycin did not alter atorvastatin exposure.

Clinical evidence

(a) Pharmacokinetic studies

Studies of the pharmacokinetic interactions of macrolides with the statins are summarised in 'Table 30.5', p.1349. The extent of the interaction (if any) varies between drug pairs, as described in the sub-sections below.

1. Atorvastatin. **Azithromycin** does not alter the pharmacokinetics of atorvastatin. **Erythromycin** increased the exposure of atorvastatin by 33%, while **clarithromycin** increased the exposure of low-dose atorvastatin by 82% with a 3-day course of the antibacterial in one study, and showed a 4.5-fold increase in high-dose atorvastatin exposure with an 8-day course of the antibacterial in another. See 'Table 30.5', p.1349 for details.

2. Fluvastatin. A single-dose of **erythromycin** did not alter the steady-state plasma concentrations of fluvastatin. However, this study does not rule out the possibility of a pharmacokinetic interaction of multiple-dose erythromycin with fluvastatin. See 'Table 30.5', p.1349 for details.

3. Lovastatin. Lovastatin exposure is increased almost 6-fold by **erythromycin**, but **roxithromycin** increased lovastatin exposure by only about 40%. See 'Table 30.5', p.1349 for details.

4. Pitavastatin. **Erythromycin** increases the exposure to pitavastatin almost 3-fold. See 'Table 30.5', p.1349 for details.

5. Pravastatin. Pravastatin exposure is increased 2-fold by **clarithromycin** and either increased by 70% or unchanged by **erythromycin**. See 'Table 30.5', p.1349 for details.

6. Rosuvastatin. **Erythromycin** decreased the exposure to rosuvastatin by 20%, but there was no change in AUC of active HMG-CoA reductase inhibitors.[1] See 'Table 30.5', p.1349 for details.

7. Simvastatin. Simvastatin exposure is increased 8- to 10-fold by **clarithromycin**, and 4- to 8-fold by **erythromycin** and **telithromycin**. Separating administration of simvastatin from telithromycin by 12 hours halves the extent of the interaction compared with simultaneous administration (4-fold versus 8.5-fold increase in AUC). See 'Table 30.5', p.1349 for details.

Table 30.5 Pharmacokinetic studies of the effect of macrolides on statins

Macrolide	*Macrolide dose*	*Statin dose*	*Change in statin exposure (AUC)*	*Refs*
Atorvastatin				
Azithromycin	500 mg daily for 3 days	10 mg daily for 8 days	No change	1
Clarithromycin	500 mg twice daily for 3 days 500 mg twice daily for 8 days	10 mg daily for 8 days 80 mg daily for 8 days	82% increase 4.5-fold increase	1 2
Erythromycin	500 mg four times daily for 11 days	10 mg single dose on day 7	33% increase	3
Fluvastatin				
Erythromycin	500 mg single dose	40 mg daily	No change	4
Lovastatin				
Erythromycin	500 mg three times daily for 7 days	40 mg daily for 14 days	5.7-fold increase	5
Roxithromycin	300 mg four times daily for 6 days	80 mg single dose	42% decrease lactone 42% increase acid	6
Pitavastatin				
Erythromycin	500 mg four times daily for 6 days	4 mg single dose on day 4	2.8-fold increase	7
Pravastatin				
Clarithromycin	500 mg twice daily for 8 days	40 mg daily for 8 days	Twofold increase	2
Erythromycin	500 mg three times daily for 7 days Not stated	40 mg daily for 14 days Not stated	No change 70% increase	5 8
Rosuvastatin				
Erythromycin	500 mg four times daily for 7 days	80 mg single dose on day 4	20% decrease	9
Simvastatin				
Clarithromycin	500 mg twice daily for 8 days	40 mg daily for 8 days	Tenfold increase 12-fold increase acid	2
	500 mg twice daily for 7 days	40 mg single dose	Eightfold increase 14-fold increase acid	10
Erythromycin	500 mg three times daily for 7 days	40 mg single dose	6.2-fold increase 3.9-fold increase acid	11
Telithromycin	800 mg daily for 5 days	40 mg single dose with the 4th dose of telithromycin	8.5-fold increase 9.4-fold increase acid	12
	800 mg daily for 5 days	40 mg single dose 12 hours after the 4th dose of telithromycin	Fourfold increase 4.3-fold increase acid	12

1. Amsden GW, Kuye O, Wei GCG. A study of the interaction potential of azithromycin and clarithromycin with atorvastatin in healthy volunteers. *J Clin Pharmacol* (2002) 42, 442– 7.
2. Jacobson TA. Comparative pharmacokinetic interaction profiles of pravastatin, simvastatin, and atorvastatin when coadministered with cytochrome P450 inhibitors. *Am J Cardiol* (2004) 94, 1140– 6.
3. Siedlik PH, Olson SC, Yang B-B, Stern RH. Erythromycin coadministration increases plasma atorvastatin concentrations. *J Clin Pharmacol* (1999) 39, 501– 4.
4. Lescol (Fluvastatin sodium). Novartis Pharmaceuticals Corp. US Prescribing information, October 2006.
5. Bottorff MB, Behrens DH, Gross A, Markel M. Differences in metabolism of lovastatin and pravastatin as assessed by CYP3A inhibition with erythromycin. *Pharmacotherapy* (1997) 17, 184.
6. Bucher M, Mair G, Kees F. Effect of roxithromycin on the pharmacokinetics of lovastatin in volunteers. *Eur J Clin Pharmacol* (2002) 57, 787– 91.
7. Livalo (Pitavastatin). Kowa Pharmaceuticals America, Inc. US Prescribing information, August 2009.
8. Lipostat (Pravastatin sodium). Bristol-Myers Squibb Pharmaceuticals Ltd. UK Summary of product characteristics, July 2010.
9. Cooper KJ, Martin PD, Dane AL, Warwick MJ, Raza A, Schneck DW. The effect of erythromycin on the pharmacokinetics of rosuvastatin. *Eur J Clin Pharmacol* (2003), 59, 51– 6.
10. Montay G, Chevalier P, Guimart C, Guillaume M, Shi J, Bhargava V. Effects of clarithromycin on the pharmacokinetics of simvastatin. *Intersci Conf Antimicrob Agents Chemother* (2003) 43, 38.
11. Kantola T, Kivistö KT, Neuvonen PJ. Erythromycin and verapamil considerably increase serum simvastatin and simvastatin acid concentrations. *Clin Pharmacol Ther* (1998) 64, 177– 82.
12. Montay G, Chevalier P, Guimart C, Boudraa Y, Guillaume M, Shi J, Bhargava V. A 12-hour dosing interval reduces pharmacokinetic interaction between telithromycin and simvastatin. *Intersci Conf Antimicrob Agents Chemother* (2003) 43, 38.

(b) Case reports

In a review of the FDA spontaneous reports of statin-associated rhabdomyolysis covering the period November 1997 to March 2000, macrolides (unspecified) were potentially implicated in cases of rhabdomyolysis seen with various statins. They were implicated in 13 of 73 cases with atorvastatin, 11 of 40 cases with lovastatin, 6 of 71 cases with pravastatin, and in 10 of 215 cases with simvastatin.[2]

In a review of the WHO adverse drug reaction database from 2000 to July 2008, there were 22 cases of rhabdomyolysis in patients taking **simvastatin** and **azithromycin**, and 18 cases in patients taking **atorvastatin** and **azithromycin** , for which the statin and azithromycin were the sole reported drugs in 4 and 6 cases, respectively. The authors calculated that this was two to three times greater than the expected number of cases.[3]

A population-based cohort study of 144 336 patients aged over 65 years taking a statin (**atorvastatin**, **simvastatin**, or **lovastatin**) and prescribed **azithromycin**, **clarithromycin**, or **erythromycin**, found that, compared with azithromycin (68 478 patients), the use of erythromycin or clarithromycin (75 858 patients) was associated with a 2-fold higher risk of hospitalisation with rhabdomyolysis within 30 days of prescription of the macrolide (relative risk 2.17, range 1.04 to 4.53).[4] Another similar study of 104 041 patients aged over 66 years taking **fluvastatin**, **pravastatin**, or **rosuvastatin** and prescribed **azithromycin** (52 518 patients) or **clarithromycin** (51 523 patients), found that the risk of admission with rhabdomyolysis within 30 days of co-prescription was 2-folder higher with clarithromycin, when compared with azithromycin (relative risk 2.27, range 0.86 to 5.96).[5]

1. Atorvastatin. A 34-year-old man who had been taking atorvastatin 40 mg daily with lamivudine, efavirenz, and lopinavir boosted with ritonavir without problem for about a year developed rhabdomyolysis 8 days after starting **clarithromycin** 500 mg twice daily and cefuroxime.[6] Another case has been described in which a patient taking atorvastatin and clarithromycin also developed acute neuropathy.[7] For another case of rhabdomyolysis in a patient taking atorvastatin when given esomeprazole, to which **clarithromycin** might have also contributed, see *Atorvastatin* in 'Statins + Drugs that affect gastric pH', p.1333.

2. Lovastatin. A 51-year-old man who had been taking lovastatin 40 mg daily for 5 years developed muscle aches and fever one day after finishing a 5-day course of **azithromycin** 250 mg daily. His creatine kinase concentrations were elevated and he was diagnosed as having rhabdomyolysis. This patient was also taking multiple medications including diltiazem, the role of which cannot be excluded.[8]

A 76-year-old woman who had been taking lovastatin 40 mg daily for 5 years developed muscle pain and weakness 2 days after completing a 10-day course of **clarithromycin** 500 mg twice daily. Later, when hospitalised, she was found to have elevated creatine kinase concentrations and was diagnosed as having acute rhabdomyolysis.[8] Another case report describes rhabdomyolysis, which developed in a patient taking lovastatin 40 mg daily shortly after completing a 2-week course of **clarithromycin** 500 mg three times daily. This patient had also recently started taking gemfibrozil, which might have played a part in the interaction,[9] see 'Statins + Fibrates; Gemfibrozil', p.1338.

A 73-year-old man who had been taking lovastatin 20 mg daily for 7 years developed multiple organ toxicity (rhabdomyolysis, acute renal failure, pancreatitis, livedo reticularis, and increased aminotransferase concentrations) after taking 1.5 g of **erythromycin** on 6 occasions over 2 weeks for endocarditis prophylaxis for dental procedures.[10] Three other cases of rhabdomyolysis attributed to an interaction between lovastatin and **erythromycin** have been reported,[11-13] although high doses of lovastatin (60 and 80 mg daily)[12,13] and other interacting drugs (ciclosporin[13] and diltiazem[12]) might have contributed to the effects seen in two of the cases.

3. Simvastatin. For a case of rhabdomyolysis in a patient taking simvastatin and nefazodone to which **azithromycin** might also have contributed, see 'Statins + Nefazodone', p.1351.

A case report describes a 77-year-old woman taking simvastatin 20 mg daily who developed myopathy 3 days after stopping a 14-day course of **clarithromycin** 500 mg twice daily.[14] Other reports describe[12] further cases of rhabdomyolysis in patients taking simvastatin,[15-23] which in some cases occurred within days of the **clarithromycin** being started. In all but one of these cases, the patients also had other factors that could have contributed to the reaction including high-dose simvastatin,[15,16,20,21] hypothyroidism,[22] and other possible interacting drugs (amiodarone,[18] ciclosporin,[17,19] or colchicine[15]). One case, in a patient with psychiatric illness, was initially mistaken as neuroleptic malignant syndrome.[21] Another case is unusual in that the patient took simvastatin with **clarithromycin** 250 mg twice daily for 3 months without problems, and only developed symptoms one month after the clarithromycin dose was increased to 500 mg twice daily.[23]

An 83-year-old man receiving multiple medication, who had been taking high-dose simvastatin 80 mg daily for at least 5 years, developed rhabdomyolysis about 2 weeks after he completed a 14-day course of **erythromycin** 500 mg four times daily (given intravenously for 2 days then orally for 10 days) for atypical pneumonia.[20] Two other cases describe rhabdomyolysis in patients taking simvastatin after taking a 4-week course of **erythromycin**,[24] and a few days after starting a 10-day course.[25]

A 73-year-old woman, who had been stable for 6 months while taking a combination of gemfibrozil 600 mg twice daily, simvastatin 80 mg daily and diltiazem, developed muscular weakness and myalgia 7 days after starting **roxithromycin**. All drugs were stopped, and initially she developed myoglobinuria and had a further elevation in her creatine kinase concentration, but this normalised over the following 18 days. She was discharged after 6 weeks, by which time she had regained full strength.[26] The contribution of roxithromycin to this case is uncertain.

Mechanism

Some macrolides inhibit CYP3A4, by which lovastatin, simvastatin and, to some extent, atorvastatin are metabolised. Hence the concurrent use of a macrolide that inhibits CYP3A4 increases the concentrations of these statins, leading in some instances to toxicity (myopathy and rhabdomyolysis). No interaction via this mechanism would be expected with rosuvastatin as it is minimally metabolised. See 'Lipid regulating drugs', p.1309, for a more detailed discussion of statin metabolism. Azithromycin (and possibly **dirithromycin** and **spiramycin**) would not be expected to interact via this mechanism as these macrolides do not appear to inhibit CYP3A4 to any great extent.

However, clarithromycin increased the exposure to pravastatin, and erythromycin increased pitavastatin exposure, and neither of these statins are metabolised by CYP3A4, so there must be other mechanism(s) involved. One possibility is inhibition of organic anion transporting polypeptides (OATPs), because there is *in vitro* evidence[27] that some macrolides (clarithromycin, erythromycin, telithromycin, and roxithromycin, but not azithromycin) might inhibit pravastatin uptake by inhibition of OATP1B1 and 1B3. Further study is needed.

Importance and management

The interaction between the macrolides and the statins is established and of clinical importance, although not all drug pairs have been studied. The outcome of concurrent use differs depending on the drug pair used, and the differing risks and management of the various drug pairs are discussed below. See also *Muscle and liver toxicity*, under 'Lipid regulating drugs', p.1309, for further guidance on monitoring, and risk factors for muscle toxicity.

Lovastatin or Simvastatin

The macrolides that inhibit CYP3A4 (clarithromycin, erythromycin, and telithromycin) markedly increase the concentrations of statins extensively metabolised by CYP3A4 (i.e. lovastatin and simvastatin).This would be expected to increase the risk of rhabdomyolysis, and the manufacturers of lovastatin and simvastatin contra-indicate the concurrent use of these macrolides (clarithromycin, erythromycin, and telithromycin), and state that the statin must be temporarily withdrawn if they are required.[28-30] This advice would seem prudent.

Atorvastatin

The pharmacokinetic interaction between clarithromycin, erythromycin, or telithromycin and atorvastatin is not as marked as that with simvastatin or lovastatin, but as the cases illustrate, adverse interactions are possible. The manufacturers of atorvastatin therefore recommend that the concurrent use of clarithromycin, erythromycin, or telithromycin should be undertaken only if the benefits outweigh the risks, and that lower doses of atorvastatin should be considered.[31,32] In addition, for clarithromycin specifically, they advise caution with the use of atorvastatin at doses of greater than 20 mg daily.[31,32] Note that the manufacturers of telithromycin specifically contra-indicate the concurrent use of atorvastatin, and state that the statin must be temporarily withdrawn if telithromycin is required.[33,34]

Pravastatin

Pravastatin exposure is moderately increased by clarithromycin and possibly slightly increased by erythromycin, and some potential cases of myopathy or rhabdomyolysis have been identified with pravastatin and macrolides in adverse event databases. Some caution would therefore seem appropriate if any patient taking pravastatin is given clarithromycin or erythromycin. The US manufacturer specifically recommends that the dose of pravastatin be limited to 40 mg daily when used with clarithromycin.[35] As pravastatin is not metabolised by CYP3A4, inhibition of CYP3A4 is not the mechanism for this interaction. Therefore, until more is understood about the potential mechanism and the effect of different macrolides, it might be prudent to extend this caution to any macrolide. Note that the UK manufacturer of telithromycin specifically advises monitoring in patients taking pravastatin.[33]

Pitavastatin

Because the exposure of pitavastatin was moderately increased by erythromycin, the manufacturer recommends that the dose of pitavastatin should be limited to 1 mg daily (the lowest available dose) when taken with erythromycin.[36] As pitavastatin is not metabolised by CYP3A4, inhibition of CYP3A4 is not the mechanism for this interaction. Therefore, until more is understood about the potential mechanism and the effect of different macrolides, it would be prudent to extend this caution to any macrolide.

Other statins

Neither **rosuvastatin** nor **fluvastatin** were affected by erythromycin in pharmacokinetic studies, and therefore an increased risk of rhabdomyolysis with these statins and erythromycin, and therefore probably other macrolides, seems unlikely. Nevertheless, the UK manufacturer of telithromycin specifically advises monitoring in patients taking fluvastatin and rosuvastatin,[33] although the US manufacturer states that an interaction with statins not metabolised by CYP3A4 will not occur.[34]

1. Cooper KJ, Martin PD, Dane AL, Warwick MJ, Raza A, Schneck DW. The effect of erythromycin on the pharmacokinetics of rosuvastatin. *Eur J Clin Pharmacol* (2003), 59, 51–6.
2. Omar MA, Wilson JP. FDA adverse event reports on statin-associated rhabdomyolysis. *Ann Pharmacother* (2002) 36, 288–95.
3. Strandell J, Bate A, Hägg S, Edwards IR. Rhabdomyolysis a result of azithromycin and statins: an unrecognized interaction. *Br J Clin Pharmacol* (2009) 68, 427–34.
4. Patel AM, Shariff S, Bailey DG, Juurlink DN, Gandhi S, Mamdani M, Gomes T, Fleet J, Hwang J, Garg AX. Statin toxicity from macrolide antibiotic coprescription: a population-based cohort study. *Ann Intern Med* (2013) 158, 869–76.
5. Li DQ, Kim R, McArthur E, Fleet J, Gailey DG, Juurlink D, Shariff SZ, Gomes T, Mamdani M, Gandhi S, Dixon S, Garg AX. Risk of adverse events among older adults following co-prescription of clarithromycin and statins not metabolized by cytochrome P450 3A4. *CMAJ* (2015) 187, 174–80.
6. Mah Ming JB, Gill MJ. Drug-induced rhabdomyolysis after concomitant use of clarithromycin, atorvastatin, and lopinavir/ritonavir in a patient with HIV. *AIDS Patient Care STDS* (2003) 17, 207–10.
7. Fadini GP, Manzato E, Crepaldi C, de Kreutzenberg S, Tiengo A, Avogaro A. Two cases of statin-induced rhabdomyolysis associated with mononeuropathy. *Clin Drug Investig* (2010) 30, 347–50.
8. Grunden JW, Fisher KA. Lovastatin-induced rhabdomyolysis possibly associated with clarithromycin and azithromycin. *Ann Pharmacother* (1997) 31, 859–63.
9. Landesman KA, Stozek M, Freeman NJ. Rhabdomyolysis associated with the combined use of hydroxymethylglutaryl-coenzyme A reductase inhibitors with gemfibrozil and macrolide antibiotics. *Conn Med* (1999) 63, 455–7.
10. Wong PWK, Dillard TA, Kroenke K. Multiple organ toxicity from addition of erythromycin to long-term lovastatin therapy. *South Med J* (1998) 91, 202–5.
11. Spach DH, Bauwens JE, Clark CD, Burke WG. Rhabdomyolysis associated with lovastatin and erythromycin use. *West J Med* (1991) 154, 213–15.
12. Ayanian JZ, Fuchs CS, Stone RM. Lovastatin and rhabdomyolysis. *Ann Intern Med* (1988) 109, 682–3.
13. Corpier CL, Jones PH, Suki WN, Lederer ED, Quinones MA, Schmidt SW, Young JB. Rhabdomyolysis and renal injury with lovastatin use. Report of two cases in cardiac transplant recipients. *JAMA* (1988) 260, 239–41.
14. Wagner J, Suessmair C, Pfister H-W. Rhabdomyolysis caused by co-medication with simvastatin and clarithromycin. *J Neurol* (2009) 256, 1182–3.
15. Lee AJ, Maddix DS. Rhabdomyolysis secondary to a drug interaction between simvastatin and clarithromycin. *Ann Pharmacother* (2001) 35, 26–31.
16. Kahri AJ, Valkonen MM, Vuoristo MKE, Pentikäinen PJ. Rhabdomyolysis associated with concomitant use of simvastatin and clarithromycin. *Ann Pharmacother* (2004) 38, 719.
17. Valero R, Rodrigo E, Zubimendi JA, Arias M. Rabdomiolisis secundaria a interacción de estatinas con macrólidos en un paciente con trasplante renal. *Nefrologia* (2004) 24, 382–3.
18. Chouhan UM, Chakrabarti S, Millward LJ. Simvastatin interaction with clarithromycin and amiodarone causing myositis. *Ann Pharmacother* (2005) 39, 1760–1.
19. Meier C, Stey C, Brack T, Maggiorini M, Risti B, Krähenbühl S. Rhabdomyolyse bei mit Simvastatin und Ciclosporin behandelten Patienten: Rolle der Aktivität des Cytochrom-P450-Enzymsystems der Leber. *Schweiz Med Wochenschr* (1995) 125, 1342–6.
20. Molden E, Andersson KS. Simvastatin-associated rhabdomyolysis after coadministration of macrolide antibiotics in two patients. *Pharmacotherapy* (2007) 27, 603–7.
21. Neuroleptic malignant syndrome or a statin drug reaction? A case report. *Clin Neuropharmacol* (2009) 32, 348–9.
22. Arnold C, Lamy N, Hagmann N. Faiblesse et douleurs musculaires généralisées chez une patiente de 88 ans: avez-vous pensé aux médicaments? *Praxis (Bern 1994)* (2010) 99, 1507–11.
23. Page SR, Yee KC. Rhabdomyolysis in association with simvastatin and dosage increment in clarithromycin. *Intern Med J* (2014) 44, 690–3.
24. Campbell G, Jayakumar U, McCracken S, Bene J. A cautionary tale: delayed onset rhabdomyolysis due to erythromycin/simvastatin interaction. *Age Ageing* (2007) 36, 597.
25. Fallah A, Deep M, Smallwood D, Hughes P. Life-threatening rhabdomyolysis following the interaction of commonly prescribed medications. *Australas Med J* (2013) 6, 112–4.
26. Huynh T, Cordato D, Yang F, Choy T, Johnstone K, Bagnall F, Hitchens N, Dunn R. HMG CoA reductase-inhibitor-related myopathy and the influence of drug interactions. *Intern Med J* (2002) 32, 486–90.
27. Seithel A, Eberl S, Singer K, Auge D, Heinkele G, Wolf NB, Dörje F, Fromm MF, König J. The influence of macrolide antibiotics on the uptake of organic anions and drugs mediated by OATP1B1 and OATP1B3. *Drug Metab Dispos* (2007) 35, 779–86.
28. Mevacor (Lovastatin). Merck & Co., Inc. US Prescribing information, February 2014.
29. Zocor (Simvastatin). Merck Sharp & Dohme Ltd. UK Summary of product characteristics, June 2015.
30. Zocor (Simvastatin). Merck & Co., Inc. US Prescribing information, March 2015.
31. Lipitor (Atorvastatin calcium). Pfizer Inc. US Prescribing information, March 2015.
32. Lipitor (Atorvastatin calcium trihydrate). Pfizer Ltd. UK Summary of product characteristics, March 2015.
33. Ketek (Telithromycin). Sanofi. UK Summary of product characteristics, November 2012.

34. Ketek (Telithromycin). Sanofi-Aventis. US Prescribing information, January 2015.
35. Pravachol (Pravastatin sodium). Bristol-Myers Squibb Company. US Prescribing information, August 2013.
36. Livalo (Pitavastatin). Kowa Pharmaceuticals America, Inc. US Prescribing information, October 2013.

Statins + Monoclonal antibodies; Tocilizumab

Tocilizumab moderately reduces simvastatin exposure in patients with rheumatoid arthritis. Other statins might be similarly affected.

Clinical evidence

In a pharmacokinetic study, 12 patients with rheumatoid arthritis, taking methotrexate and folic acid, were given single 40-mg doses of simvastatin on days 1, 15, and 43, with a single 10-mg/kg infusion of tocilizumab on day 8. On day 15, the AUC of simvastatin and its active metabolite, simvastatin acid, were decreased by 57% and 39%, respectively, and the maximum plasma concentrations were decreased by 57% and 41%, respectively. This effect was maintained at day 43 but was smaller. The pharmacokinetics of tocilizumab were not affected.[1]

Mechanism

In vitro data has found that increased interleukin-6 concentrations, as found in patients with rheumatoid arthritis, appear to reduce CYP3A4 expression and thus decrease overall CYP3A4 activity, which would be expected to result in an increase in the exposure to CYP3A4 substrates, such as simvastatin.[1] Tocilizumab is an interleukin-6 inhibitor, which has been shown in *in-vitro* studies to reverse the suppression of cytochrome P450 isoenzymes (including CYP3A4, by which simvastatin is principally metabolised), caused by interleukin. As a result the activity of CYP3A4 increases, leading to an increase in simvastatin metabolism and a decrease in its exposure.

Importance and management

The interaction between tocilizumab and statins is limited to one study, which suggests that tocilizumab moderately decreases the exposure to simvastatin. However, the authors note that because simvastatin exposure on day 1 was higher in the rheumatoid arthritis patients than in healthy subjects (based on historical data), the decreases seen at both day 15 and day 43 resulted in exposure close to that seen in healthy subjects given simvastatin alone.[1] Nevertheless, a reduction in efficacy is a possibility and it would therefore seem prudent to monitor patients accordingly and consider increasing the simvastatin dose on concurrent use with tocilizumab. **Atorvastatin** and **lovastatin** are also metabolised by CYP3A4, although this is more important for lovastatin than atorvastatin, and so they would be expected to interact similarly.

Note that as tocilizumab has a long half-life, any clinically relevant effect on cytochrome P450 isoenzymes is likely to persist for up to several weeks after it has been stopped.[2]

1. Schmitt C, Kuhn B, Zhang X, Kivitz AJ, Grange S. Disease-drug-drug interaction involving tocilizumab and simvastatin in patients with rheumatoid arthritis. *Clin Pharmacol Ther* (2011) 89, 735–40. Correction. ibid., (2011) 90, 479.
2. RoActemra (Tocilizumab). Roche Products Ltd. Summary of product characteristics, April 2014.

Statins + Nefazodone

Nefazodone has been implicated in cases of muscle toxicity and rhabdomyolysis in patients taking simvastatin, lovastatin, and pravastatin, but the case involving pravastatin has been disputed.

Clinical evidence

(a) Lovastatin

In a review of the FDA spontaneous reports of statin-associated rhabdomyolysis, covering the period November 1997 to March 2000, nefazodone was potentially implicated in 2 cases of rhabdomyolysis involving lovastatin.[1]

(b) Pravastatin

A 74-year-old man taking atenolol, aspirin and pravastatin had his treatment with citalopram replaced by nefazodone 50 mg twice daily. Because the possibility of an interaction was suspected, his plasma creatine kinase levels were monitored and were found to be 877 units/L (reference range 0 to 190 units/L) at 36 hours. Lactate dehydrogenase, aspartate aminotransferase and alanine aminotransferase were all slightly elevated and this was interpreted as indicating muscle toxicity. Nefazodone was withdrawn and although creatine kinase levels were falling, they were still above the reference range when pravastatin was withdrawn 14 days later. Pravastatin was subsequently re-introduced, and then venlafaxine 75 mg twice daily was added without problems.[2] However, the diagnosis of muscle toxicity has been questioned, and, because pravastatin levels were not measured, the possibility of an interaction has also been questioned.[3]

(c) Simvastatin

A 44-year-old man who had uneventfully taken simvastatin 40 mg daily for 19 weeks developed 'tea-coloured' urine, initially misdiagnosed as a urinary tract infection, a month after starting to take nefazodone 100 mg twice daily. One month later he also complained of severe myalgias of the thighs and calves, and was found to have muscle weakness and tenderness. Laboratory tests confirmed a diagnosis of rhabdomyolysis and myositis. He was asymptomatic within 3 weeks of stopping both drugs, and remained problem-free 5 weeks after restarting simvastatin 40 mg daily.[4] A further case of rhabdomyolysis has been reported in a 72-year-old man taking simvastatin, which developed 6 weeks after nefazodone was started (2 weeks after a dose increment). He recovered with rehydration after the nefazodone was stopped.[5] Two other similar cases have also been reported.[6,7] In the first, a patient stabilised on nefazodone for 8 years who had taken simvastatin 20 mg daily for 9 months with a dose increase to 40 mg daily about one month before symptoms of arm and leg weakness developed.[7] In the second, a recent simvastatin dose increase from 40 to 80 mg daily and recently starting **azithromycin** were possible contributing factors.[6] A review of the FDA spontaneous reports of statin-associated rhabdomyolysis, covering the period November 1997 to March 2000, nefazodone was potentially implicated in 2 cases of rhabdomyolysis involving simvastatin.[1] Similarly, in a review of adverse reactions to statins in the Swedish Adverse Drug Reactions Advisory Committee until September 2006, there is a brief note that one case of confirmed rhabdomyolysis occurred in a patient taking simvastatin and nefazodone.[8]

Mechanism

Uncertain. The suggestion is that nefazodone (an inhibitor of CYP3A4, an enzyme involved in the metabolism of simvastatin) caused a marked increase in the serum levels of simvastatin with accompanying toxicity.[4] The same mechanism might also account for the interaction with lovastatin, but does not explain the case with pravastatin, and the reason for this possible case is less unclear. See, 'Lipid regulating drugs', p.1309, for a more detailed discussion of statin metabolism.

Importance and management

Information about interactions between nefazodone and the statins seems to be limited to these reports, but they are in line with the way lovastatin, and simvastatin are known to interact with other CYP3A4 inhibitors. The manufacturers of lovastatin and simvastatin contraindicate concurrent use.[9-11] Some caution is probably prudent with **atorvastatin**, as it is also metabolised by CYP3A4, although to a lesser extent than simvastatin or lovastatin, and an atorvastatin dose reduction should be considered. Patients given atorvastatin with nefazodone should have the advice to report any signs of myopathy and possible rhabdomyolysis (i.e. otherwise unexplained muscle pain, tenderness or weakness or dark coloured urine) specifically reinforced. If myopathy does occur, the statin should be stopped immediately. See also *Muscle and liver toxicity,* under 'Lipid regulating drugs', p.1309, for further guidance on monitoring, and risk factors for muscle toxicity.

Other statins seem unlikely to interact. Note that in 2003 nefazodone was withdrawn in many countries because of cases of liver toxicity.

1. Omar MA, Wilson JP. FDA adverse event reports on statin-associated rhabdomyolysis. *Ann Pharmacother* (2002) 36, 288–95.
2. Alderman CP. Possible interaction between nefazodone and pravastatin. *Ann Pharmacother* (1999) 33, 871.
3. Bottorf MB. Comment: possible interaction between nefazodone and pravastatin. *Ann Pharmacother* (2000) 34, 538.
4. Jacobson RH, Wang P, Glueck CJ. Myositis and rhabdomyolysis associated with concurrent use of simvastatin and nefazodone. *JAMA* (1997) 277, 296.
5. Thompson M, Samuels S. Rhabdomyolysis with simvastatin and nefazodone. *Am J Psychiatry* (2002) 159, 1067.
6. Skrabal MZ, Stading JA, Monaghan MS. Rhabdomyolysis associated with simvastatin-nefazodone therapy. *South Med J* (2003) 96, 1034–5.
7. Karnik NS, Maldonado JR. Antidepressant and statin interactions: a review and case report of simvastatin and nefazodone-induced rhabdomyolysis and transaminitis. *Psychosomatics* (2005) 46. 565–8.
8. Hedenmalm K, Alvan G, Öhagen P, Dahl M-L. Muscle toxicity with statins. *Pharmacoepidemiol Drug Safety* (2010) 19, 223–31.
9. Mevacor (Lovastatin). Merck & Co., Inc. US Prescribing information, February 2014.
10. Zocor (Simvastatin). Merck Sharp & Dohme Ltd. UK Summary of product characteristics, June 2015.
11. Zocor (Simvastatin). Merck & Co., Inc. US Prescribing information, March 2015.

Statins + Nicotinic acid (Niacin)

The risk of muscle toxicity might possibly be increased in patients taking a statin with nicotinic acid, but there appear to be only isolated reports of rhabdomyolysis attributed to an interaction between these drugs. Moreover, there is evidence that the risk of myopathy after taking lovastatin with nicotinic acid or simvastatin and nicotinic acid does not exceed that of lovastatin or simvastatin alone, although there is also evidence of an increased risk of myopathy after the use of simvastatin with nicotinic acid specifically in Chinese patients.

Clinical evidence

(a) Lovastatin

A 43-year-old man taking high-dose lovastatin 40 mg twice daily developed rhabdomyolysis, which was attributed to the addition of nicotinic acid, titrated up to 2.5 g daily.[1] A similar reaction occurred in a 54-year-old man taking lovastatin 120 mg daily [greater than the recommended maximum dose] and nicotinic acid 3 g daily,[2] as well as in a 53-year-old man with a heart transplant taking multiple medications including ciclosporin, nicotinic acid 1.5 g daily and high-dose lovastatin 40 mg twice daily.[3] Myositis has also been briefly reported in a patient taking lovastatin and nicotinic acid.[1]

A combined preparation of lovastatin and nicotinic acid is marketed (*Advicor*, USA), and in a 52-week study investigating efficacy and tolerability, none of the 814 patients experienced drug-induced myopathy (myalgia and elevated creatine kinase levels greater than 10 times the upper limit of normal), although 7 patients were withdrawn from the study due to elevated creatine kinase levels.[4] A similar study reported that the risk of adverse events with extended-release nicotinic acid and lovastatin did not exceed the risks associated with the individual drug components; discontinuation of treatment due to muscle ache occurred in 2 of 57 patients (4%) taking nicotinic acid 1 g with lovastatin 20 mg, in none of 57 patients taking nicotinic acid 2 g with lovastatin 40 mg, in 1 of 61 patients (2%) taking nicotinic acid alone, and in 4 of 61 patients (7%) taking lovastatin alone.[5] Furthermore, a review of the use of extended-release niacin with lovastatin found that myalgia, which was reported in 3% of patients, tended to be associated with higher initial doses of statins.[6] In a review of the FDA spontaneous reports of statin-associated rhabdomyolysis covering the period November 1997 to March 2000, nicotinic acid was identified as a potentially interacting drug in 1 of 40 cases for lovastatin.[7] However, a later study using the FDA adverse event reporting system (1999 to March 2005), found no evidence of a clinically relevant adverse drug interaction between extended-release nicotinic acid and lovastatin, and the rate of serious adverse event reports associated with the combination was similar to that of lovastatin or extended-release nicotinic acid alone.[8]

(b) Simvastatin

In an single-dose study, the concurrent administration of simvastatin 20 mg and extended-release nicotinic acid 2 g slightly increased the AUC of simvastatin by 40% and increased the AUC of simvastatin acid by 60%.[9,10] Whether a similar effect would be seen in a multiple-dose study is unknown.

The HDL-atherosclerosis treatment study (HATS) found that the incidence of adverse effects and abnormal laboratory findings in patients taking simvastatin (mean dose 13 mg daily) with nicotinic acid (mean dose 2.4 g daily) for 3 years was similar to that in patients who received placebo: symptoms of fatigue, nausea and/or muscle aches occurred in 9% versus 5% of patients, and creatine phosphokinase levels greater than twice the upper limit of normal occurred in 3% versus 4% of patients, respectively.[11] Similarly, in analysis of safety data from clinical studies of extended-release nicotinic acid with laropiprant, there was no evidence that this preparation alone or in combination with simvastatin had adverse effects on muscle.[12] Nevertheless, the manufacturers note that, in an ongoing, double-blind, randomised cardiovascular outcomes study, an independent safety monitoring committee identified that the incidence of myopathy was higher in Chinese compared with non-Chinese patients taking simvastatin 40 mg concurrently with lipid-modifying doses of nicotinic acid 2 g with laropiprant 40 mg (difference not stated).[9,10,13]

In a review of the FDA spontaneous reports of statin-associated rhabdomyolysis covering the period November 1997 to March 2000, nicotinic acid was identified as a potentially interacting drug in 2 of 215 cases for simvastatin.[7]

(c) Other statins

In contrast to the use of lovastatin and simvastatin, there do not appear to be any published reports of myopathy occurring with nicotinic acid and any other statin. Indeed, the manufacturers of **fluvastatin**[14] and **pravastatin**[15] report clinical studies in which nicotinic acid was given with the statin and myopathy was not observed. Furthermore, nicotinic acid does not alter the bioavailability of **fluvastatin**[16] or **pravastatin**.[17]

In a review of the FDA spontaneous reports of statin-associated rhabdomyolysis covering the period November 1997 to March 2000, nicotinic acid was identified as a potentially interacting drug in 1 of 71 cases for **pravastatin**. Nicotinic acid was not identified as an interacting drug in any reports for **atorvastatin** or **fluvastatin**.[7]

Mechanism

Unknown. Additive muscle toxicity has been suggested. The finding that the risk was limited to Chinese patients in one study suggests that genetic factors might be involved.

Importance and management

The reports describing an adverse interaction between nicotinic acid and a statin are isolated and it is by no means certain that nicotinic acid contributed to what happened. For example, in one case, ciclosporin could have been a contributory factor (consider also 'Statins + Ciclosporin', p.1327) and myopathy is known to occur with lovastatin alone,[18] with a reported incidence of 0.1%. Furthermore, in a report covering recommendations to healthcare professionals regarding the safety of nicotinic acid, it was proposed that, on the basis of almost two decades of clinical evidence, the use of nicotinic acid with a statin does not potentiate statin-related myopathic reactions. In addition, it was suggested that isolated case reports of myopathy, including rhabdomyolysis, that were associated with the concurrent use of nicotinic acid and a statin might have been related to other drug interactions or possibly hepatic toxicity from earlier forms of nicotinic acid resulting in increased peripheral blood statin levels.[19] However, the latest data suggest that the risk of myopathy with the combination could be increased in Chinese patients.

Note that, in general, all the statin manufacturers advise caution on the use of statins with lipid-lowering doses of nicotinic acid. The potential benefits and risks and should carefully weighed and patients should be monitored for any signs and symptoms of muscle pain, tenderness, or weakness, particularly during the initial months of concurrent use and when the dose of either drug is increased. Patients should be told to report otherwise unexplained muscle pain, tenderness or weakness or dark coloured urine). See also *Muscle and liver toxicity,* under 'Lipid regulating drugs', p.1309, for further guidance on monitoring, and risk factors for muscle toxicity.

Some manufacturers give specific dose recommendations for the use of statins with nicotinic acid as follows.

- For **lovastatin**, in the US, the manufacturer recommends caution in patients taking nicotinic acid in daily doses of 1 g or more.[20]
- For **simvastatin**, the US manufacturer recommends avoiding the 80 mg daily dose (and recommend caution with doses greater than 20 mg daily) in Chinese patients taking nicotinic acid in daily doses of 1 g or more,[10] whereas the UK manufacturer does not recommend that Chinese patients take simvastatin with nicotinic acid in doses of 1 g or more, and they extend this recommendation to all Asian patients.[9] The US manufacturer of **nicotinic acid** recommends caution with doses of nicotinic acid of 1 g or more on the concurrent use of simvastatin.[21]
- The US manufacturers of **atorvastatin**[22] and **pitavastatin**[23] also suggest that the lowest statin dose should be used, or a statin dose reduction should be considered. The US manufacturers of **fluvastatin**,[14] **pravastatin**,[15] and **rosuvastatin**[24] advise caution on concurrent use with doses of nicotinic acid of 1 g or more. The US manufacturer of **nicotinic acid** recommends caution with doses of nicotinic acid of 1 g or more on the concurrent use of these statins.[21]

Also note that although no interaction has been shown with **acipimox** and statins, the manufacturer recommends caution on their concurrent use.[25] This is because **acipimox** is an analogue of nicotinic acid, and so might be expected to share its interactions.

1. Reaven P, Witztum JL. Lovastatin, nicotinic acid and rhabdomyolysis. *Ann Intern Med* (1988) 109, 597–8.
2. Hill MD, Bilbao JM. Case of the month: February 1999 – 54 year old man with severe muscle weakness. *Brain Pathol* (1999) 9, 607–8.
3. Norman DJ, Illingworth DR, Munson J, Hosenpud J. Myolysis and acute renal failure in a heart-transplant recipient receiving lovastatin. *N Engl J Med* (1988) 318, 46–7.
4. Kashyap ML, McGovern ME, Berra K, Guyton JR, Kwiterovich PO, Harper WL, Toth PD, Favrot LK, Kerzner B, Nash SD, Bays HE, Simmons PD. Long-term safety and efficacy of a once-daily niacin/lovastatin formulation for patients with dyslipidaemia. *Am J Cardiol* (2002) 89, 672–8.
5. Hunninghake DB, McGovern ME, Koren M, Brazg R, Murdock D, Weiss S, Pearson T. A dose-ranging study of a new, once-daily, dual-component drug product containing niacin extended-release and lovastatin. *Clin Cardiol* (2003) 26, 112–18.
6. Yim BT, Chong PH. Niacin-ER and lovastatin treatment of hypercholesterolemia and mixed dyslipidemia. *Ann Pharmacother* (2003) 37, 106–15.
7. Omar MA, Wilson JP. FDA adverse event reports on statin-associated rhabdomyolysis. *Ann Pharmacother* (2002) 36, 288–95.
8. Alsheikh-Ali AA, Karas RH. The safety of niacin in the US Food and Drug Administration adverse event reporting database. *Am J Cardiol* (2008) 101 (8A), 9B–13B.
9. Zocor (Simvastatin). Merck Sharp & Dohme Ltd. UK Summary of product characteristics, June 2015.
10. Zocor (Simvastatin). Merck & Co., Inc. US Prescribing information, March 2015.
11. Zhao X-Q, Morse JS, Dowdy AA, Heise N, DeAngelis D, Frohlich J, Chait A, Albers JJ, Brown BG. Safety and tolerability of simvastatin plus niacin in patients with coronary artery disease and low high-density lipoprotein cholesterol (The HDL Atherosclerosis Treatment Study). *Am J Cardiol* (2004) 93, 307–12.
12. McKenney J, Bays H, Koren M, Ballantyne CM, Paolini JF, Mitchel Y, Betteridge A, Kuznetsova O, Sapre A, Sisk CM, Maccubbin D. Safety of extended-release niacin/laropiprant in patients with dyslipidemia. *J Clin Lipidol* (2010) 4, 105–112.e1..
13. Tredaptive (Nicotinic acid with Laropripant). Merck Sharp & Dohme, Ltd. UK Summary of product characteristics, April 2012.
14. Lescol (Fluvastatin sodium). Novartis Pharmaceuticals Corp. US Prescribing information, October 2012.
15. Pravachol (Pravastatin sodium). Bristol-Myers Squibb Company. US Prescribing information, August 2013.
16. Smith HT, Jokubaitis LA, Troendle AJ, Hwang DS, Robinson WT. Pharmacokinetics of fluvastatin and specific drug interactions. *Am J Hypertens* (1993) 6, 375S–382S.
17. ER Squibb. Data on file. A report on the effect of nicotinic acid alone and in the presence of aspirin on the bioavailability of SQ 31,000 in healthy male subjects (Protocol No 27, 201-6). 1987.
18. Bilheimer DW. Long term clinical tolerance of lovastatin (mevinolin) and simvastatin (epistatin). An overview. *Drug Invest* (1990) 2 (Suppl 2), 58–67.
19. Guyton JR, Bays HE. Safety considerations with niacin therapy. *Am J Cardiol* (2007) 99 (Suppl), 22C–31C.
20. Mevacor (Lovastatin). Merck & Co., Inc. US Prescribing information, February 2014.
21. Niaspan (Niacin). Abbott Laboratories. US Prescribing information, April 2015.
22. Lipitor (Atorvastatin calcium). Pfizer Inc. US Prescribing information, March 2015.
23. Livalo (Pitavastatin). Kowa Pharmaceuticals America, Inc. US Prescribing information, October 2013.
24. Crestor (Rosuvastatin calcium). AstraZeneca. US Prescribing information, August 2013.
25. Olbetam (Acipimox). Pharmacia Ltd. UK Summary of product characteristics, November 2009.

Statins + NNRTIs

Delavirdine is expected to increase atorvastatin, fluvastatin, simvastatin and lovastatin exposure. This expectation is supported by a case of rhabdomyolysis, which developed in a patient taking atorvastatin and delavirdine.

Efavirenz slightly to moderately reduces atorvastatin, simvastatin, and pravastatin exposure, and tended to attenuate their cholesterol-lowering effect. Nevirapine is predicted to interact similarly. Etravirine slightly lowers atorvastatin exposure and is predicted to lower simvastatin and lovastatin exposure, whereas etravirine is predicted to increase fluvastatin concentrations. Rilpivirine does not alter atorvastatin exposure and slightly increases the exposure to its metabolites.

Clinical evidence, mechanism, importance and management

(a) Delavirdine

An isolated case report describes a 63-year-old HIV-positive man, who had been taking **atorvastatin** 20 mg daily with indinavir, lamivudine, and stavudine, and who was admitted to hospital 2 months after indinavir was replaced with delavirdine. He had a one-month history of malaise, muscle pain, vomiting, and dark urine. Laboratory tests confirmed a diagnosis of rhabdomyolysis, and he was found to have acute renal failure. All drugs were withheld, and he gradually recovered over the following month. It was suggested that delavirdine inhibited the metabolism of **atorvastatin**,[1] probably by CYP3A4. The manufacturer of delavirdine reports that it might increase the plasma concentrations of **atorvastatin**. They advise caution, due to the risk of rhabdomyolysis, and suggest using the lowest possible dose of **atorvastatin** with careful monitoring.[2] The same advice is given for **fluvastatin**,[2] which is metabolised by

CYP2C9, an isoenzyme known to be inhibited by delavirdine. See *Muscle and liver toxicity*, under 'Lipid regulating drugs', p.1309, for further guidance on monitoring, and risk factors for muscle toxicity.

Simvastatin and **lovastatin** are metabolised in a similar way to **atorvastatin**, and would therefore be expected to interact to a similar, if not greater, extent. For a case report of rhabdomyolysis in a patient taking delavirdine and atazanavir, shortly after switching from atorvastatin 40 mg daily (which he had been taking without problems) to high-dose simvastatin 80 mg daily and after also starting amiodarone, see 'Statins + HIV-protease inhibitors', p.1345. The manufacturer of delavirdine recommends that it should not be used concurrently with either **simvastatin** or **lovastatin**.[2]

(b) Efavirenz

In an open-label study, 42 healthy subjects were given efavirenz 600 mg daily for 15 days, with **atorvastatin** 10 mg daily, **simvastatin** 40 mg daily, or **pravastatin** 40 mg daily for the last 4 days. Efavirenz moderately reduced the AUC of simvastatin acid by 58% (HMG-CoA reductase activity reduced by 60%), slightly reduced the AUC of **atorvastatin** and its active metabolites by 35 to 45% (HMG-CoA reductase activity reduced by 35%), and slightly reduced the AUC of **pravastatin** by about 40%. The pharmacokinetics of efavirenz were not changed. In this short study, decreases in LDL-cholesterol were attenuated when efavirenz was given with all the statins, with the attenuation for **simvastatin** reaching statistical significance.[3] However, in a small retrospective review, **simvastatin** at a dose of just 20 mg daily reduced lipid concentrations in 13 patients taking an efavirenz-based antiretroviral regimen, although about 30% fewer patients achieved target cholesterol-lowering goals than in a control group of men without HIV infection.[4]

The reduced exposure to **atorvastatin** and **simvastatin** were expected, as efavirenz induces CYP3A4, by which **simvastatin**, and to a lesser extent **atorvastatin**, are metabolised. The reasons for the reduction in **pravastatin** exposure are less clear, as it is not notably metabolised by cytochrome P450 isoenzymes.

It would seem prudent to monitor the lipid profile of patients taking efavirenz and any of these statins, bearing in mind that a dose adjustment of the statin might be required. The UK manufacturer predicts that **rosuvastatin** will not be affected by efavirenz because it is largely excreted unchanged in the faeces,[5] but given that **pravastatin** was affected, and the mechanism for this effect is unknown, the lack of interaction with **rosuvastatin** needs confirmation.

(c) Etravirine

In a study in which 16 healthy subjects were given etravirine 800 mg twice daily for 13 days with **atorvastatin** 40 mg daily on days 8 to 11, the pharmacokinetics of etravirine were unaffected, but the AUC of **atorvastatin** was slightly decreased, by 37%, and the AUC of its active hydroxy metabolite was slightly raised, by 27%.[6] These effects probably occur because etravirine is a weak inducer of CYP3A4 by which **atorvastatin** is partially metabolised. The manufacturers reasonably predict that the plasma concentrations of other statins metabolised by CYP3A4 [i.e. **lovastatin** and **simvastatin**] might be similarly reduced.[7,8] Conversely, etravirine is a weak inhibitor of CYP2C9 by which **fluvastatin** is metabolised. The manufacturers therefore predict that **fluvastatin** plasma concentrations might be increased by etravirine.[7,8] The manufacturers recommend monitoring the concurrent use of etravirine and any of these statins, and adjusting the dose according to clinical response. However, the effect seen with atorvastatin is probably too small to be of any clinical relevance.

The manufacturers state that **pravastatin** concentrations are not expected to be affected by etravirine.[7,8] In the US they also predict that **rosuvastatin** will not be affected by etravirine,[7] whereas the UK manufacturers suggest that either increased or decreased plasma concentrations are possible because rosuvastatin is a substrate of CYP3A4 and CYP2C9, respectively.[8] However, a clinically relevant pharmacokinetic interaction by these mechanisms seems highly unlikely, as less than 10% of **rosuvastatin** is metabolised. In the US they predict that increased **pitavastatin** concentrations might occur with etravirine, because pitavastatin is a substrate of CYP2C9.[7] However, an interaction by this mechanism is also unlikely because pitavastatin is only marginally metabolised by CYP2C9.

(d) Nevirapine

Nevirapine is an inducer of CYP3A4 and would therefore be predicted to interact with **atorvastatin** and **simvastatin** in a similar way to efavirenz,[3] see under *Efavirenz*, above.

(e) Rilpivirine

The manufacturers report that, in a study in 16 subjects, supratherapeutic doses of rilpivirine (150 mg daily) increased the maximum concentration of atorvastatin 40 mg daily by 35% and reduced its minimum concentration by 15%, but the AUC was unaffected. Rilpivirine increased the AUC of the active 2-hydroxy metabolite by 39%, and that of the active 4-hydroxy metabolite by 23%. These small changes in the concentrations of atorvastatin and its metabolites are of no clinical relevance, and are likely to be even less with usual therapeutic doses of rilpivirine. Atorvastatin caused a negligible 10% decrease in the AUC and minimum concentration of rilpivirine, which is not clinically relevant. Therefore no dose adjustment of either drug is necessary on concurrent use.[9,10]

1. Castro JG, Gutierrez L. Rhabdomyolysis with acute renal failure probably related to the interaction of atorvastatin and delavirdine. *Am J Med* (2002) 112, 505.
2. Rescriptor (Delavirdine mesylate). ViiV Healthcare. US Prescribing information, August 2012.
3. Gerber JG, Rosenkranz SL, Fichtenbaum CJ, Vega JM, Yang A, Alston BL, Brobst SW, Segal Y, Aberg JA. Effect of efavirenz on the pharmacokinetics of simvastatin, atorvastatin, and pravastatin: results of AIDS Clinical Trials Group 5108 study. *J Acquir Immune Defic Syndr* (2005) 39, 307–12.
4. Rahman AP, Eaton SA, Nguyen ST, Bain AM, Payne KD, Bedimo R, Busti AJ. Safety and efficacy of simvastatin for the treatment of dyslipidemia in human immunodeficiency virus-infected patients receiving efavirenz-based highly active antiretroviral therapy. *Pharmacotherapy* (2008) 28, 913–9.
5. Sustiva Film-coated Tablets (Efavirenz). Bristol-Myers Squibb Pharmaceutical Ltd. UK Summary of product characteristics, March 2014.
6. Schöller-Gyüre M, Kakuda TN, De Smedt G, Woodfall B, Bollen S, Peeters M, Vandermeulen K, Hoetelmans RM. Pharmacokinetic interaction between the non-nucleoside reverse transcriptase inhibitor (NNRTI) TMC125 and atorvastatin in HIV-negative volunteers. 4th IAS Conference on HIV Pathogenesis, Treatment & Prevention, Sydney, July 2007. Abstract WEPEA106.
7. Intelence (Etravirine). Tibotec, Inc. US Prescribing information, August 2012.
8. Intelence (Etravirine). Janssen-Cilag Ltd. UK Summary of product characteristics, July 2012.
9. Edurant (Rilpivirine hydrochloride). Janssen-Cilag Ltd. UK Summary of product characteristics, November 2011.
10. Edurant (Rilpivirine hydrochloride). Tibotec Pharmaceuticals. US Prescribing information, August 2012.

Statins + NS5A inhibitors

Daclatasvir appears to slightly increase the exposure to rosuvastatin, and might interact similarly with other statins. Ledipasvir (with sofosbuvir) might interact similarly. Rosuvastatin and pravastatin do not appear to alter the pharmacokinetics of ombitasvir.

Clinical evidence

(a) Daclatasvir

The UK manufacturer briefly reports that, in a study in healthy subjects, daclatasvir 60 mg daily increased the AUC and maximum concentration of a single 10-mg dose of **rosuvastatin** by 58% and 2-fold, respectively.[1]

(b) Ombitasvir

1. Pravastatin. The UK and US manufacturers briefly report that, in a study in 12 healthy subjects, pravastatin 10 mg daily had no effect on the pharmacokinetics of ombitasvir 25 mg daily (in a fixed-dose combination with paritaprevir boosted with ritonavir, given with and without dasabuvir).[2,3]

2. Rosuvastatin. The UK and US manufacturers briefly report that, in a study in 11 healthy subjects, rosuvastatin 5 mg daily had no effect on the pharmacokinetics of ombitasvir 25 mg daily (in a fixed-dose combination with paritaprevir boosted with ritonavir, given with and without dasabuvir).[2,3]

Mechanism

Multiple uptake transporters, such as organic anion transporting polypeptide OATP1B1, breast cancer resistance protein (BCRP), and P-glycoprotein, are involved in the clearance of statins; rosuvastatin is a substrate for OATP1B1 and BCRP which are said to be inhibited by daclatasvir,[1] and hence concurrent use results in increased rosuvastatin exposure.

Importance and management

Evidence for an interaction between the statins and NS5A inhibitors is limited to that with **daclatasvir** and rosuvastatin, but an interaction between these two drugs would seem to occur, although further evidence is ideally required to confirm this. Daclatasvir appears to cause a slight increase in rosuvastatin exposure, and the UK manufacturer advises caution if used concurrently.[1] They extend this advice to **atorvastatin**, **fluvastatin**, **simvastatin**, **pitavastatin**, and **pravastatin**.[1] However, note that fluvastatin and simvastatin are mostly metabolised (by CYP2C9 and CYP3A4, respectively), and might not be expected to be affected in the same way as the other statins. Until more is known, it would seem prudent for patients to be monitored closely for statin adverse effects, and in practice this probably means monitoring for muscle toxicity and rhabdomyolysis (see Muscle and liver toxicity, under 'Lipid regulating drugs', p.1309 for further guidance on monitoring and the risk factors for muscle toxicity with statins).

Ledipasvir has been shown to be an inhibitor of the drug transporter proteins BCRP and P-glycoprotein *in vitro*,[4] and is predicted to greatly increase the exposure to rosuvastatin, resulting in a risk of myopathy, including rhabdomyolysis.[4,5] The UK manufacturer of ledipasvir (with sofosbuvir) contraindicates concurrent use,[4] whereas the US manufacturer does not recommend the combination.[5] Further, the UK manufacturer predicts that pravastatin might be similarly affected and advises monitoring with possible pravastatin dose adjustment, and does not exclude the possibility of an interaction with other statins (drugs not stated) for which it says a statin dose reduction should be considered and monitoring for statin adverse effects should be undertaken.[4] In contrast, the US manufacturer states that no interaction occurs with pravastatin and no dose adjustments are necessary.[5] In the absence of evidence of an interaction, and based on the known statin interactions, and the effects of increased statin exposure, some caution on concurrent use with ledipasvir (with sofosbuvir) would seem prudent as would monitoring for muscle toxicity, as described above for *daclatasvir*.

Pravastatin and rosuvasatin do not appear to alter the pharmacokinetics of **ombitasvir** (in a fixed-dose combination with paritaprevir boosted with ritonavir, given with and without dasabuvir), and no ombitasvir dose adjustment is necessary on concurrent use.

Note that, as a general rule, patients taking statins should be specifically reminded to report any signs of myopathy and possible rhabdomyolysis (such as otherwise unexplained muscle pain, tenderness, or weakness, or dark coloured urine). If myopathy does occur, the statin should be stopped immediately.

1. Daklinza (Daclatasvir dihydrochloride). Bristol-Myers Squibb Pharmaceutical Ltd. UK Summary of product characteristics, September 2014.
2. Viekira Pak (Ombitasvir, paritaprevir, ritonavir co-packaged with dasabuvir sodium monohydrate). AbbVie Inc. US Prescribing information, December 2014.
3. Viekirax (Ombitasvir, paritaprevir, ritonavir). AbbVie Ltd. UK Summary of product characteristics, January 2015.
4. Harvoni (Ledipasvir, sofosbuvir). Gilead Sciences Ltd. UK Summary of product characteristics, November 2014.
5. Harvoni (Ledipasvir, sofosbuvir). Gilead Sciences, Inc. US Prescribing information, March 2015.

Statins + Orlistat

Orlistat has no clinically relevant effect on the pharmacokinetics of atorvastatin, pravastatin or simvastatin.

Clinical evidence, mechanism, importance and management

(a) Atorvastatin

In a crossover study, 32 healthy subjects were given atorvastatin 20 mg daily for 6 days, with and without orlistat 120 mg three times daily for 6 days. Orlistat did not alter the pharmacokinetics of atorvastatin.[1] No atorvastatin dose adjustment is therefore necessary on concurrent use.

(b) Pravastatin

In a placebo-controlled, crossover study in 24 subjects with mild hypercholesterolaemia, orlistat 120 mg three times daily did not alter the pharmacokinetics, or lipid-lowering effects, of pravastatin 40 mg daily, when both drugs were given for 6 days.[2] A review includes brief details of an earlier comparative study in two groups of healthy subjects given pravastatin, either with orlistat or placebo. After 10 days there was no difference in the pravastatin AUC between the groups, but the maximum serum concentration did show a tendency to be higher (amount not stated) in the orlistat group.[3] No pravastatin dose adjustment is therefore necessary on concurrent use.

(c) Simvastatin

In a placebo-controlled, crossover study in 29 healthy subjects, orlistat 120 mg three times daily had no effect on the pharmacokinetics of simvastatin or simvastatin acid after administration of a single 80-mg dose of simvastatin.[4] No simvastatin dose adjustment is therefore necessary on concurrent use.

1. Zhi J, Moore R, Kanitra L, Mulligan TE. Pharmacokinetic evaluation of the possible interaction between selected concomitant medications and orlistat at steady state in healthy subjects. *J Clin Pharmacol* (2002) 42, 1011–19.
2. Oo CY, Akbari B, Lee S, Nichols G, Hellmann CP. Effect of orlistat, a novel anti-obesity agent, on the pharmacokinetics and pharmacodynamics of pravastatin in patients with mild hypercholesterolaemia. *Clin Drug Invest* (1999) 17, 217–23.
3. Guerciolini R. Mode of action of orlistat. *Int J Obes* (1997) 21 (Suppl 3), S12–S23.
4. Zhi J, Moore R, Kanitra L, Mulligan TE. Effects of orlistat, a lipase inhibitor, on the pharmacokinetics of three highly lipophilic drugs (amiodarone, fluoxetine, and simvastatin) in healthy volunteers. *J Clin Pharmacol* (2003) 43, 428–34.

Statins + Phenytoin

A number of isolated case reports describe a reduction in the cholesterol-lowering effect of simvastatin, fluvastatin and atorvastatin in patients taking phenytoin. The concurrent use of phenytoin and fluvastatin increases the exposure to both drugs.

Clinical evidence

A 50-year-old woman taking **simvastatin** 10 mg daily had her antiepileptic medication changed from sodium valproate to phenytoin 325 mg daily. Over the following 3 months her total cholesterol rose from 9.4 mmol/L to 15.99 mmol/L. The dose of **simvastatin** was gradually increased to 40 mg daily without an appreciable reduction in her cholesterol levels. Despite further changes (to **fluvastatin** 40 mg daily, then to **atorvastatin** 40 mg daily) her cholesterol level remained above 10 mmol/L. Finally phenytoin was discontinued and her cholesterol dropped to 6.24 mmol/L with **atorvastatin** 80 mg daily.[1] Similarly, a 78-year-old woman, who had been stable on multiple drugs including **simvastatin** 40 mg and phenytoin 300 mg daily for several years, was admitted to hospital after she inadvertently omitted her diuretic and mistakenly took extra phenytoin for a week: her phenytoin levels and also her cholesterol levels were found to be raised. The phenytoin was withheld and the cholesterol levels decreased gradually along with the reduction in phenytoin levels.[2] A further case describes a 61-year-old man taking long-term phenytoin and phenobarbital who had negligible improvement in lipid profiles while taking **atorvastatin** 40 mg for 8 weeks then 80 mg daily, even with the addition of ezetimibe 10 mg daily and nicotinic acid (niacin), titrated up to 2 g daily. His phenytoin was discontinued and 2 months later his LDL-cholesterol levels had decreased by about 50%.[3]

The addition of phenytoin 300 mg daily to **fluvastatin** 40 mg daily *increased* the maximum concentration and AUC of **fluvastatin** by 27% and 40%, respectively, and increased the maximum concentration and AUC of phenytoin by 5% and 20%, respectively.[4]

Mechanism

It seems possible that phenytoin induced the metabolism of simvastatin and atorvastatin by CYP3A4, so that they were cleared more quickly and were therefore less effective. Fluvastatin is a minor inhibitor of CYP2C9, which would explain the very slight increase in phenytoin exposure on concurrent use, but the finding of increased fluvastatin exposure is unexplained.

Importance and management

Evidence for an interaction between phenytoin and atorvastatin or simvastatin currently appears to be limited to these few reports and their general relevance remains unclear. However, if lipid levels remain elevated in a patient taking phenytoin, it might be worth considering switching to a statin that is not appreciably metabolised by the cytochrome P450 enzyme system (see *Statins*, under 'Lipid regulating drugs', p.1309).

The slight increase in fluvastatin exposure seen with phenytoin is not likely to be clinically important. Similarly, the very slight alteration in phenytoin levels caused by fluvastatin seems unlikely to be clinically relevant.

1. Murphy MJ, Dominiczak MH. Efficacy of statin therapy: possible effect of phenytoin. *Postgrad Med J* (1999) 75, 359–60.
2. Tan KM, Kelly JG, McGarry K. Statins and phenytoin interact – a case history. *Br J Clin Pharmacol* (2008) 65, 147–8.
3. Khandwala HM. Lipid lowering inefficacy of high-dose statin therapy due to concurrent use of phenytoin. *South Med J* (2006) 99, 1385–7.
4. Lescol (Fluvastatin sodium). Novartis Pharmaceuticals Corp. US Prescribing information, October 2012.

Statins + Phosphodiesterase type-5 inhibitors

Reports describe myalgia with the concurrent use of sildenafil and atorvastatin, rosuvastatin, or pravastatin; and tadalafil and pravastatin or simvastatin. The pharmacokinetics of atorvastatin and sildenafil do not appear to be altered by concurrent use, and tadalafil does not alter lovastatin pharmacokinetics.

Clinical evidence

(a) Atorvastatin

In a placebo-controlled, crossover study in 24 healthy subjects, the pharmacokinetics of **sildenafil** (single 100-mg dose) and atorvastatin (10 mg daily for 7 days) were unchanged by concurrent use.[1]

In a clinical study in which 131 men taking **sildenafil** 100 mg as needed for erectile dysfunction were randomised to atorvastatin 40 mg daily or placebo for 12 weeks, no patient had an increase in creatine kinase or a serious adverse event, although 3% of those taking atorvastatin reported myalgia. This incidence is not outside the limits of that expected for atorvastatin alone, although the study design did not allow assessment of this. Erectile function improved in the atorvastatin group compared with placebo.[2]

(b) Lovastatin

In a study in 16 healthy subjects, **tadalafil** 20 mg daily for 14 days did not affect the pharmacokinetics of a 40-mg dose of lovastatin.[3]

(c) Pravastatin

A report describes a 59-year-old man who presented with fatigue, and bilateral knee and intermittent left elbow pain, for which a cause could not be identified on medical consultation, and which did not respond to rest and regular NSAIDs. The patient had been taking multiple medications including pravastatin without problems for several years previously, and realised that he had only developed the current symptoms shortly after starting to take **tadalafil** daily. He decided to stop taking the tadalafil, and 3 days later the symptoms had resolved and he was able to resume his normal activities.[4]

(d) Rosuvastatin

Rhabdomyolysis was diagnosed in a 66-year-old man who had been taking rosuvastatin 10 mg daily for 5 months who presented with severe muscle pain and weakness, reddish-brown discoloration of urine, and maintained penile erection after beginning the use of as-needed **sildenafil**. Creatine kinase was increased at 18 386 units/L on admission, decreasing to 544 units/L after 9 days.[5]

(e) Simvastatin

A report describes a 76-year-old man who had been taking simvastatin 10 mg daily for 3 years who had experienced severe muscle aches, particularly in the lower part of his legs and feet, which had started within 10 hours of taking a single 50-mg dose of **sildenafil** and had resolved over the following 3 days. Although he was asymptomatic and showed no muscle tenderness or swelling at the time of examination, his creatine kinase concentration was marginally increased (406 units/L). There was also a mild elevation of blood urea nitrogen and an increase in creatinine and potassium concentrations. A tentative diagnosis of rhabdomyolysis was made, there being no other obvious identifiable cause for the myalgia. Both simvastatin and sildenafil were stopped, and he made a full recovery.[6] Note that this case does not fit the usual classifications for myopathy or rhabdomyolysis, see Muscle and liver toxicity, under 'Lipid regulating drugs', p.1309.

A further report describes a 48-year-old man who had been taking simvastatin 20 mg daily for 8 days who presented with severe muscle aches in the upper and lower extremities, weakness in the pelvic and shoulder girdle regions, and maintained penile erection, all of which had started within 3 hours of taking a single dose (not stated) of **tadalafil**. His creatine kinase concentration was marginally increased (210 to 444 units/L over 4 days). The symptoms resolved 5 days after cessation of both simvastatin and tadalafil.[7]

Mechanism

No pharmacokinetic interaction would be anticipated between sildenafil or tadalafil and lovastatin or atorvastatin. The reasons for the cases of myalgia are not known, although inhibition of CYP3A4 leading to increased statin concentrations and statin-induced myopathy has been proposed,[4] however, the phosphodiesterase type-5 inhibitors are not known to inhibit CYP3A4, by which atorvastatin, lovastatin, and simvastatin (but not pravastatin) are metabolised. Statins might increase the vasodilatation caused by phosphodiesterase type-5 inhibitors via a nitric oxide-mediated mechanism,[2,5] and could thereby potentiate the effect of these drugs on erectile function.

Importance and management

Evidence for an interaction between statins and the phosphodiesterase type-5 inhibitors is largely limited to case reports, but no pharmacokinetic interaction appears to occur when sildenafil or tadalafil are used with atorvastatin or lovastatin. The cases of muscle pain reported with sildenafil and atorvastatin, rosuvastatin, or simvastatin; and tadalafil and pravastatin or simvastatin are unexplained, and as such no broad generalisations can be made based on such slim evidence. Therefore, no special precautions currently seem necessary on concurrent use. Note that, daily atorvastatin has been tried with some success as an adjunct to as-needed sildenafil in men with erectile dysfunction not responding to sildenafil alone.[2]

1. Chung M, DiRico A, Calcagni A, Messig M, Scott R. Lack of a drug interaction between sildenafil and atorvastatin. *J Clin Pharmacol* (2000) 40, 1057.
2. Dadkhah F, Safarinejad MR, Asgari MA, Hosseini SY, Lashay A, Amini E. Atorvastatin improves the response to sildenafil in hypercholesterolemic men with erectile dysfunction not initially responsive to sildenafil. *Int J Impot Res* (2010) 22, 51–60.
3. Ring BJ, Patterson BE, Mitchell MI, Vandenbranden M, Gillespie J, Bedding AW, Jewell H, Payne CD, Forgue ST, Eckstein J, Wrighton SA, Phillips DL. Effect of tadalafil on cytochrome P450 3A4-mediated clearance: studies in vitro and in vivo. *Clin Pharmacol Ther* (2005) 77, 63–75.
4. Pujalte GG, Acosta L. Bilateral knee and intermittent elbow pain in a competitive archer/hunter: phosphodiesterase-5-inhibitor-statin interaction? *Clin J Sport Med* (2014) 24, e52–3.
5. Pennisi G, Vacante M, Russo C, Malaguarnera M. Rhabdomyolysis induced by rosuvastatin and sildenafil. *South Med J* (2010) 103, 1052–4.
6. Gutierrez CA. Sildenafil-simvastatin interaction: possible cause of rhabdomyolysis? *Am Fam Physician* (2001) 63, 636–7.
7. Gargante MP, Vacante M, Russo C, Malaguarnera M. Myopathy with concurrent tadalafil and simvastatin. *Case Rep Med* (2009). Epub.

Statins + Ranolazine

Ranolazine slightly increases simvastatin exposure. Other statins that are similarly metabolised might also be affected. A couple of cases of rhabdomyolysis have been reported for simvastatin in which ranolazine could have been a contributing factor.

Clinical evidence

In an open-label study, **simvastatin** 80 mg daily was given with ranolazine 1 g twice daily for 4 days. **Simvastatin** had no effect on the pharmacokinetics of ranolazine, but ranolazine increased the AUCs of simvastatin acid and simvastatin lactone by 40 to 60%, respectively.[1]

A 63-year-old man with chronic kidney disease taking high-dose **simvastatin** 80 mg daily developed rhabdomyolysis after additionally starting ranolazine 500 mg daily.[2] Another case report[3] describes rhabdomyolysis in a patient taking **simvastatin** 40 mg daily and ciclosporin, which occurred 2 months after the patient also started taking diltiazem and ranolazine 500 mg daily, both of which could have been contributing factors (see also 'Statins + Calcium-channel blockers; Diltiazem or Verapamil', p.1325).

Mechanism

Simvastatin is a substrate of CYP3A4, of which ranolazine is an inhibitor. Concurrent use can therefore increase the levels of simvastatin and its active metabolite. Note that **lovastatin** is also predominantly metabolised by CYP3A4 and **atorvastatin** is metabolised, in part, by CYP3A4, and might therefore be similarly affected.

Importance and management

Evidence for a pharmacokinetic interaction between the statins and ranolazine appears to be limited to this one study, but an interaction appears to be established. The increased simvastatin levels seen appear to be slight to moderate; however, they might be clinically relevant in some patients, as the case report appears to indicate. In the US, the recommended maximum daily dose of simvastatin in patients also taking ranolazine is 20 mg.[4] All patients taking statins should be warned about the symptoms of myopathy and told to report muscle pain or weakness. It would be prudent to reinforce this advice if patients given simvastatin, lovastatin, and possibly atorvastatin, are also given ranolazine.

1. Jerling M, Huan B-L, Leung K, Chu N, Abdallah H, Hussein Z. Studies to investigate the pharmacokinetic interactions between ranolazine and ketoconazole, diltiazem or simvastatin during combined administration in healthy subjects. J Clin Pharmacol. (2005) 45, 422–33.
2. Hylton AC, Ezekiel TO. Rhabdomyolysis in a patient receiving ranolazine and simvastatin. *Am J Health-Syst Pharm* (2010) 67, 1829–31.
3. Rifkin SI. Multiple drug interactions in a renal transplant patient leading to simvastatin-induced rhabdomyolysis: a case report. *Medscape J Med* (2008) 10, 264.
4. Zocor (Simvastatin). Merck & Co., Inc. US Prescribing information, March 2015.

Statins + Retinoids

Alitretinoin, taken orally, might very slightly decrease the exposure to simvastatin.

Clinical evidence, mechanism, importance and management

In a pharmacokinetic study in 18 healthy subjects, oral **alitretinoin** 30 mg once daily for 14 days very slightly reduced the AUC of a single 40 mg dose of **simvastatin** by 16% and reduced its maximum level by 23%. Single-dose simvastatin had no effect on **alitretinoin** pharmacokinetics.[1] The reason for the very slight reduction in **simvastatin** exposure is unknown, but is not of any clinical consequence. Therefore, no simvastatin dose adjustment seems likely to be necessary on the concurrent use of oral alitretinoin from a pharmacokinetic perspective. However, note that oral retinoids such as alitretinoin commonly increase triglyceride and cholesterol levels, and might therefore be expected to decrease the efficacy of statins (they should not be used in patients with uncontrolled hyperlipidaemia and discontinued if this develops during therapy). Nevertheless, statins might have a role in treating the adverse effects of retinoids on lipids if the oral retinoid is considered essential.[2]

1. Schmitt-Hoffmann AH, Roos B, Sauer J, Spickermann J, Maares J, Schoetzau A, Meyer I. Pharmacokinetic interactions between alitretinoin and ketoconazole or simvastatin or ciclosporin A. *Clin Exp Dermatol* (2011) 36 (Suppl 2), 24–8.
2. Beach RA, McQueen M, Wismer J. Novel management of isotretinoin-induced hypertriglyceridemia in an adolescent with severe acne. *Clin Pediatr (Phila)* (2009) 48, 551–4.

Statins + Rifampicin (Rifampin)

The effect of rifampicin on the statins appears to differ depending on the timing of administration and the duration of concurrent use.

For atorvastatin, steady-state rifampicin markedly reduces exposure when administration is separated, but slightly increases exposure when both drugs are given simultaneously; whereas, single-dose rifampicin markedly increases exposure.

For pravastatin, single-dose rifampicin moderately increases exposure when both drugs are given simultaneously but slightly lowers exposure when administration is separated, although effects are variable.

For simvastatin, steady-state rifampicin markedly to very markedly lowers exposure when administration is separated.

For rosuvastatin, steady-state rifampicin has no effect on exposure when administration is separated, although the effects are variable.

Steady-state rifampicin appears to slightly to moderately reduce fluvastatin exposure, and slightly increase steady-state pitavastatin exposure.

Clinical evidence

(a) Atorvastatin

In a study, 10 healthy subjects were given rifampicin 600 mg daily for 5 days with a single 40-mg dose of atorvastatin on day 6, about 17 hours after the last dose of rifampicin. Rifampicin markedly *decreased* the AUC of atorvastatin by 80% and decreased the AUCs of its two active metabolites by 43% and 81%, respectively. The reduction in the AUC of atorvastatin ranged from 61 to 88%.[1] Conversely, in a similar study in which the dose of atorvastatin was given at the same time as the last dose of rifampicin, the AUC of atorvastatin was slightly *increased* by 30%, with a 2.7-fold increase in its maximum concentration.[2]

Furthermore, in two other studies, a *single-dose* of intravenous or oral rifampicin markedly *increased* the AUC of a single dose of atorvastatin given *simultaneously* (about sevenfold increase).[3,4] In one of the studies, the extent of the effect varied by genotype for the gene encoding the OATP1B1 transporter.[4]

(b) Fluvastatin

The US manufacturer briefly mentions that, in a study, rifampicin 600 mg daily for 6 days reduced the AUC and maximum concentration of fluvastatin 20 mg daily by 53% and 42%, respectively.[5] Another review also mentions that pretreatment with rifampicin reduced the AUC of fluvastatin by 51%.[6]

(c) Pitavastatin

In a study in healthy subjects, concurrent administration of rifampicin 600 mg daily and pitavastatin 4 mg daily for 5 days slightly *increased* the pitavastatin AUC by 29% with a 2-fold increase in its maximum concentration. The AUC of rifampicin was negligibly reduced by 15%.[7] It is not known if administration in this study was separated or simultaneous.

(d) Pravastatin

In a study, 10 healthy subjects were given rifampicin 600 mg daily for 5 days with a single 40-mg dose of pravastatin on day 6, about 17 hours after the last dose of rifampicin. Rifampicin slightly reduced the AUC of pravastatin by 31%; however, there were large interindividual differences in the results, with 3 subjects having an *increase* in AUC.[8] Conversely, in another study, a *single* 600-mg dose of rifampicin moderately *increased* the AUC of a single 20-mg dose of pravastatin given *simultaneously* (about 2.3-fold increase).[9]

(e) Rosuvastatin

In a study, 18 healthy subjects were given rifampicin 450 mg daily for 6 days with a single 20-mg dose of rosuvastatin on day 7, about 12 hours after the last dose of rifampicin. Rifampicin did not alter the mean AUC of rosuvastatin; however, there was large interindividual variation, with 3 subjects having an increase in the AUC of rosuvastatin of more than 50% and 3 subjects having a decrease in the AUC of rosuvastatin of more than 50%.[10]

(f) Simvastatin

In a study, 10 healthy subjects were given rifampicin 600 mg daily for 5 days with a single 40-mg dose of simvastatin on day 6, about 17 hours after the last dose of rifampicin. Rifampicin markedly to very markedly reduced the AUCs of simvastatin and simvastatin acid by 87% and 93%, respectively. The reduction in AUC of simvastatin ranged from 82 to 97%.[11]

Mechanism

Rifampicin is a known potent inducer of CYP3A4 by which lovastatin and simvastatin, and to a lesser extent atorvastatin, are metabolised, and a moderate inducer of

CYP2C9, by which fluvastatin is partially metabolised. Multiple-dose rifampicin would therefore be expected to reduce the levels of these statins, as has been seen in studies with separate administration. However, rifampicin also has effects on drug transporter proteins, such as OATP, and it seems that this might account for its interaction with statins that are not greatly metabolised by cytochrome P450 isoenzymes, such as pitavastatin, pravastatin and rosuvastatin. It might also explain the difference between simultaneous and separate administration of rifampicin and some statins, and the difference in the effect of multiple-dose and single-dose rifampicin on the statins. Therefore, for atorvastatin, when this statin is given 17 hours after multiple-dose rifampicin its levels are markedly reduced (cytochrome P450 induction), but, when it is given simultaneously with multiple-dose rifampicin its levels are slightly increased (OATP inhibition and cytochrome P450 induction), and when it is given simultaneously with single-dose rifampicin, its levels are very markedly increased (OATP inhibition). This suggests that, for multiple-dose rifampicin, inhibition of OATP (probably OATP1B1) is the rate-limiting step in the elimination of atorvastatin when administration is simultaneous.

As the available data for simvastatin and rosuvastatin are for multiple-dose rifampicin with single-dose statin administration separated by 12 or 17 hours, further study is needed to assess the effect of simultaneous administration, and for single-dose rifampicin administration.

Importance and management

Evidence for an interaction between rifampicin and the statins appears to be limited to the pharmacokinetic studies cited, in which the direction and extent of the pharmacokinetic interaction appears variable for some statins, and appears to depend on whether concurrent administration is simultaneous or separated, and whether rifampicin is given as a single-dose or to steady state.

For **atorvastatin**, it appears that if the statin is given at the same time as rifampicin when rifampicin is already at steady state, a clinically relevant pharmacokinetic interaction does not occur, and no atorvastatin dose adjustment appears to be necessary. However, if administration is separated by 17 hours when rifampicin is at steady state, atorvastatin exposure is markedly reduced, and reduced efficacy might be expected. For this reason, the manufacturers recommend that, if rifampicin is required, then atorvastatin should be taken at the same time as rifampicin, and its efficacy should be monitored.[2,12] This advice seems prudent when rifampicin is at steady state. However, given the marked increase in atorvastatin exposure with single-dose rifampicin given simultaneously with atorvastatin, some caution might be appropriate for the first few days of multiple-dose rifampicin (before cytochrome P450 induction is maximal) or for when rifampicin is used for meningococcal prophylaxis (just 2 days administration) or once monthly as is recommended for leprosy. In these situations, even though the increase in atorvastatin exposure might be short-lived, because it is marked, it might be appropriate to separate the administration of rifampicin and atorvastatin, particularly with high-dose atorvastatin. Alternatively, atorvastatin could be withheld for a couple of days.

Similarly, for **pitavastatin**, there is evidence that the concurrent use of multiple-dose rifampicin slightly increases pitavastatin exposure. In general, the degree of increase seen would not be expected to be clinically relevant. Nevertheless, the manufacturer limits the maximum pitavastatin dose to 2 mg daily when it is taken with rifampicin.[7]

For **pravastatin**, the slight decrease in pravastatin exposure with separate administration at steady-state rifampicin appears unlikely to be clinically important; however, given the variability in effect, some caution might be appropriate. Similarly, the twofold increase in pravastatin exposure with single-dose simultaneous rifampicin administration is probably not clinically important because it will be short lived.

For **simvastatin** and **rosuvastatin**, the only available pharmacokinetic data are for separate administration when rifampicin is at steady state, and it is currently unclear what would happen if administration were simultaneous, or if a single dose of rifampicin was given. For separate administration with steady-state rifampicin, it is likely that a simvastatin dose increase would be required to maintain efficacy, because of the marked pharmacokinetic interaction seen. For rosuvastatin, the effects were variable, and, at present, the best approach would be to monitor efficacy and safety if concurrent use was required.

For **fluvastatin**, the pharmacokinetic study showed a slight to moderate reduction in fluvastatin exposure with steady-state rifampicin, therefore, it would be prudent to monitor for reduced efficacy, or for a possible increase in toxicity, on concurrent use.

1. Backman JT, Luurila H, Neuvonen M, Neuvonen PJ. Rifampin markedly decreases and gemfibrozil increases the plasma concentrations of atorvastatin and its metabolites. *Clin Pharmacol Ther* (2005) 78, 154–67.
2. Lipitor (Atorvastatin calcium). Pfizer Inc. US Prescribing information, March 2015.
3. Lau YY, Huang Y, Frassetto L, Benet LZ. Effect of OATP1B transporter inhibition on the pharmacokinetics of atorvastatin in healthy volunteers. *Clin Pharmacol Ther* (2007) 81, 194–204.
4. He Y-J, Zhang W, Chen Y, Guo D, Tu J-H, Xu L-Y, Tan Z-R, Chen B-L, Li Z, Zhou G, Yu B-N, Kirchheiner J, Zhou H-H. Rifampicin alters atorvastatin plasma concentration on the basis of *SLCO1B1* 521T>C polymorphism. *Clin Chim Acta* (2009) 405, 49–52.
5. Lescol (Fluvastatin sodium). Novartis Pharmaceuticals Corp. US Prescribing information, October 2012.
6. Jokubaitis LA. Updated clinical safety experience with fluvastatin. *Am J Cardiol* (1994) 73, 18D–24D.
7. Livalo (Pitavastatin). Kowa Pharmaceuticals America, Inc. US Prescribing information, October 2013.
8. Kyrklund C, Backman JT, Neuvonen M, Neuvonen PJ. Effect of rifampicin on pravastatin pharmacokinetics in healthy subjects. *Br J Clin Pharmacol* (2004) 57, 181–7.
9. Deng S, Chen X-P, Cao D, Yin T, Dai Z-Y, Luo J, Tang L, Li Y-J. Effects of a concomitant single oral dose of rifampicin on the pharmacokinetics of pravastatin in a two-phase, randomized, single-blind, placebo-controlled, crossover study in healthy Chinese male subjects. *Clin Ther* (2009) 31, 1256–63.
10. Zhang W, Deng S, Chen X-P, Zhou G, Xie H-T, He F-Y, Cao D, Li Y-J, Zhou H-H. Pharmacokinetics of rosuvastatin when coadministered with rifampicin in healthy males: a randomized, single-blind, placebo-controlled, crossover study. *Clin Ther* (2008) 30, 1283–9.
11. Kyrklund C, Backman JT, Kivistö KT, Neuvonen M, Laitila J, Neuvonen PJ. Rifampin greatly reduces plasma simvastatin and simvastatin acid concentrations. *Clin Pharmacol Ther* (2000) 68, 592–7.
12. Lipitor (Atorvastatin calcium trihydrate). Pfizer Ltd. UK Summary of product characteristics, March 2015.

Statins + Rupatadine

It has been suggested that rupatadine could exacerbate the muscle toxicity caused by the statins.

Clinical evidence, mechanism, importance and management

The UK manufacturer of rupatadine[1] reports that in clinical studies asymptomatic rises in creatine phosphokinase levels have occurred. As rupatadine is a substrate of the cytochrome P450 isoenzyme CYP3A4, by which some of the statins are also metabolised, the manufacturer advises caution on concurrent use, on the basis that the risk of interactions is unknown. However, it seems unlikely that a pharmacokinetic interaction will result in muscle disorders, because muscle disorders are usually due to a several fold rise in the levels of the statin, which is unlikely to occur as a result of competition for metabolism by the same isoenzyme. For more information on the metabolism of individual statins, and monitoring for muscle disorders, see under 'Lipid regulating drugs', p.1309).

1. Rupafin (Rupatadine fumarate). GlaxoSmithKline UK. UK Summary of product characteristics, December 2009.

Statins + Sirolimus

The concurrent use of atorvastatin and sirolimus does not alter the pharmacokinetics of either drug. However, a case report describes a patient who developed elevated sirolimus levels after atorvastatin was started. There is limited evidence to suggest a higher incidence of myopathy in transplant patients taking statins and sirolimus; and an isolated report describes a fatal case of rhabdomyolysis in a patient taking sirolimus and given simvastatin, and a case of rhabdomyolysis in a patient taking sirolimus and given fluvastatin.

Clinical evidence

(a) Pharmacokinetics

In a study in healthy subjects given **atorvastatin** 20 mg daily for 15 days, the concurrent use of sirolimus 2 mg daily for the last 5 days had no effect on the pharmacokinetics of atorvastatin. Similarly, there was no difference in sirolimus pharmacokinetics when taken with atorvastatin, when compared with a single dose of sirolimus taken alone.[1] For a single-dose study showing a lack of pharmacokinetic interaction of **atorvastatin** with the related drug everolimus, see 'Statins + Everolimus', p.1334.

In contrast to these pharmacokinetic studies, there is a case report that suggests a rise in sirolimus levels in a patient given **atorvastatin**. This patient, who had undergone a pancreatic islet transplant and who had been stable taking sirolimus 8 to 11 mg daily for 5 months, developed raised cholesterol and triglyceride levels, and so atorvastatin (dose not stated) was started. Six weeks later the trough sirolimus level was 20.5 nanograms/mL (target 7 to 10 nanograms/mL) and so the sirolimus dose was reduced. Further reductions were subsequently needed, and 3 months after the atorvastatin was started the sirolimus dose had been halved.[2]

(b) Rhabdomyolysis and myopathy

The US manufacturer notes that in clinical studies up to 90% of patients taking sirolimus required treatment for hyperlipidaemias with fibrates or statins, of whom up to half failed to achieve target lipid levels. They state that, during the concurrent use of sirolimus and statins, the incidence of myalgia was 6.7%, the incidence of raised creatine phosphokinase kinase levels was 3% and the incidence of rhabdomyolysis was less than 1%.[3] In one published retrospective analysis of 98 patients taking statins (53% **atorvastatin** and 38% **pravastatin**) who were switched from ciclosporin to sirolimus, creatine phosphokinase levels were routinely monitored and the incidence of raised levels doubled after the switch (from 20 to 40 patients). However, most of these cases were asymptomatic elevations in the patients taking **pravastatin**.[4]

A report describes a fatal case of rhabdomyolysis in a patient with persistent liver transplant rejection taking tacrolimus who was additionally given sirolimus and then developed hyperlipidaemia for which he was prescribed **simvastatin** 10 mg daily. About one month later, he then developed rhabdomyolysis with worsening renal failure.[5] A kidney transplant patient taking ciclosporin, mycophenolate mofetil and steroids for 2 years was switched from ciclosporin to sirolimus when she underwent surgery for a meningioma. She then started taking **fluvastatin** 80 mg daily and 2 weeks later developed sepsis, rhabdomyolysis and acute renal failure (creatine phosphokinase, 15 138 units/L) and required dialysis for 2 days.[6]

Mechanism

The reason for the isolated case in which the patient required reduced doses of sirolimus while taking atorvastatin is unknown. Myopathy and rhabdomyolysis are rare adverse effects of statins alone, and it is currently unclear if the risk of these adverse effects is higher in patients taking sirolimus, although there is some limited evidence to suggest it might be. Note that the incidence of these adverse effects is related to the statin dose, and higher statin doses can be used with sirolimus in an attempt to try to achieve target lipid levels.

Importance and management

The findings of the pharmacokinetic study suggest that no dose adjustments of either atorvastatin or sirolimus would be needed on concurrent use. The case report is at odds with this, and appears to be the only evidence of an interaction and so its general relevance seems likely to be small.

Statins are commonly required to treat sirolimus-induced hyperlipidaemias, and limited evidence suggests that the incidence of myopathy might possibly be increased on concurrent use. Regular testing of creatine phosphokinase has been mandated by some for the combination.[4] However, the US manufacturer of sirolimus states that patients given statins should undergo the routine monitoring for rhabdomyolysis usually required for these drugs.[3] That is, as a general rule, any patient given a statin should be advised to report any signs of myopathy and possible rhabdomyolysis (i.e. otherwise unexplained muscle pain, tenderness or weakness or dark coloured urine). If myopathy does occur, the statin should be stopped immediately. See also *Muscle and liver toxicity*, under 'Lipid regulating drugs', p.1309, for further guidance on monitoring and risk factors for muscle toxicity

1. Zimmerman JJ, Harper D, Speth JT, Frunicillo RJ, Getsy J. Potential pharmacokinetic interactions between sirolimus and atorvastatin. European Society for Organ Transplantation. 10th ESOT Congress, Lisbon, 2001, Abstract 145.
2. Barshes NR, Goodpastor SE, Goss JA, DeBakey ME. Sirolimus-atorvastatin drug interaction in the pancreatic islet transplant recipient. *Transplantation* (2003) 76, 1649–50.
3. Rapamune (Sirolimus). Wyeth Pharmaceuticals Inc. US Prescribing information, December 2012.
4. Aliabadi AZ, Mahr S, Dunkler D, Grömmer M, Zimpfer D, Wolner E, Grimm M, Zuckermann AO. Safety and efficacy of statin therapy in patients switched from cyclosporine A to sirolimus after cardiac transplantation. *Transplantation* (2008) 86, 1771–6.
5. Dopazo C, Bilbao I, Lázaro JL, Sapisochin G, Caralt M, Blanco L, Castells L, Charco R. Severe rhabdomyolysis and acute renal failure secondary to concomitant use of simvastatin with rapamycin plus tacrolimus in liver transplant patient. *Transplant Proc* (2009) 41, 1021–4.
6. Basic-Jukic N, Kes P, Bubic-Filipi L, Vranjican Z. Rhabdomyolysis and acute kidney injury secondary to concomitant use of fluvastatin and rapamycin in a renal transplant recipient. *Nephrol Dial Transplant* (2010) 25, 2036.

Statins + St John's wort (*Hypericum perforatum*)

St John's wort moderately decreases the exposure to simvastatin and reduces its lipid-lowering effect. Similarly, St John's wort reduces the lipid-lowering effect of atorvastatin. An isolated report unexpectedly describes reduced rosuvastatin efficacy during the use of St John's wort. St John's wort does not alter the pharmacokinetics of pravastatin.

Clinical evidence

In a placebo-controlled, crossover study, 16 healthy subjects took St John's wort 300 mg three times daily for 14 days. On day 14 **simvastatin** 10 mg was given to 8 subjects and **pravastatin** 20 mg was given to the other 8 subjects. St John's wort did not affect the plasma concentration of **pravastatin**, but it tended to reduce the AUC of **simvastatin** and moderately reduce the AUC of its active metabolite, simvastatin acid, by 62%.[1]

In a crossover study in 24 patients with hypercholesterolaemia taking long-term **simvastatin** 10 to 40 mg daily (an average dose of 20.8 mg daily), St John's wort (*Movina*) 300 mg twice daily for 4 weeks, raised the levels of total cholesterol from 4.56 mmol/L (pre-treatment) to 5.08 mmol/L and LDL-cholesterol from 2.30 mmol/L to 2.72 mmol/L. The authors equate the magnitude of the increased LDL-cholesterol levels to a halving of the effect of **simvastatin**.[2]

In a similar study by the same authors, 16 patients with hypercholesterolaemia taking long-term **atorvastatin** 10 to 40 mg daily (an average dose of 14.4 mg daily), were given St John's wort (*Movina*) 300 mg twice daily for 4 weeks. St John's wort raised the levels of total cholesterol from 4.76 mmol/L (pre-treatment) to 5.1 mmol/L and LDL-cholesterol from 2.39 mmol/L to 2.66 mmol/L. The levels of **atorvastatin** were not measured in this study. The authors equate the magnitude of the increased LDL-cholesterol levels to a loss of one-third of the effect of **atorvastatin**. No adverse effects were reported.[3]

A case report describes a 59-year-old man who was taking **rosuvastatin** 10 mg daily with satisfactory lipid levels. Six months later, a routine blood test indicated that his total cholesterol had risen from 4.27 mmol/L to 6.1 mmol/L. On questioning he said that he had been taking a supplement containing St John's wort 600 mg daily. He stopped taking the supplement, and 4 months later his cholesterol levels had reduced to about the former level.[4]

Mechanism

St John's wort is a weak inducer of CYP3A4, by which simvastatin, and to a lesser extent atorvastatin, are metabolised; however, this on its own does not seem sufficient to explain the reduction in statin efficacy seen. Rosuvastatin is less than 10% metabolised, so a reduction in its metabolism seems unlikely, and the case report is therefore unexplained. A lack of a pharmacokinetic interaction with pravastatin is as expected.

Importance and management

Although the evidence is limited, it appears that St John's wort can reduce the efficacy of atorvastatin and simvastatin, which appears to result in a clinically relevant increase in total cholesterol and LDL-cholesterol levels, depending on the patients baseline result and medical history. It might be prudent to consider an interaction if lipid-lowering targets are not met, and advise the patient to stop taking St John's wort or adjust the dose of the statin, as needed.

No pharmacokinetic interaction would be expected with pravastatin as it is not metabolised by CYP3A4, and this was demonstrated in the study above. Similarly, no pharmacokinetic interaction would be expected with rosuvastatin, but the case report adds a note of caution. Bear it in mind in the event of an unexpected response to treatment.

1. Sugimoto K, Ohmori M, Tsuruoka S, Nishiki K, Kawaguchi A, Harada K, Arakawa M, Sakomoto K, Masada M, Miyamori I, Fujimura A. Different effects of St John's wort on the pharmacokinetics of simvastatin and pravastatin. *Clin Pharmacol Ther* (2001) 70, 518–24.
2. Eggertsen R, Andreasson Å, Andrén L. Effects of treatment with a commercially available St John's Wort product (Movina®) on cholesterol levels in patients with hypercholesterolemia treated with simvastatin. *Scand J Prim Health Care* (2007) 25, 154–9.
3. Andrén L, Andreasson Å, Eggertsen R. Interaction between a commercially available St. John's wort product (Movina) and atorvastatin in patients with hypercholesterolemia. *Eur J Clin Pharmacol* (2007) 63, 913–16.
4. Gordon RY, Becker DJ, Rader DJ. Reduced efficacy of rosuvastatin by St John's wort. *Am J Med* (2009) 122, e1–e2.

Statins + Suxamethonium (Succinylcholine)

In one study, the concurrent use of suxamethonium in patients taking statins resulted in higher myoglobin plasma concentrations than in patients not taking statins.

Clinical evidence, mechanism, importance and management

A prospective study in 67 patients scheduled for elective surgery assessed the effect of suxamethonium 1.5 mg/kg over 5 seconds in patients who were taking statins for at least 3 months (37 patients) and those who were not taking statins (30 patients). The aim was to determine whether suxamethonium increases the plasma concentrations of myoglobin, potassium, and creatine kinase in patients taking statin more than in those not taking statins; and if suxamethonium-induced postoperative muscle pain is aggravated in patients taking statin. The statins included were **atorvastatin, lovastatin, simvastatin**, and **pravastatin**. No additional muscle relaxants were given until the neuromuscular block had resolved. The study found that myoglobin plasma concentrations 20 minutes after suxamethonium was given were about 34% higher in patients taking statins than in those not taking statins. Nevertheless, this increase was not felt to be clinically relevant. Potassium and creatine kinase concentrations, and muscle pain was not different between the groups. The authors concluded that the effect of suxamethonium given to patients taking statins is likely to be small and of limited clinical importance.[1]

1. Turan A, Mendoza ML, Gupta S, You J, Gottlieb A, Chu W, Saager L, Sessler DI. Consequences of succinylcholine administration to patients using statins. *Anesthesiology* (2011) 115, 28–35.

Statins + Tacrolimus

An isolated case report attributes rhabdomyolysis to an interaction between tacrolimus and simvastatin. Tacrolimus does not alter atorvastatin pharmacokinetics.

Clinical evidence, mechanism, importance and management

In a pharmacokinetic study in 13 healthy subjects given **atorvastatin** 40 mg daily for 4 days, the short-term use of tacrolimus (two doses of 62.5 micrograms/kg given 12 hours apart) did not alter the pharmacokinetics of **atorvastatin** or its metabolites. This was in contrast to the marked increase in atorvastatin exposure seen with ciclosporin, which was used as a positive control,[1] see also 'Statins + Ciclosporin', p.1327.

A 51-year-old woman, who was taking tacrolimus after a kidney transplant, started taking **simvastatin** 10 mg daily following a stroke. After 5 months the dose was increased to 20 mg daily, and fusidic acid was started for osteomyelitis. Muscle pain developed 2 weeks later, and after a further 3 weeks she was admitted to hospital, at which point her creatine kinase level was found to be 24 000 units/mL (reference range 10 to 70 units/mL) and she had renal impairment. The **simvastatin** and fusidic acid were immediately stopped and the patient recovered over the following 2 weeks. She was later treated with a combination of **fluvastatin**, tacrolimus and fusidic acid without incident, leading the authors to suspect that the rhabdomyolysis was caused by an interaction between **simvastatin** and tacrolimus.[2] However, note that fusidic acid has been implicated in a number of cases of rhabdomyolysis with statins, including simvastatin, see 'Statins + Fusidic acid', p.1340, many of which were only reported subsequent to this case. It therefore seems equally possible that the reaction seen in this case was actually an interaction between fusidic acid and simvastatin.

For another case of fatal rhabdomyolysis in a transplant patient taking tacrolimus and sirolimus and given simvastatin, see 'Statins + Sirolimus', p.1356.

1. Lemahieu WPD, Hermann M, Asberg A, Verbeke K, Holdaas H, Vanrenterghem Y, Maes BD. Combined therapy with atorvastatin and calcineurin inhibitors: no interactions with tacrolimus. *Am J Transplant* (2005) 5, 2236–43.
2. Kotanko P, Kiristis W, Skrabal F. Rhabdomyolysis and acute renal graft impairment in a patient treated with simvastatin, tacrolimus, and fusidic acid. *Nephron* (2002) 90, 234–5.

Statins + Tyrosine kinase inhibitors

Imatinib moderately increases the exposure to simvastatin. Single-dose dasatinib negligibly increased simvastatin exposure, but multiple doses might have a greater effect. Lovastatin and, to a lesser extent, atorvastatin would be expected to be similarly affected. Other tyrosine kinase inhibitors that also inhibit CYP3A4 might interact similarly. A case of rhabdomyolysis has been described in a patient taking erlotinib and

simvastatin. The concurrent use of pazopanib and simvastatin might increase ALT concentrations.

Clinical evidence

(a) Dasatinib

The UK and US manufacturers of dasatinib briefly report that, after concurrent administration of a single 100-mg dose of dasatinib in 54 healthy subjects, the AUC and maximum plasma concentration of **simvastatin** were increased by 20% and 37%, respectively. It is possible that the effect might be greater after multiple doses of dasatinib.[1,2]

(b) Erlotinib

A 75-year-old woman who had been taking ezetimibe 10 mg daily with high-dose **simvastatin** 80 mg daily for the past 3 years developed generalised muscle pain and weakness, diagnosed as rhabdomyolysis, 6 weeks after starting erlotinib for recurrent lung cancer.[3]

(c) Imatinib

In a clinical study, 20 patients with chronic myeloid leukaemia were given a single 40-mg dose of **simvastatin** before, and on the last day of, a 7-day course of imatinib 400 mg daily. Imatinib increased the maximum serum concentration of **simvastatin** 2-fold and the AUC, 3-fold.[4]

(d) Pazopanib

The UK and US manufacturers of pazopanib report that, in a meta-analysis of clinical studies, the concurrent use of pazopanib and **simvastatin** resulted in an increase in the incidence of increased ALT concentrations, when compared to patients not taking simvastatin (27% compared with 14%). The risk with other statins is unknown due to limited data.[5,6]

Mechanism

Imatinib and dasatinib inhibit CYP3A4, by which simvastatin is metabolised. Erlotinib is not an inhibitor of CYP3A4 and so would not be expected to increase simvastatin concentrations by this mechanism. The case described above could simply be attributable to the use of too high a dose of simvastatin in an elderly patient with failing health.

Pazopanib is a weak inhibitor of CYP3A4, and has been shown to inhibit the organic anion transporting polypeptide (OATP) 1B1 *in vitro*.[5,6]

Importance and management

Imatinib

The pharmacokinetic interaction of imatinib with simvastatin is established, and the moderately increased exposure seen is likely to increase the risk of statin toxicity (myopathy and rhabdomyolysis). On the basis of a similar pharmacokinetic interaction with other moderate CYP3A4 inhibitors, such as diltiazem (see 'Statins + Calcium-channel blockers; Diltiazem or Verapamil', p.1325), the benefits of using simvastatin with imatinib should be carefully weighed against the risks in each individual, and the statin should be used at the lowest possible dose. In patients already taking statins, the dose of the statin might need to be considerably reduced if imatinib is started. The same advice would apply to **lovastatin**, as it is similarly metabolised by CYP3A4. **Atorvastatin** is less dependent on CYP3A4 metabolism and so might be also be affected, but to a lesser extent. As a general rule, in any patient given imatinib with simvastatin (or lovastatin, and probably atorvastatin), the general advice to report any signs of myopathy and possible rhabdomyolysis (i.e. otherwise unexplained muscle pain, tenderness or weakness or dark coloured urine) should be specifically reinforced. If myopathy does occur, the statin should be stopped immediately. See also *Muscle and liver toxicity*, under 'Lipid regulating drugs', p.1309, for further guidance on monitoring, and risk factors for muscle toxicity.

Pazopanib

Evidence for an interaction between simvastatin and pazopanib is limited, but the incidence of raised ALT concentrations does appear to be increased by concurrent use. The UK manufacturer of pazopanib states that patients taking pazopanib and simvastatin should be closely monitored, and if an increase in their ALT occurs, simvastatin should be stopped.[5]

As pazopanib inhibits the organic anion transporting polypeptide (OATP) 1B1 *in vitro*, the UK manufacturer states that there is a possibility that pazopanib might affect the pharmacokinetics of drugs that are substrates of this transporter,[5] and this would include a number of the statins (see 'Statins + Rifampicin (Rifampin)', p.1355). Interactions occurring via this transporter are complex, and until more is known it might be prudent to consider applying the advice given for rifampicin and statins to a possible interaction between pazopanib and these statins.

Other tyrosine kinase inhibitors

Evidence from the single-dose study with **dasatinib** suggests that it might increase simvastatin exposure, but a multiple-dose study is required to establish the magnitude and importance of this.

The relevance of **erlotinib** to the single case of rhabdomyolysis in a patient taking high-dose simvastatin is unclear, particularly as there is no obvious mechanism for a pharmacokinetic interaction.

Evidence for an interaction between **other tyrosine kinase inhibitors** and statins is lacking, but note that some other tyrosine kinase inhibitors do also inhibit CYP3A4 (see 'Table 1.9', p.11) and might therefore be predicted to increase the exposure to some statins (namely simvastatin, lovastatin, and atorvastatin).

1. Sprycel (Dasatinib monohydrate). Bristol-Myers Squibb Company. US Prescribing information, April 2014.
2. Sprycel (Dasatinib monohydrate). Bristol-Myers Squibb Pharmaceutical Ltd. UK Summary of product characteristics, November 2013.
3. Veeraputhiran M, Sundermeyer M. Rhabdomyolysis resulting from pharmacologic interaction between erlotinib and simvastatin. *Clin Lung Cancer* (2008) 9, 232–4.
4. O'Brien SG, Meinhardt P, Bond E, Beck J, Peng B, Dutreix C, Mehring G, Milosavljev S, Huber C, Capdeville R, Fischer T. Effects of imatinib mesylate (STI517, Glivec) on the pharmacokinetics of simvastatin, a cytochrome P450 3A4 substrate, in patients with chronic myeloid leukaemia. *Br J Cancer* (2003) 89, 1855–9.
5. Votrient (Pazopanib hydrochloride). GlaxoSmithKline UK. UK Summary of product characteristics, December 2013.
6. Votrient (Pazopanib hydrochloride). GlaxoSmithKline. US Prescribing information, November 2013.

Statins + Vaccines

A study suggests that influenza vaccination does not precipitate myopathy in patients taking statins, although an isolated possible case has been reported for high-dose cerivastatin. Statins appear to have minimal beneficial effects on respiratory outcomes after influenza vaccination. In short-term use, atorvastatin does not appear to affect the antibody response to hepatitis A vaccination, but might increase the antibody response to tetanus toxoid.

Clinical evidence

(a) Hepatitis A vaccine

Atorvastatin 40 mg daily for 28 days starting on the day of vaccination had no effect on the antibody response to hepatitis A vaccine in 67 healthy young subjects when compared with 56 receiving placebo.[1]

(b) Influenza vaccine

An isolated report describes a patient taking bezafibrate and a statin (switched from simvastatin 40 mg daily to high-dose cerivastatin 2 months previously), who developed rhabdomyolysis after being given an influenza vaccine. The patient developed diffuse myalgia within 24 hours of the vaccination. Initially he attributed the myalgia to the vaccination, but he developed increasing muscular weakness, and he was unable to get out of bed 3 days post vaccination.[2] In contrast, in a study in 98 outpatients receiving influenza vaccination, there was no indication that the vaccine caused clinical or laboratory evidence of myopathy in patients taking statins. Only 2 patients experienced myalgia (one of 52 taking statins and one of 46 controls). Creatine phosphokinase levels were measured in all of the patients, before and 5 to 7 days after vaccination: no statistically significant differences were identified, and all values were within the normal range.[3]

The possibility that the statins might improve the response to influenza vaccination has been studied. For example, in one cohort of patients who had received the influenza vaccine, those who were taking statins had a statistically significant minimal lower risk of influenza morbidity, which was no longer apparent after multivariate adjustment.[4] Another study concluded that there might be a slight synergism between statins and influenza vaccination in respiratory infection outcomes.[5]

(c) Tetanus toxoid

The production of anti-tetanus toxoid antibodies was threefold higher in 10 healthy subjects who received **atorvastatin** 40 mg daily for 10 days beginning 5 days before the booster vaccine when compared with 10 subjects given placebo.[6]

Mechanism

Statins are thought to have immunomodulating properties, and it has been suggested that these might enhance responses to vaccines. The case of rhabdomyolysis coincidental with influenza vaccine probably represents a chance association, and is more likely to be due to an interaction between the statin and bezafibrate (see 'Statins + Fibrates; Miscellaneous', p.1339) or to cerivastatin alone: note that severe myopathy led to the general withdrawal of cerivastatin from the market.

Importance and management

Influenza vaccines are routinely used every year in all older adults of the population in many countries (precise recommended age varies by country), which would represent a very large number of patients taking statins who also receive the vaccination. Considering this, there seems to be no evidence to suggest that there is an adverse interaction. The isolated case report of rhabdomyolysis involving cerivastatin and influenza vaccination probably represents a chance association. The current evidence for a beneficial interaction between statins and influenza vaccination suggests that any effect is minimal and probably not clinically important.

The studies of the short term effects of statins on antibody production after hepatitis A and tetanus toxoid vaccination are more to do with clinical efficacy rather than adverse interactions. However, they indicate that statins would not be expected to have negative effects on these vaccines.

1. Packard RRS, Schlegel S, Senouf D, Burger F, Sigaud P, Perneger T, Siegrist C-A, Mach F. Atorvastatin treatment and vaccination efficacy. *J Clin Pharmacol* (2007) 47, 1022–7.
2. Plotkin E, Bernheim J, Ben-Chetrit S, Mor A, Korzets Z. Influenza vaccine–a possible trigger of rhabdomyolysis induced acute renal failure due to the combined use of cerivastatin and bezafibrate. *Nephrol Dial Transplant* (2000) 15, 740–1.
3. Chazan B, Weiss R, Tabenkin H, Mines M, Raz R. Influenza vaccine does not produce myopathy in patients taking statins. *J Fam Pract* (2002) 51, 986–8.

4. Kwong JC, Li P, Redelmeier DA. Influenza morbidity and mortality in elderly patients receiving statins: a cohort study. *PLoS One* (2009) 4, e8087.
5. Fleming DM, Verlander NQ, Elliot AJ, Zhao H, Gelb D, Jehring D, Nguyen-Van-Tam JS. An assessment of the effect of statin use on the incidence of acute respiratory infections in England during winters 1998–1999 to 2005–2006. *Epidemiol Infect* (2010) 138, 1281–8.
6. Lee PY, Scumpia PO, Byars JA, Kelly KM, Zhuang H, Shuster JS, Theriaque DW, Segal MS, Reeves WH, Brantly ML. Short-term atorvastatin treatment enhances specific antibody production following tetanus toxoid vaccination in healthy volunteers. *Vaccine* (2006) 24, 4035–40.

Statins; Pravastatin + Mianserin

An isolated report describes a possible case of rhabdomyolysis, which was attributed to the long-term concurrent use of pravastatin and mianserin, triggered by a cold virus. A possible case of neuroleptic malignant syndrome occurred in a patient given pravastatin, mianserin and amoxapine.

Clinical evidence, mechanism, importance and management

An isolated report describes a 72-year-old woman taking pravastatin 20 mg daily and mianserin 10 mg daily for 2 years, who was hospitalised because of weakness in her legs that began 2 days previously, shortly after she developed a cold. She could stand, but was unable to walk unaided. Laboratory data revealed evidence of increased creatine kinase (4 400 units/L) and other serum enzymes, which the authors state suggested rhabdomyolysis. However, this case does not fit with the usual definition of rhabdomyolysis, see *Muscle and liver toxicity* under 'Lipid regulating drugs', p.1309. Within a week of stopping the pravastatin the leg weakness had disappeared and all of the laboratory results had returned to normal. The authors of the report attributed the toxicity to the long-term use of both drugs, ageing and the development of a cold.[1] However, what part these factors and/or the presence of mianserin actually played in the development of this toxicity is not known.

In another case, a patient with chronic normal pressure hydrocephalus given mianserin, **amoxapine** and pravastatin was said to develop a condition similar to neuroleptic malignant syndrome, which was attributed to a drug interaction.[2]

It seems unlikely that either of these cases are of general relevance.

1. Takei A, Chiba S. Rhabdomyolysis associated with pravastatin treatment for major depression. *Psychiatry Clin Neurosci* (1999) 53, 539.
2. Tajima Y. Unexpected drug-interaction [In Japanese]. *Rinsho Byori* (2002) 50, 133–9.

Statins; Pravastatin + Probucol

In a single-dose study in 20 healthy subjects, probucol 500 mg did not alter the pharmacokinetics of pravastatin 20 mg.[1]

1. ER Squibb. Data on file. A report on the bioavailability of pravastatin in the presence and absence of gemfibrozil or probucol in healthy male subjects (Protocol No 27, 201-18). 1988.

Statins; Rosuvastatin + Ursodeoxycholic acid (Ursodiol)

Ursodeoxycholic acid slightly increases the exposure to rosuvastatin.

Clinical evidence, mechanism, importance and management

In a crossover study in 12 healthy subjects, ursodeoxycholic acid 500 mg daily for 14 days slightly increased the AUC of rosuvastatin by 59% when a single 20-mg dose of rosuvastatin was given on day 15 (a day after the last dose of ursodeoxycholic acid). It was suggested that ursodeoxycholic acid reduced the expression of the OATP1B1 transporter protein, of which rosuvastatin is a substrate, so resulting in increased levels.[1]

The slight increase in rosuvastatin exposure seen in this study with separate administration is probably unlikely to be clinically important in most patients. However, ideally, these results should be confirmed when administration is closer together because, in clinical use, rosuvastatin is likely to be taken within a few hours of ursodeoxycholic acid.

1. He Y-J, Zhang W, Tu J-H, Kirchheiner J, Chen Y, Guo D, Li Q, Li Z-Y, Chen H, Hu D-L, Wang D, Zhou H-H. Hepatic nuclear factor 1α inhibitor ursodeoxycholic acid influences pharmacokinetics of the organic anion transporting polypeptide 1B1 substrate rosuvastatin and bilirubin. *Drug Metab Dispos* (2008) 36, 1453–6.

Statins; Simvastatin + Ciprofloxacin

An isolated report describes rhabdomyolysis when a patient taking simvastatin was given ciprofloxacin.

Clinical evidence, mechanism, importance and management

A 77-year-old woman with hypothyroidism who had been taking simvastatin 40 mg daily for the past 7 years, along with a number of other drugs, presented with severe muscle weakness and aches 5 days after starting ciprofloxacin (dose not stated) for a urinary tract infection. She was diagnosed with rhabdomyolysis, and after stopping the simvastatin and ciprofloxacin, slowly recovered.[1]

This appears to be the only published case suggesting an interaction between ciprofloxacin and simvastatin, which are both widely used drugs. There is currently no known mechanism for a pharmacokinetic interaction, because ciprofloxacin does not inhibit CYP3A4. Therefore, at present, there is insufficient evidence to implicate ciprofloxacin in this case, and its use could have been coincidental. Further study is needed to establish any interaction.

1. Sawant RD. Rhabdomyolysis due to an uncommon interaction of ciprofloxacin with simvastatin. *Can J Clin Pharmacol* (2009) 16, e78–e79.

Statins; Simvastatin + Cyproterone

An isolated report describes rhabdomyolysis in a patient taking simvastatin and given cyproterone acetate.

Clinical evidence, mechanism, importance and management

A 66-year-old man who had been taking simvastatin (dose not stated) for the past 18 months presented with myalgia, weakness and inability to walk 14 weeks after starting cyproterone acetate 100 mg three times daily for prostate cancer. He was diagnosed with rhabdomyolysis, and after stopping the simvastatin and cyproterone, slowly recovered.[1]

This appears to be the only published case suggesting an interaction of cyproterone and simvastatin, and simvastatin drug levels were not measured. The manufacturer of cyproterone acetate notes that, *in vitro*, high concentrations of cyproterone (such as those achieved with 100 mg three times daily) inhibited a variety of cytochrome P450 isoenzymes including CYP3A4,[2] and simvastatin is extensively metabolised by CYP3A4. Therefore, in the absence of *in vivo* evidence, a pharmacokinetic interaction cannot be ruled out, although there is no evidence suggesting that cyproterone is a clinically relevant inhibitor of CYP3A4.

At present, no interaction is established, and as cyproterone acetate has limited use in prostate cancer, this combination is unlikely to occur often. Because of the seriousness of the reaction, some caution might be appropriate if concurrent use is considered necessary. Note that lower doses of cyproterone acetate, as are used for its other clinical indications, would not be anticipated to interact via this mechanism.

1. Ahamed E, Bissett D. Rhabdomyolysis in prostate cancer – caution in prescribing cyproterone acetate with statins. *Clin Oncol* (2004) 16, 528–9.
2. Cyprostat (Cyproterone acetate). Bayer plc. UK Summary of product characteristics, January 2011.

Statins; Simvastatin + Laropiprant

The manufacturer briefly states that laropiprant did not have any clinically relevant effect on the pharmacokinetics of simvastatin.[1] Note that laropiprant is used as a combination product with nicotinic acid. For mention that the incidence of myopathy was higher in Chinese compared with non-Chinese patients taking simvastatin 40 mg concurrently with lipid-modifying doses of nicotinic acid with laropiprant, see 'Statins + Nicotinic acid (Niacin)', p.1351.

1. Tredaptive (Nicotinic acid with Laropripant). Merck Sharp & Dohme, Ltd. UK Summary of product characteristics, April 2012.

Statins; Simvastatin + Mipomersen

The concurrent use of simvastatin and mipomersen does not alter the pharmacokinetics of either drug.

Clinical evidence, mechanism, importance and management

In a pharmacokinetic study in 10 healthy subjects, a single 40-mg dose of simvastatin was given alone and then with the last dose of intravenous mipomersen 200 mg over 2 hours every 2 days for 4 doses. There was no difference in the AUC of mipomersen when given alone or with simvastatin. In addition, there was no difference in the AUC of simvastatin or simvastatin acid when given alone or with mipomersen, although there was a 49% reduction in the maximum level of simvastatin.[1]

This study demonstrates that no pharmacokinetic drug interaction would be expected if mipomersen and simvastatin are used concurrently.

1. Yu RZ, Geary RS, Flaim JD, Riley GC, Tribble DL, vanVliet AA, Wedel MK. Lack of pharmacokinetic interaction of mipomersen sodium (ISIS 301012), a 2'-*O*-methoxyethyl modified antisense oligonucleotide targeting apolipoprotein B-100 messenger RNA, with simvastatin and ezetimibe. *Clin Pharmacokinet* (2009) 48, 39–50.

Statins; Simvastatin + Risperidone

A schizophrenic patient taking risperidone developed rhabdomyolysis after simvastatin was started. Another patient taking simvastatin developed rhabdomyolysis when risperidone was started.

Clinical evidence

A 22-year-old patient with schizophrenia taking risperidone 4 mg daily and clonazepam 2 mg daily for about 4 weeks started taking simvastatin 10 mg daily. After about 5 days he experienced pain in his right ankle and heel, which increased in severity and spread proximally, accompanied by swelling and a rash over the affected area. In addition, his creatine phosphokinase levels were dramatically raised (12 408 units/L). Simvastatin was discontinued and rhabdomyolysis associated with an acute compartment syndrome was diagnosed, requiring emergency surgery.[1] In another case, a 76-year-old patient who had taken simvastatin 20 mg daily for 2 years developed muscle weakness, diagnosed as rhabdomyolysis, about 12 days after starting risperidone 1 mg daily. His creatine phosphokinase levels were 12 000 units/L increasing after 48 hours to 42 000 units/L. Simvastatin and risperidone were discontinued and the muscle weakness improved and creatine phosphokinase levels decreased to the normal range.[2] A further case report describes rhabdomyolysis in a patient taking simvastatin 40 mg daily that occurred shortly after he underwent allogeneic stem cell transplantation for leukaemia, to which ciclosporin and risperidone were thought to be contributory factors.[3] However, the ciclosporin alone could have caused this interaction, see 'Statins + Ciclosporin', p.1327.

Mechanism

Unknown. It was suggested that risperidone might have reduced the metabolism of simvastatin by cytochrome P450, causing an increased plasma concentration of the statin, resulting in muscle injury.[1] However, simvastatin is principally metabolised by CYP3A4 and risperidone is not known to inhibit this isoenzyme, so this mechanism is unlikely.

Importance and management

Evidence for an interaction between simvastatin and risperidone appears to be limited to these case reports, and an interaction is not established. At present, there is insufficient evidence to suggest a general caution, especially as no mechanism is known. Bear these reports in mind in the event of an unexpected response to treatment.

1. Webber MA, Mahmud W, Lightfoot JD, Shekhar A. Rhabdomyolysis and compartment syndrome with coadministration of risperidone and simvastatin. *J Psychopharmacol* (2004) 18, 432–4.
2. Patier JL, Ferrere F, Moreno-Cobo MÁ, Echaniz A. Rabdomiólisis proucida por la asociación de sinvastatina y risperidona. *Med Clin (Barc)* (2007) 29,129; 439.
3. Vives S, Batlle M, Montané E, Ribera JM. Rabdomiólisis e insuficiencia renal aguda secundaria a la interacción de simvastatina, ciclosporina A y risperidona en un paciente receptor de un trasplante alogénico de progenitors hematopoyéticos. *Med Clin (Barc)* (2008) 131, 676.

Ursodeoxycholic acid (Ursodiol) + Bile-acid binding resins

The absorption of ursodeoxycholic acid can be more than halved by the simultaneous administration of colestilan or colestyramine.

Clinical evidence

(a) Colestilan

After an overnight fast, 5 healthy subjects were given a test meal and then 200 mg of ursodeoxycholic acid alone or with 1.5 g of colestilan granules. It was found that the ursodeoxycholic acid serum levels at 30 minutes were reduced by more than 50% by colestilan in 4 out of the 5 subjects; the mean ursodeoxycholic acid level was decreased from 9.2 micromol/L to 3.4 micromol/L.[1]

(b) Colestyramine

In a study in 5 healthy subjects, the simultaneous administration of colestyramine 4 g daily with ursodeoxycholic acid reduced the fasting serum levels of ursodeoxycholic acid by about 60%. Separating administration by 5 hours tended to diminish the reduction in ursodeoxycholic acid levels (serum levels reduced by less than 40%).[2]

Mechanism

It seems likely that the bile-acid binding resins bind with ursodeoxycholic acid (a bile acid) in the intestine and thereby reduce its absorption.

Importance and management

The interactions of colestilan and colestyramine with ursodeoxycholic acid would appear to be established, and are probably clinically important: simultaneous use should be avoided. Some manufacturers of ursodeoxycholic acid advise that, should concurrent use be necessary, administration of bile-acid binding resins such as **colestipol** and colestyramine should be separated by at least 2 hours.[3,4] However, the manufacturer of **colesevelam** advises that, in the absence of a formal drug interaction study, administration of colesevelam and ursodeoxycholic acid should be separated by more than 4 hours, and that the efficacy of ursodeoxycholic acid should be monitored.[5]

1. Takikawa H, Ogasawara T, Sato A, Ohashi M, Hasegawa Y, Hojo M. Effect of colestimide on intestinal absorption of ursodeoxycholic acid in men. *Int J Clin Pharmacol Ther* (2001) 39, 558–60.
2. Rust C, Sauter GH, Oswald M, Büttner J, Kullak-Ublick GA, Paumgartner G, Beuers U. Effect of cholestyramine on bile acid pattern and synthesis during administration of ursodeoxycholic acid in man. *Eur J Clin Invest* (2000) 30, 135–9.
3. Urdox (Ursodeoxycholic acid). Wockhardt UK Ltd. UK Summary of product characteristics, November 2010.
4. Destolit (Ursodeoxycholic acid). Norgine Ltd. UK Summary of product characteristics, December 2010.
5. Cholestagel (Colesevelam hydrochloride). Sanofi. UK Summary of product characteristics, December 2014.

Ursodeoxycholic acid (Ursodiol) + Miscellaneous

Antacids are expected to reduce ursodeoxycholic acid absorption. The concurrent use of fibrates is predicted to reduce the efficacy of ursodeoxycholic acid.

Clinical evidence, mechanism, importance and management

(a) Antacids

Some antacids have been shown to adsorb bile acids *in vitro* and some manufacturers of ursodeoxycholic acid[1-3] suggest that these antacids (a number of manufacturers specifically mention aluminium-based antacids) might be expected to have the same effect *in vivo* and reduce ursodeoxycholic acid absorption. Simultaneous concurrent use should be avoided. If concurrent use is necessary, separating administration by at least 2 hours is recommended.[1,3,4]

(b) Fibrates

The manufacturers of ursodeoxycholic acid[1-4] recommend that it should not be taken with certain blood cholesterol-lowering agents (some name **clofibrate**), which might counteract its effectiveness by increasing cholesterol elimination in the bile and thus encourage gallstone formation. Note that, all fibrates increase cholesterol elimination, and would therefore be expected to interact similarly.

1. Ursofalk Capsules (Ursodeoxycholic acid). Dr. Falk Pharma UK Ltd. UK Summary of product characteristics, September 2011.
2. Urso 250/Urso Forte (Ursodeoxycholic acid). Axcan Pharma US, Inc. US Prescribing information, November 2009.
3. Destolit (Ursodeoxycholic acid). Norgine Ltd. UK Summary of product characteristics, December 2010.
4. Urdox (Ursodeoxycholic acid). Wockhardt UK Ltd. UK Summary of product characteristics, November 2010.

31

Lithium

Lithium is used in the management of mania, bipolar disorder (formerly manic depression) and recurrent depressive illnesses. Just how it exerts its beneficial effects is not known, but it might compete with sodium ions in various parts of the body, and it alters the electrolyte composition of body fluids. The dose of lithium is adjusted to give therapeutic serum concentrations of 0.4 to 1 mmol/L, although it should be noted that this is the range used in the UK, and other ranges have been quoted. Further, in the UK, levels at the lower end of the range are recommended for maintenance therapy and elderly patients: target levels of 0.8 to 1 mmol/L are recommended for acute episodes or patients who have relapsed or have subsyndromal symptoms. It is therefore important to determine an optimum level for each patient.

Lithium monitoring

Lithium is given under close supervision with regular monitoring of serum concentrations because there is a narrow margin between therapeutic concentrations and those that are toxic. Initially weekly monitoring is advised, dropping to every 3 months for those on stable regimens. It is usual to take serum lithium samples about 10 to 12 hours after the last oral dose.

Lithium adverse effects

Lithium adverse effects that are not usually considered serious include nausea, weakness, fine tremor, mild polydipsia and polyuria. If serum concentrations rise into the 1.5 to 2 mmol/L range, toxicity usually occurs, and can present as lethargy, drowsiness, coarse hand tremor, lack of coordination, muscular weakness, increased nausea and vomiting, or diarrhoea. Higher levels result in neurotoxicity, which manifests as ataxia, giddiness, tinnitus, confusion, dysarthria, muscle twitching, nystagmus, and even coma or seizures. Cardiovascular symptoms can also develop and include ECG changes and circulatory problems, and there might be a worsening of polyuria.[1-4] In addition, lithium can induce diabetes insipidus and hypothyroidism in some patients.

Lithium levels of over 2 mmol/L can be extremely dangerous and therefore require urgent attention. Chronic lithium toxicity has been reported to have a 9% mortality rate, while acute toxicity has a 25% mortality rate.[5] However, patients with chronic lithium toxicity are more likely to experience severe symptoms at lower serum lithium levels.

Factors predisposing to lithium toxicity

Risk factors for lithium toxicity include: advanced age, congestive heart failure, renal impairment and volume depletion. Some consider these to be contraindications to the use of lithium. A history of neurological illness might increase the susceptibility to lithium toxicity.[6]

Interactions

Many of the interactions involving lithium occur because of altered serum lithium concentrations. Lithium is mainly excreted by the kidney, undergoing glomerular filtration and then tubular reabsorption, and competes with sodium for this process. Therefore, drugs that affect renal excretion (e.g. thiazides, see 'Lithium + Diuretics; Thiazide and related', p.1370) or electrolyte balance (e.g. sodium compounds, see 'Lithium + Sodium compounds', p.1378) are likely to interact. Drug interactions might be an important cause of lithium neurotoxicity occurring when serum lithium levels are within the therapeutic range.[7] This tends to occur with centrally active drugs, including many antipsychotics (for example, see 'Lithium + Ziprasidone', p.1381), carbamazepine (see 'Lithium + Carbamazepine', p.1368), and a number of antidepressants (see 'Lithium + SSRIs', p.1378, and 'Lithium + Tricyclic and related antidepressants', p.1380). Virtually all of the reports of interactions are concerned with the carbonate, but sometimes lithium is given as the acetate, aspartate, chloride, citrate, gluconate, orotate or sulfate instead. There is no reason to believe that these lithium compounds will interact any differently to lithium carbonate.

1. Finley PR, Warner MD, Peabody CA. Clinical relevance of drug interactions with lithium. *Clin Pharmacokinet* (1995) 29, 172–91.
2. Camcolit (Lithium carbonate). Norgine Ltd. UK Summary of product characteristics, August 2010.
3. Lithobid (Lithium carbonate). Noven Therapeutics. US Prescribing Information, October 2011.
4. Grandjean EM, Aubry J-M. Lithium: updated human knowledge using an evidence-based approach; part III: clinical safety. *CNS Drugs* (2009) 23, 397–418.
5. Vipond AJ, Bakewell S, Telford R, Nicholls AJ. Lithium toxicity. *Anaesthesia* (1996) 51, 1156–8.
6. Chen K-P, Shen WW, Lu M-L. Implication of serum concentration monitoring in patients with lithium intoxication. *Psychiatry Clin Neurosci* (2004) 58, 25–9.
7. Emilien G, Maloteaux JM. Lithium neurotoxicity at low therapeutic doses. Hypotheses for causes and mechanism of action following a retrospective analysis of published case reports. *Acta Neurol Belg* (1996) 96, 281–93.

Lithium + ACE inhibitors

ACE inhibitors can raise lithium levels, and in some individuals two- to fourfold increases have been recorded. Cases of lithium toxicity have been reported in patients also given captopril, enalapril or lisinopril (and possibly imidapril or perindopril). One analysis found an increased relative risk for lithium toxicity requiring hospitalisation in elderly patients newly started on an ACE inhibitor.

Clinical evidence

An analysis of 10 615 elderly patients receiving lithium found that 413 (3.9%) were admitted to hospital at least once for lithium toxicity during a 10-year study period. The prescriptions for any ACE inhibitor (not specifically named) were compared between these 413 hospitalised patients and 1 651 control patients. For any use of ACE inhibitor (63 cases and 110 controls) there was an increased relative risk of hospitalisation for lithium toxicity of 1.6. When patients who had started taking an ACE inhibitor within the last month were evaluated (14 cases and 5 controls), a dramatically increased risk of lithium toxicity was found (relative risk 7.6).[1]

Studies and case reports of the interaction between lithium and specific named ACE inhibitors are outlined in the subsections below.

(a) Captopril

A patient taking lithium carbonate developed a serum lithium level of 2.35 mmol/L and toxicity (tremor, dysarthria, digestive problems) within 10 days of starting to take captopril 50 mg daily. He was restabilised on half his previous dose of lithium.[2] A retrospective study also reports a case of increased lithium levels with captopril (see under *Lisinopril*, below).

(b) Enalapril

A woman taking lithium carbonate developed signs of lithium toxicity (ataxia, dysarthria, tremor, confusion) within 2 to 3 weeks of starting to take enalapril 20 mg daily. After 5 weeks her plasma lithium levels had risen from 0.88 mmol/L to 3.3 mmol/L, and moderate renal impairment was noted.[3] No toxicity occurred when enalapril was later replaced by nifedipine.[3] Lithium toxicity following the use of enalapril, and associated in some cases with a decrease in renal function, has been seen in another 6 patients,[4-9] and a reduced lithium dose was found adequate in a further patient taking enalapril and also taking furosemide[10] (see, 'Lithium + Diuretics; Loop', p.1369). Enalapril 5 mg daily for 9 days had no effect on the mean serum lithium levels of 9 healthy male subjects. However, one subject had a 31% increase in lithium levels.[11]

A retrospective study also reports several cases of increased lithium levels with enalapril (see under *Lisinopril*, below).

(c) Imidapril

A case report describes a patient taking several drugs including lithium carbonate 400 mg daily and imidapril 5 mg daily, who developed dyspnoea and bradyarrhythmia with a lithium level of 1.68 mmol/L, which the authors noted might have been due to an interaction between these two drugs.[12] However, note that his prescribed medication also included carbamazepine (see 'Lithium + Carbamazepine', p.1368), losartan (see 'Lithium + Angiotensin II receptor antagonists', p.1363), and nitrazepam (see 'Lithium + Benzodiazepines', p.1366). The use of any of these drugs with lithium could also have contributed to the increased lithium levels seen.

(d) Lisinopril

A retrospective study of patient records identified 20 patients who were stabilised on lithium and then started taking an ACE inhibitor (13 given lisinopril, 6 given enalapril and one given captopril). Their serum lithium levels rose by an average of 35% (from 0.64 to 0.86 mmol/L) and there was a 26% decrease in lithium clearance. Signs and symptoms suggestive of toxicity (increased tremor, confusion, ataxia), necessitating a dose reduction or lithium withdrawal, developed in four (20%) of these patients. In 3 patients the development of the interaction was delayed for several weeks.[13] A woman taking lithium developed lithium toxicity and a trough serum lithium level of 3 mmol/L within 3 weeks of stopping clonidine and starting lisinopril 20 mg daily.[14] Other reports similarly describe acute lithium toxicity in 6 patients when they were given lisinopril.[8,15-19] One of them was also taking verapamil,[17] which has also been shown to interact with lithium, but not usually to raise lithium levels (see 'Lithium + Calcium-channel blockers', p.1367), and one patient experienced an increase in lithium levels on changing from fosinopril to lisinopril.[18] A case report describes raised lithium levels of 2.04 mmol/L, without any signs of lithium toxicity in a woman taking lithium 900 mg daily with lisinopril 10 mg daily. Her lithium levels fell to 1.45 mmol/L on reducing the lithium dose to 600 mg daily, but when she took this dose without lisinopril, her lithium levels were 0.86 mmol/L.[20]

(e) Perindopril

A patient taking lithium developed lithium toxicity 3 months after starting to take perindopril.[21] This patient was also taking bendroflumethiazide, which can also interact with lithium, see 'Lithium + Diuretics; Thiazide and related', p.1370.

Mechanism

Not fully understood. It has been suggested that as both ACE inhibitors and lithium cause sodium to be lost in the urine, and also ACE inhibitors reduce thirst stimulation, fluid depletion can occur. The normal compensatory reaction for fluid depletion is constriction of the efferent renal arterioles to maintain the glomerular filtration rate, but this mechanism is blocked by the ACE inhibitor. In addition, lithium and sodium ions are competitively reabsorbed, mainly in the proximal tubule, and with less sodium available, more lithium is retained. Consequently the renal excretion of lithium falls and toxicity develops.

Importance and management

The interaction between lithium and the ACE inhibitors is established, although it seems that the incidence of adverse effects as a result of this interaction is probably small. It has been suggested that concurrent use should be avoided, or only undertaken with caution and close monitoring; however, although lithium levels can rise, this is not always of clinical importance. Nevertheless, it should be noted that the risk of lithium toxicity increases when other risk factors for raised lithium levels are also present. Only captopril, enalapril, lisinopril (and possibly imidapril and perindopril) have been reported to interact, but it seems likely, given the proposed mechanism, that this interaction will occur with any other ACE inhibitor. Therefore if any ACE inhibitor is added to established lithium treatment, monitor well for symptoms of lithium toxicity and consider measuring lithium levels more frequently. This might be particularly important during the first month of concurrent use. Be alert for the need to reduce the lithium dose (possibly by between one-third to one-half).[14,16] The development of the interaction can be delayed, so monitoring lithium levels every week[14] or every two weeks[13] for several weeks has been advised.

For more information on the risk factors for lithium toxicity, symptoms of lithium adverse effects and general monitoring, see under 'Lithium', p.1361.

1. Juurlink DN, Mamdani MM, Kopp A, Rochon PA, Shulman KI, Redelmeier DA. Drug-induced lithium toxicity in the elderly: a population-based study. *J Am Geriatr Soc* (2004) 52, 794–8.
2. Pulik M, Lida H. Interaction lithium-inhibiteurs de l'enzyme de conversion. *Presse Med* (1988) 17, 755.
3. Douste-Blazy P, Rostin M, Livarek B, Tordjman E, Montastruc JL, Galinier F. Angiotensin converting enzyme inhibitors and lithium treatment. *Lancet* (1986) i, 1448.
4. Mahieu M, Houvenagel E, Leduc JJ, Choteau P. Lithium-inhibiteurs de l'enzyme conversion: une association á éviter? *Presse Med* (1988) 17, 281.
5. Drouet A, Bouvet O. Lithium et inhibiteurs de l'enzyme de conversion. *Encephale* (1990) 16, 51–2.
6. Navis GJ, de Jong PE, de Zeeuw D. Volume homeostasis, angiotensin converting enzyme inhibition, and lithium therapy. *Am J Med* (1989) 86, 621.
7. Simon G. Combination angiotensin converting enzyme inhibitor/lithium therapy contraindicated in renal disease. *Am J Med* (1988) 85, 893–4.
8. Correa FJ, Eiser AR. Angiotensin-converting enzyme inhibitors and lithium toxicity. *Am J Med* (1992) 93, 108–9.
9. Fiegler K, Liechti ME, Bodmer M, Bruggisser M. Akzidentelle Lithiumintoxikation. *Praxis (Bern 1994)* (2009) 98, 685–91.
10. Ahmad S. Sudden hypothyroidism and amiodarone-lithium combination: an interaction. *Cardiovasc Drugs Ther* (1995) 9, 827–8.
11. DasGupta K, Jefferson JW, Kobak KA, Greist JH. The effect of enalapril on serum lithium levels in healthy men. *J Clin Psychiatry* (1992) 53, 398–400.
12. Ide N, Gotou S, Mori M. [Hospital pharmacists prevented advance of lithium intoxication through pharmaceutical interventions]. *Yakugaku Zasshi* (2009) 129, 1007–11.
13. Finley PR, O'Brien JG, Coleman RW. Lithium and angiotensin-converting enzyme inhibitors: evaluation of a potential interaction. *J Clin Psychopharmacol* (1996) 16, 68–71.
14. Baldwin CM, Safferman AZ. A case of lisinopril-induced lithium toxicity. *DICP Ann Pharmacother* (1990) 24, 946–7.
15. Griffin JH, Hahn SM. Lisinopril-induced lithium toxicity. *DICP Ann Pharmacother* (1991) 25, 101.
16. Anon. ACE inhibitors and lithium toxicity. *Biol Ther Psychiatry* (1988) 11, 43.
17. Chandragiri SS, Pasol E, Gallagher RM. Lithium, ACE inhibitors, NSAIDs, and verapamil. A possible fatal combination. *Psychosomatics* (1998) 39, 281–2.
18. Meyer JM, Dollarhide A, Tuan I-L. Lithium toxicity after switch from fosinopril to lisinopril. *Int Clin Psychopharmacol* (2005) 20, 115–18.
19. Handler J. Lithium and antihypertensive medication: a potentially dangerous interaction. *J Clin Hypertens (Greenwich)* (2009) 11, 738–42.
20. Teitelbaum M. A significant increase in lithium levels after concomitant ACE inhibitor administration. *Psychosomatics* (1993) 34, 450–3.
21. Vipond AJ, Bakewell S, Telford R, Nicholls AJ. Lithium toxicity. *Anaesthesia* (1996) 51, 1156–8.

Lithium + Acetazolamide

Some evidence suggests that the excretion of lithium can be increased by the short-term use of acetazolamide. However, lithium toxicity has been seen in one patient given both drugs for a month.

Clinical evidence, mechanism, importance and management

A single-dose study in 6 subjects given oral lithium carbonate 600 mg ten hours before oral acetazolamide 500 or 750 mg found a 31% increase in the urinary excretion of lithium.[1] Another single-dose study in 7 healthy subjects given oral lithium carbonate 600 mg the evening before an intravenous dose of acetazolamide 250 mg found a 27% increase in the urinary excretion of lithium.[2] A case report describes a woman who was successfully treated for a lithium overdose with acetazolamide, intravenous fluids, sodium bicarbonate, potassium chloride and mannitol.[3]

In another patient, lithium toxicity occurred after a month of treatment with acetazolamide. Lithium levels rose from 0.8 to 5 mmol/L, although it should be noted that the later measurement was taken 8 hours post-dose.[4] See *Lithium monitoring*, under 'Lithium', p.1361, for details of lithium monitoring.

Evidence for an interaction between lithium and acetazolamide appears limited, but the information from the small studies suggests that lithium levels might be decreased by concurrent use. It might therefore be prudent to be aware of this possibility, monitoring lithium levels if an interaction is suspected.

1. Thomsen K, Schou M. Renal lithium excretion in man. *Am J Physiol* (1968) 215, 823–7.
2. Skøtt P, Hommel E, Bruun NE, Arnold-Larsen S, Parving HH. The acute effect of acetazolamide on glomerular filtration rate and proximal tubular reabsorption of sodium and water in normal man. *Scand J Clin Lab Invest* (1989) 49, 583–7.
3. Horowitz LC, Fisher GU. Acute lithium toxicity. *N Engl J Med* (1969) 281, 1369.
4. Gay C, Plas J, Granger B, Olie JP, Loo H. Intoxication au lithium. Deux interactions inédites: l'acétazolamide et l'acide niflumique. *Encephale* (1985) 11, 261–2.

Lithium + Aciclovir

An isolated case report describes lithium toxicity which was attributed to the use of high-dose intravenous aciclovir.

Clinical evidence, mechanism, importance and management

A 42-year-old woman taking lithium carbonate 450 mg twice daily developed signs of lithium toxicity 6 days after starting treatment with intravenous aciclovir 10 mg/kg, which was given every 8 hours for a severe herpes zoster infection following chemotherapy. Her serum lithium levels had risen over fourfold to 3.4 mmol/L. The reasons for this interaction are unknown but the authors of the report suggest that aciclovir might have inhibited the renal excretion of lithium.[1]

This appears to be the first and only report of this interaction, but, as the proposed mechanism fits with the way both of these drugs interact with other substances, it would seem prudent to monitor for symptoms of lithium toxicity and consider monitoring lithium levels if high-dose intravenous aciclovir is given to any patient. The report recommends measuring lithium levels every second or third day.[1] For more information on the risk factors for lithium toxicity, symptoms of lithium adverse effects and general monitoring, see under 'Lithium', p.1361.

Oral aciclovir is predicted not to interact because of its low bioavailability, and no interaction would be expected with topical aciclovir as the plasma levels achieved by this route are minimal.

1. Sylvester RK, Leitch J, Granum C. Does acyclovir increase serum lithium levels? *Pharmacotherapy* (1996) 16, 466–8.

Lithium + Amisulpride

Amisulpride does not appear to affect the pharmacokinetics of lithium. However, lithium might increase the plasma levels of amisulpride. Neuroleptic malignant syndrome has been reported in one patient taking lithium and amisulpride.

Clinical evidence

(a) Neuroleptic malignant syndrome

A case report describes neuroleptic malignant syndrome in a 31-year-old woman taking lithium 450 mg twice daily. Quetiapine 600 mg daily was replaced with amisulpride (200 mg twice daily, titrated up to 400 mg twice daily over 3 days with no adverse effects), and the patient then went on weekend leave. Neuroleptic malignant syndrome was diagnosed upon her return. Lithium and amisulpride were withdrawn, and the patient's condition improved over several days.[1]

(b) Pharmacokinetic interaction

In a placebo-controlled pharmacokinetic study in 24 healthy subjects, lithium carbonate 500 mg twice daily was given for 7 days to obtain stable lithium serum levels, and then amisulpride 100 mg twice daily was added for a further 7 days. Amisulpride appeared to have no effect on lithium pharmacokinetics.[2] In a pharmacokinetic analysis of amisulpride levels in patients with schizophrenia or schizoaffective disorder, dose-corrected amisulpride plasma levels were 80% higher in 3 patients taking lithium than in 13 patients taking amisulpride alone.[3] In a further study by the same authors, 7 patients who had been taking amisulpride 250 to 1200 mg daily for between 9 and 110 days were given lithium carbonate 450 to 1125 mg daily. Dose-corrected plasma levels of amisulpride were increased by about 8 to 56% (mean 31%) by lithium, taken for between 3 and 73 days. There was a positive correlation between the duration of lithium treatment and the increase in amisulpride levels.[4]

Mechanism

Unknown. The patient in the case report describing neuroleptic malignant syndrome had other risk factors for the development of this effect (a recent switch of antipsychotic medication, rapid upward dose titration and a previous episode of neuroleptic malignant syndrome with risperidone).

Importance and management

Evidence for a pharmacokinetic interaction between amisulpride and lithium is limited, but it appears to be established. Although the mean increase in amisulpride levels would not be expected to be clinically relevant, the authors of the study[4] suggest that increases of up to 56% could result in increased adverse effects. It would therefore seem prudent to monitor concurrent use for amisulpride adverse effects (extrapyramidal effects, insomnia, constipation) and consider reducing the amisulpride dose if these become troublesome.

The case of neuroleptic malignant syndrome appears to be an isolated report. Neuroleptic malignant syndrome can occur with amisulpride alone and the patient had other risk factors (see *Mechanism*, above). Given these factors the general relevance of this case is unclear.

1. Yasugi S, Garg V, Been G, Magoulas P. Neuroleptic malignant syndrome. *Aust N Z J Psychiatry* (2010) 44, 584.
2. Canal M, Legangneux E, van Lier JJ, van Vliet AA, Coulouvrat C. Lack of effect of amisulpride on the pharmacokinetics and safety of lithium. *Int J Neuropsychopharmacol* (2003) 6, 103–9.
3. Bergemann N, Kopitz J, Kress KR, Frick A. Plasma amisulpride levels in schizophrenia or schizoaffective disorder. *Eur Neuropsychopharmacol* (2004) 14, 245–50.
4. Bergemann N, Abu-Tair F, Kress KR, Parzer P, Kopitz J. Increase in plasma concentration of amisulpride after addition of concomitant lithium. *J Clin Psychopharmacol* (2007) 27, 546–9.

Lithium + Angiotensin II receptor antagonists

Case reports describe lithium toxicity in patients also given candesartan, losartan, valsartan, and possibly irbesartan. Other angiotensin II receptor antagonists would be expected to interact similarly.

Clinical evidence

(a) Candesartan

A 58-year-old woman taking long-term lithium for depression (stable serum lithium levels between 0.6 and 0.7 mmol/L), and unnamed calcium-channel blockers for hypertension, was additionally given candesartan 16 mg daily. She was hospitalised 8 weeks later with a 10-day history of ataxia, increasing confusion, disorientation and agitation, and was found to have a serum lithium level of 3.25 mmol/L. She recovered completely when all the drugs were stopped. She was later restabilised on her original lithium dose with a change to urapidil for her hypertension.[1]

(b) Irbesartan

A report describes a 74-year-old woman with increased lithium levels of 2.3 mmol/L and symptoms of lithium toxicity, which were associated with the use of several drugs including irbesartan, lisinopril, escitalopram, levomepromazine, furosemide and spironolactone. It was suggested that these drugs could have delayed lithium excretion or worsened neurotoxic effects. An increase in the lisinopril dose and the addition of irbesartan several weeks before admission might have contributed to the lithium toxicity.[2]

(c) Losartan

An elderly woman taking lithium carbonate developed lithium toxicity (ataxia, dysarthria, and confusion) after starting to take losartan 50 mg daily. Her serum lithium levels rose from 0.63 mmol/L to 2 mmol/L over 5 weeks. Lithium and losartan were stopped and her symptoms had disappeared 2 days later. When lithium was restarted and losartan was replaced by nicardipine, her lithium levels were restabilised at 0.77 mmol/L within 2 weeks.[3]

An investigation into the effects of losartan on renal function in 10 subjects with essential hypertension included a lithium clearance test as a means of assessing the reabsorption of sodium by the proximal tubule. A single oral dose of lithium carbonate 750 mg was given the night before the final dose of losartan 50 mg daily for one month (or before placebo, given for 15 days). A small (6.6%) decrease in the proximal fractional reabsorption of sodium was observed; this would correspond to a similarly small decrease in lithium clearance, and was not statistically significant.[4]

(d) Valsartan

A woman with a long history of bipolar disorder was taking lithium carbonate (serum levels consistently at 0.9 mmol/L) and a number of other drugs (L-tryptophan, lorazepam, glibenclamide, conjugated oestrogens and ciprofloxacin). Two weeks before being hospitalised for a manic relapse she additionally started taking valsartan 80 mg daily. While in hospital ciprofloxacin was stopped, lorazepam was replaced by zopiclone, and quetiapine was added. On day 3 of her hospitalisation her serum lithium levels were 1.1 mmol/L and she became increasingly delirious, confused and ataxic over the next week. By day 11 her serum lithium levels had risen to 1.4 mmol/L. When an interaction was suspected, the valsartan was replaced by diltiazem. She later recovered and was stabilised on her original lithium carbonate dose with lithium levels of 0.8 mmol/L.[5] A second case describes a woman taking lithium 600 mg daily who experienced an increase in lithium serum levels to 1.72 mmol/L after she started to take valsartan 80 mg daily. She had signs of lithium toxicity including ataxia, limb rigidity and falls. Previously, her lithium levels had been stable between 0.62 and 0.87 mmol/L when she took lithium in doses of 900 mg to 1.2 g daily.[6]

Mechanism

Not fully understood. It could be that, as with the ACE inhibitors, angiotensin II receptor antagonists inhibit aldosterone secretion, resulting in increased sodium loss by the renal tubules. This causes lithium retention and thus an increase in lithium levels. However, angiotensin II receptor antagonists have less effect on aldosterone than the ACE inhibitors, making a clinically significant interaction less likely. *Animal* studies show that ramipril,[7] but not losartan,[8] decreases the excretion of lithium by the kidney, which would support this idea. In addition, the investigation into the renal effects of losartan described above appears to provide some support for this idea in humans.[4]

Importance and management

Direct information about interactions between lithium and angiotensin II receptor antagonists seems to be limited to these reports, although the interaction has been predicted to occur with all drugs of this class. Such sparse evidence is not enough to recommend contraindicating the concurrent use of angiotensin II receptor antagonists with lithium, especially as an interaction is less likely than with the ACE inhibitors (see *Mechanism*, above), although some manufacturers do not recommend the combination. One report suggests weekly monitoring for the first month of concurrent use,[5] but any rise in serum lithium levels might be gradual so that toxicity could take as long as 3 to 7 weeks to develop fully. Be mindful that the lithium dose might need to be decreased.

Patients taking lithium should be aware of the symptoms of lithium toxicity and told to report them immediately should they occur. This should be reinforced when they are given angiotensin II receptor antagonists.

For more information on the risk factors for lithium toxicity, symptoms of lithium adverse effects and general monitoring, see under 'Lithium', p.1361.

1. Zwanzger P, Marcuse A, Boerner RJ, Walther A, Rupprecht R. Lithium intoxication after administration of AT_1 blockers. *J Clin Psychiatry* (2001) 62, 208–9.
2. Spinewine A, Schoevaerdts D, Mwenge GB, Swine C, Dive A. Drug-induced lithium intoxication: a case report. *J Am Geriatr Soc* (2005) 53, 360–1.
3. Blanche P, Raynaud E, Kerob D, Galezowski N. Lithium intoxication in an elderly patient after combined treatment with losartan. *Eur J Clin Pharmacol* (1997) 52, 501.
4. Fauvel JP, Velon S, Berra N, Pozet N, Madonna O, Zech P, Laville M. Effects of losartan on renal function in patients with essential hypertension. *J Cardiovasc Pharmacol* (1996) 28, 259–63.
5. Leung M, Remick RA. Potential drug interaction between lithium and valsartan. *J Clin Psychopharmacol* (2000) 20, 392–3.
6. Su Y-P, Chang C-J, Hwang T-J. Lithium intoxication after valsartan treatment. *Psychiatry Clin Neurosci* (2007) 61, 204.
7. Barthelmebs M, Grima M, Imbs J-L. Ramipril-induced decrease in renal lithium excretion in the rat. *Br J Pharmacol* (1995) 116, 2161–5.
8. Barthelmebs M, Alt-Tebacher M, Madonna O, Grima M, Imbs J-L. Absence of a losartan interaction with renal lithium excretion in the rat. *Br J Pharmacol* (1995) 116, 2166–9.

Lithium + Antibacterials

A retrospective study of patients receiving long-term lithium found that concurrent medication, including antibacterials, tended to be associated with a higher risk of elevated serum lithium levels.

Clinical evidence, mechanism, importance and management

A multicentre, retrospective study of patients receiving long-term lithium identified 51 patients with elevated serum lithium levels (greater than or equal to 1.3 mmol/L) which was at least 50% greater than the previous serum level. Fifteen patients had taken potentially interacting medication and, of these, 7 patients had taken antibacterials (6 different unnamed antibacterials). It was suggested that the underlying infection, associated fever and poor fluid intake might have contributed to the elevated lithium levels in these patients rather than the use of the antibacterial *per se*.[1]

1. Wilting I, Movig KLL, Moolenaar M, Hekster YA, Brouwers JRBJ, Heerdink ER, Nolen WA, Egberts ACG. Drug-drug interactions as a determinant of elevated lithium serum levels in daily clinical practice. *Bipolar Disord* (2005) 7, 274–80.

Lithium + Antibacterials; Co-trimoxazole or Trimethoprim

Lithium toxicity has developed in three patients also given co-trimoxazole; in two of these patients toxicity was paradoxically accompanied by a fall in lithium levels. A further report describes lithium toxicity accompanied by an increase in lithium levels in a patient given trimethoprim.

Clinical evidence, mechanism, importance and management

Two patients stable taking lithium carbonate (serum level 0.75 mmol/L) had signs of lithium toxicity (tremor, fasciculations, muscular weakness, dysarthria, apathy) within a few days of being given co-trimoxazole (dose not stated), yet their serum lithium levels were found to have fallen to about 0.4 mmol/L. Within 48 hours of withdrawing the co-trimoxazole, the signs of toxicity had gone, and their serum lithium concentrations had returned to their former level.[1] Another report very briefly states that ataxia, tremor and diarrhoea developed in a patient taking lithium and timolol when co-trimoxazole was given.[2]

A 40-year-old woman taking lithium 1.2 g daily, experienced nausea, diarrhoea, malaise, difficulty concentrating, trembling, an uncertain gait and muscle spasms after trimethoprim 300 mg daily was started; her serum lithium levels appeared to be elevated. She made a good recovery following rehydration.[3]

The mechanism for this interaction is unclear, although trimethoprim might affect the renal excretion of lithium.[3] Given the limited evidence, the general importance of this interaction is uncertain. If concurrent use is undertaken it would clearly be prudent to monitor the clinical response, as it would appear that in this situation serum level monitoring might not always be a reliable guide to toxicity. For general information on the use of antibacterials with lithium, see 'Lithium + Antibacterials', p.1364.

1. Desvilles M, Sevestre P. Effet paradoxal de l'association lithium et sulfaméthoxazol-triméthoprime. *Nouv Presse Med* (1982) 11, 3267–8.
2. Edwards IR. Medicines Adverse Reactions Committee: eighteenth annual report, 1983. *N Z Med J* (1984) 97, 729–32.
3. de Vries PL. Lithiumintoxicatie bij gelijktijdig gebruik van trimethoprim. *Ned Tijdschr Geneeskd* (2001) 145, 539–40.

Lithium + Antibacterials; Levofloxacin

An isolated case of lithium toxicity has been reported in a patient taking lithium and levofloxacin.

Clinical evidence, mechanism, importance and management

A 56-year-old man taking lithium carbonate 400 mg three times daily for a bipolar disorder was admitted to hospital with bronchitis. He was given levofloxacin 300 mg daily, and within 2 days was noted to have developed gait ataxia, dysarthria, coarse tremor, dizziness, vomiting, and confusion. Lithium toxicity was suspected, and because of the time course of the symptoms, an interaction with levofloxacin was considered responsible. Serum lithium levels were found to have risen from 0.89 mmol/L (measured 2 weeks previously) to 2.53 mmol/L, and a reduction in his renal function was noted. Both drugs were stopped and the patient recovered over the following 4 days. His lithium level was found to be 1.12 mmol/L at that time.[1]

The mechanism of this interaction between lithium and levofloxacin is unclear. Evidence for an interaction appears to be limited to this isolated case, and therefore no general conclusions can be made. For general information on the use of lithium with antibacterials, see 'Lithium + Antibacterials', p.1364.

Evidence for a possible interaction between lithium and other quinolones is lacking; however, for a report of lithium toxicity with raised lithium levels in a patient taking ciprofloxacin and nimesulide, which was attributed to the NSAID, see *Nimesulide*, under 'Lithium + NSAIDs', p.1374.

1. Takahashi H, Higuchi H, Shimizu T. Severe lithium toxicity induced by combined levofloxacin administration. *J Clin Psychiatry* (2000) 61, 949–50.

Lithium + Antibacterials; Linezolid

Two cases describe serotonin syndrome in patients taking linezolid and lithium, although in both cases other potentially interacting drugs were also taken.

Clinical evidence, mechanism, importance and management

A retrospective review of adverse events reported to the FDA in the US identified 29 cases of serotonin syndrome involving linezolid. One patient had received lithium, but they were also taking bupropion, sertraline and trazodone,[1] which have all been associated with the development of serotonin syndrome. A case report also describes a 36-year-old woman who developed serotonin syndrome after linezolid was added to her drug regimen, which included lithium. She was also taking venlafaxine, and imipramine,[2] which have both been associated with the development of serotonin syndrome.

Although the use of linezolid was implicated in both of these cases, it is unclear what part lithium had to play, although cases of serotonin syndrome have been reported when lithium is taken with other drugs affecting serotonin, see 'Lithium + SSRIs', p.1378. However, in both of the cases cited above, other drugs were also taken which are known to result in serotonin syndrome with linezolid and therefore the general significance of these cases is unclear. For more information on serotonin syndrome and its management, see 'Drugs that cause serotonin syndrome + Other drugs that cause serotonin syndrome', p.1471.

1. Lawrence KR, Adra M, Gillman PK. Serotonin toxicity associated with the use of linezolid: a review of postmarketing data. *Clin Infect Dis* (2006) 42, 1578–83.
2. Miller DG, Lovell EO. Antibiotic-induced serotonin syndrome. *J Emerg Med* (2011) 40, 25–7.

Lithium + Antibacterials; Metronidazole

The lithium levels of three patients rose, to toxic levels in two cases, after they took metronidazole.

Clinical evidence, mechanism, importance and management

A 40-year-old woman taking lithium carbonate 1.8 g daily, levothyroxine 150 micrograms daily and propranolol 60 mg daily developed signs of lithium toxicity (ataxia, rigidity, poor cognitive function, impaired co-ordination) after completing a one-week course of metronidazole 500 mg twice daily. Her serum lithium levels had risen by 46% (from 1.3 mmol/L to 1.9 mmol/L).[1] Another report describes 2 patients whose serum lithium levels rose by about 20% and 125%, 5 to 12 days, after they finished a one-week course of metronidazole 750 mg or 1 g daily, respectively, in divided doses.[2] A degree of renal impairment occurred during concurrent use and was still present 5 to 6 months later.[2] In contrast, one other patient is said to have taken both drugs together uneventfully.[1]

There seems to be no reason for avoiding the concurrent use of metronidazole and lithium, but the outcome should be well monitored. Some have recommended that a reduction in the lithium dose should be considered, especially in patients maintained at relatively high serum lithium levels.[1,2] Further, the authors of one of the reports also recommend frequent analysis of creatinine and electrolyte levels and urine osmolality in order to detect any renal problems in patients taking this combination.[2] However, given the available information, these seem highly cautious recommendations. Patients taking lithium should be aware of the symptoms of lithium toxicity and told to report them immediately should they occur. This should be reinforced when they are given metronidazole.

For general information on the use of lithium with antibacterials, see 'Lithium + Antibacterials', above.

1. Ayd FJ. Metronidazole-induced lithium intoxication. *Int Drug Ther Newslett* (1982) 17, 15–16.
2. Teicher MH, Altesman RI, Cole JO, Schatzberg AF. Possible nephrotoxic interaction of lithium and metronidazole. *JAMA* (1987) 257, 3365–6.

Lithium + Antibacterials; Spectinomycin

An isolated case report describes a patient who developed lithium toxicity when given spectinomycin.

Clinical evidence, mechanism, importance and management

A woman developed lithium toxicity (tremor, nausea, vomiting, ataxia and dysarthria) when given spectinomycin injections (dose not stated) in addition to her long-term treatment with lithium.[1] Her serum lithium levels had risen from a range of 0.8 to 1.1 mmol/L up to 3.2 mmol/L. Spectinomycin reduces urinary output, and so it was suggested that a reduction in the renal clearance of lithium led to these elevated levels. Information seems to be limited to this report, but it would seem prudent to bear this interaction in mind in any patient given both drugs.

For general comment on the use of antibacterials in patients taking lithium, see 'Lithium + Antibacterials', p.1364.

1. Conroy RW. Quoted as a personal communication by Ayd FJ. Possible adverse drug-drug interaction report. *Int Drug Ther Newslett* (1978) 13, 15.

Lithium + Antibacterials; Tetracyclines

Two isolated reports describe increased lithium levels and lithium toxicity on the concurrent use of lithium and either tetracycline or doxycycline. Two cases of pseudotumor cerebri have been reported in patients taking lithium and minocycline.

Clinical evidence

(a) Doxycycline

A man taking lithium carbonate long-term became confused within a day of starting to take doxycycline 100 mg twice daily. By the end of a week he had developed symptoms of lithium toxicity (ataxia, dysarthria, worsened tremor, fatigue). His serum lithium levels had risen from a range of 0.8 to 1.1 mmol/L up to 1.8 mmol/L: his renal function remained normal. He recovered when the doxycycline was withdrawn.[1]

(b) Minocycline

A case report describes pseudotumor cerebri in an obese 15-year-old girl taking lithium, 4 months after she started taking minocycline 75 mg twice daily for acne.[2] Another case report describes a 13-year-old girl taking lithium for bipolar disorder and minocycline (dose not stated) for acne. She had a history of menstrual irregularities and had gained 11.4 kg in weight over the preceding 3 months. She presented with pseudotumor cerebri 3 weeks after a dose increase of lithium carbonate from 900 mg daily to 1.2 g daily, and recovered when the lithium carbonate was withdrawn and replaced with valproic acid.[3]

(c) Tetracycline

An isolated report describes a woman who had been taking lithium carbonate 800 mg twice daily for 3 years, with serum levels within the range of 0.5 to 0.84 mmol/L. Within 2 days of starting to take a sustained-release form of tetracycline (*Tetrabid*) her serum lithium levels had risen to 1.7 mmol/L, and 2 days later they had further risen to 2.74 mmol/L. By then she had clear symptoms of lithium toxicity (slight drowsiness, slurring of the speech, fine tremor and thirst).[4] In contrast, 13 healthy subjects taking lithium carbonate 450 mg twice daily or 900 mg daily had only an 8% reduction in their serum lithium levels (from 0.51 to 0.47 mmol/L) when they were given tetracycline 500 mg twice daily for 7 days.[5] The incidence of adverse reactions remained largely unchanged, except for a slight increase in CNS and gastrointestinal adverse effects.

Mechanism

Not understood. One suggested reason for the increased serum lithium levels is that tetracycline (known to have nephrotoxic potential) might have adversely affected the renal clearance of lithium.[4]

Importance and management

The reports describing a possible adverse interaction between lithium and the tetracyclines are isolated and unexplained. Two reports make the point that these drugs are commonly used for acne caused by lithium,[1,6] so any common interaction resulting in raised lithium levels would be expected to have come to light by now. The case of pseudotumor cerebri also appears rare, but note that female gender, obesity, and minocycline use alone are risk factors for its development and so greater caution might be warranted in this type of patient.[2,3] The authors advise frequent enquiry about headaches and visual changes.

There would seem to be no reason for avoiding the concurrent use of lithium and tetracycline, doxycycline or minocycline, but be aware of the potential for a rare interaction. One manufacturer advises an increased frequency of lithium level monitoring when any drug that can impair renal function is given,[7] and this could be taken to include the tetracyclines, although the available data suggests that this would be a particularly cautious approach. For general comment on the use of antibacterials in patients taking lithium, see 'Lithium + Antibacterials', p.1364.

1. Miller SC. Doxycycline-induced lithium toxicity. *J Clin Psychopharmacol* (1997) 17, 54–5.
2. Jonnalagadda J, Saito E, Kafantaris V. Lithium, minocycline, and pseudotumor cerebri. *J Am Acad Child Adolesc Psychiatry* (2005) 44, 209.
3. Hexom B, Barthel RP. Lithium and pseudotumor cerebri. *J Am Acad Child Adolesc Psychiatry* (2004) 43, 247–8.
4. McGennis AJ. Lithium carbonate and tetracycline interaction. *BMJ* (1978) 2, 1183.
5. Fankhauser MP, Lindon JL, Connolly B, Healey WJ. Evaluation of lithium–tetracycline interaction. *Clin Pharm* (1988) 7, 314–17.
6. Jefferson JW. Lithium and tetracycline. *Br J Dermatol* (1982) 107, 370.
7. Camcolit (Lithium carbonate). Norgine Ltd. UK Summary of product characteristics, August 2010.

Lithium + Aripiprazole

Lithium very slightly increases the exposure to aripiprazole. A case report describes neuroleptic malignant syndrome in a patient taking aripiprazole and lithium. Another report describes dystonia in a patient taking haloperidol and lithium that occurred after haloperidol was replaced by aripiprazole.

Clinical evidence

In a study, 7 healthy subjects were given aripiprazole 30 mg daily for 5 weeks, with lithium carbonate slow-release tablets 1.2 to 1.8 g daily (to give a plasma level of 1 to 1.4 mmol/L) during weeks 3 to 5. The AUC and maximum plasma concentrations of aripiprazole were increased by 15% and 19%, respectively.[1] Results from a routine therapeutic drug monitoring service suggest that aripiprazole levels are increased by 34% by lithium.[2] An analysis from another therapeutic drug monitoring service found that in 14 patients who had taken lithium with aripiprazole, the mean concentration/dose ratio of aripiprazole was 43% higher than in 79 control patients taking aripiprazole alone. Levels of the main metabolite, dehydroaripiprazole were not affected.[3]

Moderately severe neuroleptic malignant syndrome developed in a patient with bipolar disorder within 3 weeks of starting aripiprazole (initially 5 mg daily titrated slowly up to 15 mg twice daily) and lithium, which was increased to 600 mg twice daily. The patient improved over 4 days after aripiprazole was discontinued and lithium was withheld, and after a further 3 days lithium was restarted.[4]

A 46-year-old woman with diabetes and bipolar disorder, taking haloperidol and trihexyphenidyl, developed mild muscle rigidity, tremor and bradykinesia after also taking lithium 900 mg daily for 2 days. Polyuria and polydipsia developed after a further 5 days of lithium use (serum level 0.7 mmol/L). Haloperidol was replaced by aripiprazole 10 mg daily and 3 days later she developed Pisa syndrome (manifested as tonic flexion of the trunk and persistent dystonic contraction of cervical to lumbar musculature). Lithium was discontinued and polyuria and polydipsia improved over 5 days. Aripiprazole was discontinued and the tonic trunk flexion disappeared within 3 days.[5]

Mechanism

Unknown.

Importance and management

The concurrent use of lithium and aripiprazole slightly increases the exposure to aripiprazole, but these increases are not considered to be clinically relevant. The case describing neuroleptic malignant syndrome is isolated, and as this effect can occur in response to one antipsychotic drug an interaction is not established as the cause. The dystonic reaction was probably associated with the use of aripiprazole, but the effects of haloperidol withdrawal and concurrent lithium could not be ruled out as contributing factors.[5] The concurrent use of aripiprazole and lithium is therefore not definitely responsible for these adverse reactions, and as such, no general precautions can be recommended.

1. Citrome L, Josiassen R, Bark N, Salazar DE, Mallikaarjun S. Pharmacokinetics of aripiprazole and concomitant lithium and valproate. *J Clin Pharmacol* (2005) 45, 89–93.
2. Castberg I, Spigset O. Effects of comedication on the serum levels of aripiprazole: evidence from a routine therapeutic drug monitoring service. *Pharmacopsychiatry* (2007) 40, 107–10.
3. Waade RB, Christensen H, Rudberg I, Refsum H, Hermann M. Influence of comedication on serum concentrations of aripiprazole and dehydroaripiprazole. *Ther Drug Monit* (2009) 31, 233–8.
4. Ali S, Pearlman RL, Upadhyay A, Patel P. Neuroleptic malignant syndrome with aripiprazole and lithium: a case report. *J Clin Psychopharmacol* (2006) 26, 434–6.
5. Huang Y-C, Lee Y, Lin P-Y. Reversible Pisa syndrome associated with switching from haloperidol to aripiprazole during lithium treatment. *Prog Neuropsychopharmacol Biol Psychiatry* (2009) 33, 1284–5.

Lithium + Aspirin or other Salicylates

No clinically relevant pharmacokinetic interaction appears to occur between aspirin, lysine aspirin or sodium salicylate and lithium.

Clinical evidence, mechanism, importance and management

In a steady-state study, 10 healthy women with average plasma lithium levels of 0.63 mmol/L had a 6% rise in their renal excretion of lithium when they were given aspirin 1 g four times daily for 7 days. However, no statistically significant alteration in lithium levels was found.[1]

No change in serum lithium levels was seen in 7 patients taking lithium when they were given aspirin 975 mg four times daily for 6 days.[2] Another report states that aspirin 600 mg four times daily had no effect on the absorption or renal excretion of single doses of lithium carbonate given to 6 healthy subjects.[3] Further reports describe no change in serum lithium levels with **lysine aspirin**,[4] intravenous aspirin,[5] or intravenous **sodium salicylate**.[5] However, lithium clearance was reduced by 22% by intravenous **sodium salicylate**,[5] and a study in one healthy subject found a 32% increase in mean serum lithium levels (from 0.41 to 0.54 mmol/L) after 5 days' use of oral aspirin (975 mg four times daily for 2 days, then 650 mg four times daily for 3 days).[6]

These findings suggest that the required dose of lithium is unlikely to be changed by the concurrent use of aspirin or sodium salicylate. However, note that pyrexia, for which aspirin and other related drugs may be taken, can itself alter fluid and electrolyte balance and thereby cause elevated lithium levels.

1. Reimann IW, Diener U, Frölich JC. Indomethacin but not aspirin increases plasma lithium ion levels. *Arch Gen Psychiatry* (1983) 40, 283–6.
2. Ragheb MA. Aspirin does not significantly affect patients' serum lithium levels. *J Clin Psychiatry* (1987) 48, 425.
3. Bikin D, Conrad KA, Mayersohn M. Lack of influence of caffeine and aspirin on lithium elimination. *Clin Res* (1982) 30, 249A.

4. Singer L, Imbs JL, Danion JM, Singer P, Krieger-Finance F, Schmidt M, Schwartz J. Risque d'intoxication par le lithium en cas de traitement associé par les anti-inflammatoires non stéroïdiens. *Therapie* (1981) 36, 323–6.
5. Reimann IW, Golbs E, Fischer C, Frölich JC. Influence of intravenous acetylsalicylic acid and sodium salicylate on human renal function and lithium clearance. *Eur J Clin Pharmacol* (1985) 29, 435–41.
6. Bendz H, Feinberg M. Aspirin increases serum lithium ion levels. *Arch Gen Psychiatry* (1984) 41, 310–11.

Lithium + Baclofen

The hyperkinetic symptoms of two patients with Huntington's chorea were aggravated within a few days of starting to take lithium and baclofen.

Clinical evidence, mechanism, importance and management

A patient with Huntington's chorea, taking lithium and haloperidol, was also given baclofen, and another patient taking imipramine, clopenthixol, chlorpromazine and baclofen was also given lithium. Within a few days both patients had a severe aggravation of their hyperkinetic symptoms, which disappeared within 3 days of withdrawing the baclofen.[1] Other patients with Huntington's chorea had no major changes in their mental state or movement disorders when given up to 90 mg of baclofen daily,[2,3] which suggests that an interaction with lithium could have been the cause of the hyperkinesis in these two patients. On the basis of this very limited evidence it would seem prudent to monitor the effects of concurrent use and consider stopping one of the drugs if hyperkinesis develops.

1. Andén N-E, Dalén P, Johansson B. Baclofen and lithium in Huntington's chorea. *Lancet* (1973) ii, 93.
2. Barbeau A. G.A.B.A. and Huntington's chorea. *Lancet* (1973) ii, 1499–1500.
3. Paulson GW. Lioresal in Huntington's disease. *Dis Nerv Syst* (1976) 37, 465–7.

Lithium + Benzodiazepines

Neurotoxicity and increased lithium levels were reported in several patients when clonazepam was given to patients taking lithium, and increased lithium levels have been described in one patient taking bromazepam. An isolated case of serious hypothermia has been reported during the concurrent use of lithium and diazepam. Alprazolam seems unlikely to cause a clinically important rise in lithium levels.

Clinical evidence, mechanism, importance and management

(a) Alprazolam

In 10 healthy subjects taking lithium carbonate 900 mg to 1.5 g daily, alprazolam 2 mg daily for 4 days increased the steady-state AUC of lithium by about 8% and reduced its urinary recovery from 94% to 78%. It was suggested that these changes were unlikely to be clinically significant.[1]

(b) Bromazepam

A case report describes a patient taking lithium carbonate 900 mg daily, whose lithium levels rose from 1.12 mmol/L to 1.4 mmol/L within 4 days of starting to take bromazepam 18 mg daily. His lithium dose was reduced to 500 mg daily, which resulted in his lithium level returning to its former value.[2]

(c) Clonazepam

A retrospective study of patient records revealed 5 patients with bipolar disorder, taking lithium carbonate 900 mg to 2.4 g daily, who had developed a reversible neurotoxic syndrome with ataxia, dysarthria, drowsiness and confusion when they were given clonazepam 2 to 16 mg daily. In one case clonazepam was added to their antipsychotics (chlorpromazine, perphenazine, haloperidol) and in 4 cases clonazepam replaced the antipsychotic treatment. In all cases lithium levels rose, and in two of these cases they reached toxic levels. The authors of the report suggest that the neurotoxicity was caused either by the increase in lithium levels, or by synergistic toxicity; however, the use of antipsychotics might also have increased CNS sensitivity. It was recommended that lithium levels should be measured more frequently if clonazepam is added, with the effects of concurrent use well monitored.[3]

(d) Diazepam

A patient who was described as having profound mental retardation had occasional hypothermic episodes (below 35°C) while taking lithium and diazepam, but not while taking either drug alone. After taking lithium carbonate 1 g and diazepam 30 mg daily for 17 days, the patient's temperature fell from 35.4°C to 32°C over 2 hours, and she became comatose with reduced reflexes, dilated pupils, a systolic blood pressure of 40 to 60 mmHg, a pulse rate of 40 bpm and no piloerector response.[4] The reasons for this reaction are not known. This is an isolated case and therefore no general recommendations can be made. There seems to be no evidence of this adverse interaction with any of the other benzodiazepines.

1. Evans RL, Nelson MV, Melethil S, Townsend R, Hornstra RK, Smith RB. Evaluation of the interaction of lithium and alprazolam. *J Clin Psychopharmacol* (1990) 10, 355–9.
2. Raudino F. Interazione fra benzodiazepine e livelli plasmatici di sali di litio. *Clin Ter* (1981) 98, 683–5.
3. Koczerginski D, Kennedy SH, Swinson RP. Clonazepam and lithium—a toxic combination in the treatment of mania? *Int Clin Psychopharmacol* (1989) 4, 195–9.
4. Naylor GJ, McHarg A. Profound hypothermia on combined lithium carbonate and diazepam treatment. *BMJ* (1977) 3, 22.

Lithium + Beta blockers

One study suggests that atenolol might decrease the clearance of lithium, and another study suggests that propranolol might do likewise. An isolated report describes a patient taking lithium who developed marked bradycardia after he took low-dose propranolol.

Clinical evidence

(a) Atenolol

A study in 24 hypertensive patients who had been taking atenolol 50 mg daily for more than 3 months found that atenolol reduced the renal clearance of a single 600-mg dose of lithium carbonate by 22%.[1]

(b) Propranolol

A study in lithium-treated patients with bipolar disorder found that the clearance of lithium was about 20% lower in 23 patients also taking propranolol than in 292 similar patients taking lithium alone.[2]

A 70-year-old man stable taking lithium for 16 years was started on propranolol 30 mg daily for lithium-induced tremor. Six weeks later he was hospitalised because of vomiting, dizziness, headache and a fainting episode. His pulse rate was 35 to 40 bpm and his serum lithium level was 0.3 mmol/L. When later discharged taking lithium without propranolol his pulse rate had risen to a range of 64 to 80 bpm.[3] The authors of this case report attribute the bradycardia to an interaction with lithium, as the low dose of propranolol was considered unlikely to cause bradycardia alone.

Mechanism

It has been suggested that beta blockers alter renal vascular tone, resulting in a reduction in proximal tubular fluid output, and that this might be responsible for the observed reduction in lithium clearance.[1]

Both lithium and beta blockers affect the movement of calcium across cell membranes, which could account for the decreased contraction rate of the heart muscle, and thus bradycardia.[3]

Importance and management

The clinical impact of the reduced lithium clearance observed with both atenolol and propranolol was not evaluated in the studies described above. Given the proposed mechanism, similar changes could occur with other beta blockers. However, given the extensive, successful use of beta blockers in patients taking lithium, it is likely that this effect is of minor clinical importance.

The general relevance of the case report describing bradycardia with lithium and propranolol is uncertain, but it seems possible with all beta blockers because they can all cause bradycardia. The authors of the case report suggest careful monitoring in elderly patients with atherosclerotic cardiovascular problems.[3] However, as beta blockers are used to treat lithium-induced tremor, any serious problem would be expected to have come to light by now.

1. Krusell LR, Jespersen LT, Christensen CK, Thomsen K, Pedersen OL. Proximal tubular function in essential hypertensives on beta-blocker therapy with atenolol. *Blood Pressure* (1997) 6, 166–70.
2. Schou M, Vestergaard P. Use of propranolol during lithium treatment: an enquiry and a suggestion. *Pharmacopsychiatry* (1987) 20, 131.
3. Becker D. Lithium and propranolol: possible synergism? *J Clin Psychiatry* (1989) 50, 473.

Lithium + Caffeine

The heavy consumption of caffeine-containing drinks can cause a small reduction in serum lithium levels.

Clinical evidence

In a single-dose study in 8 healthy subjects, lithium carbonate 300 mg was given 14 hours before placebo or caffeine 400 mg (given orally as 100 mg every 30 minutes). Caffeine was associated with a 29% greater decrease in plasma lithium concentration (measured one hour after completion of caffeine administration), and a 32% increase in the urinary excretion of lithium.[1] Similarly, a study in 11 psychiatric patients taking lithium 600 mg to 1.2 g daily who were also regular coffee drinkers (4 to 8 cups daily containing 70 to 120 mg of caffeine per cup), serum lithium levels *rose* by an average of 24% when the coffee was *withdrawn*, although the levels of 3 patients did not change.[2] In addition, an early single-dose study found that the intake of xanthines such as caffeine caused an increase in lithium excretion.[3]

These findings are consistent with a report of 2 patients with lithium-induced tremors that were aggravated when they stopped drinking large amounts of coffee. One of the patients had a 50% rise in lithium levels, and required a reduction in the dose of lithium from 1.5 g daily to 1.2 g daily.[4]

In contrast, a single-dose study did not find any changes in the urinary clearance of lithium in 6 subjects given caffeine 200 mg four times daily compared with a caffeine-free control period.[5]

Mechanism

It is not clear exactly how caffeine affects the excretion of lithium by the renal tubules, but other xanthines have a similar effect (see 'Lithium + Theophylline', p.1379). It has been suggested that caffeine acts as an antagonist at renal adenosine A_1 receptors, inhibiting the proximal tubular reabsorption of lithium, but maintaining the glomerular filtration rate.

Importance and management

The weight of evidence suggests that, although there is no need for those taking lithium to avoid caffeine (from caffeine-containing herbs, coffee, tea, cola drinks etc.), they should not exceed a moderate intake. In cases where a reduction in caffeine intake is desirable, it should be withdrawn cautiously. This is particularly important in those whose serum lithium levels are already high, because of the risk of toxicity. When caffeine is withdrawn it might be necessary to reduce the dose of lithium. In addition, remember that there is a caffeine-withdrawal syndrome (headache and fatigue being the major symptoms) that might worsen some of the major psychiatric disorders (such as affective and schizophrenic disorders)[2] for which lithium is given.

1. Shirley DG, Walter SJ, Noormohamed FH. Natriuretic effect of caffeine: assessment of segmental sodium reabsorption in humans. *Clin Sci* (2002) 103, 461–6.
2. Mester R, Toren P, Mizrachi I, Wolmer L, Karni N, Weizman A. Caffeine withdrawal increases lithium blood levels. *Biol Psychiatry* (1995) 37, 348–50.
3. Thomsen K, Schou M. Renal lithium excretion in man. *Am J Physiol* (1968) 215, 823–7.
4. Jefferson JW. Lithium tremor and caffeine intake: two cases of drinking less and shaking more. *J Clin Psychiatry* (1988) 49, 72–3.
5. Bikin D, Conrad KA, Mayersohn M. Lack of influence of caffeine and aspirin on lithium elimination. *Clin Res* (1982) 30, 249A.

Lithium + Calcitonins

Limited data suggest that calcitonin, both human and salmon, increases the urinary clearance of lithium.

Clinical evidence

Prompted by the occasional observation of decreased serum lithium levels in outpatients receiving calcitonin, a study was undertaken in 4 women with bipolar depression. The patients, who had been taking lithium for 10 years, were also given calcitonin (salmon) 100 units subcutaneously for three consecutive days for postmenopausal osteoporosis. It was found that their serum lithium levels fell, on average, from 0.73 mmol/L to 0.59 mmol/L. The clearance of lithium in the urine was tested in 2 of the patients, and both had increases (9.8% and 16.2%).[1] Additionally, a crossover study in 6 healthy subjects found that giving a single intravenous dose of calcitonin (human) 500 micrograms increased the urinary clearance of lithium by 54%.[2]

Mechanism

Not known. Increased renal excretion and possibly some reduced intestinal absorption of the lithium have been suggested by the authors of the first report.[1] Using inulin and lithium clearance tests, the authors of the second report concluded that calcitonin (human) has a proximal diuretic action.[2]

Importance and management

Information seems to be limited to these studies, which only lasted for up to 3 days. One study found only a small reduction in serum lithium levels, and did not assess the effect on the control of depression.[1] It seems unlikely that this interaction will be clinically important in most patients, but as some patients could be affected, monitor the outcome of concurrent use, and consider monitoring lithium levels if an interaction is suspected.

1. Passiu G, Bocchetta A, Martinelli V, Garau P, Del Zompo M, Mathieu A. Calcitonin decreases lithium plasma levels in man. Preliminary report. *Int J Clin Pharmacol Res* (1998) 18, 179–81.
2. Bachofen M, Bock H, Beglinger C, Fischer JA, Thiel G. Calcitonin, ein proximal tubular wirkendes Diuretikum: Lithium-Clearance-Messungen am Menschen. *Schweiz Med Wochenschr* (1997) 127, 747–52.

Lithium + Calcium-channel blockers

The concurrent use of lithium and verapamil can be uneventful, but neurotoxicity (ataxia, movement disorders, tremors) with unchanged lithium levels have been reported in a few patients. In addition, either reduced or increased lithium levels have occurred with verapamil. An acute parkinsonian syndrome and marked psychosis has been seen in at least one patient taking lithium and diltiazem. Reduced lithium clearance, and one possible case of increased lithium levels have been reported with nifedipine.

Clinical evidence

(a) Diltiazem

A woman stable taking lithium for several years developed marked psychosis and parkinsonism within a week of starting to take diltiazem 30 mg three times daily.[1] An acute parkinsonism syndrome developed in a 58-year-old man taking lithium and tiotixene within 4 days of starting 30 mg of diltiazem three times daily.[2] However, this report has been questioned as the symptoms could have been attributable to an adverse effect of the tiotixene, and, even if the lithium toxicity was genuine, it is thought to have been more likely due to recent increases in the lithium dose, or the use of a diuretic than diltiazem.[3]

(b) Nifedipine

In a study of patients with essential hypertension, two doses of nifedipine 20 mg did not affect single-dose lithium clearance, but nifedipine 40 to 80 mg daily for 6 and 12 weeks was found to decrease single-dose lithium clearance by 30%.[4] A man, taking lithium carbonate 1.5 g daily with a lithium level of 0.8 mmol/L, developed ataxia and dysarthria 7 days after starting to take nifedipine, initially 30 mg daily for 48 hours, then 60 mg daily. His lithium dose was reduced by 40%, but his serum lithium level first increased to 1.1 mmol/L (about 2 weeks after starting the nifedipine), before restabilising at 0.9 mmol/L.[5] In contrast, a patient taking lithium, who developed dysarthria and ataxia after verapamil was added to her treatment (see *Verapamil*, below), was subsequently well controlled while taking lithium and nifedipine 40 mg daily.[6]

(c) Verapamil

A 42-year-old woman taking lithium carbonate 900 mg daily developed toxicity (nausea, vomiting, muscular weakness, ataxia and tinnitus) within 9 days of starting to take verapamil 80 mg three times daily. Her bipolar depressive disorder improved even though her serum lithium levels remained unchanged at 1.1 mmol/L. The toxicity disappeared within 48 hours of stopping the verapamil, but her disorder worsened. The same pattern was repeated when verapamil was restarted and then withdrawn.[7] Another 3 cases of movement disorders (including ataxia, tremors and choreoathetosis) resulting from the concurrent use of lithium and verapamil have also been reported,[6,8,9] two of which had documented unchanged serum lithium levels.[6,8] In one case the patient was restabilised by halving the dose of lithium.[8]

Conversely, a patient who was stable taking lithium 900 mg to 1.2 g daily for over 8 years had a reduction in his serum lithium levels, from about 1.04 mmol/L to 0.5 mmol/L, when he was given verapamil 80 mg four times daily. He was restabilised on approximately double the dose of lithium.[10] Another patient had an increase in his lithium clearance when he took verapamil for 3 days, and he had a reduction in his serum lithium levels, from 0.61 mmol/L to 0.53 mmol/L.[10]

In addition to unchanged or decreased lithium levels with verapamil, one manufacturer notes that increased lithium levels have occurred.[11]

Two cases of bradycardia have been reported when verapamil was given to patients taking lithium. In one case the patient's heart rate returned to normal on stopping verapamil, and in the other case, the patient (who was also taking propranolol) developed asymptomatic class I atrioventricular ectopy and died following a myocardial infarction.[12]

Mechanism

Not understood. However, it has been suggested that calcium-channel blockers and lithium affect neurotransmitter production[1,2,9,13] (several pathways have been described), which results in CNS sensitivity. This produces movement disorders, which are said to mimic lithium toxicity. In most of the cases mentioned above, symptoms of toxicity were present at therapeutic lithium levels, which would support this suggested mechanism.

It is unclear whether the cases of bradycardia are attributable to an interaction between lithium and verapamil, or the effects of verapamil alone. The contribution of propranolol in the second case could also be important, see 'Beta blockers + Calcium-channel blockers; Verapamil', p.1008.

Importance and management

The neurotoxic adverse reactions cited above for lithium and **verapamil** contrast with other reports describing uneventful concurrent use.[13-15] Reports of altered serum lithium levels (both increases and decreases) have also occurred. This unpredictability emphasises the need to monitor the effects closely where it is thought appropriate to give lithium with verapamil.

Only a couple of isolated cases describe neurotoxicity with lithium and **diltiazem**, and their general relevance is uncertain, but bear them in mind in the event of an unexpected response to treatment.

Some limited data suggest that **nifedipine** might slightly reduce lithium clearance, and the clinical relevance of this is uncertain.

1. Binder EF, Cayabyab L, Ritchie DJ, Birge SJ. Diltiazem-induced psychosis and a possible diltiazem-lithium interaction. *Arch Intern Med* (1991) 151, 373–4.
2. Valdiserri EV. A possible interaction between lithium and diltiazem: case report. *J Clin Psychiatry* (1985) 46, 540–1.
3. Flicker MR, Quigley MA, Caldwell EG. Diltiazem-lithium interaction: an opposing viewpoint. *J Clin Psychiatry* (1988) 49, 325–6.
4. Bruun NE, Ibsen H, Skøtt P, Toftdahl D, Giese J, Holstein-Rathlou NH. Lithium clearance and renal tubular sodium handling during acute and long-term nifedipine treatment in essential hypertension. *Clin Sci* (1988) 75, 609–13.
5. Pinkofsky HB, Sabu R, Reeves RR. A nifedipine-induced inhibition of lithium clearance. *Psychosomatics* (1997) 38, 400–1.
6. Wright BA, Jarrett DB. Lithium and calcium channel blockers: possible neurotoxicity. *Biol Psychiatry* (1991) 30, 635–6.
7. Price WA, Giannini AJ. Neurotoxicity caused by lithium-verapamil synergism. *J Clin Pharmacol* (1986) 26, 717–19.
8. Price WA, Shalley JE. Lithium-verapamil toxicity in the elderly. *J Am Geriatr Soc* (1987) 35, 177–8.
9. Helmuth D, Ljaljevic Z, Ramirez L, Meltzer HY. Choreoathetosis induced by verapamil and lithium treatment. *J Clin Psychopharmacol* (1989) 9, 454–5.
10. Weinrauch LA, Belok S, D'Elia JA. Decreased serum lithium during verapamil therapy. *Am Heart J* (1984) 108, 1378–80.
11. Covera-HS (Verapamil hydrochloride). Pfizer Inc. US Prescribing Information, October 2011.
12. Dubovsky SL, Franks RD, Allen S. Verapamil: a new antimanic drug with potential interactions with lithium. *J Clin Psychiatry* (1987) 48, 371–2.
13. Mallinger AG, Thase ME, Haskett R, Buttenfield J, Lukenbaugh DA, Frank E, Kupfer DJ, Manji HK. Verapamil augmentation of lithium treatment improves outcome in mania unresponsive to lithium alone: preliminary findings and a discussion of therapeutic mechanisms. *Bipolar Disord* (2008) 10, 856–66.
14. Brotman AW, Farhadi AM, Gelenberg AJ. Verapamil treatment of acute mania. *J Clin Psychiatry* (1986) 47, 136–8.
15. Gitlin MJ, Weiss J. Verapamil as maintenance treatment in bipolar illness: a case report. *J Clin Psychopharmacol* (1984) 4, 341–3.

Lithium + Carbamazepine

The concurrent use of lithium and carbamazepine might increase the risk of neurotoxicity. Sinus node dysfunction has also occurred in a few patients. An isolated report describes a patient who had a marked rise in lithium levels and lithium toxicity, which was apparently caused by carbamazepine-induced renal impairment.

Clinical evidence

(a) Neurotoxicity with normal drug levels

A patient taking lithium 1.8 g daily developed severe neurotoxicity (ataxia, truncal tremors, nystagmus, limb hyperreflexia, muscle fasciculation) within 3 days of starting to take carbamazepine 600 mg daily. Blood levels of both drugs remained within the therapeutic range. The symptoms resolved when each drug was withdrawn in turn, and recurred within 3 days of restarting concurrent treatment.[1] Five patients with rapid-cycling bipolar disorder developed similar neurotoxic symptoms (confusion, drowsiness, generalised weakness, lethargy, coarse tremor, hyperreflexia, cerebellar signs) when they were given lithium carbonate with carbamazepine (doses not stated). Plasma levels of both drugs remained within the accepted range.[2] Other reports describe adverse neurological effects during the concurrent use of lithium and carbamazepine, which were also not accompanied by notable changes in lithium levels,[3-8] although in one patient raised serum levels of both drugs were seen.[9] A systematic search through the Medline database, for reports of neurotoxic adverse effects in patients taking lithium at low therapeutic concentrations, found a total of 41 cases over about 30 years from 1966. Carbamazepine had been taken concurrently in 22% of these cases, in some instances with other potentially interacting drugs.[10] Another retrospective study of 46 patients with type I bipolar disorder found benefits with the long-term concurrent use of lithium and carbamazepine, compared with lithium (31 patients) or carbamazepine (15 patients) alone. However, rates of adverse effects increased 2.5-fold compared with monotherapy, and there were particular excesses of tremor and drowsiness.[11]

In other patients the concurrent use of lithium and carbamazepine was said to be well tolerated and beneficial,[12,13] but one report suggests that the doses might need to be carefully titrated to avoid adverse effects.[14]

(b) Sinus node dysfunction

A 9-year study in a psychiatric hospital found that, of 5 patients taking lithium who developed sinus node dysfunction, 4 were also taking carbamazepine.[15]

(c) Toxic lithium levels

An isolated case report describes carbamazepine-induced acute renal failure, which resulted in a 3.5-fold rise in lithium levels and lithium toxicity 3 weeks after carbamazepine was started.[16]

Mechanism

Not understood. A paper that plotted the serum levels of lithium and carbamazepine on a two-dimensional graph did not find any evidence of synergistic toxicity.[17] Sinus node dysfunction can be caused by either lithium or carbamazepine, but this is rare. However, the effects could possibly be additive.

Importance and management

The neurotoxic interaction between lithium and carbamazepine is established, but its incidence is unknown. The incidence of severe neurotoxicity might be quite small, but increased mild adverse events such as tremor and drowsiness seem to be fairly common.[11] The authors of one paper suggest that the risk factors appear to be a history of neurotoxicity with lithium, and compromised medical or neurological function.[2] If concurrent use is undertaken, the outcome should be closely monitored. This is particularly important because neurotoxicity can develop even though the levels remain within the accepted therapeutic range. If severe neurotoxicity develops lithium should be discontinued promptly, whatever the lithium level.[10]

The manufacturers of **oxcarbazepine**[18] predict that it might interact similarly with lithium, and therefore it would seem prudent to take similar precautions to those suggested for carbamazepine.

1. Chaudhry RP, Waters BGH. Lithium and carbamazepine interaction: possible neurotoxicity. *J Clin Psychiatry* (1983) 44, 30–1.
2. Shukla S, Godwin CD, Long LEB, Miller MG. Lithium-carbamazepine neurotoxicity and risk factors. *Am J Psychiatry* (1984) 141, 1604–6.
3. Andrus PF. Lithium and carbamazepine. *J Clin Psychiatry* (1984) 45, 525.
4. Marcoux AW. Carbamazepine-lithium drug interaction. *Ann Pharmacother* (1996) 30, 547.
5. Manto M-U, Jacquy J, Hildebrand J. Cerebellar ataxia in upper limbs triggered by addition of carbamazepine to lithium treatment. *Acta Neurol Belg* (1996) 96, 316–17.
6. Ghose K. Effect of carbamazepine in polyuria associated with lithium therapy. *Pharmakopsychiatr Neuropsychopharmakol* (1978) 11, 241–5.
7. Price WA, Zimmer B. Lithium-carbamazepine neurotoxicity in the elderly. *J Am Geriatr Soc* (1985) 33, 876–7.
8. Palma J-A, Fernandez-Torron R, Gallego Perez-Larraya J. Extrapyramidal syndrome related to lithium-carbamazepine combination therapy at therapeutic serum levels. *Clin Neuropharmacol* (2010) 33, 102–3.
9. Hassan MN, Thakar J, Weinberg AL, Grimes JD. Lithium-carbamazepine interaction: clinical and laboratory observations. *Neurology* (1987) 37 (Suppl 1), 172.
10. Emilien G, Maloteaux JM. Lithium neurotoxicity at low therapeutic doses. Hypotheses for causes and mechanism of action following a retrospective analysis of published case reports. *Acta Neurol Belg* (1996) 96, 281–93.
11. Baethge C, Baldessarini RJ, Mathiske-Schmidt K, Hennen J, Berghöfer A, Müller-Oerlinghausen B, Bschor T, Adli M, Bauer M. Long-term combination therapy versus monotherapy with lithium and carbamazepine in 46 bipolar I patients. *J Clin Psychiatry* (2005) 66, 174–82.
12. Laird LK, Knox EP. The use of carbamazepine and lithium in controlling a case of chronic rapid cycling. *Pharmacotherapy* (1987) 7, 130–2.
13. Pies R. Combining lithium and anticonvulsants in bipolar disorder: a review. *Ann Clin Psychiatry* (2002) 14, 223–32.
14. Kramlinger KG, Post RM. The addition of lithium to carbamazepine. Antidepressant efficacy in treatment-resistant depression. *Arch Gen Psychiatry* (1989) 46, 794–800.
15. Steckler TL. Lithium- and carbamazepine-associated sinus node dysfunction: nine-year experience in a psychiatric hospital. *J Clin Psychopharmacol* (1994) 14, 336–9.
16. Mayan H, Golubev N, Dinour D, Farfel Z. Lithium intoxication due to carbamazepine-induced renal failure. *Ann Pharmacother* (2001) 35, 560–2.
17. McGinness J, Kishimoto A, Hollister LE. Avoiding neurotoxicity with lithium-carbamazepine combinations. *Psychopharmacol Bull* (1990) 26, 181–4.
18. Trileptal (Oxcarbazepine). Novartis Pharmaceuticals UK Ltd. UK Summary of product characteristics, April 2012.

Lithium + Cisplatin

Isolated case reports describe either a fall or no alteration in lithium levels in patients given cisplatin. However, note that cisplatin-induced renal impairment might cause an increase in lithium levels.

Clinical evidence, mechanism, importance and management

The serum lithium levels of a woman taking lithium carbonate 300 mg four times daily fell, over a period of 2 days, from 1 mmol/L to 0.3 mmol/L, and from 0.8 mmol/L to 0.5 mmol/L, on two occasions when she was given cisplatin (100 mg/m^2 intravenously over 2 hours). To prevent cisplatin-induced renal toxicity, she was also given a fluid load over a total of 24 hours, which included one litre of sodium chloride 0.9% over 4 hours, one litre of mannitol 20% over 4 hours, and one litre of dextrose 5% in sodium chloride 0.9%. Serum lithium levels returned to normal at the end of 2 days. No change in the control of the psychotic symptoms was seen.[1] A man had a transient 64% decrease in serum lithium levels, without perceptible clinical consequences, during the first of four courses of cisplatin, bleomycin, and etoposide. The effect became less pronounced during the subsequent courses.[2] It is not clear whether the reduction in serum lithium levels in these cases was due to increased renal clearance caused by the cisplatin or the sodium load, dilution from the fluid load, or a combination of all three factors.

In contrast, one patient had no clinically significant changes in her serum lithium levels when given cisplatin, but 2 months later her deteriorating renal function resulted in a rise in her serum lithium levels.[3]

None of these interactions was of particular clinical importance, but the authors of the first report pointed out that some regimens of cisplatin involve the use of higher doses (40 mg/m^2 daily) with a sodium chloride 0.9% fluid load over 5 days, and under these circumstances it would be prudent to monitor the serum lithium levels carefully. However, because cisplatin-induced renal impairment might cause an increase in lithium levels it would seem prudent to monitor the concurrent use of lithium and cisplatin in all patients.

1. Pietruszka LJ, Biermann WA, Vlasses PH. Evaluation of cisplatin-lithium interaction. *Drug Intell Clin Pharm* (1985) 19, 31–2.
2. Beijnen JH, Bais EM, ten Bokkel Huinink WW. Lithium pharmacokinetics during cisplatin-based chemotherapy: a case report. *Cancer Chemother Pharmacol* (1994) 33, 523–6.
3. Beijnen JH, Vlasveld LT, Wanders J, ten Bokkel Huinink WW, Rodenhuis S. Effect of cisplatin-containing chemotherapy on lithium serum concentrations. *Ann Pharmacother* (1992) 26, 488–90.

Lithium + Clozapine

A few patients given lithium carbonate and clozapine have experienced adverse reactions including myoclonus, neuroleptic malignant syndrome, rhabdomyolysis, seizures, delirium, and psychoses.

Clinical evidence

A review of the medical records of 44 patients taking clozapine and lithium identified 28 patients who had experienced an adverse effect, three of which were possibly associated with the drug combination: there were two reports of myoclonus and one of a grand mal seizure.[1] A retrospective study using both Medline and the spontaneous reporting system of the FDA in the US, over the period 1969 to 1994, identified 237 cases of severe neurotoxicity involving lithium, with 188 cases involving lithium with antipsychotics, and of these, 6 involved clozapine.[2,3]

Four out of 10 patients taking lithium carbonate (mean dose of 1.4 g daily) and clozapine (mean maximum dose 900 mg daily) developed reversible neurological symptoms including involuntary jerking of the limbs and tongue, facial spasm, tremor, confusion, generalised weakness, stumbling gait, leaning and falling to the right. One of them also became delirious. Serum lithium levels remained unchanged, and the problems resolved when the lithium was stopped. Three of the four had a recurrence of the symptoms when rechallenged with the drug combination.[4]

A man with poorly controlled schizophrenia, taking clozapine 750 mg daily for 6 weeks, was given lithium, initially 900 mg and then subsequently 1.2 g daily. His serum lithium level was 0.86 mmol/L. Within one week he began to experience paroxysmal jerky movements of his upper and lower extremities lasting about 30 minutes. This myoclonus resolved when both drugs were stopped, and did not recur when clozapine was restarted alone.[5] Another patient taking lithium developed neuroleptic malignant syndrome (stiffness, rigidity, tachycardia, diaphoresis, hypertension) 3 to 4 weeks after clozapine was added. The symptoms disappeared within 2 to 3 days of stopping the clozapine.[6] An elderly man also developed neuroleptic malignant syndrome 3 days after starting to take clozapine 25 mg daily. He was also taking carbamazepine, and had stopped taking lithium 3 days earlier.[7]

A number of other case reports describe adverse neurological effects in patients taking clozapine and lithium. These include neurotoxic symptoms (ataxia, coarse tremor, myoclonus, facial spasm, and increased deep tendon reflex) which developed after 3 days of concurrent use,[8] psychosis and raised lithium levels,[9] and two cases of seizures (one within 4 days of concurrent use).[10]

A case of rhabdomyolysis has been reported in a 29-year-old man with bipolar disorder receiving valproic acid 2 g daily, lithium and clozapine (titrated up from 300 mg daily to 500 mg daily over 7 to 8 weeks). Lithium 600 mg daily was started a week later, increasing to 1.2 g daily within a week. About 10 days after that, generalised muscle aches were noted, and investigations revealed a serum lithium level of 0.48 mmol/L and an elevated serum creatine kinase level (6 776 units/L). A probable diagnosis of rhabdomyolysis was reached after excluding the possibility of infection or neuroleptic malignant syndrome. The patient recovered within a week, with intravenous hydration and a reduced clozapine dose (400 mg daily).[11]

It has been suggested that lithium may help to protect patients from the adverse effects of clozapine, in particular agranulocytosis.[12] However, lithium is thought to have masked clozapine-induced agranulocytosis in a 59-year-old woman who developed leucopenia and subsequently agranulocytosis after 40 days of treatment with lithium and clozapine,[13] and two cases of reversible leukocytosis have been reported in patients taking lithium with clozapine.[14]

Mechanism

Not understood.

Importance and management

An interaction between clozapine and lithium appears to be established; however, not all patients are affected. It is not clear why some patients develop a toxic reaction when given both drugs, and others do not, and it is also not clear which patients are at risk. One group of workers suggest that lithium levels of no more than 0.5 mmol/L might give therapeutic benefits while minimising adverse effects.[4] The concurrent use of clozapine and lithium should be well monitored for adverse effects, particularly for evidence of neuroleptic malignant syndrome, which appears to be the most common adverse effect reported.

An interaction with clozapine leading to increased lithium levels is not established: there appears to be only one case report describing this effect.

Note that lithium is associated with QT prolongation, as is clozapine. See 'Drugs that prolong the QT interval + Other drugs that prolong the QT interval', p.272, for further information on the concurrent use of two or more drugs that prolong the QT interval.

1. Bender S, Linka T, Wolstein J, Gehendges S, Paulus H-J, Schall U, Gastpar M. Safety and efficacy of combined clozapine-lithium pharmacotherapy. *Int J Neuropsychopharmacol* (2004) 7, 59–63.
2. Goldman SA. Lithium and neuroleptics in combination: is there enhancement of neurotoxicity leading to permanent sequelae? *J Clin Pharmacol* (1996) 36, 951–62.
3. Goldman SA. FDA MedWatch Report: lithium and neuroleptics in combination: the spectrum of neurotoxicity. *Psychopharmacol Bull* (1996) 32, 299–309.
4. Blake LM, Marks RC, Luchins DJ. Reversible neurologic symptoms with clozapine and lithium. *J Clin Psychopharmacol* (1992) 12, 297–9.
5. Lemus CZ, Lieberman JA, Johns CA. Myoclonus during treatment with clozapine and lithium: the role of serotonin. *Hillside J Clin Psychiatry* (1989) 11, 127–30.
6. Pope HG, Cole JO, Choras PT, Fulwiler CE. Apparent neuroleptic malignant syndrome with clozapine and lithium. *J Nerv Ment Dis* (1986) 174, 493–5.
7. Müller T, Becker T, Fritze J. Neuroleptic malignant syndrome after clozapine plus carbamazepine. *Lancet* (1988) ii, 1500.
8. Lee S-H, Yang Y-Y. Reversible neurotoxicity induced by a combination of clozapine and lithium: a case report. *Zhonghua Yi Xue Za Zhi (Taipei)* (1999) 62, 184–7.
9. Hellwig B, Hesslinger B, Walder J. Tapering off clozapine in a clozapine-lithium co-medication may cause an acute organic psychosis. A case report. *Pharmacopsychiatry* (1995) 28, 187.
10. Garcia G, Crismon ML, Dorson PG. Seizures in two patients after the addition of lithium to a clozapine regimen. *J Clin Psychopharmacol* (1994) 14, 426–7.
11. Tseng KC, Hwang TJ. Rhabdomyolysis following dose increase of clozapine and combination therapy with lithium. *J Clin Psychopharmacol* (2009) 29, 398–9.
12. Kanaan RA, Kerwin RW. Lithium and clozapine rechallenge: a retrospective case analysis. *J Clin Psychiatry* (2006) 67, 756–60.
13. Valevski A, Modai I, Lahav M, Weizman A. Clozapine-lithium combined treatment and agranulocytosis. *Int Clin Psychopharmacol* (1993) 8, 63–5.
14. Palominao A, Kukoyi O, Xiong GL. Leukocytosis after lithium and clozapine combination therapy. *Ann Clin Psychiatry* (2010) 22, 205–6.

Lithium + Colony-stimulating factors

Lithium might enhance the effects of granulocyte colony-stimulating factors.

Clinical evidence

A case report describes a 33-year-old woman taking lithium carbonate 1.2 g daily who received treatment for acute myeloid leukaemia, which included the use of recombinant human granulocyte colony-stimulating factor (G-CSF). The authors of the report suggest that the percentage and number of CD34+ cells in her peripheral blood obtained by a single apheresis were higher than they usually found in patients not taking lithium.[1]

Mechanism

Leucocytosis is a recognised effect of lithium and therefore lithium could have contributed to the higher than expected number of CD34+ cells[1] following the use of G-CSF.

Importance and management

Evidence for an interaction between lithium and colony-stimulating factor is limited to one case report. The US manufacturer advises caution if **filgrastim** is given with drugs such as lithium that can potentiate the release of neutrophils.[2] However, the UK manufacturer of filgrastim notes there is no evidence that such an interaction is harmful.[3] No general precautions can therefore be recommended on the basis of this report.

1. Canales MA, Arrieta R, Hernández-García C, Bustos JG, Aguado MJ, Hernández-Navarro F. A single apheresis to achieve a high number of peripheral blood CD34$^+$ cells in a lithium-treated patient with acute myeloid leukaemia. *Bone Marrow Transplant* (1999) 23, 305.
2. Neupogen (Filgrastim). Amgen Inc. US Prescribing information, May 2012.
3. Neupogen (Filgrastim). Amgen Ltd. UK Summary of product characteristics, March 2011.

Lithium + Corticosteroids

Corticosteroids can disturb electrolyte balance, which in theory could affect serum lithium levels, but there do not appear to be any reports of clinically significant interactions. Two case reports suggest that lithium caused resistance to corticosteroid treatment in patients with Addison's disease.

Clinical evidence, mechanism, importance and management

A patient with systemic lupus erythematosus suffering from steroid-induced depression and moderate renal impairment was given lithium 600 mg daily and her depression improved. However, serum lithium levels increased from 0.4 mmol/L to 0.8 mmol/L within one week and she had an exacerbation of a finger tremor. Lithium was discontinued and then restarted at 400 mg daily, resulting in serum levels of 0.4 mmol/L. Her depression improved, and she had only a fine finger tremor. Three other patients with steroid-induced depression were also successfully treated with lithium.[1]

A case report describes a 29-year-old patient taking several drugs, including **fludrocortisone** 150 micrograms daily and **hydrocortisone** 40 mg daily for Addison's disease, and lithium carbonate 1.2 g daily for bipolar disorder. He was admitted to hospital with an Addisonian crisis and a plasma sodium level of 117 mmol/L, but this normalised (to 130 mmol/L) within 48 hours of stopping his medication and treatment with intravenous **hydrocortisone** and hypertonic fluids. Lithium levels remained within the therapeutic range. Hyponatraemia developed a second time when lithium was reinstated, and again resolved within 48 hours after stopping lithium.[2]

Another patient with Addison's disease and bipolar disorder taking **hydrocortisone** 15 mg daily and **fludrocortisone** 100 micrograms daily developed increasing tiredness, fatigue and nausea within 6 weeks of starting to take lithium carbonate 1 g daily (serum levels 0.7 to 0.9 mmol/L). She had postural hypotension and her plasma sodium level was 129 mmol/L and her plasma potassium level was 5.1 mmol/L. The dose of **hydrocortisone** was increased to 25 mg daily. Six months later lithium was stopped and her serum potassium level fell to 3.4 mmol/L and her plasma sodium level increased to 142 mmol/L. After a further 3 months, lithium 1 g daily was restarted. Plasma renin activity was markedly elevated and so the dose of **fludrocortisone** was increased in 100-microgram increments but even at a dose of 600 micrograms daily plasma renin activity remained elevated. During a metabolic balance investigation **fludrocortisone** 1 mg daily and dietary sodium supplementation were required to normalise both plasma renin activity and serum potassium levels and to counter postural hypotension. She was discharged taking lithium 1 g daily, **fludrocortisone** 600 micrograms daily and sodium supplements. When lithium was slowly withdrawn, **fludrocortisone** was also reduced to 100 micrograms daily while maintaining plasma renin activity and blood pressure within accepted ranges. It was suggested that lithium inhibits the action of fludrocortisone on the distal renal tubule.[3]

One UK manufacturer warns that drugs affecting electrolyte balance, such as corticosteroids, can alter lithium excretion and should therefore be avoided,[4] but other manufacturers do not appear to specifically mention this potential interaction. An early study in *rats* reported increased lithium clearance with **methylprednisolone**.[5]

The available evidence is insufficient to recommend routine monitoring. However, it might be prudent to consider monitoring lithium effects in patients with renal impairment, or other conditions pre-disposing to lithium toxicity, taking levels if early symptoms suggest a potential problem. For more information on the risk factors for lithium toxicity, symptoms of lithium adverse effects and general monitoring, see under 'Lithium', p.1361.

Evidence for an effect of lithium on the response to corticosteroids appears to be limited to their use in Addison's disease. If a patient with Addison's disease is started on lithium consider the possibility that larger than anticipated corticosteroid doses might be necessary.

1. Terao T. Lithium therapy for corticosteroid-induced mood disorder. *J Clin Psychiatry* (2001) 62, 57.
2. Gómez-Herreros R, Sánchez-Luengo FG, del Valle-Villagrán J, Fernández-López I. Resistencia a la fludrocortisona en paciente con enfermedad de Addison y trastorno bipolar en tratamiento con litio. *Med Clin (Barc)* (2007) 128, 397–8.
3. Stewart PM, Grieve J, Nairn IM, Padfield PL, Edwards CRW. Lithium inhibits the action of fludrocortisone on the kidney. *Clin Endocrinol (Oxf)* (1987) 27, 63–8.
4. Li-Liquid (Lithium citrate tetrahydrate). Rosemont Pharmaceuticals Ltd. UK Summary of product characteristics, July 2011.
5. Imbs JL, Singer L, Danion JM, Schmidt M, Zawilslak R. Effects of indomethacin and methylprednisolone on renal elimination of lithium in the rat. *Int Pharmacopsychiatry* (1980) 15, 143–9.

Lithium + Diuretics; Loop

The concurrent use of lithium carbonate and furosemide can be safe and uneventful, but serious lithium toxicity has been described. Bumetanide

interacts similarly. The risk of lithium toxicity with a loop diuretic is greatly increased during the first month of concurrent use.

Clinical evidence

An analysis of 10 615 elderly patients receiving lithium found that 413 patients (3.9%) were admitted to hospital at least once for lithium toxicity during a 10-year study period. The prescriptions for any loop diuretic (not specifically named) were compared between these 413 hospitalised patients and 1 651 control patients. For any use of a loop diuretic (54 cases and 71 controls) there was an increased relative risk of hospitalisation for lithium toxicity of 1.7. When patients who were newly started on a loop diuretic were analysed (12 cases and 6 controls), a dramatically increased risk of lithium toxicity within a month of initiating treatment was found (relative risk 5.5).[1] Reports relating to specific named loop diuretics are discussed below.

(a) Bumetanide

Bumetanide has been responsible for the development of lithium toxicity in 2 patients[2,3] one of whom was following a salt-restricted diet,[3] which has also been implicated in episodes of lithium toxicity, see 'Lithium + Sodium compounds', p.1378.

(b) Furosemide

Six healthy subjects stable taking lithium carbonate 300 mg three times daily (mean serum lithium levels 0.43 mmol/L) were given furosemide 40 mg daily for 14 days. Five subjects experienced some minor adverse effects, probably attributable to the furosemide, without notable changes in serum lithium levels, but one subject experienced such a marked increase in the toxic effects of lithium that she withdrew from the study after taking both drugs for only 5 days. Her serum lithium levels were found to have risen from 0.44 mmol/L to 0.71 mmol/L.[4] There are another 4 case reports of individual patients who experienced serious lithium toxicity or other adverse reactions when given lithium and furosemide.[5-8] One of the patients was also following a salt-restricted diet,[5] which has also been implicated in episodes of lithium toxicity, see 'Lithium + Sodium compounds', p.1378.

In contrast, 6 patients who had been stable taking lithium for over 6 years had no notable changes in their serum lithium levels over a 12-week period while taking furosemide 20 to 80 mg daily.[9] Other studies in healthy subjects also found no notable changes in lithium levels when furosemide 40 or 80 mg daily was given.[10,11]

Mechanism

Not fully understood. If and when a rise in serum lithium levels occurs, it might be related to the salt depletion that can accompany the use of furosemide (for a more detailed explanation see 'Lithium + Sodium compounds', p.1378). As with the thiazides (see 'Lithium + Diuretics; Thiazide and related', below), such an interaction would take a few days to develop. This may explain why one study in subjects given a single dose of lithium did not find any effect of furosemide on the urinary excretion of lithium.[12]

Importance and management

Information about an interaction between the loop diuretics and lithium seems mainly to be limited to reports regarding furosemide. The incidence of this interaction is uncertain and its development unpredictable. It would be imprudent to give furosemide to patients stable taking lithium unless the effects can be well monitored, because some patients could develop serious toxicity. Patients taking lithium should be aware of the symptoms of lithium toxicity and told to report them immediately should they occur. Consider increased monitoring of lithium levels in patients newly started on this combination. If the proposed mechanism is correct, an interaction would be anticipated with any loop diuretic and therefore it would be prudent to apply the same precautions advised for furosemide to the use of lithium with any loop diuretic.

For more information on the risk factors for lithium toxicity, symptoms of lithium adverse effects and general monitoring, see under 'Lithium', p.1361.

1. Juurlink DN, Mamdani MM, Kopp A, Rochon PA, Shulman KI, Redelmeier DA. Drug-induced lithium toxicity in the elderly: a population-based study. *J Am Geriatr Soc* (2004) 52, 794–8.
2. Kerry RJ, Ludlow JM, Owen G. Diuretics are dangerous with lithium. *BMJ* (1980) 281, 371.
3. Huang LG. Lithium intoxication with coadministration of a loop-diuretic. *J Clin Psychopharmacol* (1990) 10, 228.
4. Jefferson JW, Kalin NH. Serum lithium levels and long-term diuretic use. *JAMA* (1979) 241, 1134–6.
5. Hurtig HI, Dyson WL. Lithium toxicity enhanced by diuresis. *N Engl J Med* (1974) 290, 748–9.
6. Oh TE. Frusemide and lithium toxicity. *Anaesth Intensive Care* (1977) 5, 60–2.
7. Grau Segura E, Pinet Ogue MC, Franco Peral M. Intoxicación por sales de litio. Presentación de un caso. *Med Clin (Barc)* (1984) 83, 294–6.
8. Thornton WE, Pray BJ. Lithium intoxication: a report of two cases. *Can Psychiatr Assoc J* (1975) 20, 281–2.
9. Saffer D, Coppen A. Frusemide: a safe diuretic during lithium therapy? *J Affect Disord* (1983) 5, 289–92.
10. Crabtree BL, Mack JE, Johnson CD, Amyx BC. Comparison of the effects of hydrochlorothiazide and furosemide on lithium disposition. *Am J Psychiatry* (1991) 148, 1060–3.
11. Shalmi M, Rasmusen H, Amtorp O, Christensen S. Effect of chronic oral furosemide administration on the 24-hour cycle of lithium clearance and electrolyte excretion in humans. *Eur J Clin Pharmacol* (1990) 38, 275–80.
12. Thomsen K, Schou M. Renal lithium excretion in man. *Am J Physiol* (1968) 215, 823–7.

Lithium + Diuretics; Potassium-sparing

There is evidence that the excretion of lithium can be increased by triamterene. In contrast, lithium levels might rise if spironolactone is used: eplerenone is predicted to interact similarly. Amiloride does not appear to interact with lithium.

Clinical evidence and mechanism

(a) Amiloride

Amiloride has been found to have no notable effect on serum lithium levels when used in the treatment of lithium-induced polyuria.[1,2] Similarly, in a study to investigate the effect of amiloride on urine osmolality in 11 patients taking lithium, there was no change in the lithium plasma levels after they took amiloride 5 mg daily for 2 weeks, then 10 mg daily for 4 weeks.[3] One review briefly mentions a case report in which amiloride was successfully used as a replacement for bendroflumethiazide, which had caused lithium toxicity.[4] However, one manufacturer[5] suggests that, as a diuretic, amiloride reduces the renal clearance of lithium, thereby increasing the risk of lithium toxicity, but there appear to be no reports of toxicity to support this statement.

(b) Spironolactone

One study found that spironolactone had no statistically significant effect on the excretion of lithium,[6] whereas in another report, the use of spironolactone 100 mg daily was accompanied by a rise in serum lithium levels from 0.63 mmol/L to 0.9 mmol/L. The levels continued to rise for several days after the spironolactone was stopped.[7]

(c) Triamterene

Triamterene, given to a patient taking lithium while following a salt-restricted diet, is said to have led to a strong lithium diuresis.[8] Similarly, triamterene increased lithium excretion in 8 healthy subjects.[9]

Importance and management

Amiloride, spironolactone and triamterene have been available for a considerable time and it might have been expected that by now any serious adverse interactions with lithium would have emerged, but information is very sparse. None of the reports available gives a clear indication of the outcome of concurrent use, but some monitoring would be a prudent precaution with any potassium-sparing diuretic. No interaction study has been undertaken with lithium and **eplerenone**, but the manufacturers suggest that lithium levels should be monitored frequently if eplerenone is also given,[10,11] although, in the UK, the manufacturer advises avoidance of the combination.[11] They state that this is because raised lithium levels have occurred with related drugs such as the ACE inhibitors and diuretics. There seems to be no clear reason to avoid the use of lithium and any potassium-sparing diuretic; however, patients taking lithium with one of these diuretics should be made aware of the symptoms of lithium toxicity (see 'Lithium', p.1361) and told to report them immediately should they occur.

1. Batlle DC, von Riotte AB, Gaviria M, Grupp M. Amelioration of polyuria by amiloride in patients receiving long-term lithium therapy. *N Engl J Med* (1985) 312, 408–14.
2. Kosten TR, Forrest JN. Treatment of severe lithium-induced polyuria with amiloride. *Am J Psychiatry* (1986) 143, 1563–8.
3. Bedford JJ, Weggery S, Ellis G, McDonald FJ, Joyce PR, Leader JP, Walker RJ. Lithium-induced nephrogenic diabetes insipidus: renal effects of amiloride. *Clin J Am Soc Nephrol* (2008) 3, 1324–31.
4. Aronson JK, Reynolds DJM. ABC of monitoring drug therapy. Lithium. *BMJ* (1992) 305, 1273–6.
5. Amilamont (Amiloride hydrochloride). Rosemont Pharmaceuticals Ltd. UK Summary of product characteristics, March 2011.
6. Thomsen K, Schou M. Renal lithium excretion in man. *Am J Physiol* (1968) 215, 823–7.
7. Baer L, Platman SR, Kassir S, Fieve RR. Mechanisms of renal lithium handling and their relationship to mineralocorticoids: a dissociation between sodium and lithium ions. *J Psychiatr Res* (1971) 8, 91–105.
8. Williams, Katz, Shield eds. Recent Advances in the Psychobiology of the Depressive Illnesses. Washington DC: DHEW Publications, 1972 p 49–58.
9. Wetzels JFM, van Bergeijk JD, Hoitsma AJ, Huysmans FTM, Koene RAP. Triamterene increases lithium excretion in healthy subjects: evidence for lithium transport in the cortical collecting tubule. *Nephrol Dial Transplant* (1989) 4, 939–42.
10. Inspra (Eplerenone). Pfizer Inc. US Prescribing information, April 2008.
11. Inspra (Eplerenone). Pfizer Ltd. UK Summary of product characteristics, October 2009.

Lithium + Diuretics; Thiazide and related

Thiazide and related diuretics can cause a rapid rise in lithium levels, leading to toxicity.

Clinical evidence

A retrospective analysis of 10 615 elderly patients receiving lithium found that 413 (3.9%) were admitted to hospital at least once for lithium toxicity during a 10-year study period. The prescriptions for a thiazide-type diuretic were compared between these 413 hospitalised patients and 1 651 control patients. For any use of a thiazide diuretic (16 cases and 37 controls) there was a non-significant increased relative risk of 1.3 for hospitalisation due to lithium toxicity. When treatment for patients who were newly started on a thiazide diuretic was analysed (5 cases and 6 controls), the increased relative risk of toxicity was also non-significant (1.3). The authors considered that these findings suggest that the use of thiazide diuretics and lithium might not be as hazardous as previously thought. However, the authors also suggest that another explanation is that clinicians were aware of the potential interaction and so adjusted doses or observed patients more closely in the outpatient setting, thereby avoiding any hospitalisations for toxicity.[1]

Case reports and studies describing the effects of the concurrent use of named thiazide diuretics and lithium are outlined below.

(a) Bendroflumethiazide

A study in 22 patients, who had been taking either bendroflumethiazide 2.5 mg daily or hydroflumethiazide 25 mg daily for at least 2 months, found that these diuretics caused a 24% reduction in the urinary clearance of a single 600-mg dose of lithium carbonate.[2] A case report describes a roughly twofold increase in serum lithium levels,[3] and a case of lithium toxicity (with a roughly threefold increase in serum lithium levels) has been mentioned in a review article,[4] both after bendroflumethiazide 5 mg daily was started in patients taking lithium. In a further case, lithium toxicity, with serum lithium levels of 4.28 mmol/L was detected 3 months after the addition of bendroflumethiazide 5 mg daily.[5] However, this case was complicated by the presence of perindopril, which might also raise lithium levels, as has occurred with other ACE inhibitors, see 'Lithium + ACE inhibitors', p.1362.

In contrast to these reports, one single-dose study found that bendroflumethiazide 7.5 mg given 10 hours after lithium carbonate 600 mg had no effect on lithium clearance.[6] However, it seems unlikely that single-dose studies will detect an interaction (see *Mechanism* below).

(b) Chlorothiazide

A single 300-mg dose of lithium carbonate was given to 4 healthy subjects alone and after the use of chlorothiazide 500 mg daily for 7 days. Lithium plasma levels were increased and lithium clearance was decreased by about 26% by chlorothiazide.[7]

Lithium toxicity developed in a patient taking lithium after she was given chlorothiazide, spironolactone and amiloride.[8] Her lithium levels rose from 0.6 mmol/L to 2.2 mmol/L. A 54-year-old patient developed nephrogenic diabetes insipidus when she took lithium carbonate. The addition of chlorothiazide reduced her polyuria, but resulted in an elevation in her lithium level from 1.3 mmol/L to more than 2 mmol/L, with accompanying signs of toxicity. The patient later successfully took chlorothiazide with a reduced dose of lithium.[9]

(c) Chlortalidone

A 58-year-old woman developed lithium toxicity within 10 days of starting chlortalidone (dose unknown).[10] Her lithium levels rose from 0.8 mmol/L to 3.7 mmol/L.

(d) Hydrochlorothiazide

In a placebo-controlled study, the serum lithium levels of 13 healthy subjects taking lithium 300 mg twice daily rose by 23% (from 0.3 to 0.37 mmol/L), when they were given hydrochlorothiazide 25 mg twice daily for 5 days.[11] Similar results were found in another small study.[12] In addition to these studies at least 6 cases of lithium toxicity have been seen when hydrochlorothiazide was given to patients taking lithium.[13-17] In these cases, hydrochlorothiazide was either given with amiloride,[13-15] spironolactone[16] or triamterene,[17] which might have contributed to the toxicity. See also 'Lithium + Diuretics; Potassium-sparing', p.1370.

(e) Hydroflumethiazide

A study in 22 patients who had been taking either bendroflumethiazide 2.5 mg daily or hydroflumethiazide 25 mg daily for at least 2 months found that these diuretics caused a 24% reduction in the urinary clearance of a single 600-mg dose of lithium carbonate.[2]

(f) Indapamide

A 64-year-old man developed lithium toxicity one week after starting to take indapamide 5 mg daily.[18] His serum lithium level was 3.93 mmol/L.

Mechanism

Not fully understood. The interaction occurs even though the thiazides and related diuretics exert their major actions in the distal part of the kidney tubule whereas lithium is mainly reabsorbed in the proximal part. However, thiazide diuresis is accompanied by sodium loss which, within a few days, is compensated by retention of sodium, this time in the proximal part of the tubule. As both sodium and lithium ions are treated similarly, the increased reabsorption of sodium would include lithium as well, hence a measurable reduction in its excretion.[5,19]

Importance and management

The interaction between lithium and the thiazide and related diuretics is established, well-documented and potentially serious. The rise in serum lithium levels and the accompanying toxicity develops most commonly within about a week to 10 days,[4,7,9-11,13,17] although it has apparently been seen after 19 days[16] and even 3 months.[5] Not every patient necessarily develops a clinically important interaction, but it is not possible to predict which patients will be affected. The lack of serious cases of toxicity in the case-control study either suggests the interaction is rare, or that appropriate precautions are adopted when the combination is prescribed.[1]

Although only the diuretics named above have been implicated in this interaction, it seems likely that all thiazides and related diuretics will interact similarly. None of the thiazide or related diuretics should be given to patients taking lithium unless the serum lithium levels can be closely monitored and appropriate downward dose adjustments made. Patients taking lithium should be aware of the symptoms of lithium toxicity and told to report them immediately should they occur. For more information on the risk factors for lithium toxicity, symptoms of lithium adverse effects and general monitoring, see under 'Lithium', p.1361.

The concurrent use of lithium and thiazides, under controlled conditions, has been advocated for certain psychiatric conditions and for the control of lithium-induced nephrogenic diabetes insipidus. A successful case is described above.[9] It has been suggested that a 40 to 70% reduction in the lithium dose would be needed with doses of 0.5 to 1 g of chlorothiazide,[20,21] but it would seem sensible to base any dose adjustments on individual lithium levels.

1. Juurlink DN, Mamdani MM, Kopp A, Rochon PA, Shulman KI, Redelmeier DA. Drug-induced lithium toxicity in the elderly: a population-based study. *J Am Geriatr Soc* (2004) 52, 794–8.
2. Petersen V, Hvidt S, Thomsen K, Schou M. Effect of prolonged thiazide treatment on renal lithium clearance. *BMJ* (1974) 3, 143–5.
3. Kerry RJ, Ludlow JM, Owen G. Diuretics are dangerous with lithium. *BMJ* (1980) 281, 371.
4. Aronson JK, Reynolds DJM. ABC of monitoring drug therapy. Lithium. *BMJ* (1992) 305, 1273–6.
5. Vipond AJ, Bakewell S, Telford R, Nicholls AJ. Lithium toxicity. *Anaesthesia* (1996) 51, 1156–8.
6. Thomsen K, Schou M. Renal lithium excretion in man. *Am J Physiol* (1968) 215, 823–7.
7. Poust RI, Mallinger AG, Mallinger J, Himmelhoch JM, Neil JF, Hanin I. Effect of chlorothiazide on the pharmacokinetics of lithium in plasma and erythrocytes. *Psychopharmacol Comm* (1976) 2, 273–84.
8. Basdevant A, Beaufils M, Corvol P. Influence des diurétiques sur l'élimination rénale du lithium. *Nouv Presse Med* (1976) 5, 2085–6.
9. Levy ST, Forrest JN, Heninger GR. Lithium-induced diabetes insipidus: manic symptoms, brain and electrolyte correlates, and chlorothiazide treatment. *Am J Psychiatry* (1973) 130, 1014–18.
10. Solomon JG. Lithium toxicity precipitated by a diuretic. *Psychosomatics* (1980) 21, 425, 429.
11. Crabtree BL, Mack JE, Johnson CD, Amyx BC. Comparison of the effects of hydrochlorothiazide and furosemide on lithium disposition. *Am J Psychiatry* (1991) 148, 1060–3.
12. Jefferson JW, Kalin NH. Serum lithium levels and long-term diuretic use. *JAMA* (1979) 241, 1134–6.
13. Macfie AC. Lithium poisoning precipitated by diuretics. *BMJ* (1975) 1, 516.
14. König P, Küfferle B, Lenz G. Ein fall von Lithiumtoxikation bei therapeutischen Lithiumdosen infolge zusätzlicher Gabe eines Diuretikums. *Wien Klin Wochenschr* (1978) 90, 380–2.
15. Dorevitch A, Baruch E. Lithium toxicity induced by combined amiloride HCl-hydrochlorothiazide administration. *Am J Psychiatry* (1986) 143, 257–8.
16. Lutz EG. Lithium toxicity precipitated by diuretics. *J Med Soc New Jers* (1975) 72, 439–40.
17. Mehta BR, Robinson BHB. Lithium toxicity induced by triamterene-hydrochlorothiazide. *Postgrad Med J* (1980) 56, 783–4.
18. Hanna ME, Lobao CB, Stewart JT. Severe lithium toxicity associated with indapamide therapy. *J Clin Psychopharmacol* (1990) 10, 379–80.
19. Schwarcz G. The problem of antihypertensive treatment in lithium patients. *Compr Psychiatry* (1982) 23, 50–54.
20. Himmelhoch JM, Poust RI, Mallinger AG, Hanin I, Neil JF. Adjustment of lithium dose during lithium-chlorothiazide therapy. *Clin Pharmacol Ther* (1977) 22, 225–7.
21. Himmelhoch JM, Forrest J, Neil JF, Detre TP. Thiazide-lithium synergy in refractory mood swings. *Am J Psychiatry* (1977) 134, 149–52.

Lithium + Food

One study suggested that food might increase the absorption of slow-release lithium. The extent to which the absorption of lithium is affected by food appears to depend on the formulation given.

Clinical evidence

In a crossover study involving 30 healthy subjects, a single 24-mmol dose of slow-release lithium sulfate or lithium citrate was given after an overnight fast and after a standard meal. When lithium was given after a meal it was considered to be completely absorbed, based on urinary excretion, but when it was given after fasting, lithium absorption appeared to be reduced in some subjects.[1]

A study in 12 healthy subjects given a single dose of a sustained-release lithium carbonate matrix tablet in the fasting and non-fasting state (standardised normal meal, high fat, or high fat/high protein meals) found that maximum plasma levels of lithium were higher when given with any type of meal compared with the fasting state, but levels remained within the therapeutic range in both fasting and non-fasting conditions.[2]

Mechanism

In both the fasting and non-fasting states, lithium plasma levels remained within the therapeutic range, and any differences in the maximum plasma levels of lithium were probably due to changes in the rate of absorption,[2] which might depend on the type and properties of the matrix used in the formulation.[3] The authors of one study suggest that the apparently reduced absorption, estimated from urinary excretion, is due to a reduction in gastrointestinal transit time, as a result of the development of diarrhoea when lithium was taken without food.[1] However, note that dehydration, which can be caused by diarrhoea, might result in reduced excretion of lithium and therefore this might not have been the most appropriate measure of lithium absorption.

Importance and management

Evidence for an interaction between lithium and food appears to be limited. The authors of one study suggested that patients should be advised to take lithium in a similar manner each day with regard to food and fluid intake, and dose adjustments should then be made on the basis of serum lithium levels.[1] However, there do not appear to be any generally accepted recommendations on the timing of lithium administration with regard to food intake. Furthermore, the findings of another study suggested that, for the specific formulation of lithium carbonate tested, administration with regard to food would not be an important consideration.[2] Available lithium preparations vary in bioavailability and the dose depends on the preparation used; changing preparations involves the same precautions used when initiating treatment. Further, it is generally recommended that patients taking lithium should maintain an adequate fluid intake and avoid dietary changes that reduce or increase sodium intake (see also 'Lithium + Sodium compounds', p.1378). Therefore no general recommendations can be made regarding the administration of lithium and meals.

1. Jeppsson J, Sjögren J. The influence of food on side effects and absorption of lithium. *Acta Psychiatr Scand* (1975) 51, 285–8.
2. Gai MN, Thielemann AM, Arancibia A. Effects of three different diets on the bioavailability of a sustained release lithium carbonate matrix tablet. *Int J Clin Pharmacol Ther* (2000) 38, 320–6.
3. Gai MN, Ferj S, Garcia E, Seitz C, Thielemann AM, Andonaegui MT.Evaluation of the in vitro and in vivo performance of two sustained-release lithium carbonate matrix tablets. Effect of different diets on bioavailability. *Drug Dev Ind Pharm* (1999) 25, 131–40.

Lithium + Gabapentin

Gabapentin does not alter the pharmacokinetics of single-dose lithium in patients with normal renal function.

Clinical evidence, mechanism, importance and management

In a double-blind study, 13 patients with normal renal function were given a single 600-mg dose of lithium, either with or without gabapentin at steady state. Gabapentin did not alter the pharmacokinetics of the lithium, and no increase in adverse effects was noted. Ideally, longer-term studies are needed to confirm this lack of interaction, especially in patients with impaired renal function as both drugs are eliminated by renal excretion.[1] However, on the basis of the information from this report, no lithium dose adjustment would be expected to be necessary on concurrent use.

1. Frye MA, Kimbrell TA, Dunn RT, Piscitelli S, Grothe D, Vanderham E, Corá-Locatelli G, Post RM, Ketter TA. Gabapentin does not alter single-dose lithium pharmacokinetics. *J Clin Psychopharmacol* (1998) 18, 461–4.

Lithium + Herbal medicines

A woman developed lithium toxicity after taking a herbal diuretic remedy. A brief report describes mania in a patient taking lithium who also took St John's wort.

Clinical evidence, mechanism, importance and management

(a) Herbal diuretics

A 26-year-old woman who had been taking lithium 900 mg twice daily for 5 months, with hydroxyzine, lorazepam, propranolol, risperidone and sertraline, came to an emergency clinic complaining of nausea, diarrhoea, unsteady gait, tremor, nystagmus and drowsiness (all symptoms of lithium toxicity). Her lithium level, which had previously been stable at 1.1 mmol/L was found to be 4.5 mmol/L. For the past 2 to 3 weeks she had been taking a non-prescription herbal diuretic containing **corn silk, *Equisetum hyemale*, juniper, ovate buchu, parsley** and **bearberry**, all of which are believed to have diuretic actions. The other ingredients were bromelain, paprika, potassium and vitamin B_6.[1]

The most likely explanation for what happened is that the herbal diuretic caused the lithium toxicity. It is impossible to know which herb or combination of herbs actually caused the toxicity, or how, but this case emphasises that herbal remedies are not risk-free just because they are natural. It also underscores the need for patients to avoid self-medication without first seeking informed advice and supervision if they are taking potentially hazardous drugs like lithium.

(b) St John's wort (Hypericum perforatum)

A search of Health Canada's database of spontaneous adverse reactions identified one case in which St John's wort was suspected of inducing mania in a patient also taking lithium.[2] The reasons for this effect are unknown, although it seems likely that the symptoms could be due to the effects of both lithium and St John's wort on serotonin. No further details were given of this case.

Note that both lithium and St John's wort have serotonergic effects, and concurrent use might lead to the serotonin syndrome. Serotonin syndrome is a rare adverse effect, but because of its severity, some caution is warranted if both drugs are given. For more information on serotonin syndrome and its management, see 'Drugs that cause serotonin syndrome + Other drugs that cause serotonin syndrome', p.1471.

1. Pyevich D, Bogenschutz MP. Herbal diuretics and lithium toxicity. *Am J Psychiatry* (2001) 158, 1329.
2. Natural health products and adverse reactions. *Can Adverse React News* (2004) 14, 2–3. Available at: http://www.hc-sc.gc.ca/dhp-mps/alt_formats/hpfb-dgpsa/pdf/medeff/carn-bcei_v14n1-eng.pdf (accessed 21/10/15).

Lithium + HIV-protease inhibitors

A report describes reduced lithium concentrations in two patients when their antiretroviral regimen was changed to include atazanavir boosted with ritonavir.

Clinical evidence, mechanism, importance and management

A case report describes a 46-year-old HIV-positive man who had been taking zidovudine with lamivudine, tenofovir, **lopinavir boosted with ritonavir**, and lithium carbonate for depression. About 3 years later, while maintained on lithium carbonate 450 mg twice daily, he started taking tenofovir, lamivudine, **atazanavir boosted with ritonavir** 300/100 mg daily as part of a new HAART regimen. Three weeks later he experienced anxiety, tremors and depressed mood and his lithium concentration had fallen from 1.47 mmol/L to 0.09 mmol/L.[1] In another case, a 35-year-old HIV-positive woman with bipolar disorder, who was stable taking lithium carbonate 450 mg twice daily, experienced instability, compulsions, panic and deep depression, which started about 2 weeks after her antiretroviral regimen was changed from abacavir, lamivudine and zidovudine to abacavir and **atazanavir boosted with ritonavir** 300/100 mg. Her plasma lithium concentrations had fallen from 1.23 mmol/L to 0.13 mmol/L.[1] The authors note that, in contrast to these 2 patients who experienced worsening depression and decreased lithium concentrations when their antiretroviral therapy was switched to an **atazanavir boosted with ritonavir** regimen, a third patient taking a triple NRTI regimen had no problems with maintenance lithium concentrations.[1]

Information regarding an interaction between lithium and the HIV-protease inhibitors appears to be limited to this one report and therefore the general importance of this potential interaction is unknown. Furthermore, the mechanism for any effect is unclear. No general recommendations can therefore be made.

1. Capetti A, Landonio S, Faggion I, Rizzardini G. Drop in plasma lithium levels in 2 patients on concomitant boosted protease inhibitor regimens. *J Int Assoc Physicians AIDS Care (Chic Ill)* (2006) 5, 119–20.

Lithium + Iodides

The hypothyroid and goitrogenic effects of lithium carbonate and iodides can be additive if they are given concurrently.

Clinical evidence

A man with normal thyroid function showed evidence of hypothyroidism after 3 weeks of taking lithium carbonate 750 mg to 1.5 g daily. After a further 2 weeks, during which he was also given **potassium iodide**, the hypothyroidism became even more marked, but resolved completely within 2 weeks of the withdrawal of both drugs. This patient was studied before the potential risk of hypothyroidism with iodine was well recognised.[1] Another report also describes a case of hypothyroidism associated with the use of lithium carbonate and **potassium iodide**.[2]

In a study of the possible effects of iodide intake on thyroid function in 10 patients receiving lithium, 3 to 5 weeks use of **potassium iodide** caused hypothyroidism in 2 patients and hyperthyroidism in one. Little effect on thyroid function was seen in 5 control patients given **potassium iodide** without lithium.[3] A case of hypothyroidism involving lithium and a product containing **isopropamide iodide** with haloperidol (*Vesalium*) has also been reported.[4,5]

A study investigating the effect of augmenting radioactive iodine (^{131}I) with lithium carbonate (750 mg daily for 10 days, starting 3 days before giving ^{131}I) in the treatment of hyperthyroidism (Graves' disease or toxic nodular goitre) found no advantage with the combination after 6 months.[6] In contrast, in a similar study in patients with Graves' disease, giving lithium carbonate 900 mg daily for 12 days, starting 5 days before giving ^{131}I resulted in a more rapid conversion to a euthyroid state (60 days compared with 90 days) and a statistically significant 6% higher maintenance of the euthyroid state after 12 months.[7]

Mechanism

Lithium accumulates in the thyroid gland and blocks the release of the thyroid hormones by thyroid-stimulating hormone, and can therefore cause clinical hypothyroidism.[1,8-15] The prevalence of hypothyroidism might be higher in women, in middle age,[15] and in countries with a higher level of nutritional iodine.[16] Potassium iodide temporarily prevents the production of thyroid hormones but, as time goes on, synthesis recommences. Thus, both lithium and iodide ions can depress the production or release of the hormones and therefore have additive hypothyroid effects.

Importance and management

The pharmacological interaction of altered thyroid function with lithium and iodides would appear to be established. However, the clinical use of iodides is now very limited (mostly to the pre-operative treatment of thyrotoxicosis). It is therefore unlikely that iodides will be used in patients taking lithium. However, note that patients taking lithium are advised against the regular use of some preparations of povidone iodine, such as sprays that can be used as disinfectants for minor wounds.[17] Where countries are adopting iodisation programmes to prevent iodine deficiency, there may be an increased risk of clinical hypothyroidism in patients taking lithium.[16] Lithium-induced hypothyroidism can be treated with levothyroxine replacement.

1. Shopsin B, Shenkman L, Blum M, Hollander CS. Iodine and lithium-induced hypothyroidism. Documentation of synergism. *Am J Med* (1973) 55, 695–9.
2. Jorgensen JV, Brandrup F, Schroll M. Possible synergism between iodine and lithium carbonate. *JAMA* (1973) 223, 192–3.
3. Spaulding SW, Burrow GN, Ramey JN, Donabedian RK. Effect of increased iodide intake on thyroid function in subjects on chronic lithium therapy. *Acta Endocrinol (Copenh)* (1977) 84, 290–6.
4. Luby ED, Schwartz D, Rosenbaum H. Lithium-carbonate-induced myxedema. *JAMA* (1971) 218, 1298–9.
5. Wiener JD. Lithium carbonate-induced myxedema. *JAMA* (1972) 220, 587.
6. Oszukowska L, Knapska-Kucharska M, Makarewicz J, Lewiński A. The influence of thiamazole, lithium carbonate, or prednisone administration on the efficacy of radioiodine treatment (^{131}I) in hyperthyroid patients. Endokrynol Pol. (2010) 61, 56–61.
7. Bogazzi F, Giovannetti C, Fessehatsion R, Tanda ML, Campomori A, Compri E, Rossi G, Ceccarelli C, Vitti P, Pinchera A, Bartalena L, Martino E. Impact of lithium on efficacy of radioactive iodine therapy for Graves' disease: a cohort study on cure rate, time to cure, and frequency of increased serum thyroxine after antithyroid drug withdrawal. *J Clin Endocrinol Metab* (2010) 95, 201–8.
8. Schou M, Amdisen A, Jensen SE, Olsen T. Occurrence of goitre during lithium treatment. *BMJ* (1968) 3, 710–13.
9. Shopsin B, Blum M, Gershon S. Lithium-induced thyroid disturbance: case report and review. *Compr Psychiatry* (1969) 10, 215–23.
10. Emerson CH, Dyson WL, Utiger RD. Serum thyrotropin and thyroxine concentrations in patients receiving lithium carbonate. *J Clin Endocrinol Metab* (1973) 36, 338–46.
11. Candy J. Severe hypothyroidism — an early complication of lithium therapy. *BMJ* (1972) 3, 277.
12. Villeneuve A, Gautier J, Jus A, Perron D. Effect of lithium on thyroid in man. *Lancet* (1973) ii, 502.
13. Lloyd GG, Rosser RM, Crowe MJ. Effect of lithium on thyroid in man. *Lancet* (1973) ii, 619.
14. Bocchetta A, Bernardi F, Pedditzi M, Loviselli A, Velluzzi F, Martino E, Del Zompo M. Thyroid abnormalities during lithium treatment. *Acta Psychiatr Scand* (1991) 83, 193–8.
15. Johnston AM, Eagles JM. Lithium-associated clinical hypothyroidism: prevalence and risk factors. *Br J Psychiatry* (1999) 175, 336–9.
16. Leutgeb U. Ambient iodine and lithium-associated clinical hypothyroidism. *Br J Psychiatry* (2000) 176, 495–6.
17. Betadine Dry Powder Spray (Povidone iodine). Molnlycke Health Care. UK Summary of product characteristics, April 2006.

Lithium + Ispaghula (Psyllium)

Ispaghula slightly reduced the absorption of lithium in a study in healthy subjects. Similarly, in an isolated case, the withdrawal of ispaghula resulted in an increase in lithium levels.

Clinical evidence

A 47-year-old woman who had recently started taking lithium was found to have a blood lithium level of 0.4 mmol/L five days after an increase in her lithium dose and whilst also taking one teaspoonful of ispaghula twice daily. The ispaghula was stopped 3 days later and lithium levels measured 4 days later were found to be 0.76 mmol/L.[1] A study in 6 healthy subjects similarly found that the absorption of lithium (as measured by the urinary excretion) was reduced by about 14% by ispaghula.[2]

Mechanism

Not understood. One idea is that the absorption of the lithium from the gut is reduced by ispaghula.[1,2]

Importance and management

Information is very limited and the general importance of this interaction is uncertain, but it would seem prudent to bear this interaction in mind in patients taking lithium who are given ispaghula preparations. If an interaction is suspected consider monitoring lithium levels and, if necessary, changing to an alternative laxative. The authors of one report suggested separating the administration of the two drugs by at least an hour[2] but the effects of this do not appear to have been studied.

1. Perlman BB. Interaction between lithium salts and ispaghula husk. *Lancet* (1990) 335, 416.
2. Toutoungi M, Schulz P, Widmer J, Tissot R. Probable interaction entre le psyllium et le lithium. *Therapie* (1990) 45, 358–60.

Lithium + Lamotrigine

Lamotrigine does not appear to cause a clinically significant alteration in lithium levels. Delirium has been reported in one patient taking both drugs.

Clinical evidence, mechanism, importance and management

In a randomised, crossover study, 20 healthy men were given 2 g of anhydrous lithium gluconate (9.8 mmol of lithium) every 12 hours for 11 doses, either with or without lamotrigine 100 mg daily. It was found that the serum lithium levels were decreased by about 8% by lamotrigine, but these small changes were not considered to be clinically relevant.[1] Analysis of serum samples from 829 patients taking lamotrigine found that, in 102 patients also taking lithium, lamotrigine levels were 13% lower than in the control group of patients not taking lithium.[2]

Based on this data, lamotrigine does not appear to have a clinically relevant effect on lithium levels and therefore no lithium dose alterations are necessary on concurrent use. Furthermore, a 2002 review of the few published reports on the use of lithium with lamotrigine suggested that concurrent use appears to be well tolerated.[3] However, one woman taking lithium who had been taking lamotrigine 50 mg for 4 weeks, experienced delirium when the dose of lamotrigine was increased to 150 mg daily. The symptoms disappeared when the lamotrigine dose was reduced to 100 mg daily.[4] It is not clear whether these effects were directly caused by the concurrent use of lithium and lamotrigine. However; the author of the review considered that if cognitive adverse effects occur, it might be worth considering a reduction in the dose of either or both drugs.[3]

1. Chen C, Veronese L, Yin Y. The effects of lamotrigine on the pharmacokinetics of lithium. *Br J Clin Pharmacol* (2000) 50, 193–5.
2. Reimers A, Skogvoll E, Sund JK, Spigset O. Drug interactions between lamotrigine and psychoactive drugs: evidence from a therapeutic drug monitoring service. *J Clin Psychopharmacol* (2005) 25, 342–8.
3. Pies R. Combining lithium and anticonvulsants in bipolar disorder: a review. *Ann Clin Psychiatry* (2002) 14, 223–32.
4. Sporn J, Sachs G. The anticonvulsant lamotrigine in treatment-resistant manic-depressive illness. *J Clin Psychopharmacol* (1997) 17, 185–9.

Lithium + Mazindol

An isolated report describes a case of lithium toxicity, which was attributed to the concurrent use of mazindol.

Clinical evidence, mechanism, importance and management

A 58-year-old woman with bipolar disorder, stable taking lithium carbonate, developed signs of lithium toxicity (sluggishness, ataxia) within 3 days of starting to take mazindol 2 mg daily. After 9 days she developed twitching, limb rigidity and muscle fasciculation, and was both dehydrated and stuporous. Her serum lithium levels were found to have risen from a range of 0.4 to 1.3 mmol/L up to 3.2 mmol/L. The mazindol was stopped, and she recovered over the next 48 hours whilst being rehydrated.[1] It is not known whether this was a direct interaction between the two drugs, but the authors suggest that the anorectic effect of mazindol led to this toxicity [i.e. the reduced intake of sodium and water caused a reduction in the renal excretion of lithium]. There seem to be no other reports of interactions between lithium and other anorectic drugs confirming this possibility. This is an isolated case and its general importance is therefore uncertain. Bear it in mind in the case of an unexpected response to treatment.

1. Hendy MS, Dove AF, Arblaster PG. Mazindol-induced lithium toxicity. *BMJ* (1980) 280, 684–5.

Lithium + Methyldopa

Symptoms of lithium toxicity, not always associated with raised lithium levels, have been described in four patients and four healthy subjects when they were also given methyldopa.

Clinical evidence

A woman with manic depression, taking lithium carbonate 900 mg daily, was hospitalised for signs of manic decompensation and her lithium dose was increased to 1.8 g daily. When she was also given methyldopa 1 g daily for hypertension, she developed signs of lithium toxicity (blurred vision, hand tremors, mild diarrhoea, confusion, and slurred speech), even though her serum lithium levels were within the range of 0.5 to 0.7 mmol/L. The methyldopa was then stopped and the lithium carbonate dose reduced to 1.5 g daily. Ten days later the lithium level was 1.4 mmol/L, and the lithium dose was decreased to 900 mg daily.[1] Later the author of this report demonstrated this interaction on himself.[2] He took lithium carbonate 150 mg four times daily for a week (lithium level 0.5 mmol/L), and then added methyldopa 250 mg every 8 hours. Within 2 days, signs of lithium toxicity had clearly developed, and the following day his lithium level had increased to 0.8 mmol/L. He then stopped methyldopa, and about 36 hours later his lithium level was 0.7 mmol/L.

There are three other cases of patients who took methyldopa with lithium, and developed symptoms of lithium toxicity. In one of these cases the patient had lithium levels within the normal therapeutic range,[3] but in the other two the lithium levels increased to 1.5 mmol/L and 1.87 mmol/L.[4,5] A small study in 3 healthy subjects also found that the concurrent use of lithium and methyldopa resulted in increased confusion, sedation and dysphoria.[6]

Mechanism

Not understood. Both a central effect and an effect on renal excretion have been proposed.[3-5]

Importance and management

Information on an interaction between lithium and methyldopa appears to be limited to the reports cited, but the interaction would seem to be established. If both drugs are given then the effects should be closely monitored. Serum lithium measurements might be unreliable because symptoms of toxicity can occur even though the levels remain within the normally accepted therapeutic range.

For more information on the risk factors for lithium toxicity, symptoms of lithium adverse effects and general monitoring, see under 'Lithium', p.1361.

1. Byrd GJ. Methyldopa and lithium carbonate: suspected interaction. *JAMA* (1975) 233, 320.
2. Byrd GJ. Lithium carbonate and methyldopa: apparent interaction in man. *Clin Toxicol* (1977) 11, 1–4.
3. Osanloo E, Deglin JH. Interaction of lithium and methyldopa. *Ann Intern Med* (1980) 92, 433–4.
4. O'Regan JB. Adverse interaction of lithium carbonate and methyldopa. *Can Med Assoc J* (1976) 115, 385–6.
5. Yassa R. Lithium-methyldopa interaction. *Can Med Assoc J* (1986) 134, 141–2.
6. Walker N, White K, Tornatore F, Boyd JL, Cohen JL. Lithium-methyldopa interactions in normal subjects. *Drug Intell Clin Pharm* (1980) 14, 638–9.

Lithium + Mirtazapine

No pharmacokinetic or pharmacodynamic interactions appeared to occur between lithium and mirtazapine in one study in healthy subjects but the manufacturers predict that serotonin syndrome could occur on concurrent use.

Clinical evidence, mechanism, importance and management

In a randomised, crossover study, 12 healthy subjects were given lithium carbonate 600 mg daily or placebo for 10 days, with a single 30-mg dose of mirtazapine on day 10. The pharmacokinetics of both mirtazapine and lithium were unaltered by concurrent use. In addition, no pharmacodynamic changes, as studied by psychometric testing, were identified.[1] The UK and US manufacturers of mirtazapine warn of the potential for serotonin syndrome in patients also taking lithium.[2,3] There do not appear to be any reports of this reaction with lithium and mirtazapine, but both drugs have been associated with this rare effect, and so some caution would appear prudent. For more information on serotonin syndrome and its management, see 'Drugs that cause serotonin syndrome + Other drugs that cause serotonin syndrome', p.1471.

1. Sitsen JMA, Voortman G, Timmer CJ. Pharmacokinetics of mirtazapine and lithium in healthy male subjects. *J Psychopharmacol* (2000) 14, 172–6.
2. Zispin SolTab (Mirtazapine). Merck Sharp & Dohme Ltd. UK Summary of product characteristics, Febraury 2015.
3. RemeronSolTab (Mirtazapine). Merck Sharp & Dohme Corp. US Prescribing information, May 2012.

Lithium + Nefazodone

No pharmacokinetic interaction appears to occur between lithium and nefazodone.

Clinical evidence, mechanism, importance and management

In a study in 12 healthy subjects, nefazodone 200 mg twice daily was given alone for 5 days. After a washout period, lithium was given for 11 days, in escalating doses from 250 mg twice daily to 500 mg twice daily. When therapeutic steady-state lithium levels were achieved nefazodone 200 mg twice daily was added for 5 days. The pharmacokinetics of both nefazodone and lithium were unaltered by concurrent use, although there were some small changes in the pharmacokinetics of the metabolites of nefazodone. Concurrent use was well tolerated and no dose adjustments were considered necessary.[1]

1. Laroudie C, Salazar DE, Cosson J-P, Cheuvart B, Istin B, Girault J, Ingrand I, Decourt J-P. Pharmacokinetic evaluation of co-administration of nefazodone and lithium in healthy subjects. *Eur J Clin Pharmacol* (1999) 54, 923–8.

Lithium + NSAIDs

NSAIDs can increase lithium levels leading to toxicity, but there is great variability between different NSAIDs and also between individuals taking the same NSAID. For example, studies have found that celecoxib causes a modest 17% increase in lithium levels, yet case reports describe increases of up to 344%. Similar effects occur with other NSAIDs, and it seems likely that all NSAIDs will interact similarly. However, note that sulindac seems unique in that it is the only NSAID that has also been reported to cause a decrease in lithium levels.

Clinical evidence

A retrospective analysis of 10 615 elderly patients receiving lithium found that 413 (3.9%) were admitted to hospital at least once for lithium toxicity during a 10-year study period. The prescriptions for any NSAID were compared between these 413 hospitalised patients and 1 651 control patients. For any use of an NSAID (63 cases and 187 controls) there was no increased relative risk of hospitalisation for lithium toxicity (relative risk 1.1). Similarly, when patients who were newly started on an NSAID were analysed (4 cases and 17 controls), there was still no increased risk (relative risk 0.6). The authors considered that these findings suggest that the use of NSAIDs and lithium might not be as hazardous as previously thought, although they did suggest that another explanation could be that clinicians were aware of the potential interaction and so adjusted doses or observed patients more closely in the outpatient setting, thereby avoiding any hospitalisations for toxicity.[1]

Case reports and studies about individual, named NSAIDs are outlined in the following subsections, and 'Table 31.1', p.1375, summarises the effects of NSAIDs on lithium concentrations.

(a) Celecoxib

A 58-year-old woman, with a stable serum lithium level of between 0.5 and 0.9 mmol/L, developed renal impairment associated with severe lithium toxicity, within 5 days of starting to take celecoxib 400 mg twice daily. Her lithium level was 4 mmol/L. Of note, and a possible contributory factor, was the presence of ibuprofen, which she had taken with her lithium for several years without incident.[2]

In addition to 3 of the cases in 'Table 31.1', p.1375, in January 2003, a review of the Adverse Event Reporting System database of the FDA in the US found 2 cases of increased lithium levels and symptoms of lithium toxicity in patients who also took celecoxib.[3]

(b) Flurbiprofen

A woman who was taking lithium carbonate 600 mg twice daily, with serum levels of 0.5 to 0.9 mmol/L, started to take flurbiprofen 200 mg daily. Within 4 days she became sleepy, hypotensive, and experienced nausea and vomiting, and tremor. Her serum lithium level had risen to 1.3 mmol/L. Seven days after stopping all treatment her lithium level had fallen to 0.5 mmol/L.[4]

(c) Ibuprofen

Three patients stable taking lithium, with plasma levels of 0.7 to 0.9 mmol/L, were given ibuprofen 1.2 or 2.4 g daily for 7 days. The serum lithium levels of one patient rose from 0.8 mmol/L to 1 mmol/L and he experienced nausea and drowsiness. The two other patients, including the one taking ibuprofen 1.2 g daily, did not develop this interaction.[5] Three other case reports describe patients with symptoms of lithium toxicity that occurred within one to 7 days of them starting to take ibuprofen 1.2 g daily.[6-8] In another case, episodes of unsteadiness and tremor associated with raised lithium levels were attributed to varying use of prescribed ibuprofen 400 mg three times daily.[9]

(d) Indometacin

A case report describes lithium toxicity in a man given indometacin 50 mg every 6 hours. Three days after he started indometacin his serum creatinine was raised, and 9 days later he had symptoms of lithium toxicity and was found to have a lithium level of 3.5 mmol/L. It was suggested that indometacin caused renal impairment, which led to lithium retention and toxicity.[10] A study in 7 healthy subjects given a 200-mmol and 40-mmol sodium diet found that indometacin 50 mg three times daily for 4 doses increased the plasma concentrations of a single 400-mg dose of lithium carbonate by 20% and 26%, respectively. Indometacin reduced lithium clearance by 16% and 28%, and fractional renal lithium reabsorption increased from 71% to 75% and from 75% to 81% during the high- and low-sodium diets, respectively.[11]

(e) Ketorolac

An 80-year-old man taking haloperidol, procyclidine, clonazepam, aspirin, digoxin and lithium (serum lithium levels between 0.5 and 0.7 mmol/L) was additionally given indometacin 100 mg daily for arthritis, which was replaced, after 13 days, by ketorolac 30 mg daily. The next day his serum lithium level was 0.9 mmol/L and 6 days later it was 1.1 mmol/L. Subsequently the patient developed severe nausea and vomiting, and both drugs were stopped.[12]

(f) Mefenamic acid

Acute lithium toxicity, accompanied by a sharp deterioration in renal function, was seen in a patient taking lithium carbonate with mefenamic acid 500 mg three times daily for 2 weeks. Withdrawal of the drugs and subsequent rechallenge confirmed this interaction.[13] Another case of toxicity was seen in a patient taking lithium who was given mefenamic acid. Her renal function was impaired when the lithium was started, but it had been stable for about 6 months before the NSAID was added.[14] A brief report also mentions another case of this interaction.[15]

(g) Meloxicam

A 49-year-old woman with bipolar disorder well-controlled with lithium (levels not stated) developed lethargy, nausea, vomiting, hypersalivation, tremors, muscle weakness and confusion and renal impairment after taking meloxicam 15 mg daily for 3 days. Neurological examination identified gross facial fasciculations, irregular coarse tremors of all four extremities, ataxia, hypertonia and hyperreflexia. Serum lithium levels were greater than 5 mmol/L. She underwent haemodialysis and her lithium levels were rapidly decreased to 0.1 mmol/L, but the patient experienced long-term neurological and cognitive impairment.[16]

(h) Niflumic acid

An isolated report describes lithium toxicity in a woman who took niflumic acid (said to be three capsules daily) for 7 days with the addition of aspirin 1.5 g daily after 5 days. Her serum lithium levels rose from 0.8 mmol/L to 1.6 mmol/L.[17]

(i) Nimesulide

A 42-year-old woman taking lithium was given nimesulide 100 mg and ciprofloxacin 250 mg, both twice daily, for flank pain and dysuria. After 72 hours, she developed symptoms of lithium toxicity and the dose of lithium was reduced. After 98 hours she had vomiting, ataxia, and oliguria, and lithium levels were found to be 3.23 mmol/L (previous level 1.08 mmol/L) and her serum creatinine was raised.[18]

(j) Oxyphenbutazone

In an apparently isolated case, a 49-year-old woman is reported to have developed nausea and vomiting associated with a rise in lithium levels following the addition of oxyphenbutazone suppositories 500 mg daily. She responded well to a reduction in the lithium dose.[19]

(k) Parecoxib

The manufacturer of parecoxib states that valdecoxib, the main active metabolite of parecoxib, has been shown to cause decreases in the clearance of lithium (serum clearance reduced by 25%, renal clearance reduced by 30%), resulting in a 34% increase in exposure.[20]

(l) Piroxicam

A 56-year-old woman, taking lithium for over 9 years, with levels usually between 0.8 and 1 mmol/L, experienced lithium toxicity (unsteadiness, trembling, confusion) and was admitted to hospital on three occasions after taking piroxicam. Her serum levels on two occasions had risen to 2.7 mmol/L and 1.6 mmol/L, although in the latter instance the lithium had been withdrawn the day before the levels were taken. In a subsequent study her serum lithium levels rose from 1 mmol/L to 1.5 mmol/L after she took piroxicam 20 mg daily.[21] Two other case reports describe lithium toxicity, which occurred 4 weeks and 4 months after piroxicam was started.[22,23]

(m) Rofecoxib

A 73-year-old man, with lithium levels of between 0.6 and 0.9 mmol/L for the past 13 years, developed symptoms of lithium toxicity (serum lithium level 1.5 mmol/L) within 9 days of starting to take rofecoxib 12.5 mg daily. An interaction was strongly suspected. However, it should be noted that the patient had required his lithium dose to be successively decreased over the 13 years to maintain his lithium levels within the desired range. Captopril 6.25 mg daily had also been started during this time,[24] although it is unclear whether it had a part to play either in the lithium dose reduction or the development of an interaction. In addition to 6 of the cases in 'Table 31.1', p.1375, in January 2003, a review of the Adverse Event Reporting System database of the FDA in the US found 7 cases of increased serum lithium concentrations after the addition of rofecoxib.[3]

(n) Sulindac

1. Lithium levels reduced. A patient stable taking lithium had a fall in her serum lithium levels (from 0.65 mmol/L to 0.39 mmol/L) 2 weeks after staring to take sulindac 100 mg twice daily. Her serum lithium levels gradually increased over the next 6 weeks (to 0.71 mmol/L) and restabilised without any change in the dose of either lithium or sulindac. She needed amitriptyline for depression while the lithium levels were low, but bouts of depression had not been uncommon, even when the lithium levels were stable.[25] The serum lithium levels of another patient were approximately halved a week after his dose of sulindac was doubled to 200 mg twice daily. He continued taking both drugs, but a higher dose of lithium was needed.[25]

2. Lithium levels unaffected. Two small studies (in a total of 10 patients)[26,27] and a case report[28] found that serum lithium levels were unaffected by the use of sulindac.

3. Lithium levels increased. Two patients developed increased serum lithium levels, apparently due to the use of sulindac.[29] In one case the lithium levels rose from 1 mmol/L to 2 mmol/L after 19 days of treatment with sulindac 150 mg twice daily, and symptoms of toxicity were seen. The levels fell to 0.8 mmol/L within 5 days of stopping the sulindac. The other patient had a rise in lithium levels from 0.9 mmol/L to 1.7 mmol/L within a week of adding sulindac 150 mg twice daily. The sulindac was continued and the lithium dose was reduced from 1.8 g daily to 1.5 g daily. The serum

Table 31.1 Summary of the effects of NSAIDs on lithium levels

NSAID	*Dose*	*Subjects*	*Increase in lithium levels*	*Time to symptoms or increase in levels*	*Refs*
Celecoxib	200 to 800 mg daily	4 cases	56 to 248%	10 days to 10 weeks	1, 2
	200 mg twice daily	Study in healthy subjects	16 to 17%		3, 4
Diclofenac	75 mg daily	Case	86%	25 days	5
	75 mg twice daily	Case	About 100%	7 days	6
	50 mg three times daily	Study in 5 healthy subjects	26%	7 to 10 days	7
Flurbiprofen	200 mg twice daily	Case	44 to 160%	4 days	8
	100 mg twice daily	Placebo-controlled study in 11 otherwise healthy subjects with bipolar disorder	19%	7 days	9
Ibuprofen	1.6 to 1.8 g daily in divided doses	Studies in 11 healthy subjects and 9 subjects with bipolar disorder	12 to 67%	6 to 9 days	10, 11
Indometacin	150 mg daily	Studies in 9 healthy subjects and 6 subjects with bipolar disorder	30 to 61%	6 to 10 days	12-14
Ketoprofen	400 mg daily	Case	About 90%	3 weeks	15
Ketorolac	60 mg daily	Case	50%	3 weeks	16
	40 mg daily	Study in 5 healthy subjects	29%	5 days	17
Lornoxicam	4 mg twice daily	Study in 12 healthy subjects	20% (61% in one subject)	7 days	18
Meloxicam	15 mg daily	Study in 16 healthy subjects	21%	14 days	19
	15 mg daily	Case	Initial level not stated but therapeutic range implied; increased to greater than 5 mmol/L	3 days	20
Naproxen	220 or 250 mg three times daily	Study in 9 healthy subjects and 7 bipolar or schizoaffective disorder	0 to 42%	5 to 6 days	21, 22
Phenylbutazone	750 mg daily (suppositories)	Case	106%	36 hours	23
	100 mg three times daily	Study in 5 subjects with bipolar disorder	0 to 15%	6 days	24
Piroxicam	20 mg daily	2 cases	130 to 235%	1 to 2 months	25, 26
Rofecoxib	Not stated or 25 mg once or twice daily	7 cases	58 to 448%	6 days to about 3 months	2, 27
	50 mg [daily]	Study in 10 healthy subjects	Unstated rise in 9 subjects, of these 3 were withdrawn early with levels of 1.26 mmol/L or more	Up to 5 days	28

1. Gunja N, Graudins A, Dowsett R. Lithium toxicity: a potential interaction with celecoxib. *Intern Med J* (2002) 32, 494-5.
2. Phelan KM, Mosholder AD, Lu S. Lithium interaction with the cyclooxygenase 2 inhibitors rofecoxib and celecoxib and other non-steroidal anti-inflammatory drugs. *J Clin Psychiatry* (2003) 64, 1328-34.
3. Celebrex (Celecoxib). Pharmacia Ltd. UK Summary of product characteristics, June 2009.
4. Celebrex (Celecoxib). Pfizer Inc. US Prescribing Information, June 2009.
5. Monji A, Maekawa T, Miura T, Nishi D, Horikawa H, Nakagawa Y, Tashiro N. Interactions between lithium and non-steroidal antiinflammatory drugs. *Clin Neuropharmacol* (2002) 25, 241-2.
6. Faaij RA, Ziere G, Zietse R, van der Cammen TJM. Delirium due to a drug-drug interaction of lithium and an NSAID. *J Nutr Health Aging* (2009) 13, 275-6.
7. Reimann IW, Frölich JC. Effects of diclofenac on lithium kinetics. *Clin Pharmacol Ther* (1981) 30, 348-52.
8. Aktepe E, Özkorumak E, Kandil S. Lithium interaction with flurbiprophen: a case report. *Klinik Psikofarmakoloji Bülteni* (2007) 17, 83–6.
9. Hughes BM, Small RE, Brink D, McKenzie ND. The effect of flurbiprofen on steady-state plasma lithium levels. *Pharmacotherapy* (1997) 17, 113-20.
10. Kristoff CA, Hayes PE, Barr WH, Small RE, Townsend RJ, Ettigi PG. Effect of ibuprofen on lithium plasma and red blood cell concentrations. *Clin Pharm* (1986) 5, 51-5.
11. Ragheb M. Ibuprofen can increase serum lithium level in lithium-treated patients. *J Clin Psychiatry* (1987) 48, 161-3.
12. Ragheb M, Ban TA, Buchanan D, Frolich JC. Interaction of indomethacin and ibuprofen with lithium in manic patients under a steady-state lithium level. *J Clin Psychiatry* (1980) 41, 397-8.
13. Frölich JC, Leftwich R, Ragheb M, Oates JA, Reimann I, Buchanan D. Indomethacin increases plasma lithium. *BMJ* (1979) 1, 1115-16.
14. Reimann IW, Diener U, Frölich JC. Indomethacin but not aspirin increases plasma lithium ion levels. *Arch Gen Psychiatry* (1983) 40, 283-6.
15. Singer L, Imbs JL, Danion JM, Singer P, Krieger-Finance F, Schmidt M, Schwartz J. Risque d'intoxication par le lithium en cas de traitement associé par les anti-inflammatories non stéroïdiens. *Therapie* (1981) 36, 323-6.
16. Iyer V, Ketorolac (Toradol®) induced lithium toxicity. *Headache* (1994) 34, 442-4.
17. Cold JA, ZumBrunnen TL, Simpson MA, Augustin BG, Awad E, Jann MW. Increased lithium serum and red blood cell concentrations during ketorolac coadministration. *J Clin Psychopharmacol* (1998) 18, 33-7.
18. Ravic M, Salas-Herrera I, Johnston A, Turner P, Foley K, Rosenow D. Influence of lornoxicam a new non-steroidal anti-inflammatory drug on lithium pharmacokinetics. *Hum Psychopharmacol* (1993) 8, 289-92.
19. Türck D, Heinzel G, Luik G. Steady-state pharmacokinetics of lithium in healthy volunteers receiving concomitant meloxicam. *Br J Clin Pharmacol* (2000) 50, 197-204.
20. Chen L, Pym H. Rapid onset of neurological symptoms and lithium toxicity on starting meloxicam. *Aust N Z J Psychiatry* (2010) 21, 380.
21. Ragheb M, Powell AL. Lithium interaction with sulindac and naproxen. *J Clin Psychopharmacol* (1986) 6, 150-4.
22. Levin GM, Grum C, Eisele G. Effect of over-the-counter dosages of naproxen sodium and acetaminophen on plasma lithium concentrations in normal volunteers. *J Clin Psychopharmacol* (1998) 18, 237-40.
23. Singer L, Imbs JL, Schmidt M, Mack G, Sebban M, Danion JM. Baisse de la clearance rénale du lithium sous l'effet de la phénylbutazone. *Encephale* (1978) 4, 33-40.
24. Ragheb M. The interaction of lithium with phenylbutazone in bipolar affective patients. *J Clin Psychopharmacol* (1990) 10, 149-150.
25. Kelly CB, Cooper SJ. Toxic elevation of serum lithium concentration by non-steroidal anti-inflammatory drugs. *Ulster Med J* (1991) 60, 240-2.
26. Harrison TM, Wynne Davies D, Norris CM. Lithium carbonate and piroxicam. *Br J Psychiatry* (1986) 149, 124-5.
27. Rätz Bravo AE, Egger SS, Crespo S, Probst WL, Krähenbühl S. Lithium intoxication as a result of an interaction with rofecoxib. *Ann Pharmacother* (2004) 38, 1189-93.
28. Sajbel TA, Carter GW, Wiley RB. Pharmacokinetic effects of rofecoxib therapy on lithium. *Pharmacotherapy* (2001) 21, 380.

lithium levels fell and were 1.2 mmol/L at 37 days and 1 mmol/L at 70 days. No symptoms of lithium toxicity occurred.[29]

(o) Tiaprofenic acid

A 79-year-old woman taking lithium (as well as fosinopril, nifedipine, oxazepam and haloperidol) had a rise in her trough serum lithium levels from 0.36 mmol/L to 0.57 mmol/L within 3 days of starting to take tiaprofenic acid 200 mg three times daily. The serum lithium levels had risen to 0.65 mmol/L by the next day and, despite halving the lithium dose, were found to be 0.69 mmol/L five days later. These rises were attributed to an interaction with the tiaprofenic acid exacerbated by the fosinopril,[30] see 'Lithium + ACE inhibitors', p.1362.

Mechanism

Not understood. It has been suggested that the interacting NSAIDs inhibit the synthesis of the renal prostaglandins (PGE_2) so that the renal blood flow is reduced, thereby reducing the renal excretion of the lithium. In addition, reduced renal PGE_2 levels may be associated with increased reabsorption of sodium and lithium. However, this fails to explain why aspirin, which blocks renal prostaglandin synthesis by 65 to 70%, does not usually affect serum lithium levels, see 'Lithium + Aspirin or other Salicylates', p.1365.

Importance and management

The interaction between the NSAIDs and lithium is well established, although the incidence is unknown. The increase in serum lithium levels appears to vary between the different NSAIDs and also between individuals taking the same NSAID (see 'Table 31.1', p.1375).

The documentation of these interactions is variable and limited, and although only some NSAIDs have been shown to interact, it seems likely that they will all interact to a greater or lesser extent. What is known indicates that most NSAIDs should be avoided, especially if other risk factors are present, unless serum lithium levels can be very well monitored (initially every few days) and the dose reduced appropriately. The effects of sulindac appear to be unpredictable (serum levels raised, lowered or unchanged) so that good monitoring is still necessary. In addition, patients taking lithium should be aware of the symptoms of lithium toxicity and told to report them immediately should they occur. This should be reinforced when they are given an NSAID. For more information on the risk factors for lithium toxicity, symptoms of lithium adverse effects and general monitoring, see under 'Lithium', p.1361.

The situation with regards to single doses of NSAIDs is less clear. As many cases have demonstrated a rise in lithium levels within a matter of days, those buying non-prescription NSAIDs should be advised to only intermittently self-medicate with NSAIDs (i.e. very short-term use), or preferably to use a non-interacting alternative, such as paracetamol, see 'Lithium + Paracetamol (Acetaminophen)', below. The same advice regarding an awareness of lithium toxicity should be reinforced. If any of the predisposing conditions that increase the risk of toxicity are present it might be safer to avoid concurrent use unless monitoring can be undertaken.

1. Juurlink DN, Mamdani MM, Kopp A, Rochon PA, Shulman KI, Redelmeier DA. Drug-induced lithium toxicity in the elderly: a population-based study. *J Am Geriatr Soc* (2004) 52, 794–8.
2. Slørdal L, Samstad S, Bathen J, Spigset O. A life-threatening interaction between lithium and celecoxib. *Br J Clin Pharmacol* (2003) 55, 413–14.
3. Phelan KM, Mosholder AD, Lu S. Lithium interaction with the cyclooxygenase 2 inhibitors rofecoxib and celecoxib and other nonsteroidal anti-inflammatory drugs. *J Clin Psychiatry* (2003) 64, 1328–34.
4. Aktepe E, Özkorumak E, Kandil S. Lithium interaction with flurbiprophen: a case report. *Klin Psikofarmakoloji Bulteni* (2007) 17, 83–6.
5. Ragheb M, Ban TA, Buchanan D, Frolich JC. Interaction of indomethacin and ibuprofen with lithium in manic patients under a steady-state lithium level. *J Clin Psychiatry* (1980) 41, 397–8.
6. Bailey CE, Stewart JT, McElroy RA. Ibuprofen-induced lithium toxicity. *South Med J* (1989) 82, 1197.
7. Ayd FJ. Ibuprofen-induced lithium intoxication. *Int Drug Ther Newslett* (1985) 20, 16.
8. Khan IH. Lithium and non-steroidal anti-inflammatory drugs. *BMJ* (1991) 302, 1537–8.
9. Kelly CB, Cooper SJ. Toxic elevation of serum lithium concentration by non-steroidal anti-inflammatory drugs. *Ulster Med J* (1991) 60, 240–2.
10. Herschberg SN, Sierles FS. Indomethacin-induced lithium toxicity. *Am Fam Physician* (1983) 28, 155–7.
11. Rabelink AJ, Koomans HA, Boer WH, Dorhout Mees EJ, van Rijn HJM. Indomethacin increases renal lithium reabsorption in man. *Nephrol Dial Transplant* (1989) 4, 27–31.
12. Langlois R, Paquette D. Increased serum lithium levels due to ketorolac therapy. *Can Med Assoc J* (1994) 150, 1455–6.
13. MacDonald J, Neale TJ. Toxic interaction of lithium carbonate and mefenamic acid. *BMJ* (1988) 297, 1339.
14. Shelley RK. Lithium toxicity and mefenamic acid: a possible interaction and the role of prostaglandin inhibition. *Br J Psychiatry* (1987) 151, 847–8.
15. Honey J. Lithium-mefenamic acid interaction: Quoted by Ayd FJ. *Int Drug Ther Newslett* (1982) 17, 16.
16. Chen L, Pym H. Rapid onset of neurological symptoms and lithium toxicity on starting meloxicam. *Aust N Z J Psychiatry* (2010) 44. 95.
17. Gay C, Plas J, Granger B, Olie JP, Loo H. Intoxication au lithium. Deux interactions inédites: l'acétazolamide et l'acide niflumique. *Encephale* (1985) 11, 261–2.
18. Bocchia M, Bertola G, Morganti D, Toscano M, Colombo E. Intossicazione da litio e uso di nimesulide. *Recenti Prog Med* (2001) 92, 462.
19. Singer L, Imbs JL, Danion JM, Singer P, Krieger-Finance F, Schmidt M, Schwartz J. Risque d'intoxication par le lithium en cas de traitement associé par les anti-inflammatoires non stéroïdiens. *Therapie* (1981) 36, 323–6.
20. Dynastat (Parecoxib sodium). Pfizer Ltd. UK Summary of product characteristics, June 2013.
21. Kerry RJ, Owen G, Michaelson S. Possible toxic interaction between lithium and piroxicam. *Lancet* (1983) i, 418–19.
22. Nadarajah J, Stein GS. Piroxicam induced lithium toxicity. *Ann Rheum Dis* (1985) 44, 502.
23. Walbridge DG, Bazire SR. An interaction between lithium carbonate and piroxicam presenting as lithium toxicity. *Br J Psychiatry* (1985) 147, 206–7.
24. Lundmark J, Gunnarsson T, Bengtsson F. A possible interaction between lithium and rofecoxib. *Br J Clin Pharmacol* (2002) 53, 403–4.
25. Furnell MM, Davies J. The effect of sulindac on lithium therapy. *Drug Intell Clin Pharm* (1985) 19, 374–6.
26. Ragheb M, Powell AL. Lithium interaction with sulindac and naproxen. *J Clin Psychopharmacol* (1986) 6, 150–4.
27. Ragheb MA, Powell AL. Failure of sulindac to increase serum lithium levels. *J Clin Psychiatry* (1986) 47, 33–4.
28. Miller LG, Bowman RC, Bakht F. Sparing effect of sulindac on lithium levels. *J Fam Pract* (1989) 28, 592–3.
29. Jones MT, Stoner SC. Increased lithium concentrations reported in patients treated with sulindac. *J Clin Psychiatry* (2000) 61, 527–8.
30. Alderman CP, Lindsay KSW. Increased serum lithium concentration secondary to treatment with tiaprofenic acid and fosinopril. *Ann Pharmacother* (1996) 30, 1411–13.

Lithium + Olanzapine

Several case reports suggest that some patients taking olanzapine and lithium develop adverse reactions (neuroleptic malignant syndrome or serotonin syndrome, encephalopathy, priapism) without raised serum lithium levels. One study found no pharmacokinetic interaction between the drugs, but another analysis suggested that lithium might reduce olanzapine plasma levels.

Clinical evidence

A 16-year-old boy taking lithium 1.2 g daily, with a therapeutic serum lithium level, developed neuroleptic malignant syndrome (generalised rigidity, urinary retention, fever, tachycardia) about 2 weeks after his olanzapine dose was increased from 10 to 20 mg daily. Both drugs were stopped, and the symptoms resolved over 8 days. He had previously taken olanzapine and lithium separately without problem.[1] Other patients have similarly developed neurotoxic adverse effects after taking lithium with olanzapine, including a 59-year-old man with therapeutic lithium levels who developed encephalopathy and confusion[2] and a woman who developed serotonin syndrome after an olanzapine dose increase,[3] although in this case citalopram might have had a part to play, see 'Lithium + SSRIs', p.1378. Another case report describes sleepwalking, which started about 6 days after olanzapine was added to the patient's usual medication of lithium and valproate.[4] A further case report describes an elderly patient who had taken lithium for 7 years, developed severe delirium and extrapyramidal symptoms after the addition of olanzapine. In this case, serum lithium levels were found to be 3 mmol/L.[5]

Other case reports describe non-ketotic hyperosmolar syndrome in a non-diabetic patient taking lithium and valproic acid, which started 5 days after olanzapine was added,[6] and priapism (reversed by surgical detumescence), which occurred when a 30-year-old man took olanzapine with lithium.[7]

In an open-label study, 12 healthy subjects took a single 32.4-mmol dose of lithium with olanzapine 10 mg, and after a washout period, olanzapine 10 mg daily for 8 days, with a single 32.4-mmol dose of lithium on the last day. No pharmacokinetic interactions were detected.[8] However, an analysis of olanzapine levels in schizophrenic patients found that the concurrent use of lithium was associated with lower olanzapine plasma levels.[9]

Mechanism

Unknown, although in some cases the effects seen are known to be adverse effects of either drug alone, and so these cases might simply represent additive adverse effects.

Importance and management

The case reports described above suggest that some patients taking olanzapine and lithium might develop a pharmacodynamic interaction, most commonly resulting in neurotoxicity; however, any adverse effect appears rare. The concurrent use of lithium and olanzapine need not be avoided but be aware that there is some risk of developing adverse reactions to the combination. The presence of other serotonergic drugs (e.g. antidepressants such as SSRIs) or dopamine antagonists (e.g. antipsychotics such as haloperidol) is likely to increase the risk of an interaction.

Olanzapine does not appear to affect lithium levels, and, given that olanzapine levels were only detected to be lower in retrospective analysis, it seems that any effect on olanzapine is managed by normal dose titration. No particular action therefore appears to be necessary.

1. Berry N, Pradhan S, Sagar R, Gupta SK. Neuroleptic malignant syndrome in an adolescent receiving olanzapine-lithium combination therapy. *Pharmacotherapy* (2003) 23, 255–9.
2. Swartz CM. Olanzapine-lithium encephalopathy. *Psychosomatics* (2001) 42, 370.
3. Haslett CD, Kumar S. Can olanzapine be implicated in causing serotonin syndrome? *Psychiatry Clin Neurosci* (2002) 56, 533–5.
4. Chiu Y-H, Chen C-H, Shen WW. Somnambulism secondary to olanzapine treatment in one patient with bipolar disorder. *Prog Neuropsychopharmacol Biol Psychiatry* (2008) 32, 581–2.
5. Tuglu C, Erdogan E, Abay E. Delirium and extrapyramidal symptoms due to a lithium-olanzapine combination therapy: a case report. *J Korean Med Sci* (2005) 20, 691–4.
6. Chen PS, Yang YK, Yeh TL, Lo YC, Wang YT. Nonketotic hyperosmolar syndrome from olanzapine, lithium, and valproic acid cotreatment. *Ann Pharmacother* (2003) 37, 919–20.
7. Jagadheesan K, Thakur A, Akhtar S. Irreversible priapism during olanzapine and lithium therapy. *Aust N Z J Psychiatry* (2004) 38, 381.
8. Demolle D, Onkelinx C, Müller-Oerlinghausen B. Interaction between olanzapine and lithium in healthy male volunteers. *Therapie* (1995) 50 (Suppl), 486.
9. Bergemann N, Frick A, Parzer P, Kopitz J. Olanzapine plasma concentration, average daily dose, and interaction with co-medication in schizophrenic patients. *Pharmacopsychiatry* (2004) 37, 63–8.

Lithium + Paracetamol (Acetaminophen)

Paracetamol does not appear to alter lithium levels to a clinically relevant extent.

Clinical evidence, mechanism, importance and management

A study in 9 healthy subjects given lithium carbonate 300 mg every 12 hours to achieve steady state, followed by the addition of 650 mg of paracetamol every 6 hours for 5 days, found no evidence that paracetamol increased serum lithium levels. Six subjects had no change in lithium levels, one subject had a 0.1 mmol/L decrease, and two had a 0.1 mmol/L increase.[1] One patient whose serum lithium level doubled while taking rofecoxib was later given paracetamol without any problems.[2] Lithium dose adjustments are therefore not expected to be necessary on the concurrent use of paracetamol.

1. Levin GM, Grum C, Eisele G. Effect of over-the-counter dosages of naproxen sodium and acetaminophen on plasma lithium concentrations in normal volunteers. *J Clin Psychopharmacol* (1998) 18, 237–40.
2. Rätz Bravo AE, Egger SS, Crespo S, Probst WL, Krähenbühl S. Lithium intoxication as a result of an interaction with rofecoxib. *Ann Pharmacother* (2004) 38, 1189–93.

Lithium + Phenytoin

Symptoms of lithium toxicity (sometimes with unchanged lithium levels) have been seen in a few patients taking lithium and phenytoin, although the interaction has not been clearly demonstrated.

Clinical evidence, mechanism, importance and management

A 48-year-old man with a prefrontal leucotomy and a history of bipolar disorder and convulsions was given increasing doses of lithium carbonate and phenytoin over a period of about 4 years. Although the serum levels of both drugs remained within the therapeutic range, he eventually began to develop symptoms of lithium toxicity (thirst, polyuria, polydipsia and tremor) that disappeared when the lithium was stopped. Later, when lithium was restarted, the symptoms returned, this time abating when the phenytoin was replaced by carbamazepine. The patient then claimed that he felt normal for the first time in years.[1] Another report describes symptoms of lithium toxicity in a 26-year-old man with lithium levels within the therapeutic range. This patient was also taking phenytoin.[2]

In a further case, a 49-year-old man with depression, cluster headaches and chronic post-traumatic seizures taking phenytoin became ataxic within 3 days of starting to take lithium. He had no other toxic symptoms and his serum lithium level was 2 mmol/L.[3] However, as he only ever took lithium in the presence of phenytoin, it is not possible to say whether the effects were as a result of an interaction, or whether toxic levels would have occurred with the lithium alone. Another similar case has also been reported.[4]

Information regarding an interaction between lithium and phenytoin seems to be limited to these reports and none of them presents a clear picture of the role of phenytoin in the reactions described.[1-4] Therefore the interaction is not well established. Patients taking lithium should be aware of the symptoms of lithium toxicity and told to report them immediately should they occur. This should be reinforced when they are given phenytoin. Increased serum lithium monitoring does not appear to be of value in this situation as the interaction occurred in patients with lithium levels within the normally accepted therapeutic range.

1. MacCallum WAG. Interaction of lithium and phenytoin. *BMJ* (1980) 280, 610–11.
2. Speirs J, Hirsch SR. Severe lithium toxicity with "normal" serum concentrations. *BMJ* (1978) 1, 815–16.
3. Salem RB, Director K, Muniz CE. Ataxia as the primary symptom of lithium toxicity. *Drug Intell Clin Pharm* (1980) 14, 622–3.
4. Raskin DE. Lithium and phenytoin interaction. *J Clin Psychopharmacol* (1984) 4, 120.

Lithium + Quetiapine

Quetiapine did not appear to affect serum lithium levels in one study, and concurrent use did not increase the incidence of extrapyramidal symptoms in another study. Isolated reports describe the development of delirium in one patient and a seizure in another patient given quetiapine and lithium.

Clinical evidence

The steady-state serum lithium levels of 10 patients with schizophrenia, schizoaffective or bipolar disorder were studied before, during, and after the concurrent use of quetiapine 250 mg three times daily. Quetiapine increased the AUC and maximum serum levels of lithium by 12% and 4.5%, respectively, but this was not statistically significant. Concurrent use was well tolerated.[1]

A randomised, placebo-controlled study found that the incidence of extrapyramidal symptoms in patients receiving quetiapine with lithium was similar to that in patients receiving placebo with lithium.[2] However, case reports describe adverse effects on the concurrent use of lithium and quetiapine. In one case, a 55-year-old man with a long history of schizoaffective disorder stopped his medication and 2 months later developed psychosis, mood instability and psychomotor agitation. He was given an initial dose of quetiapine 50 mg daily which was increased over 7 days to 700 mg daily. He became sedated, but after 10 days he was still experiencing mood fluctuations, and lithium carbonate 900 mg daily was started. Two days later he became confused, disorientated with cloudy consciousness and had short-term memory disturbances, visual hallucinations and agitation. His serum lithium level was 0.6 mmol/L. Quetiapine and lithium were stopped, and he was treated with diazepam, resulting in a gradual resolution of the delirium.[3] In another case, a 20-year-old man with bipolar disorder who was given quetiapine titrated to 600 mg daily. He was also taking lithium 450 mg daily but because of low plasma levels (0.3 mmol/L), his lithium dose was increased to 900 mg daily and then to 1200 mg daily and within a week the patient's depressive symptoms improved. However, after a further 2 days he developed myoclonus and then a generalised tonic-clonic seizure. At this point his lithium level was 0.8 mmol/L. Lithium and quetiapine were stopped and his mental state improved. He was then given quetiapine 400 mg daily.[4]

Mechanism

In one case, it was noted that lithium can induce delirium when given in combination with other drugs and that this might occur when lithium levels are within the therapeutic range.[3] The reasons for the seizure are not known but it was speculated that the patient might have had high intracellular lithium levels, due to genetic factors involving the intracellular pump, which were not reflected by the therapeutic plasma level. It was also speculated that quetiapine might have increased the risk of lithium toxicity.[4]

Importance and management

Evidence for an interaction between quetiapine and lithium appears to be restricted to the two case reports, with the two studies finding no adverse interaction. Nevertheless, as adverse effects of the type described are often rare, it seems unlikely that the studies would have detected such adverse effects and therefore the isolated case reports of delirium and seizure should be borne in mind if this combination is used.

1. Potkin SG, Thyrum PT, Bera R, Carreon D, Alva G, Kalali AH, Yeh C. Open-label study of the effect of combination quetiapine/lithium therapy on lithium pharmacokinetics and tolerability. *Clin Ther* (2002) 24, 1809–23.
2. Sachs G, Chengappa KNR, Suppes T, Mullen JA, Brecher M, Devine NA, Sweitzer DE. Quetiapine with lithium or divalproex for the treatment of bipolar mania: a randomized, double-blind, placebo-controlled study. *Bipolar Disord* (2004) 6, 213–23.
3. Miodownik C, Alkatnany A, Frolova K, Lerner V. Delirium associated with lithium-quetiapine combination. *Clin Neuropharmacol* (2008) 31, 176–9.
4. Grueneberger EC, Rountree EM, Short EB, Kahn DA. Neurotoxicity with therapeutic lithium levels: a case report. *J Psychiatr Pract* (2009) 15, 60–63.

Lithium + Risperidone

There appears to be no pharmacokinetic interaction between risperidone and lithium, although a number of case reports describe adverse effects such as extrapyramidal symptoms when both drugs are given.

Clinical evidence,

In a study, 13 patients were given lithium and a conventional antipsychotic for at least 5 days before the study, and on days one and 2 of the study. On study day 3, the patients were given lithium (dose not stated) and risperidone 1 mg twice daily. The risperidone dose was increased to 2 mg twice daily on day 4 and then to 3 mg twice daily on days 5 to 9. The steady-state pharmacokinetics of lithium were not affected by the switch to risperidone and the plasma levels of risperidone and 9-hydroxyrisperidone were comparable to historical levels in subjects taking risperidone alone.[1]

A case report describes a 42-year-old woman given lithium 800 mg daily for 2 weeks for an episode of mania, who was then also given risperidone 2 mg daily increased over 2 weeks to 5 mg daily. Three days later, she experienced extrapyramidal adverse effects (an abrupt onset of abnormal peri-oral movements). Her serum lithium level was 0.7 mmol/L. Risperidone and lithium were stopped and her symptoms resolved after intravenous promethazine was given.[2]

Another case report describes a non-diabetic patient, who developed diabetic ketoacidosis 2 years after starting to take risperidone and lithium. During this acute illness he also experienced neuroleptic malignant syndrome and a myocardial infarction. However, the authors considered the diabetic symptoms to be associated with risperidone, as the patient was able to continue taking lithium alone with no recurrence of this condition, or the need for antidiabetic medication.[3]

A 50-year-old man with a schizoaffective disorder who had been taking lithium 900 mg daily was given quetiapine for worsening psychotic symptoms. The dose of lithium was increased to 1575 mg daily because of inadequate control of symptoms and low serum lithium levels (0.5 mmol/L). Symptoms of mania subsided but the patient developed catatonic symptoms (psychomotor slowing, hypomimia, slowed speech and movement) attributed to inadequate treatment and quetiapine was replaced by risperidone, which was increased to 6 mg daily. A routine EEG was normal and lithium levels were 0.9 mmol/L. About one month later, the patient experienced rigor, fever, sweating, tachycardia, hypertension and elevated creatine phosphokinase (1 204 units/L). Neuroleptic malignant syndrome was diagnosed and lithium and risperidone were stopped. Abnormalities were observed in his EEG. He was treated with lorazepam and although brain activity normalised, rigor returned. Clozapine 400 mg daily was then started and the patient quickly regained mobility and within 5 days the catatonic and psychotic symptoms noticeably improved.[4] In a further case, a man taking lithium developed somnolence, confusion, delirium, fever and a rise in creatinine phosphokinase levels when risperidone was given.[5]

A 75-year-old man with bipolar disorder taking lithium carbonate 450 mg twice daily developed encephalopathy within a few days of starting to take risperidone 2 mg daily and this resolved when both drugs were stopped.[6] Another case of encephalopathy has also been reported following the concurrent use of these drugs.[7]

Mechanism

Unknown. In one case it was suggested that neurotoxicity might occur when patients with baseline EEG abnormalities are given lithium and risperidone.[6] In one of the cases of neuroleptic malignant syndrome, dehydration was also present, which might have predisposed the patient to neuroleptic malignant syndrome.[3]

Importance and management

The general picture that emerges from these reports is that no clinically important pharmacokinetic interaction occurs if risperidone and lithium are used together, but in some rare cases, neuroleptic malignant syndrome and other neurotoxicities might occur. There seems to be no good reason for avoiding concurrent use, but the isolated case reports should be borne in mind if this combination is used.

1. Demling JH, Huang M-L, Remmerie B, Mannaert E, Sperling W. Pharmacokinetics and safety of combination therapy with lithium and risperidone. *Pharmacopsychiatry* (2006) 39, 230–1.
2. Mendhekar DN. Rabbit syndrome induced by combined lithium and risperidone. *Can J Psychiatry* (2005) 50, 369.
3. Ananth J, Johnson KM, Levander EM, Harry JL. Diabetic ketoacidosis, neuroleptic malignant syndrome, and myocardial infarction in a patient taking risperidone and lithium carbonate. *J Clin Psychiatry* (2004) 65, 724.
4. Krähenmann R, Küchenhoff B, Böker H, Schick M. Katatones dilemma unter kombinationsbehandlung mit lithium und risperidon. *Psychiatr Prax* (2010) 37, 306–9.
5. Swanson CL, Price WA, McEvoy JP. Effects of concomitant risperidone and lithium treatment. *Am J Psychiatry* (1995) 152, 1096.
6. Boora K, Xu J, Hyatt J. Encephalopathy with combined lithium-risperidone administration. *Acta Psychiatr Scand* (2008) 117, 394–5.
7. Böker H, Brandenberger M, Schopper C. Neurotoxische enzephalopathie unter kombinationsbehandlung mit lithium und risperidon bei einer patientin mit schizoaffektiver störung. *Psychiatr Prax* (2007) 34, 38–41.

Lithium + Sodium compounds

The ingestion of marked amounts of sodium can prevent the establishment or maintenance of adequate lithium levels. Conversely, dietary salt restriction can cause lithium levels to rise to toxic concentrations if the lithium dose is not reduced appropriately.

Clinical evidence

(a) Lithium response reduced by the ingestion of sodium

A 35-year-old man who started to take lithium carbonate 250 mg four times a day, had a serum lithium level of 0.5 mmol/L by the following morning. When the dose frequency was progressively increased to five, and later six times daily, his serum lithium levels did not exceed 0.6 mmol/L because, unknown to his doctor, he was also taking **sodium bicarbonate**. The patient's wife stated that he had been taking "**Soda Bic**" for years but since he started taking lithium he had been "shovelling it in". When the **sodium bicarbonate** was stopped, relatively stable serum lithium levels of 0.8 mmol/L were achieved with the initial dose of lithium carbonate.[1]

An investigation to find out why a number of inpatients were unable either to reach or maintain adequate therapeutic serum lithium levels over a period of 2 months, revealed that a clinic nurse had been giving the patients *Efferdex*, a product containing about 50% **sodium bicarbonate**, because the patients complained of nausea. The reduction in the expected serum lithium levels was as much as 40% in some cases.[2]

Other studies confirm that the serum lithium levels can fall, and the effectiveness of treatment can lessen, if the intake of sodium is increased.[3-6]

(b) Lithium response increased by sodium restriction

The serum lithium levels of 4 patients rose more rapidly and achieved a higher peak when salt was restricted to less than 10 mmol of sodium per day compared with when the patients took a **dietary salt supplement**.[7]

Mechanism

The situation is complex and not fully established, but the mechanism can be broadly described in simplistic terms. Sodium balance is controlled by the kidney; if the serum sodium is low the kidney can reabsorb more sodium to maintain the balance. The kidney excretes and reabsorbs both lithium and sodium, but it does not appear to clearly distinguish between lithium and sodium ions. Therefore, if a patient taking lithium restricts sodium intake, the kidney might reabsorb both sodium and lithium, causing a rise in serum lithium levels. A corresponding decrease in lithium levels can occur when sodium intake is supplemented.[8,9]

Importance and management

The interaction between lithium and sodium compounds is well established and clinically important. The establishment and maintenance of therapeutic serum lithium levels can be jeopardised if the intake of sodium is altered. Warn patients not to take non-prescription antacids or urinary alkalinisers without first seeking informed advice. Sodium bicarbonate comes in various guises and disguises e.g. *Alka-Seltzer* (55.8%), *Andrews Salts* (22.6%), *Eno* (46.4%), *Jaap's Health Salts* (21.3%), *Peptac* (28.8%). Substantial amounts of sodium also occur in some **urinary alkalinising agents** (e.g. *Citralka*, *Citravescent*).[10] There are many similar preparations available throughout the world. An antacid containing **aluminium/magnesium hydroxide** with simeticone has been found to have no effect on the bioavailability of lithium carbonate,[11] so that antacids of this type would appear to be safer alternatives.

Patients already stable taking lithium should not begin to limit their intake of salt unless their serum lithium levels can be monitored and suitable dose adjustments made, because their lithium levels can rise quite rapidly.

1. Arthur RK. Lithium levels and "Soda Bic". *Med J Aust* (1975) 2, 918.
2. McSwiggan C. Interaction of lithium and bicarbonate. *Med J Aust* (1978) 1, 38–9.
3. Bleiweiss H. Salt supplements with lithium. *Lancet* (1970) i, 416.
4. Demers RG, Heninger GR. Sodium intake and lithium treatment in mania. *Am J Psychiatry* (1971) 128, 100–104.
5. Baer L, Platman SR, Kassir S, Fieve RR. Mechanisms of renal lithium handling and their relationship to mineralocorticoids: a dissociation between sodium and lithium ions. *J Psychiatr Res* (1971) 8, 91–105.
6. Demers RG, Harris RL. The effect of dietary sodium on renal lithium excretion in the manic-depressive. *Dis Nerv Syst* (1972) 33, 372–5.
7. Platman SR, Fieve RR. Lithium retention and excretion: The effect of sodium and fluid intake. *Arch Gen Psychiatry* (1969) 20, 285–9.
8. Thomsen K, Schou M. Renal lithium excretion in man. *Am J Physiol* (1968) 215, 823–7.
9. Singer I, Rotenberg D. Mechanisms of lithium action. *N Engl J Med* (1973) 289, 254–60.
10. Beard TC, Wilkinson SJ, Vial JH. Hazards of urinary alkalizing agents. *Med J Aust* (1988) 149, 723.
11. Goode DL, Newton DW, Ueda CT, Wilson JE, Wulf BG, Kafonek D. Effect of antacid on the bioavailability of lithium carbonate. *Clin Pharm* (1984) 3, 284–7.

Lithium + SSRIs

The concurrent use of lithium and an SSRI can be advantageous and uneventful, but various kinds of neurotoxicities have occurred. Isolated reports describe the development of symptoms similar to those of serotonin syndrome in patients taking lithium with fluoxetine, fluvoxamine, paroxetine or possibly citalopram. In addition, increases and decreases in serum lithium levels have been seen with fluoxetine.

Clinical evidence

(a) Citalopram

In a study in 8 healthy subjects, no pharmacokinetic changes were seen when lithium 30 mmol per day (as lithium sulfate 1.98 g daily) was added to citalopram 40 mg daily.[1] Another study, in 24 patients who had previously not responded to citalopram alone, found that the concurrent use of citalopram 40 or 60 mg and lithium carbonate 800 mg daily was effective and did not increase adverse effects.[2]

(b) Fluoxetine

A woman with bipolar affective disorder, successfully maintained for 20 years on lithium carbonate 1.2 g daily, developed stiffness of her arms and legs, dizziness, unsteadiness in walking and speech difficulties within a few days of starting fluoxetine 20 mg daily. Her serum lithium levels had risen from a range of 0.75 to 1.15 mmol/L up to 1.7 mmol/L. The lithium dose was reduced to 900 mg daily and fluoxetine was withdrawn. Within 7 days, the toxic symptoms had disappeared and her lithium levels had fallen to 0.9 mmol/L.[3] Two other patients had increases in serum lithium levels of about 45% and 70% (but no lithium toxicity) about a month after starting fluoxetine 20 mg daily or 40 mg daily, respectively. The problem resolved when the lithium dose was reduced by 40% and 30%, respectively, and in the second case, when fluoxetine was withdrawn. Both patients also developed mania, either after readjustment of the lithium dose or during concurrent use.[4]

In contrast, a study in 10 healthy subjects who took a single 32.4-mmol dose of lithium acetate, either alone, with a single 60-mg dose of fluoxetine, or with fluoxetine 60 mg after pretreatment with fluoxetine 20 mg three times daily for 7 days, found no change in the distribution or elimination of lithium. Lithium levels were lower in the first 4 hours after it was taken with the single dose of fluoxetine than when it was taken alone or at fluoxetine steady-state, but all levels remained within the therapeutic range.[5] The US manufacturer of fluoxetine[6] states that the concurrent use of these two drugs has resulted in both increased and decreased serum lithium concentrations.

Toxicity (confusion, ataxia, coarse tremor, incoordination, movement disorders, fever) was seen in a patient when lithium was added to treatment with fluoxetine, although the serum lithium levels remained within the therapeutic range.[7] A woman taking clonazepam who started taking fluoxetine 20 mg then 40 mg daily, developed tremor and ataxia 6 days after lithium carbonate 100 mg increased to 400 mg daily was added. The problems resolved when the lithium and fluoxetine were withdrawn.[8] Extrapyramidal adverse effects and ataxia were seen in one patient taking lithium and fluoxetine, and dystonia occurred in another patient who was also taking carbamazepine, captopril and trimipramine.[9] The development of serotonin syndrome is also reported to have occurred in 2 patients taking lithium and fluoxetine.[10,11] Heat stroke developed in a man taking lithium and fluoxetine, which was attributed to synergistic impairment of his temperature regulatory system by the two drugs.[12] Absence seizures occurred in another patient given both drugs.[13]

(c) Fluvoxamine

A woman taking fluvoxamine became somnolent within a day of starting to take lithium. The lithium level 20 hours after the last dose was 0.2 mmol/L. She recovered when both drugs were stopped and she was discharged taking lithium alone. The excessive somnolence was considered to have been possibly caused by increased serotonin levels caused by this drug combination.[14] A 40-year-old man taking clomipramine who started taking lithium (plasma levels 0.58 to 0.74 mmol/L) only achieved a slight reduction in depressive symptoms during 2 months of treatment. Clomipramine was replaced with fluvoxamine, which was titrated to a dose of 300 mg daily and lithium was continued (plasma levels 0.61 to 0.68 mmol/L) resulting in remission of depression over the next 2 months. However, the patient experienced severe diurnal somnolence, having repeatedly fallen asleep at work, and he had needed to pull over while driving because of sleepiness. Lithium levels were not increased during the concurrent use of fluvoxamine. Even so, the dose was reduced (plasma level 0.2 mmol/L) and the dose of fluvoxamine was reduced to 200 mg daily, but somnolence persisted until lithium was discontinued. Fluvoxamine was continued without adverse effect.[15] In a third case, a woman taking long-term lithium started taking fluvoxamine 50 mg daily, increased to 200 mg daily over 10 days. She gradually developed tremor, difficulties in making fine hand movements, impaired motor coordination and hyperreflexia. Serum lithium levels remained therapeutic throughout. The reaction was interpreted as a mild form of serotonin syndrome.[16] By 1989, the CSM in the UK had received 19 reports of adverse reactions when fluvoxamine was given with lithium (5 reports of convulsions and one of hyperpyrexia).[17]

In contrast to these reports, a study in 6 patients found that lithium (dosed to achieve plasma levels of 0.3 to 0.65 mmol/L) and fluvoxamine 100 to 150 mg daily (for between 3 and 23 weeks) was safe and effective, and no adverse interaction of any kind occurred.[18] Another study in 6 patients with depression found that lithium did not affect the pharmacokinetics of fluvoxamine 100 mg daily and concurrent use was more effective than fluvoxamine alone.[19]

It would seem therefore that concurrent use can be valuable, but there is a clear need to monitor the outcome so that any problems can be quickly identified.

(d) Paroxetine

A study in 14 patients taking lithium found that tremor activity increased when paroxetine 20 to 40 mg daily was added. The greatest increments occurred approximately 3 weeks after concurrent use was started, but tremor activity was still significantly greater than baseline after 6 weeks. No patient discontinued treatment because of the increase in tremor.[20]

In a study, 17 patients with bipolar disorder taking lithium (mean level 0.86 mmol/L) were also given paroxetine in initial doses of 5 to 20 mg daily. The mean lithium level after 3 weeks of concurrent use was 0.8 mmol/L. Adverse effects in 4 patients were possibly associated with the development of serotonin syndrome, although the possibility that other drugs (perphenazine , tranylcypromine) could be implicated in 2 of the cases and worsening symptoms of panic disorder in a third patient could not be ruled out. Adverse symptoms resolved on withdrawal of paroxetine (3 patients) and lithium (1 patient).[21]

A 59-year-old woman with a long-standing bipolar disorder who had taken paroxetine 10 mg increased to 30 mg daily for 3 weeks, developed symptoms suggestive of serotonin syndrome (shivering, tremor of her arms and legs, flushed face, agitation, and some impairment of mental focussing) after lithium 400 mg daily was added.[22] Her serum lithium and paroxetine levels were found to be 0.63 mmol/L and 690 nanograms/mL, respectively (the latter being sixfold higher than the upper levels seen in other patients). The paroxetine dose was reduced to 10 mg daily, which decreased paroxetine serum levels to 390 nanograms/mL, whereupon she became symptom-free and her depression was relieved. It is not clear whether this reaction was due to an interaction as she never took the higher dose of paroxetine in the absence of lithium.

A case report describes seizures, unsteady gait and blurred speech in a patient with bipolar disorder and cystic fibrosis who was taking lithium and paroxetine: both drugs were discontinued. However, this patient was abusing oxycodone and clonazepam and was also taking a variety of anti-asthma medications (salbutamol, salmeterol, budesonide, montelukast and cromoglicate), so the exact cause of the seizures is unclear.[23]

(e) Sertraline

In a randomised, placebo-controlled study, 16 healthy subjects were given lithium 600 mg twice daily for 9 days. On day 8, half of the subjects received two 100-mg doses of sertraline 8 hours apart, while the other half received placebo. Sertraline reduced steady-state lithium levels by 1.4%, and increased the renal excretion of lithium, but neither of these changes was statistically significant. However, there was a high incidence of adverse effects (mainly tremor and nausea) on concurrent use: tremor occurred in 7 out of the 8 taking sertraline, whereas no adverse effects were reported in the placebo group.[24]

Severe priapism occurred in a patient taking lithium carbonate 600 mg daily within 2 weeks of having the dose of sertraline increased from 50 to 100 mg daily. It was not clear whether this was purely a reaction to the increased sertraline dose, although it was suggested that the effect may have been due to the serotonergic effects of both drugs.[25]

Mechanism

Not fully understood although it seems likely that many of the symptoms could be due to the effects of both lithium and the SSRIs on serotonin.

Importance and management

The concurrent use of lithium and an SSRI usually appears to be uneventful. A review of the safety of the concurrent use of lithium and an SSRI identified 503 subjects who had received the combination without any evidence of serious adverse events.[26] However, occasionally and unpredictably adverse reactions develop, and very rarely, lithium levels might rise but the precise incidence of such effect is not known. If lithium is used in conjunction with an SSRI, be alert for any evidence of adverse effects (e.g. tremor, movement disorders) or serotonin syndrome. The symptoms might include tremor, dysarthria, ataxia, or confusion. For more information on serotonin syndrome and its management, see 'Drugs that cause serotonin syndrome + Other drugs that cause serotonin syndrome', p.1471.

1. Gram LF, Hansen MGJ, Sindrup SH, Brøsen K, Poulsen JH, Aaes-Jørgensen T, Overø KF. Citalopram: interaction studies with levomepromazine, imipramine, and lithium. *Ther Drug Monit* (1993) 15, 18–24.
2. Baumann P, Souche A, Montaldi S, Baettig D, Lambert S, Uehlinger C, Kasas A, Amey M, Jonzier-Perey M. A double-blind, placebo-controlled study of citalopram with and without lithium in the treatment of therapy-resistant depressive patients: a clinical, pharmacokinetic, and pharmacogenetic investigation. *J Clin Psychopharmacol* (1996) 16, 307–14.
3. Salama AA, Shafey M. A case of severe lithium toxicity induced by combined fluoxetine and lithium carbonate. *Am J Psychiatry* (1989) 146, 278.
4. Hadley A, Cason MP. Mania resulting from lithium-fluoxetine combination. *Am J Psychiatry* (1989) 146, 1637–8.
5. Breuel H-P, Müller-Oerlinghausen B, Nickelsen T, Heine PR. Pharmacokinetic interactions between lithium and fluoxetine after single and repeated fluoxetine administration in young healthy volunteers. *Int J Clin Pharmacol Ther* (1995) 33, 415–19.
6. Prozac (Fluoxetine hydrochloride). Eli Lilly and Company. US Prescribing information, July 2014.
7. Noveske FG, Hahn KR, Flynn RJ. Possible toxicity of combined fluoxetine and lithium. *Am J Psychiatry* (1989) 146, 1515.
8. Austin LS, Arana GW, Melvin JA. Toxicity resulting from lithium augmentation of antidepressant treatment in elderly patients. *J Clin Psychiatry* (1990) 51, 344–5.
9. Coulter DM, Pillans PI. Fluoxetine and extrapyramidal side effects. *Am J Psychiatry* (1995) 152, 122–5.
10. Karle J, Bjørndal F. Serotonergt syndrom - ved kombineret behandling med litium og fluoxetin. *Ugeskr Laeger* (1995) 157, 1204–5.
11. Muly EC, McDonald W, Steffens D, Book S. Serotonin syndrome produced by a combination of fluoxetine and lithium. *Am J Psychiatry* (1993) 150, 1565.
12. Albukrek D, Moran DS, Epstein Y. A depressed workman with heatstroke. *Lancet* (1996) 347, 1016.
13. Sacristan JA, Iglesias C, Arellano F, Lequerica J. Absence seizures induced by lithium: possible interaction with fluoxetine. *Am J Psychiatry* (1991) 148, 146–7.
14. Evans M, Marwick P. Fluvoxamine and lithium: an unusual interaction. *Br J Psychiatry* (1990) 156, 286.
15. Marchesi C, Paini M, Maggini C. Severe diurnal somnolence induced by fluvoxamine-lithium combination. *Pharmacopsychiatry* (2005) 38, 145–6.
16. Öhman R, Spigset O. Serotonin syndrome induced by fluvoxamine-lithium interaction. *Pharmacopsychiatry* (1993) 26, 263–4.
17. Committee on the Safety of Medicines. *Current Problems* (1989) 26, 3. Correction. Ibid. 1989, 27, 3.
18. Hendrickx B, Floris M. A controlled pilot study of the combination of fluvoxamine and lithium. *Curr Ther Res* (1991) 49, 106–10.
19. Miljković BR, Pokrajac M, Timotijević I, Varagić V. The influence of lithium on fluvoxamine therapeutic efficacy and pharmacokinetics in depressed patients on combined fluvoxamine-lithium therapy. *Int Clin Psychopharmacol* (1997) 12, 207–12.
20. Zanielli R, Bauer M, Jobert M, Müller-Oerlinghausen B. Changes in quantitatively assessed tremor during treatment of major depression with lithium augmented by paroxetine or amitriptyline. *J Clin Psychopharmacol* (2001) 21, 190–8.
21. Fagiolini A, Buysse DJ, Frank E, Houck PR, Luther JF, Kupfer DJ. Tolerability of combined treatment with lithium and paroxetine in patients with bipolar disorder and depression. *J Clin Psychopharmacol* (2001) 21, 474–8.
22. Sobanski T, Bagli M, Laux G, Rao ML. Serotonin syndrome after lithium add-on medication to paroxetine. *Pharmacopsychiatry* (1997) 30, 106–7.
23. Munera PA, Perel JM, Asato M. Medication interaction causing seizures in a patient with bipolar disorder and cystic fibrosis. *J Child Adolesc Psychopharmacol* (2002) 12, 275–6.
24. Apseloff G, Wilner KD, von Deutsch DA, Henry EB, Tremaine LM, Gerber N, Lazar JD. Sertraline does not alter steady-state concentrations or renal clearance of lithium in healthy volunteers. *J Clin Pharmacol* (1992) 32, 643–6.
25. Mendelson WB, Franko T. Priapism with sertraline and lithium. *J Clin Psychopharmacol* (1994) 14, 434–5.
26. Hawley CJ, Loughlin PJ, Quick SJ, Gale TM, Sivakumaran T, Hayes J, McPhee S, for the Hertfordshire Neuroscience Research Group. Efficacy, safety and tolerability of combined administration of lithium and selective serotonin reuptake inhibitors: a review of the current evidence. *Int Clin Psychopharmacol* (2000) 15, 197–206.

Lithium + Theophylline

Lithium levels are reduced by 20 to 30% by the concurrent use of theophylline.

Clinical evidence

The serum lithium levels of 10 healthy subjects taking lithium carbonate 900 mg daily fell by 20 to 30%, and the urinary clearance of lithium increased by 30%, when they were given theophylline. Steady-state theophylline levels of 5.4 to 12.7 micrograms/mL were achieved, and it was noted that higher theophylline levels were strongly correlated with increased lithium clearance.[1] This study has been reported in brief elsewhere.[2]

A man taking theophylline was diagnosed with a bipolar disorder and started taking lithium while in hospital for an exacerbation of COPD. When the dose of theophylline was raised, because of a worsening in his condition, his lithium dose also had to be increased to control the emergence of manic symptoms. He received a maximum theophylline dose of 1.5 g daily, during which time he needed 2.7 g of lithium daily. When the theophylline was stopped, he only needed around 1.5 g of lithium daily to control his manic symptoms.[3] Two studies support the evidence from these cases, with the finding that lithium excretion is increased by about 50% by aminophylline or theophylline.[4,5]

Mechanism

Uncertain. Theophylline has an effect on the renal clearance of lithium: other xanthines have a similar effect, see 'Lithium + Caffeine', p.1366.

Importance and management

Information is very limited but the interaction between aminophylline or theophylline and lithium appears to be established. Depressive and manic relapses could occur if the dose of lithium is not raised appropriately when these drugs are given. Serum lithium levels should be monitored if theophylline or aminophylline is stopped, started, or if the dose is altered.

1. Perry PJ, Calloway RA, Cook BL, Smith RE. Theophylline precipitated alterations of lithium clearance. *Acta Psychiatr Scand* (1984) 69, 528–37.
2. Cook BL, Smith RE, Perry PJ, Calloway RA. Theophylline-lithium interaction. *J Clin Psychiatry* (1985) 46, 278–9.
3. Sierles FS, Ossowski MG. Concurrent use of theophylline and lithium in a patient with chronic obstructive lung disease and bipolar disorder. *Am J Psychiatry* (1982) 139, 117–18.
4. Thomsen K, Schou M. Renal lithium excretion in man. *Am J Physiol* (1968) 215, 823–7.
5. Holstad SG, Perry PJ, Kathol RG, Carson RW, Krummel SJ. The effects of intravenous theophylline infusion versus intravenous sodium bicarbonate infusion on lithium clearance in normal subjects. *Psychiatry Res* (1988) 25, 203–11.

Lithium + Topiramate

Two isolated reports describe elevated lithium levels and evidence of toxicity in patients also taking topiramate. No important pharmacokinetic interaction has been seen in healthy subjects.

Clinical evidence, mechanism, importance and management

A 42-year-old woman with type II bipolar disorder started taking lithium carbonate 1.5 g and topiramate 500 mg daily, resulting in a steady-state trough serum lithium level of 0.5 mmol/L after 10 days. She was also started taking citalopram 10 mg daily. The patient raised the topiramate dose to 800 mg daily in an attempt to lose weight, and 5 weeks later began to complain of severe anorexia, nausea, fatigue and impaired concentration. She had managed to lose 35 lb (almost 16 kg) of weight she had gained whilst taking a previous drug combination. When examined she was lethargic, with tremors, nystagmus, bradycardia and memory loss. Her trough serum lithium level had risen by 180%, to 1.4 mmol/L. The symptoms disappeared over 4 days when the lithium was stopped. Two months later she was stabilised once again on lithium carbonate 1.2 g and topiramate 500 mg daily, with a steady-state serum lithium level of 0.5 mmol/L.[1]

Another report describes a 26-year-old woman with type I bipolar disorder taking lithium 900 mg daily, whose lithium levels increased from 0.82 mmol/L to 1.24 mmol/L after topiramate 75 mg daily was given for about one week. She also developed symptoms of toxicity (worsening concentration, confusion, lethargy). Her lithium levels increased to 1.97 mmol/L over the next 4 days despite a reduction in the dose of lithium to 750 mg daily. The lithium was stopped and then restarted at 450 mg daily, which produced therapeutic lithium levels of 0.67 mmol/L. In addition, further increases in the topiramate dose over 4 weeks (from 75 mg daily to 125 mg daily), while maintaining the dose of lithium at 450 mg daily, resulted in parallel elevations of lithium levels (from 0.67 mmol/L to 0.92 mmol/L).[2]

However, a review of the pharmacokinetic interactions of topiramate reported a study in which 12 healthy subjects receiving lithium carbonate 300 mg two or three times daily (dosing frequency unclear) were given topiramate (50 mg twice daily titrated to 100 mg twice daily). The AUC of lithium was 18% lower and its clearance was 22% higher suggesting a very slight pharmacokinetic interaction. In addition, when compared with historical data, the clearance of topiramate appeared to be lower in the presence of lithium.[3]

The reasons for these reactions are not known, but topiramate is mainly eliminated by renal excretion and high doses of topiramate might competitively interfere with lithium excretion.[1] Similarly, lithium might affect topiramate clearance.[3] Some of the toxicity could have been due to the adverse effects of either drug, with the weight loss in the first case possibly disturbing the sodium excretion, which could have affected the loss of lithium in the urine.

These cases highlight the possible risk of elevated serum lithium levels especially if high doses of topiramate are used. Patients taking lithium should be aware of the symptoms of lithium toxicity and told to report them immediately should they occur. This should be reinforced when they are given topiramate. The authors of two reports suggest that lithium levels should be monitored in patients newly started on this combination and the dose of topiramate and/or lithium carefully adjusted to minimise adverse effects.[4,5]

For more information on the risk factors for lithium toxicity, symptoms of lithium adverse effects and general monitoring, see under 'Lithium', p.1361.

1. Pinninti NR, Zelinski G. Does topiramate elevate serum lithium levels? *J Clin Psychopharmacol* (2002) 22, 340.
2. Abraham G, Owen J. Topiramate can cause lithium toxicity. *J Clin Psychopharmacol* (2004) 24, 565–7.
3. Bialer M, Doose DR, Murthy B, Curtin C, Wang S-S, Twyman RE, Schwabe S. Pharmacokinetic interactions of topiramate. *Clin Pharmacokinet* (2004) 43, 763–80.
4. Chengappa KNR, Gershon S, Levine J. The evolving role of topiramate among other mood stabilizers in the management of bipolar disorder. *Bipolar Disord* (2001) 3, 215–32.
5. Pies R. Combining lithium and anticonvulsants in bipolar disorder: a review. *Ann Clin Psychiatry* (2002) 14, 223–32.

Lithium + Tricyclic and related antidepressants

The concurrent use of a tricyclic and lithium can result in adverse effects, a few of them severe. Cases of neurotoxicity, serotonin syndrome, and neuroleptic malignant syndrome have been reported.

Clinical evidence

(a) Amitriptyline

A study in 17 lithium-maintained patients found that tremor activity increased when amitriptyline 75 to 150 mg daily was added. The greatest increments occurred within about 3 weeks of concurrent use, but tremor activity was still greater than baseline after 6 weeks. No patient discontinued treatment because of the increase in tremor.[1] Seizures occurred in a patient taking amitriptyline 300 mg daily, 13 days after lithium carbonate 300 mg three times daily was started. After recovery, concurrent use was resumed, but further seizures occurred 10 days later. Her lithium levels were 0.9 mmol/L three days before this second episode. She later took amitriptyline 500 mg daily without adverse effect.[2] Another patient developed neuroleptic malignant syndrome after one week of treatment with lithium carbonate 300 mg and amitriptyline 25 mg, both three times daily. The patient had also taken chlorpromazine for one week, just before the concurrent use of lithium and amitriptyline was started.[3] A 59-year-old patient developed tremor when he doubled the doses of **trazodone** and lithium carbonate to 250 mg daily and 800 mg daily, respectively. When the doses were reduced to **trazodone** 25 mg daily and lithium 400 mg daily, and amitriptyline 75 mg daily was added, he developed serotonin syndrome (anxiety, restlessness, tremor, myoclonus, hyperreflexia, diaphoresis, rigidity and hyperthermia).[4]

No pharmacokinetic interaction was found in 10 therapy-resistant patients with major depression who were given amitriptyline and lithium for 4 weeks.[5]

(b) Amoxapine

An analysis of the spontaneous reporting system of the FDA in the US identified one case of neurotoxicity involving the use of amoxapine and lithium.[6]

(c) Clomipramine

A man with depression, taking clomipramine 175 mg, levomepromazine 25 mg and flunitrazepam 2 mg daily started taking lithium 600 mg daily. About one week later, after his dose of lithium was raised to 1 g daily, he developed serotonin syndrome (myoclonus, shivering, tremors, incoordination). Due to this reaction, and because his serum lithium levels were 1.6 mmol/L, lithium was stopped. Serotonin syndrome then abated. The clomipramine dose was reduced, but some mild symptoms remained until the clomipramine was stopped. He responded well to lithium 600 mg daily alone, without developing serotonin syndrome.[7]

(d) Doxepin

A 64-year-old man developed periods of confusion and disorientation within 2 weeks of starting to take lithium 300 mg twice daily with doxepin 100 mg at bedtime. He was admitted to hospital with urinary retention, and he was also lethargic and became confused. Despite the withdrawal of both drugs, he developed a condition similar to neuroleptic malignant syndrome (fever, muscle rigidity, changes in consciousness, autonomic dysfunction), which was successfully treated with dantrolene.[8]

(e) Nortriptyline

A 65-year-old woman developed tremor, memory difficulties, disorganised thinking and auditory hallucinations when given lithium carbonate 300 mg twice daily (lithium level 0.82 mmol/L) and nortriptyline 50 mg daily. However, because she only ever received lithium with nortriptyline, the possibility that this was an effect of lithium alone cannot be excluded.[9]

Mechanism

Not fully understood. Tremor is a relatively frequent adverse effect of both lithium and antidepressants with serotonergic properties (see 'Table 35.3', p.1472). It might be expected that the concurrent use of lithium (which is itself serotonergic) with such antidepressants will enhance not only efficacy, but also increase the incidence of adverse effects.[1,10]

Importance and management

Although the concurrent use of lithium and tricyclics and related antidepressants can be successful, some patients might, rarely, develop severe adverse effects, particularly neurotoxic adverse effects, such as seizures and symptoms similar to those of serotonin syndrome or neuroleptic malignant syndrome. It would be prudent to be alert for these on concurrent use. More commonly, tremors can develop, and this might be as a result of additive adverse effects. If tremors become troublesome it would seem prudent to review concurrent use. For more information on serotonin syndrome and its management, see 'Drugs that cause serotonin syndrome + Other drugs that cause serotonin syndrome', p.1471.

1. Zaninelli R, Bauer M, Jobert M, Müller-Oerlinghausen B. Changes in quantitatively assessed tremor during treatment of major depression with lithium augmented by paroxetine or amitriptyline. *J Clin Psychopharmacol* (2001) 21, 190–8.
2. Solomon JG. Seizures during lithium-amitriptyline therapy. *Postgrad Med* (1979) 66, 145–8.
3. Fava S, Galizia AC. Neuroleptic malignant syndrome and lithium carbonate. *J Psychiatry Neurosci* (1995) 20, 305–6.
4. Nisijima K, Shimizu M, Abe T, Ishiguro T. A case of serotonin syndrome induced by concomitant treatment with low-dose trazodone and amitriptyline and lithium. *Int Clin Psychopharmacol* (1996) 11, 289–90.
5. Jaspert A, Ebert D, Loew T, Martus P. Lithium increases the response to tricyclic antidepressant medication – no evidence of influences of pharmacokinetic interactions. *Pharmacopsychiatry* (1993) 26, 165.
6. Goldman SA. Lithium and neuroleptics in combination: is there enhancement of neurotoxicity leading to permanent sequelae? *J Clin Pharmacol* (1996) 36, 951–62.
7. Kojima H, Terao T, Yoshimura R. Serotonin syndrome during clomipramine and lithium treatment. *Am J Psychiatry* (1993) 150, 1897.
8. Rosenberg PB, Pearlman CA. NMS-like syndrome with a lithium/doxepin combination. *J Clin Psychopharmacol* (1991) 11, 75–6.
9. Austin LS, Arana GW, Melvin JA. Toxicity resulting from lithium augmentation of antidepressant treatment in elderly patients. *J Clin Psychiatry* (1990) 51, 344–5.
10. Lafferman J, Solomon K, Ruskin P. Lithium augmentation for treatment-resistant depression in the elderly. *J Geriatr Psychiatry Neurol* (1988) 1, 49–52.

Lithium + Triptans

In two cases patients taking lithium developed symptoms suggestive of serotonin syndrome after also taking sumatriptan.

Clinical evidence, mechanism, importance and management

A comprehensive literature search published in 1998 identified several cases of adverse events reported with **sumatriptan** and lithium, although in most cases other medications were also being taken. Two patients taking **sumatriptan** and lithium concurrently were identified with symptoms suggestive of serotonin syndrome, but the symptoms were mild to moderate and self-limiting. The number of patients taking lithium and **sumatriptan** was not stated, so the incidence of this effect is unknown.[1] The conclusion was reached that **sumatriptan** can be used cautiously in patients receiving lithium.[1] There seem to be no other reports of adverse reactions following the concurrent use of lithium and a triptan; however, note that, rarely, the use of lithium or a triptan with other drugs has led to serotonin syndrome. For more information about serotonin syndrome and its management, see 'Drugs that cause serotonin syndrome + Other drugs that cause serotonin syndrome', p.1471.

1. Gardner DM, Lynd LD. Sumatriptan contraindications and the serotonin syndrome. *Ann Pharmacother* (1998) 32, 33–8.

Lithium + Valproate

No clinically relevant adverse interaction appears to occur between lithium carbonate and valproate.

Clinical evidence, mechanism, importance and management

In a crossover study, 16 healthy subjects were given valproate (as valproate semisodium) or a placebo twice daily for 12 days, to which lithium carbonate 300 mg three times daily was added on days 6 to 10. The valproate serum levels and AUC rose by 12% and 11%, respectively, while the serum lithium levels were unaltered. Adverse effects were similar with both treatments. It was concluded that the concurrent use of lithium and valproate is safe.[1] A review on the efficacy of the concurrent use of lithium and an antiepileptic in bipolar disorder lists several studies in which the combination of valproate (as valproate semisodium) and lithium was used. On the whole concurrent use was considered safe and well tolerated, although a few patients discontinued treatment due to adverse effects, which included gastrointestinal symptoms and raised liver transaminases. It was, however, difficult to know if these adverse effects were due to the individual drugs or the result of an interaction. Other adverse effects that have been reported on concurrent use include tremor, cognitive impairment and alopecia.[2]

There would appear to be no reason to avoid the concurrent use of lithium and valproate, but it would be prudent to be aware that some patients might experience an increase in adverse effects.

1. Granneman GR, Schneck DW, Cavanaugh JH, Witt GF. Pharmacokinetic interactions and side effects resulting from concomitant administration of lithium and divalproex sodium. *J Clin Psychiatry* (1996) 57, 204–6.
2. Pies R. Combining lithium and anticonvulsants in bipolar disorder: a review. *Ann Clin Psychiatry* (2002) 14, 223–32.

Lithium + Venlafaxine

Symptoms similar to those of serotonin syndrome have developed in a few patients taking lithium with venlafaxine. No clinically relevant pharmacokinetic interaction usually appears to occur between lithium and venlafaxine.

Clinical evidence

In a pharmacokinetic study, 12 healthy subjects were given a single 600-mg dose of lithium carbonate on day one and day 8, with venlafaxine 50 mg every 8 hours for 7 days from day 4. The renal clearance of venlafaxine was reduced by about 50% and that of its active metabolite, *O*-desmethylvenlafaxine, was reduced by 15%. Neither of these changes was considered to be clinically relevant, as the total clearance was not affected. The maximum serum levels of the lithium were increased by about 10%, and the time to reach maximum levels was reduced by about 30 minutes, but these changes would not be expected to be clinically relevant, and the other pharmacokinetic parameters of lithium were unchanged.[1]

In an open study of 13 patients with major depression who did not respond to a 4-week course of venlafaxine 300 mg daily, lithium was added and continued for 4 weeks. After 12 days of concurrent use, 2 patients experienced symptoms of hypomania, marked nausea and trembling (considered to be a moderate form of serotonin syndrome), and had to stop lithium. Their lithium plasma levels were within the therapeutic range (0.83 mmol/L and 0.77 mmol/L on day 7). Lithium was well tolerated by most of the other patients, with trembling being the most frequent adverse effect (4 out of 11).[2] Case reports also describe the development of serotonin syndrome in patients with lithium within the therapeutic range given venlafaxine,[3-5] although one patient was thought to be unusually sensitive to serotonergic medication,[3] and another patient had elevated venlafaxine levels.[4]

Mechanism

Both venlafaxine and lithium are known to have serotonergic effects, which could be additive on concurrent use, resulting in serotonin syndrome.

Importance and management

The general picture that emerges from these reports is that normally no clinically important pharmacokinetic interaction occurs if venlafaxine and lithium are used together, but in some rare cases, serotonin syndrome might occur. The reason for the raised venlafaxine levels seen in one of the cases is unclear.[4] There seems to be no good reason for avoiding concurrent use, but be aware that an interaction is possible and monitor the outcome carefully. For more information on serotonin syndrome and its management, see 'Drugs that cause serotonin syndrome + Other drugs that cause serotonin syndrome', p.1471.

1. Troy SM, Parker VD, Hicks DR, Boudino FD, Chiang ST. Pharmacokinetic interaction between multiple-dose venlafaxine and single-dose lithium. *J Clin Pharmacol* (1996) 36, 175–81.
2. Bertschy G, Ragama-Pardos E, Aït-Ameur A, Muscionico M, Favre S, Roth L. Lithium augmentation in venlafaxine non-responders: an open study. *Eur Psychiatry* (2003) 18, 314–17.
3. Mekler G, Woggon B. A case of serotonin syndrome caused by venlafaxine and lithium. *Pharmacopsychiatry* (1997) 30, 272–3.
4. Adan-Manes J, Novalbos J, López-Rodríguez R, Ayuso-Mateos JL, Abad-Santos F. Lithium and venlafaxine interaction: a case of serotonin syndrome. *J Clin Pharm Ther* (2006) 31, 397–400.
5. Liberek C, Aubry J-M, Baud P. Manic switch and serotonin syndrome with venlafaxine-lithium-valproate association. *Therapie* (2006) 61, 531–3.

Lithium + Ziprasidone

Oral ziprasidone does not appear to alter the pharmacokinetics of lithium. However, lithium toxicity occurred in two patients after they were given intramuscular ziprasidone and neuroleptic malignant syndrome occurred in another patient taking lithium with oral ziprasidone supplemented with intramuscular ziprasidone.

Clinical evidence

A randomised, placebo-controlled study in 25 healthy subjects taking lithium carbonate 450 mg twice daily for 15 days found that ziprasidone 20 mg twice daily on days 9 to 11, followed by 40 mg twice daily on days 12 to 15, caused only a small increase in the steady-state serum lithium levels (14% compared with 11% in the placebo group). A 5% reduction in renal clearance was seen in the ziprasidone group, compared with a 9% reduction in the placebo group. These differences were neither statistically nor clinically significant.[1]

A 41-year-old man started taking lithium carbonate 2400 mg daily and chlorpromazine 600 mg daily. He had lithium levels of 1 to 1.2 mmol/L after 10 days and was stable the following week, at which point chlorpromazine was discontinued and intramuscular ziprasidone 80 mg daily was started. Two days later, the patient developed symptoms of lithium toxicity and his serum lithium level 10 hours after his last dose of lithium was 2.9 mmol/L. Both lithium and ziprasidone were stopped and lithium levels returned to normal after 5 days. Lithium was restarted at the same dose without adverse effect and with stable levels of about 1.1 mmol/L. In another patient taking lithium carbonate 1200 mg daily, serum lithium levels increased from 1 mmol/L to 1.7 mmol/L within a day of starting intramuscular ziprasidone 80 mg daily. Both drugs were stopped and adverse symptoms resolved within one day: 3 days later lithium was restarted at the same dose with steady state levels in the therapeutic range.[2] A further case report describes a patient taking lithium 450 mg twice daily, divalproex sodium, and a number of other drugs, who started to take ziprasidone 80 mg twice daily orally with intramuscular ziprasidone 20 mg as needed (5 doses were given over 4 days). He became somnolent, and was unable to walk or follow commands. His respiratory rate was increased (28 breaths/minute), his blood pressure was decreased (68/40 mmHg), and his temperature was raised (39.4°C). He also had a raised white cell count, a high urine output and an elevated lithium level of 2.07 mmol/L. Diabetes insipidus secondary to lithium was suspected and he was also diagnosed with neuroleptic malignant syndrome.[3]

Mechanism

The authors of the case describing neuroleptic malignant syndrome note that both ziprasidone and lithium (particularly in toxicity) are associated with this syndrome. Although a reaction to ziprasidone was suspected they noted that an interaction with lithium cannot be excluded.[3]

The increase in lithium levels reported in the cases was attributed to an effect on lithium clearance resulting from the rapid increase in ziprasidone levels caused by parenteral administration.[2]

Importance and management

Evidence for an interaction between lithium and ziprasidone appears to be limited to one pharmacokinetic study in healthy subjects and a series of case reports. Although oral ziprasidone did not alter the pharmacokinetics of lithium in the study, lithium toxicity occurred in three patients given intramuscular ziprasidone. Therefore it would seem prudent to be alert for early symptoms of lithium toxicity in patients given lithium with ziprasidone (particularly via the intramuscular route), and consider monitoring lithium levels should these occur. For more information on the risk factors for lithium toxicity, symptoms of lithium adverse effects and general monitoring, see under 'Lithium', p.1361.

1. Apseloff G, Mullet D, Wilner KD, Anziano RJ, Tensfeldt TG, Pelletier SM, Gerber N. The effects of ziprasidone on steady-state lithium levels and renal clearance of lithium. *Br J Clin Pharmacol* (2000) 49 (Suppl 1), 61S–64S.
2. Miodownik C, Hausmann M, Frolova K, Lerner V. Lithium intoxication associated with intramuscular ziprasidone in schizoaffective patients. *Clin Neuropharmacol* (2005) 28, 295–7.
3. Borovicka MC, Bond LC, Gaughan KM. Ziprasidone- and lithium-induced neuroleptic malignant syndrome. *Ann Pharmacother* (2006) 40, 139–42.

32

MAOIs

The intended target of the MAOIs (monoamine oxidase inhibitors) is monoamine oxidase within the brain, but monoamine oxidase is also found in other parts of the body. Particularly high concentrations occur in the gut and liver, where it acts as a protective detoxifying enzyme against tyramine and possibly other potentially hazardous amines, which exist in foods that have undergone bacterial degradation. There are at least two forms of monoamine oxidase: MAO-A metabolises (deaminates) noradrenaline (norepinephrine) and serotonin (5-HT), while MAO-B metabolises phenylethylamine. Substances such as tyramine and dopamine are metabolised by both forms of MAO.

Some MAOIs (see 'Table 32.1', below) are non-selective or non-specific, and inhibit both MAO-A and MAO-B. They are irreversible and long acting, because the return of monoamine oxidase activity depends upon the regeneration of new enzymes. As a result their effects (both beneficial and adverse) can last for 2 to 3 weeks after they have been withdrawn. Tranylcypromine differs in being a more reversible inhibitor of MAO, so the onset and disappearance of its actions are quicker than the other non-selective MAOIs. However, its effects still last for a number of weeks after withdrawal (for example, see 'MAOIs or RIMAs + Food; Tyramine-containing', p.1389), so it is, in effect, an irreversible inhibitor, and is usually classified as such. These non-selective MAOIs cause serious and potentially life-threatening hypertensive reactions if they are given with the sympathomimetics found in some cough and cold remedies (see 'MAOIs or RIMAs + Nasal decongestants and related drugs', p.1396, and with tyramine, which can be found in some foods or drinks, see 'MAOIs or RIMAs + Food; Tyramine-containing', p.1389.

Some of the more recently developed drugs with MAO inhibitory activity (see 'Table 32.1', below) interact to a lesser extent than the non-selective MAOIs. This is because they are largely selective for one of the forms of MAO. One group of these selective inhibitors targets MAO-A, and are relatively rapidly reversible; inhibition of this enzyme is responsible for their antidepressant effect. These selective MAO-A inhibitors (moclobemide, toloxatone) have been given the acronym RIMAs (Reversible Inhibitors of Monoamine oxidase A). They leave MAO-B largely uninhibited so that there is still a metabolic pathway available for the breakdown of amines, such as tyramine, that can cause a rise in blood pressure. In practical terms this means that the amount of tyramine needed to cause a hypertensive crisis is about tenfold greater than with the non-selective MAOIs (see 'MAOIs or RIMAs + Food; Tyramine-containing', p.1389).

Both non-selective MAOIs and RIMAs cause also serious and sometimes fatal serotonin syndrome when given with other serotonergic drugs such as the SNRIs (see 'MAOIs or RIMAs + SNRIs', p.1401), SSRIs (see 'MAOIs or RIMAs + SSRIs', p.1401), and tricyclics (see 'MAOIs or RIMAs + Tricyclic and related antidepressants', p.1403). However, interactions between moclobemide and SNRIs or SSRIs are usually associated with overdose. For more information on serotonin syndrome and its management, see 'Drugs that cause serotonin syndrome + Other drugs that cause serotonin syndrome', p.1471.

The selective MAOIs that specifically inhibit MAO-B are mainly used in the treatment of Parkinson's disease, and so are covered elsewhere, see 'Antiparkinsonian and related drugs', p.752. In low doses they inhibit MAO-B, leaving MAO-A largely uninhibited. However, selegiline loses some of its selectivity at doses of more than 10 mg daily and will therefore be subject to the same interactions as the non-selective MAOIs. Rasagiline is another irreversible selective inhibitor of MAO-B used for Parkinson's disease.

Some other drugs covered elsewhere in this publication also have MAOI activity. Furazolidone is an antiprotozoal with MAOI activity. Linezolid is an oxazolidinone antibacterial with weak, reversible non-selective MAOI activity. Interactions typical of MAOIs might therefore occur with these drugs.

The product information issued by manufacturers frequently contains warnings about real and alleged interactions with MAOIs. Blackwell,[1] who has done much work on the interactions of the MAOIs, has rightly pointed out that the MAOIs are among the drugs that accumulate much myth and misinformation. He notes that the MAOIs have developed such a sinister reputation that manufacturers often issue a reflexive admonition to avoid the concurrent use of MAOIs with new drugs. This means that many of the warnings about potential interactions with the MAOIs may lack a sound scientific basis. However, equally this does not mean that the proven serious life-threatening interactions that are associated with the MAOIs should be dismissed, and it should be noted that any drug with indirectly-acting sympathomimetic activity is likely to interact.

1. Blackwell B. Monoamine oxidase inhibitor interactions with other drugs. *J Clin Psychopharmacol* (1991) 11, 55–59.

Table 32.1 Monoamine oxidase inhibitors (MAOIs)[†]

Irreversible non-selective MAO-inhibitors (MAO-A and MAO-B)	*Reversible Inhibitors of MAO-A (RIMAs)*	*Irreversible inhibitors of MAO-B**
Iproniazid	Brofaromine	Rasagiline
Isocarboxazid	Moclobemide	Selegiline
Mebanazine	Toloxatone	
Nialamide		
Phenelzine		
Tranylcypromine		

*MAO-B inhibitors are used in Parkinson's disease, so are covered elsewhere

[†]Furazolidone, a non-selective MAOI used as an antiprotozoal, and linezolid, a weak, reversible non-selective MAOI, used as an antibacterial, are covered elsewhere.

MAOIs or RIMAs + Amfetamines and related drugs

The use of a non-selective MAOI with an amfetamine or an amfetamine-related drug can result in a potentially fatal hypertensive crisis and/or serotonin syndrome. Interactions have been reported for amfetamine, dexamfetamine, and metamfetamine. Interactions have also been reported with the illicit drug ecstasy (MDMA, methylenedioxymethamfetamine) when taken with phenelzine or moclobemide.

Clinical evidence

A. MAOIs

(a) Amfetamines

A 30-year-old depressed woman who was taking **phenelzine** 15 mg three times daily and trifluoperazine 2 mg at night, acquired some **dexamfetamine sulfate** tablets from a friend and took 20 mg. Within 15 minutes she complained of severe headache, which she described as if "her head was bursting". An hour later her blood pressure was 150/100 mmHg. Later she became comatose with a blood pressure of 170/100 mmHg and died. A postmortem examination revealed a brain haemorrhage.[1]

This interaction has also been reported with:

- **Amfetamine** (single intravenous or oral dose) with **phenelzine**[2,3] or **tranylcypromine**.[4]
- **Amfetamine** and **dexamfetamine** with **phenelzine**.[5,6]
- **Metamfetamine** (single intravenous dose) with **isocarboxazid**,[7,8] **phenelzine**,[7,9] or **tranylcypromine**.[7,10]

A woman who had been addicted to high-dose **dexamfetamine** with amobarbital was hospitalised and had the **dexamfetamine** with amobarbital withdrawn. Five days later she was given a single 10-mg dose of **tranylcypromine** and within an hour had a 20-minute episode of hypertension, tachycardia, headache, sweating, lacrimation and altered consciousness, which abated without treatment. She had similar attacks at 2-hourly intervals over about 5 days, which gradually became milder and shorter.[11]

Extreme hyperpyrexia, apparently without hypertension, has been described in a woman who took **tranylcypromine** and **dexamfetamine** with amobarbital. She developed progressive agitation, diaphoresis, hyperkinesis, opisthotonus, coma and convulsions, but recovered following the use of an ice bath and other supportive measures.[12,13]

(b) Ecstasy (MDMA, methylenedioxymethamfetamine)

Marked hypertension, diaphoresis, altered mental status and hypertonicity (slow forceful twisting and arching movements) occurred in one patient taking **phenelzine** with ecstasy.[14] Increased muscle tension, decorticate-like posturing (arms, wrists and fingers bent inwards and legs extended), fever, tachycardia and coma occurred in another patient taking **phenelzine**, 15 minutes after drinking juice containing ecstasy.[15] Both patients recovered.[14,15]

B. RIMAs

Four patients died after taking **moclobemide** and **ecstasy** (MDMA, methylenedioxymethamfetamine). The clinical evidence is limited, but in each case the forensic pathologist concluded that the cause of death was the combined use of these drugs and it was suggested that what happened is consistent with serotonin syndrome. Two patients had taken maximum therapeutic doses and two moderate overdoses of **moclobemide**. Note that **moclobemide** had not been prescribed to any of them. Post-mortem analysis also found the presence of **dextromethorphan** in one patient, which was thought to have contributed,[16] see also 'MAOIs or RIMAs + Dextromethorphan and related cough suppressants', p.1387, for further information on this interaction.

A similar report describes three fatal cases of serotonin syndrome in patients taking **moclobemide** with **ecstasy**; however, in two of these cases the moclobemide appeared to have been taken in overdose.[17]

Mechanism

The hypertensive reaction can be attributed to over-stimulation of the adrenergic receptors of the cardiovascular system.[18] During treatment with non-selective MAOIs, large amounts of noradrenaline (norepinephrine) accumulate at adrenergic nerve endings not only in the brain, but also within the sympathetic nerve endings, which innervate arterial blood vessels. Stimulation of these latter nerve endings by sympathomimetic amines with indirect actions causes the release of the accumulated noradrenaline and results in the massive stimulation of the receptors. An exaggerated blood vessel constriction occurs and the blood pressure rise is proportionately excessive. Intracranial haemorrhage can occur if the pressure is so high that a blood vessel ruptures.[1]

Some of the reactions may also possibly be related to serotonin syndrome. Amfetamines act by releasing serotonin (and possibly also dopamine) from neurones in the brain, so that increased stimulation of the serotonin receptors occurs. This possibly explains their mood-modifying effects. MAOIs prevent the breakdown of serotonin within the neurones so that more serotonin is available for release, and in excess this can apparently result in the toxic and even fatal serotonin syndrome. The RIMAs (such as moclobemide) appear to behave like the older non-selective MAOIs in this context.

Importance and management

The hypertensive reaction seen in patients taking an MAOI and an amfetamine is a very well-documented, serious, and potentially fatal interaction, whereas serotonin syndrome appears to be rarer. Patients taking any of the non-selective MAOIs should not normally take amfetamines, and the US manufacturers of the MAOIs specifically contraindicate concurrent use.[19-21] It would seem prudent to also avoid the use of an amfetamine for 14 days after an MAOI has been taken. However bear in mind that there have been case reports of successful and apparently safe use of dexamfetamine with MAOIs under very well controlled conditions.[22,23] Patients taking MAOIs should be warned to avoid the illicit use of amfetamines and ecstasy.

Evidence for an interaction with the RIMAs is more limited. Nevertheless, it would also be prudent to avoid the use of moclobemide with amfetamines and related drugs, although the incidence of the interactions with moclobemide is unlikely to be as great as that seen with the non-selective MAOIs. In the cases with ecstasy, it seems likely that high doses of moclobemide were used to try to enhance the actions of the ecstasy, but these cases, nevertheless, show that concurrent use is potentially life threatening.

Interactions with other central stimulants such as **diethylpropion**, **pemoline**, **phendimetrazine**, and **phenmetrazine** do not seem to have been documented, but on the basis of their known pharmacology their concurrent use with the MAOIs should probably be avoided.

Treatment

For a brief mention of the treatment of hypertensive crisis, see *Importance and Management* under 'MAOIs or RIMAs + Nasal decongestants and related drugs', p.1396. For the management of fever and other symptoms of serotonin syndrome, see 'Drugs that cause serotonin syndrome + Other drugs that cause serotonin syndrome', p.1471.

1. Lloyd JTA, Walker DRH. Death after combined dexamphetamine and phenelzine. *BMJ* (1965) 2, 168–9.
2. Tonks CM, Livingston D. Monoamineoxidase inhibitors. *Lancet* (1963) i, 1323–4.
3. Feinberg M, de Vigne J-P, Kronfol Z, Young E. Duration of action of phenelzine in two patients. *Am J Psychiatry* (1981) 138, 379–80.
4. Zeck P. The dangers of some antidepressant drugs. *Med J Aust* (1961) 2, 607–8.
5. Devabhaktuni RV, Jampala VC. Using street drugs while on MAOI therapy. *J Clin Psychopharmacol* (1987) 7, 60–1.
6. Maletzky BM. Phenelzine as a stimulant drug antagonist: a preliminary report. *Int J Addict* (1977) 12, 651–5.
7. Mason A. Fatal reaction associated with tranylcypromine and methylamphetamine. *Lancet* (1962) i, 1073.
8. Bethune HC, Burrell RH, Culpan RH. Headache associated with monoamine oxidase inhibitors. *Lancet* (1963) ii, 1233–4.
9. Dally PJ. Fatal reaction associated with tranylcypromine and methylamphetamine. *Lancet* (1962) i, 1235–6.
10. Macdonald R. Tranylcypromine. *Lancet* (1963) i, 269.
11. Hay G. Severe reaction to monoamine-oxidase inhibitor in a dexamphetamine addict. *Lancet* (1962) ii, 665.
12. Lewis E. Hyperpyrexia with antidepressant drugs. *BMJ* (1965) 1, 1671–2.
13. Kriskó I, Lewis E, Johnson JE. Severe hyperpyrexia due to tranylcypromine–amphetamine toxicity. *Ann Intern Med* (1969) 70, 559–64.
14. Smilkstein MJ, Smolinske SC, Rumack BH. A case of MAO inhibitor/MDMA interaction: agony after ecstasy. *Clin Toxicol* (1987) 25, 149–59.
15. Kaskey GB. Possible interaction between an MAOI and "Ecstasy". *Am J Psychiatry* (1992) 149, 411–2.
16. Vuori E, Henry JA, Ojanoperä I, Nieminen R, Savolainen T, Wahlsten P, Jäntti M. Death following ingestion of MDMA (ecstasy) and moclobemide. *Addiction* (2003) 98, 365–8.
17. Pilgrim JL, Gerostamoulos D, Drummer OH, Bollmann M. Involvement of amphetamines in sudden and unexpected death. *J Forensic Sci* (2009) 54, 478–85.
18. Simpson LL. Mechanism of the adverse interaction between monoamine oxidase inhibitors and amphetamine. *J Pharmacol Exp Ther* (1978) 205, 392–9.
19. Parnate (Tranylcypromine sulfate). GlaxoSmithKline. US Prescribing information, May 2010.
20. Nardil (Phenelzine sulfate). Pfizer Inc. US Prescribing information, February 2009.
21. Marplan (Isocarboxazid). Validus Pharmaceuticals, Inc. US Prescribing information, August 2007.
22. Feinberg SS. Combining stimulants with monoamine oxidase inhibitors: a review of uses and one possible additional indication. *J Clin Psychiatry* (2004) 65, 1520–4.
23. Fawcett J, Kravitz HM, Zajecka JM, Schaff MR. CNS stimulant potentiation of monoamine oxidase inhibitors in treatment-refractory depression. *J Clin Psychopharmacol* (1991) 11, 127–32.

MAOIs + Antihistamines

The alleged interaction between the MAOIs and antihistamines appears to be based on a single *animal* study, and is probably more theoretical than real. There appear to be some exceptions, based on the additional properties of some specific antihistamines (e.g. cyproheptadine).

Clinical evidence, mechanism, importance and management

A number of lists, charts and books about adverse drug interactions suggest that potentially serious interactions can occur between the MAOIs and the antihistamines. This appears to be based on a study in *rabbits* from 1972, which showed that some antihistamines (notably alkylamine antihistamines such as **chlorphenamine**, **brompheniramine**, and also **diphenhydramine**) produced a fatal hyperpyrexia, thought to be due to serotonin potentiation, when given intravenously to **phenelzine** pretreated *rabbits*.[1] This reaction was considered to be similar to that seen with pethidine (meperidine) (see 'MAOIs or RIMAs + Opioids; Pethidine (Meperidine)', p.1399, and the tricyclics (see 'MAOIs or RIMAs + Tricyclic and related antidepressants', p.1403). However, in the 20 to 30 years since the publication of this data, the manufacturers of various antihistamines did not appear to have identified any clinical reports of adverse interactions attributed to the use of any antihistamine with an MAOI,[2-5] and there appear to be no reports published in the literature. Nevertheless, the UK manufacturers of several of the sedating antihistamines (**alimemazine**, **chlorphenamine**, **diphenhydramine**) state that MAOIs may intensify the antimuscarinic effects of the antihistamines,[6-8] and some contraindicate[7] or caution[6] concurrent use, both with, and for 14 days after stopping, an MAOI. No such warning appears to be given for the non-sedating antihistamines. However, the US manufacturers of isocarboxazid and tranylcypromine contraindicate all antihistamines.[9,10]

Despite the manufacturers' statements **chlorphenamine** has been specifically mentioned by one author as being suitable for the management of rhinitis associated with the common cold in patients taking MAOIs.[11]

In general, there would appear to be no good reason to avoid the concurrent use of sedating or non-sedating antihistamines with an MAOI. However, the other properties of the antihistamines should be considered. Cyproheptadine has specific serotonin antagonist properties, and **promethazine** is a phenothiazine, and, as a result of these properties, they may interact differently, see 'MAOIs or RIMAs + Antihistamines; Cyproheptadine', below, and 'MAOIs or RIMAs + Antipsychotics', below.

1. Sinclair JG. Antihistamine-monoamine oxidase inhibitor interaction in rabbits. *J Pharm Pharmacol* (1972) 24, 955–61.
2. Novartis Consumer Healthcare UK Ltd. Personal communication, April 2010.
3. UCB Pharma. Personal communication, March 2010.
4. Glaxo Wellcome. Personal communication, December 1995.
5. Sanofi-aventis UK. Personal communication, March 2010.
6. Nytol Original Tablets (Diphenydramine hydrochloride). GlaxoSmithKline Consumer Healthcare. UK Summary of product characteristics, November 2009.
7. Piriton (Chlorphenamine maleate). GlaxoSmithKline Consumer Healthcare. UK Summary of product characteristics, May 2010.
8. Vallergan Tablets (Alimemazine). Winthrop Pharmaceuticals UK Ltd. UK Summary of product characteristics, January 2007.
9. Parnate (Tranylcypromine sulfate). GlaxoSmithKline. US Prescribing information, May 2010.
10. Marplan (Isocarboxazid). Validus Pharmaceuticals, Inc. US Prescribing information, August 2007.
11. Jenike MA. Alcohol and antihistamines not contraindicated with MAOIs? *Am J Psychiatry* (1983) 140, 1107.

MAOIs or RIMAs + Antihistamines; Cyproheptadine

Isolated reports describe delayed hallucinations and the rapid re-emergence of depression when cyproheptadine was taken with brofaromine or phenelzine.

Clinical evidence

A woman who had responded well to **brofaromine** rapidly became depressed again when she took cyproheptadine. She had to be hospitalised due to suicidal ideation, but eventually this improved, and she continued to take **brofaromine** with cyproheptadine for 6 months.[1] A man whose depression responded well to **phenelzine** 75 mg daily was given cyproheptadine 4 mg to treat associated sexual dysfunction and anorgasmia. Within 3 days of adding the cyproheptadine his depression returned, but the anorgasmia did not improve. When the cyproheptadine was stopped his depression was relieved.[2] In another case, hallucinations developed in a woman taking **phenelzine** 2 months after cyproheptadine was started.[3]

Mechanism

Brofaromine has both reversible MAO-A inhibitory and serotonin (5-HT) uptake inhibitory properties. The reversal of the effects of brofaromine was therefore attributed by the authors of one report[1] to the blockade of 5-HT receptors by cyproheptadine, which is a serotonin antagonist. It is suggested that this blockade may either lead to neurotransmitter toxicity or MAOI withdrawal, resulting in hallucinations or re-emergence of depression, as reported in two of the cases with phenelzine.

Importance and management

Information about an interaction between the MAOIs or RIMAs and cyproheptadine seems to be limited to these reports. However, cyproheptadine has also been reported to oppose the antidepressant effects of the SSRIs, see 'SSRIs + Cyproheptadine', p.1485, which suggests that the proposed mechanism is correct. It would therefore be prudent to be alert for a reduction in efficacy or an adverse response if cyproheptadine is given with any MAOI or RIMA, although note that the manufacturer of cyproheptadine actually contraindicates concurrent use with MAOIs.[4] However, there appears to be no reason why cyproheptadine cannot be used to treat serotonin syndrome occurring in a patient taking an MAOI.

The UK manufacturer of cyproheptadine also says that MAOIs prolong and intensify the antimuscarinic effects of antihistamines,[4] but there seems to be no clinical data to support this suggestion with cyproheptadine or any other antihistamine; nevertheless, concurrent use is contraindicated by some, see 'MAOIs + Antihistamines', p.1383.

1. Katz RJ, Rosenthal M. Adverse interaction of cyproheptadine with serotonergic antidepressants. *J Clin Psychiatry* (1994) 55, 314–15.
2. Zubieta JK, Demitrack MA. Depression after cyproheptadine: MAO treatment. *Biol Psychiatry* (1992) 31, 1177–8.
3. Kahn DA. Possible toxic interaction between cyproheptadine and phenelzine. *Am J Psychiatry* (1987) 144, 1242–3.
4. Periactin (Cyproheptadine hydrochloride). Merck Sharp & Dohme Ltd. UK Summary of product characteristics, November 2008.

MAOIs + Antimuscarinics

No adverse interactions between the MAOIs and antimuscarinics have been reported, although the possibility of increased antimuscarinic effects has been suggested.

Clinical evidence, mechanism, importance and management

A hyperthermic reaction has been reported in some *animals* given **tranylcypromine** or **nialamide** with **procyclidine** or **benzatropine**. It was considered that this might be due to an exaggerated dopamine response.[1] However, there do not appear to be any reports of such an interaction occurring clinically. Nevertheless, the manufacturer of **procyclidine**,[2] and some manufacturers of irreversible, non-selective MAOIs (**isocarboxazid** and **phenelzine**)[3,4] advise caution because of the possibility that the concurrent use of an antimuscarinic and an MAOI may lead to increased antimuscarinic effects. This is presumably because, in theory, inhibition of drug-metabolising enzymes by MAOIs may possibly enhance the effects of antimuscarinics.

1. Pedersen V, Nielsen IM. Hyperthermia in rabbits caused by interaction between M.A.O.I.s, antiparkinson drugs, and neuroleptics. *Lancet* (1975) i, 409–10.
2. Kemadrin (Procyclidine hydrochloride). GlaxoSmithKline UK. UK Summary of product characteristics, May 2008.
3. Isocarboxazid. Cambridge Laboratories. UK Summary of product characteristics, February 2008.
4. Nardil (Phenelzine sulfate). Archimedes Pharma UK Ltd. UK Summary of product characteristics, October 2008.

MAOIs or RIMAs + Antipsychotics

The concurrent use of MAOIs and phenothiazines is usually safe and effective. However, rarely, cases of possible neuroleptic malignant syndrome or hyperpyrexia, in some cases fatal, have been reported when MAOIs were given with chlorpromazine, levomepromazine or trifluoperazine.

Moclobemide has been given with various antipsychotics without a significant interaction, although adverse effects may be increased. However, one case describes a fatal overdose which was attributed to an interaction between moclobemide and perazine.

Clinical evidence

A. MAOIs

MAOIs and phenothiazines have been safe and effective when used together in the treatment of psychiatric conditions, particularly in the form of a preparation containing both **tranylcypromine** and **trifluoperazine**,[1-3] which is still marketed in some countries.

However, rarely, cases suggestive of neuroleptic malignant syndrome or similar have been reported. These are discussed in the sections below.

(a) Chlorpromazine

In one case, a 70-year-old woman taking **isocarboxazid** 10 mg daily and chlorpromazine 25 mg three times daily, suddenly developed dyspnoea, tachycardia, pyrexia, muscular rigidity, hypotension, and became comatose. Her condition initially improved over 24 hours, but she later died from acute renal failure as a result of rhabdomyolysis. Throughout the previous 2 years of inpatient care, the patient had received neuroleptics intermittently and had developed an unexplained toxic confusional state on 6 occasions, which suggested that neuroleptic malignant syndrome had a milder chronic course in this patient before the full acute syndrome developed.[4]

(b) Droperidol

A patient was given oral droperidol 20 mg and hyoscine 400 micrograms preoperatively, 4 days after the withdrawal of **phenelzine** and perphenazine. About 2 hours later he was observed to be pale, sweating profusely and slightly cyanosed, with a blood pressure of 75/60 mmHg and a pulse rate of 60 bpm. He was not excitable, and no changes in respiration were seen. The blood pressure gradually rose to 115/80 mmHg over the next 45 minutes, but did not return to his normal level of 160/100 mmHg for 36 hours. The same premedication was given 11 days later without any adverse effects. The response was attributed to the residual effects of **phenelzine** treatment.[5]

(c) Levomepromazine

One study mentions an unexplained fatality in a woman who suddenly developed hyperthermia and coma while taking levomepromazine and **pargyline**.[6] Another report briefly mentions a woman who developed fatal hyperthermia while taking levomepromazine and **tranylcypromine**,[7] and a fatality following the use of an unnamed MAOI/phenothiazine combination.[7]

(d) Perphenazine

One early reviewer stated that MAOIs increase the potency of phenothiazine derivatives such that their initial dose should be reduced by three-quarters. He briefly mentions a case of a patient taking long-term perphenazine who developed a Parkinson-like syndrome with extrapyramidal symptoms a few hours after starting an MAOI.[8]

(e) Prochlorperazine

A report attributes 2 cases of fatal fulminant hepatitis to an interaction between **iproniazid** and prochlorperazine.[9]

(f) Promethazine

A single report[10] describes a woman taking an MAOI who developed a severe occipital headache after taking 30 mL of a paediatric cough linctus. Initially this interaction was attributed to promethazine, but it is now known that the linctus in question contained phenylpropanolamine, which is much more likely to have been the cause.[11] See 'MAOIs or RIMAs + Nasal decongestants and related drugs', p.1396, for discussion on the interaction with phenylpropanolamine.

(g) Trifluoperazine

In another case, a woman presented with symptoms of neuroleptic malignant syndrome one week after starting **tranylcypromine** 10 mg with trifluoperazine 1 mg and immediately after doubling the dose. She was intubated and treated with dantrolene and intravenous sodium bicarbonate, and made a full recovery.[12] Interpretation of her case is complicated by the fact she had been previously taking imipramine, and was switched to tranylcypromine with trifluoperazine without a break (see also 'MAOIs or RIMAs + Tricyclic and related antidepressants', p.1403).

B. RIMAs

The manufacturer of **moclobemide** noted that in 1992 there were data available from 110 patients given **moclobemide** 150 to 400 mg daily with various antipsychotics, namely **acepromazine**, **aceprometazine**, **alimemazine**, **bromperidol**, **chlorpromazine**, **chlorprothixene**, **clothiapine**, **clozapine**, **cyamemazine**, **flupenthixol**, **fluphenazine**, **fluspirilene**, **haloperidol**, **levomepromazine**, **penfluridol**, **pipamperone**, **prothipendyl**, **sulpiride**, **thioridazine**, or **zuclopenthixol**. There was no evidence of any clinically relevant interactions, but there was some evidence that hypotension, tachycardia, sleepiness, tremor and constipation were more common, suggesting synergistic adverse effects.[13]

A fatal case of overdose with **moclobemide** and **perazine** was attributed to synergistic effects resulting in a functional cardiovascular disorder.[14]

Mechanism

Neuroleptic malignant syndrome is a rare condition associated with a reduction in dopamine activity in the brain, which has occurred with a wide variety of dopamine antagonists including the phenothiazines. It is unclear what role, if any, is played by the MAOIs in the few possible cases cited here. Note that MAOIs can cause the similar serotonin syndrome, and it is important to differentiate between the two conditions, especially because phenothiazines would aggravate neuroleptic malignant syndrome, but can successfully treat serotonin syndrome.

Importance and management

No additional precautions would normally seem to be necessary during the concurrent use of MAOIs and phenothiazines. However, bear in mind that serious, sometimes fatal, cases of neuroleptic malignant syndrome or hyperpyrexia have rarely occurred when an MAOI was given with chlorpromazine, levomepromazine or trifluoperazine. The role of the MAOI in these cases is unclear. There is also a possibility of additive hypotension with concurrent use of MAOIs and phenothiazines: consider an interaction should troublesome hypotension occur.

Note that the UK manufacturer of **promethazine** contraindicates the use of promethazine, both with and for 14 days after stopping an MAOI.[15] However, this is more likely to be due to a theoretical interaction involving the antihistamine properties of promethazine, see 'MAOIs + Antihistamines', p.1383.

Note that **chlorpromazine**[16] has serotonin antagonist activity, and been used successfully to treat serotonin syndrome occurring with MAOIs and other serotonergic drugs, but note that it should be avoided if neuroleptic malignant syndrome is a possible diagnosis, or if the patient is hypotensive.

1. Winkelman NW. Three evaluations of a monoamine oxidase inhibitor and phenothiazine combination (a methodological and clinical study). *Dis Nerv Syst* (1965) 26, 160–4.
2. Chesrow EJ, Kaplitz SE. Anxiety and depression in the geriatric and chronically ill patient. *Clin Med* (1965) 72, 1281–4.
3. Janecek J, Schiele BC, Bellville T, Anderson R. The effects of withdrawal of trifluoperazine on patients maintained on the combination of tranylcypromine and trifluoperazine. A double blind study. *Curr Ther Res* (1963) 5, 608–15.
4. Jones EM, Dawson A. Neuroleptic malignant syndrome: a case report with post-mortem brain and muscle pathology. *J Neurol Neurosurg Psychiatry* (1989) 52, 1006–9.
5. Penlington GN. Droperidol and monoamine-oxidase inhibitors. *BMJ* (1966) 1, 483–4.
6. Barsa JA, Saunders JC. A comparative study of tranylcypromine and pargyline. *Psychopharmacologia* (1964) 6, 295–8.
7. McQueen EG. New Zealand Committee on Adverse Drug Reactions: fourteenth annual report 1979. *N Z Med J* (1980) 91, 226–9.
8. Kline NS. Psychopharmaceuticals: effects and side effects. *Bull WHO* (1959) 21, 397–410.
9. Capron J-P, Gineston J-L, Opolon P, Dupas J-L, Denis J, Quénum C, Lorriaux A. Hépatite fulminante mortelle due a l'association iproniazide-prochlorpérazine: deux cas. *Gastroenterol Clin Biol* (1980) 4, 123–7.
10. Mitchell L. Psychotropic drugs. *BMJ* (1968) 1, 381.
11. Griffin JP, D'Arcy PF eds. A Manual of Adverse Drug Interactions. 2nd ed Bristol: Wright; 1979. p. 174.
12. Lappa A, Podestà M, Capelli O, Castagna A, Di Placido G, Alampi D, Semeraro F. Successful treatment of a complicated case of neuroleptic malignant syndrome. *Intensive Care Med* (2002) 28, 976–7.
13. Amrein R, Güntert TW, Dingemanse J, Lorscheid T, Stabl M, Schmid-Burgk W. Interactions of moclobemide with concomitantly administered medication: evidence from pharmacological and clinical studies. *Psychopharmacology (Berl)* (1992) 106, S24–S31.
14. Musshoff F, Varchmin-Schultheiss K, Madea B. Suicide with moclobemide and perazine. *Int J Legal Med* (1998) 111, 196–8.
15. Phenergan (Promethazine hydrochloride). Winthrop Pharmaceuticals UK Ltd. UK Summary of product characteristics, November 2008.
16. Graham PM. Successful treatment of the toxic serotonin syndrome with chlorpromazine. *Med J Aust* (1997) 166, 166–7.

MAOIs + Barbiturates

Although MAOIs can enhance and prolong the activity of barbiturates in *animals*, only a few isolated cases of adverse responses attributed to an interaction have been described.

Clinical evidence

One reviewer[1] briefly mentions that on three or four occasions patients taking an MAOI continued, without the prescriber's knowledge, to take their usual barbiturate hypnotic and thereby '...unknowingly raised their dose of barbiturate by five to ten times, and as a consequence barely managed to stagger through the day.' No details are given, so it is not known whether the barbiturate levels of these patients were measured, or whether the raised levels are only a surmise.

A patient taking **tranylcypromine** 10 mg three times daily was inadvertently given intramuscular **amobarbital sodium** 250 mg for sedation. Within one hour she became ataxic, and fell to the floor, repeatedly hitting her head. After complaining of nausea and dizziness the patient became semicomatose and remained in that state for a further 36 hours. To what extent the head trauma played a part is uncertain.[2]

A man taking **amobarbital sodium** 195 mg at night suffered severe headache, and became confused after also taking **phenelzine** 15 mg three times daily for 4 weeks. On admission to hospital he was comatose, and he had a temperature of 40°C, a blood pressure of 150/90 mmHg, tachycardia, stertorous respiration, fixed dilated pupils, exaggerated tendon reflexes and extensor plantar responses. His condition deteriorated and he died 2 hours after admission.[3] Pathology suggested a rise in intracranial pressure was responsible. The authors attributed this response to the drugs, but did not rule out a possible contribution of alcohol.[3]

Mechanism

Not known. *Animal* studies[2,4] show that MAOIs prolong the activity of barbiturates, and that this is possibly because they inhibit the metabolism of barbiturates by a mechanism independent of MAO inhibition. Whether this occurs in man as well is uncertain.

Importance and management

The evidence for an interaction between the MAOIs and the barbiturates seems to be confined to a few unconfirmed anecdotal reports with amobarbital. There is no well-documented evidence showing that concurrent use should be avoided, although some caution is clearly appropriate as the occasional patient may experience profound sedation.

For mention of successful anaesthesia including the use of thiopental in patients taking MAOIs, see 'Anaesthetics, general + MAOIs and related drugs', p.107.

1. Kline NS. Psychopharmaceuticals: effects and side effects. *Bull WHO* (1959) 21, 397–410.
2. Domino EF, Sullivan TS, Luby ED. Barbiturate intoxication in a patient treated with a MAO inhibitor. *Am J Psychiatry* (1962) 118, 941–3.
3. MacLeod I. Fatal reaction to phenelzine. *BMJ* (1965) 1, 1554.
4. Buchel L, Lévy J. Mécanisme des phénomènes de synergie du sommeil expérimental. II. Étude des associations iproniazide-hypnotiques, chez le rat et la souris. *Arch Sci Physiol (Paris)* (1965) 19, 161–79.

MAOIs or RIMAs + Benzodiazepines

Isolated case reports describe adverse reactions (chorea, severe headache, facial flushing, and severe oedema), which have been attributed to interactions between phenelzine and chlordiazepoxide, clonazepam or nitrazepam, and between isocarboxazid and chlordiazepoxide.

Evidence from clinical studies suggests that there is no interaction between moclobemide and benzodiazepines, although one study found a slight progressive worsening in driving performance.

Clinical evidence and mechanism

(a) MAOIs

1. Chlordiazepoxide. A patient with depression responded well when given **phenelzine** 15 mg and chlordiazepoxide 10 mg three times a day, but 4 to 5 months later developed choreiform movements of moderate severity, and slight dysarthria. These symptoms subsided when both drugs were withdrawn.[1] Two patients taking chlordiazepoxide and either **phenelzine** or **isocarboxazid** developed severe oedema, which was attributed to concurrent use.[2,3] A patient became unconscious and hyperreflexic, with a low blood pressure (100/60 mmHg), increased heart rate (100 bpm), and increased temperature (38.4°C) about 29 hours after taking an overdose of **phenelzine** and chlordiazepoxide.[4] Another report briefly mentions a case of prolonged coma lasting 3 days in a patient who overdosed with **phenelzine** and chlordiazepoxide.[5]

2. Clonazepam. A patient who had been taking **phenelzine** 45 mg daily for 9 years developed a severe occipital headache after taking 500 micrograms of clonazepam. A similar but milder headache occurred the next night when she again took clonazepam 500 micrograms. No blood pressure measurements were taken.[6] Another report describes facial flushing in a patient taking clonazepam, which occurred after **phenelzine** was started, and which responded to a reduction in the clonazepam dose.[7]

3. Nitrazepam. A patient taking **phenelzine** 30 mg twice daily started to take nitrazepam 5 mg at night, which was gradually increased to 15 mg at night over 2 months. He developed MAOI toxicity (excessive sweating, postural hypotension) within 10 days of increasing his dose of nitrazepam to 15 mg daily. Both drugs were stopped and he recovered after 3 days. **Phenelzine** was restarted 2 weeks later without problems. It was suggested that because the patient was a slow acetylator, metabolism of nitrazepam by *N*-acetyl transferase would have been decreased, which may have affected the metabolism of **phenelzine**, thereby increasing its levels.[8]

(b) RIMAs

A meta-analysis of 879 patients taking **moclobemide** is reported to have found that insomnia, restlessness, agitation and anxiety occurred twice as often in the 467 patients taking one or more benzodiazepines than in those not taking concurrent benzodiazepines. However, these adverse events were often already present when **moclobemide** was started, so it is suggested that the patient groups were probably different. Apart from this difference between the patient groups, there was no evidence of any relevant pharmacokinetic or pharmacodynamic interaction.[9] Another review briefly reported that no clinically relevant interaction was noted between **moclobemide** and benzodiazepines in clinical studies.[10]

In a double-blind study in depressed patients given **moclobemide** (22 subjects) or fluoxetine (19 subjects), driving performance gradually worsened over 6 weeks. Thirty-one patients were taking long-term benzodiazepines, and at the start of the study their driving was no different to the patients not taking benzodiazepines. In an attempt to suggest a possible reason for the worsening performance, various variables were assessed in a regression analysis. It was found that patients taking **moclobemide** who were also taking a benzodiazepine with nordiazepam among its metabolites (**clorazepate**, **prazepam**, **diazepam**, **cloxazolam**, **clotiazepam**) experienced a progressive worsening in their driving, whereas patients taking other benzodiazepines (**bromazepam**, **alprazolam**, **oxazepam**, **lorazepam**) tended to have no change in driving ability. It was tentatively suggested that **moclobemide** may have inhibited the metabolism of nordiazepam by the cytochrome P450 isoenzyme CYP2C19, so increasing the effect of the benzodiazepine, and worsening driving performance.[11]

Importance and management

The case reports of adverse interactions between the MAOIs or moclobemide and the benzodiazepines that are cited here appear to be isolated, and some involve drug overdoses, so it is by no means certain that all the responses were in fact due to drug interactions. Indeed, the manufacturer of moclobemide states that if patients with depression associated with excitation or agitation are first treated with moclobemide, a sedative, such as a benzodiazepine, should also be given for up to 2 to 3 weeks.[12]

No additional precautions would normally appear to be required during concurrent use, although a reminder that the benzodiazepines may affect the performance of skilled tasks, such as driving, may be appropriate when a patient's medication is changed.

1. Macleod DM. Chorea induced by tranquillisers. *Lancet* (1964) i, 388–9.
2. Goonewardene A, Toghill PJ. Gross oedema occurring during treatment for depression. *BMJ* (1977) 1, 879–80.
3. Pathak SK. Gross oedema during treatment for depression. *BMJ* (1977) 1, 1220.
4. Young S, Walpole BG. Tranylcypromine and chlordiazepoxide intoxication. *Med J Aust* (1986) 144, 166–7.
5. Denton PH, Borrelli VM, Edwards NV. Dangers of monoamine oxidase inhibitors. *BMJ* (1962) 2, 1752–3.
6. Eppel AB. Interaction between clonazepam and phenelzine. *Can J Psychiatry* (1990) 35, 647.
7. Karagianis JL, March H. Flushing reaction associated with the interaction of phenelzine and clonazepam. *Can J Psychiatry* (1991) 36, 389.
8. Harris AL, McIntyre N. Interaction of phenelzine and nitrazepam in a slow acetylator. *Br J Clin Pharmacol* (1981) 12, 254–5.
9. Amrein R, Güntert TW, Dingesmanse J, Lorscheid T, Stabl M, Schmid-Burgk W. Interactions of moclobemide with concomitantly administered medication: evidence from pharmacological and clinical studies. *Psychopharmacology (Berl)* (1992) 106, S24–S31.
10. Zimmer R, Gieschke R, Fischbach R, Gasic S. Interaction studies with moclobemide. *Acta Psychiatr Scand* (1990) 82 (Suppl 360), 84–6.
11. Ramaekers JG, Ansseau M, Muntjewerff ND, Sweens JP, O'Hanlon JF. Considering the P450 cytochrome system as determining combined effects of antidepressants and benzodiazepines on actual driving performance of depressed outpatients. *Int Clin Psychopharmacol* (1997) 12, 159–69.
12. Manerix (Moclobemide). Meda Pharmaceuticals. UK Summary of product characteristics, September 2009.

MAOIs or RIMAs + Beta-agonist bronchodilators

A patient with asthma taking phenelzine developed tachycardia and apprehension after salbutamol (albuterol) was started. Hypomania was seen in another patient with asthma taking phenelzine when inhaled isoetarine was started. A woman taking toloxatone and phenylephrine had a hypertensive crisis when she was given [oral] terbutaline.

Clinical evidence

(a) MAOIs

A report briefly describes a case of tachycardia and apprehension in a patient taking **phenelzine** when **salbutamol** (**albuterol**) was started (route of administration not stated).[1] Hypomania developed in a patient taking **phenelzine** in the few weeks after inhaled **isoetarine** 680 micrograms up to every 4 hours was started.[2]

(b) RIMAs

A 72-year old woman taking long-term levothyroxine, **toloxatone** 400 mg daily (for 2 months), and **phenylephrine** (for 3 weeks) developed episodes of hypertension, sweating, tachycardia, and headache within 3 days after starting to take [oral] **terbutaline** 10 mg daily. She was found to have extremely high plasma catecholamine concentrations. All drugs were stopped on admission to hospital and she recovered over 2 to 3 days.[3] An interaction between phenylephrine and toloxatone might have contributed to the effects seen (see 'MAOIs or RIMAs + Phenylephrine', p.1399).

Mechanism

Note that drugs with directly-acting sympathomimetic effects (of which the beta agonists are an example) do not normally interact to cause hypertension with MAOIs (for a full discussion of the interaction, see 'MAOIs or RIMAs + Inotropes and Vasopressors', p.1392). However, phenylephrine (a directly-acting sympathomimetic that has some indirect sympathomimetic effects) might have contributed to the reaction between toloxatone and terbutaline. The reaction in the patient taking phenelzine and isoetarine resulting in hypomania is not understood.

Importance and management

Evidence for an interaction between the MAOIs or RIMAs and the beta-agonist bronchodilators appears to be limited to these isolated cases, and are not consistent with the expected pharmacological effects of the combinations. The reported reactions, therefore appear to be idiosyncratic and not indicative of an interaction of general clinical importance. Nevertheless, on the basis of interactions with other sympathomimetic drugs, (when it was available) the UK manufacturer of **fenoterol (with ipratropium)** advised caution if MAOIs were also given.[4] The UK and US manufacturers of **olodaterol** also advise caution and predict that cardiovascular effects might be increased in patients taking olodaterol with MAOIs.[5,6] Similarly, the US manufacturers of **vilanterol** predict that its cardiovascular effects might be increased if given with, or within 2 weeks of stopping, MAOIs.[7,8] It would therefore seem prudent to be alert for potential cardiac effects, such as tachycardia, on concurrent use of these beta-agonist bronchodilators and MAOIs.

1. Shader RI, Greenblatt DJ. MAOIs and drug interactions—a proposal for a clearinghouse. *J Clin Psychopharmacol* (1985) 5, A17.
2. Goldman LS, Tiller JA. Hypomania related to phenelzine and isoetharine interaction in one patient. *J Clin Psychiatry* (1987) 48, 170.
3. Lefebvre H, Richard R, Noblet C, Moore N, Wolf L-M. Life-threatening pseudo-phaeochromocytoma after toloxatone, terbutaline, and phenylephrine. *Lancet* (1993) 341, 555–6.
4. Duovent UDVs (Fenoterol hydrobromide with Ipratropium bromide). Boehringer Ingelheim Ltd. UK Summary of product characteristics, January 2009.
5. Striverdi Respimat (Olodaterol hydrochloride). Boehringer Ingelheim Ltd. UK Summary of product characteristics, October 2013.
6. Striverdi Respimat (Olodaterol hydrochloride). Boehringer Ingelheim Pharmaceuticals Inc. US Prescribing information, July 2014.
7. Breo Ellipta (Fluticasone furoate with Vilanterol). GlaxoSmithKline. US Prescribing information, April 2015.
8. Anoro Ellipta (Umeclidinium with Vilanterol). GlaxoSmithKline. US Prescribing information, May 2014.

MAOIs or RIMAs + Beta blockers

Cases of bradycardia have been reported in patients taking nadolol or metoprolol with phenelzine. MAOIs commonly cause hypotension, and might reasonably be expected to have additive blood pressure-lowering effects with the beta blockers, although this was not seen with phenelzine and atenolol in one study.

In one small study, the RIMA, moclobemide increased the hypotensive effect of metoprolol.

Clinical evidence, mechanism, importance and management

(a) MAOIs

It had been claimed[1] that MAOIs should be discontinued at least 2 weeks before starting **propranolol**, but studies in *animals*[2] using **mebanazine** as a representative MAOI did not show any significant change in the cardiovascular effects of **propranolol** following the use of an MAOI. However, bradycardia of 46 to 53 bpm has been described in two patients taking **nadolol** 40 mg or **metoprolol** 150 mg daily for hypertension within 8 to 11 days of starting **phenelzine** 60 mg daily. No noticeable adverse effects were seen, but the authors recommended careful monitoring, particularly in the elderly, who may tolerate bradycardia poorly.[3]

The US manufacturers of **isocarboxazid**[4] and **tranylcypromine**[5] contraindicate concurrent use with antihypertensives (which would reasonably be expected to include the beta blockers): other manufacturers of MAOIs caution concurrent use. Some UK manufacturers of beta blockers (e.g. **pindolol** and **celiprolol**) also state that the combination of beta blockers with MAOIs is not recommended,[6,7] and add that there is a theoretical risk of hypertension if a beta blocker is given up to 14 days after stopping an MAOI,[6] whilst the manufacturers of other beta blockers (namely **acebutolol** and **bisoprolol**) suggest caution on concurrent use, on the grounds that significant hypertension may theoretically occur.[8,9]

MAOIs can cause symptomatic *hypotension*, and therefore additive blood pressure-lowering effects may occur in patients also taking beta blockers. Some manufacturers of beta blockers warn of this risk,[8,10,11] and also of a possible risk of bradycardia.[11] However, in one small study in normotensive patients with migraine, 11 patients (33%) had orthostatic hypotension when they were given **phenelzine** alone, but none of these had orthostatic hypotension when they were also given **atenolol**.[12] Despite these findings, given the known effects of both groups of drugs, it would seem prudent to monitor blood pressure (for either hypotension or hypertension) and heart rate more closely in patients taking a beta blocker with an MAOI.

(b) RIMAs

A study in 5 subjects with hypertension taking **metoprolol** found that **moclobemide** 200 mg three times daily for 2 weeks increased the hypotensive effect of **metoprolol** (systolic blood pressure 10 to 15 mmHg lower, diastolic blood pressure 5 to 10 mmHg lower).[13] Note that in this study moclobemide did not alter the blood pressure-lowering effects of hydrochlorothiazide or nifedipine, see 'Moclobemide + Hydrochlorothiazide or Nifedipine', p.1406.

The reason for this effect is not clear, but until more is known it may be prudent to be aware that **moclobemide** may possibly increase the blood pressure-lowering effects of **metoprolol**.

1. Frieden J. Propranolol as an antiarrhythmic agent. *Am Heart J* (1967) 74, 283–5.
2. Barrett AM, Cullum VA. Lack of inter-action between propranolol and mebanazine. *J Pharm Pharmacol* (1968) 20, 911–15.
3. Reggev A, Vollhardt BR. Bradycardia induced by an interaction between phenelzine and beta blockers. *Psychosomatics* (1989) 30, 106–8.
4. Marplan (Isocarboxazid). Validus Pharmaceuticals, Inc. US Prescribing information, August 2007.
5. Parnate (Tranylcypromine sulfate). GlaxoSmithKline. US Prescribing information, May 2010.
6. Visken Tablets (Pindolol). Amdipharm. UK Summary of product characteristics, January 2005.
7. Celectol (Celiprolol hydrochloride). Winthrop Pharmaceuticals UK Ltd. UK Summary of product characteristics, March 2009.
8. Cardicor (Bisoprolol hemifumarate). Merck Serono. UK Summary of product characteristics, February 2010.
9. Sectral Capsules (Acebutolol hydrochloride). Sanofi-Aventis. UK Summary of product characteristics, November 2006.
10. Atenolol Tablets. Wockhardt UK Ltd. UK Summary of product characteristics, March 2008.
11. Eucardic (Carvedilol). Roche Products Ltd. UK Summary of product characteristics, July 2007.
12. Merikangas KR, Merikangas JR. Combination monoamine oxidase inhibitor and β-blocker treatment of migraine, with anxiety and depression. *Biol Psychiatry* (1995) 38, 603–10.
13. Amrein R, Güntert TW, Dingemanse J, Lorscheid T, Stabl M, Schmid-Burgk W. Interactions of moclobemide with concomitantly administered medication: evidence from pharmacological and clinical studies. *Psychopharmacology (Berl)* (1992) 106, S24–S31.

MAOIs and related drugs + Bupropion

Although a theoretical interaction is predicted to occur between the MAOIs and bupropion, there is little clinical evidence of serious problems. Orthostatic hypotension occurred in a patient given bupropion and the MAO-B inhibitor selegiline.

Clinical evidence, mechanism, importance and management

In an uncontrolled study, 10 patients were treated for major affective disorder (8 unipolar, 2 bipolar) with bupropion in daily doses of 225 to 450 mg and an MAOI: **isocarboxazid** (1 patient), **phenelzine** (5), **tranylcypromine** (2), and the MAO-B inhibitor **selegiline** (2). Four were transferred from the MAOI to bupropion without any washout period, and the other 6 were given both drugs concurrently. No untoward cardiovascular events occurred in most patients, although one patient taking bupropion and **selegiline**, developed orthostatic hypotension. Notable weight loss occurred in two others when they were transferred from the MAOI to bupropion.[1] A review of the published literature (Medline search from 1962 to 2003) found no documented reports of hypertensive crises or fatalities when a stimulant drug (including bupropion) was cautiously added to an MAOI, although orthostatic hypotension and elevated blood pressure were reported.[2] In addition, one case report describes intraoperative hypertension with bupropion and linezolid, which has weak MAOI activity (see 'Bupropion + Linezolid', p.1469). The US manufacturer of bupropion notes that, in studies in *animals*, the acute toxicity of bupropion was enhanced by **phenelzine**.[3]

There is little clinical evidence of serious problems when MAOIs and bupropion are given together; however, both bupropion and the MAOIs might theoretically lead to an increase in catecholamines by different pathways. For this reason, the manufacturers contraindicate concurrent use and recommend that at least 14 days should elapse between stopping an irreversible MAOI and starting bupropion.[3,4] This precaution would therefore apply particularly to the non-selective MAOIs (**phenelzine, tranylcypromine, isocarboxazid** etc.). For **moclobemide**, the manufacturers advise that a 24-hour washout period is sufficient before starting bupropion.[4]

1. Abuzzahab, FS. Combination therapy: monoamino oxidase inhibitors and bupropion HCl. *Neuropsychopharmacology* (1994) 10, 74S.
2. Feinberg SS. Combining stimulants with monoamine oxidase inhibitors: a review of uses and one possible additional indication. *J Clin Psychiatry* (2004) 65, 1520–4.
3. Zyban (Bupropion hydrochloride). GlaxoSmithKline. US Prescribing information, March 2014.
4. Zyban (Bupropion hydrochloride). GlaxoSmithKline UK. UK Summary of product characteristics, November 2013.

MAOIs + Buspirone

Cases of elevated blood pressure have been reported in patients taking buspirone and either phenelzine or tranylcypromine.

Clinical evidence, mechanism, importance and management

Four cases of significant blood pressure elevation, which occurred during the use of buspirone and either **phenelzine** or **tranylcypromine**, have been reported to the Spontaneous Reporting System of the FDA in the US. One patient was a 75-year-old woman and the other 3 patients were men aged between 30 and 42 years. The report does not say how much the blood pressure rose, or how quickly, and no other details are given.[1] On the basis of this rather sparse information the manufacturers of buspirone[2,3] recommend that it should not be used concurrently with an MAOI, and the manufacturer of tranylcypromine contraindicates concurrent use and states that at least 10 days should elapse between stopping the MAOI and starting buspirone.[4]

1. Anon. BuSpar Update. *Psychiatry Drug Alert* (1987) 1, 43.
2. Buspar (Buspirone hydrochloride). Bristol-Myers Pharmaceuticals. UK Summary of product characteristics, May 2008.
3. BuSpar (Buspirone hydrochloride). Bristol-Myers Squibb Company. US Prescribing information, November 2010.
4. Parnate (Tranylcypromine sulfate). GlaxoSmithKline. US Prescribing information, May 2010.

MAOIs + Cocaine

Some reports suggest that patients taking MAOIs may experience a severe headache if they abuse cocaine. Two isolated reports describe the delayed development of hyperpyrexia, and other symptoms including coma, agitation, muscle tremors and rigidity, after patients taking phenelzine or iproniazid were given a cocaine spray during surgery.

Clinical evidence, mechanism, importance and management

The use of cocaine is generally contraindicated in patients taking MAOIs[1-4] because it is expected to interact in the same way as some of the nasal decongestants (see 'MAOIs or RIMAs + Nasal decongestants and related drugs', p.1396). This prediction is supported by a report of hypertensive reactions in 2 patients taking **phenelzine** who became drunk and used cocaine. Both experienced frightening reactions including headache, a rise in blood pressure, palpitations, and chest tightness. One required no treatment, and the other was treated with propranolol and diazepam.[5] Because this reaction was not considered as dangerous as expected, **phenelzine** has been tried as a deterrent to the abuse of cocaine: one uncontrolled study reports its use in 26 patients without mentioning any adverse reactions.[5] Another report mentions a man given **phenelzine** for cocaine abuse who experienced no reaction to the use of cocaine. He was then given **tranylcypromine**, and after 10 weeks risked sniffing cocaine, which did produce a severe occipital headache and nausea. However, after abstaining from cocaine for 10 weeks he again used cocaine, this time without any reaction.[6]

A man taking **phenelzine** 15 mg twice daily underwent vocal chord surgery. He was anaesthetised with thiopental, and later nitrous oxide and isoflurane 0.5% in oxygen. Muscle paralysis was produced with suxamethonium and gallamine. During the operation his vocal chords were sprayed with 1 mL of a 10% cocaine spray. He regained consciousness 30 minutes after the surgery and was returned to the ward, but a further 30 minutes later he was found unconscious, with generalised coarse tremors and marked muscle rigidity. His rectal temperature was 41.5°C. He was initially thought to have malignant hyperpyrexia and was treated accordingly with wet blankets, as well as with intravenous fluids and oxygen, and he largely recovered within 7 hours. However, later it seemed more likely that the reaction had been due to an adverse interaction between the **phenelzine** and cocaine, because he had been similarly and uneventfully treated with cocaine in the absence of **phenelzine** on two previous occasions.[7] In a similar case, a woman taking **iproniazid** had her trachea sprayed with 1 mL of 10% cocaine before intubation during surgery. She was also given pethidine (meperidine) 20 mg, and shortly after surgery became pyrexial, flushed, agitated and sweated profusely. She was treated with intravenous chlorpromazine.[8] In this case, the reaction could have been due to the pethidine alone (see 'MAOIs or RIMAs + Opioids; Pethidine (Meperidine)', p.1399), or both the cocaine and the pethidine. The reasons for these adverse reactions are not understood, but a delayed excitatory reaction due to increased serotonin (5-HT) concentrations has been suggested.[7]

The general importance of these cases is not known, but bear them in mind if cocaine is used by a patient taking an MAOI.

1. Nardil (Phenelzine sulfate). Archimedes Pharma UK Ltd. UK Summary of product characteristics, October 2008.
2. Nardil (Phenelzine sulfate). Pfizer Inc. US Prescribing information, February 2009.
3. Parnate (Tranylcypromine sulfate). GlaxoSmithKline. US Prescribing information, May 2010.
4. Marplan (Isocarboxazid). Validus Pharmaceuticals, Inc. US Prescribing information, August 2007.
5. Golwyn DH. Cocaine abuse treated with phenelzine. *Int J Addict* (1988) 23, 897–905.
6. Brewer C. Treatment of cocaine abuse with monoamine oxidase inhibitors. *Br J Psychiatry* (1993) 163, 815–16.
7. Tordoff SG, Stubbing JF, Linter SPK. Delayed excitatory reaction following interaction of cocaine and monoamine oxidase inhibitor (phenelzine). *Br J Anaesth* (1991) 66, 516–18.
8. Clement AJ, Benazon D. Reactions to other drugs in patients taking monoamine-oxidase inhibitors. *Lancet* (1962) 2, 197–8.

MAOIs + Dexfenfluramine or Fenfluramine

The concurrent use of MAOIs and dexfenfluramine or fenfluramine may theoretically increase the risk of serotonin syndrome. A case of headache, neck stiffness and nausea has been reported in a patient taking phenelzine with fenfluramine.

Clinical evidence, mechanism, importance and management

A woman taking **phenelzine** developed severe headache, neck stiffness and nausea within one hour of taking fenfluramine 20 mg. She then collapsed and remained stuporous for about 4 hours.[1] The authors considered this reaction to be similar to that seen with the MAOIs and amfetamines (see 'MAOIs or RIMAs + Amfetamines and related drugs', p.1383).

The manufacturer had recommended that fenfluramine should not be used in patients with a history of depression, or during treatment with antidepressants (especially the MAOIs), and there should be an interval of 3 weeks between stopping the MAOIs and starting fenfluramine.[2] The manufacturer of dexfenfluramine similarly contraindicated its use with or within 2 weeks of stopping an MAOI,[3] and advised waiting 3 weeks between stopping dexfenfluramine and starting an MAOI. This is due to the potential risk of serotonin syndrome,[4,5] which has rarely occurred with the concurrent use of two or more serotonergic drugs (for more information on this syndrome, see 'Drugs that cause serotonin syndrome + Other drugs that cause serotonin syndrome', p.1471). However, as of 1997 the UK manufacturer of dexfenfluramine and fenfluramine had found no clinical evidence of serious problems with either of these drugs when taken with MAOIs,[6] so that the published warnings about possible interactions would appear to be based on theoretical considerations.

Note that dexfenfluramine and fenfluramine have generally been withdrawn because their use was found to be associated with a high incidence of abnormal echocardiograms indicating abnormal functioning of heart valves.

1. Brandon S. Unusual effect of fenfluramine. *BMJ* (1969) 4, 557–8.
2. Ponderax Pacaps (Fenfluramine). Servier Laboratories Ltd. ABPI Compendium of Data Sheets and Summaries of Product Characteristics 1998–9, p. 1307.
3. Adifax (Dexfenfluramine). Servier Laboratories Ltd. ABPI Compendium of Data Sheets and Summaries of Product Characteristics 1998–9, p. 1302.
4. Dolan JA, Amchin J, Albano D. Potential hazard of serotonin syndrome associated with dexfenfluramine hydrochloride (Redux): Reply. *JAMA* (1996) 276, 1220–1.
5. Schenck CH, Mahowald MW. Potential hazard of serotonin syndrome associated with dexfenfluramine hydrochloride (Redux). *JAMA* (1996) 276, 1220.
6. Servier Laboratories Ltd. Personal communication, July 1997.

MAOIs or RIMAs + Dextromethorphan and related cough suppressants

Two fatal cases of hyperpyrexia and coma (symptoms similar to serotonin syndrome) have occurred in patients taking dextromethorphan with phenelzine. Three other serious reactions occurred in patients taking dextromethorphan with isocarboxazid or phenelzine. The related cough suppressant, pholcodine, is predicted to interact similarly.

Moclobemide inhibits the metabolism of dextromethorphan, and isolated cases of severe CNS reactions have occurred on concurrent use.

Clinical evidence

(a) MAOIs

A woman taking **phenelzine** 15 mg four times daily complained of nausea and dizziness before collapsing, 30 minutes after drinking about 55 mL of a cough mixture containing dextromethorphan. She remained hyperpyrexic (42°C), hypotensive (systolic blood pressure below 70 mmHg) and unconscious for 4 hours, before she had a cardiac arrest and died.[1]

A 15-year-old girl taking **phenelzine** 15 mg three times daily (as well as thioridazine, procyclidine and metronidazole) took 13 capsules of *Romilar CF* (each capsule contained dextromethorphan hydrobromide 15 mg, phenindamine tartrate 6.25 mg, phenylephrine hydrochloride 5 mg and paracetamol (acetaminophen) 120 mg). She became comatose, hyperpyrexic (about 39.4°C), had a blood pressure of 100/60 mmHg, a pulse of 160 bpm and later died of a cardiac arrest.[2] This case is complicated by the overdose and multiplicity of drugs present, particularly the phenylephrine, which may also interact, see 'MAOIs or RIMAs + Phenylephrine', p.1399.

Three other case reports describe muscle spasms or rigidity, sweating, nausea or tremor in patients who took *Robitussin DM* (dextromethorphan hydrobromide 15 mg with guaifenesin 100 mg) and **phenelzine** or **isocarboxazid**.[3-5] One patient responded to 10 mg of intravenous diazepam and oral activated charcoal within 2 hours,[4] and the symptoms of another patient gradually resolved over 19 hours.[5]

In addition to these cases, the US manufacturer of **tranylcypromine** notes that the concurrent use of MAOIs and dextromethorphan has resulted in brief episodes of psychosis or bizarre behaviour.[6] Similarly, the US manufacturer of **phenelzine** mentions one case of drowsiness and bizarre behaviour when dextromethorphan lozenges were used by a patient taking phenelzine.[7]

(b) RIMAs

In 4 healthy subjects, **moclobemide** 300 mg twice daily for 9 days markedly reduced the *O*-demethylation of dextromethorphan 20-mg every 4 hours for 7 doses.[8] The manufacturer of moclobemide notes that isolated cases of severe CNS adverse reactions have been seen in patients also taking dextromethorphan.[9]

Note that the concurrent use of dextromethorphan may have contributed to a fatality involving the illicit use of **moclobemide** and ecstasy, see 'MAOIs or RIMAs + Amfetamines and related drugs', p.1383.

Mechanism

It has been suggested[3-5] that the effects may be due to an increase in serotonin activity in the CNS, caused by both the MAOIs and dextromethorphan. Symptoms similar to serotonin syndrome (hyperpyrexia, dilated pupils, hyperexcitability and motor restlessness) have been seen in *rabbits* given dextromethorphan and **nialamide**, phenelzine or **pargyline**.[10]

Moclobemide appears to inhibit the metabolism of dextromethorphan by the cytochrome P450 isoenzyme CYP2D6, and the combination may also cause adverse CNS effects, also possibly due to additive effects on serotonin. For more information about serotonin syndrome, see 'Drugs that cause serotonin syndrome + Other drugs that cause serotonin syndrome', p.1471.

Importance and management

Despite the very limited information available, the severity of the reactions indicates that patients taking MAOIs should avoid taking dextromethorphan: concurrent use is generally contraindicated both with and within 14 days of taking an MAOI. The manufacturer of moclobemide also contraindicates the concurrent use of dextromethorphan.[9] In addition, although direct evidence appears to be generally lacking, the related cough suppressant **pholcodine**, is similarly contraindicated with and for 14 days after the use of an MAOI.[11] Patients taking an MAOI or a RIMA should be warned that many non-prescription cough preparations contain these drugs.

1. Rivers N, Horner B. Possible lethal reaction between Nardil and dextromethorphan. *Can Med Assoc J* (1970) 103, 85.
2. Shamsie JC, Barriga C. The hazards of use of monoamine oxidase inhibitors in disturbed adolescents. *Can Med Assoc J* (1971) 104, 715.
3. Nierenberg DW, Semprebon M. The central nervous system serotonin syndrome. *Clin Pharmacol Ther* (1993) 53, 84–8.
4. Sauter D, Macneil P, Weinstein E, Azar A. Phenelzine sulfate-dextromethorphan interaction: a case report. *Vet Hum Toxicol* (1991) 33, 365.
5. Sovner R, Wolfe J. Interaction between dextromethorphan and monoamine oxidase inhibitor therapy with isocarboxazid. *N Engl J Med* (1988) 319, 1671.
6. Parnate (Tranylcypromine sulfate). GlaxoSmithKline. US Prescribing information, May 2010.
7. Nardil (Phenelzine sulfate). Pfizer Inc. US Prescribing information, February 2009.
8. Härtter S, Dingemanse J, Baier D, Ziegler G, Hiemke C. Inhibition of dextromethorphan metabolism by moclobemide. *Psychopharmacology (Berl)* (1998) 135, 22–6.
9. Manerix (Moclobemide). Meda Pharmaceuticals. UK Summary of product characteristics, September 2009.
10. Sinclair JG. Dextromethorphan-monoamine oxidase inhibitor interaction in rabbits. *J Pharm Pharmacol* (1973) 25, 803–8.
11. Pavacol-D (Pholcodine). Alliance Pharmaceuticals. UK Summary of product characteristics, May 2009.

MAOIs or RIMAs + Disulfiram

An isolated report describes delirium, which occurred when a man taking lithium, disulfiram and moclobemide had his moclobemide replaced with tranylcypromine.

Clinical evidence, mechanism, importance and management

A man with disulfiram implants taking long-term lithium was switched from **moclobemide** (dose not stated) to **tranylcypromine** 10 mg twice daily. Within 2 days he became acutely delirious (agitated, disoriented, incoherent, visual hallucinations) and later subcomatose, with nystagmus and a downward gaze. He was successfully treated with haloperidol and promethazine, and recovered within 24 hours. No alcohol was detected in his blood, and serum **tranylcypromine** levels were below 50 micrograms/L, which was considered normal.[1]

The authors of this report attribute the reaction to an interaction between **tranylcypromine** and disulfiram. However, there would seem to be other possible explanations for this reaction. MAOIs have rarely been seen to interact adversely with lithium (see 'MAOIs or RIMAs + Lithium', p.1394), and there also seems potential for an interaction between **moclobemide** and **tranylcypromine** (see 'MAOIs + MAOIs or RIMAs', p.1394). This seems to be the only report of an adverse reaction between disulfiram and an MAOI, so it also seems possible that this is just an idiosyncratic reaction. However, warnings about this drug combination, based on theoretical considerations and some studies in *animals*, have previously been given, and **tranylcypromine** was considered to be the MAOI that presented the greatest risk.[2] Consequently, the US manufacturers of **tranylcypromine**[3] and **isocarboxazid**[4] recommend caution with the concurrent use of disulfiram. Note that this particular patient did not seem to have any problems while taking **moclobemide**, which is a RIMA, with **disulfiram**.

1. Blansjaar BA, Egberts TCG. Delirium in a patient treated with disulfiram and tranylcypromine. *Am J Psychiatry* (1995) 152, 296.
2. Ciraulo DA. Can disulfiram (Antabuse) be safely co-administered with the monoamine oxidase inhibitor (MAOI) antidepressants? *J Clin Psychopharmacol* (1989) 9, 315–16.
3. Parnate (Tranylcypromine sulfate). GlaxoSmithKline. US Prescribing information, May 2010.
4. Marplan (Isocarboxazid). Validus Pharmaceuticals, Inc. US Prescribing information, August 2007.

MAOIs + Doxapram

No adverse interactions have been reported between the MAOIs and doxapram, although *animal* studies suggest that an increased pressor effect is theoretically possible.

Clinical evidence, mechanism, importance and management

The UK manufacturer notes that *animal* studies have shown that the actions of doxapram may be potentiated by pretreatment with an MAOI,[1] and that the pressor effects of MAOIs and doxapram may be additive.[2] Based on this, the manufacturers advise that concurrent use should be undertaken with great care.[1,2] To date, there appear to be no clinical reports of this interaction. Nevertheless, it may be prudent to consider blood pressure monitoring in patients given doxapram while taking an MAOI.

1. Doxapram hydrochloride. Mercury Pharma Group. UK Summary of product characteristics, March 2012.
2. Doxapram hydrochloride. Bedford Laboratories. US Prescribing information, March 2007.

MAOIs + Food; Broad bean pods

A few reports describe a rapid and potentially life-threatening hypertensive reaction when patients taking MAOIs ate young broad bean pods, which contain dopa.

Clinical evidence

A 65-year-old man with hypertension taking **pargyline** 37.5 mg daily had a severe headache and palpitations on two occasions after eating whole, cooked, broad beans (presumably young broad bean pods). A controlled study in this man found that he had a rise in systolic blood pressure from 165 mmHg to 262 mmHg about 20 minutes after eating whole broad bean pods. The pods alone had the same effect, but the beans on their own had little effect.[1] A similar rise in blood pressure with bradycardia and ECG changes was also seen in two other patients taking **pargyline**, and was reversed by intravenous phentolamine. Two normotensive subjects taking **pargyline** 50 mg daily also had an increase in blood pressure (over 70 mmHg systolic in one subject) after eating bean pods.[1] Another case report describes a man taking **phenelzine** 15 mg three times daily who had a very severe headache after eating a meal including fresh, young, sliced, broad bean pods from his garden.[2] One other case has been briefly mentioned, although it was not known whether the broad beans were eaten with or without the pods.[3]

Mechanism

The pods of the broad bean (*Vicia faba*) contain dopa,[1] which is enzymatically converted in the body, firstly to dopamine and then to noradrenaline (norepinephrine), both of which are normally broken down by monoamine oxidase. In the presence of an MAOI this breakdown is suppressed, causing an increase in the total levels of dopamine and noradrenaline. Precisely how this then leads to a sharp rise in blood pressure is not clear, but either dopamine or noradrenaline, or both, directly or indirectly stimulate the alpha receptors of the cardiovascular system.

Importance and management

Although there are only a few cases of the interaction between the non-selective MAOIs and broad bean pods, the interaction would appear to be established: it is serious and potentially life-threatening. Patients should not eat young broad bean *pods* during treatment with any of these MAOIs, nor for a period of 2 to 3 weeks after their withdrawal. It should be noted that this prohibition does not apply to 'mature' broad beans (the seeds) removed from their pods, which is the more common way of eating broad beans.

1. Hodge JV, Nye ER, Emerson GW. Monoamine-oxidase inhibitors, broad beans, and hypertension. *Lancet* (1964) i, 1108.
2. Blomley DJ. Monoamine-oxidase inhibitors. *Lancet* (1964) ii, 1181–2.
3. McQueen EG. Interactions with monoamine oxidase inhibitors. *BMJ* (1975) 4, 101.

MAOIs + Food; Monosodium glutamate

Anecdotal reports have attributed hypertension in patients taking MAOIs who had eaten certain foods (soy sauce, chicken nuggets) to an interaction with monosodium glutamate. However, a small controlled study found no evidence to support this idea, and the reaction was probably related to tyramine.

Clinical evidence

Five healthy subjects were given monosodium glutamate 400 mg to 1.6 g or a placebo with or without **tranylcypromine** for at least 2 weeks. Episodes of hypertension were seen in 2 subjects taking **tranylcypromine** with both placebo and monosodium glutamate, but no changes in blood pressure or heart rate occurred that could be attributed to an interaction while taking monosodium glutamate. The largest dose of monosodium glutamate used was about twice the amount usually found in meals with a high monosodium glutamate content.[1]

There have been anecdotal reports of hypertensive reactions in patients taking MAOIs that were attributed to interactions with the monosodium glutamate contained in soy sauce[2] and chicken nuggets.[3]

Mechanism

In large amounts, monosodium glutamate alone can cause a small rise in blood pressure, and MAOIs alone very occasionally cause hypertensive episodes. However, the reactions reported with soy sauce and chicken nuggets were probably due to a high tyramine content, as high levels of tyramine have subsequently been detected in some soy sauces,[4] see 'MAOIs or RIMAs + Food; Tyramine-containing', below.

Importance and management

An interaction between monosodium glutamate *per se* and MAOIs has not been established, although it should be pointed out that the number of subjects studied was very small. It is quite possible that the anecdotal reports were due to the tyramine content of the foods, and not to monosodium glutamate, see *Mechanism*, above. In Hong Kong, patients taking MAOIs are not advised to avoid monosodium glutamate, but are instructed to avoid excessive soy sauce because of its possible high tyramine content.[4]

1. Balon R, Pohl R, Yeragani VK, Berchou R, Gershon S. Monosodium glutamate and tranylcypromine administration in healthy subjects. *J Clin Psychiatry* (1990) 51, 303–6.
2. McCabe B, Tsuang MT. Dietary consideration in MAO inhibitor regimens. *J Clin Psychiatry* (1982) 43, 178–81.
3. Pohl R, Balon R, Berchou R. Reaction to chicken nuggets in a patient taking an MAOI. *Am J Psychiatry* (1988) 145, 651.
4. Lee S, Wing YK. MAOI and monosodium glutamate interaction. *J Clin Psychiatry* (1991) 52, 43.

MAOIs or RIMAs + Food; Tyramine-containing

A potentially life-threatening hypertensive reaction can develop in patients taking non-selective MAOIs (isocarboxazid, tranylcypromine, phenelzine) who consume foods or drinks rich in tyramine. In some cases deaths from intracranial haemorrhage have occurred.

Significant amounts of tyramine occur in some aged cheeses, yeast extracts (e.g. *Marmite*) and some types of salami. Caviar, pickled herrings, and soy sauce and other foods have also been implicated in this interaction. Note that any food high in aromatic amino acids can become high in tyramine if spoilage occurs or after storage. In addition, some beers or lagers, including those low in alcohol, or wines may contain sufficient tyramine to provoke a serious hypertensive reaction.

The RIMAs (moclobemide, toloxatone) interact with tyramine to a lesser extent.

Clinical evidence

A. Reactions to foods

(a) MAOIs

A rapid, serious, and potentially fatal rise in blood pressure can occur in patients taking MAOIs who ingest tyramine from certain foods. A violent occipital headache, pounding heart, neck stiffness, flushing, sweating, nausea and vomiting may be experienced. One of the earliest recorded observations specifically linking this reaction to **cheese** was in 1963 by a pharmacist called Rowe, who wrote to Blackwell[1] after seeing the reaction in his wife who was taking *Parstelin* (**tranylcypromine** with trifluoperazine).

'After **cheese on toast**; within a few minutes face flushed, felt very ill; head and heart pounded most violently, and perspiration was running down her neck. She vomited several times, and her condition looked so severe that I dashed over the road to consult her GP. He diagnosed 'palpitations' and agreed to call if the symptoms had not subsided in an hour. In fact the severity diminished and after about 3 hours she was normal, other than a severe headache — but 'not of the throbbing kind'. She described the early part of the attack 'as though her head must burst'.

Blackwell and his colleagues[1] discuss a series of 25 early cases, and the information that led to this interaction becoming established. **Tranylcypromine** was the most frequently implicated MAOI: of 25 cases, 17 were with **tranylcypromine**, 6 with **phenelzine** and one each with **pargyline** and **mebanazine**. In addition, **cheese** was the most frequently implicated food, being named in 18 of 25 cases, with *Marmite* (**yeast** extract) in 3 and **pickled herrings** in one. Four patients had intracranial haemorrhages and one died.[1] From 1961 up to February 1964 the FDA in the US found about 500 cases of induced hypertension with **tranylcypromine** and 38 cases of cerebral vascular accidents with 21 deaths. As a result, **tranylcypromine** was withdrawn in the US, although it was later reintroduced with many restrictions, including the need to avoid **cheese** while taking the drug.[2]

In addition to reactions to **cheese**, cases of hypertensive reactions have been reported with **avocados**,[3] **beef livers**[4] and **chicken livers**,[5] **caviar**,[6] **pickled herrings**,[7] **soused herrings**,[8] **tinned fish**,[8] **tinned milk**,[1] **peanuts**,[8] **soy sauce**,[9] **miso**,[10] a **powdered protein diet supplement** (*Ever-so-slim*[11] or *Complan*[1]), **packet soup** (containing hydrolysed **yeast**),[12] **sour cream** in coffee,[8] and **New Zealand prickly spinach**[13] (*Tetragonia tetragonoides*). [Note this is not a true spinach as found in the USA or Europe.] These reactions occurred with **tranylcypromine**,[3,5-9] **phenelzine**[4,10,11,13] or unspecified MAOIs.[8,12]

In addition, case reports of reactions with **ales**, **beers** and **lagers** have been published. A man taking **phenelzine** 60 mg daily developed a typical hypertensive reaction after drinking only 14 oz (about 400 mL) of **Upper Canada lager beer on tap** (containing about 113 mg of tyramine/L).[14] In addition, **alcohol-free beer** and **lager** may have a tyramine content that is equal to ordinary beer and lager.[15,16] One patient taking **tranylcypromine** suffered an acute cerebral haemorrhage after drinking a **de-alcoholised Irish beer**,[15] hypertensive reactions occurred in three other patients taking **tranylcypromine** or **phenelzine** after drinking no more than about 375 mL of **alcohol-free beer or lager**,[16] and a further patient taking **tranylcypromine** developed a vascular headache after drinking 3 bottles of **non-alcoholic beer**.[17]

A very extensive study of 79 different brands of beer (from Canada, England, France, Germany, Holland, Ireland, Scotland, USA) found that the tyramine content of the **bottled** and **canned beers** examined was generally too low to matter (less than 10 mg/L), but 4 of 37 **beers on tap** (all 4 were lagers) contained more than enough tyramine (27 to 113 mg/L) to cause a hypertensive reaction.[14]

In an isolated report, one author[18] anecdotally noted that some patients taking MAOIs who drank whiskey became drunk more easily than expected. There seem to be no reports of hypertensive reactions in patients taking MAOIs after drinking **spirits**, and none would be expected, see under *Mechanism*, below.

(b) RIMAs

There do not appear to be any published reports of the '**cheese** reaction' with **moclobemide**. The combination of *Bovril* (**yeast** extract) 12 g and **moclobemide** 150 mg, both three times daily, was used to normalise blood pressure in a patient with severe postural hypotension as a result of central autonomic failure.[19]

A 38-year-old man collapsed with tachycardia the morning after taking an overdose of **moclobemide** and drinking half a bottle of **whisky** (more than 350 mL). He then suffered a cardiac arrest and resuscitation was unsuccessful. His blood pressure was not recorded. The authors attributed this case to an interaction between **moclobemide** and tyramine,[20] although the tyramine content of the whisky was not assessed, so any interaction is not established, especially as whisky does not usually contain tyramine.

B. Tyramine studies

Pharmacodynamic studies comparing RIMAs with MAOIs using oral tyramine sensitivity tests have revealed that only 20 to 50 mg of oral tyramine (given with a meal) is required to raise the systolic blood pressure by 30 mmHg in subjects taking **tranylcypromine** 10 mg twice daily.[21] In other studies, the pressor tyramine dose was only 8 mg in those given **tranylcypromine**.[22] Other studies have reported the pressor tyramine dose as 15 mg[23] or 33 mg[22] in those taking **phenelzine**.

In a placebo-controlled study in healthy subjects, the mean dose of oral tyramine (added to a meal) required to raise systolic blood pressure by 30 mmHg (the tyramine 30 dose) was decreased fivefold (from 1450 mg to 306 mg, range 150 to 500 mg) by **moclobemide** 200 mg three times daily. In comparison, **tranylcypromine** 10 mg twice daily decreased the tyramine 30 dose about 38-fold.[21] In another study, the tyramine 30 dose was reduced 7-fold by **moclobemide** 150 mg three times daily, 13-fold by **phenelzine** 60 mg daily, and 55-fold by **tranylcypromine** 20 mg daily. After stopping the drugs, the pressor response to tyramine normalised within 3 days for **moclobemide**, and within 30 days for **tranylcypromine**. However, the pressor response had normalised in only 2 subjects 2 to 4 weeks after they stopped **phenelzine**, and had not normalised during the 11-week study period in the other 4 subjects.[22] In a further study the tyramine 30 dose was reduced about 4-fold by **moclobemide** 100 mg three times daily and 10.3-fold by **phenelzine** 15 mg three times daily.[24] Numerous other pharmacological studies have confirmed the low increase in pressor response to tyramine with **moclobemide**.[23,25-28]

The pressor response to oral tyramine 200 mg was not altered by pre-treatment with **toloxatone** 200 mg or 400 mg three times daily in healthy subjects, although the effect of higher doses of tyramine was increased.[29] Similar results were reported in an earlier study.[30]

Mechanism

Tyramine is an indirectly-acting sympathomimetic amine, one of its actions being to release noradrenaline (norepinephrine) from the adrenergic neurones associated with blood vessels, which causes a rise in blood pressure by stimulating their constriction.[3]

Table 32.2 The tyramine-content of some drinks

	Tyramine content (mg/L)	Refs
Ales, beers and lagers		
Beer (Canada)	0 to 11.2, 27.1, 29.5, 112.9	1,2
Beer (Former Czechoslovakia)	10.4, 47 to 60	3
Beer (Germany)	1	3
Beer (Ireland)	0.5 to 4, 54	2,3
Beer (Netherlands)	1	3
Beer (UK)	0.3 to 1.34	2-4
Beer (USA)	0.7 to 4.4	2,3,5
Low-alcohol beers	0 to 10	2,6
Wines		
Chianti (Italy)		
Governo process	1.8 to 10.4, 25.4	1,5
Newer process	0.0 to 4.7	3,4,7,8
Champagne	1, 13.7 to 18	3,9
Wine, red (Canada, France, Italy, Spain, USA)	0 to 8.6 (mean 5.2)	9
Wine, white (France, Germany, Italy, Portugal, Spain, Former Yugoslavia)	0.4 to 6.5	4,5,9
Fortified wines and spirits		
Gin	0	8
Port	Less than 0.2 (undetectable)	5
Sherry	0.2 to 3.6	1,3,5,8
Vodka	0	8
Whiskey	0	8

1. Sen NP. Analysis and significance of tyramine in foods. *J Food Sci* (1969) 34, 22-6.
2. Tailor SAN, Shulman KI, Walker SE, Moss J, Gardner D. Hypertensive episode associated with phenelzine and tap beer - a reanalysis of the role of pressor amines in beer. *J Clin Psychopharmacol* (1994) 14, 5-14.
3. Da Prada M, Zürcher G, Wüthrich I, Haefely WE. On tyramine, food, beverages and the reversible MAO inhibitor moclobemide. *J Neural Transm* (1988) (Suppl 26), 31.
4. Hannah P, Glover V, Sandler M. Tyramine in wine and beer. *Lancet* (1988) i, 879.
5. Horwitz D, Lovenberg W, Engelman K, Sjoerdsma A. Monoamine oxidase inhibitors, tyramine and cheese. *JAMA* (1964) 188, 1108-10.
6. Draper R, Sandler M, Walker PL. Clinical curio: monoamine oxidase inhibitors and non-alcoholic beer. *BMJ* (1984) 289, 308.
7. Korn A, Eichler HG, Fischbach R, Gasic S. Moclobemide, a new reversible MAO inhibitor - interaction with tyramine and tricyclic antidepressants in healthy volunteers and depressive patients. *Psychopharmacology (Berl)* (1986) 88, 153-7.
8. Shulman KI, Walker SE, MacKenzie S, Knowles S. Dietary restriction, tyramine, and use of monoamine oxidase inhibitors. *J Clin Psychopharmacol* (1989) 9, 397-402.
9. Zee JA, Simard RE, L'Heureux L, Tremblay J. Biogenic amines in wines. *Am J Enol Vitic* (1983) 34, 6-9.

Normally any ingested tyramine is rapidly metabolised by the enzyme monoamine oxidase in the gut wall and liver before it reaches the general circulation. However, if the activity of the enzyme at these sites is inhibited (by the presence of an MAOI), any tyramine passes freely into the circulation, causing not just a rise in blood pressure, but a highly exaggerated rise due to the release from the adrenergic neurones of the large amounts of noradrenaline that accumulate there during inhibition of MAO.[3] This final step in the interaction is identical to that which occurs with any other indirectly-acting sympathomimetic amine in the presence of an MAOI (see 'MAOIs or RIMAs + Nasal decongestants and related drugs', p.1396).

Tyramine is formed in foods such as cheese by the bacterial degradation of milk and other proteins, firstly to tyrosine and other amino acids, and the subsequent decarboxylation of the tyrosine to tyramine. This interaction is therefore not associated with fresh foods, but with those which have been allowed to over-ripen or 'mature' in some way,[3] or if spoilage occurs. Some ales, beers and lagers in 'social' amounts also contain enough tyramine to reach the 8 to 20 mg dose needed to provoke a reaction. However, **gin**, **whisky**, **vodka** and **other spirits** do not contain significant amounts of tyramine because they are distilled, and the volumes drunk are relatively small.[31] See 'Table 32.2', above, and 'Table 32.3', above, for a list of the tyramine content of some drinks and foods.

RIMAs such as moclobemide and toloxatone selectively inhibit MAO-A, which leaves MAO-B still available to metabolise tyramine. This means that they have less effect on the tyramine pressor response than non-selective MAOIs.

Table 32.3 The tyramine-content of some foods

Food	Tyramine content (mg/kg or mg/L)	Refs
Avocado	Higher in ripe fruit, 23, 0	1-3
Banana peel	52, 65	2,4
Banana pulp	7, 0	2-4
Caviar (Iranian)	680	5
Cheese - see Table 32.4, p.1391 and Pizza toppings, below		
Country cured ham	not detectable	6
Farmer salami sausage	314	6
Genoa salami sausage	0 to 1237 (average 534)	6
Hard salami	0 to 392 (average 210)	6
Herring (pickled)	3030	7
Lebanon bologna	0 to 333 (average 224)	6
Liver-chicken	94 to 113	8
Liver-beef	0 to 274	9
Orange pulp	10	2
Pepperoni sausage	0 to 195 (average 39)	6
Pizza toppings (cheese and pepperoni)	0 to 3.6 (0 to 0.38 mg on half a medium pizza)	10
Plum, red	6	2
Sauerkraut	55	4
Soy sauce	0 to 878	4,10-12
Soya bean curd (tofu)	0.6 to 16	10
Soya beans, fermented	713	12
Soya bean paste, fermented	206	12
Smoked landjaeger sausage	396	6
Summer sausage	184	6
Tomato	4, 0	2,3
Thuringer cervelat	0 to 162	6
Yeast extracts		
Bovril	200 to 500	13
Bovril beef cubes	200 to 500	13
Bovril chicken cubes	50 to 200	13
Marmite (UK product)	500 to 3000	3,4,13
Yoghurt	0 to 4	3,4,14

1. Generali JA, Hogan LC, McFarlane M, Schwab S, Hartman CR. Hypertensive crisis resulting from avocados and a MAO inhibitor. *Drug Intell Clin Pharm* (1981) 15, 904-6.
2. Udenfriend S, Lovenberg W, Sjoerdsma A. Physiologically active amines in common fruits and vegetables. *Arch Biochem* (1959) 85, 487.
3. Da Prada M, Zürcher G, Wüthrich I, Haefely WE. On tyramine, food, beverages and the reversible MAO inhibitor moclobemide. *J Neural Transm* (1988) (Suppl 26), 31-56.
4. Shulman KI, Walker SE, MacKenzie S, Knowles S. Dietary restriction, tyramine, and the use of monoamine oxidase inhibitors. *J Clin Psychopharmacol* (1989) 9, 397-402.
5. Isaac P, Mitchell B, Grahame-Smith DG. Monoamine-oxidase inhibitors and caviar. *Lancet* (1977) ii, 816.
6. Rice S, Eitenmiller RR, Koehler PE. Histamine and tyramine content of meat products. *J Milk Food Technol* (1975) 38, 256-8.
7. Nuessle WF, Norman FC, Miller HE. Pickled herring and tranylcypromine reaction. *JAMA* (1965) 192, 726.
8. Heberg DL, Gordon MW, Glueck BC. Six cases of hypertensive crisis in patients on tranylcypromine after eating chicken livers. *Am J Psychiatry* (1966) 122, 933-5.
9. Boulton AA, Cookson B, Paulton R. Hypertensive crisis in a patient on MAOI antidepressants following a meal of beef liver. *Can Med Assoc J* (1970) 102, 1394-5.
10. Shulman KI, Walker SE. Refining the MAOI diet: tyramine content of pizzas and soy products. *J Clin Psychiatry* (1999) 60, 191-3.
11. Lee S, Wing YK. MAOI and monosodium glutamate interaction. *J Clin Psychiatry* (1991) 52, 43.
12. Da Prada M, Zürcher G. Tyramine content of preserved and fermented foods or condiments of Far Eastern cuisine. *Psychopharmacology (Berl)* (1992) 106, S32-S34.
13. Clarke A. (Bovril Ltd). Personal communication (1987).
14. Horwitz D, Lovenberg W, Engelman K, Sjoerdsma A. Monoamine oxidase inhibitors, tyramine, and cheese. *JAMA* (1964) 188, 1108-10.

Table 32.4 The tyramine-content of some cheeses
This table is principally intended to show the extent and the variation that can occur

Variety of cheese	*Tyramine content (mg/kg)*	*Approximate mg/60g portion*	*Refs*
American processed	50	3	1
Argenti	188	11	2
Blue	31 to 997	2 to 60	2-4
Boursault	1116	67	3
Brick	194	12	2
Brie	3 to 473	0.2 to 28	1,4,5
Cambozola blue vein	18	1	4
Camembert	3 to 519	0.2 to 31	1-3,5
Cheddar	8 to 1530	0.5 to 92	2-6
Cheshire	24 to 418	1.4 to 25	5
Cream cheese	undetectable (less than 0.2), 9	0 to 0.5	1,4
Cottage cheese	undetectable (less than 0.2), 5	0 to 0.3	1,5
Danish Blue	31 to 743	2 to 45	3-5
d'Oka	158, 310	9.5, 19	2
Double Gloucester	43	2.6	5
Edam	100, 214	6, 13	2
Emmental	11 to 958	0.7 to 57	1,4,5
Feta	5.8, 20, 76	0.3 to 4.6	4-6
Gorgonzola	56 to 768	3.4 to 46	4,5
Gouda	54, 95	3.2, 5.7	2
Gouda type (Canadian)	20	1.2	3
Gourmandise	216	13	3
Gruyere	64 to 516	3.8 to 31	1,4,5,7
Kashar	44 (mean of seven samples)	2.6	7
Liederkrantz	1226, 1683	74, 101	2
Limburger	44 to 416	2.6, 25	2,5
Mozzarella	17 to 410	1 to 25	3-6
Munster	87 to 110	5.2 to 6.6	2,4,5
Mycella	1340	80	3
Parmesan	4 to 290	0.2 to 17	3-5
Provolone	38	2.3	3
Red Leicester	41	2.5	5
Ricotta	0	0	4
Romano	4, 197, 238	0.2 to 14	2,3,6
Roquefort	13 to 520	0.8 to 31	2,3,5
Stilton	359 to 2170	28 to 130	1,3-5
Tulum	208 (mean of seven samples)	12.5	7
White (Turkish)	17.5 (mean of seven samples)	1	7

1. Horwitz D, Lovenberg W, Engelman K, Sjoerdsma A. Monoamine oxidase inhibitors, tyramine and cheese. *JAMA* (1964) 188, 1108-10.
2. Kosikowsky FV, Dahlberg AC. The tyramine content of cheese. *J Dairy Sci* (1948) 31, 293-303.
3. Sen NP. Analysis and significance of tyramine in foods. *J Food Sci* (1969) 34, 22-6.
4. Shulman KI, Walker SE, MacKenzie S, Knowles S. Dietary restriction, tyramine, and the use of monoamine oxidase inhibitors. *J Clin Psychopharmacol* (1989) 9, 397-402.

Continued

Table 32.4 The tyramine-content of some cheeses (continued)
This table is principally intended to show the extent and the variation that can occur

5. Da Prada M, Zürcher G, Wüthrich I, Haefely WE. On tyramine, food, beverages and the reversible MAO inhibitor moclobemide. *J Neural Transm* (1988) (Suppl 26), 31-56.
6. Shulman KI, Walker SE. Refining the MAOI diet: tyramine content of pizzas and soy products. *J Clin Psychiatry* (1999) 60, 191-3.
7. Kayaalp SO, Renda N, Kaymakcalan S, Özer A. Tyramine content of some cheeses. *Toxicol Appl Pharmacol* (1970) 16, 459-60.

Importance and management

MAOIs

The interaction between MAOIs and tyramine found in some foodstuffs is extremely well-documented, well-established and serious (fatal in some cases).

Tranylcypromine seems more likely to cause the reaction than phenelzine (see under *Tyramine studies*, above). The incidence is uncertain, but early estimates of hypertensive reactions to tranylcypromine (before restrictions in its use with indirectly-acting sympathomimetics and foods) range from 0.03% to 20%.[2,32,33] Patients taking any of the non-selective MAOIs should not eat foods or drinks reported to contain substantial amounts of tyramine. As little as 8 to 20 mg of tyramine can raise the blood pressure in patients taking tranylcypromine, and this may be present in usual portions of hard cheeses.[22] In addition, avoidance of the prohibited foods should be continued for 2 to 3 weeks after stopping the MAOI to allow full recovery of the enzymes. However, note that in one study some patients took over 11 weeks to recover from the effects of phenelzine.[22]

'Table 32.2', p.1390, summarises the reported tyramine-content of some drinks, and 'Table 32.3', p.1390, summarises the reported tyramine-content of some foods: more extensive lists have been published elsewhere.[14,31,34] These can be used as a broad general guide when advising patients, but they cannot be an absolute guide. This is because tyramine levels vary so much it is impossible to guess the amount present in any food or drink. However, old, over-ripe strong smelling cheeses with a salty, biting taste or those with characteristic holes due to fermentation should be avoided as they generally contain high levels of tyramine. Fresh cheeses made from pasteurised milk tend to have lower levels of tyramine.[35] The tyramine-content can even differ significantly within a single cheese: the centre having the lowest levels of tyramine and the rind containing the most.[35,36] There is no guarantee that patients who have uneventfully eaten these hazardous foodstuffs on many occasions may not eventually experience a full-scale hypertensive crisis, if all the many variables conspire together.[37] Similarly, alcoholic drinks are the end product of a biological fermentation process and no two batches are ever absolutely identical. For example there may be a 50-fold difference even between wines from the same grape stock.[38]

The need to plan a sensible and safe diet for those taking MAOIs is clear, and over the years attempts have been made to produce simplified, practical diets for those taking MAOIs.[39-46] A total prohibition should be imposed on the following:

- **aged cheese**;
- **yeast extracts** such as *Marmite,* and possibly also *Bovril*;
- **pickled herrings**.

A number of other foods should also be viewed with suspicion, including:

- **sauerkraut**;
- **fermented bologna**, **salami**, **pepperoni**, and **summer sausage**;
- **fermented soya beans**, **soya bean paste** and **soya bean curd (tofu)**.[43,47]

However, some foods, such as yoghurt, fresh cream and possibly chocolate are often viewed with unjustifiable suspicion. It also seems very doubtful if either cream cheese or cottage cheese represent a hazard, or processed cheese slices.[42] Whole green bananas contain up to 65 micrograms of tyramine per gram, but this is mostly in the skin as the pulp contains relatively small amounts. Although case reports have occurred with a variety of other foods, it is generally acknowledged that widespread restrictions should not be imposed on a food based solely on an unsubstantiated isolated report,[39,40,42] and that some reports could equally be attributed to spoilage.[40,48] Therefore, of perhaps more importance is the advice to only eat protein-based foods (particularly meat, fish and liver) when fresh (within their sell-by date and after correct storage).[40,42] Note that cooking does not inactivate tyramine.

Guidance regarding alcohol consumption is less clear-cut. For **ales**, **beers** and **lagers**, one report suggested that the consumption of canned or bottled beer, including de-alcoholised beer, in moderation (fewer than four bottles, 1.5 litres in a 4-hour period) is safe in patients taking MAOIs, but, to be on the cautious side, all beers on tap, including lagers should be avoided.[14] When considering wines, Chianti has developed a sinister reputation, because 400 mL of one early sample of Italian Chianti wine (see 'Table 32.2', p.1390) contained enough tyramine to reach the 8 to 20 mg threshold for causing important hypertensive reactions. However, it is claimed[49] that the newer methods that have replaced the ancient 'governo alla toscana' process result in very low levels of tyramine in today's Chianti. This seems to be borne out by the results of analyses,[31,34,38,50] two of which did not find any tyramine at all in some samples.[31,50] Some of the other wines listed in 'Table 32.2', p.1390, also contain tyramine, but patients would have to drink as much as 2 litres or more before reaching what is believed to be the threshold dose. This suggests that small or moderate amounts (1 or 2 glasses) are unlikely to be hazardous in patients taking MAOIs. **Spirits** need not be avoided or consumed cautiously due to their low content or lack of tyramine.

Note that an exaggerated hypotensive response to alcohol is also possible in patients taking MAOIs, see 'Alcohol + MAOIs or RIMAs', p.74.

Treatment of hypertensive crises

Severe hypertensive reactions require urgent immediate treatment. The drug most commonly used to control hypertensive reactions with MAOIs is phentolamine, given as a slow intravenous injection. However, the need for the patient to get to an emergency treatment centre delays treatment, and as a consequence, providing the patient with a drug they could self administer has been suggested. Sublingual nifedipine has been advocated,[51] but does not appear to have been widely adopted, perhaps because the possibility of a sudden dramatic drop in blood pressure is just as dangerous. Another similar option is a small dose of chlorpromazine.[52] However, it is advisable to refer to current guidelines on the management of hypertensive crises for up-to-date advice.

RIMAs

RIMAs are safer than the non-selective MAOIs, because they are more readily reversible and because they only inhibit MAO-A. Therefore the risk of a serious hypertensive reaction with moclobemide is very much reduced. The authors of one study calculate that the lowest amount of tyramine (150 mg) found to cause a 30 mmHg rise in systolic blood pressure with moclobemide is equivalent to that found in about 200 g of Stilton cheese or 300 g of Gorgonzola cheese, which are really excessive amounts of cheese to be eaten in a few minutes.[21] Moreover, no 'cheese reactions' appear to have been published for moclobemide. Most patients therefore do not need to follow the special dietary restrictions required with the non-selective MAOIs, but, to be on the safe side, one manufacturer of moclobemide advises all patients to avoid large amounts of tyramine-rich foods, because a few individuals may be particularly sensitive to tyramine.[53] This warning would also seem appropriate for all RIMAs. No precautions would seem necessary for the consumption of alcoholic drinks as a serious interaction between these and RIMAs is unlikely. Note that if moclobemide were given with an MAO-B inhibitor such as selegiline, it would essentially be the same as giving a non-selective MAOI, and dietary tyramine restrictions would then be required, see 'MAO-B inhibitors + Food; Tyramine-containing', p.770.

1. Blackwell B, Marley E, Price J, Taylor D. Hypertensive interactions between monoamine oxidase inhibitors and foodstuffs. *Br J Psychiatry* (1967) 113, 349–65.
2. Sadusk JF. The physician and the Food and Drug Administration. *JAMA* (1964) 190, 907–9.
3. Generali JA, Hogan LC, McFarlane M, Schwab S, Hartman CR. Hypertensive crisis resulting from avocados and a MAO inhibitor. *Drug Intell Clin Pharm* (1981) 15, 904–6.
4. Boulton AA, Cookson B, Paulton R. Hypertensive crisis in a patient on MAOI antidepressants following a meal of beef liver. *Can Med Assoc J* (1970) 102, 1394–5.
5. Hedberg DL, Gordon MW, Glueck BC. Six cases of hypertensive crisis in patients on tranylcypromine after eating chicken livers. *Am J Psychiatry* (1966) 122, 933–7.
6. Isaac P, Mitchell B, Grahame-Smith DG. Monoamine-oxidase inhibitors and caviar. *Lancet* (1977) ii, 816.
7. Nuessle WF, Norman FC, Miller HE. Pickled herring and tranylcypromine reaction. *JAMA* (1965) 192, 726–7.
8. Kelly D, Guirguis W, Frommer E, Mitchell-Heggs N, Sargant W. Treatment of phobic states with antidepressants. A retrospective study of 246 patients. *Br J Psychiatry* (1970) 116, 387–98.
9. Abrams JH, Schulman P, White WB. Successful treatment of a monoamine oxidase inhibitor-tyramine hypertensive emergency with intravenous labetalol. *N Engl J Med* (1985) 313, 52.
10. Mesmer RE. Don't mix miso with MAOIs. *JAMA* (1987) 258, 3515.
11. Zetin M, Plon L, DeAntonio M. MAOI reaction with powdered protein dietary supplement. *J Clin Psychiatry* (1987) 48, 499.
12. McQueen EG. Interactions with monoamine oxidase inhibitors. *BMJ* (1975) 4, 101.
13. Comfort A. Hypertensive reaction to New Zealand prickly spinach in a woman taking phenelzine. *Lancet* (1981) ii, 472.
14. Tailor SAN, Shulman KI, Walker SE, Moss J, Gardner D. Hypertensive episode associated with phenelzine and tap beer—a reanalysis of the role of pressor amines in beer. *J Clin Psychopharmacol* (1994) 14, 5–14.
15. Murray JA, Walker JF, Doyle JS. Tyramine in alcohol-free beer. *Lancet* (1988) i, 1167–8.
16. Thakore J, Dinan TG, Kelleher M. Alcohol-free beer and the irreversible monoamine oxidase inhibitors. *Int Clin Psychopharmacol* (1992) 7, 59–60.
17. Draper R, Sandler M, Walker PL. Clinical curio: monoamine oxidase inhibitors and non-alcoholic beer. *BMJ* (1984) 289, 308.
18. Sargant W. Interactions with monoamine oxidase inhibitors. *BMJ* (1975) 4, 101.
19. Karet FE, Dickerson JEC, Brown J, Brown MJ. Bovril and moclobemide: a novel therapeutic strategy for central autonomic failure. *Lancet* (1994) 344, 1263–5.
20. Bleumink GS, van Vliet ACM, van der Tholen A, Stricker BHC. Fatal combination of moclobemide overdose and whisky. *Neth J Med* (2003) 61, 88–90.
21. Berlin I, Zimmer R, Cournot A, Payan C, Pedarriosse AM, Puech AJ. Determination and comparison of the pressor effect of tyramine during long-term moclobemide and tranylcypromine treatment in healthy volunteers. *Clin Pharmacol Ther* (1989) 46, 344–51.
22. Bieck PR, Antonin KH. Tyramine potentiation during treatment with MAO inhibitors: brofaromine and moclobemide vs irreversible inhibitors. *J Neural Transm* (1989) (Suppl 28), 21–31.
23. Simpson GM, Gratz SS. Comparison of the pressor effect of tyramine after treatment with phenelzine and moclobemide in healthy male volunteers. *Clin Pharmacol Ther* (1992) 52, 286–91. Correction. Ibid. (1993) 53, 95.
24. Warrington SJ, Turner P, Mant TGK, Morrison P, Haywood G, Glover V, Goodwin BL, Sandler M, St John-Smith P, McClelland GR. Clinical pharmacology of moclobemide, a new reversible monoamine oxidase inhibitor. *J Psychopharmacol* (1991) 5, 82–91.
25. Korn A, Eichler HG, Fischbach R, Gasic S. Moclobemide, a new reversible MAO inhibitor – interaction with tyramine and tricyclic antidepressants in healthy volunteers and depressive patients. *Psychopharmacology (Berl)* (1986) 88, 153–7.
26. Korn A, Da Prada M, Raffesberg W, Gasic S, Eichler HG. Effect of moclobemide, a new reversible monoamine oxidase inhibitor, on absorption and pressor effect of tyramine. *J Cardiovasc Pharmacol* (1988) 11, 17–23.
27. Burgess CD, Mellsop GW. Interaction between moclobemide and oral tyramine in depressed patients. *Fundam Clin Pharmacol* (1989) 3, 47–52.
28. Audebert C, Blin O, Monjanel-Mouterde S, Auquier P, Pedarriosse AM, Dingemanse J, Durand A, Cano JP. Influence of food on the tyramine pressor effect during chronic moclobemide treatment of healthy volunteers. *Eur J Clin Pharmacol* (1992) 43, 507–12.
29. Provost J-C, Funck-Brentano C, Rovei V, D'Estanque J, Ego D, Jaillon P. Pharmacokinetic and pharmacodynamic interaction between toloxatone, a new reversible monoamine oxidase-A inhibitor, and oral tyramine in healthy subjects. *Clin Pharmacol Ther* (1992) 52, 384–93.
30. Tipton KF, Dostert P, Strolin Benedetti M, eds. Monoamine Oxidase and Disease: Pressor amines and monoamine oxidase inhibitors. London: Academic Press; 1984. p. 429–41.
31. Shulman KI, Walker SE, MacKenzie S, Knowles S. Dietary restriction, tyramine, and use of monoamine oxidase inhibitors. *J Clin Psychopharmacol* (1989) 9, 397–402.
32. Cooper AJ, Magnus RV, Rose MJ. A hypertensive syndrome with tranylcypromine medication. *Lancet* (1964) i, 527–9.
33. Anon. Hypertensive reactions to monoamine oxidase inhibitors. *BMJ* (1964) i, 578–9.
34. Da Prada M, Zürcher G, Wüthrich I, Haefely WE. On tyramine, food, beverages and the reversible MAO inhibitor moclobemide. *J Neural Transm* (1988) (Suppl 26), 31–56.
35. Da Prada M, Zürcher G, Wüthrich I, Haefely WE. On tyramine, food, beverages and the reversible MAO inhibitor moclobemide. *J Neural Transm* (1988) (Suppl 26), 31–56.
36. Price K, Smith SE. Cheese reaction and tyramine. *Lancet* (1971) i, 130–1.
37. Hutchison JC. Toxic effects of monoamine-oxidase inhibitors. *Lancet* (1964) ii, 151.
38. Hannah P, Glover V, Sandler M. Tyramine in wine and beer. *Lancet* (1988) i, 879.
39. Sullivan EA, Shulman KI. Diet and monoamine oxidase inhibitors: a re-examination. *Can J Psychiatry* (1984) 29, 707–11.
40. McCabe BJ. Dietary tyramine and other pressor amines in MAOI regimens: a review. *J Am Diet Assoc* (1986) 86, 1059–64.
41. Brown C, Taniguchi G, Yip K. The monoamine oxidase inhibitor-tyramine interaction. *J Clin Pharmacol* (1989) 29, 529–32.
42. Gardner DM, Shulman KI, Walker SE, Tailor SAN. The making of a user friendly MAOI diet. *J Clin Psychiatry* (1996) 57, 99–104.
43. Shulman KI, Walker SE. Refining the MAOI diet: tyramine content of pizzas and soy products. *J Clin Psychiatry* (1999) 60, 191–3.
44. Shulman KI, Walker SE. Clarifying the safety of the MAOI diet and pizza: reply. *J Clin Psychiatry* (2000) 61, 145–6.
45. Marcason W. What is the bottom line for dietary guidelines when taking monoamine oxidase inhibitors? *J Am Diet Assoc* (2005) 105, 163.
46. Folks DG. Monoamine oxidase inhibitors: reappraisal of dietary considerations. *J Clin Psychopharmacol* (1983) 3, 249–52.
47. Da Prada M, Zürcher G. Tyramine content of preserved and fermented foods or condiments of Far Eastern cuisine. *Psychopharmacology (Berl)* (1992) 106, S32–S34.
48. Sen NP. Analysis and significance of tyramine in foods. *J Food Sci* (1969) 34, 22–26.
49. Kalish G. Chianti myth. *The Wine Spectator* (1981) July 31st.
50. Korn A, Eichler HG, Fischbach R, Gasic S. Moclobemide, a new reversible MAO inhibitor – interaction with tyramine and tricyclic antidepressants in healthy volunteers and depressive patients. *Psychopharmacology (Berl)* (1986) 88, 153–7.
51. Fier M. Safer use of MAOIs. *Am J Psychiatry* (1991) 148, 391–2.
52. Lippman SB, Nash K. Monoamine oxidase inhibitor update. Potential adverse food and drug interactions. *Drug Safety* (1990) 5, 195–204.
53. Manerix (Moclobemide). Meda Pharmaceuticals. UK Summary of product characteristics, September 2009.

MAOIs + Ginseng

Case reports describe headache, insomnia and tremulousness, which was attributed to the concurrent use of ginseng and phenelzine.

Clinical evidence

A 64-year-old woman taking **phenelzine** [60 mg daily] developed headache, insomnia, and tremulousness after taking *Natrol High*, a product containing ginseng,[1,2] probably *Eleutherococcus senticosus* (Siberian ginseng). She had the same symptoms on another occasion after drinking a ginseng tea (type not stated), which she had used without problem before starting phenelzine.[1] Three years later, while taking **phenelzine** 45 mg daily, she experienced the same symptoms and an increase in depression 72 hours after starting to take ginseng capsules (type not stated) and a herbal tea.[2]

Another woman with depression taking ginseng (type not stated) and bee pollen experienced relief of her depression and became active and extremely optimistic when she started to take **phenelzine** 45 mg daily, but this was accompanied by insomnia, irritability, headaches and vague visual hallucinations. When the **phenelzine** was stopped and then re-started in the absence of the ginseng and bee pollen, her depression was not relieved.[3]

Mechanism

Uncertain. It seems unlikely that the bee pollen had any part to play. Note that the ginsengs have stimulant effects, and adverse effects include insomnia, nervousness, hypertension and euphoria.

Importance and management

Evidence is limited to three case reports, and the general importance of these poorly documented early cases is unclear. It may be that these cases could just represent idiosyncratic reactions, and not be due to an interaction. The data is therefore too limited to suggest any particular caution. Nevertheless, consider the possibility of an interaction in case of an unexpected response to treatment with phenelzine (or potentially any MAOI) in a patient taking any type of ginseng.

1. Shader RI, Greenblatt DJ. Phenelzine and the dream machine—ramblings and reflections. *J Clin Psychopharmacol* (1985) 5, 65.
2. Shader RI, Greenblatt DJ. Bees, ginseng and MAOIs revisited. *J Clin Psychopharmacol* (1988) 8, 235.
3. Jones BD, Runikis AM. Interaction of ginseng with phenelzine. *J Clin Psychopharmacol* (1987) 7, 201–2.

MAOIs or RIMAs + Inotropes and Vasopressors

Hypertensive crises have occurred in patients taking MAOIs and mephentermine or metaraminol. The pressor effects of adrenaline (epinephrine), isoprenaline (isoproterenol), noradrenaline (norepinephrine) and methoxamine may be unchanged or only moderately increased in patients taking MAOIs. There is limited evidence that the increase may be somewhat greater in those who show a significant hypotensive response to the MAOI.

Moclobemide does not appear to interact with isoprenaline (isoproterenol) or noradrenaline (norepinephrine).

Clinical evidence

(a) MAOIs

1. Adrenaline (Epinephrine). In a study in two healthy subjects given **phenelzine** 15 mg three times daily and two subjects given **tranylcypromine** 10 mg three times daily for 7 days, there was no significant change in the pressor response to intravenous adrenaline after treatment with the MAOI. None of these 4 subjects had a change in blood pressure or heart rate caused by the MAOI alone.[1] In another study in 3 healthy subjects given **tranylcypromine** for 8 to 14 days, the effects of intravenous adrenaline on heart rate and diastolic blood pressure were increased two to fourfold (a moderate effect), but a lesser increase in systolic pressure was seen. This study did not state the effect of the MAOI alone on blood pressure.[2]

A patient using adrenaline 1% eye drops twice daily had no increase in blood pressure or heart rate when given **tranylcypromine** 20 mg, rising to 50 mg daily.[3] Another patient taking **phenelzine** presented with severe anaphylaxis after taking two doses of flucloxacillin, and was initially treated unsuccessfully with hydrocortisone, chlorphenamine and ranitidine because of concerns about using adrenaline with MAOIs. However, as her condition worsened she was given two 100-microgram boluses of intravenous adrenaline, with rapid improvement. No adverse reaction was noted.[4]

2. Isoprenaline (Isoproterenol). In a study in two healthy subjects given **phenelzine** 15 mg three times daily and two subjects given **tranylcypromine** 10 mg three times daily for 7 days, there was no significant change in the pressor response to intravenous isoprenaline after treatment with the MAOI. However, the tachycardia caused by isoprenaline was antagonised by the MAOIs (109 bpm with the MAOI versus 127 bpm without). In another study in 3 healthy subjects given **tranylcypromine** for 8 to 14 days, the effects of intravenous isoprenaline on heart rate and diastolic blood pressure were moderately increased, but there was no enhancement of systolic pressure. This study did not state the effect of the MAOI alone on blood pressure.[2]

3. Mephentermine. Rapid and serious increases in blood pressure and tachycardia were seen when intravenous mephentermine was given to a patient taking **phenelzine**.[5] The patient made a full recovery without the need for pharmacological intervention.

4. Metaraminol. Rapid and serious increases in blood pressure and tachycardia were seen when intramuscular metaraminol was given to a patient taking **pargyline**. The rise in blood pressure and tachycardia were also accompanied by severe headache, chest pain, loss of consciousness, neck stiffness, hypertonicity of the limbs and unreactive, dilated pupils.[6] The patient made a full recovery without the need for pharmacological intervention.

5. Methoxamine. In a study in 3 patients with hypertension who had postural hypotension after being given **pheniprazine** (a formerly investigational non-selective MAOI) the dose of methoxamine was reduced by 61 to 70%, compared with that required in the absence of an MAOI. Three patients were later given **nialamide**: augmentation of the pressor response to methoxamine only occurred in the one patient who had developed postural hypotension.[7]

6. Noradrenaline (Norepinephrine). In a randomised, placebo-controlled study in 12 healthy subjects, **phenelzine** 15 mg three times daily for 7 days had no effect on the dose of intravenous noradrenaline required to raise the systolic blood pressure by 25 mmHg. In addition, **phenelzine** had no effect on the diastolic blood pressure rises and heart rate reductions seen with noradrenaline. In this study, **phenelzine** itself had no effect on blood pressure or heart rate.[8]

Similarly, in an earlier study in two healthy subjects given **phenelzine** 15 mg three times daily and two subjects given **tranylcypromine** 10 mg three times daily for 7 days, no clinically significant potentiation of the pressor effect of noradrenaline was seen, although one of the subjects taking **tranylcypromine** had a twofold increase in the pressor response in the mid-range of noradrenaline concentrations infused, but not in the upper or lower ranges. None of these 4 subjects had a change in blood pressure or heart rate caused by the MAOI alone.[1] In another study, in 3 healthy subjects given **tranylcypromine** for 8 to 14 days, the effects of intravenous noradrenaline were slightly increased. This study did not state the effect of the MAOI alone on blood pressure.[2] In a further study, one healthy subject given **phenelzine** for 8 days experienced a marked reduction in blood pressure, but had no significant changes in the pressor response to noradrenaline.[9]

In contrast, in a study in patients with hypertension who had postural hypotension after being given either **pheniprazine** (a formerly investigational non-selective MAOI; 6 patients) or **tranylcypromine** (one patient), the dose of noradrenaline required to produce a 25 mmHg rise in systolic pressure was reduced by 62 to 87%. Three patients were later given **nialamide**: augmentation of the pressor response to noradrenaline only occurred in the one patient who had developed postural hypotension.[7]

(b) RIMAs

In a randomised, placebo-controlled study in 12 healthy subjects, **moclobemide** 100 mg three times daily for 7 days had no effect on the dose of intravenous **noradrenaline (norepinephrine)** required to raise the systolic blood pressure by 25 mmHg. In addition, **moclobemide** had no effect on the diastolic blood pressure rises and heart rate reductions seen with **noradrenaline**. In this study, **moclobemide** itself had no effect on blood pressure or heart rate.[8] A review paper also briefly mentions that **moclobemide** 600 mg daily for 3 weeks had no relevant effect on the heart rate response to intravenous **isoprenaline (isoproterenol)**.[10]

Mechanism

Adrenaline (epinephrine), isoprenaline (isoproterenol), methoxamine and noradrenaline (norepinephrine) act directly on the receptors at the nerve endings that innervate arterial blood vessels to exert their pressor effects. The use of an MAOI induces the accumulation of noradrenaline within these nerve endings, but as these pressor drugs act directly, they would not be expected to stimulate the release of this stored noradrenaline, and therefore concurrent use would not be expected to alter the pressor effects of these drugs. The enhancement in pressor effects seen in those patients whose blood pressure was lowered by the MAOI might possibly be due to an increased sensitivity of the receptors, which is seen if the nerves are cut, and is also seen during temporary 'pharmacological severance'.

Mephentermine and metaraminol exert their pressor effects in a slightly different way, and have some indirect actions on the nerve endings. Therefore, the noradrenaline accumulated as a result of MAO inhibition is released, thus precipitating a dramatic effect on blood pressure. See 'MAOIs or RIMAs + Nasal decongestants and related drugs', p.1396, for further discussion on this mechanism.

Importance and management

MAOIs

The overall picture is that no clinically relevant enhancement of the effects of **adrenaline** (epinephrine), **isoprenaline** (isoproterenol), **methoxamine** or **noradrenaline** (norepinephrine) occurs in patients taking MAOIs who do not have MAOI-induced hypotension, and the authors of three of the reports cited[1-3] are in broad agreement that problems are unlikely to occur. However, the situation in patients who show a reduced blood pressure due to the use of an MAOI is less clear. One early study[7] found an increase in the pressor effects of noradrenaline and methoxamine in hypertensive patients who had developed orthostatic hypotension when taking pheniprazine or tranylcypromine. This therefore suggests that some patients may experience an increase in blood pressure on concurrent use and this possibly explains the fact that the US manufacturers of the MAOIs contraindicate these inotropes.[11-13] However, it is worth noting that there are no case reports of interactions with these drugs. Furthermore, some consider that intravenous adrenaline may be used in life-threatening situations in patients taking MAOIs, albeit with caution.[4] Others also consider that adrenaline in eye drops or adrenaline as a component of local anaesthesia in dental and other procedures may be given to patients taking MAOIs,[3,14] and that there is no justification for the continued listing of an interaction between MAOIs and local anaesthetics with vasoconstrictors in US prescribing information.[14]

The situation with **mephentermine** and **metaraminol** is slightly different due to their indirect actions and patients taking an MAOI should not normally take any sympathomimetic amine with indirect activity. The use of mephentermine and metaraminol should be avoided in patients taking an MAOI or in those who have stopped an MAOI within the previous 14 days.

There appears to be no documented interactions between the MAOIs and **dopamine** (which has both direct and indirect sympathomimetic actions). Nevertheless, one UK manufacturer of dopamine reasonably predicts that the effects and duration of action of dopamine will be potentiated. They suggest that patients who have been taking an MAOI should be given a starting dose of dopamine that is one-tenth of the usual dose.[15] There also appears to be a lack of data regarding **dopexamine** (which also has both direct and indirect sympathomimetic actions), possibly because its concurrent use with MAOIs is contraindicated.[16] Evidence regarding an interaction between the MAOIs and **dobutamine** (which has direct sympathomimetic effects only) also appears to be lacking; but as it would be expected to behave in a similar way to adrenaline, it may be prudent to apply some caution to concurrent use. However, the US manufacturers of the MAOIs contraindicate the concurrent use of any sympathomimetic (some specifically name dopamine).[11-13]

Phenylephrine may also be used as a vasopressor, and may interact with the MAOIs, although this is possibly by a different mechanism. See 'MAOIs or RIMAs + Phenylephrine', p.1399, for further information on this interaction.

RIMAs

Evidence regarding the use of the RIMA, **moclobemide**, with inotropes and vasopressors appears to be limited to two studies, which suggest that no particular precautions would be expected to be necessary on concurrent use.

1. Boakes AJ, Laurence DR, Teoh PC, Barar FSK, Benedikter LT, Prichard BNC. Interactions between sympathomimetic amines and antidepressant agents in man. *BMJ* (1973) 1, 311–15.
2. Cuthbert MF, Vere DW. Potentiation of the cardiovascular effects of some catecholamines by a monoamine oxidase inhibitor. *Br J Pharmacol* (1971) 43, 471P–472P.
3. Thompson DS, Sweet RA, Marzula K, Peredes JC. Lack of interaction of monoamine oxidase inhibitors and epinephrine in an older patient. *J Clin Psychopharmacol* (1997) 17, 322–3.
4. Fenwick MJ, Muwanga CL. Anaphylaxis and monoamine oxidase inhibitors–the use of adrenaline. *J Accid Emerg Med* (2000) 17, 143–4.
5. Stark DCC. Effects of giving vasopressors to patients on monoamine-oxidase inhibitors. *Lancet* (1962) i, 1405–6.
6. Horler AR, Wynne NA. Hypertensive crisis due to pargyline and metaraminol. *BMJ* (1965) 2, 460–1.
7. Horwitz D, Goldberg LI, Sjoerdsma A. Increased blood pressure responses to dopamine and norepinephrine produced by monoamine oxidase inhibitors in man. *J Lab Clin Med* (1960) 56, 747–53.
8. Cusson JR, Goldenberg E, Larochelle P. Effect of a novel monoamine-oxidase inhibitor, moclobemide on the sensitivity to intravenous tyramine and norepinephrine in humans. *J Clin Pharmacol* (1991) 31, 462–7.
9. Elis J, Laurence DR, Mattie H, Prichard BNC. Modification by monoamine oxidase inhibitors of the effect of some sympathomimetics on blood pressure. *BMJ* (1967) 2, 75–8.
10. Zimmer R, Gieschke R, Fischbach R, Gasic S. Interaction studies with moclobemide. *Acta Psychiatr Scand* (1990) 82 (Suppl 360), 84–6.
11. Nardil (Phenelzine sulfate). Pfizer Inc. US Prescribing information, February 2009.
12. Marplan (Isocarboxazid). Validus Pharmaceuticals, Inc. US Prescribing information, August 2007.
13. Parnate (Tranylcypromine sulfate). GlaxoSmithKline. US Prescribing information, May 2010.
14. Yagiela JA. Adverse drug interactions in dental practice: interactions associated with vasoconstrictors. Part V of a series. *J Am Dent Assoc* (1999) 130, 701–9.
15. Dopamine Sterile Concentrate (Dopamine hydrochloride). Hospira UK Ltd. UK Summary of product characteristics, April 2003.
16. Dopacard (Dopexamine hydrochloride). Cephalon Ltd. UK Summary of product characteristics, October 2007.

MAOIs or RIMAs + Levodopa

A rapid, serious, and potentially life-threatening hypertensive reaction can occur in patients taking MAOIs if they are given levodopa. An

interaction with levodopa given with carbidopa or benserazide is less likely.

No serious hypertensive reaction has been reported to occur between moclobemide and levodopa (given with benserazide).

Clinical evidence

(a) MAOIs

A patient who had been taking **phenelzine** daily for 10 days was given 50 mg of oral levodopa. In just over one hour his blood pressure had risen from 135/90 mmHg to about 190/130 mmHg, despite a 5 mg intravenous injection of phentolamine. Blood pressure continued to rise over the next 10 minutes to 200/135 mmHg, before falling after a further 4 mg injection of phentolamine. The following day the experiment was repeated with levodopa 25 mg, but no blood pressure changes were seen. Three weeks after **phenelzine** was withdrawn even 500 mg of levodopa had no hypertensive effect.[1] Similar cases of severe, acute hypertension, accompanied in most instances by flushing, throbbing and pounding in the head, neck and chest, and light-headedness have been described in other case reports and studies in which levodopa was given with **pargyline**,[2] **nialamide**,[3] **tranylcypromine**,[4] **phenelzine**,[5] or **isocarboxazid**.[1]

A study in 4 normotensive patients with parkinsonism found that the combination of levodopa and **tranylcypromine** caused an increase in blood pressure, but this reaction was inhibited by carbidopa in 3 of the patients. In the remaining patient (who was also taking trihexyphenidyl) the pressor response with levodopa and tranylcypromine (mean increase in arterial blood pressure of 40 mmHg) was only blunted (rather than abolished) by carbidopa (mean increase in arterial blood pressure of 20 mmHg).[6]

(b) RIMAs

A study in 12 healthy subjects given a single dose of levodopa with benserazide, and **moclobemide** 200 mg twice daily, found that nausea, vomiting and dizziness were increased, but no significant hypertensive reaction was seen.[7]

Mechanism

Not fully understood. Levodopa is enzymatically converted in the body, firstly to dopamine and then to noradrenaline (norepinephrine), both of which are normally broken down by monoamine oxidase. In the presence of an MAOI this breakdown is suppressed, which means that the total levels of dopamine and noradrenaline are increased. Precisely how this then leads to a sharp rise in blood pressure is not clear, but either dopamine or noradrenaline, or both, directly or indirectly stimulate the alpha-receptors of the cardiovascular system. Dopa-decarboxylase inhibitors would be expected to minimise the interaction by decreasing the peripheral metabolism of levodopa.

Importance and management

The interaction between the non-selective MAOIs (listed in 'Table 32.1', p.1382) and levodopa in the absence of a dopa-decarboxylase inhibitor is well documented, serious and potentially life-threatening. Patients should not be given levodopa in the absence of a dopa-decarboxylase inhibitor during treatment with any of these MAOIs, nor for a period of 2 to 3 weeks after their withdrawal. Note that this interaction is inhibited or decreased by the presence of dopa-decarboxylase inhibitors[6] such as carbidopa and benserazide (as in *Sinemet* and *Madopar*) so that a serious interaction is less likely to occur with these preparations. Nevertheless, the manufacturers continue to contra-indicate use, both with and for 2 weeks after an MAOI has been stopped.

No hypertensive effect appears to occur between levodopa with benserazide and moclobemide, and would therefore not be expected with any RIMA, but bear in mind that the incidence of adverse effects may be increased by their concurrent use.

1. Hunter KR, Boakes AJ, Laurence DR, Stern GM. Monoamine oxidase inhibitors and L-dopa. *BMJ* (1970) 3, 388.
2. Hodge JV. Use of monoamine-oxidase inhibitors. *Lancet* (1965) i, 764–5.
3. Friend DG, Bell WR, Kline NS. The action of L-dihydroxyphenylalanine in patients receiving nialamide. *Clin Pharmacol Ther* (1965) 6, 362–6.
4. Sharpe J, Marquez-Julio A, Ashby P. Idiopathic orthostatic hypotension treated with levodopa and MAO inhibitor: a preliminary report. *Can Med Assoc J* (1972) 107, 296–300.
5. Kassirer JP, Kopelman RI. A modern medical Descartes. *Hosp Pract* (1987) 22, 17–25.
6. Teychenne PF, Calne DB, Lewis PJ, Findley LJ. Interactions of levodopa with inhibitors of monoamine oxidase and L-aromatic amino acid decarboxylase. *Clin Pharmacol Ther* (1975) 18, 273–7.
7. Dingemanse J. An update of recent moclobemide interaction data. *Int Clin Psychopharmacol* (1993) 7, 167–80.

MAOIs or RIMAs + Lithium

Isolated cases of buccolingual-masticatory syndrome have been described following the long-term use of tranylcypromine and lithium, which did not resolve when the MAOI was stopped. Two other cases describe confusion and delirium when patients taking lithium and phenelzine had their MAOI changed to tranylcypromine.

Limited evidence suggests that no problems occur when moclobemide is given with lithium.

Clinical evidence, mechanism, importance and management

(a) MAOIs

One report describes 2 patients with bipolar affective disorder who developed a buccolingual-masticatory syndrome (a symptom of tardive dyskinesia) after taking **tranylcypromine** 30 or 40 mg daily and lithium carbonate 900 mg or 1.2 g daily for 1.5 or 3 years. These symptoms did not resolve when the **tranylcypromine** was stopped. This reaction was attributed to dopamine receptor hypersensitivity.[1]

A report describes 2 elderly patients with major depression for which they were taking lithium, unresponsive to **phenelzine** 75 or 90 mg daily and lithium (no dose stated), who subsequently showed improvement in their depressive symptoms 10 to 12 days after **phenelzine** was switched to **tranylcypromine** 40 or 60 mg daily. One patient developed mild confusion, which resolved on stopping the lithium, and moderate delirium occurred in the other patient, which was managed with a reduction in the lithium dose (no dose stated).[2]

There appear to be no other reports suggesting that the combination of MAOIs and lithium is unsafe, and the evidence for any adverse effects on concurrent use seems to be limited to these few case reports. Any interaction seems to be rare, but bear these cases in mind in the event of any unexpected response to treatment with an MAOI and lithium. Note that both the MAOIs and lithium have serotonergic effects, and concurrent use might lead to the serotonin syndrome. Serotonin syndrome is a rare adverse effect, but because of its severity, some caution is warranted if both drugs are given. For more information on serotonin syndrome and its management, see 'Drugs that cause serotonin syndrome + Other drugs that cause serotonin syndrome', p.1471.

Note also that there are a few reports of patients taking MAOIs and lithium who developed hyperpyrexia when also given tryptophan, see 'MAOIs + Tryptophan', p.1404. The role (if any) of lithium in these cases is unknown. Note too, that lithium has been used to augment antidepressants, although most of the data relate to the use of tricyclics or SSRIs.[3]

(b) RIMAs

In a study in 50 patients taking lithium, there was no evidence of any adverse interaction when **moclobemide** 150 to 675 mg daily was added, for 3 to 52 weeks.[4] Similarly, lithium augmentation was used in a small, uncontrolled study in patients taking high-dose **moclobemide** without any evidence of important adverse effects.[5] No additional precautions would therefore seem necessary if both drugs are given.

1. Stancer HC. Tardive dyskinesia not associated with neuroleptics. *Am J Psychiatry* (1979) 136, 727.
2. Stewart JT. Not all monoamine oxidase inhibitors are created equal. *J Am Geriatr Soc* (2007) 55, 1890.
3. Nelson JC. Augmentation strategies in depression 2000. *J Clin Psychiatry* (2000) 61 (Suppl 2), 13–19.
4. Amrein R, Güntert TW, Dingemanse J, Lorscheid T, Stabl M, Schmid-Burgk W. Interactions of moclobemide with concomitantly administered medication: evidence from pharmacological and clinical studies. *Psychopharmacology (Berl)* (1992) 106, S24–S31.
5. Magder DM, Aleksic I, Kennedy SH. Tolerability and efficacy of high-dose moclobemide alone and in combination with lithium and trazodone. *J Clin Psychopharmacol* (2000) 20, 394–5.

MAOIs + MAOIs or RIMAs

Strokes, fatal reactions (possibly including serotonin syndrome), hypertensive reactions and CNS disturbances have been seen when one MAOI was abruptly replaced by another, when the two MAOIs were given together, or when there was an insufficient MAOI-free interval. A case of serotonin syndrome occurred in a patient who took an overdose of moclobemide and tranylcypromine.

Clinical evidence, mechanism, importance and management

(a) MAOIs with MAOIs

A patient who had been taking **isocarboxazid** for 3.5 weeks (starting at 10 mg daily and gradually increased to 30 mg daily) was switched to **tranylcypromine** 10 mg, starting the same day, followed by 10 mg three times daily on the following day. Later that night she complained of feeling 'funny', had difficulty in talking, developed a headache, was restless, flushed, sweating, had an elevated temperature of 39.5°C, and a pulse rate of 130 bpm. She died the following day.[1] Another patient, switched, without a drug-free period, from **phenelzine** 75 mg daily (by tapering the dose by 15 mg daily until discontinued) to **tranylcypromine** (starting at 10 mg daily, increasing by 10 mg daily, until a dose of 20 mg twice daily was reached), suffered a subcortical cerebral haemorrhage on the fourth day following the morning 20-mg dose of **tranylcypromine**, which resulted in total right-sided hemiplegia.[2,3] The patient remained significantly disabled from the sequelae of her stroke.[4] A third patient experienced a mild cerebral haemorrhage, without residual problems, when she took **phenelzine** 45 mg and **tranylcypromine** 20 mg at bedtime: the MAOIs were being switched by reducing the dose of **phenelzine** and gradually increasing the dose of **tranylcypromine**. Consumption of soy sauce may have contributed to this reaction,[5] see 'MAOIs or RIMAs + Food; Tyramine-containing', p.1389, for more details. In a fourth case, **phenelzine** 45 mg daily was stopped, and then after a 2-day drug-free period **tranylcypromine** 20 mg was given, with a further 30-mg dose the next day. The patient experienced a rise in blood pressure to 240/130 mmHg, but recovered uneventfully, and a year later was successfully switched from **phenelzine** to **tranylcypromine** with a 2-week drug-free interval.[2] In another case, hypertension with severe headache, inability to walk and slurred speech, but without permanent sequelae, resulted from starting **tranylcypromine** 30 mg seven days after discontinuing **phenelzine**. **Tranylcypromine** 10 mg daily was restarted 3 days later (10 days after discontinuing the **phenelzine**) with no adverse effects, but when the dose was increased to 20 mg daily (14 days after discontinuing **phenelzine**) the patient experienced a milder version of the same symptoms.[6]

Acute CNS toxicity, hypertension, tachycardia, tremor and urinary retention occurred in a woman 48 hours after **phenelzine** was abruptly stopped and **isocarboxazid** started. In this patient, **phenelzine** was poorly tolerated causing hypertension and headache.[7]

Switching from **iproniazid** to **tranylcypromine** with trifluoperazine may have been the cause of a fatal reaction (fever, shivering, sweating, cyanosis) in a patient also given ephedrine,[8,9] which may also interact, see 'MAOIs or RIMAs + Nasal decongestants and related drugs', p.1396.

In contrast, one woman was switched directly from **phenelzine** 60 mg daily to **tranylcypromine** 20 mg daily without any obvious problems (blood pressure was slightly high, but within the usual range for this patient). She was abruptly switched directly back to **phenelzine**, again without any adverse effect.[10,11] Similarly, a review of 8 cases of patients who were switched rapidly from **tranylcypromine** to **phenelzine** (3 cases) or *vice versa* (5 cases) found that 7 patients tolerated the switch well with minimal or no adverse effects. However, the eighth patient experienced anxiety, nausea, hyperventilation, flushing, a sense of doom, and increased insomnia, which may have been a mild form of serotonin syndrome.[12]

The reasons for these reactions are not understood, but one idea is that the amfetamine-like properties of **tranylcypromine** may have had some part to play. Certainly there are cases of spontaneous rises in blood pressure and intracranial bleeding in patients given **tranylcypromine**.[13] Not all patients have experienced adverse reactions when switched from one MAOI to another,[10,12] but because of the sometimes severe reactions, it would seem prudent to have a drug-free washout period when doing so (14 days is commonly suggested as a washout period for MAOIs), and to start dosing in a conservative and step-wise manner.

(b) RIMAs with MAOIs

A patient who took an overdose of **moclobemide** and **tranylcypromine** developed serotonin syndrome. In this analysis of **moclobemide** overdoses, the risk of developing serotonin toxicity was significantly increased in patients who also took another serotonergic drug: this case with **tranylcypromine** was one of the 11 mentioned.[14]

Note that due to the half-life of moclobemide, it is sometimes recommended that a 24-hour washout period is observed when switching from moclobemide to a potentially interacting drug. A 2-week washout period is commonly advised when switching from an MAOI to a potentially interacting drug. It may be prudent to observe these washout periods in patients swapping between MAOIs and RIMAs.

1. Bazire SR. Sudden death associated with switching monoamine oxidase inhibitors. *Drug Intell Clin Pharm* (1986) 20, 954–6.
2. Gelenberg AJ. Switching MAOI. *Biol Ther Psychiatry* (1984) 7, 33 and 36.
3. Gelenberg AJ. Switching MAOI. The sequel. *Biol Ther Psychiatry* (1985) 8, 41.
4. Mattes JA. Stroke resulting from a rapid switch from phenelzine to tranylcypromine. *J Clin Psychiatry* (1998) 59, 382.
5. Anon. Switching MAOIs: part three. *Biol Ther Psychiatry* (1987) 10, 7.
6. Chandler JD. Switching MAOIs. *J Clin Psychopharmacol* (1987) 7, 438.
7. Safferman AZ, Masiar SJ. Central nervous system toxicity after abrupt monoamine oxidase inhibitor switch: a case report. *Ann Pharmacother* (1992) 26, 337–8.
8. Low-Beer GA, Tidmarsh D. Collapse after "Parstelin". *BMJ* (1963) 2, 683–4.
9. Schrire I. Collapse after "Parstelin". *BMJ* (1963) 2, 748.
10. True BL, Alexander B, Carter B. Switching monoamine oxidase inhibitors. *Drug Intell Clin Pharm* (1985) 19, 825–7.
11. True BL, Alexander B, Carter BL. Comment: switching MAO inhibitors. *Drug Intell Clin Pharm* (1986) 20, 384–5.
12. Szuba MP, Hornig-Rohan M, Amsterdam JD. Rapid conversion from one monoamine oxidase inhibitor to another. *J Clin Psychiatry* (1997) 58, 307–10.
13. Cooper AJ, Magnus RV, Rose MJ. A hypertensive syndrome with tranylcypromine medication. *Lancet* (1964) 1, 527–9.
14. Isbister GK, Hackett LP, Dawson AH, Whyte IM, Smith AJ. Moclobemide poisoning: toxicokinetics and occurrence of serotonin toxicity. *Br J Clin Pharmacol* (2003) 56, 441–50.

MAOIs + Mazindol

An isolated report describes a patient taking phenelzine who had a marked rise in blood pressure when a single dose of mazindol was given.

Clinical evidence, mechanism, importance and management

A woman taking **phenelzine** 30 mg three times daily had a rise in blood pressure from 110/60 mmHg to 200/100 mmHg within 2 hours of receiving a 10-mg test dose of mazindol. The blood pressure remained elevated for another hour, but had fallen again after a further 3 hours. The patient experienced no subjective symptoms.[1] It is uncertain whether this hypertensive reaction was the result of an interaction, or simply a direct response to the mazindol alone (the dose was large compared with the recommended dose of 2 to 3 mg daily). The general importance of this interaction is therefore uncertain. The manufacturer has advised avoiding the concurrent use of mazindol and an MAOI, and said that mazindol should not be used until 14 days after the MAOI had been stopped.[2]

1. Oliver RM. Interaction between phenelzine and mazindol: Personal communication, 1981.
2. Sanorex (Mazindol). Novartis Pharmaceuticals. Canadian Prescribing information. Compendium of Pharmaceuticals and Specialities, 2004.

MAOIs + Methyldopa

In theory, either hypertension or hypotension may occur when non-selective MAOIs are taken with methyldopa. The concurrent use of MAOIs and methyldopa may not be desirable because methyldopa can sometimes cause depression.

Clinical evidence, mechanism, importance and management

Theoretically, methyldopa might cause severe hypertension in patients taking non-selective MAOIs, by releasing catecholamines into the circulation.[1,2] On this basis, the US manufacturers of **isocarboxazid, phenelzine**, and **tranylcypromine** specifically contraindicate the concurrent use of methyldopa.[3-5] Nevertheless, there do not appear to be any reports of hypertension occurring as a result of concurrent use. In addition, MAOIs are known to have *hypotensive* effects and additional blood pressure-lowering effects have been reported in a few patients given **pargyline** (an MAOI formerly used in the treatment of hypertension) with methyldopa.[6,7] For this reason, the UK manufacturer of methyldopa contraindicates the concurrent use of MAOIs.[8] The manufacturers of most MAOIs similarly note that they may potentiate the hypotensive effects of antihypertensives: the UK manufacturer of **isocarboxazid**[9] specifically names methyldopa.

Note that the potential depressant adverse effects of methyldopa may make it an unsuitable drug for patients with depression.

1. van Rossum JM. Potential danger of monoamineoxidase inhibitors and α-methyldopa. *Lancet* (1963) i, 950–1.
2. Natarajan S. Potential danger of monoamineoxidase inhibitors and α-methyldopa. *Lancet* (1964) i, 1330.
3. Nardil (Phenelzine sulfate). Pfizer Inc. US Prescribing information, February 2009.
4. Parnate (Tranylcypromine sulfate). GlaxoSmithKline. US Prescribing information, May 2010.
5. Marplan (Isocarboxazid). Validus Pharmaceuticals, Inc. US Prescribing information, August 2007.
6. Herting RL. Monoamine oxidase inhibitors. *Lancet* (1963) i, 1324.
7. Gillespsie L, Oates JA, Crout JR, Sjoerdsma A. Clinical and chemical studies with α-methyldopa in patients with hypertension. *Circulation* (1962) 25, 281–91.
8. Methyldopa. Actavis UK Ltd. UK Summary of product characteristics, March 2007.
9. Isocarboxazid. Cambridge Laboratories. UK Summary of product characteristics, February 2008.

MAOIs or RIMAs + Methylphenidate and related drugs

The concurrent use of non-selective MAOIs with methylphenidate can result in hypertensive crisis and/or serotonin syndrome. Dexmethylphenidate is predicted to interact similarly.

Clinical evidence

In a study of the use of **phenelzine** as an antagonist to stimulants, 3 patients also took oral or intravenous methylphenidate and all three experienced moderate to severe headache.[1] A patient started taking **tranylcypromine**, then 4 days later methylphenidate was added. After 15 days of concurrent use he had a hypertensive crisis and both drugs were stopped.[2] Another case report describes an episode of symptoms consistent with serotonin syndrome in a man taking **isocarboxazid** and trazodone 2 months after the doses of these drugs were increased and methylphenidate was added. He had experienced two similar episodes 4 and 8 weeks previously, which had each resolved spontaneously over 12 hours. All three drugs have serotonergic properties and were thought to have contributed to the reaction.[3]

Conversely, a man taking **tranylcypromine** for depression was successfully treated with methylphenidate for attention deficit hyperactivity disorder (ADHD). He was given methylphenidate 2.5 mg daily, which was very gradually increased over a number of months to 45 mg daily. He took the combination for 6 months and periodic blood pressure measurements did not change significantly from baseline.[4] Another similar case of uneventful concurrent use has been described with **phenelzine** and methylphenidate,[5] and no cases of hypertensive crisis were seen in 4 patients taking **tranylcypromine** or **phenelzine** when they also took methylphenidate for periods of 6 to 30 months.[6]

Mechanism

Methylphenidate is thought to block the reuptake of noradrenaline (norepinephrine) and dopamine leading to their accumulation in the synaptic cleft. The hypertensive reaction seen with the concurrent use of MAOIs can therefore be attributed to over-stimulation of the adrenergic receptors of the cardiovascular system by the release of large amounts of noradrenaline (norepinephrine) that have accumulated in adrenergic nerve endings as a result of MAO inhibition. The possible case of serotonin syndrome may be attributable to the release of serotonin (and possibly also dopamine) from neurones in the brain, so that increased stimulation of the serotonin receptors occurs. For more detail on both of these mechanisms see 'MAOIs or RIMAs + Amfetamines and related drugs', p.1383.

Importance and management

Evidence of hypertensive crisis and possible serotonin syndrome with the concurrent use of MAOIs and methylphenidate is limited to the few cases described here. However, note that hypertensive crisis may be serious and is potentially fatal, and has been well documented for the concurrent use of MAOIs with amfetamines, (see 'MAOIs or RIMAs + Amfetamines and related drugs', p.1383). Therefore methylphenidate should not be taken either with or within 14 days of an MAOI. However, bear in mind that some cases describe concurrent and apparently safe use under well controlled conditions.

There appears to be no evidence regarding a possible interaction between MAOIs and the d-isomer of methylphenidate, **dexmethylphenidate**, but it would be prudent to suspect that a similar interaction may occur. The manufacturer of dexmethylphenidate contraindicates its use both during and for 14 days after the use of an MAOI.[7]

1. Maletzky BM. Phenelzine as a stimulant drug antagonist: a preliminary report. *Int J Addict* (1977) 12, 651–5.
2. Sherman M, Hauser GC, Glover BH. Toxic reactions to tranylcypromine. *Am J Psychiatry* (1964) 120, 1019–21.
3. Bodner RA, Lynch T, Lewis L, Kahn D. Serotonin syndrome. *Neurology* (1995) 45, 219–23.
4. Feinberg SS. Combining stimulants with monoamine oxidase inhibitors: a review of uses and one possible additional indication. *J Clin Psychiatry* (2004) 65, 1520–4.
5. Shelton Clauson A, Elliott ES, Watson BD, Treacy J. Coadministration of phenelzine and methylphenidate for treatment-resistant depression. *Ann Pharmacother* (2004) 38, 508.
6. Feighner JP, Herbstein J, Damlouji N. Combined MAOI, TCA, and direct stimulant therapy of treatment-resistant depression. *J Clin Psychiatry* (1985) 46, 206–9.
7. Focalin XR (Dexmethylphenidate hydrochloride). Novartis. US Prescribing information, December 2013.

MAOIs + Mirtazapine

The manufacturers say that two weeks should elapse between taking an MAOI and mirtazapine.

Clinical evidence, mechanism, importance and management

No serious adverse interactions have been reported between mirtazapine and the MAOIs[1] but, to be on the safe side, the manufacturers say that the concurrent use of mirtazapine and MAOIs should be avoided both during and within 2 weeks of stopping either drug.[1,2] Both mirtazapine and MAOIs have serotonergic effects, and concurrent use might lead to the serotonin syndrome. Serotonin syndrome is a rare adverse effect, but because of its severity, some caution is warranted if both drugs are given. For more information on serotonin syndrome and its management, see 'Drugs that cause serotonin syndrome + Other drugs that cause serotonin syndrome', p.1471.

Note that there is a case of delirium possibly attributed to the use of linezolid (an antibacterial with some weak MAOI activity) with mirtazapine, see 'Linezolid + SSRIs', p.328, which gives some weight to this warning.

1. Remeron (Mirtazapine). Merck Sharp & Dohme Corp. US Prescribing information, January 2014.
2. Zispin SolTab (Mirtazapine). Merck Sharp & Dohme Ltd. UK Summary of product characteristics, February 2015.

MAOIs + Modafinil

An isolated case report describes a patient who developed an acute dyskinesia and symptoms suggestive of serotonin syndrome following the use of modafinil with tranylcypromine. In theory this interaction seems possible with the use of modafinil and any MAOI. Armodafinil would be expected to interact with MAOIs in the same way as modafinil.

Clinical evidence

A case report describes a patient taking **tranylcypromine** 80 mg daily who, 3 days after starting to take modafinil 200 mg daily, became restless, confused, and developed severe choreiform movements of her limbs, lip smacking, rhythmic rapid tongue protrusions, and opisthotonus. Her temperature rose to 38°C, and remained high for 24 hours. These symptoms resolved within 48 hours of discontinuing both drugs.[1]

Mechanism

The authors of this report suggest that the dopaminergic and serotonergic effects of modafinil were augmented by tranylcypromine. The hyperthermia and confusion that the patient experienced may have been an incomplete form of serotonin syndrome.[1]

Importance and management

This appears to be the only case report of an interaction between an MAOI and modafinil, and there are two case reports describing the successful use of these drugs.[2,3] However, if the suggested mechanism is correct, an interaction could occur between modafinil and any MAOI. It would therefore seem prudent to be alert for these adverse effects if modafinil is given with an MAOI. **Armodafinil**, the *R*-isomer of modafinil, would be expected to interact in a similar way and the manufacturer of armodafinil therefore recommends caution if an MAOI is taken concurrently.[4]

1. Vytopil M, Mani R, Adlakha A, Zhu J-J. Acute chorea and hyperthermia after concurrent use of modafinil and tranylcypromine. *Am J Psychiatry* (2007) 164, 684.
2. Clemons WE, Makela E, Young J. Concomitant use of modafinil and tranylcypromine in a patient with narcolepsy: a case report. *Sleep Med* (2004) 5, 509–11.
3. Ashton AK. Modafinil augmentation of phenelzine for residual fatigue in dysthymia. *Am J Psychiatry* (2004) 161, 1716–17.
4. Nuvigil (Armodafinil). Cephalon, Inc. US Prescribing information, June 2013.

MAOIs or RIMAs + Nasal decongestants and related drugs

The use of some nasal decongestants with non-selective MAOIs can result in a potentially fatal hypertensive crisis.

The concurrent use of ephedrine and moclobemide raises blood pressure, and this has resulted in palpitations and headache.

Clinical evidence

(a) MAOIs

A study in 3 healthy subjects, given **phenelzine** 45 mg or **tranylcypromine** 30 mg daily for 5 to 14 days, found that the blood pressure rise following oral **ephedrine** 30 mg was enhanced. The maximal increase in mean arterial pressure was 22 mmHg (compared with 4 to 6 mmHg without the MAOI). A similar increase was seen up to 10 days after discontinuation of the MAOI. A similar increase in blood pressure was also seen in one of the subjects given intravenous **ephedrine** 2 mg per minute for 6 minutes.[1]

In one subject given **tranylcypromine** 30 mg daily for 20 to 30 days, **phenylpropanolamine**, given as capsules or a linctus, caused a rapid and marked rise in blood pressure to 210/140 mmHg within 2 hours, necessitating the use of phentolamine to reverse the effect.[2] Slow-release **phenylpropanolamine** caused a smaller and more gradual rise to 160/100 mmHg over 2 hours.[2] Similarly, in 3 subjects given **tranylcypromine** 30 mg daily for 8 to 14 days, the pressor effect of intravenous **phenylpropanolamine** was potentiated by about four- to fivefold (systolic) and three- to tenfold (diastolic), and the reflex bradycardia was potentiated by about 2.5- to 6-fold.[3]

Numerous case reports describe similar rapid and serious rises in blood pressure, accompanied by tachycardia, chest pains and severe occipital headache when MAOIs were given with indirectly-acting sympathomimetics. Other symptoms that have occurred include neck stiffness, flushing, sweating, nausea, vomiting, hypertonicity of the limbs, and sometimes epileptiform convulsions: fatal intracranial haemorrhage, cardiac arrhythmias and cardiac arrest have resulted.

This interaction has been reported between:

- oral **ephedrine** and **nialamide**;[4]
- oral **isometheptene mucate** and **phenelzine**;[5]
- oral **phenylpropanolamine** and **mebanazine**,[6,7] **pargyline**,[8] or **phenelzine**;[6,7,9-12]
- and oral **pseudoephedrine** and **iproniazid**.[13]

Tachycardia, agitation, hyperreflexia and *hypotension*, then pyrexia has been described in a woman who took a single *Do-Do* tablet (**ephedrine**, caffeine, theophylline) the day after stopping **phenelzine**.[14] Similarly, fatal hyperpyrexia without hypertension occurred in a man taking **tranylcypromine** with trifluoperazine when he was given oral **ephedrine**,[15] although switching his MAOI without a full washout period may have caused, or contributed to, this reaction,[16] see 'MAOIs + MAOIs or RIMAs', p.1394. A woman taking **phenelzine** developed bradycardia of 40 bpm after taking one tablet of *Sinutab* (without codeine),[17] which probably contained **pseudoephedrine**.

(b) RIMAs

No interaction was seen in subjects taking **brofaromine** 75 mg twice daily for 10 days when they were given 75 mg of slow-release **phenylpropanolamine** (*Acutrim Late Day*), but immediate-release **phenylpropanolamine** caused a 3.3-fold increase in pressor sensitivity.[18] In a study in 11 healthy subjects taking **moclobemide** 300 mg twice daily, the pressor effects of high-dose oral **ephedrine** (two doses of 50 mg with a 4-hour interval) were increased about three- to fourfold, and this resulted in an increase in palpitations and headache.[19,20]

Mechanism

The reaction can be attributed to over-stimulation of the adrenergic receptors of the cardiovascular system. During treatment with non-selective MAOIs, large amounts of noradrenaline (norepinephrine) accumulate at adrenergic nerve endings not only in the brain, but also within the sympathetic nerve endings, which innervate arterial blood vessels. Stimulation of these latter nerve endings, by sympathomimetic amines with indirect actions, causes the release of the accumulated noradrenaline and results in the massive stimulation of the receptors. An exaggerated blood vessel constriction occurs and the blood pressure rise is proportionately excessive. Intracranial haemorrhage can occur if the pressure is so high that a blood vessel ruptures.

Importance and management

MAOIs

A very well-documented, serious, and potentially fatal interaction. Patients taking an MAOI should not normally take any sympathomimetic amine with indirect activity. These include ephedrine, isometheptene mucate, phenylpropanolamine and pseudoephedrine (see 'Table 24.1', p.1050, for a list). Note that some of these nasal decongestants are also used for their pressor effects, and concurrent use for this indication is also contraindicated.

Note that ephedrine, phenylpropanolamine and pseudoephedrine are used as vasoconstrictor decongestants in numerous oral non-prescription cough, cold and influenza preparations. Isometheptene is used in non-prescription analgesic preparations for migraine. Patients taking MAOIs should be strongly warned not to take any of these drugs either with or for 2 weeks after stopping their MAOI. Also, note that serious interactions have occurred because of confusion between non-prescription products with very similar names that contain different active ingredients.[11]

The nasal decongestants **oxymetazoline** and **xylometazoline** differ in that they have direct actions (see 'Table 24.1', p.1050), and therefore seem unlikely to interact with the MAOIs to cause dramatic increases in blood pressure (see *Mechanism*, under 'MAOIs or RIMAs + Inotropes and Vasopressors', p.1392. Furthermore, some consider it is unlikely these drugs, which are given topically, will be absorbed in sufficient quantities to cause an interaction. Nevertheless, at least one UK manufacturer of oxymetazoline contraindicates its use with or within 14 days of the use of an MAOI,[21] and the US manufacturers of the MAOIs generally contraindicate the use of any sympathomimetic.[21-24]

RIMAs

Evidence for an interaction between the RIMAs, such as moclobemide and the nasal decongestants is limited, but what is known suggests that the RIMAs will interact in the same way as the MAOIs. The manufacturer of moclobemide[25] advises avoiding sympathomimetics such as ephedrine, **pseudoephedrine** and **phenylpropanolamine**. It would also be prudent to avoid moclobemide with any of the other indirectly-acting sympathomimetics (see 'Table 24.1', p.1050, for a list), although the severity of the interactions with moclobemide is unlikely to be as great as that seen with the MAOIs. For example, ephedrine and phenylephrine have been successfully and uneventfully used in the presence of moclobemide (omitted on the day of surgery) during anaesthesia to control hypotension.[26]

Treatment

Hypertensive reactions have been controlled by intravenous phentolamine, phenoxybenzamine, intramuscular chlorpromazine, labetalol or sublingual nifedipine. The manufacturers of phenelzine state that on the basis of present evidence, slow intravenous injection of phentolamine is recommended.[27,28] However, it is advisable to refer to current guidelines on the management of hypertensive crises for up-to-date advice.

1. Elis J, Laurence DR, Mattie H, Prichard BNC. Modification by monoamine oxidase inhibitors of the effect of some sympathomimetics on blood pressure. *BMJ* (1967) 2, 75–8.
2. Cuthbert MF, Greenberg MP, Morley SW. Cough and cold remedies: a potential danger to patients on monoamine oxidase inhibitors. *BMJ* (1969) 1, 404–6.
3. Cuthbert MF, Vere DW. Potentiation of the cardiovascular effects of some catecholamines by a monoamine oxidase inhibitor. *Br J Pharmacol* (1971) 43, 471P–472P.
4. Hirsch MS, Walter RM, Hasterlik RJ. Subarachnoid hemorrhage following ephedrine and MAO inhibitor. *JAMA* (1965) 194, 1259.
5. Kraft KE, Dore FH. Computerized drug interaction programs: how reliable ? *JAMA* (1996) 275, 1087.
6. Tonks CM, Lloyd AT. Hazards with monoamine-oxidase inhibitors. *BMJ* (1965) 1, 589.
7. Wright SP. Hazards with monoamine-oxidase inhibitors: a persistent problem. *Lancet* (1978) i, 284–5.
8. Jenkins LC, Graves HB. Potential hazards of psychoactive drugs in association with anaesthesia. *Can Anaesth Soc J* (1965) 12, 121–8.
9. Mason AMS, Buckle RM. "Cold" cures and monoamine-oxidase inhibitors. *BMJ* (1969) 1, 845–6.
10. Humberstone PM. Hypertension from cold remedies. *BMJ* (1969) 1, 846.
11. Harrison WM, McGrath PJ, Stewart JW, Quitkin F. MAOIs and hypertensive crises: the role of OTC drugs. *J Clin Psychiatry* (1989) 50, 64–5. Correction. Magurno JAJ, Board AW. ibid. (1990) 51, 212–3. [drug].
12. Smookler S, Bermudez AJ. Hypertensive crisis resulting from an MAO inhibitor and an over-the-counter appetite suppressant. *Ann Emerg Med* (1982) 11, 482–4.
13. Davies R. Patient medication records. *Pharm J* (1982) 228, 652.
14. Dawson JK, Earnshaw SM, Graham CS. Dangerous monoamine oxidase inhibitor interactions are still occurring in the 1990s. *J Accid Emerg Med* (1995) 12, 49–51.
15. Low-Beer GA, Tidmarsh D. Collapse after "Parstelin". *BMJ* (1963) 2, 683–4.
16. Schrire I. Collapse after "Parstelin". *BMJ* (1963) 2, 748.
17. Terry R, Kaye AH, McDonald M. Sinutab. *Med J Aust* (1975) 1, 763.
18. Gleiter CH, Mühlbauer B, Gradin-Frimmer G, Antonin KH, Bieck PR. Administration of sympathomimetic drugs with the selective MAO-A inhibitor brofaromine. Effect on blood pressure. *Drug Invest* (1992) 4, 149–54.
19. Dingemanse J. An update of recent moclobemide interaction data. *Int Clin Psychopharmacol* (1993) 7, 167–80.
20. Dingemanse J, Guentert T, Gieschke R, Stabl M. Modification of the cardiovascular effects of ephedrine by the reversible monoamine oxidase A-inhibitor moclobemide. *J Cardiovasc Pharmacol* (1996) 28, 856–61.
21. Vicks Sinex Soother (Oxymetazoline hydrochloride). Procter & Gamble (Health and Beauty Care) Ltd. UK Summary of product characteristics, November 2006.
22. Nardil (Phenelzine sulfate). Pfizer Inc. US Prescribing information, February 2009.
23. Marplan (Isocarboxazid). Validus Pharmaceuticals, Inc. US Prescribing information, August 2007.
24. Parnate (Tranylcypromine sulfate). GlaxoSmithKline. US Prescribing information, May 2010.
25. Manerix (Moclobemide). Meda Pharmaceuticals. UK Summary of product characteristics, September 2009.
26. Martyr JW, Orlikowski CEP. Epidural anaesthesia, ephedrine and phenylephrine in a patient taking moclobemide, a new monoamine oxidase inhibitor. *Anaesthesia* (1996) 51, 1150–2.
27. Nardil (Phenelzine sulfate). Archimedes Pharma UK Ltd. UK Summary of product characteristics, October 2008.
28. Nardil (Phenelzine sulfate). Pfizer Inc. US Prescribing information, February 2009.

MAOIs or RIMAs + Opioids; Dextropropoxyphene (Propoxyphene)

An isolated report describes 'leg shakes', diaphoresis, and severe hypotension when a woman taking phenelzine was given dextropropoxyphene. Another isolated report describes a marked increase in sedation when a woman was given phenelzine and dextropropoxyphene.

Moclobemide may potentiate the effects of dextropropoxyphene.

Clinical evidence, mechanism, importance and management

(a) MAOIs

A woman taking **phenelzine** 15 mg three times daily, sodium valproate, and trazodone, was given dextropropoxyphene 100 mg and paracetamol (acetaminophen) 650 mg for back pain and headache. Some 12 hours later she was admitted to hospital for leg shakes, discomfort and weakness. She was confused and anxious, and sweating intensely. The next day she became severely hypotensive (systolic blood pressure 55 to 60 mmHg) and needed large fluid volume resuscitation in intensive care. She later recovered fully.[1] Another woman taking propranolol, oestrogen-replacement therapy and **phenelzine** became very sedated and groggy, causing her to have to lie down on two occasions, both within 2 hours of taking dextropropoxyphene 100 mg and paracetamol 650 mg. She had experienced no problems when taking either paracetamol or dextropropoxyphene with paracetamol before starting **phenelzine**, and subsequently had no problems with paracetamol alone while continuing to take **phenelzine**.[2]

The mechanisms of these interactions are not understood. It appears that dextropropoxyphene may be a weak serotonin reuptake inhibitor,[3] and some of the symptoms in the first case were not unlike those seen in serotonin syndrome.

Apart from these two isolated reports, there seems to be no other clinical evidence of adverse interactions between MAOIs and dextropropoxyphene; however, some caution would seem prudent if any MAOI is given with dextropropoxyphene. One US manufacturer of dextropropoxyphene states that concurrent use is not recommended, both with and within 14 days of stopping an MAOI.[4] For more information on serotonin syndrome and its management, see 'Drugs that cause serotonin syndrome + Other drugs that cause serotonin syndrome', p.1471.

(b) RIMAs

In *animals*, the effects of dextropropoxyphene were increased by **moclobemide**.[5] On this basis, the manufacturer of **moclobemide** cautions the concurrent use of opioids, and suggests that a dose adjustment of the opioid may be needed.[6]

1. Zornberg GL, Hegarty JD. Adverse interaction between propoxyphene and phenelzine. *Am J Psychiatry* (1993) 150, 1270–1.
2. Garbutt JC. Potentiation of propoxyphene by phenelzine. *Am J Psychiatry* (1987) 144, 251–2.
3. Codd EE, Shank RP, Schupsky JJ, Raffa RB. Serotonin and norepinephrine uptake inhibiting activity of centrally acting analgesics: structural determinants and role in antinociception. *J Pharmacol Exp Ther* (1995) 274, 1263–70.
4. Darvocet A500 (Propoxyphene napsylate with Acetaminophen). Xanodyne Pharmaceuticals, Inc. US Prescribing information, November 2009.
5. Amrein R, Güntert TW, Dingemanse J, Lorscheid T, Stabl M, Schmid-Burgk W. Interactions of moclobemide with concomitantly administered medication: evidence from pharmacological and clinical studies. *Psychopharmacology (Berl)* (1992) 106, S24–S31.
6. Manerix (Moclobemide). Meda Pharmaceuticals. UK Summary of product characteristics, September 2009.

MAOIs or RIMAs + Opioids; Fentanyl and related drugs

Fentanyl has been given to patients taking MAOIs without problems, but case reports describe fatal hyperthermia in one patient and hypertension and tachycardia in another patient following concurrent use. Case reports describe the uneventful use of alfentanil, remifentanil and sufentanil in patients taking MAOIs.

Clinical evidence

A 71-year-old woman taking *Parstelin* (**tranylcypromine** with trifluoperazine) was given an intravenous test dose of fentanyl 20 micrograms and diazepam before surgery, without problems. She was then given another 20-microgram intravenous dose of fentanyl during surgery, followed by an epidural bolus infusion of fentanyl 50 micrograms 15 minutes before the end of the surgery. After surgery she was given a continuous epidural infusion of fentanyl 50 to 70 micrograms/hour for 4 days to control postoperative pain, also without problems.[1] Similarly, another report describes 2 patients who had stopped taking **phenelzine** 36 hours and 10 days before undergoing uneventful cardiac surgery using fentanyl, pancuronium and 100% oxygen.[2] Five further patients taking **tranylcypromine**, **isocarboxazid**, or **pargyline** had no adverse reactions to fentanyl given during surgery (4 cases) and/or for postoperative pain relief (3 cases).[3]

In contrast, a man taking **tranylcypromine** who received fentanyl during and after surgery developed postoperative hypertension, hyperthermia, and severe shivering, followed by resistant hypotension. He later died.[4] Another patient taking **phenelzine** who underwent cardiac surgery, with anaesthesia maintained by fentanyl and midazolam, developed hypertension and supraventricular tachycardia, which did not respond to digoxin and esmolol. About 15 minutes after stopping the fentanyl with midazolam and starting enflurane, the haemodynamics gradually improved, and analgesia was subsequently managed with ketorolac without problems.[5]

Mechanism, importance and management

Fentanyl has been used safely in a number of patients receiving MAOIs. However, a fatality due to a serotonin-like syndrome has occurred in a patient taking an MAOI and given fentanyl, and another case of hypertension and tachycardia has occurred. The authors of one of these reports considered that there was insufficient evidence to conclude that patients taking MAOIs can be given fentanyl safely, and called for all cases of concurrent use to be reported.[4] However, the manufacturers of fentanyl (patches, lozenges, injection and nasal spray) generally contraindicate or do not recommend their concurrent use with, or within 14 days of stopping, an MAOI. Note that both fentanyl and the MAOIs have serotonergic effects, and concurrent use might lead to the serotonin syndrome. Serotonin syndrome is a rare adverse effect, but because of its severity, some caution is warranted if both drugs are given. For more information on serotonin syndrome and its management, see 'Drugs that cause serotonin syndrome + Other drugs that cause serotonin syndrome', p.1471.

There seems to be little information about the use of MAOIs with other opioids used as anaesthetic adjuncts, although there are isolated cases describing safe concurrent use with **alfentanil** with tranylcypromine or phenelzine,[6,7] **remifentanil** with phenelzine[8] and **sufentanil** with tranylcypromine.[9] Nevertheless, one UK manufacturer of alfentanil contraindicates the use of alfentanil with or within 14 days of stopping an MAOI,[10] whereas at least one manufacturer of sufentanil[11] and one manufacturer of remifentanil[12] make no mention of a potential interaction.

There appear to be no clinical reports of an interaction between moclobemide and fentanyl. However, based on results from *animal* studies, the manufacturer of **moclobemide** states that it may potentiate the effects of the opioids (they name fentanyl), and therefore advises caution on their concurrent use: a dose adjustment [presumably a reduction] of the opioid may be needed.[13]

Note that fentanyl and related drugs are frequently used during surgery, and it is generally considered that MAOIs should be discontinued 2 weeks before surgery, see 'Anaesthetics, general + MAOIs and related drugs', p.107.

1. Youssef MS, Wilkinson PA. Epidural fentanyl and monoamine oxidase inhibitors. *Anaesthesia* (1988) 43, 210–12.
2. Michaels I, Serrins M, Shier NQ, Barash PG. Anesthesia for cardiac surgery in patients receiving monoamine oxidase inhibitors. *Anesth Analg* (1984) 63, 1041–4.
3. El-Ganzouri AR, Ivankovich AD, Braverman B, McCarthy R. Monoamine oxidase inhibitors: should they be discontinued preoperatively? *Anesth Analg* (1985) 64, 592–6.
4. Noble WH, Baker A. MAO inhibitors and coronary artery surgery: a patient death. *Can J Anaesth* (1992) 39, 1061–6.
5. Insler SR, Kraenzler EJ, Licina MG, Savage RM, Starr NJ. Cardiac surgery in a patient taking monoamine oxidase inhibitors: an adverse fentanyl reaction. *Anesth Analg* (1994) 78, 593–7.
6. Powell H. Use of alfentanil in a patient receiving monoamine oxidase inhibitor therapy. *Br J Anaesth* (1990) 64, 528.
7. Beresford BJ, Glick D, Dinwiddie SH. Combination propofol-alfentanil anesthesia for electroconvulsive therapy in patients receiving monoamine oxidase inhibitors. *J ECT* (2004) 20, 120–2.
8. Ure DS, Gillies MA, James KS. Safe use of remifentanil in a patient treated with the monoamine oxidase inhibitor phenelzine. *Br J Anaesth* (2000) 84, 414–16.
9. O'Hara JF, Maurer WG, Smith MP. Sufentanil-isoflurane-nitrous oxide anesthesia for a patient treated with monoamine oxidase inhibitor and tricyclic antidepressant. *J Clin Anesth* (1995) 7, 148–50.

10. Rapifen Solution for Injection or Infusion (Alfentanil hydrochloride). Janssen-Cilag Ltd. UK Summary of product characteristics, April 2013.
11. Sufenta (Sufentanil citrate). Taylor Pharmaceuticals. US Prescribing information, July 2007.
12. Ultiva (Remifentanil hydrochloride). GlaxoSmithKline UK. UK Summary of product characteristics, December 2010.
13. Manerix (Moclobemide). Meda Pharmaceuticals. UK Summary of product characteristics, September 2009.

MAOIs or RIMAs + Opioids; Miscellaneous

Hypotension (profound in one case) has been seen in a few patients given morphine and an MAOI. One case of hypotension and stupor has occurred with papaveretum. Serious adverse effects are predicted to occur with the concurrent use of other opioids (such as buprenorphine, codeine, diamorphine, dihydrocodeine, dipipanone, hydromorphone, meptazinol, methadone and oxycodone) and the MAOIs or RIMAs, although there do not appear to be any published reports of an interaction.

Clinical evidence

(a) Morphine

A study in 15 patients who had been taking either **phenelzine**, **isocarboxazid**, **iproniazid** or *Parstelin* (**tranylcypromine** with trifluoperazine) for 3 to 8 weeks, found no changes in blood pressure, pulse rate or state of awareness when test doses of up to 4 mg of intramuscular morphine were given. However, note that none of these patients had developed an interaction with test doses of up to 40 mg of pethidine (meperidine),[1] which is known to interact in some patients. One other study reported no adverse interaction in 3 patients taking **isocarboxazid** when they were given morphine premedication,[2] and a further study revealed no problems in 9 patients taking **tranylcypromine** who were given morphine for postoperative pain relief.[3] Another patient taking **phenelzine** was uneventfully treated with morphine postoperatively,[4] and 2 patients taking MAOIs, who reacted adversely to pethidine,[5,6] had not previously done so when given morphine. In an early report, intramuscular morphine was given without apparent problem to 5 patients who had developed severe headache while taking **tranylcypromine**.[7] Another author briefly noted that he knew of about 10 cases where morphine had been used in patients taking MAOIs with no adverse effects except a more prolonged morphine action.[8]

However, a patient taking **tranylcypromine** 40 mg and trifluoperazine 20 mg daily and undergoing a preoperative test with morphine, developed pin point pupils, became unconscious and unresponsive to stimuli, and had a systolic blood pressure fall from 160 to 40 mmHg after receiving a total of 6 mg of morphine intravenously. Within 2 minutes of being given naloxone 4 mg intravenously, the patient was awake and rational with a systolic blood pressure fully restored.[9] A moderate fall in blood pressure (from 140/90 mmHg to 90/60 mmHg) was seen in another patient taking an MAOI and given morphine,[10] and a brief episode of hypotension (which was treated with phenylephrine) occurred in a patient taking **phenelzine** receiving continuous epidural morphine during surgery.[3]

(b) Papaveretum

A 54-year-old woman taking **phenelzine** was given papaveretum 10 mg as premedication, and 50 minutes later she was found to be unrousable, sweating and hypotensive.[11]

Mechanism

Unclear. Both the opioids and particularly the MAOIs can lower blood pressure and it appears that in some cases the effects might be profound. Nevertheless, serious interactions between MAOIs and opioids generally only occur when the opioid has serotonergic effects: it has been suggested that morphine, codeine, and oxycodone do not possess serotonin reuptake inhibitor activity and would therefore not be expected to cause serotonin syndrome when given with MAOIs.[12] In contrast, pethidine (meperidine), tramadol, dextropropoxyphene (propoxyphene), and methadone appear to be weak serotonin reuptake inhibitors,[12] and these drugs, with the exception of methadone, have been implicated in reports of serotonin toxicity. For more information on serotonin syndrome and its management, see 'Drugs that cause serotonin syndrome + Other drugs that cause serotonin syndrome', p.1471.

Importance and management

MAOIs with morphine

Some limited evidence suggests that patients taking MAOIs who reacted adversely with pethidine (meperidine) did not do so when given morphine,[5,6] and quite a number of reports describe the safe, uneventful use of morphine and MAOIs. The few hypotensive reactions cited here[3,9,10] are of a different character to the severe reaction seen with pethidine (see 'MAOIs or RIMAs + Opioids; Pethidine (Meperidine)', p.1399), and appear to be rare. However, many manufacturers of morphine have contraindicated or do not recommend its concurrent use with, or within 2 weeks of stopping, an MAOI.[13-15] In contrast, the manufacturers of one morphine preparation note that as severe CNS excitation or depression (hypertension or hypotension) has been seen when pethidine was given with an MAOI, consideration should be given to using a reduced morphine dose in patients taking MAOIs.[16] This is more similar to the advice of one author, who suggests that the interaction can be managed by using lower initial doses of morphine, with frequent monitoring, and a gradual upward dose titration.[17]

Clearly the advice is somewhat conflicting, with some taking a more cautious approach than others. However, the balance of information seems to suggest that most patients do not experience a reaction, with only those opioids with serotonergic effects (see *Mechanism*, above) presenting a risk of a serious adverse reaction. If the decision is taken to give morphine to a patient taking an MAOI, it would seem prudent to start with a low dose, titrating to clinical response. Monitor concurrent use carefully for any signs of adverse effects.

MAOIs with other opioids

Evidence regarding the use of a number of other opioids with MAOIs is limited, and the advice given by the manufacturers regarding concurrent use is somewhat conflicting. One manufacturer of **dihydrocodeine** advises caution with or within 14 days of the use of an MAOI,[18] whereas another manufacturer states that dihydrocodeine should not be used with or within 14 days of stopping an MAOI: if concurrent use is undertaken is should be with extreme caution.[19] One manufacturer of **meptazinol** suggests that concurrent use with or within 14 days of the use of an MAOI should be avoided.[20] Some manufacturers of other opioids contraindicate concurrent use both with, and within 14 days of an MAOI. These include **buprenorphine**,[21] **codeine**,[22] **diamorphine**,[23] **dipipanone**,[24] **hydromorphone**,[25] **methadone**,[26] and **oxycodone**.[27] However, note that not all manufacturers of some of these opioids contraindicate the use of the MAOIs (e.g. codeine). For further discussion on the reasoning and possible management of any interaction, see under *MAOIs with Morphine*, above.

Severe reactions have occurred with a number of other opioids given with MAOIs. These, and the opioids used as anaesthetic adjuncts, are discussed elsewhere. Consider also:

- 'MAOIs or RIMAs + Opioids; Dextropropoxyphene (Propoxyphene)', p.1397
- 'MAOIs or RIMAs + Opioids; Fentanyl and related drugs', p.1397
- 'MAOIs or RIMAs + Opioids; Pethidine (Meperidine)', p.1399
- 'MAOIs or RIMAs + Opioids; Tramadol', p.1399

Moclobemide

There appears to be no published reports of an interaction between moclobemide and the opioids. However, the manufacturer of moclobemide states that, in *animals*, moclobemide increases the effects of opioids. They therefore advise caution on concurrent use and suggest that a dose adjustment [reduction] of the opioid may be needed.[28] One manufacturer of meptazinol[20] suggests that the concurrent use of moclobemide should be avoided. Note also that the concurrent use of pethidine with moclobemide is contraindicated, see 'MAOIs or RIMAs + Opioids; Pethidine (Meperidine)', p.1399, for further information.

1. Evans-Prosser CDG. The use of pethidine and morphine in the presence of monoamine oxidase inhibitors. *Br J Anaesth* (1968) 40, 279–82.
2. Ebrahim ZY, O'Hara J, Borden L, Tetzlaff J. Monoamine oxidase inhibitors and elective surgery. *Cleve Clin J Med* (1993) 60, 129–130.
3. El-Ganzouri AR, Ivankovich AD, Braverman B, McCarthy R. Monoamine oxidase inhibitors: should they be discontinued preoperatively? *Anesth Analg* (1985) 64, 592–6.
4. Ure DS, Gillies MA, James KS. Safe use of remifentanil in a patient treated with the monoamine oxidase inhibitor phenelzine. *Br J Anaesth* (2000) 84, 414–16.
5. Shee JC. Dangerous potentiation of pethidine by iproniazid, and its treatment. *BMJ* (1960) 2, 507–9.
6. Palmer H. Potentiation of pethidine. *BMJ* (1960) 2, 944.
7. Brown DD, Waldron DH. An unusual reaction to tranylcypromine. *Practitioner* (1962) 189, 83–6.
8. Sargant W. Interactions with monoamine oxidase inhibitors. *BMJ* (1975) 4, 101.
9. Barry BJ. Adverse effects of MAO inhibitors with narcotics reversed with naloxone. *Anaesth Intensive Care* (1979) 7, 194.
10. Jenkins LC, Graves HB. Potential hazards of psychoactive drugs in association with anaesthesia. *Can Anaesth Soc J* (1965) 12, 121–8.
11. Spencer GT, Smith SE. Dangers of monoamine oxidase inhibitors. *BMJ* (1963) 1,750.
12. Codd EE, Shank RP, Schupsky JJ, Raffa RB. Serotonin and norepinephrine uptake inhibiting activity of centrally acting analgesics: structural determinants and role in antinociception. *J Pharmacol Exp Ther* (1995) 274, 1263–70.
13. MST Continus Tablets (Morphine sulfate). Napp Pharmaceuticals Ltd. UK summary of product characteristics, December 2009.
14. Oramorph Oral Solution (Morphine sulfate). Boehringer Ingelheim. UK Summary of product characteristics, August 2009.
15. Morphgesic SR (Morphine sulfate). Amdipharm. UK Summary of product characteristics, January 2003.
16. Morphine Sulphate Injection. Wockhardt UK Ltd. UK Summary of product characteristics, September 2007.
17. Gratz SS, Simpson GM. MAOI-Narcotic interactions. *J Clin Psychiatry* (1993) 54, 439.
18. DHC Continus (Dihydrocodeine tartrate). Napp Pharmaceuticals Ltd. UK Summary of product characteristics, February 2007.
19. Paramol (Dihydrocodeine tartrate with Paracetamol). SSL International plc. UK Summary of product characteristics, June 2007.
20. Meptid Tablets (Meptazinol hydrochloride). Almirall Ltd. UK Summary of product characteristics, January 2009.
21. BuTrans (Buprenorphine transdermal patch). Napp Pharmaceuticals Ltd. UK Summary of product characteristics, November 2008.
22. Solpadol (Codeine with Paracetamol). Sanofi-Aventis. UK Summary of product characteristics, January 2009.
23. Diamorphine hydrochloride BP for Injection. Auralis Ltd. UK Summary of product characteristics, January 2010.
24. Diconal (Dipipanone hydrochloride with Cyclizine hydrochloride). Amdipharm plc. UK Summary of product characteristics, September 2003.
25. Palladone Capsules (Hydromorphone hydrochloride). Napp Pharmaceuticals Ltd. UK Summary of product characteristics, September 2008.
26. Methadone Hydrochloride Oral Solution. Rosemont Pharmaceuticals Ltd. UK Summary of product characteristics, September 2014.
27. OxyNorm Liquid (Oxycodone hydrochloride). Napp Pharmaceuticals Ltd. UK Summary of product characteristics, July 2008.
28. Manerix (Moclobemide). Meda Pharmaceuticals. UK Summary of product characteristics, September 2009.

MAOIs or RIMAs + Opioids; Pethidine (Meperidine)

The concurrent use of pethidine and an MAOI has resulted in a serious and potentially life-threatening reaction in several patients. Excitement, muscle rigidity, hyperpyrexia, flushing, sweating and unconsciousness can occur very rapidly. Respiratory depression, with hypertension or hypotension, has also been seen.

A possible case of serotonin syndrome has been seen in a patient given moclobemide and pethidine (with lithium and nortriptyline).

Clinical evidence

(a) MAOIs

Severe, rapid and potentially fatal toxic reactions, both excitatory and depressant can occur when MAOIs are given with pethidine. In one case, a woman stopped taking **iproniazid** 50 mg twice daily and about a day and a half later, almost immediately after being given pethidine 100 mg for chest pain, she became restless and incoherent, and was comatose within 20 minutes. One hour after receiving the injection she was flushed, sweating and showed Cheyne-Stokes respiration. Her pupils were dilated and unreactive. Deep reflexes could not be initiated and plantar reflexes were extensor. Her pulse rate was 82 bpm and blood pressure 156/110 mmHg. She was rousable within 10 minutes of receiving an intravenous injection of prednisolone hemisuccinate 25 mg. A very similar reaction also occurred in another patient.[1]

In another case, a woman who, unknown to her doctor, was taking **tranylcypromine**, was given pethidine 100 mg. Within minutes she became unconscious, noisy and restless, having to be held down by 3 people. Her breathing was stertorous and her pulse was impalpable. Generalised tonic spasm developed, with ankle clonus, extensor plantar reflexes, shallow respiration and cyanosis. On admission to hospital she had a pulse rate of 160 bpm, a blood pressure of 90/60 mmHg and was sweating profusely (temperature 38.3°C). Her condition gradually improved and 4 hours after admission she was conscious but drowsy. Recovery was complete the next day.[2] Several other cases of this interaction have been reported in patients taking **iproniazid**,[3-5] **pargyline**,[6,7] **phenelzine**,[8-13] and **mebanazine**.[14] Fatalities have occurred. In addition, one of 8 patients taking an MAOI and given a 5-mg test dose of pethidine experienced a drop in systolic blood pressure of 30 mmHg and a rise in pulse rate of 20 bpm.[15]

In contrast, a study in 15 patients who had been taking **phenelzine**, **isocarboxazid**, **iproniazid** or *Parstelin* (**tranylcypromine** with trifluoperazine) for 3 to 8 weeks, found no changes in blood pressure, pulse rate or state of awareness with test doses of up to 40 mg of pethidine.[16] Similarly, no major problems were noted in a retrospective review of 45 episodes of anaesthesia in patients taking **isocarboxazid** who were given pethidine as part of their premedication.[17]

(b) RIMAs

A case report describes suspected serotonin syndrome in a 73-year-old woman, given pethidine in addition to her usual treatment with **moclobemide** 750 mg daily, nortriptyline 100 mg daily and lithium 750 mg daily.[18] Note, that both lithium and the tricyclics have been implicated in cases of serotonin syndrome, and these drugs may therefore have contributed to the interaction in this case.

Mechanism

Not understood, despite the extensive studies undertaken.[19-21] The reaction has proved difficult to study in *animals*, because *mice* appear to be more sensitive to the reaction than humans. There is some evidence that pethidine is a weak serotonin reuptake inhibitor,[22] and that the reactions may be due to an increase in levels of serotonin within the brain, which results in serotonin syndrome.

Importance and management

The interaction between pethidine and the MAOIs, which was first observed in the 1950s, is based on case reports. Nevertheless, it is serious and potentially fatal. Its incidence is unknown, but it is probably quite low, because one study that attempted to produce the interaction by giving increasing test doses of pethidine to 15 patients taking various MAOIs did not provoke the interaction.[16] It might therefore be an idiosyncratic reaction. Nevertheless, it would be imprudent to give pethidine to any patient taking an MAOI: indeed concurrent use is generally contraindicated. Bear in mind that the non-selective MAOIs are all essentially irreversible so that an interaction is possible for many days after their withdrawal: it is therefore also generally advised that pethidine should not be given within 2 weeks of stopping an MAOI. For more information on serotonin syndrome and its management, see 'Drugs that cause serotonin syndrome + Other drugs that cause serotonin syndrome', p.1471.

Information regarding an interaction between moclobemide and pethidine is sparse. Nevertheless, the manufacturer of moclobemide contraindicates concurrent use.[23] As moclobemide is a reversible inhibitor of MAO-A it is unlikely to interact 24 hours after it has been stopped. Note that other RIMAs would be expected to behave in the same way as moclobemide, although evidence for this appears to be lacking.

Sensitivity test

A sensitivity test, to assess the potential for this interaction in individual patients, has been suggested,[15] but given the fact that there are many alternatives to both pethidine and an MAOI are readily available, and that a drop in systolic blood pressure of 30 mmHg has been reported even with the first step of the test dose (5 mg of pethidine)[15] it would seem prudent to avoid the combination. Furthermore, the test dose procedure is unlikely to be suitable when opioids are required in an emergency situation.

1. Shee JC. Dangerous potentiation of pethidine by iproniazid, and its treatment. *BMJ* (1960) 2, 507–9.
2. Denton PH, Borrelli VM, Edwards NV. Dangers of monoamine oxidase inhibitors. *BMJ* (1962) 2, 1752–3.
3. Clement AJ, Benazon D. Reactions to other drugs in patients taking monoamine-oxidase inhibitors. *Lancet* (1962) ii, 197–8.
4. Papp C, Benaim S. Toxic effects of iproniazid in a patient with angina. *BMJ* (1958) 2, 1070–2.
5. Mitchell RS. Fatal toxic encephalitis occurring during iproniazid therapy in pulmonary tuberculosis. *Ann Intern Med* (1955) 42, 417–24.
6. Vigran IM. Dangerous potentiation of meperidine hydrochloride by pargyline hydrochloride. *JAMA* (1964) 187, 953–4.
7. Jenkins LC, Graves HB. Potential hazards of psychoactive drugs in association with anaesthesia. *Can Anaesth Soc J* (1965) 12, 121–8.
8. Palmer H. Potentiation of pethidine. *BMJ* (1960) 2, 944.
9. Taylor DC. Alarming reaction to pethidine in patients on phenelzine. *Lancet* (1962) ii, 401–2.
10. Cocks DP, Passmore-Rowe A. Dangers of monoamine oxidase inhibitors. *BMJ* (1962) 2, 1545–6.
11. Reid NCRW, Jones D. Pethidine and phenelzine. *BMJ* (1962) 1, 408.
12. Meyer D, Halfin V. Toxicity secondary to meperidine in patients on monoamine oxidase inhibitors: a case report and critical review. *J Clin Psychopharmacol* (1981) 1, 319–21.
13. Asch DA, Parker RM. Sounding board. The Libby Zion case. One step forward or two steps backward? *N Engl J Med* (1988) 318, 771–5.
14. Anon. Death from drugs combination. *Pharm J* (1965) 195, 341.
15. Churchill-Davidson HC. Anaesthesia and monoamine oxidase inhibitors. *BMJ* (1965) 1, 520.
16. Evans-Prosser CDG. The use of pethidine and morphine in the presence of monoamine oxidase inhibitors. *Br J Anaesth* (1968) 40, 279–82.
17. Ebrahim ZY, O'Hara J, Borden L, Tetzlaff J. Monoamine oxidase inhibitors and elective surgery. *Cleve Clin J Med* (1993) 60, 129–130.
18. Gillman PK. Possible serotonin syndrome with moclobemide and pethidine. *Med J Aust* (1995) 162, 554.
19. Leander JD, Batten J, Hargis GW. Pethidine interaction with clorgyline, pargyline or 5-hydroxytryptophan: lack of enhanced pethidine lethality or hyperpyrexia in mice. *J Pharm Pharmacol* (1978) 30, 396–8.
20. Rogers KJ, Thornton JA. The interaction between monoamine oxidase inhibitors and narcotic analgesics in mice. *Br J Pharmacol* (1969) 36, 470–80.
21. Gessner PK, Soble AG. A study of the tranylcypromine-meperidine interaction: effects of *p*-chlorophenylalanine and *l*-5-hydroxytryptophan. *J Pharmacol Exp Ther* (1973) 186, 276–87.
22. Gillman PK. Monoamine oxidase inhibitors, opioid analgesics and serotonin toxicity. *Br J Anaesth* (2005) 95, 434–41.
23. Manerix (Moclobemide). Meda Pharmaceuticals. UK Summary of product characteristics, September 2009.

MAOIs or RIMAs + Opioids; Tramadol

Serotonin syndrome developed in one patient taking iproniazid and tramadol, and delirium occurred in another patient given tramadol shortly after stopping phenelzine.

A fatal case of possible serotonin syndrome occurred in a patient abusing tramadol, moclobemide and clomipramine.

Clinical evidence, mechanism, importance and management

Serotonin syndrome (myoclonus, tremor, sweating, hyperreflexia, tachycardia) developed in a patient taking **iproniazid** when tramadol was also given. When the tramadol was stopped the patient recovered within 48 hours.[1] Another single case report describes the development of severe delirium in a patient within 3 days of stopping long term treatment with **phenelzine** 45 mg daily and starting intramuscular tramadol 100 mg three times daily. The patient became anxious and confused, and developed visual hallucinations and persecutory ideation. The symptoms disappeared within 48 hours of stopping the tramadol.[2] Another report suggests that tramadol may have contributed to the development of a fatal case of serotonin syndrome in a patient abusing tramadol, **moclobemide** and clomipramine.[3]

Information is limited, but the MAOIs and tramadol are known to have serotonergic effects. One UK manufacturer of tramadol contraindicates concurrent use, with or within 14 days of stopping an MAOI,[4] whereas a US manufacturer advises great caution if tramadol is given with an MAOI.[5] In practice this means monitoring closely for signs of serotonin syndrome; for more information on this syndrome and its management, see 'Drugs that cause serotonin syndrome + Other drugs that cause serotonin syndrome', p.1471. Note that the US manufacturer of tramadol also states that concurrent use with MAOIs may increase the risk of seizures,[5] and therefore seizure potential should also be borne in mind when the combination is given.

Evidence regarding an interaction with moclobemide is extremely limited, but moclobemide is known to have serotonergic actions. A general recommendation cannot be made based on the case report, as it involved the abuse of the drugs in question, but note that the manufacturer of **moclobemide** advises caution if it is given with other drugs that affect serotonin.[6] In practice this probably means monitoring closely for signs of serotonin syndrome, see under 'Drugs that cause serotonin syndrome + Other drugs that cause serotonin syndrome', p.1471.

1. de Larquier A, Vial T, Bréjoux G, Descotes J. Syndrome sérotoninergique lors de l'association tramadol et iproniazide. *Therapie* (1999) 54, 767–8.
2. Calvisi V, Ansseau M. Confusion mentale liée à l'administration de tramadol chez une patiente sous IMAO. *Rev Med Liege* (1999) 54, 912–13.
3. Hernandez AF, Montero MN, Pla A, Villanueva E. Fatal moclobemide overdose or death caused by serotonin syndrome? *J Forensic Sci* (1995) 40, 128–30.
4. Zydol SR Tabs (Tramadol hydrochloride). Grünenthal Ltd. UK Summary of product characteristics, January 2011.
5. Ultram ER (Tramadol hydrochloride). Pricara. US Prescribing information, June 2009.
6. Manerix (Moclobemide). Meda Pharmaceuticals. UK Summary of product characteristics, September 2009.

MAOIs or RIMAs + Phenylephrine

The concurrent use of oral phenylephrine and the non-selective MAOIs can result in a potentially life-threatening hypertensive crisis. The effects of parenteral phenylephrine may be approximately doubled by MAOIs. Some interaction occurs between phenylephrine and the RIMAs moclo-

bemide or brofaromine, but the blood pressure response appears to be much smaller than that seen with the non-selective MAOIs.

Clinical evidence

(a) MAOIs

A study in 3 healthy subjects, given **phenelzine** 45 mg or **tranylcypromine** 30 mg daily for 7 days, found that the blood pressure rise following oral phenylephrine was markedly enhanced. On 2 of 3 occasions when 45 mg of phenylephrine was given orally, the rise in blood pressure became potentially disastrous and had to be reversed with phentolamine. On these two occasions the maximal increase in mean arterial pressure was 67 mmHg (compared with 1 mmHg or 11 mmHg without the MAOI). On the other occasion, the maximal increase in mean arterial pressure was 48 mmHg. The rise in blood pressure was accompanied by a severe headache. With 3 mg and 10 mg of phenylephrine, the maximal increase was 7 mmHg and 20 mmHg, respectively. After phenylephrine 3 mg was given *intravenously* over 20 minutes, the maximal increase in mean arterial pressure was 45 mmHg, compared with 23 mmHg without an MAOI.[1]

Another study describes a similar 2- to 2.5-fold increase in the pressor effects of *intravenous* phenylephrine following the use of **phenelzine** or **tranylcypromine**.[2]

A patient taking **tranylcypromine** who developed hypotension (40/0 mmHg) during surgery had an exaggerated pressor response (250/140 mmHg) when an intravenous infusion of phenylephrine 4 mg/500 mL was started.[3] However, in another report, repeated 100-microgram doses of intravenous phenylephrine were successfully used to treat hypotension in a patient taking an MAOI, without any hypertensive reaction.[4]

A case report of hypertension that was initially attributed to phenylephrine was later corrected to pseudoephedrine.[5]

(b) RIMAs

No clinically important interaction occurred in healthy subjects taking **brofaromine** 75 mg twice daily when they were given a single 2.5-mg dose of phenylephrine as nasal drops.[6] However, higher doses (exact amount not stated) did produce a blood pressure response,[6] with a maximum recorded diastolic blood pressure of 100 mmHg.

A study in 7 healthy subjects found that **moclobemide** 100 mg three times daily for one week had no effect on the increase in blood pressure induced by intravenous phenylephrine.[7] Another study reported similar results.[8] However, when **moclobemide** was given in a dose of 200 mg three times daily for up to 3 weeks the blood pressure response to infusions of phenylephrine was increased by up to 80%.[7] In one patient taking **moclobemide** (dose withheld on the morning of surgery), ephedrine and phenylephrine were used successfully and uneventfully to control hypotension during anaesthesia.[9]

A case of life-threatening hypertension[10] occurred in a patient taking **toloxatone** and phenylephrine. Oral terbutaline was also taken, and may have contributed to the effects described, see 'MAOIs or RIMAs + Beta-agonist bronchodilators', p.1386.

Mechanism

If given orally phenylephrine is used in large doses because much of it is destroyed by MAO in the gut and liver, and only a small amount gets into the general circulation. If MAO is inhibited, most of the oral dose escapes destruction and passes freely into the circulation, hence the gross enhancement of the pressor effects. Phenylephrine has mainly direct sympathomimetic activity, but it may also have some minor indirect activity as well, which would be expected to result in the release of some of the MAOI-accumulated noradrenaline (norepinephrine) at adrenergic nerve endings (see also 'MAOIs or RIMAs + Nasal decongestants and related drugs', p.1396). This might account for the increased response to phenylephrine given parenterally.

Importance and management

The interaction between the MAOIs and *oral* phenylephrine is established, serious and potentially life-threatening: concurrent use, or use within 14 days of stopping an MAOI, is generally contraindicated. Phenylephrine commonly occurs in oral non-prescription cough, cold and influenza preparations, so patients should be strongly warned about them. Whether the effects of nasal drops, nasal sprays and eye drops are also enhanced is uncertain, but it would be prudent to avoid concurrent use until they have been shown to be safe (note that one manufacturer of phenylephrine eye drops[11] contraindicates MAOIs).

The response to *parenteral* phenylephrine is also approximately doubled, and the UK manufacturer of phenylephrine injection similarly contraindicates concurrent use both with and within 14 days of stopping an MAOI.[12] However, the US manufacturer does not contraindicate concurrent use. They state that if concurrent use is essential, the initial dose should be small, and given with due caution.[13]

The few studies that are available suggest that any interaction with RIMAs is less severe than that with MAOIs, but this needs confirmation. Until more is known it would seem prudent to consider using lower doses of phenylephrine in patients taking moclobemide, and monitoring the outcome of concurrent use carefully.

Treatment

These hypertensive reactions have been controlled by intravenous phentolamine,[1] chlorpromazine, or nifedipine.[14] However, it is advisable to refer to current guidelines on the management of hypertensive crises for up-to-date advice. In the US, the manufacturers of phenelzine advise intravenous phentolamine 5 mg, given slowly to avoid excessive hypotension.[15]

1. Elis J, Laurence DR, Mattie H, Prichard BNC. Modification by monoamine oxidase inhibitors of the effect of some sympathomimetics on blood pressure. *BMJ* (1967) 2, 75–8.
2. Boakes AJ, Laurence DR, Teoh PC, Barar FSK, Benedikter L, Prichard BNC. Interactions between sympathomimetic amines and antidepressant agents in man. *BMJ* (1973) 1, 311–15.
3. Jenkins LC, Graves HB. Potential hazards of psychoactive drugs in association with anaesthesia. *Can Anaesth Soc J* (1965) 12, 121–8.
4. El-Ganzouri A, Ivankovich AD, Braverman B, Land PC. Should MAOI be discontinued preoperatively? *Anesthesiology* (1983) 59, A384.
5. Harrison WM, McGrath PJ, Stewart JW, Quitkin F. MAOIs and hypertensive crises: the role of OTC drugs. *J Clin Psychiatry* (1989) 50, 64–5. Correction. Magurno JAJ, Board AW. ibid. (1990) 51, 212–3. [drug].
6. Gleiter CH, Mühlbauer B, Gradin-Frimmer G, Antonin KH, Bieck PR. Administration of sympathomimetic drugs with the selective MAO-A inhibitor brofaromine. Effect on blood pressure. *Drug Invest* (1992) 4, 149–54.
7. Amrein R, Güntert TW, Dingemanse J, Lorscheid T, Stabl M, Schmid-Burgk W. Interactions of moclobemide with concomitantly administered medication: evidence from pharmacological and clinical studies. *Psychopharmacology (Berl)* (1992) 106, S24–S31.
8. Korn A, Eichler HG, Gasić S. Moclobemide, a new specific MAO-inhibitor does not interact with direct adrenergic agonists. The Second Amine Oxidase Workshop, Uppsala. August 1986. *Pharmacol Toxicol* (1987) 60 (Suppl I), 31.
9. Martyr JW, Orlikowski CEP. Epidural anaesthesia, ephedrine and phenylephrine in a patient taking moclobemide, a new monoamine oxidase inhibitor. *Anaesthesia* (1996) 51, 1150–2.
10. Lefebvre H, Richard R, Noblet C, Moore N, Wolf L-M. Life-threatening pseudo-phaeochromocytoma after toloxatone, terbutaline, and phenylephrine. *Lancet* (1993) 341, 555–6.
11. Minims Phenylephrine hydrochloride 10%. Bausch & Lomb UK Ltd. UK Summary of product characteristics, November 2006.
12. Phenylephrine Injection BP. Sovereign Medical. UK Summary of product characteristics, May 2009.
13. Phenylephrine hydrochloride Injection. Teva Parenteral Medicines, Inc. US Prescribing information, October 2008.
14. Golwyn DH, Weinstock RC. MAOIs, OTC drugs, and hypertensive crisis. *J Clin Psychiatry* (1990) 51, 213.
15. Nardil (Phenelzine sulfate). Pfizer Inc. US Prescribing information, February 2009.

MAOIs + Rauwolfia alkaloids or Tetrabenazine

Central excitation and possibly hypertension can occur if rauwolfia alkaloids are given to patients already taking an MAOI, but this is less likely if the rauwolfia alkaloid is given first. Theoretically, additive blood pressure lowering effects are also a possibility. The use of drugs that have the potential to cause depression, such as the rauwolfia alkaloids or tetrabenazine, is generally contraindicated in patients needing treatment for depression.

Clinical evidence

A woman with a bipolar disorder, who had been in a depressed phase for 5 years, was given **nialamide** 100 mg three times daily. Two days later **reserpine** 500 micrograms three times daily was started. The following day she became frankly hypomanic and almost immediately went into mania.[1]

In another report, a patient who started to take **tetrabenazine** 10 mg three times daily, 2 days after stopping **nialamide** 25 mg daily, which had been taken for a week, collapsed 6 hours after the first **tetrabenazine** dose, and demonstrated epileptiform convulsions, partial unconsciousness, rapid respiration and tachycardia. He recovered within 15 minutes, but 3 days later he had a similar attack, and the **tetrabenazine** was stopped.[2]

Another author states that the use of **reserpine** or **tetrabenazine** after pretreatment with **iproniazid** can lead to a temporary disturbance of affect and memory, associated with autonomic excitation, delirious agitation, disorientation and illusions of experience and recognition, which lasts for up to 3 days.[3,4]

A prolonged period of increased motor activity after starting **reserpine** ('reserpine-reversal') possibly occurred in 3 patients with schizophrenia who had taken **phenelzine** for 12 weeks, when compared with patients given **reserpine** who had not received an MAOI. Their blood pressures rose slightly and persistently, and their psychomotor activity was considerably increased, lasting in two cases throughout the 12-week period of concurrent use.[5]

Mechanism

Theoretically, reserpine could cause hypertension in patients taking non-selective MAOIs. Rauwolfia alkaloids, such as reserpine, cause adrenergic neurones to become depleted of their normal stores of noradrenaline (norepinephrine). In this way they prevent or reduce the normal transmission of impulses at the adrenergic nerve endings of the sympathetic nervous system, and thereby act as antihypertensives. As the brain also possesses adrenergic neurones, failure of transmission in the CNS could account for the sedation and depression observed with these drugs. If rauwolfia alkaloids are given to patients already taking an MAOI, large amounts of accumulated noradrenaline can be released throughout the body. In the brain, serotonin is also released. The release of these substances results in marked central excitation and hypertension. This would account for the case reports cited and the effects seen in *animals*.[6-8] These stimulant effects are sometimes called 'reserpine-reversal' because instead of the expected sedation or depression, excitation or delayed depression is seen. Note that it depends upon the order in which the drugs are given.

Importance and management

On the basis of the theoretical risk of hypertensive crisis, the US manufacturers of **isocarboxazid**[9] and **tranylcypromine**[10] contraindicate concurrent use with reserpine. Conversely, the UK manufacturer of **isocarboxazid**[11] mentions that it may potentiate the *hypotensive* effect of **reserpine** (MAOIs alone can have hypotensive effects). In addition, the use of drugs that have the potential to cause depression (such as rauwolfia alkaloids) is generally contraindicated in patients with depression. However, one report[12] suggests that if concurrent use is considered desirable, the MAOI should be given after, and not before the rauwolfia alkaloid, so that sedation rather than excitation will occur, and this advice is also given by the UK manufacturer of

tetrabenazine.[13] It would therefore be prudent to consider the possibility of hypotension, hypertension or CNS excitation if both drugs are considered essential.

1. Gradwell BG. Psychotic reactions and phenelzine. *BMJ* (1960) 2, 1018.
2. Davies TS. Monoamine oxidase inhibitors and rauwolfia compounds. *BMJ* (1960) 2, 739–40.
3. Voelkel A. Klinische Wirkung von Pharmaka mit Einfluss auf den Monoaminestoffwechsel de Gehirns. *Confin Neurol* (1958) 18, 144–9.
4. Voelkel A. Clinical experiences with amine oxidase inhibitors in psychiatry. *Ann N Y Acad Sci* (1959) 80, 680–6.
5. Esser AH. Clinical observations on reserpine reversal after prolonged MAO inhibition. *Psychiatr Neurol Neurochir* (1967) 70, 59–63.
6. Shore PA, Brodie BB. LSD-like effects elicited by reserpine in rabbits pretreated with isoniazid. *Proc Soc Exp Biol Med* (1957) 94, 433–5.
7. Chessin M, Kramer ER, Scott CC. Modification of the pharmacology of reserpine and serotonin by iproniazid. *J Pharmacol Exp Ther* (1957) 119, 453–60.
8. von Euler US, Bygdeman S, Persson N-Å. Interaction of reserpine and monoamine oxidase inhibitors on adrenergic transmitter release. *Biochim Biol Sper* (1970) 9, 215–20.
9. Marplan (Isocarboxazid). Validus Pharmaceuticals, Inc. US Prescribing information, August 2007.
10. Parnate (Tranylcypromine sulfate). GlaxoSmithKline. US Prescribing information, May 2010.
11. Isocarboxazid. Cambridge Laboratories. UK Summary of product characteristics, February 2008.
12. Natarajan S. Potential danger of monoamineoxidase inhibitors and α-methyldopa. *Lancet* (1964) i, 1330.
13. Xenazine (Tetrabenazine). Cambridge Laboratories. UK Summary of product characteristics, February 2008.

MAOIs or RIMAs + SNRIs

Serious and potentially life-threatening reactions (serotonin syndrome) can develop if venlafaxine and non-selective MAOIs (isocarboxazid, phenelzine, tranylcypromine) are given concurrently, or even sequentially if insufficient time is left in between. Desvenlafaxine, duloxetine, levomilnacipran, and milnacipran are expected to interact with the MAOIs in the same way.

Serotonin syndrome has also been reported with moclobemide and venlafaxine, but it has usually occurred during overdose. There is also a possible case with moclobemide and duloxetine.

Clinical evidence

(a) MAOIs

1. Isocarboxazid. A man with recurrent depression taking isocarboxazid 30 mg daily was also given **venlafaxine** 75 mg. After the second dose, he developed agitation, hypomania, diaphoresis, shivering, and dilated pupils. These symptoms subsided when the **venlafaxine** was stopped. A few months later, when given both drugs again, he developed myoclonic jerks and diaphoresis.[1]

2. Phenelzine. A woman who had stopped taking phenelzine 45 mg daily 7 days previously, developed sweating, lightheadedness, and dizziness within 45 minutes of taking a single 37.5-mg dose of **venlafaxine**. In the emergency department she was found to be lethargic, agitated, and extremely diaphoretic. The agitation was treated with lorazepam. One week later, after she had recovered, she again started taking the same regimen of venlafaxine without problems.[2] A man developed serotonin syndrome when he started **venlafaxine** the day after he stopped taking phenelzine,[3] and a woman developed serotonin syndrome within one hour of taking phenelzine and **venlafaxine** together.[4] Four other patients similarly developed the reaction when phenelzine was replaced by **venlafaxine.**[5]

3. Tranylcypromine. A woman who had been taking tranylcypromine for 3 weeks developed serotonin syndrome within 4 hours of inadvertently taking a single tablet of **venlafaxine**. She recovered within 24 hours, when treated with ice packs, a cooling blanket, diazepam, and dantrolene.[6] Serotonin syndrome developed in a man taking tranylcypromine within 2 hours of taking half a **venlafaxine** tablet,[7] and another case of serotonin syndrome has been described in a man taking tranylcypromine 60 mg daily who accidentally took **venlafaxine** 300 mg.[8] This case has also been published elsewhere.[9]

(b) RIMAs

A 46-year-old woman developed symptoms, which were considered to be indicative of a mild form of serotonin syndrome, shortly after taking **duloxetine** 60 mg. The previous day she had taken the last dose of a course of treatment with **moclobemide** 600 mg daily. Her symptoms included restlessness, tremor, dizziness, headache, and tics-like facial movements. On the second day of **duloxetine** treatment, her blood pressure increased to 130/90 mmHg.[10] **Duloxetine** was stopped, and **moclobemide** restarted uneventfully after a one-week washout period.[10] Note that an increase in blood pressure is a known adverse effect of **duloxetine** alone.[11]

A 32-year-old man taking **moclobemide** 20 mg twice daily and diazepam developed serotonin syndrome 40 minutes after taking a single 150-mg dose of **venlafaxine.**[12] Serotonin toxicity (serotonin syndrome) occurred in 4 patients who took an overdose of **moclobemide** with **venlafaxine** (just 150 mg in one case and 750 mg in another). In this analysis of **moclobemide** overdoses, the risk of developing serotonin toxicity was considerably increased in patients who also took another serotonergic drug (52%; 11 of 21 patients compared with 3% taking moclobemide alone). Venlafaxine was taken in 4 of the 11 cases mentioned.[13]

Mechanism

Serotonin syndrome is thought to occur because duloxetine and venlafaxine can inhibit serotonin reuptake (their antidepressant effect is related to this activity), and MAOIs and RIMAs inhibit the metabolism of serotonin. The result is an increase in the concentrations of serotonin apparently causing overstimulation of the 5-HT_{1A} receptors in the brain and spinal cord. For more information on serotonin syndrome and its management, see 'Drugs that cause serotonin syndrome + Other drugs that cause serotonin syndrome', p.1471.

Importance and management

MAOIs

The interaction between the non-selective MAOIs and **venlafaxine** is established, serious and potentially life-threatening. The manufacturers of venlafaxine note that in some cases this interaction has been fatal. They contraindicate the use of venlafaxine with and within 14 days of stopping an MAOI.[14,15] Based on the half-life of venlafaxine they state that at least 7 days should elapse between stopping venlafaxine and starting an MAOI. In one review it was suggested that a washout period of several weeks is required between stopping MAOIs such as phenelzine and initiating a second serotonergic drug such as venlafaxine.[16]

Similarly, it is recommended that **desvenlafaxine,**[17] duloxetine,[11,18,19] **levomilnacipran,**[20] and **milnacipran**[21,22] should not be given with an MAOI or within 14 days of stopping an MAOI. Based on the half-life of duloxetine, the manufacturers advise that at least 5 days should elapse between stopping duloxetine and starting an MAOI,[11,18,19] and the manufacturers of milnacipran recommend at least a 5- to 7-day gap,[21,22] while the manufacturers of desvenlafaxine[17] and levomilnacipran[20] recommend a gap of 7 days.

RIMAs

Evidence regarding an interaction between the SNRIs and RIMAs, such as moclobemide, is limited, and most cases seem to have occurred with overdoses. Nevertheless, concurrent use is generally not recommended with **venlafaxine**. The UK manufacturer of venlafaxine states that a withdrawal period shorter than 14 days may be used before starting venlafaxine [with other similar interactions with moclobemide 24 to 48 hours has been said to be adequate], but, as with MAOIs, at least 7 days should elapse between stopping venlafaxine and starting a RIMA.[14] The concurrent use of moclobemide with **duloxetine** is not recommended, but no specific advice is given regarding a washout period.[11,18] Based on other interactions with these drugs, it would seem prudent to wait for 5 days after duloxetine is stopped before starting the other drug. It has been suggested that no washout is needed after moclobemide, but others consider a 24-hour washout a prudent measure. One manufacturer of **milnacipran** also advises against the use of moclobemide, but they state that if the combination cannot be avoided, careful clinical monitoring is required, starting with the minimum recommended dose.[21]

1. Klysner R, Larsen JK, Sørensen P, Hyllested M, Pedersen BD. Toxic interaction of venlafaxine and isocarboxazide. *Lancet* (1995) 346, 1298–9.
2. Phillips SD, Ringo P. Phenelzine and venlafaxine interaction. *Am J Psychiatry* (1995) 152, 1400–1401.
3. Heisler MA, Guidry JR, Arnecke B. Serotonin syndrome induced by administration of venlafaxine and phenelzine. *Ann Pharmacother* (1996) 30, 84.
4. Weiner LA, Smythe M, Cisek J. Serotonin syndrome secondary to phenelzine-venlafaxine interaction. *Pharmacotherapy* (1998) 18, 399–403.
5. Diamond S, Pepper BJ, Diamond ML, Freitag FG, Urban GJ, Erdemoglu AK. Serotonin syndrome induced by transitioning from phenelzine to venlafaxine: four patient reports. *Neurology* (1998) 51, 274–6.
6. Hodgman M, Martin T, Dean B, Krenzelok E. Severe serotonin syndrome secondary to venlafaxine and maintenance tranylcypromine therapy. *J Toxicol Clin Toxicol* (1995) 33, 554.
7. Brubacher JR, Hoffman RS, Lurin MJ. Serotonin syndrome from venlafaxine-tranylcypromine interaction. *Vet Hum Toxicol* (1996) 38, 358–61.
8. Claassen JAHR, Gelissen HPMM. The serotonin syndrome. *N Engl J Med* (2005) 352, 2455.
9. Zonneveld AM, Hagenaars M, Voermans NC, Gelissen HPMM, Claassen JAHR. Levensbedreigend serotoninesyndroom na eenmalige toevoeging van een serotonineheropnameremmer aan een onderhoudsbehandeling met een monoamineoxidaseremmer. *Ned Tijdschr Geneeskd* (2006) 150, 1081–4.
10. Jimenez-Genchi A. Immediate switching from moclobemide to duloxetine may induce serotonin syndrome. *J Clin Psychiatry* (2006) 67, 1821–22.
11. Cymbalta (Duloxetine hydrochloride). Eli Lilly and Company Ltd. UK Summary of product characteristics, March 2014.
12. Chan BSH, Graudins A, Whyte IM, Dawson AH, Braitberg G, Duggin GG. Serotonin syndrome resulting from drug interactions. *Med J Aust* (1998) 169, 523–5.
13. Isbister GK, Hackett LP, Dawson AH, Whyte IM, Smith AJ. Moclobemide poisoning: toxicokinetics and occurrence of serotonin toxicity. *Br J Clin Pharmacol* (2003) 56, 441–50.
14. Efexor XL (Venlafaxine hydrochloride). Pfizer Ltd. UK Summary of product characteristics, December 2013.
15. Effexor XR (Venlafaxine hydrochloride). Wyeth Pharmaceuticals Inc. US Prescribing information, March 2014.
16. Mason PJ, Morris VA, Balcezak TJ. Serotonin syndrome. Presentation of 2 cases and review of the literature. *Medicine* (2000) 79, 201–9.
17. Pristiq (Desvenlafaxine succinate). Wyeth Pharmaceuticals Inc. US Prescribing information, July 2014.
18. Yentreve (Duloxetine hydrochloride). Eli Lilly and Company Ltd. UK Summary of product characteristics, October 2013.
19. Cymbalta (Duloxetine hydrochloride). Eli Lilly and Company. US Prescribing information, July 2014.
20. Fetzima (Levomilnacipran hydrochloride). Forest Pharmaceuticals, Inc. US Prescribing information, July 2014.
21. Ixel (Milnacipran hydrochloride). Pierre Fabre Médicament. French Summary of product characteristics, February 2003.
22. Savella (Milnacipran hydrochloride). Forest Pharmaceuticals, Inc. US Prescribing information, November 2013.

MAOIs or RIMAs + SSRIs

A number of case reports describe serotonin syndrome in patients given SSRIs with MAOIs or moclobemide: some have been fatal.

Clinical evidence

A. MAOIs

(a) Fluoxetine

A very high incidence (25 to 50%) of adverse effects occurred in 12 patients taking fluoxetine 10 to 100 mg daily with either **phenelzine** 30 to 60 mg daily or **tranylcypromine** 10 to 140 mg daily, and in 6 other patients who started one of these

MAOIs 10 days or more after stopping fluoxetine. There were mental changes such as hypomania, racing thoughts, agitation, restlessness, and confusion. The physical symptoms included myoclonus, hypertension, tremor, teeth chattering, and diarrhoea.[1] A detailed review of cases reported to the manufacturers described 8 acute cases, 7 of them fatal, in patients given fluoxetine with either **tranylcypromine** or **phenelzine**.[2] Uncontrollable shivering, teeth chattering, double vision, nausea, confusion, and anxiety developed in a woman given **tranylcypromine** after stopping fluoxetine. The problem resolved within a day of stopping the **tranylcypromine**, and did not recur when fluoxetine was tried again 6 weeks later.[3]

A number of other reports describe similar reactions in patients given fluoxetine and **tranylcypromine**,[3-8] some occurring up to 6 weeks after the SSRI was stopped,[6] and several resulting in fatalities.[3,7]

(b) Sertraline

A man taking **tranylcypromine** and clonazepam was also given sertraline 25 to 50 mg daily. Within 4 days he began to experience chills, increasing confusion, sedation, exhaustion, unsteadiness, and incoordination. Other symptoms included impotence, urinary hesitancy, and constipation. These problems rapidly resolved when the sertraline was stopped and the **tranylcypromine** dose was reduced from 30 to 20 mg daily.[9]

A woman with a major depressive disorder taking lithium, thioridazine, doxepin, and **phenelzine** was also given sertraline 100 mg daily for worsening depression. Within 3 hours she became semi-comatose, with a temperature of 41°C, a heart rate of 154 bpm, and symptoms of rigidity and shivering. She was treated with diazepam, midazolam, ice packs, and dantrolene.[10] Two other similar cases, involving the use of sertraline with **isocarboxazid**[11] and **phenelzine**[12] have been reported. The latter case was fatal.[12] Another case of mild serotonin syndrome (managed with cyproheptadine) occurred in a woman who took a single dose of sertraline 11 days after stopping **isocarboxazid**.[13]

B. RIMAs

(a) Citalopram

A 34-year-old man who had been taking **moclobemide** 100 mg every 8 hours for several months was switched to citalopram 20 mg daily without a washout period. One hour later, he became agitated and had involuntary movements of the legs, which progressed to generalised rigidity. His heart rate was 100 bpm, but all other vital signs were normal. He was treated with benzodiazepines and recovered uneventfully.[14]

(b) Fluoxetine

A placebo-controlled study in 18 healthy subjects found that the use of fluoxetine 20 mg with **moclobemide** 100 to 600 mg daily for 9 days did not appear to result in an adverse interaction.[15] Other studies in healthy subjects and patients similarly found no evidence of serotonin syndrome.[16,17]

A post-marketing analysis found that at least 30 patients switched from fluoxetine to **moclobemide** within one week had experienced no adverse effects.[15,18] However, 3 patients have developed serotonin syndrome[19-21] and one developed agitation and confusion[22] following the use of **moclobemide** and fluoxetine. Furthermore, a study suggests that the combination might cause a high rate of adverse effects (insomnia, dizziness, nausea and headache).[19]

(c) Fluvoxamine

When 13 of 22 healthy subjects given fluvoxamine 100 mg daily for 9 days were also given **moclobemide**, in increasing doses of 50 to 400 mg daily from days 7 to 10, no serious adverse reactions occurred. Any adverse effects were mild to moderate (some increase in headaches, fatigue, dizziness, all of which can occur with both drugs alone) and there was no evidence of serotonin syndrome.[15,23] An open study in 6 depressed patients given **moclobemide** 225 to 800 mg daily and fluvoxamine 50 to 200 mg daily found a notable improvement in depression. Insomnia was the commonest adverse effect (treated with trazodone) but none of the patients showed any evidence of serotonin syndrome.[24] Similar results were found in other studies.[17,25]

(d) Paroxetine

An open 6-week study in 19 patients with major depression taking paroxetine (or fluoxetine) 20 mg daily, to which **moclobemide** up to 600 mg daily was added, indicated that these combinations were possibly effective.[26] An extension of this study with 50 patients is reported elsewhere.[19] However, a range of adverse effects occurred in some patients, the clearest one being insomnia, and serotonin syndrome was seen in one patient.[19,26] Conversely, serotonin syndrome was not seen in another study, where low initial doses and gradual up-titration of both paroxetine and **moclobemide** was used.[17] Two possible cases of mild serotonin syndrome occurred in women taking **moclobemide** within 2 to 24 hours of also starting paroxetine,[27] and a case report describes serotonin syndrome in a patient who was changed from paroxetine to moclobemide without an adequate washout period. She had taken her last dose of paroxetine in the morning, started taking moclobemide at lunchtime, and serotonin syndrome had developed a few hours after her second dose taken at dinnertime. However, as this patient was also taking **selegiline**, it is difficult to attribute the interaction to moclobemide and paroxetine alone.[28]

(e) Sertraline

In one study, 31 severely ill patients were given **moclobemide** 35 to 800 mg daily with SSRIs, including sertraline 25 to 100 mg daily, initially using lower than usual starting doses of both drugs, and then gradually titrating them upwards. The other SSRIs used were fluoxetine, fluvoxamine and paroxetine. There was no evidence of serotonin syndrome.[17] An open study in 5 patients with depression given **moclobemide** 150 to 600 mg daily and sertraline 25 to 200 mg daily found improvements ranging from minimal to complete remission. Insomnia was the most common adverse effect (treated with trazodone), but none of the patients showed any evidence of serotonin syndrome.[24] However, a fatality has been reported with an overdose of **moclobemide**, sertraline, and pimozide, with blood concentrations suggesting that none of the drugs individually would have been fatal.[29]

(f) Unspecified SSRIs

Serotonin toxicity (serotonin syndrome) occurred in 5 patients who took an overdose of **moclobemide** with an SSRI (specific drugs not mentioned). In this analysis of **moclobemide** overdoses, the risk of developing serotonin toxicity was considerably increased in patients who also took another serotonergic drug (52% (11 of 21 patients), compared with 3% taking moclobemide alone). Of the 11 patients mentioned, 5 patients were taking SSRIs.[30]

Mechanism

MAO-A is involved in the metabolism of serotonin, so the concurrent use of MAOIs or RIMAs with SSRIs can lead to excessive serotonin concentrations, and result in serotonin syndrome. For more information on serotonin syndrome and its management, see 'Drugs that cause serotonin syndrome + Other drugs that cause serotonin syndrome', p.1471.

Importance and management

MAOIs

The interaction between the SSRIs and MAOIs is reasonably well documented and established. Severe, sometimes fatal interactions (serotonin syndrome or similar) have occurred when MAOIs were given with fluoxetine or sertraline. The incidence appears to be low, possibly as the concurrent use of an MAOI and an SSRI is contraindicated.

MAOIs should not be given with SSRIs, and at least 2 weeks should elapse between stopping any MAOI and starting any SSRI to allow for the effects of the MAOI to diminish. Moreover, the manufacturers of each SSRI give guidance on the appropriate intervals that should be left between stopping the SSRI and starting an MAOI; that is, 7 days for sertraline,[31] citalopram,[32] **escitalopram**,[33] fluvoxamine[34] or paroxetine[35] (14 days in the US for citalopram, escitalopram, sertraline, paroxetine, and **vilazodone**[36-40]) and at least 5 weeks for fluoxetine,[41,42] with an even longer interval if long-term or high-dose fluoxetine has been used.[41]

RIMAs

The RIMAs (such as moclobemide) also have serotonergic effects, and so they are unlikely to be any safer than the non-selective MAOIs with regard to interactions with SSRIs. The few cases of serotonin syndrome cited with therapeutic doses of this combination confirm that it is not necessarily safe. The combination can be particularly problematic in overdose, and negates the generally benign course of moclobemide overdose alone.

The concurrent use of moclobemide and an SSRI is contraindicated.[43] Because the effects of moclobemide are readily reversible, only one day need elapse between stopping moclobemide and starting an SSRI. However, when stopping an SSRI and starting moclobemide, the same intervals are required as for the non-selective MAOIs (see above).

1. Feighner JP, Boyer WF, Tyler DL, Neborsky RJ. Adverse consequences of fluoxetine-MAOI combination therapy. *J Clin Psychiatry* (1990) 51, 222–5.
2. Beasley CM, Masica DN, Heiligenstein JH, Wheadon DE, Zerbe RL. Possible monoamine oxidase inhibitor — serotonin uptake inhibitor interaction: fluoxetine clinical data and preclinical findings. *J Clin Psychopharmacol* (1993) 13, 312–20.
3. Sternbach H. Danger of MAOI therapy after fluoxetine withdrawal. *Lancet* (1988) ii, 850–1.
4. Ooi, TK. The serotonin syndrome. *Anaesthesia* (1991) 46, 507–8.
5. Spiller HA, Morse S, Muir C. Fluoxetine ingestion: A one year retrospective study. *Vet Hum Toxicol* (1990) 32, 153–5.
6. Coplan JD, Gorman JM. Detectable levels of fluoxetine metabolites after discontinuation: an unexpected serotonin syndrome. *Am J Psychiatry* (1993) 150, 837.
7. Kline SS, Mauro LS, Scala-Barnett DM, Zick D. Serotonin syndrome versus neuroleptic malignant syndrome as a cause of death. *Clin Pharm* (1989) 8, 510–14.
8. Miller F, Friedman R, Tanenbaum J, Griffin A. Disseminated intravascular coagulation and acute myoglobinuric renal failure: a consequence of the serotonergic syndrome. *J Clin Psychopharmacol* (1991) 11, 277–9.
9. Bhatara VS, Bandettini FC. Possible interaction between sertraline and tranylcypromine. *Clin Pharm* (1993) 12, 222–5.
10. Graber MA, Hoehns TB, Perry PJ. Sertraline-phenelzine drug interaction: a serotonin syndrome reaction. *Ann Pharmacother* (1994) 28, 732–5.
11. Brannan SK, Talley BJ, Bowden CL. Sertraline and isocarboxazid cause a serotonin syndrome. *J Clin Psychopharmacol* (1994) 14, 144–5.
12. Keltner N. Serotonin syndrome: a case of fatal SSRI/MAOI interaction. *Perspect Psychiatr Care* (1994) 30, 26–31.
13. Lappin RI, Auchincloss EL. Treatment of the serotonin syndrome with cyproheptadine. *N Engl J Med* (1994) 331, 1021–2.
14. Gumà M, Clemente F, Segura A, Costa J. Síndrome serotoninérgico: moclobemida y citalopram. *Med Clin (Barc)* (1999) 113, 677–8.
15. Dingemanse J. An update of recent moclobemide interaction data. *Int Clin Psychopharmacol* (1993) 7, 167–80.
16. Dingemanse J, Wallnöfer A, Gieschke R, Guentert T, Amrein R. Pharmacokinetic and pharmacodynamic interactions between fluoxetine and moclobemide in the investigation of development of the "serotonin syndrome". *Clin Pharmacol Ther* (1998) 63, 403–13.
17. Bakish D, Hooper CL, West DL, Miller C, Blanchard A, Bashir F. Moclobemide and specific serotonin re-uptake inhibitor combination treatment of resistant anxiety and depressive disorders. *Hum Psychopharmacol* (1995) 10, 105–9.
18. Dingemanse J, Guentert TW, Moritz E, Eckernas S-A. Pharmacodynamic and pharmacokinetic interactions between fluoxetine and moclobemide. *Clin Pharmacol Ther* (1993) 53, 178.
19. Hawley CJ, Quick SJ, Ratnam S, Pattinson HA, McPhee S. Safety and tolerability of combined treatment with moclobemide and SSRIs: a systematic study of 50 patients. *Int Clin Psychopharmacol* (1996) 11, 187–91.
20. Benazzi F. Serotonin syndrome with moclobemide-fluoxetine combination. *Pharmacopsychiatry* (1996) 29, 162.
21. Liebenberg R, Berk M, Winkler G. Serotonergic syndrome after concomitant use of moclobemide and fluoxetine. *Hum Psychopharmacol* (1996) 11, 146–7.
22. Chan BSH, Graudins A, Whyte IM, Dawson AH, Braitberg G, Duggin GG. Serotonin syndrome resulting from drug interactions. *Med J Aust* (1998) 169, 523–5.

23. Wallnöfer A, Guentert TW, Eckernäs SA, Dingemanse J. Moclobemide and fluvoxamine co-administration: a prospective study in healthy volunteers to investigate the potential development of the 'serotonin syndrome'. *Hum Psychopharmacol* (1995) 10, 25–31.
24. Joffe RT, Bakish D. Combined SSRI-moclobemide treatment of psychiatric illness. *J Clin Psychiatry* (1994) 55, 24–5.
25. Ebert D, Albert R, May A, Stosiek I, Kaschka W. Combined SSRI-RIMA treatment in refractory depression. Safety data and efficacy. *Psychopharmacology (Berl)* (1995) 119, 342–4.
26. Hawley CJ, Ratnam S, Pattinson HA, Quick SJ, Echlin D. Safety and tolerability of combined treatment with moclobemide and SSRIs: a preliminary study of 19 patients. *J Psychopharmacol* (1996) 10, 241–5.
27. Graudins A, Stearman A, Chan B. Treatment of the serotonin syndrome with cyproheptadine. *J Emerg Med* (1998) 16, 615–19.
28. Wu M-L, Deng J-F. Serotonin toxicity caused by moclobemide too soon after paroxetine-selegiline. *J Chin Med Assoc* (2009) 72, 446–9.
29. McIntyre IM, King CV, Staikos V, Gall J, Drummer OH. A fatality involving moclobemide, sertraline, and pimozide. *J Forensic Sci* (1997) 42, 951–3.
30. Isbister GK, Hackett LP, Dawson AH, Whyte IM, Smith AJ. Moclobemide poisoning: toxicokinetics and occurrence of serotonin toxicity. *Br J Clin Pharmacol* (2003) 56, 441–50.
31. Lustral (Sertraline hydrochloride). Pfizer Ltd. UK Summary of product characteristics, March 2015.
32. Cipramil Tablets (Citalopram hydrobromide). Lundbeck Ltd. UK Summary of product characteristics, July 2015.
33. Cipralex Tablets (Escitalopram oxalate). Lundbeck Ltd. UK Summary of product characteristics, September 2013.
34. Faverin (Fluvoxamine maleate). BGP Products Ltd. UK Summary of product characteristics, August 2015.
35. Seroxat (Paroxetine hydrochloride hemihydrate). GlaxoSmithKline UK. UK Summary of product characteristics, November 2013.
36. Zoloft (Sertraline hydrochloride). Pfizer Inc. US Prescribing information, August 2014.
37. Celexa (Citalopram hydrobromide). Forest Pharmaceuticals, Inc. US Prescribing information, July 2014.
38. Lexapro (Escitalopram oxalate). Forest Pharmaceuticals, Inc. US Prescribing information, July 2014.
39. Paxil Tablets and Suspension (Paroxetine hydrochloride). GlaxoSmithKline. US Prescribing information, December 2012.
40. Viibryd (Vilazodone hydrochloride). Forest Pharmaceuticals, Inc. US prescribing information, April 2014.
41. Prozac (Fluoxetine hydrochloride). Eli Lilly and Company Ltd. UK Summary of product characteristics, October 2014.
42. Prozac (Fluoxetine hydrochloride). Eli Lilly and Company. US Prescribing information, July 2014.
43. Manerix (Moclobemide). Meda Pharmaceuticals. UK Summary of product characteristics, November 2013.

MAOIs or RIMAs + Trazodone

Isolated cases of serotonin syndrome have been reported in patients receiving trazodone and MAOIs or moclobemide. A small number of reports describe the successful use of low-dose trazodone with phenelzine or moclobemide for depression and insomnia.

Clinical evidence

(a) MAOIs

A case report describes a patient taking trazodone 50 mg daily and **isocarboxazid** 20 mg daily, who developed symptoms of serotonin syndrome and was hospitalised 2 months after dose increases to trazodone 150 mg daily and isocarboxazid 30 mg daily, and the addition of methylphenidate.[1] Note that the concurrent use of non-selective MAOIs with methylphenidate can result in hypertensive crisis and/or serotonin syndrome, see 'MAOIs or RIMAs + Methylphenidate and related drugs', p.1395, and so an interaction with trazodone in this case is by no means established. Another case report describes the successful use of **phenelzine** and trazodone 300 mg daily for the treatment of depression.[2]

(b) RIMAs

A case report describes the development of serotonin syndrome after the abrupt replacement of trazodone by **moclobemide**,[3] whereas several other reports describe the successful use of low-dose trazodone (up to 200 mg daily) to treat MAOI-induced insomnia.[4-6] In addition, one placebo-controlled study in 7 patients reported the successful use of low-dose trazodone 50 mg daily for one week in patients taking **brofaromine** 150 to 250 mg daily. No symptoms indicative of serotonin syndrome were reported on concurrent use.[7]

Mechanism

Trazodone has serotonergic effects, which might be additive with those of the MAOIs. Therefore concurrent use might therefore lead to serotonin syndrome. However, at low doses, trazodone has been reported to act mostly as a serotonin antagonist, with little of the serotonin agonist effects that develop at higher doses, and therefore the risk of serotonin syndrome might be less.[5,7]

Importance and management

Evidence for an interaction between the MAOIs or RIMAs and trazodone is limited, with the balance of the evidence with RIMAs being for favourable concurrent use if the dose of trazodone is low (200 mg daily or less). The UK manufacturer of trazodone states that possible interactions with MAOIs have occasionally been reported. They also note that although some clinicians prescribe trazodone with an MAOI, they do not recommend concurrent use.[8] They state that trazodone should not be given within 2 weeks of stopping an MAOI and MAOIs should not be taken within one week of stopping trazodone.[8] For more information on serotonin syndrome and its management, see 'Drugs that cause serotonin syndrome + Other drugs that cause serotonin syndrome', p.1471.

No specific advice appears to have been given for **moclobemide**, but, because of its half-life, a 24-hour washout is usually considered appropriate when starting potentially interacting drugs in patients who have been taking moclobemide.

1. Bodner RA, Lynch T, Lewis L, Kahn D. Serotonin syndrome. *Neurology* (1995) 45, 219–23.
2. Zetin M. Combined use of trazodone and phenelzine in depression: case report. *J Clin Psychiatry* (1984) 45, 182–3.
3. Zivanović O, Till E. Serotonin syndrome – a case account. *Med Pregl* (1992) 45, 116–8.
4. Nierenberg AA, Keck PE. Management of monoamine oxidase inhibitor-associated insomnia with trazodone. *J Clin Psychopharmacol* (1989) 9, 42–5.
5. Jacobsen FM. Low-dose trazodone as a hypnotic in patients treated with MAOIs and other psychotropics: a pilot study. *J Clin Psychiatry* (1990) 51, 298–302.
6. Magder DM, Aleksic I, Kennedy SH. Tolerability and efficacy of high-dose moclobemide alone and in combination with lithium and trazodone. *J Clin Psychopharmacol* (2000) 20, 394–5.
7. Haffmans PMJ, Vos MS. The effects of trazodone on sleep disturbances induced by brofaromine. *Eur Psychiatry* (1999) 14, 167–71.
8. Molipaxin Capsules (Trazodone hydrochloride). Sanofi-Aventis. UK Summary of product characteristics, August 2009.

MAOIs or RIMAs + Tricyclic and related antidepressants

Toxic and sometimes fatal reactions (serotonin syndrome or similar) have been reported in patients taking either MAOIs or RIMAs with tricyclic antidepressants and related drugs.

Clinical evidence

A. MAOIs

The toxic reactions that occur when the tricyclics are given with MAOIs have included (with variations) sweating, flushing, hyperpyrexia, restlessness, excitement, tremor, muscle twitching and rigidity, convulsions and coma.

One illustrative example is the case of a woman who had been taking **tranylcypromine** 10 mg twice daily for about 3 weeks, who stopped taking it 3 days before she took a single tablet of **imipramine**. Within a few hours she complained of an excruciating headache, and soon afterwards lost consciousness and started to convulse. The toxic reactions manifested were a temperature of 40.6°C, pulse rate of 120 bpm, severe extensor rigidity, carpal spasm, opisthotonos and cyanosis. She was treated with amobarbital and phenytoin, and her temperature was reduced with alcohol-ice-soaked towels. The treatment was effective and she recovered.[1]

In another illustrative case, a patient was given **imipramine** 75 mg daily for 7 weeks with the addition of lithium for the last 3 weeks. These drugs were discontinued and after a one-week washout he started **tranylcypromine**, which was gradually increased to 50 mg twice daily. After 2 weeks at this dose, he received a single 225-mg dose of **imipramine** in error. Four hours later his condition deteriorated rapidly. He was agitated, confused, with severe rigidity, myoclonic jerks, hyperthermia, hypertension and tachycardia, and 2 hours later had a cardiac and respiratory arrest. He was resuscitated and given midazolam, pancuronium, dantrolene sodium, and a cooling mattress. The following day he had a sudden fall in blood pressure, and was eventually pronounced brain dead, and artificial respiration was terminated.[2]

Similar reactions have been recorded with oral therapeutic doses of:

- **amitriptyline** with **phenelzine**;[3,4]
- **clomipramine** with **phenelzine**[5,6] or **tranylcypromine** (with or without trifluoperazine);[7-9]
- **desipramine** with **phenelzine**;[10]
- **imipramine** with **iproniazid**;[11] **isocarboxazid**,[11] **pargyline**,[12] **phenelzine**[13-15] or **tranylcypromine**.[11,16]

There have been a number of fatalities.[7,8,10,17] Reactions have also occurred when intramuscular **imipramine** was given with **phenelzine**.[18-20] In some instances the drugs were not taken together, but were substituted without a washout period in between.[5,16] In some other reports there was an overdose of one or both drugs,[21-24] and/or the presence of other potentially interacting drugs.[22,23] There are many more reports of these interactions than are listed here: those published before 1977 have been extensively reviewed elsewhere.[15,25,26]

Drugs that are related to the tricyclics appear to interact with the MAOIs in the same way. A case report describes hypertension (blood pressure 180/125 mm/Hg) in a patient who took **mianserin** 2 weeks after stopping **tranylcypromine**. The blood pressure normalised when the **mianserin** was stopped.[27] One patient who safely took **mianserin** with **tranylcypromine** as part of a study died suddenly while continuing to take the drugs after the study period.[28] This patient was also taking methyldopa, which may have contributed to the interaction, see 'MAOIs + Methyldopa', p.1395.

In contrast, there are a number of other uncontrolled studies[28-31] and reviews[25,26] describing the beneficial use of an MAOI with a tricyclic antidepressant or **mianserin**.[28] In addition, one study has reported switching 178 patients from tricyclics to MAOIs with a washout period of 4 days or less. Of these patients, 63 were given the MAOI while still being tapered from the tricyclic, all without any apparent problems.[32] A study in 60 patients given **isocarboxazid** and **mianserin** found a faster onset of antidepressant activity than would have been expected from either drug alone, and did not identify any drug interactions. The authors state that subsequently 120 patients were given the combination without any notable adverse effects.[33]

B. RIMAs

(a) Amitriptyline

Two small studies in healthy subjects and patients found no problems when **moclobemide** was given with, or 24 hours after, amitriptyline;[34,35] or when amitriptyline was given immediately after **moclobemide**.[34] However, a patient taking amitriptyline and clomipramine developed symptoms of serotonin syndrome within 30 minutes of taking a 300-mg dose of **moclobemide**, and died.[36]

Only a minor and clinically unimportant change in the pharmacokinetics of amitriptyline occurs in patients given **toloxatone**.[37]

(b) Clomipramine

A small study in healthy subjects found no problems when **moclobemide** was given 24 hours after clomipramine.[35] However, serotonin syndrome occurred in 3 patients when clomipramine was replaced by **moclobemide** without a washout period[38,39] or with only a 24-hour washout period;[40] and in another patient when **moclobemide** was replaced by clomipramine after only 12 hours.[41] A fatal case of serotonin syndrome occurred in a patient taking clomipramine and amitriptyline, with symptoms manifesting within 30 minutes of the patient taking a 300-mg dose of **moclobemide.**[36]

(c) Desipramine

A small single-dose study in healthy subjects found no problems when **moclobemide** was given with desipramine.[34]

(d) Doxepin

Serotonin toxicity (serotonin syndrome) occurred in a patient who took an overdose of **moclobemide** and doxepin. In this analysis of **moclobemide** overdoses, the risk of developing serotonin toxicity was significantly increased in patients who also took another serotonergic drug, of which this case with doxepin was one of the 11 mentioned.[42]

(e) Imipramine

Serotonin syndrome occurred in a patient who had been taking **moclobemide** for about one month and imipramine (50 mg at night increased to 200 mg at night) for about 17 days.[43]

(f) Maprotiline

One study found a non-significant 25% rise in the serum levels of maprotiline (a tetracyclic antidepressant) in 6 patients also taking **moclobemide**. No serious toxic reactions were reported.[44]

(g) Trimipramine

One study found a 39% rise in serum trimipramine levels in 15 patients also taking **moclobemide**. No serious toxic reactions were reported.[44]

Mechanism

Not understood. One idea is that both the MAOIs and the tricyclics and related drugs cause grossly elevated monoamine levels (serotonin, noradrenaline (norepinephrine)) in the brain, which 'spill-over' into areas not concerned with mood elevation. It might be related to, or the same as serotonin syndrome (for a further description of this syndrome see under 'Drugs that cause serotonin syndrome + Other drugs that cause serotonin syndrome', p.1471). Of the tricyclics, clomipramine in particular is a potent inhibitor of serotonin uptake. Less likely suggestions are that the MAOIs inhibit the metabolism of the tricyclic antidepressants, or that active and unusual metabolites of the tricyclic antidepressants are produced.[25]

Importance and management

An established and fairly common interaction, but serious and life-threatening occurrences seem rare. If concurrent use is to be avoided, the following guidelines[45] are recommended:

- A tricyclic antidepressant should *not* be started until 2 weeks after treatment with an MAOI has been stopped (3 weeks if starting clomipramine or imipramine);
- An MAOI should *not* be started until at least 7 to 14 days after a tricyclic or related antidepressant has been stopped (3 weeks in the case of clomipramine or imipramine);
- Moclobemide has a short duration of action so no treatment-free period is required after it has been stopped before starting a tricyclic antidepressant. (Note that some recommend waiting 24 hours);[41]
- Moclobemide should *not* be started until at least one week after a tricyclic antidepressant has been stopped.

No detailed clinical work has been done to find out precisely what sets the scene when the interaction does occur, but some general empirical guidelines have been suggested so that it can, as far as possible, be avoided if concurrent treatment is thought appropriate:[14,15,25,26,46]

- Treatment with both types of drug should only be undertaken by those well aware of the problems and who can undertake adequate supervision.
- Only patients refractory to all other types of treatment should be considered.
- Tranylcypromine, phenelzine, clomipramine, and possibly imipramine, appear to be high on the list of drugs that have interacted adversely. Giving clomipramine with tranylcypromine is particularly dangerous. Amitriptyline, trimipramine and isocarboxazid are possibly safer.
- Drugs should be given orally, not parenterally.
- It has been suggested that small doses should be given initially, increasing the levels of each drug, one at a time, over a period of 2 to 3 weeks to levels generally about half those used for each one individually.

Although information is limited, it seems that **mianserin** (and therefore possibly **maprotiline**) will interact similarly. It would therefore seem advisable to follow the same precautions if these tetracyclic antidepressants are given with MAOIs.

For more information on serotonin syndrome and its management, see 'Drugs that cause serotonin syndrome + Other drugs that cause serotonin syndrome', p.1471.

1. Brachfeld J, Wirtshafter A, Wolfe S. Imipramine-tranylcypromine incompatibility. Near-fatal toxic reaction. *JAMA* (1963) 186, 1172–3.
2. Otte W, Birkenhager TK, van den Broek WW. Fatal interaction between tranylcypromine and imipramine. *Eur Psychiatry* (2003) 18, 264–5.
3. Heyland D, Sauvé M. Neuroleptic malignant syndrome without the use of neuroleptics. *Can Med Assoc J* (1991) 145, 817–19.
4. Teas GA. Toxic delirium resulting from combination antidepressant therapy. *Am J Psychiatry* (1981) 138, 1127.
5. Stern TA, Schwartz JH, Shuster JL. Catastrophic illness associated with the combination of clomipramine, phenelzine, and chlorpromazine. *Ann Clin Psychiatry* (1992) 4, 81–5.
6. Pascual J, Combarros O, Berciano J. Partial status epilepticus following single low dose of clorimipramine in a patient on MAO-inhibitor treatment. *Clin Neuropharmacol* (1987) 10, 565–7.
7. Beaumont G. Drug interactions with clomipramine (Anafranil). *J Int Med Res* (1973) 1, 480–4.
8. Tackley RM, Tregaskis B. Fatal disseminated intravascular coagulation following a monoamine oxidase inhibitor/tricyclic interaction. *Anaesthesia* (1987) 42, 760–3.
9. Gillman PK. Successful treatment of serotonin syndrome with chlorpromazine. *Med J Aust* (1996) 165, 345–6.
10. Bowen LW. Fatal hyperpyrexia with antidepressant drugs. *BMJ* (1964) 2, 1465–6.
11. Ayd FJ. Toxic somatic and psychopathological reactions to antidepressant drugs. *J Neuropsychiatr* (1961) 2 (Suppl 1), S119–S122.
12. McCurdy RL, Kane FJ. Transient brain syndrome as a non-fatal reaction to combined pargyline imipramine treatment. *Am J Psychiatry* (1964), 121, 397–8.
13. Howarth E. Possible synergistic effects of the new thymoleptics in connection with poisoning. *J Ment Sci* (1961) 107, 100–103.
14. Graham PM, Potter JM, Paterson JW. Combination monoamine oxidase inhibitor/tricyclic antidepressant interaction. *Lancet* (1982) ii, 440.
15. Schuckit M, Robins E, Feighner J. Tricyclic antidepressants and monoamine oxidase inhibitors. Combination therapy in the treatment of depression. *Arch Gen Psychiatry* (1971) 24, 509–14.
16. Grantham J, Neel W, Brown RW. Toxicity reversed. Reversal of imipramine-monoamine oxidase inhibitor induced toxicity by chlorpromazine. *J Kans Med Soc* (1964) 65, 279–80.
17. Wright SP. Hazards with monoamine-oxidase inhibitors: a persistent problem. *Lancet* (1978) i, 284–5.
18. Hills NF. Combining the antidepressant drugs. *BMJ* (1965) 1, 859.
19. Lockett MF, Milner G. Combining the antidepressant drugs. *BMJ* (1965) 1, 921.
20. Singh H. Atropine-like poisoning due to tranquillizing agents. *Am J Psychiatry* (1960) 117, 360–1.
21. Davies G. Side-effects of phenelzine. *BMJ* (1960) 2, 1019.
22. Nierenberg DW, Semprebon M. The central nervous system serotonin syndrome. *Clin Pharmacol Ther* (1993) 53, 84–8.
23. Richards GA, Fritz VU, Pincus P, Reyneke J. Unusual drug interactions between monoamine oxidase inhibitors and tricyclic antidepressants. *J Neurol Neurosurg Psychiatry* (1987) 50, 1240–1.
24. Stanley B, Pal NR. Fatal hyperpyrexia with phenelzine and imipramine. *BMJ* (1964) 2, 1011.
25. Ponto LB, Perry PJ, Liskow BI, Seaba HH. Drug therapy reviews: tricyclic antidepressant and monoamine oxidase inhibitor combination therapy. *Am J Hosp Pharm* (1977) 34, 954–61.
26. Ananth J, Luchins D. A review of combined tricyclic and MAOI therapy. *Compr Psychiatry* (1977) 18, 221–30.
27. Bottlender R, Erfurth A, Hoff P, Möller H-J. Mianserin-induzierte hypertonie 2 wochen nach absetzen von tranylcypromin. *Nervenarzt* (1997) 68, 591–2.
28. Graham PM. Combined minaserin (sic) and tranylcypromine. *Br J Psychiatry* (1988) 153, 415–17.
29. Gander GA. The clinical value of monoamine oxidase inhibitors and tricyclic antidepressants in combination. *Int Congr Ser* (1966) 122, 336–43.
30. Gander DR. Treatment of depressive illnesses with combined antidepressants. *Lancet* (1965) ii, 107–9.
31. Berlanga C. Ortego-Soto HA. A 3-year follow-up of a group of treatment-resistant depressed patients with a MAOI/tricyclic combination. *J Affect Disord* (1995) 34, 187–92.
32. Kahn D, Silver JM, Opler LA. The safety of switching rapidly from tricyclic antidepressants to monoamine oxidase inhibitors. *J Clin Psychopharmacol* (1989) 9, 198–202.
33. Riise IS, Holm P. Concomitant isocarboxazid/mianserin treatment of major depressive disorder. *J Affect Disord* (1984) 6, 175–9.
34. Korn A, Eichler HG, Fischbach R, Gasic S. Moclobemide, a new reversible MAO inhibitor – interaction with tyramine and tricyclic antidepressants in healthy volunteers and depressive patients. *Psychopharmacology (Berl)* (1986) 88, 153–7.
35. Dingemanse J, Kneer J, Fotteler B, Groen H, Peeters PAM, Jonkman JHG. Switch in treatment from tricyclic antidepressants to moclobemide: a new generation monoamine oxidase inhibitor. *J Clin Psychopharmacol* (1995) 15, 41–8.
36. Kuisma MJ. Fatal serotonin syndrome with trismus. *Ann Emerg Med* (1995) 26, 108.
37. Vandel S, Bertschy G, Perault MC, Sandoz M, Bouquet S, Chakroun R, Guibert S, Vandel B. Minor and clinically non-significant interaction between toloxatone and amitriptyline. *Eur J Clin Pharmacol* (1993) 44, 97–9.
38. Spigset O, Mjorndal T, Lovheim O. Serotonin syndrome caused by a moclobemide-clomipramine interaction. *BMJ* (1993) 306, 248.
39. Chan BSH, Graudins A, Whyte IM, Dawson AH, Braitberg G, Duggin GG. Serotonin syndrome resulting from drug interactions. *Med J Aust* (1998) 169, 523–5.
40. Dardennes RM, Even C, Ballon N, Bange F. Serotonin syndrome caused by a clomipramine–moclobemide interaction. *J Clin Psychiatry* (1998) 59, 382–3.
41. Gillman PK. Serotonin syndrome – clomipramine too soon after moclobemide? *Int Clin Psychopharmacol* (1997) 12, 339–42.
42. Isbister GK, Hackett LP, Dawson AH, Whyte IM, Smith AJ. Moclobemide poisoning: toxicokinetics and occurrence of serotonin toxicity. *Br J Clin Pharmacol* (2003) 56, 441–50.
43. Brodribb TR, Downey M, Gilbar PJ. Efficacy and adverse effects of moclobemide. *Lancet* (1994) 343, 475–6.
44. König F, Wolfersdorf M, Löble M, Wößner S, Hauger B. Trimipramine and maprotiline plasma levels during combined treatment with moclobemide in therapy-resistant depression. *Pharmacopsychiatry* (1997) 30, 125–7.
45. Joint Formulary Committee. *British National Formulary.* 69 ed. London: BMJ Group and Pharmaceutical Press; 2015. p. 259, 260.
46. Katona CLE, Barnes TRE. Pharmacological strategies in depression. *Br J Hosp Med* (1985) 34, 168–71.

MAOIs + Tryptophan

A number of patients have developed severe behavioural and neurological signs of toxicity (some similar to serotonin syndrome) after taking MAOIs with tryptophan. Fatalities have occurred.

Clinical evidence

A man taking **phenelzine** 90 mg daily developed behavioural and neurological toxicity within 2 hours of being given 6 g of tryptophan.[1] He was shivering and sweating, his psychomotor retardation disappeared and he became jocular, fearful, and moderately labile. His neurological signs included bilateral Babinski signs (abnormal plantar reflexes), hyperreflexia, rapid horizontal ocular oscillations, shivering of the jaw, trunk and limbs, mild dysmetria and ataxia. The situation resolved on withdrawal of the drugs.[1]

Similar symptoms have been reported in other studies and cases. In an early study, giving tryptophan 20 to 50 mg/kg to 7 patients with hypertension who were taking an MAOI, produced neurological effects, including alcohol-like intoxication, drowsiness, hyperreflexia and clonus.[2] Similar symptoms and also sweating, flushing and paraesthesias were seen in 5 patients who were given tryptophan 30 mg/kg orally with **pargyline** or **isocarboxazid**.[3] In another study, in 14 depressed patients taking various MAOIs, 4 patients had muscular jactitation (jerking or twitching) and hyperreflexia when they were also given tryptophan 2.5 to 5 g three times daily, and in 2 patients this was severe enough to discontinue the tryptophan.[4] Other reports describe similar symptoms when patients taking **phenelzine**[5,6] or **tranylcypromine**[7] were given tryptophan.

One patient taking **tranylcypromine** and lithium had transient episodes of hyperthermia and other symptoms of neurological toxicity when the dose of tryptophan was increased to 2 g at night. He had a total of about 12 of these episodes over several weeks before tryptophan was stopped and the episodes ceased.[8] Malignant hyperpyrexia occurred in a patient taking **phenelzine** and tryptophan,[9] and fatal malignant hyperpyrexia occurred in two patients taking **phenelzine**, tryptophan and lithium.[10,11] Another patient who had been taking **tranylcypromine** for 2 weeks developed serious hyperpyrexia and muscular rigidity 2 days after starting tryptophan 6 g daily: she had discontinued levodopa with carbidopa one month previously.[12] Tryptophan may have contributed to a fatal case of serotonin syndrome in a patient switched from fluoxetine to **tranylcypromine**.[13]

Hypomania without neurological symptoms has occurred in 2 patients when tryptophan was added to **phenelzine** or **tranylcypromine**,[14] and delirium or disorientation, (sometimes with neurological symptoms) has occurred in 8 patients taking **tranylcypromine** within 2 to 4 days of starting tryptophan, or within one day of increasing the dose of tryptophan.[15] A further patient also experienced delirium within hours of tryptophan being added to her **phenelzine** treatment.[16]

Mechanism

Not understood. The reactions appear to be related to serotonin syndrome, which can occur with two or more serotonergic drugs. MAOIs might inhibit the metabolism of serotonin, formed from tryptophan, so resulting in its accumulation.[3,9]

Importance and management

Information on the interaction between MAOIs and tryptophan seems to be confined to the reports listed. Concurrent use can be effective in the treatment of depression,[17] but occasionally and unpredictably severe and even life-threatening toxicity occurs. The authors of one of the reports detailed above[1] recommend that patients taking MAOIs should start treatment with a low dose of tryptophan (500 mg). This should be gradually increased while monitoring the mental status of the patient for changes suggesting hypomania, and neurological changes, including ocular oscillations and upper motor neurone signs. For more information on serotonin syndrome and its management, see 'Drugs that cause serotonin syndrome + Other drugs that cause serotonin syndrome', p.1471.

Note that products containing tryptophan for the treatment of depression were withdrawn in many countries because of a possible association with the development of an eosinophilia-myalgia syndrome. However, because the syndrome appeared to have been associated with tryptophan from one manufacturer, tryptophan preparations were reintroduced in the UK in 1994 for restricted use.[18]

1. Thomas JN, Rubin EH. Case report of a toxic reaction from a combination of tryptophan and phenelzine. *Am J Psychiatry* (1984) 141, 281–3.
2. Oates JA, Sjoerdsma A. Neurological effects of tryptophan in patients receiving a monoamine oxidase inhibitor. *Neurology* (1960) 10, 1076–8.
3. Hodge JV, Oates JA, Sjoerdsma A. Reduction of the central effects of tryptophan by a decarboxylase inhibitor. *Clin Pharmacol Ther* (1964) 5, 149–55.
4. Pare CMB. Potentiation of monoamine-oxidase inhibitors by tryptophan. *Lancet* (1963) 2, 527–8.
5. Glassman AH, Platman SR. Potentiation of monoamine oxidase inhibitor by tryptophan. *J Psychiatr Res* (1969) 7, 83–8.
6. Levy AB, Bucher P, Votolato N. Myoclonus, hyperreflexia and diaphoresis in patients on phenelzine-tryptophan combination treatment. *Can J Psychiatry* (1985) 30, 434–6.
7. Baloh RW, Dietz J, Spooner JW. Myoclonus and ocular oscillations induced by l-tryptophan. *Ann Neurol* (1982) 11, 95–7.
8. Price WA, Zimmer B, Kucas P. Serotonin syndrome: a case report. *J Clin Pharmacol* (1986) 26, 77–8.
9. Kim SY, Mueller PD. Life-threatening interaction between phenelzine and L-tryptophan. *Vet Hum Toxicol* (1989) 31, 370.
10. Staufenberg EF, Tantam D. Malignant hyperpyrexia syndrome in combined treatment. *Br J Psychiatry* (1989) 154, 577–8.
11. Brennan D, MacManus M, Howe J, McLoughlin J. 'Neuroleptic malignant syndrome' without neuroleptics. *Br J Psychiatry* (1988) 152, 578–9.
12. Parsa MA, Rohr T, Ramirez LF, Meltzer HY. Neuroleptic malignant syndrome without neuroleptics. *J Clin Psychopharmacol* (1990) 10, 437–8.
13. Kline SS, Mauro LS, Scala-Barnett DM, Zick D. Serotonin syndrome versus neuroleptic malignant syndrome as a cause of death. *Clin Pharm* (1989) 8, 510–14.
14. Goff DC. Two cases of hypomania following the addition of l-tryptophan to a monoamine oxidase inhibitor. *Am J Psychiatry* (1985) 142, 1487–8.
15. Pope HG, Jonas JM, Hudson JI, Kafka MP. Toxic reactions to the combination of monoamine oxidase inhibitors and tryptophan. *Am J Psychiatry* (1985) 142, 491–2.
16. Alvine G, Black DW, Tsuang D. Case of delirium secondary to phenelzine/l-tryptophan combination. *J Clin Psychiatry* (1990) 51, 311.
17. Nelson JC. Augmentation strategies in depression 2000. *J Clin Psychiatry* (2000) 61 (Suppl 2), 13–19.
18. Committee on Safety of Medicines/Medicines Control Agency. L-Tryptophan (Optimax): limited availability for resistant depression. *Current Problems* (1994) 20, 2.

MAOIs + Xanthines

Isolated reports suggest that the CNS stimulant effects of caffeine may possibly be increased by the MAOIs. Another isolated report describes the development of tachycardia and apprehension in a patient taking phenelzine after she also took a cough syrup, containing choline theophyllinate.

Clinical evidence

(a) Caffeine

One reviewer briefly mentions that a patient who normally drank 10 or 12 cups of **coffee** daily, without adverse effects, experienced extreme jitteriness while taking an MAOI, which subsided when the **coffee** consumption was reduced to 2 or 3 cups a day. The same reaction was also said to have occurred in other patients taking MAOIs who drank **tea** or a **cola drink**, which both contain caffeine.[1] This reviewer also mentions another patient taking an MAOI, who claimed that a single cup of **coffee** taken in the morning kept him jittery all day and up the entire night; a reaction that occurred on three separate occasions.[1] In another report, a woman taking **phenelzine** experienced a severe headache with a slight blood pressure rise on two occasions after drinking **cola** containing 35 to 55 mg of caffeine.[2] Similarly, a brief mention is made of 2 patients taking **phenelzine** who experienced extreme restlessness, agitation, tremor, and insomnia after starting to drink large quantities of **diet cola**. This was attributed to an interaction between **phenelzine** and aspartame,[3] but could equally well be attributed to an interaction with caffeine, or indeed a reaction to caffeine alone. A woman who took a *Do-Do* tablet (containing ephedrine, caffeine, and **theophylline**) the day after stopping **phenelzine** developed severe adverse effects, including agitation.[4] Although ephedrine was the most likely cause of many of the effects (see 'MAOIs or RIMAs + Nasal decongestants and related drugs', p.1396) a contribution from the **caffeine** and **theophylline** cannot be ruled out.

(b) Theophylline

A woman with agoraphobia, taking **phenelzine** 45 mg daily, developed tachycardia, palpitations and apprehension lasting for about 4 hours after she had taken a cough syrup containing choline theophyllinate and guaifenesin. The symptoms recurred when she was again given the cough syrup, and yet again when given choline theophyllinate, but not when she was given guaifenesin.[5]

Mechanism

Unknown. Caffeine alone can cause headache, tachycardia, and jitteriness, and individuals vary in their susceptibility to these effects. The effects of caffeine, theophylline, and theobromine in *rats* were enhanced by MAOIs.[6]

Importance and management

Apart from these few reports, the literature appears to be otherwise silent about an interaction between the MAOIs and the xanthines. Whether this reflects their mildness and unimportance, or their rarity, is not clear. There would seem to be no need for any additional precautions in patients taking MAOIs who are given xanthine bronchodilators (such as **theophylline** or **aminophylline**) or consume caffeine-containing foods, beverages or pharmaceuticals. However, it would seem prudent to bear these case reports in mind should a patient taking an MAOI develop signs of caffeine-related adverse effects (such as jitteriness, headache, restlessness, insomnia). If this occurs, advise patients to decrease their caffeine intake, perhaps by using decaffeinated alternatives. Remember also that some non-prescription medicines contain caffeine. Note that some manufacturers of isocarboxazid, phenelzine and tranylcypromine recommend avoiding or contraindicate excessive amounts of tea and coffee,[7] or caffeine in any form,[8-10] but this seems overly cautious.

1. Kline NS. Psychopharmaceuticals: effects and side-effects. *Bull WHO* (1959) 21, 397–410.
2. Pakes GE. Phenelzine-cola headache. *Am J Hosp Pharm* (1979) 36, 736.
3. Shader RI, Greenblatt DJ. Phenelzine and the dream machine—ramblings and reflections. *J Clin Psychopharmacol* (1985) 5, 65.
4. Dawson JK, Earnshaw SM, Graham CS. Dangerous monoamine oxidase inhibitor interactions are still occurring in the 1990s. *J Accid Emerg Med* (1995) 12, 49–51.
5. Shader RI, Greenblatt DJ. MAOIs and drug interactions—a proposal for a clearinghouse. *J Clin Psychopharmacol* (1985) 5, A17.
6. Berkowitz BA, Spector S, Pool W. The interaction of caffeine, theophylline and theobromine with monoamine oxidase inhibitors. *Eur J Pharmacol* (1971) 16, 315–21.
7. Nardil (Phenelzine sulfate). Archimedes Pharma UK Ltd. UK Summary of product characteristics, October 2008.
8. Marplan (Isocarboxazid). Validus Pharmaceuticals, Inc. US Prescribing information, August 2007.
9. Nardil (Phenelzine sulfate). Pfizer Inc. US Prescribing information, February 2009.
10. Parnate (Tranylcypromine sulfate). GlaxoSmithKline. US Prescribing information, May 2010.

MAOIs; Phenelzine + Cloral hydrate

A case of fatal hyperpyrexia and another case of serious hypertension have been linked to interactions between cloral hydrate and phenelzine, but in both cases there are other plausible explanations for the reactions seen.

Clinical evidence, mechanism, importance and management

A woman taking **phenelzine** 15 mg three times daily was found in bed deeply comatose with marked muscular rigidity, twitching down one side and a temperature of 41°C. She died without regaining consciousness. A post mortem failed to establish the cause of death, but it subsequently came to light that she had started drinking whisky, and she had access to cloral hydrate, of which she may have taken a fatal dose.[1] Another patient taking **phenelzine** 15 mg three times daily and cloral hydrate to aid sleep, developed an excruciating headache followed by nausea, photophobia and a substantial rise in blood pressure.[2] This latter reaction is similar to the 'cheese reaction' (see 'MAOIs or RIMAs + Food; Tyramine-containing', p.1389), but at the time the authors of the report were unaware of this type of reaction and so did not find out if any tyramine-rich foods had been eaten on the day of the attack.[2]

There is no clear evidence that either of these adverse reactions was due to an interaction between **phenelzine** and cloral hydrate, and there do not seem to be any other reports to suggest that an interaction between these drugs is likely.

1. Howarth E. Possible synergistic effects of the new thymoleptics in connection with poisoning. *J Ment Sci* (1961) 107, 100–103.
2. Dillon H, Leopold RL. Acute cerebro-vascular symptoms produced by an antidepressant. *Am J Psychiatry* (1965) 121, 1012–14.

MAOIs; Phenelzine + Erythromycin

A woman taking phenelzine developed severe hypotension and fainting shortly after she started a course of erythromycin.

Clinical evidence, mechanism, importance and management

A woman taking phenelzine 15 mg daily experienced three syncopal episodes 4 days after starting to take erythromycin 250 mg four times daily for pneumonia. When admitted to hospital her supine systolic blood pressure was only 70 mmHg. When she sat up, it was unrecordable. Although she was not dehydrated, she was given 4 litres of sodium chloride 0.9%, without any effect on her blood pressure. Within 24 hours of stopping the phenelzine her blood pressure had returned to normal.[1] The reasons for this severe hypotensive reaction are not known, but it was suggested that erythromycin may have caused rapid gastric emptying, which resulted in a very rapid absorption of phenelzine (described by the author as rapid dumping into the blood stream), which resulted in the adverse effect of hypotension.[1] This seems to be the first and only report of this interaction, and so its general importance is uncertain. It seems likely to be small.

1. Bernstein AE. Drug interaction. *Hosp Community Psychiatry* (1990) 41, 806–7.

MAOIs; Phenelzine + Sulfafurazole (Sulfisoxazole)

An isolated report describes a patient taking phenelzine who developed weakness and ataxia after also taking sulfafurazole.

Clinical evidence, mechanism, importance and management

A woman who had been taking phenelzine 15 mg three times daily for about 3 weeks complained of weakness, ataxia, vertigo, tinnitus, muscle pains, and paraesthesia within 7 days of starting to take sulfafurazole 1 g four times daily. These adverse effects continued until the 10-day sulfonamide course was completed, and did not occur again in the following 8 weeks.[1] The reasons for this reaction are not understood, but as these adverse effects are a combination of the adverse effects of both drugs, it seems possible that a mutual interaction (perhaps saturation of the acetylating mechanisms in the liver) was responsible. This appears to be an isolated report and its general significance is unknown.

1. Boyer WF, Lake CR. Interaction of phenelzine and sulfisoxazole. *Am J Psychiatry* (1983) 140, 264–5.

Moclobemide + Cimetidine

Cimetidine increases the levels of moclobemide.

Clinical evidence, mechanism, importance and management

In a study in 8 healthy subjects, cimetidine 200 mg five times daily for 2 weeks increased the maximum plasma levels of a single 100-mg dose of moclobemide by 39% and reduced its clearance by 52%.[1] The probable reason for this effect is that cimetidine (a well-recognised non-specific inhibitor of cytochrome P450) reduces the metabolism of the moclobemide. The authors of this study suggest that as moclobemide is usually well-tolerated, no dose adjustment is necessary, but concurrent use should be monitored.[1] Note that one manufacturer of moclobemide recommends that moclobemide should be started at the lowest therapeutic dose in patients taking cimetidine, with the dose of moclobemide titrated as required. If cimetidine is given to a patient taking stable doses of moclobemide, the dose of the moclobemide should be reduced by 50% and adjusted as necessary.[2]

1. Schoerlin M-P, Mayersohn M, Hoevels B, Eggers H, Dellenbach M, Pfefen J-P. Cimetidine alters the disposition kinetics of the monoamine oxidase-A inhibitor moclobemide. *Clin Pharmacol Ther* (1991) 49, 32–8.
2. Manerix (Moclobemide). Meda Pharmaceuticals. UK Summary of product characteristics, September 2009.

Moclobemide + Hydrochlorothiazide or Nifedipine

Moclobemide does not appear to cause orthostatic hypotension in patients taking nifedipine or hydrochlorothiazide.

Clinical evidence, mechanism, importance and management

A study in 7 subjects taking **hydrochlorothiazide** and 6 subjects taking **nifedipine** found that the addition of moclobemide did not cause orthostatic hypotension.[1] No particular precautions would therefore appear to be necessary on concurrent use.

1. Amrein R, Güntert TW, Dingemanse J, Lorscheid T, Stabl M, Schmid-Burgk W. Interactions of moclobemide with concomitantly administered medication: evidence from pharmacological and clinical studies. *Psychopharmacology (Berl)* (1992) 106, S24–S31.

Moclobemide + Omeprazole

Omeprazole moderately increases the AUC of moclobemide in most patients. Similarly, moclobemide moderately increases the AUC of omeprazole.

Clinical evidence

In a study in 8 healthy subjects who were extensive metabolisers of CYP2C19 (that is, those with normal activity of this isoenzyme), omeprazole 40 mg daily for 7 days increased the AUC of a single 300-mg dose of moclobemide 2.2-fold. This increase led to an AUC that was still lower than that seen in 8 healthy subjects who were poor metabolisers of CYP2C19 (those with little or no activity of this isoenzyme) given moclobemide alone. Omeprazole had no appreciable effect on the pharmacokinetics of moclobemide in the poor metaboliser group.[1] A single-dose study in the same subjects also found that, in the extensive metabolisers, a 300-mg dose of moclobemide increased the AUC and maximum plasma concentration of omeprazole 40 mg 2.1-fold and 1.7-fold, respectively, and the production of omeprazole sulfone was similarly increased. The pharmacokinetics of omeprazole and omeprazole sulfone were not altered in the poor metabolisers.[2]

Mechanism

Moclobemide is an inhibitor of CYP2C19, which is the major pathway by which omeprazole is metabolised. Activity of this isoenzyme is genetically determined, and therefore some subjects have normal activity (extensive metabolisers) whereas other subjects have little or no activity (poor metabolisers). Extensive metabolisers normally metabolise omeprazole to 5-hydroxyomeprazole by CYP2C19: inhibition of this isoenzyme means that these subjects will become more dependent on other pathways, such as CYP3A4, which metabolises omeprazole to omeprazole sulfone. Hence in extensive metabolisers, moclobemide increases the concentrations of omeprazole sulfone, and the concentrations of 5-hydroxyomeprazole are reduced. Poor metabolisers do not usually metabolise omeprazole by CYP2C19, and so are unaffected by the addition of a CYP2C19 inhibitor, such as moclobemide.

Omeprazole is also an inhibitor of CYP2C19, by which moclobemide is extensively metabolised, and therefore concurrent use leads to an increase in moclobemide exposure in extensive metabolisers.

Importance and management

The pharmacokinetic interaction between omeprazole and moclobemide is established, but its clinical relevance is unclear. Both drugs are relatively safe, and therefore increased exposure is generally likely to be well tolerated. However, if the adverse effects of either drug become troublesome consider an interaction as a possible cause. Note that the effect of moclobemide on omeprazole might be of more importance if drugs that inhibit CYP3A4 are also given, as both pathways of metabolism will be blocked.

1. Yu K-S, Yim D-S, Cho J-Y, Park SS, Park JY, Lee K-H, Jang I-J, Yi S-Y, Bae K-S, Shin S-G. Effect of omeprazole on the pharmacokinetics of moclobemide according to the genetic polymorphism of CYP2C19. *Clin Pharmacol Ther* (2001) 69, 266–73.
2. Cho J-Y, Yu K-S, Jang I-J, Yang B-H, Shin S-G, Yim D-S. Omeprazole hydroxylation is inhibited by a single dose of moclobemide in homozygotic EM genotype for CYP2C19. *Br J Clin Pharmacol* (2002) 53, 393–7.

Moclobemide + Valproate

Valproic acid has no clinically significant effect on the pharmacokinetics of moclobemide.

Clinical evidence, mechanism, importance and management

In a drug interaction study in patients with depression, moclobemide 150 mg three times daily was given alone (6 patients) or with **valproic acid** 500 mg twice daily (7 patients) for 5 weeks. **Valproic acid** had no clinically significant effect on the pharmacokinetics of moclobemide. No serious adverse effects were reported with concurrent use and no clinically significant changes in blood pressure or heart rate occurred.[1] No particular precautions would therefore be expected to be necessary on concurrent use.

1. Rakic Ignjatovic A, Milijkovic B, Todorovic D, Timotijevic I, Pokrajac M. Moclobemide monotherapy vs. Combined therapy with valproic acid or carbamazepine in depressive patients: a pharmacokinetic interaction study. *Br J Clin Pharmacol* (2008) 67, 199–208.

33

Nutritional agents, Supplements and Vitamins

This section covers the interactions where there is documented evidence that a drug alters the efficacy of nutritional agents, dietary supplements and vitamins. Information on the effects of these substances on other drugs is covered in the relevant section for that drug.

Agalsidase + Miscellaneous

Agalsidase alfa and agalsidase beta are unlikely to interact with other drugs by mechanisms involving cytochrome P450.[1] The UK manufacturers suggest that agalsidase alfa and agalsidase beta should not be given with amiodarone, chloroquine, gentamicin [and therefore probably any aminoglycoside], or monobenzone due to a theoretical risk of inhibition of intra-cellular alpha-galactosidase activity.[1,2] This would be expected to reduce the efficacy of agalsidase.

1. Replagal (Agalsidase alfa). Shire Human Genetic Therapies. UK Summary of product characteristics, October 2008.
2. Fabrazyme (Agalsidase beta). Genzyme Therapeutics. UK Summary of product characteristics, February 2008.

Amygdalin + Ascorbic acid (Vitamin C)

Vitamin C may enhance the hydrolysis of amygdalin resulting in toxic levels of cyanide.

Clinical evidence

A patient with bladder cancer, who was taking several vitamin preparations, including high-dose vitamin C, and other complementary medicines in addition to her prescribed medicines, became unwell and complained of dizziness 2.5 hours after the first dose of amygdalin 3 g. She then developed tachycardia, seizures and severe lactic acidosis, and required intubation and ventilation. Cyanide poisoning was diagnosed and she recovered after being given activated charcoal and intravenous hydroxocobalamin 5 g over 30 minutes.[1]

Mechanism

There appear to be no reports of serious cyanide toxicity with doses of amygdalin up to 6 g daily. Hydrolysis of amygdalin can produce up to 6% hydrogen cyanide so a dose of 3 g could possibly produce up to 180 mg of cyanide, which is above the estimated potentially lethal dose of 50 to 100 mg. Amygdalin is hydrolysed in the presence of beta-glucosidases, which are not usually present in the upper gastrointestinal tract to any extent. However, hydrolysis of amygdalin in the gut is enhanced by ascorbic acid and it was considered likely that the high doses of vitamin C (more than 3 g daily) taken by the patient resulted in sufficient hydrolysis of amygdalin to produce toxic levels of cyanide.[1] In addition, body stores of cysteine, which facilitate cyanide detoxification, are depleted by vitamin C.[1,2]

Importance and management

Although this appears to be the only clinical report of this interaction, cyanide poisoning associated with amygdalin has been reported. It would therefore seem prudent to avoid the concurrent use of vitamin C. **Laetrile**, which is a product consisting mainly of amygdalin, would be expected to interact similarly with vitamin C.

1. Bromley J, Hughes BGM, Leong DCS, Buckley NA. Life-threatening interaction between complementary medicines: cyanide toxicity following ingestion of amygdalin and vitamin C. *Ann Pharmacother* (2005) 39, 1566–9.
2. Basu TK. High-dose ascorbic acid decreases detoxification of cyanide derived from amygdalin (laetrile): studies in guinea pigs. *Can J Physiol Pharmacol* (1983) 61, 1426–30.

Ascorbic acid (Vitamin C) + Salicylates

Aspirin might reduce the absorption of ascorbic acid by about one-third. Serum salicylate levels do not appear to be affected by ascorbic acid.

Clinical evidence, mechanism, importance and management

In a study in healthy subjects, the rise in plasma ascorbic acid levels over 3 hours was about one-third lower when a single 500-mg dose of ascorbic acid was given with **aspirin** 900 mg, when compared with ascorbic acid alone, and the urinary excretion of ascorbic acid was about 50% lower.[1] In another well-controlled study in healthy subjects, levels of ascorbic acid in the gastric mucosa, plasma and urine on day 7 were not significantly different when ascorbic acid 480 mg three times daily was given with **aspirin** 800 mg three times daily, when compared with ascorbic acid alone. However, aspirin 800 mg three times daily, given without ascorbic acid supplementation, reduced ascorbic acid levels.[2] There is some pharmacodynamic evidence that, in healthy subjects, ascorbic acid attenuates gastric mucosal lesions seen with **aspirin**.[3]

Another study, in 9 healthy subjects, found that ascorbic acid 1 g three times daily did not significantly affect the serum salicylate levels in response to **choline salicylate**.[4]

The clinical importance of the possible decrease in ascorbic acid levels is uncertain. It has been suggested that the normal physiological requirement of 30 to 60 mg of ascorbic acid daily may need to be increased to 100 to 200 mg daily in the presence of long-term **aspirin** therapy.[1]

1. Basu TK. Vitamin C-aspirin interactions. *Int J Vitam Nutr Res* (1982) 23 (Suppl), 83–90.
2. Schulz H-U, Schürer M, Krupp S, Dammann H-G, Timm J, Gessner U. Effects of acetylsalicylic acid on ascorbic acid concentrations in plasma, gastric mucosa, gastric juice and urine – a double-blind study in healthy subjects. *Int J Clin Pharmacol Ther* (2004) 42, 481–7.
3. Konturek PC, Kania J, Hahn EG, Konturek JW. Ascorbic acid attenuates aspirin-induced gastric damage: role of inducible nitric oxide synthase. *J Physiol Pharmacol* (2006) 57 (Suppl 5), 125–36.
4. Hansten PD, Hayton WL. Effect of antacid and ascorbic acid on serum salicylate concentration. *J Clin Pharmacol* (1980) 24, 326–31.

Betacarotene + Colchicine

The desired effect of betacarotene supplementation may be reduced in those taking colchicine.

Clinical evidence

Divided doses of colchicine 1.9 mg to 3.9 mg daily reduced the serum levels of betacarotene 10 000 units daily (about 6 mg) in 5 obese subjects. Levels returned to normal when colchicine was stopped.[1] However, in another study, long-term use of colchicine 1 mg to 2 mg daily for 3 years had no effect on the serum levels of diet-derived carotene in 12 patients with familial Mediterranean fever.[2]

Mechanism

The mechanism is unclear. Colchicine causes reversible malabsorption in the gastrointestinal tract by disturbing epithelial cell function and inhibiting cell proliferation. It also lowered the serum levels of cholesterol in the first study. All these factors could have an effect on the absorption of betacarotene, which largely takes place in the gastrointestinal mucosa and whose distribution is dependent on the presence of lipoproteins.

Importance and management

The evidence for a possible interaction between betacarotene and colchicine is limited to two relatively old studies. While supplemental betacarotene absorption appears to be reduced, betacarotene ingested as part of the normal diet appears to be unaffected. Based on these two findings, and the fact that there is large interindividual variation in betacarotene absorption, it is difficult to recommend a clinical course of action other than to be aware that the desired effect of betacarotene supplementation may be reduced in those taking colchicine.

1. Race TF, Paes IC, Faloon WW. Intestinal malabsorption induced by oral colchicine. Comparison with neomycin and cathartic agents. *Am J Med Sci* (1970) 259, 32–41.
2. Ehrenfeld M, Levy M, Sharon P, Rachmilewitz D, Eliakim M. Gastrointestinal effects of long-term colchicine therapy in patients with recurrent polyserositis (familial Mediterranean fever). *Dig Dis Sci* (1982) 27, 723–7.

Betacarotene + Proton pump inhibitors

The desired effect of betacarotene supplementation may be reduced in those taking proton pump inhibitors.

Clinical evidence

In a study in 10 healthy subjects the AUC of a single 120-mg dose of betacarotene was halved by pretreatment with **omeprazole** 20 mg twice daily for 7 days.[1]

Mechanism

The exact mechanism is unclear. Betacarotene is absorbed in the small intestine by a simple passive-diffusion process. It has been suggested that omeprazole may retard this diffusion,[1] and that delayed gastric emptying may also contribute.[2]

Importance and management

Evidence for an interaction between betacarotene and omeprazole is limited, and as there is large interindividual variability in betacarotene absorption, the true bioavailability of the carotenoid can vary greatly even before omeprazole is taken. Coupled with the fact that betacarotene is a normal part of the healthy diet, it is very difficult to assess the true clinical importance of this interaction. Be aware that the desired effect of betacarotene supplements may be reduced or abolished by the concurrent use of omeprazole. If the suggested mechanism is correct, other proton pump inhibitors are likely to affect betacarotene absorption similarly.

1. Tang G, Serfaty-Lacrosniere C, Ermelinda Camilo M, Russell RM. Gastric acidity influences the blood response to a β-carotene dose in humans. *Am J Clin Nutr* (1996) 64, 622–6.
2. Øster-Jørgensen E, Rasmussen L. Blood response to a β-carotene dose. *Am J Clin Nutr* (1998) 67, 349–53.

Calcitriol + Miscellaneous

Calcitriol might increase the serum concentrations of calcium and phosphate in patients taking preparations containing these substances or drugs that increase their serum concentrations (e.g. vitamin D). Corticosteroids might oppose the effect of calcitriol. Colestyramine is predicted to reduce the absorption of calcitriol.

Clinical evidence, mechanism, importance and management

Calcitriol might increase serum calcium and phosphate concentrations. As a result, the UK and US manufacturers of calcitriol advise against the concurrent use of pharmacological [treatment] doses of **vitamin D** and its derivatives, to avoid possible additive effects resulting in hypercalcaemia.[1,2] The uncontrolled intake of additional **calcium supplements** should also be avoided.[1,2] The UK and US manufacturers also note that **corticosteroids** might antagonise the increased absorption of calcium by calcitriol.[1,2] Due to the effect of **colestyramine** on the absorption of fat-soluble vitamins, the manufacturers predict that the intestinal absorption of calcitriol might be impaired on concurrent use.[1,2]

1. Rocaltrol (Calcitriol). Roche Products Ltd. UK Summary of product characteristics, June 2012.
2. Rocaltrol (Calcitriol). Validus Pharmaceuticals LLC. US Prescribing information, August 2010.

Calcitriol + Phosphate binders

Sevelamer carbonate, but not lanthanum carbonate, reduces the exposure to calcitriol.

Clinical evidence, mechanism, importance and management

In a crossover study, 41 healthy subjects were given a single 1-microgram dose of calcitriol at lunchtime alone, with **lanthanum carbonate** 1 g three times daily for one day, and with **sevelamer carbonate** 2.4 g three times daily for one day. **Lanthanum carbonate** had no effect on the AUC or maximum serum concentration of calcitriol, but doubled the time to reach the maximum serum concentration. In contrast, **sevelamer carbonate** reduced the AUC and maximum serum concentration of calcitriol by 57% and 19%, respectively, but had no effect on the time to reach the maximum serum concentration. The authors suggest that **sevelamer carbonate** binds to calcitriol, reducing its bioavailability.[1] The general relevance of this difference between lanthanum carbonate and sevelamer carbonate is not clear, but the authors of the study suggest that the findings might be important in patients with chronic kidney disease who need vitamin D supplementation.[1] The UK manufacturer of sevelamer carbonate advises that, when giving any other oral drug for which a reduction in the bioavailability could have a clinically significant effect on safety or efficacy, the drug should be given at least one hour before or 3 hours after sevelamer.[2] This would seem prudent if calcitriol is given with sevelamer carbonate, and routine monitoring of the effect of calcitriol should determine if this sufficiently manages the interaction.

1. Pierce D, Hossack S, Poole L, Robinson A, Van Heusen H, Martin P, Smyth M. The effect of sevelamer carbonate and lanthanum carbonate on the pharmacokinetics of oral calcitriol. *Nephrol Dial Transplant* (2011) 26, 1615–21.
2. Renvela (Sevelamer carbonate). Genzyme Therapeutics. UK Summary of product characteristics, December 2011.

Calcium compounds + Corticosteroids

It is unknown whether, or to what extent, corticosteroids reduce calcium absorption from calcium supplements.

Clinical evidence, mechanism, importance and management

Corticosteroids taken systemically, or inhaled at high doses, are well-known to cause osteoporosis. A number of mechanisms are involved in this adverse effect, one of which is reduced intestinal absorption of dietary calcium by the corticosteroids.[1] For example, in one controlled study in healthy subjects, oral beclometasone capsules reduced dietary calcium absorption, as assessed by a 12% reduction in the strontium absorption test.[2] However, there appears to be no evidence that corticosteroids reduce the absorption of calcium compounds given in pharmacological doses, nor, if this should this occur, that the extent is clinically relevant. Nevertheless, a number of UK manufacturers of calcium supplements state that reduced absorption might occur on the concurrent use of corticosteroids, and state that it might be necessary to increase the dose of calcium. The 2010 American College of Rheumatology recommendations state that all patients starting treatment with glucocorticoids should have a daily calcium intake of 1.2 to 1.5 g,[3] which can be achieved with standard doses of calcium supplements without the need to increase the dose. More importantly, patients requiring long-term systemic corticosteroids should have their risk of osteoporosis evaluated and other appropriate non-pharmacological and pharmacological measures taken to minimise this.[1,3]

Note that any possible interaction between corticosteroids and calcium is not relevant to calcium compounds taken as antacids or as phosphate binders, where their efficacy is not dependent on calcium absorption.

1. den Uyl D, Bultink IE, Lems WF. Advances in glucocorticoid-induced osteoporosis. *Curr Rheumatol Rep* (2011) 13, 233–40.
2. Smith BJ, Phillips PJ, Pannall PR, Cain HJ, Leckie WJ. Effect of orally administered beclomethasone dipropionate on calcium absorption from the gut in normal subjects. *Thorax* (1993) 48, 890–3.
3. Grossman JM, Gordon R, Ranganath VK, Deal C, Caplan L, Chen W, Curtis JR, Furst DE, McMahon M, Patkar NM, Volkmann E, Saag KG. American College of Rheumatology 2010 recommendations for the prevention and treatment of glucocorticoid-induced osteoporosis. *Arthritis Care Res (Hoboken)* (2010) 62, 1515–26.

Calcium compounds + Proton pump inhibitors

A study in elderly women found that omeprazole reduced the absorption of calcium from a single dose of calcium carbonate under fasting conditions. However, in another study, omeprazole did not affect the absorption of calcium from a test meal that included milk and cheese. Other proton pump inhibitors may have similar effects.

Clinical evidence

In a double-blind study, 18 elderly women (mean age 76 years) were given a multivitamin preparation containing vitamin D 400 units daily and either omeprazole 20 mg daily or placebo for 7 days and then again with calcium carbonate (elemental calcium 500 mg) after an overnight fast. Calcium supplements had been withheld for one week before the study. The fractional absorption of the single calcium carbonate dose was decreased by about 60% by omeprazole (from 9.1% with placebo to 3.5% with omeprazole).[1]

In contrast, in another study, higher 40-mg doses of omeprazole did not affect the absorption of calcium from food (535 mg from a test meal including milk and cheese).[2]

Mechanism

In vitro, calcium carbonate disintegration and dissolution is pH dependent, decreasing from 96% at pH 1 to 23% at pH 6.1.[3] Therefore increases in pH due to omeprazole could reduce calcium absorption. However, calcium absorption is dependent on other factors such as food, calcium dose and subject age. Calcium absorption in women decreases with increasing age.[4]

Importance and management

The study in elderly women found reduced calcium absorption in the presence of omeprazole. Other proton pump inhibitors might be expected to act similarly, as the mechanism appears to relate to gastric pH. However, another study found that omeprazole did not affect calcium absorption from food. Therefore factors that may influence calcium absorption other than gastric pH, including patient age, calcium dose, and food must also be considered when assessing the possibility of an interaction. More study is needed to assess the clinical relevance of this potential interaction.

1. O'Connell MB, Madden DM, Murray AM, Heaney RP, Kerzner LJ. Effects of proton pump inhibitors on calcium carbonate absorption in women: a randomized crossover trial. *Am J Med* (2005) 118, 778–81.
2. Serfaty-Lacrosniere C, Wood RJ, Voytko D, Saltzman JR, Pedrosa M, Sepe TE, Russell RR. Hypochlorhydria from short-term omeprazole treatment does not inhibit intestinal absorption of calcium, phosphorus, magnesium or zinc from food in humans. *J Am Coll Nutr* (1995) 14, 364–8.
3. Jelleff Carr C, Shangraw RF. Nutritional and pharmaceutical aspects of calcium supplementation. *Am Pharm* (1987) S27, 49–50, 54–7.
4. Ensrud KE, Duong T, Cauley JA, Heaney RP, Wolf RL, Harris E, Cummings SR, for the Study of Osteoporotic Fractures Research Group. Low fractional calcium absorption increases the risk for hip fracture in women with low calcium intake. *Ann Intern Med* (2000) 132, 345–53.

Cannabis + Disulfiram

Two isolated case reports describe hypomanic-like reactions when patients taking disulfiram used cannabis, whereas no unusual interaction with the combination was seen in other subjects.

Clinical evidence, mechanism, importance and management

A man with a 10-year history of drug abuse (alcohol, amfetamines, cocaine, cannabis) taking disulfiram 250 mg daily, experienced a hypomanic-like reaction (euphoria, hyperactivity, insomnia, irritability) on two occasions, associated with the concurrent use of cannabis. The patient said that he felt as though he had been taking amfetamine.[1] One other similar case has been reported.[2] The reason for this reaction is not understood.

In a randomised study in alcohol-dependent subjects who had previously used cannabis, no unusual interaction effects were found in a group of 11 subjects receiving disulfiram and smoking cannabis twice weekly for 4 weeks.[3] Therefore the interaction described in the two case reports would not appear to be of general significance.

1. Lacoursiere RB, Swatek R. Adverse interaction between disulfiram and marijuana: a case report. *Am J Psychiatry* (1983) 140, 243–4.
2. Mackie J, Clark D. Cannabis toxic psychosis while on disulfiram. *Br J Psychiatry* (1994) 164, 421.
3. Rosenberg CM, Gerrein JR, Schnell C. Cannabis in the treatment of alcoholism. *J Stud Alcohol* (1978) 39, 1955–8.

Cannabis + Nicotine

The effects of transdermal nicotine and cannabis smoking on increasing the heart rate are additive, and nicotine increased the stimulant effect of cannabis. Combined use might increase the addictive potential of both drugs.

Clinical evidence

In a study in 20 healthy subjects who smoked either a low-dose or high-dose cannabis cigarette 4 hours after the application of a placebo or a 21 mg nicotine patch, nicotine enhanced the maximum increase in heart rate seen with cannabis. The increase in heart rate for nicotine alone was between 10 and 15 bpm, for cannabis alone 32 and 42 bpm, for women and men, respectively, and for the combination, 45 and 58 bpm, respectively. In addition, the duration of tachycardia after smoking the low-dose cannabis was prolonged by 30 minutes by nicotine, but was not changed after the high-dose cannabis. Nicotine increased the subjective stimulant effects of cannabis, but the reported duration of effects of cannabis were shortened by nicotine. Plasma levels of nicotine and Δ^9-tetrahydrocannabinol (THC) did not differ on concurrent use. The cannabis cigarettes were standardised to 1.99% THC (low dose) and 3.51% THC (high dose).[1]

Mechanism

Unknown. The additive effect on heart rate may be due to sympathetic activity of both drugs, and might also involve cannabinoid receptors.[1]

Importance and management

Cannabis is often smoked with tobacco. The findings of the clinical study show that transdermal nicotine has additive effects with cannabis on heart rate, and increased the stimulant effect of cannabis. The clinical significance of these findings is uncertain.

1. Penetar DM, Kouri EM, Gross MM, McCarthy EM, Rhee CK, Peters EN, Lukas SE. Transdermal nicotine alters some of marihuana's effects in male and female volunteers. *Drug Alcohol Depend* (2005) 79, 211–23.

Evening primrose oil + Phenothiazines

Although seizures have occurred in a few schizophrenics taking phenothiazines and evening primrose oil, no adverse effects were seen in others, and there appears to be no firm evidence that evening primrose oil should be avoided by those at risk of seizures.

Clinical evidence

Twenty-three patients were enrolled in a placebo-controlled study of evening primrose oil in schizophrenia. During the treatment phase, patients were given 8 capsules of *Efamol* in addition to their normal medication. Seizures developed in 3 patients, one during treatment with placebo. The other two patients were taking evening primrose oil, one was receiving **fluphenazine decanoate** 50 mg once every 2 weeks and the other **fluphenazine decanoate** 25 mg once every 2 weeks with **thioridazine**, which was later changed to **chlorpromazine**.[1] In another study, 3 long-stay hospitalised schizophrenics were taking evening primrose oil. Their schizophrenia became much worse and all 3 patients showed EEG evidence of temporal lobe epilepsy.[2]

In contrast, no seizures or epileptiform events were reported in a crossover study of 48 patients (most of them schizophrenics) taking **phenothiazines** when they were given evening primrose oil for 4 months.[3] Concurrent use was also apparently uneventful in another study in schizophrenic patients.[4]

Mechanism

Not understood. One suggestion is that evening primrose oil possibly increases the well-recognised epileptogenic effects of the phenothiazines, rather than having an epileptogenic action of its own.[1] Another idea is that it might unmask temporal lobe epilepsy.[1,2]

Importance and management

The interaction between phenothiazines and evening primrose oil is not well established, nor is its incidence known, but clearly some caution is appropriate during concurrent use, because seizures may develop in a few individuals. There seems to be no way of identifying the patients at particular risk. The extent to which the underlying disease condition might affect what happens is also unclear.

No interaction between antiepileptics and evening primrose oil has been established and the reports cited above[1,2] appear to be the sole basis for the suggestion that evening primrose oil should be avoided by epileptics. No seizures appear to have been reported in patients taking evening primrose oil in the absence of phenothiazines. One review,[5] analysing these two reports, goes as far as suggesting that formularies should now remove seizures or epilepsy as an adverse effect of evening primrose oil because the evidence for the seizures clearly point to the phenothiazines taken. Moreover, the manufacturers of *Epogam*, an evening primrose oil preparation, claim that it is known to have improved the control of epilepsy in patients previously uncontrolled with conventional antiepileptic drugs, and other patients are said to have had no problems during concurrent treatment.[6]

1. Holman CP, Bell AFJ. A trial of evening primrose oil in the treatment of chronic schizophrenia. *J Orthomol Psychiatry* (1983) 12, 302–4.
2. Vaddadi KS. The use of gamma-linolenic acid and linoleic acid to differentiate between temporal lobe epilepsy and schizophrenia. *Prostaglandins Med* (1981) 6, 375–9.
3. Vaddadi KS, Courtney P, Gilleard CJ, Manku MS, Horrobin DF. A double-blind trial of essential fatty acid supplementation in patients with tardive dyskinesia. *Psychiatry Res* (1989) 27, 313–23.
4. Vaddadi KS, Horrobin DF. Weight loss produced by evening primrose oil administration in normal and schizophrenic individuals. *IRCS Med Sci* (1979) 7, 52.
5. Puri BK. The safety of evening primrose oil in epilepsy. Prostaglandins Leukot Essent Fatty Acids. (2007) 77, 101–3.
6. Scotia Pharmaceuticals Ltd. Personal Communication, January 1991.

Folic acid + Antacids or H_2-receptor antagonists

Aluminium/magnesium hydroxide-containing antacids, cimetidine and ranitidine probably do not have a clinically relevant effect on the absorption of folic acid.

Clinical evidence, mechanism, importance and management

In a well-controlled study in healthy subjects, taking two 30 mL doses of an **aluminium/magnesium hydroxide** antacid (*Mylanta II*) one hour and three hours after a single 200-microgram dose of folic acid caused a small 15% reduction in folic acid absorption (from about 51% to 43%). Two doses of **cimetidine** 300 mg (5 hours before and simultaneously with the folic acid), caused a reduction of about 8% in folic acid absorption, and two doses of **ranitidine** 150 mg (the night before and 5 hours before the folic acid) caused about a 6% decrease (not statistically significant).[1]

Drugs that increase the gastrointestinal pH might reduce folic acid absorption since the optimal pH for active intestinal transport of folic acid is about 6. It is possible that in the pH range of physiological significance, folate binds to aluminium hydroxide.

The reduction in folate absorption in this study was small and unlikely to be clinically relevant. It is possible that an individual taking **aluminium antacids** long-term and with marginal dietary folate might become folate deficient.

As neither **cimetidine** nor **ranitidine** caused a significant reduction in the absorption of folic acid, it is unlikely that other H_2-receptor antagonists would interact, although there is no published data to confirm this.

1. Russell RM, Golner BB, Krasinski SD, Sadowski JA, Suter PM, Braun CL. Effect of antacid and H_2 receptor antagonists on the intestinal absorption of folic acid. *J Lab Clin Med* (1988) 112, 458–63.

Folic acid + Sulfasalazine

Sulfasalazine can reduce the absorption of folic acid.

Clinical evidence, mechanism, importance and management

The absorption of folic acid was reduced by about one-third (from 65% to 44.5%) in patients with ulcerative and granulomatous colitis, when compared with healthy subjects, and even further reduced (down to 32%) when sulfasalazine was taken.[1] Another study confirmed that serum folate levels are lower in patients with ulcerative colitis taking sulfasalazine, and that the mechanism was an impairment of folate absorption brought about by sulfasalazine.[2] Sulfasalazine is also known to interfere with folate metabolism.

It is well established that sulfasalazine is, rarely, associated with blood dyscrasias due to folate deficiency and also other haematological toxicities, and consequently regular blood counts are recommended to detect this. The effects of folate deficiency (e.g. macrocytosis, pancytopenia) can be normalised by giving folic acid or folinic acid.

1. Franklin JL, Rosenberg IH. Impaired folic acid absorption in inflammatory bowel disease: effects of salicylazosulfapyridine (Azulfidine). *Gastroenterology* (1973) 64, 517–25.
2. Halsted CH, Gandhi G, Tamura T. Sulfasalazine inhibits the absorption of folates in ulcerative colitis. *N Engl J Med* (1981) 305, 1513–17.

Iron compounds + Antacids

The absorption of iron and the expected haematological response to iron can be reduced by the concurrent use of antacids.

Clinical evidence

(a) Iron compounds

A study in healthy subjects who were mildly iron-deficient (due to blood donation or menstruation) found that about 5 mL of *Mylanta II* (**aluminium/magnesium hydroxide** with simeticone) had little effect on the absorption of 10 or 20 mg of **ferrous sulfate** at 2 hours. However, **sodium bicarbonate** 1 g almost halved the absorption of **ferrous sulfate**.[1] Another study in healthy iron-replete subjects found that an antacid containing **aluminium/magnesium hydroxide** and **magnesium carbonate** reduced the absorption of **ferrous sulfate** and **ferrous fumarate** (both containing 100 mg of ferrous iron) by 37% and 31%, respectively.[2] Poor absorption of iron during the use of **sodium bicarbonate** and **aluminium hydroxide** has been described elsewhere.[3,4] One study did not find that the absorption of **ferrous sulfate** (iron 10 mg/kg) was affected by doses of **magnesium hydroxide** (5 mg for every 1 mg of iron) when the doses were given 30 minutes apart.[5] However, it has been suggested that, in this study, iron absorption was not measured for a sufficient period to fully rule out a reduction in absorption.[6]

Oral iron did not produce the expected rise in haemoglobin levels in patients taking non-absorbable alkalis such as **magnesium trisilicate**, and therefore a study was undertaken in 9 patients. Each patient was given 5 mg of isotopically labelled **ferrous sulfate** after a 35-g dose of **magnesium trisilicate**. The **magnesium** reduced the absorption of iron by an average of 70 to 88%, the reduction being small in some patients. However, in one individual iron absorption was reduced from 67% to 5%.[7]

(b) Iron polymaltose

In a study in patients with iron-deficiency anaemia, erythrocyte uptake of iron did not differ when oral iron polymaltose (equivalent to 100 mg of iron) was given alone or with **aluminium hydroxide** 600 mg (10 mL *Amphojel*). Iron polymaltose is a complex of ferric hydroxide with isomaltose.[8]

Mechanism

Uncertain. One suggestion is that magnesium sulfate changes ferrous sulfate into less easily absorbed salts, or increases its polymerisation.[7] Carbonates possibly cause the formation of poorly soluble iron complexes.[3] Aluminium hydroxide is believed to precipitate iron as the hydroxide and ferric ions can become intercalated into the aluminium hydroxide crystal lattice,[9] leaving less available for absorption.

Importance and management

Information is limited and difficult to assess because of the many variables (e.g. different dosages ranging from very small to those mimicking overdose, and a mix of subjects and patients). However, a reasonable 'blanket precaution' to achieve maximal absorption would be to separate the administration of iron preparations and antacids as much as possible to avoid admixture in the gut. This may not prove to be necessary with some preparations. For example, iron polymaltose does not appear to be affected by aluminium hydroxide.

Consider also 'Iron compounds + Calcium compounds', p.1412, for the effects of calcium compounds, some of which may be used as antacids.

1. O'Neil-Cutting MA, Crosby WH. The effect of antacids on the absorption of simultaneously ingested iron. *JAMA* (1986) 255, 1468–70.
2. Ekenved G, Halvorsen L, Sölvell L. Influence of a liquid antacid on the absorption of different iron salts. *Scand J Haematol* (1976) 28 (Suppl), 65–77.
3. Benjamin BI, Cortell S, Conrad ME. Bicarbonate-induced iron complexes and iron absorption: one effect of pancreatic secretions. *Gastroenterology* (1967) 35, 389–96.
4. Rastogi SP, Padilla F, Boyd CM. Effect of aluminum hydroxide on iron absorption. *J Arkansas Med Soc* (1976) 73, 133–4.
5. Snyder BK, Clark RF. Effect of magnesium hydroxide administration on iron absorption after a supratherapeutic dose of ferrous sulfate in human volunteers: a randomized controlled trial. *Ann Emerg Med* (1999) 33, 400–405.
6. Wallace KL, Curry SC, LoVecchio F, Raschke RA. Effect of magnesium hydroxide on iron absorption after ferrous sulfate. *Ann Emerg Med* (1999) 34, 685–6.
7. Hall GJL, Davis AE. Inhibition of iron absorption by magnesium trisilicate. *Med J Aust* (1969) 2, 95–6.
8. Potgieter MA, Potgieter JH, Venter C, Venter JL, Geisser P. Effect of oral aluminium hydroxide on iron absorption from iron(III)-hydroxide polymaltose complex in patients with iron deficiency anemia. *Arzneimittelforschung* (2007) 57, 392–400.
9. Coste JF, De Bari VA, Keil LB, Needle MA. *In-vitro* interactions of oral hematinics and antacid suspensions. *Curr Ther Res* (1977) 22, 205–15.

Iron compounds + Beverages

Reduced iron absorption has been reported with beverages high in polyphenolics such as cocoa, coffee, tea, pennyroyal tea and peppermint tea. Chamomile tea, green tea and rooibos tea do not appear to significantly affect iron absorption.

Clinical evidence

(a) Chamomile

A study in 13 healthy subjects found that chamomile tea (an infusion of *Matricaria chamomilla*) sweetened with panela (an unrefined cane sugar sweetener containing fructose) did not affect the absorption of iron from an iron-fortified bread, when compared with the absorption of iron from the bread alone. The tannin content of the chamomile tea was reported to be 24.5 mg in 100 mL.[1]

(b) Cocoa

In a study in 10 healthy subjects[2] a 275 mL serving of cocoa beverage reduced the absorption of radiolabelled iron from a 50 g bread roll by about 70%. In this study, the inhibitory effect of cocoa beverage on iron absorption was only slightly less that of black tea (Assam tea, *Camellia sinensis* L.).

(c) Coffee

In a series of studies in healthy subjects, drinking 200 mL of coffee with various test meals containing radiolabelled iron resulted in a 39% to 83% reduction in the absorption of iron. No decrease was observed if the coffee was drunk one hour before the meal, but when the coffee was given one hour after the meal the reduction was the same as taking it simultaneously with the meal. With one meal, the effect of coffee was about half that of tea.[3] In another study, a 275 mL serving of instant coffee reduced the absorption of radiolabelled iron from a 50 g bread roll, and this was not affected by milk.[2]

A controlled study among pregnant women in Costa Rica found that coffee consumption was associated with reductions in the haemoglobin levels and haematocrits of the mothers during pregnancy, and of their babies shortly after birth, despite the fact that the women were taking ferric sulfate 200 mg and 500 micrograms of folate daily. The babies also had a slightly lower birth weight (3189 g versus 3310 g). Almost a quarter of the mothers were considered to have iron-deficiency anaemia (haemoglobin levels of less than 11 g/dL), compared with none among the control group of non-coffee drinkers. Levels of iron in breast milk were reduced by about one-third. The coffee drinkers drank more than 450 mL of coffee daily, equivalent to more than 10 g of ground coffee.[4]

In a randomised study in Guatemalan infants, discontinuing coffee intake in those given an iron supplement led to a greater increase in serum ferritin than continuing coffee consumption (median 891 mL weekly). However, discontinuing coffee had no effect on changes in haemoglobin.[5]

(d) Pennyroyal

In a study in 9 healthy subjects, a 275 mL serving of pennyroyal tea reduced the absorption of iron in a 50 g bread roll by about 70%. The tea was prepared by adding 300 mL of boiling water to 3 g of the herbal tea, then infusing for 10 minutes before straining and serving. In this study, the inhibitory effect of pennyroyal tea on iron absorption was modestly less than that of black tea (Assam tea, *Camellia sinensis* L.).[2]

(e) Peppermint tea

In a study in 9 healthy subjects a 275 mL serving of peppermint tea reduced the absorption of iron from a 50 g bread roll by about 85%. The tea was prepared by adding 300 mL of boiling water to 3 g of the herb tea, then infusing for 10 minutes before straining and serving.[2] In this study, the inhibitory effect of peppermint tea on iron absorption was equivalent to that of black tea (Assam tea, *Camellia sinensis* L.).

(f) Rooibos

In a parallel group study in healthy subjects, mean iron absorption after ingestion of radiolabelled iron 16 mg with a beverage was 7.25% with rooibos tea, 1.7% with tea, and 9.34% with water.[6]

(g) Tea

1. Black tea. There is little data on the effect of tea on the absorption of iron from supplements. One case report describes an impaired response to iron, given to correct iron-deficiency anaemia, in a patient drinking 2 litres of black tea daily. The patient recovered when the black tea was stopped. This report did not specify whether the black tea was tea without milk, or black (fermented) tea.[7]

Some short-term controlled studies show a marked reduction in the absorption of dietary non-haem iron with black (fermented) tea beverage, some of which are cited for information.[2,3,8,9] In one of these, in a series of studies in healthy subjects, a 275 mL serving of black (fermented, Assam) tea reduced the absorption of radiolabelled iron from a 50 g bread roll by 79 to 94%. The tea was prepared by adding 300 mL of boiling water to 3 g of Assam tea, then infusing for 10 minutes before straining and serving. Milk added to the tea had very little effect on the reduction in iron absorption.[2] A study found that 150 mL of black tea reduced the absorption of radiolabelled iron from a test meal by 59% in 10 women with iron deficiency anaemia and by 49% in 10 control subjects without anaemia. When the quantity of tea was increased to 300 mL iron absorption was reduced by about 66% in both groups.[10]

Whether these reductions in iron absorption are important in the development of iron deficiency anaemia is less clear. Various epidemiological studies have looked at the correlation between tea consumption and iron deficiency in different populations. In one review of 16 of these studies, tea consumption did not influence iron status in people with adequate iron stores (as is common in the West), but there seemed to be a negative association between tea consumption and iron status in people with marginal iron status.[11] Another report describes no change in the absorption of a single dose of iron (2 to 15.8 mg/kg) in 10 iron-deficient children when the iron was given with 150 mL of tea (type unspecified) instead of water.[12]

2. Green tea. A study found that green tea extract (37 mg catechins) showed a modest 26% reduction in iron absorption,[13] and another study, of pure epigallocatechin gallate 150 mg and 300 mg, found only a 14% and 27% reduction in iron absorption, respectively.[14] A study in 4 elderly patients with iron deficiency anaemia and 11 control patients found no evidence that green tea inhibited the absorption of iron from sodium ferrous citrate.[15] Another study in pregnant women with iron deficiency anaemia reported a slightly higher resolution rate for anaemia in patients taking green tea.[16]

Note that tea has been used with some success in reducing iron accumulation and the frequency of phlebotomy in patients with iron overload syndromes.[17]

Mechanism

Tannins found in tea and polyphenolics found in cocoa, coffee, pennyroyal and peppermint tea are thought to form insoluble complexes with non-haem iron and thus reduce its absorption.[12] Chamomile tea and rooibos tea, which appear not to interact, contain much lower levels of tannins than black tea.

Importance and management

The general importance of these findings is uncertain, but be aware that black tea consumption may contribute to iron-deficiency anaemia. However, it has been suggested that no restrictions are required in healthy patients not at risk of iron deficiency.[18] Conversely, the suggestion is that patients at risk of iron deficiency (which would include those requiring iron supplements) should be advised to avoid tea with meals and for one hour after eating.[18] Note that tea is not generally considered to be a suitable drink for babies and children, because of its effects on iron absorption. Milk does not attenuate the effect of black (fermented) teas on iron absorption.

Other teas and beverages that may have similar effects to black tea appear to include cocoa, coffee, pennyroyal tea and peppermint tea.

Other teas that appear to have minimal interactions with iron include chamomile tea, green tea, and rooibos tea.

1. Olivares M, Pizarro F, Hertrampf E, Fuenmayor G, Estévez E. Iron absorption from wheat flour: effects of lemonade and chamomile infusion. *Nutrition* (2007) 23, 296–300.
2. Hurrell RF, Reddy M, Cook JD. Inhibition of non-haem iron absorption in man by polyphenolic-containing beverages. *Br J Nutr* (1999) 81, 289–95.
3. Morck TA, Lynch SR, Cook JD. Inhibition of food iron absorption by coffee. *Am J Clin Nutr* (1983) 37, 416–20.
4. Muñoz LM, Lönnerdal B, Keen CL, Dewey KG. Coffee consumption as a factor in iron deficiency anemia among pregnant women and their infants in Costa Rica. *Am J Clin Nutr* (1988) 48, 645–51.
5. Dewey KG, Romero-Abal ME, Quan de Serrano J, Bulux J, Peerson JM, Eagle P, Solomons NW. Effects of discontinuing coffee intake on iron status of iron-deficient Guatemalan toddlers: a randomized intervention study. *Am J Clin Nutr* (1997) 66, 168–76.
6. Hesseling PB, Klopper JF, van Heerden PD. The effect of rooibos tea on iron absorption [In Afrikaans]. *S Afr Med J* (1979) 55, 631–2.
7. Mahlknecht U, Weidmann E, Seipelt G. Black tea delays recovery from iron-deficiency anaemia. *Haematologica* (2001) 86, 559.
8. Disler PB, Lynch SR, Charlton RW, Torrance JD, Bothwell TH, Walker RB, Mayet F. The effect of tea on iron absorption. *Gut* (1975) 16, 193–200.
9. Rossander L, Hallberg L, Björn-Rasmussen E. Absorption of iron from breakfast meals. *Am J Clin Nutr* (1979) 32, 2484–9.
10. Thankachan P, Walczyk T, Muthayya S, Kurpad AV, Hurrell RF. Iron absorption in young Indian women: the interaction of iron status with the influence of tea and ascorbic acid. *Am J Clin Nutr* (2008) 87, 881–6.
11. Temme EHM, Van Hoydonck PGA. Tea consumption and iron status. *Eur J Clin Nutr* (2002) 56, 379–86.
12. Koren G, Boichis H, Keren G. Effects of tea on the absorption of pharmacological doses of an oral iron preparation. *Isr J Med Sci* (1982) 18, 547.
13. Samman S, Sandström B, Bjørndal Toft M, Bukhave K, Jensen M, Sørensen SS, Hansen M. Green tea or rosemary extract added to foods reduces nonheme-iron absorption. *Am J Clin Nutr* (2001) 73, 607–12.
14. Ullmann U, Haller J, Bakker GCM, Brink EJ, Weber P. Epigallocatechin gallate (EGCG) (TEAVIGO) does not impair non-haem-iron absorption in man. *Phytomedicine* (2005) 12, 410–415.
15. Kubota K, Sakuri T, Nakazato K, Shirakura T. Effect of green tea on iron absorption in elderly patients with iron deficiency anaemia [in Japanese]. *Nippon Ronen Igakkai Zasshi* (1990) 27, 555–8.
16. Mitamura T, Kitazono M, Yoshimura O, Yakushiji M. The influence of green tea upon the improvement of iron deficiency anemia with pregnancy treated by sodium ferrous citrate [in Japanese]. *Nippon Sanka Fujinka Gakkai Zasshi* (1989) 41, 688–94.
17. Kaltwasser JP, Werner E, Schalk K, Hansen C, Gottschalk R, Seidl C. Clinical trial on the effect of regular tea drinking on iron accumulation in genetic haemochromatosis. *Gut* (1998) 43, 699–704.
18. Nelson M, Poulter J. Impact of tea drinking on iron status in the UK: a review. *J Hum Nutr Diet* (2004) 17, 43–54.

Iron compounds + Calcium compounds

Calcium carbonate and calcium acetate (in large doses) modestly reduce the absorption of iron from ferrous sulfate.

Clinical evidence, mechanism, importance and management

In a single-dose study in 23 fasting healthy subjects,[1] the bioavailability of iron from **ferrous sulfate** 200 mg was reduced by 27% by **calcium acetate** 2.7 g, and by 19% by **calcium carbonate** 3 g.

A study in healthy subjects who were mildly iron-deficient (due to blood donation or menstruation) found that **calcium carbonate** 500 mg reduced the absorption of 10 or 20 mg of **ferrous sulfate** by two-thirds. Conversely, iron absorption from a multivitamin and mineral preparation was little affected by whether or not the tablet contained 200 mg of calcium (as **calcium carbonate**).[2]

It was suggested that calcium may form insoluble complexes with iron, so reducing its absorption.

The evidence is limited, but in general it appears that large doses of calcium compounds (500 mg of calcium or more) may reduce the absorption of iron; this would be expected to be clinically relevant. Ideally the findings of the study using calcium in phosphate-binding doses need replicating clinically, that is, in an appropriate patient group taking the calcium compounds long-term with meals. Nevertheless, a reasonable 'blanket precaution' to achieve maximal absorption would be to separate the administration of iron preparations and calcium as much as possible to avoid admixture in the gut. It would also seem prudent to monitor the response to iron. If the response is inadequate in those using calcium as a phosphate binder, an alternative may be to use sevelamer, which does not appear to affect iron absorption, see 'Iron compounds + Sevelamer', p.1413.

1. Pruchnicki MC, Coyle JD, Hoshaw-Woodard S, Bay WH. Effect of phosphate binders on supplemental iron absorption in healthy subjects. *J Clin Pharmacol* (2002) 42, 1171–6.
2. O'Neil-Cutting MA, Crosby WH. The effect of antacids on the absorption of simultaneously ingested iron. *JAMA* (1986) 255, 1468–70.

Iron compounds or Vitamin B_{12} + Chloramphenicol

In addition to the serious and potentially fatal bone marrow depression that can occur with chloramphenicol, it may also cause a milder, reversible bone marrow depression, which can oppose the treatment of anaemias with iron or vitamin B_{12}.

Clinical evidence

Two patients receiving **iron dextran** for iron-deficiency anaemia and also given oral chloramphenicol 3 g daily, did not have the expected haematological response to the iron.[1] Four patients receiving vitamin B_{12} for pernicious anaemia were all similarly refractory to **iron dextran** until chloramphenicol (52 to 60 mg/kg for 3 to 7 days) was withdrawn.[1]

Mechanism

Chloramphenicol can cause two forms of bone marrow depression. One is serious and irreversible, and can result in fatal aplastic anaemia, whereas the other is probably unrelated, milder and reversible, and appears to occur at chloramphenicol serum levels of 25 micrograms/mL or more. This occurs because chloramphenicol can inhibit protein synthesis, the first sign of which is a fall in the reticulocyte count, which reflects inadequate red cell maturation. This response to chloramphenicol has been seen in healthy individuals,[2] a series of patients with liver disease,[3] and in anaemic patients[1] receiving iron dextran or vitamin B_{12}.

Importance and management

An established interaction of clinical importance. The authors of one study recommend that chloramphenicol dosages of 25 to 30 mg/kg are usually adequate for treating infections without running the risk of elevating serum levels to 25 micrograms/mL or more, which is when this type of marrow depression can occur.[4] Monitor the effects of using iron or vitamin B_{12} together with chloramphenicol. A preferable alternative would be to use a different antibacterial. Note that chloramphenicol should not be used in patients with pre-existing bone-marrow depression or blood dyscrasias.

1. Saidi P, Wallerstein RO, Aggeler PM. Effect of chloramphenicol on erythropoiesis. *J Lab Clin Med* (1961) 57, 247–56.
2. Jiji RM, Gangarosa EJ, de la Macorra F. Chloramphenicol and its sulfamoyl analogue. Report of reversible erythropoietic toxicity in healthy volunteers. *Arch Intern Med* (1963) 111, 116–28.
3. McCurdy PR. Chloramphenicol bone marrow toxicity. *JAMA* (1961) 176, 588–93.
4. Scott JL, Finegold SM, Belkin GA, Lawrence JS. A controlled double-blind study of the hematologic toxicity of chloramphenicol. *N Engl J Med* (1965) 272, 1137–42.

Iron compounds + Colestyramine

Early *animal* studies found that colestyramine binds with ferrous sulfate in the gut and reduces its absorption, but iron deficiency was not seen in one small long-term clinical study.

Clinical evidence, mechanism, importance and management

In vitro studies have found that colestyramine binds with iron, and in *rats* this was found to halve the absorption of a single 100-microgram dose of **ferrous sulfate**,[1] and to significantly decrease serum iron and tissue iron stores with prolonged colestyramine use (in the absence of iron supplementation).[2] However, in 18 children, the prolonged use (1 to 2.5 years) of colestyramine did not change serum iron levels.[3]

Evidence is extremely limited, but it might suggest that no special precautions are required on concurrent use. Nevertheless, it is often advised to avoid other drugs for one hour before or 4 to 6 hours after colestyramine to minimise the possibility of interactions.

1. Thomas FB, McCullough F, Greenberger NJ. Inhibition of the intestinal absorption of inorganic and hemoglobin iron by cholestyramine. *J Lab Clin Med* (1971) 78, 70–80.
2. Thomas FB, Salsburey D, Greenberger NJ. Inhibition of iron absorption by cholestyramine. Demonstration of diminished iron stores following prolonged administration. *Am J Dig Dis* (1972) 17, 263–9.
3. West RJ, Lloyd JK. The effect of cholestyramine on intestinal absorption. Gut. (1975) 16, 93–8.

Iron compounds + H_2-receptor antagonists

Apart from a brief and unconfirmed report alleging that cimetidine reduced the response to ferrous sulfate, there appears to be no other evidence that H_2-receptor antagonists reduce the absorption of iron to a clinically relevant extent. Iron causes only a small and clinically irrelevant reduction in the serum levels of cimetidine and famotidine.

Clinical evidence, mechanism, importance and management

(a) Effect on iron

A brief report describes 3 patients taking **cimetidine** 1 g and **ferrous sulfate** 600 mg daily, whose ulcers healed after 2 months but whose anaemia and altered iron metabolism persisted. When the **cimetidine** was reduced to 400 mg daily the blood picture resolved satisfactorily within a month, without an alteration in the iron dose.[1] The author of the report attributed this response to the **cimetidine**-induced rise in gastric pH, which reduced the absorption of the iron. However, this suggested mechanism was subsequently disputed, as medicinal iron is already in the most absorbable form, Fe^{2+}, and so does not need an acidic environment to aid absorption.[2] A study in patients with iron deficiency, or iron-deficiency anaemia, found that the concurrent use of **famotidine**, **nizatidine**, or **ranitidine**, did not affect their response to 2.4 g of **iron succinyl-protein complex** (equivalent to 60 mg of iron twice daily).[3] No special precautions would seem necessary on concurrent use.

(b) Effect on H_2-receptor antagonists

In a series of three studies, healthy subjects were given **cimetidine** 300 mg with **ferrous sulfate** 300 mg, either as a tablet or a solution. The reductions in the AUC and the maximum serum levels of **cimetidine** were small (less than 16%). In the third experiment they were given **famotidine** 40 mg with **ferrous sulfate** 300 mg (as a tablet). Again, the AUC and maximum serum level reductions were also very small (10% or less). These small reductions are almost certainly due to the formation of a weak complex between the iron and these H_2-receptor antagonists.[4] An *in vitro* study with **ranitidine** found that, while it also binds with iron, it forms a very weak complex, and is less likely to bind than **cimetidine** or **famotidine**.[4] It was concluded that no clinically relevant interaction occurs between **ferrous sulfate** and any of these H_2-receptor antagonists.[4]

1. Esposito R. Cimetidine and iron-deficiency anaemia. *Lancet* (1977) ii, 1132.
2. Rosner F. Cimetidine and iron absorption. *Lancet* (1978) i, 95.
3. Bianchi FM, Cavassini GB, Leo P. Iron protein succinylate in the treatment of iron deficiency: Potential interaction with H_2-receptor antagonists. *Int J Clin Pharmacol Ther Toxicol* (1993) 31, 209–17.
4. Partlow ES, Campbell NRC, Chan SC, Pap KM, Granberg K, Hasinoff BB. Ferrous sulfate does not reduce serum levels of famotidine or cimetidine after concurrent ingestion. *Clin Pharmacol Ther* (1996) 59, 389–93.

Iron compounds + Neomycin

Neomycin may alter the absorption of iron.

Clinical evidence, mechanism, importance and management

A study in 6 patients found that neomycin markedly reduced the absorption of iron ($iron^{59}$ as **ferrous citrate**) in 4 patients, but increased its absorption in the other 2 patients who initially had low serum iron levels. None of the patients were anaemic at any time.[1] The importance of this is uncertain, but consider this possible interaction if the response to iron is poor.

1. Jacobson ED, Chodos RB, Faloon WW. An experimental malabsorption syndrome induced by neomycin. *Am J Med* (1960) 28, 524–33.

Iron compounds + Proton pump inhibitors

Omeprazole may impair the absorption of iron from oral iron compounds and vegetable sources of iron. Other proton pump inhibitors may interact similarly.

Clinical evidence

Two patients with iron deficiency anaemia as a result of erosive gastritis failed to show an improvement in their haemoglobin levels over 6 months while they were taking both an oral iron supplement and **omeprazole**. In both cases the authors report that other causes of treatment failure, such as occult gastrointestinal bleeding, were ruled out by clinical and laboratory tests. **Omeprazole** was stopped for 2 months and the patients continued to take the same dose of **ferrous sulfate**, with a noted improvement in both the haemoglobin and mean corpuscular volume (MCV). In one of these patients, serum iron levels were measured over the 2 hours after ingestion of ferrous sulfate 975 mg, both while they were taking omeprazole and 2 months after stopping omeprazole. A marked improvement in iron levels was noted after stopping omeprazole, suggesting that the iron absorption was improved.[1]

In another study in 7 patients with hereditary haemochromatosis, **omeprazole** 20 mg or **lansoprazole** 30 mg daily for 7 days suppressed the absorption of non-haem iron (iron of vegetable source) from a test meal.[2]

Mechanism

Hypochlorhydria induced by omeprazole or lansoprazole may impair the absorption of iron from oral iron preparations.[1]

Importance and management

Omeprazole does not appear to cause iron deficiency anaemia in patients with normal iron status; however, it is possible that it slows the improvement in anaemia that is expected when oral iron supplements are given to patients who are already anaemic. Although evidence for an interaction is limited, if the mechanism is correct, it would apply to all proton pump inhibitors. Bear these reports in mind should a patient taking a proton pump inhibitor fail to respond to oral iron therapy. Further study is needed.

1. Sharma VR, Brannon MA, Carloss EA. Effect of omeprazole on oral iron replacement in patients with iron deficiency anemia. *South Med J* (2004) 97, 887–9.
2. Hutchinson C, Geissler CA, Powell JJ, Bomford A. Proton pump inhibitors suppress absorption of dietary non-haem iron in hereditary haemochromatosis. *Gut* (2007) 56, 1291–5.

Iron compounds + Sevelamer

Sevelamer does not appear to affect the absorption of iron from ferrous sulfate to a clinically relevant extent.

Clinical evidence, mechanism, importance and management

In a single-dose study in 23 fasting healthy subjects,[1] the bioavailability of iron from **ferrous sulfate** 200 mg was reduced by a modest 10% by sevelamer 2.8 g. This study suggests that sevelamer is unlikely to have a clinically relevant effect on iron absorption; however, the findings need replicating in an appropriate patient group taking sevelamer long-term with meals.

1. Pruchnicki MC, Coyle JD, Hoshaw-Woodard S, Bay WH. Effect of phosphate binders on supplemental iron absorption in healthy subjects. *J Clin Pharmacol* (2002) 42, 1171–6.

Iron compounds + Vitamin E substances

Vitamin E impaired the response to iron in a group of anaemic children.

Clinical evidence, mechanism, importance and management

A group of 26 anaemic children aged 7 to 40 months were given **iron dextran** 5 mg/kg daily for 3 days. Vitamin E 200 units daily was also given to 9 of the children, starting 24 hours before the **iron dextran** and continued for a total of 4 days. It was noted that after 6 days, those taking vitamin E had a reticulocyte response of only 4.4%, compared with 14.4% in the patients not given vitamin E. The vitamin E group also had reduced haemoglobin levels and a lower haematocrit. The reasons are not understood. Check for any evidence of a reduced haematological response in anaemic patients given iron and vitamin E. The authors of the report point out that this dosage of vitamin E was well above the recommended daily dietary intake.[1]

1. Melhorn DK, Gross S. Relationships between iron-dextran and vitamin E in iron deficiency anemia in children. *J Lab Clin Med* (1969) 74, 789–802.

Melatonin + Caffeine

Caffeine increases the levels of both endogenous and orally administered melatonin.

Clinical evidence

In a crossover study, 12 healthy subjects were given a single 200-mg dose of caffeine (equivalent to one large or two small cups of coffee), 1 hour before and 1 and 3 hours after a single 6-mg oral dose of melatonin. Caffeine increased the average AUC and maximum levels of melatonin by 120% and 137%, respectively, although the half-life of melatonin was not significantly affected. The interaction was less pronounced in smokers (6 subjects) than in non-smokers (6 subjects).[1] In a similar study, taking caffeine 12 or 24 hours before melatonin did not affect the melatonin levels, although 2 subjects had raised melatonin levels when caffeine was taken 12 hours, but not 24 hours, before melatonin.[2]

In 12 healthy subjects given a single 200-mg dose of caffeine, taken in the evening, *endogenous*, nocturnal melatonin levels were found to be increased, and the AUC of melatonin was increased by 32%.[3]

Mechanism

Caffeine is thought to reduce the metabolism of melatonin by competing for metabolism by the cytochrome P450 isoenzyme CYP1A2.[1-3]

Importance and management

The interaction between caffeine and melatonin appears to be established. Melatonin is produced by the pineal gland in the body and is also available as a supplement in some parts of the world; however, the effects of long-term use of this supplement are unknown. From the above studies, it appears that caffeine significantly increases the levels of single doses of supplementary melatonin, however the long-term effects of caffeine on multiple doses of melatonin do not appear to have been studied. Melatonin can cause drowsiness when taken on its own, so patients who take melatonin should be advised that this effect may be increased (because of increased melatonin levels) if they also take caffeine, including that from beverages. This increased drowsiness may oppose the stimulating effect of caffeine, or alternatively caffeine may diminish the sedating effects of melatonin; the outcome of concurrent use does not appear to have been studied.

1. Härtter S, Nordmark A, Rose D-M, Bertilsson L, Tybring G, Laine K. Effects of caffeine intake on the pharmacokinetics of melatonin, a probe drug for CYP1A2 activity. *Br J Clin Pharmacol* (2003) 56, 679–682.
2. Härtter S, Korhonen T, Lundgren S, Rane A, Tolonen A, Turpeinen M, Laine K. Effect of caffeine intake 12 or 24 hours prior to melatonin intake and *CYP1A2*1F* polymorphism on CYP1A2 phenotyping by melatonin. *Basic Clin Pharmacol Toxicol* (2006) 99, 300–4.
3. Ursing C, Wikner J, Brismar K, Röjdmark S. Caffeine raises the serum melatonin level in healthy subjects: an indication of melatonin metabolism by cytochrome P450 (CYP)1A2. *J Endocrinol Invest* (2003) 26, 403–6.

Melatonin + Fluvoxamine

Fluvoxamine markedly increases the levels of endogenous and orally administered melatonin.

Clinical evidence

In a study in 5 healthy subjects, a single 50-mg dose of fluvoxamine taken 3 hours before a single 5-mg oral dose of melatonin markedly increased the average AUC and maximum levels of melatonin by 17-fold and 12-fold, respectively, although the half-life of melatonin was not significantly affected. The interaction was more pronounced in the one subject who was of a CYP2D6-poor metaboliser phenotype (meaning that this patient was lacking or totally deficient in this isoenzyme). All subjects reported marked drowsiness after melatonin intake that was even more pronounced when fluvoxamine was also given.[1]

Similarly, fluvoxamine 75 mg raised the levels of oral melatonin 5 mg by about 20-fold and significantly improved the sleep behaviour of a 51-year-old insomniac.[2]

In another study in 7 healthy subjects, fluvoxamine 50 mg doubled the maximum serum levels and excretion of endogenous melatonin and increased the AUC by about threefold.[3]

Mechanism

Previous studies had shown that fluvoxamine increased endogenous melatonin levels. This study demonstrates that this is likely to be via a pharmacokinetic mechanism. Fluvoxamine is known to be a potent inhibitor of the cytochrome P450 isoenzyme CYP1A2, by which melatonin is metabolised.

Importance and management

Evidence is limited, but an interaction between fluvoxamine and melatonin would appear to be established. Melatonin is produced by the pineal gland in the body, and is also available as a supplement; however, the effects of long-term use of this supplement are unknown. From the above study, it appears that fluvoxamine markedly increases the levels of single doses of supplementary melatonin, however the long-term effects of fluvoxamine on multiple doses of melatonin do not appear to have been studied. Be aware that excessive drowsiness and related adverse effects may occur on concurrent use. Note that one UK manufacturer advises that the combination should be avoided.[4] Other inhibitors of CYP1A2 may interact similarly (although to a lesser extent as fluvoxamine is currently the most potent CYP1A2 inhibitor in clinical use). The UK manufacturer specifically mentions the **quinolones**.[4] Of the quinolones in common usage, ciprofloxacin is an example of a clinically important CYP1A2 inhibitor.

Note that this effect would not be expected with other SSRIs, as these are not CYP1A2 inhibitors.

1. Härtter S, Grözinger M, Weigmann H, Röschke J, Hiemke C. Increased bioavailability of oral melatonin after fluvoxamine coadministration. *Clin Pharmacol Ther* (2000) 67, 1–6.
2. Grözinger M, Härtter S, Wang X, Röschke J, Hiemke C. Fluvoxamine strongly inhibits melatonin metabolism in a patient with low-amplitude melatonin profile. *Arch Gen Psychiatry* (2000) 57, 812.
3. von Bahr C, Ursing C, Yasui N, Tybring G, Bertilsson L, Röjdmark S. Fluvoxamine but not citalopram increases serum melatonin in healthy subjects - an indication that cytochrome P450 CYP1A2 and CYP2C19 hydroxylate melatonin. *Eur J Clin Pharmacol* (2000) 56, 123–7.
4. Circadin (Melatonin). Flynn Pharma Ltd. UK Summary of product characteristics, August 2011.

Melatonin + Miscellaneous

Alcohol may reduce the effects of melatonin on sleep. The concurrent use of imipramine and melatonin may lead to increased CNS effects. Cimetidine slightly increases melatonin levels. Psoralens are predicted to increase melatonin levels.

Clinical evidence, mechanism, importance and management

(a) Alcohol

The manufacturer of melatonin briefly notes that alcohol reduces the effectiveness of melatonin on sleep, and that it should not be taken with melatonin.[1] Given the known effects of alcohol on sleep, if melatonin is being taken to improve quality of sleep then this is sensible advice.

(b) Cimetidine

In a single-dose controlled study, cimetidine 800 mg increased the plasma concentration of melatonin after a 2 mg oral dose (magnitude not stated), whereas the plasma levels of cimetidine were unaffected. The pharmacodynamics of melatonin were not affected.[2] Cimetidine is a weak inhibitor of the cytochrome P450 isoenzyme CYP1A2, by which melatonin is principally metabolised. Therefore concurrent use results in raised melatonin levels. However, as cimetidine is a weak CYP1A2 inhibitor, the pharmacokinetic interaction would be unlikely to be clinically relevant. Nevertheless, the manufacturer recommends caution.[1] Be aware of a possible interaction if there is an increase in the adverse effects of melatonin (e.g. irritability, dry mouth, dizziness) on concurrent use. Other H_2-receptor antagonists are unlikely to interact as they are not known to have enzyme-inhibiting effects.

(c) Psoralens

The manufacturer briefly notes that **methoxsalen** and **5-methoxypsoralen** inhibit the metabolism of melatonin and increases its levels (magnitude not stated).[1] Note that 5-methoxypsoralen has been shown to increase endogenous melatonin levels (one study is cited as an example[3]).

Psoralens are potent inhibitors of the cytochrome P450 isoenzyme CYP1A2 by which melatonin is principally metabolised, and therefore concurrent use may be expected to raise melatonin levels. The manufacturer of melatonin recommends caution on concurrent use,[1] which seems prudent as the adverse effects of melatonin may be increased. Any interaction would only apply to these psoralens used orally, and not when they are used topically. Be aware of a possible interaction if there is an increase in the adverse effects of melatonin (e.g. irritability, dry mouth, dizziness) in patients also taking psoralens.

(d) Tricyclics

In a single-dose controlled study, there was no pharmacokinetic interaction between melatonin 2 mg and **imipramine** 75 mg. However, there was a possible pharmacodynamic interaction, with increased feelings of tranquillity and difficulty in performing tasks (undefined) when compared with **imipramine** alone.[1,2] This may potentially occur with all tricyclics. Patients should be warned of a possible additive effect.

1. Circadin (Melatonin). Flynn Pharma Ltd. UK Summary of product characteristics, August 2011.
2. EMEA Assessment report for Circadin. Procedure No. EMEA/H/C/695. 2007. Available at: http://www.ema.europa.eu/docs/en_GB/document_library/EPAR_-_Scientific_Discussion/human/000695/WC500026808.pdf (accessed 21/10/15).
3. Souetre E, Salvati E, Belugou JL, Krebs B, Darcourt G. 5-Methoxypsoralen as a specific stimulating agent of melatonin secretion in humans. *J Clin Endocrinol Metab* (1990) 71, 670–4.

Melatonin + Oestrogens

Oestrogens, from oral combined hormonal contraceptives, appear to increase melatonin levels.

Clinical evidence

In a clinical study, the AUC and maximum level of a single 6-mg dose of melatonin was about 4 times higher in subjects taking a an oral combined hormonal contraceptive than those not taking this type of contraceptive. Melatonin alone did not significantly affect alertness in this study, and no reduced alertness was noted in those taking oral contraceptives. The contraceptives being used by the women included **ethinylestradiol** with either cyproterone acetate, desogestrel, drospirenone or gestodene. There did not appear to be any obvious differences between these contraceptives, but the numbers of women taking each were too small for this to be conclusive.[1]

Mechanism

Ethinylestradiol is a moderate inhibitor of the cytochrome P450 isoenzyme CYP1A2, by which melatonin is principally metabolised.

Importance and management

Women taking oral combined hormonal contraceptives may have higher levels of melatonin after using supplements. Although in the study cited, this did not decrease alertness, it would be prudent to bear in mind the possibility of increased drowsiness. One UK manufacturer extends this caution to **hormone replacement therapy**,[2] although it is unclear whether the oestrogens used for HRT will have the same effect as ethinylestradiol.

1. Hilli J, Korhonen T, Turpeinen M, Hokkanen J, Mattila S, Laine K. The effect of oral contraceptives on the pharmacokinetics of melatonin in healthy subjects with CYP1A2 g.-163C>A polymorphism. *J Clin Pharmacol* (2008) 48, 986–94.
2. Circadin (Melatonin). Flynn Pharma Ltd. UK Summary of product characteristics, August 2011.

Melatonin + Tobacco

Tobacco smoking reduces melatonin levels.

Clinical evidence, mechanism, importance and management

In a study in 8 tobacco smokers, the AUC of a single 25-mg dose of melatonin was almost threefold higher when the melatonin was taken after 7 days of smoking abstinence than when taken while smoking.[1]

Constituents of tobacco smoke are minor to moderate inducers of the cytochrome P450 isoenzyme CYP1A2, by which melatonin is principally metabolised.

The finding of this study suggests that melatonin might not be as effective in smokers. Be aware of this possibility, and consider trying an increased melatonin dose if it is not effective in a smoker.

1. Ursing C, von Bahr C, Brismar K, Röjdmark S. Influence of cigarette smoking on melatonin levels in man. *Eur J Clin Pharmacol* (2005) 61, 197–201.

Nicotine + Grapefruit juice

Grapefruit slightly inhibits the metabolism and increases the renal clearance of oral nicotine.

Clinical evidence, mechanism, importance and management

In a single-dose pharmacokinetic study in healthy subjects, administration of oral nicotine 2 mg with full-strength and half-strength grapefruit juice reduced the AUC of conitine (a metabolite of nicotine) by 15% and 2.5%, respectively. Conversely, the renal clearance of nicotine was increased. It was suggested that grapefruit juice inhibits the cytochrome P450 isoenzyme CYP2A6, which is responsible for the metabolism of oral nicotine to cotinine.[1]

The changes seen here were small and unlikely to be clinically relevant. Note that nicotine is not usually given by the oral route as in this study: replacement therapy is by the buccal route (chewing gum or sublingual tablets), or the transdermal route.

1. Hukkanen J, Jacob P, Benowitz NL. Effect of grapefruit juice on cytochrome P450 2A6 and nicotine renal clearance. *Clin Pharmacol Ther* (2006) 80, 522–30.

Nicotine + Tranylcypromine

Tranylcypromine inhibits the metabolism of oral nicotine.

Clinical evidence, mechanism, importance and management

A brief report describes a study in smokers in which low-dose tranylcypromine 2.5 mg three times daily increased plasma levels of oral nicotine by about 75%, but did not affect subcutaneous nicotine. Tranylcypromine inhibits the cytochrome P450 isoenzyme CYP2A6, which is responsible for the metabolism of oral nicotine to cotinine. Inhibiting this step leads to raised nicotine levels.[1]

Note that nicotine is not usually given orally. The clinical relevance of this finding to buccal formulations of nicotine replacement therapy (chewing gum and sublingual tablets) is unknown, but it seems likely to be small.

1. Fernandes LC, Tyndale RF, Sellers EM. Tranylcypromine (TCP) inhibition of nicotine metabolism. *Drug Alcohol Depend* (2002) 66 (Suppl 1) S54–S55.

Nicotine + Vasopressin

A case report described marked hypotension and bradycardia in a young woman during surgery, which was attributed to the combined effects of a vasopressin injection and nicotine from a transdermal patch.

Clinical evidence

A 22-year-old woman in good health was anaesthetised for surgery with nitrous oxide/oxygen and isoflurane. Twenty minutes after induction she was given an injection of 0.2 units of vasopressin into the cervix. Within seconds she developed severe hypotension and bradycardia, and over the next 30 minutes blood pressures as low as 70/35 mmHg and heart rates as low as 38 bpm were recorded. She was given atropine and adrenaline (epinephrine), and eventually made a full recovery. This patient was wearing a transdermal nicotine patch.[1]

Mechanism

The circulatory collapse was attributed by the authors to the combined effects of the injected vasopressin and the nicotine from the transdermal patch. Both of these drugs can increase cardiac afterload and cause coronary artery vasoconstriction, which the authors suggest may have decreased the blood supply to the heart and resulted in cardiac depression.[1]

Importance and management

This is an isolated report and any interaction between nicotine and vasopressin is therefore not well established. Nevertheless the recommendation of the authors seems sensible, namely that nicotine patches should be removed the night before or 24 hours before surgery, and that patients should be asked to avoid smoking before surgery to make sure that nicotine levels are minimal. More study is needed.

1. Groudine SB, Morley JN. Recent problems with paracervical vasopressin: a possible synergistic reaction with nicotine. *Med Hypotheses* (1996) 47, 19–21.

Paricalcitol + Miscellaneous

Ketoconazole raises paricalcitol concentrations; other potent CYP3A4 inhibitors are predicted to interact similarly. The use of paricalcitol

increases the risks of raised calcium, phosphate, aluminium, or magnesium concentrations in patients taking drugs containing these substances, or drugs that raise the concentrations of these substances (e.g. vitamin D).

Clinical evidence, mechanism, importance and management

(a) CYP3A4 inhibitors

In a study in healthy subjects, **ketoconazole** 200 mg twice daily for 5 days did not significantly alter the maximum concentrations of paricalcitol, but the AUC of paricalcitol was doubled, and its half-life was prolonged from 9.8 hours to 17 hours.[1,2] On the basis of this interaction the US manufacturer predicts that other potent inhibitors of the cytochrome P450 isoenzyme CYP3A4 will interact similarly. They specifically name the HIV-protease inhibitors **atazanavir**, **indinavir**, **nelfinavir**, **ritonavir** and **saquinavir**; the azole antifungals **itraconazole** and **voriconazole**; and the macrolides **clarithromycin** and **telithromycin**. The US manufacturer recommends close monitoring if any of these drugs is given to a patient taking paricalcitol,[2] and recommend monitoring intact parathyroid hormone and calcium concentrations if drugs such as **ketoconazole** are started or stopped.[2]

(b) Other drugs

Paricalcitol use may lead to increased calcium and phosphate concentrations. The UK manufacturer therefore warns that the concurrent use of **calcium-** or **phosphate-containing substances** may increase this risk. They specifically advise against the concurrent use of **phosphate-containing substances** with paricalcitol.[1] In addition the concurrent use of **vitamin D** may increase the risk of hypercalcaemia, and should therefore be avoided where possible. The UK manufacturer also advises that the use of **aluminium-** and **magnesium-containing substances** (e.g. **antacids**, phosphate binders) should be avoided with paricalcitol because raised blood concentrations of these substances may occur.[1] However, note that patients with renal impairment are highly likely to be taking these drugs and having serum electrolyte concentrations frequently monitored. Furthermore the US manufacturer[2] does not advise against their concurrent use.

1. Zemplar Soft Capsules (Paricalcitol). Abbott Laboratories Ltd. UK Summary of product characteristics, January 2012.
2. Zemplar Injection (Paricalcitol). Abbott Laboratories. US Prescribing information, January 2009.

Paricalcitol + Omeprazole

The pharmacokinetics of paricalcitol are not affected by omeprazole.

Clinical evidence, mechanism, importance and management

A randomised study in 25 healthy subjects found that a single 40-mg dose of omeprazole, taken 2 hours before a single 16-microgram dose of paricalcitol, had no significant effects on the pharmacokinetics of paricalcitol. No increase in adverse effects was noted and the combination was reported to be well tolerated. No paricalcitol dosage adjustments are therefore necessary if omeprazole is also given.[1]

1. Palaparthy R, Pradhan RS, Chan J, Rieser M, Chira T, Galitz L, Awni W, Williams LA. Effect of omeprazole on the pharmacokinetics of paricalcitol in healthy subjects. *Biopharm Drug Dispos* (2007) 28, 65–71.

St John's wort (*Hypericum perforatum*) + Cimetidine

Cimetidine does not significantly alter the metabolism of the constituents of St John's wort hypericin and pseudohypericin.

Clinical evidence, mechanism, importance and management

A placebo-controlled study in healthy subjects taking St John's wort (*LI160, Lichtwer Pharma*) 300 mg three times daily found that, apart from a modest 25% increase in the AUC of pseudohypericin, cimetidine 1 g daily (in divided doses) did not significantly affect the pharmacokinetics of either the hypericin or pseudohypericin constituents of St John's wort. The available evidence therefore suggests that cimetidine is unlikely to affect the dose requirements of St John's wort.[1]

1. Johne A, Perloff ES, Bauer S, Schmider J, Mai I, Brockmöller J, Roots I. Impact of cytochrome P-450 inhibition by cimetidine and induction by carbamazepine on the kinetics of hypericin and pseudohypericin in healthy volunteers. *Eur J Clin Pharmacol* (2004) 60, 617–22.

St John's wort (*Hypericum perforatum*) + Loperamide

Delirium occurred in a woman taking St John's wort and valerian when she took loperamide.

Clinical evidence, mechanism, importance and management

A 39-year-old woman with a history of depression was hospitalised in a state of delirium. She had been taking St John's wort and valerian for 6 months (products and doses not stated) and had recently taken loperamide for diarrhoea.[1]

The authors speculated that this was an interaction between St John's wort and loperamide attributed to the MAO inhibitory activity of St John's wort, analogous to the interaction between non-selective MAOIs and pethidine (meperidine), see 'MAOIs or RIMAs + Opioids; Pethidine (Meperidine)', p.1399. However, St John's wort is not thought to act as an MAOI inhibitor, for example, it does not usually cause a hypertensive reaction with tyramine-rich food (see 'St John's wort (*Hypericum perforatum*) + Tyramine', p.1415.

This appears to be an isolated report, and its findings cannot be generalised.

1. Khawaja IS, Marotta RF, Lippmann S. Herbal medicines as a factor in delirium. *Psychiatr Serv* (1999) 50, 969–70.

St John's wort (*Hypericum perforatum*) + Tyramine

An isolated report describes a patient taking St John's wort who experienced a hypertensive crisis after consuming tyramine-rich food and drink.

Clinical evidence, mechanism, importance and management

A man who had taken a St John's wort supplement for 7 days (preparation and dose not stated) was admitted to hospital with confusion and disorientation. He was unable to recall events after eating aged cheeses and pouring a glass of red wine 8 hours earlier. On examination he had a pulse rate of 115 bpm, a respiratory rate of 16 breaths per minute and his blood pressure was 210/140 mmHg. He was given intravenous phentolamine and oral labetalol and his blood pressure decreased to 160/100 mmHg after 2 hours and the delirium also resolved. Extensive laboratory investigations did not find any cause for the hypertension and delirium.

It was suggested that the time scale of starting to regularly take St John's wort and the onset of delirium and hypertension after the consumption of tyramine-rich food and drink was suggestive of hypertension associated with MAOIs (see also 'MAOIs or RIMAs + Food; Tyramine-containing', p.1389). Although St John's wort is a potent inhibitor of monoamine oxidase, this effect has not been demonstrated at recommended doses. It was concluded that the hypertensive crisis in this patient may have been mediated by monoamine oxidase inhibition, but there was also a possibility of another, as yet unknown, pharmacological action of St John's wort being involved.[1] Given the widespread use of St John's wort this case would seem to be unusual, and there is currently little grounds for suggesting any dietary restriction in those taking St John's wort.

1. Patel S, Robinson R, Burk M. Hypertensive crisis associated with St. John's wort. *Am J Med* (2002) 112, 507–8.

Tyramine + Cimetidine

A woman taking cimetidine experienced a severe headache and hypertension when she drank *Bovril* and ate some cheese.

Clinical evidence, mechanism, importance and management

A 77-year-old woman with hiatus hernia, who had been taking cimetidine 400 mg four times daily for 3 years, experienced a severe frontal headache and hypertension, which appeared to be related to the ingestion of a cup of *Bovril* and some English cheddar cheese, both of which can contain substantial amounts of tyramine.[1] Although the authors point out the similarity between this reaction and that seen in patients taking MAOIs who eat tyramine-rich foods (see 'MAOIs or RIMAs + Food; Tyramine-containing', p.1389), there is no satisfactory explanation for what occurred. They note that the patient was also taking salbutamol (another sympathomimetic) but rule out any contribution from this drug.

This is an isolated report and there is no reason why in general patients taking cimetidine should avoid tyramine-rich foods.

1. Griffin MJJ, Morris JS. MAOI-like reaction associated with cimetidine. *Drug Intell Clin Pharm* (1987) 21, 219.

Vitamin A (Retinol) + Neomycin

Neomycin can markedly reduce the absorption of vitamin A (retinol) from the gut.

Clinical evidence, mechanism, importance and management

In a study in 5 healthy subjects, neomycin 2 g markedly reduced the absorption of a test dose of vitamin A. It is suggested that this was due to a direct chemical interference between the neomycin and bile in the gut, which disrupted the absorption of fats and fat-soluble vitamins.[1] The extent to which long-term treatment with neomycin (or other aminoglycosides) would impair the treatment of vitamin A deficiency has not been determined.

1. Barrowman JA, D'Mello A, Herxheimer A. A single dose of neomycin impairs absorption of vitamin A (Retinol) in man. *Eur J Clin Pharmacol* (1973) 5, 199–201.

Vitamin B_{12} + Miscellaneous

Neomycin, colchicine, aminosalicylic acid and H_2-receptor antagonists can reduce the absorption of vitamin B_{12} from the gut, but no interaction is likely when B_{12} is given by injection.

Clinical evidence, mechanism, importance and management

Neomycin causes a generalised malabsorption syndrome, which has been shown[1] to reduce the absorption of vitamin B_{12}. **Colchicine** has also been shown to decrease B_{12} absorption.[1] **Aminosalicylic acid** reduces vitamin B_{12} absorption for reasons that are not understood, but which are possibly related to a mild generalised malabsorption syndrome.[2] A review of the literature[3] suggests that H_2-receptor antagonists (such as **cimetidine** and **ranitidine**) can also reduce vitamin B_{12} absorption, primarily because they reduce gastric acid production. The acid is needed to aid the release of B_{12} from dietary protein sources. There is therefore a possibility that on long-term use patients could become vitamin B_{12} deficient.

Within the context of adverse drug interactions, none of these findings is normally likely to be clinically important, because for anaemia, vitamin B_{12} should be given parenterally, both for convenience and to avoid well-established problems with absorption.

1. Faloon WW, Chodos RB. Vitamin B_{12} absorption studies using colchicine, neomycin and continuous 57Co B_{12} administration. *Gastroenterology* (1969) 56, 1251.
2. Palva IP, Rytkönen U, Alatulkkila M, Palva HLA. Drug-induced malabsorption of vitamin B_{12}. V. Intestinal pH and absorption of vitamin B_{12} during treatment with para-aminosalicylic acid. *Scand J Haematol* (1972) 9, 5–7.
3. Force RW, Nahata MC. Effect of histamine H_2-receptor antagonists on vitamin B_{12} absorption. *Ann Pharmacother* (1992) 26, 1283–6.

Vitamin D substances + Antiepileptics; Enzyme-inducing

The long-term use of carbamazepine, phenytoin, phenobarbital, or primidone can disturb vitamin D and calcium metabolism and may result in osteomalacia. There are a few reports of patients taking vitamin D supplements who responded poorly to vitamin replacement while taking phenytoin or barbiturates. Serum phenytoin levels are not altered by vitamin D.

Clinical evidence

A 16-year-old with grand mal epilepsy and idiopathic hypoparathyroidism did not adequately respond to **alfacalcidol** 10 micrograms daily and calcium 6 to 12 g daily, apparently because **phenytoin** 200 mg and **primidone** 500 mg daily were also being taken. However, when **dihydrotachysterol** 0.6 to 2.4 mg daily was given normal calcium levels were achieved.[1]

Other reports describe patients whose response to usual doses of vitamin D was poor, because of the concurrent use of **phenytoin** and **phenobarbital** or **primidone**.[2-4] Other reports clearly show low serum calcium levels,[5,6] low serum vitamin D levels,[7] osteomalacia,[6] and bone structure alterations[5,7] in the presence of **phenytoin**. **Carbamazepine** may have similar effects, but the evidence is less conclusive.[8,9]

A controlled study in 151 epileptic patients taking **phenytoin** and calcium found that the addition of 2000 units of **vitamin D_2** daily over a 3-month period had no significant effect on serum **phenytoin** levels.[10]

Mechanism

The enzyme-inducing effects of phenytoin and other antiepileptics increases the metabolism of the vitamin D, thereby reducing its effects and disturbing calcium metabolism.[3] In addition, phenytoin may possibly reduce the absorption of calcium from the gut.[1]

Importance and management

The disturbance of calcium metabolism by phenytoin and other enzyme-inducing antiepileptics is very well established, but there are only a few reports describing a poor response to vitamin D. The effects of concurrent treatment should be well monitored. Those who need vitamin D supplements may possibly need greater than usual doses.

1. Rubinger D, Korn-Lubetzki I, Feldman S, Popovtzer MM. Delayed response to 1 α-hydroxycholecalciferol therapy in a case of hypoparathyroidism during anticonvulsant therapy. *Isr J Med Sci* (1980) 16, 772–4.
2. Asherov J, Weinberger A, Pinkhas J. Lack of response to vitamin D therapy in a patient with hypoparathyroidism under anticonvulsant drugs. *Helv Paediatr Acta* (1977) 32, 369–73.
3. Chan JCM, Oldham SB, Holick MF, DeLuca HF. 1-α-Hydroxyvitamin D_3 in chronic renal failure. A potent analogue of the kidney hormone, 1,25-dihydroxycholecalciferol. *JAMA* (1975) 234, 47–52.
4. Maclaren N, Lifshitz F. Vitamin D-dependency rickets in institutionalized, mentally retarded children on long term anticonvulsant therapy. II. The response to 25-hydroxycholecalciferol and to vitamin D_2. *Pediatr Res* (1973) 7, 914–22.
5. Mosekilde L, Melsen F. Anticonvulsant osteomalacia determined by quantitative analyses of bone changes. Population study and possible risk factors. *Acta Med Scand* (1976) 199, 349–55.
6. Hunter J, Maxwell JD, Stewart DA, Parson V, Williams R. Altered calcium metabolism in epileptic children on anticonvulsants. *BMJ* (1971) 4, 202–4.
7. Hahn TJ, Avioli LV. Anticonvulsant osteomalacia. *Arch Intern Med* (1975) 135, 997–1000.
8. Voudris KA, Attilakos A, Katsarou E, Garoufi A, Dimou S, Skardoutsou A, Mastroyianni S. Early alteration in bone metabolism in epileptic children receiving carbamazepine monotherapy owing to the induction of hepatic drug-metabolizing enzymes. *J Child Neurol* (2005) 20, 513–16.
9. O'Hare JA, Duggan B, O'Driscoll D, Callaghan N. Biochemical evidence for osteomalacia with carbamazepine therapy. *Acta Neurol Scand* (1980) 62, 282–6.
10. Christiansen C, Rødbro P. Effect of vitamin D2 on serum phenytoin. A controlled therapeutical trial. *Acta Neurol Scand* (1974) 50, 661–4.

Vitamin D substances; Alfacalcidol + Danazol

An isolated report describes hypercalcaemia when a woman taking alfacalcidol also took danazol.

Clinical evidence, mechanism, importance and management

A woman with idiopathic hypoparathyroidism, treated with alfacalcidol, developed hypercalcaemia when she was given danazol 400 mg daily for endometriosis. She needed a reduction in the dosage of alfacalcidol from 4 micrograms daily to 0.75 micrograms daily. When the danazol was stopped 6 months later, the alfacalcidol dosage was raised to 4 micrograms daily and she remained normocalcaemic.[1] The reasons for this interaction are not understood. Its general importance is limited as this appears to be an isolated case.

1. Hepburn NC, Abdul-Aziz LAS, Whiteoak R. Danazol-induced hypercalcaemia in alphacalcidol-treated hypoparathyroidism. *Postgrad Med J* (1989) 65, 849–50.

Vitamin K substances + Antibacterials

Seven patients in intensive care did not respond to intravenous vitamin K for hypoprothrombinaemia while receiving gentamicin and clindamycin.

Clinical evidence, mechanism, importance and management

Some patients, particularly those in intensive care who are not eating, can quite rapidly develop acute vitamin K deficiency, which leads to prolonged prothrombin times and possibly bleeding.[1,2] This can normally be controlled by giving vitamin K parenterally. However, one report describes seven such patients, all with normal liver function, who unexpectedly did not respond to intravenous **phytomenadione**. Examination of their records found that all seven were receiving **gentamicin** and **clindamycin**.[2] Just why, or if, these two antibacterials might have opposed the effects of intravenous vitamin K is not understood.

1. Ham JM. Hypoprothrombinaemia in patients undergoing prolonged intensive care. *Med J Aust* (1971) 2, 716–18.
2. Rodriguez-Erdmann F, Hoff JV, Carmody G. Interaction of antibiotics with vitamin K. *JAMA* (1981) 246, 937.

Vitamins + Orlistat

Orlistat decreases the absorption of supplemental betacarotene and vitamin E. There is some evidence to suggest that some patients may have low vitamin D levels while taking orlistat, even if they are also taking multivitamins.

Clinical evidence

Studies in healthy subjects have found that about two-thirds of a supplemental dose of **betacarotene**[1] and roughly half the dose of **vitamin E (α-tocopherol)**[2] was absorbed in the presence of orlistat, while the absorption of **vitamin A** was not affected.[2] In the first study, betacarotene was given within about 30 minutes of the orlistat,[1] whereas in the second, the vitamin supplement was given at the same time as orlistat.[2] In another study, 17 obese adolescents were given orlistat 120 mg three times daily with meals and a daily multivitamin (containing **vitamins A, D, E, and K**) to be taken at night. Levels of **vitamins A, E** and **K** were not significantly altered over 6 months of orlistat use, but **vitamin D** concentrations dropped after the first month, but had returned to baseline by 3 months. Three subjects (all African-Americans) required additional **vitamin D** supplementation, but all had a low dietary intake of **vitamin D**.[3,4]

Mechanism

Orlistat reduces dietary fat absorption by inhibiting gastrointestinal lipase. Consequently, it reduces the absorption of fat soluble vitamins.

Importance and management

An established interaction. To maximise vitamin absorption, the manufacturers recommend that any multivitamin preparation should be taken at least 2 hours before or after orlistat, such as at bedtime.[5,6] The US manufacturer suggests that patients taking orlistat should be advised to take multivitamins, because of the possibility of reduced vitamin levels.[6] Note that the authors of the study in adolescents suggest that monitoring of vitamin D may be required, even if multivitamins are given.[3]

1. Zhi J, Melia AT, Koss-Twardy SG, Arora S, Patel IH. The effect of orlistat, an inhibitor of dietary fat absorption, on the pharmacokinetics of β-carotene in healthy volunteers. *J Clin Pharmacol* (1996) 36, 152–9.
2. Melia AT, Koss-Twardy SG, Zhi J. The effect of orlistat, an inhibitor of dietary fat absorption, on the absorption of vitamins A and E in healthy volunteers. *J Clin Pharmacol* (1996) 36, 647–53.
3. McDuffie JR, Calis KA, Booth SL, Uwaifo GI, Yanovski JA. Effects of orlistat on fat-soluble vitamins in obese adolescents. *Pharmacotherapy* (2002) 22, 814–22.
4. McDuffie JR, Calis KA, Uwaifo GI, Sebring NG, Fallon EM, Hubbard VS, Yanovski JA. Three-month tolerability of orlistat in adolescents with obesity-related comorbid conditions. *Obes Res* (2002) 10, 642–50.
5. Xenical (Orlistat). Roche Products Ltd. UK Summary of product characteristics, April 2014.
6. Xenical (Orlistat). Roche Pharmaceuticals. US Prescribing information, December 2013.

Zinc compounds + Iron compounds

Some studies suggest that giving iron with zinc may reduce the bioavailability of iron and/or zinc, but other studies suggest that combined supplementation is of value in reducing deficiencies of these micronutrients.

Clinical evidence

In a study, 549 Indonesian infants were given dietary supplementation from age 6 months until age 12 months with either iron 10 mg (as **ferrous sulfate**), zinc

10 mg (as **zinc sulfate**), iron 10 mg plus zinc 10 mg, or placebo. After supplementation, the iron group and the iron plus zinc groups had haemoglobin levels of 11.9 g/dL and 11.5 g/dL respectively and serum ferritin of 46.5 micrograms/L and 32.3 micrograms/L respectively. The haemoglobin level in the group receiving zinc and iron was not significantly different from that of the placebo group. Zinc levels were lower in infants given zinc with iron than in those given zinc alone, but this difference was not found to be significant. It was concluded that supplementation with iron plus zinc was less effective than single supplements in improving iron and zinc status.[1] Similar conclusions were reached in another study using the same doses of iron and zinc.[2] A further study in 784 infants aged 4 to 7 months given iron 10 mg or zinc 10 mg alone or combined, or placebo, daily for 6 months found that haemoglobin levels were increased by about 2.3 g/dL and 2.1 g/dL when given alone or with zinc, respectively, and zinc levels were increased by 10.3 micromol/L and 8 micromol/L when given alone or with iron, respectively. Although combined iron and zinc supplements had a positive effect on iron status, iron was found to have a negative effect on zinc status in these infants.[3] Similar conclusions were reached from pooled results from 4 studies in 2468 infants given iron 10 mg and/or zinc 10 mg daily for 6 months.[4]

In a study in 14 healthy subjects, iron 500 micrograms (as **ferrous sulfate** solution) was given alone or with zinc 590 micrograms (as **zinc sulfate**) on day 1, and iron 10 mg was given alone or with zinc 11.71 mg on day 14. At the lower doses, zinc did not affect iron bioavailability, but at the higher doses, iron bioavailability was reduced by 56%.[5]

Another study in ileostomy patients given zinc 12 mg alone, with iron 100 mg or 400 mg (as **ferrous gluconate**) on three consecutive days, found zinc absorption was 44% when given alone and significantly decreased to 26% and 23% when given with iron 100 mg or 400 mg, respectively.[6]

Mechanism

One study suggests that iron affects zinc absorption in a dose-dependent manner.[6] Reduced bioavailability of iron supplements when given with zinc may depend on the total amount of both iron and zinc in the intestine, as at high doses, but not low doses, zinc appears to affect iron bioavailability.[5] In some studies in infants and children, it has been suggested that the age of the child and initial serum zinc status may partly explain differences in reported effects.[7,8] Iron supplementation may have a greater effect on haemoglobin levels in boys than in girls.[4]

Importance and management

Iron and zinc deficiencies are global problems and they often co-exist.[1,9] Some studies suggest that giving zinc with iron may not improve iron status as much as iron given alone,[1,2,4,5,7] while others suggest zinc status may be negatively affected if it is given with iron.[1,3,6] Even so, some studies found that giving combined iron and zinc was beneficial, even if not optimal.[2-4,7] One study suggests that zinc supplementation has a positive effect on growth if low haemoglobin levels and iron status is also corrected.[10] It has been suggested that supplementation programmes that provide iron and zinc together are an efficient way to provide both micronutrients, provided the benefits of individual supplementation are not lost, but more study is needed before such programmes can be established.[9]

1. Lind T, Lönnerdal B, Stenlund H, Ismail D, Seswandhana R, Ekström E-C, Persson L-Å. A community-based randomized controlled trial of iron and zinc supplementation in Indonesian infants: interactions between iron and zinc. *Am J Clin Nutr* (2003) 77, 883–90.
2. Dijkhuizen MA, Wieringa FT, West CE, Martuti S, Muhilal. Effects of iron and zinc supplementation in Indonesian infants on micronutrient status and growth. *J Nutr* (2001) 131, 2860–5.
3. Berger J, Ninh NX, Khan NC, Nhien NV, Lien DK, Trung NQ, Khoi HH. Efficacy of combined iron and zinc supplementation on micronutrient status and growth in Vietnamese infants. *Eur J Clin Nutr* (2006) 60, 443–54.
4. Wieringa FT, Berger J, Dijkhuizen MA, Hidayat A, Ninh NX, Utomo B, Wasantwisut E, Winichagoon P, for the SEAMTIZI (South-East Asia Multi-country Trial on Iron and Zinc supplementation in Infants) Study Group. Combined iron and zinc supplementation in infants improved iron and zinc status, but interactions reduced efficacy in a multicountry trial in southeast Asia. *J Nutr* (2007) 137, 466–71.
5. Olivares M, Pizarro F, Ruz M. New insights about iron bioavailability inhibition by zinc. *Nutrition* (2007) 23, 292–5.
6. Troost FJ, Brummer R-JM, Dainty JR, Hoogewerff JA, Bull VJ, Saris WHM. Iron supplements inhibit zinc but not copper absorption in vivo ileostomy subjects. *Am J Clin Nutr* (2003) 78, 1018–23.
7. Lind T, Persson L-Å, Lönnerdal B. Conflicting evidence of iron and zinc interactions in humans: does iron affect zinc absorption? Reply. *Am J Clin Nutr* (2003) 76, 1226–7.
8. Wieringa FT, Dijkhuizen MA, West CE. Iron and zinc interactions. *Am J Clin Nutr* (2004) 80, 787–8.
9. Fischer Walker C, Kordas K, Stoltzfus RJ, Black RE. Interactive effects of iron and zinc on biochemical and functional outcomes in supplementation trials. *Am J Clin Nutr* (2005) 82, 5–12.
10. Fahmida U, Rumawas JS, Utomo B, Patmonodewo S, Schultink W. Zinc-iron, but not zinc alone supplementation, increased linear growth of stunted infants with low haemoglobin. *Asia Pac J Clin Nutr* (2007) 16, 301–9.

Zinc sulphate + Calcium compounds

Calcium compounds reduce the absorption of zinc.

Clinical evidence, mechanism, importance and management

Elemental calcium, in doses of 600 mg (either as **calcium carbonate** or **calcium citrate**), was given to 9 healthy women with a single 20-mg oral dose of zinc sulphate.[1] The AUC of zinc was reduced by 72% by **calcium carbonate** and by 80% by **calcium citrate**. The reason for this interaction is not understood, nor is the clinical importance of this interaction known, but it would seem prudent to separate the administration of zinc from the administration of any calcium compound. Two to three hours separation is often sufficient to achieve maximal absorption with interactions like this. More study of this interaction is needed to confirm the extent and to determine if separation of the doses is an adequate precaution.

1. Argiratos V, Samman S. The effect of calcium carbonate and calcium citrate on the absorption of zinc in healthy female subjects. *Eur J Clin Nutr* (1994) 48, 198–204.

34

Respiratory drugs

This section includes the diverse drugs that are principally used in the management of asthma and chronic obstructive pulmonary disease (COPD), with the exception of the corticosteroids, which are covered elsewhere.

(a) Antimuscarinic (Anticholinergic) bronchodilators

The parasympathetic nervous system is involved in the regulation of bronchomotor tone and antimuscarinic drugs have bronchodilator properties. Ipratropium bromide and other antimuscarinic bronchodilators used in COPD are listed in 'Table 34.1', p.1419. A wide range of drugs have antimuscarinic adverse effects. Enhanced antimuscarinic effects occur when drugs with these properties are given concurrently, see 'Antimuscarinics + Antimuscarinics', p.754. However, these interactions do not usually occur with drugs such as ipratropium, given by inhalation.

(b) Beta$_2$-agonist bronchodilators

Salbutamol and terbutaline are examples of short-acting beta agonists that selectively stimulate the beta$_2$ receptors in the bronchi causing bronchodilation. They are used in the treatment of asthma and the management of COPD. Long-acting beta$_2$ agonists such as salmeterol are used in patients with asthma who also require anti-inflammatory drugs. 'Table 34.1', p.1419, lists the beta$_2$ agonists available. The beta$_2$ agonists represent a significant improvement on isoprenaline (isoproterenol), which also stimulates beta$_1$ receptors in the heart, and on ephedrine, which also stimulates alpha receptors. The beta$_2$ agonists can cause hypokalaemia, which can be increased by the concurrent use of other potassium-depleting drugs, see 'Beta-agonist bronchodilators + Potassium-depleting drugs', p.1422.

(c) Leukotriene antagonists

Montelukast and zafirlukast block the effects of cysteinyl leukotrienes, which cause effects such as airways oedema, bronchoconstriction and inflammation. The leukotriene antagonists are used in the treatment of asthma, either alone, or with inhaled corticosteroids. They should not be used to relieve an acute asthma attack. Both drugs are metabolised in the liver by the cytochrome P450 isoenzymes such as CYP3A4 and CYP2C9 (montelukast) and CYP2C9 (zafirlukast). Zafirlukast is thought to inhibit CYP2C9 and CYP3A4, and this is thought to be the mechanism for its interaction with warfarin, see 'Coumarins + Leukotriene antagonists', p.443. There is therefore a possibility that interactions could occur with other drugs that undergo metabolism by these isoenzymes but clinical evidence of this varies.

(d) Phosphodiesterase type-4 inhibitors

Phosphodiesterase type-4 inhibition results in the suppression of a number of inflammatory cell functions that are involved in respiratory disease states such as asthma and COPD. Drugs that inhibit this process include roflumilast. Roflumilast is metabolised by CYP3A4 and CYP1A2, and therefore might be subject to interactions with other drugs that are inducers or inhibitors of these enzymes.

(e) Xanthines

The main xanthines used in medicine are theophylline and aminophylline, the latter generally being preferred when greater water solubility is needed (e.g. in the formulation of injections). Xanthines are given in the treatment of asthma because they relax the bronchial smooth muscle. In an attempt to improve upon theophylline, various different derivatives have been made, such as diprophylline and enprofylline. 'Table 34.1', p.1419, lists these xanthines. Theophylline is metabolised by cytochrome P450 isoenzymes in the liver, principally CYP1A2, to demethylated and hydroxylated products. Many drugs interact with theophylline by inhibition or potentiation of its metabolism. In addition, the metabolism of theophylline is affected by gender, smoking, liver and cardiac disease, viral infections and genetic differences in CYP1A2 function. Theophylline has a narrow therapeutic range, and small increases in serum levels can result in toxicity. Moreover, symptoms of serious toxicity such as convulsions and arrhythmias can occur before minor symptoms suggestive of toxicity. Within the context of interactions, aminophylline generally behaves like theophylline, because it is a complex of theophylline with ethylenediamine.

Caffeine is also a xanthine and it is principally used as a central nervous system stimulant, increasing wakefulness, and mental and physical activity. It is most commonly taken in the form of tea, coffee, cola drinks ('*Coke*') and cocoa. 'Table 34.2', p.1419, lists the usual caffeine content of these drinks. Caffeine is also included in hundreds of non-prescription analgesic preparations with aspirin, codeine and/or paracetamol, but whether it enhances the analgesic effect is debatable. Caffeine is also used to assess the activity of CYP1A2 and can usefully demonstrate altered liver function, notably from drugs, as well as disease states.

Caffeine, like theophylline, also undergoes extensive hepatic metabolism, principally by CYP1A2, and interacts with many drugs, but it has a wider therapeutic range. However, other xanthines are likely to interact differently (e.g. diprophylline does not undergo hepatic metabolism), so it should not be assumed that they all share common interactions. Note though, that all xanthines can potentiate hypokalaemia caused by other drugs and that the toxic effects of different xanthines are additive.

Table 34.1 Respiratory drugs

Group	*Drugs*
Antimuscarinics (Anticholinergics)	Aclidinium, Ipratropium bromide, Oxitropium, Tiotropium, Umeclidinium bromide
Beta-2 adrenoreceptor agonists	Short-acting: Bambuterol, Clenbuterol, Fenoterol, Levosalbutamol (Levalbuterol), Pirbuterol, Procaterol, Reproterol, Salbutamol (Albuterol), Terbutaline, Tulobuterol Long-acting: Arformoterol, Formoterol, Olodaterol, Salmeterol, Vilanterol
Leukotriene antagonists and inhibitors	Montelukast, Pemirolast, Pranlukast, Zafirlukast
Lipoxygenase inhibitors	Zileuton
Mast cell stabilisers	Nedocromil sodium, Sodium cromoglicate Ketotifen, Pemirolast
PDE-4 Inhibitors	Roflumilast
Xanthine derivatives	Aminophylline, Choline theophyllinate, Diprophylline, Doxofylline, Theophylline
Other respiratory drugs	Ephedrine, Isoprenaline (Isoproterenol), Orciprenaline

Table 34.2 Caffeine-containing foods

Source	*Caffeine-content*	*Caffeine-content of foods*
Coffee	Coffee beans 1 to 2%[1]	Up to 100 mg/100 mL, decaffeinated up to about 3 mg/100 mL.[1] Instant coffee, 75 mg per cup and 100 mg per mug.[3] Can range from 210 to 340 mg/L,[4] or 21 to 120 mg per serving.[5] Brewed coffee, 100 mg per cup.[5] Ground coffee, 15 to 254 mg per serving.[5] Filter coffee, between 105 and 215 mg/L,[4] or up to 140 mg per mug.[3]
Chocolate		Plain chocolate, up to 50 mg in 50 g.[3] Milk chocolate, up to 25 mg in 50 g.[3] Chocolate bars, between 110 and 710 mg/kg.[4] Chocolate milk drinks, between 8 and 20 mg/L.[4] Chocolate powdered drinks, between 5.5 and 41 mg/L.[4]
Cola drinks		Up to 40 mg per drink;[3] 69 mg/L (range 33 to 213 mg/L).[4] Decaffeinated cola drinks less than 0.2 mg/L.[4]
Energy drinks		Guarana- and caffeine-containing energy drinks, average 269 mg/L (range 122 to 234 mg/L).[4]
Guarana*	2.5 to 7%[2]	Guarana-containing energy drinks, around 180 mg/L.[4]
Maté (Paraguay tea)	0.2 to 2%[1]	
Tea	1 to 5%[3]	Up to 60 mg/100 mL,[1] caffeine content appears to vary with form (bags, loose tea, instant tea etc.); between 102 and 326 mg/L,[4] or 1 to 90 mg per serving.[5]

* Note that guarana contains guaranine (which is known to be identical to caffeine) as well as small quantities of other xanthines.

1. Sweetman SC, editor. Martindale: The complete drug reference. 36th ed. London: Pharmaceutical Press; 2009 p. 2415.
2. Houghton P. Herbal products 7. Guarana. *Pharm J* (1995) 254, 435-6.
3. Food Standards Agency. Eating while you are pregnant. Available at http://www.food.gov.uk/multimedia/pdfs/publication/eatingwhilepregnant1209.pdf (accessed 20/10/15).
4. Ministry for Agriculture, Fisheries and Foods and UK Department of Health. Survey of caffeine and other methylxanthines in energy drinks and other caffeine-containing products (updated). Number 144, March 1998.
5. Food Standards Agency. Survey of caffeine levels in hot beverages, April 2004. Available at http://tna.europarchive.org/20110116113217/http://www.food.gov.uk/news/newsarchive/2004/apr/caffeinelevels (accessed 20/10/15).

Anti-asthma drugs + Areca (Betel nuts)

The chewing of betel nuts may worsen the symptoms of asthma.

Clinical evidence

A study of a possible interaction with betel nuts was prompted by the observation that the severe asthma of two Bangladeshi patients appeared to have been considerably worsened by chewing betel nuts. One out of 4 other patients with asthma who regularly chewed betel nuts developed severe bronchoconstriction (a 30% fall in FEV_1) on two occasions when given betel nuts to chew, and all 4 patients said that prolonged betel nut chewing induced coughing and wheezing. A double-blind study found that the inhalation of **arecoline** (the major constituent of the nut) caused bronchoconstriction in 6 of 7 asthmatics, and one of 6 healthy control subjects.[1] A study in patients with asthma who regularly chewed betel nuts found that 4 patients had a mean increase in their FEV_1 of 10 to 25%, whereas 11 patients had significant falls in their FEV_1 of 11 to 25%. Interestingly, 5 of the patients who did not think chewing betel nut affected their asthma experienced a reduction in their FEV_1.[2]

A survey in 61 patients with asthma found that 22 of the 34 patients who still chewed betel nuts, either for occasional use or regularly, reported that it worsened their asthma.[3]

Mechanism

Betel nut 'quids' consist of areca nut (*Areca catechu*) wrapped in betel vine leaf (*Piper betle*) and smeared with a paste of burnt (slaked) lime. It is chewed for the euphoric effects of the major constituent, arecoline, a cholinergic alkaloid, which appears to be absorbed through the mucous membrane of the mouth. Arecoline has identical properties to pilocarpine and normally has only mild systemic cholinergic properties; however asthmatic subjects seem to be particularly sensitive to the bronchoconstrictor effects of this alkaloid and possibly other substances contained in the nut.

Importance and management

Direct evidence appears to be limited to the above reports, but the interaction seems to be established. It would not normally appear to be a serious interaction, but patients with asthma should be encouraged to avoid betel nuts. This is a drug-disease interaction rather than a drug-drug interaction.

1. Taylor RFH, Al-Jarad N, John LME, Conroy DM, Barnes NC. Betel-nut chewing and asthma. *Lancet* (1992) 339, 1134–6.
2. Sekkadde Kiyingi K, Saweri A. Betel nut chewing causes bronchoconstriction in some asthma patients. *P N G Med J* (1994) 37, 90–9.
3. Kiyingi KS. Betel-nut chewing may aggravate asthma. *P N G Med J* (1991) 34, 117–21.

Anti-asthma drugs + Beta blockers

Non-cardioselective beta blockers oppose the bronchodilator effects of beta-agonist bronchodilators, and higher doses might be required to reverse bronchospasm. Although even cardioselective beta blockers (e.g. atenolol) can sometimes cause acute bronchospasm in patients with asthma they do not generally inhibit the bronchodilator effect of beta-agonist bronchodilators.

Clinical evidence

(a) Cardioselective beta blockers

A review of 29 studies (including 19 single-dose studies) on the use of cardioselective beta blockers in patients with reversible airway disease indicated that in patients with mild to moderate disease, the short-term use of cardioselective beta blockers does not cause significant adverse respiratory effects. Information on the effects in patients with more severe or less reversible disease, or on the frequency or severity of acute exacerbations was not available.[1] Another review indicated that when low doses of cardioselective beta blockers are given to patients with mild, intermittent or persistent asthma, or moderate persistent asthma, and heart failure or myocardial infarction, the benefits of treatment outweigh the risks. However, it was considered that further study is required to establish long-term safety, and also that beta blockers should be avoided in severe persistent asthma.[2] A review of patients with asthma or COPD taking a cardioselective beta blocker (2 810 patients) or a non-selective beta blocker (287) found no significant difference in admissions to hospital or in length of stay in these patients when compared with 5 293 patients with asthma or COPD receiving other cardiovascular medicines.[3]

The cardioselective beta blockers would not be expected to affect the beta receptors in the bronchi, but bronchospasm can sometimes occur following their use by patients with asthma and others with obstructive airways diseases, particularly if high doses are used. Deterioration of asthma was reported in a patient taking oral **betaxolol** with **theophylline** and **pranlukast**, although **betaxolol** is considered to be highly cardioselective and less likely to cause pulmonary adverse effects than other cardioselective beta blockers.[4] Further, a study in 544 patients with asthma and glaucoma found that those treated with topical beta blockers (78.5%) were more likely to attend emergency departments or require hospitalisation for asthma-related problems, than those not treated with beta blockers. Most were treated with non-cardioselective beta blockers (mainly timolol), but 169 were treated with **betaxolol**. The number of hospitalisation days per 100 years of antiglaucoma treatment was increased to about 22 in patients using **betaxolol** or **timolol** eye drops, compared with a mean of 10 days for those treated with non-beta blocker topical antiglaucoma drugs. Emergency department visits were also increased, when compared with those using non-beta blocker preparations.[5]

No adverse pharmacodynamic interaction normally occurs between beta-agonist bronchodilators and cardioselective beta blockers. This has been demonstrated in studies with:

- **Atenolol** with **salbutamol (albuterol)** inhalation.[6,7]
- **Celiprolol** in patients with asthma with **isoprenaline (isoproterenol)**, or **salbutamol**,[6,8,9] or **terbutaline** infusion or inhalation.[10]
- **Metoprolol** in patients with asthma at rest with **isoprenaline** infusion.[11,12]

In contrast, another study found that the increase in forced expiratory volume (FEV) with a **terbutaline** inhalation and infusion was reduced by about 300 mL by **atenolol** and **metoprolol**. The authors considered that this would be clinically relevant in severe asthma.[13] Another study in 12 patients with mild asthma found that single doses of **celiprolol** 200 mg or **nebivolol** 5 mg reduced the FEV_1 by 272 mL and 193 mL, respectively, when compared with placebo. Increasing inhalation of **salbutamol** to a total dose of 800 micrograms reversed these reductions but did not restore the FEV_1 back to its initial value. None of these changes was considered to be clinically significant by the authors.[14]

Fifteen patients with mild to moderate COPD and airways hyperresponsiveness were given **celiprolol** 200 mg daily, **metoprolol** 100 mg daily or **propranolol** 80 mg daily for 4 days. **Propranolol** significantly reduced the FEV_1 and increased airways hyperresponsiveness, when compared with placebo, whereas **metoprolol** only increased airways hyperresponsiveness. **Celiprolol** had no significant effects on pulmonary function. The bronchodilating effects of a single 12-microgram dose of **formoterol** were significantly reduced by **propranolol**, but not by **metoprolol** or **celiprolol**.[9]

(b) Non-selective beta blockers

Non-selective beta blockers (e.g. **propranolol**) are contraindicated in patients with asthma because they can cause bronchospasm, reduce lung ventilation and may possibly precipitate a severe asthmatic attack in some subjects. An example of the danger is illustrated by a patient with asthma who developed fatal status asthmaticus after taking just one dose of **propranolol**.[15] Another case report describes a patient with bronchial asthma receiving **salbutamol** who collapsed and died after taking three 20-mg **propranolol** tablets, which had been supplied in error instead of 20-mg prednisone tablets.[16] The manufacturer of **propranolol** notes that from 1965 to 1996, the CSM in the UK had received 51 reports of bronchospasm due to **propranolol**, 13 of them fatal, and 5 of them in patients who had a history of asthma, bronchospasm or wheeze.[17] The non-cardioselective beta blockers **oxprenolol**[7] and **propranolol**[6,7,10-12] oppose the effects of bronchodilators such as **isoprenaline (isoproterenol)**,[6,11,12] **salbutamol (albuterol)**,[6,7] and **terbutaline**.[10] Eye drops containing the non-selective beta blockers **timolol**[5,18,19] and **metipranolol**[20] have been reported to precipitate acute bronchospasm. In patients with heart failure taking **carvedilol**, 3 of 12 with concurrent asthma had wheezing requiring **carvedilol** withdrawal. In contrast, only one of 31 patients with COPD had wheezing.[21]

Mechanism

Non-selective beta blockers such as propranolol block $beta_2$ receptors in the bronchi, so that the normal bronchodilation, which is under the control of the sympathetic nervous system, is reduced or abolished. As a result the bronchoconstriction of asthma can be made worse. Cardioselective beta blockers on the other hand, preferentially block $beta_1$ receptors in the heart, with less effect on the $beta_2$ receptors, so that $beta_2$ stimulating bronchodilators, such as isoprenaline (isoproterenol), salbutamol (albuterol) and terbutaline, continue to have bronchodilator effects.

Importance and management

Non-cardioselective beta blockers (see 'Table 22.1', p.999) might oppose the bronchodilator effects of beta-agonist bronchodilators, and higher doses might be required to reverse bronchospasm. However, note that their use should be avoided in patients with asthma and those with COPD, whether given systemically or as eye drops, because serious and life-threatening bronchospasm can occur.

Cardioselective beta blockers do not generally inhibit the bronchodilator effects of beta-agonist bronchodilators. They are also generally safer in those with asthma or COPD, but they are not entirely free from risk, particularly when given in high dose, and their usage in such patients has been the subject of much debate. In 1996, the position of the CSM in the UK[22] was that cardioselective beta blockers should not be given to patients with a history of asthma and/or bronchospasm, but subsequent reviews[1,23] recommended that cardioselective beta blockers should not be withheld from patients with mild to moderate reversible airway disease, although this suggestion has been questioned,[24] particularly as there are no studies to suggest the safety of cardioselective beta blockers in patients with exacerbations of asthma,[25] and even a highly cardioselective drug such as betaxolol can cause bronchospasm.[4] More recently the 2005 Cochrane review concluded that cardioselective beta blockers did not produce any significant adverse respiratory effects, and it recommended that cardioselective beta blockers should not be withheld from patients with COPD.[26] Further reviews and guidelines have reached the same conclusions.[27-29] Cardioselective beta blockers can therefore be used in patients with mild to moderate asthma or COPD, but it would seem prudent to initiate them at a low dose and monitor the outcome closely. They should not be used in active asthma or reactive airway disease.[29]

1. Salpeter S, Ormiston T, Salpeter EE. Cardioselective β-blockers in patients with reversible airway disease: a meta-analysis. *Ann Intern Med* (2002) 137, 715–25.
2. Self T, Soberman JE, Bubla JM, Chafin CC. Cardioselective beta-blockers in patients with asthma and concomitant heart failure or history of myocardial infarction: when do benefits outweigh risks? *J Asthma* (2003) 40, 839–45.

3. Barnett MJ, Milavetz G, Kaboli PJ. β-blocker therapy in veterans with asthma or chronic obstructive pulmonary disease. *Pharmacotherapy* (2005) 25, 1550–9.
4. Miki A, Tanaka Y, Ohtani H, Sawada Y. Betaxolol-induced deterioration of asthma and a pharmacodynamic analysis based on β-receptor occupancy. *Int J Clin Pharmacol Ther* (2003) 41, 358–64.
5. Kaiserman I, Fendyur A, Vinker S. Topical beta blockers in asthmatic patients-is it safe? *Curr Eye Res* (2009) 34, 517–22.
6. Doshan HD, Rosenthal RR, Brown R, Slutsky A, Applin WJ, Caruso FS. Celiprolol, atenolol and propranolol: a comparison of pulmonary effects in asthmatic patients. *J Cardiovasc Pharmacol* (1986) 8 (Suppl 4), S105–S108.
7. Fogari R, Zoppi A, Tettamanti F, Poletti L, Rizzardi G, Fiocchi G. Comparative effects of celiprolol, propranolol, oxprenolol, and atenolol on respiratory function in hypertensive patients with chronic obstructive lung disease. *Cardiovasc Drugs Ther* (1990) 4, 1145–50.
8. Pujet JC, Dubreuil C, Fleury B, Provendier O, Abella ML. Effects of celiprolol, a cardioselective beta-blocker, on respiratory function in asthmatic patients. *Eur Respir J* (1992) 5, 196–200.
9. Van der Woude HJ, Zaagsma J, Postma DS, Winter TH, Van Hulst M, Aalbers R. Detrimental effects of β-blockers in COPD: A concern for nonselective β-blockers. *Chest* (2005) 127, 818–24.
10. Matthys H, Doshan HD, Rühle K-H, Applin WJ, Braig H, Pohl M. Bronchosparing properties of celiprolol, a new β_1, α_2 blocker, in propranolol-sensitive asthmatic patients. *J Cardiovasc Pharmacol* (1986) 8 (Suppl 4), S40–S42.
11. Thiringer G, Svedmyr N. Interaction of orally administered metoprolol, practolol and propranolol with isoprenaline in asthmatics. *Eur J Clin Pharmacol* (1976) 10, 163–70.
12. Johnsson G, Svedmyr N, Thiringer G. Effects of intravenous propranolol and metoprolol and their interaction with isoprenaline on pulmonary function, heart rate and blood pressure in asthmatics. *Eur J Clin Pharmacol* (1975) 8, 175–80.
13. Löfdahl C-G, Svedmyr N. Cardioselectivity of atenolol and metoprolol. A study in asthmatic patients. *Eur J Respir Dis* (1981) 62, 396–404.
14. Cazzola M, Noschese P, D'Amato M, D'Amato G. Comparison of the effects of single oral doses of nebivolol and celiprolol on airways in patients with mild asthma. *Chest* (2000) 118, 1322–6.
15. Anon. Beta-blocker caused death of asthmatic. *Pharm J* (1991) 247, 185.
16. Spitz DJ. An unusual death in an asthmatic patient. *Am J Forensic Med Pathol* (2003) 24, 271–2.
17. Fallowfield JM, Marlow HF. Propranolol is contraindicated in asthma. *BMJ* (1996) 313, 1486.
18. Charan NB, Lakshminarayan S. Pulmonary effects of topical timolol. *Arch Intern Med* (1980) 140, 843–4.
19. Jones FL, Ekberg NL. Exacerbation of obstructive airway disease by timolol. *JAMA* (1980) 244, 2730.
20. Vinti H, Chichmanian RM, Fournier JP, Pesce A, Taillan B, Fuzibet JG, Cassuto JP, Dujardin P. Accidents systémiques des bêta-bloquants en collyres. A propos de six observations. *Rev Med Interne* (1989) 10, 41–4.
21. Kotlyar E, Keogh AM, Macdonald PS, Arnold RH, McCaffrey DJ, Glanville AR. Tolerability of carvedilol in patients with heart failure and concomitant chronic obstructive pulmonary disease or asthma. *J Heart Lung Transplant* (2002), 21, 1290–5.
22. Committee on Safety of Medicines/Medicines Control Agency. Reminder: Beta-blockers contraindicated in asthma. *Current Problems* (1996) 22, 2.
23. Salpeter SR, Ormiston TM. Use of β-blockers in patients with reactive airway disease. *Ann Intern Med* (2003) 139, 304.
24. Shulan DJ, Katlan M, Lavsky-Shulan M. Use of β-blockers in patients with reactive airway disease. *Ann Intern Med* (2003) 139, 304.
25. Epstein PE. Fresh air and β-blockade. *Ann Intern Med* (2002) 137, 766–7.
26. Salpeter S, Ormiston T, Salpeter E. Cardioselective beta-blockers for chronic obstructive pulmonary disease (review). Available in: The Cochrane Database of Systematic Reviews; Issue 4. Chichester: John Wiley; 2005 (accessed 22/08/07).
27. Le Jemtel TH, Padeletti M, Jelic S. Diagnostic and therapeutic challenges in patients with coexistent chronic obstructive pulmonary disease and chronic heart failure. *J Am Coll Cardiol* (2007) 49, 171–80.
28. Antman EM, Anbe DT, Armstrong PW, Bates ER, Green LA, Hand M, Hochman JS, Krumholz HM, Kushner FG, Lamas GA, Mullany CJ, Ornato JP, Pearle DL, Sloan MA, Smith SC, Alpert JS, Anderson JL, Faxon DP, Fuster V, Gibbons RJ, Gregoratos G, Halperin JL, Hiratzka LF, Hunt SA, Jacobs AK. ACC/AHA guidelines for the management of patients with ST-elevation myocardial infarction. A report of the American College of Cardiology/American Heart Association Task Force on Practice Guidelines (Writing committee to revise the 1999 guidelines for the management of patients with acute myocardial infarction). *J Am Coll Cardiol* (2004) 44, E1–E212. Available at: http://circ.ahajournals.org/content/110/5/588.full.pdf+html (accessed 22/10/15).
29. Antman EM, Hand M, Armstrong PW, Bates ER, Green LA, Halasyamani LK, Hochman JS, Krumholz HM, Lamas GA, Mullany CJ, Pearle DL, Sloan MA, Smith SC, Anbe DT, Kushner FG, Ornato JP, Pearle DL, Sloan MA, Jacobs AK, Adams CD, Anderson JL, Buller CE, Creager MA, Ettinger SM, Halperin JL, Hunt SA, Lytle BW, Nishimura R, Page RL, Riegel B, Tarkington LG, Yancy CW. 2007 focused update of the ACC/AHA 2004 guidelines for the management of patients with ST-elevation myocardial infarction: a report of the American College of Cardiology/American Heart Association Task Force on Practice Guidelines. *J Am Coll Cardiol* (2008) 51, 210–47.

Beta-agonist bronchodilators + Antimuscarinics

Acute angle-closure glaucoma and increased intra-ocular pressure have developed in several patients given nebulised ipratropium and salbutamol (albuterol). Increased intra-ocular pressure has also been reported in a patient using an ipratropium metered-dose inhaler with nebulised salbutamol.

The concurrent use of vilanterol and umeclidinium does not appear to alter the pharmacokinetics of either drug to a clinically relevant extent. The concurrent use of olodaterol and tiotropium does not appear to alter the exposure to either drug.

Clinical evidence

(a) Olodaterol

The US manufacturer briefly reports that concurrent use of olodaterol and **tiotropium** for 21 days had no effect on the exposure of either drug.[1]

(b) Salbutamol (albuterol)

Five patients with an acute exacerbation of COPD, given nebulised **ipratropium** and salbutamol, developed acute angle-closure glaucoma, four of them within one to 36 hours of starting treatment. Two of the patients had a history of angle-closure glaucoma.[2] Seven other similar cases of acute angle-closure glaucoma due to the concurrent use of salbutamol and **ipratropium** are reported elsewhere.[3-7] An increase in intra-ocular pressure has also been reported in other patients given both drugs by nebuliser.[8] One case of acute angle-closure glaucoma has been reported in a patient given inhaled **ipratropium**, via a metered-dose inhaler, and nebulised salbutamol.[9]

(c) Vilanterol

In a crossover study, 14 healthy volunteers were given a single 500-microgram dose of inhaled **umeclidinium** and a single 50-microgram dose of inhaled vilanterol. When compared with giving each drug alone, the maximum plasma concentration of umeclidinium was increased by 30%, but its AUC was unaffected. The AUC of vilanterol was increased by 39%, but its maximum plasma concentration was unaffected. However, note that there was large inter-subject variability.[10]

Mechanism

The reaction seen on the concurrent use of salbutamol and ipratropium appears to occur because the antimuscarinic action of ipratropium causes semi-dilatation of the pupil, partially blocking the flow of aqueous humour from the posterior to the anterior chamber, thereby causing anterior bowing of the iris and obstructing the drainage angle. Salbutamol increases the production of aqueous humour, therefore exacerbating the situation. An additional factor that might contribute is the route of administration: higher concentrations of both drugs are achieved by using a nebuliser, and some drug could escape round the edge of the mask and have a direct action on the eye.[2]

Importance and management

An interaction between ipratropium and **salbutamol** is established but uncommon. It appears to occur mainly in patients receiving salbutamol and ipratropium by nebuliser and in those already predisposed to angle-closure glaucoma. The authors of the first report[2] advise care in the placing of the nebuliser mask to avoid the escape of droplets. The use of goggles[8,11] and continuing the application of any glaucoma treatment is also effective.[8] It has been suggested that, if possible, the simultaneous administration of nebulised salbutamol and ipratropium should be avoided in patients predisposed to angle-closure glaucoma.[2] Although there seems to be no evidence regarding an interaction between other beta-agonist bronchodilators with ipratropium, given the suspected mechanism of the interaction, similar precautions to those given for salbutamol would seem warranted.

The changes in the exposure to **vilanterol** and umeclidinium seen would not be expected to be clinically relevant. No pharmacokinetic interaction appears to occur on the concurrent use of **olodaterol** and tiotropium. Therefore no dose adjustments of either of these beta-agonist bronchodilators or either of these antimuscarinics appear necessary on concurrent use.

1. Striverdi Respimat (Olodaterol hydrochloride). Boehringer Ingelheim Pharmaceuticals Inc. US Prescribing information, July 2014.
2. Shah P, Dhurjon L, Metcalfe T, Gibson JM. Acute angle closure glaucoma associated with nebulised ipratropium bromide and salbutamol. *BMJ* (1992) 304, 40–1.
3. Packe GE, Cayton RM, Mashoudi N. Nebulised ipratropium bromide and salbutamol causing closed-angle glaucoma. *Lancet* (1984) ii, 691.
4. Reuser T, Flanagan DW, Borland C, Bannerjee DK. Acute angle closure glaucoma occurring after nebulized bronchodilator treatment with ipratropium bromide and salbutamol. *J R Soc Med* (1992) 85, 499–500.
5. Fernández-Barrientos Y, Jiménez-Santos M, Martínez-de-la-Casa JM, Méndez-Hernández C, García Feijoó J. Bloqueo angular agudo tras broncodilatadores nebulizados. *Arch Soc Esp Oftalmol* (2006) 81, 657–60.
6. De Saint Jean M, Bourcier T, Borderie V, Moldovan M, Touzeau O, Laroche L. Glaucome aigu par fermeture de l'angle après un traitement par aérosols de bromure d'ipratropium et de salbutamol. *J Fr Ophtalmol* (2000) 23, 603–5.
7. Mulpeter KM, Walsh JB, O'Connor M, O'Connell F, Burke C. Ocular hazards of nebulized bronchodilators. *Postgrad Med J* (1992) 68, 132–3.
8. Kalra L, Bone M. The effect of nebulized bronchodilator therapy on intraocular pressures in patients with glaucoma. *Chest* (1988) 93, 739–41.
9. Hall SK. Acute angle-closure glaucoma as a complication of combined β-agonist and ipratropium bromide therapy in the emergency department. *Ann Emerg Med* (1994) 23, 884–7.
10. Kelleher DL, Mehta RS, Jean-Francois BM, Preece AF, Blowers J, Crater GD, Thomas P. Safety, tolerability, pharmacodynamics and pharmacokinetics of umeclidinium and vilanterol alone and in combination: a randomized crossover trial. *PLoS One* (2012) 7, e50716.
11. Humphreys DM. Acute angle closure glaucoma associated with nebulised ipratropium bromide and salbutamol. *BMJ* (1992) 304, 320.

Beta-agonist bronchodilators + Drugs that inhibit CYP3A4 and/or P-glycoprotein

Ketoconazole very markedly increases the exposure to inhaled salmeterol, and appears to slightly increase the exposure to inhaled olodaterol and vilanterol. Other potent CYP3A4 inhibitors are expected to interact similarly. Erythromycin, fluconazole, or verapamil do not appear to affect the exposure to salmeterol, olodaterol, or vilanterol, respectively. Other moderate CYP3A4 inhibitors are expected to interact similarly. Inhibitors of P-glycoprotein are not expected to affect the exposure to vilanterol.

Clinical evidence

(a) Olodaterol

The US manufacturer briefly reports that concurrent use of oral **ketoconazole** 400 mg daily and olodaterol by inhalation (dose not stated) for 14 days increased the maximum plasma concentration and initial AUC of olodaterol by 66% and 68%, respectively.[1] In another study oral **fluconazole** 400 mg daily for 14 days had no effect on the exposure to inhaled olodaterol.[1]

(b) Salmeterol

The US manufacturer of salmeterol reports a study in which 20 healthy subjects were given oral **ketoconazole** 400 mg daily and salmeterol 50 micrograms by inhalation twice daily for 7 days. Concurrent use increased the maximum plasma concentration and AUC of salmeterol by 40% and 16-fold, respectively. Two subjects were withdrawn from the study after they developed prolonged QT intervals and one subject was withdrawn after experiencing palpitations. Potassium concentrations were not affected by concurrent use.[2]

In another study in 13 healthy subjects, **erythromycin** 500 mg three times daily was given with salmeterol 50 micrograms by inhalation twice daily for 6 days. Concurrent use resulted in a small increase in salmeterol exposure, which was not statistically significant.[2,3] Potassium concentrations were not affected by concurrent use but heart rate was increased by a modest 3.6 bpm.[2]

(c) Vilanterol

In a crossover study in 18 healthy subjects, given oral **ketoconazole** 400 mg daily for 11 days with inhaled fluticasone furoate/vilanterol trifenatate 200/25 micrograms once daily on days 5 to 11, the AUC of vilanterol increased by 65%. Potassium concentrations and heart rate were not affected by concurrent use.[4] In the same study, 18 healthy subjects were also given ketoconazole 400 mg daily for 6 days with a single-dose of inhaled vilanterol 25 micrograms on day 5. Both the AUC and maximum plasma concentration of vilanterol were increased by about 90%.[4]

In a randomised study in 15 healthy subjects, oral **verapamil** 240 mg daily for 5 days had no effect on the pharmacokinetics of inhaled vilanterol 25 micrograms daily (given in a combination preparation with inhaled umeclidinium 500 micrograms daily).[5]

Mechanism

Ketoconazole is a potent inhibitor of CYP3A4, by which olodaterol, salmeterol, and vilanterol are metabolised, and concurrent use can therefore increase their exposure. Moderate inhibitors of CYP3A4 such as erythromycin, fluconazole, and verapamil are also expected to increase the exposure to these beta-agonist bronchodilators, but to a lesser extent. Ketoconazole and verapamil also inhibit P-glycoprotein by which olodaterol and vilanterol are transported, and they might be expected to also increase the exposure to olodaterol and vilanterol by this mechanism.

Importance and management

Evidence for an interaction between salmeterol and **ketoconazole** appears to be limited to this one study from the manufacturer, but it is consistent with the known metabolism of these drugs and therefore an interaction seems to be established. Although salmeterol is given by inhalation, 90% of the drug is said to be swallowed, therefore this interaction would be expected to result in systemic effects. Salmeterol is not usually associated with QT prolongation at the recommended doses; and where QT prolongation has been seen, it is usually at doses above 300 micrograms.[6] However, a 16-fold increase in exposure with ketoconazole means that the lowest doses of salmeterol are likely to exceed this threshold, and the clinical importance of this is supported by the finding of QT prolongation in two patients in the study. The UK and US manufacturers of salmeterol therefore state that the concurrent use of ketoconazole should be avoided,[2,3] and this seems prudent. It would also seem prudent to avoid other potent CYP3A4 inhibitors (for a list see 'Table 1.9', p.11).

Ketoconazole also appears to increase the exposure to vilanterol and olodaterol, but the increases seen are slight and therefore unlikely to be clinically relevant. No dose adjustments would be expected to be necessary on concurrent use, however, the US manufacturers of vilanterol advise caution with the concurrent use of potent CYP3A4 inhibitors. Note that they name **conivaptan** and **nefazodone** as potent CYP3A4 inhibitors,[7,8] but they are generally considered to be moderate. For a list of potent CYP3A4 inhibitors see 'Table 1.9', p.11.

Information about an interaction with moderate CYP3A4 inhibitors appears to be limited to the studies when **erythromycin**, **fluconazole**, or **verapamil** were given with salmeterol, olodaterol, or vilanterol, respectively. However the lack of effect on the exposure to these beta-agonist bronchodilators suggests that a clinically relevant interaction would not be expected to occur with moderate CYP3A4 inhibitors. For a list of moderate CYP3A4 inhibitors, see 'Table 1.9', p.11.

Verapamil is also a P-glycoprotein inhibitor, and its lack of effect on the exposure to vilanterol suggests that other P-glycoprotein inhibitors might not have a clinically relevant effect on vilanterol exposure. For a list of P-glycoprotein inhibitors, see 'Table 1.12', p.14.

1. Striverdi Respimat (Olodaterol hydrochloride). Boehringer Ingelheim Pharmaceuticals Inc. US Prescribing information, July 2014.
2. Serevent Diskus (Salmeterol xinafoate). GlaxoSmithKline. US Prescribing information, February 2015.
3. Serevent Evohaler (Salmeterol xinafoate). GlaxoSmithKline UK. UK Summary of product characteristics, July 2014.
4. Kempsford R, Allen A, Bal J, Rubin D, Tombs L. The effect of ketoconazole on the pharmacokinetics and pharmacodynamics of inhaled fluticasone furoate and vilanterol trifenatate in healthy subjects. *Br J Clin Pharmacol* (2013) 75, 1478–87.
5. Mehta R, Kelleher D, Preece A, Hughes S, Crater G. Effect of verapamil on systemic exposure and safety of umeclidinium and vilanterol: a randomized and open-label study. *Int J Chron Obstruct Pulmon Dis* (2013) 8, 159–67.
6. Cazzola M, Testi R, Matera MG. Clinical pharmacokinetics of salmeterol. *Clin Pharmacokinet* (2002) 41, 19–30.
7. Breo Ellipta (Fluticasone furoate and Vilanterol). GlaxoSmithKline. US Prescribing information, April 2015.
8. Anoro Ellipta (Umeclidinium and Vilanterol). GlaxoSmithKline. US Prescribing information, May 2014.

Beta-agonist bronchodilators + Potassium-depleting drugs

Beta agonists (e.g. fenoterol, salbutamol (albuterol), terbutaline) can cause hypokalaemia. This can be increased by other potassium-depleting drugs such as amphotericin B, the corticosteroids, diuretics (e.g. bendroflumethiazide, furosemide) and theophylline. Hypokalaemia may increase the risk of serious cardiac arrhythmias.

Clinical evidence

(a) Corticosteroids

1. Hypokalaemia. The hypokalaemic effects of beta$_2$ agonists may be increased by corticosteroids. The serum potassium levels of 24 healthy subjects were reduced when they were given either **salbutamol (albuterol)** 5 mg or **fenoterol** 5 mg by nebuliser over 30 minutes. The reduction in potassium levels was greater after they also took **prednisone** 30 mg daily for a week. The greatest reduction (from 3.75 mmol/L to 2.78 mmol/L) was found 90 minutes after **fenoterol** and **prednisone** were taken. The ECG effects observed included ectopic beats and transient T wave inversion, but no significant ECG disturbances were noted.[1]

2. Pharmacokinetics. A study in 28 healthy subjects found that the pharmacokinetics of a single 1.28-mg dose of **budesonide** and a single 36-microgram dose of **formoterol** were unaltered when each drug was given together (by separate inhalers). In a similar study by the same authors, it was found that when these drugs were given together in the same inhaler (*Symbicort*, **budesonide** 1.28 mg and **formoterol** 36 micrograms per dose), the AUC of **formoterol** was 20% lower, when compared with administration by separate inhalers.[2] However, this difference is unlikely to be clinically relevant.

When 28 healthy subjects received **salmeterol** 100 micrograms, **fluticasone** 500 micrograms, or the two drugs together twice daily for 11 days, no pharmacokinetic interaction was noted.[3]

(b) Diuretics

1. Bendroflumethiazide. In a study, 10 healthy subjects were given bendroflumethiazide 5 mg daily. After 7 days the serum potassium levels were reduced by 0.71 mmol/L. When 100 micrograms to 2 mg of inhaled **salbutamol (albuterol)** was also given, the potassium levels were reduced by 1.06 mmol/L (to 2.72 mmol/L). ECG changes consistent with hypokalaemia and hypomagnesaemia were seen.[4] In another study the same authors found that the addition of bendroflumethiazide 5 mg daily to inhaled **salbutamol** 2 mg further reduced serum potassium levels by 0.4 mmol/L (to 2.92 mmol/L). This reduction was abolished by the addition of triamterene 200 mg (serum potassium 3.43 mmol/L) or spironolactone 100 mg (serum potassium 3.53 mmol/L), whereas triamterene 50 mg only attenuated the effect of bendroflumethiazide (serum potassium 3.1 mmol/L). ECG effects in response to giving **salbutamol** with bendroflumethiazide were also reduced by the addition of triamterene or spironolactone.[5] In another similar study by the same authors, the addition of 24 mmol of potassium daily did not alter the hypokalaemia or ECG changes caused by the concurrent use of bendroflumethiazide and **salbutamol**. The use of triamterene attenuated the ECG changes in some subjects.[6]

2. Furosemide. The serum potassium levels of 15 healthy subjects were measured after they were given inhaled **terbutaline** 5 mg with either placebo, furosemide 40 mg daily, or furosemide 40 mg with triamterene 50 mg daily for 4 days. With **terbutaline** alone the potassium levels were reduced by 0.53 mmol/L; when furosemide was also given they were reduced by 0.75 mmol/L; and after furosemide and triamterene were also given they were reduced by 0.59 mmol/L. These lower potassium levels were reflected in some ECG (T wave) changes.[7]

(c) Theophylline

The concurrent use of **salbutamol (albuterol)** or **terbutaline** and theophylline can cause an additional reduction in serum potassium levels: other beta$_2$ agonists are expected to interact similarly, see 'Theophylline + Beta-agonist bronchodilators', p.1437.

Mechanism

The use of two or more drugs with hypokalaemic adverse effects results in additive potassium-depleting effects.

Importance and management

An interaction between beta-agonist bronchodilators and drugs that can cause hypokalaemia is established. The CSM in the UK[8] advises that, as potentially serious hypokalaemia may result from the use of a beta$_2$ agonist, particular caution is required in severe asthma, as this effect may be potentiated by theophylline and its derivatives, corticosteroids, diuretics, and by hypoxia. Potassium levels should therefore be closely monitored in patients with severe asthma. Drugs such as **amphotericin B**, which commonly cause severe hypokalaemia, are likely to present a similar risk. Hypokalaemia may result in cardiac arrhythmias in patients with ischaemic heart disease and may also affect the response of patients to drugs such as the digitalis glycosides and antiarrhythmics.

Hypokalaemia on the concurrent use of a beta$_2$ agonist and a thiazide or loop diuretic (see 'Table 26.1', p.1117, for a list) may be reduced or even abolished by the addition of a potassium-sparing diuretic, such as spironolactone or triamterene.

1. Taylor DR, Wilkins GT, Herbison GP, Flannery EM. Interaction between corticosteroid and β-agonist drugs. Biochemical and cardiovascular effects in normal subjects. *Chest* (1992) 102, 519–24.
2. Eklund A, Tronde A, Johannes-Hellberg I, Gillen M, Borgström L. Pharmacokinetics of budesonide and formoterol administered via a series of single-drug and combination inhalers: four open-label, randomized, crossover studies in healthy adults. *Biopharm Drug Dispos* (2008) 29, 382–95.
3. Kirby S, Falcoz C, Daniel MJ, Milleri S, Squassante L, Ziviani L, Ventresca GP. Salmeterol and fluticasone propionate given as a combination. *Eur J Clin Pharmacol* (2001) 56, 781–91.
4. Lipworth BJ, McDevitt DG, Struthers AD. Prior treatment with diuretic augments the hypokalemic and electrocardiographic effects of inhaled albuterol. *Am J Med* (1989) 86, 653–7.

5. Lipworth BJ, McDevitt DG, Struthers AD. Hypokalemic and ECG sequelae of combined beta-agonist/diuretic therapy. Protection by conventional doses of spironolactone but not triamterene. *Chest* (1990) 98, 811–15.
6. Lipworth BJ, McDevitt DG, Struthers AD. Electrocardiographic changes induced by inhaled salbutamol after treatment with bendrofluazide: effects of replacement therapy with potassium, magnesium and triamterene. *Clin Sci (Lond)* (1990) 78, 255–9.
7. Newnham DM, McDevitt DG, Lipworth BJ. The effects of frusemide and triamterene on the hypokalaemic and electrocardiographic responses to inhaled terbutaline. *Br J Clin Pharmacol* (1991) 32, 630–2.
8. Committee on Safety of Medicines. β_2 agonists, xanthines and hypokalaemia. *Current Problems* (1990) 28.

Caffeine + Allopurinol

Allopurinol may invalidate the results of studies using caffeine as a probe drug to determine acetylator status or CYP1A2 activity.

Clinical evidence, mechanism, importance and management

A study in 2 healthy subjects found that allopurinol 300 or 600 mg daily inhibited the metabolism of the caffeine metabolite, 1-methylxanthine, to 1-methyluric acid.[1] In another study, in 6 healthy subjects given paraxanthine (1,7-dimethylxanthine), the major metabolite of caffeine, allopurinol increased the excretion of 1-methylxanthine and decreased the excretion of 1-methyluric acid.[2] In a study in 21 healthy subjects given a single 200-mg dose of caffeine, allopurinol 300 mg daily for 8 days altered the levels of urinary caffeine metabolites. In particular, the metabolic ratio used to determine whether people are fast or slow acetylators was substantially changed. In addition, the caffeine metabolite ratio used to express the activity of CYP1A2 was not stable when allopurinol was used.[3] Thus, allopurinol may invalidate the results of acetylator phenotyping and testing CYP1A2 activity with the urinary caffeine test. This interaction is of relevance to research rather than clinical practice.

1. Grant DM, Tang BK, Campbell ME, Kalow W. Effect of allopurinol on caffeine disposition in man. *Br J Clin Pharmacol* (1986) 21, 454–8.
2. Lelo A, Kjellen G, Birkett DJ, Miners JO. Paraxanthine metabolism in humans: determination of metabolic partial clearances and effects of allopurinol and cimetidine. *J Pharmacol Exp Ther* (1989) 248, 315–9.
3. Fuchs P, Haefeli WE, Ledermann HR, Wenk M. Xanthine oxidase inhibition by allopurinol affects the reliability of urinary caffeine metabolic ratios as markers for *N*-acetyltransferase 2 and CYP1A2 activities. *Eur J Clin Pharmacol* (1999) 54, 869–76.

Caffeine + Antiepileptics

Phenytoin moderately increases the clearance of caffeine, and possibly invalidates the caffeine breath test. Carbamazepine might interact similarly but evidence is conflicting. The concurrent use of valproate and caffeine does not appear to affect the pharmacokinetics of either drug.

Clinical evidence

In a study, the clearance of caffeine was 2.4-fold higher and its half-life was reduced by about 50% in patients with epilepsy taking **phenytoin**, when compared with healthy subjects not taking any medication. In the same study, there were no significant differences in caffeine pharmacokinetics between healthy subjects and patients taking **carbamazepine** or **valproic acid**.[1] Conversely, **carbamazepine** was considered to have induced the metabolism of caffeine in 5 children with epilepsy, as assessed by the caffeine breath test.[2]

In a study in 5 healthy subjects, caffeine was reported to reduce the AUC and maximum plasma level of **carbamazepine** by 32% and 41%, respectively. In this study, caffeine had no effect on the pharmacokinetics of **sodium valproate**.[3]

Mechanism

Phenytoin acts as an enzyme inducer, thereby increasing the metabolism of caffeine by CYP1A2 and, lowering its levels. Carbamazepine possibly has the same effect.

It has been suggested that the reduction in carbamazepine levels was because the methylxanthines, such as caffeine, are metabolised by the same isoenzymes as carbamazepine;[3] however, note that interactions as a result of this mechanism are not generally clinically relevant.

Importance and management

Evidence for an interaction between caffeine and the enzyme-inducing antiepileptics is limited, but what is known suggests that phenytoin, and possibly carbamazepine, may increase the metabolism of caffeine. However, the clinical relevance of this effect is unclear: it seems likely that it is mostly of experimental interest as phenytoin (and therefore probably also carbamazepine) might invalidate the caffeine breath test.

Note that caffeine is used as a probe substrate to assess the activity of drugs on CYP1A2. The study with phenytoin therefore suggests that this drug is a moderate inducer of CYP1A2. Carbamazepine might have similar effects but this is not established.

The interaction whereby caffeine reduces carbamazepine levels is also not established and requires further study.

1. Wietholtz H, Zysset T, Kreiten K, Kohl D, Büchsel R, Matern S. Effect of phenytoin, carbamazepine, and valproic acid on caffeine metabolism. *Eur J Clin Pharmacol* (1989) 36, 401–6.
2. Parker AC, Pritchard P, Preston T, Choonara I. Induction of CYP1A2 activity by carbamazepine in children using the caffeine breath test. *Br J Clin Pharmacol* (1998) 45, 176–8.
3. Vaz J, Kulkarni C, Joy D, Joseph T. Influence of caffeine on pharmacokinetic profile of sodium valproate and carbamazepine in normal healthy volunteers. *Indian J Exp Biol* (1998) 36, 112–14.

Caffeine + Antifungals

Fluconazole and terbinafine cause a slight reduction in the clearance of caffeine. Ketoconazole and posaconazole do not appear to have a clinically relevant effect on the pharmacokinetics of caffeine.

Clinical evidence, mechanism, importance and management

A study in 6 young subjects (average age 24 years) given **fluconazole** 400 mg daily for 10 days and 5 elderly subjects (average age 69 years) given **fluconazole** 200 mg daily for 10 days found that **fluconazole** reduced the plasma clearance of caffeine by an average of 25% (32% in the young and 17% in the elderly).[1]

In a single-dose study in 8 healthy subjects, **terbinafine** 500 mg and **ketoconazole** 400 mg decreased the clearance of caffeine by 21% and 10%, respectively, and increased its half-life by 31% and 16%, respectively.[2]

In a study in 12 healthy subjects, **posaconazole** 200 mg daily for 10 days did not affect the pharmacokinetics of a single 200-mg dose of caffeine.[3]

It seems unlikely that the slight reduction in caffeine clearance seen with fluconazole, ketoconazole and terbinafine, will have a clinically important effect. Therefore caffeine may be used with fluconazole, ketoconazole, posaconazole or terbinafine without any particular precautions.

1. Nix DE, Zelenitsky SA, Symonds WT, Spivey JM, Norman A. The effect of fluconazole on the pharmacokinetics of caffeine in young and elderly subjects. *Clin Pharmacol Ther* (1992) 51, 183.
2. Wahlländer A, Paumgartner G. Effect of ketoconazole and terbinafine on the pharmacokinetics of caffeine in healthy volunteers. *Eur J Clin Pharmacol* (1989) 37, 279–83.
3. Wexler D, Courtney R, Richards W, Banfield C, Lim J, Laughlin M. Effect of posaconazole on cytochrome P450 enzymes: a randomized, open-label, two-way crossover study. *Eur J Pharm Sci* (2004) 21, 645–53.

Caffeine + Artemisinin derivatives

Artemisinin, artenimol and artemotil reduce the metabolism of caffeine, whereas artemether and artesunate do not appear to affect the metabolism of caffeine.

Clinical evidence, mechanism, importance and management

A study in 7 healthy subjects found that a single 500-mg dose of **artemisinin** reduced the clearance of a single 136.5-mg dose of caffeine by 35%. The metabolism of caffeine to one of its major metabolites, paraxanthine (1,7-dimethylxanthine), was reduced by 66%.[1]

Another study, in 15 healthy subjects given **artemisinin** 500 mg daily for 5 days, found that the metabolism of a single 100-mg dose of caffeine to paraxanthine was reduced by 73%. As part of this study, 14 subjects were given **dihydroartemisinin [artenimol]** 60 mg daily for 5 days, and 15 subjects were given intramuscular **artemotil** 100 mg daily for 5 days. The metabolism of a single 100-mg dose of caffeine to paraxanthine was reduced by 27% by **dihydroartemisinin [artenimol]** and 30% by **artemotil**. There was no significant change in the metabolism of caffeine when 15 subjects were given **artemether** 100 mg daily for 5 days, or **artesunate** 100 mg daily for 5 days.[2] It was suggested that **artemisinin**, **dihydroartemisinin [artenimol]** and **artemotil** inhibit the metabolism of caffeine by CYP1A2 in the liver.[1,2]

Although it appears that artemisinin, artenimol and artemotil might reduce the metabolism of caffeine and therefore increase the risk of caffeine adverse effects, there is too little information to advise patients taking artemisinin derivatives to completely avoid caffeine-containing beverages (e.g. tea, coffee, cola drinks) or medicines that are formulated with caffeine (such as some analgesics). However, it would seem prudent to bear this interaction in mind if the adverse effects of caffeine (headache, insomnia, jitteriness) become troublesome.

1. Bapiro TE, Sayi J, Hasler JA, Jande M, Rimoy G, Masselle A, Masimirembwa CM. Artemisinin and thiabendazole are potent inhibitors of cytochrome P450 1A2 (CYP1A2) activity in humans. *Eur J Clin Pharmacol* (2005) 61, 755–61.
2. Asimus S, Elsherbiny D, Hai TN, Jansson B, Huong NV, Petzold MG, Simonsson USH, Ashton M. Artemisinin antimalarials moderately affect cytochrome P450 enzyme activity in healthy subjects. *Fundam Clin Pharmacol* (2007) 21, 307–16.

Caffeine + Cimetidine

Cimetidine slightly decreases the clearance of caffeine.

Clinical evidence, mechanism, importance and management

In a study in 5 subjects, cimetidine 1 g daily for 6 days increased the half-life of a single 300-mg dose of caffeine by about 70% and reduced its clearance.[1] In another study, cimetidine 1.2 g daily for 4 days increased the half-life of caffeine by 45% in 6 smokers and by 96% in 6 non-smokers. Caffeine clearance was reduced by 31% in the smokers and by 42% in the non-smokers.[2] A further study found that the half-life of caffeine was increased by 59% and its clearance decreased by 40% by cimetidine.[3] Conversely, in a study in children, cimetidine was not found to affect caffeine metabolism, as assessed by the caffeine breath test.[4]

The changes seen in some studies probably occurred because cimetidine, a well-known non-specific enzyme inhibitor, reduced the metabolism of caffeine in the liver, by CYP1A2, resulting in its accumulation.

Any increased caffeine effects are normally unlikely to be of much importance in most people, but they might have a small part to play in exaggerating the undesirable effects of caffeine from (e.g. tea, coffee, cola drinks) and some medicines, such as some analgesics, which are sometimes formulated with caffeine. If these become troublesome, advise patients to reduce their caffeine intake.

Note that caffeine is used as a probe substrate to assess the activity of drugs on CYP1A2. This study therefore suggests that cimetidine is a weak inhibitor of CYP1A2.

1. Broughton LJ, Rogers HJ. Decreased systemic clearance of caffeine due to cimetidine. *Br J Clin Pharmacol* (1981) 12, 155–9.
2. May DC, Jarboe CH, VanBakel AB, Williams WM. Effects of cimetidine on caffeine disposition in smokers and nonsmokers. *Clin Pharmacol Ther* (1982) 31, 656–61.
3. Beach CA, Gerber N, Ross J, Bianchine JR. Inhibition of elimination of caffeine by cimetidine in man. *Clin Res* (1982) 30, 248A.
4. Parker AC, Pritchard P, Preston T, Dalzell AM, Choonara I. Lack of inhibitory effect of cimetidine on caffeine metabolism in children using the caffeine breath test. *Br J Clin Pharmacol* (1997) 43, 467–70.

Caffeine + Class I antiarrhythmics

Mexiletine and propafenone slightly to moderately reduce the clearance of caffeine, whereas lidocaine, flecainide and tocainide do not appear to affect caffeine clearance. Caffeine does not alter the levels of mexiletine.

Clinical evidence

(a) Mexiletine

In a study in 7 patients with cardiac arrhythmias taking long-term mexiletine 600 mg daily the clearance of caffeine was found to be reduced by 48%.[1] In a parallel study by the same authors, in 5 healthy subjects given a single 200-mg dose of mexiletine, the clearance of a single 366-mg dose of caffeine was reduced by 57%, and its elimination half-life was prolonged from about 4 hours to 7 hours. The clearance of mexiletine was not affected by caffeine.[1] A preliminary report of this study also noted that fasting caffeine levels were almost sixfold higher during the mexiletine treatment period (1.99 micrograms/mL compared with 0.35 micrograms/mL).[2]

Another study in 14 healthy subjects found that caffeine 100 mg four times daily, for 2 days before and 2 days after a single 200-mg dose of mexiletine, did not cause any clinically significant changes in the plasma levels of mexiletine. Caffeine levels were not affected by mexilitine.[3]

(b) Propafenone

In a single-dose study in 8 healthy subjects, the clearance of a 300-mg dose of caffeine was reduced by 35% and the half-life of caffeine was extended from 3.82 hours to 5.9 hours when propafenone 300 mg was given.[4]

(c) Other antiarrhythmics

In a study in 7 healthy subjects, single doses of **lidocaine** 200 mg, **flecainide** 100 mg and **tocainide** 500 mg had no effect on the clearance of a single 366-mg dose of caffeine.[2]

Mechanism

It seems likely that mexiletine and propafenone inhibit the hepatic metabolism of caffeine by CYP1A2, leading to a reduction in its clearance.

Importance and management

A pharmacokinetic interaction between caffeine and **mexiletine** appears to be established, but its clinical importance is uncertain. Some of the adverse effects of mexiletine might be partially due to caffeine retention.[1] It has also been suggested that the caffeine test for liver function might be impaired by mexiletine.[1] The clinical significance of the interaction with **propafenone** is less clear, as no details on the clinical state of the subjects was recorded.[4] Be alert for possible adverse effects of caffeine (jitteriness, headache, insomnia) in patients also taking mexiletine or propafenone and advise them to reduce caffeine intake if these become troublesome: caffeine is commonly found in drinks (e.g. tea, coffee, cola drinks) and medicines that are formulated with caffeine (such as some analgesics).

Flecainide, **lidocaine** and **tocainide** do not appear to affect the pharmacokinetics of caffeine, and so no additional precautions seem necessary with caffeine use.

1. Joeres R, Klinker H, Heusler H, Epping J, Richter E. Influence of mexiletine on caffeine elimination. *Pharmacol Ther* (1987) 33, 163–9.
2. Joeres R, Richter E. Mexiletine and caffeine elimination. *N Engl J Med* (1987) 317, 117.
3. Labbé L, Abolfathi Z, Robitaille NM, St-Maurice F, Gilbert M, Turegon J. Stereoselective disposition of the antiarrhythmic agent mexiletine during the concomitant administration of caffeine. *Ther Drug Monit* (1999) 21, 191–9.
4. Michaud V, Mouksassi MS, Labbé L, Bélanger P-M, Ferron LA, Gilbert M, Grech-Bélanger O, Turgeon J. Inhibitory effects of propafenone on the pharmacokinetics of caffeine in humans. *Ther Drug Monit* (2006) 28, 779–83.

Caffeine + Disulfiram

Disulfiram slightly to modestly reduces the clearance of caffeine, which might complicate the withdrawal from alcohol.

Clinical evidence

A study in 10 healthy subjects and 11 recovering alcoholics found that disulfiram 250 or 500 mg daily reduced the clearance of caffeine by about 30%, but a few of the alcoholics had a more than 50% reduction.[1] In a study, 7 healthy subjects were given disulfiram 250 mg daily for 11 days, followed by a single 100-mg dose of caffeine. Disulfiram reduced the caffeine to paraxanthine ratio (a measure of caffeine metabolism) by 34%.[2]

Mechanism

Disulfiram appears to decrease the *N*-demethylation of caffeine by CYP1A2, which results in increased caffeine levels.

Importance and management

An interaction between disulfiram and caffeine is established. The concurrent use of disulfiram seems likely to result in raised caffeine levels, at least in some patients, which can cause irritability, insomnia and anxiety, similar to the symptoms of alcohol withdrawal. As coffee consumption is often particularly high among recovering alcoholics, there is the risk that they may turn to alcohol to calm themselves down. To avoid this possible complication it might be wise for recovering alcoholics not to drink too many caffeine-containing drinks (e.g. coffee, tea or cola drinks) or to drink decaffeinated products. Note also that caffeine can also be found in some formulations of medicines (such as analgesics).

Note that caffeine is used as a probe substrate to assess the activity of drugs on CYP1A2. These studies therefore suggest that disulfiram is generally a weak inhibitor of CYP1A2, although it may be a moderate inhibitor in some.

1. Beach CA, Mays DC, Guiler RC, Jacober CH, Gerber N. Inhibition of elimination of caffeine by disulfiram in normal subjects and recovering alcoholics. *Clin Pharmacol Ther* (1986) 39, 265–70.
2. Frye RF, Branch RA. Effect of chronic disulfiram administration on the activities of CYP1A2, CYP2C19, CYP2D6, CYP2E1, and N-acetyltransferase in healthy human subjects. *Br J Clin Pharmacol* (2002) 53, 155–62.

Caffeine + Food

Foods such as broccoli and green beans increase the rate of metabolism of caffeine.

Clinical evidence, mechanism, importance and management

In a study in 9 healthy subjects, the metabolism of caffeine, measured by the appearance of metabolites in the urine, was increased after the ingestion of 500 g of **green beans** or **broccoli** daily for 10 days.[1] Caffeine is metabolised by CYP1A2 and some foodstuffs are known to induce the activity of this isoenzyme, resulting in an increased rate of metabolism of substrates such as caffeine. However, this finding is unlikely to be of clinical significance, as caffeine and green vegetables are commonly ingested as part of the diet, and the amount of green vegetables given was quite large.

1. Vistisen K, Loft S, Poulsen HE. Cytochrome P450 1A2 activity in man measured by caffeine metabolism: effect of smoking, broccoli and exercise. *Adv Exp Med Biol* (1991) 283, 407–11.

Caffeine + Grapefruit juice

Grapefruit juice slightly reduces the clearance of caffeine but has no effect on its overall exposure.

Clinical evidence, mechanism, importance and management

In a study in 12 healthy subjects, 1.2 litres of grapefruit juice decreased the clearance of caffeine from coffee by 23% and prolonged its half-life by 31%, but these changes were not considered clinically relevant.[1] A crossover study in 6 healthy subjects given caffeine 3.3 mg/kg found that multiple doses of grapefruit juice (equivalent to 6 glasses) had no statistically significant effect on the AUC of caffeine, although interindividual variability in these results was seen. No changes in ambulatory blood pressure (systolic and diastolic) or heart rate were seen.[2] These studies suggest that grapefruit has no clinically relevant effect on the pharmacokinetics of caffeine.

Note that caffeine is used as a probe substrate to assess the activity of drugs and other substances on CYP1A2. This study therefore suggests that grapefruit juice has no clinically relevant effect on CYP1A2 activity.

1. Fuhr U, Klittich K, Staib AH. Inhibitory effect of grapefruit juice and the active component, naringenin on CYP1A2 dependent metabolism of caffeine in man. *Br J Clin Pharmacol* (1993) 35, 431–6. [Title corrected by erratum].
2. Maish WA, Hampton EM, Whitsett TL, Shepard JD, Lovallo WR. Influence of grapefruit juice on caffeine pharmacokinetics and pharmacodynamics. *Pharmacotherapy* (1996) 16, 1046–52.

Caffeine + Hormonal contraceptives or HRT

The clearance of caffeine is slightly to moderately reduced in women taking oral combined hormonal contraceptives or HRT.

Clinical evidence

(a) Hormonal contraceptives

In a study in 9 women taking low-dose oral combined hormonal contraceptives for at least 3 months, the clearance of a single 162-mg dose of caffeine was about 40% lower and its half-life prolonged (7.9 hours compared with 5.4 hours), when compared with 9 other women not taking a contraceptive.[1] This finding was confirmed in three other studies,[2-4] which found that caffeine elimination was prolonged, from 4 to 6 hours before the use of oral combined hormonal contraceptives, to about 9 hours by the end of the first cycle, and to about 11 hours by the end of the third cycle.[3,4] A further controlled study found that there was little difference between the effects of two oral combined hormonal contraceptives (**ethinylestradiol** 30 micrograms with **gestodene** 75 micrograms or **levonorgestrel** 125 micrograms) on caffeine: both reduced the clearance of caffeine by a little over 50%, but its maximum serum levels were unchanged.[5] A study in 7 women similarly found that the use of an oral combined hormonal contraceptive containing **ethinylestradiol** propanesulfonate 3 mg and **norethisterone** acetate 10 mg per menstrual cycle (*Deposiston*) prolonged the half-life of caffeine from 4.9 hours to 8 hours.[6]

A review of the bone mineral content of 263 users of depot **medroxyprogesterone** found that the women who reported a high caffeine intake (over 200 mg daily) had a lower spinal bone mineral content than the women who reported no caffeine intake. However, there was no statistically significant difference in bone mineral density between the two groups.[7]

(b) HRT

In one study, 12 healthy postmenopausal women were given a single 200-mg dose of caffeine after taking **estradiol** for 8 weeks, titrated to give **estradiol** plasma concentrations of 50 to 150 picograms/mL. The metabolism of caffeine was reduced by 29%. However, if the data for 2 subjects who were found to have taken extra caffeine during the study period are excluded, the reduction in caffeine metabolism was even greater (average reduction of 38%).[8]

Mechanism

Oestrogens appear to inhibit CYP1A2, the isoenzyme by which caffeine is metabolised.[8,9] Therefore concurrent use can lead to prolonged caffeine elimination.

Importance and management

The pharmacokinetic interaction between caffeine and oestrogen-containing hormonal contraceptives or HRT is established; however, given the lack of reports of adverse effects, it is probably of limited clinical importance. Some women taking these hormonal contraceptives or HRT who take caffeine-containing medicines (such as some analgesics) or caffeine-containing drinks (e.g. tea, coffee, cola drinks) may find that the adverse effects of caffeine (headache, jitteriness, insomnia), are increased and prolonged. If these become troublesome, advise those affected to reduce their caffeine intake. Note that, when combined hormonal contraceptives are administered cyclically, the interaction with caffeine will be cyclical (greatest after the first week of administration (at steady state), and least during the week of no active contraception).

Caffeine is used as a probe substrate to assess the activity of drugs on CYP1A2. These studies therefore suggest that ethinylestradiol is generally a weak to moderate inhibitor of CYP1A2.

The effect of depot medroxyprogesterone in patients with a high caffeine intake (over 200 mg daily) on bone mineral content seems unlikely to be of clinical significance as bone mineral density was not affected.

1. Abernethy DR, Todd EL. Impairment of caffeine clearance by chronic use of low-dose oestrogen-containing oral contraceptives. *Eur J Clin Pharmacol* (1985) 28, 425–8.
2. Patwardhan RV, Desmond PV, Johnson RF, Schenker S. Impaired elimination of caffeine by oral contraceptive steroids. *J Lab Clin Med* (1980) 95, 603–8.
3. Meyer FP, Canzler E, Giers H, Walther H. Langzeituntersuchung zum Einfluß von Non-Ovlon auf die Pharmakokinetik von Coffein im intraindividuellen Vergleich. *Zentralbl Gynakol* (1988) 110, 1449–54.
4. Rietveld EC, Broekman MMM, Houben JJG, Eskes TKAB, van Rossum JM. Rapid onset of an increase in caffeine residence time in young women due to oral contraceptive steroids. *Eur J Clin Pharmacol* (1984) 26, 371–3.
5. Balogh A, Klinger G, Henschel L, Börner A, Vollanth R, Kuhnz W. Influence of ethinylestradiol-containing combination oral contraceptives with gestodene or levonorgestrel on caffeine elimination. *Eur J Clin Pharmacol* (1995) 48, 161–6.
6. Meyer FP, Canzler E, Giers H, Walther H. Zeitverlauf der hemmung der coffeinelimination unter dem einfluß des oralen depotkontrazeptivum Deposiston®. *Zentralbl Gynakol* (1991) 113, 297–302.
7. Wetmore CM, Ichikawa L, LaCroix AZ, Ott SM, Scholes D. Association between caffeine intake and bone mass among young women: potential effect modification by depot medroxyprogesterone acetate use. *Osteoporos Int* (2008) 19, 519–27.
8. Pollock BG, Wylie M, Stack JA, Sorisio DA, Thompson DS, Kirshner MA, Folan MM, Condifer KA. Inhibition of caffeine metabolism by estrogen replacement therapy in postmenopausal women. *J Clin Pharmacol* (1999) 39, 936–40.
9. Shelepova T, Nafziger AN, Victory J, Kashuba ADM, Rowland E, Zhang Y, Sellers E, Kearns G, Leeder JS, Gaedigk A, Bertino JS. Effect of a triphasic oral contraceptive on drug-metabolizing enzyme activity as measured by the validated Cooperstown 5+1 cocktail. *J Clin Pharmacol* (2005) 45, 1413–21.

Caffeine + Idrocilamide

Oral idrocilamide markedly reduces the clearance of caffeine, which can lead to caffeine toxicity.

Clinical evidence

The possibility that caffeine intake might have had some part to play in the development of psychiatric disorders seen in patients taking idrocilamide, prompted a pharmacokinetic study in 4 healthy subjects. While taking oral idrocilamide 400 mg three times daily the half-life of caffeine (150 to 200 mg of caffeine from one cup of coffee) was prolonged from about 7 hours to 59 hours. The overall clearance of caffeine was decreased by 88%.[1,2]

Mechanism

Idrocilamide appears to inhibit CYP1A2 by which caffeine is metabolised, leading to its accumulation.

Importance and management

Evidence is limited but the interaction appears to be established. Patients taking oral idrocilamide should probably avoid or minimise their intake of caffeine, including caffeine-containing drinks (e.g. tea, coffee, cola drinks), otherwise caffeine adverse effects (headache, insomnia, jitteriness) may develop. Some medicines are formulated with caffeine (such as some analgesics), so these should also be used with care. The effects of topical idrocilamide on caffeine metabolism are unknown.

Note that caffeine is used as a probe substrate to assess the activity of drugs on CYP1A2. This study therefore suggests that idrocilamide is a potent inhibitor of CYP1A2. For a list of CYP1A2 substrates, see 'Table 1.2', p.5.

1. Brazier JL, Descotes J, Lery N, Ollagnier M, Evreux J-C. Inhibition by idrocilamide of the disposition of caffeine. *Eur J Clin Pharmacol* (1980) 17, 37–43.
2. Evreux JC, Bayere JJ, Descotes J, Lery N, Ollagnier M, Brazier JL. Les accidents neuro-psychiques de l'idrocilamide: conséquence d'une inhibition due métabolisme de la caféine? *Lyon Med* (1979) 241, 89–91.

Caffeine + Kava

An aqueous kava extract appeared to inhibit the metabolism of caffeine in one study, whereas another controlled study using kava root extract found no interaction.

Clinical evidence, mechanism, importance and management

In a study in 6 subjects (3 of whom smoked tobacco) who regularly took 7 to 27 g of kavalactones weekly as an aqueous kava extract, the metabolic ratio of caffeine was increased twofold when kava was withheld for 30 days, which suggested that kava inhibits CYP1A2, which is the principal isoenzyme involved in the metabolism of caffeine.[1] Furthermore, in a study in 12 non-smoking, healthy subjects given kava root extract 1 g twice daily for 28 days before receiving a single 100-mg dose of oral caffeine, no statistically significant change in the metabolic ratio of caffeine was noted.[2]

From the controlled study, it seems unlikely that kava root extract affects the metabolism of caffeine. It is possible that, in the first study, the effect of tobacco smoke, the lack of standardisation of kava intake and the small patient numbers might have influenced the results. Further study is needed to confirm this.

1. Russman S, Lauterburg BH, Barguil Y, Choblet E, Cabalion P, Rentsch K, Wenk M. Traditional aqueous kava extracts inhibit cytochrome P450 1A2 in humans: protective effect against environmental carcinogens? *Clin Pharmacol Ther* (2005) 77, 451–4.
2. Gurley BJ, Gardner SF, Hubbard MA, Williams DK, Gentry WB, Khan IA, Shah A. In vivo effects of goldenseal, kava kava, black cohosh, and valerian on human cytochrome P450 1A2, 2D6, 2E1, and 3A4/5 phenotypes. *Clin Pharmacol Ther* (2005) 77, 415–26.

Caffeine + Menthol

Menthol modestly delays caffeine maximum levels.

Clinical evidence, mechanism, importance and management

A crossover study in 11 healthy subjects found that a single 100-mg dose of menthol taken with coffee containing 200 mg of caffeine increased the time to maximum caffeine levels by about 30 minutes. The increase in the maximum level and AUC of caffeine was not statistically significant, and there were no statistically significant effects on the half-life of caffeine. It was thought that menthol reduced the rate of caffeine absorption; however, this does not appear to have affected the overall exposure to caffeine.[1] The clinical importance of this delay in caffeine maximum levels is not clear but it is seems likely to be limited.

Note that caffeine is used as a probe substrate to assess the activity of drugs and other substances on CYP1A2. This study therefore suggests that menthol has no clinically relevant effect on CYP1A2 activity.

1. Gelal A, Guven H, Balkan D, Artok L, Benowitz NL. Influence of menthol on caffeine disposition and pharmacodynamics in healthy female volunteers. *Eur J Clin Pharmacol* (2003) 59, 417–22.

Caffeine + Modafinil

The effects of modafinil on caffeine do not appear to have been studied. However, the *R*-isomer of modafinil, armodafinil, does not appear to affect the pharmacokinetics of caffeine.

Clinical evidence, mechanism, importance and management

In a study, 24 healthy subjects were given a single 200-mg dose of caffeine before and after taking **armodafinil** 250 mg daily for at least 22 days. There were no clinically significant changes in the pharmacokinetics of caffeine, and the combination was well tolerated.[1] No particular precautions regarding caffeine intake would therefore be expected to be needed in patients taking armodafinil. The effects of modafinil on caffeine metabolism do not appear to have been studied.

1. Darwish M, Kirby M, Robertson P, Hellriegel ET. Interaction profile of armodafinil with medications metabolized by cytochrome P450 enzymes 1A2, 3A4 and 2C19 in healthy subjects. *Clin Pharmacokinet* (2008) 47, 61–74.

Caffeine + Nicotine

Caffeine may increase some of the stimulant effects of nicotine, and under certain conditions, some of the cardiovascular effects of caffeine

and nicotine may be additive. Caffeine appears to cause a small, if any, rise in nicotine levels.

Clinical evidence

In a placebo-controlled study in 10 healthy non-smokers, a single 250-mg intravenous dose of caffeine increased resting blood pressure and reduced heart rate, whereas nicotine 4 mg (given as chewing gum) increased both blood pressure and heart rate. When given together, the effects of caffeine with nicotine on blood pressure were additive, resulting in an increase in blood pressure of 10.8/12.4 mmHg. However, during physical and mental stress (standing up and mental arithmetic, respectively) the cardiovascular effects were less than additive.[1] In contrast, a study in 20 non-smokers found that nicotine 2 or 4 mg (given as a chewing gum) increased heart rate and subjective effects but these effects were not influenced by oral caffeine 75 or 150 mg.[2]

In a study in 21 smokers who regularly drank one to six cups of coffee daily, a 50-mg caffeine tablet increased self-ratings of stimulated, alert and jittery at various doses of nicotine chewing gum (0.25 mg, 0.5 mg and 1 mg) when compared with nicotine gum alone.[3] In a placebo-controlled study, 12 healthy subjects were given nicotine 1 or 2 mg with caffeine 50 or 100 mg, both as a chewing gum. Both nicotine and caffeine alone increased energy expenditure; however, adding caffeine 50 mg to nicotine 1 mg had almost double the effect of increasing the nicotine dose from 1 to 2 mg. Similar effects were seen in both smokers and non-smokers. No adverse effects were reported with nicotine 1 mg either alone or given with caffeine.[4] In another similar study by the same authors, caffeine enhanced the appetite-suppressant effects of nicotine.[5] In another study in 13 smokers who regularly drank at least one cup of coffee daily, pre-treatment with oral caffeine 2.5 or 5 mg/kg (added to 180 mL of decaffeinated coffee) did not alter the subjects ability to discriminate between nasal nicotine and placebo, and did not alter the amount of caffeine they self-administered during a period of smoking cessation. Caffeine pre-treatment caused a minor dose-related increase in nicotine levels (maximum 21%).[6] In a study in 12 smokers, two doses of caffeine 150 mg (given in a decaffeinated cola drink before and during smoking) had no effect on the plasma levels of nicotine achieved by smoking 5 cigarettes.[7]

Mechanism

Not understood.

Importance and management

The interaction between caffeine and nicotine appears to be established but the effects of concurrent use are less certain, although the effects of caffeine and nicotine on blood pressure may be additive under certain conditions. Caffeine may boost some of the stimulant effects of nicotine (energy consumption, appetite suppression, and also its adverse effects, such as jitteriness), but it only appears to cause a small, if any, rise in nicotine levels. Bear the potential for this increase in effects in mind should a patient receiving nicotine replacement therapy and also taking medicines formulated with caffeine (such as some analgesics) or consuming caffeine-containing drinks (e.g. tea, coffee, cola drinks) develop troublesome nicotine-related adverse effects.

Note that smoking tobacco has been reported to increase the metabolism of caffeine, see 'Caffeine + Tobacco', p.1428.

1. Smits P, Temme L, Thien T. The cardiovascular interaction between caffeine and nicotine in humans. *Clin Pharmacol Ther* (1993) 54, 194–204.
2. Blank MD, Kleykamp BA, Jennings JM, Eissenberg T. Caffeine's influence on nicotine's effects in nonsmokers. *Am J Health Behav* (2007) 31, 473–83.
3. Duka T, Tasker R, Russell K, Stephens DN. Discriminative stimulus properties of nicotine at low doses: the effects of caffeine preload. *Behav Pharmacol* (1998) 9, 219–29.
4. Jessen AB, Toubro S, Astrup A. Effect of chewing gum containing nicotine and caffeine on energy expenditure and substrate utilization in men. *Am J Clin Nutr* (2003) 77, 1442–7.
5. Jessen A, Buemann B, Toubro S, Skovgaard IM, Astrup A. The appetite-suppressant effect of nicotine is enhanced by caffeine. *Diabetes Obes Metab* (2005) 7, 327–33.
6. Perkins KA, Fonte C, Stolinski A, Blakesley-Ball R, Wilson AS. The influence of caffeine on nicotine's discriminative stimulus, subjective, and reinforcing effects. *Exp Clin Psychopharmacol* (2005) 13, 275–81.
7. Gilbert DG, Dibb WD, Plath LC, Hiyane SG. Effects of nicotine and caffeine, separately and in combination, on EEG topography, mood, heart rate, cortisol, and vigilance. *Psychopharmacology (Berl)* (2000) 37, 583–95.

Caffeine + Psoralens

Oral methoxsalen and 5-methoxypsoralen moderately reduce the clearance of caffeine. Topical methoxsalen does not affect the clearance of caffeine.

Clinical evidence

In a study in 5 patients with psoriasis, a single 1.2-mg/kg oral dose of **methoxsalen** (8-methoxypsoralen), given one hour before a single 200-mg oral dose of caffeine, reduced the clearance of caffeine by 69%. The elimination half-life of caffeine over the period from 2 to 16 hours after taking the **methoxsalen** increased tenfold (from 5.6 hours to 57 hours).[1] In a similar study, 8 patients with psoriasis were given caffeine 200 mg with or without **5-methoxypsoralen** 1.2 mg/kg. The AUC of caffeine was increased about threefold by **5-methoxypsoralen** and there was a 66% decrease in its clearance.[2]

A study in patients receiving PUVA therapy (**methoxsalen** either orally, in 4 patients, or topically as a bath in 7 patients, plus UVA) found that the clearance of a single 150-mg dose of caffeine was considerably reduced in the patients given oral **methoxsalen** but not altered in those given topical **methoxsalen**.[3]

Mechanism

Methoxsalen and 5-methoxypsoralen inhibit the metabolism of caffeine by CYP1A2 in the liver, thereby moderately reducing caffeine clearance.[2,3]

Importance and management

An interaction between caffeine and oral methoxsalen and 5-methoxypsoralen appears to be established, but its clinical consequences are uncertain. However, it seems possible that the adverse effects of caffeine could be increased. In excess, caffeine (including that from tea, coffee and cola drinks) can cause jitteriness, headache and insomnia. If these effects develop in a patient receiving methoxsalen or 5-methoxypsoralen it may be prudent to advise them to decrease their caffeine intake. Note that some medicines, such as some analgesics, are formulated with caffeine, so these should also be used with care. Topical methoxsalen does not appear to interact with caffeine.

Note that caffeine is used as a probe substrate to assess the activity of drugs on CYP1A2. These studies therefore suggest that methoxsalen and 5-methoxypsoralen are moderate inhibitors of CYP1A2; however, it appears that topical methoxsalen is not absorbed to an extent sufficient to result in a systemic effect on CYP1A2. For a list of CYP1A2 substrates, see 'Table 1.2', p.5.

1. Mays DC, Camisa C, Cheney P, Pacula CM, Nawoot S, Gerber N. Methoxsalen is a potent inhibitor of the metabolism of caffeine in humans. *Clin Pharmacol Ther* (1987) 42, 621–6.
2. Bendriss EK, Bechtel Y, Bendriss A, Humbert P, Paintaud G, Megnette J, Agache P, Bechtel PR. Inhibition of caffeine metabolism by 5-methoxypsoralen in patients with psoriasis. *Br J Clin Pharmacol* (1996) 41, 421–4.
3. Tantcheva-Poór I, Servera-Llaneras M, Scharffetter-Kochanek K, Fuhr U. Liver cytochrome P450 CYP1A2 is markedly inhibited by systemic but not by bath PUVA in dermatological patients. *Br J Dermatol* (2001) 144, 1127–32.

Caffeine + Quinolones

Enoxacin markedly increases caffeine levels. Pipemidic acid interacts to a lesser extent, and ciprofloxacin, norfloxacin and pefloxacin interact less still. Fleroxacin, lomefloxacin, ofloxacin, rufloxacin, and trovafloxacin appear not to interact with caffeine.

Clinical evidence

The effects of various quinolones on the pharmacokinetics of caffeine[1-13] are summarised in 'Table 34.3', p.1427. In one of these studies, **ciprofloxacin** and **fleroxacin** were found to cause a greater increase in caffeine levels in women than in men; however, this difference in effect was not significant when the results were normalised for body weight.[13]

Mechanism

It would seem that the metabolism (*N*-demethylation) of caffeine is markedly reduced by some quinolones (notably enoxacin) resulting in greater levels and possibly greater effects. Other quinolones have either a much smaller effect or no effect at all. The quinolones that interact appear to inhibit CYP1A2 by which caffeine is metabolised.[14]

Importance and management

A pharmacokinetic interaction between caffeine and some quinolones is established. Based on the results of two studies,[15] the relative potencies of the quinolones as inhibitors of caffeine elimination (on a scale of 100 to 0) have been determined as follows: enoxacin 100, pipemidic acid 29, ciprofloxacin 11, norfloxacin 9 and ofloxacin 0. From further studies, clinafloxacin appears to be similar to enoxacin (profound effect), pefloxacin appears to be similar to norfloxacin (to which it is metabolised; modest effect), and fleroxacin, lomefloxacin, rufloxacin, and trovafloxacin appear to behave like ofloxacin (no clinically relevant effect). Note that the strength of the effect appears to vary with the dose of the quinolone used.

Patients taking **enoxacin** might be expected to experience an increase in the effects of caffeine (headache, jitteriness, restlessness, insomnia) if, for example, they continue to drink their usual amounts of caffeine-containing drinks (tea, coffee, cola drinks, etc.) or take medicines (such as some analgesics) that are formulated with caffeine. They should be warned to cut out or reduce their intake of caffeine if this occurs. The authors of one report suggest that patients with hepatic disorders, cardiac arrhythmias or latent epilepsy should avoid caffeine if they take enoxacin for one week or more.[1] The effects of **pipemidic acid** on the metabolism of caffeine are less than those of enoxacin, but it would still seem prudent to bear the possibility of an interaction in mind should the adverse effects of caffeine become troublesome. Similar precautions are probably warranted with **ciprofloxacin**, **norfloxacin** and **pefloxacin**, although note that their effects on caffeine metabolism in some studies appeared to be of little clinical relevance. **Fleroxacin**, **lomefloxacin**, **ofloxacin**, **rufloxacin**, and **trovafloxacin** do not interact.

Note that caffeine can be used as a probe substrate for the activity of CYP1A2: those quinolones that have the greatest effect on caffeine are the most potent CYP1A2 inhibitors (e.g. enoxacin), those that have modest effects are moderate CYP1A2 inhibitors (e.g. ciprofloxacin), and those that have little or no effect on caffeine metabolism (e.g. ofloxacin) are unlikely to have a clinically relevant effect on other CYP1A2 substrates.

1. Staib AH, Stille W, Dietlein G, Shah PM, Harder S, Mieke S, Beer C. Interaction between quinolones and caffeine. *Drugs* (1987) 34 (Suppl 1), 170–4.
2. Carbó M, Segura J, De la Torre R, Badenas JM, Camí J. Effect of quinolones on caffeine disposition. *Clin Pharmacol Ther* (1989) 45, 234–40.
3. Harder S, Staib AH, Beer C, Papenburg A, Stille W, Shah PM. 4-Quinolones inhibit biotransformation of caffeine. *Eur J Clin Pharmacol* (1988) 35, 651–6.
4. Stille W, Harder S, Mieke S, Beer C, Shah PM, Frech K, Staib AH. Decrease of caffeine elimination in man during co-administration of 4-quinolones. *J Antimicrob Chemother* (1987) 20, 729–34.
5. Healy DP, Schoenle JR, Stotka J, Polk RE. Lack of interaction between lomefloxacin and caffeine in normal volunteers. *Antimicrob Agents Chemother* (1991) 35, 660–4.
6. Peloquin CA, Nix DE, Sedman AJ, Wilton JH, Toothaker RD, Harrison NJ, Schentag JJ. Pharmacokinetics and clinical effects of caffeine alone and in combination with oral enoxacin. *Rev Infect Dis* (1989) II (Suppl 5), S1095.

Table 34.3 Effect of quinolones on caffeine pharmacokinetics in healthy subjects

Quinolone[*]	*Daily caffeine intake*[†]	*Change in AUC*	*Change in clearance*	*Refs*
Ciprofloxacin				
100 mg twice daily	230 mg	+17%		1
250 mg twice daily	220 to 230 mg	+57%	–33%	1-3
500 mg twice daily	230 mg	+58%		1
500 mg twice daily	100 mg three times daily	+127%	–49%	4
500 mg twice daily	100 mg three times daily	+101% women +80% men	–53% women –47% men	5
750 mg (3 x 12-hourly doses)	100 mg	+59%	–45%	6
Clinafloxacin				
400 mg twice daily	200 mg		–84%	7
Enoxacin				
100 mg twice daily	230 mg	+138%		1
200 mg twice daily	230 mg	+176%		1
400 mg twice daily	220 to 230 mg	+346%	–78%	1-3
400 mg twice daily	200 mg daily	+370%	–79%	8
400 mg twice daily	183 mg daily	+472%	–83%	9
Fleroxacin				
400 mg daily	100 mg three times daily	+20% women No change in men	–10% in women No change in men	5
Lomefloxacin				
400 mg daily	200 mg daily	No change	No change	10
Norfloxacin				
200 mg twice daily	230 mg	+16%		1
800 mg twice daily	350 mg	+52%	–35%	11
Ofloxacin				
200 mg twice daily	220 to 230 mg	No change	No change	1-3
Pefloxacin				
400 mg twice daily	183 mg daily	+88%	–47%	9
Pipemidic acid				
400 mg twice daily	230 mg	+179%		1
800 mg twice daily	350 mg	+119%	–63%	11
Rufloxacin				
400 mg (single dose)	200 mg	–18%	No change	12
Trovafloxacin				
200 mg daily	183 mg daily	+17%		13

*Unless otherwise stated quinolones were given for 3 to 5 days.
†Unless otherwise stated caffeine was given as a single dose.

1. Harder S, Staib AH, Beer C, Papenburg A, Stille W, Shah PM. 4-Quinolones inhibit biotransformation of caffeine. *Eur J Clin Pharmacol* (1988) 35, 651-6.
2. Staib AH, Stille W, Dietlein G, Shah PM, Harder S, Mieke S, Beer C. Interaction between quinolones and caffeine. *Drugs* (1987) 34 (Suppl 1), 170-4.
3. Stille W, Harder S, Mieke S, Beer C, Shah PM, Frech K, Staib AH. Decrease of caffeine elimination in man during co-administration of 4-quinolones. *J Antimicrob Chemother* (1987) 20, 729-34.
4. Nicolau DP, Nightingale CH, Tessier PR, Fu Q, Xuan D-W, Esguerra EM, Quintiliani R. The effect of fleroxacin and ciprofloxacin on the pharmacokinetics of multiple dose caffeine. *Drugs* (1995) 49 (Suppl 2), 357-9.
5. Kim M-Y, Nightingale CH, Nicolau DP. Influence of sex on the pharmacokinetic interaction of fleroxacin and ciprofloxacin with caffeine. *Clin Pharmacokinet* (2003), 42, 985–96.
6. Healy DP, Polk RE, Kanawati L, Rock DT, Mooney ML. Interaction between oral ciprofloxacin and caffeine in normal volunteers. *Antimicrob Agents Chemother* (1989) 33, 474-8.
7. Randinitis EJ, Koup JR, Rausch G, Vassos AB. Effect of (CLX) administration on the single-dose pharmacokinetics of theophylline and caffeine. *Intersci Conf Antimicrob Agents Chemother* (1998) 38, 6.
8. Peloquin CA, Nix DE, Sedman AJ, Wilton JH, Toothaker RD, Harrison NJ, Schentag JJ. Pharmacokinetics and clinical effects of caffeine alone and in combination with oral enoxacin. *Rev Infect Dis* (1989) II (Suppl 5), S1095.
9. Kinzig-Schippers M, Fuhr U, Zaigler M, Dammeyer J, Rüsing G, Labedzki A, Bulitta J, Sörgel F. Interaction of pefloxacin and enoxacin with the human cytochrome P450 enzyme CYP1A2. *Clin Pharmacol Ther* (1999) 65, 262-74.
10. Healy DP, Schoenle JR, Stotka J, Polk RE. Lack of interaction between lomefloxacin and caffeine in normal volunteers. *Antimicrob Agents Chemother* (1991) 35, 660-4.
11. Carbó M, Segura J, De la Torre R, Badenas JM, Camí J. Effect of quinolones on caffeine disposition. *Clin Pharmacol Ther* (1989) 45, 234-40.
12. Cesana M, Broccali G, Imbimbo BP, Crema A. Effect of single doses of rufloxacin on the disposition of theophylline and caffeine after single administration. *Int J Clin Pharmacol Ther Toxicol* (1991) 29, 133-8.
13. LeBel M, Teng R, Dogolo LC, Willavize S, Friedman HL, Vincent J. The influence of steady-state trovafloxacin on the steady-state pharmacokinetics of caffeine in healthy subjects. *Pharm Res* (1996) 13 (Suppl 9), S434.

7. Healy DP, Polk RE, Kanawati L, Rock DT, Mooney ML. Interaction between oral ciprofloxacin and caffeine in normal volunteers. *Antimicrob Agents Chemother* (1989) 33, 474–8.
8. Nicolau DP, Nightingale CH, Tessier PR, Fu Q, Xuan D-w, Esguerra EM, Quintiliani R. The effect of fleroxacin and ciprofloxacin on the pharmacokinetics of multiple dose caffeine. *Drugs* (1995) 49 (Suppl 2), 357–9.
9. LeBel M, Teng R, Dogolo LC, Willavize S, Friedman HL, Vincent J. The influence of steady-state trovafloxacin on the steady-state pharmacokinetics of caffeine in healthy subjects. *Pharm Res* (1996) 13 (Suppl 9), S434.
10. Randinitis EJ, Koup JR, Rausch G, Vassos AB. Effect of (CLX) administration on the single-dose pharmacokinetics of theophylline and caffeine. *Intersci Conf Antimicrob Agents Chemother* (1998) 38, 6.
11. Cesana M, Broccali G, Imbimbo BP, Crema A. Effect of single doses of rufloxacin on the disposition of theophylline and caffeine after single administration. *Int J Clin Pharmacol Ther Toxicol* (1991) 29, 133–8.
12. Kinzig-Schippers M, Fuhr U, Zaigler M, Dammeyer J, Rüsing G, Labedzki A, Bulitta J, Sörgel F. Interaction of pefloxacin and enoxacin with the human cytochrome P450 enzyme CYP1A2. *Clin Pharmacol Ther* (1999) 65, 262–74.
13. Kim M-Y, Nightingale CH, Nicolau DP. Influence of sex on the pharmacokinetic interaction of fleroxacin and ciprofloxacin with caffeine. *Clin Pharmacokinet* (2003), 42, 985–96.
14. Fuhr U, Wolff T, Harder S, Schymanski P, Staib AH. Quinolone inhibition of cytochrome P450-dependent caffeine metabolism in human liver microsomes. *Drug Metab Dispos* (1990) 18, 1005–10.
15. Barnett G, Segura J, de la Torre R, Carbó M. Pharmacokinetic determination of relative potency of quinolone inhibition of caffeine disposition. *Eur J Clin Pharmacol* (1990) 39, 63–9.

Caffeine + SSRIs

The clearance of caffeine is markedly reduced by fluvoxamine and although an increase in the stimulant and adverse effects of caffeine would be expected, this was not demonstrated in one study. Caffeine might cause a slight reduction in the bioavailability of fluvoxamine. A possible case of serotonin syndrome has been attributed to the concurrent use of paroxetine and caffeine.

Clinical evidence

(a) Fluvoxamine

In a randomised, crossover study, 8 healthy subjects were given fluvoxamine 50 mg daily for 4 days and then 100 mg daily for a further 8 days, with a single 200-mg oral dose of caffeine given both before and on day 8 of fluvoxamine use. Fluvoxamine reduced the total clearance of caffeine by about 80% (from 107 mL/minute to 21 mL/minute) and increased its half-life from 5 hours to 31 hours. Specifically, the clearance of caffeine by *N*3-, *N*1- and *N*7-demethylation was decreased.[1] Another study in 30 patients found a positive correlation between plasma fluvoxamine and plasma caffeine levels, suggesting that the interaction is dose-related.[2] A further study found that low, sub-therapeutic doses of fluvoxamine 10 or 20 mg daily were sufficient to markedly inhibit caffeine metabolism.[3] A study in 7 subjects found that fluvoxamine 100 mg twice daily for 4 doses increased the maximum levels of a single 250-mg dose of caffeine by 40%, and increased the AUC and half-life of caffeine 12.7-fold and 10-fold, respectively. However, this did not result in an increase in caffeine-related adverse effects, and none of the subjects felt they were more alert with the combination than with either drug alone.[4]

A study in 12 healthy subjects (6 smokers and 6 non-smokers) found that caffeine 150 mg twice daily for 11 days reduced the AUC of a single 50-mg dose of fluvoxamine taken on day 8, by about 24% but the plasma concentration of fluvoxamine was not affected.[5]

(b) Paroxetine

A case report describes a patient who took amoxapine 200 mg, paroxetine 20 mg, and a preparation containing 4.8 g of caffeine. She became restless and incoherent, with a raised temperature, pulse rate, and respiratory rate; diaphoresis, myoclonus and mild muscle rigidity. Her symptoms resolved when she was given dantrolene and diazepam. The authors of the report attributed these symptoms to serotonin syndrome.[6]

Mechanism

Fluvoxamine is a potent inhibitor of CYP1A2, which is the principal enzyme concerned with the metabolism of caffeine. As a result caffeine clearance is reduced and therefore it accumulates.[1-3]

The case of serotonin syndrome is unexplained, but the authors of the report suggest that large doses of caffeine may promote serotonin activity.[6]

Importance and management

The increase in caffeine levels that occurs with **fluvoxamine** is established. There are no reports of caffeine toxicity arising from this interaction and one study[4] found no increase in the pharmacodynamic effects or adverse effects of caffeine despite a large increase in the levels. However, an increase in the stimulant and adverse effects of caffeine (headache, jitteriness, restlessness, insomnia) may be possible in susceptible patients if they continue to consume large amounts of caffeine-containing drinks (tea, coffee, cola drinks, etc.) or take medicines formulated with caffeine (such as some analgesics). They should be warned to reduce their caffeine intake if problems develop. It has been suggested that some of the adverse effects of fluvoxamine (i.e. nervousness, restlessness and insomnia) could in fact be caused by caffeine toxicity. However, a preliminary study, as well as the study reported above,[4] found that caffeine intake had a limited effect on the frequency of adverse effects of fluvoxamine.[7] The clinical significance of the change in the AUC of fluvoxamine with caffeine intake is unclear. This slight decrease is unlikely to be important in most patients.

Note that caffeine is used as a probe substrate to assess the activity of drugs on CYP1A2. These studies therefore suggest that fluvoxamine is a potent inhibitor of CYP1A2. For a list of CYP1A2 substrates, see 'Table 1.2', p.5.

There appears to be only one isolated case of serotonin syndrome attributed to an interaction between **paroxetine** and caffeine; the authors of the report suggest that the large dose of caffeine was a contributing factor.[6] However, the patient was also taking amoxapine, and serotonin syndrome has been reported in a number of patients taking tricyclics with SSRIs (see 'Tricyclic and related antidepressants + SSRIs', p.1515). Therefore an effect of caffeine is not established, and as such, no general recommendations can be made on the basis of this case.

1. Jeppesen U, Loft S, Poulsen HE, Brøsen K. A fluvoxamine-caffeine interaction study. *Pharmacogenetics* (1996) 6, 213–222.
2. Yoshimura R, Ueda N, Nakamura J, Eto S, Matsushita M. Interaction between fluvoxamine and cotinine or caffeine. *Neuropsychobiology* (2002) 45, 32–5.
3. Christensen M, Tybring G, Mihara K, Yasui-Furokori N, Carrillo JA, Ramos SI, Andersson K, Dahl M-L, Bertilsson L. Low daily 10-mg and 20-mg doses of fluvoxamine inhibit the metabolism of both caffeine (cytochrome P4501A2) and omeprazole (cytochrome P4502C19). *Clin Pharmacol Ther* (2002) 71, 141–52.
4. Culm-Merdek KE, von Moltke LL, Harmatz JS, Greenblatt DJ. Fluvoxamine impairs single-dose caffeine clearance without altering caffeine pharmacodynamics. *Br J Clin Pharmacol* (2005) 60, 486–93.
5. Fukasawa T, Yasui-Furukori N, Suzuki A, Ishii G, Inoue Y, Tateishi T, Otani K. Effects of caffeine on the kinetics of fluvoxamine and its major metabolite in plasma after a single oral dose of the drug. *Ther Drug Monit* (2006) 28, 308–11.
6. Shioda K, Nisijima K, Nishida S, Kato S. Possible serotonin syndrome arising from an interaction between caffeine and serotonergic antidepressants. *Hum Psychopharmacol Clin Exp* (2004) 19, 353–4.
7. Spigset O. Are adverse drug reactions attributed to fluvoxamine caused by concomitant intake of caffeine? *Eur J Clin Pharmacol* (1998) 54, 665–6.

Caffeine + Tiabendazole

Tiabendazole slightly increases the exposure to caffeine.

Clinical evidence, mechanism, importance and management

A study in 7 healthy subjects found that a single 500-mg dose of tiabendazole reduced the clearance of caffeine by 66% and increased its half-life and AUC by 140% and 57%, respectively. The metabolism of caffeine to one of its major metabolites, paraxanthine, was reduced by 92%.[1]

It appears that tiabendazole inhibits the metabolism of caffeine by CYP1A2 in the liver. Although evidence for an interaction between caffeine and tiabendazole is limited, it seems possible that some patients taking tiabendazole may develop caffeine adverse effects (headache, restlessness, insomnia, and jitteriness). If these become troublesome, patients should be advised to minimise their intake of caffeine-containing beverages (e.g. tea, coffee, cola drinks) or medicines formulated with caffeine (such as analgesics).

Note that caffeine is used as a probe substrate to assess the activity of drugs on CYP1A2. This study therefore suggests that tiabendazole is possibly a weak inhibitor of CYP1A2.

1. Bapiro TE, Sayi J, Hasler JA, Jande M, Rimoy G, Masselle A, Masimirembwa CM. Artemisinin and thiabendazole are potent inhibitors of cytochrome P450 1A2 (CYP1A2) activity in humans. *Eur J Clin Pharmacol* (2005) 61, 755–61.

Caffeine + Tobacco

Tobacco smoking increases the rate of caffeine metabolism.

Clinical evidence

A review of smoking and the concurrent intake of coffee found that ex-smokers consumed more coffee than non-smokers but consumed less coffee than smokers.[1] In a study in healthy subjects, the metabolism of caffeine, measured by urinary metabolites, was found to be increased in those subjects who smoked, compared with those who were non-smokers.[2] Mathematical modelling of caffeine plasma levels in smokers and non-smokers confirmed that after adjustment for caffeine intake, the plasma levels of caffeine in non-smokers were two- to threefold higher than in those subjects who smoked.[3] A study in 12 otherwise healthy smokers found that on stopping smoking the metabolism of caffeine was reduced by about 36%.[4]

Mechanism

Smoking tobacco induces the activity of CYP1A2, the principal isoenzyme by which caffeine is metabolised, resulting in an increase in the rate of caffeine metabolism.

Importance and management

There are many studies on the concurrent use of caffeine (mainly as coffee) and smoking. Several studies, including those noted above[2-4] have assessed the effect of smoking on the metabolism of caffeine, and they suggest that caffeine levels are decreased during smoking and may increase on stopping smoking. A review of reports of nicotine withdrawal, caffeine withdrawal and caffeine toxicity suggests that reported nicotine withdrawal symptoms may be a mixture of nicotine withdrawal and caffeine toxicity.[1] As the levels of caffeine may rise, albeit modestly, in those who stop smoking, it would seem prudent to bear the possibility of an interaction in mind. If the adverse effects of caffeine (headache, jitteriness, insomnia) become troublesome, advise patients to decrease their caffeine intake. Caffeine is commonly ingested from caffeine-containing drinks (tea, coffee, cola drinks, etc.) and is present in medicines (such as some analgesics) that are formulated with caffeine.

Note that the use of nicotine replacement therapy may also exacerbate the adverse effects of caffeine, see 'Caffeine + Nicotine', p.1425.

1. Swanson JA, Lee JW, Hopp JW. Caffeine and nicotine: a review of their joint use and possible interactive effects in tobacco withdrawal. *Addict Behav* (1994) 19, 229–56.

2. Vistisen K, Loft S, Poulsen HE. Cytochrome P450 1A2 activity in man measured by caffeine metabolism: effect of smoking, broccoli and exercise. *Adv Exp Med Biol* (1991) 283, 407–11.
3. de Leon J, Diaz FJ, Rogers T, Browne D, Dinsmore L, Ghosheh OH, Dwoskin LP, Crooks PA. A pilot study of plasma caffeine concentrations in a US sample of smoker and nonsmoker volunteers. *Prog Neuropsychopharmacol Biol Psychiatry* (2003) 27, 165–71.
4. Faber MS, Fuhr U. Time response of cytochrome P450 1A2 activity on cessation of heavy smoking. *Clin Pharmacol Ther* (2004) 76, 178–84.

Caffeine + Venlafaxine

Venlafaxine does not have a clinically relevant effect on the pharmacokinetics of caffeine.

Clinical evidence, mechanism, importance and management

In a study in 15 healthy subjects, venlafaxine 37.5 mg twice daily for 3 days then 75 mg twice daily for 4 days did not affect the AUC or clearance of caffeine 200 mg daily (equivalent to about 3 cups of coffee). A slight but statistically significant decrease in the half-life, from 6.1 hours to 5.5 hours, was noted, but this would not be expected to be of clinically relevance.[1] On the basis of this study, no particular precautions are needed with the use of caffeine in a patient taking venlafaxine.

Note that caffeine is used as a probe substrate to assess the activity of drugs on CYP1A2. This study therefore suggests that venlafaxine has no clinically relevant effect on CYP1A2 activity.

1. Amchin J, Zarycranski W, Taylor KP, Albano D, Klockowski PM. Effect of venlafaxine on CYP1A2-dependent pharmacokinetics and metabolism of caffeine. *J Clin Pharmacol* (1999) 39, 252–9.

Caffeine + Verapamil

Verapamil slightly reduces the clearance of caffeine.

Clinical evidence, mechanism, importance and management

In a study in 6 healthy subjects, verapamil 80 mg three times daily for 2 days decreased the total clearance of a single 200-mg dose of caffeine by 25%, and increased its half-life by 25% (from 4.6 hours to 5.8 hours).[1] These changes are small, and any increased caffeine effects are normally unlikely to be of much importance in most people, but they might have a small part to play in exaggerating the undesirable effects of caffeine from (e.g. tea, coffee, cola drinks) and some medicines, such as some analgesics, which are sometimes formulated with caffeine. If these become troublesome, advise patients to reduce their caffeine intake.

Note that caffeine is used as a probe substrate to assess the activity of drugs on CYP1A2. This study therefore suggests that verapamil is possibly a weak inhibitor of CYP1A2.

1. Nawoot S, Wong D, Mays DC, Gerber N. Inhibition of caffeine elimination by verapamil. *Clin Pharmacol Ther* (1988) 43, 148.

Doxofylline + Miscellaneous

Limited evidence suggests that erythromycin may increase the exposure to doxofylline. Digoxin initially raises, then lowers doxofylline levels, but its bronchodilator effects do not appear to be significantly affected. Allopurinol and lithium carbonate do not appear to affect the pharmacokinetics of doxofylline.

Clinical evidence, mechanism, importance and management

(a) Digoxin

In a comparative study in 9 patients taking doxofylline 800 mg daily, digoxin 500 micrograms daily was given to 5 patients. It was found that digoxin *increased* the serum levels of doxofylline by 50% on the first day of treatment (level taken 3 hours after administration) but then *reduced* doxofylline levels by about 30% at steady-state (day 30). Nevertheless, the bronchodilating effects of doxofylline were little different between the two groups. It was concluded that concurrent use is normally safe and effective, but the initial doxofylline dose should be chosen to avoid too high a serum level on the first day, and pulmonary function should be well monitored.[1]

(b) Other drugs

Healthy subjects were given doxofylline 400 mg three times daily, either alone, or with **allopurinol** 100 mg daily, **erythromycin** 400 mg three times daily or **lithium carbonate** 300 mg three times daily. None of the pharmacokinetic parameters measured, including the maximum serum levels, were altered by any of these drugs apart from the AUC of doxofylline, which was raised by about 40% by **allopurinol**, by 70% by **erythromycin**, and by 35% by **lithium carbonate**. Only the **erythromycin** result was statistically significant.[2] The clinical relevance of these changes is uncertain, and the mechanism by which they occur is not understood. Until the situation is much clearer it would be prudent to check the outcome of adding **erythromycin** to established treatment with doxofylline, being alert for evidence of increased effects.

1. Provvedi D, Rubegni M, Biffignandi P. Pharmacokinetic interaction between doxofylline and digitalis in elderly patients with chronic obstructive bronchitis. *Acta Ther* (1990) 16, 239–46.
2. Harning R, Sekora D, O'Connell K, Wilson J. A crossover study of the effect of erythromycin, lithium carbonate, and allopurinol on doxofylline pharmacokinetics. *Clin Pharmacol Ther* (1994) 55, 158.

Leukotriene antagonists + Gemfibrozil

Gemfibrozil moderately increases the exposure to montelukast, but does not appear to affect the pharmacokinetics of zafirlukast.

Clinical evidence

(a) Montelukast

In a placebo-controlled study, 10 healthy subjects were given gemfibrozil 600 mg twice daily for 3 days, with a single 10-mg dose of montelukast on day 3. Gemfibrozil increased the AUC and maximum plasma concentration of montelukast 4.5-fold and by 50%, respectively, and prolonged its half-life 3-fold. Some patients had up to 7-fold increases in the AUC of montelukast.[1] In a similar placebo-controlled crossover study, 11 healthy subjects were given gemfibrozil 600 mg twice daily for 5 days, with a single 10-mg dose of montelukast on day 3. Gemfibrozil increased the AUC of montelukast 4.3-fold and prolonged its half-life 2.1-fold, when compared with montelukast given alone.[2]

(b) Zafirlukast

In a placebo-controlled study in 10 healthy subjects, gemfibrozil 600 mg twice daily for 5 days had no effect on the pharmacokinetics of a single 20-mg dose of zafirlukast given on day 3.[3]

Mechanism

Montelukast is primarily metabolised by CYP2C8, and gemfibrozil is an inhibitor of this isoenzyme. Concurrent use therefore increases montelukast exposure. Montelukast has also been said to be a substrate for the organic anion transporting polypeptide, OATP2B1, which has been reported to be inhibited *in vitro* by gemfibrozil. However, the authors of the study suggest that inhibition of OATP2B1 is unlikely to result in changes in montelukast exposure of the magnitude seen, as gemfibrozil only weakly inhibits this polypeptide.[1]

The lack of effect of gemfibrozil on the pharmacokinetics of zafirlukast suggests that CYP2C8 is not involved in the metabolism of zafirlukast.[3]

Importance and management

An interaction between gemfibrozil and montelukast would seem to be established and is likely to be clinically important. The evidence suggests that gemfibrozil causes a moderate increase in montelukast exposure, and concurrent use should therefore be monitored for an increase in montelukast adverse effects (abdominal pain, headache; and hyperkinesia in young children). Consider reducing the dose of montelukast should any adverse effects occur in patients also taking gemfibrozil: the authors of one study suggest a dose reduction of 50 to 80% might be required.[1]

No zafirlukast dose adjustment is needed on the concurrent use of gemfibrozil.

1. Karonen T, Filppula A, Laitila J, Niemi M, Neuvonen PJ, Backman JT. Gemfibrozil markedly increases the plasma concentrations of montelukast: a previously unrecognized role for CYP2C8 in the metabolism of montelukast. *Clin Pharmacol Ther* (2010) 88, 223–30.
2. Karonen T, Neuvonen PJ, Backman JT. CYP2C8 but not CYP3A4 is important in the pharmacokinetics of montelukast. *Br J Clin Pharmacol* (2012) 73, 257–67.
3. Karonen T, Neuvonen PJ, Backman JT. The CYP2C8 inhibitor gemfibrozil does not affect the pharmacokinetics of zafirlukast. *Eur J Clin Pharmacol* (2011) 67, 151–5.

Leukotriene antagonists; Montelukast + Anti-asthma drugs

An isolated report describes severe oedema in a patient taking oral prednisone and montelukast, but studies suggest that the concurrent use of montelukast and prednisolone or prednisone is clinically beneficial and well-tolerated. High-dose montelukast does not appear to interact adversely with salbutamol (albuterol).

Clinical evidence, mechanism, importance and management

(a) Beta$_2$ agonists

A study in patients with moderately severe asthma found no adverse interactions when **salbutamol (albuterol)** was given with high-dose montelukast 100 mg or 250 mg, with or without inhaled corticosteroids.[1] The British Thoracic Society guidelines suggest that a leukotriene antagonist can be used as an add-on therapy in patients using short-acting inhaled beta$_2$ agonists in certain circumstances.[2]

(b) Corticosteroids

A study in healthy subjects (55 taking montelukast and 36 taking placebo) found that the plasma profiles of oral **prednisone** 20 mg and of intravenous **prednisolone** 250 mg were unaffected by montelukast 200 mg daily for 6 weeks.[3] Other studies in patients using inhaled and/or oral corticosteroids have found that concurrent use is beneficial and well tolerated.[4-6]

However, an isolated report describes a case of marked peripheral oedema possibly linked to the use of **prednisone** and montelukast. A 23-year-old patient with severe allergic and exercise-induced asthma and rhinoconjunctivitis, taking salmeterol and fluticasone by inhalation and oral cetirizine, was given **prednisone** 40 mg daily for one week then 20 mg daily for a further week. When **prednisone** was stopped, severe asthma recurred and he was given **prednisone** 60 mg daily for one week then 40 mg daily for a further week with montelukast 10 mg daily. After 10 days he developed severe peripheral oedema, gaining 13 kg in weight. Renal and cardiovascular function were normal. **Prednisone** was stopped and the asthma was controlled by continued montelukast and the excess weight was lost as the oedema resolved. The patient had good tolerance of both **prednisone** and montelukast alone. The reason for this adverse reaction is unclear, but it was suggested that corticosteroid-induced renal tubular sodium and fluid retention may have occurred when montelukast was also given.[7]

This isolated report is probably of limited general relevance. Usually, no additional precautions appear to be needed if these drugs are used concurrently, and the British Thoracic Society guidelines suggest that a leukotriene antagonist can be used as an add-on therapy to inhaled steroids in certain circumstances.[2]

1. Merck Sharp & Dohme. Data on file. Botto A, Kundu S, Reiss T: a double-blind, placebo-controlled, 3-period, crossover study to investigate the bronchodilating ability of oral doses of MK-0476 and to investigate the interaction with inhaled albuterol in moderately severe asthmatic patients (Protocol 006). 1996.
2. British Thoracic Society and Scottish Intercollegiate Guidelines Network. British guideline on the management of asthma, October 2014. Available at: http://www.sign.ac.uk/pdf/SIGN141.pdf (accessed 21/10/15).
3. Merck Sharp & Dohme. Data on file. Noonan T, Shingo S, Kundu S, Reiss TF: a double-blind, placebo-controlled, parallel-group study in healthy male volunteers to investigate the safety and tolerability of 6 weeks of administration of MK-0476, and in subgroups, the effect of 6 weeks of administration of MK-0476 on the single dose pharmacokinetics of po and iv theophylline and corticosteroids. 1995.
4. Dahlén S-E, Malmström K, Nizankowska E, Dahlén B, Kuna P, Kowalski M, Lumry WR, Picado C, Stevenson DD, Bousquet J, Pauwels R, Holgate ST, Shahane A, Zhang J, Reiss TF, Szczeklik A. Improvement of aspirin-intolerant asthma by montelukast, a leukotriene antagonist. *Am J Respir Crit Care Med* (2002) 165, 9–14.
5. Knorr B, Matz J, Bernstein JA, Nguyen H, Seidenberg BC, Reiss TF, Becker A, for the Pediatric Montelukast Study Group. Montelukast for chronic asthma in 6- to 14-year-old children. A randomized, double-blind trial. *JAMA* (1998) 279, 1181–6.
6. Phipatanakul W, Greene C, Downes SJ, Cronin B, Eller TJ, Schneider LC, Irani A-M. Montelukast improves asthma control in asthmatic children maintained on inhaled corticosteroids. *Ann Allergy Asthma Immunol* (2003) 91, 49–54.
7. Geller M. Marked peripheral edema associated with montelukast and prednisone. *Ann Intern Med* (2000) 132, 924.

Leukotriene antagonists; Montelukast + Antiepileptics; Enzyme-inducing

Phenobarbital slightly reduces the exposure to montelukast. Phenytoin is predicted to interact similarly.

Clinical evidence, mechanism, importance and management

In a study, montelukast 10 mg was given to 14 healthy subjects before and after they took **phenobarbital** 100 mg daily for 14 days. It was found that **phenobarbital** reduced the AUC and the maximum serum levels of the montelukast by 38% and 20%, respectively, but these effects are slight, and it was concluded that no montelukast dose adjustment is needed.[1] The reason for these reductions is almost certainly because phenobarbital induces CYP3A4, one of the isoenzymes involved in the metabolism of montelukast, so that its metabolism is increased. The manufacturer therefore advises caution if montelukast is given with inducers of CYP3A4, such as **phenytoin** and **phenobarbital**, especially in children.[2] It would seem prudent to extend this caution to **fosphenytoin** and **primidone**, which are metabolised to phenytoin and phenobarbital, respectively. However, there does not appear to be any clinical evidence to suggest that the montelukast dose needs adjustment in the presence of any of these drugs.

1. Holland S, Shahane A, Rogers JD, Porras A, Grasing K, Lasseter K, Pinto M, Freeman A, Gertz B, Amin R. Metabolism of montelukast (M) is increased by multiple doses of phenobarbital (P). *Clin Pharmacol Ther* (1998) 63, 231.
2. Singulair (Montelukast sodium). Merck Sharp & Dohme Ltd. UK Summary of product characteristics, June 2010.

Leukotriene antagonists; Montelukast + Antihistamines

Desloratadine had no effect on the pharmacokinetics of montelukast in a single-dose study. No increase in adverse effects appears to occur on the concurrent use of montelukast and loratadine.

Clinical evidence, mechanism, importance and management

In a crossover study in 22 healthy subjects, **desloratadine** did not alter the pharmacokinetics of a single 10-mg dose of montelukast.[1] An analysis of safety data from 19 studies in which subjects were given montelukast and **loratadine** found that the rate of adverse effects in those given the combination was similar to those given placebo, or either drug alone.[2]

No particular precautions would therefore seem necessary on the concurrent use of montelukast with desloratadine or loratadine.

1. Cingi C, Toros SZ, Ince I, Ertugay CK, Gurbuz MK, Cakli H, Erdogmus N, Karasulu E, Kaya E. Does desloratadine alter the serum levels of montelukast when administered in a fixed-dose combination? *Laryngoscope* (2013) 123, 2610–4.
2. Prenner BM, Lu S, Danzig MR. Safety of fixed-dose loratadine/montelukast in subjects with allergic rhinitis. Allergy Asthma Proc. (2010) 31, 493–8.

Leukotriene antagonists; Montelukast + Azoles

Fluconazole reduces the exposure to montelukast. Itraconazole appears to have no effect on the pharmacokinetics of montelukast.

Clinical evidence

(a) Fluconazole

In a crossover study, 12 healthy subjects were given fluconazole 50 mg or 150 mg daily for 7 days with a single 10-mg dose of montelukast on day 7. Fluconazole 50 mg and 150 mg reduced the AUC of montelukast by 39% and 31%, and its maximum plasma concentration by 45% and 38%, respectively.[1]

(b) Itraconazole

In a crossover study, 11 healthy subjects were given itraconazole 100 mg daily (first dose 200 mg) for 5 days, with a single 10-mg dose of montelukast on day 3. Itraconazole did not alter the pharmacokinetics of montelukast, when compared with montelukast given alone.[2]

Mechanism

Fluconazole is an inhibitor of CYP3A4 and CYP2C9, but it appears that CYP2C8 is primarily responsible for the metabolism of montelukast, with CYP3A4 having only a minor role.[2] Further study is needed to determine the exact mechanism for this interaction.

Importance and management

An interaction between montelukast and fluconazole is limited to one study. The small reduction in the exposure to montelukast seen does not appear to be clinically relevant, however the authors[1] suggest that concurrent use might lead to montelukast treatment failure. It would seem prudent to be aware of the potential for a decrease in the efficacy of montelukast on concurrent use of fluconazole.

No montelukast dose adjustment would seem necessary on concurrent use with itraconazole.

1. Hegazy SK, Mabrouk MM, Elsisi AE, Mansour NO. Effect of clarithromycin and fluconazole on the pharmacokinetics of montelukast in human volunteers. *Eur J Clin Pharmacol* (2012) 68, 1275–80.
2. Karonen T, Neuvonen PJ, Backman JT. CYP2C8 but not CYP3A4 is important in the pharmacokinetics of montelukast. *Br J Clin Pharmacol* (2012) 73, 257–67.

Leukotriene antagonists; Montelukast + Clarithromycin

Clarithromycin increases the exposure to montelukast

Clinical evidence, mechanism, importance and management

In a crossover study, 12 healthy subjects were given clarithromycin 1 g daily for 3 days with a single 10-mg dose of montelukast on day 3. Clarithromycin increased the AUC and maximum plasma concentration of montelukast 2.4-fold and 1.7-fold, respectively.[1]

Clarithromycin is a potent CYP3A4 inhibitor, but it appears that CYP2C8 is primarily responsible for the metabolism of montelukast, with CYP3A4 having only a minor role.[2] Further study is needed to determine the exact mechanism for this interaction.

The interaction between montelukast and clarithromycin is limited to this one study, but the moderate increase in montelukast exposure suggests it is likely to be clinically relevant. It would therefore be prudent to monitor concurrent use for an increase in montelukast adverse effects (abdominal pain, headache; and hyperkinesia in young children), and consider reducing the dose of montelukast should any adverse effects occur.

1. Hegazy SK, Mabrouk MM, Elsisi AE, Mansour NO. Effect of clarithromycin and fluconazole on the pharmacokinetics of montelukast in human volunteers. *Eur J Clin Pharmacol* (2012) 68, 1275–80.
2. Karonen T, Neuvonen PJ, Backman JT. CYP2C8 but not CYP3A4 is important in the pharmacokinetics of montelukast. *Br J Clin Pharmacol* (2012) 73, 257–67.

Leukotriene antagonists; Montelukast + Grapefruit juice and other fruit juices

Grapefruit juice increased montelukast exposure in one single-dose study, but not in another. Orange juice had no effect on the pharmacokinetics of montelukast in a single-dose study.

Clinical evidence, mechanism, importance and management

A study in 22 healthy subjects found that simultaneous administration of 250 mL of **grapefruit juice** increased the AUC and mean plasma concentration of a single 10-mg dose of montelukast about 1.4-fold.[1] In a study of 24 adolescents and young adults with asthma,[2] neither concentrated **grapefruit juice** nor **orange juice** had any effect on the pharmacokinetics of a single 10-mg dose of montelukast (relative to a *Gatorade* control).

Evidence for an interaction between montelukast and **grapefruit juice** is limited and somewhat conflicting. A small increase in montelukast exposure was seen in one study, but because of the known problems of possible variability of constituents between batches of grapefruit juice, an increase in montelukast adverse effects on concurrent use cannot be ruled out. No montelukast dose adjustment would seem necessary, but bear an interaction in mind should an increase in montelukast adverse effects occur.

Evidence for an interaction between montelukast and **orange juice** is limited to a small study and the minor decrease in exposure to montelukast would seem unlikely to be clinically relevant.

1. Cingi C, Toros SZ, Gürbüz MK, Ince I, Cakli H, Erdogmus N, Karasulu E, Kaya E. Effect of grapefruit juice on bioavailability of montelukast. *Laryngoscope* (2013) 123, 816–9.
2. Mougey EB, Lang JE, Wen X, Lima JJ. Effect of citrus juice and SLCO2B1 genotype on the pharmacokinetics of montelukast. J Clin Pharmacol. (2011) 51, 751–60.

Leukotriene antagonists; Montelukast + Rifampicin (Rifampin)

Rifampicin is predicted to reduce montelukast levels.

Clinical evidence, mechanism, importance and management

The manufacturer of montelukast advise caution if it is given with inducers of CYP3A4, such as rifampicin, especially in children.[1] This is because montelukast is partly metabolised by this isoenzyme, and phenobarbital, another inducer of CYP3A4, has been found to reduce the AUC and serum levels of montelukast (see 'Leukotriene antagonists; Montelukast + Antiepileptics; Enzyme-inducing', p.1430). However, there is currently no clinical evidence to suggest that the montelukast dose needs adjustment in patients taking inducers of CYP3A4, such as rifampicin.

1. Singulair (Montelukast sodium). Merck Sharp & Dohme Ltd. UK Summary of product characteristics, June 2010.

Leukotriene antagonists; Zafirlukast + Aspirin

Aspirin 650 mg four times daily is reported to have resulted in a mean 45% increase in the plasma levels of zafirlukast 40 mg daily. No further details are available.[1,2] The clinical importance of this interaction awaits assessment but it seems likely to be small.

1. Accolate (Zafirlukast). AstraZeneca Pharmaceuticals LP. US Prescribing information, February 2011.
2. Accolate (Zafirlukast). AstraZeneca UK Ltd. UK Summary of product characteristics, February 2011.

Leukotriene antagonists; Zafirlukast + Macrolides

Zafirlukast levels are decreased by erythromycin. Zafirlukast does not affect the pharmacokinetics of azithromycin or clarithromycin.

Clinical evidence, mechanism, importance and management

(a) Azithromycin or Clarithromycin

A study in 12 healthy subjects found that zafirlukast 20 mg twice daily, taken for 12 days, did not affect the pharmacokinetics of single 500-mg doses of azithromycin or clarithromycin.[1] *In vitro*, zafirlukast has been reported to inhibit CYP3A4, the isoenzyme by which these macrolides are metabolised; however, it appears that a clinically relevant interaction does not occur *in vivo*. No dose adjustments of azithromycin or clarithromycin are therefore needed if zafirlukast is also given.

(b) Erythromycin

A study in 11 patients with asthma found that erythromycin 500 mg three times daily for 5 days *reduced* the mean plasma level of zafirlukast 40 mg by about 40%.[2,3] This reduction in levels could reduce its efficacy. Until more is known, if erythromycin is given to patients taking zafirlukast, be alert for a reduced response to zafirlukast.

1. Garey KW, Peloquin CA, Godo PG, Nafziger AN, Amsden GW. Lack of effect of zafirlukast on the pharmacokinetics of azithromycin, clarithromycin and 14-hydroxyclarithromycin in healthy volunteers. *Antimicrob Agents Chemother* (1999) 43, 1152–5.
2. Accolate (Zafirlukast). AstraZeneca Pharmaceuticals LP. US Prescribing information, February 2011.
3. Accolate (Zafirlukast). AstraZeneca UK Ltd. UK Summary of product characteristics, February 2011.

Leukotriene antagonists; Zafirlukast + Miscellaneous

Zafirlukast is predicted to increase the levels of a number of CYP3A4 substrates (e.g. dihydropyridine calcium-channel blockers).

Clinical evidence, mechanism, importance and management

Because of the apparent *in vitro* effect of zafirlukast on CYP3A4, the US manufacturer of zafirlukast advises appropriate clinical monitoring when substrates of CYP3A4 are given with zafirlukast: they name **ciclosporin** and **dihydropyridine calcium-channel blockers**.[1] However, clinical studies show that zafirlukast does not affect the pharmacokinetics of the CYP3A4 substrate terfenadine (see 'Table 39.2', p.1600), and therefore it would appear that any effect of zafirlukast on CYP3A4 is not clinically relevant.

1. Accolate (Zafirlukast). AstraZeneca Pharmaceuticals LP. US Prescribing information, February 2011.

Leukotriene antagonists; Zafirlukast + Tobacco

The UK manufacturer notes that the clearance of zafirlukast might be increased by 20% in patients who smoke.[1] This probably occurs because tobacco smoke can induce liver enzymes, which may increase the metabolism of zafirlukast. The clinical significance of this interaction is unclear, but it seems likely to be small.

1. Accolate (Zafirlukast). AstraZeneca UK Ltd. UK Summary of product characteristics, February 2011.

Omalizumab + Miscellaneous

The UK manufacturer of omalizumab states that clinical studies found no evidence to suggest that the safety of omalizumab was altered when it was used with inhaled or oral corticosteroids, inhaled short-acting and long-acting beta$_2$ agonists, leukotriene modifiers [presumably leukotriene antagonists], theophylline or oral antihistamines.[1]

1. Xolair (Omalizumab). Novartis Pharmaceuticals UK Ltd. UK Summary of product characteristics, November 2010.

Pirfenidone + Antacids

Aluminium/magnesium hydroxide (with simeticone)-containing antacids do not appear to affect the pharmacokinetics of pirfenidone.

Clinical evidence, mechanism, importance and management

In a crossover study in 16 healthy subjects, a single 801-mg dose of pirfenidone was given either alone or with an **aluminium/magnesium hydroxide** (with **simeticone**) antacid (*Mylanta Maximum Strength*) in both the fed and fasted state.[1] There were no changes in the pharmacokinetics of pirfenidone. There would therefore appear to be no reason to avoid the concurrent use of pirfenidone and this type of antacid.

1. Rubino CM, Bhavnani SM, Ambrose PG, Forrest A, Loutit JS. Effect of food and antacids on the pharmacokinetics of pirfenidone in older healthy adults. *Pulm Pharmacol Ther* (2009) 22, 279–85.

Pirfenidone + Food

Food reduces the maximum plasma concentration of pirfenidone but not the overall exposure.

Clinical evidence, mechanism, importance and management

In a study in 16 healthy subjects, administration of a single 801-mg dose of pirfenidone with food resulted in a 50% lower maximum plasma concentration than in the fasted state, but the AUC was about 80 to 85% of that seen in the fasted stated. The rate of absorption was also slower in the fed state. It was also observed that there was a lower incidence of central nervous system and gastrointestinal adverse effects in the fed subjects.[1] Pirfenidone should therefore be administered with food to reduce the incidence of dizziness and nausea.[2]

1. Rubino CM, Bhavnani SM, Ambrose PG, Forrest A, Loutit JS. Effect of food and antacids on the pharmacokinetics of pirfenidone in older healthy adults. *Pulm Pharmacol Ther* (2009) 22, 279–85.
2. Esbriet (Pirfenidone). Roche Products Ltd. UK Summary of product characteristics, September 2015.

Pirfenidone + Miscellaneous

Smoking reduces the exposure to pirfenidone, and other inducers of CYP1A2 are predicted to interact similarly. Fluvoxamine and ciprofloxacin increase the exposure to pirfenidone, and other potent and moderate inhibitors of CYP1A2 are predicted to interact similarly. Potent inhibitors of other isoenzymes involved in the metabolism of pirfenidone, such as CYP2C9, CYP2C19, and CYP2D6 might also increase the exposure to pirfenidone.

Clinical evidence, mechanism, importance and management

(a) CYP1A2 inducers

The UK manufacturer briefly notes that, in a phase 1 study, exposure to pirfenidone in smokers was 50% lower than that in non-smokers.[1] Pirfenidone is primarily metabolised by CYP1A2, which is known to be induced by smoking, so that metabolism of pirfenidone in smokers might be greater than in non-smokers. The manufacturer therefore advises that smoking should be avoided and that patients should be encouraged to stop smoking before and during treatment with pirfenidone.[1] In addition, they advise that other potent CYP1A2 inducers should be avoided. The concurrent use of moderate inducers of CYP1A2 (the manufacturer names **omeprazole**) might theoretically result in reduced plasma pirfenidone concentrations.[1] Other drugs that are potent inducers of CYP1A2 and other isoenzymes involved in the metabolism of pirfenidone (the manufacturer names **rifampicin**) should be avoided as concurrent use is predicted to result in a sizeable reduction in plasma pirfenidone concentrations.[1] However, note that omeprazole is not a known inducer of CYP1A2 and rifampicin generally only has weak inducing effects on CYP1A2. For a list of CYP1A2 inducers, see 'Table 1.2', p.5. Omeprazole is a weak to moderate inhibitor of CYP2C19, see *CYP2C19 inhibitors* below.

(b) CYP1A2 inhibitors

The UK manufacturer of pirfenidone briefly notes that, in a phase 1 study, **fluvoxamine** caused a 4-fold increase in the exposure to pirfenidone in non-smokers.[1] Fluvoxamine is a known potent inhibitor of CYP1A2, which is the principle isoenzyme involved in the metabolism of pirfenidone, and so concurrent use reduces its metabolism, resulting in increased exposure. The concurrent use of fluvoxamine and pirfenidone is therefore contraindicated.[1] The manufacturer also notes that fluvoxamine has inhibitory effects on other isoenzymes involved in the metabolism of pirfenidone and they name CYP2C9, CYP2C19, and CYP2D6 (although fluvoxamine does not usually affect CYP2D6). They state that the concurrent use of pirfenidone with other drugs that inhibit CYP1A2 and one or more of these isoenzymes should also be avoided.[1] Other potent inhibitors of CYP1A2 (see 'Table 1.2', p.5 for a list) are expected to increase the exposure to pirfenidone, and the manufacturer states that if concurrent use is unavoidable, the dose of pirfenidone should be reduced to 801 mg daily and the patient monitored for an increase in adverse effects.[1]

The UK manufacturer of pirfenidone briefly notes that **ciprofloxacin** 750 mg increased the AUC of pirfenidone by 81%. If concurrent use of this dose of ciprofloxacin is unavoidable, they recommend reducing the dose of pirfenidone to 1 602 mg daily. Pirfenidone should be used with caution in patients taking lower doses of ciprofloxacin or other moderate inhibitors of CYP1A2 (the manufacturer names **amiodarone** and **propafenone**), and they also recommend that the consumption of **grapefruit juice** should be avoided due to inhibition of CYP1A2.[1] However, note that amiodarone and grapefruit juice are not known to have clinically relevant effects on this isoenzyme, and propafenone is generally considered to be a weak inhibitor. For a list of known CYP1A2 inhibitors, see 'Table 1.2', p.5.

(c) CYP2C9 inhibitors

The UK manufacturer of pirfenidone states that special care should be exercised if CYP1A2 inhibitors are used concurrently with potent inhibitors of one or more of the other isoenzymes involved in the metabolism of pirfenidone, such as CYP2C9, and they name **amiodarone** and **fluconazole**.[1] Note that the effects of both of these drugs on CYP2C9 are generally considered to be weak to moderate. For a list of CYP2C9 inhibitors, see 'Table 1.5', p.7. Fluconazole in low doses (100 mg daily) is also a potent inhibitor of CYP2C19, see below.

(d) CYP2C19 inhibitors

The UK manufacturer of pirfenidone states that special care should be exercised if CYP1A2 inhibitors are used concurrently with potent inhibitors of one or more of the other isoenzymes involved in the metabolism of pirfenidone, such as CYP2C19, and they name **chloramphenicol**. Note that chloramphenicol is not generally considered to cause clinically relevant inhibition of this isoenzyme. For a list of known CYP2C19 inhibitors, see 'Table 1.6', p.8.

(e) CYP2D6 inhibitors

The UK manufacturer of pirfenidone states that special care should be exercised if CYP1A2 inhibitors are used concurrently with potent inhibitors of one or more of the other isoenzymes involved in the metabolism of pirfenidone, such as CYP2D6, and they name **fluoxetine** and **paroxetine**.[1] For a list of known CYP2D6 inhibitors, see 'Table 1.7', p.9.

1. Esbriet (Pirfenidone). Roche Products Ltd. UK Summary of product characteristics, September 2015.

Roflumilast + Antacids

Aluminium/magnesium hydroxide-containing antacids do not appear to affect the pharmacokinetics of roflumilast or its active metabolite.

Clinical evidence, mechanism, importance and management

In a study, 30 healthy subjects were given a single 500-microgram dose of roflumilast alone, with, or 2 hours before, 30 mL of an **aluminium/magnesium hydroxide**-containing antacid (*Maalox*). There were no changes in the pharmacokinetics of roflumilast or its active metabolite, roflumilast *N*-oxide.[1] There would therefore appear to be no reason to avoid the concurrent use of roflumilast and this type of antacid.

1. Nassr N, Lahu G, Hünnemeyer A, von Richter O, Knoerzer D, Reutter F, Zech K, Hermann R. Magnesium hydroxide/aluminium hydroxide-containing antacid does not affect the pharmacokinetics of the targeted phosphodiesterase 4 inhibitor roflumilast. *J Clin Pharmacol* (2007) 47, 660–6.

Roflumilast + Beta-agonist bronchodilators

No pharmacokinetic interaction appears to occur between roflumilast and inhaled salbutamol (albuterol), and no interaction has been reported on the concurrent use of roflumilast and inhaled formoterol.

Clinical evidence, mechanism, importance and management

In a study, 12 healthy subjects were given oral roflumilast 500 micrograms daily, inhaled **salbutamol** (**albuterol**) 200 micrograms three times daily, or both drugs together, for 7 days. The pharmacokinetics of roflumilast and its active metabolite, roflumilast *N*-oxide, were not significantly altered by **salbutamol**, and the pharmacokinetics of inhaled salbutamol were not significantly affected by roflumilast.[1] Therefore, no dose adjustments of either drug appear to be necessary on the concurrent use of roflumilast and inhaled salbutamol.

The UK manufacturer of roflumilast briefly states that no interactions have been reported on the concurrent use of inhaled **formoterol**.[2]

1. Bethke TD, Giessmann T, Westphal K, Weinbrenner A, Hauns B, Hauschke D, David M, Lahu G, Zech K, Hermann R, Siegmund W. Roflumilast, a once-daily oral phosphodiesterase 4 inhibitor, lacks relevant pharmacokinetic interactions with inhaled salbutamol when co-administered in healthy subjects. *Int J Clin Pharmacol Ther* (2006) 44, 572–9.
2. Daxas (Roflumilast). Takeda UK Ltd. UK Summary of product characteristics, August 2013.

Roflumilast + Budesonide

The concurrent use of roflumilast and inhaled budesonide does not appear to affect the pharmacokinetics of either drug.

Clinical evidence, mechanism, importance and management

In a crossover study, 12 healthy subjects were given oral roflumilast 500 micrograms daily for 7 days, inhaled budesonide 800 micrograms twice daily for 7 days, or both drugs together. Budesonide did not affect the pharmacokinetics of roflumilast measured on day 7, and there were no significant changes in the pharmacokinetics of budesonide. There was, however, a wide variation in parameters between subjects.[1] No dose adjustments of either roflumilast or inhaled budesonide are therefore expected to be necessary on concurrent use.

1. Hermann R, Siegmund W, Giessmann T, Westphal K, Weinbrenner A, Hauns B, Reutter F, Lahu G, Zech K, Bethke TD. The oral, once-daily phosphodiesterase 4 inhibitor roflumilast lacks relevant pharmacokinetic interactions with inhaled budesonide. *J Clin Pharmacol* (2007) 47, 1005–13.

Roflumilast + Cimetidine

Cimetidine increased the exposure to roflumilast and its active metabolite, roflumilast *N*-oxide, and increased its phosphodiesterase type-4 inhibitory effect.

Clinical evidence

In a crossover study, 16 healthy subjects were given a single 500-microgram oral dose of roflumilast alone, and after taking oral cimetidine 400 mg twice daily for 8 days. The AUC and maximum plasma levels of roflumilast were increased by 85% and 46%, respectively. The AUC of its active metabolite, roflumilast *N*-oxide, was increased by 44%, whereas the maximum plasma levels of roflumilast *N*-oxide were reduced by 4%. These changes resulted in an increase in the total phosphodiesterase type-4 inhibitory activity of roflumilast (that is, the combined effect of roflumilast and its active metabolite, roflumilast *N*-oxide) of 47%; however, no serious or unexpected adverse effects were reported.[1]

Mechanism

Roflumilast is metabolised to its active metabolite, roflumilast *N*-oxide, by CYP1A2 and CYP3A4. Roflumilast *N*-oxide is in turn metabolised by CYP3A4, and, to a lesser extent, by CYP2C19. Cimetidine is a weak inhibitor of these isoenzymes and therefore, concurrent use increases the exposure to both roflumilast and roflumilast *N*-oxide, which results in an increase in the total phosphodiesterase type-4 inhibition.

Importance and management

Evidence for an interaction between roflumilast and cimetidine appears to be limited to this study, which only gave a single dose of roflumilast. However, as the total phosphodiesterase type-4 inhibitory activity of roflumilast was increased by nearly 50% it is possible that, with multiple doses of roflumilast, some patients might develop roflumilast adverse effects (e.g. nausea, diarrhoea, headache). If these persist, or are particularly troublesome, if possible, reduce the roflumilast dose. Alternatively, consider replacing cimetidine with an alternative treatment, such as another H_2-receptor antagonist (other H_2-receptor antagonists are not associated with enzyme inhibitory effects); however, note that the concurrent use of roflumilast with these drugs has not been studied and so the presence of an interaction cannot entirely be ruled out.

1. Böhmer GM, Gleiter CH, Mörike K, Nassr N, Walz A, Lahu G. No dose adjustment on coadministration of the PDE4 inhibitor roflumilast with a weak CYP3A, CYP1A2, and CYP2C19 inhibitor: an investigation using cimetidine. *J Clin Pharmacol* (2011) 51, 594–602.

Roflumilast + Combined hormonal contraceptives

Combined hormonal contraceptives do not appear to have a clinically relevant effect on the pharmacodynamic effects of roflumilast.

Clinical evidence, mechanism, importance and management

The UK manufacturer of roflumilast briefly reports that, in an interaction study, the concurrent use of an oral combined hormonal contraceptive (**ethinylestradiol** with **gestodene**) increased the total phosphodiesterase type-4 inhibitory effect of roflumilast (i.e. the combined effect of roflumilast and its active metabolite, roflumilast *N*-oxide) by 17%.[1] Although the available data from this study is limited, this slight increase in the pharmacodynamic effect of roflumilast would not be expected to be clinically relevant, therefore no dose adjustment is necessary.

1. Daxas (Roflumilast). Takeda UK Ltd. UK Summary of product characteristics, August 2013.

Roflumilast + Erythromycin

Erythromycin inhibits the metabolism of roflumilast to its active *N*-oxide metabolite but this does not appear to affect the total phosphodiesterase type-4 inhibitory effects to a clinically relevant extent.

Clinical evidence

In a study, 18 healthy subjects were given a single 500-mg dose of erythromycin (as ethylsuccinate) alone or on day 11 of taking roflumilast 500 micrograms daily for

11 days. Erythromycin had no effect on the pharmacokinetics of roflumilast and its active metabolite, roflumilast *N*-oxide, and there were no clinically significant changes in the pharmacokinetics of erythromycin. In addition, vital signs, ECG and laboratory parameters were not altered to a clinically relevant extent by concurrent use.[1]

In a crossover study, 15 healthy subjects were given a single 500-microgram dose of roflumilast before and on day 7 of taking erythromycin 500 mg three times daily. Erythromycin increased the maximum levels and AUC of roflumilast by 40% and 70%, respectively. The AUC of the active metabolite, roflumilast *N*-oxide, was unchanged, but its maximum levels were decreased by 34%, and the time to maximum levels was delayed. However, the total phosphodiesterase type-4 inhibitory effects of roflumilast and its *N*-oxide metabolite were only increased by 9%, and the incidence of clinically relevant adverse effects was not increased by concurrent use.[2]

Mechanism

Roflumilast is metabolised by CYP1A2 and CYP3A4 to its active metabolite roflumilast *N*-oxide. Roflumilast *N*-oxide is in turn metabolised by CYP3A4, and probably to a lesser extent by CYP2C19. Drugs that are inhibitors of CYP3A4, such as erythromycin, inhibit the metabolism of roflumilast thereby increasing roflumilast levels and reducing the formation of its active metabolite. However, as the metabolism of the active metabolite is also inhibited, its overall exposure is unchanged. The total phosphodiesterase type-4 inhibition is the combined effects of both roflumilast and its *N*-oxide, and this appears to be only slightly affected by erythromycin.

Importance and management

Evidence for an interaction between roflumilast and erythromycin is limited to one single-dose study and one multiple-dose study, but a pharmacokinetic interaction with multiple-dose erythromycin appears to be established. However, as the overall phosphodiesterase type-4 inhibition caused by roflumilast and its active *N*-oxide metabolite appears to be unchanged, these pharmacokinetic changes are not considered clinically relevant. No roflumilast dose adjustments are therefore expected to be necessary on concurrent use.

1. Hauns B, Huennemeyer A, Siegmund W, Waitzinger J, Hermann R, Zech K, Bethke TD. Pharmacokinetics of the selective PDE4 inhibitor roflumilast and its active metabolite roflumilast N-oxide are not affected by concomitant budesonide, salbutamol or erythromycin. *J Allergy Clin Immunol* (2004) 113 (Suppl), S222.
2. Lahu G, Huennemeyer A, Herzog R, McCracken N, Hermann R, Elmlinger M, Zech K. Effect of repeated dose of erythromycin on the pharmacokinetics of roflumilast and roflumilast N-oxide. *Int J Clin Pharmacol Ther* (2009) 47, 236–45.

Roflumilast + Fluvoxamine

The exposure to roflumilast and its active metabolite, roflumilast *N*-oxide, is increased by fluvoxamine, resulting in an overall increase in its total phosphodiesterase inhibitory effects.

Clinical evidence

In a crossover study, 14 healthy subjects were given a single 500-microgram dose of roflumilast alone, or after they had taken fluvoxamine 50 mg daily for 8 days. Fluvoxamine increased the AUC of roflumilast and its active metabolite, roflumilast *N*-oxide, 2.6-fold and by 50%, respectively. In addition, the maximum plasma levels of roflumilast *N*-oxide decreased by 20%. There was an overall increase of 59% in total phosphodiesterase type-4 inhibitory activity (that is, the total activity of roflumilast and its *N*-oxide metabolite) but there were no clinically relevant changes in laboratory measurements, blood pressure, pulse or ECG, nor were there any serious or unexpected adverse effects.[1]

Mechanism

Roflumilast is metabolised by CYP1A2 and CYP3A4 to its active metabolite roflumilast *N*-oxide. Roflumilast *N*-oxide is in turn metabolised by CYP3A4, and probably to a lesser extent by CYP2C19. Fluvoxamine inhibits CYP1A2 and CYP2C19, and therefore concurrent use increases the exposure to both roflumilast and roflumilast *N*-oxide.

Importance and management

Evidence for an interaction between roflumilast and fluvoxamine appears to be limited to this study. Nevertheless, the increases in the levels of roflumilast and its active metabolite would be expected to be generally relevant as they resulted in increases in the overall phosphodiesterase type-4 inhibition. Although concurrent use might increase the efficacy of roflumilast, it seems possible that some patients might also develop roflumilast adverse effects (e.g. nausea, diarrhoea, headache). If these persist, or are particularly troublesome, if possible, reduce the roflumilast dose. Alternatively, consider replacing fluvoxamine with other suitable treatments, which might include other SSRIs. However, note that there appears to be no direct information regarding the concurrent use of roflumilast and other SSRIs. Furthermore, note that roflumilast is associated with an increased risk of psychiatric disorders including depression,[2] and therefore its use in those requiring antidepressants should be carefully considered.

1. von Richter O, Lahu G, Huennemeyer A, Herzog R, Zech K, Hermann R. Effect of fluvoxamine on the pharmacokinetics of roflumilast and roflumilast *N*-oxide. *Clin Pharmacokinet* (2007) 46, 613–22.
2. Daxas (Roflumilast). Takeda UK Ltd. UK Summary of product characteristics, August 2013.

Roflumilast + Food

Food delays and reduces the maximum levels of roflumilast, but does not affect its overall bioavailability, or the pharmacokinetics of its active metabolite to a clinically relevant extent.

Clinical evidence, mechanism, importance and management

In a crossover study in 12 healthy subjects, a single 500-microgram dose of roflumilast was given after an overnight fast, or within 5 minutes of a high-fat, high-calorie breakfast. Food delayed the maximum plasma levels of roflumilast (from one hour to 2 hours), and its maximum plasma levels were reduced by 40%. However, the AUC of roflumilast and the pharmacokinetics of its active metabolite, roflumilast *N*-oxide, were not altered to a clinically relevant extent.[1] Therefore roflumilast may be taken with or without food.

1. Hauns B, Hermann R, Hünnemeyer A, Herzog R, Hauschke D, Zech K, Bethke TD. Investigation of a potential food effect on the pharmacokinetics of roflumilast, an oral once-daily phosphodiesterase 4 inhibitor, in healthy subjects. *J Clin Pharmacol* (2006) 46, 1146–53.

Roflumilast + Ketoconazole

Ketoconazole inhibits the metabolism of roflumilast to its active *N*-oxide metabolite but does not affect the overall phosphodiesterase type-4 inhibitory activity to a clinically relevant extent.

Clinical evidence

In a study, 24 healthy subjects were given roflumilast 500 micrograms daily for 11 days, with a single 200-mg dose of ketoconazole on day 11. Ketoconazole increased the AUC of roflumilast by 34%, but its maximum plasma levels were unaffected. The AUC of the active metabolite, roflumilast *N*-oxide, was reduced by 12% by ketoconazole, and its maximum plasma levels were reduced by 20%. The total phosphodiesterase-4 inhibitory activity of roflumilast and its active metabolite was unaltered, suggesting that these changes were not clinically relevant.[1]

In a related crossover study, 16 healthy subjects were given ketoconazole 200 mg twice daily, with single 500-microgram dose of roflumilast when ketoconazole steady-state levels were achieved. Ketoconazole increased the AUC and maximum plasma levels of roflumilast by 99% and 23%, respectively. The maximum plasma levels of the active metabolite, roflumilast *N*-oxide were reduced by 38% by ketoconazole, and its half-life was prolonged from 9.6 hours to 21.5 hours. However, the total phosphodiesterase-4 inhibitory activity of roflumilast and its active metabolite was only slightly increased, and no clinically relevant adverse effects were seen, suggesting that these changes are not clinically relevant.[1]

Mechanism

Roflumilast is metabolised to its active metabolite, roflumilast *N*-oxide, by CYP1A2 and CYP3A4, and it is thought that the clearance of roflumilast *N*-oxide is also reliant on CYP3A4. Ketoconazole, an inhibitor of CYP3A4, therefore reduces the formation of the active metabolite, decreasing its levels, but also reduces roflumilast clearance, increasing its exposure. However, the total phosphodiesterase type-4 inhibition is the combined effects of both roflumilast and its *N*-oxide, and this was only slightly increased by ketoconazole.

Importance and management

Evidence for an interaction between roflumilast and ketoconazole is limited to the related studies described above. A pharmacokinetic interaction would appear to be established; however, as the overall phosphodiesterase type-4 inhibition by roflumilast and its active *N*-oxide metabolite appears to be unchanged, the pharmacokinetic changes do not appear to be clinically relevant. No roflumilast dose adjustments are therefore expected to be necessary if it is given with ketoconazole.

1. Lahu G, Huennemeyer A, von Richter O, Hermann R, Herzog R, McCracken N, Zech K. Effect of single and repeated doses of ketoconazole on the pharmacokinetics of roflumilast and roflumilast N-oxide. *J Clin Pharmacol* (2008) 48, 1339–49.

Roflumilast + Montelukast

No pharmacokinetic interaction appears to occur between roflumilast and montelukast.

Clinical evidence, mechanism, importance and management

In a study, 24 healthy subjects were given roflumilast 500 micrograms daily with montelukast 10 mg daily for 9 days. Compared with the use of either drug alone, concurrent use did not result in any clinically relevant changes in the pharmacokinetics of roflumilast or montelukast.[1] No dose adjustments would therefore be expected to be necessary on their concurrent use.

1. Böhmer GM, Nassr N, Wenger M, Hünnemeyer A, Lahu G, Templin S, Gleiter CH, Hermann R. The targeted oral, once-daily phosphodiesterase 4 inhibitor roflumilast and the leukotriene receptor antagonist montelukast do not exhibit significant pharmacokinetic interactions. *J Clin Pharmacol* (2009) 49, 389–97.

Roflumilast + Quinolones

Enoxacin increases the exposure to roflumilast and its active metabolite, roflumilast *N*-oxide, and increases its phosphodiesterase type-4 inhibitory effect. It seems possible that some other quinolones might interact similarly.

Clinical evidence

In a study, 19 healthy subjects were given a single 500-microgram oral dose of roflumilast alone, and on day 6 of a 12-day course of oral enoxacin 400 mg twice daily. Enoxacin increased the AUC, maximum plasma levels, and half-life of roflumilast by 56%, 20%, and 25%, respectively. The AUC and half life of the active metabolite, roflumilast *N*-oxide, were increased by 22% and 52%, respectively, whereas its maximum plasma levels were reduced by 14%. The time to maximum plasma concentration was halved for roflumilast, and doubled for roflumilast *N*-oxide. These changes resulted in an increase in total phosphodiesterase type-4 inhibitory activity (that is, the total effect of roflumilast and its *N*-oxide metabolite) of about 25%. One adverse effect (headache) was reported as severe, but this had resolved without further intervention at the end of the study.[1]

Mechanism

Roflumilast is metabolised to its active metabolite, roflumilast *N*-oxide, by CYP1A2 and CYP3A4. Enoxacin is a potent inhibitor of CYP1A2, and thus increases the exposure to roflumilast. However, the metabolism of roflumilast to roflumilast *N*-oxide by CYP3A4 will continue. Exposure to roflumilast *N*-oxide is increased via the effect (i.e. its production by CYP3A4 occurs more slowly than its metabolism by CYP3A4 and CYP2C19).

Importance and management

Evidence for an interaction between roflumilast and enoxacin appears to be limited to this study. Nevertheless, the increases in the levels of roflumilast and its active metabolite would not be expected to be generally relevant as they resulted in only slight increases in the overall phosphodiesterase type-4 inhibition. However, as this study only used a single dose of roflumilast it seems possible that some patients might develop roflumilast adverse effects (e.g. nausea, diarrhoea, headache) when given multiple doses of roflumilast. If these persist, or are particularly troublesome, if possible, reduce the roflumilast dose. Alternatively, consider replacing enoxacin with another suitable antibacterial, which might include one of the other quinolones. However, note that some quinolones also inhibit CYP1A2, although to a lesser extent than enoxacin (e.g. **ciprofloxacin**) and might therefore affect the metabolism of roflumilast. For a more detailed discussion of the relative CYP1A2 inhibitory potencies of various quinolones, see 'Caffeine + Quinolones', p.1426.

1. Lahu G, Nassr N, Herzog R, Elmlinger M, Ruth P, Hinder M, Huennemeyer A. Effect of steady-state enoxacin on single-dose pharmacokinetics of roflumilast and roflumilast N-oxide. *J Clin Pharmacol* (2011) 51, 586–93.

Roflumilast + Rifampicin (Rifampin) and other enzyme inducers

Rifampicin increases the metabolism of roflumilast to its active metabolite, roflumilast *N*-oxide, but decreases the overall bioavailability of roflumilast *N*-oxide and might reduce its therapeutic effects. Other enzyme inducers (e.g. carbamazepine) are predicted to interact similarly.

Clinical evidence, mechanism, importance and management

In a study, 15 healthy subjects were given a single 500-microgram dose of roflumilast alone or after taking rifampicin 600 mg daily for 8 days. Rifampicin reduced the AUC and maximum plasma levels of roflumilast by 79% and 68%, respectively. In addition, the AUC of the active metabolite, roflumilast *N*-oxide, was reduced by 56%, while its maximum plasma levels were increased by 30%. The total phosphodiesterase type-4 inhibitory activity (that is, the combined activity of roflumilast and its *N*-oxide metabolite) was reduced by 58%.[1]

Rifampicin induces the activity of CYP3A4, and, to a lesser extent, CYP1A2, which are involved in the metabolism of both roflumilast and roflumilast-*N*-oxide, leading to an increase in the clearance of both the drug and its metabolite. It is probable that the dose of roflumilast will need to be increased in patients also taking rifampicin. The UK manufacturer[2] of roflumilast predicts that other inducers of cytochrome P450 might also increase the metabolism of roflumilast and its active metabolite: they name **carbamazepine, phenobarbital** and **phenytoin**; however, note that as **fosphenytoin** is a prodrug of phenytoin, and **primidone** is metabolised to phenobarbital, they would also be expected to interact in the same way.

If a patient taking roflumilast is given any of these enzyme inducers it would seem prudent to be aware of the likely decrease in its efficacy and consider increasing the dose of roflumilast, according to clinical need.

1. Nassr N, Huennemeyer A, Herzog R, von Richter O, Hermann R, Koch M, Duffy K, Zech K, Lahu G. Effects of rifampicin on the pharmacokinetics of roflumilast and roflumilast-N-oxide in healthy subjects. *Br J Clin Pharmacol* (2009) 68, 580–7.
2. Daxas (Roflumilast). Takeda UK Ltd. UK Summary of product characteristics, August 2013.

Roflumilast + Sildenafil

The UK manufacturer of roflumilast briefly reports that no interaction has been seen between roflumilast and sildenafil.[1] There appear to be no published data regarding this; however, it would seem that no particular precautions are necessary on the concurrent use of roflumilast and sildenafil.

1. Daxas (Roflumilast). Takeda UK Ltd. UK Summary of product characteristics, August 2013.

Roflumilast + Theophylline

Theophylline slightly increases the exposure to roflumilast, but roflumilast has no effect on the exposure to theophylline.

Clinical evidence, mechanism, importance and management

In a crossover study in 24 healthy subjects, theophylline 375 mg twice daily for 5 days increased the AUC of roflumilast 500 micrograms daily by 28%, but had no effect on the exposure to its active metabolite, roflumilast *N*-oxide. The exposure to theophylline was also unaffected.[1] Despite this only slight increase in roflumilast exposure, due to a lack of clinical data on concurrent use, the UK manufacturer does not recommend concurrent use.[2] In contrast, the US manufacturer advises that no roflumilast dose adjustment is necessary on concurrent use.[3]

1. Böhmer G, Gleiter CH, Hünnemeyer A, Lahu G, Bethke TD. Study investigating pharmacokinetic interaction between theophylline and roflumilast in healthy adults. *Int J Clin Pharmacol Ther* (2011) 49, 451–60.
2. Daxas (Roflumilast). Takeda UK Ltd. UK Summary of product characteristics, August 2013.
3. Daliresp (Roflumilast). Forest Pharmaceuticals, Inc. US Prescribing information, September 2014.

Roflumilast + Tobacco

Smoking tobacco has a minimal effect on the pharmacokinetics and pharmacodynamic effects of roflumilast.

Clinical evidence

In a parallel-group study, the effect of smoking (defined as more than 18 cigarettes/day for at least 2 years) on the pharmacokinetics of a single 500-microgram dose of roflumilast was studied. There were no differences in the pharmacokinetics of roflumilast between the smokers (12 subjects) and the non-smokers (12 subjects).[1] Further, the US manufacturer of roflumilast reports that the AUC of roflumilast in the smokers was 13% lower than in the non-smokers, and the AUC of the active *N*-oxide metabolite was 17% higher in the non-smokers than in the smokers. Maximum plasma concentrations were no different between the groups.[2] In a population pharmacokinetic modelling study, the total phosphodiesterase type-4 inhibitory activity (that is, the combined inhibitory activity of roflumilast and its *N*-oxide metabolite) in smokers was found to be about 19% lower than in non-smokers.[3]

Mechanism

Roflumilast is metabolised to its active metabolite, roflumilast *N*-oxide, by CYP1A2 and CYP3A4. The polycyclic hydrocarbons present in tobacco smoke act as inducers of CYP1A2, thereby enhancing the rate at which roflumilast is converted to roflumilast *N*-oxide. However, the CYP3A4 and CYP2C19-mediated metabolism of roflumilast *N*-oxide remains unaffected. As a result, the overall effect of CYP1A2 induction is likely to be minimal.[4]

Importance and management

Evidence for a pharmacokinetic interaction between roflumilast and smoking is limited, but suggests that any effect is negligible at best. Furthermore, the reduction in total phosphodiesterase type-4 inhibitory activity in smokers would not be expected to be clinically important. No roflumilast dose adjustments would appear to be necessary in smokers.

1. Bethke T, Hünnemeyer A, Hauns B, Diedrich A, Baumgartner A, Eichberger C, Drollmann A, Hartmann M, Neuhäuser M, David M, Zech K, Wurst W. Smoking has no effect on the pharmacokinetics of roflumilast, a new, orally active, selective PDE4 inhibitor. European Respiratory Society Annual Congress, Berlin, 2001. Abstract 1061. Available at: http://www.ers-education.org/events/international-congress/berlin-2001.aspx?idParent=29601 (accessed 21/10/15).
2. Daliresp (Roflumilast). Nycomed GmbH. US Prescribing information, September 2014.
3. Lahu G, Hünnemeyer A, Diletti E, Elmlinger M, Ruth P, Zech K, McCracken N, Facius A. Population pharmacokinetic modelling of roflumilast and roflumilast *N*-oxide by total phosphodiesterase-4 inhibitory activity and development of a population pharmacodynamic-adverse event model. *Clin Pharmacokinet* (2010) 49, 589–606.
4. Giembycz MA, Field SK. Roflumilast: first phosphodiesterase 4 inhibitor approved for treatment of COPD. *Drug Des Devel Ther* (2010) 4, 147–58.

Terbutaline + Magnesium sulfate

Subcutaneous terbutaline and intravenous magnesium sulfate do not appear to interact adversely.

Clinical evidence, mechanism, importance and management

In a study, 8 healthy adults were given two 250-microgram subcutaneous doses of terbutaline 30 minutes apart, with and without intravenous magnesium sulfate 4 g in 250 mL of sodium chloride 0.9%, given over the same 30-minute period.[1] Most of the effects of terbutaline, such as those on respiratory rate, blood pressure, glucose and calcium levels, were found to be moderately increased by magnesium sulfate at 60 minutes, but these changes were all considered to be small. The authors concluded that there does not appear to be any reason to avoid the concurrent use of terbutaline and magnesium sulfate, for example in the emergency treatment of asthma and other conditions.

1. Skorodin MS, Freebeck PC, Yetter B, Nelson JE, Van de Graaff WB, Walsh JM. Magnesium sulfate potentiates several cardiovascular and metabolic actions of terbutaline. *Chest* (1994) 105, 701–5.

Theophylline + Aciclovir

Preliminary evidence suggests that aciclovir can increase the levels of theophylline.

Clinical evidence

Prompted by a case of increased theophylline adverse effects in a patient given aciclovir, a study was carried out in 5 healthy subjects who were given a single 320-mg dose of theophylline (as 400 mg of aminophylline) before and with the sixth dose of aciclovir 800 mg five times daily for 2 days. The AUC of theophylline was increased by 45% and its total body clearance was reduced by 30% by aciclovir.[1]

Mechanism

Uncertain, but the authors of the study suggest that aciclovir inhibits the metabolism of theophylline, resulting in accumulation.[1]

Importance and management

The evidence for an interaction between theophylline or aminophylline and aciclovir appears to be limited to this isolated report, and an interaction is not established. However, be alert for an increase in the adverse effects of theophylline (nausea, headache, tremor) if aciclovir is added to established treatment, and consider monitoring theophylline levels. Further study is needed to confirm an interaction.

1. Maeda Y, Konishi T, Omoda K, Takeda Y, Fukuhara S, Fukuzawa M, Ohune T, Tsuya T, Tsukiai S. Inhibition of theophylline metabolism by aciclovir. *Biol Pharm Bull* (1996) 19, 1591–5.

Theophylline + Allopurinol

Allopurinol slightly increased the exposure to theophylline in one study, but other studies have not found this effect.

Clinical evidence

In a study in 12 healthy subjects, allopurinol 300 mg twice daily for 14 days increased the half-life of a single 5-mg/kg oral dose of theophylline by 25%, and increased its AUC by 27%.[1] Similar increases were seen when a second dose of theophylline was given 28 days after starting the allopurinol.[1] However, in two other studies allopurinol 300 mg daily for 7 days did not have any effect on the pharmacokinetics of theophylline, following a single 5-mg/kg intravenous dose of aminophylline.[2,3] Similarly, in a study in 4 subjects, steady-state theophylline levels were not affected by allopurinol 100 mg three times daily. However, there was an alteration in the proportion of different urinary theophylline metabolites: methyluric acid decreased and methylxanthine increased.[3]

The peak plasma levels of theophylline 450 mg daily rose by 38% in a patient who took allopurinol for 3 days.[4] Another case report describes a patient taking theophylline 240 mg four times daily who experienced a grand mal seizure one day after starting allopurinol 100 mg three times daily. His theophylline levels were, however, elevated at 59 mg/L the day before starting allopurinol, and rose further to 86 mg/L the day after starting allopurinol. It is unclear whether the allopurinol was implicated in this case as the patient demonstrated slow metabolism of theophylline upon rechallenge.[5]

Mechanism

Uncertain. Allopurinol, a xanthine oxidase inhibitor, can block the conversion of methylxanthine to methyluric acid, but this had no effect on theophylline levels in two studies. It has also been suggested that allopurinol inhibits the oxidative metabolism of theophylline by the liver.[4]

Importance and management

Evidence for an interaction between aminophylline or theophylline and allopurinol appears to be limited to two case reports and the studies in healthy subjects and generally appears to be of limited clinical importance. Nevertheless, it would seem prudent to check for any signs of theophylline adverse effects (headache, nausea, tremor) on concurrent use, particularly in situations where the metabolism of the theophylline may already be reduced (other drugs or diseases). If theophylline adverse effects become troublesome, monitor its levels and adjust the aminophylline or theophylline dose accordingly.

1. Manfredi RL, Vesell ES. Inhibition of theophylline metabolism by long-term allopurinol administration. *Clin Pharmacol Ther* (1981) 29, 224–9.
2. Vozeh S, Powell JR, Cupit GC, Riegelman S, Sheiner LB. Influence of allopurinol on theophylline disposition in adults. *Clin Pharmacol Ther* (1980) 27, 194–7.
3. Grygiel JJ, Wing LMH, Farkas J, Birkett DJ. Effects of allopurinol on theophylline metabolism and clearance. *Clin Pharmacol Ther* (1979) 26, 660–7.
4. Barry M, Feeley J. Allopurinol influences aminophenazone elimination. *Clin Pharmacokinet* (1990) 19, 167–9.
5. Jacobs MH, Senior RM. Theophylline toxicity due to impaired theophylline degradation. *Am Rev Respir Dis* (1974) 110, 342–5.

Theophylline + Alosetron

Alosetron does not have a clinically relevant effect on the pharmacokinetics of theophylline.

Clinical evidence, mechanism, importance and management

In a placebo-controlled study, 10 healthy women were given alosetron 1 mg twice daily for 16 days with oral theophylline 200 mg twice daily from day 8 to day 16. No clinically relevant changes in the pharmacokinetics of theophylline were seen, and concurrent use was well tolerated. The effect of theophylline on alosetron pharmacokinetics was not measured but the authors of the report say that no metabolic interaction seems likely.[1] No dose adjustments would therefore appear to be needed if these drugs are used together. There appears to be no direct evidence regarding aminophylline, but as it is metabolised to theophylline, no adverse interaction would be expected with alosetron.

1. Koch KM, Ricci BM, Hedayetullah NS, Jewell D, Kersey KE. Effect of alosetron on theophylline pharmacokinetics. *Br J Clin Pharmacol* (2001) 52, 596–600.

Theophylline + Amiodarone

An isolated case report describes an elderly man who developed raised theophylline levels and toxicity when he was given amiodarone.

Clinical evidence, mechanism, importance and management

An 86-year-old man taking furosemide, digoxin, domperidone and sustained-release theophylline developed signs of theophylline toxicity when amiodarone 600 mg daily was given. After 9 days his serum theophylline levels had doubled, from about 16.8 mg/L to 35 mg/L. The toxicity disappeared when the theophylline was stopped.[1]

The reason for this adverse reaction is not understood but it has been suggested that amiodarone may reduce the metabolism of the theophylline by the liver.[1] This is an isolated case and its general importance is uncertain. More study is needed.

Note that amiodarone can cause thyroid dysfunction, which may affect aminophylline and theophylline requirements, see also 'Theophylline + Thyroid hormones and Antithyroid drugs', p.1462.

1. Soto J, Sacristán JA, Arellano F, Hazas J. Possible theophylline-amiodarone interaction. *DICP Ann Pharmacother* (1990) 24, 1115.

Theophylline + Antacids

Aluminium or magnesium hydroxide-containing antacids do not appear to affect the extent of absorption of theophylline, although they may increase the rate of absorption of some sustained-release theophylline or aminophylline preparations.

Clinical evidence, mechanism, importance and management

In a study in 12 healthy subjects, there was no difference in the steady-state maximum serum concentrations or AUC of theophylline (given as *Nuelin-Depot* or *Theodur*) when an antacid containing **aluminium/magnesium hydroxide** and **magnesium carbonate** (*Novalucid*) was given. However, the antacid caused a faster absorption of theophylline from *Nuelin-Depot*, which resulted in greater fluctuations in the serum levels. It was considered that the adverse effects of theophylline might be increased in those patients with serum levels at the top of the range.[1] Similar results have been found in single-dose studies when aminophylline (as *Aminophyllin*),[2] or theophylline (as *Slo-Phyllin Gyrocaps*,[3] *Somophyllin CRT*,[4] and *Theo-Dur*[5]) was given with **aluminium/magnesium hydroxide** antacids, and in multiple dose studies in patients when aminophylline (as *Aminophyllin*[6]) or theophylline (as *Armophylline*,[7] or *Theodur*[6]) was given with **aluminium/magnesium hydroxide** antacids. However, in contrast, administration of 30 mL of an **aluminium/magnesium hydroxide** antacid (*Maalox*) four times daily did not affect the trough levels of theophylline in a patient taking *Theo-Dur* 400 mg three times daily.[8]

In general no particular precautions seem to be necessary if antacids are given with these theophylline or aminophylline preparations. Care should be taken extrapolating this information to other modified-release preparations of theophylline and aminophylline. If an interaction is suspected, consider separating the doses, although note that the exact period by which the doses need to be separated might vary between products: 2 to 3 hours is often sufficient with other antacid interactions.

1. Myhre KI, Walstad RA. The influence of antacid on the absorption of two different sustained-release formulations of theophylline. *Br J Clin Pharmacol* (1983) 15, 683–7.
2. Arnold LA, Spurbeck GH, Shelver WH, Henderson WM. Effect of an antacid on gastrointestinal absorption of theophylline. *Am J Hosp Pharm* (1979) 36, 1059–62.
3. Shargel L, Stevens JA, Fuchs JE, Yu ABC. Effect of antacid on bioavailability of theophylline from rapid and timed-release drug products. *J Pharm Sci* (1981) 70, 599–602.
4. Ferrari M, Olivieri M, Romito D, Biasin C, Barozzi E, Bassetti S. Influence of gastric pH changes on pharmacokinetic of a sustained-release formulation of theophylline. *Riv Eur Sci Med Farmacol* (1991) 13, 269–74.
5. Darzentas LJ, Stewart RB, Curry SH, Yost RL. Effect of antacid on bioavailability of a sustained-release theophylline preparation. *Drug Intell Clin Pharm* (1983) 17, 555–7.
6. Reed RC, Schwartz HJ. Lack of influence of an intensive antacid regimen on theophylline bioavailability. *J Pharmacokinet Biopharm* (1984) 12, 315–331.
7. Muir JF, Peiffer G, Richard MO, Benhamou D, Andrejak M, Hary L, Moore N. Lack of effect of magnesium-aluminium hydroxide on the absorption of theophylline given as a pH-dependent sustained release preparation. *Eur J Clin Pharmacol* (1993) 44, 85–8.
8. Fernandes E, Melewicz FM. Antacids and theophylline-ranitidine interaction. *Ann Intern Med* (1984) 101, 279.

Theophylline + Anticholinesterases; Centrally acting

Tacrine reduces theophylline clearance. Donepezil does not appear to affect the pharmacokinetics of theophylline.

Clinical evidence, mechanism, importance and management

(a) Donepezil

An open-label, crossover study in 12 healthy subjects found that donepezil 5 mg daily for 10 days had no statistically significant effects on the pharmacokinetics of theophylline.[1] Therefore, no theophylline dose adjustments are considered necessary on concurrent use. There appears to be no direct evidence regarding aminophylline, but as it is metabolised to theophylline, no adverse interaction would be expected with donepezil.

(b) Tacrine

In a study, healthy subjects were given theophylline 158 mg alone or while taking tacrine 20 mg every 6 hours. Tacrine reduced the clearance of theophylline by 50%. It was suggested that tacrine inhibits the metabolism of theophylline by CYP1A2 in the liver.[2] It would seem prudent to be alert for theophylline adverse effects (such as headache, nausea, and tremor) in patients also given tacrine, reducing the theophylline dose if necessary to avoid toxicity. More study of this interaction is needed in patients given multiple doses of both drugs. There appears to be no direct evidence regarding aminophylline, but as it is metabolised to theophylline, it seems likely that it will be similarly affected by tacrine.

1. Tiseo PJ, Foley K, Friedhoff LT. Concurrent administration of donepezil HCl and theophylline; assessment of pharmacokinetic changes following multiple-dose administration in healthy volunteers. *Br J Clin Pharmacol* (1998) 46 (Suppl 1), 35–9.
2. deVries TM, Siedlik P, Smithers JA, Brown RR, Reece PA, Posvar EL, Sedman AJ, Koup JR, Forgue ST. Effect of multiple-dose tacrine administration on single-dose pharmacokinetics of digoxin, diazepam, and theophylline. *Pharm Res* (1993) 10 (10 Suppl), S-333.

Theophylline + Antihistamines and related drugs

Azelastine, cetirizine, ketotifen, and mizolastine do not appear to affect the pharmacokinetics of theophylline to a clinically relevant extent. Theophylline does not appear to affect the pharmacokinetics of cetirizine to a clinically relevant extent.

Clinical evidence, mechanism, importance and management

(a) Azelastine

In a study in 10 subjects with bronchial asthma, azelastine 2 mg twice daily had no clinically relevant effect on the clearance of theophylline 300 mg twice daily. However, one patient had a 21% increase and another patient had a 25% decrease in clearance.[1] These changes are generally unlikely to be clinically significant. There appears to be no direct evidence regarding aminophylline, but as it is metabolised to theophylline, no clinically relevant interaction would be expected with azelastine.

(b) Cetirizine

A single 240-mg dose of *intravenous* theophylline was given to 6 healthy subjects after they had taken cetirizine 10 mg twice daily for 3.5 days. There was no change in theophylline pharmacokinetics, but the half-life of cetirizine was decreased by 19%. This change in cetirizine pharmacokinetics was not considered to be clinically relevant.[2] There appears to be no direct evidence regarding aminophylline, but as it is metabolised to theophylline, no clinically relevant interaction would be expected with cetirizine.

(c) Ketotifen

Two studies, one in healthy adults[3] and one in asthmatic children,[4] found that ketotifen did not affect the pharmacokinetics of a single oral dose of either theophylline[3] or aminophylline.[4] It was suggested that concurrent use might actually decrease the CNS adverse effects of each drug.[3] Another crossover study was conducted in asthmatic patients sensitive to at least one commonly inhaled allergen who received ketotifen or placebo twice daily for 12 weeks. Patients received aminophylline from week 5 and week 9, which was dose adjusted to give either low theophylline levels (1 to 10 mg/L) for 4 weeks or high theophylline levels (10 to 20 mg/L) for 4 weeks. An indicator of disease control, the combined symptom score and inhaler use, indicated that the bronchodilating action of aminophylline had been potentiated by ketotifen, but there was no statistically significant effect on theophylline levels.[5] No particular precautions therefore seem necessary if theophylline or aminophylline are given with ketotifen.

(d) Mizolastine

In 17 healthy subjects, mizolastine 10 mg daily had virtually no effect on the steady-state pharmacokinetics of theophylline, although a 13% increase in mean trough level and an 8% increase in the AUC was seen. These changes were not considered clinically relevant.[6] There appears to be no direct evidence regarding aminophylline, but as it is metabolised to theophylline, no clinically relevant interaction would be expected with mizolastine.

1. Asamoto H, Kokura M, Kawakami A, Sasaki Y, Fujii H, Sawano T, Iso S, Ooishi T, Horiuchi Y, Ohara N, Kitamura Y, Morishita H. Effect of azelastine on theophylline clearance in asthma patients. *Arerugi* (1988) 37, 1033–7.
2. Hulhoven R, Desager JP, Harvengt C. Lack of clinically relevant interaction of cetirizine on theophylline disposition in healthy subjects: a placebo-controlled study. *Am J Ther* (1995) 2, 71–4.
3. Matejcek M, Irwin P, Neff G, Abt K, Wehrli W. Determination of the central effects of the asthma prophylactic ketotifen, the bronchodilator theophylline, and both in combination: an application of quantitative electroencephalography to the study of drug interactions. *Int J Clin Pharmacol Ther Toxicol* (1985) 23, 258–66.
4. Garty M, Scolnik D, Danziger Y, Volovitz B, Ilfeld DN, Varsano I. Non-interaction of ketotifen and theophylline in children with asthma an acute study. *Eur J Clin Pharmacol* (1987) 32, 187–9.
5. Hendy MS, Burge PS, Stableforth DE. Effect of ketotifen on the bronchodilating action of aminophylline. *Respiration* (1986) 49, 296–9.
6. Pinquier JL, Salva P, Deschamps C, Ascalone V, Costa J. Effect of mizolastine, a new non sedative H1 antagonist on the pharmacokinetics of theophylline. *Therapie* (1995) 50 (Suppl), 148.

Theophylline + Aspirin or NSAIDs

Aspirin, nimesulide and piroxicam do not appear to alter the pharmacokinetics theophylline.

Clinical evidence

(a) Aspirin

In 8 elderly patients (aged 60 to 81 years) with COPD, enteric-coated aspirin 650 mg daily for 4 weeks had no effect on the steady-state serum levels of theophylline.[1]

(b) Nimesulide

Nimesulide 100 mg twice daily for 7 days did not affect lung function in 10 patients with COPD taking slow-release theophylline 200 mg twice daily, although there was a slight fall in theophylline levels, which was not clinically relevant. The pharmacokinetics of nimesulide were unchanged by theophylline.[2]

(c) Piroxicam

In a study in 6 healthy subjects, piroxicam 20 mg daily for 7 days had no effect on the pharmacokinetics of theophylline (given as a single 6-mg/kg intravenous dose of aminophylline).[3]

(d) Rofecoxib

In a placebo-controlled study, 36 healthy subjects were given rofecoxib 12.5 mg, 25 mg or 50 mg daily for 7 days, with a single 300-mg dose of theophylline given on day 7. There were no significant changes in the maximum plasma levels of theophylline. However, rofecoxib 12.5 mg, 25 mg or 50 mg, increased the AUC of theophylline by 38%, 51% and 60%, respectively, and increased its half-life by 40%, 59% and 64%, respectively.

Mechanism

Rofecoxib inhibits CYP1A2, the isoenzyme by which theophylline is metabolised.[4] Therefore concurrent use decreases theophylline metabolism, leading to the increased levels seen.

Importance and management

Evidence for an interaction between theophylline and the NSAIDs appears to be limited to the studies cited. The increased theophylline levels seen with rofecoxib suggests that dose reductions of theophylline (and probably aminophylline) would be necessary if patients were also given rofecoxib; however, given the range of NSAIDs available, it would probably be better to use a non-interacting alternative (rofecoxib is the only NSAID known to inhibit CYP1A2 to a clinically relevant extent). However, note that rofecoxib was generally withdrawn worldwide in 2004 because of its cardiovascular adverse effects; this study is included for completeness.

Apart from checking that the patient is not sensitive to aspirin or any other NSAID there would seem to be no reason for avoiding aspirin or piroxicam in patients taking theophylline (or probably aminophylline).

1. Daigneault EA, Hamdy RC, Ferslew KE, Rice PJ, Singh J, Harvill LM, Kalbfleisch JH. Investigation of the influence of acetylsalicylic acid on the steady state of long-term therapy with theophylline in elderly male patients with normal renal function. *J Clin Pharmacol* (1994) 34, 86–90.
2. Auteri A, Blardi P, Bruni F, Domini L, Pasqui AL, Saletti M, Verzuri MS, Scaricabarozzi I, Vargui G, Di Perri T. Pharmacokinetics and pharmacodynamics of slow-release theophylline during treatment with nimesulide. *Int J Clin Pharmacol Res* (1991) 11, 211–7.
3. Maponga C, Barlow JC, Schentag JJ. Lack of effect of piroxicam on theophylline clearance in healthy volunteers. *DICP Ann Pharmacother* (1990) 24, 123–6.
4. Bachmann K, White D, Jauregui L, Schwartz JI, Agrawal NGB, Mazenko R, Larson PJ, Porras AG. An evaluation of the dose-dependent inhibition of CYP1A2 by rofecoxib using theophylline as a CYP1A2 probe. *J Clin Pharmacol* (2003) 43, 1082–90.

Theophylline + Azoles

Studies have found that fluconazole and ketoconazole do not affect theophylline levels to a clinically relevant extent. However, an isolated report describes a rise in serum theophylline levels due to fluconazole, and another describes falls in theophylline levels in three patients taking ketoconazole.

Clinical evidence

(a) Fluconazole

A crossover study in 5 healthy subjects found that fluconazole 100 mg given every 12 hours for 7 doses caused a 16% decrease in the clearance of a single 300-mg oral dose of aminophylline, which was not statistically significant.[1] Another study in 10 healthy subjects found that fluconazole 100 mg daily for one week had no effect on the serum levels of theophylline 150 mg twice daily.[2] In 9 subjects who took fluconazole

400 mg daily for 10 days, the clearance of a single 6-mg/kg oral dose of theophylline was reduced by 13%.[3] In contrast, a brief, isolated report states that one of 2 patients given theophylline and fluconazole had a rise (amount not specified) in their serum theophylline levels.[4]

(b) Ketoconazole

No clinically relevant changes in the pharmacokinetics of a single 3-mg/kg intravenous dose of theophylline (given as aminophylline) were seen in 12 healthy subjects who took a single 400-mg dose of ketoconazole, or in 4 subjects who took ketoconazole 400 mg daily for 5 days.[5] Similar results were found in another study in 10 healthy subjects who took ketoconazole 200 mg daily for 7 days.[6] In 6 healthy subjects ketoconazole 400 mg daily for 6 days increased the half-life of a single 250-mg oral dose of theophylline by 22%, but had no effect on its clearance.[7] In contrast, a case report describes a man whose serum theophylline levels fell sharply, from about 16.5 mg/L to 9 mg/L (reference range 10 to 20 mg/L), over the 2 hours immediately after taking 200 mg of ketoconazole. A less striking fall was seen in 2 other patients.[8]

Mechanism

Fluconazole and ketoconazole (and the other azoles) appear to have minimal effects on CYP1A2, which is concerned with the oxidative metabolism of theophylline.[1,7] It is not clear why a few individuals had some changes in theophylline levels.

Importance and management

Information regarding a possible interaction between theophylline and the azoles seem to be limited to these reports. Neither fluconazole nor ketoconazole usually appears to interact with aminophylline or theophylline to a clinically relevant extent. However, it seems that very occasionally some changes occur, so consider this interaction as a possible cause if theophylline levels adverse effects (headache, nausea, tremor) develop, or if there is any evidence to suggest that theophylline is less effective. In this case, monitor theophylline levels and adjust the dose of theophylline or aminophylline accordingly.

1. Konishi H, Morita K, Yamaji A. Effect of fluconazole on theophylline disposition in humans. *Eur J Clin Pharmacol* (1994) 46, 309–12.
2. Feil RA, Rindone JP, Morrill GB, Habib MP. Effect of low-dose fluconazole on theophylline serum concentrations in healthy volunteers. *J Pharm Technol* (1995) 11, 267–9.
3. Foisy MM, Nix D, Middleton E, Kotas T, Symonds WT. The effects of single dose fluconazole (SD FLU) versus multiple dose fluconazole (MD FLU) on the pharmacokinetics (PK) of theophylline (THL) in young healthy volunteers. *Intersci Conf Antimicrob Agents Chemother* (1995) 39, 7.
4. Tett S, Carey D, Lee H-S. Drug interactions with fluconazole. *Med J Aust* (1992) 156, 365.
5. Brown MW, Maldonado AL, Meredith CG, Speeg KV. Effect of ketoconazole on hepatic oxidative drug metabolism. *Clin Pharmacol Ther* (1985) 37, 290–7.
6. Heusner JJ, Dukes GE, Rollins DE, Tolman KG, Galinsky RE. Effect of chronically administered ketoconazole on the elimination of theophylline in man. *Drug Intell Clin Pharm* (1987) 21, 514–17.
7. Naline E, Sanceaume M, Pays M, Advenier C. Application of theophylline metabolite assays to the exploration of liver microsome oxidative function in man. *Fundam Clin Pharmacol* (1988) 2, 341–51.
8. Murphy E, Hannon D, Callaghan B. Ketoconazole—theophylline interaction. *Ir Med J* (1987) 80, 123–4.

Theophylline + Barbiturates

The clearance of theophylline is increased by phenobarbital, pentobarbital, and possibly secobarbital. Other barbiturates would be expected to interact similarly.

Clinical evidence

(a) Pentobarbital

A single case report describes a man receiving intravenous aminophylline who had a 95% rise in the clearance of theophylline after he was given high-dose intravenous pentobarbital.[1] In healthy subjects pentobarbital 100 mg daily for 10 days increased the clearance of oral theophylline by a mean of 40% and reduced the AUC by 26%, although there were marked intersubject differences in the findings.[2]

(b) Phenobarbital

In 7 children aged 6 to 12 years with asthma, phenobarbital (2 mg/kg daily to a maximum of 60 mg) for 19 days reduced the mean steady-state serum theophylline levels by 30%, and increased the clearance by 35% (range 12 to 71%).[3] In contrast, two earlier studies (one by the same group of authors) found no significant change in the pharmacokinetics of theophylline, in children with asthma given phenobarbital 2 mg/kg daily, 16 mg three times daily or 32 mg three times daily.[4,5]

In healthy adult subjects given phenobarbital, the mean theophylline clearance, from a single intravenous dose of aminophylline, was increased by 34%.[6] In another study the clearance of theophylline was increased by 17% when phenobarbital was given for 2 weeks, although this was not statistically significant.[7]

The effects of phenobarbital can be additive with the effects of phenytoin and smoking: one patient required 4 g of theophylline daily to maintain therapeutic serum levels and to control her asthma.[8]

One retrospective study found that premature infants needed a higher dose of intravenous aminophylline for neonatal apnoea when they were given phenobarbital,[9] but a later prospective study did not confirm this.[10] A study in one set of newborn twins given intravenous aminophylline found that the serum theophylline levels of the twin given phenobarbital were about half those of the twin not given phenobarbital.[11] In a more recent study, in 50 premature infants with apnoea treated with theophylline, phenobarbital increased theophylline clearance and reduced its half-life.[12]

(c) Secobarbital

The clearance of theophylline increased 4.4-fold over a 4-week period in a child given periodic doses of secobarbital and regular doses of **phenobarbital**.[13]

Mechanism

The barbiturates are potent non-specific liver-enzyme inducers, which appear to increase the metabolism of theophylline by the liver, thereby increasing its clearance.

Importance and management

The interaction between theophylline and the barbiturates is established, moderately well documented, and of clinical importance. Patients given phenobarbital or pentobarbital might need above-average doses of theophylline or aminophylline to achieve and maintain adequate theophylline levels. Concurrent use should therefore be monitored and appropriate dose increases made. Direct information about a possible interaction between aminophylline or theophylline and the other barbiturates seems to be lacking; however, as all of the barbiturates can cause liver enzyme induction, they might, to a greater or lesser extent, be expected to interact similarly.

Note that theophylline itself can cause seizures, although mostly in overdose, and should be used with caution in patients with epilepsy.

1. Gibson GA, Blouin RA, Bauer LA, Rapp RP, Tibbs PA. Influence of high-dose pentobarbital on theophylline pharmacokinetics: A case report. *Ther Drug Monit* (1985) 7, 181–4.
2. Dahlqvist R, Steiner E, Koike Y, von Bahr C, Lind M, Billing B. Induction of theophylline metabolism by pentobarbital. *Ther Drug Monit* (1989) 11, 408–10.
3. Saccar CL, Danish M, Ragni MC, Rocci ML, Greene J, Yaffe SJ, Mansmann HC. The effect of phenobarbital on theophylline disposition in children with asthma. *J Allergy Clin Immunol* (1985) 75, 716–9.
4. Goldstein EO, Eney RD, Mellits ED, Solomon H, Johnson G. Effect of phenobarbital on theophylline metabolism in asthmatic children. *Ann Allergy* (1977) 39, 69.
5. Greene J, Danish M, Ragni M, Lecks H, Yaffe S. The effect of phenobarbital upon theophylline elimination kinetics in asthmatic children. *Ann Allergy* (1977) 39, 69.
6. Landay RA, Gonzalez MA, Taylor JC. Effect of phenobarbital on theophylline disposition. *J Allergy Clin Immunol* (1978) 62, 27–9.
7. Piafsky KM, Sitar DS, Ogilvie RI. Effect of phenobarbital on the disposition of intravenous theophylline. *Clin Pharmacol Ther* (1977) 22, 336–9.
8. Nicholson JP, Basile SA, Cury JD. Massive theophylline dosing in a heavy smoker receiving both phenytoin and phenobarbital. *Ann Pharmacother* (1992) 26, 334–6.
9. Yazdani M, Kissling GE, Tran TH, Gottschalk SK, Schuth CR. Phenobarbital increases the theophylline requirement of premature infants being treated for apnea. *Am J Dis Child* (1987) 141, 97–9.
10. Kandrotas RJ, Cranfield TL, Gal P, Ransom J, Weaver RL. Effect of phenobarbital administration on theophylline clearance in premature neonates. *Ther Drug Monit* (1990) 12, 139–43.
11. Delgado E, Carrasco JM, García B, Pérez E, García Lacalle C, Bermejo T, De Juana P. Interacción teofilina-fenobarbital en un neonato. *Farm Clin* (1996) 13, 142–5.
12. Islam SI, Ali AS, Sheikh AA, Fida NM. Pharmacokinetics of theophylline in preterm neonates during the first month of life. *Saudi Med J* (2004) 25, 459–65.
13. Paladino JA, Blumer NA, Maddox RR. Effect of secobarbital on theophylline clearance. *Ther Drug Monit* (1983) 5, 135–9.

Theophylline + BCG vaccine

BCG vaccination might reduce the clearance of theophylline.

Clinical evidence, mechanism, importance and management

Two weeks after 12 healthy subjects were vaccinated with 0.1 mL of BCG vaccine, the clearance of a single 128-mg dose of theophylline (as choline theophyllinate) was reduced by 21% and the theophylline half-life was prolonged by 14% (range 10% reduction to 47% increase).[1]

Theophylline levels are unlikely to be affected to a clinically relevant extent in most patients given the BCG vaccine. However, as only a single dose of theophylline was given, it seems possible that the occasional patient might develop some signs of theophylline toxicity. Nevertheless, no action is necessary as any interaction seems likely to resolve spontaneously.

There appears to be no direct evidence regarding aminophylline, but as it is metabolised to theophylline, no clinically relevant interaction would generally be expected in patients given BCG vaccination.

1. Gray JD, Renton KW, Hung OR. Depression of theophylline elimination following BCG vaccination. *Br J Clin Pharmacol* (1983) 16, 735–7.

Theophylline + Beta-agonist bronchodilators

The concurrent use of aminophylline or theophylline and beta-agonist bronchodilators is a useful option in the management of asthma and COPD, but potentiation of some adverse reactions can occur, the most serious being hypokalaemia and tachycardia, particularly with high-dose theophylline. Some patients might have a reduction in their theophylline levels if given oral or intravenous salbutamol (albuterol) or intravenous isoprenaline (isoproterenol).

Clinical evidence

(a) Fenoterol

A study in 12 patients with chronic airways disease found that oral fenoterol 2.5 mg three times daily did not affect the steady-state level of sustained-release theophylline 10.1 mg/kg twice daily.[1] A study in 6 healthy subjects found that the fall in plasma potassium levels seen after inhalation of three doses of 600 micrograms of fenoterol, given over one hour, was not exacerbated by a 7-mg/kg infusion of theophylline.[2] A study in 8 healthy subjects found that the addition of sustained-release theophylline to inhaled fenoterol 600 and 800 micrograms increased the heart rate (from 9.1 bpm to 15.8 bpm) and systolic blood pressure (from 9 mmHg to 23.5 mmHg). Theophylline levels were not affected.[3]

(b) Formoterol

In a single-dose study, 8 healthy subjects were given oral doses of theophylline 375 mg and formoterol 144 micrograms. Concurrent use caused no significant pharmacokinetic interaction, but a significantly greater drop in the potassium level was seen, when compared with either drug given alone.[4]

(c) Isoprenaline (Isoproterenol)

An infusion of isoprenaline increased the clearance of theophylline (given as intravenous aminophylline) by a mean of 19% in 6 children with status asthmaticus and respiratory failure. Two of the children had increases in clearance of greater than 30%.[5] Another study, in 12 patients with status asthmaticus, found that an isoprenaline infusion (mean maximum rate 0.77 micrograms/kg per minute) caused a mean fall in serum theophylline levels of almost 6 micrograms/mL.[6] The levels rose again when isoprenaline was stopped.[6] A critically ill patient receiving intravenous aminophylline, phenytoin and nebulised terbutaline had a 4.5-fold increase in theophylline clearance when an isoprenaline infusion and intravenous methylprednisolone were added to the regimen.[7]

(d) Orciprenaline (Metaproterenol)

In a study in 6 healthy subjects, oral orciprenaline 20 mg every 8 hours or inhaled orciprenaline 1.95 mg every 6 hours for 3 days had no effect on the pharmacokinetics of theophylline (given as a single intravenous dose of aminophylline).[8] This confirms a previous finding in asthmatic children, in whom it was shown that oral orciprenaline did not alter steady-state serum theophylline levels.[9]

(e) Salbutamol (Albuterol)

1. Effects on heart rate or potassium levels. In healthy subjects, pretreatment with oral theophylline for 9 days significantly increased the hypokalaemia and tachycardia caused by an infusion of salbutamol (4 micrograms/kg loading dose then 8 micrograms/kg for an hour).[10] In one study in 9 patients with COPD, a potentially dangerous additive increase in heart rate of about 35 to 40% was seen when infusions of aminophylline and salbutamol were given.[11] Similarly, the heart rate was significantly higher in 15 children with asthma given single doses of oral theophylline and salbutamol (109 bpm) when compared with a control group given oral theophylline alone (91 bpm).[12] However, another study in 18 patients with COPD and heart disease found that neither the occurrence nor the severity of arrhythmias seemed to be changed when oral theophylline was given with inhaled salbutamol.[13] One report describes a 10-year-old girl given theophylline and salbutamol who had a respiratory arrest, possibly related to hypokalaemia.[14]

2. Effects on theophylline levels. In a study in 10 healthy subjects, theophylline clearance was increased by a mean of 14%, and in 3 cases by greater than 30%, when salbutamol was given orally, but no changes in clearance were seen when salbutamol was given by inhalation.[15] Another study reported a 25% reduction in serum theophylline levels in 10 patients who took oral salbutamol 16 mg.[16] A child aged 19 months given intravenous theophylline was also given an infusion of salbutamol; theophylline clearance was increased and the theophylline dose needed to be increased threefold to compensate.[17] These reports contrast with another study in 8 healthy subjects, which found no change in the steady-state pharmacokinetics of oral theophylline when oral salbutamol was also given.[18] Peak flow readings were decreased in 15 children (aged 5 to 13 years) given single doses of oral salbutamol and theophylline, but theophylline levels were not significantly decreased.[12]

(f) Terbutaline

In a study in 7 healthy subjects, pretreatment with oral theophylline for at least 4 days significantly increased the fall in serum potassium levels and rises in blood glucose levels, pulse rate, and systolic blood pressure caused by an infusion of terbutaline.[19] A study in children given slow-release formulations of both theophylline and terbutaline found no increases in reported adverse effects and simple additive effects on the control of their asthma.[20]

Oral terbutaline decreased serum theophylline levels by about 10% in 6 patients with asthma, and the control of asthma was improved.[21] Another study in children with asthma found that terbutaline elixir 75 micrograms/kg three times daily reduced the steady-state serum levels of theophylline by 22%, but the symptoms of cough and wheeze improved.[22] In a study in 9 healthy subjects, the mean half-life of theophylline (given as a single 6-mg/kg dose of intravenous aminophylline) was not significantly altered after oral terbutaline 5 mg was given three times daily for 4 days, although some subjects had an increase in theophylline clearance, and some a decrease.[23] Yet another study found no changes in the pharmacokinetics of aminophylline in children with asthma given terbutaline;[24] a study in 12 healthy adults found no clinically significant changes in the pharmacokinetics of terbutaline and theophylline when both drugs were given orally for 7 days,[25] and a study in 8 healthy subjects given subcutaneous terbutaline 250 micrograms at 0, 0.5, 4.5 and 5 hours after a single 7-mg/kg dose of oral theophylline similarly found no change in theophylline pharmacokinetics.[26]

(g) Unspecified beta$_2$ agonists

In 1990, the CSM in the UK noted that, of 26 reports they had on record of hypokalaemia with unnamed xanthines or beta$_2$ agonists, 9 occurred in patients receiving both groups of drugs. In 5 of these 9 cases, the hypokalaemia had no clinical consequence. However, in 2 cases it resulted in cardiorespiratory arrest, in one case confusion, and in a further case intestinal pseudo-obstruction.[27]

Mechanism

Beta$_2$ agonists can cause hypokalaemia, particularly when they are given parenterally or by nebulisation. Aminophylline and theophylline can also cause hypokalaemia, and this is a common feature of theophylline toxicity. The potassium-lowering effects of both these groups of drugs are additive. The reason for the reduction in theophylline levels with some beta agonists is not known.

Importance and management

The concurrent use of aminophylline or theophylline and beta$_2$ agonist bronchodilators is beneficial, but the reports outlined above illustrate some of the disadvantages and adverse effects that have been identified. In particular, it has been suggested that the use of intravenous beta$_2$ agonists in acutely ill patients receiving theophylline may be hazardous because of the risk of profound hypokalaemia and cardiac arrhythmias.[10,19] Monitoring serum potassium in these situations was suggested.[19] Moreover, the CSM in the UK particularly recommends monitoring potassium levels in patients with severe asthma as the hypokalaemic effects of beta$_2$ agonists can be potentiated by theophylline and its derivatives, corticosteroids, diuretics and hypoxia.[27]

1. Lucena MI, Almagro J, Rius F, Sanchez de la Cuesta F. Bronchodilator effect and serum theophylline level after combined treatment with fenoterol and theophylline in reversible chronic airflow obstruction. *Eur J Clin Pharmacol* (1988) 35, 669–71.
2. Deenstra M, Haalboom JRE, Struyvenberg A. Decrease of plasma potassium due to inhalation of beta-2-agonists: absence of an additional effect of intravenous theophylline. *Eur J Clin Invest* (1988) 18, 162–5.
3. Flatt A, Burgess C, Windom H, Beasley R, Purdie G, Crane J. The cardiovascular effects of inhaled fenoterol alone and during treatment with oral theophylline. *Chest* (1989) 96, 1317–20.
4. van den Berg BTJ, Derks MGM, Koolen MGJ, Braat MCP, Butter JJ, van Boxtel CJ. Pharmacokinetic/pharmacodynamic modelling of the eosinopenic and hypokalemic effects of formoterol and theophylline combination in healthy men. *Pulm Pharmacol Ther* (1999) 12, 185–92.
5. Hemstreet MP, Miles MV, Rutland RO. Effect of intravenous isoproterenol on theophylline kinetics. *J Allergy Clin Immunol* (1982) 69, 360–4.
6. O'Rourke PP, Crone RK. Effect of isoproterenol on measured theophylline levels. *Crit Care Med* (1984) 12, 373–5.
7. Griffith JA, Kozloski GD. Isoproterenol-theophylline interaction: possible potentiation by other drugs. *Clin Pharm* (1990) 9, 54–7.
8. Conrad KA, Woodworth JR. Orciprenaline does not alter theophylline elimination. *Br J Clin Pharmacol* (1981) 12, 756–7.
9. Rachelefsky GS, Katz RM, Mickey MR, Siegel SC. Metaproterenol and theophylline in asthmatic children. *Ann Allergy* (1980) 45, 207–12.
10. Whyte KF, Reid C, Addis GJ, Whitesmith R, Reid JL. Salbutamol induced hypokalaemia: the effect of theophylline alone and in combination with adrenaline. *Br J Clin Pharmacol* (1988) 25, 571–8.
11. Georgopoulos D, Wong D, Anthonisen NR. Interactive effects of systemically administered salbutamol and aminophylline in patients with chronic obstructive pulmonary disease. *Am Rev Respir Dis* (1988) 138, 1499–1503.
12. Dawson KP, Fergusson DM. Effects of oral theophylline and oral salbutamol in the treatment of asthma. *Arch Dis Child* (1982) 57, 674–6.
13. Poukkula A, Korhonen UR, Huikuri H, Linnaluoto M. Theophylline and salbutamol in combination in patients with obstructive pulmonary disease and concurrent heart disease: effect on cardiac arrhythmias. *J Intern Med* (1989) 226, 229–34.
14. Epelbaum S, Benhamou PH, Pautard JC, Devoldere C, Kremp O, Piussan C. Arrêt respiratoire chez une enfant asthmatique traitée par bêta-2-mimétiques et théophylline. Rôle possible de l'hypokaliémie dans les décès subits des asthmatiques. *Ann Pediatr (Paris)* (1989) 36, 473–5.
15. Amitai Y, Glustein J, Godfrey S. Enhancement of theophylline clearance by oral albuterol. *Chest* (1992) 102, 786–9.
16. Terra Filho M, Santos SRCJ, Cukier A, Verrastro C, Carvalho-Pinto RM, Fiss E, Vargas FS.Efeitos dos agonistas beta-2-adrenérgicos por via oral, sobre os níveis séricos de teofilina. *Rev Hosp Clin Fac Med Sao Paulo* (1991) 46, 170–2.
17. Amirav I, Amitai Y, Avital A, Godfrey S. Enhancement of theophylline clearance by intravenous albuterol. *Chest* (1988) 94, 444–5.
18. McCann JP, McElnay JC, Nicholls DP, Scott MG, Stanford CF. Oral salbutamol does not affect theophylline kinetics. *Br J Pharmacol* (1986) 89 (Proc Suppl), 715P.
19. Smith SR, Kendall MJ. Potentiation of the adverse effects of intravenous terbutaline by oral theophylline. *Br J Clin Pharmacol* (1986) 21, 451–3.
20. Chow OKW, Fung KP. Slow-release terbutaline and theophylline for the long-term therapy of children with asthma: A latin square and factorial study of drug effects and interactions. *Pediatrics* (1989) 84, 119–25.
21. Garty MS, Keslin LS, Ilfeld DN, Mazar A, Spitzer S, Rosenfeld JB. Increased theophylline clearance by terbutaline in asthmatic adults. *Clin Pharmacol Ther* (1988) 43, 150.
22. Danziger Y, Garty M, Volwitz B, Ilfeld D, Varsano I, Rosenfeld JB. Reduction of serum theophylline levels by terbutaline in children with asthma. *Clin Pharmacol Ther* (1985) 37, 469–71.
23. Lombardi TP, Bertino JS, Goldberg A, Middleton E, Slaughter RL. The effects of a beta-2 selective adrenergic agonist and a beta-nonselective antagonist on theophylline clearance. *J Clin Pharmacol* (1987) 27, 523–9.
24. Wang Y, Yin A, Yu Z. Effects of bricanyl on the pharmacokinetics of aminophylline in asthmatic patients [In Chinese]. *Zhongguo Yiyuan Yaoxue Zazhi* (1992) 12, 389–90.
25. Jonkman JHG, Borgström L, van der Boon WJV, de Noord OE. Theophylline – terbutaline, a steady state study on possible pharmacokinetic interactions with special reference to chronopharmacokinetic aspects. *Br J Clin Pharmacol* (1988) 26, 285–93.
26. Snidow J, Stephens M, Self T, Stewart C, Bobo L, Pieper JA. Acute effects of short-term subcutaneous terbutaline on theophylline disposition. *Eur J Clin Pharmacol* (1987) 32, 191–3.
27. Committee on Safety of Medicines. β_2-Agonists, xanthines and hypokalaemia. *Current Problems* (1990) 28.

Theophylline + Beta blockers

Non-cardioselective beta blockers, such as nadolol and propranolol, should not be given to patients with asthma because they can cause bronchospasm. The concurrent use of theophylline and cardioselective beta blockers such as atenolol, bisoprolol or metoprolol is not contra-indicated, but some caution is still appropriate.

Propranolol reduces the clearance of theophylline. Atenolol, bisoprolol, metoprolol and nadolol do not affect the pharmacokinetics of theophylline to a clinically relevant extent.

Clinical evidence

(a) Pharmacokinetics

A study in 8 healthy subjects (5 of whom smoked 10 to 30 cigarettes daily) found that the clearance of a single 5.7- to 6.4-mg/kg dose of theophylline (as intravenous aminophylline) was reduced by 37% by **propranolol** 40 mg every 6 hours, when compared with theophylline alone. **Metoprolol** 50 mg every 6 hours did not alter the clearance in the group as a whole, but the smokers had an 11% reduction in clearance.[1] Another study in 7 healthy subjects found that the steady-state plasma clearance of theophylline was reduced by 30% by **propranolol** 40 mg every 8 hours, and by 52% by **propranolol** 240 mg every 8 hours.[2] Further, a study in 5 healthy subjects who had received **propranolol** 60 mg every 8 hours for 3 days found that the half-life of theophylline (given as a single 6-mg/kg dose of intravenous aminophylline) was prolonged by 59%.[3] However, yet another study found no significant pharmacokinetic interaction between theophylline and **propranolol**.[4] Three other studies found that the cardioselective beta blockers **atenolol** 50 to 150 mg,[5,6] and **bisoprolol** 10 mg,[7] and the non-selective beta blocker **nadolol** 80 mg[5] did not affect the pharmacokinetics of theophylline.

(b) Pharmacodynamics

Beta blockers, particularly those that are not cardioselective, can cause bronchoconstriction, which opposes the bronchodilatory effects of theophylline. See 'Anti-asthma drugs + Beta blockers', p.1420, for mention of a patient whose asthma deteriorated when taking betaxolol with theophylline and pranlukast.

In a study in 8 healthy subjects, both **propranolol** 40 mg every 6 hours and **metoprolol** 50 mg every 6 hours prevented the mild inotropic effect seen with theophylline alone.[8] An infusion of **propranolol** reduced the hypokalaemia and tachycardia that occurred after a theophylline overdose.[9,10] **Esmolol** has been used similarly.[11]

Mechanism

It has been suggested that propranolol possibly affects the clearance of theophylline by inhibiting its metabolism (demethylation and hydroxylation).[2,12]

Importance and management

The risk of severe, possibly even fatal bronchospasm when beta blockers are taken by patients with asthma would seem to be far more important than any pharmacokinetic interaction with theophylline. For more detailed advice on the use of beta blockers in patients with respiratory disease, see 'Anti-asthma drugs + Beta blockers', p.1420. Bronchospasm can occur with beta blockers given by any route of administration, even topically as eye drops. Cardioselective beta blockers have less effect on the airways, but can still cause bronchoconstriction. See 'Table 22.1', p.999, for details of the selectivity of beta blockers.

1. Conrad KA, Nyman DW. Effects of metoprolol and propranolol on theophylline elimination. *Clin Pharmacol Ther* (1980) 28, 463–7.
2. Miners JO, Wing LMH, Lillywhite KJ, Robson RA. Selectivity and dose-dependency of the inhibitory effect of propranolol on theophylline metabolism in man. *Br J Clin Pharmacol* (1985) 20, 219–23.
3. Lombardi TP, Bertino JS, Goldberg A, Middleton E, Slaughter RL. The effects of a beta-2 selective adrenergic agonist and a beta-nonselective antagonist on theophylline clearance. *J Clin Pharmacol* (1987) 27, 523–9.
4. Minton NA, Turner J, Henry JA. Pharmacodynamic and pharmacokinetic interactions between theophylline and propranolol during dynamic exercise. *Br J Clin Pharmacol* (1995) 40, 521P.
5. Corsi CM, Nafziger AN, Pieper JA, Bertino JS. Lack of effect of atenolol and nadolol on the metabolism of theophylline. *Br J Clin Pharmacol* (1990) 29, 265–8.
6. Cerasa LA, Bertino JS, Ludwig EA, Savliwala M, Middleton E, Slaughter RL. Lack of effect of atenolol on the pharmacokinetics of theophylline. *Br J Clin Pharmacol* (1988) 26, 800–802.
7. Warrington SJ, Johnston A, Lewis Y, Murphy M. Bisoprolol: Studies of potential interactions with theophylline and warfarin in healthy volunteers. *J Cardiovasc Pharmacol* (1990) 16 (Suppl 5), S164–S168.
8. Conrad KA, Prosnitz EH. Cardiovascular effects of theophylline. Partial attenuation by beta-blockade. *Eur J Clin Pharmacol* (1981) 21, 109–114.
9. Kearney TE, Manoguerra AS, Curtis GP, Ziegler MG. Theophylline toxicity and the beta-adrenergic system. *Ann Intern Med* (1985) 102, 766–9.
10. Amin DN, Henry JA. Propranolol administration in theophylline overdose. *Lancet* (1985) i, 520–1.
11. Seneff M, Scott J, Freidman B, Smith M. Acute theophylline toxicity and the use of esmolol to reverse cardiovascular instability. *Ann Emerg Med* (1990) 19, 671–3.
12. Greenblatt DJ, Franke K, Huffman DH. Impairment of antipyrine clearance in humans by propranolol. *Circulation* (1978) 57, 1161–4.

Theophylline + Caffeine

The consumption of caffeine-containing beverages can raise theophylline levels. Similarly, removal of caffeine-containing foods from the diet might reduce the half-life of theophylline.

Clinical evidence

Caffeine can decrease the clearance of theophylline by 18 to 29%, prolong its half-life by up to 44% and increase its average serum levels by up to 23%.[1-3] In addition, plasma caffeine levels were increased about twofold when theophylline was given, and this might have caused the headaches and nausea reported in 2 subjects who did not usually drink coffee.[2] In these studies, caffeine was given in the form of tablets[1,2] or as 2 to 7 cups of instant coffee.[3] Another study found that, when 4 healthy subjects removed methylxanthines from their diet, the half-life of theophylline was reduced from 9.8 hours to 7 hours.[4]

Mechanism

Unknown. It has been suggested that as theophylline and caffeine are both metabolised by CYP1A2 and a proportion of caffeine is converted to theophylline, saturation of theophylline metabolism or competition for metabolism by CYP1A2 may occur.[3] However, note that interactions by substrate competition are rarely clinically relevant.

Importance and management

An interaction between caffeine and theophylline is reasonably well studied and established. There would, however, seem to be no good reason for patients taking theophylline to avoid caffeine (in coffee, tea, cola drinks, medications, etc.), but if otherwise unexplained adverse effects occur, it might be worth checking if caffeine is responsible. Removal of caffeine from the diet might have a modest effect on theophylline levels, but the clinical relevance of this is unclear. There appears to be no direct evidence regarding aminophylline, but as it is metabolised to theophylline, it would be expected to interact similarly.

1. Loi CM, Jue SG, Bush ED, Crowley JJ, Vestal RE. Effect of caffeine dose on theophylline metabolism. *Clin Res* (1987) 35, 377A.
2. Jonkman JHG, Sollie FAE, Sauter R, Steinijans VW. The influence of caffeine on the steady-state pharmacokinetics of theophylline. *Clin Pharmacol Ther* (1991) 49, 248–55.
3. Sato J, Nakata H, Owada E, Kikuta T, Umetsu M, Ito K. Influence of usual intake of dietary caffeine on single-dose kinetics of theophylline in healthy human subjects. *Eur J Clin Pharmacol* (1993) 44, 295–8.
4. Monks TJ, Caldwell J, Smith RL. Influence of methylxanthine-containing foods on theophylline metabolism and kinetics. *Clin Pharmacol Ther* (1979) 26, 513–24.

Theophylline + Calcium-channel blockers

Most studies suggest that diltiazem, felodipine, nifedipine and verapamil can cause some slight or negligible changes in the pharmacokinetics of theophylline, but this does not appear to affect the control of asthma. However, there are isolated case reports of unexplained theophylline toxicity in two patients given nifedipine and two patients given verapamil. Isradipine does not appear to interact with theophylline.

Clinical evidence

(a) Diltiazem

In a study in 9 healthy subjects, diltiazem 90 mg twice daily for 10 days reduced the clearance of theophylline (given as a single 6-mg/kg dose of aminophylline) by 21% and increased its half-life from 6.1 hours to 7.5 hours.[1] A 12% fall in the clearance of a single 5-mg/kg oral dose of theophylline was found when healthy subjects were given diltiazem 90 mg three times daily.[2] A further study in 9 healthy subjects given diltiazem 60 mg three times daily for 3 days found that the half-life of a single 200-mg dose of theophylline was increased from 7.58 hours to 8.59 hours and the clearance was reduced by 9%.[3] In 8 patients with asthma or COPD, diltiazem 60 mg three times daily for 5 days reduced the clearance of steady-state theophylline (given as a continuous infusion of aminophylline 12 mg/kg per day) by 22% and increased its half-life from 5.7 hours to 7.5 hours.[4]

Conversely, other studies found no significant changes in peak steady-state theophylline levels in 18 patients with asthma given diltiazem 240 to 480 mg daily for 7 days,[5] or in 7 healthy subjects given diltiazem 120 mg twice daily for 7 days.[6] Similarly, there was no statistically significant change in the half-life or clearance of theophylline (given as a single 250-mg intravenous dose of aminophylline) in healthy subjects given diltiazem 120 mg three times daily for 6 days.[7] One study found that the pharmacokinetics of a single 5-mg/kg intravenous dose of theophylline (given as aminophylline), were unaffected by diltiazem 60 mg given four times daily. However, in an extension of this study, the reduction in theophylline half-life and the increase in theophylline clearance caused by rifampicin 600 mg daily (see 'Theophylline + Rifamycins and/or Isoniazid', p.1458), were slightly attenuated by diltiazem.[8]

(b) Felodipine

In a study in 10 healthy subjects, felodipine 5 mg every 8 hours for 4 days reduced the plasma AUC of theophylline (given as theophylline aminopropanol) by 18%, but had no effect on its metabolic or renal clearance.[9]

(c) Isradipine

A crossover study in 11 healthy subjects found that isradipine 2.5 or 5 mg every 12 hours for 6 days had no significant effect on the pharmacokinetics of a single 5-mg/kg dose of aminophylline oral solution.[10]

(d) Nifedipine

In one study in 8 patients with asthma, slow-release nifedipine 20 mg twice daily reduced the mean steady-state theophylline levels by 30%, from 9.7 mg/L to 6.8 mg/L. Levels fell by 50%, 56%, and 64% in three of the patients, but no changes in the control of the asthma (as measured by peak flow determinations and symptom scores) were seen.[11] However, many other studies have found no changes, or only slight changes, in the pharmacokinetics of theophylline (given as oral theophylline or as intravenous lysine theophylline[12] or aminophylline[13]) in healthy subjects[6,12-14] or patients with asthma[5,15,16] given nifedipine. The control of the asthma was unchanged by nifedipine.[15,16] A study found that the combined use of slow-release theophylline and nifedipine improved pulmonary function and blood pressure control.[17]

In contrast, there are 2 case reports of patients who developed theophylline toxicity (theophylline levels raised to 30 mg/L and 41 mg/L, respectively), apparently due to the addition of nifedipine.[18,19] In one case, toxicity recurred on rechallenge, and resolved when the theophylline dose was reduced by 60%.[19] During a Swan Ganz catheter study of patient response to nifedipine for pulmonary hypertension, 2 patients developed serious nifedipine adverse effects, which responded to intravenous aminophylline.[20]

(e) Verapamil

In one study in 5 patients with asthma, verapamil 80 mg every 6 hours for 2 days had no effect on the pharmacokinetics of theophylline (given as aminophylline 200 mg every 6 hours) and no effect on their spirometry (FVC, FEV_1, FEF_{25-75}).[21] Similarly, a study in healthy subjects found that verapamil 80 mg every 8 hours had no effect on the steady-state levels of sustained-release theophylline 3 mg/kg per day.[22] In contrast, numerous other studies in healthy subjects (given intravenous or oral aminophylline or theophylline) have found negligible to slight reductions in theophylline clearance, of 8 to 23% with verapamil 40 to 120 mg taken every 6 to 8 hours.[2,7,14,23-25] One study found that the extent of reduction in clearance depended on the verapamil dose.[25]

An isolated report describes a woman taking digoxin and sustained-release theophylline who developed signs of toxicity (tachycardia, nausea, vomiting) after starting to take verapamil 80 mg, increased to 120 mg, every 8 hours. Her serum theophylline levels doubled over a 6-day period. Theophylline was later successfully reintroduced at one-third of the original dose.[26] Another isolated report describes a patient who needed a 50% reduction in their theophylline dose while taking verapamil 120 mg daily.[27]

Mechanism

It has been suggested that diltiazem and verapamil can, to a limited extent, decrease the metabolism of theophylline, possibly by inhibiting CYP1A2 in the liver.[28] Similarly, nifedipine might alter the hepatic metabolism of theophylline,[14] or it might increase the volume of distribution of theophylline.[12,13] Felodipine possibly reduces theophylline absorption.[9]

Importance and management

Evidence for an interaction between theophylline or aminophylline and the calcium-channel blockers is adequately documented but the results are not entirely consistent. However, the overall picture is that diltiazem, felodipine, nifedipine and verapamil do not usually have a clinically relevant effect on theophylline pharmacokinetics. However, very occasionally and unpredictably, theophylline levels have risen enough to cause toxicity in patients given nifedipine (2 case reports) or verapamil (2 case reports), and therefore, with these particular calcium-channel blockers, it would be prudent to consider the possibility of an interaction in the case of otherwise unexplained theophylline adverse effects (headache, nausea, tremor). Should these adverse effects remain troublesome, monitor theophylline levels and adjust the aminophylline or theophylline dose accordingly.

1. Nafziger AN, May JJ, Bertino JS. Inhibition of theophylline elimination by diltiazem therapy. *J Clin Pharmacol* (1987) 27, 862–5.
2. Sirmans SM, Pieper JA, Lalonde RL, Smith DG, Self TH. Effect of calcium channel blockers on theophylline disposition. *Clin Pharmacol Ther* (1988) 44, 29–34.
3. Ohashi K, Sakamoto K, Sudo T, Tateishi T, Fujimura A, Shiga T, Ebihara A. Effects of diltiazem and cimetidine on theophylline oxidative metabolism. *J Clin Pharmacol* (1993) 33, 1233–7.
4. Soto J, Sacristan JA, Alsar MJ. Diltiazem treatment impairs theophylline elimination in patients with bronchospastic airway disease. *Ther Drug Monit* (1994) 16, 49–52.
5. Christopher MA, Harman E, Hendeles L. Clinical relevance of the interaction of theophylline with diltiazem or nifedipine. *Chest* (1989) 95, 309–13.
6. Smith SR, Haffner CA, Kendall MJ. The influence of nifedipine and diltiazem on serum theophylline concentration-time profiles. *J Clin Pharm Ther* (1989) 14, 403–8.
7. Abernethy DR, Egan JM, Dickinson TH, Carrum G. Substrate-selective inhibition by verapamil and diltiazem: differential disposition of antipyrine and theophylline in humans. *J Pharmacol Exp Ther* (1988) 244, 994–9.
8. Adebayo GI, Akintonwa A, Mabadeje AFB. Attenuation of rifampicin-induced theophylline metabolism by diltiazem/rifampicin coadministration in healthy volunteers. *Eur J Clin Pharmacol* (1989) 37, 127–31.
9. Bratel T, Billing B, Dahlqvist R. Felodipine reduces the absorption of theophylline in man. *Eur J Clin Pharmacol* (1989) 36, 481–5.
10. Perreault MM, Kazierad DJ, Wilton JH, Izzo JL. The effect of isradipine on theophylline pharmacokinetics in healthy volunteers. *Pharmacotherapy* (1993) 13, 149–53.
11. Smith SR, Wiggins J, Stableforth DE, Skinner C, Kendall MJ. Effect of nifedipine on serum theophylline concentrations and asthma control. *Thorax* (1987) 42, 794–6.
12. Jackson SHD, Shah K, Debbas NMG, Johnston A, Peverel-Cooper CA, Turner P. The interaction between i.v. theophylline and chronic oral dosing with slow release nifedipine in volunteers. *Br J Clin Pharmacol* (1986) 21, 389–92.
13. Adebayo GI, Mabadeje AFB. Effect of nifedipine on antipyrine and theophylline disposition. *Biopharm Drug Dispos* (1990) 11, 157–64.
14. Robson RA, Miners JO, Birkett DJ. Selective inhibitory effects of nifedipine and verapamil on oxidative metabolism: effects on theophylline. *Br J Clin Pharmacol* (1988) 25, 397–400.
15. Garty M, Cohen E, Mazar A, Ilfeld DN, Spitzer S, Rosenfeld JB. Effect of nifedipine and theophylline in asthma. *Clin Pharmacol Ther* (1986) 40, 195–8.
16. Yilmaz E, Canberk A, Eroğlu L. Nifedipine alters serum theophylline levels in asthmatic patients with hypertension. *Fundam Clin Pharmacol* (1991) 5, 341–5.
17. Spedini C, Lombardi C. Long-term treatment with oral nifedipine plus theophylline in the management of chronic bronchial asthma. *Eur J Clin Pharmacol* (1986) 31, 105–6.
18. Parrillo SJ, Venditto M. Elevated theophylline blood levels from institution of nifedipine therapy. *Ann Emerg Med* (1984) 13, 216–17.
19. Harrod CS. Theophylline toxicity and nifedipine. *Ann Intern Med* (1987) 106, 480.
20. Kalra L, Bone MF, Ariaraj SJP. Nifedipine-aminophylline interaction. *J Clin Pharmacol* (1988) 28, 1056–7.
21. Gotz VP, Russell WL. Effect of verapamil on theophylline disposition. *Chest* (1987) 92, 75S.
22. Rindone JP, Zuniga R, Sock JA. The influence of verapamil on theophylline serum concentrations. *Drug Metabol Drug Interact* (1989) 7, 143–7.
23. Nielsen-Kudsk JE, Buhl JS, Johannessen AC. Verapamil-induced inhibition of theophylline elimination in healthy humans. *Pharmacol Toxicol* (1990) 66, 101–3.
24. Gin AS, Stringer KA, Welage LS, Wilton JH, Matthews GE. The effect of verapamil on the pharmacokinetic disposition of theophylline in cigarette smokers. *J Clin Pharmacol* (1989) 29, 728–32.
25. Stringer KA, Mallet J, Clarke M, Lindenfeld JA. The effect of three different oral doses of verapamil on the disposition of theophylline. *Eur J Clin Pharmacol* (1992) 43, 35–8.
26. Burnakis TG, Seldon M, Czaplicki AD. Increased serum theophylline concentrations secondary to oral verapamil. *Clin Pharm* (1983) 2, 458–61.
27. Bangura L, Malesker MA, Dewan NA. Theophylline and verapamil: Clinically significant drug interaction. *J Pharm Technol* (1997) 13, 241–3.
28. Fuhr U, Woodcock BG, Siewert M. Verapamil and drug metabolism by the cytochrome P450 isoform CYP1A2. *Eur J Clin Pharmacol* (1992) 42, 463–4.

Theophylline + Cannabis

Smoking cannabis appears to increase the clearance of theophylline.

Clinical evidence, mechanism, importance and management

One study found that tobacco or cannabis smoking caused similar higher total clearances of theophylline (given as oral aminophylline) than occurred in non-smokers (about 74 mL/kg per hour compared with 52 mL/kg per hour), and that clearance was even higher (93 mL/kg per hour) in those who smoked both.[1] A later analysis by the same authors, of factors affecting theophylline clearance, found that smoking two or more joints of cannabis weekly was associated with a higher total clearance of theophylline than non-use (82.9 mL/kg per hour versus 56.1 mL/kg per hour).[2] A study in which 16 of 49 healthy subjects admitted to smoking cannabis in the months before taking a single 4-mg/kg oral dose of theophylline found that cannabis use did not have a significant effect on the pharmacokinetics of theophylline. Their use was considered not to exceed normal social use of one joint per week.[3]

Both tobacco and cannabis smoke contain polycyclic hydrocarbons, which act as inducers of CYP1A2, the isoenzyme by which theophylline is metabolised, and therefore theophylline might be cleared more quickly in those who smoke these substances (consider also 'Theophylline + Tobacco', p.1462).

Evidence for an effect of smoking cannabis on theophylline levels is limited, but be alert for the need to increase the theophylline dose in regular cannabis users. Note also that irregular cannabis use might cause fluctuations in theophylline levels. An additional problem in interpreting this interaction is that the quantity of interacting constituent might vary between different sources of cannabis, and between different batches from the same source.

There appears to be no direct evidence regarding aminophylline, but as it is metabolised to theophylline, it seems likely that it will be similarly affected by cannabis.

1. Jusko WJ, Schentag JJ, Clark JH, Gardner M, Yurchak AM. Enhanced biotransformation of theophylline in marihuana and tobacco smokers. *Clin Pharmacol Ther* (1978) 24, 406–10.
2. Jusko WJ, Gardner MJ, Mangione A, Schentag JJ, Koup JR, Vance JW. Factors affecting theophylline clearances: age, tobacco, marijuana, cirrhosis, congestive heart failure, obesity, oral contraceptives, benzodiazepines, barbiturates, and ethanol. *J Pharm Sci* (1979) 68, 1358–66.
3. Gardner MJ, Tornatore KM, Jusko WJ, Kanarkowski R. Effects of tobacco smoking and oral contraceptive use on theophylline disposition. *Br J Clin Pharmacol* (1983) 16, 271–80.

Theophylline + Carbamazepine

Case reports suggest that carbamazepine might moderately increase theophylline clearance. Another single case report and a pharmacokinetic study suggest that carbamazepine exposure might be slightly reduced by theophylline.

Clinical evidence

(a) Theophylline levels reduced

An 11-year-old girl with asthma was stable for 2 months taking theophylline and phenobarbital until the phenobarbital was replaced by carbamazepine. The asthma worsened, her theophylline serum levels became subtherapeutic and the half-life of the theophylline was reduced from 5.25 hours to 2.75 hours. Asthmatic control was restored, and the half-life returned to pre-treatment levels 3 weeks after carbamazepine was replaced by ethotoin.[1] Another report noted that the clearance of theophylline in an adult patient was doubled by carbamazepine 600 mg daily.[2]

(b) Carbamazepine levels reduced

The trough carbamazepine levels of a 10-year-old girl were roughly halved when she was given theophylline for 2 days, and she experienced a grand mal seizure. Her serum theophylline levels were also unusually high at 26 mg/L for the 5 mg/kg dose she was taking, so it may be that the convulsions were as much due to this as to the fall in carbamazepine levels.[3]

A single-dose pharmacokinetic study in healthy subjects found that the AUC and maximum plasma levels of carbamazepine were reduced by 31% and 45%, respectively, by oral aminophylline.[4]

Mechanism

Not established. It has been suggested that each drug increases the liver metabolism and clearance of the other drug, resulting in a reduction in their effects,[1,3] but the exact pathway for this effect is unclear. It has also been suggested that aminophylline interferes with the absorption of carbamazepine.[4]

Importance and management

Information regarding an interaction between theophylline or aminophylline and carbamazepine seems to be limited to the reports cited. The increase in theophylline clearance is only moderate, and the evidence available is from case reports; however, theophylline has a narrow therapeutic range and therefore these changes might be clinically relevant. It would therefore be prudent to be alert for any reduction in the effects of theophylline when carbamazepine is also given, taking theophylline levels and increasing the aminophylline or theophylline dose as necessary.

The reduction in carbamazepine clearance caused by theophylline is not established, as the available evidence comes from a case report and a single dose study. Furthermore, the effects on carbamazepine exposure were slight. However, carbamazepine has a narrow therapeutic range, and so, until more is known it might be prudent to be aware that carbamazepine levels could be reduced by aminophylline (and possibly theophylline). If both drugs are given, take carbamazepine levels and increase the carbamazepine dose as necessary.

Note that theophylline should be used with caution in patients with epilepsy as it can cause seizures, although this is usually a sign of toxicity.

1. Rosenberry KR, Defusco CJ, Mansmann HC, McGeady SJ. Reduced theophylline half-life induced by carbamazepine therapy. *J Pediatr* (1983) 102, 472–4.
2. Reed RC, Schwartz HJ. Phenytoin-theophylline-quinidine interaction. *N Engl J Med* (1983) 308, 724–5.
3. Mitchell EA, Dower JC, Green RJ. Interaction between carbamazepine and theophylline. *N Z Med J* (1986) 99, 69–70.
4. Kulkarni C, Vaz J, David J, Joseph T. Aminophylline alters pharmacokinetics of carbamazepine but not that of sodium valproate — a single dose pharmacokinetic study in human volunteers. *Indian J Physiol Pharmacol* (1995) 39, 122–6.

Theophylline + Cephalosporins

Ceftibuten and cefalexin do not appear to affect the pharmacokinetics of theophylline to a clinically relevant extent. Cefaclor has been implicated in two cases of theophylline toxicity in children, but studies in adult subjects found no pharmacokinetic interaction.

Clinical evidence, mechanism, importance and management

In a study in 12 healthy subjects, **ceftibuten** 200 mg twice daily for 7 days had no clinically significant effect on the pharmacokinetics of a single intravenous dose of theophylline.[1] A study in 9 healthy adults given a single 5-mg/kg intravenous dose of aminophylline found that **cefalexin** 500 mg, then 250 mg every 6 hours for 48 hours, had no statistically significant effect on the pharmacokinetics of theophylline.[2]

A case report[3] suggested that **cefaclor** might have been responsible for the development of theophylline toxicity in 2 children. However, a single-dose study[4] and a steady-state study[5] in healthy adults found that **cefaclor** 250 mg three times daily for 8 and 9 days, respectively, had no effect on the pharmacokinetics of oral or intravenous theophylline. Although the pharmacokinetics of theophylline differ in adults and children, a clinically relevant interaction with **cefaclor** seems unlikely.

No theophylline or aminophylline dose adjustments seem to be necessary with any of these antibacterials. However, note that acute infections *per se* can alter theophylline pharmacokinetics.[6]

1. Bachmann K, Schwartz J, Jauregui L, Martin M, Nunlee M. Failure of ceftibuten to alter single dose theophylline clearance. *J Clin Pharmacol* (1990) 30, 444–8.
2. Pfeifer HJ, Greenblatt DJ, Friedman P. Effects of three antibiotics on theophylline kinetics. *Clin Pharmacol Ther* (1979) 26, 36–40.
3. Hammond D, Abate MA. Theophylline toxicity, acute illness, and cefaclor administration. *DICP Ann Pharmacother* (1989) 23, 339–40.
4. Bachmann K, Schwartz J, Forney RB, Jauregui L. Impact of cefaclor on the pharmacokinetics of theophylline. *Ther Drug Monit* (1986) 8, 151–4.
5. Jonkman JHG, van der Boon WJV, Schoenmaker R, Holtkamp A, Hempenius J. Clinical pharmacokinetics of theophylline during co-treatment with cefaclor. *Int J Clin Pharmacol Ther Toxicol* (1986) 24, 88–92.
6. Renton KW. Cytochrome P450 regulation and drug biotransformation during inflammation and infection. *Curr Drug Metab* (2004) 5, 235–43.

Theophylline + Clopidogrel and related drugs

Ticlopidine reduces the clearance of theophylline. Clopidogrel does not appear to affect the pharmacokinetics of theophylline.

Clinical evidence, mechanism, importance and management

(a) Clopidogrel

In a study in 12 healthy subjects, clopidogrel 75 mg daily for 10 days did not alter the steady-state pharmacokinetics of theophylline.[1] Therefore no theophylline dose adjustment is expected to be necessary on the concurrent use of these two drugs. There appears to be no direct evidence regarding aminophylline, but as it is metabolised to theophylline, a similar lack of adverse interaction would be expected with clopidogrel.

(b) Ticlopidine

In a study in 10 healthy subjects, ticlopidine 250 mg twice daily for 10 days reduced the clearance of a single 5-mg/kg oral dose of theophylline by 37% and increased its half-life by 44%, from about 8.5 hours to 12 hours.[2] Ticlopidine is an inhibitor of CYP1A2, the isoenzyme which metabolises theophylline in the liver, and therefore concurrent use leads to a reduction in theophylline clearance. Information is limited, nevertheless, it would seem prudent to check for any signs of theophylline adverse effects (headache, nausea, tremor) on concurrent use, particularly in situations where the metabolism of the theophylline may already be reduced (other drugs or diseases), and monitor theophylline levels accordingly.

There appears to be no direct evidence regarding aminophylline, but as it is metabolised to theophylline, it seems likely that it will be similarly affected by ticlopidine.

1. Caplain H, Thebault J-J, Necciari J. Clopidogrel does not affect the pharmacokinetics of theophylline. *Semin Thromb Hemost* (1999) 24, 65–8.
2. Colli A, Buccino G, Cocciolo M, Parravicini R, Elli GM, Scaltrini G. Ticlopidine-theophylline interaction. *Clin Pharmacol Ther* (1987) 41, 358–62.

Theophylline + Codeine

Codeine does not affect the extent of theophylline absorption from a sustained-release preparation.

Clinical evidence, mechanism, importance and management

A study in 6 healthy subjects found that codeine 30 mg prolonged the oral to caecal transit time of a single 500-mg dose of sustained-release theophylline (*Theo-Dur*). The mean amount of theophylline left to be absorbed from the colon was reduced from 58% to 33%, but the time to 90% absorption of theophylline was not affected to a statistically significant extent (7.1 hours compared with 8.5 hours). Therefore codeine does not appear to have a clinically relevant effect on the rate or extent of absorption of theophylline from a sustained-release preparation[1] and no particular precautions are necessary on their concurrent use.

1. Sommers DK, Meyer EC, Van Wyk M, Moncrieff J, Snyman JR, Grimbeek RJ. The influence of codeine, propantheline and metoclopramide on small bowel transit and theophylline absorption from a sustained-release formulation. *Br J Clin Pharmacol* (1992) 33, 305–8.

Theophylline + Corticosteroids

Theophylline and corticosteroids have established roles in the management of asthma and their concurrent use is not uncommon. There are isolated reports of increases in theophylline levels (sometimes associated with toxicity) when oral or parenteral corticosteroids are given, but other reports show no changes. Both theophylline and corticosteroids can cause hypokalaemia, which may be additive.

Clinical evidence

(a) Betamethasone

The elimination half-life of theophylline (given as an intravenous loading dose of aminophylline 10 mg/kg), followed after 24 hours by maintenance doses of intravenous aminophylline or oral aminophylline or theophylline 2 to 3 mg/kg every 12 hours) was no different in premature infants who had been exposed to betamethasone *in utero* than in those who had not, although the exposed neonates had a wider range of theophylline metabolites indicating greater hepatic metabolism.[1,2]

(b) Dexamethasone

In one study it was briefly mentioned that theophylline did not appear to affect dexamethasone metabolism.[3]

(c) Hydrocortisone

Three patients with status asthmaticus and relatively stable serum concentrations of theophylline were given a 500-mg intravenous bolus of hydrocortisone followed 6 hours later by 200 mg of hydrocortisone given every 2 hours for 3 doses. In each case the serum theophylline levels rose from about 20 mg/L to between 30 and 50 mg/L. At least 2 of the patients complained of nausea and headache.[4] In contrast, 7 healthy subjects given sustained-release theophylline had no significant change in steady-state theophylline clearance when they were given a single 33-mg/kg dose of intravenous hydrocortisone, although there was a trend towards increased clearance.[5] Intravenous bolus doses of hydrocortisone 500 mg or 1 g did not affect theophylline levels in patients taking choline theophyllinate 400 mg every 12 hours for 8 days.[6]

(d) Methylprednisolone

An 88% increase in the clearance of a single dose of intravenous aminophylline was seen in one of 3 healthy subjects pretreated with oral methylprednisolone. There was no significant change in clearance in the other 2 subjects.[7] Another study in 10 children (aged 2 to 6 years) with status asthmaticus found that intramuscular methylprednisolone tended to increase the half-life of theophylline (given as oral aminophylline or theophylline).[8] A further study also reported that when intravenous aminophylline was given to 16 children taking corticosteroids (route and type not specified) the theophylline half-life was prolonged from 5 hours to 6.2 hours, and the clearance was reduced by about one-third, when compared with 10 children not taking corticosteroids.[9] Similarly, 7 healthy subjects given sustained-release theophylline had no significant change in steady-state theophylline clearance when they were given a single 1.6-mg/kg dose of intravenous methylprednisolone, although there was a trend towards increased clearance.[5] For a report of lower than expected theophylline levels, attributed to gold therapy, in patients taking methylprednisolone, auranofin and theophylline, see 'Theophylline + Gold', p.1444.

(e) Prednisone or Prednisolone

A study in 6 healthy subjects found that a single 20-mg oral dose of prednisone had no significant effect on the pharmacokinetics of a single 200-mg oral dose of aminophylline.[10] The pharmacokinetics of a single 5.6-mg/kg intravenous dose of aminophylline was unchanged in 9 patients with chronic airflow obstruction when they were given prednisolone 20 mg daily for 3 weeks.[11]

Mechanism

Not understood.

Importance and management

The concurrent use of theophylline or aminophylline and corticosteroids is common and therapeutically valuable, whereas the few reported interactions of theophylline or aminophylline with oral or parenteral corticosteroids are poorly documented and their clinical importance is difficult to assess because both increases, small decreases and no changes in theophylline levels have been seen. It is also questionable whether the results of studies in healthy subjects can validly be extrapolated to patients with status asthmaticus. From the study data available, it would seem that, in general, a clinically relevant pharmacokinetic interaction is unlikely to occur. There do not appear to be any data on the effect of *inhaled* corticosteroids on the clearance of theophylline.

Both theophylline and corticosteroids can cause hypokalaemia, and the possibility that this may be potentiated by concurrent use should be considered.

1. Jager-Roman E, Doyle PE, Thomas D, Baird-Lambert J, Cvejic M, Buchanan N. Increased theophylline metabolism in premature infants after prenatal betamethasone administration. *Dev Pharmacol Ther* (1982) 5, 127–35.
2. Baird-Lambert J, Doyle PE, Thomas D, Jager-Roman E, Cvejic M, Buchanan N. Theophylline metabolism in preterm neonates during the first weeks of life. *Dev Pharmacol Ther* (1984) 7, 239–44.
3. Brooks SM, Sholiton LJ, Werk EE, Altenau P. The effects of ephedrine and theophylline on dexamethasone metabolism in bronchial asthma. *J Clin Pharmacol* (1977) 17, 308.
4. Buchanan N, Hurwitz S, Butler P. Asthma—a possible interaction between hydrocortisone and theophylline. *S Afr Med J* (1979) 56, 1147–8.
5. Leavengood DC, Bunker-Soler AL, Nelson HS. The effect of corticosteroids on theophylline metabolism. *Ann Allergy* (1983) 50, 249–51.

6. Tatsis G, Orphanidou D, Douratsos D, Mellissinos C, Pantelakis D, Pipini E, Jordanoglou J. The effect of steroids on theophylline absorption. *J Int Med Res* (1991) 19, 326–9.
7. Squire EN, Nelson HS. Corticosteroids and theophylline clearance. *N Engl Reg Allergy Proc* (1987) 8, 113–15.
8. De La Morena E, Borges MT, Garcia Rebollar C, Escorihuela R. Efecto de la metil-prednisolona sobre los niveles séricos de teofilina. *Rev Clin Esp* (1982) 167, 297–300.
9. Elvey SM, Saccar CL, Rocci ML, Mansmann HC, Martynec DM, Kester MB. The effect of corticosteroids on theophylline metabolism in asthmatic children. *Ann Allergy* (1986) 56, 520.
10. Anderson JL, Ayres JW, Hall CA. Potential pharmacokinetic interaction between theophylline and prednisone. *Clin Pharm* (1984) 3, 187–9.
11. Fergusson RJ, Scott CM, Rafferty P, Gaddie J. Effect of prednisolone on theophylline pharmacokinetics in patients with chronic airflow obstruction. *Thorax* (1987) 42, 195–8.

Theophylline + Co-trimoxazole

Co-trimoxazole (trimethoprim with sulfamethoxazole) does not alter the pharmacokinetics of theophylline.

Clinical evidence, mechanism, importance and management

In a study in 6 healthy subjects, co-trimoxazole (trimethoprim with sulfamethoxazole) 960 mg twice daily for 8 days had no effect on the pharmacokinetics of theophylline 250 mg, given as a single 341-mg intravenous dose of aminophylline.[1] Another study, in 8 healthy subjects, found that co-trimoxazole 960 mg twice daily for 5 days had no effect on the pharmacokinetics of a single 267-mg oral dose of theophylline.[2] No theophylline or aminophylline dose adjustments would therefore seem to be necessary if these drugs are given concurrently. However, note that acute infections *per se* can alter theophylline pharmacokinetics.[3]

1. Jonkman JHG, Van Der Boon WJV, Schoenmaker R, Holtkamp AH, Hempenius J. Lack of influence of co-trimoxazole on theophylline pharmacokinetics. *J Pharm Sci* (1985) 74, 1103–4.
2. Lo KF, Nation RL, Sansom LN. Lack of effect of co-trimoxazole on the pharmacokinetics of orally administered theophylline. *Biopharm Drug Dispos* (1989) 10, 573–80.
3. Renton KW. Cytochrome P450 regulation and drug biotransformation during inflammation and infection. *Curr Drug Metab* (2004) 5, 235–43.

Theophylline + Dextropropoxyphene (Propoxyphene)

Dextropropoxyphene does not alter theophylline clearance.

Clinical evidence, mechanism, importance and management

In a study in 6 healthy subjects, pre-treatment with dextropropoxyphene 65 mg every 8 hours for 5 days did not alter the total plasma clearance of steady-state theophylline 125 mg every 8 hours. There was a small reduction in the formation of the hydroxylated metabolite of theophylline, but this was not expected to be clinically relevant.[1] There would seem to be no need to avoid concurrent use or to take particular precautions.

There appears to be no direct evidence regarding aminophylline, but as it is metabolised to theophylline, no adverse interaction would be expected with dextropropoxyphene.

1. Robson RA, Miners JO, Whitehead AG, Birkett DJ. Specificity of the inhibitory effect of dextropropoxyphene on oxidative drug metabolism in man: effects on theophylline and tolbutamide disposition. *Br J Clin Pharmacol* (1987) 23, 772–5.

Theophylline + Disulfiram

Disulfiram causes a negligible to slight decrease in the clearance of theophylline.

Clinical evidence

After 20 recovering alcoholics took disulfiram 250 mg daily for one week, the clearance of a 5-mg/kg intravenous dose of theophylline was decreased by a mean of about 21% (range 15 to 30%). Those taking disulfiram 500 mg daily had a mean decrease of 33% (range 22 to 50%). Smoking appeared to have no important effects on the extent of this interaction. None of the patients were reported to have any significant liver disease, such as cirrhosis, which may also affect theophylline metabolism.[1]

Mechanism

Disulfiram is a weak inhibitor of CYP1A2, the isoenzyme primarily involved in the metabolism of theophylline, thereby reducing its clearance.

Importance and management

Information regarding an interaction between theophylline and disulfiram appears to be limited to this study, which found that, even at higher doses of disulfiram the effects were only slight. However, because theophylline has a narrow therapeutic range it would seem that in some patients this could result in a clinically important interaction. Therefore it would seem prudent to check for any signs of theophylline adverse effects (headache, nausea, and tremor) on concurrent use, particularly in situations where the metabolism of the theophylline may already be reduced (other drugs or diseases) and monitor theophylline levels accordingly. Note that the extent of this interaction appears to depend upon the dose of disulfiram used; higher doses present a greater risk. As aminophylline is metabolised to theophylline, it would be expected to interact with disulfiram in a similar way.

1. Loi C-M, Day JD, Jue SG, Bush ED, Costello P, Dewey LV, Vestal RE. Dose-dependent inhibition of theophylline metabolism by disulfiram in recovering alcoholics. *Clin Pharmacol Ther* (1989) 45, 476–86.

Theophylline + Diuretics

Furosemide is reported to increase, decrease or to have no effect on theophylline levels. Both theophylline and diuretics can cause hypokalaemia, which might be additive. An isolated case describes severe hyponatraemia and syndrome of inappropriate secretion of antidiuretic hormone in a premature neonate receiving chlorothiazide, spironolactone and theophylline.

Clinical evidence

In 8 patients with asthma the mean peak serum level of a 300-mg dose of sustained-release theophylline was reduced by 41% (from 12.14 mg/L to 7.16 mg/L) by a single 25-mg oral dose of **furosemide**.[1] A crossover study in 12 healthy subjects did not find any change in steady-state plasma theophylline levels when two 20-mg doses of oral **furosemide** were given 4 hours apart, although the overall renal clearance of theophylline was reduced.[2] However, 10 patients with asthma, chronic bronchitis or emphysema, receiving a continuous maintenance infusion of aminophylline, had a 21% rise in their serum theophylline levels (from 13.7 mg/L to 16.6 mg/L) 4 hours after being given a 40-mg intravenous dose of **furosemide** over 2 minutes.[3]

Four premature neonates, two given oral and two given intravenous theophylline with **furosemide** had a fall in their steady-state serum theophylline levels from 8 mg/L down to 2 to 3 mg/L when **furosemide** was given within 30 minutes of the theophylline.[4] A randomised, placebo-controlled study in 24 infants receiving ECMO (extracorporeal membrane oxygenation) found that theophylline 2 mg/kg enhanced the response to diuresis with **furosemide** 1 mg/kg. If the response were maintained over a 24-hour period an extra 110 mL/kg of fluid would have been lost.[5]

A case of severe hyponatraemia and syndrome of inappropriate secretion of antidiuretic hormone has been reported in a pre-term neonate who received theophylline, as aminophylline (maintenance dose 4 mg/kg every 12 hours), and then started to receive **chlorothiazide** 25 mg/kg every 12 hours and **spironolactone** 1 mg/kg every 12 hours. His sodium level was restored by the intravenous administration of 3% sodium chloride.[6]

Mechanism

Not understood, although in theory furosemide could increase the renal excretion of theophylline, which could explain the reduced levels. The thiazides, spironolactone and theophylline[7] have each been reported to cause hyponatraemia, and therefore the low sodium levels might have occurred as a result of the additive effects of these drugs.

Importance and management

Information regarding an interaction between furosemide and aminophylline or theophylline is limited and the outcome of concurrent use is inconsistent and uncertain. More study is needed to assess the clinical relevance of the effects of theophylline and furosemide on diuresis. However, note that theophylline clearance can be reduced by some conditions such as chronic heart failure or pulmonary oedema. Theophylline clearance could therefore be increased when the health of the patient is improved, possibly through the use of furosemide.[8] Whatever the reason for the effects seen, if both drugs are used, be aware of the potential for changes in theophylline levels. Consider measuring theophylline levels, and make appropriate theophylline or aminophylline dose adjustments as necessary.

Direct information about other loop diuretics appears to be lacking. However; the manufacturer of **torasemide** notes that it might potentiate the action of theophylline,[9] but there appears to be no published data supporting this suggestion.

Theophylline, the loop diuretics and thiazides can cause hypokalaemia, and the possibility that this might be additive on concurrent use should be considered.

The general relevance of the isolated case describing hyponatraemia with aminophylline, chlorothiazide and spironolactone is unclear.

1. Carpentiere G, Marino S, Castello F. Furosemide and theophylline. *Ann Intern Med* (1985) 103, 957.
2. Jänicke U-A, Krüdewagen B, Schulz A, Gundert-Remy U. Absence of a clinically significant interaction between theophylline and furosemide. *Eur J Clin Pharmacol* (1987) 33, 487–91.
3. Conlon PF, Grambau GR, Johnson CE, Weg JG. Effect of intravenous furosemide on serum theophylline concentration. *Am J Hosp Pharm* (1981) 38, 1345–7.
4. Toback JW, Gilman ME. Theophylline-furosemide inactivation? *Pediatrics* (1983) 71, 140–1.
5. Lochan SR, Adeniyi-Jones S, Assadi FK, Frey BM, Marcus S, Baumgart S. Coadministration of theophylline enhances diuretic response to furosemide in infants during extracorporeal membrane oxygenation: a randomized controlled pilot study. *J Pediatr* (1998) 133, 86–9.
6. Srinivasan K, Patole SK, Whitehall JS. Severe hyponatremia in a neonate – an unusual association. *Indian Pediatr* (2001) 38, 1410–12.
7. Liberopoulos EN, Alexandridis GH, Christidis DS, Elisaf MS. SIADH and hyponatremia with theophylline. *Ann Pharmacother* (2002) 36, 1180–2.
8. Nakagawa RS. Theophylline-furosemide interaction? *Am J Hosp Pharm* (1982) 39, 242.
9. Torem (Torasemide). Meda Pharmaceuticals. UK Summary of product characteristics, September 2009.

Theophylline + Dobutamine

A man taking theophylline developed marked tachycardia when he was given dobutamine.

Clinical evidence, mechanism, importance and management

A patient with asthma taking sustained-release theophylline 150 mg twice daily, digoxin and spironolactone was anaesthetised for an aortic valve replacement with fentanyl, midazolam and pipecuronium. Following induction, intubation, and ventilation with 100% oxygen, his systolic blood pressure fell from 120 mmHg to 80 mmHg, and his heart rate slowed from 70 bpm to 50 bpm. Dobutamine was given at a dose of

5 micrograms/kg per minute, and after 2 to 3 minutes his heart rate rose to 150 bpm and his systolic blood pressure rose to 190 mmHg. The authors of the report[1] attributed the tachycardia to an interaction between dobutamine and theophylline, and suggested that the interaction was possibly as a result of a synergistic increase in cyclic AMP levels in cardiac muscle and/or theophylline-induced potentiation of catecholamine action. They advised the careful titration of dobutamine in any patient with asthma taking theophylline, particularly if a slow-release preparation is being used. However, more study of this apparent interaction is needed as this appears to be the only report, and so its general importance is unknown.

1. Baraka A, Darwish R, Rizkallah P. Excessive dobutamine-induced tachycardia in the asthmatic cardiac patient: possible potentiation by theophylline therapy. *J Cardiothorac Vasc Anesth* (1993) 7, 641–2.

Theophylline + Doxapram

Doxapram pharmacokinetics are unchanged by theophylline in premature infants, but agitation and increased muscle activity may occur in adults.

Clinical evidence, mechanism, importance and management

Intravenous theophylline does not affect the pharmacokinetics of doxapram given to treat apnoea in premature infants, and no adjustment of the dose of doxapram is needed in the presence of theophylline.[1] However, the manufacturers of doxapram state that the concurrent use of doxapram and aminophylline might cause agitation, muscle fasciculation and hyperactivity. Care should therefore be taken if these drugs are used together.[2]

1. Jamali F, Coutts RT, Malek F, Finer NN, Peliowski A. Lack of a pharmacokinetic interaction between doxapram and theophylline in apnea of prematurity. *Dev Pharmacol Ther* (1991) 16, 78–82.
2. Doxapram hydrochloride. Mercury Pharma Group. UK Summary of product characteristics, March 2012.

Theophylline + Duloxetine

Duloxetine causes a negligible increase in the exposure to theophylline.

Clinical evidence, mechanism, importance and management

In a study in 28 healthy subjects, duloxetine 60 mg was given twice daily for 4 days, and with a single 197.5-mg intravenous dose of theophylline (given as aminophylline 250 mg) on day 5. Duloxetine increased the AUC of theophylline by 20% in the women who participated in the study, but no statistically significant increase in the AUC of theophylline was seen in the men. Overall, the AUC of theophylline was increased by 13%.[1] However, these increases would not be expected to be clinically relevant and no dose adjustment of theophylline or aminophylline is likely to be required if duloxetine is also given.

1. Lobo ED, Bergstrom RF, Reddy S, Quinlan T, Chappell J, Hong Q, Ring B, Knadler MP. *In vitro* and *in vivo* evaluations of cytochrome P450 1A2 interactions with duloxetine. *Clin Pharmacokinet* (2008) 47, 191–202.

Theophylline + Enoximone

Aminophylline possibly reduces the beneficial cardiovascular effects of enoximone. Theoretically, milrinone would be expected to interact similarly.

Clinical evidence, mechanism, importance and management

An experimental study into the mechanism of action of enoximone in 14 patients with ischaemic or idiopathic dilative cardiomyopathy found that pretreatment with intravenous aminophylline 7 mg/kg given over 15 minutes reduced the beneficial haemodynamic effects of intravenous enoximone 1 mg/kg given over 15 minutes.[1] This appears to occur because each drug competes for inhibition of cAMP-specific phosphodiesterases in cardiac and vascular smooth muscle. **Milrinone**, another phosphodiesterase inhibitor similar to enoximone, would be expected to interact in the same way. However, there are, at present, no published reports of a possible interaction with milrinone, and no case reports of a problem occurring with the concurrent use of either drug with theophylline or aminophylline. The clinical importance of this study therefore awaits evaluation.

1. Morgagni GL, Bugiardini R, Borghi A, Pozzati A, Ottani F, Puddu P. Aminophylline counteracts the hemodynamic effects of enoximone. *Clin Pharmacol Ther* (1990) 47, 140.

Theophylline + Ephedrine

Some data suggest that an increased frequency of adverse effects occurs when ephedrine is given with theophylline.

Clinical evidence, mechanism, importance and management

A double-blind, randomised study in 23 children aged 4 to 14 years found that when ephedrine was given with theophylline (in a ratio of 25 mg ephedrine to 130 mg theophylline), the number of adverse reactions increased significantly, when compared with each drug taken separately. Moreover, the combination was no more effective than theophylline alone and was associated with insomnia (14 patients), nervousness (13 patients) and gastrointestinal complaints (18 patients), including vomiting (12 patients). The serum theophylline levels were unchanged by ephedrine.[1] A previous study by the same authors in 12 children with asthma given ephedrine and aminophylline found similar results.[2] In contrast, a later study suggested that ephedrine 25 mg every 8 hours given with aminophylline did produce improvements in spirometry and no adverse effects were seen. However, it was calculated that the theophylline dose used was about half that used in the previous study.[3]

In the treatment of asthma, ephedrine has been largely superseded by more selective sympathomimetics, which have fewer adverse effects. Ephedrine is still an ingredient of a number of non-prescription cough and cold remedies, when it may be combined with theophylline (e.g. *Do-Do ChestEze*). Patients taking theophylline or aminophylline requiring ephedrine should be advised to report any adverse effects.

1. Weinberger M, Bronsky E, Bensch GW, Bock GN, Yecies JJ. Interaction of ephedrine and theophylline. *Clin Pharmacol Ther* (1975) 17, 585–92.
2. Weinberger MM, Bronsky EA. Evaluation of oral bronchodilator therapy in asthmatic children. *J Pediatr* (1974) 84, 421–7.
3. Tinkelman DG, Avner SE. Ephedrine therapy in asthmatic children. Clinical tolerance and absence of side effects. *JAMA* (1977) 237, 553–7.

Theophylline + Flutamide

The manufacturer of flutamide noted that cases of increased theophylline plasma levels have been reported in patients taking these two drugs together. They suggested the reason for this is that flutamide and theophylline are both metabolised by CYP1A2.[1] Note that interactions by this mechanism are rarely clinically relevant.

1. Drogenil (Flutamide). Schering-Plough Ltd. UK Summary of product characteristics, August 2007.

Theophylline + Food

The effect of food on the pharmacokinetics of theophylline is variable. In general it appears that fat or fibre in food has no effect on theophylline absorption. High-protein diets decrease the half-life of theophylline, whereas high-carbohydrate diets might increase, or have no effect on the half-life of theophylline. Clinically relevant reductions in theophylline levels have been seen in some patients given enteral feeds or total parenteral nutrition.

Clinical evidence

(a) Food

The bioavailability of theophylline from sustained-release preparations has been shown to be reduced,[1,2] increased,[1,3,4] or unaffected[5-12] when theophylline was given immediately after breakfast. In one study, when sustained-release theophylline was given after food, the bioavailability of theophylline was increased by 10%, its trough level was increased by 0.7 mg/L, and the time to reach maximum plasma levels was increased from 8.6 hours to 11.4 hours.[4] Dose dumping, leading to signs of theophylline toxicity, was seen in 3 children with asthma who were given a dose of sustained-release theophylline (*Uniphyllin*) immediately after breakfast.[7] The fat content[11,13,14] or fibre content[15] of meals does not seem to affect theophylline absorption to a clinically relevant extent. High-protein meals appear to decrease the half-life of theophylline.[16,17] In one study high-carbohydrate meals increased the half-life of theophylline,[17] while in another study a high-carbohydrate meal had no effect on the half-life of a single 350-mg dose of sustained-release theophylline, but the maximum plasma levels were increased by 56%. There was no overall effect on the extent of absorption.[18] There was no difference in theophylline metabolism in one study when patients were changed from a high-carbohydrate/low-protein diet to a high-protein/low-carbohydrate diet.[19] One study found that changing from a high-protein to a high-carbohydrate meal had an effect on the metabolism of theophylline similar to that of cimetidine, and that the effects of the meal change and cimetidine were additive.[20] The effects of spicy food have been studied, but the clinical significance of the changes are uncertain.[21]

(b) Enteral feeds

A patient with COPD had a 53% reduction in his serum theophylline levels accompanied by bronchospasm when he was fed continuously through a nasogastric tube with *Osmolite*. The interaction occurred with both theophylline tablets (*Theo-Dur*) and liquid theophylline, but not when the theophylline was given intravenously as aminophylline. It was also found that the interaction could be avoided by interrupting feeding one hour either side of the oral liquid theophylline dose.[22] Conversely, hourly administration of 100 mL of *Osmolite* did not affect the extent of theophylline absorption from a slow-release preparation (*Slo-bid Gyrocaps*) in healthy subjects, although the rate of absorption was slowed.[23] Similarly, in healthy subjects, hourly administration of 100 mL of *Ensure* for 10 hours did not affect the rate or extent of absorption of theophylline from *Theo-24* tablets.[24]

(c) Parenteral nutrition

An isolated report describes an elderly woman given intravenous aminophylline who had a reduction in her serum theophylline levels (from 16.3 mg/L to 6.3 mg/L) when the amino acid concentration of her parenteral nutrition regimen was increased from 4.25% to 7%.[25] A study in 7 patients with malnutrition (marasmus-kwashiorkor) found only a small, probably clinically irrelevant increase in the elimination of a single intravenous dose of theophylline when they were fed intravenously.[26]

Mechanism

Not fully understood. As with any sustained-release formulation, the presence of food in the gut can alter the rate or extent of drug absorption by altering gastrointestinal transit time. It has been suggested that high-protein diets stimulate liver enzymes thereby increasing the metabolism of theophylline and hastening its clearance. High-carbohydrate diets might have the opposite effect. CYP1A2 (the principal enzyme involved in the metabolism of theophylline) is known to be induced by chemicals contained in cruciferous vegetables[27] or formed by the action of high temperatures or smoke on meat.[28] This suggestion is supported by a study in which charcoal-grilled (broiled) beef decreased the half-life of theophylline by an average of 22%.[29] Further, high doses of daidzein, the principal isoflavone in soybeans, might inhibit CYP1A2 resulting in an increase in theophylline levels and half-life of about 33% and 41%, respectively.[30]

Importance and management

Interactions between theophylline and food have been thoroughly studied but there seems to be no consistent pattern in the way the absorption of different aminophylline or theophylline preparations is affected. Be alert for any evidence of an inadequate response that might be related to food intake. Avoid switching between different preparations, and monitor the effects if this is necessary. Consult the product literature for any specific information on food and encourage patients to take their theophylline consistently in relation to meals where this is considered necessary. Advise patients not to make major changes in their diet without consultation. Monitor the effects of both enteral and parenteral nutrition, as aminophylline or theophylline dose adjustments might be required.

1. Karim A, Burns T, Wearley L, Streicher J, Palmer M. Food-induced changes in theophylline absorption from controlled-release formulations. Part I. Substantial increased and decreased absorption with Uniphyl tablets and Theo-Dur Sprinkle. *Clin Pharmacol Ther* (1985) 38, 77–83.
2. Lohmann A, Dingler E, Sommer W. Influence of food on the bioavailability of theophylline from a sustained-release theophylline preparation. *Arzneimittelforschung* (1991) 41, 732–4.
3. Vaughan L, Milavetz G, Hill M, Weinberger M, Hendeles L. Food-induced dose-dumping of Theo-24, a 'once-daily' slow-release theophylline product. *Drug Intell Clin Pharm* (1984) 18, 510.
4. Arkinstall WW, Hopkinson M, Rivington RN, Calcutt L, Aitken T, Stewart JH. The clinical significance of food-induced changes in the absorption of theophylline from Uniphyl tablets. *J Allergy Clin Immunol* (1988) 82, 155–64.
5. Johansson Ö, Lindberg T, Melander A, Wåhlin-Boll E. Different effects of different nutrients on theophylline absorption in man. *Drug Nutr Interact* (1985) 3, 205–11.
6. Sips AP, Edelbroek PM, Kulstad S, de Wolff FA, Dijkman JH. Food does not effect bioavailability of theophylline from Theolin Retard. *Eur J Clin Pharmacol* (1984) 26, 405–7.
7. Steffensen G, Pedersen S. Food induced changes in theophylline absorption from a once-a-day theophylline product. *Br J Clin Pharmacol* (1986) 22, 571–7.
8. Ürmös I, Grézal G, Balogh Nemes K, Szállási T, Drabant S, Csörgo M, Klebovich I. Food interaction study of a new theophylline (Egifilin) 200 and 400 mg retard tablet in healthy volunteers. *Int J Clin Pharmacol Ther* (1997) 35, 65–70.
9. González MA, Straughn AB. Effect of meals and dosage-form modification on theophylline bioavailability from a 24-hour sustained-release delivery system. *Clin Ther* (1994) 16, 804–14.
10. Boner AL, Sette L, Messori A, Plebani M, Vallone G, Martini N. Effect of food on the bioavailability of a slow-release theophylline formulation. *J Clin Pharm Ther* (1988) 13, 77–81.
11. Pabst G, Weber W, Müller M, Barkworth MF. Ungtersuchung von nahrungsbedingten veränderungen der theophyllin-resorption. *Arzneimittelforschung* (1998) 48, 569–73.
12. Boner AL, Bennati D, Valletta EA, Plebani M, Stevens MT, Scott JCV. Evaluation of the effect of food on the absorption of sustained-release theophylline and comparison of two methods for serum theophylline analysis. *J Clin Pharmacol* (1986) 26, 638–42.
13. Thebault JJ, Aiache JM, Mazoyer F, Cardot JM. The influence of food on the bioavailability of a slow release theophylline preparation. *Clin Pharmacokinet* (1987) 13, 267–72.
14. Lefebvre RA, Belpaire FM, Bogaert MG. Influence of food on steady state serum concentrations of theophylline from two controlled-release preparations. *Int J Clin Pharmacol Ther Toxicol* (1988) 26, 375–9.
15. Fassihi AR, Dowse R, Robertson SSD. Effect of dietary cellulose on the absorption and bioavailability of theophylline. *Int J Pharmaceutics* (1989) 50, 79–82.
16. Kappas A, Anderson KE, Conney AH, Alvares AP. Influence of dietary protein and carbohydrate on antipyrine and theophylline metabolism in man. *Clin Pharmacol Ther* (1976) 20, 643–53.
17. Feldman CH, Hutchinson VE, Pippenger CE, Blumenfeld TA, Feldman BR, Davis WJ. Effect of dietary protein and carbohydrate on theophylline metabolism in children. *Pediatrics* (1980) 66, 956–62.
18. Su Y-M, Cheng T-P, Wen C-Y. Study on the effect of food on the absorption of theophylline. *J Chin Med Assoc* (2003) 66, 715–21.
19. Thompson PJ, Skypala I, Dawson S, McAllister WAC, Turner Warwick M. The effect of diet upon serum concentrations of theophylline. *Br J Clin Pharmacol* (1983) 16, 267–70.
20. Anderson KE, McCleery RB, Vesell ES, Vickers FF, Kappas A. Diet and cimetidine induce comparable changes in theophylline metabolism in normal subjects. *Hepatology* (1991) 13, 941–6.
21. Bouraoui A, Toumi A, Bouchahcha S, Boukef K, Brazier JL. Influence de l'alimentation épicée et piquante sur l'absorption de la théophylline. *Therapie* (1986) 41, 467–71.
22. Gal P, Layson R. Interference with oral theophylline absorption by continuous nasogastric feedings. *Ther Drug Monit* (1986) 8, 421–3.
23. Bhargava VO, Schaaf LJ, Berlinger WG, Jungnickel PW. Effect of an enteral nutrient formula on sustained-release theophylline absorption. *Ther Drug Monit* (1989) 11, 515–19.
24. Plezia PM, Thornley SM, Kramer TH, Armstrong EP. The influence of enteral feedings on sustained-release theophylline absorption. *Pharmacotherapy* (1990) 10, 356–61.
25. Ziegenbein RC. Theophylline clearance increase from increased amino acid in a CPN regimen. *Drug Intell Clin Pharm* (1987) 21, 220–1.
26. Cuddy PG, Bealer JF, Lyman EL, Pemberton LB. Theophylline disposition following parenteral feeding of malnourished patients. *Ann Pharmacother* (1993) 27, 846–51.
27. Pantuck EJ, Pantuck CB, Garland WA, Min BH, Wattenberg LW, Anderson KE, Kappas A, Conney AH. Stimulatory effect of Brussels sprouts and cabbage on human drug metabolism. *Clin Pharmacol Ther* (1979) 25, 88–95.
28. Kleman MI, Overvik E, Poellinger L, Gustafsson JA. Induction of cytochrome P4501A isoenzymes by heterocyclic amines and other food-derived compounds. *Princess Takamatsu Symp* (1995) 23, 163–71.
29. Kappas A, Alvares AP, Anderson KE, Pantuck EJ, Pantuck CB, Chang R, Conney AH. Effect of charcoal-broiled beef on antipyrine and theophylline metabolism. *Clin Pharmacol Ther* (1979) 23, 445–50.
30. Peng W-X, Li H-D, Zhou H-H. Effect of daidzein on CYP1A2 activity and pharmacokinetics of theophylline in healthy volunteers. *Eur J Clin Pharmacol* (2002) 59, 237–41.

Theophylline + Gold

Gold has been reported to reduce theophylline levels but evidence is limited.

Clinical evidence, mechanism, importance and management

A review of theophylline serum levels in 6 steroid-dependent patients with asthma who were taking methylprednisolone and gold (**auranofin**) and had also taken theophylline for at least 3 months, found that the actual theophylline levels were lower than the predicted levels, and that the levels were all below 10 mg/L. No information was provided regarding the control of asthma in these patients.[1] The authors of this review suggested that the gastrointestinal adverse effects and protein binding of **auranofin** might have altered the absorption and distribution of theophylline. However, note that a possible effect of methylprednisolone on theophylline clearance cannot be ruled out (see also, 'Theophylline + Corticosteroids', p.1441).

An interaction between theophylline and gold is not established as the theophylline levels were only reduced compared with those predicted using two different pharmacokinetic tools. The clinical relevance of any interaction is also unclear, as these 'low' levels were identified retrospectively. The evidence available is too limited to warrant any general precautions. There appears to be no direct evidence regarding aminophylline, but as it is metabolised to theophylline, it seems possible that it could be similarly affected by gold.

1. Falcão AC, Rocha MJ, Almeida AM, Caramona MM. Theophylline pharmacokinetics with concomitant steroid and gold therapy. *J Clin Pharm Ther* (2000) 25, 191–5.

Theophylline + Grapefruit and other fruit juices

Grapefruit and kinnow (mandarin) juice do not alter the pharmacokinetics of theophylline to a clinically relevant extent.

Clinical evidence, mechanism, importance and management

(a) Grapefruit juice

In one study, 12 healthy subjects were given a single 200-mg oral dose of theophylline solution (*Euphyllin*) diluted in either 100 mL of grapefruit juice or water, followed by another 900 mL of juice or water over the next 16 hours. The pharmacokinetics of theophylline were found to be unchanged by grapefruit juice.[1] Another study, in 10 healthy subjects who took a single 300-mg dose of sustained-release theophylline (*Theobid*) with 300 mL of water or grapefruit juice, found that although grapefruit juice lowered the plasma levels of theophylline between one and 4 hours after the dose, the AUC of theophylline was not changed, nor were there any other statistically significant pharmacokinetic changes.[2]

Theophylline is principally metabolised by CYP1A2 in the liver and the authors of the first study had previously shown that grapefruit juice had a small effect on the pharmacokinetics of caffeine which is also metabolised by CYP1A2 (see 'Caffeine + Grapefruit juice', p.1424). They also found that, *in vitro*, one of the constituents of grapefruit juice, naringenin, inhibited CYP1A2. Therefore, an interaction was theoretically possible. However, the pharmacokinetic studies suggest that no clinically relevant interaction occurs between theophylline and grapefruit juice, and therefore there would seem to be no reason why patients taking theophylline should avoid grapefruit juice. There appears to be no direct evidence regarding aminophylline, but as it is metabolised to theophylline, no clinically relevant interaction would be expected with grapefruit juice.

(b) Kinnow (mandarin) juice

In a study, 10 healthy subjects took a single 300-mg dose of sustained-release theophylline (*Theobid*) with 300 mL of water or kinnow juice. The maximum plasma levels and AUC of theophylline were not different between the two groups. The maximum plasma theophylline levels were 9.54 mg/L and 8.43 mg/L when taken with water and kinnow juice, respectively. The plasma level of theophylline taken with kinnow juice was lower at every time point than when taken with water, but this difference was only statistically significant between one and 4 hours after the start of the study.[3] However, this change would not be expected to be of clinical significance, and therefore there would seem to be no reason why patients taking theophylline should avoid kinnow juice.

1. Fuhr U, Maier A, Keller A, Steinijans VW, Sauter R, Staib AH. Lacking effect of grapefruit juice on theophylline pharmacokinetics. *Int J Clin Pharmacol Ther* (1995) 33, 311–14.
2. Gupta MC, Garg SK, Badyal D, Malhotra S, Bhargava VK. Effect of grapefruit juice on the pharmacokinetics of theophylline in healthy male volunteers. *Methods Find Exp Clin Pharmacol* (1999) 21, 679–82.
3. Gupta MC, Garg SK, Bhargava VK. Influence of kinnow juice on the pharmacokinetics of sustained release theophylline in healthy male volunteers. *Indian J Physiol Pharmacol* (2000) 44, 323–8.

Theophylline + Griseofulvin

Griseofulvin does not appear to affect the pharmacokinetics of theophylline to a clinically relevant extent.

Clinical evidence, mechanism, importance and management

In a study in 12 healthy subjects, griseofulvin 500 mg daily for 8 days reduced the half-life of theophylline (after a single oral dose of aminophylline 300 mg) from 6.6 hours to 5.7 hours, and increased the clearance of two of its metabolites. However, these changes are far too small to be of any clinical relevance.[1] No aminophylline or theophylline dose adjustments would therefore appear to be needed on the concurrent use of griseofulvin.

1. Rasmussen BB, Jeppesen U, Gaist D, Brøsen K. Griseofulvin and fluvoxamine interactions with the metabolism of theophylline. *Ther Drug Monit* (1997) 19, 56–62.

Theophylline + H_2-receptor antagonists

Cimetidine raises theophylline levels and toxicity can develop. However, the interaction is negligible with low-dose cimetidine. Although there are some contrasting reports, in general, famotidine, nizatidine, ranitidine and roxatidine do not appear to interact with theophylline.

Clinical evidence

(a) Cimetidine

A number of case reports describe increased theophylline levels, including many that were toxic, in patients (adults and children) given oral or intravenous aminophylline or theophylline with cimetidine.[1-6] A few cases describe serious adverse effects such as seizures.[3,4]

In a large number of pharmacokinetic studies healthy subjects were given oral or intravenous aminophylline or theophylline[7-16] and patients were given oral or intravenous theophylline[17-21] with oral cimetidine 800 mg to 1.2 g daily in divided doses for 4 to 10 days. It was clearly shown that cimetidine prolonged the theophylline half-life by about 30 to 65% and reduced theophylline clearance by about 20 to 40%. Steady-state serum theophylline levels were raised about one-third.[17,18,21] One of these studies[21] has also been published elsewhere.[22] The effect of cimetidine was maximal in 3 days in the one study assessing this.[17] The extent of the interaction did not differ between cimetidine 1.2 g daily and 2.4 g daily in one study,[10] although two further studies found that cimetidine 800 mg daily had less effect than cimetidine 1.2 g daily.[12,23] A study investigating low-dose cimetidine (200 mg twice daily) found only a 12% decrease in theophylline clearance.[24]

Two studies found that the effect of cimetidine on theophylline pharmacokinetics did not differ between young and elderly subjects,[12,25] whereas another study found that inhibition of theophylline metabolism was more pronounced in the elderly.[23] The inhibitory effects of cimetidine on theophylline metabolism did not differ between smokers and non-smokers in one study,[26] but were more pronounced in smokers in another.[27] In a further study the effects of cimetidine on theophylline were not affected by gender.[23] Three studies found that the inhibitory effects of cimetidine and ciprofloxacin on theophylline metabolism were additive.[25,28,29] For further information on the effect of ciprofloxacin on the pharmacokinetics of theophylline, see 'Theophylline + Quinolones', p.1455.

Three studies found that intravenous cimetidine also inhibited the clearance of theophylline (given as intravenous aminophylline or sustained-release theophylline).[30-32] In one of these, oral and intravenous cimetidine reduced theophylline clearance to the same extent, but when clearance was corrected for the lower bioavailability of oral cimetidine, oral cimetidine resulted in a greater inhibition than intravenous cimetidine.[30] Another study found that the effects of a continuous 50-mg/hour infusion of cimetidine were similar to those of an intermittent infusion of 300 mg every 6 hours.[31]

In contrast, a further study in healthy subjects found no clinically important interaction between intravenous aminophylline and an intravenous cimetidine infusion, but the aminophylline was given only 12 hours after starting cimetidine, which might have been insufficient for cimetidine to have had an effect.[33] Similarly, a subsequent study in 18 critically ill patients given a continuous 50-mg/hour intravenous infusion of cimetidine and low-dose aminophylline 10.8 mg/hour for just 48 hours found no clinically important interaction.[34]

(b) Famotidine

In a study in 10 healthy subjects, famotidine 40 mg twice daily for 5 days had no effect on the pharmacokinetics of theophylline (given as intravenous aminophylline).[14] In another study, 16 patients with bronchial asthma or COPD found that famotidine 20 mg twice daily for at least 3 days did not affect the clearance of theophylline.[35] Two further studies also found no interaction between intravenous theophylline and famotidine 20 or 40 mg twice daily for 4 or 9 days in patients with COPD.[20,36] In a post-marketing surveillance study, it was noted that 4 patients with asthma taking theophylline had also taken famotidine 40 mg daily for 4 to 8 weeks without any problems.[37] In contrast, in a patient with COPD and liver impairment, the AUC and serum levels of an intravenous dose of theophylline were raised by 78% and the clearance was halved by famotidine 40 mg daily for 8 days.[38] A later study by the same authors, in 7 patients with COPD who were similarly treated, but with normal liver function, found that the AUC of theophylline was increased by 56% and its clearance was reduced by 35% by famotidine.[39]

(c) Nizatidine

A study in 17 patients with COPD found that nizatidine 150 mg twice daily for a month had no effect on the steady-state pharmacokinetics of theophylline.[21] However, up to the end of August 1989 there were 6 reports of apparent interactions in the Spontaneous Adverse Drug Reaction Database of the FDA in the US. Four patients taking theophylline developed elevated serum theophylline levels, with symptoms of toxicity in at least one case, when given nizatidine. The problems resolved when either both drugs, or just nizatidine were stopped.[40]

(d) Ranitidine

Many studies in healthy subjects (given intravenous aminophylline or oral theophylline)[10,11,15,41-43] and patients (given sustained-release theophylline)[18,21,44-47] have found that ranitidine does not affect the pharmacokinetics of theophylline, even in daily doses far in excess of those used clinically (up to 4.2 g of ranitidine daily).[41] However, there are 7 reports describing a total of 10 patients, who developed theophylline toxicity when given ranitidine with sustained-release theophylline[48-53] or intravenous aminophylline.[54] The validity of a number of these reports has been questioned,[55-58] with the authors subsequently modifying some.[59,60]

(e) Roxatidine

Roxatidine 150 mg daily did not affect the clearance of theophylline.[61] Similarly, in 9 healthy subjects, roxatidine 150 mg twice daily did not significantly change the pharmacokinetics of a single 250-mg intravenous dose of aminophylline.[62]

Mechanism

Cimetidine is an enzyme inhibitor that reduces the metabolism (predominantly *N*-demethylation)[63] of theophylline by CYP1A2 in the liver, thereby raising its levels. Famotidine, nizatidine and ranitidine do not have enzyme-inhibiting effects so that it is not clear why they sometimes appear to affect theophylline levels.

Importance and management

The interaction between theophylline or aminophylline and cimetidine is very well documented (not all the references being listed here), very well established and clinically important. Theophylline serum levels normally rise by about one-third, but much greater increases have been seen in individual patients. Monitor theophylline levels closely: note that in one study the peak effect was reached in 3 days. Initial theophylline dose reductions of 30 to 50% have been suggested to avoid toxicity.[4] Alternatively, use one of the other H_2-receptor antagonists, or consider changing to a proton pump inhibitor, see 'Theophylline + Proton pump inhibitors', p.1454. The effect of low-dose cimetidine (200 mg twice daily) is unlikely to be clinically relevant. The situation with famotidine, nizatidine and ranitidine is not totally clear. They would not be expected to interact because they are not enzyme inhibitors like cimetidine, but very occasionally and unpredictably they appear to do so. Nevertheless, the general picture is that normally no theophylline or aminophylline dose adjustments are needed if these H_2-receptor antagonists,[56] or roxatidine are given with aminophylline or theophylline.

Note that some of the symptoms of theophylline toxicity, such as nausea, vomiting and abdominal pain, are similar to those of gastrointestinal ulceration. If a patient taking theophylline presents with these symptoms, it would seem prudent to monitor theophylline levels.

1. Weinberger MM, Smith G, Milavetz G, Hendeles L. Decreased theophylline clearance due to cimetidine. *N Engl J Med* (1981) 304, 672.
2. Campbell MA, Plachetka JR, Jackson JE, Moon JF, Finley PR. Cimetidine decreases theophylline clearance. *Ann Intern Med* (1981) 95, 68–9.
3. Lofgren RP, Gilbertson RA. Cimetidine and theophylline. *Ann Intern Med* (1982) 96, 378.
4. Bauman JH, Kimelblatt BJ, Carracio TR, Silverman HM, Simon GI, Beck GJ. Cimetidine-theophylline interaction. Report of four patients. *Ann Allergy* (1982) 48, 100–102.
5. Fenje PC, Isles AF, Baltodano A, MacLeod SM, Soldin S. Interaction of cimetidine and theophylline in two infants. *Can Med Assoc J* (1982) 126, 1178.
6. Uzzan D, Uzzan B, Bernard N, Caubarrere I. Interaction médicamenteuse de la cimétidine et de la théophylline. *Nouv Presse Med* (1982) 11, 1950.
7. Jackson JE, Powell JR, Wandell M, Bentley J, Dorr R. Cimetidine decreases theophylline clearance. *Am Rev Respir Dis* (1981) 123, 615–17.
8. Roberts RK, Grice J, Wood L, Petroff V, McGuffie C. Cimetidine impairs the elimination of theophylline and antipyrine. *Gastroenterology* (1981) 81, 19–21.
9. Reitberg DP, Bernhard H, Schentag JJ. Alteration of theophylline clearance and half-life by cimetidine in normal volunteers. *Ann Intern Med* (1981) 95, 582–5.
10. Powell JR, Rogers JF, Wargin WA, Cross RE, Eshelman FN. Inhibition of theophylline clearance by cimetidine but not ranitidine. *Arch Intern Med* (1984) 144, 484–6.
11. Ferrari M, Angelini GP, Barozzi E, Olivieri M, Penna S, Accardi R. A comparative study of ranitidine and cimetidine effects on theophylline metabolism. *G Ital Mal Torace* (1984) 38, 31–4.
12. Cohen IA, Johnson CE, Berardi RR, Hyneck ML, Achem SR. Cimetidine-theophylline interaction: effects of age and cimetidine dose. *Ther Drug Monit* (1985) 7, 426–34.
13. Mulkey PM, Murphy JE, Shleifer NH. Steady-state theophylline pharmacokinetics during and after short-term cimetidine administration. *Clin Pharm* (1983) 2, 439–41.
14. Lin JH, Chremos AN, Chiou R, Yeh KC, Williams R. Comparative effect of famotidine and cimetidine on the pharmacokinetics of theophylline in normal volunteers. *Br J Clin Pharmacol* (1987) 24, 669–72.
15. Adebayo GI. Effects of equimolar doses of cimetidine and ranitidine on theophylline elimination. *Biopharm Drug Dispos* (1989) 10, 77–85.
16. Ohashi K, Sakamoto K, Sudo T, Tateishi T, Fujimura A, Shiga T, Ebihara A. Effects of diltiazem and cimetidine on theophylline oxidative metabolism. *J Clin Pharmacol* (1993) 33, 1233–7.
17. Vestal RE, Thummel KE, Musser B, Mercer GD. Cimetidine inhibits theophylline clearance in patients with chronic obstructive pulmonary disease: A study using stable isotope methodology during multiple oral dose administration. *Br J Clin Pharmacol* (1983) 15, 411–18.
18. Boehning W. Effect of cimetidine and ranitidine on plasma theophylline in patients with chronic obstructive airways disease treated with theophylline and corticosteroids. *Eur J Clin Pharmacol* (1990) 38, 43–5.
19. Roberts RK, Grice J, McGuffie C. Cimetidine-theophylline interaction in patients with chronic obstructive airways disease. *Med J Aust* (1984) 140, 279–80.
20. Bachmann K, Sullivan TJ, Reese JH, Jauregui L, Miller K, Scott M, Yeh KC, Stepanavage M, King JD, Schwartz J. Controlled study of the putative interaction between famotidine and theophylline in patients with chronic obstructive pulmonary disease. *J Clin Pharmacol* (1995) 35, 529–35.
21. Bachmann K, Sullivan TJ, Mauro LS, Martin M, Jauregui L, Levine L. Comparative investigation of the influence of nizatidine, ranitidine, and cimetidine on the steady-state pharmacokinetics of theophylline in COPD patients. *J Clin Pharmacol* (1992) 32, 476–82.
22. Bachmann KA, Sullivan TJ, Jauregui L, Reese J, Miller K, Levine L. Drug interactions of H_2-receptor antagonists. *Scand J Gastroenterol* (1994) 29 (Suppl 206), 14–19.
23. Seaman JJ, Randolph WC, Peace KE, Frank WO, Dickson B, Putterman K, Young MD. Effects of two cimetidine dosage regimens on serum theophylline levels. *Postgrad Med* (1985) 78, 47–53.
24. Nix DE, Di Cicco RA, Miller AK, Boyle DA, Boike SC, Zariffa N, Jorkasky DK, Schentag JJ. The effect of low-dose cimetidine (200 mg twice daily) on the pharmacokinetics of theophylline. *J Clin Pharmacol* (1999) 39, 855–65.
25. Loi C-M, Parker BM, Cusack BJ, Vestal RE. Aging and drug interactions.III. Individual and combined effects of cimetidine and ciprofloxacin on theophylline metabolism in healthy male and female non-smokers. *J Pharmacol Exp Ther* (1997) 280, 627–37.
26. Cusack BJ, Dawson GW, Mercer GD, Vestal RE. Cigarette smoking and theophylline metabolism: effects of cimetidine. *Clin Pharmacol Ther* (1985) 37, 330–6.
27. Grygiel JJ, Miners JO, Drew R, Birkett DJ. Differential effects of cimetidine on theophylline metabolic pathways. *Eur J Clin Pharmacol* (1984) 26, 335–40.
28. Davis RL, Quenzer RW, Kelly HW, Powell JR. Effect of the addition of ciprofloxacin on theophylline pharmacokinetics in subjects inhibited by cimetidine. *Ann Pharmacother* (1992) 26, 11–13.
29. Loi C-M, Parker BM, Cusack BJ, Vestal RE. Individual and combined effects of cimetidine and ciprofloxacin on theophylline metabolism in male nonsmokers. *Br J Clin Pharmacol* (1993) 36, 195–200.

30. Cremer KF, Secor J, Speeg KV. Effect of route of administration on the cimetidine-theophylline drug interaction. *J Clin Pharmacol* (1989) 29, 451–6.
31. Gutfeld MB, Welage LS, Walawander CA, Wilton JH, Harrison NJ. The influence of intravenous cimetidine dosing regimens on the disposition of theophylline. *J Clin Pharmacol* (1989) 29, 665–9.
32. Krstenansky PM, Javaheri S, Thomas JP, Thomas RL. Effect of continuous cimetidine infusion on steady-state theophylline concentration. *Clin Pharm* (1989) 8, 206–9.
33. Gaska JA, Tietze KJ, Rocci ML, Vlasses PH. Theophylline pharmacokinetics: effect of continuous versus intermittent cimetidine IV infusion. *J Clin Pharmacol* (1991) 31, 668–72.
34. Mojtahedzadeh M, Sadray S, Hadjibabaie M, Fasihi M, Rezaee S. Determination of theophylline clearance after cimetidine infusion in critically ill patients. *J Infus Nurs* (2003) 26, 234–8.
35. Asamoto H, Kokura M, Kawakami A, Sawano T, Sasaki Y, Kohara N, Kitamura Y, Oishi T, Morishita H. Effect of famotidine on theophylline clearance in asthma and COPD patients. *Arerugi* (1987) 36, 1012–17.
36. Verdiani P, DiCarlo S, Baronti A. Famotidine effects on theophylline pharmacokinetics in subjects affected by COPD. Comparison with cimetidine and placebo. *Chest* (1988) 94, 807–10.
37. Chichmanian RM, Mignot G, Spreux A, Jean-Girard C, Hofliger P. Tolérance de la famotidine. Étude due réseau médecins sentinelles en pharmacovigilance. *Therapie* (1992) 47, 239–43.
38. Dal Negro R, Turco P, Pomari C, Trevisan F. Famotidina e teofillina: interferenza farmacocinetica cimetidino-simile? *G Ital Mal Torace* (1988) 42, 185–6.
39. Dal Negro R, Pomari C, Turco P. Famotidine and theophylline pharmacokinetics. An unexpected cimetidine-like interaction in patients with chronic obstructive pulmonary disease. *Clin Pharmacokinet* (1993) 24, 255–8.
40. Shinn AF. Unrecognized drug interactions with famotidine and nizatidine. *Arch Intern Med* (1991) 151, 810–14.
41. Kelly HW, Powell JR, Donohue JF. Ranitidine at very large doses does not inhibit theophylline elimination. *Clin Pharmacol Ther* (1986) 39, 577–81.
42. McEwen J, McMurdo MET, Moreland TA. The effects of once-daily dosing with ranitidine and cimetidine on theophylline pharmacokinetics. *Eur J Drug Metab Pharmacokinet* (1988) 13, 201–5.
43. Kehoe WA, Sands CD, Long LF, Lan HH, Harralson AF, Shin HT, Jones DW. Effect of ranitidine on theophylline metabolism in healthy Koreans living in China. *Ann Pharmacother* (1996) 30, 133–7.
44. Seggev JS, Barzilay M, Schey G. No evidence for interaction between ranitidine and theophylline. *Arch Intern Med* (1987) 147, 179–80.
45. Zarogoulidis K, Economidis D, Paparoglou A, Pneumaticos I, Sevastou P, Tsopouridis A, Papaioanou A. Effect of ranitidine on theophylline plasma levels in patients with COPD. *Eur Respir J* (1988) 1 (Suppl 2), 195S.
46. Pérez-Blanco FJ, Huertas González JM, Morata Garcia de la Puerta IJ, Saucedo Sánchez R. Interacción de ranitidina con teofilina. *Rev Clin Esp* (1995) 195, 359–60.
47. Cukier A, Vargas FS, Santos SRCJ, Donzella H, Terra-Filho M, Teixeira LR, Light RW. Theophylline-ranitidine interaction in elderly COPD patients. *Braz J Med Biol Res* (1995) 28, 875–9.
48. Fernandes E, Melewicz FM. Ranitidine and theophylline. *Ann Intern Med* (1984) 100, 459.
49. Gardner ME, Sikorski GW. Ranitidine and theophylline. *Ann Intern Med* (1985) 102, 559.
50. Roy AK, Cuda MP, Levine RA. Induction of theophylline toxicity and inhibition of clearance rates by ranitidine. *Am J Med* (1988) 85, 525–7.
51. Dietemann-Molard A, Popin E, Oswald-Mammosser M, Colas des Francs V, Pauli G. Intoxication à la théophylline par interaction avec la ranitidine à dose élevée. *Presse Med* (1988) 17, 280.
52. Skinner MH, Lenert L, Blaschke TF. Theophylline toxicity subsequent to ranitidine administration: a possible drug-drug interaction. *Am J Med* (1989) 86, 129–32.
53. Hegman GW, Gilbert RP. Ranitidine-theophylline interaction — fact or fiction? *DICP Ann Pharmacother* (1991) 25, 21–5.
54. Murialdo G, Piovano PL, Costelli P, Fonzi S, Barberis A, Ghia M. Seizures during concomitant treatment with theophylline and ranitidine: a case report. *Ann Ital Med Int* (1990) 5, 413–17.
55. Muir JG, Powell JR, Baumann JH. Induction of theophylline toxicity and inhibition of clearance rates by ranitidine. *Am J Med* (1989) 86, 513–14.
56. Kelly HW. Comment: ranitidine does not inhibit theophylline metabolism. *Ann Pharmacother* (1991) 25, 1139.
57. Williams DM, Figg WD, Pleasants RA. Comment: ranitidine does not inhibit theophylline metabolism. *Ann Pharmacother* (1991) 25, 1140.
58. Dobbs JH, Smith RN. Ranitidine and theophylline. *Ann Intern Med* (1984) 100, 769.
59. Roy AK. Induction of theophylline toxicity and inhibition of clearance rates by ranitidine. *Am J Med* (1989) 86, 513.
60. Hegman GW. Comment: ranitidine does not inhibit theophylline metabolism. *Ann Pharmacother* (1991) 25, 1140–41.
61. Labs RA. Interaction of roxatidine acetate with antacids, food and other drugs. *Drugs* (1988) 35 (Suppl 3), 82–9.
62. Yoshimura N, Takeuchi H, Ogata H, Ishioka T, Aoi R. Effects of roxatidine acetate hydrochloride and cimetidine on the pharmacokinetics of theophylline in healthy subjects. *Int J Clin Pharmacol Ther Toxicol* (1989) 27, 308–12.
63. Naline E, Sanceaume M, Pays M, Advenier C. Application of theophylline metabolite assays to the exploration of liver microsome oxidative function in man. *Fundam Clin Pharmacol* (1988) 2, 341–51.

Theophylline + HIV-protease inhibitors

Ritonavir slightly reduces the exposure to theophylline. Indinavir causes a negligible increase in the exposure to theophylline.

Clinical evidence, mechanism, importance and management

(a) Indinavir

A study in 12 healthy subjects given a single 250-mg oral dose of theophylline before and after indinavir 800 mg three times daily for 5 days found an 18% increase in the AUC of theophylline, which was not considered to be clinically significant.[1] No theophylline dose adjustments would therefore be expected to be necessary on the concurrent use of indinavir.

(b) Ritonavir

In a placebo-controlled study, 27 subjects taking theophylline 3 mg/kg every 8 hours were given ritonavir 300 mg increased to 500 mg twice daily for 10 days. Ritonavir reduced the AUC of theophylline by 43% and reduced its maximum and minimum steady-state concentrations by 32% and 57%, respectively. The interaction achieved its maximal effect 6 days after starting ritonavir.[2] Ritonavir is an inducer of CYP1A2, the principal isoenzyme by which theophylline is metabolised, and therefore concurrent use leads to an increase in theophylline metabolism, and a reduction in its concentrations. Although the reduction in exposure is slight, theophylline has a narrow therapeutic range, and it therefore seems possible that the efficacy of theophylline could be reduced. Monitor theophylline concentrations if ritonavir is started and be alert for the need to increase the theophylline dose. There appears to be no direct evidence regarding aminophylline, but as it is metabolised to theophylline, it seems likely that it will be similarly affected by ritonavir.

1. Mistry GC, Laurent A, Sterrett AT, Deutsch PJ. Effect of indinavir on the single-dose pharmacokinetics of theophylline in healthy subjects. *J Clin Pharmacol* (1999) 39, 636–42.
2. Hsu A, Granneman GR, Witt G, Cavanaugh JH, Leonard J. Assessment of multiple doses of ritonavir on the pharmacokinetics of theophylline. 11th Int Conf AIDS, Vancouver, 1996. Mo.B.1200.

Theophylline + Hormonal contraceptives

The clearance of theophylline is slightly reduced in women taking oral combined hormonal contraceptives, but no toxicity has been reported.

Clinical evidence

The total plasma clearance of a single 4-mg/kg oral dose of aminophylline was about 30% lower in 8 women taking an oral combined hormonal contraceptive (**ethinylestradiol** with **norgestrel**, *Ovral*) than in 8 other women not taking hormonal contraceptives.[1] The theophylline half-life was also prolonged by about 30%, from 7.34 hours to 9.79 hours. Similar results were found in other studies in subjects given intravenous or oral aminophylline and oral combined hormonal contraceptives (**ethinylestradiol** with **norgestrel**, *Ovral* and **mestranol** with **etynodiol diacetate**, *Ovulen* or unnamed products).[2,3] In contrast, no statistically significant differences were seen in the pharmacokinetics of theophylline (given as intravenous aminophylline) in 10 adolescent women (15 to 18 years) taking oral low-dose combined or sequential hormonal contraceptives (**ethinylestradiol** with **norethisterone**), when compared with age matched controls.[4] However, in the same women the clearance of oral theophylline was found to be reduced by 33% after they took an oral triphasic combined hormonal contraceptive (**ethinylestradiol** with **norethisterone**) for 3 to 4 months.[5] In a retrospective analysis of factors affecting theophylline clearance, the use of oral hormonal contraceptives was associated with a reduced theophylline clearance in women who smoked.[6]

Mechanism

It seems that the oestrogenic component of the contraceptive inhibits the metabolism of theophylline by CYP1A2 in the liver, thereby reducing its clearance.

Importance and management

A pharmacokinetic interaction between theophylline or aminophylline and combined hormonal contraceptives is established, but there seem to be no reports of theophylline toxicity resulting from concurrent use. Any interaction seems likely to be slight, although as theophylline has a narrow therapeutic range it seems possible that some women taking combined hormonal contraceptives might need less aminophylline or theophylline than those not taking these contraceptives. If theophylline adverse effects (headache, nausea, tremor) occur, consider the possibility of an interaction, monitor theophylline levels, and adjust the theophylline or aminophylline dose accordingly. Note that it has been proposed that the effects may be more apparent with long-term, high-dose contraceptive use.[1,4]

1. Tornatore KM, Kanarkowski R, McCarthy TL, Gardner MJ, Yurchak AM, Jusko WJ. Effect of chronic oral contraceptive steroids on theophylline disposition. *Eur J Clin Pharmacol* (1982) 23, 129–34.
2. Roberts RK, Grice J, McGuffie C, Heilbronn L. Oral contraceptive steroids impair the elimination of theophylline. *J Lab Clin Med* (1983) 101, 821–5.
3. Gardner MJ, Tornatore KM, Jusko WJ, Kanarkowski R. Effects of tobacco smoking and oral contraceptive use on theophylline disposition. *Br J Clin Pharmacol* (1983) 16, 271–80.
4. Koren G, Chin TF, Correia J, Tesoro A, MacLeod S. Theophylline pharmacokinetics in adolescent females following coadministration of oral contraceptives. *Clin Invest Med* (1985) 8, 222–6.
5. Long DR, Roberts EA, Brill-Edwards M, Quaggin S, Correia J, Koren G, MacLeod SM. The effect of the oral contraceptive Ortho 7/7/7® on theophylline (T) clearance in non-smoking women aged 18–22. *Clin Invest Med* (1987) 10 (4 Suppl B), B59.
6. Jusko WJ, Gardner MJ, Mangione A, Schentag JJ, Koup JR, Vance JW. Factors affecting theophylline clearances: age, tobacco, marijuana, cirrhosis, congestive heart failure, obesity, oral contraceptives, benzodiazepines, barbiturates, and ethanol. *J Pharm Sci* (1979) 68, 1358–66.

Theophylline + Idrocilamide

Idrocilamide (given orally) can moderately reduce the clearance of theophylline.

Clinical evidence, mechanism, importance and management

In a study in 6 healthy subjects, oral idrocilamide 600 mg daily for 3 days then 1.2 g for 4 days increased the half-life of a single dose of theophylline 2.5-fold (from 8.5 hours to 21.6 hours) and reduced its clearance by 67%.[1] This is due to a reduction in the metabolism of theophylline by CYP1A2 in the liver, which is inhibited by idrocilamide. Although the effects of idrocilamide were moderate, theophylline has a narrow therapeutic range, and therefore the concurrent use of theophylline and oral idrocilamide should be closely monitored, anticipating the need to reduce the theophylline dose. There appears to be no direct evidence regarding aminophylline, but as it is metabolised to theophylline it seems likely to be similarly affected by idrocilamide. The effects of topical idrocilamide on theophylline metabolism are unknown.

1. Lacroix C, Nouveau J, Hubscher Ph, Tardif D, Ray M, Goulle JP. Influence de l'idrocilamide sur le metabolisme de la theophylline. *Rev Pneumol Clin* (1986) 42, 164–6.

Theophylline + Imipenem

Seizures developed in three patients taking aminophylline or theophylline when they were given imipenem.

Clinical evidence, mechanism, importance and management

Two patients receiving intravenous aminophylline developed seizures within 11 to 56 hours of starting treatment with intravenous imipenem 500 mg every 6 to 8 hours. Seizures developed in a third patient taking theophylline after imipenem had been given for 6 days. In all 3 patients, seizures occurred 2 to 3 hours after a dose of imipenem. Theophylline serum levels appeared to be unchanged.[1] In an analysis of data from 1 754 patients who had received imipenem in dose-ranging studies, 3% had seizures, and imipenem was judged to be associated with one-third of these cases. However, the concurrent use of theophylline or aminophylline was not found to be a significant risk factor for the development of seizures with imipenem.[2] The general importance of these cases is therefore uncertain.

1. Semel JD, Allen N. Seizures in patients simultaneously receiving theophylline and imipenem or ciprofloxacin or metronidazole. *South Med J* (1991) 84, 465–8.
2. Calandra G, Lydick E, Carrigan J, Weiss L, Guess H. Factors predisposing to seizures in seriously ill infected patients receiving antibiotics: experience with imipenem/cilastatin. *Am J Med* (1988) 84, 911–18.

Theophylline + Influenza vaccines

In general, influenza vaccines (whole-virion, split-virion and surface antigen) do not appear to interact with theophylline; however, there are three reports describing rises in theophylline levels in a few patients (some to toxic levels), which were attributed to the use of an influenza vaccine.

Clinical evidence

(a) Evidence of no interaction

In 12 patients with asthma, the mean steady-state serum theophylline levels were not altered by a trivalent split-virion influenza vaccine (*Fluzone*), although one patient had an increase in levels (see *Evidence of an interaction*, below). Levels were measured before vaccination and one, 3, 7 and 14 days after vaccination.[1] Theophylline levels were unchanged in 5 patients with COPD when they were given 0.5 mL of influenza vaccine (*Fluogen*).[2] Similarly, no evidence of a rise in theophylline levels was found in a number of other studies in both adults and children, receiving maintenance theophylline or aminophylline, and given various trivalent split-virion vaccines[3-6] including *Fluzone*,[7] *Fluogen*,[8-10] *Influvac*,[11] *Mutagrip*.[12] In addition, no change in the pharmacokinetics of theophylline (given as oral aminophylline) was found after the use of a whole-virion vaccine in healthy adults.[13] No evidence of serious theophylline toxicity was seen in 119 elderly patients taking maintenance theophylline and given an unspecified influenza vaccine.[14]

(b) Evidence of an interaction

Three patients who had been taking oral choline theophyllinate 200 mg (equivalent to 128 mg of theophylline) every 6 hours for at least 7 days had a rise in their serum theophylline levels of 219%, 89%, and 85%, respectively, within 12 to 24 hours of receiving 0.5 mL of trivalent split-virion influenza vaccine (*Fluogen*). In some cases effects persisted for up to 72 hours, and two patients had signs of theophylline toxicity. A subsequent study in 4 healthy subjects found that the same dose of vaccine more than doubled the half-life of theophylline, from 3.3 hours to 7.3 hours, and halved its clearance.[15]

A 15-year-old girl had a rise in her theophylline levels from 20 mg/L to 34 mg/L (with no sign of toxicity) within 5 hours of being given a trivalent split-virion vaccine.[16] In a study where 11 of 12 patients had no increase in theophylline levels after vaccination with *Fluzone*, one woman had a rise in levels (from 10 mg/L to 24.5 mg/L) accompanied by headaches and palpitations.[1]

In 8 healthy subjects the clearance of theophylline (given as choline theophyllinate) was reduced by 25% one day after influenza vaccination (trivalent influenza vaccine, *Fluogen*). Theophylline metabolism had returned to pre-vaccination levels 7 days later.[17]

A patient with COPD taking sustained-release theophylline 300 mg twice daily (theophylline levels between 7 and 12 mg/L) developed nausea and palpitations the day after he received a trivalent influenza vaccination (*Fluogen*). His theophylline level was increased to 26 [mg/L]. His dose was reduced to 200 mg twice daily and the adverse effects resolved. However, a few days later his COPD had become symptomatic and the theophylline level was found to be subtherapeutic, so the dose was raised to 300 mg twice daily, as before.[18]

Mechanism

Uncertain. If an interaction occurs, it has been suggested it is probably due to inhibition of the liver enzymes concerned with the metabolism of theophylline, possibly secondary to interferon production, resulting in theophylline accumulation in the body.[15,17] One suggestion is that vaccine contaminants, which are potent interferon-inducing agents, might be responsible (rather than the vaccine itself), so that an interaction would seem to be less likely with modern highly-purified subunit vaccines.[19] In one study where an interaction occurred, an increase in serum interferon levels was detected,[17] whereas, in two of the studies showing no interaction, no interferon production was detected.[10,13] Influenza infection *per se* can result in decreased theophylline clearance and theophylline toxicity.[20]

Importance and management

A very thoroughly investigated interaction, the weight of evidence being that no adverse interaction normally occurs between aminophylline or theophylline and any type of influenza vaccine in children, adults or the elderly. Even so, given the occasional and unexplained reports of an interaction[1,15,16,18] it would seem prudent to consider monitoring concurrent use for signs of theophylline toxicity (headache, nausea, tremor), taking theophylline levels if necessary; however, note that problems are very unlikely to arise now that purer vaccines are available (see *Mechanism*, above). Note that any rise in theophylline levels seems likely to be transient.

1. Fischer RG, Booth BH, Mitchell DQ, Kibbe AH. Influence of trivalent influenza vaccine on serum theophylline levels. *Can Med Assoc J* (1982) 126, 1312–13.
2. Britton L, Ruben FL. Serum theophylline levels after influenza vaccine. *Can Med Assoc J* (1982) 126, 1375.
3. Stults BM, Hashisaki PA. Influenza vaccination and theophylline pharmacokinetics in patients with chronic obstructive lung disease. *West J Med* (1983) 139, 651–4.
4. Gomolin IH, Chapron DJ, Luhan PA. Lack of effect of influenza vaccine on theophylline levels and warfarin anticoagulation in the elderly. *J Am Geriatr Soc* (1985) 33, 269–72.
5. Feldman CH, Rabinowitz A, Levison M, Klein R, Feldman BR, Davis WJ. Effects of influenza vaccine on theophylline metabolism in children with asthma. *Am Rev Respir Dis* (1985) 131 (4 Suppl), A9.
6. Bryett KA, Levy J, Pariente R, Gobert P, Falquet JCV. Influenza vaccine and theophylline metabolism. Is there an interaction? *Acta Ther* (1989) 15, 49–58.
7. Goldstein RS, Cheung OT, Seguin R, Lobley G, Johnson AC. Decreased elimination of theophylline after influenza vaccination. *Can Med Assoc J* (1982) 126, 470.
8. San Joaquin VH, Reyes S, Marks MI. Influenza vaccination in asthmatic children on maintenance theophylline therapy. *Clin Pediatr (Phila)* (1982) 21, 724–6.
9. Bukowskyj M, Munt PW, Wigle R, Nakatsu K. Theophylline clearance. Lack of effect of influenza vaccination and ascorbic acid. *Am Rev Respir Dis* (1984) 129, 672–5.
10. Grabowski N, May JJ, Pratt DS, Richtsmeier WJ, Bertino JS, Sorge KF. The effect of split virus influenza vaccination on theophylline pharmacokinetics. *Am Rev Respir Dis* (1985) 131, 934–8.
11. Winstanley PA, Tjia J, Back DJ, Hobson D, Breckenridge AM. Lack of effect of highly purified subunit influenza vaccination on theophylline metabolism. *Br J Clin Pharmacol* (1985) 20, 47–53.
12. Jonkman JHG, Wymenga ASC, de Zeeuw RA, van der Boon WVJ, Beugelink JK, Oosterhuis B, Jedema JN. No effect of influenza vaccination on the theophylline pharmacokinetics as studied by ultraviolet spectrophotometry, HPLC, and EMIT assay methods. *Ther Drug Monit* (1988) 10, 345–8.
13. Hannan SE, May JJ, Pratt DS, Richtsmeier WJ, Bertino JS. The effect of whole virus influenza vaccination on theophylline pharmacokinetics. *Am Rev Respir Dis* (1988) 137, 903–6.
14. Patriarca PA, Kendal AP, Stricof RL, Weber JA, Meissner MK, Dateno B. Influenza vaccination and warfarin or theophylline toxicity in nursing-home residents. *N Engl J Med* (1983) 308, 1601–2.
15. Renton KW, Gray JD, Hall RI. Decreased elimination of theophylline after influenza vaccination. *Can Med Assoc J* (1980) 123, 288–90.
16. Walker S, Schreiber L, Middelkamp JN. Serum theophylline levels after influenza vaccination. *Can Med Assoc J* (1981) 125, 243–4.
17. Meredith CG, Christian CD, Johnson RF, Troxell R, Davis GL, Schenker S. Effects of influenza virus vaccine on hepatic drug metabolism. *Clin Pharmacol Ther* (1985) 37, 396–401.
18. Hamdy RC, Micklewright M, Beecham VF, Moore SW. Influenza vaccine may enhance theophylline toxicity. A case report and review of the literature. *J Tenn Med Assoc* (1995) 88, 463–4.
19. Winstanley PA, Back DJ, Breckenridge AM. Inhibition of theophylline metabolism by interferon. *Lancet* (1987) ii, 1340.
20. Kraemer MJ, Furukawa CT, Koup JR, Shapiro GG, Pierson WE, Bierman CW. Altered theophylline clearance during an influenza B outbreak. *Pediatrics* (1982) 69, 476–80.

Theophylline + Interferons

Theophylline clearance is reduced by some interferons, but the extent of the interaction varies greatly, with different types of interferon having slightly different effects.

Clinical evidence

(a) Interferon alfa

A study in 9 subjects (5 with stable chronic active hepatitis B and 4 healthy subjects) found that 20 hours after being given a single 9- or 18-million unit intramuscular injection of interferon (recombinant human interferon alfa A), the clearance of theophylline (given as intravenous aminophylline) was approximately halved (range 33 to 81%) in 8 of the 9 subjects. The mean theophylline elimination half-life was increased from 6.3 hours to 10.7 hours (range from 1.5- to sixfold increases). In the healthy subjects, theophylline clearance was noted to have returned to its former value 4 weeks after the study.[1] Another study, in 11 healthy subjects given interferon alfa (*Roferon-A*) 3 million units daily for 3 days, found that the terminal half-life and AUC of theophylline (given as aminophylline) were only increased by 10 to 15%, with a similar decrease in clearance.[2] In 7 patients with cancer, interferon alfa (*Intron-A*) 3 million units given three times a week for 2 weeks decreased the clearance of a single 150-mg oral dose of theophylline by 33%.[3]

(b) Interferon beta

In a study, 7 patients with chronic hepatitis C receiving interferon beta 3 to 9 million - units daily for 8 weeks were given a single 250-mg dose of intravenous aminophylline. Interferon beta reduced the clearance of theophylline by 26% (range 6 to 57%) and increased the elimination half-life by 39% (range 27 to 139%), but had no statistically significant effect on the volume of distribution, although there was wide inter-patient variability.[4]

(c) Peginterferon alfa

In a study in 14 healthy male subjects who received peginterferon alfa-2a for 4 weeks, there was a 33% increase in the AUC of a single dose of theophylline.[5]

Mechanism

Interferon alfa and peginterferon appear to inhibit CYP1A2 in the liver, the main isoenzyme concerned with the metabolism of theophylline, leading to a reduction in theophylline clearance. Interferon beta also appears to interact by the same mechanism. However, one study, in which the activity of CYP1A2 was determined in

14 patients with active hepatitis C after receiving interferon alfa and ribavirin for 4 weeks, did not find any significant change in CYP1A2 activity.[6]

Importance and management

Direct information regarding an interaction between theophylline or aminophylline and interferons appears to be limited to these reports, and so far there appear to be no reports of theophylline toxicity. However, as theophylline has a narrow therapeutic range, and the pharmacokinetic changes seen in some patients were moderate, it seems possible that some patients could experience an adverse interaction. It would therefore be prudent to monitor the concurrent use of an interferon and aminophylline or theophylline closely for adverse effects (nausea, headaches, tremor), taking theophylline levels and adjusting the theophylline or aminophylline dose if necessary. Patients with enhanced metabolism (e.g. smokers) are predicted to be most at risk.[1] The manufacturers of peginterferon alfa-2a suggest that the interaction with theophylline might not be maximal until after more than 4 weeks of concurrent use.[7]

1. Williams SJ, Baird-Lambert JA, Farrell GC. Inhibition of theophylline metabolism by interferon. *Lancet* (1987) ii, 939–41.
2. Jonkman JHG, Nicholson KG, Farrow PR, Eckert M, Grasmeijer G, Oosterhuis B, De Noorde OE, Guentert TW. Effects of α-interferon on theophylline pharmacokinetics and metabolism. *Br J Clin Pharmacol* (1989) 27, 795–802.
3. Israel BC, Blouin RA, McIntyre W, Shedlofsky SI. Effects of interferon-α monotherapy on hepatic drug metabolism in cancer patients. *Br J Clin Pharmacol* (1993) 36, 229–35.
4. Okuno H, Takasu M, Kano H, Seki T, Shiozaki Y, Inoue K. Depression of drug-metabolising activity in the human liver by interferon-β. *Hepatology* (1993) 17, 65–9.
5. Sy S, Algranti NE, Patel IH, Modi M. Cytochrome P450 (CYP)-mediated drug interactions are unlikely with peginterferon alpha-2a (PEG-IFN) except for CYP1A2. *Hepatology* (1999) 30, 193A.
6. Becquemont L, Chazouilleres O, Serfaty L, Poirier JM, Broly F, Jaillon P, Poupon R, Funck-Brentano C. Effect of interferon α-ribavirin bitherapy on cytochrome P450 1A2 and 2D6 and *N*-acetyltransferase-2 activities in patients with chronic active hepatitis C. *Clin Pharmacol Ther* (2002) 71, 488–95.
7. Pegasys (Peginterferon alfa-2a). Roche Products Ltd. UK Summary of product characteristics, October 2013.

Theophylline + Ipriflavone

An isolated report describes increased theophylline levels in a patient given ipriflavone.

Clinical evidence, mechanism, importance and management

The theophylline serum levels of a patient with COPD, taking sustained-release theophylline 300 mg twice daily, rose from 9.5 mg/L to 17.3 mg/L when ipriflavone 600 mg daily was taken for about 4 weeks. No symptoms of toxicity occurred. The theophylline serum levels returned to roughly the initial level when the ipriflavone was stopped, and rose again when it was restarted.[1] *In vitro* studies with human liver microsomes suggest that ipriflavone can inhibit CYP1A2,[2,3] which would reduce the metabolism of theophylline and increase its levels.

Although so far only one case of this interaction has been reported, the *in vitro* studies suggest that it would be prudent to monitor the theophylline levels of any patient given ipriflavone, making any dose reductions as necessary.

Aminophylline does not appear to have been studied, but as it is metabolised to theophylline, a similar interaction seems likely.

1. Takahashi J, Kawakatsu K, Wakayama T, Sawaoka H. Elevation of serum theophylline levels by ipriflavone in a patient with chronic obstructive pulmonary disease. *Eur J Clin Pharmacol* (1992) 43, 207–8.
2. Monostory K, Vereczkey L. The effect of ipriflavone and its main metabolites on theophylline biotransformation. *Eur J Drug Metab Pharmacokinet* (1996) 21, 61–6.
3. Monostory K, Vereczkey L, Lévai F, Szatmári I. Ipriflavone as an inhibitor of human cytochrome P450 enzymes. *Br J Pharmacol* (1998) 123, 605–10.

Theophylline + Leukotriene antagonists

Montelukast does not appear to affect the pharmacokinetics of theophylline. Pemirolast reduces the rate but not the extent of theophylline absorption. Zafirlukast has no effect on theophylline levels, although isolated cases of a rise in theophylline levels have been reported on concurrent use. Zafirlukast levels are modestly reduced by theophylline, but this does not appear to be clinically important.

Clinical evidence

(a) Montelukast

In a study in 16 healthy subjects, the pharmacokinetics of a single intravenous dose of theophylline were not affected to a clinically relevant extent by montelukast 10 mg daily for 10 days. However, when the subjects were given montelukast 200 mg and 600 mg daily, the AUC of theophylline was reduced by 43% and 66%, respectively. These doses are 20- and 60-fold higher than the usual 10 mg daily dose,[1] and therefore the clinical relevance of these effects is unclear.

(b) Pemirolast

In a study in 7 healthy subjects, oral pemirolast 10 mg twice daily for 4 days did not affect the steady-state serum levels or clearance of theophylline (*Theo-Dur*) 100 mg twice daily. Pemirolast increased the time to reach maximum theophylline levels, but this was not considered clinically significant.[2]

(c) Zafirlukast

In a study in 13 patients with asthma, when zafirlukast 80 mg daily was given with a single 6-mg/kg dose of a theophylline oral liquid, the mean serum levels of zafirlukast were reduced by 30%, but the serum theophylline levels remained unchanged.[3] In another study in 16 healthy children, zafirlukast 20 mg daily did not affect the pharmacokinetics of a single 16-mg/kg oral dose of sustained-release theophylline.[3] In contrast, an isolated report describes a 15-year-old girl with asthma taking sustained-release theophylline 300 mg twice daily (as well as inhaled fluticasone, salbutamol (albuterol) and salmeterol, and oral prednisolone) who became nauseous shortly after zafirlukast (dose not stated) was started. An increase in her theophylline level from 11 mg/L to 24 mg/L was noted. The theophylline was stopped, and later attempts to reintroduce theophylline at lower doses resulted in the same dramatic increases in serum theophylline levels.[4] The manufacturer of zafirlukast has received a limited number of reports of patients experiencing increased theophylline levels, with or without clinical signs or symptoms of theophylline toxicity, after the addition of zafirlukast. No further details are available.[3,5]

Mechanism

Not understood.

Importance and management

Information about the interaction between theophylline and montelukast seems to be limited. The study cited indicates that when using normal clinical doses of montelukast no dose adjustments of either drug are needed. Similarly, no adverse pharmacokinetic interaction appears to occur between pemirolast and theophylline.

No adverse pharmacokinetic interaction appears to occur between zafirlukast and theophylline: the published case involving zafirlukast is of doubtful general significance, and as further details of the reports made to the company are unavailable, their clinical significance cannot be assessed.

As aminophylline is metabolised to theophylline, a similar lack of pharmacokinetic interaction would be expected with these leukotriene antagonists.

1. Malmstrom K, Schwartz J, Reiss TF, Sullivan TJ, Reese JH, Jauregui L, Miller K, Scott M, Shingo S, Peszek I, Larson P, Ebel D, Hunt TL, Huhn RD, Bachmann K. Effect of montelukast on single-dose theophylline pharmacokinetics. *Am J Ther* (1998) 5, 189–95.
2. Hasegawa T, Takagi K, Nadai M, Ogura Y, Nabeshima T. Kinetic interaction between theophylline and a newly developed anti-allergic drug, pemirolast potassium. *Eur J Clin Pharmacol* (1994) 46, 55–8.
3. Accolate (Zafirlukast). AstraZeneca Pharmaceuticals LP. US Prescribing information, February 2011.
4. Katial RK, Stelzle RC, Bonner MW, Marino M, Cantilena LR, Smith LJ. A drug interaction between zafirlukast and theophylline. *Arch Intern Med* (1998) 158, 1713–5.
5. AstraZeneca UK. Personal communication, March 2009.

Theophylline + Loperamide

Loperamide delays the absorption of theophylline from a sustained-release preparation.

Clinical evidence, mechanism, importance and management

A study in 12 healthy subjects, on the effects of altering the transit time of drugs through the small intestine, found that high-dose loperamide (8 mg every 6 hours for a total of 8 doses) decreased the rate, but not the extent, of absorption of a single 600-mg dose of sustained-release theophylline (*Theo-24*). The maximum serum theophylline levels were reduced from 4.6 mg/L to 3.2 mg/L, and the peak level occurred at 20 hours instead of 11 hours. One suggested reason for these effects is that loperamide inhibits the movement of the gut, thereby decreasing the dissolution rate of the *Theo-24* pellets.[1] More study is needed to establish the clinical significance of this interaction in patients receiving long-term theophylline, and to establish if aminophylline is similarly affected.

1. Bryson JC, Dukes GE, Kirby MG, Heizer WD, Powell JR. Effect of altering small bowel transit time on sustained release theophylline absorption. *J Clin Pharmacol* (1989) 29, 733–8.

Theophylline + Macrolides

Troleandomycin moderately decreases theophylline clearance, and theophylline toxicity has been seen in some patients. Azithromycin, clarithromycin, dirithromycin, josamycin, midecamycin, rokitamycin, roxithromycin, spiramycin, and telithromycin normally only cause small changes in theophylline levels or do not interact at all; however, there are unexplained and isolated case reports of theophylline toxicity with josamycin and clarithromycin.

Clinical evidence

(a) Azithromycin

In an analysis of the safety data from clinical studies of azithromycin, there was no evidence that the plasma levels of theophylline were affected in patients given both drugs.[1] Similarly, no adverse effects were reported in another clinical study of patients taking azithromycin and theophylline.[2] Azithromycin 250 mg twice daily did not affect the clearance or serum theophylline levels in patients with asthma.[3] However, a 68-year-old man had a marked but transient fall in his serum theophylline level when azithromycin was withdrawn, and this was confirmed on rechallenge.[4] The same authors conducted a study in 4 healthy subjects given azithromycin 500 mg on day one then 250 mg daily for 4 days and sustained-release theophylline 200 mg twice daily. Theophylline levels were slightly elevated during the use of azithromycin, and a transient drop occurred 5 days after azithromycin was stopped.[5]

(b) Clarithromycin

In a study in 10 elderly patients with COPD, clarithromycin 250 mg twice daily for 7 days had no effect on the steady-state serum theophylline levels.[6] Similarly, two other studies found that clarithromycin had little or no effect on theophylline pharmacokinetics.[3,7] Another study in healthy subjects given clarithromycin 500 mg twice daily for 4 days found a 17% increase in the AUC and an 18% increase in the maximum plasma levels of theophylline, but this was not considered to be clinically relevant.[8] In two clinical studies in patients with an acute bacterial exacerbation of chronic bronchitis the number of patients requiring an adjustment in theophylline dose was similar when those who took clarithromycin were compared with those who took ampicillin.[9,10] However, there are isolated reports of possible theophylline toxicity in patients taking clarithromycin, including a case that resulted in rhabdomyolysis with renal failure requiring haemodialysis.[11,12] For a report of theophylline toxicity in a patient also taking clarithromycin and levofloxacin, see 'Theophylline + Quinolones', p.1455.

(c) Dirithromycin

In one study, 13 healthy subjects had a fall in their steady-state trough theophylline level of 18%, and a fall in their peak serum level of 26% while taking dirithromycin 500 mg daily for 10 days, although this was not considered clinically relevant.[13] No statistically significant changes in theophylline pharmacokinetics were seen in 14 patients with COPD who were given dirithromycin 500 mg daily for 10 days.[14] This is supported by a similar single-dose study in 12 healthy subjects.[15]

(d) Erythromycin

Erythromycin can markedly increase theophylline levels, see also 'Theophylline + Macrolides; Erythromycin', p.1450.

(e) Josamycin

Five studies in patients (both adults and children)[16-18] or healthy subjects[19] found no clinically significant changes in serum theophylline levels when josamycin was given, but a small rise in theophylline levels was described in one study in children.[20] Another study reported a 23% reduction in the levels of theophylline (given as intravenous aminophylline) in 5 patients with particularly severe respiratory impairment, but no statistically significant effect was found in 5 other patients with less severe disease.[21] However, an isolated report describes theophylline toxicity in a 80-year-old man who was given josamycin.[22]

(f) Midecamycin

In one study, 18 children with asthma had a slight decrease in serum theophylline levels when they were given midecamycin 40 mg/kg daily for 10 days for a bronchopulmonary infection, but no changes were seen in 5 healthy adult subjects.[23]

Similarly, no significant changes in serum theophylline levels were seen in 20 patients taking slow-release theophylline (*Theo-dur*) 300 mg twice daily, or intravenous theophylline 4 mg/kg three times daily, when they were given midecamycin 1.2 g daily for 10 days.[24] A number of other studies confirm the absence of a clinically important interaction between oral or intravenous theophylline or intravenous aminophylline and midecamycin in children and adults.[25-28]

(g) Rokitamycin

Two studies, in 12 adults with COPD and 11 elderly patients taking theophylline, found no statistically significant changes in serum theophylline levels when they were given rokitamycin 600 to 800 mg daily for a week.[29,30]

(h) Roxithromycin

One study in 12 healthy subjects and another in 16 patients with COPD found only minor increases in steady-state theophylline levels, which were not considered clinically relevant, when they were given roxithromycin 150 mg twice daily.[31,32] Another study in 5 healthy subjects similarly found that roxithromycin 300 mg twice daily did not affect the pharmacokinetics of theophylline.[33] However, further study in 14 patients with asthma reported an increase in serum theophylline levels in those who were given roxithromycin 150 mg twice daily, but as the rise was not quantified it is difficult to assess the clinical relevance of this finding.[3]

(i) Spiramycin

A study in 15 patients with asthma taking theophylline found that spiramycin 1 g twice daily for at least 5 days had no statistically significant effect on their steady-state serum theophylline levels.[34]

(j) Telithromycin

A study in 24 healthy subjects given theophylline found that telithromycin 800 mg daily for 4 days did not have a clinically relevant effect on theophylline exposure.[35]

(k) Troleandomycin

In a series of 8 patients with severe chronic asthma, troleandomycin 250 mg four times daily caused an average reduction in the clearance of theophylline (given as intravenous aminophylline) of 50%. One patient had a theophylline-induced seizure after 10 days, with a serum theophylline level of 43 mg/mL (reference range 10 to 20 mg/L). The theophylline half-life in this patient had increased from 4.6 hours to 11.3 hours.[36] Other studies in healthy subjects[23,37] and patients[18] given oral theophylline with troleandomycin have also found reductions in theophylline clearance and large rises in serum theophylline levels and half-life, even at low troleandomycin doses.[38]

Mechanism

It is believed that troleandomycin forms inactive cytochrome P450-metabolite complexes within the liver, the effect of which is to reduce the metabolism (*N*-demethylation and 8-hydroxylation)[37] of theophylline (which are mediated by CYP1A2). As a result, the clearance of theophylline is reduced, and its levels increased. Clarithromycin, josamycin, midecamycin, and roxithromycin are thought to rarely form these complexes, and azithromycin, dirithromycin, rokitamycin and spiramycin are not thought to inactivate cytochrome P450.[39]

Importance and management

The interaction between theophylline and troleandomycin is established and well documented. If troleandomycin is given, monitor the levels of theophylline closely and adjust the dose as necessary: reductions of 25 to 50% might be needed.[38,40]

The situation with roxithromycin is uncertain as one of four studies suggested an interaction, but the magnitude of the effect was not quantified; however, the majority of the available evidence suggests that an interaction is unlikely. Alternative macrolides that usually interact very slightly or not at all are azithromycin, clarithromycin, dirithromycin, josamycin, midecamycin, rokitamycin, spiramycin and telithromycin. However, note that isolated case reports have described theophylline toxicity with clarithromycin and josamycin, so it would seem prudent to consider an interaction if theophylline adverse effects (headache, nausea, tremor) develop, and monitor theophylline levels accordingly. In the case of azithromycin, care should be taken in adjusting the dose based on theophylline levels taken after about 5 days of concurrent use, as they may only be a reflection of a transient decrease. In addition, note that acute infection *per se* may alter theophylline pharmacokinetics.[41]

1. Hopkins S. Clinical toleration and safety of azithromycin. *Am J Med* (1991) 91 (Suppl 3A), 40S–45S.
2. Davies BI, Maesen FPV, Gubbelmans R. Azithromycin (CP-62,993) in acute exacerbations of chronic bronchitis: an open, clinical, microbiological and pharmacokinetic study. *J Antimicrob Chemother* (1989) 23, 743–51.
3. Rhee YK, Lee HB, Lee YC. Effects of erythromycin and new macrolides on the serum theophylline level and clearance. *Allergy* (1998) 53 (Suppl 43), 142.
4. Pollak PT, Slayter KL. Reduced serum theophylline concentrations after discontinuation of azithromycin: evidence for an usual interaction. *Pharmacotherapy* (1997) 17, 827–9.
5. Pollack PT, MacNeil DM. Azithromycin-theophylline inhibition-induction interaction. *Clin Pharmacol Ther* (1999) 65, 144.
6. Gaffuri-Riva V, Crippa F, Guffanti EE. Theophylline interaction with new quinolones and macrolides in COPD patients. *Am Rev Respir Dis* (1991) 143, A498.
7. Gillum JG, Israel DS, Scott RB, Climo MW, Polk RE. Effect of combination therapy with ciprofloxacin and clarithromycin on theophylline pharmacokinetics in healthy volunteers. *Antimicrob Agents Chemother* (1996) 40, 1715–16.
8. Ruff F, Chu S-Y, Sonders RC, Sennello LT. Effect of multiple doses of clarithromycin (C) on the pharmacokinetics (Pks) of theophylline (T). *Intersci Conf Antimicrob Agents Chemother* (1990) 30, 213.
9. Bachand RT. Comparative study of clarithromycin and ampicillin in the treatment of patients with acute bacterial exacerbations of chronic bronchitis. *J Antimicrob Chemother* (1991) 27 (Suppl A), 91–100.
10. Aldons PM. A comparison of clarithromycin with ampicillin in the treatment of outpatients with acute bacterial exacerbation of chronic bronchitis. *J Antimicrob Chemother* (1991) 27 (Suppl A), 101–8.
11. Abbott Labs. Personal communication, February 1995.
12. Shimada N, Omuro H, Saka S, Ebihara I, Koide H. A case of acute renal failure with rhabdomyolysis caused by the interaction of theophylline and clarithromycin. *Nippon Jinzo Gakkai Shi* (1999) 41, 460–3.
13. Bachmann K, Nunlee M, Martin M, Sullivan T, Jauregui L, DeSante K, Sides GD. Changes in the steady-state pharmacokinetics of theophylline during treatment with dirithromycin. *J Clin Pharmacol* (1990) 30, 1001–5.
14. Bachmann K, Jauregui L, Sides G, Sullivan TJ. Steady-state pharmacokinetics of theophylline in COPD patients treated with dirithromycin. *J Clin Pharmacol* (1993) 33, 861–5.
15. McConnell SA, Nafziger AN, Amsden GW. Lack of effect of dirithromycin on theophylline pharmacokinetics in healthy volunteers. *J Antimicrob Chemother* (1999) 43, 733–6.
16. Ruff F, Prosper M, Pujet JC. Théophylline et antibiotiques. Absence d'interaction avec la josamycine. *Therapie* (1984) 39, 1–6.
17. Jiménez Baos R, Casado de Frías E, Cadórniga R, Moreno M. Estudio de posibles interaccinones entre josamicina y teofilina en niños. *Rev Farmacol Clin Exp* (1985) 2, 345–8.
18. Brazier JL, Kofman J, Faucon G, Perrin-Fayolle M, Lepape A, Lanoue R. Retard d'élimination de la théophylline dû á la troléandomycine. Absence d'effet de la josamycine. *Therapie* (1980) 35, 545–9.
19. Selles JP, Panis G, Jaber H, Bres J, Armando P. Influence of josamycine on theophylline kinetics. 13th International Congress on Chemotherapy, Vienna, Aug 28–Sept 2 1983. 15–20.
20. Vallarino G, Merlini M, Vallarino R. Josamicina e teofillinici nella patologia respiratoria pediatrica. *G Ital Chemioter* (1982) 29 (Suppl 1), 129–33.
21. Bartolucci L, Gradoli C, Vincenzi V, Iapadre M, Valori C. Macrolide antibiotics and serum theophylline levels in relation to the severity of the respiratory impairment: a comparison between the effects of erythromycin and josamycin. *Chemioterapia* (1984) 3, 286–90.
22. Barbare JC, Martin F, Biour M. Surdosage en théophylline at anomalies des tests hépatiques associés à la prise de josamycine. *Therapie* (1990) 45, 357–58.
23. Lavarenne J, Paire M, Talon O. Influence d'un nouveau macrolide, la midécamycine, sur les taux sanguins de théophylline. *Therapie* (1981) 36, 451–6.
24. Rimoldi R, Bandera M, Fioretti M, Giorcelli R. Miocamycin and theophylline blood levels. *Chemioterapia* (1986) 5, 213–16.
25. Principi N, Onorato J, Giuliani MG, Vigano A. Effect of miocamycin on theophylline kinetics in children. *Eur J Clin Pharmacol* (1987) 31, 701–4.
26. Couet W, Ingrand I, Reigner B, Girault J, Bizouard J, Fourtillan JB. Lack of effect of ponsinomycin on the plasma pharmacokinetics of theophylline. *Eur J Clin Pharmacol* (1989) 37, 101–4.
27. Dal Negro R, Turco P, Pomari C, de Conti F. Miocamycin doesn't affect theophylline serum levels in COPD patients. *Int J Clin Pharmacol Ther Toxicol* (1988) 26, 27–9.
28. Principi N, Onorato J, Giuliani M, Viganó A. Effect of miocamycin on theophylline kinetics in asthmatic children. *Chemioterapia* (1987) 6 (Suppl 2), 339–40.
29. Ishioka T. Effect of a new macrolide antibiotic, 3'-O-propionyl-leucomycin A5 (Rokitamycin), on serum concentrations of theophylline and digoxin in the elderly. *Acta Ther* (1987) 13, 17–23.
30. Cazzola M, Matera MG, Paternò E, Scaglione F, Santangelo G, Rossi F. Impact of rokitamycin, a new 16-membered macrolide, on serum theophylline. *J Chemother* (1991) 3, 240–4.
31. Saint-Salvi B, Tremblay D, Surjus A, Lefebvre MA. A study of the interaction of roxithromycin with theophylline and carbamazepine. *J Antimicrob Chemother* (1987) 20 (Suppl B), 121–9.
32. Bandera M, Fioretti M, Rimoldi R, Lazzarini A, Anelli M. Roxithromycin and controlled release theophylline, an interaction study. *Chemioterapia* (1988) 7, 313–16.
33. Hashiguchi K, Niki Y, Soejima R. Roxithromycin does not raise serum theophylline levels. *Chest* (1992) 102, 653–4.
34. Debruyne D, Jehan A, Bigot M-C, Lechevalier B, Prevost J-N, Moulin M. Spiramycin has no effect on serum theophylline in asthmatic patients. *Eur J Clin Pharmacol* (1986) 30, 505–7.
35. Bhargava V, Leroy B, Shi J, Montay G. Effect of telithromycin on the pharmacokinetics of theophylline in healthy volunteers. *Intersci Conf Antimicrob Agents Chemother* (2002) 42, 28.
36. Weinberger M, Hudgel D, Spector S, Chidsey C. Inhibition of theophylline clearance by troleandomycin. *J Allergy Clin Immunol* (1977) 59, 228–31.

37. Naline E, Sanceaume M, Pays M, Advenier C. Application of theophylline metabolite assays to the exploration of liver microsome oxidative function in man. *Fundam Clin Pharmacol* (1988) 2, 341–51.
38. Kamada AK, Hill MR, Brenner AM, Szefler SJ. Effect of low-dose troleandomycin on theophylline clearance: implications for therapeutic drug monitoring. *Pharmacotherapy* (1992) 12, 98–102.
39. Periti P, Mazzei T, Mini E, Novelli A. Pharmacokinetic drug interactions of macrolides. *Clin Pharmacokinet* (1992) 23, 106–31. Correction. ibid. (1993) 24, 70.
40. Eitches RW, Rachelefsky GS, Katz RM, Mendoza GR, Siegel SC. Methylprednisolone and troleandomycin in treatment of steroid-dependent asthmatic children. *Am J Dis Child* (1985) 139, 264–8.
41. Renton KW. Cytochrome P450 regulation and drug biotransformation during inflammation and infection. *Curr Drug Metab* (2004) 5, 235–43.

Theophylline + Macrolides; Erythromycin

Theophylline clearance can be reduced by erythromycin. In some cases this has led to raised theophylline levels, and toxicity has developed in a few patients. Erythromycin exposure might be reduced by theophylline.

Clinical evidence

(a) Effect on theophylline

In a study in 12 patients with COPD, given oral aminophylline 4 mg/kg every 6 hours, the concurrent use of erythromycin stearate 500 mg every 6 hours for 2 days increased the peak serum theophylline levels by 28% and reduced its clearance by 22%. Only one patient developed clinical signs of toxicity, although the authors suggested that this could have been because the other patients had low theophylline levels (11 mg/L) to start with and they might not have been studied for long enough to detect the full effect of the erythromycin.[1] Several single-dose studies in healthy subjects or adults with asthma given aminophylline or theophylline have demonstrated this interaction[2-6] and multiple-dose studies with aminophylline have also shown that erythromycin alters theophylline pharmacokinetics.[7,8] A multiple-dose study in children with asthma found a 40% rise in the levels of theophylline (given as intravenous aminophylline).[9] There was often wide inter-subject variability, and not all patients demonstrated the interaction.[1,4,6-9]

In addition to the studies, there are several case reports where erythromycin was thought to have caused previously therapeutic theophylline levels to rise to toxic levels. In 3 cases the theophylline level rose twofold, with accompanying symptoms of toxicity,[10-12] and in one case the patient developed a fatal cardiac arrhythmia.[13] Toxic theophylline levels of 41 mg/L have also been reported in one patient 3 days after a 6-day course of erythromycin was finished, although this patient did not have any clinical signs or symptoms or theophylline toxicity.[14]

Several studies in both healthy adults,[15-18] and adults with COPD[5,19] did not demonstrate any clinically significant interaction, although two of these studies did find a reduction in the clearance of theophylline in some subjects.[15,19]

(b) Effect on erythromycin

In a study in 6 healthy subjects given erythromycin 500 mg every 8 hours, a single 250-mg intravenous dose of theophylline almost halved the peak serum levels of erythromycin and reduced the AUC_{0-8} by 38%.[6] Another pharmacokinetic study found that serum erythromycin levels fell by more than 30% when intravenous theophylline was given with oral erythromycin.[8] Other studies using intravenous erythromycin found no significant pharmacokinetic changes when theophylline was given: the renal clearance of erythromycin was increased, but this did not affect the overall clearance.[18,20]

Mechanism

The mechanism for the effects of erythromycin on theophylline levels is not fully understood. It seems most likely that erythromycin inhibits the metabolism of theophylline by the liver, resulting in a reduction in its clearance and a rise in its levels. The human organic anion transporter (OAT) 2 in the liver may also be involved in this interaction.[21] The reduction in erythromycin levels might be caused by theophylline affecting the absorption of oral erythromycin.[18]

Importance and management

The effects of erythromycin on theophylline and aminophylline are established (but still debated) and well documented. Not all the reports are referenced here. The interaction seems independent of which erythromycin salt is used. Although the pharmacokinetic effects on theophylline are variable, some patients have developed theophylline toxicity, and therefore it would seem prudent to monitor theophylline levels and anticipate the need to reduce the aminophylline or theophylline dose. Not all patients will develop this interaction but remember it can take several days (most commonly 2 to 7 days) to manifest itself. Some patients might have a high theophylline level but no clinical signs or symptoms, therefore do not rely on symptoms alone to monitor for toxicity.[14] Limited evidence suggests that levels return to normal 2 to 7 days after stopping erythromycin.[10-12,14] There are many factors, such as smoking,[3,19] which also affect theophylline pharmacokinetics, and which might play a role in altering the significance of the interaction in different patients. Other patients particularly at risk are those taking high doses of theophylline (20 mg/kg or more). Ideally, use a non-interacting antibacterial if possible. However, where concurrent treatment cannot be avoided, it has been suggested that the dose of theophylline should be reduced by 25% in patients with levels in the 15 to 20 mg/L range,[1,2,22] but little dose adjustment is probably needed for those with theophylline levels at the lower end of the range, (below 15 mg/L) unless adverse effects [nausea, headache, tremor] appear.[1,4] In practice erythromycin can probably be safely started with theophylline, with the levels monitored after 48 hours and appropriate dose adjustments then made.

The reduction in erythromycin exposure caused by theophylline is not well documented, but what is known suggests that it might be clinically important. Be alert for any evidence of an inadequate response to erythromycin and increase the dose or change the antibacterial if necessary. Intravenous erythromycin does not appear to be affected.

1. Reisz G, Pingleton SK, Melethil S, Ryan PB. The effect of erythromycin on theophylline pharmacokinetics in chronic bronchitis. *Am Rev Respir Dis* (1983) 127, 581–4.
2. Prince RA, Wing DS, Weinberger MM, Hendeles LS, Riegelman S. Effect of erythromycin on theophylline kinetics. *J Allergy Clin Immunol* (1981) 68, 427–31.
3. May DC, Jarboe CH, Ellenburg DT, Roe EJ, Karibo J. The effects of erythromycin on theophylline elimination in normal males. *J Clin Pharmacol* (1982) 22, 125–30.
4. Zarowitz BJM, Szefler SJ, Lasezkay GM. Effect of erythromycin base on theophylline kinetics. *Clin Pharmacol Ther* (1981) 29, 601–5.
5. Richer C, Mathieu M, Bah H, Thuillez C, Duroux P, Giudicelli J-F. Theophylline kinetics and ventilatory flow in bronchial asthma and chronic airflow obstruction: Influence of erythromycin. *Clin Pharmacol Ther* (1982) 31, 579–86.
6. Iliopoulou A, Aldhous ME, Johnston A, Turner P. Pharmacokinetic interaction between theophylline and erythromycin. *Br J Clin Pharmacol* (1982) 14, 495–9.
7. Branigan TA, Robbins RA, Cady WJ, Nickols JG, Ueda CT. The effects of erythromycin on the absorption and disposition kinetics of theophylline. *Eur J Clin Pharmacol* (1981) 21, 115–20.
8. Paulsen O, Höglund P, Nilsson L-G, Bengtsson H-I. The interaction of erythromycin with theophylline. *Eur J Clin Pharmacol* (1987) 32, 493–8.
9. LaForce CF, Miller MF, Chai H. Effect of erythromycin on theophylline clearance in asthmatic children. *J Pediatr* (1981) 99, 153–6.
10. Cummins LH, Kozak PP, Gillman SA. Erythromycin's effect on theophylline blood level. *Pediatrics* (1977) 59, 144–5.
11. Cummins LH, Kozak PP, Gillman SA. Theophylline determinations. *Ann Allergy* (1976) 37, 450–51.
12. Green JA, Clementi WA. Decrease in theophylline clearance after the administration of erythromycin to a patient with obstructive lung disease. *Drug Intell Clin Pharm* (1983) 17, 370–2.
13. Andrews PA. Interactions with ciprofloxacin and erythromycin leading to aminophylline toxicity. *Nephrol Dial Transplant* (1998) 13, 1006–8.
14. Wiggins J, Arbab O, Ayres JG, Skinner C. Elevated serum theophylline concentration following cessation of erythromycin treatment. *Eur J Respir Dis* (1986) 68, 298–300.
15. Pfeifer HJ, Greenblatt DJ, Friedman P. Effects of three antibiotics on theophylline kinetics. *Clin Pharmacol Ther* (1979) 26, 36–40.
16. Kelly SJ, Pingleton SK, Ryan PB, Melethil S. The lack of influence of erythromycin on plasma theophylline levels. *Chest* (1980) 78, 523.
17. Maddux MS, Leeds NH, Organek HW, Hasegawa GR, Bauman JL. The effect of erythromycin on theophylline pharmacokinetics at steady state. *Chest* (1982) 81, 563–5.
18. Pasic J, Jackson SHD, Johnston A, Peverel-Cooper CA, Turner P, Downey K, Chaput de Saintonge DM. The interaction between chronic oral slow-release theophylline and single-dose intravenous erythromycin. *Xenobiotica* (1987) 17, 493–7.
19. Stults BM, Felice-Johnson J, Higbee MD, Hardigan K. Effect of erythromycin stearate on serum theophylline concentration in patients with chronic obstructive lung disease. *South Med J* (1983) 76, 714–18.
20. Hildebrandt R, Möller H, Gundert-Remy U. Influence of theophylline on the renal clearance of erythromycin. *Int J Clin Pharmacol Ther Toxicol* (1987) 25, 601–4.
21. Kobayashi Y, Sakai R, Ohshiro N, Ohbayashi M, Kohyama N, Yamamoto T. Possible involvement of organic anion transporter 2 on the interaction of theophylline with erythromycin in the human liver. *Drug Metab Dispos* (2005) 33, 619–22.
22. Aronson JK, Hardman M, Reynolds DJM. ABC of monitoring drug therapy. Theophylline. *BMJ* (1992) 305, 1355–8.

Theophylline + Mebendazole and related drugs

Theophylline clearance can be moderately reduced by tiabendazole and toxicity has developed as a result of this interaction. Albendazole and mebendazole do not appear to affect the pharmacokinetics of aminophylline.

Clinical evidence

(a) Albendazole

A study in 6 healthy subjects found that the pharmacokinetics of a single dose of intravenous aminophylline were unaffected by a single 400-mg dose of albendazole.[1]

(b) Mebendazole

A study in 6 healthy subjects found that the pharmacokinetics of a single dose of intravenous aminophylline were unaffected by mebendazole 100 mg twice daily for 3 days.[1] The absence of a significant interaction was reported in another similar study using the same mebendazole dose.[2]

(c) Tiabendazole

An elderly man taking prednisone, furosemide, terbutaline and orciprenaline was switched from oral to intravenous aminophylline, giving a stable serum level of 21 mg/L after 48 hours. When he was also given tiabendazole 4 g daily for 5 days, for persistence of a *Strongyloides stercoralis* infestation, he developed theophylline toxicity (severe nausea) and his serum levels were found to be 46 mg/L. Three months previously, he had taken tiabendazole 3 g daily for 3 days without any symptoms of toxicity (no theophylline levels were measured).[3] The theophylline levels of another patient rose from 15 mg/L to 22 mg/L when he was given tiabendazole 1.8 g twice daily for 3 days, despite a theophylline dose reduction of one-third, made in anticipation of the interaction. Theophylline levels were still elevated 2 days after the tiabendazole was stopped, and the theophylline dose was further reduced. Levels returned to normal after 5 days, and the theophylline dose was eventually increased again.[4]

A retrospective study of patients given theophylline and tiabendazole found that 9 out of 40 (23%) had developed elevated serum theophylline levels and of those 9 patients, 5 experienced significant toxicity, with 3 requiring hospitalisation. The other 31 patients did not have theophylline levels taken.[5] A further report describes a patient receiving intravenous aminophylline who had an increase in theophylline levels from 18 mg/L to 26 mg/L within 2 days of starting tiabendazole 1.5 g twice daily.[2] The authors of this report then studied 6 healthy subjects who received a single dose of aminophylline before and while taking tiabendazole 1.5 g twice daily for 3 days. Three of the subjects had to discontinue the study because of severe nausea, vomiting or dizziness. In the remaining three, tiabendazole had striking effects on the pharmacokinetics of aminophylline; the half-life increased from 6.7 hours to 18.6 hours, the clearance fell by 66% and the elimination rate constant decreased by 65%.[2]

Mechanism

Tiabendazole inhibits the metabolism of theophylline by CYP1A2 in the liver, thereby raising its levels. The nausea and vomiting might have been due to the adverse effects of both theophylline and tiabendazole.

Importance and management

The interaction between theophylline or aminophylline and tiabendazole is established and of clinical importance. Although theophylline clearance is only moderately reduced by tiabendazole, theophylline has a narrow therapeutic range, and therefore the interaction results in notable increases in theophylline levels, which has led to toxicity in some cases. Monitor theophylline levels and reduce the theophylline or aminophylline dose accordingly: a 50% dose reduction in the theophylline dose has been suggested.[4] Alternatively, where practical, stop aminophylline or theophylline for 2 to 3 days while giving the tiabendazole.[5] Albendazole and mebendazole do not appear to interact with theophylline (given as aminophylline), and so may be suitable alternative anthelmintics depending on the condition being treated.

1. Adebayo GI, Mabadeje AFB. Theophylline disposition — effects of cimetidine, mebendazole and albendazole. *Aliment Pharmacol Ther* (1988) 2, 341–6.
2. Schneider D, Gannon R, Sweeney K, Shore E. Theophylline and antiparasitic drug interactions. A case report and a study of the influence of thiabendazole and mebendazole on theophylline pharmacokinetics in adults. *Chest* (1990) 97, 84–7.
3. Sugar AM, Kearns PJ, Haulk AA, Rushing JL. Possible thiabendazole-induced theophylline toxicity. *Am Rev Respir Dis* (1980) 122, 501–3.
4. Lew G, Murray WE, Lane JR, Haeger E. Theophylline—thiabendazole drug interaction. *Clin Pharm* (1989) 8, 225–7.
5. German T, Berger R. Interaction of theophylline and thiabendazole in patients with chronic obstructive lung disease. *Am Rev Respir Dis* (1992) 145, A807.

Theophylline + Methoxsalen

Oral methoxsalen increases the exposure to theophylline. Topical methoxsalen would not be expected to interact.

Clinical evidence, mechanism, importance and management

In a single-dose study in 3 healthy subjects, a 1.2-mg/kg oral dose of methoxsalen increased the AUC of a single 600-mg dose of theophylline (given one hour later) 1.7-fold, 2.1-fold and 2.7-fold, in the 3 subjects, respectively.[1] Methoxsalen inhibits CYP1A2, the isoenzyme involved in the metabolism of theophylline in the liver.[2] Although information is limited, an interaction between theophylline and oral methoxsalen appears to be established. Theophylline levels should be monitored on the concurrent use of oral methoxsalen, and the theophylline dose adjusted accordingly. An interaction between theophylline and topical methoxsalen (such as PUVA) seems unlikely, as caffeine, which is similarly metabolised, does not interact (see 'Caffeine + Psoralens', p.1426).

There appears to be no direct evidence regarding aminophylline, but as it is metabolised to theophylline, it seems likely that it will be similarly affected by methoxsalen.

1. Apseloff G, Shepard DR, Chambers MA, Nawoot S, Mays DC, Gerber N. Inhibition and induction of theophylline metabolism by 8-methoxypsoralen. *In vivo* study in rats and humans. *Drug Metab Dispos* (1990) 18, 298–303.
2. Tantcheva-Poór I, Servera-Llaneras M, Scharffetter-Kochanek K, Fuhr U. Liver cytochrome P450 CYP1A2 is markedly inhibited by systemic but not by bath PUVA in dermatological patients. *Br J Dermatol* (2001) 144, 1127–32.

Theophylline + Metoclopramide

Metoclopramide does not appear to affect the extent of absorption of theophylline from a sustained-release preparation.

Clinical evidence, mechanism, importance and management

In a study in 8 healthy subjects, a single 10-mg dose of metoclopramide taken 20 minutes before a 600-mg dose of sustained-release theophylline (*Theo-Dur*), caused a 15% reduction in the bioavailability of theophylline, which was not statistically significant. However, adverse effects (nausea, headache, tremors, CNS stimulation) were seen more often in those taking metoclopramide than in those taking placebo, possibly because metoclopramide caused an earlier rise in theophylline levels, and because some of the adverse effects of these two drugs might be additive.[1] A later study in 12 healthy subjects found that metoclopramide 15 mg every 6 hours had no effect on the rate or extent of absorption of a 600-mg dose of sustained-release theophylline (*Theo-24*).[2] A similar lack of interaction was found in another study using *Theo-Dur*.[3] There would seem to be no reason for avoiding concurrent use.

1. Steeves RA, Robinson JD, McKenzie MW, Justus PG. Effects of metoclopramide on the pharmacokinetics of a slow-release theophylline product. *Clin Pharm* (1982) 1, 356–60.
2. Bryson JC, Dukes GE, Kirby MG, Heizer WD, Powell JR. Effect of altering small bowel transit time on sustained release theophylline absorption. *J Clin Pharmacol* (1989) 29, 733–8.
3. Sommers DK, Meyer EC, Van Wyk M, Moncrieff J, Snyman JR, Grimbeek RJ. The influence of codeine, propantheline and metoclopramide on small bowel transit and theophylline absorption from a sustained-release formulation. *Br J Clin Pharmacol* (1992) 33, 305–8.

Theophylline + Metronidazole

Metronidazole does not affect the pharmacokinetics of theophylline, but an isolated report describes seizures in a patient taking theophylline, metronidazole and ciprofloxacin.

Clinical evidence, mechanism, importance and management

In a study in 5 women taking metronidazole 250 mg three times a day for trichomoniasis, there were no changes in the pharmacokinetics of theophylline, given as a single intravenous dose of aminophylline.[1] Another study in 10 healthy subjects confirmed this finding.[2] However, an acutely ill elderly woman taking theophylline had a generalised seizure while taking metronidazole and ciprofloxacin, despite her theophylline level being within the therapeutic range (10 to 20 mg/L).[3] As both ciprofloxacin and, more rarely, metronidazole are associated with seizures, it is possible that the seizures were not related to theophylline use[3] and the general significance of this isolated case is unknown. Although the evidence is limited, no theophylline or aminophylline dose adjustments would seem to be necessary on the concurrent use of metronidazole. However, note that acute infection *per se* might alter theophylline pharmacokinetics.[4]

1. Reitberg DP, Klarnet JP, Carlson JK, Schentag JJ. Effect of metronidazole on theophylline pharmacokinetics. *Clin Pharm* (1983) 2, 441–4.
2. Adebayo GI, Mabadeje AFB. Lack of inhibitory effect of metronidazole on theophylline disposition in healthy subjects. *Br J Clin Pharmacol* (1987) 24, 110–13.
3. Semel JD, Allen N. Seizures in patients simultaneously receiving theophylline and imipenem or ciprofloxacin or metronidazole. *South Med J* (1991) 84, 465–8.
4. Renton KW. Cytochrome P450 regulation and drug biotransformation during inflammation and infection. *Curr Drug Metab* (2004) 5, 235–43.

Theophylline + Mexiletine or Tocainide

Theophylline levels are increased by mexiletine and toxicity may occur. Tocainide does not appear to affect the clearance of theophylline to a clinically relevant extent.

Clinical evidence

(a) Mexiletine

A man developed theophylline toxicity within a few days of starting to take mexiletine 200 mg three times daily. His serum theophylline level rose from 15.3 mg/L to 25 mg/L, but fell to 14.2 mg/L, and the symptoms of toxicity resolved, when the theophylline dose was reduced by two-thirds.[1]

Other case reports describe 1.5- to threefold increases in theophylline serum levels (accompanied by clear signs of toxicity in some instances) in a total of 10 patients who were given mexiletine.[2-7] Theophylline dose reductions of 50% were required in 3 cases,[2,6] although 2 of the patients that did not require dose reductions had initial theophylline levels below the therapeutic range.[3] In another report, the arrhythmia of one patient was aggravated even at therapeutic serum theophylline levels, and mexiletine was discontinued.[4]

In a study in 15 healthy subjects, mexiletine 200 mg three times daily for 5 days reduced the clearance of a single 5-mg/kg intravenous dose of theophylline by 46% in women and 40% in men. The theophylline half-life was prolonged by 96% (from 7.4 to 14.5 hours) in women and 71% (from 8.7 to 14.9 hours) in men.[8] Two further studies in healthy subjects given theophylline with mexiletine for 5 days found a reduction in the steady-state theophylline clearance of about 45%, and an increase in its AUC of about 60%.[9,10]

(b) Tocainide

In a study, 8 healthy subjects were given tocainide 400 mg every 8 hours for 7 days, with a single 5-mg/kg intravenous dose of theophylline on day 5. The clearance of theophylline was decreased by about 10% and its half-life slightly prolonged (from 9.7 hours to 10.4 hours), but these changes were not thought to be large enough to warrant altering theophylline doses.[11]

Mechanism

Mexiletine inhibits the metabolism (demethylation) of theophylline by the liver, thereby increasing its effects.[8,10,12] It has been suggested that the interaction is due to competitive inhibition of CYP1A2.[13] However note that interactions by substrate competition are rarely clinically relevant.

Importance and management

The interaction between theophylline and mexiletine is established and of clinical importance. Monitor theophylline levels and reduce the theophylline dose as necessary to prevent the development of toxicity: it has been suggested that 50% dose reductions may be necessary.[8]

A clinically relevant interaction is not expected between theophylline and tocainide.

There appears to be no direct evidence regarding aminophylline, but as it is metabolised to theophylline, it seems likely that it will be similarly affected by mexiletine, but no clinically relevant interaction would be expected with tocainide.

1. Katz A, Buskila D, Sukenik S. Oral mexiletine-theophylline interaction. *Int J Cardiol* (1987) 17, 227–8.
2. Stanley R, Comer T, Taylor JL, Saliba D. Mexiletine-theophylline interaction. *Am J Med* (1989) 86, 733–4.
3. Ueno K, Miyai K, Seki T, Kawaguchi Y. Interaction between theophylline and mexiletine. *DICP Ann Pharmacother* (1990) 24, 471–2.

4. Kessler KM, Interian A, Cox M, Topaz O, De Marchena EJ, Myerburg RJ. Proarrhythmia related to a kinetic and dynamic interaction of mexiletine and theophylline. *Am Heart J* (1989) 117, 964–6.292
5. Kendall JD, Chrymko MM, Cooper BE. Theophylline-mexiletine interaction: a case report. *Pharmacotherapy* (1992) 12, 416–18.
6. Inafuku M, Suzuki T, Ohtsu F, Hariya Y, Nagasawa K, Yoshioka Y, Nakahara Y, Hayakawa H. The effect of mexiletine on theophylline pharmacokinetics in patients with bronchial asthma. *J Cardiol* (1992) 22, 227–33.
7. Ellison MJ, Lyman DJ, San Miguel E. Threefold increase in theophylline serum concentration after addition of mexiletine. *Am J Emerg Med* (1992) 10, 506–8.
8. Loi C-M, Wei X, Vestal RE. Inhibition of theophylline metabolism by mexiletine in young male and female nonsmokers. *Clin Pharmacol Ther* (1991) 49, 571–80.
9. Stoysich AM, Mohiuddin SM, Destache CJ, Nipper HC, Hilleman DE. Influence of mexiletine on the pharmacokinetics of theophylline in healthy volunteers. *J Clin Pharmacol* (1991) 31, 354–7.
10. Hurwitz A, Vacek JL, Botteron GW, Sztern MI, Hughes EM, Jayaraj A. Mexiletine effects on theophylline disposition. *Clin Pharmacol Ther* (1991) 50, 299–307.
11. Loi C-M, Wei X, Parker BM, Korrapati MR, Vestal RE. The effect of tocainide on theophylline metabolism. *Br J Clin Pharmacol* (1993) 35, 437–40.
12. Ueno K, Miyai K, Kato M, Kawaguchi Y, Suzuki T. Mechanism of interaction between theophylline and mexiletine. *DICP Ann Pharmacother* (1991) 25, 727–30.
13. Nakajima M, Kobayashi K, Shimada N, Tokudome S, Yamamoto T, Kuroiwa Y. Involvement of CYP1A2 in mexiletine metabolism. *Br J Clin Pharmacol* (1998) 46, 55–62.

Theophylline + Moracizine

Moracizine slightly increases theophylline clearance.

Clinical evidence

In a study, 12 healthy subjects were given a single oral dose of aminophylline and a sustained-release theophylline preparation (*TheoDur*). After they took moracizine 250 mg three times daily for 2 weeks, the AUCs of theophylline were reduced by 32% and 36%, respectively, the clearance was increased by 44% and 66%, respectively, and the elimination half-life was decreased by 33% and 20%, respectively.[1]

Mechanism

Uncertain. Moracizine is an enzyme inducer and appears to increase the metabolism of theophylline.[1] In contrast, *in vitro* and *animal* data show moracizine to be an inhibitor of CYP1A2, which is the main isoenzyme involved in the metabolism of theophylline.[2] This would, in theory, be expected to lead to raised theophylline levels, but as these studies illustrate, *in vitro* findings do not always translate in to clinically relevant effects.

Importance and management

Information regarding an interaction between theophylline and moracizine seems to be limited to this study. The clinical importance of this interaction has not been assessed, and the changes in clearance were only slight. Nevertheless, theophylline has a narrow therapeutic range and therefore it would seem prudent to monitor the effects of concurrent use to ensure theophylline remains effective. Be alert for the need to adjust the theophylline dose. There appears to be no direct evidence regarding aminophylline, but as it is metabolised to theophylline, it would be expected to interact similarly with moracizine.

1. Pieniaszek HJ, Davidson AF, Benedek IH. Effect of moricizine on the pharmacokinetics of single-dose theophylline in healthy subjects. *Ther Drug Monit* (1993) 15, 199–203.
2. Konishi H, Morita K, Minouchi T, Yamaji A. Moricizine, an antiarrhythmic agent, as a potent inhibitor of hepatic microsomal CYP1A. *Pharmacology* (2002) 66, 190–8.

Theophylline + Nefazodone

Nefazodone does not appear to affect the pharmacokinetics or pharmacodynamic effects of theophylline.

Clinical evidence, mechanism, importance and management

In a study in patients with COPD, nefazodone 200 mg twice daily for 7 days had no effect on the pharmacokinetics or pharmacodynamics of theophylline 600 mg to 1.2 g daily, nor was there any effect on their FEV_1 values.[1] No theophylline dose adjustment would therefore seem to be necessary if both drugs are used. There appears to be no direct evidence regarding aminophylline, but as it is metabolised to theophylline, no adverse interaction would be expected with nefazodone.

1. Dockens RC, Rapoport D, Roberts D, Greene DS, Barbhaiya RH. Lack of an effect of nefazodone on the pharmacokinetics and pharmacodynamics of theophylline during concurrent administration in patients with chronic obstructive airways disease. *Br J Clin Pharmacol* (1995) 40, 598–601.

Theophylline + Non-prescription theophylline products

Patients taking theophylline should not take other medications containing theophylline (some of which are non-prescription products) unless the total dose of theophylline can be adjusted appropriately.

Clinical evidence, mechanism, importance and management

A patient taking theophylline developed elevated serum theophylline levels of 35.7 micrograms/mL while taking *Quinamm* for leg cramps (a formulation containing quinine 260 mg and aminophylline 195 mg).[1] Another case report describes a patient taking theophylline, who increased her intake of *Franol Plus*, which contained theophylline and ephedrine. Theophylline levels measured on admission to hospital were 64 mg/L.[2] These case reports highlight the need to avoid the inadvertent intake of additional doses of theophylline if toxicity is to be avoided. Note that non-prescription preparations containing theophylline are available in many countries. For example, some cough and cold preparations contain theophylline (e.g. in the UK, *Do-Do ChestEze*). Patients should be warned.

1. Shane R. Potential toxicity of theophylline in combination with Quinamm. *Am J Hosp Pharm* (1982) 39, 40.
2. Thompson PJ, Hay JG. Dangers of compound drugs and intravenous aminophylline. *Lancet* (1982) 2, 1228.

Theophylline + Olanzapine

The concurrent use of theophylline and olanzapine does not appear to affect the pharmacokinetics of either drug.

Clinical evidence, mechanism, importance and management

A study in 18 healthy subjects given olanzapine 5 mg on day one, 7.5 mg on day 2 and then 10 mg daily for 7 days found no statistically significant changes in the pharmacokinetics of theophylline (given as a single 350-mg intravenous dose of aminophylline). The pharmacokinetics of olanzapine also appeared to be unchanged by theophylline.[1] No dose adjustments of either aminophylline or theophylline would appear to be necessary on concurrent use.

1. Macias WL, Bergstrom RF, Cerimele BJ, Kassahun K, Tatum DE, Callaghan JT. Lack of effect of olanzapine on the pharmacokinetics of a single aminophylline dose in healthy men. *Pharmacotherapy* (1998) 18, 1237–48.

Theophylline + Ozagrel

Ozagrel does not appear to alter the pharmacokinetics of theophylline.

Clinical evidence, mechanism, importance and management

Ozagrel 200 mg twice daily was given to 4 patients with asthma who were also taking sustained-release theophylline. After 24 weeks the ozagrel was stopped without any clinically significant effect on the pharmacokinetics of theophylline. Similarly, in another 8 patients with bronchial asthma, there were no statistically significant differences in the pharmacokinetics of theophylline (given as a single infusion of aminophylline) before and after taking ozagrel 200 mg twice daily for 7 days.[1] No theophylline or aminophylline dose adjustments would therefore seem to be needed on the concurrent use of ozagrel.

1. Kawakatsu K, Kino T, Yasuba H, Kawaguchi H, Tsubata R, Satake N, Oshima S. Effect of ozagrel (OKY-046), a thromboxane synthetase inhibitor, on theophylline pharmacokinetics in asthmatic patients. *Int J Clin Pharmacol Ther Toxicol* (1990) 28, 158–63.

Theophylline + Penicillins

Ampicillin, with or without sulbactam, amoxicillin, and ticarcillin with clavulanic acid do not alter the pharmacokinetics of theophylline.

Clinical evidence, mechanism, importance and management

A retrospective study in asthmatic children aged 3 months to 6 years found that the mean half-life of theophylline did not differ between those children given **ampicillin** and those not given ampicillin.[1] The pharmacokinetics of theophylline 8.5 mg/kg daily were not altered in 12 adult patients with COPD when they were given **ampicillin** 1 g with **sulbactam** 500 mg every 12 hours for 7 days.[2] A study in 9 healthy adult subjects found that **amoxicillin** 750 mg daily for 9 days did not affect the pharmacokinetics of theophylline 540 mg twice daily.[3,4] In a study in 12 patients with acute exacerbations of COPD, twice daily intramuscular **ticarcillin** 1 g with **clavulanic acid** 200 mg did not affect the steady-state pharmacokinetics of theophylline 600 mg daily, given as a sustained-release preparation.[5]

No theophylline dose adjustment would therefore seem to be necessary on the concurrent use of these antibacterials and theophylline. There appears to be no direct evidence regarding aminophylline, but as it is metabolised to theophylline, no adverse interaction would be expected with these penicillins. However, note that acute infections *per se* can alter theophylline pharmacokinetics.[6]

1. Kadlec GJ, Ha LT, Jarboe CH, Richards D, Karibo JM. Effect of ampicillin on theophylline half-life in infants and young children. *South Med J* (1978) 71, 1584.
2. Cazzola M, Santangelo G, Guidetti E, Mattina R, Caputi M, Girbino G. Influence of sulbactam plus ampicillin on theophylline clearance. *Int J Clin Pharmacol Res* (1991) 11, 11–15.
3. Jonkman JHG, van der Boon WJV, Schoenmaker R, Holtkamp A, Hempenius J. Lack of effect of amoxicillin on theophylline pharmacokinetics. *Br J Clin Pharmacol* (1985) 19, 99–101.
4. Jonkman JHG, van der Boon WJV, Schoenmaker R, Holtkamp AH, Hempenius J. Clinical pharmacokinetics of amoxycillin and theophylline during cotreatment with both medicaments. *Chemotherapy* (1985) 31, 329–35.
5. Matera MG, Cazzola M, Lampa E, Santangelo G, Paizis G, Vinciguerra A, Rossi F. Clinical pharmacokinetics of theophylline during co-treatment with ticarcillin plus clavulanic acid in patients suffering from acute exacerbation of chronic bronchitis. *J Chemother* (1993) 5, 233–6.
6. Renton KW. Cytochrome P450 regulation and drug biotransformation during inflammation and infection. *Curr Drug Metab* (2004) 5, 235–43.

Theophylline + Pentoxifylline

Pentoxifylline appears to raise theophylline levels.

Clinical evidence, mechanism, importance and management

In a study in 9 healthy subjects given sustained-release theophylline (*TheoDur*) 200 or 300 mg twice daily for 7 days, pentoxifylline 400 mg three times daily increased the mean trough steady-state serum theophylline level by 30%. However, the change in levels ranged from a 13% decrease to a 95% increase. Subjects complained of insomnia, nausea, diarrhoea and tachycardia more frequently while taking both drugs, although this did not reach statistical significance.[1] The mechanism of this interaction is not understood, although note that pentoxifylline is also a xanthine derivative. Patients taking theophylline with pentoxifylline should be monitored for theophylline adverse effects (headache, nausea, tremor). If an interaction is suspected, monitor theophylline levels and adjust the theophylline dose, if necessary. More study is needed to clarify this highly variable interaction.

There appears to be no direct evidence regarding aminophylline, but as it is metabolised to theophylline, it seems likely that it will be similarly affected by pentoxifylline and therefore similar precautions to those advised with theophylline would seem appropriate; however, note that one UK manufacturer[2] of aminophylline injection contraindicates the concurrent use of xanthine derivatives (they name pentoxifylline), while others advise against its use with other xanthine medications.[3]

1. Ellison MJ, Horner RD, Willis SE, Cummings DM. Influence of pentoxifylline on steady-state theophylline serum concentrations from sustained-release formulations. *Pharmacotherapy* (1990) 10, 383–6.
2. Aminophylline Injection. Hameln Pharmaceuticals Ltd. UK Summary of product characteristics, July 2010.
3. Aminophylline. Goldshield plc. UK Summary of product characteristics, August 2009.

Theophylline + Phenylpropanolamine

Phenylpropanolamine moderately reduces the clearance of theophylline.

Clinical evidence, mechanism, importance and management

In a study in 8 healthy subjects, a single 150-mg oral dose of phenylpropanolamine decreased the clearance of theophylline (given as a single 4-mg/kg intravenous dose of aminophylline one hour after the phenylpropanolamine) by 50%.[1] Although the reduction in theophylline clearance is moderate, theophylline has a narrow therapeutic range, and therefore it would be expected to result in some increase in serum theophylline levels, but so far no studies of this potentially clinically important interaction seem to have been undertaken in patients. Until more is known, it would seem prudent to be alert for evidence of theophylline adverse effects (headache, nausea, tremor) if phenylpropanolamine is given. There appears to be no direct evidence regarding aminophylline, but as it is metabolised to theophylline, it seems possible that it could be similarly affected by phenylpropanolamine.

1. Wilson HA, Chin R, Adair NE, Zaloga GP. Phenylpropanolamine significantly reduces the clearance of theophylline. *Am Rev Respir Dis* (1991) 143, A629.

Theophylline + Phenytoin

Phenytoin increases the clearance of theophylline, but the magnitude of effect reported varies widely. Limited evidence suggests that theophylline might also reduce phenytoin exposure.

Clinical evidence

(a) Reduced phenytoin serum levels

A preliminary report noted that the seizure frequency of a woman with epilepsy taking phenytoin 100 mg four times daily increased when she was given intravenous theophylline, and then later oral theophylline. Her serum phenytoin levels had more than halved, from 15.7 mg/L to around 5 to 8 mg/L. An increase in the phenytoin dose to 200 mg three times daily raised her serum phenytoin levels to only 7 to 11 mg/L until the drugs were given one to 2 hours apart. The patient then developed phenytoin toxicity with a serum level of 33 mg/L. A subsequent single-dose study in 4 healthy subjects confirmed that higher serum levels of both drugs were achieved when theophylline and phenytoin were given 2 hours apart rather than simultaneously.[1] Another study in 7 healthy subjects found that the AUC of a single 400-mg dose of phenytoin was reduced by 21% when it was given at the same time as a single 7.5-mg/kg dose of theophylline, compared with a reduction of 7% when the same doses were given 2 hours apart.[2] A later preliminary study (by some of the same authors) in 14 subjects found that after 2 weeks of concurrent use, the mean serum phenytoin levels of 5 of the subjects rose by 40% and the mean levels of the group as a whole rose by about 27% when the theophylline was stopped. Urinary concentrations of a phenytoin metabolite were raised.[3]

(b) Reduced theophylline serum levels

The observation that a patient taking phenytoin had lower than expected theophylline levels prompted a study in 10 healthy subjects. After taking phenytoin for 10 days the clearance of theophylline (after a single intravenous dose of aminophylline) was increased by 73%, and both its AUC and half-life were reduced by about 50%.[4] Another study in 6 healthy subjects found that after taking phenytoin 300 mg daily for 3 weeks the mean clearance of theophylline (after a single intravenous dose of aminophylline) was increased by 45% (range 31 to 65%).[5] Similar results were found in a further study.[6] Other reports on individual asthmatic patients have shown that phenytoin can increase the clearance of theophylline by between about 30% and 3.5-fold.[7-9] Another study[10] and a case report[11] found that the reduction in theophylline levels caused by phenytoin can be additive with the effects of smoking (consider also 'Theophylline + Tobacco', p.1462). A subsequent study found that the extent of phenytoin-induced metabolism of theophylline was not affected by age, despite an age-related reduction in theophylline metabolism.[12]

Mechanism

It seems probable that phenytoin, a known enzyme inducer, increases the metabolism of theophylline by CYP1A2 in the liver, thereby increasing its clearance. It has been suggested that theophylline either impairs phenytoin absorption or induces phenytoin metabolism, but neither suggestion seem likely.

Importance and management

The effect of phenytoin on theophylline is established and of clinical importance. Patients given both drugs should be monitored to confirm that theophylline remains effective. Ideally theophylline levels should be measured to confirm that they remain within the therapeutic range, and the aminophylline or theophylline dose adjusted accordingly. Theophylline dose increases of up to 50% or more may be required.[13] Conversely, if phenytoin is stopped, patients should be monitored for signs of theophylline toxicity (nausea, headache, tremor) and theophylline levels should be checked, with the aminophylline or theophylline dose adjusted if necessary.

Note that **fosphenytoin** is a prodrug of phenytoin and would therefore be expected to reduce theophylline levels in a similar way to phenytoin.

The effect of theophylline on phenytoin is not established and the documentation is limited. It may be prudent to monitor phenytoin levels and consider a phenytoin dose increase, if necessary. Separating the doses by 2 hours appears to minimise any interaction. Note that theophylline itself can cause seizures, although mostly in overdose, and should be used with caution in patients with epilepsy.

1. Fincham RW, Schottelius DD, Wyatt R, Hendeles L, Weinberger M. Phenytoin-theophylline interaction; a case report. In: Wada JA, Perry JK, eds. Advances in Epileptology: New York: Raven Press; 1980 p. 505.
2. Hendeles L, Wyatt R, Weinberger M, Schottelius D, Fincham R. Decreased oral phenytoin absorption following concurrent theophylline administration. *J Allergy Clin Immunol* (1979) 63, 156.
3. Taylor JW, Hendeles L, Weinberger M, Lyon LW, Wyatt R, Riegelman S. The interaction of phenytoin and theophylline. *Drug Intell Clin Pharm* (1980) 14, 638.
4. Marquis J-F, Carruthers SG, Spence JD, Brownstone YS, Toogood JH. Phenytoin-theophylline interaction. *N Engl J Med* (1982) 307, 1189–90.
5. Miller M, Cosgriff J, Kwong T, Morken DA. Influence of phenytoin on theophylline clearance. *Clin Pharmacol Ther* (1984) 35, 666–9.
6. Adebayo GI. Interaction between phenytoin and theophylline in healthy volunteers. *Clin Exp Pharmacol Physiol* (1988) 15, 883–7.
7. Sklar SJ, Wagner JC. Enhanced theophylline clearance secondary to phenytoin therapy. *Drug Intell Clin Pharm* (1985) 19, 34–6.
8. Reed RC, Schwartz HJ. Phenytoin-theophylline-quinidine interaction. *N Engl J Med* (1983) 308, 724–5.
9. Landsberg K, Shalansky S. Interaction between phenytoin and theophylline. *Can J Hosp Pharm* (1988) 41, 31–2.
10. Crowley JJ, Cusack BJ, Jue SG, Koup JR, Vestal RE. Cigarette smoking and theophylline metabolism: effects of phenytoin. *Clin Pharmacol Ther* (1987) 42, 334–40.
11. Nicholson JP, Basile SA, Cury JD. Massive theophylline dosing in a heavy smoker receiving both phenytoin and phenobarbital. *Ann Pharmacother* (1992) 26, 334–6.
12. Crowley JJ, Cusack BJ, Jue SG, Koup JR, Park BK, Vestal RE. Aging and drug interactions. II. Effect of phenytoin and smoking on the oxidation of theophylline and cortisol in healthy men. *J Pharmacol Exp Ther* (1988) 245, 513–23.
13. Slugg PH, Pippenger CE. Theophylline and its interactions. *Cleve Clin Q* (1985) 52, 417–24.

Theophylline + Pneumococcal vaccine

Pneumococcal vaccination does not appear to affect the pharmacokinetics of theophylline.

Clinical evidence, mechanism, importance and management

In a study in 6 healthy subjects, the pharmacokinetics of oral theophylline 250 mg three times daily for 10 days were unaltered both the day after and one week after they received 0.5 mL of a pneumococcal vaccine.[1] Based on this study, and the fact that pneumococcal vaccination is routinely undertaken in patients with chronic respiratory disease, and no adverse effects appear to have been reported, no particular precautions are needed on concurrent use. There appears to be no direct evidence regarding aminophylline, but as it is metabolised to theophylline, no adverse interaction would be expected with pneumococcal vaccines.

1. Cupit GC, Self TH, Bekemeyer WB. The effect of pneumococcal vaccine on the disposition of theophylline. *Eur J Clin Pharmacol* (1988) 34, 505–7.

Theophylline or Diprophylline + Probenecid

Theophylline pharmacokinetics are unaffected by probenecid, but diprophylline levels can be raised by probenecid.

Clinical evidence

(a) Diprophylline

A study in 12 healthy subjects found that the half-life of a single 20-mg/kg oral dose of diprophylline was doubled (from 2.6 to 4.9 hours) and its clearance approximately halved by probenecid 1 g, which resulted in raised serum diprophylline levels.[1]

(b) Theophylline

A study in 7 healthy subjects found that probenecid 1 g given 30 minutes before a 5.6-mg/kg oral dose of aminophylline had no significant effect on the pharmacokinetics of theophylline.[2]

Mechanism

Diprophylline is largely excreted unchanged by the kidneys, and probenecid inhibits its renal tubular secretion.[3] Theophylline is largely cleared by hepatic metabolism, and would therefore not be expected to be affected by probenecid.

Importance and management

Based on the findings of this single-dose study, it would seem to be prudent to monitor diprophylline levels if probenecid is started or stopped. No theophylline or aminophylline dose adjustments are likely to be needed in patients also taking probenecid.

1. May DC, Jarboe CH. Effect of probenecid on dyphylline elimination. *Clin Pharmacol Ther* (1983) 33, 822–5.
2. Chen TWD, Patton TF. Effect of probenecid on the pharmacokinetics of aminophylline. *Drug Intell Clin Pharm* (1983) 17, 465–6.
3. Nadai M, Apichartpichean R, Hasegawa T, Nabeshima T. Pharmacokinetics and the effect of probenecid on the renal excretion mechanism of diprophylline. *J Pharm Sci* (1992) 81, 1024–7.

Theophylline + Propafenone

Two isolated reports describe raised theophylline levels, with symptoms of toxicity, when two patients were given propafenone.

Clinical evidence

In a 71-year-old man, propafenone 150 mg daily raised the levels of sustained-release theophylline 300 mg twice daily from a range of 10.2 to 12.8 mg/L, up to 19 mg/L, and signs of theophylline toxicity developed. The day after propafenone was withdrawn the level fell to 10.8 mg/L. When the propafenone was later restarted the theophylline levels rose to 17.7 mg/L within one week, but fell when the theophylline dose was reduced by one-third.[1]

In another report, a 63-year-old man had a marked reduction in the clearance of sustained-release theophylline and a rise in his theophylline levels from 10.8 mg/L to a maximum of 20.3 mg/L over 7 days when he took propafenone 150 mg every 8 hours, increasing to 300 mg every 8 hours. Theophylline was discontinued.[2]

Mechanism

Uncertain. Propafenone appears to reduce the metabolism of theophylline by CYP1A2 the liver, thereby increasing its levels. However, propafenone is usually considered to be a weak inhibitor of this isoenzyme, so it is unclear why these two patients developed such large increases in their theophylline levels.

Importance and management

Evidence for an interaction between theophylline and propafenone appears to be limited to these two case reports, which are an insufficient basis for recommending monitoring in all patients. If a patient taking theophylline is given propafenone, and theophylline adverse effects (nausea, headache, tremor) develop, it would be prudent to consider an interaction as a possible cause. Controlled studies are needed to further investigate this potential interaction.

There appears to be no direct evidence regarding aminophylline, but as it is metabolised to theophylline, it would be expected to interact similarly with propafenone.

1. Lee BL, Dohrmann ML. Theophylline toxicity after propafenone treatment: evidence for drug interaction. *Clin Pharmacol Ther* (1992) 51, 353–5.
2. Spinler SA, Gammaitoni A, Charland SL, Hurwitz J. Propafenone-theophylline interaction. *Pharmacotherapy* (1993) 13, 68–71.

Theophylline + Propantheline

Propantheline does not appear to affect the absorption of theophylline from a sustained-release preparation.

Clinical evidence, mechanism, importance and management

A study in 6 healthy subjects found that propantheline 30 mg did not affect the rate or extent of absorption of a single 500-mg dose of sustained-release theophylline (*Theo-Dur*).[1] No particular precautions would seem to be necessary on the concurrent use of propantheline and theophylline.

1. Sommers DK, Meyer EC, Van Wyk M, Moncrieff J, Snyman JR, Grimbeek RJ. The influence of codeine, propantheline and metoclopramide on small bowel transit and theophylline absorption from a sustained-release formulation. *Br J Clin Pharmacol* (1992) 33, 305–8.

Theophylline + Proton pump inhibitors

Omeprazole, lansoprazole, dexlansoprazole, pantoprazole and rabeprazole do not appear to have a clinically relevant effect on the pharmacokinetics of theophylline.

Clinical evidence

(a) Dexlansoprazole

In a placebo-controlled study, 19 healthy subjects were given a single 400-mg intravenous dose of aminophylline (equivalent to theophylline 315 mg) on day 8 of a 9 day course of modified-release dexlansoprazole 90 mg daily. It was found that dexlansoprazole had no effect on the pharmacokinetics of theophylline.[1]

(b) Lansoprazole

In a study in 14 healthy subjects, lansoprazole 60 mg daily for 9 days caused only a very slight 13% reduction in the AUC of theophylline.[2] Other studies have also shown little or no change in theophylline pharmacokinetics on the concurrent use of lansoprazole.[3-7]

(c) Omeprazole

The changes in the half-life and clearance of theophylline caused by omeprazole were found to be small and clinically unimportant in two studies,[8,9] and no changes in the steady-state pharmacokinetics of theophylline were found in other studies.[6,10,11] One study found that omeprazole produced an 11% increase in the clearance of theophylline in poor metabolisers of omeprazole (i.e. those with low levels of CYP2C19 and therefore higher levels of omeprazole),[12] but this seems unlikely to be clinically significant.

(d) Pantoprazole

A crossover study in 8 healthy subjects found that intravenous pantoprazole 30 mg daily had no clinically important effect on the pharmacokinetics of theophylline given by infusion. No clinically relevant changes in blood pressure, heart rate, ECG and routine clinical laboratory parameters were seen.[13] Other studies have also found no significant change in theophylline pharmacokinetics when pantoprazole was given.[5,6]

(e) Rabeprazole

In a placebo-controlled study in 25 healthy subjects, a single 250-mg oral dose of theophylline was given before and after rabeprazole 20 mg daily for 7 days. No significant changes in the pharmacokinetics of theophylline were seen.[14,15]

Mechanism

It has been suggested that lansoprazole possibly induces CYP1A2, the isoenzyme by which theophylline is metabolised, to a small extent.[2]

Importance and management

The potential for an interaction between theophylline and the proton pump inhibitors seems to have been well studied. What is known suggests that no clinically relevant interaction occurs between omeprazole, lansoprazole, dexlansoprazole, pantoprazole or rabeprazole and theophylline, and therefore no theophylline dose adjustment would seem necessary on concurrent use.

There appears to be no direct evidence regarding aminophylline, but as it is metabolised to theophylline, no clinically relevant pharmacokinetic interaction would be expected with any of these proton pump inhibitors.

1. Vakily M, Lee RD, Wu J, Gunawardhana L, Mulford D. Drug interaction studies with dexlansoprazole modified release (TAK-390MR), a proton pump inhibitor with a dual delayed-release formulation. Results of four randomized, double-blind, crossover, placebo-controlled, single-centre studies. *Clin Drug Invest* (2009) 29, 35–50.
2. Granneman GR, Karol MD, Locke CS, Cavanaugh JH. Pharmacokinetic interaction between lansoprazole and theophylline. *Ther Drug Monit* (1995) 17, 460–4.
3. Kokufu T, Ihara N, Sugioka N, Koyama H, Ohta T, Mori S, Nakajima K. Effects of lansoprazole on pharmacokinetics and metabolism of theophylline. *Eur J Clin Pharmacol* (1995) 48, 391–5.
4. Ko J-W, Jang I-J, Shin S-G, Flockhart DA. Effect of lansoprazole on theophylline clearance in extensive and poor metabolizers of cytochrome P450 2C19. *Clin Pharmacol Ther* (1998) 63, 217.
5. Pan WJ, Goldwater DR, Zhang Y, Pilmer BL, Hunt RH. Lack of a pharmacokinetic interaction between lansoprazole or pantoprazole and theophylline. *Aliment Pharmacol Ther* (2000) 14, 345–52.
6. Dilger K, Zheng Z, Klotz U. Lack of drug interaction between omeprazole, lansoprazole, pantoprazole and theophylline. *Br J Clin Pharmacol* (1999) 48, 438–44.
7. Ko J-W, Jang I-J, Shin J-G, Nam S-K, Shin S-G, Flockhart DA. Theophylline pharmacokinetics are not altered by lansoprazole in CYP2C19 poor metabolizers. *Clin Pharmacol Ther* (1999) 65, 606–14.
8. Oosterhuis B, Jonkman JHG, Andersson T, Zuiderwijk PBM. No influence of single intravenous doses of omeprazole on theophylline elimination kinetics. *J Clin Pharmacol* (1992) 32, 470–5.
9. Sommers De K, van Wyk M, Snyman JR, Moncrieff J. The effects of omeprazole-induced hypochlorhydria on absorption of theophylline from a sustained-release formulation. *Eur J Clin Pharmacol* (1992) 43, 141–3.
10. Taburet AM, Geneve J, Bocquentin M, Simoneau G, Caulin C, Singlas E. Theophylline steady state pharmacokinetics is not altered by omeprazole. *Eur J Clin Pharmacol* (1992) 42, 343–5.
11. Pilotto A, Franceschi M, Lagni M, Fabrello R, Fortunato A, Meggiato T, Soffiati G, Oliani G, Di Mario F. The effect of omeprazole on serum concentrations of theophylline, pepsinogens A and C, and gastrin in elderly duodenal ulcer patients. *Am J Ther* (1995) 2, 43–6.
12. Cavuto NJ, Sukhova N, Hewett J, Balian JD, Woosley RL, Flockhart MD. Effect of omeprazole on theophylline clearance in poor metabolizers of omeprazole. *Clin Pharmacol Ther* (1995) 57, 215.
13. Schulz H-U, Hartmann M, Steinijans VW, Huber R, Lührmann B, Bliessath H, Wurst W. Lack of influence of pantoprazole on the disposition kinetics of theophylline in man. *Int J Clin Pharmacol Ther Toxicol* (1991) 29, 369–75.
14. Humphries TJ, Nardi RV, Spera AC, Lazar JD, Laurent AL, Spanyers SA. Coadministration of rabeprazole sodium (E3810) does not effect the pharmacokinetics of anhydrous theophylline or warfarin. *Gastroenterology* (1996) 110 (Suppl), A138.
15. Humphries TJ, Nardi RV, Lazar JD, Spanyers SA. Drug-drug interaction evaluation of rabeprazole sodium: a clean/expected slate? *Gut* (1996) 39 (Suppl 3), A47.

Theophylline + Pyrantel

An isolated case report describes increased theophylline levels when a child was also given pyrantel.

Clinical evidence

An 8-year-old boy with status asthmaticus was given intravenous aminophylline and then switched to sustained-release oral theophylline on day 3, at which point his serum theophylline level was 15 mg/L. On day 4 he was given a single 160-mg dose of pyrantel (for an *Ascaris lumbricoides* infection) at the same time as his second theophylline dose. About 2.5 hours later his serum theophylline level was 24 mg/L, and a further 1.5 hours later it had risen to 30 mg/L. No further theophylline was given and no symptoms of theophylline toxicity occurred. The patient was discharged later in the day without theophylline.[1]

Mechanism

Not understood. The authors of the report suggest that pyrantel inhibited the liver enzymes concerned with the metabolism of theophylline, thereby increasing its levels.[1] However, this is unlikely as the interaction occurred so rapidly. They also suggest that pyrantel might have increased drug release from the sustained-release theophylline preparation (dose dumping).

Importance and management

Information is limited to this single case report: no general conclusions can be based on such slim evidence. As the increase in theophylline levels was very rapid, it would seem prudent to bear the possibility of an interaction in mind should theophylline adverse effects (headache, nausea, tremor) occur. If an interaction is suspected, monitor theophylline levels and adjust the dose accordingly.

There appears to be no direct evidence regarding aminophylline, but as it is metabolised to theophylline, it seems possible that it could be similarly affected by pyrantel.

1. Hecht L, Murray WE, Rubenstein S. Theophylline-pyrantel pamoate interaction. *DICP Ann Pharmacother* (1989) 23, 258.

Theophylline + Pyridoxal

There is no evidence of an adverse interaction if pyridoxal (a vitamin B_6 substance) and theophylline are taken concurrently. A beneficial reduction in theophylline-induced hand tremor has been reported in one study.

Clinical evidence, mechanism, importance and management

In a placebo-controlled study, 15 young healthy adults were given sustained-release theophylline (*Theo-Dur*) for 4 weeks (dose adjusted to give plasma levels of 10 mg/L) with a vitamin B_6 supplement containing pyridoxal hydrochloride 15 mg daily. A variety of psychomotor and electrophysiological tests and self-report questionnaires were unable to distinguish between the effects of the placebo or the vitamin B_6 supplement, except that the hand tremor induced by theophylline tended to be reduced.[1] In another study by the same research group, 15 healthy subjects (smoking status not indicated) took pyridoxal 15 mg daily for 2 weeks before starting, and when also taking, sustained-release theophylline (*Theo-Dur*), 5 mg/kg daily for one week increased to 8 mg/kg daily for the next 3 weeks. This resulted in theophylline levels of 7.6 to 9.9 [mg/L]. Supplementation with pyridoxal did not prevent theophylline-induced reductions in pyridoxine 5-phosphate levels, as an indicator of vitamin B_6 status, although these did not drop below the normal reference range.[2]

There would seem to be no reason for avoiding concurrent use of theophylline and pyridoxal and it may even have some advantage.

1. Bartel PR, Ubbink JB, Delport R, Lotz BP, Becker PJ. Vitamin B-6 supplementation and theophylline-related effects in humans. *Am J Clin Nutr* (1994) 60, 93–9.
2. Delport R, Ubbink JB, Vermaak WJH, Becker PJ. Theophylline increases pyridoxal kinase activity independently from vitamin B6 nutritional status. *Res Commun Chem Pathol Pharmacol* (1993) 79, 325–33.

Theophylline + Quinine

Quinine negligibly reduces theophylline exposure and theophylline negligibly increases quinine exposure.

Clinical evidence, mechanism, importance and management

In a study in 19 healthy subjects given quinine sulfate 648 mg three times daily for 7 days with a single 300-mg oral dose of theophylline, the AUC of theophylline was reduced by 10%. In addition, the AUC of quinine AUC was increased by 14%.[1] In another study in healthy subjects given quinine sulfate 200 mg alone, or as quinine sulfate 260 mg formulated with theophylline, there was no difference in the dose-adjusted AUC of quinine between the formulations.[2]

The negligible pharmacokinetic interaction seen between quinine and theophylline is not clinically important. Despite such a small effect, the US manufacturer of quinine states that with concurrent use of theophylline or aminophylline, patients should be monitored closely for quinine adverse effects and should have their theophylline concentrations monitored frequently.[1] Given the available data, this seems overly cautious.

1. Qualaquin (Quinine sulfate). AR Scientific Inc. US Prescribing information, April 2011.
2. Fuder H, Herzog R, Vaupel W, Wetzelsberger N, Lücker PW. Study on the absolute bioavailability of quinine and theophylline from tablets after single dose oral administration as compared to intravenous infusion in healthy male non-smoking volunteers. *Methods Find Exp Clin Pharmacol* (1994) 16, 651–60.

Theophylline + Quinolones

Theophylline concentrations can be increased in most patients by enoxacin. Pipemidic acid and clinafloxacin probably interact similarly. Theophylline concentrations can also be increased in some patients by ciprofloxacin, and possibly pefloxacin. Norfloxacin, ofloxacin, pazufloxacin, or prulifloxacin normally cause a much smaller increase in theophylline concentrations. However, serious toxicity has been seen in few patients given norfloxacin. Fleroxacin, flumequine, gatifloxacin, gemifloxacin, levofloxacin, lomefloxacin, moxifloxacin, nalidixic acid, rufloxacin, sparfloxacin, and trovafloxacin appear not to interact with theophylline.

Clinical evidence

A. Pharmacokinetic studies

The effects of the quinolones on the pharmacokinetics of theophylline in clinical studies in healthy subjects or patients are listed in 'Table 34.4', p.1456.

B. Case reports

(a) Ciprofloxacin

There are numerous cases that describe the interaction between ciprofloxacin and theophylline or aminophylline, which commonly report large increases in serum theophylline concentrations (of 32 to 478%), often associated with toxicity.[1-11] From 1987 to 1988, the CSM in the UK had received 8 reports of clinically important adverse interactions between these two drugs, with one fatal case.[1] By 1991, the FDA in the US had received 39 reports of the interaction, with three deaths.[9]

In a case-control study in patients aged 66 years or over, and taking theophylline continuously, the risk of hospitalisation for theophylline toxicity was almost doubled in those who had received a prescription for ciprofloxacin in the 14 days before hospitalisation (adjusted odds ratio 1.86).[12]

An elderly woman taking theophylline developed toxic serum concentrations and died shortly after starting to take ciprofloxacin.[7] Seizures, associated with toxic concentrations of theophylline, were described in a number of the case reports.[5,9-11,13] Seizures have also occurred when ciprofloxacin was used with theophylline or aminophylline, even when theophylline concentrations were within the therapeutic range (10 to 20 mg/L).[9,14,15] Ciprofloxacin and toxic concentrations of theophylline are both known to cause seizures independently. It was suggested that, in the case of seizures, there may be a pharmacodynamic interaction between theophylline and the fluoroquinolones as well as a pharmacokinetic interaction.[9] In each case seizures began within 1 to 7 days of starting the combination and were reported as being either partial or grand mal. The addition of clarithromycin does not appear to increase the effects of ciprofloxacin on theophylline.[16]

(b) Clinafloxacin

The apparently stable serum theophylline concentrations of a 78-year-old man with steroid-dependent COPD were approximately doubled after he received intravenous clinafloxacin 200 mg every 12 hours for 5 days. Two theophylline doses were withheld, and then the dose was reduced from 300 mg every 8 hours to 200 mg every 8 hours. Within another 5 days his serum theophylline concentrations had returned to his previous steady-state level.[17]

(c) Enoxacin

Some patients in early studies of enoxacin experienced adverse effects (serious nausea and vomiting, tachycardia, seizures)[18,19] and this was found to be associated with unexpectedly high plasma theophylline concentrations.[18,20]

(d) Levofloxacin

Levofloxacin has not notably altered the pharmacokinetics of theophylline in studies, see 'Table 34.4', p.1456. However, a 59-year-old man developed theophylline toxicity 7 days and 5 days after starting clarithromycin and levofloxacin, respectively. His theophylline clearance decreased by about 40% when compared with the value before starting these drugs and so the theophylline dose was reduced. After stopping levofloxacin, the theophylline concentration decreased, and the theophylline clearance returned to its initial value. Clarithromycin was continued.[21]

(e) Norfloxacin

No clinically significant changes in theophylline concentrations occurred in a patient given norfloxacin who subsequently had marked changes when given ciprofloxacin.[3] This report and the studies in 'Table 34.4', p.1456 contrast with the records of the FDA in the US, which describe 3 patients (up to 1989)[22] and 9 patients (up to 1991)[9] who experienced increases in theophylline concentrations ranging from 64 to 171% (mean 103%) when they were given norfloxacin. Three patients developed seizures, and one died.[9]

(f) Pefloxacin

An isolated report describes convulsions in a patient, which were attributed to the use of theophylline with pefloxacin.[23] A brief report notes that 43 patients who were given pefloxacin 400 mg twice daily and theophylline did not report any unwanted drug effects.[24]

Mechanism

The interacting quinolones appear to inhibit the metabolism of theophylline by CYP1A2 in the liver. The extent of the interaction varies between the quinolones, as they affect CYP1A2 to different extents. There is some evidence that the concurrent use of theophylline and quinolones might amplify the epileptogenic activity of the quinolones.[9,25]

Importance and management

Theophylline concentrations

The interaction between **enoxacin** and theophylline is well documented, well established and of clinical importance. Enoxacin slightly to moderately increases the exposure to theophylline. Toxicity can develop rapidly (within 2 to 3 days) unless the theophylline dose is reduced. It has therefore been suggested that, when enoxacin

Table 34.4 Effect of quinolones on theophylline pharmacokinetics

Quinolone (daily dose)	*Increase in theophylline concentration*	*Increase in AUC*	*Decrease in clearance*	*Refs*
Ciprofloxacin 600 to 1500 mg	17 to 113%	22 to 52%	18 to 55%	1–12
Clinafloxacin 400 to 800 mg			46 to 69%	13
Enoxacin 600 to 1200 mg	43 to 243%	71 to 268%	42 to 74%	1,2,10,14–21
Fleroxacin 400 mg	No significant change	up to 8%	up to 6%	22–25
Flumequine 1200 mg	No significant change	No significant change	No significant change	26
Gatifloxacin 400 mg	No significant change	No significant change	No significant change	27,28
Gemifloxacin 320 mg	No significant change	No significant change		29
Levofloxacin 300 to 1000 mg	No significant change	No significant change	No significant change	30–32
Lomefloxacin 400 to 800 mg	No significant change	No significant change	No significant change	5,33–37
Moxifloxacin 200 to 400 mg	No significant change	No significant change	No significant change	38
Nalidixic acid 1000 to 2000 mg	No significant change	No significant change	No significant change	1,6,12
Norfloxacin 600 to 800 mg	up to 22%	up to 17%	up to 15%	6,18,39–42
Ofloxacin 800 mg	up to 10%	up to 10%	up to 12%	1,2,18,41,43–45
Pazufloxacin 500 mg	up to 27%	up to 33%	25%	46
Pefloxacin 400 to 800 mg	17 to 93%	19 to 53%	29%	1,2,10
Pipemidic acid 800 to 1500 mg	71%	76 to 79%	49%	2,33
Prulifloxacin 600 mg	No significant change	16%	15%	47
Rufloxacin 200 to 400 mg	No significant change	No significant change	No significant change	48,49
Sparfloxacin 200 to 400 mg	No significant change	No significant change	No significant change	50–53
Trovafloxacin 200 to 300 mg	No significant change	up to 8%	No significant change	54,55

1. Wijnands WJA, Vree TB, van Herwaarden CLA. The influence of quinolone derivatives on theophylline clearance. *Br J Clin Pharmacol* (1986) 22, 677-83.
2. Niki Y, Soejima R, Kawane H, Sumi M, Umeki S. New synthetic quinolone antibacterial agents and serum concentration of theophylline. *Chest* (1987) 92, 663-9.
3. Nix DE, DeVito JM, Whitbread MA, Schentag JJ. Effect of multiple dose oral ciprofloxacin on the pharmacokinetics of theophylline and indocyanine green. *J Antimicrob Chemother* (1987) 19, 263-9.
4. Schwartz J, Jauregui L, Lettieri J, Bachmann K. Impact of ciprofloxacin on theophylline clearance and steady-state concentrations in serum. *Antimicrob Agents Chemother* (1988) 32, 75-7.
5. Robson RA, Begg EJ, Atkinson HC, Saunders DA, Frampton CM. Comparative effects of ciprofloxacin and lomefloxacin on the oxidative metabolism of theophylline. *Br J Clin Pharmacol* (1990) 29, 491-3.
6. Prince RA, Casabar E, Adair CG, Wexler DB, Lettieri J, Kasik JE. Effect of quinolone antimicrobials on theophylline pharmacokinetics. *J Clin Pharmacol* (1989) 29, 650-4.
7. Batty KT, Davis TME, Ilett KF, Dusci LJ, Langton SR. The effect of ciprofloxacin on theophylline pharmacokinetics in healthy subjects. *Br J Clin Pharmacol* (1995) 39, 305-11.
8. Gillum JG, Israel DS, Scott RB, Climo MW, Polk RE. Effect of combination therapy with ciprofloxacin and clarithromycin on theophylline pharmacokinetics in healthy volunteers. *Antimicrob Agents Chemother* (1996) 40, 1715-16.
9. Bachman KA, Schwartz JI, Jauregui L. Predicting the ciprofloxacin-theophylline interaction from single plasma theophylline measurements. *Br J Clin Pharmacol* (1988) 26, 191–4.
10. Wijnands WJA, Vree TB, Baars AM, van Herwaarden CLA. Steady-state kinetics of the quinolone derivatives ofloxacin, enoxacin, ciprofloxacin and pefloxacin during maintenance treatment with theophylline. *Drugs* (1987) 34 (Suppl 1), 159–69.
11. Loi C-M, Parker BM, Cusack BJ, Vestal RE. Aging and drug interactions. III. Individual and combined effects of cimetidine and ciprofloxacin on theophylline metabolism in healthy male and female nonsmokers. *J Pharmacol Exp Ther* (1997) 280, 627–37.
12. Chyrek-Borowska S, Siergiejko Z, Michalska I, Szymański W. Wpływ ofloksacyny, cyprofloksacyny I kwasu nalidyksynowego na stężenie teofiliny w surowicy chorych leczonych preparatami metyloksantyn. *Pneumonol Alergol Pol* (1992) 60, s36–39.
13. Randinitis EJ, Alvey CW, Koup JR, Rausch G, Abel R, Bron NJ, Hounslow NJ, Vassos AB, Sedman AJ. Drug interactions with clinafloxacin. *Antimicrob Agents Chemother* (2001) 45, 2543-52.
14. Wijnands WJA, Vree TB, van Herwaarden CLA. Enoxacin decreases the clearance of theophylline in man. *Br J Clin Pharmacol* (1985) 20, 583-8.
15. Beckmann J, Elsäßer W, Gundert-Remy U, Hertrampf R. Enoxacin - a potent inhibitor of theophylline metabolism. *Eur J Clin Pharmacol* (1987) 33, 227-30.
16. Takagi K, Hasegawa T, Yamaki K, Suzuki R, Watanabe T, Satake T. Interaction between theophylline and enoxacin. *Int J Clin Pharmacol Ther Toxicol* (1988) 26, 288-92.
17. Rogge MC, Solomon WR, Sedman AJ, Welling PG, Koup JR, Wagner JG. The theophylline-enoxacin interaction: II. Changes in the disposition of theophylline and its metabolites during intermittent administration of enoxacin. *Clin Pharmacol Ther* (1989) 46, 420-8.
18. Sano M, Kawakatsu K, Ohkita C, Yamamoto I, Takeyama M, Yamashina H, Goto M. Effects of enoxacin, ofloxacin and norfloxacin on theophylline disposition in humans. *Eur J Clin Pharmacol* (1988) 35, 161-5.

Continued

Table 34.4 Effect of quinolones on theophylline pharmacokinetics (continued)

19. Sörgel F, Mahr G, Granneman GR, Stephan U, Nickel P, Muth P. Effects of 2 quinolone antibacterials, temafloxacin and enoxacin, on theophylline pharmacokinetics. *Clin Pharmacokinet* (1992) 22 (Suppl 1), 65-74.
20. Wijnands WJA, Vree TB, van Herwaarden CLA. The effect of the 4-quinolone enoxacin on plasma theophylline concentrations. *Pharm Weekbl Sci* (1986) 8, 42–5.
21. Rogge MC, Solomon WR, Sedman AJ, Welling PG, Toothaker RD, Wagner JG. The theophylline-enoxacin interaction: I. Effect of enoxacin dose size on theophylline disposition. *Clin Pharmacol Ther* (1988) 44, 579–87.
22. Niki Y, Tasaka Y, Kishimoto T, Nakajima M, Tsukiyama K, Nakagawa Y, Umeki S, Hino J, Okimoto N, Yagi S, Kawane H, Soejima R. Effect of fleroxacin on serum concentration of theophylline. *Chemotherapy (Tokyo)* (1990) 38, 364-71.
23. Seelmann R, Mahr G, Gottschalk B, Stephan U, Sörgel F. Influence of fleroxacin on the pharmacokinetics of theophylline. *Rev Infect Dis* (1989) 11 (Suppl 5), S1100.
24. Soejima R, Niki Y, Sumi M. Effect of fleroxacin on serum concentrations of theophylline. *Rev Infect Dis* (1989) 11 (Suppl 5), S1099.
25. Parent M, St-Laurent M, LeBel M. Safety of fleroxacin coadministered with theophylline to young and elderly volunteers. *Antimicrob Agents Chemother* (1990) 34, 1249-53.
26. Lacarelle B, Blin O, Auderbert C, Auquier P, Karsenty H, Horriere F, Durand A. The quinolone, flumequine, has no effect on theophylline pharmacokinetics. *Eur J Clin Pharmacol* (1994) 46, 477-8.
27. Stahlberg HJ, Göhler K, Guillaume M, Mignot A. Effects of gatifloxacin (GTX) on the pharmacokinetics of theophylline in healthy young volunteers. *J Antimicrob Chemother* (1999) 44 (Suppl A), 136.
28. Niki Y, Hashiguchi K, Miyashita N, Nakajima M, Matsushima T. Influence of gatifloxacin, a new quinolone antibacterial, on pharmacokinetics of theophylline. *J Infect Chemother* (1999) 5, 156–162.
29. Davy M, Allen A, Bird N, Rost KL, Fuder H. Lack of effect of gemifloxacin on the steady-state pharmacokinetics of theophylline in healthy volunteers. *Chemotherapy* (1999) 45, 478-84.
30. Niki Y, Hashiguchi K, Okimoto N, Soejima R. Quinolone antimicrobial agents and theophylline. *Chest* (1992) 101, 881.
31. Okimoto N, Niki Y, Soejima R. Effect of levofloxacin on serum concentration of theophylline. *Chemotherapy (Tokyo)* (1992) 40, 68-74.
32. Gisclon LG, Curtin CR, Fowler CL, Williams RR, Hafkin B, Natarajan J. Absence of a pharmacokinetic interaction between intravenous theophylline and orally administered levofloxacin. *J Clin Pharmacol* (1997) 37, 744-50.
33. Staib AH, Harder S, Fuhr U, Wack C. Interaction of quinolones with the theophylline metabolism in man: investigations with lomefloxacin and pipemidic acid. *Int J Clin Pharmacol Ther Toxicol* (1989) 27, 289-93.
34. Nix DE, Norman A, Schentag JJ. Effect of lomefloxacin on theophylline pharmacokinetics. *Antimicrob Agents Chemother* (1989) 33, 1006-8.
35. Wijnands GJA, Cornel JH, Martea M, Vree TB. The effect of multiple-dose oral lomefloxacin on theophylline metabolism in man. *Chest* (1990) 98, 1440-4.
36. LeBel M, Vallé F, St-Laurent M. Influence of lomefloxacin on the pharmacokinetics of theophylline. *Antimicrob Agents Chemother* (1990) 34, 1254-6.
37. Kuzuya T, Takagi K, Apichartpichean R, Muraoka I, Nadai M, Hasegawa T. Kinetic interaction between theophylline and a newly developed quinolone, NY-198. *J Pharmacobiodyn* (1989) 12, 405-9.
38. Stass H, Kubitza D. Lack of pharmacokinetic interaction between moxifloxacin, a novel 8-methoxyfluoroquinolone, and theophylline. *Clin Pharmacokinet* (2001) 40 (Suppl 1) 63–70.
39. Bowles SK, Popovski Z, Rybak MJ, Beckman HB, Edwards DJ. Effect of norfloxacin on theophylline pharmacokinetics at steady state. *Antimicrob Agents Chemother* (1988) 32, 510-12.
40. Sano M, Yamamoto I, Ueda J, Yoshikawa E, Yamashina H, Goto M. Comparative pharmacokinetics of theophylline following two fluoroquinolones co-administration. *Eur J Clin Pharmacol* (1987) 32, 431-2.
41. Ho G, Tierney MG, Dales RE. Evaluation of the effect of norfloxacin on the pharmacokinetics of theophylline. *Clin Pharmacol Ther* (1988) 44, 35–8.
42. Davis RL, Kelly HW, Quenzer RW, Standefer J, Steinberg B, Gallegos J. Effect of norfloxacin on theophylline metabolism. *Antimicrob Agents Chemother* (1989) 33, 212-4.
43. Gregoire SL, Grasela TH, Freer JP, Tack KJ, Schentag JJ. Inhibition of theophylline clearance by coadministered ofloxacin without alteration of theophylline effects. *Antimicrob Agents Chemother* (1987) 31, 375-8.
44. Al-Turk WA, Shaheen OM, Othman S, Khalaf RM, Awidi AS. Effect of ofloxacin on the pharmacokinetics of a single intravenous theophylline dose. *Ther Drug Monit* (1988) 10, 160-3.
45. Fourtillan JB, Granier J, Saint-Salvi B, Salmon J, Surjus A, Tremblay D, Vincent du Laurier M, Beck S. Pharmacokinetics of ofloxacin and theophylline alone and in combination. *Infection* (1986) 14 (Suppl 1), S67-S69.
46. Niki Y, Watanabe S, Yoshida K, Miyashita N, Nakajima M, Matsushima T. Effect of pazufloxacin mesilate on the serum concentration of theophylline. *J Infect Chemother* (2002) 8, 33–6.
47. Fattore C, Cipolla G, Gatti G, Bartoli A, Orticelli G, Picollo R, Millerioux L, Ciotolli GB, Perucca E. Pharmacokinetic interactions between theophylline and prulifloxacin in healthy volunteers. *Clin Drug Invest* (1998) 16, 387-92.
48. Cesana M, Broccali G, Imbimbo BP, Crema A. Effect of single doses of rufloxacin on the disposition of theophylline and caffeine after single administration. *Int J Clin Pharmacol Ther Toxicol* (1991) 29, 133-8.
49. Kinzig-Schippers M, Fuhr U, Cesana M, Müller C, Staib AH, Rietbrock S. Sörgel F. Absence of effect of rufloxacin on theophylline pharmacokinetics in steady state. *Antimicrob Agents Chemother* (1998) 42, 2359-64.
50. Takagi K, Yamaki K, Nadai M, Kuzuya T, Hasegawa T. Effect of a new quinolone, sparfloxacin, on the pharmacokinetics of theophylline in asthmatic patients. *Antimicrob Agents Chemother* (1991) 35, 1137-41.
51. Okimoto N, Niki Y, Sumi M, Nakagawa Y, Soejima R. Effect of sparfloxacin on plasma concentration of theophylline. *Chemotherapy (Tokyo)* (1991) 39 (Suppl 4), 158-60.
52. Mahr G, Seelmann R, Gottschalk B, Stephan U, Sörgel F. No effect of sparfloxacin (SPFX) on the metabolism of theophylline (THE) in man. *Intersci Conf Antimicrob Agents Chemother* (1990) 30, 296.
53. Yamaki K, Miyatake H, Taki F, Suzuki R, Takagi K, Satake T. Studies on sparfloxacin (SPFX) against respiratory tract infections and its effect on theophylline pharmacokinetics. *Chemotherapy (Tokyo)* (1991) 39 (Suppl 4), 280-5.
54. Dickens GR, Wermeling D, Vincent J. Phase I pilot study of the effects of trovafloxacin (CP-99,219) on the pharmacokinetics of theophylline in healthy men. *J Clin Pharmacol* (1997) 37, 248-52.
55. Vincent J, Teng R, Dogolo LC, Willavize SA, Friedman HL. Effect of trovafloxacin, a new fluoroquinolone antibiotic, on the steady-state pharmacokinetics of theophylline in healthy volunteers. *J Antimicrob Chemother* (1997) 39 (Suppl B), 81-6.

is given, the dose of theophylline should be reduced by 50%,[20,26-28] although reductions of 75% might possibly be necessary for those with high theophylline clearances.[28] Alterations in the theophylline dose should be based on careful monitoring of theophylline concentrations. New steady-state serum theophylline concentrations are achieved within about 2 to 3 days of starting and stopping enoxacin.[28,29]

Similarly, the interaction of **ciprofloxacin** with theophylline is well documented, well established and of clinical importance, but the effect is less than that of enoxacin. Ciprofloxacin slightly increases theophylline exposure. Although problems do not develop in all patients taking theophylline and ciprofloxacin, the risk seems greatest in the elderly.[12,30] Nevertheless, it would be prudent to be alert for this interaction in any patient. Some recommend an initial reduction in theophylline dose, in the order of 30 to 50% when ciprofloxacin is started.[9,31,32] However, as a proportion of patients will not require a dose reduction, others suggest that the dose should be modified based on the theophylline concentration on day 2 of ciprofloxacin use.[11,26,33-35]

Direct information about **clinafloxacin** and **pipemidic acid** is more limited, but they also appear to cause a considerable increase in theophylline concentrations, similar in magnitude to that of ciprofloxacin, and therefore it would seem prudent to take the same precautions suggested for the concurrent use of ciprofloxacin and theophylline.

Be alert for the adverse effects of theophylline (headache, nausea, tremor) if **norfloxacin**, **ofloxacin**, **pazufloxacin**, or **pefloxacin** are used because theophylline concentrations might possibly increase to a small extent (10 to 22%), but these antibacterials normally appear to be much less likely to cause clinically relevant interactions than enoxacin, ciprofloxacin, clinafloxacin, and pipemidic acid. However, be aware that norfloxacin has caused large increases in theophylline concentrations on some occasions.[9,22] If theophylline adverse effects develop, monitor theophylline concentrations and adjust the dose accordingly.

Fleroxacin, **flumequine**, **gatifloxacin**, **gemifloxacin**, **levofloxacin**, **lomefloxacin**, **moxifloxacin**, **nalidixic acid**, **rufloxacin**, **sparfloxacin**, and **trovafloxacin** do not appear to affect theophylline pharmacokinetics to a clinically relevant extent, and no particular precautions seem necessary with these drugs. However, note that acute infection *per se* can alter theophylline pharmacokinetics.[36]

There appears to be limited direct evidence regarding **aminophylline**, but as it is metabolised to theophylline, it seems likely that it will be similarly affected by the quinolones.

Seizure threshold

The manufacturers of some quinolones include a warning in their product literature about the risk of combining theophylline [and therefore probably aminophylline] with quinolones because of their potential additive effects on reducing the seizure threshold. Convulsions have been reported with theophylline and ciprofloxacin, norfloxacin, or pefloxacin. With some of these cases it is difficult to know whether what happened was due to increased theophylline concentrations, to patient pre-disposition, to potential additive effects on the seizure threshold, or to all three factors combined. However, the literature suggests that seizures attributed to concurrent use are relatively rare, so that the general warning about the risks with all quinolones might possibly be an overstatement.

1. Bem JL, Mann RD. Danger of interaction between ciprofloxacin and theophylline. *BMJ* (1988) 296, 1131.
2. Thomson AH, Thomson GD, Hepburn M, Whiting B. A clinically significant interaction between ciprofloxacin and theophylline. *Eur J Clin Pharmacol* (1987) 33, 435–6.
3. Richardson JP. Theophylline toxicity associated with the administration of ciprofloxacin in a nursing home patient. *J Am Geriatr Soc* (1990) 38, 236–8.
4. Duraski RM. Ciprofloxacin-induced theophylline toxicity. *South Med J* (1988) 81,1206.
5. Holden R. Probable fatal interaction between ciprofloxacin and theophylline. *BMJ* (1988) 297, 1339.

6. Rybak MJ, Bowles SK, Chandraseker PH, Edwards DJ. Increased theophylline concentrations secondary to ciprofloxacin. *Drug Intell Clin Pharm* (1987) 21, 879–81.
7. Paidipaty B, Erickson S. Ciprofloxacin-theophylline drug interaction. *Crit Care Med* (1990) 18, 685–6.
8. Spivey JM, Laughlin PH, Goss TF, Nix DE. Theophylline toxicity secondary to ciprofloxacin administration. *Ann Emerg Med* (1991) 20, 1131–4.
9. Grasela TH, Dreis MW. An evaluation of the quinolone-theophylline interaction using the Food and Drug Administration spontaneous reporting system. *Arch Intern Med* (1992) 152, 617–621.
10. Schlienger RG, Wyser C, Ritz R, Haefeli WE. Der klinisch-pharmakologische fall (4). Epileptischer Anfall als unerwünschte Arzneimittelwirkung bei Theophyllinintoxikation. *Schweiz Rundsch Med Prax* (1996) 85, 1407–12.
11. Andrews PA. Interactions with ciprofloxacin and erythromycin leading to aminophylline toxicity. *Nephrol Dial Transplant* (1998) 13, 1006–8.
12. Antoniou T, Gomes T, Mamdani MM, Juurlink DM. Ciprofloxacin-induced theophylline toxicity: a population-based study. *Eur J Clin Pharmacol* (2011) 67, 521–6.
13. Karki SD, Bentley DW, Raghavan M. Seizure with ciprofloxacin and theophylline combined therapy. *DICP Ann Pharmacother* (1990) 24, 595–6.
14. Semel JD, Allen N. Seizures in patients simultaneously receiving theophylline and imipenem or ciprofloxacin or metronidazole. *South Med J* (1991) 84, 465–8.
15. Bader MB. Role of ciprofloxacin in fatal seizures. *Chest* (1992) 101, 883–4.
16. Gillum JG, Israel DS, Scott RB, Climo MW, Polk RE. Effect of combination therapy with ciprofloxacin and clarithromycin on theophylline pharmacokinetics in healthy volunteers. *Antimicrob Agents Chemother* (1996) 40, 1715–16.
17. Matuschka PR, Vissing RS. Clinafloxacin-theophylline drug interaction. *Ann Pharmacother* (1995) 29, 378–80.
18. Wijnands WJA, van Herwaarden CLA, Vree TB. Enoxacin raises plasma theophylline concentrations. *Lancet* (1984) ii, 108–9.
19. Davies BI, Maesen FPV, Teengs JP. Serum and sputum concentrations of enoxacin after single oral dosing in a clinical and bacteriological study. *J Antimicrob Chemother* (1984) 14 (Suppl C), 83–9.
20. Wijnands WJA, Vree TB, van Herwaarden CLA. Enoxacin decreases the clearance of theophylline in man. *Br J Clin Pharmacol* (1985) 20, 583–8.
21. Nakamura H, Ohtsuka T, Enomoto H, Hasegawa A, Kawana H, Kuriyama T, Ohmori S, Kitada M. Effect of levofloxacin on theophylline clearance during theophylline and clarithromycin combination therapy. *Ann Pharmacother* (2001) 35, 691–3.
22. Green L, Clark J. Fluoroquinolones and theophylline toxicity: norfloxacin. *JAMA* (1989) 262, 2383.
23. Conri C, Lartigue MC, Abs L, Mestre MC, Vincent MP, Haramburu F, Constans J. Convulsions chez une malade traitée par péfloxacine et théophylline. *Therapie* (1990) 45, 358.
24. Maesen FPV, Teengs JP, Baur C, Davies BI. Quinolones and raised plasma concentrations of theophylline. *Lancet* (1984) ii, 530.
25. Segev S, Rehavi M, Rubinstein E. Quinolones, theophylline, and diclofenac interactions with the γ-aminobutyric acid receptor. *Antimicrob Agents Chemother* (1988) 32, 1624–6.
26. Wijnands WJA, Vree TB, van Herwaarden CLA. The influence of quinolone derivatives on theophylline clearance. *Br J Clin Pharmacol* (1986) 22, 677–83.
27. Takagi K, Hasegawa T, Yamaki K, Suzuki R, Watanabe T, Satake T. Interaction between theophylline and enoxacin. *Int J Clin Pharmacol Ther Toxicol* (1988) 26, 288–92.
28. Koup JR, Toothaker RD, Posvar E, Sedman AJ, Colburn WA. Theophylline dosage adjustment during enoxacin coadministration. *Antimicrob Agents Chemother* (1990) 34, 803–7.
29. Rogge MC, Solomon WR, Sedman AJ, Welling PG, Koup JR, Wagner JG. The theophylline-enoxacin interaction: II. Changes in the disposition of theophylline and its metabolites during intermittent administration of enoxacin. *Clin Pharmacol Ther* (1989) 46, 420–8.
30. Raoof S, Wollschlager C, Khan FA. Ciprofloxacin increases serum levels of theophylline. *Am J Med* (1987) 82 (Suppl 4A), 115–18.
31. Robson RA, Begg EJ, Atkinson HC, Saunders DA, Frampton CM. Comparative effects of ciprofloxacin and lomefloxacin on the oxidative metabolism of theophylline. *Br J Clin Pharmacol* (1990) 29, 491–3.
32. Prince RA, Casabar E, Adair CG, Wexler DB, Lettieri J, Kasik JE. Effect of quinolone antimicrobials on theophylline pharmacokinetics. *J Clin Pharmacol* (1989) 29, 650–4.
33. Nix DE, DeVito JM, Whitbread MA, Schentag JJ. Effect of multiple dose oral ciprofloxacin on the pharmacokinetics of theophylline and indocyanine green. *J Antimicrob Chemother* (1987) 19, 263–9.
34. Schwartz J, Jauregui L, Lettieri J, Bachmann K. Impact of ciprofloxacin on theophylline clearance and steady-state concentrations in serum. *Antimicrob Agents Chemother* (1988) 32, 75–7.
35. Batty KT, Davis TME, Ilett KF, Dusci LJ, Langton SR. The effect of ciprofloxacin on theophylline pharmacokinetics in healthy subjects. *Br J Clin Pharmacol* (1995) 39, 305–11.
36. Renton KW. Cytochrome P450 regulation and drug biotransformation during inflammation and infection. *Curr Drug Metab* (2004) 5, 235–43.

Theophylline + Ramelteon

The concurrent use of theophylline and ramelteon does not appear to cause a clinically relevant alteration in the pharmacokinetics of either drug.

Clinical evidence, mechanism, importance and management

A well controlled study in 36 healthy subjects who took ramelteon 32 mg daily with theophylline 300 mg daily found that the pharmacokinetics of theophylline were not altered to a clinically relevant extent by ramelteon. The exposure to ramelteon was increased by 40% by theophylline, but the authors considered that, as this drug has a wide therapeutic margin, the increase seen was not expected to be clinically significant.[1]

There appears to be no information about an interaction with aminophylline, but it would be expected to interact in much the same way as theophylline.

1. Tolbert D, Karim A, Johnson J, Cao C, Zhao Z, Sainati SM. Two-period crossover study to assess the drug interaction between ramelteon (TAK-375) and theophylline in healthy adults. *Sleep* (2004) 27, A48.

Theophylline + Repaglinide

Repaglinide does not have a clinically relevant effect the pharmacokinetics of theophylline.

Clinical evidence, mechanism, importance and management

In a study in 14 healthy subjects, repaglinide 2 mg three times daily for 4 days did not have a statistically significant effect on the steady-state pharmacokinetics of theophylline, although the peak plasma theophylline concentration was slightly reduced.[1] These changes would not be expected to be clinically relevant and no theophylline dose adjustments would appear to be necessary on the concurrent use with repaglinide.

There appears to be no direct evidence regarding aminophylline, but as it is metabolised to theophylline, no adverse interaction would be expected with repaglinide.

1. Hatorp V, Thomsen MS. Drug interaction studies with repaglinide: repaglinide on digoxin or theophylline pharmacokinetics and cimetidine on repaglinide pharmacokinetics. *J Clin Pharmacol* (2000) 40, 184–92.

Theophylline + Ribavirin

Ribavirin does not alter theophylline levels.

Clinical evidence, mechanism, importance and management

In a study in 13 healthy subjects, oral ribavirin 200 mg every 6 hours had no effect on the plasma levels of theophylline (given as immediate or sustained-release aminophylline). Similarly, in a study in 6 children with influenza and asthma, ribavirin 10 mg/kg daily did not affect plasma theophylline levels.[1] No theophylline or aminophylline dose adjustments therefore seem to be necessary on concurrent use of ribavirin.

1. Fraschini F, Scaglione F, Maierna G, Cogo R, Furcolo F, Gattei R, Borghi C, Palazzini E. Ribavirin influence on theophylline plasma levels in adult and children. *Int J Clin Pharmacol Ther Toxicol* (1988) 26, 30–2.

Theophylline + Rifamycins and/or Isoniazid

Rifampicin (rifampin) reduces theophylline exposure, whereas rifabutin appears to have little effect. Isoniazid can decrease or increase theophylline clearance and might increase theophylline levels. An isolated report describes theophylline toxicity one month after a patient started to take theophylline with isoniazid. Isoniazid and rifampicin increased theophylline clearance during the initial few days of tuberculosis treatment in one study, but there is some evidence that it decreases it within 4 weeks in another.

Clinical evidence

(a) Isoniazid

Theophylline toxicity has been described in one patient receiving isoniazid 5 mg/kg daily and theophylline, and this subsequently recurred on re-challenge.[1] In 7 healthy subjects, high-dose isoniazid (10 mg/kg daily) for 10 days increased the AUC_{0-6} of theophylline by only 8%. Theophylline was given as an intravenous infusion of aminophylline and its plasma levels after 6 hours were 22% higher (about 10.5 mg/L compared with 8.7 mg/L). Five subjects also had an increase in the half-life and AUC of isoniazid, but these changes were not statistically significant.[2] Another study in 13 healthy subjects found that isoniazid 400 mg daily for 2 weeks reduced the mean clearance of theophylline (given as intravenous aminophylline) by 21%.[3]

However, another study in 4 healthy subjects given isoniazid 300 mg daily for 6 days found that the clearance of oral theophylline was increased by 16%, but no consistent changes were seen in any of the other pharmacokinetic parameters measured.[4]

(b) Rifabutin

In a study in 11 healthy subjects, rifabutin 300 mg daily for 12 days reduced the AUC of a single 5-mg/kg dose of theophylline by 6%, whereas its half-life and clearance were not affected.[5]

(c) Rifampicin (Rifampin)

In a study in 7 healthy subjects, rifampicin 600 mg daily for one week reduced the AUC of theophylline (given as sustained-release aminophylline 450 mg) by 18%. A parallel study in another 8 healthy subjects given the same dose of rifampicin found that the metabolic clearance of theophylline (given as intravenous aminophylline 5 mg/kg) was increased by 45%.[6]

Similarly, other studies in healthy subjects given oral or intravenous theophylline or intravenous aminophylline and rifampicin 300 to 600 mg daily for 6 to 14 days found 25 to 82% rises in theophylline clearance, and 19 to 31% decreases in its half-life.[5,7-12] A 61% fall in the 5-hour post-dose serum levels of theophylline (given as choline theophyllinate) occurred in a 15-month-old boy when he was given a 4-day course of rifampicin 20 mg/kg daily as meningitis prophylaxis.[13]

(d) Antimycobacterials in combination

A study in patients taking a combination of **isoniazid**, **rifampicin**, **ethambutol** and **pyrazinamide** for pulmonary tuberculosis with intravenous aminophylline 7.35 mg/kg daily for 7 days found that the clearance of theophylline progressively increased, and was 53% faster on day 7.[14] In contrast, in an earlier study by the same authors, after 4 weeks of the same antimycobacterials (isoniazid, rifampicin, ethambutol with or without pyrazinamide) the theophylline clearance in patients receiving long-term theophylline was about 35% slower than in a control group of similar patients not taking antimycobacterials.[15] A single report describes unexpectedly *high* serum theophylline levels 4 days after theophylline 300 mg twice daily was started in an alcoholic patient with hepatic impairment who had started to take **rifampicin** and **isoniazid** 2 weeks previously.[16]

Mechanism

Rifampicin is a known liver enzyme inducer, which has some effect on CYP1A2, by which theophylline is metabolised. Concurrent use increases the metabolism of theophylline, thereby increasing its clearance and reducing its levels. It has been suggested that isoniazid inhibits the metabolism of theophylline by the liver, thereby reducing its clearance and increasing its plasma levels.

With combined therapy, it was suggested that the effects of rifampicin might be more apparent during the initial 7 days, but that by week 4 the effect of isoniazid might predominate, because of its reduced inactivation by rifampicin combined with a reduction in the effect of rifampicin as a result of auto-induction of its own metabolism.[15] High theophylline levels in the isolated case might have been due to liver impairment brought about by the combined use of rifampicin and isoniazid, or alcoholism.[16]

Importance and management

The interaction between aminophylline or theophylline and **rifampicin** is established. Theophylline levels and therefore its therapeutic effects are likely to be reduced during concurrent use, and this effect can usually be detected within 36 hours.[13] The wide range of increases in clearance that have been reported (25 to 82%) and the large inter-subject variation make it difficult to predict the increase in theophylline dose required, but in some instances a twofold increase might be needed.[8] Monitor theophylline levels if rifampicin is started or stopped and adjust the aminophylline or theophylline dose accordingly.

The effects of **rifabutin** are considerably smaller than those of rifampicin, with the one available study showing no significant interaction. On the basis of this, no theophylline or aminophylline dose adjustments appear to be necessary on concurrent use.

The reason for the inconsistent results with **isoniazid** alone is not understood, nor is this interaction well established. It has been suggested that it might take 3 to 4 weeks for any clinically significant increase in theophylline levels to occur.[1] However, if enzyme inhibition was the cause of an interaction, the effects would be expected more rapidly than this. All of the studies cited covered a period of only 6 to 14 days, whereas the case report describes the effects over a period up to 55 days.[1] It has also been suggested that the dose of isoniazid could be important, with the clearance of theophylline being unaffected by usual doses of isoniazid, but reduced by higher doses.[17] The outcome of concurrent isoniazid and theophylline use is therefore uncertain and possibly affected by other antimycobacterials, but it would clearly be prudent to be alert for any evidence of changes in theophylline levels and adverse effects (headache, nausea, tremor) if isoniazid is given.

Isoniazid and rifampicin are usually taken as part of a combination regimen in the treatment of tuberculosis. There is some evidence that, in the short-term, concurrent use of these drugs will decrease theophylline levels, but that theophylline levels might increase during long-term use. However this requires confirmation. Patients taking theophylline with a combined anti-tubercular regimen including isoniazid and rifampicin should have their theophylline levels closely monitored and the dose adjusted according to the response, bearing in mind that these changes might occur over a longer period of time, as reported in the case with isoniazid.

1. Torrent J, Izquierdo I, Cabezas R, Jané F. Theophylline-isoniazid interaction. *DICP Ann Pharmacother* (1989) 23, 143–5.
2. Höglund P, Nilsson L-G, Paulsen O. Interaction between isoniazid and theophylline. *Eur J Respir Dis* (1987) 70, 110–16.
3. Samigun, Mulyono, Santoso B. Lowering of theophylline clearance by isoniazid in slow and rapid acetylators. *Br J Clin Pharmacol* (1990) 29, 570–3.
4. Thompson JR, Burckart GJ, Self TH, Brown RE, Straughn AB. Isoniazid-induced alterations in theophylline pharmacokinetics. *Curr Ther Res* (1982) 32, 921–5.
5. Gillum JG, Sesler JM, Bruzzese VL, Israel DS, Polk RE. Induction of theophylline clearance by rifampin and rifabutin in healthy male volunteers. *Antimicrob Agents Chemother* (1996) 40, 1866–9.
6. Powell-Jackson PR, Jamieson AP, Gray BJ, Moxham J, Williams R. Effect of rifampicin administration on theophylline pharmacokinetics in humans. *Am Rev Respir Dis* (1985) 131, 939–40.
7. Straughn AB, Henderson RP, Lieberman PL, Self TH. Effect of rifampin on theophylline disposition. *Ther Drug Monit* (1984) 6, 153–6.
8. Robson RA, Miners JO, Wing LMH, Birkett DJ. Theophylline-rifampicin interaction: non-selective induction of theophylline metabolic pathways. *Br J Clin Pharmacol* (1984) 18, 445–8.
9. Löfdahl CG, Mellstrand T, Svedmyr N. Increased metabolism of theophylline by rifampicin. *Respiration* (1984) 46 (Suppl 1), 104.
10. Hauser AR, Lee C, Teague RB, Mullins C. The effect of rifampin on theophylline disposition. *Clin Pharmacol Ther* (1983) 33, 254.
11. Boyce EG, Dukes GE, Rollins DE, Sudds TW. The effect of rifampin on theophylline kinetics. *J Clin Pharmacol* (1986) 26, 696–9.
12. Rao S, Singh SK, Narang RK, Rajagopalan PT. Effect of rifampicin on theophylline pharmacokinetics in human beings. *J Assoc Physicians India* (1994) 42, 881–2.
13. Brocks DR, Lee KC, Weppler CP, Tam YK. Theophylline-rifampin interaction in a pediatric patient. *Clin Pharm* (1986) 5, 602–4.
14. Ahn HC, Lee YC. The clearance of theophylline is increased during the initial period of tuberculosis treatment. *Int J Tuberc Lung Dis* (2003) 7, 587–91.
15. Ahn HC, Yang JH, Lee HB, Rhee YK, Lee YC. Effect of combined therapy of oral anti-tubercular agents on theophylline pharmacokinetics. *Int J Tuberc Lung Dis* (2000) 4, 784–7.
16. Dal Negro R, Turco P, Trevisan F, De Conti F. Rifampicin-isoniazid and delayed elimination of theophylline: a case report. *Int J Clin Pharmacol Res* (1988) 8, 275–7.
17. Thompson JR, Self TH. Theophylline and isoniazid. *Br J Clin Pharmacol* (1990) 30, 909.

Theophylline + Ropinirole

The concurrent use of theophylline and ropinirole does not affect the pharmacokinetics of either drug.

Clinical evidence, mechanism, importance and management

In a study, 12 patients with parkinsonism were given ropinirole, increased from 0.5 mg to 2 mg three times daily over 28 days, then continued for a further 19 days. The pharmacokinetics of theophylline (given as a single intravenous dose of aminophylline) were assessed before ropinirole was started, and again on day 27. The pharmacokinetics of ropinirole were then assessed before, during, and after the use of oral controlled-release theophylline twice daily for 13 days (dose titrated to achieve plasma levels in the range 8 to 15 mg/L). In both cases it was found that the concurrent use of aminophylline or theophylline and ropinirole did not alter the pharmacokinetics of either drug, and concurrent use was well tolerated.[1]

Based on the results of the studies, there would appear to be no need to adjust the dose of either theophylline or aminophylline in patients also taking ropinirole.

1. Thalamas C, Taylor A, Brefel-Courbon C, Eagle S, Fitzpatrick K, Rascol O. Lack of pharmacokinetic interaction between ropinirole and theophylline in patients with Parkinson's disease. *Eur J Clin Pharmacol* (1999) 55, 299–303.

Theophylline + SSRIs

The exposure to theophylline can be rapidly increased by fluvoxamine. Citalopram, fluoxetine, paroxetine and sertraline seem unlikely to interact with theophylline.

Clinical evidence

(a) Citalopram

In a study in 13 healthy subjects, citalopram 40 mg daily for 21 days (to achieve steady-state) did not affect the pharmacokinetics of a single 300-mg oral dose of theophylline.[1]

(b) Fluoxetine

In a study in 8 healthy subjects, the pharmacokinetics of theophylline were unchanged when they were given a 6-mg/kg infusion of aminophylline over 30 minutes, 8 hours after a single 40-mg dose of fluoxetine.[2]

(c) Fluvoxamine

The effect of fluvoxamine on theophylline pharmacokinetics has been characterised in several studies in healthy subjects. In the first study, the AUC of theophylline (given as a single 442-mg oral dose of aminophylline) was increased almost threefold, the clearance was reduced by 62% and the half-life was prolonged from 7.4 hours to 32.1 hours by fluvoxamine 50 mg daily for 3 days then 100 mg daily for 13 days.[3] In a second study, the clearance of theophylline (given as a single 300-mg oral dose of aminophylline) was reduced by about 70% and the half-life was increased from 6.6 hours to 22 hours by fluvoxamine 50 to 100 mg daily for 7 days.[4] In a further study in 9 healthy subjects, the half-life of a single 250-mg dose of theophylline given on day 8 of the study, was increased from 7.6 hours to 19.2 hours when the subjects took fluvoxamine 50 mg on day one, and 75 mg daily for the following 8 days. The AUC of theophylline increased by 138% and the clearance was reduced by 59%.[5] This interaction was shown to be reduced in patients with mild and severe liver cirrhosis (Child class A and C, respectively), whereas the clearance of a single 4-mg/kg dose of theophylline elixir was reduced by 62%, 52%, and 11% in healthy subjects, patients with mild cirrhosis, and patients with severe cirrhosis, respectively. The half-life of theophylline was increased by 13.6 hours in healthy subjects compared with 10.5 hours in patients with mild cirrhosis and one hour in patients with severe cirrhosis, demonstrating the reduced metabolic capabilities of the cirrhotic liver.[6]

A number of case reports have described fluvoxamine-induced theophylline toxicity. Agitation and tachycardia (120 bpm) developed in an 83-year-old man taking theophylline 600 mg daily (*Theostat*) about a week after he started to take fluvoxamine 100 mg daily. His serum theophylline levels were found to have risen from under 15 mg/L to 40 mg/L.[7] A 70-year-old man similarly developed theophylline toxicity, with theophylline levels of about 32 mg/L (reference range 10 to 20 mg/L), when fluvoxamine was added. Subsequently the theophylline concentrations were found to parallel a number of changes in the fluvoxamine dose.[8] The clearance of theophylline in an 84-year-old man was approximately halved while he was taking fluvoxamine.[9] An 11-year-old boy complained of headaches, tiredness and vomiting within a week of starting to take fluvoxamine. His serum theophylline levels were found to have doubled from 14.2 mg/L to 27.4 mg/L.[10] A 78-year-old woman became nauseous within 2 days of starting to take fluvoxamine 50 mg daily, and by day 6, when the fluvoxamine was stopped, her serum theophylline levels were found to have increased about threefold. She had a seizure, became comatose, and developed supraventricular tachycardia (200 bpm) requiring intravenous digoxin and verapamil. She recovered uneventfully.[11] A patient taking fluvoxamine 100 mg daily developed nausea, vomiting, confusion, reduced sleep and a poor appetite 5 days after she began to take theophylline 300 mg twice daily for COPD. Her theophylline level was found to be 25.9 mg/L.[12]

Mechanism

Fluvoxamine is a potent inhibitor of CYP1A2 in the liver, by which theophylline is metabolised. Concurrent use therefore results in raised theophylline levels and, sometimes, toxicity. This metabolic function, and hence interaction, appears to be severely reduced in patients with severe cirrhosis, probably due to reduced hepatic expression of CYP1A2 and reduced uptake of fluvoxamine.[6] The other SSRIs, citalopram, fluoxetine, **paroxetine** and **sertraline** only weakly inhibited CYP1A2 *in vitro*, and consequently would not be expected to interact.[13,14]

Importance and management

The interaction between **fluvoxamine** and aminophylline or theophylline is established and clinically important. The CSM in the UK advise that concurrent use should usually be avoided, but that if this is not possible, the theophylline [or aminophylline] dose should be reduced by half when fluvoxamine is added and theophylline levels should be monitored.[15] There is evidence to suggest that the extent of this interaction is markedly reduced in patients with liver cirrhosis, particularly severe Child class C, despite higher levels of fluvoxamine,[6] although caution should still be applied with concurrent use in this patient group as they are more likely to already have high levels of theophylline due to reduced metabolism. There is good evidence to suggest that fluvoxamine is the only SSRI likely to interact (because it is the only one that affects CYP1A2 to a clinically relevant extent). This would seem to be borne out by the studies with citalopram and fluoxetine, and the lack of case reports in the literature describing problems with any of the other SSRIs.

1. Møller SE, Larsen F, Pitsiu M, Rolan PE. Effect of citalopram on plasma levels of oral theophylline. *Clin Ther* (2000) 22, 1494–1501.
2. Mauro VF, Mauro LS, Klions HA. Effect of single dose fluoxetine on aminophylline pharmacokinetics. *Pharmacotherapy* (1994) 14, 367.
3. Donaldson KM, Wright DM, Mathlener IS, Harry JD. The effect of fluvoxamine at steady state on the pharmacokinetics of theophylline after a single dose in healthy male volunteers. *Br J Clin Pharmacol* (1994) 37, 492P.
4. Rasmussen BB, Jeppesen U, Gaist D, Brøsen K. Griseofulvin and fluvoxamine interactions with the metabolism of theophylline. *Ther Drug Monit* (1997) 19, 56–62.
5. Yao C, Kunze KL, Kharasch ED, Wang Y, Trager WF, Ragueneau I, Levy RH. Fluvoxamine-theophylline interaction: gap between in vitro and in vivo inhibition constants towards cytochrome P4501A2. *Clin Pharmacol Ther* (2001) 70, 415–24.
6. Orlando R, Padrini R, Perazzi M, De Martin S, Piccoli P, Palatini P. Liver dysfunction markedly decreases the inhibition of cytochrome P450 1A2-mediated theophylline metabolism by fluvoxamine. *Clin Pharmacol Ther* (2006) 79, 489–99.
7. Diot P, Jonville AP, Gerard F, Bonnelle M, Autret E, Breteau M, Lemarie E, Lavandier M. Possible interaction entre théophylline et fluvoxamine. *Therapie* (1991) 46, 170–71.
8. Thomson AH, McGovern EM, Bennie P, Caldwell G, Smith M. Interaction between fluvoxamine and theophylline. Pharm J (1992) 249, 137. Correction. ibid. (1992) 249, 214.
9. Puranik A, Fitzpatrick R, Ananthanarayanan TS. Monitor serum theophylline. *Care Elder* (1993) 5, 237.
10. Sperber AD. Toxic interaction between fluvoxamine and sustained release theophylline in an 11-year-old boy. *Drug Safety* (1991) 6, 460–2.
11. van den Brekel AM, Harrington L. Toxic effects of theophylline caused by fluvoxamine. *Can Med Assoc J* (1994) 151, 1289–90.
12. DeVane CL, Markowitz JS, Hardesty SJ, Mundy S, Gill HS. Fluvoxamine-induced theophylline toxicity. *Am J Psychiatry* (1997) 154, 1317–18.
13. Brøsen K, Skjelbo E, Rasmussen BB, Poulsen HE, Loft S. Fluvoxamine is a potent inhibitor of cytochrome P4501A2. *Biochem Pharmacol* (1993) 45, 1211–14.
14. Rasmussen BB, Mäenpää J, Pelkonen O, Loft S, Poulsen HE, Lykkesfeldt J, Brøsen K. Selective serotonin reuptake inhibitors and theophylline metabolism in human liver microsomes: potent inhibition by fluvoxamine. *Br J Clin Pharmacol* (1995) 39, 151–9.
15. Committee on Safety of Medicines/Medicines Control Agency. Fluvoxamine increases plasma theophylline levels. *Current Problems* (1994) 20, 12.

Theophylline + St John's wort (*Hypericum perforatum*)

A patient needed a large increase in the dose of theophylline while taking St John's wort. In contrast, no pharmacokinetic interaction was found in a two-week study in healthy subjects.

Clinical evidence

A study in 12 healthy subjects found that a standardised preparation of St John's wort 300 mg (hypericin 0.27%) three times daily for 15 days had no significant effects on the plasma level of a single 400-mg oral dose of theophylline.[1]

However, an isolated case describes a woman, previously stable for several months taking theophylline 300 mg twice daily, who was found to need a large increase in her theophylline dose (to 800 mg twice daily) to achieve serum levels of 9.2 mg/L. Two months previously she had started to take 300 mg of a St John's wort supplement (hypericin 0.3%) each day. When she stopped taking the St John's wort, her serum theophylline levels doubled within a week to 19.6 mg/L and her theophylline dose was consequently reduced. This patient was also taking a whole spectrum of other drugs (amitriptyline, furosemide, ibuprofen, inhaled triamcinolone, morphine, potassium, prednisone, salbutamol (albuterol), valproic acid, zafirlukast and zolpidem) and was also a smoker. No changes in the use of these drugs or altered compliance were identified that might have offered an alternative explanation for the changed theophylline requirements.[2]

Mechanism

Uncertain. It has been suggested that treatment with St John's wort for 15 days was unlikely to induce the isoenzymes sufficiently to cause changes in plasma theophylline.[1] This is supported by studies in which the use of St John's wort for 4 weeks,[3] but not 2 weeks,[4] modestly increased the paraxanthine/caffeine ratio, used as a measure of CYP1A2 activity. The patient in the case report had been taking St John's wort for 2 months, although at a lower dose, therefore differences in duration of treatment might be one reason for the discrepancy.

Importance and management

Direct information about an apparent interaction between theophylline and St John's wort appears to be limited. Despite the isolated case report describing a large decrease in theophylline levels, no pharmacokinetic interaction was noted in healthy subjects, and mechanistic studies suggest a modest interaction at most. Furthermore most clinically significant interactions reported with St John's wort are mediated by CYP3A4. Until further evidence is available to confirm the absence of an interaction, it would be prudent to be aware of the possibility if theophylline adverse effects (headache, nausea, tremor) develop. In 2000, the CSM in the UK recommended that patients taking theophylline should not take St John's wort. In those patients already taking the combination, the St John's wort should be stopped and the theophylline dose monitored and adjusted if necessary.[5,6] However, this guidance was issued before the pharmacokinetic study that suggests that an interaction is generally unlikely.

There appears to be no direct evidence regarding aminophylline, but as it is metabolised to theophylline, no clinically relevant interaction would generally be expected with St John's wort.

1. Morimoto T, Kotegawa T, Tsutsumi K, Ohtani Y, Imai H, Nakano S. Effect of St John's wort on the pharmacokinetics of theophylline in healthy volunteers. *J Clin Pharmacol* (2004) 44, 95–101
2. Nebel A, Schneider BJ, Baker RK, Kroll DJ. Potential metabolic interaction between St John's wort and theophylline. *Ann Pharmacother* (1999) 33, 502.
3. Gurley BJ, Gardner SF, Hubbard MA, Williams DK, Gentry WB, Cui Y, Ang CYW. Cytochrome P450 phenotypic ratios for predicting herb-drug interactions in humans. *Clin Pharmacol Ther* (2002) 72, 276–287.
4. Wang Z, Gorski JC, Hamman MA, Huang S-M, Lesko LJ, Hall SD. The effects of St John's wort (*Hypericum perforatum*) on human cytochrome P450 activity. *Clin Pharmacol Ther* (2001) 70, 317–326.
5. Committee on Safety of Medicines (UK). Message from Professor A Breckenridge (Chairman of CSM) and Fact Sheet for Health Care Professionals, 29th February 2000.
6. Committee on Safety of Medicines/Medicines Control Agency. Reminder: St John's wort (*Hypericum perforatum*) interactions. *Current Problems* (2000) 26, 6–7.

Theophylline + Succimer

A single case report describes a reduction in the theophylline levels of a man given succimer.

Clinical evidence, mechanism, importance and management

A 65-year-old man with COPD and chronic lead intoxication was given a 19-day course of lead chelation with succimer. His theophylline level was found to be reduced from about 11 mg/L to 7 mg/L on day 6 and remained at this level until about 9 days after the course of succimer was completed, when it returned to pretreatment levels. His clinical status did not alter despite these changes; possibly because he was also taking prednisone.[1] The reason for these alterations is not understood, although as succimer is known to chelate heavy metals, it seems possible that theophylline might have been chelated, resulting in a reduction in its levels.

The general importance of this isolated case is unknown, but given that succimer is known to chelate some substances it would seem prudent to monitor the situation closely if succimer is added to established treatment with theophylline or aminophylline.

1. Harchelroad F. Pharmacokinetic interaction between dimercaptosuccinic acid (DMSA) and theophylline (THEO). *Vet Hum Toxicol* (1994) 36, 376.

Theophylline + Sucralfate

Two studies found that sucralfate caused only negligible changes in theophylline pharmacokinetics, but another study suggests that the absorption of sustained-release theophylline is reduced by sucralfate.

Clinical evidence, mechanism, importance and management

In a study in 8 healthy subjects, no clinically important changes occurred in the absorption of a single 5-mg/kg dose of an oral immediate-release theophylline preparation given at the same time as sucralfate 1 g four times daily, although a slight 5% decrease in the AUC was detected.[1] Another study found that sucralfate 1 g four times daily reduced the AUC of a single dose of a sustained-release theophylline preparation (*Theodur*) by 9% (timing of the theophylline dose in relation to the sucralfate dose not noted).[2] In contrast, another group of workers found that when sucralfate 1 g was given 30 minutes before a 350 mg dose of sustained-release theophylline (*PEG capsules*), the AUC of theophylline was reduced by 40%.[3]

Many patients are given sustained-release theophylline preparations, but neither of these studies clearly shows what is likely to happen in clinical practice if sucralfate is also given. It would be prudent to be alert for any evidence of a reduced response to theophylline on the concurrent use of sucralfate. Usually, separating the administration of sucralfate from other drugs by 2 hours is considered sufficient to avoid interactions that occur by reduced absorption.[4] However, the study showing decreased theophylline absorption did not examine the effect of separating the doses. Further study is needed, both to establish the effects of sucralfate on theophylline, and to establish if an interaction occurs with aminophylline preparations.

1. Cantral KA, Schaaf LJ, Jungnickel PW, Monsour HP. Effect of sucralfate on theophylline absorption in healthy volunteers. *Clin Pharm* (1988) 7, 58–61.
2. Kisor DF, Livengood B, Vieira-Fattahi S, Sterchele JA. Effect of sucralfate administration on the absorption of sustained released theophylline. *Pharmacotherapy* (1990) 10, 253.
3. Fleischmann R, Bozler G, Boekstegers P. Bioverfügbarkeit von Theophylline unter Ulkustherapeutika. *Verh Dtsch Ges Inn Med* (1984) 90, 1876–9.
4. Antepsin Suspension (Sucralfate). Chugai Pharma UK Ltd. UK Summary of product characteristics, September 2013.

Theophylline + Sulfinpyrazone

Sulfinpyrazone causes a negligible increase in the clearance of theophylline.

Clinical evidence, mechanism, importance and management

In a study in 6 healthy subjects, the total clearance of theophylline 125 mg every 8 hours for 4 days was increased by 22% (range 9 to 42%) when they were given sulfinpyrazone 200 mg every 6 hours.[1] This appeared to be the sum of an increase in the metabolism of theophylline in the liver and a decrease in its renal clearance.

Information seems to be limited to this study. The resulting reduction in theophylline levels would not be expected to be clinically relevant.

Aminophylline, which is metabolised to theophylline, would be expected to be similarly affected.

1. Birkett DJ, Miners JO, Attwood J. Evidence for a dual action of sulphinpyrazone on drug metabolism in man: theophylline-sulphinpyrazone interaction. *Br J Clin Pharmacol* (1983) 15, 567–9.

Theophylline + Tadalafil

The concurrent use of tadalafil and theophylline does not affect the pharmacokinetics of either drug, although it might slightly increase heart rate.

Clinical evidence, mechanism, importance and management

A placebo-controlled study in 17 healthy subjects given oral theophylline (to achieve steady-state levels of about 12 mg/L) found that the concurrent use of tadalafil 10 mg daily for 7 days did not affect the pharmacokinetics of either drug. Concurrent use resulted in a small increase of 3.5 bpm in the heart rate, but this was not considered to be clinically relevant in the healthy subjects.[1]

As theophylline is a non-selective phosphodiesterase inhibitor and tadalafil inhibits phosphodiesterase type-5, some additive effects could theoretically occur. On this basis, although the UK manufacturer states that this interaction was not clinically relevant in this particular study, they advise that the potential for additive effects should be considered when both drugs are used concurrently.[2] Nevertheless, most conditions where a 3.5 bpm increase in heart rate is possibly of clinical relevance (e.g. uncontrolled arrhythmias) are contraindications to the use of tadalafil.

There appears to be no direct evidence regarding aminophylline, but as it is metabolised to theophylline, it seems likely that it will interact with tadalafil in the same way.

1. Eli Lilly and Company. Personal communication, March 2003.
2. Cialis (Tadalafil). Eli Lilly and Company Ltd. UK Summary of product characteristics, March 2013.

Theophylline + Tamsulosin

The concurrent use of tamsulosin and theophylline does not affect the pharmacokinetics of either drug.

Clinical evidence, mechanism, importance and management

In a study, 10 healthy subjects were given tamsulosin 400 micrograms daily for 2 days then 800 micrograms on the following 5 days, with a single 5-mg/kg dose of intravenous theophylline one hour after the last dose of tamsulosin. The pharmacokinetics of theophylline and tamsulosin were not affected by concurrent use.[1] The safety of concurrent use was considered acceptable and dose adjustments were not considered necessary.[1]

There appears to be no direct evidence regarding aminophylline, but as it is metabolised to theophylline, no adverse interaction would be expected with tamsulosin.

1. Miyazawa Y, Starkey LP, Forrest A, Schentag JJ, Kamimura H, Swarz H, Ito Y. Effects of the concomitant administration of tamsulosin (0.8 mg/day) on the pharmacokinetic and safety profile of theophylline (5 mg/kg): a placebo-controlled evaluation. *J Int Med Res* (2002) 30, 34–43.

Theophylline + Teicoplanin

The concurrent use of theophylline and teicoplanin does not affect the pharmacokinetics of either drug.

Clinical evidence, mechanism, importance and management

Clinical studies in 20 patients with COPD found that teicoplanin 200 mg twice daily and aminophylline 240 mg twice daily (both given as intravenous infusions) had no significant effect on the steady-state pharmacokinetics of either teicoplanin or theophylline (derived from aminophylline).[1] No dose adjustment of either drug is likely to be necessary on concurrent use.

1. Angrisani M, Cazzola M, Loffreda A, Losasso C, Lucarelli C, Rossi F. Clinical pharmacokinetics of teicoplanin and aminophylline during cotreatment with both medicaments. *Int J Clin Pharmacol Res* (1992) 12, 165–71.

Theophylline + Terbinafine

Terbinafine causes a negligible increase in the exposure to theophylline.

Clinical evidence, mechanism, importance and management

In a randomised, crossover study, 12 healthy subjects were given a single 5-mg/kg oral dose of theophylline before and after taking terbinafine 250 mg daily for 3 days. The AUC and half-life of theophylline were increased by 16% and 23%, respectively, and the theophylline clearance was reduced by 14%.[1] It was suggested that this is due to the inhibitory effect of terbinafine on the activity of CYP1A2, the main isoenzyme involved in the metabolism of theophylline.[1] The changes seen were negligible, but the study periods only lasted 3 days so that the effects of longer concurrent use are uncertain; nevertheless, a clinically significant interaction seems unlikely. There appears to be no direct evidence regarding aminophylline, but as it is metabolised to theophylline, no clinically relevant interaction would be expected.

1. Trépanier EF, Nafziger AN, Amsden GW. Effect of terbinafine on theophylline pharmacokinetics in healthy volunteers. *Antimicrob Agents Chemother* (1998) 42, 695–7.

Theophylline + Tetracyclines

Theophylline levels and/or clearance can be very slightly increased or very slightly decreased by doxycycline and tetracycline, although one case report described theophylline toxicity in a patient given tetracycline while taking theophylline. In another case report, minocycline appeared to increase theophylline levels.

Clinical evidence

(a) Doxycycline

A study in 10 patients with asthma given doxycycline 100 mg twice daily on day one and then 100 mg daily for 4 days found that the mean serum theophylline level was not significantly altered. However, there was large inter-individual variation, with 4 subjects having rises in theophylline levels of more than 20% (range 24 to 31%) and 2 having decreases of 22% and 33%.[1] However, fluctuations of this size are not unusual with theophylline. Another study in 8 healthy subjects given doxycycline 100 mg daily for 7 days with theophylline 350 mg twice daily did not find any statistically significant changes in theophylline pharmacokinetics.[2]

(b) Minocycline

The serum theophylline levels of a 70-year-old woman with normal liver function increased from 9.8 mg/L to 15.5 mg/L after she was given minocycline 100 mg twice daily by infusion for 6 days. Her serum theophylline level was 10.9 mg/L fourteen - days after the minocycline was stopped.[3]

(c) Tetracycline

A patient with COPD developed signs of theophylline toxicity after taking tetracycline 250 mg four times daily for 8 days. After 10 days of tetracycline her serum theophylline levels had risen from about 13 mg/L to 30.8 mg/L. Both drugs were stopped, and after 24 hours her theophylline level had reduced to 12.4 mg/L. A later rechallenge in this patient confirmed that the tetracycline was responsible for the raised theophylline levels.[4]

In an earlier study in 8 healthy subjects, tetracycline 250 mg four times daily for 7 days did not affect the mean pharmacokinetics of theophylline (given as a single intravenous dose of aminophylline), although there was large inter-individual variation. Four subjects had a decrease in clearance of over 15%, (32% in one subject), and conversely, one subject had a 21% increase in clearance.[5] Other studies in subjects and patients given tetracycline for shorter periods have not found evidence of a clinically relevant interaction. A study in 9 healthy adults given a single 5-mg/kg intravenous dose of aminophylline found that tetracycline 250 mg every 6 hours for 48 hours had no statistically significant effect on theophylline pharmacokinetics.[6] Five non-smoking patients with COPD or asthma had an average 14% rise in serum theophylline levels and an 11% decrease in its clearance after 5 days of treatment with tetracycline 250 mg four times daily. However, when a sixth patient was included (a smoker) the results were no longer statistically significant.[7]

Mechanism

Not understood. Inhibition of theophylline metabolism and clearance by the tetracyclines has been suggested.[4]

Importance and management

Information regarding an interaction between theophylline and the tetracyclines seems to be limited. Two isolated reports describe increased theophylline levels with minocycline and tetracycline; however, controlled studies with tetracycline and doxycycline have not found any clinically relevant changes in theophylline pharmacokinetics. It has been suggested that a clinically important interaction might possibly only occur in a few patients.[1,4] It would therefore seem prudent to bear this possibility in mind should any unexpected change in theophylline levels or adverse effects (headache, nausea, tremor) occur. There seems to be no evidence of adverse interactions with any of the other tetracyclines. There appears to be no direct evidence regarding aminophylline, but as it is metabolised to theophylline, it seems likely that it will be similarly affected by the tetracyclines.

Note that acute infections *per se* can alter theophylline pharmacokinetics.[8]

1. Seggev JS, Shefi M, Schey G, Farfel Z. Serum theophylline concentrations are not affected by coadministration of doxycycline. *Ann Allergy* (1986) 56, 156–7.
2. Jonkman JHG, van der Boon WJV, Schoenmaker R, Holtkamp A, Hempenius J. No influence of doxycycline on theophylline pharmacokinetics. *Ther Drug Monit* (1985) 7, 92–4.
3. Kawai M, Honda A, Yoshida H, Goto M, Shimokata T. Possible theophylline-minocycline interaction. *Ann Pharmacother* (1992) 26, 1300–1.
4. McCormack JP, Reid SE, Lawson LM. Theophylline toxicity induced by tetracycline. *Clin Pharm* (1990) 9, 546–9.
5. Mathis JW, Prince RA, Weinberger MM, McElnay JC. Effect of tetracycline hydrochloride on theophylline kinetics. *Clin Pharm* (1982) 1, 446–8.
6. Pfeifer HJ, Greenblatt DJ, Friedman P. Effects of three antibiotics on theophylline kinetics. *Clin Pharmacol Ther* (1979) 26, 36–40.
7. Gotz VP, Ryerson GG. Evaluation of tetracycline on theophylline disposition in patients with chronic obstructive airways disease. *Drug Intell Clin Pharm* (1986) 20, 694–7.
8. Renton KW. Cytochrome P450 regulation and drug biotransformation during inflammation and infection. *Curr Drug Metab* (2004) 5, 235–43.

Theophylline + Thyroid hormones and Antithyroid drugs

Thyroid dysfunction can modestly affect theophylline requirements. Isolated cases of theophylline toxicity have been reported in patients being treated for hypothyroidism.

Clinical evidence

The theophylline elimination rate constant after a single intravenous dose of aminophylline was found to be greater in hyperthyroid patients (0.155 h^{-1}) than in euthyroid (0.107 h^{-1}) or hypothyroid patients (0.060 h^{-1}); some other pharmacokinetic parameters were also changed.[1] The authors concluded that thyroid dysfunction might modestly alter theophylline requirements. It is therefore also likely that drug-induced changes in the thyroid status, such as those caused by amiodarone (see 'Thyroid hormones + Amiodarone', p.1523), could also alter the amount of theophylline needed to maintain therapeutic levels.

(a) Antithyroid compounds

The serum theophylline level of a patient with asthma was found to have doubled, from 15.2 mg/L to 30.9 mg/L, accompanied by toxicity, 3 months after treatment for hyperthyroidism with **radioactive iodine** (^{131}I). At this point the patient was hypothyroid, and after treatment with levothyroxine was started, his serum theophylline returned to approximately the same level as before radioactive iodine treatment (13.9 mg/L).[2] Another patient with Graves' disease, treated with a combination of **thiamazole (methimazole)** 10 mg three times daily and Lugol's solution (**iodine** and **potassium iodide**) and taking theophylline 500 mg twice daily (*TheoDur*), had a theophylline level of 4.7 mg/L before radioactive iodine therapy. His level increased to 13.6 mg/L seven months after thyroid ablation.[3] In 5 hyperthyroid patients the clearance of theophylline was reduced by 20% and its half-life was increased, from 4.6 hours to 5.9 hours, when they were given **carbimazole** 45 mg and propranolol 60 mg daily. In this study, a single intravenous dose of aminophylline was given before the treatment of thyrotoxicosis and after the euthyroid state had been achieved.[4] Note that propranolol has been reported to reduce the clearance of theophylline but should generally be avoided in patients with respiratory disease; see 'Theophylline + Beta blockers', p.1438, for more information.

(b) Thyroid hormones

One week after starting to take theophylline 1 g daily, a patient who was hypothyroid (serum thyroxine 1.4 micrograms/dL, reference range 4 to 11 micrograms/dL) developed severe theophylline toxicity, manifested by ventricular fibrillation (from which he was successfully resuscitated) and repeated seizures over 24 hours. His serum theophylline level was 34.7 mg/L. After 2 months of treatment with thyroid hormones, which increased his serum thyroxine levels to 4.3 micrograms/dL, his serum theophylline level was 13.2 mg/L, 10 days after reinstitution of the same dose of theophylline.[5]

Mechanism

Thyroid status may affect the rate at which theophylline is metabolised: in hyperthyroidism theophylline metabolism is increased, whereas in hypothyroidism it is decreased.

Importance and management

It is established that changes in thyroid status may affect how the body handles theophylline (including that derived from aminophylline). Monitor the effects and anticipate the possible need to begin to reduce the theophylline dose if treatment for hyperthyroidism is started (e.g. with radioactive iodine, carbimazole, thiamazole, **propylthiouracil**, etc.). Similarly, anticipate the possible need to increase the theophylline dose if treatment is started for hypothyroidism (e.g. with levothyroxine). Stabilisation of the thyroid status may take weeks or even months to achieve so that if monitoring of the theophylline dose is considered necessary, it will need to extend over the whole of this period. This monitoring would also apply to drug-induced thyroid dysfunction.

1. Pokrajac M, Simić D, Varagić VM. Pharmacokinetics of theophylline in hyperthyroid and hypothyroid patients with chronic obstructive pulmonary disease. *Eur J Clin Pharmacol* (1987) 33, 483–6.
2. Johnson CE, Cohen IA. Theophylline toxicity after iodine 131 treatment for hyperthyroidism. *Clin Pharm* (1988) 7, 620–2.
3. Bauman JH, Teichman S, Wible DA. Increased theophylline clearance in a patient with hyperthyroidism. *Ann Allergy* (1984) 52, 94–6.
4. Vozeh S, Otten M, Staub J-J, Follath F. Influence of thyroid function on theophylline kinetics. *Clin Pharmacol Ther* (1984) 36, 634–40.
5. Aderka D, Shavit G, Garfinkel D, Santo M, Gitter S, Pinkhas J. Life-threatening theophylline intoxication in a hypothyroidic patient. *Respiration* (1983) 44, 77–80.

Theophylline + Tobacco

Tobacco smokers, and non-smokers heavily exposed to tobacco smoke, may need more theophylline than non-smokers to achieve the same therapeutic benefits, because the theophylline is cleared more quickly. This may also occur in those who chew tobacco or take snuff but not if they chew nicotine gum.

Clinical evidence

A study found that the mean half-life of theophylline (given as a single oral dose of aminophylline) was 4.3 hours in a group of tobacco smokers (20 to 40 cigarettes daily) compared with 7 hours in a group of non-smokers, and that theophylline clearance was higher (mean increase 126%) and more variable in the smokers.[1] Almost identical results were found in an earlier study,[2] and a number of later studies in subjects given oral or intravenous theophylline or aminophylline confirm these findings.[3-8] The ability of smoking to increase theophylline clearance occurs irrespective of gender,[3,6] and in the presence of congestive heart failure or liver impairment.[7] The effects of ageing on the induction of theophylline metabolism by tobacco smoking is less clear. One study has found that in both young subjects (less than 30 years old) and elderly subjects (more than 67 years old) smoking decreased the half-life and increased the clearance of theophylline, when compared with non-smokers. The effect was greater in the young subjects.[4] However, another study found no difference in the pharmacokinetics of theophylline between asthmatic and otherwise healthy smokers and non-smokers aged over 65 years.[9] A similar high clearance of theophylline (given as intravenous aminophylline) has been seen in a patient who chewed tobacco (1.11 mL/kg per minute compared with the more usual 0.59 mL/kg per minute).[10] The half-life of theophylline (given as intravenous aminophylline) in passive smokers (non-smokers regularly exposed to tobacco smoke in the air they breathe, for 4 hours a day in this study) is reported to be shorter than in non-smokers (6.93 hours compared with 8.69 hours).[11] The clearance of theophylline (given as intravenous aminophylline) in asthmatic children exposed to passive tobacco smoke was also found to be greater (1.36 mL/kg per minute compared with 0.09 mL/kg per minute) and their steady-state serum theophylline levels were lower than in similar children not exposed to passive smoking.[12]

In one study, 3 of 4 patients who stopped smoking for 3 months (confirmed by serum thiocyanate levels) had a longer theophylline half-life, but only 2 had a slight decrease in theophylline clearance.[1] In another study, ex-smokers who had stopped heavy smoking 2 years previously had values for theophylline clearance and half-life that were intermediate between non-smokers and current heavy smokers.[3] In another study, 7 hospitalised smokers who abstained from smoking for 7 days had a 36% increase in theophylline half-life and a 38% decrease in clearance (although clearance after abstinence was still higher than values usually found in non-smokers).[13]

Mechanism

Tobacco smoke contains polycyclic hydrocarbons, which act as inducers of CYP1A2, and this results in a more rapid clearance of theophylline. Both the *N*-demethylation and 8-hydroxylation of theophylline (both of which are mediated by CYP1A2) are induced.[14] Ageing appears to offset the effects of smoking on theophylline metabolism.[9]

Importance and management

An established interaction of clinical importance. Heavy smokers (20 to 40 cigarettes daily) may need a much greater aminophylline or theophylline dose than non-smokers,[1] and increased doses are likely for those who chew tobacco or take snuff,[10] but not for those who chew nicotine gum.[13,15] In patients who stop smoking, a reduction in the theophylline dose of up to 25 to 33% may be needed after one week,[13] but full normalisation of hepatic function appears to take many months or even years.[1,3] Investigators of the possible interactions of aminophylline and theophylline with other drugs should take smoking habits into account when selecting their subjects.[6,11,12] Note that the effects of cannabis (see 'Theophylline + Cannabis', p.1440), may be additive with those of tobacco smoking.

1. Hunt SN, Jusko WJ, Yurchak AM. Effect of smoking on theophylline disposition. *Clin Pharmacol Ther* (1976) 19, 546–51.
2. Jenne J, Nagasawa H, McHugh R, MacDonald F, Wyse E. Decreased theophylline half-life in cigarette smokers. *Life Sci* (1975) 17, 195–8.
3. Powell JR, Thiercelin J-F, Vozeh S, Sansom L, Riegelman S. The influence of cigarette smoking and sex on theophylline disposition. *Am Rev Respir Dis* (1977) 116, 17–23.
4. Cusack B, Kelly JG, Lavan J, Noel J, O'Malley K. Theophylline kinetics in relation to age: the importance of smoking. *Br J Clin Pharmacol* (1980) 10, 109–14.
5. Jusko WJ, Schentag JJ, Clark JH, Gardner M, Yurchak AM. Enhanced biotransformation of theophylline in marihuana and tobacco smokers. *Clin Pharmacol Ther* (1978) 24, 406–10.
6. Jennings TS, Nafziger AN, Davidson L, Bertino JS. Gender differences in hepatic induction and inhibition of theophylline pharmacokinetics and metabolism. *J Lab Clin Med* (1993) 122, 208–16.
7. Harralson AF, Kehoe WA, Chen J-D. The effect of smoking on theophylline disposition in patients with hepatic disease and congestive heart failure. *J Clin Pharmacol* (1996) 36, 862.
8. Gardner MJ, Tornatore KM, Jusko WJ, Kanarkowski R. Effects of tobacco smoking and oral contraceptive use on theophylline disposition. *Br J Clin Pharmacol* (1983) 16, 271–80.
9. Samaan S, Fox R. The effect of smoking on theophylline kinetics in healthy and asthmatic elderly males. *J Clin Pharmacol* (1989) 29, 448–50.
10. Rockwood R, Henann N. Smokeless tobacco and theophylline clearance. *Drug Intell Clin Pharm* (1986) 20, 624–5.
11. Matsunga SK, Plezia PM, Karol MD, Katz MD, Camilli AE, Benowitz NL. Effects of passive smoking on theophylline clearance. *Clin Pharmacol Ther* (1989) 46, 399–407.
12. Mayo PR. Effect of passive smoking on theophylline clearance in children. *Ther Drug Monit* (2001) 23, 503–5.
13. Lee BL, Benowitz NL, Jacob P. Cigarette abstinence, nicotine gum, and theophylline disposition. *Ann Intern Med* (1987) 106, 553–5.
14. Grygiel J, Birkett DJ. Cigarette smoking and theophylline clearance and metabolism. *Clin Pharmacol Ther* (1981) 30, 491–6.
15. Benowitz NL, Lee BL, Jacob P. Nicotine gum and theophylline metabolism. *Biomed Pharmacother* (1989) 43, 1–3.

Theophylline + Trimetazidine

Trimetazidine does not appear to alter the pharmacokinetics of theophylline.

Clinical evidence, mechanism, importance and management

In a study in 13 healthy subjects, trimetazidine 20 mg twice daily, taken for at least 14 days, did not alter the pharmacokinetics of a single 375-mg dose of theophylline.[1]

These results suggest that no theophylline dose adjustment is likely to be needed in patients given trimetazidine, but this needs confirmation in multiple-dose studies.

There appears to be no direct evidence regarding aminophylline, but as it is metabolised to theophylline, a similar lack of adverse interaction with trimetazidine would be expected.

1. Edeki TI, Johnston A, Campbell DB, Ings RMJ, Brownsill R, Genissel P, Turner P. An examination of the possible pharmacokinetic interaction of trimetazidine with theophylline, digoxin and antipyrine. *Br J Clin Pharmacol* (1989) 26, 657P.

Theophylline + Vidarabine

An isolated case report describes a woman taking aminophylline who had a rise in her theophylline levels when she started to take vidarabine.

Clinical evidence, mechanism, importance and management

A woman taking aminophylline oral liquid developed elevated serum theophylline levels (an increase from 14 mg/L to 24 mg/L) four days after starting to take vidarabine 400 mg daily for herpes zoster. She was also being treated with ampicillin, gentamicin, clindamycin and digoxin, for congestive heart failure, chronic pulmonary disease and suspected sepsis.[1] It was suggested that hypoxanthine arabinoside, the principal metabolite of vidarabine, raised theophylline levels by competing for metabolism by xanthine oxidase. The general significance of this case is uncertain. Until more is known, it would seem prudent to bear this interaction in mind if a patient taking aminophylline or theophylline develops theophylline adverse effects (nausea, headache, and tremor) when given vidarabine. If this occurs, monitor theophylline levels and adjust the dose accordingly.

1. Gannon R, Sullman S, Levy RM, Grober J. Possible interaction between vidarabine and theophylline. *Ann Intern Med* (1984) 101, 148–9.

Theophylline + Zileuton

Zileuton increases the exposure to theophylline and increases the incidence of adverse effects.

Clinical evidence

In a placebo-controlled study, 13 healthy subjects were given 200 mg of theophylline (*Slo-Phyllin*) four times daily for 5 days with zileuton 800 mg twice daily. Zileuton increased the mean steady-state peak serum levels of theophylline by 73% (from 12 mg/L to 21 mg/L), increased its AUC by 92%, and halved its apparent plasma clearance. During the use of zileuton the incidence of adverse effects (headache, gastrointestinal effects) increased, which was attributed to theophylline toxicity: this caused 3 of the original 16 subjects to withdraw from the study.[1]

Mechanism

Zileuton appears to inhibit the metabolism of theophylline by CYP1A2 in the liver, resulting in an increase in theophylline exposure.

Importance and management

Information is limited but an interaction between theophylline and zileuton appears to be established and of clinical importance. Concurrent use need not be avoided but be alert for theophylline adverse effects (headache, nausea, tremor), and if required, monitor theophylline levels and reduce the dose of theophylline as necessary. The report cited above suggests that a typical asthma patient might initially need the theophylline dose to be halved, and this dose reduction is recommended by the US manufacturers.[2] Similarly, the initial dose of theophylline should be reduced if it is given to a patient already taking zileuton, and adjusted according to theophylline levels.[2] This is based on the results of a study in over 1000 patients taking zileuton 600 mg four times daily without apparent problems when this course of action was followed.[1] There appears to be no direct evidence regarding aminophylline, but as it is metabolised to theophylline, it seems likely that it will be similarly affected by zileuton.

1. Granneman GR, Braeckman RA, Locke CS, Cavanaugh JH, Dubé LM, Awni WM. Effect of zileuton on theophylline pharmacokinetics. *Clin Pharmacokinet* (1995) 29 (Suppl 2), 77–83.
2. Zyflo CR (Zileuton). Cornerstone Therapeutics Inc. US Prescribing information, November 2011.

Umeclidinium + Verapamil

Verapamil slightly increases the exposure to inhaled umeclidinium.

Clinical evidence, mechanism, importance and management

In a randomised study in 16 healthy subjects, oral verapamil 240 mg daily for 5 days had no effect on the maximum concentration of inhaled umeclidinium 500 micrograms daily, but did increase the AUC by 39%. A similar effect was seen in another group of patients given the same dose of verapamil with inhaled umeclidinium and vilanterol in a combination preparation.[1] Umeclidinium is a substrate for P-glycoprotein, which is inhibited by verapamil. The slight increase in exposure to umeclidinium is unlikely to be clinically relevant and therefore no dose adjustment would seem necessary on concurrent use with verapamil or other P-glycoprotein inhibitors. See 'Table 1.12', p.14 for a list of clinically relevant P-glycoprotein inhibitors.

1. Mehta R, Kelleher D, Preece A, Hughes S, Crater G. Effect of verapamil on systemic exposure and safety of umeclidinium and vilanterol: a randomized and open-label study. *Int J Chron Obstruct Pulmon Dis* (2013) 8, 159–67.

35

SSRIs, Tricyclics and related antidepressants

The development of the tricyclic antidepressants arose out of work carried out on phenothiazine compounds related to chlorpromazine. The earlier molecules possessed two benzene rings joined by a third ring of carbon atoms, with sometimes a nitrogen, and had antidepressant activity, hence their name. Some of the later antidepressants have one, two or even four rings. 'Table 35.1', below, lists the common tricyclic and tetracyclic antidepressants, the selective serotonin reuptake inhibitors (SSRIs), the serotonin and noradrenaline reuptake inhibitors (SNRIs), and a number of other drugs that are also used for depression. For interactions involving MAOIs (monoamine oxidase inhibitors), see 'MAOIs', p.1382.

Many of the antidepressants are either inhibitors or substrates of CYP2D6. Interactions via CYP2D6 are complicated by genetic polymorphism with some individuals having little or no activity of this isoenzyme (poor metabolisers). See 'Genetic factors in drug metabolism', p.8, for further information.

Table 35.1 SSRIs, Tricyclics and related antidepressants

Group	*Drugs*
SNRIs (Serotonin and noradrenaline reuptake inhibitors)	Desvenlafaxine, Duloxetine, Levomilnacipran, Milnacipran, Venlafaxine
SSRIs (Selective serotonin reuptake inhibitors)	Citalopram, Escitalopram, Fluoxetine, Fluvoxamine, Paroxetine, Sertraline, Vilazodone
Tetracyclic antidepressants	Maprotiline, Mianserin
Tricyclic antidepressants	Amineptine, Amitriptyline, Amoxapine, Butriptyline, Clomipramine, Desipramine, Dibenzepin, Dosulepin, Doxepin, Imipramine, Lofepramine, Melitracen, Nortriptyline, Opipramol, Protriptyline, Trimipramine
Other antidepressants	Agomelatine, Iprindole, Mirtazapine, Nefazodone, Reboxetine, Trazodone, Viloxazine, Vortioxetine

SNRIs

Antidepressants in this group include desvenlafaxine (the major active metabolite of venlafaxine), duloxetine, levomilnacipran (an enantiomer of milnacipran), milnacipran, and venlafaxine. They inhibit both serotonin and noradrenaline reuptake but with differing selectivity. Milnacipran blocks serotonin and noradrenaline reuptake approximately equally, but duloxetine and to a greater extent venlafaxine have selectivity for serotonin and so might be expected to share the pharmacodynamic interactions of the SSRIs, see below. Duloxetine and venlafaxine are reported to weakly inhibit dopamine reuptake. They are also reported to have no appreciable affinity for histaminergic, muscarinic, or adrenergic receptors and, compared with the tricyclics, appear to lack troublesome sedative and antimuscarinic effects.

Duloxetine is a moderate inhibitor of CYP2D6 and is a substrate for CYP1A2 and so can interact with drugs that affect these isoenzymes. Venlafaxine, a CYP2D6 substrate, can interact with CYP2D6 inhibitors and to a more minor extent with CYP3A4 inhibitors. In contrast desvenlafaxine is not metabolised by CYP2D6, though CYP3A4 is involved to a minor extent. Milnacipran, however, does not appear to interact with cytochrome P450 isoenzymes, whereas levomilnacipran is affected by potent CYP3A4 inhibitors.

SSRIs

These antidepressants act on neurones in a similar way to the tricyclics (see below) but they selectively inhibit the reuptake of serotonin (5-hydroxytryptamine or 5-HT). This can lead to adverse effects such as serotonin syndrome, see 'Drugs that cause serotonin syndrome + Other drugs that cause serotonin syndrome', p.1471. The SSRIs have fewer antimuscarinic effects than the tricyclics and are also less sedative and cardiotoxic. However, they have been associated with bleeding disorders and so caution is advised if they are given with drugs known to affect platelet function.

SSRIs interact with other drugs mainly as a result of their inhibitory activity on cytochrome P450 isoenzymes in the liver; fluoxetine and paroxetine are potent inhibitors of CYP2D6, and fluvoxamine inhibits CYP1A2 and CYP2C19, but citalopram and sertraline are less likely to have any clinical effect, see 'Table 35.2', p.1465. Note that some SSRIs, such as fluoxetine, have a very long half-life and so interactions can still occur after the drug has been discontinued

Tricyclic and related antidepressants

The tricyclic antidepressants inhibit the activity of the 'uptake' mechanism by which some chemical transmitters (serotonin (5-HT) or noradrenaline (norepinephrine)) re-enter nerve endings in the CNS. In this way they increase the concentrations of the chemical transmitter in the receptor area. If depression represents some inadequacy in transmission between the nerves in the brain, increasing the amount of transmitter might go some way towards reversing this by improving transmission. Tricyclics vary in the extent that they block the reuptake of these transmitters, for example clomipramine is more selective for serotonergic transmission and imipramine is more selective for noradrenergic transmission. However, the use of all tricyclics should generally be avoided with MAOIs because of the risk of the serotonin syndrome, see 'MAOIs or RIMAs + Tricyclic and related antidepressants', p.1403.

The tricyclics also have varying degrees of antimuscarinic (sometimes referred to as anticholinergic or atropine-like) activity and can cause dry mouth, blurred vision, constipation, urinary retention, and an increase in ocular pressure. They might also cause postural hypotension, sedation, and seizures in certain individuals.

Mianserin and maprotiline are tetracyclic antidepressants, which have actions similar to those of the tricyclic antidepressants. However, while the tetracyclics are more sedating, their antimuscarinic effects are less marked. Maprotiline inhibits the reuptake of noradrenaline (norepinephrine) and has weak affinity for central adrenergic (α_1) receptors. Mianserin does not prevent the peripheral reuptake of noradrenaline; it blocks presynaptic adrenergic (α_2) receptors and increases the turnover of brain noradrenaline. It is also an antagonist of serotonin receptors in some parts of the brain.

All tricyclic antidepressants, mianserin and maprotiline are metabolised by CYP2D6 to some extent and so might be affected by inhibitors of this isoenzyme. See 'Table 35.2', p.1465, for more detail on the metabolism of individual tricyclics.

Other antidepressant drugs

(a) Agomelatine

Agomelatine is a melatonin receptor agonist at MT_1 and MT_2 receptors, and a serotonin receptor antagonist at $5\text{-}HT_{2C}$ receptors, but does not affect monoamine uptake. Agomelatine does not appear to induce or inhibit cytochrome P450 isoenzymes, however it is metabolised primarily by CYP1A2 and can interact with drugs which inhibit, or induce this isoenzyme.

(b) Mirtazapine

Mirtazapine is a piperazinoazepine and an analogue of mianserin. It is a presynaptic adrenergic α_2-antagonist that increases central noradrenergic and serotonergic transmission. It is a potent inhibitor of histamine (H_1) receptors and this accounts for its sedative properties. It has little antimuscarinic activity.

(c) Nefazodone and Trazodone

Nefazodone is a phenylpiperazine structurally related to trazodone. Both nefazodone and trazodone block the reuptake of serotonin at presynaptic neurones and block α_1-adrenoceptors, but have no apparent effect on dopamine. Unlike trazodone, nefazodone blocks the reuptake of noradrenaline. Compared to the tricyclics, neither drug has notable antimuscarinic effects, but trazodone has marked sedative properties.

Trazodone is a substrate for CYP3A4 and its plasma concentrations might be affected by inhibitors or inducers of this isoenzyme. Nefazodone is an inhibitor of CYP3A4 and therefore it will inhibit the metabolism of drugs by this route. For a list of CYP3A4 substrates, see 'Table 1.10', p.12. Note that, nefazodone has largely been withdrawn due to adverse hepatic effects.

(d) Reboxetine

Reboxetine is a potent inhibitor of noradrenaline reuptake. It has a weak effect on serotonin reuptake and no notable affinity for muscarinic receptors. Reboxetine is a substrate for CYP3A4 and its plasma concentrations can be increased by inhibitors of this isoenzyme.

(e) Vortioxetine

Vortioxetine is an inhibitor of serotonin reuptake and also acts as a serotonin antagonist at 5-HT_3 receptors, and as a serotonin agonist at 5-HT_{1A} receptors. Extensively metabolised by cytochrome P450 isoenzymes, vortioxetine is primarily metabolised by CYP2D6 and its plasma concentrations can be affected by inhibitors or inducers of this isoenzyme.

Table 35.2 Summary of the main effects of antidepressant drugs with cytochrome P450 isoenzymes

Antidepressant drug		*Isoenzyme*			
		Substrate (demonstrated clinically)	Substrate (theoretical)	Inhibits (demonstrated clinically)	Inhibits (theoretical)
Agomelatine		CYP1A2			
Bupropion		CYP2B6		CYP2D6 (potent)	
Mirtazapine			CYP1A2, CYP2D6, CYP3A4		
Nefazodone				CYP3A4 (moderate to potent)	
Reboxetine		CYP3A4			
Trazodone		CYP3A4			
Vortioxetine		CYP2D6	CYP2A6, CYP2B6, CYP2C8, CYP2C9, CYP2C19, CYP3A4		
SNRIs	**Desvenlafaxine**		CYP3A4	CYP2D6 (weak - at a dose of 400 mg)	
SNRIs	**Duloxetine**	CYP1A2, CYP2D6		CYP2D6 (moderate)	
SNRIs	**Levomilnacipran**	CYP3A4	CYP2C8, CYP2C19, CYP2D6		
SNRIs	**Milnacipran**	None			
SNRIs	**Venlafaxine**	CYP2D6	CYP3A4		
SSRIs	**Citalopram**	CYP2C19	CYP2D6, CYP3A4	CYP2D6 (weak)	
SSRIs	**Escitalopram**			CYP2D6 (weak)	
SSRIs	**Fluoxetine**		CYP2D6	CYP2D6 (moderate to potent)	CYP2C9, CYP3A4 (weak)
SSRIs	**Fluvoxamine**		CYP2D6; other metabolic pathways also appear to be involved	CYP1A2 (potent), CYP2C19 (potent), CYP3A4 (weak)	CYP2C9 (weak)
SSRIs	**Paroxetine**		CYP2D6	CYP2D6 (potent)	
SSRIs	**Sertraline**		CYP3A4, CYP2D6 (minor) and possibly other pathways	CYP2D6 (weak)	
SSRIs	**Vilazodone**	CYP3A4			CYP2C8
Tetracyclics	**Maprotiline**		CYP2D6		
Tetracyclics	**Mianserin**		CYP2D6		
Tricyclics	**Amitriptyline**	CYP1A2, CYP2D6	CYP3A4, CYP2C19		
Tricyclics	**Clomipramine**	CYP2D6, CYP1A2	CYP3A4, CYP2C19		
Tricyclics	**Desipramine**	CYP2D6			
Tricyclics	**Dosulepin**		CYP2D6 and possibly other pathways		
Tricyclics	**Doxepin**		CYP2D6, CYP1A2 (minor), CYP3A4 (minor)		
Tricyclics	**Imipramine**	CYP1A2, CYP2D6	CYP3A4, CYP2C19		
Tricyclics	**Nortriptyline**	CYP2D6			
Tricyclics	**Trimipramine**	CYP2D6	Possibly other pathways		

Agomelatine + Duloxetine

A report describes akathisia in a patient taking duloxetine after agomelatine was added.

Clinical evidence, mechanism, importance and management

A case report describes the development of akathisia in a 29-year-old woman taking duloxetine 120 mg daily. Symptoms began 3 days after trazodone 200 mg (which had failed to improve sleep quality) was switched to agomelatine 25 mg [daily]. The patient had unpleasant sensations in her legs, inner restlessness, and a constant urge to move, which grew worse at night. After 1 week the dose of agomelatine was increased to 50 mg [daily], and the following day the restlessness increased dramatically, so the agomelatine was stopped. Her symptoms resolved over the next 3 days, although some restlessness was reported by the patient until discharge. The authors suggest that noradrenergic overstimulation due to concurrent use of duloxetine and agomelatine was a possible cause of the akathisia.[1] The general clinical relevance of this case is unclear.

1. Imboden C, Hatzinger M. Agomelatine-induced akathisia with concomitant duloxetine medication: a case report. *Pharmacopsychiatry* (2012) 45, 162–3.

Agomelatine + Miscellaneous

Fluvoxamine appears to very markedly increase the exposure to agomelatine; other potent inhibitors of CYP1A2 are predicted to interact similarly. Oestrogens appear to increase the exposure to agomelatine, and other moderate inhibitors of CYP1A2 are predicted to interact similarly. Tobacco smoking appears to reduce the exposure to agomelatine. Rifampicin is predicted to reduce the exposure to agomelatine. Food does not appear to affect the pharmacokinetics of agomelatine.

Clinical evidence, mechanism, importance and management

(a) CYP1A2 inducers and inhibitors

The UK manufacturer of agomelatine notes that in a study, **fluvoxamine** (dose not specified) increased the exposure to agomelatine (dose not specified) 60-fold.[1] Agomelatine is metabolised primarily by CYP1A2, and **fluvoxamine** is a potent inhibitor of CYP1A2 meaning that it very markedly increases exposure to agomelatine. The manufacturer therefore contraindicates the concurrent use of potent CYP1A2 inhibitors with agomelatine,[1] see 'Table 1.2', p.5 for a list. Note that they additionally name **ciprofloxacin**, but this is generally considered a moderate inhibitor of CYP1A2.

The UK manufacturer also notes that in 800 patients who received agomelatine and **oestrogens** (unspecified), the exposure to agomelatine was increased several fold.[1] Oestrogens appear to be CYP1A2 inhibitors, and therefore have the potential to increase agomelatine exposure, as seen in these patients. While no specific concern was raised, the manufacturer advises caution when moderate CYP1A2 inhibitors are taken with agomelatine,[1] see 'Table 1.2', p.5 for a list. Note that they additionally name **propranolol**, but it is not known to be a clinically relevant inhibitor of CYP1A2.

Further, **tobacco smoke** is a known inducer of CYP1A2 and the UK manufacturer of agomelatine briefly notes that smoking, especially heavy smoking (15 or more cigarettes daily) decreased the exposure to agomelatine.[1] No specific advice is given and the effects of other CYP1A2 inducers do not appear to have been studied, although they might be expected to decrease agomelatine exposure. See 'Table 1.2', p.5 for a list of CYP1A2 inducers.

(b) CYP2C9 and CYP2C19 inducers and inhibitors

CYP2C9 and CYP2C19 are involved in the metabolism of agomelatine, albeit to a limited extent, but the UK manufacturer[1] advises that the effect of **fluvoxamine** on agomelatine exposure (see under *CYP12A inducers and inhibitors* above) might also be due, in part, to its inhibitory effect on CYP2C9; fluvoxamine is a weak inhibitor of CYP2C9. They also note that **rifampicin** induces both of these isoenzymes and might therefore decrease agomelatine exposure.

(c) Food

The UK manufacturer of agomelatine briefly notes that the rate of absorption and the bioavailability of agomelatine are not altered by a standard or high-fat meal. They therefore advise that agomelatine can be taken with or without food.[1]

1. Valdoxan (Agomelatine). Servier Laboratories Ltd. UK Summary of Product Characteristics, June 2014.

Antidepressants + Methylthioninium chloride (Methylene blue)

Numerous case reports and two retrospective studies describe serotonergic symptoms in patients given methylthioninium chloride who were also taking a serotonergic antidepressant.

Clinical evidence

In 2009, the MHRA issued a drug safety update on the potential CNS toxicity of methylthioninium chloride when it is used in association with serotonergic drugs. This was based on 33 cases of CNS toxicity after the use of methylthioninium chloride: 28 of these are reported in the literature and 5 have been reported directly to the MHRA. In 32 of these cases, a serotonergic drug (such as an **SSRI**, **clomipramine**, or **venlafaxine**) had also been taken. In all but one patient, methylthioninium chloride was used as a visualising agent in thyroid or parathyroid surgery. In the other patient it was used to manage uncontrolled hypotension during cardiac surgery.[1] In 2011 the FDA issued a similar communication, based on similar reports to its adverse event reporting system.[2]

A systematic review of the Medline database (from 1950 to September 2008) and PsychInfo a database of psychology literature, (from 1960 to September 2008) for reports of acute confusional state, neuropsychiatric complications or autonomic instability [suggestive of serotonin syndrome], after the use of methylthioninium chloride, identified 26 of the 28 patients cited by the MHRA. All but one of these patients had taken a serotonergic drug and for all of these patients, the authors concluded that serotonin syndrome was a possible diagnosis. The antidepressants involved were **bupropion**, **clomipramine**, **mirtazapine**, **venlafaxine**, and the SSRIs, **citalopram**, **escitalopram**, **fluoxetine**, and **paroxetine**.[3] Note, that this review also included 2 retrospective case series that described a total of 325 patients who had been given methylthioninium chloride during parathyroid surgery. Of these 325 patients, 17 of the 45 patients taking a serotonergic drug had a reaction, compared with no reactions in the 280 patients who were not taking a serotonergic drug.

Further case reports describe serotonin toxicity in patients taking **clomipramine**,[4] **duloxetine**,[5] **paroxetine**,[6] and **venlafaxine**,[7] after they were given methylthioninium chloride during parathyroid surgery, which in one case proved fatal.[7] Other reports describe serotonin syndrome in patients taking **escitalopram** and **trazadone**,[8] and **paroxetine**,[9] and given methylthioninium chloride during cardiac and pelvic surgery, respectively. In the latter case, just 1 mg/kg of methylthioninum chloride was given.[9]

Mechanism

Not fully understood. Direct toxicity from methylthioninium chloride has been suggested, but is felt to be an unlikely explanation.[3] A more favoured explanation is that the concurrent use of methylthioninium chloride with a serotonergic drug (such as an SSRI, SNRI, or some tricyclic and related antidepressants) could lead to an excess of serotonin, either because methylthioninium chloride inhibits MAO-A (which is involved in the metabolism of serotonin),[10] or because *in vitro*, methylthioninium chloride inhibited the function of the serotonin reuptake transporter.[11] Excessive serotonin can result in symptoms of serotonin syndrome.

Importance and management

Evidence for an interaction between serotonergic antidepressants and methylthioninium chloride is from a relatively small number of cases; however, an interaction would seem to be established, the outcome of which is potentially serious. The MHRA therefore advises that methylthioninium chloride should be avoided in patients taking drugs that enhance serotonergic transmission, and they specifically name the SSRIs, clomipramine, and venlafaxine. They state that if concurrent use is necessary, the lowest possible dose of methylthioninium chloride should be given and the patient closely monitored for signs of CNS toxicity for up to 4 hours after administration.[1] However this advice has been contested in one report which suggests that methylthioninium chloride at doses as low as 1 mg/kg might be sufficient to inhibit MAO-A.[12] One case report describing serotonin syndrome at this dose[9] provides some support for this suggestion.

In contrast, the FDA advises that if methylthioninium chloride is to be given, serotonergic drugs should be stopped at least 2 weeks before (5 weeks for fluoxetine). In an emergency situation, they advise that the benefit of methylthioninium chloride be weighed against the risk of serotonin toxicity, and if no alternative is available, the serotonergic drug should be stopped if methylthioninium chloride is to be used. The patient should then be closely monitored for symptoms of CNS toxicity for 2 weeks (5 weeks for fluoxetine), or until 24 hours after the last methylthioninium chloride dose (whichever is first). They also advise that treatment with serotonergic drugs should not be started or resumed until 24 hours after the last dose of methylthioninium chloride.[2] For a list of serotonergic drugs, see 'Table 35.3', p.1472, and for more information on serotonin syndrome and its management, see 'Drugs that cause serotonin syndrome + Other drugs that cause serotonin syndrome', p.1471.

1. Medicines and Healthcare Products Regulatory Agency and the Commission on Human Medicines. Methylthioninium chloride (methylene blue): update on CNS toxicity with serotonergic drugs. *Drug Safety Update* (2009) 2, 3. Available at: http://webarchive.nationalarchives.gov.uk/20141205150130/http://www.mhra.gov.uk/home/groups/pl-p/documents/publication/con043810.pdf (accessed 02/09/15).
2. FDA. Drug Safety Communication: Serious CNS reactions possible when methylene blue is given to patients taking certain psychiatric medications. July 26, 2011. Available at: http://www.fda.gov/Drugs/DrugSafety/ucm263190.htm (accessed 02/09/15).
3. Ng BKW, Cameron AJD. The role of methylene blue in serotonin syndrome: a systematic review. *Psychosomatics* (2010) 51, 194–200.
4. Héritier Barras AC, Walder B, Seeck M. Serotonin syndrome following methylene blue infusion: a rare complication of antidepressant therapy. *J Neurol Neurosurg Psychiatry* (2010) 81, 1412–13.
5. Rowley M, Riutort K, Shapiro D, Casler J, Festic E, Freeman WD. Methylene blue-associated serotonin syndrome: a 'green' encephalopathy after parathyroidectomy. *Neurocrit Care* (2009) 11, 88–93.
6. Stanford SC, Stanford BJ, Gillman PK. Risk of severe serotonin toxicity following co-administration of methylene blue and serotonin reuptake inhibitors: an update on a case report of post-operative delirium. *J Psychopharmacol* (2010) 24, 1433–8.
7. Top WM, Gillman PK, de Langen CJ, Kooy A. Fatal methylene blue associated serotonin toxicity. *Neth J Med* (2014) 72, 179–81.
8. Grubb KJ, Kennedy JL, Bergin JD, Groves DS, Kern JA. The role of methylene blue in serotonin syndrome following cardiac transplantation: a case report and review of the literature. *J Thorac Cardiovasc Surg* (2012) 144, e113–6.
9. Schwiebert C, Irving C, Gillman PK. Small doses of methylene blue, previously considered safe, can precipitate serotonin toxicity. *Anaesthesia* (2009) 64, 924.
10. Ramsay RR, Dunford C, Gillman PK. Methylene blue and serotonin toxicity: inhibition of monoamine oxidase A (MAO A) confirms a theoretical prediction. *Br J Pharmacol* (2007) 152, 946–51.
11. Oz M, Isaev D, Lorke DE, Hasan M, Petroianu G, Shippenberg TS. Methylene blue inhibits function of the 5-HT transporter. *Br J Pharmacol* (2012) 166, 168–76.
12. Gillman PK. CNS toxicity involving methylene blue: the exemplar for understanding and predicting drug interactions that precipitate serotonin toxicity. *J Psychopharmacol* (2011) 25, 429–36.

Bupropion + Antiepileptics; Enzyme-inducing

Carbamazepine causes a large decrease in the exposure to bupropion and increases the exposure to its active metabolite hydroxybupropion. Phenobarbital (and therefore probably primidone) and phenytoin (and therefore fosphenytoin) would be expected to interact similarly.

Clinical evidence

In a study in 12 patients with major affective disorders, **carbamazepine** at steady-state decreased the maximum concentration and AUC of a single 150-mg dose of bupropion by 87% and 90%, respectively, when compared with placebo. The AUC and maximum concentration of the major active metabolite, hydroxybupropion, were increased by 50% and 71%, respectively.[1] Two patients with bipolar illness who received bupropion at a variety of doses (450 to 600 mg daily and 400 to 525 mg daily) had undetectable bupropion plasma concentrations while taking **carbamazepine** but their hydroxybupropion concentrations were greatly increased.[2]

Mechanism

Bupropion is metabolised to its major active metabolite, hydroxybupropion, primarily by CYP2B6. The decrease in bupropion, and increase in hydroxybupropion, exposure seen in the study, would therefore suggest the induction of CYP2B6 by carbamazepine. However, data to support such induction is limited to an *in vitro* study,[3] and further research to elucidate the mechanism is needed.

Importance and management

Evidence for an interaction between bupropion and carbamazepine is limited, but a pharmacokinetic interaction appears to be established. However, the overall clinical importance of the changes described is uncertain. Bear in mind the possibility of reduced efficacy and/or increased toxicity (due to increased hydroxybupropion concentrations) on concurrent use, and consider adjusting the bupropion dose accordingly. The same advice would also seem appropriate with **phenytoin** (and therefore **fosphenytoin**) and **phenobarbital** (and therefore **primidone**), which would be expected to interact similarly, but clinical studies to confirm this appear to be lacking.

Note that bupropion causes dose-related seizures and is contraindicated in patients with seizure disorders.

1. Ketter TA, Jenkins JB, Schroeder DH, Pazzaglia PJ, Marangell LB, George MS, Callahan AM, Hinton ML, Chao J, Post RM. Carbamazepine but not valproate induces bupropion metabolism. *J Clin Psychopharmacol* (1995) 15, 327–33.
2. Popli AP, Tanquary J, Lamparella V, Masand PS. Bupropion and anticonvulsant drug interactions. *Ann Clin Psychiatry* (1995) 7, 99–101.
3. Dickmann LJ, Isoherranen N. Quantitative prediction of CYP2B6 induction by estradiol during pregnancy: potential explanation for increased methadone clearance during pregnancy. *Drug Metab Dispos* (2013) 41, 270–4.

Bupropion + Antiparkinsonian drugs

A small number of case reports associate the development of neurologic symptoms with concurrent use of bupropion and amantadine.

Clinical evidence

A review of the records of 8 nursing home patients receiving bupropion, found that of 6 who also received prophylactic **amantadine** for influenza, 3 developed confusion and neurologic symptoms within a week of concurrent use. Two patients required hospitalisation and in all cases symptoms resolved within 72 hours of discontinuing bupropion and amantadine. One patient subsequently received bupropion at their previous dose with no recurrence of symptoms.[1] A case report describes a 75-year-old man with Parkinsonism and depression who was started on bupropion 75 mg twice daily following a course of ECT. Concurrent medications included haloperidol, **amantadine**, and benztropine, and after 3 days of treatment with bupropion the patient experienced visual and auditory hallucinations and became disorientated, agitated and unsteady resulting in a fall. Bupropion was discontinued and the patient's symptoms resolved over the next 4 days.[2]

Mechanism

Bupropion inhibits the reuptake of dopamine, and amantadine has dopamine agonist activity. The authors of the reports suggest that the symptoms seen on concurrent use of bupropion and amantadine resulted from dopaminergic overdrive.[1,2] Further, ECT has been associated with dopaminergic effects and an increase in dopamine receptor sensitivity,[3] and this might have played a part in one of the cases. However further study is required to establish the mechanism behind the effects seen.

Importance and management

Evidence for an interaction between bupropion and antiparkinsonian drugs is limited to a few case reports, and an interaction is not established. The UK and US manufacturers state that the concurrent use of bupropion and **levodopa** or **amantadine** should be undertaken with caution because limited clinical data suggest a higher incidence of undesirable effects (nausea, vomiting, excitement, restlessness, postural tremor) in patients given bupropion with either drug.[4,5]

The case reports with amantadine add some weight to this advice, but there appears to be a lack of published data with levodopa. Some caution, and close monitoring would seem appropriate if concurrent use is required, and patients should be given small initial bupropion doses, which are increased gradually.

1. Trappler B, Miyashiro AM. Bupropion-amantadine-associated neurotoxicity. *J Clin Psychiatry* (2000) 61, 61–2.
2. Liberzon I, Dequardo JR, Silk KR. Bupropion and delirium. *Am J Psychiatry* (1990) 147, 1689–90.
3. Rudorfer MV, Manji HK, Potter WZ. Bupropion, ECT, and dopaminergic overdrive. Am J Psychiatry. (1991)148, 1101–2.
4. Zyban (Bupropion hydrochloride). GlaxoSmithKline UK. UK Summary of product characteristics, November 2013.
5. Zyban (Bupropion hydrochloride). GlaxoSmithKline. US Prescribing information, March 2014.

Bupropion + Benzodiazepines and related drugs

Visual hallucinations have been seen in one patient given zolpidem with bupropion. Bupropion appears to antagonise the impairment of function and the sedative effects induced by diazepam.

Clinical evidence, mechanism, importance and management

A crossover study in 12 healthy subjects given a single 2.5- or 5-mg dose of **diazepam**, a single 100-mg dose of bupropion, a combination of both, or placebo assessed the effects on both objective (e.g. auditory vigilance, blood pressure) and subjective (e.g. drowsiness) measures. **Diazepam** 5 mg impaired performance in the auditory vigilance test and increased the rating of subjective effects, when compared with placebo. Unexpectedly, the combination of bupropion with **diazepam** appeared to result in function similar to that seen with placebo or bupropion alone.[1] A report describes visual hallucinations lasting 3 to 4 hours when a 17-year-old boy who had been taking bupropion 450 mg daily for one month and **zolpidem** 5 to 10 mg daily for about 6 months increased his **zolpidem** dose to 60 mg.[2] Note that the recommended dose of **zolpidem** is 10 mg daily and that **zolpidem** itself can cause psychiatric adverse effects such as hallucinations.

An interaction is not established, and the study suggests that bupropion might antagonise the functional impairment and drowsiness associated with diazepam use. Bupropion is contraindicated during abrupt withdrawal from any drug known to be associated with seizures on withdrawal, particularly benzodiazepines and benzodiazepine-like drugs.[3,4]

1. Hamilton MJ, Bush M, Smith P, Peck AW. The effects of bupropion, a new antidepressant drug, and diazepam, and their interaction in man. *Br J Clin Pharmacol* (1982) 14, 791–7.
2. Elko CJ, Burgess JL, Robertson WO. Zolpidem-associated hallucinations and serotonin reuptake inhibition: a possible interaction. *Clin Toxicol* (1998) 36, 195–203.
3. Zyban (Bupropion hydrochloride). GlaxoSmithKline UK. UK Summary of product characteristics, November 2013.
4. Zyban (Bupropion hydrochloride). GlaxoSmithKline. US Prescribing information, March 2014.

Bupropion + Carbimazole

A report describes acute liver failure in a patient taking bupropion and carbimazole.

Clinical evidence, mechanism, importance and management

A 41-year-old man treated for hyperthyroidism with carbimazole 15 mg daily and propranolol 10 mg daily for 5 years received a 10-day course of bupropion 150 mg daily to aid smoking cessation. Ten weeks after completing the course of bupropion he was admitted to hospital with severe jaundice, nausea, dyspepsia, lethargy, and epigastric discomfort persisting for 5 days. The only other medication he had taken was paracetamol (acetaminophen) 500 mg to 1 g daily for up to 2 days, about 2 weeks before admission. Both carbimazole and propranolol were discontinued. He developed acute liver failure and a rapid deterioration of renal function, complicated by sepsis and coagulopathy. Liver biopsy showed evidence of non-specific drug-induced acute liver injury. The patient died 19 days after the onset of symptoms.[1]

Both bupropion and carbimazole can cause liver damage. In this case the hepatotoxicity was attributed to bupropion or a combined toxic effect of bupropion and carbimazole. The potential for serious hepatotoxicity should be borne in mind if bupropion is given with other hepatotoxic drugs.

1. Khoo A-L, Tham L-S, Lee K-H, Lim G-K. Acute liver failure with concurrent bupropion and carbimazole therapy. *Ann Pharmacother* (2003) 37, 220–3.

Bupropion + Cimetidine

Cimetidine does not appear to affect the pharmacokinetics of bupropion.

Clinical evidence, metabolism, importance and management

In a crossover study in 24 healthy subjects, a single 800-mg dose of cimetidine had no effect on the pharmacokinetics of a single 300-mg dose of bupropion (sustained release preparation).[1] Note that a study using multiple-doses of cimetidine would be preferable in order to draw more definitive conclusions. However, given the lack of other evidence, no interaction would appear to occur and no bupropion dose adjustment would seem necessary on concurrent use.

1. Kustra R, Corrigan B, Dunn J, Duncan B, Hsyu P-H. Lack of effect of cimetidine on the pharmacokinetics of sustained-release bupropion. *J Clin Pharmacol* (1999) 39, 1184–8.

Bupropion + Clopidogrel and related drugs

Clopidogrel and ticlopidine cause a small increase in bupropion exposure, and a small decrease in the exposure to its active metabolite, hydroxybupropion. Prasugrel causes a minor decrease in the exposure to bupropion and hydroxybupropion.

Clinical evidence

(a) Clopidogrel

A study in healthy subjects given clopidogrel 75 mg daily for 4 days found that the AUC of a single 150-mg dose of bupropion was increased by 60% and the AUC of its active metabolite, hydroxybupropion, was decreased by 52%.[1]

(b) Prasugrel

In a study in 30 healthy subjects, prasugrel, given as a 60-mg loading dose, then 10 mg daily for 10 days, increased the AUC of a single 150-mg dose of bupropion given on day 7 by just 18% and decreased the AUC of its active metabolite, hydroxybupropion, by 23%.[2]

(c) Ticlopidine

A study in healthy subjects given ticlopidine 250 mg twice daily for 4 days found that the AUC of a single 150-mg dose of bupropion was increased by 85% and the AUC of its active metabolite, hydroxybupropion, was decreased by 84%.[1]

Mechanism

Bupropion is metabolised by CYP2B6, which can be inhibited by clopidogrel and ticlopidine.[1,3] Concurrent use therefore decreases bupropion metabolism and increases its exposure. The effect of prasugrel on this isoenzyme appears to be less as it only produces a minimal increase in bupropion exposure.

Importance and management

The pharmacokinetic interactions between bupropion and **clopidogrel** or **ticlopidine** are established, but the clinical relevance of the increase in bupropion exposure and decrease in hydroxybupropion exposure is unclear. Until more is known about this interaction it would seem prudent to monitor concurrent use for any alterations in bupropion adverse effects (lightheadedness, gastrointestinal effects) and/or efficacy, adjusting the dose if necessary.

The minimal increase in bupropion exposure caused by **prasugrel** is unlikely to be clinically relevant.

1. Turpeinen M, Tolonen A, Uusitalo J, Jalonen J, Pelkonen O, Laine K. Effect of clopidogrel and ticlopidine on cytochrome P450 2B6 activity as measured by bupropion hydroxylation. *Clin Pharmacol Ther* (2005) 77, 553–9.
2. Farid NA, Payne CD, Ernest CS, Li YG, Winters KJ, Salazar DE, Small DS. Prasugrel, a new thienopyridine antiplatelet drug, weakly inhibits cytochrome P450 2B6 in humans. *J Clin Pharmacol* (2008) 48, 53–9.
3. Richter T, Mürdter TE, Heinkele G, Pleiss J, Tatzel S, Schwab M, Eichelbaum M, Zanger UM. Potent mechanism-based inhibition of human CYP2B6 by clopidogrel and ticlopidine. *J Pharmacol Exp Ther* (2004) 308, 189–97.

Bupropion + Corticosteroids

A patient taking bupropion had a seizure after being given an intra-articular injection of methylprednisolone.

Clinical evidence, mechanism, importance and management

A case report describes a patient taking bupropion, who experienced a severe, prolonged seizure 24 hours after receiving intra-articular **methylprednisolone** 30 mg for subacromial bursitis.[1] The author notes that there could be a risk of seizures in patients taking bupropion who are given prophylactic oral steroids.[1] This is consistent with the manufacturers' suggestion that systemic steroids could increase the risk of seizures. See 'Bupropion + Miscellaneous', p.1470, for a further discussion of the risk of seizures with bupropion.

1. White P. Interaction of intra-articular steroids and bupropion. *Clin Radiol* (2002) 57, 235.

Bupropion + Food

The absorption of bupropion does not appear to be affected by food.

Clinical evidence, mechanism, importance and management

The UK and US manufacturers of bupropion note that, in studies in healthy subjects, administration with food increased the maximum concentration of bupropion by 11 to 35% and the AUC by 16 to 19%.[1-3] They also state that the this is not considered to be clinically relevant,[2,3] and advise that bupropion can be taken without regard to food.[1-3]

1. Zyban (Bupropion hydrochloride). GlaxoSmithKline UK. UK Summary of product characteristics, November 2013.
2. Zyban (Bupropion hydrochloride). GlaxoSmithKline. US Prescribing information, March 2014.
3. Wellbutrin SR (Bupropion hydrochloride). GlaxoSmithKline. US Prescribing information, April 2014.

Bupropion + Guanfacine

A grand mal seizure in a child, which was attributed to an interaction between bupropion and guanfacine, was later identified as being more probably due to a bupropion overdose.

Clinical evidence, mechanism, importance and management

A 10-year-old girl, being treated for attention deficit hyperactivity disorder, was prescribed increasing doses of bupropion, up to 100 mg three times daily, to which guanfacine, initially 500 micrograms twice daily then 500 micrograms three times daily, was added. Ten days later she had a grand mal seizure, which the author of the report attributed to an interaction between the two drugs.[1,2] This was challenged in subsequent correspondence.[3] Furthermore, 2 years later the author of the original report wrote to say that he had now discovered that the girl had in fact taken 500 mg of bupropion and 5 mg of guanfacine before the seizure took place, so that what happened was much more likely to have been due to an overdose of the bupropion (which is known to cause seizures) than to an interaction with guanfacine.[4]

1. Tilton P. Bupropion and guanfacine. *J Am Acad Child Adolesc Psychiatry* (1998) 37, 682–3.
2. Tilton P. Seizure associated with bupropion and guanfacine. *J Am Acad Child Adolesc Psychiatry* (1999) 38, 3.
3. Namerow LB. Seizure associated with bupropion and guanfacine. *J Am Acad Child Adolesc Psychiatry* (1999) 38, 2.
4. Tilton P. Seizure after guanfacine plus bupropion: correction. *J Am Acad Child Adolesc Psychiatry* (2000) 39, 1341.

Bupropion + HIV-protease inhibitors

Ritonavir, both at doses used to boost the concentrations of other HIV-protease inhibitors and at higher doses, *decreases* bupropion exposure. Lopinavir and tipranavir, both boosted with ritonavir, interact similarly. This is the opposite effect to that which was originally predicted. Nelfinavir has no effect on bupropion exposure.

Clinical evidence

(a) Lopinavir

In a study in healthy subjects, lopinavir boosted with ritonavir 400/100 mg twice daily for 2 weeks *decreased* the AUC and maximum concentration of bupropion, after a single 100-mg dose of the sustained-release formulation, by 57%. The AUC of its active metabolite, hydroxybupropion, was also decreased by 50%. The pharmacokinetics of lopinavir boosted with ritonavir were unchanged by the single dose of bupropion.[1]

(b) Nelfinavir

In a study in 9 healthy subjects, nelfinavir 1.25 g twice daily for 14 days had no effect on the AUC or clearance of a single 150-mg dose of bupropion.[2]

(c) Ritonavir

In a crossover study in 7 healthy subjects, ritonavir 200 mg twice daily for 2 days, had no effect on the AUC and maximum concentration of a single 75-mg dose of bupropion given with the third ritonavir dose. The pharmacokinetics of the active metabolite, hydroxybupropion, were also unaffected.[3] Similar results were seen in another study in 9 healthy subjects given ritonavir up to 400 mg twice daily for 14 days and a single 150-mg dose of bupropion.[2] In contrast, in a study in 13 healthy subjects, ritonavir 200 mg three times daily for 1 day, then 300 mg twice daily for 6 days, followed by 400 mg twice daily for 11 days, *decreased* the AUC of a single 150-mg dose of bupropion given on day 3 and day 17 by 16% and 33%, respectively, and decreased the AUC of hydroxybupropion by 31% and 57%, respectively.[4] Similarly, in another study in 19 healthy subjects, ritonavir 100 mg twice daily for 22 days decreased the AUC of a single 150-mg dose of extended-release bupropion by 22%, with a similar decrease in the AUC of hydroxybupropion. Furthermore, in 22 healthy subjects, a higher dose of ritonavir (300 mg twice daily titrated to 600 mg twice daily over 22 days) decreased the AUC of bupropion and hydroxybupropion, by 66% and 78%, respectively.[5]

A retrospective study identified 10 HIV-positive patients who had taken bupropion 150 mg once or twice daily together with **nelfinavir**, ritonavir, or efavirenz for 3 weeks to 2 years (median 8 months). No seizures had occurred in these patients (predicted if a large increase in bupropion concentrations had occurred), but note that the number of patients was small. The 2 patients who received ritonavir were given 100 mg twice daily.[6]

(d) Tipranavir

The UK manufacturer of tipranavir briefly reports that tipranavir boosted with ritonavir 500/200 mg twice daily decreased the AUC and maximum plasma concentration of bupropion 150 mg twice daily by 56% and 51%, respectively. The pharmacokinetics of tipranavir were not affected by bupropion.[7]

Mechanism

Early *in vitro* data[8] indicated that nelfinavir and ritonavir are capable of inhibiting CYP2B6, which is the isoenzyme primarily involved in bupropion metabolism. It was therefore predicted that these drugs would cause an *increase* in bupropion concentrations,[8] with an increased risk of seizures. However, subsequent *in vitro* evidence[9] shows that ritonavir strongly *induces* CYP2B6. Note that it is possible for drugs to be shown to be both inhibitors and inducers of the same isoenzyme, as the studies require different methodologies. In addition, enzyme induction takes longer to become apparent than enzyme inhibition (as the enzyme has to be produced), and so would not have been apparent after just 2 days of ritonavir in the study[3] above. Clinical studies are then required to show what happens *in vivo*. In the clinical studies, at steady-state, ritonavir alone, and used to boost other HIV-protease inhibitors, decreased bupropion exposure suggesting it induces CYP2B6. This effect is not apparent during the first few days of ritonavir administration. This is not the first interaction where ritonavir has caused the opposite effect to that which was originally predicted, other examples being methadone (see 'Opioids; Methadone + HIV-protease inhibitors', p.182), and contraceptives (see 'Combined hormonal contraceptives + HIV-protease inhibitors', p.1177). Nelfinavir appears not to alter the metabolism of bupropion.

Importance and management

At steady-state, ritonavir alone, and lopinavir and tipranavir, both boosted with ritonavir, decrease the concentrations of bupropion and its active metabolite, hydroxybupropion. The decreases seen are likely to be clinically important. In patients taking ritonavir, or lopinavir or tipranavir, both boosted with ritonavir, it would seem prudent to start bupropion at the recommended starting dose and titrate to effect. Nevertheless, the UK and US manufacturers of bupropion state that the recommended dose should not be exceeded.[10,11] Although only lopinavir and tipranavir boosted with ritonavir have been studied, it seems likely that other HIV-protease inhibitors boosted with ritonavir will interact similarly.

The small study with nelfinavir showed that it has no effect on the pharmacokinetics of bupropion and that no dose adjustment is necessary on concurrent use.

1. Hogeland GW, Swindells S, McNabb JC, Kashuba AD, Yee GC, Lindley CM. Lopinavir/ritonavir reduces bupropion plasma concentrations in healthy subjects. *Clin Pharmacol Ther* (2007) 81, 69–75.
2. Kirby BJ, Collier AC, Kharasch ED, Dixit V, Desai P, Whittington D, Thummel KE, Unadkat JD. Complex drug interactions of HIV protease inhibitors 2: In vivo induction and in vitro to in vivo correlation of induction of cytochrome P450 1A2, 2B6, and 2C9 by ritonavir or nelfinavir. *Drug Metab Dispos* (2011) 39, 2329–37.
3. Hesse LM, Greenblatt DJ, von Moltke LL, Court MH. Ritonavir has minimal impact on the pharmacokinetic disposition of a single dose of bupropion administered to human volunteers. *J Clin Pharmacol* (2006) 46, 567–76.
4. Kharasch ED, Mitchell D, Coles R, Blanco R. Rapid clinical induction of hepatic cytochrome P4502B6 activity by ritonavir. *Antimicrob Agents Chemother* (2008) 52, 1663–9.
5. Park J, Vousden M, Brittain C, McConn DJ, Iavarone L, Ascher J, Sutherland SM, Muir KT. Dose-related reduction in bupropion plasma concentrations by ritonavir. *J Clin Pharmacol* (2010) 50, 1180–7.
6. Park-Wyllie LY, Antoniou T. Concurrent use of bupropion with CYP2B6 inhibitors, nelfinavir, ritonavir and efavirenz: a case series. *AIDS* (2003) 17, 638–40.
7. Aptivus Soft Capsules (Tipranavir). Boehringer Ingelheim Limited. UK Summary of product characteristics, February 2014.
8. Hesse LM, von Moltke LL, Shader RI, Greenblatt DJ. Ritonavir, efavirenz, and nelfinavir inhibit CYP2B6 activity in vitro: potential drug interactions with bupropion. *Drug Metab Dispos* (2001) 29, 100–102.
9. Faucette SR, Wang H, Hamilton GA, Jolley SL, Gilbert D, Lindley C, Yan B, Negishi M, LeCluyse EL. Regulation of CYP2B6 in primary human hepatocytes by prototypical inducers. *Drug Metab Dispos* (2004) 32, 348–58.
10. Zyban (Bupropion hydrochloride). GlaxoSmithKline UK. UK Summary of product characteristics, November 2013.
11. Zyban (Bupropion hydrochloride). GlaxoSmithKline. US Prescribing information, March 2014.

Bupropion + Hormonal contraceptives or HRT

HRT and, to a lesser extent, an oral combined hormonal contraceptive decreased the exposure to hydroxybupropion in one study.

Clinical evidence

In a three-way crossover study in 12 healthy women, a single 150-mg dose of sustained-release bupropion was given alone or on day 10 of treatment with menopausal hormone replacement therapy (**estradiol/levonorgestrel** 2 mg/250 micrograms; *Cyclabil*) or an oral combined hormonal contraceptive (**ethinylestradiol/desogestrel** 30/150 micrograms; *Marvelon*) for 10 days. The HRT decreased the AUC of the major active metabolite, hydroxybupropion, by 47% and increased the AUC of the metabolite hydrobupropion by 64%, but the AUC of bupropion was unchanged. The AUC of hydroxybupropion was also decreased by the hormonal contraceptive, but to a lesser extent (31%), the AUC of bupropion was decreased by 19% but the AUC of hydrobupropion was not affected.[1]

Mechanism

Bupropion is extensively metabolised to hydroxybupropion (the major active metabolite) by CYP2B6, and this study suggests that HRT and, to a lesser extent, oral contraceptives might inhibit CYP2B6 activity. Which of the constituents were principally responsible for this effect is unknown.

Importance and management

Evidence for an interaction between bupropion and hormonal contraceptives or HRT is limited to one study and a pharmacokinetic interaction is not established. In addition, the clinical effect of the small decrease in exposure to the major active metabolite, hydroxybupropion, and corresponding lack of effect on bupropion exposure with HRT has not been assessed. Until more is known about the consequences of altering the ratio of hydroxybupropion to bupropion, it might be prudent to be alert for changes in adverse effects and/or efficacy when bupropion is used with HRT.

The lesser effects of the combined oral contraceptive are unlikely to be clinically relevant.

1. Palovaara S, Pelkonen O, Uusitalo J, Lundgren S, Laine K. Inhibition of cytochrome P450 2B6 activity by hormone replacement therapy and oral contraceptive as measured by bupropion hydroxylation. *Clin Pharmacol Ther* (2003) 74, 326–33.

Bupropion + Lamotrigine

Bupropion does not alter the pharmacokinetics of lamotrigine. Hypomania has been reported in a patient taking bupropion and lamotrigine.

Clinical evidence, mechanism, importance and management

A crossover study in 12 healthy subjects found that steady-state bupropion 150 mg twice daily did not affect the pharmacokinetics of a single 100-mg dose of lamotrigine.[1]

A 23-year-old patient with a DSM-IV diagnosis of major depression taking bupropion 400 mg daily had an improvement in mood when she was also given lamotrigine 25 mg at night, and there was further improvement in mood, decreased anxiety and increased energy when lamotrigine was increased to 50 mg daily for 3 weeks. However, when the dose of lamotrigine was increased to 75 mg daily she reported decreased sleep, increased energy, mood lability, and increased spending, which was diagnosed as hypomania. The symptoms resolved over about 2 weeks when the lamotrigine dose was reduced to 50 mg at bedtime.

Antidepressants in high doses or in combination can induce hypomania and in this case the effect was attributed to a potentiation of the effects of bupropion, caused by lamotrigine.[2] The general relevance of this single case is uncertain.

Note that bupropion causes dose-related seizures and is contraindicated in patients with seizure disorders.

1. Odishaw J, Chen C. Effects of steady-state bupropion on the pharmacokinetics of lamotrigine in healthy subjects. *Pharmacotherapy* (2000) 20, 1448–53.
2. Margolese HC, Beauclair L, Szkrumelak N, Chouinard G. Hypomania induced by adjunctive lamotrigine. *Am J Psychiatry* (2003) 160, 183–4.

Bupropion + Linezolid

A report describes intraoperative hypertension in a patient taking bupropion and linezolid.

Clinical evidence, mechanism, importance and management

A report describes severe intermittent intraoperative hypertension in a 57-year-old man undergoing surgical removal of an infected vascular bypass graft. He was taking maintenance bupropion (dosage not stated) and linezolid, which had been started 24 hours previously for treatment of a resistant gram-positive infection.[1] Linezolid is known to have weak reversible MAOI properties, and might therefore interact with bupropion in a similar way to that predicted for non-selective MAOIs, see 'MAOIs and related drugs + Bupropion', p.1387. This report introduces a note of caution and it would seem prudent to avoid the combination where possible, but if both drugs are given together to closely monitor the patient's blood pressure. However, the US manufacturer of bupropion contraindicates the concurrent use of linezolid unless alternatives to linezolid are not available and the benefits outweigh the risk of a hypertensive reaction, in which case bupropion should be stopped and linezolid given. The patient should then be monitored for 2 weeks or until 24 hours after linezolid is stopped. Bupropion can be restarted 24 hours after the last linezolid dose.[2]

1. Marcucci C, Sandson NB, Dunlap JA. Linezolid-bupropion interaction as possible etiology of severe intermittent intraoperative hypertension? *Anesthesiology* (2004) 101, 1487–8.
2. Zyban (Bupropion hydrochloride). GlaxoSmithKline. US Prescribing information, March 2014.

Bupropion + Methylphenidate

Case reports describe grand mal seizures in one patient and myocardial infarction in another, which were associated with the concurrent use of bupropion and methylphenidate.

Clinical evidence, mechanism, importance and management

(a) Seizures

A 14-year-old boy taking methylphenidate 60 mg daily was also given bupropion 200 mg increased to 300 mg daily. The patient experienced grand mal seizures 4 weeks after the dosage increase, but remained seizure-free once the bupropion was discontinued.[1] The authors note that bupropion alone could have been the cause of the seizures, but that methylphenidate might have been a contributory factor. Note that the manufacturers of bupropion list stimulants as drugs that increase the risk of seizures with bupropion (see 'Bupropion + Miscellaneous', p.1470) and this case adds weight to that warning.

(b) Myocardial ischaemia

A report describes acute myocardial infarction in a 16-year-old boy who was taking methylphenidate 30 mg twice daily for attention-deficit hyperactivity disorder, bupropion 100 mg twice daily for depression, and sustained-release erythromycin 999 mg daily for acne (duration of each not noted). It was proposed that the erythromycin might have caused increased concentrations of bupropion leading to a hyperadrenergic state and this, together with the sympathetic effects of the methylphenidate, resulted in excessive vasospasm, leading to myocardial damage.[2] However, there is no clear known mechanism by which erythromycin (a CYP3A4 and P-glycoprotein inhibitor) would increase bupropion concentrations (a CYP2B6 substrate).

1. Ickowicz A. Bupropion-methylphenidate combination and grand mal seizures. *Can J Psychiatry* (2002) 47, 790–1.
2. George AK, Kunwar AR, Awasthi A. Acute myocardial infarction in a young male on methylphenidate, bupropion, and erythromycin. *J Child Adolesc Psychopharmacol* (2005) 15, 693–5.

Bupropion + Miscellaneous

Bupropion is predicted to have additive effects if given with other drugs that can also lower the seizure threshold. Bupropion can increase the exposure of drugs that are substrates of CYP2D6.

Clinical evidence, mechanism, importance and management

(a) CYP2B6 substrates

The UK manufacturer advises caution if bupropion is used with drugs that are substrates of CYP2B6 (like itself) and lists the antineoplastics **cyclophosphamide** and **ifosfamide**.[1] However, there is no clinical evidence that pharmacokinetic interactions occur due to competition between two drugs that are both substrates of the same isoenzyme if given together, and it is not usual to issue cautions solely on this basis.

(b) CYP2D6 substrates

Bupropion is an inhibitor of CYP2D6, and has been shown to increase the concentrations of a number of CYP2D6 substrates including desipramine (see 'Tricyclic antidepressants + Bupropion', p.1504), which can used as a probe substrate to assess the activity of drugs on CYP2D6. Note that CYP2D6 shows genetic polymorphism, with about 10% of the population having low activity of CYP2D6 (poor metabolisers). Therefore, pharmacokinetic interactions between CYP2D6 inhibitors and CYP2D6 substrates are often less important than might initially be supposed, because a potent inhibitor of this isoenzyme will effectively be changing a person who is an extensive metaboliser into a poor metaboliser (i.e. any change is still within the range of the existing population). An interaction is likely to be important when an extensive metaboliser is on established treatment with a CYP2D6 substrate that has a narrow therapeutic window, and then starts a CYP2D6 inhibitor. Bupropion should therefore be used with some caution with drugs that are known substrates of CYP2D6, particularly those with a narrow therapeutic window. For a list of CYP2D6 substrates, see 'Table 1.7', p.9. Note that the UK and US manufacturers of bupropion also name **haloperidol**. The recommendation is that if any of these drugs are added to treatment with bupropion, doses at the lower end of the range should be used. If bupropion is added to existing treatment, decreased dosages should be considered.[1,2]

Note also, that tamoxifen, which is converted by CYP2D6 to the active metabolite endoxifen, might be less effective when given with inhibitors of CYP2D6 such as bupropion, see 'Tamoxifen + SSRIs and other CYP2D6 inhibitors', p.712 for further details.

(c) Drugs that can lower the seizure threshold

There is a small dose-related risk of seizures with bupropion. At a daily dose of 300 mg of the sustained-release formulation the risk is 0.1%, which increases to 0.4% at a dose of 450 mg of the immediate-release formulation, and increases 10-fold between doses of 450 and 600 mg daily.[2] The UK and US manufacturers caution the use of other drugs that lower the seizure threshold, the concern being that these drugs might further increase the risk of seizures. They list **antipsychotics**, antidepressants, systemic steroids, and **theophylline**.[1,2] In some cases seizures have been seen when bupropion is given with these drugs, see 'SSRIs + Bupropion', p.1485, 'Tricyclic antidepressants + Bupropion', p.1504, and 'Bupropion + Corticosteroids', p.1468. The UK manufacturers additionally list **antimalarials**, **tramadol**, **quinolones**, and **sedating antihistamines**. A maximum dose of 150 mg of bupropion should be considered for patients prescribed such drugs.[1]

Caution is also urged with regard to circumstances that can lower the seizure threshold, including the use of **anorectics** or **stimulants** (one case seen with methylphenidate, see 'Bupropion + Methylphenidate', p.1469),[1,2] the excessive use of **sedatives**, and addiction to **cocaine** or **opiates**.[2]

1. Zyban (Bupropion hydrochloride). GlaxoSmithKline UK. UK Summary of product characteristics, November 2013.
2. Zyban (Bupropion hydrochloride). GlaxoSmithKline. US Prescribing information, March 2014.

Bupropion + NNRTIs

Efavirenz moderately decreases bupropion exposure. Nevirapine might interact similarly.

Clinical evidence

In a pharmacokinetic study in 13 healthy subjects, efavirenz 600 mg once daily for 13 to 15 days decreased the AUC of a single 150-mg dose of slow-release bupropion by 55% without changing the AUC of its metabolite, hydroxybupropion. There was a 2.3-fold increase in the AUC ratio of hydroxybupropion to bupropion.[1]

A retrospective study identified 10 HIV-positive patients who had taken bupropion 150 mg once or twice daily together with **nelfinavir**, **ritonavir**, or **efavirenz** for 3 weeks to 2 years (median 8 months). No seizures had occurred in these patients (predicted if a large increase in bupropion concentrations had occurred), but note that the number of patients was small.[2]

Mechanism

Bupropion is metabolised to its major active metabolite, hydroxybupropion, primarily by CYP2B6. The pharmacokinetic study therefore suggests that efavirenz induces CYP2B6 resulting in decreased bupropion exposure. This confirms some *in vitro* data showing induction,[3] but is in contrast to earlier *in vitro* data[4] which indicated that efavirenz inhibited CYP2B6. Note that it is possible for drugs to be shown to be both inhibitors and inducers of the same isoenzyme *in vitro* as the studies require different methodologies. Clinical studies are then required to show what happens *in vivo*.

Importance and management

Evidence for an interaction between bupropion and efavirenz is based on a study, and a pharmacokinetic interaction would seem to be established. The moderate decrease in bupropion exposure by efavirenz is likely to be clinically important. It would therefore be sensible to bear in mind the possibility of reduced bupropion efficacy in any patient taking efavirenz, and to titrate the bupropion dose as necessary (without exceeding the maximum dose). Of the other NNRTIs, **nevirapine** might also be an inducer of CYP2B6, and therefore some caution on concurrent use might be appropriate.

1. Robertson SM, Maldarelli F, Natarajan V, Formentini E, Alfaro RM, Penzak SR. Efavirenz induces CYP2B6-mediated hydroxylation of bupropion in healthy subjects. *J Acquir Immune Defic Syndr* (2008) 49, 513–19.
2. Park-Wyllie LY, Antoniou T. Concurrent use of bupropion with CYP2B6 inhibitors, nelfinavir, ritonavir and efavirenz: a case series. *AIDS* (2003) 17, 638–40.
3. Faucette SR, Zhang T-C, Moore R, Sueyoshi T, Omiecinski CJ, LeCluyse EL, Negishi M, Wang H. Relative activation of human pregnane X receptor versus constitutive androstane receptor defines distinct classes of CYP2B6 and CYP3A4 inducers. *J Pharmacol Exp Ther* (2007) 320, 72–80.
4. Hesse LM, von Moltke LL, Shader RI, Greenblatt DJ. Ritonavir, efavirenz, and nelfinavir inhibit CYP2B6 activity in vitro: potential drug interactions with bupropion. *Drug Metab Dispos* (2001) 29, 100–102.

Bupropion + Pseudoephedrine

A report describes acute myocardial ischaemia associated with bupropion and pseudoephedrine in a recent tobacco smoker.

Clinical evidence, mechanism, importance and management

A 21-year-old man presented to a hospital emergency department with severe chest pain radiating into both arms and between the shoulder blades, diaphoresis, and shortness of breath. This was diagnosed as an acute myocardial infarction, and it was concluded that this was due to acute myocardial ischaemia apparently brought on by the combined use of pseudoephedrine (9 tablets of 30 mg taken over the previous 3 days), bupropion for smoking cessation (started in the previous 72 hours), and **nicotine** from tobacco (he had smoked 25 cigarettes daily). The authors of the report postulate that all these drugs acted on the alpha receptors of the coronary arteries to cause vasospasm and acute ischaemia. He had also been taking erythromycin for 3 days (which is not thought to be related to the interaction), and had previously taken pseudoephedrine alone on numerous occasions without problems. He recovered fully.[1]

No general conclusions can be drawn from this case, but some warning might be appropriate for patients who are at risk of coronary ischaemia. For comment on the use of nicotine with bupropion, see 'Bupropion + Tobacco or Nicotine', p.1471.

1. Pederson KJ, Kuntz DH, Garbe GJ. Acute myocardial ischemia associated with ingestion of bupropion and pseudoephedrine in a 21-year-old man. *Can J Cardiol* (2001) 17, 599–601.

Bupropion + Rifampicin (Rifampin)

Rifampicin moderately decreases the AUC of both bupropion and its active metabolite, hydroxybupropion.

Clinical evidence

In a controlled study in 16 healthy subjects, rifampicin 600 mg daily for 10 days caused a 67% decrease in the AUC of a single 150-mg dose of bupropion given on day 8. Bupropion clearance was increased 3-fold, and the elimination half-life was decreased from 15.9 hours to 8.2 hours. The AUC of the main active metabolite, hydroxybupropion, was also decreased (by about 75%), but its maximum concentration was *increased* by about 75%. There was no difference in the effect of rifampicin on bupropion between the 9 subjects who were ethnically Chinese and the 9 who were white European, after adjusting for body-weight.[1] In another study in 9 healthy subjects, rifampicin 600 mg daily for 14 days increased the clearance of a single 150-mg dose of bupropion by 66% and decreased the AUC by 40%.[2] A study in 35 healthy Korean subjects given a single 150-mg dose of extended release bupropion before and after rifampicin 600 mg daily for 7 days, found differences in the extent of the effect of rifampicin on the metabolism of bupropion to its active metabolite hydroxybupropion, according to the genotype of the subjects. The difference in the AUC ratio of hydroxybupropion to bupropion before and after rifampicin was similar (212 to 228%) across all subjects, with the exception of 4 subjects who had variant genotypes for both CYP2B6 and the pregnane X receptor. In these 4 subjects it was only 58%, indicating a reduction in the rifampicin-induced metabolism of bupropion in these subjects.[3]

Other studies have found that rifampicin has a greater effect on the *S*-enantiomer of bupropion and the *S,S*-hydroxyl bupropion metabolite than on the other enantiomers.[4,5]

Mechanism

Rifampicin induces CYP2B6, which is responsible for the hydroxylation of bupropion, and also the metabolism of hydroxybupropion. One study suggests that the rifampicin-induced metabolism of bupropion might be decreased in those subjects who have variant genotypes for both CYP2B6 and the pregnane X receptor.[3]

Importance and management

Evidence for a pharmacokinetic interaction between bupropion and rifampicin would seem to be established. Although the clinical relevance of the interaction has not been directly assessed, the observed moderate decrease in the exposure to bupropion and its main active metabolite, hydroxybupropion, would be anticipated to reduce its efficacy.

It would therefore be sensible to bear in mind the possibility of reduced bupropion efficacy in any patient taking rifampicin, and to titrate the bupropion dose as necessary (without exceeding the maximum dose). Note that it appears that genetic polymorphism could affect the extent of this interaction, although the clinical importance of this needs to be established by further study.

1. Loboz KK, Gross AS, Williams KM, Liauw WS, Day RO, Blievernicht JK, Zanger UM, McLachlan AJ. Cytochrome P450 2B6 activity as measured by bupropion hydroxylation: effect of induction by rifampin and ethnicity. *Clin Pharmacol Ther* (2006) 80, 75–84.
2. Kirby BJ, Collier AC, Kharasch ED, Dixit V, Desai P, Whittington D, Thummel KE, Unadkat JD. Complex drug interactions of HIV protease inhibitors 2: in vivo induction and in vitro to in vivo correlation of induction of cytochrome P450 1A2, 2B6, and 2C9 by ritonavir or nelfinavir. *Drug Metab Dispos* (2011) 39, 2329–37.
3. Chung JY, Cho JY, Lim HS, Kim JR, Yu KS, Lim KS, Shin SG, Jang IJ. Effects of pregnane x receptor (*NR1I2*) and CYP2B6 genetic polymorphisms on the induction of bupropion hydroxylation by rifampin. *Drug Metab Dispos* (2011) 39, 92–7.
4. Kharasch ED, Mitchell D, Coles R. Stereoselective bupropion hydroxylation as an in vivo phenotypic probe for cytochrome P4502B6 (CYP2B6) Activity. *J Clin Pharmacol* (2008) 48, 464–74.
5. Xu H, Loboz KK, Gross AS, McLachlan AJ. Stereoselective analysis of hydroxybupropion and application to drug interaction studies. *Chirality* (2007) 19, 163–70.

Bupropion + St John's wort (*Hypericum perforatum*)

St John's wort causes a minor decrease in the exposure to bupropion. A single case describes dystonia when bupropion was started in a patient taking HRT and St John's wort. A case of mania was attributed to the use of St John's wort in a patient taking bupropion.

Clinical evidence, mechanism, importance and management

(a) Pharmacokinetic effects

In an open, two-phase pharmacokinetic study in 18 healthy subjects, St John's wort 325 mg three times daily for 14 days, decreased the AUC of a single 150-mg dose of bupropion by about 16% and increased its clearance by about 20%. The AUC and clearance of the active metabolite, hydroxybupropion, were unaffected, but its half-life was decreased by about 18%.[1] The reason for this effect is unclear as bupropion is principally metabolised by CYP2B6, which is not known to be affected by St John's wort. Similarly, the clinical consequences of this interaction are not known, and require further study.

(b) Other effects

1. Dystonia. A 58-year-old woman taking St John's wort 300 mg daily and menopausal HRT (estradiol with medroxyprogesterone) developed acute facial dystonia 4 days after starting bupropion 150 mg daily for smoking cessation. She was treated with a variety of drugs, and over a couple of weeks the spasm-free interval lengthened, and by 5 months the dystonia resolved completely and all medications were withdrawn without recurrence of the dystonia.[2] Dystonia is a rare adverse effect of bupropion alone, and the authors suggested that the combination of bupropion with St John's wort led to additive effects on serotonin reuptake inhibition, making dopaminergic adverse effects such as dystonia more likely.[2] Note also that one HRT preparation has been shown to inhibit the metabolism of bupropion to hydroxybupropion (see 'Bupropion + Hormonal contraceptives or HRT', p.1469), so it could be hypothesised that there might also be a pharmacokinetic element to this case.

From a single case report like this, is it impossible to establish an interaction. Bear this case in mind in the event of similar adverse effects.

2. Mania. A report very briefly mentions that St John's wort was suspected of inducing mania in one patient who was also taking bupropion.[3] No other details were given, and no general conclusions can be drawn from this report.

1. Lei H-P, Yu X-Y, Xie H-T, Li H-H, Fan L, Dai L-L, Chen Y, Zhou H-H. Effect of St. John's wort supplementation on the pharmacokinetics of bupropion in healthy male Chinese volunteers. *Xenobiotica* (2010) 40, 275–81.
2. Milton JC, Abdulla A. Prolonged oro-facial dystonia in a 58 year old female following therapy with bupropion and St John's wort. *Br J Clin Pharmacol* (2007) 64, 717–18.
3. Griffiths J, Jordan S, Pilan K. Natural health products and adverse reactions. *Can Adverse React News* (2004) 14 (1), 2–3.

Bupropion + Tobacco or Nicotine

Neither nicotine nor tobacco smoking alter the pharmacokinetics of bupropion. However, combined use of bupropion and nicotine replacement therapy appears to increase the risk of hypertension.

Clinical evidence, mechanism, importance and management

(a) Nicotine

Nicotine transdermal patches are reported not to affect the pharmacokinetics of bupropion or its metabolites.[1] The UK and US manufacturers of bupropion state that limited data suggest that giving up smoking is more easily achieved if bupropion is taken while using a nicotine transdermal system, but a higher rate of treatment-emergent hypertension has been noted on concurrent use.[1,2] They recommend weekly monitoring to check for any evidence of a blood pressure increase.[1] The same warning would also seem to be applicable to the use of nicotine in any other form (buccal or nasal).

For a report of acute myocardial ischaemia attributed to combined use of bupropion, nicotine (from smoking) and pseudoephedrine, see 'Bupropion + Pseudoephedrine', p.1470.

(b) Tobacco

In a pharmacokinetic study, there was no difference in the pharmacokinetics of bupropion (given as a single 150-mg sustained release tablet) and its major metabolites between subjects who were tobacco smokers and those who were non-smokers.[3] Similarly, in a study in adolescents, there was no difference in the pharmacokinetics of bupropion or hydroxybupropion between 37 smokers and 38 non-smokers when given a single 150-mg dose of sustained release bupropion.[4]

This suggests that there is no need to alter the dose of bupropion based on smoking status.

1. Zyban (Bupropion hydrochloride). GlaxoSmithKline UK. UK Summary of product characteristics, November 2013.
2. Zyban (Bupropion hydrochloride). GlaxoSmithKline. US Prescribing information, March 2014.
3. Hsyu PH, Singh A, Giargiari TD, Dunn JA, Ascher JA, Johnston JA. Pharmacokinetics of bupropion and its metabolites in cigarette smokers versus nonsmokers. *J Clin Pharmacol* (1997) 37, 737–43.
4. Stewart JJ, Berkel HJ, Parish RC, Simar MR, Syed A, Bocchini JA Jr, Wilson JT, Manno JE. Single-dose pharmacokinetics of bupropion in adolescents: effects of smoking status and gender. *J Clin Pharmacol* (2001) 41, 770–8.

Bupropion + Valproate

Valproate appears to increase the exposure to hydroxybupropion, the major active metabolite of bupropion. Evidence from one case suggests that high-dose bupropion might increase valproate concentrations. Hallucinations have been reported in a patient taking both drugs.

Clinical evidence, mechanism, importance and management

In a study in 5 patients with major affective disorders, the AUC of hydroxybupropion, the major active metabolite of bupropion, almost doubled when a single 150-mg dose of bupropion was given with valproate at steady-state, but the pharmacokinetics of bupropion itself and its two other less active metabolites were unaffected.[1] A case report describes an increase in valproate concentrations of almost 30% after bupropion was started and increased to 450 mg daily.[2] Visual and auditory hallucinations were reported in a patient taking bupropion when valproate was substituted for lithium. The hallucinations stopped when bupropion was withdrawn.[3]

The UK manufacturer recommends caution when using drugs that may inhibit bupropion metabolism, and they name valproate.[4] The case report suggests that valproate concentrations might be increased by bupropion, but an effect is not established. Awareness of the possibility of increased adverse effects of both drugs would seem appropriate on concurrent use.

Note that bupropion causes dose-related seizures and is contraindicated in patients with seizure disorders.

1. Ketter TA, Jenkins JB, Schroeder DH, Pazzaglia PJ, Marangell LB, George MS, Callahan AM, Hinton ML, Chao J, Post RM. Carbamazepine but not valproate induces bupropion metabolism. *J Clin Psychopharmacol* (1995) 15, 327–33.
2. Popli AP, Tanquary J, Lamparella V, Masand PS. Bupropion and anticonvulsant drug interactions. *Ann Clin Psychiatry* (1995) 7, 99–101.
3. Filteau M-J, Leblanc J, Lefrançoise S, Demers M-F. Visual and auditory hallucinations with the association of bupropion and valproate. *Can J Psychiatry* (2000) 45, 198–9.
4. Zyban (Bupropion hydrochloride). GlaxoSmithKline UK. UK Summary of product characteristics, November 2013.

Drugs that cause serotonin syndrome + Other drugs that cause serotonin syndrome

The concurrent use of more than one serotonergic drug increases the risk of serotonin syndrome.

Clinical evidence, mechanism, importance and management

In the 1950s a serious and life-threatening toxic reaction was reported in patients taking iproniazid (an MAOI) when they were given pethidine (meperidine). For further information about this interaction, see under 'MAOIs or RIMAs + Opioids; Pethidine (Meperidine)', p.1399. The reasons were then not understood and even now we do not have the full picture. What happened is thought to have been due to over-stimulation of 5-HT_{2A} receptors and possibly other serotonin receptors (e.g. 5-HT_{1A}) in the central nervous system (in the brain stem and spinal cord in particular) due to the combined effects of these two drugs. It can occur exceptionally after taking only one drug, which causes over-stimulation of these serotonin receptors, but much more usually it develops when two or more drugs (so-called serotonergic or serotomimetic drugs) act in concert. The effects might also be dose related. It is suggested that the serious toxic effects (rigidity, hyperthermia) are mediated by the 5-HT_{2A} receptors.[1]

The characteristic symptoms (now known as serotonin syndrome or serotonin toxicity) fall into three main areas, namely altered mental status (agitation, confusion, mania), autonomic dysfunction (diaphoresis, diarrhoea, fever, shivering) and neuromuscular abnormalities (clonus, hyperreflexia, incoordination, myoclonus, tremor). These are part of the 'Sternbach diagnostic criteria' named after Dr Harvey Sternbach who drew up this list of clinical features and who suggested that at least three of them need to be seen before classifying this toxic reaction as serotonin syndrome rather than neuroleptic malignant syndrome.[2] However, the criteria given were a proposal, which has been further developed by other workers in an attempt to improve the sensitivity of the diagnosis; this is known as the Hunter Serotonin Toxicity Criteria.[3] This system uses a smaller more specific set of clinical features, particularly clonus, agitation, diaphoresis, tremor and hyperreflexia, which are said to be more specific to serotonin toxicity. Note that conditions such as anticholinergic toxicity and neuroleptic malignant syndrome are easily confused with serotonin toxicity. In the case of neuroleptic malignant syndrome, the symptoms of bradykinesia and extrapyramidal rigidity differ from those of serotonin toxicity where hyperkinesias, hyperreflexia, and clonuses

Table 35.3 Drugs associated with serotonin syndrome

Drug	*Mechanism for effect*	*Examples*
Amfetamines	Increased serotonin release	MAOIs or RIMAs + Amfetamines and related drugs, p.1383 Amfetamines and related drugs + SSRIs, p.216
Dapoxetine	Inhibition of serotonin metabolism	Dapoxetine + Miscellaneous, p.1534
Dexfenfluramine, Fenfluramine	Increased serotonin release	MAOIs + Dexfenfluramine or Fenfluramine, p.1387
Dextromethorphan	Increased serotonin release	MAOIs or RIMAs + Dextromethorphan and related cough suppressants, p.1387 SSRIs + Dextromethorphan, p.1566
Linezolid	Inhibition of serotonin metabolism	Linezolid + SSRIs, p.328 Linezolid + SNRIs, p.328 Linezolid + Tricyclic antidepressants, p.329
Lithium	Increased post-synaptic receptor response	Note that cases with lithium are usually associated with multiple potentially serotonergic drugs or other contributing factors. Lithium + Antibacterials; Linezolid, p.1364 Lithium + Venlafaxine, p.1381 Lithium + Tricyclic and related antidepressants, p.1380 Lithium + SSRIs, p.1378 Lithium + Triptans, p.1380
MAO-B inhibitors (Selegiline, Rasagiline)	Inhibition of serotonin metabolism	MAO-B inhibitors + SSRIs or SNRIs, p.772
MAOIs	Inhibition of serotonin metabolism	Note that cases with MAOIs can be life-threatening in nature. MAOIs or RIMAs + Amfetamines and related drugs, p.1383 MAOIs + Dexfenfluramine or Fenfluramine, p.1387 MAOIs or RIMAs + Dextromethorphan and related cough suppressants, p.1387 MAOIs or RIMAs + Opioids; Fentanyl and related drugs, p.1397 MAOIs or RIMAs + Opioids; Pethidine (Meperidine) , p.1399 MAOIs or RIMAs + Opioids; Tramadol, p.1399 MAOIs or RIMAs + SNRIs, p.1401 MAOIs or RIMAs + SSRIs, p.1401
Methylthioninium chloride (Methylene blue)	Inhibition of serotonin metabolism	Antidepressants + Methylthioninium chloride (Methylene blue), p.1466
Mirtazapine	Increased serotonin release	Mirtazapine + SSRIs, p.1474 SNRIs; Venlafaxine + Mirtazapine , p.1482
Opioids*		MAOIs or RIMAs + Opioids; Dextropropoxyphene (Propoxyphene), p.1397 MAOIs or RIMAs + Opioids; Fentanyl and related drugs, p.1397 MAOIs or RIMAs + Opioids; Pethidine (Meperidine), p.1399 MAOIs or RIMAs + Opioids; Tramadol, p.1399 SSRIs + Opioids, p.1492
Pethidine (Meperidine), Tramadol	Increased serotonin release	
Dextropropoxyphene (Propoxyphene), Fentanyl, Methadone, Pentazocine, Pethidine (Meperidine), Tramadol See also Dextromethorphan, above.	Inhibition of serotonin uptake	
Sibutramine	Inhibition of serotonin uptake	SSRIs + Sibutramine, p.1495
SNRIs	Inhibition of serotonin uptake	Linezolid + SNRIs, p.328 MAO-B inhibitors + SSRIs or SNRIs, p.772 SNRIs; Venlafaxine + Mirtazapine, p.1482 SNRIs; Venlafaxine + Trazodone, p.1484 SNRIs + SSRIs, p.1478
SSRIs See also Dapoxetine, above.	Inhibition of serotonin uptake	SSRIs + Tryptophan, p.1497 Linezolid + SSRIs, p.328 SSRIs + Dextromethorphan, p.1566 MAOIs or RIMAs + SSRIs, p.1401
St John's wort (*Hypericum perforatum*)	Inhibition of serotonin uptake	SNRIs + St John's wort (*Hypericum perforatum*) , p.1479 SSRIs + St John's wort (*Hypericum perforatum*) , p.1496
Trazodone	Inhibition of serotonin uptake	MAOIs or RIMAs + Trazodone, p.1403 SNRIs; Venlafaxine + Trazodone, p.1484
Tricyclic antidepressants* Clomipramine, Imipramine	Inhibition of serotonin uptake	Tricyclic antidepressants + SNRIs, p.1514 Tricyclic and related antidepressants + SSRIs, p.1515
Triptans	Increased serotonin concentrations	Triptans + SSRIs or SNRIs, p.648 Triptans + MAOIs, p.646
Tryptophan	Increased serotonin production	MAOIs + Tryptophan, p.1404
Vortioxetine	Inhibition of serotonin uptake	

List not exhaustive
*Often all drugs of this class are associated with this effect, but, based on their pharmacology only the named examples are expected to have serotonergic effects.

predominate. In addition the onset of serotonin toxicity is usually rapid and within a few hours of the first dose of the offending drug, whereas neuroleptic malignant syndrome has a more gradual and insidious onset.

The most serious manifestations of serotonin syndrome appear to be related to the use of MAOIs or MAOI-like drugs, which inhibit serotonin metabolism. The syndrome can develop shortly after one serotonergic drug is added to another, or even if one is replaced by another without allowing a long enough washout period in between, and the problem usually resolves within about 24 hours if both drugs are withdrawn and supportive measures given. Most patients recover uneventfully, but there have been a few fatalities.

Following the first report of this syndrome, many other cases have been described involving tryptophan and MAOIs, the tricyclic antidepressants and MAOIs, and, more recently, the SSRIs, but other serotonergic drugs have also been involved and the list continues to grow. Those drugs commonly associated with serotonin toxicity, with a definable mechanism for increased serotonin concentrations are listed in 'Table 35.3', p.1472, along with examples of cases where serotonin syndrome was said to have developed as a result of their concurrent use. Many other drugs have been suggested to cause serotonin syndrome, but in the absence of a reasonable body of evidence, or a reasonable underlying mechanism for such an effect, these have not been included.

It is still not at all clear why many patients can take two, or sometimes several serotonergic drugs together without problems, while a very small number develop this potentially serious toxic reaction, but it certainly suggests that there are other factors involved that have yet to be identified. The full story is likely to be much more complex than just the simple additive effects of two drugs, and although in some instances a pharmacokinetic interaction potentially contributes, see 'Tricyclic and related antidepressants + SSRIs', p.1515, this seems unlikely to be the only additional factor involved.

It is important to recognise the possibility of serotonin toxicity early, as the patient's condition can rapidly deteriorate. Potentially precipitating drugs should be stopped, bearing in mind that if extended-release preparations or drugs with a long half-life (such as fluoxetine) have been taken the patient might take longer to respond to this action. The mainstay of treatment is supportive care and the intensity of further therapy depends on the severity of the condition. Agitated patients might benefit from the use of a benzodiazepine. Patients might also benefit from the administration of serotonin antagonists (5-HT_{2A}-receptor antagonists) such as cyproheptadine or chlorpromazine, but note that some suggest that chlorpromazine should not be given if the patient is hypotensive. Propranolol, bromocriptine, and dantrolene have also been used, but these are no longer recommended. Because of the potential severity of the condition, a poison-control centre, clinical pharmacology service or medical toxicologist should be consulted for up-to-date advice.[4]

1. Isbister GK, Buckley NA, Whyte IM. Serotonin toxicity: a practical approach to diagnosis and treatment. *Med J Aust* (2007) 187, 361–5.
2. Sternbach H. The serotonin syndrome. *Am J Psychiatry* (1991) 148, 705–13.
3. Dunkley EJC, Isbister GK, Sibbritt D, Dawson AH, Whyte IM. The Hunter Serotonin toxicity criteria: simple and accurate diagnostic decision rules for serotonin toxicity. *Q J Med* (2003) 96, 635–43.
4. Boyer EW, Shannon M. The serotonin syndrome. *N Engl J Med* (2005) 352, 1112–20.

Mirtazapine + Antiepileptics; Enzyme-inducing

Carbamazepine and phenytoin can decrease the exposure to mirtazapine. Other enzyme-inducing antiepileptics would be expected to interact similarly. Carbamazepine and phenytoin pharmacokinetics are unaffected by mirtazapine.

Clinical evidence

(a) Carbamazepine

In a placebo-controlled study, healthy subjects were given carbamazepine (at steady state) with mirtazapine for 7 days. It was found that carbamazepine decreased the AUC and maximum plasma concentration of mirtazapine by 63% and 44%, respectively, and increased the maximum concentration (but not the AUC) of the metabolite, demethylmirtazapine. Another related study found that mirtazapine did not affect the pharmacokinetics of carbamazepine.[1] In a study in 46 patients with unipolar depression given mirtazapine 45 mg daily for 2 weeks, the addition of carbamazepine for 3 weeks (dose adjusted to achieve target concentrations) in 10 of these patients decreased the concentration of mirtazapine by 47%.[2]

(b) Phenytoin

A study in 9 healthy subjects given phenytoin 200 mg daily for 17 days, with mirtazapine 15 mg daily for 2 days from day 11, and then 30 mg daily for 5 days, found that mirtazapine had no effect on the steady-state pharmacokinetics of phenytoin.[3] In a second associated study, 8 healthy subjects were given mirtazapine 15 mg daily for 2 days then 30 mg daily for 15 days with phenytoin 200 mg daily on days 8 to 17. It was found that phenytoin decreased the AUC and maximum plasma concentration of mirtazapine by 47% and 33%, respectively.[3]

Mechanism

Mirtazapine is metabolised by CYP1A2, CYP2D6, and CYP3A4, and it is likely that carbamazepine and phenytoin induce its metabolism by these routes, resulting in the decreased exposure seen in the studies.

Importance and management

The pharmacokinetic interactions between mirtazapine and carbamazepine or phenytoin would appear to be established. Although the clinical relevance of the slight to moderate decreases in exposure to mirtazapine has not been established, it would not be unexpected for decreases of this magnitude to result in reduced efficacy in some patients. Monitor concurrent use carefully. The UK manufacturers of mirtazapine advise that if carbamazepine, phenytoin, or other drugs that induce drug metabolism (such as **rifampicin (rifampin)**) are given with mirtazapine, the mirtazapine dose might have to be increased. Further, if treatment with an inducer is stopped, the mirtazapine dose might have to be reduced.[4] Although not specifically named, **fosphenytoin**, **phenobarbital**, and **primidone** can also induce cytochrome P450 isoenzymes, and they therefore might interact similarly.

Note that, as with other antidepressants, the use of mirtazapine should be carefully considered in patients taking these drugs for epilepsy, because of the possible increased risk of seizures.

1. Sitsen JMA, Maris FA, Timmer CJ. Drug-drug interaction studies with mirtazapine and carbamazepine in healthy male subjects. *Eur J Drug Metab Pharmacokinet* (2001) 26, 109–21.
2. Schüle C, Baghai TC, Eser D, Nothdurfter C, Rupprecht R. Lithium but not carbamazepine augments antidepressant efficacy of mirtazapine in unipolar depression: an open-label study. *World J Biol Psychiatry* (2009) 10, 390–9.
3. Spaans E, van den Heuvel MW, Schnabel PG, Peeters PAM, Chin-Kon-Sung UG, Colbers EPH, Sitsen JMA. Concomitant use of mirtazapine and phenytoin: a drug-drug interaction study in healthy male subjects. *Eur J Clin Pharmacol* (2002) 58, 423–9.
4. Zispin SolTab (Mirtazapine). Merck Sharp & Dohme Ltd. UK Summary of product characteristics, February 2015.

Mirtazapine + Benzodiazepines

The sedative effects of mirtazapine are increased by the benzodiazepines.

Clinical evidence, mechanism, importance and management

A single-dose study in 12 healthy subjects found that the pharmacokinetics of mirtazapine 15 mg and **diazepam** 15 mg were not affected by concurrent use. However, **diazepam** further impaired the action of mirtazapine on objectively measured skill performance: the combined actions were mostly additive. The effects seen were of similar magnitude to those found when amitriptyline 50 mg was given with diazepam 15 mg.[1]

Mirtazapine has prominent sedative effects and these are likely to be additive with those of diazepam and any other benzodiazepine.

This additive pharmacodynamic interaction is expected. Caution is required on concurrent use, particularly on starting treatment, and patients should be advised to avoid driving or operating machinery if feeling drowsy (note that this caution would apply to either drug used alone). Note that the US manufacturer actually recommends that patients taking mirtazapine avoid the use of diazepam and similar drugs, but this is probably overly cautious.[2]

1. Mattila M, Mattila MJ, Vrijmoed-de Vries M, Kuitunen T. Actions and interactions of psychotropic drugs on human performance and mood: single doses of ORG 3770, amitriptyline and diazepam. *Pharmacol Toxicol* (1989) 65, 81–8.
2. Remeron (Mirtazapine). Merck Sharp & Dohme Corp. US Prescribing information, January 2014.

Mirtazapine + Cimetidine

Cimetidine slightly increases the exposure to mirtazapine.

Clinical evidence, mechanism, importance and management

In a placebo-controlled, crossover study in 12 healthy subjects, cimetidine 800 mg twice daily was given for 14 days, with mirtazapine 30 mg added at night on days 6 to 12. Cimetidine increased the AUC and maximum plasma concentration of mirtazapine by 54% and 22%, respectively: minimum and average mirtazapine plasma concentrations, at steady state, were increased by 61% and 54%, respectively. The pharmacokinetics of the demethyl metabolite of mirtazapine were little affected. Mirtazapine did not affect the pharmacokinetics of cimetidine.[1]

Mechanism

It seems likely that cimetidine, a non-specific enzyme inhibitor, decreases the metabolism of mirtazapine.

Importance and management

This pharmacokinetic interaction between cimetidine and mirtazapine would appear to be established, but the clinical effect of the slight increase in exposure to mirtazapine does not appear to have been assessed. The authors suggested that the clinical relevance of this interaction is probably limited because of the variability of plasma mirtazapine concentrations in patients.[1] Nevertheless, the UK and US manufacturers advise that the mirtazapine dose might need to be reduced during concurrent use and increased when cimetidine is stopped.[2,3] Monitor for an increase in mirtazapine adverse effects (oedema, drowsiness, headache) when starting cimetidine.

1. Sitsen JMA, Maris FA, Timmer CJ. Concomitant use of mirtazapine and cimetidine: a drug-drug interaction study in healthy male subjects. *Eur J Clin Pharmacol* (2000) 56, 389–94.
2. Zispin SolTab (Mirtazapine). Merck Sharp & Dohme Ltd. UK Summary of product characteristics, February 2015.
3. Remeron (Mirtazapine). Merck Sharp & Dohme Corp. US prescribing information, January 2014.

Mirtazapine + CYP3A4 inhibitors

Ketoconazole appears to slightly increase the exposure to mirtazapine. Other potent CYP3A4 inhibitors might be expected to interact similarly.

Clinical evidence, mechanism, importance and management

The UK manufacturer of mirtazapine notes that **ketoconazole** increased the maximum plasma concentration and AUC of mirtazapine by about 40% and 50%, respectively.[1]

Mirtazapine is extensively metabolised by CYP3A4, which is thought to be responsible for the formation of the *N*-demethyl and *N*-oxide metabolites. Ketoconazole is a potent inhibitor of CYP3A4, and concurrent use increases mirtazapine exposure.

This pharmacokinetic interaction would appear to be established, but the clinical effect of slightly increasing the exposure to mirtazapine has not been assessed. Until more is known, some caution might be appropriate. Note that the UK manufacturer of mirtazapine advises caution and that a decrease in the dose of mirtazapine might be needed when potent inhibitors of CYP3A4 are also given,[1] see 'Table 1.9', p.11 for a list. Note that they also name **erythromycin**, and **nefazodone**,[1] but these are generally considered moderate CYP3A4 inhibitors.

1. Zispin SolTab (Mirtazapine). Merck Sharp & Dohme Ltd. UK Summary of product characteristics, February 2015.

Mirtazapine + SSRIs

In a pharmacokinetic study, paroxetine negligibly increased the exposure to mirtazapine, but mirtazapine did not affect the pharmacokinetics of paroxetine. A case report describes a large increase in the concentration of mirtazapine in a patient taking fluvoxamine. A couple of isolated reports describe possible serotonin syndrome when mirtazapine was used with fluoxetine and fluvoxamine, and a possible case was reported in a study with paroxetine. Two cases of manic symptoms in patients taking fluoxetine when mirtazapine was started, restless legs syndrome in 3 patients taking fluoxetine and mirtazapine, and a case of hypomania associated with the concurrent use of mirtazapine and sertraline, have been reported.

Clinical evidence

(a) Escitalopram

For a report of bleeding associated with the combined use of escitalopram, mirtazapine and venlafaxine, see 'SNRIs + SSRIs', p.1478.

(b) Fluoxetine

An isolated report describes a case of possible serotonin syndrome in a 75-year-old woman when fluoxetine 20 mg daily was discontinued and mirtazapine 30 mg daily started soon afterwards (exact interval not stated).[1] Symptoms including dizziness, headache, nausea, dry mouth, anxiety, agitation, suicidal ideas, and difficulty in walking occurred within hours of the first dose of mirtazapine. Symptoms worsened until mirtazapine was discontinued on day 5, after which an improvement was noticed. Fluoxetine was restarted on day 7. It has been suggested that this case is more consistent with fluoxetine-withdrawal syndrome, with the mirtazapine worsening the symptoms of anxiety.[2] Two other case reports describe the development of manic symptoms in patients taking fluoxetine, when mirtazapine was started.[3,4] A 66-year-old woman developed mania and delusions when she was switched from fluoxetine 20 mg daily to mirtazapine 30 mg daily without a washout period. The mirtazapine was discontinued, and valproate and risperidone started. Symptoms subsided over the following 2 weeks.[3] The second case describes a 48-year old woman taking fluoxetine 40 mg daily, who entered a manic state 7 weeks after mirtazapine 30 mg daily was added to her treatment, and which persisted for 3 weeks after the fluoxetine was stopped.[4]

Restless legs syndrome occurred in 3 patients taking fluoxetine and mirtazapine as part of a study of major depression with insomnia. Symptoms were bothersome paraesthesias and jerks in both lower extremities, with exacerbation at night, and relief upon movement. Treatment with mirtazapine was discontinued and symptoms ceased after 2 days.[5]

(c) Fluvoxamine

A 26-year-old woman with a 12-year history of anorexia nervosa, taking fluvoxamine 200 mg daily, developed symptoms consistent with serotonin syndrome (tremors, restlessness, twitching, flushing, diaphoresis, nausea) about 4 days after starting mirtazapine 30 mg daily.[6] It has been suggested that this case is not consistent with serotonin syndrome, and that the adverse effects were attributable to an increase in mirtazapine concentration, possibly caused by fluvoxamine.[2]

A 17-year-old boy taking mirtazapine 30 mg daily experienced increased anxiety when fluvoxamine 100 mg daily was also given. His mirtazapine concentration was increased 3-fold. In a second patient, a 43-year-old woman taking mirtazapine 15 mg daily, the addition of fluvoxamine 50 mg daily resulted in a 4-fold increase in mirtazapine concentration, accompanied by mood improvements.[7]

(d) Paroxetine

A crossover study in 21 healthy subjects given mirtazapine 30 mg daily, paroxetine 40 mg daily, or a combination of both, for 9 days, found that paroxetine increased the AUC of mirtazapine by 17%. Mirtazapine did not alter the pharmacokinetics of paroxetine. The results of psychometric assessments suggested that concurrent use of mirtazapine and paroxetine did not alter cognitive function, or cause major changes in mood or sleep, compared with the use of either drug alone. One subject developed serotonin syndrome after receiving mirtazapine for 9 days followed by mirtazapine with paroxetine for 9 days, and then paroxetine alone. The symptoms rapidly resolved after paroxetine was stopped.[8]

(e) Sertraline

A woman taking sertraline 250 mg daily was also given mirtazapine 15 mg daily because of inadequately controlled depression. Within 4 days she developed hypomanic symptoms and she stopped taking the mirtazapine. The hypomania resolved within 3 days but her depression then recurred.[9]

Mechanism

Mirtazapine is metabolised mainly by CYP1A2, CYP2D6, and CYP3A4. These isoenzymes (particularly CYP1A2) are inhibited by fluvoxamine, and so concurrent use might therefore increase mirtazapine concentrations. Paroxetine is an inhibitor of CYP2D6, and this appeared to have little effect on mirtazapine exposure.

The SSRIs and mirtazapine affect serotonin transmission, and combined use of serotonergic drugs has rarely caused the symptoms described as serotonin syndrome. It has been suggested that serotonin toxicity with mirtazapine is unlikely, because it has 5-HT_2-blocking effects,[2] but several reports suggest serotonin syndrome might be associated with the combined use of mirtazapine and an SSRI.

Importance and management

Evidence for a pharmacokinetic interaction between mirtazapine and the SSRIs is limited; with one study finding a negligible increase in mirtazapine exposure with **paroxetine**, and a case report of a patient whose mirtazapine concentration was greatly increased while taking **fluvoxamine**. Further, the clinical implications of concurrent use are not firmly established. Descriptions of patients experiencing symptoms suggestive of serotonin syndrome exist for **fluoxetine**, **fluvoxamine**, and **paroxetine**, indicating that the combined use of mirtazapine and the SSRIs can lead to serotonin syndrome. However, whether two of these cases are consistent with serotonin syndrome has been disputed.[2] Nevertheless, these and other reports of anxiety, hypomania, and the development of manic symptoms highlight the need for some caution during concurrent use. One manufacturer of mirtazapine briefly notes that, from postmarketing experience, it appears that serotonin syndrome occurs very rarely in patients taking mirtazapine alone. They recommend caution if combination with an SSRI is required, and close monitoring for symptoms of serotonin syndrome, with discontinuation of mirtazapine if this occurs.[10] It is worth noting that NICE guidelines in the UK state that augmenting SSRIs with mirtazapine might be beneficial in the treatment of depression.[11] For more information on serotonin syndrome and its management, see 'Drugs that cause serotonin syndrome + Other drugs that cause serotonin syndrome', p.1471.

1. Benazzi F. Serotonin syndrome with mirtazapine-fluoxetine combination. *Int J Geriatr Psychiatry* (1998) 13, 495–6.
2. Isbister GK, Dawson AH, Whyte IM. Comment: serotonin syndrome induced by fluvoxamine and mirtazapine. *Ann Pharmacother* (2001) 35, 1674–5.
3. Liu CC, Liang KY, Liao SC. Antidepressant-associated mania: soon after switch from fluoxetine to mirtazapine in an elderly woman with mixed depressive features. *J Psychopharmacol* (2009) 23, 220–2.
4. Ng B. Mania associated with mirtazapine augmentation of fluoxetine. *Depress Anxiety* (2002) 15, 46–7.
5. Prospero-Garcia KA, Torres-Ruiz A, Ramirez-Bermudez J, Velazquez-Moctezuma J, Arana-Lechuga Y, Teran-Perez G. Fluoxetine-mirtazapine interaction may induce restless legs syndrome: report of 3 cases from a clinical trial. *J Clin Psychiatry* (2006) 67, 1820.
6. Demers JC, Malone M. Serotonin syndrome induced by fluvoxamine and mirtazapine. *Ann Pharmacother* (2001) 35, 1217–20.
7. Anttila SAK, Rasanen I, Leinonen EVJ. Fluvoxamine augmentation increases serum mirtazapine concentrations three- to fourfold. *Ann Pharmacother* (2001) 35, 1221–3.
8. Ruwe FJL, Smulders RA, Kleijn HJ, Hartmans HLA, Sitsen JMA. Mirtazapine and paroxetine: a drug-drug interaction study in healthy subjects. *Hum Psychopharmacol* (2001) 16, 449–59.
9. Soutullo CA, McElroy SL, Keck PE. Hypomania associated with mirtazapine augmentation of sertraline. *J Clin Psychiatry* (1998) 59, 320.
10. Zispin SolTab (Mirtazapine). Merck Sharp and Dohme Ltd. UK Summary of product characteristics, February 2015.
11. National Institute for Clinical Excellence. Antidepressant treatment in adults. (issued September 2014). Available at: http://pathways.nice.org.uk/pathways/depression (accessed 28/10/15).

Mirtazapine + Tricyclic antidepressants

The concurrent use of mirtazapine with amitriptyline might have a minor effect on the maximum concentration of both drugs, but not on their exposure.

Clinical evidence

In a crossover study involving 24 healthy subjects, mirtazapine 15 mg, increasing to 30 mg daily, **amitriptyline** 25 mg, increasing to 75 mg daily or both drugs were given for periods of 9 days. **Amitriptyline** increased the maximum plasma concentration of mirtazapine, in male subjects only, by 36%. Mirtazapine increased the maximum plasma concentration of **amitriptyline** in male subjects by 23%, but in female subjects the maximum plasma concentration was *decreased* by 23%. Other pharmacokinetic parameters of amitriptyline and mirtazapine (AUC, minimum concentration, time to maximum concentration) and their main metabolites nortriptyline and demethylmirtazapine were not affected by concurrent use. The authors note that concurrent use had no consistent effects on blood pressure, heart rate, and ECG, although they note that four subjects developed postural hypotension.[1]

Mechanism

The pharmacokinetic changes were suggested to be due to differences in rates of absorption of the drugs, since the maximum concentrations were minimally altered, but the AUCs were not. Mirtazapine has alpha-blocking activity, and can therefore cause hypotension. Amitriptyline can also cause hypotension. Therefore postural hypotension might have developed as a result of the additive effects of the two drugs.

Importance and management

Evidence for an interaction between mirtazapine and amitriptyline appears to be limited to this one study. Although the changes in maximum concentrations here were statistically significant, they are minor, and there were no changes in the exposure to the drugs. These changes are therefore unlikely to be clinically relevant. There is no pharmacokinetic reason to adjust the dose of either of these drugs on concurrent use.

Note that mirtazapine and the tricyclics, **clomipramine** and **imipramine**, have serotonergic effects, and their concurrent use might lead to the serotonin syndrome. Serotonin syndrome is a rare adverse effect, but because of its severity, some caution is warranted if both drugs are given. For more information on serotonin syndrome and its management, see 'Drugs that cause serotonin syndrome + Other drugs that cause serotonin syndrome', p.1471.

1. Sennef C, Timmer CJ, Sitsen JMA. Mirtazapine in combination with amitriptyline: a drug-drug interaction study in healthy subjects. *Hum Psychopharmacol* (2003) 18, 91–101.

Nefazodone + Antidepressants

A report describes a woman who developed marked and acute hypotension and weakness when desipramine, fluoxetine, and venlafaxine were replaced by nefazodone. Other cases describe serotonin syndrome in patients given nefazodone together, or sequentially, with another serotonergic drug (amitriptyline, paroxetine, St John's wort, or trazodone). There is no pharmacokinetic interaction between desipramine and nefazodone.

Clinical evidence, mechanism, importance and management

Note that, due to adverse hepatic effects nefazodone has been widely withdrawn from the market.

(a) MAOIs

When more widely available, the US manufacturer stated that nefazodone should not be used with an MAOI or within 2 weeks of discontinuing treatment with an MAOI. Conversely at least one week should be allowed after stopping nefazodone before starting an MAOI.[1] There appears to be no direct clinical evidence that an adverse interaction occurs.

(b) Reboxetine

Nefazodone is predicted to increase the plasma concentrations of reboxetine, see 'Reboxetine + CYP3A4 inducers or inhibitors', below.

(c) SSRIs

Anecdotal evidence has suggested that patients who are switched from an SSRI to nefazodone might tolerate nefazodone poorly. Nevertheless, in a 12-week, open study involving 26 patients with depression, nefazodone 100 to 600 mg daily was equally well tolerated in 13 patients who had discontinued an SSRI within 1 to 4 weeks as in 13 patients who had received no antidepressant treatment for the previous 6 months. However, the patients who had recent exposure to an SSRI (within the previous 4 weeks) were given a washout period of 4 to 5 days for short half-life SSRIs or 7 days for **fluoxetine** before starting nefazodone.[2] Cases with specific SSRIs are discussed in the subsections below.

1. Fluoxetine. A woman with a one-year history of DSM-IV major depressive disorder and panic disorder was given daily doses of **desipramine** 75 mg, fluoxetine 20 mg, **venlafaxine** 37.5 mg, **clonazepam** 3 mg, and **valproate** 400 mg with no adverse effects, except a dry mouth and sexual difficulties.[3] The first three drugs were stopped and replaced by nefazodone 100 mg twice daily, started about 12 hours later. Within an hour of the first dose she felt very weak and her blood pressure was found to have fallen to only 90/60 mmHg (normally 120/90 mmHg). On waking the next day she had severe weakness, unsteady gait, pale, cool and sweaty skin, and paraesthesia. During the day she took two further 100 mg doses of nefazodone and her condition persisted and worsened with continuing hypotension. The nefazodone was discontinued and by the following day the weakness had improved, disappearing over the next few days. Within a week nefazodone 200 mg daily was reintroduced without problems.

The US manufacturer of nefazodone noted that nefazodone did not alter the pharmacokinetics of fluoxetine, but fluoxetine increased the AUC of the metabolites of nefazodone up to 6-fold.[1] When nefazodone 200 mg twice daily was given to patients who had been taking fluoxetine for 7 days, adverse effects (including headache and nausea) were increased. The US manufacturer advised allowing a washout period of at least one week (more might be needed depending on dose and individual patient characteristics) to minimise these effects.[1] It therefore seems likely that fluoxetine was the interacting drug, but it is impossible to rule out a contribution from the other drugs.

2. Paroxetine. A woman had her nefazodone withdrawn after about 6 months of treatment, tapering over the last fortnight to 75 mg every 12 hours. Within a day she started taking paroxetine 20 mg daily and valproic acid, and was admitted the next day with muscle rigidity, uncoordinated muscle tremors, flailing arms and twitching legs, diaphoresis, and agitation. This was identified as serotonin syndrome. Rechallenge with paroxetine 7 days later was uneventful.[4]

(d) St John's wort (Hypericum perforatum)

An elderly patient taking nefazodone 100 mg twice daily, developed symptoms similar to serotonin syndrome within 3 days of starting to take St John's wort 300 mg three times daily. The symptoms included nausea, vomiting, and restlessness. She was asked to stop both medications, but continued the St John's wort and her symptoms gradually improved over a one-week period.[5]

(e) Trazodone

A woman taking irbesartan for hypertension was also given nefazodone at an initial dose of 200 mg daily, followed by 400 mg daily for about 5 weeks. Four days after the dose was increased to 500 mg daily, and trazodone 25 to 50 mg daily was also added as a hypnotic, she was admitted to hospital with a blood pressure of 240/120 mmHg. She was confused, had difficulty concentrating and had numbness on the right side of her lips, nose, and right-hand fingers, flushed pruritic skin, nausea, and loose stools. On examination she was restless, hyperreflexic, and diaphoretic. Nefazodone and trazodone were discontinued, and she recovered after treatment with labetalol, clonidine, amlodipine, and an increased irbesartan dose.[6] Although trazodone is used with other serotonergic drugs, it is important to be aware that this might lead to the potentially fatal serotonin syndrome. See 'Drugs that cause serotonin syndrome + Other drugs that cause serotonin syndrome', p.1471 for further details on the development and management of this syndrome.

The UK and US manufacturers of trazodone state that *in vitro* drug metabolism studies suggest that there is a potential for drug interactions when trazodone is given with a potent CYP3A4 inhibitor. There might be substantial increases in trazodone concentrations, with the potential for adverse effects, and a lower dose of trazodone should be considered.[7,8] The UK manufacturer specifically mentions nefazodone, and suggests avoidance of the combination where possible,[7] however note that nefazodone is generally considered to be a moderate inhibitor of CYP3A4.

(f) Tricyclic antidepressants

1. Amitriptyline. A woman who had been taking amitriptyline 10 mg at night and thioridazine developed serotonin syndrome after taking half a tablet of nefazodone (strength unspecified).[9]

2. Desipramine. In a study in healthy subjects, desipramine titrated to 75 mg daily did not change the pharmacokinetics of nefazodone titrated to 150 mg twice daily, but the AUC of the nefazodone metabolite, meta-chlorophenylpiperazine, was increased by 40%. There was no change in the pharmacokinetics of desipramine or its metabolite. No specific dose adjustments were said to be required on concurrent use.[10]

1. Nefazodone hydrochloride. Watson Laboratories Inc. US Prescribing information, June 2004.
2. Mischoulon D, Opitz G, Kelly K, Fava M, Rosenbaum JF. A preliminary open study of the tolerability and effectiveness of nefazodone in major depressive disorder: comparing patients who recently discontinued an SSRI with those on no recent antidepressant treatment. *Depress Anxiety* (2004) 19, 43–50.
3. Benazzi F. Dangerous interaction with nefazodone added to fluoxetine, desipramine, venlafaxine, valproate and clonazepam combination therapy. *J Psychopharmacol* (1997) 11, 190–1.
4. John L, Perreault MM, Tao T, Blew PG. Serotonin syndrome associated with nefazodone and paroxetine. *Ann Emerg Med* (1997) 29, 287–9.
5. Lantz MS, Buchalter E, Giambanco V. St. John's wort and antidepressant drug interactions in the elderly. *J Geriatr Psychiatry Neurol* (1999) 12, 7–10.
6. Margolese HC, Chouinard G. Serotonin syndrome from addition of low-dose trazodone to nefazodone. *Am J Psychiatry* (2000) 157, 1022.
7. Molipaxin (Trazodone hydrochloride). Zentiva. UK Summary of product characteristics, August 2013.
8. Trazodone hydrochloride. Apotex Inc. US Prescribing information, August 2014.
9. Chan BSH, Graudins A, Whyte IM, Dawson AH, Braitberg G, Duggin GG. Serotonin syndrome resulting from drug interactions. *Med J Aust* (1998) 169, 523–5.
10. Khan AY, Preskorn SH, Horst WD. Coadministration of nefazodone and desipramine: a pharmacokinetic interaction study. *JPMA* (2007) 57, 230–5.

Nefazodone + Cimetidine

No pharmacokinetic interaction occurs between nefazodone and cimetidine.

Clinical evidence, mechanism, importance and management

In a study, 18 healthy subjects were given cimetidine 300 mg four times daily and nefazodone 200 mg every 12 hours for a week. Concurrent use did not affect the steady-state pharmacokinetics of either drug. Therefore no dose adjustments would seem to be necessary if both drugs are used concurrently.[1]

Note that nefazodone has been withdrawn in many countries because of cases of liver toxicity.

1. Barbhaiya RH, Shukla UA, Greene DS. Lack of interaction between nefazodone and cimetidine: a steady state pharmacokinetic study in humans. *Br J Clin Pharmacol* (1995) 40, 161–5.

Reboxetine + CYP3A4 inducers or inhibitors

Ketoconazole slightly increases the exposure to reboxetine. Other CYP3A4 inhibitors are expected to interact similarly. Low reboxetine concentrations have been reported in two patients also taking carbamazepine and phenobarbital. Other CYP3A4 inducers might interact similarly.

Clinical evidence

In a crossover study, 11 healthy subjects were given **ketoconazole** 200 mg daily for 5 days with a single 4-mg dose of reboxetine taken on the second day. The AUCs of the enantiomers of reboxetine were increased by 58% and 43%, without appreciably altering the maximum concentrations. Their clearance was decreased by 34% and 24%.[1]

A case report describes reboxetine concentrations that were lower than expected (by comparison with historical controls) in two patients, one receiving **carbamazepine** (with concurrent olanzapine, clonazepam, alprazolam, and buspirone) and one receiving **phenobarbital** (with concurrent clozapine and clonazepam).[2]

Mechanism

Reboxetine is metabolised principally by CYP3A4, of which ketoconazole is an inhibitor. Concurrent use therefore decreases reboxetine metabolism and increases its exposure. Carbamazepine and phenobarbital are inducers of CYP3A4, and they would therefore be expected to increase reboxetine metabolism and decrease its exposure.

Importance and management

A pharmacokinetic interaction between reboxetine and ketoconazole would appear to be established, but it would be useful to confirm the magnitude at steady-state concentrations of reboxetine. Note also that the reboxetine was given on day 2 of a 5-day course of ketoconazole and its inhibitory effects will not have been maximal after only 24 hours. The clinical relevance of an increase in the AUC of reboxetine of about 50% is unknown. The authors of the paper suggest that a reduction in reboxetine dose should be considered.[1] However, the UK manufacturer states that because reboxetine has a narrow therapeutic index, inhibition of metabolism is of major concern, and therefore inhibitors of CYP3A4 should not be given with reboxetine.[3] For a list of CYP3A4 inhibitors see 'Table 1.9', p.11. Note that they name **erythromycin**, **fluvoxamine**, and **nefazodone** as potent inhibitors, but erythromycin and nefazodone are generally considered moderate, and fluvoxamine as weak. This seems an overly cautious approach, especially given that available data suggest that patients with hepatic impairment have a 2-fold higher AUC,[4] and the recommendation in this situation is just for a halving of the starting dose of reboxetine.[3] The effect of steady-state ketoconazole (and other inhibitors) might be greater than that seen in the study, but a reduced reboxetine dose would seem acceptable, with appropriate titration based on efficacy and adverse effects.

The case reports involving carbamazepine and phenobarbital appear to be the only ones reported, and do not wholly confirm an interaction as reboxetine concentrations were not measured in the absence of these enzyme inducers. However, the UK manufacturer of reboxetine advises that on the basis of such reports, other CYP3A4 inducers might act similarly, but makes no recommendations.[3] Nevertheless, in light of these cases, and in view of the fact that CYP3A4 inhibitors are known to increase reboxetine exposure, it would seem prudent to monitor the efficacy of treatment with reboxetine in patients receiving a known inducer of CYP3A4, and consider increasing the dose if necessary. For a list of CYP3A4 inducers, see 'Table 1.9', p.11.

1. Herman BD, Fleishaker JC, Brown MT. Ketoconazole inhibits the clearance of the enantiomers of the antidepressant reboxetine in humans. *Clin Pharmacol Ther* (1999) 66, 374–9.
2. Helland A, Spigset O. Low serum concentrations of reboxetine in 2 patients treated with CYP3A4 inducers. *J Clin Psychopharmacol* (2007) 27, 308–10.
3. Edronax (Reboxetine). Pfizer Ltd. UK Summary of product characteristics, July 2013.
4. Fleishaker JC. Clinical pharmacokinetics of reboxetine, a selective norepinephrine reuptake inhibitor for the treatment of patients with depression. *Clin Pharmacokinet* (2000) 39, 413–27.

Reboxetine + Miscellaneous

Hypokalaemia might occur if reboxetine is used with potassium-depleting diuretics. Food does not appear to alter the absorption of reboxetine. Concurrent use of reboxetine with MAOIs, including linezolid and methylthioninium chloride, is predicted to have the potential to cause a tyramine-like effect [hypertensive crisis].

Clinical evidence, mechanism, importance and management

(a) Diuretics

The UK manufacturer of reboxetine briefly notes that hypokalaemia might occur if reboxetine is used with **potassium-depleting diuretics**.[1]

(b) Food

The UK manufacturer of reboxetine notes that the extent of the absorption of reboxetine is not affected by food, but it is delayed.[1] Reboxetine can be taken without regard to food.

(c) MAOIs

The UK manufacturer of reboxetine advises the avoidance of MAOIs, including **linezolid** and **methylthioninium chloride**, because of the potential risk of a tyramine-like effect [hypertensive crisis].[1]

1. Edronax (Reboxetine). Pfizer Ltd. UK Summary of product characteristics, July 2013.

Reboxetine + Quinidine

Quinidine does not appear to alter the pharmacokinetics of reboxetine.

Clinical evidence, mechanism, importance and management

In a study in 8 healthy subjects who were of the CYP2D6 extensive metaboliser phenotype (that is, they had normal activity of this isoenzyme), quinidine (dose not stated) did not alter the pharmacokinetics of reboxetine 1 mg.[1]

This study suggests that reboxetine is not a substrate of CYP2D6, of which quinidine is an inhibitor. No dose adjustment of reboxetine is likely to be needed if quinidine or other CYP2D6 inhibitors (see 'Table 1.7', p.9 for a list) are also given.

1. Rocchetti M, Pellizzoni C, Poggesi I, Davies DS, Wilkins MR, Hirokawa K, Dostert P, Benedetti MS. Genetic polymorphism and reboxetine metabolism. 1st Congress of the European Association for Clinical Pharmacology and Therapeutics. *Therapie* (1995) (Suppl.), Abstract 80.

Reboxetine + SSRIs

The concurrent use of fluoxetine and reboxetine does not appear to alter the pharmacokinetics of either drug.

Clinical evidence, mechanism, importance and management

In a placebo-controlled study in healthy subjects given reboxetine 4 mg twice daily and **fluoxetine** 20 mg daily for 8 days, there were no differences in the pharmacokinetics of either drug, when compared with another group of subjects given each drug alone.[1] In this study, combined use did not alter oral temperature and the Digit Symbol Substitution Test, which were used as possible indicators of serotonergic adverse effects. There do not appear to be any published cases of serotonin syndrome in patients taking SSRIs and reboxetine.

As reboxetine is metabolised principally by CYP3A4, and **fluoxetine** has only minor CYP3A4 inhibitory activity (see 'Benzodiazepines and related drugs + SSRIs', p.838), the lack of effect seen in the study is not unexpected. Further, reboxetine is not a substrate of CYP2D6 (see 'Reboxetine + Quinidine', above) of which fluoxetine is a potent inhibitor. No dose adjustments for either drug would appear necessary on concurrent use. Based on this evidence, and the known interaction potential of the other SSRIs, no pharmacokinetic interaction would be anticipated with these drugs either. Nevertheless, the manufacturer of reboxetine includes **fluvoxamine** as an example of a potent inhibitor of CYP3A4, and consequently recommends that its concurrent use with reboxetine should be avoided.[2] This appears to be overly cautious, because clinically fluvoxamine only appears to have weak effects on this isoenzyme.

1. Fleishaker JC, Herman BD, Pearson LK, Ionita A, Mucci M. Evaluation of the potential pharmacokinetic/pharmacodynamic interaction between fluoxetine and reboxetine in healthy volunteers. *Clin Drug Invest* (1999) 18, 141–50.
2. Edronax (Reboxetine). Pfizer Ltd. UK Summary of product characteristics, July 2013.

SNRIs + Antihypertensives

Two case reports describe the development of hypertension when desvenlafaxine and venlafaxine were started in patients whose blood pressure was previously well controlled with antihypertensives.

Clinical evidence

(a) Desvenlafaxine

A 62-year-old woman whose blood pressure was well controlled (122/82 mmHg) with **losartan** 50 mg daily and **hydrochlorothiazide** 12.5 mg daily was found to have had an increase in her blood pressure to 200/120 mmHg, 2 weeks after starting desvenlafaxine 50 mg daily. Desvenlafaxine was stopped, escitalopram, buspirone, and clonazepam were started, and within 2 weeks her blood pressure had returned to the normal range.[1]

(b) Venlafaxine

A 53-year-old woman who had her blood pressure well-controlled (130/80 mmHg) while taking **captopril** 25 mg daily and had a low-salt diet, was found to have had an increase in her arterial blood pressure to 180/110 mmHg after she started taking venlafaxine (25 mg daily titrated to 100 mg daily) for depression. It was suggested that the effects of venlafaxine on noradrenaline might have antagonised the efficacy of **captopril**.[2]

For mention of the effects of **propranolol** on venlafaxine exposure and the effects of venlafaxine on **metoprolol** exposure, see 'Beta blockers + Venlafaxine', p.1024.

Mechanism

Venlafaxine and desvenlafaxine are known to cause dose-related hypertension, which can be sustained. Use with antihypertensives might reverse or reduce their effects.

Importance and management

Evidence is limited to case reports and is based on a possible reversal or reduction of the effects of antihypertensives by the SNRIs. Note that all SNRIs used alone can cause hypertension, and as a result general warnings about this exist. The manufacturers of desvenlafaxine,[3] levomilnacipran,[4] milnacipran,[5] and venlafaxine,[6,7] advise that hypertension should be controlled before initiation of treatment. These manufacturers, and the manufacturers of **duloxetine**, also advise that blood pressure should be monitored regularly in all patients.[3-9] If sustained increases in blood pressure occur, some advise considering reducing the SNRI dose, or stopping the SNRI altogether.[3-5,7,8] If concurrent use of an antihypertensive is necessary in patients taking any of these drugs, consideration should be given to this interaction and patients monitored accordingly. Dose adjustments might be necessary.

1. Munoli RN, Praharaj SK, Bhandary RP, Selvaraj AG. Desvenlafaxine-induced worsening of hypertension. *J Neuropsychiatr Clin Neurosci* (2013) 25, E29–30.
2. Sucar DD. Interação medicamentosa de venlafaxina com captopril. *Rev Bras Psiquiatr* (2000) 22, 134–7.
3. Pristiq (Desvenlafaxine succinate). Wyeth Pharmaceuticals Inc. US Prescribing information, July 2014.
4. Fetzima (Levomilnacipran hydrochloride). Forest Pharmaceuticals Inc. US Prescribing information, July 2014.
5. Savella (Milnacipran hydrochloride). Forest Pharmaceuticals Inc. US Prescribing information, November 2013.
6. Efexor XL (Venlafaxine hydrochloride). Pfizer Ltd. UK Summary of product characteristics, December 2013.
7. Effexor XR (Venlafaxine hydrochloride). Wyeth Pharmaceuticals Inc. US Prescribing information, March 2014.
8. Cymbalta (Duloxetine hydrochloride). Eli Lilly and Company Ltd. UK Summary of product characteristics, March 2014.
9. Cymbalta (Duloxetine hydrochloride). Eli Lilly and Company. US Prescribing information, July 2014.

SNRIs + Azoles

Voriconazole slightly increases the exposure to venlafaxine and to its active metabolite *O*-desmethylvenlafaxine; a greater increase was seen in one CYP2D6 poor metaboliser. Ketoconazole negligibly increased the exposure to venlafaxine and *O*-desmethylvenlafaxine in patients who were extensive metabolisers, and slightly to moderately increased exposure in some CYP2D6 poor metabolisers. Ketoconazole appears to slightly increase the exposure to levomilnacipran and desvenlafaxine.

Clinical evidence

(a) Desvenlafaxine

The US manufacturer of desvenlafaxine notes that in a study, **ketoconazole** 200 mg twice daily increased the AUC and maximum concentration of a single 400-mg dose of desvenlafaxine by about 43% and 8%, respectively.[1]

(b) Levomilnacipran

The US manufacturer of levomilnacipran briefly notes that in a study, **ketoconazole** (dose not specified) increased the AUC and maximum concentration of levomilnacipran (dose not specified) about 1.5-fold.[2]

(c) Venlafaxine

1. Ketoconazole. In a study in 14 healthy subjects, all of whom were CYP2D6 extensive metabolisers (that is, they had with normal CYP2D6 activity), ketoconazole 100 mg twice daily for 2 days increased the AUC of venlafaxine and *O*-desmethylvenlafaxine by 21% and 23%, respectively when a single dose of venlafaxine was given on day 2. However, in 6 poor metabolisers (that is, those with low CYP2D6 activity), the response was inconsistent, with 3 out of 6 having increases in venlafaxine AUC of 81%, 126%, and 206%, respectively, and the other 3 showing little or no change.[3] In these 6 subjects, the mean increase was 70%, and the AUC of *O*-desmethylvenlafaxine was also increased (mean 33%).[3,4]

2. Voriconazole. In a crossover study in 12 healthy subjects, the AUC of a single 75-mg dose of venlafaxine given one hour after the last dose of voriconazole 400 mg twice daily for one day and 200 mg twice daily for another day, was unchanged. Similarly, the AUC of the active metabolite, *O*-desmethylvenlafaxine was also unchanged. However the combined AUC for venlafaxine and *O*-desmethylvenlafaxine was increased by 31%. In one subject who was a CYP2D6 poor metaboliser (that is, they had low CYP2D6 activity), the AUC of venlafaxine was 9-fold higher after voriconazole than the mean AUC achieved by the other 11 subjects. Further, the AUC of venlafaxine in this subject was increased almost 2-fold when compared with venlafaxine given alone, and *O*-desmethylvenlafaxine was undetectable. The combined AUC for venlafaxine and *O*-desmethylvenlafaxine was 1.9-fold higher in this subject than in the other 11 subjects. In three subjects who were CYP2D6 ultrarapid metabolisers (that is, they had greater than normal CYP2D6 activity) the AUC of venlafaxine when given alone was about half that of the CYP2D6 extensive metabolisers (that is, those with normal CYP2D6 activity), and voriconazole had similar effects on the pharmacokinetics of venlafaxine as in the extensive metabolisers.[5]

Mechanism

Levomilnacipran is principally metabolised by CYP3A4 and to a minor extent by other isoenzymes.[2] Ketoconazole is an inhibitor of CYP3A4 and thus concurrent use increases the exposure to levomilnacipran. Desvenlafaxine is also metabolised by CYP3A4, though to a minor extent, and as expected, it is less affected by ketoconazole. Venlafaxine is metabolised to the inactive metabolite *N*-desmethylvenlafaxine by CYP3A4. This metabolic route is minor in comparison to the metabolism of venlafaxine to *O*-desmethylvenlafaxine by CYP2D6, but it can assume more importance if CYP2D6 is lacking.[6] Inhibitors of CYP3A4, such as ketoconazole and voriconazole might have a greater effect on the exposure of venlafaxine and *O*-desmethylvenlafaxine in CYP2D6 poor metabolisers than in extensive metabolisers. The studies cited offer some weight to this suggestion.

Importance and management

Evidence for an interaction between **venlafaxine** and the azoles is limited to one study with ketoconazole and one with voriconazole, but a pharmacokinetic interaction is established. The negligible to slight increases in exposure to both venlafaxine and its active metabolite, *O*-desmethylvenlafaxine (which have equipotent activity), seen in extensive metabolisers given ketoconazole or voriconazole, respectively, are probably unlikely to be clinically relevant. However, the clinical relevance of the larger increases in exposure to venlafaxine and *O*-desmethylvenlafaxine seen in some poor metabolisers is not clear. Further, it appears that it is the combined exposure to both venlafaxine and *O*-desmethylvenlafaxine that is important, and data on the effects of ketoconazole and voriconazole on this are lacking; that from one poor metaboliser given voriconazole suggests that the effect on this combined AUC is greater than in extensive metabolisers, but requires confirmation in other studies. It is important to remember, that exposure to venlafaxine is already increased in poor metabolisers prior to administration of an interacting drug. However, because CYP2D6 metaboliser status is usually unknown in clinical practice, the UK and US manufacturers advise caution with concurrent use of CYP3A4 inhibitors.[4,6] The possibility of an increase in venlafaxine adverse effects should be borne in mind. Some caution would also seem prudent with drug combinations that inhibit both CYP3A4 and CYP2D6 (see under *CYP2D6 inhibitors* in 'SNRIs; Venlafaxine + Miscellaneous', p.1482), as this situation is analogous to giving a CYP3A4 inhibitor to a known CYP2D6 poor metaboliser.

Ketoconazole appears to slightly increase exposure to **levomilnacipran**, and as a result the US manufacturer advises that the dose should not exceed 80 mg daily when ketoconazole is administered concurrently. Bear in mind the possibility of increased adverse effects. Other potent inhibitors of CYP3A4 are predicted to interact similarly,[2] for a list of known clinically relevant potent CYP3A4 inhibitors, see 'Table 1.9', p.11.

Ketoconazole caused a slight increase in the exposure to high-dose **desvenlafaxine**, and the US manufacturer advises that this is not clinically relevant.[1] No interaction would be expected between desvenlafaxine and other CYP3A4 inhibitors, and no dose adjustments would seem necessary on concurrent use with any such drugs.

1. Pristiq (Desvenlafaxine succinate). Wyeth Pharmaceutical Inc. US Prescribing information, July 2014.
2. Fetzima (Levomilnacipran hydrochloride). Forest Pharmaceuticals Inc. US Prescribing information, July 2014.
3. Lindh JD, Annas A, Meurling L, Dahl M-L, AL-Shurbaji A. Effect of ketoconazole on venlafaxine plasma concentrations in extensive and poor metabolisers of debrisoquine. *Eur J Clin Pharmacol* (2003) 59, 401–6.
4. Effexor XR (Venlafaxine hydrochloride). Wyeth Pharmaceuticals Inc. US Prescribing information, March 2014.
5. Hynninen VV, Olkkola KT, Bertilsson L, Kurkinen K, Neuvonen PJ, Laine K. Effect of terbinafine and voriconazole on the pharmacokinetics of the antidepressant venlafaxine. *Clin Pharmacol Ther* (2008) 83, 342–8.
6. Efexor XL(Venlafaxine hydrochloride). Pfizer Ltd. UK Summary of product characteristics, December 2013.

SNRIs + H_2-receptor antagonists

Cimetidine slightly increases venlafaxine exposure. Duloxetine is predicted to be similarly affected. Famotidine did not alter the absorption of duloxetine.

Clinical evidence, mechanism, importance and management

(a) Duloxetine

The metabolism of duloxetine is decreased by CYP1A2 inhibitors and it is recommended that potent inhibitors of CYP1A2 should be avoided (see under fluvoxamine in 'SNRIs + SSRIs', p.1478). The US manufacturer of duloxetine specifically mentions **cimetidine** as an inhibitor of this enzyme.[1] However, **cimetidine** is a much weaker CYP1A2 inhibitor than fluvoxamine, and the UK manufacturer does not mention a possible interaction with **cimetidine**.[2] Any pharmacokinetic interaction between **cimetidine** and duloxetine is probably unlikely to be clinically important, but, until more is known, it might be prudent to beware of an increase in duloxetine adverse effects if **cimetidine** is also given.

The UK and US manufacturers report that **famotidine** had no effect on the rate or extent of absorption of a single 40-mg dose of duloxetine.[1,2] Duloxetine is formulated with a gastric-resistant coating, and this finding suggests that H_2-receptor antagonists do not lead to an earlier release of duloxetine.[1] **Famotidine** might therefore be a suitable alternative to **cimetidine** in patients taking duloxetine.

(b) Venlafaxine

In a study in 18 healthy subjects, **cimetidine** 800 mg daily for 5 days decreased the oral clearance of venlafaxine 50 mg every 8 hours by 40%, and increased its AUC by 62%. It had no effect on the formation or elimination of the major active metabolite of venlafaxine, *O*-desmethylvenlafaxine (ODV). However, the exposure to venlafaxine and ODV combined was found to be increased by only 13%. Thus the overall pharmacological activity of the two was only minimally increased by **cimetidine**[3] and no venlafaxine dose adjustments are necessary on concurrent use.[4] However, the US manufacturer of venlafaxine suggests that patients with pre-existing hypertension, the elderly and those with hepatic impairment might possibly show a more pronounced effect, and they recommend that such patients should be monitored more closely for venlafaxine adverse effects.[4]

1. Cymbalta (Duloxetine hydrochloride). Eli Lilly and Company. US Prescribing information, July 2014.
2. Cymbalta (Duloxetine hydrochloride). Eli Lilly and Company Ltd. UK Summary of product characteristics, March 2014.
3. Troy SM, Rudolph R, Mayersohn M, Chiang ST. The influence of cimetidine on the disposition kinetics of the antidepressant venlafaxine. *J Clin Pharmacol* (1998) 38, 467–74.
4. Effexor XR (Venlafaxine hydrochloride). Wyeth Pharmaceuticals Inc. US Prescribing information, March 2014.

SNRIs + Propafenone

Two reports describe hallucinations and other psychoses in patients taking venlafaxine and propafenone. Duloxetine is predicted to increase the exposure to propafenone.

Clinical evidence, mechanism, importance and management

(a) Duloxetine

Based on data for desipramine (see 'Tricyclic antidepressants + SNRIs', p.1514), duloxetine is a moderate inhibitor of CYP2D6 and is therefore predicted to increase the exposure to other drugs predominantly metabolised by CYP2D6, such as propafenone. Because propafenone has a narrow therapeutic window, the manufacturers recommend that the concurrent use of duloxetine and propafenone should be approached with caution.[1,2]

(b) Venlafaxine

A 67-year-old woman with bipolar disorder taking venlafaxine 300 mg daily, experienced symptoms of paranoia, visual hallucinations, and marked confusion about

2 weeks after starting propafenone 600 mg daily for intermittent atrial fibrillation. Serum concentrations of venlafaxine had increased from 85 to 520 nanograms/mL (upper limit of reference range 150 nanograms/mL) and concentrations of the metabolite *O*-desmethylvenlafaxine had increased but were still within the normal range. Venlafaxine was stopped for a few days then restarted at the lower dose of 75 mg daily and her mental condition (diagnosed as organic psychosis) improved. However, as she also had orthostatic hypotension her propafenone dose was subsequently reduced to 300 mg daily, which necessitated dose adjustments of venlafaxine because of a large drop in serum concentration. When propafenone was again increased to 600 mg daily the venlafaxine had to be reduced to 50 mg daily.[3] Another case of visual hallucinations and psychomotor agitation occurred in a woman taking propafenone when her dose of sustained-release venlafaxine was increased from 75 to 150 mg daily.[4]

The reasons for the interaction are not known, but venlafaxine is partly metabolised by CYP2D6 and propafenone is an inhibitor of this isoenzyme. However, this mechanism usually results in a decrease in *O*-desmethylvenlafaxine concentrations, and is generally of no clinical consequence, see 'SNRIs; Venlafaxine + Miscellaneous', p.1482. Information is limited to these two case reports, and their importance is unclear.

1. Cymbalta (Duloxetine hydrochloride). Eli Lilly and Company. US Prescribing information, July 2014.
2. Cymbalta (Duloxetine hydrochloride). Eli Lilly and Company Ltd. UK Summary of product characteristics, March 2014.
3. Pfeffer F, Grube M. An organic psychosis due to a venlafaxine-propafenone interaction. *Int J Psychiatry Med* (2001) 31, 427–32.
4. Gareri P, De Fazio P, Gallelli L, De Fazio S, Davoli A, Seminara G, Cotroneo A, De Sarro G. Venlafaxine-propafenone interaction resulting in hallucinations and psychomotor agitation. *Ann Pharmacother* (2008) 42, 434–8.

SNRIs + SSRIs

Fluvoxamine markedly increases duloxetine exposure. Paroxetine causes a slight increase in the exposure to duloxetine, and fluoxetine is predicted to interact similarly. The pharmacokinetics of milnacipran are not altered by fluoxetine, and other SSRIS would be expected not to interact.

The concurrent use of the SNRIs and SSRIs might increase the risk of serotonin syndrome. Concurrent use has also led to adverse effects such as blurred vision, constipation, and rarely, bleeding events or hypomania.

Clinical evidence

(a) Duloxetine

1. Pharmacokinetics. A crossover study in 14 male smokers found that **fluvoxamine** 100 mg daily caused a 5.6-fold increase in the AUC of a single 60-mg dose of duloxetine and a 2.4-fold increase in duloxetine maximum concentrations.[1] Similar increases in the exposure to duloxetine were found in 15 healthy subjects who were known CYP2D6 poor metabolisers (that is those with lower than normal activity of this isoenzyme) when they were given **fluvoxamine** 50 to 100 mg daily and duloxetine 40 mg twice daily.[2] A retrospective review of 13 patients with mild to severe depression, found that in 8 patients receiving duloxetine 30 mg daily (at steady state), the addition of **fluvoxamine** 25 mg daily increased the duloxetine minimum plasma concentrations approximately 3-fold on average. Note however, that the range for this effect was 50% up to 6-fold, meaning that the reliability of this result is questionable.[3] In healthy subjects, the concurrent use of **paroxetine** 20 mg daily and duloxetine 40 mg daily increased the AUC of duloxetine at steady state by about 60%.[4]

2. Serotonin syndrome. An 85-year-old man with a history of bipolar disorder and depression taking **fluoxetine** 30 mg daily, was switched to duloxetine 20 mg daily [without any washout]. A week later the patient presented at the emergency department with a 5-day history of muscle spasms, back stiffness, abdominal discomfort, and nausea. He was admitted and diagnosed with serotonin syndrome. Duloxetine was discontinued and symptoms resolved over the next few days.[5]

(b) Milnacipran

1. Pharmacokinetics. In a pharmacokinetic study in 12 healthy subjects given milnacipran 50 mg twice daily for seven doses alone, and then immediately after **fluoxetine** 20 mg daily for 3 weeks, fluoxetine had no effect on the pharmacokinetics of milnacipran.[6]

Fluoxetine has a very long half-life, and this study simulated the situation where fluoxetine is stopped and milnacipran started without a washout period.

2. Serotonin syndrome. A 57-year-old woman developed a measles-like rash and serotonin syndrome 9 days after milnacipran was started and titrated up to 50 mg twice daily. Her regular medications included **fluoxetine**, **doxepin**, and **tramadol**. The patient had been instructed to decrease her fluoxetine dose from 40 mg daily to 20 mg daily on day 7 of milnacipran but had not done so. Milnacipran, fluoxetine, and tramadol were discontinued and the patient's symptoms were managed with diphenhydramine, hydralazine, methylprednisolone, paracetamol (acetaminophen), and promethazine. Symptoms of serotonin toxicity resolved by the next morning and the rash cleared 4 days after the milnacipran was discontinued.[7]

(c) Venlafaxine

1. Antimuscarinic adverse effects. A woman taking **fluoxetine** 20 mg and clonazepam 1 mg daily developed blurred vision, dry mouth, constipation, dizziness, insomnia, and a hand tremor within a week of starting to take venlafaxine 37.5 mg daily. These symptoms worsened by the second week and persisted until the venlafaxine was stopped.[8-10] Several other patients (aged between 21 and 70 years) taking **fluoxetine** developed antimuscarinic adverse effects (including constipation, blurred vision, urinary retention, or dry mouth) within 2 to 10 days of starting venlafaxine.[9-11] One patient that only developed urinary retention had some prostate enlargement and had previously had some moderate urinary problems while taking **fluoxetine** and nortriptyline.[9,11]

2. Haemorrhages. A 60-year-old man experienced haemorrhages from his nose and rectum one week after venlafaxine 150 mg daily and mirtazapine 15 mg daily were given with **escitalopram** 20 mg daily. The bleeding progressively worsened during the following 3 weeks and then the patient reduced the doses to **escitalopram** 15 mg, mirtazapine 7.5 mg and venlafaxine 100 mg daily, and the bleeding decreased over the following week. He continued weekly tapering of the medications and the bleeding progressively decreased until it stopped when the doses were **escitalopram** 5 mg, mirtazapine 7.5 mg, and venlafaxine 37.5 mg daily. Previous treatments with these three drugs used alone had not caused haemorrhages.[12] Note that SSRIs and SNRIs alone have been associated with bleeding events.

3. Hypomania. A 31-year-old woman with recurrent unipolar depression developed a hypomanic episode the day after **paroxetine** 20 mg daily was stopped and venlafaxine 75 mg daily was started. The hypomania subsided as the dose of venlafaxine was gradually reduced to 18.75 mg daily.[13]

4. Serotonin syndrome. A 21-year-old woman whose long-term treatment with **paroxetine** was stopped a week before starting venlafaxine (37.5 mg daily for 5 days then 75 mg daily for 2 days) developed vomiting, dizziness, incoordination, anxiety, and electric shock sensations in her arms and legs within 3 days of starting venlafaxine. She stopped venlafaxine after 7 days of treatment, but symptoms persisted for 5 days until she was treated with cyproheptadine.[14]

Other similar cases resulting in serotonin syndrome have been reported in a 75-year-old man who stopped **sertraline** and started venlafaxine 48 hours later, although symptoms took 14 days to develop,[15] and in a 39-year-old woman, who stopped **fluoxetine** and started venlafaxine.[16] This patient was also taking trazodone. Further reports of serotonin syndrome have been described in patients taking venlafaxine with other potentially serotonergic drugs, see 'Tricyclic antidepressants + SNRIs', p.1514, 'SSRIs + Bupropion', p.1485, 'SNRIs + St John's wort (*Hypericum perforatum*)', p.1479, 'SNRIs; Venlafaxine + Opioids', p.1482, and 'SNRIs; Venlafaxine + Trazodone', p.1484.

Mechanism

Duloxetine is metabolised principally by CYP1A2, but also by CYP2D6. Fluvoxamine is an inhibitor of CYP1A2 and paroxetine is an inhibitor of CYP2D6. Therefore the concurrent use of these SSRIs decreases duloxetine metabolism and increases its exposure. Venlafaxine is metabolised, in part, by CYP2D6, which fluoxetine inhibits. Concurrent use might therefore increase venlafaxine concentrations, leading to some of the adverse effects described in the cases. Paroxetine probably interacts similarly. The case of bleeding was thought to be due to the combined drugs causing an increase in serotonin concentrations.

Importance and management

A pharmacokinetic interaction between the SSRIs and **duloxetine** would appear to be established, although the effects vary depending on the inhibitory potential of the SSRI on the isoenzymes involved in duloxetine metabolism. Although the clinical relevance of the marked increases in exposure to duloxetine with fluvoxamine (a potent CYP1A2 inhibitor) has not been assessed, the UK and US manufacturers consider that the effect is so great that the combination should be avoided.[17,18] This seems a prudent precaution. The increase in exposure to duloxetine seen with paroxetine 20 mg daily (a potent inhibitor of CYP2D6) is probably not clinically relevant, but the US manufacturer notes that greater increases would be expected with higher doses.[18] Other SSRIs also inhibit CYP2D6 (notably fluoxetine which is a potent CYP2D6 inhibitor), and would therefore be expected to interact similarly. Some caution on concurrent use would seem sensible.

Information about the adverse antimuscarinic effects due to an interaction between fluoxetine and **venlafaxine** seems to be limited to the reports cited, all by the same author. The incidence is not known, but if venlafaxine and fluoxetine are given concurrently, be alert for any evidence of increased antimuscarinic adverse effects (such as dry mouth, blurred vision, and urinary retention). It might be necessary to withdraw one or other of the two drugs.

The pharmacokinetics of **milnacipran** were not affected by fluoxetine, and because it is not appreciably metabolised, no interaction would be expected with other SSRIs.

There appear to be few case reports describing serotonin syndrome in patients given an SSRI and an SNRI. However, in general, concurrent use should be undertaken with caution, as both classes of drug affect serotonin, and increased serotonin concentrations can precipitate serotonin syndrome. For more information on serotonin syndrome and its management, see 'Drugs that cause serotonin syndrome + Other drugs that cause serotonin syndrome', p.1471.

1. Lobo ED, Bergstrom RF, Reddy S, Quinlan T, Chappell J, Hong Q, Ring B, Knadler MP. In vitro and in vivo evaluations of cytochrome P450 1A2 interactions with duloxetine. *Clin Pharmacokinet* (2008) 47, 192–202.
2. Small D, Loghin C, Lucas R, Knadler MP, Zhang L, Chappell J, Bergstrom R, Callaghan JT. Pharmacokinetic evaluation of combined duloxetine and fluvoxamine dosing in CYP2D6 poor metabolizers. *Clin Pharmacol Ther* (2005) 77, P37.
3. Paulzen M, Finkelmeyer A, Grözinger M. Augmentative effects of fluvoxamine on duloxetine plasma levels in depressed patients. *Pharmacopsychiatry* (2011) 44, 317–23.
4. Skinner MH, Kuan H-Y, Pan A, Sathirakul K, Knadler MP, Gonzales CR, Yeo KP, Reddy S, Lim M, Ayan-Oshodi M, Wise SD. Duloxetine is both an inhibitor and a substrate of cytochrome P4502D6 in healthy volunteers. *Clin Pharmacol Ther* (2003) 73, 170–7.
5. Liu PT, Argento V, Skudlarska B, Blagodatny M. Serotonin syndrome in an octogenarian after switch from fluoxetine to duloxetine. *J Am Geriatr Soc* (2009) 57, 2384–5.

6. Puozzo C, Hermann P, Chassard D. Lack of pharmacokinetic interaction when switching from fluoxetine to milnacipran. *Int Clin Psychopharmacol* (2006) 21, 153–8.
7. Huskey AM, Thomas CC, Waddell JA. Occurrence of milnacipran-associated morbilliform rash and serotonin toxicity. *Ann Pharmacother* (2013) 47, e32.
8. Benazzi F. Severe anticholinergic side effects with venlafaxine-fluoxetine combination. *Can J Psychiatry* (1997) 42, 980–1.
9. Benazzi F. Venlafaxine-fluoxetine interaction. *J Clin Psychopharmacol* (1999) 19, 96–8.
10. Benazzi F. Venlafaxine drug-drug interactions in clinical practice. *J Psychiatry Neurosci* (1998) 23, 181–2.
11. Benazzi F. Urinary retention with venlafaxine-fluoxetine combination. *Hum Psychopharmacol* (1998) 13, 139–40.
12. Benazzi F. Hemorrhages during escitalopram–venlafaxine–mirtazapine combination treatment of depression. *Can J Psychiatry* (2005) 50, 184.
13. Krol DGH, Nolen WA. Acute stemmingsomslag naar hypomanie bij een patiënte met een unipolaire depressie direct na starten van venlafaxine. *Tijdschr Psychiatr* (2006) 48, 405–8.
14. Chan BSH, Graudins A, Whyte IM, Dawson AH, Braitberg G, Duggin GG. Serotonin syndrome resulting from drug interactions. *Med J Aust* (1998) 169, 523–5.
15. Perry NK. Venlafaxine-induced serotonin syndrome with relapse following amitriptyline. *Postgrad Med J* (2000) 76, 254–6.
16. Bhatara VS, Magnus RD, Paul KL, Preskorn SH. Serotonin syndrome induced by venlafaxine and fluoxetine: a case study in polypharmacy and potential pharmacodynamic and pharmacokinetic mechanisms. *Ann Pharmacother* (1998) 32, 432–6.
17. Cymbalta (Duloxetine hydrochloride). Eli Lilly and Company Ltd. UK Summary of product characteristics, March 2014.
18. Cymbalta (Duloxetine hydrochloride). Eli Lilly and Company. US Prescribing information, July 2014.

SNRIs + St John's wort (*Hypericum perforatum*)

Serotonin syndrome has been reported in one patient taking venlafaxine and St John's wort. Other SNRIs might interact similarly.

Clinical evidence

An interaction between **venlafaxine** and St John's wort was reported to the Centre Régional de Pharmacovigilance de Marseille involving a 32-year-old man who had been taking **venlafaxine** 250 mg daily for several months. He started taking St John's wort at a dose of 200 drops 3 times daily (usual dose up to 160 drops daily) and on the third day felt faint and anxious, and had symptoms of diaphoresis, shivering, and tachycardia. The St John's wort was stopped and his symptoms resolved in 3 days without altering the dose of **venlafaxine**.[1] A search of Health Canada's database of spontaneous adverse reactions for the period 1998 to 2003 also found one case of suspected serotonin syndrome as a result of an interaction between **venlafaxine** and St John's wort.[2]

Mechanism

A pharmacodynamic interaction might occur between St John's wort and venlafaxine because they can both inhibit the reuptake of serotonin. Serotonin syndrome has been seen with St John's wort alone,[3] and so additive serotonergic effects appear to be the explanation for what occurred in the cases described here.

Importance and management

Information appears to be limited to these reports with **venlafaxine**. However, they suggest that **desvenlafaxine**, **duloxetine**, **levomilnacipran**, and **milnacipran** would be expected to interact similarly. Serotonin syndrome is a rare adverse effect, but because of its severity, some caution is warranted if both St John's wort and a SNRI are given. For more information on serotonin syndrome and its management, see 'Drugs that cause serotonin syndrome + Other drugs that cause serotonin syndrome', p.1471.

1. Prost N, Tichadou L, Rodor F, Nguyen N, David JM, Jean-Pastor MJ. Interaction millepertuis-venlafaxine. *Presse Med* (2000) 29, 1285–6.
2. Griffiths J, Jordan S, Pilan K. Natural health products and adverse reactions. *Can Adverse React News* (2004) 14 (1), 2–3.
3. Demott K. St. John's wort tied to serotonin syndrome. *Clin Psychiatry News* (1998) 26, 28.

SNRIs; Desvenlafaxine + Miscellaneous

It is predicted that the concurrent use of a diuretic and desvenlafaxine might increase the risk of hyponatraemia. Food does not appear to affect the pharmacokinetics of desvenlafaxine. Desvenlafaxine does not appear to have a clinically relevant effect on the pharmacokinetics of tamoxifen.

Clinical evidence, mechanism, importance and management

(a) Diuretics

The US manufacturer of desvenlafaxine briefly notes that hyponatraemia has occurred in patients receiving SNRIs, and warns that patients also taking diuretics might have a greater risk of developing hyponatraemia.[1]

(b) Food

The US manufacturer of desvenlafaxine notes that in a study, administration with a high-fat meal (800 to 1 000 calories) increased the maximum concentration of desvenlafaxine by about 16% while the AUC was similar to that seen under fasting conditions.[1] These changes are unlikely to be clinically relevant and thus desvenlafaxine can be taken with or without food.

(c) Tamoxifen

The US manufacturer of desvenlafaxine briefly notes that the pharmacokinetics of tamoxifen (dose not stated) were not affected by desvenlafaxine 100 mg daily, and no dose adjustment is necessary on concurrent use.[1]

1. Pristiq (Desvenlafaxine succinate). Wyeth Pharmaceuticals Inc. US Prescribing information, July 2014.

SNRIs; Duloxetine + Miscellaneous

Potent inhibitors of CYP1A2 and CYP2D6 are predicted to increase duloxetine exposure. Duloxetine is predicted to increase the concentrations of drugs that are substrates of CYP2D6. The absorption of duloxetine is not affected by antacids.

Clinical evidence, mechanism, importance and management

(a) Antacids

Aluminium/magnesium-containing antacids had no effect on the rate or extent of absorption of a single 40-mg dose of duloxetine.[1-3] Duloxetine is formulated with a gastric-resistant coating, but this finding suggests that antacids do not lead to an earlier release of duloxetine.[3] No separation of administration would appear to be necessary on concurrent use.

(b) CYP1A2 Inhibitors

On the basis that fluvoxamine, a potent inhibitor of CYP1A2, markedly increases duloxetine exposure (see 'SNRIs + SSRIs', p.1478), the manufacturers of duloxetine predict that other potent inhibitors of CYP1A2 will have the same effect, and suggest that their concurrent use with duloxetine should be avoided.[1-3] This seems a prudent precaution. For a list of clinically relevant potent CYP1A2 inhibitors, see 'Table 1.2', p.5. Note that the manufacturers additionally name **ciprofloxacin**, but this is generally considered a moderate CYP1A2 inhibitor.

(c) CYP2D6

1. Inhibitors. On the basis that paroxetine, a potent inhibitor of CYP2D6, slightly increases duloxetine exposure (see 'SNRIs + SSRIs', p.1478), the US manufacturer of duloxetine suggests that other potent CYP2D6 inhibitors will interact similarly.[3] The clinical relevance of any interaction is unknown, but is probably minor as CYP2D6 is not the major route of duloxetine metabolism. For a list of clinically relevant potent CYP2D6 inhibitors, see 'Table 1.7', p.9.

2. Substrates. Based on data for desipramine, which can be used as a probe substrate to assess the activity of drugs on CYP2D6, duloxetine is a moderate inhibitor of CYP2D6 (see 'Tricyclic antidepressants + SNRIs', p.1514). The manufacturers of duloxetine therefore advise caution if it is given with drugs that are predominantly metabolised by CYP2D6 and have a narrow therapeutic index.[1-3] For a list of CYP2D6 substrates see 'Table 1.7', p.9. Note that use with **thioridazine** (withdrawn in the UK) is contraindicated in the US because of the risk of arrhythmias with elevated concentrations of this drug.[3] CYP2D6 shows genetic polymorphism, and inhibition of this isoenzyme turns extensive metabolisers (that is, those with normal CYP2D6 activity) into poor metabolisers (that is, those with lower than normal CYP2D6 activity). The situation when inhibition of CYP2D6 metabolism is likely to matter most is when a patient stable taking a CYP2D6 substrate is then given duloxetine.

1. Cymbalta (Duloxetine hydrochloride). Eli Lilly and Company Ltd. UK Summary of product characteristics, March 2014.
2. Yentreve (Duloxetine hydrochloride). Eli Lilly and Company Ltd. UK Summary of product characteristics, October 2013.
3. Cymbalta (Duloxetine hydrochloride). Eli Lilly and Company. US Prescribing information, July 2014.

SNRIs; Duloxetine + Tobacco

Smoking appears to slightly decrease duloxetine concentrations.

Clinical evidence

A study in 23 patients taking duloxetine found that the mean duloxetine serum concentration in 8 **smokers** was 64% lower than in 15 **non-smokers** (24.3 nanograms/mL versus 67.8 nanograms/mL). This was despite the use of higher doses of duloxetine in smokers than non-smokers (mean 90.5 mg versus 84 mg). In a subgroup of 10 patients (4 smokers and 6 non-smokers), serum duloxetine concentrations were examined again, later during treatment. At this point the difference in duloxetine concentrations between smokers and non-smokers was less, but this was attributed to a much higher dose in smokers than non-smokers (mean 112.5 mg versus 95 mg).[1] The UK and US manufacturers briefly note that population pharmacokinetic studies have shown that **smokers** have almost 50% lower plasma concentrations of duloxetine, when compared with **non-smokers**,[2] or a 33% lower AUC.[3]

Mechanism

Tobacco smoke contains polycyclic hydrocarbons, which induce CYP1A2, by which duloxetine is metabolised. Smoking therefore increases duloxetine metabolism and lower concentrations result.

Importance and management

The limited evidence for a pharmacokinetic interaction between duloxetine and tobacco suggests that smoking decreases duloxetine concentrations. The clinical importance of these findings has not been evaluated, but is probably minor. The US manufacturer of duloxetine specifically states that dosage modifications are not recommended for smokers.[3]

1. Fric M, Pfuhlmann B, Laux G, Riederer P, Distler G, Artmann S, Wohlschläger M, Liebmann M, Deckert J. The influence of smoking on the serum level of duloxetine. *Pharmacopsychiatry* (2008) 41, 151–55.
2. Cymbalta (Duloxetine hydrochloride). Eli Lilly and Company Ltd. UK Summary of product characteristics, March 2014.
3. Cymbalta (Duloxetine hydrochloride). Eli Lilly and Company. US Prescribing information, July 2014.

SNRIs; Levomilnacipran + Miscellaneous

The concurrent use of a diuretic and levomilnacipran might increase the risk of hyponatraemia. Food does not appear to alter levomilnacipran concentrations.

Clinical evidence, mechanism, importance and management

(a) Diuretics

The US manufacturer of levomilnacipran briefly notes that hyponatraemia has occurred in patients receiving SNRIs, and warns that patients also taking diuretics might have a greater risk of developing hyponatraemia.[1]

(b) Food

The US manufacturer of levomilnacipran briefly notes that administration with food did not affect levomilnacipran concentrations.[1] Levomilnacipran can therefore be taken with or without food.

1. Fetzima (Levomilnacipran hydrochloride). Forest Pharmaceuticals Inc. US Prescribing information, July 2014.

SNRIs; Milnacipran + Miscellaneous

The manufacturers of milnacipran contraindicate its use with digitalis glycosides and MAO-B inhibitors such as selegiline and rasagiline. They also warn against concurrent use with clonidine and sympathomimetics such as adrenaline (epinephrine) or noradrenaline (norepinephrine). They suggest careful monitoring with lithium because of the risk of serotonin syndrome.

Clinical evidence, mechanism, importance and management

(a) Cardiovascular drugs

1. Clonidine. The manufacturer of milnacipran advises against the use of milnacipran with clonidine or related drugs because milnacipran might reduce the antihypertensive action of clonidine due to antagonism at the adrenergic receptors, in a way analogous to the tricyclic antidepressants (see 'Clonidine and related drugs + Tricyclic and related antidepressants', p.1057).[1]

Note that this caution is not given for the other available SNRIs, duloxetine and venlafaxine.

2. Digitalis glycosides. The manufacturer of milnacipran contraindicates its use with digitalis glycosides (such as digoxin) because of the risk of potentiating haemodynamic effects, particularly when given parenterally.[1]

3. Inotropes and Vasopressors. The manufacturer of milnacipran advises against the concurrent use of parenteral adrenaline (epinephrine) or noradrenaline (norepinephrine) because of the possible risk of hypertensive crisis with cardiac arrhythmias. This is because milnacipran inhibits noradrenaline re-uptake, see also 'Tricyclic and related antidepressants + Inotropes and Vasopressors', p.1510. They also advise caution if adrenaline or noradrenaline are used as vasoconstrictors in subcutaneous or gingival injections. In this case they recommend that, in adults, the dose of adrenaline should be limited to less than 100 micrograms in 10 minutes or 300 micrograms in one hour.[1]

Note that this caution is not given for the other available SNRIs, duloxetine and venlafaxine.

(b) Lithium

The manufacturer of milnacipran recommends regular clinical monitoring if milnacipran is given with lithium, because of the risk of serotonin syndrome.[1] Cases of serotonin syndrome have been reported with lithium and the SNRI, venlafaxine, see 'Lithium + Venlafaxine', p.1381. Serotonin syndrome is a rare adverse effect, but because of its severity, some caution is warranted if both drugs are given. For more information on serotonin syndrome and its management, see 'Drugs that cause serotonin syndrome + Other drugs that cause serotonin syndrome', p.1471.

(c) MAO-B inhibitors

The manufacturer of milnacipran contraindicates its use with selective monoamine oxidase type B inhibitors (selegiline and rasagiline) because of the risk of hypertensive crisis. They say that there should be 2 weeks between stopping the MAO-B inhibitor and starting milnacipran and at least one week between stopping milnacipran and starting the MAO-B inhibitor.[1] Note that, the more usual concern with the use of these drugs is the risk of serotonin syndrome, see 'MAO-B inhibitors + SSRIs or SNRIs', p.772.

1. Ixel (Milnacipran hydrochloride). Pierre Fabre Médicament. French Summary of product characteristics, February 2003.

SNRIs; Venlafaxine + Amfetamines

Lisdexamfetamine negligibly increased the exposure to venlafaxine. Venlafaxine did not alter the exposure to the active metabolite of lisdexamfetamine, dexamfetamine. A case of serotonin syndrome has been attributed to the concurrent use of dexamfetamine and venlafaxine.

Clinical evidence

(a) Pharmacokinetics

In a randomised study, healthy subjects were given either **lisdexamfetamine** (a prodrug of dexamfetamine) titrated to 70 mg daily over 15 days, or extended-release venlafaxine titrated to 225 mg daily over 15 days, followed by both drugs together for 15 days. In the 37 subjects initially given venlafaxine alone, there was a 13% increase in venlafaxine exposure and no difference in the exposure to the active metabolite, *O*-desmethylvenlafaxine, on concurrent use with lisdexamfetamine. Total combined exposure to venlafaxine and *O*-desmethylvenlafaxine was not altered. The exposure to dexamfetamine when lisdexamfetamine was given alone or in combination with venlafaxine (40 subjects) did not differ.[1]

(b) Serotonin syndrome

A 32-year-old patient taking **dexamfetamine** 5 mg three times daily for adult attention deficit hyperactivity disorder (ADHD) presented with marked agitation, anxiety, shivering, and tremor 2 weeks after also starting to take venlafaxine 75 to 150 mg daily. Other symptoms included generalised hypertonia, hyperreflexia, frequent myoclonic jerking, tonic spasm of the orbicularis oris muscle, and sinus tachycardia. His symptoms resolved completely when both drugs were withdrawn and cyproheptadine, to a total dose of 32 mg over 3 hours, was given. Dexamfetamine was restarted after 3 days.[2] This patient had a second episode of serotonin syndrome when citalopram was given with the dexamfetamine, see 'Amfetamines and related drugs + SSRIs', p.216.

Mechanism

The authors of the case of serotonin syndrome suggest that the combination of serotonin re-uptake blockade and either presynaptic release of serotonin or monoamine oxidase inhibition by dexamfetamine could cause increased serotonin in the CNS, and be the reason for the effects seen.

Importance and management

Evidence for an interaction between venlafaxine and lisdexamfetamine is limited, but the study suggests that no clinically relevant pharmacokinetic interaction occurs. The general relevance of the case of serotonin syndrome is unclear. For more information on serotonin syndrome and its management, see 'Drugs that cause serotonin syndrome + Other drugs that cause serotonin syndrome', p.1471.

1. Ermer J, Haffey MB, Richards C, Lasseter K, Roesch B, Purkayastha J, Corcoran M, Harlin B, Martin P. An open-label investigation of the pharmacokinetic profiles of lisdexamfetamine dimesylate and venlafaxine extended-release, administered alone and in combination, in healthy adults. *Clin Drug Investig* (2013) 33, 243–54.
2. Prior FH, Isbister GK, Dawson AH, Whyte IM. Serotonin toxicity with therapeutic doses of dexamphetamine and venlafaxine. *Med J Aust* (2002) 176, 240–1.

SNRIs; Venlafaxine + Atomoxetine

A case report describes dyskinesia and dysarthria associated with the concurrent use of venlafaxine and atomoxetine.

Clinical evidence, mechanism, importance and management

An 18-year-old woman with attention deficit hyperactivity disorder, panic attacks and generalised anxiety was given venlafaxine, initially 37.5 mg daily, increasing to 225 mg daily, to which atomoxetine 18 mg daily was added. The atomoxetine dose was subsequently increased to 40 mg daily. After 3 weeks of concurrent use (and 5 days after the last dose increase) she presented with tremors, abnormal facial movements and a speech disturbance, which resolved after both medications were discontinued. It was suggested that a pharmacodynamic interaction, resulting from excess synaptic noradrenaline, might have occurred. Furthermore, the patient was a poor metaboliser of CYP2D6 (meaning she lacked or had low levels of this isoenzyme), and it was suggested that a pharmacokinetic interaction might also have occurred;[1] both drugs are substrates for CYP2D6. The manufacturer recommends caution when atomoxetine is given with other drugs that affect noradrenaline, because of the potential for additive or synergistic pharmacological effects.[2] Although this is an isolated case it adds weight to the manufacturers caution. Bear these symptoms in mind if both drugs are given, and consider an interaction if they occur.

1. Bond GR, Garro AC, Gilbert DL. Dyskinesias associated with atomoxetine in combination with other psychoactive drugs. *Clin Toxicol* (2007) 45, 182–5.
2. Strattera (Atomoxetine hydrochloride). Eli Lilly and Company Ltd. UK Summary of product characteristics, October 2012.

SNRIs; Venlafaxine + Bupropion

Bupropion might increase the plasma concentration of venlafaxine, and decrease that of its active metabolite. In two patients, this pharmacokinetic interaction increased serotonergic adverse effects.

Clinical evidence

Bupropion increased the minimum plasma concentration of venlafaxine about 2.5-fold and decreased the minimum plasma concentration of its active metabolite, *O*-desmethylvenlafaxine, about 2.3-fold in 7 patients who had been given venlafaxine alone for a minimum of 6 weeks and then with sustained-release bupropion 150 mg daily for a further 8 weeks.[1] A case series describes 3 patients taking high-dose venlafaxine (225 to 375 mg daily) who had increases in steady-state concentrations of venlafaxine on starting bupropion 150 or 300 mg daily. In 2 of the patients this led to serotonergic adverse effects (tension, agitation, insomnia) requiring bupropion to be stopped or the venlafaxine dose to be reduced.[2]

Mechanism

Bupropion is an inhibitor of CYP2D6, which is responsible for the metabolism of venlafaxine to *O*-desmethylvenlafaxine, and would therefore be expected to increase the exposure to venlafaxine.

Importance and management

Evidence for an interaction between venlafaxine and bupropion is limited, but appears to be established. However, because venlafaxine and *O*-desmethylvenlafaxine are considered equipotent as antidepressants, any change in their ratio should not affect clinical efficacy.[3] The US manufacturer of venlafaxine therefore states that no venlafaxine dose adjustment is necessary on the concurrent use of CYP2D6 inhibitors,[3] such as bupropion. However, the case series suggests that in some instances, the increase in venlafaxine concentrations with bupropion might be sufficient to cause adverse effects. Therefore it might be prudent to be alert for any indication of increased venlafaxine adverse effects (e.g. nausea, insomnia, dry mouth) in patients also taking bupropion.

For a report of worsening symptoms of serotonin syndrome when venlafaxine was given with bupropion and sertraline, see 'SSRIs + Bupropion', p.1485.

1. Kennedy SH, McCann SM, Masellis M, McIntyre RS, Raskin J, McKay G, Baker GB. Combining bupropion SR with venlafaxine, paroxetine, or fluoxetine: a preliminary report on pharmacokinetic, therapeutic, and sexual dysfunction effects. *J Clin Psychiatry* (2002) 63, 181–6.
2. Paslakis G, Gilles M, Deuschle M. Clinically relevant pharmacokinetic interaction between venlafaxine and bupropion: a case series. *J Clin Psychopharmacol* (2010) 30, 473–4.
3. Effexor XR (Venlafaxine hydrochloride). Wyeth Pharmaceuticals Inc. US Prescribing information, March 2014.

SNRIs; Venlafaxine + Co-amoxiclav

A case of serotonin syndrome has been attributed to the concurrent use of venlafaxine and co-amoxiclav.

Clinical evidence, mechanism, importance and management

A 56-year-old man taking venlafaxine 37.5 mg twice daily for 10 months was given a course of co-amoxiclav (**amoxicillin** with **clavulanate**) 375 mg three times daily to treat gingivitis and a dental abscess. Within 3 hours of a dose of co-amoxiclav he developed tingling in the tip of his tongue, intense paraesthesia in the fingers, severe abdominal cramps, profuse diarrhoea, cold sweats, tremor, and uncontrollable shivering. He was also agitated and frightened, but not confused. The symptoms lasted for 6 hours and were initially assumed to be due to gastroenteritis. However, 2 months later while still taking venlafaxine, he developed identical symptoms after a single dose of co-amoxiclav, which was then diagnosed as serotonin syndrome. The patient had taken co-amoxiclav without problem when not taking venlafaxine, and after the second episode, continued venlafaxine without further episodes of serotonin syndrome.[1]

The reason for this effect is unclear. It is probable that many patients have received both venlafaxine and co-amoxiclav without adverse effects, so the general importance of this report is unknown, but it seems likely to be small.

1. Connor H. Serotonin syndrome after single doses of co-amoxiclav during treatment with venlafaxine. *J R Soc Med* (2003) 96, 233–4.

SNRIs; Venlafaxine + Co-trimoxazole

A report describes severe hand tremor and an increase in venlafaxine concentrations in a patient taking venlafaxine and lithium carbonate when co-trimoxazole was added.

Clinical evidence

A case report describes the development of severe bilateral resting tremor of the hands in a 46-year-old woman taking extended-release venlafaxine 112.5 mg daily and lithium carbonate 675 mg daily, 4 days into a 5-day course of co-trimoxazole (sulfamethoxazole with trimethoprim) 960 mg twice daily. Her lithium concentration was therapeutic at 0.8mmol/L, as it had been previously, however her serum concentration of the venlafaxine active moiety (venlafaxine and *O*-desmethylvenlafaxine) had increased almost 30% from 344 to 444 nanograms/L. Within 4 days of stopping co-trimoxazole, the tremor resolved and the serum concentration of the venlafaxine active moiety decreased to 358 nanograms/L. The patient was found to be an extensive metaboliser of CYP2D6 (that is, she had normal activity of CYP2D6), and an intermediate metaboliser of CYP2C19 (she had reduced activity of CYP2C19). It was noted *prior* to the addition of co-trimoxazole that her venlafaxine serum concentration was 2-fold higher than expected at a dose of 112.5 mg daily; this was attributed to her being a CYP2C19 intermediate metaboliser.[1]

Mechanism

Venlafaxine is primarily metabolised to *O*-desmethylvenlafaxine by CYP2D6; however, *in vitro* studies[2] have shown that CYP2C9 and CYP2C19 are also involved, to a lesser extent, in the metabolism of venlafaxine to both *N*-desmethylvenlafaxine and *O*-desmethylvenlafaxine. The authors of the case[1] comment that her intermediate CYP2C19 metaboliser status and the addition of co-trimoxazole, which can inhibit CYP2C9, had an additive effect on the venlafaxine serum concentration.

Importance and management

Evidence for an interaction between venlafaxine and co-trimoxazole is limited to a case report. The authors of the case suggest that the tremor was likely due to a pharmacokinetic and pharmacodynamic interaction, although they also note that it might have occurred as a side effect of co-trimoxazole.[1] Nevertheless, a mechanism for a pharmacokinetic interaction is not established, and as such the general clinical relevance of this report is unclear.

1. Geber C, Ostad Haji E, Schlicht K, Hiemke C, Tadić A. Severe tremor after co-trimoxazole-induced elevation of venlafaxine serum concentrations in a patient with major depressive disorder. *Ther Drug Monit* (2013) 35, 279–82.
2. Fogelman SM, Schmider J, Venkatakrishnan K, vonn Moltke LL, Harmatz JS, Shader RI, Greenblatt DJ. O- and N-demethylation of venlafaxine in vitro by human liver microsomes and by microsomes from cDNA-transfected cells: effect of metabolic inhibitors and SSRI antidepressants. *Neuropsychopharmacology* (1999) 20, 480–90.

SNRIs; Venlafaxine + Disulfiram

A case describes a hypertensive crisis associated with the use of venlafaxine and disulfiram.

Clinical evidence, mechanism, importance and management

A report describes a hypertensive crisis associated with a low dose of venlafaxine (75 mg daily). It was suggested that the concurrent use of disulfiram might have increased the toxicity of venlafaxine by interfering with its metabolism via CYP3A4. However, disulfiram predominantly inhibits CYP2E1 and has not been reported to notably affect CYP3A4. Note that disulfiram can provoke hypertension through its interaction with alcohol; however the authors state they found no evidence of a reaction with alcohol in this patient.[1] As a single, unexplained case, its general relevance is probably small.

1. Khurana RN, Baudendistel TE. Hypertensive crisis associated with venlafaxine. *Am J Med* (2003) 115, 676–7.

SNRIs; Venlafaxine + Jujube (*Ziziphus jujuba*)

A report describes an acute serotonin reaction when venlafaxine was given with a Chinese herbal remedy, jujube (sour date nut).

Clinical evidence, mechanism, importance and management

A 40-year-old woman with intermittent depression took jujube 500 mg daily (**sour date nut**; **suanzaoren**; *Ziziphus jujuba*), prescribed by a traditional Chinese healer, for several weeks, with minor improvement. She was then prescribed venlafaxine 37.5 mg daily by a psychiatrist, but approximately one hour after taking the first dose of venlafaxine with the jujube she became agitated, restless, nauseated, dizzy, and ataxic, and subsequently collapsed. She had symptoms of a severe acute serotonin reaction with some anaphylactic features, which improved over the following 8 hours. She stopped taking the jujube and subsequently took venlafaxine 150 mg daily for one month without adverse effects.[1] This highlights the need for physicians to ask patients about the use of herbal medicines and to advise their discontinuation before prescribing other drugs if there is any possibility of an interaction.

1. Stewart DE. Venlafaxine and sour date nut. *Am J Psychiatry* (2004) 161, 1129–30.

SNRIs; Venlafaxine + Metoclopramide

Two cases of serotonin syndrome have been attributed to the concurrent use of metoclopramide and venlafaxine.

Clinical evidence, mechanism, importance and management

A 32-year-old woman with depression who had been taking venlafaxine 225 mg daily in divided doses for 3 years was admitted to hospital after a fall. She developed a movement disorder and a period of unresponsiveness after being given a 10-mg intravenous dose of metoclopramide. After a second dose of metoclopramide the symptoms recurred and were associated with confusion, agitation, fever, diaphoresis, tachypnoea, tachycardia, and hypertension. The symptoms were consistent with serotonin syndrome, with a serious extrapyramidal movement disorder. The venlafaxine was withheld and she was given diazepam. The symptoms resolved over the next two days, after which she continued to take venlafaxine.[1] In another case, a 42-year-old woman in remission from breast cancer, who had been taking venlafaxine (dose not specified), started vomiting and took metoclopramide. On admission to hospital the following day, she was vomiting and anxious, and a head CT scan showed a frontal lesion. Intravenous fluids and metoclopramide were given and she was admitted with presumed metastatic disease and anxiety. Subsequent examination revealed a diagnosis of serotonin syndrome, which on discontinuation of venlafaxine and metoclopramide resolved within 24 hours.[2]

Information regarding an interaction between venlafaxine and metoclopramide seems to be limited to these reports, and their general relevance is unclear.

1. Fisher AA, Davis MW. Serotonin syndrome caused by selective serotonin reuptake-inhibitors–metoclopramide interaction. *Ann Pharmacother* (2002) 36, 67–71.
2. Attar-Herzberg D, Apel A, Gang N, Dvir D, Mayan H. The serotonin syndrome: initial misdiagnosis. *Isr Med Assoc J* (2009) 11, 367–70.

SNRIs; Venlafaxine + Mirtazapine

Several cases of serotonin syndrome have been reported in patients taking venlafaxine with mirtazapine.

Clinical evidence, mechanism, importance and management

A case report describes a 79-year-old man taking a number of drugs, including mirtazapine 30 mg daily and extended-release venlafaxine 225 mg daily who presented with a one to 2 week history of symptoms including agitation, confusion, myoclonic jerks, and hyperreflexia. Within 24 hours of stopping these drugs (and quetiapine and donepezil, which he was also taking) his symptoms were either improved or completely resolved.[1] Serotonin syndrome occurred in a patient given extended-release venlafaxine 75 mg daily and mirtazapine 30 mg daily during cross-tapering of the two drugs (reducing mirtazapine dose and starting venlafaxine).[2] Another report describes serotonin syndrome in an 85-year-old woman taking venlafaxine 150 mg daily and mirtazapine 30 mg daily. Her symptoms resolved on discontinuation of mirtazapine but recurred when mirtazapine was restarted.[3] A further case occurred when tramadol was given to a patient taking venlafaxine and mirtazapine.[4]

For a report of haemorrhages associated with the use of mirtazapine, venlafaxine, and escitalopram, see 'SNRIs + SSRIs', p.1478.

These cases show that serotonin syndrome might occur on the concurrent use of venlafaxine and mirtazapine. As this syndrome is potentially fatal, some caution is warranted if both drugs are given. For more information about serotonin syndrome and its management, see 'Drugs that cause serotonin syndrome + Other drugs that cause serotonin syndrome', p.1471.

1. Poeschla BD, Bartle P, Hansen KP. Serotonin syndrome associated with polypharmacy in the elderly. *Gen Hosp Psychiatry* (2011) 33, e9–e11.
2. Dimellis D. Serotonin syndrome produced by a combination of venlafaxine and mirtazapine. *World J Biol Psychiatry* (2002) 3, 167.
3. Decoutere L, De Winter S, Vander Weyden L, Spriet I, Schrooten M, Tournoy J, Fagard K. A venlafaxine and mirtazapine-induced serotonin syndrome confirmed by de- and re-challenge. *Int J Clin Pharmacol* (2012) 34, 686–8.
4. Houlihan DJ. Serotonin syndrome resulting from coadministration of tramadol, venlafaxine, and mirtazapine. *Ann Pharmacother* (2004) 38, 411–13.

SNRIs; Venlafaxine + Miscellaneous

The metabolism of venlafaxine to its active metabolite is inhibited by CYP2D6 inhibitors such as diphenhydramine, melperone, and thioridazine, but as venlafaxine and its active metabolite are equipotent, this is not considered clinically relevant. Venlafaxine modestly inhibits the metabolism of dextromethorphan, a CYP2D6 substrate.

Clinical evidence, mechanism, importance and management

(a) CYP2D6 inhibitors

Venlafaxine is primarily metabolised to its active metabolite *O*-desmethylvenlafaxine by the cytochrome P450 isoenzyme CYP2D6.[1,2] Pharmacokinetic studies show that the metabolism of venlafaxine is reduced by the CYP2D6 inhibitors **diphenhydramine**,[3] **melperone**,[4] and bupropion (see 'SNRIs; Venlafaxine + Bupropion', p.1480) in patients who are CYP2D6 extensive metabolisers (i.e. have normal levels of this isoenzyme).[3] However, the concurrent use of these inhibitors with venlafaxine would produce plasma levels of venlafaxine similar to those seen in patients who are genetically CYP2D6 poor metabolisers (about 5 to 10% of the general population), and venlafaxine and *O*-desmethylvenlafaxine are equipotent, therefore no dosage adjustment is necessary.[2] Venlafaxine is also metabolised by CYP3A4 (see 'SNRIs + Azoles', p.1477, and this metabolic pathway becomes more important when CYP2D6 is inhibited. Therefore, the UK manufacturer recommends that venlafaxine should only be used with both a CYP2D6 inhibitor and a CYP3A4 inhibitor if strictly indicated.[1]

(b) CYP2D6 substrates

In a pharmacokinetic study in 26 healthy subjects, venlafaxine, titrated to 75 mg twice daily for 4 weeks modestly inhibited the metabolism of a single 30-mg dose of **dextromethorphan**, as assessed by the molar ratio of dextromethorphan to dextrorphan in urine.[5] In another similar study venlafaxine titrated to 75 mg twice daily for 8 days did not affect the metabolism of **dextromethorphan**.[6] This suggests that venlafaxine has a minor to modest ability to inhibit the cytochrome P450 isoenzyme CYP2D6, and is generally unlikely to have a clinically relevant pharmacokinetic interaction with most CYP2D6 substrates. Note that both **dextromethorphan** and the venlafaxine have serotonergic effects, and concurrent use might lead to the serotonin syndrome. Serotonin syndrome is a rare adverse effect, but because of its severity, some caution is warranted if both drugs are given. For more information on serotonin syndrome and its management, see 'Drugs that cause serotonin syndrome + Other drugs that cause serotonin syndrome', p.1471.

A case study reports higher than expected trough plasma levels of venlafaxine and lower than expected levels of *O*-desmethylvenlafaxine in a patient also taking propranolol and **mianserin** amongst other drugs.[7] The authors suggested that these drugs might have competitively inhibited the metabolism of venlafaxine by CYP2D6. However, neither of these drugs is known to inhibit CYP2D6, and, although they are both substrates for CYP2D6, combining substrates of an isoenzyme is not usually known to cause clinically relevant pharmacokinetic interactions. Moreover, the addition of the CYP2D6 inhibitor **thioridazine** further increased the venlafaxine levels in this case, suggesting that CYP2D6 was available for inhibition. Even if a pharmacokinetic interaction with propranolol or mianserin were to be confirmed, as mentioned above, an alteration in the ratio of venlafaxine to *O*-desmethylvenlafaxine is not considered clinically relevant.

1. Efexor (Venlafaxine hydrochloride). Wyeth Pharmaceuticals. UK Summary of product characteristics, March 2008.
2. Effexor XR (Venlafaxine hydrochloride). Wyeth Pharmaceuticals Inc. US Prescribing information, March 2014.
3. Lessard E, Yessine MA, Hamelin BA, Gauvin C, Labbé L, O'Hara G, LeBlanc J, Turgeon J. Diphenhydramine alters the disposition of venlafaxine through inhibition of CYP2D6 activity in humans. *J Clin Psychopharmacol* (2001) 21, 175–84.
4. Grözinger M, Dragicevic A, Hiemke C, Shams M, Müller MJ, Härtter S. Melperone is an inhibitor of the CYP2D6 catalyzed O-demethylation of venlafaxine. *Pharmacopsychiatry* (2003) 36, 3–6.
5. Amchin J, Ereshefsky L, Zarycranski W, Taylor K, Albano D, Klockowski PM. Effect of venlafaxine versus fluoxetine on metabolism of dextromethorphan, a CYP2D6 probe. *J Clin Pharmacol* (2001) 41, 443–51.
6. Alfaro CL, Lam YWF, Simpson J, Ereshefsky L. CYP2D6 inhibition by fluoxetine, paroxetine, sertraline, and venlafaxine in a crossover study: intraindividual variability and plasma concentration correlations. *J Clin Pharmacol* (2000) 40, 58–66.
7. Eap CB, Bertel-Laubscher R, Zullino D, Amey M, Baumann P. Marked increase of venlafaxine enantiomer concentrations as a consequence of metabolic interactions: a case report. *Pharmacopsychiatry* (2000) 33, 112–15.

SNRIs; Venlafaxine + Opioids

A few cases of serotonin syndrome have been reported when tramadol was given with venlafaxine; one patient was also receiving mirtazapine. Fatal seizures occurred in an alcoholic man receiving a number of drugs, including tramadol and venlafaxine. One case of serotonin syndrome has been reported in a patient taking methadone and venlafaxine.

Clinical evidence

(a) Methadone

A 53-year-old woman taking olanzapine 5 mg daily and methadone 50 mg daily, and who had been started on extended release venlafaxine 75 mg daily within the past 5 weeks, was admitted to hospital after she developed increasing tremor, diarrhoea, sweating, insomnia, and hallucinations over the preceding 2 weeks. Serotonin syndrome was suspected and olanzapine and venlafaxine stopped. Her symptoms resolved after treatment, and she was discharged 3 days later.[1] Note that the patient had stopped fluoxetine during a previous admission, 5 weeks earlier, and a contribution from this cannot be ruled out.

(b) Tramadol

A 47-year-old man who had been stable taking venlafaxine 300 mg daily and mirtazapine 30 mg daily for 4 months was given tramadol, titrated to 300 mg daily over 4 weeks, without adverse effects. However, about 7 weeks after increasing the dose of tramadol to 400 mg daily he experienced agitation, confusion, severe shivering, diaphoresis, myoclonus, hyperreflexia, mydriasis, and tachycardia. His symptoms resolved over 36 hours after all medications were discontinued and did not recur when venlafaxine and mirtazapine were restarted without tramadol.[2] A 65-year-old woman who had been taking venlafaxine 100 mg daily for 3 weeks, developed symptoms of serotonin syndrome 3 days after tramadol 300 mg daily was started. The symptoms resolved completely 3 days after venlafaxine withdrawal, when tramadol was also withdrawn. No symptoms occurred on rechallenge with venlafaxine alone, 2 weeks later.[3] Another report describes a 68-year-old woman who had been taking venlafaxine retard 150 mg (among other medications) for almost 2 years with no adverse effects, who developed probable serotonin syndrome about one month after tramadol 150 mg daily was started.[4] A 36-year-old alcoholic died after developing seizures while taking tramadol and several other drugs, including venlafaxine, trazodone, and quetiapine, all of which interact with the neurotransmitter serotonin. It was thought that the combination of these drugs and alcohol withdrawal lowered the seizure threshold.[5]

Mechanism

Opioids such as methadone and tramadol are known to cause serotonin syndrome, as is venlafaxine. Combinations of these drugs might therefore have additive effects.

Importance and management

Evidence for an interaction between venlafaxine and opioids is limited to case studies, but based on the known effects of all of these drugs and their potential for serotonin syndrome, some caution would seem appropriate when venlafaxine is used with opioids such as tramadol or methadone. For more information on serotonin syndrome and its management, see 'Drugs that cause serotonin syndrome + Other drugs that cause serotonin syndrome', p.1471.

See *Serotonin syndrome*, under 'Additive or synergistic interactions', p.15, for further details on the development and management of this syndrome.

1. Dvir Y, Smallwood P. Serotonin syndrome: a complex but easily avoidable condition. *Gen Hosp Psychiatry* (2008) 30, 284–7.
2. Houlihan DJ. Serotonin syndrome resulting from coadministration of tramadol, venlafaxine, and mirtazapine. *Ann Pharmacother* (2004) 38, 411–13.
3. Anon. Venlafaxine + tramadol: serotonin syndrome. *Prescrire Int* (2004) 13, 57.

4. Albiñana Pérez MS, Cea Pereira L, Bilbao Salcedo J, Rodríguez Penín I. Posible syndrome serotoninérgico relacionado con la administración de venlafaxina y tramadol. *Farm Hosp* (2012) 36, 548.
5. Ripple MG, Pestaner JP, Levine BS, Smialek JE. Lethal combination of tramadol and multiple drugs affecting serotonin. *Am J Forensic Med Pathol* (2000) 21, 370–4.

SNRIs; Venlafaxine + Orphenadrine

An acute cutaneous reaction occurred on two occasions when a woman taking venlafaxine took orphenadrine with paracetamol.

Clinical evidence

A 55-year-old woman, who had been taking extended-release venlafaxine 225 mg daily for about 5 months, developed an extensive rash (diffuse and erythematous) accompanied by pruritus, sweating, hot flushes, and agitation. The reaction was initially attributed to the extended-release venlafaxine, and the patient was switched to immediate-release venlafaxine 150 mg day, which she had received in the past without problems. However, 3 months later she presented with a less severe case of the cutaneous reaction, and it transpired that she had taken a non-prescription product containing orphenadrine 35 mg and paracetamol 450 mg on both occasions.[1]

Mechanism

Results of skin testing suggested that the adverse effect was not a type I hypersensitivity reaction to orphenadrine or paracetamol. Early *in vitro* data for orphenadrine suggests that it can inhibit CYP2D6 and CYP3A4, and the authors thought that combined inhibition of these isoenzymes might have been responsible. This seems possible, see 'SNRIs; Venlafaxine + Miscellaneous', p.1482.

Importance and management

Evidence for an interaction between venlafaxine and orphenadrine is limited, and no general precautions can be issued on the basis of a single case report. Nevertheless, bear the possibility of an interaction in mind in the event of an adverse reaction to the concurrent use of these two drugs.

1. Papadimitriou GN, Theleritis CG, Papageorgiou CC, Kalogeromitros D, Syrigou E, Gregoriou S, Rabavilas AD. Acute adverse cutaneous reaction after the concomitant use of venlafaxine and orphenadrine citrate plus paracetamol in a depressed patient. *J Eur Acad Dermatol Venereol* (2006) 20, 1019.

SNRIs; Venlafaxine + Oxycodone

A case report describes the death of a CYP2D6 and CYP2C19 poor metaboliser who had high venlafaxine concentrations.

Clinical evidence, mechanism, importance and management

A case report describes a 34-year-old man taking venlafaxine 150 mg twice daily (among other medications) in whom a fatal interaction possibly involving venlafaxine, oxycodone, and ethanol was attributed to poor metaboliser status. The subject was found to have unusually high venlafaxine concentrations when compared with those seen in subjects in other studies who received venlafaxine 300 mg daily.[1] Venlafaxine is metabolised to *O*-desmethylvenlafaxine, its major active metabolite, by CYP2D6, and to *N*-desmethylvenslafaxine a minor, less active metabolite, by CYP3A4. *In vitro* studies have shown that CYP2C9 and CYP2C19 are also involved to a lesser extent in the metabolism of venlafaxine to both *N*-desmethylvenlafaxine and *O*-desmethylvenlafaxine.[2] The subject was found to be both a CYP2D6 and CYP2C19 poor metaboliser (that is, he had lower than normal activity of both of these isoenzymes). The authors also noted other factors indicating the subject might have had reduced activity of CYP3A4 also, but this was not assessed by genotyping. It therefore appears that the increase in venlafaxine concentrations was due to reduced metabolism in this patient. The authors note that venlafaxine is more cardiotoxic than its metabolite *O*-desmethylvenlafaxine, and that the increase in concentrations, combined perhaps with the CNS depressant effects of oxycodone and ethanol, might be responsible for the death of the subject.

As metaboliser status is rarely known in practice, the general clinical relevance of this case is unclear. Note that the patient was also taking haloperidol and quetiapine, both of which can increase the QT interval which might lead to torsades de pointes.

1. Jornil J, Nielsen TS, Rosendal I, Ahlner J, Zackrisson AL, Boel LW, Brock B. A poor metabolizer of both CYP2C19 and CYP2D6 identified by mechanistic pharmacokinetic simulation in a fatal drug poisoning case involving venlafaxine. *Forensic Sci Int* (2013) 226, e26–31.
2. Fogelman SM, Schmider J, Venkatakrishnan K, von Moltke LL, Harmatz JS, Shader RI, Greenblatt DJ. O- and N-demethylation of venlafaxine in vitro by human liver microsomes and by microsomes from cDNA-transfected cells: effect of metabolic inhibitors and SSRI antidepressants. *Neuropsychopharmacology* (1999) 20, 480–90.

SNRIs; Venlafaxine + Reboxetine

A case of serotonin syndrome has been described in a patient taking venlafaxine, reboxetine, and maprotiline.

Clinical evidence, mechanism, importance and management

A case report describes a 50-year-old man with a history of alcohol abuse and liver disease, taking venlafaxine, maprotiline, and reboxetine, who developed serotonin syndrome. His symptoms resolved when all medications were stopped.[1]

The general clinical relevance of this case is unclear, however as both venlafaxine and reboxetine when given alone can cause serotonin syndrome, it is possible that the patient experienced additive effects.

For more information on serotonin syndrome and its management, see 'Drugs that cause serotonin syndrome + Other drugs that cause serotonin syndrome', p.1471.

1. Bertolín-Guillén JM, Climent-Díaz B, Navarré-Gimeno A. Serotonin syndrome due to association of venlafaxine, maprotiline and reboxetine. *Eur Psychiatry* (2004) 19, 456–7.

SNRIs; Venlafaxine + Sibutramine

The use of venlafaxine with sibutramine might lead to serotonin syndrome.

Clinical evidence, mechanism, importance and management

A letter mentions a case of serotonin syndrome, that developed in a woman given venlafaxine and sibutramine (no further details given), both of which are serotonergic drugs.[1] The UK and US manufacturers of venlafaxine caution against its use with other serotonergic drugs,[2,3] but in addition, the UK manufacturer of venlafaxine specifically advises against its use with weight-loss drugs.[2] Note that sibutramine has been largely withdrawn due to the risk of serious cardiovascular effects. When available, the UK and US manufacturers advised that it should not be given with other serotonergic drugs,[4,5] or only undertaken with appropriate monitoring.[5]

Note that reports of serotonin syndrome are generally rare. If both drugs are given together it would seem prudent to monitor the outcome closely. For more information about serotonin syndrome and its management, see 'Drugs that cause serotonin syndrome + Other drugs that cause serotonin syndrome', p.1471.

1. Trakas K, Shear NH. Serotonin syndrome risk with antiobesity drug. *Can J Clin Pharmacol* (2000) 7, 216.
2. Efexor XL (Venlafaxine hydrochloride). Pfizer Ltd. UK Summary of product characteristics, December 2013.
3. Effexor XR (Venlafaxine hydrochloride). Wyeth Pharmaceuticals Inc. US Prescribing information, March 2014.
4. Reductil (Sibutramine hydrochloride monohydrate). Abbott Laboratories Ltd. UK Summary of product characteristics, December 2009.
5. Meridia (Sibutramine hydrochloride monohydrate). Abbott Laboratories. US Prescribing information, January 2010.

SNRIs; Venlafaxine + Terbinafine

Terbinafine moderately increases the exposure to venlafaxine, but only negligibly increases the total combined exposure of venlafaxine and its active metabolite.

Clinical evidence

In a randomised, crossover study, 12 healthy subjects were given a single 75-mg dose of venlafaxine, alone or after taking terbinafine 250 mg daily for 4 days. The AUC and maximum plasma concentration of venlafaxine were increased 4.9-fold and 2.7-fold, respectively, and the half-life of venlafaxine was also increased from 5.1 hours to 8.6 hours. The AUC and maximum plasma concentration of the active metabolite of venlafaxine, *O*-desmethylvenlafaxine, were decreased by 43% and 67%, respectively, and the half-life of this metabolite was almost doubled. Total combined exposure to venlafaxine and *O*-desmethylvenlafaxine was increased by 22%.[1]

Mechanism

Terbinafine inhibits CYP2D6, which is involved in the metabolism of venlafaxine to *O*-desmethylvenlafaxine. Concurrent use therefore increases exposure to venlafaxine.

Importance and management

Evidence for an interaction between venlafaxine and terbinafine is limited to this study, but a pharmacokinetic interaction is established. However, the moderate increase in the exposure to venlafaxine is probably not clinically important because the combined exposure to venlafaxine and *O*-desmethylvenlafaxine (which are both active and equipotent) was only negligibly increased, suggesting that overall no adverse effects would be expected. However, this was a single-dose study, and so could not assess the potential for venlafaxine accumulation in the presence of terbinafine. Therefore, until more is known, it might be prudent to be alert for any indication of increased venlafaxine adverse effects (e.g. nausea, insomnia, dry mouth) in patients also taking terbinafine.

1. Hynninen V-V, Olkkola KT, Bertilsson L, Kurkinen K, Neuvonen PJ, Laine K. Effect of terbinafine and voriconazole on the pharmacokinetics of the antidepressant venlafaxine. *Clin Pharmacol Ther* (2008) 83, 342–8.

SNRIs; Venlafaxine + Thiamazole

A case report describes a patient taking venlafaxine who developed akathisia and abnormal movements after thiamazole was started.

Clinical evidence, mechanism, importance and management

A case report describes a 53-year-old woman taking venlafaxine 150 mg daily (among other medications) who was started on thiamazole 20 mg daily for hypothyroidism, which was then increased to 30 mg daily after a month. Eight weeks after starting thiamazole, the patient presented with akathisia and abnormal movements of the upper extremities. As akathisia is a recognised adverse effect of venlafaxine, the dose was decreased to 112.5 mg daily. Two weeks later the abnormal movements had subsided, but the patient still exhibited occasional rocking motions and so the venlafaxine dose was further decreased to 75 mg daily. Four weeks later all symptoms had resolved and the patient's mood remained stable. The authors propose a number of hypotheses for the symptoms seen, largely based on the potential effects of the patient's thyroid status on the metabolism of venlafaxine (thyroid status can affect the metabolism of other drugs, for example see 'Theophylline + Thyroid hormones and Antithyroid drugs', p.1462), and the possibility that she was a CYP2D6 poor metaboliser (that is, she had lower than normal activity of this isoenzyme which is involved in the metabolism of venlafaxine).[1] The general clinical relevance of this single case is unclear.

1. Ng J, Sansone RA, McDonald S. Akathisia and abnormal movements of the upper extremities with venlafaxine and methimazole. *Gen Hosp Psychiatry* (2009) 31, 388–390.

SNRIs; Venlafaxine + Tobacco

The serum concentration of O-desmethylvenlafaxine, an active metabolite of venlafaxine, appears to be reduced by tobacco smoking.

Clinical evidence, mechanism, importance and management

A retrospective review of therapeutic drug monitoring results in German patients taking venlafaxine found that in 87 patients who were smokers, the dose-corrected concentration of the active metabolite, O-desmethylvenlafaxine, was 21% lower than that observed in 140 non-smokers. The dose-corrected combined concentration of venlafaxine and O-desmethylvenlafaxine was also 21% lower in the smokers than in the non-smokers. The mean daily dose and the dose-corrected concentration of venlafaxine did not differ between groups.[1] A similar study in Swedish patients found that the dose-corrected concentration of O-desmethylvenlafaxine in 58 patients who were smokers was 22% lower than that observed in 83 non-smokers.[2] These minor changes are unlikely to be clinically important.

1. Unterecker S, Hiemke C, Greiner C, Haen E, Jabs B, Deckert J, Pfuhlmann B. The effect of age, sex, smoking and co-medication on serum levels of venlafaxine and O-desmethylvenlafaxine under naturalistic conditions. *Pharmacopsychiatry* (2012) 45, 229–35.
2. Reis M, Lundmark J, Björk H, Bengtsson F. Therapeutic drug monitoring of racemic venlafaxine and its main metabolites in an everyday clinical setting. *Ther Drug Monit* (2002) 24, 545–53.

SNRIs; Venlafaxine + Trazodone

Cases of serotonin syndrome have been reported in patients taking venlafaxine with trazodone.

Clinical evidence, mechanism, importance and management

A 50-year-old HIV-positive man, who was taking methadone for opioid dependence, developed signs of serotonin syndrome 18 days after starting to take extended-release venlafaxine (dose increased to 225 mg daily over 7 days) and trazodone 100 mg at bedtime. His clinical status improved rapidly over 24 hours when all medications were discontinued. Serotonin syndrome was thought to have been precipitated by the combination of venlafaxine and trazodone, both of which inhibit the reuptake of serotonin, but methadone might have also been a contributing factor. The patient was not taking any concurrent medication for his HIV infection.[1]

In another report, a 69-year-old woman with major depression failed to respond to monotherapy with various drugs and was then given fluoxetine, trazodone, buspirone, and zolpidem. After a partial response at 2 months, she was additionally given venlafaxine 37.5 mg twice daily. On the next day she developed fever, tremor, muscle cramping, diarrhoea, ataxia, irritability, and altered consciousness, which was interpreted as serotonin syndrome. She was admitted, all medication was withdrawn, and the symptoms gradually resolved over 3 days. She then developed a full-blown manic episode.[2] Fluoxetine is known to have serotonergic effects, and might have contributed to the development of serotonin syndrome in this case.

For a case of serotonin syndrome in a patient taking trazodone, that developed when venlafaxine was abruptly switched for fluoxetine, see 'SNRIs + SSRIs', p.1478.

These cases show that serotonin syndrome might occur with concurrent use of venlafaxine and trazodone. Serotonin syndrome is a rare adverse effect, but because of its severity, some caution is warranted if both drugs are given. For more about serotonin syndrome and its management, see 'Drugs that cause serotonin syndrome + Other drugs that cause serotonin syndrome', p.1471.

1. McCue RE, Joseph M. Venlafaxine- and trazodone-induced serotonin syndrome. *Am J Psychiatry* (2001) 158, 2088–9.
2. Liau C-H, Shen WW, Su K-P. Venlafaxine-associated serotonin syndrome and manic episode in a geriatric depressive patient. *Psychiatry Clin Neurosci* (2006) 60, 121–2.

SSRIs + Ayahuasca

A man taking fluoxetine experienced symptoms of serotonin syndrome after drinking the psychoactive beverage ayahuasca, which contains monoamine oxidase-inhibiting harmala alkaloids.

Clinical evidence, mechanism, importance and management

A 36-year-old man who was taking **fluoxetine** 20 mg daily for mild depression participated in a religious ceremony using ayahuasca (also known as caapi, daime, hoasca, natema, yage) which is a psychoactive beverage characteristically containing harmala alkaloids (primarily harmine and harmaline) derived from the vine *Banisteriopsis caapi*. One hour after drinking 100 mL of ayahuasca he experienced tremors, sweating, shivering, and confusion. His condition deteriorated over the next few hours with gross motor tremors and severe nausea and vomiting, but he rapidly recovered 4 hours later, with no treatment.

The harmala alkaloids are capable of blocking the enzymatic activity of MAO for several hours, and consequently inhibit the metabolic breakdown of neurotransmitters. There is, therefore, the potential for serotonin syndrome to develop with the concurrent use of SSRIs and ayahuasca.[1]

1. Callaway JC, Grob CS. Ayahuasca preparations and serotonin reuptake inhibitors: a potential combination for severe adverse interactions. *J Psychoactive Drugs* (1998) 30, 367–9.

SSRIs + Azoles

Itraconazole slightly increases the exposure to paroxetine. The pharmacokinetics of citalopram (and therefore probably escitalopram) were not affected by a single-dose of ketoconazole. Cases of serotonin syndrome have been reported in patients taking citalopram with fluconazole, and escitalopram with miconazole. A patient taking fluoxetine developed anorexia when itraconazole was started.

Clinical evidence

(a) Pharmacokinetics

1. Citalopram. In a placebo-controlled, single-dose, crossover study in 18 healthy subjects, **ketoconazole** 200 mg did not affect the pharmacokinetics of citalopram 40 mg.[1] However note that a single-dose of ketoconazole will not have produced steady state concentrations and thus will not have had maximal effect on drug metabolising enzymes. Multiple-doses might therefore have a greater effect.

2. Paroxetine. In a crossover study in 13 healthy subjects, **itraconazole** 100 mg twice daily for 6 days increased the AUC of a single 20-mg dose of paroxetine given on day 6 by 55% and decreased its clearance by 36%.[2]

(b) Serotonin syndrome and other adverse effects

1. Citalopram. Two case reports describe life-threatening serotonin toxicity in patients with cancer whose medications included citalopram (20 and 40 mg daily) and **fluconazole** (200 and 100 mg daily, respectively). In both cases, citalopram was stopped but fluconazole continued, and symptoms resolved after 72 hours.[3] However, note that both of these cases are complicated by the use of other drugs which have also been shown to interact with citalopram: esomeprazole in one patient, see 'Proton pump inhibitors + SSRIs', p.1154, and methylthioninium chloride in the other, see 'Antidepressants + Methylthioninium chloride (Methylene blue)', p.1466.

2. Escitalopram. A case report describes an 88-year-old woman who developed serotonin syndrome 48 hours after she was started on escitalopram 5 mg daily and buccal **miconazole** 50 mg daily. She was hospitalised, and both drugs were stopped. Her symptoms resolved within 3 days.[4]

3. Fluoxetine. A man taking fluoxetine 20 mg daily, diazepam, and several anti-asthma drugs (salbutamol (albuterol), salmeterol, budesonide, theophylline) was given **itraconazole** 200 mg daily for allergic bronchopulmonary aspergillosis. Within 1 to 2 days he developed anorexia without nausea. He stopped the **itraconazole** after a week, and the anorexia resolved 1 to 2 days later.[5]

Mechanism

The azoles inhibit CYP3A4 to different degrees, and fluconazole also inhibits CYP2C19 and CYP2C9. Citalopram is metabolised by CYP2C19, with some involvement of CYP3A4 and CYP2D6, and thus its concentrations might be expected to be increased on concurrent use. The apparent absence of an interaction between ketoconazole and citalopram might be due to the use of a single-dose of ketoconazole as mentioned above, and a study to assess the effect of multiple-doses is needed. Paroxetine and fluoxetine do not appear to be primarily metabolised by CYP3A4, thus the reason for the increase in paroxetine exposure, and the case of anorexia with fluoxetine, when given with itraconazole is unclear. The mechanism for an interaction between miconazole and escitalopram is also unclear.

Importance and management

An interaction between the azoles and the SSRIs is not established. In a single-dose study, ketoconazole did not alter exposure to citalopram, however, this needs confirmation in a multiple-dose study. It appears that itraconazole might slightly increase the exposure to paroxetine. However, an increase in paroxetine exposure of this magnitude is probably not likely to be clinically important in most patients. The relevance of the two case reports of serotonin syndrome with citalopram and fluconazole is questionable given that the patients were also taking other drugs known to interact with citalopram. It is also worth noting that serotonin syndrome has been observed when SSRIs are used alone. However, note that as citalopram is known to cause a dose-dependent increase in the QT interval, in 2012 the FDA advised that the maximum dose of citalopram in patients taking a CYP2C19 inhibitor [which would include fluconazole] should be 20 mg daily because concurrent use can lead to increased citalopram concentrations and increase the risk of QT interval prolongation and Torsade de pointes.[6] Until more is known it would seem prudent to bear the possibility of an interaction in mind in the event of an increase in adverse effects.

1. Gutierrez M, Abramowitz W. Lack of effect of a single dose of ketoconazole on the pharmacokinetics of citalopram. *Pharmacotherapy* (2001) 21, 163–8.
2. Yasui-Furukori N, Saito M, Niioka T, Inoue Y, Sato Y, Kaneko S. Effect of itraconazole on pharmacokinetics of paroxetine: the role of gut transporters. *Ther Drug Monit* (2007) 29, 45–8.
3. Levin TT, Cortes-Ladino A, Weiss M, Palomba ML. Life-threatening serotonin toxicity due to a citalopram-fluconazole drug interaction: case reports and discussion. *Gen Hosp Psychiatry* (2008) 30, 372–7.

4. Baptista G, Eiden C, Monguillot P, Philibert C, Jeandel C. Serotonin syndrome during treatment with low dose of escitalopram associated with miconazole mucoadhesive tablet: a suspected drug interaction. *Int Psychogeriatr* (2012) 24, 845–7.
5. Black PN. Probable interaction between fluoxetine and itraconazole. *Ann Pharmacother* (1995) 29, 1048–9.
6. FDA. Drug safety communication: Revised recommendations for Celexa (citalopram hydrochloride) related to a potential risk of abnormal heart rhythms with high doses. March 28, 2012. Available at: http://www.fda.gov/Drugs/DrugSafety/ucm297391.htm (accessed 25/09/15).

SSRIs + Barbiturates

Paroxetine appears not to increase the psychomotor effects of amobarbital. Phenobarbital and primidone might decrease the exposure to paroxetine. Two cases of hepatotoxicity have been reported when paroxetine was given with a barbiturate.

Clinical evidence, mechanism, importance and management

In a small study in 7 healthy subjects, **phenobarbital** 100 mg daily for 14 days caused decreases of 10 to 86% in the AUC of paroxetine in 6 subjects, and a 57% *increase* in one subject. Overall, the paroxetine AUC was decreased by 25% and the elimination half-life was decreased by 38%, although these differences were not statistically significant.[1]

Phenobarbital is a well-known enzyme inducer, and these data suggest that it might decrease the exposure to paroxetine in some patients, but the clinical relevance of the changes seen is uncertain. Bear the possibility of a pharmacokinetic interaction in mind if the efficacy of paroxetine is reduced on starting phenobarbital, and adjust the paroxetine dose as necessary. **Primidone** is metabolised to phenobarbital and would be expected to interact similarly.

The sedative effects and impairment of psychomotor performance caused by **amobarbital** 100 mg were not increased by paroxetine 30 mg in 12 subjects.[2] This suggests that no adverse pharmacodynamic interaction occurs.

Two cases of hepatitis in young women were considered to be caused by the concurrent use of *Atrium* (a barbiturate complex) and paroxetine, which are both rarely associated with hepatotoxicity.[3] The relevance of these cases is uncertain.

Note that the SSRIs can cause seizures and so they should be used with caution in patients given barbiturates for epilepsy. This warning is emphasised by an isolated report describing a tonic clonic seizure in a woman taking paroxetine who was anaesthetised with methohexital. See 'Anaesthetics, general + SSRIs', p.111.

1. Greb WH, Buscher G, Dierdorf H-D, Köster FE, Wolf D, Mellows G. The effect of liver enzyme inhibition by cimetidine and enzyme induction by phenobarbitone on the pharmacokinetics of paroxetine. *Acta Psychiatr Scand* (1989) 80 (Suppl 350), 95–8.
2. Cooper SM, Jackson D, Loudon JM, McClelland GR, Raptopoulos P. The psychomotor effects of paroxetine alone and in combination with haloperidol, amylobarbitone, oxazepam, or alcohol. *Acta Psychiatr Scand* (1989) 80 (Suppl 350), 53–55.
3. Cadranel J-F, Di Martino V, Cazier A, Pras V, Bachmeyer C, Olympio P, Gonzenbach A, Mofredj A, Coutarel P, Devergie B, Biour M. *Atrium* and paroxetine-related severe hepatitis. *J Clin Gastroenterol* (1999) 28, 52–5.

SSRIs + Bupropion

There are isolated reports of serotonin syndrome, hypersexuality, psychosis, mania, and seizures associated with the use of bupropion and an SSRI. Bupropion caused a small increase in citalopram concentrations, but limited evidence suggests that the plasma concentrations of fluoxetine and paroxetine are not altered by bupropion.

Clinical evidence

(a) Citalopram

In a study in 28 healthy subjects, the addition of sustained-release bupropion 300 mg daily to citalopram 40 mg daily resulted in a 39% increase in the AUC of citalopram and a 30% increase in its maximum concentration.[1]

(b) Fluoxetine

Bupropion had no effect on the minimum concentrations of fluoxetine or norfluoxetine in a study in 5 patients who had been given fluoxetine (dose not stated) alone for a minimum of 6 weeks and then with sustained-release bupropion 150 mg daily for a further 8 weeks.[2]

The day after stopping fluoxetine 60 mg daily, a 41-year-old man started taking bupropion 75 mg and later 100 mg three times daily. After 10 days he became edgy and anxious and after 12 days he developed myoclonus. After 14 days he became severely agitated and psychotic, with delirium and hallucinations. His behaviour returned to normal 6 days after the bupropion was stopped.[3] Another patient taking lithium carbonate for bipolar disorder developed anxiety, panic, and eventually mania a little over a week after stopping fluoxetine and starting bupropion.[4]

A review briefly mentions an unpublished case of a patient who had a grand mal seizure after being given fluoxetine and bupropion 300 mg daily.[5]

A 35-year-old woman taking fluoxetine 40 mg daily was given low-dose bupropion (100 mg daily) to treat fluoxetine-induced sexual dysfunction. Despite a good initial response, hypersexuality developed, and so the bupropion was stopped.[6]

(c) Paroxetine

Bupropion had no effect on the minimum concentrations of paroxetine in a study in 4 patients who had been given paroxetine alone for a minimum of 6 weeks and then with sustained-release bupropion 150 mg daily for a further 8 weeks.[2]

(d) Sertraline

A 62-year-old woman taking therapeutic doses of bupropion and sertraline experienced upper extremity tremor, clumsiness, and gait difficulties, fluctuating symptoms of confusion, forgetfulness, and alternating agitation and lethargy, which started after a few days on this regimen. **Venlafaxine** was then added and the clinical picture worsened with deterioration of mental status, hallucinations, insomnia, myoclonic jerks, postural and balance difficulties, incoordination, and incontinence. The medications were discontinued and the symptoms, which were indicative of serotonin syndrome, gradually resolved.[7]

Another case describes spontaneous orgasm with the combined use of bupropion and sertraline. Bupropion had been successfully used to treat SSRI-induced impaired sexual function, but after 6 weeks of concurrent use she experienced a sudden-onset, spontaneous orgasm; this occurred again on rechallenge with bupropion.[8]

Mechanism

Several mechanisms have been proposed. Bupropion inhibits CYP2D6, by which some SSRIs are predominantly metabolised (see 'Table 35.2', p.1465), so might increase their plasma concentrations and the risk of toxicity. One study did find a small increase in citalopram concentrations; however, another small study unexpectedly found no changes in the plasma concentrations of fluoxetine or paroxetine when given with bupropion.[2] An *in vitro* study demonstrated that several SSRIs (paroxetine, sertraline, norfluoxetine, and fluvoxamine) could inhibit CYP2B6, the isoenzyme involved in bupropion hydroxylation,[9] and in one of the cases described above it was suggested that residual fluoxetine might have inhibited the metabolism of bupropion, leading to toxic concentrations.[3] A pharmacodynamic mechanism has also been proposed. Bupropion can cause seizures and SSRIs can further lower the seizure threshold, see 'Bupropion + Miscellaneous', p.1470.

Importance and management

Information is limited, but what is known suggests that if concurrent or sequential use of bupropion and an SSRI is thought appropriate, the patient should be closely monitored and reduced doses should be considered. The manufacturers recommend that drugs that are metabolised by CYP2D6, particularly those with a narrow therapeutic range, should be given with bupropion with caution, and initiated at the lower end of the dose range. If bupropion is given to a patient already taking a drug metabolised by CYP2D6, the need to decrease the dose of that drug should be considered.[10,11] They specifically name paroxetine,[10,11] and the US manufacturer additionally names fluoxetine and sertraline.[11] In addition, the manufacturers advise caution if bupropion is given with antidepressants that lower the seizure threshold[10,11] and, in this situation, the UK manufacturer says that consideration should be given to reducing the dose of bupropion to a maximum of 150 mg daily for smoking cessation.[10]

1. GlaxoSmithKline. Data on file. A randomized, crossover, 3-period, 2-way interaction study to evaluate potential drug interactions between Wellbutrin XL® and citalopram in healthy volunteers (Study WXL103104). 2005. Available at: http://www.gsk-clinicalstudyregister.com/ (accessed 21/10/15).
2. Kennedy SH, McCann SM, Masellis M, McIntyre RS, Raskin J, McKay G, Baker GB. Combining bupropion SR with venlafaxine, paroxetine, or fluoxetine: a preliminary report on pharmacokinetic, therapeutic, and sexual dysfunction effects. *J Clin Psychiatry* (2002) 63, 181–6.
3. van Putten T, Shaffer I. Delirium associated with bupropion. *J Clin Psychopharmacol* (1990) 10, 234.
4. Zubieta JK, Demitrack MA. Possible bupropion precipitation of mania and a mixed affective state. *J Clin Psychopharmacol* (1991) 11, 327–8.
5. Ciraulo DA, Shader RI. Fluoxetine drug-drug interactions.II. *J Clin Psychopharmacol* (1990) 10, 213–17.
6. Chollet CAS, Andreatini R. Effect of bupropion on sexual dysfunction induced by fluoxetine: a case report of hypersexuality. *J Clin Psychiatry* (2003) 64, 1268–9.
7. Munhoz RP. Serotonin syndrome induced by a combination of bupropion and SSRIs. *Clin Neuropharmacol* (2004) 27, 219–22.
8. Grimes JB, Labbate LA. Spontaneous orgasm with the combined use of bupropion and sertraline. *Biol Psychiatry* (1996) 40, 1184–5.
9. Hesse LM, Venkatakrishnan K, Court MH, von Moltke LL, Duan SX, Shader RI, Greenblatt DJ. CYP2B6 mediates the in vitro hydroxylation of bupropion: potential drug interactions with other antidepressants. *Drug Metab Dispos* (2000) 28, 1176–83.
10. Zyban (Bupropion hydrochloride). GlaxoSmithKline UK. UK Summary of product characteristics, November 2013.
11. Zyban (Bupropion hydrochloride). GlaxoSmithKline. US Prescribing information, March 2014.

SSRIs + Cyproheptadine

Several reports suggest that cyproheptadine can oppose the antidepressant effects of fluoxetine, and another describes the same effect with paroxetine.

Clinical evidence

(a) Fluoxetine

Three men with depression complained of anorgasmia when taking fluoxetine. When this was treated with cyproheptadine their depressive symptoms returned, decreasing again when cyproheptadine was stopped.[1] Two women also complained of anorgasmia within 1 to 3 months of starting to take fluoxetine 40 to 60 mg daily for bulimia nervosa. When cyproheptadine was added to treat the anorgasmia, the urge to binge on food returned in both of them and one experienced increased depression. These symptoms resolved 4 to 7 days after stopping cyproheptadine.[2] A woman successfully treated with fluoxetine 40 mg daily had a re-emergence of her depressive symptoms on two occasions within 36 hours of starting to take cyproheptadine.[3] In a further case, a woman who responded well to fluoxetine 20 mg daily for depression had a recurrence of her depression after she began to take cyproheptadine for migraine. Increasing the dose of fluoxetine to 40 mg daily controlled the depressive symptoms while cyproheptadine was continued for migraine.[4] In contrast, no exacerbation of depression was seen in a study in which both cyproheptadine and fluoxetine were used in 2 patients.[5]

(b) Paroxetine

A woman taking paroxetine 20 mg daily for depression relapsed and worsened, and developed confusion and psychotic symptoms, within 2 days of starting to take cyproheptadine 2 mg twice daily for anorgasmia.[6] The psychotic symptoms resolved 2 days after stopping cyproheptadine.

Mechanism

Although the mechanism is not fully understood, it has been suggested that because cyproheptadine is a serotonin antagonist it blocks or opposes the serotonergic effects of these SSRIs.[1-3,6]

Importance and management

Direct information about this interaction appears to be limited to these reports, although cyproheptadine has also been found to oppose the antidepressant effects of MAOIs (see 'MAOIs or RIMAs + Antihistamines; Cyproheptadine', p.1384). One study suggests that not every patient is affected.[5] If concurrent use is thought appropriate, the patient should be closely monitored for evidence of a reduced antidepressant response.

Because of its serotonin antagonist effects, cyproheptadine has been used to treat serotonin syndrome, including cases resulting from the use of SSRIs. See 'Drugs that cause serotonin syndrome + Other drugs that cause serotonin syndrome', p.1471 for further details on the development and management of this syndrome.

1. Feder R. Reversal of antidepressant activity of fluoxetine by cyproheptadine in three patients. *J Clin Psychiatry* (1991) 52, 163–4.
2. Goldbloom DS, Kennedy SH. Adverse interaction of fluoxetine and cyproheptadine in two patients with bulimia nervosa. *J Clin Psychiatry* (1991) 52, 261–2.
3. Katz RJ, Rosenthal M. Adverse interaction of cyproheptadine with serotonergic antidepressants. *J Clin Psychiatry* (1994) 55, 314–15.
4. Boon F. Cyproheptadine and SSRIs. *J Am Acad Child Adolesc Psychiatry* (1999) 38, 112.
5. McCormick S, Olin J, Brotman AW. Reversal of fluoxetine-induced anorgasmia by cyproheptadine in two patients. *J Clin Psychiatry* (1990) 51, 383–4.
6. Christensen RC. Adverse interaction of paroxetine and cyproheptadine. *J Clin Psychiatry* (1995) 56, 433–4.

SSRIs + Food

Food slightly increases the exposure to vilazodone. Paroxetine exposure appears to be slightly decreased by the consumption of large volumes of milk. The pharmacokinetics of citalopram, escitalopram, fluoxetine, fluvoxamine, paroxetine, and sertraline are not altered by food.

Clinical evidence, mechanism, importance and management

(a) Citalopram

The UK and US manufacturers of citalopram briefly note that its absorption is not affected by food intake and that it can be taken without regard to food.[1,2]

(b) Escitalopram

A randomised crossover study in 17 healthy subjects given a single 20-mg dose of escitalopram followed by a standardised high-fat breakfast (1000 calories, 50% fat) or a single 20-mg dose of escitalopram in the fasted state, found that administration with food did not affect the pharmacokinetics of escitalopram.[3] Escitalopram can be taken without regard to food.

(c) Fluoxetine

The UK and US manufacturers of fluoxetine briefly note that food intake does not affect the bioavailability of fluoxetine,[4,5] although its absorption might be delayed by 1 to 2 hours, however this is probably not clinically relevant.[5] Fluoxetine can be taken with or without food.

(d) Fluvoxamine

A crossover study in 12 healthy subjects found that the pharmacokinetics of a single 50-mg dose of fluvoxamine taken 15 minutes before a standardised breakfast were no different to when it was taken in the fasted state.[6] Fluvoxamine can be taken without regard to food.

(e) Paroxetine

A study in healthy subjects found that the pharmacokinetics of a single 30-mg dose of paroxetine were not altered by high- or low-fat food, when compared with the fasting state. A 40% decrease in exposure was seen when paroxetine was taken with one litre of **milk**,[7] but it would seem unlikely that many people would drink such a large amount regularly, at the same time as taking paroxetine, and so this interaction is unlikely to be generally relevant. The US manufacturer of paroxetine states that it can be taken with or without food,[8] however the UK manufacturer recommends it be taken with food.[9]

(f) Sertraline

In a randomised crossover study, 24 healthy subjects were given a single 100-mg dose of sertraline either after a 6 hour fast, or 30 minutes after a standardised meal (35% fat). The maximum plasma concentration of sertraline was 25% higher after food than in the fasting state and was achieved more rapidly (5.4 versus 7.9 hours). However the AUC was not altered by administration with food, and 12 to 24 hours after administration the plasma concentrations of all subjects were similar.[10] Sertraline can be taken without regard to food.

(g) Vilazodone

The US manufacturer of vilazodone briefly notes that when it was given in the fasted state, the AUC and maximum plasma concentration were decreased by about 50% and 60%, respectively, when compared with when vilazodone was given with food. They therefore advise that vilazodone should be taken with food to avoid the possibility of reduced efficacy in some patients.[11]

1. Cipramil Tablets (Citalopram hydrobromide). Lundbeck Ltd. UK Summary of product characteristics, July 2015.
2. Celexa (Citalopram hydrobromide). Forest Pharmaceuticals, Inc. US Prescribing information, July 2014.
3. Søgaard B, Mengel H, Rao N, Larsen F. The pharmacokinetics of escitalopram after oral and intravenous administration of single and multiple doses to healthy subjects. *J Clin Pharmacol* (2005) 45, 1400–6.
4. Prozac (Fluoxetine hydrochloride). Eli Lilly and Company Ltd. UK Summary of product characteristics, October 2014.
5. Prozac (Fluoxetine hydrochloride). Eli Lilly and Company. US Prescribing information, July 2014.
6. Van Harten J, Van Bemmel P, Dobrinska MR, Ferguson RK, Raghoebar M. Bioavailability of fluvoxamine given with and without food. Biopharm Drug Dispos. (1991) 12, 571–6.
7. Greb WH, Brett MA, Buscher G, Dierdorf H-D, von Schrader HW, Wolf D, Mellows G, Zussman BD. Absorption of paroxetine under various dietary conditions and following antacid intake. *Acta Psychiatr Scand* (1989) 80 (Suppl 350), 99–101.
8. Paxil Tablets and Suspension (Paroxetine hydrochloride). GlaxoSmithKline. US Prescribing information, December 2012.
9. Seroxat (Paroxetine hydrochloride hemihydrate). GlaxoSmithKline. UK Summary of product characteristics, August 2015.
10. Ronfeld RA, Wilner KD, Baris BA. Sertraline. Chronopharmacokinetics and the effect of coadministration with food. *Clin Pharmacokinet* (1997) 32 (Suppl 1), 50–5.
11. Viibryd (Vilazodone hydrochloride). Forest Pharmaceuticals, Inc. US Prescribing information, March 2015.

SSRIs + Grapefruit juice

Grapefruit juice slightly increases the exposure to fluvoxamine, and there is a case report of adverse effects attributed to this pharmacokinetic interaction. Sertraline exposure is moderately increased by grapefruit juice. Excessive consumption of grapefruit caused symptoms similar to serotonin syndrome in a patient taking fluoxetine and trazodone.

Clinical evidence

(a) Fluoxetine

A 57-year-old HIV-positive man had been receiving indinavir, stavudine, and lamivudine, as well as other medications including fluoxetine 20 mg daily and trazodone 200 mg daily. He complained of dizziness, mild confusion, diarrhoea, visual changes, and a general feeling of being "out of sorts" for approximately one month. On further questioning it was found that the patient had been having one grapefruit each morning but had increased his consumption to 3 per day. His symptoms resolved when he stopped eating grapefruit.[1]

(b) Fluvoxamine

A randomised, placebo-controlled, crossover study in 10 healthy subjects found that 250 mL of grapefruit juice three times daily for 6 days increased the AUC of a single 75-mg dose of fluvoxamine by 60% and increased its maximum plasma concentration by 33%.[2]

A 75-year-old woman taking fluvoxamine 150 mg at night experienced palpitations when on holiday in Florida. When she returned home the palpitations stopped. The only change identified was that she drank grapefruit juice daily while in Florida. She had previously experienced palpitations when taking a higher dose of fluvoxamine (200 mg at night).[3]

(c) Sertraline

In a crossover study, 8 healthy subjects were given 250 mL of regular strength grapefruit juice three times daily for 5 days with a single 75-mg dose of sertraline on day 6. Grapefruit juice increased the AUC and maximum plasma concentration of sertraline 2-fold and by 66%, respectively.[4] Another study in 5 patients taking sertraline 50 to 75 mg daily found that the concurrent use of grapefruit juice for one week increased the minimum concentration of sertraline by almost 50%.[5]

Mechanism

Grapefruit juice is an inhibitor of CYP3A4 and sertraline is partially metabolised by this isoenzyme. Therefore grapefruit juice would be expected to reduce the metabolism of sertraline. This has been demonstrated *in vitro*; grapefruit juice inhibited the formation of desmethylsertraline in a dose-dependent manner.[5] Fluoxetine and fluvoxamine are not appreciably metabolised by CYP3A4, but grapefruit juice also inhibits other isoenzymes that could affect the metabolism of SSRIs, especially if the patient is also a CYP2D6 poor metaboliser (that is, has lower than normal activity of this isoenzyme).[2,3] Note that this might have been the case with the subjects included in one study.[4]

Importance and management

The pharmacokinetic interactions between grapefruit juice and fluvoxamine and sertraline would appear to be established. Grapefruit juice moderately increases the exposure to sertraline, although further study is needed to confirm this as both studies were in a small group of patients. The slight increase in fluvoxamine exposure seen would not usually be considered to be clinically relevant. However, the fluvoxamine dose given in the study was at the lower end of the recommended licensed dose, and given the case report of an interaction with a higher dose, the possibility of a greater increase in fluvoxamine exposure with multiple, higher doses cannot be ruled out. In addition, given the isolated report of an interaction between grapefruit and fluoxetine, until more is known about the mechanism for this effect, the possibility of an interaction with grapefruit juice should be borne in mind, especially if unusual amounts of grapefruit have been consumed. Note that the UK manufacturer of sertraline advises avoiding the concurrent use of sertraline and grapefruit juice.[6]

1. DeSilva KE, Le Flore DB, Marston BJ, Rimland D. Serotonin syndrome in HIV-infected individuals receiving antiretroviral therapy and fluoxetine. *AIDS* (2001) 15, 1281–5.
2. Hori H, Yoshimura R, Ueda N, Eto S, Shinkai K, Sakata S, Ohmori O, Terao T, Nakamura J. Grapefruit juice-fluvoxamine interaction. Is it risky or not? *J Clin Psychopharmacol* (2003) 23, 422–4.
3. Wiens A. How does grapefruit juice affect psychotropic medications? *J Psychiatry Neurosci* (2000) 25, 198.
4. Ueda N, Yoshimura R, Umene-Nakano W, Ikenouchi-Sugita A, Hori H, Hayashi K, Kodama Y, Nakamura J. Grapefruit juice alters plasma sertraline levels after single ingestion of sertraline in healthy volunteers. *World J Biol Psychiatry* (2009) 10, 832–5.
5. Lee AJ, Chan WK, Harralson AF, Buffum J, Bui B-CC. The effects of grapefruit juice on sertraline metabolism: an in vitro and in vivo study. *Clin Ther* (1999) 21, 1890–9.
6. Lustral (Sertraline hydrochloride). Pfizer Ltd. UK Summary of product characteristics, March 2015.

SSRIs + H_2-receptor antagonists

The exposure to citalopram, escitalopram, paroxetine, and sertraline is slightly increased by cimetidine.

Clinical evidence

(a) Citalopram

1. Pharmacokinetics. In a study, 12 healthy subjects were given citalopram 40 mg daily for 21 days and then for the next 8 days they were also given **cimetidine** 400 mg twice daily. **Cimetidine** caused a 29% decrease in the oral clearance of citalopram, a 39% increase in its maximum serum concentrations, and a 43% increase in its AUC. Some changes in the renal clearance of the citalopram metabolites were also seen.[1]

2. Serotonin syndrome. A case report describes a 75-year-old man with Alzheimer's disease and behavioural disturbances, taking citalopram, donepezil, quetiapine, and ticlopidine who was admitted to hospital with gastric bleeding due to an ulcer and started on **cimetidine**. Five weeks later the patient was re-admitted with what was thought to be serotonin syndrome. Citalopram and cimetidine were discontinued, and symptoms were fully resolved a week later.[2]

(b) Escitalopram

In a controlled study in 16 healthy subjects, **cimetidine** 400 mg twice daily for 5 days increased the AUC of escitalopram by about 70% when a single 20-mg dose of escitalopram was given on day 4. There was also a 22% increase in the maximum plasma concentration of escitalopram.[3]

(c) Paroxetine

In a study in 10 healthy subjects, **cimetidine** 200 mg four times daily for 8 days did not affect the mean pharmacokinetic values or bioavailability of a single 30-mg dose of paroxetine. However, in 2 subjects the AUC of paroxetine was increased by 55% and 81%, respectively.[4] Another study in 11 healthy subjects found that **cimetidine** 300 mg three times daily increased the AUC of paroxetine 30 mg daily by about 50% after one week of concurrent use.[5]

(d) Sertraline

In a randomised, crossover study, 12 healthy subjects were given either **cimetidine** 800 mg or a placebo at bedtime for 8 days, with a single 100-mg dose of sertraline on day 2. **Cimetidine** increased the AUC of sertraline by 50%, increased its maximum serum concentrations by 24%, and prolonged its half-life by 26%.[6]

Mechanism

Cimetidine is known to inhibit the activity of some of the isoenzymes involved in the metabolism of the SSRIs (e.g. CYP2C19, CYP2D6, and CYP3A4) and might therefore increase their exposure on concurrent use. Further study is required to establish the specific isoenzymes involved.

Importance and management

The pharmacokinetic interactions between cimetidine and citalopram, escitalopram, paroxetine, and sertraline are established. However, the slight increases seen in their exposure would not be expected to be clinically relevant in most patients because the SSRIs are usually well tolerated, have a wide therapeutic range, and there are large pharmacokinetic variations between individual subjects.[1,3]. The general relevance of the case of serotonin syndrome with citalopram is unclear as it is complicated by other factors related to the patient's comorbidities. Nevertheless, as citalopram has been reported to cause small dose-related increases in the QT interval, the FDA in the US[7] advises that the dose of citalopram should be limited to 20 mg daily in those patients also taking cimetidine. In addition, the results from the paroxetine study suggest that individual patients could experience greater increases in the exposure to the SSRI. Therefore it would seem prudent to bear the possibility of an interaction in mind should any SSRI adverse effects (such as dry mouth, nausea, diarrhoea, dyspepsia, tremor, ejaculatory delay, sweating) occur, and to consider reducing the SSRI dose if these become troublesome.

If the suggested mechanism of interaction is true, one of the other H_2-receptor antagonists that lack enzyme inhibitory activity, such as ranitidine or famotidine, might be a non-interacting alternative to cimetidine, but this needs confirmation.

1. Priskorn M, Larsen F, Segonzac A, Moulin M. Pharmacokinetic interaction study of citalopram and cimetidine in healthy subjects. *Eur J Clin Pharmacol* (1997) 52, 241–2.
2. Talarico G, Tosto G, Pietracupa S, Piacentini E, Canavelli M, Lenzi GL, Bruno G. Serotonin toxicity: a short review of the literature and two case reports involving citalopram. *Neurol Sci* (2011) 32, 507–9.
3. Malling D, Poulsen MN, Søgaard B. The effect of cimetidine or omeprazole on the pharmacokinetics of escitalopram in healthy subjects. *Br J Clin Pharmacol* (2005) 60, 287–90.
4. Greb WH, Buscher G, Dierdorf H-D, Köster FE, Wolf D, Mellows G. The effect of liver enzyme inhibition by cimetidine and enzyme induction by phenobarbitone on the pharmacokinetics of paroxetine. *Acta Psychiatr Scand* (1989) 80 (Suppl 350), 95–8.
5. Bannister SJ, Houser VP, Hulse JD, Kisicki JC, Rasmussen JGC. Evaluation of the potential for interactions of paroxetine with diazepam, cimetidine, warfarin, and digoxin. *Acta Psychiatr Scand* (1989) 80 (Suppl 350), 102–6.
6. Invicta Pharmaceuticals. Data on file. Phase 1 study to assess the potential of cimetidine to alter the disposition of sertraline in normal, healthy male volunteers (Study 050-019). 1991.
7. FDA Drug Safety communication: Abnormal heart rhythms associated with high doses of Celexa (citalopram hydrochloride). August 24, 2011. Available at: http://www.fda.gov/Drugs/DrugSafety/ucm269086.htm (accessed 03/09/15).

SSRIs + HIV-protease inhibitors

Darunavir boosted with ritonavir slightly decreases paroxetine and sertraline exposure. Fosamprenavir boosted with ritonavir slightly decreases paroxetine exposure. Paroxetine does not appear to alter the exposure of darunavir or fosamprenavir, both boosted with ritonavir, and sertraline does not appear to alter darunavir concentrations, whereas fluoxetine negligibly increased the exposure of ritonavir in one study. Two cases of serotonin syndrome have been attributed to the use of fluoxetine and ritonavir.

Clinical evidence

(a) Darunavir

In a pharmacokinetic study, the AUC and minimum concentration of **paroxetine** were decreased by 39% and 37%, respectively, when **paroxetine** 20 mg daily and darunavir boosted with ritonavir 400/100 mg twice daily were given concurrently. The AUC and minimum concentration of darunavir were unaffected on concurrent use.[1,2]

In a very similar study using the same dose of darunavir boosted with ritonavir, the AUC and minimum concentration of **sertraline** 50 mg daily were decreased by 49% without any effect on darunavir concentrations.[1,2] Note that the dose of darunavir used in these studies (400 mg twice daily) is less than that recommended (600 mg twice daily).[1,2] For a case report describing serotonin syndrome in a patient with reduced activity of CYP2C19, CYP2D6, and CYP3A4, and taking **escitalopram**, esomeprazole, and darunavir boosted with ritonavir, see 'Proton pump inhibitors + SSRIs', p.1154.

(b) Fosamprenavir

In a pharmacokinetic study in healthy subjects, the AUC and maximum concentration of **paroxetine** were decreased by 54% and 50%, respectively, when **paroxetine** 20 mg daily and fosamprenavir boosted with ritonavir 700/100 mg twice daily were given together for 10 days. The pharmacokinetics of fosamprenavir and ritonavir did not differ from historical control values.[3]

(c) Ritonavir

In a single-dose study involving 18 healthy subjects, no statistically significant pharmacokinetic changes were seen when ritonavir 600 mg was given at the same time as **escitalopram** 20 mg.[4] These findings need confirmation with multiple doses, because the effects of ritonavir on drug metabolising enzymes would not have been maximal before **escitalopram** was given.

In a study, ritonavir 600 mg was given to 16 healthy subjects before and after they took **fluoxetine** 30 mg twice daily for 8 days. The maximum plasma concentration of ritonavir was unaffected, but its AUC increased by 19%. These changes were not considered large enough to warrant changing the dose of ritonavir.[5] The study was criticised for not achieving steady-state before assessing the pharmacokinetics and thus possibly underestimating the interaction.[6] However, the authors state that **fluoxetine** concentrations were equivalent to those seen at steady-state, and multiple dosing of ritonavir is likely to induce its own metabolism, so if anything, the interaction would be lessened at steady-state.[7]

Two cases of serotonin syndrome were attributed to adding ritonavir to established **fluoxetine** treatment. One of these patients later tolerated **saquinavir** boosted with ritonavir when the **fluoxetine** dose was halved, and in the other **nelfinavir** was substituted for ritonavir.[8] Another case of serotonin syndrome developed in a patient taking **fluoxetine** and trazodone when ritonavir was added, see 'Trazodone + HIV-protease inhibitors', p.1499.

Mechanism

It has been assumed that ritonavir would increase the concentrations of SSRIs that are substrates for CYP2D6 (e.g. fluoxetine, paroxetine, sertraline) due to the inhibitory effect of ritonavir on this isoenzyme.[9] However, low-dose ritonavir used as a pharmacokinetic booster with other HIV-protease inhibitors actually *decreases* paroxetine and sertraline concentrations. The mechanism is not known.

Importance and management

The pharmacokinetic interaction showing an unexpected decrease in **paroxetine** and **sertraline** exposure with low-dose ritonavir, when given to boost darunavir and fosamprenavir, is established. Although the clinical relevance of these decreases is not certain, it would be prudent to anticipate some reduction in the efficacy of these SSRIs when starting these HIV-protease inhibitors, and to monitor the clinical effect and increase the SSRI dose as necessary. Whether other SSRIs would be affected similarly is unknown, but **fluoxetine** would be expected to be. Moreover, whether other HIV-protease inhibitors boosted with ritonavir interact similarly is unknown, but it would be prudent to expect that they might also decrease the exposure of these SSRIs. Despite this, the UK manufacturer of ritonavir states that it will *increase* the concentrations of fluoxetine, paroxetine, and sertraline.[9] In addition, the US manufacturer of **tipranavir**[10] also predicts that tipranavir boosted with ritonavir will result in an *increase* in the concentrations of these SSRIs. However, given the unexpected outcome with ritonavir, the outcome of any interaction between these SSRIs and tipranavir is as yet unknown.

The available data for ritonavir alone and darunavir and fosamprenavir, both boosted with ritonavir, suggest that the pharmacokinetics of these HIV-protease inhibitors are not affected to a clinically relevant extent by fluoxetine, sertraline, or paroxetine. This suggests that there are no pharmacokinetic concerns regarding antiviral efficacy or adverse effects.

Although there is a study suggesting **escitalopram** concentrations are not affected by ritonavir, the findings of this study are questionable as it used simultaneous single doses. The general relevance of the few cases of serotonin syndrome is also uncertain.

1. Prezista (Darunavir ethanolate). Janssen-Cilag Ltd. UK Summary of product characteristics, March 2014.
2. Prezista (Darunavir ethanolate). Janssen Pharmaceuticals, Inc. US Prescribing information, April 2014.
3. van der Lee MJ, Blenke AAM, Rongen GA, Verwey-van Wissen CPWGM, Koopmans PP, Pharo C, Burger DM. Interaction study of the combined use of paroxetine and fosamprenavir-ritonavir in healthy subjects. *Antimicrob Agents Chemother* (2007) 51, 4098–104.
4. Gutierrez, MM, Rosenberg J, Abramowitz W. An evaluation of the potential for pharmacokinetic interaction between escitalopram and the cytochrome P450 3A4 inhibitor ritonavir. *Clin Ther* (2003) 25, 1200–10.
5. Ouellet D, Hsu A, Qian J, Lamm JE, Cavanaugh JH, Leonard JM, Granneman GR. Effect of fluoxetine on the pharmacokinetics of ritonavir. *Antimicrob Agents Chemother* (1998) 42, 3107–12.
6. Bellibas SE. Ritonavir-fluoxetine interaction. *Antimicrob Agents Chemother* (1999) 43, 1815.
7. Ouellet D, Hsu A. Ritonavir-fluoxetine interaction. *Antimicrob Agents Chemother* (1999) 43, 1815.
8. DeSilva KE, Le Flore DB, Marston BJ, Rimland D. Serotonin syndrome in HIV-infected individuals receiving antiretroviral therapy and fluoxetine. *AIDS* (2001) 15, 1281–5.
9. Norvir Film-coated Tablets (Ritonavir). AbbVie Ltd. UK Summary of product characteristics, March 2014.
10. Aptivus (Tipranavir). Boehringer Ingelheim Pharmaceuticals, Inc. US Prescribing information, April 2014.

SSRIs + 5-HT$_3$-receptor antagonists

Fluvoxamine markedly increases alosetron exposure. Alosetron does not alter fluoxetine exposure. Symptoms similar to serotonin syndrome have been reported in one patient taking paroxetine and ondansetron. A patient taking sertraline and dolasetron also developed symptoms similar to serotonin syndrome, but subsequently took sertraline and ondansetron without problems. A report describes failure of ondansetron antiemetic prophylaxis in 3 patients taking fluoxetine, and a case-control study suggests that antiemetic prophylaxis with ondansetron and aprepitant might be less effective in patients taking an SSRI.

Clinical evidence

(a) Fluoxetine

A study in 12 healthy subjects found that **alosetron** 1 mg twice daily for 15 days had no effect on the pharmacokinetics of a single 20-mg dose of fluoxetine other than a median 3-hour delay in the time to reach the maximum concentrations of both *S*- and *R*-fluoxetine.[1]

A case series describes 3 patients receiving cancer chemotherapy in whom antiemetic prophylaxis with **ondansetron** failed while they were taking fluoxetine. In each case, fluoxetine was stopped and ondansetron was partially or completely effective the following day. One of the patients had been taking fluoxetine long-term, whereas the other two had received fluoxetine for one and three weeks, respectively.[2]

(b) Fluvoxamine

The US manufacturer[3] of **alosetron** states that fluvoxamine (50 mg daily increased to 200 mg daily for 16 days) increased the AUC of alosetron about 6-fold and prolonged its half-life about 3-fold, when a single 1-mg dose of alosetron was given on day 16.

(c) Paroxetine

A possible case of serotonin syndrome (or possibly neuroleptic malignant syndrome) was reported in a 49-year-old woman who developed postoperative delirium. She had been taking paroxetine 30 mg daily up to 2 days before surgery and was given **ondansetron** 4 mg during surgery and morphine during and after surgery. Approximately one hour after leaving theatre she became agitated and confused. She also displayed uncontrolled limb movements, brisk reflexes, ankle clonus, abnormal ocular function, hypertension, pyrexia, and increased creatinine kinase. The delirium did not respond to naloxone, diazepam, or flumazenil, and lasted for nearly 2 days.[4]

(d) Sertraline

A 49-year-old woman who had been taking **sertraline** for some time without incident, was premedicated with **dolasetron** 100 mg before receiving her first cycle of adjuvant chemotherapy for breast cancer. Shortly afterwards she developed symptoms of profound agitation and elation, but with an overwhelming desire to commit suicide, and was disoriented. The symptoms resolved within hours without pharmacological intervention. Three weeks later she received the same medications except that **ondansetron** was substituted for **dolasetron** and she experienced no adverse effects. The author concluded that a variant of serotonin syndrome might rarely be seen when 5-HT$_3$-receptor antagonists and SSRIs are given together.[5]

(e) Various SSRIs

In a retrospective case-control study in chemonaive patients receiving **ondansetron** and **aprepitant** as antiemetic prophylaxis, 59.1% of patients also taking an SSRI (**citalopram** 2 patients, **escitalopram** 3 patients, **fluoxetine** 4 patients, **paroxetine** 2 patients, **sertraline** 2 patients) or an SNRI (**venlafaxine** 9 patients) experienced at least one episode of grade 1 acute vomiting, compared with 22.7% of patients not taking an SSRI or SNRI (odds ratio 4.72). Grade 2 acute vomiting occurred in 41.2% of patients taking an SSRI or SNRI, compared with 5.9% of patients not taking an SSRI or SNRI (odds ratio 5.07).[6]

Mechanism

Several explanations for the agitation and delirium, involving the disruption of serotonergic and/or dopaminergic transmission, have been suggested.[4] There has been some debate about whether inhibition of CYP2D6 was another possible mechanism with the paroxetine case, but this seems unlikely.[4,7]

The increase in alosetron exposure probably occurs because fluvoxamine is a potent inhibitor of CYP1A2, the isoenzyme by which alosetron is metabolised.

Regarding the failure of antiemetic prophylaxis, a pharmacodynamic interaction at the 5-HT3 receptor has been proposed,[6] and it has been suggested that accumulation of serotonin as a result of the use of SSRIs might overcome the blockade by 5-HT$_3$-receptor antagonists, such as ondansetron, reducing their efficacy.[2] However, as fluoxetine has such a long half-life, any such effect is unlikely to be reversed as rapidly as stated in the case series on stopping fluoxetine. Further research is needed.

Importance and management

Evidence for an interaction between the SSRIs and 5-HT$_3$-receptor antagonists is limited and not established. A small number of cases of serotonin syndrome arising in patients given a SSRI with a 5-HT$_3$-receptor antagonist have been reported, but no general recommendations can be made from such a small data set. Nevertheless, it would be prudent to bear in mind the possibility of serotonin syndrome if similar adverse effects occur. For more information on serotonin syndrome and its management, see 'Drugs that cause serotonin syndrome + Other drugs that cause serotonin syndrome', p.1471.

The marked increase in alosetron exposure caused by fluvoxamine, a potent CYP1A2 inhibitor, is likely to be clinically important, and the US manufacturer of alosetron therefore contraindicates concurrent use.[3] They also state that moderate inhibitors of CYP1A2 should also be avoided, as they have not been studied, and they name the **quinolones**. Note however, that the quinolones inhibit CYP1A2 to varying extents and some have no effect at all. For a list of CYP1A2 inhibitors, see 'Table 1.2', p.5. If concurrent use is considered necessary, it would be prudent to monitor for alosetron adverse effects (such as constipation, abdominal discomfort, nausea) and to reduce the alosetron dose accordingly.

Alosetron does not appear to have a clinically relevant effect on the pharmacokinetics of fluoxetine, and so no dose adjustment of fluoxetine is likely to be necessary on concurrent use.

The report of failure of ondansetron prophylaxis in 3 patients taking fluoxetine, and the retrospective case-control study, suggest that antiemetic prophylaxis with ondansetron alone, or with aprepitant, might be less effective in patients taking an SSRI or **SNRI**. Until more is known, bear the possibility of an interaction in mind in cases of otherwise unexplained reduced antiemetic efficacy in patients also taking an SSRI or **SNRI**.

1. D'Souza DL, Dimmitt DC, Robbins DK, Nezamis J, Simms L, Koch KM. Effect of alosetron on the pharmacokinetics of fluoxetine. *J Clin Pharmacol* (2001) 41, 455–8.
2. Koriech OM. Fluoxetine treatment comprises the antiemetic efficacy of ondansetron in cancer patients. *Clin Oncol (R Coll Radiol)* (1995) 7, 371–2.
3. Lotronex (Alosetron hydrochloride). Prometheus Laboratories, Inc. US Prescribing information, March 2014.
4. Stanford BJ, Stanford SC. Postoperative delirium indicating an adverse drug interaction involving the selective serotonin reuptake inhibitor, paroxetine? *J Psychopharmacol* (1999) 13, 313–17.
5. Sorscher SM. Probable serotonin syndrome variant in a patient receiving a selective serotonin reuptake inhibitor and a 5-HT$_3$ receptor antagonist. *J Psychopharmacol* (2002) 16, 191.
6. Mir O, Durand JP, Boudou-Rouquette P, Giroux J, Coriat R, Cessot A, Ropert S, Goldwasser F, Gaillard R. Interaction between serotonin reuptake inhibitors, 5-HT3 antagonists, and NK1 antagonists in cancer patients receiving highly emetogenic chemotherapy: a case-control study. *Support Care Cancer* (2012) 20, 2235–9.
7. Palmer JL. Postoperative delirium indicating an adverse drug interaction involving the selective serotonin reuptake inhibitor, paroxetine? *J Psychopharmacol* (2000) 14, 186–8.

SSRIs + Interferons

In one patient taking paroxetine and trazodone, depression recurred when interferon alfa was given. Another patient taking interferon alfa developed a manic episode when citalopram and quetiapine were added. Peginterferon alfa 2-b appeared to decrease the half-life of fluoxetine in a patient with hepatitis C.

Clinical evidence

(a) Citalopram

A case report describes a 33-year-old woman with hepatitis C who developed depression during treatment with **peginterferon alfa**, and was started on citalopram 20 mg daily and quetiapine 25 mg at night. Two weeks later the patient experienced a manic episode. Citalopram was stopped and interferon withheld for a week while quetiapine was increased to 150 mg at night. The manic symptoms resolved and the patient completed 6 months of treatment with interferon at half, and then at full dose, while quetiapine was continued.[1] SSRIs have been used to try to treat depression caused by interferon alfa. In a study, 28 out of 100 patients treated with **peginterferon alfa-2b** and ribavirin who developed clinically relevant interferon-induced depression were randomised to citalopram 20 mg daily or placebo. The study was terminated early because citalopram proved superior to placebo within 4 weeks.[2]

(b) Fluoxetine

In a study in 19 patients with chronic hepatitis C, the pharmacokinetics of a single 40-mg dose of fluoxetine were unaltered after 2 months of treatment with **peginterferon alfa-2b** (1 microgram/kg weekly) and **ribavirin**, except for a decrease in the fluoxetine half-life from 47.3 to 33.23 hours.[3]

(c) Paroxetine

A 31-year-old woman, whose mood and other depressive symptoms improved during treatment with **paroxetine** 50 mg daily and trazodone 50 mg at night, was later found to have essential thrombocythaemia. After unsuccessful treatment with dipyridamole, she was given **interferon alfa**, stabilised at 3 million units three times weekly. After 3 months her depressive symptoms returned, and worsened over a period of 6 months, despite increased doses of trazodone and cognitive therapy. **Interferon alfa** was discontinued and replaced by hydroxycarbamide, and then anagrelide. After a good response to a course of ECT, her depressive symptoms were controlled by **paroxetine** 50 mg daily and trazodone 150 mg at night.[4] SSRIs have been used to try to prevent depression caused by interferon alfa. For example, in one study, 9 of 20 patients taking high-dose **interferon alfa** developed depression, compared with just 2 of 18 patients also given **paroxetine** (10 mg daily titrated up to 40 mg daily started 2 weeks before the interferon).[5]

Mechanism

Unknown. Interferon commonly causes depression, and in one case report it was suggested that this might be due to the capacity of interferon to impair serotonin synthesis, by inducing enzymes that degrade the serotonin precursor tryptophan.[4] Interferon therapy can cause mania, and in the case in which mania occurred in a patient taking citalopram and interferon alfa, the author suggests that the risk of mania might be increased by the addition of an antidepressant.[1] The decrease in fluoxetine half-life seen with interferon alfa 2-b suggests that it might induce the metabolism of fluoxetine in patients with chronic hepatitis. It has been proposed that this might be due to an improvement in liver function related to the use of the interferon.[3]

Importance and management

A pharmacokinetic interaction between SSRIs and interferon is not established and further research is needed. However a pharmacodynamic interaction might occur. It seems possible that interferon might reduce the antidepressant efficacy of the SSRIs. The general relevance of the case of mania attributed to citalopram is unclear. The possible pharmacodynamic interaction, and the use of SSRIs for the prevention and treatment of interferon-induced depression mean it would seem prudent to closely monitor the response to antidepressant therapy in patients with interferon-induced depression, which would identify a poor or manic response.

1. Beckwith AR. The precipitation of mania by citalopram in a patient with interferon-induced depression. *Psychosomatics* (2008) 49, 362–3.
2. Kraus MR, Schäfer A, Schöttker K, Keicher C, Weissbrich B, Hofbauer I, Scheurlen M. Therapy of interferon-induced depression in chronic hepatitis C with citalopram: a randomised, double-blind, placebo-controlled study. *Gut* (2008) 57, 531–6.
3. Furlanut M, Soardo G, Donnini D, Sechi L, Franceschi L. Fluoxetine disposition in patients with chronic hepatitis C treated with interferon-α. *Clin Pharmacokinet* (2010) 49, 767–72.
4. McAllister-Williams RH, Young AH, Menkes DB. Antidepressant response reversed by interferon. *Br J Psychiatry* (2000) 176, 93.
5. Musselman DL, Lawson DH, Gumnick JF, Manatunga AK, Penna S, Goodkin RS, Greiner K, Nemeroff CB, Miller AH. Paroxetine for the prevention of depression induced by high-dose interferon alfa. *N Engl J Med* (2001) 344, 961–6.

SSRIs + Lysergide (LSD)

Three patients with a history of lysergide (LSD) abuse experienced a new onset or worsening of the LSD flashback syndrome when given fluoxetine, paroxetine, or sertraline. Grand mal convulsions occurred when one patient taking LSD was given fluoxetine. In contrast, one study found that SSRIs reduced or eliminated the subjective responses to LSD.

Clinical evidence

An 18-year-old girl with depression, panic, and anxiety disorders, and with a long history of illicit drug abuse experienced a 15-hour LSD flashback within 2 days of starting to take **sertraline** 50 mg daily. Another flashback lasting a day occurred when the **sertraline** was replaced by **paroxetine**. No further flashbacks occurred when the SSRIs were stopped. A 17-year-old boy with depression, also with a long history of illicit drug abuse (including LSD), began to experience LSD flashbacks 2 weeks after starting to take **paroxetine**. His father, a chronic drug abuser, had taken both **fluoxetine** and **paroxetine** for depression and had also reported new onset of a flashback syndrome.[1] Another report describes a patient taking **fluoxetine**, who developed grand mal convulsions, which were tentatively attributed to the concurrent use of LSD.[2] In contrast, a retrospective study found that 28 of 32 subjects (88%) who took LSD and who had taken an SSRI (**fluoxetine**, **paroxetine**, or **sertraline**) or trazodone for more than 3 weeks had a subjective decrease or virtual elimination of their responses to LSD. However, another subject who had taken **fluoxetine** for only one week had an increased response to LSD.[3]

Mechanism

Not understood. Lysergide increases serotonin in the brain, and one suggestion is that when the serotonin re-uptake is blocked in the brain, there is an increased stimulation of 5-HT$_1$ and 5-HT$_2$ receptors.[1] Changes in brain catecholamine systems might also be involved.[3]

Importance and management

Information is very limited and conflicting. The authors of the first report suggest that patients who are given SSRIs should be warned about the possibility of flashback or hallucinations if they have a known history of LSD use.

1. Markel H, Lee A, Holmes RD, Domino EF. Clinical and laboratory observations. LSD flashback syndrome exacerbated by selective serotonin reuptake inhibitor antidepressants in adolescents. *J Pediatr* (1994) 125, 817–9.
2. Picker W, Lerman A, Hajal F. Potential interaction of LSD and fluoxetine. *Am J Psychiatry* (1992) 149, 843–4.
3. Bonson KR, Buckholtz JW, Murphy DL. Chronic administration of serotonergic antidepressants attenuates the subjective effects of LSD in humans. *Neuropsychopharmacology* (1996) 14, 425–36.

SSRIs + Macrolides

A case report describes a man who developed apparent acute fluoxetine toxicity while taking clarithromycin. Other reports describe the development of serotonin syndrome in patients taking erythromycin with sertraline, and clarithromycin with citalopram or paroxetine.

Clinical evidence

(a) Citalopram

The Canadian regulatory authorities briefly mention a case of serotonin syndrome and QT prolongation, which occurred when **clarithromycin** was taken with citalopram for 4 days.[1]

(b) Fluoxetine

A 53-year-old-man taking fluoxetine 80 mg and nitrazepam 10 mg at bedtime for depression and insomnia was given **clarithromycin** 250 mg twice daily for a respiratory infection. Within a day he started to become increasingly confused, and after 3 days was admitted to hospital with a diagnosis of psychosis and delirium. When no organic cause for the delirium could be found, all his medications were stopped, and **erythromycin** was started. His mental state returned to normal after 36 hours. Once the antibacterial course had finished, the fluoxetine and nitrazepam were restarted and no further problems occurred.[2]

(c) Paroxetine

A very brief report describes serotonin syndrome (acute ocular clonus, akathisia, and fever) in a 39-year-old woman, which developed 5 days after she had *stopped* paroxetine 10 mg twice daily and 4 doses after she had started **clarithromycin** 500 mg twice daily.[3]

(d) Sertraline

A 12-year-old boy with severe obsessive-compulsive disorder and simple phobia, responded to sertraline 12.5 mg daily, titrated over 12 weeks to 37.5 mg daily. Five weeks later, he was given **erythromycin** 200 mg twice daily for an infection, and 4 days later he began to feel mildly nervous. Over the next 10 days his nervousness grew, culminating in panic, restlessness, irritability, agitation, paraesthesias, tremulousness, decreased concentration, and confusion. The symptoms abated within 72 hours of stopping both drugs.[4]

Mechanism

The effects seen in the case with fluoxetine were attributed to fluoxetine toxicity, and that with sertraline and paroxetine to serotonin syndrome. In these two cases, the authors suggested that erythromycin and clarithromycin (known inhibitors of CYP3A4), reduced the metabolism of the SSRIs, thereby increasing their serum concentrations and precipitating the observed toxicity.[2,4] However, these SSRIs do not appear to be primarily metabolised by this isoenzyme, although CYP3A4 does have some involvement in sertraline metabolism.

Importance and management

Evidence for an interaction between the SSRIs and the macrolides is from case reports only, and the relationship between the drug use and the development of the adverse effects is tenuous in some. Furthermore the proposed mechanism for the interaction is not established. The general relevance of these isolated reports is therefore unknown. However, be aware that some SSRIs and macrolides have been associated with prolongation of the QT interval, see 'Drugs that prolong the QT interval + Other drugs that prolong the QT interval', p.272.

1. Canadian Adverse Drug Reaction Monitoring Programme. Citalopram (Celexa) and clarithromycin (Biaxin): interaction. *Can Adverse Drug React News* (2000) 10, 7.
2. Pollak PT, Sketris IS, MacKenzie SL, Hewlett TJ. Delirium probably induced by clarithromycin in a patient receiving fluoxetine. *Ann Pharmacother* (1995) 29, 486–8.
3. Jaber BL, Lobon LF, Madias NE. The serotonin syndrome complicating co-prescription of paroxetine and clarithromycin. *Am J Med* (2006) 119, e3.
4. Lee DO, Lee CD. Serotonin syndrome in a child associated with erythromycin and sertraline. *Pharmacotherapy* (1999) 19, 894–6.

SSRIs + Methylphenidate

Hallucinations have been reported in two patients taking methylphenidate with fluoxetine, and one taking methylphenidate with sertraline. One report describes serotonin syndrome and manic switch in a patient taking methylphenidate with paroxetine. Two further reports describe

serotonin syndrome in one patient and a seizure in another when methylphenidate was taken with sertraline. In contrast a case report describes improvement of the symptoms of serotonin syndrome in a patient taking paroxetine on the days she also took methylphenidate.

Clinical evidence

(a) Fluoxetine

Visual and tactile hallucinations occurred when a 10-year-old boy was started on fluoxetine 10 mg daily and methylphenidate controlled release (*OROS* osmotic release oral system) 18 mg daily. Four days later, 3 hours after taking his medication, he experienced intense hallucinations believing a car was heading toward him and feeling the sensation of insects crawling on his face. He experienced a similar, less severe episode the next day, after which his mother discontinued the medications, and no further episodes occurred. Methylphenidate was later reintroduced at the same dose, without recurrence of the hallucinations, and after two weeks, mirtazapine 15 mg daily was successfully added.[1] Another case report describes a 14-year-old girl who developed visual and auditory hallucinations while taking fluoxetine 20 mg daily and methylphenidate 20 mg daily. The hallucinations stopped when methylphenidate was discontinued and recurred on rechallenge.[2]

(b) Paroxetine

A report describes serotonin syndrome and manic switch after an 18-year-old boy with major depression received paroxetine 20 mg daily and methylphenidate 10 mg daily for a month. Manic symptoms presented 3 days prior to admission, and (because symptoms persisted) his mother made him take a second dose of both medications 2 hours after his regular dose on the day he was admitted. Paroxetine and methylphenidate were discontinued and within 24 hours symptoms due to serotonin syndrome had resolved, however manic symptoms persisted. Valproate and risperidone were started and lithium and quetiapine later added due to poor response. Six weeks later symptoms had improved sufficiently for the patient to be managed at a day clinic.[3] In contrast, another case report describes a 20-year-old woman who experienced intermittent diarrhoea, weakness, sweating, and mild somnolence while treated with paroxetine for two years. She then started methylphenidate and found that the symptoms subsided on the days she took methylphenidate. When she stopped taking methylphenidate the symptoms worsened, particularly the somnolence, and 10 days later she was admitted (with what was diagnosed as serotonin syndrome after a retrospective review). Paroxetine was stopped and all symptoms resolved within 2 days.[4]

(c) Sertraline

A 61-year-old man with major depression was prescribed sertraline 50 mg daily without response. Three months later the dose was increased to 100 mg daily and methylphenidate 2.5 mg daily was started. His symptoms improved and the dose of methylphenidate was increased to 2.5 mg twice daily and then 5 mg twice daily. After several days at the higher dose, the patient experienced visual hallucinations and confusion. The methylphenidate was discontinued and a day later the psychosis resolved. He was maintained on sertraline 100 mg daily and his mood and motivation remained good.[5] Another case describes the development of serotonin syndrome in a 62-year-old woman taking sertraline 100 mg daily without response, who was prescribed methylphenidate 10 mg daily to augment sertraline. Symptoms developed 5 days after the addition of methylphenidate and resolved within 10 days of all medication being stopped.[6] A further report describes a tonic-clonic seizure in a 13-year-old boy after he had been taking sertraline 25 to 50 mg daily and methylphenidate 80 mg daily for about 2 weeks. He had no history of seizure and had been receiving methylphenidate without significant adverse effects for about 10 months before the seizure and following discontinuation of the sertraline experienced no further seizures.[7]

Mechanism

Unknown. Methylphenidate can lower the seizure threshold in individuals with, and rarely without, a history of convulsions or EEG abnormalities.[8] SSRIs can also lower the convulsive threshold. Additive effects might possibly account for the case in which a seizure occurred, however the patient had been taking both medications for 10 months, and it is quite possible that the seizure was not associated.

Importance and management

Evidence for an interaction between the SSRIs and methylphenidate is limited to case reports, and is not established. In contrast to the cases of adverse effects described above, a beneficial increase in effects has been reported with methylphenidate and SSRIs (**fluoxetine**, **paroxetine**, **sertraline**) without important adverse effects.[9,10] Note also, that in one case report methylphenidate appeared to improve the symptoms associated with serotonin syndrome.[4]

The general relevance of these cases is likely to be small, especially when set in the context of beneficial concurrent use. However, if adverse CNS effects become troublesome, it might be worth considering this interaction as a possible cause: in both cases the adverse effects resolved when one of the drugs was withdrawn.

1. Coskun M, Zoroglu S. Tactile and visual hallucinations in a child with methylphenidate and fluoxetine combination. *J Clin Psychopharmacol* (2008) 28, 723–5.
2. Abali O, Mukkades NM. Metilfenidat tedavisi ile ortaya çikan varsanılar: olgu sunumu. *Klin Psikofarmakoloji Bulteni* (2007) 17, 195–7.
3. Park YM, Jung YK. Manic switch and serotonin syndrome induced by augmentation of paroxetine with methylphenidate in a patient with major depression. *Prog Neuropsychopharmacol Biol Psychiatry* (2010) 34, 719–20.
4. Attar-Herzberg D, Apel A, Gang N, Dvir D, Mayan H. The serotonin syndrome: initial misdiagnosis. *Isr Med Assoc J* (2009) 11, 367–70.
5. McGlohn SE, Bostwick JM. Sertraline with methylphenidate in an ICU patient. *Psychosomatics* (1995) 36, 584–5.
6. Ishii M, Tatsuzawa Y, Yoshino A, Nomura S. Serotonin syndrome induced by augmentation of SSRI with methylphenidate. *Psychiatry Clin Neurosci* (2008) 62, 246.
7. Feeney DJ, Klykylo WM. Medication-induced seizures. *J Am Acad Child Adolesc Psychiatry* (1997) 36, 1018–19.
8. Equasym (Methylphenidate hydrochloride). Shire Pharmaceuticals Ltd. UK Summary of product characteristics, February 2014.
9. Gammon GD, Brown TE. Fluoxetine and methylphenidate in combination for treatment of attention deficit disorder and comorbid depressive disorder. *J Child Adolesc Psychopharmacol* (1993) 3, 1–10.
10. Stoll AL, Pillay SS, Diamond L, Workum SB, Cole JO. Methylphenidate augmentation of serotonin selective reuptake inhibitors: a case series. *J Clin Psychiatry* (1996) 57, 72–6.

SSRIs + Metoclopramide

There are two reports of serotonin syndrome in patients taking sertraline when they were also given metoclopramide and one in a patient taking fluoxetine and metoclopramide. A few reports describe extrapyramidal symptoms in patients given fluoxetine, fluvoxamine, paroxetine, or sertraline with metoclopramide. Fluoxetine slightly increases metoclopramide exposure.

Clinical evidence

A regional pharmacovigilance centre in France reported 4 cases of extrapyramidal adverse effects linked to the concurrent use of an SSRI (unnamed) and metoclopramide.[1]

(a) Fluoxetine

In a pharmacokinetic study in 24 healthy subjects, fluoxetine 60 mg daily for 9 days increased the AUC of metoclopramide by 89% when a single 20-mg dose of metoclopramide was given with the last dose of fluoxetine. The dose of fluoxetine chosen in this study was anticipated to result in the same plasma concentrations as the usual therapeutic dose of 20 mg given long-term.[2]

A 19-year-old girl taking fluoxetine developed abdominal pain, vomiting, and diarrhoea for which she started taking metoclopramide. The following day she was admitted to hospital with suspected gastroenteritis; both medications were stopped and symptoms improved within 24 hours. A retrospective review of this case considered that she had in fact experienced serotonin syndrome.[3] Two patients developed extrapyramidal symptoms while taking fluoxetine and metoclopramide.[4,5] Another case of dyskinesia occurred in a women taking fluoxetine 20 mg daily a day after starting metoclopramide.[6]

(b) Fluvoxamine

A 14-year-old boy taking fluvoxamine 50 mg daily for anorexia nervosa was, after day 7, given metoclopramide 10 mg three times daily. On the third day of concurrent use he developed acute movement disorders, including acute dystonia, jaw rigidity, horizontal nystagmus, uncontrolled tongue movements, and dysarthria. The boy had taken the same dose of metoclopramide alone on other occasions without experiencing extrapyramidal reactions.[7] Another report described extrapyramidal reactions in 2 women taking fluvoxamine within hours of starting metoclopramide.[6]

(c) Paroxetine

A report describes extrapyramidal reactions in 2 women taking paroxetine 20 mg daily within hours of starting metoclopramide 20 mg six-hourly.[6] In one case, this resolved on withdrawal of metoclopramide and treatment with biperiden.[6]

(d) Sertraline

A woman with gastro-oesophageal reflux, controlled with metoclopramide 15 mg four times daily, developed symptoms consistent with a mandibular dystonia (periauricular pain, jaw tightness, the sensation of her teeth clenching and grinding) 2 days after starting sertraline 50 mg daily. A 50-mg dose of diphenhydramine resolved the problem within 30 minutes, but the same symptoms recurred the next day, 8 hours after taking sertraline. The symptoms were relieved by 2 mg of oral benzatropine.[8] Dystonia occurred in another woman taking metoclopramide 3 days after starting sertraline 50 mg daily and resolved on stopping sertraline.[6]

A patient who had been taking sertraline 100 mg daily started taking metoclopramide 10 mg four times daily for nausea. After 24 hours his symptoms had worsened and he developed malaise, cardiac arrhythmia, visual hallucinations, diaphoresis, sialosis, hyperreflexia, and tremor. Serotonin syndrome was diagnosed and his symptoms improved with cyproheptadine.[9] Another patient taking sertraline 100 mg daily for depression over an 18-month period developed agitation, dysarthria, diaphoresis, and a movement disorder within 2 hours of receiving a single 10-mg intravenous dose of metoclopramide. The symptoms, diagnosed as serotonin syndrome with a serious extrapyramidal movement disorder, resolved within 6 hours of treatment with diazepam.[10]

Mechanism

Both the SSRIs and metoclopramide can cause extrapyramidal reactions; metoclopramide by blocking dopamine D_2 receptors in the basal ganglia, and the SSRIs by inhibition of dopamine neurotransmission; their effects might be additive.[7,8] There might be a pharmacokinetic component to the interaction with some SSRIs, since metoclopramide is partially metabolised by CYP2D6 and fluoxetine and paroxetine are inhibitors of this isoenzyme. Note that fluvoxamine and sertraline have little effect on CYP2D6. Disruption of serotonergic and/or dopaminergic transmission on concurrent use might contribute to serotonin syndrome or serotonin syndrome-like effects.[10].

Importance and management

Information on an interaction between the SSRIs and metoclopramide seems to be limited to these reports, but they highlight the fact that care should be taken if two drugs with the potential to cause the same adverse effects are used together. The slight increase in metoclopramide exposure with fluoxetine is probably unlikely to be generally clinically relevant, but bear it in mind should increased adverse effects occur.

1. Anon. Extrapyramidal reactions to SSRI antidepressant + neuroleptic combinations. *Prescrire Int* (2004) 13, 57.
2. Vlase L, Leucuta A, Farcau D, Nanulescu M. Pharmacokinetic interaction between fluoxetine and metoclopramide in healthy volunteers. *Biopharm Drug Dispos* (2006) 27, 285–9.
3. Attar-Herzberg D, Apel A, Gang N, Dvir D, Mayan H. The serotonin syndrome: initial misdiagnosis. *Isr Med Assoc J* (2009) 11, 367–70.
4. Coulter DM, Pillans PI. Fluoxetine and extrapyramidal side effects. *Am J Psychiatry* (1995) 152, 122–5.
5. Fallon BA, Liebowitz MR. Fluoxetine and extrapyramidal symptoms in CNS lupus. *J Clin Psychopharmacol* (1991) 11, 147–8.
6. Netherlands Pharmacovigilance Centre. A combination of metoclopramide and selective serotonin reuptake inhibitors: additional extrapyramidal effects? March 2005. Available at: www.lareb.nl/Signalen/kwb_2005_1_metoc (accessed 03/09/15).
7. Palop V, Jimenez MJ, Catalán C, Martínez-Mir I. Acute dystonia associated with fluvoxamine-metoclopramide. *Ann Pharmacother* (1999) 33, 382.
8. Christensen RC, Byerly MJ. Mandibular dystonia associated with the combination of sertraline and metoclopramide. *J Clin Psychiatry* (1996) 57, 596.
9. Vandemergel X, Beukinga I, Nève P. Syndrome sérotoninergique secondaire à la prise de sertraline et de metoclopramide. *Rev Med Brux* (2000) 3, 161–3.
10. Fisher AA, Davis MW. Serotonin syndrome caused by selective serotonin reuptake-inhibitors–metoclopramide interaction. *Ann Pharmacother* (2002) 36, 67–71.

SSRIs + Nasal decongestants

A case report describes serotonin syndrome associated with the use of sertraline and etilefrine, and another report describes adverse effects associated with the use of fluoxetine and phenylpropanolamine.

Clinical evidence, mechanism, importance and management

(a) Etilefrine

A case of serotonin syndrome was reported in a 39-year-old woman taking sertraline 50 mg daily for 3 months, after taking one 25 mg dose of etilefrine. Her symptoms resolved within about 12 hours with supportive treatment. Etilefrine was stopped and sertraline re-started 48 hours later, when the patient was asymptomatic. At 6-months follow-up no further complications had occurred.[1] The clinical relevance of this is unclear.

(b) Phenylpropanolamine

A 16-year-old girl with an eating disorder, taking **fluoxetine** 20 mg daily, developed vague medical complaints of dizziness, 'hyper' feelings, diarrhoea, palpitations, and a reported weight loss of about 6.5 kg within 2 weeks. The author of the report suggested that these effects might have been the result of an interaction with phenylpropanolamine (1 to 2 capsules of *Dexatrim* daily), which the patient was surreptitiously taking, associated with a restricted food and fluid intake.[2] The clinical relevance of this report is unclear.

1. Martínez Hernanz A, Pérez Sales P. Síndrome serotoninérgico por sertralina y etilefrina: una interacción no descrita. *Psiquis (Mexico)* (2001) 2, 222–4.
2. Walters AM. Sympathomimetic-fluoxetine interaction. *J Am Acad Child Adolesc Psychiatry* (1992) 31, 565–6.

SSRIs + NNRTIs

Efavirenz appears to slightly decrease sertraline exposure, but not paroxetine exposure. Paroxetine and sertraline, and probably also fluoxetine, do not appear to alter efavirenz concentrations. Serotonin syndrome occurred in a woman taking fluoxetine when efavirenz was added.

There is limited evidence that nevirapine might decrease fluoxetine plasma concentrations, but it appears not to affect fluvoxamine concentrations. Limited evidence also suggests that fluoxetine has no effect on nevirapine concentrations, but fluvoxamine might modestly increase them.

Fluoxetine appears to increase delavirdine minimum concentrations. Etravirine does not appear to affect paroxetine concentrations, and paroxetine does not appear to affect etravirine concentrations.

Clinical evidence

(a) Delavirdine

The US manufacturer of delavirdine briefly notes that population pharmacokinetic data from efficacy studies showed that, in 36 patients receiving **fluoxetine** (varying doses) and delavirdine (200 mg to 400 mg three times daily), delavirdine minimum concentrations were increased by about 50%.[1]

(b) Efavirenz

1. Fluoxetine. A case of serotonin syndrome in a woman taking fluoxetine coincided with the start of a new antiretroviral regimen including efavirenz. Symptoms resolved when the fluoxetine dose was halved.[2] A preliminary report of a retrospective population pharmacokinetic analysis, notes that use of SSRIs (including fluoxetine) in 17 patients, did not appear to alter efavirenz pharmacokinetics, when compared with data from patients not taking SSRIs (317 patients).[3]

2. Paroxetine. The US manufacturer of efavirenz notes that there was no change in the pharmacokinetics of either paroxetine or efavirenz when paroxetine 20 mg daily and efavirenz 600 mg daily were given together for 14 days.[4] A preliminary report of a retrospective population pharmacokinetic analysis, notes that SSRIs (including paroxetine) in 17 patients, did not appear to alter efavirenz pharmacokinetics, when compared with data from patients not taking SSRIs (317 patients).[3]

3. Sertraline. In one study, sertraline 50 mg daily for 14 days had no effect on the pharmacokinetics of efavirenz 600 mg daily; however, the sertraline AUC was decreased by 39% and the minimum concentration was decreased by 46% when given with efavirenz.[4,5] A preliminary report of a retrospective population pharmacokinetic analysis, notes that SSRIs (including sertraline) in 17 patients did not appear to alter efavirenz pharmacokinetics, when compared with data from patients not taking SSRIs (317 patients).[3]

(c) Etravirine

A preliminary report of a randomised crossover study in 16 HIV-negative subjects given etravirine 800 mg twice daily for 14 days, with **paroxetine** 20 mg daily on days 8 to 14, found that there was no change in the pharmacokinetics of either paroxetine or etravirine when compared with each drug given alone.[6]

(d) Nevirapine

1. Fluoxetine. In a pharmacokinetic-modelling study in 173 HIV-positive patients taking a nevirapine-containing regimen, there was little difference in nevirapine clearance (10% decrease) between 7 patients also taking fluoxetine and the rest of the group. In addition, the median plasma concentrations of fluoxetine and its active metabolite norfluoxetine tended to be lower in these 7 patients than in another control group of 17 patients without HIV infection taking fluoxetine, but this only reached statistical significance when the plasma concentrations of fluoxetine and norfluoxetine were combined (46% lower).[7]

2. Fluvoxamine. In a pharmacokinetic-modelling study in 173 HIV-positive patients taking a nevirapine-containing regimen, the apparent clearance of nevirapine was 34% lower in 7 patients also taking fluvoxamine, and this appeared to be dependent on the dose of fluvoxamine. The median plasma concentration of fluvoxamine did not differ between these 7 patients and a control group of 29 patients without HIV infection taking fluvoxamine.[7]

Mechanism

Delavirdine is metabolised primarily by CYP3A4, however *in vitro* data suggest it might also be metabolised by CYP2D6. As fluoxetine is an inhibitor of CYP2D6, this might account for the increase in delavirdine concentrations seen on concurrent use. The case of serotonin syndrome in the patient taking efavirenz and fluoxetine was attributed to increased fluoxetine concentrations caused by efavirenz.[2] However, note that paroxetine, which is similarly metabolised, is not affected by efavirenz. Sertraline, unlike fluoxetine and paroxetine, is in part metabolised by CYP3A4, of which efavirenz is an inducer. Concurrent use therefore causes a decrease in sertraline concentrations. It was suggested that the lower concentrations of fluoxetine and norfluoxetine seen with nevirapine might be due to induction of CYP3A4 by nevirapine, while the decreased clearance of nevirapine seen with fluvoxamine might be due to inhibition of CYP3A4 by fluvoxamine.[7] However note that fluoxetine is not a known substrate of CYP3A4; further evidence is needed.

Importance and management

The available information suggests that **efavirenz** concentrations are unaffected by SSRIs (paroxetine, sertraline, fluoxetine), therefore no change in virologic efficacy would be anticipated, and no efavirenz dose adjustments are likely to be needed. Paroxetine pharmacokinetics are unaffected by efavirenz and no dose adjustment is necessary on concurrent use. Sertraline exposure is slightly decreased by efavirenz and minimum concentrations are decreased, but as SSRIs are generally considered to have a wide therapeutic margin, such a small decrease in exposure would not be expected to affect efficacy. In cases of an otherwise unexplained reduction in sertraline efficacy or suspected withdrawal symptoms, bear the possibility of an interaction in mind and consider increasing the sertraline dose. The general relevance of the case of serotonin syndrome is uncertain, but it introduces a note of caution about concurrent use.

No dose adjustment of either paroxetine or **etravirine** would appear to be needed on concurrent use.

Delavirdine plasma concentrations appear to be increased by fluoxetine, which might increase adverse effects. Cautious monitoring for an increase in the adverse effects of delavirdine would seem to be prudent if concurrent use is necessary.

The findings of the pharmacokinetic-modelling study with **nevirapine** are preliminary, and require confirmation in a controlled study, nevertheless, they provide some evidence that fluoxetine concentrations might be decreased by nevirapine. Monitoring fluoxetine efficacy might be prudent. They also suggest that nevirapine concentrations might be modestly increased by fluvoxamine, therefore it might be prudent to monitor for nevirapine adverse effects. More study is needed.

1. Rescriptor (Delavirdine mesylate). ViiV Healthcare. US Prescribing information, August 2012.
2. DeSilva KE, Le Flore DB, Marston BJ, Rimland D. Serotonin syndrome in HIV-infected individuals receiving antiretroviral therapy and fluoxetine. *AIDS* (2001) 15, 1281–5.
3. Ruiz NM, Labriola DF, Fiske WD, Joshi AS, Manion DJ, Villano SA. Efavirenz plasma levels are unaffected in patients receiving selective serotonin reuptake inhibitors. 40th Interscience Conference on Antimicrobial Agents and Chemotherapy, Toronto, 2000. Abstract 1635.
4. Sustiva (Efavirenz). Bristol-Myers Squibb Company. US Prescribing information, May 2014.
5. Sustiva Film-coated Tablets (Efavirenz). Bristol-Myers Squibb Pharmaceutical Ltd. UK Summary of product characteristics, March 2014.

6. Schöller-Gyüre M, Kakuda TN, Bollen S, De Smedt G, Woodfall B, Peeters M, Vandermeulen K, Hoetelmans RM. No pharmacokinetic interaction between TMC125 (etravirine; ETR) and paroxetine in HIV-negative volunteers. 11th European AIDS Conference, Madrid, October 2007. Abstract P4.3/01. Available at: http://medadvocates.org/resources/conferences/11th_eacs/etravirine/jd123036%20scholler%20final.pdf (accessed 25/09/2015).
7. De Maat MMR, Huitema ADR, Mulder JW, Meenhorst PL, van Gorp ECM, Mairuhu ATA, Beijnen JH. Drug interaction of fluvoxamine and fluoxetine with nevirapine in HIV-1-infected individuals. *Clin Drug Invest* (2003) 23, 629–37.

SSRIs + Opioids

Symptoms of serotonin syndrome have been reported with opioids including fentanyl, hydromorphone, oxycodone, pentazocine, pethidine (meperidine), and possibly also morphine, when these opioids were given with an SSRI.

Paroxetine does not alter the pharmacokinetics of oxycodone, but does decrease the exposure to its metabolite, oxymorphone, although most evidence suggests that this does not alter the analgesic effect. Fluoxetine reduced the analgesic effects of morphine in one study and of oxycodone in one case. Fluoxetine and paroxetine are predicted to reduce the analgesic efficacy of codeine.

Clinical evidence

(a) Codeine

Fluoxetine and **paroxetine** (potent CYP2D6 inhibitors) are predicted to decrease the metabolism of codeine to morphine and thereby possibly reduce its analgesic efficacy (see also 'Opioids; Codeine and related drugs + Quinidine', p.194). There is no evidence for this, although on this basis, **fluoxetine** has been tried for the treatment of codeine dependence. In one small pilot study, **fluoxetine** 20 mg daily reduced codeine use by 30 to 100%,[1] but in a later small controlled study by the same research group, although there was a reduction in codeine use, this did not differ from placebo.[2]

(b) Fentanyl

A 65-year-old woman taking **citalopram**, rabeprazole, tolterodine, and **hydrocodone** developed probable serotonin syndrome while hospitalised and within 24 hours of starting transdermal fentanyl 25 micrograms/hour. Fentanyl was discontinued, and all signs and symptoms resolved over the next few days, and did not recur when **oxycodone** was started.[3] Two similar reports describe serotonin syndrome which occurred 48 hours after **citalopram** and **paroxetine** were started in patients using a fentanyl patch. The symptoms resolved after both fentanyl and the SSRI were stopped.[4] Two other reports describe patients who developed serotonin syndrome[5] or toxicity[6] after receiving parenteral fentanyl and **paroxetine**. In the case of serotonin syndrome, the patient was taking a number of potentially causative drugs, including **paroxetine** and fentanyl, but all symptoms resolved within 36 hours of their cessation and with supportive treatment.[5] In the case of serotonin toxicity, the patient was stabilised on **paroxetine** and underwent surgery, during and after which she received fentanyl. She developed symptoms suggestive of serotonin toxicity (a vague affectation, intermittent agitation, bilateral hyperreflexia, inducible clonus, and hypertension), all of which completely resolved 24 hours after fentanyl was stopped. She had previously stopped paroxetine on the morning of surgery.[6] A report describes two cases of serotonin syndrome in patients undergoing surgery. In the first case, a 46-year-old woman taking **sertraline** 50 mg daily and cetirizine 10 mg daily developed symptoms suggestive of serotonin syndrome after receiving fentanyl 50 micrograms along with midazolam and propofol at the start of surgery. In the second case, a 59-year-old woman taking **escitalopram** received fentanyl 250 micrograms and **morphine** during 3 hours in theatre. Following surgery she was transferred to ICU due to hypoxia and respiratory acidosis, and the following morning she developed symptoms of serotonin syndrome. Propofol was started and the patient reintubated. After a toxicology consultation, propofol was stopped and the patient managed with lorazepam and cyproheptadine. Symptoms resolved over the next 3 days and the patient made a full recovery.[7] Note that this patient was on a large number of other drugs, many of which are potentially causative drugs, including **oxycodone**. For mention of another case of serotonin syndrome in a patient taking fentanyl and escitalopram with oxycodone, see under *Oxycodone*, below.

(c) Hydrocodone

Visual hallucinations occurred in a 90-year-old woman taking hydrocodone when her antidepressant was changed from **citalopram** 10 mg daily to **escitalopram** 10 mg daily. The hallucinations stopped after her hydrocodone was discontinued because of improvement in pain control. The patient had previously taken **paroxetine** and the same dose of hydrocodone, without experiencing hallucinations or other serotonin-related symptoms.[8]

(d) Hydromorphone

An 81-year-old woman who had been taking **fluoxetine** 20 mg daily along with other medication for several years, developed abnormal movements, confusion, incoherent speech, sweating, facial redness, tremor, hyperreflexia, and muscle spasm 2 days after starting to take hydromorphone 12 mg daily. The symptoms resolved within 2 weeks of stopping **fluoxetine** (the hydromorphone was continued).[9]

(e) Methadone

The SSRIs, particularly fluvoxamine, can increase methadone concentrations, see 'SSRIs + Opioids; Methadone', p.1493.

(f) Morphine

A placebo-controlled study in 35 patients found that the preoperative use of **fluoxetine** 10 mg daily for 7 days reduced the analgesic effect of intravenous morphine given for postoperative dental pain.[10] In contrast, a crossover study in 15 healthy subjects found that a single 60-mg dose of **fluoxetine** minimally improved (by 3 to 8%) the analgesic effect (as assessed by dental electrical stimulation) of morphine sulfate in doses tailored to produce and maintain steady-state plasma concentrations of 15, 30, and 60 nanograms/mL for 60 minutes. Plasma concentrations of morphine were not affected by **fluoxetine**, and morphine was found not to affect plasma concentrations of **fluoxetine** or its metabolite, norfluoxetine. The subjects experienced less nausea and drowsiness while taking both drugs, but the psychomotor and respiratory depressant effects of morphine were not altered.[11]

A patient experienced postoperative delirium which lasted for nearly 2 days and included agitation, confusion, uncontrolled limb movements, abnormal ocular function, hypertension, pyrexia, brisk reflexes, ankle clonus, and increased creatinine kinase. She had been taking **paroxetine** before surgery, and during surgery she was given morphine and ondansetron.[12]

(g) Oxycodone

1. Pharmacokinetic studies and analgesic effects. In a study, 20 patients with chronic pain (all CYP2D6 extensive or ultrarapid metabolisers, that is, they had normal, or higher than normal, isoenzyme activity, respectively) stable taking oxycodone, were given **paroxetine** 20 mg daily for 7 days. **Paroxetine** increased the dose-adjusted AUC of oxycodone by 19% and that of the metabolite, noroxycodone, 2-fold, but decreased the AUC of the metabolite, oxymorphone, by 67%. However, despite these pharmacokinetic changes, paroxetine had no effect on the use of rescue morphine or oxycodone analgesia (as assessed using visual analogue scales for pain intensity or pain relief).[13] Similar findings were reported in two placebo-controlled studies in healthy subjects given a single 10-mg oral dose[14] or a single 0.1-mg/kg intravenous dose[15] of oxycodone: **paroxetine** pretreatment decreased the AUC of oxymorphone by 44% or 66%, respectively, and increased the AUC of noroxycodone by 68% or 70%, respectively, but had no effect on pain scores, as assessed by the cold pressor test.[14,15] In another study in 12 healthy subjects who were all CYP2D6 extensive metabolisers, pretreatment with **paroxetine** 20 mg for just 3 doses had no effect on the pharmacokinetics of a single 0.2-mg/kg oral dose of oxycodone, or its metabolite, noroxycodone, but did decrease the maximum plasma concentration of its metabolite, oxymorphone, by 38%. However, in contrast, in this study, pretreatment with paroxetine blunted oxycodone-induced miosis and the analgesic effect of oxycodone, as assessed using the cold pressor test: this effect was greatest at 2-hours post-oxycodone and reduced over time.[16]

A man with advanced multiple sclerosis found that when he began to take **fluoxetine** 20 mg daily for depression he needed to increase his analgesic dose of oxycodone (for painful muscle spasms) about 4-fold, from 65 to 75 mg daily to about 250 to 275 mg daily.[17]

2. Serotonin syndrome. A bone-marrow transplant recipient taking, among other drugs, **sertraline** 50 mg daily, ciclosporin 75 mg daily, and oxycodone 10 mg as needed, developed severe tremors and visual hallucinations. This coincided with him taking oxycodone 200 mg over 48 hours for severe pain. An adverse reaction to ciclosporin was initially suspected (although serum concentrations were not high), and this was temporarily discontinued along with the oxycodone. The visual hallucinations decreased but the tremors continued, and did not lessen until **sertraline** was discontinued and cyproheptadine given. It was concluded that the patient was experiencing a form of serotonin syndrome as a result of increased opioid use while taking an SSRI.[18] Serotonin syndrome also occurred in a 66-year-old man taking oxycodone 120 mg daily and intranasal **fentanyl** 200 micrograms up to four times daily when **escitalopram** 5 mg daily was added to his treatment. Most symptoms resolved within 2 days, but blurred vision persisted.[19] Two other cases describe probable serotonin syndrome in elderly patients taking **sertraline** or **escitalopram** and extended-release oxycodone. In both cases symptoms of serotonin syndrome (agitation, increased muscle tone, ataxia, tremor, and/or myoclonic jerks) occurred after increasing the opioid dose.[8] Another case of severe serotonergic symptoms including confusion, nausea, fever, shivering, agitation, clonus, hyperreflexia, hypertonia, and tachycardia occurred in a 70-year-old woman taking **fluvoxamine** 200 mg daily when she started taking oxycodone 40 mg twice daily. Discontinuation of these two drugs resulted in resolution of her symptoms over 48 hours.[20]

(h) Pentazocine

A placebo-controlled study in 35 patients found that **fluoxetine** 10 mg daily for 7 days preoperatively did not appear to reduce the analgesic effects of pentazocine 45 mg given intravenously for postoperative dental pain.[10]

A man who had been taking **fluoxetine** 20 mg daily, later increased to 40 mg daily, was given a single 100-mg oral dose of pentazocine (*Talwin Nx* containing pentazocine 50 mg and naloxone 500 micrograms) for a severe headache. Within 30 minutes he complained of lightheadedness, anxiety, nausea, and paraesthesias of the hands. He was diaphoretic, flushed, and ataxic, and had a mild tremor of his arms. His blood pressure was 178/114 mmHg, heart rate 62 bpm, and respiration 16 breaths per minute. He was given intramuscular diphenhydramine 50 mg and recovered over the following 4 hours.[21]

(i) Pethidine (Meperidine)

A 43-year-old man who had been taking **fluoxetine** approximately every other day experienced symptoms of serotonin syndrome immediately after receiving pethidine 50 mg intravenously for an endoscopic procedure.[22] A 44-year-old woman taking **citalopram** 20 mg daily increased to 40 mg daily, transdermal **fentanyl**, and intravenous **hydromorphone** or oral **hydrocodone** with paracetamol (as needed), promethazine, gatifloxacin, zolpidem, and lansoprazole, developed symptoms suggestive of serotonin syndrome within 10 hours of starting pethidine by patient controlled analgesia (PCA) for breakthrough pain (total dose over 8 hours was 230 mg). Once pethidine was stopped, the symptoms resolved.[23]

(j) Tramadol

Serotonin syndrome has occurred in a number of patients taking SSRIs with tramadol, see 'SSRIs + Opioids; Tramadol', p.1494.

Mechanism

Oxycodone is principally metabolised by CYP3A4, and to a lesser extent, by CYP2D6. Paroxetine inhibits CYP2D6 so that the metabolism of oxycodone to the metabolite, oxymorphone, is decreased. However, the pharmacokinetic studies show that while exposure to oxymorphone is decreased by paroxetine, the pharmacokinetics of oxycodone itself are not affected. Furthermore, the effects of oxycodone (including analgesia) do not generally appear to be reduced by the concurrent use of paroxetine, suggesting that perhaps the pharmacological activity of oxycodone is not related to the metabolite oxymorphone (which has generally been considered the active metabolite). Further study is required.

The metabolism of codeine, hydrocodone, and similar opioids might also be affected by SSRIs that are potent CYP2D6 inhibitors, such as fluoxetine and paroxetine. See also 'Opioids; Codeine and related drugs + Quinidine', p.194, for further discussion of this mechanism.

Buprenorphine and morphine are not metabolised by CYP2D6, so their metabolism would not be expected to be affected by paroxetine or fluoxetine.

It has been suggested that the reason for the reduced morphine analgesia might have something to do with the initial effects of SSRIs on serotonergic neurotransmission.[11] Serotonin syndrome seems to develop unpredictably in some patients given two or more serotonergic drugs, in this case, opioids and SSRIs.

Importance and management

Adverse interactions between SSRIs and the opioids named above seem rare, and there is little evidence to suggest that they cannot be used together safely and effectively. However, the possibility of serotonin syndrome or serotonin toxicity should be considered in patients experiencing altered mental status, autonomic dysfunction, and neuromuscular adverse effects while receiving these drugs. For more information on serotonin syndrome and its management, see 'Drugs that cause serotonin syndrome + Other drugs that cause serotonin syndrome', p.1471.

Pharmacokinetic studies show that paroxetine does not affect the pharmacokinetics of **oxycodone**, and despite decreases in exposure to the metabolite oxymorphone, also does not generally affect oxycodone analgesia. No oxycodone dose adjustment would appear to be necessary, but if an insufficient analgesic response is seen in a patient receiving this combination, consider an interaction as a possible cause. The evidence suggesting that fluoxetine might decrease **morphine** or oxycodone analgesia is limited and insufficient to suggest any change in practice. Similarly, if a patient does not seem to respond well to either of these opioids, consider an interaction as a possible cause. Although there is no evidence for reduced analgesic efficacy of **codeine** with paroxetine and fluoxetine, on the basis of the limited data with quinidine, which is also a potent CYP2D6 inhibitor, this would seem to be a possibility, see 'Opioids; Codeine and related drugs + Quinidine', p.194. Note that any interaction would only occur in those of extensive or ultrarapid CYP2D6 phenotype, and not in patients who are CYP2D6 poor metabolisers, in whom codeine might not be effective anyway. Monitor for a reduced response to codeine in patients taking fluoxetine or paroxetine, and consider using an alternative analgesic. Other SSRIs do not inhibit CYP2D6 to the same extent (see 'Table 1.7', p.9) and would therefore seem unlikely to interact similarly.

1. Romach MK, Otton SV, Somer G, Tyndale RF, Sellers EM. Cytochrome P450 2D6 and treatment of codeine dependence. *J Clin Psychopharmacol* (2000) 20, 43–5.
2. Fernandes LC, Kilicarslan T, Kaplan HL, Tyndale RF, Sellers EM, Romach MK. Treatment of codeine dependence with inhibitors of cytochrome P450 2D6. *J Clin Psychopharmacol* (2002) 22, 326–9.
3. Ailawadhi S, Sung K-W, Carlson LA, Baer MR. Serotonin syndrome caused by interaction between citalopram and fentanyl. *J Clin Pharm Ther* (2007) 32, 199–202.
4. Attar-Herzberg D, Apel A, Gang N, Dvir D, Mayan H. The serotonin syndrome: initial misdiagnosis. *Isr Med Assoc J* (2009) 11, 367–70.
5. Gollapudy S, Kumar V, Dhamee MS. A case of serotonin syndrome precipitated by fentanyl and ondansetron in a patient receiving paroxetine, duloxetine and bupropion. *J Clin Anesth* (2012) 24, 251–2.
6. Rang ST, Field J, Irving C. Serotonin toxicity caused by an interaction between fentanyl and paroxetine. *Can J Anesth* (2008) 55, 521–5.
7. Kirschner R, Donovan JW. Serotonin syndrome precipitated by fentanyl during procedural sedation. *J Emerg Med* (2010) 38, 477–80.
8. Gnanadesigan N, Espinoza RT, Smith R, Israel M, Reuben DB. Interaction of serotonergic antidepressants and opioid analgesics: is serotonin syndrome going undetected? *J Am Med Dir Assoc* (2005) 6, 265–9.
9. Anon. Fluoxetine + hydromorphone: serotonin syndrome? *Prescrire Int* (2004) 13, 57.
10. Gordon NC, Heller PH, Gear RW, Levine JD. Interactions between fluoxetine and opiate analgesia for postoperative dental pain. *Pain* (1994) 58, 85–8.
11. Erjavec MK, Coda BA, Nguyen Q, Donaldson G, Risler L, Shen DD. Morphine-fluoxetine interactions in healthy volunteers: analgesia and side effects. *J Clin Pharmacol* (2000) 40, 1286–95.
12. Stanford BJ, Stanford SC. Postoperative delirium indicating an adverse drug interaction involving the selective serotonin reuptake inhibitor, paroxetine? *J Psychopharmacol* (1999) 13, 313–17.
13. Lemberg KK, Heiskanen TE, Neuvonen M, Kontinen VK, Neuvonen PJ, Dahl M-L. Kalso EA. Does co-administration of paroxetine change oxycodone analgesia: an interaction study in chronic pain patients. *Scand J Pain* (2010) 1, 24–33.
14. Grönlund J, Saari TI, Hagelberg NM, Neuvonen PJ, Olkkola KT, Laine K. Exposure to oral oxycodone is increased by concomitant inhibition of CYP2D6 and 3A4 pathways, but not by inhibition of CYP2D6 alone. *Br J Clin Pharmacol* (2010) 70, 78–87.
15. Grönlund J, Saari TI, Hagelberg NM, Neuvonen PJ, Laine K, Olkkola KT. Effect of inhibition of cytochrome P450 enzymes 2D6 and 3A4 on the pharmacokinetics of intravenous oxycodone: a randomized, three-phase, crossover, placebo-controlled study. *Clin Drug Investig* (2011) 31, 143–53.
16. Kummer O, Hammann F, Moser C, Schaller O, Drewe J, Krähenbühl S. Effect of the inhibition of CYP3A4 or CYP2D6 on the pharmacokinetics and pharmacodynamics of oxycodone. *Eur J Clin Pharmacol* (2011) 67, 63–71.
17. Otton SV, Wu D, Joffe RT, Cheung SW, Sellers EM. Inhibition by fluoxetine of cytochrome P450 2D6 activity. *Clin Pharmacol Ther* (1993) 53, 401–9.
18. Rosebraugh CJ, Flockhart DA, Yasuda SU, Woosley RL. Visual hallucination and tremor induced by sertraline and oxycodone in a bone marrow transplant patient. *J Clin Pharmacol* (2001) 41, 224–7.
19. Reich M, Lefebvre-Kuntz D. Antidépresseurs sérotonergiques et antalgiques opiacés: une association parfois «douloureuse». À propos d'un cas clinique. *L'Encephale* (2010) 36 (Suppl 2), D119–23.
20. Karunatilake H, Buckley NA. Serotonin syndrome induced by fluvoxamine and oxycodone. *Ann Pharmacother* (2006) 40, 155–7.
21. Hansen TE, Dieter K, Keepers GA. Interaction of fluoxetine and pentazocine. *Am J Psychiatry* (1990) 147, 949–50.
22. Tissot TA. Probable meperidine-induced serotonin syndrome in a patient with a history of fluoxetine use. *Anesthesiology* (2003) 98, 1511–12.
23. Altman EM, Manos GH. Serotonin syndrome associated with citalopram and meperidine. *Psychosomatics* (2007) 48, 361–3.

SSRIs + Opioids; Methadone

Methadone plasma concentrations might be increased by fluvoxamine. Sertraline, paroxetine, and possibly fluoxetine, might also increase methadone concentrations, albeit to a lesser extent.

Clinical evidence

(a) Fluoxetine

Methadone 30 to 100 mg daily and fluoxetine 20 mg daily were given to 9 patients (two of them also taking fluvoxamine). Although there were possible compliance problems with some of the patients, the methadone concentration-to-dose ratio of the group as a whole was not altered by the addition of the fluoxetine.[1] This is consistent with the results of two other studies, which found that fluoxetine did not appear to alter the methadone plasma concentrations of patients treated for cocaine dependence.[2,3] However, the plasma samples for 7 of the 9 patients in the first study[1] were subsequently analysed to measure the *S*- and *R*-enantiomers of methadone separately. This analysis revealed that fluoxetine 20 mg daily increased the concentration-to-dose ratio of the active *R*-methadone by 33%, without changing either the total or inactive *S*-methadone concentration-to-dose ratios.[4] Moreover, a patient taking methadone developed opioid toxicity when given fluoxetine (with ciprofloxacin), see 'Quinolones + Opioids; Methadone', p.352.

(b) Fluvoxamine

Five patients taking maintenance doses of methadone were given fluvoxamine. Two of them had an increase of about 20% in the methadone plasma-to-dose ratio, while the other 3 had 40 to 100% increases in the methadone plasma-to-dose ratio (suggesting increased methadone plasma concentrations). One of them developed asthenia, marked drowsiness, and nausea, which disappeared when both drug doses were reduced.[5] A subsequent analysis of the enantiomers of methadone revealed that fluvoxamine increased the concentrations of both *R*- and *S*-methadone.[4] A report describes one patient who was unable to maintain adequate methadone concentrations, despite a daily dose of 200 mg, and experienced withdrawal symptoms until fluvoxamine was added.[6] Another patient taking methadone 70 mg daily and diazepam 2 mg twice daily was admitted to hospital with an acute exacerbation of asthma and intractable cough 3 weeks after starting fluvoxamine 100 mg daily. Blood gas measurements indicated severe hypoxaemia and hypercapnia. The symptoms resolved when the methadone dose was reduced to 50 mg daily and diazepam was gradually withdrawn, at which point methadone concentrations fell by about 23% (from 262 to 202 nanograms/mL).[7]

(c) Paroxetine

Paroxetine 20 mg daily increased steady-state methadone concentrations by 35% in 10 patients taking maintenance doses of methadone. Both *R*- and *S*-methadone concentrations were increased in the 8 patients who were CYP2D6 extensive metabolisers (that is, those with normal isoenzyme activity), but in the 2 patients who were poor metabolisers (that is, those with lower than normal activity of this isoenzyme) only the *S*-methadone concentrations were increased. Apart from one patient who reported feeling high during the first night after starting paroxetine, no symptoms of over-medication or toxicity were noted.[8]

(d) Sertraline

A placebo-controlled study in 31 methadone-maintained patients with depression found that sertraline increased the methadone concentration-to-dose ratio by 26%, whereas patients taking placebo had a 16% decrease in this ratio after 6 weeks of concurrent use, but by 12 weeks the ratios had shifted towards baseline values. Adverse effects were similar in both groups.[9] A 31-year-old woman taking methadone 230 mg daily was found to have a prolonged QT interval after sertraline 50 mg daily was added to her medications, although she was asymptomatic. The QT interval returned to normal when the methadone and sertraline were stopped and her methadone was replaced with morphine.[10]

Mechanism

Fluvoxamine, and to a lesser extent fluoxetine, paroxetine, and sertraline, can inhibit the metabolism of methadone (possibly by CYP3A4,[11] CYP2D6,[11,12] and/or CYP1A2[4]) thereby allowing it to accumulate in the body.

Importance and management

Information regarding an interaction between fluvoxamine and methadone is limited, but it indicates that the effects of starting or stopping fluvoxamine should be monitored in patients taking methadone, being alert for the need to adjust the methadone dose. Although the increase in methadone plasma concentrations with sertraline and paroxetine, and possibly also fluoxetine, is unlikely to have clinical effects in most patients, the possibility should be borne in mind, especially if high doses of methadone are being used. Note that methadone alone can prolong the QT interval in high doses, and this effect has also been associated with some SSRIs, see 'Drugs that prolong the QT interval + Other drugs that prolong the QT interval', p.272.

Both methadone and the SSRIs have serotonergic effects, and concurrent use might lead to the serotonin syndrome. Serotonin syndrome is a rare adverse effect, but because of its severity, some caution is warranted if both methadone and a SSRI are given. For more information on serotonin syndrome and its management, see 'Drugs that cause serotonin syndrome + Other drugs that cause serotonin syndrome', p.1471.

1. Bertschy G, Eap CB, Powell K, Baumann P. Fluoxetine addition to methadone in addicts: pharmacokinetic aspects. *Ther Drug Monit* (1996) 18, 570–2.
2. Batki SL, Manfredi LB, Jacob P, Jones RT. Fluoxetine for cocaine dependence in methadone maintenance: quantitative plasma and urine cocaine-benzoylecgonine concentrations. *J Clin Psychopharmacol* (1993) 13, 243–50.
3. Baño MD, Agujetas M, M, López ML, Tena T, Rodríguez A, Lora-Tamayo C, Guillén JL. Eficacia de la fluoxetina (FX) en el tratamiento de la adicción a cocaína en pacientes en mantenimiento con metadona y su interacción en los niveles plasmáticos. *Actas Esp Psiquiatr* (1999) 27, 321–4.
4. Eap CB, Bertschy G, Powell K, Baumann P. Fluvoxamine and fluoxetine do not interact in the same way with the metabolism of the enantiomers of methadone. *J Clin Psychopharmacol* (1997) 17, 113–17.
5. Bertschy G, Baumann P, Eap CB, Baettig D. Probable metabolic interaction between methadone and fluvoxamine in addict patients. *Ther Drug Monit* (1994) 16, 42–5.
6. DeMaria PA, Serota RD. A therapeutic use of the methadone fluvoxamine drug interaction. *J Addict Dis* (1999) 18, 5–12.
7. Alderman CP, Frith PA. Fluvoxamine-methadone interaction. *Aust N Z J Psychiatry* (1999) 33, 99–101.
8. Begré S, von Bardeleben U, Ladewig D, Jaquet-Rochat S, Cosendai-Savary L, Golay KP, Kosel M, Baumann P, Eap CB. Paroxetine increases steady-state concentrations of (R)-methadone in CYP2D6 extensive but not poor metabolizers. *J Clin Psychopharmacol* (2002) 22, 211–15.
9. Hamilton SP, Nunes EV, Janal M, Weber L. The effect of sertraline on methadone plasma levels in methadone-maintenance patients. *Am J Addict* (2000) 9, 63–9.
10. Piguet V, Desmeules J, Ehret G, Stoller R, Dayer P. QT interval prolongation in patients on methadone with concomitant drugs. *J Clin Psychopharmacol* (2004) 24, 446–8.
11. Iribarne C, Picart D, Dréano Y, Berthou F. In vitro interactions between fluoxetine or fluvoxamine and methadone or buprenorphine. *Fundam Clin Pharmacol* (1998) 12, 194–9.
12. Wang J-S, DeVane CL. Involvement of CYP3A4, CYP2C8, and CYP2D6 in the metabolism of (*R*)- and (*S*)-methadone in vitro. *Drug Metab Dispos* (2003) 31, 742–7.

SSRIs + Opioids; Tramadol

Paroxetine and escitalopram might decrease the exposure to a metabolite of tramadol. The concurrent use of tramadol and an SSRI might increase both the risk of seizures and serotonin syndrome. One patient developed hallucinations when taking tramadol with paroxetine. Two patients have developed mania with serotonin syndrome while taking tramadol with fluoxetine or paroxetine.

Clinical evidence

The CSM in the UK has publicised 27 reports of convulsions and one of worsening epilepsy with tramadol, a reporting rate of 1 in 7 000 patients. Some of the patients were given doses well in excess of those recommended, and some were taking an SSRI (5 patients), which are known to reduce the convulsive threshold.[1] Similarly, of 124 seizure cases associated with tramadol reported to the FDA in the US, 20 included the concurrent use of SSRIs.[2]

The Australian Adverse Drug Reaction Advisory Committee has stated that tramadol might cause serotonin syndrome, particularly when it is used at high doses or in combination with other drugs increasing serotonin concentrations; of 20 reported cases of serotonin syndrome associated with tramadol, 16 were taking potentially interacting medicines including an SSRI.[3] Cases of serotonin syndrome with specific SSRIs are discussed in the subsections below.

(a) Citalopram

A 70-year-old woman who had been taking citalopram 10 mg daily for 3 years developed tremors, restlessness, fever, confusion, and visual hallucinations after starting to take tramadol 50 mg daily for pain relief following an operation. Her symptoms stopped after tramadol was stopped. However, she continued to take citalopram and one year later she developed identical symptoms after taking tramadol 20 mg daily. Citalopram is metabolised by CYP2C19 and tramadol is *O*-demethylated by CYP2D6 and the patient was found to be deficient in both these isoenzymes, suggesting that her metabolising capacity of both pathways was reduced.[4] Another case report describes a 78-year-old woman taking citalopram (dose not stated) who presented with confusion after a recent fall and starting tramadol for pain. Examination after deterioration on admission to hospital, found that she was tachycardic, had global myoclonus, increased tone, hyperreflexia, and bilateral upgoing plantars. Serotonin syndrome was diagnosed and alternative diagnoses excluded. Symptoms resolved on discontinuation of citalopram and tramadol.[5] A similar case occurred in a 62-year-old man taking citalopram 40 mg daily and bupropion 150 mg twice daily who presented to hospital 3 days after starting tramadol 50 mg three times daily, with tremors, diaphoresis, and anxiety. Serotonin syndrome was diagnosed, all three medications were stopped, and diazepam and labetalol were used to manage the symptoms which resolved within 48 hours. The patient was restarted on antidepressant medications at a lower dose (not stated) and titrated as an outpatient.[6] A further case describes galactorrhoea in a 34-year-old woman taking citalopram 40 mg daily, tramadol 37.5 mg daily, and alprazolam, 7 days after the citalopram dose had been increased from 20 mg daily. Her prolactin concentration was found to be 2-fold higher than the normal upper limit. The citalopram and tramadol were stopped and residual galactorrhoea was still present 7 days later, but prolactin concentrations were within the normal range. The patient self-medicated with tramadol for 3 days and her prolactin concentration rose. On rechallenge with citalopram [without tramadol], her galactorrhoea worsened.[7] Whether this report represents an interaction or simply an adverse effect is unclear.

(b) Escitalopram

A placebo-controlled, crossover study in 15 healthy subjects given escitalopram 20 mg daily with tramadol 150 mg, found that the median AUC of the tramadol metabolite, (+)-*O*-desmethyltramadol, was decreased by 29% by escitalopram. This decrease in AUC did not reduce the analgesic effect, as assessed by the cold pressor test.[8]

(c) Fluoxetine

A 44-year-old woman with a long history of opioid analgesic dependence (tramadol average dose of 400 mg daily) was started on fluoxetine 20 mg daily. She independently increased her fluoxetine dose to 80 mg daily over several weeks and experienced unrest, increasing nausea and vomiting, and headache. Eight weeks later she was admitted to hospital as a psychiatric emergency, with disorientation, confusion, and visual hallucinations. She also had continuous tremor and an ataxic, unsteady gait. Shortly prior to admission she had also increased her tramadol dose to 800 mg. Clinical investigation revealed mydriasis and hyperreflexia, low grade fever, increased creatine phosphokinase and ALT, and a fluoxetine serum concentration of 1065 nanograms/mL. Serotonin syndrome was diagnosed and the fluoxetine stopped. Gradual withdrawal of tramadol and other supportive therapies resolved the psychiatric symptoms within 6 days, and by day 26 all symptoms had disappeared and the fluoxetine concentrations had fallen to 293 nanograms/mL.[9] Two other case reports describe the development of serotonin syndrome in women taking fluoxetine within about 3 to 4 weeks of tramadol being started.[10,11] For another case of serotonin syndrome in a patient taking fluoxetine and tramadol with milnacipran and doxepin, see 'SNRIs + SSRIs', p.1478.

(d) Paroxetine

A placebo-controlled, crossover study in 16 healthy subjects found that pretreatment with paroxetine 20 mg daily for 3 days increased the AUC of tramadol by about 35%, and decreased the AUCs of the *O*-demethylated metabolites of tramadol by 40 to 67%. The analgesic effect of tramadol was reduced, but not abolished.[12] In another placebo-controlled, crossover study, 10 healthy subjects who were CYP2D6 extensive metabolisers (that is, they had normal isoenzyme activity), were given single 10-, 20-, 30-, and 50-mg doses of paroxetine at bedtime, and a single 50-mg dose of tramadol the following morning. Paroxetine caused a dose-dependent reduction in the production of the tramadol metabolite, (+)-*O*-desmethyltramadol.[13]

A case report describes a man who had been taking paroxetine 20 mg daily for 4 months without problems developed shivering, diaphoresis, and myoclonus, and became subcomatose within 12 hours of taking tramadol 100 mg. This was diagnosed as serotonin syndrome. Tramadol was stopped, the paroxetine dose halved and he became conscious within a day. The other symptoms gradually disappeared over the next week.[14] Similar reactions have occurred in a 78-year-old woman taking paroxetine 20 mg daily, 3 days after starting tramadol 50 mg three times daily,[15] and in an 85-year-old woman taking both drugs.[16] A further case describes the abrupt onset of serotonin syndrome and mania in a 53-year-old woman who was taking paroxetine 20 mg and tramadol 200 mg, after she independently increased her dose of both paroxetine and tramadol (to 4 tablets daily, exact dose not stated). Manic symptoms persisted after the resolution of other symptoms of serotonin syndrome (within one week).[17] A tetraparetic patient with chronic pain developed nightmares and hallucinations 56 days after starting to take tramadol, paroxetine, and dosulepin, which only stopped when the drugs were withdrawn.[18]

(e) Sertraline

A 42-year-old woman was admitted to intensive care with atypical chest pain, sinus tachycardia, confusion, psychosis, sundowning [increased agitation, activity, and negative behaviours, which happen late in the day or evening], agitation, diaphoresis, and tremor. She was taking a large number of drugs, including sertraline and tramadol. She was diagnosed as having serotonin syndrome, attributed to an increase in the dose of tramadol (from 150 mg daily to 300 mg daily in increments of 50 mg every 2 to 3 days), and an increased sertraline dose (original amounts not stated but 100 mg daily when the adverse events developed). The tramadol had been started 3 weeks previously and she had been taking the sertraline for a year.[19] Other case reports describe serotonin syndrome in an 88-year-old woman taking sertraline and tramadol,[20] and in a 55-year-old man taking sertraline who was suspected of abusing tramadol.[21] In a further report, serotonin syndrome occurred after the first dose of sertraline 50 mg in a 75-year-old woman who had been taking tramadol 50 mg daily for 3 days. The concentration of serotonin (5-hydroxytryptamine) in her CSF was found to be elevated to 38.5 nanograms/mL (reference value less than 10 picograms/mL).[22]

Mechanism

Tramadol can rarely cause seizures and SSRIs can reduce the seizure threshold, thus if both are taken together the risk is increased. Serotonin syndrome seems to develop unpredictably in some patients given two or more serotonergic drugs (in this case, tramadol and SSRIs).

Paroxetine is a CYP2D6 inhibitor, the isoenzyme by which tramadol is metabolised, which results in reduced formation of its *O*-demethylated metabolites. The reduction in these metabolites can result in reduced analgesia as the opioid effect of tramadol is thought to be mediated mainly by (+)-*O*-desmethyltramadol.[12] Escitalopram is only a weak inhibitor of CYP2D6, and the reduction in exposure to (+)-*O*-desmethyltramadol seen in one study did not result in a reduction in analgesic effect.[8]

Importance and management

Because of the possible increased risk of seizures, tramadol should be used with caution in patients taking drugs such as the SSRIs, which can lower the seizure threshold. The concurrent use of tramadol and an SSRI can also lead to an increase in serotonin-associated effects, which can include serotonin syndrome. Note, that 2 cases of mania with serotonin syndrome have also been reported.[10,17] However, the relatively few reported cases of serotonin syndrome or other reactions due to an interaction between an SSRI and tramadol need to be set in the wider context of apparently uneventful and advantageous use in other patients,[12,23,24] although some have suggested that the incidence of serotonin syndrome could be underreported.[25] There would seem to be little reason for totally avoiding the concurrent use of the SSRIs and tramadol but it would clearly be prudent to monitor the outcome closely. For more information on serotonin syndrome and its management, see 'Drugs that cause serotonin syndrome + Other drugs that cause serotonin syndrome', p.1471.

Tramadol analgesia might possibly be altered by paroxetine and potentially by other SSRIs that inhibit CYP2D6, such as fluoxetine, but perhaps not by weak inhibitors such as escitalopram. For a list of CYP2D6 inhibitors by potency, see 'Table 1.7', p.9. Bear the potential for this interaction in mind should a patient taking these SSRIs have a reduced response to tramadol, and adjust the dose of tramadol as necessary.

1. Committee on Safety of Medicines/Medicines Control Agency. In focus–tramadol. *Current Problems* (1996) 22, 11.
2. Kahn LH, Alderfer RJ, Graham DJ. Seizures reported with tramadol. *JAMA* (1997) 278, 1661.
3. Adverse Drug Reactions Advisory Committee (ADRAC). Tramadol – four years' experience. *Aust Adverse Drug React Bull* (2003) 22, 2.
4. Mahlberg R, Kunz D, Sasse J, Kirchheiner J. Serotonin syndrome with tramadol and citalopram. *Am J Psychiatry* (2004) 161, 1129.
5. Peacock LE, Wright F. Serotonin syndrome secondary to tramadol and citalopram. *Age Ageing* (2011) 40, 528. Epub.
6. Shahani L. Tramadol precipitating serotonin syndrome in a patient on antidepressants. *J Neuropsychiatr Clin Neurosci* (2012) 24, E52.
7. Bondolfi G, Rubin C, Bryois C, Eap CB. Galactorrhoea induced by a pharmacodynamic interaction between citalopram, alprazolam and tramadol: a case report. *Therapie* (1997) 52, 76–7.
8. Noehr-Jensen L, Zwisler ST, Larsen F, Sindrup SH, Damkier PM, Brosen K. Escitalopram is a weak inhibitor of the CYP2D6-catalyzed O-demethylation of (+)-tramadol but does not reduce the hypoalgesic effect in experimental pain. *Clin Pharmacol Ther* (2009) 86, 626–33.
9. Lange-Asschenfeldt C, Weigmann H, Hiemke C, Mann K. Serotonin syndrome as a result of fluoxetine in a patient with tramadol abuse: plasma level-correlated symptomatology. *J Clin Psychopharmacol* (2002) 22, 440–1.
10. Gonzalez-Pinto A, Imaz H, De Heredia JL, Gutierrez M, Micó JA. Mania and tramadol-fluoxetine combination. *Am J Psychiatry* (2001) 158, 964–5.
11. Kesavan S, Sobala GM. Serotonin syndrome with fluoxetine plus tramadol. *J R Soc Med* (1999) 92, 474–5.
12. Laugesen S, Enggaard TP, Pedersen RS, Sindrup SH, Brøsen K. Paroxetine, a cytochrome P450 2D6 inhibitor, diminishes the stereoselective *O*-demethylation and reduces the hypoalgesic effect of tramadol. *Clin Pharmacol Ther* (2005) 77, 312–23.
13. Nielsen AG, Pedersen RS, Noehr-Jensen L, Damkier P, Brosen K. Two separate dose-dependent effects of paroxetine: mydriasis and inhibition of tramadol's O-demethylation via CYP2D6. *Eur J Clin Pharmacol* (2010) 66, 655–60.
14. Egberts ACG, ter Borgh J, Brodie-Meijer CCE. Serotonin syndrome attributed to tramadol addition to paroxetine therapy. *Int Clin Psychopharmacol* (1997) 12, 181–182.
15. Lantz MS, Buchalter EN, Giambanco V. Serotonin syndrome following the administration of tramadol with paroxetine. *Int J Geriatr Psychiatry* (1998) 13, 343–5.
16. Llinares-Tello F, Escrivá-Moscardó S, Martínez-Pastor F, Martínez-Mascaraque P. Probable síndrome serotoninérgico relacionado con la administración de paroxetina y tramadol. *Med Clin (Barc)* (2007) 128, 438.
17. John AP, Koloth R. Severe serotonin toxicity and manic switch induced by combined use of tramadol and paroxetine. *Aust N Z J Psychiatry* (2007) 41, 192–3.
18. Devulder J, De Laat M, Dumoulin K, Renson A, Rolly G. Nightmares and hallucinations after long term intake of tramadol combined with antidepressants. *Acta Clin Belg* (1996) 51, 184–6.
19. Mason BJ, Blackburn KH. Possible serotonin syndrome associated with tramadol and sertraline coadministration. *Ann Pharmacother* (1997) 31, 175–7.
20. Sauget D, Franco PS, Amaniou M, Mazere J, Dantoine T. Possible syndrome sérotoninergique induit par l'association de tramadol à de la sertraline chez une femme âgée. *Therapie* (2002) 57, 309–10.
21. Nayyar N. Serotonin syndrome associated with sertraline, trazodone and tramadol abuse. *Indian J Psychiatry* (2009) 51, 68.
22. Mittino D, Mula M, Monaco F. Serotonin syndrome associated with tramadol-sertraline coadministration. *Clin Neuropharmacol* (2004) 27, 150–1.
23. Fanelli J, Montgomery C. Use of the analgesic tramadol in antidepressant potentiation. *Psychopharmacol Bull* (1996) 32, 442.
24. Barkin RL. Alternative dosing for tramadol aids effectiveness. *Formulary* (1995) 30, 542–3.
25. Freeman WD, Chabolla DR. 36-Year-old woman with loss of consciousness, fever, and tachycardia. *Mayo Clin Proc* (2005) 80, 667–70.

SSRIs + Rifampicin (Rifampin)

A few cases describe a decrease in the efficacy of citalopram and sertraline after rifampicin was started. Paroxetine is predicted to be similarly affected, as might other SSRIs.

Clinical evidence

A 34-year-old man, with a long-standing history of anxiety disorder, taking **sertraline** 200 mg at bedtime, reported that the medication was no longer working well. He was experiencing a significant amount of anxiety, excessive worry, and poor energy. He additionally reported feeling "spaced out" and having dizziness exacerbated by movement, lethargy, and insomnia. He had started taking rifampicin 300 mg twice daily and co-trimoxazole 7 days earlier and it was found that his **sertraline** and *N*-desmethylsertraline concentrations were only 39% and 46%, respectively, of the concentrations achieved when he was not taking rifampicin and co-trimoxazole. He later experienced similar symptoms when the **sertraline** dose was tapered so that paroxetine could be substituted.[1] A 55-year-old man taking **citalopram** 40 to 60 mg daily also reported a decrease in therapeutic efficacy (increased crying and panic attacks) after starting rifampicin 600 mg twice daily. His condition improved when the rifampicin was stopped.[2] Similarly, a 27-year-old woman taking **citalopram** 20 mg daily developed gastrointestinal symptoms, anxiety, agitation, and tachycardia 5 days after starting rifampicin 600 mg daily with doxycycline 100 mg twice daily for brucellosis. Propranolol 20 mg twice daily was started and the citalopram dose increased to 40 mg daily, after which the symptoms gradually improved. Propranolol was tapered off and the patient remained stable on the brucellosis treatment and citalopram 40 mg daily.[3]

Mechanism

Both sertraline and citalopram are metabolised by cytochrome P450 isoenzymes including CYP3A4, of which rifampicin is a known inducer. It would therefore appear that rifampicin induced the metabolism of these two drugs resulting in decreased plasma concentrations.

Importance and management

Evidence for an interaction between the SSRIs and rifampicin is limited to a few reports, but as rifampicin is a well-known, potent enzyme inducer, clinicians should be aware that rifampicin might decrease citalopram or sertraline plasma concentrations leading to decreased efficacy or symptoms of SSRI withdrawal. In theory, rifampicin could affect other SSRIs metabolised by other cytochrome P450 isoenzymes, but there appear to be no reports of this. The UK manufacturer of **paroxetine** suggests that dose adjustment on starting or stopping enzyme inducing drugs such as rifampicin should be guided by clinical effect (tolerability and efficacy), and they suggest that no initial anticipatory dose adjustment is necessary.[4] Until more is known this would seem to be a sensible approach with rifampicin and any SSRI.

1. Markowitz JS, DeVane CL. Rifampin-induced selective serotonin reuptake inhibitor withdrawal syndrome in a patient treated with sertraline. *J Clin Psychopharmacol* (2000) 20, 109–10.
2. Kukoyi O, Argo TR, Carnaham RM. Exacerbation of panic disorder with rifampin therapy in a patient receiving citalopram. *Pharmacotherapy* (2005) 25, 435–7.
3. Khalili H, Dashti-Khavidaki S, Amini S, Mousavi M. Recurrence of panic attacks after brucellosis treatment - highly probable citalopram and rifampin drug interaction. J Clin Psychopharmacol. (2012) 32, 842–4.
4. Seroxat (Paroxetine hydrochloride hemihydrate). GlaxoSmithKline UK. UK Summary of product characteristics, August 2015.

SSRIs + Sibutramine

Two case reports suggest that the concurrent use of sertraline or citalopram with sibutramine might cause serotonin syndrome.

Clinical evidence, mechanism, importance and management

A 43-year-old woman taking **citalopram** 40 mg daily was also given sibutramine 10 mg daily. Within a few hours of taking the first dose of sibutramine she developed racing thoughts, hyperactivity, psychomotor agitation, shivering, and diaphoresis, which continued for the 3 days that she continued to take sibutramine. The authors suggested that one of the reasons for the hypomania might have been serotonin syndrome, which could have been caused by the use of two drugs with serotonergic action.[1] A letter briefly mentions another possible case of serotonin syndrome, following the use of sibutramine and **sertraline**.[2] Note that sibutramine has been largely withdrawn due to the risk of serious cardiovascular effects. When it was available, the manufacturers advised that concurrent use of any other drug with serotonergic actions should be avoided[3] where possible, or only undertaken with appropriate monitoring.[4] For more information about serotonin syndrome and its management, see 'Drugs that cause serotonin syndrome + Other drugs that cause serotonin syndrome', p.1471.

1. Benazzi F. Organic hypomania secondary to sibutramine-citalopram interaction. *J Clin Psychiatry* (2002) 63, 165.
2. Trakas K, Shear NH. Serotonin syndrome risk with antiobesity drug. *Can J Clin Pharmacol* (2000) 7, 216.
3. Reductil (Sibutramine hydrochloride monohydrate). Abbott Laboratories Ltd. UK Summary of product characteristics, December 2009.
4. Meridia (Sibutramine hydrochloride monohydrate). Abbott Laboratories. US Prescribing information, January 2010.

SSRIs + SSRIs

A report describes an adverse reaction (hypertension, tachycardia, fever, auditory hallucinations, and confusion) in a man when he started sertraline within a day of stopping fluoxetine. A small study found that the concurrent use of citalopram and fluvoxamine greatly increased citalopram plasma concentrations: escitalopram will be similarly affected. Note that combining more than one SSRI is unusual, and would be expected to increase the risk of adverse effects.

Clinical evidence

(a) Citalopram or Escitalopram with Fluvoxamine

A study in 7 patients with depression who had not responded to treatment with citalopram 40 mg daily for 3 weeks, found that the addition of fluvoxamine (50 mg increased to 100 mg daily for another 3 weeks) increased *R*-citalopram concentrations almost 2-fold and *S*-citalopram concentrations 3-fold. Six of the 7 patients showed clinical improvement. None of the patients developed serotonin syndrome, and no changes in vital signs or ECGs were seen.[1] This study shows that the concentrations of escitalopram, the *S*-isomer of citalopram, will also be increased by fluvoxamine.

(b) Fluoxetine with Sertraline

One of 16 healthy subjects who began to take sertraline 50 mg daily on the day after stopping a 2-week trial of fluoxetine 20 mg daily, rapidly developed hypertension, tachycardia, fever, auditory hallucinations, and confusion. Most of these symptoms disappeared 48 hours after stopping the sertraline, but the confusion took a week to subside.[2] The other 15 subjects had no clinically important adverse effects. This subject was later found to have a history of psychosis so the picture is a little confused, but the rapid abatement of the symptoms when the sertraline was stopped suggests that they were due either to the sertraline alone, or to an interaction with the residual fluoxetine.

Mechanism

Fluvoxamine increases citalopram concentrations, with a greater effect on *S*-citalopram (escitalopram), possibly by inhibiting CYP2C19. Fluoxetine has a very long half-life, and might therefore have contributed to the adverse effects seen when switching to sertraline in the case described. Combining drugs with serotonergic actions such as two SSRIs is likely to have additive effects.

Importance and management

There is very little information on combining SSRIs because this is not a usual therapeutic strategy. It is likely that combining two SSRIs will have additive effects. Some SSRI manufacturers include other SSRIs in the list of serotonergic drugs that would increase the risk of serotonergic adverse effects (including the rare serotonin syndrome) on concurrent use. On this basis they advise caution or avoidance of concurrent use. Some caution would seem prudent. The one study with fluvoxamine and citalopram highlights the fact that there might be a pharmacokinetic component to the interaction between some SSRIs, which would intensify any effects.

On the basis of the possible interaction, it is also not clear whether a washout period is needed if switching between two SSRIs, particularly when the first has a long half-life, such as fluoxetine. A decision on this will depend on the severity of the depression in the particular patient being treated. The UK and US manufacturers of sertraline imply caution when they state that there is limited experience regarding the optimal timing of switching from one SSRI to another,[3,4] and further that the duration of a washout period has not yet been established.[4]

For further details on the development and management of serotonin syndrome, see 'Drugs that cause serotonin syndrome + Other drugs that cause serotonin syndrome', p.1471.

1. Bondolfi G, Chautems C, Rochat B, Bertschy G, Baumann P. Non-response to citalopram in depressive patients: pharmacokinetic and clinical consequences of a fluvoxamine augmentation. *Psychopharmacology (Berl)* (1996) 128, 421–5.
2. Rosenblatt JE, Rosenblatt NC. How long a hiatus between discontinuing fluoxetine and beginning sertraline? *Curr Affect Illn* (1992) 11, 2.
3. Lustral (Sertraline hydrochloride). Pfizer Ltd. UK Summary of product characteristics, March 2015.
4. Zoloft (Sertraline hydrochloride). Pfizer Inc. US Prescribing information, August 2014.

SSRIs + St John's wort (*Hypericum perforatum*)

Cases of severe sedation, mania, and serotonin syndrome have been reported in patients taking St John's wort with SSRIs.

Clinical evidence

(a) Citalopram

A brief case report describes serotonin syndrome in a woman who had been taking citalopram 20 mg daily for 2 months, three weeks after she also started taking St John's wort. She presented to hospital extremely agitated with unusual behaviour and was expressing suicidal thoughts. On admission, she was perspiring and complained of nausea and abdominal discomfort, with a tachycardia of 120 beats per minute and fluctuating blood pressure.[1] No further details are given.

(b) Fluoxetine

For a report of hypomania when St John's wort, ginkgo biloba, and melatonin were added to treatment with fluoxetine and buspirone, see 'Buspirone + St John's wort (*Hypericum perforatum*)', p.846.

For a report of serotonin syndrome when eletriptan, fluoxetine, and St John's wort were used together, see 'Triptans + St John's wort (*Hypericum perforatum*)', p.649.

(c) Paroxetine

In one report, a woman stopped taking paroxetine 40 mg daily after 8 months, and 10 days later started to take 600 mg of St John's wort powder daily. No problems occurred until the next night when she took a single 20-mg dose of paroxetine because she thought it might help her sleep. The following day at noon she was found still to be in bed, rousable but incoherent, groggy and slow moving and almost unable to get out of bed. Two hours later she still complained of nausea, weakness, and fatigue, but her vital signs and mental status were normal. Within 24 hours all symptoms had resolved.[2]

(d) Sertraline

Four elderly patients taking sertraline developed symptoms characteristic of serotonin syndrome within 2 to 4 days of also taking St John's wort 300 mg, either two or three times daily. The symptoms included dizziness, nausea, vomiting, headache, anxiety, confusion, restlessness, and irritability. Two patients were treated with oral cyproheptadine 4 mg either two or three times daily, and the symptoms of all patients resolved within a week. They later resumed treatment with sertraline without problems.[3] A search of Health Canada's database of spontaneous adverse reactions from 1998 to 2003 found 2 cases of suspected serotonin syndrome as a result of an interaction between sertraline and St John's wort.[4]

Mania developed in a 28-year-old man, who continued to take St John's wort against medical advice while also receiving sertraline 50 mg daily for depression; he was also receiving testosterone replacement post-orchidectomy.[5]

Mechanism

A pharmacodynamic interaction might occur between St John's wort and SSRIs because they can both inhibit the reuptake of 5-hydroxytryptamine (serotonin).[6] Serotonin syndrome has been seen with St John's wort alone,[7] and so additive serotonergic effects appear to be the explanation for what occurred in the cases described here.

Importance and management

Information appears to be limited to these reports, but interactions between SSRIs and St John's wort would seem to be established. The incidence is not known but it is probably small, nevertheless because of the potential severity of the reaction it would seem prudent to avoid concurrent use. The CSM in the UK advised that St John's wort should be stopped if patients are taking an SSRI because of the risk of increased serotonergic effects and an increased incidence of adverse reactions.[8]

For more information on serotonin syndrome and its management, see 'Drugs that cause serotonin syndrome + Other drugs that cause serotonin syndrome', p.1471.

1. Witharana D, Pollard A, Vaughan J. Continuing awareness of serotonin syndrome needed. *Pharm J* (2007) 278, 487.
2. Gordon JB. SSRIs and St. John's wort: possible toxicity? *Am Fam Physician* (1998) 57, 950–3.
3. Lantz MS, Buchalter E, Giambanco V. St. John's wort and antidepressant drug interactions in the elderly. *J Geriatr Psychiatry Neurol* (1999) 12, 7–10.
4. Griffiths J, Jordan S, Pilon K. Natural health products and adverse reactions. *Can Adverse React News* (2004) 14 (1), 2–3.
5. Barbenel DM, Yusufi B, O'Shea D, Bench CJ. Mania in a patient receiving testosterone replacement post-orchidectomy taking St John's wort and sertraline. *J Psychopharmacol* (2000) 14, 84–6.
6. Izzo AA. Drug interactions with St. John's wort (Hypericum perforatum): a review of the clinical evidence. *Int J Clin Pharmacol Ther* (2004) 42, 139–48.
7. Demott K. St. John's wort tied to serotonin syndrome. *Clin Psychiatry News* (1998) 26, 28.
8. Committee on Safety of Medicines (UK). Message from Professor A Breckenridge (Chairman of CSM) and Fact Sheet for Health Care Professionals, 29th February 2000. Available at: http://www.mhra.gov.uk/home/groups/comms-ic/documents/websiteresources/con019563.pdf (accessed 03/09/15).

SSRIs + Terbinafine

Terbinafine moderately increases exposure to paroxetine. Some other SSRIs might interact similarly.

Clinical evidence

In a crossover study, 12 healthy subjects were given a single 20-mg dose of paroxetine alone and after taking terbinafine 125 mg daily for 6 days. Terbinafine increased the AUC and maximum plasma concentration of paroxetine 2.5-fold and 86%, respectively, and the half-life of paroxetine was also increased by 48% (from about 15 hours to 23 hours).[1]

Mechanism

Terbinafine inhibits CYP2D6, the isoenzyme by which paroxetine is metabolised. Concurrent use therefore decreases paroxetine metabolism and increases its exposure.

Importance and management

Information appears to be limited to one study, but the results are consistent with the way both drugs are known to interact. Be aware that paroxetine exposure might be increased if terbinafine is also given, and consider a dose reduction if adverse effects become troublesome. Note that many of the SSRIs are metabolised, at least in part, by CYP2D6 (see 'Table 35.2', p.1465), and so might interact similarly, although the clinical relevance of these potential interactions is unknown.

1. Yasui-Furukori N, Saito M, Inoue Y, Niioka T, Sato Y, Tsuchimine S, Kaneko S. Terbinafine increases the plasma concentration of paroxetine after a single oral administration of paroxetine in healthy subjects. *Eur J Clin Pharmacol* (2007) 63, 51–6.

SSRIs + Tobacco

Smoking has minimal effects on fluvoxamine pharmacokinetics. It is unclear whether smoking has any effect on citalopram pharmacokinetics, or the pharmacokinetics of other SSRIs.

Clinical evidence

(a) Citalopram

In a pharmacokinetic study in adolescent patients (under 21 years of age), there was a clear dose-concentration relationship for citalopram and its metabolite, desmethylcitalopram, in the 9 non-smokers, whereas no such relationship was seen in the 10 smokers.[1]

(b) Fluvoxamine

A comparative study in 12 smokers and 12 non-smokers given single 50-mg oral doses of fluvoxamine found that smoking decreased the fluvoxamine AUC and maximum serum concentrations by about 30%.[2] A study in Japanese patients stabilised on fluvoxamine (mean dose 109.4 mg daily) found that the steady-state concentration-to-dose ratio in the 6 smokers was about 50% lower than in the 26 non-smokers.[3] A similar study, also in Japanese patients, found that heavy smoking (20 or more cigarettes a day) decreased the steady-state fluvoxamine concentration by about 60% in patients taking fluvoxamine 50 mg daily when compared with non-smokers. There was also a trend toward a lower fluvoxamine concentration in those taking fluvoxamine 100 mg daily and who were smokers, but this did not reach statistical significance. However smoking did not appear to alter the fluvoxamine concentration in those taking fluvoxamine 150 or 200 mg.[4] Another study in Japanese patients taking fluvoxamine 200 mg daily found no difference in the steady-state plasma concentrations of fluvoxamine and its metabolite (fluvoxamino acid) between 34 non-smokers and 15 smokers.[5]

Mechanism

Unclear. Tobacco smoke is a known inducer of CYP1A2, but fluvoxamine and citalopram are not known substrates for this isoenzyme (rather, fluvoxamine is a known inhibitor), and therefore further study is required to establish the reason for the effects seen in smokers.

Importance and management

Evidence for an interaction between the SSRIs and tobacco smoke is limited. It appears that an interaction with fluvoxamine might occur and that it might produce a greater decrease in the fluvoxamine concentrations achieved with lower doses of fluvoxamine, but not higher doses. The overall pharmacokinetic effect of smoking is probably at most minimal; however, how a sudden withdrawal from heavy smoking would affect fluvoxamine pharmacokinetics has not been investigated. It is unclear whether smoking has any effect on citalopram pharmacokinetics.

1. Reis M, Olsson G, Carlsson B, Lundmark J, Dahl ML, Walinder J, Ahlner J, Bengtsson F. Serum levels of citalopram and its main metabolites in adolescent patients treated in a naturalistic clinical setting. *J Clin Psychopharmacol* (2002) 22, 406–13.
2. Spigset O, Carleborg L, Hedenmalm K, Dahlqvist R. Effect of cigarette smoking on fluvoxamine pharmacokinetics in humans. *Clin Pharmacol Ther* (1995) 58, 399–403.
3. Katoh Y, Uchida S, Kawai M, Takei N, Mori N, Kawakami J, Kagawa Y, Yamada S, Namiki N, Hashimoto H. Effects of cigarette smoking and cytochrome P450 2D6 genotype on fluvoxamine concentration in plasma of Japanese patients. *Biol Pharm Bull* (2010) 33, 285–8.
4. Suzuki Y, Sugai T, Fukui N, Watanabe J, Ono S, Inoue Y, Ozdemir V, Someya T. CYP2D6 genotype and smoking influence fluvoxamine steady-state concentration in Japanese psychiatric patients: lessons for genotype-phenotype association study design in translational pharmacogenetics. *J Psychopharmacol* (2011) 25, 908–14.
5. Gerstenberg G, Aoshima T, Fukasawa T, Yoshida K, Takahashi H, Higuchi H, Murata Y, Shimoyama R, Ohkubo T, Shimizu T, Otani K. Effects of the CYP 2D6 genotype and cigarette smoking on the steady-state plasma concentrations of fluvoxamine and its major metabolite fluvoxamino acid in Japanese depressed patients. *Ther Drug Monit* (2003) 25, 463–8.

SSRIs + Tryptophan

Central and peripheral toxicity developed in five patients taking high doses of fluoxetine when they were given tryptophan, which was attributed to serotonin syndrome. Adverse effects have occurred on combined use of paroxetine and tryptophan.

Clinical evidence

(a) Fluoxetine

Five patients taking fluoxetine 50 to 100 mg daily (high doses) for at least 3 months developed a number of reactions including central toxicity (agitation, restlessness, aggressive behaviour, worsening of obsessive-compulsive disorders) and peripheral toxicity (abdominal cramps, nausea, diarrhoea) within a few days of starting to take tryptophan 1 to 4 g daily. These symptoms disappeared when the tryptophan was stopped. Some of the patients had taken tryptophan in the absence of fluoxetine without problems.[1]

Conversely, in a placebo-controlled study involving 30 patients with depression, the use of tryptophan 1 g daily titrated to 4 g daily during the initial 8 weeks of treatment with fluoxetine 20 mg daily was beneficial and well-tolerated. No cases of serotonin syndrome occurred.[2]

(b) Paroxetine

The US manufacturer of paroxetine notes that adverse experiences, consisting primarily of headache, nausea, sweating, and dizziness, have been reported when paroxetine was taken with tryptophan.[3]

Mechanism

Tryptophan is a precursor of serotonin (5-hydroxytryptamine) and the authors of the fluoxetine cases point out that the symptoms resemble serotonin syndrome, which occurs when serotonin concentrations are increased.[1] The reaction appears to be dose related. It is likely to occur with any SSRI.

Importance and management

The cases with fluoxetine appear to be the only ones published, nevertheless, they demonstrate the potential for additive adverse effects. Serotonin syndrome is a rare adverse effect, but because of its severity, some caution is warranted if both tryptophan and fluoxetine or other SSRIs are given; the UK manufacturer of paroxetine additionally mentions the serotonin precursor **oxitriptan** [L-5-hydroxytryptophan].[4] If tryptophan is used to augment the initial response to SSRIs, the SSRI should be started at a low dose, with tryptophan gradually introduced, starting with a low dose. Patients should be closely monitored for adverse effects.[2] For more information on serotonin syndrome and its management, see 'Drugs that cause serotonin syndrome + Other drugs that cause serotonin syndrome', p.1471.

1. Steiner W, Fontaine R. Toxic reaction following the combined administration of fluoxetine and L-tryptophan: five case reports. *Biol Psychiatry* (1986) 21, 1067–71.
2. Levitan RD, Shen J-H, Jindal R, Driver HS, Kennedy SH, Shapiro CM. Preliminary randomized double-blind placebo-controlled trial of tryptophan combined with fluoxetine to treat major depressive disorder: antidepressant and hypnotic effects. *J Psychiatry Neurosci* (2000) 25, 337–46.
3. Paxil Tablets and Suspension (Paroxetine hydrochloride). GlaxoSmithKline. US Prescribing information, December 2012.
4. Seroxat (Paroxetine hydrochloride hemihydrate). GlaxoSmithKline. UK Summary of product characteristics, August 2015.

SSRIs; Citalopram + Irinotecan

A report attributes a case of rhabdomyolysis to the use of citalopram and irinotecan.

Clinical evidence, mechanism, importance and management

A 74-year-old man who had been taking citalopram for 2 months developed rhabdomyolysis after undergoing initial treatment for gastrointestinal cancer with irinotecan. All medications were discontinued, but the rhabdomyolysis was exacerbated upon restarting the citalopram for depression. The citalopram was discontinued and he improved over the next 5 days.[1]

The authors suggested that concentrations of citalopram might have increased because irinotecan might inhibit CYP3A4, and the cytochrome system might also have been compromised by the malignancy,[1] however the patient was also taking **simvastatin**, which is well known to be associated with a risk of rhabdomyolysis. An interaction between citalopram and irinotecan is therefore not established, and speculatively, this seems more likely to be a case of simvastatin adverse effects.

1. Richards S, Umbreit JN, Fanucchi MP, Giblin J, Khuri F. Selective serotonin reuptake inhibitor-induced rhabdomyolysis associated with irinotecan. South Med J 92003) 96, 1031–3.

SSRIs; Citalopram + Topiramate

A report attributes a case of serotonin syndrome to the use of citalopram and topiramate.

Clinical evidence, mechanism, importance and management

A 65-year-old woman with mild cognitive impairment, taking topiramate 50 mg daily for migraine, was started on citalopram 20 mg daily for depression. Three days later the patient was admitted to hospital with restlessness, confusion, irritability, fever, tremors, myoclonus, and hyperreflexia. Serotonin syndrome was thought to be the cause; citalopram and topiramate were stopped and within a few days the symptoms resolved.[1] Citalopram is metabolised by CYP2C19 with some involvement of CYP3A4 and CYP2D6. Topiramate is a weak inducer of CYP3A4 and might inhibit CYP2C19. The authors suggest that topiramate decreased the metabolism of citalopram resulting in serotonin syndrome in this patient,[1] but this requires confirmation. As such the general relevance of this case is unknown.

1. Talarico G, Tosto G, Pietracupa S, Piacentini E, Canavelli M, Lenzi GL, Bruno G. Serotonin toxicity: a short review of the literature and two case reports involving citalopram. *Neurol Sci* (2011) 32, 507–9.

SSRIs; Escitalopram + HCV-protease inhibitors

Boceprevir and telaprevir minimally decrease the exposure to escitalopram, but simeprevir has no effect. Escitalopram minimally decreases the exposure to simeprevir, but has no effect on the pharmacokinetics of boceprevir or telaprevir.

Clinical evidence, mechanism, importance and management

(a) Boceprevir

In a study in 10 healthy subjects, boceprevir 800 mg three times daily for 5 days decreased the AUC and maximum plasma concentration of a single 10-mg dose of escitalopram by 21% and 19%, respectively. Escitalopram had no effect on the pharmacokinetics of boceprevir.[1] These very small changes would not be expected to be clinically relevant, and no dose adjustment would appear necessary on the concurrent use of boceprevir and escitalopram.

(b) Simeprevir

In a study, 18 healthy subjects were given escitalopram 10 mg daily for 7 days with simeprevir 150 mg daily for 7 days. Escitalopram decreased the AUC of simeprevir by 25%, and the maximum and minimum concentrations by 20% and 32%, respectively. Simeprevir did not affect the pharmacokinetics of escitalopram.[2,3] The mechanism behind this interaction is unknown, but such small changes would not be expected to be clinically important, and the UK and US manufacturers of simeprevir advise that no dose adjustment is needed on concurrent use of simeprevir and escitalopram.[2,3]

(c) Telaprevir

In a study, 13 healthy subjects were given escitalopram 10 mg daily for 7 days with telaprevir 750 mg three times daily for 14 days. Telaprevir decreased the AUC of escitalopram by 35%, and the maximum and minimum plasma concentrations by 30%, and 42%, respectively. Escitalopram had no effect on the pharmacokinetics of telaprevir.[4,5] The mechanism for this interaction is unknown and the clinical relevance of these reductions is unclear, although note that the SSRIs have a wide therapeutic margin. However, until more is known, it would seem prudent to bear the possibility of an interaction in mind should escitalopram appear to be less effective, and to consider increasing the escitalopram dose if necessary.[4,5]

1. Hulskotte EGJ, Gupta S, Xuan F, van Zutven MGJA, O'Mara E, Galitz L, Wagner JA, Butterton JR. Co-administration of the HCV protease inhibitor boceprevir has no clinically meaningful effect on the pharmacokinetics of the selective serotonin reuptake inhibitor escitalopram. Hep Dart 2011, Hawaii, December 2011. Abstract 121.
2. Olysio (Simeprevir sodium). Janssen Cilag Ltd. UK Summary of product characteristics, May 2014.
3. Olysio (Simeprevir sodium). Janssen Products, LP. US Prescribing information, November 2014.
4. Incivo (Telaprevir). Janssen-Cilag Ltd. UK Summary of product characteristics, July 2014.
5. Incivek (Telaprevir). Vertex Pharmaceuticals, Inc. US Prescribing information, October 2013.

SSRIs; Fluoxetine + Aminoglutethimide

Evidence from one case suggests that the effects of fluoxetine are increased by aminoglutethimide.

Clinical evidence, mechanism, importance and management

A patient with severe obsessive-compulsive disorder, resistant to clomipramine combined with SSRIs, improved when given fluoxetine 40 mg daily and aminoglutethimide 250 mg four times daily. Over a four-and-a-half year period, whenever attempts were made to reduce the dosage of either drug, the patient started to relapse.[1] The evidence suggests that aminoglutethimide has a potentiating effect on fluoxetine. However, more study is needed to confirm the efficacy and safety of this drug combination in other patients.

1. Chouinard G, Bélanger M-C, Beauclair L, Sultan S, Murphy BEP. Potentiation of fluoxetine by aminoglutethimide, an adrenal steroid suppressant, in obsessive-compulsive disorder resistant to SSRIs: a case report. *Prog Neuropsychopharmacol Biol Psychiatry* (1996) 20, 1067–79.

SSRIs; Fluoxetine + Cannabinoids

A report describes mania when a patient taking fluoxetine smoked cannabis.

Clinical evidence, mechanism, importance and management

A 21-year-old woman with a 9-year history of bulimia and depression started taking fluoxetine 20 mg daily. A month later, about 2 days after smoking two 'joints' of **cannabis (marijuana)**, she experienced a persistent sense of well-being, increased energy, hypersexuality, and pressured speech. These symptoms progressed into grandiose delusions, for which she was hospitalised. Her mania and excitement were controlled with lorazepam and perphenazine, and she largely recovered after about 8 days. The reasons for this reaction are not understood but the authors of the report point out that one of the active components of cannabis, **dronabinol (Δ9-tetrahydrocannabinol)** is, like fluoxetine, a potent inhibitor of serotonin uptake. Thus a synergistic effect on central serotonergic neurones might have occurred.[1] This seems to be the first and only report of an apparent adverse interaction between cannabis and fluoxetine. The patient had only started fluoxetine 4 weeks before the manic episode, and was still suffering 'hyper' feelings over a month after smoking the cannabis. The symptoms only resolved when the fluoxetine was withdrawn, and so an interaction is by no means established. Note however that the manufacturers of **dronabinol**,[2] and **nabilone**,[3,4] advise caution on concurrent use with other psychoactive drugs, such as SSRIs, due to the risk of additive or synergistic CNS effects.

1. Stoll AL, Cole JO, Lukas SE. A case of mania as a result of fluoxetine-marijuana interaction. *J Clin Psychiatry* (1991) 52, 280–1.
2. Marinol (Dronabinol). AbbVie Inc. US Prescribing information, February 2013.
3. Nabilone Capsules. Meda Pharmaceuticals Ltd. UK Summary of product characteristics, June 2009.
4. Cesamet (Nabilone). Meda Pharmaceuticals Inc. US Prescribing information, April 2011.

SSRIs; Fluoxetine + Orlistat

Orlistat does not appear to affect the pharmacokinetics of fluoxetine.

Clinical evidence, mechanism, importance and management

The pharmacokinetics of a single 40-mg oral dose of fluoxetine (a lipophilic drug) were not affected by orlistat 120 mg three times daily in healthy subjects.[1] Therefore, no fluoxetine dose adjustments appear to be needed on the concurrent use of orlistat.

1. Zhi J, Moore R, Kanitra L, Mulligan TE. Effects of orlistat, a lipase inhibitor, on the pharmacokinetics of three highly lipophilic drugs (amiodarone, fluoxetine, and simvastatin) in healthy volunteers. *J Clin Pharmacol* (2003) 43, 428–35.

SSRIs; Fluvoxamine + Clindamycin

A man taking fluvoxamine developed severe orofacial dyskinesia two - days after starting to take clindamycin.

Clinical evidence, mechanism, importance and management

A 32-year-old man with a major depressive episode was admitted to hospital 10 days after starting fluvoxamine 100 mg daily for 10 days. The fluvoxamine dose was increased to 200 mg daily, and after 4 weeks his mood was stabilised. Two days after starting clindamycin 300 mg daily for a furuncle, severe orofacial dyskinesia developed, which disappeared after he was given intravenous biperiden. The fluvoxamine concentration taken at this time was actually below the usual therapeutic range.[1]

The authors speculated that the time course of events suggests that clindamycin might have contributed to the dyskinesia. However, there is no known mechanism for an interaction. Clindamycin would not be expected to alter the pharmacokinetics of fluvoxamine, and the fluvoxamine blood concentration appears to confirm this. Clindamycin is also not known to cause extrapyramidal adverse effects.

Based on this single case, no general advice can be given, but bear it in mind in case of a similar unexpected reaction.

1. Jakob F, Wolf J. EPMS under antidepressive therapy with fluvoxamine and concomitant antibiotic therapy with clindamycin. *Pharmacopsychiatry* (2007) 40, 129.

SSRIs; Fluvoxamine + Enoxacin

Enoxacin might minimally increase fluvoxamine concentrations, but does not appear to affect its exposure.

Clinical evidence, mechanism, importance and management

In a placebo-controlled study, 10 healthy subjects were given enoxacin 100 mg twice daily for 11 days, with a single 50-mg dose of fluvoxamine on the eighth day. Enoxacin increased the plasma concentrations of fluvoxamine at 2 and 3 hours, by 59% and 51%, respectively, with a 14% increase in the maximum plasma concentration. There was no change in the AUC or elimination half-life of fluvoxamine, or in the pharmacokinetics of the active metabolite of fluvoxamine, fluvoxamino acid. Sleepiness was increased from 30 minutes to 4 hours, but there was no change in the digit symbol substitution test or adverse effects.[1]

It was suggested[1] that enoxacin slightly inhibits the metabolism of fluvoxamine by CYP1A2; however fluvoxamine is not known to be metabolised by this route, rather, it is a potent CYP1A2 inhibitor itself. Additionally, given the lack of effect on fluvoxamine exposure, inhibition of CYP1A2 would seem unlikely, but the exact mechanism is not known.

The interpretation of this study is difficult. The minor change in just the maximum concentration of fluvoxamine would be very unlikely to be clinically relevant, and is unlikely to explain an increase in sleepiness. Further study is necessary, with multiple doses of fluvoxamine. Until more is known, bear the possibility of an interaction in mind in the event of increased sleepiness with enoxacin.

1. Kunii T, Fukasawa T, Yasui-Furukori N, Aoshima T, Suzuki A, Tateishi T, Inoue Y, Otani K. Interaction study between enoxacin and fluvoxamine. *Ther Drug Monit* (2005) 27, 349–53.

SSRIs; Paroxetine + Antacids

Aluminium hydroxide minimally decreases paroxetine absorption.

Clinical evidence, mechanism, importance and management

In a study in healthy subjects, *Aludrox* (aluminium hydroxide) 15 mL twice daily increased the absorption of a single 30-mg dose of paroxetine by about 12%, and increased its maximum plasma concentration by 14%.[1] These changes are unlikely to be clinically important. No particular precautions would seem to be necessary on concurrent use.

1. Greb WH, Brett MA, Buscher G, Dierdorf H-D, von Schrader HW, Wolf D, Mellows G, Zussman BD. Absorption of paroxetine under various dietary conditions and following antacid intake. *Acta Psychiatr Scand* (1989) 80 (Suppl 350), 99–101.

SSRIs; Paroxetine + Aprepitant

The concurrent use of paroxetine and aprepitant appears to slightly decrease the exposure to both drugs.

Clinical evidence, mechanism, importance and management

The US manufacturer of aprepitant notes that the concurrent use of paroxetine 20 mg daily and aprepitant 85 or 170 mg daily decreased the AUC of both drugs by about 25%, and decreased the maximum serum concentrations by about 20%.[1] These changes are unlikely to be clinically important. A clinically relevant interaction with **fosaprepitant** (which is rapidly metabolised to aprepitant) seems unlikely.

1. EMEND Capsules (Aprepitant). Merck & Co., Inc. US Prescribing information, August 2014.

SSRIs; Vilazodone + Miscellaneous

Carbamazepine appears to slightly decrease the exposure to vilazodone. Other potent CYP3A4 inducers might interact similarly. Ketoconazole appears to slightly increase the exposure to vilazodone. Other CYP3A4 inhibitors might interact similarly. The concurrent use of a diuretic and vilazodone might increase the risk of hyponatraemia. *In vitro* data suggests that vilazodone might increase the concentrations of CYP2C8 substrates.

Clinical evidence, mechanism, importance and management

(a) CYP2C8 substrates

The US manufacturer of vilazodone notes that *in vitro* studies suggest vilazodone might inhibit the metabolism of CYP2C8 substrates leading to an increase in their concentration.[1] However, they also note that this has not been tested *in vivo*, and as predictions made on the basis of *in vitro* effects do not always mirror what happens in clinical use, further study is required to establish the relevance of this, if any, in practice.

(b) CYP3A4 inducers and inhibitors

The US manufacturer of vilazodone briefly notes that in a study, **carbamazepine** decreased the exposure to vilazodone by about 45%.[1] Carbamazepine is a potent inducer of CYP3A4, by which vilazodone is primarily metabolised, hence concurrent use decreases its exposure. The manufacturer advises that if a potent CYP3A4 inducer is used for more than 14 days, consideration should be given to increasing the vilazodone dose up to 2-fold over 1 to 2 weeks, but not exceeding the maximum dose of 80 mg daily. Once the CYP3A4 inducer is stopped, the vilazodone dose should be reduced to the original dose within 14 days.[1] See 'Table 1.9', p.11, for a list of potent CYP3A4 inducers.

The US manufacturer also briefly notes that in a study, **ketoconazole** increased vilazodone exposure by about 50%. Ketoconazole is a potent inhibitor of CYP3A4, hence concurrent use increases its exposure. The manufacturer advises that if a potent CYP3A4 inhibitor is given concurrently, the dose of vilazodone should not exceed 20 mg daily.[1] Moderate inhibitors of CYP3A4 would also be expected to increase vilazodone exposure, but to a lesser extent than potent inhibitors. If vilazodone is given with a moderate CYP3A4 inhibitor, it would seem prudent to be alert for an increase in vilazodone adverse effects, and to adjust the dose if necessary. See 'Table 1.9', p.11, for a list of clinically relevant CYP3A4 inhibitors.

(c) Diuretics

The US manufacturer of vilazodone briefly notes that hyponatraemia has occurred in patients receiving SNRIs, and warns that patients also taking diuretics might have a greater risk of developing hyponatraemia.[1]

1. Viibryd (Vilazodone hydrochloride). Forest Pharmaceuticals, Inc. US Prescribing information, March 2015.

Tianeptine + Oxazepam

A study in healthy subjects given tianeptine 12.5 mg and oxazepam 10 mg both three times daily found no significant changes in the pharmacokinetics of either drug.[1]

1. Toon S, Holt BL, Langley SJ, Mullins FGP, Rowland M, Halliday MS, Salvadori C, Delalleau B. Pharmacokinetic and pharmacodynamic interaction between the antidepressant tianeptine and oxazepam at steady-state. *Psychopharmacology (Berl)* (1990) 101, 226–32.

Trazodone + Azoles

It appears that ketoconazole might inhibit the metabolism of trazodone. It is predicted that itraconazole and voriconazole might interact similarly, while fluconazole and posaconazole might also do so, but to a lesser extent.

Clinical evidence, mechanism, importance and management

An *in vitro* study found that **ketoconazole** inhibited the metabolism of trazodone to its principal active metabolite, *m*-chlorophenylpiperazine, and was of similar potency to ritonavir in this regard.[1]

Trazodone is a substrate for CYP3A4 and inhibitors of this enzyme such as **ketoconazole** might inhibit its metabolism, leading to substantial increases in trazodone plasma concentrations with the potential for adverse effects,[2-4] as has been shown for ritonavir, see 'Trazodone + HIV-protease inhibitors', below.

On the basis of the available data, the FDA in the US, and the UK and US manufacturers of trazodone recommend that a lower dose should be considered if it is given with a potent CYP3A4 inhibitor,[2-4] which would include **itraconazole**, **ketoconazole**, and **voriconazole**. However, the UK manufacturer also suggests that the combination should be avoided, where possible.[4] The US manufacturer specifically warns that the risk of arrhythmias might be increased by concurrent use.[2] **Fluconazole** and **posaconazole**, both moderate CYP3A4 inhibitors, might also inhibit the metabolism of trazodone, but to a lesser extent. Nevertheless, some caution on concurrent use would seem sensible.

1. Zalma A, von Moltke LL, Granda BW, Harmatz JS, Shader RI, Greenblatt DJ. In vitro metabolism of trazodone by CYP3A: inhibition by ketoconazole and human immunodeficiency viral protease inhibitors. *Biol Psychiatry* (2000) 47, 655–61.
2. Trazodone hydrochloride. Apotex Inc. US Prescribing information, August 2014.
3. Lewis-Hall FC. Bristol-Myers Squibb Company. Letter to healthcare professionals, April 2004.
4. Molipaxin (Trazodone hydrochloride).Zentiva. UK Summary of product characteristics, August 2013.

Trazodone + Ginkgo (*Ginkgo biloba*)

Coma developed in an elderly patient with Alzheimer's disease after she took trazodone with ginkgo.

Clinical evidence

An 80-year-old woman with Alzheimer's disease became comatose a few days after starting low-dose trazodone 20 mg twice daily and ginkgo biloba. The patient woke immediately after being given flumazenil 1 mg intravenously.[1]

Mechanism

Unknown. The authors suggested that ginkgo flavonoids increased the metabolism of trazodone to its active metabolite, 1-(m-chlorophenyl)piperazine (mCPP) by inducing CYP3A4. The increased concentrations of the metabolite were thought to have enhanced the release of GABA (gamma-amino butyric acid). In addition, it was suggested that the ginkgo flavonoids produced a subclinical increase in GABA via a direct effect on the benzodiazepine binding site of the GABA receptor. It was proposed that flumazenil might have blocked the direct effect of the flavonoids, thus causing the GABA activity to fall below that required to have a clinical effect.[1] However, note that clinically relevant CYP3A4 induction by gingko has not been seen with the conventional CYP3A4 probe substrate midazolam.

Importance and management

Evidence for an interaction between ginkgo and trazodone appears to be limited to this case, from which no general conclusions can be drawn. Bear this interaction in mind in case of an unexpected response to concurrent use.

1. Galluzzi S, Zanetti O, Binetti G, Trabucchi M, Frisoni GB. Coma in a patient with Alzheimer's disease taking low dose trazodone and ginkgo biloba. *J Neurol Neurosurg Psychiatry* (2000) 68, 679–80.

Trazodone + Food

Food decreased the maximum concentration of immediate-release trazodone and increased the maximum concentration of extended-release trazodone, but did not alter the overall exposure to either formulation.

Clinical evidence, mechanism, importance and management

A crossover study in 8 healthy subjects given a single 100-mg trazodone capsule following an overnight fast, or after a standardised (unspecified) breakfast, found that food decreased the maximum concentration of trazodone by 22% and increased the time to maximum concentration by 51%, but did not affect the AUC.[1] In a randomised crossover study in 34 healthy subjects, a single 300-mg trazodone extended-release caplet was given following an overnight fast, or after a high-fat, high-calorie (991.6 kcal) standardised breakfast. Food increased the maximum concentration of trazodone by 86%, but did not alter the time to maximum concentration or the AUC.[2] The overall absorption of trazodone (AUC) was unaffected by food, but the maximum concentration might be decreased or increased, depending on formulation. The UK and US manufacturers of immediate-release trazodone advise that the dose should be taken after food,[3] or after a light meal or snack.[4] Further, the UK manufacturer advises that administration after a meal might reduce adverse effects.[3]

1. Nilsen OG, Dale O. Single dose pharmacokinetics of trazodone in healthy subjects. Pharmacol Toxicol. (1992) 71, 150–3.
2. Karhu D, Gossen ER, Mostert A, Cronjé T, Fradette C. Safety, tolerability and pharmacokinetics of once-daily trazodone extended-release caplets in healthy subjects. *Int J Clin Pharmacol Ther* (2011) 49, 730–43.
3. Molipaxin (Trazodone hydrochloride). Zentiva. UK Summary of product characteristics, August 2013.
4. Trazodone hydrochloride. Apotex Inc. US Prescribing information, August 2014.

Trazodone + Haloperidol

Low-dose haloperidol does not alter the pharmacokinetics of trazodone to a clinically relevant extent.

Clinical evidence, mechanism, importance and management

Nine depressed patients who had been taking trazodone 150 to 300 mg at bedtime for 2 to 19 weeks were given haloperidol 4 mg daily for a week. Plasma trazodone concentrations were not notably changed, but the concentrations of its active metabolite (*m*-chlorophenylpiperazine) were increased by 18% (from 78 to 92 nanograms/mL).[1] This small increase is unlikely to be clinically relevant, and no trazodone dose adjustment is needed on concurrent use with low-dose haloperidol. The effect of high-dose haloperidol on the pharmacokinetics of trazodone is not known, but some caution might be appropriate.

1. Mihara K, Otani K, Ishida M, Yasui N, Suzuki A, Ohkubo T, Osanai T, Kaneko S, Sugawara K. Increases in plasma concentration of m-chlorophenylpiperazine, but not trazodone, with low-dose haloperidol. *Ther Drug Monit* (1997) 19, 43–5.

Trazodone + HIV-protease inhibitors

Ritonavir moderately increases the exposure to trazodone. Other potent CYP3A4 inhibitors are predicted to have a similar effect. A possible case of serotonin syndrome has been seen in a patient taking ritonavir and multiple serotonergic drugs, including trazodone.

Clinical evidence

A randomised, placebo-controlled study in 10 healthy subjects found that short-term exposure to low-dose **ritonavir** (200 mg twice daily for 2 days) decreased the clearance of a single 50-mg dose of trazodone by 52%. The AUC of trazodone increased 2.4-fold, whereas its mean maximum plasma concentration increased by just 34%.[1] Symptoms of serotonin syndrome occurred in an HIV-positive patient taking antiretrovirals and other drugs, including fluoxetine, lithium, and trazodone, when **ritonavir** was added. The symptoms resolved on discontinuing the trazodone and halving the **ritonavir** dose.[2] Serotonin syndrome has also been seen in a patient taking trazodone, fluoxetine, **indinavir**, and excessive amounts of grapefruit, see 'SSRIs + Grapefruit juice', p.1486.

Mechanism

An *in vitro* study demonstrated that the metabolism of trazodone to its principal active metabolite, *m*-chlorophenylpiperazine (mCPP), was inhibited by ritonavir, which is an inhibitor of CYP3A4 (by which trazodone is metabolised). Indinavir, **saquinavir**, and **nelfinavir** also inhibited mCPP formation.[3]

Importance and management

Although data are limited, what is available suggests that a pharmacokinetic interaction between ritonavir and trazodone is established and likely to be clinically important, with the potential for increased adverse effects. The FDA in the US, and the UK and US manufacturers of trazodone therefore recommend that a lower dose of trazodone should be considered if it is given with potent CYP3A4 inhibitors, such as ritonavir or the other HIV-inhibitors boosted with ritonavir.[4-6]. However, the UK manufacturer also suggests that the combination should be avoided where possible.[5] The US manufacturer specifically warns that the risk of arrhythmias might be increased by concurrent use.[6] See 'Table 1.9', p.11 for a list of clinically relevant potent CYP3A4 inhibitors, but note that the UK manufacturer additionally names **nefazodone** as a potent CYP3A4 inhibitor,[5] but it is generally considered a moderate inhibitor.

1. Greenblatt DJ, von Moltke LL, Harmatz JS, Fogelman SM, Chen G, Graf JA, Mertzanis P, Byron S, Culm KE, Granda BW, Daily JP, Shader RI. Short-term exposure to low-dose ritonavir impairs clearance and enhances adverse effects of trazodone. *J Clin Pharmacol* (2003) 43, 414–22.
2. DeSilva KE, Le Flore DB, Marston BJ, Rimland D. Serotonin syndrome in HIV-infected individuals receiving antiretroviral therapy and fluoxetine. *AIDS* (2001) 15, 1281–5.
3. Zalma A, von Moltke LL, Granda BW, Harmatz JS, Shader RI, Greenblatt DJ. In vitro metabolism of trazodone by CYP3A: inhibition by ketoconazole and human immunodeficiency viral protease inhibitors. *Biol Psychiatry* (2000) 47, 655–61.
4. Lewis-Hall FC. Bristol-Myers Squibb Company. Letter to healthcare professionals, April 2004.
5. Molipaxin (Trazodone hydrochloride). Zentiva. UK Summary of product characteristics, August 2013.
6. Trazodone hydrochloride. Apotex Inc. US Prescribing information, August 2014.

Trazodone + Lysergide (LSD)

A retrospective study found that 28 of 32 subjects (88%) who took LSD and who had taken an SSRI or trazodone for more than 3 weeks had a subjective decrease or virtual elimination of their responses to LSD.[1] The reason for this effect is not understood. Lysergide increases serotonin in the brain, and one suggestion is that when the serotonin re-uptake is blocked in the brain, there is an increased stimulation of 5-HT$_1$ and 5-HT$_2$ receptors.

1. Bonson KR, Buckholtz JW, Murphy DL. Chronic administration of serotonergic antidepressants attenuates the subjective effects of LSD in humans. *Neuropsychopharmacology* (1996) 14, 425–36.

Trazodone + Macrolides

Clarithromycin moderately increases exposure to trazodone. Telithromycin, erythromycin, and roxithromycin are also likely to increase trazodone exposure, though the extent might differ.

Clinical evidence

In a crossover study in 10 healthy subjects, **clarithromycin** 500 mg (4 doses over 32 hours) increased the AUC and maximum concentration of a single 50-mg dose of trazodone 2-fold and by 35%, respectively. Further, the clearance was decreased by 46%, and the elimination half-life was almost doubled.[1]

Mechanism

Clarithromycin is an inhibitor of CYP3A4, of which trazodone is a substrate, thus concurrent use can increase the exposure to trazodone.

Importance and management

Evidence for an interaction between trazodone and the macrolides is limited to one study with **clarithromycin** but this is consistent with the disposition of trazodone and the well-known effects of clarithromycin on other similarly metabolised drugs. Thus an interaction would seem to be established and the moderate increase in exposure to trazodone is likely to be clinically important, and might result in increased adverse effects. The FDA in the US and the UK and US manufacturers of trazodone recommend that a lower dose should be considered if it is given with potent CYP3A4 inhibitors,[2-4] such as clarithromycin or **telithromycin**. However, the UK manufacturer also suggests that the combination should be avoided, where possible.[2] The US manufacturer specifically warns that the risk of arrhythmias might be increased by concurrent use.[3] Note that the UK manufacturer additionally names **erythromycin** as a potent CYP3A4 inhibitor,[2] but this is generally considered a moderate inhibitor and so would be expected to have a smaller effect than clarithromycin. **Roxithromycin** is only a weak CYP3A4 inhibitor and would therefore be expected to only have a minor effect on trazodone exposure. With concurrent use of erythromycin or roxithromycin, it would seem prudent to be aware of this interaction, to be alert for any increase in adverse effects such as sedation, and to reduce the trazodone dose as necessary. If starting trazodone in a patient taking one of these two macrolides it would seem sensible to start with a low dose and to increase cautiously.

1. Farkas D, Volak LP, Harmatz JS, von Moltke LL, Court MH, Greenblatt DJ. Short-term clarithromycin administration impairs clearance and enhances pharmacodynamic effects of trazodone but not of zolpidem. *Clin Pharmacol Ther* (2009) 85, 644–50.
2. Molipaxin (Trazodone hydrochloride). Zentiva. UK Summary of product characteristics, August 2013.
3. Trazodone hydrochloride. Apotex Inc. US Prescribing information, August 2014.
4. Lewis-Hall FC. Bristol-Myers Squibb Company. Letter to healthcare professionals, April 2004.

Trazodone + NNRTIs; Delavirdine

Delavirdine is predicted to increase the plasma concentration of trazodone.

Clinical evidence, mechanism, importance and management

On the basis of the interaction between trazodone and ritonavir (see 'Trazodone + HIV-protease inhibitors', p.1499), the US manufacturer of delavirdine predicts that, as it is also a CYP3A4 inhibitor, concurrent use might increase the plasma concentration of trazodone. They therefore recommend caution, and that a lower dose of trazodone should be considered.[1] However, note that ritonavir is a well-known potent inhibitor of CYP3A4, and while delavirdine does appear to inhibit CYP3A4, the potency of its effect is difficult to classify due to a lack of clinical data. Until more is known, it would seem sensible to bear the possibility of increased adverse effects in mind if delavirdine and trazodone are used concurrently.

1. Rescriptor (Delavirdine mesylate). ViiV Healthcare. US Prescribing information, August 2012.

Trazodone + Pseudoephedrine

A report describes a woman taking trazodone who developed a toxic reaction when she took pseudoephedrine.

Clinical evidence, mechanism, importance and management

A report describes a woman who had been taking trazodone 250 mg daily for 2 years who took two doses of a non-prescription medicine containing pseudoephedrine. Within 6 hours she experienced dread, anxiety, panic, confusion, depersonalisation, and the sensation that parts of her body were separating. None of these symptoms had been experienced in the past when she was taking either preparation alone.[1] The reasons for this reaction are not understood, and no general conclusions can be drawn.

1. Weddige RL. Possible trazodone-pseudoephedrine toxicity: a case report. *Neurobehav Toxicol Teratol* (1985) 7, 204.

Trazodone + SSRIs

Trazodone and fluoxetine have been used concurrently with advantage, but some patients have developed increased adverse effects. Fluoxetine might increase trazodone concentrations, whereas citalopram has little effect on trazodone concentrations. Possible serotonin syndrome has been reported in patients taking trazodone with paroxetine or trazodone with fluoxetine. Hepatotoxicity was seen in a patient taking paroxetine, trazodone, and cloral hydrate.

Clinical evidence

(a) Citalopram

In a study using data from trazodone therapeutic drug monitoring, the trazodone concentration-to-dose ratio was 28% higher in 41 patients taking trazodone with citalopram than in 40 patients taking trazodone alone, but this difference was not statistically significant.[1]

(b) Fluoxetine

In a controlled study, 27 patients were given trazodone 100 mg daily alone for one week, and then randomised to receive fluoxetine 20 mg daily, pindolol 7.5 mg daily, or placebo for 4 weeks. Fluoxetine increased trazodone concentrations by 43% at 2 weeks and 65% at 4 weeks compared with baseline values, whereas pindolol and placebo had no effect.[2] Similarly, a patient taking trazodone had a 31% increase in the trazodone plasma concentration corrected for dose (suggesting increased trazodone concentrations) when fluoxetine 40 mg daily was added. She became sedated and developed an unstable gait.[3] In another study, the trazodone concentration-to-dose ratio was 28% higher in 16 patients taking trazodone with fluoxetine than in 40 patients taking trazodone alone, but this difference was not statistically significant.[1]

A man with traumatic brain injury showed new-onset dysarthria and speech blocking when fluoxetine was added to trazodone. His speech returned to normal when the fluoxetine was stopped.[4] A 39-year-old HIV-positive man taking multiple antiviral and antibacterial drugs experienced bilateral hand tremor while receiving trazodone 50 mg at bedtime, which worsened when the dose of trazodone was increased to 100 mg and fluoxetine 20 mg daily was added. The trazodone and fluoxetine were discontinued and the tremor completely disappeared after 7 days without specific treatment for myoclonus.[5]

Five out of 16 patients taking fluoxetine stopped taking trazodone 25 to 75 mg, which was given for insomnia, because of excessive sedation the next day.[6] Three out of 8 patients had improvement in sleep and depression when given both drugs but the other 5 were either unaffected or had intolerable adverse effects (headaches, dizziness, daytime sedation, fatigue).[7] However, another report described advantageous concurrent use in 6 patients without an increase in adverse effects.[8] A case report describes delirium and a tonic clonic seizure in a 71-year-old woman taking fluoxetine 20 mg and trazodone 100 mg (recently increased from 50 mg) which was attributed to serotonin syndrome.[9] For another case describing serotonin syndrome, which developed in a patient taking fluoxetine, trazodone, and buspirone when venlafaxine was added, see 'SNRIs; Venlafaxine + Trazodone', p.1484.

(c) Paroxetine

A case report describes a 29-year-old woman with depression taking trazodone 200 mg daily for the past 3 months. In order to improve her depressive symptoms her trazodone dose was reduced to 50 mg daily and 2 weeks later, paroxetine 20 mg daily was added. Within 24 hours she developed symptoms including agitation and sweating, which was described as serotonin syndrome and her drugs were stopped. She recovered with supportive measures.[10] Another case report describes a 49-year-old taking **cloral hydrate** 250 mg daily (for 22 days), paroxetine 20 mg daily (for 18 days), and trazodone 50 mg daily (for 8 days) who developed fever, vomiting, and a maculopapular rash. The medications were stopped and fluvoxamine and mianserin started. Hepatic dysfunction, eosinophilia, and pneumonitis were noted. The patient's renal function also deteriorated and fluvoxamine and mianserin were stopped. Hepatic and renal function continued to deteriorate and high-dose steroids were started. The rash resolved after 4 days, pneumonitis after 7 days, and renal function after 10 days. His liver function tests did not improve until 7 days after his regular medications had been stopped (4 days after starting steroids) and returned to normal after 6 weeks.[11]

(d) Sertraline

For a case describing serotonin syndrome in a patient taking trazodone who received escalating doses of sertraline and risperidone, see 'Risperidone + SSRIs', p.887.

Mechanism

It appears that the plasma concentrations of trazodone can be increased due to inhibition of its metabolism via cytochrome P450 isoenzymes by fluoxetine and/or its metabolite, norfluoxetine.[2] Trazodone is a substrate for CYP3A4 and, although fluoxetine is a weak inhibitor of this isoenzyme, norfluoxetine is a moderate inhibitor.[5] *In vitro* data suggest that citalopram has little inhibitory effect on CYP3A4.[1] Serotonin syndrome seems to develop unpredictably in some patients given two or more serotonergic drugs.

Importance and management

These cases and studies suggest that the concurrent use of trazodone and fluoxetine can be useful and uneventful but it would seem prudent to monitor the outcome for any evidence of increased adverse effects. Citalopram would not be expected to have a pharmacokinetic interaction with trazodone. However, the cases with fluoxetine suggest that a pharmacodynamic interaction (leading to adverse effects such as dysarthria, tremor, and sedation) might be possible. A similar case is described with paroxetine, but as this patient was not given an SSRI alone, it is not possible to definitively attribute this reaction to an interaction. A few cases of possible serotonin syndrome have been reported with trazodone and fluoxetine, paroxetine, or sertraline, suggesting that a degree of caution would be prudent on their concurrent use. As SSRIs as a group can be associated with serotonin syndrome, the same caution would seem appropriate for all SSRIs in combination with trazodone. For more information on serotonin syndrome and its management, see 'Drugs that cause serotonin syndrome + Other drugs that cause serotonin syndrome', p.1471. The relevance of the case of hepatotoxicity in a patient taking paroxetine, trazodone and cloral hydrate is unclear.

1. Prapotnik M, Waschgler R, König P, Moll W, Conca A. Therapeutic drug monitoring of trazodone: are there pharmacokinetic interactions involving citalopram and fluoxetine? *Int J Clin Pharmacol Ther* (2004) 42, 120–4.
2. Maes M, Westenberg H, Vandoolaeghe E, Demedts P, Wauters A, Neels H, Meltzer HY. Effects of trazodone and fluoxetine in the treatment of major depression: therapeutic pharmacokinetic and pharmacodynamic interactions through formation of meta-chlorophenylpiperazine. *J Clin Psychopharmacol* (1997) 17, 358–64.
3. Aranow RB, Hudson JI, Pope HG, Grady TA, Laage TA, Bell IR, Cole JO. Elevated antidepressant plasma levels after addition of fluoxetine. *Am J Psychiatry* (1989) 146, 911–13.
4. Patterson DE, Braverman SE, Belandres PV. Speech dysfunction due to trazodone-fluoxetine combination in traumatic brain injury. *Brain Inj* (1997) 11, 287–91.
5. Darko W, Guharoy R, Rose F, Lehman D, Pappas V. Myoclonus secondary to the concurrent use of trazodone and fluoxetine. *Vet Hum Toxicol* (2001) 43, 214–5.
6. Metz A, Shader RI. Adverse interactions encountered when using trazodone to treat insomnia associated with fluoxetine. *Int Clin Psychopharmacol* (1990) 5, 191–4.
7. Nierenberg AA, Cole JO, Glass L. Possible trazodone potentiation of fluoxetine: a case series. *J Clin Psychiatry* (1992) 53, 83–5.
8. Swerdlow NR, Andia AM. Trazodone-fluoxetine combination for treatment of obsessive-compulsive disorder. *Am J Psychiatry* (1989) 146, 1637.
9. Amir I, Dano M, Joffe A. Recurrent toxic delirium in a patient treated with SSRIs: is old age a risk factor? *Isr J Psychiatry Relat Sci* (1997) 34, 119–21.
10. Reeves RR, Bullen JA. Serotonin syndrome produced by paroxetine and low-dose trazodone. *Psychosomatics* (1995) 36, 159–60.
11. Azaz-Livshits T, Hershko A, Ben-Chetrit E. Paroxetine associated hepatotoxicity: a report of 3 cases and a review of the literature. *Pharmacopsychiatry* (2002) 35, 112–5.

Trazodone + Tryptophan

A case report describes the development of anorexia, psychosis, and hypomania in a patient taking trazodone and tryptophan.

Clinical evidence, mechanism, importance and management

A case report describes the effective use of trazodone 100 mg and tryptophan 500 mg, both three times weekly, with daily clonazepam, in a woman with schizophrenia and congenital defects. However, the patient stopped eating, lost 4.5 kg in weight over 3 weeks, developed signs of psychosis or hypomania, and soon afterwards became drowsy and withdrawn. When the drugs were withdrawn the aggressive behaviour restarted, but she responded again to lower doses of trazodone and tryptophan, although the signs of psychosis re-emerged.[1] This single case probably has little general relevance.

Note that both trazodone and tryptophan have serotonergic effects, and concurrent use might lead to the serotonin syndrome. Serotonin syndrome is a rare adverse effect, but because of its severity, some caution is warranted if both drugs are given. For more information on serotonin syndrome and its management, see 'Drugs that cause serotonin syndrome + Other drugs that cause serotonin syndrome', p.1471.

1. Patterson BD, Srisopark MM. Severe anorexia and possible psychosis or hypomania after trazodone-tryptophan treatment of aggression. *Lancet* (1989) i, 1017.

Tricyclic antidepressants + ACE inhibitors

Limited evidence from two patients suggests that enalapril may increase the effects of clomipramine, resulting in adverse effects. The concurrent use of tricyclic antidepressants and ACE inhibitors may possibly enhance the risk of postural hypotension.

Clinical evidence

Two patients taking **enalapril** (one taking 20 mg daily and the other taking 20 mg five times weekly) were given **clomipramine** for depression. The **clomipramine** dose of one of them was increased from 25 to 50 mg, and 10 days later he became euphoric and exalted. The problem resolved when the **clomipramine** dose was reduced to 25 mg again. The other patient had been stable taking **enalapril** for over a year when **clomipramine** and disulfiram 400 mg daily were added. Within 2 weeks he developed confusion, irritability and insomnia. These adverse effects diminished when the **clomipramine** dosage was reduced to 50 mg daily.[1]

Mechanism

The ratio of clomipramine to its metabolite (desmethylclomipramine) is normally less than 1, but both of these patients demonstrated a ratio of more than 1. This suggests that the normal metabolism (demethylation) of the clomipramine was inhibited, thus allowing the clomipramine to accumulate and its toxic effects to manifest themselves. In the second patient the disulfiram may also have had a minor additional enzyme inhibitory effect.[1]

Importance and management

Information regarding an interaction between clomipramine and enalapril is limited to these two cases and the interaction is not firmly established. More study is needed. There seems to be nothing documented about adverse effects from the concurrent use of the other ACE inhibitors and tricyclic antidepressants, although tricyclic antidepressants may cause postural hypotension, which could be more severe in the presence of ACE inhibitors.

1. Toutoungi M. Potential effect of enalapril on clomipramine metabolism. *Hum Psychopharmacol* (1992) 7, 347–9.

Tricyclic antidepressants + Ademetionine

A severe reaction, diagnosed as serotonin syndrome, developed in a woman taking ademetionine shortly after her clomipramine dosage was increased.

Clinical evidence, mechanism, importance and management

An elderly woman with a major affective disorder was given intramuscular ademetionine 100 mg daily and **clomipramine** 25 mg daily for 10 days. The **clomipramine** dose was then increased to 75 mg daily and, about 2 to 3 days later, she became progressively agitated, anxious, and confused. On admission to hospital she was stuporous, with a pulse rate of 130 bpm, a respiratory rate of 30 breaths per minute, and she had diarrhoea, myoclonus, generalised tremors, rigidity, hyperreflexia, shivering, profound diaphoresis, and dehydration. Her temperature rose from 40.5°C to 43° C. She had no infection, and was diagnosed with serotonin syndrome. The drugs were withdrawn and she was given dantrolene 50 mg intravenously every 6 hours for 48 hours. She made a complete recovery.[1] The reason for this severe adverse reaction is not understood, although there appears to be a connection between ademetionine and serotonin in the brain.[1,2] Another possibility is that serotonin syndrome was simply triggered by the large increase in the clomipramine dose. The UK manufacturer states that **clomipramine** should be used with caution in elderly patients as they generally show a stronger response to it; doses should be increased slowly from 10 mg daily to around 30 to 75 mg daily over about 10 days.[3]

An interaction is therefore not established; however, as both ademetionine and the tricyclics have serotonergic effects, concurrent use might lead to the serotonin syndrome. Serotonin syndrome is a rare adverse effect, but because of its severity, some caution is warranted if both drugs are given. For more information on serotonin syndrome and its management, see 'Drugs that cause serotonin syndrome + Other drugs that cause serotonin syndrome', p.1471.

1. Iruela LM, Minguez L, Merino J, Monedero G. Toxic interaction of *S*-adenosylmethionine and clomipramine. *Am J Psychiatry* (1993) 150, 522.
2. Young SN. Clinical nutrition: 3. The fuzzy boundary between nutrition and psychopharmacology. *Can Med Assoc J* (2002) 166, 205–9.
3. Anafranil (Clomipramine hydrochloride). Novartis Pharmaceuticals UK Ltd. UK Summary of product characteristics, January 2014.

Tricyclic antidepressants + Amfetamines

No pharmacokinetic interaction was reported in children receiving dexamfetamine and desipramine, but concurrent use of amfetamines and tricyclics might increase the risk of cardiovascular adverse effects.

Clinical evidence, mechanism, importance and management

A retrospective review in children and adolescents taking either **desipramine** alone, or with a stimulant, indicated the absence of a clinically significant interaction between **desipramine** and **dexamfetamine** in 4 children who received both drugs; pharmacokinetic parameters for desipramine were similar in each group.[1]

The US manufacturers of **dexamfetamine** and **benzfetamine**, state that amfetamines might enhance the activity of the tricyclics.[2,3] Further, the US manufacturer of **dexamfetamine** states that **dexamfetamine** with **desipramine** or **protriptyline**, and possibly other tricyclics, causes striking and sustained increases in the concentrations of **dexamfetamine** in the brain, and that cardiovascular effects can be potentiated.[2] The UK manufacturer of dexamfetamine gives a similar warning.[4]

The clinical relevance of these warnings is unclear. It might be prudent to carefully consider the risks of using the combination of an amfetamine and a tricyclic in patients with pre-existing cardiovascular disorders.

Note that some tricyclics (see 'Table 35.3', p.1472) and the amfetamines have serotonergic effects, and concurrent use might lead to the serotonin syndrome. Serotonin syndrome is a rare adverse effect, but because of its severity, some caution is warranted if both drugs are given. For more information on serotonin syndrome and its management, see 'Drugs that cause serotonin syndrome + Other drugs that cause serotonin syndrome', p.1471.

1. Cohen LG, Prince J, Biederman J, Wilens T, Faraone SV, Whitt S, Mick E, Spencer T, Meyer MC, Polisner D, Flood JG. Absence of effect of stimulants on the pharmacokinetics of desipramine in children. *Pharmacotherapy* (1999) 19, 746–52.
2. Dexedrine (Dextroamphetamine sulfate). Amedra Pharmaceuticals, LLC. US Prescribing information, October 2013.
3. Didrex (Benzphetamine hydrochloride). Pfizer, Inc. US Prescribing information, August 2010.
4. Dexamfetamine sulphate tablets. Auden McKenzie (Pharma Division) Ltd. UK Summary of product characteristics. March 2010.

Tricyclic antidepressants + Amiodarone

An isolated case of orobuccal dyskinesia was reported in a woman taking amitriptyline after starting amiodarone.

Clinical evidence, mechanism, importance and management

An 82-year-old woman, who had been taking **amitriptyline** 50 mg daily for about a year for insomnia, presented to hospital with garbled speech one month after starting amiodarone for atrial fibrillation. She was taking numerous other drugs including alendronate, aspirin, bumetanide, transdermal lidocaine, oxycodone, pantoprazole, simvastatin, tiagabine, tizanidine, and tolterodine. Stroke was excluded, and her dyskinesia nearly completely resolved within a couple of days of stopping **amitriptyline**, implicating the tricyclic. It was concluded that amiodarone had inhibited the metabolism of **amitriptyline** resulting in increased **amitriptyline** concentrations and in the orobuccal dyskinesia.[1] **Amitriptyline** is thought to be metabolised by CYP2D6, and amiodarone appears to inhibit this isoenzyme. However, dyskinesias with tricyclic antidepressants are rare and not a usual dose-related adverse effect. It is not possible to conclude from this one case whether a drug interaction occurred. Bear the possibility in mind in the event of a similar outcome on the concurrent use of amiodarone and a tricyclic.

Note that amiodarone is known to prolong the QT interval, and this rarely also occurs with tricyclic antidepressants (mostly in overdose), so bear in mind the possibility of additive QT prolongation, see 'Drugs that prolong the QT interval + Other drugs that prolong the QT interval', p.272 for further information.

1. Pawar PS, Woo DA. Extrapyramidal symptoms with concomitant use of amitriptyline and amiodarone in an elderly patient. *Am J Geriatr Pharmacother* (2010) 8, 595–8.

Tricyclic antidepressants + Aspirin

In one study the incidence and severity of adverse effects increased when aspirin was given with imipramine.

Clinical evidence, mechanism, importance and management

A study in 20 patients with depression, given **imipramine** in their usual dose of 75 mg twice daily for 5 days, found that when aspirin 500 mg twice daily was added for a further 2 days, the incidence and range of adverse effects increased by 52% and 56%, respectively, with adverse effects described as severe increasing 2.5-fold. The degree of binding of **imipramine** to plasma proteins decreased by 12% when aspirin was given, and it was suggested that the increase in the amount of 'free' (and pharmacologically active) **imipramine** in the plasma manifested as an increase in adverse effects.[1]

Information about this interaction seems to be limited to this report, which was only short-term, so the effects of long-term concurrent use are unclear.

Note that it has been suggested that tricyclic antidepressants might increase the risk of gastrointestinal bleeding with aspirin or NSAIDs,[2] similar to the SSRIs (see 'Antiplatelet drugs + SSRIs or SNRIs', p.780), but information on this appears to be limited. More study is needed.

1. Juárez-Olguín H, Jung-Cook H, Flores-Pérez J, Asseff IL. Clinical evidence of an interaction between imipramine and acetylsalicylic acid on protein binding in depressed patients. *Clin Neuropharmacol* (2002) 25, 32–6.
2. Go MF. Drug injury in the upper gastrointestinal tract: nonsteroidal anti-inflammatory drugs. *Gastrointest Endosc Clin N Am* (2006) 16, 83–97.

Tricyclic and related antidepressants + Azoles; Fluconazole

Fluconazole has increased amitriptyline and nortriptyline levels in a number of cases. Mental changes, syncope, and a prolonged QTc interval have also been seen when fluconazole was given with a tricyclic.

Clinical evidence

(a) Amitriptyline

A man with AIDS given fluconazole 200 mg daily and amitriptyline 25 mg then 50 mg three times daily developed mental changes and visual hallucinations within 3 days of concurrent use. His serum amitriptyline level was found to be 724 nanograms/mL (reference range 150 to 250 nanograms/mL). His confusion resolved within 4 days of stopping the amitriptyline, at which point the levels had fallen to 270 nanograms/mL. Two similar cases were described in this report, in one case in a patient with renal impairment.[1]

A woman taking amitriptyline 100 mg twice daily, isosorbide mononitrate and metoprolol became lethargic, drowsy and confused 4 days after starting fluconazole 100 mg daily. She was found to have elevated serum levels of amitriptyline plus its metabolite nortriptyline of 956 nanograms/mL (patient's usual range 150 to 250 nanograms/mL) and a prolonged QTc interval. At first, an amitriptyline overdose was suspected. The patient was intubated, but she became delirious, agitated and disorientated. She recovered over the next 24 hours and the amitriptyline level had fallen to 190 nanograms/mL after 4 days. It was concluded that the amitriptyline toxicity was due to an interaction with fluconazole.[2]

Other reports similarly describe increased amitriptyline levels when fluconazole was given; in a child who developed syncope as a result[3] and in a 57-year-old woman who developed QT prolongation (although hypokalaemia and the use of sertraline, which can increase serum tricyclic levels, may have contributed to this effect).[4]

(b) Nortriptyline

An elderly woman taking nortriptyline 75 mg daily and other drugs (ciclosporin, morphine, metoclopramide, bumetanide as well as an unnamed antibacterial) was given fluconazole (loading dose of 200 mg, followed by 100 mg daily). After concurrent use for 13 days her trough serum nortriptyline levels had risen by 70% (from 149 nanograms/mL to 252 nanograms/mL).[5]

Mechanism

Not understood, but it has been suggested that the fluconazole inhibits the cytochrome P450 isoenzymes CYP2C9, CYP2C19, CYP3A4 and possibly CYP2D6, some of which are concerned with the metabolism of these tricyclics.[1,3] Concurrent use therefore decreases the metabolism of the tricyclic and its level rises. However, note that fluconazole does not inhibit CYP2D6 to a clinically relevant extent, and only tends to inhibit CYP3A4 in doses of 200 mg daily or more. Therefore other conditions must be necessary for an interaction to occur.

Importance and management

Information about an interaction between the tricyclics and fluconazole seems to be limited to these case reports, which, bearing in mind the widespread use of these drugs, would suggest that clinically relevant interactions are uncommon. The evidence suggests that other factors (such as renal impairment and other potentially interacting medications) may be necessary before this interaction occurs. Bear this possible interaction in mind if tricyclic adverse effects become troublesome.

1. Newberry DL, Bass SN, Mbanefo CO. A fluconazole/amitriptyline drug interaction in three male adults. *Clin Infect Dis* (1997) 24, 270–1.
2. Duggal HS. Delirium associated with amitriptyline/fluconazole drug. *Gen Hosp Psychiatry* (2003) 25, 297–8.
3. Robinson RF, Nahata MC, Olshefski RS. Syncope associated with concurrent amitriptyline and fluconazole therapy. *Ann Pharmacother* (2000) 34, 1406–9.
4. Dorsey ST, Biblo LA. Prolonged QT interval and torsades de pointes caused by the combination of fluconazole and amitriptyline. *Am J Emerg Med* (2000) 18, 227–9.
5. Gannon RH, Anderson ML. Fluconazole-nortriptyline drug interaction. *Ann Pharmacother* (1992) 26, 1456–7.

Tricyclic antidepressants + Azoles; Ketoconazole

Ketoconazole does not affect the pharmacokinetics of desipramine, and has only modest effects on the pharmacokinetics of amitriptyline and imipramine.

Clinical evidence, mechanism, importance and management

A placebo-controlled study in 8 healthy subjects found that ketoconazole 200 mg every 12 hours for 3 doses decreased the mean apparent oral clearance of **amitriptyline** 50 mg by 26% and increased its AUC by about 24%.[1] Similarly, two groups of 6 healthy subjects were given a single 100-mg dose of either **imipramine** or **desipramine** alone, and then again on day 10 of a 14-day course of ketoconazole 200 mg daily. It was found that ketoconazole caused the oral clearance of **imipramine** to fall by 17%, its half-life to rise by 15% and the AUC of the desipramine metabolite to fall by 9%. No significant changes in the pharmacokinetics of **desipramine** were seen.[2]

Ketoconazole inhibits the metabolism of the cytochrome P450 isoenzyme CYP3A4, which has only a minor role in the metabolism of amitriptyline and imipramine, and hence the changes seen are small. Desipramine is not metabolised by CYP3A4 and is therefore unaffected by ketoconazole.

These modest changes would not be expected to be clinically significant and therefore no dose adjustments would appear necessary if ketoconazole is used with these drugs. Information about other tricyclics seems to be lacking, but as they share similar metabolic routes to the tricyclics studied, no clinically relevant interaction would be expected.

1. Venkatakrishnan K, Schmider J, Harmatz JS, Ehrenberg BL, von Moltke LL, Graf JA, Mertzanis P, Corbett KE, Rodriguez MC, Shader RI, Greenblatt DJ. Relative contribution of CYP3A to amitriptyline clearance in humans: in vitro and in vivo studies. *J Clin Pharmacol* (2001) 41, 1043–54.
2. Spina E, Avenoso A, Campo GM, Scordo MG, Caputi AP, Perucca E. Effect of ketoconazole on the pharmacokinetics of imipramine and desipramine in healthy subjects. *Br J Clin Pharmacol* (1997) 43, 315–8.

Tricyclic antidepressants + Baclofen

An isolated report describes a patient with multiple sclerosis taking baclofen, who was unable to stand within a few days of starting to take nortriptyline, and later imipramine.

Clinical evidence, mechanism, importance and management

A man with multiple sclerosis, who was taking baclofen 10 mg four times a day to relieve spasticity, complained of leg weakness and was unable to stand within 6 days of starting to take **nortriptyline** 50 mg at bedtime. His muscle tone returned 48 hours after stopping the **nortriptyline**. Two weeks later he was given **imipramine** 75 mg daily and once again his muscle tone was lost.[1]

The reason for this reaction is not understood, although it has been suggested that effects on GABA-receptors may be involved.[2]

The UK manufacturer of baclofen warns that the effect of baclofen might be potentiated by tricyclic antidepressants, resulting in pronounced muscular hypotonia.[2] However, this case report appears to be the only documentation to suggest that a clinically relevant interaction occurs.

Both the tricyclics and baclofen have antimuscarinic effects, which might be additive on concurrent use (see 'Antimuscarinics + Antimuscarinics', p.754).

1. Silverglat MJ. Baclofen and tricyclic antidepressants: possible interaction. *JAMA* (1981) 246, 1659.
2. Lioresal Tablets (Baclofen). Novartis Pharmaceuticals UK Ltd. UK Summary of product characteristics, February 2013.

Tricyclic and related antidepressants + Barbiturates or Phenytoin

The plasma levels of amitriptyline, imipramine, nortriptyline and mianserin can be reduced by the barbiturates. A reduced therapeutic response would be expected. The tricyclics also lower the convulsive threshold and may be inappropriate for patients with convulsive disorders.

Clinical evidence

A comparative study in 5 pairs of twins given **nortriptyline** found that the twins also taking unnamed barbiturates had considerably lower steady-state plasma **nortriptyline** levels.[1]

Similar observations have been made in patients and healthy subjects taking **nortriptyline** with **amobarbital**[2,3] or **pentobarbital**,[4] and **protriptyline** with **amobarbital sodium**.[5] Another patient had a reduction in blood **imipramine** levels of about 50% (and loss of antidepressant control) within 2 weeks of starting to take about 400 mg of **butalbital** daily.[6]

A comparative study in 6 epileptics and 6 healthy subjects found that **phenytoin** with either **phenobarbital** or carbamazepine markedly reduced the AUC of a single 30-mg dose of **mianserin**.[7,8]

Mechanism

The barbiturates are potent liver enzyme inducers and may therefore increase the metabolism and clearance of the tricyclic antidepressants and mianserin from the body.

Importance and management

The interaction between tricyclic antidepressants or mianserin and barbiturates is established. By no means has every drug pair been studied but as the barbiturates as a whole are potent liver enzyme inducers one should be alert for this interaction with any of them. Some reduction in the effects of the antidepressant would be expected, but the general clinical importance is uncertain. Note that the tricyclics and mianserin lower the convulsive threshold and may therefore be inappropriate for patients with epilepsy.

Tricyclic antidepressants may increase the duration of barbiturate anaesthesia, see 'Anaesthetics, general and/or Neuromuscular blockers + Tricyclic and related antidepressants', p.112.

1. Alexanderson B, Price Evans DA, Sjöqvist F. Steady-state plasma levels of nortriptyline in twins: influence of genetic factors and drug therapy. *BMJ* (1969) 4, 764–8.
2. Burrows GD, Davies B. Antidepressants and barbiturates. *BMJ* (1971) 4, 113.
3. Silverman G, Braithwaite R. Interaction of benzodiazepines with tricyclic antidepressants. *BMJ* (1972) 4, 111.
4. Steiner E, Koike Y, Lind M, von Bahr C. Increased nortriptyline metabolism after treatment with pentobarbital in man. *Acta Pharmacol Toxicol (Copenh)* (1986) 59 (Suppl 4), 91.
5. Moody JP, Whyte SF, MacDonald AJ, Naylor GJ. Pharmacokinetic aspects of protriptyline plasma levels. *Eur J Clin Pharmacol* (1977) 11, 51–6.
6. Garey KW, Amsden GW, Johns CA. Possible interaction between imipramine and butalbital. *Pharmacotherapy* (1997) 17, 1041–2.
7. Nawishy S, Hathway N, Turner P. Interactions of anticonvulsant drugs with mianserin and nomifensine. *Lancet* (1981) ii, 871–2.
8. Richens A, Nawishy S, Trimble M. Antidepressant drugs, convulsions and epilepsy. *Br J Clin Pharmacol* (1983) 15, 295S–298S.

Tricyclic antidepressants + Benzodiazepines and related drugs

The concurrent use of tricyclic antidepressants and benzodiazepines is not uncommon and normally appears to be uneventful. However, concurrent use has led to adverse effects (e.g. drowsiness, incoordination). One study found that diazepam may increase the risks of carrying out complex tasks (e.g. driving) if added to amitriptyline, and this seems possible with any benzodiazepine and tricyclic.

Clinical evidence

(a) Amitriptyline

1. Chlordiazepoxide. Clinical studies in large numbers of patients have found that the incidence of adverse reactions while taking amitriptyline and chlordiazepoxide was no greater than might have been expected with either of the drugs used alone,[1-3] but a few adverse reports have been documented. A depressed patient taking amitriptyline 150 mg and chlordiazepoxide 40 mg daily became confused, forgetful and uncoordinated. He acted as though he was drunk.[4] Two other patients taking amitriptyline and chlordiazepoxide experienced drowsiness, memory impairment, slurring of the speech and an inability to concentrate. Both were unable to work and one described himself as feeling drunk.[5] Four patients taking *Limbitrol* (a combination preparation containing chlordiazepoxide and amitriptyline) are reported to have experienced some manifestations of toxicity (delusions, confusion, agitation, disorientation, dry mouth, blurred vision).[6] Some of these effects seem to arise from increased CNS depression (possibly additive) and/or an increase in the antimuscarinic adverse effects of the tricyclic.

2. Diazepam. A study found an increase in amitriptyline levels when diazepam was given.[7] In contrast, two studies suggested that diazepam did not affect amitriptyline levels.[3,8] However, other studies found that the addition of diazepam to amitriptyline 50 to 75 mg further reduced attention and the performance of a number of psychomotor tests.[9,10]

3. Nitrazepam or Oxazepam. A study of the effects of nitrazepam and oxazepam on the steady-state plasma levels of amitriptyline did not find any interactions.[3]

(b) Clomipramine

One study suggested that **alprazolam** does not affect clomipramine levels.[11]

(c) Desipramine

1. Clonazepam. An isolated report describes a patient taking desipramine 300 mg daily whose serum desipramine levels were halved when he was given clonazepam 3 mg daily and rose again when the clonazepam was withdrawn.[12]

2. Zolpidem. Visual hallucinations have been seen in one patient given zolpidem and desipramine.[13]

(d) Imipramine

1. Alprazolam. Population pharmacokinetic data suggests that alprazolam raises imipramine levels by about 20 to 30%.[14]

2. Zaleplon. A single 75-mg dose of imipramine had no effect on the pharmacokinetics of zaleplon 20 mg, and psychomotor tests showed only short term additive effects lasting 1 to 2 hours.[15]

3. Zolpidem. A single-dose study using zolpidem 20 mg and imipramine 75 mg found no effect on the pharmacokinetics of either drug. However, imipramine increased the sedative effects of zolpidem, and anterograde amnesia was seen.[16]

(e) Nortriptyline

Studies on the effects of **alprazolam**, **chlordiazepoxide**, **diazepam**, **nitrazepam** and **oxazepam** on the steady-state plasma levels of nortriptyline have found no interactions.[3,17,18]

(f) Trimipramine

In a study, when 10 healthy subjects were given **zopiclone** and trimipramine for a week there was no statistically significant change in the bioavailability of either drug.[19]

Mechanism

Uncertain. Additive CNS depression and increased antimuscarinic effects are a possibility with some combinations.

Importance and management

There seems to be no reason for avoiding the concurrent use of benzodiazepines and tricyclics although the advantages and disadvantages of such use remain the subject of debate. Other combinations of tricyclic antidepressants and benzodiazepines would be expected to behave in the same way as those described here. Some patients will possibly experience increased drowsiness and inattention, particularly with the more sedative antidepressants such as amitriptyline, especially during the first few days, and this may be exaggerated by benzodiazepines. Driving risks may therefore be increased: patients should be warned.

1. Haider I. A comparative trial of Ro 4–6270 and amitriptyline in depressive illness. *Br J Psychiatry* (1967) 113, 993–8.
2. General Practitioner Clinical Trials. Chlordiazepoxide with amitriptyline in neurotic depression. *Practitioner* (1969) 202, 437–40.
3. Silverman G, Braithwaite RA. Benzodiazepines and tricyclic antidepressant plasma levels. *BMJ* (1973) 3, 18–20.
4. Kane FJ, Taylor TW. A toxic reaction to combined Elavil-Librium therapy. *Am J Psychiatry* (1963) 119, 1179–80.
5. Abdou FA. Elavil-Librium combination. *Am J Psychiatry* (1964) 120, 1204.
6. Beresford TP, Feinsilver DL, Hall RCW. Adverse reactions to a benzodiazepine-tricyclic antidepressant compound. *J Clin Psychopharmacol* (1981) 1, 392–4.
7. Dugal R, Caille G, Albert J-M, Cooper SF. Apparent pharmacokinetic interaction of diazepam and amitriptyline in psychiatric patients: a pilot study. *Curr Ther Res* (1975) 18, 679–87.
8. Otani K, Nordin C, Bertilsson L. No interaction of diazepam on amitriptyline disposition in depressed patients. *Ther Drug Monit* (1987) 9, 120–2.
9. Patat A, Klein MJ, Hucher M, Granier J. Acute effects of amitriptyline on human performance and interactions with diazepam. *Eur J Clin Pharmacol* (1988) 35, 585–92.
10. Moskowitz H, Burns M. The effects on performance of two antidepressants, alone and in combination with diazepam. *Prog Neuropsychopharmacol Biol Psychiatry* (1988) 12, 783–92.
11. Carson SW, Wright CE, Millikin SP, Lyon J, Chambers JH. Pharmacokinetic evaluation of the combined administration of alprazolam and clomipramine. *Clin Pharmacol Ther* (1992) 51, 154.
12. Deicken RF. Clonazepam-induced reduction in serum desipramine concentration. *J Clin Psychopharmacol* (1988) 8, 71–3.
13. Elko CJ, Burgess JL, Robertson WO. Zolpidem-associated hallucinations and serotonin reuptake inhibition: a possible interaction. *J Toxicol Clin Toxicol* (1998) 36, 195–203.
14. Grasela TH, Antal EJ, Ereshefsky L, Wells BG, Evans RL, Smith RB. An evaluation of population pharmacokinetics in therapeutic trials. Part II. Detection of a drug-drug interaction. *Clin Pharmacol Ther* (1987) 42, 433–41.
15. Darwish M. Overview of drug interaction studies with zaleplon. Poster presented at 13th Annual Meeting of Associated Professional Sleep Studies (APSS), Orlando, Florida, June 23rd, 1999.
16. Sauvanet JP, Langer SZ, Morselli PL, eds. Imidazopyridines in Sleep Disorders. New York: Raven Press; 1988 p. 165–73.
17. Bertilsson L, Åberg-Wistedt A, Lidén A, Otani K, Spina E. Alprazolam does not inhibit the metabolism of nortriptyline in depressed patients or inhibit the metabolism of desipramine in human liver microsomes. *Ther Drug Monit* (1988) 10, 231–3.
18. Gram LF, Overø KF, Kirk L. Influence of neuroleptics and benzodiazepines on metabolism of tricyclic antidepressants in man. *Am J Psychiatry* (1974) 131, 863.
19. Caille G, Du Souich P, Spenard J, Lacasse Y, Vezina M. Pharmacokinetic and clinical parameters of zopiclone and trimipramine when administered simultaneously to volunteers. *Biopharm Drug Dispos* (1984) 5, 117–25.

Tricyclic and related antidepressants + Beta blockers

Propranolol increased imipramine levels in two children and maprotiline levels in isolated cases. Labetalol has been found to increase imipramine levels in adults. Amitriptyline does not appear to affect the pharmacokinetics of atenolol or metoprolol.

Clinical evidence

(a) Amitriptyline

A placebo-controlled study in 6 healthy subjects found that amitriptyline 75 mg daily did not affect the pharmacokinetics of **atenolol** 100 mg daily or **metoprolol** 100 mg twice daily, given for 2 weeks.[1]

(b) Imipramine

1. Labetalol. In a study in 13 healthy subjects, labetalol 200 mg every 12 hours for 4 days, increased the AUC of a single 100-mg dose of imipramine by 53%, when compared with a placebo. The maximum plasma level of imipramine increased by 28%.[2]

2. Propranolol. A 9-year-old boy was given propranolol for the control of anger and aggression, and imipramine for stress and depression. When his imipramine dose was raised from 60 to 80 mg daily and his propranolol dose was also raised, from 360 to 400 mg daily, his levels of imipramine plus its metabolite, desipramine rose sharply, from a total of 139 nanograms/mL to 469 nanograms/mL. Reducing the imipramine dose to 60 mg and raising the propranolol dose to 440 mg daily only reduced the total imipramine/desipramine levels to 426 nanograms/mL. Another imipramine dose reduction, to 40 mg, and an increase in the propranolol dose to 480 mg daily resulted in a final total imipramine/desipramine level of 207 nanograms/mL. No significant adverse effects or heart block occurred.[3]

A 9-year-old girl taking imipramine 75 mg daily with a total imipramine/desipramine level of 260 nanograms/mL, had a marked rise to 408 nanograms/mL within 3 days of starting to take propranolol 10 mg three times daily. Two days after stopping the imipramine, her desipramine level (imipramine not measured) had fallen from 382 nanograms/mL to 222 nanograms/mL.[3]

(c) Maprotiline

A patient experienced maprotiline toxicity (dizziness, hypotension, dry mouth, blurred vision, etc.) after taking **propranolol** 120 mg daily for 2 weeks. His trough maprotiline levels had risen by 40%. The levels fell and the adverse effects disappeared when the **propranolol** was withdrawn.[4] Another patient taking **propranolol** 120 mg daily began to experience visual hallucinations and psychomotor agitation within a few days of starting to take maprotiline 200 mg daily.[5] A further patient taking haloperidol, benzatropine, triamterene, hydrochlorothiazide and **propranolol** became disorientated, agitated and uncooperative, with visual hallucinations and incoherent speech, within a week of starting to take maprotiline 150 mg daily. These symptoms disappeared when all the drugs were withdrawn. Reintroduction of the antihypertensive drugs with haloperidol and desipramine proved effective and uneventful.[6]

Mechanism

Uncertain. The suggestion is that the affected drugs compete for metabolism (hydroxylation) by the same cytochrome P450 isoenzymes (particularly CYP2D6) in the liver.[2,3] Atenolol is mainly renally excreted and would therefore not be affected in this way. It has also been suggested that propranolol (and therefore possibly other beta blockers) reduces the blood flow to the liver so that the metabolism of maprotiline is reduced, leading to its accumulation in the body.

Importance and management

Information about an interaction between the beta blockers and tricyclic antidepressants or maprotiline seems to be limited to these studies and case reports. The authors of one of the reports[5] say that simultaneous use is inadvisable, but on the basis of these few cases, and with no further information, this seems over-cautious. In general it would seem that any interaction does not lead to adverse effects in most patients (the studies suggest the increase in tricyclic levels is modest). However, if adverse effects (e.g. dry mouth, blurred vision and urinary retention) occur it would seem prudent to consider an interaction as a possible cause, decreasing the antidepressant dose as appropriate.

1. Kirch W, Spahn H, Kitteringham NR, Hutt HJ, Mutschler E, Ohnhaus EE. Interaction between the β-adrenoceptor blockers metoprolol and atenolol with amitriptyline and their effects on oxidative liver metabolism. *Br J Clin Pharmacol* (1984) 17, 65S–68S.
2. Hermann DJ, Krol TF, Dukes GE, Hussey EK, Danis M, Han Y-H, Powell JR, Hak LJ. Comparison of verapamil, diltiazem, and labetalol on the bioavailability and metabolism of imipramine. *J Clin Pharmacol* (1992) 32, 176–83.
3. Gillette DW, Tannery LP. Beta blocker inhibits tricyclic metabolism. *J Am Acad Child Adolesc Psychiatry* (1994) 33, 223–4.
4. Tollefson G, Lesar T. Effect of propranolol on maprotiline clearance. *Am J Psychiatry* (1984) 141, 148–9.
5. Saiz-Ruiz J, Moral L. Delirium induced by association of propranolol and maprotiline. *J Clin Psychopharmacol* (1988) 8, 77–8.
6. Malek-Ahmadi P, Tran T. Propranolol and maprotiline toxic interaction. *Neurobehav Toxicol Teratol* (1985) 7, 203.

Tricyclic antidepressants + Bupropion

Bupropion may increase the levels of the tricyclic antidepressants, including desipramine, imipramine, and nortriptyline. Adverse effects including confusion, lethargy and unsteadiness have been reported with nortriptyline and bupropion. Seizures occurred in two patients given clomipramine or trimipramine and bupropion.

Clinical evidence

A pharmacokinetic study in healthy subjects found that bupropion doubled the maximum plasma levels of **desipramine** and increased its AUC fivefold. The effect was present for at least 7 days after the last dose of bupropion.[1,2] Another study in a 64-year-old woman taking **imipramine** 150 to 200 mg daily found that when bupropion 225 mg daily was added, there was a fourfold rise in the plasma levels of imipramine and its metabolite desipramine, but no problems were reported. A comparison of the estimated clearances of imipramine and its main metabolite desipramine were: **imipramine** 1.7 mL/minute and desipramine 1.7 mL/minute without bupropion; and imipramine 0.73 mL/minute and desipramine 0.31 mL/minute with bupropion.[3]

An 83-year-old woman taking **nortriptyline** 75 mg at night had a plasma **nortriptyline** level of 96 nanograms/mL, but when sustained-release bupropion 150 mg twice daily was added she became unsteady, confused and lethargic and her plasma nortriptyline level increased by about 200% (to 274 nanograms/mL). The increased plasma **nortriptyline** level and toxicity occurred again when she was rechallenged with bupropion.[4]

A report describes a seizure when **trimipramine** 100 mg daily was taken with bupropion 150 mg twice daily. The addition of bupropion resulted in a substantial increase in the plasma levels of **trimipramine** into the 'toxic' range. The patient was later successfully treated with lower doses of both drugs (**trimipramine** 50 mg at night and bupropion 150 mg daily).[5] Another case report describes prolonged seizure activity after the concurrent use of bupropion 300 mg daily and **clomipramine** 25 mg daily, which persisted even after discontinuation of both drugs.[6]

Mechanism

In vitro studies[1,2] have shown that both bupropion and its active metabolite, hydroxybupropion, are inhibitors of CYP2D6, the isoenzyme involved in the metabolism of these tricyclics. Therefore concurrent use decreases the metabolism of the tricyclics and their levels rise.

Importance and management

Although clinical evidence for an interaction between the tricyclics and bupropion is limited, the rise in tricyclic levels is in line with the way both drugs are known to interact, and therefore an interaction would seem to be established. It would be prudent to be alert for increased tricyclic adverse effects if bupropion is also given, reducing the tricyclic dose as necessary.

Note that bupropion is predicted to increase the risk of seizures with tricyclics, and this effect is dose-related. See 'Bupropion + Miscellaneous', p.1470.

1. Zyban (Bupropion hydrochloride). GlaxoSmithKline UK. UK Summary of product characteristics, November 2013.
2. Zyban (Bupropion hydrochloride). GlaxoSmithKline. US Prescribing information, March 2014.
3. Shad MU, Preskorn SH. A possible bupropion and imipramine interaction. *J Clin Psychopharmacol* (1997) 17, 118–19.
4. Weintraub D. Nortriptyline toxicity secondary to interaction with bupropion sustained-release. *Depress Anxiety* (2001) 13, 50–2.
5. Enns MW. Seizure during combination of trimipramine and bupropion. *J Clin Psychiatry* (2001) 62, 476–7.
6. Shin Y-W, Erm TM, Choi EJ, Kim SY. A case of prolonged seizure activity after combined use of bupropion and clomipramine. *Clin Neuropharmacol* (2004) 27, 192–4.

Tricyclic antidepressants + Calcium-channel blockers

Diltiazem and verapamil can increase plasma imipramine levels, possibly accompanied by undesirable ECG changes. Two isolated reports describe increased nortriptyline and trimipramine levels in two patients given diltiazem.

Clinical evidence

(a) Imipramine

In a study, 12 healthy subjects were given a 7-day course of **verapamil** 120 mg every 8 hours and 13 healthy subjects were given a 7-day course of **diltiazem** 90 mg every 8 hours. The AUCs of a single 100-mg dose of imipramine given on day 4 were increased by 15% by **verapamil**, and by 30% by **diltiazem**. One hour after taking imipramine (2 hours after taking the calcium-channel blockers), the average PR interval was greater than 200 milliseconds, which represented first-degree heart block. Two subjects developed second-degree heart block after taking imipramine with **verapamil**.[1]

(b) Nortriptyline

A diabetic patient taking **nifedipine**, glipizide and aspirin started taking nortriptyline, and, at the same time, the **nifedipine** was replaced by **diltiazem**, initially 180 mg daily, then raised to 240 mg daily after a week. Several changes in the nortriptyline dosage were made over a 4-week period because its plasma levels became unexpectedly high (the ratio of plasma nortriptyline to its dosage were approximately doubled), which was attributed to the use of **diltiazem**.[2]

(c) Trimipramine

A depressed woman taking trimipramine 125 mg daily developed high plasma trimipramine levels of 546 micrograms/L while taking **diltiazem** 60 mg three times daily. Two weeks later the trimipramine levels reached 708 micrograms/L, despite a reduction in the trimipramine dose to 75 mg daily. She showed no toxicity and her ECG was normal.[3]

Mechanism

It has been suggested that diltiazem and verapamil increase the bioavailability of imipramine by decreasing its clearance. The ECG changes appear to result from the increased imipramine levels and the additive effects of both drugs on the atrioventricular conduction time. Diltiazem may similarly affect nortriptyline and trimipramine.

Importance and management

Information appears to be limited to these reports so that the general clinical importance of each of these interactions is uncertain. However it would seem prudent to be alert for evidence of increases in the adverse effects of the tricyclic antidepressants if diltiazem or verapamil is added. The evidence of heart block with imipramine and verapamil is of particular concern. Note that it has also been suggested that the postural hypotension that may occur in patients taking tricyclics could be exacerbated by the use of antihypertensives. Patients should be warned.

1. Hermann DJ, Krol TF, Dukes GE, Hussey EK, Danis M, Han Y-H, Powell JR, Hak LJ. Comparison of verapamil, diltiazem, and labetalol on the bioavailability and metabolism of imipramine. *J Clin Pharmacol* (1992) 32, 176–83.
2. Krähenbühl S, Smith-Gamble V, Hoppel CL. Pharmacokinetic interaction between diltiazem and nortriptyline. *Eur J Clin Pharmacol* (1996) 49, 417–19.
3. Cotter PA, Raven PW, Hudson M. Asymptomatic tricyclic toxicity associated with diltiazem. *Ir J Psychol Med* (1996) 13, 168–9.

Tricyclic antidepressants + Cannabis

Case reports describe tachycardia when patients taking tricyclic antidepressants smoked cannabis. Hypertension and drowsiness might occur when cannabinoids are used with tricyclics.

Clinical evidence

A 21-year-old woman taking **nortriptyline** 30 mg daily experienced marked tachycardia (an increase from 90 to 160 bpm) after smoking a cannabis cigarette. It was controlled with propranolol.[1] A 26-year-old man complained of restlessness, dizziness, and tachycardia (120 bpm) after smoking cannabis while taking **imipramine** 25 mg twice daily.[2] Four adolescents aged 15 to 18 years, taking tricyclic antidepressants for attention-deficit hyperactivity disorder, experienced transient cognitive changes, delirium, and tachycardia after smoking cannabis.[3]

Mechanism

Increased heart rates are well-documented adverse effects of both the tricyclic antidepressants and cannabis, and what occurred was probably due to the additive beta-adrenergic and antimuscarinic effects of the tricyclics, in combination with the beta-adrenergic effect of the cannabis.

Importance and management

Evidence for an interaction between cannabis and tricyclics appears to be limited. The manufacturer of **dronabinol**, a cannabinoid, notes that hypertension and drowsiness as well as tachycardia have been reported when cannabinoids have been used with tricyclics.[4] It would therefore seem that an interaction is established.

If concurrent use is undertaken, it would be prudent to be alert for these adverse effects, taking particular caution in those with underlying cardiac disease, which might make these effects more problematic.

1. Hillard JR, Vieweg WVR. Marked sinus tachycardia resulting from the synergistic effects of marijuana and nortriptyline. *Am J Psychiatry* (1983) 140, 626–7.
2. Kizer KW. Possible interaction of TCA and marijuana. *Ann Emerg Med* (1980) 9, 444.
3. Wilens TE, Biederman J, Spencer TJ. Case study: adverse effects of smoking marijuana while receiving tricyclic antidepressants. *J Am Acad Child Adolesc Psychiatry* (1997) 36, 45–8.
4. Marinol (Dronabinol). AbbVie Inc. US Prescribing information, February 2013.

Tricyclic and related antidepressants + Carbamazepine

The serum levels of amitriptyline, desipramine, doxepin, imipramine, nortriptyline and mianserin can be reduced (halved or more) by carbamazepine. In contrast, raised clomipramine levels have been seen in patients taking carbamazepine. An isolated report describes carbamazepine toxicity in a patient shortly after she started to take desipramine.

Clinical evidence

(a) Carbamazepine levels increased

A woman receiving long-term treatment with carbamazepine developed toxicity (nausea, vomiting, blurred vision with visual hallucinations, slurred speech, ataxia) within 6 days of starting to take **desipramine** daily (3 days at 150 mg daily). Her carbamazepine levels were found to have doubled from 7.7 micrograms/mL to 15 micrograms/mL.[1]

(b) Tricyclic levels increased

A study confirming the value of carbamazepine and **clomipramine** in the treatment of post-herpetic neuralgia found that carbamazepine appeared to raise both clomipramine plasma levels and those of its major metabolite (desmethylclomipramine).[2]

(c) Tricyclic levels reduced

A study found that carbamazepine reduced the serum levels of **nortriptyline** by 58% and of **amitriptyline** plus its metabolite, nortriptyline, by 60% in 8 psychiatric patients. In 17 other patients carbamazepine reduced serum **doxepin** levels by 54% and reduced the levels of doxepin plus its metabolite, nordoxepin, by 55%.[3] A retrospective study of very large numbers of patients confirmed that carbamazepine approximately halves the serum levels of **amitriptyline** and **nortriptyline**.[4] An elderly woman needed her **nortriptyline** dosage to be increased from 75 to 150 mg daily to achieve effective antidepressant serum levels when carbamazepine 500 to 600 mg daily was added.[5]

A study in 36 children (aged 5 to 16 years) with attention-deficit disorder taking **imipramine**, or **imipramine** and carbamazepine for 1 to 6 months, found that even though the **imipramine** dosage was significantly higher in the combined treatment group, the plasma levels were significantly lower; and the total plasma antidepressant levels were about half of those found in the children not taking carbamazepine.[6] A study[7] in 6 healthy subjects found that carbamazepine 200 mg twice daily for a month increased the apparent oral clearance of a single 100-mg dose of **desipramine** (given on day 24) by 31% and shortened its half-life from 22.1 hours to 17.8 hours. A patient given **desipramine** and carbamazepine is reported to have had exceptionally low serum desipramine levels and cardiac complaints, which may have been due to the presence of increased levels of the hydroxy metabolite of desipramine.[8]

A study in 13 patients with endogenous depression (DSM-III-R) taking **imipramine**, which confirmed that carbamazepine reduced the total serum levels of imipramine and desipramine, found that levels of the pharmacologically active free drugs remained unchanged.[9,10] Moreover 10 of the patients demonstrated a positive therapeutic response (greater than a 50% decrease in the Hamilton Depression Rating Scale) and a reduction in adverse drug reactions.[9]

A comparative study in 6 epileptics and 6 healthy subjects showed that phenytoin with either phenobarbital or carbamazepine markedly reduced the plasma levels of a single dose of **mianserin**.[11,12] The mean half-life of **mianserin** was reduced by 75% (from 16.9 hours to 4.8 hours) and the AUC was reduced by 86%. Another study in 4 patients found that carbamazepine reduced serum **mianserin** levels by 70%.[13] In another study 12 patients taking **mianserin** 60 mg daily were also given carbamazepine 400 mg daily for 4 weeks. Average plasma levels of total *S*-mianserin (the more potent enantiomer) and total *R*-mianserin were reduced by about 45% in the presence of carbamazepine.[14]

Mechanism

It seems likely that the carbamazepine (a recognised enzyme-inducing drug) increases the metabolism and loss of these tricyclics and mianserin from the body, thereby reducing their serum levels. The reason for the increased serum carbamazepine and clomipramine levels is not understood, although it has been suggested that both drugs may compete for hydroxylation by the hepatic microsomal enzyme system.[1,2] In addition, they both share a similar 3-ringed structure, and carbamazepine has been reported to interfere with an assay (serum fluorescence-polarised immunoassay) for tricyclic antidepressants, resulting in false positive results.[15]

Importance and management

The reduction in the serum levels of amitriptyline, desipramine, doxepin, imipramine, nortriptyline and mianserin caused by the interaction with carbamazepine appears to be established but the clinical importance is very much less certain. Evidence from one study,[9] that achieved a beneficial response in patients taking tricyclics and carbamazepine, suggests that it is possibly not necessary to increase the tricyclic dosage to accommodate this interaction. The fact that a retrospective study found that increased imipramine doses were being given to those taking carbamazepine suggests that this interaction will be naturally accounted for. If carbamazepine is added to treatment with any of these tricyclics or mianserin, be aware that the dose of the tricyclic may need to be titrated up to achieve the desired therapeutic response. One study suggests that the dose of mianserin may need to be approximately doubled if carbamazepine 400 mg daily is added.[14]

Remember too that the tricyclics and mianserin can lower the convulsive threshold and should therefore be used with caution in patients with epilepsy.

1. Lesser I. Carbamazepine and desipramine: a toxic reaction. *J Clin Psychiatry* (1984) 45, 360.
2. Gerson GR, Jones RB, Luscombe DK. Studies on the concomitant use of carbamazepine and clomipramine for the relief of post-herpetic neuralgia. *Postgrad Med J* (1977) 53 (Suppl 4), 104–9.
3. Leinonen E, Lillsunde P, Laukkanen V, Ylitalo P. Effects of carbamazepine on serum antidepressant concentrations in psychiatric patients. *J Clin Psychopharmacol* (1991) 11, 313–18.
4. Jerling M, Bertilsson L, Sjöqvist F. The use of therapeutic drug monitoring data to document kinetic drug interactions: an example with amitriptyline and nortriptyline. *Ther Drug Monit* (1994) 16, 1–12.
5. Brøsen K, Kragh-Sørensen P. Concomitant intake of nortriptyline and carbamazepine. *Ther Drug Monit* (1993) 15, 258–60.
6. Brown CS, Wells BG, Cold JA, Froemming JH, Self TH, Jabbour JT. Possible influence of carbamazepine on plasma imipramine concentrations in children with attention deficit hyperactivity disorder. *J Clin Psychopharmacol* (1990) 10, 359–62.
7. Spina E, Avenoso A, Campo GM, Caputi AP, Perucca E. The effect of carbamazepine on the 2-hydroxylation of desipramine. *Psychopharmacology (Berl)* (1995) 117, 413–16.
8. Baldessarini RJ, Teicher MH, Cassidy JW, Stein MH. Anticonvulsant cotreatment may increase toxic metabolites of antidepressants and other psychotropic drugs. *J Clin Psychopharmacol* (1988) 8, 381–2.
9. Szymura-Oleksiak J, Wyska E, Wasieczko A. Effects of carbamazepine coadministration on free and total serum concentrations of imipramine and its metabolites. *Eur J Clin Pharmacol* (1997) 52 (Suppl) A141.
10. Szymura-Oleksiak J, Wyska E, Wasieczko A. Pharmacokinetic interaction between imipramine and carbamazepine in patients with major depression. *Psychopharmacology (Berl)* (2001) 154, 38–42.
11. Nawishy S, Hathway N, Turner P. Interactions of anticonvulsant drugs with mianserin and nomifensine. *Lancet* (1981) ii, 871–2.
12. Richens A, Nawishy S, Trimble M. Antidepressant drugs, convulsions and epilepsy. *Br J Clin Pharmacol* (1983) 15, 295S–298S.
13. Leinonen E, Lillsunde P, Laukkanen V, Ylitalo P. Effects of carbamazepine on serum antidepressant concentrations in psychiatric patients. *J Clin Psychopharmacol* (1991) 11, 313–18.
14. Eap CB, Yasui N, Kaneko S, Baumann P, Powell K, Otani K. Effects of carbamazepine coadministration on plasma concentrations of the enantiomers of mianserin and of its metabolites. *Ther Drug Monit* (1999) 21, 166–70.
15. Saidinejad M, Law T, Ewald MB. Interference by carbamazepine and oxcarbazepine with serum- and urine-screening assays for tricyclic antidepressants. *Pediatrics* (2007) 120, e504–e509.

Tricyclic antidepressants + Cinacalcet

Cinacalcet causes a large increase in the levels of the tricyclic antidepressants.

Clinical evidence

A study in 14 healthy subjects found that cinacalcet 90 mg daily significantly increased the AUC and maximum plasma concentration of a single 50-mg dose of **desipramine** 3.6-fold and 1.8-fold, respectively, and the half-life of **desipramine** was approximately doubled.[1]

Mechanism

Cinacalcet is a potent inhibitor of the cytochrome P450 isoenzyme CYP2D6, by which desipramine is predominantly metabolised. Concurrent use therefore decreases desipramine metabolism, resulting in the raised levels seen.

Importance and management

An interaction between cinacalcet and desipramine is established, and would be expected to be clinically significant. Dose reductions of desipramine are likely to be needed if cinacalcet is also given. If starting desipramine in a patient taking cinacalcet it would seem prudent to start at the lowest dose and titrate upwards carefully. If both drugs are given, monitor closely for adverse effects such as dry mouth, urinary retention and constipation.

There seems to be no evidence regarding other tricyclics, but as they are, in general, predominantly metabolised by CYP2D6, they would be expected to interact similarly. Therefore the same precautions suggested for desipramine would be advisable.

Note that, the tricyclics have been associated with QT prolongation, most usually when their levels are high, and this interaction may therefore increase the risk of this effect. See 'Drugs that prolong the QT interval + Other drugs that prolong the QT interval', p.272, for further discussion on QT prolongation.

1. Harris RZ, Salfi M, Posvar E, Hoelscher D, Padhi D. Pharmacokinetics of desipramine HCl when administered with cinacalcet HCl. *Eur J Clin Pharmacol* (2007) 63, 159–63.

Tricyclic antidepressants + Cobicistat

Cobicistat slightly increases the exposure to single-dose desipramine. Other tricyclics are expected to interact similarly.

Clinical evidence

In a pharmacokinetic study in 8 healthy subjects, cobicistat 150 mg daily slightly increased the AUC and maximum plasma concentration of a single 50-mg dose of desipramine by 65% and 24%, respectively.[1]

Mechanism

Desipramine is a probe substrate of CYP2D6, and this shows that cobicistat is a weak inhibitor of CYP2D6.

Importance and management

The evidence for an interaction between cobicistat (usually given with elvitegravir as a pharmacokinetic booster) and tricyclic antidepressants is limited to the study with desipramine above. The US manufacturer of elvitegravir boosted with cobicistat (in a fixed-dose combination also including emtricitabine and tenofovir disoproxil fumarate) states that the plasma concentrations of the tricyclic antidepressants (they name **amitriptyline**, desipramine, **imipramine**, and **nortriptyline**) might be increased on concurrent use. They recommend careful dose titration of the tricyclic antidepressants with monitoring for antidepressant response.[1] However, the slight increase seen in desipramine exposure is probably not generally clinically relevant. Until more is known, some caution might be appropriate on concurrent use.

1. Stribild (Elvitegravir, cobicistat, emtricitabine, tenofovir disoproxil fumarate). Gilead Sciences, Inc. US Prescribing information, August 2012.

Tricyclic antidepressants + Colestyramine

Colestyramine causes a modest decrease in the plasma concentration of imipramine. A case report suggests that the plasma concentration of doxepin might be decreased by colestyramine, and *in vitro* evidence suggests that amitriptyline, desipramine, and nortriptyline are also likely to be similarly affected.

Clinical evidence

Six patients with depression taking **imipramine** 75 to 150 mg, usually twice daily, were given colestyramine 4 g three times daily for 5 days. The plasma concentration of **imipramine** decreased by an average of 23% (range 11 to 30%) and the plasma concentration of desipramine (the major metabolite) was also decreased, although this was less consistent and said not to be statistically significant. The effect of these decreased plasma concentrations on the control of the depression was not assessed.[1]

A man whose depression was controlled with **doxepin** relapsed within a week of starting to take colestyramine 6 g twice daily. Within 3 weeks of increasing the dosage separation of the two drugs from 4 to 6 hours, his combined serum concentration of antidepressant (i.e. **doxepin** plus the metabolite *n*-desmethyldoxepin) had increased from 39 to 81 nanograms/mL and his depression had improved. Decreasing the colestyramine to a single 6-g dose daily, separated from the **doxepin** by 15 hours, resulted in a further increase in his serum of antidepressant concentration, to 117 nanograms/mL, which was accompanied by relief of his depression.[2]

Mechanism

It seems almost certain that these tricyclics become bound to the colestyramine (an anion-exchange resin) within the gut, thereby decreasing their absorption. An *in vitro* study[3] with simulated gastric fluid found that, at pH 1, **amitriptyline**, **desipramine**, doxepin, imipramine, and **nortriptyline** were approximately 79 to 90% bound by colestyramine: at pH 4 they were 36 to 48% bound and at pH 6.5 they were 62 to 76% bound. In an earlier study,[4] binding of these tricyclics at pH 1 had ranged from 76 to 100%.

Importance and management

The interaction between imipramine and colestyramine is established, but of uncertain clinical importance because the decrease in the plasma concentration of imipramine seen in the study was only modest (23%) and the effects were not measured. The single case involving doxepin[2] was unusual because the patient had an abnormal gastrointestinal tract (hemigastrectomy with pyloroplasty and chronic diarrhoea). Nevertheless, given the way colestyramine is generally known to interact, it would seem prudent to be alert for any evidence of a decreased antidepressant response if colestyramine is given with any tricyclic. A simple way of minimising any interaction is to separate administration, and it is usually suggested that other drugs should be given one hour before or 4 to 6 hours after colestyramine.

1. Spina E, Avenoso A, Campo GM, Caputi AP, Perucca E. Decreased plasma concentrations of imipramine and desipramine following cholestyramine intake in depressed patients. *Ther Drug Monit* (1994) 16, 432–4.

2. Geeze DS, Wise MG, Stigelman WH. Doxepin-cholestyramine interaction. *Psychosomatics* (1988) 29, 233–6.
3. Bailey DN. Effect of pH changes and ethanol on the binding of tricyclic antidepressants to cholestyramine in simulated gastric fluid. *Ther Drug Monit* (1992) 14, 343–6.
4. Bailey DN, Coffee JJ, Anderson B, Manoguerra AS. Interactions of tricyclic antidepressants with cholestyramine in vitro. *Ther Drug Monit* (1992) 14, 339–42.

Tricyclic and related antidepressants + Co-trimoxazole

In isolated cases the efficacy of tricyclic antidepressants and viloxazine appears to have been reduced by co-trimoxazole.

Clinical evidence, mechanism, importance and management

Four patients taking tricyclic antidepressants (**imipramine**, **clomipramine**, **dibenzepin**) and one taking **viloxazine** relapsed into depression when they took co-trimoxazole (trimethoprim with sulfamethoxazole) for 2 to 9 days.[1] Another patient taking alprazolam and **imipramine** for 5 years for panic disorder, and who had not had panic attacks for several months, developed insomnia, anxiety, and panic attacks within 6 days of starting to take co-trimoxazole. The panic attacks stopped when she stopped taking co-trimoxazole.[2]

The reason for the reduction in the efficacy of treatment is not known. In the second case, one possibility was that co-trimoxazole, which might cause nervousness, had exacerbated the panic disorder.[2] These seem to be the only reports of a possible interaction between these drugs so that the general importance is uncertain. It seems likely to be small.

1. Brion S, Orssaud E, Chevalier JF, Plas J, Waroquaux O. Interaction entre le cotrimoxazole et les antidépresseurs. *Encephale* (1987) 13, 123–6.
2. Zealberg JJ, Lydiard RB, Christie S. Exacerbation of panic disorder in a woman treated with trimethoprim-sulfamethoxazole. *J Clin Psychopharmacol* (1991) 11, 144–5.

Tricyclic antidepressants + Cyclobenzaprine

Episodes of fainting in a patient might have been due to increased concentrations of nortriptyline, which were thought to have been caused by cyclobenzaprine.

Clinical evidence, mechanism, importance and management

A patient taking multiple medications, including citalopram, **nortriptyline** 100 mg at bedtime for pain and insomnia, and cyclobenzaprine 60 to 80 mg daily for pain, reported light-headedness and fainting episodes. Toxicology screens also found he had taken cocaine. Serum concentrations of **nortriptyline** of 406 nanograms/mL (therapeutic range 50 to 150 nanograms/mL) were found. The **nortriptyline** dose was halved to 50 mg daily and then discontinued; serum concentrations of 631 nanograms/mL and 400 nanograms/mL were found after 3 and 4 weeks, respectively. The episodes of syncope/presyncope only stopped when cyclobenzaprine was also discontinued.

Due to the complexities of the case, various causes including arrhythmias, cardiac ischaemia, seizures, orthostasis and anxiety were considered. The patient had previously experienced syncopal episodes attributed to misuse of prescription drugs, apparently including **nortriptyline**. It was considered that the symptoms could have been due to increased serum concentrations of **nortriptyline** in the presence of cyclobenzaprine, as well as to effects of cyclobenzaprine.[1]

While taking both drugs the patient experienced considerable fluctuations in his serum concentrations of **nortriptyline**, which might have been due to an interaction with cyclobenzaprine. However, cyclobenzaprine is structurally related to the tricyclic antidepressants and is known to interfere with certain assays for tricyclics; indeed, as a serum concentration of **nortriptyline** was reported as 378 nanograms/mL, several months after nortriptyline had been discontinued, and a re-evaluation using a high-performance liquid chromatographic (HPLC) assay revealed the patient's nortriptyline concentration to be 0, an interference of cyclobenzaprine with the assay method is possible in this case.[1]

This is an isolated case, with many complicating factors, so an interaction is by no means established.

Both the tricyclics and cyclobenzaprine have antimuscarinic effects, which might be additive on concurrent use (see 'Antimuscarinics + Antimuscarinics', p.754).

1. Rosenlicht NZ, Riley-Lazo KP. Interactions of cyclobenzaprine and tricyclic antidepressants. *J Clin Psychiatry* (2005) 66, 134–5.

Tricyclic antidepressants + Disulfiram

Disulfiram modestly increases the exposure to imipramine and desipramine. The concurrent use of amitriptyline and disulfiram has been reported to cause a therapeutically useful increase in the effects of disulfiram, but 'organic brain syndrome' has been seen in two patients.

Clinical evidence, mechanism, importance and management

It has been noted that **amitriptyline** increases the effects of both disulfiram and citrated **calcium carbimide** without any increase in adverse effects.[1] A study in two men found that disulfiram 500 mg daily increased the AUC of **imipramine** (12.5 mg given intravenously after an overnight fast) by about 30%, and of **desipramine** 12.5 mg given intravenously in one subject by a similar amount.[2] Maximum plasma concentrations were also increased.

The suggested reason for this increase in tricyclic exposure is that disulfiram inhibits the metabolism of the antidepressants by the liver. The increase in tricyclic exposure is modest and would not normally be expected to lead to an increase in adverse effects. However, a case report describes a man taking disulfiram who, when given **amitriptyline**, complained of dizziness, visual and auditory hallucinations, and who became disorientated to person, place, and time. A similar reaction was seen in another patient.[3]

It seems unlikely that most patients will experience a clinically relevant interaction. Nevertheless, the case reports introduce a note of caution. If tricyclic adverse effects (e.g. dry mouth, urinary retention, constipation) become troublesome, it would seem worth considering this interaction as a possible cause.

1. MacCallum WAG. Drug interactions in alcoholism treatment. *Lancet* (1969) i, 313.
2. Ciraulo DA, Barnhill J, Boxenbaum H. Pharmacokinetic interaction of disulfiram and antidepressants. *Am J Psychiatry* (1985) 142, 1373–4.
3. Maany I, Hayashida M, Pfeffer SL, Kron RE. Possible toxic interaction between disulfiram and amitriptyline. *Arch Gen Psychiatry* (1982) 39, 743–4.

Tricyclic antidepressants + Fenfluramine

It has been said that the concurrent use of tricyclics and fenfluramine is safe and effective; however, others have suggested that, as fenfluramine can cause depression, it should be avoided in patients with a history of depression.

Clinical evidence, mechanism, importance and management

Exacerbation of depression has been seen in some patients given fenfluramine,[1] and several cases of withdrawal depression have been seen in patients taking amitriptyline and fenfluramine following episodes of severe depression.[2] The UK manufacturers did advise that fenfluramine should not be used in patients with a history of depression or in those being treated with antidepressants.[3] On the other hand, it has been also claimed that fenfluramine could be used safely and effectively with tricyclic antidepressants.[4,5] One report described an increase in the plasma concentration of amitriptyline when fenfluramine 60 mg daily was given to patients taking amitriptyline 150 mg daily.[6]

Some tricyclics (see 'Table 35.3', p.1472) and fenfluramine have serotonergic effects, and concurrent use might lead to the serotonin syndrome. Serotonin syndrome is a rare adverse effect, but because of its severity, some caution is warranted if both drugs are given. For more information on serotonin syndrome and its management, see 'Drugs that cause serotonin syndrome + Other drugs that cause serotonin syndrome', p.1471.

Note that fenfluramine was widely withdrawn in 1997 because its use was found to be associated with a high incidence of abnormal echocardiograms indicating abnormal functioning of heart valves.

1. Gaind R. Fenfluramine (Ponderax) in the treatment of obese psychiatric out-patients. *Br J Psychiatry* (1969) 115, 963–4.
2. Harding T. Fenfluramine dependence. *BMJ* (1971) 3, 305.
3. ABPI Data Sheet Compendium, 1998–99 p 1307. Datapharm publications, London.
4. Pinder RM, Brogden RN, Sawyer PR, Speight TM, Avery GS. Fenfluramine: a review of its pharmacological properties and therapeutic efficacy in obesity. *Drugs* (1975) 10, 241–323.
5. Mason EC. Servier Laboratories Ltd. Personal Communication, February 1976.
6. Gunne L-M, Antonijevic S, Jonsson J. Effect of fenfluramine on steady state plasma levels of amitriptyline. *Postgrad Med J* (1975) 51 (Suppl 1), 117.

Tricyclic antidepressants + Flupentixol and related drugs

Flupentixol did not appear to inhibit the metabolism of imipramine in two patients but high levels of imipramine and its metabolite, desipramine, were found in another patient. In a retrospective study, zuclopenthixol did not seem to affect serum concentrations of tricyclic antidepressants.

Clinical evidence

A study using oral ^{14}C-**imipramine** found that flupentixol 3 to 6 mg daily did not decrease the total urinary excretion of radioactivity in 2 patients, suggesting that the metabolism of **imipramine** was not affected by flupentixol.[1] However, there is an isolated report of very high plasma levels of **imipramine** and its metabolite desipramine in a patient with schizophrenia who was given flupentixol decanoate 40 mg intramuscularly every 2 weeks and **imipramine** 150 mg daily. It was suggested that this may have resulted from competitive inhibition of liver enzymes.[2]

Using data from a drug monitoring database, the steady-state concentration/dose ratios for **amitriptyline** and/or **nortriptyline** in 50 patients also taking zuclopenthixol were compared with 206 patients taking amitriptyline and 444 patients taking nortriptyline but not taking potentially interacting drugs. Zuclopenthixol did not appear to affect **amitriptyline** or **nortriptyline** serum concentrations under routine therapeutic drug monitoring.[3]

Mechanism

Zuclopenthixol and flupentixol are partly metabolised by the cytochrome P450 isoenzyme CYP2D6. Many of the tricyclics are also metabolised by this isoenzyme, but this does not appear to lead to an interaction.

Importance and management

The interaction between flupentixol and imipramine is an isolated case and its general significance is unknown. The studies with flupentixol and zuclopenthixol suggest that, in general, a clinically significant pharmacokinetic interaction does not occur with the tricyclics. Nevertheless, the manufacturer of both flupentixol and zuclopenthixol has suggested that the metabolism of tricyclic antidepressants may be inhibited by these drugs.[4,5] Note that zuclopenthixol, flupentixol and the tricyclic antidepressants have some antimuscarinic activity, which may lead to a pharmacological interaction, see 'Antipsychotics + Antimuscarinics', p.805.

1. Gram LF, Overø KF. Drug interaction: inhibitory effect of neuroleptics on metabolism of tricyclic antidepressants in man. *BMJ* (1972) 1, 463–5.
2. Cook PE, Dermer SW, Cardamone J. Imipramine-flupenthixol decanoate interaction. *Can J Psychiatry* (1986) 31, 235–7.
3. Linnet K. Comparison of the kinetic interactions of the neuroleptics perphenazine and zuclopenthixol with tricyclic antidepressives. *Ther Drug Monit* (1995) 17, 308–11.
4. Depixol Tablets (Flupentixol dihydrochloride). Lundbeck Ltd. UK Summary of product characteristics, November 2008.
5. Clopixol Tablets (Zuclopenthixol dihydrochloride). Lundbeck Ltd. UK Summary of product characteristics, March 2009.

Tricyclic antidepressants + Food

Limited evidence suggests that very high-fibre diets can decrease the serum concentrations of doxepin and desipramine, and therefore decrease their effects. The bioavailability of amitriptyline might be affected by food. An isolated report describes urticaria attributed to a possible drug-food interaction between clomipramine and cod.

Clinical evidence, mechanism, importance and management

Three patients had no response to **doxepin** or **desipramine** and had decreased serum tricyclic antidepressant concentrations while taking very high-fibre diets (wheat bran, wheat germ, oat bran, rolled oats, sunflower seeds, coconut shreds, raisins, bran muffins). When the diet was changed or stopped, the serum tricyclic antidepressant concentrations increased and the depression was relieved.[1] The reasons for this effect are not known. This interaction might possibly provide an explanation for otherwise unaccountable relapses or inadequate responses to tricyclic antidepressant treatment.

Another study in 12 healthy subjects found that breakfast had no effect on the bioavailability of a 50-mg dose of **imipramine**, or on its maximum concentration or the time to taken to reach the maximum concentration.[2] A study in 9 healthy subjects given a single 25-mg dose of **amitriptyline** in the fasting state, and with a standardised breakfast, found that there were no consistent changes in the bioavailability of **amitriptyline** or its main metabolite nortriptyline. Similar results were found in a parallel study in which the same subjects were given a single 25-mg dose of **nortriptyline**. However, there were large interindividual changes in the AUC of **amitriptyline** after food, ranging from an increase of 94% to a decrease of about 40%. The largest food-related **amitriptyline** AUC *increases* occurred among the subjects with the lowest fasting AUC values and the only major food-related *decrease* occurred in the subject with the largest fasting AUC. It was concluded that for an individual patient, the timing of **amitriptyline** administration in relation to food intake should be standardised to avoid large variations in drug concentrations.[3]

An isolated report describes a severe generalised urticaria that occurred after the ingestion of **cod** by a 33-year-old woman treated with **clomipramine** 100 mg daily. Clomipramine was gradually discontinued and the rash improved. Her antidepressant was changed to paroxetine and she then ate cod without developing any adverse effects. Furthermore, rechallenge with **clomipramine** did not induce any adverse events, but when she was rechallenged with **clomipramine** and cod, the urticaria was again observed. Ingestion of other fish during **clomipramine** treatment did not induce an effect.[4] This appears to be an isolated report. Its general relevance is therefore probably small.

1. Stewart DE. High-fiber diet and serum tricyclic antidepressant levels. *J Clin Psychopharmacol* (1992) 12, 438–40.
2. Abernethy DR, Divoll M, Greenblatt DJ, Shader RI. Imipramine pharmacokinetics and absolute bioavailability: effect of food. *Clin Res* (1983) 31, 626A.
3. Liedholm H, Lidén A. Food intake and the presystemic metabolism of single doses of amitriptyline and nortriptyline. *Fundam Clin Pharmacol* (1998) 12, 636–42.
4. Gallelli L, De Fazio S, Corace E, De Sarro G, Garcia CS, De Fazio P. Generalised urticaria in a young woman treated with clomipramine and after ingestion of codfish. *Pharmacopsychiatry* (2006) 39, 154–6.

Tricyclic antidepressants + Furazolidone

An isolated report describes the development of toxic psychosis, hyperactivity, sweating, and hot and cold flushes when a woman taking amitriptyline also took furazolidone and diphenoxylate with atropine.

Clinical evidence, mechanism, importance and management

A depressed woman taking conjugated oestrogens 1.25 mg daily and **amitriptyline** 75 mg daily, was also given furazolidone 300 mg daily and diphenoxylate with atropine sulfate. Two days later she began to experience blurred vision, profuse perspiration followed by alternate chills and hot flushes, restlessness, motor activity, persecutory delusions, auditory hallucinations, and visual illusions. The symptoms cleared within a day of stopping the furazolidone.[1] The reasons for this reaction are not understood but the authors point out that furazolidone has MAO-inhibitory properties, and that the symptoms were similar to those seen when the tricyclic antidepressants and MAOIs interact. However the MAO-inhibitory activity of furazolidone normally develops over several days. Whether the concurrent use of atropine and **amitriptyline** (both of which have antimuscarinic activity) had some part to play in the reaction is uncertain. No firm conclusions can be drawn from this slim evidence, but clinicians should be aware of this case when considering the concurrent use of any tricyclic antidepressant and furazolidone.

1. Aderhold RM and Muniz CE. Acute psychosis with amitriptyline and furazolidone. *JAMA* (1970) 213, 2080.

Tricyclic antidepressants + Grapefruit juice

Grapefruit juice did not appear to have a clinically significant effect on the concentrations of amitriptyline or clomipramine in one study. However, an isolated report describes increased clomipramine concentrations when two children were also given grapefruit juice.

Clinical evidence, mechanism, importance and management

A study in 6 patients given **clomipramine** 112.5 to 225 mg daily found that grapefruit juice 250 mL increased the mean plasma concentrations of **clomipramine** and its metabolite, desmethylclomipramine, by 4.5% and 10.5%, respectively. In another 7 patients taking **amitriptyline** 100 to 150 mg daily grapefruit juice did not affect the plasma concentrations of the tricyclic.[1] However, an isolated report describes an 8-year-old boy with Tourette's syndrome and obsessive-compulsive disorder who had minimal improvement when taking **clomipramine** 25 mg three times daily for 3 months. He was additionally given 250 mL of frozen concentrate grapefruit juice with each dose of **clomipramine** and, after 3 days, his minimum blood concentration of clomipramine had increased from 73 nanograms/mL to 198 nanograms/mL and those of the desmethylclomipramine had increased from 144 nanograms/mL to 233 nanograms/mL, and a clinical improvement was seen. Plasma concentrations of **clomipramine** were also increased in a 13-year-old girl, with an autistic spectrum disorder, when grapefruit juice was added to each dose of clomipramine, but no clinical improvement was seen.[2]

The studies (and the known metabolic pathways of the tricyclics, see 'Table 35.2', p.1465) suggest that an interaction with grapefruit juice is unlikely. The reason for the increased clomipramine concentrations in the children is unclear. Dose adjustments of the tricyclics would generally not be expected to be necessary in those who drink grapefruit juice.

1. Vandel P, Regina W, Reix I, Vandel S, Sechter D, Bizouard P. Faut-il contre-indiquer le jus de pamplemousse? Une approche en psychiatrie. *Encephale* (1999) 25, 67–71.
2. Oesterheld J, Kallepalli BR. Grapefruit juice and clomipramine: shifting metabolic ratios. *J Clin Psychopharmacol* (1997) 17, 62–3.

Tricyclic antidepressants + H_2-receptor antagonists

Cimetidine can raise the plasma levels of amitriptyline, desipramine, doxepin, imipramine and nortriptyline. Other tricyclic antidepressants are expected to interact similarly. Ranitidine does not appear to interact with the tricyclics.

Clinical evidence

(a) Amitriptyline

A group of healthy subjects took **cimetidine** 300 mg every 6 hours for 4 days, with a single 25-mg dose of amitriptyline on day 3. The peak plasma levels and the AUC of amitriptyline were raised by 37% and 80%, respectively, but the levels of nortriptyline (a metabolite of amitriptyline) were reduced.[1]

Another study by the same authors found that **ranitidine** does not interact with amitriptyline.[2]

(b) Desipramine

In a study in 8 patients, **cimetidine** 1 g daily for 4 days raised the plasma levels of desipramine 100 to 250 mg daily by 51%, and raised the levels of its hydroxylated metabolite (2-hydroxydesipramine) by 46%.[3] Another study suggests that this interaction does not occur in those individuals who have low levels or are completely lacking CYP2D6.[4]

(c) Doxepin

A study in 10 healthy subjects given a single 100-mg oral dose of doxepin 12 hours after starting to take **cimetidine** 300 mg every 6 hours found that the peak plasma level and AUC of doxepin were raised by 28% and 31%, respectively.[5]

In another study, **cimetidine** 600 mg twice daily was found to double the steady-state plasma levels of doxepin 50 mg daily, whereas **ranitidine** 300 mg daily had no effect on doxepin levels.[6] A patient taking doxepin complained that the normally mild adverse effects (urinary hesitancy, dry mouth and decreased visual acuity) became incapacitating when he also took **cimetidine**. His serum doxepin levels were found to be elevated in the presence of cimetidine.[7]

(d) Imipramine

In 12 healthy subjects, **cimetidine** 300 mg every 6 hours for 3 days raised the peak plasma levels and the AUC of a single 100-mg dose of imipramine by 65% and 172%, respectively. After taking **ranitidine** 150 mg twice daily for 3 days the pharmacokinetics of imipramine were unaltered.[8] These findings with **cimetidine** confirm those of previous studies.[9,10]

There are case reports of patients taking imipramine who developed severe antimuscarinic adverse effects (dry mouth, urine retention, blurred vision), associated with very marked rises in serum imipramine levels, when they also took **cimetidine**.[11,12]

(e) Nortriptyline

In a study in 6 healthy subjects, **cimetidine** 300 mg four times daily for 2 days did not affect the peak plasma levels of nortriptyline, but its AUC was increased by 20%.[9]

A case report describes a patient whose serum nortriptyline levels were raised about one-third while taking **cimetidine**.[13] Another patient complained of abdominal pain and distension (but no other antimuscarinic adverse effects) when taking nortriptyline and **cimetidine**.[14]

Mechanism

Cimetidine is a non-specific enzyme inhibitor, which reduces the metabolism of the tricyclic antidepressants, and may also reduce the hepatic clearance of these drugs. This results in a rise in their plasma levels. Ranitidine does not interact because it is not an enzyme inhibitor.

Importance and management

The interactions of the tricyclics with cimetidine are well established, well documented and of clinical importance. The incidence is uncertain but most patients could be affected. Those taking amitriptyline, desipramine, doxepin, imipramine or nortriptyline who are given cimetidine should be warned that adverse effects such as dry mouth, urinary retention, blurred vision, constipation, tachycardia, and postural hypotension may be more likely to occur. Other tricyclic antidepressants would be expected to be similarly affected. If symptoms are troublesome reduce the dosage of the antidepressant (33 to 50% has been suggested) or replace the cimetidine with ranitidine, which does not appear to interact. Other H_2-receptor antagonists that do not cause enzyme inhibition (e.g. **famotidine** and **nizatidine**) would also not be expected to interact. Note that if cimetidine is discontinued, decreases in plasma levels of the tricyclic antidepressants may occur, which could result in loss of therapeutic efficacy.

Note that, the tricyclics have been associated with QT prolongation, most usually when their levels are high, and this interaction may therefore increase the risk of this effect. See 'Drugs that prolong the QT interval + Other drugs that prolong the QT interval', p.272, for further discussion on QT prolongation.

1. Curry SH, DeVane CL, Wolfe MM. Cimetidine interaction with amitriptyline. *Eur J Clin Pharmacol* (1985) 29, 429–33.
2. Curry SH, DeVane CL, Wolfe MM. Lack of interaction of ranitidine with amitriptyline. *Eur J Clin Pharmacol* (1987) 32, 317–20.
3. Amsterdam JD, Brunswick DJ, Potter L, Kaplan MJ. Cimetidine-induced alterations in desipramine plasma concentrations. *Psychopharmacology (Berl)* (1984) 83, 373–5.
4. Steiner E, Spina E. Differences in the inhibitory effect of cimetidine on desipramine metabolism between rapid and slow debrisoquin hydroxylators. *Clin Pharmacol Ther* (1987) 42, 278–82.
5. Abernethy DR, Todd EL. Doxepin-cimetidine interaction: increased doxepin bioavailability during cimetidine treatment. *J Clin Psychopharmacol* (1986) 6, 8–12.
6. Sutherland DL, Remillard AJ, Haight KR, Brown MA, Old L. The influence of cimetidine versus ranitidine on doxepin pharmacokinetics. *Eur J Clin Pharmacol* (1987) 32, 159–64.
7. Brown MA, Haight KR, McKay G. Cimetidine-doxepin interaction. *J Clin Psychopharmacol* (1985) 5, 245–7.
8. Wells BG, Pieper JA, Self TH, Stewart CF, Waldon SL, Bobo L, Warner C. The effect of ranitidine and cimetidine on imipramine disposition. *Eur J Clin Pharmacol* (1986) 31, 285–90.
9. Henauer SA, Hollister LE. Cimetidine interaction with imipramine and nortriptyline. *Clin Pharmacol Ther* (1984) 35, 183–7.
10. Abernethy DR, Greenblatt DJ, Shader RI. Imipramine-cimetidine interaction: impairment of clearance and enhanced absolute bioavailability. *J Pharmacol Exp Ther* (1984) 229, 702–705.
11. Shapiro PA. Cimetidine-imipramine interaction: case report and comments. *Am J Psychiatry* (1984) 141, 152.
12. Miller DD, Macklin M. Cimetidine-imipramine interaction: a case report. *Am J Psychiatry* (1983) 140, 351–2.
13. Miller DD, Sawyer JB, Duffy JP. Cimetidine's effect on steady-state serum nortriptyline concentrations. *Drug Intell Clin Pharm* (1983) 17, 904–5.
14. Lerro FA. Abdominal distention syndrome in a patient receiving cimetidine-nortriptyline therapy. *J Med Soc New Jers* (1983) 80, 631–2.

Tricyclic antidepressants + Haloperidol and related drugs

Serum desipramine levels can be increased by haloperidol. This may have caused a grand mal seizure in one case but toxic reactions appear to be uncommon. Desipramine and bromperidol appear not to interact.

Clinical evidence

(a) Bromperidol

When 13 patients with schizophrenia taking bromperidol 12 to 24 mg daily for 1 to 20 weeks were also given **desipramine** 50 mg daily for a week, bromperidol plasma levels remained unchanged and no adverse clinical events were seen.[1]

(b) Haloperidol

1. Desipramine. A comparative study in patients taking similar doses of desipramine (2.5 to 2.55 mg/kg) found that the two patients also taking haloperidol had steady-state plasma desipramine levels that were more than double those of 15 other patients not taking haloperidol (255 nanograms/mL compared with 110 nanograms/mL).[2]

A case report describes a patient who had a grand mal seizure when taking desipramine with haloperidol. Her serum desipramine levels were unusually high, at 610 nanograms/mL.[3]

2. Imipramine. The urinary excretion of a test dose of ^{14}C-imipramine given to two patients with schizophrenia patients was reduced by about 35 to 40% when they took haloperidol 12 to 20 mg daily.[4] The plasma metabolite levels of ^{14}C-nortriptyline of another patient with schizophrenia fell when haloperidol 16 mg daily was taken, whereas the plasma levels of unchanged nortriptyline rose.[5]

Mechanism

Haloperidol reduces the metabolism of the tricyclic antidepressants, thereby reducing their clearance, which results in a rise in their plasma levels.

Importance and management

The interaction between the tricyclic antidepressants and haloperidol is established though its documentation is sparse. Concurrent use is common whereas adverse reactions are not, but be aware that serum desipramine levels may be elevated. This may have been the cause of the grand mal seizure in the case cited.[3] Imipramine appears to interact similarly. Monitor the outcome if haloperidol is added to established treatment with tricyclic antidepressants.

Note that bromperidol and haloperidol prolong the QT-interval, and this effect has been seen with tricyclics, usually in overdose, see 'Drugs that prolong the QT interval + Other drugs that prolong the QT interval', p.272. Also, the concurrent use of antipsychotics and drugs with antimuscarinic effects, including tricyclic antidepressants, has led to severe adverse effects, see also, 'Antipsychotics + Antimuscarinics', p.805.

1. Suzuki A, Otani K, Ishida M, Yasui N, Kondo T, Mihara K, Kaneko S, Inoue Y. No interaction between desipramine and bromperidol. *Prog Neuropsychopharmacol Biol Psychiatry* (1996) 20, 1265–71.
2. Nelson JC, Jatlow PI. Neuroleptic effect on desipramine steady-state plasma concentrations. *Am J Psychiatry* (1980) 137, 1232–4.
3. Mahr GC, Berchou R, Balon R. A grand mal seizure associated with desipramine and haloperidol. *Can J Psychiatry* (1987) 32, 463–4.
4. Gram LF, Overø KF. Drug interaction: inhibitory effect of neuroleptics on metabolism of tricyclic antidepressants in man. *BMJ* (1972) 1, 463–5.
5. Gram LF, Overø KF, Kirk L. Influence of neuroleptics and benzodiazepines on metabolism of tricyclic antidepressants in man. *Am J Psychiatry* (1974) 131, 863–6.

Tricyclic and related antidepressants + HIV-protease inhibitors

Ritonavir increases desipramine exposure and is predicted to also increase the concentrations of other tricyclic antidepressants. A case report describes potentially life-threatening cardiac conduction problems and antimuscarinic effects when ritonavir and other HIV-protease inhibitors were given with maprotiline.

Clinical evidence

(a) Desipramine

A study in 15 healthy subjects found that **lopinavir boosted with ritonavir** 400/100 mg twice daily modestly reduced the maximum plasma concentration of a single 100-mg dose of desipramine by 23%, but the AUC was unaffected. These results were not statistically significant.[1]

The preliminary report of a study in 14 healthy subjects given a single 100-mg dose of desipramine before and after they took **ritonavir** 500 mg twice daily for 10 days, notes that **ritonavir** increased the AUC of desipramine 2.5-fold and nearly doubled the half-life. The maximum plasma concentrations were also increased by 22%.[2] Another study in 13 healthy subjects, found that **ritonavir** 100 mg twice daily for 14 days increased the AUC of a single 50-mg dose of desipramine by 26% and prolonged the half-life by 30%. However, there was considerable interindividual variability in desipramine pharmacokinetic parameters, both with and without ritonavir; in the presence of ritonavir 12 of 13 subjects had an increase in the AUC of desipramine ranging from 4 to 71%.[3]

(b) Maprotiline

A report describes a 32-year-old man with AIDS taking low-dose maprotiline 50 mg daily and fluconazole 200 mg daily, who experienced severe hypotension, cardiac conduction problems and other symptoms such as dry mouth, constipation and dysuria, 8 weeks after starting a combination of antiretroviral drugs including **ritonavir** 400 mg twice daily, **saquinavir**, **indinavir**, **amprenavir** and stavudine. The serum concentrations of maprotiline reached 1.5 mmol/L (reference range 0.3 to 1 mmol/L). Clinical and electrical abnormalities disappeared within 72 hours of stopping the maprotiline, antiretroviral drugs and fluconazole.[4]

Mechanism

The tricyclic antidepressants and maprotiline are metabolised, at least in part by CYP2D6. Ritonavir is a known inhibitor of this isoenzyme, and therefore concurrent use decreases the metabolism of the tricyclics, leading to an increase in their concentrations. **Tipranavir** appears to be the only other HIV-protease inhibitor that also affects this isoenzyme to a clinically relevant extent, see 'Table 21.2', p.894.

Importance and management

An interaction between desipramine and ritonavir appears to be established. However, its clinical relevance appears to depend on the dose of ritonavir used, with the studies suggesting that higher doses of ritonavir (500 mg twice daily) have a moderate effect on desipramine concentrations, which might require a dose reduction. In contrast, when ritonavir is given as a pharmacokinetic enhancer (i.e. at a dose of 100 mg twice daily), the effects are slight and unlikely to require dose adjustments of the tricyclic. Because of the increased concentrations seen, it would seem prudent to monitor for increased tricyclic adverse effects (e.g. dry mouth, urinary retention, constipation) in any patient given ritonavir (regardless of dose). It might be prudent to consider starting desipramine at a low dose in patients taking ritonavir 500 mg twice daily, increasing the dose slowly.

There seems to be little information regarding other tricyclics, but as they are all metabolised, at least in part, by CYP2D6, similar precautions to those suggested for desipramine would seem prudent.

Other HIV-protease inhibitors, with the exception of tipranavir, would not be expected to interact by this mechanism. However, the manufacturer of nelfinavir suggests that, as it is primarily metabolised by CYP3A4 and CYP2C19, drugs that could inhibit CYP2C19 (including amitriptyline and imipramine) might be expected to reduce the conversion of nelfinavir to its major active metabolite M8, and increase plasma nelfinavir concentrations. However, limited clinical data suggests this is unlikely to be clinically important.[5] Furthermore, these tricyclics are not usually considered to be inhibitors of these isoenzymes. A clinically relevant interaction therefore seems unlikely.

1. Bertz R, Foit C, Chiu Y-L, Bernstein B, Boller S, Owen JR, Williams L, Ji Q, Renz C, Hsu A, Granneman GR, Sun E. Multiple-dose Kaletra (lopinavir/ritonavir) does not affect the pharmacokinetics of the CYP2D6 probe, desipramine. 9th Conference on Retroviruses and Opportunistic Infections, Seattle WA, February 2002. Abstract 433-W. Available at: http://archive-org.com/page/747829/2012-11-25/http://retroconference.org/2002/Abstract/13452.htm (accessed 21/10/15).
2. Bertz RI, Cao G, Cavanaugh JH, Hsu A, Granneman GR, Leonard JM. Effect of ritonavir on the pharmacokinetics of desipramine. 11th International Conference on AIDS, Vancouver, 1996. Abstract Mo.B.1201.
3. Aarnoutse RE, Kleinnijenhuis J, Koopmans PP, Touw DJ, Wieling J, Hekster YA, Burger DM. Effect of low-dose ritonavir (100 mg twice daily) on the activity of cytochrome P450 2D6 in healthy volunteers. *Clin Pharmacol Ther* (2005) 78, 664 –74.
4. Hocqueloux L, Gallien S, Bornstain C, Molina J-M. Quadricyclic antidepressant overdosage in a patient with AIDS under mega-highly active antiretroviral therapy. *Arch Intern Med* (2001) 161, 2260–1.
5. Viracept (Nelfinavir mesilate). Roche Products Ltd. UK Summary of product characteristics, June 2012.

Tricyclic and related antidepressants + Inotropes and Vasopressors

Patients taking tricyclic antidepressants show a grossly exaggerated response (hypertension, cardiac arrhythmias, etc.) to parenteral noradrenaline (norepinephrine), adrenaline (epinephrine) and to a lesser extent to phenylephrine. Case reports suggest that this interaction only occurs rarely with local anaesthetics containing these vasoconstrictors. Evidence for or against a similar interaction with mianserin and maprotiline is sparse.

Case reports describe reduced action of ephedrine in patients taking tricyclic antidepressants or mianserin.

Clinical evidence

(a) Adrenaline (Epinephrine) or Noradrenaline (Norepinephrine)

The effects of intravenous infusions of noradrenaline were increased about ninefold, and of adrenaline about threefold, in 6 healthy subjects who had been taking **protriptyline** 60 mg daily for 4 days.[1,2]

Similarly, the pressor effects of intravenous infusions of noradrenaline were increased four to eightfold, and of adrenaline two to fourfold in 4 healthy subjects who had been taking **imipramine** 75 mg daily for 5 days. Some potentiation of adrenaline-induced tachycardia occurred in one subject and striking changes in heart rhythm occurred in all 4 subjects.[3]

Five patients taking **nortriptyline**, **desipramine** or other unnamed tricyclic antidepressants experienced adverse reactions, some of them severe (throbbing headache, chest pain) following the injection of *Xylestesin* (lidocaine with 1:25 000 noradrenaline) during dental treatment.[4] Several episodes of marked increases in blood pressure, dilated pupils, intense malaise, violent but transitory tremor, and palpitations have been reported in patients taking unnamed tricyclic antidepressants when they were given local anaesthetics containing adrenaline or noradrenaline for dental treatment.[5]

There are other reports describing this interaction between:

- adrenaline with **amitriptyline**[6] and **nortriptyline**;[7]
- noradrenaline with **amitriptyline**,[8,9] **clomipramine**,[10] **desipramine**,[8,9] **imipramine**[8,10,11] and **protriptyline**.[9]

In contrast, in 5 healthy subjects taking **maprotiline**[12] and 5 patients with depression taking **mianserin**,[13] the pressor response to noradrenaline remained largely unchanged. However, a case report describes a 71-year-old woman who had been taking **mianserin** long-term who developed hypotension, following spinal anaesthesia and general anaesthesia, which was refractory to multiple boluses of ephedrine. However, her blood pressure increased excessively following a small dose of adrenaline.[14]

(b) Ephedrine

An elderly woman taking **amitriptyline** 75 mg daily developed hypotension (70 mmHg systolic) during subarachnoid anaesthesia, but her blood pressure rose only minimally when she was given intravenous boluses of ephedrine totalling 90 mg.[15] Similarly, in another patient receiving long-term **amitriptyline**, hypotension occurred during combined general and epidural anaesthesia, which was refractory to high doses of ephedrine, but control was achieved with noradrenaline.[16] Other reports describe hypotension refractory to ephedrine in patients receiving long-term **imipramine** and **lofepramine**,[17] or **mianserin**.[14]

(c) Isoprenaline (Isoproterenol)

In a study in 4 healthy subjects who had been taking **imipramine** 75 mg daily for 5 days, there were no noticeable or consistent changes in the response of blood pressure to isoprenaline and no abnormalities of heart rhythm were seen, but in one of the subjects there was a potentiation of isoprenaline-induced tachycardia.[3]

A case report describes a 30-year old woman with asthma who died due to aspiration of gastric contents in response to a cardiac arrhythmia following the use of an isoprenaline aerosol whilst taking **amitriptyline**; she was also taking other drugs including theophylline, ephedrine and phenobarbital.[18]

(d) Phenylephrine

The pressor effects of intravenous infusions of phenylephrine were increased two to threefold in 4 healthy subjects who had been taking **imipramine** 75 mg daily for 5 days.[3]

(e) Tyramine

The pressor response to tyramine was inhibited in 20 patients taking **clomipramine**,[19] and in patients (number not stated) taking **amitriptyline** 150 mg.[20] In 5 healthy subjects taking **maprotiline**, the pressor response to tyramine was reduced threefold.[12] The tyramine-response was unchanged by **mianserin**.[20-22]

Mechanism

The tricyclics and some related antidepressants block or inhibit the uptake of noradrenaline into adrenergic neurones. Thus the most important means by which noradrenaline is removed from the adrenoceptor area is inactivated and the concentration of noradrenaline outside the neurone can rise. If more noradrenaline (or one of the other directly-acting alpha or alpha/beta agonists i.e. adrenaline, phenylephrine) is then given, the adrenoceptors of the cardiovascular system concerned with raising blood pressure and/or cardiac rate and rhythm become grossly stimulated by this superabundance of amines, and the normal response becomes exaggerated. Mianserin, unlike the tricyclics, does not prevent the peripheral uptake of noradrenaline, and this may explain why it appears to interact somewhat differently in some cases.

Tyramine, and to some extent ephedrine, exerts its effects on blood pressure by causing the release of noradrenaline from adrenergic neurones. In the presence of a tricyclic antidepressant, the uptake of these amines into adrenergic neurones is partially or totally prevented and the noradrenaline-releasing effects are therefore blocked.[19] Consequently the effects of these drugs (and therefore probably other indirectly-acting sympathomimetics) might be expected to be reduced by tricyclic antidepressants.

For a categorisation of sympathomimetic drugs, see 'Table 24.1', p.1050.

Importance and management

A well documented, well established and potentially serious interaction. The parenteral use of noradrenaline, adrenaline, phenylephrine or any other sympathomimetic amines with predominantly direct activity should be avoided in patients taking tricyclic antidepressants. If these inotropes must be used, the rate and amount injected must be very much reduced to accommodate the exaggerated responses that will occur. Evidence for a similar interaction with maprotiline and mianserin is sparse, but maprotiline is known to have the same effects on noradrenaline as the tricyclics, and a case report describes a similar interaction between adrenaline and mianserin, so some caution seems prudent.

The situation where adrenaline or noradrenaline are used with a local anaesthetic for surface or infiltration anaesthesia, or nerve block is less clear. The cases cited are all from the 1960s or 1970s, and the preparations concerned contained concentrations of adrenaline or noradrenaline several times greater than those used currently. However, it should be noted that preparations such as *Xylocaine* with adrenaline still carry a caution about their use with tricyclic antidepressants.[23] Anecdotal evidence suggests that local anaesthetics containing sympathomimetics are, in practice, commonly used in patients receiving tricyclic antidepressants,[24] so the scarcity of reports, especially recent ones, would add weight to the argument that the interaction is only rarely significant. However, it would still seem advisable to be aware of the potential for interaction. Aspiration has been recommended to avoid inadvertent intravenous administration. **Felypressin** has been shown to be a safe alternative.[25-27] If an adverse interaction occurs it can be controlled by the use of an alpha-receptor blocker, such as phentolamine.

Phenylephrine can be absorbed systemically from the eye and one manufacturer has contraindicated the use of phenylephrine eye drops in patients receiving tricyclic antidepressants, or within several days or their discontinuation, because the pressor response to adrenergic agents and the risk of cardiac arrhythmia may be potentiated.[28] However, it does not seem to have been established whether the response to oral doses or nasal drops containing phenylephrine is enhanced by the presence of a tricyclic. Nevertheless, some caution seems prudent.

The effects of indirectly-acting sympathomimetics are expected to be reduced by tricyclic antidepressants, but there appear to be only a few reports of reduced efficacy of ephedrine, which has mixed indirect and direct sympathomimetic actions.

1. Svedmyr N. The influence of a tricyclic antidepressive agent (protriptyline) on some of the circulatory effects of noradrenaline and adrenaline in man. *Life Sci* (1968) 7, 77–84.
2. Svedmyr N. Potentieringsrisker vid tillförsel av katekolaminer till patienter som behandlas med tricykliska antidepressiva medel. *Lakartidningen* (1968) 65 (Suppl 1), 72–6.
3. Boakes AJ, Laurence DR, Teoh PC, Barar FSK, Benedikter LT, Prichard BNC. Interactions between sympathomimetic amines and antidepressant agents in man. *BMJ* (1973) 1, 311–15.
4. Boakes AJ, Laurence DR, Lovel KW, O'Neil R, Verrill PJ. Adverse reactions to local anaesthetic/vasoconstrictor preparations. A study of the cardiovascular responses to Xylestesin and Hostacain-with-Noradrenaline. *Br Dent J* (1972) 133, 137–40.
5. Dam WH. Personal communication cited by Kristoffersen MB. Antidepressivas potensering af katekolaminvirkning. *Ugeskr Laeger* (1969) 131, 1013–14.
6. Siemkowicz E. Hjertestop efter amitriptylin og adrenalin. *Ugeskr Laeger* (1975) 137, 1403–4.

7. Persson G, Siwers B. The risk of potentiating effect of local anaesthesia with adrenalin in patients treated with tricyclic antidepressants. *Swed Dent J* (1975) 68, 9–18.
8. Fischbach R, Harrer G, Harrer H. Verstärkung der Noradrenalin-Wirkung durch Psychopharmaka beim Menschen. *Arzneimittelforschung* (1966) 16, 263–5.
9. Mitchell JR, Cavanaugh JH, Arias L, Oates JA. Guanethidine and related agents. III. Antagonism by drugs which inhibit the norepinephrine pump in man. *J Clin Invest* (1970) 49, 1596–1604.
10. Borg K-O, Johnsson G, Jordö L, Lundborg P, Rönn O, Welin-Fogelberg I. Interaction studies between three antidepressant drugs (zimelidine, imipramine and chlorimipramine) and noradrenaline in healthy volunteers and some pharmacokinetics of the drugs studied. *Acta Pharmacol Toxicol (Copenh)* (1979) 45, 198–205.
11. Gershon S, Holmberg G, Mattsson E, Mattsson N, Marshall A. Imipramine hydrochloride. Its effects on clinical, autonomic and psychological functions. *Arch Gen Psychiatry* (1962) 6, 96–101.
12. Briant RH, George CF. The assessment of potential drug interactions with a new tricyclic antidepressant drug. *Br J Clin Pharmacol* (1974) 1, 113–18.
13. Ghose K. Studies on the interaction between mianserin and noradrenaline in patients suffering from depressive illness. *Br J Clin Pharmacol* (1977) 4, 712–14.
14. Takeguchi Y, Miyamoto Y, Sone T, Kato H. Severe hypotension during anesthesia in a patient on long-term antidepressant therapy. *Masui* (2003) 52, 284–7.
15. Serle DG. Amitriptyline and ephedrine in subarachnoid anaesthesia. *Anaesth Intensive Care* (1985) 13, 214.
16. Boada S, Solsona B, Papaceit J, Saludes J, Rull M. Hipotensión por bloqueo simpático refractaria a efedrina en una paciente en tratamiento crónico con antidepresivos tricíclicos. *Rev Esp Anestesiol Reanim* (1999) 46, 364–6.
17. Takakura K, Nagaya M, Mori M, Koga H, Yoshitake S, Noguchi T. Refractory hypotension during combined general and epidural anaesthesia in a patient on tricyclic antidepressants. *Anaesth Intensive Care* (2006) 34, 111–14.
18. Kadar D. Amitriptyline and isoproterenol: fatal drug combination. *Can Med Assoc J* (1975) 112, 556–7.
19. Mulgirigama LD, Pare CMB, Turner P, Wadsworth J, Witts DJ. Tyramine pressor responses and plasma levels during tricyclic antidepressant therapy. *Postgrad Med J* (1977) 53 (Suppl 4), 30–4.
20. Ghose K, Coppen A, Turner P. Autonomic actions and interactions of mianserin hydrochloride (Org. GB 94) and amitriptyline in patients with depressive illness. *Psychopharmacology (Berl)* (1976) 49, 201–4.
21. Coppen A, Ghose K, Swade C, Wood K. Effect of mianserin hydrochloride on peripheral uptake mechanisms for noradrenaline and 5-hydroxytryptamine in man. *Br J Clin Pharmacol* (1978) 5, 13S–17S.
22. Coppen AJ, Ghose K. Clinical and pharmacological effects of treatment with a new antidepressant. *Arzneimittelforschung* (1976) 26, 1166–7.
23. Xylocaine 1% and 2% with Adrenaline (Lidocaine with Adrenaline). AstraZeneca UK Ltd. UK Summary of product characteristics, September 2006.
24. Brown RS, Lewis VA. More on the contraindications to vasoconstrictors in dentistry. *Oral Surg Oral Med Oral Pathol* (1993) 76, 2–3.
25. Aellig WH, Laurence DR, O'Neil R, Verrill PJ. Cardiac effects of adrenaline and felypressin as vasoconstrictors in local anaesthesia for oral surgery under diazepam sedation. *Br J Anaesth* (1970) 42, 174–6.
26. Goldman V, Astrom A, Evers H. The effect of a tricyclic antidepressant on the cardiovascular effects of local anaesthetic solutions containing different vasoconstrictors. *Anaesthesia* (1971) 26, 91.
27. Perovic J, Terzic M, Todorovic L. Safety of local anaesthesia induced by prilocaine with felypressin in patients on tricyclic antidepressants. *Bull Group Int Rech Sci Stomatol Odontol* (1979) 22, 57–62.
28. Minims Phenylephrine Hydrochloride 10%. Bausch & Lomb UK Ltd. UK Summary of product characteristics, November 2006.

Tricyclic antidepressants + Macrolides

Troleandomycin increases the plasma levels of imipramine, and an isolated report suggests that josamycin may possibly increase amitriptyline levels. Erythromycin may possibly raise clomipramine levels, but was not found to interact with other tricyclic antidepressants in one study.

Clinical evidence, mechanism, importance and management

(a) Erythromycin

Erythromycin 250 mg four times daily for 6 days was found not to affect the tricyclic antidepressant levels of 8 patients taking **desipramine**, **imipramine**, **doxepin**, or **nortriptyline**.[1] Behavioural changes have been reported in a 15-year-old patient when erythromycin was added to a regimen of **clomipramine** and risperidone,[2] resulting in symptoms compatible with serotonin syndrome, although mental confusion and autonomic instability were absent.[3] It was suggested that erythromycin increased **clomipramine** levels by inhibiting its metabolism by the cytochrome P450 isoenzyme CYP3A4.[4] **Clomipramine** levels may also have been raised by competition with risperidone for metabolism by CYP2D6.

In general, no interaction would be expected between the tricyclics and erythromycin; the isolated report seems unlikely to be of general significance.

(b) Josamycin

A patient taking **amitriptyline** had a marked increase in the total serum levels of **amitriptyline** and its metabolite, nortriptyline, after taking josamycin but no toxicity was reported. It was suggested that josamycin had inhibited **amitriptyline** metabolism.[5] This is an isolated case and although its general significance is unknown, it seems likely to be small.

(c) Troleandomycin

A study in 9 healthy Chinese men found that when they were given troleandomycin 250 mg daily for 2 days before a single 100-mg oral dose of **imipramine**, the AUC of the **imipramine** was increased by 59% and its oral clearance was reduced by 30%. It is thought that troleandomycin inhibits the *N*-demethylation of **imipramine** by inhibiting the cytochrome P450 isoenzyme subfamily CYP3A.[6] The clinical importance of this interaction is uncertain, but it may be prudent to be alert for increased antimuscarinic adverse effects (e.g. dry mouth, blurred vision, urinary retention) if troleandomycin is given to a patient taking imipramine.

1. Amsterdam JD, Maislin G. Effect of erythromycin on tricyclic antidepressant metabolism. *J Clin Psychopharmacol* (1991) 11, 203–6.
2. Fisman S, Reniers D, Diaz P. Erythromycin interaction with risperidone or clomipramine in an adolescent. *J Child Adolesc Psychopharmacol* (1996) 6, 133–8.
3. Fisman S, Diaz P. Erythromycin and clomipramine: Noncompetitive inhibition of demethylation. Reply. *J Child Adolesc Psychopharmacol* (1996) 6, 213.
4. Oesterheld JR. Erythromycin and clomipramine: Noncompetitive inhibition of demethylation. *J Child Adolesc Psychopharmacol* (1996) 6, 211–12.
5. Sánchez Romero A, Calzado Solaz C. Posible interacción entre josamicina y amitriptilina. *Med Clin (Barc)* (1992) 98, 279.
6. Wang J-S, Wang W, Xie H-G, Huang S-L, Zhou H-H. Effect of troleandomycin on the pharmacokinetics of imipramine in Chinese: the role of CYP3A. *Br J Clin Pharmacol* (1997) 44, 195–8.

Tricyclic antidepressants + Maprotiline

An isolated case describes severe, reversible hepatitis associated with the concurrent use of maprotiline and opipramol.

Clinical evidence, mechanism, importance and management

A patient who had been taking opipramol 150 mg daily for 2 months developed a progressive fatigue syndrome while taking opipramol 100 mg daily and maprotiline 75 mg daily for a further 2 months. Six weeks later he was found to have a marked elevation of liver enzymes and jaundice. Liver enzymes decreased upon cessation of the antidepressants, and normalised completely within 2 months.[1]

It was thought that the concurrent use of both drugs had led to the hepatotoxicity seen: both maprotiline and the tricyclic antidepressants have been associated with hepatotoxicity.

The general relevance of this isolated case is unclear, but it serves as a reminder of the risks of using two potentially hepatotoxic drugs at the same time.

Both the tricyclics and maprotiline have antimuscarinic effects, which might be additive on concurrent use (see 'Antimuscarinics + Antimuscarinics', p.754).

1. Braun JS, Geiger R, Wehner H, Schäffer S, Berger M. Hepatitis caused by antidepressive therapy with maprotiline and opipramol. *Pharmacopsychiatry* (1998) 31, 152–5.

Tricyclic antidepressants + Methylphenidate and related drugs

Methylphenidate can increase the plasma concentration and rate of response to imipramine and other tricyclic antidepressants. This has led to both increased beneficial and adverse effects. No significant pharmacokinetic interaction has been reported between desipramine and methylphenidate. An isolated report describes a blood dyscrasia in a child given methylphenidate and imipramine.

Clinical evidence

A study in 'several patients' found a dramatic increase in the plasma concentration of **imipramine** and its active metabolite, desipramine, when they took methylphenidate. In one patient taking **imipramine** 150 mg daily, the use of methylphenidate 20 mg daily increased the plasma concentration of imipramine from 100 nanograms/mL to 700 nanograms/mL and increased the plasma concentration of desipramine from 200 nanograms/mL to 850 nanograms/mL over a period of 16 days. Clinical improvement occurred in several of the patients.[1] Similar effects have been described in other reports.[2-5] It seems that elevation of drug plasma concentrations takes several days to occur, and several days to wear off.[3]

In contrast, a retrospective review in children and adolescents taking either **desipramine** alone, or with a stimulant, indicated the absence of a clinically significant interaction between **desipramine** and methylphenidate in 25 children who received both drugs; pharmacokinetic parameters for desipramine were similar in each group.[6] In one patient taking **desipramine** 250 mg daily, the concurrent use of methylphenidate 40 mg daily resulted in a small decrease in the serum concentration of **desipramine**, but a marked improvement in mood.[7] However, a further report describes more frequent adverse effects in 10 paediatric patients taking methylphenidate with **desipramine** than with methylphenidate alone, but the plasma concentration of desipramine was not particularly increased.[8]

A study of the combined use of tricyclic antidepressants (**desipramine, imipramine, nortriptyline, doxepin**) with methylphenidate 5 to 15 mg twice daily was undertaken in 20 of 41 patients with depression who responded to a test dose of methylphenidate. Combined use accelerated the antidepressant response to tricyclics with 6 of 20 patients responding after one week and 10 of 16 patients responding after 2 weeks. Adverse effects included insomnia, dizziness, hypotension, and dry mouth. Methylphenidate was discontinued after less than 2 weeks of concurrent use in 3 patients because of increased anxiety, irritability, and hypomania.[9]

An uncontrolled case series in 50 patients with treatment-resistant depression included four patients taking a tricyclic with methylphenidate. In one patient taking **nortriptyline** 250 mg, starting methylphenidate 20 mg daily doubled the serum concentration of nortriptyline from 0.54 to 1.06 micromol/L, and he developed tricyclic adverse effects, including dry mouth and constipation. Concurrent use of methylphenidate 10 mg daily in a second patient led to a small increase in the serum concentration of **dosulepin** 150 mg. No noticeable increases in the tricyclic serum concentrations were seen in two other patients taking unspecified tricyclics.[10]

A report describes a 9-year-old boy and a 15-year-old boy who exhibited severe behavioural problems until the **imipramine** and methylphenidate that they were taking were stopped.[11] Another case report describes the development of oculogyric crisis in a 10-year-old girl after the addition of **imipramine** to treatment with methylphenidate and valproic acid.[12] Three patients taking tricyclic antidepressants and with labile blood pressure experienced hypertensive episodes when methylphenidate was also given. They responded to withdrawal of methylphenidate and two patients had further hypertensive episodes when rechallenged with methylphenidate.[13] An isolated report describes leucopenia, anaemia, eosinophilia, and thrombocytosis in a 10-year-old child when **imipramine** and methylphenidate were given.[14]

Mechanism

In vitro experiments with human liver slices indicate that methylphenidate inhibits the metabolism of imipramine, resulting in increased blood concentrations.[3] The accelerated response to tricyclic antidepressants might also be partly due to increased serum concentrations in the presence of methylphenidate, although the adverse effects observed were not entirely consistent with increased plasma concentrations of tricyclics.[9] The blood dyscrasia might have been due to the rare additive effects of both drugs.[14]

Importance and management

Evidence is somewhat conflicting, but in general, the combination of methylphenidate and tricyclic antidepressants might result in some therapeutic improvement including, in some patients, an accelerated response. This might be partially because of the very large increase in the blood concentration of the antidepressant due to methylphenidate, but might also be due to an additional effect on mood attributable to methylphenidate. Concurrent use might cause adverse effects sufficiently severe to necessitate withdrawal of methylphenidate, but it is not certain whether this can solely be attributed to increases in the serum concentrations of the tricyclic antidepressants. It has been suggested that the concurrent use of methylphenidate and tricyclics in children and adolescents can be undesirable, due to case reports of adverse behavioural effects.[11] If concurrent use is deemed necessary it would seem prudent to monitor for adverse tricyclic effects (e.g. dry mouth, blurred vision, urinary retention) and adjust the dose of the tricyclic as necessary, particularly when methylphenidate is started or stopped. If this is not effective it might be necessary to withdraw one or both drugs.

The US manufacturer of **dexmethylphenidate**, the d-isomer of methylphenidate, notes the interaction of methylphenidate and states that dose reductions of tricyclics (they name **clomipramine**, desipramine, and imipramine) might be required.[15] Although they make no direct recommendation for the use of dexmethylphenidate with tricyclics, until more is known, it might be prudent to follow the same precautions given for methylphenidate.

1. Dayton PG, Perel JM, Israili ZH, Faraj BA, Rodewig K, Black N, Goldberg LI. Studies with methylphenidate: drug interactions and metabolism. In Sellers EM, ed. Clinical Pharmacology of Psychoactive Drugs.Toronto: Alcoholism and Drug Addiction Research Foundation; 1975 p. 183–202.
2. Cooper TB, Simpson GM. Concomitant imipramine and methylphenidate administration: a case report. *Am J Psychiatry* (1973) 130, 721.
3. Wharton RN, Perel JM, Dayton PG, Malitz S. A potential clinical use for methylphenidate with tricyclic antidepressants. *Am J Psychiatry* (1971) 127, 1619–25.
4. Zeidenberg P, Perel JM, Kanzler M, Wharton RN, Malitz S. Clinical and metabolic studies with imipramine in man. *Am J Psychiatry* (1971) 127, 1321–6.
5. Cooper TB, Simpson GM. Concomitant imipramine and methylphenidate administration: a case report. *Am J Psychiatry* (1973) 130, 721.
6. Cohen LG, Prince J, Biederman J, Wilens T, Faraone SV, Whitt S, Mick E, Spencer T, Meyer MC, Polisner D, Flood JG. Absence of effect of stimulants on the pharmacokinetics of desipramine in children. *Pharmacotherapy* (1999) 19, 746–52.
7. Drimmer EJ, Gitlin MJ, Gwirtsman HE. Desipramine and methylphenidate combination treatment for depression: case report. *Am J Psychiatry* (1983) 140, 241–2.
8. Pataki CS, Carlson GA, Kelly KL, Rapport MD, Biancaniello TM. Side effects of methylphenidate and desipramine alone and in combination in children. *J Am Acad Child Adolesc Psychiatry* (1993) 32, 1065–72.
9. Gwirtsman HE, Szuba MP, Toren L, Feist M. The antidepressant response to tricyclics in major depressives is accelerated with adjunctive use of methylphenidate. *Psychopharmacol Bull* (1994) 30, 157–64.
10. Parker G, Brotchie H. Do the old psychostimulant drugs have a role in managing treatment-resistant depression? *Acta Psychiatr Scand* (2010) 121, 308–14.
11. Grob CS, Coyle JT. Suspected adverse methylphenidate-imipramine interactions in children. *J Dev Behav Pediatr* (1986) 7, 265–7.
12. Tahiroglu AY, Avci A. Polypharmacy and EPS in a child; a case report. *Psychopharmacol Bull* (2007) 40, 129–33.
13. Flemenbaum A. Hypertensive episodes after adding methylphenidate (Ritalin) to tricyclic antidepressants. *Psychosomatics* (1972) 13, 265–8.
14. Burke MS, Josephson A, Lightsey A. Combined methylphenidate and imipramine complication. *J Am Acad Child Adolesc Psychiatry* (1995) 34, 403–4.
15. Focalin XR (Dexmethylphenidate hydrochloride). Novartis. US Prescribing information, December 2013.

Tricyclic antidepressants + Mirabegron

Mirabegron moderately increases the exposure to desipramine. Other tricyclics and drugs that are also metabolised by CYP2D6 are expected to interact similarly.

Clinical evidence

In a phase I study in 28 healthy subjects given a single 50-mg dose of desipramine before and on day 14 of an 18-day course of mirabegron 100 mg daily, the AUC and maximum plasma concentration of desipramine were increased 3.4-fold and by 79%, respectively.[1]

Mechanism

Mirabegron is an inhibitor of CYP2D6, by which desipramine is metabolised. Concurrent use therefore decreases its metabolism resulting in increased exposure.

Importance and management

Evidence for an interaction between desipramine and mirabegron is limited to this study, but a pharmacokinetic interaction is established and likely to be clinically important. The moderate increase in desipramine exposure seen might result in an increase in antimuscarinic adverse effects (such as dry mouth, urinary retention, constipation). It would therefore seem prudent to monitor for such effects on concurrent use, and consider reducing the desipramine dose if they become troublesome. All tricyclic antidepressants are metabolised by CYP2D6 to some extent, therefore they are expected to interact similarly on concurrent use with mirabegron.

Note that desipramine can be used as a probe substrate to assess the activity of drugs on CYP2D6. This study therefore suggests that mirabegron is a moderate inhibitor of this isoenzyme. Other drugs that are also substrates of CYP2D6 might be expected to interact similarly, and some caution on concurrent use would seem prudent. For a list of CYP2D6 substrates see 'Table 1.7', p.9.

1. Krauwinkel W, Dickinson J, Schaddelee M, Meijer J, Tretter R, van de Wetering J, Strabach G, van Gelderen M. The effect of mirabegron, a potent and selective β_3-adrenoceptor agonist, on the pharmacokinetics of CYP2D6 substrates desipramine and metoprolol. *Eur J Drug Metab Pharmacokinet* (2014) 39, 43–52.

Tricyclic antidepressants + Modafinil

The blood concentration of clomipramine was reported to be increased by modafinil in one patient. However, a study found that the concurrent use of modafinil and clomipramine did not affect the pharmacokinetics of either drug. Armodafinil would be expected to interact in a similar way to modafinil.

Clinical evidence

In a placebo-controlled, crossover study, 18 patients were given a single 50-mg dose of **clomipramine** on day 1 and modafinil 200 mg daily on days 1 to 3. No pharmacokinetic changes were found to have occurred with either of the two drugs.[1] However, a single case report describes a patient taking **clomipramine** 75 mg daily who had an increase in her blood concentration of **clomipramine** and its metabolite, desmethylclomipramine, when modafinil 200 mg was added.[2]

Mechanism

Clomipramine is metabolised by CYP2D6 and possibly CYP2C19. It was suggested that the patient in the case report was a poor metaboliser of CYP2D6 (that is, she had low activity of this isoenzyme), so that CYP2C19 might play a greater role in clomipramine metabolism. Modafinil is a weak inhibitor of CYP2C19 and, in poor metabolisers of CYP2D6, additional inhibition of CYP2C19 by modafinil might result in an increase in clomipramine concentrations.

Importance and management

Information about an interaction between the tricyclic antidepressants and modafinil appears to be limited to one study and a case report with clomipramine. Information about other tricyclic antidepressants is lacking, but the UK and US manufacturers of modafinil state that other CYP2D6 poor metabolisers (about 7 to 10% of the Caucasian population) might possibly also show increased tricyclic antidepressant exposure in the presence of modafinil.[3,4] Therefore monitoring the concurrent use of all tricyclic antidepressants with modafinil would seem to be a prudent precaution, as lower doses of tricyclic antidepressants might be required in those patients deficient in CYP2D6.[3,4] **Armodafinil**, the *R*-isomer of modafinil, would be expected to interact in a similar way, and the US manufacturer of armodafinil recommends that a reduction in the armodafinil dose might be required if clomipramine is taken concurrently.[5]

Note that not all tricyclic antidepressants are metabolised in the same way, and only those affected by CYP2C19 would be expected to be affected, see 'Table 35.2', p.1465, for more information on the metabolism of the tricyclics.

1. Wong YN, Gorman S, Simcoe D, McCormick GC, Grebow P. A double-blind placebo-controlled crossover study to investigate the kinetics and acute tolerability of modafinil and clomipramine alone and in combination in healthy male volunteers. Association of Professional Sleep Societies meeting, San Francisco, June 1997, Abstract 117.
2. Grözinger M, Härtter S, Hiemke C, Griese E-U, Röschke J. Interaction of modafinil and clomipramine as comedication in a narcoleptic patient. *Clin Neuropharmacol* (1998) 21, 127–9.
3. Provigil (Modafinil). Cephalon, Inc. US Prescribing information, October 2010.
4. Provigil (Modafinil). Cephalon (UK) Ltd. UK Summary of product characteristics, August 2013.
5. Nuvigil (Armodafinil). Cephalon, Inc. US Prescribing information, June 2013.

Tricyclic antidepressants + Nasal decongestants

The effects of pseudoephedrine and other related drugs are predicted to be altered by the tricyclic antidepressants; however, there appears to be a lack of reported cases.

Clinical evidence, mechanism, importance and management

Some manufacturers of pseudoephedrine-containing products suggest that its activity might be diminished or enhanced by tricyclic antidepressants. There is some concern that concurrent use may lead to a rise in blood pressure.[1,2] In practice, the efficacy of ephedrine (which has similar effects mixed indirect and direct action on adrenergic neurones to pseudoephedrine) is diminished by tricyclics, when it is given as a vasopressor, see 'Tricyclic and related antidepressants + Inotropes and Vasopressors', p.1510. Therefore a similar reduction in effect would be expected when these drugs are given as nasal decongestants.

Furthermore, one manufacturer[2] warns of an increased risk of arrhythmias on concurrent use, but this effect only appears to have been seen with intravenous adrenaline, and even then, rarely.

1. Adult Meltus Dry Coughs with Congestion (Dextromethorphan hydrobromide and Pseudoephedrine hydrochloride). SSL International plc. UK Summary of product characteristics, January 2007.
2. Boots Cold & Flu Relief with Ibuprofen (Ibuprofen and Pseudoephedrine hydrochloride). Boots Company PLC. UK Summary of product characteristics, May 2004.

Tricyclic and related antidepressants + Oestrogens

There is limited evidence suggesting that oestrogens can sometimes affect the therapeutic response to imipramine, and also cause imipramine toxicity. Tricyclic-induced akathisia was attributed to the concurrent use of conjugated oestrogens in three patients. Maprotiline levels are not affected by hormonal contraceptives

Clinical evidence

A study in women taking **imipramine** 150 mg daily for primary depression found that those given **ethinylestradiol** 25 or 50 micrograms [daily] for one week had a greater improvement than those given **imipramine** alone. However, after 2 weeks, those given **ethinylestradiol** 50 micrograms daily had less improvement than other women given only 25 micrograms of **ethinylestradiol** [daily] or a placebo.[1] In an earlier associated study 5 patients taking **imipramine** 150 mg and **ethinylestradiol** 50 micrograms daily developed signs of **imipramine** toxicity (severe lethargy (4 patients), hypotension (4), coarse tremor (2), mild depersonalisation (2)) that was dealt with by halving the **imipramine** dose.[1] Similarly, in a case report, long-standing **imipramine** toxicity was relieved in a woman taking **imipramine** 100 mg daily when her dose of **conjugated oestrogens**, which she had increased to 7.5 mg daily, was reduced to 625 micrograms daily.[2] In another report, akathisia in 3 patients was attributed to an interaction between **conjugated oestrogens** in usual doses of 1.25 mg daily and **amitriptyline**, **clomipramine** or **doxepin**.[3]

A study found that oral contraceptives increased the absolute bioavailability of **imipramine** by 60%.[4] Several studies have shown that plasma **clomipramine** levels were raised or remained unaffected by the concurrent use of oestrogen-containing contraceptives; however, they were unable to confirm that tricyclic antidepressant toxicity occurs more often in those taking oral contraceptives than those who are not.[5-8]

A study in women found that, over a 28-day period, the use of oral hormonal contraceptives did not significantly affect the steady-state blood levels of **maprotiline** 75 mg given at night, nor was its therapeutic effectiveness changed.[9]

Mechanism

Among the possible reasons for these effects are that the oestrogens increase the bioavailability of imipramine,[4] by inhibiting its metabolism.[10] Other tricyclic antidepressants might be similarly affected.

Importance and management

These interactions are inadequately established. There is no obvious reason for avoiding concurrent use, but it would seem reasonable to be alert for any evidence of toxicity and/or lack of response to tricyclic antidepressant treatment in those taking oestrogens in any form. One study suggested that the imipramine dosage should be reduced by about one-third,[4] but given the lack of confirmatory data it would seem prudent to only adjust tricyclic doses according to response.

1. Prange AJ, Wilson IC, Alltop LB. Estrogen may well affect response to antidepressant. *JAMA* (1972) 219, 143–4.
2. Khurana RC. Estrogen-imipramine interaction. *JAMA* (1972) 222, 702–3.
3. Krishnan KRR, France RD, Ellinwood EH Jr. Tricyclic-induced akathisia in patients taking conjugated estrogens. *Am J Psychiatry* (1984) 141, 696–7.
4. Abernethy DR, Greenblatt DJ, Shader RI. Imipramine disposition in users of oral contraceptive steroids. *Clin Pharmacol Ther* (1984) 35, 792–7.
5. Beaumont G. Drug interactions with clomipramine (Anafranil). *J Int Med Res* (1973) 1, 480–84.
6. Gringras M, Beaumont G, Grieve A. Clomipramine and oral contraceptives: an interaction study — clinical findings. *J Int Med Res* (1980) 8 (Suppl 3), 76–80.
7. Luscombe DK, Jones RB. Effects of concomitantly administered drugs on plasma levels of clomipramine and desmethylclomipramine in depressive patients receiving clomipramine therapy. *Postgrad Med J* (1977) 53 (Suppl 4), 77.
8. John VA, Luscombe DK, Kemp H. Effects of age, cigarette smoking and the oral contraceptive on the pharmacokinetics of clomipramine and its desmethyl metabolite during chronic dosing. *J Int Med Res* (1980) 8 (Suppl 3), 88–95.
9. Luscombe DK. Interaction studies: the influence of age, cigarette smoking and the oral contraceptive on blood concentrations of maprotiline. In 'Depressive Illness — Far Horizons?' McIntyre JNM (ed), Cambridge Med Publ, Northampton 1982, p 61–2.
10. Somani SM, Khurana RC. Mechanism of estrogen-imipramine interaction. *JAMA* (1973) 223, 560.

Tricyclic antidepressants + Orlistat

Orlistat does not appear to affect the plasma levels of clomipramine or desipramine in patients, or the pharmacokinetics of amitriptyline in healthy subjects.

Clinical evidence, mechanism, importance and management

A preliminary study in patients who had been taking psychotropic drugs long-term found no clinically relevant changes in plasma levels of **clomipramine** (3 patients) or **desipramine** (1 patient) when they were given orlistat over an 8-week period.[1] A study in 20 healthy subjects found that orlistat 120 mg three times daily for 6 days did not affect the pharmacokinetics of **amitriptyline** 25 mg three times daily.[2]

Although evidence is limited no particular precautions seem likely to be necessary on concurrent use.

1. Hilger E, Quiner S, Ginzel I, Walter H, Saria L, Barnas C. The effect of orlistat on plasma levels of psychotropic drugs in patients with long-term psychopharmacotherapy. *J Clin Psychopharmacol* (2002) 22, 68–70.
2. Zhi J, Moore R, Kanitra L, Mulligan TE. Pharmacokinetic evaluation of the possible interaction between selected concomitant medications and orlistat at steady state in healthy subjects. *J Clin Pharmacol* (2002) 42, 1011–19.

Tricyclic antidepressants + Oxybutynin

Oxybutynin reduced the blood levels of clomipramine in one patient. Both tricyclics and oxybutynin have antimuscarinic effects, which would be expected to be additive on concurrent use.

Clinical evidence, mechanism, importance and management

An elderly woman had **clomipramine** and desmethylclomipramine blood levels of 405 and 50 nanograms/mL, respectively, after taking clomipramine 25 mg daily and fluvoxamine 100 mg daily for 18 days. Within one week of starting oxybutynin 5 mg daily, the levels of **clomipramine** and desmethylclomipramine had fallen to 133 nanograms/mL and less than 25 nanograms/mL, respectively, and remained low during a further week of concurrent treatment.[1]

It has been suggested that **clomipramine** levels may be reduced because oxybutynin is an inducer of cytochrome P450 isoenzymes, which could increase the metabolism of clomipramine, and therefore reduce it levels.[1] However, oxybutynin does not usually act in this way.

This appears to be the only report of an interaction, the mechanism of which is not fully clear. It is therefore of unknown general significance. However, note that both tricyclic antidepressants and oxybutynin have antimuscarinic effects, which may be additive on concurrent use. Consider 'Antimuscarinics + Antimuscarinics', p.754, for more on this potential interaction.

1. Grözinger M, Härtter S, Hiemke C, Röschke J. Oxybutynin enhances the metabolism of clomipramine and dextrorphan possibly by induction of a cytochrome P450 isoenzyme. *J Clin Psychopharmacol* (1999) 19, 287–9.

Tricyclic antidepressants + Propafenone

An isolated report describes markedly raised serum desipramine levels in a patient who also took propafenone.

Clinical evidence

A man with major depression responded well to **desipramine** 175 mg daily with serum desipramine levels in the range of 500 to 1000 nanomol/L. When he was treated for paroxysmal atrial fibrillation with digoxin 250 micrograms daily, and propafenone 150 mg twice daily and 300 mg at night, he developed markedly elevated serum **desipramine** levels (2092 nanomol/L) and toxicity (dry mouth, sedation, shakiness) while taking desipramine 150 mg daily. The adverse effects resolved when the **desipramine** was stopped for 5 days, but when it was restarted at 75 mg daily his serum desipramine levels were still raised, at 1130 nanomol/L.[1]

Mechanism

Propafenone is an inhibitor of the cytochrome P450 isoenzyme CYP2D6, by which desipramine is predominantly metabolised. Concurrent use therefore decreases desipramine metabolism and results in an increase in its levels.

Importance and management

This appears to be the only report of an interaction between desipramine and propafenone, but it is in line with the way both drugs are known to interact. An interaction would therefore seem to be established, although its general importance is uncertain. It would seem prudent to be alert for signs of desipramine toxicity in any patient also given propafenone. Reduce the desipramine dosage appropriately. Other tricyclic antidepressants might be expected to be similarly affected as they are also metabolised, at least in part, by CYP2D6.

Note that, the tricyclics have been associated with QT prolongation, most usually when their levels are high, and this interaction may therefore increase the risk of this effect. See 'Drugs that prolong the QT interval + Other drugs that prolong the QT interval', p.272, for further discussion on QT prolongation.

1. Katz MR. Raised serum levels of desipramine with the antiarrhythmic propafenone. *J Clin Psychiatry* (1991) 52, 432–3.

Tricyclic antidepressants + Quinidine or Quinine

Quinidine can reduce the clearance of desipramine, imipramine, nortriptyline and trimipramine, and quinine can reduce the clearance of desipramine, thereby increasing their plasma levels.

Clinical evidence

(a) Quinidine

In a study in 5 healthy subjects quinidine 50 mg given one hour before a single 50-mg dose of **nortriptyline** increased the **nortriptyline** AUC fourfold, and increased the half-life from 14.2 hours to 44.7 hours.[1] The clearance fell by 65%. A single-dose study in healthy subjects found that quinidine 200 mg daily reduced the clearance of **imipramine** 100 mg and **desipramine** 100 mg by 30% and 85%, respectively.[2] A further study in 2 healthy subjects similarly found that quinidine 50 mg almost doubled the half-life of a single 75-mg dose of **trimipramine**, which was reflected in some waking EEG changes.[3]

In healthy subjects given quinidine 800 mg daily for 2 days, the urinary excretion of 2-hydroxydesipramine from a single 25-mg dose of **desipramine** was reduced by 97% and 68%, respectively in subjects with normal levels and low levels of [CYP2D6].[4]

(b) Quinine

Quinine 750 mg daily for 2 days reduced the urinary excretion of 2-hydroxydesipramine from a single 25-mg dose of **desipramine** in those with normal levels of [CYP2D6] by 56% but had no significant effect on the clearance in those with low levels of [CYP2D6].[4]

Mechanism

Quinidine reduces the metabolism (hydroxylation) of these tricyclic antidepressants, by inhibiting the cytochrome P450 isoenzyme CYP2D6, and thereby reduces their loss from the body.[5,6] Quinine inhibits the metabolism of desipramine to a lesser extent than quinidine, as it is a less potent inhibitor of CYP2D6.

Importance and management

An interaction between quinidine and the tricyclics appears to be established. It would be expected to be clinically relevant with nortriptyline, and possibly desipramine, but probably not with imipramine. This is due to differences in the way the tricyclics are metabolised (see "Drugs that prolong the QT interval + Other drugs that prolong the QT interval', p.272, for further discussion on QT prolongation.

Information about the effect of quinine on tricyclics is very limited, but the effects are smaller than those of quinidine and therefore less likely to result in clinically significant adverse effects.

1. Ayesh R, Dawling S, Widdop B, Idle JR, Smith RL. Influence of quinidine on the pharmacokinetics of nortriptyline and desipramine in man. *Br J Clin Pharmacol* (1988) 25, 140P–141P.
2. Brøsen K, Gram LF. Quinidine inhibits the 2-hydroxylation of imipramine and desipramine but not the demethylation of imipramine. *Eur J Clin Pharmacol* (1989) 37, 155–60.
3. Eap CB, Laurian S, Souche A, Koeb L, Reymond P, Buclin T, Baumann P. Influence of quinidine on the pharmacokinetics of trimipramine and on its effect on the waking EEG of healthy volunteers. A pilot study on two subjects. *Neuropsychobiology* (1992) 25, 214–20.
4. Steiner E, Dumont E, Spina E, Dahlqvist R. Inhibition of desipramine 2-hydroxylation by quinidine and quinine. *Clin Pharmacol Ther* (1988) 43, 577–81.
5. Pfandl B, Mörike K, Winne D, Schareck W, Breyer-Pfaff U. Stereoselective inhibition of nortriptyline hydroxylation in man by quinidine. *Xenobiotica* (1992) 22, 721–30.
6. Von Moltke LL, Greenblatt DJ, Cotreau-Bibbo MM, Duan SX, Harmatz JS, Shader RI. Inhibition of desipramine hydroxylation *in vitro* by serotonin-reuptake-inhibitor antidepressants, and by quinidine and ketoconazole: a model system to predict drug interactions *in vivo*. *J Pharmacol Exp Ther* (1994) 268, 1278–83.

Tricyclic antidepressants + Rifampicin (Rifampin)

In three patients a marked reduction in nortriptyline and amitriptyline levels occurred when rifampicin was given.

Clinical evidence

A man with tuberculosis needed to take 175-mg doses of **nortriptyline** to achieve therapeutic serum levels while taking isoniazid 300 mg, rifampicin 600 mg, pyrazinamide 1.5 g and pyridoxine 25 mg daily. Three weeks after stopping the antitubercular drugs, the patient suddenly became drowsy and his **nortriptyline** serum levels were found to have risen from 193 nanomol/L to 562 nanomol/L, and later to 671 nanomol/L. It was then found possible to maintain his **nortriptyline** serum levels in the range of 150 to 500 nanomol/L with only 75 mg of **nortriptyline** daily.[1]

A woman taking **amitriptyline** and fluoxetine had a marked fall in her plasma **amitriptyline** levels when she took rifampicin 600 mg, isoniazid 200 mg and ethambutol 1.2 g daily. When these antitubercular drugs were stopped, her **amitriptyline** plasma levels rose.[2] In a further case, in a 43-year-old woman, the serum levels of **nortriptyline** 50 mg daily were not detectable when rifampicin 600 mg daily was given. Increasing the dose of **nortriptyline** to 75 mg daily failed to produce detectable serum levels. Two weeks after discontinuation of rifampicin, **nortriptyline** levels increased.[3]

Mechanism

It seems highly probable that rifampicin (a well recognised and potent enzyme inducer) increased the metabolism of nortriptyline and amitriptyline by the liver thereby reducing their levels.

Importance and management

Information about the interaction between tricyclic antidepressants and rifampicin seems to be limited to just these three reports, which is a little surprising since both have been widely used for a considerable time. This suggests that generally this interaction may have limited clinical importance. However, bear this interaction in mind if patients taking rifampicin seem unresponsive to treatment with tricyclics. Increase the tricyclic dosage if necessary, and remember to readjust the dose if rifampicin is stopped.

1. Bebchuk JM, Stewart DE. Drug interaction between rifampin and nortriptyline: a case report. *Int J Psychiatry Med* (1991) 21, 183–7.
2. Bertschy G, Vandel S, Perault MC. Un cas d'interaction métabolique: amitriptyline, fluoxétine, antituberculeux. *Therapie* (1994) 49, 509–12.
3. Self T, Corley CR, Nabhan S, Abell T. Case report: interaction of rifampin and nortriptyline. *Am J Med Sci* (1996) 311, 80–1.

Tricyclic antidepressants + SNRIs

The use of duloxetine or venlafaxine with the tricyclics is expected to increase the risk of serotonin syndrome: cases have been seen with venlafaxine. Increased antimuscarinic adverse effects, movement disorders and seizures have also been reported. Venlafaxine and duloxetine appear to increase the levels of desipramine or its 2-hydroxydesipramine metabolite. Other tricyclics are expected to interact similarly.

Clinical evidence

(a) Duloxetine

In a study in healthy subjects, duloxetine 60 mg twice daily increased the AUC of a single 50-mg dose of **desipramine** 2.9-fold.[1]

(b) Venlafaxine

A 74-year-old man taking venlafaxine 150 mg daily and thioridazine had his treatment changed to daily doses of venlafaxine 75 mg, **desipramine** 50 mg, haloperidol 500 micrograms and alprazolam 250 micrograms. Within 5 days he exhibited severe antimuscarinic adverse effects (acute confusion, delirium, stupor, urinary retention and paralytic ileus). This was attributed to an interaction between the venlafaxine and **desipramine**.[2] Similarly, a 75-year-old man taking haloperidol, alprazolam and venlafaxine developed urinary retention and became delirious when he also took **desipramine**.[3] Similar effects have been seen in other cases involving **nortriptyline** 20 mg daily[4] and **clomipramine** 150 mg daily.[3]

A 69-year-old man with bipolar disorder, who had been taking venlafaxine up to 337.5 mg daily, thioridazine 25 mg at night, and sodium valproate 1.2 g daily for several months with no adverse motor symptoms, experienced extrapyramidal effects 3 to 4 days after the venlafaxine was gradually replaced by **nortriptyline** 50 mg daily. Symptoms persisted despite withdrawal of thioridazine, but improved on reduction of the **nortriptyline** dosage to 20 mg daily.[5]

A 25-year-old woman taking venlafaxine 150 mg daily and **trimipramine** 50 mg daily for depression developed seizures within 11 days of the **trimipramine** dose being increased to 100 mg daily. Both drugs were stopped and the patient had no further seizures.[6]

There is also a report of the serotonin syndrome occurring in a 21-year-old patient when **amitriptyline** 10 mg at night was added to the range of medications she was receiving, which included venlafaxine 37.5 mg daily, pethidine (meperidine) 400 mg daily and fluconazole 200 mg daily.[7] There are two other reports of the serotonin syndrome in patients who had discontinued venlafaxine 3 days and 2 weeks, respectively, before starting **amitriptyline**.[8,9]

Venlafaxine has only slight effects on the metabolism of **imipramine** to desipramine (AUC and maximum concentrations increased by 35%),[10,11] but the AUC of another metabolite, 2-hydroxydesipramine, is increased 4.5-fold by venlafaxine 75 mg twice daily.[11]

Mechanism

Not fully established. It has been suggested that venlafaxine can inhibit the metabolism of these tricyclics by the cytochrome P450 isoenzyme CYP2D6, leading to an increase in their serum levels and a marked increase in their antimuscarinic adverse effects.[3] However, studies indicate that venlafaxine is a relatively weak inhibitor of CYP2D6.[10] Nevertheless, it does appear to have some effect on the metabolism of desipramine.

The other effects (seizures, antimuscarinic effects, serotonin syndrome) seem likely to have occurred due to the additive effects of the venlafaxine and tricyclic.

Importance and management

Information regarding an interaction between the tricyclics and SNRIs appears to be sparse, mainly coming from case reports, although an interaction resulting in raised tricyclic levels appears to be established. It would therefore seem prudent to monitor for antimuscarinic adverse effects (dry mouth, urinary retention, constipation) in any patient given the combination and consider reducing the dose of the tricyclic if adverse effects become troublesome.

There only appears to be one case report describing serotonin syndrome with venlafaxine and amitriptyline, and this particular case is complicated by the presence of fluconazole, which can increase amitriptyline levels (see 'Tricyclic and related antidepressants + Azoles; Fluconazole', p.1502), and pethidine (meperidine), which has also been implicated in cases of serotonin syndrome. Nevertheless, both the tricyclics and the SNRIs have been associated with this effect, and so some caution would seem warranted. For more information on serotonin syndrome and its management, see 'Drugs that cause serotonin syndrome + Other drugs that cause serotonin syndrome', p.1471.

1. Skinner MH, Kuan H-Y, Pan A, Sathirakul K, Knadler MP, Gonzales CR, Yeo KP, Reddy S, Lim M, Ayan-Oshodi M, Wise SD. Duloxetine is both an inhibitor and a substrate of cytochrome P4502D6 in healthy volunteers. *Clin Pharmacol Ther* (2003) 73, 170–7.
2. Benazzi F. Anticholinergic toxic syndrome with venlafaxine-desipramine combination. *Pharmacopsychiatry* (1998) 31, 36–7.
3. Benazzi F. Venlafaxine drug-drug interactions in clinical practice. *J Psychiatry Neurosci* (1998) 23, 181–2.
4. Benazzi F. Venlafaxine-fluoxetine-nortriptyline interaction. *J Psychiatry Neurosci* (1997) 22, 278–9.
5. Conforti D, Borgherini G, Fiorellini Bernardis LA, Magni G. Extrapyramidal symptoms associated with the adjunct of nortriptyline to a venlafaxine-valproic acid combination. *Int Clin Psychopharmacol* (1999) 14, 197–8.

6. Schlienger RG, Klink MH, Eggenberger C, Drewe J. Seizures associated with therapeutic doses of venlafaxine and trimipramine. *Ann Pharmacother* (2000) 34, 1402–5.
7. Dougherty JA, Young H, Shafi T. Serotonin syndrome induced by amitriptyline, meperidine, and venlafaxine. *Ann Pharmacother* (2002) 36, 1647–8.
8. McDaniel WW. Serotonin syndrome: early management with cyproheptadine. *Ann Pharmacother* (2001) 35, 870–3.
9. Perry NK. Venlafaxine-induced serotonin syndrome with relapse following amitriptyline. *Postgrad Med J* (2000) 76, 254–6.
10. Efexor (Venlafaxine hydrochloride). Wyeth Pharmaceuticals. UK Summary of product characteristics, March 2008.
11. Effexor XR (Venlafaxine hydrochloride). Wyeth Pharmaceuticals Inc. US Prescribing information, March 2014.

Tricyclic and related antidepressants + SSRIs

The concentrations of the tricyclic antidepressants can be increased by the SSRIs, but the extent varies greatly, from 20% to 10-fold: fluvoxamine, fluoxetine, and paroxetine appear to have the greatest effects. Tricyclic toxicity has been seen in a number of cases. Tricyclics might increase the concentrations of citalopram and possibly fluvoxamine, but the importance of this is unclear. There are several case reports of serotonin syndrome following concurrent, and even sequential, use of the SSRIs and tricyclics.

One study suggested that there was no clinically important pharmacokinetic interaction between fluoxetine and mianserin.

Clinical evidence

(a) Citalopram

In one study[1] citalopram caused a 47% increase in the AUC of desipramine (the primary metabolite of **imipramine**), and a reduction in the concentrations of the subsequently formed metabolite of desipramine (2-hydroxydesipramine) after a single 100-mg oral dose of **imipramine**. In contrast, 5 patients taking **amitriptyline, clomipramine** or **maprotiline** had no changes in their plasma tricyclic antidepressant concentrations when citalopram 20 to 60 mg daily was also given.[2] In another general study, in which 18 patients were given citalopram and tricyclic antidepressants, the serum concentrations of citalopram were doubled in those receiving **clomipramine**; pooled results for all the tricyclics showed a 44% increase in serum citalopram concentrations.[3] An increase of this size is of doubtful clinical importance with citalopram. In 2 patients the plasma concentrations of **clomipramine** 100 mg daily remained stable when the dose was reduced to 75 mg daily and citalopram 40 mg daily was started.[4,5] One had elevated concentrations of desmethylclomipramine[4] and the other had elevated concentrations of the active metabolite, 8-hydroxydesmethylclomipramine.[5]

A case report describes elevated **desipramine** concentrations in a patient taking paroxetine that resolved when the patient was switched to citalopram.[6]

(b) Escitalopram

Escitalopram 20 mg daily for 21 days increased the maximum serum concentrations of a single 50-mg dose of **desipramine** by 40% and increased the AUC 2-fold, respectively.[7]

(c) Fluoxetine

Four patients given **desipramine** 300 mg, **imipramine** 150 mg or **nortriptyline** 100 mg, each daily, had 2- to 4-fold increases in plasma tricyclic antidepressant concentrations within 1 to 2 weeks of starting fluoxetine 10 to 60 mg daily. Two of them developed antimuscarinic adverse effects (constipation, urinary hesitancy).[8] A report describes extremely high concentrations and prolonged elimination of **imipramine** following overdose with "a handful" of **imipramine** tablets in a patient taking fluoxetine 20 mg daily.[9]

Controlled studies have also found large increases in the exposure to tricyclics in patients taking fluoxetine. In one, the exposure to desipramine was increased 4.8-fold (range 2.5 to 6.3-fold) by the concurrent use of fluoxetine.[10] A number of other reports and studies clearly confirm that sizeable increases occur in the concentrations of **amitriptyline**,[11-14] **clomipramine**,[12,15] **desipramine**,[16-24] **imipramine**,[12,20-22,25,26] **nortriptyline**[18,19,27-29] and possibly **protriptyline**,[30] accompanied by toxicity, if fluoxetine is added without reducing the dose of the tricyclic antidepressant. Delirium and seizures have also been described,[21,31] and a death has been attributed to chronic **amitriptyline** toxicity caused by fluoxetine.[32] The pharmacokinetics of fluoxetine appear not to be affected by **amitriptyline**.[14]

A migraine-like stroke developed in a woman 48 hours after her long-standing treatment with fluoxetine 100 mg daily was abruptly changed to **clomipramine** 200 mg daily.[33]

A study involving 34 patients found that the combination of fluoxetine 20 mg daily and **mianserin** 30 mg daily was superior to fluoxetine and placebo in the acute treatment of major depression, and no major adverse effects were reported. However, 12 patients did not complete 6 weeks of treatment, and of these, 2 dropped out because of adverse effects (dizziness and sedation) after one and 3 weeks, respectively. After 4 weeks of treatment, headache and increased body weight occurred more frequently in those taking both drugs than in those taking fluoxetine alone. **Mianserin** had no effect on fluoxetine plasma concentrations and the plasma concentration of mianserin was similar to that previously reported.[34]

(d) Fluvoxamine

The **amitriptyline** plasma concentrations of 8 patients rose (range 15 to 233%) when they were also given fluvoxamine 100 to 300 mg daily. Even larger rises in plasma **clomipramine** concentrations occurred (up to 8-fold) in four other patients given fluvoxamine 100 to 300 mg daily. The tricyclic doses remained the same or were slightly lower. No toxicity was seen.[35-37]

A number of other reports and studies confirm that increases occur in the concentrations of **amitriptyline**,[38-41] **clomipramine**,[38-43] **desipramine**,[44-47] **imipramine**,[38,39,44-48] **maprotiline**[38] and **trimipramine**[49] in the presence of fluvoxamine. This interaction seems severe with **clomipramine** (a 10-fold rise in one case)[43] and mild with **desipramine**.[46,47] One study also suggested that fluvoxamine concentrations may be raised by tricyclics.[38] An isolated report describes worsening depression in a patient taking **dosulepin** 75 mg daily and **mianserin** within 24 hours of replacing the **dosulepin** with fluvoxamine 75 mg daily. The symptoms continued during the next day but were reversed within a day of fluvoxamine being replaced with **dosulepin**.[50]

(e) Paroxetine

A study in 17 healthy subjects taking **desipramine** 50 mg daily found that when they were also given paroxetine 20 mg daily for 10 days the maximum plasma concentration of the **desipramine** increased 4.6-fold, the minimum plasma concentration increased 6.1-fold and the AUC increased 5.2-fold. About a 10-fold increase in the maximum plasma concentrations and AUC of the paroxetine also occurred.[51] Another study found a 5-fold decrease in **desipramine** clearance in the presence of paroxetine 20 mg daily.[52] Paroxetine has also been shown to increase the concentrations of **clomipramine**,[53] **desipramine**,[6] **imipramine**,[54,55] and **trimipramine**.[56] This resulted in a variety of adverse effects including dizziness,[53] confusion,[6] sedation[56] and memory impairment.[56]

A 21-year-old man developed serotonin syndrome when he took one tablet of paroxetine only one day after stopping **desipramine**, which he had taken for 5 days. He recovered after treatment with cyproheptadine.[57] A woman taking paroxetine 30 mg daily developed serotonin syndrome (tachycardia, delirium, bizarre movements, myoclonus) within 2 hours of taking a single 50-mg dose of **imipramine**. She recovered when treated with intravenous fluids, sedation and cyproheptadine.[58]

(f) Sertraline

In 9 healthy subjects, sertraline 50 mg daily increased the maximum plasma concentrations of **desipramine** 50 mg daily by 31% at steady-state, and increased the AUC by 23%.[10] A later related study in 17 healthy subjects by the same group of workers found that, using the same drug doses, sertraline increased the **desipramine** maximum plasma concentrations by 44%, the minimum concentrations by 19% and the AUC by 37%. The maximum plasma concentrations and AUC of the sertraline were increased about 2-fold.[51] Other studies have found that sertraline increases **desipramine**,[59-62] **imipramine**,[59] and **nortriptyline**[63] concentrations, but it has also been suggested that sertraline has no effect on **imipramine** concentrations.[64,65]

A woman who had been taking sertraline 50 mg daily (as well as morphine sulfate and pericyazine) developed serotonin syndrome within 3 days of starting to take **amitriptyline** 75 mg daily. She recovered when all of the psychotropic drugs were withdrawn.[66]

Mechanism

Fluoxetine, paroxetine, and to a lesser extent sertraline and citalopram, inhibit CYP2D6, which is involved in the metabolism of the tricyclic antidepressants. Hence these SSRIs cause tricyclic concentrations to rise. Fluvoxamine causes a similar effect, probably by inhibiting metabolism through CYP1A2 and possibly other isoenzymes. The elevated concentrations of 8-hydroxydesmethylclomipramine during concurrent clomipramine and citalopram administration in one patient may have been due to the inhibition of glucuronidation by citalopram.[5] The interaction is likely to vary depending on the various routes of metabolism of the tricyclics, and the various cytochrome P450 isoenzymes inhibited by the SSRIs. See 'Table 35.2', p.1465, for information on the metabolic routes of the tricyclics and the inhibitory potential of the SSRIs.

Serotonin syndrome possibly develops because both the tricyclics and SSRIs affect serotonin transmission, which may result in increased serotonin concentrations.

Importance and management

The interactions of the SSRIs and tricyclic antidepressants are established and of clinical importance. The SSRIs increase tricyclic concentrations, with fluvoxamine, fluoxetine and paroxetine apparently having the greatest effects. The increased tricyclic concentrations can be beneficial.[38,41,67] However, it has been suggested that patients given fluoxetine should have their tricyclic dose reduced to one-quarter.[20] Similar recommendations have been made with fluvoxamine (reduction in tricyclic dose to one-third)[44] and sertraline.[68] It would also seem prudent to consider a dose reduction of the tricyclic if paroxetine is added. Some suggest that a small initial dose of the SSRI should also be used.[68]

Patients taking any combination of tricyclic and SSRI should be monitored for adverse effects (e.g. dry mouth, sedation, confusion) with tricyclic concentrations monitored where possible. Remember that the active metabolite of fluoxetine has a half-life of 7 to 15 days, and so any interaction may persist for some time after the fluoxetine is withdrawn,[69-71] and may occur on sequential use. The manufacturer of clomipramine also recommends avoidance of drugs that can cause an accumulation of clomipramine and they advise a washout period of 2 to 3 weeks before and after treatment with fluoxetine.[72]

Serotonin syndrome seems to occur rarely but patients and prescribers should be aware of the symptoms so that prompt action can be taken if problems occur. For more about the serotonin syndrome and its management, see 'Drugs that cause serotonin syndrome + Other drugs that cause serotonin syndrome', p.1471.

1. Gram LF, Hansen MG, Sindrup SH, Brøsen K, Poulsen JH, Aaes-Jørgensen T, Overø KF. Citalopram: interaction studies with levomepromazine, imipramine and lithium. *Ther Drug Monit* (1993) 15, 18–24.

2. Baettig D, Bondolfi G, Montaldi S, Amey M, Baumann P. Tricyclic antidepressant plasma levels after augmentation with citalopram: a case study. *Eur J Clin Pharmacol* (1993) 44, 403–5.
3. Leinonen E, Lepola U, Koponen H, Kinnunen I. The effect of age and concomitant treatment with other psychoactive drugs on serum concentrations of citalopram measured with a nonenantioselective method. *Ther Drug Monit* (1996) 18, 111–17.
4. Haffen E, Vandel P, Broly F, Vandel S, Sechter D, Bizouard P, Bechtel PR. Citalopram: an interaction study with clomipramine in a patient heterozygous for CYP2D6 genotype. *Pharmacopsychiatry* (1999) 32, 232–4.
5. Haffen E, Vandel P, Bonin B, Vandel S. Citalopram pharmacokinetic interaction with clomipramine. UDP-glucuronosyltransferase inhibition? A case report. *Therapie* (1999) 54, 768–70.
6. Ashton AK. Lack of desipramine toxicity with citalopram. *J Clin Psychiatry* (2000) 61, 144.
7. Lexapro (Escitalopram oxalate). Forest Pharmaceuticals Inc. US Prescribing information, July 2014.
8. Aranow RB, Hudson JI, Pope HG, Grady TA, Laage TA, Bell IR, Cole JO. Elevated antidepressant plasma levels after addition of fluoxetine. *Am J Psychiatry* (1989) 146, 911–13.
9. Rosenstein DL, Takeshita J, Nelson JC. Fluoxetine-induced elevation and prolongation of tricyclic levels in overdose. *Am J Psychiatry* (1991) 148, 807.
10. Preskorn SH, Alderman J, Chung M, Harrison W, Messig M, Harris S. Pharmacokinetics of desipramine coadministered with sertraline or fluoxetine. *J Clin Psychopharmacol* (1994) 14, 90–8.
11. March JS, Moon RL, Johnston H. Fluoxetine-TCA interaction. *J Am Acad Child Adolesc Psychiatry* (1990) 29, 985–6.
12. Vandel S, Bertschy G, Bonin B, Nezelof S, François TH, Vandel B, Sechter D, Bizouard P. Tricyclic antidepressant plasma levels after fluoxetine addition. *Neuropsychobiology* (1992) 25, 202–7.
13. Bertschy G, Vandel S, Perault MC. Un cas d'interaction métabolique: amitriptyline, fluoxétine, anti-tuberculeux. *Therapie* (1994) 49, 509–12.
14. El-Yazigi A, Chaleby K, Gad A, Raines DA. Steady-state kinetics of fluoxetine and amitriptyline in patients treated with a combination of these drugs as compared with those treated with amitriptyline alone. *J Clin Pharmacol* (1995) 35, 17–21.
15. Balant-Gorgia AE, Ries C, Balant LP. Metabolic interaction between fluoxetine and clomipramine: A case report. *Pharmacopsychiatry* (1996) 29, 38–41.
16. Bell IR, Cole JO. Fluoxetine induces elevation of desipramine level and exacerbation of geriatric nonpsychotic depression. *J Clin Psychopharmacol* (1988) 8, 447–8.
17. Goodnick PJ. Influence of fluoxetine on plasma levels of desipramine. *Am J Psychiatry* (1989) 146, 552.
18. Vaughan DA. Interaction of fluoxetine with tricyclic antidepressants. *Am J Psychiatry* (1988) 145, 1478.
19. von Ammon Cavanaugh S. Drug-drug interactions of fluoxetine with tricyclics. *Psychosomatics* (1990) 31, 273–6.
20. Westermeyer J. Fluoxetine-induced tricyclic toxicity: extent and duration. *J Clin Pharmacol* (1991) 31, 388–92.
21. Preskorn SH, Beber JH, Faul JC, Hirschfeld RMA. Serious adverse effects of combining fluoxetine and tricyclic antidepressants. *Am J Psychiatry* (1990) 147, 532.
22. Bergstrom RF, Peyton AL, Lemberger L. Quantification and mechanism of the fluoxetine and tricyclic antidepressant interaction. *Clin Pharmacol Ther* (1992) 51, 239–48.
23. Nelson JC, Mazure CM, Bowers MB, Jatlow PI. A preliminary, open study of the combination of fluoxetine and desipramine for rapid treatment of major depression. *Arch Gen Psychiatry* (1991) 48, 303–7.
24. Wilens TE, Biederman J, Baldessarini RJ, McDermott SP, Puopolo PR, Flood JG. Fluoxetine inhibits desipramine metabolism. *Arch Gen Psychiatry* (1992) 49, 752.
25. Faynor SM, Espina V. Fluoxetine inhibition of imipramine metabolism. *Clin Chem* (1989) 35, 1180.
26. Hahn SM, Griffin JH. Comment: fluoxetine adverse effects and drug interactions. *DICP Ann Pharmacother* (1991) 25, 1273–4.
27. Kahn DG. Increased plasma nortriptyline concentration in a patient cotreated with fluoxetine. *J Clin Psychiatry* (1990) 51, 36.
28. Schraml F, Benedetti G, Hoyle K, Clayton A. Fluoxetine and nortriptyline combination therapy. *Am J Psychiatry* (1989) 146, 1636–7.
29. Downs JM, Downs AD, Rosenthal TL, Deal N, Akiskal HS. Increased plasma tricyclic antidepressant concentrations in two patients concurrently treated with fluoxetine. *J Clin Psychiatry* (1989) 50, 226–7.
30. Paul K-L, Bhatara VS. Anticholinergic delirium possibly associated with protriptyline and fluoxetine. *Ann Pharmacother* (1997) 31, 1260–1.
31. Sternbach H. Fluoxetine-clomipramine interaction. *J Clin Psychiatry* (1995) 56, 171–2.
32. Preskorn SH, Baker B. Fatality associated with combined fluoxetine-amitriptyline therapy. *JAMA* (1997) 277, 1682.
33. Molaie M. Serotonin syndrome presenting with migraine like stroke. *Headache* (1997) 37, 519–21.
34. Dam J, Ryde L, Svejsø J, Lauge N, Lauritsen B, Bech P. Morning fluoxetine plus evening mianserin versus morning fluoxetine plus evening placebo in the acute treatment of major depression. *Pharmacopsychiatry* (1998) 31, 48–54.
35. Vandel S, Bertschy G, Allers G. Fluvoxamine tricyclic antidepressant interaction. *Therapie* (1990) 45, 21.
36. Bertschy G, Vandel S, Vandel B, Allers G, Vomat R. Fluvoxamine-tricyclic antidepressant interaction. An accidental finding. *Eur J Clin Pharmacol* (1991) 40, 119–120.
37. Bertschy G, Vandel S, Nezelof S, Bizouard P, Bechtel P. L'interaction fluvoxamine-antidépresseurs tricycliques. *Therapie* (1993) 48, 63–4.
38. Härtter S, Wetzel H, Hammes E, Hiemke C. Inhibition of antidepressant demethylation and hydroxylation by fluvoxamine in depressed patients. *Psychopharmacology (Berl)* (1993) 110, 302–8.
39. Szegedi A, Wetzel H, Leal M, Härtter S, Hiemke C. Combination treatment with clomipramine and fluvoxamine: drug monitoring, safety, and tolerability data. *J Clin Psychiatry* (1996) 57, 257–64.
40. Vandel S, Bertschy G, Baumann P, Bouquet S, Bonin B, Francois T, Sechter D, Bizouard P. Fluvoxamine and fluoxetine: Interaction studies with amitriptyline, clomipramine and neuroleptics in phenotyped patients. *Pharmacol Res* (1995) 31, 347–53.
41. Vandel P, Bonin B, Bertschy G, Baumann P, Bouquet S, Vandel S, Sechter D, Bizouard P. Observations of the interaction between tricyclic antidepressants and fluvoxamine in poor metabolisers of dextromethorphan and mephenytoin. *Therapie* (1997) 52, 74–6.
42. Conus P, Bondolfi G, Eap CB, Macciardi F, Baumann P. Pharmacokinetic fluvoxamine-clomipramine interaction with favorable therapeutic consequences in therapy-resistant depressive patient. *Pharmacopsychiatry* (1996) 29, 108–110.
43. Roberge C, Lecordier-Maret F, Beljean-Leymarie M, Heriault F, Starace J. Major drug interaction between fluvoxamine and clomipramine: about a case report. *J Pharm Clin* (1998) 17, 117–19.
44. Spina E, Campo GM, Avenoso A, Pollicino MA, Caputi AP. Interaction between fluvoxamine and imipramine/desipramine in four patients. *Ther Drug Monit* (1992) 14, 194–6.
45. Maskall DD, Lam RW. Increased plasma concentration of imipramine following augmentation with fluvoxamine. *Am J Psychiatry* (1993) 150, 1566.
46. Spina E, Pollicino AM, Avenso A, Campo GM, Caputi AP. Fluvoxamine-induced alterations in plasma concentrations of imipramine and desipramine in depressed patients. *Int J Clin Pharmacol Res* (1993) 13, 167–71.
47. Spina E, Pollicino AM, Avenoso A, Campo GM, Perucca E, Caputi AP. Effect of fluvoxamine on the pharmacokinetics of imipramine and desipramine in healthy subjects. *Ther Drug Monit* (1993) 15, 243–6.
48. Xu Z-H, Huang S-L, Zhou H-H. Inhibition of imipramine *N*-demethylation by fluvoxamine in Chinese young men. *Acta Pharmacol Sin* (1996) 17, 399–402.
49. Seifritz E, Holsboer-Trachsler E, Hemmeter U, Eap CB, Baumann P. Increased trimipramine plasma levels during fluvoxamine comedication. *Eur Neuropsychopharmacol* (1994) 4, 15–20.
50. Sato K, Yoshida K, Higuchi H, Shimizu T. Rapid worsening of depressive symptoms in a patient with depression after switching from a TCA to an SSRI. *J Neuropsychiatr Clin Neurosci* (2002) 14, 357.
51. Alderman J, Preskorn SH, Greenblatt DJ, Harrison W, Penenberg D, Allison J, Chung M. Desipramine pharmacokinetics when coadministered with paroxetine or sertraline in extensive metabolizers. *J Clin Psychopharmacol* (1997) 17, 284–91.
52. Brøsen K, Hansen JG, Nielsen KK, Sindrup SH, Gram LF. Inhibition by paroxetine of desipramine metabolism in extensive but not in poor metabolizers of sparteine. *Eur J Clin Pharmacol* (1993) 44, 349–55.
53. Skjelbo EF, Brøsen K. Interaktion imellem paroxetin og clomipramin som mulig årsag til indlæggelse på medicinsk afdeling. *Ugeskr Laeger* (1998) 160, 5665–6.
54. Albers LJ, Reist C, Helmeste D, Vu R, Tang SW. Paroxetine shifts imipramine metabolism. *Psychiatry Res* (1996) 59, 189–96.
55. Yoon YR, Shim JC, Shin JG, Shon JH, Kim YH, Cha IJ. Drug interaction between paroxetine and imipramine. Kor Soc Pharmacol Meeting, Seoul, S Korea, October 1997, p168.
56. Leinonen E, Koponen HJ, Lepola U. Paroxetine increases serum trimipramine concentration. A report of two cases. *Hum Psychopharmacol* (1995) 10, 345–7.
57. Chan BSH, Graudins A, Whyte IM, Dawson AH, Braitberg G, Duggin GG. Serotonin syndrome resulting from drug interactions. *Med J Aust* (1998) 169, 523–5.
58. Weiner AL, Tilden FF, McKay CA. Serotonin syndrome: case report and review of the literature. *Conn Med* (1997) 61, 717–21.
59. Kurtz DL, Bergstrom RF, Goldberg MJ, Cerimele BJ. The effect of sertraline on the pharmacokinetics of desipramine and imipramine. *Clin Pharmacol Ther* (1997) 62, 145–56.
60. Zussman BD, Davie CC, Fowles SE, Kumar R, Lang U, Wargenau M, Sourgens H. Sertraline, like other SSRIs, is a significant inhibitor of desipramine metabolism in vivo. *Br J Clin Pharmacol* (1995) 39, 550P–551P.
61. Lydiard RB, Anton RF, Cunningham T. Interactions between sertraline and tricyclic antidepressants. *Am J Psychiatry* (1993) 150, 1125–6.
62. Barros J, Asnis G. An interaction of sertraline and desipramine. *Am J Psychiatry* (1993) 150, 1751.
63. Solai LK, Mulsant BH, Pollock BG, Sweet RA, Rosen J, Yu K, Reynolds CF. Effect of sertraline on plasma nortriptyline levels in depressed elderly. *J Clin Psychiatry* (1997) 58, 440–3.
64. Erikson SM, Carson SW, Grimsley S, Carter JG, Kumar A, Jann MW. Effect of sertraline on steady-state serum concentrations of imipramine and its metabolites. *Pharmacotherapy* (1994) 14, 368.
65. Jann MW, Carson SW, Grimsley SR, Erikson S, Kumar A, Carter JG. Effects of sertraline upon imipramine pharmacodynamics. *Clin Pharmacol Ther* (1995) 57, 207.
66. Alderman CP, Lee PC. Comment: serotonin syndrome associated with combined sertraline-amitriptyline treatment. *Ann Pharmacother* (1996) 30, 1499–1500.
67. Wetzel H, Härtter A, Szegedi A, Hammes E, Leal M, Hiemke C. Fluvoxamine co-medication to tricyclic antidepressants: metabolic interactions, clinical efficiency and side-effects. *Pharmacopsychiatry* (1993) 26, 211.
68. Eiber R, Escande M. Associations et interactions: les antidépresseurs tricycliques et les inhibiteurs spécifiques de la recapture de la sérotonine. *Encephale* (1999) 25, 584–9.
69. Downs JM, Dahmer SK. Fluoxetine and elevated plasma levels of tricyclic antidepressants. *Am J Psychiatry* (1990) 147, 1251.
70. Skowron DM, Gutierrez MA, Epstein S. Precaution with titrating nortriptyline after the use of fluoxetine. *DICP Ann Pharmacother* (1990) 24, 1008.
71. Müller N, Brockmöller J, Roots I. Extremely long plasma half-life of amitriptyline in a woman with the cytochrome P450IID6 29/29-kilobase wild-type allele — a slowly reversible interaction with fluoxetine. *Ther Drug Monit* (1991) 13, 533–6.
72. Anafranil (Clomipramine hydrochloride). Novartis Pharmaceuticals UK Ltd. UK Summary of product characteristics, January 2014.

Tricyclic antidepressants + St John's wort (*Hypericum perforatum*)

The plasma levels of amitriptyline, and its active metabolite, nortriptyline, are modestly reduced by St John's wort.

Clinical evidence

Twelve depressed patients were given **amitriptyline** 75 mg twice daily and St John's wort extract (*Lichtwer Pharma, Berlin*) 900 mg daily for at least 14 days. The AUC_{0-12} of the **amitriptyline** was reduced by about 22% and the AUC of nortriptyline (its metabolite) was reduced by about 41%.[1]

Mechanism

Not fully understood. St John's wort is known to induce the activity of the cytochrome P450 isoenzyme CYP3A4, which is a minor route of metabolism of the tricyclic antidepressants. However, the tricyclics are predominantly metabolised by CYP2D6, so an effect on CYP3A4 is unlikely to lead to a clinically relevant reduction in their levels. Induction of P-glycoprotein by St John's wort may also contribute; however, the extent of its involvement in the transport of the tricyclics is unclear.

Importance and management

The evidence for an interaction is limited to this study, and based on the minor reduction in amitriptyline levels seen, it seems unlikely that a clinically significant reduction in efficacy would occur. Other tricyclics would be expected to interact similarly.

Both the tricyclics and St John's wort are antidepressants, but whether concurrent use is beneficial or safe is not known, and it was not assessed in this study. Further study is needed. However, note that some tricyclics (see 'Table 35.3', p.1472) and St John's wort have serotonergic effects, and concurrent use might lead to the serotonin syndrome. Serotonin syndrome is a rare adverse effect, but because of its severity, some caution is warranted if both drugs are given. For more information on serotonin syndrome and its management, see 'Drugs that cause serotonin syndrome + Other drugs that cause serotonin syndrome', p.1471.

1. Johne A, Schmider J, Brockmöller J, Stadelmann AM, Störmer E, Bauer S, Scholler G, Langheinrich M, Roots I. Decreased plasma levels of amitriptyline and its metabolites on comedication with an extract from St. John's wort (*Hypericum perforatum*). *J Clin Psychopharmacol* (2002) 22, 46–54.

Tricyclic antidepressants + Sucralfate

Sucralfate causes a modest decrease in the absorption of amitriptyline.

Clinical evidence, mechanism, importance and management

When 6 healthy subjects took a single 75-mg dose of **amitriptyline** with a single 1-g dose of sucralfate, the AUC of the amitriptyline was decreased by 50%.[1] This reduction probably occurred because sucralfate decreased the absorption of amitriptyline from the gut. There seems to be nothing documented about other tricyclics, but they would be expected to interact similarly.

If sucralfate is given to a patient taking any tricyclic antidepressant it would seem prudent to monitor to confirm that the therapeutic effects of the antidepressant are not lost. It is generally recommended that other drugs should be given at least 2 hours before or after sucralfate to avoid a decrease in bioavailability.[2,3]

1. Ryan R, Carlson J, Farris F. Effect of sucralfate on the absorption and disposition of amitriptyline in humans. *Fedn Proc* (1986) 45, 205.
2. Antepsin Suspension (Sucralfate). Chugai Pharma UK Ltd. UK Summary of product characteristics, September 2013.
3. Carafate Suspension (Sucralfate). Aptalis Pharma US, Inc. US Prescribing information, March 2013.

Tricyclic antidepressants + Temsirolimus

Temsirolimus did not alter desipramine pharmacokinetics in a single-dose study.

Clinical evidence, mechanism, importance and management

In a single-dose study in healthy subjects, the pharmacokinetics of oral desipramine 50 mg were unaffected by intravenous temsirolimus 25 mg given at the same time.[1] On the basis of this study, the manufacturer does not anticipate that a pharmacokinetic interaction will occur when temsirolimus is given at this dose with drugs that are substrates of the cytochrome P450 isoenzyme CYP2D6.[2,3] For a list of CYP2D6 substrates, see 'Table 1.7', p.9. However, simultaneous dosing of these two drugs would not have allowed for maximal hepatic enzyme inhibition, so a multiple-dose study or single-dose study where desipramine was given on day 2 or 3 after intravenous temsirolimus would provide more proof of a lack of interaction. Furthermore, based on *in vitro* studies in human liver microsomes, plasma concentrations reached after a 175 mg dose of temsirolimus might inhibit CYP2D6 and therefore caution is advised when temsirolimus is given at this dose with other drugs metabolised by CYP2D6 and that have a narrow therapeutic index.[3]

1. Boni J, Abbas R, Leister C, Burns J, Jordan R, Hoffmann M, DeMaio W, Hug B. Disposition of desipramine, a sensitive cytochrome P450 2D6 substrate, when coadministered with intravenous temsirolimus. *Cancer Chemother Pharmacol* (2009) 64, 263–70.
2. Torisel (Temsirolimus). Wyeth Pharmaceuticals Inc. US Prescribing information, October 2014.
3. Torisel (Temsirolimus). Pfizer Ltd. UK Summary of product characteristics, October 2013.

Tricyclic antidepressants + Terbinafine

Terbinafine moderately increases the AUC of desipramine. Case reports describe increases in the serum concentrations of amitriptyline, desipramine, imipramine, and nortriptyline, with associated toxicity, in patients additionally given oral terbinafine.

Clinical evidence

(a) Amitriptyline

A 37-year-old woman who had been taking amitriptyline 75 mg daily, valproate and olanzapine for 3 years, developed extreme dryness of the mouth, nausea and dizziness shortly after starting to take terbinafine 250 mg daily. Serum concentrations of amitriptyline and its metabolite nortriptyline rose from just under 400 nanomol/L to over 1800 nanomol/L. Terbinafine was stopped, and the amitriptyline dose reduced to 25 mg daily, but the amitriptyline and nortriptyline concentrations did not return to baseline for several months. The patient had normal activity of CYP2D6.[1]

(b) Desipramine

In a pharmacokinetic study, terbinafine 250 mg daily for 21 days caused a 4.9-fold increase in the AUC of a single 50-mg dose of desipramine, and increased its maximum concentrations 1.9-fold. The AUC of desipramine was still more than double that at baseline, 4 weeks after stopping desipramine. The healthy subjects used in this study were extensive CYP2D6 metabolisers (that is, they had normal activity of this isoenzyme), which is the most common phenotype.[2]

A case report describes a 3.5-fold increase in desipramine concentrations, with associated toxicity (dizziness, ataxia, incoordination, and difficulty swallowing), in a 52-year-old man taking desipramine 350 mg daily, which occurred within 2 to 3 weeks of him starting to take terbinafine. The desipramine was stopped for a few days and restarted at a dose of just 50 mg daily, which gave similar serum concentrations to those seen before terbinafine was started. When the terbinafine was stopped, the dose of desipramine needed to be gradually titrated up to the initial amount.[3]

(c) Imipramine

A 51-year-old man who had been taking lithium carbonate and varying doses of imipramine 150 to 200 mg daily for 10 years was also given oral terbinafine 250 mg daily for onychomycosis. About a week later he complained of dizziness, muscle twitching and excessive mouth dryness. His serum imipramine concentrations, measured 5 days later, had risen from his usual range of 100 to 200 nanograms/mL up to 530 nanograms/mL. Within 10 days of reducing his daily imipramine dose from 200 to 75 mg daily, his serum concentrations had fallen to 229 nanograms/mL. His liver function was normal.[4]

(d) Nortriptyline

A report describes a large increase in the serum concentrations of nortriptyline (about doubled) accompanied by evidence of toxicity (fatigue, vertigo, loss of energy and appetite, and falls) in a 74-year-old man taking nortriptyline 125 mg daily, roughly 14 days after he started to take terbinafine 250 mg daily. His symptoms responded to a dose reduction to 75 mg of nortriptyline daily. His serum concentrations were similarly elevated when he was later rechallenged with terbinafine. His liver function was normal.[5] The same authors reported a similar case in a woman who had been taking nortriptyline and terbinafine for one month before she showed signs of an interaction. A later rechallenge with terbinafine confirmed the interaction.[6]

Mechanism

Terbinafine is an inhibitor of CYP2D6, which is the principal enzyme involved in the metabolism of many tricyclics. Terbinafine can have a very prolonged half-life, so an interaction might occur or continue for a number of weeks after stopping the drug.

Importance and management

Although there are only a few case reports an interaction appears to be confirmed, and the increase in the concentrations of tricyclic antidepressant in the presence of terbinafine appears to be clinically important. It would seem prudent to monitor for tricyclic adverse effects (such as dry mouth, blurred vision and urinary retention) if terbinafine is also given, and consider reducing the dose of the tricyclic if these become troublesome. Tricyclic concentrations may return to normal only slowly after discontinuation of terbinafine.[1,2,6] It is also suggested that there might be a risk of clinically important interactions if these drugs are given within 3 months of stopping terbinafine.[1]

Note that, the tricyclics have been associated with QT prolongation, most usually when their concentrations are high, and this interaction might therefore increase the risk of this effect. See 'Drugs that prolong the QT interval + Other drugs that prolong the QT interval', p.272, for further discussion on QT prolongation.

1. Castberg I, Helle J, Aamo TO. Prolonged pharmacokinetic drug interaction between terbinafine and amitriptyline. *Ther Drug Monit* (2005) 27, 680–2.
2. Madani S, Barilla D, Cramer J, Wang Y, Paul C. Effect of terbinafine on the pharmacokinetics and pharmacodynamics of desipramine in healthy volunteers identified as cytochrome P450 2D6 (CYP2D6) extensive metabolizers. *J Clin Pharmacol* (2002) 42, 1211–18.
3. O'Reardon JP, Hetznecker JM, Rynn MA, Baldassano CF, Szuba MP. Desipramine toxicity with terbinafine. *Am J Psychiatry* (2002) 159, 492. Erratum ibid. 1076.
4. Teitelbaum ML, Pearson VE. Imipramine toxicity and terbinafine. *Am J Psychiatry* (2001) 158, 2086.
5. van der Kuy P-HM, Hooymans PM, Verkaaik AJB. Nortriptyline intoxication induced by terbinafine. *BMJ* (1998) 316, 441.
6. van der Kuy P-HM, van den Heuvel HA, Kempen RW, Vanmolkot LML. Pharmacokinetic interaction between nortriptyline and terbinafine. *Ann Pharmacother* (2002) 36, 1712–14.

Tricyclic antidepressants + Thyroid hormones

The antidepressant response to imipramine, amitriptyline, and possibly other tricyclics can be accelerated by the use of thyroid hormones. However, isolated cases of paroxysmal atrial tachycardia, thyrotoxicosis, and hypothyroidism have occurred on concurrent use with imipramine.

Clinical evidence, mechanism, importance and management

The addition of **liothyronine** 25 micrograms daily was found to increase the speed and efficacy of **imipramine** in relieving depression.[1] Similar results have been described in other studies with **desipramine**[2] or **amitriptyline**[3] but the reasons are not understood. One possible explanation is that the patients had overt or subclinical hypothyroidism, which after correction with **liothyronine** allowed them to overcome an impaired response to tricyclic antidepressants.[4] Other suggestions are that small alterations in thyroid hormone concentrations might result in alterations in cerebral function[5] and that thyroid hormones might increase receptor sensitivity to neurotransmitters such as serotonin (5-hydroxytryptamine, 5-HT).[6]

However, adverse reactions have also been seen when thyroid hormones were given with tricyclics. A patient being treated for both hypothyroidism and depression with **thyroid** 60 mg and **imipramine** 150 mg daily complained of dizziness and nausea. She was found to have developed paroxysmal atrial tachycardia.[7] A 10-year-old girl with congenital hypothyroidism, well controlled with desiccated **thyroid** 150 mg daily, developed severe thyrotoxicosis after taking **imipramine** 25 mg daily for 5 months for enuresis. The problem disappeared when the **imipramine** was withdrawn.[8] It has been suggested that desipramine (the active metabolite of imipramine) might inhibit the uptake of T3 into the brain by inhibiting monocarboxylate transporter 8 (a thyroid hormone plasma membrane transport protein)[9], resulting in increased serum T3 concentrations, which could explain the adverse effects seen in the case reports. However this needs confirmation in a clinical study.

The interaction between thyroid hormones and tricyclics is normally advantageous,[6] in which **liothyronine** appears to have a significantly greater antidepressant-potentiating effect than **levothyroxine**.[5] There would seem to be no good reason, generally speaking, for avoiding concurrent use unless problems arise.

1. Wilson IC, Prange AJ, McClane TK, Rabon AM, Lipton MA. Thyroid-hormone enhancement of imipramine in nonretarded depressions. *N Engl J Med* (1970) 282, 1063–7.
2. Extein I. Case reports of L-triiodothyronine potentiation. *Am J Psychiatry* (1982) 139, 966–7.
3. Wheatley D. Potentiation of amitriptyline by thyroid hormone. *Arch Gen Psychiatry* (1972) 26, 229–33.
4. Berlin I, Corruble E. Thyroid hormones and antidepressant response. *Am J Psychiatry* (2002) 159, 1441.
5. Joffe RT, Singer W. A comparison of triiodothyronine and thyroxine in the potentiation of tricyclic antidepressants. *Psychiatry Res* (1990) 32, 241–51.
6. Altshuler LL, Bauer M, Frye MA, Gitlin MJ, Mintz J, Szuba MP, Leight KL, Whybrow PC. Does thyroid supplementation accelerate tricyclic antidepressant response? A review and meta-analysis of the literature. *Am J Psychiatry* (2001) 158, 1617–22.
7. Prange AJ. Paroxysmal auricular tachycardia apparently resulting from combined thyroid-imipramine treatment. *Am J Psychiatry* (1963) 119, 994–5.
8. Colantonio LA, Orson JM. Triiodothyronine thyrotoxicosis. Induction by desiccated thyroid and imipramine. *Am J Dis Child* (1974) 128, 396–7.
9. Roth S, Kinne A, Schweizer U. The tricyclic antidepressant desipramine inhibits T3 import into primary neurons. *Neurosci Lett* (2010) 478, 5–8.

Tricyclic and related antidepressants + Tobacco

Smoking tobacco decreases the plasma concentrations of amitriptyline, clomipramine, desipramine, imipramine, and nortriptyline, but this does not appear to result in a clinically significant interaction. The blood concentration of maprotiline is not affected by smoking tobacco.

Clinical evidence

Two studies found no difference between the steady-state plasma concentrations of **nortriptyline** in tobacco smokers and non-smokers,[1,2] but others have found that smoking tobacco decreases the plasma concentrations of **amitriptyline**, **clomipramine**,[3] **desipramine**, **imipramine**,[4] and **nortriptyline**.[5] For example a 25% decrease in the plasma concentration of **nortriptyline** was found in one study,[5] and a 45% decrease in the total concentration of **imipramine** and its metabolite, desipramine, was found in another.[4] Smoking has no effect on the efficacy or the blood concentration of **maprotiline**.[6,7]

Mechanism

The probable reason for the decreased plasma concentrations of the tricyclics is that some of the components of tobacco smoke are enzyme inducers, which increase the metabolism of these antidepressants by the liver.

Importance and management

The interactions between tobacco smoke and the tricyclics are established, but it might wrongly be concluded from the figures quoted that smokers need higher doses of the tricyclics to control their depression. Some evidence suggests that the plasma concentration of free (and pharmacologically active) nortriptyline is greater in smokers than non-smokers (10.2% compared with 7.4%), which probably offsets the decrease in total plasma concentration.[5] Thus the apparently lower plasma concentration in smokers might be as therapeutically effective as the higher concentration in non-smokers, so that there is probably no need to increase the dosage to accommodate this interaction.

1. Norman TR, Burrows GD, Maguire KP, Rubinstein G, Scoggins BA, Davies B. Cigarette smoking and plasma nortriptyline levels. *Clin Pharmacol Ther* (1977) 21, 453–6.
2. Alexanderson B, Price Evans DA, Sjöqvist F. Steady-state plasma levels of nortriptyline in twins: influence of genetic factors and drug therapy. *BMJ* (1969) 4, 764–8.
3. John VA, Luscombe DK, Kemp H. Effects of age, cigarette smoking and the oral contraceptive on the pharmacokinetics of clomipramine and its desmethyl metabolite during chronic dosing. *J Int Med Res* (1980) 8 (Suppl 3), 88–95.
4. Perel JM, Hurwic MJ, Kanzler MB. Pharmacodynamics of imipramine in depressed patients. *Psychopharmacol Bull* (1975) 11, 16–18.
5. Perry PJ, Browne JL, Prince RA, Alexander B, Tsuang MT. Effects of smoking on nortriptyline plasma concentrations in depressed patients. *Ther Drug Monit* (1986) 8, 279–84.
6. Luscombe DK. Interaction studies: the influence of age, cigarette smoking and the oral contraceptive on blood concentrations of maprotiline. In 'Depressive Illness — Far Horizons?' McIntyre JNM (ed), Cambridge Med Publ, Northampton 1982, p 61–2.
7. Holman RM. Maprotiline and cigarette smoking: an interaction study: clinical findings. In 'Depressive Illness — Far Horizons?' McIntyre JNM (ed), Cambridge Med Publ, Northampton 1982, p 66–7.

Tricyclic antidepressants + Valproate

Amitriptyline and nortriptyline plasma levels can be increased by sodium valproate and valpromide. Status epilepticus, tremulousness and/or sleep disturbances have been attributed to elevated clomipramine or nortriptyline levels in patients taking valproate or valproic acid. Valproate pharmacokinetics may be modestly affected by amitriptyline.

Clinical evidence

(a) Amitriptyline

In one study, 15 healthy subjects were given a single 50-mg dose of amitriptyline 2 hours after taking the ninth dose of valproate semisodium 500 mg every 12 hours. The maximum plasma levels and AUC of amitriptyline were raised by 19% and 30%, respectively. The corresponding values for the nortriptyline metabolite were 28% and 55%, respectively.[1] Similarly, in 10 patients taking amitriptyline 125 mg daily, the use of valpromide 600 mg daily for 10 days caused a 50% rise in the mean steady-state plasma levels of amitriptyline and a 65% rise in the levels of the nortriptyline metabolite, when compared with 10 similar patients taking amitriptyline alone.[2,3]

A study in 6 patients with depression found that amitriptyline 100 mg daily for 3 weeks produced a 43% increase in the volume of distribution and a 16% increase in the plasma half-life of a single 400-mg intravenous dose of sodium valproate. The AUC and total body clearance of valproate were not significantly changed.[4]

(b) Clomipramine

An epileptic patient who had been seizure-free for 3 years while taking valproic acid developed a prolonged episode of status epilepticus 12 days after starting to take clomipramine 75 mg daily. The clomipramine serum level 7 hours after the last dose was 342 nanograms/mL (usual levels 68 to 272 nanograms/mL). The seizure was attributed to the elevated clomipramine levels.[5] Similarly, a patient taking clomipramine 150 mg daily, suffered feelings of numbness and sleep disturbances attributed to elevated serum levels of clomipramine and desmethylclomipramine, caused by valproate 1 to 1.4 g daily. Halving the dose of clomipramine restored serum concentrations to therapeutic levels.[6]

(c) Desipramine

A woman taking valproic acid, tiotixene and desipramine developed elevated and potentially toxic serum desipramine levels (a rise from 259 nanograms/mL to 324 nanograms/mL) at the end of a 3-month period during which valproic acid was gradually withdrawn and replaced by clorazepate. The authors of the report attributed this reaction to the valproic acid withdrawal.[7]

(d) Nortriptyline

One patient developed grossly elevated nortriptyline plasma levels (393 nanograms/mL, about threefold higher than the therapeutic range) and evidence of toxicity (tremulousness of hands and fingers) about one week after starting to take valproate 750 mg to 1 g daily. The toxicity rapidly disappeared when both drugs were stopped. Another patient, with bipolar disorder, also developed elevated nortriptyline plasma levels, attributed to the addition of valproate, and his rate of mood cycling increased.[8]

Mechanism

Uncertain. Inhibition of the metabolism of these tricyclics by valproate has been suggested.[5,6,8]

Importance and management

Information seems to be limited to these reports, and an interaction is not established. However, if tricyclic adverse effects (e.g. dry mouth, urinary retention, constipation) develop in patients also taking valproate it would be prudent to consider an interaction as a possible cause.

The occurrence of status epilepticus in one patient reinforces the fact that the tricyclics can lower the convulsive threshold and should therefore be used with caution in patients with epilepsy.

1. Wong SL, Cavanaugh J, Shi H, Awni WM, Granneman GR. Effects of divalproex sodium on amitriptyline and nortriptyline pharmacokinetics. *Clin Pharmacol Ther* (1996) 60, 48–53.
2. Bertschy G, Vandel S, Jounet JM, Allers G. Interaction valpromide-amitriptyline. Augmentation de la biodisponibilité de l'amitriptyline et de la nortriptyline par le valpromide. *Encephale* (1990) 16, 43–5.
3. Vandel S, Bertschy G, Jounet JM, Allers G. Valpromide increases the plasma concentrations of amitriptyline and its metabolite nortriptyline in depressive patients. *Ther Drug Monit* (1988) 10, 386–9.
4. Pisani F, Primerano G, D'Agostino AA, Spina E, Fazio A. Valproic acid-amitriptyline interaction in man. *Ther Drug Monit* (1986) 8, 382–3.
5. DeToledo JC, Haddad H, Ramsay RE. Status epilepticus associated with the combination of valproic acid and clomipramine. *Ther Drug Monit* (1997) 19, 71–3.
6. Fehr C, Gründer G, Hiemke C, Dahmen N. Increase in serum clomipramine concentrations caused by valproate. *J Clin Psychopharmacol* (2000) 20, 493–4.
7. Joseph AB, Wroblewski BA. Potentially toxic serum concentrations of desipramine after discontinuation of valproic acid. *Brain Inj* (1993) 7, 463–5.
8. Fu C, Katzman M, Goldbloom DS. Valproate/nortriptyline interaction. *J Clin Psychopharmacol* (1994) 14, 205–6.

Tricyclic antidepressants + Yohimbine

Low-dose yohimbine can decrease dry mouth and orthostatic hypotension associated with tricyclic antidepressants. Amitriptyline and clomipramine can increase yohimbine plasma concentrations.

Clinical evidence

In a study, 12 patients with orthostatic hypotension associated with **clomipramine** 150 mg daily for 2 to 7 days were given oral yohimbine 4 mg three times daily. Yohimbine appeared to decrease the orthostatic hypotension and induced a significant increase in blood pressure at a dose not usually associated with changes in blood pressure. However, the plasma concentration of yohimbine measured 2 hours after dosing was much greater than that seen in healthy subjects not taking **clomipramine** and appeared to correlate with the plasma concentration of desmethylclomipramine but not with that of **clomipramine**.[1]

Another study found that low-dose yohimbine 4 mg significantly increased the salivary volume for 3 hours in 10 patients with depression taking **amitriptyline** or **clomipramine**, but had no effect on salivary volume in healthy subjects not taking tricyclics. The plasma concentration of yohimbine after 90 minutes was 72.7 nanograms/mL in the patients taking the tricyclics, compared with 18.7 nanograms/mL in healthy subjects not taking tricyclics.[2]

Mechanism

Not fully understood. A pharmacodynamic interaction might occur, involving α_2-adrenoceptor inhibition by yohimbine and inhibition of noradrenaline (norepinephrine) reuptake by the tricyclic antidepressant. A pharmacokinetic interaction might occur as yohimbine and tricyclic antidepressants are both hydroxylated by hepatic enzymes. An interaction could also occur due to decreased first pass hepatic clearance of yohimbine.

Importance and management

The usefulness of this interaction in the treatment of antidepressant-associated dry mouth and hypotension is uncertain. Yohimbine is chemically similar to reserpine and might increase anxiety; the US manufacturer of yohimbine warns that it should not be used in conjunction with mood-modifying drugs such as antidepressants.[3] If concurrent use is undertaken it would be prudent to be aware that the plasma concentration of yohimbine might be increased, and be alert for adverse effects that might occur as a result of this.

1. Lacomblez L, Bensimon G, Isnard F, Diquet B, Lecrubier Y, Puech AJ. Effect of yohimbine on blood pressure in patients with depression and orthostatic hypotension induced by clomipramine. *Clin Pharmacol Ther* (1989) 45, 241–51.
2. Bagheri H, Picault P, Schmitt L, Houin G, Berlan M, Montastruc JL. Pharmacokinetic study of yohimbine and its pharmacodynamic effects on salivary secretion in patients treated with tricyclic antidepressants. *Br J Clin Pharmacol* (1994) 37, 93–6.
3. Yocon (Yohimbine hydrochloride). Glenwood, LLC. US Prescribing information, March 2009.

Tricyclic antidepressants; Amitriptyline + Ethchlorvynol

Transient delirium has been attributed to the concurrent use of amitriptyline and ethchlorvynol,[1] but no details were given and there appear to be no other reports confirming this alleged interaction. Its general relevance is therefore probably small.

1. Hussar DA. Tabular compilation of drug interactions. *Am J Pharm* (1969) 141, 109–56.

Tricyclic antidepressants; Desipramine + Febuxostat

Febuxostat does not affect the pharmacokinetics of desipramine.

Clinical evidence, mechanism, importance and management

A placebo-controlled crossover study in 18 subjects, febuxostat 120 mg daily modestly increased the total exposure to a single 25-mg oral dose of desipramine. The maximum plasma concentration and AUC of desipramine were increased by 14% and 12%, respectively.[1] The incidence of adverse events was similar for both treatment regimens.

The pharmacokinetic changes are too small to be clinically relevant and therefore no desipramine dosage adjustment is necessary in patients also given febuxostat.

1. Khosravan R, Erdman K, Vernillet L, Wu JT, Joseph-Ridge N, Umeda S, Mulford D. Effect of febuxostat on pharmacokinetics of desipramine, a CYP2D6 substrate, in healthy subjects. *Clin Pharmacol Ther* (2005) 77, P43.

Tricyclic antidepressants; Doxepin + Tamoxifen

An isolated report describes a reduction in doxepin serum levels, which was attributed to the use of tamoxifen.

Clinical evidence, mechanism, importance and management

A 79-year-old woman with a long history of bipolar disorder, which was stabilised with lithium carbonate and doxepin 200 mg at bedtime, was given tamoxifen 20 mg daily after a mastectomy for breast cancer. It was noted that her total blood levels of doxepin and its major metabolite were reduced by about 25% over the next 11 months. The control of her depression remained unchanged. The reasons for this apparent interaction are not known.[1] The manufacturer of tamoxifen has another undetailed and isolated report of a possible interaction.[2]

These appears to be the only reports of an interaction between a tricyclic antidepressant and tamoxifen so that their general importance is not known. The evidence is too sparse to warrant recommending any particular precautions.

1. Jefferson JW. Tamoxifen-associated reduction in tricyclic antidepressant levels in blood. *J Clin Psychopharmacol* (1995) 15, 223–4.
2. Zeneca, Personal communication. November 1995.

Tricyclic antidepressants; Imipramine + Vinpocetine

Vinpocetine does not appear to affect imipramine levels.

Clinical evidence, mechanism, importance and management

In 18 healthy subjects the steady-state plasma levels of imipramine 25 mg three times daily were unaffected by vinpocetine 10 mg three times daily, when both drugs were taken together for 10 days.[1] No imipramine dose adjustments are therefore likely be necessary if vinpocetine is also given. There seems to be nothing documented about any of the other tricyclic antidepressants.

1. Hitzenberger G, Schmid R, Braun W, Grandt R. Vinpocetine therapy does not change imipramine pharmacokinetics in man. *Int J Clin Pharmacol Ther Toxicol* (1990) 28, 99–104.

Vortioxetine + Bupropion

Bupropion moderately increases the exposure to vortioxetine, however vortioxetine does not affect the pharmacokinetics of bupropion.

Clinical evidence

In a study, healthy subjects were given vortioxetine 10 mg daily on days 1 to 14, vortioxetine 10 mg daily with bupropion 75 mg twice daily on days 5 to 17, and vortioxetine 10 mg daily with bupropion 150 mg twice daily on days 18 to 28. Bupropion increased the maximum concentration of vortioxetine 2.1-fold and its AUC 2.3-fold. In another group of healthy subjects given bupropion 75 mg twice daily on days 1 to 3, bupropion 150 mg twice daily on days 4 to 14, and bupropion 150 mg twice daily with vortioxetine 10 mg daily on days 15 to 28, vortioxetine did not affect the maximum concentration or the AUC of bupropion.[1]

Mechanism

Vortioxetine is metabolised primarily by CYP2D6 to an inactive metabolite,[1] and bupropion is an inhibitor of CYP2D6. Concurrent use therefore decreases the metabolism of vortioxetine, and increases its exposure.

Importance and management

Evidence for an interaction between bupropion and vortioxetine is limited to the studies cited, but a pharmacokinetic interaction would seem to be established, and the resulting moderate increase in vortioxetine exposure is likely to be clinically important. The US manufacturer advises that the dose of vortioxetine should be reduced by half when it is given with bupropion, or other potent CYP2D6 inhibitors[2] (see 'Table 1.7', p.9 for as list). They also advise that the vortioxetine dose should be increased to the original dose when bupropion is stopped.[2] The pharmacokinetics of bupropion are not affected by vortioxetine and so no bupropion dose adjustment is needed on concurrent use.

1. Chen G, Lee R, Højer AM, Buchbjerg JK, Serenko M, Zhao Z. Pharmacokinetic drug interactions involving vortioxetine (Lu AA21004), a multimodal antidepressant. *Clin Drug Investig* (2013) 33, 727–36.
2. Brintellix (Vortioxetine hydrobromide). Takeda Pharmaceuticals America, Inc. US Prescribing information, September 2013.

Vortioxetine + Azoles

Fluconazole and ketoconazole slightly increase the exposure to vortioxetine. Other azoles might be expected to interact similarly.

Clinical evidence

(a) Fluconazole

A randomised study in 16 healthy subjects found that fluconazole 200 mg daily for 7 days, increased the AUC of a single 10-mg dose of vortioxetine by 46%, but had no effect on the maximum concentration.[1]

(b) Ketoconazole

A randomised study in 17 healthy subjects that ketoconazole 400 mg daily for 7 days, increased the maximum concentration and AUC of a single 10-mg dose of vortioxetine by 31% and 83%, respectively.[1]

Mechanism

Vortioxetine is extensively metabolised by cytochrome P450 isoenzymes, primarily by CYP2D6 to an inactive metabolite, but many other isoenzymes are said to be involved.[1] Fluconazole is an inhibitor of CYP2C19, CYP2C9, and CYP3A4 and ketoconazole is an inhibitor of CYP3A4. Any, or all of these might be involved in increasing the exposure of vortioxetine in the studies.

Importance and management

Evidence for an interaction between vortioxetine and the azoles is limited to the studies with fluconazole and ketoconazole, but a pharmacokinetic interaction would appear to be established. Nevertheless, the exact mechanism behind this is yet to be elucidated, and the increases in exposure seen with both of these azoles were only slight, suggesting that the interaction is not likely to be clinically relevant. The authors of the studies suggest that the drugs can be used together without alteration of the vortioxetine dose.[1] However, further data are required from longer-term concurrent use to confirm this. Until more is known, it would seem prudent, to monitor patients for an increase in vortioxetine adverse effects. Other azoles, such as **itraconazole**, **posaconazole**, and **voriconazole**, are known to inhibit isoenzymes thought to be involved in the metabolism of vortioxetine, and these might be expected to also increase the exposure to vortioxetine, but to differing extents. Until more is known, it might be prudent to follow similar advice as for ketoconazole.

1. Chen G, Lee R, Højer AM, Buchbjerg JK, Serenko M, Zhao Z. Pharmacokinetic drug interactions involving vortioxetine (Lu AA21004), a multimodal antidepressant. *Clin Drug Investig* (2013) 33, 727–36.

Vortioxetine + Omeprazole

No pharmacokinetic interaction appears to occur between vortioxetine and single-dose omeprazole.

Clinical evidence, mechanism, importance and management

Two studies in healthy subjects given a single 40-mg dose of omeprazole alone, then vortioxetine 10 mg daily alone for 14 days, and then with a single 40-mg dose of omeprazole on day 15, found no changes in the pharmacokinetics of either drug.[1] However, it is unlikely that a single-dose of omeprazole (a CYP2C19 inhibitor) would have resulted in any change in the pharmacokinetics of vortioxetine because this would not be sufficient to inhibit the isoenzyme and alter the pharmacokinetics. A multiple-dose study is required to completely exclude an interaction. Nevertheless, as CYP2C19 does not appear to be the only isoenzyme involved in the metabolism of vortioxetine, it would seem unlikely that inhibition of CYP2C19 by omeprazole in isolation would result in any clinically relevant effect on vortioxetine exposure. No dose adjustments would therefore seem necessary on concurrent use of omeprazole and vortioxetine.

1. Chen G, Lee R, Højer AM, Buchbjerg JK, Serenko M, Zhao Z. Pharmacokinetic drug interactions involving vortioxetine (Lu AA21004), a multimodal antidepressant. *Clin Drug Investig* (2013) 33, 727–36.

Vortioxetine + Rifampicin (Rifampin) and other enzyme inducers

Rifampicin moderately decreases the exposure to vortioxetine. Other potent cytochrome P450 isoenzyme inducers might be expected to interact similarly.

Clinical evidence

In study in 14 healthy subjects, **rifampicin** 600 mg daily for 11 days decreased the AUC of a single 20-mg dose of vortioxetine given on the final day by 72%, and decreased its maximum concentration by 51%.[1]

Mechanism

Vortioxetine is extensively metabolised by cytochrome P450 isoenzymes, primarily by CYP2D6 to an inactive metabolite, but many other isoenzymes are said to be involved.[1] Rifampicin is a well-known, non-specific, cytochrome P450 isoenzyme inducer and therefore decreases vortioxetine exposure on concurrent use.

Importance and management

Evidence for an interaction between **rifampicin** and vortioxetine is limited to one study, but a pharmacokinetic interaction would appear to be established, and the moderate decrease in vortioxetine exposure is likely to be clinically relevant. The US manufacturer recommends that if rifampicin, or other potent cytochrome P450 isoenzyme inducers (they name **carbamazepine** and **phenytoin** (and therefore **fosphenytoin**)) are to be taken for more than 14 days, consideration should be given to increasing the vortioxetine dose, but to not more than three times the original dose, and not exceeding the maximum recommended dose. The dose should be reduced to the original dose within 14 days of stopping the inducer.[2] This advice could reasonably be applied to the potent cytochrome P450 isoenzyme inducer, **phenobarbital** (and therefore **primidone**).

1. Chen G, Lee R, Højer AM, Buchbjerg JK, Serenko M, Zhao Z. Pharmacokinetic drug interactions involving vortioxetine (Lu AA21004), a multimodal antidepressant. *Clin Drug Investig* (2013) 33, 727–36.
2. Brintellix (Vortioxetine hydrobromide). Takeda Pharmaceuticals America, Inc. US Prescribing information, September 2013.

36
Thyroid hormones

This section covers the interactions where there is documented evidence that a drug alters or potentially alters the efficacy of thyroid hormones. The mechanism for this can be pharmacokinetic (altered absorption or metabolism) or pharmacodynamic (when the drug in question alters thyroid function).

Regulation of thyroid hormones

The thyroid gland produces two hormones called tri-iodothyronine (T3) and thyroxine (levothyroxine or T4). Production of these hormones is dependent on iodine. They are largely bound to plasma proteins and once released T4 is converted to T3. Secretion of these hormones is controlled by a negative feedback system, regulated by thyrotrophin-releasing hormone (TRH) and thyroid-stimulating hormone (TSH), so that when unbound T3 and T4 concentrations decrease, TRH is secreted by the hypothalamus which in turn stimulates the production and release of TSH. The increased concentrations of TSH result in the increased production and release of both T3 and T4. As concentrations of thyroid hormones increase, so the concentrations of TSH decrease.

Diagnosis of hyper- and hypothyroidism is achieved by measuring concentrations of unbound T3 or T4 and circulating TSH. Hyperthyroidism is characterised by high concentrations of unbound T3 or T4 and low concentrations of TSH, whereas hypothyroidism is characterised by low concentrations of unbound T3 or T4 and high concentrations of TSH. In general, the aim of treatment is to restore the balance of hormones with the main marker of treatment efficacy being normal TSH concentrations.

Drugs and thyroid function

Many drugs are known to alter thyroid function and could therefore affect disease control, see 'Table 36.1', p.1522, for a list: note that this list is not exhaustive. These are often described as drug interactions, but are, more accurately, drug-disease interactions and are therefore not the subject of specific monographs. In general, the risk of an adverse effect will be dependent on how common altered thyroid function is with the drug, and the circumstances under which the drug is being used. As a general recommendation, consider increasing the frequency of thyroid function monitoring if these drugs are given to patients with thyroid dysfunction.

Table 36.1 Drugs known to alter thyroid function

Drug	*Proposed mechanism by which thyroid function affected*	*Further information**
Alemtuzumab	Associated with development of antithyroid antibodies	Might be associated with hypothyroidism or hyperthyroidism, or both (particularly in patients treated with alemtuzumab for multiple sclerosis)
Anabolic steroids	Reduction in thyroid-binding globulin	
Asparaginase	Reduction in thyroid-binding globulin	
Bexarotene	Reduction in TSH secretion and possibly interferes with thyroid hormone metabolism	Hypothyroidism develops rapidly and can be treated with thyroid hormones
Bromocriptine and related dopamine agonists	Reduction in TSH secretion	
Corticosteroids (Glucocorticoids)	Reduction in TSH secretion and a reduction in thyroid-binding globulin	Have been used in symptomatic subacute thyroiditis
Dexamethasone (greater than 4 mg daily)	Reduction in peripheral conversion of thyroxine to T3 by inhibition of 5-deiodinase	
Dopamine	Reduction in TSH secretion	In doses greater than or equal to 1 microgram/kg per minute
Dopamine antagonists (e.g. Metoclopramide)	Increase in TSH secretion	
Fluorouracil	Increase in thyroid-binding globulin	
Furosemide	Displaces thyroid hormones from protein-binding sites	In doses greater than 80 mg intravenously
Heparin	Displaces thyroid hormones from protein-binding sites	
Interferon alfa	Associated with development of antithyroid microsomal antibodies	Might be associated with transient hypothyroidism or hyperthyroidism, or both
Interleukin-2	Thyroiditis	Occurs in about 20% of patients (transient and painless)
Lithium	Reduction in thyroid hormone secretion	
Mercaptopurine	Reduction in thyroid hormone synthesis or secretion	Interferes with organic iodine binding
Mitotane	Increase in thyroid-binding globulin	
Nicotinic acid	Reduction in thyroid-binding globulin	
NSAIDs (Fenmates, Phenylbutazone)	Displaces thyroid hormones from protein-binding sites	
Opioids (Diamorphine, Methadone)	Increase in thyroid-binding globulin	
Radiographic contrast media (iodine-containing)	Reduction in thyroid hormone synthesis or secretion	
Salicylates	Displaces thyroid hormones from protein-binding sites	In doses greater than 2 g daily
Sodium nitroprusside	Reduction in thyroid hormone synthesis or secretion	Effect caused by the thiocyanate metabolite
Somatostatin analogues (e.g. Octreotide)	Reduction in TSH secretion	Effects transient. Some sources suggest an effect only occurs with doses greater than 100 micrograms per day
Soya isoflavones	Reduction in thyroid hormone synthesis or secretion	
Sulfonamides	Reduction in thyroid hormone synthesis or secretion	
Tamoxifen	Increase in thyroid-binding globulin	
Tolbutamide	Reduction in thyroid hormone synthesis or secretion	
Tobacco	Reduction in thyroid hormone synthesis or secretion	Effect might be caused by the thiocyanate component of tobacco smoke

*In general, if an interaction is suspected, monitor thyroid function and adjust the thyroid hormone dose accordingly

Thyroid hormones + Amiodarone

Patients taking levothyroxine for hypothyroidism might develop elevated TSH concentrations or overt hypothyroidism if they are also given amiodarone.

Clinical evidence

A patient with hypothyroidism who was euthyroid while taking **levothyroxine** 75 micrograms daily had an increase in TSH, up to 20 to 30 mU/L within about 10 weeks of starting amiodarone (initially 800 mg daily, reduced to 200 mg daily). The thyroxine/T3 ratio decreased by 33%. She developed fatigue, weakness, cold intolerance, and hyponatraemia. **Levothyroxine** was gradually increased to 112 micrograms daily, and amiodarone was maintained at 200 mg daily. Her TSH concentration decreased to 4.2 mU/L and the symptoms of hypothyroidism resolved.[1] Similar increases in TSH were reported when two other patients taking stable doses of **levothyroxine** started taking amiodarone.[1,2]

In a study investigating the effect of amiodarone and **levothyroxine** treatment, 5 patients were given **levothyroxine** 300 micrograms daily for 16 days, with amiodarone 400 mg daily from day 10 to day 16. When compared with a control group taking **levothyroxine** alone, there was a decrease in serum T3 concentrations and an increase in reverse-T3 concentrations. This suggests that amiodarone interferes with thyroid hormone metabolism, possibly leading to hypothyroidism, even in the presence of **levothyroxine**.[3]

Mechanism

Amiodarone has complex effects on thyroid function and can cause hypothyroidism or hyperthyroidism in some euthyroid patients. Its effects are primarily attributed to its high iodine content, but amiodarone and its desethyl metabolite have direct cytotoxic effects on the thyroid gland.[4] Amiodarone also alters the serum concentrations of thyroid hormones. Basal-serum TSH concentrations increase when amiodarone is started, but generally decrease to normal after about 3 months of treatment. Amiodarone reduces the peripheral conversion of thyroxine to T3 which results in an increase in thyroxine, a modest decrease in T3, and a decrease in reverse-T3 clearance.

Importance and management

Amiodarone is a well-known cause of hypothyroidism or hyperthyroidism, and thyroid function should be regularly assessed when it is used. Particular care is required in patients with thyroid dysfunction, in whom amiodarone use might not be appropriate. The UK manufacturer of amiodarone[5] contraindicates its use in patients with current or previous thyroid dysfunction, although levothyroxine can be used to manage amiodarone-induced hypothyroidism.[5,6] It would be prudent for patients taking levothyroxine or **liothyronine** and amiodarone to have their thyroid function very closely monitored. Note that, if amiodarone is discontinued, its effects will persist for a very long time due to its prolonged half-life (mean of 53 days).

1. Figge J, Dluhy RG. Amiodarone-induced elevation of thyroid stimulating hormone in patients receiving levothyroxine for primary hypothyroidism. *Ann Intern Med* (1990) 113, 553–5.
2. Sanmartí A, Lucas A, Castellanos JM, Foz M. Modificaciones en las concentraciones de hormonas tiroideas en un paciente tiroidectomizado en tratamiento con levotiroxina y amiodarona. *Med Clin (Barc)* (1989) 93, 195.
3. Burger A, Dinichert D, Nicod P, Jenny M, Lemarchand-Béraud T, Vallotton MB. Effect of amiodarone on serum triiodothyronine, reverse triiodothyronine, thyroxin, and thyrotropin. A drug influencing peripheral metabolism of thyroid hormones. *J Clin Invest* (1976) 58, 255–9.
4. Padmanabhan H. Amiodarone and thyroid dysfunction. *South Med J* (2010) 103, 922–30.
5. Cordarone X (Amiodarone hydrochloride). Zentiva. UK Summary of product characteristics, April 2014.
6. Cordarone (Amiodarone hydrochloride). Wyeth Pharmaceuticals Inc. US Prescribing information, December 2014.

Thyroid hormones + Androgens

A study suggests that patients with hypothyroidism might require levothyroxine dose reductions if they are given fluoxymesterone or methyltestosterone. Liothyronine is expected to be similarly affected.

Clinical evidence

In a study, 11 women with metastatic, hormone-dependent breast cancer were given **fluoxymesterone** 10 mg twice daily. After 4 weeks of treatment, 7 women (who had no evidence of thyroid disease) had decreased serum concentrations of total thyroxine and thyroxine-binding globulin, but their calculated free thyroxine index and measured free hormone concentrations were unchanged. These patients remained asymptomatic 6 to 12 weeks after **fluoxymesterone** was discontinued, with serum concentrations returning to baseline. In contrast the other 4 women, whose primary hypothyroidism of 5 to 20 years duration was stabilised with **levothyroxine**, developed hyperthyroidism after starting **fluoxymesterone** 10 mg twice daily. Their serum free thyroxine concentrations increased and their TSH concentrations decreased. **Levothyroxine** dose reductions of between 25 and 50% were required to maintain a euthyroid state.[1]

A 39-year-old man, who had been taking **levothyroxine** (125 micrograms daily) for 4 years following a subtotal thyroidectomy, developed hyperthyroidism on 2 separate occasions after using high-dose intramuscular **methyltestosterone** for muscle-building. The man's twin brother, who did not have thyroid disease and who had also been using methyltestosterone, had normal concentrations of TSH, free thyroxine, and T3, but reduced concentrations of thyroxine-binding globulin and total thyroid hormones. Four months after discontinuing methyltestosterone, thyroid function tests had returned to within normal limits in both twins.[2]

Mechanism

The exact mechanism of this interaction is not known, but studies have reported a decrease in the binding capacity of thyroxine-binding globulin and an increase in the binding of thyroxine-binding prealbumin after the short-term use of androgens.[3,4]

Importance and management

Evidence for an interaction between fluoxymesterone[1] or methyltestosterone[2] and levothyroxine appears to be limited to these studies. However, what is known suggests that patients with thyroid dysfunction who are taking levothyroxine might need dose adjustments to remain euthyroid if fluoxymesterone or methyltestosterone is started. Evidence regarding possible interactions of both **liothyronine** and other androgens appears to be lacking, but it would seem reasonable to expect them to interact in the same way. Therefore if any patient with thyroid dysfunction taking a thyroid hormone is given an androgen, it would be prudent to be alert for symptoms of hyperthyroidism and to monitor thyroid function (some have suggested monitoring within 6–8 weeks of starting the androgen[5]). The dose of the thyroid hormone should be adjusted accordingly.

1. Arafah BM. Decreased levothyroxine requirement in women with hypothyroidism during androgen therapy for breast cancer. *Ann Intern Med* (1994) 121, 247–51.
2. Krysiak R, Okopien B. Methyltestosterone-induced transient hyperthyroidism in a hypothyroid patient. *Acta Clin Belg* (2013) 68, 65–7.
3. Braverman LE, Ingbar SH. Effects of norethandrolone on the transport in serum and peripheral turnover of thyroxine. *J Clin Endocrinol Metab* (1967) 28, 389–96.
4. Braverman LE, Socolow EL, Woeber KA, Ingbar SH. Effect of norethandrolone on the metabolism of 125-I-labeled thyroxine-binding prealbumin. *J Clin Endocrinol Metab* (1968) 28, 831–5.
5. Tahboub R, Arafah BM. Sex steroids and the thyroid. *Best Pract Res Clin Endocrinol Metab* (2009) 23, 769–80.

Thyroid hormones + Antacids

Several reports describe reduced levothyroxine effects in patients given aluminium-containing antacids. Magnesium-containing antacids might have a similar effect.

Clinical evidence

A man with hypothyroidism corrected with **levothyroxine** 150 micrograms daily developed high serum TSH concentrations (an increase from 1.1 mU/L up to 36 mU/L) while taking an **aluminium/magnesium hydroxide** antacid (*Silain-Gel*), and on two subsequent occasions when rechallenged. The reasons are not understood. Although he remained asymptomatic throughout,[1] the increase in the TSH concentrations indicated that the dose of **levothyroxine** had become insufficient in the presence of the antacid. A subsequent study by the same authors confirmed this finding. Five hypothyroid patients taking stable doses of **levothyroxine** were also given the same **aluminium/magnesium hydroxide** antacid (*Silain-Gel*) 4 times daily, for periods of 2 or 4 weeks, with the antacid and **levothyroxine** dose separated by at least 2 hours. Serum TSH concentrations increased during periods of antacid treatment from 2.62 mU/L to 7.19 mU/L.[2] Two similar cases have also been reported, where the presence of an **aluminium/magnesium**-containing antacid or **magnesium oxide** reduced the response to **levothyroxine**. One patient required four times her normal dose of **levothyroxine**.[3]

Mechanism

In vitro studies using crushed *Silain-Gel* tablets (aluminium hydroxide 80 mg with magnesium hydroxide 33 mg) or *Maalox* suspension 0.9 mL (aluminium hydroxide 40 mg with magnesium hydroxide 36 mg) found a non-specific adsorption or complexing of levothyroxine to aluminium hydroxide, the extent of which might depend on the specific preparation (in the study, 10.5% and 22.2% for the suspension and tablets, respectively).[2] Another *in vitro* study found that the adsorption of levothyroxine increased to about 52% as the amount of aluminium increased to 200 mg in the sample.[3] Magnesium hydroxide[2] and magnesium oxide[3] were reported not to adsorb levothyroxine to any extent *in vitro*, although the isolated case report[3] suggests that magnesium oxide might adsorb levothyroxine.

Importance and management

The general importance of the interaction between levothyroxine and aluminium-containing antacids is not known, but if an interaction is suspected, it might be prudent to monitor thyroid function and adjust the levothyroxine dose accordingly. Alternatively consider the possibility of using a different antacid, although note that magnesium-containing antacids might interact similarly; as might calcium-containing antacids, see 'Thyroid hormones + Calcium compounds', p.1524.

1. Sperber AD, Liel Y. Evidence for interference with the intestinal absorption of levothyroxine sodium by aluminum hydroxide. *Arch Intern Med* (1991) 152, 183–4.
2. Liel Y, Sperber AD, Shany S. Nonspecific intestinal adsorption of levothyroxine by aluminium hydroxide. *Am J Med* (1994) 97, 363–5.
3. Mersebach H, Rasmussen ÅK, Kirkegaard L, Feldt-Rasmussen U. Intestinal adsorption of levothyroxine by antacids and laxatives: case stories and *in vitro* experiments. *Pharmacol Toxicol* (1999) 84, 107–9.

Thyroid hormones + Barbiturates

A case report describes thyrotoxicosis when a patient taking levothyroxine reduced her dose of secobarbital with amobarbital. Phenobarbital might reduce endogenous thyroxine concentrations in euthyroid patients.

Clinical evidence

An elderly woman taking **levothyroxine** 300 micrograms daily for hypothyroidism complained of severe breathlessness within a week of reducing her nightly dose of

Tuinal (**secobarbital** 100 mg with **amobarbital** 100 mg) from two capsules to one capsule. She was subsequently found to be thyrotoxic. She became symptom-free when the dose of the **levothyroxine** was halved.[1]

In a retrospective analysis of 223 euthyroid children started on antiepileptic drugs, the 33 children taking **phenobarbital** had reduced average serum free thyroxine concentrations after 1 and 6 months, but this reduction did not persist at 12 months. Average serum TSH concentrations increased progressively (from 2.81 to 3.70 mU/L) throughout the 12-month study period.[2]

Mechanism

The reason for this effect is not known, but **phenobarbital** has been shown to reduce the serum concentrations of *endogenous* thyroid hormones in some studies,[3] and it seems possible that in the case report secobarbital and amobarbital acted in the same way. This effect has also been seen with other enzyme-inducing drugs, for example see 'Thyroid hormones + Phenytoin', p.1528.

Importance and management

The general importance of the interaction between levothyroxine and the barbiturates is unknown, but the lack of reports suggest that it is small. Be alert for any evidence of changes in thyroid status if barbiturates are added or withdrawn from patients taking levothyroxine. Monitor thyroid function if an interaction is suspected, and adjust the levothyroxine dose accordingly. Although the possibility of a similar interaction with **liothyronine** does not appear to have been studied, it would seem prudent to be alert for a similar reduction in its effect in the presence of barbiturates.

1. Hoffbrand BI. Barbiturate/thyroid-hormone interaction. *Lancet* (1979) ii, 903–4.
2. Yilmaz Ü, Yilmaz TS, Akinci G, Korkmaz HA, Tekgül H. The effect of antiepileptic drugs on thyroid function in children. *Seizure* (2014) 23, 29–35.
3. Ohnhaus EE, Studer H. A link between liver microsomal enzyme activity and thyroid hormone metabolism in man. *Br J Clin Pharmacol* (1983) 15, 71–6.

Thyroid hormones + Bile-acid binding resins

The absorption levothyroxine from the gut is reduced by the concurrent use of colestyramine. Colesevelam also decreases levothyroxine absorption, and colestipol and colestilan seem likely to interact similarly. There is no direct evidence regarding liothyronine, but these bile acid binding resins might also reduce its absorption.

Clinical evidence

(a) Colesevelam

In a single-dose study, 6 healthy subjects were given a large dose of **levothyroxine** (1000 micrograms) at the same time as colesevelam 3.75 g. Colesevelam decreased the serum thyroxine AUC_{0-6} by 96%.[1] Another study similarly found that colesevelam 3.75 g given at the same time as levothyroxine, decreased the AUC_{0-48} of a 600-microgram dose of **levothyroxine** by 22%. Separating the doses by 4 hours resulted in no change in the serum thyroxine AUC.[2]

(b) Colestilan

In vitro studies showed a high binding potential between colestilan and levothyroxine,[3] however, there appear to be no reports published in the literature confirming an interaction.

(c) Colestipol

A study in patients with atherosclerosis, taking colestipol and nicotinic acid for one year, found reductions in total serum thyroxine and thyroxine-binding globulin, but these changes were considered benign as the patients remained euthyroid.[4]

(d) Colestyramine

A patient with hypothyroidism, taking **levothyroxine**, had a reduction in his basal metabolic rate when given colestyramine: this prompted a further study in two similar patients taking **thyroid extract** 60 mg daily or **levothyroxine** 100 micrograms daily, and 5 healthy subjects. Colestyramine 4 g four times daily reduced the absorption of Iodine-131 labelled **levothyroxine**, the amount recovered in the faeces being roughly doubled. One of the patients had a worsening of her hypothyroidism. Giving the **levothyroxine** 4 to 5 hours after the colestyramine reduced but did not completely prevent the interaction.[5] Another report describes a patient taking **levothyroxine** whose TSH concentrations increased when colestyramine was taken, and decreased again when it was stopped, indicating impaired **levothyroxine** absorption.[6]

Two case reports describe the use of colestyramine to achieve a more rapid return to normal thyroid function in patients who had become hyperthyroid while taking **levothyroxine**,[7] and in a case of **levothyroxine** overdose.[8] A further case report describes a patient taking **levothyroxine** and colestyramine, who only became euthyroid when the **levothyroxine** was taken in the morning, and the colestyramine was taken at night.[9]

Mechanism

Colestyramine, colestipol, colesevelam, and possibly colestilan bind to levothyroxine in the gut, thereby reducing its absorption. As levothyroxine probably also undergoes enterohepatic recirculation, continued contact with these bile-acid binding resins is possible and separating administration might not entirely eliminate the interaction. Colestyramine and colestipol also appear to reduce the levels of *endogenous* thyroxine.[10,11]

Importance and management

The interaction between levothyroxine and colestyramine appears to be established (although the documentation is very limited) and the reduced thyroxine concentrations that result are of clinical importance. The interaction can be minimised by separating the doses by 4 to 6 hours, but some case results suggest that this might only diminish the extent of the interaction (see *Mechanism*, above). Therefore the outcome should be monitored so that any necessary thyroid hormone dose adjustments can be made. Colestipol appears to interact in a similar way to colestyramine, and similar precautions would therefore seem prudent if it is given with levothyroxine.

Colesevelam also appears to interact in a similar way to colestyramine. The US manufacturer states that levothyroxine should be given at least 4 hours before colesevelam,[12] and the UK manufacturer of colesevelam advises that it should be given at least 4 hours before or 4 hours after any interacting drug.[13] Colestilan is predicted to interact in a similar way to colestyramine, consequently, the UK manufacturer of colestilan advises that any interacting drug should be given at least 1 hour before, or 3 hours after, taking colestilan.[3]

Data regarding **liothyronine** appears to be limited; nevertheless, *in vitro* tests[5] show that it interacts with colestyramine in a similar way to levothyroxine and therefore, until more is known, similar precautions to those advised for levothyroxine would seem prudent, with this and other bile-acid binding resins.

1. Weitzman SP, Ginsburg KC, Carlson HE. Colesevelam hydrochloride and lanthanum carbonate interfere with the absorption of levothyroxine. *Thyroid* (2009) 19, 77–79.
2. Brown KS, Armstrong IC, Wang A, Walker JR, Noveck RJ, Swearingen D, Allison M, Kissling JC, Kisicki J, Salazar DE. Effect of the bile acid sequestrant colesevelam on the pharmacokinetics of pioglitazone, repaglinide, estrogen estradiol, norethindrone, levothyroxine, and glyburide. *J Clin Pharmacol* (2010) 50, 554–65.
3. BindRen (Colestilan). Mitsubishi Tanabe Pharma Europe Ltd. UK Summary of product characteristics, August 2013.
4. Cashin-Hemphill L, Spencer CA, Nicoloff JT, Blankenhorn DH, Nessim SA, Chin HP, Lee NA. Alterations in serum thyroid hormonal indices with colestipol-niacin therapy. *Ann Intern Med* (1987) 107, 324–9.
5. Northcutt RC, Stiel JN, Hollifield JW, Stant EG. The influence of cholestyramine on thyroxine absorption. *JAMA* (1969) 208, 1857–61.
6. Harmon SM, Seifert CF. Levothyroxine-cholestyramine interaction reemphasized. *Ann Intern Med* (1991) 115, 658–9.
7. Shakir KMM, Michaels RD, Hays JH, Potter BB. The use of bile acid sequestrants to lower serum thyroid hormones in iatrogenic hyperthyroidism. *Ann Intern Med* (1993) 118, 112–13.
8. de Luis DA, Dueñas A, Martin J, Abad L, Cuellar L, Aller R. Light symptoms following a high-dose intentional *L*-thyroxine ingestion treated with cholestyramine. *Horm Res* (2002) 57, 61–3.
9. Rosenberg R. Malabsorption of thyroid hormone with cholestyramine administration. *Conn Med* (1994) 58, 109.
10. Kaykhaei MA, Shams M, Sadegholvad A, Dabbaghmanesh MH, Omrani GR. Low doses of cholestyramine in the treatment of hyperthyroidism. *Endocrine* (2008) 34, 52–5.
11. Hagag P, Nissenbaum H, Weiss M. Role of colestipol in the treatment of hyperthyroidism. *J Endocrinol Invest* (1998) 21, 725–31.
12. Welchol (Colesevelam hydrochloride). Daiichi Sankyo, Inc. US Prescribing information, January 2014.
13. Cholestagel (Colesevelam hydrochloride). Sanofi. UK Summary of product characteristics, December 2014.

Thyroid hormones + Bulk-forming laxatives

A study found that polycarbophil calcium or ispaghula had no effect on levothyroxine absorption. In contrast, another study found that dietary fibre reduced levothyroxine exposure.

Clinical evidence, mechanism, importance and management

A study in 8 healthy subjects found that neither **polycarbophil calcium** 1 g nor **ispaghula** 3.4 g affected the absorption of a single 600-microgram dose of **levothyroxine**.[1]

A study in 2 patients and 2 healthy subjects, given a single 200-microgram dose of **levothyroxine**, found that 10.2 g of **dietary fibre** from bran lowered the average increase in serum **levothyroxine** by about 80% and 75%, in the patients and subjects respectively, and reduced the AUC of **levothyroxine** by roughly 70 to 90% and 65 to 80%, respectively.[2]

Evidence for an interaction between levothyroxine and bulk-forming laxatives is limited, but the effects seen might be expected to affect **levothyroxine** requirements. Until more is known, if an interaction is suspected, it might be prudent to monitor thyroid function and adjust the levothyroxine dose accordingly.

1. Chiu AC, Sherman SI. Effects of pharmacological fiber supplements on levothyroxine absorption. *Thyroid* (1998) 8, 667–71.
2. Benvenga S, Bartolone L, Pappalardo MA, Russo A, Lapa D, Giorgianni G, Saraceno G, Trimarchi F. Altered intestinal absorption of L-thyroxine caused by coffee. *Thyroid* (2008) 18, 293–301.

Thyroid hormones + Calcium compounds

The efficacy of levothyroxine can be reduced by calcium carbonate. Calcium acetate and calcium citrate reduced levothyroxine absorption in pharmacokinetic studies.

Clinical evidence

(a) Calcium acetate

A retrospective study identified 67 patients taking **levothyroxine** and a phosphate binder (calcium carbonate, calcium acetate, or sevelamer). The TSH concentrations were 5- to 6-fold higher in patients taking calcium carbonate or sevelamer (both thought to reduce **levothyroxine** efficacy) than calcium acetate, and the effects became more pronounced over time.[1] This study suggests that calcium acetate has little effect on the efficacy of **levothyroxine.**

In a single-dose pharmacokinetic study, which compared three different calcium compounds in 8 healthy subjects, giving calcium acetate (500 mg elemental calcium) at the same time as a large 1000-microgram dose of **levothyroxine** reduced the thyroxine AUC by about 25% compared with when levothyroxine was given alone.[2]

(b) Calcium carbonate

In a study, 20 patients with hypothyroidism were given **levothyroxine**, to which calcium carbonate 1.2 g daily was then added for 3 months. While taking the calcium carbonate their mean free thyroxine concentrations decreased from 16.7 picomol/L to 15.4 picomol/L and increased again to 18 picomol/L when it was stopped. The mean total thyroxine concentrations over the same period were about 118 nanomol/L, 111 nanomol/L, and 120 nanomol/L, respectively, and the mean TSH concentrations were 1.6 mU/L, 2.7 mU/L, and 1.4 mU/L, respectively.[3] In a single-dose pharmacokinetic study in 7 healthy subjects, giving calcium carbonate 2 g at the same time as a large 1000-microgram dose of **levothyroxine**, reduced the total thyroxine absorption over 6 hours from a mean thyroxine AUC of 220,551 microgram-min (without calcium carbonate) to 164,993 microgram-min (with calcium carbonate).[4] In a later single-dose pharmacokinetic study, which compared 3 different calcium compounds in 8 healthy subjects, giving calcium carbonate (500 mg elemental calcium) at the same time as a large 1000-microgram dose of **levothyroxine** reduced the thyroxine AUC by about 21% compared with when levothyroxine was given alone.[2]

A woman with thyroid cancer taking **levothyroxine** 125 micrograms daily to suppress serum TSH concentrations had a reduced response (fatigue, weight gain) when she took *Tums* containing calcium carbonate for the prevention of osteoporosis. She often took the two together. Over a 5-month period her serum TSH concentrations increased from 0.08 mU/L to 13.3 mU/L. Within 3 weeks of stopping the calcium carbonate, her serum TSH concentrations had decreased to 0.68 mU/L.[5] Other reports have described 5 patients who had elevations in their TSH concentrations while taking calcium carbonate with **levothyroxine**. All concentrations returned to normal when administration was separated by about 4 hours,[5-7] or in one case when the calcium supplementation was stopped.[8]

(c) Calcium citrate

In a single-dose pharmacokinetic study, which compared three different calcium compounds in 8 healthy subjects, giving calcium citrate (500 mg elemental calcium) at the same time as a large 1000-microgram dose of **levothyroxine** reduced the thyroxine AUC by about 19% compared with when levothyroxine was given alone.[2]

(d) Unspecified calcium compounds

A large retrospective population analysis of patients taking long-term **levothyroxine** found that oral calcium (unspecified compounds) increased serum TSH concentrations.[9]

Mechanism

In vitro studies indicate that levothyroxine is adsorbed onto calcium carbonate when the pH is low (as in the stomach), which would reduce the amount available for absorption.[3] Other calcium compounds are likely to have a similar effect.

Importance and management

An interaction between levothyroxine and calcium carbonate is established, but seems to be of limited clinical importance. The study cited[3] shows that the mean reduction in the absorption of levothyroxine is quite small, but the case reports[5,6] show that some individuals can experience a reduction in the absorption that is clinically important. As it is impossible to predict which patients are likely to be clinically affected, the cautious approach would be to advise all patients to separate the doses of the two preparations by at least 4 hours to avoid admixture in the gut. This interaction would be expected to occur with calcium carbonate in any form but it is not known whether other thyroid hormone preparations interact in the same way as levothyroxine.

Pharmacokinetic studies have shown that calcium acetate and calcium citrate can affect the absorption of levothyroxine but the clinical relevance of this in patients regularly taking thyroid hormones is not known. It might be prudent to advise patients to separate the doses of levothyroxine and the calcium acetate or calcium citrate by at least 4 hours in the case of an unexpected response to levothyroxine treatment.

1. Diskin CJ, Stokes TJ, Dansby LM, Radcliff L, Carter TB. Effect of phosphate binders upon TSH and L-thyroxine dose in patients on thyroid replacement. *Int Urol Nephrol* (2007) 39, 599–602.
2. Zamfirescu I, Carlson HE. Absorption of levothyroxine when coadministered with various calcium formulations. *Thyroid* (2011) 21, 483–6.
3. Singh N, Singh PN, Hershmann JM. Effect of calcium carbonate on the absorption of levothyroxine. *JAMA* (2000) 283, 2822–25.
4. Singh N, Weisler SL, Hershman JM. The acute effect of calcium carbonate on the intestinal absorption of levothyroxine. *Thyroid* (2001) 11, 967–971.
5. Schneyer CR. Calcium carbonate and reduction of levothyroxine efficacy. *JAMA* (1998) 279, 750.
6. Butner LE, Fulco PP, Feldman G. Calcium carbonate-induced hypothyroidism. *Ann Intern Med* (2000) 132, 595.
7. Csako G, McGriff NJ, Rotman-Pikielny P, Sarlis NJ, Pucino F. Exaggerated levothyroxine malabsorption due to calcium carbonate supplementation in gastrointestinal disorders. *Ann Pharmacother* (2001) 35, 1578–83.
8. Mazokopakis EE, Giannakopoulos TG, Starakis IK. Interaction between levothyroxine and calcium carbonate. *Can Fam Physician* (2008) 54, 39.
9. Irving SA, Vadiveloo T, Leese GP. Drugs that interact with levothyroxine: an observational study from the Thyroid Epidemiology, Audit and Research Study (TEARS). *Clin Endocrinol (Oxf)* (2015) 82, 136–41.

Thyroid hormones + Carbamazepine

Clinical hypothyroidism can occur in patients taking levothyroxine when they are given carbamazepine.

Clinical evidence

In a study, when 10 patients whose hypothyroidism was stabilised with **levothyroxine** were given carbamazepine, there was a minor decrease of about 10 to 15% in free thyroxine, and a decrease of 15 to 25% in total thyroxine, with a consequent increase in TSH concentrations. In 3 of the 10 patients, the TSH concentration increased to over 5 mU/L, requiring treatment adjustment. In a control group of 19 patients with no thyroid disorder, similar changes in thyroxine concentrations caused just a small non-statistically significant increase in TSH concentrations.[1] Similar findings were reported in another study when 5 children taking stable doses of **levothyroxine** were given carbamazepine. In this study, 2 children had greatly increased TSH concentrations, and all 5 children had their **levothyroxine** dose increased to restore pretreatment thyroid function.[2] Another study in 9 patients taking **levothyroxine** found that thyroxine and T3 concentrations were reduced after they had been taking carbamazepine for 3 weeks, but there was no change in TSH concentrations.[3]

A prospective study in patients with epilepsy found that free thyroxine concentrations were decreased during carbamazepine treatment but were reversed after the carbamazepine was stopped.[4]

In a retrospective analysis of 223 euthyroid children started on antiepileptic drugs, the 36 children taking carbamazepine had reduced average serum free thyroxine concentrations after 1, 6, and 12 months, and increased average serum TSH concentrations at months 1 and 6, but the increase was not statistically significant after 12 months.[5]

Mechanism

Carbamazepine can increase the metabolism of endogenous thyroid hormones, thereby reducing their plasma concentrations, but this rarely results in hypothyroidism in euthyroid patients. However, in patients taking levothyroxine replacement therapy, the decrease appears more likely to be clinically relevant.[1] This effect has also been seen with other enzyme-inducing drugs, see 'Thyroid hormones + Barbiturates', p.1523.

Importance and management

Although the evidence is limited, an interaction between levothyroxine and carbamazepine is established. The available evidence suggests that some patients taking levothyroxine might require an increase in dose when they start carbamazepine. Be alert for this effect if both drugs are given, and monitor thyroid function if an interaction is suspected: adjust the levothyroxine dose accordingly. Also be alert for changes in levothyroxine dose requirements if carbamazepine treatment is stopped.

Given the proposed mechanism of the interaction with levothyroxine, it seems likely that **liothyronine** might be similarly affected by carbamazepine, but this does not appear to have been studied. Nevertheless, it might be prudent to consider similar precautions to those suggested for levothyroxine.

1. 1. Simko J, Horacek J. Carbamazepine and risk of hypothyroidism: a prospective study. *Acta Neurol Scand* (2007) 116, 317–21.
2. De Luca F, Arrigo T, Pandullo E, Siracusano MF, Benvenga S, Trimarchi F. Changes in thyroid function tests induced by 2 month carbamazepine treatment in L-thyroxine-substituted hypothyroid children. *Eur J Pediatr* (1986) 145, 77–9.
3. Aanderud S, Myking OL, Strandjord RE. The influence of carbamazepine on thyroid hormones and thyroxine binding globulin in hypothyroid patients substituted with thyroxine. *Clin Endocrinol (Oxf)* (1981) 15, 247–52.
4. Lossius MI, Taubøll E, Mowinckel P, Gjerstad L. Reversible effects of antiepileptic drugs on thyroid hormones in men and women with epilepsy: a prospective randomized double-blind withdrawal study. *Epilepsy Behav* (2009) 16, 64–8.
5. Yilmaz Ü, Yilmaz TS, Akinci G, Korkmaz HA, Tekgül H. The effect of antiepileptic drugs on thyroid function in children. *Seizure* (2014) 23, 29–35.

Thyroid hormones + Chloroquine with Proguanil

A case report describes a reduction in the control of hypothyroidism in a patient taking levothyroxine when chloroquine and proguanil antimalarial prophylaxis was given.

Clinical evidence, mechanism, importance and management

A case report describes a woman with stable hypothyroidism taking **levothyroxine** 125 micrograms daily, who was given antimalarial prophylaxis with chloroquine 100 mg daily and proguanil 200 mg daily for 2 months. At a routine monitoring appointment 4 weeks later, she was noted to have a TSH concentration of 44.8 mU/L. No change was made to her **levothyroxine** dose and the increase in her TSH concentration resolved within one week of stopping both chloroquine and proguanil at the end of the required period of prophylaxis. A subsequent course of prophylaxis with the same antimalarial regimen produced a similar effect, with the TSH concentration increasing from 3.2 mU/L to 54.7 mU/L. This increase resolved within 4 weeks of stopping the antimalarials.[1]

This appears to be the only published report of an interaction between **levothyroxine** and the combination of chloroquine and proguanil, and its general importance is unclear, especially as no action appeared to be necessary to manage the effects of the interaction. This interaction might have more relevance to other indications for chloroquine, where it is used long-term, but more study is needed to establish this. However, until more is known, bear this case report in mind should a patient taking

levothyroxine and either proguanil and/or chloroquine experience an unexpected decrease in the control of their hypothyroidism.

1. Munera Y, Hugues FC, Le Jeunne C, Pays JF. Interaction of thyroxine sodium with antimalarial drugs. *BMJ* (1997) 314, 1593.

Thyroid hormones + Chromium compounds

Chromium picolinate decreases levothyroxine absorption.

Clinical evidence, mechanism, importance and management

In a single-dose study in 7 healthy subjects, giving a large dose of **levothyroxine** (1000 micrograms) at the same time as chromium picolinate 1 mg resulted in a 17% decrease in the AUC_{0-6} of thyroxine.[1] This preliminary evidence suggests that, until more is known, it would be prudent to be alert for symptoms of hypothyroidism during concurrent use. If such symptoms occur, monitor thyroid function, and adjust the dose of the **levothyroxine** accordingly. Separation of administration might minimise any interaction, but this needs confirmation.

1. John-Kalarickal J, Pearlman G, Carlson HE. New medications which decrease levothyroxine absorption. *Thyroid* (2007) 17, 763–5.

Thyroid hormones + Ciprofloxacin

A case report describes unexplained hypothyroidism in patients taking levothyroxine who had also been taking ciprofloxacin. A case of Stevens-Johnson syndrome was attributed to high concentrations of ciprofloxacin, which, it was suggested, might have been caused by levothyroxine.

Clinical evidence, mechanism, importance and management

(a) Effect on ciprofloxacin

A 66-year-old woman, taking **levothyroxine** 150 micrograms daily after total thyroidectomy, developed Stevens-Johnson syndrome 10 days after starting ciprofloxacin 1 g daily. The patient was also found to be hyperthyroid and so the dose of **levothyroxine** was reduced. The ciprofloxacin was stopped and the patient gradually improved over the following 18 days: all symptoms had resolved after 40 days. The authors comment that high drug doses and slow metabolism are risk factors for the development of Stevens-Johnson syndrome, as is the use of ciprofloxacin. They suggest that **levothyroxine** might have inhibited the metabolism of ciprofloxacin, leading to high plasma ciprofloxacin concentrations; however, ciprofloxacin concentrations were not measured,[1] and levothyroxine is not known to inhibit the isoenzymes involved in the metabolism of ciprofloxacin. More study is therefore needed to establish an interaction as this effect might have been due to ciprofloxacin alone.

(b) Effect on levothyroxine

An 80-year-old patient with advanced thyroid cancer taking **levothyroxine** 125 micrograms daily was given oral ciprofloxacin 750 mg twice daily and intravenous dicloxacillin for osteomyelitis complicating a fracture. After 4 weeks of treatment she complained of increasing tiredness, and her TSH was found to be 10 times the upper limit of the reference range. Increasing the **levothyroxine** dose to 200 micrograms daily did not have any effect on TSH, so the dose was returned to 125 micrograms. The ciprofloxacin was then stopped, and her thyroid function tests rapidly normalised.[2]

Another woman, with stable thyroid function, taking **levothyroxine** 150 micrograms daily, had a more than 10-fold increase in TSH concentrations after taking ciprofloxacin 500 mg twice daily for 3 weeks.[2] When the administration of **levothyroxine** and ciprofloxacin was separated by 6 hours, the thyroid function tests normalised, which suggests that concurrent dosing somehow reduces the absorption of **levothyroxine**.

In a single-dose study in 8 healthy subjects, giving ciprofloxacin 750 mg at the same time as a large dose (1000 micrograms) of **levothyroxine** reduced the thyroxine AUC by 39%.[3]

This interaction is not established. Nevertheless it might be prudent to consider the possibility of an interaction if otherwise unexplained hypothyroidism occurs in a patient taking levothyroxine and ciprofloxacin.

1. Cholongitas E, Georgousaki C, Spyrou S, Katsogridakis K, Dasenaki M. Stevens-Johnson syndrome related to ciprofloxacin, possibly enhanced by overadministration of levothyroxine. *Dermatol Online J* (2009) 15, 16.
2. Cooper JG, Harboe K, Frost SK, Skadberg Ø. Ciprofloxacin interacts with thyroid replacement therapy. *BMJ* (2005) 330, 1002.
3. Goldberg AS, Tirona RG, Asher LJ, Kim RB, Van Uum SHM. Ciprofloxacin and rifampicin have opposite effects on levothyroxine absorption. *Thyroid* (2013) 23, 1374–78.

Thyroid hormones + Coffee

Coffee can reduce the absorption of levothyroxine.

Clinical evidence

A patient with hypothyroidism due to Hashimoto's thyroiditis had normal serum TSH concentrations when she took **levothyroxine** 100 micrograms with water an hour before breakfast. However, she became hypothyroid when she took the same dose of **levothyroxine** with a double espresso coffee, followed by a second coffee 5 to 10 minutes later. Her TSH returned to normal when she took **levothyroxine** with water, 30 minutes before coffee. Further, TSH increased again when she took **levothyroxine** with one cup of espresso or water, followed by a cup of espresso 1 to 5 minutes later.[1] The authors also report seven other similar cases.[1] The same authors also conducted a study in 6 of these 8 patients and 9 healthy subjects, in which a single 200-microgram dose of **levothyroxine** was given with coffee, water, or water followed 60 minutes later by coffee. The effect of coffee only occurred if it was taken at the same time as **levothyroxine**. In patients and healthy subjects, concurrent coffee lowered the average increase in serum **levothyroxine** by 36% and 29%, respectively and the **levothyroxine** AUC by 36% and 27%, respectively when compared with water. The time of the maximum incremental rise in **levothyroxine** was delayed by coffee (by 50 minutes and 43 minutes respectively).[1]

In an open-label crossover study, a patient taking **levothyroxine** tablets for hypothyroidism had uncontrolled TSH concentrations (24–34 mU/L) whilst reportedly consuming coffee at the same time as levothyroxine. Her TSH concentrations decreased insufficiently (to 22.4 mU/L) when coffee was consumed 20 minutes after taking levothyroxine, but decreased more noticeably (to 5.8 mU/L) when coffee was consumed 60 minutes after levothyroxine. When the patient was switched to the same dose of levothyroxine given as a *soft gel capsule* (containing levothyroxine dissolved in glycerin), and coffee was taken 60 minutes afterwards, the TSH concentration became very low (0.06 mU/L) and the patient experienced symptoms of hyperthyroidism.[2] In the same study, 7 patients taking **levothyroxine** tablets for TSH suppression, had uncontrolled TSH concentrations reportedly because of concurrent coffee consumption, and were switched to the *soft gel capsule* formulation of levothyroxine. The average TSH concentrations of the 7 patients did not differ whether coffee was consumed at the same time as levothyroxine *soft gel capsules*, or 60 minutes afterwards.[2]

A 6-month observational study in 54 patients taking **levothyroxine** *liquid* for hypothyroidism, found that TSH, free thyroxine, and free T3 concentrations did not alter when the patients switched from consuming coffee with, or within a few minutes of, taking levothyroxine liquid, to taking levothyroxine 30 minutes before breakfast (with or without coffee).[3]

Mechanism

Coffee appears to interfere with the intestinal absorption of levothyroxine. An *in vitro* study[1] found that coffee can sequester levothyroxine. Any effect of coffee on the absorption of levothyroxine might differ between levothyroxine formulations. It has been suggested that formulations which do not require dissolution (such as an oral solution or soft gel capsule) are absorbed faster and are less affected by coffee than a tablet.[2-4]

Importance and management

Evidence regarding an interaction between levothyroxine and coffee is limited, but it does indicate that coffee (espresso in both the study and the case report) reduces the absorption of levothyroxine. The interaction appears to be avoided by taking levothyroxine with water and not drinking coffee for at least 60 minutes afterwards. Some suggest that patients should be counselled to avoid caffeine-containing liquids for at least 30 minutes after taking levothyroxine.[5] However, given that it is widely recommended that patients take levothyroxine in the morning, it seems probable that many patients do take levothyroxine with coffee. Therefore, based on the available evidence, unless hypothyroidism is proving difficult to manage, no particular precautions are warranted.

1. Benvenga S, Bartolone L, Pappalardo MA, Russo A, Lapa D, Giorgianni G, Saraceno G, Trimarchi F. Altered intestinal absorption of L-thyroxine caused by coffee. *Thyroid* (2008) 18, 293–301.
2. Vita R, Saraceno G, Trimarchi F, Benvenga S. A novel formulation of L-thyroxine (L-T4) reduces the problem of L-T4 malabsorption by coffee observed with traditional tablet formulations. *Endocrine* (2013) 43, 154–60.
3. Cappelli C, Pirola I, Gandossi E, Formenti A, Castellano M. Oral liquid levothyroxine treatment at breakfast: a mistake? *Eur J Endocrinol* (2013) 170, 95–9.
4. Vita R, Fallahi P, Antonelli A, Benvenga S. The administration of L-thyroxine as soft gel capsule or liquid solution. *Expert Opin Drug Deliv* (2014) 11, 1103–11.
5. Joint Formulary Committee. *British National Formulary.* 70 ed. London: BMJ Group and Pharmaceutical Press; 2015. p.665.

Thyroid hormones + Ezetimibe

Ezetimibe does not appear to alter levothyroxine absorption.

Clinical evidence, mechanism, importance and management

In a single-dose study in 7 healthy subjects, giving a large dose of **levothyroxine** (1000 micrograms) at the same time as ezetimibe 10 mg did not alter the AUC_{0-6} of thyroxine.[1] Similarly, in another single-dose study in 10 healthy subjects, ezetimibe 10 mg did not affect the AUC of serum thyroxine in response to a single 600-microgram dose of **levothyroxine**.[2]

These findings suggest that levothyroxine requirements are unlikely to change in patients taking ezetimibe.

1. John-Kalarickal J, Pearlman G, Carlson HE. New medications which decrease levothyroxine absorption. *Thyroid* (2007) 17, 763–5.
2. Ananthakrishnan S, Braverman LE, Levin RM, Magnani B, Pearce EN. The effect of famotidine, esomeprazole, and ezetimibe on levothyroxine absorption. *Thyroid* (2008) 18, 493–8.

Thyroid hormones + Grapefruit juice

A case report describes hypothyroidism in a patient taking levothyroxine and drinking large amounts of grapefruit juice. However, a pharmaco-

kinetic study did not find a clinically relevant interaction between levothyroxine and grapefruit juice.

Clinical evidence

A 36-year-old woman, with previously stable thyroid function taking **levothyroxine** 100 micrograms daily and drinking large amounts of grapefruit juice (specific volumes not stated), had a very high TSH concentration even after an increase in her **levothyroxine** dose to 150 micrograms daily. When she was advised to drink less grapefruit juice, her TSH decreased to within the normal range.[1] This case prompted a crossover study in 10 healthy subjects, which found that grapefruit juice caused an 11% reduction in the maximal increase in thyroxine after a single 600-microgram dose of **levothyroxine**. In this study, normal-strength grapefruit juice 200 mL was taken three times a day for 2 days, then on the third day, grapefruit juice 200 mL was taken one hour before, simultaneously with, and one hour after, **levothyroxine**.[1]

Mechanism

Uncertain, but grapefruit juice might reduce the OATP1A2-mediated uptake of levothyroxine.[2]

Importance and management

Evidence of an interaction between levothyroxine and grapefruit juice is limited. The single-dose pharmacokinetic study established that grapefruit juice appears to have only small effects on thyroxine concentrations in those taking levothyroxine, which suggests that a clinically relevant interaction is unlikely. In the absence of further information, no particular precautions are required, but consider the possibility of an interaction in the event of an unexpected decrease in the response to levothyroxine.

1. Lilja JJ, Laitinen K, Neuvonen PJ. Effects of grapefruit juice on the absorption of levothyroxine. *Br J Clin Pharmacol* (2005) 60, 337–41.
2. Bailey DG. Fruit juice inhibition of uptake transport: a new type of food–drug interaction. *Br J Clin Pharmacol* (2010) 70, 645–55.

Thyroid hormones + H_2-receptor antagonists

Cimetidine, but not ranitidine or famotidine, causes a small reduction in the absorption of levothyroxine.

Clinical evidence, mechanism, importance and management

In a study in 10 women with simple goitre, **cimetidine** 400 mg, given 90 minutes before a single capsule of **levothyroxine**, reduced absorption of **levothyroxine** over the first 4 hours by about 21%.

A single 300-mg dose of **ranitidine** was found not to affect the absorption of **levothyroxine** in a matched group of 10 women.[1] Similarly, in a study in 10 healthy subjects, **famotidine** 20 mg twice daily for one week did not affect the AUC of serum thyroxine in response to a single 600-microgram dose of **levothyroxine**.[2]

A large retrospective population analysis of patients taking long-term **levothyroxine** found that unspecified H_2-receptor antagonists had no effect on serum TSH concentrations.[3]

The reason for the reduction in **levothyroxine** absorption with **cimetidine** is not understood, and its clinical importance awaits assessment, but the magnitude of the effect is small, and therefore it seems unlikely to be generally relevant.

1. Jonderko G, Jonderko K, Marcisz CZ, Kotulska A. Effect of cimetidine and ranitidine on absorption of [^{125}I] levothyroxine administered orally. *Acta Pharmacol Sin* (1992) 13, 391–4.
2. Ananthakrishnan S, Braverman LE, Levin RM, Magnani B, Pearce EN. The effect of famotidine, esomeprazole, and ezetimibe on levothyroxine absorption. *Thyroid* (2008) 18, 493–8.
3. Irving SA, Vadiveloo T, Leese GP. Drugs that interact with levothyroxine: an observational study from the Thyroid Epidemiology, Audit and Research Study (TEARS). *Clin Endocrinol (Oxf)* (2015) 82, 136–41.

Thyroid hormones + HIV-protease inhibitors

Case reports suggest that HIV-protease inhibitors boosted with ritonavir increase levothyroxine requirements. Nelfinavir might interact similarly. The situation with indinavir is less clear, with no effect, a reduction and an increase in levothyroxine requirements reported in different cases; the outcome seems likely to depend on the other antiretrovirals given.

Clinical evidence

(a) Indinavir

A 36-year-old HIV-positive woman taking **levothyroxine** 750 micrograms daily (following partial thyroid gland destruction for Graves' disease) was given stavudine, lamivudine, and indinavir. After about 7 weeks she presented with symptoms of hyperthyroidism (including nervousness, palpitations, and weight loss). Her serum TSH was low and serum thyroxine was high. After stepped dose decreases her thyroid function was finally stabilised with **levothyroxine** 120 micrograms daily.[1] See also *Nelfinavir* and *Ritonavir-based regimens*, below.

(b) Nelfinavir

In a woman, a 4-week course of antiretroviral prophylaxis, including 2 weeks of **indinavir** then 2 weeks of nelfinavir, tended to reduce the efficacy of **levothyroxine** 125 micrograms daily. She was fatigued and had elevated TSH concentrations (6.2 mU/L at day 12 and 17.4 mU/L at day 27) and hypercholesterolaemia, which resolved after the antiretroviral drugs were stopped.[2] For a case where hypothyroidism did not improve on switching from lopinavir boosted with ritonavir to nelfinavir, see *Ritonavir-based regimens*, below.

(c) Ritonavir-based regimens

An HIV-positive man, taking **levothyroxine** for autoimmune thyroiditis, developed an enlarged thyroid gland and marked lethargy about a month after his antiretrovirals were changed to include stavudine, lamivudine, **saquinavir** 400 mg twice daily, and ritonavir 600 mg twice daily. It became necessary to double his maintenance dose of **levothyroxine** to re-stabilise him. When the ritonavir and **saquinavir** were withdrawn and replaced by **indinavir**, the patient was able to go back to the original dose of **levothyroxine**.[3] In another HIV-positive female patient, taking zidovudine, lamivudine, and **lopinavir boosted with ritonavir**, **levothyroxine** was started after a total thyroidectomy and post-surgical radioiodine therapy. However, abnormal thyroid function persisted despite an increase in the **levothyroxine** dose to 225 micrograms daily. The antiretrovirals were withdrawn and thyroid function normalised. However, when the same antiretroviral regimen was restarted 8 months later because of a reduced CD4 cell count, hypothyroidism recurred within a month. A switch to **nelfinavir** did not normalise thyroid function, and the patient was eventually stabilised on a combination of three NRTIs.[4]

Mechanism

Uncertain. Ritonavir *increases* the activity of the glucuronyltransferases, which are concerned with the metabolism (conjugation) of levothyroxine, and might therefore reduce its effect. Conversely, indinavir might *reduce* the activity of glucuronyltransferases.

Importance and management

Direct information about an interaction between HIV-protease inhibitors and levothyroxine seems limited. Whether or not an interaction occurs seems to depend on the individual HIV-protease inhibitor, how it affects glucuronidation, and how much remaining thyroid function a patient has.[2] Until more is known about this interaction it would seem prudent to monitor thyroid function more closely if a HIV-protease inhibitor is given to a patient with pre-existing hypothyroidism.

1. Lanzafame M, Trevenzoli M, Faggian F, Marcati P, Gatti F, Carolo G, Concia E. Interaction between levothyroxine and indinavir in a patient with HIV infection. *Infection* (2002) 30, 54–5.
2. Nerad JL, Kessler HA. Hypercholesterolemia in a health care worker receiving thyroxine after post-exposure prophylaxis for human immunodeficiency virus infection. *Clin Infect Dis* (2001) 32, 1635–6.
3. Tseng A, Fletcher D. Interaction between ritonavir and levothyroxine. *AIDS* (1998) 12, 2235–6.
4. Touzot M, Le Beller C, Touzot F, Louet AL, Piketty C. Dramatic interaction between levothyroxine and lopinavir/ritonavir in a HIV-infected patient. *AIDS* (2006) 20, 1210–2.

Thyroid hormones + Iron compounds

Ferrous sulfate reduces the effects of levothyroxine in patients with treated hypothyroidism.

Clinical evidence

In a study, 14 patients with primary hypothyroidism taking stable doses of **levothyroxine** had an increase in TSH concentrations from 1.6 mU/L to 5.4 mU/L when given **ferrous sulfate** 300 mg daily for 12 weeks. The symptoms of hypothyroidism in 9 patients worsened.[1] In another report, a woman with hypothyroidism taking a stable dose of **levothyroxine** had a very marked increase in TSH concentrations when she took **ferrous sulfate**. Her **levothyroxine** dose needed to be increased from 175 micrograms daily to 200 micrograms daily.[2] Another similar report is described, in which a pregnant woman required an increase in her **levothyroxine** dose (from 150 micrograms daily to 250 micrograms daily) while taking **ferrous sulfate** 325 mg three times daily with meals and levothyroxine at bedtime. When the ferrous sulfate was stopped after delivery, she had symptoms of hyperthyroidism, and required a reduction in her levothyroxine dose to the original level. When the ferrous sulfate was restarted 12 weeks postpartum, the same interaction occurred.[3] In a further report, a 95-year-old woman treated successfully with **levothyroxine** 75 micrograms daily for many years experienced a recurrence of hypothyroidism with elevated serum TSH when she was given **ferrous sulfate** 80 mg daily (*Tardyferon*).[4]

A large retrospective population analysis of patients taking long-term **levothyroxine** found that oral iron (salt unspecified) increased median serum TSH concentrations by 0.36 mU/L over 6 months.[5]

Mechanism

The addition of iron to levothyroxine *in vitro* was found to produce a poorly soluble purple iron-levothyroxine complex. This might also occur in the gut,[1] leading to a reduction in the absorption of levothyroxine.

Importance and management

Information is limited to these reports but the interaction between ferrous sulfate and levothyroxine appears to be clinically important. Be alert for this effect if both drugs are given, and monitor thyroid function if an interaction is suspected: adjust the levothyroxine dose accordingly. Although it has been suggested that the doses of ferrous sulfate and levothyroxine should be separated by 2 hours or more, on the assumption that reduced absorption accounts for this interaction,[1] one case report suggests that this might not prevent the interaction.[3] The same precautions would seem appropriate with any other iron compound.

1. Campbell NRC, Hasinoff BB, Stalts H, Rao B, Wong NCW. Ferrous sulfate reduces thyroxine efficacy in patients with hypothyroidism. *Ann Intern Med* (1992) 117, 1010–3.

2. Schlienger JL. Accroissement des besoins en thyroxine par le sulfate de fer. *Presse Med* (1994) 23, 492.
3. Shakir KMM, Chute JP, Aprill BS, Lazarus AA. Ferrous sulfate-induced increase in requirement for thyroxine in a patient with primary hypothyroidism. *South Med J* (1997) 90, 637–9.
4. Fiaux E, Kadri K, Levasseur C, Le Guillou C, Chassagne P. Hypothyroïdie secondaire à une interaction médicamenteuse entre lévothyroxine et sels de fer. *Rev Med Interne* (2010) 31, e4–e5.
5. Irving SA, Vadiveloo T, Leese GP. Drugs that interact with levothyroxine: an observational study from the Thyroid Epidemiology, Audit and Research Study (TEARS). *Clin Endocrinol (Oxf)* (2015) 82, 136–41.

Thyroid hormones + Lanthanum

Lanthanum carbonate decreases levothyroxine absorption.

Clinical evidence, mechanism, importance and management

In a single-dose study, 6 healthy subjects were given a large dose of **levothyroxine** (1000 micrograms) at the same time as lanthanum carbonate 500 mg. Lanthanum decreased the serum thyroxine AUC_{0-6} by about 40%.[1]

The interaction between **levothyroxine** and lanthanum appears to be established (although the documentation is very limited) and the reduced thyroxine exposure that results seems likely to be of clinical importance.

The UK and US manufacturers of lanthanum carbonate advise that thyroid replacement therapy [presumably levothyroxine and possibly **liothyronine**] should not be taken within 2 hours of lanthanum, and that closer monitoring of TSH concentrations is recommended during concurrent use[2,3] so that any necessary dose adjustments can be made.

1. Weitzman SP, Ginsburg KC, Carlson HE. Colesevelam hydrochloride and lanthanum carbonate interfere with the absorption of levothyroxine. *Thyroid* (2009) 19, 77–79.
2. Fosrenol (Lanthanum carbonate hydrate). Shire Pharmaceuticals Ltd. UK Summary of product characteristics, March 2013.
3. Fosrenol (Lanthanum carbonate hydrate). Shire US Inc. US Prescribing information, September 2014.

Thyroid hormones + Oestrogens

Oral HRT (conjugated oestrogens) appears to increase the requirement for levothyroxine in some patients. A similar effect might therefore be expected with oral combined hormonal contraceptives, which include oestrogens.

Clinical evidence

In 25 postmenopausal women taking stable doses of **levothyroxine** (for hypothyroidism or TSH suppression), the addition of HRT (**conjugated oestrogens** 0.625 mg daily with or without **medroxyprogesterone acetate** 5 mg daily for 12 days each month) decreased serum free thyroxine concentrations and increased TSH concentrations. The changes in TSH were clinically important in 10 of the 25 women, requiring increased doses of **levothyroxine**, although only one woman had symptoms of hypothyroidism.[1] A large retrospective population analysis of patients taking long-term **levothyroxine** found that unspecified oestrogens increased serum TSH concentrations.[2]

Mechanism

Oestrogens increase thyroxine binding-globulin. In women with normal thyroid function this does not alter free thyroxine concentrations or TSH concentrations,[1,3] as the thyroxine secretion can increase to accommodate the changes. However, in women with hypothyroidism, who cannot compensate for the increased thyroxine binding, decreased free thyroxine and therefore increased TSH can result. One cross-over study found that oral HRT (conjugated oestrogens) had a greater effect on thyroxine concentrations and thyroxine-binding globulin than transdermal HRT (**ethinylestradiol**), which had minimal effects on these markers of thyroid function. Thyroxine binding-globulin is synthesised in the liver, and it is suggested that oral oestrogens increase this synthesis more than transdermal oestrogens because higher concentrations of oestrogen are present in the liver following oral dosing: an oral dose of oestrogen undergoes first-pass metabolism in the liver whereas transdermal oestrogens do not.[4]

Importance and management

Although these studies appear to be the only evidence of an interaction between levothyroxine and oestrogens, it would be prudent to monitor thyroid function several months after starting or stopping oral conjugated oestrogens to check levothyroxine requirements. This potential interaction should not affect the management and dosing of patients already taking HRT and newly started on levothyroxine, as the levothyroxine dose is usually adjusted according to thyroid function tests and clinical improvement of symptoms. Theoretically, the interaction should not apply to transdermal HRT (see *Mechanism*, above), but this requires confirmation.

The interaction is predicted to occur in any patient taking oral oestrogens, including combined hormonal contraceptives (although there do not appear to be any published studies in patients taking thyroid replacement therapy). Nevertheless, it has been suggested that all patients taking levothyroxine and oral oestrogens should have their thyroid function assessed 6–8 weeks after starting or stopping the oestrogen.[5] However, one could argue that if a clinically important interaction between levothyroxine and oral combined hormonal contraceptives were to occur, it would have come to light by now.

The effects of oestrogens on **liothyronine** do not appear to have been studied, but it would be expected to be affected in the same way as levothyroxine, although it has a lower affinity for thyroxine-binding globulin. Nevertheless, it would be advisable to follow the same precautions advised for levothyroxine.

1. Arafah BM. Increased need for thyroxine in women with hypothyroidism during estrogen therapy. *N Engl J Med* (2001) 344, 1743–9.
2. Irving SA, Vadiveloo T, Leese GP. Drugs that interact with levothyroxine: an observational study from the Thyroid Epidemiology, Audit and Research Study (TEARS). *Clin Endocrinol (Oxf)* (2015) 82, 136–41.
3. Ågren UM, Anttila M, Mäenpää-Liukko K, Rantala M-L, Rautiainen H, Sommer WF, Mommers E. Effects of a monophasic combined oral contraceptive nomegestrol acetate and 17β-oestradiol in comparison to one containing levonorgestrel and ethinylestradiol on markers of endocrine function. *Eur J Contracept Reprod Health Care* (2011) 16, 458–67.
4. Shifren JL, Desindes S, McIlwain M, Doros G, Mazer NA. A randomized, open-label, crossover study comparing the effects of oral versus transdermal estrogen therapy on serum androgens, thyroid hormones, and adrenal hormones in naturally menopausal women. *Menopause* (2007) 14, 985–94.
5. Tahboub R, Arafah BM. Sex steroids and the thyroid. *Best Pract Res Clin Endocrinol Metab* (2009) 23, 769–80.

Thyroid hormones + Orlistat

A woman taking levothyroxine developed symptoms of hypothyroidism when she started to take orlistat.

Clinical evidence

A case report describes a woman taking stable doses of **levothyroxine** 250 micrograms daily after a thyroidectomy, who started to take orlistat. Within 2 weeks she had developed signs of hypothyroidism (tiredness, lethargy, cold intolerance): her free thyroxine concentration was found to be 7 picomol/L, and her TSH concentration was 73.6 mU/L. Two weeks after stopping orlistat, and increasing the dose of **levothyroxine** to 300 [micrograms] daily, her symptoms improved, and 4 weeks later her thyroxine and TSH concentrations had normalised.[1]

Mechanism

It is suggested that orlistat might have bound to levothyroxine in the gastrointestinal tract, thus reducing its bioavailability.[1]

Importance and management

Evidence for an interaction between levothyroxine and orlistat is limited, but the result of concurrent use, probably as a result of reduced absorption, is consistent with the way both drugs are known to interact with other substances. Some manufacturers of levothyroxine and orlistat recommend that the administration of levothyroxine and orlistat should be separated by at least 4 hours.[2,3] It would be prudent to monitor the response to concurrent use, to confirm that this is effective.

1. Madhava K, Hartley A. Hypothyroidism in thyroid carcinoma follow-up: orlistat may inhibit the absorption of thyroxine. *Clin Oncol* (2005) 17, 492–3.
2. Synthroid (Levothyroxine sodium). Abbott Laboratories. US Prescribing information, June 2011.
3. Xenical (Orlistat). Roche Pharmaceuticals. US Prescribing information, December 2013.

Thyroid hormones + Phenytoin

Clinical hypothyroidism can occur when patients taking a stable dose of levothyroxine start to take phenytoin, and probably also fosphenytoin. Correction of hypothyroidism with levothyroxine does not appear to affect the pharmacokinetics of phenytoin. However, a case report describes a patient with phenytoin toxicity who also had hypothyroidism despite taking levothyroxine. Liothyronine would be expected to interact similarly.

Clinical evidence

A patient with a 27-year history of epilepsy, who was taking phenytoin 400 mg daily and carbamazepine 500 mg twice daily, and who had also been taking **levothyroxine** 250 micrograms daily for 4 years reduced to 200 micrograms daily 6 weeks previously, developed dysarthria, visual disturbance, incoordination, and mobility problems. Her blood carbamazepine concentration was within the therapeutic range, but her phenytoin concentration was greatly elevated at 43 [micrograms/mL] (therapeutic range 10 to 20 [micrograms/mL]), her free thyroxine concentration was low and her TSH concentration was increased, indicating phenytoin toxicity and hypothyroidism. Phenytoin was temporarily withdrawn. After 12 days her phenytoin concentration decreased to about 12 [micrograms/mL] and she was discharged, taking **levothyroxine** 100 micrograms daily, phenytoin 300 mg daily, carbamazepine, and lamotrigine. Three weeks later she was euthyroid and symptom-free.[1]

A study in 7 patients found that the pharmacokinetics of phenytoin were unchanged by **levothyroxine**. The pharmacokinetics of phenytoin were assessed in the hypothyroid state and after the patients had been euthyroid for 4 to 11 months.[2]

In a study, 6 patients whose hypothyroidism was stabilised with **levothyroxine** were given phenytoin 350 mg daily for 14 days. Phenytoin appeared to slightly reduce the intestinal absorption of **levothyroxine** and to increase the metabolism of thyroxine. Total and free serum concentrations of thyroxine and T3 were decreased and there was an associated increase in TSH.[3]

A case report describes a patient with hypothyroidism taking stable doses of **levothyroxine** 150 micrograms daily for 4 years, who developed hypothyroidism when given phenytoin 300 mg daily. Doubling the **levothyroxine** dose effectively controlled the hypothyroidism. Later this interaction was confirmed when stopping and restarting phenytoin produced the same effect.[4]

Mechanism

Phenytoin can induce the metabolism of endogenous thyroid hormones, thereby reducing their plasma concentrations, but this rarely results in hypothyroidism in euthyroid patients. However, in patients taking levothyroxine replacement therapy, the decrease appears more likely to be clinically relevant.[5] In addition, it has been suggested[6] that as phenytoin can reduce thyroid hormone concentrations there might be a resultant decrease in the activity of the enzymes involved in the metabolism of phenytoin.

Importance and management

Although the evidence is limited, the interaction between levothyroxine and phenytoin is established. The available evidence suggests that some patients taking levothyroxine might require an increase in dose when they start phenytoin (and therefore probably its prodrug, **fosphenytoin**). Be alert for this effect if both drugs are given, and monitor thyroid function if an interaction is suspected, adjusting the levothyroxine dose accordingly. This effect has been seen with other enzyme-inducing drugs, for example see 'Thyroid hormones + Barbiturates', p.1523.

Given the proposed mechanism of the interaction with levothyroxine, it seems likely that **liothyronine** could be similarly affected by phenytoin, but this does not appear to have been studied. Nevertheless, it would seem prudent to undertake the same precautions given for levothyroxine, if phenytoin or fosphenytoin is started.

The case of hypothyroidism and phenytoin toxicity is of unknown general relevance, particularly as studies have not found phenytoin metabolism to be altered by thyroid function.[2]

1. Betteridge T, Fink J. Phenytoin toxicity and thyroid dysfunction. *N Z Med J* (2009) 122, 102–4.
2. Mølholm Hansen J, Skovsted L, Kampmann JP, Lumholtz BI, Siersbæk-Nielsen K. Unaltered metabolism of phenytoin in thyroid disorders. *Acta Pharmacol Toxicol (Copenh)* (1978) 42, 343–6.
3. Faber J, Lumholtz IB, Kirkegaard C, Poulsen S, Jørgensen PH, Siersbaek-Nielsen K, Friis T. The effects of phenytoin (diphenylhydantoin) on the extrathyroidal turnover of thyroxine, 3,5,3'-triiodothyronine, 3,3',5'-triiodothyronine, and 3',5'-diiodothyronine in man. *J Clin Endocrinol Metab* (1985) 61, 1093–9.
4. Blackshear JL, Schultz AL, Napier JS, Stuart DD. Thyroxine replacement requirements in hypothyroid patients receiving phenytoin. *Ann Intern Med* (1983) 99, 341–2.
5. Simko J, Horacek J. Carbamazepine and risk of hypothyroidism: a prospective study. *Acta Neurol Scand* (2007) 116, 317–21.
6. Sarich TC, Wright JM. Hypothyroxinemia and phenytoin toxicity: a vicious circle. *Drug Metabol Drug Interact* (1996) 13, 155–60.

Thyroid hormones + Piracetam

A case report describes behavioural changes in a 10-year-old boy with hypothyroidism after piracetam was introduced.

Clinical evidence, mechanism, importance and management

A 10-year-old boy with a learning disorder, who was taking a stable dose of **levothyroxine** (150 micrograms daily) for secondary hypothyroidism, developed marked behavioural changes when he was given piracetam (4.8 g daily in divided doses). Piracetam was stopped and over the next 3 days the boy's behaviour returned to his usual disposition. The same behaviour pattern recurred on 2 subsequent occasions when piracetam was reintroduced, followed by recovery when piracetam was stopped.[1] It is unclear whether the adverse effects were due to piracetam itself or to an interaction with levothyroxine.

This is an isolated report and its general relevance is therefore unknown, but it would be prudent to bear the possibility of an interaction in mind should these adverse events occur with the concurrent use of levothyroxine and piracetam.

1. Waters B, Resnick M, Simeon J, Trites R, Fiedorowicz C. An adverse reaction to piracetam in an hypothyroid 10 year old boy. *Prog Neuropsychopharmacol* (1980) 4, 207–9.

Thyroid hormones + Polystyrene sulfonate

A woman taking levothyroxine for hypothyroidism relapsed when she took sodium polystyrene sulfonate. Calcium polystyrene sulfonate would be expected to interact similarly.

Clinical evidence

A woman taking **levothyroxine** 150 micrograms daily for hypothyroidism, following a total thyroidectomy, later developed renal impairment and required dialysis. She was also taking digoxin, clofibrate, calcium carbonate, ferrous sulfate, nicotinic acid, folic acid, and magnesium sulfate. Because of persistent hyperkalaemia she started taking sodium polystyrene sulfonate 15 g daily (at the same time as the **levothyroxine**). After 6 months, she developed lethargy, a hoarse voice, facial fullness, and weight gain (all symptoms of hypothyroidism). These symptoms resolved within 6 weeks of increasing the **levothyroxine** dose to 200 micrograms daily and separating its administration from the sodium polystyrene sulfonate by 10 hours.[1]

Mechanism

Sodium polystyrene sulfonate is a cation-exchange resin that is used to bind potassium ions in exchange for sodium. An *in vitro* study found that when levothyroxine 200 micrograms was dispersed in 100 mL water with 15 g sodium polystyrene sulfonate, the concentration of the levothyroxine at pH 2 decreased by 93% and at pH 7 by 98%.[1] This drop in concentration would be expected to occur in the gut as well, thereby reducing the amount of levothyroxine available for absorption. Calcium polystyrene sulfonate would be expected to interact similarly.

Importance and management

Information about an interaction between levothyroxine and polystyrene sulfonates seems to be limited to this study, but it would appear to be of general importance. Separate the doses of levothyroxine and polystyrene sulfonates as much as possible (10 hours was effective in the case reported) and monitor thyroid function to confirm that this is effective.

1. McLean M, Kirkwood I, Epstein M, Jones B, Hall C. Cation-exchange resin and inhibition of intestinal absorption of thyroxine. *Lancet* (1993) 341, 1286.

Thyroid hormones + Proton pump inhibitors

The efficacy of levothyroxine might be decreased by omeprazole and lansoprazole. Pantoprazole and esomeprazole did not appear to interact in this way in short-term studies.

Clinical evidence

In a randomised, crossover study in 20 healthy subjects, pretreatment with **pantoprazole** 40 mg daily for one week had no effect on the AUCs of TSH or thyroxine after a single 4-micrograms/kg dose of **levothyroxine**.[1] Similarly, in a study in 10 healthy subjects, **esomeprazole** 40 mg daily for one week did not affect the AUC of serum thyroxine in response to a single 600-microgram dose of **levothyroxine**.[2]

In contrast, in a non-randomised study in 10 women with multi-nodular goitre and gastro-oesophageal reflux disease, taking a stable dose of **levothyroxine** to suppress thyroid growth, **omeprazole** 40 mg daily for at least 6 months caused a variable increase in TSH concentrations (median 1.7 mU/L versus 0.1 mU/L before treatment). At that time, the dose of **levothyroxine** was increased to suppress TSH concentrations: this required a median dose of **levothyroxine** of 2.16 micrograms/kg, compared with 1.58 micrograms/kg before starting **omeprazole** (a 37% increase).[3] Similarly, in a retrospective analysis of 37 patients who had been taking stable doses of levothyroxine for at least 6 months and had then taken **lansoprazole** 30 mg daily for at least 2 months, the mean TSH concentrations were increased (by about 0.7 mU/L).[4]

A large retrospective population analysis of patients taking long-term **levothyroxine** found that unspecified proton pump inhibitors increased serum TSH concentrations.[5] Similarly, an observational study in patients taking **levothyroxine** for hypothyroidism found that unspecified proton pump inhibitors increased TSH concentrations initially, followed by a decrease, which the authors postulated was due to adjustments in levothyroxine dose.[6] A prospective observational cohort study in 24 patients taking a proton pump inhibitor (**omeprazole**, **pantoprazole**, **lansoprazole**, or **esomeprazole**) and **levothyroxine** tablets found that TSH concentrations were lower after patients were switched to the same dose of a levothyroxine oral solution. Some of the patients subsequently developed symptoms of hyperthyroidism and required dose reduction of the levothyroxine oral solution.[7]

Mechanism

A decrease in gastric acidity might decrease levothyroxine absorption. Supporting this is the finding that in patients with impaired gastric acid secretion, the required dose of levothyroxine was 22 to 34% higher than in patients free of gastric disease.[3] However, this effect could be due to the disease rather than gastric acid *per se*.[8] Any effect of proton pump inhibitors on the absorption of levothyroxine might differ between levothyroxine formulations. It has been suggested that formulations which do not require dissolution (such as oral solutions) are absorbed faster, and are less affected by decreased gastric acidity, than tablets.[7]

Importance and management

An interaction between levothyroxine and the proton pump inhibitors is not established. The studies with pantoprazole and esomeprazole did not reveal a change in levothyroxine absorption, whereas the study in patients who had been taking omeprazole for 6 months suggested that patients might need a small increase in levothyroxine dose, and the retrospective analysis with lansoprazole showed an even smaller increase in TSH. The population analysis and the observational study in patients taking levothyroxine found that TSH concentrations were increased by proton pump inhibitors, but these studies did not examine which specific proton pump inhibitors were taken or the clinical outcomes for individuals. Bear in mind the possibility of an interaction if a patient starting a proton pump inhibitor shows signs of reduced levothyroxine efficacy. Any interaction can take several months to develop. Further study is needed to establish an interaction.

1. Dietrich JW, Gieselbrecht K, Holl RW, Boehm BO. Absorption kinetics of levothyroxine is not altered by proton-pump inhibitor therapy. *Horm Metab Res* (2006) 38, 57–9.
2. Ananthakrishnan S, Braverman LE, Levin RM, Magnani B, Pearce EN. The effect of famotidine, esomeprazole, and ezetimibe on levothyroxine absorption. *Thyroid* (2008) 18, 493–8.
3. Centanni M, Gargano L, Canettieri G, Viceconti N, Franchi A, Delle Fave G, Annibale B. Thyroxine in goiter, Helicobacter pylori infection, and chronic gastritis. *N Engl J Med* (2006) 354, 1787–95.
4. Sachmechi I, Reich DM, Aninyei M, Wibowo F, Gupta G, Kim PJ. Effect of proton pump inhibitors on serum thyroid-stimulating hormone level in euthyroid patients treated with levothyroxine for hypothyroidism. *Endocr Pract* (2007) 13, 345–9.
5. Irving SA, Vadiveloo T, Leese GP. Drugs that interact with levothyroxine: an observational study from the Thyroid Epidemiology, Audit and Research Study (TEARS). *Clin Endocrinol (Oxf)* (2015) 82, 136–41.
6. Trifirò G, Parrino F, Sultana J, Giorgianni F, Ferrajolo C, Bianchini E, Medea G, Benvenga S, Cricelli I, Cricelli C, Lapi F. Drug interactions with levothyroxine therapy in patients with hypothyroidism: observational study in General Practice. *Clin Drug Investig* (2015) 35, 187–95.
7. Vita R, Saraceno G, Trimarchi F, Benvenga S. Switching levothyroxine from the tablet to the oral solution formulation corrects the impaired absorption of levothyroxine induced by proton-pump inhibitors. *J Clin Endocrinol Metab* (2014) 99, 4481–6.
8. Dietrich JW, Boehm BO. Thyroxine in goiter, H. pylori infection, and gastritis. *N Engl J Med* (2006) 355, 1177.

Thyroid hormones + Raloxifene

Two patients developed increased levothyroxine requirements after taking raloxifene for a number of months.

Clinical evidence

A 79-year-old woman taking **levothyroxine** 150 micrograms daily developed elevated TSH concentrations and symptoms of hypothyroidism within 2 to 3 months of starting to take raloxifene 60 mg daily. Over the next 6 months the **levothyroxine** dose was progressively increased to 300 micrograms daily without normalising her TSH concentration. This patient took raloxifene early in the morning, at the same time as **levothyroxine**. Subsequently, separating the dose of raloxifene and **levothyroxine** by 12 hours led to a reduction in her TSH concentration. In a single-dose study in this patient, serum thyroxine concentrations were reduced when **levothyroxine** 1000 micrograms was given with raloxifene 60 mg, and separating the doses of raloxifene and **levothyroxine** by 12 hours was found to reduce TSH concentrations.[1] Another very similar case has been reported in a 47-year-old woman, which also resolved on separating administration of the **raloxifene** and **levothyroxine** by 12 hours.[2]

Mechanism

It appears that raloxifene reduces the absorption of levothyroxine, but the mechanism for this is not known.

Importance and management

The interaction between levothyroxine and raloxifene is not established, but the similar outcomes in both case reports suggest that an interaction might occur. Further study is needed, but until then it would be prudent to monitor for otherwise unexplained symptoms of hypothyroidism. If an interaction is suspected, monitor thyroid function and try separating administration by 12 hours before increasing the levothyroxine dose.

1. Siraj ES, Gupta MK, Reddy SSK. Raloxifene causing malabsorption of levothyroxine. *Arch Intern Med* (2003) 163, 1367–70.
2. Garwood CL, Van Schepen KA, McDonough RP, Sullivan AL. Increased thyroid-stimulating hormone levels associated with concomitant administration of levothyroxine and raloxifene. *Pharmacotherapy* (2006) 26, 881–5.

Thyroid hormones + Rifampicin (Rifampin)

Two case reports suggest that rifampicin might reduce the effects of thyroid hormones. However, in a single-dose study, rifampicin increased the exposure to thyroxine.

Clinical evidence

A woman with Turner's syndrome, who had undergone a total thyroidectomy and who was taking **levothyroxine** 100 micrograms daily, had a large decrease in serum thyroxine concentrations and free thyroxine index with a dramatic increase in TSH concentrations when given rifampicin. However, no symptoms of clinical hypothyroidism developed, and the decrease in serum thyroxine occurred before starting rifampicin, which could reflect the clinical picture of an acute infection.[1] Another case describes a *decrease* in TSH concentrations when rifampicin was discontinued.[2]

In a single-dose study in 8 healthy subjects, giving rifampicin 600 mg at the same time as a large dose (1000 micrograms) of **levothyroxine** increased the thyroxine AUC by 25%.[3]

Mechanism

A possible reason for the changes seen in the case reports is that rifampicin, a well-known, non-specific, enzyme inducer, can increase the metabolism of many drugs and thereby reduce their effects. Rifampicin has been found to reduce endogenous serum thyroxine concentrations in healthy subjects[4] and possibly in patients.[2] Note that, other enzyme inducers have, rarely, also been seen to interact in this way, see 'Thyroid hormones + Phenytoin', p.1528. The authors of the single-dose study[3] noted that the increased thyroxine exposure seen with a single-dose of rifampicin was unexpected. As rifampicin has effects on drug transporter proteins, the authors speculated that transporters such as OATP or P-glycoprotein might have been involved, however, this requires further investigation.

Importance and management

There seem to be no reports of clinically relevant adverse effects in patients given thyroid hormones and rifampicin, and the evidence for this interaction is by no means conclusive. Although rifampicin can affect thyroid hormones, it appears that healthy individuals can compensate for this. As hypothyroid patients might not be able to compensate in the same way, bear this interaction in mind if thyroid function tests are unexpectedly altered when rifampicin is given to a patient taking **levothyroxine**. If symptoms of hypothyroidism develop, monitor thyroid hormone concentrations, and adjust the dose of levothyroxine accordingly. It would seem prudent to take similar precautions in patients given **liothyronine** and rifampicin.

The clinical relevance of the increase in thyroxine exposure seen with a single dose of rifampicin is unknown, but bear this in mind if there is an unexpected response to treatment.

1. Isley WL. Effect of rifampin therapy on thyroid function tests in a hypothyroid patient on replacement L-thyroxine. *Ann Intern Med* (1987) 107, 517–18.
2. Nolan SR, Self TH, Norwood JM. Interaction between rifampin and levothyroxine. *South Med J* (1999) 92, 529–31.
3. Goldberg AS, Tirona RG, Asher LJ, Kim RB, Van Uum SHM. Ciprofloxacin and rifampicin have opposite effects on levothyroxine absorption. *Thyroid* (2013) 23, 1374–78.
4. Ohnhaus EE, Studer H. A link between liver microsomal enzyme activity and thyroid hormone metabolism in man. *Br J Clin Pharmacol* (1983) 15, 71–6.

Thyroid hormones + Sevelamer

Sevelamer decreases the response to levothyroxine.

Clinical evidence

A 62-year-old haemodialysis patient with chronic tubulointerstitial nephritis, taking amlodipine, enalapril, esomeprazole, paracetamol, vitamin B, and sevelamer 3200 mg daily at breakfast, was given **levothyroxine** for hypothyroidism in a dose gradually increased to 150 micrograms daily, also with breakfast. After 3 months, clinical response was inadequate and her TSH was 196 mU/L. Three weeks after starting to take **levothyroxine** 175 micrograms at night, rather than in the morning, and at least 4 hours after any other medicine, TSH concentrations had decreased to 19 mU/L. However, 9 months later after hospitalisation for arteriovenous fistula problems, during which time she was again given **levothyroxine** with her other medicines in the morning, her TSH concentration increased to 76 mU/L. **Levothyroxine** was then changed back to a night-time dose and the TSH concentration rapidly normalised.[1] A similar case of hypothyroidism occurred in a 55-year-old haemodialysis patient who had been taking sevelamer 800 mg with breakfast at the same time as **levothyroxine** 100 micrograms. He also took sevelamer 1200 mg with his lunch and dinner. The dose of levothyroxine was increased to 150 micrograms daily in the morning but his TSH concentration remained high, however, once the patient started taking levothyroxine at night, 2 hours after dinner, his TSH concentration returned to within the normal range.[2]

In another case report, a 26 year old patient taking long-term **levothyroxine** 150 micrograms every morning was experiencing symptoms of hypothyroidism and had an increased TSH (650 mU/L). She had been taking sevelamer carbonate for 18 months, at a dose of 800 mg three times a day, with the first dose taken in the morning. The patient did not respond to progressively increased levothyroxine doses. However, when the sevelamer doses were rearranged so that the first dose was taken 4 hours after levothyroxine, her symptoms improved, and her TSH concentrations decreased to 5.7 mU/L after 15 days.[3] In a single-dose study in 7 healthy subjects, giving a large dose of **levothyroxine** (1000 micrograms) at the same time as sevelamer hydrochloride 800 mg resulted in a decrease of about 50% in the $AUC_{0\text{-}6}$ of thyroxine.[4] A retrospective study identified 67 patients who were taking **levothyroxine** and a phosphate binder (calcium carbonate, calcium acetate, or sevelamer hydrochloride). The TSH concentrations were significantly higher in patients taking sevelamer than calcium acetate, and the difference was greater over time. In addition, patients taking sevelamer required higher **levothyroxine** doses than those taking either of the calcium compounds.[5]

Mechanism

It seems likely that sevelamer binds with levothyroxine leaving less available for absorption.

Importance and management

Evidence for an interaction between sevelamer and levothyroxine is limited, but the available data suggests that sevelamer decreases the absorption of levothyroxine, and that this could result in increased dose requirements. The UK manufacturer of sevelamer notes that there have been post-marketing reports of increased TSH concentrations in patients given sevelamer with levothyroxine, and recommends closer monitoring of TSH concentrations in such patients,[6,7] which seems prudent. The authors of the case reports also note that hypothyroidism has been reported when levothyroxine has been taken at the same time as sevelamer and suggest that maximum possible separation of administration can minimise any interaction.[1-3] Where there is a potential risk of decreased absorption, it is generally recommended that other drugs should be avoided for at least 1 hour before, or 3 hours after, sevelamer.

1. Arnadottir M, Johannesson AJ. Phosphate binders and timing of levothyroxine administration. *Nephrol Dial Transplant* (2008) 23, 420.
2. Granata A, Floccari F, Gallieni M. Levothyroxine and sevelamer: listen to the patient. *Endocr Pract* (2011) 17, 961–2.
3. Iovino M, Iovine N, Petrosino A, Giagulli VA, Licchelli B, Guastamacchia E, Triggiani V. Sevelamer carbonate markedly reduces levothyroxine absorption. *Endocr Metab Immune Disord Drug Targets* (2014) 14, 206–9.
4. John-Kalarickal J, Pearlman G, Carlson HE. New medications which decrease levothyroxine absorption. *Thyroid* (2007) 17, 763–5.
5. Diskin CJ, Stokes TJ, Dansby LM, Radcliff L, Carter TB. Effect of phosphate binders upon TSH and L-thyroxine dose in patients on thyroid replacement. *Int Urol Nephrol* (2007) 39, 599–602.
6. Renagel (Sevelamer hydrochloride). Sanofi. UK Summary of product characteristics, February 2015.
7. Renvela (Sevelamer carbonate). Sanofi. UK Summary of product characteristics, March 2014.

Thyroid hormones + Simeticone

A case report describes a poor response to levothyroxine for the control of congenital hypothyroidism in an infant given simeticone.

Clinical evidence, mechanism, importance and management

A case report describes an infant with congenital hypothyroidism whose thyroid function did not respond adequately to increasing doses of **levothyroxine** (given as crushed tablets in water). **Levothyroxine** was gradually increased, from 50 micrograms daily at diagnosis (13 days old) to 75 micrograms daily at 12 weeks, because TSH concentrations remained too high (although free thyroxine concentrations were within normal range by week 6). At 12 weeks, it was discovered that, since week 5, the infant had been given simeticone-containing infant colic drops (*Infacol*), 0.5 mL before each feed. The colic drops were stopped and, 2 weeks later, TSH and free thyroxine concentrations were within the normal range. After 4 weeks the levothyroxine dose was decreased to 50 micrograms daily, whilst maintaining normal TSH concentrations.[1]

It has been suggested that simeticone might interfere with the intestinal absorption of levothyroxine, but this has not been confirmed. This case appears to be the only published report of a possible interaction between levothyroxine and simeticone. Until more is known, if concurrent use of simeticone-containing colic drops and levothyroxine is necessary in an infant, it would be prudent to monitor thyroid function frequently and adjust the dose of **levothyroxine** accordingly. The general relevance of this possible interaction to other simeticone preparations (e.g. combinations with antacids), or in other age groups, is not known.

1. Balapatabendi M, Harris D, Shenoy SD. Drug interaction of levothyroxine with infant colic drops. *Arch Dis Child* (2011) 96, 888–9.

Thyroid hormones + SSRIs

A study suggests that the effects of levothyroxine can be opposed by sertraline in some patients, but another study suggests that neither fluoxetine nor sertraline affect thyroid function in patients taking levothyroxine.

Clinical evidence

Nine patients with hypothyroidism taking **levothyroxine** were noted to have elevated TSH concentrations (indicating a decrease in the efficacy of their treatment), when they were also taking **sertraline**. Two other patients with thyroid cancer, whose TSH concentrations had been deliberately depressed, developed TSH concentrations in the normal range while taking **sertraline**. None of the patients showed any signs of hypothyroidism at the time, and all of them had been taking the same dose of **levothyroxine** for at least 6 months. TSH concentrations of up to almost 17 mU/L (reference range given as 0.3 to 5 mU/L) were seen in some patients. The **levothyroxine** doses were increased by 11 to 50%, until the TSH concentrations were back to normal. The authors of this report state that they know of three other patients whose TSH concentrations were unaltered by **sertraline**.[1] Similarly, the manufacturers of sertraline state that a review of their early-alert safety database to the end of July 1997 had identified 14 cases of hypothyroidism where a possible relation to sertraline could not be excluded. Seven of the patients were also taking **levothyroxine**.[2]

In contrast, in a prospective study in 57 patients with depression (28 with hypothyroidism treated with levothyroxine and 29 with normal thyroid function), neither **fluoxetine** 20 mg daily nor **sertraline** 50 mg daily for 90 days had a clinically relevant effect on thyroid function in either group of patients.[3]

Mechanism

Unknown.

Importance and management

Evidence for an interaction between levothyroxine and **sertraline** is conflicting. The reasons for the conflicting results are not clear, but they could be a reflection of differing degrees of hypothyroidism in the patients studied.[4] Any interaction appears rare, but if an interaction is suspected, it would seem prudent to monitor thyroid function and adjust the levothyroxine dose accordingly. Limited evidence suggests that **fluoxetine** does not interact with levothyroxine, and evidence for other SSRIs appears to be lacking. More study is needed.

1. McCowen KC, Spark R. Elevated serum thyrotropin in thyroxine-treated patients with hypothyroidism given sertraline. *N Engl J Med* (1997) 337, 1010–11.
2. Clary CM, Harrison WM. Elevated serum thyrotropin in thyroxine-treated patients with hypothyroidism given sertraline. *N Engl J Med* (1997) 337, 1011.
3. de Carvalho GA, Bahls S-C, Boeving A, Graf H. Effects of selective serotonin reuptake inhibitors on thyroid function in depressed patients with primary hypothyroidism or normal thyroid function. *Thyroid* (2009) 19, 691–7.
4. McCowen KC, Garber JR. Effect of SSRI antidepressants on l-thyroxine requirements. *Thyroid* (2010) 20, 937.

Thyroid hormones + Statins

Isolated cases describe patients taking levothyroxine who became either hypo- or hyperthyroid after taking lovastatin. Other reports describe reduced levothyroxine efficacy in patients taking simvastatin.

Clinical evidence, mechanism, importance and management

(a) Lovastatin

A 54-year-old man with diabetes taking **levothyroxine** 150 micrograms daily for Hashimoto's thyroiditis, and a number of other drugs (gemfibrozil, clofibrate, propranolol, diltiazem, quinidine, aspirin, dipyridamole, insulin) started taking lovastatin 20 mg daily. Weakness and muscle aches (with a normal creatinine phosphokinase) developed within 2 to 3 days, and over a 27-day period he lost 10% of his body weight. His serum thyroxine concentrations increased from about 145 nanomol/L to 350 nanomol/L. The author of the report suggested that the lovastatin might have displaced the thyroid hormones from their binding sites, thereby increasing their effects and causing the patient's acute thyrotoxic state. It was suggested that he did not have any cardiac symptoms because of his pre-existing drug regimen.[1]

In contrast, a woman with goitrous hypothyroidism due to Hashimoto's thyroiditis, which was being treated with **levothyroxine** 125 micrograms daily, developed evidence of hypothyroidism (elevated TSH) on two occasions while taking lovastatin 20 or 60 mg daily. No clinical signs of hypothyroidism developed, apart from some increased fatigue, and possibly an increased sensitivity to insulin. The author suggested that lovastatin might have influenced the absorption or clearance of **levothyroxine**.[2]

When the second report[2] was published, the manufacturers of lovastatin reported that at that time (August 1989) more than 1 million patients had taken lovastatin, and hypothyroidism had only been reported in 3 patients.[3] It seems that any interaction is a very rare event and consequently unlikely to happen in most patients. No special precautions would therefore seem to be necessary on concurrent use.

(b) Simvastatin

A 75-year-old woman who had been taking a stable dose of **levothyroxine** 800 micrograms weekly for many years had a gradual increase in TSH concentrations and increasing tiredness after starting to take simvastatin 10 mg daily. After 4 months the **levothyroxine** dose was increased to 900 micrograms weekly, but the patient's symptoms had not improved in 2 weeks and the simvastatin was stopped. The patient's symptoms gradually resolved, and the dose of levothyroxine was reduced back to the previous level.[4]

Another patient, who had recently started taking **levothyroxine** 50 micrograms daily because of increasing TSH concentrations, was given simvastatin 10 mg daily. The TSH concentration continued to increase, so the simvastatin was stopped, and the TSH concentration decreased to the normal range within 4 weeks without the need for an alteration in the **levothyroxine** dose. This patient was subsequently given **pravastatin** without a change in thyroid status.[4] A further report describes an 85-year-old taking **levothyroxine** 100 micrograms daily who developed muscle pain, lower limb weakness, rhabdomyolysis, and hypothyroidism about 2 weeks after her dose of simvastatin was increased to 80 mg daily. Simvastatin was discontinued and the patient's TSH concentration decreased to normal within 4 weeks without modifying her dose of **levothyroxine**.[5]

The authors conclude that any interaction must be extremely rare given the frequent use of simvastatin and **levothyroxine**.[4,5] Moreover, a cross sectional study in 41 patients receiving levothyroxine, found that giving simvastatin 20 mg daily for 3 months had no statistically significant effect on serum TSH or free thyroxine concentrations, and none of the patients experienced any symptoms of hypothyroidism.[6] No particular precautions would appear to be required on concurrent use.

(c) Unspecified statins

A large retrospective population analysis of 1149 patients stable taking long-term **levothyroxine**, found that unspecified statins decreased the median serum TSH concentration from 1.62 to 1.45 mU/L after 6 months.[7] This analysis did not examine which specific statins were taken, and the clinical relevance of the decrease in TSH is unknown.

1. Lustgarten BP. Catabolic response to lovastatin therapy. *Ann Intern Med* (1988) 109, 171–2.
2. Demke DM. Drug interaction between thyroxine and lovastatin. *N Engl J Med* (1989) 321, 1341–2.
3. Gormley GJ, Tobert JA. Drug interaction between thyroxine and lovastatin. *N Engl J Med* (1989) 321, 1342.
4. Kisch E, Segall HS. Interaction between simvastatin and L-thyroxine. *Ann Intern Med* (2005) 143, 547.
5. Kiernan TJ, Rochford M, McDermott JH. Simvastatin induced rhabdomyolysis and an important clinical link with hypothyroidism. Int J Cardiol. (2007) 119, 374–6.
6. Abbasinazari M, Nakhjavani M, Gogani S. The effects of simvastatin on the serum concentrations of thyroid stimulating hormone and free thyroxine in hypothyroid patients treated with levothyroxine. *Iran J Med Sci* (2011) 36, 80–83.
7. Irving SA, Vadiveloo T, Leese GP. Drugs that interact with levothyroxine: an observational study from the Thyroid Epidemiology, Audit and Research Study (TEARS). *Clin Endocrinol (Oxf)* (2015) 82, 136–41.

Thyroid hormones + Sucralfate

Sucralfate might reduce levothyroxine absorption, but not all studies have found this effect.

Clinical evidence

A woman with hypothyroidism did not respond to **levothyroxine**, despite taking 4.8 micrograms/kg daily, while taking sucralfate (dose not stated). Her response remained inadequate (TSH concentrations high, thyroxine concentrations low) even when the **levothyroxine** was taken 2.5 hours after the sucralfate. However, when **levothyroxine** was taken 4.5 hours before the sucralfate, the thyroxine and TSH concentrations gradually became normal.[1] Similarly, a single-dose study in healthy subjects found that giving a large dose of **levothyroxine** (1000 micrograms) with the last dose of sucralfate (five 1-g doses given every 6 hours), resulted in a 72% reduction in **levothyroxine** absorption, and a delay of 2 hours in reaching maximum absorption. Separating the doses by 8 hours avoided this effect.[2] Conversely, in 10 patients whose hypothyroidism was managed with stable doses of **levothyroxine**, giving sucralfate 1 g daily for 6 weeks at the same time as **levothyroxine** did not alter the concentrations of thyroxine or TSH.[3] Another placebo-controlled study similarly found that sucralfate had little effect on the absorption of **levothyroxine**, with just a minor decrease in serum thyroxine concentrations seen (about 94 nanomol/L with sucralfate versus about 105 nanomol/L with placebo).[4]

Mechanism

An *in vitro* study suggests that sucralfate binds strongly to levothyroxine, and it is presumed that this can also occur in the gut, thereby reducing levothyroxine absorption.[1]

Importance and management

An interaction between levothyroxine and sucralfate is not established, and the findings of the studies are somewhat contradictory. Nevertheless, it might be prudent not to take sucralfate until a few hours after levothyroxine. Patients should be advised accordingly and the response well monitored.

1. Havrankova J, Lahaie R. Levothyroxine binding by sucralfate. *Ann Intern Med* (1992) 117, 445–6.
2. Sherman SI, Tielens ET, Ladenson PW. Sucralfate causes malabsorption of L-thyroxine. *Am J Med* (1994) 96, 531–5.
3. Khan F, Jeanniton E, Renedo M. Does sucralfate impede levothyroxine therapy? *Ann Intern Med* (1993) 118, 317.
4. Campbell JA, Schmidt BA, Bantle JP. Sucralfate and the absorption of L-thyroxine. *Ann Intern Med* (1994) 121, 152.

Thyroid hormones + Tyrosine kinase inhibitors

Imatinib appears to cause hypothyroidism in thyroidectomy patients taking levothyroxine. A possible case of hypothyroidism has also occurred in a patient taking levothyroxine and sunitinib.

Clinical evidence

(a) Imatinib

A retrospective analysis of 11 patients with thyroid cancer taking **levothyroxine** found that 8 patients who had previously undergone a total thyroidectomy developed markedly elevated TSH concentrations and were clinically hypothyroid after taking imatinib. Despite a mean 3-fold increase in the dose of **levothyroxine**, hypothyroidism was reversed in only 3 patients. Thyroid function tests normalised on discontinuing imatinib. Conversely, no effect on thyroid function was seen in the 3 patients who had not had their thyroid gland removed.[1] In another report by the same authors, a woman taking **levothyroxine** following a thyroidectomy remained euthyroid when restarting imatinib. In this case the **levothyroxine** dose was immediately increased from 175 micrograms daily to 300 micrograms daily.[2] Another case report describes a 59-year-old woman who was euthyroid on **levothyroxine** after a subtotal thyroidectomy, but who became hypothyroid after starting imatinib and required a levothyroxine dose increase.[3]

(b) Sunitinib

A patient taking **levothyroxine** who was unable to tolerate imatinib[2] (see *Imatinib*, above), started taking sunitinib 5 months later. She was given sunitinib 50 mg daily for 4 weeks of a 6-week cycle. After 3 days her TSH concentrations increased, with normal free thyroxine and T3 concentrations, and the **levothyroxine** dose was increased to 300 micrograms daily. However, the TSH concentrations did not return to normal, and, additionally, haematological toxicity occurred. When her blood counts recovered, she was given a reduced dose of sunitinib 37.5 mg with **levothyroxine** 300 micrograms daily for the second cycle. On this cycle she remained euthyroid without serious haematological toxicity.[2]

Mechanism

Uncertain. The authors of the retrospective analysis suggest that imatinib might increase the clearance of thyroxine and T3 by inducing glucuronyltransferases (UGTs).[1] Patients who have undergone a thyroidectomy cannot respond to these changes and therefore become hypothyroid.

Importance and management

Interpretation of the cases cited is complicated by the possibility of the effects seen being a result of a drug-disease interaction between the tyrosine kinase inhibitor and thyroid disease, rather than a true drug-drug interaction, as a large number of the tyrosine kinase inhibitors are known to cause thyroid dysfunction themselves.[4] Whether this effect is a class effect, remains to be established. Nevertheless, the occurrence of imatinib-induced hypothyroidism in thyroidectomy patients taking levothyroxine would seem to be established. TSH concentrations should be more closely monitored in thyroidectomy patients taking levothyroxine if they are given imatinib, anticipating the need to increase the levothyroxine dose. The authors of the retrospective analysis suggest that, in thyroidectomy patients, the dose of levothyroxine should be doubled before starting imatinib.[1] Note that toxicity of imatinib (fatigue and periorbital oedema) might be indistinguishable from symptoms of hypothyroidism.[2] Although evidence is limited, similar precautions seem warranted for sunitinib.

1. de Groot JWB, Zonnenberg BA, Plukker JTM, van Der Graaf WTA, Links TP. Imatinib induces hypothyroidism in patients receiving levothyroxine. *Clin Pharmacol Ther* (2005) 78, 433–8.
2. de Groot JWB, Links TP, van der Graaf WTA. Tyrosine kinase inhibitors causing hypothyroidism in a patient on levothyroxine. *Ann Oncol* (2006) 17, 1719–20.
3. de Diego García P, Trincado Aznar P, Playán Usón J, Albero Gamboa R. Levothyroxine therapy and imatinib. *Endocrinol Nutr* (2008) 55, 304–7.
4. Brown RL. Tyrosine kinase inhibitor-induced hypothyroidism: incidence, etiology, and management. *Target Oncol* (2011) 6, 217–26.

37

Urological drugs

The drug classes used for various genito-urinary disorders are summarised in 'Table 37.1', below. The main groups of drugs included in this chapter are the urinary antimuscarinics and the phosphodiesterase type-5 inhibitors, along with various individual drugs. Note that, where the interaction involves these drugs affecting other drugs, the interaction is generally covered elsewhere.

Antimuscarinics

The main pharmacodynamic interaction of antimuscarinic drugs is an increased risk of antimuscarinic effects (e.g. dry mouth, constipation, confusion) when used with other drugs with antimuscarinic properties. Many drugs have antimuscarinic adverse effects, which may not be readily appreciated from their clinical uses, see 'Table 18.2', p.754, for a list. Some of the newer antimuscarinics used for incontinence have greater selectivity for the M_3 muscarinic receptors of the bladder. However, it is not established whether this results in a clinically relevant difference in the incidence of antimuscarinic adverse effects or antimuscarinic drug interactions.

Some of the urinary antimuscarinics, including darifenacin, solifenacin, and tolterodine, are principally metabolised by the cytochrome P450 isoenzyme system, or, in the case of fesoterodine, its main active metabolite is metabolised by these isoenzymes. Therefore clinically important pharmacokinetic drug interactions can occur with these drugs, due to an alteration in their metabolism.

Phosphodiesterase type-5 inhibitors

The main concern regarding the phosphodiesterase type-5 (PDE5) inhibitors has centred around their cardiovascular adverse effects. Therefore the possible risks of their use in patients with cardiovascular disease, and their drug interactions with drugs used in cardiovascular disease have been particularly studied. Important interactions occur with nitrates, see 'Phosphodiesterase type-5 inhibitors + Nitrates', p.1545, and also alpha blockers, see 'Phosphodiesterase type-5 inhibitors + Alpha blockers', p.1538. All the phosphodiesterase type-5 inhibitors are metabolised, to a greater or lesser extent, by CYP3A4, and therefore clinically relevant drug interactions can occur with drugs that induce or inhibit this route of metabolism.

Table 37.1 Classification of urological drugs

Group	*Drugs*
Drugs for benign prostatic hyperplasia	
Alpha blockers	See Alpha blockers, p.89
Anti-androgens	Dutasteride, Finasteride
Drugs for urinary incontinence	
Antimuscarinics and/or Antispasmodics	Darifenacin, Fesoterodine, Flavoxate, Imidafenacin, Oxybutynin, Propiverine, Solifenacin, Tolterodine, Trospium
Beta-3 adrenoceptor agonists	Mirabegron
SNRIs	Duloxetine, covered under SSRIs, Tricyclics and related antidepressants, p.1464
Drugs for nocturnal enuresis in children	
Tricyclic antidepressants	Imipramine, covered under SSRIs, Tricyclics and related antidepressants, p.1464
Vasopressin analogues	Desmopressin
Drugs for erectile dysfunction	
Dopaminergic agonists	Apomorphine, covered under Antiparkinsonian and related drugs, p.752
Muscle relaxants	Papaverine
Phosphodiesterase type-5 inhibitors	Avanafil, Sildenafil, Tadalafil, Vardenafil
Prostaglandins	Alprostadil
Others	Phentolamine, Yohimbine
Drugs for premature ejaculation	
Short-acting SSRIs	Dapoxetine

Alprostadil + Miscellaneous

Some manufacturers state that the concurrent use of intracavernosal alprostadil with other drugs used for erectile dysfunction increases the risk of prolonged erections. The concurrent use of alprostadil with antihypertensives, alpha blockers, and drugs causing vasodilation, such as the nitrates, may theoretically increase the risk of hypotension. Nasal decongestants and anorectics might theoretically reduce the efficacy of alprostadil. Clinical experience suggests that alprostadil, given by infusion, does not interact with 'penicillin', gentamicin, dopamine, isoprenaline (isoproterenol), furosemide, or digoxin.

Clinical evidence, mechanism, importance and management

A. Erectile dysfunction

(a) Appetite suppressants and decongestants

Some manufacturers state that, theoretically, sympathomimetics (such as **nasal decongestants** and **anorectics**[1]) might diminish the effect of alprostadil for erectile dysfunction.[1,2]

(b) Other drugs for erectile dysfunction

Prolonged priapism occurred in a man who, because of an inadequate response to a single 100-mg dose of **sildenafil**, used an intracavernosal injection of alprostadil 15 micrograms about one hour after taking the **sildenafil**.[3] Two other similar cases are described, one in a man who took **sildenafil** 100 mg and then, 90 minutes later, used 0.25 mL of intracavernosal *Trimix* (**papaverine**, **phentolamine** and alprostadil), and another in a man who took **tadalafil** 20 mg and then used *Trimix* 18 hours later.[3] Note that tadalafil has a half-life of 17.5 hours.[3] Some manufacturers state that smooth muscle relaxants, such as **papaverine**, and other drugs used to induce erections such as **alpha-blocking drugs** [e.g. intracavernosal **phentolamine**] or the phosphodiesterase type-5 inhibitors, such as **sildenafil**, should not be used concurrently with intracavernosal alprostadil because of the risk of priapism.[2,4] This recommendation does not appear to have been made for alprostadil for urethral application.[1,5]

(c) Vasodilating drugs

Alprostadil can rarely cause hypotension.[1,2,4] Some manufacturers state that there is a theoretical risk of hypotensive symptoms if alprostadil is used with vasodilating medications,[1,2,4] or antihypertensives,[2,5] and that this might be more common in the elderly.[1] Vasodilating medications would include the **alpha blockers** and the **nitrates**. One manufacturer states that, as the concurrent use of vasoactive drugs (not named) has not been studied, concurrent use is not recommended. They also state that, in clinical studies, the concurrent use of antihypertensives (not named) had no effect on the efficacy or safety of alprostadil.[6]

B. Neonatal congenital heart defects

The manufacturers of intravenous alprostadil note that there are no known drug interactions between alprostadil infusion and other drugs commonly given to neonates with congenital heart defects, including antibacterials such as **penicillin** (sic) or **gentamicin**, vasopressors, such as **dopamine** or **isoprenaline (isoproterenol)**, diuretics such as **furosemide**, and **digoxin**.[7,8]

1. Muse (Alprostadil). Meda Pharmaceuticals. UK Summary of product characteristics, November 2009.
2. Caverject Dual Chamber Injection (Alprostadil). Pharmacia Ltd. UK Summary of product characteristics, April 2010.
3. McMahon CG. Priapism associated with concurrent use of phosphodiesterase inhibitor drugs and intracavernous injection therapy. *Int J Impot Res* (2003) 15, 383–4.
4. Viridal Duo (Alprostadil). UCB Pharma Ltd. UK Summary of product characteristics, January 2010.
5. Muse (Alprostadil). Vivus Inc. US Prescribing information, August 2003.
6. Caverject Impulse (Alprostadil). Pharmacia & Upjohn Company. US Prescribing information, September 2006.
7. Prostin VR Sterile Solution (Alprostadil). Pharmacia Ltd. UK Summary of product characteristics, January 2008.
8. Prostin VR Paediatric (Alprostadil), Pharmacia & Upjohn Company. US Prescribing information, April 2006.

Dapoxetine + Miscellaneous

Ketoconazole, a CYP3A4 inhibitor, doubles the exposure to dapoxetine, and other CYP3A4 inhibitors are predicted to interact with dapoxetine similarly. Fluoxetine, a CYP2D6 inhibitor, also almost doubles the exposure to dapoxetine. Additive serotonergic effects may occur if dapoxetine is given with other drugs with serotonergic effects, such as the MAOIs, other SSRIs, and triptans.

Dapoxetine has no clinically relevant effect on the pharmacokinetics of desipramine, glibenclamide (glyburide), midazolam, omeprazole; nevertheless the manufacturer suggests that a clinically relevant interaction may still occur with other drugs metabolised similarly to midazolam and desipramine that have a narrow therapeutic window.

Dapoxetine does not affect the pharmacokinetics or anticoagulant effects of a single-dose of warfarin; nevertheless, the manufacturers do not exclude the possibility of an interaction with the long-term use of warfarin. No pharmacokinetic interaction occurs with alcohol; however, concurrent use is predicted increase the risk of adverse effects such as dizziness and orthostatic hypotension.

Clinical evidence, mechanism, importance and management

(a) Alcohol

In a single-dose, crossover study in 20 healthy men, the pharmacokinetics of dapoxetine 60 mg and its metabolites were not altered by alcohol 0.5 g/kg given 30 minutes after the dapoxetine. Concurrent use did not appear to alter the effects of alcohol on cognitive function, although there was a high degree of variability between subjects, precluding definitive assessment. Somnolence was the most common adverse effect, and was more common on concurrent use than with either drug alone (30% compared with 13% for dapoxetine and 9.5% for alcohol).[1] However, the manufacturer states that concurrent use might increase the risk and severity of alcohol-related adverse reactions, such as dizziness, drowsiness, slow reflexes or altered judgement. In addition, they state that concurrent use may increase the risk of syncope and thereby increase the risk of accidental injury. For this reason, they advise that patients taking dapoxetine should avoid drinking alcohol.[2]

(b) CYP2C9 substrates

Dapoxetine 60 mg daily for 6 days had no effect on the pharmacokinetics of a single 5-mg dose of **glibenclamide** (glyburide).[2] Glibenclamide is a known substrate of CYP2C9 and this study therefore suggests that dapoxetine is unlikely to affect the pharmacokinetics of drugs that are substrates of this isoenzyme. For a list of CYP2C9 substrates, see 'Table 1.5', p.7. Consider also *Warfarin*, below.

(c) CYP2C19 substrates

Dapoxetine 60 mg daily for 6 days had no effect on the metabolism of a single 40-mg dose of **omeprazole**.[2] Omeprazole is a known substrate of CYP2C19 and this study therefore suggests that no pharmacokinetic interaction would be expected between dapoxetine and omeprazole or other CYP2C19 substrates. For a list of CYP2C19 substrates, see 'Table 1.6', p.8.

(d) CYP2D6 inhibitors

The manufacturer states that **fluoxetine** 60 mg daily for 7 days increased the AUC of a single 60-mg dose of dapoxetine by 88% and increased its maximum concentration by 50%. The manufacturer estimates that this may double the AUC of the total active drug (dapoxetine and its metabolite desmethyldapoxetine).[2]

Dapoxetine is a substrate of CYP2D6, an isoenzyme that shows genetic polymorphism. Inhibition of CYP2D6 may increase the concentrations of dapoxetine in CYP2D6 extensive metabolisers (that is, those with normal concentrations of this isoenzyme) to those seen in CYP2D6 poor metabolisers (that is, those deficient or lacking in CYP2D6), and may increase the incidence and severity of dose-dependent adverse effects such as syncope and orthostatic hypotension.[2] For this reason, the manufacturer recommends caution when increasing the dose of dapoxetine to 60 mg in patients taking potent CYP2D6 inhibitors, as this may lead to an increase in adverse effects.[2] For a list of inhibitors of CYP2D6 see 'Table 1.7', p.9.

Note that dapoxetine is an SSRI and the concurrent use of dapoxetine with other SSRIs, such as **fluoxetine**, is generally not clinically indicated. See *Other drugs with serotonergic effects*, below). **Fluoxetine** was used in this pharmacokinetic study solely because it is a recommended CYP2D6 inhibitor for drug interaction studies.

(e) CYP2D6 substrates

Dapoxetine 60 mg daily for 6 days slightly increased the AUC of a single 50-mg dose of **desipramine** (by 19%).[2] This shows that dapoxetine slightly inhibits CYP2D6 when given at the maximum recommended dose (60 mg) and the maximum recommended frequency (once every 24 hours). This increase is not clinically relevant; therefore important pharmacokinetic interactions are unlikely with any drugs that are CYP2D6 substrates. Nevertheless, the manufacturer contraindicates the concurrent use of dapoxetine both with and for 14 days after stopping **thioridazine**. Furthermore, **thioridazine** should not be given for at least 7 days after stopping dapoxetine. They state that this is because dapoxetine may increase **thioridazine** concentrations and therefore increase the risk of QTc prolongation.[2] This is a cautious approach. However, note that **thioridazine** has been withdrawn in many countries because of its cardiovascular adverse effects.

(f) CYP3A4 inhibitors

The manufacturer reports that, in a study, **ketoconazole** 200 mg twice daily for 7 days increased the AUC of a single 60-mg dose of dapoxetine by 99% and increased its maximum concentration by 35%. Dapoxetine is metabolised, in part, by CYP3A4. Therefore, the manufacturer estimates that potent inhibitors of CYP3A4 may double the AUC of the total active drug (dapoxetine and its metabolite desmethyldapoxetine).

The clinical relevance of these increases has not been assessed; however, an important adverse reaction of dapoxetine is syncope or orthostatic hypotension, and this is dose-related. The manufacturer therefore takes a cautious approach and contraindicates the use of dapoxetine in patients taking potent CYP3A4 inhibitors: they specifically name **ketoconazole**, **itraconazole**, **nefazodone**, **telithromycin**, and the HIV-protease inhibitors, **ritonavir**, **saquinavir**, **nelfinavir**, and **atazanavir**.[2] However, if the patient is known to be a CYP2D6 extensive metaboliser (which is generally unlikely), a 30-mg dose may be used.

There does not appear to be any published data regarding the concurrent use of dapoxetine with moderate CYP3A4 inhibitors; nevertheless, the manufacturer predicts that they may also cause clinically relevant increases in the exposure to dapoxetine and its active metabolite. They therefore state that the maximum dose of dapoxetine should be limited to 30 mg in patients taking moderate CYP3A4 inhibitors, and they specifically name **erythromycin**, **clarithromycin**, **fluconazole**, **aprepitant**, **verap-**

amil, **diltiazem** and the HIV-protease inhibitors, **amprenavir** and **fosamprenavir**).[2] However, if the patient is known to be a CYP2D6 extensive metaboliser (which is generally unlikely), a 60-mg dose may be used.

For a list of CYP3A4 inhibitors, see 'Table 1.9', p.11.

(g) CYP3A4 substrates

The manufacturer reports that, in a study, dapoxetine 60 mg daily for 6 days slightly decreased the AUC of a single 8-mg dose of midazolam by 20%.[2] This shows that dapoxetine is a weak inducer of CYP3A4 when given at its maximum recommended dose (60 mg) and frequency (once every 24 hours).This is unlikely to be clinically relevant for midazolam and most CYP3A4 substrates, but the manufacturer cautiously notes that it could be clinically relevant with drugs extensively metabolised by CYP3A4 with a narrow therapeutic margin.[2] However, they do not give any examples. For a list of CYP3A4 substrates, see 'Table 1.10', p.12.

(h) Food

In a study in 27 healthy subjects, a high-fat meal slightly reduced the maximum concentration of dapoxetine by 11%, without affecting overall absorption (AUC), when compared with the fasting state.[3] These modest effects are unlikely to be clinically relevant, therefore dapoxetine can be taken without regard to the timing of meals.[2]

(i) Nitrates

Dapoxetine alone can cause syncope and orthostatic hypotension. The manufacturer therefore recommends caution when it is given with drugs that can cause vasodilation,[2] such as the nitrates, because of a possibility of an increase in these adverse effects.

(j) Other drugs with serotonergic effects

Dapoxetine is a short-acting SSRI, and therefore has serotonergic effects. The concurrent use of SSRIs and MAOIs has resulted in serious, sometimes fatal, reactions (serotonin syndrome or similar), see 'MAOIs or RIMAs + SSRIs', p.1401. Consequently, the manufacturer of dapoxetine contraindicates concurrent use with MAOIs, both during and for 14 days after stopping the MAOI, and an MAOI should not be started for at least 7 days after stopping dapoxetine.[2] Similarly, serotonin syndrome is said to have occurred with use of SSRIs and **tryptophan**, **tramadol**, **triptans**, **linezolid**, other **SSRIs**, **SNRIs**, **lithium**, and **St John's wort**. For a list of drugs suspected to have serotonergic effects, see 'Table 35.3', p.1472. The manufacturer notes that, as well as the possible risk of serotonin syndrome, some recreational drugs might increase the risk of arrhythmias and hyperthermia if used with dapoxetine, and they name **ketamine**, **ecstasy** (see 'Amfetamines and related drugs + SSRIs', p.216), and **lysergide** (LSD) (see 'SSRIs + Lysergide (LSD)', p.1489). For this reason, the manufacturer of dapoxetine states that it should not be used in patients taking these or any other serotonergic medicinal or herbal products, either during or within 14 days of discontinuing the serotonergic drug. They also advise that serotonergic drugs should not be started for at least 7 days after stopping dapoxetine.[2] This seems a cautious approach. For more information about serotonin syndrome and its management, see 'Drugs that cause serotonin syndrome + Other drugs that cause serotonin syndrome', p.1471.

(k) Warfarin

Dapoxetine 60 mg daily for 6 days had no effect on the pharmacokinetics of a single 25-mg dose of warfarin, nor did it affect the INR or prothrombin time in response to warfarin.[2] This study suggests that dapoxetine is unlikely to interact with warfarin; however, a similar lack of interaction has been seen in studies with warfarin and other serotonergic drugs, but rarely, isolated cases of bleeding have occurred, possibly as a result of the serotonergic effects of these drugs affecting platelet function (see 'Coumarins and related drugs + SSRIs', p.469). Therefore, the manufacturer recommends caution in patients taking warfarin because of the lack of data with long-term warfarin.[2]

1. Modi NB, Dresser M, Desai D, Edgar C, Wesnes K. Dapoxetine has no pharmacokinetic or cognitive interactions with ethanol in healthy male volunteers. *J Clin Pharmacol* (2007) 47, 315–22.
2. Priligy (Dapoxetine hydrochloride). Janssen–Cilag AB. Swedish Summary of product characteristics, February 2010.
3. Dresser MJ, Kang D, Staehr P, Gidwani S, Guo C, Mulhall JP, Modi NB. Pharmacokinetics of dapoxetine, a new treatment for premature ejaculation: impact of age and effects of a high-fat meal. *J Clin Pharmacol* (2006) 46, 1023–9.

Dapoxetine + Phosphodiesterase type-5 inhibitors

In single doses, sildenafil negligibly increased exposure to dapoxetine, but tadalafil had no effect on the pharmacokinetics of dapoxetine. Theoretically, syncope and orthostatic hypotension could be more common if a phosphodiesterase type-5 inhibitor is given with dapoxetine.

Clinical evidence, mechanism, importance and management

A single-dose, crossover study in 22 healthy men found that when **sildenafil** 100 mg was given with dapoxetine 60 mg there was a 19% increase in the dapoxetine AUC. In the same patients, **tadalafil** 20 mg did not alter the pharmacokinetics of dapoxetine. Furthermore, when compared with historical data, it appeared that dapoxetine did not affect the pharmacokinetics of these phosphodiesterase type-5 inhibitors.[1]

On the basis of this study, no clinically relevant pharmacokinetic interaction is anticipated between single doses of dapoxetine and **sildenafil** or **tadalafil**. However, the phosphodiesterase type-5 inhibitors (including **vardenafil** and **avanafil**) and dapoxetine can cause syncope and orthostatic hypotension, and this might be additive on concurrent use. The UK manufacturer of dapoxetine therefore advises against its concurrent use with phosphodiesterase type-5 inhibitors.[2]

1. Dresser MJ, Desai D, Gidwani S, Seftel AD, Modi NB. Dapoxetine, a novel treatment for premature ejaculation, does not have pharmacokinetic interactions with phosphodiesterase-5 inhibitors. *Int J Impot Res* (2006) 18, 104–10.
2. Priligy (Dapoxetine hydrochloride). A. Menarini Farmaceutica Internazionale SRL. UK Summary of product characteristics, December 2013.

Desmopressin + Erythromycin

Erythromycin does not affect the absorption of desmopressin given orally.

Clinical evidence, mechanism, importance and management

In a study, 18 healthy subjects were given erythromycin 250 mg four times daily for 3 days, with a 400-microgram oral dose of desmopressin one hour after the final dose of erythromycin. When compared with desmopressin alone, the time to peak desmopressin levels was reduced from 1.3 hours to 0.9 hours by erythromycin, but other pharmacokinetic parameters were not affected, suggesting the erythromycin did not affect gastrointestinal motility sufficiently to affect total desmopressin absorption.[1]

This study suggests that no pharmacokinetic interaction of clinical relevance would be expected if erythromycin is given to patients receiving oral desmopressin.

1. Callréus T, Lundahl J, Höglund P, Bengtsson P. Changes in gastrointestinal motility influence the absorption of desmopressin. *Eur J Clin Pharmacol* (1999) 55, 305–9.

Desmopressin + Food

Food reduces the absorption of oral desmopressin. Buccal desmopressin may interact similarly.

Clinical evidence, mechanism, importance and management

In a study in healthy subjects, a standardised meal decreased the AUC of a 400-microgram dose of oral desmopressin by about 40% when the tablets were given either at the same time as the meal or 1.5 hours after the meal, when compared with the fasting state. The maximum level of desmopressin was reduced by about 50% and there was an increase in the time to maximum level from 1 hour to 1.5 hours. However, the meal did not significantly alter the pharmacodynamic effect of desmopressin (urine production and osmolality).[1] A preliminary report of this study has been published elsewhere.[2]

Despite the finding of a lack of pharmacodynamic effect, the UK manufacturer of desmopressin considers that the effect of food could be clinically important, particularly with lower doses of desmopressin. They suggest that if a reduction in efficacy is noted, then the effect of food should be considered before increasing the dose.[3] They also apply this advice to the buccal tablets,[4] for which the majority is absorbed in the stomach after being swallowed in saliva, with a small amount absorbed through the buccal mucosa.[5] If problems occur, it may be prudent to advise patients to take oral or buccal desmopressin tablets consistently with respect to food.

1. Rittig S, Jensen AR, Jensen KT, Pedersen EB. Effect of food intake on the pharmacokinetics and antidiuretic activity of oral desmopressin (DDAVP) in hydrated normal subjects. *Clin Endocrinol (Oxf)* (1998) 48, 235–41.
2. Rittig S, Jensen AR, Jensen KT, Pedersen EB. Desmopressin tablet treatment: factors influencing gastrointestinal absorption. *Scand J Urol Nephrol* (1997) 183 (Suppl), 51–2.
3. Desmotabs (Desmopressin acetate). Ferring Pharmaceuticals Ltd. UK Summary of product characteristics, May 2008.
4. DesmoMelt (Desmopressin oral lyphosilate). Ferring Pharmaceuticals Ltd. UK Summary of product characteristics, October 2009.
5. Personal communication. Ferring Pharmaceuticals Ltd, May 2010.

Desmopressin + Loperamide

Loperamide may markedly increase the absorption of oral desmopressin.

Clinical evidence

In a study, 18 healthy subjects were given a 400-microgram oral dose of desmopressin as immediate-release tablets, either alone or after three doses of loperamide 4 mg, given 24 hours, 12 hours and 1 hour before the desmopressin. Loperamide increased the AUC and peak plasma levels of desmopressin 3.1-fold and 2.3-fold, respectively, and the time to peak desmopressin plasma levels was increased from 1.3 hours to 2 hours, whereas the elimination half-life was unaltered.[1]

Mechanism

The authors of the study suggest that loperamide increases the absorption of desmopressin by slowing gastrointestinal motility. Other mechanisms such as reduced pancreatic secretion or reduced enzymatic degradation of desmopressin in the intestine were also suggested, but considered less likely as desmopressin clearance was not significantly affected.[1]

Importance and management

Evidence for an interaction between loperamide and desmopressin appears to be limited to one study. Increased desmopressin absorption could lead to a prolonged duration of action, and if fluid intake is not restricted in such a situation, there could be an increased risk of water intoxication and/or hyponatraemia.[1] It would therefore be prudent to increase the monitoring of the effects of oral desmopressin in any patient also given loperamide, reducing the desmopressin dose or dose frequency as necessary. However, note that in primary nocturnal enuresis, the indication for loperamide (diarrhoea) is a reason to temporarily stop desmopressin.[2-4]

Although the effect of loperamide on sublingual formulations of desmopressin has not been studied, until more is known, the same precautions should be applied. However, as the loperamide interacts by an effect on the gut, no interaction would be expected with intranasal or parenteral desmopressin.

1. Callréus T, Lundahl J, Höglund P, Bengtsson P. Changes in gastrointestinal motility influence the absorption of desmopressin. *Eur J Clin Pharmacol* (1999) 55, 305–9.
2. Desmotabs (Desmopressin acetate). Ferring Pharmaceuticals Ltd. UK Summary of product characteristics, May 2008.
3. Committee on Safety of Medicines/Medicines Control Agency. Hyponatraemic convulsions in patients with enuresis treated with vasopressin. *Current Problems* (1996) 22, 4.
4. DDAVP Tablets (Desmopressin acetate). Sanofi-Aventis U.S. LLC. US Prescribing information, July 2007.

Desmopressin + Miscellaneous

The effects of any drug that can cause water retention or hyponatraemia (e.g. tricyclic antidepressants, SSRIs, chlorpromazine, carbamazepine, and NSAIDs) may be additive with those of desmopressin. This may lead to water overload and/or hyponatraemia. An isolated report describes reduced desmopressin requirements with lamotrigine.

Clinical evidence

(a) Carbamazepine

In a retrospective analysis of 103 children with cranial diabetes insipidus, major complications (symptomatic water overload) or asymptomatic hyponatraemia were seen in 33 children. In patients taking desmopressin with carbamazepine, major complications were more common than in those not receiving carbamazepine (33% versus 10%).[1]

(b) Imipramine

A 10-year-old boy who had been receiving intranasal desmopressin for 7 months for primary nocturnal enuresis had a hyponatraemic convulsion a few weeks after imipramine 25 mg at night was added.[2]

(c) Lamotrigine

Two children with cranial diabetes insipidus treated with desmopressin had gradually decreased desmopressin requirements after starting lamotrigine in incremental doses. In one of the cases, the dose of desmopressin subsequently needed *increasing* by 25 to 50 micrograms as the lamotrigine dose was *reduced* in 50 mg decrements.[3]

(d) NSAIDs

In a study in 5 patients with central diabetes insipidus, three 50-mg doses of **indometacin** (given in a 24-hour period) further increased the urinary osmolality in response to intranasal desmopressin 7.5 micrograms twice daily for 3 days.[4] In another study, in 6 patients with neurogenic diabetes insipidus, indometacin 25 mg four times daily for 3 days increased the urinary osmolality in response to a single 0.5-microgram subcutaneous injection of desmopressin, when compared with desmopressin alone.[5] Similarly, in healthy women, **indometacin** pre-treatment enhanced the reduction in urine flow rate seen with desmopressin, but this occurred during the first 60 minutes and appeared to be inhibited at later time points.[6] In another study in healthy subjects, the antidiuretic effect of desmopressin 2 micrograms was not altered by **piroxicam** (20 mg on day 1 then 10 mg daily for 3 days) although it was slightly lower in females and slightly higher in males.[7] This study also found no differences in the pharmacokinetics of desmopressin when given alone and with steady-state **piroxicam**.

A case report describes a 55-year-old woman with von Willebrand's disease who went into a hyponatraemic coma after she had received desmopressin (dose not stated) given as prophylaxis for bleeding before dental surgery and **ibuprofen** (dose not stated) as an analgesic. Because she had previously received desmopressin without any complications, this reaction was attributed to an additive effect with the **ibuprofen**.[8]

Mechanism

Additive water retentive effects may occur.

Importance and management

Any drug that is known to induce the syndrome of inappropriate antidiuretic hormone secretion (SIADH) has the potential to have additive effects with desmopressin. This increases the risk of water retention and/or hyponatraemia. Examples include carbamazepine, **chlorpromazine**, the **SSRIs** and the **tricyclic antidepressants**, such as imipramine. Other drugs that can cause water retention, such as the NSAIDs, might also increase the risk of fluid overload and hyponatraemia. The increased risk may well be small, with severe complications being rare. However, it would be prudent to exercise caution on concurrent use,[9,10] with more frequent monitoring of serum sodium.

The case report with lamotrigine suggests that it might interact similarly.

1. Rizzo V, Albanese A, Stanhope R. Morbidity and mortality associated with vasopressin replacement therapy in children. *J Pediatr Endocrinol Metab* (2001) 14, 861–7.
2. Hamed M, Mitchell H, Clow DJ. Hyponatraemic convulsion associated with desmopressin and imipramine treatment. *BMJ* (1993) 306, 1169.
3. Mewasingh L, Aylett S, Kirkham F, Stanhope R. Hyponatraemia associated with lamotrigine in cranial diabetes insipidus. *Lancet* (2000) 356, 656.
4. Düsing R, Herrmann R, Glänzer K, Vetter H, Overlack A, Kramer HJ. Renal prostaglandins and water balance: studies in normal volunteer subjects and in patients with central diabetes insipidus. *Clin Sci (Lond)* (1981) 61, 61–7.
5. Moses AM, Moses LK, Notman DD, Springer J. Antidiuretic responses to injected desmopressin, alone and with indomethacin. *J Clin Endocrinol Metab* (1981) 52, 910–13.
6. Agnoli GC, Borgatti R, Cacciari M, Lenzi P, Marinelli M, Stipo L. Low-dose desmopressin infusion: renal action in healthy women in moderate salt retention and depletion, and interactions with prostanoids. *Prostaglandins Leukot Essent Fatty Acids* (2002) 67, 263–73.
7. Odeberg JM, Callréus T, Lundin S, Roth EB, Höglund P. A pharmacokinetic and pharmacodynamic study of desmopressin: evaluating sex differences and the effect of pre-treatment with piroxicam, and further validation of an indirect response model. *J Pharm Pharmacol* (2004) 56, 1389–98.
8. García EBG, Ruitenberg A, Madretsma GS, Hintzen RQ. Hyponatraemic coma induced by desmopressin and ibuprofen in a woman with von Willebrand's disease. *Haemophilia* (2003) 9, 232–4.
9. Desmotabs (Desmopressin acetate). Ferring Pharmaceuticals Ltd. UK Summary of product characteristics, May 2008.
10. DDAVP Tablets (Desmopressin acetate). Sanofi-Aventis U.S. LLC. US Prescribing information, July 2007.

Dutasteride + Colestyramine

The absorption of dutasteride was not affected when it was given one hour before colestyramine.

Clinical evidence, mechanism, importance and management

In a study in 12 healthy subjects, the absorption of dutasteride 5 mg was not affected when it was given one hour before a single 12-g dose of colestyramine.[1,2] No additional precautions seem necessary if this dosing interval is observed, which is in accordance with the general recommendation that other drugs are given one hour before or 4 to 6 hours after colestyramine.

1. GlaxoSmithKline. Personal communication, August 2003.
2. Avodart (Dutasteride). GlaxoSmithKline. US Prescribing information, October 2012.

Dutasteride + Miscellaneous

Preliminary evidence suggests that diltiazem and verapamil, moderate CYP3A4 inhibitors, cause moderate increases in dutasteride levels. Other moderate CYP3A4 inhibitors would be expected to interact similarly, and more potent CYP3A4 inhibitors would be expected to have a greater effect. No clinically relevant interaction appears to occur between dutasteride and amlodipine.

Clinical evidence, mechanism, importance and management

(a) Amlodipine

In a population pharmacokinetic analysis it was found that the use of amlodipine (4 subjects) was not associated with any significant change in the clearance of dutasteride.[1]

(b) CYP3A4 inhibitors

In a population pharmacokinetic analysis, it was found that **diltiazem** (5 subjects) and **verapamil** (6 subjects) were associated with a 44% and 37% decrease in dutasteride clearance, respectively,[1] and an 80% and 60% increase in its serum levels, respectively.[2] The changes were thought to be due to the inhibitory effect of **diltiazem** and **verapamil** on CYP3A4. Dutasteride has a wide safety margin, so these moderate changes are not thought to be clinically relevant.[1,2] However, in the UK, the manufacturers warn that potent CYP3A4 inhibitors (they name **indinavir**, **itraconazole**, **ketoconazole**, **nefazodone** and **ritonavir**) may cause a clinically relevant increase in dutasteride levels, and so they suggest reducing the dosing frequency if increased dutasteride adverse effects occur in the presence of these drugs.[2] The US manufacturer similarly recommends caution on the long-term use of potent CYP3A4 inhibitors, and they name **ritonavir** as an example. They also predict that **cimetidine** and **ciprofloxacin** may increase dutasteride levels by inhibiting CYP3A4.[1] However, note that **cimetidine** only weakly inhibits this isoenzyme, and ciprofloxacin does not generally appear to have a clinically relevant inhibitory effect on CYP3A4, and therefore clinically relevant interactions seem unlikely.

1. Avodart (Dutasteride). GlaxoSmithKline. US Prescribing information, October 2012.
2. Avodart (Dutasteride). GlaxoSmithKline UK. UK Summary of product characteristics, March 2010.

Finasteride + St John's wort (*Hypericum perforatum*)

St John's wort moderately reduces the exposure to finasteride.

Clinical evidence

An open study in 12 healthy men given 5 mg finasteride directly into the intestine via a catheter, found that St. John's wort (*Movina*) 300 mg twice daily (equivalent to hyperforin 4%) for 14 days reduced the maximum plasma concentration and AUC of finasteride by 34% and 58%, respectively. The clearance of finasteride was increased almost 2.5-fold. The AUC of the finasteride metabolite, carboxy-finasteride, remained largely unaffected but the maximum plasma concentration was increased by 62%.[1]

A patient with BPH controlled with finasteride had an increase in his serum prostate-specific antigen (PSA) concentration when St John's wort 900 mg (containing 4% hyperforin) daily was started. St John's wort was stopped and PSA concentrations gradually returned to baseline. Urological tests showed no changes in disease status.[2,3]

Mechanism

Finasteride is primarily metabolised by CYP3A4 in the liver, which is known to be induced by St. John's wort, and this most likely leads to the reduction in exposure seen.

Importance and management

The study and case report seem to be the only clinical evidence of the effects of St John's wort on finasteride. However, the moderate reduction in finasteride exposure seen in the study suggests that it is possible that finasteride will be less effective in those taking St John's wort. There is insufficient evidence to suggest that St John's wort should be avoided in patients taking finasteride. Nevertheless, it would seem prudent to bear the potential for reduced efficacy in mind, especially in patients taking finasteride for BPH.

1. Lundahl A, Hedeland M, Bondesson U, Knutson L, Lennernäs H. The effect of St. John's wort on the pharmacokinetics, metabolism and biliary excretion of finasteride and its metabolites in healthy men. *Eur J Pharm Sci* (2009) 36, 433–43.
2. Lochner S. Interaktionen zwischen Johanniskrautextrakt und Finasterid? *Med Monatsschr Pharm* (2010) 33, 307.
3. Lochner S. Personal communication, July 2012.

Mirabegron + Food

Food modestly decreases the exposure to mirabegron.

Clinical evidence, mechanism, importance and management

In a crossover study, healthy subjects were given a single 50- or 100-mg dose of mirabegron after an overnight fast, 30 minutes after a high-fat breakfast or 30 minutes after a low-fat breakfast. The maximum concentration and AUC of mirabegron were decreased by 45% and 17%, respectively, in the 50-mg group when given after the high-fat breakfast, compared with the fasted state. When given after the low-fat breakfast they were decreased by 75% and 51%, respectively, compared with the fasted state. In the 100-mg group, the maximum concentration and AUC were decreased by 39% and 18%, respectively, after the high-fat breakfast, and by 64% and 47%, respectively, after the low-fat breakfast, when compared with the fasted state. These changes were all considered to be of a magnitude that would be clinically important, however, based on the results of a number of phase 3 studies in which mirabegron was administered irrespective of food contents and intake [and was efficacious], it was considered that the effects of food seen in this study are of little importance when mirabegron is used clinically.[1] As a result, mirabegron can be administered without regard to food.

1. Lee J, Zhang W, Moy S, Kowalski D, Kerbusch V, van Gelderen M, Sawamoto T, Grunenberg N, Keirns J. Effects of food intake on the pharmacokinetic properties of mirabegron oral controlled-absorption system: a single-dose, randomized, crossover study in healthy subjects. *Clin Ther* (2013) 35, 333–41.

Mirabegron + Ketoconazole and other CYP3A4 inhibitors

Ketoconazole slightly increases mirabegron exposure. Other CYP3A4 and/or P-glycoprotein inhibitors might be expected to interact similarly.

Clinical evidence

In a phase I study in 23 healthy subjects given a single 100-mg dose of mirabegron before, and on day 4 of a 9-day course of ketoconazole 400 mg daily, the AUC and maximum plasma concentration of mirabegron were increased by 81% and 45%, respectively.[1]

Mechanism

Ketoconazole is an inhibitor of CYP3A4 and P-glycoprotein, by which mirabegron is partly metabolised, and transported, respectively. Concurrent use therefore increases its exposure. The exact role of each of these mechanisms is not clear without further study.

Importance and management

Evidence for an interaction between ketoconazole and mirabegron is limited to this study, but a pharmacokinetic interaction is established. As the increase in mirabegron exposure was only slight, this suggests that mirabegron is not a sensitive CYP3A4 substrate and no dose adjustment or additional monitoring would seem necessary on concurrent use with ketoconazole, or other CYP3A4 and/or P-glycoprotein inhibitors. However, note that the UK manufacturer does not recommend the use of mirabegron in patients with severe renal impairment, or moderate hepatic impairment, and who are also receiving potent CYP3A4 inhibitors. They also recommend that the dose of mirabegron is reduced to 25 mg daily in patients with mild to moderate renal impairment, or mild hepatic impairment, and who are also receiving potent CYP3A4 inhibitors.[2] For a list of potent CYP3A4 inhibitors, see 'Table 1.9', p.11.

1. Lee J, Moy S, Meijer J, Krauwinkel W, Sawamoto T, Kerbusch V, Kowalski D, Roy M, Marion A, Takusagawa S, van Gelderen M, Keirns J. Role of cytochrome P450 isoenzymes 3A and 2D6 in the in vivo metabolism of mirabegron, a β_3-adrenoceptor agonist. *Clin Drug Investig* (2013) 33, 429–40.
2. Betmiga (Mirabegron). Astellas Pharma Ltd. UK Summary of product characteristics, November 2014.

Mirabegron + Miscellaneous

Mirabegron slightly increases digoxin exposure and might increase its effects. Other P-glycoprotein substrates might be similarly affected. No interaction occurs between mirabegron and ethinyloestradiol, levonorgestrel, metformin, solifenacin, tamsulosin, or warfarin.

Clinical evidence, mechanism, importance and management

(a) Combined oral contraceptives

The US manufacturer briefly notes that in a study, mirabegron 100 mg had little or no effect on the maximum concentrations and AUC of **ethinylestradiol** 30 micrograms and **levonorgestrel** 150 micrograms, when given as a once daily combined hormonal contraceptive.[1] No dose adjustments are therefore necessary on concurrent use.[1,2]

(b) Digoxin and other P-glycoprotein substrates

The UK and US manufacturers briefly note that in a study, mirabegron 100 mg increased the maximum concentration and AUC of a single 250 microgram dose of digoxin by 29% and 27%, respectively.[1,2] Mirabegron inhibits P-glycoprotein, of which digoxin is a substrate, and therefore its exposure increases. It would therefore seem prudent to start digoxin at the lowest dose possible in patients already receiving mirabegron, and then monitor and titrate according to effect as usual, bearing in mind that a smaller dose than expected might be required. In patients already taking digoxin who are started on mirabegron, it would seem prudent to monitor digoxin concentrations more closely, being alert for signs of increased effects (such as bradycardia) and the need to adjust the digoxin dose.

The UK manufacturer also advises that mirabegron has the potential to increase the exposure of other sensitive P-glycoprotein substrates, and names **dabigatran**.[2] If dabigatran is given concurrently with mirabegron it would seem prudent to monitor for signs of increased effects (such as bleeding, bruising, or anaemia), adjusting the dose as necessary, and discontinuing mirabegron if severe bleeding occurs. For a list of other P-glycoprotein substrates, see 'Table 1.12', p.14.

(c) Metformin

The US manufacturer briefly notes that in a study, mirabegron 160 mg had little or no effect on the maximum concentration and AUC of metformin 500 mg twice daily. The maximum concentration and AUC of mirabegron were decreased by about 25%.[1] No dose adjustments are therefore necessary on concurrent use.[1,2]

(d) Solifenacin

The US manufacturer briefly notes that in a study, mirabegron 100 mg increased the maximum concentration and AUC of a single 10-mg dose of solifenacin by about 25%. The maximum concentration and AUC of mirabegron were not notably altered.[1] No dose adjustments are therefore necessary on concurrent use, however the UK and US manufacturers advise that mirabegron should be used with caution in patients taking antimuscarinics because of the risk of urinary retention, which has been reported in such patients post-marketing.[1,2].

(e) Tamsulosin

The US manufacturer briefly notes that in a study, mirabegron 100 mg increased the maximum concentration and AUC of a single 400-microgram dose of tamsulosin by about 60%. The maximum concentration and AUC of mirabegron were not notably altered. No dose adjustments are therefore necessary on concurrent use, however the UK and US manufacturers advise that mirabegron should be used with caution in patients taking antimuscarinics or those with bladder obstruction, because of the risk of urinary retention, which has been reported in such patients post-marketing.[1,2].

(f) Warfarin

The US manufacturer briefly notes that in a study, mirabegron 100 mg increased the maximum concentration and AUC of *S*- and *R*-warfarin by about 4% and about 9% after a single 25-mg dose of warfarin. No effect on INR or prothrombin time was seen.[1] No dose adjustment is therefore necessary on concurrent use.[1,2]

1. Myrbetriq (Mirabegron). Astellas Pharma US, Inc. US Prescribing information, February 2014.
2. Betmiga (Mirabegron). Astellas Pharma Ltd. UK Summary of product characteristics, November 2014.

Mirabegron + Rifampicin (Rifampin) and other CYP3A4 inducers

Rifampicin slightly decreases mirabegron exposure. Other inducers of CYP3A4 and/or P-glycoprotein might be expected to interact similarly.

Clinical evidence

In a phase I study in 24 healthy subjects given a single 100-mg dose of mirabegron before, and on day 8 of a 10-day course of rifampicin (rifampin) 600 mg daily, the AUC and maximum plasma concentration of mirabegron were decreased by 35% and 44%, respectively.[1]

Mechanism

Rifampicin is a well-known, non-specific enzyme inducer, having effects on CYP3A4 and uridine diphospho glucuronosyltransferase (UGT) which are both involved in the metabolism of mirabegron. Rifampicin also induces P-glycoprotein by which mirabegron is transported. Concurrent use therefore decreases its exposure. The exact role of each of these mechanisms is not clear without further study.

Importance and management

Evidence for an interaction between rifampicin and mirabegron is limited to this study, but a pharmacokinetic interaction is established. As the decrease in mirabegron exposure was only slight, no dose adjustment or additional monitoring would seem necessary on concurrent use with rifampicin or other inducers of CYP3A4 and/or P-glycoprotein.

1. Lee J, Moy S, Meijer J, Krauwinkel W, Sawamoto T, Kerbusch V, Kowalski D, Roy M, Marion A, Takusagawa S, van Gelderen M, Keirns J. Role of cytochrome P450 isoenzymes 3A and 2D6 in the in vivo metabolism of mirabegron, a β_3-adrenoceptor agonist. *Clin Drug Investig* (2013) 33, 429–40.

Papaverine + Diazepam

Two men given normal test doses of papaverine for the investigation of impotence had prolonged erections, which were attributed to the concurrent use of diazepam.

Clinical evidence, mechanism, importance and management

Undesirably prolonged erections (duration of 5 hours and 6 hours) occurred in 2 patients who had been given 5 or 10 mg of diazepam intravenously for anxiety before a 60-mg intracavernosal injection of papaverine.[1] Papaverine acts by relaxing the arterioles that supply the corpora so that the pressure rises. The increased pressure in the corpora compresses the trabecular venules so that the pressure continues to maintain the erection. Diazepam also relaxes smooth muscle and it would seem that this effect can be additive with the effects of papaverine. The authors of the report suggest that caution is warranted with the choice of papaverine dose in patients taking anxiolytics (i.e. use less) although these two cases involving diazepam seem to be the only ones reported.[1]

1. Vale JA, Kirby RS, Lees W. Papaverine, benzodiazepines, and prolonged erections. *Lancet* (1991) 337, 1552.

Phosphodiesterase type-5 inhibitors + Alpha blockers

Postural hypotension might occur if doses of sildenafil, tadalafil, or vardenafil at the higher end of the therapeutic range are given at the same time as doxazosin or terazosin. The effect might not be as great with some of the other alpha blockers (such as tamsulosin and alfuzosin). Avanafil appears to have a similar effect on standing systolic blood pressure when given with doxazosin or tamsulosin.

Clinical evidence

(a) Avanafil

The US manufacturer briefly reports that, in a randomised crossover study in 24 healthy male subjects, mean standing systolic blood pressure was decreased by 2.5 mmHg after **doxazosin** 8 mg daily was given for 11 days with a single 200-mg dose of avanafil on days 8 and 11, and by 3.6 mmHg after **tamsulosin** 400 micrograms daily was given for 11 days with a single 200-mg dose of avanafil on days 8 and 11, when compared with placebo. Three of the subjects in the doxazosin group, and two of the subjects in the tamsulosin group, had a standing systolic blood pressure of less than 85 mmHg. There were no cases of syncope in either group.[1]

(b) Sildenafil

Retrospective analysis of pooled data from various clinical studies that included patients taking non-nitrate antihypertensives, such as the alpha blockers, suggested that the adverse effect profile, blood pressure, and heart rate were not sufficiently different between those also given sildenafil and those also given placebo to be clinically important.[2,3] However, the US manufacturer of sildenafil notes that, in specific interaction studies, when sildenafil 100 mg was given simultaneously with **doxazosin** 4 mg after at least 14 consecutive daily doses of **doxazosin**, severe postural hypotension (starting at 35 minutes and lasting 8 hours) occurred in one of 4 subjects with BPH, and two others had mild dizziness. Two of the subjects had a standing systolic blood pressure of less than 85 mmHg. This did not occur in a further 17 subjects who, as a result of these effects, were given a lower dose of sildenafil 25 mg. In two other studies in men with BPH, 2 of 19 patients and 3 of 20 patients had a standing systolic blood pressure of less than 85 mmHg after receiving 14 days of **doxazosin** then a single dose of sildenafil 50 mg or 100 mg given at the same time as **doxazosin**.[4]

A case report describes a patient with intermittent Wolff-Parkinson-White syndrome taking **doxazosin** 1 mg daily for mild hypertension who developed palpitations and chest pain one hour after taking sildenafil 50 mg and drinking 1.5 L of beer. He had atrial fibrillation (which failed to respond to direct-current (DC) conversion, but reverted spontaneously after 4 hours) and severe hypotension lasting 16 hours, for which he was given a dopamine infusion. The authors considered that the hypotension might have been caused by an interaction between the alcohol, **doxazosin**, and sildenafil.[5]

In a well-controlled study, 22 healthy subjects took **silodosin** 8 mg daily for 21 days, with a single 100-mg dose of sildenafil on day 7, 14 or 21. When compared with placebo, the mean maximum decrease in supine blood pressure occurred one hour post-dose and was 7.9/4.7 mmHg. There were no clinically relevant changes in orthostatic blood pressure or heart rate, and no orthostatic hypotension occurred.[6]

In 16 patients with BPH who had been taking **tamsulosin** 400 micrograms daily for 9 to 14 days, a single 100-mg dose of sildenafil caused a mean 14 mmHg decrease in arterial pressure, compared with a decrease of 11 mmHg with sildenafil alone. Tamsulosin alone did not change arterial blood pressure.[7] One patient was excluded from the analysis because he developed clinically important decreases in peripheral vascular resistance and notable hypotension during the tilt test. His arterial pressure was 100/80 mmHg with **tamsulosin** alone, 75/50 mmHg with sildenafil alone (test stopped at 5 minutes), and 60/45 mmHg with the combination (test stopped at 90 seconds).[8]

(c) Tadalafil

In a well-controlled study in 18 healthy subjects, a single 20-mg dose of tadalafil was given at the same time as **doxazosin** 8 mg following a minimum of 7 days of pretreatment with **doxazosin** 8 mg daily. The blood-pressure lowering effects of doxazosin were increased: the mean maximum systolic decreases for the combination were 19.6 mmHg when lying and 27.8 mmHg when standing, which was 3.6 mmHg and 9.8 mmHg greater than when doxazosin was given with placebo. Five of the subjects had a standing systolic blood pressure of less than 85 mmHg. Some of the subjects felt dizzy, but none of them fainted.[9]

Conversely, only a small (3.2 mmHg and 1.7 mmHg) additional drop in blood pressure was seen when tadalafil 10 or 20 mg was given 2 hours after **tamsulosin** 400 micrograms. Note that the 2-hour difference was used so that the maximum plasma concentrations of each drug would coincide. None of the subjects had a standing systolic blood pressure of less than 85 mmHg.[9] In a placebo-controlled study, 17 healthy subjects were given extended-release **alfuzosin** 10 mg daily, with a single 20-mg oral dose of tadalafil on day 7. The additional blood pressure-lowering effect of the tadalafil was small (2.1 mmHg systolic supine and 4.3 mmHg systolic standing). One of the subjects had a decrease in standing systolic blood pressure to less than 85 mmHg. No syncope or severe adverse events were reported. Note that the doses were separated in such a way that the maximum plasma concentrations of each drug would coincide.[10]

The above studies used single doses of tadalafil. In another two studies in healthy subjects, tadalafil 5 mg daily was given alone and then either **doxazosin** (titrated from 1 mg daily to 4 mg daily) or **tamsulosin** 400 micrograms daily were added. The mean maximum additional decrease in standing systolic blood pressure on adding the alpha blocker was similar (0.5 mmHg with doxazosin 4 mg and 0.9 mmHg for tamsulosin). Standing systolic blood pressure of less than 85 mmHg occurred in 1 of 37 subjects receiving doxazosin and none of 35 subjects receiving tamsulosin.[11]

In a well-controlled study, 22 healthy subjects took **silodosin** 8 mg daily for 21 days, with a single 20-mg dose of tadalafil on day 7, 14 or 21. When compared with placebo, the mean maximum decrease in standing blood pressure occurred 12 hours post-dose and was 8.5/4 mmHg. There were no clinically relevant changes in orthostatic blood pressure or heart rate, and no orthostatic hypotension occurred.[6]

(d) Vardenafil

The manufacturers of vardenafil have conducted several placebo-controlled, randomised, crossover studies, in patients with BPH and in healthy subjects taking alpha blockers, to assess the effects of the concurrent use of vardenafil on blood pressure. Vardenafil 5 mg was given to 21 patients taking **terazosin** 5 or 10 mg daily. Vardenafil given simultaneously caused notable hypotension in one patient (blood pressure 80/60 mmHg) and 5 patients experienced a decrease in standing systolic blood pressure of greater than 30 mmHg (compared with only 2 patients in the placebo group). When vardenafil was given 6 hours after the alpha blocker no adverse effects were reported.[12] Vardenafil 10 or 20 mg was also given to healthy subjects taking **terazosin** 10 mg daily, either simultaneously with the terazosin or separated by 6 hours. Due to clinically important hypotension in most of the subjects given the drugs simultaneously, this arm of the study was halted.[12]

Vardenafil 5 mg was given to 21 patients taking **tamsulosin** 400 micrograms daily. Vardenafil given simultaneously caused notable hypotension in 2 patients (systolic blood pressure less than 85 mmHg) and 2 patients experienced a decrease in systolic blood pressure of greater than 30 mmHg (compared with only one patient in the placebo group). When vardenafil was given 6 hours after the alpha blocker notable hypotension still occurred in 2 patients and one experienced postural hypotension of greater than 30 mmHg.[12] Larger doses of vardenafil (10 then 20 mg) given to 23 patients with BPH taking **tamsulosin** 400 or 800 micrograms resulted in mean additional decreases in supine systolic blood pressure of 4.5 mmHg and 4 mmHg, respectively, when compared with placebo. A decrease in standing systolic blood pressure of greater than 30 mmHg occurred in one patient, and 3 patients became dizzy, but no patient had a systolic blood pressure of less than 85 mmHg.[12,13] When vardenafil 10 or 20 mg was given to 20 healthy subjects taking **tamsulosin** 400 micrograms daily, 7 subjects became dizzy.[12] Vardenafil (single 5- and 10–mg doses) was given to 24 patients with BPH taking **alfuzosin** 10 mg daily for at least 4 weeks. When vardenafil was given 4 hours after the alpha blocker a decrease in standing systolic blood pressure of greater than 30 mmHg occurred in one patient, and 3 patients became dizzy (compared with one taking placebo), but no patient had a systolic blood pressure of less than 85 mmHg.[12]In a crossover study, 37 patients stable taking controlled-release **doxazosin** 4 mg or 8 mg daily were given a single 10-mg dose of vardenafil. The maximum decrease in blood pressure compared with placebo was 6.6/4.6 mmHg.[14] In a study of the effect of vardenafil on blood pressure in normotensive men with erectile dysfunction, three patients had fainting episodes after their first dose of vardenafil 10 mg. Two of these were taking **doxazosin** for BPH.[15]

Mechanism

Phosphodiesterase type-5 inhibitors cause mild to moderate vasodilatation of vascular smooth muscle in veins and arteries, and so can lower blood pressure. This could be additive or synergistic with the orthostatic hypotension that can occur with alpha blockers.

Importance and management

The interactions between the phosphodiesterase type-5 inhibitors and the alpha blockers are established, and concurrent use requires caution. The risk of symptomatic hypotension is reduced if the patient taking an alpha blocker is haemodynamically stable before the phosphodiesterase type-5 inhibitor is started, and if it is started at the lowest recommended dose. The risk could also be minimised if administration is separated so that the maximum concentrations of the two drugs do not coincide. If an alpha blocker is required in a patient already using a phosphodiesterase type-5 inhibitor, extra caution is required, particularly with alpha blockers well-known to be associated with first-dose hypotension, such as immediate-release alfuzosin, prazosin, and terazosin. This effect appears to occur less frequently with modified-release alfuzosin and tamsulosin, and possibly silodosin, although evidence for silodosin is limited. Patients should be warned of the risks of taking an alpha blocker with a phosphodiesterase type-5 inhibitor and advised what to do in the event of postural hypotensive symptoms (i.e. lie down, raise the legs, and, when recovered, get up slowly). However, note that the UK manufacturer of **tadalafil** states that the concurrent use of tadalafil and doxazosin is not recommended,[16,17] and the US manufacturer states that the combined use of tadalafil and alpha blockers is not recommended for treating benign prostatic hyperplasia.[18]

Note that the combination of sildenafil and doxazosin has been used for erectile dysfunction refractory to sildenafil monotherapy.[19]

1. Stendra (Avanafil). Vivus, Inc. US Prescribing information, January 2015.
2. Zusman RM, Prisant LM, Brown MJ. Effect of sildenafil citrate on blood pressure and heart rate in men with erectile dysfunction taking concomitant antihypertensive medication. *J Hypertens* (2000) 18, 1865–9.
3. Böhm M, Burkart M, Baumann G. Sildenafil is well tolerated by erectile dysfunction patients taking antihypertensive medications, including those on multidrug regimens. *Curr Drug Saf* (2007) 2, 5–8.
4. Viagra (Sildenafil citrate). Pfizer Inc. US Prescribing information, March 2015.
5. Hayashi K, Minezaki KK, Narukawa M, Ookubo M, Mitsuhashi T, Shimada K. Atrial fibrillation and continuous hypotension induced by sildenafil in an intermittent WPW syndrome patient. *Jpn Heart J* (1999) 40, 827–30.
6. MacDiarmid SA, Hill LA, Volinn W, Hoel G. Lack of pharmacodynamic interaction of silodosin, a highly selective α1a-adrenoceptor antagonist, with the phosphodiesterase-5 inhibitors sildenafil and tadalafil in healthy men. *Urology* (2010) 75, 520–5.
7. Nieminen T, Tammela TLJ, Kööbi T, Kähönen M. The effects of tamsulosin and sildenafil in separate and combined regimens on detailed hemodynamics in patients with benign prostatic enlargement. *J Urol (Baltimore)* (2006) 176, 2551–6.
8. Hypotensive potential of sildenafil and tamsulosin during orthostasis. *Clin Drug Investig* (2006) 26, 667–71.
9. Kloner RA, Jackson G, Emmick JT, Mitchell MI, Bedding A, Warner MR, Pereira A. Interaction between the phosphodiesterase 5 inhibitor, tadalafil and 2 α-blockers, doxazosin and tamsulosin in healthy normotensive men. *J Urol (Baltimore)* (2004) 172, 1935–40.
10. Giuliano F, Kaplan SA, Cabanis M-J, Astruc B. Hemodynamic interaction study between the alpha$_1$-blocker alfuzosin and the phosphodiesterase-5 inhibitor tadalafil in middle-aged healthy male subjects. *Urology* (2006) 67, 1199–1204.
11. Guillaume M, Lonsdale F, Darstein C, Jimenez MC, Mitchell MI. Hemodynamic interaction between a daily dosed phosphodiesterase 5 inhibitor, tadalafil, and the α-adrenergic blockers, doxazosin and tamsulosin, in middle-aged healthy male subjects. *J Clin Pharmacol* (2007) 47, 1303–10.
12. Levitra (Vardenafil hydrochloride). Bayer HealthCare Pharmaceuticals Inc. US prescribing information, April 2014.
13. Auerbach SM, Gittelman M, Mazzu A, Cihon F, Sundaresan P, White WB. Simultaneous administration of vardenafil and tamsulosin does not induce clinically significant hypotension in patients with benign prostatic hyperplasia. *Urology* (2004) 64, 998–1003; discussion 1003–4.
14. Ng C-F, Wong A, Cheng C-W, Chan ES-Y, Wong H-M, Hou S-M. Effect of vardenafil on blood pressure profile of patients with erectile dysfunction concomitantly treated with doxazosin gastrointestinal therapeutic system for benign prostatic hyperplasia. *J Urol (Baltimore)* (2008) 180, 1042–6.
15. Pomara G, Morelli G, Pomara S, Taddei S, Ghiadoni L, Dinelli N, Travaglini F, Dicuio M, Mondaini N, Salvetti A, Selli C. Cardiovascular parameter changes in patients with erectile dysfunction using pde-5 inhibitors: a study with sildenafil and vardenafil. *J Androl* (2004) 25, 625–9.
16. Cialis (Tadalafil). Eli Lilly and Company Ltd. UK Summary of product characteristics, March 2013.
17. Adcirca (Tadalafil). Eli Lilly and Company Ltd. UK Summary of product characteristics, May 2013.
18. Cialis (Tadalafil). Eli Lilly and Company. US Prescribing information, April 2014.
19. De Rose AF, Giglio M, Traverso P, Lantieri P, Carmignani G. Combined oral therapy with sildenafil and doxazosin for the treatment of non-organic erectile dysfunction refractory to sildenafil monotherapy. *Int J Impot Res* (2002) 14, 50–3.

Phosphodiesterase type-5 inhibitors + Antacids

Aluminium/magnesium hydroxide-containing antacids do not have a clinically relevant effect on the absorption of sildenafil, tadalafil or vardenafil.

Clinical evidence, mechanism, importance and management

(a) Sildenafil

In a single-dose study in 12 healthy subjects, the bioavailability of sildenafil was not affected by single 30-mL doses of an **aluminium/magnesium hydroxide** antacid.[1] Therefore, no additional precautions are needed if these drugs are used together

(b) Tadalafil

A randomised, crossover study in 12 healthy subjects found that 20 mL of *Maalox* (**aluminium/magnesium hydroxide**) reduced the mean maximum serum level of a single 10-mg dose of tadalafil by 30%. Although peak tadalafil levels were delayed by 2.5 hours, the total amount of tadalafil absorbed was unchanged. None of the changes caused were considered to be clinically relevant, and there would appear to be no reason for avoiding concurrent use.[2]

(c) Vardenafil

In a crossover study, 12 healthy subjects were given a single 20-mg dose of vardenafil with 10 mL of an **aluminium/magnesium hydroxide** antacid (*Maalox 70*). The bioavailability of vardenafil was not significantly altered by the antacid, therefore no additional precautions are needed if these drugs are used together.[3]

1. Wilner K, Laboy L, LeBel M. The effects of cimetidine and antacid on the pharmacokinetic profile of sildenafil citrate in healthy male volunteers. *Br J Clin Pharmacol* (2002) 53, 31S–36S.
2. Eli Lilly and Company. Personal communication, March 2003.
3. Rohde G, Wensing G, Sachse R. The pharmacokinetics of vardenafil, a new selective PDE5 inhibitor, are not affected by the antacid, Maalox 70. *Pharmacotherapy* (2001) 21, 1254.

Phosphodiesterase type-5 inhibitors + Antihypertensives

No interactions appear to occur between avanafil, sildenafil, tadalafil, or vardenafil and most other antihypertensive drugs. The exceptions might be diltiazem and verapamil, which theoretically might inhibit the metabolism of the phosphodiesterase type-5 inhibitors.

Potentially serious interactions with phosphodiesterase type-5 inhibitors and alpha blockers or nitrates are discussed in 'Phosphodiesterase type-5 inhibitors + Alpha blockers', p.1538 and 'Phosphodiesterase type-5 inhibitors + Nitrates', p.1545.

Clinical evidence

(a) Avanafil

The UK and US manufacturers briefly report that **amlodipine** 5 mg daily increased the maximum plasma concentration and AUC of a single 200-mg dose of avanafil by about 22 to 28% and 60 to 70%, respectively. There was no effect of avanafil on the pharmacokinetics of amlodipine.[1,2] They also report that in a study to determine the effect of a single 200-mg dose of avanafil with **amlodipine** (5 mg daily) and **enalapril** (20 mg daily) on blood pressure, concurrent use of enalapril and avanafil resulted in a decrease in supine blood pressure of about 2/3 mmHg, and use of amlodipine with avanafil resulted in a decrease of about 1/-1 mmHg.[1,2]

(b) Sildenafil

In a study in 8 hypertensive men taking one to five antihypertensives (**amlodipine** (5 patients), a **diuretic** (4 patients), an **ACE inhibitor** (3 patients), an **angiotensin II receptor antagonist** (2 patients), **diltiazem** (1 patient)), a single 50-mg dose of sildenafil decreased the systolic blood pressure by a mean maximum of 24 mmHg, compared with only 6 mmHg for placebo. One patient had a blood pressure decrease of 48/23 mmHg, but none complained of hypotensive symptoms.[3] Three retrospective analyses of pooled data from various clinical studies suggest that patients taking one or more non-nitrate antihypertensives (**ACE inhibitors**, alpha blockers, **angiotensin II receptor antagonists, beta blockers, calcium-channel blockers, diuretics**) had no important difference in blood pressure or heart rate when given sildenafil, when compared with those taking antihypertensives and placebo,[4] and that the incidence of adverse events related to blood pressure decreases, such as dizziness, did not differ between the two groups.[4-6] In a placebo-controlled study in patients with hypertension stabilised with two or more antihypertensives (including **diuretics, calcium-channel blockers, ACE inhibitors, beta blockers**, alpha blockers, **angiotensin II receptor antagonists**), the occurrence of adverse events potentially related to hypotensive effects (dizziness, hypotension, labile blood pressure, vertigo) was less than 4% in those given sildenafil.[7] Note that combined use with alpha blockers may be especially likely to induce hypotensive events, see 'Phosphodiesterase type-5 inhibitors + Alpha blockers', p.1538.

The UK and US manufacturers report that, in population pharmacokinetic analysis, there was no effect on sildenafil pharmacokinetics in those taking **ACE inhibitors, calcium-channel blockers** and **thiazide** and **related diuretics**,[8,9] whereas the AUC of the less potent active metabolite of sildenafil was increased by 62% by **loop** and **potassium-sparing diuretics** and 2-fold by **non-selective beta blockers**.[9] Furthermore, in population pharmacokinetic analysis of patients with pulmonary hypertension, there appeared to be an increase in sildenafil exposure when it was taken with **beta blockers** (none named) in combination with CYP3A4 substrates (none named).[10,11]

The pharmacokinetics of **amlodipine** were not altered in 16 patients taking **amlodipine** 5 or 10 mg daily when they took a single 100-mg dose of sildenafil 2 hours after their morning dose of amlodipine. Blood pressure was decreased by an additional 8/7 mmHg by sildenafil, when compared with placebo.[12]

A case report describes a patient taking **diltiazem** 30 mg three times daily who underwent coronary angiography 48 hours after taking sildenafil 50 mg, and who developed profound and persistent hypotension (blood pressure 90/60 mmHg) after receiving sublingual nitrate for pain related to angina during the procedure.[13] It was suggested that **diltiazem** might have inhibited the metabolism of sildenafil so that it interacted with the nitrate,[13,14] although the timescale for this interaction has been disputed.[15] Another patient taking **diltiazem** developed posterior ischaemic optic neuropathy after taking three capsules of a Chinese herbal medicine: each capsule was subsequently found to contain about 32 mg of sildenafil. After 6 weeks his visual acuity improved in one eye to enable him to count fingers, and in the other eye he could detect hand movements. The authors suggest that **diltiazem** inhibited the metabolism of sildenafil and thereby contributed to the development of this adverse effect, which was likely due to sildenafil-induced hypotension.[16] A further case report describes a 77-year-old man who developed sudden bilateral hearing loss with intermittent tinnitus after taking sildenafil 20 mg three times daily for 1 day for pulmonary hypertension. He was also taking **furosemide** 20 to 40 mg daily and **diltiazem** 120 mg daily. Prior to initiation of sildenafil the patient had received a 10 day course of high-dose furosemide (60 mg IV twice daily for 5 days, followed by 120 mg orally twice daily for 5 days). The patient had no previous history of ototoxicity with furosemide. Discontinuation of furosemide resulted in self-reported improvement in hearing within days, and discontinuation of sildenafil then resulted in self-reported hearing loss returning to normal. The authors suggest that the risk of drug-induced ototoxicity with phosphodiesterase type-5 inhibitors might be increased with concurrent high-dose loop diuretics, and CYP3A4 inhibitors such as diltiazem which can increase the exposure to phosphodiesterase type-5 inhibitors.[17]

(c) Tadalafil

Placebo-controlled studies in patients taking **enalapril**, **metoprolol**, or **bendroflumethiazide**, found that the addition of a 10-mg dose of tadalafil did not have a clinically relevant effect on blood pressure or heart rate.[18] Similar results were seen in a study in patients taking **amlodipine** and given tadalafil 20 mg.[18] In another study in patients taking unnamed **angiotensin II receptor antagonists** (alone or in combination with **thiazides**, **calcium-channel blockers**, or **beta blockers**[19]), tadalafil 20 mg lowered the mean blood pressure by 8/4 mmHg more than placebo.[20] About twice as many patients taking tadalafil had a potentially clinically relevant decrease in blood pressure, when compared with those taking the antihypertensives alone, although no potential hypotensive symptoms (e.g. dizziness) occurred.[18]

In phase III studies in patients taking antihypertensives (**ACE inhibitors**, **calcium-channel blockers**, **thiazide diuretics**, **beta blockers**, **angiotensin II receptor antagonists**, alpha blockers, and **loop diuretics**) blood pressure was similar in those given tadalafil and those given placebo. There was no difference in the number of patients with a potentially clinically relevant decrease in systolic blood pressure (greater than 30 mmHg), and there was a similar incidence of dizziness.[18]

In a study 8 healthy subjects took a single 20-mg dose of tadalafil alone, or 2 hours before a single 5-mg sublingual dose of **nitrendipine**. Both treatments slightly lowered blood pressure (by about 2 mmHg and 3 mmHg) with no statistically significant difference between them. There were no episodes of clinically relevant hypotension.[21]

(d) Vardenafil

The preliminary report of a randomised, crossover study in 22 patients with hypertension stabilised by slow-release **nifedipine** 30 or 60 mg daily, given a single 20-mg dose of vardenafil, or placebo notes that vardenafil had no effect on the pharmacokinetics of **nifedipine**, but did cause a further decrease in supine blood pressure of about 6/5 mmHg. Heart rate was increased by 4 bpm.[22] The US manufacturer briefly notes that **nifedipine** did not alter vardenafil concentrations.[23]

The UK manufacturer states that, although not specifically studied, population pharmacokinetic analysis has suggested that **ACE inhibitors**, **beta blockers**, and **diuretics** have no effect on vardenafil pharmacokinetics.[24]

Mechanism

Phosphodiesterase type-5 inhibitors cause mild to moderate vasodilatation of vascular smooth muscle in veins and arteries, and so can lower blood pressure. This effect might be additive with the effects of antihypertensive drugs.

It should be noted that some calcium-channel blockers (e.g. **diltiazem**, **verapamil**) are known to inhibit CYP3A4, by which avanafil, sildenafil, tadalafil, and vardenafil are metabolised, and so these calcium-channel blockers have the potential to increase phosphodiesterase type-5 inhibitor exposure.

Importance and management

A small, additional decrease in blood pressure might be anticipated when phosphodiesterase type-5 inhibitors are used in patients taking antihypertensives such as beta blockers, ACE inhibitors, calcium-channel blockers, and diuretics. This effect rarely appears to result in clinically important adverse effects,[25] but consider also whether the patient's underlying cardiovascular disease would make resumption of sexual activity high-risk: poorly controlled hypertension and unstable or refractory angina are categorised as high-risk.[25]

There are no established pharmacokinetic interactions between phosphodiesterase type-5 inhibitors and ACE inhibitors, beta blockers, and dihydropyridine calcium-channel blockers. There are some preliminary data suggesting a small increase in exposure to sildenafil with loop and potassium-sparing diuretics and non-selective beta blockers, but the manufacturer does not consider this to be clinically relevant.[9] Note that some consider that the precautions required for alpha blockers (see 'Phosphodiesterase type-5 inhibitors + Alpha blockers', p.1538) should also be applied to the beta blockers that also have alpha blocker activity, such as **carvedilol** and **labetalol**.[25]

Although there appears to be no pharmacokinetic data on the effects of **diltiazem** or **verapamil** given with phosphodiesterase type-5 inhibitors, on the basis that other moderate CYP3A4 inhibitors (such as erythromycin) inhibit the metabolism of avanafil, sildenafil, tadalafil, and vardenafil (see 'Phosphodiesterase type-5 inhibitors + Macrolides', p.1544), increased effects might be predicted. A lower starting dose of these phosphodiesterase type-5 inhibitors might therefore be appropriate in any patient also given diltiazem or verapamil. Note that the UK and US manufacturers of avanafil give specific dosing advice for use with all moderate CYP3A4 inhibitors (which therefore incudes diltiazem and verapamil), see 'Phosphodiesterase type-5 inhibitors + Macrolides', p.1544 for details.

For information on interactions between phosphodiesterase type-5 inhibitors and nitrates, see 'Phosphodiesterase type-5 inhibitors + Nitrates', p.1545.

1. Spedra (Avanafil). A. Menarini Farmaceutica Internazionale SRL. UK Summary of product characteristics, January 2015.
2. Stendra (Avanafil). Vivus, Inc. US Prescribing information, January 2015.
3. Mahmud A, Hennessy M, Feely J. Effect of sildenafil on blood pressure and arterial wave reflection in treated hypertensive men. *J Hum Hypertens* (2001) 15, 707–13.
4. Zusman RM, Prisant LM, Brown MJ. Effect of sildenafil citrate on blood pressure and heart rate in men with erectile dysfunction taking concomitant antihypertensive medication. *J Hypertens* (2000) 18, 1865–9.
5. Kloner RA, Brown M, Prisant LM, Collins M, for the Sildenafil Study Group. Effect of sildenafil in patients with erectile dysfunction taking antihypertensive therapy. *Am J Hypertens* (2001) 14, 70–3.
6. Böhm M, Burkart M, Baumann G. Sildenafil is well tolerated by erectile dysfunction patients taking antihypertensive medications, including those on multidrug regimens. *Curr Drug Saf* (2007) 2, 5–8.
7. Pickering TG, Shepherd AMM, Puddey I, Glasser DB, Orazem J, Sherman N, Mancia G. Sildenafil citrate for erectile dysfunction in men receiving multiple antihypertensive agents: a randomized controlled trial. *Am J Hypertens* (2004) 17, 1135–42.
8. Viagra (Sildenafil citrate). Pfizer Ltd. UK Summary of product characteristics, June 2015.
9. Viagra (Sildenafil citrate). Pfizer Inc. US Prescribing information, March 2015.
10. Revatio Tablets (Sildenafil citrate). Pfizer Ltd. UK Summary of product characteristics, April 2015.
11. Revatio (Sildenafil citrate). Pfizer Inc. US Prescribing information, April 2015.
12. Webb DJ, Freestone S, Allen MJ, Muirhead GJ. Sildenafil citrate and blood-pressure–lowering drugs: results of drug interaction studies with an organic nitrate and a calcium antagonist. *Am J Cardiol* (1999) 83, 21C–28C.
13. Khoury V, Kritharides L. Diltiazem-mediated inhibition of sildenafil metabolism may promote nitrate-induced hypotension. *Aust N Z J Med* (2000) 30, 641–2.
14. Kiritharides L. Diltiazem-mediated inhibition of sildenafil metabolism may promote nitrate-induced hypotension. Reply. *Intern Med J* (2001) 31, 374–5.
15. Howes L. Diltiazem-mediated inhibition of sildenafil metabolism may promote nitrate-induced hypotension. *Intern Med J* (2001) 31, 373.
16. Su DH-W, Ang P-S, Tow SL-C. Bilateral posterior ischaemic optic neuropathy associated with use of sildenafil. *J Neuroophthalmol* (2008) 28, 75.
17. Skeith L, Yamashita C, Mehta S, Farquhar D, Kim RB. Sildenafil and furosemide associated ototoxicity: consideration of drug-drug interactions, synergy, and broader clinical relevance. *J Popul Ther Clin Pharmacol* (2013) 20, e128–31.
18. Kloner RA, Mitchell M, Emmick JT. Cardiovascular effects of tadalafil in patients on common antihypertensive therapies. *Am J Cardiol* (2003) 92 (Suppl), 47M–57M.
19. Cialis (Tadalafil). Eli Lilly and Company Ltd. UK Summary of product characteristics, March 2013.
20. Cialis (Tadalafil). Eli Lilly and Company. US Prescribing information, April 2014.
21. Park J-W, Leithäuser B, Jung F. Sublingual application of liquid nitrendipine does not result in critical hypotension in healthy volunteers under phosphodiesterase-5 inhibition. *Clin Hemorheol Microcirc* (2008) 39, 323–8.
22. Rohde G, Jordaan PJ. Influence of vardenafil on blood pressure and pharmacokinetics in hypertensive patients on nifedipine therapy. 31st Annual Meeting of the American College of Clinical Pharmacology, San Francisco, California, 2002.
23. Levitra (Vardenafil hydrochloride). Bayer HealthCare Pharmaceuticals Inc. US Prescribing information, April 2014.
24. Levitra (Vardenafil hydrochloride). Bayer plc. UK Summary of product characteristics, April 2014.
25. Kostis JB, Jackson G, Rosen R, Barrett-Connor E, Billups K, Burnett AL, Carson C, Cheitlin M, Debusk R, Fonseca V, Ganz P, Goldstein I, Guay A, Hatzichristou D, Hollander JE, Hutter A, Katz S, Kloner RA, Mittleman M, Montorsi F, Montorsi P, Nehra A, Sadovsky R, Shabsigh R. Sexual dysfunction and cardiac risk (the Second Princeton Consensus Conference). *Am J Cardiol* (2005) 96, 313–21.

Phosphodiesterase type-5 inhibitors + Azoles

Ketoconazole very markedly increases avanafil and vardenafil exposure, moderately increases tadalafil exposure, and probably also increases sildenafil exposure. Itraconazole and other azoles that are potent CYP3A4 inhibitors, such as voriconazole, are predicted to interact similarly. Fluconazole, miconazole, and posaconazole might also increase the exposure to these phosphodiesterase type-5 inhibitors.

Clinical evidence

(a) Avanafil

The UK and US manufacturers briefly note that, in a study in 15 healthy males, **ketoconazole** 400 mg daily increased the AUC and maximum concentration of a single 50-mg dose of avanafil about 13-fold and 3-fold, respectively.[1,2]

(b) Sildenafil

The UK and US manufacturers of sildenafil state that population data from clinical studies suggests that **ketoconazole** decreases the clearance of sildenafil,[3,4] without increasing the incidence of adverse effects.[3]

(c) Tadalafil

In a randomised study in 12 healthy subjects, **ketoconazole** 200 mg daily increased the AUC of a single 10-mg dose of tadalafil 2-fold, and **ketoconazole** 400 mg daily increased the AUC of a single 20-mg dose of tadalafil 4-fold, with only a minor increase in the maximum plasma concentration of tadalafil (15% and 22%, respectively).[5,6]

A case report describes a 56-year-old man who was taking **itraconazole** 400 mg daily for 7 days each month. Within a few hours of his first 10-mg dose of tadalafil he developed priapism, which lasted for more than 4 hours. The same reaction occurred when he took tadalafil during the following month. He had seemingly previously taken sildenafil with **itraconazole** without adverse effect.[7] Another case report describes a patient taking tadalafil 20 mg for erectile dysfunction who developed sclerosing lymphangitis of the penis after the third dose of **fluconazole** 300 mg once weekly.[8]

(d) Vardenafil

The UK and US manufacturers of vardenafil state that, in a study in healthy subjects, **ketoconazole** 200 mg daily increased the AUC of a 5-mg dose of vardenafil 10-fold, and increased its maximum plasma concentration 4-fold.[9,10]

Mechanism

Avanafil, sildenafil, tadalafil, and vardenafil are all principally metabolised by CYP3A4, and avanafil, sildenafil, and vardenafil are also metabolised to a minor extent by CYP2C9. Ketoconazole and itraconazole are potent inhibitors of CYP3A4, and therefore they inhibit avanafil, sildenafil, tadalafil, and vardenafil metabolism, which leads to an increase in their exposure. Fluconazole is a moderate inhibitor of CYP3A4 and is also a potent inhibitor of CYP2C9, and so it would also increase the exposure of these phosphodiesterase type-5 inhibitors, although the role of this potential interaction in the case of sclerosing lymphangitis with tadalafil is uncertain.

Importance and management

Information about the interaction between the phosphodiesterase type-5 inhibitors and ketoconazole or itraconazole is limited for some drug pairs, but what is known suggests that they behave in line with the predicted metabolic effects.

On the basis of the very marked effect of ketoconazole and another potent CYP3A4 inhibitor, ritonavir (see 'Phosphodiesterase type-5 inhibitors + HIV-protease inhibitors', p.1543) on **avanafil** exposure, the UK manufacturer contraindicates its concurrent use with potent CYP3A4 inhibitors,[2] and the US manufacturer does not recommend their concurrent use.[1] See 'Table 1.9', p.11 for a list of known clinically important CYP3A4 inhibitors. Note that they additionally name **nefazodone** and **indinavir**, but these are generally considered to be moderate CYP3A4 inhibitors. **Fluconazole** is a moderate CYP3A4 inhibitor and its effects on avanafil exposure are predicted to be similar to those seen with another moderate CYP3A4 inhibitor, erythromycin. See *Importance and management* in 'Phosphodiesterase type-5 inhibitors + Macrolides', p.1544 for dosing advice. Note also that fluconazole potently inhibits CYP2C9, by which avanafil is also minimally metabolised and so involvement of this pathway in any interaction cannot be ruled out.

When used for erectile dysfunction, the UK and US manufacturers of **sildenafil** recommend that a low starting dose (25 mg) should be considered if ketoconazole or itraconazole are used concurrently.[3,4] When used for pulmonary hypertension, the manufacturers state that the concurrent use of sildenafil with ketoconazole or itraconazole is contraindicated in the UK,[11] or not recommended in the US.[12]

When used for erectile dysfunction, the UK manufacturer of **tadalafil** advises caution[5] and the US manufacturer advises that the "as needed" dose of tadalafil should not exceed 10 mg in a 72-hour period, and that the daily dose should not exceed 2.5 mg daily in patients taking potent CYP3A4 inhibitors such as ketoconazole and itraconazole.[6] However, note that a 10 mg dose of tadalafil has caused priapism in one patient taking itraconazole. For benign prostatic hyperplasia, the US manufacturer advises that the tadalafil dose should not exceed 2.5 mg daily.[6] For pulmonary hypertension, the UK and US manufacturers state that the concurrent use of tadalafil with ketoconazole or itraconazole should be avoided.[13,14]

The UK manufacturer of **vardenafil** advises avoiding the concurrent use of ketoconazole and itraconazole in all patients, and specifically contraindicates concurrent use in patients over 75 years of age.[9] In contrast, the US manufacturer recommends that the dose of vardenafil should not exceed 5 mg in 24 hours when used with ketoconazole or itraconazole 200 mg daily, or 2.5 mg in 24 hours with ketoconazole or itraconazole 400 mg daily.[10]

For all of these phosphodiesterase type-5 inhibitors, similar advice would apply if **posaconazole** and **voriconazole** (which are all also clinically important inhibitors of CYP3A4) are given concurrently. Voriconazole also inhibits CYP2C9 which is involved to a minor extent in the metabolism of avanafil, sildenafil, and vardenafil, and so involvement of this pathway in any interaction cannot be ruled out. **Fluconazole**, a potent CYP2C9 inhibitor, might also affect the exposure to sildenafil and vardenafil. Note that at maximum doses, **miconazole** oral gel is sufficiently absorbed to have systemic effects, including inhibition of CYP3A4 and CYP2C9, and so might also interact with these phosphodiesterase type-5 inhibitors in the same way.

1. Stendra (Avanafil). Vivus, Inc. US Prescribing information, January 2015.
2. Spedra (Avanafil). A. Menarini Farmaceutica Internazionale SRL. UK Summary of product characteristics, January 2015.
3. Viagra (Sildenafil citrate). Pfizer Ltd. UK Summary of product characteristics, June 2015.
4. Viagra (Sildenafil citrate). Pfizer Inc. US Prescribing information, March 2015.
5. Cialis (Tadalafil). Eli Lilly and Company Ltd. UK Summary of product characteristics, March 2013.
6. Cialis (Tadalafil). Eli Lilly and Company. US Prescribing information, April 2014.
7. Galatti L, Fioravanti A, Salvo F, Polimeni G, Giustini SE. Interaction between tadalafil and itraconazole. *Ann Pharmacother* (2005) 39, 200.
8. Guarneria C, Polimeni G. Sclerosing lymphangitis of the penis after coadministration of tadalafil and fluconazole. *Clin Exp Dermatol* (2009) 34, e225–e226.
9. Levitra (Vardenafil hydrochloride). Bayer plc. UK Summary of product characteristics, April 2014.
10. Levitra (Vardenafil hydrochloride). Bayer HealthCare Pharmaceuticals Inc. US prescribing information April 2014.
11. Revatio Tablets (Sildenafil citrate). Pfizer Ltd. UK Summary of product characteristics, April 2015.
12. Revatio (Sildenafil citrate). Pfizer Inc. US Prescribing information, April 2015.
13. Adcirca (Tadalafil). Eli Lilly and Company. US Prescribing information, April 2015.
14. Adcirca (Tadalafil). Eli Lilly and Company Ltd. UK Summary of product characteristics, May 2013.

Phosphodiesterase type-5 inhibitors + Endothelin receptor antagonists

Bosentan moderately decreases sildenafil exposure, and slightly decreases tadalafil exposure. Bosentan exposure is moderately increased by sildenafil, but is not affected by tadalafil. No pharmacokinetic interaction occurs between ambrisentan and sildenafil or tadalafil, or between macitentan and sildenafil.

Clinical evidence

(a) Ambrisentan

1. Sildenafil. A crossover study in 19 healthy subjects found that sildenafil 20 mg three times daily for 7 days did not alter the pharmacokinetics of a single 10-mg dose of ambrisentan. Ambrisentan 10 mg daily for 7 days increased the maximum concentration of a single 20-mg dose of sildenafil by 13%, with no notable effects on its other pharmacokinetic parameters. No additive or synergistic reduction in blood pressure was noted.[1]

2. Tadalafil. In a crossover study in 23 healthy subjects, tadalafil 40 mg daily for 8 days decreased the AUC of a single 10-mg dose of ambrisentan given on day 6, by about 12%. Maximum plasma concentrations of ambrisentan were similar in the presence and absence of tadalafil. The pharmacokinetics of tadalafil were not affected by concurrent use with ambrisentan.[2]

(b) Bosentan

1. Sildenafil. In 10 patients with pulmonary hypertension, bosentan 62.5 mg twice daily for one month decreased the AUC of a single 100-mg dose of sildenafil by 53% and increased its clearance 2.3-fold. After a second month of bosentan, at an increased dose of 125 mg twice daily, the AUC of a single 100-mg dose of sildenafil was decreased by 69%, and the clearance increased 3.4-fold. The AUC of the primary metabolite, desmethylsildenafil, was also decreased in a dose-dependent manner by bosentan.[3] In another well-controlled study in healthy subjects, the concurrent use of bosentan 125 mg twice daily and sildenafil 80 mg three times daily for 6 days decreased the AUC of sildenafil by 63% and increased the AUC of bosentan by 50%, when compared with either drug given alone.[4]

In contrast, in a small study in Japanese patients with pulmonary hypertension, pretreatment with bosentan (dose not stated) did not alter the AUC of a single 50-mg dose of sildenafil in 4 patients, when compared with another 4 patients who did not receive pre-treatment with bosentan. However the AUC of the primary sildenafil metabolite, desmethylsildenafil, was 57% lower in the group pre-treated with bosentan.[5] Furthermore, a population pharmacokinetic analysis in 46 paediatric Japanese patients with pulmonary hypertension suggested that the pharmacokinetics of bosentan were not affected by sildenafil.[6]

2. Tadalafil. In a well-controlled study in healthy subjects, the concurrent use of tadalafil 40 mg daily and bosentan 125 mg twice daily for 10 days decreased the AUC of tadalafil by 41%. There was also a 13% increase in the AUC of bosentan, which was not statistically significant.[7]

(c) Macitentan

A crossover study in 12 healthy male subjects given **sildenafil** 20 mg three times daily for 3 days (followed by 20 mg daily on day 4) with macitentan 10 mg daily (after a 30 mg loading dose on day 1), found that the maximum concentration and AUC of sildenafil were increased by 26% and 15%, respectively, although the change in AUC was not statistically significant. The pharmacokinetics of macitentan were unaffected.[8]

Mechanism

Bosentan induces CYP3A4, by which sildenafil and tadalafil are principally metabolised. The mechanism by which sildenafil increases bosentan exposure is unknown, but might, in part, involve inhibition of organic anion transporting polypeptides (OATP).[9]

Importance and management

The pharmacokinetic interactions of **bosentan** with sildenafil and tadalafil are established and potentially clinically important. The efficacy of sildenafil and tadalafil might be reduced in patients taking bosentan, and should be monitored, particularly when these phosphodiesterase type-5 inhibitors are given for erectile dysfunction. Note that concurrent use does not appear to be uncommon in clinical studies of the use of phosphodiesterase inhibitors and endothelin receptor antagonists for pulmonary hypertension. In addition, sildenafil might increase the effects of bosentan, therefore patients should be monitored for signs of bosentan adverse effects such as flushing, headache, and oedema. Tadalafil is unlikely to affect bosentan exposure.

No dose adjustment of either drug is required on the concurrent use of **ambrisentan** and either sildenafil or tadalafil. Similarly, no dose adjustments are required if **macitentan** and sildenafil are given concurrently.

1. Spence R, Mandagere A, Dufton C, Venitz J. Pharmacokinetics and safety of ambrisentan in combination with sildenafil in healthy volunteers. *J Clin Pharmacol* (2008) 48, 1451–9.
2. Spence R, Mandagere A, Harrison B, Dufton C, Boinpally R. No clinically relevant pharmacokinetic and safety interactions of ambrisentan in combination with tadalafil in healthy volunteers. *J Pharm Sci* (2009) 98, 4962–74.
3. Paul GA, Gibbs JSR, Boobis AR, Abbas A, Wilkins MR. Bosentan decreases the plasma concentration of sildenafil when coprescribed in pulmonary hypertension. *Br J Clin Pharmacol* (2005) 60, 107–12.
4. Burgess G, Hoogkamer H, Collings L, Dingemanse J. Mutual pharmacokinetic interactions between steady-state bosentan and sildenafil. *Eur J Clin Pharmacol* (2008) 64, 43–50.
5. Hatano M, Yao A, Kinugawa K, Hirata Y, Nagai R. Acute effect of sildenafil is maintained in pulmonary arterial hypertension patients chronically treated with bosentan. *Int Heart J* (2011) 52, 233–9.
6. Taguchi M, Ichida F, Hirono K, Miyawaki T, Yoshimura N, Nakamura T, Akita C, Nakayama T, Saji T, Kato Y, Horiuchi I, Hashimoto Y. Pharmacokinetics of bosentan in routinely treated Japanese pediatric patients with pulmonary arterial hypertension. *Drug Metab Pharmacokinet* (2011) 26, 280–7.
7. Wrishko RE, Dingemanse J, Yu A, Darstein C, Phillips DL, Mitchell MI. Pharmacokinetic interaction between tadalafil and bosentan in healthy male subjects. *J Clin Pharmacol* (2008) 48, 610–18.
8. Sidharta PN, van Giersbergen PL, Woltz M, Dingemanse J. Investigation of mutual pharmacokinetic interactions between macitentan, a novel endothelin receptor antagonist, and sildenafil in healthy subjects. *Br J Clin Pharmacol* (2014) 78, 1035–42.
9. Treiber A, Schneiter R, Häusler S, Stieger B. Bosentan is a substrate of human OATP1B1 and OATP1B3: inhibition of hepatic uptake as the common mechanism of its interactions with cyclosporin A, rifampicin, and sildenafil. *Drug Metab Dispos* (2007) 35, 1400–7.

Phosphodiesterase type-5 inhibitors + Food

Food appears to delay the absorption of avanafil, sildenafil, and vardenafil, but not tadalafil; however, the amount absorbed does not appear to be affected.

Clinical evidence

(a) Avanafil

The UK and US manufacturers of avanafil briefly note that in a study, the time to reach maximum concentration was delayed by about 1.25 hours and its mean maximum concentration was 39% lower, when given with a high-fat meal, compared with the fasted state. However, there was no change in the AUC of avanafil.[1,2]

(b) Sildenafil

In a crossover study in 33 healthy subjects given a single 100-mg dose of sildenafil, the maximum plasma concentration of sildenafil was 29% lower when it was taken after a high-fat breakfast, when compared with after an overnight fast. In addition, the maximum plasma concentration of sildenafil was delayed, from about one hour to 2 hours. However, there was no change in the AUC of sildenafil.[3]

(c) Tadalafil

In a study in 18 healthy subjects there were no differences in the pharmacokinetics of a single 20-mg dose of tadalafil taken after a 10-hour fast, or after a high-fat breakfast.[4]

(d) Vardenafil

In a study in 22 healthy subjects given a single 20-mg dose of vardenafil, the time to reach the maximum plasma concentration was increased from one hour to 2 hours, and its maximum plasma concentration was decreased by 18% when it was given with a high-fat breakfast, when compared with after an overnight fast. However, there was no difference in the AUC of vardenafil. Conversely, there was no difference in any of the pharmacokinetic parameters of vardenafil when it was taken with a moderate-fat evening meal, when compared with taking it on an empty stomach (6 hours after lunch and 4 hours before an evening meal).[5]

Mechanism

It is likely that the delay in absorption of avanafil, sildenafil, and vardenafil is due to delayed gastric emptying in the presence of food.

Importance and management

Food has no clinically relevant effect on the overall absorption of avanafil, sildenafil, tadalafil, or vardenafil. Although, when compared with fasting, there was a delay in time to maximum plasma concentration of avanafil, sildenafil, and vardenafil when they were given after a high-fat meal, it is unclear whether this results in a clinically relevant effect on the time to the onset of activity of on-demand doses for erectile dysfunction. Note that a moderate-fat evening meal did not delay the onset of action of vardenafil. Nevertheless, it might be prudent for patients to be aware that timing of avanafil, sildenafil, and vardenafil in relation to meals might alter the time to the onset of action for erectile dysfunction (faster on an empty stomach, slower with meals). Any effect of food is unlikely to be clinically relevant if sildenafil is taken regularly for pulmonary hypertension.

1. Spedra (Avanafil). A. Menarini Farmaceutica Internazionale SRL. UK Summary of product characteristics, January 2015.
2. Stendra (Avanafil). Vivus, Inc. US Prescribing information, January 2015.
3. Nichols DJ, Muirhead GJ, Harness JA. Pharmacokinetics of sildenafil citrate after single oral doses in healthy male subjects: absolute bioavailability, food effects and dose proportionality. *Br J Clin Pharmacol* (2002) 52 (Suppl 1), 5S–12S.
4. Forgue ST, Patterson BE, Bedding AW, Payne CD, Phillips DL, Wrishko RE, Mitchell MI. Tadalafil pharmacokinetics in healthy subjects. *Br J Clin Pharmacol* (2006) 61, 280–8.
5. Rajagopalan P, Mazzu A, Xia C, Dawkins R, Sundaresan P. Effect of high-fat breakfast and moderate-fat evening meal on the pharmacokinetics of vardenafil, an oral phosphodiesterase-5 inhibitor for the treatment of erectile dysfunction. *J Clin Pharmacol* (2003) 43, 260–7.

Phosphodiesterase type-5 inhibitors + Grapefruit and other fruit juices

Grapefruit juice negligibly increases the exposure of sildenafil. Avanafil, tadalafil, and vardenafil are predicted to be similarly affected. Unexpectedly, pomelo juice decreased the exposure of sildenafil.

Clinical evidence

(a) Grapefruit juice

In a study, 250 mL of grapefruit juice was given to 24 healthy subjects, both one hour before and with a 50-mg dose of **sildenafil**. There was a 23% increase in the AUC of **sildenafil**, but the maximum plasma concentration was not changed. Inter-individual variation in **sildenafil** pharmacokinetics was also increased by grapefruit juice.[1] A further report describes one patient who experienced a 2.7-fold increase in the AUC of **sildenafil** after taking a single 25-mg dose of **sildenafil** with 250 mL of grapefruit juice.[2]

(b) Pomelo juice

In a crossover study, when 6 healthy fasting subjects took a single 50-mg dose of **sildenafil** with 250 mL of pomelo (*Citrus grandis*) juice, the maximum plasma concentration and AUC of **sildenafil** were *decreased* by 37% and 40%, respectively, when compared with water.[3]

Mechanism

Grapefruit juice inhibits CYP3A4, predominantly in the gut wall. Sildenafil is predominantly metabolised by CYP3A4 and has only moderate oral bioavailability; nevertheless, it appears that its exposure is not usually appreciably increased by grapefruit juice. Pomelo is related to grapefruit and therefore was predicted to interact similarly; however, it had the opposite effect. The mechanism whereby it decreased sildenafil exposure is unknown.

Importance and management

A pharmacokinetic study indicates that grapefruit juice interacts with **sildenafil**, but that the effect is minor, and unlikely to be clinically important in most patients. Nevertheless, the authors suggest that the combination is best avoided due to the increased inter-individual variability in sildenafil pharmacokinetics.[1] The case report describing a much greater increase in sildenafil exposure does give some weight to this advice. However, note that when used for erectile dysfunction, reduced doses of sildenafil are permitted with much more potent inhibitors of CYP3A4 than grapefruit juice (such as itraconazole, see 'Phosphodiesterase type-5 inhibitors + Azoles', p.1540). The UK manufacturer of sildenafil for pulmonary arterial hypertension states that no sildenafil dose adjustment is needed with grapefruit juice, although they do not recommend concurrent use.[4] It might still be prudent to be alert for sildenafil adverse effects and avoid grapefruit juice if these become troublesome.

The UK and US manufacturers of **tadalafil** predict that grapefruit juice will increase its concentrations,[5-7] and the UK manufacturer advises caution on their concurrent use.[5] It might therefore be prudent to be alert for tadalafil adverse effects and avoid grapefruit juice if these become troublesome.

The UK and US manufacturers of **avanafil**[8,9] and **vardenafil**[10,11] also predict that grapefruit juice will increase their exposures, and the advice of the UK manufacturers is to avoid the combinations.[8,10] For avanafil, this should be for 24 hours prior to taking a dose.[8]

The decreased sildenafil exposure seen in the pomelo juice study was unexpected, particularly because pomelo juice has increased the bioavailability of ciclosporin, another CYP3A4 substrate (see 'Ciclosporin + Grapefruit and other fruit juices', p.1229). It seems possible that other mechanisms are therefore involved. Until more is known, consider the possibility that sildenafil might be less effective if taken with pomelo juice.

1. Jetter A, Kinzig-Schippers M, Walchner-Bonjean M, Hering U, Bulitta J, Schreiner P, Sörgel F, Fuhr U. Effects of grapefruit juice on the pharmacokinetics of sildenafil. *Clin Pharmacol Ther* (2002) 71, 21–9.
2. Sheu M-T, Wu A-B, Yeh G-C, Hsia A, Ho H-O. Development of a liquid chromatographic method for bioanalytical applications with sildenafil. *J Chromatogr B Analyt Technol Biomed Life Sci* (2003) 791, 255–62.
3. Al-Ghazawi MA, Tutunji MS, AbuRuz SM. The effects of pummelo juice on pharmacokinetics of sildenafil in healthy adult male Jordanian volunteers. *Eur J Clin Pharmacol* (2010) 66, 159–63.
4. Revatio Tablets (Sildenafil citrate). Pfizer Ltd. UK Summary of product characteristics, April 2015.
5. Cialis (Tadalafil). Eli Lilly and Company Ltd. UK Summary of product characteristics, March 2013.
6. Cialis (Tadalafil). Eli Lilly and Company. US Prescribing information, April 2014.
7. Adcirca (Tadalafil). Eli Lilly and Company. US Prescribing information, April 2015.
8. Spedra (Avanafil). A. Menarini Farmaceutica Internazionale SRL. UK Summary of product characteristics, January 2015.
9. Stendra (Avanafil). Vivus, Inc. US Prescribing information, January 2015.
10. Levitra (Vardenafil hydrochloride). Bayer plc. UK Summary of product characteristics, April 2014.
11. Levitra (Vardenafil hydrochloride). Bayer HealthCare Pharmaceuticals Inc. US prescribing information, April 2014.

Phosphodiesterase type-5 inhibitors + H_2-receptor antagonists

Sildenafil exposure is modestly increased by cimetidine. No clinically relevant interaction appears to occur when nizatidine is given with tadalafil and when cimetidine or ranitidine is given with vardenafil.

Clinical evidence, mechanism, importance and management

(a) Sildenafil

In a study in 10 healthy subjects, **cimetidine** 800 mg daily for 4 days increased the AUC of a single 50-mg dose of sildenafil given on day 3 by 56%, when compared with 10 healthy subjects given sildenafil and placebo.[1] In addition, the manufacturers state that population pharmacokinetic analysis revealed a reduced clearance of sildenafil in patients taking CYP3A4 inhibitors, including **cimetidine**.[2,3] It has been suggested that these changes occur because **cimetidine** is a non-specific cytochrome P450 inhibitor,[2] with some minor effects on CYP3A4, which decreases the metabolism of sildenafil, leading to an increase in its exposure. Although the effects of this interaction are modest, the UK manufacturers of sildenafil for erectile dysfunction state that, although no increase in adverse effects was seen, a starting dose of 25 mg of sildenafil should be considered.[3] This seems a cautious approach. Furthermore, the UK manufacturer of sildenafil for pulmonary arterial hypertension[4] and the US manufacturer of sildenafil for erectile dysfunction[2] do not advise a sildenafil dose reduction in those taking **cimetidine**.

(b) Tadalafil

In a single-dose, crossover study in 12 healthy subjects, **nizatidine** 300 mg reduced the mean maximum serum levels of tadalafil 10 mg by 14%, but other pharmacokinetic parameters, including the extent of absorption, were largely unchanged. This suggests that changes in gastric pH are unlikely to alter the absorption of tadalafil.[5] These changes are not clinically relevant, and there would appear to be no reason for avoiding concurrent use.

(c) Vardenafil

In a crossover study, 10 healthy subjects were given a single 20-mg dose of vardenafil after they had taken **cimetidine** 400 mg twice daily for 3 days, **ranitidine** 150 mg twice daily for 3 days or with no pre-treatment. **Cimetidine** slightly increased the relative bioavailability of vardenafil (by about 12%, not considered clinically relevant), while **ranitidine** had no effect. It was concluded that changes in gastric pH do not alter the absorption of vardenafil.[6] No special precautions appear to be necessary during concurrent use.

1. Wilner K, Laboy L, LeBel M. The effects of cimetidine and antacid on the pharmacokinetic profile of sildenafil citrate in healthy male volunteers. *Br J Clin Pharmacol* (2002) 53, 31S–36S.
2. Viagra (Sildenafil citrate). Pfizer Inc. US Prescribing information, March 2015.
3. Viagra (Sildenafil citrate). Pfizer Ltd. UK Summary of product characteristics, June 2015.
4. Revatio Tablets (Sildenafil citrate). Pfizer Ltd. UK Summary of product characteristics, April 2015.
5. Eli Lilly and Company. Personal communication, March 2003.
6. Rohde G, Wensing G, Unger S, Sachse R. The pharmacokinetics of vardenafil, a new selective PDE5 inhibitor, is minimally affected by coadministration with cimetidine or ranitidine. *Pharmacotherapy* (2001) 21, 1254.

Phosphodiesterase type-5 inhibitors + HIV-protease inhibitors

Sildenafil exposure is moderately increased by indinavir, saquinavir, and darunavir boosted with ritonavir; and very markedly increased by ritonavir. A fatal heart attack occurred in a man taking ritonavir and saquinavir when he also took sildenafil. Vardenafil exposure is very markedly increased by indinavir and ritonavir, and avanafil exposure is very markedly increased by ritonavir. Increases in the concentrations of these phosphodiesterase type-5 inhibitors are predicted to occur with other HIV-protease inhibitors. Ritonavir and tipranavir boosted with ritonavir moderately increase tadalafil exposure, but at steady-state, these HIV-protease inhibitors had little effect on tadalafil pharmacokinetics. Priapism occurred in a patient after tadalafil was taken at the same time as ritonavir.

The phosphodiesterase type-5 inhibitors do not appear to alter the pharmacokinetics of the HIV-protease inhibitors.

Clinical evidence

A. Avanafil

The UK and US manufacturers briefly report that, in a study, **ritonavir** 600 mg twice daily increased the AUC and maximum concentration of a single 50-mg dose of avanafil 13-fold and 2-fold, respectively.[1,2]

B. Sildenafil

(a) Darunavir

In a crossover study in 16 healthy subjects, the pharmacokinetics of a 100-mg dose of sildenafil given alone were compared with those of a 25-mg dose of sildenafil given on day 7 of an 8-day course of darunavir boosted with ritonavir 400/100 mg twice daily. Despite the 4-fold lower sildenafil dose given with darunavir boosted with ritonavir, the AUC of sildenafil was similar in both arms of the study, although the AUC of the principal metabolite of sildenafil, *N*-desmethylsildenafil, was decreased by 95% when sildenafil was taken with darunavir boosted with ritonavir. The pharmacokinetics of darunavir and ritonavir were similar to those of historical controls suggesting single-dose sildenafil does not alter their pharmacokinetics.[3]

(b) Fosamprenavir

In a patient taking fosamprenavir boosted with ritonavir 700/100 mg twice daily, and sildenafil 20 mg three times daily for pulmonary hypertension, the maximum concentration of sildenafil was found to be 515.4 nanograms/mL and 406 nanograms/mL, 2 hours after the morning and afternoon doses on one day, respectively. The authors note that values greater than 500 nanograms/mL have been reported to be associated with adverse effects, but the patient reported no such problems.[4]

(c) Indinavir

A study in 6 HIV-positive patients found that sildenafil 25 mg did not alter the plasma concentrations of indinavir. However, the sildenafil AUC was about 4.4-fold higher than the AUC in historical control patients taking sildenafil (data normalised to a 25 mg dose) without indinavir.[5] Similarly, another study in just 2 HIV-positive patients found that sildenafil 25 mg did not affect the pharmacokinetics of indinavir.[6] For a case report describing higher sildenafil concentrations in a patient taking indinavir and lopinavir boosted with ritonavir, see *Lopinavir*, below.

(d) Lopinavir

A case report describes a patient taking lopinavir boosted with ritonavir 666/166 mg daily and **indinavir** 1200 mg daily in whom sildenafil was given in increasing doses for pulmonary hypertension, with careful monitoring of plasma concentrations. In this patient, the plasma-concentration-time curves for sildenafil, over 8 hours after a dose, were almost identical for 25 mg once daily, 25 mg twice daily, and 25 mg three times daily, the only difference being a higher residual concentration (minimum concentration) as the dose interval was shortened. This patient had no adverse effects or changes in systolic blood pressure, but did show a clinical improvement in his condition. The pharmacokinetics of sildenafil in this patient were then compared with those obtained in 3 healthy subjects who were given a single 50-mg dose of sildenafil. The maximum plasma concentration in both the healthy subjects and the patient was similar, but the AUC (normalised to dose) in the patient was 2- to almost 3-fold higher and the elimination half-life was extended from 1.9 hours to up to 3.1 hours.[7] In a patient taking lopinavir with ritonavir 400/100 mg twice daily, and sildenafil 20 mg three times daily for pulmonary hypertension, the maximum concentration of sildenafil was found to be 655.2 nanograms/mL and 370.5 nanograms/mL, 2 hours after the morning and afternoon doses on one day, respectively. The authors note that values greater than 500 nanograms/mL have been reported to be associated with adverse effects, but the patient reported no such problems.[4]

(e) Nelfinavir

A study in 5 HIV-positive patients found that sildenafil 25 mg did not affect the pharmacokinetics of nelfinavir.[6]

(f) Ritonavir

In a randomised, placebo-controlled study, 28 healthy subjects were given sildenafil 100 mg before and after taking ritonavir for 7 days (300 mg, 400 mg, and 500 mg twice daily on days 1, 2, and 3 to 7, respectively). It was found that the AUC of sildenafil was increased 11-fold and its maximum serum concentrations were increased 3.9-fold by ritonavir, but the steady-state concentrations of ritonavir remained unchanged. Despite the increase in sildenafil concentrations, the incidence and severity of the sildenafil adverse effects were not increased, which the authors attribute to the adverse effect profile of sildenafil being related more to the maximum concentration than the AUC.[8] However, note that this kind of study is not powered to assess differences in incidence of adverse effects, and there was a trend for them to be increased with the combination.

A study in 2 HIV-positive patients found that sildenafil 25 mg did not affect the pharmacokinetics of ritonavir (given with saquinavir).[6]

(g) Saquinavir

1. Saquinavir boosted with ritonavir. A 47-year-old man, with no cardiovascular risk factors apart from smoking, had a myocardial infarction when he took sildenafil 25 mg while he was also taking ritonavir 400 mg twice daily and saquinavir 400 mg twice daily. One hour after the ninth dose (used over the previous 12 weeks), he had an onset of severe chest pain, and died about one day later.[9]

A study in 2 HIV-positive patients found that sildenafil 25 mg did not affect the pharmacokinetics of saquinavir boosted with ritonavir.[6]

2. Unboosted saquinavir. In a randomised, placebo-controlled study, 28 healthy subjects were given sildenafil 100 mg before and after taking saquinavir 1.2 g three times daily for 7 days. It was found that the AUC of sildenafil was increased 3.1-fold and its maximum serum concentrations were increased 2.4-fold, but the incidence and severity of the sildenafil adverse effects, and the steady-state concentrations of saquinavir, remained unchanged.[8]

C. Tadalafil

(a) Fosamprenavir

A patient taking fosamprenavir boosted with ritonavir 1400/200 mg twice daily took two doses of tadalafil 10 mg (given to him by an acquaintance) at the same time as the ritonavir (accidentally at first), and experienced priapism on both occasions, which did not hinder urinary flow and resolved spontaneously. When advised to stop the tadalafil, no further episodes of priapism occurred.[10]

(b) Ritonavir

The UK and US manufacturers of tadalafil note that ritonavir 200 mg twice daily (duration not stated) increased the AUC of a single 20-mg dose of tadalafil 2.2-fold, without affecting its maximum serum concentrations.[11-13] However, they state that a higher ritonavir dose of 500 mg or 600 mg twice daily at steady state increased the AUC of a single 20-mg dose of tadalafil by only 32%, and *decreased* its maximum concentration by 30%.[11,13]

(c) Tipranavir

In a crossover study in 17 healthy subjects, the first dose of tipranavir boosted with ritonavir 500/200 mg twice daily (given for 11 days) increased the AUC of a single 10-mg dose of tadalafil given on day 1, 2.3-fold. However, no change in tadalafil exposure occurred after a further single 10-mg dose was given on day 9, when concentrations of tipranavir boosted with ritonavir were at steady-state.[14]

D. Vardenafil

When a single 10-mg dose of vardenafil was given with **indinavir** 800 mg three times daily, the AUC of vardenafil was increased 16-fold, and its maximum plasma concentration was increased 7-fold.[15,16] Moreover, **ritonavir** 600 mg twice daily produced a 49-fold increase in the AUC of vardenafil, and prolonged its half-life to 26 hours.[16]

Mechanism

HIV-protease inhibitors inhibit the activity of CYP3A4 (to varying extents, see 'Antivirals', p.893), the isoenzyme by which avanafil, sildenafil, and vardenafil are metabolised. This results in an increase in their exposure.

Tadalafil is also metabolised by CYP3A4; however, steady-state ritonavir, or tipranavir boosted with ritonavir appear to unexpectedly have only minimal effects on its exposure, and therefore the involvement of other mechanisms in this interaction cannot be ruled out.

Importance and management

Information about interactions between the phosphodiesterase type-5 inhibitors and HIV-protease inhibitors appears to be limited to the studies and cases cited, but the pharmacokinetic interactions are established and of clinical importance, with varying degrees of severity.

Avanafil

As ritonavir very markedly increased avanafil exposure, their concurrent use is contraindicated by the UK manufacturer,[2] and not recommended by the US manufacturer.[1] This recommendation would also apply to the concurrent use of all **HIV-protease inhibitors boosted with ritonavir** with avanafil.

Sildenafil for erectile dysfunction

When single doses of sildenafil are used for erectile dysfunction, the UK manufacturer states that the concurrent use of **ritonavir** is not advised.[17] In this situation, if the decision is taken to use sildenafil in a patient taking ritonavir, the dose of sildenafil should not exceed a single 25-mg dose in a 48-hour period,[8,17,18] but note that the fatality described above[9] occurred despite the use of this dose. This dose advice would also apply to **HIV-protease inhibitors boosted with ritonavir.**

For **saquinavir**, the UK and US manufacturers of sildenafil for erectile dysfunction recommend that a low starting dose of sildenafil 25 mg should be considered.[8,17,18] However, note that the UK manufacturer of saquinavir contraindicates the concurrent use of saquinavir boosted with ritonavir and sildenafil because of a possible increased risk of QT prolongation.[19] Consider also 'Drugs that prolong the QT interval + Other drugs that prolong the QT interval', p.272.

The authors of the **indinavir** study suggest that a starting dose of 12.5 mg might be more appropriate for erectile dysfunction in those taking indinavir, and that the maximum dose frequency should be reduced to once or twice weekly.[5]

Direct evidence for **other HIV-protease inhibitors** is lacking but they would be expected to increase sildenafil exposure to a greater or lesser extent (see *Mechanism*, above) and, in the absence of any specific information, it would seem consistent, in those with erectile dysfunction, to follow the broad principle of starting with a low sildenafil dose at reduced frequency.

Sildenafil for pulmonary hypertension

Because of the very marked increase in exposure, the concurrent use of **ritonavir** and sildenafil for pulmonary hypertension is not recommended by the US manufacturer,[20] and is contraindicated by the UK manufacturer.[21] This would include ritonavir used with other HIV-protease inhibitors as a pharmacokinetic enhancer, as the FDA in the US contraindicates all **HIV-protease inhibitors** with sildenafil for this indication.[22] Nevertheless, a single case describes the successful use of sildenafil for pulmonary hypertension with HIV-protease inhibitors boosted with ritonavir.[7]

Note that the advice regarding the use of **saquinavir** is mixed. Concurrent use is contraindicated by the FDA,[22] whereas, the UK manufacturer of sildenafil for pulmonary hypertension states that, in patients taking saquinavir, a downward reduction of the oral sildenafil dose to 20 mg twice daily[21] or a downward reduction of the intravenous sildenafil dose to 10 mg twice daily, should be considered.[23] However, note that the UK manufacturer of saquinavir contraindicates the concurrent use of saquinavir boosted with ritonavir and sildenafil because of a possible increased risk of QT prolongation.[19] Consider also 'Drugs that prolong the QT interval + Other drugs that prolong the QT interval', p.272.

Tadalafil

The US manufacturer of tadalafil for erectile dysfunction advises that the 'as needed' dose should not exceed 10 mg every 72 hours and the daily dose should not exceed 2.5 mg daily in patients taking **ritonavir**,[11] whereas the UK manufacturer simply advises caution on concurrent use.[12] For pulmonary hypertension, the UK manufacturer of tadalafil does not recommend the concurrent use of ritonavir.[24] However, the US manufacturer advises that tadalafil can be started at a lower dose of 20 mg daily in those taking ritonavir for at least one week, and increased to the usual dose of 40 mg daily if tolerated. In those already taking tadalafil and starting ritonavir, they recommended stopping tadalafil at least 24 hours before starting ritonavir, and then restarting tadalafil at least one week later, at a dose of 20 mg daily, increasing to 40 mg daily if tolerated.[13] For benign prostatic hyperplasia, the US manufacturer recommends that the daily dose of tadalafil should not exceed 2.5 mg daily in patients taking **ritonavir**.[11]

Similar dose adjustments are recommended for **tipranavir boosted with ritonavir**[25,26] and might be expected to apply to all **HIV-protease inhibitors boosted with ritonavir**. In the absence of specific information, it is probably prudent to exercise caution in patients taking any HIV-protease inhibitor and tadalafil. However, note that the UK manufacturer of **saquinavir** contraindicates the concurrent use of saquinavir boosted with ritonavir and tadalafil because of a possible increased risk of QT prolongation.[19]

Vardenafil

Due to the very marked increase in exposure, the UK manufacturer of vardenafil[15] contraindicates its use with **ritonavir**, whereas the US manufacturer states that the dose of vardenafil should not exceed 2.5 mg in 72 hours.[16] Until more is known, it would be prudent to apply this advice to all **HIV-protease inhibitors boosted with ritonavir** (but see also, *saquinavir*, below).

The US manufacturers of **nelfinavir** advise that the dose of vardenafil should not exceed 2.5 mg in 24 hours.[27]

The advice regarding the use of some **unboosted HIV-protease inhibitors** varies. The UK manufacturer of vardenafil[15] contraindicates its use with **indinavir**, whereas the US manufacturer states that the dose of vardenafil should not exceed 2.5 mg in 24 hours.[16]

The US manufacturer of **fosamprenavir**[28] states that the dose of vardenafil should not exceed 2.5 mg in 24 hours. Similarly, the US manufacturer of vardenafil recommends that the dose of vardenafil should not exceed 2.5 mg in 24 hours when used with **atazanavir** or **saquinavir**. However, the UK manufacturer of saquinavir contraindicates the concurrent use of **saquinavir boosted with ritonavir** with vardenafil because of a possible increased risk of QT prolongation.[19] Consider also 'Drugs that prolong the QT interval + Other drugs that prolong the QT interval', p.272.

1. Stendra (Avanafil). Vivus, Inc. US Prescribing information, January 2015.
2. Spedra (Avanafil). A. Menarini Farmaceutica Internazionale SRL. UK Summary of product characteristics, January 2015.
3. Sekar V, Lefebvre E, De Marez T, De Pauw M, De Paepe E, Vangeneugden T, Hoetelmans RMW. Effect of repeated doses of darunavir plus low-dose ritonavir on the pharmacokinetics of sildenafil in healthy male subjects. Phase I randomized, open-label, two-way crossover study. *Clin Drug Invest* (2008) 28, 479–85.
4. Chinello P, Cicalini S, Pichini S, Pacifici R, Tempestilli M, Petrosillo N. Sildenafil plasma concentrations in two HIV patients with pulmonary hypertension treated with ritonavir-boosted protease inhibitors. *Curr HIV Res* (2012) 10, 162–4.
5. Merry C, Barry MG, Ryan M, Tjia JF, Hennessy M, Eagling V, Mulcahy F, Back DJ. Interaction of sildenafil and indinavir when co-administered to HIV positive patients. AIDS (Hagerstown) 1999, 13, F101–F107.
6. Bratt G, Ståhle L. Sildenafil does not alter nelfinavir pharmacokinetics. *Ther Drug Monit* (2003) 25, 240–2.
7. Aschmann YZ, Kummer O, Linka A, Wenk M, Azzola A, Bodmer M, Krähenbühl S, Haschke M. Pharmacokinetics and pharmacodynamics of sildenafil in a patient treated with human immunodeficiency virus protease inhibitors. *Ther Drug Monit* (2008) 30, 130–4.
8. Muirhead GJ, Wulff MB, Fielding A, Kleinermans D, Buss N. Pharmacokinetic interactions between sildenafil and saquinavir/ritonavir. *Br J Clin Pharmacol* (2000) 50, 99–107.
9. Hall MCS, Ahmad S. Interaction between sildenafil and HIV-1 combination therapy. *Lancet* (1999) 353, 2071–2.
10. Loulergue P, Gaillard R, Mir O. Interaction involving tadalafil and CYP3A4 inhibition by ritonavir. *Scand J Infect Dis* (2011) 43, 239–40.
11. Cialis (Tadalafil). Eli Lilly and Company. US Prescribing information, April 2014.
12. Cialis (Tadalafil). Eli Lilly and Company Ltd. UK Summary of product characteristics, March 2013.
13. Adcirca (Tadalafil). Eli Lilly and Company. US Prescribing information, April 2015.
14. Garraffo R, Lavrut T, Ferrando S, Durant J, Rouyrre N, MacGregor TR, Sabo JP, Dellamonica P. Effect of tipranavir/ritonavir combination on the pharmacokinetics of tadalafil in healthy volunteers. *J Clin Pharmacol* (2011) 51, 1071–8.
15. Levitra (Vardenafil hydrochloride). Bayer plc. UK Summary of product characteristics, April 2014.
16. Levitra (Vardenafil hydrochloride). Bayer HealthCare Pharmaceuticals Inc. US prescribing information, April 2014.
17. Viagra (Sildenafil citrate). Pfizer Ltd. UK Summary of product characteristics, June 2015.
18. Viagra (Sildenafil citrate). Pfizer Inc. US Prescribing information, March 2015.
19. Invirase (Saquinavir mesilate). Roche Products Ltd. UK Summary of product characteristics, May 2014.
20. Revatio (Sildenafil citrate). Pfizer Inc. US Prescribing information, April 2015.
21. Revatio Tablets (Sildenafil citrate). Pfizer Ltd. UK Summary of product characteristics, April 2015.
22. FDA. New label information affecting all approved protease inhibitors for the treatment of HIV. Available at: https://aidsinfo.nih.gov/news/863/new-label-information-affecting-all-approved-protease-inhibitors-for-treatment-of-hiv (accessed 15/10/15).
23. Revatio Injection (Sildenafil citrate). Pfizer Ltd. UK Summary of product characteristics, October 2014.
24. Adcirca (Tadalafil). Eli Lilly and Company Ltd. UK Summary of product characteristics, May 2013.
25. Aptivus Soft Capsules (Tipranavir). Boehringer Ingelheim Ltd. UK Summary of product characteristics, June 2015.
26. Aptivus (Tipranavir). Boehringer Ingelheim Pharmaceuticals, Inc. US Prescribing information, March 2015.
27. Viracept (Nelfinavir mesylate). Agouron Pharmaceuticals, Inc. US Prescribing information, May 2013.
28. Lexiva (Fosamprenavir calcium). ViiV Healthcare. US Prescribing information, April 2013.

Phosphodiesterase type-5 inhibitors + Macrolides

Erythromycin moderately increases avanafil, sildenafil, and vardenafil exposure, and is predicted to similarly affect tadalafil exposure. Single-dose clarithromycin moderately increases sildenafil exposure and is predicted to increase avanafil, tadalafil, and vardenafil exposure. Azithromycin does not alter sildenafil exposure.

Clinical evidence

(a) Avanafil

The UK and US manufacturers briefly note that, in a study in 15 healthy males, **erythromycin** 500 mg twice daily increased the AUC and maximum concentration of a single 200-mg dose of avanafil 3.6-fold and 2-fold, respectively.[1,2]

(b) Sildenafil

In a study in 24 healthy subjects, **erythromycin** 500 mg twice daily for 5 days was found to increase the AUC of a single 100-mg dose of sildenafil almost 3-fold.[3] In the same study, **azithromycin** 500 mg daily for 3 days had no effect on the pharmacokinetics of sildenafil.[3] In a single-dose study in 12 healthy subjects, **clarithromycin** 500 mg increased the AUC of sildenafil 50 mg 2.3-fold, and increased its maximum concentration 2.4-fold when the sildenafil was taken 2 hours after the **clarithromycin**. It is possible that if clarithromycin had been given to steady-state, a greater effect would have been seen.[4]

(c) Vardenafil

In a study in healthy subjects, **erythromycin** 500 mg three times daily increased the AUC of a single 5-mg dose of vardenafil 4-fold, and increased its maximum plasma concentration 3-fold.[5,6]

Mechanism

Avanafil, sildenafil, and vardenafil are all metabolised by CYP3A4. The macrolides are inhibitors of this isoenzyme (to varying extents) and therefore inhibit avanafil, sildenafil, and vardenafil metabolism. This leads to increased exposure of the phosphodiesterase type-5 inhibitors. Azithromycin does not usually act as a CYP3A4 inhibitor and therefore does not interact with sildenafil.

Importance and management

A pharmacokinetic interaction between the macrolides and phosphodiesterase type-5 inhibitors would seem to be established on the basis that, although most of the studies concern the use of sildenafil, the other phosphodiesterase type-5 inhibitors are metabolised similarly and therefore their exposures would also be expected to be increased. These interactions are predicted to result in both increased efficacy and an increased incidence of phosphodiesterase type-5 inhibitor adverse effects.

Clarithromycin and telithromycin are potent CYP3A4 inhibitors and, because of the effects of the other potent CYP3A4 inhibitors, such as ketoconazole and ritonavir (see 'Phosphodiesterase type-5 inhibitors + Azoles', p.1540 and 'Phosphodiesterase type-5 inhibitors + HIV-protease inhibitors', p.1543, respectively), their concurrent use with **avanafil** is contraindicated.[1,2] Erythromycin moderately increased avanafil exposure, and as a result the UK manufacturer advises that on concurrent use, the dose of avanafil should not exceed 100 mg with an interval of at least 48 hours between doses,[2] while the US manufacturer advises that the dose of avanafil should not exceed 50 mg with an interval of at least 24 hours between doses.[1] The manufacturers extend their advice to all moderate CYP3A4 inhibitors, see 'Table 1.9', p.11 for a list. Note that the UK manufacturer additionally names **amprenavir** and **fosamprenavir**,[2] but as these are only given with ritonavir and as such they are generally considered to be potent CYP3A4 inhibitors (see also 'Phosphodiesterase type-5 inhibitors + HIV-protease inhibitors', p.1543).

The UK and US manufacturers recommend that a low starting dose of **sildenafil** 25 mg should be considered in patients with erectile dysfunction taking CYP3A4 inhibitors such as erythromycin.[7,8] For pulmonary hypertension, the UK manufacturer states that a reduction of the sildenafil dose to 20 mg twice daily orally or 10 mg twice daily intravenously should be considered with erythromycin, and 20 mg daily orally or 10 mg daily intravenously with clarithromycin or telithromycin.[9,10] Azithromycin does not appear to affect the pharmacokinetics of sildenafil and therefore might provide a non-interacting alternative in some patients.

On the basis of the effects of other CYP3A4 inhibitors, such as ketoconazole (see 'Phosphodiesterase type-5 inhibitors + Azoles', p.1540), the UK and US manufacturers of **tadalafil** advise caution with concurrent use of erythromycin and clarithromycin as adverse effects might be increased in some patients.[11,12]

The UK manufacturer of **vardenafil** states that dose adjustments might be necessary in patients taking erythromycin or clarithromycin, and recommends that the dose of vardenafil should not exceed 5 mg.[5] However, note, they name clarithromycin as a moderate CYP3A4 inhibitor (like erythromycin), but it is generally considered to be a potent inhibitor of this isoenzyme, and therefore concurrent use with vardenafil might result in even greater increases in exposure. Concurrent use with potent CYP3A4 inhibitors is not recommended, and is contraindicated in patients over 75 years.[5] The US manufacturer similarly recommends that the dose of vardenafil should not exceed 5 mg in 24 hours for erythromycin, but further restricts the dose to 2.5 mg in 24 hours in patients taking clarithromycin.[6]

1. Stendra (Avanafil). Vivus, Inc. US Prescribing information, January 2015.
2. Spedra (Avanafil). A. Menarini Farmaceutica Internazionale SRL. UK Summary of product characteristics, January 2015.
3. Muirhead GJ, Faulkner S, Harness JA, Taubel J. The effects of steady-state erythromycin and azithromycin on the pharmacokinetics of sildenafil citrate in healthy volunteers. *Br J Clin Pharmacol* (2002) 53, 37S–43S.
4. Hedaya MA, El-Afify DR, El-Maghraby GM. The effect of ciprofloxacin and clarithromycin on sildenafil oral bioavailability in human volunteers. *Biopharm Drug Dispos* (2006) 27, 103–10.
5. Levitra (Vardenafil hydrochloride). Bayer plc. UK Summary of product characteristics, April 2014.
6. Levitra (Vardenafil hydrochloride). Bayer HealthCare Pharmaceuticals Inc. US Prescribing information, April 2014.
7. Viagra (Sildenafil citrate). Pfizer Ltd. UK Summary of product characteristics, June 2015.
8. Viagra (Sildenafil citrate). Pfizer Inc. US Prescribing information, March 2015.
9. Revatio Tablets (Sildenafil citrate). Pfizer Ltd. UK Summary of product characteristics, April 2015.
10. Revatio Injection (Sildenafil citrate). Pfizer Ltd. UK Summary of product characteristics, October 2014.
11. Cialis (Tadalafil). Eli Lilly and Company Ltd. UK Summary of product characteristics, March 2013.
12. Cialis (Tadalafil). Eli Lilly and Company. US Prescribing information, April 2014.

Phosphodiesterase type-5 inhibitors + Nitrates

Phosphodiesterase type-5 inhibitors potentiate the hypotensive effects of nitrates, which might result in potentially serious hypotension or even precipitate myocardial infarction. There appears to be no direct evidence regarding the use of nicorandil and the phosphodiesterase type-5 inhibitors, but it is thought that they are likely to interact in the same way.

Clinical evidence

(a) Avanafil

The US manufacturer briefly describes a randomised crossover study in healthy men, which found that 28% of subjects who received a single 400-microgram dose of sublingual **glyceryl trinitrate** after a single 200-mg dose of avanafil had a decrease in standing systolic blood pressure of 30 mmHg or more, compared with 15% of subjects who received placebo (relevant timings of respective doses not stated).[1]

(b) Sildenafil

1. Glyceryl trinitrate (Nitroglycerin). In a placebo-controlled study in 15 men with angina, taking sublingual glyceryl trinitrate 500 micrograms one hour *before* a single 50-mg dose of sildenafil caused a mean blood pressure fall of about 36/21 mmHg, compared with a fall of 26/11 mmHg when glyceryl trinitrate was given before placebo. Individual blood pressure falls as great as 84 mmHg (systolic) and 34 mmHg (diastolic) were seen.[2]

Further studies have evaluated the effect of giving glyceryl trinitrate *after* sildenafil. In one study, 33 healthy subjects and 20 patients with angina were given glyceryl trinitrate 400 micrograms sublingually at various time points after a single 100-mg dose of sildenafil to evaluate the duration of the haemodynamic interaction. In the group of patients, the hypotensive reaction to glyceryl trinitrate was still greater after sildenafil than after placebo 8 hours after sildenafil was taken (the last time point tested in this group), whereas in the healthy subjects, the increased hypotensive reaction was most apparent at one hour and had almost disappeared by 4 hours.[3] In a study of multiple-dose sildenafil, 12 healthy subjects took sildenafil 25 mg three times daily or placebo for 13 doses, with a step-wise infusion of glyceryl trinitrate (2.5 micrograms/minute increased to 40 micrograms/minute) started one hour after the tenth dose of sildenafil. They were also given a single 500-microgram dose of sublingual glyceryl trinitrate one hour after the last dose of sildenafil. Sildenafil halved the dose of intravenous glyceryl trinitrate required to cause a greater than 25 mmHg fall in systolic blood pressure (32.5 micrograms versus 71.7 micrograms). With the sublingual glyceryl trinitrate, the fall in systolic blood pressure was more than four times greater after taking sildenafil than after placebo, and more of the subjects removed the glyceryl trinitrate tablet because of symptomatic hypotension or a fall in systolic blood pressure of greater than 25 mmHg (11 versus 4).[4]

Conversely, a placebo-controlled, randomised study in 32 men with stable coronary artery disease suggested that 45 minutes after a single 100-mg dose of sildenafil had been given, it was possible to cautiously give intravenous glyceryl trinitrate, starting at a low dose and slowly increasing to a maximum of 160 micrograms/minute. Sildenafil caused an additional reduction in blood pressure of about 4 to 6 mmHg, when compared with placebo. In general, when compared with placebo, the dose of nitrate tolerated was lower in the presence of sildenafil, and despite this, hypotension was more common.[5] Similarly, in a limited and preliminary study it was reported that no blood pressure alteration was seen when a small dose of glyceryl trinitrate (amount not specified) was given as a transdermal patch while subjects were taking 50 mg of sildenafil. In addition, the beneficial effects of the glyceryl trinitrate on the radial artery pressure waveform were approximately doubled, and persisted for up to 8 hours.[6]

A postmarketing report from the FDA for the period late March to July 1998 briefly lists 69 fatalities in patients who had taken sildenafil. These were mostly in middle-aged and elderly men (average age 64 years), 12 of whom had also taken glyceryl trinitrate or a nitrate medication, but it is not clear what part (if any) the nitrates played in the deaths.[7]

2. Isosorbide dinitrate. In a double-blind, placebo-controlled study in 16 men with angina, the fall in blood pressure seen when taking isosorbide dinitrate 20 mg twice daily was approximately doubled by a single 50-mg dose of sildenafil (mean blood pressure fall of 44/26 mmHg with sildenafil, compared with 22/13 mmHg with placebo). The decrease was greatest from about 1 to 3 hours after dosing, and was still apparent at 6 hours.[2]

(c) Tadalafil

In a single-dose, placebo-controlled study, 51 patients with chronic stable angina were given tadalafil 5 mg, 10 mg or a placebo, followed 2 hours later by 400 micrograms of sublingual **glyceryl trinitrate**. Although tadalafil caused little additional decrease in blood pressure to that seen with **glyceryl trinitrate**, a potentially clinically important blood pressure reduction (standing systolic blood pressure less than 85 mmHg) was seen in 13 and 11 of the patients when given tadalafil 5 and 10 mg, respectively, compared with one patient in the placebo group.[8,9] In a similar study in 45 patients taking long-term oral **isosorbide mononitrate**, single-dose tadalafil 5 or 10 mg had minimal effects on the decrease in blood pressure caused by the nitrate, but again, more patients had a standing systolic blood pressure of less than 85 mmHg when receiving tadalafil 10 mg than placebo (6 versus 0).[8,9] Another similar single-dose study in 48 healthy subjects compared the effects of tadalafil 10 mg, sildenafil 50 mg, and placebo, in combination with 400 micrograms of sublingual **glyceryl trinitrate**. Again, it was found that the presence of the tadalafil had minimal effects on the mean maximum decreases in blood pressure, but it was noted that 23 patients given tadalafil and 23 given sildenafil had a standing systolic blood pressure of 85 mmHg or less following the use of the nitrate, compared with 12 in the placebo group.[9,10] In a further study, a haemodynamic interaction between tadalafil 20 mg daily for 7 days and a single 400-microgram dose of sublingual **glyceryl trinitrate** was seen when the **glyceryl trinitrate** was given 4, 8 and 24 hours after the last dose of tadalafil, and was not seen at 48, 72 and 96 hours. Note that no time points between 24 and 48 hours were examined.[11]

An analysis of the rates of serious cardiovascular adverse events (mortality, myocardial infarction, thrombotic strokes) in clinical studies involving tadalafil indicated that adverse events were no more frequent than in the general population of men with erectile dysfunction.[9]

(d) Vardenafil

A single 400-microgram dose of sublingual **glyceryl trinitrate** (**nitroglycerin**) given to 18 healthy subjects 1 to 24 hours after a single 10-mg dose of vardenafil was found to be no different to placebo in causing changes in seated heart rate and blood pressure.[12,13] However, a single 20-mg dose of vardenafil did potentiate the blood pressure-lowering effects (about an 8 mmHg additional drop in systolic blood pressure compared with placebo) and increases in heart rate seen with **sublingual nitrates** (400 micrograms) taken 1 and 4 hours after the vardenafil. These effects were not seen when the nitrate was taken 24 hours after the vardenafil dose.[12,14]

Mechanism

Sexual stimulation causes the endothelium of the penis to release nitric oxide (NO), which in turn activates guanylate cyclase to increase the production of cyclic guanosine monophosphate (cGMP). This relaxes the blood vessel musculature of the corpus cavernosum thus allowing it to fill with blood and cause an erection. The erection ends when the guanosine monophosphate is removed by an enzyme (type 5 cGMP phosphodiesterase, or PDE5). Avanafil, sildenafil, tadalafil, and vardenafil inhibit this enzyme thereby increasing and prolonging the effects of the cyclic guanosine monophosphate. Because this vasodilation is usually fairly localised (these drugs are highly selective for PDE5) it normally only causes mild to moderate falls in blood pressure (on average about 10 mmHg) with mild headache or flushing. Nitrates increase the production of cyclic guanosine monophosphate, and when phosphodiesterase type-5 inhibitors (PDE5 inhibitors) are taken concurrently, cyclic guanosine monophosphate accumulates and high levels of nitric oxide enter the circulation. This markedly increases systemic vasodilation and hence causes the hypotensive effect.

Importance and management

The interaction between phosphodiesterase type-5 inhibitors and nitrates is established, clinically important, potentially serious, and even possibly fatal. The use of phosphodiesterase type-5 inhibitors with organic nitrates of any form is generally considered contraindicated because of the risk of precipitating serious hypotension, or even myocardial infarction.[15] If nitrate administration is medically essential, for sildenafil, a 24-hour separation is considered adequate,[16] whereas nitrates can be given 12 hours after the last dose of avanafil,[1] but should not be given for at least 48 hours after the last dose of tadalafil because this has a long elimination half-life.[17-19] The US manufacturer of vardenafil states that a suitable time interval between dosing of vardenafil and nitrates has not been determined.[14] The ACC/AHA Expert consensus document provides a useful list of many of the organic nitrates available, which include glyceryl trinitrate (nitroglycerin), isosorbide mononitrate, isosorbide dinitrate, sodium nitroprusside (see 'Sodium nitroprusside + Miscellaneous', p.1075), and illicit substances such as **amyl nitrite**.[16] However, the use of some nitrate donors might be beneficial in the setting of pulmonary hypertension, see 'Phosphodiesterase type-5 inhibitors; Sildenafil + Nitric oxide', p.1547.

If patients develop angina during sexual activity after taking a phosphodiesterase type-5 inhibitor they should discontinue sexual activity, relax for 5 to 10 minutes, and if the pain persists seek emergency care, informing medical personnel that they have taken a phosphodiesterase type-5 inhibitor. In the event of myocardial infarction, usual therapies can be given, with the exception of organic nitrates.[20] Note that, in the study where glyceryl trinitrate infusions were successfully given to patients who had taken sildenafil, the patients had stable heart disease, and the suggestion of this being a usable combination might not be applicable to patients experiencing episodes of acute cardiac disease.

There is no known antidote to the phosphodiesterase type-5 interaction with nitrates. Important hypotension should be managed by placing the patient in the Trendelenburg position (that is, laid flat on their back, with their feet higher than their head) and giving intravenous fluids and alpha agonists such as phenylephrine. It has also been suggested that, if hypotension is refractory, intra-aortic balloon counter-pulsation should be used.[20]

An interaction between **nicorandil** and the phosphodiesterase type-5 inhibitors does not appear to have been studied, but because part of its vasodilatory actions are mediated by the release of nitric oxide (like conventional nitrates), the UK manufacturer of nicorandil contraindicates its use with all phosphodiesterase type-5 inhibitors.[21]

1. Stendra (Avanafil). Vivus, Inc. US Prescribing information, January 2015.
2. Webb DJ, Muirhead G, Wulff M, Sutton A, Levi R, Dinsmore WW. Sildenafil citrate potentiates the hypotensive effects of nitric oxide donor drugs in male patients with stable angina. *J Am Coll Cardiol* (2000) 36, 25–31.
3. Oliver JJ, Kerr DM, Webb DJ. Time-dependent interactions of the hypotensive effects of sildenafil citrate and sublingual glyceryl trinitrate. *Br J Clin Pharmacol* (2009) 67, 403–12.
4. Webb DJ, Freestone S, Allen MJ, Muirhead GJ. Sildenafil citrate and blood-pressure-lowering drugs: results of drug interaction studies with an organic nitrate and a calcium antagonist. *Am J Cardiol* (1999) 83, 21C–28C.
5. Parker JD, Bart BA, Webb DJ, Koren MJ, Siegel RL, Wang H, Malhotra B, Jen F, Glue P. Safety of intravenous nitroglycerin after administration of sildenafil citrate to men with coronary artery disease: a double-blind, placebo-controlled, randomized, crossover trial. *Crit Care Med* (2007) 35, 1863–8.
6. O'Rourke M, Jiang X-J. Sildenafil/nitrate interaction. *Circulation* (2000) 101, e90.
7. FDA (US Food and Drug Administration) postmarketing information sildenafil citrate (Viagra): Postmarketing safety of sildenafil citrate (Viagra). Reports of death in Viagra users received from marketing (late March) through July 1998. August 27th 1998.
8. Kloner RA, Emmick J, Bedding A, Humen D. Pharmacodynamic interactions between tadalafil and nitrates. *Int J Impot Res* (2002) 14 (Suppl 3) S29.
9. Kloner RA, Mitchell M, Emmick J. Cardiovascular effects of tadalafil. *Am J Cardiol* (2003) 92 (Suppl) 37M–46M.
10. Kloner RA, Mitchell MI, Bedding A, Emmick J. Pharmacodynamic interactions between tadalafil and nitrates compared with sildenafil. *J Urol (Baltimore)* (2002) 167 (Suppl) 176–7.
11. Kloner RA, Hutter AM, Emmick JT, Mitchell MI, Denne J, Jackson G. Time course of the interaction between tadalafil and nitrates. *J Am Coll Cardiol* (2003) 42, 1855–60.
12. Levitra (Vardenafil hydrochloride). Bayer plc. UK Summary of product characteristics, April 2014.
13. Mazzu AL, Nicholls AJ, Zinny M. Vardenafil, a new selective PDE-5 inhibitor, interacts minimally with nitroglycerin in healthy middle-aged male subjects. *Int J Impot Res* (2001) 13 (Suppl 5) S64.
14. Levitra (Vardenafil hydrochloride). Bayer HealthCare Pharmaceuticals Inc. US Prescribing information, April 2014.
15. Viagra (Sildenafil). Pfizer Inc. Dear Doctor letter, May 1998.
16. ACC/AHA Expert consensus document. Use of sildenafil (Viagra) in patients with cardiovascular disease. *J Am Coll Cardiol* (1999) 33, 273–82.
17. Cialis (Tadalafil). Eli Lilly and Company Ltd. UK Summary of product characteristics, March 2013.
18. Cialis (Tadalafil). Eli Lilly and Company. US Prescribing information, April 2014.
19. Adcirca (Tadalafil). Eli Lilly and Company. US Prescribing information, April 2015.
20. Kostis JB, Jackson G, Rosen R, Barrett-Connor E, Billups K, Burnett AL, Carson C, Cheitlin M, Debusk R, Fonseca V, Ganz P, Goldstein I, Guay A, Hatzichristou D, Hollander JE, Hutter A, Katz S, Kloner RA, Mittleman M, Montorsi F, Montorsi P, Nehra A, Sadovsky R, Shabsigh R. Sexual dysfunction and cardiac risk (the Second Princeton Consensus Conference). Am J Cardiol. (2005) 96, 313–21.
21. Ikorel (Nicorandil). Zentiva. UK Summary of product characteristics, November 2014.

Phosphodiesterase type-5 inhibitors + Rifampicin (Rifampin) and other CYP3A4 inducers

Rifampicin markedly decreases tadalafil exposure, and is predicted to interact similarly with avanafil, sildenafil, and vardenafil. Other CYP3A4 inducers are likely to interact similarly.

Clinical evidence

The US manufacturer briefly reports that in a study, rifampicin 600 mg daily decreased the AUC and maximum plasma concentration of a single 10-mg dose of **tadalafil** by 88% and 46%, respectively.[1]

Mechanism

Rifampicin (rifampin) induces the activity of CYP3A4, the principal enzyme concerned with the metabolism of tadalafil and concurrent use results in decreased exposure.

Importance and management

The pharmacokinetic interaction between rifampicin and tadalafil is established, and will almost certainly occur with **avanafil**, **sildenafil**, and **vardenafil**, which are metabolised in a similar way. It seems unlikely that standard doses of these phosphodiesterase type-5 inhibitors would be as effective as usual in patients taking rifampicin. However, if a patient taking rifampicin is given a phosphodiesterase type-5 inhibitor for **erectile dysfunction**, the interaction seems unlikely to be particularly problematic, as the dose of the phosphodiesterase type-5 inhibitor is titrated according to efficacy and tolerability. Nevertheless, it would be prudent to be aware of this interaction as it seems possible that even the maximum recommended doses of these phosphodiesterase type-5 inhibitors will be ineffective. Furthermore, it would be prudent to monitor efficacy in a patient taking a phosphodiesterase type-5 inhibitor who is subsequently started on rifampicin, as it seems likely that previously effective doses will become ineffective. However, note that the UK and US manufacturers of **avanafil** specifically do not recommend concurrent use.[2,3]

The interaction with rifampicin seems likely to be of importance in patients taking sildenafil or tadalafil for **pulmonary hypertension**, or taking tadalafil for **BPH**, where regular doses are given. For sildenafil, the UK manufacturer states that sildenafil efficacy should be closely monitored, with the sildenafil dose adjusted as necessary.[4] For tadalafil for pulmonary hypertension, the UK and US manufacturers do not recommend the concurrent use of rifampicin,[5,6] and for BPH they predict that efficacy might be reduced but give no specific advice.[1,7] It would therefore seem prudent that in these patients, the efficacy is monitored and consideration given to adjusting the tadalafil dose accordingly.

Some, but not all, of the manufacturers of phosphodiesterase type-5 inhibitors predict that other CYP3A4 inducers (see 'Table 1.9', p.11 for a list) will interact similarly; the UK and US manufacturers of **avanafil** specifically do not recommend concurrent use.[2,3] Until more is known, if other CYP3A4 enzyme inducers are given to a patient taking sildenafil, tadalafil, or vardenafil, it would seem prudent to follow the advice given here for rifampicin.

1. Cialis (Tadalafil). Eli Lilly and Company. US Prescribing information, April 2014.
2. Spedra (Avanafil). A. Menarini Farmaceutica Internazionale SRL. UK Summary of product characteristics, January 2015.
3. Stendra (Avanafil). Vivus, Inc. US Prescribing information, January 2015.
4. Revatio Tablets (Sildenafil citrate). Pfizer Ltd. UK Summary of product characteristics, April 2015.
5. Adcirca (Tadalafil). Eli Lilly and Company. US Prescribing information, April 2015.
6. Adcirca (Tadalafil). Eli Lilly and Company Ltd. UK Summary of product characteristics, May 2013.
7. Cialis (Tadalafil). Eli Lilly and Company Ltd. UK Summary of product characteristics, March 2013.

Phosphodiesterase type-5 inhibitors; Avanafil + Miscellaneous

Avanafil does not appear to alter the pharmacokinetics of desipramine or omeprazole.

Clinical evidence, mechanism, importance and management

(a) Desipramine

The US manufacturer briefly notes that, in a study in 20 healthy male subjects, a single 200-mg dose of avanafil increased the AUC and maximum plasma concentration of a single 50-mg dose of desipramine (taken 2 hours before) by 5.7% and 5.2%, respectively.[1] Such minor changes in the pharmacokinetics of desipramine are not likely to be clinically important.

Note that desipramine can be used as a probe substrate to assess the activity of drugs on CYP2D6. This study therefore suggests that avanafil does not inhibit this isoenzyme to a clinically relevant extent.

(b) Omeprazole

The US manufacturer briefly notes that, in a study in 19 healthy male subjects, a single 200-mg dose of avanafil increased the AUC and maximum plasma concentration of omeprazole 40 mg daily for 8 days by 5.9% and 8.6%, respectively.[1] Such minor changes in the pharmacokinetics of omeprazole are not likely to be clinically important.

Note that omeprazole can be used as a probe substrate to assess the activity of drugs on CYP2C19. This study therefore suggests that avanafil does not inhibit this isoenzyme to a clinically relevant extent.

1. Stendra (Avanafil). Vivus, Inc. US Prescribing information, January 2015.

Phosphodiesterase type-5 inhibitors; Sildenafil + Antidepressants

Retrospective analysis of clinical study data suggested that SSRIs and tricyclic antidepressants did not alter sildenafil pharmacokinetics. However, in one pharmacokinetic study, fluvoxamine was found to modestly increase the levels and vascular effects of sildenafil.

Clinical evidence

The manufacturer notes that population pharmacokinetic analysis of clinical study data indicate that inhibitors of CYP2D6, such as **SSRIs** and **tricyclic antidepressants**, do not have any effect on the pharmacokinetics of sildenafil.[1,2] However, in a placebo-controlled study in healthy subjects, pre-treatment with **fluvoxamine** 50 mg daily for

3 days then 100 mg daily for 6 days increased the AUC of sildenafil 50 mg by 40%. This resulted in an increase in the vascular effects of sildenafil.[3]

Mechanism

Sildenafil is principally metabolised by CYP3A4, and to a lesser extent by CYP2C9. Fluvoxamine probably raises sildenafil levels by inhibition of both of these isoenzymes. Grouping all SSRIs and tricyclics together in a retrospective analysis would not be a sensitive enough technique to have picked up this modest effect of fluvoxamine.

Importance and management

The increases in sildenafil levels with fluvoxamine are modest, and the authors concluded that they do not suggest a large clinically relevant interaction. Nevertheless, they suggest it may be prudent to consider a 25-mg starting dose of sildenafil in patients taking fluvoxamine.[3] This seems sensible. Although retrospective analyses of clinical study data are useful to identify potentially important drug interactions, they are not sensitive enough to rule out interactions, and should not replace prospective pharmacokinetic studies.

1. Viagra (Sildenafil citrate). Pfizer Ltd. UK Summary of product characteristics, June 2015.
2. Viagra (Sildenafil citrate). Pfizer Inc. US Prescribing information, March 2015.
3. Hesse C, Siedler H, Burhenne J, Riedel K-D, Haefeli WE. Fluvoxamine affects sildenafil kinetics and dynamics. *J Clin Psychopharmacol* (2005) 25, 589–92.

Phosphodiesterase type-5 inhibitors; Sildenafil + Cannabis

Myocardial infarction has been reported in a man who had smoked cannabis and taken sildenafil.

Clinical evidence

A 41-year old man with no history of cardiac disease experienced a myocardial infarction after smoking cannabis and recreationally taking a tablet of sildenafil (strength not specified). Later tests showed that he had no evidence of inducible ischaemia.[1]

Mechanism

Myocardial infarction is a rare adverse effect of sildenafil alone. It was suggested that the metabolism of sildenafil by CYP3A4 might be inhibited by constituents of cannabis such as cannabidiol, thereby increasing the risk of adverse events. However, in clinical studies, oral cannabis did not alter levels of other CYP3A4 substrates.

Importance and management

An interaction between sildenafil and cannabis is not established. The vasodilatory effects of sildenafil necessitate caution in its use in patients with cardiovascular disease: myocardial infarction has rarely been associated with its use. The contribution of an interaction between sildenafil and cannabis to this case is unclear.

1. McLeod AL, McKenna CJ, Northridge DB. Myocardial infarction following the combined recreational use of Viagra® and cannabis. *Clin Cardiol* (2002) 25, 133–4.

Phosphodiesterase type-5 inhibitors; Sildenafil + Cocaine

An isolated report describes fatal acute aortic dissection possibly associated with the use of cocaine and sildenafil.

Clinical evidence, mechanism, importance and management

A 42-year-old man developed chest pain radiating to his back 2 hours after sniffing cocaine and one hour after taking sildenafil 50 mg. The chest pain subsided spontaneously but he developed severe pain in his right groin and leg and became pale and sweaty. His blood pressure and heart rate were increased (160/100 mmHg and 92 bpm, respectively), his respiration rate was 16 breaths/minute, and an ECG showed occasional isolated ventricular beats. A CT scan and transoesophageal cardiac ultrasonography revealed an aortic dissection in the descending aorta. He was closely monitored and given intravenous glyceryl trinitrate, labetalol, metoprolol, captopril and ranitidine, but died 12 days later.[1]

Cardiovascular complications including aortic dissection have been reported with cocaine.[1] There is also an isolated report of aortic dissection after sildenafil use, in a patient who was taking a number of other medicines including isosorbide mononitrate.[2] It was suggested that acute dissection in the reported case probably coincided with the expected peak levels of sildenafil, but after the time period of 30 minutes when the cardiovascular effects of cocaine usually occur. However, the patient's heavy smoking and hypertension may also be factors in this case. It was further suggested that, in cases where acute aortic dissection is associated with cocaine, vasodilatation due to the concurrent use of sildenafil could reduce organ perfusion and aggravate injury due to hypovolaemia and ischaemia.[1]

This is an isolated case, and it is not clear if it is generally applicable.

1. Famularo G, Polchi S, Di Bona G, Manzara C. Acute aortic dissection after cocaine and sildenafil abuse. *J Emerg Med* (2001) 21, 78–9.
2. Nachtnebel A, Stöllberger C, Ehrlich M, Finsterer J. Aortic dissection after sildenafil-induced erection. *South Med J* (2006) 99, 1151–2.

Phosphodiesterase type-5 inhibitors; Sildenafil + Dihydrocodeine

An isolated report describes two men taking sildenafil who had prolonged erections following orgasm while also taking dihydrocodeine.

Clinical evidence, mechanism, importance and management

Two men, successfully using 100-mg doses of sildenafil for erectile dysfunction, experienced prolonged erections after orgasm while also taking dihydrocodeine 30 to 60 mg every 6 hours for soft tissue injuries. One of them had two erections lasting 4 hours and 5 hours, and this did not occur on subsequent occasions when the dihydrocodeine was stopped. The other patients had 2- to 3-hour erections on three occasions during the first week of dihydrocodeine use, but no problems over the next 2 weeks while continuing to take the dihydrocodeine.[1] The reasons for this effect are not understood.

Priapism associated with sildenafil use is rare, and there appear to be no other reports about an interaction between sildenafil and dihydrocodeine. Excessively prolonged erections can have serious consequences, and patients are advised to seek immediate medical assistance in the event of an erection lasting longer than 4 hours.

1. Goldmeier D, Lamba H. Prolonged erections produced by dihydrocodeine and sildenafil. *BMJ* (2002) 324, 1555.

Phosphodiesterase type-5 inhibitors; Sildenafil + Ecstasy

The abuse of sildenafil and ecstasy (MDMA, methylenedioxymethamfetamine) has been reported to result in serious headache and priapism requiring emergency treatment.

Clinical evidence, mechanism, importance and management

A journalist's account, based purely on anecdotal reports, claims that the illicit use of sildenafil with ecstasy (MDMA, methylenedioxymethamfetamine) causes "hammerheading" because of the pounding headache and the prolonged and painful penile erections that require emergency medical treatment.[1] The report does not say how much of each of these drugs is taken to produce these adverse effects. The outcome can clearly be unpleasant and painful, and the priapism is potentially serious. Until further information is available it may be prudent to avoid concurrent use.

1. Breslau K, Peraino K, Fantz A. The 'sextasy' craze. Newsweek, June 3, 2002, 30.

Phosphodiesterase type-5 inhibitors; Sildenafil + Nitric oxide

The concurrent use of sildenafil and inhaled nitric oxide might have beneficial effects in pulmonary hypertension, but systemic vasodilation and hypotension are possible.

Clinical evidence

In a study in 15 infants at risk of pulmonary hypertension after corrective cardiac surgery, the concurrent use of intravenous sildenafil and inhaled nitric oxide augmented the pulmonary vasodilator effects of inhaled nitric oxide. However, significant systemic hypotension occurred, which, along with a decrease in oxygenation, was considered sufficiently detrimental for the study to be stopped early.[1] In contrast, in a study in 35 neonates with persistent pulmonary hypertension, the use of intravenous sildenafil in the 29 patients already receiving inhaled nitric oxide increased oxygenation and caused no clinically relevant changes in blood pressure or heart rate in the majority of patients, although in 2 cases treatment-related hypotension required discontinuation of sildenafil.[2] Beneficial combined use has also been described in adult patients with severe hypoxaemia caused by pulmonary hypertension: a few references are cited as examples.[3,4] In a placebo-controlled study in 29 infants, the use of enteral sildenafil to prevent rebound hypertension during weaning from inhaled nitric oxide, did not result in any difference in blood pressure between the sildenafil group and the placebo group: the benefit of sildenafil was such that the study was stopped early.[5]

Mechanism

Patients with pulmonary arterial hypertension are thought to have deficiencies in endogenous nitric oxide. Inhaled nitric oxide is therefore used, and causes some pulmonary-specific vasodilatory effects. Phosphodiesterase type-5 inhibitors also increase the activity of endogenous nitric oxide by inhibiting the breakdown of cyclic guanosine monophosphate (cGMP). When given in combination, sildenafil augments and prolongs the effects of inhaled nitric oxide, in the same way as other nitric oxide donors, see 'Phosphodiesterase type-5 inhibitors + Nitrates', p.1545. As sildenafil is not pulmonary specific, systemic vasodilation and hypotension is possible.

Importance and management

In contrast to the situation in erectile dysfunction, where the interaction between phosphodiesterase type-5 inhibitors and nitrates is unwanted and potentially serious, in pulmonary hypertension, the same pharmacodynamic interaction might prove to be clinically useful.[4] Nevertheless, a reduction in systemic blood pressure due to sildenafil might be detrimental, and could outweigh any benefits in some patient groups.[1] The manufacturers of sildenafil for pulmonary artery hypertension contraindicates its use with any nitric oxide donor,[6,7] although in specialist paediatric units, sildenafil may be used to aid weaning from nitric oxide.[8]

Note that **nitric oxide** is not to be confused with the anaesthetic **nitrous oxide**, which is not a nitric oxide donor.

1. Stocker C, Penny DJ, Brizard CP, Cochrane AD, Soto R, Shekerdemian LS. Intravenous sildenafil and inhaled nitric oxide: a randomised trial in infants after cardiac surgery. *Intensive Care Med* (2003) 29, 1996–2003.
2. Steinhorn RH, Kinsella JP, Pierce C, Butrous G, Dilleen M, Oakes M, Wessel DL. Intravenous sildenafil in the treatment of neonates with persistent pulmonary hypertension. *J Pediatr* (2009) 155, 841–7.
3. Bigatello LM, Hess D, Dennehy KC, Medoff BD, Hurford WE. Sildenafil can increase the response to inhaled nitric oxide. *Anesthesiology* (2000) 92, 1827–9.
4. Lepore JJ, Maroo A, Bigatello LM, Dec GW, Zapol WM, Bloch KD, Semigran J. Hemodynamic effects of sildenafil in patients with congestive heart failure and pulmonary hypertension: combined administration with inhaled nitric oxide. *Chest* (2005) 127, 1647–53.
5. Namachivayam P, Theilen U, Butt WW, Cooper SM, Penny DJ, Shekerdemian LS. Sildenafil prevents rebound pulmonary hypertension after withdrawal of nitric oxide in children. *Am J Respir Crit Care Med* (2006) 174, 1042–7.
6. Revatio Tablets (Sildenafil citrate). Pfizer Ltd. UK Summary of product characteristics, April 2015.
7. Revatio (Sildenafil citrate). Pfizer Inc. US Prescribing information, April 2015.
8. Paediatric Formulary Committee. *BNF for Children* 2015–2016. London: BMJ Group, Pharmaceutical Press, and RCPCH Publications; 2015. p.87.

Phosphodiesterase type-5 inhibitors; Sildenafil + Treprostinil

There is no pharmacokinetic interaction between sildenafil and treprostinil.

Clinical evidence, mechanism, importance and management

In a crossover study in 18 healthy subjects, sildenafil 20 mg three times daily did not affect the pharmacokinetics of treprostinil 1 mg twice daily, when each was given for 4.5 days. Similarly, treprostinil did not affect the pharmacokinetics of sildenafil.[1] No dose adjustments are therefore necessary on concurrent use.

1. Gotzkowsky SK, Kumar P, Mottola D, Laliberte K. Lack of a pharmacokinetic interaction between treprostinil diolamine and sildenafil in healthy adult volunteers. *J Cardiovasc Pharmacol* (2013) 61, 444–51.

Urinary antimuscarinics + CYP3A4 inhibitors; Moderate

Erythromycin and fluconazole (both moderate CYP3A4 inhibitors) cause a moderate increase in darifenacin exposure. Other moderate CYP3A4 inhibitors are predicted to interact similarly. Moderate CYP3A4 inhibitors might also be expected to increase the exposure of fesoterodine, solifenacin, tolterodine, and oxybutynin: this effect has been seen with fluconazole and fesoterodine.

Clinical evidence

(a) Darifenacin

The UK and US manufacturers of darifenacin note that, in a study in healthy subjects, **erythromycin** 500 mg daily increased the steady-state AUC of darifenacin 30 mg daily by 95%.[1-3] **Fluconazole** 200 mg then 100 mg daily had a similar effect, causing an 84% increase in the steady-state AUC of darifenacin 30 mg daily.[1,2]

(b) Fesoterodine

In a crossover study, 26 healthy subjects were given a single 8-mg dose of fesoterodine, alone or with a single 200-mg dose of **fluconazole**. **Fluconazole** increased the AUC and maximum plasma concentration of 5-hydroxymethyltolterodine (the active metabolite of fesoterodine) by 27% and 19%, respectively.[4]

Mechanism

Erythromycin and fluconazole are moderate inhibitors of CYP3A4, by which darifenacin is principally metabolised. Fesoterodine is a prodrug and is rapidly converted to its more active metabolite, 5-hydroxymethyltolterodine, which is partially metabolised by CYP3A4. Therefore concurrent use leads to an increase in darifenacin and 5-hydroxymethyltolteridone exposure.

Solifenacin, oxybutynin, and tolterodine are also metabolised by CYP3A4 and might also be expected to be affected by erythromycin and fluconazole, but, based on the way potent CYP3A4 inhibitors interact with these urinary antimuscarinics (see 'Urinary antimuscarinics + CYP3A4 inhibitors; Potent', below) the magnitude of any interaction would be expected to be slight to moderate at worst.

Importance and management

The pharmacokinetic interaction between darifenacin and erythromycin or fluconazole is established, but the clinical relevance of the increase in **darifenacin** exposure has not been assessed. The UK manufacturer[3] recommends an initial dose of darifenacin 7.5 mg daily in those taking moderate CYP3A4 inhibitors, increasing the dose to 15 mg daily if it is well tolerated, whereas the US manufacturer[1] states that dose adjustments are not required on the concurrent use of moderate CYP3A4 inhibitors. If darifenacin is given with a moderate CYP3A4 inhibitor, bear in mind the possibility of an interaction if antimuscarinic adverse effects (dry mouth, constipation, drowsiness) are increased. For a list of clinically relevant moderate CYP3A4 inhibitors, see 'Table 1.9', p.11. Note that **verapamil**, which is a moderate CYP3A4 inhibitor, also inhibits P-glycoprotein, and the UK manufacturer of darifenacin[3] suggests that the concurrent use of P-glycoprotein inhibitors should be avoided.

The slight increase in the exposure to 5-hydroxymethyltolterodine (the active metabolite of **fesoterodine**) is unlikely to be clinically important. Other urinary antimuscarinics would be expected to interact similarly, and it appears unlikely that a clinically relevant interaction would occur in the majority of patients taking **fesoterodine**, **solifenacin**, **tolterodine**, or **oxybutynin** with a moderate CYP3A4 inhibitor. However, until more is known about the clinical outcome of concurrent use, it may be prudent to bear in mind the possibility of an interaction if an increase in antimuscarinic adverse effects (dry mouth, constipation, drowsiness) occurs. For a list of clinically relevant moderate CYP3A4 inhibitors, see 'Table 1.9', p.11. Note that the UK manufacturer of fesoterodine[5] additionally mentions amprenavir and fosamprenavir (which have also sometimes been considered to be potent inhibitors). The manufacturers of oxybutynin also mention miconazole.[6]

The situation for **tolterodine** is less clear because the manufacturers consider erythromycin,[7,8] and miconazole[7] to be potent CYP3A4 inhibitors: the UK manufacturer[8] does not recommend concurrent use, and the US manufacturer[7] recommends that the dose of tolterodine should be reduced to 1 mg twice daily. However, erythromycin does not appear to be a potent inhibitor of CYP3A4 in clinical use (for example, the increase in darifenacin exposure with erythromycin above was about 9-fold less than that with ketoconazole, a known potent CYP3A4 inhibitor).

1. Enablex (Darifenacin hydrobromide). Novartis. US Prescribing information, January 2010.
2. Skerjanec A. The clinical pharmacokinetics of darifenacin. *Clin Pharmacokinet* (2006) 45, 325–50.
3. Emselex (Darifenacin hydrobromide). Novartis Pharmaceuticals UK Ltd. UK Summary of product characteristics, December 2011.
4. Malhotra B, Dickins M, Alvey C, Jumadilova Z, Li X, Duczynski G, Gandelman K. Effects of the moderate CYP3A4 inhibitor, fluconazole, on the pharmacokinetics of fesoterodine in healthy subjects. *Br J Clin Pharmacol* (2011) 72, 263–9.
5. Toviaz (Fesoterodine fumarate). Pfizer Ltd. UK Summary of product characteristics, October 2010.
6. Ditropan XL (Oxybutynin chloride). Ortho-McNeil-Janssen Pharmaceuticals, Inc. US Prescribing information, July 2009.
7. Detrol (Tolterodine tartrate). Pharmacia & Upjohn Company. US Prescribing information, March 2008.
8. Detrusitol (Tolterodine tartrate). Pharmacia Ltd. UK Summary of product characteristics, February 2009.

Urinary antimuscarinics + CYP3A4 inhibitors; Potent

Ketoconazole (a potent CYP3A4 inhibitor) very markedly increases darifenacin exposure and markedly increases fesoterodine and solifenacin exposure. Other potent CYP3A4 inhibitors are expected to interact similarly. Itraconazole and ketoconazole increase the exposure to oxybutynin, but do not alter the concentrations of its active metabolite. Itraconazole modestly increases the exposure to imidafenacin. Ketoconazole can markedly increase tolterodine exposure, but only in those who have low concentrations or are lacking CYP2D6.

Clinical evidence

(a) Darifenacin

In a study in 16 healthy subjects, **ketoconazole** 400 mg daily for 6 days caused a marked tenfold increase in the steady-state AUC of darifenacin 30 mg daily.[1] The UK manufacturer[2] also notes that **ketoconazole** 400 mg caused a fivefold increase in the steady-state AUC of a 7.5-mg dose of darifenacin: a greater, tenfold increase was seen in CYP2D6 poor metabolisers (that is, those with low concentrations or lacking this isoenzyme).

(b) Fesoterodine

In a crossover study in 18 healthy subjects, a single 8-mg dose of fesoterodine was given alone and then on day 5 of a 6-day course of **ketoconazole** 200 mg twice daily. **Ketoconazole** increased the AUC of the active metabolite of fesoterodine, 5-hydroxymethyltolterodine, 2.5-fold in CYP2D6 poor metabolisers (that is, those with low concentrations or lacking this isoenzyme) and 2.3-fold in CYP2D6 extensive metabolisers (that is, those with normal concentrations of this isoenzyme).[3] However, the overall extent of exposure (AUC and maximum concentration) to 5-hydroxymethyltolterodine was about twofold higher in poor metabolisers when compared with extensive metabolisers. **Ketoconazole** increased fesoterodine exposure in extensive metabolisers to a concentration similar to that seen in poor metabolisers not taking **ketoconazole**.[3]

(c) Imidafenacin

In a study in 10 healthy subjects, **itraconazole** 200 mg daily for 9 days increased the maximum plasma concentrations and AUC of a single 100-microgram dose imidafenacin given on day 8 by 30% and 75%, respectively.[4]

(d) Oxybutynin

In a study, a single 5-mg dose of oxybutynin was given to 10 healthy subjects after they had taken **itraconazole** 200 mg daily or placebo for 4 days. The peak serum concentrations and AUC of oxybutynin were increased twofold, while the pharmacokinetics of the active metabolite of oxybutynin were unchanged. The sum of the oxybutynin and its metabolite concentrations was on average about 13% higher than with placebo. No increase in adverse effects was seen.[5] **Ketoconazole** also increases oxybutynin concentrations about 2-fold.[6,7]

(e) Solifenacin

In a crossover study[8] in healthy subjects, **ketoconazole** 200 mg daily for 20 days caused a twofold increase in the AUC of a single 10-mg dose of solifenacin given on day 7. Moreover, the manufacturer notes that a higher dose of **ketoconazole** (400 mg daily) increased the AUC of solifenacin about threefold.[9,10]

(f) Tolterodine

A study in 8 healthy subjects who were CYP2D6 poor metabolisers (that is, those with low amounts or lacking this isoenzyme) found that after taking **ketoconazole** 200 mg daily for 4 days the clearance of a single 2-mg dose of tolterodine was reduced by 61% and its AUC was increased 2.5-fold.[11] In a subsequent multiple-dose study, 6 of the original subjects were given tolterodine 1 mg twice daily (half of the usual dose). **Ketoconazole** 200 mg daily caused a 2.1-fold increase in the AUC of tolterodine, and a 2.2-fold increase in the AUC of the active moiety (unbound tolterodine plus metabolite).[11]

Mechanism

Darifenacin is primarily metabolised by CYP3A4 and CYP2D6, and imidafenacin and solifenacin are principally metabolised by CYP3A4. Ketoconazole and itraconazole are known, potent inhibitors of CYP3A4 and concurrent use therefore increases the concentrations of these urinary antimuscarinics to varying extents. Oxybutynin is also metabolised by CYP3A4, but most of the pharmacological activity of oxybutynin is attributed to a metabolite, the formation of which does not appear to be dependent on CYP3A4,[5] and therefore the sum of oxybutynin and its active metabolite is largely unchanged by these azoles.

Fesoterodine is a prodrug and is rapidly converted to its more active metabolite, 5-hydroxymethyltolterodine, which is primarily metabolised by CYP2D6 and CYP3A4. Ketoconazole, an inhibitor of CYP3A4, may therefore increase the concentrations of 5-hydroxymethyltolterodine.

Although tolterodine is normally metabolised to its active metabolite by CYP2D6, in those with low amounts of this isoenzyme (about 5 to 10% of the population), metabolism by CYP3A4 becomes more important and therefore in these patients an increase in its concentrations can occur if CYP3A4 inhibitors, such as ketoconazole, are also given.

Importance and management

Established pharmacokinetic interactions. The very marked increase in **darifenacin** exposure caused by ketoconazole is of concern. The UK manufacturer contraindicates the concurrent use of ketoconazole and other potent CYP3A4 inhibitors,[2] whereas the US manufacturer recommends that the daily dose of darifenacin is limited to 7.5 mg (half the usual dose), both with ketoconazole and other potent inhibitors of CYP3A4.[12] It may be prudent to assess antimuscarinic adverse effects (such as dry mouth, constipation, drowsiness) in patients given darifenacin with a potent CYP3A4 inhibitor, and to withdraw the drug if it is not tolerated.

As a result of the increase in exposure seen with ketoconazole, the manufacturers of **fesoterodine** recommend that its maximum dose should be restricted to 4 mg daily when it is given with potent CYP3A4 inhibitors.[13,14] In the UK, fesoterodine is contraindicated in patients taking potent CYP3A4 inhibitors who also have moderate to severe hepatic or renal impairment.[13]

For **oxybutynin**, the available evidence suggests that the pharmacokinetic interaction with itraconazole is only of minor importance,[5] but note that this was only a single-dose study and it might therefore not necessarily reflect the full picture in practice. Moreover, some manufacturers recommend caution if oxybutynin is given with itraconazole or ketoconazole,[6,7] and, until more is known this might be prudent, both with these drugs and other potent CYP3A4 inhibitors. Consider the possibility of an interaction if antimuscarinic effects (such as dry mouth, constipation, drowsiness) are increased.

For **solifenacin**, the UK and US manufacturers recommend that its daily dose is limited to 5 mg if it is given with ketoconazole or other potent CYP3A4 inhibitors.[9,10] In addition, in the UK, in patients with severe renal impairment or moderate hepatic impairment, the concurrent use of solifenacin and potent CYP3A4 inhibitors is contraindicated.[9] Note that high concentrations of solifenacin cause a small increase in the QT interval, see 'Drugs that prolong the QT interval + Other drugs that prolong the QT interval', p.272.

For **tolterodine**, the UK manufacturer[15] considers that the twofold increase in concentrations represents a risk of overdose in CYP2D6 poor metabolisers. Consequently, they do not recommend the use of potent CYP3A4 inhibitors with tolterodine in any patient (note that metaboliser status is rarely known), especially those with risk factors for QT-prolongation (see also 'Drugs that prolong the QT interval + Other drugs that prolong the QT interval', p.272). However, the US manufacturer[16] recommends that the dose of tolterodine should be reduced to 1 mg twice daily in patients also taking drugs that are potent inhibitors of CYP3A4. It may be prudent to assess antimuscarinic adverse effects (such as dry mouth, constipation, drowsiness) in these patients, and to reduce the dose further or withdraw the drug if it is not tolerated.

Potent inhibitors of CYP3A4 include the azoles, many of the HIV-protease inhibitors, and some macrolides. Note that there is some difference in opinion as to whether or not clarithromycin is a potent or moderate CYP3A4 inhibitor. Its interaction with midazolam (a drug used to assess the potency of effect of other drugs on CYP3A4), would suggest it is a potent inhibitor (see 'Benzodiazepines and related drugs + Macrolides', p.827).

1. Skerjanec A. The clinical pharmacokinetics of darifenacin. *Clin Pharmacokinet* (2006) 45, 325–50.
2. Emselex (Darifenacin hydrobromide). Novartis Pharmaceuticals UK Ltd. UK Summary of product characteristics, December 2011.
3. Malhotra B, Sachse R, Wood N. Evaluation of drug–drug interactions with fesoterodine. *Eur J Clin Pharmacol* (2009) 65, 551–60.
4. Ohno T, Nakayama K, Nakade S, Kitagawa J, Ueda S, Miyabe H, Miyata Y, Ohnishi A. Effect of itraconazole on the pharmacokinetics of imidafenacin in healthy subjects. *J Clin Pharmacol* (2008) 48, 330–4.
5. Lukkari E, Juhakoski A, Aranko K, Neuvonen PJ. Itraconazole moderately increases serum concentrations of oxybutynin but does not affect those of the active metabolite. *Eur J Clin Pharmacol* (1997) 52, 403–6.
6. Ditropan XL (Oxybutynin chloride). Ortho-McNeil-Janssen Pharmaceuticals, Inc. US Prescribing information, July 2009.
7. Lyrinel XL (Oxybutynin hydrochloride). Janssen-Cilag Ltd. UK Summary of product characteristics, April 2009.
8. Swart PJ, Krauwinkel WJJ, Smulders RA, Smith NN. Pharmacokinetic effect of ketoconazole on solifenacin in healthy volunteers. *Basic Clin Pharmacol Toxicol* (2006) 99, 33–6.
9. Vesicare (Solifenacin succinate). Astellas Pharma Ltd. UK Summary of product characteristics, November 2009.
10. VESIcare (Solifenacin succinate). GlaxoSmithKline. US Prescribing information, November 2008.
11. Brynne N, Forslund C, Hallén B, Gustafsson LL, Bertilsson L. Ketoconazole inhibits the metabolism of tolterodine in subjects with deficient CYP2D6 activity. *Br J Clin Pharmacol* (1999) 48, 564–72.
12. Enablex (Darifenacin hydrobromide). Novartis. US Prescribing information, January 2010.
13. Toviaz (Fesoterodine fumarate). Pfizer Ltd. UK Summary of product characteristics, October 2010.
14. Toviaz (Fesoterodine fumarate). Pfizer Inc. US Prescribing information, September 2010.
15. Detrusitol (Tolterodine tartrate). Pharmacia Ltd. UK Summary of product characteristics, February 2009.
16. Detrol (Tolterodine tartrate). Pharmacia & Upjohn Company. US prescribing information, March 2008.

Urinary antimuscarinics + Food

Food might modestly reduce the absorption of controlled-release trospium, and might modestly increase the absorption of immediate-release tolterodine and one formulation of controlled-release oxybutynin. Food does not affect the pharmacokinetics of some other controlled-release oxybutynin preparations, or controlled-release darifenacin controlled-release tolterodine, or immediate-release fesoterodine and solifenacin.

Clinical evidence, mechanism, importance and management

(a) Darifenacin

The manufacturer briefly notes that food had no effect on the steady-state pharmacokinetics of extended-release darifenacin, and the tablets may be taken with or without food.[1,2]

(b) Fesoterodine

In a study in 16 healthy subjects, the AUC and maximum plasma levels of the active metabolite of fesoterodine, 5- hydroxymethyltolterodine, were slightly increased by about 19% when a single 8-mg dose of fesoterodine was given after a high-fat breakfast compared with the fasted state.[3] In another similar study, in 24 healthy subjects, the AUC and maximum plasma levels of 5-hydroxymethyltolterodine were increased by 12% and 29%, respectively, in the fed state, when compared with the fasted state.[4] These slight changes are not expected to be clinically relevant, and fesoterodine may be given without regard to food.

(c) Oxybutynin

In a crossover study in 50 healthy subjects, the pharmacokinetics of a single 15-mg dose of slow-release oxybutynin (*Ditropan XL*) did not differ when taken after a high-fat breakfast when compared with fasting.[5] Similarly, the manufacturer notes that the absorption of a prolonged-release formulation of oxybutynin (*Lyrinel XL*) was unaffected by food.[6] However, in another crossover study, in 23 healthy subjects who were given a single 10-mg dose of controlled-release oxybutynin (*Cystrin*) after a high-fat breakfast or an overnight fast, there was no change in the AUC of oxybutynin but the maximum plasma levels of oxybutynin and its metabolite, *N*-desethyloxybutynin, were increased about twofold. The decrease in saliva secretion was greater when taken after food (40% versus 20%), but there was no difference in the incidence of adverse events.[7] Similar results were found in another study in 31 healthy subjects.[8]

The relevance of the increase in exposure to oxybutynin from one formulation, *Cystrin*, when taken with food is likely to be small, but the authors suggest that if adverse effects are troublesome, then it could be taken half- to one-hour before food.[8] Some other formulations of controlled-release oxybutynin (*Ditropan XL*, *Lyrinel XL*) may be taken with or without food.

(d) Solifenacin

In a crossover study in 23 healthy subjects, food did not affect the pharmacokinetics of solifenacin 10 mg, taken within 5 minutes of a high-fat, high-calorie breakfast, when compared with the fasted state.[9] Solifenacin may be taken with or without food.

(e) Tolterodine

In a crossover study in 23 healthy subjects (all CYP2D6 extensive metabolisers; that is, those with normal levels of this isoenzyme) a single 2-mg dose of immediate-release tolterodine was given alone, or after a standard breakfast. The AUC and maximum plasma levels of tolterodine were increased by 53% and 49%, respectively, but the levels of the active metabolite, 5-hydroxymethyl, were not affected, and there was no difference in incidence of antimuscarinic adverse effects, such as dry mouth.[10] In another crossover study, in 17 healthy subjects, there was no change in the maximum level or AUC of tolterodine when a single 8-mg dose of extended-release tolterodine [presumed to be *Detrusitol XL*[11]] was taken under fasting conditions and after a high-fat breakfast.[12] These preparations of tolterodine may therefore be taken without regard to food.

(f) Trospium

Giving trospium extended-release capsules immediately after a high fat-content meal reduced the AUC and maximum plasma levels of trospium by 35% and 60%, respectively. The reduction in trospium exposure with food is modest and probably not clinically relevant; nevertheless, the manufacturer recommends that trospium should be taken on an empty stomach at least one hour before a meal.[13,14]

1. Enablex (Darifenacin hydrobromide). Novartis. US Prescribing information, January 2010.
2. Emselex (Darifenacin hydrobromide). Novartis Pharmaceuticals UK Ltd. UK Summary of product characteristics, December 2011.

3. Malhotra B, Sachse R, Wood N. Influence of food on the pharmacokinetic profile of fesoterodine. *Int J Clin Pharmacol Ther* (2009) 47, 384–390.
4. Malhotra B, Guan Z, Wood N, Gandelman K. Pharmacokinetic profile of fesoterodine. *Int J Clin Pharmacol Ther* (2008) 46, 556–63.
5. Sathyan G, Hu W, Gupta SK. Lack of effect of food on the pharmacokinetics of an extended-release oxybutynin formulation. *J Clin Pharmacol* (2001) 41, 187–92.
6. Lyrinel XL (Oxybutynin hydrochloride). Janssen-Cilag Ltd. UK Summary of product characteristics, April 2009.
7. Lukkari E, Castrèn-Kortekangas P, Juhakoski A, Löyttyniemi E, Aranko K, Neuvonen PJ. Effect of food on the bioavailability of oxybutynin from a controlled release tablet. *Eur J Clin Pharmacol* (1996) 50, 221–3.
8. Lukkari E, Aranko K, Juhakoski A, Hakonen T, Neuvonen PJ. Effect of time interval between food and drug ingestion on the absorption of oxybutynin from a controlled-release tablet. *Pharmacol Toxicol* (1997) 81, 31–34.
9. Uchida T, Krauwinkel WJ, Mulder H, Smulders RA. Food does not affect the pharmacokinetics of solifenacin, a new muscarinic receptor antagonist: results of a randomized crossover trial. *Br J Clin Pharmacol* (2004) 58, 4–7.
10. Olsson B, Brynne N, Johansson C, Arnberg H. Food increases the bioavailability of tolterodine but not effective exposure. *J Clin Pharmacol* (2001) 41, 298–304.
11. Detrusitol XL (Tolterodine tartrate). Pharmacia Ltd. UK Summary of product characteristics, September 2010.
12. Olsson B, Szamosi J. Food does not influence the pharmacokinetics of a new extended release formulation of tolterodine for once daily treatment of patients with overactive bladder. *Clin Pharmacokinet* (2001) 40, 135–43.
13. Regurin XL (Trospium chloride). Speciality European Pharma. UK Summary of product characteristics, November 2008.
14. Sanctura XR (Trospium chloride). Allergan Inc. US Prescribing information, September 2009.

Urinary antimuscarinics + Rifampicin (Rifampin) and other CYP3A4 inducers

Rifampicin, a CYP3A4 inducer, markedly reduces the exposure to the active metabolite of fesoterodine. Other CYP3A4 inducers would be expected to interact similarly. Darifenacin and solifenacin levels are also predicted to be reduced by CYP3A4 inducers.

Clinical evidence

In a study in 12 healthy subjects, a single 8-mg dose of **fesoterodine** was given on day 7 of an 8-day course of rifampicin 600 mg daily. The AUC and maximum plasma levels of the active metabolite of fesoterodine, 5-hydroxymethyltolterodine, were reduced by about 78% and 72%, respectively, with no difference between CYP2D6 poor metabolisers (that is, those with low levels or lacking this isoenzyme) and CYP2D6 extensive metabolisers (that is, those with normal levels of this isoenzyme).[1]

Mechanism

Fesoterodine is a pro-drug and is rapidly converted to 5-hydroxymethyltolterodine, which is primarily metabolised by CYP2D6 and CYP3A4, of which rifampicin is a potent inducer. **Solifenacin** and **darifenacin** are principally metabolised by CYP3A4, and would be expected to be similarly affected by rifampicin.

Importance and management

The clinical relevance of the marked reduction in the levels of the active metabolite of **fesoterodine** by rifampicin has not been assessed, but reduced efficacy would be expected. In the UK, the manufacturer does not recommend the concurrent use of fesoterodine with rifampicin or other CYP3A4 inducers: they specifically name **carbamazepine, phenobarbital, phenytoin, St John's wort**.[2] However, note that the potency of the enzyme-inducing effect of these drugs varies and thus the magnitude of their effect on fesoterodine metabolism will also vary. The US manufacturer notes that reduced levels of the active metabolite of fesoterodine may occur on the concurrent use of CYP3A4 inducers, but states that no fesoterodine dose adjustments are recommended.[3] If concurrent use is necessary, until the clinical relevance of this interaction is known, it would seem prudent to closely monitor the efficacy of fesoterodine.

The efficacy of **darifenacin** and **solifenacin** is also expected to be reduced by CYP3A4 inducers: the manufacturers name **barbiturates, carbamazepine, phenytoin, rifampicin** and **St John's wort**.[4-6] For a list of CYP3A4 inducers, see 'Table 1.9', p.11.

1. Malhotra B, Sachse R, Wood N. Evaluation of drug–drug interactions with fesoterodine. *Eur J Clin Pharmacol* (2009) 65, 551–60.
2. Toviaz (Fesoterodine fumarate). Pfizer Ltd. UK Summary of product characteristics, October 2010.
3. Toviaz (Fesoterodine fumarate). Pfizer Inc. US Prescribing information, September 2010.
4. Vesicare (Solifenacin succinate). Astellas Pharma Ltd. UK Summary of product characteristics, November 2009.
5. VESIcare (Solifenacin succinate). GlaxoSmithKline. US Prescribing information, November 2008.
6. Emselex (Darifenacin hydrobromide). Novartis Pharmaceuticals UK Ltd. UK Summary of product characteristics, December 2011.

Urinary antimuscarinics + SSRIs or SNRIs

Fluoxetine causes a slight increase in the total AUC of tolterodine and its active metabolite. Duloxetine increases the maximum levels of tolterodine by 64%. Paroxetine, a CYP2D6 inhibitor, causes a small increase in darifenacin levels; other CYP2D6 inhibitors (e.g. quinidine) are therefore also expected to increase the levels of darifenacin.

Clinical evidence

(a) Darifenacin

The manufacturers note that, in a study, **paroxetine** 20 mg daily increased the steady-state AUC of darifenacin 30 mg daily by 33%.[1,2]

(b) Tolterodine

1. Duloxetine. In a placebo-controlled, crossover study, 14 healthy subjects were given duloxetine 40 mg twice daily and tolterodine 2 mg twice daily for 5 days. Duloxetine increased the steady-state AUC of tolterodine by 71% and increased its maximum level by 64%. However, duloxetine had no effect on the pharmacokinetics of 5-hydroxymethyl-tolterodine, the active metabolite of tolterodine.[3]

2. Fluoxetine. In a study, 13 psychiatric patients with symptoms of urinary incontinence were given tolterodine 2 mg twice daily for 5 doses, followed by fluoxetine 20 mg daily for 3 weeks, and then both drugs together for a further 3 days. Nine of the 13 patients completed the study; the other 4 withdrew during the fluoxetine phase because of fluoxetine-related adverse effects. In the 7 patients that were CYP2D6 extensive metabolisers (that is, those with normal levels of this isoenzyme) fluoxetine caused a 4.8-fold increase in the AUC of tolterodine and a minor reduction in its active and equipotent metabolite. In contrast, fluoxetine increased the AUC of tolterodine by only about 25% in the 2 patients that were CYP2D6 poor metabolisers (that is, those lacking or totally deficient in this isoenzyme). These changes in AUC represent an increase of about 25% in active moiety (unbound tolterodine plus metabolite) for both poor and extensive metabolisers, a change within normal variation.[4]

Mechanism

Duloxetine, fluoxetine and paroxetine are inhibitors of CYP2D6, by which tolterodine is metabolised therefore concurrent use decreases the metabolism of tolterodine, leading to the increased levels seen. Darifenacin is also metabolised by this isoenzyme, but only in part, and therefore its levels are more modestly raised by CYP2D6 inhibitors such as fluoxetine.

Importance and management

Darifenacin

The minor pharmacokinetic interaction between paroxetine and darifenacin is unlikely to be clinically relevant, and no dose adjustments are recommended by the US manufacturer of darifenacin in the presence of CYP2D6 inhibitors.[1] However, the UK manufacturer recommends that the dose of darifenacin should be started at 7.5 mg daily and, if well tolerated, titrated to 15 mg daily in the presence of CYP2D6 inhibitors including paroxetine, **terbinafine** and **quinidine**.[2] This seems a cautious approach. For a list of CYP2D6 inhibitors, see 'Table 1.7', p.9.

Tolterodine

The increases in tolterodine levels with duloxetine and fluoxetine are not considered to be clinically relevant, and no routine dose adjustment of tolterodine is considered to be necessary. However, if CYP3A4 inhibitors are also being taken, this interaction could be important. For further information, see 'Urinary antimuscarinics + CYP3A4 inhibitors; Potent', p.1548.

1. Enablex (Darifenacin hydrobromide). Novartis. US Prescribing information, January 2010.
2. Emselex (Darifenacin hydrobromide). Novartis Pharmaceuticals UK Ltd. UK Summary of product characteristics, December 2011.
3. Hua TC, Pan A, Chan C, Poo YK, Skinner MH, Knadler MP, Gonzales CR, Wise SD. Effect of duloxetine on tolterodine pharmacokinetics in healthy volunteers. *Br J Clin Pharmacol* (2004) 57, 652–6.
4. Brynne N, Svanström C, Åberg-Wistedt A, Hallén B, Bertilsson L. Fluoxetine inhibits the metabolism of tolterodine—pharmacokinetic implications and proposed clinical relevance. *Br J Clin Pharmacol* (1999) 48, 553–63.

Urinary antimuscarinics; Darifenacin + Miscellaneous

The concurrent use of darifenacin and drugs such as the bisphosphonates may increase the risk of oesophagitis. Cimetidine causes a small increase in darifenacin levels. High-dose darifenacin increases the levels of imipramine, a CYP2D6 substrate, and is therefore predicted to increase the levels of other CYP2D6 substrates such as flecainide and thioridazine. Ciclosporin may raise darifenacin levels, but good evidence for this is lacking. Darifenacin does not significantly affect the pharmacokinetics of midazolam

Clinical evidence, mechanism, importance and management

(a) Bisphosphonates

Darifenacin causes dyspepsia in more than 10% of patients. The UK manufacturers therefore advise caution with the use of drugs that can exacerbate oesophagitis, and they name the bisphosphonates.[1] Patients taking both drugs should have a low tolerance for reporting dyspeptic symptoms.

(b) Ciclosporin

The UK manufacturers of darifenacin state that the use of ciclosporin should be avoided with darifenacin because ciclosporin is a potent inhibitor of P-glycoprotein.[1] However, they give no clinical evidence for this interaction and the US manufacturers do not make any mention of P-glycoprotein.[2] Until more is known, bear in mind the possibility of an interaction if antimuscarinic adverse effects (dry mouth, constipation, drowsiness) are increased.

(c) Cimetidine

The manufacturers note that, in a study in healthy subjects, cimetidine 800 mg twice daily increased the steady-state AUC of darifenacin 30 mg daily by 34%.[2,3] Cimetidine is a non-specific inhibitor of cytochrome P450 isoenzymes, in particular CYP3A4 and CYP2D6, by which darifenacin is metabolised. This modest change in darifenacin exposure is unlikely to be clinically relevant. However, the UK manufacturer states that, in the presence of cimetidine, the dose of darifenacin should be started at 7.5 mg daily and, if well tolerated, titrated to 15 mg daily.[1] This seems a cautious approach.

(d) CYP2D6 substrates

The US manufacturer notes that, in a study in healthy subjects, steady-state darifenacin 30 mg daily increased the AUC of **imipramine** by 70% and increased the AUC of its active metabolite, desipramine, 2.6-fold.[3] Because of these changes, the manufacturers recommend caution if darifenacin is given with **tricyclic antidepressants**; it would seem prudent to monitor concurrent use for tricyclic adverse effects (e.g. sedation, constipation, dry mouth). The manufacturers also recommend caution if darifenacin is given with other CYP2D6 substrates that have a narrow therapeutic window, and specifically name **flecainide** and **thioridazine**.[1,2] See 'Table 1.7', p.9, for a list of known CYP2D6 substrates.

Note that both the tricyclics and darifenacin have antimuscarinic effects, which might be additive on concurrent use (see 'Antimuscarinics + Antimuscarinics', p.754).

(e) Midazolam

The manufacturers note that, in a study in healthy subjects, darifenacin 30 mg daily increased the AUC of a single 7.5-mg dose of midazolam by 17%.[1-3] This change is not clinically important.

1. Emselex (Darifenacin hydrobromide). Novartis Pharmaceuticals UK Ltd. UK Summary of product characteristics, December 2011.
2. Enablex (Darifenacin hydrobromide). Novartis. US Prescribing information, January 2010.
3. Skerjanec A. The clinical pharmacokinetics of darifenacin. *Clin Pharmacokinet* (2006) 45, 325–50.

Urinary antimuscarinics; Tolterodine + Miscellaneous

Tolterodine does not alter the metabolism of debrisoquine, omeprazole or caffeine.

Clinical evidence, mechanism, importance and management

In a pharmacokinetic study in 12 healthy men, tolterodine 4 mg twice daily for 6 days had no effect on debrisoquine hydroxylation (a measure of CYP2D6 activity), omeprazole hydroxylation (a measure of CYP2C19 activity) or sulphoxidation (a measure of CYP3A4 activity) or caffeine demethylation (a measure of CYP1A2 activity), after single doses of **debrisoquine** 10 mg, **omeprazole** 20 mg and **caffeine** 100 mg.[1] This shows that tolterodine has no clinically relevant effect on these isoenzymes, and is therefore unlikely to alter the pharmacokinetics of drugs that are substrates for CYP2D6, CYP2C19, CYP3A4 and CYP1A2.

For mention that **omeprazole** slightly increases the maximum level of tolterodine from a controlled-release preparation, see 'Enteric-coated, delayed-release preparations + Drugs that affect gastric pH', p.1569.

1. Brynne N, Böttiger Y, Hallén B, Bertilsson L. Tolterodine does not affect the human *in vivo* metabolism of the probe drugs caffeine, debrisoquine and omeprazole. *Br J Clin Pharmacol* (1999) 47, 145–50.

Urinary antimuscarinics; Trospium + Miscellaneous

Bile-acid binding resins are expected to reduce the absorption of trospium. Overall, antacids do not appear to affect the absorption of trospium, but increases and decreases in absorption have been seen.

Clinical evidence, mechanism, importance and management

(a) Antacids

The US manufacturer briefly mentions that, in a pharmacokinetic study in 11 healthy subjects, the mean AUC of **trospium** from extended-release capsules was comparable when given with and without an antacid containing **aluminium hydroxide** and **magnesium carbonate**. However, 5 individuals had either an increase or decrease in trospium exposure (amount not stated) in presence of antacid. They state that the clinical relevance of these findings is not known.[1] One UK manufacturer of an extended-release formulation of trospium briefly states that antacids had no effect on the oral bioavailability of trospium.[2]

(b) Bile-acid binding resins

The UK manufacturer notes that an interaction between trospium and **colestyramine** or **colestipol** cannot be excluded and advises that these products are not given simultaneously.[2] The usual recommendation to avoid an interaction is to give other drugs one hour before or 4 to 6 hours after taking colestyramine, and one hour before or 4 hours after taking colestipol.

1. Sanctura XR (Trospium chloride). Allergan Inc. US Prescribing information, September 2009.
2. Regurin XL (Trospium chloride). Speciality European Pharma. UK Summary of product characteristics, November 2008.

Yohimbine + Glyceryl trinitrate (Nitroglycerin)

No significant hypotensive interaction occurred in healthy subjects given yohimbine and a glyceryl trinitrate infusion.

Clinical evidence, mechanism, importance and management

In a placebo-controlled study, 16 healthy male subjects were given a single 7.7-mg oral dose of yohimbine tartrate (as NMI 861; yohimbine plus l-arginine glutamate) followed by a step-wise infusion of glyceryl trinitrate, starting at 2.5 micrograms/minute and then doubled every 15 minutes until symptomatic hypotension or a sustained decrease in systolic blood pressure of greater than 25 mmHg occurred, or until a maximum dose of 40 micrograms/minute had been reached, at which point the infusion was stopped. There was no significant difference in the hypotensive response to intravenous glyceryl trinitrate given with yohimbine or placebo.[1]

1. Kernohan AFB, McIntyre M, Hughes DM, Tam SW, Worcel M, Reid JL. An oral yohimbine/l-arginine combination (NMI 861) for the treatment of male erectile dysfunction: a pharmacokinetic, pharmacodynamic and interaction study with intravenous nitroglycerine in healthy male subjects. *Br J Clin Pharmacol* (2005) 59, 85–93.

38

Miscellaneous drugs

This sections deals with interactions where the affected drug does not fall in to the therapeutic classifications or drug groups used to define the other sections in this publication.

Abiraterone + Miscellaneous

Abiraterone increases the exposure to dextromethorphan, a CYP2D6 substrate, and is predicted to affect the metabolism of other CYP2D6 substrates. Abiraterone does not affect the exposure to theophylline. Potent inhibitors of CYP3A4 (such as ketoconazole) are predicted to increase the exposure to abiraterone, and potent inducers of CYP3A4 (such carbamazepine) are predicted to reduce abiraterone exposure. Food increases the bioavailability of abiraterone.

Clinical evidence, mechanism, importance and management

(a) CYP1A2 substrates

The US manufacturer states that abiraterone inhibits CYP1A2 *in vitro*. However, they also briefly report that, in a study, abiraterone 1 g daily (given with prednisone 5 mg twice daily) had no effect on the exposure to a single 100-mg dose of **theophylline**, a CYP1A2 probe substrate.[1] Therefore, a clinically relevant interaction with other CYP1A2 substrates seems unlikely to occur. For a list of CYP1A2 substrates, see 'Table 1.2', p.5.

(b) CYP2D6 substrates

The manufacturers briefly report that, in a drug interaction study, abiraterone 1 g daily (given with prednisone 5 mg twice daily) increased the AUC and maximum concentration of a single 30-mg dose of **dextromethorphan** 2.9-fold and 2.8-fold, respectively. The AUC of the active metabolite of dextromethorphan, dextrorphan, was increased by about 30%.[1,2]

Dextromethorphan is a probe substrate for CYP2D6, and the results of this study show that abiraterone moderately inhibits CYP2D6. On this basis the manufacturers predict that abiraterone could increase the exposure to other drugs that are substrates of CYP2D6, which might increase their adverse effects. The US manufacturer therefore advises avoiding concurrent use of abiraterone and CYP2D6 substrates that also have a narrow therapeutic margin (and they name **thioridazine**), but if an alternative cannot be used, they advise caution and consideration of a dose reduction for the CYP2D6 substrate.[1] The UK manufacturer similarly advises caution and a dose reduction with CYP2D6 substrates, in particular for drugs with a narrow therapeutic index, and they name the antiarrhythmics **flecainide** and **propafenone**; the antipsychotics **haloperidol** and **risperidone**; the beta blockers **metoprolol** and **propranolol**; **desipramine**; and **venlafaxine**.[2] Such precautions would seem prudent. For a list of CYP2D6 substrates, see 'Table 1.7', p.9.

Note that the UK manufacturer also advises caution on the use of abiraterone with some opioid analgesics, such as **codeine**, that are metabolised by CYP2D6 to their active metabolite. Inhibition of this route of metabolism could lead to a reduction in the concentrations of the active metabolite, and a subsequent reduction in the analgesic effect of codeine.[2] Note that CYP2D6 is subject to genetic polymorphism and this could affect individual susceptibility to this interaction, see 'Opioids; Codeine and related drugs + Quinidine', p.194. The manufacturer also gives similar advice for **oxycodone** and **tramadol**;[2] however, note that inhibition of the metabolism of oxycodone to oxymorphone by CYP2D6 would not be expected to cause a clinically relevant reduction in the analgesic effects of oxycodone (see 'Opioids; Codeine and related drugs + Quinidine', p.194), and the efficacy of tramadol has been shown to be unaffected by inhibition of CYP2D6, (see 'Opioids + Quinidine', p.194).

(c) CYP3A4 inducers or inhibitors

The manufacturers state that abiraterone is a substrate of CYP3A4 *in vitro*. They therefore predict that drugs that induce or inhibit CYP3A4 might increase the concentrations of abiraterone and increase the risk of adverse effects. As the outcome of concurrent use of these drugs with abiraterone has not been studied in healthy subjects or patients, the manufacturers advise avoiding, or if this is not possible, they advise caution, on the concurrent use of abiraterone with potent inhibitors of CYP3A4: they name the azoles **itraconazole**, **ketoconazole** and **voriconazole**; the macrolides **clarithromycin** and **telithromycin**; and the HIV-protease inhibitors **atazanavir**, **indinavir**, **nelfinavir**, **ritonavir**, and **saquinavir**.[1,2] If both drugs are necessary, it would seem prudent to monitor for an increase in abiraterone adverse effects such as hypokalaemia, hypertension, and peripheral oedema. The manufacturers also predict that potent inducers of CYP3A4 will lower abiraterone concentrations, and they name **carbamazepine**, **phenytoin** (and therefore consider **fosphenytoin**), **phenobarbital** (and therefore consider **primidone**), **rifampicin**, **rifabutin**, and **rifapentine**.[1,2] If both drugs are necessary, monitor for a reduction in the efficacy of abiraterone.

(d) Food

The manufacturers briefly report that, in a study, a low-fat meal (containing 7% fat with 300 calories) increased the AUC and maximum concentration of abiraterone about fivefold and sevenfold, respectively, when compared with the fasted state. A high-fat meal (containing 57% fat with 825 calories) increased the AUC and maximum concentration of abiraterone about 10-fold and 17-fold, respectively, when compared with the fasted state. They therefore advise that abiraterone is taken on an empty stomach at least one hour before and at least 2 hours after food.[1,2]

1. Zytiga (Abiraterone acetate). Centocor Ortho Biotech, Inc. US Prescribing information, April 2011.
2. Zytiga (Abiraterone acetate). Janssen-Cilag Ltd. UK Summary of product characteristics, September 2011.

Acamprosate + Miscellaneous

Naltrexone modestly increases the rate and extent of acamprosate absorption. There is no pharmacokinetic interaction between acamprosate and alcohol or diazepam. Disulfiram does not alter the pharmacokinetics of acamprosate, and acamprosate does not alter the pharmacokinetics of imipramine or naltrexone. The combination of acamprosate and barbiturates, meprobamate, or oxazepam does not appear to increase the risk of adverse effects.

Clinical evidence, mechanism, importance and management

(a) Alcohol

In studies in healthy subjects, the pharmacokinetics of both alcohol and acamprosate were unchanged by concurrent use.[1]

(b) Disulfiram

In a study in 12 healthy subjects, disulfiram 500 mg daily for 7 days did not alter the plasma levels of acamprosate 666 mg three times daily.[1]

(c) Naltrexone

In a study in 24 healthy subjects, the concurrent use of naltrexone 50 mg daily and acamprosate 2 g daily for 7 days modestly increased the rate and extent of absorption of acamprosate, as indicated by a 33% increase in its maximum level, a 33% reduction in the time to maximum level, and a 25% increase in its AUC. There was no change in naltrexone pharmacokinetics.[2] Similarly, an increase in acamprosate levels was seen in a study into the use of acamprosate and naltrexone in alcohol-dependent subjects.[3] No particular adverse events were identified on concurrent use,[2,3] suggesting that the drugs may be used together without dose adjustment.

(d) Other drugs

A 15-day study in 591 patients, to assess the effects of the concurrent use of acamprosate with other drugs commonly used in the management of alcohol withdrawal, found no evidence of additional adverse effects when **meprobamate**, **oxazepam**, or the barbiturate complex **tetrabamate**, which includes **phenobarbital**, were also given.[4] Other studies found that acamprosate caused no clinically relevant changes in **imipramine** pharmacokinetics, and the pharmacokinetics of both **diazepam** and acamprosate were unchanged by concurrent use.[1]

No special precautions would therefore appear to be needed if any of these drugs is given with acamprosate.

1. Saivin S, Hulot T, Chabac S, Potgieter A, Durbin P, Houin G. Clinical pharmacokinetics of acamprosate. *Clin Pharmacokinet* (1998) 35, 331–45.
2. Mason BJ, Goodman AM, Dixon RM, Hameed MHA, Hulot T, Wesnes K, Hunter JA, Boyeson MG. A pharmacokinetic and pharmacodynamic drug interaction study of acamprosate and naltrexone. Neuropsychopharmacology. (2002) 27, 596–606.
3. Johnson BA, O'Malley SS, Ciraulo DA, Roache JD, Chambers RA, Sarid-Segal O, Couper D. Dose-ranging kinetics and behavioral pharmacology of naltrexone and acamprosate, both alone and combined, in alcohol-dependent subjects. *J Clin Psychopharmacol* (2003) 23, 281–93.
4. Aubin HJ, Lehert P, Beaupère B, Parot P, Barrucand D. Tolerability of the combination of acamprosate with drugs used to prevent alcohol withdrawal syndrome. *Alcoholism* (1995) 31, 25–38.

Allopurinol + Aluminium hydroxide

Three haemodialysis patients did not respond to allopurinol while taking aluminium hydroxide. Separating the doses by 3 hours appeared to solve this.

Clinical evidence

Three patients receiving haemodialysis, taking 5.7 g of aluminium hydroxide daily and allopurinol 300 mg daily for high phosphate and uric acid levels, had no reduction in their hyperuricaemia until the aluminium hydroxide was given 3 hours before the allopurinol, whereupon their uric acid levels fell by 40 to 65%. When one patient returned to taking both preparations together, her uric acid levels began to rise.[1]

Mechanism

Not understood. Antacids are well known to reduce the absorption of a number of drugs, but this is the only evidence of this possibly occurring with allopurinol.

Importance and management

Information seems to be limited to this anecdotal report. If allopurinol is not effective in patients with renal impairment taking large doses of aluminium, consider the possibility of an interaction. Try separating the administration of these two drugs by 3 hours or more. The effects of lower doses of aluminium and the effects in patients with normal renal function do not appear to have been studied.

1. Weissman I, Krivoy N. Interaction of aluminum hydroxide and allopurinol in patients on chronic hemodialysis. *Ann Intern Med* (1987) 107, 787.

Allopurinol + Iron compounds

No adverse interaction occurs if iron and allopurinol are given concurrently.

Clinical evidence, mechanism, importance and management

Some early *animal* studies, where allopurinol was given in very large doses, suggested that allopurinol might have an inhibitory effect on the release of iron from hepatic stores. It was feared that this might result in hepatic iron overload. This led the manufacturers of allopurinol in some countries to issue a warning about their concurrent use.[1] However, subsequent research suggests that no special precautions are needed.[1-3]

1. Ascione FJ. Allopurinol and iron. *JAMA* (1975) 232, 1010.
2. Emmerson BT. Effects of allopurinol on iron metabolism in man. *Ann Rheum Dis* (1966) 25, 700–703.
3. Davis PS, Deller DJ. Effect of a xanthine-oxidase inhibitor (allopurinol) on radioiron absorption in man. *Lancet* (1966) ii, 470–2.

Allopurinol + Tamoxifen

A single case report describes allopurinol hepatotoxicity in a man given tamoxifen.

Clinical evidence, mechanism, importance and management

An elderly man who had been taking allopurinol 300 mg daily for 12 years developed fever and marked increases in his serum levels of lactic dehydrogenase and alkaline phosphatase within a day of starting to take tamoxifen 10 mg twice daily.[1] He rapidly recovered when the allopurinol was stopped. The reasons for the reaction are not understood, but the authors suggested that the increased hepatotoxic effect may have resulted from tamoxifen inhibiting allopurinol metabolism, thereby increasing the serum levels of allopurinol and its metabolite. The general importance of this isolated report is not known.

1. Shah KA, Levin J, Rosen N, Greenwald E, Zumoff B. Allopurinol hepatotoxicity potentiated by tamoxifen. *N Y State J Med* (1982) 82, 1745–6.

Allopurinol + Thiazide diuretics

Severe allergic reactions to allopurinol have developed a few patients with renal impairment who were also taking thiazide diuretics.

Clinical evidence, mechanism, importance and management

Most patients tolerate allopurinol very well, but life-threatening hypersensitivity reactions (e.g. rash, vasculitis, hepatitis, eosinophilia, progressive renal impairment) develop very occasionally with doses of 200 to 400 mg of allopurinol daily.[1] A report of six such hypersensitivity reactions found that all of the reported cases were associated with pre-existing renal impairment, and in half of these, the patients were also taking thiazide diuretics.[1] Another report describes two patients who developed a hypersensitivity vasculitis while taking allopurinol and **hydrochlorothiazide**.[2] The excretion of oxipurinol (the major metabolite of allopurinol) is reduced in renal impairment, but studies indicate that, in healthy subjects with normal renal function, thiazide diuretics such as **hydrochlorothiazide** do not appear to affect either the plasma levels of oxipurinol or its excretion.[3-5] Furthermore, allopurinol does not appear to affect **hydrochlorothiazide** pharmacokinetics.[5] However, another study found that the effects of allopurinol on pyrimidine metabolism were enhanced by the use of thiazides (i.e. they potentially increase hyperuricaemia, which may lead to renal damage).[6] Some caution is therefore appropriate if both drugs are used, particularly if renal function is impaired, but more study is needed to confirm this possible interaction.

1. Hande KR, Noone RM, Stone WJ. Severe allopurinol toxicity. Description and guidelines for prevention in patients with renal insufficiency. *Am J Med* (1984) 76, 47–56.
2. Young JL, Boswell RB, Nies AS. Severe allopurinol hypersensitivity. Association with thiazides and prior renal compromise. *Arch Intern Med* (1974) 134, 553–8.
3. Hande KR. Evaluation of a thiazide-allopurinol drug interaction. *Am J Med Sci* (1986) 292, 213–16.
4. Löffler W, Landthaler R, de Vries JX, Walter-Sack I, Ittensohn A, Voss A, Zöllner N. Interaction of allopurinol and hydrochlorothiazide during prolonged oral administration of both drugs in normal subjects. I. Uric acid kinetics. *Clin Investig* (1994) 72, 1071–5.
5. de Vries JX, Voss A, Ittensohn A, Walter-Sack I, Löffler W, Landthaler R, Zöllner N. Interaction of allopurinol and hydrochlorothiazide during prolonged oral administration of both drugs in normal subjects. II. Kinetics of allopurinol, oxipurinol, and hydrochlorothiazide. *Clin Investig* (1994) 72, 1076–81.
6. Wood MH, O'Sullivan WJ, Wilson M, Tiller DJ. Potentiation of an effect of allopurinol on pyrimidine metabolism by chlorothiazide in man. *Clin Exp Pharmacol Physiol* (1974) 1, 53–8.

Allopurinol + Uricosuric drugs

Probenecid and benzbromarone increase the renal excretion of oxipurinol, the active metabolite of allopurinol. Theoretically, the use of uricosuric drugs with allopurinol could lead to uric acid precipitation in the kidneys and therefore maintenance of a high urine output is recommended when allopurinol is given by injection. Probenecid markedly increases the serum levels of allopurinol riboside, which may be advantageous in some circumstances.

Clinical evidence, mechanism, importance and management

(a) Allopurinol

Probenecid appears to increase the renal excretion of the active metabolite of allopurinol, oxipurinol,[1] while allopurinol is thought to inhibit the metabolism of **probenecid**.[2] One study suggested that allopurinol can increase the half-life and raise the serum levels of **probenecid** by about 50% and 20%, respectively.[2] However, a subsequent randomised study in 11 healthy subjects found that allopurinol 150 mg twice daily did not affect the pharmacokinetics of **probenecid** 500 mg twice daily when both drugs were given together for 7 days. This study also found that the mean plasma oxipurinol AUC and maximum levels were approximately halved when **probenecid** was added to allopurinol.[3] In another study, **benzbromarone** lowered the AUC of oxipurinol by about 40%, but did not affect allopurinol levels.[4]

It has been suggested that the use of allopurinol and **probenecid** might lead to an increase in the excretion of uric acid, which could result in the precipitation of uric acid in the kidneys. Conversely, increased renal excretion of oxipurinol might decrease the efficacy of allopurinol. However, the clinical importance of these mutual interactions seems to be minimal. No problems were reported in two studies in patients given 100 to 600 mg of allopurinol and 500 mg to 2.5 g of **probenecid** daily for between 8 and 16 weeks,[5] and the concurrent use of allopurinol and **probenecid**[3] or **benzbromarone**[4] was more effective in lowering uric acid levels than allopurinol alone. Nevertheless, the UK manufacturer of allopurinol recommends that the significance of any reduction in efficacy, which may occur when uricosuric drugs are given with allopurinol, should be assessed in each case.[6] For allopurinol injection, the US manufacturer recommends that, to help prevent renal precipitation of urates in patients receiving concurrent uricosuric drugs, a fluid intake sufficient to give a urinary output of at least 2 litres daily, and the maintenance of neutral or slightly alkaline urine, are desirable.[7]

(b) Allopurinol riboside

A study in 3 healthy subjects found that **probenecid** halved the clearance, increased the peak plasma levels and AUC, and extended the half-life of allopurinol riboside.[8] In some circumstances such an interaction may be advantageous as there is some evidence that the cure rate of American trypanosomiasis (Chagas' disease) and cutaneous leishmaniasis is better when the two drugs are used together.[8,9]

1. Elion GB, Yü T-F, Gutman AB, Hitchings GH. Renal clearance of oxipurinol, the chief metabolite of allopurinol. *Am J Med* (1968) 45, 69–77.
2. Horwitz D, Thorgeirsson SS, Mitchell JR. The influence of allopurinol and size of dose on the metabolism of phenylbutazone in patients with gout. *Eur J Clin Pharmacol* (1977) 12, 133–6.
3. Stocker SL, Williams KM, McLachlan AJ, Graham GG, Day RO. Pharmacokinetic and pharmacodynamic interaction between allopurinol and probenecid in healthy subjects. *Clin Pharmacokinet* (2008) 47, 111–8.
4. Müller FO, Schall R, Groenewoud G, Hundt HKL, van der Merwe JC, van Dyk M. The effect of benzbromarone on allopurinol/oxypurinol kinetics in patients with gout. *Eur J Clin Pharmacol* (1993) 44, 69–72.
5. Yü T-F, Gutman AB. Effect of allopurinol (4-hydroxypyrazolo(3,4-d)pyrimidine) on serum and urinary uric acid in primary and secondary gout. *Am J Med* (1964) 37, 885–98.
6. Zyloric (Allopurinol). GlaxoSmithKline UK. UK Summary of product characteristics, September 2006.
7. Aloprim (Allopurinol sodium). Bedford Laboratories. US Prescribing information, June 2004.
8. Were JBO, Shapiro TA. Effects of probenecid on the pharmacokinetics of allopurinol riboside. *Antimicrob Agents Chemother* (1993) 37, 1193–6.
9. Saenz RE, Paz HM, Johnson CM, Marr JJ, Nelson DJ, Pattishall KH, Rogers MD. Treatment of American cutaneous leishmaniasis with orally administered allopurinol riboside. *J Infect Dis* (1989) 160, 153–8.

Amifampridine + Miscellaneous

Amifampridine is predicted to increase the effects of the anticholinesterases. Drugs with antimuscarinic effects are predicted to reduce the efficacy of amifampridine. Drugs that lower the seizure threshold may

increase the risk of seizures with amifampridine. Drugs that are enzyme inhibitors (e.g. ketoconazole) or inducers (e.g. carbamazepine) are predicted to affect the concentrations of amifampridine. The concurrent use of neuromuscular blockers with amifampridine might reduce the effects of both drugs. The effect of food on the pharmacokinetics of amifampridine is unknown.

Clinical evidence, mechanism, importance and management

(a) Anticholinesterases

Amifampridine prolongs neuromuscular depolarisation and this leads to an increase in the release of acetylcholine into the neuromuscular junction. The manufacturer therefore states that concurrent use with an anticholinesterase might lead to an increase in the effects of both drugs.[1] It would seem prudent to bear the possibility of an interaction in mind should an increase in cholinergic adverse effects (such as nausea, vomiting, blurred vision, drowsiness) occur. See 'Table 11.1', p.365, for a list of anticholinesterases.

(b) Antimuscarinics

Amifampridine prolongs neuromuscular depolarisation and this leads to an increase in the release of acetylcholine into the neuromuscular junction. The manufacturer therefore predicts that the concurrent use of amifampridine and antimuscarinics (which block the actions of acetylcholine) might reduce the efficacy of both drugs and they caution concurrent use. They name the **tricyclics**, some **antihistamines**, **antimuscarinics** (see 'Table 18.2', p.754, for a list), atropine-like **antispasmodics**, **phenothiazines**, **disopyramide** and **clozapine**.[1]

Note that the tricyclics and phenothiazines may also increase the risk of seizures with amifampridine, see *Drugs that lower the seizure threshold*, below. Note also that **clozapine**, **disopyramide**, some phenothiazines, and some tricyclics are predicted to increase the risk of QT prolongation with amifampridine, see 'Drugs that prolong the QT interval + Other drugs that prolong the QT interval', p.272, for further information on the concurrent use of two or more drugs that prolong the QT interval.

(c) Drugs that lower the seizure threshold

Amifampridine might increase the risk of seizures: this effect is dose-dependent. The manufacturer therefore states that the risks of using other drugs that lower the seizure threshold should be considered carefully. They name the **tricyclics**, **SSRIs**, **phenothiazines** and **butyrophenones**, **mefloquine**, **bupropion** and **tramadol**. Note that amifampridine is contraindicated in patients with epilepsy.[1]

Note that some tricyclics, some phenothiazines and some butyrophenones are also associated with an increased risk of QT interval prolongation, see 'Drugs that prolong the QT interval + Other drugs that prolong the QT interval', p.272, for further information on the concurrent use of two or more drugs that prolong the QT interval. Some of these drugs also have antimuscarinic adverse effects, see *Antimuscarinics*, above.

(d) Enzyme inhibitors or inducers

The manufacturer of amifampridine states that the mechanism of the metabolism and elimination of amifampridine is unknown. There is also no data regarding the potential for amifampridine to interact with cytochrome P450, although they do state that elimination might be mainly by the kidneys, suggesting any interaction could be limited. Nevertheless, because of the lack of data, the manufacturer of amifampridine advises caution on the concurrent use of enzyme inhibitors (they name **cimetidine** and **ketoconazole**) or inducers (they name the **barbiturates**, **carbamazepine** and **rifamycins**). They advise monitoring patients for increased amifampridine adverse effects (such as paraesthesias, nausea and diarrhoea) or a reduction in the efficacy of amifampridine, and adjusting the dose of amifampridine as necessary.[1]

(e) Food

The manufacturer notes that the effect of food on the absorption of amifampridine has not been studied; however they advise that amifampridine should be taken with food.[1]

(f) Neuromuscular blockers

Amifampridine prolongs neuromuscular depolarisation and the manufacturer therefore predicts that concurrent use with a non-depolarising muscle relaxant or with a depolarising muscle relaxant might decrease the efficacy of both drugs.[1] It would be prudent to bear the possibility of an interaction in mind should a loss of efficacy of amifampridine or the muscle relaxant occur. See 'Table 5.2', p.98, for a list of neuromuscular blockers.

(g) Other drugs

The manufacturer of amifampridine states that there is no data regarding the route of metabolism of amifampridine or the potential for amifampridine to interact with cytochrome P450. As the potential for an interaction between amifampridine and other drugs cannot be ruled out, they caution its use with other drugs that are metabolised or actively secreted: concurrent use should be monitored and dose adjustments of the affected drug made if necessary. They specifically contraindicate the concurrent use of amifampridine with drugs that have a narrow therapeutic margin.[1]

1. Firdapse (Amifampridine phosphate). BioMarin Europe Ltd. UK Summary of product characteristics, December 2009.

Apremilast + Combined hormonal contraceptives

No pharmacokinetic interaction occurs between apremilast and ethinylestradiol or norgestimate.

Clinical evidence, mechanism, importance and management

The UK and US manufacturers briefly note that in a study, there was no pharmacokinetic interaction between apremilast and **ethinylestradiol** or **norgestimate**, when given as an oral combined hormonal contraceptive.[1,2] No dose adjustments are therefore necessary on concurrent use.[1,2]

1. Otezla (Apremilast). Celgene Ltd. UK Summary of product characteristics, January 2015.
2. Otezla (Apremilast). Celgene Corporation. US Prescribing information, December 2014.

Apremilast + Ketoconazole and other CYP3A4 inhibitors

Ketoconazole slightly increases apremilast exposure. Other potent CYP3A4 inhibitors might be expected to interact similarly.

Clinical evidence

In a study in 18 healthy subjects, ketoconazole 400 mg daily for 5 days increased the AUC of a single 20-mg dose of apremilast by 36%.[1]

Mechanism

Ketoconazole is a potent inhibitor of CYP3A4, by which apremilast is partly metabolised. Concurrent use therefore increases apremilast exposure.

Importance and management

Evidence for an interaction between ketoconazole and apremilast is limited to this study, but a pharmacokinetic interaction would seem to be established. However, as the increase in apremilast exposure is only slight, it is unlikely to be clinically relevant. No dose adjustment or additional monitoring would seem necessary on concurrent use with ketoconazole or other CYP3A4 inhibitors.

1. Liu Y, Zhou S, Wan Y, Wu A, Palmisano M. The impact of co-administration of ketoconazole and rifampicin on the pharmacokinetics of apremilast in healthy volunteers. *Br J Clin Pharmacol* (2014) 78, 1050–7.

Apremilast + Methotrexate

No pharmacokinetic interaction occurs between apremilast and methotrexate.

Clinical evidence, mechanism, importance and management

In a study in 15 patients with rheumatoid and psoriatic arthritis who were stable taking methotrexate 7.5 to 20 mg once weekly, apremilast 30 mg twice daily for 6 days had no effect on the pharmacokinetics of methotrexate.[1] Similarly, the pharmacokinetics of apremilast were not affected. No dose adjustments are therefore necessary on concurrent use.

1. Liu Y, Zhou S, Nissel J, Wu A, Lau H, Palmisano M. The pharmacokinetic effect of coadministration of apremilast and methotrexate in individuals with rheumatoid arthritis and psoriatic arthritis. *Clin Pharmacol Drug Dev* (2014) 3, 456–65.

Apremilast + Rifampicin (Rifampin) and other CYP3A4 inducers

Rifampicin moderately decreases apremilast exposure. Other potent inducers of CYP3A4 might be expected to interact similarly.

Clinical evidence

In a study in 20 healthy subjects, rifampicin 600 mg daily for 14 days decreased the AUC and maximum plasma concentration of a single 30-mg dose of apremilast by 72% and 43%, respectively.[1]

Mechanism

Rifampicin is a potent inducer of CYP3A4, by which apremilast is partly metabolised. Concurrent use therefore decreases apremilast exposure.

Importance and management

Evidence for an interaction between rifampicin and apremilast is limited to this study, but a pharmacokinetic interaction would seem to be established. The decrease in apremilast exposure is moderate, hence the UK and US manufacturers advise that concurrent use of rifampicin and other potent CYP3A4 inducers is not recommended due to a possible reduction in the clinical effect of apremilast.[2,3] Note that the UK manufacturer includes **St John's wort** as a potent inducer, but it is generally considered as moderate. For a list of other potent CYP3A4 inducers, see 'Table 1.9', p.11.

1. Liu Y, Zhou S, Wan Y, Wu A, Palmisano M. The impact of co-administration of ketoconazole and rifampicin on the pharmacokinetics of apremilast in healthy volunteers. *Br J Clin Pharmacol* (2014) 78, 1050–7.

2. Otezla (Apremilast). Celgene Ltd. UK Summary of product characteristics, January 2015.
3. Otezla (Apremilast). Celgene Corporation. US Prescribing information, December 2014.

Ataluren + Miscellaneous

Ataluren might increase the risk of nephrotoxicity with intravenous aminoglycosides. Ataluren exposure is predicted to be increased by inhibitors of BCRP, and decreased by inducers of UGT1A9. Ataluren is predicted to increase the exposure of drugs that are metabolised by UGT1A9 or transported by OATP1B3, OAT1, and OAT3. There appears to be no pharmacokinetic interaction between ataluren and systemic corticosteroids.

Clinical evidence, mechanism, importance and management

(a) Aminoglycosides

The manufacturer briefly reports that in a clinical trial in cystic fibrosis patients, the concurrent use of ataluren and intravenous aminoglycosides resulted in a number of cases of increased creatinine concentrations. In all cases this resolved on stopping the aminoglycoside, or interrupting or stopping the ataluren. They suggest that ataluren might potentiate the nephrotoxic effects of aminoglycosides and therefore contra-indicate concurrent use. If the aminoglycoside is necessary, ataluren should be stopped during treatment and should not be restarted until 2 days after the last dose of the aminoglycoside. Further, the patient should be well hydrated. Use of other **nephrotoxic drugs** (e.g. **vancomycin**) is also not recommended, but if such a combination is unavoidable careful monitoring of renal function is advised.[1]

(b) Breast cancer resistance protein (BCRP) inhibitors

In vitro, ataluren is a substrate of the drug transporter, breast cancer resistance protein (BCRP).[1] Inhibitors of this drug transporter could increase the exposure to ataluren, and the manufacturer therefore advises caution on concurrent use with drugs that are inhibitors of BCRP (they name **ciclosporin**).[1] However, note that predictions made on the basis of *in vitro* effects do not always mirror what happens in clinical use. Hence further study is required to establish the relevance, if any, in practice.

(c) Corticosteroids

The manufacturer briefly reports that concurrent use of corticosteroids (**deflazacort**, **prednisone**, or **prednisolone**) with ataluren did not affect the plasma concentrations of ataluren or the corticosteroid.[1]

Note however that blood pressure should be monitored every 6 months, or more frequently if necessary, in patients taking ataluren and systemic corticosteroids since both drugs can cause hypertension and concurrent use is likely to exacerbate this effect.[1]

(d) UDP-glucuronosyltransferase inducers

Ataluren is metabolised by glucuronidation, mainly by the glucuronosyltransferase, UGT1A9, in the liver and intestine. Inducers of this enzyme could decrease the exposure to ataluren, and the manufacturer advises caution on concurrent use with such drugs (they name **mycophenolate**).[1]

(e) Other drugs

In vitro, ataluren is an inhibitor of UGT1A9, the organic anion transporting polypeptide, OATP1B3, and the organic anion transporters, OAT1 and OAT3. The manufacturer therefore advises caution when ataluren is given with drugs that are substrates of these because of the risk of increases in exposure [and hence adverse effects] of these drugs. They specifically name **aciclovir**, **bumetanide**, **captopril**, **ciprofloxacin**, **furosemide**, the statins **atorvastatin**, **pravastatin**, **pitavastatin**, and **rosuvastatin**, **oseltamivir**, and **valsartan**.[1] Note that predictions made on the basis of *in vitro* effects do not always mirror what happens in clinical use. Hence further study is required to establish the relevance, if any, in practice.

1. Translarna (Ataluren). PTC Therapeutics International Limited. European Prescribing information, July 2014.

Baclofen + Ibuprofen

A man developed baclofen toxicity when given ibuprofen.

Clinical evidence, mechanism, importance and management

An isolated report describes a 64-year-old man taking baclofen 20 mg three times daily, who developed baclofen toxicity (confusion, disorientation, bradycardia, blurred vision, hypotension and hypothermia) after taking 8 doses of ibuprofen 600 mg three times daily. It appeared that the toxicity was caused by ibuprofen-induced acute renal impairment leading to baclofen accumulation.[1] Renal impairment is a relatively rare adverse effect of ibuprofen. The general importance of this interaction is likely to be very small. There appears to be no information about baclofen and other NSAIDs, and little reason for avoiding concurrent use.

1. Dahlin PA, George J. Baclofen toxicity associated with declining renal clearance after ibuprofen. *Drug Intell Clin Pharm* (1984) 18, 805–8.

Baclofen + Miscellaneous

Common adverse effects of baclofen include hypotension, sedation and somnolence. Bear the possibility of additive effects in mind when baclofen is used with antihypertensives or drugs causing sedation.[1]

1. Lioresal Tablets (Baclofen). Novartis Pharmaceuticals UK Ltd. UK Summary of product characteristics, February 2013.

Baclofen + Tizanidine

No pharmacokinetic interaction appears to occur between baclofen and tizanidine.

Clinical evidence, mechanism, importance and management

In a randomised, three-period study, 15 healthy subjects were given baclofen 10 mg three times daily and tizanidine 4 mg three times daily, together and alone, for 7 consecutive doses. There was no change in the steady-state AUC or maximum level of tizanidine or baclofen when given together. The only change that was statistically significant was a 27% increase in the renal clearance of one tizanidine metabolite, but this was not considered clinically relevant.[1] No changes in the doses of either drug are therefore likely to be needed if they are taken concurrently.

1. Shellenberger MK, Groves L, Shah J, Novak GD. A controlled pharmacokinetic evaluation of tizanidine and baclofen at steady state. *Drug Metab Dispos* (1999) 27, 201–4.

Benzbromarone + Chlorothiazide

Benzbromarone lowers uric acid levels in patients taking chlorothiazide, without affecting diuretic activity.[1,2]

1. Heel RC, Brogden RN, Speight TM, Avery GS. Benzbromarone: a review of its pharmacological properties and therapeutic use in gout and hyperuricaemia. *Drugs* (1977) 14, 349–66.
2. Gross A, Giraud V. Über die Wirkung von Benzbromaron auf Urikämie und Urikosurie. *Med Welt* (1972) 23, 133–6.

Betahistine + Antihistamines

Betahistine is predicted to antagonise the effects of antihistamines.

Clinical evidence, mechanism, importance and management

On theoretical grounds, betahistine is expected to antagonise the effects of the antihistamines, because betahistine is an analogue of histamine.[1] However, there appears to be only one, isolated, unconfirmed, very brief case report of an interaction, which describes a patient whose labyrinthine symptoms (vertigo, dizziness, nausea and vomiting) were controlled by betahistine, and whose symptoms returned during the concurrent use of terfenadine and other unspecified drugs.[2] The general relevance of this interaction is unclear.

1. Serc (Betahistine). Solvay Healthcare Ltd. UK Summary of product characteristics, October 2006.
2. Beeley L, Cunningham H, Brennan A. *Adverse Drug React Bull* (1993) 36, 28.

Bisphosphonates + Aminoglycosides

Severe hypocalcaemia occurred in three patients taking sodium clodronate when they were given netilmicin or amikacin. Theoretically, additive calcium lowering effects could occur with any bisphosphonate and aminoglycoside combination.

Clinical evidence

A 62-year-old woman with multiple myeloma was given **sodium clodronate** 2.4 g daily for osteolysis and bone pain. After 7 days she developed grand mal seizures, and her serum calcium was found to be 1.72 mmol/L (reference range 2.25 to 2.6 mmol/L). Despite daily calcium infusions her calcium remained low. The authors state that symptomatic hypocalcaemia with clodronate is rare, and attributed the dramatic response in this patient to an interaction with a course of **netilmicin** given 5 days earlier for septicaemia.[1]

A 69-year-old man with prostate cancer had been taking **sodium clodronate** 2.4 g daily for bone pain for 13 months, and serum calcium levels had always remained within the reference range. After being admitted with febrile neutropenia following a course of chemotherapy, the clodronate was withdrawn and he was given intravenous **amikacin** and ceftazidime. After 7 days he became unconscious, and developed spontaneous twitching movements in his arms and legs. His calcium was found to be 1.39 mmol/L and he was diagnosed with hypocalcaemic tetany. He was given calcium infusions, and his serum calcium returned to normal over the next 12 hours.[2]

A further case report describes a 50-year-old patient taking **clodronate** 1.6 g daily, who developed febrile neutropenia for which he was given **amikacin** and ampicillin. Five days after starting **amikacin** his calcium began to fall and, despite stopping the clodronate and supplementing with calcium 8 g daily, his calcium level stabilised at just 1.65 mmol/L. The patient subsequently died from aspergillus pneumonia.[3]

Mechanism

Not fully understood, but one suggestion is that any fall in blood calcium levels brought about by the use of clodronate is normally balanced to some extent by the excretion of parathyroid hormone, which raises blood calcium levels. However, the aminoglycoside antibacterials can damage the kidneys, not only causing the loss of calcium, but of magnesium as well. Any hypomagnesaemia inhibits the activity of the parathyroid gland, so that the normal homoeostatic response to hypocalcaemia is reduced or even abolished.[1,2] Clodronate itself can sometimes be nephrotoxic.

Importance and management

Direct information seems to be limited to these three reports. Biochemical hypocalcaemia is believed to occur in about 10% of patients taking bisphosphonates,[4] but symptomatic hypocalcaemia is said to be rare.[2] It seems therefore that the addition of the aminoglycoside in these cases precipitated severe clinical hypocalcaemia. The authors of these reports therefore advise care if bisphosphonates are given with aminoglycosides, and recommend close monitoring of calcium and magnesium levels.[1-3] They also point out that the renal loss of calcium and magnesium can continue for weeks after aminoglycosides are stopped, and that bisphosphonates can also persist in bone for weeks.[1,2] This means that the interaction is potentially possible whether the drugs are given concurrently or sequentially. Note also that some manufacturers advise caution on the concurrent use of other drugs that cause nephrotoxicity, as concurrent use may lead to an increase in bisphosphonate levels; this would reasonably be expected to include the aminoglycosides.

1. Pedersen-Bjergaard U, Myhre J. Severe hypoglycaemia (sic) after treatment with diphosphonate and aminoglycoside. *BMJ* (1991) 302, 295.
2. Mayordomo JI, Rivera F. Severe hypocalcaemia after treatment with oral clodronate and aminoglycoside. *Ann Oncol* (1993) 4, 432–5.
3. Bondiau PY, Peyrade F, Creisson A, Pivot X, Lagrange JL, Thyss A. Hypocalcémie sévère après traitment par diphosphonates et aminoglycosides. *Presse Med* (1994) 23, 816.
4. Jodrell DI, Iveson TJ, Smith IE. Symptomatic hypocalcaemia after treatment with high-dose aminohydroxypropylidene diphosphonate. *Lancet* (1987) i, 622.

Bisphosphonates + Aspirin or NSAIDs

The concurrent use of alendronate and naproxen increased the incidence of gastric mucosal damage in a small pharmacological study, and increased the risk of upper gastrointestinal disorders in a case-control study. However, two analyses of placebo-controlled studies found no increased risk of gastrointestinal damage with the combination. There was no increased risk of gastrointestinal adverse effects in patients taking NSAIDs who were given risedronate.

Indometacin raises tiludronate bioavailability, whereas aspirin and diclofenac do not appear to affect the pharmacokinetics of tiludronate. NSAIDs may exacerbate the renal impairment sometimes seen with clodronate; zoledronate is predicted to interact similarly.

Clinical evidence, mechanism, importance and management

(a) Alendronate

In a short-term endoscopy study in 26 healthy subjects, gastric mucosal damage developed in 8% of those given alendronate alone, in 12% of those given **naproxen** alone, and 38% of those given both drugs.[1] In a case-control study,[2] the risk of having an acid-related upper gastrointestinal disorder with alendronate was increased by the concurrent use of NSAIDs (relative risk 1.7). However, retrospective analysis of data from a very large long-term placebo-controlled study found no evidence that the risk of upper gastrointestinal adverse effects with concurrent use of NSAIDs and alendronate was any greater than with NSAIDs and placebo.[3] Note that this finding has been questioned,[4] and some of the issues responded to.[5] Similarly, in a retrospective analysis of a 12-week placebo-controlled study, in those taking regular NSAIDs (about half of the patients) there was no difference in the incidence of upper gastrointestinal adverse events between those given alendronate and those given placebo. The most commonly used NSAIDs in this study were **aspirin**, **celecoxib**, **rofecoxib**, **ibuprofen** and **naproxen**.[6]

Alendronate is commonly known to be associated with oesophageal adverse effects, and there are strict dosing instructions to minimise this risk.[7] It may also cause local irritation of the stomach, although its potential to cause gastric ulcers is not considered established.[3,7]

The interpretation of these data has been debated. Some consider that alendronate should not be given to patients taking NSAIDs,[4] while others urge caution in their use together.[1,2] However, some consider that there is no evidence that alendronate adds to the known gastrointestinal toxicity of NSAIDs.[5] The UK manufacturer issues no caution about the concurrent use of NSAIDs with alendronate.[7] The US manufacturer states that alendronate can be used with NSAIDs, but that caution is required.[8] It would seem sensible to monitor the concurrent use of alendronate and NSAIDs carefully.

(b) Clodronate

The manufacturer notes that patients receiving NSAIDs with clodronate have developed renal impairment, although a synergistic action has not been established.[9] Clodronate alone may cause renal impairment, and the manufacturer suggests that renal function should be assessed before giving clodronate.[9] This would seem particularly important in those taking NSAIDs.

(c) Ibandronate

The manufacturer notes that the incidence of upper gastrointestinal adverse events in patients taking NSAIDs or aspirin did not differ between those receiving ibandronate and those receiving placebo in a large clinical osteoporosis study.[10] In this study, 62% of patients were taking aspirin or NSAIDs. Nevertheless, the manufacturers recommend that, since both bisphosphonates and NSAIDs are associated with gastrointestinal irritation, caution should be taken during concurrent use.[10,11]

(d) Risedronate

In a pooled analysis of phase III osteoporosis studies of risedronate, there was no increased risk of upper gastrointestinal adverse events in those also receiving aspirin and/or NSAIDs (63% of patients).[12] Similarly, in a retrospective analysis of a 2-year placebo-controlled study, in those regularly taking NSAIDs (about two-thirds of patients) there was no difference in the incidence of upper gastrointestinal adverse events between those given risedronate and those given placebo.[13] A similar lack of difference in incidence of gastrointestinal adverse effects was also seen in a once-weekly risedronate study.[14] This suggests that no special precautions are likely to be necessary on concurrent use.

(e) Tiludronate

Single-dose studies in 12 healthy subjects found that **diclofenac** 25 mg and aspirin 600 mg had no significant effect on the pharmacokinetics of tiludronate when taken at the same time. When taken 2 hours after tiludronate, aspirin decreased the AUC of tiludronate by about 50% and diclofenac increased it by about 50%, but neither of these changes was statistically significant.[15] On the other hand, **indometacin** 50 mg increased the maximum serum concentration and the AUC of tiludronate about twofold when these drugs were taken together, but not when they were given 2 hours apart.[15] For this reason the manufacturers advise that **indometacin** and tiludronate should be given 2 hours apart.[16,17] The US manufacturer also advises that aspirin should not be taken within 2 hours of tiludronate,[17] but the reason for this is unclear.

(f) Zoledronate

Although there appears to be no direct evidence regarding the use of zoledronate with NSAIDs, one US manufacturer[18] states that caution is warranted on the concurrent use of nephrotoxic drugs, and specifically names the NSAIDs. Consider also, *Clodronate*, above.

1. Graham DY, Malaty HM. Alendronate and naproxen are synergistic for development of gastric ulcers. *Arch Intern Med* (2001) 161, 107–110.
2. Ettinger B, Pressman A, Schein J. Clinic visits and hospital admissions for care of acid-related upper gastrointestinal disorders in women using alendronate for osteoporosis. *Am J Manag Care* (1998) 4, 1377–82.
3. Bauer DC, Black D, Ensrud K, Thompson D, Hochberg M, Nevitt M, Musliner T, Freedholm D, for the Fracture Intervention Trial Research Group. Upper gastrointestinal tract safety profile of alendronate. *Arch Intern Med* (2000) 160, 517–25.
4. Rothschild BM. Alendronate and nonsteroidal anti-inflammatory drug interaction safety is not established. *Arch Intern Med* (2000) 160, 1702.
5. Bauer DC, for the Fracture Intervention Trial Research Group. Alendronate and nonsteroidal anti-inflammatory drug interaction safety is not established: a reply. *Arch Intern Med* (2000) 160, 2686.
6. Cryer B, Miller P, Petruschke RA, Chen E, Geba GP, de Papp AE. Upper gastrointestinal tolerability of once weekly alendronate 70 mg with concomitant non-steroidal anti-inflammatory drug use. *Aliment Pharmacol Ther* (2005) 21, 599–607.
7. Fosamax Once Weekly (Alendronate sodium). Merck Sharp & Dohme Ltd. UK Summary of product characteristics, October 2008.
8. Fosamax (Alendronate sodium). Merck & Co. Inc. US Prescribing information, June 2009.
9. Bonefos Capsules (Sodium clodronate). Schering Health Care Ltd. UK Summary of product characteristics, June 2013.
10. Boniva (Ibandronate sodium). Roche Therapeutics Inc. US Prescribing information, January 2011.
11. Bonviva Film-Coated Tablets (Ibandronic sodium monohydrate). Roche Products Ltd. UK Summary of product characteristics, July 2011.
12. Taggart H, Bolognese MA, Lindsay R, Ettinger MP, Mulder H, Josse RG, Roberts A, Zippel H, Adami S, Ernst TF, Stevens KP. Upper gastrointestinal tract safety of risedronate: a pooled analysis of 9 clinical trials. *Mayo Clin Proc* (2002) 77, 262–70. Correction: *ibid.*, 601.
13. Adami S, Pavelka K, Cline GA, Hosterman MA, Barton IP, Cohen SB, Bensen WG. Upper gastrointestinal tract safety of daily oral risedronate in patients taking NSAIDs: a randomized, double-blind, placebo-controlled trial. *Mayo Clin Proc* (2005) 80, 1278–85.
14. Actonel Once a Week (Risedronate sodium). Warner Chilcott UK Ltd. UK Summary of product characteristics, February 2013.
15. Sanofi Winthrop. Data on file. June 1996.
16. Skelid (Disodium tiludronate). Sanofi-Aventis. UK Summary of product characteristics, November 2008.
17. Skelid (Tiludronate disodium). Sanofi-Aventis US. US Prescribing information, April 2006.
18. Reclast (Zoledronic acid). Novartis. US Prescribing information, January 2010.

Bisphosphonates + Miscellaneous

Ranitidine has no clinically significant effect on the pharmacokinetics of ibandronate, nor is there any pharmacokinetic interaction with hormone replacement therapy or tamoxifen. Melphalan and prednisolone have been given uneventfully with ibandronate. The risk of hypocalcaemia is predicted to be increased if loop diuretics are given with bisphosphonates, but a loop diuretic has been reported not to alter the calcium-lowering effect of pamidronate.

Clinical evidence, mechanism, importance and management

(a) Diuretics

Loop diuretics alone have been used to treat hypercalcaemia, so their effect might be additive with that of bisphosphonates used to treat hypercalcaemia. One US manufacturer of **zoledronic acid** advises caution on the concurrent use of loop diuretics because of an increased risk of hypocalcaemia.[1] In contrast, one UK manufacturer of **zoledronic acid**[2] and one manufacturer of **ibandronate**[3] note that, in clinical studies, no clinically significant interactions appeared to occur in patients also given diuretics, and the US manufacturer of **pamidronate** states that a loop diuretic had no effect on the calcium-lowering action of **pamidronate**.[4] Whether a clinically relevant interaction occurs is therefore unclear. However, note that calcium levels should be monitored in patients given bisphosphonates and therefore any interaction is likely to be identified by routine monitoring.

(b) HRT

The UK manufacturer of **ibandronate** briefly notes that, in a pharmacokinetic study in postmenopausal women, **ibandronate** did not interact with hormone replacement therapy.[5]

(c) Melphalan with prednisolone

The UK manufacturer of **ibandronate** briefly notes that no interaction was seen when **ibandronate** was given with melphalan and prednisolone in patients with multiple myeloma.[5]

(d) Ranitidine

The US manufacturer of ibandronate reports that in a study, healthy subjects were given ranitidine 25 mg intravenously 90 and 15 minutes before a single 10-mg oral dose of **ibandronate**, with a further 25-mg dose of ranitidine 30 minutes after taking **ibandronate**. Ranitidine slightly increased the oral bioavailability of **ibandronate** by 20%.[6] This increase is not considered to be clinically relevant[6] and no dose adjustment of ibandronate is needed on concurrent use.[5]

(e) Tamoxifen

The UK manufacturer of **ibandronate** briefly notes that, in a pharmacokinetic study in postmenopausal women, **ibandronate** did not interact with tamoxifen.[5]

1. Zometa (Zoledronic acid). Novartis. US Prescribing information, January 2010.
2. Zometa (Zoledronic acid). Novartis Pharmaceuticals UK Ltd. UK Summary of product characteristics, January 2010.
3. Bondronat Film-Coated Tablets (Ibandronate sodium monohydrate). Roche Products Ltd. UK Summary of product characteristics, July 2011.
4. Aredia (Pamidronate disodium). Novartis. US Prescribing information, November 2008.
5. Bonviva Film-Coated Tablets (Ibandronic sodium monohydrate). Roche Products Ltd. UK Summary of product characteristics, July 2011.
6. Boniva (Ibandronate sodium). Roche Therapeutics Inc. US Prescribing information, January 2011.

Bisphosphonates + Polyvalent cations

The oral absorption of bisphosphonates is reduced by food and polyvalent cations, including aluminium/magnesium hydroxide, bismuth and other antacids, calcium-rich foods, calcium supplements, iron preparations, magnesium-containing laxatives and milk.

Clinical evidence

(a) Alendronate

In pharmacokinetic studies, taking alendronate either 60 or 30 minutes before a standardised breakfast reduced its bioavailability by 40%, when compared with taking it 2 hours before breakfast. Taking alendronate with breakfast markedly reduced its bioavailability by more than 85%, as did taking alendronate 2 hours after breakfast. Both **black coffee** and **orange juice** reduced alendronate bioavailability by about 60%.[1]

(b) Clodronate

In a randomised study in 31 healthy subjects, the AUC of clodronate was reduced to 10% of the optimum level when it was taken with breakfast. Delaying administration until 2 hours after breakfast only slightly improved the AUC (34% of optimum). The best AUC was achieved when clodronate was given 2 hours before breakfast, although the AUC one hour before breakfast was similar (91% of optimum).[2]

(c) Ibandronate

The manufacturer notes that the extent of absorption of ibandronate is impaired when it is taken with food or beverages (other than plain water). Bioavailability is reduced by about 90% when ibandronate is given with a standard breakfast, when compared with the bioavailability seen in fasted subjects. The manufacturers say that there is no meaningful reduction in bioavailability when ibandronic acid is taken 60 minutes before a meal[3] or the first food of the day.[4]

(d) Risedronate

The absorption of risedronate 30 mg, taken 30 minutes before breakfast, was reduced by 55%, when compared with the fasting state (no food or drink for 10 hours before or for 4 hours after dosing). Administration one hour before breakfast reduces absorption by 30%, when compared with the fasting state. Administration 2 hours after dinner (evening meal) results in similar absorption to administration 30 minutes before breakfast.[5,6] The manufacturer says that risedronate is clinically effective when taken at least 30 minutes before breakfast.[5]

(e) Tiludronate

In a study in 12 healthy subjects the maximum serum levels and AUC of tiludronate were halved when *Maalox* (**aluminium/magnesium hydroxide**) was taken one hour before tiludronate, but the bioavailability was only slightly affected when *Maalox* was taken 2 hours after tiludronate.[7]

Mechanism

The bisphosphonates can form complexes with a number of polyvalent metallic ions (e.g. Al^{3+}, Ca^{2+}, Fe, Mg^{2+}), which can impair their absorption.

Importance and management

Established and important interactions. Bisphosphonates should be prevented from coming into contact with a range of preparations such as **antacids** (containing **aluminium, bismuth, calcium, magnesium**), laxatives (containing magnesium), **iron preparations** and calcium or other **mineral supplements**. **Food**, in particular **milk** and **dairy products**, contain calcium, and may also impair absorption.

Recommendations on the timing of administration of bisphosphonates in relation to food and other drugs vary slightly between products.

- The manufacturers of **alendronate**[8,9] suggest that, in order to avoid absorption interactions, patients should take alendronate after an overnight fast at least 30 minutes before taking any other drug or food, and that alendronate should be taken with plain (not mineral) water only.
- The manufacturers of **clodronate**[10] suggest leaving one hour between the administration of food and clodronate.
- The manufacturers of **etidronate**[11,12] recommend it is given on an empty stomach at least 2 hours from any food, particularly that containing polyvalent cations (as listed above), and from medicines containing these cations.
- The manufacturers of **ibandronate**[3,4,13] recommend it is taken with plain water on an empty stomach (overnight fast of at least 6 hours) at least 30 minutes[13] to one hour[4] before the first food or drink (other than water) of the day, or any other medications.
- The manufacturers of **risedronate**[5,14] recommend it is taken with water at least 30 minutes before the first food or drink of the day. Alternatively, they say it should be given at least 2 hours from any food or drink at any other time of the day, and at least 30 minutes before going to bed.
- The manufacturers of **tiludronate**[15,16] recommend that it is taken with water on an empty stomach (at least 2 hours before or after meals). In addition, they recommend that administration of tiludronate and antacids or calcium compounds should be separated by 2 hours.

1. Gertz BJ, Holland SD, Kline WF, Matuszewski BK, Freeman A, Quan H, Lasseter KC, Mucklow JC, Porras AG. Studies of the oral bioavailability of alendronate. *Clin Pharmacol Ther* (1995) 58, 288–98.
2. Laitinen K, Patronen A, Harju P, Löyttyniemi E, Pylkkänen L, Kleimola T, Perttunen K. Timing of food intake has a marked effect on the bioavailability of clodronate. *Bone* (2000) 27, 293–6.
3. Boniva (Ibandronate sodium). Roche Therapeutics Inc. US Prescribing information, January 2011.
4. Bonviva Film-Coated Tablets (Ibandronic sodium monohydrate). Roche Products Ltd. UK Summary of product characteristics, July 2011.
5. Actonel (Risedronate sodium). Procter & Gamble Pharmaceuticals Inc. US Prescribing information, April 2008.
6. Mitchell DY, Heise MA, Pallone KA, Clay ME, Nesbitt JD, Russell DA, Melson CW. The effect of dosing regimen on the pharmacokinetics of risedronate. *Br J Clin Pharmacol* (1999) 48, 536–42.
7. Sanofi Winthrop. Data on file. June 1996.
8. Fosamax Once Weekly (Alendronate sodium). Merck Sharp & Dohme Ltd. UK Summary of product characteristics, October 2008.
9. Fosamax (Alendronate sodium). Merck & Co. Inc. US Prescribing information, June 2009.
10. Bonefos Capsules (Sodium clodronate). Schering Health Care Ltd. UK Summary of product characteristics, June 2013.
11. Didronel (Etidronate disodium). Procter & Gamble Pharmaceuticals UK Ltd. UK Summary of product characteristics, October 2006.
12. Didronel (Etidronate disodium). Procter & Gamble Pharmaceuticals. US Prescribing information, October 2007.
13. Bondronat Film-Coated Tablets (Ibandronate sodium monohydrate). Roche Products Ltd. UK Summary of product characteristics, July 2011.
14. Actonel 30 mg Film Coated Tablets (Risedronate sodium). Warner Chilcott UK Ltd. UK Summary of product characteristics, February 2013.
15. Skelid (Disodium tiludronate). Sanofi-Aventis. UK Summary of product characteristics, November 2008.
16. Skelid (Tiludronate disodium). Sanofi-Aventis US. US Prescribing information, April 2006.

Bisphosphonates + Thalidomide

The pharmacokinetics of zoledronate are not affected by thalidomide. It is uncertain if thalidomide increases the risk of osteonecrosis of the jaw caused by bisphosphonates.

Clinical evidence

(a) Renal function and pharmacokinetics

Acute renal failure (a marked rise in creatinine levels with hypocalcaemia) occurred in 2 of 16 patients with myeloma who had their bisphosphonate treatment switched from **pamidronate** to **zoledronate**. Both of these patients were also taking thalidomide, which was speculated to possibly have contributed to the renal impairment.[1] However, in a sub-study of a controlled clinical study, there was no evidence of renal impairment, and no difference in serum creatinine levels between 12 patients receiving thalidomide and 12 patients not receiving thalidomide, for up to 16 infusions of **zoledronate**. In this study, intravenous zoledronic acid 4 mg every 4 weeks with alternate day prednisolone was given, with or without thalidomide 200 mg daily, for up to 16 months. Moreover, the zoledronic acid pharmacokinetics during the first and second infusions did not differ between 12 patients randomised to receive thalidomide and 12 patients not receiving thalidomide. The subjects in this study were patients with multiple myeloma with no disease progression 6 weeks after autologous stem-cell transplantation and conditioning with melphalan.[2]

(b) Osteonecrosis of the jaw

In a retrospective analysis of 28 cases of osteonecrosis of the jaw occurring in 254 patients given **pamidronate** or **zoledronate**, **zoledronate** was associated with a much higher risk than **pamidronate**, and a multivariate model revealed that the concurrent use of thalidomide increased the risk of osteonecrosis of the jaw 2.4-fold.[3] Similarly, in another review of 35 cases of **pamidronate** or **zoledronate**-associated osteonecrosis of the jaw, although no statistical analysis was carried out, concurrent use of thalidomide was frequent (46% of cases), leading the authors to suggest that the possible link should be further investigated.[4] Conversely, in a cohort of 259 patients with multiple myeloma who had all received treatment with **zoledronate**, thalidomide and dexamethasone, just 9 (6.6%) developed osteonecrosis of the jaw, which was stated to be comparable to the incidence previously reported for zoledronic acid alone.[5]

Mechanism

Uncertain. Thalidomide can rarely affect renal function, and was suggested to possibly interact with zoledronate. The antiangiogenic activity of thalidomide might increase the risk of osteonecrosis with bisphosphonates.

Importance and management

No interaction is established, and the data from the controlled study suggest that the combination of thalidomide and zoledronate has no greater risk of renal impairment than zoledronate alone. Thalidomide does not alter the pharmacokinetics of zoledronate. Further study is needed to ascertain if thalidomide increases the risk of osteonecrosis of the jaw seen with bisphosphonates.

1. Jones SG, Dolan G, Lengyel K, Myers B. Severe increase in creatinine with hypocalcaemia in thalidomide-treated myeloma patients receiving zoledronic acid infusions. *Br J Haematol* (2002) 119, 576–7.
2. Spencer A, Roberts A, Kennedy N, Ravera C, Cremers S, Bilic S, Neeman T, Copeman M, Schran H, Lynch K. Renal safety of zoledronic acid with thalidomide in patients with myeloma: a pharmacokinetic and safety sub-study. *BMC Clin Pharmacol* (2008) 8, 2.
3. Zervas K, Verrou E, Teleioudis Z, Vahtsevanos K, Banti A, Mihou D, Krikelis D, Terpos E. Incidence, risk factors and management of osteonecrosis of the jaw in patients with multiple myeloma: a single-centre experience in 303 patients. *Br J Haematol* (2006) 134, 620–3.
4. Pozzi S, Marcheselli R, Sacchi S, Baldini L, Angrilli F, Pennese E, Quarta G, Stelitano C, Caparotti G, Luminari S, Musto P, Natale D, Broglia C, Cuoghi A, Dini D, Di Tonno P, Leonardi G, Pianezze G, Pitini V, Polimeno G, Ponchio L, Masini L, Musso M, Spriano M, Pollastri G; Gruppo Italiano Studio Linfomi. Bisphosphonate-associated osteonecrosis of the jaw: a review of 35 cases and an evaluation of its frequency in multiple myeloma patients. *Leuk Lymphoma* (2007) 48, 56–64.
5. Tosi P, Zamagni E, Cangini D, Tacchetti P, Di Raimondo F, Catalano L, D'Arco A, Ronconi S, Cellini C, Offidani M, Perrone G, Ceccolini M, Brioli A, Tura S, Baccarani M, Cavo M. Osteonecrosis of the jaws in newly diagnosed multiple myeloma patients treated with zoledronic acid and thalidomide-dexamethasone. *Blood* (2006)108, 3951–2.

Bisphosphonates; Alendronate + Phosphates

An isolated report describes a patient taking alendronate, who developed hypocalcaemic tetany after receiving two doses of oral *Fleet Phospho-Soda* (monobasic sodium phosphate with dibasic sodium phosphate).

Clinical evidence

A patient with Crohn's disease taking a 5-aminosalicylate (unnamed) and prednisone developed mild osteoporosis and was given alendronate 10 mg daily. About 18 months later she underwent elective bowel surgery, receiving 2 doses of oral *Fleet Phospho-Soda* (monobasic sodium phosphate with dibasic sodium phosphate) 2 hours apart before surgery. About 6 hours postoperatively she developed paraesthesia of her extremities and perioral region, hypophosphataemia, and hypocalcaemic tetany. She recovered after treatment with intravenous calcium gluconate 2 g over 30 minutes. Her serum calcium, phosphate and magnesium levels were low, and she was therefore given calcitriol and further calcium supplements.[1]

Mechanism

Hypocalcaemia in this patient was probably due to several factors, including disease of the terminal ileum and a history of diarrhoea, which could have resulted in calcium malabsorption and relative vitamin D deficiency. *Fleet Phospho-Soda* also causes hypocalcaemia, which is usually accompanied by hyperphosphataemia. The authors of the report suggest that alendronate was also a factor in the development of hypocalcaemia, and further, that the hypophosphataemia was possibly linked to high parathyroid hormone levels preoperatively.[1]

Importance and management

The authors of this isolated case advise care if phosphate-based oral laxatives are given to patients taking bisphosphonates, especially in patients with intestinal malabsorption syndromes.[1]

However, this appears to be the only report of hypocalcaemic tetany associated with the use of bisphosphonates and *Fleet Phospho-Soda*. It has also been noted that the patient's low magnesium levels could result in tetany.[2] Long-term prednisone treatment, which decreases calcium absorption, may also be involved. Further, the 2 doses of *Fleet-Phospho-Soda* were given 2 hours apart, rather than at the recommended interval of 10 to 12 hours. Other authors, in considering these factors, suggest that patients taking bisphosphonates are not at increased risk of hypocalcaemic tetany if they are given *Fleet Phospho-Soda*.[2]

1. Campisi P, Badhwar V, Morin S, Trudel JL. Postoperative hypocalcemic tetany caused by Fleet® Phospho®-Soda preparation in a patient taking alendronate sodium. *Dis Colon Rectum* (1999) 42, 1499–501.
2. Francis MD, Caswell M. Patients on bisphosphonates should not be at increased risk for hypocalcemic-induced tetany when given Fleet® Phospho-Soda®. *Dis Colon Rectum* (2003) 46, 1717–18.

Brimonidine or Latanoprost + NSAIDs

The intraocular pressure-lowering effect of brimonidine eye drops might be reduced by oral indometacin. The reduction in intraocular pressure by latanoprost eye drops was not significantly reduced by oral indometacin, slightly reduced by bromfenac eye drops, but enhanced by oral nimesulide and diclofenac eye drops.

Clinical evidence

In a double-blind study, 20 patients with open-angle glaucoma or ocular hypertension received treatment for their right eye with either latanoprost 0.005% eye drops in the morning and drug-free vehicle in the evening or with brimonidine 0.2% eye drops in the morning and evening. One week later treatment was started for the left eye with the opposite regimen to that used in the right eye. After another week the patients were given oral **indometacin** 25 mg four times daily for 2 weeks. Compared with pretreatment values, the intraocular pressure reduction with brimonidine alone was 14%, which fell to a non-significant 11% reduction when **indometacin** was given. Compared with pretreatment values the intraocular pressure with latanoprost alone was 25%, and this was not significantly altered when **indometacin** was given. Peripheral retinal microcirculation was increased by 23% with latanoprost, but not significantly affected by brimonidine. When **indometacin** was also given the effect of latanoprost became non-significant, and in the case of brimonidine, was reduced to a value lower than that measured before brimonidine was given. **Indometacin** did not affect visual function parameters.[1]

In another study, 11 healthy subjects were given latanoprost 0.005% eye drops daily, in both eyes for 8 weeks, with **bromfenac** eye drops put in one eye twice daily between weeks 4 and 6. After a 4-week washout period, **bromfenac** was again given for 2 weeks to the same eyes as before. Bromfenac alone did not affect intraocular pressure, but was found to significantly inhibit the intraocular pressure-lowering effects of latanoprost. At week 6, latanoprost reduced intraocular pressure by about 23% to 52%, but in those eyes also treated with **bromfenac** the reduction was between about 7% and 35%.[2] In a further similar study in patients with glaucoma, **bromfenac** eye drops twice daily for 12 weeks slightly attenuated the reduction in intraocular pressure seen with latanoprost eye drops (maximum difference 1.08 mmHg).[3]

In contrast to these studies, other researchers have found that 2 hours after a single 100-mg oral dose of **nimesulide**, the intraocular pressure in patients whose glaucoma was controlled by latanoprost was further reduced by about 3 mmHg.[4] Another study in patients with glaucoma found that 5 weeks of **diclofenac** 0.1% eye drops enhanced the intraocular pressure reducing effect of latanoprost eye drops: after one week intraocular pressure was reduced by 4.1 mmHg, compared with a 0.67 mmHg in those given placebo.[5]

Mechanism

Brimonidine might reduce intraocular pressure by decreasing aqueous inflow and increasing uveoscleral outflow. The latter effect is thought to occur by stimulation of endogenous prostaglandin $F_{2\alpha}$ formation.[1] Latanoprost is a synthetic analogue of dinoprost (prostaglandin $F_{2\alpha}$) which also reduces intraocular pressure by increasing uveoscleral outflow. It is also reported to induce endogenous prostaglandins.[2] NSAIDs, such as indometacin and bromfenac, might possibly antagonise this action by inhibiting the induction of endogenous prostaglandins by suppressing cyclo-oxygenase activity. However, it has also been suggested that the expression of prostaglandin receptors in ocular tissue may be up-regulated in the presence of prostaglandin inhibitors such as NSAIDs, resulting in a greater response to prostaglandin analogues.[4,5]

Importance and management

The reduction in the intraocular pressure-lowering effect of brimonidine with oral indometacin might be of clinical importance.[1] If intraocular pressure is not adequately reduced in patients receiving brimonidine for the treatment of glaucoma, consider an oral NSAID as the possible cause.

The situation with latanoprost is unclear. Both a small reduction, no effect, and an enhanced effect have been seen with various NSAIDs (some oral and some eye drops). Until more is known, additional monitoring might be appropriate when an oral or ocular NSAID is stopped or started in a patient stabilised on latanoprost.

1. Sponsel WE, Paris G, Trigo Y, Pena M, Weber A, Sanford K, McKinnon S. Latanoprost and brimonidine: therapeutic and physiologic assessment before and after oral nonsteroidal anti-inflammatory therapy. *Am J Ophthalmol* (2002) 133, 11–18.
2. Kashiwagi K, Tsukahara S. Effect of non-steroidal anti-inflammatory ophthalmic solution on intraocular pressure reduction by latanoprost. *Br J Ophthalmol* (2003) 87, 297–301.
3. Chiba T, Kashiwagi K, Chiba N, Tsukahara S. Effect of non-steroidal anti-inflammatory ophthalmic solution on intraocular pressure reduction by latanoprost in patients with primary open angle glaucoma or ocular hypertension. *Br J Ophthalmol* (2006) 90, 314–17.
4. Costagliola C, Parmeggiani F, Caccavale A, Sebastiani A. Nimesulide oral administration increases the intraocular pressure-lowering effect of latanoprost in patients with primary open-angle glaucoma. *Am J Ophthalmol* (2006) 141, 379–81.
5. Costagliola C, Parmeggiani F, Antinozzi PP, Caccavale A, Cotticelli L, Sebastiani A. The influence of diclofenac ophthalmic solution on the intraocular pressure-lowering effect of topical 0.5% timolol and 0.005% latanoprost in primary open-angle glaucoma patients. *Exp Eye Res* (2005) 81, 610–15.

Charcoal, activated + Miscellaneous

Small doses of activated charcoal appear to have little effect on the absorption of ciprofloxacin and oral contraceptives (administration separated), and only modestly reduces nizatidine and amlodipine absorption. Case reports describe the lack of efficacy of mitobronitol and

reduced serum phenobarbital levels in the presence of small doses of activated charcoal.

Clinical evidence, mechanism, importance and management

The use of activated charcoal, in a usual dose of 50 g, to reduce the absorption of drugs and poisons after acute overdose is well established, as is repeated doses of activated charcoal to enhance the elimination of some drugs taken in overdose after they have been absorbed. Studies and references supporting these therapeutic uses of activated charcoal are not reviewed here. Activated charcoal is also included in various remedies used for gastrointestinal disorders such as flatulence or diarrhoea. Doses in these instances are very much lower (1 to 2 g daily) than those used in the treatment of poisoning, and there seems to be little reported about the effects of these doses on the absorption of other drugs.

In a study in 8 healthy subjects, a formulation of small spherical activated charcoal particles (*Kremezin* 2-g *granules*), used to adsorb uraemic toxins in renal disease, hardly affected the bioavailability of **amlodipine** 5 mg when both drugs were given together, after a meal. The maximum amlodipine plasma concentration was reduced by 16%, but the AUC_{0-72} was decreased by only 7% (not statistically significant). In one subject the AUC was reduced by 26%, but even this would not be expected to be clinically significant.[1]

In one single-dose study in healthy subjects, **nizatidine** absorption was reduced by about 30% when it was taken one hour before activated charcoal 2 g.[2] In another single-dose study in 6 subjects, taking activated charcoal 1 g soon after ciprofloxacin 500 mg, had little effect on the pharmacokinetics of **ciprofloxacin** 500 mg (AUC reduced by 10%).[3]

In one case report, an antiemetic complementary remedy containing activated charcoal was thought to be the cause of a lack of effect of **mitobronitol** 125 mg used to treat primary thrombocythaemia in one patient.[4] In another case report,[5] activated charcoal 2 g three times daily was given with **phenobarbital** and enteral nutrition via a gastric fistula tube. The charcoal appeared to reduce the absorption of **phenobarbital** (serum level 4.3 mg/L, compared with a previous level of 24.8 mg/L). Giving the activated charcoal at least one hour apart from the **phenobarbital** resulted in an increase in serum levels to about 16 to 18 mg/L.

In a study in 9 healthy subjects, activated charcoal 5 g four times daily was taken for 3 days, mid-cycle, with the first daily dose taken 3 hours after the morning dose of a **combined oral contraceptive** (ethinylestradiol with norethisterone or gestodene), had no effect on the pharmacokinetics of the contraceptive steroids,[6] and ovulation (assessed by hormone measurements and ultrasonography) did not occur.[7] The authors concluded that repeated charcoal treatment, given 3 hours after and at least 12 hours before a **combined oral contraceptive**, can be used to treat diarrhoea in women taking **combined oral contraceptives**.[6,7]

1. Tanaka C, Ohtani H, Tsujimoto M, Ohdo S, Taniguchi M, Mizooku Y, Saitoh Y, Kimura M, Uchimaru H, Irie S, Sawada Y. Effects of dosing interval on the pharmacokinetic interaction between oral small spherical activated charcoal and amlodipine in humans. *J Clin Pharmacol* (2007) 47, 904–8.
2. Knadler MP, Bergstrom RF, Callaghan JT, Obermeyer BD, Rubin A. Absorption studies of the H_2-blocker nizatidine. *Clin Pharmacol Ther* (1987) 42, 514–20.
3. Torre D, Sampietro C, Rossi S, Bianchi W, Maggiolo F. Ciprofloxacin and activated charcoal: pharmacokinetic data. *Rev Infect Dis* (1989) 11 (Suppl 5), S1015–S1016.
4. Windrum P, Hull DR, Morris TCM. Herb-drug interactions. *Lancet* (2000) 355, 1019–20.
5. Tanaka C, Yagi H, Sakamoto M, Koyama Y, Ohmura T, Ohtani H, Sawada Y. Decreased phenobarbital absorption with charcoal administration for chronic renal failure. *Ann Pharmacother* (2004) 38, 73–6.
6. Elomaa K, Ranta S, Tuominen J, Lähteenmäki P. The possible role of enterohepatic cycling on bioavailability of norethisterone and gestodene in women using combined oral contraceptives. *Contraception* (2001) 63, 13–8.
7. Elomaa K, Ranta S, Tuominen J, Lähteenmäki P. Charcoal treatment and risk of escape ovulation in oral contraceptive users. *Hum Reprod* (2001) 16, 76–81.

Chlorzoxazone + Disulfiram

Disulfiram increases the plasma concentrations of chlorzoxazone.

Clinical evidence

In a pharmacokinetic study in 6 healthy subjects, a single 500-mg dose of disulfiram markedly inhibited the metabolism of a single 750-mg dose of chlorzoxazone (clearance reduced by 85%, half-life increased from 0.92 to 5.1 hours, and a twofold increase in peak plasma concentrations).[1]

In a pharmacokinetic study, 7 healthy subjects were given disulfiram 250 mg daily for 11 days with a single 250-mg dose of chlorzoxazone 3 days before disulfiram was started, then again on day 2 and day 11. On day 2 and day 11 disulfiram reduced chlorzoxazone clearance by 90% and 89%, respectively, and increased the maximum plasma concentrations of chlorzoxazone 7.9-fold and 7.4-fold, respectively.[2] Further data from this study are presented elsewhere.[3]

Mechanism

Disulfiram is a potent inhibitor of CYP2E1, by which chlorzoxazone is metabolised. Concurrent use therefore leads to reduced chlorzoxazone clearance and increased plasma concentrations. Note that chlorzoxazone is used as a probe substrate in evaluating the effects of drugs on CYP2E1, see 'Table 1.8', p.10.

Importance and management

The pharmacokinetic interaction between chlorzoxazone and disulfiram is established. No increased adverse effects were seen in the above studies while using these single doses, but an increase in chlorzoxazone toxicity (sedation, headache, nausea) would be expected with multiple doses. Be alert for the need to reduce the chlorzoxazone dose if disulfiram is given concurrently.

1. Kharasch ED, Thummel KE, Mhyre J, Lillibridge JH. Single-dose disulfiram inhibition of chlorzoxazone metabolism: a clinical probe for P450 2E1. *Clin Pharmacol Ther* (1993) 53, 643–50.
2. Frye RF, Tammara B, Cowart TD, Bramer SL. Effect of disulfiram-mediated CYP2E1 inhibition on the disposition of vesnarinone. *J Clin Pharmacol* (1999) 39, 1177–83.
3. Frye RF, Branch RA. Effect of chronic disulfiram administration on the activities of CYP1A2, CYP2C19, CYP2D6, CYP2E1, and N-acetyltransferase in healthy human subjects. *Br J Clin Pharmacol* (2002) 53, 155–62.

Chlorzoxazone + Isoniazid

Isoniazid reduces the clearance of chlorzoxazone. The adverse effects of chlorzoxazone could be increased in some patients (particularly slow acetylators of isoniazid) if they also take isoniazid.

Clinical evidence

Five out of 10 healthy slow acetylators of isoniazid experienced an increase in the adverse effects of a 750-mg dose of chlorzoxazone (sedation, headache, nausea) after taking isoniazid 300 mg daily for 7 days. These symptoms disappeared within 2 days of withdrawing the isoniazid.[1] Pharmacokinetic analysis found that the clearance of chlorzoxazone was reduced by 56% when given on the last day of isoniazid use, then increased by 56% when given 2 days after stopping isoniazid.[1] Similar findings were reported in another study in slow acetylators of isoniazid. In this study, chlorzoxazone clearance was reduced by 78% when subjects had taken isoniazid 300 mg daily for 14 days, at which point the isoniazid was stopped. Two days later chlorzoxazone clearance was increased by 58%, and it had returned to normal 2 weeks later.[2] Rapid acetylators of isoniazid also had a 60% reduction in chlorzoxazone clearance on the last day of isoniazid use, but did not have any increase 2 days later.[2]

Mechanism

Isoniazid appears to cause a dual interaction. During administration, it inhibits the activity of CYP2E1, the isoenzyme involved in the metabolism of chlorzoxazone. Shortly after stopping isoniazid, the metabolism of chlorzoxazone is increased, possibly because of induction of CYP2E1, although this effect was only evident in the slow acetylators.[1,2]

Importance and management

The increase in chlorzoxazone levels with isoniazid is established, and occurs in both slow and fast acetylators of isoniazid, although the increase in levels is slightly greater in slow acetylators. In practical terms this means that it might be necessary to reduce the chlorzoxazone dose in some patients if they take isoniazid. Monitor concurrent use carefully. The rebound increase in chlorzoxazone clearance in slow acetylators on stopping isoniazid was short-lived and is probably of little clinical importance.

1. Zand R, Nelson SD, Slattery JT, Thummel KE, Kalhorn TF, Adams SP, Wright JM. Inhibition and induction of cytochrome P4502E1-catalyzed oxidation by isoniazid in humans. *Clin Pharmacol Ther* (1993) 54, 142–9.
2. O'Shea D, Kim RB, Wilkinson GR. Modulation of CYP2E1 activity by isoniazid in rapid and slow *N*-acetylators. *Br J Clin Pharmacol* (1997) 43, 99–103.

Cinacalcet + Food

Cinacalcet absorption is increased by food.

Clinical evidence

In a pharmacokinetic study in 29 healthy subjects, the AUC of cinacalcet was raised by 68% when a single 90-mg dose of cinacalcet was taken within 5 minutes of finishing a high-fat, high-calorie breakfast, when compared with the fasted state (10 hours). Similarly, a low-fat, low-calorie breakfast increased the AUC of cinacalcet by 50%. Food had no effect on the elimination half-life of cinacalcet.[1]

Mechanism

Food increases the rate and extent of absorption of cinacalcet, independently of the fat content. Possible mechanisms include increased gastric residence time or decreased presystemic metabolism.[1]

Importance and management

An established pharmacokinetic interaction. Cinacalcet should be taken with food or shortly after a meal[2,3] to maximise absorption.

1. Padhi D, Salfi M, Harris RZ. The pharmacokinetics of cinacalcet are unaffected following consumption of high-and low-fat meals. *Am J Ther* (2007) 14, 235–40.
2. Mimpara (Cinacalcet). Amgen Ltd. UK Summary of product characteristics, March 2009.
3. Sensipar (Cinacalcet). Amgen Inc. US Prescribing information, December 2008.

Cinacalcet + Ketoconazole and other CYP3A4 inhibitors

Ketoconazole causes about a twofold increase in cinacalcet exposure, and is therefore likely to increase cinacalcet adverse effects. Other potent CYP3A4 inhibitors are predicted to affect cinacalcet in the same way as ketoconazole.

Clinical evidence

In a pharmacokinetic study in 20 healthy subjects, the AUC and maximum level of cinacalcet were raised about twofold when a single 90-mg dose of cinacalcet was given on day 5 of a 7-day course of ketoconazole 200 mg twice daily. The median elimination half-life of cinacalcet was slightly increased and its clearance reduced by 65%. This resulted in an increase in the proportion of subjects reporting a treatment-related adverse event (42% versus 21%).[1]

Mechanism

Cinacalcet is extensively metabolised, in part by the cytochrome P450 isoenzyme CYP3A4, of which ketoconazole is a potent inhibitor. Ketoconazole therefore increases cinacalcet levels. The lack of change in elimination half-life suggests that the interaction principally resulted in an increase in the bioavailability of cinacalcet.

Importance and management

The pharmacokinetic interaction is established and likely to be clinically important. Cinacalcet treatment is monitored by measuring parathyroid hormone and serum calcium levels, and these should be closely monitored when ketoconazole is started or stopped, anticipating the need to adjust the cinacalcet dosage accordingly. Other potent CYP3A4 inhibitors would be predicted to interact similarly, and the manufacturers specifically mention **itraconazole**, **voriconazole**, **telithromycin**, **ritonavir** and **erythromycin**[2,3] (although note that erythromycin is sometimes considered to be a moderate CYP3A4 inhibitor).

On the basis that a potent CYP3A4 inhibitor caused just a twofold increase in AUC, weak to moderate CYP3A4 inhibitors would be unlikely to cause clinically relevant increases in cinacalcet levels.

1. Harris RZ, Salfi M, Sullivan JT, Padhi D. Pharmacokinetics of cinacalcet hydrochloride when administered with ketoconazole. *Clin Pharmacokinet* (2007) 46, 495–501.
2. Mimpara (Cinacalcet). Amgen Ltd. UK Summary of product characteristics, March 2009.
3. Sensipar (Cinacalcet). Amgen Inc. US Prescribing information, December 2008.

Cinacalcet + Miscellaneous

Potent CYP1A2 inhibitors (e.g. fluvoxamine, ciprofloxacin) are predicted to increase cinacalcet levels. Tobacco smoking induces CYP1A2 and is associated with lower cinacalcet levels. Rifampicin is predicted to reduce cinacalcet levels, because of its CYP3A4-inducing effects. Calcium carbonate, pantoprazole and sevelamer do not alter cinacalcet pharmacokinetics, and cinacalcet does not alter midazolam pharmacokinetics.

Clinical evidence, mechanism, importance and management

(a) Calcium carbonate

In a single-dose study in healthy subjects, the AUC of cinacalcet 100 mg was not changed by calcium carbonate 1.5 g.[1,2]

(b) CYP1A2 inducers and inhibitors

Cinacalcet is extensively metabolised, in part by the cytochrome P450 isoenzyme CYP1A2. The UK manufacturer notes that the clearance of cinacalcet was 36 to 38% higher in **smokers** than non-smokers, and that tobacco smoking induces CYP1A2. They suggest that the cinacalcet dose might need to be adjusted if a patient starts or stops smoking. Moreover, although the effect of CYP1A2 inhibitors such as **fluvoxamine** and **ciprofloxacin** on cinacalcet has not been studied, the manufacturer suggests that cinacalcet dose adjustment might be needed if these potent inhibitors are started or stopped.[3] Until more is known, it would be prudent to increase monitoring of parathyroid hormone and serum calcium levels in these situations.

(c) Midazolam

The manufacturers report that cinacalcet 90 mg daily for 5 days did not affect the pharmacokinetics of a single 2-mg oral dose of midazolam given on day 5, when compared with the pharmacokinetics of midazolam alone.[2,3]

(d) Pantoprazole

In a study in healthy subjects, the AUC of a single 90-mg dose of cinacalcet was not changed by pantoprazole 80 mg daily for 3 days.[1,2]

(e) Rifampicin (Rifampin)

Cinacalcet is extensively metabolised, in part by the cytochrome P450 isoenzyme CYP3A4. On the basis that the CYP3A4 inhibitor ketoconazole causes clinically relevant increases in cinacalcet levels (see 'Cinacalcet + Ketoconazole and other CYP3A4 inhibitors', p.1559), rifampicin, a CYP3A4 inducer, is predicted to decrease levels of cinacalcet.[3] It would be prudent to monitor cinacalcet efficacy if rifampicin is required, anticipating the need to increase the dose.

(f) Sevelamer

In a study in healthy subjects, the AUC of a single 90-mg dose of cinacalcet was not changed when it was given with the first dose of sevelamer 2.4 g three times daily for 2 days.[1,2]

1. Padhi D, Harris R, Salfi M, Yates W, Hansen J, Flynn J, Sullivan JT. Cinacalcet HCl absorption in study subjects is not affected by coadministration of medications commonly prescribed to chronic kidney disease (CKD) patients (pantoprazole, sevelamar [sic] HCl, and calcium carbonate). *J Am Soc Nephrol* (2003) 14, 461A.
2. Sensipar (Cinacalcet). Amgen Inc. US Prescribing information, December 2008.
3. Mimpara (Cinacalcet). Amgen Ltd. UK Summary of product characteristics, March 2009.

CNS depressants + CNS depressants

The concurrent use of two or more drugs that are CNS depressants can increase drowsiness and reduce alertness. These drugs include alcohol (even in small amounts), antidepressants, antiemetics, antiepileptics, antihistamines, antipsychotics, anxiolytics, barbiturates, hypnotics, opioid analgesics, and skeletal muscle relaxants. This increases the risk of accidents when driving or handling other potentially dangerous machinery, and may make the performance of everyday tasks more difficult and hazardous.

Clinical evidence, mechanism, importance and management

Many drugs have the propensity to cause depression of the central nervous system, resulting in drowsiness, sedation, respiratory depression and at the extreme, death. If more than one CNS depressant is taken, their effects may be additive. It is not uncommon for patients, particularly the elderly, to be taking numerous drugs (and possibly alcohol as well). Such patients are therefore at risk of cumulative CNS depression ranging from mild drowsiness through to a befuddled stupor, which can make the performance of the simplest everyday task more difficult or even impossible. The importance of this will depend on the context: it may considerably increase the risk of accident in the kitchen, at work, in a busy street, driving a car, or handling other potentially dangerous machinery where alertness is at a premium. It has been estimated that as many as 600 traffic accident fatalities each year in the UK can be attributed to the sedative effects of psychoactive drugs.[1] In a Spanish study of fatal road traffic accidents, blood samples were analysed from 9.7% of drivers killed in road accidents over a 10-year period. Of these drivers, medicines were detected in 4.7% (269 cases), and of these **benzodiazepines** were the most common (73%). Other drugs present in 6% to 12% of cases included **antidepressants**, **analgesics**, **antiepileptics**, **barbiturates** and **antihistamines**. Of the benzodiazepine cases, almost three quarters had another substance detected, mainly illicit drugs (cocaine, **opioids**, or cannabis) or **alcohol**. Only 7.7% had taken **benzodiazepines** or another medicinal drug alone.[2] **Alcohol** almost certainly makes things worse, particularly in the elderly.[3]

An example of the lethal effects of combining an **antihistamine**, a **benzodiazepine** and **alcohol** is briefly mentioned in the monograph 'Alcohol + Antihistamines', p.54. A less spectacular but socially distressing example is that of a woman accused of shoplifting while in a confused state arising from the combined sedative effects of *Actifed*, a *Beechams Powder* and *Dolobid* (containing **triprolidine**, **salicylamide** and **diflunisal**, respectively).[4]

Few, if any, well-controlled studies have investigated the cumulative or additive detrimental effects of CNS depressants (except with **alcohol**), but the following is a list of some of the groups of drugs that to a greater or lesser extent possess CNS depressant activity, which therefore might be expected to interact in this way: **alcohol**, **opioids**, **antiepileptics**, **antidepressants**, **antihistamines**, **antiemetics**, **antipsychotics**, **anxiolytics** and **hypnotics**. Some of the interactions of **alcohol** with these drugs are dealt with in individual monographs.

1. Anon. Sedative effects of drugs linked to accidents. *Pharm J* (1994) 253, 564.
2. Carmen del Río M, Gómez J, Sancho M, Alvarez FJ. Alcohol, illicit drugs and medicinal drugs in fatally injured drivers in Spain between 1991 and 2000. *Forensic Sci Int* (2002) 127, 63–70.
3. Gerbino PP. Complications of alcohol use combined with drug therapy in the elderly. *J Am Geriatr Soc* (1982) 30 (11 Suppl), S88–S93.
4. Herxheimer A, Haffner BD. Prosecution for alleged shoplifting: successful pharmacological defence. *Lancet* (1982) i, 634.

Colchicine + Azoles

Ketoconazole increases the exposure to colchicine. Other azoles would be expected to interact similarly.

Clinical evidence

In a study in 24 healthy subjects, **ketoconazole** 200 mg twice daily for 5 days, increased the AUC and maximum concentration of a single 600-microgram dose of colchicine 2.9-fold and by 89%, respectively.[1]

Mechanism

Ketoconazole is a known potent inhibitor of CYP3A4 and also inhibits P-glycoprotein, both of which are involved in the metabolism of colchicine and hence concurrent use increases the exposure to colchicine. Other azoles also inhibit CYP3A4, and so would also be expected to interact similarly. Any effect would be more notable in patients with renal impairment, in whom colchicine clearance is already reduced.

Importance and management

Information regarding the interaction between colchicine and azoles is limited to the pharmacokinetic study with ketoconazole, but given the increase in colchicine exposure seen and the case reports of serious toxicity reported with other less potent CYP3A4 inhibitors (such as erythromycin, see 'Colchicine + Macrolides', p.1562), it might be predicted that ketoconazole and other azoles could provoke acute colchicine toxicity, at the least in pre-disposed individuals. Until more information is available, if any patient is given colchicine with an azole, monitor for signs of colchicine toxicity (such as nausea, vomiting, diarrhoea, myopathy, and pancytopenia) and anticipate the need to reduce the colchicine dose.

The US manufacturer makes specific recommendations for colchicine dose reductions in patients taking potent CYP3A4 inhibitors (they name ketoconazole and

itraconazole), and moderate CYP3A4 inhibitors (they name **fluconazole**), or if they have stopped taking them within 2 weeks of starting colchicine. See 'Colchicine + Macrolides', p.1562, for further details. Note that **voriconazole** is a potent CYP3A4 inhibitor and **posaconazole** is a moderate CYP3A4 inhibitor, and as such the relevant dosing information might be equally applied to these azoles.

Note that patients with renal or hepatic impairment have a greater risk of developing colchicine toxicity, and for this reason the manufacturers of colchicine contraindicate the concurrent use of potent CYP3A4 inhibitors in such patients.[2,3]

1. Terkeltaub RA, Furst DE, DiGiacinto JL, Kook KA, Davis MW. Novel evidence-based colchicine dose-reduction algorithm to predict and prevent colchicine toxicity in the presence of cytochrome P450 3A4/P-glycoprotein inhibitors. *Arthritis Rheum* (2011) 63, 226 Erratum ibid. (2011) 63, 3521
2. Colchicine. Wockhardt UK Ltd. UK Summary of product characteristics, June 2010.
3. Colcrys (Colchicine). Takeda Pharmaceuticals America, Inc. US Prescribing information, November 2012.

Colchicine + Calcium-channel blockers

Diltiazem and verapamil increase the exposure to colchicine. Colchicine toxicity has been seen in one patient after colchicine was given to a patient taking verapamil.

Clinical evidence

(a) Diltiazem

In a study in 20 healthy subjects, extended-release diltiazem 240 mg daily for 7 days increased the AUC and maximum concentration of a single 600-microgram dose of colchicine by 27% and 29%, respectively.[1]

(b) Verapamil

In a study in 24 healthy subjects, extended-release verapamil 240 mg daily for 5 days increased the AUC and maximum concentration of a single 600-microgram dose of colchicine by 88% and 30%, respectively.[1]

An 83-year-old man who was taking slow-release verapamil 120 mg daily for tachyarrhythmia, as well as furosemide, aspirin, ambroxol and theophylline, took colchicine 2 mg over a 2-day period for acute gout, with diclofenac for pain. He had muscle weakness in his limbs and 4 days later became immobile. On admission to hospital he had flaccid tetraparesis (weakness of all four extremities). A diagnosis of colchicine-induced neuromyopathy was made after excessive concentrations of colchicine were found in his serum and CSF. The serum half-life was increased 8-fold (from a reference value of 34 hours to 272 hours) and the CSF:serum ratio was increased to about 50%, much higher than the expected ratio of less than 10%. At follow up 40 days later he had partially recovered and colchicine was not detectable in his serum. Usual features of colchicine-induced neuropathy, such as high cumulative dose, long-term treatment, or renal impairment were not found.[2]

Mechanism

Diltiazem and verapamil are both moderate inhibitors of CYP3A4, the isoenzyme involved in the metabolism of colchicine, and therefore increase its exposure. In addition, verapamil is an inhibitor of P-glycoprotein which is also involved in the metabolism of colchicine and might explain why verapamil causes a larger increase in colchicine exposure than diltiazem. More specifically, inhibition of P-glycoprotein at the blood-brain barrier might have resulted in the increased colchicine accumulation in the CSF seen in the case report.[2] Any effect would be more notable in patients with renal impairment, in whom colchicine clearance is already reduced.

Importance and management

Information regarding the interaction between colchicine and diltiazem or verapamil is limited, but is consistent with that seen with other inhibitors of CYP3A4 and P-glycoprotein. As seen in the verapamil case report, it can provoke acute colchicine toxicity, at the very least in pre-disposed individuals. Until more information is available, if any patient is given colchicine with diltiazem or verapamil, monitor for signs of colchicine toxicity (such as nausea, vomiting, diarrhoea, myopathy, and pancytopenia), particularly in patients with pre-existing hepatic or renal impairment. Additionally, anticipate the need to reduce the colchicine dose.

The US manufacturer makes specific recommendations for colchicine dose reductions in patients taking moderate CYP3A4 inhibitors (they name diltiazem and verapamil), or if they have stopped taking these drugs within 2 weeks of starting colchicine. See 'Colchicine + Macrolides', p.1562, for further details.

1. Terkeltaub RA, Furst DE, DiGiacinto JL, Kook KA, Davis MW. Novel evidence-based colchicine dose-reduction algorithm to predict and prevent colchicine toxicity in the presence of cytochrome P450 3A4/P-glycoprotein inhibitors. *Arthritis Rheum* (2011) 63, 226 Erratum ibid. (2011) 63, 3521.
2. Tröger U, Lins H, Scherrmann J-M, Wallesch C-W, Bode-Böger SM. Tetraparesis associated with colchicine is probably due to inhibition by verapamil of the P-glycoprotein efflux pump in the blood-brain barrier. *BMJ* (2005) 331, 613. Correction. ibid., (2006) 332, 882.

Colchicine + Digoxin

Isolated cases of myopathy and rhabdomyolysis have been attributed to the concurrent use of colchicine and digoxin.

Clinical evidence

The FDA in the US reports that several cases of myopathy and/or rhabdomyolysis have occurred in patients taking colchicine and also taking digoxin.[1] However, published evidence for an interaction appears to be limited, and only three cases of colchicine myopathy, where the patient was also taking digoxin, have been identified. In one report, a 59-year-old man was admitted to hospital with rhabdomyolysis one month after starting colchicine 600 micrograms twice daily for repeated attacks of gout. On admission he was also taking indometacin 25 to 50 mg four times daily as needed to treat the gout attack, as well as his regular medications, which included digoxin 250 micrograms and verapamil 240 mg daily. He was also found to have mild renal impairment. The colchicine was stopped and his creatine phosphokinase concentrations and muscle strength returned to normal within several weeks. Note that in this case, the patients' digoxin concentration was found to be subtherapeutic.[2]

Another report describes a 73-year-old man with deteriorating renal function, taking digoxin 125 micrograms daily, who developed rhabdomyolysis 6 weeks after his colchicine dose was increased to 1.5 mg daily. The colchicine was stopped and his muscle power returned to normal after 2 weeks.[3] The third report describes a 58-year-old man with a history of renal impairment, taking digoxin 125 micrograms daily, who developed rhabdomyolysis 2 days after starting colchicine 3 mg daily.[4]

In a study in 2 healthy subjects taking digoxin 250 micrograms daily, *ColBenemid* (probenecid 500 mg with colchicine 500 micrograms) twice daily for 3 days had no effect on plasma digoxin concentrations.[5]

Mechanism

Both colchicine and digoxin are substrates for P-glycoprotein; however, it is unclear if competition for this transporter could have been responsible for the colchicine toxicity seen. Colchicine alone can, rarely, cause myopathy, and the effects seen could potentially have been adverse drug reactions.

Importance and management

Evidence for an interaction between colchicine and digoxin is limited to these cases and the possible mechanism for an interaction is unknown. In all three cases, the myopathy could have been caused by colchicine alone, particularly as predisposing factors such as renal impairment were present. It seems likely that this, as well as other factors including recent colchicine initiation,[2,4] a recent dose increase,[3] high doses[4] and the concurrent use of verapamil,[2] which is a known P-glycoprotein inhibitor (see 'Colchicine + Miscellaneous', p.1563) were responsible. Nevertheless, the US manufacturer of colchicine suggests careful monitoring of patients taking colchicine with digoxin, especially during the initiation of treatment, being alert for signs of muscle pain, tenderness or weakness.[6] Based on the published evidence this advice seems overly cautious, and standard monitoring of colchicine treatment would seem sufficient.

Very limited evidence suggests that colchicine does not affect digoxin concentrations.

1. FDA Information for healthcare professionals: new safety information for colchicine (marketed as Colcrys). July 30th 2009. Available at: http://www.fda.gov/Drugs/DrugSafety/PostmarketDrugSafetyInformationforPatientsandProviders/DrugSafetyInformationforHeathcareProfessionals/ucm174315.htm (accessed 21/10/15).
2. Dawson TM, Starkebaum G. Colchicine induced rhabdomyolysis. *J Rheumatol* (1997) 24, 2045–6.
3. Chattopadhyay I, Shetty HG, Routledge PA, Jeffery J. Colchicine induced rhabdomyolysis. *Postgrad Med J* (2001) 77, 191–2.
4. Debie K, Conraads V, Vrints C. Colchicine-induced rhabdomyolysis in a patient with chronic heart failure. *Acta Cardiol* (2003) 58, 561–2.
5. Jaillon P, Weissenburger J, Cheymol G, Graves P, Marcus F. Les effets du probénécide sur la concentration plasmatique à l'équilibre de digoxine. *Therapie* (1980) 35, 655–6.
6. Colcrys (Colchicine). Takeda Pharmaceuticals America, Inc. US Prescribing information, November 2012.

Colchicine + Grapefruit and other fruit juices

Grapefruit juice is predicted to increase the exposure to colchicine, although one study found no interaction. A case of colchicine toxicity has been reported in a child who consumed large quantities of grapefruit juice. Seville orange juice appears to slightly decrease the exposure to colchicine.

Clinical evidence and mechanism

(a) Grapefruit juice

In a study in 21 healthy subjects, 240 mL of undiluted grapefruit juice twice daily for 4 days had no effect on the AUC or maximum concentration of a single 600-microgram dose of colchicine.[1]

An 8-year-old girl who was stable taking colchicine 2 mg daily for familial Mediterranean fever, developed multi-organ failure due to colchicine toxicity 2 months after she started to drink one litre of grapefruit juice daily. She was admitted to hospital with fever, recurrent vomiting, severe abdominal pain, and a sore throat. She was also found to be tachycardic and hypotensive, and the following day developed congestive heart failure which required circulatory support in intensive care. She subsequently developed pancytopenia on day 3 of admission, when the colchicine was stopped. These symptoms began to resolve 6 days after admission to hospital, but she developed alopecia, atonic falls, and weakness during the second week of her hospital stay. The falls and weakness resolved within a few days.[2]

(b) Other fruit juices

In a study in 23 healthy subjects, 240 mL of **Seville orange juice** twice daily for 4 days decreased the AUC and maximum concentration of a single 600-microgram dose of colchicine by 23% and 24%, respectively, and increased its time to maximum concentration by one hour.[1]

Mechanism

Colchicine is metabolised by CYP3A4 and is also a substrate for P-glycoprotein. Grapefruit juice is known to be a weak inhibitor of CYP3A4, mostly affecting intestinal activity, but its effect on P-glycoprotein is less well-established. An *in vitro* study found that grapefruit juice increased colchicine absorption, and the authors suggest that this is predominantly due to intestinal P-glycoprotein inhibition, rather than CYP3A4 inhibition. They also report that the major constituents of grapefruit juice, 6,7-dihydroxybergamottin, naringen, and naringenin, had a similar effect.[3]

The mechanism for the decrease in colchicine exposure by Seville orange juice is unknown. The authors of the study suggest that Seville orange juice might contain an as yet unknown constituent that is not present in grapefruit juice, which might have been responsible for the difference in the interaction outcomes. They also suggest that it is possible that the interaction might be mediated by OATP.[1]

Importance and management

An interaction between colchicine and grapefruit juice is not established. The evidence is limited and the only published pharmacokinetic study unexpectedly found that no interaction occurred, although the case report suggests that some individuals might be affected. However, as grapefruit juice inhibits CYP3A4, the US manufacturer predicts that it will increase colchicine concentrations and recommends that the dose of colchicine be reduced in patients who drink grapefruit juice.[4] See 'Colchicine + Macrolides', below, for detailed recommendations on colchicine dose adjustment in these patients; however, note that as the effect of grapefruit juice is likely to vary with different batches of the juice, it might be prudent to avoid grapefruit juice altogether.

The slight decrease in colchicine exposure reported with Seville orange juice would not be expected to be of clinical relevance in most patients. However, it might be prudent to bear the possibility of an interaction in mind in patients who might be predisposed to colchicine toxicity, such as those with renal impairment, who develop otherwise unexplained colchicine adverse effects.

1. Wason S, DiGiacinto JL, Davis MW. Effects of grapefruit and Seville orange juices on the pharmacokinetic properties of colchicine in healthy subjects. *Clin Ther* (2012) 34, 2161–73.
2. Goldbart A, Press J, Sofer S, Kapelushnik J. Near fatal acute colchicine intoxication in a child. A case report. *Eur J Pediatr* (2000) 159, 895–7.
3. Dahan A, Amidon GL. Grapefruit juice and its constituents augment colchicine intestinal absorption: potential hazardous interaction and the role of P-glycoprotein. *Pharm Res* (2009) 26, 883–92.
4. Colcrys (Colchicine). Takeda Pharmaceuticals America, Inc. US Prescribing information, November 2012.

Colchicine + HIV-protease inhibitors

Ritonavir increases the exposure to colchicine. Other HIV-protease inhibitors are predicted to interact similarly.

Clinical evidence

In a study in 18 healthy subjects, **ritonavir** 100 mg twice daily for 5 days increased the AUC and maximum concentration of a single 600-microgram dose of colchicine about 2.7-fold and 3.5-fold, respectively.[1] The US guidelines on the treatment of HIV infection briefly report that **ritonavir** 100 mg twice daily increased the AUC and maximum concentration of colchicine (dose not stated) nearly 4-fold and 2.9-fold, respectively.[2]

Mechanism

Ritonavir is a known potent inhibitor of CYP3A4, the isoenzyme involved in the metabolism of colchicine, and therefore concurrent use increases colchicine exposure. Other HIV-protease inhibitors also inhibit CYP3A4 and so would also be expected to interact similarly. In addition, as colchicine is also a substrate for P-glycoprotein, which can be affected by some HIV-protease inhibitors, colchicine exposure might be further altered by concurrent use, see 'Table 1.12', p.14. Any effect would be more notable in patients with renal impairment, in whom colchicine clearance is already reduced.

Importance and management

Information regarding the interaction between colchicine and HIV-protease inhibitors is limited to the pharmacokinetic studies with ritonavir, but given the moderate increases in colchicine exposure reported, and the case reports of serious toxicity with other less potent CYP3A4 inhibitors (such as erythromycin, see 'Colchicine + Macrolides', below), ritonavir and the other HIV-protease inhibitors would be expected to have the potential to provoke acute colchicine toxicity, at the least in predisposed individuals. Until more information is available, if any patient is given colchicine with a HIV-protease inhibitor, monitor for signs of colchicine toxicity (such as nausea, vomiting, diarrhoea, myopathy, and pancytopenia), and anticipate the need to reduce the colchicine dose.

The US manufacturer makes specific recommendations for colchicine dose reductions in patients taking potent CYP3A4 inhibitors (they name the HIV-protease inhibitors, with the exception of unboosted amprenavir and fosamprenavir) or moderate CYP3A4 inhibitors (they name unboosted **amprenavir** and **fosamprenavir**), or if they have stopped taking these drugs within 2 weeks of starting colchicine. See 'Colchicine + Macrolides', below, for further details.

Note that patients with renal or hepatic impairment have a greater risk of developing colchicine toxicity, and for this reason the manufacturers of colchicine contraindicate the concurrent use of potent CYP3A4 inhibitors in such patients.[3,4]

1. Terkeltaub RA, Furst DE, DiGiacinto JL, Kook KA, Davis MW. Novel evidence-based colchicine dose-reduction algorithm to predict and prevent colchicine toxicity in the presence of cytochrome P450 3A4/P-glycoprotein inhibitors. *Arthritis Rheum* (2011) 63, 226 Erratum ibid. (2011) 63, 3521
2. Panel on Antiretroviral Guidelines for Adults and Adolescents. Guidelines for the use of antiretroviral agents in HIV-1-infected adults and adolescents. US Department of Health and Human Services (April 2015). 1–288. Available at: https://aidsinfo.nih.gov/contentfiles/lvguidelines/adultandadolescentgl.pdf (accessed 20/09/15).
3. Colchicine. Wockhardt UK Ltd. UK Summary of product characteristics, June 2010.
4. Colcrys (Colchicine). Takeda Pharmaceuticals America, Inc. US Prescribing information, November 2012.

Colchicine + Macrolides

Clarithromycin moderately increases, and azithromycin slightly increases, the exposure to single-dose colchicine. Telithromycin would be expected to interact similarly. Several case reports describe acute life-threatening colchicine toxicity, some of which were fatal, caused by the concurrent use of erythromycin or clarithromycin.

Clinical evidence

(a) Azithromycin

In a study in 21 healthy subjects, azithromycin (a single 500-mg dose followed by 250 mg daily for 4 days), increased the AUC and maximum concentration of a single 600-microgram dose of colchicine by 43% and 11%, respectively.[1]

A heart and lung transplant patient taking azithromycin 250 mg daily for lung transplant bronchiolitis, developed multi-organ failure and rhabdomyolysis 8 days after stopping colchicine, taken as 1 mg three times daily on day one, 1 mg twice daily on day 2, and 1 mg daily for 6 days, for acute gout.[2] He was also taking ciclosporin and pravastatin which could have contributed to the interaction, see 'Ciclosporin + Colchicine', p.1223, and 'Statins + Colchicine', p.1330.

(b) Clarithromycin

In a study in 23 healthy subjects, clarithromycin 250 mg twice daily for 7 days increased the AUC and maximum concentration of a single 600-microgram dose of colchicine 3.4-fold and 3-fold, respectively.[1]

In a patient who had been taking colchicine 1.5 mg daily for 6 years, signs of acute colchicine toxicity developed 4 days after a 7-day course of clarithromycin 1 g daily, amoxicillin, and omeprazole was started for *H. pylori*-associated gastritis. The colchicine dose was reduced to 500 micrograms daily and then, after recovery, gradually increased slowly back to 1.5 mg daily.[3] In another case, a 67-year-old man receiving CAPD, who was taking colchicine 500 micrograms twice daily, was admitted with symptoms of colchicine toxicity (including pancytopenia) 4 days after starting a course of clarithromycin 500 mg twice daily for an upper respiratory tract infection. All drugs were stopped and supportive treatment given, but he later died from multi-organ failure.[4]

These case reports led to a retrospective study of patients who had taken colchicine and clarithromycin as inpatients. Of 116 patients given the drugs, 88 had received them concurrently and 28 received them sequentially. Nine of the concurrent group died (compared with only one of the sequential group), and of the nine, five had pancytopenia, and six had renal impairment. In the 88 patients receiving the drugs concurrently, longer overlapping therapy increased the relative risk of death 2.16-fold, the presence of renal impairment increased the risk 9.1-fold, and the development of pancytopenia increased the risk 23.4-fold.[5]

Three further cases of fatal agranulocytosis, presumed to result from the use of colchicine with clarithromycin, have been reported,[6,7] and 2 other cases describe colchicine toxicity during clarithromycin use in patients with renal impairment.[8] A patient who had been taking clarithromycin 500 mg twice daily for 2 days for a tooth abscess, and who increased his colchicine dose from 1 mg daily to 12 mg daily to treat a gout flare, developed colchicine toxicity 3 days later, resulting in multi-organ failure, neutropenia, and thrombocytopenia. The patient died 3 days after admission.[9] Two cases of rhabdomyolysis have been reported, one occurred 3 days after a patient taking colchicine 600 micrograms daily started to take clarithromycin 500 mg twice daily,[10] the other 9 days after a patient taking colchicine 600 micrograms twice daily started clarithromycin 500 mg twice daily.[11] In another case, a 73-year-old man with chronic renal impairment, who was stable taking colchicine 500 micrograms daily, developed neuromyopathy a few days after completing a 10-day course of clarithromycin (dose not stated).[12] This patient was also taking simvastatin, which could have contributed to the interaction, see 'Statins + Colchicine', p.1330.

(c) Erythromycin

A 29-year-old woman with familial Mediterranean fever and amyloidosis, who was taking long-term colchicine 1 mg daily, developed acute and life-threatening colchicine toxicity (fever, diarrhoea, myalgia, pancytopenia, and later, alopecia) 16 days after starting to take erythromycin 2 g daily. This patient had both cholestasis and renal impairment, factors that would be expected to reduce colchicine clearance and therefore predispose her to colchicine toxicity. Colchicine concentrations increased from below 12.6 nanograms/mL to 22 nanograms/mL after the addition of erythromycin.[13]

Mechanism

Clarithromycin is a potent inhibitor and erythromycin is a moderate inhibitor of CYP3A4, and both macrolides inhibit P-glycoprotein. CYP3A4 and P-glycoprotein are involved in the metabolism and transport of colchicine and therefore concurrent use results in increased colchicine exposure and the adverse effects seen. Telithromycin is also a potent CYP3A4 inhibitor, and would be expected to have a similar effect. Azithromycin does not generally inhibit CYP3A4 to any clinically relevant extent, but is a P-glycoprotein inhibitor and so also increases colchicine exposure. Note, that any effect would be more notable in patients with renal impairment, in whom colchicine clearance is already reduced.

Importance and management

Information regarding the interaction between colchicine and the macrolides is largely limited to case reports with azithromycin, erythromycin, and clarithromycin, but given the increases in exposure to a single-dose of colchicine reported in the few available pharmacokinetic studies, it would seem that these macrolides can provoke acute colchicine toxicity, at the least, in pre-disposed individuals. A greater increase in colchicine exposure might occur with multiple dosing of colchicine, or higher macrolide doses. Other macrolides do not appear to have been studied. However, until more information is available, if any patient is given colchicine with a macrolide, monitor for signs of colchicine toxicity (such as nausea, vomiting, diarrhoea, myopathy, and pancytopenia) and anticipate the need to reduce the colchicine dose.

The US manufacturer of colchicine[14] makes the following specific recommendations for reducing the colchicine dose in patients taking **potent CYP3A4 inhibitors**, or if they have stopped taking such drugs within 2 weeks of starting colchicine, and they specifically name **clarithromycin** and **telithromycin**:

- For the treatment of gout, the dose of colchicine should be reduced to a single dose of 600 micrograms, with a further 300-microgram dose one hour later. The dose should not be repeated within 3 days;
- For gout prophylaxis, the dose of colchicine should be reduced to 300 micrograms daily (if the initial dose was 600 micrograms twice daily) or on alternate days (if the initial dose was 600 micrograms daily);
- For familial Mediterranean fever, a maximum total daily dose of colchicine 600 micrograms (which can be given as 300 micrograms twice daily) is recommended.

Note that patients with renal or hepatic impairment have a greater risk of developing colchicine toxicity, and for this reason the manufacturers of colchicine[14,15] specifically contraindicate the concurrent use of potent CYP3A4 inhibitors (see 'Table 1.9', p.11, for examples) in these patients.

The US manufacturer of colchicine[14] also advises the following dose reductions in patients taking **moderate CYP3A4 inhibitors**, or if they have stopped taking such drugs within 2 weeks of starting colchicine, and they specifically name **erythromycin**:

- For the treatment of gout, the dose of colchicine should be reduced to a single dose of 1.2 mg. The dose should not be repeated within 3 days;
- For gout prophylaxis, the dose of colchicine should be reduced to 300 micrograms twice daily or 600 micrograms daily (if the initial dose was 600 micrograms twice daily) or 300 micrograms daily (if the initial dose was 600 micrograms daily);
- For familial Mediterranean fever, a maximum total daily dose of colchicine 1.2 mg (which can be given as 600 micrograms twice daily) is recommended.

No specific advice is given for **azithromycin**, and given that the pharmacokinetic study showed only a slight increase in colchicine exposure, and the case report was complicated by concurrent use of other drugs known to have important effects on colchicine concentrations themselves, a clinically important interaction of the magnitude seen with other more potent CYP3A4 inhibitors might not be expected. However, as azithromycin is a P-glycoprotein inhibitor, it would seem prudent to monitor for signs of colchicine toxicity (such as nausea, vomiting, diarrhoea, myopathy, and pancytopenia), particularly in patients with pre-existing hepatic or renal impairment, and to anticipate the need to reduce the colchicine dose.

1. Terkeltaub RA, Furst DE, DiGiacinto JL, Kook KA, Davis MW. Novel evidence-based colchicine dose-reduction algorithm to predict and prevent colchicine toxicity in the presence of cytochrome P450 3A4/P-glycoprotein inhibitors. *Arthritis Rheum* (2011) 63, 226 Erratum ibid. (2011) 63, 3521.
2. Bouquié R, Deslandes G, Renaud C, Dailly E, Haloun A, Jolliet P. Colchicine-induced rhabdomyolysis in a heart/lung transplant patient with concurrent use of cyclosporin, pravastatin, and azithromycin. *J Clin Rheumatol* (2011) 17, 28–30.
3. Rollot F, Pajot O, Chauvelot-Moachon L, Nazal EM, Kélaïdi C, Blanche P. Acute colchicine intoxication during clarithromycin administration. *Ann Pharmacother* (2004) 38, 2074–7.
4. Dogukan A, Oymak FS, Taskapan H, Güven M, Tokgoz B, Utas C. Acute fatal colchicine intoxication in a patient on continuous ambulatory peritoneal dialysis (CAPD). Possible role of clarithromycin administration. *Clin Nephrol* (2001) 55, 181–2.
5. Hung IFN, Wu AKL, Cheng VCC, Tang BSF, To KW, Yeung CK, Woo PCY, Lau SKP, Cheung BMY, Yuen KY. Fatal interaction between clarithromycin and colchicine in patients with renal insufficiency: a retrospective study. *Clin Infect Dis* (2005) 41, 291–300.
6. Cheng VCC, Ho PL, Yuen KY. Two probable cases of serious drug interaction between clarithromycin and colchicine. *South Med J* (2005) 98, 811–13.
7. Huynh-Do U. In den gärten der Medea. *Ther Umsch* (2006) 63, 783–7.
8. Akdag I, Ersoy A, Kahveciogiu S, Gullulu M, Dilek K. Acute colchicine intoxication during clarithromycin administration in patients with chronic renal failure. *J Nephrol* (2006) 19, 515–17.
9. Izquierdo Pajuelo MJ, Jiménez Delgado JD, Rangel Mayoral JF, Liso Rubio, FJ. Interacción mortal entre colchicina y claritromicina. *Farm Hosp* (2010) 34, 309–10.
10. McKinnell J, Tayek JA. Short term treatment with clarithromycin resulting in colchicine-induced rhabdomyolysis. *J Clin Rheumatol* (2009) 15, 303–5.
11. Kim JB, Kim S, Lee T, Lee YS, Cho YS, Moon HB, Kim YG, Kim TB.Colchicine-induced rhabdomyolysis caused by interaction with clarithromycin in a patient with Behçet disease. *J Clin Rheumatol* (2013) 19, 108–9.
12. van der Velden W, Huussen J, ter Laak H, de Sévaux R. Colchicine-induced neuromyopathy in a patient with chronic renal failure: the role of clarithromycin. *Neth J Med* (2008) 66, 204–6.
13. Caraco Y, Putterman C, Rahamimov R, Ben-Chetrit E. Acute colchicine intoxication - possible role of erythromycin administration. *J Rheumatol* (1992) 19, 494–6.
14. Colcrys (Colchicine). Takeda Pharmaceuticals America, Inc. US Prescribing information, November 2012.
15. Colchicine. Wockhardt UK Ltd. UK Summary of product characteristics, June 2010.

Colchicine + Miscellaneous

Drugs that inhibit P-glycoprotein, such as quinidine and ranolazine, are predicted to increase the exposure to colchicine. The CYP3A4 inhibitor aprepitant is also predicted to interact similarly.

Clinical evidence, mechanism, importance and management

(a) Aprepitant

Colchicine is a CYP3A4 substrate and drugs that inhibit its metabolism by this route can increase its exposure and cause toxicity. The US manufacturer of colchicine recommends that the colchicine dose is reduced in patients taking **moderate CYP3A4 inhibitors**, or if they have stopped taking them within 2 weeks of starting colchicine, and they name aprepitant: see 'Colchicine + Macrolides', p.1562, for further details. The pro-drug of aprepitant, **fosaprepitant**, also inhibits CYP3A4 and so might be expected to interact similarly.

(b) P-glycoprotein inhibitors

Colchicine is a substrate for P-glycoprotein and drugs that inhibit this transporter can increase its exposure, which can lead to toxicity. The manufacturers of colchicine[1,2] therefore recommend that the colchicine dose is reduced or treatment is interrupted in patients with normal renal or hepatic function who are also taking P-glycoprotein inhibitors, and they specifically include **quinidine**[1] and **ranolazine**[2] in this advice. For the more detailed advice, given by the US manufacturer, for dose reductions in patients receiving P-glycoprotein inhibitors with colchicine, see 'Ciclosporin + Colchicine', p.1223. The manufacturers also contraindicate the concurrent use of colchicine and P-glycoprotein inhibitors in patients with renal or hepatic impairment.[1,2] For a list of drugs that inhibit P-glycoprotein, see 'Table 1.12', p.14.

1. Colchicine. Wockhardt UK Ltd. UK Summary of product characteristics, June 2010.
2. Colcrys (Colchicine). Takeda Pharmaceuticals America, Inc. US Prescribing information, November 2012.

Contrast media + Phenothiazines

Two isolated case reports describe epileptiform reactions in two patients when metrizamide was used for lumbar myelography in the presence of chlorpromazine or dixyrazine. No such cases appear to have been reported for intrathecal iohexol: nevertheless, the manufacturer of iohexol advises the avoidance of phenothiazines and other drugs that lower seizure threshold when iohexol is used intrathecally. Phenothiazines should also be avoided if iomeprol is required, and also if iopamidol is used for neuroradiological procedures.

Clinical evidence

A patient receiving long-term treatment with **chlorpromazine** 75 mg daily had a grand mal seizure three-and-a-half hours after being given **metrizamide** (16 mL of 170 mg iodine per mL by the lumbar route). He had another seizure 5 hours later.[1] One out of 34 other patients demonstrated epileptogenic activity on an EEG when given **metrizamide** for lumbar myelography. The patient was taking **dixyrazine** 10 mg three times daily.[2] However, a clinical study in 26 patients given **levomepromazine** for the relief of lumbago-sciatic pain found no evidence of an increased risk of seizures after they were given **metrizamide** for myelography.[3]

Mechanism

Intrathecal metrizamide or iohexol alone are rarely associated with seizures. Theoretically, this risk might be increased in patients taking other drugs that lower the seizure threshold, such as the phenothiazines.

Importance and management

The case report with intrathecal metrizamide led to the advice to stop phenothiazines before giving this contrast agent.[4] Intrathecal iohexol has also rarely been associated with seizures, and consequently the US manufacturer recommends that drugs that lower the seizure threshold, especially phenothiazines, are not recommended for use with iohexol by this route.[5] They should be stopped 48 hours before the procedure and not restarted until at least 24 hours after the procedure. The manufacturer of **iomeprol** gives the same advice.[6] However, the manufacturer of **iopamidol** advises that stopping phenothiazines is only necessary during neuroradiological use; the phenothiazine should be stopped 48 hours before the procedure and not restarted until at least 12 hours after the procedure has finished.[7] This advice specifically includes phenothiazines used for their antiemetic properties, for example, prochlorperazine. Although this risk is theoretical this would seem to be a prudent precaution. This advice does not apply to other routes of iohexol administration.[5]

1. Hindmarsh T, Grepe A and Widen L. Metrizamide-phenothiazine interaction. Report of a case with seizures following myelography. *Acta Radiol Diagnosis* (1975) 16, 129–34.
2. Hindmarsh T. Lumbar myelography with meglumine iocarmate and metrizamide. *Acta Radiol Diagnosis* (1975) 16, 209–22.
3. Standnes B, Oftedal S-I, Weber H. Effect of levomepromazine on EEG and on clinical side effects after lumbar myelography with metrizamide. *Acta Radiol Diagnosis* (1982) 23, 111–14.
4. Fedutes BA, Ansani NT. Seizure potential of concomitant medications and radiographic contrast media agents. *Ann Pharmacother* (2003) 37, 1506–10.
5. Omnipaque (Iohexol). GE Healthcare Inc. US Prescribing information, September 2007.
6. Iomeron (Iomeprol). Bracco UK Ltd. UK Summary of product characteristics, September 2008.
7. Niopam (Iopamidol). Bracco UK Ltd. UK Summary of product characteristics, July 2005.

Contrast media + Rifampicin (Rifampin)

Rifampicin may impair the biliary excretion of contrast media.

Clinical evidence, mechanism, importance and management

The manufacturers of rifampicin advise that tests involving contrast media visualisation of the gall bladder should be undertaken before the morning dose of rifampicin, given orally[1,2] or before the daily dose of rifampicin given parenterally,[3] as the biliary excretion of contrast media may be impaired.

1. Rifater Tablets (Rifampicin, Isoniazid and Pyrazinamide). Sanofi-Aventis. UK Summary of product characteristics, March 2009.
2. Rifadin (Rifampicin). Sanofi-Aventis US LLC. US Prescribing information, March 2007.
3. Rifadin for Infusion (Rifampicin). Sanofi-Aventis. UK Summary of product characteristics, March 2009.

Contrast media; Iopanoic acid + Colestyramine

A single report describes poor radiographic visualisation of the gall bladder due to an interaction between iopanoic acid and colestyramine within the gut.

Clinical evidence, mechanism, importance and management

The cholecystogram of a man with post-gastrectomy syndrome taking colestyramine, who was given oral iopanoic acid as an X-ray contrast medium, suggested that he had an abnormal and apparently collapsed gall bladder. A week after stopping the colestyramine a repeat cholecystogram gave excellent visualisation of a gall bladder of normal appearance.[1] The same effects have been observed experimentally in *dogs*.[1] This effects probably occurs because colestyramine binds with the iopanoic acid in the gut so that little is absorbed and little is available for secretion in the bile, hence the poor visualisation of the gall bladder.

On the basis of reports about other drugs that similarly bind to colestyramine, it seems probable that this interaction could be avoided if the administration of iopanoic acid and colestyramine were to be separated as much as possible (note that it is usually recommended that other drugs are given 1 hour before or 4 to 6 hours after colestyramine). Whether other oral acidic X-ray contrast media bind in a similar way to colestyramine is uncertain, but this possibility should be considered.

1. Nelson JA. Effect of cholestyramine on telepaque oral cholecystography. *Am J Roentgenol Radium Ther Nucl Med* (1974) 122, 333–4.

Cyclobenzaprine + Food

Food does not have a clinically relevant effect on the pharmacokinetics of modified-release cyclobenzaprine

Clinical evidence, mechanism, importance and management

In a randomised, crossover study, 15 healthy subjects were given a single 30-mg dose of modified-release cyclobenzaprine, either in the fasted state, or with a high-fat meal. When compared with the fasted state, food increased the exposure of cyclobenzaprine by 20%, which was not statistically significant.[1] In a study, 12 healthy subjects were given a single 20-mg dose of modified-release cyclobenzaprine with a high-fat meal. The AUC and maximum concentration of cyclobenzaprine were increased by 11% and 47%, respectively, compared with the fasted state. However, there was considerable individual variation in the effects of food in this study.[2] These modest effects on cyclobenzaprine exposure are unlikely to be clinically relevant and cyclobenzaprine can be taken without regard to meals.

1. Darwish M, Xie F. Effect of food on the pharmacokinetics of once-daily cyclobenzaprine extended-release 30 mg: a randomized, open-label, crossover, single-centre study. Clin Drug Investig. (2009) 29,145–52.
2. Gai MN, Costa E, Arancibia A. Bioavailability of a controlled-release cyclobenzaprine tablet and influence of a high fat meal on bioavailability. *Int J Clin Pharmacol Ther* (2009) 47, 269–74.

Cyclobenzaprine + Fluoxetine and Droperidol

A patient taking cyclobenzaprine and fluoxetine developed torsade de pointes and ventricular fibrillation when droperidol was also taken.

Clinical evidence

A 59-year-old woman who had been taking fluoxetine and cyclobenzaprine long-term, and who had a prolonged baseline QTc interval of 497 milliseconds, was given droperidol before surgery on her Achilles tendon. During the surgery she developed torsade de pointes, which progressed to ventricular fibrillation. On the first postoperative day after the cyclobenzaprine had been withdrawn, her QTc interval had decreased towards normal (440 milliseconds).[1]

Mechanism

The authors suggested that fluoxetine might have raised cyclobenzaprine serum levels by inhibition of cytochrome P450 (possibly CYP3A4, which is involved in the metabolism of cyclobenzaprine), and as a result the patient's QTc interval was prolonged. Cyclobenzaprine can cause arrhythmias, particularly in high doses. Therefore the addition of droperidol, which is known to prolong the QT interval, might have further extended the QTc interval and precipitated the torsade de pointes.

Importance and management

This is an isolated report, nevertheless, it is possible that a pharmacokinetic interaction occurs between cyclobenzaprine and fluoxetine, and that additive QT prolonging effects occur with cyclobenzaprine and droperidol, see also 'Drugs that prolong the QT interval + Other drugs that prolong the QT interval', p.272. Some caution would be appropriate on concurrent use.

1. Michalets EL, Smith LK, Van Tassel ED. Torsade de pointes resulting from the addition of droperidol to an existing cytochrome P450 drug interaction. *Ann Pharmacother* (1998) 32, 761–5.

Cyclobenzaprine + Serotonergic drugs

Two cases of possible serotonin syndrome have been described in patients given cyclobenzaprine while taking serotonergic drugs (phenelzine in one case, and duloxetine with bupropion in the other).

Clinical evidence

A 70-year-old woman who had been taking **phenelzine** 15 mg four times daily for several years underwent surgery for an infected hip replacement. She was taking cefazolin and, for pain, paracetamol and **oxycodone**. Six days later she started to take cyclobenzaprine 10 mg three times daily for muscle spasm. After the third dose she became confused, agitated, febrile and tachycardic. Cyclobenzaprine and oxycodone were stopped, with no improvement in her condition. Eventually a diagnosis of serotonin syndrome was suspected, and phenelzine was also stopped. She recovered over the subsequent 3 days.[1]

In a similar case, a 53-year-old man taking **duloxetine**, pregabalin, **bupropion** and oxycodone or hydromorphone as needed, underwent orthopaedic surgery and was given cyclobenzaprine 10 mg three times daily. Five days after surgery he became tachycardic and markedly agitated, and developed excessive sweating; he eventually required sedation and intubation. Cyclobenzaprine and duloxetine were stopped, and he was treated with cyproheptadine (a serotonin antagonist), and recovered over the following 2 days.[1]

Mechanism

The concurrent use of serotonergic drugs can, rarely, precipitate serotonin syndrome (see under 'Drugs that cause serotonin syndrome + Other drugs that cause serotonin syndrome', p.1471). Cyclobenzaprine is structurally related to the tricyclic antidepressants and might therefore have serotonergic effects, which could be additive with known serotonergic drugs.

Importance and management

These cases illustrate the potential for serotonin syndrome to develop when multiple drugs with serotonergic effects (such as the MAOIs, some opioids, the SNRIs) are given together. Although case reports for cyclobenzaprine are generally lacking, based on the way tricyclics (which are related to cyclobenzaprine) are known to interact with MAOIs, it would seem prudent to avoid the concurrent use of cyclobenzaprine and MAOIs: note that the US manufacturer of cyclobenzaprine[2] contraindicates concurrent use.

1. Keegan MT, Brown DR, Rabinstein AA. Serotonin syndrome from the interaction of cyclobenzaprine with other serotoninergic drugs. *Anesth Analg* (2006) 103, 1466–8.
2. Amrix (Cyclobenzaprine hydrochloride). Cephalon Inc. US Prescribing information, December 2008.

Dantrolene + Metoclopramide

Metoclopramide increases the exposure to dantrolene.

Clinical evidence, mechanism, importance and management

A study in paraplegics and quadriplegics with spinal cord injuries found that a single 10-mg intravenous dose of metoclopramide increased the AUC and maximum plasma level of a single 100-mg oral dose of dantrolene by 52% (12 patients assessed) and 72% (13 patients assessed), respectively. The reasons for this effect are not known, although it was suggested that absorption might have been affected. The clinical relevance of this interaction is uncertain but the authors of the study suggest that patients should be well monitored if metoclopramide is added or withdrawn from patients who are taking dantrolene.[1]

1. Gilman TM, Segal JL, Brunnemann SR. Metoclopramide increases the bioavailability of dantrolene in spinal cord injury. *J Clin Pharmacol* (1996) 36, 64–71.

Dantrolene + Oestrogens

The concurrent use of dantrolene and oestrogens might increase the risk of hepatotoxicity.

Clinical evidence, mechanism, importance and management

Dantrolene can cause hepatotoxicity, and risk factors include female gender, age over 30 years, and concurrent use of other hepatotoxic drugs.[1,2] The manufacturers also state that dantrolene-related hepatotoxicity appears to be more common in those also taking oestrogens.[1,2] The US manufacturer specifically notes that the risk of hepatotoxicity is in women over 35 years and states that, while a definitive interaction has not been established, caution is recommended on concurrent use.[2] In practice, this means that patients should be advised to seek medical advice if they develop symptoms such as generalised itching, yellowing of the eyes or skin, weight loss, nausea, or vomiting.

1. Dantrium Capsules (Dantrolene sodium). SpePharm UK Ltd. UK Summary of product characteristics, January 2012.
2. Dantrium Capsules (Dantrolene sodium). JHP Pharmaceuticals. US Prescribing information, October 2009.

Dextromethorphan + Amiodarone

Amiodarone can modestly reduce the clearance of dextromethorphan.

Clinical evidence

A study in 8 patients with cardiac arrhythmias found that amiodarone (1 g daily for 10 days followed by 200 to 400 mg daily for a mean duration of 76 days) changed their excretion of dextromethorphan 40 mg and its metabolite. The amount of unchanged dextromethorphan in the urine rose by nearly 150%, whereas the amount of its metabolite (dextrorphan) fell by about 25%.[1] All patients were of extensive CYP2D6 metaboliser phenotype (that is, they had normal levels of this isoenzyme) before amiodarone, and the effect of the amiodarone was modest (did not change them into pseudo-poor metabolisers, that is, those lacking or deficient in this isoenzyme).[1]

Mechanism

In vitro studies using liver microsomes have shown that amiodarone inhibits the metabolism (*O*-demethylation) of dextromethorphan by inhibiting the cytochrome P450 isoenzyme CYP2D6 within the liver.[1] This will occur in extensive metabolisers, but not poor metabolisers of this isoenzyme, see 'Genetic factors in drug metabolism', p.8, for further discussion of metaboliser phenotypes.

Importance and management

Information seems to be limited to this study. The implications are that amiodarone might interfere with the results of phenotyping if dextromethorphan is used to determine CYP2D6 activity. The extent of the interaction is unlikely to be clinically relevant in patients taking dextromethorphan, since this drug has a wide therapeutic index and its dose is not individually titrated.

1. Funck-Brentano C, Jacqz-Aigrain E, Leenhardt A, Roux A, Poirier J-M, Jaillon P. Influence of amiodarone on genetically determined drug metabolism in humans. *Clin Pharmacol Ther* (1991) 50, 259–66.

Dextromethorphan + Bupropion

Bupropion may reduce the metabolism of dextromethorphan in some patients.

Clinical evidence, mechanism, importance and management

In a study in 21 subjects who were quitting smoking and were CYP2D6 extensive metabolisers (that is, those with normal levels of this isoenzyme), 6 of 13 subjects who received bupropion 150 mg daily for 3 days and then twice daily for 14 days had metabolic ratios of dextromethorphan 30 mg similar to those seen in poor metabolisers (that is, those lacking or deficient in this isoenzyme): the metabolism of dextromethorphan to dextrorphan was substantially reduced. No such change was seen in the 8 subjects who received placebo.[1]

This suggests that bupropion can inhibit the cytochrome P450 isoenzyme CYP2D6, and is sufficiently potent an inhibitor to change up to half of extensive metabolisers into 'pseudo' poor metabolisers.

It has been suggested that care should be taken when initiating or discontinuing bupropion in patients taking CYP2D6 substrates, due to the possibility of raised levels.[1] Dextromethorphan is used as a probe substrate for CYP2D6, and is generally considered to have a wide therapeutic range and its dose is not individually titrated; therefore, the interaction with bupropion is unlikely to be clinically relevant. Nevertheless, it is possible that some extensive metaboliser patients might become more sensitive to the adverse effects of dextromethorphan while taking bupropion.

1. Kotlyar M, Brauer LH, Tracy TS, Hatsukami DK, Harris J, Bronars CA, Adson DE. Inhibition of CYP2D6 activity by bupropion. *J Clin Psychopharmacol* (2005) 25, 226–9.

Dextromethorphan + Celecoxib

Celecoxib modestly increases the plasma levels of dextromethorphan.

Clinical evidence, mechanism, importance and management

The manufacturers of celecoxib note that the plasma levels of dextromethorphan have been increased by 136% in the presence of celecoxib. Celecoxib inhibits the cytochrome P450 isoenzyme CYP2D6 and thus inhibits the metabolism of dextromethorphan by this isoenzyme.[1]

Dextromethorphan is used as a probe substrate for CYP2D6, and is generally considered to have a wide therapeutic range and its dose is not individually titrated; therefore, its interaction with celecoxib is unlikely to be clinically relevant. However, based on this pharmacokinetic interaction, the manufacturers of celecoxib suggest that caution should be observed with drugs that have a narrow therapeutic margin and are known to be predominantly metabolised by CYP2D6. They mention tricyclics, SSRIs, neuroleptics, and anti-arrhythmics, although not all drugs in these classes are important CYP2D6 substrates (for a list of CYP2D6 substrates, see 'Table 1.7', p.9). They say that the dose of CYP2D6 substrates may need to be decreased on starting celecoxib and increased on stopping it.[1] However, celecoxib is a very moderate CYP2D6 inhibitor when compared with the known potent CYP2D6 inhibitors cinacalcet and quinidine, and therefore any interactions with celecoxib as a result of this mechanism would, at worst, only be expected to be of only modest clinical relevance. So far there appear to be no direct clinical reports of any problems with concurrent use.

1. Celebrex (Celecoxib). Pfizer Ltd. UK Summary of product characteristics, January 2013.

Dextromethorphan + Cinacalcet

Cinacalcet very markedly increases dextromethorphan levels.

Clinical evidence

In a pharmacokinetic study in 23 healthy subjects who were extensive CYP2D6 metabolisers (that is, those with normal levels of this isoenzyme), the AUC of a single 30-mg dose of dextromethorphan was very markedly increased (by 11.4-fold) when given on day 8 of cinacalcet 50 mg daily for 8 days.[1]

Mechanism

In vitro, cinacalcet is a potent inhibitor of the cytochrome P450 isoenzyme CYP2D6, comparable to the well-known potent CYP2D6 inhibitor quinidine. This human study with the CYP2D6 probe substrate dextromethorphan confirms that cinacalcet is a clinically important CYP2D6 inhibitor.

Importance and management

A pharmacokinetic interaction between cinacalcet and dextromethorphan is established. However, dextromethorphan has a wide therapeutic range, and its dose is not individually titrated, so the interaction with cinacalcet is unlikely to be generally clinically relevant. Nevertheless, it is possible that some extensive metaboliser patients might become more sensitive to the adverse effects of dextromethorphan while taking cinacalcet.

Dextromethorphan is also used as a probe substrate for CYP2D6. These results therefore also suggest that cinacalcet will increase the levels of drugs that are substrates for CYP2D6. However, this will occur only in individuals who are extensive metabolisers. Poor metabolisers lack or have low levels of CYP2D6, and would not be affected. The effect of cinacalcet on CYP2D6 is likely to be important for CYP2D6 substrates that have a narrow therapeutic window. For a list of drugs that are CYP2D6 substrates, see 'Table 1.7', p.9.

1. Nakashima D, Takama H, Ogasawara Y, Kawakami T, Nishitoba T, Hoshi S, Uchida E, Tanaka H. Effect of cinacalcet hydrochloride, a new calcimimetic agent, on the pharmacokinetics of dextromethorphan: in vitro and clinical studies. *J Clin Pharmacol* (2007) 47, 1311–19.

Dextromethorphan + Grapefruit and other fruit juices

Grapefruit juice and the juice of the bitter orange increase the absorption of dextromethorphan.

Clinical evidence, mechanism, importance and management

In a study, 11 healthy subjects were given single 30-mg doses of dextromethorphan at bedtime, followed by 200 mL of water, 200 mL of grapefruit juice (prepared by diluting 1 part of 100% pure frozen concentrate, *Minute Maid*, with 3 parts water) or 200 mL of freshly-squeezed juice of the bitter orange. Measurement of the amount of dextromethorphan and its metabolites in the urine indicated that the bioavailability of dextromethorphan was increased by more than fivefold by grapefruit juice and by more than fourfold by bitter orange juice. Dextromethorphan levels were still raised 3 days later, indicating a sustained effect of the juices.

It was suggested that these fruit juices increased the absorption of dextromethorphan through the gut wall by inhibiting the cytochrome P450 isoenzyme CYP3A and P-glycoprotein.[1] The authors did not report any adverse effects of the increased exposure to dextromethorphan in these subjects, and dextromethorphan is generally considered to have a wide therapeutic range and the dose is not individually titrated. Therefore, the interaction with these fruit juices is probably unlikely to be clinically relevant. Note that, bitter orange is a different species to oranges that are usually consumed as part of the diet, and these results are not applicable to conventional orange juice.

1. Di Marco MP, Edwards DJ, Wainer IW, Ducharme MP. The effect of grapefruit juice and seville orange juice on the pharmacokinetics of dextromethorphan: the role of gut CYP3A and P-glycoprotein. *Life Sci* (2002) 71, 1149–60.

Dextromethorphan + HIV-protease inhibitors

Darunavir and tipranavir, both boosted with ritonavir, increase dextromethorphan exposure.

Clinical evidence

(a) Darunavir

In a study in healthy subjects, darunavir boosted with ritonavir 600/100 mg twice daily for 7 days increased the AUC of a single 30-mg dose of dextromethorphan 2.7-fold without increasing the AUC of the metabolite dextrorphan.[1]

(b) Tipranavir

In a study in 23 healthy subjects, the first dose of tipranavir boosted with ritonavir 500/200 mg twice daily increased the AUC of a single dose of dextromethorphan

2.9-fold, and by steady-state the AUC of dextromethorphan had increased 5.9-fold. Of the 23 subjects, 22 were CYP2D6 extensive metabolisers (that is, those with normal isoenzyme activity), and 6 of these became like poor metabolisers after receiving tipranavir boosted with ritonavir.[2]

Mechanism

Dextromethorphan is a probe substrate for CYP2D6 and ritonavir is a known inhibitor of this isoenzyme. The studies here show that darunavir boosted with ritonavir moderately inhibits CYP2D6 and that tipranavir boosted with ritonavir potently inhibits CYP2D6.

Importance and management

Dextromethorphan is used as a probe substrate for CYP2D6, and is generally considered to have a wide therapeutic range and its dose is not individually titrated; therefore its interaction with darunavir or tipranavir, both boosted with ritonavir, is unlikely to be clinically relevant. However, based on this pharmacokinetic interaction, tipranavir boosted with ritonavir in particular is likely to have a clinically relevant interaction with some CYP2D6 substrates. For a list of CYP2D6 substrates, see 'Table 1.7', p.9.

1. Sekar V, Spinosa-Guzman S, Meyvisch P, Stevens T, De Pauw M, Vangeneugden T, Hoetelmans R. Cocktail study to investigate the in-vivo drug interaction potential of darunavir coadministered with low-dose ritonavir (DRV/r; RTV) on cytochrome P450 enzymes 2D6, 2C9 and 2C19. 5th International Workshop on Clinical Pharmacology of HIV, New Orleans, April 2008, P23.
2. Dumond JB, Vourvahis M, Rezk NL, Patterson KB, Tien H-C, White N, Jennings SH, Choi SO, Li J, Wagner MJ, La-Beck NM, Drulak M, Sabo JP, Castles MA, Macgregor TR, Kashuba ADM. A phenotype-genotype approach to predicting CYP450 and P-glycoprotein drug interactions with the mixed inhibitor/inducer tipranavir/ritonavir. *Clin Pharmacol Ther* (2010) 87, 735–42.

Dextromethorphan + Methadone

An isolated report describes dextromethorphan-induced delirium, which was attributed to an interaction with methadone.

Clinical evidence

An 83-year-old patient with a 5-month history of hypersomnia and confusion noticed a great improvement in her symptoms on stopping a cough medicine containing dextromethorphan 30 mg with guaifenesin 600 mg twice daily. The cough medicine had been prescribed for a pneumonia-related cough 5 months previously and had not been discontinued. She was also taking a variety of other medications including methadone for pain related to spinal stenosis, escitalopram, metoclopramide, metolazone, and warfarin.[1]

Mechanism

Dextromethorphan is a probe substrate for CYP2D6, an enzyme which shows polymorphism. Methadone is an inhibitor of CYP2D6 *in vitro*,[2] but there is little clinical evidence that it acts as a CYP2D6 inhibitor *in vivo*. In the case of the elderly woman, it was suggested that methadone had reduced dextromethorphan metabolism resulting in dextromethorphan-induced delirium.[1] However, it is also possible that this case was solely due to the long-term use of dextromethorphan. Of the other drugs this patient was taking, escitalopram is a weak inhibitor of CYP2D6 and might have a slight effect on dextromethorphan exposure. In addition, the CYP2D6 metaboliser status of this patient is unknown: if she was a poor metaboliser then CYP2D6 inhibitors would have no additional effect on dextromethorphan exposure.

Importance and management

The case report described here does not prove that a pharmacokinetic interaction occurs between methadone and dextromethorphan, and further study is needed. Note that dextromethorphan has been tried in patients taking methadone maintenance therapy to reduce tolerance to methadone because of its activity as an antagonist of NMDA. In one such study, dextromethorphan was titrated to 240 mg daily for 6 weeks, and no problems were reported.[3]

Note that both methadone and dextromethorphan have serotonergic effects, and concurrent use might lead to the serotonin syndrome. Serotonin syndrome is a rare adverse effect, but because of its severity, some caution is warranted if both drugs are given. For more information on serotonin syndrome and its management, see 'Drugs that cause serotonin syndrome + Other drugs that cause serotonin syndrome', p.1471.

1. Lotrich FE, Rosen J, Pollock BG. Dextromethorphan-induced delirium and possible methadone interaction. *Am J Geriatr Pharmacother* (2005) 3, 17–20.
2. Wu D, Otton SV, Sproule BA, Busto U, Inaba T, Kalow W, Sellers EM. Inhibition of human cytochrome P450 2D6 (CYP2D6) by methadone. *Br J Clin Pharmacol* (1993) 35, 30–4.
3. Salehi M, Zargar A, Ramezani MA. Effects of dextromethorphan on reducing methadone dosage in opium addicts undergoing methadone maintenance therapy: a double blind randomized clinical trial. *J Res Med Sci* (2011) 16, 1354–60.

Dextromethorphan + Quinidine

Quinidine markedly increases the plasma levels of dextromethorphan in those who have normal levels of CYP2D6. This effect is maximal at low doses of quinidine (25 to 30 mg).

Clinical evidence

In a study, 6 subjects with normal levels of CYP2D6 (extensive metabolisers) were given dextromethorphan 60 mg twice daily. Steady-state plasma dextromethorphan levels averaged only 12 nanograms/mL. However, after being given quinidine 75 mg twice daily for a week, then a single 60-mg dose of dextromethorphan, their plasma levels of dextromethorphan were over threefold higher, at 38 nanograms/mL.[1] Some of the patients given the combination had an increase in dextromethorphan adverse effects (nervousness, tremors, restlessness, dizziness, shortness of breath, confusion etc).[1] Similarly, other pharmacokinetic studies have found increases in dextromethorphan levels in extensive CYP2D6 metabolisers, but not in those totally lacking or deficient in this isoenzyme (poor metabolisers).[2-4] In a dose-ranging study, quinidine 25 to 30 mg daily produced maximal increases in dextromethorphan levels, with higher doses producing no further increases, and lower doses producing smaller increases.[5] In one experimental study of citric acid-induced cough, quinidine increased the cough-suppressant effect of dextromethorphan.[6,7]

Mechanism

Quinidine inhibits the oxidative metabolism of dextromethorphan by the cytochrome P450 isoenzyme CYP2D6 to dextrorphan, effectively making extensive metabolisers of CYP2D6 into the poor metaboliser phenotype, see 'Genetic factors in drug metabolism', p.8, for further discussion of metaboliser phenotypes.

Importance and management

An established interaction. Dextromethorphan is used as a probe substrate for CYP2D6, and is generally considered to have a wide therapeutic range, and its dose is not individually titrated; therefore, the interaction with quinidine is unlikely to be clinically relevant. Nevertheless, it is possible that some extensive metabolisers of CYP2D6 might become more sensitive to the adverse effects of dextromethorphan if they are taking quinidine. This effect is maximal at low doses of quinidine (25 to 30 mg).

Low-dose quinidine has been given with dextromethorphan to sustain therapeutic levels of dextromethorphan and thereby try and improve its efficacy in various neurological disorders (dextromethorphan is an *N*-methyl-D-aspartate antagonist, which means it can affect pain transmission), and a fixed dose combination is available.

1. Zhang Y, Britto MR, Valderhaug KL, Wedlund PJ, Smith RA. Dextromethorphan: enhancing its systemic availability by way of low-dose quinidine-mediated inhibition of cytochrome P4502D6. *Clin Pharmacol Ther* (1992) 51, 647–55.
2. Schadel M, Wu D, Otton SV, Kalow W, Sellers EM. Pharmacokinetics of dextromethorphan and metabolites in humans: influence of CYP2D6 phenotype and quinidine inhibition. *J Clin Psychopharmacol* (1995) 15, 263–9.
3. Desmeules JA, Oestreicher MK, Piguet V, Allaz A-F, Dayer P. Contribution of cytochrome P-4502D6 phenotype to the neuromodulatory effects of dextromethorphan. *J Pharmacol Exp Ther* (1999) 288, 607–12.
4. Capon DA, Bochner F, Kerry N, Mikus G, Danz C, Somogyi AA. The influence of CYP2D6 polymorphism and quinidine on the disposition and antitussive effect of dextromethorphan in humans. *Clin Pharmacol Ther* (1996) 60, 295–307.
5. Pope LE, Khalil MH, Berg JE, Stiles M, Yakatan GJ, Sellers EM. Pharmacokinetics of dextromethorphan after single or multiple dosing in combination with quinidine in extensive and poor metabolizers. *J Clin Pharmacol* (2004) 44, 1132–42.
6. Abdul Manap R, Wright CE, Gregory A, Rostami-Hodjegan A, Meller ST, Kelm GR, Lennard MS, Tucker GT, Morice AH. The antitussive effect of dextromethorphan in relation to CYP2D6 activity. *Br J Clin Pharmacol* (1999) 48, 382–7.
7. Moghadamnia AA, Rostami-Hodjegan A, Abdul-Manap R, Wright CE, Morice AH, Tucker GT. Physiologically based modelling of inhibition of metabolism and assessment of relative potency of drug and metabolite: dextromethorphan vs. dextrorphan using quinidine inhibition. *Br J Clin Pharmacol* (2003) 56, 57–67.

Dextromethorphan + Reboxetine

Reboxetine does not appear to alter dextromethorphan pharmacokinetics.

Clinical evidence, mechanism, importance and management

In a study in 10 healthy subjects who were of the CYP2D6 extensive metaboliser phenotype (that is, those with normal activity of this isoenzyme), the pharmacokinetics of a single 30-mg dose of dextromethorphan were not affected by reboxetine 8 mg daily for one week.[1] In another study in 26 healthy subjects given reboxetine 6 mg daily with a single 30-mg dose of dextromethorphan on day 11, reboxetine did not alter the dextromethorphan concentrations achieved by extensive, intermediate, or poor CYP2D6 metabolisers, when compared with those seen with dextromethorphan given alone.[2]

Dextromethorphan is used as a probe drug to assess the activity of drugs on CYP2D6. These studies therefore suggest that reboxetine is not an inducer or inhibitor of CYP2D6, and dose adjustments are not likely to be needed when substrates of this isoenzyme are given with reboxetine. However CYP2D6 poor metaboliser status alone might lead to higher dextromethorphan concentrations.

1. Avenoso A, Facciolà G, Scordo MG, Spina E. No effect of the new antidepressant reboxetine on CYP2D6 activity in healthy volunteers. *Ther Drug Monit* (1999) 21, 577–9.
2. Kuhn UD, Kirsch M, Merkel U, Eberhardt AM, Wenda B, Maurer I, Härtter S, Hiemke C, Volz HP, Balogh A. Reboxetine and cytochrome P450 – comparison with paroxetine treatment in humans. *Int J Clin Pharmacol Ther* (2007) 45, 36–46.

Dextromethorphan + SSRIs

Paroxetine and fluoxetine considerably increase dextromethorphan concentrations, whereas fluvoxamine and sertraline have lesser effects.

A few reports describe the development of a serotonin-like syndrome in patients taking citalopram, fluoxetine, or paroxetine when they took dextromethorphan. In some of these cases, other serotonergic drugs

might have contributed. Another report describes hallucinations in a woman taking fluoxetine and dextromethorphan.

Clinical evidence

(a) Citalopram

A man who had been taking citalopram 30 mg, nefazodone 600 mg, and long-acting oxycodone 10 mg at bedtime without problems, started taking a cough syrup containing dextromethorphan and within a day he began to experience fatigue, lethargy, jitteriness, and headache. He stopped taking the dextromethorphan and his symptoms gradually disappeared over several hours.[1] A case of serotonin syndrome occurred a couple of days after taking dextromethorphan (*Night and Day* capsules) in a 46-year-old man who had been taking citalopram 40 mg daily and methadone 70 mg daily for 2 years.[2] A further case describes a 20-year-old man admitted to hospital and subsequently diagnosed with serotonin syndrome, after he was found to have a therapeutic concentration of citalopram and supratherapeutic concentrations of dextromethorphan and **chlorphenamine**.[3] It has been suggested that chlorphenamine, which has been shown to inhibit serotonin reuptake, might have contributed in this case.[4]

(b) Fluoxetine

In a pharmacokinetic study in healthy subjects given fluoxetine 20 mg daily for 4 weeks, the ratio of dextromethorphan to its metabolite, dextrorphan, in urine increased 17-fold, after a single 30-mg dose of dextromethorphan was given.[5] Another study using fluoxetine 60 mg daily for 8 days found a similar effect (18-fold increase in the ratio).[6] In a study in 14 healthy subjects given fluoxetine 20 mg daily for 28 days and a single 30-mg dose of dextromethorphan on days 7, 14, 21, and 28, the mean CYP2D6 inhibition half-life was 6.9 days, but the inhibitory effects remained for 42 days after the fluoxetine was stopped. In this study, the ratio of dextromethorphan to its metabolite, dextrorphan, in urine increased 55-fold but there was large interindividual variability.[7]

A woman who had been taking fluoxetine 20 mg daily for 17 days took about 10 mL of a cough syrup containing dextromethorphan, and a further dose the next morning, with the next dose of fluoxetine. Within 2 hours vivid hallucinations developed (bright colours, distortions of shapes and sizes), which lasted 6 to 8 hours. The patient said they were similar to her past experience with LSD 12 years earlier.[8]

(c) Fluvoxamine

In a pharmacokinetic study in healthy subjects given fluvoxamine 150 mg daily for 4 weeks, the ratio of dextromethorphan to its metabolite, dextrorphan, in urine increased about 2-fold (median), after a single 30-mg dose of dextromethorphan.[9]

(d) Paroxetine

In a pharmacokinetic study in healthy subjects given paroxetine 20 mg daily for 8 days, the ratio of dextromethorphan to its metabolite, dextrorphan, in urine increased 35-fold, after a single 30-mg dose of dextromethorphan was given.[6] A 10-fold increase in the ratio of dextromethorphan to dextrorphan was seen in another study using just a single 20-mg dose of paroxetine.[10] In a study in 13 healthy subjects given paroxetine 20 mg daily for 10 days and a single 30-mg dose of dextromethorphan on days 5 and 10, the mean CYP2D6 inhibition half-life was 2.9 days, and the inhibitory effects remained for 5 days after the paroxetine was stopped. In this study, the ratio of dextromethorphan to its metabolite, dextrorphan, in urine increased 8.6-fold.[7]

A man with multiple medical problems was admitted to hospital as an emergency, mainly because he was vomiting blood. He was taking diazepam, diltiazem, glyceryl trinitrate, paroxetine, piroxicam, ranitidine, and ticlopidine. Four days previously he had begun to take *Nyquil*, a non-prescription remedy for colds, containing dextromethorphan, pseudoephedrine, paracetamol (acetaminophen), and doxylamine. After two days he developed shortness of breath, nausea, headache, and confusion, and on admission he was also diaphoretic, tremulous, tachycardic, and hypertensive. Later he became rigid. The eventual diagnosis was that he was suffering from serotonin syndrome, attributed to an interaction between paroxetine and dextromethorphan in the presence of vascular disease. He was successfully treated with lorazepam 16 mg intravenously over 1 hour. The bleeding was thought to be from a small prepyloric ulcer.[11]

The authors of this report very briefly describe another patient taking paroxetine who developed symptoms consistent with serotonin syndrome within a few hours of taking a non-prescription cough remedy containing dextromethorphan and guaifenesin. She needed intensive care treatment.[12]

(e) Sertraline

In a pharmacokinetic study in healthy subjects, sertraline 100 mg daily for 8 days did not have a statistically significant effect on the ratio of dextromethorphan to its metabolite, dextrorphan, in urine, after a single 30-mg dose of dextromethorphan was given.[6] In a study in 12 healthy subjects given sertraline 50 mg daily for 3 days followed by 100 mg daily for 10 days, and a single 30-mg dose of dextromethorphan on days 5 and 10, the mean CYP2D6 inhibition half-life was 3 days, and the inhibitory effects remained for 5 days after the sertraline was stopped. In this study, the ratio of dextromethorphan to its metabolite, dextrorphan, in urine increased 15.6-fold, but there was large interindividual variability.[7]

Mechanism

Fluoxetine and paroxetine are inhibitors of CYP2D6, by which dextromethorphan is metabolised, resulting in increased dextromethorphan concentrations. Fluvoxamine and sertraline have much less effect on CYP2D6. Whether an increase in dextromethorphan concentrations has any bearing on the likely development of serotonin syndrome remains to be seen.

The symptoms that developed with citalopram or paroxetine and dextromethorphan were attributed by the authors of the reports to serotonin syndrome caused by the additive effects of the SSRIs and dextromethorphan on serotonin transmission.

Importance and management

Evidence for an interaction between the SSRIs and dextromethorphan is from a number of studies and a pharmacokinetic interaction is established. Paroxetine and fluoxetine are potent inhibitors of CYP2D6 and have considerable effects on dextromethorphan concentrations, whereas fluvoxamine and sertraline have minimal effects. However, this pharmacokinetic interaction will occur only in individuals who are CYP2D6 extensive metabolisers (that is, those with normal activity of this isoenzyme). Poor metabolisers have reduced CYP2D6 activity, and would not be affected. At the most, maximal inhibition of CYP2D6 therefore increases dextromethorphan concentrations in extensive metabolisers to those already seen in poor metabolisers. Dextromethorphan is generally considered to have a wide therapeutic range and the dose is not individually titrated; therefore, the interaction with paroxetine and fluoxetine is unlikely to be clinically relevant in terms of common adverse effects of dextromethorphan. Nevertheless, it is possible that some extensive metaboliser patients might become more sensitive to the adverse effects of dextromethorphan while taking paroxetine or fluoxetine. One study also showed that the duration of the inhibitory effect of fluoxetine was far longer in one group of subjects (42 days) than in 2 other groups taking paroxetine or sertraline (5 days each). This highlights the importance of bearing in mind the half-life of individual SSRIs when stopping them and starting a CYP2D6 substrate. Moreover, it is unclear what effect these pharmacokinetic interactions have on the development of serotonin syndrome, if any. So far, these few reports seem to be the only cases of serotonin syndrome being attributed to an interaction between an SSRI and dextromethorphan. However, it has been suggested that the incidence of mild serotonin excess (as seen in the case with citalopram) might be more common than is known.[1] The general importance of this apparent interaction is therefore very uncertain. The SSRIs are now very widely prescribed and dextromethorphan is a relatively common ingredient of non-prescription medicines. More study is therefore needed to establish this apparent interaction, but in the meantime, it seems unlikely that any general precautions are needed in patients taking SSRIs who use dextromethorphan-containing products.

On the basis of the difference in pharmacokinetic interaction between SSRIs and dextromethorphan, it had been predicted that sertraline and fluvoxamine might be less likely to cause serotonin syndrome with dextromethorphan than paroxetine and fluoxetine.[12,13] In considering this possibility, it should be noted that cases of serotonin syndrome have been reported with citalopram, which is not a potent CYP2D6 inhibitor. However in one of the citalopram case reports,[3] it appears that the patient might have been abusing dextromethorphan. Note that serotonin syndrome has been described in a patient prescribed dextromethorphan alone.[14] Serotonin syndrome is a rare adverse effect, but because of its severity, some caution might be warranted if both dextromethorphan and an SSRI are given. For more information on serotonin syndrome and its management, see 'Drugs that cause serotonin syndrome + Other drugs that cause serotonin syndrome', p.1471.

1. Ener RA, Meglathery SB, Van Decker WA, Gallagher RM. Serotonin syndrome and other serotonergic disorders. *Pain Med* (2003) 4, 63–74.
2. Cameron C. Serotonin syndrome precipitated by an over-the-counter cold remedy. *Aust Prescriber* (2006) 29, 71.
3. Schwartz AR, Pizon AF, Brooks DE. Dextromethorphan-induced serotonin syndrome. *Clin Toxicol* (2008) 46, 771–3.
4. Karamanakos PN, Panteli ES. Comment on "Dextromethorphan-induced serotonin syndrome". *Clin Toxicol* (2008) 46, 1101.
5. Amchin J, Ereshefsky L, Zarycranski W, Taylor K, Albano D, Klockowski PM. Effect of venlafaxine versus fluoxetine on metabolism of dextromethorphan, a CYP2D6 probe. *J Clin Pharmacol* (2001) 41, 443–51.
6. Alfaro CL, Lam YW, Simpson J, Ereshefsky L. CYP2D6 inhibition by fluoxetine, paroxetine, sertraline, and venlafaxine in a crossover study: intraindividual variability and plasma concentration correlations. *J Clin Pharmacol* (2000) 40, 58–66.
7. Liston HL, DeVane CL, Boulton DW, Risch SC, Markowitz JS, Goldman J. Differential time course of cytochrome P450 2D6 enzyme inhibition by fluoxetine, sertraline, and paroxetine in healthy volunteers. J Clin Psychopharmacol. (2002) 22, 169–73.
8. Achamallah NS. Visual hallucinations after combining fluoxetine and dextromethorphan. *Am J Psychiatry* (1992) 149, 1406.
9. Kashuba AD, Nafziger AN, Kearns GL, Leeder JS, Gotschall R, Rocci ML, Kulawy RW, Beck DJ, Bertino JS. Effect of fluvoxamine therapy on the activities of CYP1A2, CYP2D6, and CYP3A as determined by phenotyping. *Clin Pharmacol Ther* (1998) 64, 257–68.
10. Wilner KD, Demattos SB, Anziano RJ, Apseloff G, Gerber N. Ziprasidone and the activity of cytochrome P450 2D6 in healthy extensive metabolizers. *Br J Clin Pharmacol* (2000) 49, (Suppl 1), 43S–47S.
11. Skop BP, Finkelstein JA, Mareth TR, Magoon MR, Brown TM. The serotonin syndrome associated with paroxetine, an over-the-counter cold remedy, and vascular disease. *Am J Emerg Med* (1994) 12, 642–4.
12. Skop BP, Brown TM, Mareth TR. The serotonin syndrome associated with paroxetine. *Am J Emerg Med* (1995) 13, 606–7.
13. Harvey AT, Burke M. Comment on: The serotonin syndrome associated with paroxetine, an over-the-counter-cold remedy, and vascular disease. *Am J Emerg Med* (1995) 13, 605–6.
14. Kinoshita H, Ohkubo T, Yasuda M, Yakushiji F. Serotonin syndrome induced by dextromethorphan (Medicon) administered at the conventional dose. *Geriatr Gerontol Int* (2011) 11, 1212.

Dextromethorphan + Tyrosine kinase inhibitors

Pazopanib increases the concentration of dextromethorphan. There is no pharmacokinetic interaction between sorafenib and dextromethorphan.

Clinical evidence

(a) Sorafenib

In a phase I/II pharmacokinetic study in 18 patients with advanced melanoma, sorafenib 400 mg twice daily for 28 days did not alter the pharmacokinetics of a single 30-mg dose of dextromethorphan.[1]

(b) Pazopanib

In a pharmacokinetic study in patients with cancer, pazopanib 800 mg daily for 17 days, increased the ratio of dextromethorphan to dextrorphan concentrations in the urine after oral administration of a single 30-mg dose of dextromethorphan, by 33 to 64%.[2]

Mechanism

In vitro studies show that sorafenib,[3] and pazopanib,[4] inhibit CYP2D6, by which dextromethorphan is metabolised.

Importance and management

No pharmacokinetic interaction occurs between sorafenib and dextromethorphan, and no special precautions are necessary on concurrent use. Pazopanib caused a small increase in the dextromethorphan concentration, but as dextromethorphan has a wide therapeutic range, and its dose is not individually titrated, this would not be expected to be clinically important. Note that dextromethorphan can be used as a probe substrate to assess the activity of drugs on CYP2D6, and the study with sorafenib therefore suggests that it is not a clinically relevant inhibitor of CYP2D6. The situation with pazopanib is not established (although the authors suggested that it is only a weak inhibitor of CYP2D6[2]); however, the US manufacturer of pazopanib states that use with CYP2D6 substrates that have a narrow therapeutic range is not recommended.[4] For a list of known, clinically relevant CYP2D6 substrates, see 'Table 1.7', p.9.

Information about an interaction between other tyrosine kinase inhibitors and dextromethorphan is lacking.

1. Flaherty KT, Lathia C, Frye RF, Schuchter L, Redlinger M, Rosen M, O'Dwyer PJ. Interaction of sorafenib and cytochrome P450 isoenzymes in patients with advanced melanoma: a phase I/II pharmacokinetic interaction study. *Cancer Chemother Pharmacol* (2011) 68, 1111–8.
2. Goh BC, Reddy NJ, Dandamudi UB, Laubscher KH, Peckham T, Hodge JP, Suttle AB, Arumugham T, Xu Y, Xu C-F, Lager J, Dar MM, Lewis LD. An evaluation of the drug interaction potential of pazopanib, an oral vascular endothelial growth factor receptor tyrosine kinase inhibitor, using a modified Cooperstown 5 +1 cocktail in patients with advanced solid tumours. *Clin Pharmacol Ther* (2010) 88, 652–9.
3. Nexavar (Sorafenib tosylate). Bayer HealthCare Pharmaceuticals Inc. US Prescribing information, November 2013.
4. Votrient (Pazopanib hydrochloride). GlaxoSmithKline. US Prescribing information, November 2013.

Disulfiram + Celecoxib

An isolated report describes encephalopathy and polyneuropathy which developed in an elderly patient taking disulfiram when she was also given celecoxib and citalopram.

Clinical evidence, mechanism, importance and management

An elderly patient with chronic alcoholism who had been taking disulfiram 400 mg daily for 4 months, was given citalopram 20 mg daily and celecoxib. She became apathetic and confused and also developed ataxia, and was found to have vascular encephalopathy and polyneuropathy. Encephalopathy and polyneuropathy may occur with disulfiram alone, but the authors suggest that it is rare, and only usually occurs in overdose. It was suggested that in this case an interaction between either celecoxib or citalopram and disulfiram may have resulted in toxic levels of disulfiram, or that disulfiram had inhibited citalopram and/or celecoxib metabolism and increased their levels. In addition, some of the central effects may have been due to additive effects of the individual drugs.[1]

This appears to be an isolated case, and an interaction is by no means established. No general conclusions can therefore be drawn.

1. Berger A, Pategay N, Vogt N. Encéphalopathie aiguë et polyneuropathie au disulfiram: toxicité propre et interactions. Acute encephalopathy and polyneuropathy secondary to disulfiram administration: self toxicity and interactions. *Therapie* (2002) 57, 505–7.

Eltrombopag + HIV-protease inhibitors

No clinically relevant pharmacokinetic interaction appears to occur between lopinavir boosted with ritonavir and eltrombopag.

Clinical evidence, mechanism, importance and management

In a phase I, crossover study in 40 healthy subjects, **lopinavir boosted with ritonavir** 400/100 mg twice daily for 14 days reduced the AUC of a single 100-mg dose of eltrombopag by 17%. The pharmacokinetics of **lopinavir** and **ritonavir** were not affected by eltrombopag. The incidence of serious adverse effects did not increase on concurrent use. The authors of the study concluded that no eltrombopag dose adjustment was needed on the concurrent use of **lopinavir boosted with ritonavir**.[1] Despite this, the UK manufacturer of eltrombopag advises caution and recommends close monitoring of platelet counts in patients given **lopinavir boosted with ritonavir**, to ensure that eltrombopag remains effective.[2] However, this appears to be overly-cautious and changes of this magnitude would not be expected to be clinically relevant. There appears to be no information about the concurrent use of other HIV-protease inhibitors with eltrombopag.

1. Wire MB, McLean HB, Pendry C, Theodore D, Park JW, Peng B. Assessment of the pharmacokinetic interaction between eltrombopag and lopinavir-ritonavir in healthy adult subjects. *Antimicrob Agents Chemother* (2012) 56, 2846–51.
2. Revolade (Eltrombopag olamine). Novartis Pharmaceuticals UK Ltd. UK Summary of product characteristics, May 2015.

Eltrombopag + Miscellaneous

Eltrombopag is expected to affect the levels of substrates of the breast cancer receptor protein (such as topotecan), substrates of UDP-glucuronyltransferase (such as the opioids) and substrates of the organic anion transporter (such as methotrexate).The concurrent use of eltrombopag and other drugs that are used for treating idiopathic thrombocytopenic purpura (such as corticosteroids and immunoglobulins) may result in platelet counts that are higher than is desirable. The levels of eltrombopag are predicted to be raised by CYP1A2 and CYP2C8 inhibitors, and reduced by inducers of these isoenzymes. Eltrombopag does not affect the pharmacokinetics of caffeine, flurbiprofen, midazolam, or omeprazole.

Clinical evidence, mechanism, importance and management

(a) CYP1A2 inducers or inhibitors

The US manufacturer of eltrombopag states that *in vitro* studies indicate that the cytochrome P450 isoenzyme CYP1A2 is involved in the metabolism of eltrombopag. However, the clinical relevance of the effects of CYP1A2 inhibitors (they name **ciprofloxacin** and **fluvoxamine**) and CYP1A2 inducers (they name **tobacco** and **omeprazole**) on the pharmacokinetics of eltrombopag is unknown. If concurrent use is undertaken, the manufacturer states that patients should be monitored for an increase in eltrombopag effects (e.g. peripheral oedema, muscle spasm, insomnia, nausea) or a reduction in its efficacy.[1]

(b) CYP2C8 inducers or inhibitors

The US manufacturer of eltrombopag states that *in vitro* studies indicate that the cytochrome P450 isoenzyme CYP2C8 is involved in the metabolism of eltrombopag. However, the clinical relevance of the effects of CYP2C8 inhibitors (they name **gemfibrozil** and **trimethoprim**) and CYP2C8 inducers (they name **rifampicin (rifampin)**) on the pharmacokinetics of eltrombopag is unknown. If concurrent use is undertaken, the manufacturer states that patients should be monitored for an increase in eltrombopag effects (e.g. peripheral oedema, muscle spasm, insomnia, nausea) or a reduction in its efficacy.[1] Note that eltrombopag is also predicted to decrease rifampicin exposure see under *Organic anion transporter substrates*, below.

(c) Methotrexate and Topotecan

Topotecan and methotrexate are substrates for breast cancer resistance protein (BCRP), and the UK manufacturer of eltrombopag advises caution on concurrent use,[2] presumably because eltrombopag is an inhibitor of this drug transporter and may therefore increase topotecan and methotrexate levels. Note that methotrexate is also a substrate for the organic anion transporter OATP1B1, see under *Organic anion transporter substrates*, below.

(d) Organic anion transporter substrates

Eltrombopag is an inhibitor of the organic anion transporter OATP1B1. The manufacturers of eltrombopag therefore predict that the concurrent use of substrates of this transporter may result in an increase in their exposure. They name **methotrexate**,[1,2] **benzylpenicillin**, **nateglinide**, **repaglinide** and **rifampicin (rifampin)**.[1] The US manufacturer advises that patients taking eltrombopag should be monitored for an increase in the adverse effects of these substrates, and that a dose reduction should be considered, if necessary.[1] Note that rifampicin is also predicted to decrease eltrombopag exposure, see under *CYP2C8 inducers or inhibitors*, above. Note that methotrexate is also a substrate for breast cancer receptor protein (BCRP) and eltrombopag may increase its exposure by this mechanism, see under *Topotecan*, above.

(e) UDP-glucuronyltransferase substrates

The US manufacturer[1] of eltrombopag states that *in vitro* studies demonstrate that eltrombopag is an inhibitor of several UDP-glucuronyltransferases; however, the clinical significance of this has not been studied. They therefore advise monitoring in patients given eltrombopag and a substrate of UDP-glucuronyltransferase: they name **paracetamol (acetaminophen)**, the **opioids** and **NSAIDs**.[1] The clinical relevance of this prediction is unknown, but bear the possibility in mind should an increase in the adverse effects of these drugs occur.

(f) Other drugs

The UK manufacturer of eltrombopag states that, in clinical studies, eltrombopag was given with other drugs used for the treatment of idiopathic thrombocytopenic purpura, such as **azathioprine**, **corticosteroids**, **danazol**, intravenous **immunoglobulin** and **anti-D immunoglobulin**. However, concurrent use may result in a greater increase in platelet counts and they therefore advise close monitoring to ensure that platelet counts remain within the desired range.[2]

A study in 24 healthy subjects investigated the effect of eltrombopag on probe substrates for cytochrome P450 isoenzymes. Eltrombopag 75 mg dose was given on days 3 to 9, with single 5-mg doses of **midazolam** (a CYP3A4 substrate) on days 1 and 8 and single doses of **caffeine** 100 mg (a CYP1A2 substrate), **flurbiprofen** 50 mg (a CYP2C9 substrate), and **omeprazole** 20 mg (a CYP2C19 substrate) on days 2 and 9. Eltrombopag had no clinically significant effect on the metabolism of these probe substrates, and therefore a clinically significant interaction with other substrates of CYP1A2, CYP2C9, CYP2C19 and CYP3A4 would not be expected.[3]

1. Promacta (Eltrombopag olamine). GlaxoSmithKline. US Prescribing information, December 2011.
2. Revolade (Eltrombopag olamine). Novartis Pharmaceuticals UK Ltd. UK Summary of product characteristics, May 2015.

3. Jenkins J, Williams D, Deng Y, Collins DA, Kitchen VS. Eltrombopag. An oral thrombopoietin receptor agonist, has no impact on the pharmacokinetic profile of probe drugs for cytochrome P450 isoenzymes CYP3A4, CYP1A2, CYP2C9, CYP2C19 in healthy men: a cocktail analysis. *Eur J Clin Pharmacol* (2010) 66, 67–76.

Eltrombopag + Polyvalent cations

Aluminium- and magnesium-containing antacids reduce the bioavailability of eltrombopag. Other antacids or supplements containing polyvalent cations would be expected to interact similarly. High-calcium foods appear to decrease the exposure to eltrombopag whereas low-calcium foods (both high fat and low fat) do not affect eltrombopag exposure.

Clinical evidence

(a) Antacids

In a single-dose, crossover study, 25 healthy subjects were given a 75-mg dose of eltrombopag (as a tablet) with a 30-mL dose of an antacid containing **aluminium hydroxide** and **magnesium carbonate**. The antacid reduced the AUC and maximum concentration of eltrombopag by about 70%, when compared with dosing in the fasted state.[1]

(b) Foods

In a crossover study, a single 50-mg dose of eltrombopag (as a tablet) was given to 16 healthy subjects after an overnight fast or with a high-fat, high-calcium breakfast. The AUC and maximum concentration of eltrombopag were 59% and 65% lower, respectively, in the presence of a high-fat, high-calcium breakfast, when compared with the fasting state.[1]

A study by the same authors in healthy subjects found that taking a single 75-mg dose of eltrombopag (as a tablet) one hour before a high-fat, low-calcium meal, at the same time as a high-fat, low-calcium meal, or at the same time as a low-fat, low-calcium meal did not affect the pharmacokinetics of eltrombopag (24 or 25 subjects assessed), when compared with the fasted state.[1]

Mechanism

Eltrombopag is known to chelate with a number of polyvalent cations (such as magnesium), which can reduce its absorption.

Importance and management

Polyvalent cations, including those found in foods, decrease the absorption of eltrombopag to a clinically relevant extent. The manufacturers of eltrombopag state that eltrombopag should be taken at least 4 hours before or after antacids, foods or other products (e.g. mineral supplements) containing polyvalent cations such as **aluminium**, **calcium**, **iron**, **magnesium**, **selenium** and **zinc**.[2,3]

1. Williams DD, Peng B, Bailey CK, Wire MB, Deng Y, Park JW, Collins DA. Kapsi SG, Jenkins JM. Effects of food and antacids on the pharmacokinetics of eltrombopag in healthy adult subjects: two single-dose, open-label, randomized-sequence, crossover studies. *Clin Ther* (2009) 31, 764–76.
2. Promacta (Eltrombopag olamine). GlaxoSmithKline. US Prescribing Information, December 2011.
3. Revolade (Eltrombopag olamine). Novartis Pharmaceuticals UK Ltd. UK Summary of product characteristics, May 2015.

Enteric-coated, delayed-release preparations + Drugs that affect gastric pH

Theoretically, enteric-coated, delayed-release preparations may possibly dissolve prematurely if they are taken at the same time as antacids. This has been seen with some preparations, but not others. Release characteristics are likely to depend on the specific coating, and the manufacturers advice should be followed.

Clinical evidence

(a) Antacid

A placebo-controlled, crossover study in 21 healthy subjects, found that when extended-release **oxybutynin** 10 mg (*Ditropan XL*) was given at the same time as *Maalox* 20 mL (**aluminium/magnesium hydroxide** and **simeticone**) there was no change in the pharmacokinetics of **oxybutynin** or its metabolite.[1]

In an identical study in 23 healthy subjects, *Maalox* increased the maximum plasma level of a single 4-mg dose of extended-release **tolterodine** (*Detrol LA*) by 50%, but did not change the time to maximum level, elimination half-life, or AUC of **tolterodine**.[1]

(b) Omeprazole

In a placebo-controlled, crossover study in 39 healthy subjects, pre-treatment with omeprazole 20 mg daily for 4 days did not alter the pharmacokinetics of extended-release **oxybutynin** 10 mg [*Ditropan XL*]. The metabolites of **oxybutynin** were similarly unaffected. Pre-treatment with omeprazole increased the maximum plasma level of a single 4-mg dose of extended release **tolterodine** [*Detrol LA*] by 38%, but did not change the time to maximum level, elimination half-life, or AUC of **tolterodine**.[2]

The bioavailability of enteric-coated preparations of aspirin, diclofenac, and ketoprofen are unaffected by omeprazole, see 'NSAIDs or Aspirin + Proton pump inhibitors', p.156.

Mechanism

A marked rise in pH caused by antacids might cause premature dissolution of the coating of preparations formulated to prevent release of the contents until they reach the more alkaline conditions within the small intestine. Other types of delayed release preparations that have release characteristics independent of pH, such as those based on the osmotic principle, would not be expected to be affected.

Importance and management

Traditionally, it has been considered that drugs formulated with enteric coatings to resist gastric acid, or formulated as delayed-release preparations, should not be given with antacids. Accelerated drug release from a delayed-release product (dose dumping) might lead to increased adverse effects and lack of efficacy for the duration of the dose interval. The evidence above for extended-release tolterodine suggests that an antacid did cause a faster release of tolterodine from this product, but whether the 50% increase in the maximum level is sufficient to cause an increase in adverse effects is not known. Pre-treatment with omeprazole caused a smaller 38% increase in maximum tolterodine levels. The extended-release oxybutynin product was not affected by antacid or omeprazole, which was not unexpected because release from this product is osmotically driven and pH independent.

Release characteristics are likely to depend on the specific coating, and therefore no general advice can be given. The manufacturers' advice should be followed.

1. Sathyan G, Dmochowski RR, Appell RA, Guo C, Gupta SK. Effect of antacid on the pharmacokinetics of extended-release formulations of tolterodine and oxybutynin. *Clin Pharmacokinet* (2004) 43, 1059–68.
2. Dmochowski R, Chen A, Sathyan G, MacDiarmid S, Gidwani S, Gupta S. Effect of the proton pump inhibitor omeprazole on the pharmacokinetics of extended-release formulations of oxybutynin and tolterodine. *J Clin Pharmacol* (2005) 45, 961–8.

Ethylene dibromide + Disulfiram

The very high incidence of malignant tumours in *rats* exposed to both ethylene dibromide and disulfiram is the basis of the recommendation that concurrent exposure to these compounds should be avoided.

Clinical evidence, mechanism, importance and management

Research conducted to establish the occupational safety of exposure to ethylene dibromide found that the incidence of malignant tumours in *rats* exposed to 20 ppm ethylene dibromide (7 hours daily, 5 days weekly), while receiving a diet containing 0.05% disulfiram by weight, was very high.[1,2] The reasons for this effect are not understood. In addition to the precautions needed to protect workers from the toxic effects of ethylene dibromide, it has been strongly recommended that disulfiram should not be given to those who may be exposed to this compound.[2] This information is also summarised in another report.[3]

1. Plotnick HB. Carcinogenesis in rats of combined ethylene dibromide and disulfiram. *JAMA* (1978) 239, 1609.
2. Anon. Ethylene dibromide and disulfiram toxic interaction. National Institute for Occupational Safety and Health Current Intelligence Bulletin. *US Department of Health, Education and Welfare Publication* (1978) No 78–145.
3. Stein HP, Bahlman LJ, Leidel NA, Parker JC, Thomas AW, Millar JD. Ethylene dibromide and disulfiram toxic interaction. *Am Ind Hyg Assoc J* (1978) 39, A35–A37.

Fampridine (Dalfampridine) + Food

Food does not appear to affect the exposure to single-dose fampridine.

Clinical evidence, mechanism, importance and management

In a crossover study, 28 healthy subjects were given a single 10-mg dose of extended-release fampridine, either following a 12-hour fast or a high-fat meal. The AUC of fampridine was not affected by food, but the maximum plasma concentration was increased by 23%.[1]. The UK manufacturer of fampridine states that, as food increases the maximum concentration of fampridine, and there is a direct correlation between fampridine maximum concentrations and dose-related adverse effects, fampridine should be taken without food.[2] However, changes of this magnitude seem generally unlikely to be clinically relevant, and the US manufacturer states that fampridine can be taken with or without food.[3].

1. Henney HR, Faust B, Blight AR. Effect of food on the single-dose pharmacokinetics and tolerability of dalfampridine extended-release tablets in healthy volunteers. *Am J Health-Syst Pharm* (2011) 68, 2148–54.
2. Fampyra (Fampridine). Biogen Idec Ltd. UK Summary of product characteristics, July 2014.
3. Ampyra (Dalfampridine). Acorda Therapeutics, Inc. US Prescribing information, January 2014.

Fampridine (Dalfampridine) + Miscellaneous

Cimetidine, an inhibitor of organic cation transporter 2, is predicted to inhibit the renal excretion of fampridine. Substrates of this transporter, such as metformin, are also predicted to affect fampridine renal clearance. Drugs that lower the seizure threshold might increase the risk of

seizures with fampridine. No pharmacokinetic interaction appears to occur between fampridine and baclofen or interferon beta.

Clinical evidence, mechanism, importance and management

(a) Baclofen

The US manufacturer of fampridine notes that a population analysis indicates that baclofen does not affect fampridine pharmacokinetics.[1] The UK manufacturer also states that no pharmacokinetic interaction was seen on concurrent use.[2] Therefore, no dose adjustment of either drug is needed on concurrent use.

(b) Drugs that lower the seizure threshold

The UK manufacturer of fampridine briefly notes that because fampridine increases seizure risk, it should be used with caution when any factors which might lower the seizure threshold are present.[2] It would therefore seem prudent to carefully consider the risk of using a drug that might lower the seizure threshold with fampridine. This might include drugs such as **tricyclics**, **SSRIs**, **phenothiazines** and **butyrophenones**, **mefloquine**, **bupropion**, and **tramadol**.

(c) Inhibitors and substrates of organic cation transporter 2

The UK manufacturer states that fampridine is a substrate for the renal organic cation transporter 2, and about 60% is excreted by this mechanism. They therefore contraindicate the concurrent use of fampridine with drugs that inhibit this transporter (they name **cimetidine**),[2] presumably because the resulting reduction in fampridine clearance could lead to an increase in its adverse effects. In addition, they predict that substrates of organic cation transporter 2 might affect fampridine clearance and they advise caution on concurrent use: they name **carvedilol**, **metformin**, and **propranolol** as examples.[2] Until more is known, it would seem prudent to monitor concurrent use for an increase in fampridine adverse effects (such as insomnia, balance disorders, and tremor).

(d) Interferon beta

The US manufacturer of fampridine states that an 8 million unit dose of interferon beta-1b, given subcutaneously, had no effect on the pharmacokinetics of fampridine.[1] The UK manufacturer also states that no pharmacokinetic interaction was seen on concurrent use.[2] Therefore, no dose adjustment of either drug appears to be needed on concurrent use.

1. Ampyra (Dalfampridine). Acorda Therapeutics, Inc. US Prescribing information, January 2014.
2. Fampyra (Fampridine). Biogen Idec Ltd. UK Summary of product characteristics, July 2014.

Febuxostat + Miscellaneous

Febuxostat might increase azathioprine and mercaptopurine exposure. Low-dose febuxostat does not appear to affect the pharmacokinetics of theophylline, but high-dose febuxostat might increase the exposure to theophylline. The concurrent use of colchicine or hydrochlorothiazide and febuxostat does not affect the pharmacokinetics of either drug to a clinically relevant extent. Food and antacids do not affect the absorption of febuxostat to a clinically relevant extent. Febuxostat does not appear to interact with warfarin.

Clinical evidence, mechanism, importance and management

(a) Antacids

In a randomised, crossover study, 24 healthy subjects were given febuxostat 80 mg either alone, or with an **aluminium/magnesium hydroxide** antacid. Although the antacid delayed (by one hour) and reduced (by 32%) the maximum plasma concentration of febuxostat, the AUC was only reduced by 15%.[1] This slight reduction is not considered to be clinically relevant, and so no dose adjustment of febuxostat is likely to be needed on concurrent use.

(b) Azathioprine or Mercaptopurine

Azathioprine and mercaptopurine are known to be metabolised by xanthine oxidase, of which febuxostat is an inhibitor. Allopurinol, also a xanthine oxidase inhibitor, is known to increase exposure to these drugs (see 'Thiopurines + Allopurinol', p.720) leading to toxicity. As the concurrent use of febuxostat and azathioprine or mercaptopurine has not been studied, concurrent use is contraindicated[2] or not recommended.[3] If the concurrent use of febuxostat is considered essential, it would seem prudent to reduce the dose of azathioprine or mercaptopurine and monitor closely for haematological toxicity. Note that, with allopurinol, dose reductions do not always prevent the development of haematological toxicity.

(c) Colchicine

In a study, the concurrent use of colchicine 600 micrograms twice daily and febuxostat 40 or 120 mg daily caused slight changes in the maximum concentrations and AUCs of both drugs, but these changes were less than 20%, and were not considered to be clinically relevant. No dose adjustment of either drug is therefore needed on concurrent use.[2]

(d) Food

In a randomised, crossover study, healthy subjects were given febuxostat, as either a single 40-mg dose (23 subjects), a single 120-mg dose (19 subjects), or 80 mg daily for 6 days (23 subjects), when fasting, or with a meal. Although food decreased the maximum plasma concentrations of febuxostat (maximum 46% during multiple dosing) the absorption (AUC) and the effects of febuxostat on uric acid concentrations were not affected to a clinically relevant extent.[1] Febuxostat can therefore be taken without regard to meals.

(e) Hydrochlorothiazide

In a single-dose study, healthy subjects were given febuxostat 80 mg with hydrochlorothiazide 50 mg. Compared with the use of either drug alone, concurrent use did not affect the pharmacokinetics of either drug to a clinically relevant extent.[4] No dose adjustment of either drug is therefore needed on concurrent use, although note that hydrochlorothiazide and other **thiazide** diuretics can exacerbate gout and so some caution is warranted if both drugs are given.

(f) Theophylline

In a crossover study in 24 healthy subjects febuxostat 80 mg daily for 7 days did not affect the pharmacokinetics of a single 400-mg dose of theophylline given on day 5. However, there was an alteration in the concentration of urinary theophylline metabolites: methyluric acid decreased by 95% and methylxanthine increased 400-fold, although neither metabolite has any pharmacological activity.[5] Theophylline is known to be metabolised, in part, by xanthine oxidase, of which febuxostat is an inhibitor. The US manufacturer of febuxostat states that the long-term safety of exposure to methylxanthine is unknown and recommend caution with concurrent use.[2] The UK manufacturer states that no special caution is advised when febuxostat 80 mg daily is given with theophylline, but notes that no data are available for febuxostat 120 mg.[3] The authors of the original study suggest that a higher dose of febuxostat might increase theophylline exposure.[5] Therefore if theophylline, or **aminophylline**, are given with high-dose febuxostat, it might be prudent to check for any signs of theophylline adverse effects (headache, nausea, tremor). If theophylline adverse effects are troublesome, monitor concentrations and adjust the dose accordingly.

(g) Warfarin

In a study in healthy subjects, febuxostat 80 mg daily did not affect the pharmacokinetics of warfarin, or alter the INR in response to warfarin. Furthermore, *in vitro* data suggests that febuxostat does not inhibit CYP2C9, the major isoenzyme involved in the metabolism of warfarin.[2] No dose adjustments are needed if patients taking warfarin are given febuxostat.

1. Khosravan R, Grabowski B, Wu J-T, Joseph-Ridge N, Vernillet L. Effect of food or antacid on pharmacokinetics and pharmacodynamics of febuxostat in healthy subjects. *Br J Clin Pharmacol* (2007) 65, 355–63.
2. Uloric (Febuxostat). Takeda Pharmaceuticals America, Inc. US Prescribing information, March 2013.
3. Adenuric (Febuxostat). A. Menari Pharma UK S.R.L. UK Summary of product characteristics, February 2014.
4. Grabowski B, Khosravan R, Wu, J-T, Vernillet L, Lademacher C. Effect of hydrochlorothiazide on the pharmacokinetics and pharmacodynamics of febuxostat, a non-purine selective inhibitor of xanthine oxidase. *Br J Clin Pharmacol* (2010) 70, 57–64.
5. Tsai M, Wu JT, Gunawardhana L, Naik H. The effects of xanthine oxidase inhibition by febuxostat on the pharmacokinetics of theophylline. *Int J Clin Pharmacol Ther* (2012) 50, 331–7.

Fingolimod + Atropine

Atropine appears to reverse the bradycardic effects of fingolimod.

Clinical evidence, mechanism, importance and management

Fingolimod is known to be cause bradycardia, with a maximal effect around 4 to 5 hours after initiation. A randomised, placebo-controlled study was therefore designed to see if atropine could prevent or reverse this reduction in heart rate. In this study, 24 healthy subjects were given a single 5-mg dose of fingolimod with an intravenous atropine infusion (titrated to achieve a heart rate of 110 to 120 bpm or to a maximum total atropine dose of 2 mg). The atropine infusion was given either 5 minutes before (12 subjects) or 4 hours after (12 subjects) the fingolimod dose. Bradycardia started within 1 to 2 hours of starting fingolimod, and this was prevented when atropine was given at the same time as fingolimod. Giving atropine 4 hours after fingolimod also reversed the bradycardia seen with fingolimod alone. Atropine had no clinically relevant effect on the pharmacokinetics of fingolimod or its active metabolite, fingolimod phosphate. Concurrent use was well tolerated, and no clinically relevant adverse effects on blood pressure or ECG changes occurred. Therefore it would appear that atropine could be used to prevent or reverse the heart rate reduction in response to fingolimod.[1]

1. Kovarik JM, Slade A, Riviere G-J, Neddermann D, Maton S, Hunt TL, Schmouder RL. The ability of atropine to prevent and reverse the negative chronotropic effect of fingolimod in healthy subjects. *Br J Clin Pharmacol* (2008) 66, 199–206.

Fingolimod + Ciclosporin

No clinically relevant pharmacokinetic interaction appears to occur between fingolimod and ciclosporin.

Clinical evidence, mechanism, importance and management

In a randomised, crossover study, 12 patients with psoriasis were given ciclosporin 200 mg twice daily for 8 days, with a single 1-mg dose of fingolimod on day 5. The maximum concentration of fingolimod, and its AUC over the time period assessed were not affected by ciclosporin. Also, with the exception of the trough concentration, which was increased by 11%, the steady-state pharmacokinetics of ciclosporin were not altered by fingolimod.[1] The concurrent use of fingolimod and ciclosporin does not appear to affect the pharmacokinetics of either drug to a clinically relevant extent, and therefore no dose adjustments appear necessary on concurrent use. However, note that the UK manufacturer of fingolimod contraindicates the concurrent use of other immunosuppressive treatments, see 'Fingolimod + Miscellaneous', below.

1. Kovarik JM, Schmouder R, Barilla D, Büche M, Rouilly M, Berthier S, Wang Y, Van Saders C, Mayer T, Gottlieb AB. FTY720 and cyclosporine: evaluation for a pharmacokinetic interaction. *Ann Pharmacother* (2004) 38, 1153–8.

Fingolimod + Combined hormonal contraceptives

Fingolimod does not appear to affect the exposure to ethinylestradiol and levonorgestrel from an oral combined hormonal contraceptive.

Clinical evidence, mechanism, importance and management

In a pharmacokinetic study in 31 healthy subjects, fingolimod 0.5 mg daily for 2 weeks did not affect the exposure to **ethinylestradiol** (30 micrograms daily) and **levonorgestrel** (150 micrograms daily), given as an oral combined hormonal contraceptive. The pharmacokinetics of fingolimod were unaltered.[1] The UK and US manufacturers of fingolimod state that, although there are no studies on the concurrent use of fingolimod and hormonal contraceptives containing other progestogens, fingolimod is not expected to affect the exposure to these progestogens. Note that as fingolimod is teratogenic, the manufacturers advise that women of child-bearing potential given fingolimod should use adequate contraceptive measures [not specified] during, and for 2 months after stopping, fingolimod.[2,3]

1. David OJ, Ocwieja M, Meiser K, Emotte C, Jakab A, Wemer J, den Daas I, Schmouder R. Pharmacokinetics of fingolimod (FTY720) and a combined oral contraceptive coadministered in healthy women: drug-drug interaction study results. *Int J Clin Pharmacol Ther* (2012) 50, 540–4.
2. Gilenya (Fingolimod hydrochloride). Novartis Pharmaceuticals UK Ltd. UK Summary of product characteristics, February 2015.
3. Gilenya (Fingolimod hydrochloride). Novartis. US Prescribing information, May 2015.

Fingolimod + Drugs that prolong the QT interval

Fingolimod alone does not appear to cause QT prolongation. However, fingolimod can cause bradycardia, and this might increase the risk of QT prolongation if it is given with drugs that prolong the QT interval.

Clinical evidence, mechanism, importance and management

In a randomised, placebo-controlled study in 60 healthy subjects, doses of fingolimod of up to 5 mg did not prolong the QT interval.[1] However, fingolimod can cause clinically relevant bradycardia, and this is a known risk factor for torsade de pointes in the presence of QT-prolonging drugs. The US and UK manufacturers therefore contraindicate the concurrent use of fingolimod and **class Ia antiarrhythmics** (such as **quinidine** or **procainamide**) or **class III antiarrhythmics** (such as **amiodarone** or **sotalol**).[2,3] For a list of class Ia and class III antiarrhythmics, see 'Table 9.1', p.260. In addition, the UK manufacturer[3] also recommends avoiding the concurrent use of fingolimod with drugs that might prolong the QT interval in patients with additional risk factors for QT prolongation, such as hypokalaemia and heart failure, see 'Drugs that prolong the QT interval + Other drugs that prolong the QT interval', p.272. The US manufacturer advises overnight continuous ECG monitoring after the first dose of fingolimod if it is given to patients taking QT-prolonging drugs with a known risk of torsade de pointes, and they specifically name **citalopram**, **chlorpromazine**, **haloperidol**, **methadone**, and **erythromycin**.[2] However, a retrospective analysis of 3 300 patients with multiple sclerosis monitored for at least 6 hours after their first dose of fingolimod, found that those taking **SSRIs**, including **citalopram** and **escitalopram** (which have been associated with QT-interval prolongation), did not have a higher incidence of QTc interval or heart rate changes than those treated with fingolimod alone.[4] Although retrospective analyses of clinical study data are useful to identify potentially important drug interactions, they are not sensitive enough to rule out interactions, and should not replace prospective pharmacokinetic studies.

1. Schmouder R, Serra D, Wang Y, Kovarik JM, DiMarco J, Hunt TL, Bastien M-C. FTY720: placebo-controlled study of the effect on cardiac rate and rhythm in healthy subjects. *J Clin Pharmacol* (2006) 56, 895–904.
2. Gilenya (Fingolimod hydrochloride). Novartis. US Prescribing information, May 2015.
3. Gilenya (Fingolimod hydrochloride). Novartis Pharmaceuticals UK Ltd. UK Summary of product characteristics, February 2015.
4. Bermel RA, Hashmonay R, Meng X, Randhawa S, von Rosenstiel P, Sfikas N, Kantor D. Fingolimod first-dose effects in patients with relapsing multiple sclerosis concomitantly receiving selective serotonin-reuptake inhibitors. *Mult Scler Relat Disord* (2015) 4, 273–80.

Fingolimod + Food

Food does not appear to affect the exposure to fingolimod.

Clinical evidence, mechanism, importance and management

In a randomised, crossover study, 14 healthy subjects were given a single 1-mg dose of fingolimod, either in the fasted state or immediately after a high-fat breakfast. When compared with fasting, food had no effect on the maximum plasma levels or AUC of fingolimod.[1] Therefore, fingolimod may be taken without regard to meals.

1. Kovarik JM, Schmouder R, Barilla D, Wang Y, Kraus G. Single-dose FTY720 pharmacokinetics, food effect, and pharmacological responses in healthy subjects. *Br J Clin Pharmacol* (2004) 57, 586–91.

Fingolimod + Isoprenaline (Isoproterenol)

Isoprenaline appears to reverse the bradycardic effects of fingolimod.

Clinical evidence, mechanism, importance and management

In a randomised, placebo-controlled study, 14 healthy subjects were given a single 5-mg dose of fingolimod with intravenous isoprenaline (titrated to achieve a heart rate of 100 to 120 bpm or a maximum infusion rate of 5 micrograms per minute), given as four 30 minute infusions at 3, 4, 5 and 6 hours after fingolimod was given.[1] Isoprenaline reversed the reduction in heart rate induced by fingolimod; however, 41% more isoprenaline was required to reach the target heart rate in the presence of fingolimod, when compared with isoprenaline given alone. In this study, isoprenaline had no effect on the pharmacokinetics of fingolimod or its active metabolite, fingolimod phosphate. Concurrent use was generally well tolerated. It would therefore appear that isoprenaline could be used to prevent or reverse the heart rate reduction in response to fingolimod.[1]

1. Kovarik JM, Riviere G-J, Neddermann D, Maton S, Hunt TL, Schmouder RL. A mechanistic study to assess whether isoproterenol can reverse the negative chronotropic effect of fingolimod. *J Clin Pharmacol* (2008) 48, 303–10.

Fingolimod + Ketoconazole

Ketoconazole slightly increases the exposure to fingolimod. Exposure to the active metabolite of fingolimod is also increased.

Clinical evidence, mechanism, importance and management

In a crossover study, 22 healthy subjects were given ketoconazole 200 mg twice daily for 9 days, with a single 5-mg dose of fingolimod on day 4. Ketoconazole increased the AUC_{0-120} and maximum plasma concentration of fingolimod by 41% and 23% respectively. In addition, the AUC_{0-120} of the active metabolite, fingolimod phosphate, was increased by nearly 70%.[1] It was suggested that ketoconazole might have inhibited the hydroxylation of fingolimod by CYP4F2, leading to the increased exposure seen, although the authors state that this might not be the sole mechanism.[1]

The clinical relevance of this increase in the exposure to fingolimod and its active metabolite is unclear; however, until more is known, it would seem prudent to bear the possibility of an interaction in mind if fingolimod adverse effects (such as back pain, diarrhoea, and bradycardia) occur on concurrent use, adjusting the fingolimod dose as necessary. Other azoles are predicted to interact similarly, see 'Fingolimod + Miscellaneous', below.

1. Kovarik JM, Dole K, Riviere G-J, Pommier F, Maton S, Jin Y, Lasseter KC, Schmouder RL. Ketoconazole increases fingolimod blood levels in a drug interaction via CYP4F2 inhibition. *J Clin Pharmacol* (2009) 49, 212–18.

Fingolimod + Miscellaneous

Carbamazepine decreases the exposure to fingolimod, and other potent CYP3A4 inducers are predicted to act similarly. CYP3A4 inhibitors are predicted to increase fingolimod exposure. Additive bradycardia is predicted to occur if fingolimod is given with other drugs that can cause bradycardia (such as digoxin). Amantadine, amitriptyline, baclofen, corticosteroids, fluoxetine, gabapentin, modafinil, oxybutynin, paroxetine, and pregabalin do not appear to affect the pharmacokinetics of fingolimod.

Clinical evidence, mechanism, importance and management

(a) Cytochrome P450 inducers

Fingolimod appears to be principally metabolised by CYP4F2, although CYP3A4 might also be involved.[1,2] The UK and US manufacturers of fingolimod report that **carbamazepine** 600 mg twice daily given with a single 2-mg dose of fingolimod, decreased the AUC of both fingolimod and its metabolite, fingolimod-phosphate, by about 40%.[1,2] Carbamazepine is a potent inducer of CYP3A4, therefore other potent inducers of this isoenzyme might similarly reduce fingolimod exposure, see 'Table 1.9', p.11 for a list. Note that the manufacturers name **efavirenz** and **St John's wort** as potent inducers of CYP3A4, but they are generally considered to be moderate inducers. The clinical relevance of this interaction is not known, but bear it in mind if the response to fingolimod is not as expected on concurrent use of a CYP3A4 inducer. However, the UK manufacturers of fingolimod recommend avoiding the concurrent use of St John's wort.[1]

(b) Cytochrome P450 inhibitors

The UK manufacturer of fingolimod[1] predicts that CYP3A4 inhibitors might increase fingolimod exposure. However, although a slight increase in fingolimod exposure has been seen with ketoconazole, a known potent CYP3A4 inhibitor, this is probably not due to CYP3A4 inhibition, see 'Fingolimod + Ketoconazole', above. Nevertheless, until more is known, it would seem prudent to bear the possibility of an interaction in mind if fingolimod adverse effects (such as back pain, diarrhoea, and bradycardia) occur on concurrent use of a CYP3A4 inhibitor, adjusting the fingolimod dose as necessary. For a list of clinically relevant CYP3A4 inhibitors, see 'Table 1.9', p.11.

(c) Drugs that can cause bradycardia

The UK manufacturer of fingolimod predicts that drugs that cause bradycardia (they name **digoxin**, **ivabradine**, **anticholinesterases**, and **pilocarpine**) might exacerbate fingolimod-induced bradycardia and therefore they advise against initiating fingolimod in patients taking these drugs.[1] This is presumably based on the effects of giving fingolimod with other drugs that cause bradycardia, such as the beta blockers, see 'Beta blockers + Fingolimod', p.1010. If concurrent use is unavoidable, extended monitoring, including overnight ECG monitoring, is recommended after the first dose of fingolimod.[1,2] Note that the maximum effect of fingolimod on heart rate usually resolves within one month of starting treatment.[1,2]

(d) Immunosuppressants

The UK manufacturer of fingolimod contraindicates the concurrent use of other immunosuppressive treatments due to an increased risk of opportunistic infections.[1] Due to the long half-life of **natalizumab** (2 to 3 months), **mitoxantrone**, and **teriflunomide**, the UK and US manufacturers of fingolimod advise caution when switching from these drugs to fingolimod.[1,2]

(e) Vaccines

As with other immunosuppressants, fingolimod is expected to reduce the response to vaccines during, and for up to 2 months after stopping, fingolimod.[1,2] In addition, the concurrent use of fingolimod with live vaccines should be avoided, during and for 2 months after stopping fingolimod, as it can increase the risk of systemic infections.[2] See 'Immunosuppressants + Vaccines', p.1264, for more general information on the use of vaccines in immunosuppressed patients.

(f) Other drugs

The US manufacturer reports that, in a population pharmacokinetic evaluation, predose concentrations of fingolimod and its active metabolite, fingolimod phosphate, were not affected to a clinically relevant extent when it was given to patients with multiple sclerosis taking **fluoxetine** or **paroxetine** (both CYP2D6 inhibitors), **amantadine**, **amitriptyline**, **baclofen**, **corticosteroids**, **gabapentin**, **modafinil**, **oxybutynin** or **pregabalin**.[2]

1. Gilenya (Fingolimod hydrochloride). Novartis Pharmaceuticals UK Ltd. UK Summary of product characteristics, February 2015.
2. Gilenya (Fingolimod hydrochloride). Novartis. US Prescribing information, May 2015.

Glucagon + Beta blockers

The blood glucose-elevating effects of glucagon may be reduced by propranolol and possibly other beta blockers.

Clinical evidence, mechanism, importance and management

In a study in 5 healthy subjects the blood glucose-elevating effect of glucagon was reduced in the presence of **propranolol**.[1] Blood glucose levels increased by about 45% in the presence of glucagon, but when **propranolol** was also given the increase was only about 15%. The reason for this effect is uncertain, but one suggestion is that the **propranolol** inhibits the effects of the catecholamines that are released by glucagon. If this mechanism is correct, it seems possible that other beta blockers may interact in the same way as **propranolol**. However, the clinical importance of the interaction is uncertain. Note that glucagon may be used for treating beta blocker poisoning.

1. Messerli FH, Kuchel O, Tolis G, Hamet P, Frayasse J, Genest J. Effects of β-adrenergic blockage on plasma cyclic AMP and blood sugar responses to glucagon and isoproterenol in man. *Int J Clin Pharmacol Biopharm* (1976) 14, 189–94.

Histamine + Miscellaneous

Although there appears to be no published data regarding the interactions of histamine, a number of effects can be predicted based on the known actions of other drugs (e.g. effects reduced by the antihistamines) or based on the behaviour of endogenous histamine.

Clinical evidence, mechanism, importance and management

There appears to be no data published regarding the interactions of histamine; however, the manufacturers predict that a number of interactions may occur, based on the known effects of histamine.

Histamine may be used as a control response in skin testing for hypersensitivity and the manufacturers therefore reasonably suggest that the concurrent use of **antihistamines**[1,2] (including **antipsychotics** with histamine blocking properties)[1] may inhibit the response to histamine. The length of the suppression of the response is said to vary, from 24 hours with short-acting antihistamines such as **chlorphenamine**, to 40 days, with long-acting antihistamines such as astemizole.[2] Other drugs that are predicted to affect the response to histamine given as a skin test include **dopamine**, parenteral **ephedrine**, the **tricyclic antidepressants** (effect said to last for a few weeks) and oral **terbutaline** (and therefore presumably other **beta agonist bronchodilators** given orally). Beta agonist bronchodilators given by inhalation, **theophylline** and **sodium cromoglycate** are said not to affect the response to histamine given as a skin test.[2]

In contrast, **propranolol** is said to increase the skin sensitivity to histamine.[2] Furthermore, if histamine is given systemically it is advised that **beta blockers** and other **antihypertensives** are used with caution as they may worsen the effects of histamine on blood pressure (hypotension is a very common adverse effect of histamine). The use of **clonidine** is specifically contraindicated.[1]

H_2-receptor antagonists with an imidazole structure (**cimetidine** is named) are contraindicated,[1] because of their structural similarity to histamine, and systemic **corticosteroids** are also contraindicated[1] (although note that short-acting corticosteroids are said not to affect the response to histamine given for skin testing[2]).

Other drugs that may interact with systemic histamine[1] include the **MAOIs**, **antimalarials** and **antitrypanosomal drugs**, which are said to alter the metabolism of endogenous histamine; and **neuromuscular blockers**, **opioids** and **X-ray contrast media**, which can induce the release of endogenous histamine.

1. Ceplene (Histamine dihydrochloride). Meda Pharmaceuticals. UK Summary of product characteristics, October 2008.
2. Histatrol (Histamine phosphate). Alk-Abelló, Inc. US Prescribing information, June 2002.

Icatibant + Miscellaneous

ACE inhibitors might oppose the effects of icatibant. Pharmacokinetic drug interactions involving cytochrome P450 isoenzymes are not expected.

Clinical evidence, mechanism, importance and management

(a) ACE inhibitors

As icatibant is a selective bradykinin antagonist, concurrent use of ACE inhibitors, which can increase bradykinin concentrations, could oppose the effects of icatibant and reduce its efficacy. This has not been formally studied, but the UK manufacturer notes that ACE inhibitors are contraindicated in hereditary angioedema (the licensed indication for icatibant) due to possible enhancement of bradykinin concentrations.[1] Further, the US manufacturer states that icatibant might attenuate the antihypertensive effect of ACE inhibitors.[2]

(b) Cytochrome P450 enzyme system

In vitro studies show that icatibant is not a cytochrome P450 substrate, and does not inhibit or induce the major cytochrome P450 isoenzymes involved in drug metabolism.[1,2] Pharmacokinetic drug interactions involving this metabolic pathway are not expected.

1. Firazyr (Icatibant acetate). Shire Human Genetic Therapies. UK Summary of product characteristics, April 2014.
2. Firazyr (Icatibant acetate). Shire Orphan Therapies, Inc. US Prescribing information, August 2013.

Idebenone + Miscellaneous

There appears to be no clinically important pharmacokinetic interaction between idebenone and amitriptyline, donepezil, fluvoxamine, or lithium. However, food increases the bioavailability of idebenone.

Clinical evidence, mechanism, importance and management

(a) Donepezil

The manufacturer of idebenone reports that no significant pharmacokinetic interaction was seen between donepezil 5 mg daily and idebenone 360 mg three times daily for 14 days.[1] No dose adjustment of either drug would therefore be expected to be necessary on their concurrent use.

(b) Food

In a crossover study, 14 healthy subjects were given single 150-mg or 750-mg doses of idebenone when fasting or after a fat-rich meal. Food increased the maximum plasma levels and AUC of idebenone up to fivefold.[2] The manufacturer of idebenone[1] therefore advises that idebenone should be taken with food, to maximise absorption.

(c) Other drugs

A number of pharmacokinetic studies have assessed the potential of idebenone (as a single 120-mg dose, or 120 mg three times daily) to interact with other drugs. The concurrent use of idebenone and single doses of **amitriptyline** 75 mg, **fluvoxamine** 100 mg and **lithium** 2252 mg had no significant pharmacokinetic effect on either drug.[1] Therefore no dose adjustments would appear to be necessary on the concurrent use of idebenone and any of these drugs.

1. Catena (Idebenone). Santhera Pharmaceuticals Ltd. Canadian Prescribing information, July 2008.
2. Kutz K, Drewe J, Vankan P. Pharmacokinetic properties and metabolism of idebenone. *J Neurol* (2009) 256 (Suppl 1), 31–5.

Iron chelators + Ascorbic acid (Vitamin C)

High-dose vitamin C may cause cardiac disorders in some patients given desferrioxamine (deferoxamine). Other iron chelators are expected to interact similarly.

Clinical evidence, mechanism, importance and management

Vitamin C is given with iron chelators to patients with iron overload because it mobilises iron stores and thus promotes the excretion of iron. One study in 11 patients with thalassaemia noted that a striking deterioration in left ventricular function occurred when the patients were given 500 mg of vitamin C with intramuscular **desferrioxamine** (deferoxamine). In most patients left ventricular function returned to normal when the vitamin C was stopped.[1] For this reason it has been suggested that vitamin C should be used with **desferrioxamine** with caution,[2] only where there is a demonstrated need,[3] and in the lowest possible dose.[1] The manufacturers of **desferrioxamine** recommend that a maximum daily dose of 200 mg of vitamin C should be used in adults, that vitamin C should not be given within the first month of **desferrioxamine** treatment, that cardiac function should be monitored during combined use, and that vitamin C should not be given to those with cardiac failure.[4,5]

The UK manufacturers of **deferasirox** note that, although concurrent use with vitamin C has not been formally studied, doses of vitamin C up to 200 mg daily were allowed in clinical studies of **deferasirox** without adverse consequences.[6]

The manufacturer of **deferiprone** advise caution with the use of vitamin C, based on the way desferrioxamine is expected to interact.[7] It would therefore seem prudent to follow similar precautions to those advised with the other iron chelators.

1. Henry W. Echocardiographic evaluation of the heart in thalassemia major. *Ann Intern Med* (1979) 91, 892–4.
2. Cohen A, Cohen IJ, Schwartz E. Scurvy and altered iron stores in thalassemia major. *N Engl J Med* (1981) 304, 158–60.
3. Nienhuis AW. Vitamin C and iron. *N Engl J Med* (1981) 304, 170–1.
4. Desferal Vials (Desferrioxamine mesilate). Novartis Pharmaceuticals UK Ltd. UK Summary of product characteristics, August 2006.
5. Desferal Vials (Deferoxamine mesylate). Novartis. US Prescribing information, November 2007.
6. Exjade (Deferasirox). Novartis Pharmaceuticals UK Ltd. UK Summary of product characteristics, December 2011.
7. Ferriprox Tablets (Deferiprone). Swedish Orphan Biovitrum Ltd. UK Summary of product characteristics, September 2010.

Iron chelators + Food

Food, but not apple or orange juice, increases the bioavailability of deferasirox. Food does not appear to affect the absorption of deferiprone.

Clinical evidence, mechanism, importance and management

In single-dose studies in healthy subjects, giving **deferasirox** 30 minutes before a high-fat breakfast, 30 minutes before a standard breakfast, or with a standard breakfast modestly increased the AUC by 18%, 29% and 31%, respectively, when compared with the fasted state. In a further study in 12 patients with iron overload, giving **deferasirox** 5 minutes before a high-fat breakfast increased the AUC by 62% when compared with the fasted state. Nevertheless the concentration of iron-**deferasirox** complex in the plasma was unaffected by timing in relation to food.[1] However, the manufacturer recommends that, to limit variability, **deferasirox** is taken on an empty stomach at least 30 minutes before food.[2,3]

In a further study, the AUC of **deferasirox** was not significantly different when the tablets for oral suspension were dispersed in water, orange juice, or apple juice.[4] Therefore, any of these drinks is suitable for dispersing **deferasirox** tablets.[2,3]

Food does not appear to decrease the absorption of **deferiprone**.[5]

1. Galanello R, Piga A, Cappellini MD, Forni GL, Zappu A, Origa R, Dutreix C, Belleli R, Ford JM, Rivière G-J, Balez S, Alberti D, Séchaud R. Effect of food, type of food, and time of food intake on deferasirox bioavailability: recommendations for an optimal deferasirox administration regimen. *J Clin Pharmacol* (2008) 48, 428–35.
2. Exjade (Deferasirox). Novartis Pharmaceuticals UK Ltd. UK Summary of product characteristics, December 2011.
3. Exjade (Deferasirox). Novartis. US Prescribing information, September 2012.
4. Séchaud R, Dutreix C, Balez S, Pommier F, Dumortier T, Morisson S, Brun E. Relative bioavailability of deferasirox tablets administered without dispersion and dispersed in various drinks. *Int J Clin Pharmacol Ther* (2008) 46, 102–8.
5. Ferriprox Tablets (Deferiprone). Swedish Orphan Biovitrum Ltd. UK Summary of product characteristics, September 2010.

Iron chelators + Miscellaneous

The use of deferasirox and deferiprone with aluminium antacids is not recommended. Rifampicin (rifampin) reduces the exposure to deferasirox: carbamazepine, phenobarbital, phenytoin, and ritonavir are predicted to interact similarly. Colestyramine also reduces deferasirox exposure.

Deferasirox decreases the levels of midazolam and increases the levels of repaglinide and theophylline. Other drugs that have similar routes of metabolism are also expected to be affected (e.g. ciclosporin, paclitaxel, tizanidine).

Bisphosphonates, corticosteroids, and NSAIDs (including analgesic dose aspirin) may increase the risk of gastrointestinal ulceration with deferasirox. Deferasirox may increase the risk of bleeding with anticoagulants. Deferiprone can cause neutropenia and agranulocytosis, which may be exacerbated by other drugs with this effect.

Clinical evidence, mechanism, importance and management

(a) Aluminium-containing antacids

Although concurrent use has not been formally studied, the manufacturer recommends that **deferasirox** is not taken with aluminium-containing antacids.[1,2] **Deferasirox** has a lower affinity for aluminium than for iron, but theoretically aluminium might reduce the efficacy of **deferasirox**. Similar precautions are advised with **deferiprone**.[3]

(b) Colestyramine

In a study in healthy subjects, **colestyramine** reduced the AUC of a single dose of **deferasirox** by 45%. Therefore, the US manufacturer advises avoiding concurrent use. If both drugs must be given, the manufacturers advise giving consideration to increasing the dose of deferasirox to 30 mg/kg and monitoring ferritin levels and the clinical response to guide further dose adjustments.[2]

(c) CYP1A2 substrates

In a study in healthy subjects repeated doses of **deferasirox** 30 mg/kg daily increased the AUC a single 120-mg dose of theophylline by 84%, without affecting peak **theophylline** levels.[1] However, with multiple doses of **theophylline**, some **theophylline** accumulation would be expected. The UK manufacturer therefore states that the concurrent use of **theophylline** [and probably also **aminophylline**] and **deferasirox** should be avoided.[1] If both drugs are given it would seem prudent to anticipate the need for a dose reduction and monitor **theophylline** levels closely. On the basis of this study, they also advise against the concurrent use of deferasirox with other CYP1A2 substrates that have a narrow therapeutic margin: **clozapine** and **tizanidine** are specifically named. See 'Table 1.2', p.5, for a list of clinically relevant CYP1A2 substrates.

(d) CYP2C8 substrates

In a study in 24 healthy subjects, **deferasirox** 30 mg/kg daily for 4 days increased the AUC of a single 500-microgram dose of **repaglinide** 2.3-fold and increased its maximum levels by about 60%. In addition, deferasirox caused a slight increase in the blood-glucose lowering effects of **repaglinide**.[4] The UK manufacturers advise against concurrent use.[1] If both drugs are given, the manufacturers advise monitoring blood-glucose levels closely and giving consideration to reducing the **repaglinide** dose.[1,2] On the basis of this study, caution is advised with other CYP2C8 substrates, and **paclitaxel** is specifically named.[1,2] See 'Table 1.4', p.6, for a list of clinically relevant CYP2C8 substrates.

(e) CYP3A4 substrates

In a study in 22 healthy subjects, **deferasirox** 30 mg/kg daily for 5 days decreased the mean AUC and peak levels of a single 5-mg dose of **midazolam** by 10% and 21%, respectively.[4] Changes of this magnitude would not be expected to be clinically relevant. However, the manufacturers cautiously suggest that the effect may be greater in a clinical setting, and so advise caution if **deferasirox** is given with **midazolam**, or other substrates of CYP3A4 (they name **ciclosporin** (**cyclosporine**), **ergotamine**, **hormonal contraceptives** and **simvastatin**).[1,2]

(f) UGT enzyme inducers

In a study in 20 healthy subjects, **rifampicin** (**rifampin**) 600 mg daily for 9 days reduced the AUC of a single 30-mg/kg dose of **deferasirox** by 45%.[4] The mechanism for this interaction was thought to be UGT induction, and therefore caution is warranted with other drugs said to induce this enzyme, such as **carbamazepine**, **phenobarbital** [and therefore probably **primidone**], **phenytoin** [and therefore **fosphenytoin**] and **ritonavir**. The manufacturers recommend that the efficacy of **deferasirox** (serum ferritin levels and clinical response) should be monitored if any of these drugs is started or stopped, and the dose of **deferasirox** adjusted if necessary.[1,2]

(g) Other drugs

The manufacturers of **deferasirox** advise that caution is warranted in patients taking analgesic-dose **aspirin**, **bisphosphonates**, **corticosteroids** or **NSAIDs**. This is because **deferasirox** has caused gastrointestinal ulceration, which may be additive with these drugs. Furthermore, they advise caution with **anticoagulants** as the use of **deferasirox** may increase the risk of bleeding.[1,2]

The manufacturer of **deferiprone** advises that **deferiprone** has been shown to cause neutropenia, including agranulocytosis, therefore **deferiprone** is contraindicated with drugs that are known to be associated with these effects.[3]

1. Exjade (Deferasirox). Novartis Pharmaceuticals UK Ltd. UK Summary of product characteristics, December 2011.
2. Exjade (Deferasirox). Novartis. US Prescribing information, September 2012.
3. Ferriprox Tablets (Deferiprone). Swedish Orphan Biovitrum Ltd. UK Summary of product characteristics, September 2010.
4. Skerjanec A, Wang J, Maren K, Rojkjaer L. Investigation of the pharmacokinetic interactions of deferasirox, a once-daily oral iron chelator, with midazolam, rifampin and repaglinide in healthy volunteers. *J Clin Pharmacol* (2010) 50, 205–13.

Iron chelators + Phenothiazines

Prochlorperazine caused unconsciousness in two patients receiving desferrioxamine (deferoxamine).

Clinical evidence, mechanism, importance and management

The use of prochlorperazine in 2 patients receiving **desferrioxamine** (deferoxamine) resulted in unconsciousness for 48 to 72 hours. It was suggested that the drug combination resulted in increased removal of iron from the central nervous system, thereby impairing noradrenergic and serotonergic systems.[1] It has also been suggested that **desferrioxamine**-induced damage of the retina may be more likely in the presence of phenothiazines.[2] It would seem wise to avoid the concurrent use of **desferriox-**

amine and prochlorperazine. The manufacturer[3] of chlorpromazine predicts that a similar interaction may occur with chlorpromazine, but there seems to be no direct evidence of adverse interactions with chlorpromazine or any other phenothiazine. In addition, there appears to be no evidence of an interaction between the phenothiazines and other iron chelators.

1. Blake DR, Winyard P, Lunec J, Williams A, Good PA, Crewes SJ, Gutteridge JMC, Rowley D, Halliwell B, Cornish A, Hider RC. Cerebral and ocular toxicity induced by desferrioxamine. *Q J Med* (1985) 56, 345–55.
2. Pall H, Blake DR, Good PA, Wynyard P, Williams AC. Copper chelation and the neuro-ophthalmic toxicity of desferrioxamine. *Lancet* (1986) ii, 1279.
3. Largactil (Chlorpromazine hydrochloride). Sanofi-Aventis. UK Summary of product characteristics, March 2009.

Ivacaftor + Miscellaneous

Ketoconazole markedly increases the exposure to ivacaftor, and fluconazole moderately increases the exposure to ivacaftor. Other moderate and potent CYP3A4 inhibitors are predicted to interact similarly. Rifampicin (rifampin) markedly decreases the exposure to ivacaftor: other potent CYP3A4 inducers are predicted to interact similarly. Ivacaftor slightly increases the exposure to midazolam; other sensitive CYP3A4 substrates might be similarly affected.

Ivacaftor exposure is increased by fat-containing foods. Ivacaftor increases the exposure to digoxin and, theoretically, ivacaftor might increase the exposure to other drugs that are substrates of P-glycoprotein and increase the exposure to drugs that are substrates of CYP2C9 (such as warfarin).

Ivacaftor does not increase the exposure to desipramine or rosiglitazone, and the concurrent use of an oral combined hormonal contraceptive and ivacaftor does not affect the exposure to either drug. Ciprofloxacin does not affect the exposure to ivacaftor.

Clinical evidence, mechanism, importance and management

(a) Ciprofloxacin

The UK and US manufacturers of ivacaftor briefly note that ciprofloxacin had no effect on exposure to ivacaftor.[1,2]

(b) Combined hormonal contraceptives

In a drug interaction study 22 healthy women were given an oral combined hormonal contraceptive with ivacaftor 150 mg twice daily for 28 days.[3,4] There was no change in the exposure to ivacaftor,[1] and no clinically relevant increase in the exposure to the contraceptive hormones, norethisterone and ethinylestradiol.[1,2,4] No adjustment of the contraceptive or ivacaftor is therefore considered necessary on concurrent use.

(c) CYP2C9 substrates

In vitro studies indicate that ivacaftor might inhibit CYP2C9,[1,2] an isoenzyme important in **warfarin** metabolism. Although clinical data appears to be lacking, until more is known the UK and US manufacturers recommend monitoring the INR on the concurrent use of ivacaftor and **warfarin**.[1,2] The US manufacturers also suggest monitoring with other CYP2C9 substrates, but do not specifically name any.[1] For a list of clinically relevant CYP2C9 substrates, see 'Table 1.5', p.7.

(d) CYP3A4 inducers

In a drug interaction study, 24 healthy subjects were given ivacaftor 150 mg before and after taking **rifampicin (rifampin)** 600 mg daily for 10 days. Rifampicin decreased the exposure to ivacaftor by 89% and decreased the exposure to its active metabolite by 75%.[2] Ivacaftor is principally metabolised by CYP3A.[1,2] Rifampicin is a potent inducer of CYP3A4 and therefore concurrent use results in a marked decrease in ivacaftor exposure. The UK and US manufacturers of ivacaftor[1,2] therefore do not recommend concurrent use with potent inducers of CYP3A (see 'Table 1.9', p.11, for a list for clinically relevant CYP3A4 inducers). Note that the manufacturers consider **St John's wort** and **rifabutin** to be potent inducers of CYP3A.

If concurrent use is unavoidable, it seems likely that the dose of ivacaftor will need to be greatly increased to achieve efficacy, although this does not appear to have been studied. Monitor the outcome closely, expecting a loss of efficacy.

(e) CYP3A4 inhibitors

In a drug interaction study, 24 healthy subjects were given ivacaftor 150 mg before and after taking **ketoconazole** 400 mg daily for 10 days.[3] **Ketoconazole** increased ivacaftor exposure 8.5-fold.[2] A similar study, with **fluconazole** 400 mg as a loading dose, and then 200 mg daily for 9 days,[3] found that **fluconazole** increased ivacaftor exposure 3-fold.[2]

Ivacaftor is principally metabolised by CYP3A.[1,2] Ketoconazole is a potent inhibitor of CYP3A4 and concurrent use therefore results in a marked increase in ivacaftor exposure, whereas fluconazole, a moderate CYP3A4 inhibitor, causes a moderate increase in ivacaftor exposure.

The UK and US manufacturers of ivacaftor[1,2] recommend that the dose frequency of ivacaftor be reduced to twice a week when given with **potent CYP3A inhibitors**; and to once daily when given with **moderate CYP3A inhibitors** (see 'Table 1.9', p.11, for a list of clinically relevant CYP3A4 inhibitors). Note that the manufacturers consider **posaconazole** a potent inhibitor of CYP3A, but it is generally considered to be a moderate inhibitor of this isoenzyme.

Although grapefruit juice is a weak CYP3A4 inhibitor, the UK and US manufacturers state that patients taking ivacaftor should avoid food containing grapefruit, presumably because of the potential variability in the effect of grapefruit juice (see Grapefruit juice, under 'Drug-food interactions', p.16). They also apply this advice to the use of Seville (bitter) oranges, which are also known to inhibit CYP3A4.

(f) CYP3A4 substrates

A drug interaction study in 24 healthy subjects found that multiple doses of ivacaftor 150 mg twice daily increased the exposure to a single 2-mg dose of **midazolam** by 54%.[2-4] This indicates that ivacaftor is a weak CYP3A4 inhibitor. The UK and US manufacturers of ivacaftor therefore advise caution and monitoring for benzodiazepine adverse effects on concurrent use, and further apply this caution to the use of **alprazolam**, **diazepam**, and **triazolam**.[1,2] However, note that **diazepam** is not a particularly sensitive substrate for CYP3A4 and therefore a clinically relevant interaction would not be expected.

The manufacturers also suggest caution with other CYP3A substrates and some monitoring would seem prudent with those with a narrow therapeutic index. For a list of sensitive CYP3A4 substrates, see 'Table 1.10', p.12.

(g) Desipramine

A drug interaction study in 24 healthy subjects found that multiple doses of ivacaftor 150 mg twice daily did not affect exposure to a single 50-mg dose of desipramine.[3,4] Therefore, no adjustment of the desipramine dose is likely to be needed in patients also given ivacaftor. This study also indicates that ivacaftor is unlikely to affect the metabolism of other CYP2D6 substrates by this mechanism.

(h) Food

Fat-containing foods were found to increase the exposure to ivacaftor around 2- to 4-fold.[1,2] The UK and US manufacturers recommend that ivacaftor be taken with fat containing food (they name eggs, butter, nuts, peanut butter, cheese, and whole-milk dairy products).[1,2]

(i) P-glycoprotein substrates

In vitro studies indicate that ivacaftor might inhibit P-glycoprotein[1,2] A drug interaction study in 20 healthy subjects found that multiple doses of ivacaftor 150 mg twice daily increased the exposure to a single 250-microgram dose of **digoxin** by 32% and increased the maximum concentration by 23%.[4] The UK and US manufacturers advise caution with the use of ivacaftor in patients given P-glycoprotein substrates (they name **digoxin**, **ciclosporin**, and **tacrolimus**). Until more is known it would be prudent to be alert for increased adverse effects if ivacaftor is given with these drugs, monitoring drug concentrations, and adjusting doses if necessary. For a list of clinically relevant P-glycoprotein substrates, see 'Table 1.12', p.14.

(j) Rosiglitazone

A drug interaction study in 24 healthy subjects found that multiple doses of ivacaftor 150 mg twice daily did not affect the exposure to a single 4-mg dose of rosiglitazone.[3,4] Therefore, no rosiglitazone dose adjustment is likely to be needed in patients also given ivacaftor. This study also indicates that ivacaftor is unlikely to affect the metabolism of other CYP2C8 substrates by this mechanism.

1. Kalydeco (Ivacaftor). Vertex Pharmaceuticals Inc. US Prescribing information, March 2015.
2. Kalydeco (Ivacaftor). Vertex Pharmaceuticals UK Ltd. UK Summary of product characteristics, December 2014.
3. European Medicines Agency. CHMP assessment report for Kalydeco. Procedure No. EMEA/H/C/002494//0000. Available at: http://www.ema.europa.eu/docs/en_GB/document_library/EPAR_-_Public_assessment_report/human/002494/WC500130766.pdf (accessed 05/10/15).
4. Robertson SM, Luo X, Dubey N, Li C, Chavan AB, Gilmartin GS, Higgins M, Mahnke L. Clinical drug-drug interaction assessment of ivacaftor as a potential inhibitor of cytochrome P450 and P-glycoprotein. *J Clin Pharmacol* (2015) 55, 56-62.

Laropiprant + Clarithromycin

Clarithromycin slightly increases laropiprant exposure.

Clinical evidence

In a randomised, crossover study in 8 healthy subjects, clarithromycin 500 mg twice daily for 7 days was given with a single 40-mg dose of laropiprant on day 5. Clarithromycin increased the AUC and maximum plasma levels of laropiprant by 39% and 46%, respectively.[1]

Mechanism

Clarithromycin probably inhibits the metabolism of laropiprant by CYP3A4, which plays a minor route in its metabolism. The effect is not via inhibition of P-glycoprotein, because laropiprant is not a substrate for this transporter.

Importance and management

Although clarithromycin causes a slight increase in the exposure to laropiprant, this is not expected to be clinically important. Therefore no laropiprant dose adjustments would seem necessary on concurrent use. Note that laropiprant is only available as a combination product with nicotinic acid.

1. Wang Y-H, Schwartz JI, Luo W-L, James P, Desai R, Wenning LA, Wagner JA, Lai E. Effects of multiple doses of clarithromycin on the pharmacokinetics of laropiprant in healthy subjects. *Cardiovasc Ther* (2011) 29, 140–45.

Laropiprant + Miscellaneous

Laropiprant does not alter the pharmacokinetics of simvastatin or midazolam but does increase the exposure to the active hydroxy metabolite of midazolam. Laropiprant is predicted to inhibit the glucuronidation of zidovudine.

Clinical evidence, mechanism, importance and management

(a) Midazolam

The UK manufacturer reports that multiple doses of laropiprant 40 mg did not alter the pharmacokinetics of midazolam. As midazolam is a probe substrate of CYP3A4, the lack of effect of laropiprant on the pharmacokinetics of midazolam indicates that laropiprant is neither an inducer nor an inhibitor of CYP3A4. However, laropiprant increased the AUC and maximum plasma concentration of the active metabolite of midazolam, 1'-hydroxymidazolam, by 98% and 59%, respectively. *In vitro* data suggest that laropiprant is an inhibitor of UGT2B4 and UGT2B7, by which 1'-hydroxymidazolam is predominantly metabolised.[1] It therefore seems likely that the increase in 1'-hydroxymidazolam exposure is due to inhibition of its glucuronidation by laropiprant. Although the clinical relevance of the slight to moderate increase in 1'-hydroxymidazolam exposure has not been assessed, the UK manufacturer of laropiprant advises caution in patients given midazolam, as an increase in its sedative effects could occur.[1] The degree of sedation will depend on the individual patient and drug combination; however, warn all patients of the potential effects, and advise caution with driving or undertaking other skilled tasks.

(b) Zidovudine

The UK manufacturer states that clinical and *in vitro* data show that laropiprant is an inhibitor of UGT2B4 and UGT2B7. They therefore predict that laropiprant might increase the concentrations of drugs that are predominantly metabolised by this route, such as zidovudine, and advise caution on their concurrent use.[1] Until more is known, bear the possibility of an interaction in mind if laropiprant is given with zidovudine. However, note that, as yet there are no clinically important interactions with zidovudine known to occur by inhibition of its glucuronidation, see 'NRTIs; Zidovudine + Drugs that inhibit glucuronidation', p.985.

1. Tredaptive (Nicotinic acid with Laropiprant). Merck Sharp & Dohme Ltd. UK Summary of product characteristics, April 2012.

Lasofoxifene + Azoles

Ketoconazole increases the exposure to lasofoxifene whereas fluconazole does not affect the pharmacokinetics of lasofoxifene.

Clinical evidence

(a) Fluconazole

In a study, one group of 15 healthy postmenopausal women were given a single 250-microgram dose of lasofoxifene alone and a second group were given the same dose of lasofoxifene on day 2 of a 20-day course of fluconazole 400 mg daily. There was no difference in the pharmacokinetics of lasofoxifene in the two groups, suggesting that fluconazole does not affect the pharmacokinetics of lasofoxifene.[1]

(b) Ketoconazole

In a study, one group of 15 healthy postmenopausal women were given a single 250-microgram dose of lasofoxifene alone and a second group were given the same dose of lasofoxifene on day 2 of a 20-day course of ketoconazole 400 mg daily. Ketoconazole increased the AUC and maximum plasma concentration of lasofoxifene by 20% and 11%, respectively.[1]

Mechanism

Lasofoxifene is partially metabolised by CYP3A4, of which ketoconazole is a potent inhibitor. Concurrent use therefore decrease lasofoxifene metabolism resulting in the increased exposure see. Fluconazole is also an inhibitor of CYP3A4, but it does not affect lasofoxifene metabolism, presumably because other routes of metabolism compensate.

Importance and management

Evidence for an interaction between lasofoxifene and the azoles appears to be limited to one study involving fluconazole and ketoconazole. The increase in lasofoxifene exposure with ketoconazole is negligible and unlikely to be clinically relevant. No lasofoxifene dose adjustment would therefore appear to be necessary if it is given with ketoconazole or fluconazole.

1. Ouellet D, Bramson C, Roman D, Remmers AE, Randinitis E, Milton A, Gardner M. Effects of three cytochrome P450 inhibitors, ketoconazole, fluconazole, and paroxetine, on the pharmacokinetics of lasofoxifene. *Br J Clin Pharmacol* (2006) 63, 59–66.

Lasofoxifene + Miscellaneous

CYP3A4 inducers (e.g. carbamazepine) are predicted to increase lasofoxifene clearance. Lasofoxifene bioavailability might be decreased by proton pump inhibitors. Paroxetine caused a slight increase in lasofoxifene exposure. No clinically relevant changes in lasofoxifene pharmacokinetics occur with colestyramine. Lasofoxifene does not alter the pharmacokinetics of chlorzoxazone or dextromethorphan, or affect the metabolism of methylprednisolone.

Clinical evidence, mechanism, importance and management

(a) Chlorzoxazone

In a study in 18 healthy postmenopausal women, lasofoxifene (a 4-mg loading dose then 500 micrograms daily for 4 days) had no effect on the pharmacokinetics of a single 250-mg dose of chlorzoxazone given on day 4.[1] This suggests that chlorzoxazone dose adjustments are unlikely to be needed if lasofoxifene is also given. Note that chlorzoxazone is used as a probe substrate in evaluating the effects of drugs on CYP2E1, and this study therefore suggests that lasofoxifene is unlikely to affect the pharmacokinetics of CYP2E1 substrates (see 'Table 1.8', p.10, for a list).

(b) CYP3A4 inducers

Lasofoxifene is partially metabolised by CYP3A4. When it was available, the manufacturer predicted that inducers of this isoenzyme and glucuronyltransferases (e.g. **phenytoin**, **carbamazepine**, **barbiturates** and **St John's wort**) might increase lasofoxifene clearance,[2] which could result in a decrease in its efficacy. It might therefore be prudent to monitor for lasofoxifene efficacy in the presence of these drugs and consider increasing the lasofoxifene dose, if appropriate. Note that the potent CYP3A4 *inhibitor*, ketoconazole, has only slight effects on lasofoxifene exposure (see 'Lasofoxifene + Azoles', above) and therefore this predicted interaction with CYP3A4 inducers would not be expected to be clinically relevant. However, ideally this requires confirmation in a pharmacokinetic study.

(c) Dextromethorphan

In a study in 18 healthy postmenopausal women, lasofoxifene (a 4-mg loading dose followed by 500 micrograms daily for 4 days) had no effect on the pharmacokinetics of a single 30-mg oral dose of dextromethorphan given on day 5.[1] This suggests that dextromethorphan dose adjustments are unlikely to be needed if lasofoxifene is also given. Note that dextromethorphan is used as a probe substrate in evaluating the effects of drugs on CYP2D6, and this study therefore suggests that lasofoxifene is unlikely to affect the pharmacokinetics of CYP2D6 substrates (see 'Table 1.7', p.9, for a list).

(d) Paroxetine

In a randomised study, 10 healthy postmenopausal women were given paroxetine 30 mg daily for 21 days with a single 250 microgram-dose of lasofoxifene on day 8. Paroxetine increased the AUC and maximum plasma concentration of lasofoxifene by 35% and 18%, respectively, and increased its half-life from 168 hours to 202 hours.[3] It is likely that these changes occurred because lasofoxifene is partially metabolised by CYP2D6, of which paroxetine is an moderate inhibitor. However, these changes are unlikely to be clinically relevant as the increase in exposure is slight.

(e) Other drugs

Lasofoxifene solubility is pH-dependent. In view of the lack of data available, when it was available, the manufacturer advised caution when lasofoxifene is given with **proton pump inhibitors**,[2] as a reduction in solubility could alter lasofoxifene bioavailability and theoretically decrease efficacy. The manufacturer stated that the concurrent use of systemic **oestrogens** or **HRT** has not been studied with lasofoxifene and their concurrent use with lasofoxifene is therefore not recommended. **Colestyramine** was reported to have no clinically relevant effect on lasofoxifene pharmacokinetics. Lasofoxifene was reported not to affect the metabolism of **methylprednisolone**,[2] and therefore, no methylprednisolone dose adjustment is expected to be necessary on their concurrent use.

1. Moller RA, Fisher JM, Taylor AE, Kolluri S, Gardner MJ, Obach RS, Walsky RL. Effects of steady-state lasofoxifene on CYP2D6- and CYP2E1-mediated metabolism. *Ann Pharmacother* (2006) 40, 32–7.
2. Fablyn (Lasofoxifene tartrate). Pfizer Ltd. European Summary of product characteristics, February 2009. Available at: http://www.ema.europa.eu/docs/en_GB/document_library/EPAR_-_Product_Information/human/000977/WC500020092.pdf (accessed 21/10/15).
3. Ouellet D, Bramson C, Roman D, Remmers AE, Randinitis E, Milton A, Gardner M. Effects of three cytochrome P450 inhibitors, ketoconazole, fluconazole, and paroxetine, on the pharmacokinetics of lasofoxifene. *Br J Clin Pharmacol* (2006) 63, 59–66.

Memantine + Antidiabetics

The concurrent use of glibenclamide (glyburide) with metformin and memantine does not appear to affect the pharmacokinetics of these drugs.

Clinical evidence, mechanism, importance and management

In a study in 21 healthy subjects who took glibenclamide (glyburide) 1.25 mg with metformin 250 mg twice daily for 6 days, the administration of a single 20-mg dose of memantine did not result in any changes in the pharmacokinetics of any of the three drugs. Memantine did not reduce the glucose-lowering effects of either antidiabetic drug.[1] Evidence is limited, but dose adjustments would not appear to be necessary on concurrent use.

1. Rao N, Chou T, Ventura D, Abramowitz W. Investigation of the pharmacokinetic and pharmacodynamic interactions between memantine and glyburide/metformin in healthy young subjects: a single-center, multiple-dose, open-label study. *Clin Ther* (2005) 27, 1596–1606.

Memantine + Co-trimoxazole

A single case report describes myoclonus and confusion, which developed when a patient took memantine and co-trimoxazole or trimethoprim.

Clinical evidence, mechanism, importance and management

A 78-year-old woman who was taking memantine 15 mg daily in two divided doses took co-trimoxazole (trimethoprim 160 mg with sulfamethoxazole 800 mg) twice daily for 5 days for a urinary tract infection. During the course of treatment she developed significant upper extremity muscle twitching, confusion and agitation. These symptoms diminished on stopping the co-trimoxazole. The patient experienced a second, similar episode when she started to take trimethoprim 100 mg daily as prophylaxis for urinary tract infections. In light of a similar report of an interaction between the related drug, amantadine, and co-trimoxazole (see 'Amantadine + Co-trimoxazole', p.753) the authors of this report considered it was likely that the patient's symptoms were due to an interaction between memantine and trimethoprim.[1] Note that the patient was also taking a number of drugs, including hydrochlorothiazide, which has been suggested to reduce memantine renal excretion, see 'Memantine + Miscellaneous', below, for details.

1. Moellentin D, Picone C, Leadbetter E. Memantine-induced myoclonus and delirium exacerbated by trimethoprim. *Ann Pharmacother* (2008) 42, 443–7.

Memantine + Miscellaneous

The use of memantine, an NMDA antagonist, with other NMDA antagonists, such as amantadine, ketamine and dextromethorphan is predicted to increase the risk of adverse effects. Memantine is predicted to interact with other drugs eliminated by the same renal secretion mechanism, but no important interaction was seen with hydrochlorothiazide and triamterene.

Clinical evidence, mechanism, importance and management

(a) Interactions involving cytochrome P450 isoenzymes

The results of *in vitro* studies indicate that memantine is not likely to cause interactions by inducing or inhibiting the major cytochrome P450 isoenzymes involved in drug metabolism (CYP1A2, CYP2C9, CYP3A4).[1,2] However, an *in vitro* study has demonstrated that memantine may inhibit CYP2B6 at clinically relevant concentrations.[3] **Cyclophosphamide** and **ifosfamide** are substrates of this isoenzyme, but there are few other drugs that are metabolised by this route. No metabolic interaction as a result of this mechanism appears to have been described.[3] In addition, memantine is not significantly metabolised by the cytochrome P450 enzyme system, and is therefore not expected to undergo interactions as a result of this mechanism.[1]

(b) Other drugs eliminated by renal tubular secretion

Memantine is predicted to interact with other drugs that use the same renal cationic transport system leading to increased levels of memantine and/or the other drug. The manufacturer lists **cimetidine**, **ranitidine**, **hydrochlorothiazide**, metformin, **nicotine**, **procainamide**, **quinidine**, **quinine** and **triamterene** as possible examples.[1,2] However, in an interaction study, the concurrent use of memantine and **hydrochlorothiazide** with **triamterene** did not result in any change in the steady-state AUC of memantine or **triamterene**, and the AUC of **hydrochlorothiazide** showed a modest *reduction* of about 20%.[1] This degree of change is unlikely to be clinically relevant. Furthermore, a study with metformin found no interaction (see 'Memantine + Antidiabetics', p.1575). Therefore, a clinically important interaction as a result of this mechanism seems unlikely.

(c) Other NMDA antagonists

Memantine is chemically related to **amantadine**, and the manufacturer advises that concurrent use should be avoided[2] or undertaken with caution[1] because of the increased risk of adverse CNS-related drug reactions such as psychosis.[2] Although there are no data, an increased risk is also predicted for **ketamine** and **dextromethorphan**, which are also NMDA antagonists. Avoidance of,[2] or caution with,[1] concurrent use is advised.

(d) Warfarin

The manufacturer of memantine notes that, although no causal relationship has been established, isolated cases of INR increases have been reported in patients taking warfarin. They suggest close monitoring of anticoagulant effects if both drugs are given.[1,2]

(e) Other drugs

Memantine might modify the effects of antispasmodic drugs such as **dantrolene** or **baclofen** and dosage adjustment might be required.[2] Memantine is predicted to enhance the effects of **antimuscarinics**, **levodopa** and dopaminergic (**dopamine agonist**) drugs.[2] Memantine is predicted to reduce the effects of **barbiturates** and **antipsychotics**.[2]

1. Namenda (Memantine hydrochloride). Forest Pharmaceuticals, Inc. US Prescribing information, April 2007.
2. Ebixa (Memantine hydrochloride). Lundbeck Ltd. UK Summary of product characteristics, July 2009.
3. Micuda S, Mundlova L, Anzenbacherova E, Anzenbacher P, Chladek J, Fuksa L, Martinkova J. Inhibitory effects of memantine on human cytochrome P450 activities: prediction of in vivo drug interactions. *Eur J Clin Pharmacol* (2004) 60, 583–9.

Memantine + Urinary alkalinisers

Drugs that increase the pH of the urine (e.g. sodium bicarbonate, carbonic anhydrase inhibitors) may reduce the elimination of memantine.

Clinical evidence, mechanism, importance and management

In 12 healthy subjects, the clearance of memantine 10 mg daily was markedly reduced by about 80% when the urine was alkaline (pH 8) compared with acidic urine (pH 5). The maximum plasma memantine levels were not affected by the urinary pH, but the bioavailability of memantine was increased by almost 20%.[1] This might be expected to lead to memantine accumulation and an increase in adverse effects. Drugs that could interact via this mechanism include **sodium bicarbonate** and **carbonic anhydrase inhibitors**[2] [such as **acetazolamide**]. The clinical relevance of these findings does not appear to have been established. Consider the possibility of an interaction if patients taking memantine with a urinary alkaliniser develop memantine adverse effects (e.g. dizziness, headache, constipation).

1. Freudenthaler S, Meineke I, Schreeb K-H, Boakye E, Gundert-Remy U, Gleiter CH. Influence of urine pH and urinary flow on the renal excretion of memantine. *Br J Clin Pharmacol* (1998) 46, 541–6.
2. Namenda (Memantine hydrochloride). Forest Pharmaceuticals, Inc. US Prescribing information, April 2007.

Metyrapone + Miscellaneous

The results of the metyrapone test for Cushing's syndrome are unreliable in patients taking cyproheptadine or phenytoin. The manufacturer also states that barbiturates, antidepressants, some hormones, and antipsychotics may influence the results of the metyrapone test. Metyrapone may reduce the metabolism of paracetamol (acetaminophen).

Clinical evidence

(a) Cyproheptadine

In 9 a study in healthy subjects, pretreatment with cyproheptadine 4 mg every 6 hours, 2 days before and throughout a standard metyrapone test (750 mg every 4 hours for 6 doses), reduced the metyrapone-induced urinary 17-hydroxycorticosteroid response by 32%, and also reduced the serum 11-deoxycortisol response.[1]

(b) Paracetamol (Acetaminophen)

In a randomised study, 8 healthy subjects were given metyrapone 750 mg one hour before and 3 hours after a single 1-g dose of paracetamol. Metyrapone decreased the glucuronidation of paracetamol from about 52% to 36% of the dose. Although the formation of other metabolites were increased, overall paracetamol excretion in the urine was decreased from about 75% to 69%.[2]

(c) Phenytoin

A study in 5 healthy subjects and 3 patients taking phenytoin 300 mg found that serum metyrapone levels 4 hours after taking a regular 750-mg dose were very low, when compared with those of a control group (6.5 micrograms/100 mL versus 48.2 micrograms/100 mL). The response to metyrapone (i.e. the fall in circulating glucocorticoids) is related to serum levels and was therefore proportionately lower.[3] Other reports confirm that the urinary steroid response to metyrapone is subnormal in patients taking phenytoin.[4,5]

Doubling the dose of metyrapone from 750 mg every 4 hours to every 2 hours has been shown to give results similar to those in subjects not taking phenytoin.[3]

Mechanism

Phenytoin is a potent liver enzyme inducer that increases the metabolism of metyrapone, thereby reducing its effects.[3,6]

Importance and management

The results of metyrapone tests for Cushing's syndrome will be unreliable in patients taking cyproheptadine and phenytoin, and therefore these should be withdrawn before the test; the US manufacturer advises 2 weeks.[7] The UK manufacturer also states that **barbiturates**, antidepressants (they name **amitriptyline**) and antipsychotics (they name **chlorpromazine**), hormones that affect the hypothalamo-pituitary-adrenal axis (the US manufacturers name **oestrogens**[7]), and **antithyroid drugs** may influence the results of the test. They recommend that, if any of these drugs cannot be withdrawn before the test, the necessity of carrying out the metyrapone test should be reviewed.[8]

In addition, the US manufacturer notes that metyrapone inhibits the glucuronidation of paracetamol, and may therefore increase paracetamol toxicity.[7] However, one study suggests that the extent may be modest, and, as metyrapone is usually only given for 24 hours, the clinical relevance of this effect seems small.

1. Plonk J, Feldman JM, Keagle D. Modification of adrenal function by the anti-serotonin agent cyproheptadine. *J Clin Endocrinol Metab* (1976) 42, 291–5.
2. Galinsky RE, Nelson EB, Rollins DE. Pharmacokinetic consequences and toxicologic implications of metyrapone-induced alterations of acetaminophen elimination in man. *Eur J Clin Pharmacol* (1987) 33, 391–6.
3. Meikle AW, Jubiz W, Matsukura S, West CD, Tyler FH. Effect of diphenylhydantoin on the metabolism of metyrapone and release of ACTH in man. *J Clin Endocrinol Metab* (1969) 29, 1553–8.

4. Krieger DT. Effect of diphenylhydantoin on pituitary-adrenal interrelations. *J Clin Endocrinol Metab* (1962) 22, 490–3.
5. Werk EE, Thrasher K, Choi Y, Sholiton LJ. Failure of metyrapone to inhibit 11-hydroxylation of 11-deoxycortisol during drug therapy. *J Clin Endocrinol Metab* (1967) 27, 1358–60.
6. Jubiz W, Levinson RA, Meikle AW, West CD, Tyler FH. Absorption and conjugation of metyrapone during diphenylhydantoin therapy: mechanism of the abnormal response to oral metyrapone. *Endocrinology* (1970) 86, 328–31.
7. Metopirone (Metyrapone). Novartis. US Prescribing information, August 2005.
8. Metopirone (Metyrapone). Alliance Pharmaceuticals. UK Summary of product characteristics, February 2005.

Mifepristone + Aspirin or NSAIDs

Theoretically NSAIDs might reduce the efficacy of mifepristone, and combined use is often not recommended. However, evidence from two studies with naproxen and diclofenac suggests no reduction in mifepristone efficacy.

Clinical evidence

(a) Mifepristone

In a study in women undergoing surgical first-trimester termination of pregnancy, patients received mifepristone 100 mg 48 hours and 36 hours before surgery for cervical ripening. There was no difference in the cervical softening effect between 13 women randomised to receive **naproxen** (500 mg given 60, 48, 36, 24 and 12 hours before the procedure) and 15 women randomised to receive placebo.[1]

(b) Mifepristone and misoprostol

Women undergoing second trimester medical terminations of pregnancy were given oral mifepristone 600 mg on day one, then 36 to 48 hours later, intravaginal misoprostol 800 micrograms. Starting 3 hours later, misoprostol 400 micrograms was given orally every 3 hours until expulsion, up to a maximum of nine oral doses of misoprostol. The women were randomised to receive a single dose of either paracetamol 1 g with dihydrocodeine 20 mg (n=38) or **diclofenac** 100 mg (n=36), given at the time of the intravaginal dose of misoprostol. The use of **diclofenac** did not increase either the time required for termination, or the amount of misoprostol needed.[2]

Mechanism

Mifepristone is thought to work by increasing prostaglandin production. Theoretically NSAIDs could reduce this, and therefore reduce the efficacy of mifepristone.

Importance and management

Because of theoretical concerns of antagonistic effects, NSAID analgesics, including **aspirin**, have been avoided in protocols for medical termination of pregnancy. However, the limited available evidence suggests that this might not be necessary.

For more information about the use of vaginal prostaglandins with NSAIDs, see under 'NSAIDs or Aspirin + Prostaglandins', p.156.

1. Rådestad A, Bygdeman M. Cervical softening with mifepristone (RU 486) after pretreatment with naproxen. A double-blind randomized study. *Contraception* (1992) 45, 221–7.
2. Fiala C, Swahn ML, Stephansson O, Gemzell-Danielsson K. The effect of non-steroidal anti-inflammatory drugs on medical abortion with mifepristone and misoprostol at 13-22 weeks gestation. *Hum Reprod* (2005) 20, 3072–7.

Mifepristone + Miscellaneous

Mifepristone is predicted to inhibit the metabolism of CYP3A4 substrates. Mifepristone is a CYP3A4 substrate, and its levels are therefore predicted to be affected by inducers and inhibitors of this isoenzyme.

Clinical evidence, mechanism, importance and management

In vitro study has found that mifepristone is an inhibitor of the cytochrome P450 isoenzyme CYP3A4.[1] The manufacturers therefore advise caution when mifepristone is given to patients taking CYP3A4 substrates (the US manufacturers specifically note CYP3A4 substrates with a narrow therapeutic index) as an increase in the levels of the substrate may result.[2,3] The clinical relevance of this prediction is unclear, and published reports describing an interaction between CYP3A4 substrates and mifepristone appear to be lacking.

Mifepristone is also a CYP3A4 substrate, and the US manufacturer predicts that its levels may be raised by inhibitors of this isoenzyme (they name **itraconazole, ketoconazole, erythromycin** and **grapefruit juice**) and lowered by inducers of this isoenzyme (they name **carbamazepine, dexamethasone, phenobarbital, phenytoin, rifampicin (rifampin)** and **St John's wort** (*Hypericum perforatum*)). However, the clinical relevance of these predictions is unclear (particularly with dexamethasone, which, unlike the other drugs named, does not usually cause clinically relevant interactions by this mechanism), and published reports describing an interaction between these drugs and mifepristone appear to be lacking.

See 'Table 1.9', p.11, for a list of CYP3A4 inducers and inhibitors, and 'Table 1.10', p.12, for a list of CYP3A4 substrates.

1. He K, Woolf TF, Hollenberg PF. Mechanism-based inactivation of cytochrome P-450-3A4 by mifepristone (RU486). *J Pharmacol Exp Ther* (1999) 288, 791–7.
2. Mifegyne (Mifepristone). Exelgyn Laboratories. UK Summary of product characteristics, May 2008.
3. Mifeprex (Mifepristone). Danco Laboratories, LLC. US Prescribing information, April 2009.

Nitisinone + Miscellaneous

Nitisinone is metabolised by CYP3A4 and therefore inhibitors or inducers of this isoenzyme are predicted to affect nitisinone metabolism. The effect of food on the pharmacokinetics of nitisinone is unknown.

Clinical evidence, mechanism, importance and management

(a) CYP3A4 inducers or inhibitors

In vitro studies suggest that nitisinone is metabolised by the cytochrome P450 isoenzyme CYP3A4.[1,2] The UK manufacturers therefore predict that inhibitors or inducers of CYP3A4 (none specified) may affect the levels of nitisinone, and that the dose of nitisinone may need to be adjusted on concurrent use.[1] There appear to be no published reports of an interaction; however, there is brief mention of a patient who developed increased nitisinone plasma levels after stopping **phenobarbital**,[2] a CYP3A4 inducer: the magnitude of the increase is not stated. This supports the predicted interaction, and therefore, until clinical data is available, it may be prudent to bear the possibility of an interaction in mind if inhibitors or inducers of CYP3A4 are also given. See 'Table 1.9', p.11, for a list of CYP3A4 inducers and inhibitors.

(b) Food

The manufacturers of nitisinone state that the effect of food on the pharmacokinetics of nitisinone has not been studied.[1,3] The UK manufacturer notes that, as nitisinone has been given with food in efficacy studies, if a patient starts to take nitisinone with food, this may be continued as it is maintained.[1] However, the US manufacturer advises that, as there are no data on the effects of food on the pharmacokinetics of nitisinone, it should be taken at least one hour before or 2 hours after food.[3]

1. Orfadin (Nitisinone). Swedish Orphan International Ltd. UK Summary of product characteristics, August 2007.
2. Ofradin. EPAR - Scientific discussion. Available at: http://www.ema.europa.eu/docs/en_GB/document_library/EPAR_-_Scientific_Discussion/human/000555/WC500049192.pdf (accessed 21/10/15).
3. Orfadin (Nitisinone). Swedish Orphan International AB. US Prescribing information, January 2010.

Oxiracetam + Miscellaneous

Limited evidence suggests that the half-life of oxiracetam might be shorter in patients taking carbamazepine with valproate or clobazam. Oxiracetam probably does not affect sodium valproate, carbamazepine or clobazam levels.

Clinical evidence, mechanism, importance and management

Oxiracetam 800 mg twice daily for 14 days did not affect the serum levels of **sodium valproate**, **carbamazepine**, or **clobazam** and their metabolites in 3 patients with epilepsy taking **carbamazepine** and **valproate** and one patient taking **carbamazepine** and **clobazam**.[1] However, it was noted that the oxiracetam half-life was 2.8 to 7.56 hours,[1] which tended to be shorter than that seen in a previous study in healthy subjects who had been given oxiracetam 2 g (half-life of 5.6 to 11.7 hours).[2] The clinical relevance of this finding is uncertain, but the authors suggest that it may be necessary to raise the oxiracetam dose or to give the oxiracetam more frequently in the presence of these drugs.[1]

1. van Wieringen A, Meijer JWA, van Emde Boas W, Vermeij TAC. Pilot study to determine the interaction of oxiracetam with antiepileptic drugs. *Clin Pharmacokinet* (1990) 18, 332–8.
2. Perucca E, Albrici A, Gatti G, Spalluto R, Visconti M, Crema A. Pharmacokinetics of oxiracetam following intravenous and oral administration in healthy volunteers. *Eur J Drug Metab Pharmacokinet* (1984) 9, 267–74.

Oxygen; hyperbaric + Miscellaneous

It has been suggested, but not confirmed, that because increased levels of carbon dioxide in the tissues can increase the 'sensitivity' to oxygen-induced convulsions, carbonic anhydrase inhibitors, such as acetazolamide, are contraindicated in those given hyperbaric oxygen, because they cause carbon dioxide to persist in the tissues. It has been suggested that hyperbaric oxygen should not be given during opioid or barbiturate withdrawal because the convulsive threshold of such patients is already low.[1]

1. Gunby P. HBO can interact with preexisting patient conditions. *JAMA* (1981) 246, 1177–8.

Parathyroid hormones + Alendronate

There is some evidence that alendronate may reduce the anabolic effects of parathyroid hormone, so the combination may not be as effective as parathyroid hormone alone.

Clinical evidence

In a study, postmenopausal women with low mineral density at the hip or spine were given either **human recombinant parathyroid hormone** 100 micrograms daily, alendronate 10 mg daily, or both treatments for 12 months. All patients received calcium and vitamin D supplementation. Bone mineral density at the spine increased in all groups: however, volumetric density of trabecular bone at the spine was increased the most in patients taking parathyroid hormone alone (about twice that found in either of the other groups). Parathyroid hormone alone had greater effects on bone formation than parathyroid hormone with alendronate, and bone resorption decreased in those taking parathyroid hormone with alendronate or alendronate alone.[1]

In another study, men with low bone density were given either alendronate 10 mg daily, subcutaneous **teriparatide** 40 micrograms daily, or both. Alendronate was given for 30 months and parathyroid hormone was started at month 6. Bone mineral density at the lumbar spine and femoral neck increased significantly more in patients receiving parathyroid hormone alone than in patients receiving parathyroid hormone with alendronate, or alendronate alone.[2]

A further study in postmenopausal women found that the previous use of alendronate prevented **teriparatide**-induced increases in bone mineral density, especially in the first 6 months.[3] However, in another study, women who had received alendronate for at least one year were randomised to continue with alendronate alone, or to receive additional cyclical or daily **teriparatide**. Both daily and cyclical treatment with teriparatide in addition to alendronate increased spinal bone mass density more than alendronate alone.[4]

Mechanism

Alendronate may attenuate parathyroid-induced stimulation of bone formation.[2] It has been suggested it is the inhibition of overall bone turnover rather than inhibition of bone resorption by alendronate that impairs the anabolic activity of parathyroid hormone.[5]

Importance and management

The reports suggest that if parathyroid hormone or teriparatide is to be given for osteoporosis, it might be preferable to use them alone and not with alendronate, and possibly not with any other bisphosphonate. However, many patients with osteoporosis may already be receiving a bisphosphonate, and more study is required to establish the optimal regimens for starting parathyroid hormone and discontinuing the bisphosphonate in such patients.[5] Subsequent research suggests that the addition of parathyroid hormone to alendronate is more effective than no treatment, and that patients discontinuing parathyroid hormone do better if they are then given alendronate.[6]

1. Black DM, Greenspan SL, Ensrud KE, Palermo L, McGowan JA, Lang TF, Garnero P, Bouxsein ML, Bilezikian JP, Rosen CJ, for the PaTH Study Investigators. The effects of parathyroid hormone and alendronate alone or in combination in postmenopausal osteoporosis. *N Engl J Med* (2003) 349, 1207–15.
2. Finkelstein JS, Hayes A, Hunzelman JL, Wyland JJ, Lee H, Neer RM. The effects of parathyroid hormone, alendronate, or both in men with osteoporosis. *N Engl J Med* (2003) 349, 1216–26.
3. Ettinger B, San Martin J, Crans G, Pavo I. Differential effects of teriparatide on BMD after treatment with raloxifene or alendronate. *J Bone Miner Res* (2004) 19, 745–51.
4. Cosman F, Nieves J, Zion M, Woelfert L, Luckey M, Lindsay R. Daily and cyclic parathyroid hormone in women receiving alendronate. N Engl J Med. (2005) 353, 566–75.
5. Khosia S. Parathyroid hormone plus alendronate—a combination that does not add up. *N Engl J Med* (2003) 349, 1277–9.
6. Black DM, Bilezikian JP, Ensrud KE, Greenspan SL, Palermo L, Hue T, Lang TF, McGowan JA, Rosen CJ; for the PaTH Study Investigators. One year of alendronate after one year of parathyroid hormone (1-84) for osteoporosis. *N Engl J Med* (2005) 353, 555–65.

Parathyroid hormones; Teriparatide + Miscellaneous

The clinical effects of teriparatide are not significantly affected by furosemide, hormone replacement therapy, hydrochlorothiazide, or raloxifene.

Clinical evidence, mechanism, importance and management

(a) Furosemide

A study in 28 subjects (9 healthy subjects and 17 subjects with mild to moderate renal impairment) found that furosemide 20 to 100 mg had no clinically significant effect on the response to teriparatide.[1]

(b) Hormone replacement therapy

The effects of teriparatide on serum and urine calcium levels, and teriparatide adverse effects, are not affected by the concurrent use of hormone replacement therapy.[2]

(c) Hydrochlorothiazide

A study in 20 healthy subjects found that although hydrochlorothiazide 25 mg caused a minor reduction in the urinary excretion of calcium, the serum calcium response to a 40-microgram dose of teriparatide was unaffected.[1]

(d) Raloxifene

In a study, postmenopausal women were given subcutaneous teriparatide 20 micrograms daily for 18 months. The expected teriparatide-induced increases in bone mineral density were not affected by previous treatment with raloxifene.[3] Similarly, the manufacturer states that the effects of teriparatide on serum and urine calcium levels, and teriparatide adverse effects, are not affected by raloxifene.[2]

1. Forteo (Teriparatide). Eli Lilly and Company. US Prescribing information, March 2012.
2. Forsteo (Teriparatide). Eli Lilly and Company Ltd. UK Summary of product characteristics, July 2011.
3. Ettinger B, San Martin J, Crans G, Pavo I. Differential effects of teriparatide on BMD after treatment with raloxifene or alendronate. *J Bone Miner Res* (2004) 19, 745–51.

Pasireotide + Miscellaneous

Pasireotide might decrease ciclosporin exposure and have additive effects with other drugs that affect heart rate. Pasireotide concentrations might be increased by P-glycoprotein inhibitors such as verapamil.

Clinical evidence, mechanism, importance and management

(a) Ciclosporin

Pasireotide might decrease ciclosporin exposure. It would therefore seem prudent to monitor ciclosporin concentrations on concurrent use, adjusting the dose of ciclosporin as necessary.[1] Ciclosporin might also increase pasireotide concentrations, see *P-glycoprotein inhibitors*, below.

(b) Drugs that cause bradycardia

Bradycardia is a common adverse effect of pasireotide, and this effect seems most likely to be of importance in those with pre-existing cardiac disease, particularly if they are taking other drugs that affect heart rate, such as a **beta blocker** or a calcium-channel blocker (**verapamil** or **diltiazem**). The manufacturer therefore advises that heart rate should be monitored, particularly at the start of concurrent use. They also suggest monitoring with anticholinergics and specifically name **ipratropium bromide** and **oxybutynin**.[1] If bradycardia develops consider adjusting the dose of, for example, the beta blocker, according to clinical need. **Verapamil** might also increase pasireotide concentrations, see *P-glycoprotein inhibitors*, below.

(c) P-glycoprotein inhibitors

In vitro, pasireotide has been shown to be a substrate of P-glycoprotein and therefore the manufacturers predict that potent P-glycoprotein inhibitors (they name **ciclosporin, clarithromycin, ketoconazole**, and **verapamil**), will increase pasireotide concentrations.[1] Until more is known it would seem prudent to monitor for pasireotide adverse effects (such as abdominal pain, diarrhoea, and myalgia), reducing the pasireotide dose if these become particularly troublesome.

See also *Ciclosporin*, above, and, for the effects of verapamil, *Drugs that cause bradycardia*, above.

1. Signifor (Pasireotide diaspartate). Novartis Pharmaceuticals UK Ltd. UK Summary of product characteristics, April 2012.

Penicillamine + Antacids

The absorption of penicillamine can be reduced by 30 to 40% if antacids containing aluminium/magnesium hydroxide are taken at the same time. This does not occur with sodium bicarbonate.

Clinical evidence

In a study in 6 healthy fasting subjects, *Maalox-plus* (**aluminium/magnesium hydroxide, simeticone**) 30 mL reduced the absorption of a single 500-mg dose of penicillamine by one-third.[1] Another similar study found that 30 mL of *Aludrox* (**aluminium/magnesium hydroxide**) reduced the absorption of penicillamine by about 40%.[2] In contrast, a single 7.06-g dose of **sodium bicarbonate** had little effect on the absorption of penicillamine (non-significant 15% reduction in AUC).[2]

Mechanism

The most likely explanation is that the penicillamine forms less soluble chelates with magnesium and aluminium ions in the gut, which reduces its absorption.[2]

Importance and management

The interaction between penicillamine and aluminium and magnesium-containing antacids is established, and might be of clinical importance. If maximal absorption is needed the administration of the two drugs should be separated to avoid mixing in the gut. Two to three hours has been found enough for most other drugs that have reduced absorption in the presence of aluminium/magnesium hydroxide antacids. Sodium bicarbonate does not interact and therefore the timing of the doses does not need to be adjusted in patients taking penicillamine.

1. Osman MA, Patel RB, Schuna A, Sundstrom WR, Welling PG. Reduction in oral penicillamine absorption by food, antacid and ferrous sulphate. *Clin Pharmacol Ther* (1983) 33, 465–70.
2. Ifan A, Welling PG. Pharmacokinetics of oral 500-mg penicillamine: effect of antacids on absorption. *Biopharm Drug Dispos* (1986) 7, 401–5.

Penicillamine + Disease-modifying antirheumatic drugs

Penicillamine plasma levels are increased by chloroquine and an increase in penicillamine toxicity is possible. Penicillamine should not be used with gold.

Clinical evidence, mechanism, importance and management

(a) Chloroquine or Hydroxychloroquine

Studies in which chloroquine was given to patients taking penicillamine found that giving both drugs was more effective, less effective, or indistinguishable from giving penicillamine alone. However, in some instances penicillamine toxicity was reported to be increased by chloroquine.[1] A pharmacokinetic study in patients with rheumatoid arthritis taking penicillamine 250 mg daily found that a single 250-mg dose of chloroquine phosphate increased the AUC of penicillamine by 34%, and raised its peak plasma levels by about 55%.[1] It therefore seems possible that any increased toxicity is a reflection of increased plasma penicillamine levels. Be alert for evidence of toxicity if both drugs are used. Note that the US manufacturer states that penicillamine should not be used in patients who are receiving antimalarials (which would include chloroquine and hydroxychloroquine) because these drugs are also associated with serious haematological effects.[2]

(b) Gold

There is some evidence that using gold with penicillamine may increase the risk of adverse effects, and the manufacturer says that they should not be used together.[2,3] In addition, patients who have had an adverse reaction to gold may be at a greater risk of serious adverse reactions to penicillamine,[2,3] and caution is recommended.[3]

1. Seideman P, Lindström B. Pharmacokinetic interactions of penicillamine in rheumatoid arthritis. *J Rheumatol* (1989) 16, 473–4.
2. Cuprimine (Penicillamine). Merck & Co., Inc. US Prescribing information, October 2004.
3. Distamine (Penicillamine). Alliance Pharmaceuticals. UK Summary of product characteristics, June 2010.

Penicillamine + Food

Food can reduce the absorption of penicillamine by as much as a half.

Clinical evidence

In a study in healthy subjects, the presence of food reduced the plasma levels of penicillamine 500 mg by about 50%. The total amount absorbed was similarly reduced.[1,2] These figures are in good agreement with previous findings.[3]

Mechanism

Uncertain. One suggestion is that food delays gastric emptying so that the penicillamine is exposed to more prolonged degradation in the stomach.[2] Another idea is that the protein in food reduces penicillamine absorption.

Importance and management

An established interaction. If maximal effects are required the penicillamine should be taken at least 30 minutes before food.

1. Schuna A, Osman MA, Patel RB, Welling PG, Sundstrom WR. Influence of food on the bioavailability of penicillamine. *J Rheumatol* (1983) 10, 95–7.
2. Osman MA, Patel RB, Schuna A, Sundstrom WR, Welling PG. Reduction in oral penicillamine absorption by food, antacid and ferrous sulphate. *Clin Pharmacol Ther* (1983) 33, 465–70.
3. Bergstrom RF, Kay DR, Harkcom TM, Wagner JG. Penicillamine kinetics in normal subjects. *Clin Pharmacol Ther* (1981) 30, 404–13.

Penicillamine + Iron compounds

The absorption of penicillamine can be reduced as much as two-thirds by oral iron compounds.

Clinical evidence

In a study in 5 healthy subjects, **ferrous iron** 90 mg (as *Fersamal*) reduced the absorption of penicillamine 250 mg by about two-thirds (using the cupruretic effects of penicillamine as a measure).[1]

A two-thirds reduction in the absorption of penicillamine 500 mg has been described in 6 other subjects who were also given **ferrous sulfate** 300 mg.[2] Other studies confirm this interaction.[3,4] There is also evidence that the withdrawal of iron from patients stabilised on penicillamine can lead to the development of toxicity (nephropathy) unless the penicillamine dosage is reduced.[5]

Mechanism

It is believed that the iron and penicillamine form a chemical complex or chelate within the gut, which is less easily absorbed.

Importance and management

An established and clinically important interaction. For maximal absorption give iron at least 2 hours after penicillamine. This should reduce their admixture in the gut.[1] Only ferrous sulfate and fumarate have been studied but other iron compounds would be expected to interact similarly. Do not withdraw iron suddenly from patients stabilised on penicillamine because the marked increase in absorption that follows may precipitate penicillamine toxicity. The toxic effects of penicillamine seem to be dependent on the size of the dose and are possibly also related to the rate at which the dosage is increased.[5]

1. Lyle WH. Penicillamine and iron. *Lancet* (1976) ii, 420.
2. Osman MA, Patel RB, Schuna A, Sundstrom WR, Welling PG. Reduction in oral penicillamine absorption by food, antacid, and ferrous sulphate. *Clin Pharmacol Ther* (1983) 33, 465–70.
3. Lyle WH, Pearcey DF, Hui M. Inhibition of penicillamine-induced cupruresis by oral iron. *Proc R Soc Med* (1977) 70 (Suppl 3), 48–9.
4. Hall ND, Blake DR, Alexander GJM, Vaisey C, Bacon PA. Serum SH reactivity: a simple assessment of D-penicillamine absorption? *Rheumatol Int* (1981) 1, 39–41.
5. Harkness JAL, Blake DR. Penicillamine nephropathy and iron. *Lancet* (1982) ii, 1368–9.

Penicillamine + Miscellaneous

An isolated report describes penicillamine-induced breast enlargement in a woman taking an oral combined hormonal contraceptive. This might also have occurred when penicillamine was given with a corticosteroid or cimetidine.

Clinical evidence, mechanism, importance and management

A woman with Wilson's disease began to develop dark facial hair about 10 months after starting to take penicillamine 1.25 to 1.5 g daily. After 20 months her testosterone levels were found to be slightly raised, and so she was given an oral **combined hormonal contraceptive**, but within a month her breasts began to enlarge and become more tender. After a further 6 months the penicillamine was replaced by trientine hydrochloride.[1] The reasons are not understood, but the authors of the report suggest that the penicillamine was the prime cause of the macromastia, but it possibly needed the presence of a 'second trigger' (i.e. the contraceptive) to set things in motion.[1]

There are 12 other cases of macromastia and gynaecomastia on record associated with the use of penicillamine. In some of these cases the second trigger may possibly have been a **corticosteroid** or **cimetidine**.[1] Macromastia appears to be an unusual adverse effect of penicillamine and there would seem to be no general reason for patients taking penicillamine to avoid hormonal contraceptives.

1. Rose BI, LeMaire WJ, Jeffers LJ. Macromastia in a woman treated with penicillamine and oral contraceptives. *J Reprod Med* (1990) 35, 43–5.

Penicillamine + NSAIDs

Indometacin slightly increases penicillamine levels. The use of penicillamine and an NSAID might increase the risk of renal damage.

Clinical evidence, mechanism, importance and management

Indometacin has been found to increase the AUC of penicillamine by 26% and the peak plasma levels by about 22%.[1] The UK manufacturer notes that use of NSAIDs may increase the risk of renal damage with penicillamine.[2] The US manufacturer specifically recommends avoiding **oxyphenbutazone** or **phenylbutazone** because these drugs are also associated with serious haematological and renal effects.[3] Urinalysis for detection of haematuria or proteinuria should be regularly carried out in patients taking penicillamine.[2,3] Be alert for evidence of toxicity if NSAIDs and penicillamine are used together.

1. Seideman P, Lindström B. Pharmacokinetic interactions of penicillamine in rheumatoid arthritis. *J Rheumatol* (1989) 16, 473–4.
2. Distamine (Penicillamine). Alliance Pharmaceuticals. UK Summary of product characteristics, June 2010.
3. Cuprimine (Penicillamine). Merck & Co., Inc. US Prescribing information, October 2004.

Phenylephrine + Paracetamol (Acetaminophen)

Phenylephrine exposure appears to be modestly increased by paracetamol.

Clinical evidence

In an analysis of 4 randomised, crossover studies in 90 healthy subjects given a single dose of paracetamol 1 g with phenylephrine 10 mg (*Sudafed*), the phenylephrine AUC and maximum plasma concentration were about 2-fold and up to 4-fold higher, respectively, when compared with phenylephrine 10 mg given alone. However there was large inter-individual variability. When phenylephrine 5 mg was given with 1 g paracetamol (*Maxiclear*), the phenylephrine exposure was comparable with that of a 10-mg dose of phenylephrine given alone.[1]

Mechanism

The authors of this study suggest that as paracetamol and phenylephrine both undergo similar, extensive, capacity-limited first-pass metabolism, the metabolism of phenylephrine is reduced due to saturation of the metabolic pathway by paracetamol, thereby increasing phenylephrine exposure.[1] Further study is needed to determine the exact mechanism.

Importance and management

An interaction between phenylephrine and paracetamol is limited to this single study, and its clinical relevance is uncertain. Phenylephrine and paracetamol are widely used together for the treatment of symptoms of common colds and influenza, and any serious problem would be expected to have come to light by now. No particular precautions seem necessary on concurrent use, but until more is known, bear this potential interaction in mind in the case of increased phenylephrine adverse effects.

1. Atkinson HC, Stanescu I, Salem II, Potts AL, Anderson BJ. Increased bioavailability of phenylephrine by co-administration of acetaminophen: results of four open-label, crossover pharmacokinetic trials in healthy volunteers. *Eur J Clin Pharmacol* (2015) 71, 151–8. Correction. ibid., 771–2.

Phenylpropanolamine + Indinavir

A report describes a hypertensive crisis when a patient taking indinavir was also given phenylpropanolamine.

Clinical evidence, mechanism, importance and management

A 28-year-old woman was prescribed HIV-prophylaxis following a needle stick injury. She was initially given zidovudine, indinavir and lamivudine, but after one week stavudine was substituted for zidovudine as she was experiencing nausea and vomiting. Six hours after taking *Tavist-D* (clemastine with phenylpropanolamine) for a sinus complaint she had a feeling of chest tightness associated with difficulty in breathing, and shortly afterwards she experienced left-sided upper extremity weakness, followed by a severe right-sided temporal headache. Her blood pressure was 220/120 mmHg, but returned to normal within 4 hours, and the neurological deficit resolved over the next 8 hours. However, 12 hours later, the same neurological deficit recurred, although no increase in blood pressure was noted. The neurological deficit was thought to be due to reversible cerebral vasoconstriction, secondary to phenylpropanolamine toxicity. She was treated with nimodipine 60 mg every 4 hours and aspirin 325 mg daily, and her symptoms did not recur.[1]

The patient had been taking phenylpropanolamine intermittently for several years without any adverse reaction and it was thought that the recent addition of the HIV prophylaxis potentiated the effect of the phenylpropanolamine.[1] It seems likely that the indinavir was responsible for the interaction as it is a potent enzyme inhibitor.

This is an isolated report and its general significance is not known, but it would be prudent to be alert for this interaction in patients taking both drugs. Note that phenylpropanolamine is no longer available in the US and UK and its use has been restricted in many other countries.

1. Khurana V, de la Fuente M, Bradley TP. Hypertensive crisis secondary to phenylpropanolamine interacting with triple-drug therapy for HIV prophylaxis. *Am J Med* (1999) 106, 118–19.

Phenylpropanolamine + Indometacin

An isolated report describes a patient taking phenylpropanolamine who developed serious hypertension after taking a single dose of indometacin, but a controlled study in other subjects did not find any evidence of an adverse interaction.

Clinical evidence

A woman who had been taking phenylpropanolamine 85 mg daily for several months as an appetite suppressant, developed a severe bifrontal headache within 15 minutes of taking indometacin 25 mg. Thirty minutes later her systolic blood pressure was 210 mmHg and her diastolic blood pressure was unrecordable. A later study in this patient confirmed that neither drug on its own caused this response, but when they were taken together the blood pressure rose to a maximum of 200/150 mmHg within about 30 minutes of taking the indometacin, and was associated with bradycardia. Her blood pressure was rapidly reduced by phentolamine.[1]

In contrast, a controlled study in 14 healthy young women found no evidence that sustained-release indometacin 75 mg twice daily, given with sustained-release phenylpropanolamine 75 mg daily, caused a rise in blood pressure.[2]

Mechanism

Not understood.

Importance and management

Direct information seems to be limited to these reports. They suggest that an adverse hypertensive response is unlikely in most individuals given these drugs. However, note that phenylpropanolamine alone has been associated with severe hypertension and has been implicated in causing stroke.[3] It is therefore no longer available in the US and UK and its use has been restricted in many other countries.

1. Lee KY, Beilin LJ, Vandongen R. Severe hypertension after ingestion of an appetite suppressant (phenylpropanolamine) with indomethacin. *Lancet* (1979) i, 1110–11.
2. McKenney JM, Wright JT, Katz GM, Goodman RP. The effect of phenylpropanolamine on 24–hour blood pressure in normotensive subjects administered indomethacin. *DICP Ann Pharmacother* (1991) 25, 234–9.
3. Brust JCM. Editorial comment: over-the-counter cold remedies and stroke. *Stroke* (2003) 34, 1673.

Polystyrene sulfonate + Antacids

The concurrent use of some antacids with sodium polystyrene sulfonate can result in metabolic alkalosis. Use with aluminium hydroxide has resulted in intestinal obstruction. Calcium polystyrene sulfonate is said to interact similarly.

Clinical evidence, mechanism, importance and management

A man with hyperkalaemia developed metabolic alkalosis when given 30 g of sodium polystyrene sulfonate with **magnesium hydroxide** 30 mL three times daily.[1] Alkalosis has also been described in a study in a number of patients given this cation exchange resin with *Maalox* (**magnesium/aluminium hydroxide**) and **calcium carbonate**.[2]

The suggested reason is that the breakdown of the **magnesium hydroxide** usually requires equal amounts of bicarbonate and hydrogen ions, and so does not cause any acid-base disturbance. However, when sodium polystyrene sulfonate is given, it binds the **magnesium**, while the hydroxide is neutralised by the hydrogen ions. This results in a relative excess of bicarbonate ions, which are absorbed, leading to metabolic alkalosis.

This interaction appears to be established. Concurrent use should be undertaken with caution and serum electrolytes should be closely monitored. Giving the resin rectally as an enema can avoid the problem. Calcium polystyrene sulfonate is said to interact similarly.[3]

In addition to alkalosis, the manufacturer also notes that concurrent use of **aluminium hydroxide** and the resins has resulted in intestinal obstruction due to 'concretions' of **aluminium hydroxide**.[3,4] Caution is advised.

1. Fernandez PC, Kovnat PJ. Metabolic acidosis reversed by the combination of magnesium and a cation-exchange resin. *N Engl J Med* (1972) 286, 23–4.
2. Schroeder ET. Alkalosis resulting from combined administration of a 'nonsystemic' antacid and a cation-exchange resin. *Gastroenterology* (1969) 56, 868–74.
3. Calcium resonium (Calcium polystyrene sulfonate). Sanofi-Aventis. UK Summary of product characteristics, April 2009.
4. Resonium A (Sodium polystyrene sulfonate). Sanofi-Aventis. UK Summary of product characteristics, April 2009.

Polystyrene sulfonate + Sorbitol

Potentially fatal colonic necrosis may occur if sodium polystyrene sulfonate is given as an enema with sorbitol. Calcium polystyrene sulfonate may interact similarly.

Clinical evidence

Five patients with uraemia developed severe colonic necrosis after being given enemas containing sodium polystyrene sulfonate and sorbitol for the treatment of hyperkalaemia. Four of the 5 patients died as a result. Associated studies in uraemic *rats* found that all of them died over a 2-day period after being given enemas of sodium polystyrene sulfonate with sorbitol. Extensive haemorrhage and transmural necrosis developed. No deaths occurred when enemas without sorbitol were given.[1] A number of other similar cases have been reported, a few of which are cited.[2-4] In one retrospective analysis, intestinal necrosis occurred in 2 of 117 patients (1.7%) who had received sodium polystyrene sulfonate within one week of surgery, and in both of these cases it had been given in sorbitol. Conversely, of 862 patients who did not receive sodium polystyrene sulfonate, none developed intestinal necrosis.[5]

Mechanism

Not understood.

Importance and management

Information is limited and the interaction between sorbitol and polystyrene sulfonate is not firmly established; nevertheless, its seriousness indicates that sodium polystyrene sulfonate should not be given as an enema in aqueous vehicles containing sorbitol. Note that the manufacturers advise against the concurrent use of both *oral* and rectal sorbitol with sodium or calcium polystyrene sulfonate, because of the risk of colonic necrosis.[6,7]

1. Lillemoe KD, Romolo JL, Hamilton SR, Pennington LR, Burdick JF, Williams GM. Intestinal necrosis due to sodium polystyrene (Kayexalate) in sorbitol enemas: clinical and experimental support for the hypothesis. *Surgery* (1987) 101, 267–72.
2. Rashid A, Hamilton SR. Necrosis of the gastrointestinal tract in uremic patients as a result of sodium polystyrene sulfonate (Kayexalate) in sorbitol: an underrecognized condition. *Am J Surg Pathol* (1997) 21, 60–9.
3. Rogers FB, Li SC. Acute colonic necrosis associated with sodium polystyrene sulfonate (Kayexalate) enemas in a critically ill patient: case report and review of the literature. *J Trauma* (2001) 51, 395–7.
4. Kelsey PB, Chen S, Lauwers GY. Case records of the Massachusetts General Hospital. Weekly clinicopathological exercises. Case 37-2003. A 79-year-old man with coronary artery disease, peripheral vascular disease, end-stage renal disease, and abdominal pain and distention. *N Engl J Med* (2003) 349, 2147–55.
5. Gerstman BB, Kirkman R, Platt R. Intestinal necrosis associated with postoperative orally administered sodium polystyrene sulfonate in sorbitol. *Am J Kidney Dis* (1992) 20, 159–61.
6. Resonium A (Sodium polystyrene sulfonate). Sanofi-Aventis. UK Summary of product characteristics, April 2009.
7. Calcium resonium (Calcium polystyrene sulfonate). Sanofi-Aventis. UK Summary of product characteristics, April 2009.

Prostacyclins + Miscellaneous

The concurrent use of iloprost, epoprostenol, and treprostinil with an antiplatelet drug might increase the risk of bleeding.

Clinical evidence, mechanism, importance and management

The manufacturer of iloprost notes that as it inhibits platelet aggregation, there is a possibility of an increased risk of bleeding if it is given with anticoagulants or with other antiplatelet drugs, and they advise caution on concurrent use: they name **aspirin**, **clopidogrel**, **ticlopidine**, **NSAIDs**, **heparin** and the glycoprotein IIb/IIIa-receptor antagonists, **abciximab**, **eptifibatide**, and **tirofiban**.[1] It would also seem prudent to apply similar caution to the use of **prasugrel** in patients given iloprost. Other prostacyclins that affect platelet aggregation (such as **epoprostenol** and **treprostinil**) have the potential to interact similarly. Consider also, 'Glycoprotein IIb/IIIa-receptor antagonists + Antiplatelet drugs', p.796.

1. Ventavis (Iloprost trometamol). Bayer plc. UK Summary of product characteristics, July 2011.

Pseudoephedrine + Antacids or Antidiarrhoeals

Kaolin does not appear to interact significantly with pseudoephedrine. Aluminium hydroxide may possibly cause a more rapid onset of pseudoephedrine.

Clinical evidence

In a single-dose, crossover study in 6 healthy subjects, 30 mL of **aluminium hydroxide gel** did not affect the total amount of a single 60-mg dose of pseudoephedrine absorbed over 24 hours, but the rate of absorption was significantly increased during the first 3 hours.[1] Conversely, 30 mL of a 30% suspension of **kaolin** reduced the amount of a single 60-mg dose of pseudoephedrine absorbed by just 10%. The rate of absorption was also decreased.[1]

Mechanism

The increased rate of absorption of pseudoephedrine seen with aluminium hydroxide is probably also due to pH rises, which favour the formation of the lipid-soluble absorbable form of pseudoephedrine. The reduced absorption with kaolin is probably due to adsorption of the pseudoephedrine onto the surface of the kaolin.

Importance and management

Aluminium hydroxide may possibly cause a more rapid onset of pseudoephedrine activity (but this needs confirmation). Any interaction seems unlikely to be clinically significant. Similarly, the effects of kaolin on pseudoephedrine absorption are small and unlikely to be clinically important.

For the effect of sodium bicarbonate on pseudoephedrine and ephedrine, see 'Pseudoephedrine and related drugs + Urinary acidifiers or alkalinisers', below.

1. Lucarotti RL, Colaizzi JL, Barry H, Poust RI. Enhanced pseudoephedrine absorption by concurrent administration of aluminium hydroxide gel in humans. *J Pharm Sci* (1972) 61, 903–5.

Pseudoephedrine and related drugs + Caffeine

Phenylpropanolamine can raise blood pressure and in some cases this may be further increased by caffeine. Combined use has resulted in hypertensive crises in a few individuals. Ephedrine may interact similarly. Phenylpropanolamine can markedly raise plasma caffeine levels, and isolated reports describe the development of acute psychosis when caffeine was given with phenylpropanolamine or ephedrine.

Clinical evidence

(a) Ephedrine

1. Clinical studies. In a single-dose, randomised study, 15 healthy subjects were given ephedrine 25 mg, caffeine 200 mg, both drugs together, or placebo. An assessment of systolic blood pressure found that ephedrine had no significant effect, caffeine caused a 9.1 mmHg increase, and the use of both drugs resulted in an 11.7 mmHg increase. Caffeine alone did not increase heart rate, but both ephedrine and ephedrine plus caffeine caused heart rate increases of roughly 11%. Subjective tests suggested that there was no significant difference in feelings of headache, chest pain, heart pounding or shortness of breath between the treatments. There was no significant pharmacokinetic interaction between the drugs.[1] Another randomised study, investigating the combination of ephedrine 20 mg and caffeine 200 mg, both three times daily, compared with either drug alone, or placebo, for weight loss, did not find any significant hypertensive effects with the combination, although the authors suggested that this may have been due to the favourable effects of weight loss on blood pressure. However, one patient was withdrawn due to a rise in blood pressure, to 185/125 mmHg.[2]

Numerous other clinical studies have investigated the haemodynamic effects of combinations of ephedrine or ephedra with caffeine or caffeine-containing herbs, some showing increases in heart rate and blood pressure and others not. However, none of these compared the combination with either constituent alone, so it is not possible to assess the possibility of an interaction from these reports.

2. Case reports. A review of reports from the FDA in the US revealed that several patients have experienced severe adverse effects (subarachnoid haemorrhage, cardiac arrest, hypertension, tachycardia and neurosis) after taking dietary supplements containing ephedrine or **ephedra** alkaloids with caffeine.[3] However, it is not possible to definitively say that these effects were the result of an interaction because none of the patients took either drug separately. Similarly, a meta-analysis assessing the safety of ephedra or ephedrine and caffeine found a two- to threefold increase in the risk of adverse events (including psychiatric symptoms and palpitations) with ephedra or ephedrine, but it was concluded that it was not possible to assess the contribution of caffeine to these events.[4]

Two episodes of acute psychosis occurred in a 32-year-old man after he took *Vigueur fit* tablets (containing **ephedra** alkaloids and caffeine), *Red Bull* (containing caffeine) and alcohol. He had no previous record of aberrant behaviour despite regularly taking 6 to 9 tablets of *Vigueur fit* daily (about twice the recommended dose). However, on this occasion, over a 10-hour period, he consumed 3 or 4 bottles of *Red Bull* (containing about 95 mg of caffeine per 250-mL bottle) and enough alcohol to reach a blood-alcohol level of about 335 mg%. No more episodes occurred after he stopped taking the *Vigueur fit* tablets. **Ephedra** alkaloids (ephedrine and **pseudoephedrine**) may cause psychosis and it appears that their effects may be exaggerated by an interaction with caffeine and alcohol.[5]

(b) Phenylpropanolamine

In a placebo-controlled study, the mean blood pressure of 16 healthy subjects rose by 11/12 mmHg after they took caffeine 400 mg, by 12/13 mmHg after they took phenylpropanolamine 75 mg, and by 12/11 mmHg when both drugs were taken. Phenylpropanolamine 150 mg caused a greater rise of 36/18 mmHg. One of the subjects had a hypertensive crisis after taking phenylpropanolamine 150 mg and again 2 hours after taking caffeine 400 mg. This needed antihypertensive treatment.[6] The same group of workers describe a similar study in which the AUC of caffeine 400 mg increased by more than threefold, and the mean peak caffeine concentration increased almost fourfold (from 2.1 to 8 micrograms/mL) after phenylpropanolamine 75 mg was given.[7] Additive increases in blood pressure are described in another report.[8]

Mania with psychotic delusions occurred in a healthy woman (who normally drank 7 to 8 cups of **coffee** daily) within 3 days of her starting to take a phenylpropanolamine-containing decongestant. She recovered within a week of stopping both the **coffee** and the phenylpropanolamine.[9]

Mechanism

Ephedrine and caffeine may cause catecholamine release and an increase in intracellular calcium release which leads to vasoconstriction. Myocardial ischaemia may occur as a result of this vasoconstriction (in the coronary artery), and this may result in myocardial necrosis and cell death.

Importance and management

Fairly well established interactions. These studies illustrate the potential hazards of these drugs, even in normal healthy individuals. However, it has to be said that there seem to be few reports of adverse interactions, which is perhaps surprising bearing in mind that coffee/caffeine is very widely used and ephedrine and phenylpropanolamine have also been widely available without prescription. One possible explanation for this could be that these interactions may go unrecognised or be attributed to one drug only e.g. phenylpropanolamine, whereas caffeine has also been taken either as part of the preparation[3,10] or in beverages (often not reported). Nevertheless, serious adverse events have been reported with caffeine and phenylpropanolamine or dietary supplements containing ephedra alkaloids (sometimes called ma huang) and therefore these preparations may pose a serious health risk to some users.[3] The risk may be affected by individual susceptibility, the additive stimulant effects of caffeine, the variability in the contents of alkaloids in non-prescription dietary supplements, or pre-existing medical conditions,[3] including compromised cardiac function,[1] and hypertension, or obesity and old age.[6]

Note that, phenylpropanolamine is no longer available in the US and UK and its use has been restricted in many other countries. In addition, because of the associated health risks, the FDA bans combinations of caffeine with ephedrine or pseudoephedrine, and also bans herbal products containing ephedra. As a result of this, many manufacturers replaced ephedra with bitter orange (*Citrus aurantium*), which contains a similar sympathomimetic alkaloid (synephrine). Evidence shows that these products are no safer than ephedra products when used in a similar way. It would be prudent to avoid using herbal products containing combinations of bitter orange and caffeine or caffeine-containing herbs, especially in patients with risk factors such as heart conditions, diabetes, thyroid disease, or hypertension.

1. Haller CA, Jacob P, Benowitz NL. Enhanced stimulant and metabolic effects of combined ephedrine and caffeine. *Clin Pharmacol Ther* (2004) 75, 259–73.
2. Astrup A, Breum L, Toubro S, Hein P, Quaade F. The effect and safety of an ephedrine/caffeine compound compared to ephedrine, caffeine and placebo in obese subjects on an energy restricted diet. A double blind trial. *Int J Obes Relat Metab Disord* (1992) 16, 269–77.
3. Haller CA, Benowitz NL. Adverse cardiovascular and central nervous system events associated with dietary supplements containing ephedra alkaloids. *N Engl J Med* (2000) 343, 1833–8.
4. Shekelle PG, Hardy ML, Morton SC, Maglione M, Mojica WA, Suttorp MJ, Rhodes SL, Jungvig L, Gagné J. Efficacy and safety of ephedra and ephedrine for weight loss and athletic performance: a meta-analysis. *JAMA* (2003) 280, 1537–45.
5. Tormey WP, Bruzzi A. Acute psychosis due to the interaction of legal compounds – ephedra alkaloids in 'Vigueur Fit' tablets, caffeine in 'Red Bull' and alcohol. *Med Sci Law* (2001) 41, 331–6.
6. Lake CR, Zaloga G, Bray J, Rosenberg D, Chernow B. Transient hypertension after two phenylpropanolamine diet aids and the effects of caffeine: a placebo-controlled follow-up study. *Am J Med* (1989) 86, 427–32.
7. Lake CR, Rosenberg DB, Gallant S, Zaloga G, Chernow B. Phenylpropanolamine increases plasma caffeine levels. *Clin Pharmacol Ther* (1990) 47, 675–85.
8. Brown NJ, Ryder D, Branch RA. A pharmacodynamic interaction between caffeine and phenylpropanolamine. *Clin Pharmacol Ther* (1991) 50, 363–71.
9. Lake CR. Manic psychosis after coffee and phenylpropanolamine. *Biol Psychiatry* (1991) 30, 401–4.
10. Lake CR, Gallant S, Masson E, Miller P. Adverse drug effects attributed to phenylpropanolamine: a review of 142 case reports. *Am J Med* (1990) 89, 195– 208.

Pseudoephedrine and related drugs + Urinary acidifiers or alkalinisers

Alkalinisation of the urine (e.g. by sodium bicarbonate) causes retention of ephedrine and pseudoephedrine by the kidneys, leading to the possible development of toxicity (tremors, anxiety, insomnia, tachycardia). Acidification of the urine (e.g. with ammonium chloride) has the opposite effect.

Clinical evidence

(a) Ephedrine

When the urine was made acidic (pH of about 5) with **ammonium chloride**, the excretion of ephedrine in the urine of 3 healthy subjects was two- to fourfold higher than when the urine was made alkaline (pH of about 8) with **sodium bicarbonate**.[1]

(b) Pseudoephedrine

A patient with renal tubular acidosis and persistently alkaline urine developed unexpected toxicity (cachexia and personality changes) when given therapeutic doses (not stated) of pseudoephedrine for 2.5 months. She was found to have a very prolonged pseudoephedrine half-life of 50 hours (10 times expected). Therefore 8 subjects (adults and children) were studied, to establish the possible effects of changing the urinary pH on pseudoephedrine elimination. When the urinary pH was adjusted using **ammonium chloride** or **sodium bicarbonate**, within the approximate range of 5.7 to 7.8, the half-life of a single dose of pseudoephedrine (about 5 mg/kg) was found to increase from 1.9 hours at the lowest pH to 21 hours at the highest pH.[2]

This confirms an earlier study, in which it was found that at a urinary pH of 8, the half-life of pseudoephedrine was 16, 9.2, and 15 hours in 3 subjects, respectively. At a urinary pH of about 5, the half-life was 4.8, 3, and 6.4 hours, respectively.[3] **Sodium bicarbonate** was given to raise urinary pH and **ammonium chloride** to lower urinary pH.

Another study in 6 healthy subjects found that **sodium bicarbonate** 5 g initially increased the excretion rate of a single 60-mg dose of pseudoephedrine, but as the urinary pH increased the excretion of pseudoephedrine was reduced.[4]

Mechanism

Ephedrine and pseudoephedrine are basic drugs, which are mainly excreted unchanged in the urine. In acidic urine, most of the drug is ionised in the tubular filtrate and unable to diffuse passively back into the circulation, and is therefore lost in the urine. In alkaline urine, these drugs mostly exist in lipid-soluble forms, which are reabsorbed.

The increased rate of absorption of pseudoephedrine seen with sodium bicarbonate is probably also due to pH rises, which favour the formation of the lipid-soluble absorbable form of pseudoephedrine.

Importance and management

The interaction between ephedrine or pseudoephedrine and urinary alkalinisers are established but reports of adverse reactions in patients appear to be rare. Be aware that any increase in the adverse effects of these drugs (tremor, anxiety, insomnia, tachycardia, etc.) could be due to drug retention brought about by this interaction. **Acetazolamide** also makes the urine alkaline and would be expected to interact with ephedrine and pseudoephedrine in the same way as sodium bicarbonate.

Acidification of the urine with ammonium chloride increases the loss of ephedrine and pseudoephedrine in the urine and could be exploited in cases of drug overdosage.

1. Wilkinson GR, Beckett AH. Absorption, metabolism and excretion of the ephedrines in man. I. The influence of urinary pH and urine volume output. *J Pharmacol Exp Ther* (1968) 162, 139–47.
2. Brater DC, Kaojarern S, Benet LZ, Lin ET, Lockwood T, Morris RC, McSherry EJ, Melmon KL. Renal excretion of pseudoephedrine. *Clin Pharmacol Ther* (1980) 28, 690–4.
3. Kuntzman RG, Tsai I, Brand L, Mark LC. The influence of urinary pH on the plasma half-life of pseudoephedrine in man and dog and a sensitive assay for its determination in human plasma. *Clin Pharmacol Ther* (1971) 12, 62–7.
4. Lucarotti RL, Colaizzi JL, Barry H, Poust RI. Enhanced pseudoephedrine absorption by concurrent administration of aluminium hydroxide gel in humans. *J Pharm Sci* (1972) 61, 903–5.

PUVA + Metoclopramide

Metoclopramide does not appear to affect the pharmacokinetics of methoxsalen.

Clinical evidence, mechanism, importance and management

In a study, 6 healthy subjects were given a single 25-mg/m^2 dose of **methoxsalen** and a single 10-mg dose of metoclopramide with a standard breakfast, followed by a 4-hour period during which no further food or drink was taken. Metoclopramide increased the intersubject variation in the pharmacokinetics of **methoxsalen**, but overall, its pharmacokinetics were not significantly altered.[1] It would therefore appear that metoclopramide can be given with **methoxsalen** without the need for a **methoxsalen** dose adjustment.

1. Studer-Sachsenberg EM, Piletta P-A, Fathi M, Saurat J-H, Salomon D. Influence of metoclopramide on the pharmacokinetics of 8-methoxypsoralen. *Dermatology* (1997) 195, 81–3.

PUVA + Miscellaneous

Two case reports describe photosensitivity in patients taking methoxsalen and undergoing PUVA, one in a patient taking rue (*Ruta graveolens*) and another in a patient who ate large amounts of celery soup.

Clinical evidence, mechanism, importance and management

A 35-year-old woman taking **methoxsalen** and undergoing PUVA for psoriasis unexpectedly developed increased photosensitivity. Over the previous weekend and on the morning of therapy she had been drinking a concoction of **rue** (***Ruta graveolens***).[1] This plant naturally contains 5-methoxypsoralen so it would appear that a pharmacodynamic interaction occurred, which resulted in the photosensitivity.

The authors note that other herbal products contain photosensitising substances (e.g. those containing members of the **Umbelliferae** family; such as **celery**, or ***Chlorella*** species), and so suggest that patients undergoing PUVA should be warned about the potential interactions.[1] This warning appears justified by the case of a woman taking **methoxsalen** and undergoing PUVA, who developed photosensitivity after eating a large quantity of soup containing **celery**, parsnip and parsley.[2]

1. Puig L. Pharmacodynamic interaction with phototoxic plants during PUVA therapy. *Br J Dermatol* (1997) 136, 973–4.
2. Boffa MJ, Gilmour E, Ead RD. Celery soup causing severe phototoxicity during PUVA therapy. *Br J Dermatol* (1996) 135, 330–45.

PUVA + Phenytoin

Methoxsalen levels can be markedly reduced by phenytoin. This resulted in the failure of PUVA for psoriasis in one patient.

Clinical evidence, mechanism, importance and management

A patient with epilepsy did not respond to treatment for psoriasis with PUVA (12 treatments of **methoxsalen** 30 mg given orally and ultraviolet A irradiation) while taking phenytoin 250 mg daily. **Methoxsalen** serum levels were normal in the absence of phenytoin, but abnormally low while taking phenytoin,[1] due, it is suggested, to the enzyme-inducing effects of phenytoin. This appears to be the only report of an interaction but it should be borne in mind in any patient given both drugs, as it could potentially lead to serious erythema and blistering if the phenytoin dose is reduced during therapy, as **methoxsalen** levels rise and therefore photosensitivity caused by the **methoxsalen** may be increased.

1. Staberg B, Hueg B. Interaction between 8-methoxypsoralen and phenytoin. Consequence for PUVA therapy. *Acta Derm Venereol* (1985) 65, 553–5.

Radiopharmaceuticals + Colchicine

An isolated case report describes an unexpected imaging result, thought to be due to colchicine interfering with the uptake of [18F]-methylcholine.

Clinical evidence, mechanism, importance and management

Colchicine has been reported to interfere with the uptake of [18F]-methylcholine when used to image prostate cancer. A patient taking colchicine 500 micrograms daily for gout prophylaxis had no evidence of active uptake of [18F]-methylcholine into relevant organs. It was suspected that the colchicine had interfered with this uptake, and so the patient was asked to stop colchicine for 2 weeks. When the scan was repeated, [18F]-methylcholine uptake into organs was normal.[1]

Choline is an amino acid which undergoes anabolic and catabolic metabolism. It is incorporated into phosphatidylcholine in the anabolic pathway. The authors suggest that colchicine increased the breakdown of phosphatidylcholine, which interfered with the anabolic pathway for the uptake of [18F]-methylcholine. They therefore recommend that colchicine should be stopped for 48 hours before [18F]-methylcholine PET or CT scans.[1] However, this appears to be the only published report of an interaction with [18F]-methylcholine, and so its general relevance is unknown. The advice to stop colchicine seems overly-cautious, although it would seem prudent to bear the possibility of an interaction in mind should a patient taking colchicine and undergoing a [18F]-methylcholine PET or CT scan have an unexpected scan result.

1. Roef MJ, van der Poel H, van der Laken CJ, Vogel WV. Colchicine must be stopped before imaging with [18F]-methylcholine PET/CT. *Nucl Med Commun* (2010) 31, 1075–7.

Raloxifene + Fenofibrate

An isolated report describes cholestasis in a patient taking raloxifene, shortly after fenofibrate was added.

Clinical evidence, mechanism, importance and management

A case report describes a 60-year-old woman who had been taking raloxifene 60 mg daily for 3 years, who developed dark urine 14 days after starting to take fenofibrate 250 mg daily. Her liver function was normal before she started to take fenofibrate, and she had no family history of liver dysfunction. Both drugs were stopped, and 2 days later she was admitted with jaundice. Her liver enzymes were considerably increased, imaging showed cholelithiasis with no other pathological findings, and a liver biopsy found hepatocellular cholestasis. Her liver enzymes decreased, but 21 months later, they were still higher than before fenofibrate was started. The authors of the report suggest that the liver dysfunction was due to an interaction between raloxifene and fenofibrate, rather than an adverse effect of fenofibrate or raloxifene, because the picture presented was not consistent with the liver injuries reported with either drug in other cases.[1] However, the mechanism for this is not known. This is an isolated report, and as such the general clinical relevance is probably small.

1. Lucena MI, Andrade RJ, Vicioso L, González FJ, Pachkoria K, García-Muñoz B. Prolonged cholestasis after raloxifene and fenofibrate interaction: a case report. *World J Gastroenterol* (2006) 12, 5244–6.

Raloxifene + Miscellaneous

The absorption of raloxifene is reduced by colestyramine and predicted to be reduced by colestipol. No clinically relevant changes in raloxifene

pharmacokinetics occur with aluminium/magnesium hydroxide, amoxicillin, ampicillin or calcium carbonate. Raloxifene does not alter digoxin or methylprednisolone levels. Oral antibacterials, antihistamines, aspirin, benzodiazepines, H_2-receptor antagonists, ibuprofen or paracetamol (acetaminophen) were used in clinical studies without any obvious effect on raloxifene levels. Smoking does not appear to alter the efficacy of raloxifene.

Clinical evidence, mechanism, importance and management

(a) Ampicillin and Amoxicillin

Ampicillin is reported to reduce the maximum serum levels of raloxifene by 28% and the extent of the absorption by 14% without affecting the elimination rate.[1] This is thought to be because ampicillin reduces the number of enteric bacteria and so reduces enterohepatic recycling of raloxifene. These small changes are unlikely to be clinically relevant. In another clinical efficacy study, there was no discernible difference in the plasma levels of raloxifene when it was taken with amoxicillin.[1]

(b) Antacids

The manufacturer of raloxifene reports that an antacid containing **aluminium/magnesium hydroxide**, given 1 hour before and 2 hours after raloxifene, had no effect on its absorption. Also, no interaction was seen with **calcium carbonate**.[2] There would therefore appear to be no reason for avoiding the concurrent use of these antacids and raloxifene.

(c) Colestyramine

The manufacturer reports that colestyramine reduced the absorption of raloxifene by about 60% due to an interruption in enterohepatic cycling.[1] It is recommended that these two drugs should not be used concurrently.[1,3] The manufacturers also predict that **colestipol** will interact similarly.[1,3]

(d) Digoxin

Raloxifene is reported not to affect the steady-state AUC of digoxin, while the maximum serum levels of digoxin were increased by less than 5%.[3]

(e) Methylprednisolone

Steady state raloxifene had no effect on the pharmacokinetics of a single oral dose of methylprednisolone.[1,3]

(f) Tobacco

Retrospective analysis of data from a placebo-controlled study of raloxifene found that raloxifene was equally effective in current tobacco smokers as non-smokers, although smokers had a lower baseline bone mineral density.[4]

(g) Miscellaneous

Data from clinical efficacy studies revealed no clinically relevant differences in the plasma levels of raloxifene when stratified according to concurrent drug use. These drugs included **oral antibacterials** (not named), **antihistamines** (not named), **aspirin**, **benzodiazepines** (not named), **H_2-receptor antagonists** (not named), NSAIDs (**ibuprofen**, **naproxen**), and **paracetamol (acetaminophen)**.[3] There would therefore appear to be no reason for avoiding the concurrent use of any of these drugs with raloxifene.

1. Evista (Raloxifene hydrochloride). Eli Lilly and Company. US Prescribing information, October 2008.
2. Eli Lilly and Company Limited. Personal communication, September 1998.
3. Evista (Raloxifene hydrochloride). Daiichi Sankyo UK Ltd. UK Summary of product characteristics, August 2003.
4. Chapurlat RD, Ewing SK, Bauer DC, Cummings SR. Influence of smoking on the antiosteoporotic efficacy of raloxifene. *J Clin Endocrinol Metab* (2001) 86, 4178–82.

Regadenoson + Methylxanthines

Methylxanthines (such as theophylline and caffeine) are expected to reduce the vasodilating effects of regadenoson, although one study found that caffeine did not interfere with the effects of regadenoson in radionuclide cardiac imaging. Aminophylline reduces the gastrointestinal adverse effects of regadenoson, when compared with placebo, and it has been shown to reduce the duration of vasodilation seen with regadenoson.

Clinical evidence

(a) Aminophylline

In a randomised study in 248 patients given intravenous aminophylline 75 mg or placebo 2 minutes after regadenoson, the incidence of diarrhoea and abdominal discomfort was 50% lower in those given aminophylline (124 patients) than in those given placebo (124 patients). The incidence of diarrhoea specifically, was 70% lower in the aminophylline group than in the placebo group, but the incidence of abdominal discomfort was no different between the groups.[1] The US manufacturer of regadenoson also notes that post-marketing experience includes reports of abdominal pain, occasionally severe, and musculoskeletal pain, a few minutes after giving regadenoson, and that aminophylline can reduce the severity.[2] The UK manufacturer briefly notes that a slow intravenous injection of aminophylline 100 mg has been shown to reduce the duration of vasodilation seen with regadenoson 400 micrograms in patients undergoing cardiac catheterisation.[3]

(b) Caffeine

In a study, 41 healthy subjects were given a single 200-mg dose of caffeine (as a capsule) 2 hours before they were given regadenoson as part of a positron emission tomography (PET) cardiac imaging scan. No difference in myocardial blood flow was found either at rest or when stress was induced with regadenoson between those who took placebo and those who were given caffeine. However, the heart rate increase in response to regadenoson was reduced by 20 bpm in those who took caffeine, when compared with placebo. No difference in blood pressure or the incidence of adverse effects was found between the two groups.[4]

Mechanism

Methylxanthines, such as theophylline and caffeine, are adenosine receptor antagonists, and are therefore expected to reduce the vasodilatory effects of regadenoson, which is a selective adenosine A_2-receptor agonist. However, one study suggests that modest caffeine intake might not interfere with the effects of regadenoson during radionuclide myocardial imaging. Nevertheless, the authors state that this needs further confirmation in patients and with higher caffeine doses.[4] The authors of the study with aminophylline suggest that it attenuates the adverse effects of regadenoson.[1]

Importance and management

Evidence for a pharmacodynamic interaction between methylxanthines and regadenoson is limited to two studies with aminophylline and caffeine, both of which suggest no adverse outcome. In fact, in the case of aminophylline, the authors of the aminophylline study go so far as to say that the results support the routine use of intravenous aminophylline to reduce the frequency and severity of regadenoson adverse effects.[1] Although the UK and US manufacturers of regadenoson advise that intravenous aminophylline can be given to reduce excessive and/or persistent regadenoson adverse effects,[2,3] the UK manufacturer states that because aminophylline can prolong a seizure, or cause multiple seizures (due to its proconvulsant effects), giving aminophylline solely for the purpose of stopping a seizure induced by regadenoson is not recommended.[3] The US manufacturer similarly advises against such use.[2] The UK and US manufacturers also give more general advice about the use of methylxanthines, as follows: **theophylline** [and therefore aminophylline] and other xanthine-containing products such as **tea** and **coffee** [as well as **chocolate** and **cola drinks**] should be avoided for at least 12 hours before regadenoson is given as part of radionuclide myocardial imaging.[2,3]

1. Doukky R, Morales Demori R, Jain S, Kiriakos R, Mwansa V, Calvin JE. Attenuation of the side effect profile of regadenoson: a randomized double-blinded placebo-controlled study with aminophylline in patients undergoing myocardial perfusion imaging. "The ASSUAGE trial". *J Nucl Cardiol* (2012) 19, 448–57.
2. Lexiscan (Regadenoson). Astellas Pharma US, Inc. US Prescribing information, July 2014.
3. Rapiscan (Regadenoson). Rapidscan Pharma Solutions EU Ltd. UK Summary of product characteristics, June 2014.
4. Gaemperli O, Schepis T, Koepfli P, Siegrist PT, Fleischman S, Nguyen P, Olmsted A, Wang W, Lieu H, Kaufmann PA. Interaction of caffeine with regadenoson-induced hyperemic myocardial blood flow as measured by positron emission tomography: a randomized, double-blind, placebo-controlled crossover trial. *J Am Coll Cardiol* (2008) 51, 328–9.

Regadenoson + Miscellaneous

Dipyridamole is predicted to alter the effects of regadenoson. ACE inhibitors, angiotensin II receptor antagonists, beta blockers, calcium-channel blockers, cardiac glycosides, and nitrates do not appear to alter the efficacy of regadenoson.

Clinical evidence, mechanism, importance and management

(a) Dipyridamole

Regadenoson is a selective adenosine A_2-receptor agonist, and as dipyridamole increases the plasma concentrations of adenosine by inhibiting its uptake into cells, the cardiac effects of regadenoson might be altered by concurrent use. The UK and US manufacturers therefore advise that dipyridamole should be avoided, if possible, for at least 2 days before giving regadenoson.[1,2] Note also, that regadenoson can cause transient ischaemic attacks and, post-marketing, it has been reported to cause stroke.[1,2]

(b) Other drugs

The UK and US manufacturers report that, in clinical studies, **ACE inhibitors**, **angiotensin II receptor antagonists**, **beta blockers**, **calcium-channel blockers**, **cardiac glycosides**, and **nitrates** did not affect the efficacy or safety of regadenoson in patients taking these drugs.[1,2] Therefore, no additional precautions seem to be necessary on concurrent use. However, note that regadenoson can cause clinically important increases in blood pressure, which is some cases can result in hypertensive crisis. The risk might be increased in patients with uncontrolled hypertension and therefore the UK manufacturer advises that consideration should be given to delaying giving regadenoson until blood pressure is well controlled.[2]

1. Lexiscan (Regadenoson). Astellas Pharma US, Inc. US Prescribing information, July 2014.
2. Rapiscan (Regadenoson). Rapidscan Pharma Solutions EU Ltd. UK Summary of product characteristics, June 2014.

Retinoids + Food

Fatty foods increase the absorption of acitretin, alitretinoin, etretinate, and isotretinoin.

Clinical evidence

(a) Acitretin

In a study in 18 healthy subjects the absorption of acitretin was increased by 90% and its maximum plasma concentrations were increased by 70% when acitretin 50 mg was taken with a standard breakfast. The breakfast consisted of two poached eggs, two slices of toast, two pats of margarine, and 8 oz (about 240 mL) of skimmed milk.[1]

(b) Alitretinoin

In a randomised, crossover study in 29 healthy subjects, the AUC and maximum plasma concentration of alitretinoin were increased about 4-fold when a single 40-mg dose of alitretinoin was taken with a standard breakfast. The breakfast consisted of fried eggs, bacon, fried potato, toast with butter, and whole milk.[2]

(c) Etretinate

Studies have found that high-fat meals and **milk** cause about a 2- to 5-fold increase in the absorption of **etretinate**, when compared with high-carbohydrate meals or when fasting.[3,4]

(d) Isotretinoin

In a study in 20 healthy subjects the AUC of a single 80-mg dose of isotretinoin was increased by 40%, 70%, and 90% when taken one hour before a standard breakfast, during breakfast, and one hour after breakfast, respectively, when compared with the same dose of isotretinoin taken 4 hours before breakfast.[5] In a pharmacokinetic study in 57 healthy subjects, isotretinoin in a capsule formulation with lipids, was found to be bioequivalent to a standard capsule formulation when given with a standard high-fat meal (50 g fat). However, when given after an overnight fast, the AUC and maximum concentration of isotretinoin were about 2-fold higher with the lipid formulation than with the standard formulation.[6]

Mechanism

It is thought that, because these retinoids are lipid soluble, they are absorbed into the lymphatic system by becoming incorporated into the bile-acid micelles of the fats in the food. In this way, losses due to first-pass liver metabolism and gut wall metabolism are minimised, and bioavailability is increased.

Importance and management

The interactions between retinoids and foods are established and of clinical importance. The UK and US manufacturers of acitretin recommend taking it with meals[7,8] or with milk.[7] Most of the manufacturers of isotretinoin recommend taking it with food,[9,10] although some manufacturers of isotretinoin capsules that are formulated with lipids state that it may be taken without regard for food.[11] The UK manufacturer of oral **alitretinoin**[12] recommends taking it with food, and, on the basis of these interactions, the UK manufacturer of oral **tretinoin** also recommends administration with food.[13] Similar recommendations were made with etretinate when it was available.[14]

1. McNamara PJ, Jewell RC, Jensen BK, Brindley CJ. Food increases the bioavailability of acitretin. *J Clin Pharmacol* (1988) 28, 1051–5.
2. Schmitt-Hoffmann AH, Roos B, Sauer J, Schleimer M, Kovācs P, Stoeckel K, Maares J. Influence of food on the pharmacokinetics of oral alitretinoin (9-cis retinoic acid). *Clin Exp Dermatol* (2011) 36 (Suppl 2), 18–23.
3. DiGiovanna JJ, Cross EG, McClean SW, Ruddel ME, Gantt G, Peck GL. Etretinate: effect of milk intake on absorption. *J Invest Dermatol* (1984) 82, 636–40.
4. Colburn WA, Gibson DM, Rodriguez LC, Buggé CJL, Blumenthal HP. Effect of meals on the kinetics of etretinate. *J Clin Pharmacol* (1985) 25, 583–9.
5. Colburn WA, Gibson DM, Wiens RE, Hanigan JJ. Food increases the bioavailability of isotretinoin. *J Clin Pharmacol* (1983) 23, 534–9.
6. Webster GF, Leyden JJ, Gross JA. Comparative pharmacokinetic profiles of a novel isotretinoin formulation (isotretinoin-Lidose) and the innovator isotretinoin formulation: a randomized, 4-treatment, crossover study. *J Am Acad Dermatol* (2013) 69, 762–7.
7. Neotigason (Acitretin). Actavis UK Ltd. UK Summary of product characteristics, February 2015.
8. Soriatane (Acitretin). Stiefel Labs, Inc. US Prescribing information, May 2015.
9. Roaccutane (Isotretinoin). Roche Products Ltd. UK Summary of product characteristics, January 2012.
10. Accutane (Isotretinoin). Roche Laboratories Inc. US Prescribing information, November 2008.
11. Absorica (isotretinoin). Ranbaxy Laboratories Inc. US Prescribing information, August 2014.
12. Toctino (Alitretinoin). Basilea Pharmaceutica. UK Summary of product characteristics, July 2014.
13. Vesanoid (Tretinoin). Roche Products Ltd. UK Summary of product characteristics, May 2015.
14. Tigason (Etretinate). Roche Products Ltd. ABPI Datasheet Compendium, 1993–1994, p.1347–9.

Retinoids + HIV-protease inhibitors

Symptoms of retinoid toxicity and reduced plasma concentrations of retinoic acid occurred in a patient who took isotretinoin with indinavir and ritonavir. HIV-protease inhibitors are predicted to inhibit the metabolism of alitretinoin.

Clinical evidence, mechanism, importance and management

An HIV-positive patient taking oral isotretinoin 50 mg daily for severe acne developed signs of retinoid toxicity after starting to take **indinavir** 800 mg daily, **ritonavir** 600 mg daily, zidovudine 600 mg daily, and lamivudine 300 mg daily. However, plasma concentrations of 4-oxo retinoic acids and non-oxidised retinoic acids were *decreased*. Since HIV-protease inhibitors such as **indinavir** and **ritonavir** are inhibitors of the cytochrome P450 isoenzyme CYP3A4, this finding was not expected. Oxidative metabolism of retinoic acid is reduced by other CYP3A4 inhibitors with resultant increases in plasma retinoic acid.[1] It was suggested that the symptoms of retinoid toxicity and reduced plasma retinoid concentrations may have resulted from increased cellular uptake of retinoids and this may be associated with modulation of retinoic acid signalling by HIV-protease inhibitors[1,2]

The clinical relevance of this case is unclear, but bear it in mind in the event of unexpected toxicity on concurrent use.

The UK manufacturers of alitretinoin note that, although the concurrent use of HIV-protease inhibitors have not been studied, other drugs that inhibit CYP3A4 (such as ketoconazole) raise **alitretinoin** concentrations.[3] It may therefore be prudent to be alert for an increase in the adverse effects of **alitretinoin** if HIV-protease inhibitors are also being taken.

1. Sass JO, Padberg J. Human isotretinoin metabolism during indinavir therapy. *AIDS Res Hum Retroviruses* (2000) 16, 1451–2.
2. Lenhard JM, Weiel JE, Paulik MA, Furfine ES. Stimulation of vitamin A_1 acid signaling by the HIV protease inhibitor indinavir. *Biochem Pharmacol* (2000) 59, 1063–8.
3. Toctino (Alitretinoin). Basilea Pharmaceutica. UK Summary of product characteristics, July 2014.

Retinoids + Tetracyclines

The development of pseudotumour cerebri (benign intracranial hypertension) has been associated with the concurrent use of acitretin, etretinate, isotretinoin, or topical tretinoin with a tetracycline. Other retinoids are expected to interact similarly.

Clinical evidence, mechanism, importance and management

The concurrent use of **isotretinoin** and a tetracycline has resulted in the development of pseudotumour cerebri (i.e. a clinical picture of cranial hypertension with headache, dizziness and visual disturbances). By 1983, the FDA in the US had received reports of 10 patients with pseudotumour cerebri and/or papilloedema associated with the use of **isotretinoin**. Four had retinal haemorrhages, and 5 of the 10 were also taking a tetracycline.[1] The manufacturers also have similar reports on file of 3 patients given **isotretinoin** and either **minocycline** or **tetracycline**.[2] The same reaction has been seen in a patient given **etretinate** with **minocycline**,[3] and a patient given **doxycycline** with topical **tretinoin** gel;[4] although in this latter case, neither drug was given alone, and so an interaction is not established.

Both retinoids and tetracyclines alone can cause increased intracranial pressure, and they might have an additive effect when used together.

The manufacturers of **acitretin**,[5,6] oral **alitretinoin**,[7] **isotretinoin**[8] and oral **tretinoin**[9] contraindicate their use with tetracyclines, or advise avoiding the concurrent use of tetracyclines.[10]

1. Anon. Adverse effects with isotretinoin. *FDA Drug Bull* (1983) 13, 21–3.
2. Shalita AR, Cunningham WJ, Leyden JJ, Pochi PE, Strauss JS. Isotretinoin treatment of acne and related disorders: an update. *J Am Acad Dermatol* (1983) 9, 629–38.
3. Viraben R, Mathieu C, Fonton B. Benign intracranial hypertension during etretinate therapy for mycosis fungoides. *J Am Acad Dermatol* (1985) 13, 515–17.
4. Tabibian JH, Gutierrez MA. Doxycycline-induced pseudotumor cerebri. South Med J. (2009) 102, 310–11.
5. Neotigason (Acitretin). Actavis UK Ltd. UK Summary of product characteristics, February 2015.
6. Soriatane (Acitretin). Stiefel Labs, Inc. US Prescribing information, May 2015.
7. Toctino (Alitretinoin). Basilea Pharmaceutica. UK Summary of product characteristics, July 2014.
8. Roaccutane (Isotretinoin). Roche Products Ltd. UK Summary of product characteristics, January 2012.
9. Vesanoid (Tretinoin). Roche Products Ltd. UK Summary of product characteristics, May 2015.
10. Accutane (Isotretinoin). Roche Laboratories Inc. US Prescribing information, November 2008.

Retinoids + Vitamin A (Retinol)

A condition similar to vitamin A (retinol) overdosage may occur if oral retinoids such as acitretin, alitretinoin, isotretinoin or tretinoin are given with vitamin A.

Clinical evidence, mechanism, importance and management

Combined treatment with **isotretinoin** and vitamin A may result in a condition similar to overdosage with vitamin A. Signs and symptoms of hypervitaminosis A include skin changes (yellowing, dryness, alopecia), anorexia, vomiting, neuropsychiatric effects, raised intracranial pressure, and musculoskeletal effects, including premature fusion of the epiphyseal discs in children (which is irreversible). Concurrent use should therefore be avoided or very closely monitored.

The manufacturers of **acitretin** say that the concurrent use of high-dose vitamin A should be avoided: in the UK[1] they advise no more than 4000 to 5000 units of vitamin A daily, which is the recommended daily allowance, and in the US[2] they advise doses of no more than the minimum recommended daily allowance. Similarly, the manufacturers of oral **alitretinoin**,[3] **isotretinoin**[4,5] and oral **tretinoin**[6,7] say that vitamin A should be avoided.

1. Neotigason (Acitretin). Actavis UK Ltd. UK Summary of product characteristics, June 2011.
2. Soriatane (Acitretin). Stiefel Labs, Inc. US Prescribing information, May 2015.
3. Toctino (Alitretinoin). Basilea Pharmaceutica. UK Summary of product characteristics, July 2014.
4. Roaccutane (Isotretinoin). Roche Products Ltd. UK Summary of product characteristics, January 2012.
5. Accutane (Isotretinoin). Roche Laboratories Inc. US Prescribing information, November 2008.
6. Vesanoid (Tretinoin). Roche Products Ltd. UK Summary of product characteristics, May 2015.
7. Vesanoid (Tretinoin). Roche Laboratories Inc. US Prescribing information, July 2008.

Ritodrine + Miscellaneous

Supraventricular tachycardia developed in a woman given ritodrine when she was also given glycopyrronium (glycopyrrolate), and tachycardia has been reported in two patients when atropine was used with ritodrine. Hypertension has been reported when cyclopropane was given to patients who had recently received ritodrine. The abuse of cocaine does not appear to increase the incidence of adverse effects in patients given ritodrine. Hypokalaemia is a known adverse effect of ritodrine and this effect may be additive with other drugs that lower potassium levels.

Clinical evidence, mechanism, importance and management

(a) Antimuscarinics

A case report describes premature labour in a 39-year-old woman who was 28 weeks pregnant, which was arrested with an intravenous infusion of ritodrine hydrochloride. Two weeks later, while she was receiving the maximum dose of ritodrine (300 micrograms/minute), her uterine contractions began again and she was scheduled for an emergency caesarean section. The ritodrine was discontinued 40 minutes before the operation. It was noted in the operating room that she had copious oral secretions so she was given 100% oxygen by mask and 200 micrograms of intravenous **glycopyrronium (glycopyrrolate)**. Shortly afterwards she developed a supraventricular tachycardia (a rise in heart rate from 80 up to 180 bpm), which was converted to sinus tachycardia of 130 bpm when she was given intravenous propranolol 500 micrograms, in divided doses over several minutes.[1] Two other patients given intravenous ritodrine 6 mg over 3 minutes developed tachyarrhythmias when they were premedicated with **atropine**.[2]

The reason for these reactions is not understood. Ritodrine alone has been responsible for tachyarrhythmias and one possible explanation for this interaction is that the effects of ritodrine and the antimuscarinic drug were additive.

Information is very limited and the interaction is not well established but some caution is clearly appropriate if both drugs are used. The authors of the first report advise avoidance. Arrhythmias have occurred when other sympathomimetics have been given with antimuscarinics, see 'Inotropes and Vasopressors + Antimuscarinics', p.1064.

(b) Cocaine

A study in 51 pregnant patients given ritodrine for premature labour found no evidence of an increase in adverse effects in 17 of the patients who had been abusing cocaine.[3]

(c) Cyclopropane

In an analysis of 43 women who had a caesarean section under cyclopropane anaesthesia, all of the 6 who had previously been given ritodrine developed unacceptably high blood pressure (185/103 mmHg) after cyclopropane was started. Arrhythmias were reported in two of these patients.[4]

(d) Drugs that lower potassium

Ritodrine is a beta$_2$ agonist, and in common with other drugs of this class, may lower potassium levels. These effects may be additive with other drugs that are known to lower potassium levels, such as **amphotericin B**, the **corticosteroids**, **loop** or **thiazide diuretics**, consider 'Beta-agonist bronchodilators + Potassium-depleting drugs', p.1422, and **theophylline**, consider 'Theophylline + Beta-agonist bronchodilators', p.1437.

1. Simpson JI, Giffin JP. A glycopyrrolate-ritodrine drug-drug interaction. *Can J Anaesth* (1988) 35, 187–9.
2. Sheybany S, Murphy JF, Evans D, Newcombe RG, Pearson JF. Ritodrine in the management of fetal distress. *Br J Obstet Gynaecol* (1982) 89, 723–6.
3. Darby MJ, Mazdisnian F. Does recent cocaine use increase the risk of side effects with β-adrenergic tocolysis? *Am J Obstet Gynecol* (1991) 164, 377.
4. Johannsen G. Ritodrine and cyclopropane interaction. *Anaesthesia* (1980) 35, 84–85.

Romiplostim + Miscellaneous

The combination of romiplostim and other drugs that are used to treat idiopathic thrombocytopenic purpura may result in platelet counts that are higher than is desirable.

Clinical evidence, mechanism, importance and management

The manufacturers state that no drug interaction studies have been undertaken with romiplostim.[1,2] The UK manufacturer states that, in clinical studies, romiplostim was given with other drugs used to treat idiopathic thrombocytopenic purpura, such as **azathioprine**, **corticosteroids**, **danazol**, intravenous **immunoglobulin**, and **anti-D immunoglobulin**. However, concurrent use may result in a greater increase in platelet counts, and they therefore recommend close monitoring to ensure that platelet counts remain within the desired range. They also note that when patients are given romiplostim, the doses of **azathioprine**, **corticosteroids**, and **danazol** and may need to be reduced or the drug stopped. Platelet counts should be closely monitored during dose adjustments of these drugs to avoid an undesirable reduction in the platelet count.[1]

1. Nplate (Romiplostim). Amgen Ltd. UK Summary of product characteristics, January 2010.
2. Nplate (Romiplostim). Amgen Inc. US Prescribing information, August 2008.

Sapropterin + Miscellaneous

Drugs that affect folate metabolism (such as methotrexate and trimethoprim) are predicted to reduce sapropterin exposure. Sapropterin is predicted to cause hypotension and other vasodilators that affect nitric oxide metabolism or effects (such as minoxidil, the nitrates, and phosphodiesterase type-5 inhibitors) might increase this effect. The concurrent use of levodopa and sapropterin has been reported to cause convulsions, excitability, and irritability. Food increases the absorption of sapropterin.

Clinical evidence, mechanism, importance and management

(a) Drugs that affect the metabolism or effects of nitric oxide

Sapropterin is a synthetic form of tetrahydrobiopterin, which is a co-factor for nitric oxide synthetase. It can therefore increase vasodilatation and cause hypotension. The UK and US manufacturers of sapropterin predict that it will have similar effects, and therefore advise caution if it is given with other drugs that cause vasodilatation by altering nitric oxide metabolism or effects, such as **glyceryl trinitrate**, **isosorbide dinitrate**, **sodium nitroprusside**, **molsidomine** (which are nitric oxide donors), **phosphodiesterase type-5 inhibitors**, and **minoxidil**.[1,2] However, the US manufacturer notes that, in *animal* studies, the concurrent use of sapropterin with a **phosphodiesterase type-5 inhibitor** had no effect on blood pressure.[1] Until clinical evidence becomes available, caution would be appropriate.

(b) Folate antagonists

Folate antagonists inhibit the enzyme dihydropteridine reductase and thereby reduce the regeneration of tetrahydrobiopterin by this enzyme. Sapropterin is a synthetic form of tetrahydrobiopterin, and the manufacturer predicts that it will be metabolised in a similar way to tetrahydrobiopterin.[2] The UK and US manufacturers of sapropterin therefore advise caution on the concurrent use of drugs that inhibit folate metabolism, such as **methotrexate**[1,2] and **trimethoprim**.[2] Until more is known, this would seem prudent.

(c) Food

In a randomised, crossover study in 30 healthy subjects, a high-calorie breakfast (about 1 000 calories) increased the maximum plasma concentration and AUC of a single 10-mg/kg dose of sapropterin (rounded to the nearest 100 mg to avoid breaking tablets) by 25% and 35%, respectively.[3] The US manufacturer also reports that, in a study, a high-fat, high-calorie meal increased the maximum plasma concentration and AUC of *dissolved* sapropterin tablets by 84% and 87%, respectively, although there was wide inter-subject variation.[1] The UK and US manufacturers advise that sapropterin should be taken with food, preferably at the same time each day, to increase absorption.[1,2]

(d) Levodopa

The US manufacturer notes that, in a 10-year postmarketing survey of sapropterin for a different indication, 3 patients with underlying neurological disorders who took levodopa and sapropterin experienced convulsions, exacerbation of convulsions, over-stimulation, or irritability.[1] The UK and US manufacturers of sapropterin therefore advise caution on the concurrent use of levodopa.[1,2]

1. Kuvan (Sapropterin dihydrochloride). BioMarin Pharmaceutical Inc. US Prescribing information, December 2007.
2. Kuvan (Sapropterin dihydrochloride). Merck Serono. UK Summary of product characteristics, June 2010.
3. Musson DG, Kramer WG, Foehr ED, Bieberdorf FA, Hornfeldt CS, Kim SS, Dorenbaum A. Relative bioavailability of sapropterin from intact and dissolved sapropterin dihydrochloride tablets and the effects of food: a randomized, open-label, crossover study in healthy adults. *Clin Ther* (2010) 32, 338–46.

Sodium oxybate + Miscellaneous

Additive CNS depressant effects are predicted when sodium oxybate is given with other CNS depressant drugs, and concurrent use of sedative hypnotics should be avoided. In theory, sodium oxybate may interact with valproate, phenytoin and ethosuximide. No pharmacokinetic interaction occurs with omeprazole, protriptyline, zolpidem or modafinil, but a pharmacodynamic interaction cannot be ruled out. Food markedly delays and modestly reduces the absorption of sodium oxybate.

Clinical evidence, mechanism, importance and management

(a) Antiepileptics

The UK manufacturer suggests that, as sodium oxybate is metabolised by gamma hydroxybutyrate dehydrogenase there is a potential risk of an interaction with drugs that induce or inhibit this enzyme. They name **valproate**, **phenytoin** and **ethosuximide**.[1] However, there do not appear to be any *in vivo* studies to confirm this prediction and its clinical relevance is unclear.

See also *Barbiturates*, below.

(b) CNS depressants

Sodium oxybate is the sodium salt of **gamma hydroxybutyrate** (GHB), a CNS depressant substance with well known abuse potential. When used clinically it is predicted to have additive effects with other CNS depressants and the manufacturers specifically say it should not be used with these.[1,2]

1. Antidepressants. The manufacturer notes that there was no pharmacokinetic interaction between sodium oxybate and **protriptyline**, but that the possibility of a pharmacodynamic interaction was not assessed.[1,2] The UK manufacturer states that the rate of adverse effects was increased when sodium oxybate was given with **tricyclic antidepressants**.[1]

2. Barbiturates. The UK manufacturer specifically contraindicates the use of sodium oxybate in patients taking barbiturates.[1]

3. Benzodiazepines and related hypnotics. The manufacturer states that sodium oxybate should not be given in combination with sedative hypnotics,[1,2] and the UK manufacturer specifically advises against the concurrent use of benzodiazepines because of the possibility of an increased risk of respiratory depression.[1]

The manufacturer notes that there was no pharmacokinetic interaction between sodium oxybate and **zolpidem**, but that the possibility of a pharmacodynamic interaction was not assessed,[1] and cannot be ruled out.[2]

4. Opioids. The UK manufacturer specifically contraindicates the use of sodium oxybate in patients taking opioids.[1]

(c) Food

In a study in 34 healthy subjects, giving 4.5 g of sodium oxybate solution after a high-fat meal delayed the time to maximum level from 0.75 hours to 2 hours, and reduced the maximum level by 58% and the AUC by 35%, when compared with the fasted state.[3] The first dose of sodium oxybate should be taken at least 2 to 3 hours after the evening meal, and patients should always try to keep the same timing of dosing in relation to meals.[1,2]

(d) Modafinil and other CNS stimulants

The manufacturer notes that there was no pharmacokinetic interaction between sodium oxybate and **modafinil**, but that the possibility of a pharmacodynamic interaction was not assessed.[1,2] Case reports describe an anxiety and depression in patients taking modafinil when sodium oxybate was added. The symptoms disappeared when sodium oxybate or modafinil was stopped or the sodium oxybate dose reduced.[4,5] Although concurrent use is common (about 80% of patients in clinical studies of sodium oxybate were also taking CNS stimulants[1]) consider the possibility of an interaction if psychiatric adverse effects develop on concurrent use. The reports suggest that withdrawal of either drug should stop these symptoms.

Armodafinil, the *R*-isomer of modafinil, would be expected to behave in the same way.

(e) Proton pump inhibitors

In a crossover study in 44 healthy subjects, pretreatment with **omeprazole** 40 mg daily for 5 days did not alter the pharmacokinetics of a single 3-g dose of sodium oxybate. There was no difference in the frequency and severity of adverse events.[6] No sodium oxybate dose adjustment is therefore expected to be needed in patients taking proton pump inhibitors.[1]

1. Xyrem (Sodium oxybate). UCB Pharma Ltd. UK Summary of product characteristics, April 2011.
2. Xyrem (Sodium oxybate). Jazz Pharmaceuticals, Inc. US Prescribing information, November 2005.
3. Borgen LA, Okerholm R, Morrison D, Lai A. The influence of gender and food on the pharmacokinetics of sodium oxybate oral solution in healthy subjects. *J Clin Pharmacol* (2003) 43, 59–65.
4. Rossetti AO, Heinzer RC, Tafti M, Buclin T. Rapid occurrence of depression following addition of sodium oxybate to modafinil. *Sleep Med* (2010) 11, 500–1.
5. Ortega-Albás JJ, López-Bernabé R, Serrano AL, Díaz JR. Sodium oxybate and modafinil: a good combination? *Sleep Med* (2010) 11, 957.
6. Borgen LA, Morrison D, Lai A. The effect of omeprazole on the bioavailability of sodium oxybate. *Clin Pharmacol Ther* (2004) 75, P21.

Somatropin + Miscellaneous

Somatropin is predicted to increase the clearance of drugs metabolised by CYP3A4 (such as ciclosporin). Somatropin may reduce the efficacy of insulin.

Clinical evidence, mechanism, importance and management

(a) Antidiabetics

Somatropin may cause hyperglycaemia and increase the risk of insulin resistance. The manufacturers therefore advise that patients with diabetes should be monitored when they are given somatropin; they specifically note that the dose of **insulin** may need adjusting.[1,2] One manufacturer reasonably states that antidiabetic therapy may need adjusting.[3] Patients should be advised to monitor blood glucose levels more frequently on concurrent use, and their antidiabetics should be adjusted if necessary.

(b) CYP3A4 substrates

Some manufacturers of somatropin report a study in patients with growth hormone deficiency, which found that somatropin may increase the clearance of drugs that are metabolised by cytochrome P450 isoenzymes, in particular CYP3A4. They therefore predict that somatropin may increase the clearance of these drugs and reduce their levels: they name **sex hormones**, **antiepileptics**, and **ciclosporin**.[1-3] However, note that, although ciclosporin and many **oestrogens** and **testosterone** are metabolised by CYP3A4 there appears to be little evidence to suggest that many antiepileptics are metabolised to a clinically relevant extent by this route: the exception appears to be **carbamazepine**, see 'Carbamazepine + Azoles', p.568. There does not appear to be any reports of an interaction, and therefore the clinical significance of this prediction is unknown. Until clinical data are available, it would seem prudent to bear the possibility of an interaction in mind should the efficacy of these drugs be reduced in a patient given somatropin. One manufacturer states that monitoring is advisable.[1]

1. Saizen (Somatropin). Merck Serono. UK Summary of product characteristics, April 2009.
2. NutropinAq (Somatropin). Ipsen Ltd. UK Summary of product characteristics, July 2009.
3. Genotropin (Somatropin). Pharmacia Ltd. UK Summary of product characteristics, March 2009.

Strontium ranelate + Miscellaneous

Foods and calcium compounds markedly reduce the absorption of strontium ranelate, whereas aluminium and magnesium antacids only slightly reduce strontium ranelate absorption. Strontium ranelate is predicted to reduce the absorption of the quinolones and the tetracyclines. Vitamin D does not affect strontium ranelate bioavailability.

Clinical evidence, mechanism, importance and management

(a) Antacids

The manufacturer notes that **aluminium/magnesium hydroxide** slightly reduced the absorption of strontium ranelate (AUC decreased by 20 to 25%) when given either at the same time or 2 hours before the strontium. However, when the antacid was given 2 hours *after* strontium, absorption was barely affected.[1] Therefore, the manufacturers recommend that antacids should be taken 2 hours after strontium ranelate. However, because it is also recommended that strontium ranelate is taken at bedtime, they say that, if this is impractical, concurrent intake is acceptable.[1] Note that **calcium**-containing antacids would have a greater effect, see *Foods and Calcium compounds* below, and concurrent intake would not be recommended.

(b) Foods and Calcium compounds

The manufacturer notes that food, milk, dairy products, and calcium supplements reduce the bioavailability of strontium ranelate by about 60 to 70%, when compared with administration 3 hours after a meal.[1] This is because divalent cations such as calcium form complexes with strontium ranelate, preventing its absorption. Therefore, strontium ranelate should not be taken within 2 hours of eating, or presumably within 2 hours of any calcium compound. The manufacturer recommends that strontium ranelate should be taken at bedtime, at least 2 hours after eating.[1]

(c) Quinolones and Tetracyclines

The manufacturer predicts that strontium will complex with quinolones and tetracyclines, preventing their absorption. Because of this, they recommend that when treatment with quinolones or tetracyclines is required, treatment with strontium ranelate should be temporarily suspended.[1]

(d) Vitamin D

The manufacturer notes that vitamin D supplements had no effect on strontium ranelate bioavailability.[1]

1. Protelos (Strontium ranelate). Servier Laboratories Ltd. UK Summary of product characteristics, January 2008.

Sugammadex + Miscellaneous

Sugammadex might slightly reduce progestogen exposure from oral hormonal contraceptives. Toremifene and intravenous fusidic acid are predicted to displace vecuronium or rocuronium from sugammadex, and so result in recurrence of the neuromuscular blockade, or delay in recovery. Drugs with neuromuscular blocking activity might reduce the effectiveness of sugammadex. Cases of QT prolongation have been seen in patients who have received sugammadex with sevoflurane or propofol.

Clinical evidence, mechanism, importance and management

No pharmacokinetic drug interaction studies have been conducted with sugammadex, and interactions have been predicted on the basis of the binding affinity of sugammadex and other drugs.

(a) Anaesthetics

The manufacturer of sugammadex notes that a few cases of QTc interval prolongation have been reported in patients who have received sugammadex and **sevoflurane** or **propofol**. Details of the other drugs given during the period of anaesthesia were not given.[1] Note that sugammadex alone does not appear to prolong the QTc interval to a clinically relevant extent.[1]

(b) Fusidic acid

The manufacturer of sugammadex predicts intravenous fusidic acid might cause some displacement of vecuronium or rocuronium from the sugammadex complex, and may delay recovery. Consideration may be given to using a further dose of sugammadex.[1] The importance of this potential interaction requires confirmation. Until further data are available these recommendations should be followed.

(c) Hormonal contraceptives

The manufacturer predicts that the AUC of progestogens might be reduced (by 34%, an amount they say is similar to the decrease seen when a hormonal contraceptive is taken 12 hours late) when patients also receive a single bolus dose of sugammadex, and that the effect on the estrogen will be lower. This is based on the fact that sugammadex might bind progestogens in the blood, so lowering the free plasma concentrations. They advise that the same precautions should be followed as for when one daily dose of the oral hormonal contraceptive is missed.[1] For non-oral hormonal contraceptives, they advise that patients should use an additional non-hormonal contraceptive method for the next 7 days, and also follow the specific product guidelines.[1]

Even if this predicted pharmacokinetic interaction is proved, it is difficult to envisage that a 34% reduction in AUC of a progestogen on a single day when the woman has undergone surgery will be clinically relevant, even for oral progestogen-only contraceptives, and especially for parenteral progestogen-only contraceptives and the levonorgestrel IUD. Note that combined hormonal contraceptives are usually discontinued before major surgery or surgery involving prolonged immobilisation of a lower limb, because of the increased risk of thrombosis.

(d) Neuromuscular blocking drugs

Sugammadex is used therapeutically to reverse the activity of **rocuronium** or **vecuronium**. If further neuromuscular blockade is required within 24 hours of giving sugammadex, a non-steroidal neuromuscular blocking agent should be used.[1] Examples of non-steroidal neuromuscular blocking agents (that is, benzylisoquinolinium type neuromuscular blocking agents) are given in 'Table 5.2', p.98.

The manufacturer states that, if other drugs that potentiate the neuromuscular blocking effect of **rocuronium** or **vecuronium** are given in the post-operative period (after reversal of the effects of **rocuronium** or **vecuronium** with sugammadex) there is the possibility of recurrence of blockade, and a further dose of sugammadex may be required.[1]

(e) Toremifene

The manufacturer of sugammadex predicts that toremifene might displace vecuronium or rocuronium from the sugammadex complex. This may result in a delayed recovery following neuromuscular blockade if toremifene has been given on the same day.[1] The importance of this potential interaction requires confirmation.

1. Bridion (Sugammadex sodium). Organon Laboratories Ltd. UK Summary of product characteristics, June 2010.

Sulfinpyrazone + NSAIDs

A brief report suggests that the uricosuric effects of sulfinpyrazone are not opposed by the concurrent use of flufenamic acid, meclofenamic acid or mefenamic acid.[1,2] However, note that sulfinpyrazone can cause gastric bleeding and inhibit platelet aggregation, effects that might be additive with NSAIDs.

Consider also 'Uricosuric drugs + Aspirin or other Salicylates', p.1590.

1. Latham BA, Radcliff F, Robinson RG. The effect of mefenamic acid and flufenamic acid on plasma uric acid levels. *Ann Phys Med* (1966) 8, 242–3.
2. Robinson RG, Radcliff FJ. The effect of meclofenamic acid on plasma uric acid levels. *Med J Aust* (1972) 1, 1079–80.

Sulfinpyrazone + Probenecid

Probenecid reduces the urinary excretion of sulfinpyrazone, but the overall uric acid clearance remains unaltered.

Clinical evidence, mechanism, importance and management

A study in 8 patients with gout found that although probenecid inhibited the renal tubular excretion of sulfinpyrazone, reducing it by about 75%, the maximal uric acid clearance was about the same as when either drug was given alone.[1] There would therefore seem to be no advantage in using these drugs together. The possibility of an increase in the adverse effects of sulfinpyrazone, caused by this reduction in excretion, does not seem to have been studied.

1. Perel JM, Dayton PG, Snell MM, Yü TF, Gutman AB. Studies of interactions among drugs in man at the renal level: probenecid and sulphinpyrazone. *Clin Pharmacol Ther* (1969) 10, 834–40.

Testosterone + Miscellaneous

Dutasteride and finasteride increase the levels of oral testosterone. Food has little effect on the absorption of oral testosterone.

Clinical evidence, mechanism, importance and management

In a pharmacokinetic study in healthy men, **dutasteride** 500 micrograms daily for 6 days increased the AUC of testosterone and testosterone enanthate given as single oral doses of 200 mg, 400 mg and 800 mg on days 4, 5 and 6 of dutasteride administration. The increases in testosterone AUC ranged from 42% with the 200 mg dose to 2.6-fold with the 800 mg dose. Moreover, **dutasteride** attenuated the increase in serum dihydrotestosterone seen with oral testosterone. In this study, subjects had their endogenous testosterone temporarily suppressed by the injection of the GnRH antagonist acyline.[1]

In a similar subsequent study, **finasteride** 5 mg daily increased AUC of testosterone 400 mg 2.3-fold. **Food** caused a slight non-significant decrease in testosterone levels, when compared with the fasting state.[2]

Testosterone is poorly bioavailable by the oral route, and is rapidly metabolised to dihydrotestosterone by 5-alpha reductase. By inhibiting this enzyme, dutasteride and finasteride reduce the formation of dihydrotestosterone and increase testosterone levels.[1,2]

These studies suggest that the 5-alpha reductase inhibitors might be useful in increasing testosterone oral bioavailability for oral replacement therapy.[1,2]

1. Amory JK, Bremner WJ. Oral testosterone in oil plus dutasteride in men: a pharmacokinetic study. *J Clin Endocrinol Metab* (2005) 90, 2610–7.
2. Amory JK, Page ST, Bremner WJ. Oral testosterone in oil: pharmacokinetic effects of 5α reduction by finasteride or dutasteride and food intake in men. *J Androl* (2006) 27, 72–8.

Tizanidine + Antihypertensives

Tizanidine is predicted to increase the effects of antihypertensive drugs and a number of case reports describe severe hypotension in patients taking tizanidine with lisinopril. The US manufacturer of tizanidine advises against the use of antihypertensives that are related to tizanidine (e.g. clonidine).

Clinical evidence

A 10-year-old child taking **lisinopril** developed severe hypotension within a week of starting to take tizanidine.[1] Similarly, a 48-year-old stroke patient taking **amlodipine**, **nimodipine**, **lisinopril**, and **labetalol**, which had been added sequentially to control hypertension, had a dramatic reduction in blood pressure (from 130/85 mmHg to 66/42 mmHg) within 2 hours of her first dose of tizanidine 2 mg. She was given dopamine to maintain her blood pressure, and tizanidine and all the antihypertensives were withdrawn. Later **labetalol**, **amlodipine**, **nimodipine** and tizanidine were successfully resumed without producing similar problems.[2] In a third case, an 85-year-old man taking multiple drugs including **lisinopril** 40 mg daily was given tizanidine 2 mg three times daily for chronic back pain. After the third dose of tizanidine, he complained of weakness and was found to have severe hypotension (blood pressure 60/32 mmHg) and bradycardia (heart rate 37 bpm) He was given intravenous fluids, and several drugs, including tizanidine and **lisinopril**, were discontinued. Within 24 hours his blood pressure had increased to 158/70 mmHg and his heart rate was 65 bpm. At discharge, all medication except tizanidine was restarted and after 2 weeks he had experienced no further symptoms.[3]

Mechanism

Tizanidine is a centrally acting α_2-adrenergic agonist structurally related to clonidine and can cause dose-related hypotension (66% of patients given a single 8-mg dose of tizanidine had a 20% reduction in blood pressure). This can result in bradycardia, dizziness or light-headedness, and rarely syncope. The antihypertensive effects of tizanidine are said to be less than one-tenth of those of clonidine.[4] Nevertheless, these effects are expected to be additive with other antihypertensive drugs. However, in the cases with lisinopril, it was suggested that ACE inhibition, combined with the alpha-agonist effects of tizanidine prevented the usual sympathetic response to hypotension (that is, it was not thought to be due to simple additive hypotensive effects).[1,2]

Importance and management

Tizanidine alone can cause hypotension, an effect that is usually minimised by titration of the dose. Patients should be warned about this effect. Because of this, the manufacturers state that tizanidine might increase the effects of antihypertensive drugs, including **diuretics**, and recommend caution on concurrent use.[4,5] This is a prudent precaution. The US manufacturer additionally states that tizanidine (an α_2-adrenergic agonist that is structurally related to clonidine) should not be used with other α_2-adrenergic agonists [e.g. **clonidine**, **methyldopa**].[4] The UK manufacturer also states that the concurrent use of **beta blockers** may potentiate bradycardia and hypotension.[5] This seems a reasonable prediction, as this effect has been seen with clonidine, see 'Clonidine and related drugs + Beta blockers', p.1056.

1. Johnson TR, Tobias JD. Hypotension following the initiation of tizanidine in a patient treated with an angiotensin converting enzyme inhibitor for chronic hypertension. *J Child Neurol* (2000) 15, 818–19.
2. Kao C-D, Chang J-B, Chen J-T, Wu Z-A, Shan D-E, Liao K-K. Hypotension due to interaction between lisinopril and tizanidine. *Ann Pharmacother* (2004) 38, 1840–43.
3. Publow SW, Branam DL. Hypotension and bradycardia associated with concomitant tizanidine and lisinopril therapy. *Am J Health-Syst Pharm* (2010) 67, 1606–10.
4. Zanaflex (Tizanidine hydrochloride). Acorda Therapeutics, Inc. US Prescribing information, April 2008.
5. Zanaflex (Tizanidine hydrochloride). Cephalon Ltd. UK Summary of product characteristics, April 2010.

Tizanidine + Cranberry juice

Cranberry juice does not affect the pharmacokinetics of tizanidine.

Clinical evidence

In a randomised, crossover study in 10 healthy subjects, 200 mL of cranberry juice three times daily for 10 days had no effect on the pharmacokinetics of a single 1-mg oral dose of tizanidine, taken on day 5. In this study, the cranberry juice used was a concentrate (*Kontiomehu sokeroitu karpalomehu*) diluted 1 to 4 with tap water before use.[1]

Mechanism

This study suggests that cranberry juice has no clinically relevant effect on CYP1A2 activity.

Importance and management

Although the evidence is limited to this particular study, there appears to be no need for any special precautions when taking cranberry juice with tizanidine.

Tizanidine is used as a probe drug for CYP1A2 activity, and therefore these results also suggest that a pharmacokinetic interaction between cranberry juice and other CYP1A2 substrates is unlikely.

1. Lilja JJ, Backman JT, Neuvonen PJ. Effects of daily ingestion of cranberry juice on the pharmacokinetics of warfarin, tizanidine, and midazolam – probes of CYP2C9, CYP1A2, and CYP3A4. *Clin Pharmacol Ther* (2007) 81, 833–9.

Tizanidine + CYP1A2 inhibitors

Fluvoxamine causes a very marked increase in tizanidine exposure with a consequent increase in hypotensive and sedative effects. Similarly, ciprofloxacin markedly increases tizanidine exposure and adverse effects. Combined hormonal contraceptives moderately increase tizanidine levels and might increase its adverse effects; mexiletine has similar effects. Other inhibitors of CYP1A2 are predicted to interact similarly.

Clinical evidence

(a) Ciprofloxacin

In a placebo-controlled, crossover study in 10 healthy subjects, ciprofloxacin 500 mg twice daily for 3 days markedly increased the AUC of a single 4-mg dose of tizanidine tenfold and increased its maximum level sevenfold, without significantly affecting its half-life. The hypotensive and sedative effects of tizanidine were also markedly increased by ciprofloxacin.[1]

A case report describes a 45-year-old Japanese woman with multiple sclerosis, taking tizanidine 3 mg daily, who had a reduction in blood pressure (from 124/88 mmHg to 102/74 mmHg) and heart rate (from 86 bpm to 58 bpm) shortly after starting to take ciprofloxacin 400 mg daily. After 2 days she complained of drowsiness and her blood pressure was 92/54 mmHg.[2] Retrospective analysis revealed 8 patients who had taken tizanidine with ciprofloxacin. In 7 of these patients, the mean reduction in blood pressure on starting ciprofloxacin was 21.3/15.4 mmHg, and the heart rate reduction was 14.9 bpm. Adverse effects attributable to tizanidine occurred in three of the patients.[2]

(b) Fluvoxamine

In a placebo-controlled, crossover study in 10 healthy subjects, fluvoxamine 100 mg daily for 4 days very markedly increased the AUC of a single 4-mg dose of tizanidine 33-fold and increased its maximum level 12-fold. The elimination half-life of tizanidine was prolonged from 1.5 hours to 4.3 hours. The hypotensive and sedative effects of tizanidine were also markedly increased by fluvoxamine, with all of the 10 subjects somnolent and dizzy for 3 to 6 hours.[3]

A case report describes a 70-year-old Japanese woman who started taking tizanidine 3 mg daily 15 days after starting fluvoxamine (100 mg increased to 150 mg daily). Her heart rate dropped from about 85 bpm to a range of 56 to 60 bpm. After tizanidine was stopped, the symptoms improved immediately.[4] Retrospective analysis revealed 23 patients who had taken tizanidine with fluvoxamine. Of these patients, 6 had adverse effects including low heart rate, dizziness, drowsiness and hypotension. The patients with adverse effects were, on average, older and taking higher doses of fluvoxamine and tizanidine than those without adverse effects.[4] In a later retrospective analysis by the same researchers, of 11 patients who had been taking tizanidine and fluvoxamine together, the mean reduction in blood pressure was 13/7.8 mmHg, and the heart rate reduction was 15.5 bpm.[2]

(c) Hormonal contraceptives

In a study in 15 healthy women taking an oral combined hormonal contraceptive (**gestodene**, with **ethinylestradiol** 20 micrograms in 12 subjects and **ethinylestradiol** 30 micrograms in 3 subjects), the AUC of a single 4-mg dose of tizanidine was 3.9-fold higher than in 15 healthy women not taking a hormonal contraceptive. The elimination half-life of tizanidine was unchanged. In addition, the maximum blood pressure-lowering effect of tizanidine was greater in the hormonal contraceptive users (29/21 mmHg) than in non-users (17/13 mmHg).[5] The manufacturer also notes that retrospective analysis of population pharmacokinetic data found that the clearance of tizanidine is about 50% lower in women taking oral contraceptives.[6,7]

(d) Mexiletine

In a study, 12 healthy subjects (5 smokers and 7 non-smokers) were given tizanidine 2 mg before and after taking mexiletine 50 mg three times daily for 5 doses. Mexiletine increased the AUC_{0-5} and maximum levels of tizanidine 3.6-fold and 3.1-fold, respectively; there appeared to be no difference in these findings in the smokers and non-smokers. Tizanidine alone reduced blood pressure and this effect was enhanced by mexiletine. The frequency of drowsiness was also increased by concurrent use (3 patients versus 10 patients).[8] The same researchers also undertook a retrospective review which identified 15 patients taking mexiletine and tizanidine. Concurrent use reduced blood pressure by 12/9 mmHg more than in patients taking mexiletine alone, and the incidence of drowsiness appeared to be increased, with one patient discontinuing concurrent use because of this.[8]

Mechanism

Tizanidine is a substrate of CYP1A2, and undergoes substantial metabolism by this route. Ciprofloxacin appears to inhibit mainly the presystemic metabolism of tizanidine by this isoenzyme, leading to increased absorption, as reflected by the increase in maximum level without a change in elimination half-life. Fluvoxamine inhibited both the presystemic metabolism of tizanidine and the elimination phase. Fluvoxamine, which is a known moderate inhibitor of CYP1A2, has the most marked effect. The contraceptive steroids and mexiletine are weaker inhibitors of CYP1A2 by comparison.

Importance and management

A pharmacokinetic interaction between tizanidine and drugs that inhibit CYP1A2 is well established, and clinically important. The common adverse effects of tizanidine, such as hypotension and sedation, are dose-related, and consequently the manufacturers recommend starting with a low dose of tizanidine (2 or 4 mg) in patients taking these drugs, carefully titrating to the usual maximum of 24 mg daily, and not exceeding 36 mg daily.[6,7] This represents a maximum 18-fold variation in dose. **Fluvoxamine** increases the exposure to tizanidine by a mean of 33-fold, which, broadly speaking, changes a 2 mg dose into a 66 mg dose, which is far higher than the maximum recommended dose. For this reason, the authors of one of the studies conclude that the combination is potentially hazardous and should be avoided,[3] and the manufacturers contraindicate the combination.[6,7] Given the available data this is sensible advice. Note that other **SSRIs** are generally not considered to inhibit CYP1A2, see 'Theophylline + SSRIs', p.1459, and might therefore be suitable alternatives to fluvoxamine.

For **ciprofloxacin**, there is a marked tenfold increase in exposure to tizanidine, with a consequent increase in adverse effects. Some authors recommend caution if both drugs are necessary,[1] whereas others suggest that this combination should be avoided.[2] The manufacturers contraindicate the combination.[6,7] If ciprofloxacin is considered the most appropriate antibacterial to use in a patient already taking tizanidine, anticipate the need to reduce the tizanidine dose before starting ciprofloxacin, and closely monitor adverse effects: starting ciprofloxacin could cause marked hypotension, bradycardia, and sedation. Note that the manufacturers also recommend that the use of tizanidine with **enoxacin** and **norfloxacin** should generally be avoided, or undertaken with caution. However, note that enoxacin is usually considered a more potent inhibitor of CYP1A2 than ciprofloxacin, whereas norfloxacin only has modest effects on CYP1A2. Other quinolones can also inhibit CYP1A2, to varying degrees, see 'Table 34.4', p.1456.

For **combined hormonal contraceptives**, the increase in exposure to tizanidine is a more moderate fourfold. The manufacturer states that a clinical response or adverse effects might occur at lower doses of tizanidine in patients taking oral contraceptives,[6] and that during dose titration, individual doses should be reduced. Care is needed.[7] Similar precautions seem warranted with **mexiletine**.

In addition, the manufacturers also recommend that the use of tizanidine with other inhibitors of CYP1A2 should generally be avoided, or used with caution, and they specifically mention **aciclovir**, **amiodarone**, **cimetidine**, **famotidine**, **propafenone**, **ticlopidine**, **verapamil** and **zileuton**.[6,7] However, note that some of these drugs have not been shown to have clinically relevant effects on this isoenzyme. For a list of clinically relevant CYP1A2 inhibitors, see 'Table 1.2', p.5.

1. Granfors MT, Backman JT, Neuvonen M, Neuvonen PJ. Ciprofloxacin greatly increases concentrations and hypotensive effect of tizanidine by inhibiting its cytochrome P450 1A2-mediated presystemic metabolism. *Clin Pharmacol Ther* (2004) 76, 598–606.
2. Momo K, Homma M, Kohda Y, Ohkoshi N, Yoshizawa T, Tamaoka A. Drug interaction of tizanidine and ciprofloxacin: case report. *Clin Pharmacol Ther* (2006) 80, 717–9.
3. Granfors MT, Backman JT, Neuvonen M, Ahonen J, Neuvonen PJ. Fluvoxamine drastically increases concentrations and effects of tizanidine: a potentially hazardous interaction. *Clin Pharmacol Ther* (2004) 75, 331–41.
4. Momo K, Doki K, Hosono H, Homma M, Kohda Y. Drug interaction of tizanidine and fluvoxamine. *Clin Pharmacol Ther* (2004) 76, 509–10.
5. Granfors MT, Backman JT, Laitila J, Neuvonen PJ. Oral contraceptives containing ethinyl estradiol and gestodene markedly increase plasma concentrations and effects of tizanidine by inhibiting cytochrome P450 1A2. *Clin Pharmacol Ther* (2005) 78, 400–11.
6. Zanaflex (Tizanidine hydrochloride). Cephalon Ltd. UK Summary of product characteristics, April 2010.
7. Zanaflex (Tizanidine hydrochloride). Acorda Therapeutics, Inc. US Prescribing information, April 2008.
8. Momo K, Homma M, Osaka Y, Inomata S, Tanaka M, Kohada Y. Effects of mexiletine, a CYP1A2 inhibitor, on tizanidine pharmacokinetics and pharmacodynamics. *J Clin Pharmacol* (2010) 50, 331–7.

Tizanidine + Food

Food has a minor effect on tizanidine pharmacokinetics: it increases the maximum concentration and AUC of tizanidine tablets, but decreases the maximum concentration and increases the AUC of tizanidine capsules. Giving the capsule contents with apple sauce resulted in a minor increase in the AUC and the maximum plasma concentrations of tizanidine.

Clinical evidence

In a single-dose, randomised, crossover study in 81 healthy subjects, the absorption of tizanidine *capsules* was equivalent to that of *tablets* in fasted subjects. When the *tablets* were taken with food, the mean maximum concentration of tizanidine was increased by about 25%, and the median time to peak plasma concentration increased from about one hour to one hour and 25 minutes, and the extent of absorption was increased by about 30%. Conversely, when the *capsules* were taken with food, the maximum concentration of tizanidine decreased by about 15%, the median time to peak plasma concentration increased from one hour to 3 hours, and the extent of absorption increased by just 10%.[1] Similar findings were reported in another smaller study.[2]

In a randomised, crossover study, 27 healthy subjects were given tizanidine 6 mg *capsules* swallowed whole in a fasted state or with the contents mixed with 30 mL of apple sauce. Giving the capsule contents in apple sauce resulted in a 14% and 17%

increase in the tizanidine AUC and the maximum plasma concentration, respectively, when compared with giving an intact capsule while fasting.[3]

Mechanism

Not known.

Importance and management

Tizanidine tablets appear to be bioequivalent to tizanidine capsules when taken *without* food. The effect of food on tizanidine appears to be complex and differs between the tablet and capsule formulations, which do not appear to be bioequivalent when taken *with* food. The available data suggest that giving tizanidine capsules or tablets with food delays the onset of effects and slightly increases the bioavailability, whereas food causes a small increase in the maximum tizanidine concentration from tablets and a small decrease in the maximum tizanidine concentration from capsules. However, these small differences seem unlikely to be generally clinically relevant. Nevertheless, the US manufacturer states that the differences between fed and fasted state and between the formulations might alter the onset of effect and the risk of adverse effects. They advise caution when switching from one formulation to another and recommend that patients should be advised to take their formulation in a consistent manner in relation to timing of food. In addition, they state that care is required if switching from taking the capsule intact to mixing its contents with apple sauce.[4]

1. Shah J, Wesnes KA, Kovelesky RA, Henney HR. Effects of food on the single-dose pharmacokinetics/pharmacodynamics of tizanidine capsules and tablets in healthy volunteers. *Clin Ther* (2006) 28, 1308–17.
2. Henney HR, Shah J. Relative bioavailability of tizanidine 4-mg capsule and tablet formulations after a standardized high-fat meal: a single-dose, randomized, open-label, crossover study in healthy subjects. *Clin Ther* (2007) 29, 661–9.
3. Henney HR, Fitzpatrick A, Stewart J, Runyan JD. Relative bioavailability of tizanidine hydrochloride capsule formulation compared with capsule contents administered in applesauce: a single-dose, open-label, randomized, two-way, crossover study in fasted healthy adult subjects. *Clin Ther* (2008) 30, 2263–71.
4. Zanaflex (Tizanidine hydrochloride). Acorda Therapeutics, Inc. US Prescribing information, April 2008.

Tizanidine + Miscellaneous

The sedative effects of tizanidine and other sedative drugs and alcohol are additive. Increased bradycardia might occur if digoxin is given with tizanidine. No interaction occurs with paracetamol (acetaminophen).

Clinical evidence, mechanism, importance and management

(a) CNS depressants

One of the most common adverse effects of tizanidine is somnolence or drowsiness (occurring in up to 50% of patients[1]) for which reason the manufacturers warn about the possibility of increased sedation with other **sedative drugs**, and **alcohol**.[2,3] In addition to additive sedative effects, **alcohol** increased the AUC of tizanidine by about 20% and increased its maximum concentration by 15%, which was associated with an increase in the adverse effects of tizanidine.[3] Patients should be warned that concurrent use might increase drowsiness, and be advised to avoid driving and related skilled tasks if affected.

(b) Digoxin

Tizanidine alone can cause bradycardia.[2,3] The UK manufacturer predicts that the concurrent use of digoxin might potentiate bradycardia and therefore advises caution if both drugs are given.[2]

(c) Paracetamol (Acetaminophen)

A review briefly mentions that, in a single-dose study in 20 healthy subjects, no clinically relevant interaction occurred between 650 mg of paracetamol and 4 mg of tizanidine.[1]

1. Wagstaff AJ, Bryson HM. Tizanidine. A review of its pharmacology, clinical efficacy and tolerability in the management of spasticity associated with cerebral and spinal disorders. *Drugs* (1997) 53, 435–52.
2. Zanaflex (Tizanidine hydrochloride). Cephalon Ltd. UK Summary of product characteristics, April 2010.
3. Zanaflex (Tizanidine hydrochloride). Acorda Therapeutics, Inc. US Prescribing information, April 2008.

Tizanidine + NSAIDs

Celecoxib and tolfenamic acid do not appear to affect the pharmacokinetics or pharmacodynamics of tizanidine. Rofecoxib (now withdrawn) caused a very marked increase in the exposure to tizanidine.

Clinical evidence

(a) Celecoxib

In a placebo-controlled, crossover study in 12 healthy subjects, celecoxib 200 mg twice daily for 4 days had no effect on the pharmacokinetics of a single 2-mg dose of tizanidine given on the morning of day 4. Also, the pharmacodynamic effects of tizanidine were not altered by celecoxib.[1]

(b) Rofecoxib

In a placebo-controlled, crossover study in 9 healthy subjects, rofecoxib 25 mg daily for 4 days very markedly increased the AUC of a single 4-mg dose of tizanidine 13.6-fold and increased the maximum level 6.1-fold. The hypotensive and sedative effects of tizanidine were also increased by rofecoxib. There was no evidence of QT prolongation in this study.[2]

A case report describes an otherwise healthy 59-year-old woman, who developed sinus bradycardia (30 bpm) with chest pain and acute right heart failure while taking tizanidine, diclofenac and rofecoxib. This resolved promptly after stopping the medication.[3]

(c) Tolfenamic acid

In a placebo-controlled, crossover study in 10 healthy subjects, tolfenamic acid 200 mg three times daily for 3 days had no effect on the pharmacokinetics of a single 4-mg dose of tizanidine given on day 3. The only change was a slight 13% decrease in the plasma levels of the secondary metabolite of tizanidine, M4. The pharmacodynamic effects of tizanidine were not altered by tolfenamic acid.[4]

Mechanism

Tizanidine is a substrate of CYP1A2, and undergoes substantial presystemic metabolism by this isoenzyme. Rofecoxib, an inhibitor of CYP1A2, decreases both the presystemic metabolism of tizanidine, and its elimination phase.[5] Despite *in vitro* evidence of CYP1A2 inhibition,[1,4] neither celecoxib nor tolfenamic acid appear to alter the pharmacokinetics of tizanidine *in vivo*.

Importance and management

The pharmacokinetic interaction of rofecoxib with tizanidine is well established, and the combination should be avoided. However, note that rofecoxib was generally withdrawn worldwide in 2004 because of its cardiovascular adverse effects, but the interaction is included here for completeness.

Neither celecoxib nor tolfenamic acid interact with tizanidine, so no particular precautions are required if these NSAIDs are given to patients taking tizanidine.

1. Karjalainen MJ, Neuvonen PJ, Backman JT. Celecoxib is a CYP1A2 inhibitor in vitro but not in vivo. *Eur J Clin Pharmacol* (2008) 64, 511–19.
2. Backman JT, Karjalainen MJ, Neuvonen M, Laitila J, Neuvonen PJ. Rofecoxib is a potent inhibitor of cytochrome P450 1A2: studies with tizanidine and caffeine in healthy subjects. *Br J Clin Pharmacol* (2006) 62, 345–57.
3. Kick A, Bertoli R, Moschovitis G, Caduff Janosa P, Cerny A. Extreme Sinusbradykardie (30/min) mit akuter Rechtsherzbelastung unter Tizanidin (Sirdalud®): Mögliche Arzneimittelinteraktion mit rofecoxib (Vioxx®). *Med Klin* (2005) 100, 213–16.
4. Karjalainen MJ, Neuvonen PJ, Backman JT. Tolfenamic acid is a potent CYP1A2 inhibitor in vitro but does not interact in vivo: correction for protein binding is needed for data interpretation. *Eur J Clin Pharmacol* (2007) 63, 829–36.
5. Karjalainen MJ, Neuvonen PJ, Backman JT. Rofecoxib is a potent, metabolism-dependent inhibitor of CYP1A2: implications for in vitro prediction of drug interactions. *Drug Metab Dispos* (2006) 34, 2091–6.

Tizanidine + Rifampicin (Rifampin)

Rifampicin moderately decreases tizanidine exposure.

Clinical evidence, mechanism, importance and management

In a placebo-controlled, crossover study in 10 healthy subjects, pre-treatment with rifampicin 600 mg daily for 5 days moderately reduced the AUC and peak level of a single 4-mg dose of tizanidine given on day 6 by 54% and 51%, respectively, without altering its half-life. In addition, rifampicin attenuated the reduction in blood pressure seen with tizanidine (10/9 mmHg with rifampicin and 17/13 mmHg with placebo).[1]

Rifampicin appears to be only a weak to moderate inducer of CYP1A2, by which tizanidine is extensively metabolised.[1]

Although rifampicin moderately reduces tizanidine exposure, the clinical relevance of this is unclear. However, bearing in mind that the dose of tizanidine is titrated according to response, this interaction seems unlikely to be clinically important. Note that a small increase in dose might be required if rifampicin is given to those taking established doses of tizanidine.

1. Backman JT, Granfors MT, Neuvonen PJ. Rifampicin is only a weak inducer of CYP1A2-mediated presystemic and systemic metabolism: studies with tizanidine and caffeine. *Eur J Clin Pharmacol* (2006) 62, 451–61.

Trientine + Miscellaneous

Trientine can possibly chelate with iron thereby reducing its absorption. On theoretical grounds a similar chelation interaction may occur with calcium, magnesium or zinc compounds, and mineral supplements.

Clinical evidence, mechanism, importance and management

(a) Iron compounds

Trientine is a copper-chelating agent used for Wilson's disease. One of the adverse effects of trientine is that it can cause iron deficiency, probably because it chelates with iron in the gut and thereby reduces its absorption. It is usual to resolve this iron deficiency, where necessary, by giving an iron supplement. The manufacturers suggest that the iron supplement should be given at a different time of the day from trientine to minimise their admixture in the gut.[1,2] A separation of at least 2 hours is recommended.[2]

(b) Other mineral supplements and antacids

Trientine may be inactivated by binding with metallic ions in the gastrointestinal tract. The UK manufacturer states that there is no evidence that **calcium** or **magnesium antacids** alter the efficacy of trientine, but it is good practice to separate their administration.[1] In fact, a study reported by the manufacturer of a **zinc** compound found that, in patients with Wilson's disease taking **zinc** 50 mg three times daily and trientine 250 mg four times daily resulted in only a mild interaction, which only produced slight alterations in copper excretion.[3] Nevertheless, the US manufacturer states that, in general, mineral supplements should not be given with trientine. They say that it is important that trientine is taken at least one hour before or after any other drug or **milk**, and at least one hour before or 2 hours after meals.[2]

1. Trientine dihydrochloride. Univar Ltd. UK Summary of product characteristics, July 2003.
2. Syprine (Trientine hydrochloride). Merck & Co., Inc. US Prescribing information, May 2007.
3. Wilzin (Zinc acetate dihydrate). Orphan Europe (UK) Ltd. UK Summary of product characteristics, October 2004.

Uricosuric drugs + Aspirin or other Salicylates

The uricosuric effects of high doses of aspirin or other salicylates and uricosuric drugs such as benzbromarone, probenecid and sulfinpyrazone are not additive as might be expected but are mutually antagonistic. Low-dose, enteric-coated aspirin appears not to interact with probenecid.

Clinical evidence

(a) Benzbromarone

In a study in 6 subjects with gout,[1] a single 160-mg dose of benzbromarone increased the percent ratio of urate to creatinine clearance by 371% at its peak (i.e. benzbromarone increases urate clearance). However, when the same dose of benzbromarone was given with a single 600-mg dose of aspirin, the peak ratio of urate to creatinine clearance with benzbromarone 160 mg was reduced by about 75% (i.e. aspirin reduces the effect of benzbromarone on urate clearance). In another study aspirin, in divided doses of 650 mg, up to a total of 5.2 g daily, was given to 29 healthy subjects taking benzbromarone 40 to 80 mg daily. The urate lowering effects of benzbromarone were most affected by aspirin 2.7 g; benzbromarone reduced the urate levels by 60%, but in the presence of aspirin 2.7 g the levels were only reduced by 48%.[2]

(b) Probenecid

A study found that the average urinary uric acid excretion in 24 hours was 673 mg with a single 3-g daily dose of probenecid, 909 mg with a 6-g daily dose of **sodium salicylate**, but only 114 mg when both drugs were given.[3] Similar antagonism has been seen in other studies in patients given aspirin 2.6 to 5.2 g daily.[4-6] No antagonism is seen until serum salicylate levels of 50 to 100 mg/L are reached.[6] Therefore no interaction would be expected with low, antiplatelet-dose aspirin. This was confirmed by a crossover study in 11 patients with gouty arthritis, regularly taking probenecid, which found that enteric-coated aspirin 325 mg daily, taken either with probenecid or 6 hours after probenecid, had no effect on serum urate levels or on the 24-hour urate excretion.[7]

(c) Sulfinpyrazone

When **sodium salicylate** 6 g was given with sulfinpyrazone 600 mg daily to one patient the average urinary uric acid excretion in 24 hours was 30 mg, whereas when each drug was used alone in the same doses the average 24-hour urinary excretion was 281 mg for **sodium salicylate** and 527 mg for sulfinpyrazone.[3] A later study in 5 men with gout, given sulfinpyrazone for about an hour (300 mg bolus followed by a 10 mg/minute infusion), found that the addition of **sodium salicylate** (3 g bolus followed by a 10 to 20 mg/minute infusion) virtually abolished uricosuria. When the drugs were given in the reverse order to 3 other patients the same result was seen.[8]

In another study, the uricosuria caused by sulfinpyrazone 400 mg daily was found to be completely abolished by aspirin 3.5 g.[9] In 5 healthy subjects the clearance of a single 400-mg dose of sulfinpyrazone was modestly increased by 12 to 27% by four doses of aspirin 325 mg, given over 24 hours.[10]

Mechanism

Not fully understood. Uricosuric drugs compete successfully with salicylate for secretion by the kidney tubules so that salicylate excretion is reduced, but the salicylate blocks the inhibitory effect of uricosuric drugs on the tubular reabsorption of uric acid causing the uric acid to accumulate within the body.[8]

Importance and management

Well established and clinically important interactions. Regular administration of anti-inflammatory doses of aspirin and other salicylates antagonises the effects of uricosuric drugs such as benzbromarone, probenecid, and sulfinpyrazone, and should generally be avoided in those with hyperuricaemia or gout. Serum salicylate levels of 50 to 100 mg/L are necessary before this interaction occurs. Doses of aspirin as low as 700 mg can cause an appreciable fall in uric acid excretion,[9] but the effects of an occasional small dose are probably of little practical importance. Low-dose aspirin (325 mg or less daily) does not seem to interact.

Note that sulfinpyrazone can cause gastric bleeding and inhibit platelet aggregation; effects that might be additive with those of aspirin.

1. Sinclair DS, Fox IH. The pharmacology of hypouricemic effect of benzbromarone. *J Rheumatol* (1975) 2, 437–45.
2. Sorensen LB, Levinson DJ. Clinical evaluation of benzbromarone. *Arthritis Rheum* (1976) 19, 183–90.
3. Seegmiller JE, Grayzel AI. Use of the newer uricosuric agents in the management of gout. *JAMA* (1960) 173, 1076–80.
4. Pascale LR, Dubin A, Hoffman WS. Therapeutic value of probenecid (Benemid®) in gout. *JAMA* (1952) 149, 1188–94.
5. Gutman AB, Yü TF. Benemid (*p*-di-*n*-propylsulfamyl-benzoic acid) as uricosuric agent in chronic gouty arthritis. *Trans Assoc Am Physicians* (1951) 64, 279–88.
6. Pascale LR, Dubin A, Bronsky D, Hoffman WS. Inhibition of the uricosuric action of Benemid by salicylate. *J Lab Clin Med* (1955) 45, 771–7.
7. Harris M, Bryant LR, Danaher P, Alloway J. Effect of low dose daily aspirin on serum urate levels and urinary excretion in patients receiving probenecid for gouty arthritis. *J Rheumatol* (2000) 27, 2873–6.
8. Yu TF, Dayton PG, Gutman AB. Mutual suppression of the uricosuric effects of sulfinpyrazone and salicylate: a study in interactions between drugs. *J Clin Invest* (1963) 42, 1330–9.
9. Kersley GD, Cook ER, Tovey DCJ. Value of uricosuric agents and in particular of G.28 315 in gout. *Ann Rheum Dis* (1958) 17, 326–33.
10. Buchanan MR, Endrenyi L, Giles AR, Rosenfeld J. The effect of aspirin on the pharmacokinetics of sulfinpyrazone in man. *Thromb Res* (1983) (Suppl 4), 145–52.

Vaccines + Chloroquine and related drugs

Chloroquine reduces the antibody response to live oral cholera vaccine and to intradermal human diploid rabies vaccine. Hydroxychloroquine might also reduce the antibody response to intradermal human diploid rabies vaccine. Chloroquine does not appear to alter the antibody response to tetanus, diphtheria, measles, poliomyelitis, oral typhoid (live), or BCG vaccines.

Clinical evidence, mechanism, importance and management

(a) Cholera vaccine

A study in healthy subjects found that chloroquine reduced the vibriocidal antibody titre of *Vibrio cholerae* CVD103-HgR live oral vaccine in the 30 subjects who received both treatments. The seroconversion rate fell from 91% in subjects who received the live oral cholera vaccine alone to 67% in those who were also given two doses of chloroquine diphosphate 250 mg, 7 days apart. It was suggested that concurrent use should be avoided, and chloroquine prophylaxis started no sooner than 8 days after vaccination.[1]

(b) Rabies vaccine

In a study, 51 healthy subjects were given intradermal rabies vaccine 0.1 mL on days 0, 7, and 28. Of these subjects, 26 were also given chloroquine base 300 mg weekly, starting 9 days before the first dose of vaccine until day 48. The other 25 subjects not given chloroquine served as controls. The mean neutralising antibody titre for the chloroquine group was significantly lower than that for the control group on days 28, 49, and 105. The results indicate that chloroquine, in the doses used for malaria prophylaxis, can reduce the antibody response to primary immunisation with intradermal human diploid rabies vaccine.[2] Another study similarly found that chloroquine prophylaxis was associated with poor antibody response to this vaccine.[3] One manufacturer of chloroquine advises against the use of pre-exposure intradermal human diploid rabies vaccine in patients taking chloroquine prophylaxis. When vaccinating against rabies with this vaccine, they recommend giving the vaccine before starting chloroquine, to avoid reducing the effectiveness of the vaccine.[4]

The manufacturers of **hydroxychloroquine** note that it might also reduce the antibody response to primary immunisation with intradermal human diploid rabies vaccine.[5]

(c) Typhoid vaccine

A study in healthy subjects investigated the use of chloroquine with a combination of cholera and *oral* typhoid vaccine (Ty21a vaccine strain). Cholera and typhoid vaccines had previously been shown not to affect each other, and the addition of chloroquine did not significantly reduce the serum antibody response to these vaccines. The authors therefore concluded that chloroquine could be given at the same time as *oral* typhoid vaccine without reducing its efficacy.[1] Similarly, a study (unpublished) suggests that the use of chloroquine with pyrimethamine and sulfadoxine did not alter the immune response to oral typhoid vaccine.[6]

(d) Yellow fever vaccine

A study in 50 healthy subjects found chloroquine phosphate 500 mg, given weekly for 4 weeks, did not affect the antibody titre of a single dose of yellow fever 17D vaccine.[7] Another study also reported that chloroquine does not adversely affect the antibody response to yellow fever vaccine.[8]

(e) Other vaccines

Chloroquine has does not appear to alter the immune response to tetanus, diphtheria, measles, oral poliomyelitis, or BCG vaccines.[6,9,10]

1. Kollaritsch H, Que JU, Kunz C, Wiedermann G, Herzog C, Cryz SJ. Safety and immunogenicity of live oral cholera and typhoid vaccines administered alone or in combination with antimalarial drugs, oral polio vaccine, or yellow fever vaccine. *J Infect Dis* (1997) 175, 871–5.
2. Pappaioanou M, Fishbein DB, Dreesen DW, Schwartz IK, Campbell GH, Sumner JW, Patchen LC, Brown WJ. Antibody response to preexposure human diploid-cell rabies vaccine given concurrently with chloroquine. *N Engl J Med* (1986) 314, 280–4.
3. Taylor DN, Wasi C, Bernard K. Chloroquine prophylaxis associated with a poor antibody response to human diploid cell rabies vaccine. *Lancet* (1984) i, 1405.
4. Avloclor (Chloroquine phosphate). AstraZeneca UK Ltd. UK Summary of product characteristics, July 2010.
5. Plaquenil (Hydroxychloroquine sulfate). Sanofi-Aventis. UK Summary of product characteristics, July 2010.
6. Wolfe MS, Precautions with oral live typhoid (Ty 21a) vaccine. *Lancet* (1990) 336, 631–2.
7. Barry M, Patterson JE, Tirrell S, Cullen MR, Shope RE. The effect of chloroquine prophylaxis on yellow fever vaccine antibody response: comparison of plaque reduction neutralization test and enzyme-linked immunosorbent assay. *Am J Trop Med Hyg* (1991) 44, 79–82.
8. Tsai TF, Bolin RA, Lazuick JS, Miller KD. Chloroquine does not adversely affect the antibody response to yellow fever vaccine. *J Infect Dis* (1986) 154, 726–7.
9. Greenwood BM. Chloroquine prophylaxis and antibody response to immunisation. *Lancet* (1984) ii, 402–3.
10. Bradley-Moore AM, Greenwood BM, Bradley AK, Bartlett A, Bidwell DE, Voller A, Craske J, Kirkwood BR, Gilles HM. Malaria chemoprophylaxis with chloroquine in young Nigerian children. II. Effect on the immune response to vaccination. *Ann Trop Med Parasitol* (1985) 79, 563–73.

Vaccines + Proguanil

Proguanil, but not proguanil with atovaquone, appears to reduce the effectiveness of live oral typhoid vaccine. Note that the capsular polysaccharide typhoid vaccine for injection would not be affected. Atovaquone with proguanil did not alter the efficacy of cholera vaccine.

Clinical evidence, mechanism, importance and management

(a) Cholera vaccine

In a placebo-controlled study, 330 children were given a cholera vaccine (*Vibrio cholerae* CVD103-HgR) 3 weeks after starting a 12-week course of atovaquone with proguanil (for malaria prophylaxis) or placebo. Atovaquone with proguanil was found to be effective and did not alter the immunogenicity of the cholera vaccine.[1]

(b) Typhoid vaccine

In a study in 30 healthy subjects, the anti-*Salmonella typhi* lipopolysaccharide antibody response was reduced when proguanil was given both with, and 7 days after, oral typhoid vaccine (live attenuated *S. typhi* Ty21a strain).[2]

In a placebo-controlled study, 330 children were given an oral typhoid vaccine (live attenuated *S typhi* Ty21a strain) 3 weeks after starting a 12-week course of atovaquone with proguanil (for malaria prophylaxis) or placebo. Atovaquone with proguanil was found to be effective and did not alter the immunogenicity of the oral typhoid vaccine.[1]

The WHO has stated that proguanil should be stopped from 3 days before until 3 days after receiving live oral typhoid vaccine (Ty21a strain).[3] The UK manufacturers similarly recommend an interval of at least 3 days between the last dose of live oral typhoid vaccine (Ty21a strain) and the first dose of antimalarial prophylaxis. However, they also state that malaria prophylaxis with the fixed dose combination of atovaquone and proguanil may be given concurrently with the vaccine.[4] The US manufacturer says that proguanil should only be given if 10 days or more have elapsed since the final dose of live oral typhoid vaccine.[5] Note that this advice does not apply to the capsular polysaccharide typhoid vaccine for injection, because this does not contain live organisms.

1. Faucher J-F, Binder R, Missinou MA, Matsiegui P-B, Gruss H, Neubauer R, Lell B, Que JU, Miller GB, Kremsner PG. Efficacy of atovaquone/proguanil for malaria prophylaxis in children and its effect on the immunogenicity of live oral typhoid and cholera vaccines. *Clin Infect Dis* (2002) 35, 1147–54.
2. Kollaritsch H, Que JU, Kunz C, Wiedermann G, Herzog C, Cryz SJ. Safety and immunogenicity of live oral cholera and typhoid vaccines administered alone or in combination with antimalarial drugs, oral polio vaccine, or yellow fever vaccine. *J Infect Dis* (1997) 175, 871–5.
3. WHO. International Travel and Health; Vaccine-preventable diseases and vaccines. Geneva: WHO, 2012. Available at: http://www.who.int/ihr/publications/ith/en/ (accessed 21/10/15).
4. Vivotif (Oral typhoid vaccine). Masta Ltd. UK Summary of product characteristics, March 2005.
5. Vivotif (Typhoid vaccine live oral Ty21a). Berna Products. US Prescribing information, August 2006.

Vaccines; Cholera + Vaccines; Yellow fever

The efficacy of cholera and yellow fever vaccines do not appear to be affected by concurrent administration.

Clinical evidence, mechanism, importance and management

A study in healthy subjects found that yellow fever vaccine did not affect the vibriocidal antibody titre of *Vibrio cholerae* CVD103-HgR live oral vaccine, when both vaccines were given at the same time.[1] Another retrospective study of subjects who had been given cholera vaccine alone or with yellow fever vaccine found that the rates of seroconversion and antibody titres after yellow fever vaccine was not affected by concurrent administration.[2]

1. Kollaritsch H, Que JU, Kunz C, Wiedermann G, Herzog C, Cryz SJ. Safety and immunogenicity of live oral cholera and typhoid vaccines administered alone or in combination with antimalarial drugs, oral polio vaccine, or yellow fever vaccine. *J Infect Dis* (1997) 175, 871–5.
2. Poveda J-D, Raccurt CP, Le Fur R, M'Bailara L, Malvy JMD, Le Bras M, Saliou P, Fleury HJA. L'effet inhibiteur de la vaccination anticholérique simultanée ou rapprochée sur l'immunisation contre la fièvre jaune est-il réel ou supposé? Résultats d'une étude rétrospective. *Bull Soc Pathol Exot Filiales* (1990) 83, 529–35.

Vaccines; Typhoid + Antibacterials

Live oral typhoid vaccine should not be given to patients taking antibacterials, or within three days of their use. Note that this advice does not apply to the capsular polysaccharide typhoid vaccine for injection.

Clinical evidence, mechanism, importance and management

The manufacturer notes that sulfonamides and antibacterials may be active against the vaccine organism (live attenuated *Salmonella typhi,* Ty21a strain), and could therefore prevent multiplication and reduce the immune response achieved.[1,2] Note that this has been shown with some antimalarials such as proguanil, see 'Vaccines + Proguanil', above.

It would be prudent to avoid the concurrent use of antibacterials and the live oral typhoid vaccine. The WHO recommends that antibacterial drugs should be stopped from 3 days before to 3 days after receiving live oral typhoid vaccine (Ty21a strain).[3] Similarly, the UK manufacturers and Department of Health recommend that vaccination with live oral typhoid vaccine should not start within 3 days of completing treatment with antibacterials, nor should antibacterials be given within 3 days of receiving the last dose of vaccine.[1,4]

These precautions do not apply to the capsular polysaccharide typhoid vaccine for parenteral use, because this does not contain live organisms.

1. Vivotif (Oral typhoid vaccine). Masta Ltd. UK Summary of product characteristics, March 2005.
2. Vivotif (Typhoid vaccine live oral Ty21a). Berna Products. US Prescribing information, August 2006.
3. WHO. International travel and health; Vaccine-preventable diseases and vaccines. Geneva: WHO, 2012. Available at: http://www.who.int/ith/en/ (accessed 21/10/15).
4. Department of Health. Immunisation Against Infectious Disease (updated 28th August 2015): "The Green Book". Available at: https://www.gov.uk/government/collections/immunisation-against-infectious-disease-the-green-book (accessed 21/10/15).

Vaccines; Typhoid + Mefloquine

Some sources suggest that mefloquine should not be given at the same time as oral attenuated live typhoid vaccine, whereas others suggest that concurrent administration is acceptable. Note that this advice does not apply to the capsular polysaccharide typhoid vaccine for injection.

Clinical evidence

An *in vitro* study found that mefloquine killed a significant amount of *S.typhi* (Ty21a vaccine strain), which suggested that concurrent administration could possibly reduce the efficacy of the vaccine.[1] A study in healthy subjects investigated the use of mefloquine with a combination of cholera and oral typhoid vaccine (Ty21a vaccine strain). Cholera and typhoid vaccines had previously been shown not to affect each other, and the addition of mefloquine did not significantly reduce the serum antibody response to these vaccines. The authors therefore concluded that mefloquine could be given at the same time as oral typhoid vaccine without reducing its efficacy.[2]

Mechanism

Oral typhoid vaccine requires active replication of the attenuated *Salmonella typhi* strain in the ileum for the development of immunity. Mefloquine is thought to have some antibacterial effect, which may diminish the amount of *S. typhi* present, and therefore reduce the immune response produced by the vaccine.[2,3]

Importance and Management

As mefloquine is rapidly absorbed it has been suggested that by 8 hours after a dose, the levels of mefloquine will be insufficient to inhibit live oral typhoid vaccine.[4] Based on the results of the above study the US manufacturers note that mefloquine can be given at the same time as oral typhoid vaccine.[2,5] The UK manufacturers of the oral typhoid vaccine recommend separating the dose of oral typhoid vaccine and mefloquine by at least 12 hours.[6] However, the manufacturers of mefloquine say that immunisation with vaccines such as oral typhoid should be completed at least 3 days before the first dose of mefloquine.[7,8] The UK Department of Health say that mefloquine can be given 12 hours before or after vaccination with oral typhoid vaccine.[9] It would therefore seem acceptable to separate administration by 12 hours. Note that this advice does not apply to the capsular polysaccharide typhoid vaccine for injection.

1. Horowitz H, Carbonaro CA. Inhibition of *Salmonella typhi* oral vaccine strain Ty21a, by mefloquine and chloroquine. *J Infect Dis* (1992) 166, 1462–4.
2. Kollaritsch H, Que JU, Kunz C, Wiedermann G, Herzog C, Cryz SJ. Safety and immunogenicity of live oral cholera and typhoid vaccines administered alone or in combination with antimalarial drugs, oral polio vaccine, or yellow fever vaccine. *J Infect Dis* (1997) 175, 871–5.
3. Brachman PS, Metchock B, Kozarsky PE. Effects of antimalarial chemoprophylactic agents on the viability of the Ty21a typhoid vaccine strain. *Clin Infect Dis* (1992) 15, 1057–8.
4. Cryz SJ. Post-marketing experience with live oral Ty21a vaccine. *Lancet* (1993) 341, 49–50.
5. Vivotif (Typhoid vaccine live oral Ty21a). Berna Products. US Prescribing information. August 2006.
6. Vivotif (Oral typhoid vaccine). Masta Ltd. UK Summary of product characteristics. March 2005.
7. Lariam (Mefloquine hydrochloride). Roche Products Ltd. UK Summary of product characteristics, November 2011.
8. Lariam (Mefloquine hydrochloride). Roche Pharmaceuticals. US Prescribing information, September 2008.
9. Department of Health. Immunisation Against Infectious Disease (updated 11th September 2013): "The Green Book". Available at: https://www.gov.uk/government/publications/green-book-the-complete-current-edition (accessed 25/09/13).

Varenicline + Amfetamines

The effectiveness of varenicline as a smoking-cessation aid was reduced in a patient taking amfetamine with dexamfetamine.

Clinical evidence

An 18-year-old man taking **amfetamine** with **dexamfetamine** (*Adderall*) 30 mg twice daily on work days for attention deficit hyperactivity disorder (ADHD) started taking varenicline 500 micrograms daily as an aid to smoking cessation. By day 2 he noted a reduced urge to smoke: he had not taken **amfetamine** with **dexamfetamine** for 3 days before starting varenicline. On day 4, he restarted the amfetamines, but at a reduced dose of 30 mg daily because of a diminishing supply, and the varenicline dose was increased to 500 micrograms twice daily. He stopped smoking on day 8, when the varenicline was increased to 1 mg twice daily. He subsequently obtained a new prescription for **amfetamine** with **dexamfetamine**, which he started on day 23 at his full dose of 30 mg *twice* daily, and within 24 hours he noticed that varenicline 1 mg twice daily was not working as effectively. Within 48 hours he started smoking again. Subsequently, on starting a second course of varenicline while taking **amfetamine** with **dexamfetamine** 30 mg twice daily, he stopped smoking for only one day.[1]

Mechanism

Varenicline reduces the rewarding effects of nicotine by preventing nicotine-induced stimulation of alpha$_4$/beta$_2$ nicotinic acetylcholine receptors and subsequent dopamine release. Amfetamine may decrease varenicline efficacy by increasing mesolimbic dopamine levels. It has been suggested that other drugs that increase dopamine levels may also reduce the efficacy of varenicline.[1]

Importance and management

Evidence for an interaction seems to be limited to this case report, the general relevance of which is unclear. However, the case does suggest that the use of amfetamines may diminish the efficacy of varenicline, which may make it a less desirable choice in patients taking amfetamines who wish to use varenicline as an aid to smoking cessation.

1. Whitley HP, Moorman KL. Interference with smoking-cessation effects of varenicline after administration of immediate-release amphetamine-dextroamphetamine. *Pharmacotherapy* (2007) 27, 1440–5.

Vasopressin antagonists + Diuretics; Loop, Thiazide and related

The concurrent use of tolvaptan and furosemide or hydrochlorothiazide does not appear to affect the pharmacokinetics or pharmacodynamics of either drug to a clinically relevant extent. Furosemide does not appear to alter the pharmacokinetics of conivaptan. However, the concurrent use of vasopressin antagonists and diuretics might increase the risk of dehydration and hypovolaemia.

Clinical evidence

(a) Conivaptan

The US manufacturer briefly reports that the pharmacokinetics of oral conivaptan 20 to 40 mg daily were not altered by **furosemide** up to 80 mg daily.[1]

(b) Tolvaptan

In a single-dose, randomised, crossover study in 6 healthy subjects given tolvaptan 30 mg, **furosemide** 80 mg or both drugs together, there were no differences in the pharmacokinetics of **furosemide**, but the AUC of tolvaptan was very slightly increased, by 24%.[2] However, there were no changes in the pharmacodynamics of either drug. In the same study, a further 6 healthy subjects were given tolvaptan 30 mg, **hydrochlorothiazide** 100 mg or both drugs together. There were no differences found in the pharmacokinetics or pharmacodynamics of either drug.[2] Furthermore, the concurrent use of tolvaptan and either **furosemide** or **hydrochlorothiazide** did not result in a greater 24-hour urinary volume than tolvaptan alone, suggesting that the diuretic effect of these drugs was not additive.[2]

Mechanism

Unknown.

Importance and management

The very slight increase in tolvaptan exposure caused by furosemide did not result in an increased diuretic effect. Therefore no clinically important pharmacokinetic interaction would be expected if vasopressin antagonists are given with loop diuretics, such as furosemide, or thiazide diuretics, such as hydrochlorothiazide. However, note that vasopressin antagonists induce copious and prolonged water loss which can result in dehydration and hypovolaemia, particularly in volume-depleted patients taking diuretics. For this reason, the US manufacturers state that caution is warranted on concurrent use.[3]

1. Vaprisol (Conivaptan hydrochloride). Astellas Pharma US, Inc. US Prescribing information, February 2011.
2. Shoaf SE, Bramer SL, Bricmont P, Zimmer CA. Pharmacokinetic and pharmacodynamic interaction between tolvaptan, a non-peptide AVP antagonist, and furosemide or hydrochlorothiazide. *J Cardiovasc Pharmacol* (2007) 50, 213–22.
3. Samsca (Tolvaptan). Otsuka America Pharmaceutical Inc. US Prescribing information, February 2012.

Vasopressin antagonists + Ketoconazole and other CYP3A4 inhibitors

Ketoconazole (a potent CYP3A4 inhibitor) moderately increases the exposure to tolvaptan and markedly increases the exposure to conivaptan. Other potent CYP3A4 inhibitors (such as clarithromycin and ritonavir) are likely to interact similarly. Grapefruit juice also increases the exposure to oral tolvaptan.

Clinical evidence

(a) Grapefruit juice

In a crossover study in 20 healthy subjects, 240 mL of grapefruit juice increased the maximum plasma concentration and AUC of a single 60-mg dose of **tolvaptan** by 86% and 56%, respectively. However, the increase in concentration was only seen at 16-hours post-dose, and the **tolvaptan** elimination half-life was unaffected. No increase in **tolvaptan** adverse effects was reported.[1]

(b) Ketoconazole

1. Tolvaptan. In a placebo-controlled study, 17 healthy subjects were given a single 30-mg dose of tolvaptan before and on day 2 of a 3-day course of ketoconazole 200 mg daily. Ketoconazole increased the AUC and maximum plasma concentration of tolvaptan 3.5-fold and 5.3-fold, respectively, although some patients had increases above 7-fold. Despite these changes, concurrent use only slightly increased urinary output, by about 30% over 24 hours, when compared with the placebo group. No ECG changes, or changes in vital signs or clinical laboratory measurements was reported, and no severe adverse effects occurred.[2]

2. Conivaptan. The US manufacturer of conivaptan reports that ketoconazole 200 mg increased the maximum plasma concentrations and AUC of oral conivaptan 10 mg 4-fold and 11-fold, respectively.[3]

Mechanism

Ketoconazole is a potent inhibitor of hepatic CYP3A4, the isoenzyme by which tolvaptan and conivaptan are predominantly metabolised. Concurrent use therefore decreases the metabolism of tolvaptan and conivaptan, and increases their exposure. However, the overall effect of increased tolvaptan exposure on the urinary excretion rate is less than expected for an increase in exposure of this magnitude, as this pathway becomes saturated. Grapefruit juice is also an inhibitor of CYP3A4 in the intestine.

Importance and management

Tolvaptan

The clinical relevance of the moderate increase in tolvaptan exposure with ketoconazole has not been directly assessed, but an increase in tolvaptan effects would be expected. The US manufacturer of tolvaptan contraindicates the concurrent use of ketoconazole and other potent CYP3A4 inhibitors, because there is no data to suggest a suitable dose adjustment for safe concurrent use. They specifically name **itraconazole**; the macrolides **clarithromycin** and **telithromycin**; the HIV-protease inhibitors **indinavir**, **nelfinavir**, **ritonavir**, and **saquinavir**, and **nefazodone**.[4] In addition, they also state that moderate CYP3A4 inhibitors, such as **aprepitant**, **diltiazem**, **erythromycin**, **fluconazole**, and **verapamil**, should generally be avoided.[4] In the UK, the manufacturer simply advises caution with any CYP3A4 inhibitor.[5] In addition, both the UK and US manufacturers state that the use of **grapefruit juice** should be avoided in patients taking tolvaptan.[4,5] If a CYP3A4 inhibitor is considered essential in a patient taking tolvaptan, monitor for an increase in adverse effects, such as dry mouth, thirst, and increased frequency of urination, and, ideally monitor fluid and electrolyte status. If possible, reduce the dose of tolvaptan, according to clinical response.

Conivaptan

The clinical relevance of the marked increase in conivaptan exposure with ketoconazole has not been directly assessed, but an increase in conivaptan effects would be expected. The US manufacturer of conivaptan[3] contraindicates the concurrent use of ketoconazole and other potent CYP3A inhibitors: they specifically name **clarithromycin**, **itraconazole**, and the HIV-protease inhibitors **indinavir** and **ritonavir**, which are, specifically CYP3A4 inhibitors. For a list of CYP3A4 inhibitors, see 'Table 1.9', p.11. If a CYP3A4 inhibitor is considered essential in a patient taking conivaptan, monitor for an increase in adverse effects, such as dry mouth, thirst, and increased frequency of urination, and, ideally monitor fluid and electrolyte status. If possible, reduce the dose of conivaptan, according to clinical response.

1. Shoaf SE, Mallikaarjun S, Bricmont P. Effect of grapefruit juice on the pharmacokinetics of tolvaptan, a non-peptide arginine vasopressin antagonist, in healthy subjects. *Eur J Clin Pharmacol* (2012) 68, 207–11.
2. Shoaf SE, Bricmont P, Mallikaarjun S. Effects of CYP3A4 inhibition and induction on the pharmacokinetics and pharmacodynamics of tolvaptan, a non-peptide AVP antagonist in healthy subjects. *Br J Clin Pharmacol* (2012) 73, 579–87.
3. Vaprisol (Conivaptan hydrochloride). Astellas Pharma US, Inc. US Prescribing information, February 2011.
4. Samsca (Tolvaptan). Otsuka America Pharmaceutical Inc. US Prescribing information, February 2012.
5. Samsca (Tolvaptan). Otsuka Pharmaceuticals (UK) Ltd. UK Summary of product characteristics, April 2012.

Vasopressin antagonists + Miscellaneous

The risk of hyperkalaemia with tolvaptan is increased by the concurrent use of drugs known to increase serum potassium concentrations, such as ACE inhibitors, angiotensin II receptor antagonists, and potassium-sparing diuretics. Conivaptan increases the exposure to amlodipine, midazolam, and simvastatin, and tolvaptan increases lovastatin levels, but lovastatin does not alter tolvaptan exposure. P-glycoprotein inhibitors, such as ciclosporin, are predicted to increase tolvaptan exposure. Captopril does not alter the pharmacokinetics of conivaptan. Tolvaptan and conivaptan do not alter the pharmacokinetics of warfarin to a clinically relevant extent.

Clinical evidence, mechanism, importance and management

(a) ACE inhibitors

The US manufacturer reports that **captopril** 25 mg did not alter the pharmacokinetics of **conivaptan** 20 to 40 mg daily.[1] For the effects of concurrent use on serum potassium concentrations see, *Potassium-sparing drugs*, below.

(b) Amlodipine

The US manufacturer states that oral **conivaptan** 40 mg twice daily doubled the AUC and half-life of amlodipine. They advise that the concurrent use of CYP3A substrates, which would include amlodipine, should be avoided for at least one week after **conivaptan** is given.[1]

(c) Midazolam

The US manufacturer notes that **conivaptan** 40 mg daily increased the AUC of intravenous midazolam 1 mg and oral midazolam 2 mg 2-fold and 3-fold, respectively. They advise that concurrent use of CYP3A substrates should be avoided for at least one week after **conivaptan** is given.[1]

Note that midazolam can be used as a probe substrate to assess the activity of drugs on CYP3A4. This study therefore suggests that conivaptan is a moderate inhibitor of CYP3A4. For a list of CYP3A4 substrates, see 'Table 1.10', p.12.

(d) P-glycoprotein inhibitors

The US manufacturer states that as **tolvaptan** is a substrate of P-glycoprotein. P-glycoprotein inhibitors would be expected to increase **tolvaptan** exposure: they name **ciclosporin**. They therefore advise that the dose of **tolvaptan** might need to be reduced if ciclosporin or other P-glycoprotein inhibitors are also given.[2] Until more is known, it would seem prudent to monitor concurrent use for an increase in **tolvaptan** adverse effects (such as dry mouth, thirst and increased frequency of urination), and adjust the tolvaptan dose if necessary. For a list of drugs that inhibit P-glycoprotein, see 'Table 1.12', p.14.

(e) Potassium-sparing drugs

Tolvaptan can increase serum potassium concentrations.[2,3] The US manufacturer notes that, in clinical studies, the incidence of hyperkalaemia was about 1 to 2% higher in patients who had taken tolvaptan with **ACE inhibitors**, **angiotensin II receptor antagonists** and **potassium-sparing diuretics** than when any of these drugs were given with placebo. They therefore recommend monitoring serum potassium concentration on the concurrent use of tolvaptan and any of these drugs.[2] On this basis, the same precautions would also seem prudent in patients taking **potassium supplements**.

(f) Statins

1. Lovastatin. Exposure to **tolvaptan** is not affected by lovastatin; however, **tolvaptan** increased the plasma concentration of lovastatin and its active metabolite by 40% and 30%, respectively.[2] This is because **tolvaptan** is a weak CYP3A4 inhibitor,[2] by which lovastatin is metabolised. The increase in lovastatin concentration is probably not clinically relevant.

2. Simvastatin. The manufacturer reports that **conivaptan** 30 mg daily increased the AUC of simvastatin 3-fold. They also note that two cases of rhabdomyolysis were reported during clinical studies in patients taking a concurrent statin metabolised by CYP3A4. Based on this, they advise that the concurrent use of CYP3A substrates, which would include simvastatin, should be avoided for at least one week after **conivaptan** is given.[1]

(g) Warfarin

The manufacturers briefly note that **tolvaptan** does not alter the pharmacokinetics of warfarin to a clinically relevant extent.[2,3] The US manufacturer reports that **conivaptan** 40 mg daily for 4 days increased the AUC and maximum plasma concentration of a single 25-mg dose of warfarin by 14% and 17%, respectively; however, the prothrombin times and INR were unaltered.[1] These small increases are unlikely to be clinically important. Therefore, no warfarin dose adjustment would be expected to be needed on the concurrent use of **tolvaptan** or **conivaptan**.

1. Vaprisol (Conivaptan hydrochloride). Astellas Pharma US, Inc. US Prescribing information, February 2011.
2. Samsca (Tolvaptan). Otsuka America Pharmaceutical Inc. US Prescribing information, February 2012.
3. Samsca (Tolvaptan). Otsuka Pharmaceuticals (UK) Ltd. UK Summary of product characteristics, April 2012.

Vasopressin antagonists + Rifampicin (Rifampin) and other CYP3A4 inducers

Rifampicin, a CYP3A4 inducer, markedly reduces the exposure to tolvaptan. Other CYP3A4 inducers (such as carbamazepine and phenytoin) might interact similarly. Conivaptan might also be similarly affected by CYP3A4 inducers.

Clinical evidence

In a study, 15 healthy subjects were given a single 240-mg dose of tolvaptan 2 days before and on day 7 of an 8-day course of rifampicin 600 mg daily. Rifampicin decreased the AUC and maximum plasma concentration of tolvaptan by 83% and 87%, respectively. Concurrent use had no initial effect on the urinary excretion rate and only reduced the mean daily urine volume by about 30% in the first 12 hours, despite the large reduction in tolvaptan exposure. At 24 hours post-dose, the urinary excretion rate and urine volume in response to tolvaptan were about halved in the subjects also given rifampicin, when compared with a placebo group given tolvaptan alone.[1] Note that the tolvaptan dose used in this study is four times the maximum licensed daily dose.

Mechanism

Rifampicin is a potent CYP3A4 inducer, by which tolvaptan is primarily metabolised. It would therefore appear that rifampicin induces the metabolism of tolvaptan, resulting in reduced plasma concentrations.

Importance and management

Although evidence for an interaction between **tolvaptan** and rifampicin is limited to one study, an interaction would appear to be established. The reduction in tolvaptan exposure seen with rifampicin reduces its effectiveness. The UK and US manufacturers predict that other CYP3A4 inducers are likely to interact similarly, and they name the **barbiturates**.[2,3] The US manufacturer of tolvaptan also names **carbamazepine**, **phenytoin** (and therefore also consider **fosphenytoin**), **rifabutin**, **rifapentine**, and **St John's wort**.[2] Because of the potency of the effect of rifampicin, the US manufacturer states that concurrent use should be avoided, or, if concurrent use is necessary, the dose of tolvaptan might need to be increased.[2] The UK manufacturer simply advises caution on concurrent use.[3] Therefore if tolvaptan is given with a CYP3A4 inducer, it would seem prudent to monitor the outcome of concurrent use, being alert for a reduction in tolvaptan efficacy, and increase the dose of tolvaptan as necessary. For a list of CYP3A4 inducers, see 'Table 1.9', p.11.

Note that **conivaptan** is also a substrate for CYP3A4 and *ketoconazole*, a potent CYP3A4 *inhibitor*, has been reported to markedly *increase* its exposure, see 'Vasopressin antagonists + Ketoconazole and other CYP3A4 inhibitors', p.1592. It would therefore seem possible that potent CYP3A4 inducers could decrease conivaptan exposure, although there does not appear to be any published data regarding such an effect. Nevertheless, until more is known, it would seem prudent to be aware of the possibility of a reduction in conivaptan efficacy if CYP3A4 inducers are also taken.

1. Shoaf SE, Bricmont P, Mallikaarjun S. Effects of CYP3A4 inhibition and induction on the pharmacokinetics and pharmacodynamics of tolvaptan, a non-peptide AVP antagonist in healthy subjects. *Br J Clin Pharmacol* (2012) 73, 579–87.
2. Samsca (Tolvaptan). Otsuka America Pharmaceutical Inc. US Prescribing information, February 2012.
3. Samsca (Tolvaptan). Otsuka Pharmaceuticals (UK) Ltd. UK Summary of product characteristics, April 2012.

Vasopressin antagonists; Tolvaptan + Food

Food does not affect the pharmacokinetics of tolvaptan

Clinical evidence, mechanism, importance and management

In a randomised, crossover study, 46 healthy subjects were given a single 30-mg dose of tolvaptan, either in the fasted state, or immediately after a high-fat meal or a Japanese standard meal. When compared with the fasted state, food had no clinically relevant effect on the pharmacokinetics of tolavaptan.[1] Therefore, tolvaptan can be taken without regard to meals.

1. Shoaf SE, Kim SR, Bricmont P, Mallikaarjun S. Pharmacokinetics and pharmacodynamics of single-dose oral tolvaptan in fasted and non-fasted states in healthy Caucasian and Japanese male subjects. *Eur J Clin Pharmacol* (2012) 68,1595–603.

Vinpocetine + Antacids

In a study in 18 healthy subjects, aluminium/magnesium hydroxide gel, one sachet four times daily, had no significant effect on the serum levels of vinpocetine 20 mg three times daily.[1] No special precautions seem necessary if these drugs are taken together.

1. Lohmann A, Grobara P, Dingler E. Investigation of the possible influence of the absorption of vinpocetine with concomitant application of magnesium-aluminium-hydroxide gel. *Arzneimittelforschung* (1991) 41, 1164–7.

39

Archived monographs

The monographs in this section include those drugs for which use has fallen into decline, usually as a result of their toxic adverse effects. These monographs are kept for completeness and are no longer systematically maintained, and have been moved to this section to distinguish them from the rest of the publication which is routinely, systematically, revised and updated.

9-Aminocamptothecin + Antiepileptics; Enzyme-inducing

Carbamazepine, phenobarbital, and phenytoin can lower the levels of 9-aminocamptothecin.

Clinical evidence, mechanism, importance and management

A study in 59 patients with glioblastoma multiforme or recurrent high grade astrocytomas found that the steady-state plasma levels of 9-aminocamptothecin were reduced to about one third in 29 of the patients also taking antiepileptics (**carbamazepine**, **phenobarbital**, **phenytoin**, sodium valproate). The incidence of myelosuppression was greater in those not taking antiepileptics.[1] A further study also found that the clearance of 9-aminocamptothecin was increased by **carbamazepine** and **phenytoin**.[2] The reason for the reduced 9-aminocamptothecin levels is not known, but it seems likely that it was due to the enzyme-inducing activity of **carbamazepine**, **phenobarbital** and **phenytoin**. These results suggest that higher than usual doses of 9-aminocamptothecin are possibly needed in the presence of these antiepileptics. **Fosphenytoin** and **primidone**, which are metabolised to phenytoin and phenobarbital, respectively, would be expected to interact similarly.

NOTE. The reader is cautioned that this monograph is included purely for archival purposes, and is no longer subject to systematic revision and update.

1. Grossman SA, Hochberg F, Fisher J, Chen T-L, Kim L, Gregory R, Grochow LB, Piantadosi S. Increased 9-aminocamptothecin dose requirements in patients on anticonvulsants. *Cancer Chemother Pharmacol* (1998) 42, 118–26.
2. Minami H, Lad TE, Nicholas MK, Vokes EE, Ratain MJ. Pharmacokinetics and pharmacodynamics of 9-aminocamptothecin infused over 72 hours in phase II studies. *Clin Cancer Res* (1999) 5, 1325–30.

Aminoglutethimide + Digoxin and related drugs

The clearance of digitoxin is markedly increased by aminoglutethimide.

Clinical evidence, mechanism, importance and management

The clearance of **digitoxin** was increased by a mean of 109% in 5 patients who took aminoglutethimide (250 mg four times a day in 4 patients, and 125 mg twice daily in one patient).[1,2] The likely reason for this effect is that aminoglutethimide increases the metabolism of **digitoxin** by the liver.

This increase in clearance would be expected to be clinically important, but this does not appear to have been assessed. Check that patients do not become under-digitalised during concurrent use. No interaction would be expected with **digoxin** because it is largely excreted unchanged in the urine and therefore metabolism by the liver has little part to play in its clearance.

NOTE. The reader is cautioned that this monograph is included purely for archival purposes, and is no longer subject to systematic revision and update.

1. Lønning PE, Kvinnsland S and Bakke OM. Effect of aminoglutethimide on antipyrine, theophylline and digitoxin disposition in breast cancer. *Clin Pharmacol Ther* (1984) 36, 796–802.
2. Lønning PE. Aminoglutethimide enzyme induction: pharmacological and endocrinological implications. *Cancer Chemother Pharmacol* (1990) 26, 241–4.

Aminoglutethimide + Medroxyprogesterone or Megestrol

Aminoglutethimide reduces the plasma levels of medroxyprogesterone and megestrol given orally. Intravenous medroxyprogesterone acetate does not appear to be affected.

Clinical evidence

(a) Medroxyprogesterone acetate

In a study in 6 postmenopausal women with breast cancer, aminoglutethimide 250 mg two to four times daily approximately halved the plasma levels of oral medroxyprogesterone acetate 500 mg three times daily.[1] Another study in postmenopausal women found that aminoglutethimide 250 mg four times daily reduced medroxyprogesterone levels by 63% after oral administration, but did not appear to affect its levels after intravenous administration.[2] In another study in 6 women with advanced breast cancer, it was found that as the dose of aminoglutethimide was gradually reduced from 250 mg twice daily and finally withdrawn, the plasma levels of oral medroxyprogesterone steadily climbed to three times the initial level, although the dose remained constant at a total of 800 mg daily.[3]

(b) Megestrol

In a study in 6 postmenopausal women, aminoglutethimide 250 mg four times daily reduced the serum levels of megestrol 160 mg daily by 78%.[2]

Mechanism

The most likely reason for this interaction is that aminoglutethimide acts as an enzyme inducer, increasing the metabolism of the progestogens, thereby decreasing their levels. When the aminoglutethimide is withdrawn, the enzyme induction ceases, and the progestogen level rises. The fact that the interaction did not appear to occur with intravenous administration suggests that aminoglutethimide might be principally affecting presystemic metabolism.

Importance and management

The interaction between aminoglutethimide and oral medroxyprogesterone or megestrol appears to be established and is possibly clinically important. A 50% reduction in the plasma levels of medroxyprogesterone and megestrol should be expected on the concurrent use of aminoglutethimide, and this may reduce the adrenal suppressive effect of these progestogens.[1] The authors of one report[3] state that to achieve adequate plasma medroxyprogesterone acetate levels in breast cancer (above 100 nanograms/mL) in the presence of aminoglutethimide 125 or 250 mg twice daily, a dose of medroxyprogesterone acetate 800 mg daily is probably necessary. This is double the usual recommended dose for this condition.

Note that limited data suggest that *intravenous* medroxyprogesterone does not appear to be affected by aminoglutethimide. It therefore seems unlikely that depot medroxyprogesterone acetate will be affected, although the UK manufacturer includes the possibility of the interaction in their product information.[4] However, if the mechanism for the aminoglutethimide interaction is correct (enzyme induction), this suggests that depot medroxyprogesterone would be unlikely to be affected, as there is no evidence that it interacts with enzyme inducers, see 'Progestogen-only contraceptives; Injections + Enzyme inducers', p.1199.

NOTE. The reader is cautioned that this monograph is included purely for archival purposes, and is no longer subject to systematic revision and update.

1. Van Deijk WA, Blijham GH, Mellink WAM, Meulenberg PMM. Influence of aminoglutethimide on plasma levels of medroxyprogesterone acetate: its correlation with serum cortisol. *Cancer Treat Rep* (1985) 69, 85–90.
2. Lundgren S, Lønning PE, Aakvaag A, Kvinnsland S. Influence of aminoglutethimide on the metabolism of medroxyprogesterone acetate and megestrol acetate in postmenopausal patients with advanced breast cancer. *Cancer Chemother Pharmacol* (1990) 27, 101–5.
3. Halpenny O, Bye A, Cranny A, Feely J, Daly PA. Influence of aminoglutethimide on plasma levels of medroxyprogesterone acetate. *Med Oncol Tumor Pharmacother* (1990) 7, 241–7.
4. Depo-Provera (Medroxyprogesterone acetate). Pfizer Ltd. UK Summary of product characteristics, September 2012.

Aminoglutethimide + Miscellaneous

Danazol may reduce the efficacy of aminoglutethimide. Aminoglutethimide markedly increases tamoxifen clearance and reduces its serum levels, whereas tamoxifen does not affect aminoglutethimide levels. A single case report describes hyponatraemia, which occurred after a patient had taken aminoglutethimide and bendroflumethiazide for 10 months.

Clinical evidence, mechanism, importance and management

(a) Danazol

In a randomised study, giving danazol with aminoglutethimide in women with breast cancer reduced the response rate compared with the use of aminoglutethimide alone. It was suggested that danazol suppresses sex hormone-binding globulin leading to increased free estradiol, which counteracts the estradiol suppressive effect of aminoglutethimide.[1] However, note that danazol is not usually considered to possess oestrogenic effects. Nevertheless, because of the serious therapeutic implications of such an interaction, danazol should probably not be given with aminoglutethimide.

(b) Diuretics

A woman who had been taking **bendroflumethiazide** 10 mg daily and potassium chloride 578 mg for several years for hypertension and mild cardiac decompensation, was given aminoglutethimide 1 g daily and hydrocortisone 60 mg daily for breast cancer. After 10 months of treatment she was hospitalised with severe hyponatraemia, which resolved when all the drugs were withdrawn. No clinically important change in electrolytes occurred over 3 months when the aminoglutethimide and hydrocortisone were used alone, but serum sodium fell again when the diuretic was restarted. The serum sodium levels were subsequently maintained by the addition of fludrocortisone 100 micrograms daily.[2] The hyponatraemia was thought to be caused by the combined inhibitory effect of aminoglutethimide on aldosterone production (which normally retains sodium in the body) and the sodium loss caused by the diuretic. Plasma electrolytes should be monitored when aminoglutethimide is used, and this would seem particularly important if it is given with any diuretic, as they all have the potential to reduce sodium levels.

(c) Tamoxifen

In 6 menopausal women with breast cancer, aminoglutethimide 250 mg four times daily for 6 weeks markedly reduced the serum levels of tamoxifen 20 to 80 mg daily and most of its metabolites. The clearance of the tamoxifen was increased 3.2-fold and the tamoxifen AUC was reduced by 73% (range 56 to 80%). Tamoxifen did not alter the pharmacokinetics of aminoglutethimide.[3] It is likely that aminoglutethimide, an enzyme inducer, increases the metabolism of tamoxifen by the liver, thereby increasing its loss from the body. It was originally hypothesised that the combination of an oestrogen antagonist, such as tamoxifen, and an aromatase inhibitor should provide additional benefit in the treatment of hormone-dependent cancers; however, no clinical studies have found this to be so. The pharmacokinetic interaction described above may partly explain this. Based on this evidence, these drugs should not be used concurrently.

NOTE. The reader is cautioned that this monograph is included purely for archival purposes, and is no longer subject to systematic revision and update.

1. Dowsett M, Murray RML, Pitt P, Jeffcoate SL. Antagonism of aminoglutethimide and danazol in the suppression of serum free oestradiol in breast cancer patients. *Eur J Cancer Clin Oncol* (1985) 21, 1063–8.
2. Bork E, Hansen M. Severe hyponatremia following simultaneous administration of aminoglutethimide and diuretics. *Cancer Treat Rep* (1986) 70, 689–90.
3. Lien EA, Anker G, Lønning PE, Solheim E, Ueland PM. Decreased serum concentrations of tamoxifen and its metabolites induced by aminoglutethimide. *Cancer Res* (1990) 50, 5851–7.

Table 39.1 Summary of the effect of azoles and macrolides on the pharmacokinetics of astemizole and terfenadine and the associated cardiovascular effects

Antihistamine (Oral unless specified)	*Azole or Macrolide (Oral unless specified)*	*Duration of combined use (days)*	*Subjects*	*Cmax increase*†	*AUC increase*	*Effect on QTc*	*Refs*
Azoles							
Astemizole 10 mg single dose	Itraconazole 200 mg twice daily	Single dose	12 healthy subjects	No clinically relevant change	82%	No clinically relevant change	1
Terfenadine 60 mg twice daily	Fluconazole 200 mg daily	6	6 healthy subjects		No change terfenadine 34% terfenadine acid metabolite	No clinically relevant change	2
Terfenadine 60 mg twice daily	Fluconazole 800 mg daily	7	Note - 6 subjects previously found to have measurable terfenadine levels at steady state		52% terfenadine 5% terfenadine acid metabolite	Increase	3
Terfenadine 120 mg single dose	Itraconazole 200 mg daily	Single dose	6 healthy subjects	Terfenadine 25%, 115%, 156% in the 3 subjects who had measurable levels before itraconazole	30% terfenadine acid metabolite	Mean increase of 27 milliseconds when compared with terfenadine alone	4
Terfenadine 120 mg single dose	Ketoconazole 400 mg daily	Single dose	12 healthy subjects	Greater than or equal to 170% terfenadine ↓71% terfenadine acid metabolite	Not measured	Prolongation by 10 to 20 milliseconds	5, 6
Terfenadine 60 mg twice daily	Ketoconazole 200 mg twice daily	4 to 7	6 healthy subjects	Below 5 to 7 nanograms/mL. Marked interindividual variability; an 11-fold increase in terfenadine level was observed in one subject.	57% terfenadine acid metabolite	Mean increase of 74 milliseconds when compared with terfenadine alone	7
Macrolides							
Astemizole 30 mg single dose	Dirithromycin 500 mg daily	Single dose of antihistamine	18 healthy subjects	No clinically relevant change	36%	No change	8
Astemizole 200 micrograms/kg daily	Erythromycin 50 mg/kg per day	14	10 patients aged 5 to 12 years	Not studied	Not studied	No significant change with Bazett's correction	9
Terfenadine 60 mg twice daily	Azithromycin 500 mg, then 250 mg daily	5	30 healthy subjects	Terfenadine undetectable No change in terfenadine acid metabolite	No change in terfenadine acid metabolite	No change	10, 11
Terfenadine 60 mg twice daily	Clarithromycin 500 mg twice daily	7	6 healthy subjects	4 of 6 subjects with measurable terfenadine levels 110% terfenadine acid metabolite	156% terfenadine acid metabolite	Mean increase of 20 milliseconds when compared with terfenadine alone	10
Terfenadine 60 mg twice daily	Clarithromycin 500 mg twice daily	5	14 healthy subjects	2 of 14 subjects with measurable terfenadine levels 119% terfenadine acid metabolite	181% terfenadine acid metabolite	Not studied	12
Terfenadine 60 mg twice daily	Dirithromycin 500 mg daily	10	6 healthy subjects	No clinically relevant change in terfenadine acid metabolite	No clinically relevant change in terfenadine acid metabolite	No change	13
Terfenadine 60 mg twice daily	Erythromycin 500 mg three times daily	7	9 subjects	3 of 9 subjects with measurable terfenadine levels 107% terfenadine acid metabolite	170% terfenadine acid metabolite	64 milliseconds in the 3 subjects with measurable terfenadine levels. No significant change in the other 6 subjects	14

†Note that terfenadine levels are normally undetectable

Continued

Table 39.1 Summary of the effect of azoles and macrolides on the pharmacokinetics of astemizole and terfenadine and the associated cardiovascular effects (continued)

Antihistamine (Oral unless specified)	*Azole or Macrolide (Oral unless specified)*	*Duration of combined use (days)*	*Subjects*	*Cmax increase*†	*AUC increase*	*Effect on QTc*	*Refs*
Macrolides							
Terfenadine 60 mg twice daily	Erythromycin 500 mg three times daily	7	6 healthy subjects	3 of 6 subjects with measurable terfenadine levels 87% terfenadine acid metabolite	109% terfenadine acid metabolite	Mean increase of 34 milliseconds	10
Terfenadine 60 mg twice daily	Erythromycin 333 mg three times daily	7		22% terfenadine acid metabolite	42% terfenadine acid metabolite	Mean increase of 4 to 10 milliseconds with erythromycin alone. No further increase with terfenadine	5, 15
Terfenadine 1 mg/kg twice daily	Erythromycin 50 mg/kg per day	14	10 patients aged 5 to 12 years	Not studied	Not studied	No significant change with Bazett's correction	9

†Note that terfenadine levels are normally undetectable

1. Lefebvre RA, Van Peer A, Woestenborghs R. Influence of itraconazole on the pharmacokinetics and electrocardiographic effects of astemizole. *Br J Clin Pharmacol* (1997) 43, 319–22.
2. Honig PK, Wortham DC, Zamani K, Mullin JC, Conner DP, Cantilena LR. The effect of fluconazole on the steady-state pharmacokinetics and electrographic pharmacodynamics of terfenadine in humans. *Clin Pharmacol Ther* (1993) 53, 630–6.
3. Cantilena LR, Sorrels S, Wiley T, Wortham D. Fluconazole alters terfenadine pharmacokinetics and electrocardiographic pharmacodynamics. *Clin Pharmacol Ther* (1995) 57, 185.
4. Honig PK, Wortham DC, Hull R, Zamani K, Smith JE, Cantilena LR. Itraconazole affects single-dose terfenadine pharmacokinetics and cardiac repolarization pharmacodynamics. *J Clin Pharmacol* (1993) 33, 1201–6.
5. Mathews DR, McNutt B, Okerholm R, Flicker M, McBride G. Torsades de pointes occurring in association with terfenadine use. *JAMA* (1991) 266, 2375–6.
6. Eller MG, Okerholm RA. Pharmacokinetic interaction between terfenadine and ketoconazole. *Clin Pharmacol Ther* (1991) 49, 130.
7. Honig PK, Wortham DC, Zamani K, Conner DP, Mullin JC, Cantilena LR. Terfenadine-ketoconazole interaction. Pharmacokinetic and electrocardiographic consequences. *JAMA* (1993) 269, 1513–18.
8. Bachmann K, Sullivan TJ, Reese JH, Jauregui L, Miller K, Scott M, Stotka J, Harris J. A study of the interaction between dirithromycin and astemizole in healthy adults. *Am J Ther* (1997) 4, 73–9.
9. Delgado LF, Pferferman A, Solé D, Naspitz CK. Evaluation of the potential cardiotoxicity of the antihistamines terfenadine, astemizole, loratadine, and cetirizine in atopic children. *Ann Allergy Asthma Immunol* (1998) 80, 333–7.
10. Honig PK, Wortham DC, Zamani K, Cantilena LR. Comparison of the effect of the macrolide antibiotics erythromycin, clarithromycin and azithromycin on terfenadine steady-state pharmacokinetics and electrocardiographic parameters. *Drug Invest* (1994) 7, 148–56.
11. Harris S, Hilligoss DM, Colangelo PM, Eller M, Okerholm R. Azithromycin and terfenadine: lack of drug interaction. *Clin Pharmacol Ther* (1995) 58, 310–15.
12. Gustavson LE, Blahunka KS, Witt GF, Harris SI, Palmer RN. Evaluation of the pharmacokinetic drug interaction between terfenadine and clarithromycin. *Pharm Res* (1993) 10 (10 Suppl), S-311.
13. Goldberg MJ, Ring B, DeSante K, Cerimele B, Hatcher B, Sides G, Wrighton S. Effect of dirithromycin on human CYP3A in vitro and on pharmacokinetics and pharmacodynamics of terfenadine in vivo. *J Clin Pharmacol* (1996) 36, 1154–60.
14. Honig PK, Woosley RL, Zamani K, Conner DP, Cantilena LR. Changes in the pharmacokinetics and electrocardiographic pharmacodynamics of terfenadine with concomitant administration of erythromycin. *Clin Pharmacol Ther* (1992) 52, 231–8.
15. Eller M, Russell T, Ruberg S, Okerholm R, McNutt B. Effect of erythromycin on terfenadine metabolite pharmacokinetics. *Clin Pharmacol Ther* (1993) 53, 161.

Aminoglutethimide + Theophylline

Aminoglutethimide increases the clearance of theophylline.

Clinical evidence, mechanism, importance and management

Aminoglutethimide 250 mg four times a day increased the clearance of sustained-release theophylline 200 mg twice daily by 18 to 43% in 3 patients.[1] Theophylline clearance was assessed before starting aminoglutethimide as well as during weeks 2 to 12 of concurrent use.

It seems probable that aminoglutethimide, a known enzyme inducer, increases the metabolism of theophylline by the liver, thereby decreasing its levels.

The clinical importance of this increased metabolism is uncertain, but it seems likely that the effects of theophylline would be reduced to some extent. It would seem prudent to monitor the effects of concurrent use for theophylline adverse effects (headache, nausea and tremor) and, if necessary, take theophylline levels. Increase the theophylline dose accordingly. Note that, aminophylline is metabolised to theophylline and would be expected to be similarly affected by aminoglutethimide.

NOTE. The reader is cautioned that this monograph is included purely for archival purposes, and is no longer subject to systematic revision and update.

1. Lønning PE, Kvinnsland S, Bakke OM. Effect of aminoglutethimide on antipyrine, theophylline and digitoxin disposition in breast cancer. *Clin Pharmacol Ther* (1984) 36, 796–802.

Astemizole or Terfenadine + CYP3A4 inhibitors

Astemizole and terfenadine are metabolised by CYP3A4. Drugs that inhibit this isoenzyme, such as the azoles, some macrolides, nefazodone and the HIV-protease inhibitors raise the concentrations of these antihistamines, which can result in life-threatening arrhythmias; this has been seen in a number of cases.

Grapefruit juice also raises terfenadine concentrations, but does not appear to alter the pharmacokinetics of astemizole.

Clinical evidence

A. Azoles

Pharmacokinetic studies with **fluconazole**, **itraconazole** and **ketoconazole** have shown increased exposure to astemizole and terfenadine. Details of these studies are summarised in 'Table 39.1', p.1596.

The subsections below include additional data from case reports or other studies.

(a) Astemizole

A 63-year old woman developed torsade de pointes and was found to have a prolonged QT interval after taking astemizole and **ketoconazole**. These two drugs were withdrawn and she was successfully treated with a temporary pacemaker, magnesium sulphate and lidocaine. She was later discharged with a normal ECG.[1]

(b) Terfenadine

1. Itraconazole. A 26-year-old woman taking terfenadine 60 mg twice daily began to have fainting episodes on the third evening after starting to take itraconazole 100 mg twice daily for vaginitis. When admitted to hospital the next morning her ECG showed a QT interval of 580 milliseconds and her heart rate was 67 bpm. Several episodes of torsade de pointes were recorded, and she fainted during two of them. No arrhythmias were seen 20 hours after the last itraconazole dose, and her QT interval returned to normal after 3 days. She was found to have terfenadine concentrations of 28 nanograms/mL in the first sample of serum taken (normally less than 5 nanograms/mL) and she still had concentrations of 12 nanograms/mL about 60 hours after taking the last tablet.[2,3] Two other similar cases have been reported,[4,5] and the FDA has received four well-documented cases of severe cardiac complications due to this interaction.[6]

2. Ketoconazole. A 39-year-old woman taking terfenadine 60 mg twice daily developed a number of episodes of syncope and light-headedness, preceded by palpitations, dyspnoea and diaphoresis, within 2 days of starting to take ketoconazole 200 mg twice daily. ECG monitoring revealed torsade de pointes and a QTc interval of 655 milliseconds. Her terfenadine serum concentrations were 57 nanograms/mL (concentrations expected to be 10 nanograms/mL or less). Other drugs being taken were cefaclor (stopped 3 to 4 days before the problems started) and medroxyprogesterone acetate. She had taken terfenadine and cefaclor on two previous occasions in the absence of ketoconazole without problems.[7,8] Other cases of an interaction between terfenadine and ketoconazole have also been reported.[9,10]

3. Oxiconazole. A 25-year-old woman complained of palpitations and chest pain radiating down her left arm, and was also found to be having frequent ventricular premature beats in a pattern of bigeminy. On questioning it turned out that she was taking terfenadine and using topical oxiconazole for ringworm on her arm. Both drugs were stopped and her symptoms disappeared the following week.[11]

B. Grapefruit juice

(a) Astemizole

In a study in 12 healthy subjects the steady-state pharmacokinetics of astemizole 30 mg daily for 4 days, then 10 mg daily for the next 20 days, were unaffected by 200 mL of grapefruit juice given every 4 hours.[12]

(b) Terfenadine

Terfenadine 60 mg was given to 6 healthy subjects every 12 hours for 14 days, simultaneously with 240 mL of double-strength grapefruit juice every 12 hours for the final 7 days. Terfenadine was only detectable in the plasma when grapefruit juice was taken. The mean QTc interval was found to have risen from 420 to 434 milliseconds,[13] which is not of a magnitude usually considered to be clinically significant. The effects on the AUC were less pronounced in a further 6 subjects who took the grapefruit juice 2 hours after the terfenadine.[13] Several other reports confirm these pharmacokinetic findings, although some did not find any changes in the QTc interval.[14-16]

C. HIV-protease inhibitors

Nelfinavir 750 mg every 8 hours for 5 days raised the concentrations of a single 60-mg dose of terfenadine from less than 5 nanograms/mL to a range of 5 to 15 nanograms/mL. The pharmacokinetics of **nelfinavir** were unaffected.[17] This rise in terfenadine concentrations is predicted to prolong the QT interval, and to increase the risk of torsade de pointes.

D. Macrolides

Pharmacokinetic studies with **erythromycin** and **clarithromycin** have shown increased exposure to astemizole and/or terfenadine. One study with **dirithromycin** and astemizole, showed an increase in the AUC of astemizole, but no effect on the pharmacokinetics of terfenadine was seen in another study. **Azithromycin** did not affect the pharmacokinetics of terfenadine in one study. Details of these studies are summarised in 'Table 39.1', p.1596.

The subsections below include additional data from case reports or other studies.

(a) Astemizole

An 87-year-old woman collapsed suddenly in her kitchen 4 days after starting to take astemizole 10 mg daily and **erythromycin** twice daily (dose unknown). An ECG showed her to be having multiple episodes of torsade de pointes, the longest of which lasted 17 seconds. Her QTc was 720 milliseconds and she was mildly hypokalaemic. She was given a temporary pacemaker and when she was eventually discharged with a normal sinus rhythm, her QTc had fallen to 475 milliseconds.[18] A second case report describes a 30-year-old woman who took astemizole 10 mg twice daily with **erythromycin** 250 mg every 6 hours for 3 days and developed syncope, which was shown to be due to torsade de pointes.[19] This patient was known to have congenital long QT syndrome, and had previously experienced syncope when taking astemizole, and therefore in this case an interaction is not established.

(b) Terfenadine

1. Erythromycin. An 18-year-old girl who was taking terfenadine 60 mg twice daily and erythromycin 250 mg every 6 hours, fainted while at school and, when later hospitalised, was seen to have repeated episodes of ventricular tachycardia and ventricular fibrillation requiring resuscitation. Later she was also noted to have torsade de pointes. Her QTc interval was found to be prolonged at 630 milliseconds. The drugs were withdrawn and 9 days later, after a period in intensive care, she was discharged symptom-free with a normal QTc interval.[20] A further case describes a 63-year-old man who had taken terfenadine 240 mg each day and erythromycin 2 g each day for 3 days, and subsequently experienced three syncopal episodes in one day. An ECG showed a prolonged QT interval and torsade de pointes, which resolved after intravenous magnesium sulphate was given.[21]

In contrast, a retrospective report found no documented cardiac adverse events in 92 patients who had received erythromycin and terfenadine.[22]

2. Troleandomycin. A woman taking terfenadine 60 mg three times daily developed torsade de pointes and a prolonged QTc interval when troleandomycin 500 mg three times daily was added. She recovered when both were stopped, but again developed a significantly prolonged QTc interval when both were restarted.[23]

E. Nefazodone

(a) Astemizole

The manufacturers of nefazodone and astemizole noted that an *in vitro* study suggests that nefazodone may increase astemizole concentrations.[24,25]

(b) Terfenadine

In a randomised, placebo-controlled study, healthy subjects were given nefazodone 300 mg twice daily and terfenadine 60 mg twice daily, alone and in combination. Nefazodone increased the AUC of terfenadine about fivefold, which was associated with a mean increase in the QTc interval of 42.4 milliseconds. This was considered to result in a clinically significant increase in the risk of torsade de pointes.[26]

Mechanism

Astemizole and terfenadine are known to be metabolised by the cytochrome P450 isoenzyme CYP3A4. The azoles, some macrolides, nefazodone and the HIV-protease inhibitors are known inhibitors of this isoenzyme, but vary in the strength of their effect. Grapefruit juice may also inhibit CYP3A4, but exerts its effect mainly on intestinal CYP3A4. The concurrent use of astemizole or terfenadine and these CYP3A4 inhibitors therefore leads to increased antihistamine concentrations. High serum concentrations of astemizole and terfenadine (but not its metabolites) block cardiac potassium channels leading to prolongation of the QT interval, which may precipitate the development of torsade de pointes (see 'Table 15.2', p.629).

Importance and management

The interactions of astemizole and terfenadine with CYP3A4 inhibitors (namely the azoles, some macrolides, nefazodone and the HIV-protease inhibitors) are established and clinically important. Much of the evidence for particular pairs of these antihistamines and CYP3A4 inhibitors is indirect and from the reports above it seems that only a very few individuals develop a clinically important adverse interaction, but identifying them in advance is not often practical or possible. The incidence of an interaction is probably low, but because of the potential severity and unpredictability of this interaction, the concurrent use of astemizole and terfenadine was contraindicated with all azoles and all macrolides (except azithromycin and astemizole) in all patients. The UK manufacturer of terfenadine extended this contraindication to the concurrent use of topical azoles and macrolides.[27] Similarly, the use of other CYP3A4 inhibitors, including grapefruit juice, nefazodone and the HIV-protease inhibitors, was also contraindicated.

Because of the risks of raised terfenadine and astemizole concentrations, the manufacturers of many other drugs known to inhibit CYP3A4, even weakly, often still include contraindications for the concurrent use of these antihistamines. For a list of clinically relevant CYP3A4 inhibitors, see 'Table 1.9', p.11, but note that this list may not include every drug contraindicated for use with these antihistamines.

NOTE. The reader is cautioned that this monograph is included purely for archival purposes, and is no longer subject to systematic revision and update.

1. Tsai W-C, Tsai L-M, Chen J-H. Combined use of astemizole and ketoconazole resulting in torsade de pointes. *J Formos Med Assoc* (1977) 96, 144–6.
2. Pohjola-Sintonen S, Viitasalo M, Toivonen L, Neuvonen P. Torsades de pointes after terfenadine-itraconazole interaction. *BMJ* (1993) 306, 186.
3. Pohjola-Sintonen S, Viitasalo M, Toivonen L, Neuvonen P. Itraconazole prevents terfenadine metabolism and increases risk of torsades de pointes ventricular tachycardia. *Eur J Clin Pharmacol* (1993) 45, 191–3.
4. Crane JK, Shih H-T. Syncope and cardiac arrhythmia due to an interaction between itraconazole and terfenadine. *Am J Med* (1993) 95, 445–6.
5. Romkes JH, Froger CL, Wever EFD, Westerhof PW. Wegrakingen tijdens simultaan gebruik van terfenadine en itraconazol. *Ned Tijdschr Geneeskd* (1997) 141, 950–3.
6. Honig PK, Wortham DC, Hull R, Zamani K, Smith JE, Cantilena LR. Itraconazole affects single-dose terfenadine pharmacokinetics and cardiac repolarization pharmacodynamics. *J Clin Pharmacol* (1993) 33, 1201–6.
7. Monahan BP, Ferguson CL, Killeavy ES, Lloyd BK, Troy J, Cantilena LR. Torsades de pointes occurring in association with terfenadine use. *JAMA* (1990) 264, 2788–90.
8. Cantilena LR, Ferguson CL, Monahan BP. Torsades de pointes occurring in association with terfenadine use. *JAMA* (1991) 266, 2375–6.
9. Zimmermann M, Duruz H, Guinand O, Broccard O, Levy P, Lacatis D, Bloch A. Torsades de pointes after treatment with terfenadine and ketoconazole. *Eur Heart J* (1992) 13, 1002–3.
10. Peck CC, Temple R, Collins JM. Understanding consequences of concurrent therapies. *JAMA* (1993) 269, 1550–2.
11. Griffith JS. Interaction between terfenadine and topical antifungal agents. *Am Fam Physician* (1995) 51, 1396–7.
12. Janssen-Cilag Ltd. Data on file (Study AST-BEL-7 + Amendment). 1995.
13. Benton RE, Honig PK, Zamani K, Cantilena LR, Woosley RL. Grapefruit juice alters terfenadine pharmacokinetics, resulting in prolongation of repolarization on the electrocardiogram. *Clin Pharmacol Ther* (1996) 59, 383–8.
14. Honig PK, Wortham DC, Lazarev A, Cantilena LR. Grapefruit juice alters the systemic bioavailability and cardiac repolarization of terfenadine in poor metabolizers of terfenadine. *J Clin Pharmacol* (1996) 36, 345–51.
15. Clifford CP, Adams DA, Murray S, Taylor GW, Wilkins MR, Boobis AR, Davies DS. The cardiac effects of terfenadine after inhibition of its metabolism by grapefruit juice. *Eur J Clin Pharmacol* (1997) 52, 311–15.
16. Rau SE, Bend JR, Arnold JMO, Tran LT, Spence JD, Bailey DG. Grapefruit juice–terfenadine single-dose interaction: magnitude, mechanism, and relevance. *Clin Pharmacol Ther* (1997) 61, 401–9.
17. Kerr B, Yuep G, Daniels R, Quart B, Kravcik S, Sahai J, Anderson R. Strategic approach to nelfinavir mesylate (NFV) drug interactions involving CYP3A metabolism. 6th European Conference on Clinical Aspects and Treatment of HIV-infection, Hamburg, October 11–15th 1997. Abstracts.
18. Goss JE, Ramo BW, Blake K. Torsades de pointes associated with astemizole (Hismanal) therapy. *Arch Intern Med* (1993) 153, 2705.
19. Hsieh M-H, Chen S-A, Chiang C-E, Tai C-T, Lee S-H, Wen Z-C, Chang M-S. Drug induced torsades de pointes in one patient with congenital long QT syndrome. *Int J Cardiol* (1996) 54, 85–8.
20. Biglin KE, Faraon MS, Constance TD, Lieh-Lai M. Drug-induced torsades de pointes: a possible interaction of terfenadine and erythromycin. *Ann Pharmacother* (1994) 28, 282.
21. Gully C, Riem R. Torsades de pointes imputables à l'association terfenadine-érythromycine. *Ann Med Interne (Paris)* (1994) 145, 257–8.
22. Schoenwetter WF, Kelloway JS, Lindgren D. A retrospective evaluation of potential cardiac side-effects induced by concurrent use of terfenadine and erythromycin. *J Allergy Clin Immunol* (1993) 91, 259.
23. Fournier P, Pacouret G, Charbonnier B. Une nouvelle cause de torsades de pointes: association terfénadine et troléandomycine. *Ann Cardiol Angeiol (Paris)* (1993) 42, 249–52.
24. Hismanal (Astemizole). Janssen-Cilag Ltd. UK Summary of product characteristics, June 1998.
25. Robinson DS, Roberts DL, Smith JM, Stringfellow JC, Kaplita SB, Seminara JA, Marcus RN. The safety profile of nefazodone. *J Clin Psychiatry* (1996) 57 (Suppl 2), 31–8.
26. Abernethy DR, Barbey JT, Franc J, Brown KS, Feirrera I, Ford N, Salazar DE. Loratadine and terfenadine interaction with nefazodone; both antihistamines are associated with QTc prolongation. *Clin Pharmacol Ther* (2001) 69; 96–103.
27. Histafen (Terfenadine). Approved Prescription Services Ltd. UK Summary of product characteristics, December 1999.

Astemizole or Terfenadine + Drugs that prolong the QT interval

Astemizole and terfenadine may prolong the QT interval, particularly if their levels are raised: their effects may be additive with those of other drugs that can also prolong the QT interval.

Clinical evidence, mechanism, importance and management

See 'Drugs that prolong the QT interval + Other drugs that prolong the QT interval', p.272, for a further discussion on the concurrent use of drugs that prolong the QT interval.

(a) Quinine

In a study, 12 healthy subjects were given astemizole 30 mg daily for 4 days followed by 10 mg daily for the next 20 days. The steady-state pharmacokinetics of astemizole were then assessed after the subjects took quinine 20 mg every 4 hours for 12 hours (a total of 80 mg quinine), and after a single 430-mg dose of quinine. The smaller dose of quinine caused only a slight increase in the maximum plasma levels and AUC of astemizole, but the larger, single dose of quinine resulted in a transient threefold increase in the maximum plasma levels and AUC of astemizole and particularly desmethylastemizole, a metabolite of astemizole that causes QT prolongation.[1]

Case reports illustrate the clinical relevance of these findings. In one case,a patient who had been taking astemizole 10 mg daily for 10 months with fluoxetine, alprazolam, isradipine, and diuretics with potassium had a syncopal episode one hour after taking the first dose of quinine sulphate 260 mg for leg cramp. The ECG showed recurrent episodes of torsade de pointes with a QT interval of greater than 680 milliseconds. The only electrolyte abnormality was slight hypomagnesaemia. Intravenous magnesium was given and the patient's QT interval shortened to 420 milliseconds over 3 days.[2] The manufacturers have on record two other case reports[3] of cardiac arrhythmias possibly attributable to an interaction between astemizole and quinine. The mechanism responsible for these effects is uncertain. One suggestion is that the interaction is not primarily due to inhibition of the metabolism of astemizole by the quinine, but rather to a transient quinine-induced displacement of both astemizole and its metabolite from its tissue binding sites.[1]

Information is very limited, but on the basis of the evidence cited above the manufacturer of astemizole contraindicated the concurrent use of quinine in order to avoid the risk of cardiac arrhythmias.[4] The larger single 430-mg dose of quinine used in the study cited approached the dose used for the treatment of malaria, whereas the smaller dose of 80 mg was equivalent to the amount contained in 2 litres of a quinine-containing soft drink.[1] There would therefore appear to be less risk associated with moderate quantities of quinine-containing drinks.

(b) Quinolones

In a single-dose, placebo-controlled study in 8 healthy subjects, **sparfloxacin** 400 mg increased the QT interval by 14 milliseconds, **terfenadine** 60 mg increased the QT interval by 7.5 milliseconds (not statistically significant), and the combination caused an increase of 24.7 milliseconds. The effects of the combination in this study were shown to be purely additive.[5]

Similarly, in a placebo-controlled study 22 patients were given **sparfloxacin** 400 mg on day one and 200 mg on days 2 to 4 with terfenadine 60 mg twice daily for 7 doses. The increase in the QT interval when the two drugs were given together was additive, and no pharmacokinetic interaction was found.[6]

As the effects of therapeutic doses of terfenadine on the QT interval are minimal, any additional effect with **sparfloxacin** would be small. Nevertheless, because torsade de pointes can cause sudden death, the combination of two drugs with the potential to prolong the QT interval is generally considered to be contraindicated. Note that the UK manufacturer of terfenadine specifically contraindicated **sparfloxacin**.[7]

Other quinolones that cause QT prolongation include **gatifloxacin** and **moxifloxacin**, see 'Table 9.2', p.273, and it would also be prudent to avoid use of antihistamines that prolong the QT interval (e.g. astemizole and terfenadine) with these quinolones.

(c) Sotalol

A 71-year-old woman with a history of atrial fibrillation, which had been successfully treated with sotalol 80 mg twice daily for the past 8 months (QT interval at restoration of sinus rhythm of 430 milliseconds), was admitted to hospital with chemotherapy-induced febrile neutropenia. She was given terfenadine 60 mg twice daily, and 7 days later developed experienced light-headedness. The following day she had several brief episodes of dizziness, and an ECG showed repeated self-limiting episodes of torsade de pointes with a prolonged QT interval of 660 milliseconds. On one occasion she required resuscitation. Both drugs were stopped and no further episodes of arrhythmia occurred 72 hours after temporary pacing was discontinued.[8]

It seems likely that the adverse effects in this patient resulted from the additive effects of both drugs on the QT interval, which can lead to the development of torsade de pointes. This case confirms a previous mention of the possibility of this interaction.[9]

Although this seems to be the first report of this interaction, it is consistent with the known pharmacology of both drugs. Torsade de pointes is potentially life threatening, and therefore the concurrent use of these two drugs should generally be avoided.

(d) Other drugs that prolong the QT interval

A review of data on the use of five non-sedating antihistamines (including astemizole and terfenadine) from the UK General Practice Research Database found an overall relative risk of ventricular arrhythmias of 4.2 compared with non-use. However, it did not identify a higher risk of ventricular arrhythmias with terfenadine than with the other non-sedating antihistamines. The relative risk of developing a ventricular arrhythmia was highest during astemizole use (19). Within the data used for this study there were no cases of ventricular arrhythmias in patients taking terfenadine and inhibitors of the cytochrome P450 isoenzyme CYP3A4.[10] The authors concluded that the absolute risk of ventricular arrhythmias with the use of one of these drugs alone was quite small. However, in the presence of other drugs that prolong the QT interval, the risk may be larger. A retrospective review of a cohort of 14 638 patients with urinary incontinence diagnosed between January 1991 and June 1995, identified a significant association between the use of non-sedating antihistamines (terfenadine and astemizole) with drugs that are CYP3A4 inhibitors and the incidence of ventricular arrhythmias, with an adjusted relative risk of 5.47. This combination was also shown to carry a significant risk of sudden death (relative risk 21.5).[11]

The manufacturers of astemizole[4] and terfenadine[7] contraindicated the concurrent use of any other drugs that prolongs the QT interval (for a list, see 'Table 9.2', p.273). However, the primary risk of QT prolongation and torsade de pointes with astemizole and terfenadine appears to be from drugs that significantly inhibit their metabolism such as CYP3A4 inhibitors, see 'Astemizole or Terfenadine + CYP3A4 inhibitors', p.1597..

NOTE. The reader is cautioned that this monograph is included purely for archival purposes, and is no longer subject to systematic revision and update.

1. Janssen-Cilag Ltd. Data on file (Study AST-BEL-7 + Amendment). 1995.
2. Martin ES, Rogalski K, Black JN. Quinine may trigger torsades de pointes during astemizole therapy. *Pacing Clin Electrophysiol* (1997) 20, 2024–5.
3. Janssen-Cilag Ltd. Personal Communication, May 1997.
4. Hismanal (Astemizole). Janssen-Cilag Ltd. UK Summary of product characteristics, June 1998.
5. Akhtar M, Saha N, Roy A, Pillai KK. Effect of sparfloxacin and terfenadine combination on QT-intervals at various RR-intervals. *Indian J Pharmacol* (2002) 34, 264–8.
6. Morganroth J, Hunt T, Dorr MB, Magner D, Talbot GH. The effect of terfenadine on the cardiac pharmacodynamics of sparfloxacin. *Clin Ther* (1999) 21, 1514–24.
7. Histafen (Terfenadine). Approved Prescription Services Ltd. UK Summary of product characteristics, December 1999.
8. Feroze H, Suri R, Silverman DI. Torsades de pointes from terfenadine and sotalol given in combination. *Pacing Clin Electrophysiol* (1996) 19, 1519–21.
9. Woosley RL, Chen Y, Freiman JP, Gillis RA. Mechanism of the cardiotoxic actions of terfenadine. *JAMA* (1993) 269, 1532–6.
10. De Abajo FJ, García Rodríguez AL. Risk of ventricular arrhythmias associated with nonsedating antihistamine drugs. *Br J Clin Pharmacol* (1999) 47, 307–13.
11. Wang PS, Levin R, Zhao SZ, Avorn J. Urinary antispasmodic use and risks of ventricular arrhythmia and sudden death in older patients. *J Am Geriatr Soc* (2002) 50, 117–24.

Astemizole or Terfenadine + Miscellaneous

In many countries astemizole and terfenadine have been withdrawn from the market, or are only available for restricted use because of their potential to cause torsade de pointes, especially when serum levels are elevated. This can lead to cardiac arrest and sudden death. Many of their interactions, and their importance and management, are summarised in 'Table 39.2', p.1600. Consider also 'Astemizole or Terfenadine + CYP3A4 inhibitors', p.1597, and 'Astemizole or Terfenadine + Drugs that prolong the QT interval', above.

Bretylium + Miscellaneous

The pressor effects of adrenaline (epinephrine) and noradrenaline (norepinephrine) are increased in the presence of bretylium. Amfetamine and protriptyline antagonise the blood pressure lowering effect of bretylium.

Clinical evidence

(a) Adrenaline (Epinephrine) or Noradrenaline (Norepinephrine)

In 4 healthy subjects, a dose of bretylium sufficient to produce postural hypotension enhanced the pressor effect of noradrenaline. A similar effect was found with adrenaline.[1]

(b) Amfetamine

When 7 patients with hypertension taking bretylium 600 mg to 4 g daily were given a single 25-mg dose of amfetamine, 6 patients had a rise in blood pressure.[2]

(c) Protriptyline

An experimental study found that protriptyline can return blood pressure to normal in patients taking bretylium, without reducing its antiarrhythmic efficacy.[3]

Mechanism

Animal studies have shown that bretylium reduces blood pressure via its blocking effects on adrenergic neurones similar to guanethidine.[4,5] Bretylium therefore enhances the effects of directly-acting sympathomimetics such as noradrenaline (norepinephrine), and is antagonised by drugs with indirect sympathomimetic activity such as the amfetamines and the tricyclic antidepressants.

Importance and management

Although documentation is limited, based on the known pharmacology of bretylium, these interactions would appear to be established. The use of bretylium is limited to the short-term control of ventricular arrhythmias. In this situation, if directly-acting sympathomimetics such as noradrenaline (norepinephrine) are required to reverse bretylium-induced hypotension, this should be undertaken with caution because their effects may be enhanced.

Table 39.2 Summary of the interactions of Astemizole and Terfenadine

Interacting drugs	*Reported effects*	*Action*	*Refs*
Astemizole			
Alcohol	Three studies have found that astemizole does not interact with alcohol.	As some patients may experience drowsiness with non-sedating antihistamines all patients should be advised to be alert to the possibility of drowsiness if they have not taken the drug before. Any drowsiness would be apparent after the first few doses.	1-3
Calcium-channel blockers	See under *Terfenadine*, below.		
Diazepam	Astemizole did not enhance the effects of diazepam in one study.	None.	4
Terbinafine	No adverse interactions reported in a large post-marketing survey of patients taking terbinafine and other drugs, including astemizole.	None.	5
Terfenadine			
Alcohol	One study found that terfenadine alone did not affect psychomotor skills, nor did it alter the adverse effects of alcohol. Another study had similar findings. However, a later study found that terfenadine slowed brake reaction times in the laboratory when given either alone or with alcohol.	As some patients may experience drowsiness with non-sedating antihistamines all patients should be advised to be alert to the possibility of drowsiness if they have not taken the drug before. Any drowsiness would be apparent after the first few doses.	6-8
Atorvastatin	Atorvastatin caused some small to moderate changes in the pharmacokinetics of terfenadine and its metabolite fexofenadine, but without affecting the QT interval.	None.	9
Buspirone	Terfenadine had no significant effects on the pharmacokinetics or pharmacodynamics of buspirone in one study.	None.	10
Calcium-channel blockers: Diltiazem Lercanidipine Nicardipine Nifedipine Verapamil	An isolated report describes severe angina in a patient taking nifedipine 10 mg three times daily when she took terfenadine 60 mg for seasonal allergy. A second patient taking verapamil 80 mg three times daily also experienced adverse effects (including severe headache and confusion) after taking a single 60-mg dose of terfenadine.	Verapamil, diltiazem, and to a lesser extent nicardipine are inhibitors of CYP3A4, but there appear to be no other reports of interactions with terfenadine or astemizole (both substrates of CYP3A4). Of all the calcium-channel blockers, only the UK manufacturer of lercanidipine advises caution during the concurrent use of terfenadine and astemizole; however, lercanidipine does not appear to inhibit CYP3A4, and therefore an interaction, at least by this mechanism, seems unlikely.	11, 12
Carbamazepine	Carbamazepine toxicity, attributed to the use of terfenadine, has been described in one case report. A total carbamazepine serum level of 8.9 mg/L was within the reference range, but free carbamazepine levels were almost three times the upper limit of normal.	None. Interaction not established.	13
Diazepam	The concurrent use of diazepam and terfenadine had no effect on psychomotor performance in one study.	None.	6
Docetaxel	The manufacturers of docetaxel state that *in vitro* studies have shown that the metabolism of docetaxel can be modified by drugs that are metabolised by CYP3A4, and they name terfenadine.	None. Clinically relevant pharmacokinetic drug interactions do not usually occur between drugs that just share the same metabolic route.	14
Flecainide	It has been suggested that the concurrent use of terfenadine and flecainide may increase the risk of ventricular arrhythmias.	Terfenadine can cause QT prolongation, but usually only when its levels are raised; however flecainide is not known to affect their metabolism. There appear to be no published reports of an interaction between these drugs, and therefore an interaction is not established.	15
H_2-receptor antagonists: Cimetidine Ranitidine	Cimetidine or ranitidine do not affect the pharmacokinetics of terfenadine. An isolated case of torsade de pointes was reported in a patient taking terfenadine, cimetidine, chlorphenamine and co-proxamol (paracetamol (acetaminophen) and dextropropoxyphene (propoxyphene)).	None with terfenadine and ranitidine. Unclear with terfenadine and cimetidine, not enough evidence to advise avoidance, but some caution is warranted because of the case report of torsade de pointes.	16-18
Montelukast	Montelukast did not affect the pharmacokinetics of terfenadine, or its effects on the QTc interval in one study.	None.	19
Paracetamol (Acetaminophen)	Torsade de pointes occurred in a patient taking terfenadine with large doses of paracetamol (acetaminophen) and amitriptyline in an isolated report.	Unlikely to be clinically important, especially at therapeutic doses of paracetamol.	20
Phenytoin	Terfenadine had no effect on the pharmacokinetics of phenytoin in one study.	None.	21

Continued

Table 39.2 Summary of the interactions of Astemizole and Terfenadine (continued)

Interacting drugs	*Reported effects*	*Action*	*Refs*
SSRIs: Fluoxetine Paroxetine	Two case reports describe cardiotoxicity (including prolonged QT interval) in patients taking terfenadine and fluoxetine. Fluoxetine and paroxetine do not appear to affect the pharmacokinetics of terfenadine.	Avoid. The concurrent use of terfenadine and citalopram, fluoxetine, fluvoxamine and paroxetine was contraindicated. Interaction with sertraline unlikely.	22-27
Terbinafine	No adverse interactions reported in a large post-marketing survey of patients taking terbinafine and other drugs, including terfenadine. Concurrent use well-tolerated in a study.	None.	5, 28
Theophylline	Terfenadine did not affect the pharmacokinetics of theophylline in three studies.	None.	29-31
Venlafaxine	Venlafaxine did not affect terfenadine pharmacokinetics in one study.	None.	32
Zafirlukast	A study in 16 healthy men found that terfenadine reduced the mean maximum plasma levels and AUC of zafirlukast by 70% and 60%, respectively. Another study found that the AUC of terfenadine and the QTc interval were not significantly increased on concurrent use.	If both drugs are given be alert for a reduced response to zafirlukast.	33, 34
Zileuton	Zileuton caused a modest increase in terfenadine levels seen in one study, without an increase in the QT interval.	Avoid. Zileuton is contraindicated due to risk of torsade de pointes as a result of raised terfenadine levels.	22, 35

1. Hindmarch I, Bhatti JZ. Psychomotor effects of astemizole and chlorpheniramine, alone and in combination with alcohol. *Int Clin Psychopharmacol* (1987) 2, 117–19.
2. Bateman DN, Chapman PH, Rawlins MD. Lack of effect of astemizole on ethanol dynamics or kinetics. *Eur J Clin Pharmacol* (1983) 25, 567–8.
3. Moser L, Plum H, Bückmann M. Interaktionen eines neuen Antihistaminikums mit Diazepam und Alkohol. *Med Welt* (1984) 35, 296–9.
4. Moser L. Die wirkung von astemizol auf die psychophysischen leistungen. *Z Hautkr* (1985) 60, 56–8.
5. Hall M, Monka C, Krupp P, O'Sullivan D. Safety of oral terbinafine. Results of a postmarketing surveillance study in 25 884 patients. *Arch Dermatol* (1997) 133, 1213–19.
6. Moser L, Hüther KJ, Koch-Weser J, Lundt PV. Effects of terfenadine and diphenhydramine alone or in combination with diazepam or alcohol on psychomotor performance and subjective feelings. *Eur J Clin Pharmacol* (1978) 14, 417–23.
7. O'Hanlon JF. Antihistamines and driving performance: The Netherlands. *J Respir Dis* (1988) (Suppl), S12–S17.
8. Bhatti JZ, Hindmarch I. The effects of terfenadine with and without alcohol on an aspect of car driving performance. *Clin Exp Allergy* (1989) 19, 609–11.
9. Stern RH, Smithers JA, Olson SC. Atorvastatin does not produce a clinically significant effect on the pharmacokinetics of terfenadine. *J Clin Pharmacol* (1998) 38, 753–7.
10. Lamberg TS, Kivistö KT, Neuvonen PJ. Lack of effect of terfenadine on the pharmacokinetics of the CYP3A4 substrate buspirone. *Pharmacol Toxicol* (1999) 84, 165–9.
11. Falkenberg HM. Possible interaction report. *Can Pharm J* (1988) 121, 294.
12. Zanidip (Lercanidipine hydrochloride). Recordati Pharmaceuticals Ltd. UK Summary of product characteristics, October 2004.
13. Hirschfeld S, Jarosinski P. Drug interaction of terfenadine and carbamazepine. *Ann Intern Med* (1993) 118, 907–8.
14. Taxotere (Docetaxel trihydrate). Sanofi-Aventis. UK Summary of product characteristics, December 2009.
15. Tambocor (Flecainide acetate). Meda Pharmaceuticals. UK Summary of product characteristics, December 2009.
16. Eller MG, Okerhold RA. Effect of cimetidine on terfenadine and terfenadine metabolite pharmacokinetics. *Pharm Res* (1991) 8 (10 Suppl), S-297.
17. Honig PK, Wortham DC, Zamani K, Conner DP, Mullin JC, Cantilena LR. Effect of concomitant administration of cimetidine and ranitidine on the pharmacokinetics and electrocardiographic effects of terfenadine. *Eur J Clin Pharmacol* (1993) 45, 41–6.
18. Ng PW, Chan WK, Chan TYK. Torsade de pointes during concomitant use of terfenadine and cimetidine. *Aust N Z J Med* (1996) 26, 120–1.
19. Holland S, Gertz B, DeSmet M, Michiels N, Larson P, Freeman A, Keymeulen B. Montelukast (MON) has no effect on terfenadine (T) pharmacokinetics (PK) or QTc. *Clin Pharmacol Ther* (1998) 63, 232.
20. Matsis PP, Easthope RN. Torsades de pointes ventricular tachycardia associated with terfenadine and paracetamol self medication. *N Z Med J* (1994) 107, 402–403.
21. Coniglio AA, Garnett WR, Pellock JH, Tsidonis O, Hepler CD, Serafin R, Small RE, Driscoll SM, Karnes HT. Effect of acute and chronic terfenadine on free and total serum phenytoin concentrations in epileptic patients. *Epilepsia* (1989) 30, 611–16.
22. Histafen (Terfenadine). Approved Prescription Services Ltd. UK Summary of product characteristics, December 1999.
23. Swims MP. Potential terfenadine-fluoxetine interaction. *Ann Pharmacother* (1993) 27, 1404–5.
24. Marchiando RJ, Cook MD, Jue SG. Probable terfenadine-fluoxetine-associated cardiac toxicity. *Ann Pharmacother* (1995) 29, 937–8.
25. Bergstrom RF, Goldberg MJ, Cerimele BJ, Hatcher BL. Assessment of the potential for a pharmacokinetic interaction between fluoxetine and terfenadine. *Clin Pharmacol Ther* (1997) 62, 643–51.
26. Martin DE, Zussman BD, Everitt DE, Benincosa LJ, Etheredge RC, Jorkasky DK. Paroxetine does not affect the cardiac safety and pharmacokinetics of terfenadine in healthy adult men. *J Clin Psychopharmacol* (1997) 17, 451–9.
27. Committee on Safety of Medicines/Medicines Control Agency. Sertraline and terfenadine. *Current Problems* (1998) 24, 4.
28. Robbins B, Chang C-T, Cramer JA, Garreffa S, Hafkin B, Hunt TL, Meligeni J. Safe coadministration of terbinafine and terfenadine: a placebo-controlled crossover study of pharmacokinetic and pharmacodynamic interactions in healthy volunteers. *Clin Pharmacol Ther* (1996) 59, 275–83.
29. Brion N, Naline E, Beaumont D, Pays M, Advenier C. Lack of effect of terfenadine on theophylline pharmacokinetics and metabolism in normal subjects. *Br J Clin Pharmacol* (1989) 27, 391–5.
30. Luskin SS, Fitzsimmons WE, MacLeod CM, Luskin AT. Pharmacokinetic evaluation of the terfenadine-theophylline interaction. *J Allergy Clin Immunol* (1989) 83, 406–11.
31. Fitzsimmons WE, Luskin SS, MacLeod CM, Luskin AT. Single-dose study of the effect of terfenadine on theophylline absorption and disposition. *Ann Allergy* (1989) 62, 213–14.
32. Amchin J, Zarycranski W, Taylor K, Albano D, Klockowski PM. Effect of venlafaxine on the pharmacokinetics of terfenadine. *Psychopharmacol Bull* (1998) 34, 383–9.
33. Suttle AB, Birmingham BK, Vargo DL, Wilkinson LA, Morganroth J. Pharmacokinetics of zafirlukast and terfenadine after coadministration to healthy men. *J Clin Pharmacol* (1997) 37, 870.
34. Vargo DL, Suttle AB, Wilkinson LA, Thyrum PT, Tschan JH, Morganroth J. Effect of zafirlukast on QTc and area under the curve of terfenadine in healthy men. *J Clin Pharmacol* (1997) 37, 870.
35. Awni WM, Cavanaugh JH, Leese P, Kasier J, Cao G, Locke CS, Dube LM. The pharmacokinetic and pharmacodynamic interaction between zileuton and terfenadine. *Eur J Clin Pharmacol* (1997) 52, 49–54.

Bretylium is no longer used for the treatment of hypertension, therefore the interactions with amfetamines and tricyclics are unlikely to be of much general relevance.

NOTE. The reader is cautioned that this monograph is included purely for archival purposes, and is no longer subject to systematic revision and update.

1. Laurence DR, Nagle RE. The interaction of bretylium with pressor agents. *Lancet* (1961) i, 593–4.
2. Wilson R, Long C. Action of bretylium antagonised by amphetamine. *Lancet* (1960) ii, 262.
3. Woosley RL, Reele SB, Roden DM, Nies AS, Oates JA. Pharmacological reversal of hypotensive effect complicating antiarrhythmic therapy with bretylium. *Clin Pharmacol Ther* (1982) 32, 313–21.
4. Day MD. Effect of sympathomimetic amines on the blocking action of guanethidine, bretylium and xylocholine. *Br J Pharmacol* (1962) 18, 421–39.
5. Boura ALA, Green AF. Comparison of bretylium and guanethidine: tolerance and effects on adrenergic nerve function and responses to sympathomimetic amines. *Br J Pharmacol* (1962) 19, 13–41.

Bucolome + Miscellaneous

Bucolome increases the anticoagulant effects of warfarin by inhibiting its metabolism and inhibits the metabolism of losartan to its active metabolite, E-3174.

Clinical evidence

(a) Losartan

A study in 6 healthy subjects found that bucolome 300 mg daily for one week increased the peak plasma levels and AUC of a single dose of losartan 25 mg by 79% and 67%, respectively. Peak plasma levels and the AUC of E-3174, the active metabolite of losartan, were decreased by 83%.[1]

(b) Warfarin

A study in Japanese patients stabilised on warfarin found that the addition of bucolome 300 mg daily increased the INR of 21 patients by 50% despite a 58% reduction in the warfarin dose, when compared with another group of 34 patients taking warfarin and not taking bucolome.[2] In another 7-day study, 25 Japanese patients with heart disease taking warfarin and bucolome 300 mg daily were compared with another control group of 30 patients taking warfarin alone. It was found that bucolome had no effect on the serum levels of *R*-warfarin but both the serum levels of *S*-warfarin and the prothrombin times rose. These changes were complete within 7 days.[3] In one analysis, the daily dose of warfarin was found to be about 40% lower in 78 patients taking bucolome, when compared with 99 patients not taking bucolome, although the thrombotest values were lower in those also taking bucolome (suggesting greater anticoagulation). Bucolome appeared to reduce the between patient variation in intrinsic hepatic clearance of warfarin.[4] A patient who had been taking warfarin with bucolome for 18 days developed gross haematuria. He was found to have an intraluminal ureteral haematoma and an excessively prolonged prothrombin time, and was treated with intravenous vitamin K.[5]

Mechanism

In vitro studies show that the bucolome can inhibit the metabolism of the more potent enantiomer *S*-warfarin by CYP2C9, thereby reducing its clearance and increasing its effects.[2] Similarly, bucolome appears to inhibit the metabolism of losartan to E-3174 by CYP2C9.[1]

Importance and management

The clinical importance of this effect of bucolome on losartan metabolism is not known, but, because the exposure to the active metabolite is markedly reduced, a reduced therapeutic effect of losartan seems possible. Until more is known it would be prudent to monitor blood pressure if bucolome is given to patients taking losartan.

Information on an interaction between bucolome and warfarin appears to be limited to the reports cited here but the interaction would seem to be established and clinically important. Monitor the INR closely if both drugs are given. A reduced warfarin dose (the study[3] cited above suggests a 30 to 60% reduction) is likely to be needed to avoid excessive anticoagulation and possible bleeding. Note that bucolome is sometimes used with warfarin to enhance its therapeutic effect.[4] Based on the mechanism of action, **acenocoumarol** and **phenprocoumon** would be expected to be similarly affected.

NOTE. The reader is cautioned that this monograph is included purely for archival purposes, and is no longer subject to systematic revision and update.

1. Kobayashi M, Takagi M, Fukumoto K, Kato R, Tanaka K, Ueno K. The effect of bucolome, a CYP2C9 inhibitor, on the pharmacokinetics of losartan. *Drug Metab Pharmacokinet* (2008) 23, 115–19.
2. Takahashi H, Kashima T, Kimura S, Murata N, Takaba T, Iwade K, Abe T, Tainaka H, Yasumori T, Echizen H. Pharmacokinetic interaction between warfarin and a uricosuric agent, bucolome: application of in vitro approaches to predicting in vivo reduction of (S)-warfarin clearance. *Drug Metab Dispos* (1999) 27, 1179–86.
3. Matsumoto K, Ishida S, Ueno K, Hashimoto H, Takada M, Tanaka K, Kamakura S, Miyatake K, Shibakawa M. The stereoselective effects of bucolome on the pharmacokinetics and pharmacodynamics of racemic warfarin. *J Clin Pharmacol* (2001) 41, 459–64.
4. Osawa M, Hada N, Matsumoto K, Hasegawa T, Kobayashi D, Morimoto Y, Yamaguchi M, Kanamoto I, Nakagawa T, Sugibayashi K. Usefulness of coadministration of bucolome in warfarin therapy: pharmacokinetic and pharmacodynamic analysis using outpatient prescriptions. *Int J Pharm* (2005) 293, 43–9.
5. Murosaki N, Senoh H, Takemoto M. Intraluminal ureteral hematoma complicating anticoagulant therapy [In Japanese]. *Nippon Hinyokika Gakkai Zasshi* (2005) 96, 564–7.

Carbenoxolone + Antacids

There is some evidence to suggest that antacids may possibly reduce the bioavailability of carbenoxolone liquid.

Clinical evidence, mechanism, importance and management

In a study in 6 healthy subjects, the bioavailability of carbenoxolone in a liquid formulation was found to be approximately half that of carbenoxolone in granular and capsule formulations when each preparation was given with an **aluminium/magnesium hydroxide** antacid.[1] The extent to which antacids might reduce the ulcer-healing effects of carbenoxolone liquid seems not to have been assessed, but consider the possibility of a reduction in its efficacy if an antacid is also given.

NOTE. The reader is cautioned that this monograph is included purely for archival purposes, and is no longer subject to systematic revision and update.

1. Crema F, Parini J, Visconti M, Perucca E. Effetto degli antiacidi sulla biodisponibilità del carbenoxolone. *Farmaco (Prat)* (1987) 42, 357–64.

Carbenoxolone + Antihypertensives

Carbenoxolone causes fluid retention and raises blood pressure in some patients. This may be expected to oppose the effects of antihypertensive drugs. The potassium-depleting effects of carbenoxolone and diuretics such as the thiazides or loop diuretics can be additive. Both spironolactone and amiloride can oppose the ulcer-healing effects of carbenoxolone.

Clinical evidence, mechanism, importance and management

(a) Antihypertensives, general

In a study, 5 out of 10 patients taking carbenoxolone 300 mg daily, and 2 out of 10 patients taking carbenoxolone 150 mg daily, had a rise in their diastolic blood pressure of 20 mmHg or more.[1] Other reports[2-8] confirm that hypertension and fluid retention occur in patients taking carbenoxolone, with the reported incidence of hypertension varying from as low as 4%[8] to as high as 50%,[7] and fluid retention occurring in 0%[2] to 46%[7] of patients.

The reason for the blood pressure rise is that carbenoxolone has mineralocorticoid-like activity and therefore causes sodium and water retention.

There appear to be few direct reports of adverse interactions between antihypertensives and carbenoxolone. However, patients taking carbenoxolone should have regular checks on their weight and blood pressure, and carbenoxolone should be used with caution, if at all, in those with cardiac disease such as hypertension or congestive heart failure.

For a discussion of case reports of hypokalaemia with the concurrent use of diuretics and carbenoxolone, see *Diuretics*, below.

(b) Diuretics

Isolated reports describe hypokalaemia in patients given carbenoxolone and a loop or thiazide diuretic. For example, rhabdomyolysis and acute tubular necrosis associated with severe hypokalaemia has been reported in a patient given carbenoxolone and **chlortalidone**, without a potassium supplement.[9] Another case report describes laryngospasm and stridor secondary to hypokalaemia and alkalosis in a patient taking long-term **furosemide** and a carbenoxolone-containing antacid (*Pyrogastrone*).[10]

Thiazide diuretics have been used to control the oedema and hypertension caused by carbenoxolone. However, if these or other potassium-depleting diuretics (see 'Table 26.1', p.1117) are used it should be remembered that the potassium-losing effects of carbenoxolone and the diuretic may be additive, and therefore a potassium supplement may be needed to prevent hypokalaemia. Note that **spironolactone**[3] and **amiloride**[11] are best avoided with carbenoxolone because they oppose its ulcer-healing effects. Nevertheless, there is a case report of the successful use of **spironolactone** (an aldosterone antagonist) in a patient with carbenoxolone-associated hypertension and hypokalaemia.[12]

Possible alternatives to carbenoxolone are the H_2-receptor antagonists, or the proton pump inhibitors, which do not appear to interact with antihypertensives.

NOTE. The reader is cautioned that this monograph is included purely for archival purposes, and is no longer subject to systematic revision and update.

1. Turpie AGG, Thomson TJ. Carbenoxolone sodium in the treatment of gastric ulcer with special reference to side-effects. *Gut* (1965) 6, 591.
2. Bank S, Marks IN. Maintenance carbenoxolone sodium in the prevention of gastric ulcer recurrence. In: Baron A, Sullivan S, eds. Carbenoxolone Sodium: London: Butterworths; 1970. p. 103–16.
3. Doll R, Langman MJS, Shawdon HH. Treatment of gastric ulcer with carbenoxolone: antagonistic effect of spironolactone. *Gut* (1968) 9, 42–5.
4. Montgomery RD, Cookson JB. Comparative trial of carbenoxolone and a deglycyrrhizinated liquorice preparation (Caved-S). *Clin Trials J* (1972) 9, 33–5.
5. Langman MJS, Knapp DR, Wakley EJ. Treatment of chronic gastric ulcer with carbenoxolone and gefarnate: a comparative trial. *BMJ* (1973) 3, 84–6.
6. Horwich L, Galloway R. Treatment of gastric ulceration with carbenoxolone sodium: clinical and radiological evaluation. *BMJ* (1965) 2, 1274–7.
7. Fraser PM, Doll R, Langman MJS, Misiewicz JJ, Shawdon HH. Clinical trial of a new carbenoxolone analogue (BX-24), zinc sulphate, and vitamin A in the treatment of gastric ulcer. *Gut* (1972) 13, 459–63.
8. Montgomery RD. Side effects of carbenoxolone sodium: a study of ambulant therapy of gastric ulcer. *Gut* (1967) 8, 148–50.
9. Descamps C, Vandenbroucke JM, van Ypersele de Strihou C. Rhabdomyolysis and acute tubular necrosis associated with carbenoxolone and diuretic treatment. *BMJ* (1977) 1, 272.
10. Sarkar SK. Stridor due to drug-induced hypokalaemic alkalosis. *J Laryngol Otol* (1987) 101, 197–8.
11. Reed PI, Lewis SI, Vincent-Brown A, Holdstock DJ, Gribble RJN, Murgatroyd RE, Baron JH. The influence of amiloride on the therapeutic and metabolic effects of carbenoxolone in patients with gastric ulcer. *Scand J Gastroenterol* (1980) 15 (Suppl 65), 51–5.
12. Celi FS, D'Erasmo E, Oddo CM, Aliberti G. Carbenoxolone and hypokalaemic hypertension: case report. *Riv Eur Sci Med Farmacol* (1988) 10, 383–4.

Carbenoxolone + Phenytoin

In a study in 4 healthy subjects a single 100-mg dose of phenytoin had no significant effect on the half-life of a single 100-mg dose of carbenoxo-

lone.[1] This limited evidence would seem to suggest that phenytoin is unlikely to alter the effects of carbenoxolone.

NOTE. The reader is cautioned that this monograph is included purely for archival purposes, and is no longer subject to systematic revision and update.

1. Thornton PC, Papouchado M, Reed PI. Carbenoxolone interactions in man - preliminary report. *Scand J Gastroenterol* (1980) 15 (Suppl 65), 35–9.

Carbenoxolone + Sulfonylureas

Chlorpropamide appears to reduce the levels of carbenoxolone, whereas tolbutamide does not appear to have any significant effect on the pharmacokinetics of carbenoxolone.

Clinical evidence, mechanism, importance and management

In a study in 4 healthy subjects, a single 500-mg dose of **tolbutamide** had no significant effect on the half-life of a single 100-mg dose of carbenoxolone, whereas a single 250-mg dose of **chlorpropamide** delayed the absorption of carbenoxolone and reduced its plasma levels in 6 patients taking carbenoxolone 100 mg three times daily.[1] The limited evidence suggests that tolbutamide would not be expected to alter the effects of carbenoxolone; however, the clinical relevance of the interaction with chlorpropamide is uncertain.

NOTE. The reader is cautioned that this monograph is included purely for archival purposes, and is no longer subject to systematic revision and update.

1. Thornton PC, Papouchado M, Reed PI. Carbenoxolone interactions in man - preliminary report. *Scand J Gastroenterol* (1980) 15 (Suppl 65), 35–9.

Ciclosporin + Muromonab-CD3

Muromonab-CD3 appears to increase ciclosporin blood concentrations, and there is an increased risk of reactivation of viral infections on their concurrent use.

Clinical evidence, mechanism, importance and management

In the preliminary report of a retrospective review, when 5 mg of muromonab-CD3 was given daily for 10 days to 10 kidney transplant patients to treat acute rejection, their ciclosporin minimum concentrations on day 8 were higher than before the muromonab-CD3 was started, despite a 50% reduction in the ciclosporin dose. When the muromonab-CD3 was withdrawn, the ciclosporin dose needed to be increased again.[1] The US manufacturer formerly noted that there is an increased risk of reactivation of cytomegalovirus when an immunosuppressive regimen including ciclosporin is used after an anti-lymphocyte antibody such as muromonab-CD3.[2]

The reasons for the increase in ciclosporin concentrations are not understood. Muromonab-CD3 augments the immunosuppressant effects of ciclosporin and consequently increases the risk of infection and reactivation of viral infections. Note that the authors of the first study say that ciclosporin doses are routinely reduced before use of muromonab-CD3 to avoid over-immunosuppression, and therefore the relevance of their retrospective findings on ciclosporin concentrations is uncertain.

NOTE. The reader is cautioned that this monograph is included purely for archival purposes, and is no longer subject to systematic revision and update.

1. Vrahnos D, Sanchez J, Vasquez EM, Pollak R, Maddux MS. Cyclosporine levels during OKT3 treatment of acute renal allograft rejection. *Pharmacotherapy* (1991) 11, 278.
2. Orthoclone OKT3 (Muromonab-CD3). Ortho Biotech. US Prescribing information, November 2004.

Clofibrate + Miscellaneous

Combined hormonal contraceptives appear to increase the clearance of clofibrate, and rifampicin (rifampin) might reduce the plasma levels of the active metabolite of clofibrate. Probenecid appears to increase the levels of clofibric acid, the active metabolite of clofibrate. Colestyramine and colestipol do not alter the pharmacokinetics of clofibrate

The use of clofibrate in patients with nephrotic syndrome taking furosemide has sometimes led to marked diuresis with severe and disabling adverse muscular effects.

Clofibrate appears to slightly reduce ibuprofen exposure.

Clinical evidence, mechanism, importance and management

(a) Bile-acid binding resins

In a study in 24 healthy subjects **colestipol** 10 g daily did not alter the pharmacokinetics of clofibrate 500 mg daily, when both drugs were given at the same time, for 6 days.[1] Similarly, in a study in 6 patients, **colestyramine** 4 g four times daily had no effect on the fasting plasma levels, urinary and faecal excretion, or the half-life of clofibrate 1 g twice daily. In this study, the morning and evening doses of **colestyramine** were taken at the same time as the clofibrate.[2] The findings of these studies show that there is no need to separate administration of clofibrate from **colestipol** or **colestyramine**.

(b) Combined hormonal contraceptives

A comparative study in men, women, and women taking oral combined hormonal contraceptives found that the clearance of clofibrate was 48% higher in those taking combined hormonal contraceptives, compared with women not taking these contraceptives, apparently due to an increase in clofibrate glucuronidation.[3] Another study found that 21 women taking oral hormonal contraceptives had a 25% higher urinary excretion of clofibric acid glucuronide compared with women not taking oral contraceptives.[4] A couple of early case reports describe increased cholesterol levels in two women with familial hypercholesterolaemia taking clofibrate when they were also given a high-dose oral combined hormonal contraceptive (ethinylestradiol 50 micrograms with norethisterone or norgestrel).[5,6]

Combined hormonal contraceptives are known inducers of glucuronidation, a route by which many of the fibrates are metabolised. Combined hormonal contraceptives are also known to be associated with some adverse effects on plasma lipids, which can depend on the progestogen used. Both of these effects might contribute to attenuation of the benefits of fibrates.

Although the evidence is indirect, it appears that combined hormonal contraceptives might reduce clofibrate exposure. Neither of the pharmacokinetic studies addressed the question of whether concurrent use might reduce clofibrate efficacy, but it would seem prudent to be aware that this could be possible. Note also that combined hormonal contraceptives themselves can have adverse effects on serum lipids, which might also attenuate the benefit of fibrates. Further, bear in mind that the indications for fibrates might be a contraindication to the use of combined hormonal contraceptives if other risk factors for arterial disease are present.

(c) Diuretics

Three patients with hyperlipoproteinaemia secondary to nephrotic syndrome, taking **furosemide** 80 to 500 mg daily, developed severe muscle pain, low lumbar backache, stiffness, and general malaise with pronounced diuresis, within 3 days of starting to take clofibrate 1 to 2 g daily. Similarly, a patient taking **bendroflumethiazide** 10 mg daily developed adverse muscle effects within 3 days of starting to take clofibrate 2 g daily. Of these 4 patients, 3 had documented raised serum transaminase levels or creatine phosphokinase levels, and 3 were also taking **spironolactone** 75 or 100 mg daily. Two other patients had raised levels of serum transaminases or creatine phosphokinase while taking clofibrate with **furosemide**. Further study in 4 of the 6 patients discussed above and 4 healthy controls, found that free serum clofibrate was substantially higher in the patients, and this correlated with low serum albumin. Urinary clofibrate excretion was markedly delayed.[7]

The reason for these findings is not understood. The marked diuresis may have been due to competition and displacement of furosemide by clofibrate from its plasma protein binding sites. Clofibrate occasionally causes muscle toxicity, which could have been exacerbated by the urinary loss of sodium and potassium and the increase in the half-life of clofibrate.

The clinical documentation for an interaction between diuretics and clofibrate seems to be limited to these reports. In the case of clofibrate and furosemide it appears to be a combination of a drug-drug interaction, with or without a drug-disease interaction (clofibrate with nephrotic syndrome). The authors of one report[7] suggest that serum proteins and renal function should be checked before giving clofibrate to any patient. If serum albumin is low, the total daily dose of clofibrate should not exceed 500 mg for each 1 g per 100 mL of the albumin concentration. However, note that this guidance dates from the 1970s.

(d) Ibuprofen

In a pharmacokinetic study, 12 healthy subjects were given a single 400-mg dose of ibuprofen alone and then after pretreatment with clofibrate 1 g twice daily for 7 days. The AUC of *R*-ibuprofen was reduced by 69% and the AUC of *S*-ibuprofen was reduced by 32%, with a 239% and 61% increase in clearance of *R*-ibuprofen and *S*-ibuprofen, respectively. Analysis showed that the clearance of *R*-ibuprofen by inversion to *S*-ibuprofen was increased, as well as clearance by other mechanisms.[8] *S*-ibuprofen is primarily responsible for the therapeutic effect of ibuprofen, and it seems unlikely that the slight reduction in the levels of this active enantiomer seen with clofibrate will be clinically relevant.

(e) Probenecid

A pharmacokinetic study in 4 healthy subjects taking clofibrate 500 mg every 12 hours found that probenecid 500 mg every 6 hours for 7 days almost doubled the steady-state levels of clofibric acid, the active metabolite of clofibrate, from 72 mg/L to 129 mg/L, and raised the free clofibric acid levels from 2.5 mg/L to 9.1 mg/L. The suggested reason is that probenecid reduces the renal clearance of clofibrate and clofibric acid glucuronide and/or that it inhibits glucuronidation.[9] The clinical importance of this interaction is uncertain, but it may be prudent to be alert for increased clofibrate adverse effects (e.g. gastrointestinal disturbances, headache, fatigue) and review treatment if these become a problem. There appears to be no information about other fibrates and probenecid, but other fibrates also undergo glucuronidation.

(f) Rifampicin (Rifampin)

In a study in 5 healthy subjects, the steady-state plasma levels of the active metabolite of clofibrate, clofibric acid, were reduced by 35% after they took rifampicin 600 mg daily for 7 days.[10] This reduction in clofibric acid levels appears to occur because its metabolism by the liver and/or the kidneys is increased.[10] On the basis of this study it would seem prudent to monitor serum lipid levels of patients taking clofibrate if rifampicin is added, and to increase the clofibrate dose if necessary. More study is needed to establish this interaction.

NOTE. The reader is cautioned that this monograph is included purely for archival purposes, and is no longer subject to systematic revision and update.

1. DeSante KA, DiSanto AR, Albert KS, Weber DJ, Welch RD, Vecchio TJ. The effect of colestipol hydrochloride on the bioavailability and pharmacokinetics of clofibrate. *J Clin Pharmacol* (1979) 19, 721–25.
2. Sedaghat A, Ahrens EH. Lack of effect of cholestyramine on the pharmacokinetics of clofibrate in man. *Eur J Clin Invest* (1975) 5, 177–85.

3. Miners JO, Robson RA, Birkett DJ. Gender and oral contraceptive steroids as determinants of drug glucuronidation: effects on clofibric acid elimination. *Br J Clin Pharmacol* (1984) 18, 240–43.
4. Liu H-F, Magdalou J, Nicolas A, Lafaurie C, Siest G. Oral contraceptives stimulate the excretion of clofibric acid glucuronide in women and female rats. *Gen Pharmacol* (1991) 22, 393–7.
5. Smith RBW, Prior IAM. Oral-contraceptive opposition to hypocholesterolaemic action of clofibrate. *Lancet* (1968) 1, 750–1.
6. Robertson-Rintoul J. Raised serum-lipids and oral contraceptives. *Lancet* (1972) 2, 1320–21.
7. Bridgman JF, Rosen SM, Thorp JM. Complications during clofibrate treatment of nephrotic-syndrome hyperlipoproteinaemia. *Lancet* (1972) ii, 506–9.
8. Scheuerer S, Hall SD, Williams KM, Geisslinger G. Effect of clofibrate on the chiral inversion of ibuprofen in healthy volunteers. *Clin Pharmacol Ther* (1998) 64, 168–76.
9. Veenendaal JR, Brooks PM, Meffin PJ. Probenecid-clofibrate interaction. *Clin Pharmacol Ther* (1981) 29, 351–8.
10. Houin G, Tillement J-P. Clofibrate and enzymatic induction in man. *Int J Clin Pharmacol Ther Toxicol* (1978) 16, 150–4.

Glutethimide + Miscellaneous

Compared with either drug alone, the use of glutethimide with alcohol results in greater impairment in some psychomotor tests, but improvement in others. Glutethimide might potentiate and prolong the analgesic effect of codeine and might also to worsen psychomotor performance in smokers more than in non-smokers. The anticoagulant effects of warfarin and ethyl biscoumacetate can be decreased by glutethimide.

Clinical evidence, mechanism, importance and management

(a) Alcohol

In a series of studies, blood-alcohol concentrations were raised by 11% by glutethimide, while plasma and urinary glutethimide concentrations were reduced.[1] Neither glutethimide nor alcohol alone impaired reaction times, but the combination did. However, in two other tests (tracking efficacy and finger tapping) impairment was greatest after glutethimide alone and reduced by the presence of alcohol.[2] In contrast, a later study found that glutethimide did not subjectively or objectively impair the performance of a number of psychomotor skill tests related to driving, and did not interact with alcohol given the morning after the glutethimide dose.[1] Both drugs are CNS depressants and their effects would be expected to be additive.

The information is limited and somewhat contradictory; nevertheless, patients should be warned about the probable results of taking glutethimide and alcohol together. Driving, handling dangerous machinery, or undertaking any task needing alertness and full co-ordination, is likely to be made more difficult and hazardous. There is no evidence of a hangover effect, which could result in an interaction with alcohol the next day.[1]

(b) Codeine

A study in *animals* suggested that glutethimide might potentiate and prolong the analgesic effect of codeine by increasing the plasma concentration of its morphine metabolite.[3] Glutethimide given with codeine can produce a euphoric state and might be addictive; seizures and psychosis have been reported.[4] Two studies have reported 21 deaths associated with concurrent use.[5,6] Given the wide availability of alternative hypno-sedatives, it would seem prudent to choose a safer alternative.

(c) Tobacco smoking

A study in 7 subjects found that glutethimide appeared to worsen psychomotor performance in smokers more than in non-smokers, possibly due to an increase in glutethimide absorption.[7] However there would seem to be no need for particular caution if smokers take glutethimide.

(d) Warfarin and related drugs

Ten subjects stabilised on warfarin, with average prothrombin times of 18.8 seconds, had a mean reduction of 2.7 seconds in their prothrombin times after they took glutethimide 500 mg at bedtime for 4 weeks.[8,9] Other studies have shown that up to 1 g of glutethimide daily for one to 3 weeks reduced the half-life of single-dose warfarin by between one-third to one-half.[10,11] Conversely, an unexplained report describes a paradoxical increase in prothrombin times and severe bruising in a patient stabilised on warfarin who took 3.5 g of glutethimide over a 5-day period.[12]

Glutethimide 500 or 750 mg daily for 10 days has been found to reduce the half-life of single-dose **ethyl biscoumacetate** by about one-third,[13,14] whereas in contrast, an early study in 25 patients taking **ethyl biscoumacetate** found no evidence of an interaction.[15]

Glutethimide is a liver enzyme inducer, which increases the metabolism and clearance of the anticoagulants from the body, thereby reducing their effects.[8-11,13,14] There is no obvious explanation for the reports finding no interaction or increased effects.

The interaction of glutethimide with warfarin is established, while the interaction with **ethyl biscoumacetate** is uncertain. Information about both interactions is limited and there seems to be nothing documented about any other anticoagulant. However, it would be prudent to monitor the effect of adding glutethimide to patients taking any coumarin, being alert for the need to increase the anticoagulant dose. Other interactions due to enzyme induction can take several weeks to develop fully and persist after withdrawal, so good monitoring and dose adjustment should continue until anticoagulant stability is confirmed. The benzodiazepines might be useful non-interacting alternatives, see 'Coumarins + Benzodiazepines and related drugs', p.412.

NOTE. The reader is cautioned that this monograph is included purely for archival purposes, and is no longer subject to systematic revision and update.

1. Saario I, Linnoila M. Effect of subacute treatment with hypnotics, alone or in combination with alcohol, on psychomotor skills related to driving. *Acta Pharmacol Toxicol (Copenh)* (1976) 38, 382–92.
2. Mould GP, Curry SH, Binns TB. Interactions of glutethimide and phenobarbitone with ethanol in man. *J Pharm Pharmacol* (1972) 24, 894–9.
3. Popa D, Loghin F, Imre S, Curea E. The study of codeine-gluthetimide [sic] pharmacokinetic interaction in rats. *J Pharm Biomed Anal* (2003) 32, 867–77.
4. Shamoian CA. Codeine and glutethimide: euphoretic, addicting combination. *N Y State J Med* (1975) 75, 97–9.
5. Bender FH, Cooper JV, Dreyfus R. Fatalities associated with an acute overdose of glutethimide (Doriden) and codeine. *Vet Hum Toxicol* (1988) 30, 332–3.
6. Bailey DN, Shaw RF. Blood concentrations and clinical findings in nonfatal and fatal intoxications involving glutethimide and codeine. *J Toxicol Clin Toxicol* (1985-1986) 23, 557–70.
7. Crow JW, Lain P, Bochner F, Shoeman DW, Azarnoff DL. Glutethimide and 4-OH glutethimide: pharmacokinetics and effect on performance in man. *Clin Pharmacol Ther* (1977) 22, 458–64.
8. Udall JA. Clinical implications of warfarin interactions with five sedatives. *Am J Cardiol* (1975) 35, 67–71.
9. Udall JA. Warfarin interactions with chloral hydrate and glutethimide. *Curr Ther Res* (1975) 17, 67–74.
10. Corn M. Effect of phenobarbital and glutethimide on biological half-life of warfarin. *Thromb Diath Haemorrh* (1966) 16, 606–12.
11. MacDonald MG, Robinson DS, Sylwester D, Jaffe JJ. The effects of phenobarbital, chloral betaine, and glutethimide administration on warfarin plasma levels and hypoprothrombinemic responses in man. *Clin Pharmacol Ther* (1969) 10, 80–4.
12. Taylor PJ. Hemorrhage while on anticoagulant therapy precipitated by drug interaction. *Ariz Med* (1967) 24, 697–9.
13. van Dam FE, Gribnau-Overkamp MJH. The effect of some sedatives (phenobarbital, gluthetimide, chlordiazepoxide, chloral hydrate) on the rate of disappearance of ethyl biscoumacetate from the plasma. *Folia Med Neerl* (1967) 10, 141–5.
14. van Dam FE, Overkamp M, Haanen C. The interaction of drugs. *Lancet* (1966) ii, 1027.
15. Grilli H. Gluthetimida y tiempo de protrombina. Su aplicación en la terapéutica anticoagulante. *Prensa Med Argent* (1959) 46, 2867–9.

Guanadrel + Digoxin

Guanadrel did not affect the pharmacokinetics of a single dose of digoxin in one study.

Clinical evidence, mechanism, importance and management

In 13 healthy subjects, guanadrel 10 mg orally every 12 hours for 8 days did not affect the pharmacokinetics of a single 1-mg intravenous dose of digoxin given on day 3. One subject experienced a 10-minute episode of asymptomatic second-degree heart block (Wenckebach) 3 hours after the dose of digoxin. The reason for this effect was not clear.[1] Note that the digoxin dose in this study was high and was given intravenously. There seem to be no other reports of adverse interactions between digoxin and guanadrel. No digoxin dose adjustment is likely to be required on concurrent use.

NOTE. The reader is cautioned that this monograph is included purely for archival purposes, and is no longer subject to systematic revision and update.

1. Wright CE, Andreadis NA. Digoxin pharmacokinetics when administered concurrently with guanadrel sulfate. *Drug Intell Clin Pharm* (1986) 20, 465.

Halofantrine + Antacids

Magnesium carbonate halves the maximum plasma levels of halofantrine. Aluminium hydroxide and magnesium trisilicate seem less likely to interact.

Clinical evidence

A single-dose study in healthy subjects found that **magnesium carbonate** 1 g reduced the maximum plasma levels of halofantrine 500 mg by almost 50%. The AUC was also reduced by 28%, but this was not statistically significant. The active metabolite of halofantrine, which is equally potent, was similarly affected.[1]

Mechanism

Magnesium carbonate might decrease the absorption of halofantrine. An *in vitro* study showed that the halofantrine adsorptive capacity of various antacids was highest for magnesium carbonate, intermediate for **aluminium hydroxide**, and least for **magnesium trisilicate**.[1]

Importance and management

The pharmacokinetic interaction between halofantrine and magnesium carbonate appears to be established. Its clinical importance does not seem to have been assessed, but the authors note that the clinical efficacy of halofantrine is related to peak levels, and therefore they consider that magnesium carbonate might affect antimalarial efficacy.[1] One way to minimise the interaction is to separate the dosages of halofantrine and magnesium carbonate as much as possible (at least 2 to 3 hours has worked with other drugs that interact with antacids in this way) to reduce admixture in the gut. There do not appear to be any studies to see if other antacids behave similarly, but the *in vitro* data with aluminium hydroxide and magnesium trisilicate (see Mechanism, above) suggest that they are less likely to interact.[1]

NOTE. The reader is cautioned that this monograph is included purely for archival purposes, and is no longer subject to systematic revision and update.

1. Aideloje SO, Onyeji CO, Ugwu NC. Altered pharmacokinetics of halofantrine by an antacid, magnesium carbonate. *Eur J Pharm Biopharm* (1998) 46, 299–303.

Halofantrine + Miscellaneous

Halofantrine prolongs the QT interval and therefore should not be used with other drugs that can prolong the QT interval because of the

increased risk of cardiac arrhythmias. The concurrent and sequential use of halofantrine and mefloquine markedly increased the risk of clinically important increases in the QT interval.

Pyrimethamine/sulfadoxine and tetracycline have been shown to increase halofantrine levels. *In vitro* studies suggest that diltiazem, erythromycin, ketoconazole, mefloquine, quinine, and quinidine might also increase the toxicity of halofantrine. Fatty food markedly increases halofantrine levels. Grapefruit juice has a similar effect.

Clinical evidence, mechanism, importance and management

(a) CYP3A4 inhibitors

A study in *animals* found that **ketoconazole** roughly doubled the AUC of halofantrine and inhibited its metabolism to the equipotent metabolite, desbutylhalofantrine.[1] **Ketoconazole** markedly inhibited the metabolism of halofantrine by CYP3A4 *in vitro*.[2,3] It has been suggested that the rise in halofantrine levels could reasonably be expected to increase toxicity.[2,3] Other CYP3A4 inhibitors, such as **diltiazem** and **erythromycin**, also inhibited the metabolism of halofantrine *in vitro*,[3] which is in line with their known clinical effects on other CYP3A4 substrates. It would therefore seem prudent to be cautious if any of these drugs, or other known CYP3A4 inhibitors (see 'Table 1.9', p.11, for a list), are given with halofantrine, as raised halofantrine levels may increase its adverse cardiac effects, see *Drugs that prolong the QT interval*, below. *In vitro* studies[2,3] also found that **quinine** and **quinidine** had moderate inhibitory effects on halofantrine metabolism by CYP3A4, but note that these drugs are not known to be clinically significant inhibitors of this isoenzyme. Probably of more importance is the potential for additive cardiac effects, see *Drugs that prolong the QT interval*, below.

(b) Drugs that prolong the QT interval

Halofantrine, in therapeutic doses, can prolong the QT interval in the majority of patients, causing ventricular arrhythmias in a very small number. By 1993, worldwide, 14 cases of cardiac arrhythmias associated with halofantrine had been reported, and 8 patients were known to have died. In order to reduce the likelihood of arrhythmias, in 1994 the CSM in the UK advised that halofantrine should not be taken with drugs that may induce arrhythmias. They named **chloroquine**, **mefloquine**, **quinine**, **tricyclic antidepressants**, **antipsychotics**, **certain antiarrhythmics**, **terfenadine** and **astemizole**, as well as drugs causing electrolyte disturbances.[4] Although not listed, it would seem prudent to avoid other drugs that prolong the QT interval. For a list, see 'Table 9.2', p.273.

Animal studies found that although **mefloquine** alone did not significantly alter the QTc interval, it enhanced the effects of halofantrine by increasing blood levels.[5] Similarly, a study in patients with malaria found that the risk of clinically relevant QT prolongation was increased twofold when halofantrine was used after **mefloquine** failure (7 of 10 patients), when compared with use as primary treatment (18 of 51 patients). However, the authors note that their population had longer baseline QT intervals than the average population, which may have made them more susceptible to the effects of halofantrine[6] The manufacturers of **mefloquine**[7,8] contraindicate the concurrent use of halofantrine, and the sequential use of halofantrine after **mefloquine** treatment.

(c) Food

A study in 6 healthy subjects found that the maximum plasma levels and AUC of a single 250-mg dose of halofantrine were increased by about 6.6-fold and 2.9-fold, respectively, when given with a **fatty meal** rather than in a fasting state. The AUC of the metabolite desbutylhalofantrine was also increased.[9] *Animal* data suggest that **fats** may reduce the presystemic metabolism of halofantrine.[1] As this is likely to increase the risk of halofantrine-induced arrhythmias (see *Drugs that prolong the QT interval*, above), halofantrine should not be taken with **meals**, but should be taken on an empty stomach.[4]

(d) Grapefruit juice or Orange juice

A crossover study in 12 healthy subjects given halofantrine 500 mg with 250 mL of either water, orange juice or grapefruit juice (standard strength), found that grapefruit juice increased the AUC and peak plasma levels of halofantrine by 2.8-fold and 3.2-fold, respectively. The QTc interval increased by 17 milliseconds with halofantrine, and by 31 milliseconds when grapefruit juice was also given. Orange juice did not affect the pharmacokinetics or pharmacodynamics of halofantrine.[10] These data suggest that grapefruit juice should be avoided by patients taking halofantrine due to the increased risk of arrhythmias.[10]

(e) Pyrimethamine/Sulfadoxine

In a preliminary study in healthy subjects, pyrimethamine/sulfadoxine (*Fansidar*) raised the AUC_{0-6} and peak plasma levels of halofantrine by about 60%, without changing the overall AUC. This might lead to an increased incidence of arrhythmias,[11] see *Drugs that prolong the QT interval*, above.

(f) Tetracyclines

A study in 8 healthy subjects found that **tetracycline** 500 mg twice daily for 7 days increased the maximum plasma levels, AUC and elimination half-life of a single 500-mg dose of halofantrine by 146%, 99%, and 73%, respectively. Increases in the major metabolite of halofantrine also occurred in the presence of **tetracycline**.[12] As both halofantrine and **tetracycline** are excreted into the bile, competition for this elimination route may result in increased plasma levels. There may be an increased risk of halofantrine toxicity if it is used with higher doses of tetracycline.[12]

NOTE. The reader is cautioned that this monograph is included purely for archival purposes, and is no longer subject to systematic revision and update.

1. Khoo S-M, Porter CJH, Edwards GA, Charman WN. Metabolism of halofantrine to its equipotent metabolite, desbutylhalofantrine, is decreased when orally administered with ketoconazole. *J Pharm Sci* (1998) 87, 1538–41.
2. Baune B, Furlan V, Taburet AM, Farinotti R. Effect of selected antimalarial drugs and inhibitors of cytochrome P-450 3A4 on halofantrine metabolism by human liver microsomes. *Drug Metab Dispos* (1999) 27, 565–8.
3. Baune B, Flinois JP, Furlan V, Gimenez F, Taburet AM, Becquemont L, Farinotti R. Halofantrine metabolism in microsomes in man: major role of CYP 3A4 and CYP 3A5. *J Pharm Pharmacol* (1999) 51, 419–26.
4. Committee on Safety of Medicines/Medicines Control Agency. Cardiac arrhythmias with halofantrine (Halfan). *Current Problems* (1994) 20, 6.
5. Lightbown ID, Lambert JP, Edwards G, Coker SJ. Potentiation of halofantrine-induced QTc prolongation by mefloquine: correlation with blood concentrations of halofantrine. *Br J Pharmacol* (2001) 132, 197–204.
6. Nosten F, ter Kuile FO, Luxemburger C, Woodrow C, Kyle DE, Chongsuphajaisiddhi T, White NJ. Cardiac effects of antimalarial treatment with halofantrine. *Lancet* (1993) 341, 1054–6.
7. Lariam (Mefloquine hydrochloride). Roche Products Ltd. UK Summary of product characteristics, November 2011.
8. Lariam (Mefloquine hydrochloride). Roche Pharmaceuticals. US Prescribing information, September 2008.
9. Milton K, Edwards G, Ward SA, Orme ML'E, Breckenridge AM. Pharmacokinetics of halofantrine in man: effects of food and dose size. *Br J Clin Pharmacol* (1989) 28, 71–7.
10. Charbit B, Becquemont L, Lepère B, Peytavin G, Funck-Brentano C. Pharmacokinetic and pharmacodynamic interaction between grapefruit juice and halofantrine. *Clin Pharmacol Ther* (2002) 72, 514–23.
11. Hombhanje FW. Effect of a single dose of Fansidar™ on the pharmacokinetics of halofantrine in healthy volunteers: a preliminary report. *Br J Clin Pharmacol* (2000) 49, 283–4.
12. Bassi PU, Onyeji CO, Ukponmwan OE. Effects of tetracycline on the pharmacokinetics of halofantrine in healthy volunteers. *Br J Clin Pharmacol* (2004) 58, 52–5.

Idoxuridine + Miscellaneous

The topical solution of idoxuridine, *Herpid*, contains the solvent dimethyl sulfoxide as an absorption enhancer. This can increase the absorption of many substances, and therefore no other topical medications should be used concurrently on the same areas as *Herpid*.[1]

NOTE. The reader is cautioned that this monograph is included purely for archival purposes, and is no longer subject to systematic revision and update.

1. Herpid (Idoxuridine). Astellas Pharma Ltd. UK Summary of product characteristics, January 2008.

Mecamylamine + Alcohol

Mecamylamine appears to reduce some of the effects of alcohol, without affecting blood-alcohol levels.

Clinical evidence, mechanism, importance and management

In a crossover study in 22 healthy subjects, a single 7.5- to 12.5-mg dose of mecamylamine reduced the levels of alcohol (0.7 or 0.8 g/kg) by about 14% (estimated from graph), and reduced the pleasurable and stimulant effects of alcohol.[1] A placebo-controlled study in 27 healthy subjects given a single 7.5- or 15-mg dose of mecamylamine with alcohol 0.8 g/kg found that none of the physiological effects of mecamylamine or alcohol, or blood-alcohol levels, were affected by concurrent use. Mecamylamine reduced the stimulant effects of alcohol and reduced the desire for more alcohol; this effect appeared greater in men.[2]

These studies suggest that mecamylamine can safely be given with alcohol; however, the manufacturer of a formerly available US preparation of mecamylamine warned that alcohol might enhance its hypotensive effect,[3] an effect common to the use of alcohol with many antihypertensive drugs, see 'Alcohol + Antihypertensives', p.55.

NOTE. The reader is cautioned that this monograph is included purely for archival purposes, and is no longer subject to systematic revision and update.

1. Blomqvist O, Hernandez-Avila CA, Van Kirk J, Rose JE, Kranzler HR. Mecamylamine modifies the pharmacokinetics and reinforcing effects of alcohol. *Alcohol Clin Exp Res* (2002) 26, 326–31.
2. Chi H, de Wit H. Mecamylamine attenuates the subjective stimulant-like effects of alcohol in social drinkers. *Alcohol Clin Exp Res* (2003) 27, 780–86.
3. Inversine (Mecamylamine). Targacept, Inc. US Prescribing information, July 2002.

Mequitazine + Miscellaneous

An isolated case describes torsade de pointes, possibly due to the use of spiramycin with mequitazine. Mequitazine does not affect the pharmacokinetics of theophylline.

Clinical evidence, mechanism, importance and management

(a) Spiramycin

A 21-year-old woman with congenital long QT syndrome had several syncopal attacks, at least one of which was caused by torsade de pointes. This was attributed to the concurrent use of mequitazine and spiramycin over a 2-day period. The problem resolved when the drugs were withdrawn.[1] This isolated case is of unknown general importance.

(b) Theophylline

In a study in 7 patients with asthma, the steady-state pharmacokinetics of theophylline were not significantly affected when mequitazine 6 mg daily was given for 3 weeks.[2]

There appears to be no direct evidence regarding aminophylline, but as it is metabolised to theophylline, no adverse interaction would be expected with mequitazine.

(c) Other drugs

Note that mequitazine is a phenothiazine that has been used as a sedating antihistamine. It would therefore be expected to share the general interactions of these classes of drugs.

NOTE. The reader is cautioned that this monograph is included purely for archival purposes, and is no longer subject to systematic revision and update.

1. Verdun F, Mansourati J, Jobic Y, Bouquin V, Munier S, Guillo P, Pagès Y, Boschat J, Blanc J-J. Torsades de pointes sous traitement par spiramycine et méquitazine. À propos d'un cas. *Arch Mal Coeur Vaiss* (1997) 90, 103–6.
2. Hasegawa T, Takagi K, Kuzuya T, Nadai M, Apichartpichean R, Muraoka I. Effect of mequitazine on the pharmacokinetics of theophylline in asthmatic patients. *Eur J Clin Pharmacol* (1990) 38, 255–8.

Methaqualone + Alcohol

The CNS depressant effects of alcohol are increased by the concurrent use of methaqualone with or without diphenhydramine.

Clinical evidence

(a) Methaqualone

A retrospective study of drivers arrested for driving under the influence of drugs and/or alcohol found that, generally speaking, those with blood methaqualone levels of 1 mg/L or less had no symptoms of sedation, whereas those with levels above 2 mg/L demonstrated staggering gait, drowsiness, incoherence and slurred speech. These effects were increased if the drivers had also been drinking alcohol. The authors state that the levels of methaqualone needed for driving skills to become impaired are considerably lowered by alcohol, but no precise measure of this is presented in the paper.[1]

(b) Methaqualone with diphenhydramine

A double-blind study in 12 healthy subjects given two *Mandrax* tablets (methaqualone 250 mg with diphenhydramine 25 mg) found that the resulting sedation and reduction in cognitive skills were enhanced by alcohol 0.5 g/kg. Residual amounts of a single dose of *Mandrax* continued to interact for as long as 72 hours. Methaqualone blood levels are also raised by regular moderate amounts of alcohol.[2] Similar effects on sedation were seen in another study.[3]

Mechanism

Alcohol, methaqualone and diphenhydramine are all CNS depressants, the effects of which can be additive. A hangover can occur because the elimination half-life of methaqualone is long (10 to 40 hours).

Importance and management

The interaction between methaqualone and alcohol is an established interaction of importance. Those taking either methaqualone or methaqualone with diphenhydramine should be warned that handling machinery, driving a car, or any other task requiring alertness and full coordination, will be made more difficult and hazardous if they drink alcohol. Levels of alcohol below the legal driving limit with normal amounts of methaqualone could cause considerable sedation. Patients should also be told that a significant interaction can possibly occur the following day, because methaqualone has a long half-life.

Note that methaqualone has been withdrawn from the market in many countries because of problems of abuse.

NOTE. The reader is cautioned that this monograph is included purely for archival purposes, and is no longer subject to systematic revision and update.

1. McCurdy HH, Solomons ET, Holbrook JM. Incidence of methaqualone in driving-under-the-influence (DUI) cases in the State of Georgia. *J Anal Toxicol* (1981) 5, 270–4.
2. Roden S, Harvey P, Mitchard M. The effect of ethanol on residual plasma methaqualone concentrations and behaviour in volunteers who have taken Mandrax. *Br J Clin Pharmacol* (1977) 4, 245–7.
3. Saario I, Linnoila M. Effect of subacute treatment with hypnotics, alone or in combination with alcohol, on psychomotor skills related to driving. *Acta Pharmacol Toxicol (Copenh)* (1976) 38, 382–92.

Methaqualone + Coumarins

Methaqualone may cause a very small and clinically unimportant reduction in the anticoagulant effects of warfarin.

Clinical evidence, mechanism, importance and management

The average prothrombin time of 10 patients stabilised on **warfarin** was 20.9 seconds before, 20.4 seconds during, and 19.6 seconds after taking methaqualone 300 mg at bedtime for 4 weeks.[1] The plasma **warfarin** levels of another patient were unaffected by methaqualone, although there was some evidence that enzyme induction had occurred.[2] Methaqualone has some enzyme-inducing effects so that any small changes in prothrombin times reflect a limited increase in the metabolism and clearance of **warfarin**, but these appear to be too small to be of clinical significance.[2,3] No special precautions seem to be necessary.

NOTE. The reader is cautioned that this monograph is included purely for archival purposes, and is no longer subject to systematic revision and update.

1. Udall JA. Clinical implications of warfarin interactions with five sedatives. *Am J Cardiol* (1975) 35, 67–71.
2. Whitfield JB, Moss DW, Neale G, Orme M, Breckenridge A. Changes in plasma γ-glutamyl transpeptidase activity associated with alterations in drug metabolism in man. *BMJ* (1973) 1, 316–18.
3. Nayak RK, Smyth RD, Chamberlain AP, Polk A, DeLong AF, Herczeg T, Chemburkar PB, Joslin RS, Reavey-Cantwell NH. Methaqualone pharmacokinetics after single- and multiple-dose administration in man. *J Pharmacokinet Biopharm* (1974) 2, 107–21.

Moracizine + Miscellaneous

Cimetidine slightly increases the exposure to moracizine, but moracizine does not affect the pharmacokinetics of cimetidine. A pharmacokinetic interaction occurs between moracizine and diltiazem resulting in increased systemic availability of moracizine and decreased systemic availability of diltiazem. There seems to be no adverse interaction between moracizine and low-dose propranolol.

Clinical evidence, mechanism, importance and management

(a) Cimetidine

In a study in 8 healthy subjects, cimetidine 300 mg four times daily for 7 days halved the clearance of a single 500-mg dose of moracizine and increased both its half-life and AUC by 39%. Moracizine is reported not to affect the pharmacokinetics of cimetidine. It is believed that these pharmacokinetic changes occur because cimetidine, a well-known, non-specific enzyme inducer, reduces moracizine metabolism by the liver.[1] Despite the increase in plasma moracizine concentrations, the PR and QRS intervals were not further prolonged. It has been suggested that this effect might occur because some of the metabolites of moracizine, whose production is inhibited by cimetidine, could also be pharmacologically active.

Concurrent use should be closely monitored for moracizine adverse effects (e.g. dizziness, abdominal pain, blurred vision), but measuring plasma moracizine levels is likely be of limited value because of the potential effects of the moracizine metabolites.

(b) Diltiazem

After 16 healthy subjects took both diltiazem 60 mg and moracizine 250 mg every 8 hours for 7 days, the maximum plasma concentration of moracizine was increased by 89%, the AUC was increased by 121%, and clearance was decreased by 54%. In addition, the maximum plasma concentration and AUC of diltiazem decreased by 36% and its clearance was increased by 52%. The AUCs for the diltiazem metabolites were not affected. No clinically important changes in ECG parameters were seen. However, the frequency of adverse events (e.g. headache, dizziness, paraesthesia) was greater on concurrent use (76%) than with either drug alone (54% and 45% for moracizine and diltiazem, respectively).[2]

Diltiazem is known to inhibit the cytochrome P450 enzyme system and probably reduces the rate of metabolism of moracizine, while moracizine increases that of diltiazem. The clinical importance of this interaction is not known. However, particular caution is advised if diltiazem and moracizine are given concurrently, in light of the increase in adverse events. Dose adjustments might also be required to obtain optimum therapeutic responses.[2]

(c) Propranolol

In controlled studies, the efficacy and tolerability of the combination of propranolol and moracizine was compared with either drug alone in patients with ventricular arrhythmias. The combination was well tolerated, with no evidence of any adverse interactions, nor any beneficial interactions. However, the dose of propranolol used was fairly low at 120 mg daily.[3,4]

NOTE. The reader is cautioned that this monograph is included purely for archival purposes, and is no longer subject to systematic revision and update.

1. Biollaz J, Shaheen O, Wood AJJ. Cimetidine inhibition of ethmozine metabolism. *Clin Pharmacol Ther* (1985) 37, 665–8.
2. Shum L, Pieniaszek HJ, Robinson CA, Davidson AF, Widner PJ, Benedek IH, Flamenbaum W. Pharmacokinetic interactions of moricizine and diltiazem in healthy volunteers. *J Clin Pharmacol* (1996) 36, 1161–8.
3. Pratt CM, Butman SM, Young JB, Knoll M, English LD. Antiarrhythmic efficacy of Ethmozine® (moricizine HCl) compared with disopyramide and propranolol. *Am J Cardiol* (1987) 60, 52F–58F.
4. Butman SM, Knoll ML, Gardin JM. Comparison of ethmozine to propranolol and the combination for ventricular arrhythmias. *Am J Cardiol* (1987) 60, 603–7.

Nefazodone + Loratadine

There is some evidence from one study that the concurrent use of nefazodone and loratadine increases the QT interval.

Clinical evidence, mechanism, importance and management

A randomised, placebo-controlled study in healthy subjects found that when they were given nefazodone 300 mg twice daily with loratadine 20 mg daily, the loratadine AUC was increased by 39%. Similarly, the QTc interval was increased by 21.6 milliseconds by concurrent use, which was about half the increase seen with terfenadine 60 mg twice daily given with the same dose of nefazodone (see also 'Astemizole or Terfenadine + Miscellaneous', p.1599). Neither nefazodone or loratadine alone prolonged the QTc interval.[1]

The findings for loratadine in this study were unexpected, as this antihistamine was considered to have no clinically relevant effect on the QT interval (but see also 'Table 15.2', p.629). The use of the Bazett formula to calculate QTc has been questioned,[2] but this is the most commonly used formula, and any overestimation would also apply to terfenadine.

This appears to be the only study to have directly compared loratadine with terfenadine, and although it shows that loratadine at twice the recommended dose has half the QT-prolonging effect of terfenadine (at the maximum recommended dose), it nevertheless raises questions about the cardiac safety of loratadine.[2,3] Further study is needed.

NOTE. The reader is cautioned that this monograph is included purely for archival purposes, and is no longer subject to systematic revision and update.

1. Abernethy DR, Barbey JT, Franc J, Brown KS, Feirrera I, Ford N, Salazar DE. Loratadine and terfenadine interaction with nefazodone; both antihistamines are associated with QTc prolongation. *Clin Pharmacol Ther* (2001) 69; 96–103.
2. Barbey JT. Loratadine/nefazodone interaction. *Clin Pharmacol Ther* (2002) 71, 403.
3. Abernethy DR. Reply. *Clin Pharmacol Ther* (2002) 71, 403.

Phenformin + Miscellaneous

Phenformin has been largely withdrawn worldwide because it was associated with a high incidence of lactic acidosis. It's interactions from when it was available are summarised here.

Clinical evidence, mechanism, importance and management

(a) Alcohol

A controlled study in 5 ketosis-resistant patients with type 2 diabetes taking phenformin 50 to 100 mg daily found that the equivalent of about 85 mL (3 oz) of whiskey greatly increased their blood lactate and lactate-pyruvate concentrations. Two of them had blood-lactate concentrations of more than 50 mg%, and one of these patients had previously experienced nausea, weakness, and malaise while taking phenformin and alcohol.[1] The ingestion of alcohol is described in other reports as having preceded the onset of phenformin-induced lactic-acidosis.[2-4] Some patients have complained that alcohol tastes metallic. The reasons for the increased blood lactate concentrations are not clear, but one suggestion is that they might possibly be related to the competitive demands for isoenzymes by the reactions that convert alcohol to acetaldehyde, and lactate to pyruvate.[1] A study in healthy subjects found that moderate alcohol consumption both improves insulin action, without affecting non-insulin mediated glucose uptake, and decreases lactate clearance. The increase in blood lactate with alcohol is therefore mainly due to inhibition of clearance. Alcohol did not appear to notably affect beta-cell function.[5]

(b) Colestipol

In a randomised study in 12 diabetic patients with elevated serum cholesterol concentrations, the concurrent use of phenformin and a sulfonylurea (**chlorpropamide**, **tolbutamide**, or **tolazamide**) in 4 patients, inhibited the normal hypocholesterolaemic effects of colestipol 5 g three times daily. The control of diabetes was not affected by the colestipol.[6]

(c) Diuretics, thiazide and related

A long-term study in 53 patients with type 2 diabetes found that **chlorothiazide** 500 mg or 1 g daily or **trichlormethiazide** 4 or 8 mg daily caused a mean increase in blood glucose concentrations from about 6.7 mmol/L to 7.8 mmol/L, but only 7 patients needed a change in their treatment. The oral antidiabetics used included **phenformin**.[7]

(d) Maprotiline

An elderly diabetic woman taking glibenclamide (glyburide) and phenformin developed hypoglycaemia when given **maprotiline**. She was restabilised on half the dose of **glibenclamide** and **phenformin**.[8]

(e) Prazosin

According to the UK manufacturer of prazosin, no interaction would be expected between prazosin and phenformin.[9]

(f) Tetracyclines

There are at least 6 cases on record of lactic-acidosis in patients taking phenformin that were apparently precipitated by the concurrent use of tetracycline.[10-13] Where still available, concurrent use of phenformin with tetracyclines should be avoided.

(g) Warfarin

Haematuria occurred in a patient taking warfarin 3 months after phenformin was started. Her prothrombin values were normal.[14] Phenformin might have increased fibrinolysis to the point where it was additive with the effects of the warfarin. In general no interaction would be expected with warfarin.

NOTE. The reader is cautioned that this monograph is included purely for archival purposes, and is no longer subject to systematic revision and update.

1. Johnson HK, Waterhouse C. Relationship of alcohol and hyperlactatemia in diabetic subjects treated with phenformin. *Am J Med* (1968) 45, 98–104.
2. Davidson MB, Bozarth WR, Challoner DR, Goodner CJ. Phenformin, hypoglycemia and lactic acidosis. Report of an attempted suicide. *N Engl J Med* (1966) 275, 886–8.
3. Gottlieb A, Duberstein J, Geller A. Phenformin acidosis. *N Engl J Med* (1962) 267, 806–9.
4. Schaffalitzky de Muckadell OB, Køster A, Jensen SL. Fenformin-alkohol interaktion. *Ugeskr Laeger* (1973) 135, 925–7.
5. Avogaro A, Watanabe RM, Gottardo L, de Kreutzenberg S, Tiengo A, Pacini G. Glucose tolerance during moderate alcohol intake: insights on insulin action from glucose/lactate dynamics. *J Clin Endocrinol Metab* (2002) 87, 1233–8.
6. Bandisode MS, Boshell BR. Hypocholesterolemic activity of colestipol in diabetes. *Curr Ther Res* (1975) 18, 276–84.
7. Kansal PC, Buse J, Buse MG. Thiazide diuretics and control of diabetes mellitus. *South Med J* (1969) 62, 1374–9.
8. Zogno MG, Tolfo L, Draghi E. Hypoglycemia caused by maprotiline in a patient taking oral antidiabetics. *Ann Pharmacother* (1994) 28, 406.
9. Hypovase (Prazosin hydrochloride). Pfizer Ltd. UK Summary of product characteristics, June 2009.
10. Aro A, Korhonen T, Halinen M. Phenformin-induced lacticacidosis precipitated by tetracycline. *Lancet* (1978) 1, 673–4.
11. Tashima CK. Phenformin, tetracycline, and lactic acidosis. *BMJ* (1971) 4, 557–8.
12. Blumenthal SA, Streeten DHP. Phenformin-related lactic acidosis in a thirty-year-old man. *Ann Intern Med* (1976) 84, 55–6.
13. Phillips PJ, Pain RW. Phenformin, tetracycline and lactic acidosis. *Ann Intern Med* (1977) 86, 111.
14. Hamblin TJ. Interaction between warfarin and phenformin. *Lancet* (1971) ii, 1323.

Pirenzepine + Antacids

The bioavailability of pirenzepine is increased by aluminium/magnesium hydroxide with calcium carbonate and decreased by aluminium/magnesium hydroxide with simeticone.

Clinical evidence, mechanism, importance and management

In a study in 20 healthy subjects, the AUC of a single 50-mg dose of pirenzepine was reduced by about 30% by 30 mL of *Mylanta II* (**aluminium/magnesium hydroxide** and **simeticone**). The antacid reduced the peak plasma levels of pirenzepine by about 45%.[1] Another study in 10 healthy subjects found that the AUC of a single 50-mg dose of pirenzepine was *increased* by almost 25% by 10 mL of an antacid (*Trigastril*, **aluminium/magnesium hydroxide** and **calcium carbonate**).[2] In practical terms these modest changes in bioavailability are probably too small to be clinically relevant.

NOTE. The reader is cautioned that this monograph is included purely for archival purposes, and is no longer subject to systematic revision and update.

1. Matzek KM, MacGregor TR, Keirns JJ, Vinocur M. Effect of food and antacids on the oral absorption of pirenzepine in man. *Int J Pharmaceutics* (1986) 28, 151–5.
2. Vergin H, Herrlinger C, Gugler R. Effect of an aluminium-hydroxide containing antacid on the oral bioavailability of pirenzepine. *Arzneimittelforschung* (1989) 39, 520–3.

Pirenzepine + Cimetidine

The pharmacokinetics of pirenzepine and cimetidine are not affected when both drugs are given together, but pirenzepine increases the cimetidine-induced reduction in gastric acid secretion, which is an apparently advantageous interaction.[1]

NOTE. The reader is cautioned that this monograph is included purely for archival purposes, and is no longer subject to systematic revision and update.

1. Jamali F, Mahachai V, Reilly PA, Thomson ABR. Lack of pharmacokinetic interaction between cimetidine and pirenzepine. *Clin Pharmacol Ther* (1985) 38, 325–30.

Pirenzepine + Food

Food slightly reduces the bioavailability of pirenzepine.

Clinical evidence, mechanism, importance and management

In a study in 20 healthy subjects, the AUC of a single 50-mg dose of pirenzepine was reduced by about 30% when it was taken half-an-hour before food, or with food. Peak plasma levels were reduced by about 30% and 45%, respectively, and the time to achieve peak levels was also reduced.[1] In practical terms this modest change in bioavailability is probably too small to be clinically relevant. The authors of this report suggest taking pirenzepine with food because compliance is better if dosing is associated with a convenient daily ritual.[1]

NOTE. The reader is cautioned that this monograph is included purely for archival purposes, and is no longer subject to systematic revision and update.

1. Matzek KM, MacGregor TR, Keirns JJ, Vinocur M. Effect of food and antacids on the oral absorption of pirenzepine in man. *Int J Pharmaceutics* (1986) 28, 151–5.

Pirenzepine + Theophylline

Pirenzepine does not appear to alter the pharmacokinetics of theophylline.

Clinical evidence, mechanism, importance and management

In 5 healthy subjects, pirenzepine 50 mg twice daily for 5 days had no effect on the pharmacokinetics of theophylline (given as aminophylline 6.5 mg/kg, intravenously).[1] This would suggest that no theophylline or aminophylline dose adjustments are likely to be needed on concurrent use.

NOTE. The reader is cautioned that this monograph is included purely for archival purposes, and is no longer subject to systematic revision and update.

1. Sertl K, Rameis H, Meryn S. Pirenzepin does not alter the pharmacokinetics of theophylline. *Int J Clin Pharmacol Ther Toxicol* (1987) 25, 15–17.

Pirmenol + Miscellaneous

Rifampicin markedly increases the clearance of pirmenol. Cimetidine does not affect the pharmacokinetics of pirmenol.

Clinical evidence, mechanism, importance and management

(a) Cimetidine

In a study in 8 healthy subjects, cimetidine 300 mg four times daily for 8 days had no effect on the pharmacokinetics of a single 150-mg oral dose of pirmenol.[1] No pirmenol dose adjustment would therefore be needed on concurrent use.

(b) Rifampicin (Rifampin)

In a study in 12 healthy subjects, rifampicin 600 mg daily for 14 days, increased the clearance of a single 150-mg dose of pirmenol sevenfold, and decreased the AUC by 83%.[2] The probable reason for these pharmacokinetic changes is that rifampicin, a well-known, non-specific enzyme inducer, increases the hepatic metabolism of pirmenol. Monitor concurrent use closely and anticipate the need to increase the dose of pirmenol. However, note that, with such a marked reduction in pirmenol exposure it is possible that dose increases will be ineffective, and alternative anti-arrhythmics should be considered.

NOTE. The reader is cautioned that this monograph is included purely for archival purposes, and is no longer subject to systematic revision and update.

1. Stringer KA, Lebsack ME, Cetnarowski-Cropp AB, Goldfarb AL, Radulovic LL, Bockbrader HN, Chang T, Sedman AJ. Effect of cimetidine administration on the pharmacokinetics of pirmenol. *J Clin Pharmacol* (1992) 32, 91–4.
2. Stringer KA, Cetnarowski AB, Goldfarb AB, Lebsack ME, Chang TS, Sedman AJ. Enhanced pirmenol elimination by rifampin. *J Clin Pharmacol* (1988) 28, 1094–7.

Rauwolfia alkaloids + Digoxin and related drugs

The concurrent use of digitalis glycosides and rauwolfia alkaloids is usually uneventful, but the incidence of arrhythmias appears to be increased, particularly in those with atrial fibrillation. Excessive bradycardia and syncope have also been described.

Clinical evidence

Three patients taking digoxin and either **reserpine** or whole root ***Rauwolfia serpentina*** developed arrhythmias, namely atrial tachycardia with 4:1 Wenckebach irregular block, ventricular bigeminy and tachycardia, and atrial fibrillation. A large number of other patients were given both drugs without problems.[1]

The incidence of premature ventricular systoles was roughly doubled in patients taking digoxin and **rauwolfia** compared with a similar group taking **rauwolfia** alone.[2] **Reserpine** reduced the tolerated dose of **acetylstrophanthidin** in 15 patients with congestive heart failure; 8 out of 9 patients with atrial fibrillation developed ECG abnormalities, including complete heart block and ventricular ectopics, during acute digitalisation following **reserpine** use, compared with only one of 9 patients not taking **reserpine**.[3]

A case report describes a man taking digoxin 250 micrograms and 375 micrograms on alternate days and **reserpine** 25 micrograms daily, who developed sinus bradycardia and carotid sinus supersensitivity. He was hospitalised because of syncope, which resolved when the **reserpine** was withdrawn.[4]

Mechanism

Not understood. A possible explanation is that because the rauwolfia alkaloids deplete the neurotransmitter from the sympathetic nerve supply to the heart, the parasympathetic vagal supply (i.e. heart slowing) has full rein. Digitalis also reduces heart rate which in the presence of the rauwolfia becomes excessive. In this situation the rate could become so slow that ectopic foci, which would normally be swamped by a faster, more normal beat, begin to fire, leading to the development of arrhythmias. Syncope could also result from the combination of bradycardia and the hypotensive effects of reserpine.

Importance and management

Although the evidence suggests that not all patients taking digitalis glycosides and a rauwolfia alkaloid develop an interaction, some caution is advisable. One group of authors warn that arrhythmias must be anticipated. Particular risk of arrhythmias seems to occur in patients with atrial fibrillation, and in digitalised patients given reserpine parenterally, because of the sudden release of catecholamines that takes place.[4]

NOTE. The reader is cautioned that this monograph is included purely for archival purposes, and is no longer subject to systematic revision and update.

1. Dick HLH, McCawley EL, Fisher WA. Reserpine-digitalis toxicity. *Arch Intern Med* (1962) 109, 503–6.
2. Schreader CJ, Etzl MM. Premature ventricular contractions due to rauwolfia therapy. *JAMA* (1956) 162, 1256.
3. Lown B, Ehrlich L, Lipschultz B, Blake J. Effect of digitalis in patients receiving reserpine. *Circulation* (1961) 24, 1185–91.
4. Bigger JT, Strauss HC. Digitalis toxicity: drug interactions promoting toxicity and the management of toxicity. *Semin Drug Treat* (1972) 2, 147–77.

Repirinast + Theophylline

Repirinast does not affect the pharmacokinetics of theophylline.

Clinical evidence, mechanism, importance and management

In 10 patients with asthma given a single dose of aminophylline, repirinast 300 mg daily had no effect on the pharmacokinetics of theophylline.[1] Another study in 7 patients with asthma found that repirinast (dose unclear) for 3 weeks had no effect on the pharmacokinetics of theophylline 400 to 800 mg, given in two divided doses.[2] No aminophylline or theophylline dose adjustments would therefore be expected to be necessary in the presence of repirinast.

NOTE. The reader is cautioned that this monograph is included purely for archival purposes, and is no longer subject to systematic revision and update.

1. Nagata M, Tabe K, Houya I, Kiuchi H, Sakamoto Y, Yamamoto K, Dohi Y. The influence of repirinast, an anti-allergic drug, on theophylline pharmacokinetics in patients with bronchial asthma. *Nihon Kyobu Shikkan Gakkai Zasshi* (1991) 29, 413–19.
2. Takagi K, Kuzuya T, Horiuchi T, Nadai M, Apichartpichean R, Ogura Y, Hasegawa T. Lack of effect of repirinast on the pharmacokinetics of theophylline in asthmatic patients. *Eur J Clin Pharmacol* (1989) 37, 301–3.

Rofecoxib + Opioids

Rofecoxib does not appear to affect the pharmacokinetics of tramadol and can modestly affect perioperative morphine requirements.

Clinical evidence, mechanism, importance and management

Analysis of data from a study in patients receiving stable doses of celecoxib or **rofecoxib**, found that the clearance of **tramadol** (given with paracetamol) did not differ between the coxibs.[1] **Tramadol** is metabolised by CYP2D6 and CYP3A4; rofecoxib (when available) was not known to inhibit CYP2D6 or CYP3A4, and so would not be expected to interact with tramadol.

In a study, patients given preoperative and postoperative rofecoxib, or placebo, found that rofecoxib reduced **morphine** requirements and pain scores. In another group of patients given placebo preoperatively and **rofecoxib** postoperatively, rofecoxib did not notably affect **morphine** requirements or pain scores at 24 hours after the operation compared to those given placebo pre-and postoperatively, but did show improvement at 48 hours and 72 hours after the operation. However, preoperative rofecoxib was considered to provide only modest benefit and possibly offered little benefit over early postoperative administration.[2]

NOTE. The reader is cautioned that this monograph is included purely for archival purposes, and is no longer subject to systematic revision and update.

1. Punwani NG. Tramadol pharmacokinetics and its possible interactions with cyclooxygenase 2-selective nonsteroidal anti-inflammatory drugs. *Clin Pharmacol Ther* (2004) 75, 363–5.
2. Riest G, Peters J, Weiss M, Pospiech J, Hoffmann O, Neuhäuser M, Beiderlinden M, Eikermann M. Does perioperative administration of rofecoxib improve analgesia after spine, breast and orthopaedic surgery? *Eur J Anaesthesiol* (2006) 23, 219–26.

Sitaxentan + Miscellaneous

Sitaxentan has been withdrawn worldwide due to reports of fatal liver toxicity. When available, sitaxentan was found to slightly increase the exposure to combined hormonal contraceptives and sildenafil, and to increase the anticoagulant effects of warfarin. Ciclosporin was found to greatly increase the plasma concentration of sitaxentan, whilst omeprazole slightly increased its exposure. Atorvastatin was predicted to increase concentrations of sitaxentan.

Sitaxentan had no effect on the pharmacokinetics of ciclosporin, digoxin, nifedipine, omeprazole, ketoconazole, fluconazole, or simvastatin, and fluconazole, ketoconazole, nelfinavir, and pravastatin had no effect on the pharmacokinetics of sitaxentan.

Clinical evidence, mechanism, importance and management

(a) Ciclosporin

The UK manufacturer reported that sitaxentan did not alter ciclosporin concentrations, but ciclosporin did increase the minimum concentrations of sitaxentan 6-fold. They suggested that this might have been via inhibition of OATP by ciclosporin, and the concurrent use of sitaxentan and ciclosporin was contraindicated.[1]

(b) Combined hormonal contraceptives

The UK manufacturer reported that sitaxentan increased the AUC of **norethisterone** by 47%, and increased the AUC of **ethinylestradiol** by 59%, when given as an oral combined hormonal contraceptive (ethinylestradiol 35 micrograms with norethisterone 1 mg). The efficacy of the contraceptive, as measured by FSH, LH, and progesterone concentrations, was unaffected.[1] How sitaxentan increased contraceptive steroid concentrations was unclear, but it could cause some inhibition of CYP2C9 and CYP3A4/5 which is partly involved in their metabolism.[1] The increase in ethinylestradiol exposure seen might have been equivalent to changing a 30 microgram preparation to a 50 microgram preparation, with the potential to increase its adverse effects. The manufacturer specifically noted that the increase in exposure to oestrogen might theoretically have increased the risk of venous thromboembolism, and, in women who smoke, they recommended that prophylaxis of venous thromboembolism with vitamin K antagonists should be considered, as is traditionally used in pulmonary arterial hypertension.[1] It was therefore considered prudent to use a low-dose oral combined hormonal contraceptive (20 microgram dose of ethinylestradiol) and to monitor for increased contraceptive adverse effects, such as nausea and breast tenderness.

(c) CYP3A4 inhibitors

The UK manufacturer of sitaxentan briefly reported that the concurrent use of **fluconazole** and sitaxentan did not affect the pharmacokinetics of either drug. Similarly, the concurrent use of **ketoconazole** and sitaxentan did not affect the pharmacokinetics of either drug.[1] No dose adjustment was necessary on the concurrent use with either of these drugs.

(d) Digoxin

The UK manufacturer of sitaxentan noted that it did not alter the pharmacokinetics of digoxin.[1] No digoxin dose adjustments were therefore expected to be needed if sitaxentan was also given.

(e) HIV-protease inhibitors

The UK manufacturer of sitaxentan briefly reported that, in a clinical interaction study, nelfinavir, an OATP inhibitor, did not cause any clinically relevant changes in the plasma concentrations of sitaxentan.[1] No sitaxentan dose adjustment was necessary with **nelfinavir**. Although nothing was known about the effect of HIV-protease inhibitors boosted with ritonavir on sitaxentan, *in vitro*, **ritonavir** inhibited sitaxentan hepatic uptake,[2] and so some caution was considered appropriate on concurrent use.

(f) Nifedipine

Sitaxentan did not alter the clearance of nifedipine (given as three 10 mg doses),[1] but the UK manufacturer stated that, because the dose of nifedipine was small, a greater effect with larger doses could not be ruled out.[1] However, note that sitaxentan did not affect the pharmacokinetics of other CYP3A4 substrates such as sildenafil (see under *sildenafil*, below) to a clinically relevant extent, and so an interaction at any nifedipine dose seemed unlikely.

(g) Omeprazole

The UK manufacturer briefly reported that, in a study, omeprazole (a CYP2C19 substrate and inhibitor) was found to increase the AUC of sitaxentan by 30%, which was not considered to be clinically important.[1]

(h) Sildenafil

In a study in 22 healthy subjects, the AUC and maximum plasma concentration of a single 100-mg dose of sildenafil were increased by 28% and 18%, respectively, by sitaxentan 100 mg daily for 7 days. Furthermore, sitaxentan did not alter the pharmacokinetics of the active metabolite of sildenafil.[3] On this basis, sitaxentan appeared to be a weak inhibitor of CYP3A4 and therefore had only slight effects on sildenafil exposure, meaning that the dose of sildenafil did not need to be adjusted if sitaxentan was also given.

(i) Statins

The UK manufacturer stated that, in a clinical interaction study, **pravastatin** had no clinically relevant effect on sitaxentan concentrations,[1] but they predicted that **atorvastatin** might have increased sitaxentan concentrations.[1] Both atorvastatin and pravastatin are OATP inhibitors, although pravastatin inhibits this transporter only weakly. As pravastatin had no effect on the concentration of sitaxentan, no dose adjustment was expected to be needed on concurrent use. Whether atorvastatin could increase the concentration of sitaxentan, as predicted, remained to be established; however, it was suggested that patients requiring both drugs should be closely monitored for sitaxentan adverse effects (headache, flushing, oedema). Sitaxentan does not affect CYP3A4 to a clinically relevant extent,[1] and was therefore not expected to affect the concentration of **simvastatin**.

(j) Warfarin

The UK manufacturer noted that sitaxentan increased the exposure to *S*-warfarin 2.4-fold: patients receiving warfarin tended to require lower doses of warfarin to achieve therapeutic INR values in the presence of sitaxentan.[1] Also, in the STRIDE-2 study in patients with pulmonary arterial hypertension, the average warfarin dose after 18 weeks of the concurrent use of sitaxentan 50 mg or 100 mg daily was 2.8 mg daily and 2.1 mg daily, respectively, compared with 3.7 mg in a placebo group. However, the number of patients taking sitaxentan with an INR of more than 3.5 was similar to the placebo group. Note that in this study an initial warfarin dose reduction of 80% was used in patients randomised to sitaxentan or placebo.[4] Sitaxentan was reported to inhibit CYP3A4 and CYP2C9, which are involved in the metabolism of *R*-warfarin and *S*-warfarin, respectively.[1] Therefore, concurrent use decreased the metabolism of warfarin, resulting in increased anticoagulant effects, meaning that smaller warfarin doses were necessary to avoid over-anticoagulation. The manufacturers also predicted that **acenocoumarol**, **phenprocoumon**, and **fluindione** (and therefore presumably other indanediones) would interact similarly to warfarin. They advised that if patients taking sitaxentan were to be started on one of these anticoagulants, they should be started on the lowest possible dose (for example 0.5 mg warfarin daily[5]) with small dose increases (0.5 mg daily was suggested[5]) in order to reach the target INR. If sitaxentan was to be started in a patient already taking an anticoagulant, the dose of the anticoagulant was to be reduced; the Australian manufacturer recommended a warfarin dose reduction of 80%.[5] Close monitoring of the INR was recommended in all patients taking both drugs.[1,5]

NOTE. The reader is cautioned that this monograph is included purely for archival purposes, and is no longer subject to systematic revision and update.

1. Thelin (Sitaxentan sodium). Pfizer Ltd. UK Summary of product characteristics, July 2010.
2. Hartman JC, Brouwer K, Mandagere A, Melvin L, Gorczynski R. Evaluation of the endothelin receptor antagonists ambrisentan, darusentan, bosentan, and sitaxsentan as substrates and inhibitors of hepatobiliary transporters in sandwich-cultured human hepatocytes. *Can J Physiol Pharmacol* (2010) 88, 682–91.
3. Stavros F, Kramer WG, Wilkins MR. The effects of sitaxentan on sildenafil pharmacokinetics and pharmacodynamics in healthy subjects. *Br J Clin Pharmacol* (2010) 69, 23–6.
4. Barst RJ, Langleben D, Badesch D, Frost A, Lawrence EC, Shapiro S, Naeije R, Galie N, on behalf of the STRIDE-2 study group. Treatment of pulmonary arterial hypertension with the selective endothelin-A receptor antagonist sitaxsentan. *J Am Coll Cardiol* (2006) 47, 2049–56.
5. Thelin (Sitaxentan sodium). Pfizer Australia Pty Ltd. Australian Prescribing information, July 2009.

Tacrine + Miscellaneous

In many countries tacrine has been withdrawn from the market due to hepatotoxicity effects. The risk of adverse effects, including bradycardia, might be increased if tacrine is given with amiodarone. Cimetidine possibly increases the effects of tacrine. Fluvoxamine markedly increases tacrine exposure, and increases its adverse effects. A small study suggests that HRT can increase the exposure of tacrine. An isolated report described movement disorders when haloperidol was given with tacrine. An isolated report describes a woman taking tacrine who became delirious when she also started to take ibuprofen. Enoxacin possibly increases the effects of tacrine. Smoking tobacco reduces the exposure of tacrine. Tacrine does not appear to affect the pharmacokinetics of diazepam. Memantine does not appear to attenuate the anticholinesterase effects of tacrine. Quinidine does not affect the metabolism of tacrine.

Clinical evidence, mechanism, importance and management

(a) Amiodarone

The effects of tacrine on concurrent use with amiodarone do not appear to have been studied, but as for other centrally-acting anticholinesterases (see 'Anticholinesterases; Centrally acting + Amiodarone', p.366), it would also be expected to slow the heart rate, and therefore might have additive effects with amiodarone.

(b) Cimetidine

In a study in 10 healthy, elderly subjects, cimetidine 300 mg four times daily for 2 days decreased the clearance of a single 40-mg dose of tacrine by 30%, and increased its AUC and maximum plasma concentration by 39% and 35%, respectively.[1] The US manufacturer of tacrine stated that cimetidine increased the AUC and the maximum plasma concentration of tacrine by about 64% and 54%, respectively.[2] The reason for these changes is not established, but it seems probable that cimetidine (a well-recognised liver enzyme inhibitor) reduces the metabolism of tacrine by CYP1A2. An increase in both the beneficial effects and possibly adverse effects of tacrine (nausea, vomiting, diarrhoea) seems possible: one patient had to be withdrawn from the study mentioned above due to nausea and vomiting.[1] If the suggested mechanism of interaction is correct, the other H_2-receptor antagonists would not be expected to interact in this way.

(c) Diazepam

In a small study, tacrine 20 mg every 6 hours did not affect the pharmacokinetics of a single 2-mg dose of diazepam, when compared with diazepam alone.[3] No diazepam dose adjustments would seem necessary if tacrine is also given.

(d) Fluvoxamine

Fluvoxamine is an inhibitor of CYP1A2, the main isoenzyme involved in the metabolism of tacrine. An *in vitro* study showed that fluvoxamine is a potent inhibitor of tacrine metabolism, and it was therefore predicted that fluvoxamine might dramatically increase tacrine plasma concentrations in patients.[4] This prediction was confirmed in a placebo-controlled study in 13 healthy subjects who had an 8-fold increase in the mean AUC of a single 40-mg dose of tacrine after taking fluvoxamine 100 mg for 6 days. A very large increase in the AUC of the hydroxylated metabolites of tacrine, and an 8-fold decrease in the clearance of tacrine were also seen. No subjects had any adverse effects when they took tacrine after placebo, but 5 had adverse effects (nausea, vomiting, sweating, and diarrhoea) when they took tacrine after fluvoxamine.[5] Another pilot study in one individual found that the total clearance of tacrine was reduced about 10-fold and its half-life increased 10-fold by fluvoxamine 100 mg daily.[6] A further study by the same authors, in 18 healthy subjects, found that the clearance of tacrine was reduced by about 85% by fluvoxamine 50 or 100 mg.[7] It is likely that standard tacrine doses will be poorly tolerated in the presence of fluvoxamine because of cholinergic adverse effects, and a decrease in tacrine dose is probably necessary.[7] Other SSRIs such as **fluoxetine**, **paroxetine**, or **sertraline** may be suitable alternatives, as they seem unlikely to inhibit tacrine metabolism (they do not inhibit CYP1A2 to a clinically relevant extent).

(e) Haloperidol

An isolated report describes an 87-year-old man with dementia, who started taking haloperidol 5 mg daily for symptoms of agitation and paranoia. Doses of greater than 5 mg were noted to cause extrapyramidal symptoms. After 10 days, tacrine 10 mg four times daily was added. Within 72 hours he developed severe parkinsonian symptoms, which resolved within 8 hours of stopping both drugs.[8] Another isolated report describes a woman taking haloperidol 10 mg daily who similarly developed a disabling parkinsonian syndrome within one week of starting tacrine 10 mg four times daily.[9] One possible reason is that the haloperidol blocked the dopamine receptors in striatum, thereby increasing striatal acetylcholine activity, which was further increased by the tacrine.[10] It is not clear whether patients given other dopamine receptor blocking drugs and tacrine would similarly show this reaction.

(f) HRT

Observational results from a multicentre study of women with Alzheimer's disease receiving tacrine or placebo suggested that women receiving HRT (**conjugated oestrogens**, **estradiol**, or **estrone sulfate**) and tacrine performed better on both cognitive and clinical assessments than women receiving tacrine alone or placebo. However, the subgroup of patients receiving HRT was not randomised and these patients were somewhat younger and better educated.[11] Following these observations, a randomised, crossover, placebo-controlled study was undertaken in 10 healthy women who were given HRT (**estradiol** 2 mg with **levonorgestrel** 250 micrograms daily) with a single 40-mg dose of tacrine on day 10. The HRT increased the mean tacrine AUC by 60%, increased the maximum plasma concentration of tacrine by 46%, and reduced the tacrine clearance by 31%. The AUC of one individual was increased 3-fold. These pharmacokinetic changes are thought to occur because HRT reduces the metabolism of tacrine to its main metabolite (1-hydroxytacrine) by CYP1A2.[12] The importance of this interaction is uncertain, but increased tacrine concentrations would be expected to increase its adverse effects. Therefore it would seem prudent to be alert for the need to use a smaller tacrine dose in patients given HRT.

(g) Ibuprofen

A 71-year-old woman with diabetes and probable Alzheimer's disease developed delirium while taking tacrine 40 mg four times daily. The symptoms included delusions, hallucinations, and fluctuating awareness. She was also bradycardic, diaphoretic, and dizzy.[13] She was eventually stabilised with tacrine 20 mg four times daily, and continued this for 8 months without problems, but became delirious again 2 weeks after starting to take ibuprofen 600 mg daily. The delirium resolved when both drugs were withdrawn. The reasons for this reaction are unknown. This is the first and only report of this apparent interaction and its general importance is probably small, especially as the patient had previously experienced delirium with tacrine alone.

(h) Memantine

An *in vitro* study in *rats* suggested that memantine does not attenuate the anticholinesterase effects of tacrine at therapeutic concentrations.[14]

(i) Other drugs that affect acetylcholine

The effects of tacrine, a centrally-acting anticholinesterase inhibitor, are expected to be additive with those of other anticholinesterases (e.g. neostigmine) and cholinergics (e.g. pilocarpine). The effects of tacrine and drugs with antimuscarinic effects are expected to be antagonistic, but case reports have described the opposite effect (see 'Anticholinesterases; Centrally acting + Other drugs that affect acetylcholine', p.369).

(j) Quinidine

In a study in 11 healthy subjects, quinidine 83 mg every 8 hours did not affect the clearance of a single 40-mg dose of tacrine.[15] As quinidine inhibits CYP2D6 in the liver, it was concluded that CYP2D6 does not have an important role to play in the metabolism of tacrine. No tacrine dose adjustments would be expected to be necessary if quinidine is also given.

(k) Quinolones

In vitro studies with human and *rat* liver microsomes found that **enoxacin**, a specific inhibitor of CYP1A2, greatly inhibited all known routes by which tacrine is metabolised.[16] A reasonable conclusion to be drawn from this is that the effects of tacrine (both beneficial and adverse) would be increased by **enoxacin**, but this interaction does not appear to have been studied in patients or healthy subjects. The same study also suggested that **enoxacin** possibly inhibits the production of the hepatotoxic metabolites of tacrine.[17]

Other quinolones vary in the extent to which they inhibit CYP1A2 (see 'Theophylline + Quinolones', p.1455), so that any interaction with other quinolones would be expected to reflect this variation.

(l) Tobacco

A comparative study in 7 tobacco smokers and 4 non-smokers found that the AUC of a single 40-mg dose of tacrine in the smokers was about 10% of that in the non-smokers. The elimination half-life in the smokers was also reduced, to about two-thirds of that in non-smokers. The increase in tacrine metabolism in smokers is thought to occur because some of the components of tobacco smoke increase the activity of CYP1A2 in the liver, by which tacrine is metabolised.[18] In practical terms it would appear that smokers are likely to need larger doses of tacrine than non-smokers, although this needs confirmation in multiple-dose studies.

For a brief mention of the effects of smoking in patients with Alzheimer's disease and dementia, see 'Anticholinesterases; Centrally acting + Tobacco', p.370.

NOTE. The reader is cautioned that this monograph is included purely for archival purposes, and is no longer subject to systematic revision and update.

1. Forgue ST, Reece PA, Sedman AJ, deVries TM. Inhibition of tacrine oral clearance by cimetidine. *Clin Pharmacol Ther* (1996) 59, 444–9.
2. Cognex (Tacrine hydrochloride). Sciele Pharma, Inc. US Prescribing information, June 2006.
3. deVries TM, Siedlik P, Smithers JA, Brown RR, Reece PA, Posvar EL, Sedman AJ, Koup JR, Forgue ST. Effect of multiple-dose tacrine administration on single-dose pharmacokinetics of digoxin, diazepam, and theophylline. *Pharm Res* (1993) 10 (10 Suppl), S-333.
4. Becquemont L, Le Bot MA, Riche C, Beaune P. Influence of fluvoxamine on tacrine metabolism in vitro: potential implication for the hepatotoxicity in vivo. *Fundam Clin Pharmacol* (1996) 10, 156–7.
5. Becquemont L, Ragueneau I, Le Bot MA, Riche C, Funck-Brentano C, Jaillon P. Influence of the CYP1A2 inhibitor fluvoxamine on tacrine pharmacokinetics in humans. *Clin Pharmacol Ther* (1997) 61, 619–27.
6. Larsen JT, Hansen LL, Brøsen K. Tacrine-fluvoxamine interaction study in healthy volunteers. *Eur J Clin Pharmacol* (1997) 52 (Suppl), A136.
7. Larsen JT, Hansen LL, Spigset O, Brøsen K. Fluvoxamine is a potent inhibitor of tacrine metabolism in vivo. *Eur J Clin Pharmacol* (1999) 55, 375–82.
8. McSwain ML, Forman LM. Severe parkinsonian symptom development on combination treatment with tacrine and haloperidol. *J Clin Psychopharmacol* (1995) 15, 284.
9. Maany I. Adverse interaction of tacrine and haloperidol. *Am J Psychiatry* (1996) 153, 1504.
10. Zhao Q, Xie C, Pesco-Koplowitz L, Jia X, Parier J-L. Pharmacokinetic and safety assessments of concurrent administration of risperidone and donepezil. *J Clin Pharmacol* (2003) 43, 180–6.
11. Schneider LS, Farlow MR, Henderson VW, Pogoda JM. Effects of estrogen replacement therapy on response to tacrine in patients with Alzheimer's disease. *Neurology* (1996) 46, 1580–4.
12. Laine K, Palovaara S, Tapanainen P, Manninen P. Plasma tacrine concentrations are significantly increased by concomitant hormone replacement therapy. *Clin Pharmacol Ther* (1999) 66, 602–8.
13. Hooten WM, Pearlson G. Delirium caused by tacrine and ibuprofen interaction. *Am J Psychiatry* (1996) 153, 842.
14. Wenk GL, Quack G, Moebius H-J, Danysz W. No interaction of memantine with anticholinesterase inhibitors approved for clinical use. *Life Sci* (2000) 66, 1079–83.
15. deVries TM, O'Connor-Semmes RL, Guttendorf RJ, Reece PA, Posvar EL, Sedman AJ, Koup JR, Forgue ST. Effect of cimetidine and low-dose quinidine on tacrine pharmacokinetics in humans. *Pharm Res* (1993) 10 (10 Suppl), S-337.
16. Madden S, Woolf TF, Pool WF, Park BK. An investigation into the formation of stable, protein-reactive and cytotoxic metabolites from tacrine *in vitro*. Studies with human and rat liver microsomes. *Biochem Pharmacol* (1993) 46, 13–20.
17. Madden S, Woolf TF, Pool WF, Park BK. An investigation into the formation of stable, protein-reactive and cytotoxic metabolites from tacrine *in vitro*. Studies with human and rat liver microsomes. *Biochem Pharmacol* (1993) 46, 13–20.
18. Welty D, Pool W, Woolf T, Posvar E, Sedman A. The effect of smoking on the pharmacokinetics and metabolism of Cognex® in healthy volunteers. *Pharm Res* (1993) 10 (10 Suppl), S-334.

Tegaserod + Combined hormonal contraceptives

Tegaserod does not alter the pharmacokinetics or ovulation suppressant effect of an oral combined hormonal contraceptive containing ethinylestradiol with levonorgestrel.

Clinical evidence, mechanism, importance and management

In a placebo-controlled study in healthy women taking a triphasic, oral combined hormonal contraceptive (**ethinylestradiol** with **levonorgestrel**), tegaserod 6 mg twice daily for a complete cycle had no effect on the AUC of **ethinylestradiol** and caused an 8% decrease in the AUC of **levonorgestrel**, which would not be expected to be clinically relevant. In addition, no ovulation occurred as assessed by progesterone levels.[1,2]

This study suggests that tegaserod is unlikely to alter the efficacy of combined hormonal contraceptives (oral, patch and vaginal ring), and so no additional contraceptive precautions are likely to be necessary on concurrent use.

NOTE. The reader is cautioned that this monograph is included purely for archival purposes, and is no longer subject to systematic revision and update.

1. Zhou H, Walter YH, Hubert M, Ma P, Osborne S, Appel-Dingemanse A, McLeod JF. Tegaserod (HTF 919) does not decrease the effectiveness of an oral contraceptive when coadministered to healthy female subjects. *Gastroenterology* (2000) 118, A1207.
2. Appel-Dingemanse S. Clinical pharmacokinetics of tegaserod, a serotonin 5-HT_4 receptor partial agonist with promotile activity. *Clin Pharmacokinet* (2002) 41, 1021–42.

Tegaserod + Digoxin

Tegaserod reduces digoxin exposure.

Clinical evidence, mechanism, importance and management

A study in 12 healthy subjects given tegaserod 6 mg twice daily for 5 days found that the time to peak levels of a single 1-mg dose of digoxin, given on day 4, was reduced by 30 minutes, and the mean AUC and maximum plasma concentrations were reduced by 12% and 15%, respectively.[1] Changes of this magnitude are unlikely to be clinically relevant.

NOTE. The reader is cautioned that this monograph is included purely for archival purposes, and is no longer subject to systematic revision and update.

1. Zhou H, Horowitz A, Ledford PC, Hubert M, Appel-Dingemanse S, Osborne S, McLeod JF. The effects of tegaserod (HTF 919) on the pharmacokinetics and pharmacodynamics of digoxin in healthy subjects. *J Clin Pharmacol* (2001) 41, 1131–9.

Tegaserod + Omeprazole

The delay in gastric emptying that may be caused by omeprazole could be prevented by tegaserod.

Clinical evidence, mechanism, importance and management

In a placebo-controlled study in 39 healthy male subjects, omeprazole 20 mg twice daily was found to slightly increase the half-life for gastric emptying by about 22%, and increased gastric retention time at 60 and 120 minutes after a test meal by about 10%. When tegaserod 6 mg three times daily was added for 14 days, tegaserod largely prevented the delayed gastric emptying seen with omeprazole alone.[1] No significant adverse effects were reported in this study.[1] The clinical relevance of this effect is uncertain.

NOTE. The reader is cautioned that this monograph is included purely for archival purposes, and is no longer subject to systematic revision and update.

1. Tougas G, Earnest DL, Chen Y, Vanderkoy C, Rojavin M. Omeprazole delays gastric emptying in healthy volunteers: an effect prevented by tegaserod. *Aliment Pharmacol Ther* (2005) 22, 59–65.

Tegaserod + Theophylline

Tegaserod does not appear to alter the pharmacokinetics of theophylline.

Clinical evidence, mechanism, importance and management

In a study in 18 healthy subjects, the pharmacokinetics of a single 600-mg dose of controlled-release theophylline were unchanged when it was given with three doses of tegaserod 6 mg (the first was given about 24 hours before the theophylline, the second simultaneously, and the third 12 hours later).[1] No theophylline dose adjustments would therefore appear necessary on concurrent use. There appears to be no direct evidence regarding aminophylline, but as it is metabolised to theophylline, no adverse interaction would be expected with tegaserod.

NOTE. The reader is cautioned that this monograph is included purely for archival purposes, and is no longer subject to systematic revision and update.

1. Zhou H, Khalilieh S, Svendsen K, Pommier F, Osborne S, Appel-Dingemanse S, Lasseter K, McLeod JF. Tegaserod coadministration does not alter the pharmacokinetics of theophylline in healthy subjects. *J Clin Pharmacol* (2001) 41, 987–93.

Tocainide + Miscellaneous

A report describes a tonic-clonic seizure in a man during the period when his medication was being changed from intravenous lidocaine to oral tocainide. Rises in urinary pH (e.g. with some antacids, diuretics or alkaline salts) can slightly reduce the clearance of tocainide. Cimetidine slightly reduces the exposure to tocainide but ranitidine does not appear to interact. Phenobarbital does not appear to alter the pharmacokinetics of tocainide, however. rifampicin (rifampin) decreases the exposure to tocainide.

Clinical evidence, mechanism, importance and management

(a) Antacids or urinary alkalinisers

The preliminary findings of a study suggested that when 5 healthy subjects took an unnamed antacid the resultant rise in urinary pH reduced the total clearance of tocainide by 28% and increased its AUC by 33%.[1] Tocainide is a weak base so alkalinisation of the urine increases the number of non-ionised molecules available for passive reabsorption, reducing urinary loss and increasing tocainide exposure.

This would appear to be an established interaction of uncertain, but probably limited, clinical importance. There seem to be no reports of adverse reactions in patients as a result of this interaction, but be alert for any evidence of increased tocainide adverse effects (such as nausea, tremor, hypotension) if other drugs are given that can raise the urinary pH (such as **sodium bicarbonate** and **acetazolamide**). Reduce the tocainide dose if necessary. See 'Quinidine + Antacids or Urinary alkalinisers', p.293, for a list of antacids and their effect on urinary pH.

(b) H_2-receptor antagonists

In a preliminary report of a study in 11 healthy subjects, 4 days of treatment with **cimetidine** (dose not stated) had a small effect on the pharmacokinetics of tocainide 500 mg given intravenously over 15 minutes, which was not considered to be clinically important.[2] In another study, in 7 healthy subjects, **cimetidine** 300 mg four times daily for 2 days reduced the AUC of a single 400-mg oral dose of tocainide by about one-third.[2] The reasons for these slight changes and their clinical importance are uncertain, but be alert for evidence of a reduced response to tocainide in the presence of **cimetidine**. **Ranitidine** 150 mg twice daily does not affect the pharmacokinetics of tocainide.[3]

(c) Lidocaine

An elderly man taking furosemide and co-trimoxazole experienced a tonic-clonic seizure while his medication was being changed from intravenous lidocaine to oral tocainide, although the serum levels of both antiarrhythmics remained within their therapeutic ranges. The patient became progressively agitated and disorientated about 8 hours after starting oral tocainide 600 mg every 6 hours while still receiving lidocaine 2 mg/minute intravenously. About one hour later he had a seizure. The patient subsequently tolerated each drug separately, at concentrations similar to those that preceded the seizure, without problems.[4] A study in *animals*[5] found that tocainide reduces the lidocaine serum levels at which seizures occur by about 45%. Tocainide is no longer widely available, but the US manufacturer previously noted that the concurrent use of lidocaine and tocainide might cause an increased incidence of adverse effects, including CNS adverse reactions such as seizures, because the two drugs have similar pharmacodynamic effects.[6] Great care must therefore be used if tocainide is given during systemic lidocaine use. Note that the manufacturer of one topical lidocaine preparation advises that, although the systemic absorption of topical lidocaine is low, the possible risk of additive systemic toxicity occurring in patients also receiving tocainide cannot be ruled out.[7]

(d) Phenobarbital

In a study in 6 healthy subjects, phenobarbital 100 mg daily for 15 days did not alter the AUC of a single 600-mg dose of tocainide. In addition, the percentage of the dose excreted unchanged in the urine and as the glucuronide metabolite did not differ.[8] Phenobarbital at this dose does not appear to alter the metabolism of tocainide. No tocainide dose adjustment appears to be necessary if phenobarbital is also given.

(e) Rifampicin (Rifampin)

In a study in 8 healthy subjects, rifampicin 300 mg twice daily for 5 days reduced the AUC of a single 600-mg oral dose of tocainide by almost 30% and similarly reduced the half-life, from 13.2 hours to 9.4 hours.[9] Information is limited to this study, but the effect seen is consistent with the well-known enzyme-inducing effects of rifampicin. The interaction would therefore seem to be established, but such a slight reduction in tocainide exposure suggests that its clinical importance is probably minor. Be alert for any evidence of a reduction in tocainide serum levels and effects if rifampicin is also given. Increase the tocainide dose as necessary.

NOTE. The reader is cautioned that this monograph is included purely for archival purposes, and is no longer subject to systematic revision and update.

1. Meneilly GP, Scavone JM, Meneilly GS, Wei JY. Tocainide: pharmacokinetic alterations during antacid-induced urinary alkalinization. *Clin Pharmacol Ther* (1987) 41, 178.
2. Price BA, Holmes GI, Antonello J, Yeh KC, Demetriades J, Irvin JD, McMahon FG. Intravenous tocainide (T) maintains safe therapeutic levels when administered concomitantly with cimetidine (C). *Clin Pharmacol Ther* (1987), 41, 237.
3. North DS, Mattern AL, Kapil RP, Lalonde RL. The effect of histamine-2 receptor antagonists on tocainide pharmacokinetics. *J Clin Pharmacol* (1988) 28, 640–3.
4. Forrence E, Covinsky JO, Mullen C. A seizure induced by concurrent lidocaine-tocainide therapy — Is it just a case of additive toxicity? *Drug Intell Clin Pharm* (1986) 20, 56–9.
5. Schuster MR, Paris PM, Kaplan RM, Stewart RD. Effect on the seizure threshold in dogs of tocainide/lidocaine administration. *Ann Emerg Med* (1987) 16, 749–51.
6. Tonocard (Tocainide). AstraZeneca. US Prescribing information, September 2000.
7. Versatis Medicated Plaster (Lidocaine). Grunenthal Ltd. UK Summary of product characteristics, December 2011.
8. Elvin AT, Lalka D, Stoeckel K, du Souich P, Axelson JE, Golden LH, McLean AJ. Tocainide kinetics and metabolism: effects of phenobarbital and substrates of glucuronyl transferase. *Clin Pharmacol Ther* (1980) 28, 652–8.
9. Rice TL, Patterson JH, Celestin C, Foster JR, Powell JR. Influence of rifampin on tocainide pharmacokinetics in humans. *Clin Pharm* (1989) 8, 200–205.

Troleandomycin + Opioids

Troleandomycin does not alter the pharmacokinetics of methadone, but does reduce the clearance of alfentanil, and might reduce the metabolism of fentanyl when given transmucosally. An isolated report describes signs of dextromoramide overdose after starting troleandomycin.

Clinical evidence, mechanism, importance and management

(a) Dextromoramide

A man taking dextromoramide developed signs of overdose (a morphine-like coma, mydriasis, and depressed respiration) 3 days after he started to take troleandomycin for a dental infection. He recovered when given naloxone. A possible explanation for this effect is that troleandomycin reduced the metabolism of dextromoramide, thereby increasing its serum concentrations and effects.[1] The general importance of this interaction is uncertain but concurrent use should be well monitored.

(b) Fentanyl and related drugs

A study in 9 healthy subjects given troleandomycin 500 mg orally found that the clearance of intravenous **alfentanil** 20 micrograms/kg was reduced by almost 70%, when compared with placebo.[2] Similar results were found in another study.[3] A further study found that oral troleandomycin (500 mg starting 105 minutes before an **alfentanil** infusion then 250 mg every 6 hours for 3 doses) reduced the clearance of **alfentanil** by 88%.[4] This study found that troleandomycin only reduced intravenous **fentanyl** clearance by 39%. In another study in 12 healthy subjects, maximum **fentanyl** concentrations and maximum miosis following oral transmucosal fentanyl 10 micrograms/kg were minimally affected by oral troleandomycin (500 mg given about 3 hours before and 9 hours after the opioid), but **fentanyl** metabolism, elimination, and duration of effects were greatly affected (**fentanyl** AUC increased by 77%; norfentanyl AUC decreased by 36%; AUC_{0-10} of miosis increased by 53%).[5] Troleandomycin inhibits CYP3A4 and has also been reported to inhibit CYP3A5. Fentanyl is metabolised by CYP3A4, but is a high-extraction drug (see 'Changes in first-pass metabolism', p.4), and so is more affected by changes in hepatic blood flow than effects on the isoenzymes responsible for its metabolism. Note that alterations in intestinal or hepatic CYP3A activity also appear to have little influence on oral transmucosal fentanyl absorption and onset of effect; however, a large proportion (approximately 75%) is swallowed and its systemic clearance can be decreased by CYP3A inhibitors.[5,6] Alfentanil appears to be metabolised by multiple CYP3A enzymes (including CYP3A4 and CYP3A5),[7] and is a low-extraction drug meaning that it is more affected by CYP3A inhibitors than fentanyl. Hence concurrent use of CYP3A inhibitors decreases alfentanil clearance.

(c) Methadone

A randomised, crossover study in 12 healthy subjects found that troleandomycin did not affect the pharmacokinetics of oral or intravenous methadone. Troleandomycin caused only a small reduction in methadone *N*-demethylation after oral methadone, suggesting only a small role for CYP3A4 in human methadone metabolism.[8]

NOTE. The reader is cautioned that this monograph is included purely for archival purposes, and is no longer subject to systematic revision and update.

1. Carry PV, Ducluzeau R, Jourdan C, Bourrat Ch, Vigneau C, Descotes J. De nouvelles interactions avec les macrolides? *Lyon Med* (1982) 248, 189–90.
2. Kharasch ED, Russell M, Mautz D, Thummel KE, Kunze KL, Bowdle A, Cox K. The role of cytochrome P450 3A4 in alfentanil clearance: implications for interindividual variability in disposition and perioperative drug interactions. *Anesthesiology* (1997) 87, 36–50.
3. Kharasch ED, Walker A, Hoffer C, Sheffels P. Intravenous and oral alfentanil as in vivo probes for hepatic and first-pass cytochrome P450 3A activity: non-invasive assessment by use of pupillary miosis. *Clin Pharmacol Ther* (2004) 76, 452–66.

4. Ibrahim AE, Feldman J, Karim A, Kharasch ED. Simultaneous assessment of drug interactions with low- and high-extraction opioids. Application to parecoxib effects on the pharmacokinetics and pharmacodynamics of fentanyl and alfentanil. *Anesthesiology* (2003) 98, 853–61.
5. Kharasch ED, Whittington D, Hoffer C. Influence of hepatic and intestinal cytochrome P4503A activity on the acute disposition and effects of oral transmucosal fentanyl citrate. *Anesthesiology* (2004) 101, 729–37.
6. Actiq (Fentanyl citrate lozenge). Teva Pharmaceuticals Ltd. UK Summary of product characteristics, June 2015.
7. Klees TM, Sheffels P, Dale O, Kharasch ED. Metabolism of alfentanil by cytochrome P4503A (CYP3A) enzymes. *Drug Metab Dispos* (2005) 33, 303–11.
8. Kharasch ED, Hoffer C, Whittington D, Sheffels P. Role of hepatic and intestinal cytochrome P450 3A and 2B6 in the metabolism, disposition, and miotic effects of methadone. *Clin Pharmacol Ther* (2004) 76, 250–69.

Viloxazine + Carbamazepine and related drugs

Viloxazine can increase carbamazepine levels and toxicity has been seen. Viloxazine does not appear to alter oxcarbazepine levels.

Clinical evidence

(a) Carbamazepine

The serum carbamazepine levels of 7 patients rose by 50% (from 8.1 micrograms/mL to 12.1 micrograms/mL) after they took viloxazine 100 mg three times daily for 3 weeks.[1] Signs of mild toxicity (dizziness, ataxia, fatigue, drowsiness) developed in 5 of the 7 patients. These symptoms disappeared and the serum carbamazepine levels fell when viloxazine was withdrawn.[1] Another report found a 2.5-fold increase in serum carbamazepine levels in one patient that occurred within 2 weeks of starting viloxazine 300 mg daily.[2] Another report found an average 55% rise in plasma carbamazepine levels and toxicity in 4 of 7 patients also taking viloxazine.[3] Yet another patient developed choreoathetosis and increased serum carbamazepine levels, which were attributed to the use of viloxazine.[4]

In one study, the pharmacokinetics of a single dose of viloxazine were reported to be unaffected by carbamazepine,[5] but in the case report cited above, which was at steady-state, the viloxazine levels were found to be reduced by carbamazepine.[2]

(b) Oxcarbazepine

In 6 patients with simple or partial seizures the steady-state serum levels of oxcarbazepine (average dose 1.5 g daily) were unaffected by the addition of viloxazine 100 mg twice daily for 10 days. No adverse effects were seen.[6]

Mechanism

Uncertain. What is known suggests that viloxazine inhibits the metabolism of carbamazepine, thereby reducing its clearance and raising its serum levels.

Importance and management

Information seems to be limited to the reports cited. If concurrent use is undertaken, serum carbamazepine levels should be monitored closely and suitable dose reductions made as necessary to avoid possible toxicity. No dose adjustment seems to be necessary with oxcarbazepine.

NOTE. The reader is cautioned that this monograph is included purely for archival purposes, and is no longer subject to systematic revision and update.

1. Pisani F, Narbone MC, Fazio A, Crisafulli P, Primerano G, Amendola D'Angostino A, Oteri G, Di Perri R. Effect of viloxazine on serum carbamazepine levels in epileptic patients. *Epilepsia* (1984) 25, 482–5.
2. Odou P, Geronimi-Ferret D, Degen P, Robert H. Viloxazine-carbamazépine. Double interaction dangereuse? A propos d'un cas. *J Pharm Clin* (1996) 15, 157–60.
3. Pisani F, Fazio A, Oteri G, Perucca E, Russo M, Trio R, Pisani B, Di Perri R. Carbamazepine-viloxazine interaction in patients with epilepsy. *J Neurol Neurosurg Psychiatry* (1986) 49, 1142–5.
4. Mosquet B, Starace J, Madelaine S, Simon JY, Lacotte J, Moulin M. Syndrome choréo-athétosique sous carbamazépine et viloxazine. *Therapie* (1994) 49, 513–14.
5. Pisani F, Fazio A, Spina E, Artesi C, Pisani B, Russo M, Trio R, Perucca E. Pharmacokinetics of the antidepressant drug viloxazine in normal subjects and in epileptic patients receiving chronic anticonvulsant treatment. *Psychopharmacology (Berl)* (1986) 90, 295–8.
6. Pisani F, Fazio A, Oteri G, Artesi C, Xiao B, Perucca E, Di Perri R. Effects of the antidepressant drug viloxazine on oxcarbazepine and its hydroxylated metabolites in patients with epilepsy. *Acta Neurol Scand* (1994) 90, 130–2.

Viloxazine + Coumarins and related drugs

A single report describes three cases where viloxazine possibly increased the anticoagulant effects of acenocoumarol and fluindione.

Clinical evidence

An 82-year-old woman with angina, hypertension and atrial fibrillation, who was taking **acenocoumarol**, molsidomine and flunitrazepam, had a rise in her INR from 3.3 to 7.9 when she started to take viloxazine (dose not stated) for depression. Five days after stopping the viloxazine her INR had fallen to 2.6. This report also briefly describes two other cases where viloxazine possibly caused an increase in the anticoagulant effects of **acenocoumarol** and **fluindione**.[1]

Mechanism

Not understood. The authors of the report suggest that viloxazine possibly inhibits cytochrome P450 within the liver, resulting in a reduction in the metabolism of the anticoagulants.[1]

Importance and management

Information seems to be limited to this report so that its general importance is uncertain. Be alert for the need to reduce the dose of acenocoumarol and fluindione if viloxazine is added to established anticoagulant treatment. Take the same precautions with any of the other coumarin or indanedione anticoagulants, but so far there seems to be no direct evidence that they interact.

NOTE. The reader is cautioned that this monograph is included purely for archival purposes, and is no longer subject to systematic revision and update.

1. Chiffoleau A, Delavaud P, Spreux A, Fialip J, Kergueris MF, Chichmanian RM, Lavarenne J, Bourin M, Larousse C. Existe-t-il une interaction métabolique entre la viloxazine et les antivitamines K? *Therapie* (1993) 48, 492–3.

Viloxazine + Phenytoin

Viloxazine can raise phenytoin levels, and signs of toxicity have developed in some patients. Phenytoin does not appear to affect the pharmacokinetics of viloxazine.

Clinical evidence

The serum phenytoin levels of 10 patients with epilepsy rose by 37% (from 18.8 micrograms/mL to 25.7 micrograms/mL) over the 3 weeks following the addition of viloxazine 150 to 300 mg daily. The increase ranged from 7 to 94%. Signs of toxicity (ataxia, nystagmus) developed in 4 of the patients 12 to 16 days after starting viloxazine. Their serum phenytoin levels had risen to between 32.3 and 41 micrograms/mL. When viloxazine was withdrawn the symptoms disappeared and phenytoin levels fell.[1] The pharmacokinetics of viloxazine were unaffected by phenytoin.[2]

Mechanism

Uncertain. What is known suggests that viloxazine inhibits the metabolism of phenytoin, thereby reducing its clearance and raising its serum levels.

Importance and management

Information seems to be limited to the reports cited. If concurrent use is undertaken, serum phenytoin levels should be monitored closely and suitable dose reductions made as necessary to avoid possible toxicity.

NOTE. The reader is cautioned that this monograph is included purely for archival purposes, and is no longer subject to systematic revision and update.

1. Pisani F, Fazio A, Artesi C, Russo M, Trio R, Oteri G, Perucca E, Di Perri R. Elevation of plasma phenytoin by viloxazine in epileptic patients: a clinically significant interaction. *J Neurol Neurosurg Psychiatry* (1992) 55, 126–7.
2. Pisani F, Fazio A, Spina E, Artesi C, Pisani B, Russo M, Trio R, Perucca E. Pharmacokinetics of the antidepressant drug viloxazine in normal subjects and in epileptic patients receiving chronic anticonvulsant treatment. *Psychopharmacology (Berl)* (1986) 90, 295–8.

Viloxazine + Theophylline

Viloxazine increases theophylline levels and toxicity may occur.

Clinical evidence

A study in 8 healthy subjects given a single 200-mg dose of theophylline suggested that pretreatment with viloxazine 100 mg three times daily for 3 days increased the AUC_{0-24} of theophylline by 47%, increased its maximum serum concentration, and reduced its clearance.[1]

An elderly woman hospitalised for respiratory failure and treated with a variety of drugs including theophylline, developed acute theophylline toxicity (a grand mal seizure) 2 days after starting to take viloxazine 200 mg daily. Her serum theophylline levels had increased threefold (from about 10 mg/L to 28 mg/L), but the levels fell when viloxazine was withdrawn.[2] Nausea and vomiting, associated with raised serum theophylline levels, occurred in another patient also taking viloxazine. Theophylline was stopped, and then reintroduced at 25% of the original dose. The theophylline level subsequently became subtherapeutic when viloxazine was stopped.[3] A further case report describes an elderly man who had a marked rise in his serum theophylline levels to toxic concentrations (55.3 mg/L) when viloxazine, 100 mg then 300 mg daily, was started.[4]

Mechanism

It is suggested that viloxazine antagonises the metabolism of theophylline by the liver, thereby reducing its clearance and resulting in an increase in its serum levels.

Importance and management

Information regarding an interaction between theophylline and viloxazine seems to be limited to these reports but it would appear to be a clinically important interaction. Theophylline levels should be well monitored if viloxazine is added, anticipating the need to reduce the dose. There appears to be no direct evidence about aminophylline, but it would be prudent to expect it to interact with viloxazine in the same way as theophylline.

NOTE. The reader is cautioned that this monograph is included purely for archival purposes, and is no longer subject to systematic revision and update.

1. Perault MC, Griesemann E, Bouquet S, Lavoisy J, Vandel B. A study of the interaction of viloxazine with theophylline. *Ther Drug Monit* (1989) 11, 520–2.
2. Laaban JP, Dupeyron JP, Lafay M, Sofeir M, Rochemaure J, Fabiani P. Theophylline intoxication following viloxazine induced decrease in clearance. *Eur J Clin Pharmacol* (1986) 30, 351–3.
3. Thomson AH, Addis GJ, McGovern EM, McDonald NJ. Theophylline toxicity following coadministration of viloxazine. *Ther Drug Monit* (1988) 10, 359–60.
4. Vial T, Bertholon P, Lafond P, Pionchon C, Grangeon C, Bruel M, Antoine JC, Ollagnier M, Evreux JC. Surdosage en théophylline secondaire à un traitement par viloxazine. *Rev Med Interne* (1994) 15, 696–8.

Index

All of the pairs of drugs included in the text of this book which are known to interact or not are listed in this index. They may also be listed under the group names if two or more members of the group interact, **but you should always look up the names of both individual drugs and their groups to ensure that you have access to all the information in this book**. You can possibly get a lead on the way unlisted drugs behave if you look up those which are related, but bear in mind that none of them are indentical and any conclusions reached should only be tentative.